# ABPI COMPENDIUM OF DATA SHEETS

# AND

# SUMMARIES OF PRODUCT CHARACTERISTICS

# 1998–99

**With The Code of Practice for the
Pharmaceutical Industry**

Datapharm Publications Limited
12 Whitehall, London SW1A 2DY

**Responsibility for Data Sheets and Summaries of Product Characteristics**

The data sheets and summaries of product characteristics in this Compendium are prepared independently by each participating company and each proof is checked and the text confirmed as correct by the participant concerned. Neither Datapharm Publications Limited nor The Association of the British Pharmaceutical Industry (ABPI) gives any guarantee whatsoever as to the accuracy of the information contained in the data sheets or summaries of product characteristics and accepts no liability whatsoever in respect of any loss, damage or expense arising from any such information or for any error or omission in the data sheets or summaries of product characteristics and in particular (but without prejudice to the generality of the foregoing) shall not be liable for any consequential damages or expenses or any loss of profit or any liability to third parties incurred by anyone relying on the information contained in the data sheets and summaries of product characteristics appearing in this Compendium.

Published by Datapharm Publications Limited

Compiled by Gillian Walker BSc, MRPharmS

ISBN 0 907102 16 6
ISSN 1364–5005

Typeset, printed and bound in Great Britain
by William Clowes Limited, Beccles and London

# THE COMPENDIUM

This is the second edition of the Compendium in which summaries of product characteristics (SPCs) appear. New requirements came into effect in 1995 replacing data sheets with SPCs for new products and those products coming up for licence renewal. There will be a period of about five years during which data sheets will coexist with SPCs and this edition of the Compendium reflects that fact.

Both data sheets and SPCs are prepared by the individual companies concerned and, in consequence, vary somewhat in style, but all follow either the requirements laid down by 'The Medicines (Data Sheet) Regulations 1972' (for data sheets) or the European Commission's Committee for Proprietary Medicinal Products (CPMP) Note for Guidance (for SPCs).

Participation in the Compendium is open to all companies supplying medicinal products intended for use under medical supervision.

Data sheets and SPCs are intended for members of the medical and pharmaceutical professions and are written with them in mind. Any member of the public who reads them should bear in mind the need to take professional advice before making any decision affecting his or her own medication based upon their contents.

## DATE OF PREPARATION
The data sheets included in this Compendium were finalised during the third quarter of 1997 and the Compendium itself was published in January 1998. Summaries of product characteristics have individual dates of approval/revision.

## REVISED DATA SHEETS/SPCs
Individual participating companies may issue loose leaf data sheets/summaries of product characteristics (SPCs) which supersede those included in this Compendium.

It is advisable to retain any such revised data sheets/SPCs which are received and to indicate that fact on the corresponding data sheets or SPCs in the Compendium.

## LEGAL CATEGORY
The following abbreviations are used under the heading 'Legal category' in data sheets and summaries of product characteristics in the Compendium.

GSL A preparation which is included in the General Sale List.

P A pharmacy sale medicine which can be sold only from a retail pharmacy.

POM A prescription only medicine.

CD A preparation controlled by the Misuse of Drugs Act 1971 and Regulations. The CD is followed by (Sch 1), (Sch 2), (Sch 3), (Sch 4) or (Sch 5) depending on the schedule to the Misuse of Drugs Regulations 1985, as amended, in which the preparation is included.

*Doctors are reminded that certain of the particulars must be in their own handwriting on prescriptions for preparations coming within Schedule 2 and Schedule 3 (except phenobarbitone) to the Misuse of Drugs Regulations 1985, as amended.*

## SYMBOLS AND ABBREVIATIONS
An asterisk (*) by the name of a product indicates that the name is a trade mark. The company symbols which appear in certain participants' sections are also trade marks.

An inverted triangle (▼) by the name of a product indicates that that product is newly introduced and there are special requirements as to the reporting of adverse reactions (see page iv).

OP in the 'Package quantities' section of a data sheet indicates that the pack is an 'original pack'.

## FURTHER INFORMATION
The regulations which relate to data sheets restrict the scope of the material which may be given under the heading 'Further information' and require insertion of the word 'Nil' in any data sheet where there is no entry under that heading. Companies are, of course, none the less always willing to provide additional information on their products upon request.

**Enquiries should be directed to the companies concerned. Addresses and telephone numbers are provided in the Directory of Participants in the coloured section at the end of the Compendium.**

# The reporting of adverse reactions

Any drug may produce unwanted or unexpected adverse reactions. Detection and recording of these is of vital importance. Doctors† are urged to help by reporting adverse reactions to:

Medicines Control Agency
CSM Freepost
London SW8 5BR
(0800 731 6789)

Suspected adverse reactions to *any* therapeutic agent should be reported, including drugs (those taken for *self-medication* as well as those *prescribed*), blood products, vaccines, X-ray contrast media, dental or surgical materials, intra-uterine devices, and contact lens fluids.

† Hospital pharmacists may also report suspected reactions; a demonstration scheme will also allow community pharmacists within the CSM's Monitoring Centres in Cardiff, Birmingham, Liverpool and Newcastle to report suspected reactions. All pharmacists must discuss the particular case with the patient's doctor before sending a yellow card report. Whilst it is not recommended for a report to be made against the advice of the patient's doctor, the pharmacist may wish to exercise professional judgement in sending such a report.

## Newer drugs marked ▼

Doctors are asked to report *all* suspected reactions (i.e. any adverse or any unexpected event, however minor, which could conceivably be attributed to the drug). Reports should be made despite uncertainty about a causal relationship, irrespective of whether the reaction is well recognised, and even if other drugs have been given concurrently.

## Established drugs

Doctors are asked to report *all* serious suspected reactions including those that are fatal, life-threatening, disabling, incapacitating, or which result in or prolong hospitalisation; they should be reported even if the effect is well recognised.

Examples include anaphylaxis, blood disorders, endocrine disturbances, effects on fertility, haemorrhage from any site, renal impairment, jaundice, ophthalmic disorders, severe CNS effects, severe skin reactions, reactions in pregnant women, and any drug interactions. Reports of serious adverse reactions are required to enable risk/benefit ratios to be compared with other drugs of a similar class. For established drugs doctors are asked not to report well known, relatively minor side-effects, such as dry mouth with tricyclic antidepressants, constipation with opioids, or nausea with digoxin.

## Special problems

*(i) Delayed drug effects* Doctors are reminded that some reactions (e.g., the development of cancers, chloroquine retinopathy and retroperitoneal fibrosis) may become manifest months or years after drug exposure. Please report any suspicion of such an association.

*(ii) Drugs in the elderly* Doctors are asked to be particularly alert to the possibility of adverse reactions when drugs are given to the elderly.

*(iii) Congenital abnormalities* When an infant is born with a congenital abnormality or there is a malformed aborted fetus, doctors are asked to consider the possibility that this might be an adverse reaction to a drug and to report all drugs (including self-medication) taken by the mother during pregnancy.

*(iv) Adverse reactions to vaccines* Doctors are asked to report all suspected reactions to both new and established vaccines. The balance between risks and benefits needs to be kept under continuous review.

## Yellow Cards

Prepaid Yellow Cards for reporting are available from the above address and forms for doctors are also included at the back of the Compendium.

A 24-hour Freefone service is available to all parts of the United Kingdom. For advice and information on adverse reactions contact the National Yellow Card Information Service at the Medicines Control Agency on 0800 7316789. Outside office hours a telephone-answering machine will take messages.

The following regional centres also collect data:

| | |
|---|---|
| CSM Mersey | CMS Wales |
| Freepost | Freepost |
| Liverpool L3 3AB | Cardiff CF4 1ZZ |
| (0151 794 8113) | (01222 744181 Direct Line) |
| | |
| CSM Northern | CSM West |
| Freepost | Midlands |
| Newcastle upon | Freepost |
| Tyne | Birmingham |
| NE1 1BR | B18 7BR |
| (0191-232 1525 Direct Line) | |

*The above statement and the symbols marking certain products have been included in the Compendium at the request of the Medicines Control Agency.*

*The individual companies concerned would find it helpful to be informed by practitioners of any adverse reactions to their products which are reported.*

# Contents

v

# Contents

# Abbott Laboratories Limited
Queenborough
Kent ME11 5EL

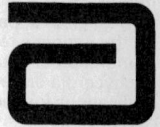

## CALCIJEX*

**Presentation** Calcijex (calcitriol injection) is a sterile, isotonic, clear, aqueous solution for intravenous injection. It is available in 1 ml ampoules each containing calcitriol (1 microgram/ml or 2 micrograms/ml).

**Uses** Calcijex is indicated in the management of hypocalcaemia in patients undergoing dialysis for chronic renal failure. It has been shown to significantly reduce elevated parathyroid hormone (PTH) levels. Reduction of PTH has been shown to result in an improvement in renal osteodystrophy.

*Actions:* Calcitriol is the active form of vitamin D$_3$ (cholecalciferol). It is produced in the kidney from the vitamin D metabolite 25-hydroxyvitamin D$_3$ (calcifediol). A vitamin D-resistant state may exist in uremic patients because of the failure of the kidney to adequately produce the active compound, calcitriol.

The known sites of action of calcitriol are intestine, bone, kidney and parathyroid gland. Calcitriol is the most active known form of vitamin D$_3$ in stimulating intestinal calcium absorption. In bone, calcitriol, in conjunction with parathyroid hormone, stimulates resorption of calcium; and in the kidney, calcitriol increases the tubular reabsorption of calcium. *In-vitro* and *in-vivo* studies have shown that calcitriol directly suppresses secretion and synthesis of PTH by the parathyroids.

Calcitriol when administered by bolus injection is rapidly available in the blood stream. Vitamin D metabolites are known to be transported in blood, bound to specific plasma proteins. The pharmacological activity of an administered dose of calcitriol lasts approximately 3 to 5 days.

**Dosage and administration** The optimal dose of Calcijex must be carefully determined for each patient.

The recommended initial dose of Calcijex is 0.50 µg (approximately 0.01 µg/kg) administered three times weekly, approximately every other day. If a satisfactory response in the biochemical parameters and clinical manifestations of the disease state is not observed, the dose may be increased by 0.25 to 0.50 µg increments at two to four week intervals. During this titration period, serum calcium and phosphorus levels should be obtained at least twice weekly, and if hypercalcaemia is noted, the drug should be immediately discontinued until normocalcaemia ensues. Most patients undergoing haemodialysis respond to doses of between 0.5 and 3.0 µg three times weekly.

Parenteral drug products such as Calcijex should be inspected visually for particulate matter prior to administration. Although calcitriol itself is a colourless, crystalline compound, the sodium ascorbate added as an antioxidant in Calcijex is white or very faintly yellow, and can turn yellow as it combines with oxygen.

Calcijex should be drawn up into a plastic 1 ml tuberculin syringe and administered as a bolus dose intravenously at the end of dialysis. It may be administered through the catheter at the end of haemodialysis.

The effectiveness of Calcijex therapy is predicted on the assumption that each patient is receiving an adequate and appropriate daily intake of calcium. To ensure that each patient receives an adequate daily intake of calcium, the physician should either prescribe a calcium supplement, or instruct the patient in proper dietary measures. Patients should be informed of the symptoms of hypercalcaemia (see *Side-effects*).

*Use in children:* Safety and efficacy of Calcijex in children have not been established.

*Use in pregnancy and lactation:* There are no adequate and well-controlled studies in pregnant women. Calcijex should be used during pregnancy only if the potential benefit justifies the potential risk to the foetus.

It is not known whether this drug is excreted in human milk. Because of the potential for serious adverse reaction in nursing infants due to calcitriol, breast feeding cannot be recommended.

### Contra-indications, warnings, etc

*Contra-indications:* Calcijex should not be given to patients with hypercalcaemia or evidence of vitamin D toxicity.

Calcijex injection should not be given to patients with previous hypersensitivity to calcitriol or any of its excipients.

*Warnings:* Since calcitriol is the most potent metabolite of vitamin D available, vitamin D and its derivatives should be withheld during treatment.

In patients undergoing dialysis who have high serum phosphorus levels, appropriate serum phosphate binders should be used. Overdosage of any form of vitamin D is dangerous (see also *Overdosage*). Progressive hypercalcaemia due to overdosage of vitamin D and its metabolites may be so severe as to require emergency attention. Chronic hypercalcaemia can lead to generalised vascular calcification, nephrocalcinosis and other soft-tissue calcification. The serum calcium times phosphorus (Ca×P) product should not be allowed to exceed 70. Radiographic evaluation of suspect anatomical regions may be useful in the early detection of this condition.

*Precautions:* Excessive dosage of Calcijex induces hypercalcaemia, and in some instances hypercalciuria. Therefore, serum calcium and phosphorous should be determined at least twice weekly early in treatment during dosage adjustment. Should hypercalcaemia develop, the drug should be discontinued immediately.

*Renal transplantation:* The rate of bone loss can be excessive and may exceed 5% per year in the immediate post-transplant period. Recommendations for treating post-transplant bone loss with calcitriol have not been established.

*Interactions:*

Magnesium-containing antacids: Magnesium-containing antacids and Calcijex should not be used concomitantly, because such use may lead to the development of hypermagnesaemia.

Cardiac glycosides: Calcijex should be given cautiously to patients on cardiac glycosides, because hypercalcaemia in such patients may precipitate cardiac arrhythmias.

Barbiturates and anticonvulsants: Higher doses of Calcijex may be required for patients taking barbiturates or anticonvulsants as these may reduce its effects.

Corticosteroids: The effects of Calcijex may be counteracted by corticosteroids.

*Side-effects:* Adverse effects of Calcijex are, in general, similar to those encountered with excessive vitamin D intake. The early symptoms of vitamin D intoxication associated with hypercalcaemia include weakness, headache, somnolence, nausea, vomiting, dry mouth, constipation, muscle pain, bone pain and metallic taste. Late signs include polyuria, polydipsia, anorexia, weight loss, nocturia, conjunctivitis (calcific), pancreatitis, photophobia, rhinorrhea, pruritus, hyperthermia, decreased libido, elevated BUN, albuminuria, hypercholesterolaemia, elevated SGOT and SGPT, ectopic calcification, hypertension, cardiac arrhythmias and, rarely, overt psychosis.

Rare cases of hypersensitivity reactions have been reported including anaphylaxis and localised redness at the injection site.

*Overdosage:* Administration of Calcijex to patients in excess of their requirements can cause hypercalcaemia, hypercalciuria and hyperphosphataemia. High intake of calcium and phosphate concomitant with Calcijex may lead to similar abnormalities.

General treatment of hypercalcaemia (greater than 1 mg/dl above the upper limit of normal range) consists of immediate discontinuation of Calcijex therapy, institution of a low calcium diet and withdrawal of calcium supplements. Serum calcium levels should be determined daily until normocalcaemia (8.5 to 10.5 mg/dl) ensues. Hypercalcaemia usually resolves in two to seven days. When serum calcium levels have returned to within normal limits, Calcijex therapy may be reinstituted at a dose 0.5 µg less than prior therapy. Serum calcium levels should be obtained at least twice weekly after all dosage changes.

Persistent or markedly elevated serum calcium levels may be corrected by dialysis against a calcium-free dialysate.

The treatment of acute accidental overdosage of Calcijex should consist of general supportive measures. Serial serum electrolyte determinations (especially calcium), rate of urinary calcium excretion and assessment of electrocardiographic abnormalities due to hypercalcaemia should be obtained. Such monitoring is critical in patients receiving digitalis. Discontinuation of supplemental calcium and initiation of low calcium diet are also indicated in accidental overdosage. Due to the pharmacological action of calcitriol lasting only 3–5 days, further measures are probably unnecessary. However, should persistent and markedly elevated serum calcium levels occur, there are a variety of therapeutic alternatives which may be considered, depending on the patient's underlying condition. These include the use of drugs such as biphosphonates, mithramycin, calcitonin, gallium nitrate and corticosteroids as well as measures to induce an appropriate forced diuresis. The use of peritoneal dialysis and haemodialysis against a calcium-free dialysate has also been reported.

**Pharmaceutical precautions** Calcitriol is known to be adsorbed onto PVC containers and tubing. It should therefore not be infused with the dialysate during CAPD as the dose could be significantly reduced due to drug adsorption to the PVC bag and tubing. See *Dosage and Administration* for recommended dosage method.

Store at room temperature and protect from light.

Discard any unused solution immediately after use.

**Legal category** POM.

**Package quantities** Calcijex is supplied in 1 ml amber glass ampoules containing calcitriol (1 microgram/ml or 2 micrograms/ml).

**Further information** Nil.

**Product licence numbers**
| | |
|---|---|
| 1 microgram ampoule | 0037/0245 |
| 2 microgram ampoule | 0037/0246. |

## DOPAMINE HYDROCHLORIDE 400 mg in 5% DEXTROSE INJECTION
## DOPAMINE HYDROCHLORIDE 800 mg in 5% DEXTROSE INJECTION

**Qualitative and quantitative composition** Each 250 ml of the injection contains either 400 mg or 800 mg of Dopamine Hydrochloride USP, sodium metabisulphite, dextrose anhydrous or hydrous, water for injections and hydrochloric acid or sodium hydroxide.

**Pharmaceutical form** A clear, sterile solution for intravenous infusion.

**Clinical particulars**

*Therapeutic indications:* Dopamine administered intravenously is a positive myocardial inotropic agent, which also may increase mesenteric and renal blood flow plus urinary output.

Dopamine hydrochloride in 5% Dextrose is indicated for the correction of haemodynamic imbalances present in shock due to myocardial infarction, trauma, endotoxic septicaemia, open heart surgery, renal failure and chronic cardiac decompensation as in refractory congestive failure.

*Posology and method of administration:*

*Adults:* Where appropriate, restoration of the circulatory volume should be instituted or completed with a suitable plasma expander or whole blood, prior to administration of dopamine hydrochloride.

Begin infusion of dopamine hydrochloride solution at doses of 2.5 micrograms/kg/min in patients who are likely to respond to modest increments of heart force and renal perfusion.

In more seriously ill patients, begin infusion of dopamine hydrochloride at doses of 5 micrograms/kg/min and increase gradually using 5 to 10 micrograms/kg/min increments up to a rate of 20 to 50 micrograms/kg/min as needed. If doses in excess of 50 micrograms/kg/min are required, it is advisable to check urine output frequently. Should urinary flow begin to decrease in the absence of hypotension, reduction of dopamine dosage should be considered. It has been found that more than 50% of patients have ben satisfactorily maintained on doses less than 20 micrograms/kg/min.

As with all potent intravenously administered drugs, care should be taken to control the rate of infusion so as to avoid inadvertent administration of a bolus drug.

In patients who do not respond to these doses with adequate arterial pressures or urine flow, additional increments of dopamine may be given in an effort to produce an appropriate arterial pressure and central perfusion.

Dosage of dopamine should be adjusted according to the patient's response, with particular attention to dimunition of established urine flow rate, increasing tachycardia or development of new dysrhythmias as indications for decreasing or temporarily suspending the dosage.

*Children:* Safety and effectiveness in children have not been established.

*Contra-indications:* Use in patients with phaeochromocytoma.

Dextrose solution without electrolytes should not administered simultaneously with blood through the same infusion set because of the possibility that pseudo-agglutination of the red blood cells may occur.

*Special warnings and special precautions for use:* Hypovolemia should be corrected where necessary prior to treatment with dopamine.

Avoid bolus administration of the drug.

Excess administration of potassium-free solutions may result in significant hypokalaemia.

The intravenous administration of these solutions can cause a fluid and/or solute overload resulting in dilution of serum electrolyte concentrations, overhydration, congested states or pulmonary oedema.

If a disproportionate rise in diastolic pressure (i.e. a marked decrease in pulse pressure) is observed, the infusion rate should be decreased and the patient observed carefully for further evidence of predominant vasoconstriction activity, unless such an effect is desired.

Patients with a history of peripheral vascular disease should be closely monitored for any changes in colour or temperature of the skin of the extremities. If a change of skin colour or temperature occurs, and is thought to be the result of compromised circulation to the extremities, the benefits of continued dopamine infusion should be weighed against the risk of possible necrosis. These changes may be reversed by decreasing the rate or discontinuing the infusion.

Dopamine hydrochloride in 5% Dextrose injection should be infused into a large vein whenever possible to prevent the possibility of infiltration of perivascular tissue adjacent to the infusion site. Extravasation may cause necrosis and sloughing of the surrounding tissue. Ischaemia can be reversed by infiltration of the affected area with 10–15 ml of saline containing 5 to 10 mg phentolamine mesylate. A syringe with a fine hypodermic needle should be used to liberally infiltrate the ischaemic area as soon as extravasation is noted.

Dopamine should not be administered in the presence of uncorrected tachyarrythmias or ventricular fibrillation.

Dopamine hydrochloride in 5% Dextrose contains sodium metabisulphite which may cause allergic type reactions, including anaphylactic symptoms and life threatening or less severe asthmatic episodes in certain susceptible people.

Dextrose solutions should be used with caution in patients with known subclinical or overt diabetes mellitus.

*Interaction with other medicaments and other forms of interaction:* Patients who have been treated with monoamine oxidase (MAO) inhibitors prior to administration of dopamine should receive a substantially reduced dosage of the latter. The starting dose in such patients should be reduced to at least one tenth of the usual dose.

Dopamine should be used with extreme caution in patients inhaling cyclopropane or halogenated hydrocarbon anaesthetics.

*Pregnancy and lactation:* Animal studies have shown no evidence of teratogenic effects with dopamine. The drug may be used in pregnant women when, in the judgement of the physician, the expected benefits outweigh the potential risk to the foetus.

*Effects on ability to drive and use machines:* None.

*Undesirable effects:* The most frequently reported adverse reactions to dopamine have been ectopic beats, tachycardia, nausea, vomiting, anginal pain, palpitations, dyspnoea, headache, hypotension and vasoconstriction.

Very rarely reported reactions include aberrant conduction, bradycardia, piloerection, widened QRS complex, azotaemia and elevated blood pressure.

*Overdosage:* Accidental overdosage as evidenced by excessive blood pressure elevation can be controlled by dose reduction or discontinuing the administration for a short period until the patient's condition stabilises.

If these measures fail, an infusion of phentolamine mesylate should be considered.

**Pharmacological properties**

*Pharmacodynamic properties:* Dopamine is a sympathomimetic agent with both direct and indirect effects. It dilates renal and mesenteric blood vessels and increases urine output. Dopamine also stimulates beta adrenergic receptors in the myocardium.

*Pharmacodynamic properties:* Dopamine is metabolised in the liver, kidney and plasma by MAO and catechol-O-methyl transferase to inactive compounds; homovanillic acid (HVA) and 3,4-dihydroxyphenyl-acetic acid. About 25% of the dose is taken up into specialised neurosecretory vesicles where it is hydroxylated to form noradrenaline.

It has been reported that about 80% of the drug is excreted within 24 hours, primarily as HVA. A very small portion is excreted unchanged.

*Preclinical safety data:* There are no pre-clinical data of relevance to the prescriber which are additional to that already included in other sections of the SPC.

**Pharmaceutical particulars**

*List of excipients:* Dextrose; sodium metabisulphite; hydrochloric acid, and/or sodium hydroxide; water for injections.

*Incompatibilties:* Do not add sodium bicarbonate or other alkaline substances, since dopamine is inactivated in alkaline solution.

*Shelf life:* 2 years.

*Special precautions for storage:* Store away from heat and protect from freezing.

*Nature and contents of container:* A flexible, copolyester 250 ml blow moulded container or 150 ml fabricated container, within an aluminium foil overwrap.

*Instructions for use/handling:* Use only if solution is clear and container is intact. For single use only. Discard unused portion.

Other drugs should not be added to this solution.

**Marketing authorisation numbers**

| | |
|---|---|
| Dopamine 400 mg | 0037/0146 |
| Dopamine 800 mg | 0037/0147 |

**Date of approval/revision of SPC** September 1996.

**Legal category** POM.

## ENFLURANE

**Presentation** Enflurane is an inhalation anaesthetic with a pleasant ethereal odour. No additives or stabilisers are present.

**Uses** Enflurane may be used for induction and maintenance of general anaesthesia. Adequate data are not available yet to establish its full place in obstetric anaesthesia other than in caesarean section. High concentrations of enflurane may produce marked uterine relaxation.

Enflurane may be used for outpatient and dental anaesthesia in view of the rapidity of action and recovery, with stability of the cardiovascular system. Enflurane can be used in children.

*Actions:* Induction and recovery are rapid. It does not stimulate excessive salivation, tracheobronchial secretions or cause bronchial constriction. Pharyngeal and laryngeal reflexes are diminished quickly. The level of anaesthesia changes rapidly with enflurane. Tachypnoea does not usually occur. Spontaneous respiration becomes depressed as the depth of anaesthesia increases.

Enflurane provokes a 'sigh' response reminiscent of that seen with diethyl ether.

During induction there is a decrease in blood pressure followed by a return to near normal levels, which may or may not be associated with surgical stimulation.

Blood pressure tends to fall in direct relation to the depth of anaesthesia but cardiac rate and rhythm remain stable. Enflurane appears to 'sensitise' the myocardium to adrenaline in man to a lesser extent than halothane. Available data indicate that subcutaneous injections of adrenaline may be safely administered to humans in concentrations of 1:100,000 or less at a dose of 10 ml in any given 10 minute period and not more than 30 ml/hour. All the usual precautions in the use of vasoconstrictor substances must be observed.

Good muscular relaxation is obtained with enflurane, but should greater relaxation be necessary minimal doses of an intravenous muscle relaxant may be used with measures to ensure adequate ventilation.

All commonly used intravenous muscle relaxants are compatible with enflurane.

*Note:* Enflurane potentiates the effect of the non-depolarising muscle relaxants which should therefore be used in reduced dosage. Neostigmine does not reverse the direct effect of enflurane.

Enflurane produces little post-operative analgesia.

Metabolism of enflurane in the human body proceeds at a low rate; inorganic fluoride is formed but serum levels in healthy individuals have not been shown to rise to significant levels.

**Dosage and administration** Vaporisers calibrated specifically for enflurane should be used so that the concentration being delivered is known.

The inspired concentration required to achieve clinical anaesthesia depends upon the age of the patient and to a minimal extent on body temperature. The MAC value is higher in children and decreases with advancing age, falling from an average in oxygen of 2.4% in the newborn and 2.5% at puberty, to 1.9% in young adults, and 1.7% at middle age. As with other agents, lesser concentrations of enflurane are normally required to maintain surgical anaesthesia in elderly patients. MAC values increase with increasing body temperature.

*Premedication:* Drugs used for premedication should be selected for each individual patient. The use of anticholinergic drugs is a matter of choice.

*Induction:* To avoid excitement a short-acting barbiturate or other intravenous induction agent should be administered, followed by inhalation of the enflurane mixture. Enflurane and oxygen alone or oxygen-nitrous oxide mixtures may be used.

It is recommended that enflurane induction be initiated at a concentration of 0.4% and gradually increased by 0.5% increments after every few breaths until surgical anaesthesia is achieved.

The maximum inspired concentration during induction should be no more than 4.5%. High inspired concentrations should be lowered as rapidly as possible to maintenance levels to prevent overdosage, and the blood pressure carefully observed.

*Maintenance:* In conjunction with nitrous oxide, surgical levels of anaesthesia may be maintained with a 0.5%–3% concentration of enflurane. A 3% concentration should not be exceeded for maintenance during spontaneous respiration. With controlled respiration techniques, during prolonged operations, single or supplementary doses of muscle relaxants may be used if required, bearing in mind the possibility of some slight potentiation. Ventilation to maintain the carbon dioxide tension in arterial blood in the the 4.7–6.0 kPa (35–45 mmHg) range is preferred to hyper- or hypoventilation, in order to minimise the possibility of CNS excitation.

Blood pressure levels during maintenance depend on enflurane concentration in the absence of other complicating factors. Excessive decreases (unless related to hypovolaemia) may be due to depth of anaesthesia and in such instances should be corrected by reducing the inspired enflurane concentration.

*Elderly:* As with other agents, lesser concentrations of enflurane are normally required to maintain surgical anaesthesia in elderly patients.

**Contra-indications, warnings, etc**

*Contra-indications:* Known sensitivity to enflurane and in patients with known or suspected genetic susceptability to malignant hyperthermia.

*Precautions:* Enflurane should be used with caution in patients who, by virtue of medical or drug history, may be considered more susceptible to cerebral stimulation produced by this drug. Increasing depth of anaesthesia with enflurane may produce changes in the electroencephalogram characterised by high voltage, fast frequency waves progressing through spike-dome complexes alternating with periods of electrical silence to frank seizure activity patterns. The latter may or may not be associated with motor movement. Motor activity, when encountered, generally consists of twitching or 'jerks' of various muscle groups; it is self-limiting and can be terminated by lowering the anaesthetic concentration. This electroencephalographic pattern associated with deep anaesthesia may be exacerbated by hyperventilation producing low arterial carbon dioxide tension. The pattern serves as a warning that depth of anaesthesia is excessive. Cerebral blood flow and metabolism studies in normal volunteers during seizure patterns show no evidence of cerebral hypoxia, and recovery appears to be uncomplicated.

In susceptible individuals, enflurane anaesthesia may trigger a skeletal muscle hypermetabolic state and the clinical syndrome known as malignant hyperthermia. The syndrome includes non-specific features such as muscle rigidity, tachycardia, tachypnoea cyanosis, arrhythmias and unstable blood pressure.

Treatment includes discontinuing enflurane anaesthesia, administration of dantrolene sodium and supportive therapy. Renal failure may appear late and urine flow should be sustained if possible.

Since levels of anaesthesia may be altered easily and rapidly, only vaporisers which deliver a predictable output with reasonable accuracy should be used. Hypotension and respiratory exchange can serve as a guide to anaesthetic depth. With deep levels of anaesthesia, more marked hypotension and respiratory depression are encountered.

The action of non-depolarising relaxants is augmented by enflurane, so less than the usual amount of those drugs should be used.

Overdosage or unduly rapid absorption of adrenaline administered topically or by subcutaneous o submucosal injection during enflurane anaesthesia may give rise to cardiac arrhythmias (see 'Actions' section). Care must be taken to avoid intravenous injection.

Bromsulphthalein (BSP) retention is mildly raised post-operatively in some cases. There is some elevation of blood glucose and white blood cell count intra-operatively.

Enflurane has been reported to interact with dry carbon dioxide absorbents to form carbon monoxide. In order to minimise the risk of formation of carbon monoxide in rebreathing circuits and the possibility of elevated carboxyhaemoglobin levels, carbon dioxide absorbents should not be allowed to dry out.

*Use in pregnancy:* Reproduction studies have been performed in rats and rabbits. Following single and multiple maternal administrations, no evidence of teratogenicity due to enflurane was found in the developing foetuses in these species. The relevance of these studies to the human is not known. Since there is no adequate experience in pregnant women who have received the drug, safety in pregnancy has not been established.

It is not known whether enflurane is excreted in breast milk and caution should therefore be exercised when enflurane is administered to a nursing mother.

*Adverse reactions:*

1. Motor activity exemplified by movement of various muscle groups and seizures may be encountered with deep levels of enflurane anaesthesia, particularly with hyperventilation.
2. Hypotension, respiratory depression and arrhythmias have been reported.
3. Elevation of the white blood cell count has been observed. It has not been determined whether this is related to enflurane or to surgical stress.
4. A mild increase in serum glucose concentration has been observed in some normal and diabetic patients, as with other anaesthetic agents. There seems to be no contra-indication to the use of the agent in these patients for whom rapid recovery is advantageous.
5. Hepatic enzyme changes occur less frequently and to a lesser degree after multiple enflurane anaesthetics when compared with multiple exposures to halothane. While jaundice and significant hepatic enzyme increases occasionally occur after halothane anaesthesia, this is extremely rare after the administration of enflurane in the absence of complicating factors such as blood transfusion or concomitant administration of hepatotoxic drugs.
6. Increased serum inorganic fluoride levels have been found during and immediately after enflurane anaesthesia due to biodegradation of the agent. These levels normally remain well below the postulated threshold for nephrotoxicity and, after reaching a peak within eight hours of the end of the anaesthetic, rapidly return to preoperative values.

Although there is no evidence that enflurane anaesthesia adversely affects the normal or diseased kidney it may be prudent to avoid its use in cases of chronic renal failure.

*Side-effects:* Nausea, vomiting, hiccups or shivering may occur occasionally.

**Pharmaceutical precautions** Store away from heat. Keep well closed.

**Legal category** P.

**Package quantities** Enflurane is supplied in bottles of 250 ml.

**Further information** Nil.

**Product licence number** 0037/0053.

## ERYTHROCIN* 250
## ERYTHROCIN* 500

**Presentation** Erythrocin 250 and Erythrocin 500 are white, film-coated tablets containing respectively 250 mg and 500 mg of erythromycin as Erythromycin Stearate BP. They are Erythromycin Stearate Tablets BP.

**Uses** For the prophylaxis and treatment of infections caused by erythromycin-sensitive organisms.

*Clinical indications:*

1. Upper respiratory tract infections.
2. Lower respiratory tract infections.
3. Infections of the external and middle ear.
4. Skin and soft tissue infections.
5. Oral/dental infections.
6. Eye infections.
7. Genito-urinary infections.
8. Gastrointestinal and biliary infections.
9. Other infections: Osteomyelitis, diphtheria, scarlet fever.
10. Prophylaxis: pre- and post-operative, trauma, burns, rheumatic fever, infective endocarditis following dental procedures.

*Note:* Erythromycin has also proved to be of value in endocarditis and septicaemia but in these conditions initial administration of erythromycin lactobionate by the intravenous route is advised.

*Microbiology:* Erythromycin has been shown to be active in vitro against the following organisms: Staphylococci, Streptococci, *Haemophilus influenzae*, L-forms, Meningococci; *Mycoplasma pneumoniae, Legionella pneumophila, Branhamella catarrhalis, Bordetella pertussis, Corynebacterium diphtheriae* (as an adjunct to antitoxin), Neisseria, *Treponema pallidum, Chlamydia trachomatis, Chlamydia pneumoniae*, Clostridia, *Ureaplasma urealytica*, Campylobacter, *Listeria monocytogenes.*

*Note:* The majority of strains of *Haemophilus influenzae* are susceptible to the concentrations reached after ordinary doses.

**Dosage and administration**

*Adults and children over 8 years:* For mild to moderate infections 1–2 g daily in divided doses. For severe infections this may be increased to 4 g daily in divided doses. Tablets should be taken before or with meals.

*Elderly:* No special dosage recommendations.

*Children under 8 years:* Erythroped suspension is recommended.

*Period of dosing with regard to indication:* Duration of dosing should be related to the severity and site of infection, but generally lies within the range of 5–14 days. However, the duration may need to be longer in certain cases, e.g. NGU and syphilis 10–21 days or longer, chlamydial inclusion conjunctivitis up to 21 days, acne may require prolonged treatment. Prophylaxis prior to dental or surgical procedures should begin $1\frac{1}{2}$ to 2 hours before the procedure and continued every 6 hours for 8 doses.

**Contra-indications, warnings, etc**

*Contra-indications:* Known sensitivity to erythromycin. Erythromycin is contra-indicated with either astemizole or terfenadine. Erythromycin is contraindicated with ergotamine and dihydroergotamine.

*Precautions:* Erythromycin is excreted principally by the liver, so caution should be exercised in administering the antibiotic to patients with impaired hepatic function or concomitantly receiving potentially hepatotoxic agents.

The administration of erythromycin has been infrequently associated with the occurrence of reversible cholestatic jaundice.

There have been reports suggesting erythromycin does not reach the foetus in adequate concentrations to prevent congenital syphilis. Infants born to women treated during pregnancy with oral erythromycin for early syphilis should be treated with an appropriate penicillin regimen.

There have been reports that erythromycin may aggravate the weakness of patients with myasthenia gravis.

Erythromycin interferes with the fluorometric determination or urinary catecholamines.

As with other broad spectrum antibiotics, pseudomembraneous colitis has been reported rarely with erythromycin.

Rhabdomyolysis with or without renal impairment has been reported in seriously ill patients receiving erythromycin concomitantly with lovastatin.

*Interactions:* Concomitant use of erythromycin with terfenadine or astemizole is likely to result in an enhanced risk of cardiotoxicity with these drugs. The concomitant use of erythromycin with either astemizole or terfenadine is therefore contraindicated.

Erythromycin significantly alters the metabolism of terfenadine when taken concomitantly. Rare cases of serious cardiovascular adverse events including death, cardiac arrest, torsades de pointes and other ventricular arrhythmias have been observed.

Concurrent use of erythromycin and ergotamine or dihydroergotamine has been associated in some patients with acute ergot toxicity characterised by the rapid development of severe peripheral vasospasm and dysethesia.

Increases in serum concentrations of the following drugs may occur when administered concurrently with erythromycin: digoxin, warfarin, carbamazepine, phenytoin, theophylline, cyclosporin, bromocriptine, disopyramide, alfentanil, triazolam, astemizole, hexobarbitone, midazolam, terfenadine, valporate. Appropriate monitoring should be undertaken and dosage should be adjusted as necessary.

When oral erythromycin is given concurrently with theophylline, there is also a significant decrease in erythromycin serum concentrations. The decrease could result in subtherapeutic concentrations of erythromycin.

*Use in pregnancy and nursing mothers:* There is no evidence of hazard from erythromycin in human pregnancy. It has been in wide use for many years without apparent ill consequence. Animal studies have shown no hazard.

Erythromycin has been reported to cross the placental barrier in humans, but foetal plasma levels are generally low.

Erythromycin is excreted in breast milk, therefore, caution should be exercised when erythromycin is administered to a nursing mother.

*Side-effects:* Occasional side-effects such as nausea, abdominal discomfort, vomiting and diarrhoea may be experienced. Reversible hearing loss associated with doses of erythromycin usually greater than 4 g per day has been reported. Allergic reactions are rare and mild, although anaphylaxis has occurred. Skin reactions ranging from mild eruptions to erythema multiforme, Stevens-Johnson syndrome and toxic epidermal neurolysis have rarely been reported. There are no reports implicating erythromycin products with abnormal tooth development and only rare reports of damage to the blood, kidneys, liver or central nervous system.

Cardiac arrhythmias have been very rarely reported in patients receiving erythromycin therapy. There have been isolated reports of chest pain, dizziness and palpitations; however, a cause and effect relationship has not been established.

*Overdosage:* Symptoms: Hearing loss, severe nausea, vomiting and diarrhoea.

Treatment: Gastric lavage, general supportive measures.

**Pharmaceutical precautions** Keep bottle tightly closed.

**Legal category** POM.

**Package quantities** Erythrocin 250: Containers of 100, 500 tablets.

Erythrocin 500: Containers of 100 and 500 tablets.

**Further information** Erythrocin 250 and 500 contain no dyes. They contain respectively 0.07 g and 0.15 g Maize Starch BP.

**Product licence number**

Erythrocin 250 0037/5079R

Erythrocin 500 0037/5044R

## ERYTHROMID*

**Presentation** Erythromid is an white to off-white, enteric-coated, film-coated tablet containing 250 mg of Erythromycin BP. They are Erythromycin Tablets BP.

**Uses** For the prophylaxis and treatment of infections caused by erythromycin-sensitive organisms.

*Clinical indications:*

1. Upper respiratory tract infections.
2. Lower respiratory tract infections.
3. Infections of the external and middle ear.
4. Skin and soft tissue infections.
5. Oral/dental infections.
6. Eye infections.
7. Genito-urinary infections.
8. Gastrointestinal and biliary infections.
9. Other infections: Osteomyelitis, diphtheria, scarlet fever.
10. Prophylaxis: pre- and post-operative, trauma, burns, rheumatic fever, infective endocarditis following dental procedures.

*Note:* Erythromycin has also proved to be of value in endocarditis and septicaemia, but in these conditions initial administration of erythromycin lactobionate by the intravenous route is advised.

*Microbiology indications:* Erythromycin has been shown to be active in vitro against the following organisms: Staphylococci, Streptococci, *Haemophilus influenzae*, L-forms, Meningococci, *Mycoplasma pneumoniae, Legionella pneumophila, Branhamella catarrhalis, Bordetella pertussis, Corynebacterium diphtheriae* (as an adjunct to antitoxin), Neisseria, *Treponema pallidum, Chlamydia trachomatis, Chlamydia pneumoniae*, Clostridia, *Ureaplasma urealytica*, Campylobacter *Listeria Monocytogenes.*

*Note:* The majority of strains of *Haemophilus influenzae* are susceptible to the concentrations reached after ordinary doses.

**Dosage and administration**

*Adults and children over 8 years:* For mild to moderate infections 1–2 g daily in divided doses. For severe infections this may be increased to 4 g daily in divided doses. Tablets should be taken before or with meals.

*Elderly:* No special dosage recommendations.

*Children under 8 years:* Erythroped suspension is recommended.

*Period of dosing with regard to indication:* Duration of dosing should be related to the severity and site of infection, but generally lies within the range of 5–14 days. However, the duration may need to be longer in certain cases, e.g. NGU and syphilis 10–21 days or longer, chlamydial inclusion conjunctivitis up to 21 days, acne may require prolonged treatment. Prophylaxis prior to dental or surgical procedures should begin 1½ to 2 hours before the procedure and continued every 6 hours for 8 doses.

**Contra-indications, warnings, etc**
*Contra-indications:* Known sensitivity to erythromycin. Erythromycin is contra-indicated with either terfenadine or astemizole.

Erythromycin is contra-indicated with ergotamine and dihydroergotamine.

*Precautions:* Erythromycin is excreted principally by the liver, so caution should be exercised in administering the antibiotic to patients with impaired hepatic function or concomitantly receiving potentially hepatotoxic agents.

The administration of erythromycin has been infrequently associated with the occurrence of reversible cholestatic jaundice.

There have been reports suggesting erythromycin does not reach the foetus in adequate concentrations to prevent congenital syphilis. Infants born to women treated during pregnancy with oral erythromycin for early syphilis should be treated with an appropriate penicillin regimen.

There have been reports that erythromycin may aggravate the weakness of patients with myasthenia gravis.

Erythromycin interferes with the fluorometric determination or urinary catecholamines.

As with other broad spectrum antibiotics, pseudomembraneous colitis has been reported rarely with erythromycin.

Rhabdomyolysis with or without renal impairment has been reported in seriously ill patients receiving erythromycin concomitantly with lovastatin.

*Interactions:* Concomitant use of erythromycin with terfenadine or astemizole is likely to result in an enhanced risk of cardiotoxicity with these drugs. The concomitant use of erythromycin with either astemizole or terfenadine is therefore contra-indicated.

Erythromycin significantly alters the metabolism of terfenadine when taken concomitantly. Rare cases of serious cardiovascular adverse events including death, cardiac arrest, torsades de pointes and other ventricular arrhythmias have been observed.

Concurrent use of erythromycin and ergotamine or dihydroergotamine has been associated in some patients with acute ergot toxicity characterised by the rapid development of severe peripheral vasospasm and dysethesia.

Increases in serum concentrations of the following drugs may occur when administered concurrently with erythromycin: digoxin, warfarin, carbamazepine, phenytoin, theophylline, cyclosporin, bromocriptine, disopyramide, alfentanil, triazolam, astemizole, hexobarbitone, midazolam, terfenadine, valporate. Appropriate monitoring should be undertaken and dosage should be adjusted as necessary.

When oral erythromycin is given concurrently with theophylline, there is also a significant decrease in erythromycin serum concentrations. The decrease could result in subtherapeutic concentrations of erythromycin.

*Use in pregnancy and nursing mothers:* There is no evidence of hazard from erythromycin in human pregnancy. It has been in wide use for many years without apparent ill consequence. Animal studies have shown no hazard.

Erythromycin has been reported to cross the placental barrier in humans, but foetal plasma levels are generally low.

Erythromycin is excreted in breast milk, therefore, caution should be exercised when erythromycin is administered to a nursing mother.

*Side-effects:* Occasional side-effects such as nausea, abdominal discomfort, vomiting and diarrhoea may be experienced. Reversible hearing loss associated with doses of erythromycin usually greater than 4 g per day has been reported. Allergic reactions are rare and mild, although anaphylaxis has occurred extremely rarely. Skin reactions ranging from mild eruptions to erythema multiforme, Stevens-Johnson syndrome and toxic epidermal neurolysis have rarely been reported. There are no reports implicating erythromycin products with abnormal tooth development and only rare reports of damage to the blood, kidneys, liver or central nervous system.

Cardiac arrhythmias have been very rarely reported in patients receiving erythromycin therapy. There have been isolated reports of chest pain, dizziness and palpitations; however, a cause and effect relationship has not been established.

*Overdosage:* Symptoms: Hearing loss, severe nausea, vomiting and diarrhoea. Treatment: Gastric lavage, general supportive measures.

**Pharmaceutical precautions** Keep bottle tightly closed. Protect from light. Store below 25°C.

**Legal category** POM.

**Package quantities** Erythromid: Containers of 100, 500 and 1000 tablets.

**Further information** No metabolisable carbohydrate is present.

**Product licence number**
Erythromid 0037/5019R.

## ERYTHROMYCIN LACTOBIONATE

**Presentation** A sterile, white, lyophilised presentation of 1.0 g of erythromycin as erythromycin lactobionate in a vial.

When reconstituted with 20 ml Water for Injections BP provides 22 ml of solution. Deliberate overage ensures that each 20 ml of this solution contains 1.0 g of erythromycin as erythromycin lactobionate.

The solution must be further diluted prior to intravenous administration (see dosage and administration).

Erythromycin Lactobionate is not suitable for intramuscular use. It is intended for intravenous use.

**Uses**
*Clinical indications:* Erythromycin lactobionate is indicated in severe and immunocompromised cases of infections caused by sensitive organisms where high blood levels are required at the earliest opportunity or when the oral route is compromised.

1. Upper respiratory tract infections.
2. Lower respiratory tract infections.
3. Skin and soft tissue infections.
4. Oral/dental infections.
5. Gastro-intestinal and biliary infections.
6. Endocarditis.
7. Septicaemia.
8. Prophylaxis: Peri-operative secondary infection prophylaxis, severe trauma and burns secondary infection prophylaxis, endocarditis prophylaxis (dental procedures).

*Microbiology:* Erythromycin has been shown to be active in vitro against the following organisms: Staphylococci, Streptococci, *Haemophilus influenzae*, L-forms, Meningococci, *Mycoplasma pneumoniae*, *Legionella pneumophila*, *Branhamella catarrhalis*, *Bordetella pertussis*, Corynebacterium diphtheriae (as an adjunct to antitoxin), Neisseria, *Treponema pallidum*, *Chlamydia trachomatis*, *Chlamydia pneumoniae*, Clostridia, *Ureaplasma urealytica*, Campylobacter, *Listeria monocytogenes*.

**Dosage and administration**
*Recommended dosage*
*Adults, children and neonates:* Severe and immunocompromised infections, 50 mg/kg/day, preferably by continuous infusion (equivalent to 4 g per day for adults).

Mild to moderate infections (oral route compromised) 25 mg/kg/day.

*Elderly:* No special dosage recommendations.

*Recommended administration:* Continuous intravenous infusion with an erythromycin concentration of 1 mg/ml (0.1% solution) is recommended.

If required, solution strengths up to 5 mg/ml (0.5% solution) may be used, but should not be exceeded. Higher concentrations may result in pain along the vein.

Bolus injection is not recommended.

However, if it is decided to administer the daily dose as 4 doses once every 6 hours, then the erythromycin concentration should not exceed 5 mg/ml and the time of each infusion should be between 20 and 60 minutes.

Intravenous therapy should be replaced by oral administration at the appropriate time.

*Preparation of solution for intravenous administration*
*Step 1:* Inject 20 ml of Water for Injections BP into the vial and shake to dissolve contents. Do not use saline or other diluents. This will give 22 ml of solution.

20 ml of this solution will contain 1.0 g erythromycin (50 mg erythromycin/ml).

Use within 24 hours of preparation. Keep in a refrigerator between 2°C and 8°C.

This solution must be further diluted before administration, see Step 2.

Step 2: Solutions for administration are prepared with Sodium Chloride Intravenous Infusion BP 0.9% w/v (see also below).

| *Dose required* | *Volume from Step 1* | *Volume of sterile 0.9% saline* | *Total volume* | *Erythromycin concentration* |
|---|---|---|---|---|
| 1.0 g | 20 ml | 1000 ml | 1020 ml | 1.0 mg/ml |
| 500 mg | 10 ml | 500 ml | 510 ml | |
| 1.0 g | 20 ml | 500 ml | 520 ml | 1.9 mg/ml |
| 500 mg | 10 ml | 250 ml | 260 ml | |
| 1.0 g | 20 ml | 200 ml | 220 ml | 4.6 mg/ml |
| 500 mg | 10 ml | 100 ml | 110 ml | |

If, for clinical reasons, 0.9% saline is not suitable, then neutralised Glucose Intravenous Infusion BP 5% w/v may be used. Neutralised glucose solution is prepared by the addition of 5 ml of sterile 8.4% w/v sodium bicarbonate solution to each litre of Glucose Intravenous Injection BP 5% w/v.

It is necessary to buffer the glucose solution in this way because the stability of Erythromycin Lactobionate is adversely affected below pH 5.5.

To ensure potency, all solutions for administration should be used within 8 hours of preparation.

**Contra-indications, warnings, etc**
*Contra-indications:* Known sensitivity to erythromycin. Erythromycin is contra-indicated with either terfenadine or astemizole.

Erythromycin is contra-indicated with ergotamine and dihydroergotamine.

*Precautions:* Extravasation should be avoided. The injection should be slow to avoid pain along the vein. Erythromycin is excreted principally by the liver, so caution should be exercised in administering the antibiotic to patients with impaired hepatic function or concomitantly receiving potentially hepatotoxic agents.

The administration of erythromycin has been infrequently associated with the occurrence of reversible cholestatic jaundice.

There have been reports suggesting erythromycin does not reach the foetus in adequate concentrations to prevent congenital syphilis. Infants born to women treated during pregnancy with oral erythromycin for early syphilis should be treated with an appropriate penicillin regimen.

There have been reports that erythromycin may aggravate the weakness of patients with myasthenia gravis.

Erythromycin interferes with the fluorometric determination or urinary catecholamines.

As with other broad spectrum antibiotics, pseudomembraneous colitis has been reported rarely with erythromycin.

Rhabdomyolysis with or without renal impairment has been reported in seriously ill patients receiving erythromycin concomitantly with lovastatin.

*Interactions:* Concomitant use of erythromycin with terfenadine or astemizole is likely to result in an enhanced risk of cardiotoxicity with these drugs. The concomitant use of erythromycin with either astemizole or terfenadine is therefore contra-indicated.

Erythromycin significantly alters the metabolism of terfenadine when taken concomitantly. Rare cases of serious cardiovascular adverse events including death, cardiac arrest, torsades de pointes and other ventricular arrhythmias have been observed.

Concurrent use of erythromycin and ergotamine or dihydroergotamine has been associated in some patients with acute ergot toxicity characterised by the rapid development of severe peripheral vasospasm and dysethesia.

Increases in serum concentrations of the following drugs may occur when administered concurrently with erythromycin: digoxin, warfarin, carbamazepine phenytoin, theophylline, cyclosporin, bromocriptine disopyramide, alfentanil, triazolam, astemizole, hexobarbitone, midazolam, terfenadine, valporate. Appropriate monitoring should be undertaken and dosage should be adjusted as necessary.

When oral erythromycin is given concurrently wit theophylline, there is also a significant decrease ir erythromycin serum concentrations. The decrease could result in subtherapeutic concentrations of erythromycin.

*Use in pregnancy and nursing mothers:* There is nc evidence of hazard from erythromycin in humai pregnancy. It has been in wide use for many years without apparent ill consequence. Animal studie have shown no hazard.

Erythromycin has been reported to cross the placen tal barrier in humans, but foetal plasma levels ar generally low.

Erythromycin is excreted in breast milk, therefore caution should be exercised when erythromycin i administered to a nursing mother.

*Side-effects:* Occasional venous irritation has bee encountered, but if the infusion is given slowly, i dilute solution, as recommended above, pain an vessel trauma are minimised.

Occasional side-effects such as nausea, abdomina discomfort, vomiting and diarrhoea may be exper enced. Reversible hearing loss associated with dose of erythromycin usually greater than 4 g per day ha been reported. Allergic reactions are rare and milc although anaphylaxis has occurred extremely rarely Skin reactions ranging from mild eruptions to ery thema multiforme, Stevens-Johnson syndrome an toxic epidermal neurolysis have rarely been reporte There are no reports implicating erythromycin pro ucts with abnormal tooth development and only rar reports of damage to the blood, kidneys, liver c central nervous system.

Cardiac arrhythmias have been very rarely reported in patients receiving erythromycin therapy. There have been isolated reports of chest pain, dizziness and palpitations; however, a cause and effect relationship has not been established.

*Overdosage:* Symptoms: Hearing loss, severe nausea, vomiting and diarrhoea.

Treatment: General supportive measures.

**Pharmaceutical precautions** The powder is stable at room temperature.

**Legal category** POM.

**Package quantities** 1 g vials of Erythromycin Lactobionate.

**Further information** Contains no sodium. Compatibility with other IV additives has not been established.

**Product licence number** 0037/0092.

## ERYTHROPED* A

**Presentation**

*Erythroped A:* Oval, yellow film coated tablet. Each tablet contains 500 mg erythromycin as erythromycin ethylsuccinate.

**Uses** For the prophylaxis and treatment of infections caused by erythromycin sensitive organisms.

*Clinical indications:*

1. Upper respiratory tract infections
2. Lower respiratory tract infections
3. Infections of the external and middle ear
4. Skin and soft tissue infections.
5. Oral/dental infections
6. Eye infections
7. Genito-urinary infections
8. Gastrointestinal and biliary infections.
9. Other infections: Osteomyelitis, diphtheria, scarlet fever.
10. Prophylaxis: pre- and post-operative, trauma, burns, rheumatic fever, infective endocarditis following dental procedures.

*Note:* Erythromycin has also proved to be of value in endocarditis and septicaemia, but in these conditions initial administration of erythromycin lactobionate by the intravenous route is advised.

*Microbiology:* Erythromycin has been shown to be active in vitro against the following organisms: Staphylococci, Streptococci, *Haemophilus influenzae*, L-forms, Meningococci, *Mycoplasma pneumoniae*, *Legionella pneumophila*, *Branhamella catarrhalis*, *Bordetella pertussis*, *Corynebacterium diphtheriae* (as an adjunct to antitoxin), Neisseria, *Treponema pallidum*, *Chlamydia trachomatis*, *Chlamydia pneumoniae*, Clostridia, *Ureaplasma urealytica*, Campylobacter, *Listeria monocytogenes*.

*Note:* The majority of strains of *Haemophilus influenzae* are susceptible to concentrations reached after ordinary doses.

**Dosage and administration**

*Adults and children over 8 years:* For mild to moderate infections 2 g daily in divided doses. Up to 4 g daily in severe infections.

*Elderly:* No special dosage recommendations.

*Children under 8 years:* Not recommended for children under 8 years as unit doses are too large. Erythroped suspensions are recommended.

*Period of dosing with regard to indication:* Duration of dosing should be related to the severity and site of infection, but generally lies within the range of 5–14 days. However, the duration may need to be longer in certain cases, e.g. NGU and syphilis 10–21 days or longer, chlamydial inclusion conjunctivitis up to 21 days, acne may require prolonged treatment. Prophylaxis prior to dental or surgical procedures should begin 1½ to 2 hours before the procedure and continued every 6 hours for 8 doses.

**Contra-indications, warnings, etc**

*Contra-indications:* Known hypersensitivity to erythromycin. Erythromycin is contra-indicated with either astemizole or terfenadine. Erythromycin is contra-indicated with ergotamine and dihydroergotamine.

*Precautions:* Erythromycin is excreted principally by the liver, so caution should be exercised in administering the antibiotic to patients with impaired hepatic function or concomitantly receiving potentially hepatotoxic agents.

The administration of erythromycin has been infrequently associated with the occurrence of reversible cholestatic jaundice.

There have been reports suggesting erythromycin does not reach the foetus in adequate concentrations to prevent congenital syphilis. Infants born to women treated during pregnancy with oral erythromycin for early syphilis should be treated with an appropriate penicillin regimen.

There have been reports that erythromycin may aggravate the weakness of patients with myasthenia gravis.

Erythromycin interferes with the fluorometric determination or urinary catecholamines.

As with other broad spectrum antibiotics, pseudomembraneous colitis has been reported rarely with erythromycin.

Rhabdomyolysis with or without renal impairment has been reported in seriously ill patients receiving erythromycin concomitantly with lovastatin.

*Interactions:* Concomitant use of erythromycin with terfenadine or astemizole is likely to result in an enhanced risk of cardiotoxicity with these drugs. The concomitant use of erythromycin with either astemizole or terfenadine is therefore contra-indicated.

Erythromycin significantly alters the metabolism of terfenadine when taken concomitantly. Rare cases of serious cardiovascular adverse events including death, cardiac arrest, torsades de pointes and other ventricular arrhythmias have been observed.

Concurrent use of erythromycin and ergotamine or dihydroergotamine has been associated in some patients with acute ergot toxicity characterised by the rapid development of severe peripheral vasospasm and dysethesia.

Increases in serum concentrations of the following drugs may occur when administered concurrently with erythromycin: digoxin, warfarin, carbamazepine, phenytoin, theophylline, cyclosporin, bromocriptine, disopyramide, alfentanil, triazolam, astemizole, hexobarbitone, midazolam, terfenadine, valporate. Appropriate monitoring should be undertaken and dosage should be adjusted as necessary.

When oral erythromycin is given concurrently with theophylline, there is also a significant decrease in erythromycin serum concentrations. The decrease could result in subtherapeutic concentrations of erythromycin.

*Use in pregnancy and nursing mothers:* There is no evidence of hazard from erythromycin in human pregnancy. It has been in wide use for many years without apparent ill consequence. Animal studies have shown no hazard.

Erythromycin has been reported to cross the placental barrier in humans, but foetal plasma levels are generally low.

Erythromycin is excreted in breast milk, therefore, caution should be exercised when erythromycin is administered to a nursing mother.

*Side-effects:* Occasional side-effects such as nausea, abdominal discomfort, vomiting and diarrhoea may be experienced. Reversible hearing loss associated with doses of erythromycin usually greater than 4 g per day has been reported. Allergic reactions are rare and mild, although anaphylaxis has occurred. Skin reactions ranging from mild eruptions to erythema multiforme, Stevens-Johnson syndrome and toxic epidermal neurolysis have rarely been reported. There are no reports implicating erythromycin products with abnormal tooth development and only rare reports of damage to the blood, kidneys, liver or central nervous system.

Cardiac arrhythmias have been very rarely reported in patients receiving erythromycin therapy. There have been isolated reports of chest pain, dizziness and palpitations; however, a cause and effect relationship has not been established.

*Overdosage:* Symptoms: Hearing loss, severe nausea, vomiting and diarrhoea.

Treatment: Gastric lavage, general supportive measures.

**Pharmaceutical precautions** Store below 30°C.

**Legal category** POM.

**Package quantities** Erythroped A: Blister packs of 28 tablets OP.

**Further information** Dyes: Tablets contain E104 (non-azo).

Sugar content: Tablets – sugar free.

**Product licence number** 0037/0137

## ERYTHROPED* A SACHET

**Qualitative and quantitative composition** Erythromycin as erythromycin ethylsuccinate 1000 mg per sachet.

**Pharmaceutical form** Granules for reconstitution.

**Clinical particulars**

*Therapeutic indications:*

1. Upper respiratory tract infections.
2. Lower respiratory tract infections.
3. Skin and soft tissue infections.
4. Bone infections.
5. Sexually transmitted diseases.
6. Oral/dental infections.
7. Eye infections.
8. Gastro-intestinal infections.
9. Prophylaxis.

*Note:* Erythromycin has also proved to be of value in endocarditis and septicaemia but in these conditions initial administration of erythromycin lactobionate by the intravenous route is recommended.

*Microbiology:* Erythromycin has shown to be active *in vitro* against the following organisms: Staphylococci, Streptococci, *Haemophilus influenzae*, L-forms, Meningococci, *Mycoplasma pneumoniae*, *Legionella pneumophila*, *Branhamella catarrhalis*, *Bordetella pertussis*, *Corynebacterium diphtheriae* (as an adjunct to antitoxin), Neisseria, *Treponema palladium*, *Chlamydia trachomatis*, *Chlamydia pneumoniae*, Clostridia, *Ureaplasma urealytica*, Campylobacter, *Listeria monocytogenes*.

The majority of strains of *Haemophilus influenzae* are susceptible to the concentrations reached after ordinary doses.

*Posology and method of administration:* Reconstitution: Erythroped products are taken orally after being reconstituted as follows. Disperse the contents of the sachet in a little water immediately before taking.

*Adults and children over 8 years:* For mild to moderate infections 2 g/day in divided doses. For severe infections up to 4 g/day.

*Elderly:* No special dosage recommendations.

*Children aged 2–8:* For mild to moderate infections 1 g daily in divided doses.

*Infants and babies up to 2 years:* For mild to moderate infections 500 mg daily in divided doses.

For severe infections doses may be doubled.

*Period of dosing with regard to to indication:* Duration of dosing should be related to the site and severity of infection, but generally lies within the range 5–14 days. However, the duration may need to be longer in certain cases i.e. NGU and syphilis 10–21 days or longer, chlamydial inclusion conjunctivitis up to 21 days, acne may require prolonged treatment. Prophylaxis prior to dental or surgical procedures should begin 1½ to 2 hours before the procedure and continued every 6 hours for 8 doses.

*Contra-indications:* Known hypersenitivity to erythromycin. Erythromycin is contra-indicated with either astemizole or terfenadine.

Erythromycin is contra-indicated with ergotamine and dihydroergotamine.

*Special warnings and special precautions for use:* Erythromycin is excreted principally by the liver, so caution should be exercised in administering the antibiotic to patients with impaired hepatic function or concomitantly receiving potentially hepatotoxic agents. The administration of erythromycin has been frequently associated with the occurrence of reversible cholestatic jaundice.

There have been reports suggesting erythromycin does not reach the foetus in adequate concentrations to prevent congenital syphilis. Infants born to women treated during pregnancy with oral erythromycin for early syphilis should be treated with an appropriate penicillin regimen.

There have been reports that erythromycin may aggravate the weakness of patients with myasthenia gravis.

Erythromycin interferes with the fluorometric determination of urinary catecholamines.

Pseudomembraneous colitis has been reported with nearly all antibacterial agents, including macrolides, and may range in severity from mild to life-theatening.

Rhabdomyolysis with or without renal impairment has been reported in seriously ill patients receiving erythromycin concomitantly with lovastatin.

*Interaction with other medicaments and other forms of interaction:* Concomitant use of erythromycin with terfenadine or astemizole is likely to result in an enhanced risk of cardiotoxicity with these drugs. The concomitant of erythromycin with either astemizole or terfenadine is therefore contraindicated.

Erythromycin significantly alters the metabolism of terfenadine when taken concomitantly. Rare cases of serious cardiovascular adverse events including death, cardiac arrest, torsades de pointe and other ventricular arrhythmias have been observed.

Concurrent use of erythromycin and ergotamine or dihydroergotamine has been associated in some patients with acute ergot toxicity characterised by the rapid development of severe peripheral vasospasm and dysethesia.

Increases in serum concentrations of the following drugs may occur when administered concurrently with erythromycin: alfentanil, astemizole, bromocriptine, carbamazepine, cyclosporin, digoxin, dihydroergotamine, disopyramide, ergotamine, hexobarbitone, midazolam, phenytoin, terfenadine, theophylline, triazolam, valproate and warfarin. Appropriate monitoring should be undertaken and dosage should be adjusted as necessary.

When oral erythromycin is given concurrently with theophylline, there is also a significant decrease in erythromycin serum concentrations. The decrease could result in subtherapeutic concentrations of erythromycin.

*Pregnancy and lactation:* There is no evidence of hazard from erythromycin in human pregnancy. It has been in widespread use for a number of years without apparent ill consequence. Animal studies have shown no hazard.

Erythromycin has been reported to cross the placental barrier in humans, but foetal plasma levels are generally low.

Erythromycin is excreted in breast milk, therefore, caution should be exercised when erythromycin is administered to a nursing mother.

*Effects on ability to drive and to use machines:* None reported.

*Undesirable effects:* Occasional side effects such as nausea, abdominal discomfort, vomiting and diarrhoea may be experienced. Reversible hearing loss associated with doses of erythromycin usually greater than 4 g per day has been reported. Allergic reactions are rare and mild, although anaphylaxis has occurred. Skin reactions ranging from mild eruptions to erythema multiforme, Stevens-Johnson syndrome and toxic epidermal necrolysis have rarely been reported. There are no reports implicating erythromycin products with abnormal tooth development, and only rare reports of damage to the blood, kidneys, liver or central nervous system.

Cardiac arrhythmias have been very rarely reported in patients receiving erythromycin therapy. There have been isolated reports of chest pain, dizziness and palpitations, however, a cause and effect relationship has not been established.

*Overdosage:* Symptoms: Hearing loss, severe nausea, vomiting and diarrhoea.

Treatment: Gastric lavage, general supportive measures.

### Pharmacological properties

*Pharmacodynamic properties:* Erythromycin ethylsuccinate is less susceptible than erythromycin to the adverse effect of gastric acid. It is absorbed from the small intestine. It is widely distributed throughout body tissues. Little metabolism occurs and only about 5% is excreted in the urine. It is excreted principally by the liver.

*Pharmacokinetic particulars:* Peak blood levels normally occur within 1 hour of dosing of erythromycin ethylsuccinate granules. The elimination half life is approximately 2 hours. Doses may be administered 2, 3 or 4 times a day.

*Preclinical safety data:* Long-term (2 years) oral studies conducted in rats with erythromycin base did not provide evidence of tumorigenicity. Mutagenicity studies have not been conducted. There was no apparent effect on male or female fertility in rats fed erythromycin (base) at levels up to 0.25% of diet. There is no evidence of teratogenicity or any other adverse effect on reproduction in female rats fed erythromycin base (up to 0.25% of diet) prior to and during mating, during gestation and through weaning of 2 successive litters. There are, however, no adequate and well-controlled studies in pregnant women. Because animal reproduction studies are not always predictive of human response, this drug should be used in pregnancy only if it is clearly needed. Erythromycin has been reported to cross the placental barrier in humans, but foetal plasma levels are generally low.

### Pharmaceutical particulars

*List of excipients:* Dye yellow E110; sucrose; sodium citrate granular; saccharin sodium; aluminium magnesium silicate (micro); flavour, orange bramble; silicon dioxide, colloidal; surfactant, polymer 188; carmellose sodium.

*Incompatibilities:* None stated.

*Shelf life:* 36 months in sachets.

*Special precautions for storage:* Store away from heat (30°C).

*Nature and contents of container:* 14 laminate foil sachets.

*Instructions for use/handling:* Not applicable.

**Marketing authorisation number**    0037/0141.

**Date of approval/revision of SPC**    17 October 1996.

**Legal category**    POM.

## ERYTHROPED* PI and ERYTHROPED* PI SACHET
## ERYTHROPED* and ERYTHROPED* SACHET
## ERYTHROPED* FORTE and ERYTHROPED* FORTE SACHET

### Qualitative and quantitative composition

|  | Quantity mg/5 ml or sachet |
|---|---|
| Erythroped PI: Erythromycin as Erythromycin Ethylsuccinate | 125 |
| Erythroped: Erythromycin as Erythromycin Ethylsuccinate | 250 |
| Erythroped Forte: Erythromycin as Erythromycin Ethylsuccinate | 500 |

**Pharmaceutical form**    Granules for reconstitution.

### Clinical particulars

*Therapeutic indications:* For the prophylaxis and treatment of infections caused by erythromycin-sensitive organisms.

Erythromycin is highly effective in the treatment of a great variety of clinical infections.

1. Upper respiratory tract infections: Tonsilitis, peritonsillar abscess, pharyngitis, laryngitis, sinusitus, secondary infections in colds and influenza.

2. Lower respiratory tract infections: Tracheitis, acute and chronic bronchitis, pneumonia (lobar pneumonia, bronchopneumonia, primary atypical pneumonia), bronchiectasis, Legionnaire's disease.

3. Ear infection: Otitis media and otitis externa, mastoiditis.

4. Oral infections: Gingivitis, Vincent's angina.

5. Eye infections: Blepharitis.

6. Skin and soft tissue infections: Boils and carbuncles, paronychia, abscesses, pustular acne, impetigo, cellulitis, erysipelas.

7. Gastrointestinal infections: Cholecystitis, staphylococcal enterocolitis.

8. Prophylaxis: pre- and post-operative, trauma, burns, rheumatic fever.

9. Other infections: Osteomyelitis, urethritis, gonorrhoea, syphilis, lymphogranuloma venereum, diphtheria, prostatitis, scarlet fever.

*Note:* The antibiotic has also proved to be of value in endocarditis and septicaemia, but in these conditions initial administration of erythromycin lactobionate by the intravenous route is advisable.

*Microbiological indications:* Erythromycin is active against a wide variety of pathogenic organisms, gram positive cocci – staphylococci, pneumococci and streptococci (including enterococci) – meningococci, mycoplasma, L-forms, *Haemophilus influenzae*, the agents causing trachoma and lymphogranuloma venereum, chlamydia, clostridia, corynebacterium diphtheria (as an adjunct to antitoxin), neisseria, *Treponema pallidum*, bordetella.

*Note:* The majority of strains of *Haemophilus influenzae* are susceptible to the concentrations reached after ordinary doses.

*Posology and method of administration:* For oral administration.

*ERYTHROPED PI*

*Children up to 2 years of age:* 30 mg/kg/day in divided doses. For severe infections, up to 50 mg/kg/day in divided doses.

Normal doses: 125 mg four times a day or 250 mg twice daily.

*ERYTHROPED*

*Adults:* 2 g/day in divided doses. For severe infections up to 4 g/day in divided doses.

*Children:* 30 mg/kg/day in divided doses. For severe infections, up to 50 mg/kg/day in divided doses. Erythroped suspension is recommended for 2–8 year olds.

Normal dose: 250 mg four times daily or 500 mg twice daily.

*ERYTHROPED FORTE*

*Adults and children over 8 years:* 2 g/day in divided doses. For severe infections up to 4 g/day in divided doses.

**Contra-indications:** Known hypersensitivity to erythromycin. Erythromycin is contraindicated with either astemizole or terfenadine.

Erythromycin is contraindicated with ergotamine and dihydroergotamine.

*Special warnings and special precautions for use:* Erythromycin is excreted principally by the liver, so caution should be exercised in administering the antibiotic to patients with impaired hepatic function or concomitantly receiving potentially hepatotoxic agents. The administration of erythromycin has been infrequently associated with the occurrence of reversible cholestatic jaundice.

There have been reports suggesting erythromycin does not reach the foetus in adequate concentrations to prevent congenital syphilis. Infants born to women treated during pregnancy with oral erythromycin for early syphilis should be treated with an appropriate penicillin regimen. There have been reports that erythromycin may aggravate the weakness of patients with myasthenia gravis.

Erythromycin interferes with the fluorometric determination of urinary catecholamines.

As with other broad spectrum antibiotics, pseudomembranous colitis has been reported rarely with erythromycin.

Rhabdomyolysis with or without renal impairment has been reported in seriously ill patients receiving erythromycin concomitantly with lovastatin.

*Interaction with other medicaments and other forms of interaction:* Concomitant use of erythromycin with terfenadine or astemizole is likely to result in an enhanced risk of cardiotoxicity with these drugs. The concomitant use of erythromycin with either astemizole or terfenadine is therefore contraindicated.

Erythromycin significantly alters the metabolism of terfenadine when taken concomitantly. Rare cases of serious cardiovascular adverse events including death, cardiac arrest, torsades de pointes and other ventricular arrhythmias have been observed.

Concurrent use of erythromycin and ergotamine or dihydroergotamine has been associated in some patients with acute ergot toxicity characterised by the rapid development of severe peripheral vasospasm and dysesthesia.

Increases in serum concentrations of the following drugs may occur when administered concurrently with erythromycin: astemizole, terfenadine, digoxin, warfarin, carbamazepine, phenytoin, theophylline, cyclosporin, ergotamine, dihydroergotamine, hexobarbitone, bromocryptine, disopyramide, valproate, alfentanil, midazolam, and triazolam. Appropriate monitoring should be undertaken and dosage should be adjusted as necessary.

When oral erythromycin is given concurrently with theophylline, there is also a significant decrease in erythromycin serum concentrations. The decrease could result in subtherapeutic concentrations of erythromycin.

*Pregnancy and lactation:* There is no evidence of hazard from erythromycin in human pregnancy. It has been in widespread use for a number of years without apparent ill consequence. Animal studies have shown no hazard.

Erythromycin has been reported to cross the placental barrier in humans, but foetal plasma levels are generally low.

Erythromycin is excreted in breast milk, therefore, caution should be exercised when erythromycin is administered to a nursing mother.

*Effects on ability to drive and to use machines:* None reported.

*Undesirable effects:* Occasional side effects such as nausea, abdominal discomfort, vomiting and diarrhoea may be experienced. Reversible hearing loss associated with doses of erythromycin usually greater than 4 g per day has been reported. Allergic reactions are rare and mild, although anaphylaxis has occurred. Skin reactions ranging from mild eruptions to erythema multiforme, Stevens-Johnson syndrome and toxic epidermal necrolysis have rarely been reported. There are no reports implicating erythromycin products with abnormal tooth development, and only rare reports of damage to the blood, kidneys, liver or central nervous system.

Cardiac arrhythmias have been very rarely reported in patients receiving erythromycin therapy. There have been isolated reports of chest pain, dizziness and palpitations, however, a cause and effect relationship has not been established.

*Overdosage:* Symptoms: Hearing loss, severe nausea, vomiting and diarrhoea.

Treatment: Gastric lavage, general supportive measures.

### Pharmacological properties

*Pharmacodynamic properties: Anti-microbial action:* Similar to that of penicillin. It is active against most Gram positive and some Gram negative bacteria.

*Absorption and fate:* Erythromycin ethylsuccinate is less susceptible than erythromycin to the adverse effect of gastric acid. It is absorbed from the small intestine. It is widely distributed throughout body tissues. Little metabolism occurs and only about 5% is eliminated in the urine. It is excreted by the liver.

*Pharmacokinetic particulars:* Peak blood levels normally occur within 1 hour of dosing of erythromycin ethylsuccinate granules. The elimination half life is approximately 2 hours. Doses may be administered 2, 3 or 4 times a day.

*Preclinical safety data:* There are no preclinical data of relevance to the prescriber which are additional to that already included in other sections of the SPC.

### Pharmaceutical particulars

*List of excipients:* Polysorbate 80, dye yellow quinoline (E104), sodium methyl hydroxybenzoate, sodium propyl hydroxybenzoate, xanthan gum, sodium citrate powder, sugar cane white granular, titanium dioxide, flavour banana imitation entrapped No 2, flavour entrapped artificial cream.

*Incompatibilities:* None stated.

*Shelf life:* Bottles – 18 months unopened; 14 days after reconstitution. Sachets – 36 months; 18 months when included in a combination pack.

*Special precautions for storage:* Store bottle in a cool, dry place. Erythromycin suspension should be stored in a cool place and the container kept tightly closed. The suspension should be used within 14 days of dispensing. Shake well before using.

*Nature and contents of container:* White (opaque or translucent) HDPE bottles with 140 ml fill. Cap: wadless white polypropylene screw cap or white metal screw cap with waxed aluminium liner or white, child resistant closure with a low density polyethylene liner.

1, 10 or 28 laminate foil sachets. The pack size of 10 sachets contains 4 Erythroped PI sachets, 4 Erythroped sachets and 2 Erythroped Forte sachets and may also be supplied with 4 Erythroped A tablets.

*Instructions for use/handling:* Not applicable.

**Marketing authorisation numbers**

| | |
|---|---|
| Erythroped PI | 0037/0149 |
| Erythroped PI Sachet | 0037/0156 |
| Erythroped | 0037/0150 |
| Erythroped Sachet | 0037/0157 |
| Erythroped Forte | 0037/0151 |
| Erythroped Forte Sachet | 0037/0158 |

**Date of approval/revision of SPC** November 1996.

**Legal category** POM.

## ERYTHROPED* PI SF
## ERYTHROPED* SF
## ERYTHROPED* PI SF SACHET
## ERYTHROPED* SF SACHET

**Presentation** Erythromycin ethylsuccinate in the form of sugar free granules which, when reconstituted, make a banana flavour suspension. It is available in two strengths:

1. Erythroped PI SF which contains 125 mg erythromycin per sachet or 5 ml.
2. Erythroped SF, containing 250 mg erythromycin per sachet or 5 ml.

**Uses** For the prophylaxis and treatment of infections caused by erythromycin sensitive organisms.

*Clinical indications:*

1. Upper respiratory tract infections
2. Lower respiratory tract infections
3. Infections of the external and middle ear
4. Skin and soft tissue infections
5. Oral/dental infections
6. Eye infections
7. Genito-urinary infections
8. Gastrointestinal and biliary infections
9. Other infections: Osteomyelitis, diphtheria, scarlet fever
10. Prophylaxis: pre- and post-operative, trauma, burns, rheumatic fever, infective endocarditis following dental procedures

*Note:* Erythromycin has also proved to be of value in endocarditis and septicaemia, but in these conditions initial administration of erythromycin lactobionate by the intravenous route may be advisable.

*Microbiology:* Erythromycin has been shown to be active in vitro against the following organisms: Staphylococci, Streptococci, *Haemophilus influenzae*, L-forms, Meningococci, *Mycoplasma pneumoniae*, *Legionella pneumophilia*, *Branhamella catarrhalis*, *Bordetella pertussis*, *Corynebacterium diphtheriae* (as an adjunct to antitoxin), Neisseria, *Treponema pallidum*, *Chlamydia trachomatis*, *Chlamydia pneumoniae*, Clostridia, *Ureaplasma urealytica*, Campylobacter, *Listeria monocytogenes.*

*Note:* The majority of strains of *Haemophilus influenzae* are susceptible to the concentrations reached after ordinary doses.

**Dosage and administration**

*Reconstitution:* Erythroped SF products are taken orally after being reconstituted as follows:

Erythroped PI SF: Add 109 ml water to the granules contained in 140 ml bottle and shake vigorously. This will make 140 ml of the suspension, each 5 ml containing 125 mg erythromycin activity.

Erythroped SF: Add 105 ml water to the granules contained in 140 ml bottle and shake vigorously. This will make 140 ml of the suspension, each 5 ml containing 250 mg erythromycin activity.

Erythroped PI SF Sachet and Erythroped SF Sachet: Disperse the contents of the sachet in a little water immediately before taking.

*Recommended dosage*

*Infants and children up to 2 years of age:* Use Erythroped PI SF, 250 mg twice daily or 125 mg four times daily.

*Children between 2 and 8 years:* Use Erythroped SF, 500 mg twice daily or 250 mg four times daily.

In terms of mg/kg the usual childrens dose is 30 mg erythromycin/kg/day in divided doses. In very severe infections this may be increased to 50 mg erythromycin/kg/day in divided doses.

*Elderly:* No special dosage recommendation.

*Period of dosing with regard to indication:* Duration of dosing should be related to the severity and site of infection, but generally lies within the range of 5–14 days. However, the duration may need to be longer in certain cases, e.g. NGU and syphilis 10–21 days or longer, chlamydial inclusion conjunctivitis up to 21 days, acne may require prolonged treatment. Prophylaxis prior to dental or surgical procedures should begin 1½ to 2 hours before the procedure and continued every 6 hours for 8 doses.

**Contra-indications, warnings, etc**

*Contra-indications:* Known hypersensitivity to erythromycin. Erythromycin is contra-indicated with either astemizole or terfenadine.

Erythromycin is contra-indicated with ergotamine and dihydroergotamine.

*Precautions:* Erythromycin is excreted principally by the liver, so caution should be exercised in administering the antibiotic to patients with impaired hepatic function or concomitantly receiving potentially hepatotoxic agents.

The administration of erythromycin has been infrequently associated with the occurrence of reversible cholestatic jaundice.

There have been reports suggesting erythromycin does not reach the foetus in adequate concentrations to prevent congenital syphilis. Infants born to women treated during pregnancy with oral erythromycin for early syphilis should be treated with an appropriate penicillin regimen.

There have been reports that erythromycin may aggravate the weakness of patients with myasthenia gravis.

Erythromycin interferes with the fluorometric determination or urinary catecholamines.

As with other broad spectrum antibiotics, pseudomembraneous colitis has been reported rarely with erythromycin.

Rhabdomyolysis with or without renal impairment has been reported in seriously ill patients receiving erythromycin concomitantly with lovastatin.

*Interactions:* Concomitant use of erythromycin with terfenadine or astemizole is likely to result in an enhanced risk of cardiotoxicity with these drugs. The concomitant use of erythromycin with either astemizole or terfenadine is therefore contra-indicated.

Erythromycin significantly alters the metabolism of terfenadine when taken concomitantly. Rare cases of serious cardiovascular adverse events including death, cardiac arrest, torsades de pointes and other ventricular arrhythmias have been observed.

Concurrent use of erythromycin and ergotamine or dihydroergotamine has been associated in some patients with acute ergot toxicity characterised by the rapid development of severe peripheral vasospasm and dysethesia.

Increases is serum concentrations of the following drugs may occur when administered concurrently with erythromycin: digoxin, warfarin, carbamazepine, phenytoin, theophylline, cyclosporin, bromocriptine, disopyramide, alfentanil, triazolam, astemizole, hexobarbitone, midazolam, terfenadine, valporate. Appropriate monitoring should be undertaken and dosage should be adjusted as necessary.

When oral erythromycin is given concurrently with theophylline, there is also a significant decrease in erythromycin serum concentrations. The decrease could result in subtherapeutic concentrations of erythromycin.

*Use in pregnancy and nursing mothers:* There is no evidence of hazard from erythromycin in human pregnancy. It has been in wide use for many years without apparent ill consequence. Animal studies have shown no hazard.

Erythromycin has been reported to cross the placental barrier in humans, but foetal plasma levels are generally low.

Erythromycin is excreted in breast milk, therefore, caution should be exercised when erythromycin is administered to a nursing mother.

*Side-effects:* Occasional side-effects such as nausea, abdominal discomfort, vomiting and diarrhoea may be experienced. Reversible hearing loss associated with doses of erythromycin usually greater than 4 g per day has been reported. Allergic reactions are rare and mild, although anaphylaxis has occurred. Skin reactions ranging from mild eruptions to erythema multiforme, Stevens-Johnson syndrome and toxic epidermal neurolysis have rarely been reported. There are no reports implicating erythromycin products with abnormal tooth development and only rare reports of damage to the blood, kidneys, liver or central nervous system.

Cardiac arrhythmias have been very rarely reported in patients receiving erythromycin therapy. There have been isolated reports of chest pain, dizziness and palpitations; however, a cause and effect relationship has not been established.

*Overdosage:* Symptoms: Hearing loss, severe nausea, vomiting and diarrhoea. Treatment: Gastric lavage, general supportive measures.

**Pharmaceutical precautions** Erythroped SF suspensions should be stored in a cool place and the container kept tightly closed. The suspensions should be used within 7 days of dispensing. Shake well before using. Store below 30°C.

**Legal category** POM.

**Package quantities** 140 ml bottles and container of 28 single dose sachets (OP).

**Product licence numbers**

| | | |
|---|---|---|
| Erythroped PI SF | 125 mg/5 ml | 0037/0223 |
| Erythroped PI SF Sachet | 125 mg/5 ml | 0037/0226 |
| Erythroped SF | 250 mg/5 ml | 0037/0224 |
| Erythroped SF Sachet | 250 mg/5 ml | 0037/0227 |

## FERROGRAD*

**Presentation** Each red Filmtab* (film-coated tablet Abbott) contains Dried Ferrous Sulphate BP 325 mg (equivalent to 105 mg elemental iron) in a controlled release form (Gradumet*).

**Uses** For the prevention and treatment of iron-deficiency anaemia.

The Gradumet device allows controlled release of ferrous sulphate over a number of hours and reduces gastro-intestinal intolerance. The device consists of an inert plastic matrix, honeycombed by thousands of narrow passages which contain ferrous sulphate together with a water soluble channelling agent. As the tablet passes down the gastro-intestinal tract the iron is leached out. The spent matrix is finally excreted in the stools.

**Dosage and administration**

*Recommended adult oral dosage:* One tablet a day before food. As gastro intestinal intolerance is not a problem with Ferrograd, it should be given on an empty stomach when iron is most effectively absorbed.

*Children:* Not recommended for children under 12 years of age.

*Elderly:* The controlled release tablet and its inert plastic matrix may cause a safety hazard in some elderly or other patients suffering from delayed intestinal transit.

**Contra-indications, warnings, etc**

*Contra-indications:* Intestinal diverticula or any intestinal obstruction.

*Precautions:* Iron interacts with tetracyclines, magnesium trisilicate, trientine and zinc salts and absorption of all of these agents may be impaired. Ferrograd tablets should be kept out of children's reach. The controlled release tablet and its inert plastic matrix may cause a safety hazard in some elderly or other patients suffering from delayed intestinal transit.

*Pregnancy:* Ferrograd tablets are not appropriate for use during pregnancy since they do not contain folic acid.

*Side-effects:* Side-effects reported are similar to those associated with conventional oral iron preparations, ie. nausea, vomiting, abdominal pain or discomfort, diarrhoea and/or constipation, but the incidence of side-effects is less owing to the controlled release of nature of the formulation.

*Overdosage:* Symptoms: Initial symptoms of iron overdosage include nausea, vomiting, diarrhoea, abdominal pain, haematemesis, rectal bleeding, lethargy and circulatory collapse. Hyperglycaemia and metabolic acidosis may also occur. The controlled release characteristic may delay excessive absorption of iron, and thus allow more time for counter measures to be implemented. However, initial symptoms of overdosage may be absent due to the controlled release formulation. Therefore, if overdosage is suspected, treatment should be implemented immediately. In severe cases, after a latent phase, relapse may occur after 24–48 hours, manifested by hypotension, coma and hepatocellular necrosis and renal failure.

Treatment: The following steps are recommended to minimise or prevent further absorption of the medication:

*Children*

1. Administer an emetic such as syrup of ipec.
2. Emesis should be followed by gastric lavage with desferrioxamine solution (2 g/l). This should then be followed by the instillation of desferrioxamine 5 g in

50–100 ml water, to be retained in the stomach. Inducing diarrhoea in children may be dangerous and should not be undertaken in young children. Keep the patient under constant surveillance to detect possible aspiration of vomitus – maintain suction apparatus and standby emergency oxygen in case of need.

3. Unleached tablets are radio-opaque. Therefore, an abdominal x-ray should be taken to determine the number of tablets retained in the stomach following emesis and gastric lavage.

4. Severe poisoning: in the presence of shock and/ or coma with high serum iron levels (serum iron >90 μmol/l) immediate supportive measures plus i.v infusion of desferrioxamine should be instituted. Desferrioxamine 15 mg/kg body weight should be administered every hour by slow i.v infusion to a maximum 80 mg/kg/24 hours. Warning: hypotension may occur if the infusion rate is too rapid.

5. Less severe poisoning: i.m desferrioxamine 1 g 4–6 hourly is recommended.

6. Serum iron levels should be monitored throughout.

*Adults*

1. Administer an emetic.

2. Gastric lavage may be necessary to remove drug already released into the stomach. This should be undertaken using desferrioxamine solution (2 g/l). Desferrioxamine 5 g in 50–100 ml water should be introduced into the stomach following gastric emptying. Keep the patient under constant surveillance to detect possible aspiration of vomitus; maintain suction apparatus and standby emergency oxygen in case of need.

3. Unleached tablets are radio-opaque. Therefore, an abdominal x-ray of the patient should be taken to determine the number of tablets retained in the stomach following emesis and gastric lavage. The risk/benefit ratio of x-raying pregnant women must be carefully weighed but should be avoided if possible.

4. A drink of mannitol or sorbitol should be given to induce small bowel emptying.

5. Severe poisoning: in the presence of shock and/ or coma with high serum iron levels (>142 μmol/l) immediate supportive measures plus i.v infusion of desferrioxamine should be instituted. The recommended dose of desferrioxamine is 5 mg/kg/h by slow i.v infusion up to a maximum of 80 mg/kg/24 hours. Warning: hypotension may occur if the infusion rate is too rapid.

6. Less severe poisoning: i.m desferrioxamine 50 mg/kg up to a maximum dose of 4 g should be given.

7. Serum iron levels should be monitored throughout.

**Pharmaceutical precautions** Nil.

**Legal category** P.

**Package quantities** Ferrograd is supplied in 5 carton packs, each containing 30 (3×10) tablets (OP).

**Further information** Ferrograd Folic tablets are available for the prevention and treatment of anaemia in pregnancy and for the prophylaxis of megaloblastic anaemia of pregnancy.

**Product licence number** 0037/5000R.

# FERROGRAD* FOLIC

**Presentation** A two-layered (red and yellow), round, bi-convex Filmtab* (film-coated tablet Abbott). Each tablet contains Dried Ferrous Sulphate BP 325 mg (equivalent to 105 mg elemental iron) in a controlled release form (red half – Gradumet*) and 350 micrograms Folic Acid BP (yellow half).

**Uses** Ferrograd Folic is indicated:

1. For the prevention and treatment of iron-deficiency anaemia of pregnancy.

2. For the prophylaxis of megaloblastic anaemia of pregnancy.

Folic acid requirements in pregnancy can be met with supplements of between 300 and 400 micrograms daily. Without such supplements folate deficiency may develop leading to megaloblastic anaemia with attendant obstetric risks. Doses over 400 micrograms may mask undiagnosed primary $B_{12}$ deficiency. In the extremely unlikely event of this condition occurring in a pregnant woman, the safe prophylactic dose is considered to be 350 micrograms.

The Gradumet device allows controlled release of ferrous sulphate over a number of hours, and reduces gastro-intestinal intolerance. The device consists of an inert plastic matrix, honeycombed by thousands of narrow passages which contain the ferrous sulphate together with water-soluble channelling agent. As the tablet passes down the gastro-intestinal tract the iron is leached out. The spent matrix is finally excreted in the stools.

**Dosage and administration**

*Recommended adult oral dosage:* One tablet daily before food throughout pregnancy and during the first month of the puerperium.

*Children:* Not recommended for children under 12 years of age.

*Elderly:* The controlled release tablet and its inert plastic matrix may cause a safety hazard in some elderly or other patients suffering from delayed intestinal transit.

**Contra-indications, warnings, etc**

*Contra-indications:* Megaloblastic anaemia due to primary vitamin $B_{12}$ deficiency. Intestinal diverticula or any intestinal obstruction.

*Precautions:* Iron interacts with tetracyclines, magnesium trisilicate, trientine and zinc salts and absorption of all of these agents may be impaired. Ferrograd Folic tablets should be kept out of children's reach. The controlled release tablet and its inert plastic matrix may cause a safety hazard in some elderly or other patients suffering from delayed intestinal transit.

*Side-effects:* Side-effects reported are similar to those associated with conventional oral iron preparations, ie. nausea, vomiting, abdominal pain or discomfort, diarrhoea and/or constipation, but the incidence of side-effects is less owing to the controlled release nature of the formulation.

*Overdosage:* Symptoms: initial symptoms of iron overdosage include nausea, vomiting, diarrhoea, abdominal pain, haematemesis, rectal bleeding, lethargy and circulatory collapse. Hyperglycaemia and metabolic acidosis may also occur. The controlled release characteristic may delay excessive absorption of iron, and thus allow more time for counter measures to be implemented. However, initial symptoms of overdosage may be absent due to the controlled release formulation. Therefore, if overdosage is suspected, treatment should be implemented immediately. In severe cases, after a latent phase, relapse may occur after 24–48 hours, manifested by hypotension, coma and hepatocellular necrosis and renal failure.

Treatment: The following steps are recommended to minimise or prevent further absorption of the medication:

*Children*

1. Administer an emetic such as syrup of ipec.

2. Emesis should be followed by gastric lavage with desferrioxamine solution (2 g/l). This should then be followed by the instillation of desferrioxamine 5 g in 50–100 ml water, to be retained in the stomach. Inducing diarrhoea in children may be dangerous and should not be undertaken in young children. Keep the patient under constant surveillance to detect possible aspiration of vomitus – maintain suction apparatus and standby emergency oxygen in case of need.

3. Unleached tablets are radio-opaque. Therefore, an abdominal x-ray should be taken to determine the number of tablets retained in the stomach following emesis and gastric lavage.

4. Severe poisoning: in the presence of shock and/ or coma with high serum iron levels (serum iron >90 μmol/l) immediate supportive measures plus i.v infusion of desferrioxamine should be instituted. Desferrioxamine 15 mg/kg body weight should be administered every hour by slow i.v infusion to a maximum 80 mg/kg/24 hours. Warning: hypotension may occur if the infusion rate is too rapid.

5. Less severe poisoning: i.m desferrioxamine 1 g 4–6 hourly is recommended.

6. Serum iron levels should be monitored throughout.

*Adults*

1. Administer an emetic.

2. Gastric lavage may be necessary to remove drug already released into the stomach. This should be undertaken using desferrioxamine solution (2 g/l). Desferrioxamine 5 g in 50–100 ml water should be introduced into the stomach following gastric emptying. Keep the patients under constant surveillance to detect possible aspiration of vomitus; maintain suction apparatus and standby emergency oxygen in case of need.

3. Unleached tablets are radio-opaque. Therefore, an abdominal x-ray of the patient should be taken to determine the number of tablets retained in the stomach following emesis and gastric lavage. The risk/benefit ratio of x-raying pregnant women must be carefully weighed but should be avoided if possible.

4. A drink of mannitol or sorbitol should be given to induce small bowel emptying.

5. Severe poisoning: in the presence of shock and/ or coma with high serum iron levels (>142 μmol/l) immediate supportive measures plus i.v infusion of desferrioxamine should be instituted. The recommended dose of desferrioxamine is 5 mg/kg/h by slow i.v infusion up to a maximum of 80 mg/kg/24 hours. Warning: hypotension may occur if the infusion rate is too rapid.

6. Less severe poisoning: i.m desferrioxamine 50 mg/kg up to a maximum dose of 4 g should be given.

7. Serum iron levels should be monitored throughout.

**Pharmaceutical precautions** Nil.

**Legal category** P.

**Package quantities** Ferrograd Folic is supplied in 5 carton packs, each containing 30 (3×10) tablets (OP).

**Further information** Nil.

**Product licence number** 0037/5002R.

# HYTRIN* TABLETS

**Qualitative and quantitative composition** Terazosin as monohydrochloride dihydrate 1 mg, 2 mg, 5 mg or 10 mg per tablet.

**Pharmaceutical form** Round, flat bevelled tablets embossed with ⊐ logo and triangular facets on one face and plain on the other. Hytrin tablets are coloured as follows: 1 mg (white); 2 mg (yellow); 5 mg (tan); 10 mg (blue).

**Clinical particulars**

*Therapeutic indications:* Orally administered Hytrin is indicated in the treatment of mild to moderate hypertension. It may be used in combination with thiazide diuretics and/or other antihypertensive drugs or as sole therapy where other agents are inappropriate or ineffective. The hypotensive effect is most pronounced on the diastolic pressure. Although the exact mechanism of the hypotensive action of terazosin is not established, the relaxation of peripheral blood vessels appears to be produced mainly by competitive antagonism of post-synaptic alpha₁-adrenoceptors. Hytrin usually produces an initial gradual decrease in blood pressure followed by a sustained antihypertensive action.

*Posology and method of administration:*
*Adults:*

*Initial dose* – 1 mg before bedtime is the starting dose for all patients and should not be exceeded. Compliance with this initial dosage recommendation should be strictly observed to minimise potential for acute first-dose hypotensive episodes.

*Subsequent doses* – The single daily dosage may be increased by approximately doubling the dosage at weekly intervals to achieve the desired blood pressure response.

The usual maintenance dose is 2 mg to 10 mg once daily. Doses over 20 mg rarely improve efficacy and doses over 40 mg have not been studied.

*Use with thiazide diuretics and other antihypertensive agents:* When adding a thiazide diuretic or antihypertensive agent to a patient's regimen the dose of Hytrin should be reduced and retitration carried out if necessary. Caution should be observed when Hytrin is administered with thiazides or other antihypertensive agents as hypotension may develop.

*Use in renal insufficiency:* Pharmacokinetic studies indicate that patients with impaired renal function need no alteration in recommended dosage.

*Use in children:* Safety and efficacy in children has not been established.

*Use in the elderly:* Pharmacokinetic studies in the elderly indicate that no alteration in dosage recommendation is required.

*Contra-indications:* Known sensitivity to alpha-adrenoceptor antagonists.

*Special warnings and special precautions for use:* As with other alpha adrenoceptor antagonists, terazosin is not recommended in patients with a history of micturition syncope.

In clinical trials, the incidence of postural hypotension was greater in BPH patients than those with hypertension. In these cases, the incidence of postural hypotension events was greater in patients aged 65 years and over (5.6%) than those aged less than 65 years (2.6%).

If administration is discontinued for more than several days, therapy should be re-instituted using the initial dosing regimen.

*Interaction with other medicaments and other forms of interaction:* In patients receiving terazosin plus ACE inhibitors or diuretics the proportion reporting dizziness or related side effects was greater than in the total population of terazosin treated patients from clinical trials.

Caution should be observed when terazosin is administered with other antihypertensive agents, to avoid the possibility of significant hypotension. When adding terazosin to a diuretic or other antihypertensive agent, dosage reduction and retitration may be necessary.

Terazosin has been given without interaction with analgesics/anti-inflammatories, cardiac glycosides, hypoglycemics, antiarrhythmics, anxiolytics/seda tives, antibacterials, hormone/steroids and drugs used for gout.

*Pregnancy and lactation:* Although no teratogenic effects were seen in animal testing, the safety of Hytrin use during pregnancy or during lactation has not yet been established. Hytrin should not be used therefore in pregnancy unless the potential benefit outweighs the risk.

*Effects on ability to drive and use machines:* Dizziness, light-headedness or drowsiness may occur with the initial dose or in association with missed doses and subsequent reinitiation of Hytrin therapy. Patients should be cautioned about these possible adverse effects and the circumstances in which they may occur and advised to avoid driving or hazardous tasks for approximately 12 hours after initial dose or when the dose is increased.

*Undesirable effects:* Hytrin in common with other alpha-adrenoceptor antagonists may cause syncope. Syncopal episodes have occurred within 30 or 90 minutes of the intitial dose of the drug. Syncope has occasionally occurred in association with rapid dosage increases or the introduction of another antihypertensive agent.

In clinical trials in hypertension, the incidence of syncopal episodes was approximately one per cent. In most cases this was believed to be due to an excessive postural hypotensive effect although occasionally the syncopal episode has been preceded by a bout of tachycardia with heart rates of 120 to 160 beats per minute.

If syncope occurs the patient should be placed in a recumbent position and supportive treatment applied as necessary.

Dizziness, light-headedness or fainting may occur when standing up quickly from a lying or sitting position. Patients should be advised of this possibility and instructed to lie down if these symptoms appear and then sit for a few minutes before standing up to prevent their recurrence.

These adverse effects are self limiting and in most cases do not recur after the initial period of therapy or during subsequent re-titration.

*Adverse events reported with terazosin:* The most common events were asthenia, palpitations, nausea, peripheral oedema, dizziness, somnolence, nasal congestion/rhinitis and blurred vision/amblyopia.

In addition, the following have been reported: back pain; headache; tachycardia; postural hypotension; syncope; oedema; weight gain; pain in extremities; decreased Ibidio; depression; nervousness; paraesthesia; vertigo; dyspnoea; sinusitis and impotence.

Additional adverse reactions reported in clinical trials or reported during marketing experience but not clearly associated with the use of terazosin include the following: chest pain; facial oedema; fever; abdominal pain; neck pain; shoulder pain; vasodilatation; arrhythmia; constipation; diarrhoea; dry mouth; dyspepsia; flatulence; vomiting; gout; arthralgia; arthritis; joint disorders; myalgia; anxiety; insomnia; bronchitis; epistaxis; flu symptoms; pharyngitis; rhinitis; cold symptoms; pruritis; rash; increased cough; sweating; abnormal vision; conjunctivitis; tinnitus; urinary frequency; urinary tract infection and urinary incontinence primarily reported in post-menopausal women.

At least two cases of anaphylactoid reactions have been reported with the administration of terazosin.

*Post marketing experience:* Thrombocytopenia and priapism have been reported. Atrial fibrillation has been reported: however, a cause and effect relationship has not been established.

*Laboratory tests:* Small but statistically significant decreases in haemotocrit, haemoglobin, white blood cells, total protein and albumin were observed in controlled clinical trials. These laboratory findings suggest the possibility of haemodilution. Treatment with terazosin for up to 24 months had no significant effect on prostate specific antigen (PSA) levels.

*Overdosage:* Should administratioin of Hytrin lead to acute hypotension, cardiovascular support is of first importance. Restoration of blood pressure and normalisation of heart rate may be accomplished by keeping the patient in a supine position. If this measure is inadequate, shock should first be treated with volume expanders and if necessary, vasopressors could then be used. Renal function should be monitored and general supportive measures applied as required. Dialysis may not be of benefit since laboratory data indicate that terazosin is highly protein bound.

**Pharmacological properties**

*Pharmacodynamics:* Although the exact mechanism of the hypotensive action is not established, the relaxation of peripheral blood vessels' appears to be produced mainly by competitive antagonism of post-synaptic alpha-adrenoceptors. Hytrin usually produces an initial gradual decrease in blood pressure followed by a sustained antihypertensive action.

Clinical experience indicates that a 2–5% decrease in total cholesterol plasma concentration and a 3–7% decrease in the combined $LDL_c+VLDL_c$ fraction plasma concentration from pretreatment values are associated with the administration of therapeutic doses of terazosin.

In clinical trials, plasma concentrates of total cholesterol and combined low density and very low density lipoproteins were found to be slightly reduced following Hytrin administration. Additionally, the increase in total cholesterol seen with other hypertensive agents did not occur when these were used in combination with Hytrin.

*Pharmacokinetics:* The plasma concentration of the parent drug is a maximum about 1 hour post administration and declines with a half-life of approximately 12 hours. Food has little or no effect on bioavailability. Approximately 40% of the administered dose is eliminated in the urine and 60% in the faeces. The drug is highly bound to plasma proteins.

*Preclinical safety data:* Carcinogenicity: Hytrin has been shown to produce tumours in male rats when administered at a high dose over a long period of time. No such occurrences were seen in female rats or in a similar study in mice. The relevance of these findings with respect to the clinical use of the drug in man is unknown.

**Pharmaceutical particulars**

*List of excipients:* Lactose, maize starch, purified talc, magnesium stearate and purified water; quinoline yellow (E104) 2 mg tablet only; iron oxide burnt sienna (E172) 5 mg tablet only; FD&C No 2 blue (E132) 10 mg tablet only.

*Incompatibilities:* None known.

*Shelf life:* 36 months.

*Special precautions for storage:* None.

*Nature and contents of container:* Tablets in a blister original pack. Blisters are packaged in a carton with a pack insert. Starter pack: 7×1 mg + 21×2 mg tablets. Maintenance packs: 28×2 mg; 28×5 mg; 28×10 mg.

*Instructions for use/handling:* Not applicable.

**Marketing authorisation numbers**

| | |
|---|---|
| 1 mg | 0037/0159 |
| 2 mg | 0037/0160 |
| 5 mg | 0037/0161 |
| 10 mg | 0037/0162 |

**Date of approval/revision of SPC** May 1997.

**Legal category** POM.

## HYTRIN* BPH

**Presentation** Hytrin BPH (terazosin as terazosin hydrocloride) is presented as round flat bevelled tablets embossed with the logo and triangular facets on one face and plain on the other. Hytrin BPH tablets are available as follows: 1 mg white tablets; 2 mg yellow tablets; 5 mg tan tablets; and 10 mg blue tablets.

**Uses** Orally administered Hytrin BPH is indicated as a therapy for the symptomatic treatment of urinary obstruction caused by benign prostatic hyperplasia (BPH).

*Actions:* Terazosin is a selective post synaptic alpha-1-adrenoceptor antagonist. Antagonism of alpha-1-receptors on prostatic and urethral smooth muscle has been shown to improve urinary outflow and relieve urinary obstructive symptoms of BPH.

**Dosage and administration**

*Adults only:* The dose of terazosin should be adjusted according to the patient's responses. The following is a guide to its administration:

*Initial dose:* 1 mg before bedtime is the starting dose for all patients and should not be exceeded. Strict compliance with this essential dosage recommendation should be observed to minimise the potential for acute first dose hypotensive episodes (see *Postural Hypotension* below).

*Subsequent doses:* The single daily dose may be increased by approximately doubling the dose at weekly intervals to achieve the desired reduction in symptoms.

The maintenance dose is usually 5 to 10 mg once daily. Improvement in symptoms have been detected as early as two weeks after starting treatment with terazosin.

At present, there are insufficient data to suggest additional symptomatic relief with doses above 10 mg once daily.

*Use in renal insufficiency:* Pharmacokinetic studies indicate that patients with impaired renal function need no alteration in the recommended dosage.

*Use in the elderly:* Pharmacokinetic studies in the elderly indicate that no alteration in dosage recommendation is required.

*Use in children:* Use in children for BPH is not applicable.

**Contra-indications, warnings, etc**

*Contra-indications:* Known sensitivity to alpha-adrenoceptor antagonists.

*Interactions:* In patients receiving terazosin plus ACE inhibitors or diuretics the proportion reporting dizziness or related side effects was greater than in the total population of terazosin treated patients from clinical trials.

Caution should be observed when terazosin is administered with other antihypertensive agents, to avoid the possibility of significant hypotension. When adding terazosin to a diuretic or other antihypertensive agent, dosage reduction and retitration may be necessary.

Terazosin has been given without interaction with analgesics/anti-inflammatories, cardiac glycosides, hypoglycemics, antiarrhythmics, anxiolytic/sedatives, antibacterials, hormones/steroids and drugs used for gout.

*Warnings:* As with other alpha adrenoceptor antagonists, terazosin is not recommended in patients with a history of micturition syncope.

*Postural hypotension:* Postural hypotension has been reported to occur in patients receiving terazosin for the symtomatic treatment of urinary obstruction caused by BPH. In clinical trials, the incidence of postural hypotension was greater in BPH patients than those with hypertension. In these cases, the incidence of postural hypotension events was greater in patients aged 65 years and over (5.6%) than those aged less than 65 years (2.6%).

If administration is discontinued for more than several days, therapy should be re-instituted using the initial dosing regimen.

Carcinogenicity: Hytrin has been shown to produce tumours in male rats when administered at a high dose over a long period of time. No such occurences were seen in female rats or in a similar study of mice. The relevance of these findings with respect to the clinical use of the drug in man is unknown.

*Precautions:* Dizziness, light-headedness or drowsiness may occur with the initial dose or in association with missed doses and subsequent reinitiation of Hytrin therapy. Patients should be cautioned about these possible adverse effects and the circumstnces in which they may occur and advised to avoid driving or hazardous tasks for approximately 12 hours after initial dose or when the dose is increased.

*Side effects:* Hytrin in common with other alpha-adrenoceptor antagonists may cause syncope. Syncopal episodes have occurred within 30 to 90 minutes of the initial dose of the drug. Syncope has occasionally occurred in association with rapid dosage increases or the introduction of another anti-hypertensive agent.

In clincial trials in hypertension, the incidence of syncopal episodes was approximately one per cent. In most cases this was believed to be due to an excessive postural hypotensive effect although occasionally the syncopal episode has been preceded by a bout of tachycardia with heart rates of 120 to 160 beats per minute.

If syncope occurs the patient should be placed in a recumbent position and supportive treatment applied as necessary.

Dizziness, light-headedness or fainting may occur when standing up quickly from a lying or sitting position. Patients should be advised of this possibility and instructed to lie down if these symptoms appear and then sit for a few minutes before standing to prevent their recurrence.

These adverse effects are self limiting and in most cases do not recur after the initial period of therapy or during subsequent re-titration.

*Adverse events reported with terazosin:* The most common events were asthenia, palpitations, nausea, peripheral oedema, dizziness, somnolence, nasal congestion/rhinitis and blurred vision/amblyopia.

In addition, the following have been reported: back pain; headache; tachycardia; postural hypotension; syncope; oedema; weight gain; pain in extremities; decreased libido; depression; nervousness; paraesthesia; vertigo; dyspnoea; sinutitis and impotence.

Additional adverse reactions reported in clinical trials or reported during marketing experience but not clearly associated with the use of terazosin include the following: chest pain; facial oedema; fever; abdominal pain; neck pain; shoulder pain; vasodilation; arrhythmia; constipation; diarrhoea; dry mouth; dyspepsia; flatulence; vomiting; gout; arthralgia; arthritis; joint disorders; myalgia; anxiety; insomnia; bronchitis; epistaxis; flu symptoms; pharyngitis; rhinitis; cold symptoms; pruritis; rash; increased cough; sweating; abnormal vision; conjunctivitis; tinnitus; urinary frequency; urinary tract infection and urinary incontinence primarily reported in post-menopausal women.

At least two cases of anaphylactoid reactions have been reported with the administration of terazosin.

*Post marketing experience:* Thrombocytopenia and priapism have been reported. Atrial fibrillation has been reported: however, a cause and effect relationship has not been established.

*Laboratory tests:* Small but statistically significant decreases in haematocrit, haemoglobin, white blood cells, total protein and albumin were observed in controlled clinical trials. These laboratory findings suggest the possibility of haemodilution. Treatment with terazosin for up to 24 months had not significant effect on prostate specific antigen (PSA) levels.

*Use in pregnancy:* Although no teratogenic effects were seen in animal testing, the safety of Hytrin use during pregnancy or during lactation has not yet been established. Hytrin should not be used therefore in pregnancy unless the potential benefit outweighs the risk.

*Treatment of overdosage:* Should administration of terazosin lead to acute hypotension, cardiovascular support is of first importance. Restoration of blood pressure and normalisation of heart rate may be accomplished by keeping the patient in a supine position. If this measure is inadequate, shock should first be treated with volume expanders and, if necessary, vasopressors could then be used. Renal function should be monitored and general supportive measures applied as required. Dialysis may not be of benefit since laboratory data indicate that terazosin is highly protein bound.

**Pharmaceutical precautions** Nil.

**Legal category** POM.

**Package quantities** Starter Pack: Blister containing 7×1 mg + 14×2 mg + 7×5 mg.
2 mg tablets: Blister packs containing 28 tablets (OP).
5 mg tablets: Blister packs containing 28 tablets (OP).
10 mg tablets: Blister packs containing 28 tablets (OP).

**Further information** Nil.

**Product licence numbers**
1 mg tablet   0037/0234
2 mg tablet   0037/0235
5 mg tablet   0037/0236
10 mg tablet  0037/0237

## ISOFLURANE

**Presentation** Isoflurane is an inhalation anaesthetic with a mildly pungent ethereal odour. No additive or stabiliser is present.

**Uses** Inhalation anaesthesia.

*Actions:* Induction and particularly recovery are rapid. Although slight pungency may limit the rate of induction, excessive salivation and tracheobronchial secretions are not stimulated. Pharyngeal and laryngeal reflexes are diminished quickly. Levels of anaesthesia change rapidly with Isoflurane. Heart rhythm remains stable. Spontaneous respiration becomes depressed as depth of anaesthesia increases and should be closely monitored.

During induction there is a decrease in blood pressure which returns towards normal with surgical stimulation.

Blood pressure tends to fall during maintenance in direct relation to depth of anaesthesia, due to peripheral vasodilation, but cardiac rhythm remains stable. With controlled respiration and normal $PaCO_2$, cardiac output tends to be maintained despite increasing depth of anaesthesia, primarily through a rise in heart rate. With spontaneous respiration, the resulting hypercapnia may increase heart rate and cardiac output above awake levels.

Cerebral blood flow remains unchanged during light Isoflurane anaesthesia but tends to rise at deeper levels. Increases in cerebrospinal fluid pressure may be prevented or reversed by hyperventilating the patient before or during anaesthesia.

Electroencephalographic changes and convulsions are extremely rare with Isoflurane.

Isoflurane appears to sensitise the myocardium to adrenaline to an even lesser extent than enflurane. Limited data suggest that subcutaneous infiltration of up to 50 ml of 1:200,000 solution adrenaline does not induce ventricular arrhythmias in patients anaesthetised with Isoflurane.

Muscular relaxation may be adequate for some intra-abdominal operations at normal levels of anaesthesia, but should greater relaxation be required small doses of intravenous muscle relaxants may be used. All commonly used muscle relaxants are markedly potentiated by Isoflurane, the effect being most profound with non-depolarising agents. Neostigmine reverses the effects of non-depolarising muscle relaxants but has no effect on the relaxant properties of Isoflurane itself. All commonly used muscle relaxants are compatible with Isoflurane.

Isoflurane may be used for the induction and maintenance of general anaesthesia. Adequate data are not available to establish its place in pregnancy or obstetrics anaesthesia other than for caesarian section.

Relatively little metabolism of Isoflurane occurs in the human body. In the post-operative period only 0.17% of the isoflurane taken up can be recovered as urinary metabolites. Peak serum inorganic fluoride values usually average less than 5 micromol/litre and occur about four hours after anaesthesia, returning to normal levels within 24 hours. No signs of renal injury have been reported after Isoflurane administration.

**Dosage and administration** Vaporisers specially calibrated for Isoflurane should be used so that the concentration of anaesthetic delivered can be accurately controlled.

MAC values for Isoflurane vary with age. The table below indicates average MAC values for different age groups:

| Age | Average MAC value in oxygen |
| --- | --- |
| 0–1 month | 1.6% |
| 1–6 months | 1.87% |
| 6–12 months | 1.8% |
| 1–5 years | 1.6% |
| mid-twenties | 1.28% |
| mid-forties | 1.15% |
| mid-sixties | 1.05% |

*Premedication:* Drugs used for premedication should be selected for the individual patient, bearing in mind the respiratory depressant effect of Isoflurane. The use of anticholinergic drugs is a matter of choice but may be advisable for inhalation induction in paediatrics.

*Induction:* A short-acting barbiturate or other intravenous induction agent is usually administered followed by inhalation of the Isoflurane mixture. Alternatively, Isoflurane with oxygen or with an oxygen/nitrous oxide mixture may be used.

It is recommended that induction with Isoflurane be initiated at a concentration of 0.5%. Concentrations of 1.5 to 3.0% usually produce surgical anaesthesia in 7 to 10 minutes.

*Maintenance:* Surgical levels of anaesthesia may be maintained with 1.0–2.5% Isoflurane in oxygen/nitrous oxide mixtures. An additional 0.5–1.0% Isoflurane may be required when given with oxygen alone.

For caesarian section, 0.5–0.75% Isoflurane in a mixture of oxygen/nitrous oxide is suitable to maintain anaesthesia for this procedure.

Arterial pressure levels during maintenance tend to be inversely related to alveolar Isoflurane concentrations in the absence of other complicating factors. Excessive falls in blood pressure may be due to depth of anaesthesia and, in these circumstances, should be corrected by reducing the inspired Isoflurane concentration.

*Elderly:* As with other agents, lesser concentrations of Isoflurane are normally required to maintain surgical anaesthesia in elderly patients. See above for MAC values.

**Contra-indications, warnings, etc**
*Contra-indications:* Known sensitivity to Isoflurane, or history of malignant hyperpyrexia following its administration should be considered contra-indications.

*Precautions:* Since levels of anaesthesia may be altered quickly and easily with Isoflurane, only vaporisers which deliver a predictable output with reasonable accuracy, or techniques during which inspired or expired concentrations can be monitored, should be used. The degree of hypotension and respiratory depression may provide some indication of anaesthetic depth.

Clinical data demonstrate that Isoflurane may produce hepatic injury in very rare instances.

As with other halogenated agents, Isoflurane must be used with caution in patients with increased intracranial pressure. In such cases hyperventilation may be necessary.

The action of non-depolarising relaxants is markedly potentiated with Isoflurane.

Isoflurane has been reported to interact with dry carbon dioxide absorbents to form carbon monoxide. In order to minimise the risk of formation of carbon monoxide in rebreathing circuits and the possibility of elevated carboxyhaemoglobin levels, carbon dioxide absorbents should not be allowed to dry out.

*Use in pregnancy:* Reproduction studies have been carried out on animals after repeated exposure to anaesthetic concentrations of Isoflurane. Studies with the rat demonstrated no effect on fertility, pregnancy or delivery or on the viability of the offspring. No evidence of teratogenicity was revealed. Comparable experiments in rabbits produced similar negative results. The relevance of these studies to the human is not known. Safety in pregnancy has not been established. Blood losses comparable with those found following anaesthesia with other inhalation agents have been observed with isoflurane in patients undergoing induced abortion. Adequate data have not been developed to establish the safety of Isoflurane in obstetric anaesthesia, other than for caesarian section.

*Side effects:*
1. Arrhythmias have been occasionally reported.
2. Elevation of the white blood cell count has been observed, even in the absence of surgical stress.
3. Minimally raised levels of serum inorganic fluoride occur during and after Isoflurane anaesthesia, due to biodegradation of the agent. It is unlikely that the low levels of serum inorganic fluoride observed (mean 4.4 micromol/l in one study) could cause renal toxicity, as these are well below the proposed threshold levels for kidney toxicity.
4. Undesirable effects during recovery (shivering, nausea and vomiting) are minor in nature and comparable in incidence with those found with other anaesthetics.

*Overdosage:* As with other halogenated anaesthetics, hypotension and respiratory depression have been observed. Close monitoring of blood pressure and respiration is recommended. Supportive measures may be necessary to correct hypotension and respiratory depression resulting from excessively deep levels of anaesthesia.

**Pharmaceutical precautions** Store below 25°C. Keep container well closed.

**Legal category** P.

**Package quantities** Isoflurane is supplied in bottles of 250 ml.

**Further information** Nil.

**Product licence number** 0037/0115.

## KLARICID*

**Qualitative and quantitative composition** Clarithromycin 250 mg per tablet.

**Pharmaceutical form** A yellow, ovaloid film-coated tablet containing 250 mg of clarithromycin.

**Clinical particulars**
*Therapeutic indications:* Klaricid is indicated in the treatment of infections caused by one or more susceptible organisms. Indications include:

Lower respiratory tract infections for example, acute and chronic bronchitis, and pneumonia.

Upper respiratory tract infections for example, sinusitis and pharyngitis.

Klaricid is appropriate for initial therapy in community acquired respiratory infections and has been shown to be active *in vitro* against common and atypical respiratory pathogens as listed in the microbiology section.

Klaricid is also indicated in skin and soft tissue infections of mild to moderate severity.

Klaricid in the presence of acid suppression effected by omeprazole is also indicated for the eradication of *H pylori* in patients with duodenal ulcers. See *Dosage and administration* section.

Klaricid is usually active against the following organisms *in vitro*:

*Gram-positive bacteria: Staphylococcus aureus* (methicillin susceptible); *Streptococcus pyogenes* (Group A beta-haemolytic streptococci); alpha haemolytic streptococci (viridans group); *Streptococcus (Diplococcus) pneumoniae; Streptococcus agalactiae; Listeria monocytogenes.*

*Gram-negative bacteria: Haemophilus influenzae; Haemophilus parainfluenzae, Moraxella (Branhamella) catarrhalis, Neisseria gonorrhoeae; Legionella pneumophila, Bordetella pertussis, Helicobacter pylori; Campylobacter jejuni.*

*Mycoplasma: Mycoplasma pneumoniae; Ureaplasma urealyticum.*

*Other organisms: Chlamydia trachomatis; Mycobacterium avium; Mycobacterium leprae.*

*Anaerobes:* Macrolide-susceptible *Bacteroides fragilis; Clostridium perfringens; Peptococcus species; Peptostreptococcus* species; *Propionibacterium* acnes.

Clarithromycin also has bactericidal activity against several bacterial strains. These organisms include *Haemophilus influenzae, Streptococcus pneumoniae, Streptococcus pyogenes, Streptococcus agalactiae, Moraxella (Branhamella) catarrhalis, Neisseria gonorrhoeae, Helicobacter pylori* and *Campylobacter* spp.

The activity of clarithromycin against *H pylori* is greater at neutral pH than at acid pH.

*Posology and method of administration*
*Patients with respiratory tract/skin and soft tissue infections:*
*Adults:* The usual dose is 250 mg twice daily for

days although this may be increased to 500 mg twice daily for up to 14 days in severe infections.

*Children older than 12 years:* As for adults.
*Children younger than 12 years:* Use Klaricid Paediatric Suspension.

*Eradication of H pylori in patients with duodenal ulcers (Adults):*

*Dual therapy:* The usual dose of clarithromycin is 500 mg three times daily for 14 days. Klaricid (500 mg tds) may be administered with oral omeprazole 40 mg once daily. The pivotal study was conducted with omeprazole 40 mg once daily for 28 days. Supportive studies have been conducted with omeprazole 40 mg once daily for 14 days.

For further information on the dosage for omeprazole see the Astra data sheet.

*Triple therapy:* Klaricid (500 mg) twice daily should be given with amoxycillin 1000 mg twice daily and omeprazole 20 mg daily for 10 days.

*Elderly:* As for adults.

*Renal impairment:* Dosage adjustments are not usually required except in patients with severe renal impairment (creatinine clearance <30 ml/min). If adjustment is necessary, the total daily dosage should be reduced by half, e.g. 250 mg once daily or 250 mg twice daily in more severe infections.

Klaricid may be given without regard to meals as food does not affect the extent of bioavailability.

*Contra-indications:* Clarithromycin is contra-indicated in patients with known hypersensitivity to macrolide antibiotic drugs.

Clarithromycin and ergot derivates should not be co-administered.

Concomitant administration of clarithromycin and any of the following drugs is contra-indicated: cisapride, pimozide and terfenadine. Elevated cisapride, pimozide and terfenadine levels have been reported in patients receiving either of these drugs and clarithromycin concomitantly. This may result in QT prolongation and cardiac arrhythmias including ventricular tachycardia, ventricular fibrillation and Torsade de Pointes. Similar effects have been observed with concomitant administration of astemizole and other macrolides.

*Special warnings and special precautions for use:* Clarithromycin is principally excreted by the liver and kidney. Caution should be exercised in administering this antibiotic to patients with impaired hepatic or renal function.

Prolonged or repeated use of clarithromycin may result in an overgrowth of non-susceptible bacteria or fungi. If super-infection occurs, clarithromycin should be discontinued and appropriate therapy instituted.

*H pylori* organisms may develop resistance to clarithromycin in a small number of patients.

*Interaction with other medicaments and other forms of interaction:* Clarithromycin has been shown not to interact with oral contraceptives.

As with other macrolide antibiotics the use of clarithromycin in patients concurrently taking drugs metabolised by the cytochrome p450 system (e.g. warfarin, ergot alkaloids, triazolam, midazolam, disopyramide, lovastatin, phenytoin and cyclosporin) may be associated with elevations in serum levels of these other drugs.

The administration of clarithromycin to patients who are receiving theophylline has been associated with an increase in serum theophylline levels and potential theophylline toxicity.

The use of clarithromycin in patients receiving warfarin may result in potentiation of the effects of warfarin. Prothrombin time should be frequently monitored in these patients. The effects of digoxin may be potentiated with concomitant administration of Klaricid. Monitoring of serum digoxin levels should be considered.

Clarithromycin may potentiate the effects of carbamazepine due to a reduction in the rate of excretion.

Simultaneous oral administratioin of clarithromycin tablets and zidovudine to HIV infected adult patients may result in decreased steady-state zidovudine levels. This can be largely avoided by staggering the doses of Klaricid and zidovudine by 1 to 2 hours. No such reaction has been reported in children.

Although the plasma concentrations of clarithromycin and omeprazole may be increased when they are administered concurrently, no adjustment to the dosage is necessary. Increased plasma concentrations of clarithromycin may also occur when it is co-administered with Maalox or ranitidine. No adjustment to the dosage is necessary.

*Pregnancy and lactation:* The safety of clarithromycin during pregnancy and breast feeding of infants has not been established. Klaricid should thus not be used during pregnancy or lactation unless the benefit is considered to outweigh the risk. Some animal studies have suggested an embryotoxic effect, but only at dose levels which are clearly toxic to mothers. Clarithromycin has been found in milk of lactating animals and in human breast milk.

*Effects on ability to drive and use machines:* None known.

*Undesirable effects:* Clarithromycin is generally well tolerated. Side effects include nausea, dyspepsia, diarrhoea, vomiting and abdominal pain. Stomatitis, glossitis and oral monilia have been reported. Other side-effects include headache and allergic reactions ranging from urticaria and mild skin eruptions to anaphylaxis and rarely Stevens-Johnson syndrome. Taste perversion may occur. Reversible tongue discolouration has been seen in clinical trials when clarithromycin and omeprazole were given together. There have been reports of transient central nervous system side-effects including anxiety, dizziness, insomnia, hallucinations, psychosis, bad dreams and confusion, however, a cause and effect relationship has not been established. There have been reports of hearing loss with clarithromycin which is usually reversible upon withdrawal of therapy. Pseudomembranous colitis has been reported rarely with clarithromycin, and may range in severity from mild to life threatening. As with other macrolides, hepatic dysfunction (which is usually reversible) including altered liver function tests, hepatitis and cholestasis with or without jaundice, has been reported. Dysfunction may be severe and very rarely fatal hepatic failure has been reported.

*Overdosage:* Reports indicate that the ingestion of large amounts of clarithromycin can be expected to produce gastro-intestinal symptoms. One patient who had a history of bipolar disorder ingested 8 g of clarithromycin and showed altered mental status, paranoid behaviour, hypokalemia and hypoxemia. Allergic reactions accompanying overdosage should be treated by gastric lavage and supportive measures. As with other macrolides, clarithromycin serum levels are not expected to be appreciably affected by haemodialysis or peritoneal dialysis.

**Pharmaceutical properties**

*Microbiology:* Clarithromycin is a semi-synthetic derivative of erythromycin A. It exerts its antibacterial action by binding to the 50s ribosomal sub-unit of susceptible bacteria and suppresses protein synthesis. It is highly potent against a wide variety of aerobic and anaerobic gram-positive and gram-negative organisms. The minimum inhibitory concentrations (MICs) of clarithromycin are generally two-fold lower than the MICs of erythromycin.

The 14-hydroxy metabolite of clarithromycin also has antimicrobial activity. The MICs of this metabolite are equal or two-fold higher than the MICs of the parent compound, except for *H influenzae* where the 14-hydroxy metabolite is two-fold more active than the parent compound.

Klaricid is usually active against the following organisms *in vitro*:

*Gram-positive bacteria: Staphylococcus* (methicillin susceptible); *Streptococcus pyogenes* (Group A beta-hemolytic streptococci); alpha-hemolytic streptococci (viridans group); *Streptococcus (Diplococcus) pneumoniae; Streptococcus agalactiae; Listeria monocytogenes.*

*Gram-negative bacteria: Haemophilus influenzae; Haemophilus parainfluenzae; Moraxella (Branhamella) catarrhalis; Neisseria gonorrhoeae; Legionella pneumophila; Bordetella pertussis; Helicobacter pylori; Campylobacter jejuni.*

*Mycoplasma: Mycoplasma pneumoniae; Ureaplasma urealyticum.*

*Other organisms: Chlamydia trachomatis; Mycobacterium avium; Mycobacterium leprae; Mycobacterium Kansasaii; Mycobacterium chelonae; Mycobacterium fortuitum; Mycobacterium intracellulare.*

*Anaerobes:* Macrolide-susceptible *Bacteroides fragilis; Clostridium perfringens; Peptococcus* species; *Peptostreptococcus* species; *Propionibacterium* acnes.

Clarithromycin has bactericidal activity against several bacterial strains. The organisms include *Haemophilus influenzae, Streptococcus pneumoniae, Streptococcus pyogenes, Streptococcus agalactiae, Moraxella (Branhamella) catarrhalis, Neisseria gonorrhoeae* and *Helicobacter pylori* and *Campylobacter* spp.

*Pharmacokinetics: Helicobacter pylori (H pylori)* is associated with acid peptic disease including duodenal ulcer and gastric ulcer in which about 95% and 80% of patients respectively are infected with the agent. *H pylori* is also implicated as a major contribution factor in the development of gastric and ulcer recurrence in such patients.

Clarithromycin has been used in small numbers of patients in other treatment regimens. Possible kinetic interactions have not been fully investigated. These regimens include: clarithromycin plus tinidazole and omeprazole; clarithromycin plus tetracycline, bismuth subsalicylate and ranitidine; clarithromycin plus ranitidine alone.

Clinical studies using various different *H pylori* eradication regimens (including clarithromycin plus omeprazole) have shown that eradication of *H pylori* prevents ulcer recurrence.

Clarithromycin is rapidly and well absorbed from the gastro-intestinal tract after oral administration of Klaricid tablets. The microbiologically active metabolite 14-hydroxyclarithromycin is formed by first pass metabolism. Klaricid may be given without regard to meals as food does not affect the extent of bioavailability of Klaricid tablets. Food does slightly delay the onset of absorption of clarithromycin and formation of the 14-hydroxymetabolite. The pharmacokinetics of clarithromycin are non linear; however, steady-state is attained within 2 days of dosing. At 250 mg b.i.d. 15–20% of unchanged drug is excreted in the urine. With 500 mg b.i.d. daily dosing urinary excretion is greater (approximately 36%). The 14-hydroxy-clarithromycin is the major urinary metabolite and accounts for 10–15% of the dose. Most of the remainder of the dose is eliminated in the faeces, primarily via the bile. 5–10% of the parent drug is recovered from the faeces.

When clarithromycin 500 mg is given three times daily, the clarithromycin plasma concentrations are increased with respect to the 500 mg twice daily dosage.

Klaricid provides tissue concentrations that are several times higher than the circulating drug levels. Increased levels have been found in both tonsillar and lung tissue. Clarithromycin is 80% bound to plasma proteins at therapeutic levels.

Klaricid also penetrates the gastric mucus. Levels of clarithromycin in gastric mucus and gastric tissue are higher when clarithromycin is co-administered with omeprazole than when clarithromycin is administered alone.

*Preclinical safety data:* In acute mouse and rat studies, the median lethal dose was greater than the highest feasible dose for administration (5 g/kg).

In repeated dose studies, toxicity was related to dose, duration of treatment and species. Dogs were more sensitive than primates or rats. The major clinical signs at toxic doses included emesis, weakness, reduced food consumption and weight gain, salivation, dehydration and hyperactivity. In all species the liver was the primary target organ at toxic doses. Hepatotoxicity was detectable by early elevations of liver function tests. Discontinuation of the drug generally resulted in a return to or toward normal results. Other tissues less commonly affected included the stomach, thymus and other lymphoid tissues and the kidneys. At near therapeutic doses, conjunctival injection and lacrimation occurred only in dogs. At a massive dose of 400 mg/kg/day, some dogs and monkeys developed corneal opacities and/or oedema.

Fertility and reproduction studies in rats have shown no adverse effects. Teratogenicity studies in rats (Wistar (p.o.) and Sprague-Dawley (p.o. and i.v.)), New Zealand White rabbits and cynomolgous monkeys failed to demonstrate any teratogenicity from clarithromycin. However, a further similar study in Sprague-Dawley rats indicated a low (6%) incidence of cardiovascular abnormalities which appeared to be due to spontaneous expression of genetic changes. Two mouse studies revealed a variable incidence (3–30%) of cleft palate and embryonic loss was seen in monkeys but only at dose levels which were clearly toxic to the mothers.

**Pharmaceutical particulars**

*List of excipients:* Croscarmellose sodium; starch, pregelatinised; cellulose microcrystalline; quinoline yellow, E104; silica gel; povidone; stearic acid; magnesium stearate; talc.

*Tablet coating:* Hypromellose; hydroxypropylcellulose; propylene glycol; sorbitan monooleate; titanium dioxide; sorbic acid; vanillin; quinoline yellow E104.

*Incompatibilities:* None known.

*Shelf life:* The recommended shelf life is 24 months.

*Special precautions for storage:* Protect from light. Store in a dry place.

*Nature and contents of container:* 2/14 tablets in a blister pack. The blisters are packaged in a carton with a pack insert.

*Instructions for use/handling:* Not applicable.

**Marketing authorisation number** 0037/0211.

**Date of approval/revision of SPC** August 1996.

**Legal category** POM.

## KLARICID* 500

**Qualitative and quantitative composition** Clarithromycin 500 mg/tablet.

**Pharmaceutical form** A yellow, ovaloid film-coated tablet containing 500 mg of clarithromycin.

**Clinical particulars**

*Therauputic indications:* Klaricid is indicated for treatment of infections caused by susceptible organisms. Indications include:

Lower respiratory tract infections for example, acute and chronic bronchitis, and pneumonia.

Upper respiratory tract infections for example, sinusitis and pharyngitis.

Klaricid is appropriate for initial therapy in community acquired respiratory infections and has been shown to be active *in vitro* against common and atypical respiratory pathogens as listed in the microbiology section.

Klaricid is also indicated in skin and soft tissue infections of mild to moderate severity.

Klaricid in the presence of acid suppression effected by omeprazole is also indicated for the eradication of *H pylori* in patients with duodenal ulcers. See *Posology and method of administration* section.

Klaricid is usually active against the following organisms *in vitro*:

Gram-positive bacteria: *Staphylococcus aureus* (methicillin susceptible); *Streptococcus pyogenes* (Group A beta-hemolytic streptococci) alpha-hemolytic streptococci (viridans group); *Streptococcus* (*Diplococcus*) *pneumoniae*; *Streptococcus agalactiae*, *Listeria monocytogenes*.

Gram-negative bacteria: *Haemophilus influenzae*, *Haemophilus parainfluenzae*, *Moraxella (Branhamella) catarrhalis*, *Neisseria gonorrhoeae*; *Legionella pneumophila*, *Bordetella pertussis*, *Helicobacter pylori*; *Campylobacter jejuni*.

Mycoplasma: *Mycoplasma pneumoniae*; *Ureaplasma urealyticum*.

Other organisms: *Chlamydia trachomatis*; *Mycobacterium avium*; *Mycobacterium leprae*; *Mycobacterum Kansasaii*; *Mycobacterium chelonae*; *Mycobacterium fortuitum*; *Mycobacterium intracellulare*.

Anaerobes: Macrolide-susceptible *Bacteroides fragilis*; *Clostridium perfringens*; *Peptococcus* species; *Peptostreptococcus* species; *Propionibacterium acnes*.

Clarithromycin has bactericidal activity against several bacterial strains. The organisms include *Haemophilus influenzae*, *Streptococcus pneumoniae*, *Streptococcus pyogenes*, *Streptococcus agalactiae*, *Moraxella (Branhamella) catarrhalis*, *Neisseria gonorrhoeae*, *Helicobacter pylori* and *Campylobacter* spp.

The activity of clarithromycin against *Helicobacter pylori* is greater at neutral pH than at acid pH.

*Posology and method of administration*

*Patients with respiratory tract/skin and soft tissue infections*

*Adults:* The usual dose is 250 mg twice daily for 7 days although this may be increased to 500 mg twice daily for up to 14 days in severe infections.

*Children older than 12 years:* As for adults.

*Children younger than 12 years:* Use Klaricid Paediatric Suspension.

*Eradication of H pylori in patients with duodenal ulcers (Adults):*

*Triple therapy (7 days):* Klaricid (500 mg) twice daily and omeprazole 40 mg daily should be given with amoxycillin 1000 mg twice daily for 7 days.

*Triple therapy (10 days):* Klaricid (500 mg) twice daily should be given with amoxycillin 1000 mg twice daily and omeprazole 20 mg daily for 10 days.

*Dual therapy (14 days):* The usual dose of Klaricid is 500 mg three times daily for 14 days. Klaricid should be administered with oral omeprazole 40 mg once daily. The pivotal study was conducted with omeprazole 40 mg once daily for 28 days. Supportive studies have been conducted with omeprazole 40 mg once daily for 14 days.

For further information on the dosage for omeprazole see the Astra data sheet.

*Elderly:* As for adults.

*Renal impairment:* Dosage adjustments are not usually required except in patients with severe renal impairment (creatinine clearance <30 ml/min). If adjustment is necessary, the total daily dosage should be reduced by half, e.g. 250 mg once daily or 250 mg twice daily in more severe infections.

Klaricid may be given without regard to meals as food does not affect the extent of bioavailability.

*Contra-indications:* Clarithromycin is contra-indicated in patients with known hypersensitivity to macrolide antibiotic drugs.

Clarithromycin and ergot derivatives should not be co-administered.

Concomitant administration of clarithromycin and any of the following drugs is contra-indicated: cisapride, pimozide and terfenadine. Elevated cisapride, pimozide and terfenadine levels have been reported in patients receiving either of these drugs and clarithromycin concomitantly. This may result in QT prolongation and cardiac arrhythmias including ventricular tachycardia, ventricular fibrillation and Torsade de Pointes. Similar effects have been observed with concomitant administration of astemizole and other macrolides.

*Special warnings and special precautions for use:* Clarithromycin is principally excreted by the liver and kidney. Caution should be exercised in administering this antibiotic to patients with impaired hepatic or renal function.

Prolonged or repeated use of clarithromycin may result in an overgrowth of non-susceptible bacteria or fungi. If super-infection occurs, clarithromycin should be discontinued and appropriate therapy instituted.

*H pylori* organisms may develop resistance to clarithromycin in a small number of patients.

*Interaction with other medicaments and other forms of interaction:* Clarithromycin has been shown not to interact with oral contraceptives.

As with other macrolide antibiotics the use of clarithromycin in patients concurrently taking drugs metabolised by the cytochrome p450 system (e.g. warfarin, ergot alkaloids, triazolam, midazolam, disopyramide, lovastatin, phenytoin and cyclosporin) may be associated with elevations in serum levels of these other drugs.

The administration of clarithromycin to patients who are receiving theophylline has been associated with an increase in serum theophylline levels and potential theophylline toxicity.

The use of clarithromycin in patients receiving warfarin may result in potentiation of the effects of warfarin. Prothrombin time should be frequently monitored in these patients. The effects of digoxin may be potentiated with concomitant administration of Klaricid. Monitoring of serum digoxin levels should be considered.

Clarithromycin may potentiate the effects of carbamazepine due to a reduction in the rate of excretion.

Simultaneous oral administration of clarithromycin tablets and zidovudine to HIV infected adult patients may result in decreased steady-state zidovudine levels. This can be largely avoided by staggering the doses of Klaricid and zidovudine by 1–2 hours. No such reaction has been reported in children.

Although the plasma concentrations of clarithromycin and omeprazole may be increased when they are administered concurrently, no adjustment to the dosage is necessary. Increased plasma concentrations of clarithromycin may also occur when it is co-administered with Maalox or ranitidine. No adjustment to the dosage is necessary.

*Pregnancy and lactation:* The safety of clarithromycin during pregnancy and breast feeding of infants has not been established. Klaricid should thus not be used during pregnancy or lactation unless the benefit is considered to outweight the risk. Some animal studies have suggested an embryotoxic effect, but only at dose levels which are clearly toxic to mothers. Clarithromycin has been found in the milk of lactating animals and in human breast milk.

*Effects on ability to drive and use machines:* None known.

*Undesirable effects:* Clarithromycin is generally well tolerated. Side effects reported include nausea, dyspepsia, diarrhoea, vomiting and abdominal pain. Stomatitis and glossitis and oral monilia have been reported. Other side-effects include headache and allergic reactions ranging from urticaria and mild skin eruptions to anaphylaxis and rarely Stevens-Johnson syndrome. Taste perversion may occur. Reversible tongue discolouration has been seen in clinical trials when clarithromycin and omeprazole were given together. There have been reports of transient central nervous system side-effects including anxiety, dizziness, insomnia, hallucinations, psychosis, bad dreams and confusion, however, a cause and effect relationship has not been established. There have been reports of hearing loss with clarithromycin which is reversible upon withdrawal of therapy. Pseudomembranous colitis has been reported rarely with clarithromycin, and may range in severity from mild to life threatening. As with other macrolides, hepatic dysfunction (which is usually reversible) including altered liver function tests, hepatitis and cholestasis with or without jaundice, has been reported. Dysfunction may be severe and very rarely fatal hepatic failure has been reported.

*Overdosage:* Reports indicate that the ingestion of large amounts of clarithromycin can be expected to produce gastro-intestinal symptoms. One patient who had a history of bipolar disorder ingested 8 grams of clarithromycin and showed altered mental status, paranoid behaviour, hypokalemia and hypoxemia. Allergic reactions accompanying overdosage should be treated by gastric lavage and supportive measures. As with other macrolides, clarithromycin serum levels are not expected to be appreciably affected by haemodialysis or peritoneal dialysis.

**Pharmacological properties**

*Microbiology:* Clarithromycin is a semi-synthetic derivative of erythromycin A. It exerts its antibacterial action by binding to the 50s ribosomal sub-unit of susceptible bacteria and suppresses protein synthesis. It is highly potent against a wide variety of aerobic and anaerobic gram-positive and gram-negative organisms. The minimum inhibitory concentrations (MICs) of clarithromycin are generally two-fold lower than the MICs of erythromycin.

The 14-hydroxy metabolite of clarithromycin also has antimicrobial activity. The MICs of the metabolite are equal or two-fold higher than the MICs of the parent compound, except for H influenzae where the 14-hydroxy metabolite is two-fold more active than the parent compound.

Klaricid is usually active against the following organisms in vitro:

Gram-positive bacteria: *Staphylococcus aureus* (methicillin susceptible); *Streptococcus pyogenes* (Group A beta-hemolytic streptococci) alpha-hemolytic streptococci (viridans group); *Streptococcus* (*Diploococcus*) *pneumoniae*; *Streptococcus agalactiae*, *Listeria monocytogenes*.

Gram-negative bacteria: *Haemophilus influenzae*, *Haemophilus parainfluenzae*, *Moraxella (Branhamella) catarrhalis*, *Neisseria gonorrhoeae*; *Legionella pneumophila*, *Bordetella pertussis*, *Helicobacter pylori*; *Campylobacter jejuni*.

Mycoplasma: *Mycoplasma pneumoniae*; *Ureaplasma urealyticum*.

Other organisms: *Chlamydia trachomatis*; *Mycobacterium avium*; *Mycobacterium leprae*; *Mycobacterium Kansasaii*; *Mycobacterium chelonae*; *Mycobacterium fortuitum*; *Mycobacterium intracellulare*.

Anaerobes: Macrolide-susceptible *Bacteroides fragilis*; *Clostridium perfringens*; *Peptococcus* species; *Peptostreptococcus* species; *Propionibacterium acnes*.

Clarithromycin has bactericidal activity against several bacterial strains. The organisms include *Haemophilus influenzae*, *Streptococcus pneumoniae*, *Streptococcus pyogenes*, *Streptococcus agalactiae*, *Moraxella (Branhamella) catarrhalis*, *Neisseria gonorrhoeae*, *Helicobacter pylori* and *Campylobacter* spp.

*Pharmacokinetics: Helicobacter pylori* (*H. pylori*) is associated with acid peptic disease including duodenal ulcer and gastric ulcer in which about 95% and 80% of patients respectively are infected with the agent. *H. pylori* is also implicated as a major contribution factor in the development of gastritis and ulcer recurrence in such patients.

Clarithromycin has been used in small numbers of patients in other treatment regimens. Possible kinetic interactions have not been fully investigated. These regimens include: clarithromycin plus tinidazole and omeprazole; clarithromycin plus tetracycline; bismuth subsalicylate and ranitidine; clarithromycin plus ranitidine alone.

Clinical studies using various different *H. pylori* eradication regimens (including clarithromycin plus omeprazole) have shown that eradication of *H. pylori* prevents ulcer recurrence.

Clarithromycin is rapidly and well absorbed from the gastro-intestinal tract after oral administration of Klaricid tablets. The microbiologically active metabolite 14-hydroxyclarithromycin is formed by first pass metabolism. Klaricid may be given without regard to meals as food does not affect the extent of bioavailability of Klaricid tablets. Food does slightly delay the onset of absorption of clarithromycin and formation of the 14-hydroxymetabolite. The pharmacokinetics of clarithromycin are non linear; however, steady-state is attained within 2 days of dosing. At 250 mg b.i.d. 15–20% of unchanged drug is excreted in the urine. With 500 mg b.i.d. daily dosing urinary excretion is greater (approximately 36%). The 14-hydroxy-clarithromycin is the major urinary metabolite and accounts for 10–15% of the dose. Most of the remainder of the dose is eliminated in the faeces, primarily via the bile. 5–10% of the parent drug is recovered from the faeces.

When clarithromycin 500 mg is given three times daily, the clarithromycin plasma concentrations are increased with respect to the 500 mg twice daily dosage.

Klaricid provides tissue concentrations that are several times higher than the circulating drug levels. Increased levels have been found in both tonsillar and lung tissue. Clarithromycin is 80% bound to plasma proteins at therapeutic levels.

Klaricid also penetrates the gastric mucus. Levels of clarithromycin in gastric mucus and gastric tissue are higher when clarithromycin is co-administered with omeprazole than when clarithromycin is administered alone.

*Preclinical safety data:* In acute mouse and rat studies, the median lethal dose was greater than the highest feasible dose for administration (5 g/kg).

In repeated dose studies, toxicity was related to dose, duration of treatment and species. Dogs were more sensitive than primates or rats. The major clinical signs at toxic doses included emesis, weakness, reduced food consumption and weight gain, salivation, dehydration and hyperactivity. In all species the liver was the primary target organ at toxic doses. Hepatotoxicity was detectable by early elevations of liver function tests. Discontinuation of the drug generally resulted in a return to or toward normal results. Other tissues less commonly affected included the stomach, thymus and other lymphoid tissues and the kidneys. At near therapeutic doses, conjunctival injection and lacrimation occurred only in dogs. At a massive dose of 400 mg/kg/day, some dogs and monkeys developed corneal opacities and/or oedema.

Fertility and reproduction studies in rats have shown no adverse effects. Teratogenicity studies in rats (Wistar (p.o.) and Sprague-Dawley (p.o. and i.v.)), New Zealand White rabbits and cynomolgous monkeys failed to demonstrate any teratogenicity from clarithromycin. However, a further similar study in Sprague-Dawley rats indicated a low (6%) incidence of cardiovascular abnormalities which appeared to be due to spontaneous expression of genetic changes. Two mouse studies revealed a variable incidence (3–30%) of cleft palate and embryonic loss was seen in monkeys but only at dose levels which were clearly toxic to the mothers.

### Pharmaceutical particulars

*List of excipients:* Croscarmellose sodium, cellulose microcrystalline, silicon dioxide, povidone (K value 29–32), stearic acid, magnesium stearate, talc, hypromellose, hydroxypropylcellulose, propylene glycol, sorbitan monooleate, titanium dioxide, sorbic acid, vanillin, quinoline yellow (Aluminium Lake) E104.

*Incompatibilities:* None known.

*Shelf life:* The recommended shelf life is 36 months stored at room temperature (15˚ to 30˚C).

*Special precautions for storage:* Protect from light.

*Nature and contents of container:* Tablets in a blister original pack. The blisters are packaged in a carton with a pack insert.

Tablets in HDPE bottle with a pack insert.

*Instructions for use/handling:* Not applicable.

**Marketing authorisation number** 0037/0254.

**Date of approval/revision of SPC** July 1997.

**Legal category** POM.

## KLARICID* IV

**Presentation** A sterile, white to off white lyophilised powder containing 500 mg clarithromycin per vial and lactobionic acid as a solubilising agent.

When reconstituted with 10 ml Sterilised Water for Injections, each ml of the resulting solution contains 50 mg clarithromycin. This solution must be further diluted prior to intravenous administration (see dosage and administration).

**Uses** Klaricid IV is indicated whenever parenteral therapy is required for treatment of infections caused by susceptible organisms in the following conditions: Lower respiratory tract infections for example, acute and chronic bronchitis, and pneumonia; upper respiratory tract infections for example, sinusitis and pharyngitis; skin and soft tissue infections.

*Microbiology:* Clarithromycin is a semi-synthetic derivative of erythromycin A. It exerts its anti-bacterial action by binding to the 50s ribosomal sub-unit of susceptible bacteria and suppresses protein synthesis. It is highly potent against a wide variety of aerobic and anaerobic gram-positive and gram-negative organisms. The minimum inhibitory concentrations (MICs) of clarithromycin are generally two-fold lower than the MICs of erythromycin. The 14-hydroxy metabolite of clarithromycin also has anti-microbial activity. The MICs of this metabolite are equal or two-fold higher than the MICs of the parent compound, except for *H. influenzae* where the 14-hydroxy metabolite is twice as active as the parent compound.

Klaricid is usually active against the following organisms *in vitro:* Gram-positive bacteria: Staphylococcus aureus (methicillin susceptible); *Streptococcus pyogenes* (Group A beta-haemolytic streptococci); alpha-haemolytic streptococci (viridans group); *Streptococcus (Diplococcus) pneumoniae; Streptococcus agalactiae; Listeria monocytogenes.*

Gram-negative bacteria: *Haemophilus influenzae, Haemophilus parainfluenzae, Moraxella (Branhamella) catarrhalis, Neisseria gonorrhoeae; Legionella pneumophila, Bordetella pertussis, Helicobacter pylori; Campylobacter jejuni.*

*Mycoplasma: Mycoplasma pneumoniae; Ureaplasma urealyticum.*

Other Organisms: *Chlamydia trachomatis; Mycobacterium avium; Mycobacterium leprae.*

*Anaerobes:* Macrolide-susceptible *Bacteroides fragilis; Clostridium perfringens; Peptococcus* species; *Peptostreptococcus* species; *Propionibacterium acnes.*

Clarithromycin also has bactericidal activity against several bacterial strains. These organisms include *H.*

*influenzae, Streptococcus pneumoniae, Streptococcus pyogenes, Streptococcus agalactiae, Moraxella (Branhamella) catarrhalis, Neisseria gonorrhoeae* and *Campylobacter* spp.

The activity of clarithromycin against *Helicobacter pylori* is greater at neutral pH than at acid pH.

### Dosage and administration

*Recommended dosage:* Intravenous therapy may be given for 2 to 5 days and should be changed to oral clarithromycin therapy when appropriate.

*Adults:* The recommended dosage of Klaricid IV is 1.0 gram daily, divided into two 500 mg doses, appropriately diluted as described below.

*Children:* At present, there are insufficient data to recommend a dosage regimen for routine use in children.

*Elderly:* As for adults.

*Renal impairment:* In patients with renal impairment who have creatinine clearance less than 30 ml/min, the dosage of clarithromycin should be reduced to one half of the normal recommended dose.

*Recommended administration:* Klaricid IV should be administered into one of the larger proximal veins as an IV infusion over 60 minutes, using a solution concentration of about 2 mg/ml. Clarithromycin should not be given as a bolus or an intramuscular injection.

*Preparation of the solution for intravenous administration*

*Step 1:* Inject 10 ml Sterilised Water for Injections into the vial and shake to dissolve the contents. Do not use diluents containing preservatives or inorganic salts. Each ml of reconstituted solution contains 50 mg clarithromycin. Use within 24 hours. Can be stored from 5˚C up to room temperature (25˚C).

*Step 2:* Add the reconstituted product (500 mg in 10 ml Water for Injections) to 250 ml of one of the following diluents before administration: 5% dextrose in Lactated Ringer's solution, 5% dextrose, Lactated Ringer's, 5% dextrose in 0.3% sodium chloride, Normosol-M in 5% dextrose, Normosol-R in 5% dextrose, 5% dextrose in 0.45% sodium chloride, or 0.9% sodium chloride.

The final diluted product (concentration about 2 mg/ml) should be used within 6 hours if stored at room temperature (25˚C), or within 24 hours if stored at 5˚C. Compatibility with other IV additives has not been established.

### Contra-indications, warnings, etc

*Contra-indications:* Klaricid IV is contra-indicated in patients with known hypersensitivity to macrolide antibiotic drugs.

Klaricid and ergot derivatives should not be co-administered.

Concomitant administration of clarithromycin and any of the following drugs is contra-indicated: cisapride, pimozide and terfenadine. Elevated cisapride, pimozide and terfenadine levels have been reported in patients receiving either of these drugs and clarithromycin concomitantly. This may result in QT prolongation and cardiac arrhythmias including ventricular tachycardia, ventricular fibrillation and Torsade de Pointes. Similar effects have been observed with concomitant administration of astemizole and other macrolides.

*Precautions:* Clarithromycin is principally excreted by the liver and kidneys. Caution should be exercised in administering this antibiotic to patients with impaired hepatic and renal function.

Prolonged or repeated use of clarithromycin may result in an overgrowth of non-susceptible bacteria or fungi. If super-infection occurs, clarithromycin should be discontinued and appropriate therapy instituted.

*Interactions:* Clarithromycin has been shown not to interact with oral contraceptives.

As with other macrolide antibiotics, the use of clarithromycin in patients concurrently taking drugs metabolised by the cytochrome p450 system (e.g. warfarin, ergot alkaloids, triazolam, midazolam, disopyramide, lovastatin, phenytoin and cyclosporin) may be associated with elevations in serum levels of these other drugs.

The administration of Klaricid to patients who are receiving theophylline has been associated with increased serum theophylline levels and potential theophylline toxicity.

The use of Klaricid in patients receiving warfarin may result in a potentiation of the effects of warfarin. Prothrombin time should be frequently monitored in these patients. The effects of digoxin may be potentiated with concomitant administration of Klaricid. Monitoring of serum digoxin levels should be considered.

Klaricid may potentiate the effects of carbamazepine due to a reduction in the rate of excretion.

Simultaneous oral administration of clarithromycin tablets and zidovudine to HIV-infected adult patients may result in decreased steady-state zidovudine

concentrations. Since this interaction in adults is thought to be due to interference of clarithromycin with simultaneously administered oral zidovudine, this interaction should not be a problem when clarithromycin is administered intravenously.

With oral clarithromycin, the interaction can be largely avoided by staggering the doses; see data sheet for Klaricid tablets for further information.

No similar reaction has been reported in children.

*Side-effects:* The most frequently reported infusion-related adverse events in clinical studies were injection-site inflammation, tenderness, phlebitis and pain. The most common non-infusion-related adverse event reported was taste perversion.

During clinical studies with *oral* Klaricid, the drug was generally well tolerated. Side-effects included nausea, vomiting, diarrhoea, dyspepsia and abdominal pain. Stomatitis and glossitis and oral monilia have been reported. Other side-effects include headache and allergic reactions ranging from urticaria and mild skin eruptions to anaphylaxis and rarely, Stevens-Johnson syndrome. Taste perversion may occur with oral treatment. There have been reports of transient central nervous system side-effects including anxiety, dizziness, insomnia, hallucinations, psychosis, bad dreams and confusion, however, a cause and effect relationship has not been established. There have been reports of hearing loss with clarithromycin which is usually reversible upon withdrawal of therapy.

Pseudomembranous colitis has been reported rarely with clarithromycin and may range in severity from mild to life threatening. As with other macrolides, hepatic dysfunction (which is usually reversible) including altered liver function tests, hepatitis and cholestasis with or without jaundice, has been reported. Dysfunction may be severe and very rarely fatal hepatic failure has been reported.

*Use in pregnancy and lactating women:* The safety of Klaricid during pregnancy and breast feeding of infants has not been established. Clarithromycin should thus not be used during pregnancy or lactation unless the benefit is considered to outweigh the risk. Some animal studies have suggested an embryotoxic effect but only at dose levels which are clearly toxic to mothers. Clarithromycin has been found in the milk of lactating animals and in human breast milk.

*Overdosage:* There is no experience of overdosage after I.V. administration of clarithromycin. However, reports indicate that the ingestion of large amounts of clarithromycin orally can be expected to produce gastro-intestinal symptoms. Allergic reactions accompanying overdosage should be treated by gastric lavage and supportive measures.

As with other macrolides, clarithromycin serum levels are not expected to be appreciably affected by haemodialysis or peritoneal dialysis.

One patient who had a history of bipolar disorder ingested 8 grams of clarithromycin and showed altered mental status, paranoid behaviour, hypokalaemia and hypoxaemia.

**Pharmaceutical precautions** Store powder at up to 30˚C and protect from light.

**Legal category** POM.

**Package quantities** Packs of 1.

**Further information** Nil.

**Product licence number** 0037/0251.

## KLARICID* PAEDIATRIC SUSPENSION

**Qualitative and quantitative composition** Clarithromycin 125 mg/5 ml.

**Pharmaceutical form** White to off-white granules for reconstitution.

**Clinical particulars**

*Therapeutic indications:* Klaricid Paediatric Suspension is indicated for the treatment of infections caused by susceptible organisms. Indications include: Lower respiratory tract infections; upper respiratory tract infections; skin and skin structure infections; acute otitis media.

Klaricid Paediatric Suspension is usually active against the following organisms *in vitro:*

Gram-positive bacteria: *Staphylococcus aureus* (methicillin susceptible); *Streptococcus pyogenes* (Group A beta-haemolytic streptococci); alpha-haemolytic streptococci (viridans group); *Streptococcus (Diplococcus) pneumoniae; Streptococcus agalactiae; Listeria monocytogenes.*

Gram-negative bacteria: *Haemophilus influenzae, Haemophilus parainfluenzae, Moraxella (Branhamella) catarrhalis, Neisseria gonorrhoeae; Legionella pneumophila, Bordetella pertussis, Helicobacter pylori; Campylobacter jejuni.*

Mycoplasma: *Mycoplasma pneumoniae; Ureaplasma urealyticum.*

Other organisms: *Chlamydia trachomatis; Mycobacterium avium; Mycobacterium leprae; Chlamydia pneumoniae.*

Anaerobes: Macrolide-susceptible *Bacteroides fragilis; Clostridium perfringens; Peptococcus* species; *Peptostreptococcus* species; *Propionibacterium acnes.*

Klaricid Paediatric Suspension has bactericidal activity against several bacterial strains. These organisms include *H. influenzae, Streptococcus pneumoniae, Streptococcus pyogenes, Streptococcus agalactiae, Moraxella (Branhamella) catarrhalis, Neisseria gonorrhoeae, Helicobacter pylori* and *Campylobacter* species.

The activity of clarithromycin against *H. pylori* is greater at neutral pH than at acid pH.

*Posology and method of administration:* Recommended doses and dosage schedules: The usual duration of treatment is for 5 to 10 days depending on the pathogen involved and the severity of the condition. The recommended daily dosage of Klaricid Paediatric Suspension in children is given in the following table and is based on a 7.5 mg/kg b.i.d. regime. Doses up to 500 mg b.i.d. have been used in the treatment of severe infection.

**Klaricid Paediatric Suspension dosage in children**

| Dosage based on body weight (kg) | | | |
|---|---|---|---|
| Weight* (kg) | Approx. age (yrs) | Dosage (ml) bid | Dosage per 5 ml teaspoonful twice daily |
| 8–11 | 1–2 | 2.5 | ½ |
| 12–19 | 3–6 | 5 | 1 |
| 20–29 | 7–9 | 7.5 | 1½ |
| 30–40 | 10–12 | 10 | 2 |

\* Children <8 kg should be dosed on a per kg basis (approx. 7.5 mg/kg bid)

*Preparation for use:*
*100 ml bottle:* 53 ml of water should be added to the granules in the bottle and shaken to yield 100 ml of reconstituted suspension. The concentration of clarithromycin in the reconstituted suspension is 125 mg per 5 ml.
*70 ml bottle:* 37 ml of water should be added to the granules in the bottle and shaken to yield 70 ml of reconstituted suspension. The concentration of clarithromycin in the reconstituted suspension is 125 mg per 5 ml.
*Sachet:* After cutting along the dotted line, empty contents of sachet into a glass, half fill the sachet with cold water. Add to glass and stir thoroughly before taking.

*Contra-indications:* Klaricid Paediatric Suspension is contra-indicated in patients with known hypersensitivity to macrolide antibiotic drugs and other ingredients.

Klaricid Paediatric Suspension and ergot derivatives should not be co-administered.

Concomitant administration of clarithromycin and any of the following drugs is contra-indicated: cisapride, pimozide and terfenadine. Elevated cisapride, pimozide and terfenadine levels have been reported in patients receiving either of these drugs and clarithromycin concomitantly. This may result in QT prolongation and cardiac arrhythmias including ventricular tachycardia, ventricular fibrillation and Torsade de Pointes. Similar effects have been observed with concomitant administration of astemizole and other macrolides.

*Special warnings and special precautions for use:* Clarithromycin is principally excreted by the liver and kidneys. This antibiotic should not be administered to paediatric patients with hepatic or renal failure.

Prolonged or repeated use of clarithromycin may result in an overgrowth of non-susceptible bacteria or fungi. If super-infection occurs, clarithromycin should be discontinued and appropriate therapy instituted.

*Interaction with other medicaments and other forms of interaction* As with other macrolide antibiotics, the use of clarithromycin in patients concurrently taking drugs metabolized by the cytochrome P450 system (e.g. warfarin, ergot alkaloids, triazolam, midazolam, disopyramide, lovastatin, phenytoin and cyclosporin) may be associated with elevations in serum levels of these other drugs.

The administration of clarithromycin to patients who are receiving theophylline has been associated with an increase of serum theophylline levels and potential theophylline toxicity.

The use of Klaricid Paediatric Suspension in patients receiving digoxin, warfarin and carbamazepine may result in potentiation of their effects due to a reduction in the rate of excretion. Prothrombin time should be frequently monitored in patients receiving warfarin. Monitoring of serum digoxin levels should be considered.

Simultaneous oral administration of clarithromycin tablets and zidovudine to HIV-infected adult patients may result in decreased steady-state zidovudine levels. To date, this interaction does not appear to occur in paediatric HIV-infected patients taking Klaricid

Paediatric Suspension with zidovudine or dideoxyinosine.

*Pregnancy and lactation:* The safety of clarithromycin during pregnancy and breast feeding of infants has not been established. Some animal studies have suggested an embryotoxic effect, but only at dose levels which are clearly toxic to mothers. Therefore, if a patient of post-pubertal age becomes pregnant, clarithromycin should not be used during pregnancy or lactation unless the benefit outweighs the risk. Clarithromycin has been found in the milk of lactating animals and in human breast milk.

*Effects on ability to drive and use machines:* None known.

*Undesirable effects:* Clarithromycin is generally well tolerated. Side-effects reported include nausea, dyspepsia, vomiting, diarrhoea and abdominal pain. Taste perversion may occur and stomatitis and glossitis and oral monilia have been reported. Other rare side-effects include headache and allergic reactions ranging from urticaria and mild skin eruptions to anaphylaxis and rarely, Stevens-Johnson syndrome. There have been reports of transient central nervous system side-effects including anxiety, dizziness, insomnia, hallucinations, psychosis, bad dreams and confusion; however, a cause and effect relationship has not been established. There have been reports of hearing loss with clarithromycin which is usually reversible upon withdrawal of therapy. Pseudomembranous colitis has been reported rarely with clarithromycin and may range in severity from mild to life threatening. As with other macrolides, hepatic dysfunction (which is usually reversible) including altered liver function tests, hepatitis and cholestasis with or without jaundice has been reported. Dysfunction may be severe, and very rarely, fatal hepatic failure has been reported.

*Overdosage:* Reports indicate that the ingestion of large amounts of clarithromycin can be expected to produce gastro-intestinal symptoms. Allergic reactions accompanying overdosage should be treated by gastric lavage and supportive measures. One patient who had a history of bipolar disorder ingested 8 grams of clarithromycin and showed altered mental status, paranoid behaviour, hypokalaemia and hypoxemia.

**Pharmacological properties**
*Microbiology:* Clarithromycin is a semi-synthetic derivative of erythromycin A. It exerts its anti-bacterial action by binding to the 50s ribosomal sub-unit of susceptible bacteria and suppresses protein synthesis. Clarithromycin demonstrates excellent *in-vitro* activity against standard strains of clinical isolates. It is highly potent against a wide variety of aerobic and anaerobic gram-positive and gram-negative organisms. The minimum inhibitory concentrations (MICs) of clarithromycin are generally two-fold lower than the MICs of erythromycin.

The 14-(R)-hydroxy metabolite of clarithromycin formed in man by first pass metabolism also has antimicrobial activity. The MICs of this metabolite are equal or two-fold higher than the MICs of the parent compound, except for *H. influenzae* where the 14-hydroxy metabolite is two-fold more active than the parent compound. Clarithromycin is also bactericidal against several bacterial strains.

Clarithromycin is usually active against the following organisms *in vitro*: Gram-positive bacteria: *Staphylococcus aureus* (methicillin susceptible); *Streptococcus pyogenes* (Group A beta-haemolytic streptococci); alpha-haemolytic streptococci (viridans group); *Streptococcus (Diplococcus) pneumoniae; Streptococcus agalactiae; Listeria monocytogenes.*

Gram-negative bacteria: *Haemophilus influenzae, Haemophilus parainfluenzae, Moraxella (Branhamella) catarrhalis, Neisseria gonorrhoeae; Legionella pneumophila, Bordetella pertussis, Helicobacter pylori; Campylobacter jejuni.*

Mycoplasma: *Mycoplasma pneumoniae; Ureaplasma urealyticum.*

Other organisms: *Chlamydia trachomatis; Mycobacterium avium; Mycobacterium leprae; Chlamydia pneumoniae.*

Anaerobes: Macrolide-susceptible *Bacteroides fragilis; Clostridium perfringens; Peptococcus* species; *Peptostreptococcus* species; *Propionibacterium acnes.*

Clarithromycin also has bactericidal activity against several bacterial strains. These organisms include *H. influenzae, Streptococcus pneumoniae, Streptococcus pyogenes, Streptococcus agalactiae, Moraxella (Branhamella) catarrhalis, Neisseria gonorrhoeae, Helicobacter pylori* and *Campylobacter* species.

*Pharmacokinetics:* Clarithromycin is rapidly and well absorbed from the gastro-intestinal tract after oral administration. The microbiologically active 14(R)-hydroxyclarithromycin is formed by first pass metabolism. Clarithromycin, may be given without regard to meals as food does not affect the extent of bioavailability. Food does slightly delay the onset of absorption of clarithromycin and formation of the 14-

hydroxy metabolite. Although the pharmacokinetics of clarithromycin are non linear, steady state is attained within 2 days of dosing. 14-Hydroxyclarithromycin is the major urinary metabolite and accounts for 10–15% of the dose. Most of the remainder of the dose is eliminated in the faeces, primarily via the bile. 5–10% of the parent drug is recovered from the faeces.

Clarithromycin provides tissue concentrations that are several times higher than circulating drug level. Increased levels of clarithromycin have been found in both tonsillar and lung tissue. Clarithromycin penetrates into the middle ear fluid at concentrations greater than in the serum. Clarithromycin is 80% bound to plasma proteins at therapeutic levels.

Klaricid Paediatric Suspension does not contain tartrazine or other azo dyes, lactose or gluten.

*Preclinical safety data:* The acute oral LD$_{50}$ values for a clarithromycin suspension administered to 3-day old mice were 1290 mg/kg for males and 1230 mg/kg for females. The LD$_{50}$ values in 3-day old rats were 1330 mg/kg for males and 1270 mg/kg for females. For comparison, the LD$_{50}$ of orally-administered clarithromycin is about 2700 mg/kg for adult mice and about 3000 mg/kg for adult rats. These results are consistent with other antibiotics of the penicillin group, cephalosporin group and macrolide group in that the LD$_{50}$ is generally lower in juvenile animals than in adults.

In both mice and rats, body weight was reduced or its increase suppressed and suckling behaviour and spontaneous movements were depressed for the first few days following drug administration. Necropsy of animals that died disclosed dark-reddish lungs in mice and about 25% of the rats; rats treated with 2197 mg/kg or more of a clarithromycin suspension were also noted to have a reddish-black substance in the intestines, probably because of bleeding. Deaths depressed suckling behaviour or bleeding from the intestines.

Pre-weaning rats (5 days old) were administered a clarithromycin suspension formulation for two weeks at doses of 0, 15, 55 and 200 mg/kg/day. Animals from the 200 mg/kg/day group had decreased body-weight gains, decreased mean haemoglobin and haematocrit values, and increased mean relative kidney weights compared to animals from the control group. Treatment-related minimal to mild multifocal vacuolar degeneration of the intrahepatic bile duct epithelium and an increased incidence of nephritic lesions were also observed in animals from this treatment group. The 'no-toxic effect' dosage for this study was 55 mg/kg/day.

An oral toxicity study was conducted in which immature rats were administered a clarithromycin suspension (granules for suspension) for 6 weeks at daily dosages of 0, 15, 50 and 150 mg base/kg/day. No deaths occurred and the only clinical sign observed was excessive salivation for some of the animals at the highest dosage from 1 to 2 hours after administration during the last 3 weeks of treatment. Rats from the 150 mg/kg dose group had lower mean body weights during the first three weeks, and were observed to have decreased mean serum albumin values and increased mean relative liver weight compared to the controls. No treatment-related gross or microscopic histopathological changes were found. A dosage of 150 mg/kg/day produced slight toxicity in the treated rats and the 'no effect dosage' was considered to be 50 mg/kg/day.

Juvenile beagle dogs, 3 weeks of age, were treated orally daily for four weeks with 0, 30, 100, or 300 mg/kg of clarithromycin, followed by a 4-week recovery period. No deaths occurred and no change in the general condition of the animals were observed. Necropsy revealed no abnormalities. Upon histological examination, fatty deposition of centrilobular hepatocytes and cell infiltration of portal areas were observed by light microscopy and an increase in hepatocellular fat droplets was noted by electron microscopy in the 300 mg/kg dose group. The toxic dose in juvenile beagle dogs was considered to be greater than 300 mg/kg and the 'no effect dose' 100 mg/kg.

*Fertility, reproduction and teratogenicity:* Fertility and reproduction studies have shown daily dosages of 150–160 mg/kg/day to male and female rats caused no adverse effects on the oestrus cycle, fertility, parturition and number and viability of offspring. Two teratogenicity studies in both Wistar (p.o.) and Sprague-Dawley (p.o. and i.v.) rats, one study in New Zealand white rabbits and one study in cynomolgus monkeys failed to demonstrate any teratogenicity from clarithromycin.

**Pharmaceutical particulars**
*List of excipients:* Carbopol 974P, povidone K90, water purified, hydroxypropylmethylcellulose phthalate (HP-55), castor oil, acetone, ethanol, silicon dioxide, sucrose, xanthan gum, flavour – fruit punch, potassium sorbate, citric acid, titanium dioxide and maltodextrin.

*Incompatibilities:* None known.

*Shelf life: bottles:* The recommended shelf life is 24 months stored at room temperature at 15–30°C. Once reconstituted, Klaricid Paediatric Suspension should be used within 14 days.

*Sachets:* The recommended shelf life is 18 months stored at room temperature (15° to 30°C).

*Special precautions for storage:* None stated.

*Nature and contents of container:* Granules for reconstitution in a HDPE bottle. Pack sizes of 70 and 100 ml are available.

Granules for reconstitution in paper/LDPE/Al foil/ LDPE sachet. Packs of 2 sachets.

*Instructions for use/handling:* Not applicable.

**Marketing authorisation number** 0037/0264.

**Date of approval/revision of SPC** June 1996.

**Legal category** POM.

## KLARICID* XL

**Qualitative and quantitative composition** Clarithromycin 500 mg per tablet.

**Pharmaceutical form** A yellow, ovaloid tablet containing 500 mg of clarithromycin in a modified-release preparation.

**Clinical particulars**

*Therapeutic indications:* Klaricid XL is indicated for treatment of infections caused by susceptible organisms. Indications include:

Lower respiratory tract infections for example, acute and chronic bronchitis, and pneumonia.

Upper respiratory tract infections for example, sinusitis and pharyngitis.

Klaricid XL is also indicated in skin and soft tissue infections of mild to moderate severity, for example folliculitis, cellulitis and erysipelas.

*Posology and method of administration:*

*Adults:* The usual recommended dosage of Klaricid XL in adults is one 500 mg modified-release tablet daily to be taken with food. In more severe infections, the dosage can be increased to two 500 mg modified-release tablets daily. The usual duration of treatment is 7 to 14 days.

*Children older than 12 years:* As for adults.

*Children younger than 12 years:* Use Klaricid Paediatric Suspension.

Klaricid XL should not be used in patients with renal impairment (creatinine clearance less than 30 ml/ min). Klaricid immediate release tablets may be used in this patient population (see *Contra-indications*).

*Contra-indications:* Clarithromycin is contra-indicated in patients with known hypersensitivity to macrolide antibiotic drugs.

Clarithromycin and ergot derivates should not be co-administered.

As the dose cannot be reduced from 500 mg daily, Klaricid XL is contra-indicated in patients with creatinine clearance less than 30 ml/min.

Concomitant administration of clarithromycin and any of the following drugs is contra-indicated: cisapride, pimozide and terfenadine. Elevated cisapride, pimozide and terfenadine levels have been reported in patients receiving either of these drugs and clarithromycin concomitantly. This may result in QT prolongation and cardiac arrhythmias including ventricular tachycardia, ventricular fibrillation and torsade de pointes. Similar effects have been observed with concomitant administration of astemizole and other macrolides.

*Special warnings and special precautions for use:* Clarithromycin is principally excreted by the liver and kidney. Caution should be exercised in administering this antibiotic to patients with impaired hepatic or renal function.

Prolonged or repeated use of clarithromycin may result in an overgrowth of non-susceptible bacteria or fungi. If super-infection occurs, clarithromycin should be discontinued and appropriate therapy instituted.

*Interaction with other medicaments and other forms of interaction:* Clarithromycin has been shown not to interact with oral contraceptives.

As with other macrolide antibiotics the use of clarithromycin in patients concurrently taking drugs metabolised by the cytochrome P450 system (e.g. warfarin, ergot alkaloids, triazolam, midazolam, disopyramide, lovastatin, phenytoin and cyclosporin) may be associated with elevations in serum levels of these other drugs.

The administration of clarithromycin to patients who are receiving theophylline has been associated with an increase in serum theophylline levels and potential theophylline toxicity.

The use of clarithromycin in patients receiving warfarin may result in potentiation of the effects of warfarin. Prothrombin time should be frequently monitored in these patients.

The effects of digoxin may be potentiated with concomitant administration of clarithromycin. Monitoring of serum digoxin levels should be considered.

Clarithromycin may potentiate the effects of carbamazepine due to a reduction in the rate of excretion.

Interaction studies have not been conducted with Klaricid XL and zidovudine.

If concomitant administration of clarithromycin and zidovudine is reqiuired, then an immediate release formulation of clarithromycin should be used.

*Pregnancy and lactation:* The safety of clarithromycin during pregnancy and breast feeding of infants has not been established. Clarithromycin should thus not be used during pregnancy or lactation unless the benefit is considered to outweigh the risk. Some animal studies have suggested an embryotoxic effect, but only at dose levels which are clearly toxic to mothers. Clarithromycin has been found in milk of lactating animals and in human breast milk.

*Effects on ability to drive and use machines:* The medicine is unlikely to produce an effect.

*Undesirable effects:* Clarithromycin is generally well tolerated. Side effects reported include nausea, dyspepsia, diarrhoea, vomiting and abdominal pain. Stomatitis, glossitis and oral monilia have been reported. Other side-effects include headache and allergic reactions ranging from urticaria and mild skin eruptions to anaphylaxis and rarely Stevens-Johnson syndrome. Taste perversion may occur. There have been reports of transient central nervous system side-effects including anxiety, dizziness, insomnia, hallucinations, psychosis, bad dreams and confusion, however, a cause and effect relationship has not been established. Pseudomembranous colitis has been reported rarely with clarithromycin, and may range in severity from mild to life threatening. As with other macrolides, hepatic dysfunction (which is usually reversible) including altered liver function tests, hepatitis and cholestasis with or without jaundice, has been reported. Dysfunction may be severe and very rarely fatal hepatic failure has been reported. There have been reports of hearing loss with clarithromycin, which is usually reversible upon withdrawal of treatment.

*Overdosage:* Reports indicate that the ingestion of large amounts of clarithromycin can be expected to produce gastro-intestinal symptoms. One patient who had a history of bipolar disorder ingested 8 g of clarithromycin and showed altered mental status, paranoid behaviour, hypokalaemia and hypoxaemia. Allergic reactions accompanying overdosage should be treated by gastric lavage and supportive measures. As with other macrolides, clarithromycin serum levels are not expected to be appreciably affected by haemodialysis or peritoneal dialysis.

**Pharmaceutical properties**

*Microbiology:* Clarithromycin is a semi-synthetic derivative of erythromycin A. It exerts its antibacterial action by binding to the 50s ribosomal sub-unit of susceptible bacteria and suppresses protein synthesis. It is highly potent against a wide variety of aerobic and anaerobic gram-positive and gram-negative organisms. The minimum inhibitory concentrations (MICs) of clarithromycin are generally two-fold lower than the MICs of erythromycin.

The 14-hydroxy metabolite of clarithromycin also has antimicrobial activity. The MICs of this metabolite are equal or two-fold higher than the MICs of the parent compound, except for *H influenzae* where the 14-hydroxy metabolite is two-fold more active than the parent compound.

Clarithromycin is usually active against the following organisms *in vitro*:

*Gram-positive bacteria: Staphylococcus* (methicillin susceptible); *Streptococcus pyogenes* (Group A beta-hemolytic streptococci); alpha-hemolytic streptococci (viridans group); *Streptococcus (Diplococcus) pneumoniae; Streptococcus agalactiae; Listeria monocytogenes.*

*Gram-negative bacteria: Haemophilus influenza; Haemophilus parainfluenza; Moraxella (Branhamella) catarrhalis; Neisseria gonorrhoeae; Legionella pneumophila; Bordetella pertussis; Campylobacter jejuni.*

*Mycoplasma: Mycoplasma pneumoniae; Ureaplasma urealyticum.*

*Other organisms: Chlamydia trachomatis; Mycobacterium avium; Mycobacterium leprae; Mycobacterium kansasaii; Mycobacterium chelonae; Mycobacterium fortuitum; Mycobacterium intracellularis; Chlamydia pneumoniae.*

*Anaerobes: Clostridium perfringens; Peptococcus* species; *Peptostreptococcus* species; *Propionibacterium* acnes.

Clarithromycin has bactericidal activity against several bacterial strains. The organisms include *Haemophilus influenzae, Streptococcus pneumoniae, Streptococcus pyogenes, Streptococcus agalactiae, Moraxella (Branhamella) catarrhalis, Neisseria gonorrhoeae* and *Campylobacter* spp.

*Pharmacokinetics:* The kinetics of orally administered modified-release clarithromycin have been studied in adult humans and compared with clarithromycin 250 mg and 500 mg immediate release tablets. The extent of absorption was found to be equivalent when equal total daily doses were administered. The absolute bioavailability is approximately 50%. Little or no unpredicted accumulation was found and the metabolic disposition did not change in any species following multiple dosing. Based upon the finding of equivalent absorption the following *in vitro* and *in vivo* data are applicable to the modified-release formulation.

*In vitro:* Results of *in vitro* studies showed that the protein binding of clarithromycin in human plasma averaged 70% at concentrations of 0.45–4.5 mcg/ml. A decrease in binding to 41% at 45.0 mcg/ml suggested that the binding sites might become saturated, but this only occurred at concentrations far in excess of therapeutic drug levels.

*In vivo:* Clarithromycin levels in all tissues, except the central nervous system, were several times higher than the circulating drug levels. The highest concentrations were found in the liver and lung tissue, where the tissue to plasma ratios reached 10 to 20.

The pharmacokinetic behaviour of clarithromycin is non-linear. In fed patients given 500 mg clarithromycin modified-release daily, the peak steady state plasma concentration of clarithromycin and 14 hydroxy clarithromycin were 1.3 and 0.48 mcg/ml, respectively. When the dosage was increased to 1000 mg daily, these steady-state values were 2.4 mcg/ml and 0.67 mcg/ml respectively. Elimination half-lives of the parent drug and metabolite were approximately 5.3 and 7.7 hours respectively. The apparent half-lives of both clarithromycin and its hydroxylated metabolite tended to be longer at higher doses.

Urinary excretion accounted for approximately 40% of the clarithromycin dose. Faecal elimination accounts for approximately 30%.

*Preclinical safety data:* In repeated dose studies, clarithromycin toxicity was related to dose and duration of treatment. The primary target organ was the liver in all species, with hepatic lesions seen after 14 days in dogs and monkeys. Systemic exposure levels associated with this toxicity are not known but toxic mg/kg doses were higher than the dose recommended for patient treatment.

No evidence of mutagenic potential of clarithromycin was seen during a range of *in vitro* and *in vivo* tests.

Fertility and reproduction studies in rats have shown no adverse effects. Teratogenicity studies in rats (Wistar (p.o.) and Sprague-Dawley (p.o. and i.v.)), New Zealand White rabbits and cynomolgous monkeys failed to demonstrate any teratogenicity from clarithromycin. However, a further similar study in Sprague-Dawley rats indicated a low (6%) incidence of cardiovascular abnormalities which appeared to be due to spontaneous expression of genetic changes. Two mouse studies revealed a variable incidence (3–30%) of cleft palate and in monkeys embryonic loss was seen but only at dose levels which were clearly toxic to the mothers.

No other toxicological findings considered to be of relevance to the dose level recommended for patient treatment have been reported.

**Pharmaceutical particulars**

*List of excipients:* Citric acid anhydrous, sodium alginate, sodium calcium alginate, lactose, povidone K30, talc, stearic acid, magnesium stearate, methyl hydroxypropylcellulose 6 cps, polyethylene glycol 400, polyethylene glycol 800, titanium dioxide (E171), sorbic acid, quinoline yellow (dye) aluminium lake (E104).

*Incompatibilities:* None known.

*Shelf life:* The shelf life is 18 months when stored in HDPE or glass bottles and in PVC/PVdC blisters.

*Special precautions for storage:* Store between 15°C and 30°C. Protect from light.

*Nature and contents of container:* 1, 7 or 14 tablets in a blister original pack. The blisters, of PVC/PVdC, are heat sealed with 20 micron hard tempered aluminium foil and packaged in a cardboard carton with a pack insert.

*Instructions for use/handling:* Not applicable.

**Marketing authorisation number** 0037/0275.

**Date of approval/revision of SPC** November 1996.

**Legal category** POM.

## NORVIR* ▼

**Qualitative and quantitative composition** Norvir oral solution contains 80 mg of ritonavir per ml. Each Norvir capsule contains 100 mg ritonavir.

## Pharmaceutical form

   Oral solution.
   Capsules.

## Clinical particulars

*Therapeutic indications:* Norvir is indicated in combination with antiretroviral nucleoside analogue(s) for the treatment of HIV-1 infected adult patients with advanced or progressive immunodeficiency.

Clinical endpoint data are only available in patients with advanced HIV-disease. In patients with less advanced HIV-disease only data based on biological markers such as viral load and CD4 cell count are yet available. In these patients studies on the effect of ritonavir on clinical endpoints are ongoing.

See *Pharmacodynamic properties* for the results of the important studies.

*Posology and method of administration:* Norvir solution is administered orally and should preferably be ingested with food. The recommended dosage of Norvir solution is 600 mg (7.5 ml) twice daily by mouth.

The bitter taste of Norvir solution may be lessened if mixed with chocolate milk.

Norvir capsules are administered orally and should preferably be ingested with food. The recommended dosage of ritonavir capsules is 600 mg (6 capsules) twice daily by mouth.

Paediatric use: The safety and efficacy of ritonavir in children below the age of 12 have not been established.

Renal and hepatic impairment: Currently, there are no data specific to these patient populations and therefore specific dosage recommendations cannot be made. Ritonavir is principally metabolised and eliminated by the liver. Norvir should not be given to patients with severe hepatic insufficiency (see Section 4.3 contra-indications). Because ritonavir is highly protein bound it is unlikely that it will be significantly removed by haemodialysis or peritoneal dialysis.

*Contra-indications:* Patients with known hypersensitivity to ritonavir or any of its excipients. Patients with severe hepatic insufficiency.

*In vitro* and *in vivo* studies have demonstrated that ritonavir is a potent inhibitor of CYP3A- and CYP2D6-mediated biotransformations. Based primarily on literature review, ritonavir is expected to produce large increases in the plasma concentrations of the following drugs: amiodarone, astemizole, bepridil, bupropion, cisapride, clozapine, dihydroergotamine, encainide, ergotamine, flecainide, meperidine, pimozide, piroxicam, propafenone, propoxyphene, quinidine, and terfenadine. These agents have recognized risks of arrhythmias, hematologic abnormalities, seizures, or other potentially serious adverse effects. Additionally, severe ergotism, characterised by peripheral vasospasm and ischaemia of the extremities, has been associated with co-administration of ritonavir and ergotamine or dihydroergotamine. These drugs should not be co-administered with ritonavir. Ritonavir in addition is likely to produce large increases in these highly metabolized sedatives and hypnotics: alprazolam, clorazepate, diazepam, estazolam, flurazepam, midazolam, triazolam and zolpidem. Due to the potential for extreme sedation and respiratory depression from these agents, they should not be co-administered with ritonavir.

Concomitant use of ritonavir and rifabutin is contraindicated because of clinical consequences such as uveitis resulting from a multifold increase of rifabutin serum concentrations.

*Special warnings and special precautions for use:* There are no data on the pharmacokinetics and safety of ritonavir in patients with significant hepatic or renal dysfunction. Ritonavir is principally metabolized and eliminated by the liver. Therefore, caution should be exercised when administering this drug to patients with impaired hepatic function (see *Contra-indications*).

The safety and efficacy of ritonavir in children below the age of 12 have not been established. Therefore, ritonavir should be used in children below the age of 12 only when the potential benefits clearly outweigh the potential risks.

Human pharmacokinetic data for combination of Norvir with antiretroviral drugs other than zidovudine and didanosine (ddl) are not yet available. Although the clinical use of combinations with zalcitabine (ddC) and stavudine (d4T) in a relatively limited number of patients did not seem to be associated with unfavorable effects, the use of combinations of Norvir with other nucleoside analogues should be guided by cautious therapeutic and safety monitoring.

Extra monitoring is recommended when diarrhoea occurs. The relatively high frequency of diarrhoea during treatment with ritonavir may compromise the absorption and efficacy (due to decreased compliance) of ritonavir or other concurrent medications. Serious persistent vomiting and/or diarrhoea associated with ritonavir use might also compromise renal function. It is advisable to monitor renal function in patients with renal function impairment.

A pharmacokinetic study demonstrated that ritonavir extensively inhibits the metabolism of saquinavir resulting in greatly increased saquinavir plasma concentrations (see *Interactions*). Due to a lack of sufficient safety data, ritonavir should not be given concomitantly with saquinavir or other protease inhibitors.

Norvir oral solution contains 43% ethanol, therefore concomitant administration of Norvir with disulfiram or drugs with disulfiram-like reactions (e.g. metronidazole) should be avoided.

There have been reports of increased bleeding, including spontaneous skin haematomas and haemarthroses, in haemophiliac patients type A and B treated with protease inhibitors. In some patients additional factor VIII was given. In more than a half of the reported cases, treatment with protease inhibitors was continued or reintroduced if treatment had been discontinued. A causal relationship has been evoked, although the mechanism of action has not been elucidated. Haemophiliac patients should therefore be made aware of the possibility of increased bleeding.

There may be an increased risk for transaminase elevations in patients with underlying hepatitis b or c, therefore, caution should be exercised when administering ritonavir alone or in combination with other antiretrovirals to patients with pre-existing liver disease, liver enzyme abnormalities, or hepatitis.

*Interaction with other medicaments and other forms of interaction:* Refer also to *Contra-indications.*

Ritonavir has a high affinity for several cytochrome P450 (CYP) isoforms with the following ranked order: CYP3A > CYP2D6 > CYP2C9. In addition to the drugs listed in the *Contra-indications* section, the following drugs or drug classes are known or suspected to be metabolized by these same cytochrome P450 isozymes: immunosuppressants (e.g. cyclosporine, tacrolimus), macrolide antibiotics (e.g. erythromycin), various steroids (e.g. dexamethasone, prednisolone), other HIV-protease inhibitors, nonsedating antihistamines (e.g. loratidine), calcium channel antagonists, several tricyclic antidepressants (e.g. desipramine, imipramine, amitriptyline, nortriptyline), other antidepressants (e.g., fluoxetine, paroxetine, sertraline), neuroleptics (e.g. haloperidol, risperidone, thioridazine), antifungals (e.g. ketoconazole, itraconazole), morphinomimetics (e.g. methadone, fentanyl), carbamazepine, warfarin, tolbutamide. Due to the potential for significant elevation of serum levels of these drugs they should not be used concomitantly with ritonavir without a careful assessment of the potential risks and benefits. Careful monitoring of therapeutic and adverse effects is recommended when these drugs are concomitantly administered with ritonavir .

There are no pharmacokinetic data available on the concomitant use of morphine with ritonavir. On the basis of the metabolism of morphine (glucoronidation) lower levels of morphine may be expected.

Norvir increases the AUCs (area under the curve) of the following drugs when administered concomitantly:

*Clarithromycin:* because of the large therapeutic window for clarithromycin, no dosage reduction should be necessary in patients with normal renal function. For patients with renal impairment the following dosage adjustment should be considered: for creatinine clearance ($CL_{CR}$) of 30 to 60 ml/min. the clarithromycin dose should be reduced by 50%, for $CL_{CR}$ < 30 ml/min. the clarithromycin dose should be reduced by 75%. Doses of clarithromycin > 1 g/day should not be coadministered with Norvir.

*Desipramine:* dosage reduction of desipramine should be considered in patients taking the combination.

*Rifabutin and its active metabolite 25-O-desacetyl rifabutin:* concomitant use with ritonavir has resulted in a multifold increase in the AUC of rifabutin and its active metabolite 25-O-desacetyl rifabutin with clinical consequences. Therefore, the concomitant use of ritonavir and rifabutin is contraindicated. (see Section 4.3 Contra-indications).

*Saquinavir:* preliminary data derived from a few pharmacokinetic studies in patients and healthy volunteers indicate that co-administration of ritonavir 400-600 mg twice daily dosing regimens produce multifold increase in saquinavir steady state blood levels.

Norvir decreases the AUCs of the following drugs when administered concomitantly:

*Zidovudine (AZT) and ddl:* zidovudine and ddl have little if any effect on ritonavir pharmacokinetics. Ritonavir decreased the mean zidovudine AUC by approx. 25% in a study which has not been of sufficient duration to reach stady state for ritonavir. Ritonavir resulted in a reduction of the mean ddl AUC by 13% when given 2.5 hours apart from ritonavir. Dose alteration of AZT or ddl during concomitant Norvir therapy should usually not be necessary. However, dosing of ritonavir and ddl should be separated by 2.5 hours to avoid formulation incompatibilities. Human pharmacokinetic data for combination with antiretroviral drugs other than zidovudine and ddl are not yet available (see also *Special warnings and special precautions for use*).

*Ethinyl estradiol:* because concomitant administration of ritonavir with a fixed combination oral contraceptive resulted in a reduction of the ethinyl estradiol mean AUC by 41%, increased doses of oral contraceptives containing ethinyl estradiol, or alternate methods of contraception should be considered.

*Theophylline:* an increased dosage of theophylline may be required, as concomitant use with ritonavir caused an approx. 45 % decrease in the AUC of theophylline.

*Fixed combination of sulfamethoxazole/trimethoprim:* the concomitant administration of Norvir and sulfamethoxazole/trimethoprim resulted in a 20 % reduction of the sulfamethoxazole AUC and a 20% increase of the trimethoprim AUC. Dose alteration of sulfamethoxazole/trimethoprim during concomitant Norvir therapy should not be necessary.

Because ritonavir is highly protein bound, the possibility of increased therapeutic and toxic effects due to protein binding displacement of concomitant medications should be considered.

Cardiac and neurologic events have been reported when ritonavir has been co-administered with disopyramide, mexiletine, nefazadone, or fluoxetine. The possibility of drug interaction cannot be excluded.

*Use during pregnancy and lactation:* No treatment-related malformations were observed with ritonavir in either rats or rabbits. Developmental toxicity observed in rats (embryolethality, decreased fetal body weight and ossification delays and visceral changes, including delayed testicular descent) occurred mainly at a maternally toxic dosage. Developmental toxicity in rabbits (embryolethality, decreased litter size and decreased fetal weights) occurred at a maternally toxic dosage. There are no studies in pregnant women. This drug should be used during pregnancy only if the potential benefits clearly outweigh the potential risks.

It is not known whether this drug is excreted in human milk. Milk excretion has not been measured in the animal studies, however a study in rats showed some effects on offspring development during lactation which are compatible with excretion of ritonavir in milk in that species. HIV-infected women should not breast feed their infants under any circumstances to avoid transmission of HIV.

*Effects on ability to drive and use machines:* Norvir has not specifically been tested for its possible effects on the ability to drive a car or operate machines. As somnolence and dizziness are known undesirable effects, this should be taken into account when driving or using machinery.

Norvir oral solution contains 43% alcohol.

*Undesirable effects:* In clinical studies (Phase II/III), the following adverse events with possible, probable or unknown relationship to ritonavir have been reported in ≥2% of 1033 patients:

*Gastrointestinal:* Nausea (47.5%), diarrhea (44.9%), vomiting (23.6%), abdominal pain (11.6%), taste perversion (11.4%); frequently dyspepsia, anorexia, local throat irritation; occasionally flatulence, dry mouth, eructation, mouth ulcer.

*Nervous system:* circumoral paresthesia (26.6%), peripheral paresthesia (15.4%); frequently dizziness, paresthesia, hyperesthesia, somnolence; occasionally insomnia, anxiety.

*Skin:* Frequently rash; occasionally pruritus, sweating.

*Respiratory system:* occasionally pharyngitis, cough increased.

*Cardiovascular:* Frequently vasodilation.

*Others:* Asthenia (22.3%), headache (15.5%); occasionally fever, pain, hyperlipemia, myalgia, weight loss, decrease of free and total thyroxine ($T_4$) values.

Nausea, diarrhea, vomiting, asthenia, taste perversion, circumoral and peripheral paresthesia, and vasodilatation have been observed most frequently and are felt to be clearly related to ritonavir.

Allergic reactions including urticaria, mild skin eruptions, bronchospasm, and angioedema have been reported. Rare cases of anaphylaxis have been reported

There have been spontaneous reports of seizure. Hyperglycemia has been reported in individuals with and without a known history of diabetes. Cause and effect relationship has not been established.

Dehydration usually associated with gastrointestinal symptoms, and sometimes resulting in hypotension, syncope, or renal insufficiency has been reported. Syncope, orthostatic hypotension and renal insufficiency have also been reported without known dehydration.

Hepatic transaminase elevations exceeding five times the upper limit of normal, clinical hepatitis, and jaundice have occurred in patients receiving ritonavir alone or in combination with other antiretrovirals.

*Clinical chemistry:* High gamma-glutamyl transpeptidase (GGT) (12%); frequently high creatine phosphokinase (CPK), high triglycerides, high alanine transaminase (SGPT); occasionally high aspartate transaminase (SGOT), high amylase, high uric acid, low potassium, high glucose, low total calcium, high magnesium, high total bilirubin, high alkaline phosphatase.

Hypertriglyceridemia, hypercholesterolemia and hyperuricemia were clearly related to ritonavir therapy.

*Hematology:* Low white blood cell (WBC) (16%); occasionally low hemoglobin, low neutrophils, high eosinophils, high WBC, high neutrophils, high prothrombin time.

*Overdose:* Human experience of acute overdose with ritonavir is limited. One patient in clinical trials took ritonavir 1500 mg/day for two days and reported paresthesia which resolved after the dose was decreased. A case of renal failure with eosinophilia has been reported.

The signs of toxicity observed in animals (mice and rats) included decreased activity, ataxia, dyspnea and tremors.

There is no specific antidote for overdose with ritonavir. Treatment of overdose with ritonavir should consist of general supportive measures including monitoring of vital signs and observation of the clinical status of the patient. Due to the solubility characteristics and possibility of transintestinal elimination, it is proposed that management of overdose could entail gastric lavage and administration of activated charcoal. Since ritonavir is extensively metabolized by the liver and is highly protein bound, dialysis is unlikely to be beneficial in significant removal of the drug.

**Pharmacological properties**

*Pharmacodynamic properties:* Pharmaco-therapeutic group: antiviral for systemic use. ATC code: JO5A EO3.

Ritonavir is an orally active peptidomimetic inhibitor of the HIV-1 and HIV-2 aspartyl proteases. Inhibition of HIV protease renders the enzyme incapable of processing the *gag-pol* polyprotein precursor which leads to the production of HIV particles with immature morphology that are unable to initiate new rounds of infection. Ritonavir has selective affinity for the HIV protease and has little inhibitory activity against human aspartyl proteases.

*In vitro* data indicates that ritonavir is active against all strains of HIV tested in a variety of transformed and primary human cell lines. The concentration of drug that inhibits 50% and 90% of viral replication *in vitro* is approximately 0.02 μM and 0.11μM, respectively. Similar potencies were found with both AZT-sensitive and AZT-resistant strains of HIV. Studies which measured direct cell toxicity of ritonavir on several cell lines showed no direct toxicity at concentrations up to 25 μM, with a resulting *in vitro* therapeutic index of at least 1000.

*Resistance:* Ritonavir-resistant isolates of HIV-1 have been selected *in vitro*. The resistant isolates showed reduced susceptibility to ritonavir and genotypic analysis showed that the resistance was attributable primarily to specific amino acid substitutions in the HIV-1 protease at codons 82 and 84.

Susceptibility of clinical isolates to ritonavir was monitored in controlled clinical trials. Some patients receiving ritonavir monotherapy developed HIV strains with decreased susceptibility to drug. Serial genotypic and phenotypic analysis indicated that susceptibility to ritonavir declined in an ordered and stepwise fashion. Initial mutations occurred at position 82 from wildtype valine to usually alanine or phenylalanine (V82A/F). Viral strains isolated *in vivo* without a change at codon 82 did not have decreased susceptibility to ritonavir.

*Cross-resistance to other antiretrovirals:* Serial HIV isolates obtained from six patients during ritonavir therapy showed a decrease in ritonavir susceptibility *in vitro* but did not demonstrate a concordant decrease in susceptibility to saquinavir in vitro when compared to matched baseline isolates. However, isolates from two of these patients demonstrated decrease susceptibility to indinavir *in vitro* (8-fold). Cross-resistance between ritonavir and reverse transcriptase inhibitors is unlikely because of the different enzyme targets involved. One ZDV-resistant HIV isolate tested *in vitro* retained full susceptibility to ritonavir.

*Clinical pharmacodynamic data:* The effects of ritonavir (alone or combined with other antiretroviral agents) on biological markers of disease activity such as CD4 cell count and viral RNA were evaluated in several studies involving HIV-1 infected patients. The following studies are the most important.

A controlled study with ritonavir as add-on therapy in HIV-1 infected patients extensively pre-treated with nucleoside analogues and baseline CD4 cell counts ≤100 cells/μl showed a reduction in mortality and AIDS defining events. The mean average change from baseline over 16 weeks for HIV RNA levels was -0.79 $\log_{10}$ (maximum mean decrease: 1.29 $\log_{10}$ ) in the ritonavir group vs -0.01 $\log_{10}$ in the control group. The most frequently used nucleosides in this study were zidovudine, stavudine, didanosine and zalcitabine.

In a study recruiting less advanced HIV-1 infected patients (CD4 200-500 cells/μl) without previous antiretroviral therapy, ritonavir in combination with zidovudine or alone reduced viral load in plasma and increased CD4 count. The effects of ritonavir monotherapy seemed unexpectedly to be at least as large as the combination therapy, a finding which has not been explained adequately. The mean average change from baseline over 16 weeks for HIV RNA levels was –1.03 $\log_{10}$ in the ritonavir group vs -0.80 $\log_{10}$ in the ritonavir+ zidovudine group vs -0.42 $\log_{10}$ in the zidovudine group. Clinical endpoint results of this study are not yet available.

The use of ritonavir monotherapy can not be recommended because of concern about the emergence of resistance.

In an open label trial in 32 antiretroviral naive HIV-1 infected patients the combination of ritonavir with zidovudine and zalcitabine decreased the viral load (mean decrease at week 20 of -1.76 $\log_{10}$).

Studies investigating optimal combinations and the long term efficacy and safety of ritonavir are ongoing.

*Pharmacokinetic properties:* There is no parenteral formulation of ritonavir, therefore the extent of absorption and absolute bioavailability have not been determined. The pharmacokinetics of ritonavir during multiple dose regimens were studied in non-fasting HIV positive adult volunteers. Upon multiple dosing, ritonavir accumulation is slightly less than predicted from a single dose due to a time and dose-related increase in apparent clearance (Cl/F). Trough concentrations of ritonavir were observed to decrease over time, possibly due to enzyme induction, but appeared to stabilize by the end of 2 weeks. At steady state with a 600 mg bid dose, maximal concentration (Cmax ) and trough concentration (Ctrough) values of 11.2 ± 3.6 and 3.7 ± 2.6 μg/ml (mean ± SD) were observed, respectively. The half life (t1/2) of ritonavir was approximately 3 to 5 hours. The steady-state apparent clearance in patients treated with 600 mg bid has averaged 8.8 + 3.2 L/h. Renal clearance averaged less than 0.1 L/h and was relatively constant throughout the dosage range. The time to maximum concentration (Tmax) remained constant at approximately 4 hours with increasing dose.

The pharmacokinetics of ritonavir are dose-dependent: more than proportional increases in the AUC and $C_{max}$ were reported with increasing dose. Ingestion with food results in higher ritonavir exposure than ingestion in the fasted state.

No clinically significant differences in AUC or $C_{max}$ were noted between males and females. Ritonavir pharmacokinetic parameters were not statistically significantly associated with body weight or lean body mass.

The apparent volume of distribution ($V_B/F$) of ritonavir is approximately 20-40 L after a single 600 mg dose. The protein binding of ritonavir in human plasma was noted to be approximately 98-99%. Ritonavir binds to both human alpha 1-acid glycoprotein (AAG) and human serum albumin (HSA) with comparable affinities. Plasma protein binding is constant over the concentration range of 0.1-100 mg/ml.

Tissue distribution studies with $^{14}$C-labeled ritonavir in rats showed the liver, adrenals, pancreas, kidneys and thyroid to have the highest concentrations of drug. Tissue to plasma ratios of approximately 1 measured in rat lymph nodes suggests that ritonavir distributes into lymphatic tissues. Ritonavir penetrates minimally into the brain.

Ritonavir was noted to be extensively metabolized by the hepatic cytochrome P450 system, primarily isozyme CYP3A4 and to a lesser extent CYP2D6. Animal studies as well as *in vitro* experiments with human hepatic microsomes indicated that ritonavir primarily underwent oxidative metabolism. Four ritonavir metabolites have been identified in man. The isopropylthiazole oxidation metabolite (M-2) is the major metabolite and has antiviral activity similar to that of parent drug. However, the AUC of the M-2 metabolite was approximately 3% of the AUC of parent drug.

Human studies with radiolabeled ritonavir demonstrated that the elimination of ritonavir was primarily via the hepatobiliary system; approximately 86% of radiolabel was recovered from stool, part of which is expected to be unabsorbed ritonavir. In these studies renal elimination was not found to be a major route of elimination of ritonavir. This was consistent with the observations in animal studies.

*Preclinical safety data:* Repeated dose toxicity studies in animals identified major target organs as the liver, retina, thyroid gland and kidney. Hepatic changes involved hepatocellular, biliary and phagocytic elements and were accompanied by increases in hepatic enzymes. Hyperplasia of the retinal pigment epithelium (RPE) and retinal degeneration have been seen in all of the rodent studies conducted with ritonavir, but have not been seen in dogs. Ultrastructural evidence suggests that these retinal changes may be secondary to phospholipidosis. However, clinical trials revealed no evidence of drug-induced ocular changes in humans. All thyroid changes were reversible upon discontinuation of drug. Clinical investigation in humans has revealed no clinically significant alteration in thyroid function tests. Renal changes including tubular degeneration, chronic inflammation and proteinurea were noted in rats and are felt to be attributable to species-specific spontaneous disease. Furthermore, no clinically significant renal abnormalities were noted in clinical trials.

Long-term carcinogenicity studies of ritonavir in animal systems have not been completed. However, ritonavir was not found to be mutagenic or clastogenic in a battery of *in vitro* and *in vivo* assays including the Ames bacterial reverse mutation assay using *S. typhimurium* and *E. coli*, the mouse lymphoma assay, the mouse micronucleus test and chromosomal aberration assays in human lymphocytes.

**Pharmaceutical particulars**

*List of excipients:* Norvir oral solution contains: ethanol, purified water, polyoxyl 35 castor oil, propylene glycol, anhydrous citric acid, saccharin sodium, peppermint oil, creamy caramel flavour, and dye E110.

Norvir gelatine capsules contain: saturated polyglycolyzed glycerides, ethanol, polyoxyl 35 castor oil, propylene glycol, medium chain triglycerides, polysorbate 80, and anhydrous citric acid. The banding components are: gelatine and polysorbate 80. The printing ingredients are: shellac, blue 2 and titanium dioxide.

*Incompatibilities:* Norvir oral solution should not be diluted with water.

*Shelf life:* Norvir oral solution: 24 months under recommended storage conditions.

Norvir capsules: 12 months under recommended storage conditions.

*Special precautions for storage:* Norvir oral solution should be stored under refrigeration between 2°-8°C until it is dispensed to the patient. Refrigeration by the patient is not required if used within 30 days and stored below 30°C.

Norvir capsules should be stored under refrigeration between 2°-8°C at all times. Avoid exposure to freezing and excessive heat.

*Nature and contents of container:* Norvir oral solution is supplied in amber coloured multiple-dose polyethylene terephthalate (PET) bottles in a 90 ml size. Each commercial pack contains 5 bottles of 90 ml (450 ml). A dosage cup containing graduations at 3.75 ml (300 mg dose), 5 ml (400 mg dose), 6.25 ml (500 mg dose) and 7.5 ml (600 mg dose) is provided.

Norvir capsules are supplied in amber coloured high density polyethylene (HDPE) bottles containing 84 capsules. Each commercial pack contains 4 bottles of 84 capsules (336 capsules).

*Instructions for use/handling:* The dosage cup with Norvir oral solution should be cleaned immediately with hot water and dish soap after use. When cleaned immediately, drug residue is removed. The device must be dry prior to use

**Marketing authorisation numbers**

| | |
|---|---|
| Norvir oral solution | EU/1/96/016/001 |
| Norvir capsules | EU/1/96/016/002 |

**Date of approval/revision of SPC** July 1997

**Legal category** POM

## SELSUN* SUSPENSION

**Presentation** Selsun suspension is presented as a viscous yellow suspension of Selenium Sulphide BP 2.5%.

**Uses**

*Indications:* For the treatment of simple dandruff and seborrhoeic dermatitis of the scalp.

*Main pharmacological action:* Selenium sulphide appears to have a cytostatic effect on cells of the epidermis and follicular epithelium, thus reducing corneocyte production. Selsun acts as an antiseborrhoeic agent which effectively controls itching and scaling dandruff. It has activity against certain dermatophytes including *Pityrosporum orbiculare* the organism causing pityriasis versicolor (tinea versicolor).

**Dosage and administration**

*Adults and the elderly:* A liberal application should be made twice a week for the first two weeks and then once a week for the next two weeks to control condition. After this initial course of treatment Selsun should not be used more often than necessary.

*Children aged 5–14 years:* Treatment as for adults.

*Children under 5 years:* Not recommended.

**Contra-indications, warnings, etc**
*Contra-indications:* Do not allow contact with broken skin.

*Precautions:* Very few cases of hypersensitivity reactions have been reported.

Selsun should be very thoroughly rinsed from the hair before dyeing, tinting or waving the hair. It should not be applied for a period of two days before or after any of these procedures. Contact with eyes should be avoided.

*Use in pregnancy:* It is not known whether Selsun can cause foetal harm when applied to the body surfaces of a pregnant woman or can affect reproductive capacity. Its effect on the milk of a lactating woman is unknown. As with all medications, avoid during the first 3 months of pregnancy.

*Side-effects:* Increased falling out of hair may occur with active treatment of any scalp condition. Oiliness of the hair may increase following the use of Selsun.

*Overdosage*

*Topical application:* None known.

*Ingestion:* Symptoms: Nausea and vomiting. Treatment: Vomiting should be provoked or gastric lavage undertaken. General supportive measures are required. A purgative may be administered to hasten elimination.

**Pharmaceutical precautions** Store in a cool place.

**Legal category** P.

**Package quantities** Selsun suspension is available in bottles of 50, 100 and 150 ml.

**Further information** Nil.

**Product licence number** 0037/5010R.

## SEVOFLURANE ▼

**Qualitative and quantitative composition** The finished product comprises only the active ingredient sevoflurane.

**Pharmaceutical form** Sevoflurane is a nonflammable volatile liquid. Sevoflurane is administered via inhalation of the vaporised liquid.

**Clinical particulars**
*Therapeutic indications:* Sevoflurane is indicated for induction and maintenance of general anaesthesia in adult and paediatric patients for inpatient and outpatient surgery.

*Posology and method of administration:* Sevoflurane should be delivered via a vaporiser specifically calibrated for use with sevoflurane so that the concentration delivered can be accurately controlled. MAC (minimum alveolar concentration) values for sevoflurane decrease with age and with the addition of nitrous oxide. The table below indicates average MAC values for different age groups:

**Effect of age on MAC of sevoflurane**

| *Age of patient (years)* | *Sevoflurane in oxygen* | *Sevoflurane in 65% $N_2O$/ 35%$O_2$** |
|---|---|---|
| <3 | 3.3–2.6% | 2.0% |
| 3–<5 | 2.5% | Not available |
| 5–12 | 2.4% | Not available |
| 25 | 2.5% | 1.4% |
| 35 | 2.2% | 1.2% |
| 40 | 2.05% | 1.1% |
| 50 | 1.8% | 0.98% |
| 60 | 1.6% | 0.87% |
| 80 | 1.4% | 0.70% |

* In paediatric patients 60%$N_2O$/40%$O_2$ was used.

*Induction:* Dosage should be individualised and titrated to the desired effect according to the patient's age and clinical status. A short acting barbiturate or other intravenous induction agent may be administered followed by inhalation of sevoflurane. Induction with sevoflurane may be achieved in oxygen or in combination with oxygen-nitrous oxide mixtures. In adults inspired concentrations of up to 5% sevoflurane usually produce surgical anaesthesia in less than 2 minutes. In children, inspired concentrations of up to 7% sevoflurane usually produce surgical anaesthesia in less than 2 minutes.

*Maintenance:* Surgical levels of anaesthesia may be sustained with concentrations of 0.5–3% sevoflurane with or without the concomitant use of nitrous oxide.

*Elderly:* As with other inhalation agents, lesser concentrations of sevoflurane are normally required to maintain surgical anaesthesia.

*Emergence:* Emergence times are generally short following sevoflurane anaesthesia. Therefore, patients may require early post operative pain relief.

*Contra-indications:* Sevoflurane should not be used in patients with known sensitivity to sevoflurane. Sevoflurane is also contraindicated in patients with known or suspected genetic susceptibility to malignant hyperthermia.

*Special warnings and special precautions for use:* Sevoflurane should be administered only by persons trained in the administration of general anaesthesia. Facilities for maintenance of a patent airway, artificial ventilation, oxygen enrichment and circulatory resuscitation must be immediately available. Sevoflurane should be delivered via a vaporiser specifically calibrated for use with sevoflurane so that the concentration delivered can be accurately controlled. Hypotension and respiratory depression increase as anaesthesia is deepened.

During the maintenance of anaesthesia, increasing the concentration of sevoflurane produces dose-dependent decreases in blood pressure. Excessive decrease in blood pressure may be related to depth of anaesthesia and in such instances may be corrected by decreasing the inspired concentration of sevoflurane. The recovery from general anaesthesia should be assessed carefully before patients are discharged from the recovery room.

*Malignant hyperthermia:* In susceptible individuals, potent inhalation anaesthetic agents may trigger a skeletal muscle hypermetabolic state leading to high oxygen demand and the clinical syndrome known as malignant hyperthermia. Treatment includes discontinuation of triggering agents (e.g. sevoflurane), administration of intravenous dantrolene sodium, and application of supportive therapy. Renal failure may appear later, and urine flow should be monitored and sustained if possible.

Because of the small number of patients with renal insufficiency (baseline serum creatinine greater than 133 mcmol/l) studied, the safety of Sevoflurane administration in this group has not been fully established. Therefore, Sevoflurane should be used with caution in patients with renal insufficiency.

Sevoflurane produces low levels of Compound A (pentafluoroisopropenyl fluoromethyl ether (PIFE)) and trace amounts of Compound B (pentafluoromethoxy isopropyl fluoromethyl ether (PMFE)), when in direct contact with $CO_2$ absorbents. Levels of Compound A increase with: increase in canister temperature; increase in anaesthetic concentration; decrease in gas flow rate and increase more with the use of Baralyme rather than soda lime (see also '*Pharmaceutical particulars*').

In some studies in rats, nephrotoxicity was seen in animals exposed to levels of Compound A in excess of those usually seen in routine clinical practice. The mechanism of this renal toxicity in rats is unknown and its relevance to man has not been established (see '*Preclinical safety data*' for further details).

Experience with repeat exposure to sevoflurane is very limited. However, there were no obvious differences in adverse events between first and subsequent exposures.

*Interactions with other medicaments and other forms of interaction:* The action of non-depolarising muscle relaxants is markedly potentiated with sevoflurane, therefore, when administered with sevoflurane, dosage adjustments of these agents should be made.

Sevoflurane is similar to isoflurane in the sensitisation of the myocardium to the arrhythmogenic effect of exogenously administered adrenaline.

MAC values for sevoflurane decrease with the addition of nitrous oxide as indicated in the table on 'Effect of age on MAC of sevoflurane' (see '*Posology and method of administration*').

As with other agents, lesser concentrations of sevoflurane may be required following use of an intravenous anaesthetic e.g. propofol.

The metabolism of sevoflurane may be increased by known inducers of CYP2E1 (e.g. isoniazid and alcohol) but it is not inducible by barbiturates.

*Pregnancy and lactation:* With the exception of one study in Caesarean Section, there are no other studies in pregnant women, including in labour and delivery. Experience in Caesarean Section is limited to one trial in a small number of patients.

Reproduction studies have been performed in rats and rabbits at doses up to 1 MAC. No effects on male and female reproductive capabilities were observed. Reduced foetal body weights concomitant with increased skeletal variations were noted in rats only at maternally toxic concentrations. No adverse foetal effects were observed in rabbits. Sevoflurane was not teratogenic.

Therefore, sevoflurane should be used during pregnancy only if clearly needed.

It is not known whether sevoflurane is excreted in human milk therefore caution should be exercised when sevoflurane is administered to a nursing woman.

*Effects on ability to drive and use machines:* As with other agents, patients should be advised that performance of activities requiring mental alertness, such as operating hazardous machinery, may be impaired for some time after general anaesthesia.

Patients should not be allowed to drive for a suitable period after sevoflurane anaesthesia.

*Undesirable effects:* As with all potent inhaled anaesthetics, sevoflurane may cause dose-dependent cardio-respiratory depression. Most adverse events are mild to moderate in severity and are transient. Nausea and vomiting are commonly observed in the post-operative period, at a similar incidence to those found with other inhalation anaesthetics. These effects are common sequelae of surgery and general anaesthesia which may be due to the inhalational anaesthetic, other agents administered intra-operatively or post-operatively and to the patient's response to the surgical procedure.

Adverse event data are derived from controlled clinical trials conducted in the United States and Europe in over 3,200 patients. The type, severity and frequency of adverse events in sevoflurane patients were comparable to adverse events in patients treated with other inhalational anaesthetics.

The most frequent adverse events associated with sevoflurane overall were nausea (24%) and vomiting (17%). Agitation occurred frequently in children (23%). Other frequent adverse events (≥10%) associated with sevoflurane administration overall were: increased cough and hypotension.

In addition to nausea and vomiting, other frequent adverse events (≥10%) by age listings were: in adults, hypotension; in elderly, hypotension and bradycardia; in children, agitation and increased cough.

Less frequent adverse events (1–<10% overall) associated with sevoflurane administration were: agitation, somnolence, chills, bradycardia, dizziness, increased salivation, respiratory disorder, hypertension, tachycardia, laryngismus, fever, headache, hypothermia, increased SGOT.

Occasional (<1% overall) adverse events occurring during clinical trials included: arrhythmias, increased LDH, increased SGPT, hypoxia, apnoea, leukocytosis, ventricular extrasystoles, supra-ventricular extrasystoles, asthma, confusion, increased creatinine, urinary retention, glycosuria, atrial fibrillation, complete AV block, bigeminy, leucopenia.

Malignant hyperthermia and acute kidney failure have been reported very rarely.

Rare reports of post-operative hepatitis exist, but with an uncertain relationship to Sevoflurane.

As with other anaesthetic agents, cases of twitching and jerking movements with spontaneous resolution have been reported in children receiving Sevoflurane for induction of anaesthesia with an uncertain relationship to Sevoflurane.

*Laboratory findings:* Transient elevations in glucose and white blood cell count may occur as with use of other anaesthetic agents.

Occasional cases of transient changes in hepatic function tests were reported with sevoflurane.

*Overdose:* In the event of overdosage, the following action should be taken. Stop drug administration, establish a clear airway and initiate assisted or controlled ventilation with pure oxygen and maintain adequate cardiovascular function.

**Pharmacological properties**
*Pharmacodynamic properties:* Changes in the clinical effects of sevoflurane rapidly follow changes in the inspired concentration.

*Cardiovascular effects:* As with all other inhalation agents sevoflurane depresses cardiovascular function in a dose related fashion. In one volunteer study, increases in sevoflurane concentration resulted in decrease in mean arterial pressure, but there was no change in heart rate. Sevoflurane did not alter plasma noradrenaline concentrations in this study.

*Nervous system effects:* No evidence of seizure was observed during the clinical development programme.

In patients with normal intracranial pressure (ICP), sevoflurane had minimal effect on ICP and preserved $CO_2$ responsiveness. The safety of sevoflurane has not been investigated in patients with a raised ICP. In patients at risk for elevations of ICP, sevoflurane should be administered cautiously in conjunction with ICP-reducing manoeuvres such as hyperventilation.

*Pharmacokinetic properties:* The low solubility of sevoflurane in blood should result in alveolar concentrations which rapidly increase upon induction and rapidly decrease upon cessation of the inhaled agent.

In humans, <5% of the absorbed sevoflurane is metabolised. The rapid and extensive pulmonary elimination of sevoflurane minimises the amount of anaesthetic available for metabolism. Sevoflurane is defluorinated via cytochrome P450 (CYP)2E1 resulting in the production of hexafluoroisopropanol (HFIP) with release of inorganic fluoride and carbon dioxide (or a one carbon fragment). HFIP is then rapidly conjugated with glucuronic acid and excreted in the urine.

The metabolism of sevoflurane may be increased by known inducers of CYP2E1 (e.g. isoniazid and alcohol), but it is not inducible by barbiturates.

Transient increases in serum inorganic fluoride levels may occur during and after sevoflurane anaesthesia. Generally, concentrations of inorganic fluoride peak within 2 hours of the end of sevoflurane anaesthesia and return within 48 hours to preoperative levels.

*Preclinical safety data:* Animal studies have shown that hepatic and renal circulation are well maintained with sevoflurane.

Sevoflurane decreases the cerebral metabolic rate for oxygen ($CMRO_2$) in a fashion analogous to that seen with isoflurane. An approximately 50% reduction of $CMRO_2$ is observed at concentrations approaching 2.0 MAC. Animal studies have demonstrated that sevoflurane does not have a significant effect on cerebral blood flow.

In animals, sevoflurane significantly suppresses electroencephalographic (EEG) activity comparable to equipotent doses of isoflurane. There is no evidence that sevoflurane is associated with epileptiform activity during normocapnia or hypocapnia. In contrast to enflurane, attempts to elicit seizure-like EEG activity during hypopcapnia with rhythmic auditory stimuli have been negative.

Compound A was minimally nephrotoxic at concentrations of 50–114 ppm for 3 hours in a range of studies in rats. The toxicity was characterised by sporadic single cell necrosis of the proximal tubule cells. The mechanism of the renal toxicity in rats is unknown and its relevance to man has not been established. Comparable human threlolds for Compound A-related nephrotoxicty would be predicted to be 150–200 ppm. The concentrations of Compound A found in routine clinical practice are on average 19 ppm in adults (maximum 32 ppm) with use of soda lime as the $CO_2$ absorbent.

**Pharmaceutical particulars**
*List of excipients:* None.

*Incompatibilities:* Sevoflurane is chemically stable. No discernible degradation occurs in the presence of strong acids or heat. The only known degradation reaction in the clinical setting is through direct contact with $CO_2$ absorbents (soda lime and Baralyme) producing low levels of Compound A (pentafluoroisopropenyl fluoromethyl ether (PIFE)), and trace amounts of Compound B (pentafluoromethoxy isopropyl fluoromethyl ether (PMFE)).

The interaction with $CO_2$ absorbents is not unique to sevoflurane. The production of degradants in the anaesthesia circuit results from the extraction of the acidic proton in the presence of a strong base (KOH and/or NaOH) forming an alkene (Compound A) from sevoflurane, similar to formation of 2-bromo-2-chloro-1, 1-difluoro ethylene (BCDFE) from halothane. No dose adjustment or change in clinical practice is necessary when rebreathing circuits are used.

Higher levels of Compound A are obtained when using Baralyme rather than soda lime.

*Shelf life:* The recommended shelf life is 24 months.

*Special precautions for storage:* None.

*Nature and contents of container:* 100 ml and 250 ml amber glass bottles.

*Instructions for use/handling:* Sevoflurane should be administered via a vaporiser calibrated specifically for sevoflurane using a key filler system designed for sevoflurane specific vaporisers or other appropriate sevoflurane specific vaporiser filling systems.

Some halogenated anaesthetics have been reported to interact with dry carbon dioxide absorbent to form carbon monoxide. To date there is no evidence that this can occur with sevoflurane. However, in order to minimise the risk of formation of carbon monoxide in re-breathing circuits and the possibility of elevated carboxyhaemoglobin levels, carbon dioxide absorbents should not be allowed to dry out.

**Marketing authorisation number** 0037/0258.

**Date of approval/revision of SPC** March 1997.

**Legal category** POM.

## SURVANTA*

**Presentation** Survanta (Beractant) is a sterile, non-pyrogenic pulmonary surfactant intended for intratracheal use only. It is a bovine lung extract containing phospholipids, neutral lipids, fatty acids and surfactant associated proteins to which have been added dipalmitoyl phosphatidylcholine, palmitic acid and tripalmitin. The resulting composition provides:

| | |
|---|---|
| phospholipid | 25 mg/ml |
| (including 11.0–15.5 mg/ml disaturated phosphatylcholines) | |
| triglycerides | 0.5–1.75 mg/ml |
| free fatty acids | 1.4–3.5 mg/ml |
| protein | less than 1.0 mg/ml |

It is suspended in 0.9% sodium chloride (PhEur) solution

Each millilitre of Survanta contains 25 mg phospholipids. It is an off-white to light brown liquid supplied in single-use glass vials containing 8 ml (200 mg phospholipids).

**Uses** Survanta is indicated for the treatment of Respiratory Distress Syndrome (RDS) (hyaline membrane disease) in newborn premature infants with a birth weight of 700 g or greater, who are intubated and are receiving mechanical ventilation.

*Pharmacological properties:* The mode of action of Survanta is biophysical rather than biochemical i.e., it reduces surface tension and concomitantly increases lung compliance. Intratracheally administered Survanta distributes rapidly to the alveolar surfaces and stabilises the aveoli against collapse during respiration thereby increasing alveolar ventilation.

**Dosage and administration**
*Dosage in infants:* 100 mg phospholipid/kg birth weight in a volume not exceeding 4 ml/kg.

Treatment of RDS should be administered early in the course of RDS, ie: preferably less than 8 hours of age. Depending on clinical course, this dose may be repeated within 48 hours at intervals of at least 6 hours for up to 4 doses.

*Method of administration:* Survanta should be administered by intratracheal instillation (i.e. drug is conducted into the lungs via an endotracheal tube) using a 5 Fr catheter. The tip of the catheter should lie at the end of the endotracheal tube. Infants should not be intubated solely for the purpose of administering Survanta.

Survanta should be warmed to room temperature before administration (see Precautions).

Before administering Survanta in infants on mechanical ventilation, set the respiratory frequency at 60/minute-with inspiration time 0.5s and $FiO_2$ at 1.0. Inspiratory pressure needs no change at this point.

To ensure distribution of Survanta throughout the lungs, each dose is divided into fractional doses. Each dose can be administered as either two half-doses or four quarter-doses. Each fractional dose is administered with the infant in different positions as given below. Between each position the infant should be ventilated for 30 seconds.

*For four quarter-doses,* the recommended positions are:

Right Lateral Position with the head lowered (i.e. head and body slanting down at an angle of approximately 15°).
Left Lateral Position with the head lowered (i.e. head and body slanting down at an angle of approximately 15°).
Right Lateral Position with the head elevated (i.e. head and body slanting up at an angle of approximately 15°).
Left Lateral Position with the head elevated (i.e. head and body slanting up at an angle of approximately 15°).

For administration of each quarter dose, the ventilator is disconnected, the catheter inserted, the dose administered then the ventilator reconnected. Between each quarter dose the infant is ventilated for 30 seconds.

*For two half-doses,* the recommended positions are:
With the infant supine, the head and body turned approximately 45° to the right.
With the infant supine, the head and body turned approximately 45° to the left.

When two half-doses of Survanta are being administered there are 2 alternative methods of administration:

*Instillation with disconnection from the ventilator.* Each half dose is administered by disconnecting the endotracheal tube from the ventilator, inserting the catheter and administering the half dose. Between the half doses, the ventilator is reconnected for 30 seconds.

Alternatively,

*Instillation without disconnection from the ventilator (through a suction port connector).* The first half dose is administered by inserting catheter through a suction port connector without disconnection from the ventilator. There should be at least 30 seconds between the half doses during which time the catheter is retracted from the endotracheal tube but not removed from the connector. The catheter is then reinserted into the endotracheal tube and the second half dose administered. The catheter is then withdrawn completely.

*Dosage in adults:* Not applicable.

*Dosage in elderly:* Not applicable.

**Contra-indications, warnings, etc** No specific contra-indications for Survanta have been defined by the clinical studies.

*Warnings and precautions*
*Special precautions for use:* Survanta should only be administered with adequate facilities for ventilation and monitoring of babies with RDS.

Marked improvements in oxygenation may occur within minutes of the administration of Survanta. Therefore, frequent and careful monitoring of systemic oxygenation is essential to avoid hyperoxia. Following Survanta administration, monitoring of the arterial blood gases, the fraction of inspired oxygen and ventilatory change is required to ensure appropriate adjustments.

During the dosing procedure, transient episodes of bradycardia and/or oxygen desaturation have been reported. If these occur, dosing should be stopped and appropriate measures to alleviate the condition should be initiated. After stabilisation the dosing procedure should be resumed.

Survanta is stored refrigerated (2–8°C). Before administration, Survanta should be warmed by standing at room temperature for 20 minutes or warmed in the hand for 8 minutes. ARTIFICIAL WARMING METHODS SHOULD NOT BE USED. Discard each vial if not used within 8 hours of warming to room temperature. VIALS SHOULD NOT BE RETURNED TO THE REFRIGERATOR ONCE WARMED.

Each vial of Survanta is for single use. Used vials with residual drug should be discarded.

Survanta should be inspected visually for discolouration prior to administration. The colour of Survanta is off-white to light brown. Some settling may occur during storage. If this occurs, gently invert the vial several times (DO NOT SHAKE) to redisperse.

*Side-effects:* Intracranial haemorrhage has been observed in patients who received either Survanta or placebo. The incidence of intracranial haemorrhage in all patients is similar to that reported in the literature in this patient population. Pulmonary haemorrhage has been reported. No other serious adverse reactions have been reported. No antibody production to Survanta proteins has been observed.

*Overdose:* If an excessively large dose of Survanta is given, observe the infant for signs of acute airway obstruction. Treatment should be symptomatic and supportive. Rales and moist breath sounds can transiently occur after Survanta is given, and do not indicate overdosage. Endotracheal suctioning or other remedial action is not required unless clear-cut signs of airway obstruction are present.

*Incompatibilities (major):* None experienced to date, as product administration is unique.

**Pharmaceutical precautions** Survanta must be protected from light and stored under refrigeration between 2–8°C. DO NOT FREEZE. Any inadvertently frozen product should be discarded.

**Legal category** POM.

**Package quantities** Survanta is supplied in vials of 8 ml suspension. Cartons are packed with 1 vial of Survanta.

**Further information** Nil.

**Product licence number** 0037/0218.

*Trade Mark

# Alcon Laboratories (U.K.) Limited

Pentagon Park
Boundary Way
Hemel Hempstead
Hertfordshire, HP2 7UD

**Alcon**

## ALOMIDE* OPHTHALMIC SOLUTION

**Qualitative and quantitative composition** Lodoxamide trometamol 0.178% HSE (equivalent to 0.1% w/v lodoxamide).

**Pharmaceutical form** Eye drops.

### Clinical particulars

*Therapeutic indications:* Alomide Ophthalmic Solution is indicated in the treatment of non-infectious allergic conjunctivitis (vernal conjunctivitis, giant papillary conjunctivitis, and allergic-atopic conjunctivitis). The etiologic factors are unknown, but common airborne allergens and contact lenses have been implicated. Lodoxamide trometamol may be effective against other ocular diseases where type I immediate hypersensitivity (or mast cells) play a major role in the inflammatory process.

*Posology and method of administration:*
*Adults and children:* One or two drops in each eye four times a day at regular intervals. Patients should be advised that the effect of Alomide therapy is dependent upon its administration at regular intervals, as directed. Improvements in signs and symptoms in response to Alomide therapy (decreased discomfort, itching, foreign body sensation, photophobia, acute ocular pain, tearing, discharge, erythema/swelling, conjunctival redness, limbal reaction, epithelial disease, ptosis) are usually evident within a few days, but longer treatment for up to four weeks is sometimes required. Once symptomatic improvement has been established, therapy should be continued for as long as needed to sustain improvement. Patients should also be advised that instillation of eye drops in allergic conjunctivitis may cause discomfort initially and that this will decline with improvement of the disease (see *Undesirable effects*).

*Children less than 4 years:* The safety and effectiveness of Alomide in children below the age of four years have not been established.

*Elderly:* There are no special precautions to be followed in prescribing Alomide for the elderly.

If required, corticosteroids may be used concomitantly with Alomide.

*Contra-indications:* Alomide is contra-indicated in those persons who have a known hypersensitivity to lodoxamide or any component of the medicament.

*Special warnings and precautions for use:* Alomide is not for injection. The recommended frequency of administration should not be exceeded. As with all preparations containing benzalkonium chloride, users of soft (hydrophilic) contact lenses should refrain from wearing lenses while under treatment with Alomide. Lenses may be worn within a few hours of discontinuation of treatment.

*Interaction with other medicaments and other forms of interaction:* None known.

*Pregnancy and lactation:* Reproduction studies with lodoxamide trometamol administered orally to rats and rabbits in doses of 100 mg/kg/day (more than 5000 times the proposed human dose) produced no evidence of developmental toxicity. However, there are no adequate and well-controlled studies in pregnant women. Since animal reproduction studies are not always predictive of human response, Alomide should be used during pregnancy only if clearly needed.

It is not known whether lodoxamide is secreted in human milk. Because many drugs are excreted in human milk, caution should be exercised when Alomide is administered to nursing mothers.

*Effect on ability to drive and use machines:* Alomide is unlikely to affect a patient's ability to drive or to use machinery.

*Undesirable effects:* During clinical studies of Alomide, the most frequently reported ocular adverse experiences were transient burning, stinging or discomfort upon instillation, which occurred in 13% of patients. Other ocular events occurring in 1 to 5% of the patients included ocular pruritus, blurred vision, lid margin crusting, dry eye, tearing and hyperaemia. Events that occurred in less than 1% of the patients included foreign body sensation, ocular pain, discharge, ocular edema, ocular fatigue, ocular warming

sensation, lid edema, chemosis, anterior chamber cells, epitheliopathy, keratopathy/keratitis, blepharitis, sticky sensation, corneal erosion, dim vision, corneal abrasion and allergy. Non-ocular events are rare and reported at incidences below 1%; these included warm sensation, headache, nausea, stomach discomfort, dizziness, somnolence, dry nose, sneezing and rash.

*Overdose:* In the event of a topical overdose, flush from the eye with running water. Accidental overdose of an oral preparation of 120 to 180 mg of lodoxamide resulted in temporary sensation of warmth, profuse sweating, diarrhoea, light-headedness and a feeling of stomach distension; no permanent adverse effects were observed. Consideration may be given by the physician to emesis in the event of accidental ingestion.

### Pharmacological properties

*Pharmacodynamic properties:* Lodoxamide, a mast cell stabiliser inhibits the *in vivo* Type I immediate hypersensitivity reaction in animals and man.

*In vitro* studies have demonstrated the ability of lodoxamide to stabilise mast cells and prevent the antigen specific induced release of histamine. In addition, lodoxamide prevents the release of other mast cell inflammatory mediators (i.e. SRS-A, slow reacting substances of anaphylaxis also known as the peptido-leukotrienes). Lodoxamide inhibits histamine release *in vitro* by preventing the movement of calcium into the mast cell after stimulation.

*Pharmacokinetic properties:* The oral bioavailability of $^{14}$C-lodoxamide in man is 71%, approximately 87% of the absorbed drug undergoes biotransformation. The metabolic transformation of lodoxamide results from stepwise hydrolysis of the oxylamide groups to form the monoxamate and the diamine. The diamine undergoes further hydroxylation followed by conjugation to either the O-glucuronide or O-sulphate. The O-glucuronide and O-sulphate metabolites account for 79% of the biotransformed lodoxamide, with the monoxamate and diamine accounting for 5% and 3% of the excreted metabolites. Only 2.7% of the absorbed dose is recovered as unchanged drug in the urine.

*Preclinical safety data:* There are no preclinical data of relevance to the prescriber which were additional to that already included in other sections of the SPC.

### Pharmaceutical particulars

*List of excipients:* Benzalkonium chloride, mannitol, methylhydroxypropylcellulose PhEur, sodium citrate, citric acid, disodium edetate, tyloxapol sodium hydroxide and/or hydrochloric acid (to adjust pH), purified water.

*Incompatibilities:* None known.

*Shelf life:* 24 months. The contents and bottle should be discarded one month after opening the container for the first time.

*Special precautions for storage:* Store upright at room temperature.

*Nature and contents of container:* Alomide is supplied in 5 ml, 10 ml and 15 ml natural, low-density polyethylene bottles with natural, low density polyethylene dispensing plugs and tamper evident polypropylene screw caps. Only 5 ml and 10 ml are currently marketed.

*Instructions for use/handling:* The dispensing tip should not be touched with the fingers or by the conjunctiva when drops are instilled. The container should be kept tightly closed.

**Marketing authorisation number** 0649/0117.

**Date of approval/revision of SPC** 25 March 1997.

**Legal category** POM.

## BETOPTIC*

**Qualitative and quantitative composition** Betaxolol hydrochloride USP 0.56% w/v.

**Pharmaceutical form** Sterile ophthalmic solution.

### Clinical particulars

*Therapeutic indications:* Betoptic is indicated for the reduction of elevated intraocular pressure in patients with ocular hypertension and chronic open angle glaucoma.

*Posology and method of administration:*
*Adults (including the elderly):* The usual dose is one drop to be instilled into the affected eye(s) twice daily.

*Children:* Betoptic is not recommended for use in children.

*Contra-indications:* Betoptic is contra-indicated in patients with sinus bradycardia greater than a first degree block, cardiogenic shock or a history of overt cardiac failure and in patients with hypersensitivity to any component.

*Special warnings and special precautions for use:* Patients who are receiving a beta-adrenergic blocking agent orally and Betoptic should be observed for potential additive effect either on intraocular pressure or the known systemic effects of beta-blockade.

While Betoptic has demonstrated a low potential for systemic effects, it should be used with caution in patients with diabetes (especially labile diabetes) or in patients suspected of developing thyrotoxicosis.

Consideration should be given to the gradual withdrawal of beta-adrenergic blocking agents prior to general anaesthesia because of the reduced ability of the heart to respond to beta-adrenergically mediated sympathetic reflex stimuli.

Betoptic, a cardioselective beta-blocker, has produced only minimal effects in patients with reversible airway obstruction, however, caution should be exercised in the treatment of patients with a history of obstructive pulmonary disease.

In patients with angle-closure glaucoma, the immediate treatment objective is to re-open the angle by constriction of the pupil with a miotic agent, betaxolol has no effect on the pupil; therefore, Betoptic should be used with a miotic to reduce elevated intraocular pressure in angle-closure glaucoma.

This product contains benzalkonium chloride and is not recommended for use when soft contact lenses are being worn.

*Interaction with other medicaments and other forms of interaction:* Although Betoptic used alone has little or no effect on pupil size, mydriasis resulting from concomitant therapy with Betoptic and adrenaline has been reported occasionally.

Close observation of the patient is recommended when a beta blocker is administered to patients receiving catecholamine-depleting drugs such as reserpine, because of possible additive effects and the production of hypotension and/or bradycardia. Caution should be exercised in patients using concomitant adrenergic psychotropic drugs.

*Pregnancy and lactation:* Although animal studies have not demonstrated any specific hazard there are no adequate and well-controlled studies in pregnant women. Because animal studies are not always predictive of human response this drug should be used during pregnancy only if clearly indicated.

It is not known whether Betoptic is excreted in human milk, caution should therefore be exercised when Betoptic is administered to nursing mothers.

*Effects on ability to drive and use machines:* No effects on ability to drive and use machines have been reported.

*Undesirable effects:* Although Betopic is generally well tolerated, discomfort of short duration may be experienced by some patients upon instillation and occasional tearing has been reported. Rare instances of decreased corneal sensitivity, erythema, itching, corneal punctate staining, keratitis, anisocoria and photophobia have been reported.

Systemic reactions following topical administration of Betoptic (e.g. insomnia and depressive neurosis) have only rarely been reported.

*Overdosage:* A topical overdose of Betoptic may be flushed from the eye(s) with warm tap water.

### Pharmacological properties

*Pharmacodynamic properties:* Betaxolol is a cardioselective Beta$_1$ receptor blocker which, when applied topically to the eye, lowers intraocular pressure. It is thought to produce this effect by reducing the rate of production of aqueous humour.

*Clinical pharmacology:* Several studies have indicated that betaxolol may have a beneficial effect on visual function for up to 48 months in patients with chronic open-angle glaucoma and up to 60 months in patients with ocular hypertension. Moreover there is evidence that betaxolol maintains or increases ocular blood flow/perfusion.

*Pharmacokinetic properties:* Betaxolol is highly lipophylic which results in good permeation of the cornea, allowing high intraocular levels of the drug. Betaxolol is characterised by its good oral absorption, low first pass loss and a relatively long half-life of approx 16–22 hours. The elimination of Betaxolol is primarily by the renal rather than faecal route. The major metabolic pathways yield two carboxylic acid forms plus unchanged betaxolol in the urine (approx. 16% of the administered dose).

*Preclinical safety data:* There are no preclinical data of relevance to the prescriber which are additional to that already in other sections of the SPC.

### Pharmaceutical particulars

*List of excipients:* Disodium edetate, sodium chloride, benzalkonium chloride, sodium hydroxide, hydrochloric acid, purified water.

*Incompatibilities:* None known.

*Shelf life:* Unopened 36 months, after opening 28 days.

*Special precautions for storage:* Store below 25°C.

*Nature and contents of container:* 5 ml and 10 ml LDPE bottles (10 ml present in 15 ml container) with LDPE plug and white polystyrene or polypropylene cap.

*Instructions for use/handling:* Do not touch the top of the bottle to any surface as this may contaminate the contents.

**Marketing authorisation number**  0649/0097.

**Date of approval/revision of SPC**  13 August 1997.

**Legal category**  POM.

## BALANCED SALT SOLUTION ALCON BSS*

**Presentation**  A sterile physiological balanced salt solution which is isotonic to the tissues of the eye. It is a lint free solution containing essential ions for normal cell metabolism. Each ml contains Sodium Chloride PhEur 0.64%, Potassium Chloride PhEur 0.075%, Calcium Chloride PhEur 0.048%, Magnesium Chloride Hexahydrate PhEur 0.03%, Sodium Acetate PhEur 0.39%, Sodium Citrate PhEur 0.17% and Water for Injection PhEur.

**Uses**  As a physiologic irrigating solution.

**Dosage and administration**  Sufficient to produce the required irrigation.

*Administration:*

*15 ml Steri-Unit Drop-Tainer dispensers:* The adaptor plug is designed to accept an ophthalmic irrigating needle. Intra-ocular tissue may be irrigated by attaching the needle to the Steri-Unit Drop-Tainer Bottle as follows:

1. Aseptically remove the Drop-Tainer by peeling off the paper backing.
2. Snap on surgical irrigator needle. Push well to ensure it is firmly in place.
3. Test patency of the assembly.

Squeeze out several drops before inserting into the anterior chamber. The needle should be removed from the chamber prior to releasing pressure to prevent suction.

*250 ml and 500 ml bottles:*

*Note:* Use an administration set with an air inlet in the plastic spike since the bottle does not contain a separate airway tube. Follow directions of the particular administration set to be used. Flip-off plastic cap from the aluminium seal and insert spike aseptically into the bottle through the centre target area of the rubber stopper. Allow the fluid to flow and remove air from the tubing before irrigation begins.

### Contra-indications, warnings, etc

*Contra-indications:* There are no specific contra-indications for this product. When the corneal endothelium is abnormal, irrigation or any trauma may result in bullous keratopathy.

Not for intravenous infusion.

**Pharmaceutical precautions**  This solution contains no preservative and should not be re-used.

Store in a cool place. Do not freeze.

15 presentation: If the blister or paper backing is damaged or broken, sterility of the enclosed bottle cannot be assured. Open under aseptic conditions only.

250 ml and 500 ml bottles: Do not use unless product is clear and vacuum is present.

**Legal category**  P.

**Package quantities**  15 ml Steri-Unit Drop-Tainer dispenser; 250 ml and 500 ml glass infusion bottles.

**Further information**  The enclosed Steri-Unit Drop-Tainers are sterile and may be safely handled by the surgeon.

**Product licence numbers**
15 ml Steri-Unit-Drop-Tainer                    0649/0007
250 ml and 500 ml glass infusion bottle   0649/0099

## BSS PLUS*

**Presentation**  BSS Plus is a sterile 500 ml intraocular irrigating solution consisting of two separate parts for aseptic reconstitution just prior to use. Part I is a 480 ml sterile solution in a 500 ml single-dose bottle, Part II is a sterile concentrate solution in a 20 ml single-dose vial for addition to Part I. A sterile vacuum transfer device is included to facilitate correct reconstitution of the product.

Each ml of the reconstituted solution contains Sodium Chloride PhEur 7.14 mg, Potassium Chloride PhEur 0.38 mg, Calcium Chloride Dihydrate PhEur 0.154 mg, Magnesium Chloride Hexahydrate PhEur 0.2 mg, Dried Sodium Phosphate USP 0.42 mg, Sodium Bicarbonate PhEur 2.1 mg, Dextrose Anhydrous PhEur 0.92 mg, Glutathione Disulphide 0.184 mg.

The reconstituted product has a pH of approximately 7.4 and an Osmolality of approximately 305 mOsm.

**Uses**  BSS Plus is indicated for use as an irrigating solution during intraocular surgical procedures involving perfusion of the eye with relatively large volumes of perfusion fluid over a relatively long period of time (e.g. pars plana vitrectomy, phacoemulsification, extracapsular cataract extraction/lens aspiration, anterior segment reconstruction etc.)

**Dosage and administration**  Reconstitute BSS Plus just prior to use in surgery. Follow the same strict aseptic procedures in the reconstitution of BSS Plus as is used for intravenous additives.

*Reconstitution using the BSS Plus Vacuum Transfer Device:*

1. Pull the tab to remove the outer aluminium ring and dust cover from BSS Plus Part I (480 ml) bottle. Remove the blue flip-off seal from the BSS Plus Part II (20 ml) vial. Clean and disinfect the rubber stoppers on both containers by using sterile alcohol wipes.
2. Peel open a BSS Plus Vacuum Transfer Device package (as supplied) and remove the sterile transfer spike.
Note: This device is vented permitting air to enter the vial during solution transfer, thereby preventing the creation of a vacuum inside the vial. An air-inlet filter is incorporated as part of the device to maintain sterility of BSS Plus during reconstitution. DO NOT REMOVE THE AIR-INLET FILTER.
3. Remove the protector for the white plastic piercing pin.
4. Firmly grasp the device from behind the flange and insert the white piercing pin into the upright rubber stopper of the BSS Plus Part II (20 ml) vial.
5. Remove the guard from the filter needle. Firmly grasp the 20 ml vial in the palm of one hand and with thumb and index finger, hold the plastic flange against the top of the vial.
6. Invert the vial and immediately insert the filter needle into the rubber injection site of the BSS Plus Part I (480 ml) bottle.
7. Fluid will automatically transfer from the vial into the large vacuum bottle unless the filter becomes occluded or loss of vacuum occurs. NOTE: an excess volume of the Part II solution is provided in each vial which accounts for the small residual volume that will remain after transfer.
8. After solution transfer has been completed, immediately remove the needle from the BSS Plus Part I container and discard the transfer device safely.

*Alternative reconstitution method:* Solution transfer may be accomplished by using a 20 ml syringe to remove the Part II solution from the vial and transferring exactly 20 ml to the Part I bottle through the target area of the rubber stopper.

After reconstitution gently agitate the contents to mix the solution. Place a sterile safety cap over the rubber stopper of the Part I bottle if the solution is not going to be used immediately. Remove the tear-off portion of the label. Record the time and date of reconstitution and the patient's name on the bottle label.

The solution should be used according to the technique standardly employed by the operating surgeon. Use an administration set with an inlet in the plastic spike since the bottle does not contain a separate airway tube. Follow the directions for the particular administration set to be used. Insert the spike aseptically into the bottle through the centre target area of the rubber stopper. Allow the fluid to flow to remove air from the tubing before intraocular

irrigation begins. If a second bottle is necessary to complete the surgical procedure ensure that the vacuum is vented from the second bottle BEFORE attachment to the administration set.

Each unit is for single patient use only. Any remaining solution at the end of the surgical procedure should be discarded.

There are no special precautions for use in children or the elderly.

### Contra-indications, warnings, etc

*Contra-indications:* There are no specific contra-indications to the use of BSS Plus, however, contra-indications for the surgical procedure which BSS Plus is to be used should be strictly adhered to.

*Precautions:* Do not use BSS Plus until reconstituted.
Do not use Part I if it does not contain a vacuum.
Do not use additives other than Part II.
Do not use if the reconstituted solution is discoloured or contains a precipitate.
Do not use the transfer device if the packaging is opened or damaged.
Do not re-use the transfer device. Destroy after use.
Since BSS Plus is intended for intraocular irrigation it does not contain a preservative and therefore should not be reused. Discard any unused portion six hours after preparation.

*Drug interactions:* Specific drug interaction studies with BSS Plus have not been conducted. However, none of the components of BSS Plus are foreign to the eye, hence, no adverse drug interactions are envisaged.

*Adverse reactions:* There are no known adverse reactions to BSS Plus.

*Pregnancy and lactation:* There is no known or perceived hazard for use in pregnancy or lactation. Use is therefore at the discretion of the physician.

*Overdosage:* The solution has no pharmacological action and thus has no potential for overdosage. However, as with any intraocular surgical procedure, the duration of intraocular manipulation should be kept to a minimum.

**Pharmaceutical precautions**  Store at a temperature not exceeding 28°C. Do not refrigerate. The reconstituted product does not contain a preservative. Discard solution six hours after reconstitution.

**Legal category**  P.

**Package quantities**  BSS Plus is supplied in two parts for reconstitution prior to use; a 500 ml bottle containing 480 ml (Part I) and a 20 ml vial (Part II). A sterile vacuum transfer device is included to facilitate correct reconstitution of the product.

**Further information**  None of the components of BSS Plus are foreign to the eye and BSS Plus has no pharmacological action. Human *in vitro* studies have shown BSS Plus to be an effective irrigating solution for providing corneal detumescence and maintaining corneal endothelial integrity during long-term perfusion. An *in vivo* study in rabbits has shown that BSS Plus is more suitable than normal saline or Balanced Salt Solution for intravitreal irrigation because BSS Plus contains the appropriate bicarbonate, pH and ionic composition necessary for the maintenance of normal retinal electrical activity. Human *in vivo* studies have demonstrated BSS Plus to be safe and effective when used during surgical procedures such as pars plana vitrectomy, phacoemulsification, extracapsular cataract extraction/lens aspiration, anterior segment reconstruction etc.

**Product licence number**  0649/0100.

## CILOXAN*

**Presentation**  A sterile ophthalmic solution containing 0.35% w/v ciprofloxacin hydrochloride (equivalent to 0.3% w/v ciprofloxacin base) and preserved with benzalkonium chloride 0.006% w/v.

**Uses**  Ciloxan is indicated for the treatment of corneal ulcers and superficial infections of the eye and adnexa caused by susceptible strains of bacteria.

### Dosage and administration

*Adults:*

*Superficial ocular infection:* The usual dose is one or two drops in the affected eye(s) four times a day. In severe infections, the dosage for the first two days may be one or two drops every two hours during waking hours.

*Corneal ulcers:* Ciloxan must be administered in the following intervals, even during night time: On the first day, instill 2 drops into the affected eye every 15 minutes for the first six hours and then 2 drops into the affected eye every 30 minutes for the remainder of the day. On the second day, instill 2 drops in the affected eye hourly.

On the third through the fourteenth day, place two

drops in the affected eye every 4 hours. If the patient needs to be treated longer than 14 days, the dosing regimen is at the discretion of the attending physician.

For either indication a maximum duration of therapy of 21 days is recommended.

*Children:* The safety and efficacy of Ciloxan in children under the age of 1 year has not been established.

*Elderly:* There are no special prescribing instructions for the elderly.

**Contra-indications, warnings, etc**
*Contra-indications:* Hypersensitivity to any component of this medication. The use of Ciloxan is also contra-indicated in patients with hypersensitivity to other quinolones.

*Precautions:* As with other antibacterial preparations, prolonged use of ciprofloxacin may result in overgrowth of nonsusceptible organisms, including fungi. If superinfection occurs, appropriate therapy should be initiated. Whenever clinical judgement dictates, the patient should be examined with the aid of magnification, such as slit lamp biomicroscopy and, where appropriate, fluorescein staining.

Ciprofloxacin should be discontinued at the first appearance of a skin rash or any other sign of hypersensitivity reaction.

Serious and occasionally fatal hypersensitivity (anaphylactic) reactions, some following the first dose, have been reported in patients receiving systemic quinolone therapy. Some reactions were accompanied by cardiovascular collapse, loss of consciousness, tingling, pharyngeal or facial edema, dyspnea, urticaria, and itching. Only a few patients had a history of hypersensitivity reactions. Serious anaphylactic reactions require immediate emergency treatment with epinephrine and other resuscitation measures, including oxygen, intravenous fluids, intravenous antihistamines, corticosteroids, pressor amines and airway management, as clinically indicated.

During therapy, soft contact lenses should not be worn.

*Use in pregnancy:* As there are no controlled studies in pregnancy women Ciloxan should be used during pregnancy only if the potential benefit justifies the potential risk to the foetus.

*Use by nursing mothers:* Orally administered ciprofloxacin is excreted in the human milk. Excretion of ciprofloxacin into human milk following topical ophthalmic administration has not been investigated. Therefore caution should be exercised when Ciloxan is administered to nursing mothers.

*Adverse reactions:* Local burning and ocular discomfort may occur as well as itching, foreign body sensation, lid margin crusting, crystals/scales, conjunctival hyperemia and bad taste following installation. Additionally, corneal staining, keratopathy/keratitis, allergic reactions, lid edema, tearing, photophobia, corneal infiltrates, nausea and decreased vision have been reported. Hypersensitivity reactions cannot be excluded.

In patients with corneal ulcer and frequent administration of the drug white precipitates have been observed which resolved after continuous application of the Ciloxan. The precipitate does not preclude the continued use of Ciloxan nor does it adversely affect the clinical course of the ulcer or the visual outcome. The onset of the precipitate was within 24 hours to 7 days after starting therapy. Resolution of the precipitate varied from immediately to 13 days after therapy commencing.

*Drug interactions:* Specific drug interaction studies have not been conducted with ophthalmic ciprofloxacin. However, the systemic administration of some quinolones has been shown to elevate plasma concentrations of theophylline, to interfere with the metabolism of caffeine, and to enhance the effect of the oral anticoagulant, warfarin, and its derivatives. Transient elevations in serum creatinine has been reported in patients receiving cyclosporin concomitantly with systemic ciprofloxacin.

*Treatment of overdosage:* A topical overdose of Ciloxan may be flushed from the eyes with warm tap water.

**Pharmaceutical precautions** Incompatible with alkaline solutions. Keep the container tightly closed. Store at room temperature (below 25°C). Discard contents one month after opening.

**Legal category** POM.

**Package quantities** 5 ml containers.

**Further information** Ciprofloxacin has cidal and inhibitory activities against bacteria which result from an interference with DNA gyrase, an enzyme needed by the bacterium for the synthesis of DNA. Thus, vital information from the bacterial chromosomes cannot be transcribed, which causes a break-down of bacterial metabolism.

Ciprofloxacin has a very high *in vitro* activity against almost all Gram negative microorganisms including

*Pseudomonas aeruginosa.* It is also effective against Gram positive bacteria, such as staphylococci and streptococci. Anaerobes are in general less susceptible.

Resistance development against ciprofloxacin occurs infrequently. A plasmid mediated bacterial resistance does not appear to occur with the fluoroquinolone class of antibiotics.

The arthropathogenic potential of some quinolones in immature animals after oral administration is recognised. Topical ocular administration of ciprofloxacin to immature animals did not cause any arthopathy and there is no evidence that the ophthalmic dosage form has any effect on the weight bearing points.

**Product licence number** 0649/0125.

## ILUBE* EYE DROPS

**Qualitative and quantitative composition** Acetylcysteine BP 5% w/v.

**Pharmaceutical form** Sterile Ophthalmic Solution.

**Clinical particulars**
*Therapeutic indications:* Ilube Eye Drops are artificial tears with mucolytic and lubricant properties, indicated for the relief of dry eye syndromes associated with deficient tear secretion, impaired or abnormal mucus production.

*Posology and method of administration:* Ilube Eye Drops are administered by topical instillation into the conjunctival sac. The usual dose is 1 or 2 drops instilled into the affected eye three or four times daily.

*Contra-indications:* Known hypersensitivity to any component.

*Special warnings and precautions for use:* Ilube Eye Drops contain benzalkonium chloride as preservative and, therefore, should not be used to treat patients who wear soft contact lenses. Discontinue use if discomfort, increased reddening or irritation occurs and persists.

*Interactions with other medicaments and other forms of interaction:* None known.

*Pregnancy and lactation:* Not applicable.

*Effects on ability to drive and use machinery:* None known.

*Undesirable effects:* None known.

*Overdose:* None known.

**Pharmacological properties**
*Pharmacodynamic properties:* Acetylcysteine, a derivative of the naturally occurring amino acid L-cysteine, is neither an enzyme nor a detergent. Acetylcysteine has been shown to dramatically reduce the viscosity and tenacity of sputum. The liquefying action is due to the presence of a free sulphydryl group which opens up disulphide bonds present in mucus. This pharmacological action of acetylcysteine is of benefit to patients suffering from ocular mucus abnormality.

Acetylcysteine has marked mucolytic properties which reduce the viscosity and tenacity of mucus in the eyes. This combined with the emollient properties of hypromellose, ensures lubrication and soothing relief for dry eye syndrome.

*Pharmacokinetic properties:* No specific work has been carried out on the pharmacokinetic properties of acetylcysteine when used as a topical preparation for the eye. Acetylcysteine has marked mucolytic properties which reduce the viscosity and tenacity of mucus in the eye. This, combined with the emollient properties of hypromellose, ensures lubrication and soothing relief for dry eye syndromes.

*Preclinical safety data:* There are no preclinical data of relevance to the prescriber which are additional to that already included in other sections of the SPC.

**Pharmaceutical particulars**
*List of excipients:* Inactive excipients: Disodium edetate PhEur, hydroxypropylmethylcellulose USP, benzalkonium chloride BP, sodium hydroxide BP, purified water PhEur.

*Incompatibilities:* None known.

*Shelf life:* 24 months (unopened), 1 month (after first opening).

*Special precautions for storage:* Store below 25°C. Protect from light. Discard 28 days after first opening the pack.

*Nature and contents of container:* 15 ml or 10 ml amber type 1 glass bottle with polypropylene screw cap lined with a rubber wad. The bottle and cap are closed with a tamper evident shrink-sleeve (alternatively tamper evidency is provided by the presence of a sticker covering the opening edge of the outer carton). The dropper assembly comprises a rubber teat, a plastic cap and a polycarbonate pipette.

*Instructions for use/handling:* Do not touch dropper

to any surface as this may contaminate the contents. Keep tightly closed after first opening.

**Marketing authorisation number** PL 00649/0144

**Date of approval/revision of SPC** 18 June 1997

**Legal category** POM.

## IOPIDINE 0.5% OPHTHALMIC SOLUTION*

**Qualitative and quantitative composition** Iopidine 0.5% Ophthalmic Solution contains apraclonidine hydrochloride 0.5% (as base) and benzalkonium chloride 0.01% as preservative, sodium acetate (trihydrate) 0.07%, sodium chloride 0.757%, hydrochloric acid/sodium hydroxide q.s. to pH 5.3 and purified water to 100%.

**Pharmaceutical form** Iopidine 0.5% Ophthalmic Solution is a sterile, buffered isotonic ophthalmic solution.

**Clinical particulars**
*Therapeutic indications:* Iopidine 0.5% Ophthalmic Solution is indicated for short-term adjunctive therapy of chronic glaucoma in patients on maximally tolerated medical therapy who require additional IOP reduction to delay laser treatment or glaucoma surgery.

The IOP lowering efficacy of Iopidine 0.5% Ophthalmic Solution diminishes over time in most patients. Although some patients have received successful treatment with Iopidine 0.5% Ophthalmic Solution for longer periods, the benefit for most patients is less than one month.

The addition of Iopidine 0.5% Ophthalmic Solution to patients already using two aqueous suppressing drugs (i.e. beta-blockers plus carbonic anhydrase inhibitor) as part of their maximally tolerated medical therapy may not provide additional benefit. This is because Iopidine 0.5% Ophthalmic Solution is an aqueous suppressing drug and the addition of a third aqueous suppressant may not significantly reduce IOP.

*Posology and method of administration:* One drop of Iopidine 0.5% Ophthalmic Solution should be instilled into the affected eye(s) three times per day (t.i.d.). Since Iopidine 0.5% Ophthalmic Solution will be used with other ocular glaucoma therapies, an approximate five minute interval between instillation of each medication should be observed to prevent washout of the previous dose. The maximum recommended duration of therapy is one month due to loss of effect over time. However, some patients may benefit from treatment with Iopidine 0.5% Ophthalmic Solution for longer periods.

Clinical studies to establish safety and efficacy in children have not been conducted and, therefore, Iopidine 0.5% Ophthalmic Solution is not recommended for use in children.

There are no special precautions for administration to the elderly.

*Contra-indications:* Iopidine 0.5% Ophthalmic Solution is contra-indicated in patients with a history of severe or unstable and uncontrolled cardiovascular disease.

Iopidine 0.5% Ophthalmic Solution is contra-indicated in patients with hypersensitivity to any component of the formulation or to systemic clonidine and in patients receiving monoamine oxidase inhibitors, systemic sympathomimetics or tricyclic antidepressants.

Iopidine 0.5% Ophthalmic Solution is preserved with benzalkonium chloride and should not be used whilst the patient is wearing soft contact lenses.

*Special warnings and special precautions for use*
*Warnings:* For topical ophthalmic use only. Not for injection or oral ingestion. While the topical administration of Iopidine 0.5% Ophthalmic Solution had minimal effect on heart rate or blood pressure in clinical studies evaluating glaucoma patients including those with cardiovascular disease, the possibility of a vasovagal attack should be considered and caution should be exercised in patients with a history of such episodes. Iopidine 0.5% Ophthalmic Solution should be used with caution in patients with a history of angina, severe coronary insufficiency, recent myocardial infarction, overt cardiac failure, cerebrovascular disease, chronic renal failure, Raynaud's disease or thromboangiitis obliterans. Caution in and monitoring of depressed patients are advised since apraclonidine has been rarely associated with depression.

In end-stage glaucoma, if reduction in vision occurs immediately following Iopidine 0.5% Ophthalmic Solution therapy, treatment should be suspended.

*Precautions:* As with all glaucoma patients on maximally tolerated medical therapy, those who are treated with Iopidine 0.5% Ophthalmic Solution to delay surgery should have frequent follow-up examinations and treatment should be discontinued if the intraocular pressure rises significantly. The loss of effect which occurs over time in most patients appears to be an individual occurrence with a variable time of onset and should be closely monitored. Furthermore, these patients should have their visual fields evaluated periodically.

No data are available on the topical use of apraclonidine in patients with renal or hepatic failure. Systemic absorption of apraclonidine following topical administration is low, resulting in plasma levels less than 1.0 ng/ml. Nonetheless, since the structurally related compound clonidine is partly metabolized in the liver and undergoes a significant increase in half-life in patients with severe renal impairment, close monitoring of patients with impaired renal or hepatic function is advised. Close monitoring of cardiovascular parameters in patients with impaired liver function is also advised as the systemic dosage form of clonidine is partly metabolised in the liver.

Use of Iopidine 0.5% Ophthalmic Solution can result in an ocular intolerance reaction characterised wholly or in part by the symptoms of ocular hyperaemia, pruritis, discomfort, tearing, foreign body sensation, and oedema of the lids and conjunctiva. If such ocular symptoms occur, Iopidine 0.5% Ophthalmic Solution therapy should be discontinued. Also, preclinical data suggest that there may be patients who develop a contact sensitisation response with repeated use of the drug. Ocular intolerance responses are more common in patients treated for more than one month.

Discontinuation of therapy in the event of rising intraocular pressure should coincide with the initiation of alternative therapy, or pressure-relieving surgery. Since apraclonidine is a potent depressor of intraocular pressure, patients who develop an exaggerated reduction in intraocular pressure should be closely monitored.

*Interaction with other medicaments and other forms of interaction:* No drug interactions were reported in those patients who were receiving concomitant medication for glaucoma or for other ocular disorders or for any systemic disease present during clinical studies.

Although no specific drug interactions with topical glaucoma drugs or systemic medicaments were identified in clinical studies of Iopidine 0.5% Ophthalmic Solution, the possibility of an additive or potentiating effect with CNS depressants (alcohol, barbiturates, opiates, sedatives, anaethetics) should be considered. Iopidine 0.5% Ophthalmic Solution has been used as additive therapy with topical epinephrine and dipivefrin without evidence of adverse interaction. However, there is a theoretical possibility that use of Iopidine 0.5% Ophthalmic Solution in conjunction with topical sympathomimetics may give rise to a systemic pressor response and blood pressure should be checked initially in patients receiving these drug combinations.

The possibility exists for an additive or potentiating effect with CNS depressants; tricyclic antidepressants have been reported to blunt the hypotensive effect of systemic clonidine. It is not known whether or not the concurrent use of these agents with Iopidine 0.5% Ophthalmic Solution can lead to a reduction in IOP lowering effect. No data on the level of circulating catecholamines after apraclonidine withdrawal are available. Caution, however, is advised in patients taking tricyclic antidepressants which can affect the metabolism and uptake of circulating amines.

An additive hypotensive effect has been reported with the combination of systemic clonidine and neuroleptic therapy. Systemic clonidine may inhibit the production of catecholamine in response to insulin-induced hypoglycaemia and mask the signs and symptoms of hypoglycaemia.

Since apraclonidine may reduce pulse and blood pressure, caution in using drugs such as beta-blockers (ophthalmic and systemic), antihypertensives, and cardiac glycosides is advised. Patients using cardiovascular drugs concurrently with Iopidine 0.5% Ophthalmic Solution should have pulse and blood pressure frequently monitored. Caution should be exercised with simultaneous use of clonidine and other similar pharmacologic agents.

*Pregnancy and lactation:* There are no studies of Iopidine 0.5% Ophthalmic Solution in pregnant women. Iopidine 0.5% Ophthalmic Solution should be used during pregnancy only if the potential benefit to the mother justifies the potential risk to the fetus.

Animal studies have been conducted which have demonstrated an absence of teratogenic effects in rats and rabbits. Slight fetal toxicity has been observed when pregnant animals were dosed systemically with apraclonidine over the entire period of organogenesis at exposure levels (mg/kg/d) of 60 times the recommended dosage regimen for Iopidine 0.5% Ophthalmic Solution. It is not known if topically applied apraclonidine is excreted in human milk. Since many drugs are excreted in human milk, caution should be exercised when Iopidine 0.5% Ophthalmic Solution is administered to nursing women.

*Effects on ability to drive and use machines:* since clonidine-like drugs may cause drowsiness, patients so affected are advised not drive or operate machinery.

*Undesirable effects:* Use of Iopidine 0.5% Ophthalmic Solution can lead to an ocular intolerance reaction characterised wholly or in part by the symptoms of hyperaemia, pruritus, discomfort, tearing, foreign body sensation, and oedema of the lids and conjunctiva. The pattern of the reactions was thought to be allergy-like. The mean onset of these reactions was 44 days (range 1–127 days). If such ocular intolerance symptoms occur, Iopidine 0.5% Ophthalmic Solution should be discontinued.

In clinical studies, the overall discontinuation rate related to Iopidine 0.5% Ophthalmic Solution was 15%. The most commonly reported events leading to discontinuation included (in decreasing order of frequency) hyperaemia, pruritus, tearing, discomfort, lid oedema, dry mouth, and foreign body sensation.

The following adverse reactions (incidences) were reported in clinical studies of Iopidine 0.5% Ophthalmic Solution as being possibly, probably, or definitely related to therapy:

*Ocular:* Hyperaemia (13%), pruritus (10%), discomfort (6%), tearing (4%). The following adverse reactions were reported in less than 3% of the patients: lid oedema, blurred vision, foreign body sensation, dry eye, conjunctivitis, discharge, blanching. The following adverse reactions were reported in less than 1% of patients: lid margin crusting, conjunctival follicles, conjunctival oedema, oedema, abnormal vision, pain, lid disorder, keratitis, blepharitis, photophobia, corneal staining, lid erythema, blepharoconjunctivitis, irritation, corneal erosion, corneal infiltrate, keratopathy, lid scales, lid retraction.

*Nonocular: Body as a whole:* The following adverse reactions were reported in less than 3% of the patients: headache, asthenia. The following adverse reactions (incidences) were reported in less than 1% of the patients: chest pain, abnormal coordination, malaise, facial oedema.

*Cardiovasular:* The following adverse reactions were reported in less than 1% of the patients: peripheral oedema, arrhythmia. Although there were no reports of bradycardia related to Iopidine 0.5% Ophthalmic Solution from clinical studies, the possibility of its occurrence based on apraclonidine's alpha-2-adrenergic agonist effect should be considered.

*Central nervous system:* The following adverse reactions were reported in less than 1% of the patients: somnolence, dizziness, nervousness, depression, insomnia, paraesthesia.

*Digestive system:* Dry mouth (10%). The following adverse reactions were reported in less than 1% of the patients: constipation, nausea.

*Musculoskeletal:* Myalgia (0.2%).

*Respiratory system:* Dry nose (2%). The following adverse reactions were reported in less than 1% of the patients: rhinitis, dyspnea, pharyngitis, asthma.

*Skin:* The following adverse reactions were reported in less than 1% of the patients: contact dermatitis, dermatitis.

*Special senses:* Taste perversion (3%), parosmia (0.2%).

*Overdose:* Iopidine 0.5% Ophthalmic Solution may be flushed from the eyes with water. While no instances of human ingestion of Iopidine 0.5% Ophthalmic Solution are known, overdose with the oral form of clonidine has been reported to cause hypotension, transient hypertension, asthenia, vomiting, irritability, diminished or absent reflexes, lethargy, somnolence, sedation or coma, pallor, hypothermia, bradycardia, conduction defects, arrhythmias, dryness of the mouth, miosis, apnoea, respiratory depression, hypoventilation, and seizure. Treatment of a oral overdose includes supportive and symptomatic therapy; a patent airway should be maintained. Haemodialysis is of limited value, since a maximum of 5% of circulating drug is removed.

**Pharmacological properties**

*Pharmacodynamic properties:* Apraclonidine is a relatively selective alpha-2-adrenergic agonist which does not possess significant membrane stabilising (local anaesthetic) activity. When instilled into the eye, apraclonidine has the action of reducing intraocular pressure. Ophthalmic apraclonidine has minimal effect on cardiovascular parameters. Aqueous fluorophotometry studies in man suggest that the mechanism of the ocular hypotensive action of apraclonidine is related to a reduction in aqueous formation. The onset of action of apraclonidine can usually be noted within one hour and the maximum intraocular pressure reduction usually occurs three to five hours after application of a single dose.

*Pharmacokinetic properties:* Following topical ocular administration to New Zealand White rabbits, apraclonidine reached peak concentrations after two hours in the aqueous humour, iris, ciliary body and lens. The cornea exhibited the greatest concentration and peaked at the earliest time point (20 minutes). The tissue distribution of apraclonidine from highest to lowest concentration in microgram equivalents per gram of tissue was cornea, iris-ciliary body, aqueous humour, lens and vitreous humour. The elimination half-life of apraclonidine from the aqueous humour was determined to be approximately two hours.

Plasma concentration of apraclonidine following three times daily, bilateral, topical ocular dosing of Iopidine 0.5% Ophthalmic Solution to normal human volunteers was less than 1.0 ng/ml. A steady state level was attained after five days of dosing. The half-life of the drug was calculated to be eight hours.

*Preclinical safety data:* Administration of apraclonidine intravenously and via the topical ocular route to both cats and monkeys resulted in a reduced anterior segment blood flow, whereas flow to the posterior segment, i.e. retina, choroid or optic nerve head, was not affected. Chronic treatment of primates with apraclonidine hydrochloride 1.5% ocularly three times a day for one year did not result in morphologic effects which would be indicative of vasoconstriction of the anterior or posterior segments of the eye. Although ocular blood flow studies have not been conducted in humans, the animal studies provide a basis for the safe use of this drug in the treatment of chronic glaucoma.

*Acute toxicity:* Acute toxicity was evaluated intravenously and orally in rats and mice and orally in primates. The approximate oral $LD_{50}$ ranged from 5.04 mg/kg (mice) to 63.9 mg/kg (rats); no lethalities were observed in primates at 55 mg/kg. In rodents toxic signs included lethargy, hypothermia, corneal cloudiness, and haemorrhagic areas as well as distension of the gastrointestinal tract. Pronounced inhibition of gastrointestinal motility is considered the cause of mortality in mice. The reduced intestinal motility was observed in mice after intravenous administration of 0.1 mg/kg. Lethargy and disturbed defecation were found in monkeys after oral administration of 55 mg/kg. The normal human dose from ophthalmic use is 0.03 mg/kg/d in divided doses.

*Subchronic and chronic toxicity:* Rabbits tolerated apraclonidine hydrochloride solutions of 0.5%, 1% or 1.5% (2 drops t.i.d.), over a period of one month without signs of systemic toxicity. Conjunctival irritation and minimal corneal cloudiness (at 1.5%) were sporadic observations.

Rats and mice received daily oral doses of up to 1.2 mg/kg and 2 mg/kg, respectively, over a period of 13 weeks. Mortalities occurred in rats at 1.2 mg/kg/d and in mice at 1.6 mg/kg/d. Pharmacotoxic reactions included disturbed defecation and distended abdomen plus corneal cloudiness in female mice of the high-dose group. Rats in the high-dose group that died before the end of the study showed toxic effects on the immune system, but these effects were not seen in animals which survived to the end of the study. No drug-related toxic or ophthalmic findings were observed when monkeys received apraclonidine hydrochloride solutions of 0.5%, 1% and 1.5% by topical ocular administration t.i.d. for one year. Mild hepatocyte vacuolisation was observed in the group receiving the 1.5% solution.

*Local tolerance:* The topical ocular administration of apraclonidine hydrochloride solutions of 0.5%, 1% and 1.5% (2 drops instilled at 30 min intervals into one eye for 6 h) led to dose-dependent conjunctival and corneal irritation in the rabbit.

Assessment of the sensitisation potential in the guinea pig proved apraclonidine hydrochloride to be moderately sensitising.

*Mutagenic and tumorigenic potential:* Mutagenicity testing of apraclonidine hydrochloride using different standard systems all produced negative results.

Two-year long-term studies evaluating the carcinogenic potential in rats (at doses of 0.1, 0.3 and 1.0 mg/kg/d) and mice (at doses of 0.1, 0.3 and 0.6 mg/kg/d) revealed no signs of a tumorigenic potential of apraclonidine hydrochloride. After 18 months of oral treatment both species (rats from 0.3 mg/kg/d and mice from 0.6 mg/kg/d) showed an increased incidence of ocular changes (mineralisation and vascularisation of the cornea, and keratitis). In addition, renal changes (mineralisation) were found in rats from 0.3 mg/kg/d onward.

*Reproduction toxicity:* Studies performed in rats and rabbits did not suggest any teratogenic action. Slight fetal toxicity was observed in pregnant animals which during the whole period of morphogenesis were systemically exposed to 60 times the apraclonidine hydrochloride dosage proposed for treatment with Iopidine 0.5% Ophthalmic Solution.

**Pharmaceutical particulars**

*List of excipients:* Inactive excipients in Iopidine 0.5% Ophthalmic Solution are sodium acetate (trihydrate), 0.07% sodium chloride 0.757%, hydrochloric acid and/or sodium hydroxide q.s. to pH 5.3 and purified water to 100%. The solution is preserved with benzalkonium chloride 0.01%.

*Incompatibilities:* None known.

*Shelf life:* Twenty four months (unopened), one month (after bottle is opened).

*Special precautions for storage:* Store at room temperature (15–25°C). Protect from light.

*Nature and contents of container:* Iopidine 0.5% Ophthalmic Solution will be packaged as 5 ml in a 5 ml, and 10 ml in a 10 ml, white LDPE Drop-Tainer* with a natural LDPE dispensing plug and white polypropylene closure.

*Instructions for use/handling:* Do not touch dropper tip to any surface as this may contaminate the contents. If the drop of medication is not retained in the eye upon dosing for any reason, instil another drop.

**Marketing authorisation number** 0649/0132.

**Date of approval/revision of SPC** 29 December 1994.

**Legal category** POM.

## IOPIDINE* 1.0% OPHTHALMIC SOLUTION

**Qualitative and quantitative composition** Iopidine 1.0% Ophthalmic Solution contains apraclonidine hydrochloride 1.15% w/v HSE (equivalent to apraclonidine 1% w/v).

**Pharmaceutical form** Eye drops.

**Clincal particulars**

*Therapeutic indications:* Iopidine 1.0% Ophthalmic Solution is indicated to control or prevent postsurgical elevations in intraocular pressure that occur in patients after anterior segment laser surgery. (Clinical trials have been conducted in trabeculoplasty, iridotomy and capsulotomy).

*Posology and method of administration:*

*Adults:* One drop of Iopidine 1.0% Ophthalmic Solution should be instilled into the eye scheduled for operation one hour before initiating anterior segment laser surgery. A second drop should be instilled to the same eye immediately upon completion of the laser surgical procedure.

*Children:* Safety and effectiveness of Iopidine in children have not been established and therefore Iopidine 1.0% Ophthalmic Solution is not recommended for use in children.

*Elderly:* There are no special precautions for administration to the elderly.

*Contra-indications:* Iopidine 1.0% Ophthalmic Solution is contraindicated in patients with a history of severe or unstable and uncontrolled cardiovascular disease.

Iopidine 1.0% Ophthalmic Solution is contraindicated for children, for patients receiving monoamine oxidase inhibitor therapy, systemic sympathomimetic agents, tricyclic antidepressants, and for patients with hypersensitivity to any component of the preparation or to clonidine.

*Special warnings and special precautions for use:*

*Warnings:* For topical ophthalmic use only. Not for injection or oral ingestion. While the topical administration of two drops of Iopidine 1.0% Ophthalmic Solution had minimal effect on heart rate or blood pressure in clinical studies evaluating patients undergoing anterior segment laser surgery, including those with cardiovascular disease, the possibility of a vasovagal attack should be considered and caution should be exercised in patients with a history of such episodes. Iopidine 1.0% Ophthalmic Solution should be used with caution in patients with a history of angina, severe coronary insufficiency, recent myocardial infarction, overt cardiac failure, cerebrovascular disease, chronic renal failure, Raynaud's disease or thromboangiitis obliterans. Caution in and monitoring of depressed patients are advised since apraclonidine has been rarely associated with depression.

*Precautions:* No data are available on the topical use of apraclonidine in patients with renal or hepatic failure. Systemic absorption of apraclonidine following topical administration is low, resulting in plasma levels less than 1.0 ng/ml. Nonetheless, since the structurally related compound clonidine is partly metabolised in the liver and undergoes a significant increased in half-life in patients with severe renal impairment, close monitoring of patients with impaired renal or hepatic function is advised. Close monitoring of cardiovascular parameters in patients with impaired liver function is also advised as the systemic dosage form of clonidine is partly metabolised in the liver.

Since apraclonidine is a potent depressor of intraocular pressure, patients who develop an exaggerated reduction in intraocular pressure should be closely monitored.

*Interactions with other medicaments and other forms of interactions:* No drug interactions were reported in those patients who were receiving concomitant medication for glaucoma or for other ocular disorders or for any systemic disease present during clinical studies.

Although no specific drug interactions with topical glaucoma drugs or systemic medicaments were identified in clinical studies of Iopidine 1.0% Ophthalmic Solution, the possibility of an additive or potentiating effect with CNS depressants (alcohol, barbiturates, opiates, sedatives, anaesthetics) should be considered. There is a theoretical possibility that use of Iopidine 1.0% Ophthalmic Solution in conjunction with topical sympathomimetics may give rise to a systemic pressor response and blood pressure should be checked initially in patients receiving these drug combinations.

The possibility exists for an additive or potentiating effect with CNS depressants; tricyclic antidepressants have been reported to blunt the hypotensive effect of systemic clonidine. It is not known whether or not the concurrent use of these agents with Iopidine 1.0% Ophthalmic Solution can lead to a reduction in IOP lowering effect. No data on the level of circulating catecholamines after apraclonidine withdrawal are available. Caution, however, is advised in patients taking tricyclic antidepressants which can affect the metabolism and uptake of circulating amines.

An additive hypotensive effect has been reported with the combination of systemic clonidine and neuroleptic therapy. Systemic clonidine may inhibit the production of catecholamine in response to insulin-induced hypoglycaemia and mask the signs and symptoms of hypoglycaemia.

Since apraclonidine may reduce pulse and blood pressure, caution in using drugs such as beta-blockers (ophthalmic and systemic), antihypertensives, and cardiac glycosides is advised. Patients using cardiovascular drugs concurrently with Iopidine 1.0% Ophthalmic Solution should have pulse and blood pressure frequently monitored. Caution should be exercised with simultaneous use of clonidine and other similar pharmacologic agents.

*Pregnancy and lactation:* There are no well controlled studies of Iopidine 1.0% Ophthalmic Solution in pregnant women. Iopidine 1.0% Ophthalmic Solution should be used in pregnancy only if the potential benefit to the mother justifies the potential risk to the foetus.

Animal studies have been conducted which have demonstrated an absence of teratogenic effects in rats and rabbits. Embryotoxicity has been observed when pregnant rabbits were dosed orally with doses of apraclonidine (doses >1.25 mg/kg/day) that were maternally toxic, and administered over the entire period of organogenesis at exposure levels >100 times the recommended daily dosage regimen for Iopidine 1.0% Ophthalmic Solution based on a 50 kg person. It is not known if topically applied apraclonidine is excreted in human milk. Because many drugs are excreted in human milk, caution should be exercised when Iopidine 1.0% Ophthalmic Solution is administered to nursing women.

*Effects on ability to drive and use machines:* Clonidine-like drugs may cause drowsiness; patients if so affected should not drive or operate machinery.

*Undesirable effects:* The following adverse reactions (incidences) were reported in clinical studies in Iopidine 1.0% Ophthalmic Solution in laser surgery as being possible, probably, or definitely related to therapy:

*Ocular:* Ocular hyperaemia (1.3%). The following adverse reactions were reported in less than 1% of the patients: upper lid elevation, ocular inflammation, conjunctival bleeding, mydriasis.

*Nonocular:* The following adverse reactions were reported in less than 1% of the patients: irregular heart rate, nasal decongestion. The following adverse events were observed in investigational studies dosing Iopidine 1.0% Ophthalmic Solution once or twice daily for up to 28 days in nonlaser studies:

*Ocular:* Conjunctival blanching, upper lid elevation, mydriasis, burning, discomfort, foreign body sensation, dryness, itching, hypotony, blurred or dimmed vision, allergic response, conjunctival microhaemorrhage.

*Gastrointestinal:* Abdominal pain, diarrhoea, stomach discomfort, emesis.

*Cardiovascular:* Bradycardia, vasovagal attacks, palpitations, orthostatic episode.

*Central nervous system:* Insomnia, dream disturbances, irritability, decreased libido.

*Other:* Taste abnormalities, dry mouth, nasal burning or dryness, headache, heat cold sensation, chest heaviness or burning, clammy or sweaty palms, body heat sensation, shortness of breath, increased pharyngeal secretion, extremity pain or numbness, fatigue, paresthesia, pruritus not associated with rash.

*Overdose:* In the case of accidental overdose, Iopidine 1% can be removed by rinsing the eye with water. While no instances of accidental or intentional ingestion of ophthalmic apraclonidine are known, overdose with the oral form of clonidine has been reported to cause hypotension, transient hypertension, asthenia, vomiting, irritability, diminished or absent reflexes, lethargy, somnolence, sedation or coma, pallor, hypothermia, bradycardia, conduction defects, arrhythmias, dryness of the mouth, miosis, apnea, respiratory depression, hypoventilation, and seizure. Treatment of an oral overdose includes supportive and symptomatic therapy, a patent airway should be maintained. Haemodialysis is of limited value since a maximum of 5% of circulating drug is removed.

**Pharmacological properties**

*Pharmacodynamic properties:* Apraclonidine is a relatively selective alpha-2-adrenergic agonist which does not possess significant membrane stabilising (local anaesthetic) activity. When instilled into the eye, apraclonidine has the action of reducing intraocular pressure. Ophthalmic apraclonidine has minimal effect on cardiovascular parameters. Aqueous fluorophotometry studies in man suggest that the mechanism of the ocular hypotensive action of apraclonidine is related to reduction in aqueous formation. The onset of action of Iopidine 1.0% Ophthalmic Solution can usually be noted within one hour and the maximum intraocular pressure reduction usually occurs three to five hours after application of a single dose.

*Pharmacokinetic properties:* Following topical ocular administration to New Zealand albino rabbits, apraclonidine reached peak concentrations after two hours in the aqueous humor, iris, ciliary body and lens. The cornea exhibited the greatest concentration and peaked at the earliest time point (20 minutes). The tissue distribution of apraclonidine from highest to lowest concentration in microgram equivalents per gram of tissue was cornea, iris-ciliary body, aqueous humour, lens and vitreous humour. The elimination half-life of apraclonidine from the aqueous humour was determined to be approximately two hours.

Plasma concentration of apraclonidine following three times daily, bilateral, topical ocular dosing of 0.5% apraclonidine ophthalmic solution to normal human volunteers was less than 1.0 ng/ml. A steady state level was attained after five days of dosing. The systemic elimination half-life of apraclonidine was approximately 8 hours.

*Preclinical safety data:* Administration of apraclonidine intravenously and via the topical ocular route to both cats and monkeys resulted in a reduced anterior segment blood flow whereas flow to the posterior segment (i.e. retina, choroid or optic nerve head) was not affected. Chronic treatment of primates with apraclonidine hydrochloride 1.5% ocularly three times a day for one year did not result in morphological effects.

*Acute toxicity:* Acute toxicity was evaluated intravenously and orally in rats and mice and orally in primates. The approximate oral $LD_{50}$ ranged from 5.04 mg/kg (mice) to 63.9 mg/kg (rats); no lethalities were observed in primates at 55 mg/kg. In rodents toxic signs included lethargy, hypothermia, corneal cloudiness, and haemorrhagic areas as well as distension of the gastrointestinal tract. Pronounced inhibition of gastrointestinal motility is considered the cause of mortality in mice. The reduced intestinal motility was observed in mice after intravenous administration of 0.1 mg/kg. Lethargy and disturbed defecation were found in monkeys after oral administration of 55 mg/kg. The normal human dose from ophthalmic use is approximately 0.01 mg/kg/d.

*Subchronic and chronic toxicity:* Rabbits tolerated apraclonidine hydrochloride solutions of 0.5%, 1% or 1.5% (2 drops t.i.d.) over a period of one month without signs of systemic toxicity. Minimal corneal cloudiness was observed sporadically in some eyes receiving the 1.5% apraclonidine hydrochloride solution.

Rats and mice received daily oral doses of up to 1.2 mg/kg and 2 mg/kg, respectively, over a period of 13 weeks. Mortalities occurred in rats at 1.2 mg/kg/d and in mice at 1.6 mg/kg/d. Pharmacotoxic reactions included disturbed defecation and distended abdomen plus corneal cloudiness predominantly in female mice of the high-dose group. Rats in the high-dose group that died before the end of the study showed lymphocytic effects in the spleen and thymus, but these effects were not seen in animals which survived to the end of the study. No drug-related toxic or ophthalmic findings were observed when monkeys received apraclonidine hydrochloride solutions of 0.5%, 1% and 1.5% by topical ocular administration t.i.d. for one year.

*Local tolerance:* The topical ocular administration of apraclonidine hydrochloride solutions of 0.5%, 1% and 1.5% (2 drops instilled at 30 min intervals into one eye for 6 h) led to dose-dependent conjunctival and corneal irritation in the rabbit.

Assessment of the sensitisation potential in the guinea pig proved apraclonidine hydrochloride to be moderately sensitising.

*Mutagenic and tumorigenic potential:* Mutagenicity testing of apraclonidine hydrochloride using different standard systems all produced negative results.

Two-year long-term studies evaluating the carcinogenic potential in rats (at doses of 0.1, 0.3 and 1.0 mg/kg/d) and mice (at doses of 0.1, 0.3 and 0.6 mg/kg/d) revealed no signs of a carcinogenic potential of apraclonidine hydrochloride. Both species showed an increased incidence of ocular changes (mineralisation and neo-vascularisation of the cornea, and keratitis), which are considered related to the pharmacological effect of the drug in reducing the tear film. In addition, renal changes (mineralisation) were found in rats from 0.3 mg/kg/d onward.

*Reproduction toxicity:* Studies performed in rats and rabbits did not suggest any teratogenic effects of apraclonidine. Embryotoxicity has been observed when pregnant rabbits were dosed orally with doses of apraclonidine (doses >1.25 mg/kg/day) that were maternally toxic, and administered over the entire period of organogenesis at exposure levels >100 times the recommended daily dosage regimen for lopidine 1.0% Ophthalmic Solution based on a 50 kg person.

**Pharmaceutical particulars**

*List of excipients:* Inactive excipients in lopidine 1.0% Ophthalmic Solution are Sodium acetate (trihydrate), sodium chloride, hydrochloric acid and/or sodium hydroxide (to adjust pH), purified water.

*Incompatibilities:* None known.

*Shelf life:* 24 months.

*Special precautions for storage:* Store below 25°C. Protect from light.

*Nature and contents of container:* Two sealed LDPE form/fill/seal single-dose containers each containing 0.25 ml and wrapped in a foil pouch. Preservative free.

*Instructions for use/handling:* If the drop of medication is not retained in the eye upon dosing for any reason, instil another drop. Discard any unused contents immediately after use.

**Marketing authorisation number** 0649/0120.

**Date of approval/revision of SPC** 19 September 1996.

**Legal category** POM.

## ISOPTO* ALKALINE

**Qualitative and quantitative composition** Hydroxypropylmethyl Cellulose PhEur 1.0% w/v.

**Pharmaceutical form** Sterile eye drops for topical ocular administration.

**Clinical particulars**

*Therapeutic indications:* Used topically to provide tear-like lubrication for the symptomatic relief of dry eyes and eye irritation associated with deficient tear production. (Usually in cases of rheumatoid arthritis, keratoconjunctivitis sicca and xerophthalmia.) Also used as an ocular lubricant for artificial eyes.

*Posology and method of administration:*

*Adults, children and the elderly:* The dose depends on the need for lubrication. Usually one to two drops to each eye three times daily, or as prescribed.

*Contra-indications:* Hypersensitivity to any component of the product. This product contains benzalkonium chloride and should not be used when soft contact lenses are worn.

*Special warnings and special precautions for use:* If irritation persists or worsens, or headache, eye pain, vision changes or continued redness occur, discontinue use and consult a physician. To preserve sterility do not allow the dropper to touch the eye or any other surface.

*Interaction with other medicaments and other forms of interaction:* None known.

*Pregnancy and lactation:* There is insufficient evidence as to safety in pregnancy and this product should, therefore, only be used in pregnancy if it is considered essential by the physician.

*Effects on ability to drive and use machines:* May cause transient blurring of vision on instillation. Do not drive or operate hazardous machinery unless vision is clear.

*Undesirable effects:* May cause transient mild stinging or temporarily blurred vision.

*Overdose:* Not applicable.

**Pharmacological properties**

*Pharmacodynamic properties:* Hydroxylpropylmethylcellulose is an inert substance. It has no pharmacological activity.

*Pharmacokinetic properties:* Hydroxylpropylmethylcellulose is an inert substance. It has no pharmacological activity and, hence, the pharmacokinetic properties have not been studied.

*Preclinical safety data:* There are no preclinical data of relevance to the prescriber which are additional to that already included in other sections of the SPC.

**Pharmaceutical particulars**

*List of excipients:* Sodium citrate dihydrate PhEur, sodium phosphate dried USP, sodium biphosphate USP, sodium chloride PhEur, benzalkonium chloride PhEur, purified water PhEur.

*Incompatabilities:* None known.

*Shelf life:* 36 months (unopened), 1 month (after first opening).

*Special precautions for storage:* Store at a temperature not exceeding 25°C. Do not refrigerate. Keep container tightly closed. Discard 1 month after opening.

*Nature and contents of container:* Drop-Tainer – Natural Low Density Polyethylene Bottle and Plug. Polystyrene or Polypropylene cap.

*Instructions for use/handling:* Do not touch dropper tip to any surface as this may contaminate the contents. If the drop of medication is not retained in the eye upon dosing for any reason, instill another drop.

**Marketing authorisation number** 0649/5900R.

**Date of approval/revision of SPC** 29 July 1996.

**Legal category** POM.

## ISOPTO* ATROPINE

**Qualitative and quantitative composition** Atropine Sulphate PhEur 1.0% w/v.

**Pharmaceutical form** Sterile ophthalmic solution for topical ocular administration.

**Clinical particulars**

*Therapeutic indications:* Atropine is a powerful and long-acting anti-cholinergic agent used for producing cycloplegia and mydriasis. It is indicated for: Cycloplegic refraction, particularly in the determination of refraction in children below the age of six and in children with convergent strabismus.

In the treatment of iritis and uveitis to immobilise the ciliary muscle and iris and to prevent or breakdown adhesions.

*Posology and method of administration:*

*Adults and the Elderly:* For refraction, instil one drop into each eye twice daily for one or two days before examination. For uveitis, instil one or two drops into the eye(s) four times daily, or as required.

Atropine should be used with particular caution in the elderly who are prone to systemic adverse effects and to the precipitation and exacerbation of glaucoma.

*Children:* For refraction, instil one drop twice daily for one to three days before examination and one hour before examination.

*Usage in children:* Do not use during the first three months of life due to possible association with the development of amblyopia. Safety and efficacy for use in children has not been established therefore use with extreme caution.

*Contra-indications:* Glaucoma or a tendency towards glaucoma (e.g. narrow anterior chamber angle). Hypersensitivity to any component. This product contains benzalkonium chloride and should not be used when soft contact lenses are worn.

*Special warnings and special precautions for use:* To reduce systemic absorption the lacrimal sac should be compressed at the medial canthus by digital pressure for at least one minute after instillation of the drops.

Extreme caution is advised for use in childen and individuals susceptible to belladonna alkaloids because of the increased risk of systemic toxicity. Parents should be warned of the oral toxicity of this preparation for children and advised to wash their hands after use.

*Interaction with other medicaments and other forms of interaction:* The effects of anti-muscarinic agents may be enhanced by the concomitant administration of other drugs with anti-muscarinic properties such as amantadine, some anti-histamines, butyrophenones, phenothiazines and tricyclic anti-depressants.

*Pregnancy and lactation:* There is insufficient evidence as to drug safety in pregnancy and lactation, this product should not be used during pregnancy unless it is considered essential by a physician.

*Effects on ability to drive and use machines:* May cause blurred vision and sensitivity to light. Patients should be warned not to drive or engage in other hazardous activities unless vision is clear. Complete recovery from the effects of Atropine eye drops may take up to seven days.

*Undesirable effects: Local:* Increased intraocular pressure, transient stinging, and sensitivity to light secondary to pupillary dilation. Prolonged administration may lead to local irritation, hyperaemia, oedema and conjunctivitis.

*Systemic:* Systemic anti-cholinergic toxicity is manifested by dryness in the mouth, flushing, dryness of the skin, bradycardia followed by tachycardia with palpitations and arrhythmias, urinary urgency, difficulty and retention, reduction in the tone and motility of the gastrointestinal tract leading to constipation.

Vomiting, giddiness and staggering may occur, a rash may be present in children and abdominal distension in infants.

Toxic doses cause rapid respiration, hyperpyrexia and CNS stimulation or depression marked by restlessness, confusion, hallucinations and occasionally convulsions. In severe toxicity coma may lead to circulatory and respiratory failure and death.

*Overdose:* Systemic toxicity may occur following topical use, particularly in children. It is manifested by flushing and dryness of the skin (a rash may be present in children), blurred vision, a rapid and irregular pulse, fever, abdominal distention in infants, convulsions and hallucinations and the loss of neuromuscular co-ordination.

Treatment is supportive (there is no evidence that physostigmine is superior to supportive management). In infants and small children the body surface must be kept moist. If accidentally ingested, induce emesis or perform gastric lavage.

**Pharmacological properties**

*Pharmacodynamic properties:* Atropine blocks the response of the sphincter muscle to the iris and the accommodative muscle of the ciliary body to cholinergic stimulation producing pupillary dilatation – mydriasis and paralysis of accommodation – cycloplegia.

The ocular effects of topically applied atropine are prolonged accommodation and pupillary reflexes may not fully recover for 7–12 days.

*Pharmacokinetic properties:* Atropine is readily absorbed transconjunctivally and is distributed throughout the body. It is mainly metabolised in the liver and some is excreted. Unchanged in the urine.

*Preclinical safety data:* No specific preclinical studies have been conducted with Isopto Atropine. The reported, oral $LD_{50}$ in mice is 75 mg/kg and in rats is 500 mg/kg.

**Pharmaceutical particulars**

*List of excipients:* Boric acid, benzalkonium chloride, hydroxypropyl methyl cellulose, sodium hydroxide and/or hydrochloric (to adjust pH), purified water.

*Incompatibilities:* None known.

*Shelf life:* 36 months (unopened), 1 month (after first opening).

*Special precautions for storage:* Store at a temperature not exceeding 25°C away from direct sunlight. Do not refrigerate. Keep container tightly closed. Discard 1 month after opening.

*Nature and contents of container:* Drop-Tainer – natural low density polyethylene bottle and plug. Polystyrene or polypropylene cap.

*Instructions for use/handling:* Do not touch dropper tip to any surface as this may contaminate the contents. If the drop of medication is not retained in the eye upon dosing for any reason, instill another drop.

**Marketing authorisation number** 0649/5901R.

**Date of approval/revision of SPC** 23 July 1996.

**Legal category** POM.

## ISOPTO* CARBACHOL

**Qualitative and quantitative composition** Carbachol USP 3.0% w/v.

**Pharmaceutical form** Sterile eye drop for topical administration to humans.

**Clinical particulars**

*Therapeutic indications:* A directly acting miotic used for the treatment of glaucoma. May be used topically to control intraocular pressure in patients who become refractory to pilocarpine alone and in patients who are unable to tolerate pilocarpine.

*Posology and method of administration*

*Adults and the elderly:* One or two drops up to four times daily. The frequency of instillation is determined by the severity of the glaucoma and the response to treatment.

*Children:* Not recommended for use in chidlren. The safety and efficacy of use in children has not been established.

*Contra-indications:* Conditions where pupillary constriction is undesirable, e.g. acute iritis, anterior uveitis and some forms of secondary glaucoma. Hypersensitivity to any component of the preparation. This product contains benzalkonium chloride and should not be used when soft contact lenses are worn.

*Special warnings and special precautions for use:* Although systemic reactions rarely occur in the treatment of chronic simple glaucoma with the usual doses used, in the treatment of acute closed-angle glaucoma the possibility of systemic reactions must be considered because of the higher doses given. Caution is particularly advised with patients with acute heart failure, bronchial asthma, peptic ulceration, hypertension or hypotension, urinary tract obstruction, gastro-intestinal spasm, recent myocardial infarct and Parkinson's disease.

Carbachol penetrates the intact cornea poorly. To reduce the risk of systemic toxicity, use carbachol with caution in the presence of a corneal abrasion or damage to the epithelial barrier of the conjunctiva or cornea caused by topical anaesthesia or tonometry.

Retinal detachments have been caused in susceptible individuals and those with pre-existing retinal disease, therefore, fundus examination is advised in all patients prior to the initiation of therapy.

*Interaction with other medicaments and other forms of interaction:* None known.

*Pregnancy and lactation:* Safety for use in pregnancy and lactation has not been established, therefore, use only when clearly indicated.

*Effects on ability to drive and use machines:* Causes difficulty with dark adaptation, therefore, caution is necessary with night driving and when hazardous tasks are undertaken in poor illumination. May cause accommodation spasm. Patients should be advised not to drive or use machinery.

*Undesirable effects*
*Local:* Burning, itching, smarting, blurring, ciliary spasm, conjunctival vascular congestion, induced myopia, sensitisation of the lids and conjunctiva, reduced visual acuity in poor illumination, lens changes with chronic use, increased pupillary block, retinal detachments and vitreous haemorrhages.

*Systemic:* Systemic reactions following ocular use are rare but they may include hypotension, bradycardia, bronchial spasm, pulmonary oedema, salivation, sweating, nausea, vomiting, diarrhoea and lacrimation, cardiac arrhythmia, gastro-intestinal cramping, asthma, frequent urgency to urinate.

*CNS:* Browache and headache (especially in younger patients who have recently started therapy).

*Overdose:* If accidentally ingested induce emesis or perform gastric lavage. Observe for signs of toxicity (salivation, lacrimation, sweating, nausea, vomiting and diarrhoea). If these occur, therapy with anticholinergic agents, such as atropine, may be necessary.

**Pharmacological properties**
*Pharmacodynamic properties:* Carbachol is the carbamyl ester of choline, it is a parasympathomimetic agent and its pharmacological properties are similar to those of acetylcholine. Carbachol is totally resistant to hydrolysis by acetylcholinesterase or non-specific cholinesterase. Carbachol has, therefore, a two-phase physiological action, direct and indirect which is advantageous in the treatment of glaucoma. In the eye, topical administration of carbachol produces miosis and accommodative spasm, more intense and of longer duration than that produced by pilocarpine.

*Pharmacokinetic properties:* Carbachol is not lipid soluble at any pH and thus penentration of the intact corneal epithelium is poor. Hydroxypropylmethylcellulose is present in Isopto Carbachol to reduce the surface tension of the formulation and to aid penetration of carbachol across the cornea. Studies with Isopto Carbachol formulated in a hydroxypropylmethylcellulose vehicle have provided evidence of intraocular penetration as demonstrated by miotic activity in animal studies.

*Preclinical safety data:* There are no preclinical safety data of relevance to the prescriber which are not already covered by the clinical section of the SPC.

**Pharmaceutical particulars**
*List of excipients:* Benzalkonium Chloride 0.005% w/v; boric acid; sodium borate; sodium chloride; HPMC 2910; sodium hydroxide; hydrochloric acid; purified water.

*Incompatibilities:* None known.

*Shelf life:* 48 months unopened 28 days after opening.

*Special precautions for storage:* Store at 8–25°C away from direct sunlight.
Keep the container tightly closed.
Discard 1 month after opening.

*Nature and contents of container:* Drop-Tainer – Natural low density polyethylene bottle and plug. Polystyrene or polypropylene cap.

*Instructions for use/handling:* Do not touch dropper tip to any surface as this may contaminate the contents.

If the drop of medication is not retained in the eye upon dosing for any reason then instil another drop.

**Marketing authorisation number**    0649/5902R.

**Date of approval/revision of SPC**    25 January 1996.

**Legal category**    POM.

## ISOPTO* CARPINE
## 0.5%, 1.0%, 2.0%, 3.0%, 4.0%

**Presentation**    Isopto Carpine is a clear, colourless, sterile solution available in five strengths; containing 0.5, 1, 2, 3 or 4% pilocarpine hydrochloride and 0.5% hydroxypropyl methylcellulose (hypromellose), and preserved with benzalkonium chloride 0.01%.

**Uses**    Isopto Carpine is a directly-acting miotic used for the treatment of glaucoma. For topical instillation into the eye it is indicated for chronic simple glaucoma, patients may be maintained on pilocarpine as long as intraocular pressure is controlled and there is no deterioration in the visual fields. Also indicated for acute (closed angle glaucoma), pilocarpine may be used alone or in conjunction with other agents to decrease intraocular pressure prior to surgical treatment and for miosis to counter the effects of cycloplegic and mydriatic eye drops.

**Dosage and administration**    One or two drops up to four times daily or as prescribed. The frequency of instillation and concentration of drops used are determined by the severity of the glaucoma and the response to treatment.

*Usage in children:* At the discretion of the physician. Safety and efficacy of use in children has not been established.

**Contra-indications, warnings, etc**
*Contra-indications:* Contraindicated in conditions where pupillary constriction is undesirable, e.g. acute iritis, anterior uveitis and some forms of secondary glaucoma. Hypersensitivity to any components of the preparation. Patients wearing soft contact lenses should not use this preparation.

*Warnings:* For topical use only. Not for injection. Although systemic reactions rarely occur in the treatment of chronic simple glaucoma with the usual doses used, in the treatment of acute closed-angle glaucoma the possibility of systemic reactions must be considered because of the higher doses given. Caution is particularly advised with patients with acute heart failure, bronchial asthma, peptic ulceration, hypertension, urinary tract obstruction and Parkinson's disease. As with all miotics rare cases of retinal detachment have been reported when used in certain susceptible individuals and those with pre-existing retinal disease, therefore fundus examination is advised in all patients prior to the initiation of therapy. The miosis usually causes difficulty with dark adaptation, therefore, caution is necessary with night driving and when hazardous tasks are undertaken in poor illumination. May cause accommodation spasm. Patients should be advised not to drive or use machinery if vision is not clear.

*Adverse reactions:* Local: Burning, itching, smarting, blurring, ciliary spasm, conjunctival vascular congestion, induced myopia, sensitisation of the lids and conjunctiva, reduced visual acuity in poor illumination, lens changes with chronic use, increased pupillary block, retinal detachments and vitreous haemorrhages.
CNS: Browache and headache (especially in younger patients who have recently started therapy).
Systemic: Systemic reactions following ocular use are rare but they may include hypertension, tachycardia, bronchial spasm, pulmonary oedema, salivation, sweating, nausea, vomiting, diarrhoea and lacrimation.

*Overdosage:* If accidentally ingested, induce emesis or perform gastric lavage. Observe for signs of toxicity (salivation, lacrimation, sweating, nausea, vomiting and diarrhoea). If these occur, therapy with anticholinergic agents, such as atropine, may be necessary.

*Use in pregnancy:* Safety for use in pregnancy and lactation has not been established, therefore, use only when clearly indicated.

**Pharmaceutical precautions**    Isopto Carpine should be stored in a cool place away from direct sunlight. Keep the container tightly closed. The contents should be discarded one month after opening.

**Legal category**    POM.

**Package quantities**    10 ml containers.

**Further information**    Isopto Carpine eye drops are contained in an unbreakable semi-rigid, plastic dropper bottle with screw-on cap.

**Product licence numbers**
0.5%    0649/5903
1.0%    0649/5904
2.0%    0649/5905
3.0%    0649/5906
4.0%    0649/5907

## ISOPTO* FRIN 0.12%

**Presentation**    Isopto Frin is a clear, colourless sterile solution, containing Phenylephrine Hydrochloride BP 0.12% and Hydroxypropylmethylcellulose (Hypromellose) USP 0.5%, and preserved with Benzethonium Chloride USP 0.01%.

**Uses**    For the temporary relief of redness of the eye due to minor eye irritations.

**Dosage and administration**    One or two drops instilled topically into the eye up to four times a day. Isopto Frin is suitable for use by both adults and children.

**Contra-indications, warnings, etc**
*Contra-indications:* Not to be used by contact lens wearers except under medical supervision.

*Interactions:* Phenylephrine may interfere with the actions of antihypertensive agents while monoamine oxidase inhibitors and tricyclic antidepressants can exacerbate the systemic effects of phenylephrine.

*Effects on ability to drive and to use machines:* As with other eyedrops blurring of vision may occur immediately after instillation. Patients should be advised not to drive until any effects on vision have cleared.

*Warnings and precautions:* Patients being treated for high blood pressure or depression should consult their doctor before using these drops. If eye pain, changes in vision, continued redness of the eye are experienced or if the condition worsens or persists for more than 24 hours, patients should consult their doctor. Isopto Frin should not be used in patients with any eye disease or who have had eye surgery except under the advice and supervision of a doctor. Continued use of this product may increase redness of the eye. Care should be exercised in its use in small children, pressure should be put on the inner canthus of the eye for a few minutes after instillation to decrease systemic absorption through the conjunctiva. Use with caution on an inflamed eye, as hyperaemia greatly increases the rate of systemic absorption through the conjunctiva. Slight dilation of the pupil may occur in some patients. For this reason it should be used with care where narrow angle glaucoma may be present since its use may precipitate angle closure or in those with a shallow anterior chamber.

*Pregnancy Warning:* This product should only be used during pregnancy if considered essential by the physician.

*Treatment of overdose:* An overdose from a 0.12% solution of phenylephrine hydrochloride is extremely unlikely. Symptoms would however be those of acute hypertension. In such an event a quick acting adrenergic blocking agent such as 5 to 10 mg phentolamine mesylate, followed by a β-blocking agent such as 2.5 to 5 mg propranolol should be given.

**Pharmaceutical precautions**    Isopto Frin eye drops should be stored in a cool place away from direct sunlight. Keep the container tightly closed. Contents should be discarded one month after opening. If the solution changes colour or becomes cloudy, do not use.

**Legal category**    P.

**Package quantities**    10 ml containers.

**Further information**    Isopto Frin eye drops are contained in an unbreakable semi-rigid plastic dropper bottle with screw-on cap.

**Product licence number**    0649/5911.

## ISOPTO* PLAIN

**Presentation**    Isopto Plain is a sterile, clear, colourless solution containing hydroxypropyl methylcellulose (hypromellose) 0.5% and preserved with benzalkonium chloride 0.01%.

**Uses**    Isopto Plain is used topically to provide tear-like lubrication for the symptomatic relief of dry eyes and eye irritation associated with deficient tear production. (Usually in cases of rheumatoid arthritis, keratoconjunctivitis, sicca and xerophthalmia.) Also used as an ocular lubricant for artificial eyes.

**Dosage and administration**    It is suitable for use both by adults and children. The dose depends on the need for lubrication. Usually one to two drops to each eye three times daily or as prescribed.

**Contra-indications, warnings, etc**
*Contra-indications:* In those persons showing hypersensitivity to any component of the product. This product contains benzalkonium chloride and should not be used when soft contact lenses are worn.
*Warnings:* If irritation persists or worsens, or headache, eye pain, vision changes or continued redness occur, discontinue use and consult a physician. To preserve sterility do not allow the dropper to touch the eye or any other surface. This product may cause transient blurring of vision and mild stinging on instillation. Do not drive or operate hazardous machinery unless vision is clear.
*Use in pregnancy:* There is insufficient evidence as to safety in pregnancy and this product should, therefore, only be used in pregnancy if it is considered essential by the physician.

**Pharmaceutical precautions** The eye-drops should be stored in a cool place (8° to 25°C). Keep the container tightly closed. Keep out of reach of children. Discard contents one month after opening.

**Legal category** P.

**Package quantities** 10 ml containers.

**Further information** Isopto Plain eye-drops are contained in an unbreakable semi-rigid plastic dropper bottle with a screw-on cap.

**Product licence number** 0649/5920.

## LUBRI-TEARS*

**Presentation** Pale yellow, sterile ophthalmic ointment containing active ingredients: Wool Fat PhEur 10% w/w, White Soft Paraffin BP 60% w/w, Liquid Paraffin PhEur 30% w/w. No preservatives are included in the formulation.

**Uses** As adjunctive therapy to lubricate and protect the eye in conditions such as exposure keratitis, decreased corneal sensitivity, recurrent corneal erosions, keratitis sicca, ophthalmic surgery and non-ophthalmic surgery.

**Dosage and administration** Pull down the lower eye lid and place a small quantity in the conjunctival sac. Use as required. There is no variation of dosage for age.

**Contra-indications, warnings, etc**
*Contra-indications:* Hypersensitivity to the active ingredients.
*Precautions and warnings:* Application of the ointment may cause blurring of vision. Patients should be advised not to drive or operate machinery if affected.
*Use in pregnancy and lactation:* Suitable for use in pregnancy and lactation.

**Pharmaceutical precautions** Store below 30°C. To avoid contamination during use, do not allow the tube tip to touch any surface. Close the tube after each application.

**Legal category** P.

**Package quantities** Ophthalmic ointment tubes of 5 g.

**Further information** Nil.

**Product licence number** 0649/0143.

## MAXIDEX*

**Presentation** Dexamethasone 0.1% in a vehicle containing 0.5% hydroxypropyl methylcellulose (hypromellose). A sterile, isotonic, ophthalmic suspension, preserved with benzalkonium chloride 0.01%.

**Uses** Indicated for treatment of steroid responsive inflammatory conditions of the conjunctiva, cornea and anterior segment of the eye, such as: anterior uveitis, iritis, cyclitis, allergic and vernal conjunctivitis, herpes zoster keratitis, superficial punctate keratitis and non specific superficial keratitis. Also indicated for the treatment of corneal injury from chemical, radiation or thermal burns or following penetration by foreign bodies. Indicated for post-operative use to reduce inflammatory reactions and suppress graft reaction.

**Dosage and administration** The frequency of instillation of drops and the duration of treatment will vary depending upon the severity of the underlying condition and the response to treatment. Severe inflammations require one or two drops instilled into the eye every thirty to sixty minutes until a satisfactory response occurs. Subconjunctival or systemic steroid therapy should be considered if there is no response. When a favourable response has been observed reduce the dosage towards one drop every four hours.

**Contra-indications, warnings, etc**
*Contra-indications:* Contra-indicated in herpes simplex and other viral diseases of the cornea and conjunctiva, fungal disease, ocular tuberculosis, untreated purulent infections and hypersensitivity to any component of the preparation. This product should not be used when soft lenses are being worn.
*Warnings:* Topical corticosteroids should never be given for an undiagnosed red eye as inappropriate use is potentially blinding. Because of the risk of "steroid glaucoma" and cataract formation the intraocular pressure and the lens must be checked frequently during use of this preparation. To avoid the risk of enhancement of herpetic corneal disease, frequent slit-lamp examination is essential. Topical steroids may mask or enhance the activity of acute purulent eye infections. In such cases antibiotic therapy is mandatory. Persistent corneal ulceration following long-term topical steroid use may be due to fungal invasion. Topical corticosteroids are not effective in mustard gas keratitis or Skogren's keratoconjunctivitis. Patient should be warned not to drive or use hazardous machinery if vision is not clear.
*Precautions:* This product may cause transient stinging on instillation or sensitivity to bright light.
*Adverse reactions:* Topical steroid use may result in increased intraocular pressure leading to optic nerve damage, reduced visual acuity and visual field defects. Intensive or prolonged use of topical corticosteroids may lead to the formation of posterior subcapsular cataracts. In those diseases causing thinning of the cornea or sclera, perforation of the globe may occur. Viral and fungal infections may be exacerbated by steroids. Transient stinging or burning may occur on instillation of the drops. Systemic side effects may occur with extensive use.
*Use in pregnancy:* There is inadequate evidence of safety in human pregnancy. Topical administration of corticosteroids to pregnant animals can cause abnormalities of foetal development including cleft palate and intra-uterine growth retardation. There may therefore be a very small risk of such effects in the human pregnancy.
*Treatment of overdose:* Long-term intensive topical use may lead to systemic effects. Oral ingestion of the contents of one bottle (up to 10 mls) is unlikely to lead to any serious adverse effects.

**Pharmaceutical precautions** Maxidex should be stored in a cool place away from direct sunlight. Keep the container tightly closed. The contents should be discarded one month after opening. Shake well before using.

**Legal category** POM.

**Package quantities** 5 ml and 10 ml containers.

**Further information** Maxidex eye drops are contained in an unbreakable semi-rigid, plastic dropper bottle with a screw-on cap, containing 5 ml or 10 ml of the preparation. Maxidex is a highly penetrating form of dexamethasone, a 0.1% microfine suspension especially formulated to provide maximum corneal absorption.

**Product licence number** 0649/5914.

## MAXITROL* EYE DROPS

**Qualitative and quantitative composition** Dexamethasone PhEur 0.1% w/v, *Polymyxin B Sulphate PhEur 6000.0 U, *Neomycin Sulphate (as base) 3500.0 U.
*The quantity of ingredient is expressed per ml of product.

**Pharmaceutical form** White sterile suspension for topical ocular administration.

**Clinical particulars**
*Therapeutic indications:* Maxitrol Eye Drops is indicated for the short-term treatment of steroid responsive conditions of the eye when prophylactic antibiotic treatment is also required, after excluding the presence of fungal and viral disease.
*Posology and method of administration*
*Children and adults (including the elderly):* Apply one or two drops to each affected eye up to six times daily or, more frequently if required. (Severe infections may require one or two drops every 15–20 minutes initially, reducing the frequency of instillation gradually as the infection is controlled.)
*Contra-indications:* Hypersensitivity to neomycin or to any component of the preparation. (Cross-sensitivity with other aminoglycoside antibiotics may occur.) Herpes simplex and other viral diseases of the cornea and conjunctiva, fungal disease, ocular tuberculosis, untreated purulent infections. This product contains benzalkonium chloride and should not be used when soft contact lenses are worn.
*Special warning and special precautions for use:* In severe infections topical use should be supplemented with appropriate systemic treatment.

Prolonged use should be avoided as it may lead to skin sensitisation and the emergence of resistant organisms.

Neomycin may cause irreversible partial or total deafness when given systemically or when applied topically to open wounds or damaged skin. This effect is dose-related and is enhanced by renal or hepatic impairment. Although this effect has not been reported following topical ocular use the possibility should be considered when high dose topical treatment is given to small children or infants. Topical corticosteroids should never be given for an undiagnosed red eye as inappropriate use is potentially blinding.

Because of the risk of 'steroid glaucoma' and cataract formation the intraocular pressure and the lens must be checked frequently during use of this preparation.

To avoid the risk of enhancement of herpetic corneal disease, frequent slip lamp examination is essential.

Topical steroids may mask or enhance the activity of acute purulent eye infections. In such cases antibiotic therapy is mandatory. Persistent corneal ulceration following long-term topical steroid use may be due to fungal invasion.

Topical corticosteroids are not effective in mustard gas keratitis or Sjorgren's keratoconjunctivitis.

*Interaction with other medicaments and other forms of interaction:* None relevant to topical use.

*Pregnancy and lactation:* Safety for use in pregnancy and lactation has not been established. Topical administration of corticosteroids to pregnant animals can cause abnormalities of foetal development including cleft palate and intra-uterine growth with retardation. There may therefore be a very small risk of such effects in human pregnancy. Use only when it is considered essential by the physician.

*Effects on ability to drive and use machines:* May cause transient blurring of vision on instillation. Warn patients not to drive or operate hazardous machinery unless vision is clear.

*Undesirable effects:* Hypersensitivity reactions, usually of the delayed type, occur frequently with local treatment with neomycin. Irritation, burning, stinging, itching and dermatitis may occur. Topical steroid use may result in increased intraocular pressure leading to optic nerve disease, reduced visual acuity and visual field defects. Intensive or prolonged use of topical corticosteroids may lead to formation of posterior subcapsular cataracts. In those diseases causing thinning of the cornea or sclera, perforation of the globe may occur. Viral and fungal infections may be exacerbated by steroids. Systemic side effects may occur with extensive use.

*Overdose:* Long-term intensive topical use may lead to systemic effects. Oral ingestion of the contents of one bottle (up to 10 ml) is unlikely to lead to any serious adverse effects.

**Pharmacological properties**
*Pharmacodynamic properties:* Maxitrol contains dexamethasone, neomycin sulphate and polymyxin B sulphate as active constituents.

Dexamethasone is a synthetic glucocorticoid with a potent anti-inflammatory activity. The relative anti-inflammatory potency of dexamethasone is 25 times that of cortisone, but its effects on sodium and water retention, potassium loss and abnormal sugar metabolism are minimal.

Neomycin is a broad spectrum antibiotic, highly sensitive gram negative organisms include: *E. coli, Enterobactor aerogenes, K. pneumoniae,* Pasteurella, *Pr. vulgaris,* Salmonella, Shigella, *Haemophilus influenzae, Neisseria meningitidis, Vibrio cholerae,* and *Bordetella pertussis.*

Gram positive microorganisms that are inhibited include: *Bacillus anthracis, Corynebacterium diptheriae, Staph. aureus, Strep. facecalis, Listeria monocytogenes* and *M. tuberculosis. Borrelia* and *Leptospira interrogans (icterohaemorrhagiae)* are also suppressed. Strains of *Pseudomonas aeruginosa* are resitant to neomycin.

Polymyxin B sulphate is active only against gram negative bacteria and is particularly active against *Pseudomonas aeruginosa.* Other sensitive organisms are: Enterobacter, *Escherichia coli,* Klebsiella, Salmonella, Pasteurella, Bordetella and Shigella. However, protens and most strains of Neisseria, Providentia and Serratia are resistant to Polymyxin B. Most sensitive organisms are inhibited by 0.1 to 0.2 units/ml.

*Pharmacokinetic properties:* Dexamethasone, like other corticosteroids, is absorbed rapidly after oral administration and has a biological half-life of about 190 minutes. Sufficient absorption may occur after topical application to the skin and eye to produce systemic effects. Intraocular penetration of dexamethasone occurs in significant amounts and contributes to the effectiveness of dexamethasone in anterior segment inflammatory disease.

Polymyxin B sulphate is not absorbed from the gastrointestinal tract or through intact skin, although the intact corneal epithelium prevents penetration into the corneal stroma, therapeutic concentrations do enter the stroma after epithelial damage. Good stromal penetration occurs after epithelial abrasion following topical instillation, subconjunctival injection, or corneal bath. No significant polymyxin B penetration into the vitrous is demonstrable after parenteral or local administration of the drug.

Neomycin is poorly absorbed from the gastrointestinal tract and after topical administration insufficient is absorbed to produce systemic effects. Absorption has been reported to occur from wounds and inflamed skin. After absorption neomycin is rapidly excreted by the kidneys in active form.

*Preclinical safety data:* There are no preclinical data of relevance to the prescriber which are additional to that already included in other sections of the SPC.

### Pharmaceutical particulars
*List of excipients:* Sodium chloride, polysorbate 20, benzalkonium chloride, hydroxypropyl methylcellulose, hydrochloric acid/sodium hydroxide, purified water.

*Incompatibilities:* None known.

*Shelf life:* Unopened 24 months, after opening 28 days.

*Special precautions for storage:* Store at 8–25°C away from direct sunlight. Keep the container tightly closed.

*Nature and contents of container:* 5 ml and 10 ml Drop-Tainers, natural LDPE bottle and plug with a polystyrene or polypropylene cap.

*Instructions for use/handling:* Do not touch the tip of the bottle to any surface as this contaminate the contents.

**Marketing authorisation number** 0649/5915R.

**Date of approval/revision of SPC** 24 January 1996.

**Legal category** POM.

## MAXITROL* OINTMENT

**Qualitative and quantitative composition** Dexamethasone PhEur 0.1% w/w; *Polymyxin B Sulphate PhEur 6000.0 U; *Neomycin Sulphate (as base) 3500.0 U.

*The quantity of ingredient is expressed per gram of product.

**Pharmaceutical form** White to very pale yellow greasy homogeneous ointment for topical administration.

### Clinical particulars
*Therapeutic indications:* Maxitrol Ointment is indicated for the short-term treatment of steroid responsive conditions of the eye when prophylactic antibiotic treatment is also required, after excluding the presence of fungal and viral disease.

*Posology and method of administration*
*Children and adults (including the elderly):* Apply a small amount into the conjunctival sac(s) up to three or four times daily or, may be used adjunctively with drops at bedtime.

*Contra-indications:* Hypersensitivity to neomycin or to any component of the preparation. (Cross-sensitivity with other aminoglycoside antibiotics may occur.) Herpes simplex and other viral diseases of the cornea and conjunctiva, fungal disease, ocular tuberculosis, untreated purulent infections.

*Special warnings and special precautions for use:* In severe infections topical use should be supplemented with appropriate systemic treatment.

Prolonged use should be avoided as it may lead to skin sensitisation and the emergence of resistant organisms.

Neomycin may cause irreversible partial or total deafness when given systemically or when applied topically to open wounds or damaged skin. This effect is dose-related and is enhanced by renal or hepatic impairment. Although this effect has not been reported following topical ocular use the possibility should be considered when high dose topical treatment is given to small children or infants.

Topical corticosteroids should never be given for an undiagnosed red eye as inappropriate use is potentially blinding.

Because of the risk of 'steroid glaucoma' and cataract formation the intraocular pressure and the lens must be checked frequently during use of this preparation.

To avoid the risk of enhancement of herpetic corneal disease, frequent slip lamp examination is essential.

Topical steroids may mask or enhance the activity of acute purulent eye infections. In such cases antibiotic therapy is mandatory. Persistent corneal ulceration following long-term topical steroid use may be due to fungal invasion.

Topical corticosteroids are not effective in mustard gas keratitis or Sjorgren's keratoconjunctivitis.

*Interaction with other medicaments and other forms of interaction:* None relevant to topical use.

*Pregnancy and lactation:* Safety for use in pregnancy and lactation has not been established. Topical administration of corticosteroids to pregnant animals can cause abnormalities of foetal development including cleft palate and intra-uterine growth with retardation. There may therefore be a very small risk of such effects in human pregnancy. Use only when it is considered essential by the physician.

*Effects on ability to drive and use machines:* May cause transient blurring of vision on instillation. Warn patients not to drive or operate hazardous machinery unless vision is clear.

*Undesirable effects:* Hypersensitivity reactions, usually of the delayed type, occur frequently with local treatment with neomycin. Irritation, burning, stinging, itching and dermatitis may occur. Topical steroid use may result in increased intraocular pressure leading to optic nerve disease, reduced visual acuity and visual field defects. Intensive or prolonged use of topical corticosteroids may lead to formation of posterior subcapsular cataracts. In those diseases causing thinning of the cornea or sclera, perforation of the globe may occur. Viral and fungal infections may be exacerbated by steroids. Systemic side effects may occur with extensive use.

*Overdose:* Long-term intensive topical use may lead to systemic effects. Oral ingestion of the contents of one tube is unlikely to lead to any serious adverse effects.

### Pharmacological properties
*Pharmacodynamic properties:* Maxitrol contains dexamethasone, neomycin sulphate and polymyxin B sulphate as active constituents.

Dexamethasone is a synthetic glucocorticoid with a potent anti-inflammatory activity. The relative anti-inflammatory potency of dexamethasone is 25 times that of cortisone, but its effects on sodium and water retention, potassium loss and abnormal sugar metabolism are minimal.

Neomycin is a broad spectrum antibiotic, highly sensitive gram negative organisms include: *E. coli, Enterobacter aerogenes, K. pneumoniae, Pasteurella, Pr. vulgaris, Salmonella, Shigella, Haemophilus influenzae, Neisseria meningitidis, Vibrio cholerae,* and *Bordetella pertussis.*
Gram positive microorganisms that are inhibited include: *Bacillus anthracis, Corynebacterium diptheriae, Staph. aureus, Strep. facecalis, Listeria monocytogenes* and *M. tuberculosis. Borrelia* and *Leptospira interrogans (icterohaemorrhagiae)* are also suppressed. Strains of *Pseudomonas aeruginosa* are resitant to neomycin.
Polymyxin B sulphate is active only against gram negative bacteria and is particularly active against *Pseudomonas aeruginosa.* Other sensitive organisms are: *Enterobacter, Escherichia coli,* Klebsiella, Salmonella, Pasteurella, Bordetella and Shigella. However, protens and most strains of Neisseria, Providentia and Serratia are resistant to Polymyxin B. Most sensitive organisms are inhibited by 0.1 to 0.2 units/ml.

*Pharmacokinetic properties:* Dexamethasone, like other corticosteroids, is absorbed rapidly after oral administration and has a biological half-life of about 190 minutes. Sufficient absorption may occur after topical application to the skin and eye to produce systemic effects. Intraocular penetration of dexamethasone occurs in significant amounts and contributes to the effectiveness of dexamethasone in anterior segment inflammatory disease.

Polymyxin B sulphate is not absorbed from the gastrointestinal tract or through intact skin, although the intact corneal epithelium prevents penetration into the corneal stroma, therapeutic concentrations do enter the stroma after epitherlial damage. Good stromal penetration occurs after epithelial abrasion following topical instillation, subconjunctival injection, or corneal bath. No significant polymyxin B penetration into the vitreous is demonstrable after parenteral or local administration of the drug.

Neomycin is poorly absorbed from the gastrointestinal tract and after topical administration insufficient is absorbed to produce systemic effects. Absorption has been reported to occur from wounds and inflamed skin. After absorption neomycin is rapidly excreted by the kidneys in active form.

*Preclinical safety data:* There are no preclinical data of relevance to the prescriber which are additional to that already included in other sections of the SPC.

### Pharmaceutical particulars
*List of excipients:* Methylparaben, propylparaben, liquid lanolin (Lantrol), petrolatum (Penndrake No. 4).

*Incompatibilities:* None known.

*Shelf life:* Unopened 30 months, after opening 28 days.

*Special precautions for storage:* Store at 8–25°C away from direct sunlight. Keep the container tightly closed.

*Nature and contents of container:* 3.5 g metal tube with nozzle and screw cap.

*Instructions for use/handling:* Do not touch the top of the tube to any surface as this may contaminate the contents.

**Marketing authorisation number** 0649/5916R.

**Date of approval/revision of SPC** 18 January 1996.

**Legal category** POM.

## MYDRIACYL* 0.5% and 1.0%

**Qualitative and quantitative composition** Tropicamide BP 0.5% w/v and 1.0% w/v.

**Pharmaceutical form** Sterile eye drops for topical ocular administration.

### Clincal particulars
*Therapeutic indications:* Tropicamide is a short acting anticholinergic agent used as a mydriatic and cycloplegic. It is indicated for topical use for: Diagnostic purposes for fundoscopy and cycloplegic refraction. Use in pre- and post-operative states where a short acting mydriatic is required.

*Posology and method of administration:*
*Adults, elderly and children: Fundoscopy:* One or two drops of 0.5% solution instilled into the eyes 15 to 20 minutes prior to examination.

*Cycloplegic refraction:* One or two drops of 1% solution repeated after 5 minutes. If the patient is not seen within 20 to 30 minutes an additional drop may be instilled to prolong the effect.

*Use in children:* Tropicamide has been reported to be inadequate for cycloplegia in children. A more powerful cycloplegic agent, such as atropine, may be required.

*Contra-indications:* Glaucoma or a tendency towards glaucoma (e.g. Narrow anterior chamber angle). Hypersensitivity to any component. This preparation contains benzalkonium chloride and should not be used where soft contact lenses are worn.

*Special warnings and special precautions for use:* Because of the risk of precipitating angle-closure glaucoma in the elderly and others prone to raised intraocular pressure, an estimate of the depth of the angle of the anterior chamber should be made before use.

Extreme caution is advised for use in children and individuals susceptible to belladonna alkaloids because of the increased risk of systemic toxicity. Parents should be warned of the oral toxicity of this preparation for children and advised to wash their hands after use.

Use with caution in an inflamed eye as the hyperaemia greatly increases the rate of systemic absorption through the conjunctiva.

To reduce systemic absorption the lacrimal sac should be compressed at the medial canthus by digital pressure for at least one minute after instillation of the drops.

*Interaction with other medicaments and other forms of interaction:* The effect of anti-muscarinic agents may be enhanced by the concomitant administration of other drugs with anti-muscarinic properties such as amantadine, some anti-histamines, butyrophenones, phenothiazines and tricyclic anti-depressants.

*Pregnancy and lactation:* There is insufficient evidence as to drug safety in pregnancy and lactation. This product should be used during pregnancy only when it is considered essential by a physician.

*Effects on ability to drive and use machines:* May cause blurred vision and sensitivity to light. Patients should be warned not to drive or engage in other hazardous activities unless vision is clear. Complete recovery from the effects of tropicamide eyedrops may take up to six hours.

*Undesirable effects: Local:* Increased intraocular pressure, transient stinging and sensitivity to light secondary to pupillary dilation. Prolonged administration may lead to local irritation, hyperaemia, oedema and conjunctivitis.

*Systemic:* Systemic anti-cholinergic toxicity is manifested by dryness of the mouth, flushing, dryness of the skin, bradycardia followed by tachycardia with palpitations and arrhythmias, urinary urgency, difficulty and retention, reduction in the tone and motility of the gastrointestinal tract leading to constipation.

Vomiting, giddiness and staggering may occur, a rash may be present in children and abdominal distention in infants.

Psychotic reactions, behavioural disturbances and cardio-respiratory collapse may occur in children.

*Overdose:* Systemic toxicity may occur following

topical use, particularly in children, it is manifested by flushing and dryness of the skin (a rash may be present in children), blurred vision, a rapid and irregular pulse, fever, abdominal distention in infants, convulsions and hallucinations and the loss of neuro-muscular co-ordination.

Treatment is supportive (there is no evidence that physostigmine is superior to supportive management). In infants and small children the body surface must be kept moist. If accidentally ingested, induce emesis or perform gastric lavage.

### Pharmacological properties
*Pharmacodynamic properties:* Tropicamide is an anticholinergic which blocks the responses of the sphincter muscle of the iris and the ciliary muscle to cholinergic stimulation thus dilating the pupil (mydriasis). At higher concentrations (1%), tropicamide also paralyses accommodation. This preparation acts rapidly and has a relatively short duration of action.

*Pharmacokinetic properties:* Tropicamide administered topically to the human eye does not bind to tissues as firmly as does atropine. The wash out time for half recovery of carbachol responsiveness was shown to be less than 15 minutes for non-pigmented iris and 30 minutes for pigmented iris.

*Preclinical safety data:* There are no preclinical data of relevance to the prescriber which are additional to that already included in other sections of the SPC.

### Pharmaceutical particulars
*List of excipients:* Benzalkonium chloride, disodium edetate, sodium chloride, sodium hydroxide and/or hydrochloric acid (to adjust pH), purified water.

*Incompatibilities:* None known.

*Shelf life:* 36 months (unopened). 1 month (after first opening).

*Special precautions for storage:* Store at a temperature not exceeding 25°C away from direct sunlight. Do not refrigerate. Keep container tightly closed. Discard contents one month after opening.

*Nature and contents of container:* Pack size – 5 ml. Drop-Tainer – Natural Low Density Polyethylene Bottle and Plug. Polystyrene or Polypropylene cap.

*Instructions for use/handling:* Do not touch dropper tip to any surface as this may contaminate the contents.

### Marketing authorisation numbers
0.5%  0649/5917R
1.0%  0649/5918R

**Date of approval/revision of SPC** 29 July 1996.

**Legal category** POM.

## PILOGEL*

**Qualitative and quantitative composition** Pilogel contains active ingredient Pilocarpine Hydrochloride PhEur 40 mg, 4.0% w/w and Benzalkonium Chloride PhEur 0.008% w/w as preservative, Carbomer 940 3.5% w/w, Edetate Disodium PhEur 0.01% w/w, Sodium Hydroxide PhEur and/or Hydrochloric acid PhEur q.s. to pH 4.7–5.1, Purified Water PhEur to 100%.

**Pharmaceutical form** Sterile ophthalmic gel.

**Clinical particulars**
*Therapeutic indications:* Pilogel is indicated for the control of intraocular pressure in patients with ocular hypertension and chronic open-angle glaucoma. It may be used in combination with other miotics, beta-blockers, carbonic anhydrase inhibitors, sympatho-mimetics or hyperosmotic agents.

*Posology and method of administration*
*Adults:* Apply a 1.0–1.5 cm (½ inch) ribbon of gel under the lower eyelid of the eye(s) to be treated once a day at bedtime. After the gel has been instilled, close the eye, hold the lid shut and move the eye in several different directions.

*Elderly:* There are no special dosage modifications required for the elderly.

*Children:* Pilogel is not recommended for use in children.

*Contra-indications:* Miotics are contra-indicated where constriction of the pupil is undesirable such as in acute iritis, in those persons showing hypersensitivity to any of the components and in pupillary block glaucoma.

*Special warnings and special precautions for use:* For topical use only. This product contains benzalkonium chloride and is not recommended for use when soft contact lenses are worn. As with all miotics rare cases of retinal detachment have been reported when used in certain susceptible individuals and those with pre-existing retinal disease, therefore, fundus examination is advised in all patients prior to the initiation of therapy. The miosis usually causes difficulty in dark adaptation. Patients should be advised to exercise

caution in night driving and other hazardous occupations in poor illumination.

*Interaction with other medicaments and other forms of interactions:* Although clinically not proven, the miotic effects of pilocarpine may be antagonised by long term topical or systemic corticosteroid therapy, systemic anticholinergics, antihistamines, pethidine, sympathomimetics, or tricyclic antidepressants. Concomitant administration of two different miotic drugs is not recommended because of potential interdrug antagonism, and potential development of unresponsiveness to both drugs.

*Pregnancy and lactation:* There is insufficient evidence as to the drug safety in human pregnancy. This product should, therefore, only be used during pregnancy if considered essential by the physician.

*Effects on ability to drive and use machines:* Pilogel causes miosis which usually results in difficulty in dark adaptation. Patients should be advised to exercise caution in night driving and other hazardous occupations in poor illumination.

*Undesirable effects:* The following adverse reactions associated with pilocarpine therapy have been reported:

*Local:* Burning, itching, smarting, blurring, ciliary spasm, conjunctival vascular congestion, induced myopia, sensitisation of the lids and conjunctiva, reduced visual acuity in poor illumination, lens changes with chronic use, increased pupillary block, retinal detachments and vitreous haemorrhages. Ocular reactions usually occur during initiation of therapy and often will not persist with continued therapy.

*CNS:* Browache and headache, especially in younger patients who have recently started therapy.

*Systemic:* Systemic reactions following ocular use are rare but they may include hypertension, tachycardia, bronchial spasm, pulmonary oedema, salivation, sweating, nausea, vomiting, diarrhoea and lacrimation.

*Overdose:* Systemic reactions following topical administration are extremely rare. If accidentally ingested, induce emesis or perform gastric lavage. Observe for signs of toxicity (salivation, lacrimation, sweating, nausea, vomiting and diarrhoea). If these occur, therapy with anti-cholinergic agents, such as atropine, may be necessary.

**Pharmacological properties** Pilocarpine is a direct acting cholinergic parasympathomimetic agent. It acts through a direct stimulation of muscarinic receptors in the iris sphincter pupillae muscle and the ciliary muscle both of which receive parasympathetic innervation. Contraction of the sphincter pupillae muscle causes miosis (constriction of the pupil) whilst contraction of the ciliary muscle increases tension on the scleral spur, opening trabecular meshwork spaces to facilitate outflow of aqueous humor and thus lower intraocular pressure. Pilocarpine has been used as an ophthalmic medication for many years and the toxicity profile of pilocarpine has been well docmented. All the excipients used in Pilogel have been widely used in pharmaceutical preparations. In addition acute, sub-acute and chronic ocular toxicity studies have demonstrated that Pilogel has a low potential for ocular irritation and toxicity.

**Pharmaceutical particulars**
*List of excipients:* Benzalkonium chloride, Carbomer 940, edetate disodium, sodium hydroxide and/or hydrochloric acid, purified water.

*Incompatibilities:* None known.

*Shelf life:* 24 months.

*Special precaution for storage:* Store at a temperature not exceeding 25°C. Do not freeze. Avoid excessive heat. Discard product 28 days after opening. Keep out of the reach of children.

*Nature and contents of container:* Collapsible tin ophthalmic tube, lined with an epoxy phenolic lacquer and fitted with a black polyethylene cap containing 5 g.

*Instructions for use/handling:* Instructions for patients are as follows:

1. Wash your hands before using pilogel.
2. Sit down in front of a mirror so that you can see what you are doing.
3. Remove the cap from the tube.
4. Make sure the tube tip does not touch anything as this may contaminate the contents.
5. Hold the tube upside down in one hand between your fingers.
6. Using the forefinger of your other hand, gently pull down the lower eyelid of the affected eye.
7. Place the tube tip close to, but not touching, your eye and gently squeeze the tube with your fingers so that a 1 to 1.5 cm (½ inch) strip is applied into the gap between the eye and the lower lid.
8. Now release the lower eyelid, close your eye and hold the eyelids shut while moving your eye around in several different directions.

9. Repeat steps 5 to 8 above, for the other eye, if necessary.
10. Replace and tightly close the cap on the tube.

**Marketing authorisation number** 0649/0115.

**Date of approval/revision of SPC** 17 May 1995.

**Legal category** POM.

## PROVISC VISCOELASTIC SOLUTION*

**Presentation** A viscoelastic solution which is a sterile, non-pyrogenic, non-inflammatory high molecular weight fraction of sodium hyaluronate containing approximately 10.0 mg/ml dissolved in sodium chloride phosphate buffer.

**Uses** Provisc is indicated for use as a surgical aid in anterior segment surgical procedures including cataract extraction with intraocular lens (IOL) implantation.

**Dosage and administration** A cannula or needle is used to inject a sufficient amount of Provisc viscoelastic solution into the anterior chamber. The injection may be performed before or after delivery of the crystalline lens. Provisc viscoelastic preparation may also be used to coat surgical instruments and the intraocular lens prior to implantation.

Provisc can also be injected during surgery to replace any Provisc lost during surgical manipulation.

At the end of surgery, Provisc should be removed by irrigation and/or aspiration to minimise the potential for a rise in IOP. As surgical techniques for cataract extraction and IOL insertion differ the volume of Provisc required will be dependent upon the type of surgery planned. As a guide to the volumes used the anterior chamber has a volume of 0.2–0.3 ml. In surgical procedures of the anterior segment of the eye, the total amount after repeated injections will usually be less than 1 ml.

**Contra-indications, warnings, etc**
*Contra-indications:* Provisc viscoelastic solution should not be used in patients with hypersensitivity to any components in this preparation.

*Warnings:* Precautions normally associated with the surgical procedure should be observed.

Post-operative increases in intraocular pressure have been reported with sodium hyaluronate products. The IOP should be carefully monitored and appropriate therapy instituted if significant increases occur.

Remove Provisc viscoelastic solution by irrigation and/or aspiration at the close of surgery. Do not overfill the anterior chamber. As Provisc solution is obtained from microbial fementation, the physician should be aware of potential allergic risks which can occur with the injection of any biological material.

Do not re-use cannulas.

Use only if solution is clear.

Avoid trapping air bubbles.

*Undesirable effects:* Provisc viscoelastic solution is extremely well tolerated after injection into human eyes during ophthalmic surgical procedures. As with most viscoelastic ophthalmic preparations, a transient rise in intraocular pressure has been reported in some cases.

Post-operative inflammatory reactions such as hypopyon and iritis have been reported with the use of ophthalmic viscoelastic preparations, as well as incidents of corneal oedema and decompensation. Their relationship to the use of sodium hyaluronate (Provisc) has not be established.

*Use in pregnancy and lactation:* The safety and efficacy of Provisc viscoelastic solution has not been studied in pregnant women. Provisc produces its effects as a result of its mechanical properties and is removed from the eye at the end of the surgical procedure. The risks of use in surgery should be weighed against any potential benefit.

*Drug interactions:* None known.

*Treatment of overdosage:* Not applicable.

**Pharmaceutical precautions** Store in refrigerator (2–8°C). Protect from freezing. Protect from light.

**Legal category** POM.

**Package quantities** 0.55 ml.

**Product licence number** 0649/0123.

## TEARS Naturale*

**Presentation** Tears Naturale is a clear, colourless sterile solution, presented in a 15 ml Drop-Tainer Dispenser, and contains the Duasorb water soluble polymeric system Dextran 70 0.1% and Hydroxypropyl Methylcellulose (Hypromellose) USP 0.3%, and preserved with Benzalkonium Chloride PhEur 0.01% and Disodium Edetate PhEur 0.05%.

**Uses** A soothing solution for use as an artificial tear

and lubricant in the relief of dry eye syndromes associated with deficient tear secretion or deficient mucous.

**Dosage and administration**  Instill 1 or 2 drops into the eye(s), as frequently as to relieve eye irritation symptoms.

**Contra-indications, warnings, etc**

*Contra-indications:* This product contains benzalkonium chloride, and should not be used when soft contact lenses are being worn.

*Precautions:* If irritation persists, discontinue use.

**Pharmaceutical precautions**  To avoid contaminating the solution, do not let the dropper tip touch any surface. Keep the container tightly closed. Discard the contents 1 month after opening.

**Legal category**  P.

**Package quantities**  15 ml.

**Further information**  Tears Naturale eye-drops are contained in an unbreakable semi-rigid plastic dropper bottle with a screw-on cap.

**Product licence number**  0649/0031.

## TOBRALEX*

**Presentation**  A sterile, clear, colourless to very pale yellow ophthalmic solution containing Tobramycin BP 0.3% w/v, preserved with 0.01% Benzalkonium Chloride PhEur.

**Uses**  Tobralex (tobramycin) Sterile Ophthalmic Solution is a bactericidal topical antibiotic indicated in the treatment of external bacterial conditions of the eye and its appendages. The spectrum of activity covers a wide range of Gram-positive organisms and many Gram-negative organisms.

A significant bacterial population resistant to tobramycin has not yet been reported. However, there is the possibility that bacterial resistance may develop following prolonged use.

**Dosage and administration**  Adults and children: In mild to moderate cases, instil one or two drops into the affected eye every four hours. For severe infections, instil two drops into the eye hourly until there is an improvement and then reduce treatment, prior to discontinuation.

**Contra-indications, warnings, etc**

*Contra-indications:* Persons with known sensitivity to tobramycin or gentamicin.

*Warnings:* Sensitivity may occur in some patients. If so, discontinue use. Transient irritation may occur with some susceptible patients.

Tobralex ophthalmic solution is not for injection. This product contains benzalkonium chloride and should not be used when soft contact lenses are being worn.

*Precautions:* As with other antibiotics, prolonged use may result in the overgrowth of non-susceptible organisms, including fungi. If super-infection occurs, appropriate therapy should be initiated.

*Use in pregnancy:* Reproduction studies in animals at doses up to thirty-three times the normal human systemic dose have revealed no evidence of impaired fertility or harm to the foetus due to tobramycin. There are, however, no adequate and well-controlled studies in pregnant women. Because animal studies are not always predictive of human response, this drug should be used during pregnancy only if clearly needed.

*Nursing mothers:* Because of the potential for adverse reactions in nursing infants from Tobralex, a decision should be made whether to discontinue nursing the infant or discontinue the drug, taking into account the importance of the drug to the mother.

*Adverse reactions:* The most frequent adverse reactions to Tobralex Ophthalmic Solution are localized ocular toxicity and hypersensitivity, including lid itching and swelling, and conjunctival erythema. These reactions occur in less than 3% of patients treated with Tobralex. Similar reactions may occur with the topical use of other aminoglycoside antibiotics. Other adverse reactions have not been reported from Tobralex therapy, however, if topical ocular tobramycin is administered concomitantly with systemic aminoglycoside antibiotics, care should be taken to monitor the total serum concentration.

*Overdosage:* Clinically apparent signs and symptoms of an overdose of Tobralex Ophthalmic Solution (punctate keratitis, erythema, increased lacrimation, oedema and lid itching) may be similar to adverse reaction effects seen in some patients.

**Pharmaceutical precautions**  Store at 8°C to 25°C. Do not freeze. Keep the container tightly closed. Discard contents one month after opening.

Sterile until opened.

**Legal category**  POM.

**Package quantities**  5 ml.

**Further information**  Tobralex eye drops are contained in an unbreakable semi-rigid plastic dropper bottle with screw-on cap.

**Product licence number**  0649/0044.

*Trade Mark

**Allen & Hanburys**
Stockley Park West,
Uxbridge, Middlesex UB11 1BT

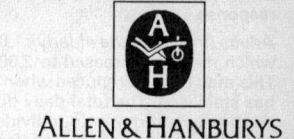

ALLEN & HANBURYS

## BECLOFORTE* DISKHALER*

**Presentation** The active ingredient is presented in a disk comprising eight regularly spaced double-foil blisters each delivering a mixture of 400 micrograms microfine beclomethasone dipropionate as the monohydrate and larger particle lactose.

The disk is intended only for use in a specific drug delivery device known as the Diskhaler. The contents of each blister are deposited into the Diskhaler device when pierced with an integral needle. The contents are then available to the patient to inhale by breath operation which allows the drug to be fully available even at low inspiratory flow rates.

Becloforte Diskhaler therefore provides reliable drug delivery for many patients.

**Uses** Beclomethasone dipropionate provides effective anti-inflammatory action in the lungs without the problems of systemic corticosteroid treatment, and offers preventive treatment of asthma.

*Therapeutic indications:*
*Adults:* Becloforte Diskhaler is indicated in the prophylactic management of severe asthma, i.e. patients with severe chronic asthma and those who are dependent on systemic corticosteroids for adequate control of symptoms. On transfer to high dose inhaled beclomethasone dipropionate, many patients who are dependent on systemic corticosteroids for adequate control of symptoms may be able to reduce significantly, or eliminate, their requirement for oral corticosteroids.

Becloforte Diskhaler is particularly useful in patients who have difficulty with co-ordinating the effective use of metered-dose inhalers.

**Dosage and administration** Becloforte Diskhaler is for inhalation use only. For optimum results Becloforte Diskhaler should be used regularly.

Patients should be given a starting dose of inhaled beclomethasone dipropionate which is appropriate for the severity of their disease. The dose may then be adjusted until control is achieved or reduced to the minimum effective dose according to individual response.

*Adults:* The minimum starting dose is 400 micrograms twice daily.

For patients who have been shown to require higher doses (greater than 800 micrograms) of beclomethasone dipropionate to control their asthma, the dosage may be increased to 800 micrograms twice daily.

*Children:* Becloforte Diskhaler is not indicated for use in children.

There is no need to adjust the dose in elderly patients or in those with hepatic or renal impairment.

**Contra-indications, warnings, etc**
*Contra-indications:* Becloforte Diskhaler is contra-indicated in patients with a history of hypersensitivity to any of its components. Special care is necessary in patients with active or quiescent pulmonary tuberculosis.

*Precautions:* Becloforte Diskhaler is not designed to relieve acute asthmatic symptoms, for which an inhaled short-acting bronchodilator is required. Patients should be advised to have such rescue medication available.

Severe asthma requires regular medical assessment, including lung-function testing, as patients are at risk of severe attacks and even death. Increasing use of bronchodilators, in particular short-acting inhaled $\beta_2$-agonists, to relieve symptoms indicates deterioration of asthma control. If patients find that short-acting relief bronchodilator treatment becomes less effective, or they need more inhalations than usual, medical attention must be sought. In this situation patients should be reassessed and consideration given to the need for increased anti-inflammatory therapy (e.g. higher doses of inhaled corticosteroids or a course of oral corticosteroids). Severe exacerbations of asthma must be treated in the normal way.

In the majority of patients no significant adrenal suppression occurs until doses of 1,500 micrograms per day are exceeded. Reduction of plasma cortisol levels has been reported in some patients who received 2,000 micrograms per day of inhaled beclomethasone dipropionate. In such patients the risks of developing adrenal suppression should be balanced against the therapeutic advantages, and precautions should be taken to provide systemic steroid cover in situations of prolonged stress. Prolonged suppression of the hypothalamic-pituitary-adrenal (HPA) axis may eventually lead to systemic effects including growth retardation in children and adolescents.

Lack of response or severe exacerbations of asthma should be treated by increasing the dose of inhaled beclomethasone dipropionate and, if necessary, by giving a systemic steroid and/or an antibiotic if there is an infection, and by use of β-agonist therapy.

*For the transfer of patients being treated with oral corticosteroids:* The transfer of oral steroid-dependent patients to inhaled beclomethasone dipropionate, and their subsequent management, needs special care as recovery from impaired adrenocortical function, caused by prolonged systemic steroid therapy, may take a considerable time.

Patients who have been treated with systemic steroids for long periods of time, or at a high dose, may have adrenocortical suppression. With these patients adrenocortical function should be monitored regularly and their dose of systemic steroid reduced cautiously.

After approximately a week, gradual withdrawal of the systemic steroid is commenced. Decrements in dosage should be appropriate to the level of maintenance systemic steroid, and introduced at not less than weekly intervals. For maintenance doses of prednisolone (or equivalent) of 10 mg daily or less, the decrements in dose should be not greater than 1 mg per day, at not less than weekly intervals. For maintenance doses of prednisolone in excess of 10 mg daily, it may be appropriate to employ cautiously, larger decrements in dose at weekly intervals.

Some patients feel unwell in a non-specific way during the withdrawal phase despite maintenance or even improvement of the respiratory function. They should be encouraged to persevere with inhaled beclomethasone dipropionate and to continue withdrawal of systemic steroid, unless there are objective signs of adrenal insufficiency.

Patients weaned off oral steroids whose adrenocortical function is impaired should carry a steroid warning card indicating that they may need supplementary systemic steroid during periods of stress, e.g. worsening asthma attacks, chest infections, major intercurrent illness, surgery, trauma, etc.

Replacement of systemic steroid treatment with inhaled therapy sometimes unmasks allergies such as allergic rhinitis or eczema previously controlled by the systemic drug. These allergies should be symptomatically treated with antihistamine and/or topical preparations, including topical steroids.

Treatment with Becloforte Diskhaler should not be stopped abruptly.

As with all inhaled corticosteroids, special care is necessary in patients with active or quiescent pulmonary tuberculosis.

*Pregnancy:* There is inadequate evidence of safety in human pregnancy. Administration of corticosteroids to pregnant animals can cause abnormalities of fetal development including cleft palate and intra-uterine growth retardation. There may therefore be a very small risk of such effects in the human fetus. It should be noted, however, that the fetal changes in animals occur after relatively high systemic exposure. Because beclomethasone dipropionate is delivered directly to the lungs by the inhaled route it avoids the high level of exposure that occurs when corticosteroids are given by systemic routes. The use of beclomethasone dipropionate in pregnancy requires that the possible benefits of the drug be weighed against the possible hazards. It should be noted that the drug has been in widespread use for many years without apparent ill consequence.

*Lactation:* No specific studies examining the transference of beclomethasone dipropionate into the milk of lactating animals have been performed. It is reasonable to assume that beclomethasone dipropionate is secreted in milk but at the dosages used for direct inhalation there is low potential for significant levels in breast milk.

The use of beclomethasone dipropionate in mothers breast feeding their babies requires that the therapeutic benefits of the drug be weighed against the potential hazards to the mother and baby.

*Side-effects:* Candidiasis of the mouth and throat (thrush) occurs in some patients, the incidence of which is increased with doses greater than 400 micrograms beclomethasone dipropionate per day. Patients with high blood levels of *Candida precipitins,* indicating a previous infection, are most likely to develop this complication. Patients may find it helpful to rinse their mouth thoroughly with water after using Becloforte Diskhaler. Symptomatic candidiasis can be treated with topical anti-fungal therapy whilst still continuing with the treatment.

In some patients inhaled beclomethasone dipropionate may cause hoarseness or throat irritation. It may be helpful to rinse the mouth out with water immediately after inhalation.

As with other inhalation therapy, paradoxical bronchospasm may occur with an immediate increase in wheezing after dosing. This responds to a fast-acting inhaled bronchodilator. The preparation should be discontinued immediately, the patient assessed and, if necessary, alternative therapy instituted.

Hypersensitivity reactions including rashes, urticaria, pruritus and erythema, and oedema of the eyes, face, lips and throat, have been reported.

*Overdosage:* Acute. Inhalation of the drug in doses in excess of those recommended may lead to temporary suppression of adrenal function. This does not necessitate emergency action being taken. In these patients treatment with beclomethasone dipropionate by inhalation should be continued at a dose sufficient to control asthma; adrenal function recovers in a few days and can be verified by measuring plasma cortisol.

Chronic. Use of inhaled beclomethasone dipropionate in daily doses in excess of 1,500 micrograms over prolonged periods may lead to some degree of adrenal suppression. Monitoring of adrenal reserve may be indicated. Treatment with inhaled beclomethasone dipropionate should be continued at a dose sufficient to control asthma.

**Pharmaceutical precautions** Whilst the disks provide a good protection to the blister contents from the effects of the atmosphere, they should not be exposed to extremes of temperature and should be stored below 30°C. A disk may be kept in the Diskhaler inhaler at all times but a blister should only be pierced immediately prior to use. Failure to observe this instruction may affect the operation of the Diskhaler.

**Legal category** POM.

**Package quantities** Becloforte Diskhaler is supplied as a carton containing 14 disks (14 x 8 blisters) together with a Diskhaler inhaler.

**Further information** Nil.

**Product licence number** 10949/0066

## BECLOFORTE* EASI-BREATHE* INHALER

**Qualitative and quantitative composition** 250 micrograms Beclomethasone Dipropionate BP per actuation. Each canister delivers 200 actuations.

**Pharmaceutical form** Aerosol.

**Clinical particulars**
*Therapeutic indications:* Beclomethasone dipropionate given by inhalation offers preventative treatment for asthma. It provides effective anti-inflammatory action in the lungs without the problems of systemic corticosteroid treatment.

Becloforte Easi-Breathe Inhaler is indicated in the prophylactic management of severe asthma in adults.

*Severe asthma:* Patients with severe chronic asthma and those who are dependent on systemic corticosteroids for adequate control of symptoms. Many patients who are dependent on systemic corticosteroids for adequate control of symptoms may be able to reduce significantly, or eliminate, their requirement for oral corticosteroids when they are transferred to high dose inhaled beclomethasone dipropionate.

*Posology and method of administration:* Becloforte Easi-Breathe Inhaler is for oral inhalation use only. The inhaler can be used alone or in combination with the Optimiser* spacer device.

Patients should be given a starting dose of inhaled beclomethasone dipropionate appropriate to the severity of their disease. Those demonstrating a need for high dose inhaled steroid therapy should start on 1,000 micrograms daily. The dose may then be adjusted until control is achieved, or reduced to the minimum effective dose according to individual response.

*Adults (including the elderly):* 1,000 micrograms daily which may be increased to 2,000 micrograms daily. This may then be reduced when the patient's asthma has stabilised. The total daily dose may be administered as two, three, or four divided doses.

Becloforte Easi-Breathe Inhaler is not recommended for children.

*Contra-indications:* Hypersensitivity to any of the components.

Special care is necessary in patients with active or quiescent pulmonary tuberculosis.

*Special warnings and special precautions for use:* Patients should be instructed in the proper use of the inhaler, and their technique checked, to ensure that the drug reaches the target areas within the lungs. They should also be made aware that Becloforte Easi-Breathe Inhaler has to be used regularly, every day, even when they are asymptomatic, for optimum benefit.

Becloforte Easi-Breathe Inhaler is not designed to relieve acute asthma symptoms for which an inhaled short-acting bronchodilator is required. Patients should be advised to have such relief medication available.

Severe asthma requires regular medical assessment, including lung-function testing, as patients are at risk of severe attacks and even death. Patients must be instructed to seek medical attention if short-acting relief bronchodilator treatment becomes less effective, or more inhalations than usual are required as this may indicate deterioration of asthma control. In this situation, patients should be assessed and the need for increased anti-inflammatory therapy (e.g. higher doses of inhaled corticosteroid or a course of oral corticosteroid) considered.

Severe exacerbations of asthma must be treated in the normal way, e.g. by increasing the dose of inhaled beclomethasone dipropionate and, if necessary, by giving a systemic steroid, and/or an antibiotic if there is an infection, and by use of β-agonist therapy.

Treatment with Becloforte Easi-Breathe Inhaler should not be stopped abruptly.

Significant adrenal suppression rarely occurs before doses of 1,500 micrograms per day of inhaled beclomethasone dipropionate are exceeded. Reduction of plasma cortisol levels has been reported in some patients taking 2,000 micrograms per day. In such patients, the risks of developing adrenal suppression should be balanced against the therapeutic advantages, and precautions taken to provide systemic steroid cover in situations of prolonged stress. Prolonged suppression of the hypothalamic-pituitary-adrenal (HPA) axis may eventually lead to systemic effects, including growth retardation in children and adolescents.

The transfer to Becloforte Easi-Breathe Inhaler of patients who have been treated with systemic steroids for long periods of time, or at a high dose, needs special care, since recovery from any adrenocortical suppression sustained may take a considerable time. Approximately one week after initiating treatment with Becloforte Easi-Breathe Inhaler, reduction of the dose of systemic steroid can be commenced.

The size of the reduction should correspond to the maintenance dose of systemic steroid. Reductions in dose of not more than 1 mg are suitable for patients receiving maintenance doses of 10 mg daily or less of prednisolone or its equivalent. Larger reductions in dose may be appropriate for higher maintenance doses. The reductions in dose should be introduced at not less than weekly intervals. Adrenocortical function should be monitored regularly as the dose of systemic steroid is gradually reduced.

Some patients feel unwell in a non-specific way during the withdrawal phase despite maintenance or even improvement of the respiratory function. They should be encouraged to persevere with inhaled beclomethasone dipropionate and to continue withdrawal of systemic steroid, unless there are objective signs of adrenal insufficiency

Patients weaned off oral steroids whose adrenocortical function is impaired should carry a steroid warning card indicating that they may need supplementary systemic steroid during periods of stress, e.g. worsening asthma attacks, chest infections, major intercurrent illness, surgery, trauma, etc.

Replacement of systemic steroid treatment with inhaled therapy sometimes unmasks allergies such as allergic rhinitis or eczema previously controlled by the systemic drug. These allergies should be symptomatically treated with antihistamine and/or topical preparations, including topical steroids.

As with all inhaled corticosteroids, special care is necessary in patients with active or quiescent pulmonary tuberculosis.

*Interaction with other medicaments and other forms of interaction:* None reported.

*Pregnancy and lactation:* There is inadequate evidence of safety in human pregnancy. Administration of corticosteroids to pregnant animals can cause abnormalities of fetal development including cleft palate and intra-uterine growth retardation. There may therefore be a very small risk of such effects in the human fetus. It should be noted, however, that the fetal changes in animals occur after relatively high systemic exposure. Becloforte Easi-Breathe Inhaler delivers the drug directly to the lungs by the inhaled route and so avoids the high level of exposure that occurs when corticosteroids are given by systemic routes.

The use of beclomethasone dipropionate in pregnancy requires that the possible benefits of the drug be weighed against the possible hazards.

No specific studies examining the transference of beclomethasone dipropionate into the milk of lactating animals have been performed. It is reasonable to assume that beclomethasone dipropionate is secreted in milk, but at the dosages used for direct inhalation there is low potential for significant levels in breast milk.

The use of beclomethasone dipropionate in mothers breast feeding their babies requires that the therapeutic benefits of the drug be weighed against the potential hazards to the mother and baby.

*Effects on the ability to drive and use machines:* None reported.

*Undesirable effects:* As with other inhalation therapy, paradoxical bronchospasm may occur with an immediate increase in wheezing after dosing. This should be treated immediately with a fast-acting inhaled bronchodilator. The Becloforte Easi-Breathe Inhaler should be discontinued immediately, the patient assessed and, if necessary, alternative therapy instituted.

Hypersensitivity reactions including rashes, urticaria, pruritus and erythema, and oedema of the eyes, face, lips and throat, have been reported.

Candidiasis of the mouth and throat (thrush) occurs in some patients, the incidence increasing with doses greater than 400 micrograms beclomethasone dipropionate per day. Patients with high blood levels of *Candida precipitins*, indicating a previous infection, are most likely to develop this complication. Patients may find it helpful to rinse their mouth thoroughly with water after using the inhaler. The Optimiser spacer can be used to reduce oropharyngeal deposition. Symptomatic candidiasis can be treated with topical anti-fungal therapy whilst still continuing with Becloforte Easi-Breathe Inhaler.

In some patients inhaled beclomethasone dipropionate may cause hoarseness or throat irritation. It may be helpful to rinse the mouth out with water immediately after inhalation. Alternatively, the Optimiser spacer can be used to reduce oropharyngeal deposition.

*Overdose:*

*Acute:* Inhalation of the drug in doses in excess of those recommended may lead to temporary suppression of adrenal function. This does not require emergency action. In these patients treatment should be continued at a dose sufficient to control asthma; adrenal function recovers in a few days and can be verified by measuring plasma cortisol.

*Chronic:* Use of inhaled beclomethasone dipropionate in daily doses in excess of 1,500 micrograms over prolonged periods may lead to some degree of adrenal suppression. Monitoring of adrenal reserve may be indicated. Treatment should be continued at a dose sufficient to control asthma.

**Pharmacological properties**

*Pharmacodynamic properties:* Beclomethasone dipropionate given by inhalation has a potent glucocorticoid anti-inflammatory action within the lungs.

*Pharmacokinetic properties:* Beclomethasone 17,21-dipropionate (BDP) administered intravenously is cleared rapidly with a half-life of approximately 30 minutes. Beclomethasone 17-monopropionate (BMP) appears rapidly in the plasma after intravenous administration of BDP and is itself cleared with a half-life again of about 30 minutes. BDP is bound to plasma proteins to the extent of 87%. Up to 14% of an intravenous dose of BDP is excreted in the urine in 96 hours, mainly as polar metabolites, a proportion of which are conjugated. Up to 64% of the dose is excreted in faeces in this time, again primarily as free and conjugated metabolites.

After inhalation about 25% of the dose reaches the lungs and is available for absorption from this site. The remainder is deposited on the delivery device or in the oropharynx. That portion deposited in the mouth or upper airways will ultimately be swallowed.

There is rapid metabolic inactivation of most of the swallowed portion of BDP during its first passage through the liver. An oral dose (4 mg) of tritium-labelled BDP was absorbed slowly with peak levels of radioactivity equivalent to 20 ng drug/ml plasma being reached 5 hours after dosing. Excretion was mainly in the faeces (35–76% of the dose in 96 hours) and primarily as polar metabolites although the presence of BDP and BMP in faeces suggested incomplete absorption of the dose. Up to 14% of the dose was excreted as polar metabolites in urine.

The lung tissue rapidly hydrolyses BDP to BMP which in turn is hydrolysed more slowly to beclomethasone. The liver also metabolises BDP and BMP and further converts it to polar metabolites.

*Preclinical safety data:* BDP has low acute oral, subcutaneous and intraperitoneal toxicity in mice and rats, and repeat dose toxicity studies showed findings characteristic of glucocorticoids, with no evidence of irritancy to the respiratory tract. The main findings, at above therapeutic doses, were depression of corticosterone levels in rats and cortisol levels in dogs. BDP is non-genotoxic, and demonstrated no oncogenic potential following combined inhalation/oral administration to rats. Susceptibility of fetuses to cleft palate, noted in the mouse organogenesis study, is considered to have no relevance for therapeutic use.

**Pharmaceutical particulars**

*List of excipients:* Oleic acid, dichlorodifluoromethane, trichlorofluoromethane.

*Incompatibilities:* None reported.

*Shelf life:* Two years when stored below 30°C.

*Special precautions for storage:* Store below 30°C.

As with most inhaled medicines in aerosol canisters, the therapeutic effect may decrease when the canister is cold.

Protect from frost and direct sunlight.

The canister should not be broken, punctured or burnt, even when apparently empty.

*Nature and contents of container:* An inhaler comprising an aluminium can fitted with a breath-operated, metering valve, actuator and dust cap. Each canister contains 200 metered actuations of 250 micrograms beclomethasone dipropionate.

*Instructions for use/handling:* The aerosol spray is inhaled through the mouth into the lungs. After shaking the inhaler, open the cap and place the mouthpiece in the mouth with the lips closed around it. Suck in slowly through the mouthpiece, this releases a spray. The inhaler can be used with the Optimiser spacer device.

For detailed instructions for use refer to the patient information leaflet in every pack.

*Marketing authorisation holder:* Glaxo Wellcome UK Ltd, trading as Allen & Hanburys, Stockley Park West, Uxbridge, Middlesex, UB11 1BT.

**Marketing authorisation number** 10949/0270.

**Date of approval/revision of SPC** December 1996.

**Legal category** POM.

## BECLOFORTE* INTEGRA*

**Presentation** Becloforte Integra is a metered-dose aerosol with an integral compact spacer device which delivers 250 micrograms Beclomethasone Dipropionate BP per actuation.

Other ingredients: Oleic acid, trichlorofluoromethane, dichlorodifluoromethane.

**Uses** Beclomethasone dipropionate given by inhalation offers preventative treatment for asthma. It provides effective anti-inflammatory action in the lungs without the problems of systemic corticosteroid treatment.

Becloforte Integra is indicated in the prophylactic management of severe asthma in adults with severe chronic asthma and those who are dependent on systemic corticosteroids for adequate control of symptoms. Many patients who are dependent on systemic corticosteroids for adequate control of symptoms may be able to reduce significantly, or eliminate, their requirement for oral corticosteroids when they are transferred to Becloforte Integra.

**Dosage and administration** Becloforte Integra is for inhalation use only.

Some patients find difficulty in co-ordinating the firing of an inhaler with inspiration and therefore fai to maximise the potential benefit offered by treatment Becloforte Integra may be used in patients who find i difficult to synchronise aerosol actuation with inspir ation of breath. Patients should inhale straight away after discharging the dose into the spacer device.

Patients should be given a starting dose of inhaled beclomethasone dipropionate appropriate to the severity of their disease. The dose may then be adjusted until control is achieved, or reduced to the minimum effective dose according to individual re sponse.

*Adults (including the elderly):* Two inhalation (500 micrograms) twice daily, or one inhalatio (250 micrograms) four times daily, is the recom mended dosage. If necessary, this may be increase to two inhalations (500 micrograms) three or fou times daily.

*Children:* Becloforte Integra is not indicated for use in children.

**Contra-indications, warnings, etc**

*Contra-indications:* Becloforte Integra is contra-indicated in patients with a history of hypersensitivity to any of the components.

Special care is necessary in patients with active or quiescent pulmonary tuberculosis.

*Precautions:* Patients should be instructed in the proper use of the inhaler to ensure that the drug reaches the target areas within the lungs. They should also be made aware that Becloforte Integra has to be used regularly, every day, even when they are asymptomatic, for optimum benefit.

Becloforte Integra is not designed to relieve acute asthma symptoms for which an inhaled short-acting bronchodilator is required. Patients should be advised to have such relief medication available. They should be instructed to seek medical advice if short-acting relief bronchodilator treatment becomes less effective, or more inhalations than usual are required. In this situation, patients should be assessed and the need for increased anti-inflammatory therapy (e.g. higher doses of inhaled corticosteroid or a course of oral corticosteroid) considered.

Severe exacerbations of asthma must be treated in the normal way, e.g. by increasing the dose of inhaled beclomethasone dipropionate and, if necessary, by giving a systemic steroid and/or an antibiotic if there is an infection, and by use of β-agonist therapy. Treatment with Becloforte Integra should not be stopped abruptly.

Significant adrenal suppression rarely occurs before doses of 1,500 micrograms per day of inhaled beclomethasone dipropionate are exceeded. Reduction of plasma cortisol levels has been reported in some patients taking 2,000 micrograms per day. In such patients, the risks of developing adrenal suppression should be balanced against the therapeutic advantages, and precautions taken to provide systemic steroid cover in situations of prolonged stress. Prolonged suppression of the hypothalamic-pituitary-adrenal (HPA) axis may eventually lead to systemic effects including growth retardation in children and adolescents.

The transfer to Becloforte Integra of patients who have been treated with systemic steroids for long periods of time, or at a high dose, needs special care, since recovery from any adrenocortical suppression sustained may take a considerable time. Approximately one week after initiating treatment with Becloforte Integra, reduction of the dose of systemic steroid can be commenced. The size and frequency of the reduction should correspond to the maintenance dose of systemic steroid. Weekly reductions in dose of 1 mg are suitable for patients receiving maintenance doses of 10 mg daily or less of prednisolone or its equivalent. Larger reductions in dose may be appropriate for higher maintenance doses of prednisolone or its equivalent. Adrenocortical function should be monitored regularly as the dose of systemic steroid is gradually reduced.

Some patients feel unwell in a non-specific way during the withdrawal phase despite maintenance or even improvement of the respiratory function. They should be encouraged to persevere with inhaled beclomethasone dipropionate and to continue withdrawal of systemic steroid, unless there are objective signs of adrenal insufficiency.

Patients weaned off oral steroids whose adrenocortical function is impaired should carry a steroid warning card indicating that they may need supplementary systemic steroid during periods of stress, e.g. worsening asthma attacks, chest infections, major intercurrent illness, surgery, trauma, etc.

Replacement of systemic steroid treatment with inhaled therapy sometimes unmasks allergies such as allergic rhinitis or eczema previously controlled by the systemic drug. These allergies should be symptomatically treated with antihistamine and/or topical preparations, including topical steroids.

As with all inhaled corticosteroids, special care is necessary in patients with active or quiescent pulmonary tuberculosis.

*Pregnancy:* There is inadequate evidence of safety in human pregnancy. Administration of corticosteroids to pregnant animals can cause abnormalities of fetal development including cleft palate and intra-uterine growth retardation. There may therefore be a very small risk of such effects in the human fetus. It should be noted, however, that the fetal changes in animals occur after relatively high systemic exposure. Becloforte Integra delivers beclomethasone dipropionate directly to the lungs by the inhaled route and so avoids the high level of exposure that occurs when corticosteroids are given by systemic routes.

The use of Becloforte Integra in pregnancy requires that the possible benefits of the drug be weighed against the possible hazards. It should be noted that the drug has been in widespread use for many years without apparent ill consequence.

*Lactation:* No specific studies examining the transference of beclomethasone dipropionate into the milk of lactating animals have been performed. It is reasonable to assume that beclomethasone dipropionate is secreted in milk, but at the dosages used for direct inhalation there is low potential for significant levels in breast milk.

The use of Becloforte Integra in mothers breast feeding their babies requires that the therapeutic benefits of the drug be weighed against the potential hazards to the mother and baby.

*Side-effects:* Candidiasis of the mouth and throat (thrush) occurs in some patients, the incidence increasing with doses greater than 400 micrograms beclomethasone dipropionate per day. Patients with high blood levels of *Candida precipitins*, indicating a previous infection, are most likely to develop this complication. Patients may find it helpful to rinse their mouth thoroughly with water after using the inhaler. Symptomatic candidiasis can be treated with topical anti-fungal therapy whilst still continuing with Becloforte Integra.

In some patients inhaled beclomethasone dipropionate may cause hoarseness or throat irritation. It may be helpful to rinse out the mouth thoroughly with water immediately after inhalation.

As with other inhalation therapy, paradoxical bronchospasm may occur with an immediate increase in wheezing after dosing. This responds to a fast-acting inhaled bronchodilator. Becloforte Integra should be discontinued immediately, the patient assessed and, if necessary, alternative therapy (e.g. Becloforte Diskhaler*) instituted.

Hypersensitivity reactions including rashes, urticaria, pruritus and erythema, and oedema of the eyes, face, lips and throat, have been reported.

*Overdosage:* Acute. Inhalation of the drug in doses in excess of those recommended may lead to temporary suppression of adrenal function. This does not require emergency action. In these patients treatment should be continued at a dose sufficient to control asthma; adrenal function recovers in a few days and can be verified by measuring plasma cortisol.

Chronic. Use of inhaled beclomethasone dipropionate in daily doses in excess of 1,500 micrograms over prolonged periods may lead to some degree of adrenal suppression. Monitoring of adrenal reserve may be indicated. Treatment should be continued at a dose sufficient to control asthma.

**Pharmaceutical precautions** Becloforte Integra should be stored at a temperature below 30°C (86°F). As with most inhaled medications in aerosol canisters, the therapeutic effect of this medication may decrease when the canister is cold.

Protect from frost and direct sunlight.

The canister should not be punctured, broken or burnt even when apparently empty.

**Legal category** POM.

**Package quantities** Becloforte Integra consists of an inhaler section providing 200 metered actuations together with an integral compact spacer device. Refill inhaler sections are also available.

**Further information** Nil.

**Product licence number** 10949/0041

## BECLOFORTE* INHALER

**Presentation** Becloforte Inhaler is a metered-dose aerosol which delivers 250 micrograms Beclomethasone Dipropionate BP (as the trichlorofluoromethane solvate) per actuation into the mouthpiece of a specially designed actuator.

**Uses** Beclomethasone dipropionate provides effective anti-inflammatory action in the lungs, without the problems of systemic corticosteroid treatment, and offers preventive treatment of asthma.

*Therapeutic indications:*

*Adults:* Becloforte Inhaler is indicated in the prophylactic management of severe asthma, i.e. patients with severe chronic asthma and those who are dependent on systemic corticosteroids for adequate control of symptoms. On transfer to high dose inhaled beclomethasone dipropionate, many patients who are dependent on systemic corticosteroids for adequate control of symptoms may be able to reduce significantly, or eliminate, their requirement for oral corticosteroids.

**Dosage and administration** Becloforte Inhaler is for inhalation use only.

Some patients find difficulty in co-ordinating the firing of the inhaler with inspiration and therefore fail to maximise the potential benefit offered by treatment. Becloforte Inhaler may be used with a Volumatic* spacer device in patients who find it difficult to synchronise aerosol actuation with inspiration of breath.

Patients should be given a starting dose of inhaled beclomethasone dipropionate which is appropriate for the severity of their disease. The dose may then be adjusted until control is achieved, or reduced to the minimum effective dose according to individual response.

Patients demonstrating a need for high dose inhaled steroid therapy should start on 1,000 micrograms daily.

*Adults:* Two inhalations (500 micrograms) twice daily, or one inhalation (250 micrograms) four times daily, is the recommended maintenance dosage. If necessary, dosage may be increased to two inhalations (500 micrograms) three or four times daily, according to response.

*Children:* Becloforte Inhaler is not indicated for use in children.

There is no need to adjust the dose in elderly patients or in those with hepatic or renal impairment.

**Contra-indications, warnings, etc**

*Contra-indications:* Becloforte Inhaler is contra-indicated in patients with a history of hypersensitivity to any of its components.

Special care is necessary in patients with active or quiescent pulmonary tuberculosis.

*Precautions:* Patients' inhaler technique should be checked to make sure that aerosol actuation is synchronised with inspiration of breath for optimum delivery of drug to the lungs.

Patients should be made aware of the prophylactic nature of therapy with Becloforte Inhaler and that, for optimum benefits, they should use it regularly, every day, even when they are asymptomatic.

Becloforte Inhaler is not designed to relieve acute asthmatic symptoms for which an inhaled short-acting bronchodilator is required. Patients should be advised to have such relief medication available. Severe asthma requires regular medical assessment, including lung-function testing, as patients are at risk of severe attacks and even death.

Increasing use of bronchodilators, in particular short-acting inhaled $\beta_2$-agonists, to relieve symptoms indicates deterioration of asthma control. If patients find that short-acting relief bronchodilator treatment becomes less effective, or they need more inhalations than usual, medical attention must be sought. In this situation patients should be reassessed and consideration given to the need for increased anti-inflammatory therapy (e.g. higher doses of inhaled corticosteroids or a course of oral corticosteroids). Severe exacerbations of asthma must be treated in the normal way.

In the majority of patients no significant adrenal suppression occurs until doses of 1,500 micrograms per day are exceeded. Reduction of plasma cortisol levels has been reported in some patients who received 2,000 micrograms per day of inhaled beclomethasone dipropionate. In such patients the risks of developing adrenal suppression should be balanced against the therapeutic advantages, and precautions should be taken to provide systemic steroid cover in situations of prolonged stress. Prolonged suppression of the hypothalamic-pituitary-adrenal (HPA) axis may eventually lead to systemic effects including growth retardation in children and adolescents.

Lack of response or severe exacerbations of asthma should be treated by increasing the dose of inhaled beclomethasone dipropionate and, if necessary, by giving a systemic steroid and/or an antibiotic if there is an infection, and by use of β-agonist therapy.

*For the transfer of patients being treated with oral corticosteroids:* The transfer of oral steroid-dependent patients to inhaled beclomethasone dipropionate, and their subsequent management, needs special care as recovery from impaired adrenocortical function, caused by prolonged systemic steroid therapy, may take a considerable time.

Patients who have been treated with systemic steroids for long periods of time, or at a high dose, may have adrenocortical suppression. With these patients adrenocortical function should be monitored regularly and their dose of systemic steroid reduced cautiously.

After approximately a week, gradual withdrawal of the systemic steroid is commenced. Reductions in dosage should be appropriate to the level of maintenance systemic steroid, and introduced at not less than weekly intervals. For maintenance doses of prednisolone, or its equivalent, of 10 mg daily or less, the reductions in dose should be not greater than 1 mg per day, at not less than weekly intervals. For maintenance doses of prednisolone in excess of 10 mg daily, it may be appropriate to employ cautiously larger reductions in dose at weekly intervals.

Some patients feel unwell in a non-specific way during the withdrawal phase despite maintenance or even improvement of the respiratory function. They should be encouraged to persevere with inhaled beclomethasone dipropionate and to continue withdrawal of systemic steroid, unless there are objective signs of adrenal insufficiency.

Patients weaned off oral steroids whose adrenocortical function is impaired should carry a steroid warning card indicating that they may need supplementary systemic steroid during periods of stress, e.g. worsening asthma attacks, chest infections, major intercurrent illness, surgery, trauma, etc.

Replacement of systemic steroid treatment with inhaled therapy sometimes unmasks allergies such as allergic rhinitis or eczema previously controlled by the systemic drug. These allergies should be symptomatically treated with antihistamine and/or topical preparations, including topical steroids.

Treatment with Becloforte Inhaler should not be stopped abruptly.

As with all inhaled corticosteroids, special care is necessary in patients with active or quiescent pulmonary tuberculosis.

*Pregnancy:* There is inadequate evidence of safety in human pregnancy. Administration of corticosteroids to pregnant animals can cause abnormalities of fetal development including cleft palate and intra-uterine growth retardation. There may therefore be a very small risk of such effects in the human fetus. It should be noted, however, that the fetal changes in animals occur after relatively high systemic exposure. Beclomethasone dipropionate is delivered directly to the lungs by the inhaled route and so avoids the high level of exposure that occurs when corticosteroids are given by systemic routes.

The use of beclomethasone dipropionate in pregnancy requires that the possible benefits of the drug be weighed against the possible hazards. It should be noted that the drug has been in widespread use for many years without apparent ill consequence.

*Lactation:* No specific studies examining the transference of beclomethasone dipropionate into the milk of lactating animals have been performed. It is reasonable to assume that beclomethasone dipropionate is secreted in milk, but at the dosages used for direct inhalation there is low potential for significant levels in breast milk.

The use of beclomethasone dipropionate in mothers breast feeding their babies requires that the therapeutic benefits of the drug be weighed against the potential hazards to the mother and baby.

*Side-effects:* Candidiasis of the mouth and throat (thrush) occurs in some patients, the incidence increases with doses greater than 400 micrograms beclomethasone dipropionate per day. Patients with high blood levels of *Candida precipitins*, indicating a previous infection, are most likely to develop this complication. Patients may find it helpful to rinse their mouth thoroughly with water after using the inhaler. Symptomatic candidiasis can be treated with topical anti-fungal therapy whilst still continuing with the Becloforte Inhaler.

In some patients inhaled beclomethasone dipropionate may cause hoarseness or throat irritation. It may be helpful to rinse out the mouth thoroughly with water immediately after inhalation. The use of the Volumatic spacer device may be considered.

As with other inhalation therapy, paradoxical bronchospasm may occur with an immediate increase in wheezing after dosing. This responds to a fast-acting inhaled bronchodilator. Becloforte Inhaler should be discontinued immediately, the patient assessed and, if necessary, alternative therapy (e.g. Becloforte Diskhaler*) instituted.

Hypersensitivity reactions including rashes, urticaria, pruritus and erythema, and oedema of the eyes, face, lips and throat, have been reported.

*Overdosage:* Acute. Inhalation of the drug in doses in excess of those recommended may lead to temporary suppression of adrenal function. This does not necessitate emergency action being taken. In these patients treatment with beclomethasone dipropionate by inhalation should be continued at a dose sufficient to control asthma; adrenal function recovers in a few days and can be verified by measuring plasma cortisol.

Chronic. Use of inhaled beclomethasone dipropionate in daily doses in excess of 1,500 micrograms over prolonged periods may lead to some degree of adrenal suppression. Monitoring of adrenal reserve may be indicated. Treatment with inhaled beclomethasone dipropionate should be continued at a dose sufficient to control asthma.

**Pharmaceutical precautions** Becloforte Inhaler should be stored at a temperature below 30°C.

As with most inhaled medications in aerosol canisters, the therapeutic effect of this medication may decrease when the canister is cold.

Protect from frost and direct sunlight.

The canister should not be punctured, broken or burnt even when apparently empty.

**Legal category** POM.

**Package quantities** Becloforte Inhaler provides 200 metered actuations.

**Further information** Nil.

**Product licence number** 10949/0065

## BECODISKS*

**Presentation:** The active ingredient is presented in a disk comprising eight regularly spaced double-foil blisters each containing either 100 micrograms or 200 micrograms of Beclomethasone Dipropionate BP, or 400 micrograms of beclomethasone dipropionate as the monohydrate, and larger particle lactose. Each dosage strength is identified in the centre of the disk as 'Becodisk 100 mcg', or 'Becodisk 200 mcg', or 'Becodisk 400 mcg' respectively.

Becodisks are intended only for use in a specific drug delivery device known as the Diskhaler*. The contents of each blister are deposited in the Diskhaler device when pierced with an integral needle. The contents are then available to the patient to inhale by breath operation which allows the drug to be fully available even at low inspiratory flow rates.

Becodisks therefore provide reliable drug delivery for many patients.

**Uses** Beclomethasone dipropionate provides effective anti-inflammatory action in the lungs, without the problems of systemic corticosteroid treatment, and offers preventive treatment of asthma.

Becodisks are particularly useful in patients who have difficulty with co-ordinating the effective use of metered-dose inhalers.

*Therapeutic indications:* Becodisks are indicated for a wide range of patients with asthma.

*Adults:* Prophylactic management in:

*mild asthma:* Patients requiring symptomatic bronchodilator asthma medication on a regular basis.

*moderate asthma:* Patients with unstable or worsening asthma despite prophylactic therapy or bronchodilator alone.

*severe asthma:* Patients with severe chronic asthma and those who are dependent on systemic corticosteroids for adequate control of symptoms. On transfer to high dose inhaled beclomethasone dipropionate, many patients who are dependent on systemic corticosteroids for adequate control of symptoms may be able to reduce significantly, or eliminate, their requirement for oral corticosteroids.

*Children:* Any child who requires prophylactic asthma medication.

**Dosage and administration** Becodisks are for inhalation use only, using a Becotide* Diskhaler. Patients should be made aware of the prophylactic nature of therapy with inhaled beclomethasone dipropionate and that it should be taken regularly every day even when they are asymptomatic. Patients should be given a starting dose of inhaled beclomethasone dipropionate which is appropriate to the severity of their disease. The dose may then be adjusted until control is achieved or reduced to the minimum effective dose according to individual response.

*Adults:* 400 micrograms twice daily is the usual starting dose. One 400 micrograms blister or two 200 micrograms blisters twice daily is the usual maintenance dose. Alternatively, 200 micrograms may be administered three or four times daily.

*Children:* 100 micrograms two, three or four times a day according to the response. Alternatively the usual starting dose of 200 micrograms twice daily may be administered.

There is no need to adjust the dose in elderly patients or in those with hepatic or renal impairment.

**Contra-indications, warnings, etc**

*Contra-indications:* Becodisks are contra-indicated in patients with a history of hypersensitivity to any of the components. Special care is necessary in patients with active or quiescent pulmonary tuberculosis.

*Precautions:* Patients should be instructed in the proper use of the Diskhaler to ensure that the drug reaches the target areas within the lungs. They should also be made aware that Becodisks have to be used regularly, every day, for optimum benefit. Patients should be made aware of the prophylactic nature of therapy with Becodisks and that they should be used regularly, even when they are asymptomatic.

Becodisks are not designed to relieve acute asthmatic symptoms for which an inhaled short-acting bronchodilator is required. Patients should be advised to have such rescue medication available.

Severe asthma requires regular medical assessment, including lung-function testing, as patients are at risk of severe attacks and even death.

Increasing use of bronchodilators, in particular short-acting inhaled $\beta_2$-agonists, to relieve symptoms indicates deterioration of asthma control. If patients find that short-acting relief bronchodilator treatment becomes less effective, or they need more inhalations than usual, medical attention must be sought. In this situation patients should be reassessed and consideration given to the need for increased anti-inflammatory therapy (e.g. higher doses of inhaled corticosteroids or a course of oral corticosteroids). Severe exacerbations of asthma must be treated in the normal way.

In the majority of patients no significant adrenal suppression occurs until the daily dose is in excess of that recommended for Becodisks (e.g. 1,500 micrograms per day). Reduction of plasma cortisol levels has been reported in some patients who received 2,000 micrograms per day of inhaled beclomethasone dipropionate. In such patients the risks of developing adrenal suppression should be balanced against the therapeutic advantages, and precautions should be taken to provide systemic steroid cover in situations of prolonged stress. Prolonged suppression of the hypothalamic-pituitary-adrenal (HPA) axis may eventually lead to systemic effects including growth retardation in children and adolescents.

Lack of response or severe exacerbations of asthma should be treated by increasing the dose of inhaled beclomethasone dipropionate and, if necessary, by giving a systemic steroid and/or antibiotic if there is an infection, and by use of β-agonist therapy.

*For the transfer of patients being treated with oral corticosteroids:* The transfer of oral steroid-dependent patients to Becodisks, and their subsequent management, needs special care as recovery from impaired adrenocortical function, caused by prolonged systemic steroid therapy, may take a considerable time.

Patients who have been treated with systemic steroids for long periods of time or at a high dose may have adrenocortical suppression. With these patients adrenocortical function should be monitored regularly and their dose of systemic steroid reduced cautiously.

After approximately a week, gradual withdrawal of the systemic steroid is commenced. Decrements in dosages should be appropriate to the level of maintenance systemic steroid, and introduced at not less than weekly intervals. For maintenance doses of prednisolone (or equivalent) of 10 mg daily or less, the decrements in dose should be not greater than 1 mg per day, at not less than weekly intervals. For maintenance doses of prednisolone in excess of 10 mg daily, it may be appropriate to employ cautiously, larger decrements in dose at weekly intervals.

Some patients feel unwell in a non-specific way during the withdrawal phase despite maintenance or even improvement of the respiratory function. They should be encouraged to persevere with the Diskhaler and withdrawal of systemic steroid continued, unless there are objective signs of adrenal insufficiency.

Patients weaned off oral steroids whose adrenocortical function is impaired should carry a steroid warning card indicating that they may need supplementary systemic steroid during periods of stress, e.g. worsening asthma attacks, chest infections, major intercurrent illness, surgery, trauma, etc.

Replacement of systemic steroid treatment with inhaled therapy sometimes unmasks allergies such as allergic rhinitis or eczema previously controlled by the systemic drug. These allergies should be symptomatically treated with antihistamine and/or topical preparations, including topical steroids.

Treatment with Becodisks should not be stopped abruptly.

As with all inhaled corticosteroids, special care is necessary in patients with active or quiescent pulmonary tuberculosis.

*Pregnancy:* There is inadequate evidence of safety in human pregnancy. Administration of corticosteroids to pregnant animals can cause abnormalities of fetal development including cleft palate and intra-uterine growth retardation. There may therefore be a very small risk of such effects in the human fetus. It should be noted, however, that the fetal changes in animals occur after relatively high systemic exposure. Because beclomethasone dipropionate is delivered directly to the lungs by the inhaled route it avoids the high level of exposure that occurs when corticosteroids are given by systemic routes.

The use of beclomethasone dipropionate in pregnancy requires that the possible benefits of the drug be weighed against the possible hazards. It should be noted that the drug has been in widespread use for many years without apparent ill consequence.

*Lactation:* No specific studies examining the transference of beclomethasone dipropionate into the milk of lactating animals have been performed. It is reasonable to assume that beclomethasone dipropionate is secreted in milk, but at the dosages used for direct inhalation there is low potential for significant levels in breast milk.

The use of beclomethasone dipropionate in mothers breast feeding their babies requires that the therapeutic benefits of the drug be weighed against the potential hazards to the mother and baby.

*Side-effects:* Candidiasis of the mouth and throat (thrush) occurs in some patients, the incidence increase with doses greater than 400 micrograms beclomethasone dipropionate per day. Patients with high blood levels of *Candida precipitins*, indicating a previous infection, are more likely to develop this complication. Some patients may find it helpful to rinse their mouth thoroughly with water after using Becodisks. Symptomatic candidiasis can be treated with topical anti-fungal therapy whilst still continuing with the treatment.

In some patients inhaled beclomethasone dipropionate may cause hoarseness or throat irritation. It may be helpful to rinse the mouth out with water immediately after inhalation.

As with other inhalation therapy, paradoxical bronchospasm may occur with an immediate increase in wheezing after dosing. This responds to a fast-acting inhaled bronchodilator. The preparation should be discontinued immediately, the patient assessed, and if necessary alternative therapy instituted.

Hypersensitivity reactions including rashes, urticaria, pruritus and erythema, and oedema of the eyes, face, lips and throat, have been reported.

*Overdosage:* Acute. Inhalation of the drug in doses in excess of those recommended may lead to temporary suppression of adrenal function. This does not necessitate emergency action being taken. In these patients treatment with beclomethasone dipropionate by inhalation should be continued at a dose sufficient to control asthma; adrenal function recovers in a few days and can be verified by measuring plasma cortisol.

Chronic. Use of inhaled beclomethasone dipropionate in daily doses in excess of 1,500 micrograms over prolonged periods may lead to some degree of adrenal suppression. Monitoring of adrenal reserve may be indicated. Treatment with inhaled beclomethasone dipropionate should be continued at a dose sufficient to control asthma.

**Pharmaceutical precautions** Whilst the disks provide a good protection to the blister contents from the effects of the atmosphere they should not be exposed to extremes of temperature and should be stored below 30°C. A disk may be kept in the Diskhaler at all times but a blister should only be pierced immediately prior to use. Failure to observe this instruction may affect the operation of the Diskhaler.

**Legal category** POM.

**Package quantities** Becodisks 100 micrograms and 200 micrograms are supplied in cartons of 14, together with a Diskhaler device. Becodisks 400 micrograms are supplied in cartons of 7 with a Diskhaler device.

**Further information** Nil.

**Product licence numbers**
Becodisks 100 micrograms 10949/0055
Becodisks 200 micrograms 10949/0056
Becodisks 400 micrograms 10949/0057

## BECONASE* AQUEOUS NASAL SPRAY

**Presentation** Beconase Aqueous Nasal Spray is a presentation of an aqueous suspension of microfine Beclomethasone Dipropionate BP delivered by a metering, atomising pump. Each 100 mg spray delivered by the nasal applicator contains 50 micrograms Beclomethasone Dipropionate BP.

**Uses** Beconase Aqueous Nasal Spray is indicated for the prophylaxis and treatment of perennial and seasonal allergic rhinitis including hayfever, and vasomotor rhinitis. Beclomethasone dipropionate has a potent, anti-inflammatory effect within the respiratory tract at doses which are not systemically active.

**Dosage and administration** Beconase Aqueous Nasal Spray is for administration by the intranasal route only.

*Adults and children:* The recommended dosage is two sprays into each nostril twice daily (400 micrograms/day). For some patients, a dosage regimen of a single spray into each nostril three or four times daily may be preferred. Total daily administration should not normally exceed eight sprays.

For full therapeutic benefit regular usage is essential. The co-operation of the patient should be sought to comply with the regular dosage schedule and it should be explained that maximum relief may not be obtained within the first few doses.

For children under six years old, there are insufficient clinical data to recommend use.

**Contra-indications, warnings, etc**
*Contra-indications:* Beconase Aqueous Nasal Spray is contra-indicated in patients with a history of hypersensitivity to any of its components.

*Precautions:* Infections of the nasal passages and paranasal sinuses should be appropriately treated but do not constitute a specific contra-indication to treatment with Beconase Aqueous Nasal Spray.

Care must be taken while transferring patients from systemic steroid treatment to Beconase Aqueous Nasal Spray if there is any reason to suppose that their adrenal function is impaired.

Systemic effects may rarely occur. These include hypothalamic-pituitary-adrenal (HPA) suppression and growth retardation in children.

Although Beconase Aqueous Nasal Spray will control seasonal allergic rhinitis in most cases, an abnormally heavy challenge of summer allergens may, in certain instances, necessitate appropriate additional therapy particularly to control eye symptoms.

*Pregnancy:* There is inadequate evidence of safety in human pregnancy. Administration of corticosteroids to pregnant animals can cause abnormalities of fetal development including cleft palate and intra-uterine growth retardation. There may therefore be a very small risk of such effects in the human fetus. It should be noted, however, that the fetal changes in animals occur after relatively high systemic exposure. Beconase Aqueous Nasal Spray delivers beclomethasone dipropionate directly to the nasal mucosa and so minimises systemic exposure.

The use of beclomethasone dipropionate should be avoided during pregnancy unless thought essential by the doctor.

*Lactation:* No specific studies examining the transference of beclomethasone dipropionate into the milk of lactating animals have been performed. It is reasonable to assume that beclomethasone dipropionate is secreted in milk, but at the dosages used for direct intranasal administration there is low potential for significant levels in breast milk.

The use of beclomethasone dipropionate in mothers breast feeding their babies requires that the therapeutic benefits of the drug be weighed against the potential hazards to the mother and baby.

*Side-effects:* Rare cases of nasal septal perforation have been reported following the use of intranasal corticosteroids.

As with other nasal sprays, dryness and irritation of the nose and throat, unpleasant taste and smell and epistaxis have been reported rarely.

Rare cases of raised intra-ocular pressure or glaucoma in association with intranasal formulations of beclomethasone dipropionate have been reported.

Hypersensitivity reactions including rashes, urticaria, pruritus and erythema, and oedema of the eyes, face, lips and throat, have been reported.

*Overdosage:* The only harmful effect that follows inhalation of large amounts of the drug over a short time period is suppression of HPA function. No special emergency action need be taken. Treatment with Beconase Aqueous Nasal Spray should be continued at the recommended dose. HPA function recovers in a day or two.

**Pharmaceutical precautions** Beconase Aqueous Nasal Spray should be protected from light and stored below 30°C. Do not refrigerate.

**Legal category** POM.

**Package quantities** Beconase Aqueous Nasal Spray is supplied in an amber glass bottle fitted with a metering, atomising pump and nasal applicator. Each bottle provides approximately 200 metered sprays in recommended use.

**Further information** Beconase Aqueous Nasal Spray is an alternative intranasal presentation of Beclomethasone Dipropionate BP to Beconase Nasal Spray and is available for those who may prefer an aqueous product.

**Product licence number** 10949/0104

## BECOTIDE* 50 EASI-BREATHE* INHALER
## BECOTIDE* 100 EASI-BREATHE* INHALER

**Qualitative and quantitative composition** 50 or 100 micrograms Beclomethasone Dipropionate BP per actuation. Each canister delivers 200 actuations.

**Pharmaceutical form** Aerosol.

**Clinical particulars**

*Therapeutic indications:* Beclomethasone dipropionate given by inhalation offers preventative treatment for asthma. It provides effective anti-inflammatory action in the lungs without the problems of systemic corticosteroid treatment.

Becotide Easi-Breathe Inhalers are indicated in the prophylactic management of mild, moderate, or severe asthma in adults or children.

*Mild asthma:* Patients requiring symptomatic bronchodilator asthma medication on a regular basis.

*Moderate asthma:* Patients with unstable or

worsening asthma despite prophylactic therapy or bronchodilator alone.

*Severe asthma:* Patients with severe chronic asthma and those who are dependent on systemic corticosteroids for adequate control of symptoms. Many patients who are dependent on systemic corticosteroids for adequate control of symptoms may be able to reduce significantly, or eliminate, their requirement for oral corticosteroids when they are transferred to high dose inhaled beclomethasone dipropionate.

*Posology and method of administration:* Becotide Easi-Breathe Inhalers are for oral inhalation use only. The inhalers can be used alone or in combination with the Optimiser* spacer device.

Patients should be given a starting dose of inhaled beclomethasone dipropionate appropriate to the severity of their disease. The dose may than be adjusted until control is achieved, or reduced to the minimum effective dose according to individual response.

*Adults (including the elderly):* The usual starting dose is 200 micrograms twice a day. In more severe cases the starting dose may need to increase to 600 to 800 micrograms per day which may then be reduced when the patient's asthma has stabilised. The total daily dose may be administered as two, three, or four divided doses.

*Children:* The usual starting dose is 100 micrograms twice a day. This may be increased to 400 micrograms per day according to the response, administered as two, three, or four divided doses.

*Conta-indications:* Hypersensitivity to any of the components.

Special care is necessary in patients with active or quiescent pulmonary tuberculosis.

*Special warnings and special precautions for use:* Patients should be instructed in the proper use of the inhaler, and their technique checked, to ensure that the drug reaches the target areas within the lungs. They should also be made aware that Becotide Easi-Breathe Inhaler has to be used regularly, every day, even when they are asymptomatic, for optimum benefit.

Becotide Easi-Breathe Inhaler is not designed to relieve acute asthma symptoms for which an inhaled short-acting bronchodilator is required. Patients should be advised to have such relief medication available.

Severe asthma requires regular medical assessment, including lung-function testing, as patients are at risk of severe attacks and even death. Patients must be instructed to seek medical attention if short-acting relief bronchodilator treatment becomes less effective, or more inhalations than usual are required as this may indicate deterioration of asthma control. In this situation, patients should be assessed and the need for increased anti-inflammatory therapy (e.g. higher doses of inhaled corticosteroid or a course of oral corticosteroid) considered.

Severe exacerbations of asthma must be treated in the normal way, e.g. by increasing the dose of inhaled beclomethasone dipropionate and, if necessary by giving a systemic steroid, and/or an antibiotic if there is an infection, and by use of β-agonist therapy.

Treatment with Becotide Easi-Breathe Inhaler should not be stopped abruptly.

Significant adrenal suppression rarely occurs before doses of 1,500 micrograms per day of inhaled beclomethasone dipropionate are exceeded. Reduction of plasma cortisol levels has been reported in some patients taking 2,000 micrograms per day. In such patients, the risks of developing adrenal suppression should be balanced against the therapeutic advantages, and precautions taken to provide systemic steroid cover in situations of prolonged stress. Prolonged suppression of the hypothalamic-pituitary-adrenal (HPA) axis may eventually lead to systemic effects, including growth retardation in children and adolescents.

The transfer to Becotide Easi-Breathe Inhaler of patients who have been treated with systemic steroids for long periods of time, or at a high dose, needs special care, since recovery from any adrenocortical suppression sustained may take a considerable time. Approximately one week after initiating treatment with Becotide Easi-Breathe Inhaler, reduction of the dose of systemic steroid can be commenced. The size of the reduction should correspond to the maintenance dose of systemic steroid. Reductions in dose of not more than 1 mg are suitable for patients receiving maintenance doses of 10 mg daily or less of prednisolone or its equivalent. Larger reductions in dose may be appropriate for higher maintenance doses. The reductions in dose should be introduced at not less than weekly intervals. Adrenocortical function should be monitored regularly as the dose of systemic steroid is gradually reduced.

Some patients feel unwell in a non-specific way during the withdrawal phase despite maintenance or even improvement of the respiratory function. They should be encouraged to persevere with inhaled beclomethasone dipropionate and to continue withdrawal of systemic steroid, unless there are objective signs of adrenal insufficiency.

Patients weaned off oral steroids whose adrenocortical function is impaired should carry a steroid warning card indicating that they may need supplementary systemic steroid during periods of stress, e.g. worsening asthma attacks, chest infections, major intercurrent illness, surgery, trauma, etc.

Replacement of systemic steroid treatment with inhaled therapy sometimes unmasks allergies such as allergic rhinitis or eczema previously controlled by the systemic drug. These allergies should be symptomatically treated with antihistamine and/or topical preparations, including topical steroids.

As with all inhaled corticosteroids, special care is necessary in patients with active or quiescent pulmonary tuberculosis.

*Interaction with other medicaments and other forms of interaction:* None reported.

*Pregnancy and lactation:* There is inadequate evidence of safety in human pregnancy. Administration of corticosteroids to pregnant animals can cause abnormalities of fetal development including cleft palate and intra-uterine growth retardation. There may therefore be a very small risk of such effects in the human fetus. It should be noted, however, that the fetal changes in animals occur after relatively high systemic exposure. Becotide Easi-Breathe Inhaler delivers the drug directly to the lungs by the inhaled route and so avoids the high level of exposure that occurs when corticosteroids are given by systemic routes.

The use of beclomethasone dipropionate in pregnancy requires that the possible benefits of the drug be weighed against the possible hazards.

No specific studies examining the transference of beclomethasone dipropionate into the milk of lactating animals have been performed. It is reasonable to assume that beclomethasone dipropionate is secreted in milk, but at the dosages used for direct inhalation there is low potential for significant levels in breast milk.

The use of beclomethasone dipropionate in mothers breast feeding their babies requires that the therapeutic benefits of the drug be weighed against the potential hazards to the mother and baby.

*Effects on the ability to drive and use machines:* None reported.

*Undesirable effects:* As with other inhalation therapy, paradoxical bronchospasm may occur with an immediate increase in wheezing after dosing. This should be treated immediately with a fast-acting inhaled bronchodilator. The Becotide Easi-Breathe Inhaler should be discontinued immediately, the patient assessed and, if necessary, alternative therapy instituted.

Hypersensitivity reactions including rashes, urticaria, pruritus and erythema, and oedema of the eyes, face, lips and throat, have been reported.

Candidiasis of the mouth and throat (thrush) occurs in some patients, the incidence increasing with doses greater than 400 micrograms beclomethasone dipropionate per day. Patients with high blood levels of *Candida precipitins*, indicating a previous infection, are most likely to develop this complication. Patients may find it helpful to rinse their mouth thoroughly with water after using the inhaler. The Optimiser spacer can be used to reduce oropharyngeal deposition. Symptomatic candidiasis can be treated with topical anti-fungal therapy whilst still continuing with Becotide Easi-Breathe Inhaler.

In some patients inhaled beclomethasone dipropionate may cause hoarseness or throat irritation. It may be helpful to rinse the mouth out with water immediately after inhalation. Alternatively, the Optimiser spacer can be used to reduce oropharyngeal deposition.

*Overdose:*

*Acute:* Inhalation of the drug in doses in excess of those recommended may lead to temporary suppression of adrenal function. This does not require emergency action. In these patients treatment should be continued at a dose sufficient to control asthma; adrenal function recovers in a few days and can be verified by measuring plasma cortisol.

*Chronic:* Use of inhaled beclomethasone dipropionate in daily doses in excess of 1,500 micrograms over prolonged periods may lead to some degree of adrenal suppression. Monitoring of adrenal reserve may be indicated. Treatment should be continued at a dose sufficient to control asthma.

**Pharmacological properties**

*Pharmacodynamic properties:* Beclomethasone dipropionate given by inhalation has a potent glucocorticoid anti-inflammatory action within the lungs.

*Phamacokinetic properties:* Beclomethasone 17,21-dipropionate (BDP) administered intravenously is cleared rapidly with a half-life of approximately 30 minutes. Belclomethasone 17-monopropionate (BMP) appears rapidly in the plasma after intravenous administration of BDP and is itself cleared with a half-life again of about 30 minutes. BDP is bound to plasma proteins to the extent of 87%. Up to 14% of an intravenous dose of BDP is excreted in the urine in 96 hours, mainly as polar metabolites, a proportion of which are conjugated. Up to 64% of the dose is excreted in faeces in this time, again primarily as free and conjugated metabolites.

After inhalation about 25% of the dose reaches the lungs and is available for absorption from this site. The remainder is deposited on the delivery device or in the oropharynx. That portion deposited in the mouth or upper airways will ultimately be swallowed.

There is rapid metabolic inactivation of most of the swallowed portion of BDP during its first passage through the liver. An oral dose (4 mg) of tritium-labelled BDP was absorbed slowly with peak levels of radioactivity equivalent to 20 ng drug/ml plasma being reached 5 hours after dosing. Excretion was mainly in the faeces (35–76% of the dose in 96 hours) and primarily as polar metabolites although the presence of BDP and BMP in faeces suggested incomplete absorption of the dose. Up to 14% of the dose was excreted as polar metabolites in urine.

The lung tissue rapidly hydrolyses BDP to BMP which in turn is hydrolysed more slowly to beclomethasone. The liver also matabolises BDP to BMP and further converts it to polar metabolites.

*Preclinical safety data:* BDP has low acute oral, subcutaneous and intraperitoneal toxicity in mice and rats, and repeat dose toxicity studies showed findings characteristic of glucocorticoids, with no evidence of irritancy to the respiratory tract. The main findings, at above therapeutic doses, were depression of corticosterone levels in rats and cortisol levels in dogs. BDP is non-genotoxic, and demonstrated no oncogenic potential following combined inhalation/oral administration to rats. Susceptibility of fetuses to cleft palate, noted in the mouse organogenesis study, is considered to have no relevance for therapeutic use.

**Pharmaceutical particulars**

*List of excipients:* Oleic acid, dichlorodifluoromethane, trichlorofluoromethane.

*Incompatibilities:* None reported.

*Shelf life:* Two years when stored below 30°C.

*Special precautions for storage:* Store below 30°C.

As with most inhaled medicines in aerosol canisters, the therapeutic effect may decrease when the canister is cold.

Protect from frost and direct sunlight.

The canister should not be broken, punctured or burnt, even when apparently empty.

*Nature and contents of container:* An inhaler comprising an aluminium can fitted with a breath-operated metering valve, actuator and dust cap. Each canister contains 200 metered actuations of 50 or 100 micrograms beclomethasone dipropionate.

*Instructions for use/handling:* The aerosol spray is inhaled through the mouth into the lungs. After shaking the inhaler, open the cap and place the mouthpiece in the mouth with the lips closed around it. Suck in slowly through the mouthpiece, this releases a spray.

The inhaler can be used with the Optimiser spacer device.

For detailed instructions for use refer to the patient information leaflet in every pack.

*Marketing authorisation holder:* Glaxo Wellcome UK Ltd, trading as Allen & Hanburys, Stockley Park West, Uxbridge, Middlesex, UB11 1BT.

**Marketing authorisation numbers**
Becotide 50 Easi-Breathe Inhaler 10949/00268
Becotide 100 Easi-Breathe Inhaler 10949/00269

**Date of approval/revision of SPC** December 1996.

**Legal category** POM.

## BECOTIDE* INHALERS

**Presentation** Becotide 50 Inhaler is a metered-dose aerosol which delivers 50 micrograms Beclomethasone Dipropionate BP per actuation into the mouthpiece of a specially designed actuator.

Becotide 100 Inhaler is a metered-dose aerosol which delivers 100 micrograms Beclomethasone Dipropionate BP per actuation into the mouthpiece of a specially designed actuator.

Becotide 200 Inhaler is a metered-dose aerosol which delivers 200 micrograms Beclomethasone Dipropionate BP per actuation into the mouthpiece of a specially designed actuator.

Other ingredients: Oleic acid, dichlorodifluoromethane and trichlorofluoromethane.

**Uses** Beclomethasone dipropionate given by inhalation offers preventative treatment for asthma. It provides effective anti-inflammatory action in the lungs without the problems of systemic corticosteroid treatment.

Becotide Inhaler is indicated for a wide range of patients with asthma.

*Therapeutic indications:*

*Adults:* Prophylactic management in:

*mild asthma:* Patients requiring intermittent symptomatic bronchodilator asthma medication on a regular basis.

*moderate asthma:* Patients with unstable or worsening asthma despite prophylactic therapy or bronchodilator alone.

*severe asthma:* Patients with severe chronic asthma and those who are dependent on systemic corticosteroids for adequate control of symptoms. On transfer to high dose inhaled beclomethasone dipropionate, many patients who are dependent on systemic corticosteroids for adequate control of symptoms may be able to reduce significantly, or eliminate, their requirement for oral corticosteroids.

*Children:* Any child who requires prophylactic asthma medication.

**Dosage and administration** Becotide Inhalers are for inhalation use only. A Volumatic* spacer device may be used in patients who find it difficult to synchronise aerosol actuation with inspiration of breath.

Patients should be given a starting dose of inhaled beclomethasone dipropionate which is appropriate for the severity of their disease. The dose may then be adjusted until control is achieved or reduced to the minimum effective dose according to individual response.

*Adults:* The usual starting dose is 200 micrograms twice a day. In more severe cases dosage may be started at, or increased to, 600 to 800 micrograms per day, and subsequently reduced when the patient's asthma has stabilised. The total daily dose may be administered as two, three or four divided doses.

*Children:* 50 to 100 micrograms, two, three or four times daily, according to the response. Alternatively, 100 micrograms or 200 micrograms twice daily may be administered. The usual starting dose is 100 micrograms twice a day.

The Babyhaler* spacer device may be used with Becotide 50 Inhaler to facilitate administration to children under 5 years of age.

Becotide 200 Inhaler is not suitable for children.

There is no need to adjust the dose in elderly patients or in those with hepatic or renal impairment.

If patients find that short-acting relief bronchodilator treatment becomes less effective or they need more inhalations than usual, medical attention must be sought.

**Contra-indications, warnings, etc**

*Contra-indications:* Becotide Inhaler is contra-indicated in patients with a history of hypersensitivity to any of its components.

Special care is necessary in patients with active or quiescent pulmonary tuberculosis.

*Precautions:* Patients should be instructed in the proper use of the inhaler to ensure that the drug reaches the target areas within the lungs. They should also be made aware that Becotide Inhaler has to be used regularly, every day, for optimum benefit. Patients should be made aware of the prophylactic nature of therapy with Becotide Inhaler and that it should be taken regularly, even when they are asymptomatic.

Becotide Inhaler is not designed to relieve acute asthma symptoms for which an inhaled short-acting bronchodilator is required. Patients should be advised to have such relief medication available.

Severe asthma requires regular medical assessment, including lung-function testing, as patients are at risk of severe attacks and even death. Increasing use of bronchodilators, in particular short-acting inhaled $\beta_2$-agonists, to relieve symptoms indicates deterioration of asthma control. If patients find that short-acting relief bronchodilator treatment becomes less effective, or they need more inhalations than usual, medical attention must be sought. In this situation patients should be reassessed and consideration given to the need for increased anti-inflammatory therapy (e.g. higher doses of inhaled corticosteroids or a course of oral corticosteroids). Severe exacerbations of asthma must be treated in the normal way.

In the majority of patients significant adrenal suppression does not occur until the daily dose is in excess of that recommended for Becotide Inhaler (e.g. 1,500 micrograms per day). Reduction of plasma cortisol levels has been reported in some patients who received 2,000 micrograms per day of inhaled beclomethasone dipropionate. In such patients the risks of developing adrenal suppression should be balanced against the therapeutic advantages, and precautions should be taken to provide systemic steroid cover in situations of prolonged stress. Prolonged suppression of the hypothalamic-pituitary-adrenal (HPA) axis may eventually lead to systemic effects including growth retardation in children and adolescents.

Lack of response or severe exacerbations of asthma should be treated by increasing the dose of inhaled beclomethasone dipropionate and, if necessary, by giving a systemic steroid and/or an antibiotic if there is an infection, and by use of β-agonist therapy.

*For the transfer of patients being treated with oral corticosteroids:* The transfer of oral steroid-dependent patients to inhaled beclomethasone dipropionate, and their subsequent management, needs special care as recovery from impaired adrenocortical function, caused by prolonged systemic steroid therapy, may take a considerable time.

Patients who have been treated with systemic steroids for long periods of time, or at a high dose, may have adrenocortical suppression. With these patients adrenocortical function should be monitored regularly and their dose of systemic steroid reduced cautiously.

After approximately a week, gradual withdrawal of the systemic steroid is commenced. Reductions in dosage should be appropriate to the level of maintenance systemic steroid, and introduced at not less than weekly intervals. For maintenance doses of prednisolone, or its equivalent, of 10 mg daily or less, the reductions in dose should be not greater than 1 mg per day, at not less than weekly intervals. For maintenance doses of prednisolone in excess of 10 mg daily, it may be appropriate to employ cautiously larger reductions in dose at weekly intervals.

Some patients feel unwell in a non-specific way during the withdrawal phase despite maintenance or even improvement of the respiratory function. They should be encouraged to persevere with inhaled beclomethasone dipropionate and to continue withdrawal of systemic steroid, unless there are objective signs of adrenal insufficiency.

Patients weaned off oral steroids whose adrenocortical function is impaired should carry a steroid warning card indicating that they may need supplementary systemic steroid during periods of stress, e.g. worsening asthma attacks, chest infections, major intercurrent illness, surgery, trauma, etc.

Replacement of systemic steroid treatment with inhaled therapy sometimes unmasks allergies such as allergic rhinitis or eczema previously controlled by the systemic drug. These allergies should be symptomatically treated with antihistamine and/or topical preparations, including topical steroids.

Treatment with Becotide Inhaler should not be stopped abruptly.

As with all inhaled corticosteroids, special care is necessary in patients with active or quiescent pulmonary tuberculosis.

*Pregnancy:* There is inadequate evidence of safety in human pregnancy. Administration of corticosteroids to pregnant animals can cause abnormalities of fetal development including cleft palate and intra-uterine growth retardation. There may therefore be a very small risk of such effects in the human fetus. It should be noted, however, that the fetal changes in animals occur after relatively high systemic exposure. Beclomethasone dipropionate is delivered directly to the lungs by the inhaled route and so avoids the high level of exposure that occurs when corticosteroids are given by systemic routes.

The use of beclomethasone dipropionate in pregnancy requires that the possible benefits of the drug be weighed against the possible hazards. It should be noted that the drug has been in widespread use for many years without apparent ill consequence.

*Lactation:* No specific studies examining the transference of beclomethasone dipropionate into the milk of lactating animals have been performed. It is reasonable to assume that beclomethasone dipropionate is secreted in milk, but at the dosages used for direct inhalation there is low potential for significant levels in breast milk.

The use of beclomethasone dipropionate in mothers breast feeding their babies requires that the therapeutic benefits of the drug be weighed against the potential hazards to the mother and baby.

*Side-effects:* Candidiasis of the mouth and throat (thrush) occurs in some patients, the incidence increases with doses greater than 400 micrograms beclomethasone dipropionate per day. Patients with high blood levels of *Candida precipitins,* indicating a previous infection, are most likely to develop this complication. Patients may find it helpful to rinse their mouth thoroughly with water after using the inhaler. Symptomatic candidiasis can be treated with topical anti-fungal therapy whilst still continuing with Becotide Inhaler.

In some patients inhaled beclomethasone dipropionate may cause hoarseness or throat irritation. It may be helpful to rinse the mouth out with water immediately after inhalation. The use of the Volumatic spacer device may be considered.

As with other inhalation therapy, paradoxical bronchospasm may occur with an immediate increase in wheezing after dosing. This responds to a fast-acting inhaled bronchodilator. The preparation should be discontinued immediately, the patient assessed and, if necessary, alternative therapy (e.g. Becodisks*) instituted.

Hypersensitivity reactions including rashes, urticaria, pruritus and erythema, and oedema of the eyes, face, lips and throat, have been reported.

*Overdosage:* Acute. Inhalation of the drug in doses in excess of those recommended may lead to temporary suppression of adrenal function. This does not necessitate emergency action being taken. In these patients treatment with beclomethasone dipropionate by inhalation should be continued at a dose sufficient to control asthma; adrenal function recovers in a few days and can be verified by measuring plasma cortisol.

Chronic. Use of inhaled beclomethasone dipropionate in daily doses in excess of 1,500 micrograms over prolonged periods may lead to some degree of adrenal suppression. Monitoring of adrenal reserve may be indicated. Treatment with inhaled beclomethasone dipropionate should be continued at a dose sufficient to control asthma.

**Pharmaceutical precautions** Becotide Inhaler should be stored at a temperature below 30°C.

As with most inhaled medications in aerosol canisters, the therapeutic effect of this medication may decrease when the canister is cold.

Protect from frost and direct sunlight.

The canister should not be punctured, broken or burnt even if it is apparently empty.

**Legal category** POM.

**Package quantities** Becotide 50 Inhaler, Becotide 100 Inhaler and Becotide 200 Inhaler provide 200 metered actuations.

**Further information** Nil.

**Product licence numbers**
Becotide 50 Inhaler 10949/0058
Becotide 100 Inhaler 10949/0059
Becotide 200 Inhaler 10949/0060

## BECOTIDE* ROTACAPS*

**Presentation** Becotide Rotacaps capsules, an alternative inhalation form of beclomethasone dipropionate to Becotide Inhaler, are especially valuable for treating patients who are unable to use pressurised inhalers effectively, or who might use them incorrectly.

Becotide Rotacaps contain a mixture of microfine beclomethasone dipropionate and large particle lactose in coloured, hard gelatin capsules. Each Rotacaps capsule contains 100 micrograms (buff/colourless), 200 micrograms (brown/colourless) or 400 micrograms (dark brown/colourless) beclomethasone dipropionate, and is marked Becotide 100, Becotide 200 or Becotide 400, respectively.

The contents of the Rotacaps capsule are inhaled using a specially developed device called a Rotahaler* inhaler which separates the capsule into halves that rotate and release the drug when the patient inhales. This breath actuation is very sensitive and so the drug is fully available even at the lowest inspiratory flow rates. The Rotahaler device is therefore a reliable drug delivery system for many patients.

**Uses** Beclomethasone dipropionate provides effective anti-inflammatory action in the lungs, without the problems of systemic corticosteroid treatment, and offers preventive treatment of asthma. Becotide Rotacaps are indicated for a wide range of patients with asthma.

*Therapeutic indications:*
*Adults:* Prophylactic management in:

*mild asthma:* Patients requiring symptomatic bronchodilator asthma medication on a regular basis.

*moderate asthma:* Patients with unstable or worsening asthma despite prophylactic therapy or bronchodilator alone.

*severe asthma:* Patients with severe chronic asthma and those who are dependent on systemic corticosteroids for adequate control of symptoms. On transfer to high dose inhaled beclomethasone dipropionate, many patients who are dependent on systemic corticosteroids for adequate control of symptoms may be able to reduce significantly, or eliminate, their requirement for oral corticosteroids.

*Children:* Any child who requires prophylactic asthma medication.

**Dosage and administration** Patients should be made aware of the prophylactic nature of therapy with inhaled beclomethasone dipropionate and that it should be taken regularly every day even when they are asymptomatic.

Becotide Rotacaps are for inhalation use only, using a Becotide Rotahaler. For optimum results Becotide Rotacaps should be used regularly. Patients should be given a starting dose of inhaled beclomethasone dipropionate which is appropriate for the severity of their disease. The dose may then be adjusted until control is achieved or reduced to the minimum effective dose according to the individual response.

*Adults:* 400 micrograms twice daily is the usual starting dose. One 400 micrograms Rotacaps capsule or two 200 micrograms Rotacaps capsules twice a day is the usual maintenance dose. Alternatively, one 200 micrograms Rotacaps capsule may be given three or four times daily.

*Children:* One 100 micrograms Rotacaps capsule two, three or four times a day, according to the response. Alternatively, the usual starting dose of 200 micrograms twice daily may be administered.

There is no need to adjust the dose in elderly patients or in those with hepatic or renal impairment.

**Contra-indications, warnings, etc**
*Contra-indications:* Becotide Rotacaps are contra-indicated in patients with a history of hypersensitivity to any of the components. Special care is necessary in patients with active or quiescent pulmonary tuberculosis.

*Precautions:* Patients should be instructed in the proper use of the Rotahaler to ensure that the drug reaches the target areas within the lungs. They should also be made aware that Becotide Rotacaps have to be used regularly, every day, for optimum benefit. They should be made aware of the prophylactic nature of therapy with inhaled beclomethasone dipropionate and that it should be taken regularly, even when they are asymptomatic.

Becotide Rotacaps are not designed to relieve acute asthmatic symptoms for which an inhaled short-acting bronchodilator is required. Patients should be advised to have such rescue medication available.

Severe asthma requires regular medical assessment, including lung-function testing, as patients are at risk of severe attacks and even death.

Increasing use of bronchodilators, in particular short-acting inhaled $\beta_2$-agonists, to relieve symptoms indicates deterioration of asthma control. If patients find that short-acting relief bronchodilator treatment becomes less effective, or they need more inhalations than usual, medical attention must be sought. In this situation patients should be reassessed and consideration given to the need for increased anti-inflammatory therapy (e.g. higher doses of inhaled corticosteroids or a course of oral corticosteroids). Severe exacerbations of asthma must be treated in the normal way.

In the majority of patients no significant adrenal suppression occurs until the daily dose is in excess of that recommended for Becotide Rotacaps (e.g. 1,500 micrograms per day). Reduction of plasma cortisol levels has been reported in some patients who received 2,000 micrograms per day of inhaled beclomethasone dipropionate. In such patients the risks of developing adrenal suppression should be balanced against the therapeutic advantages, and precautions should be taken to provide systemic steroid cover in situations of prolonged stress. Prolonged suppression of the hypothalamic-pituitary-adrenal (HPA) axis may eventually lead to systemic effects including growth retardation in children and adolescents.

Lack of response or severe exacerbations of asthma should be treated by increasing the dose of inhaled beclomethasone dipropionate and, if necessary, by giving a systemic steroid and/or antibiotic if there is an infection, and by use of β-agonist therapy.

*For the transfer of patients being treated with oral corticosteroids:* The transfer of oral steroid-dependent patients to Becotide Rotacaps, and their subsequent management, needs special care as recovery from impaired adrenocortical function, caused by prolonged systemic steroid therapy, may take a considerable time.

Patients who have been treated with systemic steroids for long periods of time, or at a high dose, may have adrenocortical suppression. With these patients adrenocortical function should be monitored regularly and their dose of systemic steroid reduced cautiously.

After approximately a week, gradual withdrawal of the systemic steroid is commenced. Decrements in dosage should be appropriate to the level of maintenance systemic steroid, and introduced at not less than weekly intervals. For maintenance doses of prednisolone, or its equivalent, of 10 mg daily or less, the decrements in dose should not be greater than 1 mg per day, at not less than weekly intervals. For maintenance doses of prednisolone in excess of 10 mg daily, it may be appropriate to employ cautiously larger decrements in dose at weekly intervals.

Some patients feel unwell in a non-specific way during the withdrawal phase despite maintenance or even improvement of the respiratory function. They should be encouraged to persevere with the Rotahaler and withdrawal of systemic steroid continued, unless there are objective signs of adrenal insufficiency.

Patients weaned off oral steroids whose adreno-cortical function is impaired should carry a steroid warning card indicating that they may need supplementary systemic steroid during periods of stress, e.g. worsening asthma attacks, chest infections, major intercurrent illness, surgery, trauma, etc.

Replacement of systemic steroid treatment with inhaled therapy sometimes unmasks allergies such as allergic rhinitis or eczema previously controlled by the systemic drug. These allergies should be symptomatically treated with antihistamine and/or topical preparations, including topical steroids.

Treatment with Becotide Rotacaps should not be stopped abruptly.

As with all inhaled corticosteroids, special care is necessary in patients with active or quiescent pulmonary tuberculosis.

*Pregnancy:* There is inadequate evidence of safety in human pregnancy. Administration of corticosteroids to pregnant animals can cause abnormalities of fetal development including cleft palate and intra-uterine growth retardation. There may therefore be a very small risk of such effects in the human fetus. It should be noted, however, that the fetal changes in animals occur after relatively high systemic exposure. Because beclomethasone dipropionate is delivered directly to the lungs by the inhaled route it avoids the high level of exposure that occurs when corticosteroids are given by systemic routes.

The use of beclomethasone dipropionate in pregnancy requires that the possible benefits of the drug be weighed against the possible hazards. It should be noted that the drug has been in widespread use for many years without apparent ill consequence.

*Lactation:* No specific studies examining the transference of beclomethasone dipropionate into the milk of lactating animals have been performed. It is reasonable to assume that beclomethasone dipropionate is secreted in milk, but at the dosages used for direct inhalation there is low potential for significant levels in breast milk.

The use of beclomethasone dipropionate in mothers breast feeding their babies requires that the therapeutic benefits of the drug be weighed against the potential hazards to the mother and baby.

*Side-effects:* Candidiasis of the mouth and throat (thrush) occurs in some patients, the incidence increases with doses greater than 400 micrograms beclomethasone dipropionate per day. Patients with high blood levels of *Candida precipitins*, indicating a previous infection, are more likely to develop this complication. Some patients may find it helpful to rinse their mouth thoroughly with water after using the Rotahaler. Symptomatic candidiasis can be treated with topical anti-fungal therapy whilst still continuing with the treatment.

In some patients inhaled beclomethasone dipropionate may cause hoarseness or throat irritation. It may be helpful to rinse the mouth out with water immediately after inhalation.

As with other inhalation therapy, paradoxical bronchospasm may occur with an immediate increase in wheezing after dosing. This responds to a fast-acting inhaled bronchodilator. The preparation should be discontinued immediately, the patient assessed and, if necessary, alternative therapy instituted.

Hypersensitivity reactions including rashes, urticaria, pruritus and erythema, and oedema of the eyes, face, lips and throat, have been reported.

*Overdosage:* Acute. Inhalation of the drug in doses in excess of those recommended may lead to temporary suppression of adrenal function. This does not necessitate emergency action being taken. In these patients treatment with beclomethasone dipropionate by inhalation should be continued at a dose sufficient to control asthma; adrenal function recovers in a few days and can be verified by measuring plasma cortisol.

Chronic. Use of inhaled beclomethasone dipropionate in daily doses in excess of 1,500 micrograms over prolonged periods may lead to some degree of adrenal suppression. Monitoring of adrenal reserve may be indicated. Treatment with inhaled beclomethasone dipropionate should be continued at a dose sufficient to control asthma.

**Pharmaceutical precautions** To keep the Rotacaps capsules in good condition it is important that they are stored in a dry place below 30°C where they will not be exposed to extremes of temperature. A convenient supply may be carried in the special container for the Rotahaler device. The Rotacaps capsules should be inserted into the Rotahaler immediately prior to use to avoid softening. Failure to observe this instruction may affect the delivery of the drug. The Rotacaps must only be used in the Rotahaler.

**Legal category** POM.

**Package quantities** Becotide Rotacaps 100 micrograms, 200 micrograms and 400 micrograms are supplied in packs of 112.

**Further information** Nil.

**Product licence numbers**
Becotide Rotacaps 100 micrograms 10949/0061
Becotide Rotacaps 200 micrograms 10949/0062
Becotide Rotacaps 400 micrograms 10949/0063

# FLIXONASE* AQUEOUS NASAL SPRAY

**Presentation** Flixonase Aqueous Nasal Spray is an aqueous suspension of microfine fluticasone propionate (0.05% w/w) for topical administration to the nasal mucosa by means of a metering, atomising spray pump. Each 100 mg of spray delivered by the nasal adaptor contains 50 micrograms of fluticasone propionate.

Other ingredients: Microcrystalline cellulose, sodium carboxymethylcellulose, dextrose, polysorbate 80, purified water, benzalkonium chloride and phenylethylalcohol.

**Uses** Flixonase Aqueous Nasal Spray is indicated for the prophylaxis and treatment of seasonal allergic rhinitis including hayfever, and perennial rhinitis. Fluticasone propionate has potent anti-inflammatory activity but when used topically on the nasal mucosa has no detectable systemic activity.

**Dosage and administration** Flixonase Aqueous Nasal Spray is for administration by the intranasal route only.

*Adults and children over 12 years of age:* For the prophylaxis and treatment of seasonal allergic rhinitis and perennial rhinitis: two sprays into each nostril once a day, preferably in the morning. In some cases two sprays into each nostril twice daily may be required. The maximum daily dose should not exceed four sprays into each nostril.

*Elderly:* The normal adult dosage is applicable.

*Children under 12 years of age:* For the prophylaxis and treatment of seasonal allergic rhinitis and perennial rhinitis in children aged 4 to 11 years a dose of one spray into each nostril once daily is recommended. In some cases one spray into each nostril twice daily may be required. The maximum daily dose should not exceed two sprays into each nostril.

For full therapeutic benefit regular usage is essential. The absence of an immediate effect should be explained to the patient as maximum relief may not be obtained until after 3 to 4 days of treatment.

**Contra-indications, warnings, etc**
*Contra-indications:* Flixonase Aqueous Nasal Spray is contra-indicated in patients with hypersensitivity to any of its ingredients.

*Precautions:* Infections of the nasal airways should be appropriately treated but do not constitute a specific contra-indication to treatment with Flixonase Aqueous Nasal Spray.

The full benefit of Flixonase Aqueous Nasal Spray may not be achieved until treatment has been administered for several days.

Care must be taken while transferring patients from systemic steroid treatment to Flixonase Aqueous Nasal Spray if there is any reason to suppose that their adrenal function is impaired.

Although Flixonase Aqueous Nasal Spray will control seasonal allergic rhinitis in most cases, an abnormally heavy challenge of summer allergens may in certain instances necessitate appropriate additional therapy, particularly to control eye symptoms.

*Pregnancy:* There is inadequate evidence of safety in human pregnancy. Administration of corticosteroids to pregnant animals can cause abnormalities of fetal development, including cleft palate and intra-uterine growth retardation. There may therefore be a very small risk of such effects in the human fetus. It should be noted, however, that the fetal changes in animals occur after relatively high systemic exposure; direct intranasal application ensures minimal systemic exposure.

As with other drugs the use of Flixonase Aqueous Nasal Spray during human pregnancy requires that the possible benefits of the drug be weighed against the possible hazards.

*Lactation:* The secretion of fluticasone propionate in human breast milk has not been investigated. Subcutaneous administration of fluticasone propionate to lactating laboratory rats produced measurable plasma levels and evidence of fluticasone propionate in the milk. However, following intranasal administration to primates, no drug was detected in the plasma, and it is therefore unlikely that the drug would be detectable in milk. When fluticasone propionate is used in breast feeding mothers the therapeutic benefits must be weighed against the potential hazards to mother and baby.

*Side-effects:* Extremely rare cases of nasal septal perforation have been reported following the use of intranasal corticosteroids, usually in patients who have had previous nasal surgery.

As with other nasal sprays, dryness and irritation of the nose and throat, unpleasant taste and smell and epistaxis have been reported.

Hypersensitivity reactions including skin rash and oedema of the face or tongue have been reported.

There have also been rare reports of anaphylaxis/anaphylactoid reactions and bronchospasm.

*Overdosage:* There are no data available on the effects of acute or chronic overdosage with Flixonase Aqueous Nasal Spray. Intranasal administration of 2 mg fluticasone propionate twice daily for seven days to healthy human volunteers had no effect on hypothalamic-pituitary-adrenal (HPA) axis function. Inhalation or oral administration of high doses of corticosteroids over a long period may lead to suppression of HPA function.

**Pharmaceutical precautions** Shake gently before use. Flixonase Aqueous Nasal Spray should be stored below 30°C.

**Legal category** POM.

**Package quantities** Flixonase Aqueous Nasal Spray is supplied in an amber glass bottle fitted with a metering, atomising pump, nasal adaptor and a dust cover. Each bottle provides approximately 120 metered sprays, when used as recommended.

**Further information** Nil.

**Product licence number** 10949/0036

# FLIXOTIDE* ACCUHALER*

**Qualitative and quantitative composition** Flixotide Accuhaler is a moulded plastic device containing a foil strip with 28 or 60 regularly placed blisters each containing a mixture of microfine fluticasone propionate (50 micrograms, 100 micrograms, 250 micrograms or 500 micrograms) and larger particle size lactose.

**Pharmaceutical form** Multi-dose dry powder inhalation device.

**Clinical particulars**

*Therapeutic indications:* Fluticasone propionate given by inhalation offers preventative treatment for asthma. At recommended doses it has a potent glucocorticoid anti-inflammatory action within the lungs, without the adverse effects observed when corticosteroids are administered systemically. In the majority of patients it has no effect on adrenal function or reserve at recommended doses.

*Adults:* Prophylactic management in:

Mild asthma: Patients requiring intermittent symptomatic bronchodilator asthma medication on a regular daily basis.

Moderate asthma: Patients with unstable or worsening asthma despite prophylactic therapy or bronchodilator alone.

Severe asthma: Patients with severe chronic asthma and those who are dependent on systemic corticosteroids for adequate control of symptoms. On introduction of inhaled fluticasone propionate many of these patients may be able to reduce significantly, or to eliminate, their requirement for oral corticosteroids.

*Children:* Any child who requires prophylactic medication, including patients not controlled on currently available prophylactic medication.

*Posology and method of administration:* Flixotide Accuhaler is for oral inhalation use only. Flixotide Accuhaler is suitable for many patients, including those who cannot use a metered-dose inhaler successfully.

Patients should be made aware of the prophylactic nature of therapy with Flixotide Accuhaler and that it should be taken regularly even when they are asymptomatic. The onset of therapeutic effect is within 4 to 7 days.

*Adults and children over 16 years:* 100 to 1,000 micrograms twice daily.

Patients should be given a starting dose appropriate to the severity of their disease. Equivalent disease control is usually obtained at half the daily dose of other currently available inhaled steroids.

Typical starting doses are:
Mild asthma: 100 to 250 micrograms twice daily.
Moderate asthma: 250 to 500 micrograms twice daily.
Severe asthma: 500 to 1,000 micrograms twice daily.

The dose should be adjusted until control is achieved or reduced to the minimum effective dose, according to the individual response.

*Children aged 4 years and over:* 50 to 100 micrograms twice daily.

The starting dose should be appropriate to the severity of the disease. The dose should be adjusted until control is achieved and then reduced to the minimum effective dose according to the individual response.

Flixotide Accuhaler 250 micrograms and Flixotide Accuhaler 500 micrograms are not suitable for use in children.

*Special patient groups:* There is no need to adjust the dose in elderly patients or in those with hepatic or renal impairment.

*Contra-indications:* Hypersensitivity to any ingredient of the preparation.

*Special warnings and special precautions for use:*
Flixotide Accuhaler is not designed to relieve acute symptoms for which an inhaled short acting bronchodilator is required. Patients should be advised to have such rescue medication available.

Severe asthma requires regular medical assessment, including lung-function testing, as patients are at risk of severe attacks and even death. Increasing use of short-acting inhaled $\beta_2$-agonists to relieve symptoms indicates deterioration of asthma control. If patients find that short-acting relief bronchodilator treatment becomes less effective, or they need more inhalations than usual, medical attention must be sought. In this situation patients should be reassessed and consideration given to the need for increased anti-inflammatory therapy (e.g. higher doses of inhaled corticosteroids or a course of oral corticosteroids). Severe exacerbations of asthma must be treated in the normal way.

Adrenal function and adrenal reserve usually remain within the normal range on inhaled fluticasone propionate. In patients taking maintenance doses of inhaled fluticasone propionate no systemic side effects (e.g. associated with suppression of hypothalamic-pituitary-adrenal [HPA] axis) have been observed in clinical trials. In particular, it is unlikely that the growth of younger patients would be stunted.

Some depression of plasma cortisol may occur in a small number of adult patients on higher doses (e.g. more than 1 mg daily).

The benefits of inhaled fluticasone propionate should minimise the need for oral steroids. However, patients transferred from other inhaled steroids, or oral steroids, remain at risk of impaired adrenal reserve for some time after transferring to inhaled fluticasone propionate. The possibility of adverse effects may persist for some time. These patients may require specialised advice to determine the extent of adrenal impairment before elective procedures. The possibility of residual impaired adrenal response should always be considered in emergency (medical or surgical) and elective situations likely to produce stress, and appropriate corticosteroid treatment considered.

Lack of response or severe exacerbations of asthma should be treated by increasing the dose of inhaled fluticasone propionate and, if necessary, by giving a systemic steroid and/or an antibiotic if there is an infection.

Replacement of systemic steroid treatment with inhaled therapy sometimes unmasks allergies such as allergic rhinitis or eczema previously controlled by the systemic drug. These allergies should be symptomatically treated with antihistamine and/or topical preparations, including topical steroids.

As with all inhaled corticosteroids, special care is necessary in patients with active or quiescent pulmonary tuberculosis.

Treatment with Flixotide Accuhaler should not be stopped abruptly.

*For the transfer of patients being treated with oral corticosteroids:* The transfer of oral steroid-dependent patients to Flixotide Accuhaler and their subsequent management needs special care as recovery from impaired adrenocortical function, caused by prolonged systemic steroid therapy, may take a considerable time.

Patients who have been treated with systemic steroids for long periods of time or at a high dose may have adrenocortical suppression. With these patients adrenocortical function should be monitored regularly and their dose of systemic steroid reduced cautiously.

After approximately a week, gradual withdrawal of the systemic steroid is commenced. Decrements in dosages should be appropriate to the level of maintenance systemic steroid, and introduced at not less than weekly intervals. For maintenance doses of prednisolone (or equivalent) of 10 mg daily or less, the decrements in dose should not be greater than 1 mg per day, at not less than weekly intervals. For maintenance doses of prednisolone in excess of 10 mg daily, it may be appropriate to employ cautiously, larger decrements in dose at weekly intervals.

Some patients feel unwell in a non-specific way during the withdrawal phase despite maintenance or even improvement of the respiratory function. They should be encouraged to persevere with inhaled fluticasone propionate and to continue withdrawal of systemic steroid, unless there are objective signs of adrenal insufficiency.

Patients weaned off oral steroids whose adrenocortical function is still impaired should carry a steroid warning card indicating that they need supplementary systemic steroid during periods of stress, e.g. worsening asthma attacks, chest infections, major intercurrent illness, surgery, trauma, etc.

*Interaction with other medicaments and other forms of interaction:* No specific drug interaction studies have been performed. However, because of the very low plasma drug concentrations achieved after inhaled dosing, there are unlikely to be any implications for displacement drug interactions.

There were no reports of suspected drug interactions in the clinical programme.

*Pregnancy and lactation:* There is inadequate evidence of safety of fluticasone propionate in human pregnancy. Administration of corticosteroids to pregnant animals can cause abnormalities of fetal development, including cleft palate and intra-uterine growth retardation. There may therefore be a very small risk of such effects in the human fetus. It should be noted, however, that the fetal changes in animals occur after relatively high systemic exposure. Because Flixotide Accuhaler delivers fluticasone propionate directly to the lungs by the inhaled route it avoids the high level of exposure that occurs when corticosteroids are given by systemic routes. Administration of fluticasone propionate during pregnancy should only be considered if the expected benefit to the mother is greater than any possible risk to the fetus.

The secretion of fluticasone propionate in human breast milk has not been investigated. Subcutaneous administration of fluticasone propionate to lactating laboratory rats produced measurable plasma levels and evidence of fluticasone propionate in the milk. However, plasma levels in humans after inhalation at recommended doses are likely to be low.

When fluticasone propionate is used in breast feeding mothers the therapeutic benefits must be weighed against the potential hazards to mother and baby.

*Effects on ability to drive and use machines:* Fluticasone propionate is unlikely to produce an effect.

*Undesirable effects:* As with other inhalation therapy, paradoxical bronchospasm may occur with an immediate increase in wheezing after dosing. This should be treated immediately with a fast-acting, inhaled bronchodilator. Flixotide Accuhaler should be discontinued immediately, the patient assessed and, if necessary, alternative therapy instituted.

Candidiasis of the mouth and throat (thrush) occurs in some patients. Such patients may find it helpful to rinse out their mouth with water after inhalation. Symptomatic candidiasis can be treated with topical anti-fungal therapy whilst still continuing with Flixotide Accuhaler.

In some patients inhaled fluticasone propionate may cause hoarseness. It may be helpful to rinse out the mouth with water immediately after inhalation.

There have been rare reports of peripheral oedema and cutaneous hypersensitivity reactions such as skin rash.

There have been very rare reports of dyspepsia and arthralgia although a causal link with fluticasone propionate has not been established.

*Overdose:*
*Acute:* Inhalation of the drug in doses in excess of those recommended may lead to temporary suppression of adrenal function. This does not necessitate emergency action being taken. In these patients treatment with fluticasone propionate by inhalation should be continued at a dose sufficient to control asthma; adrenal function recovers in a few days and can be verified by measuring plasma cortisol.

*Chronic:* Use of inhaled fluticasone propionate in daily doses in excess of 2 milligrams over prolonged periods may lead to some degree of adrenal suppression. Monitoring of adrenal reserve may be indicated. Treatment with inhaled fluticasone propionate should be continued at a dose sufficient to control asthma.

**Pharmacological properties**
*Pharmacodynamic properties:* Fluticasone propionate given by inhalation at recommended doses has a potent glucocorticoid anti-inflammatory action within the lungs, resulting in reduced symptoms and exacerbations of asthma, without the adverse effects observed when corticosteroids are administered systemically.

*Pharmacokinetic properties:* Systemic absolute bioavailability of fluticasone propionate is estimated at 12–26% of an inhaled dose, dependent on presentation. Systemic absorption occurs mainly through the lungs and is initially rapid then prolonged. The remainder of the dose may be swallowed.

Absolute oral bioavailability is negligible (<1%) due to a combination of incomplete absorption from the GI tract and extensive first-pass metabolism.

87–100% of an oral dose is excreted in the faeces, up to 75% as parent compound. There is also a non-active major metabolite.

After an intravenous dose, fluticasone propionate is extensively distributed in the body. The very high clearance rate indicates extensive hepatic clearance.

*Preclinical safety data:* Toxicology has shown only those class effects typical of potent corticosteroids, and these only at doses greatly in excess of that proposed for therapeutic use. No novel effects were identified in repeat dose toxicity tests, reproductive studies or teratology studies. Fluticasone propionate is devoid of mutagenic activity *in vitro* and *in vivo* and showed no tumorigenic potential in rodents. It is both non-irritant and non-sensitising in animal models.

**Pharmaceutical particulars**
*List of excipients:* Lactose.

*Incompatibilities:* None reported.

*Shelf life:* 18 months when stored below 30°C.

*Special precautions for storage:* Store below 30°C (86°F). Store in a dry place.

*Nature and contents of container:* The powder mix of fluticasone propionate and lactose is filled into a blister strip consisting of a formed base foil with a peelable foil laminate lid. The foil strip is contained within the Accuhaler device.

*Instructions for use/handling:* The powdered medicine is inhaled through the mouth into the lungs.

The Accuhaler device contains the medicine in individual blisters which are opened as the device is manipulated.

For detailed instructions for use refer to the Patient Information Leaflet in every pack.

**Marketing authorisation numbers**
Flixotide Accuhaler 50 micrograms 10949/0226
Flixotide Accuhaler 100 micrograms 10949/0227
Flixotide Accuhaler 250 micrograms 10949/0228
Flixotide Accuhaler 500 micrograms 10949/0229

**Date of approval/ revision of SPC** March 1997.

**Legal category** POM.

## FLIXOTIDE* DISKHALER*

**Presentation** The active ingredient is presented in a disk comprising four regularly spaced double-foil blisters each delivering a mixture of fluticasone propionate and lactose. Flixotide Diskhaler is available in four strengths containing 50 micrograms, 100 micrograms, 250 micrograms or 500 micrograms fluticasone propionate per blister.

**Uses** Fluticasone propionate given by inhalation offers preventative treatment for asthma. At recommended doses it has a potent glucocorticoid anti-inflammatory action within the lungs, without the adverse effects observed when corticosteroids are administered systemically. In the majority of patients it has no effect on adrenal function or reserve at recommended doses.

*Therapeutic indications:*
*Adults:* Prophylactic management in:

*mild asthma:* Patients requiring intermittent symptomatic bronchodilator asthma medication on a regular daily basis

*moderate asthma:* Patients with unstable or worsening asthma despite prophylactic therapy or bronchodilator alone.

*severe asthma:* Patients with severe chronic asthma and those who are dependent on systemic corticosteroids for adequate control of symptoms. On introduction of inhaled fluticasone propionate many of these patients may be able to reduce significantly, or to eliminate, their requirement for oral corticosteroids.

*Children:* Any child who requires prophylactic medication, including patients not controlled on currently available prophylactic medication.

**Dosage and administration** Flixotide Diskhaler is for oral inhalation use only. Flixotide Diskhaler is suitable for many patients, including those who cannot use a metered-dose inhaler successfully.

Patients should be made aware of the prophylactic nature of therapy with Flixotide Diskhaler and that it should be taken regularly even when they are asymptomatic. The onset of therapeutic effect is within 4 to 7 days.

*Adults and children over 16 years:* 100 to 1,000 micrograms twice daily.

Patients should be given a starting dose appropriate to the severity of their disease.

Equivalent disease control is usually obtained at half the daily dose of other currently available inhaled steroids.

Typical starting doses are:

*mild asthma:* 100 to 250 micrograms twice daily,

*moderate asthma:* 250 to 500 micrograms twice daily,

*severe asthma:* 500 to 1,000 micrograms twice daily. The dose should be adjusted until control is achieved, and then reduced to the minimum effective dose according to individual response.

*Children aged 4 and over:* 50 to 100 micrograms twice daily.

The starting dose should be appropriate to the severity of the disease. The dose should be adjusted until control is achieved, and then reduced to the minimum effective dose according to individual response.

Flixotide Diskhaler 250 micrograms and Flixotide Diskhaler 500 micrograms are not suitable for use in children.

*Special patient groups:* There is no need to adjust the dose in elderly patients or in those with hepatic or renal impairment.

### Contra-indications, warnings, etc

*Contra-indications:* Flixotide Diskhaler is contra-indicated in patients with a history of hypersensitivity to any of its components.

*Precautions:* Flixotide Diskhaler is not designed to relieve acute symptoms, for which an inhaled short-acting bronchodilator is required. Patients should be advised to have such rescue medication available.

Severe asthma requires regular medical assessment, including lung-function testing, as patients are at risk of severe attacks and even death. Increasing use of short-acting inhaled $\beta_2$-agonists to relieve symptoms indicates deterioration of asthma control. If patients find that short-acting relief bronchodilator treatment becomes less effective, or they need more inhalations than usual, medical attention must be sought. In this situation patients should be reassessed and consideration given to the need for increased anti-inflammatory therapy (e.g. higher doses of inhaled corticosteroids or a course of oral corticosteroids). Severe exacerbations of asthma must be treated in the normal way.

Adrenal function and adrenal reserve usually remain within the normal range on inhaled fluticasone propionate. In patients taking maintenance doses of inhaled fluticasone propionate no systemic side effects (e.g. associated with suppression of hypothalamic-pituitary-adrenal [HPA] axis) have been observed in clinical trials. In particular, it is unlikely that the growth of younger patients would be stunted.

Some depression of plasma cortisol may occur in a small number of adult patients on higher doses (e.g. more than 1 mg daily).

The benefits of inhaled fluticasone propionate should minimise the need for oral steroids. However patients transferred from other inhaled steroids, or oral steroids, remain at risk of impaired adrenal reserve for some time after transferring to inhaled fluticasone propionate. The possibility of adverse effects may persist for some time.

These patients may require specialised advice to determine the extent of adrenal impairment before elective procedures. The possibility of residual impaired adrenal response should always be considered in emergency (medical or surgical) and elective situations likely to produce stress, and appropriate corticosteroid treatment considered.

Lack of response or severe exacerbations of asthma should be treated by increasing the dose of inhaled fluticasone propionate and, if necessary, by giving a systemic steroid and/or an antibiotic if there is an infection.

*For the transfer of patients being treated with oral corticosteroids:* The transfer of oral steroid-dependent patients to Flixotide Diskhaler, and their subsequent management, needs special care as recovery from impaired adrenocortical function, caused by prolonged systemic steroid therapy, may take a considerable time.

Patients who have been treated with systemic steroids for long periods of time, or at a high dose, may have adrenocortical suppression. With these patients, adrenocortical function should be monitored regularly and their dose of systemic steroid reduced cautiously.

After approximately a week, gradual withdrawal of the systemic steroid is started by reducing the daily dose by 1 mg prednisolone, or its equivalent, at not less than weekly intervals. For maintenance doses of prednisolone in excess of 10 mg daily, it may be appropriate to cautiously use larger reductions in dose at weekly intervals.

Some patients feel unwell in a non-specific way during the withdrawal phase despite maintenance or even improvement of respiratory function. They should be encouraged to persevere with Flixotide Diskhaler and to continue withdrawal of systemic steroid, unless there are objective signs of adrenal insufficiency.

Patients transferred from oral steroids whose adrenocortical function is still impaired should carry a steroid warning card indicating that they need supplementary systemic steroid during periods of stress, e.g. worsening asthma attacks, chest infections, major intercurrent illness, surgery, trauma, etc.

Replacement of systemic steroid treatment with inhaled therapy sometimes unmasks allergies such as allergic rhinitis or eczema previously controlled by the systemic drug. These allergies should be symptomatically treated with antihistamine and/or topical preparations, including topical steroids.

Treatment with Flixotide Diskhaler should not be stopped abruptly.

Special care is necessary in patients with active or quiescent pulmonary tuberculosis.

*Pregnancy and lactation:* There is inadequate evidence of safety of fluticasone propionate in human pregnancy. Administration of corticosteroids to pregnant animals can cause abnormalities of fetal development, including cleft palate and intra-uterine growth retardation. There may therefore be a very small risk of such effects in the human fetus. It should be noted, however, that the fetal changes in animals occur after relatively high systemic exposure. Because fluticasone propionate is delivered directly to the lungs by the inhaled route it avoids the high level of exposure that occurs when corticosteroids are given by systemic routes. Administration of fluticasone propionate during pregnancy should only be considered if the expected benefit to the mother is greater than any possible risk to the fetus. The secretion of fluticasone propionate in human breast milk has not been investigated.

Subcutaneous administration of fluticasone propionate to lactating laboratory rats produced measurable plasma levels and evidence of fluticasone propionate in the milk. However plasma levels in humans after inhalation at recommended doses are likely to be low. When fluticasone propionate is used in breast feeding mothers the therapeutic benefits must be weighed against the potential hazards to mother and baby.

*Side-effects:* As with other inhalation therapy, paradoxical bronchospasm may occur with an immediate increase in wheezing after dosing. This should be treated immediately with a fast-acting inhaled bronchodilator. Flixotide Diskhaler should be discontinued immediately, the patient assessed and, if necessary, alternative therapy instituted.

Candidiasis of the mouth and throat (thrush) occurs in some patients. Such patients may find it helpful to rinse out their mouth with water after using the Inhaler. Symptomatic candidiasis can be treated with topical anti-fungal therapy whilst still continuing with inhaled fluticasone propionate.

In some patients inhaled fluticasone propionate may cause hoarseness. It may be helpful to rinse out the mouth with water immediately after inhalation.

There have been rare reports of peripheral oedema and cutaneous hypersensitivity reactions such as skin rash.

There have been very rare reports of dyspepsia and arthralgia although a causal link with fluticasone propionate has not been established.

*Overdosage:* Acute. Inhalation of the drug in doses in excess of those recommended may lead to temporary suppression of adrenal function. This does not necessitate emergency action being taken. In these patients treatment with fluticasone propionate by inhalation should be continued at a reduced dose to control asthma; adrenal function recovers in a few days and can be verified by measuring plasma cortisol.

Chronic. Use of inhaled fluticasone propionate in daily doses in excess of 2 mg over prolonged periods may lead to some degree of adrenal suppression. Monitoring of adrenal reserve may be indicated. Treatment with Flixotide Diskhaler should be continued at a dose sufficient to control asthma.

**Pharmaceutical precautions** Whilst the disks provide good protection to the blister contents from the effect of the atmosphere, they should not be exposed to extremes of temperature and should be stored below 30°C.

Disks may be kept in the Diskhaler at all times but a blister should only be pierced immediately prior to use. Failure to observe this instruction will affect operation of the Diskhaler.

**Legal category** POM.

**Package quantities** Flixotide Diskhaler is supplied in cartons containing 14 disks (14 x 4 blisters), together with a Diskhaler inhaler.

**Further information** Nil.

**Product licence numbers**
Flixotide Diskhaler 50 micrograms 10949/0005
Flixotide Diskhaler 100 micrograms 10949/0006
Flixotide Diskhaler 250 micrograms 10949/0007
Flixotide Diskhaler 500 micrograms 10949/0008

## FLIXOTIDE* INHALER

**Presentation** Flixotide Inhaler is a pressurised metered-dose inhaler available in four strengths delivering 25 micrograms, 50 micrograms, 125 micrograms or 250 micrograms fluticasone propionate per actuation.

Other ingredients: trichlorofluoromethane, dichlorodifluoromethane and lecithin.

**Uses** Fluticasone propionate given by inhalation offers preventative treatment for asthma. At recommended doses it has a potent glucocorticoid anti-inflammatory action within the lungs, without the adverse effects observed when corticosteroids are administered systemically.

In the majority of patients it has no effect on adrenal function or reserve at recommended doses.

*Therapeutic indications:*

*Adults:* Prophylactic management in:

*mild asthma:* Patients requiring intermittent symptomatic bronchodilator asthma medication on a regular daily basis.

*moderate asthma:* Patients with unstable or worsening asthma despite prophylactic therapy or bronchodilator alone.

*severe asthma:* Patients with severe chronic asthma and those who are dependent on systemic corticosteroids for adequate control of symptoms. On introduction of inhaled fluticasone propionate many of these patients may be able to reduce significantly or to eliminate their requirement for oral corticosteroids.

*Children:* Any child who requires prophylactic medication, including patients not controlled on currently available prophylactic medication.

**Dosage and administration** Flixotide Inhaler is for oral inhalation use only. A Volumatic* spacer device may be used in patients who find it difficult to synchronise aerosol actuation with inspiration of breath.

Patients should be made aware of the prophylactic nature of therapy with Flixotide Inhaler and that it should be taken regularly even when they are asymptomatic. The onset of therapeutic effect is within 4 to 7 days.

*Adults and children over 16 years:* 100 to 1,000 micrograms twice daily, usually as two inhalations twice daily.

Patients should be given a starting dose appropriate to the severity of their disease.

Equivalent disease control is usually obtained at half the daily dose of other currently available inhaled steroids.

Typical starting doses are:

*mild asthma:* 100 to 250 micrograms twice daily,

*moderate asthma:* 250 to 500 micrograms twice daily,

*severe asthma:* 500 to 1,000 micrograms twice daily. The dose should be adjusted until control is achieved, and then reduced to the minimum effective dose according to individual response.

*Children aged 4 and over:* 50 to 100 micrograms twice daily.

The starting dose should be appropriate to the severity of the disease. The dose should be adjusted until control is achieved, and then reduced to the minimum effective dose according to individual response.

Flixotide Inhaler 125 micrograms and Flixotide Inhaler 250 micrograms are not suitable for use in children.

*Special patient groups:* There is no need to adjust the dose in elderly patients or those with hepatic or renal impairment.

### Contra-indications, warnings, etc

*Contra-indications:* Flixotide Inhaler is contra-indicated in patients with a history of hypersensitivity to any of its components.

*Precautions:* Patients' inhaler technique should be checked regularly to make sure that inhaler actuation is synchronised with inspiration to ensure optimum delivery of the drug to the lungs.

Flixotide Inhaler is not designed to relieve acute symptoms, for which an inhaled short-acting bronchodilator is required. Patients should be advised to have such rescue medication available.

Severe asthma requires regular medical assessment, including lung-function testing, as patients are at risk of severe attacks and even death. Increasing use of short-acting inhaled $\beta_2$-agonists to relieve symptoms indicates deterioration of asthma control. If patients find that short-acting relief bronchodilator treatment becomes less effective, or they need more inhalations than usual, medical attention must be sought. In this situation patients should be reassessed and consideration given to the need for increased anti-inflammatory therapy (e.g. higher doses of inhaled corticosteroids or a course of oral corticosteroids). Severe exacerbations of asthma must be treated in the normal way.

Adrenal function and adrenal reserve usually remain within the normal range on inhaled fluticasone propionate. In patients taking maintenance doses of inhaled fluticasone propionate no systemic side effects (e.g. associated with suppression of hypothalamic-pituitary-adrenal [HPA] axis) have been observed in clinical trials. In particular, it is unlikely that the growth of younger patients would be stunted.

Some depression of plasma cortisol may occur in a small number of adult patients on higher doses (e.g. more than 1 mg daily).

The benefits of inhaled fluticasone propionate should minimise the need for oral steroids. However, patients transferred from other inhaled steroids, or oral steroids, remain at risk of impaired adrenal reserve for some time after transferring to inhaled fluticasone propionate. The possibility of adverse effects may persist for some time.

These patients may require specialised advice to determine the extent of adrenal impairment before elective procedures. The possibility of residual impaired adrenal response should always be considered in emergency (medical or surgical) and elective situations likely to produce stress, and appropriate corticosteroid treatment considered.

Lack of response or severe exacerbations of asthma should be treated by increasing the dose of inhaled fluticasone propionate and, if necessary, by giving a systemic steroid and/or an antibiotic if there is an infection.

*For the transfer of patients being treated with oral corticosteroids:* The transfer of oral steroid-dependent patients to Flixotide Inhaler, and their subsequent management, needs special care as recovery from impaired adrenocortical function, caused by prolonged systemic steroid therapy, may take a considerable time.

Patients who have been treated with systemic steroids for long periods of time, or at a high dose, may have adrenocortical suppression. With these patients adrenocortical function should be monitored regularly and their dose of systemic steroid reduced cautiously.

After approximately a week, gradual withdrawal of the systemic steroid is started by reducing the daily dose by 1 mg prednisolone, or its equivalent. For maintenance doses of prednisolone in excess of 10 mg daily, it may be appropriate to cautiously use larger reductions in dose at weekly intervals.

Some patients feel unwell in a non-specific way during the withdrawal phase despite maintenance or even improvement of respiratory function. They should be encouraged to persevere with Flixotide Inhaler and to continue withdrawal of systemic steroid, unless there are objective signs of adrenal insufficiency.

Patients transferred from oral steroids whose adrenocortical function is still impaired should carry a steroid warning card indicating that they need supplementary systemic steroid during periods of stress, e.g. worsening asthma attacks, chest infections, major intercurrent illness, surgery, trauma, etc.

Replacement of systemic steroid treatment with inhaled therapy sometimes unmasks allergies such as allergic rhinitis or eczema previously controlled by the systemic drug. These allergies should be symptomatically treated with antihistamine and/or topical preparations, including topical steroids.

Treatment with Flixotide Inhaler should not be stopped abruptly.

Special care is necessary in patients with active or quiescent pulmonary tuberculosis.

*Pregnancy and lactation:* There is inadequate evidence of safety of fluticasone propionate in human pregnancy. Administration of corticosteroids to pregnant animals can cause abnormalities of fetal development, including cleft palate and intra-uterine growth retardation. There may therefore be a very small risk of such effects in the human fetus. It should be noted, however, that the fetal changes in animals occur after relatively high systemic exposure. Because fluticasone propionate is delivered directly to the lungs by the inhaled route it avoids the high level of exposure that occurs when corticosteroids are given by systemic routes. Administration of fluticasone propionate during pregnancy should only be considered if the expected benefit to the mother is greater than any possible risk to the fetus.

The secretion of fluticasone propionate in human breast milk has not been investigated. Subcutaneous administration of fluticasone propionate to lactating laboratory rats produced measurable plasma levels and evidence of fluticasone propionate in the milk. However plasma levels in humans after inhalation at recommended doses are likely to be low. When fluticasone propionate is used in breast feeding mothers the therapeutic benefits must be weighed against the potential hazards to mother and baby.

*Side-effects:* As with other inhalation therapy, paradoxical bronchospasm may occur with an immediate increase in wheezing after dosing. This should be treated immediately with a fast-acting inhaled bronchodilator. Flixotide Inhaler should be discontinued immediately, the patient assessed and, if necessary, alternative therapy instituted.

Candidiasis of the mouth and throat (thrush) occurs in some patients. Such patients may find it helpful to rinse out their mouth with water after using the Inhaler. Symptomatic candidiasis can be treated with topical anti-fungal therapy whilst still continuing with inhaled fluticasone propionate.

In some patients inhaled fluticasone propionate may cause hoarseness. It may be helpful to rinse out the mouth with water immediately after inhalation.

There have been rare reports of peripheral oedema and cutaneous hypersensitivity reactions such as skin rash.

There have been very rare reports of dyspepsia and arthralgia although a causal link with fluticasone propionate has not been established.

*Overdosage:* Acute. Inhalation of the drug in doses in excess of those recommended may lead to temporary suppression of adrenal function. This does not necessitate emergency action being taken. In these patients treatment with fluticasone propionate by inhalation should be continued at a reduced dose to control asthma; adrenal function recovers in a few days and can be verified by measuring plasma cortisol.

Chronic. Use of inhaled fluticasone propionate in daily doses in excess of 2 mg over prolonged periods may lead to some degree of adrenal suppression. Monitoring of adrenal reserve may be indicated. Treatment with Flixotide Inhaler should be continued at a dose sufficient to control asthma.

**Pharmaceutical precautions** Flixotide Inhaler should be stored between 2°C and 30°C.

As with most inhaled medications in pressurised canisters, the therapeutic effect of this medication may decrease when the canister is cold.

Protect from frost and direct sunlight.

The canister should not be punctured, broken or burnt even when apparently empty.

**Legal category** POM.

**Package quantities** Flixotide Inhaler is a pressurised metered-dose inhaler with a specially designed actuator. Each canister provides 120 inhalations.

**Further information** Nil.

**Product licence numbers**
Flixotide Inhaler 25 micrograms 10949/0001
Flixotide Inhaler 50 micrograms 10949/0002
Flixotide Inhaler 125 micrograms 10949/0003
Flixotide Inhaler 250 micrograms 10949/0004

## SEREVENT* ACCUHALER*

**Qualitative and quantitative composition** Serevent Accuhaler is a moulded plastic device containing a foil strip with 60 regularly spaced blisters each containing 50 micrograms of salmeterol (as xinafoate) and lactose.

**Pharmaceutical form** Inhalation powder.

**Clinical particulars**

*Therapeutic indications:* Salmeterol is a selective $\beta_2$-agonist providing long-acting (usually 12 hours) bronchodilatation with a relatively slow onset (within 10–20 minutes) in reversible airways obstruction.

Serevent Accuhaler can be used to treat reversible airways obstruction in patients requiring long-term regular bronchodilator therapy, including those with asthma and with chronic obstructive pulmonary disease (COPD).

It is particularly useful in the treatment of nocturnal asthma and in the prevention of exercise-induced symptoms.

Serevent Accuhaler should not be used to treat acute asthma symptoms (see *Special warnings*).

Patients with asthma should normally also be receiving regular and adequate doses of inhaled anti-inflammatory agents (e.g. corticosteroids, and/or in children, sodium cromoglycate), or oral corticosteroids. Serevent Accuhaler is not a replacement for these treatments which should be continued at the same dose, and not stopped or reduced, when treatment with Serevent Accuhaler is initiated.

*Posology and method of administration:* Serevent Accuhaler is for inhalation use only.

Serevent Accuhaler should be used regularly. The full benefits of treatment will be apparent after several doses of the drug.

*In reversible airways obstruction such as asthma*

*Adults (including the elderly):* One inhalation (50 micrograms) twice daily, increasing to two inhalations (2 × 50 micrograms) twice daily if required.

*Children 4 years and over:* One inhalation (50 micrograms) twice daily.

The dosage or frequency of administration should only be increased on medical advice.

There are insufficient clinical data to recommend the use of Serevent Accuhaler in children under the age of four.

*In chronic obstructive pulmonary disease*

*Adults (including the elderly):* One inhalation (50 micrograms) twice daily.

*Children:* Not appropriate.

*Special patient groups:* There is no need to adjust the dose in patients with impaired renal function.

*Contra-indications:* Hypersensitivity to any ingredient of the preparation.

*Special warnings and special precautions for use:* Serevent Accuhaler should not be initiated in patients with significantly worsening or acutely deteriorating asthma.

Sudden and progressive deterioration in asthma control is potentially life-threatening and consideration should be given to starting or increasing corticosteroid therapy. Under these circumstances, daily peak flow monitoring may be advisable.

Serevent Accuhaler is not a replacement for inhaled or oral corticosteroids or sodium cromoglycate (see *Therapeutic indications*). Patients with asthma must be warned not to stop steroid therapy (and for children, sodium cromoglycate therapy), and not to reduce it without medical advice, even if they feel better on Serevent Accuhaler.

With its relatively slow onset of action Serevent Accuhaler should not be used to relieve acute asthma symptoms, for which an inhaled short-acting bronchodilator is required. Patients should be advised to have such rescue medication available.

Bronchodilators should not be the only or the main treatment in patients with severe or unstable asthma. Severe asthma requires regular medical assessment, including lung-function testing, as patients are at risk of severe attacks and even death. Physicians should consider using the maximum recommended dose of inhaled corticosteroid and/or oral corticosteroid therapy in these patients.

Increasing use of bronchodilators, in particular short-acting inhaled $\beta_2$-agonists to relieve symptoms, indicates deterioration of asthma control. The patient should be instructed to seek medical advice if short-acting relief bronchodilator treatment becomes less effective, or more inhalations than usual are required. In this situation the patient should be assessed and consideration given to the need for increased anti-inflammatory therapy (e.g. higher doses of inhaled corticosteroid or a course of oral corticosteroid). Severe exacerbations of asthma must be treated in the normal way.

Salmeterol should be administered with caution in patients with thyrotoxicosis.

Potentially serious hypokalaemia may result from $\beta_2$-agonist therapy. Particular caution is advised in acute severe asthma as this effect may be potentiated by hypoxia and by concomitant treatment with xanthine derivatives, steroids and diuretics. Serum potassium levels should be monitored in such situations.

*Interaction with other medicaments and other forms of interaction:* Both non-selective and selective β-blockers should be avoided in patients with reversible obstructive airways disease, unless there are compelling reasons for their use.

*Pregnancy and lactation:* In animal studies, some effects on the fetus, typical for a $\beta_2$-agonist, occurred at exposure levels substantially higher than those that occur with therapeutic use. Extensive experience with other $\beta_2$-agonists has provided no evidence that such effects are relevant for women receiving clinical doses. As yet, experience of the use of salmeterol during pregnancy is limited. As with any medicine, use during pregnancy should be considered only if the expected benefit to the mother is greater than any possible risk to the fetus.

Plasma levels of salmeterol after inhaled therapeutic doses are negligible, and therefore levels in milk should be correspondingly low. Nevertheless as there is limited experience of the use of salmeterol in nursing mothers, its use in such circumstances should only be considered if the expected benefit to the mother is greater than any possible risk to the infant.

Studies in lactating animals support the view that salmeterol is likely to be secreted in only very small amounts into breast milk.

*Effects on ability to drive and use machines:* None reported.

*Undesirable effects:* As with other inhalation therapy, paradoxical bronchospasm may occur with an immediate increase in wheezing and drop in peak expiratory flow rate (PEFR) after dosing. This responds to a fast-acting inhaled bronchodilator. Serevent Accuhaler should be discontinued immediately, the patient assessed, and if necessary an alternative presentation or therapy should be instituted.

The pharmacological side effects of $\beta_2$-agonist treatment, such as tremor, subjective palpitations and headache, have been reported, but tend to be transient and to reduce with regular therapy. Tachycardia may occur in some patients.

Potentially serious hypokalaemia may result from $\beta_2$-agonist therapy.

There have been reports of the following: hypersensitivity reactions such as rash and oedema including angioedema; muscle cramps; non-specific chest pain; local irritation; arthralgia.

*Overdose:* The symptoms and signs of salmeterol overdosage are tremor, headache and tachycardia. The preferred antidote for overdosage with Serevent Accuhaler is a cardioselective β-blocking agent. Cardioselective β-blocking drugs should be used with caution in patients with a history of bronchospasm.

**Pharmacological properties**

*Pharmacodynamic properties:* Salmeterol is a selective long-acting (usually 12 hour) $\beta_2$-adrenoceptor agonist with a long side-chain which binds to the exo-site of the receptor. These pharmacological properties of salmeterol offer more effective protection against histamine-induced bronchoconstriction and produce a longer duration of bronchodilatation, lasting for at least 12 hours, than recommended doses of conventional short-acting $\beta_2$-agonists. *In vitro* tests have shown that salmeterol is a potent and long-lasting inhibitor of the release from human lung, of mast cell mediators, such as histamine, leukotrienes and prostaglandin $D_2$. In man, salmeterol inhibits the early and late phase response to inhaled allergen; the latter persisting for over 30 hours after a single dose when the bronchodilator effect is no longer evident. Single dosing with salmeterol attenuates bronchial hyper-responsiveness. These properties indicate that salmeterol has additional non-bronchodilator activity, but the full clinical significance is not yet clear. The mechanism is different from the anti-inflammatory effect of corticosteroids, which should not be stopped or reduced when Serevent Accuhaler is prescribed.

Salmeterol has been studied in the treatment of conditions associated with COPD, and has shown to improve symptoms and pulmonary function, and quality of life. Salmeterol acts as a $\beta_2$-agonist on the reversible component of the disease. *In vitro* salmeterol has also been shown to increase cilial beat frequency of human bronchial epithelial cells, and also reduce a ciliotoxic effect of *Pseudomonas* toxin on the bronchial epithelium of patients with cystic fibrosis.

*Pharmacokinetic properties:* Salmeterol acts locally in the lung, therefore plasma levels are not predictive of therapeutic effects. In addition there are only limited data available on the pharmacokinetics of salmeterol because of the technical difficulty of assaying the drug in plasma due to the low plasma concentrations at therapeutic doses (approximately 200 pg/ml or less) achieved after inhaled dosing. After regular dosing with salmeterol xinafoate, xinafoic acid can be detected in the systemic circulation, reaching steady state concentrations of approximately 100 ng/ml. These concentrations are up to 1000-fold lower than steady state levels observed in toxicity studies. These concentrations in long-term regular dosing (more than 12 months) in patients with airways obstruction, have been shown to produce no ill effects.

*Preclinical safety data:* In reproduction studies in animals, some effects on the fetus, typical of a $\beta_2$-agonist, have been observed at very high doses.

Salmeterol xinafoate produced no genetic toxicity in a range of studies using either prokaryotic or eukaryotic cell systems *in vitro* or *in vivo* in the rat.

Long term studies with salmeterol xinafoate, induced class-related benign tumours of smooth muscle in the mesovarium of rats and the uterus of mice. The scientific literature and our own pharmacological studies provide good evidence that these effects are species-specific and have no relevance for clinical use.

**Pharmaceutical particulars**

*List of excipients:* Lactose.

*Incompatibilities:* None reported.

*Shelf Life:* 24 months when stored below 30°C for moderate climates.

18 months when stored below 30°C for tropical climates.

*Special precautions for storage:* Store below 30°C in a dry place.

*Nature and contents of container:* The powder mix of salmeterol xinafoate and lactose is filled into a blister strip consisting of a formed base foil with a peelable foil laminate lid. The foil strip is contained within the Accuhaler device.

*Instructions for use/handling:* The powdered medicine is inhaled through the mouth into the lungs.

The Accuhaler device contains the medicine in individual blisters which are opened as the device is manipulated.

For detailed instructions for use refer to the Patient Information Leaflet in every pack.

*Marketing authorisation holder:* Glaxo Wellcome UK Ltd, trading as Allen & Hanburys, Stockley Park West, Uxbridge, Middlesex UB11 1BT.

**Marketing authorisation number** 10949/0214

**Date of approval/revision of SPC** March 1997.

**Legal category** POM.

## SEREVENT* DISKHALER*

**Qualitative and quantitative composition** Disks comprising four regularly spaced double-foil blisters each delivering a mixture of 50 micrograms salmeterol (as xinafoate) and lactose used in a Diskhaler device.

**Pharmaceutical form** Inhalation powder.

**Clinical particulars**

*Therapeutic indications:* Salmeterol is a selective $\beta_2$-agonist providing long-acting (usually 12 hours) bronchodilatation with a relatively slow onset (within 10–20 minutes) in reversible airways obstruction.

Serevent Diskhaler can be used to treat reversible airways obstruction in patients requiring long-term regular bronchodilator therapy, including those with asthma and with chronic obstructive pulmonary disease (COPD).

It is particularly useful in the treatment of nocturnal asthma and in the prevention of exercise-induced symptoms.

Serevent Diskhaler should not be used to treat acute asthma symptoms (see *Special warnings*).

Patients with asthma should normally also be receiving regular and adequate doses of inhaled anti-inflammatory agents (e.g. corticosteroids, and/or in children, sodium cromoglycate), or oral corticosteroids. Serevent Diskhaler is not a replacement for these treatments which should be continued at the same dose, and not stopped or reduced, when treatment with Serevent Diskhaler is initiated.

*Posology and method of administration:* Serevent Diskhaler is for inhalation use only.

Serevent Diskhaler should be used regularly. The full benefits of treatment will be apparent after several doses of the drug.

*In reversible airways obstruction such as asthma:*

*Adults (including the elderly):* One blister (50 micrograms) twice daily, increasing to two blisters (2 × 50 micrograms) twice daily if required.

*Children 4 years and over:* One blister (50 micrograms) twice daily.

The dosage or frequency of administration should only be increased on medical advice.

There are insufficient clinical data to recommend the use of Serevent Diskhaler in children under the age of four.

*In chronic obstructive pulmonary disease:*

*Adults (including the elderly):* One blister (50 micrograms) twice daily.

*Children:* Not appropriate.

*Special patient groups:* There is no need to adjust the dose in patients with impaired renal function.

*Contra-indications:* Hypersensitivity to any ingredient of the preparation.

*Special warnings and special precautions for use:* Serevent Diskhaler should not be initiated in patients with significantly worsening or acutely deteriorating asthma.

Sudden and progressive deterioration in asthma control is potentially life-threatening and consideration should be given to starting or increasing corticosteroid therapy. Under these circumstances, regular peak flow monitoring may be advisable.

Serevent Diskhaler is not a replacement for inhaled or oral corticosteroids or sodium cromoglycate (see *Therapeutic indications*). Patients with asthma must be warned not to stop steroid therapy (and for children, sodium cromoglycate therapy), and not to reduce it without medical advice, even if they feel better on Serevent Diskhaler.

With its relatively slow onset of action Serevent Diskhaler should not be used to relieve acute asthma symptoms, for which an inhaled short-acting bronchodilator is required. Patients should be advised to have such rescue medication available.

Bronchodilators should not be the only or the main treatment in patients with severe or unstable asthma. Severe asthma requires regular medical assessment, including lung-function testing, as patients are at risk of severe attacks and even death. Physicians should consider using the maximum recommended dose of inhaled corticosteroid and/or oral corticosteroid therapy in these patients.

Increasing use of bronchodilators, in particular short-acting inhaled $\beta_2$-agonists to relieve symptoms, indicates deterioration of asthma control. The patient should be instructed to seek medical advice if short-acting relief bronchodilator treatment becomes less effective, or more inhalations than usual are required. In this situation the patient should be assessed and consideration given to the need for increased anti-inflammatory therapy (e.g. higher doses of inhaled corticosteroid or a course of oral corticosteroid). Severe exacerbations of asthma must be treated in the normal way.

Salmeterol should be administered with caution in patients with thyrotoxicosis.

Potentially serious hypokalaemia may result from $\beta_2$-agonist therapy. Particular caution is advised in acute severe asthma as this effect may be potentiated by hypoxia and by concomitant treatment with xanthine derivatives, steroids and diuretics. Serum potassium levels should be monitored in such situations.

*Interaction with other medicaments and other forms of interaction:* Both non-selective and selective β-blockers should be avoided in patients with reversible obstructive airways disease, unless there are compelling reasons for their use.

*Pregnancy and lactation:* In animal studies, some effects on the fetus, typical for a $\beta_2$-agonist occurred at exposure levels substantially higher than those that occur with therapeutic use. Extensive experience with other $\beta_2$-agonists has provided no evidence that such effects are relevant for women receiving clinical doses. As yet, experience of the use of salmeterol during pregnancy is limited. As with any medicine, use during pregnancy should be considered only if the expected benefit to the mother is greater than any possible risk to the fetus.

Plasma levels of salmeterol after inhaled therapeutic doses are negligible, and therefore levels in milk should be correspondingly low. Nevertheless, as there is limited experience of the use of salmeterol in nursing mothers, its use in such circumstances should only be considered if the expected benefit to the mother is greater than any possible risk to the infant.

Studies in lactating animals support the view that salmeterol is likely to be secreted in only very small amounts into breast milk.

*Effects on the ability to drive and use machines:* None reported.

*Undesirable effects:* As with other inhalation therapy, paradoxical bronchospasm may occur with an immediate increase in wheezing and drop in peak expiratory flow rate (PEFR) after dosing. This responds to a fast-acting inhaled bronchodilator. Serevent Diskhaler should be discontinued immediately, the patient assessed, and if necessary an alternative presentation or therapy should be instituted.

The pharmacological side-effects of $\beta_2$-agonist treatment, such as tremor, subjective palpitations and headache, have been reported, but tend to be transient and to reduce with regular therapy. Tachycardia may occur in some patients.

Potentially serious hypokalaemia may result from $\beta_2$-agonist therapy.

There have been reports of the following: hypersensitivity reactions such as rash and oedema including angioedema; muscle cramps; non-specific chest pain; local irritation; arthralgia.

*Overdose:* The symptoms and signs of salmeterol overdosage are tremor, headache and tachycardia. The preferred antidote for overdosage with Serevent Diskhaler is a cardioselective β-blocking agent. Cardioselective β-blocking drugs should be used with caution in patients with a history of bronchospasm.

**Pharmacological properties**

*Pharmacodynamic properties:* Salmeterol is a selective long-acting (usually 12 hours) $\beta_2$-adrenoceptor agonist with a long side-chain which binds to the exo-site of the receptor. These pharmacological properties of salmeterol offer more effective protection against histamine-induced bronchoconstriction and produce a longer duration of bronchodilatation, lasting for at least 12 hours, than recommended doses of conventional short-acting $\beta_2$-agonists. *In vitro* tests have shown that salmeterol is a potent and long-lasting inhibitor of the release from the human lung of mast cell mediators, such as histamine, leukotrienes and prostaglandin $D_2$. In man, salmeterol inhibits the early and late phase response to inhaled allergen; the latter persisting for over 30 hours after a single dose when the bronchodilator effect is no longer evident. Single dosing with salmeterol attenuates bronchial hyper-responsiveness. These properties indicate that salmeterol has additional non-bronchodilator activity, but the full clinical significance is not yet clear. The mechanism is different from the anti-inflammatory effect of corticosteroids, which should not be stopped or reduced when Serevent Diskhaler is prescribed.

Salmeterol has been studied in the treatment of conditions associated with COPD, and has been shown to improve symptoms and pulmonary function, and quality of life. Salmeterol acts as a $\beta_2$-agonist on the reversible component of the disease. *In vitro* salmeterol has also been shown to increase cilial beat frequency of human bronchial epithelial cells, and also reduce a ciliotoxic effect of *Pseudomonas* toxin on the bronchial epithelium of patients with cystic fibrosis.

*Pharmacokinetic properties:* Salmeterol acts locally in the lung, therefore plasma levels are not predictive of therapeutic effect. In addition there are only limited data available on the pharmacokinetics of salmeterol because of the technical difficulty of assaying the drug in plasma because of the very low plasma concentrations (approximately 200 pg/ml or less) achieved after inhaled dosing. After regular dosing with salmeterol xinafoate, xinafoic acid can be detected in the systemic circulation, reaching steady state concentrations of approximately 100 ng/ml. These concentrations are up to 1000-fold lower than steady state levels observed in toxicity studies. These concentrations in long term regular dosing (more than 12 months) in patients with airways obstruction, have been shown to produce no ill effects.

*Preclinical safety data:* In reproduction studies in animals, some effects on the fetus, typical of a $\beta_2$-agonist, have been observed at very high doses.

Salmeterol xinafoate produced no genetic toxicity in a range of studies using either prokaryotic or eukaryotic cell systems *in vitro* or *in vivo* in the rat.

Long-term studies with salmeterol xinafoate, induced class-related benign tumours of smooth muscle in the mesovarium of rats and the uterus of mice. The scientific literature and our own pharmacological studies provide good evidence that these effects are species-specific and have no relevance for clinical use.

**Pharmaceutical particulars**

*List of excipients:* Lactose.

*Incompatibilities:* None reported.

*Shelf life:* 2 years when stored below 25°C.

*Special precautions for storage:* Store below 25°C.

A disk may be kept in the Diskhaler device but the blisters must only be pierced immediately prior to use.

*Nature and contents of container:* A circular double-foil disk with four blisters containing the powder mix of salmeterol (as xinafoate) and lactose. The foil disk is inserted into the Diskhaler device.

The following packs are available: 14 disks alone or with a Diskhaler. 5 disks with a Diskhaler (Hospital only).

*Instructions for use/handling:* The powdered medicine is inhaled through the mouth into the lungs. The Diskhaler device is loaded with a disk which contains the medicine in individual blisters which are opened as the device is manipulated.

For detailed instructions for use refer to the Patient Information Leaflet in every pack.

*Marketing authorisation holder:* Glaxo Wellcome UK Ltd, trading as Allen & Hanburys, Stockley Park West, Uxbridge, Middlesex UB11 1BT.

**Marketing authorisation number** 10949/0069

**Date of approval/revision of SPC** March 1997.

**Legal category** POM.

## SEREVENT* INHALER

**Qualitative and quantitative composition** Each metered dose actuation delivers 25 micrograms salmeterol (as xinafoate). Each canister delivers 60/120 actuations.

**Pharmaceutical form** Pressurised metered-dose aerosol.

**Clinical particulars**

*Therapeutic indications:* Salmeterol is a selective $\beta_2$-agonist providing long-acting (usually 12 hours) bronchodilatation with a relatively slow onset (within 10–20 minutes) in reversible airways obstruction.

Serevent Inhaler can be used to treat reversible airways obstruction in patients requiring long-term regular bronchodilator therapy, including those with asthma and with chronic obstructive pulmonary disease (COPD).

It is particularly useful in the treatment of nocturnal asthma and in the prevention of exercise-induced symptoms.

Serevent Inhaler should not be used to treat acute asthma symptoms (see *Special warnings*).

Patients with asthma should normally also be receiving regular and adequate doses of inhaled anti-inflammatory agents (e.g. corticosteroids, and/or in children, sodium cromoglycate), or oral corticosteroids. Serevent Inhaler is not a replacement for these treatments which should be continued at the same dose, and not stopped or reduced, when treatment with Serevent Inhaler is initiated.

*Posology and method of administration:* Serevent Inhaler is for inhalation use only. A Volumatic* spacer device may be used in patients who find it difficult to synchronise aerosol actuation with inspiration of breath.

Serevent Inhaler should be used regularly. The full benefits of treatment will be apparent after several doses of the drug.

*In reversible airways obstruction such as asthma:*

*Adults (including the elderly):* Two inhalations (2 × 25 micrograms) twice daily, increasing to four inhalations (4 × 25 micrograms) twice daily if required.

*Children aged 4 years and over:* Two inhalations (2 × 25 micrograms) twice daily.

The dosage or frequency of administration should only be increased on medical advice.

There are insufficient clinical data to recommend the use of Serevent Inhaler in children under the age of four.

*In chronic obstructive pulmonary disease:*

*Adults (including the elderly):* Two inhalations (2 × 25 micrograms) twice daily.

*Children:* Not appropriate.

*Special patient groups:* There is no need to adjust the dose in patients with impaired renal function.

*Contra-indications:* Hypersensitivity to any ingredient of the preparation.

*Special warnings and special precautions for use:* Serevent Inhaler should not be initiated in patients with significantly worsening or acutely deteriorating asthma.

Sudden and progressive deterioration in asthma control is potentially life-threatening and consideration should be given to starting or increasing corticosteroid therapy. Under these circumstances, regular peak flow monitoring may be advisable.

Serevent Inhaler is not a replacement for inhaled or oral corticosteroids or sodium cromoglycate (see *Therapeutic indications*). Patients with asthma must be warned not to stop steroid therapy (and for children, sodium cromoglycate therapy), and not to reduce it without medical advice, even if they feel better on Serevent Inhaler.

With its relatively slow onset of action Serevent Inhaler should not be used to relieve acute asthma symptoms, for which an inhaled short-acting bronchodilator is required. Patients should be advised to have such rescue medication available.

Bronchodilators should not be the only or the main treatment in patients with severe or unstable asthma. Severe asthma requires regular medical assessment, including lung-function testing, as patients are at risk of severe attacks and even death. Physicians should consider using the maximum recommended dose of inhaled corticosteroid and/or oral corticosteroid therapy in these patients.

Increasing use of bronchodilators, in particular short-acting inhaled $\beta_2$-agonists to relieve symptoms, indicates deterioration of asthma control. The patient should be instructed to seek medical advice if short-acting relief bronchodilator treatment becomes less effective, or more inhalations than usual are required. In this sitution the patient should be assessed and consideration given to the need for increased anti-inflammatory therapy (e.g. higher doses of inhaled corticosteroid or a course of oral corticosteroid). Severe exacerbations of asthma must be treated in the normal way.

Salmeterol should be administered with caution in patients with thyrotoxicosis.

Potentially serious hypokalaemia may result from $\beta_2$-agonist therapy. Particular caution is advised in acute severe asthma as this effect may be potentiated by hypoxia and by concomitant treatment with xanthine derivatives, steroids and diuretics. Serum potassium levels should be monitored in such situations.

*Interaction with other medicaments and other forms of interaction:* Both non-selective and selective β-blockers should be avoided in patients with reversible obstructive airways disease, unless there are compelling reasons for their use.

*Pregnancy and lactation:* In animal studies, some effects on the fetus, typical for a $\beta_2$-agonist, occurred at exposure levels substantially higher than those that occur with therapeutic use. Extensive experience with other $\beta_2$-agonists has provided no evidence that such effects are relevant for women receiving clinical doses. As yet, experience of the use of salmeterol during pregnancy is limited. As with any medicine, use during pregnancy should be considered only if the expected benefit to the mother is greater than any possible risk to the fetus.

Plasma levels of salmeterol after inhaled therapeutic doses are negligible, and therefore levels in milk should be correspondingly low. Nevertheless, as there is limited experience of the use of salmeterol in nursing mothers, its use in such circumstances should only be considered if the expected benefit to the mother is greater than any possible risk to the infant.

Studies in lactating animals support the view that salmeterol is likely to be secreted in only very small amounts into breast milk.

*Effects on the ability to drive and use machines:* None reported.

*Undesirable effects:* As with other inhalation therapy, paradoxical bronchospasm may occur with an immediate increase in wheezing and drop in peak expiratory flow rate (PEFR) after dosing. This responds to a fast-acting inhaled bronchodilator, Serevent Inhaler should be discontinued immediately, the patient assessed, and if necessary an alternative presentation (e.g. Serevent Diskhaler*) or therapy should be instituted.

In a study involving 11,000 patients a very low percentage (1.1%) of patients experienced a drop of 20% or more in PEFR whilst taking Serevent Inhaler. This occurred most frequently in patients over 60 and those with a poor baseline peak flow. This drop in PEFR occurred in a similar percentage in a control group of patients taking placebo.

The pharmacological side-effects of $\beta_2$-agonist treatment, such as tremor, subjective palpitations and headache, have been reported, but tend to be transient and to reduce with regular therapy. Tachycardia may occur in some patients.

Potentially serious hypokalaemia may result from $\beta_2$-agonist therapy.

There have been reports of the following: hypersensitivity reactions such as rash and oedema including angioedema; muscle cramps; non-specific chest pain; local irritation; arthralgia.

*Overdose:* The symptoms and signs of salmeterol overdosage are tremor, headache and tachycardia. The preferred antidote for overdosage with Serevent Inhaler is a cardioselective β-blocking agent. Cardioselective β-blocking drugs should be used with caution in patients with a history of bronchospasm.

**Pharmocological properties**

*Pharmacodynamic properties:* Salmeterol is a selective long-acting (usually 12 hours) $\beta_2$-adrenoceptor agonist with a long side-chain which binds to the exo-side of the receptor. These pharmacological properties of salmeterol offer more effective protection against histamine-induced bronchoconstriction and produce a longer duration of bronchodilatation, lasting for at least 12 hours, than recommended doses of conventional short-acting $\beta_2$-agonists. *In vitro* tests have shown that salmeterol is a potent and long-lasting inhibitor of the release from the human lung of mast cell mediators, such as histamine, leukotrienes and prostaglandin $D_2$. In man, salmeterol inhibits the early and late phase response to inhaled allergen; the latter persisting for over 30 hours after a single dose when the bronchodilator effect is no longer evident. Single dosing with salmeterol attenuates bronchial hyper-responsiveness. These properties indicate that salmeterol has additional non-bronchodilator activity, but the full clinical significance is not yet clear. The mechanism is different from the anti-inflammatory effect of corticosteroids, which should not be stopped or reduced when Serevent Inhaler is prescribed.

Salmeterol has been studied in the treatment of conditions associated with COPD, and has been shown to improve symptoms and pulmonary function, and quality of life. Salmeterol acts as a $\beta_2$-agonist on the reversible component of the disease. *In vitro* salmeterol has also been shown to increase cilial beat frequency of human bronchial epithelial cells, and also reduce a ciliotoxic effect of *Pseudomonas* toxin on the bronchial epithelium of patients with cystic fibrosis.

*Pharmacokinetic properties:* Salmeterol acts locally in the lung, therefore plasma levels are not predictive of therapeutic effect. In addition there are only limited data available on the pharmacokinetics of salmeterol because of the technical difficulty of assaying the drug in plasma because of the very low plasma concentrations (approximately 200 pg/ml or less) achieved after inhaled dosing. After regular dosing with salmeterol xinafoate, xinafoic acid can be detected in the systemic circulation, reaching steady state concentrations of approximately 100 ng/ml. These concentrations are up to 1000-fold lower than steady state levels observed in toxicity studies. These concentrations in long term regular dosing (more than 12 months) in patients with airways obstruction, have been shown to produce no ill effects.

*Preclinical safety data:* In reproduction studies in animals, some effects on the fetus, typical of a $\beta_2$-agonist, have been observed at very high doses.

Salmeterol xinafoate produced no genetic toxicity

in a range of studies using either prokaryotic or eukaryotic cell systems *in vitro* or *in vivo* in the rat.

Long-term studies with salmeterol xinafoate, induced class-related benign tumours of smooth muscle in the mesovarium of rats and the uterus of mice. The scientific literature and our own pharmacological studies provide good evidence that these effects are species-specific and have no relevance for clinical use.

### Pharmaceutical particulars

*List of excipients:* Lecithin, dichlorodifluoromethane, trichlorofluoromethane.

*Incompatibilities:* None reported.

*Shelf life:* 2 years when stored below 30°C.

*Special precautions for storage:* Salmeterol Inhaler should be stored below 30°C.

Protect from frost and direct sunlight.

As with most inhaled medications in aerosol canisters, the therapeutic effect of this medication may decrease when the canister is cold.

The canister should not be broken, punctured or burnt, even when apparently empty.

*Nature and contents of container:* An inhaler comprising an aluminium alloy can fitted with a metering valve, actuator and dust cap. Each canister contains 120 (Hospital packs 60) metered actuations of 25 micrograms salmeterol (as xinafoate).

*Instructions for use/handling:* The aerosol spray is inhaled through the mouth into the lungs. After shaking the inhaler, the mouthpiece is placed in the mouth and the lips closed around it. The actuator is depressed to release a spray, which must coincide with inspiration of breath.

For detailed instructions for use refer to the Patient Information Leaflet in every pack.

*Marketing authorisation holder:* Glaxo Wellcome UK Limited, trading as Allen & Hanburys, Stockley Park West, Uxbridge, Middlesex UB11 1BT.

**Marketing authorisation number**   10949/0068

**Date of approval/revision of SPC**   March 1997.

**Legal category**   POM.

## VENTIDE* INHALER

**Presentation** Ventide Inhaler is a pressurised metered-dose inhaler which delivers 100 micrograms Salbutamol BP and 50 micrograms Beclomethasone Dipropionate BP per actuation.

Other ingredients: Oleic acid, dichlorodifluoromethane, trichlorofluoromethane.

**Uses** Salbutamol is a selective $\beta_2$-agonist providing short-acting (4-6 hour) bronchodilatation with a fast onset (within 5 minutes) in reversible airways obstruction.

Beclomethasone dipropionate given by inhalation offers effective anti-inflammatory action in the lungs without the problems of systemic corticosteroid treatment.

Ventide Inhaler is suitable for those patients who require regular doses of both drugs for treatment of reversible airways obstruction.

Ventide Inhaler is not intended for use as a first-line treatment but after the need for inhaled corticosteroid therapy has been established.

**Dosage and administration** Ventide Inhaler is for inhalation use only. A Volumatic* spacer device may be used in patients who find it difficult to synchronise aerosol actuation with inspiration of breath.

*Adults (including the elderly):* Two inhalations (200 micrograms salbutamol and 100 micrograms beclomethasone dipropionate) three or four times a day.

*Children:* One or two inhalations (100 or 200 micrograms salbutamol and 50 or 100 micrograms beclomethasone dipropionate) two, three or four times a day.

### Contra-indications, warnings, etc

*Contra-indications:* Although intravenous salbutamol, and occasionally salbutamol tablets, are used in the management of premature labour uncomplicated by conditions such as placenta praevia, ante-partum haemorrhage or toxaemia of pregnancy, inhaled salbutamol preparations are not appropriate for managing premature labour. Salbutamol preparations should not be used for threatened abortion.

Ventide Inhaler is contra-indicated in patients with a history of hypersensitivity to any of the components.

*Precautions:* Patients should be instructed in the proper use of the inhaler to ensure that the drug reaches the target area within the lungs. They should also be made aware that Ventide Inhaler must be used regularly, every day, for optimum benefit. Patients should be regularly reassessed so that their continuing need for corticosteroid therapy can also be reviewed.

Ventide Inhaler is not for use in acute attacks but for routine long-term management, so patients will require a fast- and short-acting inhaled bronchodilator to relieve acute symptoms. However, should the effect of the additional inhaled bronchodilator or the relief provided by the Ventide Inhaler last for less than three hours, patients should be advised that this may indicate that their condition is worsening and to seek medical advice, in case treatment with inhaled corticosteroid needs to be increased, or treatment with systemic corticosteroid needs to be started or increased. As there may be adverse effects associated with excessive dosing, the dosage or frequency of administration should only be increased on medical advice.

Severe asthma requires regular medical assessment, including lung-function testing, as patients are at risk of severe attacks and even death. Increasing use of short-acting inhaled $\beta_2$-agonists to relieve symptoms, indicates deterioration of asthma control. If patients find that short-acting relief bronchodilator treatment becomes less effective, or they need more inhalations than usual, medical attention must be sought.

For those patients who are steroid-dependent it is advisable to commence therapy with beclomethasone dipropionate alone.

Patients who have been weaned in the previous few months from long-term systemic corticosteroids need special consideration until the hypothalamic-pituitary-adrenal (HPA) system has recovered sufficiently to enable the patient to cope with emergencies such as trauma, surgery or infections. Such patients should carry a steroid warning card indicating that they may need supplementary systemic steroid during periods of stress, until their adrenocortical function has become normal. These patients should also be given a supply of oral steroid to use in emergency when their airways obstruction worsens.

Significant adrenal suppression rarely occurs before doses of 1,500 micrograms per day of inhaled beclomethasone dipropionate are exceeded. Reduction of plasma cortisol levels has been reported in some patients taking 2,000 micrograms per day. In such patients, the risks of developing adrenal suppression should be balanced against the therapeutic advantages, and precautions taken to provide systemic steroid cover in situations of prolonged stress. Prolonged suppression of the HPA axis may eventually lead to systemic effects, including growth retardation in children and adolescents.

As with all inhaled corticosteroids, special care is necessary in patients with active or quiescent pulmonary tuberculosis.

Salbutamol should be administered cautiously to patients suffering from thyrotoxicosis.

Salbutamol and non-selective β-blocking drugs, such as propranolol, should not normally be prescribed together.

Potentially serious hypokalaemia may result from $\beta_2$-agonist therapy, mainly from parenteral and nebulised administration. Particular caution is advised in acute severe asthma, as this effect may be potentiated by hypoxia and by concomitant treatment with xanthine derivatives, steroids and diuretics. Serum potassium levels should be monitored in such situations.

Treatment should not be stopped abruptly.

*Pregnancy:* Administration of drugs during pregnancy should only be considered if the expected benefit to the mother is greater than any possible risk to the fetus. As with the majority of drugs, there is little published evidence of the safety of salbutamol in the early stages of human pregnancy, but in animal studies there was evidence of some harmful effects on the fetus at very high dose levels.

There is inadequate evidence of safety of beclomethasone dipropionate in human pregnancy. Administration of corticosteroids to pregnant animals can cause abnormalities of fetal development including cleft palate and intra-uterine growth retardation. There may therefore be a very small risk of such effects on the human fetus. It should be noted however, that the fetal changes in animals occur after relatively high systemic exposure. Because beclomethasone dipropionate is delivered directly to the lungs by the inhaled route it avoids the high level of exposure that occurs when corticosteroids are given by systemic routes.

The use of Ventide Inhaler in pregnancy requires that the possible benefit of the drugs be weighed against the possible hazards.

*Lactation:* No specific studies examining the transference of beclomethasone dipropionate into the milk of lactating animals have been performed. It is reasonable to assume that beclomethasone dipropionate is secreted in milk, but at the dosages used for direct inhalation there is low potential for significant levels in breast milk. As salbutamol is probably also secreted in breast milk the use of Ventide Inhaler in nursing mothers should be restricted to situations where it is felt that the expected benefit to the mother is likely to outweigh any potential risk to the neonate.

*Side-effects:* As with other inhalation therapy, paradoxical bronchospasm may occur with an immediate increase in wheezing after dosing. This should be treated immediately with a fast-acting inhaled bronchodilator. Ventide Inhaler should be discontinued immediately, the patient assessed and, if necessary, alternative therapy instituted.

Hoarseness, mouth and throat irritation may occur. It may be helpful to rinse the mouth with water immediately after inhalation.

Hypersensitivity reactions, including angioedema, bronchospasm, hypotension and collapse have been reported very rarely. Rashes, urticaria, pruritus and erythema and oedema of the eyes, face, lips and throat, have also been reported.

*Salbutamol:* Salbutamol may cause a fine tremor of skeletal muscle, usually the hands are most obviously affected. This effect is dose related and is common to all β-adrenergic stimulants. Headaches have occasionally been reported. Tachycardia, with or without peripheral vasodilatation, may rarely occur.

There have been very rare reports of muscle cramps. Potentially serious hypokalaemia may result from $\beta_2$-agonist therapy.

As with other $\beta_2$-agonists, hyperactivity in children has been reported rarely.

*Beclomethasone dipropionate:* Candidiasis of the mouth and throat (thrush) occurs in some patients inhaling beclomethasone dipropionate, the incidence increases with doses greater than 400 micrograms beclomethasone dipropionate per day. Patients with high blood levels of *Candida precipitins,* indicating a previous infection, are most likely to develop this complication. Such patients may find it helpful to rinse their mouth with water after using the inhaler. The condition usually responds to topical anti-fungal therapy without discontinuing treatment with Ventide Inhaler.

*Overdosage:*
*Salbutamol:* The preferred antidote for overdosage with salbutamol is a cardioselective, β-blocking agent, but β-blocking drugs should be used with caution in patients with a history of bronchospasm. Hypokalaemia may occur following overdose with salbutamol. Serum potassium levels should be monitored.

*Beclomethasone dipropionate:* Acute. Inhalation of the drug in doses in excess of those recommended may lead to temporary suppression of adrenal function. This does not require emergency action. In these patients treatment should be continued at a dose sufficient to control asthma; adrenal function recovers in a few days and can be verified by measuring plasma cortisol.

Chronic. Use of inhaled beclomethasone dipropionate in daily doses in excess of 1,500 micrograms over prolonged periods may lead to some degree of adrenal suppression. Monitoring of adrenal reserve may be indicated. Treatment should be continued at a dose sufficient to control asthma.

**Pharmaceutical precautions** Ventide Inhaler should be stored below 30°C, protected from direct sunlight, heat and frost. The canister should not be punctured, broken or burnt even if it is apparently empty.

As with most inhaled medications in aerosol canisters, the therapeutic effect of this medication may decrease when the canister is cold.

**Legal category**   POM.

**Package quantities** Ventide Inhaler is a metered-dose aerosol with a specially designed actuator. Each canister provides 200 inhalations.

**Further information** Products containing salbutamol do not cause difficulty in micturition because, unlike sympathomimetic drugs such as ephedrine, salbutamol does not stimulate alpha-adrenoceptors.

Salbutamol products are not contra-indicated in patients under treatment with monoamine oxidase inhibitors (MAOIs).

**Product licence number**   10949/0076

## VENTIDE* ROTACAPS*
## VENTIDE* PAEDIATRIC ROTACAPS*

**Presentation** Ventide Rotacaps capsules contain a mixture of microfine salbutamol sulphate, microfine beclomethasone dipropionate and larger particle lactose in grey/colourless hard gelatin capsules. Each light grey Rotacaps capsule contains 200 micrograms salbutamol (as sulphate) plus 100 micrograms beclomethasone dipropionate. Each dark grey Rotacaps capsule contains 400 micrograms salbutamol (as sulphate) plus 200 micrograms beclomethasone dipropionate. The capsules are marked 'Ventide Paed' or 'Ventide' respectively. The contents of a capsule are inhaled using a specific drug delivery device called a Ventide Rotahaler*.

**Uses** Salbutamol is a selective $\beta_2$-agonist providing short-acting (4-6 hour) bronchodilatation with a fast onset (within 5 minutes) in reversible airways obstruction. Beclomethasone dipropionate given by inhalation offers effective anti-inflammatory action in the lungs without the problems of systemic corticosteroid treatment.

Ventide Rotacaps and Ventide Paediatric Rotacaps are suitable for those patients who require regular doses of both drugs for treatment of reversible airways obstruction.

Ventide Rotacaps and Ventide Paediatric Rotacaps are not intended for use as a first-line treatment but after the need for inhaled corticosteroid therapy has been established.

**Dosage and administration** Ventide Rotacaps and Ventide Paediatric Rotacaps are for inhalation use only, using a Ventide Rotahaler. They are suitable for many patients including those who cannot use a metered-dose inhaler successfully.

*Adults (including the elderly)*: One Ventide Rotacaps capsule (400 micrograms salbutamol and 200 micrograms beclomethasone dipropionate) three or four times a day.

*Children:* One Ventide Paediatric Rotacaps capsule (200 micrograms salbutamol and 100 micrograms beclomethasone dipropionate) two, three or four times a day.

**Contra-indications, warnings, etc**
*Contra-indications:* Although intravenous salbutamol, and occasionally salbutamol tablets, are used in the management of premature labour uncomplicated by conditions such as placenta praevia, ante-partum haemorrhage or toxaemia of pregnancy, inhaled salbutamol preparations are not appropriate for managing premature labour. Salbutamol preparations should not be used for threatened abortion.

Ventide Rotacaps and Ventide Paediatric Rotacaps are contra-indicated in patients with a history of hypersensitivity to any of the components.

*Precautions:* Patients should be instructed in the proper use of the Rotahaler device to ensure that the drug reaches the target area within the lungs. They should also be made aware that Ventide Rotacaps or Ventide Paediatric Rotacaps must be used regularly, every day, for optimum benefit. Patients should be regularly reassessed so that their continuing need for corticosteroid therapy can also be reviewed.

Ventide Rotacaps or Ventide Paediatric Rotacaps are not for use in acute attacks but for routine long-term management, so patients will require a fast- and short-acting inhaled bronchodilator to relieve acute symptoms. However, should the effect of the additional inhaled bronchodilator, or the relief provided by Ventide Rotacaps or Ventide Paediatric Rotacaps, last for less than three hours, patients should be advised that this may indicate that their condition is worsening and to seek medical advice, in case treatment with inhaled corticosteroid needs to be increased, or treatment with systemic corticosteroid needs to be started or increased. As there may be adverse effects associated with excessive dosing, the dosage or frequency of administration should only be increased on medical advice.

Severe asthma requires regular medical assessment, including lung-function testing, as patients are at risk of severe attacks and even death. Increasing use of bronchodilators, in particular short-acting inhaled $\beta_2$-agonists to relieve symptoms, indicates deterioration of asthma control. If patients find that short-acting relief bronchodilator treatment becomes less effective, or they need more inhalations than usual, medical attention must be sought.

For those patients who are steroid-dependent it is advisable to commence therapy with beclomethasone dipropionate alone.

Patients who have been weaned in the previous few months from long-term systemic corticosteroid need special consideration until the hypothalamic-pituitary-adrenal (HPA) system has recovered sufficiently to enable the patient to cope with emergencies such as trauma, surgery or infections. Such patients should carry a steroid warning card indicating that they may need supplementary systemic steroid during periods of stress, until their adrenocortical function has become normal. These patients should also be given a supply of oral steroid to use in emergency when their airways obstruction worsens.

Significant adrenal suppression rarely occurs before doses of 1,500 micrograms per day of inhaled beclomethasone dipropionate are exceeded. Reduction of plasma cortisol levels has been reported in some patients taking 2,000 micrograms per day. In such patients, the risks of developing adrenal suppression should be balanced against the therapeutic advantages, and precautions taken to provide systemic steroid cover in situations of prolonged stress. Prolonged suppression of the HPA axis may eventually lead to systemic effects, including growth retardation in children and adolescents.

As with all inhaled corticosteroids special care is necessary in patients with active or quiescent pulmonary tuberculosis.

Salbutamol should be administered cautiously to patients suffering from thyrotoxicosis.

Salbutamol and non-selective $\beta$-blocking drugs, such as propranolol, should not normally be prescribed together.

Potentially serious hypokalaemia may result from $\beta_2$-agonist therapy, mainly from parenteral and nebulised administration. Particular caution is advised in acute severe asthma, as this effect may be potentiated by hypoxia and by concomitant treatment with xanthine derivatives, steroids and diuretics. Serum potassium levels should be monitored in such situations.

Treatment should not be stopped abruptly.

*Pregnancy:* Administration of drugs during pregnancy should only be considered if the expected benefit to the mother is greater than any possible risk to the fetus. As with the majority of drugs, there is little published evidence of the safety of salbutamol in the early stages of human pregnancy, but in animal studies there was evidence of some harmful effects on the fetus at very high dose levels.

There is inadequate evidence of safety of beclomethasone dipropionate in human pregnancy. Administration of corticosteroids to pregnant animals can cause abnormalities of fetal development including cleft palate and intra-uterine growth retardation. There may therefore, be a very small risk of such effects on the human fetus. It should be noted however, that the fetal changes in animals occur after relatively high systemic exposure. Because beclomethasone dipropionate is delivered directly to the lungs by the inhaled route it avoids the high level of exposure that occurs when corticosteroids are given by systemic routes.

The use of Ventide Rotacaps in pregnancy requires that the possible benefit of the drugs be weighed against the possible hazards.

*Lactation:* No specific studies examining the transference of beclomethasone dipropionate into the milk of lactating animals have been performed. It is reasonable to assume that beclomethasone dipropionate is secreted in milk, but at the dosages used for direct inhalation there is low potential for significant levels in breast milk. As salbutamol is probably also secreted in breast milk the use of Ventide Rotacaps in nursing mothers should be restricted to situations where it is felt that the expected benefit to the mother is likely to outweigh any potential risk to the neonate.

*Side-effects:* As with other inhalation therapy, paradoxical bronchospasm may occur with an immediate increase in wheezing after dosing. This should be treated immediately with a fast-acting inhaled bronchodilator. The preparation should be discontinued immediately, the patient assessed and, if necessary, alternative therapy instituted.

Hoarseness, mouth and throat irritation may occur. It may be helpful to rinse the mouth with water immediately after inhalation.

Hypersensitivity reactions, including angioedema, bronchospasm, hypotension and collapse have been reported very rarely. Rashes, urticaria, pruritus and erythema and oedema of the eyes, face, lips and throat, have also been reported.

*Salbutamol:* Salbutamol may cause a fine tremor of skeletal muscle, usually the hands are most obviously affected. This effect is dose related and common to all $\beta$-adrenergic stimulants. Headaches have occasionally been reported. Tachycardia, with or without peripheral vasodilatation, may rarely occur.

There have been very rare reports of muscle cramps. Potentially serious hypokalaemia may result from $\beta_2$-agonist therapy.

As with other $\beta_2$-agonists, hyperactivity in children has been reported rarely.

*Beclomethasone dipropionate:* Candidiasis of the mouth and throat (thrush) occurs in some patients; the incidence increases with doses greater than 400 micrograms beclomethasone dipropionate per day. Patients with high blood levels of *Candida precipitins*, indicating a previous infection, are more likely to develop this complication. Such patients may find it helpful to rinse their mouth with water after using the Rotahaler device. The condition usually responds to topical anti-fungal therapy without discontinuing treatment with Ventide Rotacaps or Ventide Paediatric Rotacaps.

*Overdosage:*
*Salbutamol:* The preferred antidote for overdosage with salbutamol is a cardioselective, $\beta$-blocking agent, but $\beta$-blocking drugs should be used with caution in patients with a history of bronchospasm. Hypokalaemia may occur following overdose with salbutamol. Serum potassium levels should be monitored.

*Beclomethasone dipropionate:* Acute. Inhalation of the drug in doses in excess of those recommended may lead to temporary suppression of adrenal function. This does not require emergency action. In these patients treatment should be continued at a dose sufficient to control asthma; adrenal function recovers in a few days and can be verified by measuring plasma cortisol.

Chronic. Use of inhaled beclomethasone dipropionate in daily doses in excess of 1,500 micrograms over prolonged periods may lead to some degree of adrenal suppression. Monitoring of adrenal reserve may be indicated. Treatment should be continued at a dose sufficient to control asthma.

**Pharmaceutical precautions** To keep the Rotacaps capsules in good condition it is important that they are stored in a dry place, below 30°C, where they will not be exposed to extremes of temperature. A convenient supply may be carried in the special container for the Rotahaler. A capsule should only be inserted into the Rotahaler immediately prior to use. Failure to observe this instruction may affect the operation of the Rotahaler.

**Legal category** POM.

**Package quantities** Ventide Rotacaps and Ventide Paediatric Rotacaps are supplied in containers of 112.

**Further information** Products containing salbutamol do not cause difficulty in micturition because, unlike sympathomimetic drugs such as ephedrine, salbutamol does not stimulate alpha-adrenoceptors.

Salbutamol products are not contra-indicated in patients under treatment with monoamine oxidase inhibitors (MAOIs).

**Product licence numbers**
Ventide Rotacaps 10949/0077
Ventide Paediatric Rotacaps 10949/0078

## VENTODISKS*

**Presentation** Ventodisks is a dry powder inhalation device available in two strengths providing 200 micrograms or 400 micrograms salbutamol per blister. The active ingredient is presented in a disk comprising eight regularly spaced double-foil blisters each containing a mixture of microfine salbutamol (as sulphate) and larger particle lactose.

The disks are intended only for use in a specific drug delivery device known as the Ventolin* Diskhaler*.

**Uses** Salbutamol is a selective $\beta_2$-agonist providing short-acting (4-6 hour) bronchodilatation with a fast onset (within 5 minutes) in reversible airways obstruction.

Ventodisks can be used in the management of asthma, bronchospasm and/or reversible airways obstruction.

Ventodisks is particularly suitable for the relief of asthma symptoms. It should be used to relieve symptoms when they occur, and to prevent them in those circumstances recognised by the patient to precipitate an asthma attack (e.g. before exercise or unavoidable allergen exposure).

Ventodisks is particularly valuable as relief medication in mild, moderate or severe asthma, provided that reliance on it does not delay the introduction and use of regular inhaled corticosteroid therapy.

**Dosage and administration** Ventodisks is for inhalation use only, using a Ventolin Diskhaler. Ventodisks is suitable for many patients including those who cannot use a metered-dose inhaler successfully.

*Adults (including the elderly):* For the relief of acute bronchospasm 200 micrograms or 400 micrograms should be taken as a single dose. The maximum daily dose is 400 micrograms four times a day.

To prevent allergen- or exercise-induced symptoms, 400 micrograms should be taken 10-15 minutes before challenge.

*Children:* The recommended dose for relief of acute bronchospasm or before allergen exposure or exercise is 200 micrograms. The maximum daily dose is 200 micrograms four times a day.

On-demand use of Ventodisks should not exceed four times daily. Reliance on such frequent supplementary use, or a sudden increase in dose, indicates poorly controlled or deteriorating asthma (see *Precautions*).

**Contra-indications, warnings, etc**
*Contra-indications:* Although intravenous salbutamol, and occasionally salbutamol tablets, are used in the management of premature labour uncomplicated by conditions such as placenta praevia, ante-partum haemorrhage, or toxaemia of pregnancy, inhaled salbutamol preparations are not appropriate for

managing premature labour. Salbutamol preparations should not be used for threatened abortion.

Ventodisks is contra-indicated in patients with a history of hypersensitivity to any of the components.

*Precautions:* Bronchodilators should not be the only or main treatment in patients with severe or unstable asthma. Severe asthma requires regular medical assessment, including lung-function testing, as patients are at risk of severe attacks and even death. Physicians should consider using the maximum recommended dose of inhaled corticosteroid and/or oral corticosteroid therapy in these patients.

The dosage or frequency of administration should only be increased on medical advice.

Increasing use of bronchodilators, in particular short-acting inhaled β₂-agonists to relieve symptoms, indicates deterioration of asthma control. The patient should be instructed to seek medical advice if short-acting relief bronchodilator treatment becomes less effective, or more inhalations than usual are required. In this situation the patient should be assessed and consideration given to the need for increased anti-inflammatory therapy (e.g. higher doses of inhaled corticosteroid or a course of oral corticosteroid).

Severe exacerbations of asthma must be treated in the normal way.

Salbutamol should be administered cautiously to patients suffering from thyrotoxicosis.

Salbutamol and non-selective β-blocking drugs such as propranolol, should not usually be prescribed together.

Potentially serious hypokalaemia may result from β₂-agonist therapy, mainly from parenteral and nebulised administration. Particular caution is advised in acute severe asthma as this effect may be potentiated by hypoxia and by concomitant treatment with xanthine derivatives, steroids and diuretics. Serum potassium levels should be monitored in such situations.

*Pregnancy:* Administration of drugs during pregnancy should only be considered if the expected benefit to the mother is greater than any possible risk to the fetus. As with the majority of drugs, there is little published evidence of the safety of salbutamol in the early stages of human pregnancy, but in animal studies there was evidence of some harmful effects on the fetus at very high dose levels.

*Lactation:* As salbutamol is probably secreted in breast milk, its use in nursing mothers requires careful consideration. It is not known whether salbutamol has a harmful effect on the neonate, and so its use should be restricted to situations where it is felt that the expected benefit to the mother is likely to outweigh any potential risk to the neonate.

*Side-effects:* As with other inhalation therapy, paradoxical bronchospasm may occur with an immediate increase in wheezing after dosing. This should be treated immediately with an alternative presentation or a different fast-acting inhaled bronchodilator. The preparation should be discontinued immediately, the patient assessed and, if necessary, alternative therapy instituted.

Hypersensitivity reactions including angioedema, urticaria, bronchospasm, hypotension and collapse have been reported very rarely.

Potentially serious hypokalaemia may result from β₂-agonist therapy.

Ventodisks may cause a fine tremor of skeletal muscle, usually the hands are most obviously affected. This effect is dose-related and is common to all β-adrenergic stimulants.

Tachycardia, with or without peripheral vasodilatation, may rarely occur.

Headaches have occasionally been reported.

Mouth and throat irritation may occur with inhaled salbutamol.

As with other β₂-agonists hyperactivity in children has been reported rarely.

There have been very rare reports of muscle cramps.

*Overdosage:* The preferred antidote for overdosage with salbutamol is a cardioselective β-blocking agent, but β-blocking drugs should be used with caution in patients with a history of bronchospasm.

Hypokalaemia may occur following overdose with salbutamol. Serum potassium levels should be monitored.

**Pharmaceutical precautions** Whilst the disks provide a good protection to the blister contents from the effects of the atmosphere, they should not be exposed to extremes of temperature and should be stored below 30°C. A disk may be kept in the Diskhaler at all times but a blister should only be pierced immediately prior to use. Failure to observe this instruction may affect the operation of the Diskhaler.

**Legal category** POM.

**Package quantities** Ventodisks 200 micrograms and 400 micrograms are supplied in cartons containing 14 disks (14 x 8 blisters), together with a Diskhaler device.

**Further information** Ventodisks does not cause difficulty in micturition because unlike sympathomimetic drugs such as ephedrine, salbutamol does not stimulate alpha-adrenoceptors. Ventodisks is not contra-indicated in patients under treatment with monoamine oxidase inhibitors (MAOIs).

**Product licence numbers**
Ventodisks 200 micrograms 10949/0079
Ventodisks 400 micrograms 10949/0080

# VENTOLIN* ACCUHALER*

**Qualitative and quantitative composition** Ventolin Accuhaler is a plastic inhaler device containing a foil strip with 60 regularly spaced blisters each containing a mixture of 200 micrograms of microfine salbutamol (as sulphate) and larger particle lactose.

**Pharmaceutical form** Multi-dose dry powder inhalation device.

**Clinical particulars**

*Therapeutic indications:* Ventolin Accuhaler can be used in the management of asthma, bronchospasm and/or reversible airways obstruction.

Ventolin Accuhaler is particularly suitable for the relief of asthma symptoms. It should be used to relieve symptoms when they occur, and to prevent them in those circumstances recognised by the patient to precipitate an asthma attack (e.g. before exercise or unavoidable allergen exposure).

Ventolin Accuhaler is particularly valuable as relief medication in mild, moderate or severe asthma, provided that reliance on it does not delay the introduction and use of regular inhaled corticosteroid therapy.

*Posology and method of administration:* Ventolin Accuhaler is for inhalation use only. Ventolin Accuhaler is suitable for many patients including those who cannot use a metered-dose inhaler successfully.

*Adults (including the elderly):* For the relief of acute bronchospasm, 200 micrograms as a single dose. The maximum daily dose is 200 micrograms four times a day.

To prevent allergen- or exercise-induced symptoms, 200 micrograms should be taken 10-15 minutes before challenge.

*Children:* The recommended dose for relief of acute bronchospasm or before allergen exposure or exercise is 200 micrograms. The maximum daily dose is 200 micrograms four times a day.

On-demand use of Ventolin Accuhaler should not exceed four times daily. Reliance on such frequent supplementary use, or a sudden increase in dose, indicates poorly controlled or deteriorating asthma (see *Precautions*).

*Contra-indications:* Although intravenous salbutamol, and occasionally salbutamol tablets, are used in the management of premature labour uncomplicated by conditions such as placenta praevia, ante-partum haemorrhage, or toxaemia of pregnancy, inhaled salbutamol preparations are not appropriate for managing premature labour. Salbutamol preparations should not be used for threatened abortion.

Ventolin Accuhaler is contra-indicated in patients with a history of hypersensitivity to any of the components.

*Special warnings and precautions for use:* Bronchodilators should not be the only or main treatment in patients with severe or unstable asthma. Severe asthma requires regular medical assessment, including lung-function testing, as patients are at risk of severe attacks and even death. Physicians should consider using the maximum recommended dose of inhaled corticosteroid and/or oral corticosteroid therapy in these patients.

The dosage or frequency of administration should only be increased on medical advice.

Increasing use of bronchodilators, in particular short-acting inhaled β₂-agonists to relieve symptoms, indicates deterioration of asthma control. The patient should be instructed to seek medical advice if short-acting relief bronchodilator treatment becomes less effective, or more inhalations than usual are required. In this situation the patient should be assessed and consideration given to the need for increased anti-inflammatory therapy (e.g. higher doses of inhaled corticosteroid or a course of oral corticosteroid).

Severe exacerbations of asthma must be treated in the normal way.

Salbutamol should be administered cautiously to patients suffering from thyrotoxicosis.

Potentially serious hypokalaemia may result from β₂-agonist therapy, mainly from parenteral and nebulised administration. Particular caution is advised in acute severe asthma as this effect may be potentiated by hypoxia and by concomitant treatment with xanthine derivatives, steroids and diuretics. Serum

potassium levels should be monitored in such situations.

*Interaction with other medicaments and other forms of interaction:* Salbutamol and non-selective β-blocking drugs such as propranolol, should not usually be prescribed together.

*Pregnancy and lactation:*
*Pregnancy:* Administration of drugs during pregnancy should only be considered if the expected benefit to the mother is greater than any possible risk to the fetus. As with the majority of drugs, there is little published evidence of the safety of salbutamol in the early stages of human pregnancy, but in animal studies there was evidence of some harmful effects on the fetus at very high dose levels.

*Lactation:* As salbutamol is probably secreted in breast milk, its use in nursing mothers requires careful consideration. It is not known whether salbutamol has a harmful effect on the neonate, and so its use should be restricted to situations where it is felt that the expected benefit to the mother is likely to outweigh any potential risk to the neonate.

*Effects on ability to drive and use machines:* None reported.

*Undesirable effects:* As with other inhalation therapy, paradoxical bronchospasm may occur with an immediate increase in wheezing after dosing. This should be treated immediately with an alternative presentation or a different fast-acting inhaled bronchodilator. The preparation should be discontinued immediately, the patient assessed and, if necessary, alternative therapy instituted.

Hypersensitivity reactions including angioedema, urticaria, bronchospasm, hypotension and collapse have been reported very rarely.

Potentially serious hypokalaemia may result from β₂-agonist therapy.

Ventolin Accuhaler may cause a fine tremor of skeletal muscle, usually the hands are most obviously affected. This effect is dose-related and is common to all β-adrenergic stimulants.

Tachycardia, with or without peripheral vasodilatation, may rarely occur.

Headaches have occasionally been reported.

Mouth and throat irritation may occur with inhaled salbutamol.

As with other β₂-agonists hyperactivity in children has been reported rarely.

There have been very rare reports of muscle cramps.

*Overdose:* The preferred antidote for overdosage with salbutamol is a cardioselective β-blocking agent, but β-blocking drugs should be used with caution in patients with a history of bronchospasm.

Hypokalaemia may occur following overdose with salbutamol. Serum potassium levels should be monitored.

**Pharmacological properties**
*Pharmacodynamic properties:* Salbutamol is a selective β₂-adrenoceptor agonist. At therapeutic doses it acts on the β₂-adrenoceptors of bronchial muscle, with little or no action on the β₁-adrenoceptors of cardiac muscle.

Salbutamol provides short-acting (4-6 hour) bronchodilatation with a fast onset (within 5 minutes) in reversible airways obstruction.

*Pharmacokinetic properties:* Salbutamol administered intravenously has a half-life of 4 to 6 hours and is excreted partly renally, and partly by metabolism to the inactive 4'-O-sulphate (phenolic sulphate) which is also excreted primarily in the urine. The faeces are a minor route of excretion. After administration by the inhaled route between 10 and 20% of the dose reaches the lower airways. The remainder is retained in the delivery system or is deposited in the oropharynx from where it is swallowed. The fraction deposited in the airways is absorbed into the pulmonary tissues and circulation, but is not metabolised by the lung. On reaching the systemic circulation it becomes accessible to hepatic metabolism and is excreted, primarily in the urine, as unchanged drug and as the phenolic sulphate. The swallowed portion of an inhaled dose is absorbed from the gastrointestinal tract and undergoes considerable first-pass metabolism to the phenolic sulphate. Both unchanged drug and conjugate are excreted primarily in the urine. Almost all of a dose of salbutamol given intravenously orally or by inhalation is excreted within 72 hours. Salbutamol is bound to plasma proteins to the extent of 10%.

*Preclinical safety data:* In common with other potent selective β₂-receptor agonists, salbutamol has been shown to be teratogenic in mice when given subcutaneously. In a reproductive study, 9.3% of fetuses were found to have cleft palate at 2.5 mg/kg, 4 times the maximum human oral dose. In rats, treatment at the levels of 0.5, 2.32, 10.75 and 50 mg/kg/day orally throughout pregnancy resulted in no significant fetal abnormalities. The only toxic effect was an increase in neonatal mortality at the highest dose level as the result of lack of maternal care. A reproductive study in rabbits revealed cranial malformations in 37% of fetuses at 50 mg/kg/day, 78 times the maximum human oral dose.

**Pharmaceutical particulars**

*List of excipients:* Lactose.

*Incompatibilities:* None reported.

*Shelf life:* 18 months.

*Special precautions for storage:* Store below 30°C (86°F). Store in a dry place.

*Nature and contents of container:* The powder mix of salbutamol (as sulphate) and lactose is filled into a blister strip consisting of a formed base foil with a peelable foil laminate lid. The foil strip is contained within the Accuhaler device.

*Instructions for use/handling:* The powdered medicine is inhaled through the mouth into the lungs.

The Accuhaler device contains the medicine in individual blisters which are opened as the device is manipulated.

For detailed instructions for use refer to the Patient Information Leaflet in every pack.

**Marketing authorisation number**   10949/0252

**Date of approval/revision of SPC** December 1995

**Legal category** POM.

## VENTOLIN* EASI-BREATHE* INHALER

**Qualitative and quantitative composition**   100 micrograms Salbutamol BP per actuation. Each canister delivers 200 actuations.

**Pharmaceutical form**   Aerosol.

### Clinical particulars

*Therapeutic indications:* Ventolin Easi-Breathe Inhaler provides short-acting (4 to 6 hour) bronchodilatation with fast onset (within 5 minutes) in reversible airways obstruction.

It is particularly suitable for the relief and prevention of asthma symptoms. It should be used to relieve symptoms when they occur, and to prevent them in those circumstances recognised by the patient to precipitate an asthma attack (e.g. before exercise or unavoidable allergen exposure).

Ventolin Easi-Breathe Inhaler is particularly valuable as relief medication in mild, moderate or severe asthma, provided that reliance on it does not delay the introduction and use of regular inhaled corticosteroid therapy.

*Posology and method of administration:* Ventolin Easi-Breathe Inhaler is for oral inhalation use only.

*Adults (including the elderly):* For the relief of acute asthma symptoms including bronchospasm, one inhalation (100 micrograms) may be administered as a single minimum starting dose. This may be increased to two inhalations if necessary. To prevent allergen- or exercise-induced symptoms, two inhalations should be taken 10–20 minutes before challenge.

For chronic therapy, two inhalations up to four times a day.

*Children:* For the relief of acute asthma symptoms including bronchospasm, or before allergen exposure or exercise, one inhalation, or two if necessary.

For chronic therapy, two inhalations up to four times a day.

On-demand use of Ventolin Easi-Breathe Inhaler should not exceed 8 inhalations in any 24 hours. Reliance on such frequent supplementary use, or a sudden increase in dose, indicates poorly controlled or deteriorating asthma (see *Special warnings and precautions for use*).

*Contra-indications:* Although intravenous salbutamol, and occasionally salbutamol tablets, are used in the management of premature labour uncomplicated by conditions such as placenta praevia, ante-partum haemorrhage or toxaemia of pregnancy, inhaled salbutamol preparations are not appropriate for managing premature labour. Salbutamol preparations should not be used for threatened abortion.

Ventolin Easi-Breathe Inhaler is contra-indicated in patients with a history of hypersensitivity to any of the components.

*Special warnings and special precautions for use:* Patients should be instructed in the proper use of the inhaler, and their technique checked, to ensure that the drug reaches the target areas within the lungs. Bronchodilators should not be the only or main treatment in patients with severe or unstable asthma. Severe asthma requires regular medical assessment, including lung-function testing, as patients are at risk of severe attacks and even death. Physicians consider using the maximum recommended dose of inhaled corticosteroid and/or oral corticosteroid therapy in these patients.

The dosage or frequency of administration should only be increased on medical advice. If a previously effective dose of inhaled salbutamol fails to give relief lasting at least three hours, the patient should be advised to seek medical advice.

Increasing use of bronchodilators, in particular short-acting inhaled β₂-agonists, to relieve symptoms, indicates deterioration of asthma control. The patient should be instructed to seek medical advice if short-acting relief bronchodilator treatment becomes less effective, or more inhalations than usual are required. In this situation the patient should be assessed and consideration given to the need for increased anti-inflammatory therapy (e.g. higher doses of inhaled corticosteroid or a course of oral corticosteroid).

Severe exacerbations of asthma must be treated in the normal way.

Salbutamol should be administered cautiously to patients with thyrotoxicosis. Potentially serious hypokalaemia may result from β₂-agonist therapy, mainly from parenteral and nebulised administration. Particular caution is advised in acute severe asthma as this effect may be potentiated by hypoxia and by concomitant treatment with xanthine derivatives, steroids and diuretics. Serum potassium levels should be monitored in such situations.

*Interaction with other medicaments and other forms of interaction:* Salbutamol and non-selective β-blocking drugs such as propranolol, should not usually be prescribed together.

*Pregnancy and lactation:* Administration of drugs during pregnancy should only be considered if the expected benefit to the mother is greater than any possible risk to the fetus. As with the majority of drugs, there is little published evidence of the safety of salbutamol in the early stages of human pregnancy, but in animal studies there was evidence of some harmful effects on the fetus at very high dose levels.

As salbutamol is probably secreted in breast milk, its use in nursing mothers requires careful consideration. It is not known whether salbutamol has a harmful effect on the neonate, and so its use should be restricted to situations where it is felt that the expected benefit to the mother is likely to outweigh any potential risk to the neonate.

*Effects on the ability to drive and use machines:* None reported.

*Undesirable effects:* As with other inhalation therapy, paradoxical bronchospasm may occur with an immediate increase in wheezing after dosing. This should be treated immediately with an alternative presentation or a different fast-acting inhaled bronchodilator. Ventolin Easi-Breathe Inhaler should be discontinued immediately, the patient assessed and, if necessary, alternative therapy instituted.

Hypersensitivity reactions including angioedema, urticaria, bronchospasm, hypotension and collapse have been reported very rarely.

Potentially serious hypokalaemia may result from β₂-agonist therapy.

Ventolin Easi-Breathe Inhaler may cause a fine tremor of skeletal muscle, usually the hands are most obviously affected. This effect is dose-related and is common to all β-adrenergic stimulants.

Tachycardia, with or without peripheral vasodilatation, may rarely occur.

Headaches have occasionally been reported.

Mouth and throat irritation may occur with inhaled salbutamol.

As with other β₂-agonists hyperactivity in children has been reported rarely.

There have been very rare reports of muscle cramps.

*Overdose:* The preferred antidote for overdosage with salbutamol is a cardioselective β-blocking agent, but β-blocking drugs should be used with caution in patients with a history of bronchospasm.

Hypokalaemia may occur following overdose with salbutamol. Serum potassium levels should be monitored.

### Pharmacological properties

*Pharmacodynamic properties:* Salbutamol is a selective β₂-adrenoceptor agonist. At therapeutic doses it acts on the β₂-adrenoceptors of bronchial muscle providing short-acting (4–6 hour) bronchodilatation with a fast onset (within 5 minutes) in reversible airways obstruction.

*Pharmacokinetic properties:* Salbutamol administered intravenously has a half-life of 4 to 6 hours and is cleared, partly renally and partly by metabolism, to the inactive 4'-O-sulphate (phenolic sulphate) which is also excreted primarily in the urine. The faeces are a minor route of excretion.

After administration by the inhaled route between 10 and 20% of the dose reaches the lower airways. The remainder is retained in the delivery system or is deposited in the oropharynx from where it is swallowed. The fraction deposited in the airways is absorbed into the pulmonary tissues and circulation, but is not metabolised by the lung. On reaching the systemic circulation it becomes accessible to hepatic metabolism and is excreted, primarily in the urine, as unchanged drug and as the phenolic sulphate.

The swallowed portion of an inhaled dose is absorbed from the gastrointestinal tract and undergoes considerable first-pass metabolism to the phenolic sulphate. Both unchanged drug and conjugate are excreted primarily in the urine. Most of a dose of salbutamol given intravenously, orally or by inhalation is excreted within 72 hours. Salbutamol is bound to plasma proteins to the extent of 10%.

*Preclinical safety data:* In common with other potent selective β₂-agonists, salbutamol has been shown to be teratogenic in mice when given subcutaneously. In a reproductive study, 9.3% of fetuses were found to have cleft palate at 2.5 mg/kg dose. In rats, treatment at the levels of 0.5, 2.32, 10.75 and 50 mg/kg/day orally throughout pregnancy resulted in no significant fetal abnormalities. The only toxic effect was an increase in neonatal mortality at the highest dose level as the result of lack of maternal care. Reproductive studies in the rabbit at doses of 50 mg/kg/day (i.e. much higher than the normal human dose) have shown fetuses with treatment related changes; these included open eyelids (ablepharia), secondary palate clefts (palatoschisis), changes in ossification of the frontal bones of the cranium (cranioschisis) and limb flexure.

### Pharmaceutical particulars

*List of excipients:* Oleic acid, dichlorodifluoromethane, trichlorofluoromethane.

*Incompatibilities:* None reported.

*Shelf life:* Three years when stored below 30°C.

*Special precautions for storage:* Store below 30°C. Protect from frost and direct sunlight.

As with most inhaled medications in aerosol canisters, the therapeutic effect of this medication may decrease when the canister is cold.

The canister should not be broken, punctured or burnt, even when apparently empty.

*Nature and contents of container:* An inhaler comprising an aluminium can fitted with a breath-operated metering valve, actuator and dust cap. Each canister contains 200 metered actuations providing 100 micrograms Salbutamol BP.

*Instructions for use/handling:* The aerosol spray is inhaled through the mouth into the lungs. After shaking the inhaler, open the cap and place the mouthpiece in the mouth with the lips closed around it. Suck in slowly through the mouthpiece, this releases a spray.

For detailed instructions for use refer to the Patient Information Leaflet in every pack.

*Marketing authorisation holder:* Glaxo Wellcome UK Ltd, trading as Allen & Hanburys, Stockley Park West, Uxbridge, Middlesex UB11 1BT.

**Marketing authorisation number**   10949/0267.

**Date of approval/revision of SPC**   December 1996.

**Legal category**   POM.

## VENTOLIN* INHALER

**Presentation** Ventolin Inhaler is a pressurised metered-dose inhaler delivering 100 micrograms Salbutamol BP per actuation.

Other ingredients: Oleic acid, dichlorodifluoromethane, trichlorofluoromethane.

**Uses** Salbutamol is a selective β₂-agonist providing short-acting (4-6 hour) bronchodilatation with a fast onset (within 5 minutes) in reversible airways obstruction.

Ventolin Inhaler can be used in the management of asthma, bronchospasm and/or reversible airways obstruction.

Ventolin Inhaler is particularly suitable for the relief of asthma symptoms. It should be used to relieve symptoms when they occur, and to prevent them in those circumstances recognised by the patient to precipitate an asthma attack (e.g. before exercise or unavoidable allergen exposure).

Ventolin Inhaler is particularly valuable as relief medication in mild, moderate or severe asthma, provided that reliance on it does not delay the introduction and use of regular inhaled corticosteroid therapy.

**Dosage and administration** Ventolin Inhaler is for inhalation use only. A Volumatic* spacer device may be used in patients who find it difficult to synchronise aerosol actuation with inspiration of breath.

*Adults (including the elderly):* For the relief of acute bronchospasm, one or two inhalations (100 or 200 micrograms) as necessary. To prevent allergen- or exercise-induced symptoms, two inhalations should be taken 10-15 minutes before challenge.

*Children:* One or two inhalations for the relief of acute

bronchospasm, or before allergen exposure or exercise.

The Babyhaler* spacer device may be used to facilitate administration to children under 5 years of age.

On-demand use of Ventolin Inhaler should not exceed 8 inhalations in any 24 hours. Reliance on such frequent supplementary use, or a sudden increase in dose, indicates poorly controlled or deteriorating asthma (see *Precautions*).

**Contra-indications, warnings, etc**
*Contra-indications:* Although intravenous salbutamol, and occasionally salbutamol tablets, are used in the management of premature labour uncomplicated by conditions such as placenta praevia, ante-partum haemorrhage or toxaemia of pregnancy, inhaled salbutamol preparations are not appropriate for managing premature labour. Salbutamol preparations should not be used for threatened abortion.

Ventolin Inhaler is contra-indicated in patients with a history of hypersensitivity to any of the components.

*Precautions:* Patients' inhaler technique should be checked to make sure that aerosol actuation is synchronised with inspiration of breath for optimum delivery of drug to the lungs.

Bronchodilators should not be the only or main treatment in patients with severe or unstable asthma. Severe asthma requires regular medical assessment, including lung-function testing, as patients are at risk of severe attacks and even death. Physicians should consider using the maximum recommended dose of inhaled corticosteroid and/or oral corticosteroid therapy in these patients.

The dosage or frequency of administration should only be increased on medical advice.

Increasing use of bronchodilators, in particular short-acting inhaled $\beta_2$-agonists, to relieve symptoms, indicates deterioration of asthma control. The patient should be instructed to seek medical advice if short-acting relief bronchodilator treatment becomes less effective, or more inhalations than usual are required. In this situation the patient should be assessed and consideration given to the need for increased anti-inflammatory therapy (e.g. higher doses of inhaled corticosteroid or a course of oral corticosteroid).

Severe exacerbations of asthma must be treated in the normal way.

Salbutamol should be administered cautiously to patients suffering from thyrotoxicosis.

Salbutamol and non-selective $\beta$-blocking drugs such as propranolol, should not usually be prescribed together.

Potentially serious hypokalaemia may result from $\beta_2$-agonist therapy, mainly from parenteral and nebulised administration. Particular caution is advised in acute severe asthma as this effect may be potentiated by hypoxia and by concomitant treatment with xanthine derivatives, steroids and diuretics. Serum potassium levels should be monitored in such situations.

*Pregnancy:* Administration of drugs during pregnancy should only be considered if the expected benefit to the mother is greater than any possible risk to the fetus. As with the majority of drugs, there is little published evidence of the safety of salbutamol in the early stages of human pregnancy, but in animal studies there was evidence of some harmful effects on the fetus at very high dose levels.

*Lactation:* As salbutamol is probably secreted in breast milk, its use in nursing mothers requires careful consideration. It is not known whether salbutamol has a harmful effect on the neonate, and so its use should be restricted to situations where it is felt that the expected benefit to the mother is likely to outweigh any potential risk to the neonate.

*Side-effects:* As with other inhalation therapy, paradoxical bronchospasm may occur with an immediate increase in wheezing after dosing. This should be treated immediately with an alternative presentation or a different fast-acting inhaled bronchodilator. Ventolin Inhaler should be discontinued immediately, the patient assessed and, if necessary, alternative therapy instituted.

Hypersensitivity reactions including angioedema, urticaria, bronchospasm, hypotension and collapse have been reported very rarely.

Potentially serious hypokalaemia may result from $\beta_2$-agonist therapy.

Ventolin Inhaler may cause a fine tremor of skeletal muscle, usually the hands are most obviously affected. This effect is dose-related and is common to all $\beta$-adrenergic stimulants.

Tachycardia, with or without peripheral vasodilatation, may rarely occur.

Headaches have occasionally been reported.

Mouth and throat irritation may occur with inhaled salbutamol.

As with other $\beta_2$-agonists hyperactivity in children has been reported rarely.

There have been very rare reports of muscle cramps.

*Overdosage:* The preferred antidote for overdosage with salbutamol is a cardioselective $\beta$-blocking agent, but $\beta$-blocking drugs should be used with caution in patients with a history of bronchospasm.

Hypokalaemia may occur following overdose with salbutamol. Serum potassium levels should be monitored.

**Pharmaceutical precautions** Ventolin Inhaler should be stored below 30°C protected from direct sunlight, heat and frost. The canister should not be broken, punctured or burnt, even when apparently empty.

As with most inhaled medications in aerosol canisters, the therapeutic effect of this medication may decrease when the canister is cold.

**Legal category** POM.

**Package quantities** Ventolin Inhaler is a metered-dose aerosol with a specially designed actuator. Each canister provides 200 inhalations.

**Further information** Ventolin Inhaler does not cause difficulty in micturition because, unlike sympathomimetic drugs such as ephedrine, salbutamol does not stimulate alpha-adrenoceptors. Ventolin Inhaler is not contra-indicated in patients under treatment with monoamine oxidase inhibitors (MAOIs).

**Product licence number** 0045/5022R

*Product licence holder:* Allen & Hanburys Ltd, Greenford, Middlesex UB6 0HB.

## VENTOLIN* INJECTION 250 micrograms (0.25 mg) in 5 ml VENTOLIN* INJECTION 500 micrograms (0.5 mg) in 1 ml

**Qualitative and quantitative composition** Ventolin Injection 250 micrograms (0.25 mg) in 5 ml (50 micrograms/ml) is presented as ampoules of 5 ml, each containing 250 micrograms salbutamol as Salbutamol Sulphate BP in a sterile isotonic solution.

Ventolin Injection 500 micrograms (0.5 mg) in 1 ml (500 micrograms/ml) is presented as ampoules of 1 ml, each containing 500 micrograms salbutamol as Salbutamol Sulphate BP in a sterile isotonic solution.

**Pharmaceutical form** Clear, colourless or pale straw-coloured solution for injection.

**Clinical particulars**

*Therapeutic indications:* Ventolin Injection is indicated for the relief of severe bronchospasm.

*Posology and method of administration:* Ventolin Injection may be administered by the subcutaneous, intramuscular or intravenous route, under the direction of a physician.

*Adults:* Subcutaneous route: 500 micrograms (8 micrograms/kg body weight) and repeated every four hours as required.

Intramuscular route: 500 micrograms (8 micrograms/kg body weight) and repeated every four hours as required.

Intravenous route: 250 micrograms (4 micrograms/kg body weight) injected slowly. If necessary the dose may be repeated.

Ventolin Injection 250 micrograms in 5 ml (50 micrograms/ml) is a suitably dilute preparation for slow intravenous injection, but if Ventolin Injection 500 micrograms in 1 ml (500 micrograms/ml) is used, the injection may be facilitated by dilution with Water for Injections BP.

*Children:* There are insufficient data to recommend a dosage regime for routine use.

*Contra-indications:* Although intravenous salbutamol, and occasionally salbutamol tablets, are used in the management of premature labour uncomplicated by conditions such as placenta praevia, ante-partum haemorrhage or toxaemia of pregnancy, salbutamol preparations should not be used for threatened abortion.

Ventolin Injection is contra-indicated in patients with a history of hypersensitivity to any of the components.

*Special warnings and precautions for use:* Bronchodilators should not be the only or main treatment in patients with severe or unstable asthma. Severe asthma requires regular medical assessment, including lung-function testing, as patients are at risk of severe attacks and even death. Physicians should consider using the maximum recommended dose of inhaled corticosteroid and/or oral corticosteroid therapy in these patients.

The dosage or frequency of administration should only be increased on medical advice.

Patients being treated with Ventolin Injection may also be receiving short-acting inhaled bronchodilators to relieve symptoms. Increasing use of bronchodilators, in particular short-acting inhaled $\beta_2$-agonists to relieve symptoms, indicates deterioration of asthma control. The patient should be instructed to seek medical advice if short-acting relief bronchodilator treatment becomes less effective, or more inhalations than usual are required. In this situation the patient should be assessed and consideration given to the need for increased anti-inflammatory therapy (e.g. higher doses of inhaled corticosteroid or a course of oral corticosteroid).

Severe exacerbations of asthma must be treated in the normal way.

The use of Ventolin Injection in the treatment of severe bronchospasm does not obviate the requirement for corticosteroid therapy as appropriate. When practicable, administration of oxygen concurrently with Ventolin Injection is recommended. In common with other $\beta$-adrenoceptor agonists, salbutamol can induce reversible metabolic changes such as hypokalaemia and increased blood glucose levels. Diabetic patients may be unable to compensate for the increase in blood glucose and the development of ketoacidosis has been reported. Concurrent administration of corticosteroids can exaggerate this effect.

Salbutamol should be administered cautiously to patients suffering from thyrotoxicosis.

Potentially serious hypokalaemia may result from $\beta_2$-agonist therapy, mainly from parenteral and nebulised administration. Particular caution is advised in acute severe asthma as this effect may be potentiated by hypoxia and by concomitant treatment with xanthine derivatives, steroids and diuretics. Serum potassium levels should be monitored in such situations.

*Interaction with other medicaments and other forms of interaction:* Ventolin Injection should not be administered in the same syringe as any other medication.

Salbutamol and non-selective $\beta$-blocking drugs such as propranolol, should not usually be prescribed together.

*Pregnancy and lactation:* Administration of drugs during pregnancy should only be considered if the expected benefit to the mother is greater than any possible risk to the fetus. As with the majority of drugs, there is little published evidence of the safety of salbutamol in the early stages of human pregnancy, but in animal studies there was evidence of some harmful effects on the fetus at very high dose levels.

As salbutamol is probably secreted in breast milk, its use in nursing mothers requires careful consideration. It is not known whether salbutamol has a harmful effect on the neonate, and so its use should be restricted to situations where it is felt that the expected benefit to the mother is likely to outweigh any potential risk to the neonate.

*Effect on ability to drive and use machines:* None reported.

*Undesirable effects:* Hypersensitivity reactions including angioedema, urticaria, bronchospasm, hypotension and collapse have been reported very rarely.

Enhancement of physiological tremor may occur with Ventolin Injection. This effect is caused by a direct action on skeletal muscle and is common to all $\beta$-adrenergic stimulants.

Tachycardia, with or without dilatation of periphera arterioles leading to a small reduction in arteria pressure, may occur. Increases in heart rate are more likely to occur in patients with normal heart rates and these increases are dose-dependent. In patients with pre-existing sinus tachycardia, especially those in status asthmaticus, the heart rate tends to fall as the condition of the patient improves.

Headaches have occasionally been reported.

There have been very rare reports of muscle cramps.

Potentially serious hypokalaemia may result from $\beta_2$-agonist therapy.

Intramuscular use of the undiluted injection may produce slight pain or stinging.

*Overdose:* The preferred antidote for overdosage with salbutamol is a cardioselective $\beta$-blocking agent, bu $\beta$-blocking drugs should be used with caution i patients with a history of bronchospasm.

Hypokalaemia may occur following overdose wit salbutamol. Serum potassium levels should b monitored.

**Pharmacological properties**
*Pharmacodynamic properties:* Salbutamol is selective $\beta_2$-agonist providing short-acting (4-6 hour bronchodilatation with a fast onset (within 5 minutes in reversible airways obstruction.

*Pharmacokinetic properties:* Salbutamol adminis tered intravenously has a half-life of 4 to 6 hours an is cleared partly renally and partly by metabolism t the inactive 4'-0-sulphate (phenolic sulphate) which i also excreted primarily in the urine. The faeces are minor route of excretion. Most of a dose of salbutamo given intravenously, orally or by inhalation is excrete within 72 hours. Salbutamol is bound to plasm proteins to the extent of 10%.

*Preclinical safety data:* No additional preclinical safety data are included here.

**Pharmaceutical particulars**

*List of excipients:* Sodium chloride, sodium hydroxide, sulphuric acid and Water for Injections.

*Incompatibilities:* None stated.

*Shelf life:* 36 months.

*Special precautions for storage:* Store below 30°C and protect from light.

*Nature and contents of container:* Clear, neutral glass ampoules.

Ventolin Injection 250 micrograms in 5 ml is available in packs of 10.

Ventolin Injection 500 micrograms in 1 ml is available in packs of 5.

*Instructions for use/handling:* The only recommended diluents for Ventolin Injection are Water for Injections BP, Sodium Chloride Injection BP, Sodium Chloride and Dextrose Injection BP or Dextrose Injection BP.

All unused admixtures of Ventolin Injection should be discarded twenty-four hours after preparation.

**Marketing authorisation numbers**
Ventolin Injection 250 micrograms in 5 ml 10949/0083
Ventolin Injection 500 micrograms in 1 ml 10949/0084

**Date of approval/revision of SPC** October 1995.

**Legal category** POM.

## VENTOLIN* NEBULES*

**Presentation** *Ventolin Nebules 2.5 mg:* Each plastic ampoule contains 2.5 ml of a sterile 0.1% w/v solution of salbutamol (as Salbutamol Sulphate BP) in normal saline.

*Ventolin Nebules 5 mg:* Each plastic ampoule contains 2.5 ml of a sterile 0.2% w/v solution of salbutamol (as Salbutamol Sulphate BP) in normal saline.

Ventolin Nebules do not contain a preservative. The acidity of the solution is adjusted to pH4 with sulphuric acid if required.

**Uses** Salbutamol is a selective $\beta_2$-agonist providing short-acting (4-6 hour) bronchodilatation with a fast onset (within 5 minutes) in reversible airways obstruction.

Ventolin Nebules can be used in the management of asthma, bronchospasm and/or reversible airways obstruction.

Ventolin Nebules are indicated for use in the routine management of chronic bronchospasm unresponsive to conventional therapy, and in the treatment of acute severe asthma.

**Dosage and administration** Ventolin Nebules are for inhalation use only under the direction of a physician, using a suitable nebuliser.

The solution should not be injected or administered orally.

*Adults (including the elderly):* 2.5 mg to 5 mg salbutamol up to four times a day. Up to 40 mg per day can be given under strict medical supervision in hospital.

*Children:* 2.5 mg to 5 mg up to four times a day.

In infants under 18 months old the clinical efficacy of nebulised salbutamol is uncertain. As transient hypoxaemia may occur supplemental oxygen therapy should be considered.

Ventolin Nebules are intended to be used undiluted. However, if prolonged delivery time (more than 10 minutes) is required, the solution may be diluted with sterile normal saline.

**Contra-indications, warnings, etc**

*Contra-indications:* Although intravenous salbutamol, and occasionally salbutamol tablets, are used in the management of premature labour uncomplicated by conditions such as placenta praevia, ante-partum haemorrhage or toxaemia of pregnancy, inhaled salbutamol preparations are not appropriate for managing premature labour. Salbutamol preparations should not be used for threatened abortion.

Ventolin Nebules are contra-indicated in patients with a history of hypersensitivity to any of the components.

*Precautions:* Bronchodilators should not be the only or main treatment in patients with severe or unstable asthma. Severe asthma requires regular medical assessment, including lung-function testing, as patients are at risk of severe attacks and even death. Physicians should consider using the maximum recommended dose of inhaled corticosteroid and/or oral corticosteroid therapy in these patients.

Patients receiving treatment at home should seek medical advice if treatment with Ventolin Nebules becomes less effective.

The dosage or frequency of administration should only be increased on medical advice.

Patients being treated with Ventolin Nebules may also be receiving other dosage forms of short-acting inhaled bronchodilators to relieve symptoms. Increasing use of bronchodilators, in particular short-acting inhaled $\beta_2$-agonists, to relieve symptoms, indicates deterioration of asthma control. The patient should be instructed to seek medical advice if short-acting relief bronchodilator treatment becomes less effective or more inhalations than usual are required. In this situation patients should be assessed and consideration given to the need for increased anti-inflammatory therapy (e.g. higher doses of inhaled corticosteroid or a course of oral corticosteroid).

Severe exacerbations of asthma must be treated in the normal way.

Salbutamol should be administered cautiously to patients suffering from thyrotoxicosis.

Salbutamol and non-selective β-blocking drugs such as propranolol, should not usually be prescribed together.

Ventolin Nebules should be used with care in patients known to have received large doses of other sympathomimetic drugs.

Potentially serious hypokalaemia may result from $\beta_2$-agonist therapy, mainly from parenteral and nebulised administration. Particular caution is advised in acute severe asthma as this effect may be potentiated by hypoxia and by concomitant treatment with xanthine derivatives, steroids and diuretics. Serum potassium levels should be monitored in such situations.

In common with other β-adrenoceptor agonists, salbutamol can induce reversible metabolic changes such as increased blood glucose levels. Diabetic patients may be unable to compensate for the increase in blood glucose and the development of ketoacidosis has been reported. Concurrent administration of corticosteroids can exaggerate this effect.

A small number of cases of acute angle-closure glaucoma have been reported in patients treated with a combination of nebulised salbutamol and ipratropium bromide. A combination of nebulised salbutamol with nebulised anticholinergics should therefore be used cautiously. Patients should receive adequate instruction in correct administration and be warned not to let the solution or mist enter the eye.

*Pregnancy:* Administration of drugs during pregnancy should only be considered if the expected benefit to the mother is greater than any possible risk to the fetus. As with the majority of drugs, there is little published evidence of the safety of salbutamol in the early stages of human pregnancy, but in animal studies there was evidence of some harmful effects on the fetus at very high dose levels.

*Lactation:* As salbutamol is probably secreted in breast milk, its use in nursing mothers requires careful consideration. It is not known whether salbutamol has a harmful effect on the neonate, and so its use should be restricted to situations where it is felt that the expected benefit to the mother is likely to outweigh any potential risk to the neonate.

*Side-effects:* As with other inhalation therapy, paradoxical bronchospasm may occur with an immediate increase in wheezing after dosing. This should be treated immediately with an alternative presentation or a different fast-acting inhaled bronchodilator. The preparation should be discontinued immediately, the patient assessed and, if necessary, alternative therapy instituted.

Solutions which are not of neutral pH may rarely cause bronchospasm.

Hypersensitivity reactions including angioedema, urticaria, bronchospasm, hypotension and collapse have been reported very rarely.

Potentially serious hypokalaemia may result from $\beta_2$-agonist therapy.

Ventolin Nebules may cause a fine tremor of skeletal muscle, usually the hands are most obviously affected. This effect is dose-related and is common to all β-adrenergic stimulants.

Tachycardia, with or without peripheral vasodilatation, may rarely occur.

Headaches have occasionally been reported.

Mouth and throat irritation may occur with inhaled salbutamol.

As with other $\beta_2$-agonists hyperactivity in children has been reported rarely.

There have been very rare reports of muscle cramps.

*Overdosage:* The preferred antidote to overdosage with salbutamol is a cardio-selective β-blocking agent, but β-blocking drugs should be used with caution in patients with a history of bronchospasm.

Hypokalaemia may occur following overdose with salbutamol. Serum potassium levels should be monitored.

**Pharmaceutical precautions** Ventolin Nebules should be stored below 30°C. The Nebules should be protected from light after removal from the foil tray.

*Dilution:* Ventolin Nebules may be diluted with Sodium Chloride Injection BP (normal saline). Solutions in nebulisers should be replaced daily.

**Legal category** POM.

**Package quantities** Ventolin Nebules 2.5 mg and 5 mg are each available in boxes containing 20 Nebules in strips of 5.

**Further information** Ventolin Nebules do not cause difficulty in micturition because, unlike sympathomimetic drugs such as ephedrine, salbutamol does not stimulate alpha-adrenoceptors.

Ventolin Nebules are not contra-indicated in patients under treatment with monoamine oxidase inhibitors (MAOIs).

*Administration:* The nebulised solution may be inhaled through a face mask, T-piece or via an endotracheal tube. Intermittent positive pressure ventilation (IPPV) may be used but is rarely necessary. When there is a risk of anoxia through hypoventilation, oxygen should be added to the inspired air.

As many nebulisers operate on a continuous flow basis, it is likely that some nebulised drug will be released into the local environment. Ventolin Nebules should therefore be administered in a well-ventilated room, particularly in hospitals when several patients may be using nebulisers at the same time.

**Product licence numbers**
Ventolin Nebules 2.5 mg 10949/0085
Ventolin Nebules 5.0 mg 10949/0086

## VENTOLIN* RESPIRATOR SOLUTION

**Qualitative and quantitative composition** Aqueous, colourless to light yellow solution, pH 3.5, providing 5 mg/ml of salbutamol (as Salbutamol Sulphate BP).

**Pharmaceutical form** Solution for nebulisation.

**Clinical particulars**

*Therapeutic indications:* Ventolin Respirator Solution is indicated for use in the routine management of chronic bronchospasm unresponsive to conventional therapy, and in the treatment of acute severe asthma.

*Posology and method of administration:* Ventolin Respirator Solution is for inhalation use only under the direction of a physician, using a suitable nebuliser.

The solution should not be injected or administered orally.

Ventolin Respirator Solution may be administered intermittently or continuously.

Salbutamol has a duration of action of 4 to 6 hours in most patients.

*1. Intermittent administration*

*Adults:* Ventolin Respirator solution 0.5 ml (2.5 mg of salbutamol) should be diluted to a final volume of 2 ml with normal saline for injection. This may be increased to 1 ml (5 mg of salbutamol) diluted to a final volume of 2.5 ml. The resulting solution is inhaled from a suitably driven nebuliser until aerosol generation ceases. Using a correctly matched nebuliser and driving source this should take about ten minutes.

Ventolin Respirator Solution may be used undiluted for intermittent administration. For this, 2 ml of Ventolin Respirator Solution (10 mg of salbutamol) is placed in the nebuliser and the patient allowed to inhale the nebulised solution until bronchodilatation is achieved. This usually takes 3–5 minutes.

Some adult patients may require higher doses of salbutamol up to 10 mg, in which case nebulisation of the undiluted solution may continue until aerosol generation ceases.

*Children:* The same mode of administration for intermittent administration is also applicable to children. The minimum starting dosage for children under the age of twelve years is 0.5 ml (2.5 mg of salbutamol) diluted to 2 to 2.5 ml with normal saline for injection. Some children may, however, require higher doses of salbutamol up to 5 mg.

Intermittent treatment may be repeated up to four times daily.

*2. Continuous administration*

Ventolin Respirator Solution is diluted with normal saline for injection to contain 50–100 micrograms of salbutamol per ml, (1–2 ml solution made up to 100 ml with diluent). The diluted solution is administered as an aerosol by a suitably driven nebuliser. The usual rate of administration is 1–2 mg per hour.

Delivery of the aerosol may be by face mask, T-piece or via an endotracheal tube. Intermittent positive pressure ventilation (IPPV) may be used, but is rarely necessary. When there is a risk of anoxia through hypoventilation, oxygen should be added to the inspired air. In infants under 18 months the clinical efficacy of nebulised salbutamol is uncertain. As transient hypoxaemia may occur supplemental oxygen therapy should be considered.

*Contra-indications:* Hypersensitivity. Threatened abortion.

*Special warnings and precautions for use:* Bronchodilators should not be the only or main treatment in patients with severe or unstable asthma. Severe asthma requires regular medical assessment, including lung-function testing, as patients are at risk of severe attacks and even death. Physicians should consider using the maximum recommended dose of inhaled corticosteroid and/or oral corticosteroid therapy in these patients.

Patients receiving treatment at home should be warned to seek medical advice if treatment with Ventolin Respirator Solution becomes less effective. As there may be adverse effects associated with excessive dosing the dosage or frequency of administration should only be increased on medical advice.

Patients being treated with Ventolin Respirator Solution may also be receiving other dosage forms of short-acting inhaled bronchodilators to relieve symptoms.

Increasing use of bronchodilators, in particular short-acting inhaled $\beta_2$-agonists, to relieve symptoms, indicates deterioration of asthma control. The patient should be instructed to seek medical advice if short-acting relief bronchodilator treatment becomes less effective, or more inhalations than usual are required. In this situation the patient should be assessed and consideration given to the need for increased anti-inflammatory therapy (e.g. higher doses of inhaled corticosteroid or a course of oral corticosteroid).

Severe exacerbations of asthma must be treated in the normal way.

Salbutamol should be administered cautiously to patients suffering from thyrotoxicosis.

Ventolin Respirator Solution should be used with care in patients known to have received large doses of other sympathomimetic drugs.

Potentially serious hypokalaemia may result from $\beta_2$-agonist therapy, mainly from parenteral and nebulised administration. Particular caution is advised in acute severe asthma as this effect may be potentiated by hypoxia and by concomitant treatment with xanthine derivatives, steroids and diuretics. Serum potassium levels should be monitored in such situations.

In common with other β-adrenoceptor agonists, salbutamol can induce reversible metabolic changes such as increased blood glucose levels. Diabetic patients may be unable to compensate for the increase in blood glucose and the development of ketoacidosis has been reported. Concurrent administration of corticosteroids can exaggerate this effect.

A small number of cases of acute angle-closure glaucoma have been reported in patients treated with a combination of nebulised salbutamol and ipratropium bromide. A combination of nebulised salbutamol with nebulised anticholinergics should therefore be used cautiously. Patients should receive adequate instruction in correct administration and be warned not to let the solution or mist enter the eye.

*Interaction with other medicaments and other forms of interaction:* Should not normally be prescribed with non-selective β-blocking drugs such as propranolol.

*Use during pregnancy and lactation:* Administration of drugs during pregnancy should only be considered if the expected benefit to the mother is greater than any possible risk to the fetus. As with the majority of drugs, there is little published evidence of the safety of salbutamol in the early stages of human pregnancy, but in animal studies there was evidence of some harmful effects on the fetus at very high dose levels.

As salbutamol is probably secreted in breast milk, its use in nursing mothers requires careful consideration. It is not known whether salbutamol has a harmful effect on the neonate, and so its use should be restricted to situations where it is felt that the expected benefit to the mother is likely to outweigh any potential risk to the neonate.

*Effect on the ability to drive and use machines:* None reported.

*Undesirable effects:* As with other inhalation therapy, paradoxical bronchospasm may occur with an immediate increase in wheezing after dosing. This should be treated immediately with an alternative presentation or a different fast-acting inhaled bronchodilator. The preparation should be discontinued immediately, the patient assessed and, if necessary, alternative therapy instituted.

Non-isotonic solutions, or solutions which are not of neutral pH, or which contain benzalkonium chloride, may rarely cause paradoxical bronchospasm.

Hypersensitivity reactions including angioedema, urticaria, bronchospasm, hypotension and collapse have been reported very rarely.

Potentially serious hypokalaemia may result from $\beta_2$-agonist therapy.

Ventolin Respirator Solution may cause a fine tremor of skeletal muscle, usually the hands are most obviously affected. This effect is dose-related and is common to all β-adrenergic stimulants.

Tachycardia, with or without peripheral vasodilatation, may rarely occur.

Headaches have occasionally been reported.

Mouth and throat irritation may occur with inhaled salbutamol.

As with other $\beta_2$-agonists hyperactivity in children has been reported rarely.

There have been very rare reports of muscle cramps.

*Overdose:* Discontinue administration of Ventolin Respirator Solution if there are any signs of overdosage.

The preferred antidote for overdosage with salbutamol is a cardioselective β-blocking agent, but β-blocking drugs should be used with caution in patients with a history of bronchospasm.

Hypokalaemia may occur following overdose with salbutamol. Serum potassium levels should be monitored.

**Pharmacological properties**

*Pharmacodynamic properties:* Salbutamol is a selective $\beta_2$-agonist providing short-acting (4–6 hours) bronchodilatation with a fast onset (within 5 minutes) in reversible airways obstruction. At therapeutic doses it acts on the $\beta_2$-adrenoceptors of bronchial muscle. With its fast onset of action, it is particularly suitable for the management and prevention of attack in asthma.

*Pharmacokinetic properties:* Salbutamol administered intravenously has a half-life of 4 to 6 hours and is cleared partly renally and partly by metabolism to the inactive 4′-0-sulphate (phenolic sulphate) which is also excreted primarily in the urine. The faeces are a minor route of excretion. Most of a dose of salbutamol given intravenously, orally or by inhalation is excreted within 72 hours. Salbutamol is bound to plasma proteins to the extent of 10%.

After administration by the inhaled route between 10 and 20% of the dose reaches the lower airways. The remainder is retained in the delivery system or is deposited in the oropharynx from where it is swallowed. The fraction deposited in the airways is absorbed into the pulmonary tissues and circulation, but is not metabolised by the lung. On reaching the systemic circulation it becomes accessible to hepatic metabolism and is excreted, primarily in the urine, as unchanged drug and as the phenolic sulphate.

The swallowed portion of an inhaled dose is absorbed from the gastrointestinal tract and undergoes considerable first-pass metabolism to the phenolic sulphate. Both unchanged drug and conjugate are excreted primarily in the urine.

*Preclinical safety data:* No additional preclinical safety data are included here.

**Pharmaceutical particulars**

*List of excipients:* Preservative: Benzalkonium chloride. Sulphuric acid if required to adjust to pH 3.5. Purified water.

*Incompatibilities:* None known.

*Shelf life:* Unopened: 3 years. Following opening for the first time: 28 days.

*Special precautions for storage:* Store below 25°C. Protect from light. Discard any contents remaining one month after opening the bottle.

*Nature and contents of container:* Screw-capped 20 ml amber glass bottle.

*Instructions for use/handling:* Inhalation use only, using a suitable nebuliser.

As many nebulisers operate on a continuous flow basis, it is likely that nebulised drug will be released into the local environment. Ventolin Respirator Solution should therefore be administered in a well ventilated room, particularly in hospitals when several patients may be using nebulisers at the same time.

*Marketing authorisation holder:* Glaxo Wellcome UK Ltd, trading as Allen & Hanburys Stockley Park West, Uxbridge, Middlesex UB11 1BT.

**Marketing authorisation number** 10949/0244

**Date of approval/revision of SPC** July 1996.

**Legal category** POM.

## VENTOLIN* ROTACAPS*

**Presentation** Ventolin Rotacaps capsules contain a mixture of microfine salbutamol sulphate and larger particle lactose in blue/colourless hard gelatin capsules. Each Rotacaps capsule contains 200 micrograms (light blue) or 400 micrograms (dark blue) of salbutamol (as sulphate) and is marked Ventolin 200 or Ventolin 400 respectively. The contents of a Rotacaps capsule are inhaled using a specific drug delivery device called a Ventolin Rotahaler*.

**Uses** Salbutamol is a selective $\beta_2$-agonist providing short-acting (4-6 hour) bronchodilatation with a fast onset (within 5 minutes) in reversible airways obstruction.

Ventolin Rotacaps can be used in the management of asthma, bronchospasm and/or reversible airways obstruction.

Ventolin Rotacaps are particularly suitable for the relief of asthma symptoms. They should be used to relieve symptoms when they occur, and to prevent them in those circumstances recognised by the patient to precipitate an asthma attack (e.g. before exercise or unavoidable allergen exposure).

Ventolin Rotacaps are particularly valuable as relief medication in mild, moderate or severe asthma, provided that reliance on them does not delay the introduction and use of regular inhaled corticosteroid therapy.

**Dosage and administration** Ventolin Rotacaps are for inhalation use only, using a Ventolin Rotahaler. Ventolin Rotacaps are suitable for many patients including those who cannot use a metered-dose inhaler successfully.

*Adults (including the elderly):* For the relief of acute bronchospasm 200 micrograms or 400 micrograms should be taken as a single dose. The maximum daily dose is 400 micrograms four times a day. To prevent allergen- or exercise-induced symptoms, 400 micrograms should be taken 10-15 minutes before challenge.

*Children:* The recommended dose for the relief of acute bronchospasm or before allergen exposure or exercise is 200 micrograms. The maximum daily dose is 200 micrograms four times a day.

On-demand use of Ventolin Rotacaps should not exceed four times daily. Reliance on such frequent supplementary use, or a sudden increase in dose, indicates poorly controlled or deteriorating asthma (see *Precautions*).

**Contra-indications, warnings, etc**

*Contra-indications:* Although intravenous salbutamol, and occasionally salbutamol tablets, are used in the management of premature labour uncomplicated by conditions such as placenta praevia, ante-partum haemorrhage or toxaemia of pregnancy, inhaled salbutamol preparations are not appropriate for managing premature labour. Salbutamol preparations should not be used for threatened abortion.

Ventolin Rotacaps are contra-indicated in patients with a history of hypersensitivity to any of the components.

*Precautions:* Patients should be instructed in the proper use of the Rotahaler device to ensure that the drug reaches the target area within the lungs.

Bronchodilators should not be the only or main treatment in patients with severe or unstable asthma. Severe asthma requires regular medical assessment, including lung-function testing, as patients are at risk of severe attacks and even death. Physicians should consider using the maximum recommended dose of inhaled corticosteroid and/or oral corticosteroid therapy in these patients.

The dosage or frequency of administration should only be increased on medical advice.

Increasing use of bronchodilators, in particular short-acting inhaled $\beta_2$-agonists to relieve symptoms, indicates deterioration of asthma control. The patient should be instructed to seek medical advice if short-acting relief bronchodilator treatment becomes less effective, or more inhalations than usual are required. In this situation the patient should be assessed and consideration given to the need for increased anti-inflammatory therapy (e.g. higher doses of inhaled corticosteroid or a course of oral corticosteroid).

Severe exacerbations of asthma must be treated in the normal way.

Salbutamol should be administered cautiously to patients suffering from thyrotoxicosis.

Salbutamol and non-selective β-blocking drugs such as propranolol, should not usually be prescribed together.

Potentially serious hypokalaemia may result from $\beta_2$-agonist therapy, mainly from parenteral and nebulised administration. Particular caution is advised in acute severe asthma as this effect may be potentiated by hypoxia and by concomitant treatment with xanthine derivatives, steroids and diuretics. Serum potassium levels should be monitored in such situations.

*Pregnancy:* Administration of drugs during pregnancy should only be considered if the expected benefit to the mother is greater than any possible risk to the fetus. As with the majority of drugs, there is little published evidence of the safety of salbutamol in the early stages of human pregnancy, but in animal studies there was evidence of some harmful effects on the fetus at very high dose levels.

*Lactation:* As salbutamol is probably secreted in breast milk, its use in nursing mothers requires careful consideration. It is not known whether salbutamol has a harmful effect on the neonate, and so its use should be restricted to situations where it is felt that the expected benefit to the mother is likely to outweigh any potential risk to the neonate.

*Side-effects:* As with other inhalation therapy, paradoxical bronchospasm may occur with an immediate increase in wheezing after dosing. This should be treated immediately with an alternative presentation or a different fast-acting inhaled bronchodilator. The preparation should be discontinued immediately, the patient assessed and, if necessary, alternative therapy instituted.

Hypersensitivity reactions including angioedema, urticaria, bronchospasm, hypotension and collapse have been reported very rarely.

Potentially serious hypokalaemia may result from $\beta_2$-agonist therapy.

Ventolin Rotacaps may cause a fine tremor of skeletal muscle, usually the hands are most obviously affected. This effect is dose-related and is common to all β-adrenergic stimulants.

Tachycardia, with or without peripheral vasodilatation, may rarely occur.

Headaches have occasionally been reported.

Mouth and throat irritation may occur with inhaled salbutamol.

As with other $\beta_2$-agonists hyperactivity in children has been reported rarely.

There have been very rare reports of muscle cramps.

*Overdosage:* The preferred antidote for overdosage with salbutamol is a cardioselective β-blocking agent, but β-blocking drugs should be used with caution in patients with a history of bronchospasm.

Hypokalaemia may occur following overdose with salbutamol. Serum potassium levels should be monitored.

**Pharmaceutical precautions** To keep the Rotacaps capsules in good condition it is important that they are stored in a dry place below 30°C where they will not be exposed to extremes of temperature. A convenient supply may be carried in the special container for the Rotahaler device. A capsule should only be inserted in the Rotahaler immediately prior to use. Failure to observe this instruction may affect the operation of the Rotahaler.

**Legal category** POM.

**Package quantities** Ventolin Rotacaps 200 micrograms and 400 micrograms are supplied in containers of 112.

**Further information** Ventolin Rotacaps do not cause difficulty in micturition because, unlike sympathomimetic drugs such as ephedrine, salbutamol does not stimulate alpha-adrenoceptors.

Ventolin Rotacaps are not contra-indicated in patients under treatment with monoamine oxidase inhibitors (MAOIs).

**Product licence numbers**
Ventolin Rotacaps 200 micrograms 10949/0072
Ventolin Rotacaps 400 micrograms 10949/0073

# VENTOLIN* SOLUTION FOR INTRAVENOUS INFUSION
## 5 mg in 5 ml (1 mg/ml)

**Qualitative and quantitative composition** Ventolin Solution for Intravenous Infusion 5 mg in 5 ml (1 mg/ml) is presented as ampoules of 5 ml, each containing 5 mg salbutamol as Salbutamol Sulphate BP in a sterile isotonic solution.

**Pharmaceutical form** Clear, colourless or pale straw-coloured solution for intravenous infusion.

**Clinical particulars**

*Therapeutic indications:* Ventolin Solution for Intravenous Infusion should be administered under the direction of a physician. It is indicated for two distinct clinical situations:

(1) For the relief of severe bronchospasm.

(2) In the management of premature labour; to arrest uncomplicated labour between 24 and 33 weeks of gestation in patients with no medical or obstetric contra-indication to tocolytic therapy. Data suggest that the main effect of tocolytic therapy is a delay in delivery of up to 48 hours. This delay may be used to administer glucocorticoids or to implement other measures known to improve perinatal health.

*Posology and method of administration:* Ventolin Solution for Intravenous Infusion is used to prepare an infusion solution. It should not be injected undiluted. Ventolin Solution for Intravenous Infusion should not be administered in the same syringe or infusion as any other medication.

1. *In severe bronchospasm.*

*Adults:* A suitable solution for infusion providing 10 micrograms salbutamol/ml is prepared by diluting 5 ml Ventolin Solution for Intravenous Infusion to 500 ml with an infusion solution such as Sodium Chloride and Dextrose Injection BP. Other suitable diluents are Water for Injections BP, Sodium Chloride Injection BP or Dextrose Injection BP.

Infusion rates providing 3 to 20 micrograms salbutamol/minute (0.3 to 2 ml/minute of the above infusion

solution) are usually adequate. Higher doses have been used with success in patients with respiratory failure.

*Children:* There are insufficient data to recommend a dosage regime for routine use.

2. *In the management of premature labour.*

The infusion, prepared as described below, should be administered as early as possible after the diagnosis of premature labour, and after evaluation of the patient to eliminate any contra-indications to the use of salbutamol (see *Contra-indications*).

During infusion the maternal pulse rate should be monitored and the infusion rate adjusted to avoid excessive maternal heart rate (above 140 beats/minute).

It is essential that the volume of infusion fluid is kept to a minimum to control the level of hydration and so avoid the risk of maternal pulmonary oedema (see *Undesirable effects*). A controlled infusion device, preferably a syringe pump, should be used.

Infusion rates providing 10 to 45 micrograms salbutamol/minute are generally adequate to control uterine contractions. A starting rate of 10 micrograms/minute is recommended, increasing the rate at 10-minute intervals until there is evidence of patient response shown by diminution in strength, frequency or duration of contractions. Thereafter the infusion rate may be increased slowly until contractions cease. Once uterine contractions have ceased the infusion rate should be maintained at the same level for one hour and then reduced by 50% decrements at six-hourly intervals. If labour progresses despite treatment the infusion should be stopped. If contractions have been successfully inhibited by the infusion, treatment may be continued orally with Ventolin Tablets 4 mg given three or four times daily.

*Dilution:* The recommended diluent is 5% Dextrose (see precautions for use in diabetic patients).

*For use in a syringe pump:* Prepare a solution providing 200 micrograms salbutamol/ml by diluting 10 ml Ventolin Solution for Intravenous Infusion with 40 ml diluent. An infusion rate of 10 to 45 micrograms/minute is equivalent to 0.05 to 0.225 ml/minute of this solution.

*Other infusion methods:* Prepare a solution providing 20 micrograms salbutamol/ml by diluting 10 ml Ventolin Solution for Intravenous Infusion with 490 ml diluent. An infusion rate of 10 to 45 micrograms/minute is equivalent to 0.5 to 2.25 ml/minute of this solution.

*Contra-indications:* Although Ventolin Solution for Intravenous Infusion and occasionally salbutamol tablets, are used in the management of premature labour uncomplicated by conditions such as placenta praevia, ante-partum haemorrhage or toxaemia of pregnancy, salbutamol preparations should not be used for threatened abortion.

Ventolin Solution for Intravenous Infusion is contra-indicated in patients with a history of hypersensitivity to any of the components.

*Special warnings and precautions for use:* Bronchodilators should not be the only or main treatment in patients with severe or unstable asthma. Severe asthma requires regular medical assessment, including lung-function testing, as patients are at risk of severe attacks and even death. Physicians should consider using the maximum recommended dose of inhaled corticosteroid and/or oral corticosteroid therapy in these patients.

The dosage or frequency of administration should only be increased on medical advice.

Patients being treated with Ventolin Solution for Intravenous Infusion may also be receiving short-acting inhaled bronchodilators to relieve symptoms. Increasing use of bronchodilators, in particular short-acting inhaled $\beta_2$-agonists to relieve symptoms, indicates deterioration of asthma control. The patient should be instructed to seek medical advice if short-acting relief bronchodilator treatment becomes less effective, or more inhalations than usual are required. In this situation the patient should be assessed and consideration given to the need for increased anti-inflammatory therapy (e.g. higher doses of inhaled corticosteroid or a course of oral corticosteroid).

Severe exacerbations of asthma must be treated in the normal way.

The use of Ventolin Solution for Intravenous Infusion in the treatment of severe bronchospasm does not obviate the requirement for corticosteroid therapy as appropriate. When practicable, administration of oxygen concurrently with parenteral Ventolin is recommended, particularly when it is given by intravenous infusion to hypoxic patients. In common with other β-adrenoceptor agonists, salbutamol can induce reversible metabolic changes such as hypokalaemia and increased blood glucose levels. Diabetic patients may be unable to compensate for the increase in blood glucose and the development of ketoacidosis has been reported. Concurrent administration of corticosteroids can exaggerate this effect.

Therefore, diabetic patients and those concurrently receiving corticosteroids should be monitored frequently during intravenous infusion of Ventolin so that remedial steps (e.g. an increase in insulin dosage) can be taken to counter any metabolic change occurring. For these patients it may be preferable to dilute Ventolin Solution for Intravenous Infusion in Sodium Chloride Injection BP rather than in diluents containing dextrose.

Salbutamol should be administered cautiously to patients suffering from thyrotoxicosis.

Potentially serious hypokalaemia may result from $\beta_2$-agonist therapy, mainly from parenteral and nebulised administration. Particular caution is advised in acute severe asthma as this effect may be potentiated by hypoxia and by concomitant treatment with xanthine derivatives, steroids and diuretics. Serum potassium levels should be monitored in such situations.

As maternal pulmonary oedema has been reported during or following treatment of premature labour with $\beta_2$-agonists, careful attention should be given to fluid balance and cardio-respiratory function monitored. In patients being treated for premature labour by intravenous infusion of salbutamol, increases in maternal heart rate of the order of 20 to 50 beats per minute usually accompany the infusion. The maternal pulse rate should be monitored and not normally allowed to exceed a steady rate of 140 beats per minute. Maternal blood pressure may fall slightly during the infusion; the effect being greater on diastolic than on systolic pressure. Falls in diastolic pressure are usually within the range of 10 to 20 mmHg. The effect of infusion on fetal heart rate is less marked, but increases of up to 20 beats per minute may occur. In the treatment of premature labour, before Ventolin Solution for Intravenous Infusion is given to any patient with known heart disease, an adequate assessment of the patient's cardiovascular status should be made by a physician experienced in cardiology. In order to minimise the risk of hypotension associated with tocolytic therapy, special care should be taken to avoid caval compression by keeping the patient in the left or right lateral positions throughout the infusion.

*Interaction with other medicaments and other forms of interaction:* Ventolin Solution for Intravenous Infusion should not be administered in the same syringe or infusion as any other medication.

Salbutamol and non-selective β-blocking drugs such as propranolol, should not usually be prescribed together.

*Pregnancy and lactation:* Administration of drugs during pregnancy should only be considered if the expected benefit to the mother is greater than any possible risk to the fetus. As with the majority of drugs, there is little published evidence of the safety of salbutamol in the early stages of human pregnancy, but in animal studies there was evidence of some harmful effects on the fetus at very high dose levels.

As salbutamol is probably secreted in breast milk, its use in nursing mothers requires careful consideration. It is not known whether salbutamol has a harmful effect on the neonate, and so its use should be restricted to situations where it is felt that the expected benefit to the mother is likely to outweigh any potential risk to the neonate.

*Effect on ability to drive and use machines:* None reported.

*Undesirable effects:* Hypersensitivity reactions including angioedema, urticaria, bronchospasm, hypotension and collapse have been reported very rarely.

Enhancement of physiological tremor may occur with Ventolin Solution for Intravenous Infusion. This effect is caused by a direct action on skeletal muscle and is common to all β-adrenergic stimulants.

Tachycardia, with or without dilatation of peripheral arterioles leading to a small reduction in arterial pressure, may occur. Increases in heart rate are more likely to occur in patients with normal heart rates and these increases are dose-dependent. In patients with pre-existing sinus tachycardia, especially those in status asthmaticus, the heart rate tends to fall as the condition of the patient improves.

Maternal pulmonary oedema has been reported in association with use of β-agonists, including salbutamol, for the management of premature labour; in some cases this has proved fatal. Predisposing factors include fluid overload, multiple pregnancy, pre-existing cardiac disease and maternal infection. Close monitoring of the patient's state of hydration is essential. If signs of pulmonary oedema develop (e.g. cough, shortness of breath), treatment should be discontinued immediately and diuretic therapy instituted.

Headaches have occasionally been reported.

There have been very rare reports of muscle cramps.

Potentially serious hypokalaemia may result from $\beta_2$-agonist therapy.

In the management of premature labour, intravenous infusion of Ventolin has occasionally been associated with nausea, vomiting and headaches.

*Overdose:* The preferred antidote for overdosage with salbutamol is a cardioselective β-blocking agent, but β-blocking drugs should be used with caution in patients with a history of bronchospasm.

Hypokalaemia may occur following overdose with salbutamol. Serum potassium levels should be monitored.

**Pharmacological properties**
*Pharmacodynamic properties:* Salbutamol is a selective $\beta_2$-agonist which acts on the $\beta_2$-adrenoceptors of the bronchi and uterus.

*Pharmacokinetic properties:* Salbutamol administered intravenously has a half-life of 4 to 6 hours and is cleared partly renally and partly by metabolism to the inactive 4'-0-sulphate (phenolic sulphate) which is also excreted primarily in the urine. The faeces are a minor route of excretion. Most of a dose of salbutamol given intravenously, orally or by inhalation is excreted within 72 hours. Salbutamol is bound to plasma proteins to the extent of 10%.

*Preclinical safety data:* No additional preclinical safety data are included here.

**Pharmaceutical particulars**
*List of excipients:* Sodium chloride, sodium hydroxide, sulphuric acid and Water for Injections.

*Incompatibilities:* None stated.

*Shelf life:* 36 months.

*Special precautions for storage:* Store below 30°C and protect from light.

*Nature and contents of container:* Clear, neutral glass ampoules, available in boxes of 10.

*Instructions for use/handling:* Ventolin Solution for Intravenous Infusion must be diluted before use. The recommended diluents are Water for Injections BP, Sodium Chloride Injection BP, Sodium Chloride and Dextrose Injection BP and Dextrose Injection BP. (See *Posology and method of administration.*)

All unused admixtures of Ventolin Solution for Intravenous Infusion with infusion fluids should be discarded twenty-four hours after preparation.

*Marketing authorisation holder:* Glaxo Wellcome UK Ltd, trading as Allen & Hanburys, Stockley Park West, Uxbridge, Middlesex UB11 1BT.

**Marketing authorisation number** 10949/0087

**Date of approval/revision of SPC** May 1996.

**Legal category** POM.

## VENTOLIN* SYRUP

**Presentation** Salbutamol 2 mg as Salbutamol Sulphate BP in each 5 ml of a fruit-flavoured, sugar-free syrup.

Other ingredients: Water, Sodium citrate, citric acid, hydroxypropylmethylcellulose, saccharin sodium, sodium chloride, sodium benzoate and orange flavour.

**Uses** Salbutamol is a selective $\beta_2$-agonist providing short-acting (4-6 hour) bronchodilatation in reversible airways obstruction.

Ventolin Syrup can be used in the management of asthma, bronchospasm and/or reversible airways obstruction.

Ventolin Syrup is suitable for children and adults who are unable to use an inhaler device.

**Dosage and administration**
*Adults:* The minimum starting dose is 2 mg (5 ml syrup) three times a day. The usual effective dose is 4 mg (10 ml syrup) three or four times a day, which may be increased to a maximum of 8 mg (20 ml syrup) three or four times a day if adequate bronchodilatation is not obtained.

In elderly patients, or in those known to be unusually sensitive to β-adrenergic stimulant drugs, it is advisable to initiate treatment with the minimum starting dose.

*Children 2–6 years:* The minimum starting dose is 1 mg (2.5 ml syrup) three times daily. This may be increased to 2 mg (5 ml syrup) three or four times daily.

*6–12 years:* The minimum starting dose is 2 mg (5 ml syrup) three times daily. This may be increased to four times daily.

*Over 12 years:* The minimum starting dose is 2 mg (5 ml syrup) three times daily. This may be increased to 4 mg (10 ml syrup) three or four times daily.

**Contra-indications, warnings, etc**
*Contra-indications:* Although intravenous salbutamol, and occasionally salbutamol tablets, are used in the management of premature labour uncomplicated by conditions such as placenta praevia, ante-partum haemorrhage or toxaemia of pregnancy, salbutamol preparations should not be used for threatened abortion.

Ventolin Syrup is contra-indicated in patients with a history of hypersensitivity to any of the components.

*Precautions:* Bronchodilators should not be the only or main treatment in patients with severe or unstable asthma. Severe asthma requires regular medical assessment, including lung-function testing, as patients are at risk of severe attacks and even death. Physicians should consider using the maximum recommended dose of inhaled corticosteroid and/or oral corticosteroid therapy in these patients.

Patients should seek medical advice if treatment with Ventolin Syrup becomes less effective.

The dosage or frequency of administration should only be increased on medical advice.

Patients taking Ventolin Syrup may also be receiving short-acting inhaled bronchodilators to relieve symptoms. Increasing use of bronchodilators, in particular short-acting inhaled $\beta_2$-agonists to relieve symptoms, indicates deterioration of asthma control. The patient should be instructed to seek medical advice if short-acting relief bronchodilator treatment becomes less effective, or more inhalations than usual are required. In this situation the patient should be assessed and consideration given to the need for increased anti-inflammatory therapy (e.g. higher doses of inhaled corticosteroid or a course of oral corticosteroid).

Severe exacerbations of asthma must be treated in the normal way.

Salbutamol should be administered cautiously to patients suffering from thyrotoxicosis.

Salbutamol and non-selective β-blocking drugs such as propranolol, should not usually be prescribed together.

Potentially serious hypokalaemia may result from $\beta_2$-agonist therapy, mainly from parenteral and nebulised administration. Particular caution is advised in acute severe asthma as this effect may be potentiated by hypoxia and by concomitant treatment with xanthine derivatives, steroids and diuretics. Serum potassium levels should be monitored in such situations.

In common with other β-adrenoceptor agonists, salbutamol can induce reversible metabolic changes such as increased blood glucose levels. Diabetic patients may be unable to compensate for the increase in blood glucose and the development of ketoacidosis has been reported. Concurrent administration of corticosteroids can exaggerate this effect.

*Pregnancy:* Administration of drugs during pregnancy should only be considered if the expected benefit to the mother is greater than any possible risk to the fetus. However, as with the majority of drugs, there is little published evidence of the safety of salbutamol in the early stages of human pregnancy, but in animal studies there was evidence of some harmful effects on the fetus at very high dose levels.

*Lactation:* As salbutamol is probably secreted in breast milk, its use in nursing mothers requires careful consideration. It is not known whether salbutamol has a harmful effect on the neonate and so its use should be restricted to situations where it is felt that the expected benefit to the mother is likely to outweigh any potential risk to the neonate.

*Side-effects:* Hypersensitivity reactions including angioedema, urticaria, bronchospasm, hypotension and collapse have been reported very rarely.

Potentially serious hypokalaemia may result from $\beta_2$-agonist therapy.

Ventolin Syrup may cause a fine tremor of skeletal muscle, usually the hands are most obviously affected. This effect is dose-related and is common to all β-adrenergic stimulants. A few patients feel tense. This is also due to the effects on skeletal muscle and not to direct CNS stimulation.

Tachycardia, with or without peripheral vasodilatation, may rarely occur.

Headaches have occasionally been reported.

As with other $\beta_2$-agonists hyperactivity in children has been reported rarely.

There have been very rare reports of muscle cramps.

*Overdosage:* The preferred antidote for overdosage with salbutamol is a cardioselective β-blocking agent, but β-blocking drugs should be used with caution in patients with a history of bronchospasm.

Hypokalaemia may occur following overdose with salbutamol. Serum potassium levels should be monitored.

**Pharmaceutical precautions** Ventolin Syrup should be stored at a temperature not exceeding 30°C. Ventolin Syrup should be protected from light.

*Dilution:* Ventolin Syrup does not contain sugars. It may be diluted with Purified Water BP. The resulting mixture should be protected from light and used within 28 days. A 50% v/v dilution of Ventolin Syrup has been shown to be adequately preserved against microbial contamination. However, to avoid the possibility of introducing excessive microbial contamination, the Purified Water used for dilution should be recently prepared or alternatively it should be boiled and cooled immediately before use. Dilution of Ventolin Syrup with Syrup BP or Sorbitol solutions is not recommended as this may result in precipitation of the cellulose thickening agent. Admixture of Ventolin Syrup with other liquid preparations is not recommended.

**Legal category** POM.

**Package quantities** Ventolin Syrup is supplied in bottles of 150 ml.

**Further information** Ventolin Syrup preparation does not contain sugars, so it is unlikely to predispose to dental caries with long-term use. It does not contain any artificial colouring agent.

Ventolin Syrup does not cause difficulty in micturition because, unlike sympathomimetic drugs such as ephedrine, salbutamol does not stimulate alpha-adrenoceptors.

Ventolin Syrup is not contra-indicated in patients under treatment with monoamine oxidase inhibitors (MAOIs).

**Product licence number** 10949/0088

## VOLMAX* TABLETS

**Presentation** *Volmax Tablets 4 mg*: White hexagonal controlled-release tablets each containing 4 mg salbutamol as Salbutamol Sulphate BP. Printed 4 on one side.

*Volmax Tablets 8 mg:* White hexagonal controlled-release tablets each containing 8 mg salbutamol as Salbutamol Sulphate BP. Printed 8 on one side.

Other ingredients: The tablet core contains sodium chloride, silica gel, povidone, croscarmellose sodium and magnesium stearate. The outer coats contain cellulose acetate, hydroxypropylmethylcellulose and E171 (titanium dioxide). The numbers '4' or '8' are printed with E132 (indigo carmine).

The tablets consist of an outer semi-permeable membrane and an inner core containing salbutamol sulphate. There is a hole in the outer coat which allows a gradual osmotically controlled release of the drug.

**Uses** Salbutamol is a selective $\beta_2$-adrenoceptor agonist.

Volmax Tablets are indicated for the treatment of asthma, bronchospasm and/or reversible airways obstruction.

Volmax Tablets are suitable oral therapy for children and adults who are unable to use an inhaler device. In these patients the controlled-release formulation makes Volmax Tablets helpful in the management of nocturnal asthma.

**Dosage and administration** Volmax Tablets must be swallowed whole with a glass of water and not chewed or crushed.

Volmax Tablets sustain bronchodilatation over a period of 12 hours.

Adults (including the elderly): One 8 mg tablet twice daily.

Children aged 3-12 years: One 4 mg tablet twice daily.

**Contra-indications, warnings, etc**
*Contra-indications:* Although intravenous salbutamol, and occasionally salbutamol tablets, are used in the management of premature labour uncomplicated by conditions such as placenta praevia, ante-partum haemorrhage or toxaemia of pregnancy, salbutamol preparations should not be used for threatened abortion.

Volmax Tablets are contra-indicated in patients with a history of hypersensitivity to any of the components.

*Precautions:* Bronchodilators should not be the only or main treatment in patients with severe or unstable asthma. Severe asthma requires regular medical assessment, including lung-function testing, as patients are at risk of severe attacks and even death. Physicians should consider using the maximum recommended dose of inhaled corticosteroid and/or oral corticosteroid therapy in these patients.

Patients should seek medical advice if treatment with Volmax Tablets becomes less effective.

The dosage or frequency of administration should only be increased on medical advice.

Patients taking Volmax Tablets may also be receiving short-acting inhaled bronchodilators to relieve symptoms. Increasing use of bronchodilators, in particular short-acting inhaled $\beta_2$-agonists to relieve symptoms, indicates deterioration of asthma control. The patient should be instructed to seek medical advice if short-acting relief bronchodilator treatment becomes less effective, or more inhalations than usual are required. In this situation the patient should be assessed and consideration given to the need for increased anti-inflammatory therapy (e.g. higher doses of inhaled corticosteroid or a course of oral corticosteroid).

Severe exacerbations of asthma must be treated in the normal way.

Salbutamol should be administered cautiously to patients suffering from thyrotoxicosis.

Salbutamol and non-selective β-blocking drugs such as propranolol, should not usually be prescribed together.

Potentially serious hypokalaemia may result from β₂-agonist therapy, mainly from parenteral and nebulised administration. Particular caution is advised in acute severe asthma as this effect may be potentiated by hypoxia and by concomitant treatment with xanthine derivatives, steroids and diuretics. Serum potassium levels should be monitored in such situations.

In common with other β-adrenoceptor agonists, salbutamol can induce reversible metabolic changes such as increased blood glucose levels. Diabetic patients may be unable to compensate for the increase in blood glucose and the development of ketoacidosis has been reported. Concurrent administration of corticosteroids can exaggerate this effect.

*Pregnancy:* Administration of drugs during pregnancy should only be considered if the expected benefit to the mother is greater than any possible risk to the fetus. As with the majority of drugs, there is little published evidence of the safety of salbutamol in the early stages of human pregnancy, but in animal studies there was evidence of some harmful effects on the fetus at very high dose levels.

*Lactation:* As salbutamol is probably secreted in breast milk, its use in nursing mothers requires careful consideration. It is not known whether salbutamol has a harmful effect on the neonate and so its use should be restricted to situations where it is felt that the expected benefit to the mother is likely to outweigh any potential risk to the neonate.

*Side-effects:* Hypersensitivity reactions including angioedema, urticaria, bronchospasm, hypotension and collapse have been reported very rarely.

Potentially serious hypokalaemia may result from β₂-agonist therapy.

Volmax Tablets may cause a fine tremor of skeletal muscle, usually the hands are most obviously affected. This effect is common to all β-adrenergic stimulants. A few patients feel tense. This is also due to the effects on skeletal muscle and not to direct CNS stimulation.

Tachycardia, with or without peripheral vasodilatation, may rarely occur.

Headaches have occasionally been reported.

As with other β₂-agonists hyperactivity in children has been reported rarely.

There have been very rare reports of muscle cramps.

*Overdosage:* The preferred antidote for overdosage with salbutamol is a cardioselective beta-blocking agent, but β-blocking drugs should be used with caution in patients with a history of bronchospasm.

Hypokalaemia may occur following overdose with salbutamol. Serum potassium levels should be monitored.

**Pharmaceutical precautions** Volmax Tablets should be stored at a temperature not exceeding 30°C. Volmax Tablets should not be removed from their foil pack until required.

**Legal category** POM.

**Package quantities** Volmax Tablets are supplied in double-foil blisters of 14 in cartons of 56.

**Further information** Volmax Tablets do not cause difficulty in micturition because, unlike sympathomimetic drugs such as ephedrine, salbutamol does not stimulate alpha-adrenoceptors.

Volmax Tablets are not contra-indicated in patients under treatment with monoamine oxidase inhibitors (MAOIs).

**Product licence numbers**
Volmax Tablets 4 mg 10949/0089
Volmax Tablets 8 mg 10949/0090

*\*Trade Mark*

# Allergan Ltd
Coronation Road
High Wycombe
Bucks HP12 3SH

## ACULAR* ▼

**Presentation**  Clear, colourless to slightly yellow, sterile ophthalmic solution containing ketorolac trometamol 0.5% (w/v). Also contains benzalkonium chloride PhEur 0.01% (w/v) and disodium edetate PhEur 0.1% (w/v), with octoxynol 40, sodium chloride PhEur, sodium hydroxide PhEur or hydrochloric acid PhEur (to adjust pH) and purified water PhEur.

**Uses**  Acular is indicated for the prophylaxis and reduction of inflammation and associated symptoms following ocular surgery.

**Dosage and administration**  One drop instilled into the eye three times daily starting 24 hours pre-operatively and continuing for up to three weeks post-operatively.

**Contra-indications, warnings, etc**
*Contra-indications:* Acular is contra-indicated in individuals hypersensitive to any component of the medication.

The potential exists for cross-sensitivity to acetyl-salicylic acid and other non-steroidal anti-inflammatory drugs. Acular is contra-indicated in individuals who have previously exhibited sensitivities to these drugs.

Acular is contra-indicated in children and during pregnancy or lactation.

*Warnings:* It is recommended that Acular be used with caution in patients with known bleeding tendencies, patients who are receiving other medications which may prolong bleeding time, or patients with a known history of peptic ulceration.

In common with other anti-inflammatory drugs, Acular may mask signs of infection.

Acular contains benzalkonium chloride as a preservative and should not be used in patients continuing to wear soft (hydrophilic) contact lenses.

Transient blurring of vision may occur on instillation of eye drops. Do not drive or use hazardous machinery unless vision is clear.

*Use in pregnancy and lactation:* There was no evidence of teratogenicity in rats or rabbits studied at maternally-toxic doses of ketorolac. Prolongation of the gestation period and/or delayed parturition were seen in the rat. Ketorolac and its metabolites have been showed to pass into the foetus and milk of animals. Ketorolac has been detected in human milk at low levels. Safety in human pregnancy has not been established. Ketorolac is therefore contra-indicated during pregnancy, labour or delivery, or in mothers who are breast feeding.

*Adverse reactions:* The most frequent adverse events reported with the use of Acular are transient stinging and burning on instillation and other minor symptoms of ocular irritation.

Blurring and/or diminished vision have been reported with the use of Acular and other non-steroidal anti-inflammatory drugs.

None of the typical adverse reactions reported with the systemic non-steroidal anti-inflammatory agents (including ketorolac trometamol) have been observed at the doses used in topical ophthalmic therapy.

*Drug interactions:* Acular has been safely administered with systemic and ophthalmic medications such as antibiotics, sedatives, beta blockers, carbonic anhydrase inhibitors, miotics, mydriatics, cycloplegics and corticosteroids.

**Pharmaceutical precautions**  Discard any unused contents 28 days after opening the bottle. To avoid contamination do not allow dropper tip to touch any surface. Keep out of reach of children.

**Legal category**  Prescription only medicine (POM).

**Package quantities**  Acular is supplied in a plastic dropper bottle containing 5 ml.

**Further information**  Acular (ketorolac trometamol) is a non-steroidal anti-inflammatory agent demonstrating analgesic and anti-inflammatory activity. Ketorolac trometamol inhibits the cyclo-oxygenase enzyme essential for biosynthesis of prostaglandins. Acular has been shown to reduce prostaglandin levels in the aqueous humour after topical ophthalmic administration.

In pre-clinical studies Acular did not a) delay the healing of experimental corneal wounds, or b) enhance the spread of experimental ocular infections of *Candida albicans, Herpes simplex* virus type one, or *Pseudomonas aeruginosa.*

Ketorolac trometamol given systemically does not cause pupil constriction. Results from clinical studies indicate that Acular has no significant effect on intraocular pressure.

**Product licence number**  0426/0082

## ALPHAGAN* ▼

**Qualitative and quantitative composition**  Brimonidine tartrate 0.2% (equivalent to brimonidine base 0.13%).

**Pharmaceutical form**  Eye drops.

**Clinical particulars**
*Therapeutic indications:* Alphagan may be used as monotherapy for the lowering of intraocular pressure (IOP) in patients with open angle glaucoma or ocular hypertension, who are known, or thought likely to be intolerant of topical betablocker therapy and/or in whom topical betablocker therapy is contra-indicated. Alphagan may be used as adjunctive therapy when IOP is not adequately controlled by a topical beta-blocking agent.

*Posology and method of administration:* The recommended dose is one drop of Alphagan in the affected eye(s) twice daily, approximately 12 hours apart. No dosage adjustment is required for use in elderly patients.

If more than one topical ophthalmic drug is to be used, the drugs should be instilled 5–15 minutes apart.

The safety and effectiveness of Alphagan in children has not been established.

*Contra-indications:* Alphagan is contra-indicated in patients with hypersensitivity to brimonidine tartrate or any component of this medication. Alphagan is also contra-indicated in patients receiving monoamine oxidase (MAO) inhibitor therapy and patients on antidepressants which affect noradrenergic transmission (e.g. tricyclic antidepressants and mianserin).

*Special warnings and special precautions for use:* Caution should be exercised in treating patients with severe cardiovascular disease.

Alphagan should be used with caution in patients with depression, cerebral or coronary insufficiency, Raynaud's phenomenon, orthostatic hypotension or thromboangiitis obliterans.

Alphagan has not been studied in patients with hepatic or renal impairment; caution should be used in treating such patients.

The preservative in Alphagan, benzalkonium chloride, may be absorbed by soft contact lenses. Patients wearing soft (hydrophilic) contact lenses should be instructed to wait at least 15 minutes before inserting soft contact lenses after instilling Alphagan.

*Interactions:* Although specific drug interaction studies have not been conducted with Alphagan, the possibility of an additive or potentiating effect with CNS depressants (alcohol, barbiturates, opiates, sedatives, or anaesthetics) should be considered.

No data on the level of circulating catecholamines after Alphagan administration are available. Caution, however, is advised in patients taking medications which can affect the metabolism and uptake of circulating amines.

After the application of Alphagan, clinically insignificant decreases in blood pressure were noted in some patients. Caution is advised when using drugs such as antihypertensives and/or cardiac glycosides concomitantly with Alphagan.

Caution is advised when initiating (or changing the dose of) a concomitant systemic agent which may interact with alpha-adrenergic agonists or interfere with their activity i.e. sympathomimetic agents, agonists or antagonists of the adrenergic receptor.

*Pregnancy and lactation:* The safety of use during human pregnancy has not been established. Evaluation of experimental animal studies does not indicate direct or indirect harmful effects with respect to the development of the embryo or foetus, the course of gestation and peri- and postnatal development. Alphagan should be used during pregnancy only if the potential benefit to the mother justifies the potential risk to the foetus.

*Use during lactation:* It is not known if Alphagan is excreted in human milk. Caution should be exercised when administering Alphagan to nursing women, since it has been shown to be excreted in the milk of the lactating rat.

*Effects on ability to drive and use machines:* Alphagan may cause fatigue and/or drowsiness, which may impair the ability to drive or operate machinery.

*Undesirable effects:*
*Ocular effects:* The most frequently reported ocular adverse events were ocular hyperaemia, ocular burning/stinging, blurring, foreign body sensation, conjunctival follicles and ocular pruritus. Ocular allergic reaction occurred in 12.7% of subjects in clinical trials. Of these subjects, the onset of ocular allergy occurred between 3 and 9 months in the majority of patients.

Ocular events occurring occasionally included: corneal erosion/staining, photophobia, eyelid hyperaemia, ocular ache/pain, ocular dryness, tearing, eyelid oedema, conjunctival oedema, blepharitis, conjunctival blanching, ocular irritation, abnormal vision, conjunctival discharge and conjunctivitis.

*Systemic effects:* The most frequently reported systemic effects were oral dryness, headache and fatigue/drowsiness.

Occasional reports included upper respiratory symptoms, dizziness, gastrointestinal symptoms, asthenia and abnormal taste.

Rarely reported systemic events included depression, systemic allergic reaction, nasal dryness and palpitations.

*Overdose:* Ophthalmic overdose: There is no experience with the unlikely case of an overdosage via the ophthalmic route.

*Systemic overdose resulting from accidental ingestion:* No incidences of human ingestion of Alphagan are known. Oral overdoses of other alpha₂ agonists have been reported to cause symptoms such as hypotension, asthenia, vomiting, lethargy, sedation, bradycardia, arrhythmias, miosis, respiratory depression and seizure.

No clinical signs were observed at the 2 mg base/kg dose level using 0.2% of Alphagan orally in mice and rats. This dose is equivalent to a total of 15 ml of Alphagan inadvertently consumed by a 10 kg child.

**Pharmacological properties**
*Pharmacodynamic properties:* Alphagan is an alpha adrenergic receptor agonist that is 1000-fold more selective for the alpha₂ adrenoreceptor than the alpha₁ adrenoreceptor. This selectivity results in no mydriasis and the absence of vasoconstriction in microvessels associated with human retinal xenografts.

Topical administration of brimonidine decreases intraocular pressure (IOP) in humans with minimal effect on cardiovascular parameters. There are no effects on pulmonary function.

Alphagan has a rapid onset of action, with peak ocular hypotensive effect seen at two hours post dosing.

Fluorophotometric studies in animals and humans suggest that brimonidine tartrate has a dual mechanism of action. It is thought that Alphagan may lower IOP by reducing aqueous humour production and enhancing uveoscleral outflow.

*Pharmacokinetic properties:*
*General characteristics:* After ocular administration of a 0.2% solution twice daily for 10 days, plasma concentrations were low (mean Cmax was 0.06 ng/ml). There was a slight accumulation in the blood after multiple (2 times daily for 10 days) instillations. The area under the plasma concentration-time curve over 12 hours at steady state ($AUC_{0-12h}$) was 0.31 ng·hr/ml, as compared to 0.23 ng·hr/ml after the first dose. The mean apparent half-life in the systemic circulation was approximately 3 hours in humans after topical dosing.

The plasma protein binding of brimonidine after topical dosing in humans is approximately 29%.

In humans, the systemic metabolism of brimonidine is extensive undergoing primarily hepatic metabolism. *In vitro* metabolism by animal liver is mediated largely by aldehyde oxidase and cytochrome P450.

After oral administration, brimonidine and its metabolites are rapidly eliminated from systemic circulation via urinary excretion in both animals and man. A small amount of the dose is excreted as the parent drug in urine. Approximately 87% of an orally administered radioactive dose is eliminated in humans within 120 hours, with 74% found in the urine.

*Kinetics profile:* Both plasma Cmax and AUC of brimonidine increase linearly with ocular dosing.

*Characteristics in elderly patients:* The Cmax, AUC, and apparent half-life of brimonidine are similar in the elderly (subjects 65 years or older) compared with young adults, indicating that its systemic absorption and elimination are not affected by age.

*Preclinical safety data:* Alphagan has been shown to be non mutagenic and non carcinogenic in a series of animal studies.

**Pharmaceutical particulars**

*List of excipients:* Benzalkonium chloride (preservative); polyvinyl alcohol; sodium chloride; sodium citrate dihydrate; citric acid monohydrate; purified water; hydrochloric acid or sodium hydroxide to adjust pH.

*Incompatibilities:* Physical and chemical incompatibilities have not been observed.

*Shelf life:* Alphagan has a shelf life of 36 months in the unopened 5 ml container and should be used within 28 days after first opening.

*Special precautions for storage:* Alphagan should be stored at or below 25°C (77°F).

*Nature and contents of container:* White low density polyethylene dropper bottles with a 35 microlitre tip. The cap is either a conventional screw cap or a Compliance Cap (C-Cap).

*Instructions for use/handling:* None.

**Marketing authorisation number** 00426/0088

**Date of approval/revision of SPC** March 1997.

**Legal category** POM.

## BETAGAN*

**Presentation** Betagan is a clear, colourless to light yellow, sterile ophthalmic solution containing levobunolol hydrochloride 0.5% (w/v). Also contains Liquifilm* (polyvinyl alcohol USP) 1.4% (w/v), benzalkonium chloride PhEur 0.004% (w/v), disodium edetate PhEur 0.0127% (w/v), with sodium metabisulphite BP, sodium phosphate dibasic USP, potassium phosphate monobasic USP, sodium chloride PhEur and purified water PhEur.

Betagan Unit Dose is a clear, colourless to light yellow, sterile ophthalmic solution in unit dose presentation, containing levobunolol hydrochloride USP 0.5% (w/v). Also contains Liquifilm* (polyvinyl alcohol USP) 1.4% (w/v), disodium edetate PhEur 0.1% (w/v), sodium phosphate dibasic USP, potassium phosphate monobasic NF, sodium chloride PhEur and purified water PhEur.

**Uses** Betagan is indicated for the reduction of intraocular pressure in chronic open-angle glaucoma and ocular hypertension.

**Dosage and administration** The recommended adult dose is one drop of Betagan in the affected eye(s) once or twice daily.

EACH VIAL OF BETAGAN UNIT DOSE SHOULD BE USED FOR A SINGLE DOSE AND DISCARDED AFTER USE.

In common with other topical ophthalmic beta-adrenergic blocking agents, full clinical response may take several weeks to occur. Intraocular pressure should, therefore, be measured approximately four weeks after starting treatment. Because of diurnal variations in intraocular pressure satisfactory response is best determined by measuring the intraocular pressure at different times during the day.

*Use in the elderly:* The recommended dosage is suitable for use in the elderly.

*Use in children:* Betagan is not currently recommended for use in children.

*Concomitant administration:* If the patient's intraocular pressure is not satisfactory on this regimen, concomitant therapy with dipivefrin or adrenaline, and/or pilocarpine and other miotics, and/or systemically administered carbonic anhydrase inhibitors can be instituted.

**Contra-indications, warnings, etc**

*Contra-indications:* Bronchial asthma; history of bronchial asthma; chronic obstructive pulmonary disease; sinus bradycardia; second and third degree atrioventricular block; cardiac failure; cardiogenic shock; hypersensitivity to any component.

*Warnings:* As with other topically applied ophthalmic drugs, Betagan may be absorbed systemically and adverse reactions typical of oral beta-adrenoceptor blocking agents may occur.

Respiratory and cardiac reactions have been reported including, rarely, death due to bronchospasm or associated with cardiac failure.

Congestive heart failure should be adequately controlled before commencing therapy with Betagan.

In patients with a history of cardiac disease pulse rates should be monitored.

Diabetic control should be monitored during Betagan therapy in patients with labile diabetes.

Betagan contains benzalkonium chloride and should not be used in patients continuing to wear hydrophilic (soft) contact lenses.

Betagan has little or no effect on pupil size and if administered in angle-closure glaucoma, for reduction of intraocular pressure, must only be given in combination with a miotic.

*Use in pregnancy:* Betagan has not been studied in human pregnancy. It is recommended that Betagan be avoided in pregnancy.

*Use during lactation:* If treatment with Betagan during lactation is considered necessarily for the benefit of the mother, consideration should be given to the cessation of breast feeding.

*Interactions:* Use with caution in patients receiving oral beta-adrenergic blocking agents, because of the potential for additive effects on systemic blockade.

*Side effects:*

*Ocular:* Transient burning and stinging on instillation; blepharoconjunctivitis and iridocyclitis have been reported occasionally. The pharmacological and physical properties of levobunolol indicate a potential for post-instillation reduction in corneal sensitivity: this potential has not been confirmed in clinical studies with Betagan.

*Cardiovascular:* Bradycardia and hypotension have been reported occasionally.

*Respiratory:* There have been reports of dyspnoea and asthma.

*CNS:* Headache, transient ataxia and dizziness, and lethargy have been reported occasionally.

*Dermatological:* Urticaria and pruritis have been rarely reported.

*Overdosage:* There are no data available on human overdosage with Betagan, which is unlikely to occur via the ocular route. Should accidental ocular overdosage occur, flush the eye(s) with water or normal saline. If accidentally ingested, systemic symptoms may result.

The symptoms associated with systemic overdosage are most likely to be bradycardia, hypotension, bronchospasm and cardiac failure. Therapy for overdosage of a beta-adrenergic blocking agent should be instituted, such as intravenous administration of atropine sulphate 0.25 to 2 mg to induce vagal blockade. Conventional therapy for hypotension, bronchospasm, heart block and cardiac failure may be necessary.

**Pharmaceutical precautions** Betagan should be stored at or below 25°C and protected from light. Discard any unused contents 28 days after opening the bottle. Discard each unit dose vial after use. Keep out of the reach of children.

**Legal category** POM.

**Package quantities** Betagan is supplied in plastic dropper bottles containing 5 ml of 0.5% w/v solution or in a triple pack (3×5 ml bottles). Betagan Unit Dose is supplied in plastic unit-dose vials containing 0.4 ml of 0.5% w/v solution of levobunolol hydrochloride. Cartons contain 30 unit doses. The unit dose vials are packaged in foil pouches, with five unit dose vials enclosed in each foil pouch.

**Further information** In controlled clinical studies of approximately two years duration, intraocular pressure was well controlled in approximately 80% of subjects treated with Betagan 0.5% b.i.d. No significant effect on pupil size, tear production or corneal sensitivity was observed.

In a 3 month study, one drop once-a-day of Betagan 0.5% controlled intraocular pressure in 72% of subjects.

The onset of action is detected within one hour of instillation, with maximum effect seen between 2 and 6 hours. A significant decrease in intraocular pressure can be maintained for up to 24 hours following a single dose.

Diminished response after prolonged therapy has been reported in some patients.

Betagan reduces intraocular pressure with little or no effect on pupil size or accommodation, so the blurred vision and night blindness associated with miotics would not be expected and have not been reported with use of Betagan. This is particularly important in cataract patients with lens opacities who experience decreased visual acuity with pupillary constriction on miotic therapy.

**Product licence numbers**

Betagan 0426/0060
Betagan Unit Dose 0426/0072

## BOTOX* ▼

**Qualitative and quantitative composition** *Clostridium botulinum* toxin type A-haemagglutinin complex, 100 units.

**Pharmaceutical form** Powder for solution for injection.

**Clinical particulars**

*Therapeutic indications:* Botox is indicated for the symptomatic relief of blepharospasm, hemifacial spasm and idiopathic cervical dystonia (spasmodic torticollis).

*Posology and method of administration:* **Doses recommended for Botox are not interchangeable with other preparations of botulinum toxin.**

There is no difference in dose between adults and the elderly. The safety and effectiveness of Botox in children have not been demonstrated.

*Blepharospasm:* After reconstitution, Botox is injected using a sterile, 27–30 gauge needle.

Electromyographic guidance is not necessary. The initial recommended dose is 1.25–2.5 U (0.05–0.1 ml volume at each site) injected into the medial and lateral orbicularis oculi of the upper lid and the lateral orbicularis oculi of the lower lid. Additional sites in the brow area, the lateral orbicularis and in the upper facial area may also be injected if spasms here interfere with vision. In general, the initial effect of the injections is seen within three days and reaches a peak at one to two weeks post-treatment. Each treatment lasts approximately three months, following which the procedure can be repeated indefinitely. At repeat treatment sessions, the dose may be increased up to two-fold if the response from the initial treatment is considered insufficient – usually defined as an effect that does not last longer than two months. However, there appears to be little benefit obtainable from injecting more than 5.0 U per site. The intial dose should not exceed 25 U per eye. Normally no additional benefit is conferred by treating more frequently than every three months. It is rare for the effect to be permanent.

In the management of blepharospasm total dosing should not exceed 100 U every 12 weeks.

*Hemifacial spasm:* Patients with hemifacial spasm or VIIth nerve disorders should be treated as for unilateral blepharospasm, with other affected facial muscles being injected as needed. Electromyographic control may be necessary to identify affected small circumoral muscles.

*Cervical dystonia:* Several dosing regimens have been used in clinical trials for treatment of cervical dystonia with Botox. Dosing must be tailored to the individual patient based on the patient's head and neck position, location of pain, muscle hypertrophy, patient's body weight, and patient response.

In practice, the maximum total dose is not usually more than 200 U. No more than 50 U should be given at any one injection site. The dilutions suggested are indicated in the following table:

| *Diluent added* | *Resulting dose in units per 0.1 ml* |
|---|---|
| 0.5 ml | 20.0 U |
| 1.0 ml | 10.0 U |
| 2.0 ml | 5.0 U |
| 4.0 ml | 2.5 U |
| 8.0 ml | 1.25 U |

The treatment of cervical dystonia typically may include injection of Botox into the sternocleidomastoid, levator scapulae, scalene, splenius capitis, and/or the trapezius muscle(s). The muscle mass and the degree of hypertrophy are factors to be taken into consideration when selecting the appropriate dose.

The sternocleidomastoid muscle should not be injected bilaterally as there is an increased risk of adverse effects (in particular dysphagia) when bilateral injections or doses in excess of 100 U are administered to this muscle.

A 25, 27 or 30 gauge needle may be used for superficial muscles, and a 22 gauge needle may be used for deeper musculature. For cervical dystonia, localisation of the involved muscles with electromyographic guidance may be useful.

Multiple injection sites allow Botox to have more uniform contact with the innervation areas of the dystonic muscle and are especially useful in larger muscles. The optimal number of injection sites is dependent upon the size of the muscle to be chemically denervated.

*Contra-indications:* Botox is contra-indicated (a) in individuals with a known hypersensitivity to any component of the formulation; (b) when there are generalised disorders of muscle activity (e.g. myasthenia gravis); (c) when aminoglycoside antibiotics or spectinomycin are already being used or are likely to be used; (d) when there are bleeding disorders of any type, in case of anticoagulant therapy and whenever there is any reason to avoid intramuscular injections, and (e) during pregnancy or lactation.

*Special warnings and special precautions for use:* The relevant anatomy, and any alterations to the anatomy due to prior surgical procedures, must be understood

The following doses are recommended:

| Cervical dystonia classification | Muscle groupings | Total dosage; number of sites |
|---|---|---|
| *Type I* Head *rotated* toward side of shoulder elevation | Sternomastoid | 50–100 U; at least 2 sites |
| | Levator scapulae | 50 U; 1–2 sites |
| | Scalene | 25–50 U; 1–2 sites |
| | Splenius capitis | 25–75 U; 1–3 sites |
| | Trapezius | 25–100 U; 1–8 sites |
| *Type II* Head rotation only | Sternomastoid | 25–100 U; at least 2 sites if >25 U given |
| *Type III* Head *tilted* toward side of shoulder elevation | Sternomastoid | 25–100 U at posterior border; at least 2 sites if >25 U given |
| | Levator scapulae | 25–100 U; at least 2 sites |
| | Scalene | 25–75 U; at least 2 sites |
| | Trapezius | 25–100 U; 1–8 sites |
| *Type IV* Bilateral posterior cervical muscle spasm with elevation of the face | Splenius capitis and cervicis | 50–200 U; 2–8 sites, treat bilaterally (This is the total dose and not the dose for each side of the neck) |

prior to administering Botox. Extra caution should be paid in the case of injection sites close to structures such as the carotid artery and pleural apices.

The recommended dosages and frequency of administration of Botox should not be exceeded.

Adrenaline and other treatments for anaphylaxis should be available.

**Reconstituted Botox is for intramuscular injection ONLY.**

*Blepharospasm:* Reduced blinking following Botox injection of the orbicularis muscle can lead to corneal exposure, persistent epithelial defect and corneal ulceration, especially in patietns with VIIth nerve disorders. Careful testing of corneal sensation in eyes previously operated upon, avoidance of injection into the lower lid area to avoid ectropion, and vigorous treatment of any epithelial defect should be employed. This may require protective drops, ointment, bandage soft contact lenses, or closure of the eye by patching or other means.

*Cervical dystonia:* Limiting the dose injected into the sternocleidomastoid muscle to less than 100 U may decrease the occurrence of dysphagia. Patients with smaller neck muscle mass, or patients who require bilateral injections into the sternocleidomastoid muscle, have been reported to be at greater risk of dysphagia. Dysphagia is attributable to the spread of the toxin to the oesophageal musculature.

*General:* The safety and effectiveness of Botox in children have not been demonstrated.

*Interactions with other medicaments and other forms of interaction:* The effect of botulinum toxin may be potentiated by aminoglycoside antibiotics or other drugs that interfere with neuromuscular transmission e.g. tubocurarine-type muscle relaxants. Concomitant use of Botox with aminoglycosides or spectinomycin is contra-indicated. Polymyxins, tetracyclines and lincomycin should be used with caution in the Botox-treated patient. Muscle relaxants should also be used with caution, perhaps reducing the starting dose of relaxant, or using an intermediate-action drug, such as vecuronium or atracurium, rather than those with longer lasting effects.

*Pregnancy and lactation:* Botox has been shown to produce abortions and effects at daily doses of 0.125 U/kg/day and at 2 U/kg and higher in rabbits, the most sensitive species; whereas in rats and mice, no abortions or effects were observed when up to 4 U/kg of Botox were injected. Doses of 8 and 16 U/kg in rats and mice have been shown to be associated with reduced foetal body weight and/or delayed ossification of the hyoid bone, which may be reversible.

Botox is contra-indicated in pregnancy and lactation.

*Effects on the ability to drive and use machines:* Due to the nature of the disease being treated, the effects of Botox on the ability to drive or to operate machines cannot be predicted. Some of the post-therapy and/or unwanted effects may temporarily impair the ability to drive or operate machinery and consequently an affected person should avoid these tasks until faculties are fully recovered.

*Undesirable effects:* Side-effects may occur from misplaced injections of Botox temporarily paralysing nearby muscle groups. Execessive doses may cause paralysis in muscles distant to the injection site.

*Blepharospasm:* The most commonly-reported side-effects are ptosis, lacrimation, irritation (including dry eye and photophobia) and lagophthalmos. Ectropion, keratitis, diplopia and entropion have been reported rarely. Ecchymosis occurs easily in the soft eyelid tissues. This can be minimised by applying gentle pressure at the injection site immediately after the injection.

One case of angle-closure glaucoma following treatment with botulinum toxin has been reported.

*Cervical dystonia:* In an evaluation of 710 patients, dysphagia was observed in 15.8% of the patients. Other frequently reported adverse reactions were pain and soreness at the injection site (16.3%), and local weakness (12.8%). Less frequent adverse reactions (1–5%) included bruising at the injection site, general weakness, malaise and nausea.

Rare adverse events observed during clinical trials in <1% of patients with Botox injection include drowsiness, numbness, stiffness, diplopia, ptosis, headache, dyspnea, fever, and flu syndrome.

Further possible adverse events which may be associated with treatment for cervical dystonia are neck weakness and instability, head tremor, dysphonia and interference with local autonomic system functions (e.g. dry mouth) and allergic reactions such as mild fever and/or the development of a local or more generalised maculo-papular rash.

Dysphagia ranges in severity from very mild to severe, with potential for aspiration, and in rare instances may require medical intervention. It may persist for two or three weeks after injection, but has been reported in one case to last five months post-injection. Dysphagia appears to be dose-related and has been reported in clinical trials to occur less frequently with total doses below 200 U in one treatment session.

*General:* Following injection of Botox some distant muscles can show increased electrophysiologic jitter which is not associated with clinical weakness or other types of electrophysiologic abnormalities.

This product contains a small amount of human albumin.

The viral safety of the human albumin used as excipient in Botox is documentated through the several steps of its preparation. Particular care is given to the controls of the donors, to the manufacturing process and to the virus removal/inactivation process. Concerning this last point, a high margin of safety from the risk of viral transmission is got by using a combination of removal by the Cohn ethanol fractionation process and inactivation by pasteurisation (10 hours at 60°C).

Botox has not been known to transmit hepatitis or human immunodeficiency virus.

*Overdosage:* Based on reports on individual human cases of intoxication, the lethal dose for humans is estimated to be 3,000 to 30,000 U or higher after oral administration.

A case of peripheral neuropathy has been reported in a large adult male who received 1800 U of Botox intramuscularly (for neck and back spasm, and severe pain) in an 11 week period. There have not been any reported instances of systemic toxicity resulting from accidental injection or oral ingestion of Botox. Should overdosage occur, the patient should be medically supervised for several days for signs or symptoms of systemic weakness or muscle paralysis. The entire content of one vial is below the estimated dose for systemic toxicity in humans weighing 6 kg or greater.

Specific anti-toxin to botulinum toxin is only likely to be effective if given within 30 minutes of botulinum toxin injection.

**Pharmacological properties**

*Pharmacodynamic properties:* ATC class MO3A X01.

The active constituent in Botox is a protein complex derived from *Clostridium botulinum*. The protein consists of type A neurotoxin and several other proteins. Under physiological conditions it is presumed that the complex dissociates and releases the pure neurotoxin.

*Clostridium botulinum* toxin type A blocks cholinergic transport at the neuromuscular junction by preventing the release of acetylcholine. The nerve endings of the neuromuscular junction no longer respond to nerve impulses and secretion of the chemotransmitter is prevented (chemical denervation). Re-establishment of impulse transmission is by newly formed nerve endings and motor end plates.

*Pharmacokinetic properties:*

*(a) General characteristics of the active substance:* Classical absorption, distribution, biotransformation and elimination studies on the active substance have not been performed due to the extreme toxicity of botulinum toxin type A.

*(b) Characteristics in patients:* Human ADME studies have not been performed due to the nature of the product. It is believed that little systemic distribution of therapeutic doses of Botox occurs. Botox is probably metabolised by proteases and the molecular components recycled through normal metabolic pathways.

*Preclinical safety data:*

*Acute toxicity:* In monkeys receiving a single intramuscular (i.m.) injection of Botox, the No Observed Effect Level (NOEL) ranged from 4 to 24 U/kg. The i.m. $LD_{50}$ was reported to be 39 U/kg.

*Toxicity on repeated injection:* In three different studies (six months in rats; 20 weeks in juvenile monkeys; 1 year in monkeys) where the animals received i.m. injections, the NOEL was at the following respective Botox dosage levels: <4 U/kg, 8 U/kg and 4 U/kg. The main systemic effect was a transient decrease in body weight gain.

There was no indication of a cumulative effect in the animal studies when Botox was given at dosage intervals of 1 month or greater.

*Local toxicity:* Botox was shown not to cause ocular or dermal irritation, or give rise to toxicity when injected into the vitreous body in rabbits.

Allergic or inflammatory reactions in the area of the injection sites are rarely observed after Botox administration. However, formation of haematoma may occur.

*Reproduction toxicology:*

*Teratogenic effects:* When pregnant mice and rats were injected intramuscularly during the period of organogenesis, the developmental NOEL of Botox was at 4 U/kg. Reductions in ossification were observed at 8 and 16 U/kg (mice) and reduced ossification of the hyoid bone at 16 U/kg (rats). Reduced foetal body weights were observed at 8 and 16 U/kg (rats).

In a range finding study in rabbits, daily injections at dosages of 0.5 U/kg/day (days 6 to 18 of gestation), and 4 and 6 U/kg (administered on days 6 and 13 of gestation), caused death and abortions among surviving dams. External malformations were observed in one foetus each in the 0.125 U/kg/day and the 2 U/kg dosage groups. The rabbit appears to be a very sensitive species to Botox treatment.

*Impairment of fertility and reproduction:* The reproductive NOEL following i.m. injection of Botox was 4 U/kg in male rats and 8 U/kg in female rats. Higher dosages were associated with dose-dependent reductions in fertility. Provided impregnation occurred, there were no adverse effects on the numbers or viability of the embryos sired or conceived by treated male or female rats.

*Pre- and post-natal developmental effects:* In female rats, the reproductive NOEL was 16 U/kg. The developmental NOEL was 4 U/kg.

*Mutagenicity:* Botox has been evaluated and shown to be non-mutagenic in a number of *in vitro* and *in vivo* systems including the Ames test, the AS52/XPRT Mammalian Cell Forward Gene Mutation assay and the CHO test, and non-clastogenic in the mouse PCE test.

*Carcinogenicity:* No animal studies have been conducted.

*Antigenicity:* Botox showed antigenicity in mice only in the presence of adjuvant. Botox was found to be slightly antigenic in the guinea pig.

*Blood compatibility:* No haemolysis was detected up to 100 U/ml of Botox in normal human blood.

**Pharmaceutical particulars**

*List of excipients:* Human serum albumin, sodium chloride.

*Incompatibilities:* None known, other than described under *Interactions* above.

*Shelf life:* Unopened vial – 24 months. Reconstituted vial – 4 hours.

*Special precautions for storage:* Unopened vials should be stored in a freezer at or below –5°C. After reconstitution Botox may be stored in a refrigerator (2–8°C) for up to 4 hours prior to use.

*Nature and contents of containers:* Clear glass vial

with rubber stopper and tamper-proof aluminium seal, containing white powder for injection.

*Instructions for use/handling:* Botox is reconstituted prior to use with sterile unpreserved normal saline (0.9% sodium chloride for injection). It is good practice to perform vial reconstitution and syringe preparation over plastic-lined paper towels to catch any spillage. An appropriate amount of diluent (see dilution table below) is drawn up into a syringe. The exposed portion of the rubber septum of the vial is cleaned with alcohol (70%) prior to insertion of the needle. Since Botox is denatured by bubbling or similar violent agitation, the diluent should be injected gently into the vial. Discard the vial if a vacuum does not pull the diluent into the vial. Reconstituted Botox is a clear colourless to slightly yellow solution free of particulate matter. When reconstituted, Botox may be stored in a refrigerator (2–8˚C) for up to 4 hours prior to use. After this period used or unused vials should be discarded.

Dilution table

| Diluent added | Resulting dose in units per 0.1 ml |
|---|---|
| 0.5 ml | 20.0 U |
| 1.0 ml | 10.0 U |
| 2.0 ml | 5.0 U |
| 4.0 ml | 2.5 U |
| 8.0 ml | 1.25 U |

The 'unit' by which the potency of preparations of Botox is measured should be used to calculate dosages of Botox only and is not transferable to other preparations of botulinum toxin.

An injection volume of approximately 0.1 ml is recommended. A decrease or increase in the Botox dose is possible by administering a smaller or larger injection volume. The smaller the injection volume the less discomfort and less spread of toxin in the injected muscle occurs. This is of benefit in reducing effects on nearby muscles when small muscle groups are being injected.

For safe disposal, unused vials should be reconstituted with a small amount of water then autoclaved. Any used vials, syringes, and spillages etc. should be autoclaved, or the residual Botox inactivated using dilute hypochlorite solution (0.5%).

**Marketing authorisation number** PL 0426/0074.

**Date of approval/revision of SPC** 20 June 1997.

**Legal category** POM.

## LACRI-LUBE*

**Presentation** Off-white, smooth, preservative-free sterile ophthalmic ointment containing White Soft Paraffin BP 57.3% (w/w), Mineral Oil USP 42.5% (w/w) and Lanolin Alcohols NF 0.2% (w/w).

**Uses** Useful as adjunctive therapy to lubricate and protect the eye in conditions such as exposure keratitis, decreased corneal sensitivity, recurrent corneal erosions, keratitis sicca, and also in ophthalmic and non-ophthalmic surgery.

**Dosage and administration** For topical administration. Pull lower lid down to form a pocket and apply a small amount as required. There is no variation of dose for age.

**Contra-indications, warnings, etc** Do not use in patients hypersensitive to lanolin alcohols.

**Pharmaceutical precautions** Store away from heat. To avoid contamination during use, do not touch tube tip to any surface.

**Legal category** P.

**Package quantities** Lacri-Lube is available in 3.5 g and 5 g ophthalmic ointment tubes.

**Further information** Dry eye symptoms commonly persist at night – Lacri-Lube has been specifically formulated to lubricate and protect the dry eye during sleep.

Lacri-Lube can provide prophylactic ocular care during general surgical procedures as an adjunct to taping of the eyelids.

**Product licence number** 0426/0041

## LIQUIFILM* TEARS

**Presentation** Clear, colourless to slightly straw-coloured, sterile, aqueous ophthalmic solution containing Liquifilm (polyvinyl alcohol USP) 1.4% (w/v). Also contains disodium edetate PhEur 0.015% (w/v), benzalkonium chloride PhEur 0.005% (w/v) with sodium chloride PhEur, sodium phosphate PhEur and purified water PhEur.

**Uses** Liquifilm Tears is an ocular lubricant for the relief of dry eye and dry eye symptoms.

**Dosage and administration** For all ages. One or two drops administered topically to the affected eye(s) as required.

**Contra-indications, warnings, etc**
*Contra-indications:* Sensitivity to any of the components. Not for use with soft (hydrophilic) contact lenses because of the presence of benzalkonium chloride as a preservative.

*Warnings:* If irritation increases or persists, discontinue use and consult a doctor.

**Pharmaceutical precautions** Store at room temperature. Discard any unused contents 28 days after opening the bottle. To avoid contamination, do not allow dropper tip to touch any surface. Keep out of reach of children.

**Legal category** P.

**Package quantities** Liquifilm Tears is available in plastic dropper bottles containing 15 ml.

**Further information** Liquifilm Tears (polyvinyl alcohol) lowers the surface tension at the surface of the corneal epithelium, providing a lubricant layer which enhances patient comfort. Liquifilm Tears can help to restore normal tear film tonicity and to act as a wetting agent for lipid-, aqueous- and mucin-deficient eyes.

**Product licence number** 0426/0009R

## LIQUIFILM* TEARS PRESERVATIVE FREE

**Presentation** Clear, colourless to very slightly yellow, sterile, ophthalmic solution in a single-use container. Liquifilm Tears Preservative Free contains Liquifilm (polyvinyl alcohol USP) 1.4% (w/v) and povidone BP 0.6% (w/v) together with sodium chloride PhEur and purified water PhEur.

**Uses** Liquifilm Tears Preservative Free is an ocular lubricant for symptomatic relief of dry eye and symptomatic relief of eye irritation associated with deficient tear production.

**Dosage and administration** For all ages. One or two drops administered topically to the affected eye(s) as required, or as directed.

**Contra-indications, warnings, etc**
*Contra-indications:* Hypersensitivity to any components of the formulation

*Warnings:* May cause transient blurring. Do not drive or use hazardous machinery unless vision is clear. May cause transient stinging or irritation on instillation. If symptoms worsen or persist or other adverse effects occur, discontinue use and consult a doctor. In order to avoid contamination, dropper should not be allowed to touch eye or any other surface. Use immediately after opening. Do not store opened container.

**Pharmaceutical precautions** Store unopened container at room temperature. Discard container after single use as Liquifilm Tears Preservative Free contains no preservative.

**Legal category** P.

**Package quantities** Liquifilm Tears Preservative Free is available in packs of 30 units containing 0.4 ml.

**Further information** Nil.

**Product licence number** 0426/0063

## ZORAC* ▼

**Qualitative and quantitative composition** 1 g gel contains: Zorac 0.05% (tazarotene 0.5 mg) or Zorac 0.1% (tazarotene 1.0 mg).

**Pharmaceutical form** Aqueous gel.

**Clinical particulars**
*Therapeutic indications:* For the topical treatment of mild to moderate plaque psoriasis involving up to 10% body surface area.

*Posology and method of administration:* Zorac gel is available in two concentrations. Treatment with the higher concentration gel gives a faster and numerically higher response rate. Treatment with the lower concentration gel is associated with a somewhat lower incidence of local adverse events (see *Undesirable effects* and *Pharmacological properties*). The physician should choose the concentration to be used based on clinical circumstances and the principle of using the least concentration of drug to achieve the desired effect.

Individual variations with respect to efficacy and tolerability are possible. It is thus advisable for patients to consult their physician on a weekly basis when initiating therapy.

A thin film of the gel should be applied once daily in the evening; care should be taken to apply it only to areas of affected skin, avoiding application to healthy skin or in skin folds. Treatment is limited to 10% body surface area (approximately equivalent to the total skin area of one arm).

If the patient experiences more drying or irritation, an effective greasy emollient (without pharmaceutically active ingredients) can be applied to the areas of the skin to be treated to improve tolerability. Healthy skin around the psoriatic plaques can be covered by using zinc paste, for example, to prevent irritation.

Usually, the treatment period is up to 12 weeks. Clinical experience, particularly on tolerability, is available on periods of use of up to 12 months.

*Contra-indications:* Hypersensitivity to any ingredient of the medication.

Pregnancy or in women planning a pregnancy.

Breast-feeding mothers

Since there is, as yet, no clinical experience, Zorac should not be used in the treatment of psoriasis pustulosa and psoriasis exfoliativa, and the gel should not be applied to intertriginous areas, to the face, or to hair-covered scalp.

*Special warnings and special precautions for use:* Care should be taken to ensure that Zorac is applied only to psoriatic lesions, as application to normal, eczematous or inflamed skin or skin affected by other pathologies may cause irritation. Patients should be advised to wash their hands after application of the gel to avoid accidental transfer to the eyes.

If psoriatic areas on the skin of the hands are being treated, particular care should be taken to ensure that no gel is transferred to facial skin or the eyes.

If skin irritation develops, treatment with Zorac should be interrupted.

The safety of use on more than 10% of the body surface areas has not been established. There is limited experience of application to up to 20% of the body surface area.

Patients should be advised to avoid excessive exposure to UV light (including sunlight, use of a solarium, PUVA or UVB therapy) during treatment with Zorac (see *Preclinical safety data*).

No therapeutic studies using Zorac under occlusion or concomitantly with other antipsoriatic agents (including tar shampoos) have been carried out. To minimise interference with absorption and to avoid unnecessary spreading of the medication, topical application of emollients and cosmetics should not be applied within 1 hour of applying Zorac.

The safety and efficacy of Zorac have not been established in patients under the age of 18 years.

*Interactions with other medicaments and other forms of interaction:* Concomitant use of pharmaceutical and cosmetic preparations which cause irritation or have a strong drying effect should be avoided.

*Pregnancy and lactation*
*Pregnancy:* Although in animals no malformations were observed after dermal application, skeletal alterations were seen in the foetuses, which may be attributable to systemic retinoid effects. Teratogenic effects were observed after oral administration.

In view of these findings Zorac gel must not be used by pregnant women or women planning a pregnancy.

Women of childbearing potential should be informed of the potential risk and adopt adequate birth control measures when Zorac is used.

*Lactation:* Although no data are available on the excretion of tazarotene in human milk, animal data indicate that excretion into milk is possible. For that reason Zorac gel should not be used during breast feeding.

*Effects on ability to drive and use machines:* None known.

*Undesirable effects:* The most frequently reported adverse reactions in controlled clinical trials of Zorac in the treatment of psoriasis were pruritus (incidence 20–25%), burning, erythema, and irritation (10–20%), desquamation, non-specific rash, irritant contact dermatitis, skin pain, and a worsening of psoriasis (5–10%). More rarely observed were stinging and inflamed and dry skin (1–3%). The incidence of adverse reactions appears to be concentration-related and dependent on duration of use. The higher concentration gel (0.1%) may cause up to 5% more cases of severe skin irritation than the lower concentration gel (0.05%), especially during the first 4 weeks of use.

*Overdosage:* Excessive dermal use of Zorac may result in marked redness, peeling or local discomfort.

Inadvertent ingestion of Zorac is a theoretical possibility. In such a case, the signs and symptoms associated with hypervitaminosis A (severe headache, nausea, vomiting, drowsiness, irritability and pruritus) may occur. However, it is likely that these symptoms would prove to be reversible.

**Pharmacological properties** Both gels have demonstrated therapeutic effects as early as 1 week after commencement of a course of treatment. A good clinical response was seen in up to 65% of the patients after 12 weeks of treatment. The therapeutic effect of the higher concentration gel is more rapidly apparent and the efficacy more marked. In various studies in which patients were also evaluated for 12 weeks following cessation of therapy, it was found that patients continued to show a certain clinical benefit, however, no difference between the higher and lower concentrations with regard to this effect was observed.

*Pharmacodynamic properties:* Topical antipsoriatic agent (D05A).

Tazarotene, a member of the acetylenic class of retinoids, is a prodrug which is converted to its active free form, tazarotenic acid, by de-esterification in the skin area. Tazarotenic acid is the only known metabolite of tazarotene to have retinoid activity.

The active metabolite specifically regulates gene expression, thus modulating cell proliferation, hyperplasia, and differentiation in a wide range of tissues, as has been demonstrated in *in vitro* and *in vivo* trials.

The exact mechanism of action of tazarotene in psoriasis is, as yet, unknown. Improvement in psoriatic patients occurs in association with restoration of normal cutaneous morphology, and reduction of the inflammatory markers ICAM-1 and HLA-DR, and of markers of epidermal hyperplasia and abnormal differentiation, such as elevated keratinocyte transglutaminase, involucrin, and keratin 16.

*Pharmacokinetic properties:*
*(a) General characteristics*
*Absorption:* Systemic absorption is limited. Results of a pharmacokinetic study of single topical application of 0.1% $^{14}$C-tazarotene gel show that approximately 5% is absorbed when applied to normal skin under occlusion.

After a single topical application of tazarotene gel to 20% body surface area for 10 hours in healthy volunteers, tazarotene was not detectable in the plasma. Maximum plasma levels for the active metabolite tazarotenic acid of 0.3±0.2 ng/ml (for the 0.05% strength) and 0.5±0.3 ng/ml (0.1% gel) were measured after approximately 15 hours. The AUC was 40% higher for the 0.1% gel compared with the 0.05% gel. Thus, the two strengths of the gel are not strictly dose proportional with respect to systemic absorption. Repeated topical application of the 0.1% gel over 7 days led to maximum plasma levels for tazarotenic acid of 0.7±0.6 ng/ml after 9 hours.

*Biotransformation:* After dermal administration, tazarotene undergoes esterase hydrolysis to form its free acid, tazarotenic acid, and oxidative metabolism to form inactive sulphoxide and sulphone derivatives.

*Elimination:* Secondary metabolites of tazarotenic acid (the sulphoxide, the sulphone and an oxygenated derivative of tazarotenic acid) have been detected in human urine and faeces. The elimination half-life of tazarotenic acid after dermal application of tazarotene is approximately 18 hours in normal and psoriatic subjects.

After intravenous administration, the half-life of tazarotene was approximately 6 hours and that of tazarotenic acid 14 hours.

*(b) Characteristics after use in patients:* After single topical application of 0.1% $^{14}$C-tazarotene gel for 10 hours to psoriatic lesions (without occlusion), 4.5% of the dose was recovered in the stratum corneum and 2.4% in the epidermal/dermal layers. Less than 1% of the dose was absorbed systemically. More than 75% of drug elimination was completed within 72 hours.

In a small five patient study, repeated topical application of tazarotene 0.1% gel over 13 days resulted in a mean peak plasma level of tazarotenic acid of 12±8 ng/ml. these patients had psoriatic lesions on 8–18% of body surface area. In a larger 24 psoriatic patient study, tazarotene 0.05% and 0.1% gels were applied for 3 months and yielded a Cmax of 0.45±0.78 ng/ml and 0.83±1.22 ng/ml, respectively.

In a 1 year clinical study with 0.05% and 0.1% tazarotene gel, tazarotene was detected in 3 out of 112 patients at plasma concentrations below 1 ng/ml, while its active metabolite tazarotenic acid was found in 31 patients. Only four patients had plasma concentrations of tazarotenic acid greater than or equal to 1 ng/ml (maximum 2.8 ng/ml).

*Preclinical safety data:*
*Subacute/chronic toxicity:* The safety of daily dermal application of tazarotene gel was tested in mouse, rat and mini-pig over periods of up to one year. The main observation was reversible skin irritation. In the case of the mini-pig, an incomplete healing of the dermal irritation was observed after an 8 week recovery period. The rat appears to be the most sensitive species to tazarotene, as is the case with other retinoids. Here, dermal application induced severe skin reactions and clinically significant retinoid-like systemic effects. No adverse systemic effects were observed in the other species.

After oral administration of 0.025 mg/kg/day for 1 year in the cynomolgus monkey, no toxic effects were observed. At higher doses, typical symptoms of retinoid toxicity were seen.

*Reproductive toxicity:* Safety of use during pregnancy has not been established. Teratogenic and embryotoxic effects were observed after oral administration in the rat and rabbit. In dermal application studies during foetal development, skeletal alterations and decreased pup weight at birth and at the end of the lactation period were observed.

Animal tests suggest that tazarotene or its active metabolite is excreted in breast milk and passes the placenta barrier.

No effects on fertility are reported after topical application in the male and female rat.

*Mutagenicity/Carcinogenicity:* No evidence of a mutagenic potential of tazarotene has been reported in *in vitro* and *in vivo* trials.

In long term investigations of the effects of dermal and oral administration in animals, no carcinogenic effects were observed.

There was an increased incidence of photocarcinogenic effects in the hairless mouse when exposed to UV light after topical application of tazarotene.

*Local tolerability:* Tazarotene gel has a considerable irritative potential on skin in all animal species investigated.

Instillation of tazarotene gel in the eye of the rabbit resulted in irritation with marked hyperaemia of the conjunctiva, but there was no corneal damage.

### Pharmaceutical particulars

*List of excipients:* Benzyl alcohol, macrogol 400, hexylene glycol (2-methylpentane-2,4-diol), carbomer, trometamol, poloxamer 407, polysorbate 40, ascorbic acid, butyl hydroxyanisole, butyl hydroxytoluene, disodium edetate dihydrate, purified water.

*Incompatibilities:* Tazarotene is susceptible to oxidising agents and may undergo ester hydrolysis when in contact with bases.

*Shelf life:* Finished product in the unopened container: 24 months. Finished product after first opening of the container: 180 days.

*Special precautions for storage:* Zorac gel should not be stored at temperatures over 30˚C.

*Nature and contents of container:* Aluminium tube, internally lacquered, with seal and polypropylene screw cap containing a colourless to light yellow, translucent to cloudy, homogeneous gel.
Pack sizes: 30 g and 60 g.

*Instructions for use/handling:* To break the seal, use the top of the cap. Keep tube tightly closed when not in use.

**Marketing authorisation numbers**
Zorac 0.05%        PL 00426/0096
Zorac 0.1%         PL 00426/0097

**Date of approval/revision of SPC** 30 July 1997.

**Legal category** POM.

*\*Trade Mark*

# Alpha Therapeutic UK Ltd
Howlett Way
Thetford
Norfolk
IP24 1HZ

**alpha**

## ALBUTEIN* 5%

**Presentation** Albutein 5% is Albumin Solution BP 5% and each 100 ml of solution contains 5 g of human serum albumin. It is a clear, almost colourless to amber sterile aqueous solution for single dose intravenous administration.

**Uses** Albumin is a highly soluble globular protein (MW 66,500) which is important in regulating the osmotic pressure of plasma. Albutein 5% solution supplies the oncotic equivalent of approximately its own volume of normal human plasma and will increase the circulating plasma volume by an amount equal to the volume infused. The degree and duration of volume expansion depend upon the initial blood volume. The effect of infused albumin persists longer in patients with diminished blood volume than in individuals with normal blood volume. Albumin is also a transport protein and binds naturally occurring, therapeutic and toxic materials in the circulation. The binding properties of albumin may in special circumstances provide an indication for its clinical use. For such purposes, however, Albutein 20% or Albutein 25% should be used.

Albutein 5% is indicated:

1. For the treatment of hypovolaemic shock.
2. In conditions in which there is severe hypoalbuminaemia. However unless the pathologic condition responsible for the hypoalbuminaemia can be corrected, administration of albumin can afford only symptomatic or supportive relief.
3. For the treatment of burns.
4. As an adjunct in cardiopulmonary bypass procedures.

In those conditions in which the colloid requirement is high and there is less need for fluid, albumin should be administered as the 20% or 25% solutions.

**Dosage and administration** Albutein 5% is intended for intravenous administration. The total dosage will vary with the individual.

*Adults:* An initial infusion of 500 ml is suggested. This may be repeated in 15–30 minutes if the initial dose is inadequate. Additional amounts should be administered as clinically indicated.

The rate of administration should be 1–2 ml per minute in patients with slightly low or normal blood volume. In patients with shock and/or greatly reduced blood volume, Albutein 5% may be administered as rapidly as necessary.

*Children:* Dosage will vary with clinical state and body weight. A dose of one-quarter to one-half of the adult dose may be administered or dosage may be calculated on the basis of 3–5 ml per kilogram body weight.

The rate of administration should be calculated on one-quarter of the adult rate.

**Contra-indications, warnings, etc** Albutein 5% is contra-indicated in patients with severe anaemia or cardiac failure in the presence of normal or increased intravascular volume and in patients with a history of allergic reactions to albumin products.

Albutein 5% should be administered with caution to patients with low cardiac reserve. Additional fluids may be required for patients with marked dehydration. Rapid infusion may cause vascular overload with resultant pulmonary oedema. Patients should be closely monitored for signs of increased venous pressure. A rapid rise in blood pressure following infusion necessitates careful observation of injured or postoperative patients to detect and treat severed blood vessels that may not have bled at a lower pressure.

Do not use for control of haemorrhage due to deficiencies or defects in the clotting mechanism. The product is not intended for use in dialysis patients or in premature infants.

Albumin naturally binds a variety of therapeutic and toxic materials and thus administration of Albutein 5% may modify the pre-existing distribution of certain substances.

Adverse reactions are rare. However allergic or pyrogenic reactions, characterised primarily by fever and chills, nausea, vomiting, tachycardia and hypotension have been reported.

If such reactions occur the infusion should be discontinued and appropriate therapy (eg. antihistamine) or specific support treatment should be given.

Reproduction studies have not been conducted with albumin. Human albumin should be given to a pregnant woman only if clearly needed.

Administration of large quantities of albumin may require supplementation with red cell concentrates to help overcome any resulting relative anaemia.

**Pharmaceutical precautions** Do not use if the solution appears turbid or contains a deposit. Since the solution does not contain a preservative it should be used within 3 hours of penetration of the container. Discard any unused portion.

Do not administer protein hydrolysates or alcohol via the same administration set used for Albutein 5%.

Albutein 5% should be stored between 2°C and 25°C protected from light.

**Legal category** POM.

**Package quantities** Albutein 5% is supplied in:
250 ml glass vials containing 12.5 g of albumin.
500 ml glass vials containing 25.0 g of albumin.

**Further information** Albutein 5% is prepared from plasma obtained from carefully selected and rigorously screened donors. The final product is heated at 60°C for 10 hours. However as with all blood products the risk of viral transmission with this product cannot be absolutely excluded. Nevertheless there are no known cases of viral transmission resulting from the administration of Albutein 5%.

**Product licence number** 4447/0007.

## ALBUTEIN* 20%

**Presentation** Albutein 20% is Albumin Solution BP 20% and each 100 ml of solution contains 20 g of human serum albumin. It is a clear, almost colourless to amber sterile aqueous solution for single dose intravenous administration.

**Uses** Albumin is a highly soluble globular protein (MW 66,500) which is important in regulating the osmotic pressure of plasma. Albutein 20% solution supplies the oncotic equivalent of approximately 4 times its own volume of normal human plasma. It will increase the circulating plasma volume by an amount approximately 2.5 times the volume infused within 15 minutes, if the recipient is adequately hydrated. The degree and duration of volume expansion depend upon the initial blood volume. The effect of infused albumin persists longer in patients with diminished blood volume than in individuals with normal blood volume. Albumin is also a transport protein and binds naturally occurring, therapeutic and toxic materials in the circulation. The binding properties of albumin may in special circumstances provide an indication for its clinical use.

Albutein 20% is indicated:

1. For the treatment of hypovolaemic shock.
2. In conditions in which there is severe hypoalbuminaemia. However unless the pathologic condition responsible for the hypoalbuminaemia can be corrected, administration of albumin can afford only symptomatic or supportive relief.
3. For the treatment of burns.
4. As an adjunct in cardiopulmonary bypass procedures.
5. In conjunction with exchange transfusion in the treatment of neonatal hyperbilirubinaemia.

**Dosage and administration** Albutein 20% is intended for intravenous administration. The total dosage will vary with the individual.

*Adults:* An initial infusion of 100 ml is suggested. This may be repeated in 15–30 minutes if the initial dose is inadequate. Additional amounts should be administered as clinically indicated.

The rate of administration should be 1 ml per minute in patients with slightly low or normal blood volume. In patients with shock and/or greatly reduced blood volume, Albutein 20% may be administered as rapidly as necessary.

*Children:* Dosage will vary with clinical state and body

weight. Dosage may be calculated on the basis of 1 ml per kilogram body weight for Albutein 20%.

The rate of administration should be calculated on one-quarter to one-half of the adult rate.

**Contra-indications, warnings, etc** Albutein 20% is contra-indicated in patients with severe anaemia or cardiac failure in the presence of normal or increased intravascular volume and in patients with a history of allergic reactions to albumin products.

Albutein 20% should be administered with caution to patients with low cardiac reserve. Additional fluids may be required for patients with marked dehydration. Rapid infusion may cause vascular overload with resultant pulmonary oedema. Patients should be closely monitored for signs of increased venous pressure. A rapid rise in blood pressure following infusion necessitates careful observation of injured or postoperative patients to detect and treat severed blood vessels that may not have bled at a lower pressure.

Do not use for control of haemorrhage due to deficiencies or defects in the clotting mechanism. The product is not intended for use in dialysis patients or in premature infants.

Albumin naturally binds a variety of therapeutic and toxic materials and thus administration of Albutein 20% may modify the pre-existing distribution of certain substances.

Adverse reactions are rare. However allergic or pyrogenic reactions, characterised primarily by fever and chills, nausea, vomiting, tachycardia and hypotension have been reported.

If such reactions occur the infusion should be discontinued and appropriate therapy (eg. antihistamine) or specific support treatment should be given.

Reproduction studies have not been conducted with albumin. Human albumin should be given to a pregnant woman only if clearly needed.

Administration of large quantities of albumin may require supplementation with red cell concentrates to help overcome any resulting relative anaemia.

**Pharmaceutical precautions** Do not use if the solution appears turbid or contains a deposit. Since the solution does not contain a preservative it should be used within 3 hours of penetration of the container. Discard any unused portion.

Do not administer protein hydrolysates or alcohol via the same administration set used for Albutein 20%.

Albutein 20% should be stored between 2°C and 25°C protected from light.

**Legal category** POM.

**Package quantities** Albutein 20% is supplied in:
50 ml glass vials containing 10 g of albumin.
100 ml glass vials containing 20 g of albumin.

**Further Information** Albutein 20% is prepared from plasma obtained from carefully selected and rigorously screened donors. The final product is heated at 60°C for 10 hours. However as with all blood products the risk of viral transmission with this product cannot be absolutely excluded. Nevertheless there are no known cases of viral transmission resulting from the administration of Albutein 20%.

**Product licence number** 4447/0008.

## ALPHAGLOBIN*

**Qualitative and quantitative composition** Alphaglobin is available in 4 sizes containing 0.5 g, 2.5 g, 5.0 g, or 10.0 g immunoglobulin per vial.

**Pharmaceutical form** Alphaglobin is a sterile, pasteurised, 50 g/litre solution of highly purified intact human normal immunoglobulin for intravenous infusion. The solution contains an immunoglobulin G subclass distribution that approximates to the distribution found in normal plasma and contains not more than 0.05 mg/ml IgA. The product is stabilised by 5% D-sorbitol.

### Clinical particulars
*Therapeutic indications:* Alphaglobin has been used as substitution/replacement therapy in primary and secondary antibody deficiency disorders and for the

prevention and treatment of infections associated with these conditions. Alphaglobin has also been used to modify or control the individual's immune response in idiopathic thrombocytopenic purpura.

1. Replacement therapy for congenital agammaglobulinaemia and hypogammaglobulinaemia and other primary immunodeficiency syndromes including common variable immunodeficiency, severe combined immunodeficiency and Wiskott-Aldrich syndrome.
2. Replacement therapy for secondary immunodeficiency disorders.
3. Treatment of idiopathic thrombocytopenic purpura (ITP).
4. Prophylactic use in children with symptomatic HIV infection who have recurrent bacterial infections.

*Posology and method of administration:*
*Posology:* Immunodeficiency Syndromes: The usual dosage of Alphaglobin in immunodeficiency syndromes is 200 ml/kg bodyweight usually administered once a month by intravenous infusion. If the clinical response is inadequate or the level of serum IgG achieved is felt to be insufficient the dose may be increased to 300–400 mg/kg bodyweight or the infusion may be repeated more frequently than once a month.

Idiopathic Thrombocytopenic Purpura: The usual treatment regimen is 400 mg/kg bodyweight daily for 5 days. Maintenance doses of 400 mg/kg bodyweight may be given every few weeks as required to maintain the platelet count.

*Elderly*: There is no evidence to suggest that the dosage regimens used for adults are inappropriate for the elderly.

*Administration*: Alphaglobin should be infused at a rate of 0.01–0.02 ml/kg bodyweight per minute for the first thirty minutes. If the patient does not experience any discomfort the rate may be increase up to 0.07 ml/kg per minute and if tolerated subsequent infusions to the same patient may be at the higher rate. If adverse effects occur the rate should be reduced or the infusion interrupted until the symptoms subside. The infusion may then be resumed at a rate which is tolerated by the patient.

*Contra-indications*: Alphaglobin is contra-indicated in individuals with a history of anaphylactic or severe systematic response to intramuscular or intravenous immune globulin preparations.

Although only containing trace quantities of IgA, Alphaglobin, as with all blood products containing IgA, is contra-indicated in patients with selective IgA deficiency who possess antibody to IgA.

*Special warnings and special precautions for use*: Patients with agamma- or extreme hypogammaglobulinaemia who have never before received immunoglobulin therapy or whose time from last treatment is greater than 8 weeks may be at risk of developing inflammatory reactions on infusion of Alphaglobin. Such reactions appear to be related to the rate of infusion. They are manifested by a rise in temperature, chills, nausea and vomiting. Vital signs should be monitored continuously and the patient should be carefully observed throughout the infusion.

The rate of administration specified in Section relating to *Posology and method of administration* should be closely followed, at least until the physician has had sufficient experience with a given patient. Adrenaline should be available for treatment of any acute anaphylactoid reaction.

This product is prepared from pooled units of human plasma which have been individually tested and found non-reactive for hepatitis B surface antigen, antibodies to hepatitis C and antibodies to human immunodeficiency viruses HIV-1 and -2. The plasma used in the preparation of this product has also been screened for alanine aminotransferase (ALT) and each unit used in manufacture has been found to have an ALT level of less than twice the upper limit of normal for the test. Other screening procedures are used to eliminate high risk plasma donors.

The manufacturing process of Alphaglobin includes a 60°C 10 hour pasteurisation process specifically designed to inactivate any contaminating viruses. The results from *in vitro* studies on various stages of the manufacturing process including the cold ethanol fractionation, pasteurisation, polyethylene glycol precipitation and DEAE Sephadex filtration steps, indicate that considerable quantities of HIV-1 and model viruses of other blood borne infections are both inactivated and partitioned during the process.

However, despite all precautions taken by the manufacturer the risk of transmission of infection, of blood borne viruses, by intravenous immunoglobulin preparations cannot be entirely excluded.

*Interaction with other medicaments*: Alphaglobin is supplied as a sterile 5% solution. It should not be mixed with any other drugs or intravenous fluids. It should be administered by a separate intravenous line.

*Pregnancy and lactation*: Animal reproduction studies using Alphaglobin indicate that there appear to be no harmful effects to either the mother or the offspring. However, the safety of this product in pregnant women has not been established in controlled clinical trials.

Alphaglobin should, therefore, be given to pregnant women only if clearly indicated.

*Effect on ability to drive and use machines*: Not applicable.

*Undesirable effects:* Clinical investigations have confirmed that Alphaglobin is well tolerated and not likely to produce side effects when infused at the recommended rates. However, the first infusion of immunoglobulin particularly in previously untreated agamma- and hypogammaglobulinaemic patients or patients who have previously received another immunoglobulin preparation may lead to systemic side effects. Some of the effects may occur as a result of a reaction between the antibodies administered and free antigens in the blood and tissues of the patient.

Adverse reactions such as headache, chills, fever, nausea, vomiting, allergic reactions, rash, arthralgia and mild back pain may occur occasionally. As with other intravenous immune globulin preparations, Alphaglobin has been associated at high doses with rare occurrences of aseptic meningitis and haemolytic anaemia.

Rarely immunoglobulins may cause a fall in blood pressure and, in isolated cases, anaphylactic shock, even when the patient has shown no sensitivity to previous administration.

*Overdose*: Overdosage with Alphaglobin has not been reported but is unlikely to have any harmful effects.

**Pharmacological properties**
*Pharmacodynamic properties:* Alphaglobin is a high purity human immunoglobulin class G (IgG) preparation which contains antibodies against the wide spectrum of antigens to which the plasma donor population has been exposed.

Alphaglobin retains the biological functions of endogenous gammaglobulin and has very low anti-complementary activity.

*Pharmacokinetic properties:* As Alphaglobin is administered intravenously, the dose is immediately bioavailable in the circulation.

Alphaglobin has a half-life of about 46 days (range 33–65 days). This half-life may vary from patient to patient.

*Preclinical safety data*: Not applicable.

**Pharmaceutical particulars**
*List of excipients:* 5% D-sorbitol, Water for Injections.

*Incompatibilities:* Alphaglobin should not be mixed with any other drugs or intravenous fluids. It should be administered by a separate intravenous line.

*Shelf life:* The shelf life of Alphaglobin is 2 years if stored below 25°C and protected from light.

*Special precautions for storage:* Alphaglobin should be stored below 25°C and protected from light. The contents must **not** be frozen.

*Nature and contents of container:* Alphaglobin is supplied in Type II clear glass vials, 10 ml, 50 ml, 100 ml and 200 ml.

*Instructions for use/handling:* Ensure aseptic technique is used during attachment of infusion lines.

*Pharmaceutical precautions:* If large volumes are to be administered it is advisable to ensure the solution is near to body temperature prior to infusion.

Do not use after expiry date.

**Marketing authorisation number** 4447/0031

**Date of approval/revision of SPC** 1 February 1997

**Legal category** POM

## ALPHANATE*

**Qualitative and quantitative composition** Alphanate is a high purity, solvent detergent and heat treated, freeze dried human coagulation Factor VIII, PhEur.

| *Active ingredient (Nominal)* | *Specification* | *Quantity* |
|---|---|---|
| Human coagulation Factor VIII | PhEur | 250 IU/vial |
| Human coagulation Factor VIII | PhEur | 500 IU/vial |
| Human coagulation Factor VIII | PhEur | 1000 IU/vial |
| Human coagulation Factor VIII | PhEur | 1500 IU/vial |

Each container is labelled with the number of International Units of Factor VIII activity.

**Pharmaceutical form** Sterile, non-pyrogenic, white/slightly yellow lyophilisate that is reconstituted with the Water for Injections BP/PhEur diluent (PL 4447/0016) supplied with the product. For intravenous administration.

**Clinical particulars**
*Therapeutic indications*: Alphanate is indicated for the treatment and prophylaxis of bleeding in patients with moderate or severe Factor VIII deficiency due to congenital haemophilia A or acquired Factor VIII deficiency.

*Posology and method of administration:* The dose and dosing schedule for Alphanate must be adjusted according to the needs of the individual patient, taking into account the severity of the haemostatic disorder, the location and extent of the bleeding and the clinical condition.

*Posology : Factor VIII replacement therapy:* The required dosage may be estimated using the following formula as a guide:

| Body weight (kg) | × Desired increase in Factor VIII (%) | × 0.5 = | Number of Factor VIII units required (IU) |
|---|---|---|---|

*Example:*
50 kg×30%×0.5=750 IU Alphanate

This calculation is based on the empirical finding that 1 IU of Factor VIII per kg body weight raises the plasma Factor VIII activity by approximately 2% (i.e. 0.5 IU/kg required for a 1% increase in plasma Factor VIII level).

The patient's plasma Factor VIII levels should be determined and monitored during treatment with Alphanate. This is particularly important in the case of surgical procedures.

*Treatment schedules:*
Haemorrhagic Events: If not prescribed otherwise by the attending physician, the following dosage schedule is recommended. For each of the following haemorrhagic events, the Factor VIII activity should not fall below the given plasma activity level (in % of normal) over the corresponding period.

| *Haemorrhagic event* | *Therapeutically effective plasma level of Factor VIII activity* | *Period that therapeutic plasma level of Factor VIII activity should be maintained* |
|---|---|---|
| Minor haemorrhage: (Including haemorrhage into joints) | 30% | At least 1 day, depending on the severity of the haemorrhage. |
| Major haemorrhage: (Including haemorrhage into muscles; tooth extraction; mild trauma capitis; minor operations; haemorrhages in the oral cavity) | 40 – 50% | 3–4 days or until adequate wound healing has been achieved. |
| Life-threatening haemorrhage: (Including major operations; gastro-intestinal bleeding; intracranial, intra-abdominal or intra-thoracic haemorrhages; fractures) | 60 – 100% | For 7 days. Factor VIII therapy should continue for at least another 7 days until adequate healing has been achieved. |

Under certain circumstances larger amounts than those calculated will be required, especially for the initial dose.

*Prophylaxis:* For long-term prophylaxis against bleeding in patients with severe haemophilia A, Alphanate should be administered at doses of 10 to 50 IU/kg at intervals of 2 to 3 days. In some cases, especially in younger patients, shorter dosage intervals or higher doses may be necessary.

*Elderly patients:* The dosage regimens recommended for adults are appropriate for the elderly.

*Administration:* Alphanate is intended for intravenous administration only. Once reconstituted with the diluent supplied, Alphanate may be administered at a rate of no more than 10 ml/minute by injection or infusion. (For full details of reconstitution and use refer to the *Instructions for use/handling* section).

*Contra-indications:* None known.

*Special warnings and special precautions for use:* If allergic or anaphylactic reactions occur, administration should be stopped immediately. Subsequent treatment, where necessary, should follow the current specific guidelines for shock therapy.

After repeated treatment with Factor VIII concentrate, the level of inhibitor in the plasma should be determined.

Patients receiving Factor VIII concentrates should be vaccinated against hepatitis A and B.

*Interaction with other medicaments and other forms of interaction:* As Factor VIII is a constituent of normal plasma, no such interactions are anticipated.

*Pregnancy and lactation:* The safety of human coagulation Factor VIII for use in human pregnancy has not been established in controlled clinical trials. Experimental animal studies are insufficient to assess safety with respect to reproduction, development of the embryo or foetus, the course of gestation and peri- and postnatal development. Therefore, Factor VIII concentrates should only be used if clearly needed during pregnancy and lactation.

*Effects on ability to drive and use machines:* As Factor VIII is a constituent of normal plasma no effects on ability to drive or use machines are anticipated.

*Undesirable effects:*

1. Occasionally, mild reactions occur following the administration of Factor VIII concentrates. These may include allergic reactions, urticaria, fever, chills, nausea, vomiting, headache, somnolence or lethargy.
2. Very rarely, anaphylactic reactions occur following the administration of Factor VIII concentrates.
3. Patients receiving Factor VIII concentrates may develop antibodies (inhibitors) to the Factor VIII protein. In these patients, the response to Alphanate may be much less than would otherwise be expected, and larger doses are often required. The management of patients with inhibitors requires careful monitoring, especially if surgical procedures are indicated.
4. With products derived from human plasma, the transmission of infectious diseases due to the transmission of pathogens cannot be totally excluded.

This product is prepared from pooled units of human plasma derived from fully screened donors. Each unit has been individually tested and found nonreactive for hepatitis B surface antigen, antibodies to human immunodeficiency viruses (HIV-1 and -2) and antibodies to hepatitis C virus (HCV). Each unit has also been tested and found to have alanine aminotransferase (ALT) levels less than twice the upper limit of normal for the test.

The manufacturing process for Alphanate includes an organic solvent, tri-(n-butyl)-phosphate, and detergent, polysorbate-80, virus inactivation step designed to reduce the risk of transmitting infective agents. This process has been shown to be effective against a wide range of lipid-enveloped viruses. The manufacturing process also includes a heat-treatment step in which lyophilised Alphanate is heated at 80°C for 72 hours. This second inactivation step is designed to further reduce the risk of transmitting infective agents, in particular non-lipid-enveloped viruses.

As with all drugs, the risks associated with use must be weighed against the benefits of therapy.

*Overdose:* Massive doses of Factor VIII have, rarely, resulted in acute haemolytic anaemia, increased bleeding tendency or hyperfibrinogenaemia. In the case of overdose the patient should be carefully monitored and supportive treatment given.

**Pharmacological properties**
*Pharmacodynamic properties:* Factor VIII is a constituent of normal plasma as the Factor VIII/von Willebrand Factor complex and forms part of the clotting process. As a cofactor for Factor IX, it accelerates the conversion of Factor X to activated Factor X. Activated Factor X converts prothrombin into thrombin. Thrombin then converts fibrinogen into fibrin and a clot can be formed. The Factor VIII activity is greatly reduced in patients with haemophilia A or acquired Factor VIII deficiency. The administration of Factor VIII concentrates such as Alphanate to these patients therefore temporarily corrects their blood clotting mechanism and minimises the hazards of haemorrhage.

*Pharmacokinetic properties:* After injection of the product, approximately two thirds to three quarters of the Factor VIII remains in the circulation. The achieved Factor VIII activity in the plasma should be between 80–120 percent of the predicted value.

Plasma Factor VIII activity probably decreases by a two-phase exponential decay. In the initial phase, distribution between the intravascular and other compartments (body fluids) occurs with a half-life of elimination from the plasma of 3–6 hours. In the subsequent slower phase (which probably reflects the consumption of Factor VIII) the half-life varies between 8–20 hours, with an average of 12 hours. This appears to correspond to the true biological half-life.

In clinical studies, the Factor VIII half life of Alphanate was estimated at approximately 12 hours. Mean recovery was approximately 87%.

*Preclinical safety data:* As Alphanate is purified from

pooled human plasma it is considered to act in the same manner as endogenous Factor VIII. Toxicity testing is therefore of no relevance.

Immunoelectrophoretic and immunoprecipitation studies on rabbit antisera raised against Alphanate indicate that no detectable new antigenic determinants were generated by heat-treatment.

**Pharmaceutical particulars**
*List of excipients:*

| Material | Specification |
|---|---|
| Albumin | PhEur |
| Histidine | USP |
| Arginine | USP |
| Water for Injections (Diluent) | BP/PhEur |

*Incompatabilities:* Alphanate should not be mixed with other drugs before administration.

Use only approved injection/infusion sets because treatment may fail as a consequence of adsorption to the internal surface of some infusion equipment.

*Shelf life:* Lyophilised Alphanate has a shelf life of 24 months at 2–8°C. Storage at no more than 30°C for 6 months within this period is acceptable.

Reconstituted Alphanate has a shelf life of 3 hours at 25°C.

*Special precautions for storage:* Lyophilised Alphanate should be stored under refrigeration (2–8°C), protected from light. Do not freeze.

Reconstituted Alphanate should not be stored prior to administration.

*Nature and contents of containers:* Alphanate is supplied as lyophilisate in clear Type I/II glass, single dose vials with rubber stoppers and aluminium caps (bearing the lot number) with plastic flip-off top. Water for Injections diluent (5 ml for 250/500 IU/vial; 10 ml for 1000/1500 IU/vial) is provided in a separate vial.

*Instructions for use/handling:* Alphanate is for intravenous administration after reconstitution with the Water for Injections diluent provided.

Use aseptic technique during reconstitution and administration.

Usually the reconstituted solution is clear or slightly opalescent–do not use solutions which are cloudy or have deposits.

Alphanate should be used immediately after reconstitution.

Any unused solution must be discarded appropriately.

All reconstitution and administration equipment must be discarded appropriately.

*Reconstitution:* Use only the diluent and devices provided.
1. Warm diluent and concentrate vials to at least room temperature (but not above 37°C).
2. Remove plastic flip-off tops from the diluent and concentrate vials.
3. Swab the exposed rubber surfaces with alcohol. Do not leave excess cleaning agent in indentation on the stopper.
3. Remove covering from the vented filter spike. Remove plastic sheath from pointed end of vented filter spike and insert point through rubber stopper of concentrate vial. Air will be drawn through the sterile filter into the vial, thus releasing the vacuum. Leave the device inserted in the stopper.
4. Using the needle provided draw up the required volume of Water for Injections into the syringe.
5. Remove the plastic cap from the top of the vented filter spike. Insert the filled syringe into the exposed Luer end of the device. Depress the syringe plunger to transfer all the diluent into the concentrate vial. DO NOT REMOVE THE SYRINGE FROM THE VENTED FILTER SPIKE, DO NOT REMOVE THE DEVICE FROM THE STOPPER. Maintain the concentrate vial and spike/syringe assembly in the vertical position.
6. Holding the entire assembly securely, GENTLY SWIRL the diluent until all concentrate is dissolved. When the reconstitution procedure is strictly followed a few small particles may occasionally remain. The microaggregate filter built into the filter spike will retain any remaining particles, without reducing the label potency.

*Administration:* By syringe:
1. Invert the vial and withdraw the reconstituted product into the syringe via the vented filter spike with inbuilt microaggregate filter.
2. Detach the syringe from the filter spike and discard the empty concentrate vial with the filter spike attached.
3. Attach the syringe to the infusion set, expel air from the syringe and infusion set. Perform venepuncture and administer slowly.
4. If the patient is to receive more than one vial of concentrate, the infusion set will allow this to be performed with a single venepuncture.

By administration set:
1. Close clamp on the administration set. Remove the filter spike from the vial.
2. With vial upright, insert the piercing pin of the

administration set straight through the stopper centre. Do not twist or angle.
3. Immediately invert vial to automatically establish a proper fluid level in drip chamber (half full).
4. Attach infusion set, open the clamp and allow the solution to expel air from the tubing and needle, then close the clamp.
5. Perform venepuncture, release the clamp and administer slowly.

**Marketing authorisation number** 4447/0005

**Date of approval/revision of SPC** 20 September 1996

**Legal category** POM

## ALPHANINE*

**Qualitative and quantitative composition:** High purity, solvent detergent and nanofiltered human coagulation Factor IX, freeze dried in vials containing 500 IU, 1000 IU or 1500 IU (nominal sizes). Each container is labelled with the number of International Units of Factor IX activity.

**Pharmaceutical form:** Sterile, non-pyrogenic, white/ slightly yellow friable powder that is reconstituted with the Water for Injections BP/PhEur diluent (PL 4447/0016) supplied with the product. For intravenous administration only.

**Clinical particulars**
*Therapeutic indications:* For the prevention and control of bleeding in patients with Factor IX deficiency due to haemophilia B.

*Posology and method of administration:* The dose of AlphaNine for a particular patient depends upon the level of plasma Factor IX which is to be achieved. The desired plasma level of Factor IX will vary according to the patient's age and clinical condition, and as such should be decided upon by the physician, based on clinical experience. The patient's plasma Factor IX level should be determined and monitored during treatment.

The following formula provides a guide for dosage calculations:

| Body weight (kg) | $\times 1.0 \times$ | Desired increase in Factor IX (%) | = | Number of Factor IX units required |
|---|---|---|---|---|

Infusions are generally required daily.

*Contra-indications:* There are no known contra-indications to the use of AlphaNine.

*Special warnings and special precautions for use:* This product is prepared from pooled units of human plasma derived from screened donors. Each unit has been individually tested and found non-reactive for hepatitis B surface antigen, antibodies to HIV-1, HIV-2 and hepatitis C virus, and also to have an alanine amino-transferase level of less than twice the upper limit of normal for the test. Incubation in an organic solvent / detergent mixture during manufacture is designed to reduce the risk of transmitting infection with lipid-enveloped viruses. The specific viral filtration step in AlphaNine manufacture has been demonstrated to remove substantial amounts of non-lipid enveloped viruses.

However, testing methods are not yet sufficiently sensitive to detect all units of potentially infectious plasma, and no treatment during manufacture has been shown to eliminate totally the risk of viral infectivity. Therefore, despite the rigorous precautions taken by the manufacturer, it cannot be assumed that this product is totally free of viral contamination.

As with all drugs the risks associated with use must be weighed against the benefits of therapy.

Patients receiving Factor IX concentrates should be vaccinated against hepatitis A and B.

Occasionally haemophilia B sufferers develop inhibitors to Factor IX. In these patients the response to AlphaNine may be much less than would otherwise be expected and larger doses would be required. The management of patients with inhibitors requires careful monitoring, especially if surgical procedures are indicated.

AlphaNine is not suitable for the reversal of anticoagulant over-dosage.

*Interaction with other medicaments and other forms of interaction:* As Factor IX is a constituent of normal plasma, no interactions are anticipated.

*Pregnancy and lactation:* Animal reproduction studies have not been conducted with AlphaNine. AlphaNine should be given to a pregnant or lactating woman only if clearly indicated.

*Effects on ability to drive and use machines:* As Factor IX is a constituent of normal plasma, no effects on ability to drive or use machines are anticipated.

*Undesirable effects:* Occasionally, mild reactions occur following the administration of Factor IX concentrates. These may include allergic reactions, mild chills, nausea or stinging at the infusion site. Slowing the infusion rate will usually relieve the symptoms. For highly reactive individuals who require additional AlphaNine, product from a different lot should be administered.

Thrombosis or disseminated intravascular coagulation have been reported following the administration of Prothrombin Complex Concentrates (PCCs) especially to patients with liver disease or undergoing surgery. The thrombogenic potential of AlphaNine has been shown in clinical trials to be very considerably reduced from that of PCCs (data available for single doses only). However patients in high risk groups receiving AlphaNine should be closely observed for signs of intravascular coagulation.

*Overdose:* In the event of an overdose the patient should be carefully monitored and supportive treatment given.

### Pharmacological properties

*Pharmacodynamic properties:* AlphaNine is human coagulation Factor IX derived from human plasma. Its actions are understood to mimic exactly those of endogenous circulating Factor IX. The administration of AlphaNine increases the plasma levels of Factor IX, which in haemophilia B sufferers temporarily corrects their blood clotting disorder and minimises the hazards of haemorrhage.

*Pharmacokinetic properties:* Following administration by intravenous infusion, distribution of Factor IX between the intra- and extra-vascular compartments occurs resulting in equilibration. The elimination of Factor IX, which reflects its actual biological usage, then takes place. The median half life of Factor IX from AlphaNine has been estimated to be approximately 21 hours.

*Preclinical safety data:* The thrombogenic potential of purified Factor IX preparations such as AlphaNine has been examined in various animal models including the Wessler stasis rabbit model, porcine, canine and rodent models. The results have been compared with PCC preparations, which carry a known clinical risk of thromboembolic episodes. Purified Factor IX preparations have been shown to be associated with a very substantial reduction in thrombogenic activity compared with PCCs, even at doses many times higher than those which are employed in the clinical setting.

### Pharmaceutical particulars

*List of excipients:* AlphaNine is Coagulation Factor IX purified from human plasma.

The other components may be listed as follows:

| | |
|---|---|
| Dextrose | PhEur |
| Heparin | PhEur |
| Sodium hydroxide | PhEur |
| Hydrochloric acid | PhEur |

*Incompatibilities:* AlphaNine is supplied in glass vials, each with a vial of diluent (Water for Injections). No data on incompatibilities with other containers or solutions are available. It is therefore recommended that AlphaNine be reconstituted only with the diluent provided.

*Shelf life:* Lyophilised AlphaNine has a shelf life of 24 months at 2–8°C. Storage at no more than 30°C for 1 month within this period is acceptable.

Reconstituted AlphaNine has a shelf life of 3 hours at 25°C.

*Special precautions for storage:* Lyophilised AlphaNine should be stored under refrigeration (2–8°C), protected from light. Do not freeze.

*Nature and contents of container:* AlphaNine is a white/slightly yellow friable powder containing 500 IU, 1000 IU or 1500 IU of Factor IX (nominal sizes). The actual assay value is printed on the vial label. The container is Type I glass and is closed with a grey butyl rubber stopper, aluminium crimp seal (bearing the lot number) and plastic "Flip-Off" dust cover.

Each vial of AlphaNine is supplied with a separate diluent vial containing 10 ml Water for Injections (PL 4447/0016).

*Instructions for use/handling:* AlphaNine must be reconstituted with the diluent provided, before administration. AlphaNine is intended for intravenous use only and should be used within three hours of reconstitution. It is recommended that the solution be administered at less than 10 ml/minute. Aseptic technique must be employed.

Check assay value on label carefully before use.

*Reconstitution:*

1. Warm the diluent and concentrate vials to at least room temperature (but not above 37°C). This may take up to 45 minutes following removal from refrigerator, depending on the temperature of the room.
2. Remove the plastic flip-off caps from the diluent and concentrate vials.
3. Swab the exposed rubber surfaces with alcohol. Do not leave excess cleaning agent in the indentation on the stoppers.
4. Remove the covering from one end of a double-

ended needle to expose the short needle. Insert this exposed short needle through the depression in the centre of the stopper in the vial of diluent.
5. Remove the plastic cap from the upper end of the double-ended needle now seated in the stopper of the diluent vial. Holding the concentrate vial in one hand, invert the vial of diluent in the other hand and push the exposed end of the needle through the depression in the centre of the stopper, making certain that the diluent is always above the vial of concentrate. There should be enough vacuum in the vial to draw in all of the diluent.
6. Disconnect the two vials by removing the needle from the concentrate vial stopper. Swirl the concentrate vial until all concentrate is dissolved: do not shake. Reconstitution normally requires less than five minutes. When the reconstitution procedure is strictly followed a few small particles may occasionally remain. The microaggregate filter will retain particles and the labelled potency will not be reduced.

*Administration:*

1. Peel the cover from the microaggregate filter package and securely install the syringe into the exposed luer inlet of the filter using a slight clockwise twisting motion.
2. Remove the filter from the packaging. Remove the protective sleeve from the spike end of the filter using a clockwise twisting motion.
3. Pull back the plunger to aspirate sufficient air into the syringe to allow the reconstituted product to be withdrawn as described in the next step.
4. Insert the spike end of the filter into the reconstituted concentrate vial. Inject air and aspirate the reconstituted product from the vial into the syringe.
5. Remove and discard the filter from the syringe. Attach the syringe to an infusion set. Expel the air from the syringe and the infusion set. Perform venepuncture and administer slowly.
6. If the patient is to receive more than one vial of concentrate, the infusion set will allow this to be performed with a single venepuncture.
7. Discard all administration equipment after use.

*By administration set:*

1. Close the clamp on the administration set.
2. With the vial upright, insert the piercing pin straight through the stopper centre. Do not twist or angle.
3. Immediately invert the vial to automatically establish a proper fluid level in the drip chamber (half full).
4. Attach an infusion set, open the clamp and allow the solution to expel air from the tubing and needle, then close the clamp.
5. Perform venepuncture and adjust the flow, not to exceed 10 ml/minute.
6. Discard all administration equipment after use.

### Marketing authorisation numbers

| | |
|---|---|
| 500 IU/Vial | 4447/0030 |
| 1000 IU/Vial | 4447/0035 |
| 1500 IU/Vial | 4447/0036 |

**Date of approval/revision of SPC** February 1997

**Legal category** POM

## ALPHAPARIN*

### Qualitative and quantitative composition

Pre-filled syringes: Certoparin sodium 3000 IU (as anti-Xa) in 0.3 ml Water for Injections.

Ampoules: Certoparin sodium 3000 IU (as anti-Xa) and sodium chloride 1.69 mg in 0.5 ml Water for Injections.

**Pharmaceutical form** Pre-filled syringes and ampoules for subcutaneous injection.

### Clinical particulars

*Therapeutic indications:* The prophylaxis of peri- and post-operative venous thromboembolism.

*Posology and method of administration:*
*Adults:* 3000 IU per day. The first injection should be given 1 to 2 hours before surgery. Injections should then be given once daily for 7 to 10 days or until the patient is mobile. At each injection, the entire contents of the pre-filled syringe or ampoule should be administered.

*Elderly:* There is no reason, based on clinical trials, why elderly patients should require dosages other than those stated above.

*Children:* No studies have been carried out in children.

*Contra-indications:* Major bleeding disorders, bleeding ulcers of the stomach or intestine, severe hypertension (>200/120 mm Hg), hypersensitivity to heparin, subacute bacterial endocarditis, severe renal and/or hepatic dysfunction.

*Special warnings and precautions for use:* Alphaparin must not be administered by the intramuscular route.

Like heparin, this product may cause the following

misleading results: simulation of low cholesterol values in the serum; high T3 and T4 values in non-fasting patients; high blood sugar values; false positive bromsulphthalein test. It is recommended that the platelet count should be monitored before surgery, during therapy and at the end of treatment.

As the different low molecular weight heparins have differing characteristics, it is not recommended that similar preparations are given during treatment.

*Interactions with other medicaments and other forms of interaction:* As with the use of unfragmented heparin, the following interactions should be considered:

– Potentiation of effect by non-steroidal anti-inflammatory drugs as well as dicoumarols, dipyridamole, dextrans, ethacrynic acid and cytostatic agents.
– Reduction of effect by antihistamines, digitalis preparations, tetracyclines and ascorbic acid.

*Pregnancy and lactation:* A study in 60 pregnant women showed no passage of certoparin across the placenta. It is also known from unfractionated heparin and other low molecular weight heparins that they do not pass across the placenta, nor are they excreted in breast milk. Alphaparin should only be used in such patients if the theoretical advantages are considered to outweigh the potential risks.

*Effects on ability to drive and use machines:* Not applicable.

*Undesirable effects:* Minor bleeding at the injection site may be seen. In isolated cases there have been reports of hypersensitivity reactions (e.g. allergic skin reactions with swelling, pruritis or rash) at the site of injection or over the entire body. Other side effects which are associated with treatment with unfragmented heparin may also occur and include thrombocytopenia, raised liver enzymes and osteoporosis.

*Overdose:* Due to the mode of administration, overdosage is not likely to occur. Acute haemorrhage and cutaneous and mucosal bleeding would be expected. The effect of overdosage can be neutralised by slow iv injection of protamine sulphate, 1500 IU for each dose of Alphaparin. The effect on aPTT and prothrombin time is rapidly reversed, whilst the anti-Xa activity returns to normal more slowly.

### Pharmacological properties

*Pharmacodynamic properties:* Certoparin is a low molecular weight heparin with anti-thrombotic activity similar to unfractionated heparin. It has a powerful inhibitory effect on factor Xa but only a slight effect on aPTT. At the recommended doses, it does not significantly influence platelet aggregation.

*Pharmacokinetic properties:* Measured by the inhibition of factor Xa, which reaches its maximum after approximately 2 to 4 hours, subcutaneously administered certoparin is quickly absorbed. The mean half life of factor Xa inhibition is calculated to be 4.3 hours, compared with a mean half life of 2.2 hours for unfractionated heparin.

*Toxicological results:* The results of acute single dose and repeat dose toxicological studies showed that the tolerance of Alphaparin at high doses is limited only by its anticoagulant effect. The LD50 was found to be at least 30 times higher than the recommended human dose. Chronic toxicity studies revealed no toxic effect on any organ. No measurable transplacental passage was detected.

### Pharmaceutical properties

*List of excipients:*
Pre-filled syringes: Water for Injections.
Ampoules: Sodium chloride, Water for Injections.

*Incompatibilities:* Do not mix Alphaparin with other injections or infusions.

*Shelf life:* 24 months.

*Storage conditions:* Store at room temperature below 25°C.

*Nature and contents of container:*
Pre-filled syringes: PhEur type I glass syringe of 0.5 ml volume with chlorinated butyl rubber stopper and natural rubber cap.
Ampoules: PhEur type I glass ampoules of 1 ml volume.

*Instructions for use/handling:* Subcutaneous injection, usually into the peritoneal fold. With the patient supine, a fold of skin between the navel and the iliac crest should be lifted (not squeezed), the full length of the needle inserted and held vertically throughout the injection.

The injection can be administered at other sites if deemed necessary.

### Marketing authorisation numbers

| | |
|---|---|
| Pre-filled syringes | 4447/0033 |
| Ampoules | 4447/0034 |

**Date of approval/revision of SPC** November 1995.

**Legal category** POM

*Trade Mark

# Amersham International plc
Amersham Place
Little Chalfont
Buckinghamshire
United Kingdom

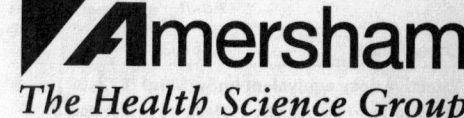

## CERETEC*
### Kit for the preparation of Technetium [⁹⁹mTc] Exametazime Injection

**Qualitative and quantitative composition** Exametazime 0.5 mg.

**Pharmaceutical form** Powder for injection.

**Clinical particulars**

*Indications:*

(i) Technetium [⁹⁹mTc] Exametazime Injection is indicated for brain scintigraphy. The product is to be used for the diagnosis of abnormalities of regional cerebral blood flow, such as those occurring following stroke and other cerebrovascular disease, epilepsy, Alzheimer's Disease and other forms of dementia, transient ischaemic attack, migraine and tumours of the brain.

(ii) Technetium [⁹⁹mTc] Exametazime Injection is also indicated for *in vitro* technetium-99m leucocyte labelling, the labelled leucocytes subsequently being re-injected and scintigraphy carried out to image the sites of localisation. This procedure may be used in the detection of sites of focal infection (e.g. abdominal abscess), in the investigation of pyrexia of unknown origin and in the evaluation of inflammatory conditions not associated with infection such as inflammatory bowel disease.

*Posology and method of administration:* The route of administration is direct intravenous injection for brain scintigraphy studies and intravenous injection of labelled leucocytes post labelling *in vitro*.

Dose for adults and the elderly:
(i) for brain scintigraphy, 350-500MBq
(ii) for *in vivo* localisation of technetium-99m-labelled leucocytes, 200MBq
Normally a once-only diagnostic procedure

Technetium [⁹⁹mTc]-Exametazime and Technetium-99m-labelled leucocytes are not recommended for administration to children.

*Contra-indications:* There are no specific contra-indications.

*Special warnings and precautions for use:* Radiopharmaceutical agents should only be used by qualified personnel with the appropriate government authorisation for the use and manipulation of radionuclides. They may be received, used and administered only by authorised persons in designated clinical settings. Their receipt, storage, use, transfer and disposal are subject to the regulations and/or appropriate licences of the local competent official organisations.

Radiopharmaceuticals should be prepared by the user in a manner which satisfies both radiation safety and pharmaceutical quality requirements. Appropriate aseptic precautions should be taken, complying with the requirements of Good Manufacturing Practice for pharmaceuticals. Normal safety precautions for the handling of blood products should be observed in the preparation and administration of labelled leucocytes.

When preparing technetium-99m-labelled leucocytes it is essential that cells are washed free of sedimentation agents before they are re-injected into the patient as materials used in cell separation may cause hypersensitivity reactions.

*Interaction with other medicaments and other forms of interaction:* No drug interactions have been reported to date.

*Pregnancy and lactation:* No data are available on the use of this product in human pregnancy. Animal reproduction studies have not been performed.

When it is necessary to administer radioactive medicinal products to women of childbearing potential, information should always be sought about pregnancy. Any woman who has missed a period should be assumed to be pregnant until proven otherwise. Where uncertainty exists it is important that radiation exposure should be the minimum consistent with achieving the desired clinical information. Alternative techniques which do not involve ionising radiation should be considered. Radionuclide procedures carried out on pregnant women also involve radiation doses to the foetus. Only imperative investigations should be carried out during preg-

nancy, when the likely benefit exceeds the risk incurred by the mother and the foetus.

Before administering a radioactive medicinal product to a mother who is breast feeding consideration should be given as to whether the investigation could be reasonably delayed until after the mother has ceased breast feeding and as to whether the most appropriate choice of radiopharmaceutical has been made, bearing in mind the secretion of activity in breast milk. If the administration is considered necessary, breast feeding should be interrupted for 12 hours and the expressed feeds discarded. Breast feeding can be restarted when the level in the milk will not result in a radiation dose to the child greater than 1 mSv.

*Effects on ability to drive and use machines:* No effects on the ability to drive or to operate machines have been reported to date.

*Undesirable effects:* A very few cases of mild hypersensitivity evidenced by the development of an urticarial erythematous rash have been reported following direct intravenous injection of the reconstituted product. A very few reports have also been received of hypersensitivity reactions, possibly anaphylactic in nature, following administration of technetium-99m-labelled leucocytes prepared using Technetium [⁹⁹mTc]-exametazime.

For each patient, exposure to ionising radiation must be justifiable on the basis of likely benefit. The activity administered must be such that the resulting radiation dose is as low as reasonably achievable bearing in mind the need to obtain the intended diagnostic result.

Exposure to ionising radiation is linked with cancer induction and a potential for development of hereditary defects. For diagnostic nuclear medicine investigations the current evidence suggests that these adverse effects will occur with low frequency because of the low radiation doses incurred.

For most diagnostic investigations using a nuclear medicine procedure the radiation dose (EDE) is less than 20 mSv. Higher doses may be justified in some clinical circumstances.

*Overdose:* In the event of the administration of a radiation overdose frequent micturition and defecation should be encouraged in order to minimise the absorbed dose to patient.

**Pharmacological properties**

*Pharmacodynamic properties:* At the chemical concentrations and activities used for diagnostic procedures technetium [⁹⁹mTc]-exametazime and technetium-99m-labelled leucocytes do not appear to exert any pharmacodynamic effects.

*Pharmacokinetic properties:*

(i) Direct intravenous injection

The technetium-99m complex of the active ingredient is uncharged, lipophilic and of sufficiently low molecular weight to cross the blood-brain barrier. It is rapidly cleared from the blood after intravenous injection. Uptake in the brain reaches a maximum of 3.5-7.0% of the injected dose within one minute of injection. Up to 15% of the cerebral activity washes out of the brain 2 minutes post injection after which there is little loss of activity for the following 24 hours except by physical decay of technetium-99m. The activity not associated with the brain is widely distributed throughout the body particularly in muscle and soft tissue. About 20% of the injected dose is removed by the liver immediately after injection and excreted through the hepatobiliary system. About 40% of the injected dose is excreted through the kidneys and urine over the 48 hours after injection resulting in a reduction in general muscle and soft tissue background.

(ii) Injection of labelled leucocytes

Technetium-99m-labelled leucocytes distribute between the marginating pools of the liver (within 5 minutes) and spleen (within about 40 minutes), and the circulating pool, (the latter represents approximately 50% of the leucocyte pool). Approximately 37% of the cell associated technetium-99m is recoverable from the circulating pool 40 minutes after injection. Technetium-99m activity is slowly eluted from the cells and is excreted partly by the kidneys

and partly via the liver into the gall bladder. This results in increasing amounts of activity being seen in the intestines.

*Preclinical safety data* There are no additional preclinical safety data of relevance for the prescriber in recognising the safety profile of the product used for the authorised indications.

*Radiation dosimetry data:* Technetium-99m disintegrates with the emission of gamma radiation with an energy of 140 keV and a half-life of 6 hours to technetium-99 which can be regarded as quasi-stable.

(i) Brain scintigraphy

According to ICRP 62 (International Commission on Radiological Protection) the estimated absorbed radiation doses to various organs following administration of technetium [⁹⁹mTc]-exametazime to adults are in the table below:

| Organ | Absorbed dose per unit activity administered (mGy/MBq) Adult |
|---|---|
| Adrenals | 5.3E–03 |
| Bladder | 2.3E–02 |
| Bone surfaces | 5.1E–03 |
| Brain | 6.8E–03 |
| Breast | 2.0E–03 |
| Gall bladder | 1.8E–02 |
| GI tract | |
| Stomach | 6.4E–03 |
| SI | 1.2E–02 |
| ULI | 1.8E–02 |
| LLI | 1.5E–02 |
| Heart | 3.7E–03 |
| Kidneys | 3.4E–02 |
| Liver | 8.6E–03 |
| Lungs | 1.1E–02 |
| Muscles | 2.8E–03 |
| Oesophagus | 2.6E–03 |
| Ovaries | 6.6E–03 |
| Pancreas | 5.1E–03 |
| Red marrow | 3.4E–03 |
| Skin | 1.6E–03 |
| Spleen | 4.3E–03 |
| Testes | 2.4E–03 |
| Thymus | 2.6E–03 |
| Thyroid | 2.6E–02 |
| Uterus | 6.6E–03 |
| Remaining organs | 3.2E–03 |

**Effective dose equivalent (mSv/MBq) 1.1E–02**

Effective Dose (E) is 4.7 mSv/500 MBq (70 kg individual).

(ii) *In vivo* localisation of technetium-99m-labelled leucocytes

The estimated absorbed radiation doses to various organs following the intravenous administration of technetium-99m-labelled leucocytes to adults given by ICRP 53 are in the table below:

| Organ | Absorbed dose per unit activity administered (mGy/MBq) Adult |
|---|---|
| Adrenals | 8.9E–03 |
| Bladder wall | 2.6E–03 |
| Bone surfaces | 1.3E–02 |
| Breast | 3.1E–03 |
| GI tract | |
| Stomach wall | 8.0E–03 |
| Small intestine | 4.9E–03 |
| ULI wall | 4.9E–03 |
| LLI wall | 3.9E–03 |
| Heart | 9.0E–03 |
| Kidneys | 9.9E–03 |
| Liver | 2.0E–02 |
| Lungs | 6.9E–03 |
| Ovaries | 4.2E–03 |
| Pancreas | 1.4E–02 |
| Red marrow | 2.2E–02 |
| Spleen | 1.5E–01 |
| Testes | 1.7E–03 |
| Thyroid | 2.4E–03 |
| Uterus | 3.8E–03 |

| Organ | Absorbed dose per unit activity administered (mGy/MBq) Adult |
|---|---|
| Other tissue | 3.4E–03 |

**Effective dose equivalent (mSv/MBq)** 1.7E–02

Effective Dose (E) is 2.2 mSv/200 MBq (70 kg individual).

## Pharmaceutical particulars

*List of excipients:* The finished product contains the following excipients: Sodium chloride BP, Stannous chloride dihydrate DAB, Nitrogen gas USP

*Incompatibilities:* There are no known incompatibilities.

*Shelf-life:* The shelf-life of the product is 26 weeks from the day of manufacture. The labelled product must be injected within 30 minutes of reconstitution.

*Special precautions for storage:* Store the unopened product at any temperature in the range 2-25˚C. Store the reconstituted product at 15-25˚C. Storage should be in acordance with national regulations for radioactive materials.

*Nature and contents of the container:* The product is supplied in a glass vial sealed with a chlorobutyl rubber closure and metal overseal.

*Instructions for use/handling:* Procedure for preparation of technetium [⁹⁹ᵐTc]exametazime for intravenous injection or *in vitro* leucocyte labelling:

Use aseptic technique throughout

(i) Place the vial in a shielding container and swab the closure with the sanitising swab provided.

(ii) Using a 10 ml syringe, inject into the shielded vial 5 ml of sterile eluate from a ⁹⁹ᵐTc generator (see notes 1–6). Before withdrawing the syringe from the vial withdraw 5 ml of gas from the space above the solution to normalise the pressure in the vial. Shake the shielded vial for 10 seconds to ensure complete dissolution of the powder.

(iii) Assay the total activity and calculate the volume to be injected or used for *in vitro* technetium-99m-leucocyte labelling.

(iv) Complete the label provided and attach to the vial.

(v) Use within a maximum of 30 minutes after reconstitution. Discard any unused material.

*Note:*

1. For the highest radiochemical purity reconstitute with freshly eluted ⁹⁹ᵐTc generator eluate.

2. Use only eluate which was eluted less than 2 hours previously from a generator which was eluted within 24 hours.

3. 0.37–1.11GBq (10–30 mCi) technetium-99m may be added to the vial.

4. Before reconstitution the generator eluate may be adjusted to the correct radioactive concentration (0.37–1.11GBq in 5 ml) by dilution with saline for injection.

5. Pertechnetate complying with the specifications prescribed by the USP and BP/PhEur monographs on Sodium Pertechnetate [⁹⁹ᵐTc] Injection should be used.

6. The pH of the prepared injection/labelling agent is in the range 9.0–9.8.

Procedure for separation of leucocytes and subsequent *in vitro* labelling with technetium [⁹⁹ᵐTc] exametazime

Use aseptic technique throughout

i) Draw 9 ml of acid-citrate-dextrose⁽ᵃ⁾ into each of two 60 ml plastic non-heparinized syringes.

ii) Withdraw 51 ml of patient's blood into each syringe, using a 19G Butterfly needle infusion set. Close the syringes with sterile hubs.

iii) Dispense 2 ml sedimentation agent⁽ᵇ⁾ into each of 5 Universal containers or tubes.

iv) Without attaching a needle to the syringes dispense 20 ml of blood into each of the 5 Universal tubes containing sedimentation agent. Dispense the remaining 20 ml of blood into a tube without sedimentation agent.

TIP To avoid bubbles and frothing run the blood gently down the sides of the tubes.

v) Mix the blood and sedimentation agent with one gentle inversion. Remove the cap of the Universal tube and burst the bubble formed at the top using a sterile needle. Replace the cap and allow the tubes to stand for 30-60 minutes for erythrocyte sedimentation to take place.

TIP The period of time for erythrocyte sedimentation depends on the patient's condition. As a guideline it should be stopped when the blood has sedimented to give approximately half the volume as sedimented red cells.

vi) Meanwhile centrifuge the tube containing 20 ml of blood and no sedimentation agent at 2000 g for 10 minutes. This will yield supernatant cell-free plasma (CFP) containing ACD which is retained, at room temperature, for use as a cell labelling and re-injection medium.

vii) When sufficient red cell sedimentation has taken place [see (v)] carefully transfer 15 ml aliquots of the cloudy straw-coloured supernatant into clean Universal tubes. Take care to avoid withdrawing any sedimented erythrocytes. The supernatant is leucocyte-rich, platelet-rich plasma [LRPRP].

TIP Do not use needles on sampling syringes to avoid unnecessary cell damage.

viii) Centrifuge the LRPRP at 150 g for 5 minutes to give supernatant, platelet-rich plasma (PRP) and a pellet of 'mixed' leucocytes.

ix) Remove as much of the PRP as possible into clean Universal tubes and further centrifuge at 2000 g for 10 minutes to give more supernatant, cell-free plasma (CFP) containing sedimentation agent. This will be used to wash the cells after labelling.

x) Meanwhile loosen the pellets of 'mixed' leucocytes by *very* gently tapping and swirling the Universal tubes. Using a syringe, without an attached needle, pool all the cells into one tube then, using the same syringe, add 1 ml of cell-free plasma containing ACD (from vi) and *gently* swirl to resuspend.

xi) Reconstitute a vial of Ceretec with 5 ml of ⁹⁹ᵐTc generator eluate containing approximately 500MBq (13.5 mCi) of ⁹⁹ᵐTcO₄⁻ (using the procedure described above).

xii) *Immediately* following reconstitution add 4 ml of the resulting technetium [⁹⁹ᵐTc] exametazime solution to the 'mixed' leucocytes in CFP (from x).

xiii) *Gently* swirl to mix and incubate for 10 minutes at room temperature.

xiv) If required, immediately spot the chromatography strips for assessment of radiochemical purity of the technetium [⁹⁹ᵐTc] exametazime, as instructed overleaf.

xv) On completion of incubation *carefully* add 10 ml of CFP containing sedimentation agent (from ix) to the cells, in order to stop labelling. Gently invert the cells to mix.

xvi) Centrifuge at 150 g for 5 minutes.

xvii) Remove and retain all of the supernatant.

TIP It is critical that all the supernatant which contains unbound technetium [⁹⁹ᵐTc] exametazime is removed at this stage. This can be best achieved using a syringe with a wide-bore [19G] needle.

xviii) Gently resuspend the technetium-99m labelled mixed leucocyte preparation in 5-10 ml of CFP containing ACD from (vi). Gently swirl to mix.

xix) Measure the radioactivity in the cells and in the supernatant from (xvii). Calculate the labelling efficiency [LE] which is defined as the activity in the cells as a percentage of the sum of the activity in the cells and the activity in the supernatant.

TIP Labelling efficiency depends on the patient's leucocyte count and will vary according to the volume of the initial blood sample. Using the volumes in (ii), a LE of about 55% might be expected.

xx) Without attaching a needle, carefully draw up the labelled cells into a plastic, non-heparinised syringe and close it with a sterile hub. Measure the radioactivity.

xxi) Labelled cells are now ready for re-injection. This should be performed without delay.

*Note*

(a) Acid-citrate-dextrose (ACD) should be made up as follows:

NIH Formula A. For 1 litre add 22 g trisodium citrate, 8 g citric acid, 22.4 g dextrose and make up to 1 litre with Water for Injections PhEur. The product should be manufactured under aseptic condition. Commercial preparations of the product are also available. The product should be stored under the conditions recommended by the manufacturer and should be used only up to the expiry date given by the manufacturer.

(b) 6% hydroxyethyl starch should be manufactured under aseptic conditions. Commercial preparations of the product are available. The product should be stored under the conditions recommended by the manufacturer and should be used only up to the expiry date given by the manufacturer.

*Radiochemical purity measurement:* Three potential radiochemical impurities may be present in the prepared exametazime injection. These are a secondary technetium [⁹⁹ᵐTc]-exametazime complex, free pertechnetate and reduced-hydrolysed-technetium-99m. A combination of two chromatographic systems is necessary for the determination of the radiochemical purity of the injection.

Test samples are applied by needle approximately 2.5cm from the bottom of two Gelman ITLC/SG strips (2.5cm x 20cm). The strips are then immediately placed in prepared ascending chromatography development tanks, one containing butan-2-one and the other 0.9% aq. sodium chloride (1cm depth fresh solvent). After a 15cm elution the strips are removed, solvent fronts marked, the strips dried and the distribution of activity determined using suitable equipment.

*Interpretation of chromatograms*

System 1 (ITLC:butan-2-one(MEK))

Secondary technetium [⁹⁹ᵐTc] exametazime complex and reduced-hydrolysed-technetium remain at the origin.

Lipophilic technetium [⁹⁹ᵐTc] exametazime complex and pertechnetate migrate at Rf 0.8-1.0.

System 2 (ITLC:0.9% sodium chloride)

Lipophilic technetium [⁹⁹ᵐTc] exametazime complex, secondary technetium [⁹⁹ᵐTc] exametazime complex and reduced-hydrolysed-Tc remain at the origin. Pertechnetate migrates at Rf 0.8-1.0.

(i) Calculate the percentage of activity due to both secondary technetium [⁹⁹ᵐTc] exametazime complex and reduced-hydrolysed-technetium[⁹⁹ᵐTc] from System 1 (A%). Calculate the percentage of activity due to pertechnetate from System 2 (B%).

(ii) The radiochemical purity (as percentage lipophilic technetium [⁹⁹ᵐTc] exametazime complex) is given by: 100-(A%+B%) where:

A% represents the level of secondary technetium [⁹⁹ᵐTc] exametazime complex plus reduced-hydrolysed technetium-99m

B% represents the level of pertechnetate.

A radiochemical purity of at least 80% may be expected provided the test samples have been taken and analysed within 30 minutes of reconstitution.

**Marketing authorisation number** 0221/0126

**Date of approval/revision of SPC** March 1995

**Legal category** POM

## METASTRON*

**Qualitative and quantitative composition** A solution of the active ingredient strontium-89 chloride, (150MBq) in 4 ml water.

*Physical characteristics:* Strontium-89 is a pure beta emitter with an energy of 1.463MeV and a half-life of 50.5 days.

**Pharmaceutical form** Sterile aqueous solution for intravenous injection.

## Clinical particulars

*Therapeutic Indications:* Metastron is indicated as an adjunct to and as an alternative to external beam radiotherapy for the palliation of pain from bone metastases secondary to prostatic carcinoma at the stage of hormone therapy failure.

*Posology and method of administration:* Metastron is an aqueous solution for intravenous injection and should be used without dilution. The recommended dose is 150MBq (4 mCi) per injection. Alternatively in particularly heavy or light framed patients a dose of 2MBq (55µCi)/kg 'fat-free' body weight may be used. This dosage is suitable for the elderly. Repeat administrations should not be performed within 3 months of the previous Metastron injection. Further administrations are not indicated in patients who have not responded to a previous administration of Metastron. The product is not for administration to children.

*Contra-indications:* Use of the product in patients with evidence of seriously compromised bone marrow, particularly low neutrophil and platelet counts, is not recommended unless the potential benefit of the treatment is considered to outweigh the risk.

Metastron should not be used as a primary treatment for cord compression secondary to spinal metastases where more rapid treatment may be necessary.

*Special warnings and precautions for use:* Special precautions, such as urinary catheterisation, should be taken following administration of Metastron to patients who are significantly incontinent to minimise risks of radioactive contamination. International guidelines for disposal of radioactive waste must be followed.

It is recommended that the haematology of patients should be monitored. In considering repeat administration of Metastron the patient's haematological response to his initial dose, his current platelet levels and any other evidence of marrow depletion should all be carefully considered.

A cytotoxic agent may be administered to a patient who has previously received Metastron provided that his haematological parameters are stable and within the normal range. An interval of 12 weeks is recommended between administration of the two therapies.

The expected time of onset of pain relief (10 to 20 days following Metastron administration) should be taken into account in patient management. It is not recommended that Metastron is administered to patients with very short life expectancies.

Care should be exercised in the pre-treatment assessment of the haematological status of patients who, for the same cause, have previously received extensive bone radiation and/or another injectable bone-seeking isotope.

It is important that written information concerning

this treatment and the associated safety precautions are given to the patient, relatives and hospital staff. Users should refer to the accompanying Patient Information.

*Interaction with other medicaments and other forms of interaction:* Calcium therapy should be discontinued at least two weeks before Metastron administration.

*Pregnancy and lactation:* Not relevant due to indication.

*Effects on ability to drive and use machines:* None known.

*Undesirable effects:* Adverse effects may include an exacerbation of pain within the first few days of administration. In clinical trials this effect was temporary and controlled with analgesics. Some degree of haematological toxicity, including thrombocytopenia and leucopenia, is to be expected following administration of Metastron. Typically platelets will be depressed by about 30% (95% confidence limits 10-55%) compared to pre-administration levels. Because of the natural progress of their disease more severe depression of platelet levels may be observed in some patients.

*Overdose:* Not applicable.

**Pharmacological properties**

*Pharmacodynamic properties:* The chemical properties of strontium enable it to imitate calcium *in vivo*, rapidly localising in proliferating bone. Strontium-89 is a beta emitter (100%), with a physical half-life of 50.5 days. The range of β-particles in tissue is 0.8cm.

*Pharmacokinetic properties:* The extent of uptake and retention of strontium-89 will depend on the metastatic involvement of the skeleton. Strontium is retained in lesions with a long biological half life compared to the physical half-life of strontium-89, whilst strontium taken up into normal bone exhibits a half life of about 14 days. The longer retention of strontium-89 in metastatic lesions enables the isotope to deliver a larger radiation dose to metastases whilst delivering a relatively small dose to bone marrow.

Strontium which is not localised in the skeleton is excreted mainly via the urine with a small amount via the faeces.

*Preclinical safety data:* The chemical toxicity of non-radioactive strontium chloride is well-documented and of little consequence, particularly in terms of the risk/benefit to the patient for whom this product is intended.

*Radiation dosimetry:* The estimated radiation doses that would be received by normal healthy adults from the intravenous administration of 1MBq of strontium-89 are given in the table below. Data are taken from the ICRP publication 'Radiation Dose to Patients from Radiopharmaceuticals' ICRP 53.

Radiation doses to normal adults from the intravenous injection of strontium-89

| Organ | Absorbed radiation dose mGy/MBq |
|---|---|
| Bone surfaces | 17.0 |
| Red bone marrow | 11.0 |
| Lower large intestine wall | 4.7 |
| Bladder wall | 1.3 |
| Testes | 0.78 |

When osseous metastases are present significantly enhanced localisation of the radiopharmaceutical will occur with correspondingly higher doses to the metastases relative to other organs.

The absorbed dose to vertebral metastases has been measured in a group of 10 patients with widely varying extends of disease*. The minimum, maximum and mean doses in this group are listed below.

Radiation dose to vertebral metastases from intravenous injection of strontium-89

| | Absorbed radiation dose mGy/MBq |
|---|---|
| Minimum | 60 |
| Maximum | 610 |
| Mean | 230 |

*Blake, G M *et al* Strontium-89 therapy: Measurement of absorbed dose to skeletal metastases. J Nucl Med 1988; 29(4), 549-557.

The effective dose equivalent (EDE) for strontium-89 is 435 mSv per 150MBq.

**Pharmaceutical particulars**

*List of excipients:* Strontium chloride and Water for Injections PhEur.

*Incompatibilities:* None.

*Shelf life:* The shelf life of the product is 28 days post the radioactivity reference date.

*Special precautions for storage:* The product should be stored at room temperature.

*Nature and contents of container:* The product is supplied in a neutral glass vial as an aqueous solution. The vial is sealed with a PTFE coated rubber closure and metal overseal.

*Instructions for use/handling:* The normal precautions for handling radioactive materials should be observed.

After use, all materials associated with the preparation and administration of radiopharmaceuticals, including any unused product and its container, should be decontaminated or treated as radioactive waste and disposed of in accordance with the conditions specified by the local competent authority. Contaminated materials must be disposed of as radioactive waste via an authorised route.

**Marketing authorisation number** 0221/0127

**Date of approval/revision of SPC** February 1993

**Legal category** POM

## MYOVIEW* ▼
## Kit for the preparation of Technetium [99mTc] Tetrofosmin Injection

**Qualitative and quantitative composition** Tetrofosmin 0.23 mg/vial

**Pharmaceutical form** Lyophilisate for injection, intended for reconstitution with 4-8 ml of sterile Sodium Pertechnetate [99mTc] Injection PhEur at a radioactive concentration not exceeding 1.1GBq/ml.

**Clinical particulars**

*Indication:* Myoview is a myocardial perfusion agent indicated as an adjunct in the diagnosis and localization of myocardial ischaemia and/or infarction.

*Posology and method of administration:* For the diagnosis and localization of myocardial ischaemia the recommended procedure involves two intravenous injections of 99mTc-tetrofosmin. For adults and the elderly 185-250MBq is given at peak exercise, followed by 500-750MBq given at rest approximately 4 hours later. The activity administered should be restricted to 1000MBq in any one day.

As an adjunct in the diagnosis and localization of myocardial infarction, one injection of 99mTc-tetrofosmin (185-250MBq) at rest is sufficient.

Myoview is not recommended for use in children or adolescents as data are not available for these age groups.

Patients should be requested to fast overnight or to have only a light breakfast on the morning of the procedure.

Planar or preferably SPECT imaging should begin no earlier than 15 minutes post-injection. There is no evidence for significant changes in myocardial concentration or redistribution of 99mTc-tetrofosmin, therefore, images may be acquired up to at least four hours post-injection. For planar imaging the standard views (anterior, LAO 40°-45°, LAO 65°-70° and/or left lateral) should be acquired.

*Contra-indications:* Myoview is contraindicated in pregnancy and in patients with known hypersensitivity to tetrofosmin.

*Special warnings and precautions for use:* Radiopharmaceutical agents should only be used by qualified personnel with the appropriate government authorisation for the use and manipulation of radionuclides. They may be received, used and administered only by authorised persons in designated clinical settings. Their receipt, storage, use, transfer and disposal are subject to the regulations and/or appropriate licences of the local competent official organisations.

Radiopharmaceuticals should be prepared by the user in a manner which satisfies both radiation safety and pharmaceutical quality requirements. Appropriate aseptic precautions should be taken, complying with the requirements of Good Manufacturing Practice for pharmaceuticals.

*Interaction with other medicaments and other forms of interaction:* The interaction of Myoview with other drugs has not been systematically investigated, however no interactions were reported in clinical studies in which Myoview was administered to patients receiving comedication. Drugs which influence myocardial function and/or blood flow, e.g. beta blockers, calcium antagonists or nitrates, can lead to false negative results in diagnosis of coronary artery disease. The results of imaging studies should always, therefore, be considered in the light of current medication.

*Pregnancy and lactation:* Myoview is contraindicated in pregnancy. Animal reproductive toxicity studies have not been performed with this product. Radionu-

clide procedures carried out on pregnant women also involve radiation doses to the foetus. Administration of 99mTc-tetrofosmin at doses of 250MBq at exercise, followed by 750MBq at rest results in an absorbed dose to the uterus of 8.1 mGy. A radiation dose above 0.5 mGy (equivalent to that exposure from annual background radiation) would be regarded as a potential risk to the foetus.

When it is necessary to administer radioactive medicinal products to women of childbearing potential, information should always be sought about pregnancy. Any woman who has missed a period should be assumed to be pregnant until proven otherwise. Where uncertainty exists it is important that radiation exposure should be the minimum consistent with achieving the desired clinical information. Alternative techniques which do not involve ionising radiation should be considered.

Before administering a radioactive medicinal product to a mother who is breast feeding consideration should be given as to whether the investigation could be reasonably delayed until the mother has ceased breast feeding and as to whether the most appropriate choice of radiopharmaceutical has been made, bearing in mind the secretion of activity in breast milk. It is not known whether 99mTc-tetrofosmin is secreted in human milk, therefore if administration is considered necessary, formula feeding should be substituted for breast feeding for at least 12 hours.

*Effects on ability to drive and use machines:* None known.

*Undesirable effects:* No serious adverse effects have been reported following 99mTc-tetrofosmin injection. A few patients experienced a feeling of bodily warmth, vomiting (12-24 hours post-injection), a transient metallic taste, disturbance of smell or a mild burning sensation in the mouth after injection. Transient rises in white blood cell counts have been reported in a small number of patients.

For each patient, exposure to ionising radiation must be justifiable on the basis of likely benefit. The activity administered must be such that the resulting radiation dose is as low as reasonably achievable bearing in mind the need to obtain the intended diagnostic result. Exposure to ionising radiation are linked with cancer induction and a potential for development of hereditary defects. For diagnostic nuclear medicine investigations the current evidence suggests that these adverse events will occur with negligible frequency because of the low radiation dose incurred.

For most diagnostic investigations using a nuclear medicine procedure the radiation dose (EDE) delivered is less than 20 mSv. Higher doses may be justified in some clinical circumstances.

*Overdose:* In cases of overdosage of radioactivity frequent micturition and defaecation should be encouraged in order to minimize radiation dosage to the patient.

**Pharmacological properties**

*Pharmacodynamic properties:* Pharmacological effects are not expected following intravenous administration of reconstituted Myoview at the recommended dosage. Studies in animals have shown that myocardial uptake of 99mTc-tetrofosmin is linearly related to coronary blood flow, confirming the effectiveness of the complex as a myocardial perfusion imaging agent.

*Pharmacokinetic properties:* 99mTc-tetrofosmin is rapidly cleared from the blood after intravenous injection; less than 5% of the administered activity remains in whole blood at 10 minutes post-injection. Uptake in the myocardium is rapid, reaching a maximum of about 1.2% of injected dose with sufficient retention to allow imaging of the myocardium by planar or SPECT techniques from 5 minutes up to 4 hours post-administration. Background tissue clearance is rapid from lung and liver and activity is reduced in these organs following exercise, with enhanced sequestration in skeletal muscle. Approximately 66% of the injected activity is excreted within 48 hours post-injection, with approximately 40% excreted in the urine and 26% in the faeces.

*Preclinical safety data:* Acute toxicity studies employing Myoview at dosage levels of approximately 1050 times the maximum human single dose failed to reveal mortality or any significant signs of toxicity in rats or rabbits. In repeated dose studies some evidence of toxicity was observed in rabbits, but only at cumulative doses exceeding 10,000 times the maximum human single dose. In rats receiving these doses there was no significant evidence of toxicity. Studies on reproductive toxicity have not been conducted. Tetrofosmin showed no evidence of mutagenic potential in *in vitro* or *in vivo* mutagenicity studies. Studies to assess the carcinogenic potential of Myoview have not been performed.

*Radiation dosimetry data:* The estimated absorbed

radiation dose to an average adult patient (70 kg) from intravenous injections of $^{99m}$Tc-tetrofosmin are listed in the table below. The values are calculated assuming urinary bladder emptying at 3.5 hour intervals.

Frequent bladder emptying should be encouraged after dosing to minimize radiation exposure.

| Organ | Absorbed radiation dose (μGy/MBq) | |
| --- | --- | --- |
| | Exercise | Rest |
| Gallbladder wall | 33.2 | 48.6 |
| Upper large intestine | 20.1 | 30.4 |
| Lower large intestine | 15.3 | 22.2 |
| Urinary bladder wall | 15.6 | 19.3 |
| Small intestine | 12.1 | 17.0 |
| Kidney | 10.4 | 12.5 |
| Salivary glands | 8.0 | 11.6 |
| Ovaries | 7.9 | 9.6 |
| Uterus | 7.3 | 8.4 |
| Bone surface | 6.2 | 5.6 |
| Thyroid | 4.3 | 5.8 |
| Pancreas | 5.0 | 5.0 |
| Stomach | 4.6 | 4.6 |
| Adrenals | 4.3 | 4.1 |
| Red Marrow | 4.1 | 4.0 |
| Heart wall | 4.1 | 4.0 |
| Spleen | 4.1 | 3.8 |
| Muscle | 3.5 | 3.3 |
| Testes | 3.4 | 3.1 |
| Liver | 3.2 | 4.2 |
| Thymus | 3.1 | 2.5 |
| Brain | 2.7 | 2.2 |
| Lungs | 2.3 | 2.1 |
| Skin | 2.2 | 1.9 |
| Breasts | 2.2 | 1.8 |
| Total body | 3.8 | 3.7 |

The effective dose equivalent (EDE) resulting from the administration of doses of reconstituted Myoview of 250MBq after exercise and 750MBq at rest is 2.15 mSv after exercise and 8.38 mSv at rest (per 70 kg individual).

Sodium Pertechnetate [$^{99m}$Tc] Injection is produced by a [$^{99}$Mo/$^{99m}$Tc] generator. [$^{99m}$Tc] Technetium disintegrates with the emission of gamma radiation (energy 141 keV) and a half-life of 6.02 hours.

## Pharmaceutical particulars

*List of excipients:* Stannous chloride dihydrate DAB, disodium sulphosalicylate, sodium D-gluconate, sodium hydrogen carbonate, Nitrogen gas USP.

*Incompatibilities:* None known, however $^{99m}$Tc-tetro-fosmin should not be mixed or diluted with any substance other than those recommended for reconstitution.

*Shelf-life:* The shelf-life of the packaged product is 26 weeks and that of the prepared injection 8 hours after reconstitution with Sodium Pertechnetate [$^{99m}$Tc] Injection PhEur.

*Special precautions for storage:* Store the product at 2-8°C before and after reconstitution.

*Nature and contents of the container:* The product is supplied in a clear glass vial sealed with a chlorobutyl rubber closure and metal overseal.

*Instructions for use/handling:* Normal safety precautions for the handling of radioactive materials should be observed in addition to the use of aseptic technique to maintain sterility of the vial contents.

Procedure for the preparation of $^{99m}$Tc-tetrofosmin:

1. Place the vial in a suitable shielding container and sanitize the rubber septum with the swab provided.

2. Using a shielded, 10 ml sterile syringe, inject the required activity of Sodium Pertechnetate [$^{99m}$Tc] Injection PhEur (appropriately diluted with 0.9% Sodium Chloride Injection BP) into the shielded vial (see Notes 1 and 2). Before removing the syringe from the vial, withdraw a volume of gas from above the solution equal to the volume of eluate added, to normalise the pressure inside the vial. Shake the vial to ensure complete dissolution of the powder.

3. Incubate at room temperature for 15 minutes.

4. During this time assay the total activity, complete the user label provided and attach it to the vial.

5. Store the reconstituted injection at 2-8°C and use within 8 hours of preparation. Dispose of any unused material and its container via an authorised route.

**Notes:**

1. The Sodium Pertechnetate [$^{99m}$Tc] Injection PhEur used for reconstitution should contain less than 5ppm aluminium.

2. The volume of diluted Sodium Pertechnetate [$^{99m}$Tc] Injection PhEur added to the vial must be in the range 4-8 ml.

3. The radioactive concentration of the diluted Sodium Pertechnetate [$^{99m}$Tc] Injection PhEur must not exceed 1.1GBq/ml when it is added to the vial.

4. The pH of the prepared injection is in the range 7.5-9.0.

*Radiochemical purity measurement:* Radiochemical purity may be checked according to the following procedure:

*Equipment and eluent:*
1. Gelman ITLC/SG strip (2cm x 20cm)
2. Ascending chromatography tank and cover
3. 35:65 v/v mixture of acetone and dichloromethane
4. 1 ml syringe with 22-25G needle
5. Suitable counting equipment

*Method:*

1. Pour the 35:65 acetone:dichloromethane mixture into the chromatography tank to a depth of 1cm and cover the tank to allow the solvent vapour to equilibrate.

2. Mark an ITLC/SG strip with a pencil line at 3cm from the bottom and, using an ink marker pen, at 15cm from the pencil line. The pencil line indicates the origin where the sample is to be applied and movement of colour from the ink line will indicate the position of the solvent front when upward elution should be stopped.

3. Cutting positions at 3cm and 12cm above the origin (Rf's 0.2 and 0.8 respectively) should also be marked in pencil.

4. Using a 1 ml syringe and needle, apply a 10-20μl sample of the prepared injection at the origin of the strip. Do not allow the spot to dry. Place the strip in the chromatography tank immediately and replace the cover. Ensure that the strip is not adhering to the walls of the tank.

**Note:** A 10-20μl sample will produce a spot with a diameter of 7-10 mm. Smaller sample volumes have been shown to give unreliable radiochemical purity values.

5. When the solvent reaches the ink line, remove the strip from the tank and allow it to dry.

6. Cut the strip into 3 pieces at the marked cutting positions and measure the activity on each using suitable counting equipment. Try to ensure similar counting geometry for each piece and minimize equipment dead time losses.

7. Calculate the radiochemical purity from:

$$\%\,^{99m}\text{Tc-tetrofosmin} = \frac{\text{Activity of centre piece}}{\text{Total activity of all 3 pieces}} \times 100$$

*Note:* Free [$^{99m}$Tc] pertechnetate runs to the top piece of the strip. $^{99m}$Tc-tetrofosmin runs to the centre piece of the strip. Reduced hydrolysed-$^{99m}$Tc and any hydrophilic complex impurities remain at the origin in the bottom piece of the strip.

Do not use material if the radiochemical purity is less than 90%.

**Marketing authorisation number** 0221/0128

**Date of approval/revision of SPC** 13 December 1993

**Legal category** POM

*Trade Mark

**Approved Prescription Services Ltd**
Brampton Road
Hampden Park
Eastbourne
East Sussex
BN22 9AG

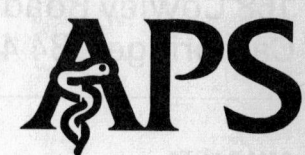

## APSTIL* TABLETS

**Presentation** Apstil is presented as pink, biconvex, film-coated tablets plain on one side and inscribed APS over a code number on the reverse. The tablets contain Diethylstilboestrol PhEur and comply with the monograph for Stilboestrol Tablets BP.

There are two strengths available: Apstil 1 mg Tablets marked 1313; and Apstil 5 mg Tablets marked 1314. The tablets also contain lactose and colours E171, E127, E110 and E132.

**Uses** Stilboestrol is a synthetic non-steroidal oestrogen hormone. It has been in use for many years. However, it has carcinogenic potential, so its use is now only justified in the management of malignant disease.

It may be used to suppress androgenic hormonal activity in the management of androgen-dependent carcinomas such as carcinoma of the prostate in males and some post-menopausal carcinomas such as breast cancer in females.

Apstil Tablets may therefore be used in:
a. Carcinoma of the prostate;
b. Metastatic post-menopausal carcinoma of the breast.

### Dosage and administration

**Adults:**
Management of prostatic carcinoma 1-3 mg daily.
Management of post-menopausal breast carcinoma 10-20 mg daily.

*Children:* Not suitable.

*The elderly:* As the conditions for which Apstil is indicated primarily occur in the elderly, the recommended dosage remains unchanged.

### Contra-indications, warnings, etc.
*Contra-indications:* Stilboestrol is contra-indicated in:
a. pregnancy–it is not suitable for pre-menopausal women;
b. children;
c. any oestrogen-dependent neoplasms especially of the genital tract;
d. pre-menopausal carcinoma of the breast;
e. endometrial hyperplasia;
f. uterine fibromyomata (fibroids);

or where there is:

g. undiagnosed vaginal bleeding;
h. a history of herpes gestationis;
i. porphyria;
j. moderate to severe hypertension;
k. severe or active liver disease;

l. a history of thrombo-embolism or conditions predisposing to it such as sickle cell anaemia, untreated polycythaemia and pulmonary hypertension;
m. hyperlipoproteinaemia;
n. any cardiovascular or cerebrovascular disorder.

*Precautions:* Care should be taken when administering Stilboestrol preparations to patients with:

a. cardiac failure;
b. hypertension;
c. diabetes;
d. epilepsy;
e. migraine;
f. depression;
g. contact lenses;
h. cholelithiasis;
i. a history of or with cholestatic jaundice from any cause e.g., jaundice of pregnancy or following the use of oral contraceptives;
j. any evidence of renal dysfunction.

During treatment with Apstil the blood pressure should be monitored at regular intervals and if hypertension develops treatment should be stopped. In addition, if surgery is contemplated or signs or symptoms of thrombosis develop treatment should also be discontinued. This is because of the significant increase in risk of deep vein thrombosis in the presence of high oestrogen activity.

In patients who suffer from diabetes, glucose tolerance may be lowered, and the need for insulin or other anti-diabetic drugs may be increased.

In thyroid disease or investigations of thyroid function, thyroid hormone binding globulin may be increased leading to increased circulating total thyroid hormone, which may lead to difficulty in interpreting thyroid function tests.

Oestrogens may antagonise diuretics and reduce the effect of anti-hypertensives.

*Pregnancy:* Apstil is NOT indicated for pre-menopausal women.

*Children:* Apstil is NOT suitable for children.

*Adverse reactions:* As high doses of stilboestrol in early pregnancy have caused vaginal carcinoma in female offspring 16-20 years later, it should not be used in pre-menopausal women.

As with other oestrogens the following hormonal disturbances may occur – fluid retention, headache, nausea and vomiting, weight gain, hypertension, breast discomfort, chloasma, skin rashes, erythema nodosum, cholelithiasis and cholestatic jaundice.

Venous thrombosis, thromboembolism and possibly cerebral and coronary thrombosis are also risks.

In women, Stilboestrol may cause an increase in the size of uterine fibromyomata, endometrial proliferation and/or an aggravation or recurrence of endometriosis and an excessive production of cervical mucous. The risk of endometrial neoplasia is increased significantly.

In both sexes the use of Stilboestrol may cause tenderness, pain, enlargement and secretion of milk like fluid from the breast. It also may aggravate corneal discomfort in patients with contact lenses and be associated with fluctuating moods (both elation and depression) and headaches including an increase in incidence of migraine.

The general metabolic effects of Stilboestrol include sodium and water retention, reduced glucose tolerance and changes in body weight (usually increases).

In men there will be some feminization, e.g. gynaecomastia and testicular atrophy, and impotence.

Other effects may be withdrawal bleeding in women and an increased incidence of cholelithiasis. In the event of prolonged usage there is an increased risk of endometrial carcinoma.

*Overdosage:* There is no specific antidote to stilboestrol. The commonest symptoms of overdosage are nausea and vomiting. Management may include gastric lavage associated with special care of plasma electrolytes and any other appropriate symptomatic relief. Should the overdose (abuse) be in female children, an oestrogen-withdrawal bleed may be induced.

**Pharmaceutical precautions** Apstil Tablets should be stored in a dry place below 25°C and protected from light.

**Legal category** POM.

**Package quantities**
Apstil Tablets 1 mg: Blister packs of 56.
Apstil Tablets 5 mg: Blister packs of 28.

**Further information** Apstil should not be used in children or young adults because it has carcinogenic potential.

In prostatic carcinoma and metastatic post-menopausal breast carcinoma, stilboestrol causes temporary disease regression in approximately 80% and 30% of patients respectively.

**Product licence numbers**
Apstil Tablets 1 mg    0289/5188R
Apstil Tablets 5 mg    0289/5189R

*\*Trade Mark*

# ASTA Medica Limited
168 Cowley Road
Cambridge CB4 4DL

ASTA MEDICA

## ANABACT*

**Presentation** A pale yellow water-based clear gel containing metronidazole 0.75% w/w for topical application.

### Uses
*Action:* Prophylaxis and treatment of anaerobic bacterial infections especially those associated with pungent odours.

*Indications:* For the treatment of malodorous fungating tumours.

### Dosage and administration
*Adults and elderly:* Clean the wound thoroughly. Apply the gel over the complete area and cover with a non-adherent dressing. Use twice daily or as directed.

*Children:* Not recommended.

### Contra-indications, warnings, etc
*Contra-indications:* Known hypersensitivity to metronidazole, Bronopol, Hydroxybenzoic acid esters, hydroxyethylcellulose or propylene glycol.

*Use in pregnancy and lactation:* The safety of metronidazole in pregnancy and lactation has not been adequately established. The gel should therefore not be used in these circumstances unless the physician considers it essential. Medication should be stopped if the patient becomes pregnant.

*Side-effects:* Dryness of the skin, itching and peeling have reported during treatment with Metronidazole Topical Gel.

*Warnings* Strong sunlight should be avoided as metronidazole is unstable under ultra-violet light.

Contact with the eyes should be avoided, but if it should occur the gel should be washed out carefully with water.

*Interactions:* Oral metronidazole has been shown to cause a Disulfiram-like reaction in a small number of patients taking concomitant alcohol. This reaction has not been reported with the topical preparation.

*Overdosage:* There are no clinical reports of overdosage.

**Pharmaceutical precautions** To be stored between 15°C-25°C. The cap should be replaced after use. To be stored away from direct sunlight.

**Legal category** POM.

**Package quantities** Tubes containing 15 g and 30 g.

**Further information**
*Ingredients:* Metronidazole, bronopol, hydroxybenzoic acid esters, hydroxyethylcellulose, propylene glycol and purified water.

**Product licence number** 12650/0002

*Product licence holder:* Bioglan Pharmaceuticals Ltd

## BRONCHODIL* AEROSOL

**Qualitative and quantitative composition** Each 0.05 ml actuation contains 0.5 mg reproterol hydrochloride.

**Pharmaceutical form** Metered dose aerosol containing 400 inhalations. Administration by inhalation.

### Clinical particulars
*Therapeutic indications:* Bronchodil, a selective beta$_2$-adrenergic stimulant is indicated for the treatment of conditions involving reversible airways obstruction, such as bronchial asthma, including that of an allergic origin, acute and chronic bronchitis and emphysema.

It is effective in the prophylaxis of acute attacks of bronchospasm.

*Posology and method of administration:* For administration by inhalation.

*Adults including elderly:* For acute attacks of bronchospasm the usual dose is 1 or 2 inhalations, repeated every 3–6 hours as required. For chronic reversible obstruction of the airways, and the prophylaxis of recurrent attacks of acute bronchospasm, the usual dose is 2 inhalations three times a day.

*Children 6-12 years:* No more than 1 inhalation every 3–6 hours for acute attacks, or three times a day for prophylaxis.

*Contra-indications:* Bronchodil is contraindicated in patients with proven allergy to any of its components.

*Special warnings and special precautions for use:* Care should be taken with patients suffering from myocardial infarction, thyrotoxicosis or phaeochromocytoma. Bronchodil should be used with caution in patients already receiving sympathomimetic agents. Exceeding the stated dose does not produce an enhanced therapeutic effect and should be avoided. Patients should be advised to seek medical advice if their prescribed dose of beta agonist becomes less effective.

*Interactions:* Bronchodil should not be prescribed with beta-blocking drugs.

Potentially serious hypokalaemia may result from beta$_2$ agonist therapy. Particular caution is advised in severe asthma as this effect may be potentiated by concomitant treatment with xanthine derivatives, steroids, diuretics and by hypoxia. It is recommended that serum potassium levels are monitored in such situations.

*Use in pregnancy and lactation:* Although no teratogenic effects have been observed in animal experiments, caution is recommended during the first trimester of pregnancy.

*Effects on ability to drive and use machines:* None.

*Other undesirable effects:* Bronchodil is generally well-tolerated but, as with other beta-adrenergic stimulants, digital tremor, palpitations, slight tachycardia and restlessness may occasionally occur.

Potentially serious hypokalaemia may result from beta$_2$ agonist therapy.

*Overdosage:* The preferred antidote for overdosage with Bronchodil Aerosol is a cardioselective beta blocking agent, but beta blocking drugs should be used with caution in patients with a history of bronchospasm.

### Pharmacological properties
*Pharmacodynamic properties:* Reproterol is a novel, selective beta$_2$-adrenergic stimulant with very little action on the cardiac receptors. It also inhibits phosphodiesterase.

*Pharmacokinetic properties:* Inhalation of 1 mg reproterol by a metered dose inhaler results in barely detectable plasma levels precluding formal pharmacokinetic studies.

*Preclinical safety data:* Not applicable.

### Pharmaceutical particulars
*Excipients:* Each 0.05 ml actuation contains: Saccharin (micronised), sorbitan trioleate, trichlorofluoromethane 11, dichlorotetrafluoroethane 114, dichlorodifluoromethane 12, dentomint.

*Incompatibilities:* None.

*Shelf life:* Three years.

*Special precautions for storage:* Do not store above 25°C.

*Nature and contents of container:* Aluminium monobloc cans closed with metered dose valves which release 0.05 ml aerosol suspension per operation of the valve. Contains 400 metered doses.

*Instructions for use and handling:* Do not attempt to open or puncture the container or expose it to temperatures above 50°C (122°F). Do not burn it even when empty.

**Marketing authorisation number** 8336/0026

**Date of approval/revision of SPC** March 1995.

**Legal category** POM.

## CYCLO-PROGYNOVA* 1 mg
## CYCLO-PROGYNOVA* 2 mg

### Qualitative and quantitative composition

*Cyclo-Progynova 1 mg*

| | |
|---|---|
| Beige tablets | 1 mg oestradiol valerate |
| Pale Brown tablets | 250 micrograms levonorgestrel |
| | 1 mg oestradiol valerate |

*Cyclo-Progynova 2 mg*

| | |
|---|---|
| White Tablets | 2 mg oestradiol valerate |
| Pale Brown Tablets | 500 micrograms norgestrel |
| | 2 mg oestradiol valerate |

**Pharmaceutical form** Sugar-coated tablets.

### Clinical particulars

*Therapeutic indications:*
*Cyclo-Progynova 1 mg and 2 mg:* Hormone replacement therapy for the treatment of the climacteric syndrome.

*Cyclo-Progynova 2 mg:* Prevention of postmenopausal osteoporosis in women considered at risk of developing fractures. Epidemiological studies suggest a number of risk factors may contribute to postmenopausal osteoporosis including:

- early menopause (either natural or surgically induced)
- family history of osteoporosis
- recent corticosteroid therapy
- thin
- a small frame
- cigarette consumption

For maximum prophylactic benefit treatment should commence as soon as possible after the menopause.

Bone mineral density measurements may help to confirm the presence of low bone mass.

*Posology and method of administration:* Cyclo-Progynova 1 mg or Cyclo-Progynova 2 mg to be taken orally at the following doses:
*Adult women:* One tablet per day for 21 days with a 7-day tablet-free interval between courses.

*Contra-indications:*

- pregnancy
- severe disturbances of liver function
- previous or existing liver tumours
- jaundice or general pruritus during a previous pregnancy
- Dubin-Johnson syndrome
- Rotor syndrome
- existing or previous thromboembolic processes
- sickle-cell anaemia
- suspected or existing hormone-dependent disorders or tumours of the uterus and breast
- undiagnosed irregular vaginal bleeding
- congenital disturbances of lipid metabolism
- a history of herpes gestationis
- otosclerosis with deterioration in previous pregnancies
- endometriosis
- severe diabetes with vascular changes
- mastopathy

*Special warnings and special precautions for use:* Before starting treatment, pregnancy must be excluded. If withdrawal bleeding fails to occur at about 28-day intervals, treatment should be stopped until pregnancy has been ruled out.

Before starting Cyclo-Progynova patients should have a thorough general medical and gynaecological examination with special emphasis on the bodyweight, blood pressure, heart, breasts, pelvic organs with an endometrial assessment if indicated, the legs and skin. Follow up examinations are recommended at least six-monthly during treatment.

Treatment should be stopped at once if migrainous or frequent and unusually severe headaches occur for the first time, or if there are other symptoms that are possible prodromata of vascular occlusion.

Treatment should also be stopped if trauma, illness or impending surgery is considered to entail a risk of thrombosis.

Treatment should be stopped at once if jaundice or pregnancy occurs, or if there is a significant rise in blood-pressure, the occurrence of thromboembolic disease or if there are exacerbations of epileptic seizures.

Pre-existing fibroids may increase in size under the influence of oestrogens. If this is observed, treatment should be discontinued.

In patients with mild chronic liver disease, liver function should be checked every 8-12 weeks.

Persistent breakthrough bleeding during treatment is an indication for endometrial assessment which may include biopsy.

Prolonged exposure to unopposed oestrogens may increase the risk of development of endometrial carcinoma. The general consensus of opinion is that the addition of 10 days progestogen towards the end of the cycle, as in Cyclo-Progynova, diminishes the possibility of such a risk, and some investigators consider that it might be protective.

At the present time there is some evidence which

suggests a slight increase in the relative risk of breast cancer in post-menopausal women receiving long-term hormone replacement therapy. A careful appraisal of the risk/benefit ratio should be undertaken before treating for longer than 5 to 10 years.

Thromboembolism has been reported in connection with oestrogen replacement therapy but there is no evidence to date that the overall incidence is increased.

Some women are predisposed to cholestasis during steroid therapy. Diseases that are known to be subject to deterioration during pregnancy (e.g. multiple sclerosis, epilepsy, diabetes, benign breast disease, hypertension, cardiac or renal dysfunction, asthma, porphyria, tetany and otosclerosis) and women with a strong family history of breast cancer should be carefully observed during treatment.

In rare cases benign, and in even rarer cases, malignant liver tumours leading in isolated cases to life-threatening intra-abdominal haemorrhage have been observed after the use of hormonal substances such as those contained in Cyclo-Progynova. If severe upper abdominal complaints, liver enlargement or signs of intra-abdominal haemorrhage occur, a liver tumour should be included in the differential diagnosis.

*Interaction with other medicaments and other forms of interaction:* Hormonal contraception should be stopped when treatment with Cyclo-Progynova is started and the patient should be advised to take non-hormonal contraceptive precautions.

Drugs which induce hepatic microsomal enzyme systems e.g. barbiturates, phenytoin, rifampicin, accelerate the metabolism of oestrogen/progestogen combinations such as Cyclo-Progynova and may reduce their efficacy.

The requirement for oral antidiabetics or insulin can change.

*Use in pregnancy and lactation:* Contra-indicated.

*Effects on ability to drive and to use machinery:* None known.

*Undesirable effects:* During the first few months of treatment, breakthrough bleeding, spotting and breast tenderness or enlargement can occur. These are usually temporary and normally disappear after continued treatment. Other symptoms known to occur are: anxiety, increased appetite, bloating, palpitations, depressive symptoms, dizziness, dyspepsia, leg pains and oedema, altered libido, headache, nausea, rashes, vomiting and altered weight.

*Overdose:* There have been no reports of ill-effects from overdosage which it is, therefore, generally unnecessary to treat. There are no specific antidotes, and treatment should be symptomatic.

**Pharmacological properties**

*Pharmacodynamic properties:* Cyclo-Progynova contains oestradiol valerate, (the valeric-acid ester of the endogenous female oestrogen, oestradiol) and the synthetic progestogen, levonorgestrel.

Oestradiol valerate provides hormone replacement during and after the climacteric. The addition of levonorgestrel in the second half of each course of tablets helps to provide good cycle control and opposes the development of endometrial hyperplasia.

*Pharmacokinetic properties:* Following oral administration to man, oestradiol valerate is split into the biologically-active oestradiol and the valerate which is rapidly degraded. Oestradiol is metabolised in the liver with the formation of sulphuric acid and glucuronic acid esters (conjugated oestrogens) which are excreted in the urine.

Levonorgestrel is similarly absorbed from the gastrointestinal tract, metabolised by the liver and excreted in the urine and faeces as glucuronide and sulphate conjugates.

*Preclinical safety data:* There are no preclinical safety data which could be of relevance to the prescriber and which are not already included in other relevant sections of the SPC.

**Pharmaceutical particulars**

*List of excipients:* Lactose, maize starch, povidone, talc, magnesium stearate (E572), sucrose, calcium carbonate (E170), polyethylene glycol 6000, montan glycol wax, titanium dioxide (E171), yellow ferric oxide (E172), red brown ferric oxide (E172), glycerin.

*Incompatibilities:* None stated.

*Shelf life:* Five years.

*Special precautions for storage:* Not applicable.

*Nature and contents of container:* Cardboard outer containing either: one circular blister pack or three circular blister packs. Each pack consists of aluminium foil and PVC and contains 21 tablets.

*Instructions for use/handling:* None stated.

**Marketing authorisation numbers**
Cyclo-Progynova 1 mg      .      .      08336/0087

Cyclo-Progynova 2 mg      .      .      08336/0088

**Date of approval/revision of SPC** April 1995

**Legal category** POM

## DIUMIDE-K* CONTINUS* Tablets

**Presentation** White and orange film-coated bi-layered tablets, bi-convex in shape embossed DK on one side. Each tablet contains Frusemide PhEur 40 mg and Potassium Chloride PhEur 600 mg (8 m Eq), the latter incorporated within a patented controlled release system.

### Uses
*Action:* Frusemide is a loop-diuretic, inhibiting resorption from the ascending loop of Henlé. Potassium chloride is present in the tablets to counteract the urinary loss of potassium induced by frusemide.

*Indications:* Diumide K Continus Tablets are indicated in patients requiring diuresis and concomitant potassium supplementation.

Indications include cardiac oedema, pulmonary oedema, hepatic oedema, renal oedema and peripheral oedema of various aetiologies.

### Dosage and administration
*Dosage:*
*Adults:* The usual adult dose is one tablet daily, normally in the morning. This may be adjusted depending on the condition.

*Children:* Diumide-K Continus Tablets are not suitable for paediatric use.

*Elderly:* Normal adult dose.

*Administration:* The tablets should be swallowed whole with water preferably prior to or during a meal. The tablets should not be chewed so as not to destroy the controlled release system constituting the potassium chloride layer.

### Contra-indications, warnings, etc
*Contra-indications:* Diumide-K Continus tablets are contra-indicated in porphyria, hyperkalaemia, precomatose states associated with liver cirrhosis, Addison's disease and concomitant administration of potassium sparing diuretics. Although the controlled release system minimises the likelihood of oesophageal ulceration, all solid forms of potassium medication are contra-indicated in the presence of obstructions in the digestive tract (e.g. resulting from compression of the oesophagus due to dilation of the left atrium or from stenosis of the gut).

*Use in pregnancy:* Specific experience is unavailable with Diumide-K Continus Tablets. Rat studies have shown the administration of frusemide (37.5-300 mg/kg twice daily) on days 6-17 of gestation produced dose related increases in wavy ribs. When providing potassium chloride during the dosing period, the incidence of wavy ribs reduced by 90% indicating that the teratogenicity was probably related to hypokalaemia.

In humans, frusemide crosses the placenta. Oral doses of 25 to 40 mg have produced peak cord serum concentrations after approximately 9 hours. Maternal and cord levels were equal at approximately 8 hours. Increased foetal urine production after maternal frusemide therapy has been observed in new-borns exposed to frusemide shortly before birth. Urinary sodium and potassium in treated neonates have been found to be significantly greater than in non exposed controls. Neonatal electrolyte disturbances may occur.

Whilst potassium chloride is a natural constituent of tissues and fluids, high or low levels can be detrimental to maternal and foetal cardiac function and serum levels should therefore be monitored closely. Frusemide has been used in pregnancy, in labour and in the puerperium in cases of excessive weight gain, oedema, hypertension and toxaemia of pregnancy with satisfactory results and with no embryofoetotoxic or teratogenic effects.

Diumide-K Continus Tablets should not be administered during the first trimester. Diuretics may reduce placental perfusion. After the first trimester, Diumide-K Continus Tablets should not be administered if the adequacy of placental perfusion is suspect.

*Nursing mothers:* Lactation may be inhibited due to maternal fluid depletion. Frusemide is excreted into breast milk, therefore Diumide-K Continus Tablets should be used with caution.

*Precautions:* Care should be exercised in patients with renal insufficiency where there is a risk of hyperkalaemia.

As with all medicines keep out of the reach of children.

*Interactions:* Care should be taken in patients being concurrently administered cardiac glycosides, hypotensive agents including ACE inhibitors and nephrotoxic antibiotics. Non-steroidal anti-inflammatory

drugs antagonise the diuretic effect. Serum lithium levels may be increased with concomitant administration.

*Side-effects:* Frusemide is generally well tolerated and the patented controlled release tablet ensures virtual absence of gastro-intestinal side-effects often associated with potassium administration.

Patients with prostatic hypertrophy or impairment of micturition have an increased risk of developing acute urinary retention.

Latent diabetes may become manifest or the insulin requirements of diabetic patients may increase.

Water and electrolyte balance may be disturbed and serum calcium levels may be reduced. Raised urea and creatinine levels may occur.

Hyperuricaemia may occur with frusemide therapy. In rare instances of allergic reaction treatment should be discontinued. Bone marrow depression and acute pancreatitis have also been reported as rare complications and therapy should be withdrawn.

*Overdosage:* Overdosage is characterised by excessive diuresis. Treatment of overdosage should be aimed at fluid replacement and correction of the resulting electrolyte imbalance.

**Pharmaceutical precautions** Store at or below 30°C.

**Legal category** POM.

**Package quantities** Cartons of 30 tablets (OP) in blister packs of 10. Containers of 250 tablets or 1000 tablets.

**Further information** Frusemide produces a rapid and sustained diuresis which lasts for approximately four hours following administration. The potassium chloride content is released from the patented controlled release tablet over a prolonged period ensuring maximum absorption and the avoidance of 'flushing out' of the potassium by the action of the diuretic.

**Product licence number** 8336/0001

## DIUREXAN* TABLETS

**Presentation** Tablets each containing 20 mg xipamide. The tablets are white, round with a bisecting score on one side and debossed A on the other, and have a diameter of 6 mm.

### Uses
*Action:* Diurexan is a diuretic and antihypertensive agent having a gentle onset of action and gradual, prolonged effect. Whereas the main diuretic activity lasts for up to 12 hours, the antihypertensive effect is evident for 24 hours or more.

*Indications:*

*Hypertension:* All grades of hypertension respond to treatment with Diurexan. It is an effective treatment on its own in mild to moderate hypertension, and may be used alone or combined with other antihypertensive agents in severe hypertension.

*Oedema:* Diurexan is indicated whenever diuretic therapy is required including congestive cardiac failure, hepatic oedema, renal oedema and peripheral oedema due to venous insufficiency.

### Dosage and administration
*Hypertension*

*Adults:* 1 tablet (20 mg) daily, as a single early morning dose. When using Diurexan in combination with other antihypertensive therapy, the same dose of 20 mg, as a single early morning dose, should be maintained.

*Children:* No dose recommended.

*Elderly:* See *Precautions.*

*Oedema*

*Adults:* In the initial phase of treatment the usual dose is 2 tablets (40 mg) daily in a single early morning dose. Depending on the patient's response, the dose may be lowered to 1 tablet daily when sufficient control of oedema has been achieved. Higher doses, up to 4 tablets daily (80 mg), may be employed in resistant cases.

*Children:* No dose recommended.

*Elderly:* See *Precautions.*

### Contra-indications, warnings, etc
*Contra-indications:* Diurexan is contra-indicated in severe electrolyte deficiency, precomatose states associated with liver cirrhosis, severe renal insufficiency, hypersensitivity to xipamide and untreated Addison's disease.

*Use in pregnancy:* Animal experiments have indicated that Diurexan is devoid of teratogenic properties or effects on fertility and reproduction. However care should be taken when treating hypertension or oedema in pregnancy as excessive use may result in hypovolaemia and reduced placental perfusion. As with all drugs, treatment should be avoided in the first trimester of pregnancy.

*Lactation:* No information is available on the excretion

of xipamide in breast milk. Treatment should be avoided in breast feeding mothers.

*Precautions:* Like other diuretics, Diurexan may induce hypokalaemia in long-term therapy. Potassium supplements may be necessary, particularly in the elderly where dietary potassium intake may be inadequate, in digitalised patients and in conditions where additional potassium loss occurs such as vomiting, diarrhoea, malnutrition, nephrosis, hepatic cirrhosis and hyperaldosteronism.

Diurexan may exacerbate gout or induce hyperuricaemia or impaired glucose metabolism in patients predisposed to these conditions. In such patients serum urate or glucose levels should be monitored. Hyperuricaemia may require concomitant use of a uricosuric agent while diabetic patients will probably require an adjustment of insulin dosage, or other hypoglycaemic agent therapy.

As with all antihypertensive agents, care should be taken in patients with severe coronary or cerebral arteriosclerosis.

An increased risk of developing urinary retention may arise in patients with prostatic hypertrophy.

*Side-effects:* Diurexan is generally well tolerated. Slight gastro-intestinal disturbances have been reported in a few cases as have episodes of mild dizziness.

Hypokalaemia and, more rarely, other electrolyte disturbances such as hyponatraemia have been reported.

*Interactions:* The dosage of other hypotensive drugs and cardiac glycosides may require adjustment when used in conjunction with Diurexan.

Diabetic patients may require an increase in their dose of insulin or oral hypoglycaemic drug.

Corticosteroids, ACTH, carbenoxolone, amphotericin and laxatives may provoke hypokalaemia.

Increased serum lithium levels may occur due to diminished urinary excretion.

*Overdosage:* Little information is available on the effects of acute overdosage with xipamide however hypotension with metabolic disturbances and electrolyte imbalances are likely. Chronic overdose may lead to a temporary increase in blood viscosity due to haemoconcentration although thromboembolic complications have not been reported. There is no specific antidote to xipamide. Gastric lavage or induced emesis may prevent further absorption. General measures should be aimed at the maintenance of blood pressure, restoration of blood volume and correction of electrolyte imbalance with appropriate intravenous infusion as required.

**Pharmaceutical precautions** Store in a cool, dry place

**Legal category** POM.

**Package quantities** Cartons of 140 tablets in blister packs of 14 tablets.

**Further information** Nil.

**Product licence number** 8336/0008

## ENDOXANA* INJECTION
## ENDOXANA* TABLETS

### Presentation
*Tablets:* White, sugar-coated tablets containing Cyclophosphamide Monohydrate BP 53.5 mg (equivalent to 50 mg anhydrous cyclophosphamide).

*Injection:* White powder for injection in vials containing Cyclophosphamide Monohydrate BP 213.8 mg, 534.5 mg or 1,069 mg (equivalent to 200 mg, 500 mg or 1,000 mg anhydrous cyclophosphamide respectively) and sodium chloride sufficient to render isotonic when diluted with water for injections using the volume recommended for each strength.

### Uses
*Action:* Cyclophosphamide is inert until activated by microsomal enzymes. This occurs mainly in the liver, producing potent alkylating cytotoxic metabolites.

*Indications:* Endoxana is a cytotoxic drug for the treatment of malignant disease. As a single agent it has successfully produced an objective remission in a wide range of malignant conditions. Endoxana is also frequently used in combination with other cytotoxic drugs, radiotherapy or surgery.

**Dosage and administration** Endoxana should only be used by clinicians experienced in the use of cancer chemotherapy.

*Dosage:* The dose, route of administration and frequency of administration should be determined by the tumour type, tumour stage, the general condition of the patient, previous cytotoxic chemotherapy and whether other chemotherapy or radiotherapy is to be administered concurrently. A guide to dosage regimens used for most indications is given below:

a. 100-300 mg daily as an oral dose. This dose may be divided.

or

b. 80-300 mg/m² as single iv dose daily.

or

c. 300-600 mg/m² as a single iv dose weekly.

or

d. 600-1500 mg/m² as a single iv dose, or short infusion at 10–20 day intervals.

With single doses of cyclophosphamide over 10 mg/kg, mesna should be given concurrently, in addition to a good fluid intake, to avoid urothelial toxicity.

Endoxana tablets should be swallowed with sufficient fluid without chewing.

*Elderly:* No specific information on the use of this product in the elderly is available. Clinical trials have included patients over 65 years and no adverse reactions specific to this age group have been reported.

*Children:* No specific information. Children have received Endoxana, no adverse reactions specific to this group have been reported.

*Administration:* Endoxana is inert until activated by enzymes in the liver. However, safe handling is required and advice is included under 'Pharmaceutical precautions'. The dry contents of a vial should be dissolved in water for injections (5 ml per 100 mg Endoxana) and used within eight hours. The pH of an aqueous solution is between 4.0 and 6.0.

Endoxana is usually given directly into the tubing of a fast running iv infusion with the patient supine. Care should be taken that extravasation does not take place, however, should it occur, no specific measures need be taken.

Endoxana injection may also be given intraperitoneally or intrapleurally, but these routes offer no therapeutic advantages over the iv route. Endoxana has been given intra-arterially and by local perfusion. These routes should be used only by clinicians experienced in these procedures.

A minimum urine output of 100 ml/hr should be maintained during therapy with conventional doses to avoid cystitis. If the larger doses are used, an output of at least this level should be maintained for 24 hours following administration, if necessary by forced diuresis. Alkalinisation of the urine is not recommended. Endoxana should be given early in the day and the bladder voided frequently. The patient should be well hydrated and maintained in fluid balance.

Mesna (Uromitexan) can be used concurrently with Endoxana to reduce urotoxic effects (for dosage see Uromitexan data sheet). If mesna (Uromitexan) is used to reduce urothelial toxicity, frequent emptying of the bladder should be avoided.

Endoxana should be avoided in patients with cystitis from any cause until it has been treated.

Anti-emetics given before and during therapy may reduce nausea and vomiting.

If the leucocyte count is below 4,000/mm³ or the platelet count is below 100,000/mm³, treatment with Endoxana should be temporarily withheld until the blood count returns to normal levels.

For oral administration an elixir may be prepared by dissolving the contents of the dry powder vials in Aromatic Elixir USP shortly before oral administration.

### Contra-indications, warnings, etc
*Contra-indications:* Endoxana should only be administered where there are facilities for regular monitoring of clinical, biochemical and haematological parameters before, during and after administration and under the direction of a specialist oncology service.

Endoxana is contra-indicated in patients with known hypersensitivity to cyclophosphamide, with acute infections, with bone marrow aplasia, or with acute urothelial toxicity from cytotoxic chemotherapy or radiation therapy.

Endoxana should not be used in the management of non-malignant disease, except for immunosuppression in life-threatening situations.

*Use in pregnancy and lactation:* Endoxana should not be used in pregnancy, especially the first trimester, unless the expected benefit is thought to outweigh the substantial risk to the foetus. Mothers should not breast-feed while being treated with Endoxana or for 36 hours after stopping treatment.

*Precautions:* Care should be exercised in patients who are elderly, debilitated, have diabetes mellitus or evidence of myelosuppression or who have recently received or are receiving concurrent treatment with radiotherapy or cytotoxic agents.

Endoxana is not recommended in patients with a plasma creatinine greater than 120μ mol/l (1.5 mg/100 ml) bilirubin greater than 17μ mol/l (1 mg/100 ml); or serum transaminases or alkaline phosphatase more than 2-3 times the upper limit of normal.

Cardiotoxicity may be induced in patients who have had or are receiving mediastinal irradiation, doxorubicin or high doses of cyclophosphamide. In such instances cyclophosphamide therapy should be stopped and appropriate treatment instituted.

Contraception in both sexes is advised during and for at least 3 months after Endoxana therapy. Patients should receive counselling with respect of subsequent pregnancies.

Endoxana may have an adverse effect on prepubertal gonads and amenorrhoea and azoospermia often occur. Appropriate counselling should be given.

*Interactions:* The following clinically significant interactions of cyclophosphamide with other drugs have been reported: allopurinol (increased incidence of bone marrow depression), sulfonylureas (enhanced hypoglycaemic effect) and suxamethonium (prolonged apnoea).

Increased myelosuppression may be seen following concurrent administration of other bone marrow depressant drugs.

*Side-effects:* During Endoxana therapy, the reticuloendothelial system is depressed, granulopoiesis and lymphopoiesis being more affected than thrombopoiesis and erythropoiesis, but this depression is reversible. When a single dose is given, the fall in the peripheral white cell count reaches its nadir within 5 to 10 days. Recovery is seen at 10-14 days following administration, with full recovery in most cases by 21-28 days. The fall in the peripheral count and the time taken to recover may increase with increasing doses of Endoxana.

Haematuria may occur during or after therapy with Endoxana. Acute sterile haemorrhagic cystitis may occur in up to 10% of patients not given mesna (Uromitexan) in conjunction with Endoxana. Late sequelae of this cystitis are bladder contracture and fibrosis.

An alteration in carbohydrate metabolism may been seen in patients on Endoxana; hyperglycaemia has been reported.

Azoospermia often occurs in men and is dose dependent. Spontaneous recovery of fertility may occur, and is also dependent on dose. Menstruation in women commonly ceases during therapy, and may be permanent, particularly in older women. Endoxana may have an adverse effect on prepubertal gonads.

Cardiotoxicity may be induced in patients who have had or are receiving mediastinal irradiation or doxorubicin. It has also been reported with high doses of cyclophosphamide. This mainly occurs as a tachyarrhythmia and may progress in severe cases to intractable heart failure. Following large doses, ECG changes and elevation of LDH, SGOT and CPK have been reported in some patients.

There is evidence that, like other alkylating agents, cyclophosphamide is a human carcinogen. In certain laboratory tests, it has been shown to be mutagenic, teratogenic and carcinogenic and as with other cytotoxic drugs there have been reports of possible drug-induced neoplasia. There is an excess risk of acute leukaemia and bladder cancer following cyclophosphamide therapy.

Anorexia, nausea, vomiting and mucosal ulceration can occur. Nausea and vomiting may be reduced by administration of an anti-emetic agent, before, during and after therapy.

Alopecia occurs to some degree in about 20% of patients receiving over 100 mg daily and is inevitable following high doses. Epilation usually commences after the first three weeks of treatment but regrowth is evident after three months in most patients even though they remain on treatment.

Cyclophosphamide therapy may lead to inappropriate secretion of anti-diuretic hormone, fluid retention and hyponatraemia, with subsequent water intoxication. Should this occur, diuretic therapy should be instigated.

*Other side-effects include:* Pigmentation of the fingernails and the skin (mainly the palms of the hands and the soles of the feet), macrocytosis, and induction of hyperglycaemia or hypoglycaemia. Pneumonitis and interstitial pulmonary fibrosis may also occur.

Side-effects have occasionally occurred after cessation of treatment.

*Overdosage:* The most serious consequences of overdosage are profound myelosuppression, haemorrhagic cystitis, and cardiotoxicity in the form of arrhythmias and severe heart failure. Myelosuppression usually recovers spontaneously. Myelosuppression may be alleviated by transfusion of red cells, platelets or white cells. Broad spectrum antibiotic cover may be necessary.

If the overdose is recognised within the first 24 hours and possibly up to 48 hours, iv mesna may be beneficial in ameliorating damage to the urinary system. Normal supportive measures such as analgesics and maintenance of fluid balance should be instituted. If, despite these measures the cystitis does not resolve, more intensive treatment may be necessary and a urological opinion should be sought. No further courses should be given until the patient has fully recovered.

Endoxana is dialysable.

*Pharmaceutical precautions*: The following protective recommendations are advised during handling due to the toxic nature of the substance.

Reconstitution and administration must be undertaken only by trained personnel. Pregnant staff and breast feeding mothers should be excluded.

Protective clothing, goggles, masks and disposable PVC or Latex gloves should be worn.

A designated area should be defined for reconstitution (preferably under a laminar-airflow system). The work surface should be protected by a disposable, plastic-backed, absorbent paper. Accidental contact with the skin or eyes should be treated immediately by copious lavage with water. Soap and water should then be used on non-mucous membranes. Spillages should be removed with dry or moist disposable towels.

Care must be taken in the disposal of all waste materials (syringes, needles and disposable towels etc). Used items should be placed in appropriate secure containers, in readiness for destruction in a chemical incinerator equipped with an after-burner.

Store below 25°C. Vials should on no account be stored above the recommended temperature as this can cause degradation of the active ingredient, identifiable by a yellow melted appearance to the vial contents. Vials containing melted material should not be used.

Endoxana injection is compatible with dextrose and saline infusion solutions. Endoxana injection is chemically stable for 6 days at room temperature in saline and 48 hours at room temperature in dextrose. As Endoxana does not contain a preservative, the above solutions should be used within eight hours unless prepared under strict aseptic technique.

**Legal category** POM.

**Package quantities** Cartons containing 10 blister packs, each of 10 x 50 mg tablets.
200 mg dry vials in packs of 10
500 mg dry vials, singles
1 g, dry vials, singles

**Further information** The dosage regimen for mesna (Uromitexan) varies according to the dose of Endoxana administered. In general, i.v. Uromitexan is given as 60% w/w of the dose of i.v. Endoxana in three equal doses of 20% at 0, 4 and 8 hours. With the higher doses of Endoxana, the dose and frequency of administration may need to be increased. Uromitexan Tablets are also available; full prescribing information for both presentations is available on the appropriate data sheet.

**Product licence numbers**

| | |
|---|---|
| 50 mg Tablets | 8336/0016 |
| 200 mg Vials | 8336/0012 |
| 500 mg Vials | 8336/0013 |
| 1,000 mg Vials | 8336/0014 |

## FERROCONTIN* CONTINUS* TABLETS

**Presentation**

Red, film-coated, bi-convex tablets, plain on one side, embossed with FC on the other side. Each tablet contains the equivalent of 100 mg ferrous iron in the form of ferrous glycine sulphate within a patented controlled release system.

**Uses**

*Indications:* Ferrocontin Continus Tablets are indicated for the treatment and prophylaxis of iron deficiency anaemia.

**Dosage and administration**

*Dosage:*

*Adults:* One tablet to be taken daily, or as directed by the physician.

*Children:* Not suitable for children under 10 years.

*Elderly:* Normal adult dose.

*Administration:* Ferrocontin Continus Tablets should be swallowed whole and not chewed.

**Contra-indications, warnings, etc**

*Contra-indications:* None.

*Use in pregnancy:* When administering ferrous sulphate to pregnant mice and rats in dosages of up to 100 times (1200 mg/kg/day) the human adult dose, no influence on survival of dams nor survival, development and appearance of foetuses and offspring was observed. Experimental studies have not been described on the use of glycine in pregnancy in laboratory animals.

There are conflicting reports on the tendency of ferrous sulphate to induce congenital malformations in the foetuses of women receiving iron containing preparations during the first trimester. Harmful effects on the foetus, the mother or the pregnancy have not been reported for the ingestion of glycine.

Ferrocontin Continus Tablets should be used with caution during the first trimester of pregnancy.

*Nursing mothers:* Iron salts are excreted into breast milk which may be of benefit when there is iron deficiency in the neonate.

*Precautions:* As with all medicines keep out of the reach of children.

*Interactions:* Absorption of levodopa and quinolones are reduced by oral iron. Tetracyclines will chelate with iron, impairing the absorption of both agents. Concurrent administration reduces the absorption of penicillamine and biphosphonates. Absorption of oral iron is reduced by concurrent zinc salts, trientine and magnesium trisilicate.

*Side-effects:* The symptoms of nausea and gastro-intestinal irritation often associated with iron therapy are unlikely to occur with Ferrocontin Continus Tablets.

*Overdosage:* Acute iron overdosage is serious and requires rapid treatment. 30 mg/kg body weight may be enough to cause symptoms of toxicity which may present in four stages.

1. Six hours after ingestion: gastrointestinal toxicity with vomiting and diarrhoea, cardiovascular toxicity with hypotension and tachycardia, metabolic effects such as acidosis and hyperglycaemia, and CNS depression from lethargy to coma.
2. Six to twenty-four hours after ingestion: temporary remission and stabilisation.
3. Recurrence of gastrointestinal toxicity with shock, metabolic acidosis, convulsions, coma, hepatic necrosis and jaundice, hypoglycaemia, coagulation disorders, oliguria or renal failure, and pulmonary oedema.
4. Several weeks after ingestion: gastrointestinal obstruction and late hepatic damage.

Patients with mild to moderate overdosage will generally recover following the first stage. Serum iron concentrations may be used to indicate the severity of overdosage.

Treatment should aim to prevent the absorption of iron from the alimentary tract by emesis or stomach lavage with 1% sodium bicarbonate. Oral and/or systemic desferrioxamine may be given for severe overdosage if necessary, according to product instructions. Fluid and electrolyte balance should be maintained and general supportive measures given as required.

Ferrous glycine sulphate will be released for absorption over some hours from tablets remaining in the intestine.

**Pharmaceutical precautions** Store in a cool dry place protected from light.

**Legal category** P.

**Package quantities** Containers of 30 (OP, child resistant) and 250 tablets.

**Further information** The amino acid-iron chelate ferrous glycine sulphate prevents oxidation to the ferric form in the gastro-intestinal tract, thus enhancing absorption. The use of a patented controlled release system optimises the bioavailability of ferrous iron and minimises the likelihood of side-effects.

**Product licence number** 8336/0004

## FERROCONTIN* FOLIC CONTINUS* TABLETS

**Presentation** Pale orange, film-coated, bi-convex tablets. Each tablet contains the equivalent of 100 mg ferrous iron in the form of ferrous glycine sulphate within a patented controlled release system and 0.5 mg folic acid BP.

**Uses**

*Indications:* Ferrocontin Folic Continus Tablets are indicated for the prophylaxis of iron and folic acid deficiencies during pregnancy.

**Dosage and administration**

*Dosage:*

*Adults:* One tablet to be taken daily, or as directed by the physician.

*Children:* Not appropriate.

*Elderly:* Not appropriate.

*Administration:* Ferrocontin Folic Continus tablets should be swallowed whole and not chewed.

**Contra-indications, warnings, etc**

*Contra-indications:* The tablets should not be given to patients with vitamin $B_{12}$ deficiency without concomitant $B_{12}$ supplementation.

*Use in pregnancy:* When administering ferrous sulphate to pregnant mice and rats in dosages of up to 100 times (1200 mg/kg/day) the human adult dose, no influence on survival of dams nor survival, development and appearance of foetuses and offspring was observed. Experimental studies have not been described on the use of glycine in pregnancy in laboratory animals.

Studies in pregnant rats have confirmed that the administration of folic acid antagonists results in embryo destruction and foetal abnormalities. Coadministration of folic acid has been shown to safeguard against these effects. Very high doses of folic acid have been shown to cause foetal abnormalities in rats.

There are conflicting reports on the tendency of ferrous sulphate to induce congenital malformations in the foetuses of women receiving iron containing preparations during the first trimester. Harmful effects on the foetus, the mother or the pregnancy have not been reported for the ingestion of glycine.

Folic acid deficiency during pregnancy and especially multiple pregnancy may lead to the appearance of foetal malformations. Imbalance in folate requiring trophoblast cells may also lead to detachment of the placenta.

Harmful effects on the foetus, the mother or the pregnancy have not been reported for the ingestion of folic acid.

Ferrocontin Folic Continus tablets should be used with caution during the first trimester of pregnancy.

*Nursing mothers:* Iron salts and folic acid are excreted into breast milk which may be of benefit when there is iron or folic acid deficiency in the neonate.

*Precautions:* As with all medicines keep out of the reach of children.

*Interactions:* Tetracyclines will chelate with iron, impairing the absorption of both agents. Concurrent administration reduces the absorption of penicillamine, zinc salts, trientine and magnesium trisilicate. Folate administration may reduce serum anticonvulsant levels.

*Side-effects:* The symptoms of nausea and gastrointestinal irritation often associated with iron therapy are unlikely to occur with Ferrocontin Folic Continus Tablets.

*Other special warnings:* The presence of pernicious anaemia is unlikely to be masked by the daily administration of 500 micrograms folic acid. However, vitamin $B_{12}$ deficiency should be excluded before commencing Ferrocontin Folic Continus.

*Overdosage:* Toxicity from the iron content will predominate. Acute iron overdosage is serious and requires rapid treatment. 30 mg/kg body weight may be enough to cause symptoms of toxicity which may present in four stages.

1. Six hours after ingestion: gastrointestinal toxicity with vomiting and diarrhoea, cardiovascular toxicity with hypotension and tachycardia, metabolic effects such as acidosis and hyperglycaemia, and CNS depression from lethargy to coma.
2. Six to twenty-four hours after ingestion: temporary remission and stabilisation.
3. Recurrence of gastrointestinal toxicity with shock, metabolic acidosis, convulsions, coma, hepatic necrosis and jaundice, hypoglycaemia, coagulation disorders, oliguria or renal failure, and pulmonary oedema.
4. Several weeks after ingestion: gastrointestinal obstruction and late hepatic damage.

Patients with mild to moderate overdosage will generally recover following the first stage. Serum iron concentrations may be used to indicate the severity of overdosage.

Treatment should aim to prevent the absorption of iron from the alimentary tract by emesis or stomach lavage with 1% sodium bicarbonate. Oral and/or systemic desferrioxamine may be given for severe overdosage if necessary, according to product instructions. Fluid and electrolyte balance should be maintained and general supportive measures given as required.

Ferrous glycine sulphate will be released for absorption over a period of hours from tablets remaining in the intestine.

**Pharmaceutical precautions** Store in a cool dry place, protected from light.

**Legal category** P.

**Package quantities** Containers of 30 (OP, child resistant) and 250 tablets.

**Further information** The amino acid-iron chelate ferrous glycine sulphate prevents oxidation to the ferric form in the gastrointestinal tract, thus enhancing absorption. The use of a patented controlled release system optimises the bioavailability of ferrous iron and minimises the likelihood of side-effects.

**Product licence number** 8336/0005

## HONVAN* INJECTION
## HONVAN* TABLETS

**Qualitative and quantitative composition**

*Honvan Injection*–300 mg fosfestrol tetrasodium BP in 5 ml solution.

*Honvan Tablets*–120 mg fosfestrol tetrasodium BP

**Pharmaceutical form** Sterile aqueous solution for injection. Film-coated tablets for oral use.

**Clinical particulars**

*Therapeutic indications:* Honvan is a synthetic oestrogen used for the treatment of prostatic carcinoma. Honvan may be used as an adjuvant to surgery, in inoperable cases and for the reduction of pain due to metastases. Patients who are resistant to conventional hormone therapy have responded to Honvan. Where acute retention has occurred the use of Honvan may reduce the need for transurethral resection.

*Posology and method of administration*

*Route of administration:* Intravenous injection.

The patient should preferably by lying down and the injection given slowly into the vein. Slow infusions are not recommended as high local cytotoxic levels may not be achieved.

*Dosage*: The dosage should be according to clinical and biochemical findings. Response to treatment with Honvan may be objectively assessed by the reduction of plasma acid phosphatase concentrations and the degree of reduction in size of the primary prostatic tumour, cutaneous, subcutaneous or lymph node metastases, bone lesions or visceral metastases. Subjective improvement may be made by the reduction of pain, improvement in urinary function and improvement in patient well-being.

*Adults:* Initial therapy: acute retention of urine and relapse: 2-4 ampoules Honvan intravenous as a single injection daily for at least five days or until a response has been obtained (seven to ten days). Maintenance: 1 ampoule intravenously one to four times weekly.

*Route of administration:* Oral.

*Dosage:* The dosage should be according to clinical and biochemical findings. Response to treatment with Honvan may be objectively assessed by the reduction of plasma acid phosphatase concentrations and the degree of reduction in size of the primary prostatic tumour, cutaneous, subcutaneous or lymph node metastases, bone lesions or visceral metastases. Subjective improvement may be made by the reduction of pain, improvement in urinary function and improvement in patient well being.

Oral maintenance therapy is usually 1-6 tablets daily in divided doses. The initial dose should be up to 2 tablets three times daily for the first week, reducing over the next two weeks to the lowest dose that will control the disease which is usually 1-3 tablets daily in divided doses.

*Oral and intravenous*

*Children:* Not recommended.

*Elderly:* No specific information on the use of this product in the elderly is available. Clinical trials have included patients over 65 and no adverse reactions specific to this group have been included.

*Contra-indications:* History of hypersensitivity to Honvan or other synthetic oestrogens.

*Special warnings and special precautions for use:* Honvan should only be administered under the direction of a specialist oncology service having facilities for the regular monitoring of clinical biochemical and haematological effects during and after administration.

Caution is advised when using Honvan in patients with poor cardiac reserve or fluid retention and in those cases concomitant diuretic therapy may be indicated. Caution is also advised for patients with active thrombophlebitis or thromboembolic disorders, cardiac failure, hypertension or cerebrovascular disease.

Particular care should be taken in patients over 70 years of age, those on long-term Honvan therapy and those having had recent surgery. Caution is also advised in patients with a history of liver disease and diabetic patients. Glucose tolerance may be impaired in the latter and their urine should be carefully monitored.

In rare cases hypersensitivity to Honvan has been noted. Honvan Injection is non-irritant to the veins and should an injection accidentally enter the paravenous tissue no specific action is necessary.

*Interaction with other medicaments and other forms of interaction:* Honvan is not known to interact with any other drugs, food or alcohol.

*Pregnancy and lactation:* Honvan should not be administered to pregnant women as oestrogens have been shown to be teratogenic to the foetus.

*Effects on ability to drive and use machines:* None known.

*Undesirable effects:* Pain in bony metastases may occur during or immediately after administration of Honvan. A burning in the perineum may occur during or immediately after i.v. injection. Perineal discomfort may be reduced by prior administration of a sedative.

Anorexia, nausea, vomiting, dizziness, fever, rigor, abdominal cramps and abdominal bloating may occur. Skin rash and disturbances of vision have been reported.

Transient rises in transferase and aspartate levels have been reported. A moderate hypophosphataemia

may occur and there may be a transient rise in alkaline phosphatase. Fluid retention and hypernatraemia have been reported, fluid retention may lead to congestive cardiac failure. There is an increased risk of pulmonary embolism, deep vein thrombosis and cerebrovascular accidents reported with oestrogens.

Androgen reduction may lead to impotence, mental disturbance and mood changes, gynaecomastia and testicular atrophy.

*Overdose:* In the event of overdosage, monitoring for fluid retention should be undertaken and in patients with cardiac disease, the administration of diuretics and digitalis should be considered.

**Pharmacological properties**

*Pharmacodynamic properties:* Fosfestrol Tetrasodium is a water soluble synthetic oestrogen which is inert. The active principle is diethylstilboestrol which becomes liberated through enzymatic cleavage as soon as it enters the body.

Diethylstilboestrol has three principal effects in man:

(i) oestrogen-like effects in hormone sensitive tissues

(ii) oestrogen-like negative feedback on the endocrine system, thereby reducing the production of male sexual hormones

(iii) at high doses indirect interference with cellular reproductive functions, i.e. some cytotoxic activity.

*Pharmacokinetic properties:* Following i.v. infusion, plasma levels of Fosfestrol Tetrasodium and DES (DES = Diethylstilboestrol) monophosphate rise steeply for 1.5 hours, thereafter more slowly. Both these compounds have short half lives, 5 minutes and 30 minutes respectively. DES appears gradually during the infusion as does DES monoglucuronide; the latter reaches greater concentration than the DES.

The main metabolites of Fosfestrol Tetrasodium are conjugates: DES monoglucuronide, DES monosulphate, DES glucuronide sulphate. Oxidative metabolism also takes place but does not play a major role.

Tetrasodium Fosfestrol→DES monophosphate→DES→conjugates and other metabolites.

These DES conjugates may also behave as pro-drugs.

The metabolism of Tetrasodium Fosfestrol after oral administration follows the same time course for DES. After oral administration, unchanged fosfestrol could not be detected. This is due to extensive first pass metabolism by phosphatase enzymes in the gut wall.

Plasma protein binding has been shown to be concentration dependent. DES is 95% protein bound.

Elimination studies show that only DES glucuronide and DES glucuronide-sulphate can be found in urine following either i.v. or oral administration. The other conjugates as well as free DES appear in the faeces.

90-95% of the dose given is trapped in the enterohepatic cycle from where it escapes over a period of 24 hours.

*Preclinical safety data:* Not relevant.

**Pharmaceutical particulars**

*List of excipients:*

*Honvan Injection:* Water for injections; sodium hydroxide, Nitrogen.

*Honvan Tablets:*

| | |
|---|---|
| Lactose | 42.74–31.86 mg |
| Maize starch | 11.20 mg |
| Talc | 4.0 mg |
| Magnesium stearate | 2.7 mg |
| Aerosil 200v | 2.0 mg |
| Gelatine | 1.0 mg |
| Lactose monohydrate | 0.98 mg |
| Eudragit NE30D | 0.23 mg |
| Polyethylene glycol 6000 | 0.23 mg |
| Carboxymethylcellulose sodium | 0.06 mg |
| Purified water | - |

*Incompatibilities:* Honvan Injection is incompatible with aqueous solutions of pH less than 7 and solutions containing calcium or magnesium ions.

*Shelf life:* 3 years.

*Special precautions for storage:* Store at up to 25°C

*Nature and contents of container:*
Injection: Clear glass ampoules in a folded cardboard box.
Tablets: PVC/PVDC–aluminium blister pack, in a folded cardboard box.

*Instructions for use and handling:* These medicines should not be handled by pregnant women.

**Marketing authorisation numbers**
Honvan Injection    8336/0048
Honvan Tablets      8336/0047

**Date of approval/revision of SPC** March 1996.

**Legal category** POM.

# MITOXANA* INJECTION

**Qualitative and quantitative composition**
1 vial of 1 g Mitoxana Injection contains 1 g of ifosfamide.
1 vial of 2 g Mitoxana Injection contains 2 g of ifosfamide.

**Pharmaceutical form** Dry powder for injection after reconstitution.

**Clinical particulars**
*Therapeutic indications:* Mitoxana is a cytotoxic drug for the treatment of malignant disease. As a single agent is has successfully produced an objective remission in a wide range of malignant conditions. Mitoxana is also frequently used in combination with other cytotoxic drugs, radiotherapy and surgery.

*Posology and method of administration:* For intravenous use as a diluted solution only–by infusion, or if solution is less than 4% by direct injection. Mitoxana should only be used by clinicians experienced in the use of cancer chemotherapy.

*Dosage:* Mitoxana should not be used without the concurrent administration of Uromitexan (mesna) to protect against urothelial toxicity that can occur with the oxazaphosphorine alkylating agents. The dose and frequency of administration should be determined by the tumour type, tumour stage, the general condition of the patient, any previous cytotoxic therapy, and whether other chemotherapy or radiotherapy is to be administered concurrently.

A guide to the dosage regimens used for most indications is given below:
(a) 8–12 g/m² equally fractionated as single daily doses over 3–5 days every 2–4 weeks.
(b) 5–6 g/m² (maximum 10 g) given as a 24 hour infusion every 3–4 weeks.

The frequency of dosage is determined by the degree of myelosuppression and the time taken to recover adequate bone marrow function. The usual number of courses given is 4, but up to 7 (6 by 24 hour infusion) courses have been given. Re-treatment has been given following relapse.

*Children:* In children, the dosage and administration should be determined by the tumour type, tumour stage, the general condition of the patient, any previous cytotoxic therapy, and whether chemotherapy or radiotherapy is to be administered concurrently. Clinical trials have involved doses of:
(a) 5 g/m² over 24 hours
(b) 9 g/m² equally fractionated as single daily doses over 5 days
(c) 9 g/m² as a continuous infusion over 72 hours - repeated at three weekly intervals.

*Elderly:* No specific information on the use of this product in the elderly is available. Clinical trials have included patients over 65 years and no adverse reactions specific to this age group have been reported.

*Administration:* Mitoxana is inert until activated by enzymes in the liver. However, safe handling is required and advice is included under Pharmaceutical Precautions. The dry contents of a vial should be dissolved in Water for Injections as follows:
1 g vial: add 12.5 ml of Water for Injections
2 g vial: add 25 ml of Water for Injections

The resultant solution of 8% of ifosfamide should not be injected directly into the vein. The solution may be:
1. diluted to less than a 4% solution and injected directly into the vein, with the patient supine.
2. infused in 5% dextrose-saline or normal saline over 30-120 mins.
3. injected directly into a fast-running infusion.
4. made up in 3 litres of dextrose-saline or normal saline and infused over 24 hours. Each litre should be given over eight hours, and should be freshly made up immediately before infusion.

Care should be taken that extravasation does not take place, however should it occur, local tissue damage is unlikely and no specific measures need be taken. Repeated intravenous injections of large doses of Mitoxana have resulted in local irritation.

Mesna (Uromitexan) should be used to prevent urothelial toxicity.

Where Mitoxana is used as an i.v. bolus, increased dosages of mesna are recommended in children, patients whose urothelium may be damaged from previous therapies and those who are not adequately protected by the standard dose of mesna.

The patient should be well hydrated and maintained in fluid balance, replacement fluids being given as necessary to achieve this. The fluid intake of patients on the intermittent regimen should be at least 2 litres in 24 hours. As Mitoxana may exert an antidiuretic effect, a diuretic may be necessary to ensure an adequate urinary output.

Urine should be sent for laboratory analysis before, and at the end of, each course of treatment, and the patient should be monitored for output and evidence of proteinuria and haematuria at regular intervals (4-hourly if possible) throughout the treatment period. The patient should be instructed to report any signs or symptoms of cystitis. Mitoxana should be avoided in patients with cystitis from any cause until it has been treated.

Antiemetics given before, during and after therapy may reduce nausea and vomiting. Oral hygiene is important.

If leucocyte count is below 4,000/mm³ or the platelet count is below 100,000/mm³, treatment with Mitoxana should be withheld until the blood count returns to normal.

There should be no signs or symptoms of urothelial toxicity or renal or hepatic impairment prior to the start of each course of Mitoxana.

*Contra-indications:* Mitoxana should only be administered when there are facilities for regular monitoring of clinical, biochemical and haematological parameters before, during and after administration and under the direction of a specialist oncology service.

Mitoxana is contra-indicated in patients with known hypersensitivity to ifosfamide, bone marrow aplasia, myelosuppression, urinary tract obstruction, acute infections including urinary tract infection, or with acute urothelial toxicity from cytotoxic chemotherapy or radiation therapy.

Mitoxana is contra-indicated in patients with renal impairment (serum creatinine greater than 120µ mol/l or 1.5 mg/100 ml) or hepatic impairment (bilirubin greater than 17µ mol/l or 1 mg/100 ml), or serum transaminases or alkaline phosphatase more than 2.5 times the upper limit of normal.

Contraception in both sexes is advised during and for at least 6 months after Mitoxana therapy. Patients should receive counselling with respect to subsequent pregnancies.

*Special warnings and special precautions for use:* Care should be exercised in patients who are elderly, debilitated, have diabetes mellitus or evidence of myelosuppression or who have recently received or are receiving concurrent treatment with radiotherapy or cytotoxic agents. Any electrolyte imbalances should be corrected before treatment is started.

Caution is necessary in patients who have previously received platinum compounds or undergone a nephrectomy.

In children, high cumulative doses of ifosfamide and continued treatment in the presence of renal tubular dysfunction may be associated with increased frequency or severity of renal damage.

Mitoxana is a potent immunuosuppressive drug and the increased risk to the patient should be borne in mind.

Amenorrhoea and azoospermia can occur. Patients should be warned of a potential risk to future progeny.

Mitoxana has been shown to be mutagenic, teratogenic and carcinogenic in laboratory tests and there is a risk of drug-induced neoplasia following long-term treatment.

*Interaction with other medicaments and other forms of interaction:* Concurrent administration of anticoagulants, especially Warfarin, can result in disturbance of anticoagulant control and an increased risk of bleeding. Concurrent administration of antidiabetic agents, sulfonylureas for instance and ifosfamide may enhance the hypoglycaemic effects of the former drugs. Theoretical interactions of ifosfamide and allopurinol resulting in an increased severity of bone marrow depression may occur. Prior treatment with enzyme inducing drugs may result in a faster metabolism of ifosfamide.

*Pregnancy and lactation:* Contraception is advised in both sexes during Mitoxana therapy and for at least six months following treatment. Patients should receive counselling with respect to subsequent pregnancies. Mothers should not breast-feed while being treated with Mitoxana as ifosfamide has been shown to be teratogenic in animals and is excreted in breast milk.

Mitoxana should not be used in pregnancy especially the first trimester, unless the expected benefit is thought to outweigh the substantial risk to the foetus.

*Effects on ability to drive and use machines:* Potential side-effects on the central nervous system may transiently impair the ability to operate machinery and motor vehicles.

*Undesirable effects:* Treatment with ifosfamide may be associated with the following dose-related, generally reversible side-effects.

Urogenital tract–Urothelial toxicity is the usual dose-limiting factor. This can be largely prevented by the concurrent administration of mesna. Urotoxicity involving the efferent urinary tract as well as the bladder can lead to haemorrhagic cystitis and dysuria.

Nephrotoxicity may occur with oliguria, raised uric acid, increased blood urea and serum creatinine and decreased creatinine clearance. Glycosuria, proteinu-ria, aminoaciduria and hyperphosphaturia which may lead to renal rickets have been reported with changes in serum proteins and electrolytes. Nephrotoxicity is usually reversible, especially in the early stages but severe cases are recorded. Delay in the diagnosis and treatment of renal toxicity may, especially in children, lead to a full picture of Fanconi's Syndrome or diabetes insipidus. Patients with pre-existing renal dysfunction and/or prior treatment with nephrotoxic drugs such as cisplatin may be predisposed to nephrotoxicity.

Haematological reactions–large doses of ifosfamide give rise to a predictable bone marrow toxicity and consequent immunosuppression. The white cell count reaches its nadir 5-10 days after commencing treatment, recovery commencing after 10-14 days and usually returning to normal within 2-3 weeks. About 30% of patients would be expected to have a fall in haemoglobin of greater than 2 g/100 ml and a white cell count less than 2000/mm³, but only 5% would be expected to have a platelet count less than 100,000/mm³. There have been only occasional reports of coagulation disorders.

Central nervous system side-effects may occur. These may present as drowsiness, confusion, disorientation, restlessness, depressive psychoses and/or hallucinations, rarely convulsions. These will rarely persist beyond 2 days, and will usually resolve spontaneously after cessation of treatment. Occasionally tonic-clonic spasms, motor unrest and emotional lability have been noted.

A severe encephalopathy occurs less frequently. The symptoms may be preceded by EEG abnormalities. Clumsiness, confusion, disorientation, logorrhoea, echolalia, perseveration, aggression and depression of conscious level have been reported. Fever and tachycardia may be present. Occasionally recovery has been incomplete with persistent psychological disturbances, coma and death.

If central nervous system toxicity is suspected, ifosfamide should be stopped and supportive therapy given. There are indications of a higher incidence of CNS effects in elderly patients and those with cerebral metastases. Special care should be taken in giving Mitoxana to patients with reduced plasma albumin levels and/or impaired kidney function.

Gastrointestinal reactions–frequently nausea and vomiting, very occasionally anorexia, diarrhoea or constipation. Nausea and vomiting may be reduced by the prior administration of an anti-emetic.

Other side-effects include: frequent but reversible alopecia, stomatitis, dermatitis, impairment of gonadal function and hypersensitivity reactions. More rarely hepatic dysfunction (including jaundice and increased liver enzyme and/or bilirubin levels), thrombophlebitis at site of injection or syndrome of inappropriate antidiuretic hormone secretion may occur.

There have been isolated reports of cardiac arrhythmia or heart failure after very high doses of ifosfamide and/or prior or concurrent treatment with anthracyclines. As is the case with cytotoxic therapy in general, treatment with ifosfamide involves the risk of secondary tumours as late sequelae.

*Overdose:* The most serious consequences of overdosage are haemorrhagic cystitis and myelosuppression. The latter usually recovers spontaneously, but until it does, administration of a broad spectrum antibiotic may be advisable. Transfusion of whole blood should be given as necessary. If the overdosage is recognised within the first 24 hours, i.v. mesna may be beneficial in ameliorating damage to the urinary system.

Normal supportive measures such as analgesics and maintenance of fluid balance should be instituted. If despite these measures the cystitis does not resolve, more intensive treatment may be necessary and a urological opinion should be sought. No further courses should be given until the patient has fully recovered.

**Pharmacological properties**

*Pharmacodynamic properties:* Mitoxana is an antineoplastic, a cytotoxic alkylating agent. It is a prodrug and shows no in vitro cytotoxic activity until activated by microsomal enzymes. The cytotoxic activity of Mitoxana (alkylation of the nucleophilic centres in the cells) is associated with the activated oxazaphosphorine ring hydroxylated at the C4 atom which interacts with DNA-DNA cross linking. This activity manifests itself by blocking the late S and early G2 phases of the cell cycle.

*Pharmacokinetic properties:* Mitoxana is rapidly absorbed from the site of administration, activation of Mitoxana is primarily in the liver by microsomal mixed function oxidases. Elimination of metabolised Mitoxana is primarily via the kidneys. The serum half-life ranges between 4–8 hours depending on the dose and dosage regimen. Over 80% of a single dose of ifosfamide was excreted in the urine within 24 hours. Approximately 80% of the dose was excreted as parent compound. Significant quantities of unchanged ifosfamide were found in the cerebrospinal fluid consistent with the high lipid solubility of the drug.

*Preclinical safety data:* Not relevant.

**Pharmaceutical particulars**

*List of excipients:* None.

*Incompatibilities:* None known.

*Shelf life:* Five years.

The reconstituted solution should be used immediately. The product does not contain a preservative, therefore microbial stability cannot be guaranteed. When prepared under strict aseptic conditions, ifosfamide is, as a 4% solution, however, chemically stable for 7 days at room temperature with Water for Injections, 0.9% saline, dextrose/saline and dextrose solutions. Ifosfamide and mesna when prepared under strict aseptic conditions at the recommended dilutions are chemically stable with:

(i) 0.9% saline and dextrose/saline solution for one week at room temperature.

(ii) Water for Injection for one week under refrigeration.

(iii) 5% dextrose solution for 24 hours at room temperature.

(iv) 0.9% saline solution for 28 days at room temperature.

*Special precautions for storage:* The vials should be stored below 25°C, protected from light.

*Nature and contents of container:* Glass injection vial with rubber closure and beading cap. Packed in a cardboard box.

*Instructions for use and handling:* The following protective recommendations are advised during handling due to the toxic nature of the substance:

Reconstitution and administration must be undertaken only by trained personnel. Pregnant staff and breastfeeding mothers should be excluded.

Protective clothing, goggles, masks and disposable PVC or latex gloves should be worn.

A designated area should be defined for reconstitution (preferably under a laminar-airflow system). The work surface should be protected by a disposable, plastic backed absorbent paper. Accidental contact with the skin or eyes should be treated immediately by copious lavage with water. Soap and water should then be used on non-mucous membranes. Spillage should be removed by dry or moist disposable towels.

Care must be taken in the disposal of all waste material (syringes, needles and disposable towels etc.) Used items should be placed in appropriate secure containers in readiness for destruction in a chemical incinerator equipped with an after-burner.

**Marketing authorisation numbers**

| | |
|---|---|
| 1 g Mitoxana Injection | 8336/0031 |
| 2 g Mitoxana Injection | 8336/0032 |

**Date of approval/revision of SPC** December 1994.

**Legal category** POM.

# PENDRAMINE*

**Presentation** Tablets each containing 125 mg or 250 mg D-penicillamine base. The 125 mg tablets are white, elongated, film coated with bisecting score on one side, and have a length of 11 mm and a width of 5.5 mm. The 250 mg tablets are white, elongated, film coated with bisecting score on one side, debossed HB on the same side, and have a length of 16 mm and a width of 7 mm.

**Uses**

*Indications:* Pendramine is indicated for the treatment of severe active rheumatoid arthritis, Wilson's disease, cystinuria, heavy metal poisoning and active chronic hepatitis.

**Dosage and administration** A guide for the dosage regimes for oral administration is given below:

*1. Severe active rheumatoid arthritis*

*Dosage:*

*Adults:* A dose of 125-250 mg daily for the initial 4 week period, before food then increasing at intervals of not less than four weeks by similar amounts. The ultimate maintenance dose will depend on the response obtained in individual patients. The usual maintenance dose is 500-750 mg in divided dosages. Improvement may not occur for some months.

A few patients may require up to 2000 mg daily to obtain benefit.

The minimum maintenance dose to achieve suppression of symptoms should be used. Treatment should be discontinued if no benefit is obtained within 12 months.

When clinical assessment shows that suppression of disease activity has been achieved, the dose should be kept at this maintenance level for six months, thereafter reducing the daily dosage by 250 mg at intervals of two or three months. Relapse may occur following withdrawal or when an inadequate dose level is reached, usually within three months, but most patients respond to further courses of Pendramine.

*Children:* 15-20 mg/kg/day is considered appropriate in the majority of cases. It is suggested that the initial dose is lower and increased at four-weekly intervals over a period of three to six months.

*Elderly:* Increased toxicity unrelated to renal function occurs in the elderly. A maximum initial dose of 50-125 mg daily for 4-8 weeks should be used, increased at intervals of not less than 4 weeks by similar amounts. The maximum recommended dose is 1000 mg daily.

*2. Wilson's disease:* D-penicillamine is a copper-chelating agent, and is most effectively used in conjunction with a low-copper diet (below 1 mg of copper per day).

*Dosage:*

*Adults:* 1500 to 2000 mg daily in divided doses, to be taken 30 minutes before food. The dose may be reduced to 750-1000 mg daily when disease control is achieved as evidenced by urinary copper excretion (Twenty-four hour urine samples should be examined at 3-monthly intervals). A dose of 2000 mg daily should not be continued for more than one year.

*Children:* Up to 20 mg per kg body weight daily in divided doses before food. Minimum dose 500 mg/day.

*Elderly:* Up to 20 mg per kg body weight daily in divided doses before food. The dosage should be adjusted to achieve disease control.

*3. Cystinuria:* Prevention and treatment of cystine stones.

*Dosage:*

*Treatment of stones:*

*Adults:* For the treatment of cystine stones, 750 mg daily in divided doses and especially at bedtime, increasing to 1500-2000 mg daily. The dose is adjusted to maintain urinary excretion of cystine below 100 mg per day. Maintain adequate fluid intake of 3 litres/day to provide a urine flow of 2 ml/min.

*Children:* Up to 30 mg per kg body weight daily in divided doses and especially at bedtime. The dose should be adjusted to maintain urine cystine levels below 100 mg/day.

*Elderly:* The minimum dose which maintains urinary excretion of cystine below 100 mg per day.

*Prophylaxis:*

*Adults:* (No history of stone formation but a cystine output in excess of 300 mg per day) 250-750 mg at night before retiring. The dose is adjusted to maintain overnight urine cystine excretion below 100 mg/day.

Fluid intake should not be less than 3 litres/day.

Safety in pregnancy is not established but if treatment is unavoidable should not exceed a dose of 1000 mg/24 hours.

*Children:* Paediatric dosage not yet established.

*Elderly:* The minimum dose required to maintain urinary excretion of cystine below 100 mg per day should be used.

*4. Heavy metal poisoning (lead)*

*Dosage:*

*Adults:* Daily oral dose of 1500-2000 mg in divided doses until urinary lead is stabilised at 0.5 mg/day.

*Children:* 20-25 mg per kg body weight daily in divided doses before food.

*Elderly:* 20 mg per kg body weight until urinary lead is stabilised at 0.5 mg/day.

*5. Active chronic hepatitis*

*Dosage:*

*Adults:* Pendramine is intended for the maintenance treatment of active chronic hepatitis. The diagnosis should be based on a history of at least three months duration with features of chronic aggressive hepatitis, with or without cirrhosis. Treatment with Pendramine should not be commenced until the disease process has been brought under control, initially by treatment with corticosteroids (e.g. 30 mg prednisone daily, sometimes with 75 mg azathioprine daily added to the regime). Disease control should be evidenced by biochemical analysis of liver function to include evaluation of serum bilirubin and transaminase activity.

Pendramine therapy should be commenced with 500 mg daily, in divided doses, increasing gradually over three months to the maintenance dose of 1250 mg daily. Concurrently, the dosage of corticosteroids should be reduced and phased out over a three-month period. Throughout therapy, liver function tests should be carried out at suitable intervals for assessment of disease status.

*Children:* Not recommended.

*Elderly:* Not recommended.

**Contra-indications, warnings, etc**

*Contra-indications:* Pendramine is contra-indicated in renal insufficiency; lupus erythematosus; hypersensitivity to D-penicillamine particularly if nephrotic syndrome or bone marrow depression has previously occurred.

*Use in pregnancy:* The safety of penicillamine in pregnancy has not been established. It has been shown to be teratogenic in rats when given in doses several times higher than those administered to humans.

*Nursing mothers:* Safety in lactation has not been established.

*Precautions:* Known sensitivity to penicillamine. Throughout pregnancy.

Penicillamine should not be used in patients who are receiving concurrent gold therapy, antimalarial or cytotoxic drugs, oxyphenbutazone or phenylbutazone since these drugs have a propensity to cause similar serious haematologic and/or renal adverse reactions.

Establish the lowest effective dose of D-penicillamine by quantitative amino acid chromatography on urine. Urine protein estimations should be carried out initially weekly for the first three months of therapy and thereafter monthly. Renal function should be assessed monthly for 6 months and 3 monthly thereafter.

The observation of proteinuria necessitates repeated quantitative estimations. Heavy or steadily increasing proteinuria or significant haematuria necessitates withdrawal of Pendramine.

With the exception of Wilson's disease patients (see later) platelet and white cell counts must be normal before commencing treatment. Because of the risk of blood dyscrasias and renal disturbances, full blood counts and urine examinations are essential during treatment. Weekly tests are recommended after each increase in dose as well as during the first eight weeks of therapy to monitor thrombocytopenia and neutropenia then monthly when dosage regimes have been stabilised.

Platelet counts below 120,000 $mm^{-3}$ or leucocyte counts below 2,500 $mm^{-3}$ necessitate withdrawal of D-penicillamine with resumption at a reduced dosage when counts return to normal. Recurrence of thrombocytopenia or leucopenia are indications for cessation of treatment.

A low platelet or white cell count is not a contra-indication to commence treatment of Wilson's disease. Treatment should be discontinued however, if a low initial count falls further and/or excessive bruising or petechial haemorrhages occur.

Allergic phenomena occurring early, unless severe, respond to cyproheptadine and temporary reductions of dose of D-penicillamine. Copper supplements may be necessary for alleviating taste impairment when treating conditions other than Wilson's disease.

In the treatment of rheumatoid arthritis, response to Pendramine is often slow and the use of existing analgesics, anti-inflammatories or steroids should be continued and later gradually withdrawn, subject to patient improvement.

*Interactions:* Concomitant oral iron therapy should not be given within 2 hours of taking penicillamine. Pendramine should not be given concurrently with iron or other heavy metals with which it may form complexes.

*Side-effects:* Both the frequency and severity of many side-effects and adverse reactions to D-penicillamine are found to be dose-related, hence the importance of initiating therapy at low doses and gradually increasing the quantity of drug given to optimum level.

Nausea and vomiting may occur.

D-penicillamine may cause allergic reactions such as urticaria and erythema accompanied by hyperpyrexia. Transient rashes and fever may occur early in therapy; if persistent, temporary withdrawal of treatment with or without a short course of steroids may be necessary. Penicillamine may be re-introduced at a lower dosage. If steroids are given, penicillamine should be reintroduced before steroid withdrawal.

A late rash, described as 'Epidermolysis Bullosa' and 'Penicillamine Dermopathy' may occur, after several months or years of therapy and may necessitate discontinuation of treatment.

Goodpastures syndrome, haemolytic anaemia and anorexia have been reported.

Other disorders of later onset and attributed to D-penicillamine are rheumatoid-like reactions, stomatitis and taste impairment. Reversible loss of taste occurs frequently. Reactions involving the appearance of thrombocytopenia, neutropenia or proteinuria may occur, particularly with higher dose levels. Less common are nephrotic syndrome and haematuria, purpura and increased skin friability due to increased collagen. Haematuria is rare, but if it occurs, treatment should be stopped immediately.

Serious complications include myasthenia gravis, pemphigus, nephrotic syndrome, Stevens-Johnson-like syndrome and lupus erythematosus. Deaths from agranulocytosis and aplastic anaemia have been recorded.

Iron deficiency may occur in menstruating women.

*Overdosage:* Treatment of overdosage is symptomatic and withdrawal of the drug is necessary if serious side effects as mentioned above occur.

**Pharmaceutical precautions** Store in a dry place below 25°C. Keep containers tightly closed.

**Legal category** POM.

**Package quantities** Tablets: 125 mg, plastic bottles of 100; 250 mg, plastic bottles of 100.

**Further information** Pendramine may be considered as an alternative to prednisone in the treatment of active chronic hepatitis when the latter drug causes complications such as diabetes, osteoporosis, etc. Occasionally, patients with rheumatoid arthritis who have responded to a particular dose begin to relapse. Most of these will respond to a dose increase which should be gradual.

**Product licence numbers**

Pendramine 125 mg 8336/0045
Pendramine 250 mg 8336/0046

## RHINOLAST* NASAL SPRAY

**Qualitative and quantitative composition** Azelastine hydrochloride 0.1% w/v.

**Pharmaceutical form** Nasal spray.

**Clinical particulars**

*Therapeutic Indications:* For the treatment of both seasonal allergic rhinitis (e.g. Hay fever) and perennial allergic rhinitis.

*Posology and method of administration:* Route of application is topical–nasal mucosa.

*Adults:* One application (0.14 ml) in each nostril twice daily (0.56 mg of azelastine hydrochloride).

*Elderly:* There have been no specific studies in the elderly.

*Children:* For children aged 5 years and older, one application (0.14 ml) in each nostril twice daily (0.56 mg of azelastine hydrochloride).

*Contra-indications:* Proven allergy against azelastine hydrochloride or benzalkonium chloride.

*Special warnings and precautions for use:* None.

*Interactions with other medicaments and other forms of interaction:* No specific interactions have been studied.

*Pregnancy and lactation:* At high oral doses in animals, 500 times the proposed oral human daily dose, foetal death, growth retardation and an increased incidence of skeletal abnormalities occurred during reproduction toxicity testing. Due to the nasal route of administration and the low dose administered, minimal systemic exposure can be expected. However as with all medicines caution should be exercised with use during pregnancy and lactation.

*Effects on ability to drive and use machines:* None.

*Undesirable effects:* Occasionally the nasal mucosa may become irritated (level of incidence 5%). A bitter taste can occur after administration (level of incidence 3%) due to incorrect method of application i.e. head tilting too far backwards.

*Overdose:* The results of animal studies show that toxic doses can product CNS symptoms, e.g. excitation, tremor, convulsions. Should these occur in humans symptomatic and supportive treatment should be instigated as there is no specific antidote. Gastric lavage is recommended if the overdose is recent.

With the nasal route of administration overdosage reactions are not anticipated.

**Pharmacological properties**

*Pharmacodynamic properties:* Azelastine, a phthalazinone derivative of novel structure, is classified as a potent long acting anti-allergic compound with particularly strong H1 antagonist properties.

Data from animal studies show that where high levels of azelastine are achieved both inhibition and release of chemical mediators (e.g. leukotriene, histamine, serotonin) involved in allergic reaction occurs.

*Pharmacokinetic properties:* After repeated nasal application (0.14 mg) into each nostril twice daily, the plasma levels of azelastine were about 0.26ng/ml. The levels of the active metabolite desmethylazelastine were detected at or below the lower limit of quantification (0.12ng/ml).

After repeated oral administration, the mean $C_{max}$ steady state plasma levels were determined giving 3.9 ng/ml for azelastine and 1.86 ng/ml for desmethylazelastine after 2.2 mg b.i.d. azelastine which represents the therapeutic oral dose for the treatment of allergic rhinitis.

Following oral administration azelastine is rapidly absorbed showing an absolute bioavailability of 81%. Food has no influence on absorption. The volume of distribution is high indicating distribution predominantly to the peripheral tissues. The level of protein binding is low, (80-95% a level too low to give concern over drug displacement reactions).

Plasma elimination half lives after a single dose of azelastine are approximately 20 hours for azelastine and about 45 hours for N desmethylazelastine (a therapeutically active metabolite). Excretion occurs mainly via the faeces. The sustained excretion of small amounts of the dose in the faeces suggest that some enterohepatic circulation may take place.

*Preclinical safety data:* Not relevant.

## Pharmaceutical particulars

*List of excipients:* Methylhydroxypropyl cellulose, sodium edetate, benzalkonium chloride, citric acid, sodium phosphate, sodium chloride, purified water.

*Incompatibilities:* None.

*Shelf life:* Three years unopened.

*Special precautions for storage:* Do not store below 8°C. Do not refrigerate.

*Nature and contents of container:*
10 ml or 20 ml polyethylene bottle with polypropylene cap and polyethylene seal.
10 ml or 20 ml glass bottle with screw closure and polypropylene seal.
10 ml or 20 ml glass bottle with pump attached.
10 ml glass bottle with pump attached, containing 5 ml aqueous solution.
10 ml polyethylene bottle with polypropylene cap and polyethylene seal, containing 5 ml aqueous solution.

*Instruction for use/handling:*

*For separate bottle and pump:* Open the bottle by unscrewing the cap. Place the spray pump nozzle in the bottle and screw the pump onto the bottle. Remove the protective cap. Before first using, squeeze down the collar several times until an even spray emerges. The Rhinolast spray is now ready to use.

*For attached pump and bottle:* Remove the protective cap. Before first using, squeeze down the collar several times until an even spray emerges. The Rhinolast spray is now ready to use.

**Marketing authorisation number** 8336/0039

**Date of approval/revision of SPC** July 1996.

**Legal category** POM.

# UROMITEXAN* INJECTION

**Presentation** Clear, glass ampoules containing a clear, colourless, aqueous solution of mesna (sodium 2-mercapto-ethanesulphonate) 400 mg in 4 ml and 1000 mg in 10 ml.

## Uses

*Action:* Mesna is a sulphydryl-containing compound which is excreted in the urine. Co-administration with oxazaphosphorine alkylating agents such as ifosfamide (Mitoxana) and cyclophosphamide (Endoxana) significantly reduces their urotoxic effects by reacting with the causal metabolites, including acrolein, in the urinary system. No reduction in the antitumour activity of these oxazaphosphorine compounds has been detected.

*Indications:* For the prophylaxis of urothelial toxicity including haemorrhagic cystitis, microhaematuria and macrohaematuria in patients treated with ifosfamide or cyclophosphamide, in doses considered to be urotoxic.

## Dosage and administration

*Dosage:* Sufficient mesna must be given to protect the patient adequately from the urotoxic effects of the oxazaphosphorine. The duration of mesna treatment should equal that of the oxazaphosphorine treatment plus the time taken for the urinary concentration of metabolites to fall to non-toxic levels. This usually occurs within 8-12 hours after the end of oxazaphosphorine treatment but may vary depending on the scheduling of the oxazaphosphorine. Urinary output should be maintained at 100 ml/hr (as required for oxazaphosphorine treatment) and the urine monitored for haematuria and proteinuria throughout the treatment period.

*Intravenous usage of mesna*

*Where ifosfamide or cyclophosphamide is used as an iv bolus:* Mesna is given by intravenous injection over 15-30 minutes at 20% of the simultaneously administered oxazaphosphorine on a weight for weight basis

(w/w). The same dose of mesna is repeated after 4 and 8 hours. The total dose of mesna is 60% (w/w) of the oxazaphosphorine dose. This is repeated on each occasion that the cytotoxic agents are used.

*e.g.*

|  | 0 hrs | 4 hrs | 8 hrs |
|---|---|---|---|
| Mitoxana/Endoxana | 2 g | - | - |
| Uromitexan | 400 mg | 400 mg | 400 mg |

If necessary the dose of mesna can be increased to 40% of the oxazaphosphorine dose given four times at three hourly intervals (0, 3, 6 and 9 hours). (Total dose = 160% (w/w) of the oxazaphosphorine dose). This larger dose is recommended in children, or in patients whose urothelium may be damaged from previous treatment with oxazaphosphorine or pelvic irradiation, or in patients who are not adequately protected by the standard dose of mesna.

*e.g.*

|  | 0 hrs | 3 hrs | 6 hrs | 9 hrs |
|---|---|---|---|---|
| Mitoxana/Endoxana | 2 g | - | - | - |
| Uromitexan | 800 mg | 800 mg | 800 mg | 800 mg |

*Where cyclophosphamide is used orally:* The same dose regimen of mesna applies as though cyclophosphamide were used as an iv bolus.

*Where ifosfamide is used as a 24-hour infusion:* Mesna can be used as a concurrent infusion. An initial 20% (w/w) of the total ifosfamide dose is given as an i.v. bolus, then an infusion of 100% (w/w) of the ifosfamide over 24 hours, followed by a further 12-hour infusion of 60% (w/w) of the ifosfamide dose. (Total mesna dose = 180% of the ifosfamide dose) (see Table 1).

The final 12-hour infusion of mesna after 24 hour infusion of ifosfamide and mesna, can be replaced by boluses at 28, 32 and 36 hours, each of 20% (w/w) of the 24 hour ifosfamide dose, or by oral mesna.

*Where ifosfamide is used as a long-term infusion:* Mesna is given initially as an i.v. bolus of 20% (w/w) of the first 24-hour ifosfamide infusion dose as the infusion starts, then as concurrent infusions of 100% (w/w) of the daily ifosfamide dose. This is followed by a further 12-hour infusion of 60% (w/w) of the *final 24 hour* dose (see Table 2).

As above, the final 12-hour infusion of mesna, after long-term infusion of ifosfamide and mesna, can be replaced by boluses each of 20% (w/w) of the 24 hour ifosfamide dose, or by oral mesna.

Mesna can be mixed in the same infusion bag as the ifosfamide.

*Oral use of mesna ampoules:* Mesna has been shown to be effective when taken orally. Compared with intravenous administration, overall availability of mesna in urine after oral administration is approximately 50%; the onset of urinary excretion is delayed by up to 2 hours and is more prolonged than following intravenous dosing.

For intermittent oxazaphosphorine therapy, oral mesna 40% (w/w) of the oxazaphosphorine dose should be given 2 hours prior to the oxazaphosphorine dose, and repeated at 2 and 6 hours. Alternatively, an initial intravenous dose of mesna 20% (w/w) of the oxazaphosphorine dose could be given with the cytotoxic dose. Additional oral mesna 40% (w/w) of the oxazaphosphorine dose can then be given at 2 and 6 hours.

*e.g.*

|  | - 2 hrs | 0 hrs | 2 hrs | 6 hrs |
|---|---|---|---|---|
| Mitoxana/Endoxana | - | 1 g iv | - | - |
| Uromitexan | 400 mg po | - | 400 mg po | 400 mg po |
|  |  | 200 mg iv | 400 mg po | 400 mg po |

Oral mesna may also be used following a 24-hour infusion of ifosfamide and mesna. The first dose of 40% (w/w) of the ifosfamide is given as the infusion is stopped, and repeated after 2 and 6 hours.

*e.g.*

|  | 0 hrs | 0-24 hrs | 24 hrs | 26 hrs | 30 hrs |
|---|---|---|---|---|---|
| Mitoxana | - | 5 g/m² infusion | - | - | - |
| Uromitexan | 1 g/m² iv | 5 g/m² infusion | 2 g/m² po | 2 g/m² po | 2 g/m² po |

If mesna is to be taken orally, it should be added to a flavoured drink such as orange juice or cola. This may be stored in the refrigerator for up to 24 hours in a sealed container.

Mesna tablets are also available for oral administration. The dose of mesna tablets is the same as for oral use of mesna injection outlined above. Further information on the use of mesna tablets can be found on a separate datasheet or from ASTA Medica Ltd.

*Elderly:* No specific information on the use of this product in the elderly is available. Clinical trials have included patients over 65 years and no adverse reactions specific to this age group have been reported.

*Children:* Because of greater frequency of micturition, children may require shorter intervals between doses. (e.g. 3 hourly, see above, under *Dosage*)

## Contra-indications, warnings, etc

*Contra-indications:* Known hypersensitivity to mesna or any thiol containing compounds.

*Use in pregnancy and lactation:* Pregnancy and lactation are contraindications for cytostatic treatment and consequently Uromitexan is not likely to be used under these circumstances.

Should an individual patient be undergoing oxazaphosphorine therapy during pregnancy then Uromitexan should be administered to this patient.

Animal studies have shown no evidence of embryotoxic or teratogenic effects of Uromitexan.

*Precautions:* As mesna counteracts only the urotoxic side-effects of oxazaphosphorines, other side-effects of cytotoxic therapy e.g. myelosuppression, nausea, vomiting, alopecia, may still be expected. No other interaction between mesna and these alkylating agents has been demonstrated.

The prevention of urotoxicity with Uromitexan should only be undertaken after medical guidance and careful consideration of the risks and benefits.

*Interactions:* There are no known in vivo interactions of mesna with other agents.

*Side-effects:* Because patients receive potent cytotoxic agents concurrently, the side-effect profile of mesna is difficult to define. However, in healthy volunteers the following side-effects occurred at single doses of 60-70 mg/kg per day: nausea, vomiting, colic, diarrhoea, headache, fatigue, limb and joint pains, depression, irritability, lack of energy, rash, hypotension and tachycardia.

In rare cases, pseudoallergic reactions (rash, pruritus, blistering of skin and mucous membranes, fever, urticarial oedema, sudden hypotension and tachycardia and a transient rise of liver transaminases) have been reported. These pseudoallergic reactions appear

**Table 1: Where ifosfamide is used as a 24-hour infusion**

|  | 0 hrs | 0-24 hrs | 24 hrs | 28 hrs | 32 hrs | 36 hrs |
|---|---|---|---|---|---|---|
| Mitoxana | - | 5 g/m² infusion | - | - | - | - |
| Uromitexan | 1 g/m² iv | 5 g/m² infusion | ← 3 g/m² infusion → | | | |
|  |  |  | 1 g/m² iv | 1 g/m² iv | 1 g/m² iv |

**Table 2: Where ifosfamide is used as a long-term infusion**

|  | Day 1 | | Day 2 | Day 3 | | Day 4 | | |
|---|---|---|---|---|---|---|---|---|
|  | 0 hrs | 0-24 hrs | 0-24 hrs | 0-24 hrs | 24 hrs | 4 hrs | 8 hrs | 12 hrs |
| Mitoxana | - | 2 g/m² infusion | 2 g/m² infusion | 2 g/m² infusion | - | - | - | - |
| Uromitexan | 0.4 g/m² iv | 2 g/m² infusion | 2 g/m² infusion | 2 g/m² infusion | ← 1.2 g/m² → infusion | | | |
|  |  |  |  |  |  | 0.4 g/m² iv | 0.4 g/m² iv | 0.4 g/m² iv |

to be more common in patients with autoimmune disorders.

*Overdosage:* Healthy volunteers given single bolus doses of 70 mg/kg mesna showed no evidence of major toxic side-effects. A specific antidote to mesna is not known.

**Pharmaceutical precautions** Protect from light, store below 30°C.

Mesna is chemically compatible with 0.9% saline for 24 hours. Mesna and ifosfamide are chemically compatible with 0.9% saline for 24 hours

Mesna is incompatible with platinum derivatives and nitrogen mustard and must not be mixed in the same infusion solution.

**Legal category** POM.

**Package quantities**
4 ml ampoules in boxes of 15.
10 ml ampoules in boxes of 15.

**Further information** There is evidence that the long-term urothelial toxicity of the oxazaphosphorines can be almost totally prevented by the concurrent administration of mesna in the appropriate dosage. Mesna only exerts this protective effect on the urinary tract and other precautionary measures recommended for the use of oxazaphosphorines are not affected and should continue to be used. A false positive test of urinary ketones (e.g. Rothera's test, N-Multistix reagent strip) may arise in patients treated with mesna. The colour is red-violet rather than violet and it will fade immediately on the addition of glacial acetic acid. A false negative or false positive reaction in the dipstick tests for erythrocytes in the urine of patients treated with mesna may occur, therefore use of urinary microscopy is recommended.

**Product licence numbers**
4 ml ampoules Uromitexan
Injection 400 mg 8336/0033
10 ml ampoules Uromitexan
Injection 1 g 8336/0033

## UROMITEXAN TABLETS*

**Presentation** White, oblong biconvex film-coated tablets containing 400 mg and 600 mg of mesna (sodium 2-mercaptoethanesulphonate).

**Uses**

*Action:* Mesna is a sulphydryl-containing compound which is excreted in the urine. Co-administration with oxazaphosphorine alkylating agents such as ifosfamide (Mitoxana) and cyclophosphamide (Endoxana) significantly reduces their urotoxic effects by reacting with the causal metabolites, including acrolein, in the urinary system. No reduction in the antitumour activity of these oxazaphosphorine compounds has been detected.

*Indications:* For the prophylaxis of urothelial toxicity including haemorrhagic cystitis, microhaematuria and macrohaematuria in patients treated with ifosfamide and cyclophosphamide, in doses considered to be urotoxic.

**Dosage and administration**

*Dosage:* Sufficient Uromitexan must be given to protect the patient adequately from the urotoxic effects of the oxazaphosphorine. The duration of Uromitexan treatment should equal that of the oxazaphosphorine treatment plus the time taken for the urinary concentration of oxazaphosphorine metabolites to fall to non-toxic levels. This usually occurs within 8-12 hours after the end of oxazaphosphorine treatment but may vary depending on the scheduling of oxazaphosphorine. When calculating the dose of Uromitexan the quantity should be rounded down to the nearest whole tablet. Urinary output should be maintained at 100 ml/hr (as required for oxazaphosphorine treatment) and the urine monitored for haematuria and proteinuria throughout the treatment period.

Compared with intravenous administration, overall availability of mesna in urine after oral administration is approximately 50%; and the onset of urinary excretion is delayed by up to 2 hours and is more prolonged than following intravenous dosing.

*For intermittent oxazaphosphorine therapy:* oral mesna 40% (w/w) of the oxazaphosphorine dose should be given 2 hours prior to, and repeated 2 hours and 6 hours after the oxazaphosphorine dose. Alternatively, an initial intravenous dose of mesna (20% (w/w) of the oxazaphosphorine dose) can be given with the cytotoxic dose, additional oral mesna 40% (w/w) of the oxazaphosphorine dose should then be given at 2 and 6 hours.

*e.g.*

| | *-2 hrs* | *0 hrs* | *2 hrs* | *6 hrs* |
|---|---|---|---|---|
| Cyclophosphamide/ Ifosfamide | - | 1 g iv | - | - |
| Uromitexan | 400 mg po | - | 400 mg po | 400 mg po |
| | | 200 mg iv | 400 mg po | 400 mg po |

*Following 24-hour infusion of ifosfamide and Uromitexan:* the first oral Uromitexan dose of 40% (w/w) of the ifosfamide dose is given as the infusion is stopped, and the same dose is repeated at 2 and 6 hours.

*e.g.*

| | *0 hrs* | *0-24 hrs* | *24 hrs* | *26 hrs* | *30 hrs* |
|---|---|---|---|---|---|
| Ifosfamide | - | 5 g/m² infusion | - | - | - |
| Uromitexan | 1 g/m² iv | 5 g/m² infusion | 2 g/m² po | 2 g/m² po | 2 g/m² |

*Following long-term infusion:* the first oral Uromitexan dose should be 40% (w/w) of the ifosfamide dose taken in the FINAL 24 HOURS, and is given as the infusion is stopped and the same dose repeated at 2 and 6 hours (see Table 1).

Higher doses of Uromitexan can be given if urothelial toxicity occurs.

*Elderly:* No specific information on the use of this product in the elderly is available. Clinical trials have included patients over 65 years and no adverse reactions specific to this age group have been reported.

*Children:* Due to increased micturition, children may require shorter intervals between doses and/or an increased number of individual doses.

*High risk patients:* Those who have had previous irradiation of the small pelvis, occurrence of cystitis during previous cyclophosphamide, ifosfamide or trofosfamide therapy, history of urinary tract lesions, may also require shorter intervals between doses and/or an increased number of doses.

**Contra-indications, warnings, etc**

*Contra-indications:* Known hypersensitivity to mesna or any thiol containing compounds.

*Use in pregnancy and lactation:* Cytostatic treatment is contra-indicated during pregnancy and lactation, and consequently Uromitexan is not likely to be used under these circumstances.

Should an individual patient be undergoing oxazaphosphorine therapy during pregnancy then Uromitexan should be administered to this patient.

Animal studies have shown no evidence of embryotoxic or teratogenic effects of Uromitexan.

*Precautions:* As Uromitexan counteracts only the urotoxic side-effects of oxazaphosphorines, other side-effects of cytotoxic therapy eg myelosuppression, nausea, vomiting, alopecia, may still be expected. No other interaction between Uromitexan and these alkylating agents has been demonstrated.

Oral Uromitexan should be replaced by i.v. Uromitexan in patients experiencing vomiting.

The prevention of urotoxicity with Uromitexan tablets should only be undertaken after medical guidance and careful consideration of the risks and benefits.

*Interactions:* There are no known in-vivo interactions of Uromitexan with other agents. There is no interaction with food.

*Side effects:* Because patients receive potent cytotoxic agents concurrently, the side-effect profile of Uromitexan is difficult to define. However, in healthy volunteers the following side effects occurred at single doses of 60-70 mg/kg per day: nausea, vomiting, colic, diarrhoea, headache, fatigue, limb and joint pains, depression, irritability, lack of energy, rash, hypotension and tachycardia.

In rare cases, pseudoallergic reactions (rash, pruritus, blistering of skin and mucous membranes, urticarial oedema, sudden hypotension, tachycardia and a transient rise of liver transaminases) have been reported. These pseudoallergic reactions appear to be more common in patients with autoimmune disorders.

*Overdosage:* Healthy volunteers given single bolus doses of 70 mg/kg Uromitexan showed no evidence of major toxic side-effects.

A specific antidote to Uromitexan is not known.

**Pharmaceutical precautions** None necessary.

**Legal category** POM.

**Package quantities** Ten tablets in a blister strip. Pack size–10 tablets.

**Further information** There is evidence that the long term urothelial toxicity of the oxazaphosphorines can be almost totally prevented by the concurrent administration of Uromitexan in the appropriate dosage. Uromitexan only exerts this protective effect on the urinary tract and other precautionary measures recommended for the use of oxazaphosphorine are not affected and should continue to be used.

A false positive test for urinary ketones (eg Rothera's test, N-Multistix reagent strip) may arise in patients treated with Uromitexan. The colour is red-violet rather than violet and it will fade immediately on the addition of glacial acetic acid.

A false positive or false negative reaction in the dipstick test for erythrocytes in the urine of patients treated with Uromitexan may occur, therefore use of urinary microscopy is recommended.

**Product licence numbers**
400 mg film coated tablets 8336/0049
600 mg film coated tablets 8336/0050

Table 1: Following long-term infusion

| | Day 1 | | Day 2 | Day 3 | Day 4 | | |
|---|---|---|---|---|---|---|---|
| | *0 hrs* | *0-24 hrs* | *0-24 hrs* | *0-24 hrs* | *24 hrs* | *26 hrs* | *30 hrs* |
| Ifosfamide | - | 2 g/m² infusion | 2 g/m² infusion | 2 g/m² infusion | - | - | - |
| Uromitexan | 0.4 g/m² iv | 2 g/m² infusion | 2 g/m² infusion | 2 g/m² infusion | 0.8 g/m² po | 0.8 g/m² po | 0.8 g/m² po |

## VIVAPRYL*

**Qualitative and quantitative composition**

Vivapryl 5 mg contain 5 mg selegiline hydrochloride per tablet

Vivapryl 10 mg contain 10 mg selegiline hydrochloride per tablet.

**Pharmaceutical form** Tablets for immediate release.

**Clinical particulars**

*Therapeutic indications:* For the treatment of Parkinson's disease or symptomatic Parkinsonism. May be used alone, in early Parkinson's disease to delay the need for levodopa (with or without decarboxylase inhibitor), or as an adjunct with levodopa (with or without decarboxylase inhibitor).

*Posology and method of administration:*

*Route of administration:* Vivapryl Tablets are intended for oral administration.

*Dosage:* 10 mg daily, either alone or as an adjunct to levodopa or levodopa/peripheral decarboxylase inhibitor. May be administered either as a single dose in the morning or in two divided doses taken at breakfast and lunch.

When Vivapryl is added to a levodopa regimen it is possible to reduce the levodopa dosage by an average of 30 per cent.

*Contra-indications:* None.

*Special warnings and special precautions for use:* As selegiline potentiates the effect of levodopa, the side-effects of levodopa might be emphasised, particularly in patients on a high dosage of levodopa. The addition of Vivapryl to maximal doses of levodopa may cause involuntary movements and/or agitation. Such side-effects disappear when the levodopa dosage is decreased. Levodopa treatment can be reduced by an average of 30 per cent when Vivapryl is added to the treatment.

*Interaction with other medicaments and other forms of interaction:* Severe, life threatening interaction with pethidine has been reported. Vivapryl should not be given in conjunction with non-specific monoamine oxidase inhibitors or fluoxetine.

*Pregnancy and lactation:* Vivapryl is indicated for Parkinsonism. This tends to be a disease of the elderly, past child bearing age. There is inadequate data to assess the effects of selegiline on pregnancy and lactation and Vivapryl should not be used in such cases.

*Effects on ability to drive and use machines:* None.

*Undesirable effects:* Hypotension and nausea have been reported as isolated symptoms. confusion or psychosis have also been reported.

*Overdose:* No specific information is available concerning clinically significant overdose of selegiline. However, since the selective inhibition of MAO-B is achieved only at the dosage range recommended (i.e. 10 mg/day), overdoses are likely to cause significant inhibition of both MAO-A and MAO-B. Consequently, the signs and symptoms of overdose may resemble those observed with marketed, non-selective MAO inhibitors. In the case of suspected overdose the patient should be kept under observation for 24-48 hours.

**Pharmacological properties**

*Pharmacodynamic properties:* Selegiline is a highly selective inhibitor of monoamine oxidase type B, an enzyme involved in the metabolic degradation of dopamine in the brain. The resultant preservation of dopamine in the basal ganglia appears to enhance the therapeutic efficacy of levodopa. Additionally, it has been shown in animals that selegiline can prevent the appearance of MPTP induced Parkinsonism. This effect may result from the inhibition of the conversion of MPTP to its putative toxic metabolite by MAO-B and has led to speculation that selegiline may alter the progression of idiopathic Parkinson's disease by reducing the generation of potentially neurotoxic substances from either endogenous or exogenous compounds.

*Pharmacokinetic properties:* Selegiline is rapidly absorbed following oral administration and distributed in the tissues. It is almost completely metabolised to form norselegiline, methamphetamine and amphetamine. Approximately 50% of an oral dose is excreted in the urine in 24 hours, mainly in the form of methamphetamine.

*Preclinical safety data:* No pre-clinical safety data has been obtained for Vivapryl, since the excipients are widely used in pharmaceutical formulation and the toxicological profile of selegiline is well known.

**Pharmaceutical particulars**

*List of excipients:* Vivapryl tablets also contain: Lactose monohydrate, microcrystalline cellulose, maize starch, citric acid and magnesium stearate.

*Incompatibilities:* None.

*Shelf life:* 2 Years.

*Special precautions for storage:* Store below 25°C, protect from heat, moisture and light, keep out of the reach of children.

*Nature and contents of container:* Vivapryl will be presented in blisters formed from approximately 20 μm thick aluminium and contained within a printed boxboard carton. Each carton will contain either 30, 60 or 100 tablets as stated on the carton.

*Instructions for use/handling:* Use as directed by the physician.

**Marketing authorisation numbers**
Vivapryl 5 mg 8336/0055
Vivapryl 10 mg 8336/0056

**Date of approval/revision of SPC** October 1995.

**Legal category** POM.

## ZAMADOL CAPSULES* ▼

**Qualitative and quantitative composition** Each capsule contains tramadol hydrochloride 50 mg.

**Pharmaceutical form** Hard gelatin capsules.

**Clinical particulars**

*Therapeutic Indications:* For the treatment and prevention of moderate to severe pain.

*Posology and method of administration:* The capsules are for oral administration. As with all analgesic drugs the dosing of Zamadol Capsules 50 mg should be adjusted depending on the severity of the pain and the individual clinical response of the patient.

The capsules should only be administered where there is a medical need for pain relief and treatment should normally be for a limited period and intermittent.

A total oral daily dose of over 400 mg is not usually necessary.

*Adults and children aged 12 years and over:* For acute pain an initial dose of 100 mg is usually required. For chronic painful conditions an initial dose of 50 mg is recommended. Subsequent doses should be 50 mg to 100 mg administered 4-6 hourly. The dose level and frequency of dosing will depend on the severity of the pain.

*Elderly patients:* Dosing as for adults but it should be noted that in a study in elderly volunteers (aged over 75 years) the elimination half-life for orally administered tramadol was increased by 17%.

*Patients with renal insufficiency:* The usual initial adult doses should be employed, but the elimination of tramadol may be prolonged in patients with renal impairment and therefore the dosage interval should be adjusted.

For creatinine clearance <30 ml/min the dosing should be increased to 12 hourly intervals.

For creatinine clearance <10 ml/min (severe renal impairment) tramadol is not recommended.

Tramadol is removed very slowly by haemodialysis or haemofiltration and therefore post-dialysis dosing to maintain analgesia is usually unnecessary.

*Patients with hepatic insufficiency:* The usual adult doses should be used, but it should be noted that elimination of tramadol may be prolonged in severe hepatic impairment and dosing should be at 12 hourly intervals.

*Children under 12 years:* Not recommended.

*Contra-indications:* Zamadol Capsules 50 mg should not be given to patients who have previously shown hypersensitivity to the product.

The product should not be administered to patients suffering from acute intoxication with hypnotics, centrally acting analgesics, opioids, psychotropic drugs or alcohol.

In common with other opioid analgesics, tramadol should not be administered to patients who are receiving monoamine oxidase inhibitors or within 2 weeks of their withdrawal.

*Special warnings and precautions for use*

*Warnings:* Zamadol Capsules 50 mg are not a suitable substitute in opioid dependent patients. The product does not suppress morphine withdrawal symptoms although it is an opioid agonist.

Tramadol has been demonstrated to have a low potential to cause physical dependence but cases of abuse and dependency have been reported.

*Precautions:* In patients with severe renal or hepatic impairment, head injury, increased intracranial pressure, or patients in shock or at risk of convulsions, Zamadol Capsules 50 mg should be used with caution.

At present Zamadol Capsules 50 mg should not be used during light planes of anaesthesia as enhanced intra-operative recall was reported in a study of the use of tramadol during anaesthesia with enflurane and nitrous oxide.

At therapeutic doses of tramadol respiratory depression has been reported infrequently. Therefore care should be taken when administering Zamadol Capsules 50 mg to patients with existing respiratory depression or to patients taking concomitant CNS depressant drugs.

*Interaction with other medicaments and other forms of interaction:* Zamadol Capsules 50 mg may potentiate the CNS depressant effects of other centrally acting drugs (including alcohol) when administered concomitantly with such drugs.

Administration of Zamadol Capsules 50 mg together with carbamazepine results in markedly decreased serum concentrations of tramadol which may reduce analgesic effectiveness and shorten the duration of action.

Changes in serum concentrations of tramadol have been associated with the simultaneous dosing with cimetidine. However, such changes are clinically insignificant and therefore no dosage adjustment for Zamadol Capsules 50 mg is recommended in patients receiving chronic cimetidine therapy.

Theoretically, tramadol could interact with noradrenaline, 5-HT or lithium due to their mechanisms of actions, and thus potentiate their antidepressant effect. However there have been no reports of such interactions.

*Pregnancy and lactation*

*Pregnancy:* Zamadol Capsules 50 mg should not be used in pregnancy as there is inadequate evidence available to assess the safety of tramadol in pregnant women.

Studies of tramadol in rats and rabbits have revealed no teratogenic effects. However, embryotoxicity was shown in the form of delayed ossification. Fertility, reproductive performance and development of offspring were unaffected.

*Lactation:* Zamadol Capsules 50 mg should not be administered during breast feeding as tramadol and its metabolites have been detected in breast milk. An infant could ingest 0.1% of the dose administered to the mother.

*Effects on ability to drive and use machines:* Zamadol Capsules 50 mg may cause drowsiness and this effect may be potentiated by alcohol and other CNS depressants. Patients should be warned not to drive or operate machinery if affected.

*Undesirable effects:* Drowsiness, somnolence, tiredness, fatigue, dizziness, headache, confusion, constipation, pruritis, hallucinations and infrequently respiratory depression have been reported. Dependence, dysphoria and epileptiform convulsions have rarely been reported.

Tachycardia, bradycardia, increase in blood pressure, orthostatic hypotension, syncope, anaphylaxis, flushing, skin rashes and diaphoresis have rarely been reported. There have been rare cases of blood dyscrasias observed with tramadol treatment but direct causality has not been confirmed.

Nausea, vomiting and occasionally dry mouth have been reported.

*Overdose:* Symptoms of tramadol overdose include vomiting, miosis, sedation, coma, seizures, cardiovascular collapse and respiratory depression. Such symptoms are typical of opioid analgesics.

Treatment of overdose requires the maintenance of the airway and cardiovascular functions. Respiratory depression may be reversed using naloxone and fits controlled with diazepam.

The treatment of acute overdose of tramadol using haemodialysis or haemofiltration alone is not sufficient or suitable due to the slow elimination of tramadol from the serum by these routes.

**Pharmacological properties**

*Pharmacodynamic properties:* Tramadol, a cyclohexanol derivative, is a centrally acting analgesic which possesses opioid agonist properties. Tramadol appears to modify the transmission of pain impulses by inhibition of monoamine reuptake. The duration of analgesia with orally administered tramadol has been shown to be 3-6 hours with maximum pain relief at 1-4 hours post-dosing. Tramadol also has an antitussive action but has no effect on gastrointestinal motility. At the recommended dosages, the effects of tramadol given orally on the respiratory and cardiovascular systems appear to be clinically insignificant.

*Pharmacokinetic properties:* Following oral dosing, tramadol is rapidly and almost completely absorbed. After oral administration as capsules or tablets, tramadol appears in the plasma within 15-45 minutes, reaching peak plasma concentrations at a mean of 2 hours. The mean oral bioavailability of tramadol is approximately 68% after single doses and increases to 90 to 100% on multiple administration.

The half-life of absorption for oral tramadol (solid dose formulation) is 0.38 ± 0.18 hours with a peak plasma concentration of 280 ± 49ng/ml 2.0 hours after oral dosing with 100 mg tramadol (solid dose formulation). Tramadol has a high tissue affinity with an apparent volume of distribution of 306 litres after oral dosing in healthy volunteers.

Tramadol undergoes hepatic metabolism with approximately 85% of an oral dose being metabolised in young healthy volunteers. Tramadol is biotransformed primarily by N- and O-demethylation and by glucuronidation of the O-demethylation products. Eleven metabolites have so far been identified in man.

Only one metabolite, O-demethyl tramadol (M1), is pharmacologically active showing analgesic activity.

The mean elimination half-life of tramadol following oral administration is 5-6 hours. Approximately 90% of an oral dose is excreted by the kidneys.

Effect of age: Tramadol pharmacokinetics show little age-dependence in volunteers up to the age of 75 years. In volunteers aged over 75 years, the terminal elimination half-life was 7.0 ± 1.6 h compared to 6.0 ± 1.5 h in young volunteers after oral administration.

Effect of hepatic or renal impairment: As both tramadol and its pharmacologically active metabolite, O-demethyl tramadol, are eliminated both metabolically and renally, the terminal half-life of elimination ($t_{\frac{1}{2}}$) may be prolonged in patients with hepatic or renal dysfunction. However, the increase in $t_{\frac{1}{2}}$ is relatively small if either excretory organ is functioning normally. In liver cirrhosis patients, the mean $t_{\frac{1}{2}}$ of tramadol was 13.3 ± 4.9 hours. In patients with renal failure (creatinine clearance < 5 mL/min) the $t_{\frac{1}{2}}$ of tramadol was 11.0 ± 3.2 hours and that of M1 was 16.9 ± 3.0 hours. Extreme values observed to date are 22.3 hours (tramadol) and 36.0 hours (M1) in liver cirrhosis patients and 19.5 hours (tramadol) and 43.2 hours (M1) in renal failure patients.

*Preclinical safety data:* The standard range of pharmacodynamic pharmacokinetic and toxicological tests have been carried out for Tramadol and the effects observed from these investigations that are relevant to the prescriber are mentioned in other sections.

**Pharmaceutical particulars**

*List of excipients:* Zamadol capsules contain: Dibasic calcium phosphate anhydrous, magnesium stearate, colloidal anhydrous silica. The capsule shell contains: Gelatin and titanium dioxide (E171).

*Incompatibilities:* No pharmaceutical incompatibilities reported.

*Shelf life:* Two years, as packaged for sale.

*Special precautions for storage:* No special requirements.

*Nature and contents of container:* White opaque PVC/PVDC and aluminium foil blister strips. Each strip contains 10 capsules. The blister strips are packed in cartons containing 100 capsules.

*Instructions for use/handling:* None.

**Marketing authorisation number** 8336/0061

**Date of approval/revision of SPC** August 1996.

**Legal category**   POM.

*\*Trade Mark*

**Astra Pharmaceuticals Limited**
Home Park
Kings Langley
Herts WD4 8DH

ASTRA

## BAMBEC* TABLETS

**Qualitative and quantitative composition** Bambuterol hydrochloride INN 10 mg; bambuterol hydrochloride INN 20 mg

**Pharmaceutical form**  Tablet.

**Clinical particulars**

*Therapeutic indications:* Management of asthma, bronchospasm and/or reversible airways obstruction.

*Posology and method of administration:* Bambec is formulated as a tablet and should be taken orally. Bambec Tablets 20 mg are effective once daily.

*Adults:* The recommended starting doses are 10-20 mg. The 10 mg dose may be increased to 20 mg if necessary after 1-2 weeks, depending on the clinical effect. In patients who have previously tolerated β-agonists well, the recommended starting as well as maintenance, dose is 20 mg.

*Children:* Until the clinical documentation has been completed, Bambec should not be used in children.

*Elderly:* Dose adjustment is not required in the elderly.

*Significant hepatic dysfunction:* Not recommended because of unpredictable conversion to terbutaline.

*Moderate to severely impaired renal function (GFR <50 ml/min):* It is recommended that the starting dose of Bambec should be halved in these patients.

*Contra-indications:* Bambec tablets are contra-indicated in patients with a history of hypersensitivity to any of their ingredients. Bambec is presently not recommended for children due to limited clinical data in this age group.

*Special warnings and special precautions for use:* Care should be taken with patients suffering from myocardial insufficiency or thyrotoxicosis.

Due to the hyperglycaemic effects of β₂-stimulants additional blood glucose measurements are recommended initially when Bambec therapy is commenced in diabetic patients. If diabetic treatment becomes less effective or shorter acting the patient's general condition should be reviewed.

Due to the positive inotropic effects of β₂-agonists these drugs should not be used in patients with hypotrophic cardiomyopathy.

β-agonists may be arrhythmogenic and this must be considered in the treatment of the individual patient. Unpredictable interindividual variation in the metabolism of bambuterol to terbutaline has been shown in subjects with liver cirrhosis. The use of another β-agonist is recommended in patients with cirrhosis and other forms of severely impaired liver function.

Potentially serious hypokalaemia may result from β₂-agonist therapy. Particular caution is advised in severe asthma as this effect may be potentiated by concomitant treatment with xanthine derivatives, steroids, diuretics and by hypoxia. It is recommended that serum potassium levels are monitored in such situations.

*Interaction with other medicaments and other forms of interaction:* Bambuterol may interact with suxamethonium (succinyl choline).

A prolongation of the muscle-relaxing effect of suxamethonium of up to 2 fold has been observed in some patients after taking Bambec 20 mg on the evening prior to surgery. The interaction is dose dependent. It is due to the fact that plasma cholinesterase, which interactivates suxamethonium, is partly, but fully reversibly, inhibited by bambuterol. In extreme situations, the interaction may result in a prolonged apnoea time which may be of clinical importance.

Bambuterol may also interact with other muscle relaxants metabolised by plasma cholinesterases.

Beta-receptor blocking agents, especially non-selective ones, may partly or totally inhibit the effect of beta-stimulants.

*Use during pregnancy:* Unless there are compelling reasons, avoid in pregnancy, lactation and women of child-bearing potential who are not taking adequate contraceptive precautions.

Although no teratogenic effects have been observed in animals after administration of bambuterol there is no experience of use in human pregnancy. Terbutaline, the active metabolite of bambuterol has been in widespread clinical use for many years and may be considered in such patients. Terbutaline should be

used with caution in the first trimester of pregnancy. Maternal β₂-agonist treatment may result in transient hypoglycaemia in pre-term new-born infants.

It is not known whether bambuterol or intermediary products pass into breast milk. Terbutaline does pass into breast milk, but an effect on the infant is unlikely at therapeutic doses.

*Effects on ability to drive and use machines:* No effects are known.

*Undesirable effects:* Side effects which have been reported e.g. tremor, headache, cramps and palpitations are all characteristics of sympathomimetic amines. The intensity of the side effects is dose dependent and the majority of these effects have reversed spontaneously within the first 1-2 weeks of treatment.

Potentially serious hypokalaemia may result from β₂-agonist therapy.

Urticaria and exanthema may occur.

*Overdosage:* No cases of overdosage with Bambec have yet been reported.

**Pharmacological properties**

*Pharmacodyamic properties:* Bambuterol is an active precursor of the selective β₂-adrenergic agonist terbutaline.

Bambuterol is the bis-dimethylcarbamate of terbutaline, and is present in the formulation as a 1:1 racemate.

Pharmacodynamic studies have shown that after oral administration of bambuterol to guinea pigs, a sustained protective effect was achieved against histamine induced bronchoconstriction. At equipotent doses, the duration of the relaxing activity was more prolonged than after plain terbutaline. Bambuterol, or the monocarbamatester, did not exert any smooth muscle relaxing properties. The bronchoprotective effects seen after oral administration of bambuterol are related to the generation of terbutaline, as were the secondary effects (effects on other organs).

Pharmacodynamic studies have been conducted in asthmatics and healthy volunteers. The effects observed were bronchodilation, tremor and increases in heart rate. The metabolic effects included a small increase in blood glucose, while the effect on serum potassium was negligible. In short-term studies on lipoprotein metabolism, an increase in HDL cholesterol, has been observed. In conclusion, all pharmacodynamic effects observed can be ascribed to the active metabolite terbutaline.

*Pharmacokinetic properties:* On average, 17.5% of an oral dose is absorbed. Approximately 70-90% of the absorption occurs in the first 24 hours.

Bambuterol is metabolised in the liver and terbutaline is formed by both hydrolysis and oxidation. After absorption from the gut, about 2/3 of terbutaline is first-pass metabolised, bambuterol escapes this first-pass metabolism. Of the absorbed amount, about 65% reaches the circulation. Bambuterol therefore has a bioavailability of about 10%. Protein binding of bambuterol is low, 40-50% at therapeutic concentrations. The terminal half-life of bambuterol after an oral dose is 9-17 hours. Studies on the effects on plasma cholinesterase showed that bambuterol inhibited activity, but that this was reversible.

All categories of subjects studies were able to form terbutaline in a predictive way except for liver cirrhotics.

*Preclinical safety data:* Bambuterol has not revealed any adverse effects which pose a risk to man at therapeutic dosages in the toxicity studies.

Bambuterol is given as a racemate: (-)-bambuterol is responsible for the pharmacodynamic effects via generation of (-)-terbutaline. (+)-bambuterol generates the pharmacodynamic inactive (+)-terbutaline. Both (+) and (-)-bambuterol are equally active as plasma cholinesterase inhibitors. This inhibition is reversible.

The toxicity studies showed that bambuterol has β₂-stimulatory effects, expressed as cardiotoxicity in dogs, and at high doses, observed in the acute toxicity studies, cholinergic effects.

There is no evidence from the preclinical safety data to indicate that bambuterol cannot be used in man for the intended indications with sufficient safety.

**Pharmaceutical particulars**

*List of excipients:* Lactose; maize starch; povidone; microcrystalline cellulose; magnesium stearate; water, purified.

*Incompatibilities:* Not applicable

*Shelf life:* 3 years.

*Special precautions for storage:* Store below 30°C.

*Nature and contents of container:* PVC blisters: 7 or 28 tablets.

*Instructions for use/handling:* Bambec should be taken once daily, shortly before bedtime.

*Marketing authorisation holder:* Astra Pharmaceuticals Ltd, Home Park, Kings Langley, Herts WD4 8DH.

**Marketing authorisation numbers**
Bambec 10 mg          0017/0313
Bambec 20 mg          0017/0314

**Date of approval/revision of SPC**   March 1995

**Legal category** POM

## BETALOC* TABLETS 50 mg and 100 mg

**Presentation**  White tablets containing either 50 mg (coded A/BB) or 100 mg (coded A/ME) metoprolol tartrate.

*Inactive ingredients:* Microcrystalline cellulose, lactose, sodium starch glycolate, colloidal silica, polyvidone, magnesium stearate.

**Uses**  In the management of hypertension and angina pectoris. Cardiac arrhythmias, especially supraventricular tachyarrhythmias.

Adjunct to the treatment of hyperthyroidism.

Early intervention with Betaloc in acute myocardial infarction reduces infarct size and the incidence of ventricular fibrillation. Pain relief may also decrease the need for opiate analgesics.

Betaloc has been shown to reduce mortality when administered to patients with acute myocardial infarction.

Prophylaxis of migraine.

**Dosage and administration**  The dose must always be adjusted to the individual requirements of the patient. The following are guidelines:

*Hypertension:* Total daily dosage Betaloc 100–400 mg to be given as a single or twice daily dose. The starting dose is 100 mg per day. This may be increased by 100 mg per day at weekly intervals. If full control is not achieved using a single daily dose, a b.d. regimen should be initiated. Combination therapy with a diuretic or other anti-hypertensive agent may also be considered.

*Angina:* Usually Betaloc 50–100 mg twice or three times daily.

*Cardiac arrhythmias:* Betaloc 50 mg b.i.d. or t.i.d. should usually control the condition. If necessary the dose can be increased up to 300 mg per day in divided doses.

Following the treatment of an acute arrhythmia with Betaloc injection, continuation therapy with Betaloc tablets should be initiated 4–6 hours later. The initial oral dose should not exceed 50 mg t.i.d.

*Hyperthyroidism:* Betaloc 50 mg four times a day. The dose should be reduced as the euthyroid state is achieved.

*Myocardial infarction:* Early intervention – to achieve optimal benefits from intravenous Betaloc, suitable patients should present within 12 hours of the onset of chest pain. Therapy should commence with 5 mg i.v. every 2 minutes to a maximum of 15 mg total as determined by blood pressure and heart rate. The second or third dose should not be given if the systolic blood pressure is <90 mmHg, the heart rate is <40 beats/min and the P-Q time is >0.26 seconds, or if there is any aggravation of dyspnoea or cold sweating. Orally, therapy should commence 15 minutes after the last injection with 50 mg every 6 hours for 48 hours. Patients who fail to tolerate the full intravenous dose should be given half the suggested oral dose.

Maintenance – The usual maintenance dose is 200 mg daily, given in divided doses.

*Migraine prophylaxis:* Betaloc 100–200 mg daily, given in divided doses.

*Elderly:* There are no special dosage requirements in otherwise healthy elderly patients.

*Significant hepatic dysfunction:* A reduction in dosage may be necessary.

**Contra-indications, warnings, etc**
*Contra-indications:* AV block. Uncontrolled heart failure. Severe bradycardia. Sick-sinus syndrome. Cardiogenic shock. Severe peripheral arterial disease. Known hypersensitivity to Betaloc or other β-blockers.

Betaloc is also contra-indicated when myocardial infarction is complicated by significant bradycardia, first degree heart block, systolic hypotension (<100 mmHg) and/or severe heart failure.

*Warnings:* Betaloc may aggravate bradycardia, symptoms of peripheral arterial circulatory disorders and anaphylactic shock.

Abrupt interruption of β-blockers is to be avoided. When possible, Betaloc should be withdrawn gradually over a period of 10 days, in diminishing doses to 25 mg daily for the last 6 days. During its withdrawal patients should be kept under close surveillance, especially those with known ischaemic heart disease.

Betaloc may be administered when heart failure has been controlled. Digitalisation and/or diuretic therapy should also be considered for patients with a history of heart failure, or patients known to have a poor cardiac reserve.

Although cardioselective β-blockers may have less effect on lung function than non-selective β-blockers, as with all β-blockers these should be avoided in patients with reversible obstructive airways disease unless there are compelling clinical reasons for their use. When administration is necessary, use of a $\beta_2$-bronchodilator (e.g. terbutaline) may be advisable in some patients.

In labile and insulin-dependent diabetes it may be necessary to adjust the hypoglycaemic therapy.

In patients with a phaeochromocytoma, an α-blocker should be given concomitantly.

In the presence of liver cirrhosis the bioavailability of Betaloc may be increased.

The administration of adrenaline to patients undergoing β-blockade can result in an increase in blood pressure and bradycardia, although this is less likely to occur with $\beta_1$-selective drugs.

Betaloc therapy must be reported to the anaesthetist prior to general anaesthesia. If withdrawal of Betaloc is considered desirable, this should if possible be completed at least 48 hours before general anaesthesia. However, in some patients it may be desirable to employ a β-blocker as premedication. By shielding the heart against the effects of stress the β-blocker may prevent excessive sympathetic stimulation provoking cardiac arrhythmias or acute coronary insufficiency. If a β-blocker is given for this purpose, an anaesthetic with little negative inotropic activity should be selected to minimise the risk of myocardial depression.

*Pregnancy:* Betaloc should not be used in pregnancy or nursing mothers unless the physician considers that the benefit outweighs the possible hazard to the foetus/infant. As with all β-blockers Betaloc may cause side-effects e.g. bradycardia, hypoglycaemia in the foetus, and in the newborn and breastfed infant. Betaloc has, however, been used in pregnancy associated hypertension under close supervision, after 20 weeks gestation. Although Betaloc crosses the placental barrier and is present in cord blood, no evidence of foetal abnormalities has been reported.

*Lactation:* The amount of Betaloc ingested via breast milk should not produce significant β-blocking effects in the neonate if the mother is treated with normal therapeutic doses.

*Interactions:* The effects of Betaloc and other antihypertensive drugs on blood pressure are usually additive, and care should be taken to avoid hypotension. However, combinations of antihypertensive drugs may often be used with benefit to improve control of hypertension.

Betaloc can reduce myocardial contractility and impair intracardiac conduction. Care should be exercised when drugs with similar activity, e.g. antiarrhythmic agents, general anaesthetics, are given concurrently. Like all other β-blockers, Betaloc should not be given in combination with verapamil since this may cause bradycardia, hypotension and asystole. Care should also be exercised when β-blockers are given in combination with sympathetic ganglion blocking agents, other β-blockers (i.e. eye drops) or MAO inhibitors. If combination treatment with clonidine is to be discontinued, Betaloc should be withdrawn several days before clonidine.

As β-blockers may affect the peripheral circulation, care should be exercised when drugs with similar activity e.g. ergotamine are given concurrently.

Betaloc will antagonise the $\beta_1$-effects of sympathomimetic agents but should have little influence on the bronchodilator effects of $\beta_2$-agonists at normal therapeutic doses. Enzyme inducing agents (e.g. rifampicin) may reduce plasma concentrations of Betaloc, whereas enzyme inhibitors (e.g. cimetidine) may increase plasma concentrations. Betaloc may impair the elimination of lignocaine.

Indomethacin may reduce the antihypertensive effect of β-blockers.

*Side-effects:* These are usually mild and infrequent. The most common appear to be lassitude, GI disturbances (nausea, vomiting or abdominal pain) and disturbances of sleep pattern. In many cases these effects have been transient or have disappeared after a reduction in dosage.

Effects related to the CNS which have been reported occasionally are dizziness and headache and rarely paraesthesia, muscle cramps, depression and decreased mental alertness. There have also been isolated reports of personality disorders.

Cardiovascular effects which have been reported occasionally are bradycardia, postural hypotension and rarely, heart failure, palpitations, cardiac arrhythmias, Raynauds phenomenon, peripheral oedema and precordial pain. There have also been isolated reports of cardiac conduction abnormalities, and gangrene in patients with pre-existing severe peripheral circulatory disorders.

Common gastro-intestinal disturbances have been described above but rarely diarrhoea or constipation also occur and there have been isolated cases of dry mouth and abnormal liver function.

Skin rashes (urticaria, psoriasiform, dystrophic skin lesions) and positive anti-nuclear antibodies (not associated with SLE) occur rarely. Isolated cases of photosensitivity, increased sweating and alopecia have been reported. Respiratory effects include occasional reports of dyspnoea on exertion and rare reports of bronchospasm and isolated cases of rhinitis.

Isolated cases of weight gain, thrombocytopenia, disturbances of vision, conjunctivitis, tinnitus and dry or irritated eyes have also been reported.

The reported incidence of skin rashes and/or dry eyes is small and in most cases the symptoms have cleared when treatment was withdrawn. Discontinuation of the drug should be considered if any such reaction is not otherwise explicable.

*Overdosage:* Poisoning due to an overdose of Betaloc may lead to severe hypotension, sinus bradycardia, atrioventricular block, heart failure, cardiogenic shock, cardiac arrest, bronchospasm, impairment of consciousness, coma, nausea, vomiting, cyanosis, hypoglycaemia and, occasionally, hyperkalaemia. The first manifestations usually appear 20 minutes to 2 hours after drug ingestion.

Treatment should include close monitoring of cardiovascular, respiratory and renal function, and blood glucose and electrolytes. Further absorption may be prevented by induction of vomiting, gastric lavage or administration of activated-charcoal if ingestion is recent. Cardiovascular complications should be treated symptomatically, which may require the use of sympathomimetic agents (e.g. noradrenaline, metaraminol), atropine or inotropic agents (e.g. dopamine, dobutamine). Temporary pacing may be required for AV block. Glucagon can reverse the effects of excessive β-blockade, given in a dose of 1–10 mg intravenously. Intravenous $\beta_2$-stimulants e.g. terbutaline may be required to relieve bronchospasm.

Betaloc cannot be effectively removed by haemodialysis.

**Pharmaceutical precautions** Store below 25°C.

**Legal category** POM

**Package quantities**
PVC/Aluminium blister strips (10 tablets per strip) in a cardboard outer, pack size 100.

**Further information** Betaloc is well absorbed after oral administration, peak plasma concentrations occurring 1.5–2 hours after dosing. The bioavailability of a single dose is approximately 50%, increasing to approximately 70% during repeated administration. The bioavailability also increases if metoprolol is given with food.

Elimination is mainly by hepatic metabolism and the average elimination half-life is 3.5 hours (range 1 to 9 hours). Rates of metabolism vary between individuals, with poor metabolisers (approximately 10%) showing higher plasma concentrations and slower elimination than extensive metabolisers. Within individuals, however, plasma concentrations are stable and reproducible.

Because of variation in rates of metabolism, the dose of Betaloc should always be adjusted to the individual requirements of the patient. As the therapeutic response, adverse effects and relative cardioselectivity are related to plasma concentration, poor metabolisers may require lower than normal doses. Dosage adjustment is not routinely required in the elderly or in patients with renal failure, but dosage may need to be reduced in patients with significant hepatic dysfunction when Betaloc elimination may be impaired.

**Product licence numbers**

| | |
|---|---|
| Tablets 50 mg | 0017/0073R |
| Tablets 100 mg | 0017/0074R |

## BETALOC* I.V. INJECTION

**Presentation**
*Ampoules:* Each ampoule of 5 ml contains 5 mg metoprolol tartrate and sodium chloride.

*Inactive ingredients:* Sodium chloride, water for injection.

**Uses** Control of tachyarrhythmias, especially supraventricular tachyarrhythmias.

Early intervention with Betaloc in acute myocardial infarction reduces infarct size and the incidence of ventricular fibrillation. Pain relief may also decrease the need for opiate analgesics.

Betaloc has been shown to reduce mortality when administered to patients with acute myocardial infarction.

**Dosage and administration** *Control of tachyarrhythmias:* Initially up to 5 mg injected i.v. at a rate of 1–2 mg per minute. The injection can be repeated at 5 minute intervals until a satisfactory response has been obtained. A total dose of 10–15 mg generally proves sufficient.

Because of the risk of a pronounced drop of blood pressure, the i.v. administration of Betaloc to patients with a systolic blood pressure below 100 mmHg should only be given with special care.

*During anaesthesia:* 2–4 mg injected slowly i.v. at induction is usually sufficient to prevent the development of arrhythmias during anaesthesia. The same dosage can also be used to control arrhythmias developing during anaesthesia. Further injections of 2 mg may be given as required to a maximum overall dose of 10 mg.

*Myocardial infarction:* Early intervention. To achieve optimal benefits from intravenous Betaloc, suitable patients should present within 12 hours of the onset of chest pain. Therapy should commence with 5 mg i.v. every 2 minutes to a maximum of 15 mg total as determined by blood pressure and heart rate. The second or third dose should not be given if the systolic blood pressure is <90 mm Hg, the heart rate is <40 beats/min and the P-Q time is >0.26 seconds, or if there is any aggravation of dyspnoea or cold sweating. Orally, therapy should commence 15 minutes after the injection with 50 mg every 6 hours for 48 hours. Patients who fail to tolerate the full intravenous dose should be given half the suggested oral dose.

*Elderly:* There are no special dosage requirements in otherwise healthy elderly patients.

*Significant hepatic dysfunction:* A reduction in dosage may be necessary.

**Contra-indications, warnings, etc**
*Contra-indications:* AV Block. Uncontrolled heart failure. Severe bradycardia. Sick-sinus syndrome. Cardiogenic shock. Severe peripheral arterial disease. Known hypersensitivity to Betaloc or other β-blockers.

Betaloc i.v. is also contra-indicated when myocardial infarction is complicated by significant bradycardia, first degree heart block, systolic hypotension (<100 mmHg) and/or severe heart failure.

*Warnings:* Betaloc i.v. may aggravate bradycardia, symptoms of peripheral arterial circulatory disorders and anaphylactic shock.

Betaloc i.v. may be administered when heart failure has been controlled. Digitalisation and/or diuretic therapy should also be considered for patients with a history of heart failure, or patients known to have a poor cardiac reserve.

Although cardioselective β-blockers may have less effect on lung function than non-selective β-blockers, as with all β-blockers these should be avoided in patients with reversible obstructive airways disease unless there are compelling clinical reasons for their use. When administration is necessary, use of a $\beta_2$-bronchodilator (e.g. terbutaline) may be advisable in some patients.

In labile and insulin-dependent diabetes it may be necessary to adjust the hypoglycaemic therapy.

In patients with a phaeochromocytoma, an α-blocker should be given concomitantly.

The administration of adrenaline to patients undergoing β-blockade can result in an increase in blood pressure and bradycardia although this is less likely to occur with $\beta_1$-selective drugs.

Betaloc i.v. therapy must be reported to the anaesthetist prior to general anaesthesia. However, in some patients it may be desirable to employ a β-blocker as premedication. By shielding the heart against the effects of stress the β-blocker may prevent excessive sympathetic stimulation provoking cardiac arrhythmias or acute coronary insufficiency. If a β-blocker is given for this purpose, an anaesthetic with little negative inotropic activity should be selected to minimise the risk of myocardial depression.

*Pregnancy:* Betaloc i.v. should not be used in pregnancy or nursing mothers unless the physician considers that the benefit outweighs the possible hazard to the foetus/infant. As with all β-blockers metoprolol may cause side-effects e.g. bradycardia, hypoglycaemia in the foetus, and in the newborn and breastfed infant. Metoprolol has, however, been used in pregnancy associated hypertension under close supervision, after 20 weeks gestation. Although Betaloc i.v. crosses the placental barrier and is present in cord blood, no evidence of foetal abnormalities has been reported.

*Lactation:* The amount of Betaloc i.v. ingested via breast milk should not produce significant β-blocking effects in the neonate if the mother is treated with normal therapeutic doses.

*Interactions:* The effects of Betaloc i.v. and other antihypertensive drugs on blood pressure are usually additive, and care should be taken to avoid hypotension.

Betaloc i.v. can reduce myocardial contractility and impair intracardiac conduction. Care should be exercised when drugs with similar activity, e.g. antiarrhythmic agents, general anaesthetics, are given concurrently. Like all other β-blockers, Betaloc i.v. should not be given in combination with verapamil since this may cause bradycardia, hypotension and asystole. Care should also be exercised when β-blockers are given in combination with sympathetic ganglion blocking agents, other β-blockers (i.e. eye drops) or MAO inhibitors.

As β-blockers may affect the peripheral circulation, care should be exercised when drugs with similar activity e.g. ergotamine are given concurrently.

Betaloc i.v. will antagonise the $\beta_1$-effects of sympathomimetic agents but should have little influence on the bronchodilator effects of $\beta_2$-agonists at normal therapeutic doses. Enzyme inducing agents (e.g. rifampicin) may reduce plasma concentrations of Betaloc, whereas enzyme inhibitors (e.g. cimetidine) may increase plasma concentrations. Betaloc i.v. may impair the elimination of lignocaine.

*Side-effects:* As in the case of other β-blockers, a marked fall in blood pressure may sometimes occur following intravenous injection of Betaloc. Other side-effects are usually mild and infrequent. The most common appear to be lassitude, GI disturbances (nausea, vomiting or abdominal pain) and disturbances of sleep pattern. In many cases these effects have been transient or have disappeared after a reduction in dosage.

Effects related to the CNS which have been reported occasionally are dizziness and headache and rarely paraesthesia, muscle cramps, depression and decreased mental alertness. There have also been isolated reports of personality disorders.

Cardiovascular effects which have been reported occasionally are bradycardia, postural hypotension and rarely, heart failure, palpitations, cardiac arrhythmias, Raynauds phenomenon, peripheral oedema and precordial pain. There have also been isolated reports of cardiac conduction abnormalities, and gangrene in patients with pre-existing severe peripheral circulatory disorders.

Common gastro-intestinal disturbances have been described above but rarely diarrhoea or constipation also occur and there have been isolated cases of dry mouth and abnormal liver function.

Skin rashes (urticaria, psoriasiform, dystrophic skin lesions) and positive anti-nuclear antibodies (not associated with SLE) occur rarely. Isolated cases of photosensitivity, increased sweating and alopecia have been reported. Respiratory effects include occasional reports of dyspnoea on exertion and rare reports of bronchospasm and isolated cases of rhinitis.

Isolated cases of weight gain, thrombocytopenia, disturbances of vision, conjunctivitis, tinnitus and dry or irritated eyes have also been reported.

The reported incidence of skin rashes and/or dry eyes is small and in most cases the symptoms have cleared when treatment was withdrawn. Discontinuation of the drug should be considered if any such reaction is not otherwise explicable.

*Overdosage:* Poisoning due to an overdose of Betaloc i.v. may lead to severe hypotension, sinus bradycardia, atrioventricular block, heart failure, cardiogenic shock, cardiac arrest, bronchospasm, impairment of consciousness, coma, nausea, vomiting, cyanosis, hypoglycaemia and, occasionally, hyperkalaemia.

Treatment should include close monitoring of cardiovascular, respiratory and renal function, and blood glucose and electrolytes. Cardiovascular complications should be treated symptomatically, which may require the use of sympathomimetic agents (e.g. noradrenaline, metaraminol), atropine or inotropic agents (e.g. dopamine, dobutamine). Temporary pacing may be required for AV block. Glucagon can reverse the effects of excessive β-blockade, given in a dose of 1–10 mg intravenously. Intravenous $\beta_2$-stimulants e.g. terbutaline may be required to relieve bronchospasm.

Betaloc i.v. cannot be effectively removed by haemodialysis.

**Pharmaceutical precautions** Protect from light. Store below 25°C.

**Legal category** POM

**Package quantities** 5×5 ml ampoules.

**Further information** Betaloc is a cardioselective $\beta_1$-receptor blocker exhibiting no intrinsic sympathomimetic activity. Elimination is mainly by hepatic metabolism and the average elimination half-life is 3.5 hours (range 1 to 9 hours). Rates of metabolism vary between individuals, with poor metabolisers (approximately 10%) showing higher plasma concentrations and slower elimination than extensive metabolisers. Within individuals, however, plasma concentrations are stable and reproducible.

**Product licence number** 0017/0072

# BETALOC* SA

**Presentation** White tablets (coded A/MD) containing 200 mg metoprolol tartrate, extended release formulation (Durules*).

*Inactive ingredients:* Sodium aluminium silicate, paraffin, magnesium stearate, ethylcellulose, hydroxypropyl methylcellulose, polyethylene glycol, titanium dioxide.

**Uses** In the management of angina pectoris and hypertension.

Prophylaxis of migraine.

**Dosage and administration** *Angina pectoris and hypertension:* One tablet daily, in the morning. In rare cases two tablets may be indicated.

*Migraine Prophylaxis:* One tablet daily, in the morning.

Betaloc SA tablets must not be chewed or crushed. They should be swallowed whole with half a glass of water.

*Elderly:* There are no special dosage requirements in otherwise healthy elderly patients.

*Significant hepatic dysfunction:* A reduction in dosage may be necessary.

**Contra-indications, warnings, etc**

*Contra-indications:* AV block. Uncontrolled heart failure. Severe bradycardia. Sick-sinus syndrome. Cardiogenic shock. Severe peripheral arterial disease. Known hypersensitivity to Betaloc SA or other β-blockers.

*Warnings:* Betaloc SA may aggravate bradycardia, symptoms of peripheral arterial circulatory disorders and anaphylactic shock.

Abrupt interruption of β-blockers is to be avoided. When possible, Betaloc SA should be withdrawn gradually over a period of 10 days. During its withdrawal patients should be kept under close surveillance, especially those with known ischaemic heart disease.

Betaloc SA may be administered when heart failure has been controlled. Digitalisation and/or diuretic therapy should also be considered for patients with a history of heart failure, or patients known to have a poor cardiac reserve.

Although cardioselective β-blockers may have less effect on lung function than non-selective β-blockers, as with all β-blockers these should be avoided in patients with reversible obstructive airways disease unless there are compelling clinical reasons for their use. When administration is necessary, use of a $\beta_2$-bronchodilator (e.g. terbutaline) may be advisable in some patients.

In labile and insulin-dependent diabetes it may be necessary to adjust the hypoglycaemic therapy.

In patients with phaeochromocytoma, an α-blocker should be given concomitantly.

In the presence of liver cirrhosis the bioavailability of Betaloc SA may be increased.

The administration of adrenaline to patients undergoing β-blockade can result in an increase in blood pressure and bradycardia although this is less likely to occur with $\beta_1$-selective drugs.

Betaloc SA therapy must be reported to the anaesthetist prior to general anaesthesia. If withdrawal of metoprolol is considered desirable, this should if possible be completed at least 48 hours before general anaesthesia. However, in some patients it may be desirable to employ a β-blocker as premedication. By shielding the heart against the effects of stress the β-blocker may prevent excessive sympathetic stimulation provoking cardiac arrhythmias or acute coronary insufficiency. If a β-blocker is given for this purpose, an anaesthetic with little negative inotropic activity should be selected to minimise the risk of myocardial depression.

*Pregnancy:* Betaloc SA should not be used in pregnancy or nursing mothers unless the physician considers that the benefit outweighs the possible hazard to the foetus/infant. As with all β-blockers metoprolol may cause side-effects e.g. bradycardia, hypoglycaemia in the foetus, and in the newborn and breastfed infant. Metoprolol has, however, been used in pregnancy associated hypertension under close supervision, after 20 weeks gestation. Although Betaloc SA crosses the placental barrier and is present in cord blood, no evidence of foetal abnormalities has been reported.

*Lactation:* The amount of metoprolol ingested via breast milk should not produce significant β-blocking effects in the neonate if the mother is treated with normal therapeutic doses.

*Interactions:* The effects of Betaloc SA and other antihypertensive drugs on blood pressure are usually additive, and care should be taken to avoid hypotension. However, combinations of antihypertensive drugs may often be used with benefit to improve control of hypertension.

Betaloc SA can reduce myocardial contractility and impair intracardiac conduction. Care should be exercised when drugs with similar activity, e.g. antiarrhythmic agents, general anaesthetics, are given concurrently. Like all other β-blockers, Betaloc SA should not be given in combination with verapamil since this may cause bradycardia, hypotension and asystole. Care should also be exercised when β-blockers are given in combination with sympathetic ganglion blocking agents, other β-blockers (i.e. eye drops) or MAO inhibitors. If combination treatment with clonidine is to be discontinued, Betaloc SA should be withdrawn several days before clonidine.

As β-blockers may affect the peripheral circulation, care should be exercised when drugs with similar activity e.g. ergotamine are given concurrently.

Betaloc SA will antagonise the $\beta_1$-effects of sympathomimetic agents but should have little influence on the bronchodilator effects of $\beta_2$-agonists at normal therapeutic doses. Enzyme inducing agents (e.g. rifampicin) may reduce plasma concentrations of Betaloc SA, whereas enzyme inhibitors (e.g. cimetidine) may increase plasma concentrations. Betaloc SA may impair the elimination of lignocaine.

Indomethacin may reduce the antihypertensive effect of β-blockers.

*Side-effects:* These are usually mild and infrequent. The most common appear to be lassitude, GI disturbances (nausea, vomiting or abdominal pain) and disturbances of sleep pattern. In many cases these effects have been transient or have disappeared after a reduction in dosage.

Effects related to the CNS which have been reported occasionally are dizziness and headache and rarely paraesthesia, muscle cramps, depression and decreased mental alertness. There have also been isolated reports of personality disorders.

Cardiovascular effects which have been reported occasionally are bradycardia, postural hypotension and rarely, heart failure, palpitations, cardiac arrhythmias, Raynauds phenomenon, peripheral oedema and precordial pain. There have also been isolated reports of cardiac conduction abnormalities, and gangrene in patients with pre-existing severe peripheral circulatory disorders.

Common gastro-intestinal disturbances have been described above but rarely diarrhoea or constipation also occur and there have been isolated cases of dry mouth and abnormal liver function.

Skin rashes (urticaria, psoriasiform, dystrophic skin lesions) and positive anti-nuclear antibodies (not associated with SLE) occur rarely. Isolated cases of photosensitivity, increased sweating and alopecia have been reported. Respiratory effects include occasional reports of dyspnoea on exertion and rare reports of bronchospasm and isolated cases of rhinitis.

Isolated cases of weight gain, thrombocytopenia, disturbances of vision, conjunctivitis, tinnitus and dry or irritated eyes have also been reported.

The reported incidence of skin rashes and/or dry eyes is small and in most cases the symptoms have cleared when treatment was withdrawn. Discontinuation of the drug should be considered if any such reaction is not otherwise explicable.

*Overdosage:* Poisoning due to an overdose of Betaloc SA may lead to severe hypotension, sinus bradycardia, atrioventricular block, heart failure, cardiogenic shock, cardiac arrest, bronchospasm, impairment of consciousness, coma, nausea, vomiting, cyanosis, hypoglycaemia and, occasionally, hyperkalaemia. The first manifestations usually appear 20 minutes to 2 hours after drug ingestion.

Treatment should include close monitoring of cardiovascular, respiratory and renal function, and blood glucose and electrolytes. Further absorption may be prevented by induction of vomiting, gastric lavage or administration of activated-charcoal if ingestion is recent. Cardiovascular complications should be treated symptomatically, which may require the use of sympathomimetic agents (e.g. noradrenaline, metaraminol), atropine or inotropic agents (e.g. dopamine, dobutamine). Temporary pacing may be required for AV block. Glucagon can reverse the effects of excessive β-blockade, given in a dose of 1–10 mg intravenously. Intravenous $\beta_2$-stimulants e.g. terbutaline may be required to relieve bronchospasm.

Metoprolol cannot be effectively removed by haemodialysis.

**Pharmaceutical precautions** Store below 25°C.

**Legal category** POM

**Package quantities** Blister strips (press through packs of thermoformed PVC) 7 tablets per strip–pack size 28.

**Further information** Administration of Betaloc SA results in a controlled release of active substance which means that the peak plasma levels are reduced. Compared to Betaloc tablets the absorption phase is prolonged and the duration of effect is extended. The substance is completely absorbed and the maximal β-blocking effect is reached after about four hours.

These factors may lead to a more convenient dosage and an improved degree of $\beta_1$-selectivity.

The effect on the pulse and blood pressure remain pronounced 24 hours after administration.

Elimination is mainly by hepatic metabolism and the average elimination half-life is 3.5 hours (range 1 to 9 hours). Rates of metabolism vary between individuals, with poor metabolisers (approximately 10%) showing higher plasma concentrations and slower elimination than extensive metabolisers. Within individuals, however, plasma concentrations are stable and reproducible.

**Product licence number** 0017/0093

## BRICANYL* INHALER
## BRICANYL* SPACER INHALER

**Presentation**
*Bricanyl Inhaler:* Metered dose aerosol delivering 0.25 mg terbutaline sulphate per actuation.

*Bricanyl Spacer Inhaler:* Metered dose aerosol with extended mouthpiece delivering 0.25 mg terbutaline sulphate per actuation.

*Bricanyl Refill Canister:* Canister containing 400 doses of terbutaline sulphate 0.25 mg. For use with the Nebuhaler or as a refill for Bricanyl Spacer Inhaler.

*Inactive ingredients:* All the above contain sorbitan trioleate and chlorofluorocarbons 11, 12 and 114.

*Nebuhaler:* 750 ml plastic cone with a one-way valve. For use in conjunction with Bricanyl refill canister.

Both the Bricanyl Spacer Inhaler and the Nebuhaler are recommended to enable patients with difficulty co-ordinating conventional aerosols to derive greater therapeutic benefit. A package insert is provided giving simple operating instructions.

**Uses** Terbutaline is a selective $\beta_2$-adrenergic agonist recommended for the relief and prevention of bronchospasm in bronchial asthma and in chronic bronchitis, emphysema and other bronchopulmonary disorders in which bronchospasm is a complicating factor.

**Dosage and administration**
*Bricanyl Inhaler: Adults and children:* Prophylaxis and relief of acute attacks: One or two inhalations as required, with a short interval between each inhalation at 6 hourly intervals. Not more than 8 inhalations should be necessary in any 24 hours, but medical advice should be sought and treatment reviewed if condition fails to improve.

*Bricanyl Spacer Inhaler: Adults and children:* Prophylaxis and relief of acute attacks: One or two inhalations as required, with a short interval between each inhalation at 6 hourly intervals. Not more than 8 inhalations should be necessary in any 24 hours, but medical advice should be sought and treatment reviewed if condition fails to improve.

*Nebuhaler: Adults and children:* The dose must always be adjusted to patient response and severity of the bronchospasm. Patients must be instructed to actuate the aerosol and breathe in slowly and deeply through the mouthpiece. Ideally two inspirations per actuation are required to empty the Nebuhaler.

*Prophylaxis and relief of acute attacks:* One or two inhalations as required, with a short interval between each inhalation at 6 hourly intervals. Not more than 8 inhalations should be necessary in any 24 hours, but medical advice should be sought and treatment reviewed if condition fails to improve.

Bricanyl via the Nebuhaler may also be used in conditions such as severe bronchospasm and severe acute asthma which are normally managed by administration of nebulised bronchodilators.

*For hospital use in acute asthma: Adults:* The initial dose should be 2 mg (8 actuations); this may be repeated up to a total dose of 8 mg in one hour. Thereafter a dose of up to 4 mg may be given four times daily.

A similar dose range may be used for domiciliary use, but patients should be warned that if either the usual relief or duration of action is diminished, they should seek medical advice immediately.

*Children over 5 years:* Dosage must be individualised but clinical studies have shown that when used for the management of acute asthma in children, the following dosages given over a 15 minute period have been as effective as equal doses administered by nebuliser.

| | |
|---|---|
| Children under 25 kg | 1.25–2.5 mg (5–10 puffs) |
| Children over 25 kg | 2.5–5.0 mg (10–20 puffs) |

*Elderly:* Dosage as for adults. Because of the difficulty experienced by many elderly patients in co-ordinating inhalation with actuation, Bricanyl Spacer Inhaler or use via the Nebuhaler will provide a more certain delivery of drug.

**Contra-indications, warnings, etc**
*Contra-indications:* Bricanyl preparations are contra-indicated in patients with a history of hypersensitivity to any of their constituents.

*Precautions:* Care should be taken with patients suffering from myocardial insufficiency or thyrotoxicosis. Due to the hyperglycaemic effects of $\beta_2$-stimulants, additional blood glucose measurements are initially recommended when Bricanyl therapy is commenced in diabetic patients. If treatment becomes less effective or shorter acting the patients general condition should be reviewed. Due to the positive inotropic effect of $\beta_2$-agonists, these drugs should not be used in patients with hypertrophic cardiomyopathy.

Potentially serious hypokalaemia may result from $\beta_2$-agonist therapy. Particular caution is advised in severe asthma as this effect may be potentiated by concomitant treatment with xanthine derivatives, steroids, diuretics and by hypoxia. It is recommended that serum potassium levels are monitored in such situations.

*Interactions:* β-blocking agents especially the non-selective ones such as propranolol may partially or totally inhibit the effect of β-stimulants. Therefore Bricanyl and non-selective β-blockers should not normally be administered concurrently. Bricanyl should be used with caution in patients receiving other sympathomimetics.

*Pregnancy and lactation:* Although no teratogenic effects have been observed in animals or in patients, Bricanyl should only be administered with caution during the first trimester of pregnancy. Terbutaline is secreted via breast milk, but effect on the infant is unlikely at therapeutic doses.

*Side-effects:* The frequency of side-effects is low at the recommended doses. Side-effects which have been recorded such as tremor, tonic cramp and palpitations are all characteristic of sympathomimetic amines. A few patients feel tense; this is also due to the effects on skeletal muscle and not to direct CNS stimulation. Whenever these side-effects have occurred the majority have usually been spontaneously reversible within the first week of treatment. Rare cases of bronchospasm have occurred. The chlorofluorocarbons used as propellants may in some asthmatics cause a fall in $FEV_1$ immediately after exposure.

Potentially serious hypokalaemia may result from $\beta_2$-agonist therapy.

*Overdose:* (i) *Possible symptoms and signs:* Headache, anxiety, tremor, tonic cramp, palpitations, arrhythmia. A fall in blood pressure sometimes occurs. Laboratory findings: hypokalaemia, hyperglycaemia and lactic acidosis sometimes occur.

(ii) *Treatment: Mild and moderate cases:* Reduce the dose.

*Severe cases:* Determination of acid-base balance, blood sugar and electrolytes. Monitoring of heart rate and rhythm and blood pressure. Metabolic changes should be corrected. A cardioselective β-blocker (e.g. metoprolol) is recommended for the treatment of arrhythmias causing haemodynamic deterioration. The β-blocker should be used with care because of the possibility of inducing bronchoconstriction. If the $\beta_2$-mediated reduction in peripheral vascular resistance significantly contributes to the fall in blood pressure, a volume expander should be given.

**Pharmaceutical precautions** Store at temperatures not exceeding 25°C.

**Legal category** POM

**Package quantities** Bricanyl Inhaler: Aerosol containing 400 metered doses.

Bricanyl Spacer Inhaler: Aerosol containing 400 metered doses complete with extended mouthpiece.

Bricanyl Refill Canister: Canister containing 400 doses.

Nebuhaler: 750 ml plastic cone with a one-way valve.

**Further information** Bricanyl is also available as Respirator Solution, Tablets, Syrup and Injection.

**Product licence number** 0017/0061R

## BRICANYL* INJECTION

**Presentation** Clear aqueous solution for injection containing 0.5 mg terbutaline sulphate per ml, sodium chloride and water for injection.

Bricanyl Injection is available in 1 ml and 5 ml ampoules. Bricanyl Injection in 1 ml ampoules is intended for subcutaneous, intramuscular or intravenous injection. Bricanyl Injection in 5 ml ampoules is intended for infusion after dilution with infusion solutions.

**Uses** 1. *For bronchodilation:* Terbutaline is a selective $\beta_2$-adrenergic agonist recommended for the relief of bronchospasm in bronchial asthma and other broncho-pulmonary disorders in which bronchospasm is a complicating factor.

2. *For the management of uncomplicated premature labour:* To arrest labour between 24 and 33 weeks of gestation in patients with no medical or obstetric contra-indication to tocolytic therapy. The main effect of tocolytic therapy is a delay in delivery of up to 48 hours; no statistically significant effect on perinatal mortality or morbidity has as yet been observed in randomised-controlled trials. The greatest benefit from tocolytic therapy is gained by using the delay in delivery to administer glucocorticoids or to implement other measures known to improve perinatal health.

**Dosage and administration** The dosage should be individual.

1. *For bronchodilation:* When a rapid therapeutic response is required, Bricanyl can be administered by any of the three standard parenteral routes: subcutaneous, intramuscular, or i.v. bolus. The preferred routes will usually be subcutaneous or intramuscular. When given as an i.v. bolus the injection must be made slowly noting patient response.

*Adults:* 0.5 ml–1 ml (0.25–0.50 mg) up to four times a day.

*Children:* 2–15 years. 0.01 mg/kg body weight to a maximum of 0.3 mg total.

| *Age* | *Average weight kg* | *(lb)* | *mg terbutaline* | *ml volume* |
|---|---|---|---|---|
| <3 | 10 | (22) | 0.1 | 0.2 |
| 3 | 15 | (33) | 0.15 | 0.3 |
| 6 | 20 | (44) | 0.2 | 0.4 |
| 8 | 25 | (55) | 0.25 | 0.5 |
| 10+ | 30+ | (66+) | 0.3 | 0.6 |

*By infusion:* 3–5 ml (1.5–2.5 mg) in 500 ml dextrose, saline or dextrose/saline given by continuous intravenous infusion at a rate of 10–20 drops (0.5–1 ml) per minute for 8 to 10 hours. A corresponding reduction in dosage should be made for children.

*Elderly:* Dosages as for adults.

2. *For the management of premature labour. Procedure:* To be administered as early as possible after the diagnosis of premature labour, and after evaluation of the patient to rule out contra-indications to the use of terbutaline (see Contra-indications).

Initially 5 microgram/min should be infused during the first 20 minutes increasing by 2.5 micrograms/min at 20 minute intervals until contractions stop. More than 10 micrograms/min should seldom be given, 20 micrograms/min should not be exceeded.

The infusion should be stopped if labour progresses despite treatment at the maximum dose. **If successful**, the infusion should continue for 1 hour at the chosen rate and then be decreased by 2.5 micrograms/min every 20 minutes to the lowest dose that produces suppression of contractions. Keep the infusion at this rate for 12 hours and then continue with oral maintenance therapy.

As an alternative, subcutaneous injections (0.25 mg) should be given four times a day for a few days before oral treatment is commenced.

Oral treatment may be continued for as long as the physician considers it desirable to prolong pregnancy.

*Special cautions for infusion:* The dose must be individually titrated with reference to suppression of contractions, increase in pulse rate and changes in blood pressure, which are limiting factors. These parameters should be carefully monitored during treatment. A maternal heart rate of more than 135 beats/min should be avoided.

Careful control of the level of hydration is essential to avoid the risk of maternal pulmonary oedema (see *Side-effects*). The volume of fluid in which the drug is administered should thus be kept to a minimum. A controlled infusion device should be used preferably a syringe pump.

*Dilution:* The recommended infusion fluid is 5% dextrose.

If a syringe pump is available, the concentration of the drug infused should be 0.1 mg/ml (10 ml Bricanyl Injection should be added to 40 ml of 5% dextrose). At this dilution, 5 micrograms/min equates with 0.05 ml/min, and 10 micrograms/min equates with 0.1 ml/min. If no syringe pump is available, the concentration of the drug should be 0.01 mg/ml (10 ml Bricanyl Injection should be added to 490 ml of 5% dextrose). At this dilution, 5 micrograms/min equates with 0.5 ml/min and 10 micrograms/min equates with 1 ml/min.

**Contra-indications, warnings, etc**
*Contra-indications:* Bricanyl preparations are contra-indicated in patients with a history of hypersensitivity to any of their constituents.

Although Bricanyl Injection and Tablets are used in the management of uncomplicated premature labour, their use in the following conditions is contra-indicated: Any condition of the mother or foetus in which prolongation of the pregnancy is hazardous e.g. severe toxaemia, ante-partum haemorrhage, intra-uterine infection, abruptio placentae, threatened abortion during the first and second trimesters or cord compression.

*Precautions:* Care should be taken with patients suffering from myocardial insufficiency or thyrotoxicosis. Due to the hyperglycaemic effects of $\beta_2$-stimulants, additional blood glucose measurements are initially recommended when Bricanyl therapy is commenced in diabetic patients. If treatment becomes less effective or shorter-acting, the patients' general condition should be reviewed.

Due to the positive inotropic effect of $\beta_2$-agonists these drugs should not be used in patients with hypertrophic cardiomyopathy.

Potentially serious hypokalaemia may result from $\beta_2$-agonist therapy. Particular caution is advised in severe asthma as this effect may be potentiated by concomitant treatment with xanthine derivatives, steroids, diuretics and by hypoxia. It is recommended that serum potassium levels are monitored in such situations.

In premature labour in a patient with known or suspected cardiac disease a physician experienced in cardiology should assess the suitability of treatment before i.v. infusion with Bricanyl.

In order to minimise the risk of hypotension associated with tocolytic therapy, special care should be taken to avoid caval compression by keeping the patient in the left or right lateral positions throughout the infusion.

*Warnings:* In treatment of premature labour, hyperglycaemia and ketoacidosis have been found in pregnant women with diabetes after treatment with $\beta_2$-stimulants. It may therefore be necessary to adjust the insulin dose when $\beta_2$-stimulants are used in the treatment.

Increased tendency to uterine bleeding has been reported in connection with Caesarean section. However, this can be effectively stopped by propranolol 1–2 mg injected intravenously.

*Interactions:* β-blocking agents especially the non-selective ones such as propranolol may partially or totally inhibit the effect of β-stimulants. Therefore Bricanyl and non-selective β-blockers should not normally be administered concurrently. Bricanyl should be used with caution in patients receiving other sympathomimetics.

*Pregnancy and lactation:* Although no teratogenic effects have been observed in animals or in patients, Bricanyl should only be administered with caution during the first trimester of pregnancy.

Terbutaline is secreted into breast milk, but effects on the infant are unlikely at therapeutic doses.

*Side-effects:* When used as a bronchodilator the frequency of side-effects is low. Side-effects which have been recorded such as tremor, tonic cramp and palpitations are all characteristics of sympathomimetic amines. A few patients feel tense; this is also due to the effects on skeletal muscle and not to direct CNS stimulation. Whenever these side-effects have occurred the majority have usually been spontaneously reversible within the first week of treatment. Urticaria and exanthema may occur.

Potentially serious hypokalaemia may result from $\beta_2$-agonist therapy.

In common with other $\beta_2$-agonists maternal pulmonary oedema has been reported in association with the use of terbutaline for the management of premature labour; in some cases this has proved fatal. Predisposing factors include fluid overload, multiple pregnancy, pre-existing cardiac disease and maternal infection. Close monitoring of the patient's state of hydration is essential. If signs of pulmonary oedema develop (e.g. cough, shortness of breath), treatment should be discontinued immediately and diuretic therapy instituted.

*Overdosage:* Possible symptoms and signs: Headache, anxiety, tremor, tonic cramp, palpitations, arrhythmia. A fall in blood pressure sometimes occurs. Laboratory findings: hypokalaemia, hyperglycaemia and lactic acidosis sometimes occur.

*Treatment:*

*(a) Mild and moderate cases:* Reduce the dose.

*(b) Severe cases:* Determination of acid-base balance, blood sugar and electrolytes. Monitoring of heart rate and rhythm and blood pressure. Metabolic changes should be corrected. A cardioselective β-blocker (e.g. metoprolol) is recommended for the treatment of arrhythmias causing haemodynamic deterioration. The β-blocker should be used with care because of the possibility of inducing bronchoconstriction. If the $\beta_2$-mediated reduction in peripheral vascular resistance significantly contributes to the fall in blood pressure, a volume expander should be given.

*(c) In preterm labour:* Pulmonary oedema: discontinue administration of Bricanyl. A normal dose of loop diuretic (e.g. frusemide) should be given intravenously.

Increased bleeding in connection with Caesarian section: Propranolol, 1–2 mg intravenously.

**Pharmaceutical precautions** Store below 25°C. Protect from light.

*Bronchodilation:* The recommended diluent is water for injection, or dextrose. Saline should be avoided due to the risk of pulmonary oedema. If saline is used the patient should be carefully monitored.

In the management of premature labour the recommended infusion fluid is 5% dextrose.

**Legal category** POM

**Package quantities** Packs of 5×1 ml ampoules and 10×5 ml ampoules.

**Further information** Nil

**Product licence number** 0017/0048R

## BRICANYL* RESPULES*
## BRICANYL* RESPIRATOR SOLUTION

**Presentation** A clear aqueous isotonic solution for nebulisation. Single dose plastic units (Respules) containing 5 mg terbutaline sulphate in 2 ml. Multidose bottles containing 100 mg terbutaline sulphate in 10 ml (10 mg/ml).

*Inactive ingredients:* Sodium chloride, sodium edetate, chlorobutanol (Respirator solution only).

**Uses** Terbutaline is a selective $\beta_2$-adrenergic agonist recommended for the relief of severe bronchospasm in bronchial asthma and in chronic bronchitis, emphysema and other bronchopulmonary disorders in which bronchospasm is a complicating factor.

**Dosage and administration** In most patients the use of terbutaline sulphate, based on the doses below, given 2–4 times daily will be sufficient to relieve bronchospasm. In acute severe asthma additional doses may be necessary.

*Bricanyl Respules:*

| | | |
|---|---|---|
| Adults: | | 1 or 2 Respules (5 or 10 mg) |
| Children: | (>25 kg) | 1 Respule (5 mg) |
| Children: | (<25 kg) | use multidose bottles. |

*Multidose bottles:*

Adults: 0.5 to 1 ml (5 to 10 mg) diluted to required nebuliser volume with sterile physiological saline.

Children: 0.2 to 0.5 ml (2 to 5 mg), see table, diluted to required nebuliser volume with sterile physiological saline.

*Table illustrating ml undiluted solution from multi-dose bottle required for administration to children*

| *Age* | *Average weight* | | *mg terbutaline* | *ml undiluted solution* |
|---|---|---|---|---|
| | *kg* | *lb* | | |
| <3 | 10 | 22 | 2.0 | 0.2 |
| 3 | 15 | 33 | 3.0 | 0.3 |
| 6 | 20 | 44 | 4.0 | 0.4 |
| 8+ | 25+ | 55+ | 5.0 | 0.5 |

*Elderly:* Dosage as for adults.

*Chronic Usage:* If Bricanyl Respirator Solution is to be used in a continuous ventilation system, a suitable dosage is 1–2 mg/hour at a dilution of 100 microgram/ml (1:100 dilution) for adults, with a pro rata reduction in dosage for children.

**Contra-indications, warnings, etc**
*Contra-indications:* Bricanyl preparations are contra-indicated in patients with a history of hypersensitivity to any of their constituents.

*Precautions:* Care should be taken with patients suffering from myocardial insufficiency or thyrotoxicosis.

Due to the hyperglycaemic effects of $\beta_2$-stimulants, additional blood glucose measurements are initially recommended when Bricanyl therapy is commenced in diabetic patients. If treatment becomes less effective or shorter acting, the patients general condition should be reviewed.

Due to the positive inotropic effect of the $\beta_2$-agonists, these drugs should not be used in patients with hypertrophic cardiomyopathy.

Potentially serious hypokalaemia may result from $\beta_2$-agonist therapy. Particular caution is advised in severe asthma as this effect may be potentiated by concomitant treatment with xanthine derivatives, steroids, diuretics and by hypoxia. It is recommended that serum potassium levels are monitored in such situations.

*Interactions:* β-blocking agents especially the non-selective ones such as propranolol may partially or totally inhibit the effect of β-stimulants. Therefore Bricanyl and non-selective β-blockers should not normally be administered concurrently. Bricanyl should be used with caution in patients receiving other sympathomimetics.

*Pregnancy:* Although no teratogenic effects have been observed in animals or in patients, Bricanyl should only be administered with caution during the first trimester of pregnancy.

*Lactation:* Terbutaline is excreted in breast milk, but effect on the infant is unlikely at therapeutic doses.

*Side-effects:* The frequency of side-effects is low. Side-effects which have been recorded, such as tremor, tonic cramps and palpitations, are all characteristic of sympathomimetic amines. A few patients feel tense; this is also due to effects on skeletal muscle and not to direct CNS stimulation. Whenever these side-effects have occurred, the majority have been spontaneously reversible within the first week of treatment. Rare cases of bronchospasm have occurred

Potentially serious hypokalaemia may result from $\beta_2$-agonist therapy.

*Overdosage:*
*(i) Possible symptoms and signs:* Headache, anxiety, tremor, tonic cramp, palpitations and arrhythmia. A fall in blood pressure sometimes occurs.

Laboratory findings: Hypokalaemia, hyperglycaemia and metabolic acidosis sometimes occur.

*(ii) Treatment:* (a) *Mild and moderate cases:* Reduce the dose.

(b) *Severe cases:* Determination of acid-base balance, blood sugar and electrolytes. Monitoring of heart rate and rhythm and blood pressure. Metabolic changes should be corrected. A cardioselective β-blocker (e.g. metoprolol) is recommended for the treatment of arrhythmias causing haemodynamic deterioration. The β-blocker should be used with care because of the possibility of inducing bronchoconstriction. If the $\beta_2$-mediated reduction in peripheral vascular resistance significantly contributes to the fall in blood pressure, a volume expander should be given.

**Pharmaceutical precautions**

| | |
|---|---|
| Bricanyl Respirator Solution: | Store below 25°C. Protect from light. |
| Bricanyl Respules: | Store below 30°C. Away from light. |

Single dose plastic units (Respules) in an opened foil envelope must be used within 3 months. Bricanyl Respules will not normally require dilution at recommended doses. The pH of Bricanyl Respules is 3–4.5.

Bricanyl Respirator Solution in multidose bottles contains preservative and may be diluted before use with sterile physiological saline. Solution in nebulisers should be replaced daily. The pH of Bricanyl Respirator Solution is 2.5–3.5.

**Legal category** POM

**Package quantities** Single dose units (Respules): Packs of 20×2 ml. (Strips of 5 units wrapped in a foil envelope).

Multidose bottles: 10 ml bottle.

**Further information** Bricanyl Respirator Solution contains 0.1 mg/ml sodium edetate, which has been shown to cause bronchoconstriction at levels above 1.2 mg/ml.

**Product licence numbers**

| | |
|---|---|
| Single dose units Respules | 0017/0228 |
| Multidose bottles | 0017/0078R |

## BRICANYL* SA

**Presentation** White tablet with engraving A/BD containing 7.5 mg Terbutaline Sulphate PhEur in a sustained-release formulation.

*Inactive ingredients:* Polyvinyl chloride, colloidal silicon dioxide, tartaric acid, ethyl cellulose, stearyl alcohol.

**Uses** Terbutaline is a selective $\beta_2$-adrenergic agonist recommended for relief and prevention of bronchospasm in bronchial asthma and in chronic bronchitis, emphysema and other bronchopulmonary disorders in which bronchospasm is a complicating factor.

**Dosage and administration**
*Adults:* 1 tablet morning and evening. The tablet may not be divided or chewed, but must be swallowed whole together with liquid.

*Elderly:* Dosage as for adults.

**Contra-indications, warnings, etc**
*Contra-indications:* Bricanyl oral preparations are contra-indicated in patients with a history of hypersensitivity to any of their constituents.

*Precautions:* Care should be taken with patients suffering from myocardial insufficiency or thyrotoxicosis. Due to the hyperglycaemic effects of $\beta_2$-stimulants, additional blood glucose measurements are initially recommended when Bricanyl therapy is commenced in diabetic patients. If treatment becomes less effective or shorter acting the patient's general condition should be reviewed.

Potentially serious hypokalaemia may result from $\beta_2$-agonist therapy. Particular caution is advised in severe asthma as this effect may be potentiated by concomitant treatment with xanthine derivatives, steroids, diuretics and by hypoxia. It is recommended that serum potassium levels are monitored in such situations.

Due to the positive inotropic effect of $\beta_2$-agonists, these drugs should not be used in patients with hypertrophic cardiomyopathy.

*Interactions:* β-blocking agents especially the non-selective ones such as propranolol may partially or totally inhibit the effect of β-stimulants. Therefore, Bricanyl oral preparations and non-selective β-blockers should not normally be administered concurrently. Bricanyl should be used with caution in patients receiving other sympathomimetics.

*Use in pregnancy and lactation:* Although no teratogenic effects have been observed in animals or in patients, terbutaline should only be administered with caution during the first trimester of pregnancy.

Terbutaline is secreted via breast milk, but effect on the infant is unlikely at therapeutic doses.

*Side-effects:* The frequency of side-effects is low at the recommended doses. Side-effects which have been recorded such as tremor, headache, tonic cramp and palpitations are all characteristic of sympathomimetic amines. A few patients feel tense; this is also due to the effects on skeletal muscle and not to direct CNS stimulation. Whenever these side-effects have occurred the majority have usually been spontaneously reversible within the first week of treatment. Urticaria and exanthema may occur. In children, sleep disturbances and disturbances of behavioural effects have been observed.

Potentially serious hypokalaemia may result from $\beta_2$-agonist therapy.

*Overdosage:*
*Possible symptoms and signs:* Headache, anxiety, tremor, tonic cramp, palpitations, arrhythmia. A fall in blood pressure sometimes occurs.

Laboratory findings: hypokalaemia, hyperglycaemia and lactic acidosis sometimes occur.

*Treatment:* (a) *Mild and moderate cases:* Reduce the dose.

(b) *Severe cases:* Gastric lavage, activated charcoal. Determination of acid-base balance, blood sugar and electrolytes. Monitoring of heart rate and rhythm and blood pressure. Metabolic changes should be corrected. A cardioselective β-blocker (e.g. metoprolol) is recommended for the treatment of arrhythmias causing haemodynamic deterioration. The β-blocker should be used with care because of the possibility of inducing bronchoconstriction. If the $\beta_2$-mediated reduction in peripheral vascular resistance significantly contributes to the fall in blood pressure, a volume expander should be given.

**Pharmaceutical precautions** No special storage conditions are necessary.

**Legal category** POM

**Package quantities** Glass bottles containing 60 tablets.

**Further information** The inactive components in Bricanyl SA form a matrix which is insoluble in the digestive juices. The empty matrix may sometimes pass through the digestive system unchanged and be excreted.

**Product licence number** 0017/0110

## BRICANYL* TABLETS
## BRICANYL* SYRUP

**Presentation**
*Bricanyl Tablets 5 mg:* Off white tablet, engraved with A/BT and scored on one side, symbol '5' on the reverse containing Terbutaline Sulphate PhEur 5 mg.

*Inactive ingredients:* Lactose, maize starch, povidone, microcrystalline cellulose, magnesium stearate.

*Bricanyl Syrup:* A clear colourless raspberry-flavoured aqueous syrup containing 0.30 mg terbutaline sulphate PhEur per ml.

*Inactive ingredients:* Citric acid, disodium edetate, ethanol, glycerol, sodium hydroxide, sorbitol, sodium benzoate, flavour raspberry, flavour lemon limette, water.

**Uses** *1. For bronchodilation:* Terbutaline is a selective $\beta_2$-adrenergic agonist recommended for the relief and prevention of bronchospasm in bronchial asthma and other bronchopulmonary disorders in which bronchospasm is a complicating factor.

*2. For the management of uncomplicated premature labour.*

**Dosage and administration**
(1) *Use in bronchospasm*
Bricanyl Tablets and Syrup have a duration of action of 7 to 8 hours. The minimum recommended dosage interval is therefore 7 hours.

*Adults:*
*Tablets:* During the first 1–2 weeks 2.5 mg (half a tablet) 3 times in a 24 hour period is recommended. The dose may then be increased to 5 mg (1 tablet) 3 times in 24 hours to achieve adequate bronchodilation.

*Syrup:* The starting dose should be 2×5 ml spoonfuls 3 times in 24 hours. The dose may then be increased to 3×5 ml spoonfuls 3 times in 24 hours if necessary.

*Elderly:* Dosage as for adults.

*Children: Tablets:* 7–15 years, the starting dose should normally be 2.5 mg (half a tablet) 2 times in 24 hours. However, in some patients, the dose may need to be increased to 2.5 mg 3 times in 24 hours.
*Syrup:* The following dosage is recommended – 0.075 mg (0.25 ml)/kg body weight 3 times in a 24 hour period e.g.

| *Body weight (kg)* | Dosage |
|---|---|
| 14 | 3.5 ml×3 |
| 16 | 4 ml×3 |
| 18 | 4.5 ml×3 |
| 20 | 5 ml×3 |
| 24 | 6 ml×3 |
| 28 | 7 ml×3 |
| 32 | 8 ml×3 |
| 36 | 9 ml×3 |
| 40 | 10 ml×3 |

(2) *Use in the management of premature labour:* Oral treatment should not be used initially in an attempt to arrest premature labour. After uterine contractions have been controlled by intravenous infusion of Bricanyl Injection, (see Bricanyl Injection data sheet) or subcutaneous injections (0.25 mg, 4 times in a 24 hour period for a few days) maintenance therapy can be continued with oral treatment (5 mg, 3 times in a 24 hour period). Oral treatment may be continued for as long as the physician considers it desirable to prolong pregnancy.

**Contra-indications, warnings, etc**
*Contra-indications:* Bricanyl oral preparations are contra-indicated in patients with a history of hypersensitivity to any of their constituents.

Although Bricanyl Injection and Tablets are used in the management of uncomplicated premature labour, their use in the following conditions is contra-indicated:

any condition of the mother or foetus in which prolongation of the pregnancy is hazardous, e.g. severe toxaemia, ante-partum haemorrhage, intra-uterine infection, abruptio placentae, threatened abortion during the first and second trimesters, or cord compression.

*Precautions:* Care should be taken with patients suffering from myocardial insufficiency or thyrotoxicosis. Due to the hyperglycaemic effects of $\beta_2$-stimulants, additional blood glucose measurements are initially recommended when Bricanyl therapy is commenced in diabetic patients. If a previously effective dosage regimen no longer gives the same symptomatic relief the patient should seek further medical advice, for reassessment of asthma therapy, as soon as possible.

Potentially serious hypokalaemia may result from $\beta_2$-agonist therapy. Particular caution is advised in severe asthma as this effect may be potentiated by concomitant treatment with xanthine derivatives, steroids, diuretics and by hypoxia. It is recommended that serum potassium levels are monitored in such situations.

Due to the positive inotropic effect of $\beta_2$-agonists, these drugs should not be used in patients with hypertrophic cardiomyopathy.

*Warnings:* During infusion treatment in pregnant women with $\beta_2$-stimulants in combination with corticosteroids a rare complication with a pathological picture resembling pulmonary oedema, has been reported.

Increased tendency to uterine bleeding has been reported in connection with Caesarian section. However, this can be effectively stopped by propranolol 1–2 mg injected intravenously.

*Interactions: β-blocking agents, especially the non-selective ones such as propranolol may partially or totally inhibit the effect of β-stimulants. Therefore Bricanyl preparations and non-selective β-blockers should not normally be administered concurrently. Bricanyl should be used with caution in patients receiving other sympathomimetics.*

*Use in pregnancy and lactation:* Although no teratogenic effects have been observed in animals or in patients, Bricanyl should only be administered with caution during the first trimester of pregnancy.

Terbutaline is secreted via breast milk, but effect on the infant is unlikely at therapeutic doses.

*Side-effects:* The frequency of side-effects is low at the recommended doses. Side-effects which have been recorded such as tremor, headache, tonic cramp and palpitations are all characteristic of sympathomimetic amines. A few patients feel tense; this is also due to the effects on skeletal muscle and not to direct CNS stimulation. Whenever these side-effects have occurred the majority have usually been spontaneously reversible within the first week of treatment. Urticaria and exanthema may occur.

In children sleep disturbances and disturbances of behavioural effects have been observed.

Potentially serious hypokalaemia may result from $\beta_2$-agonist therapy.

*Overdosage:*
*Possible symptoms and signs:* Headache, anxiety, tremor, tonic cramp, palpitations, arrhythmia. A fall in blood pressure sometimes occurs. Laboratory findings: hypokalaemia, hyperglycaemia and lactic acidosis sometimes occur.

*Treatment: (a) Mild and moderate cases:* Reduce the dose.

(b) *Severe cases:* Gastric lavage, administration of activated charcoal. Determination of acid-base balance, blood sugar and electrolytes. Monitoring of heart rate and rhythm and blood pressure. Metabolic changes should be corrected. A cardioselective β-blocker (e.g. metoprolol) is recommended for the treatment of arrhythmias causing haemodynamic deterioration. The $\beta_2$-blocker should be used with care because of the possibility of inducing bronchoconstriction. If the $\beta_2$-mediated reduction in peripheral vascular resistance significantly contributes to the fall in blood pressure, a volume expander should be given.

(c) *In preterm labour:* Pulmonary oedema: discontinue administration of Bricanyl. A normal dose of loop diuretic (e.g. frusemide) should be given intravenously.

Increased bleeding in connection with Caesarian section: Propranolol, 1–2 mg intravenously.

**Pharmaceutical precautions**

| | |
|---|---|
| Bricanyl Tablets: | Store below 25°C. |
| Bricanyl Syrup: | Store below 25°C. |

**Legal category** POM

**Package quantities**

| | |
|---|---|
| Bricanyl Tablets: | Securitainers of 100. |
| Bricanyl Syrup: | Bottles of 300 ml. |

**Further information** Bricanyl Tablets and Syrup exert a prolonged bronchodilation, in clinical trials demonstrated for up to 8 hours. Maximum plasma concentration is reached 1–4 hours after dosing.

Bricanyl oral preparations contain no colouring agents and are sugar-free.

A suitable regimen for providing eight-hourly oral administration is: on rising, in the mid-afternoon, on retiring.

**Product licence numbers**

| | |
|---|---|
| Bricanyl Tablets | 0017/0047R |
| Bricanyl Syrup | 0017/0058R |

## BRICANYL* TURBOHALER*

**Presentation** Breath-actuated metered dose powder inhaler delivering 0.5 mg terbutaline sulphate per actuation. Each inhaler contains 100 doses. Bricanyl Turbohaler is free from propellants, lubricants, preservatives, carrier substances or other additives.

**Uses** Terbutaline is a selective $\beta_2$-adrenergic agonist recommended for the relief and prevention of bronchospasm in bronchial asthma and other bronchopulmonary disorders in which bronchospasm, or reversible airways obstruction, is a complicating factor.

**Dosage and administration**
*Adults and children:* One inhalation (0.5 mg) as required. Not more than 4 inhalations should be necessary in any 24 hour period.
The duration of action of a single dose is up to 6 hours.

*Elderly:* Dosage as for adults.

**Contra-indications, warnings, etc**
*Contra-indications:* Bricanyl preparations are contra-indicated in patients with a history of sensitivity to terbutaline sulphate.

*Precautions:* Care should be used in patients suffering from myocardial insufficiency or thyrotoxicosis. Due to the hyperglycaemic effects of $\beta_2$-stimulants, additional blood glucose measurements are initially recommended when Bricanyl therapy is commenced in diabetic patients. If a previously effective dosage regimen no longer gives the same symptomatic relief the patient should seek further medical advice, for reassessment of asthma therapy, as soon as possible.
Due to the positive inotropic effect of $\beta_2$-agonists, these drugs should not be used in patients with hypertrophic cardiomyopathy.
Potentially serious hypokalaemia may result from $\beta_2$-agonist therapy. Particular caution is advised in severe asthma as this effect may be potentiated by concomitant treatment with xanthine derivatives, steroids, diuretics and by hypoxia. It is recommended that serum potassium levels are monitored in such situations.

*Use in pregnancy and lactation:* Although no teratogenic effects have been observed in animals or in patients Bricanyl should only be administered with caution during the first trimester of pregnancy.
Terbutaline is secreted via breast milk, but effect on the infant is unlikely at therapeutic doses.

*Interactions:* β-blocking agents especially the non-selective ones such as propranolol may partially or totally inhibit the effect of β-stimulants. Therefore Bricanyl preparations and non-selective β-blockers should not normally be administered concurrently. Bricanyl should be used with caution in patients receiving other sympathomimetics.

*Side-effects:* The frequency of side-effects is low. Side-effects which have been recorded such as tremor, tonic cramp and palpitations are all characteristic of sympathomimetic amines. A few patients feel tense; this is also due to the effects on skeletal muscle and not to direct CNS stimulation. Whenever these have occurred, the majority have been spontaneously reversible within the first week of treatment.
Potentially serious hypokalaemia may result from $\beta_2$-agonist therapy.

*Overdosage:* (i) *Possible symptoms and signs:* Headache, anxiety, tremor, tonic cramp, palpitations and arrhythmia. A fall in blood pressure sometimes occurs.
*Laboratory findings*: Hypokalaemia, hyperglycaemia and metabolic acidosis sometimes occur.
*(ii) Treatment: Mild and moderate cases:* Reduce the dose.
*Severe cases:* Determination of acid-base balance, blood sugar and electrolytes. Monitoring of heart rate and rhythm and blood pressure. Metabolic changes should be corrected. A cardioselective β-blocker (e.g. metoprolol) is recommended for the treatment of arrhythmias causing haemodynamic deterioration. The β-blocker should be used with care because of the possibility of inducing bronchoconstriction. If the $\beta_2$-mediated reduction in peripheral vascular resistance significantly contributes to the fall in blood pressure, a volume expander should be given.

**Pharmaceutical precautions** Store below 30°C.

**Legal category** POM

**Package quantities** Powder inhaler containing 100 doses.

**Further information** Bricanyl Turbohaler is breath-actuated and therefore there is no need to co-ordinate the release of the dose and the inhalation. Treatment with Bricanyl Turbohaler is effective even at low inspiratory flow rates, such as those present during an acute asthmatic attack.

**Product licence number** 0017/0241

## CITANEST*

**Presentation** Glass vials containing a sterile, clear, aqueous solution of prilocaine hydrochloride 5 mg(0.5%) single dose and multidose, or 10 mg(1%) multidose.

*Inactive ingredients:* Sodium chloride, sodium hydroxide. The multidose vials contain methylparahydroxybenzoate. No preservative is added to the 5 mg single dose.

**Uses** Citanest is a local anaesthetic solution for use in infiltration anaesthesia, intravenous regional anaesthesia and nerve blocks.

**Dosage and administration** The dose is adjusted according to the response of the patient and the site of administration. The lowest concentration and smallest dose producing the required effect should be given.
In children over 6 months of age the dosage can be calculated on a weight basis, up to 5 mg/kg.
The maximum dose for healthy adults should not exceed 400 mg.
Elderly or debilitated patients require smaller doses, commensurate with age and physical status.
Citanest 0.5% is a single dose vial for use on one patient during one treatment only. The remaining contents should be discarded.

**Contra-indications, warnings, etc**
*Contra-indications:* Known hypersensitivity to anaesthetics of the amide type or to any other component of the solution.
Citanest should be avoided in patients with anaemia and congenital or acquired methaemoglobinaemia.

*Precautions and warnings:* Great caution should be exercised to avoid accidental intravascular injection of this compound since it may give rise to the rapid onset of toxicity, with marked restlessness, twitching or convulsions, followed by coma with apnoea and cardiovascular collapse.
Use cautiously in the elderly, patients in poor health, in patients with epilepsy, severe or untreated hypertension, impaired cardiac conduction, severe heart disease, impaired respiratory function and in patients with liver or kidney damage, if the dose or site of administration is likely to result in high blood levels.
Facilities for resuscitation should be available when local anaesthetics are administered.
Local anaesthetics should be avoided when there is inflammation in the region of the proposed injection.

*Adverse reactions:* In common with other local anaesthetics, adverse reactions to Citanest are rare and are usually the result of excessively high blood concentrations due to inadvertent intravascular injection, excessive dosage, rapid absorption or occasionally to hypersensitivity, idiosyncrasy or diminished tolerance on the part of the patient. In such circumstances systemic effects occur involving the central nervous system and/or the cardiovascular system.
CNS reactions are excitatory and/or depressant, and may be characterised by nervousness, dizziness, blurred vision and tremors, followed by drowsiness, convulsions, unconsciousness and possibly respiratory arrest. The excitatory reactions may be very brief or may not occur at all, in which case the first manifestations of toxicity may be drowsiness, merging into unconsciousness and respiratory arrest.
Cardiovascular reactions are depressant, and may be characterised by hypotension, myocardial depression, bradycardia and possibly cardiac arrest.
Allergic reactions are extremely rare. They may be characterised by cutaneous lesions, urticaria, oedema or anaphylactoid reactions. Detection of sensitivity by skin testing is of doubtful value.
Hypotension may occur as a physiological response to central nerve blocks.
This product gives rise to methaemoglobinaemia in a dose related fashion.
Clinically significant levels of methaemoglobin may occur with cyanosis when doses of prilocaine exceed 600 mg.
Methaemoglobinaemia may occur at lower doses of prilocaine in patients suffering from anaemia, from congenital or acquired haemoglobinopathy (including methaemoglobinaemia), or in patients receiving concomitant therapy e.g. sulphonamides, known to cause such conditions. Infants are particularly susceptible, due to a lower activity of the enzyme which reduces methaemoglobin to haemoglobin.
Methaemoglobinaemia may be treated by the intravenous administration of a 1% solution of methylene blue in a dose of 1 mg/kg, over a 5 minute period.

*Use in pregnancy and lactation*: Although there is no evidence from animal studies of harm to the foetus, as with all drugs, Citanest should not be given during early pregnancy unless the benefits are considered to outweigh the risks. Prilocaine enters mothers milk but there is generally no risk of effects on the infant at recommended doses.

*Interactions:* Patients receiving concomitant sulphonamide therapy with prilocaine e.g. cotrimoxazole are at increased risk of developing methaemoglobinaemia. Prilocaine should be used with caution in patients receiving other local anaesthetics or agents structurally related to amide-type anaesthetics, since the toxic effects are additive.

*Overdosage:* Treatment of a patient with systemic toxicity consists of arresting convulsions and ensuring adequate ventilation with oxygen, if necessary by assisted or controlled ventilation (respiration). If convulsions occur they must be treated promptly by intravenous injection of thiopentone 100 to 200 mg or diazepam 5 to 10 mg. Alternatively succinylcholine 50 to 100 mg i.v. may be used providing the clinician is capable of performing endotracheal intubation and managing a fully paralysed patient. If cardiac arrest occurs effective cardiopulmonary resuscitation must be instituted. This should include external cardiac compression, artificial ventilation with oxygen, adrenaline and sodium bicarbonate.

**Pharmaceutical precautions** Single dose vial: 0.5%: Store below 25°C. Multi dose vials: 0.5%, 1.0%: Store at room temperature.

**Legal category** POM

**Package quantities**
Single dose vial: 0.5%: Packs of 5×50 ml.
Multi dose vials: 0.5%, 1.0%: Packs of 5×20 ml and packs of 5×50 ml.

**Further information** Citanest 0.5% SDV (single dose vial) is preservative free and should therefore be used on one occasion only. Citanest multidose vials contain methylhydroxybenzoate 1 mg/ml.

**Product licence numbers**

| | |
|---|---|
| 0.5% (multi-dose vial) | 0017/5047R |
| 1.0% (multi-dose vial) | 0017/5048R |
| 0.5% (single-dose vial) | 0017/0208 |

## CITANEST* 2% SOLUTION

**Presentation** Glass vials containing a sterile clear aqueous solution of Prilocaine Hydrochloride BP 20.0 mg/ml.

*Inactive ingredients:* Sodium chloride to produce an isotonic solution. No preservative is added.

**Uses** Citanest 2% is a local anaesthetic for use in infiltration anaesthesia, epidurals, nerve blocks, analgesia.

**Dosage and administration** The dose is adjusted according to the response of the patient and the site of administration.
The smallest dose to produce the required effect should be given.
In children over 6 months of age the dosage can be calculated on a weight basis up to 5 mg/kg.
The maximum dose for healthy adults should not exceed 400 mg.
Elderly or debilitated patients require smaller doses, commensurate with age and physical status.
Citanest 2% is a single dose vial for use on one patient during one treatment only. The remaining contents should be discarded.

**Contra-indications, warnings, etc**
*Contra-indications:* Known hypersensitivity to anaesthetics of the amide type or to any other component of the solution.
Citanest should be avoided in patients with anaemia or congenital or acquired methaemoglobinaemia.

*Precautions and Warnings:* Great caution should be exercised to avoid accidental intravascular injection of this compound since it may give rise to the rapid onset of toxicity, with marked restlessness, twitching or convulsions, followed by coma with apnoea and cardiovascular collapse.
Use cautiously in the elderly, patients in poor health, in patients with epilepsy, severe or untreated hypertension, impaired cardiac conduction, severe heart disease, impaired respiratory function and in patients with liver or kidney damage, if the dose or site of administration is likely to result in high blood levels.
In epidural anaesthesia, careful monitoring of the foetal heart rate is necessary and caution should be taken in patients with impaired cardiovascular function.
Facilities for resuscitation should be available when local anaesthetics are administered.
Local anaesthetics should be avoided when there is inflammation in the region of the proposed injection.

*Adverse reactions:* In common with other local anaesthetics, adverse reactions to Citanest are extremely rare and are usually the result of excessively high blood concentrations due to inadvertent intravascular injection, excessive dosage, rapid absorption or occasionally to hypersensitivity, idiosyncrasy or diminished tolerance on the part of the patient. In such circumstances systemic effects occur involving the central nervous system and/or the cardiovascular system.

CNS reactions are excitatory and/or depressant, and may be characterised by nervousness, dizziness, blurred vision and tremors, followed by drowsiness, convulsions, unconsciousness and possibly respiratory arrest. The excitatory reactions may be very brief or may not occur at all, in which case the first manifestations of toxicity may be drowsiness, merging into unconsciousness and respiratory arrest. Cardiovascular reactions are depressant, and may be characterised by hypotension, myocardial depression, bradycardia and possibly cardiac arrest.

Allergic reactions are extremely rare. They may be characterised by cutaneous lesions, urticaria, oedema or anaphylactoid reactions. Detection of sensitivity by skin testing is of doubtful value.

Hypotension may occur as a physiological response to central nerve blocks.

This product gives rise to methaemoglobinaemia in a dose related fashion.

Clinically significant levels of methaemoglobin may occur with cyanosis when doses of prilocaine exceed 600 mg.

Methaemoglobinaemia may occur at lower doses of prilocaine in patients suffering from anaemia, from congenital or acquired haemoglobinopathy (including methaemoglobinaemia), or in patients receiving concomitant therapy e.g. sulphonamides, known to cause such conditions. Infants are particularly susceptible, due to a lower activity of the enzyme which reduces methaemoglobin to haemoglobin.

Methaemoglobinaemia may be treated by the intravenous administration of a 1% solution of methylene blue in a dose of 1 mg/kg, over a 5 minute period

*Use in pregnancy and lactation:* Although there is no evidence from animal studies of harm to the foetus, as with all drugs Citanest should not be given during early pregnancy unless the benefits are considered to outweigh the risks. Prilocaine enters the mothers milk but there is generally no risk of effects on the infant at recommended doses.

*Interactions:* Patients receiving concomitant sulphonamide therapy with prilocaine e.g. cotrimoxazole are at increased risk of developing methaemoglobinaemia. Prilocaine should be used with caution in patients receiving other local anaesthetics or agents structurally related to amide-type anaesthetics, since the toxic effects are additive.

*Overdosage:* Treatment of a patient with systemic toxicity consists of arresting convulsions and ensuring adequate ventilation with oxygen, if necessary by assisted or controlled ventilation (respiration). If convulsions occur they must be treated promptly by intravenous injection of thiopentone 100 to 200 mg or diazepam 5 to 10 mg. Alternatively succinylcholine 50 to 100 mg i.v. may be used providing the clinician is capable of performing endotracheal intubation and managing a fully paralysed patient. If cardiac arrest occurs effective cardiopulmonary resuscitation must be instituted. This should include external cardiac compression, artificial ventilation with oxygen, adrenaline and sodium bicarbonate.

**Pharmaceutical precautions** Store below 25°C.

**Legal category** POM

**Package quantities** Packs of 5×10 ml single dose vials.

**Further information** Citanest 2% single dose vials is preservative free and should therefore be used on one occasion only.

**Product licence number** 0017/0090

## CITANEST* 3% WITH OCTAPRESSIN*

**Presentation** A sterile aqueous solution for dental anaesthesia containing prilocaine hydrochloride 30 mg per ml and octapressin corresponding to felypressin 0.03 I.U. per ml.
*Inactive ingredients:* sodium chloride.

**Uses** Citanest with Octapressin is a local anaesthetic solution for use in dental infiltration anaesthesia and all dental nerve block techniques.

**Dosage and administration** In normal healthy adults the usual dose is 1 to 5 ml. Children under 10 years of age require approximately 1-2 ml.

A dose of 10 ml (5 cartridges) of Citanest with Octapressin should not be exceeded.

Elderly or debilitated patients require smaller doses.

**Contra-indications, warnings, etc**
*Contra-indications:* Known hypersensitivity to anaesthetics of the amide type or to any component of the solution.

Citanest should be avoided in patients with anaemia or congenital or acquired methaemoglobinaemia.

*Precautions and warnings:* Great caution must be exercised to avoid accidental intravascular injection of this compound, since it may give rise to the rapid onset of toxicity, with marked restlessness, twitching, or convulsions, followed by coma with apnoea and cardiovascular collapse.

In common with other local anaesthetics, Citanest should be used cautiously in the elderly, patients in poor health, in patients with epilepsy, severe or untreated hypertension, impaired cardiac conduction, severe heart disease, impaired respiratory function and in patients with liver or kidney damage, if the dose or site of administration is likely to result in high blood levels.

Facilities for resuscitation should be available when local anaesthetics are administered.

Local anaesthetics should be avoided when there is inflammation in the region of the proposed injection.

*Adverse reactions:* In common with other local anaesthetics, adverse reactions to Citanest are extremely rare in dental practice and are usually the result of excessively high blood concentrations due to inadvertent intravascular injection, excessive dosage, rapid absorption or occasionally to hypersensitivity, idiosyncrasy or diminished tolerance on the part of the patient.

In such circumstances systemic effects occur involving the central nervous system and/or the cardiovascular system.

CNS reactions are excitatory and/or depressant, and may be characterised by nervousness, dizziness, blurred vision and tremors, followed by drowsiness, convulsions, unconsciousness and possibly respiratory arrest. The excitatory reactions may be brief or may not occur at all, in which case the first manifestations of toxicity may be drowsiness, merging into unconsciousness and respiratory arrest. Cardiovascular reactions are depressant, and may be characterised by hypotension, myocardial depression, bradycardia and possibly cardiac arrest.

Allergic reactions are extremely rare. They may be characterised by cutaneous lesions, urticaria, oedema or anaphylactoid reactions. Detection of sensitivity by skin testing is of doubtful value.

This product gives rise to methaemoglobinaemia in a dose related fashion.

Clinically significant levels of methaemoglobin may occur with cyanosis when doses of prilocaine exceed 600 mg.

Methaemoglobinaemia may occur at lower doses of prilocaine in patients suffering from anaemia, from congenital or acquired haemoglobinopathy (including methaemoglobinaemia), or in patients receiving concomitant therapy e.g. sulphonamides, known to cause such conditions. Infants are particularly susceptible, due to a lower activity of the enzyme which reduces methaemoglobin to haemoglobin.

Methaemoglobinaemia may be treated by the intravenous administration of a 1% solution of methylene blue in a dose of 1 mg/kg, over a 5 minute period.

*Use in pregnancy and lactation:* Although there is no evidence of harm to the foetus, as with all drugs Citanest should not be given in early pregnancy unless the benefits are considered to outweigh the risks. Prilocaine enters the mother's milk but there is generally no risk of effects on the infant at recommended doses.

*Interactions:* Patients receiving concomitant sulphonamide therapy with prilocaine e.g. cotrimoxazole are at increased risk of developing methaemoglobinaemia. The vasopressor properties of Octapressin should be borne in mind. Prilocaine should be used with caution in patients receiving other local anaesthetics or agents structurally related to amide-type anaesthetics since the toxic effects are additive.

*Overdosage:* Treatment of a patient with systemic toxicity consists of arresting convulsions and ensuring adequate ventilation with oxygen, if necessary by assisted or controlled ventilation (respiration). If convulsions occur they must be treated promptly by intravenous injection of thiopentone 100 to 200 mg or diazepam 5 to 10 mg. If cardiac arrest occurs effective cardiopulmonary resuscitation must be instituted. This should include external cardiac compression, artificial ventilation with oxygen, adrenaline and sodium bicarbonate.

**Pharmaceutical precautions** Store below 25°C.

**Legal category** POM

**Package quantities** Glass or polypropylene cartridges of 2.2 ml standard and 2.2 ml self-aspirating, in boxes of 100.

**Further information** Nil

**Product licence number** 0017/5003R

## CITANEST* 4%

**Presentation** 2.2 ml glass or polypropylene cartridge containing a colourless, sterile, clear, aqueous solution. Each millilitre contains Prilocaine Hydrochloride 40 mg.

*Inactive ingredients:* Sodium chloride, sodium hydroxide.

**Uses** Citanest 4% is a local anaesthetic solution for use in dental infiltration anaesthesia and all dental nerve block techniques.

**Dosage and administration** In normal healthy adults the usual dose is l ml to 2 ml. Children under 10 years of age require approximately 1 ml

The maximum dose of Citanest should not exceed 400 mg (5 cartridges, 10 ml) for healthy adults.

Citanest 4% is a single dose for use on one patient during one treatment only. The remaining contents should be discarded.

Elderly or debilitated patients require smaller doses.

**Contra-indications, warnings, etc**
*Contra-indications:* Known hypersensitivity to anaesthetics of the amide type or to any other component of the solution.

Citanest should be avoided in patients with anaemia or congenital or acquired methaemoglobinaemia.

*Precautions and warnings:* Great caution must be exercised to avoid accidental intravascular injection of this compound, since it may give rise to the rapid onset of toxicity, with marked restlessness, twitching, or convulsions, followed by coma with apnoea and cardiovascular collapse.

In common with other local anaesthetics, Citanest should be used cautiously in the elderly, patients in poor health, in patients with epilepsy, severe or untreated hypertension, impaired cardiac conduction, severe heart disease, impaired respiratory function and in patients with liver or kidney damage, if the dose or site of administration is likely to result in high blood levels.

Facilities for resuscitation should be available when local anaesthetics are administered. Local anaesthetics should be avoided when there is inflammation in the region of the proposed injection.

*Adverse reactions:* In common with other local anaesthetics, adverse reactions to Citanest are extremely rare in dental practice and are usually the result of excessively high blood concentrations due to inadvertent intravascular injection, excessive dosage, rapid absorption or occasionally to hypersensitivity, idiosyncrasy or diminished tolerance on the part of the patient.

In such circumstances systemic effects occur involving the central nervous system and/or the cardiovascular system.

CNS reactions are excitatory and/or depressant, and may be characterised by nervousness, dizziness, blurred vision and tremors, followed by drowsiness, convulsions, unconsciousness and possibly respiratory arrest. The excitatory reactions may be brief or may not occur at all, in which case the first manifestations of toxicity may be drowsiness, merging into unconsciousness and respiratory arrest. Cardiovascular reactions are depressant, and may be characterised by hypotension, myocardial depression, bradycardia and possibly cardiac arrest. Allergic reactions are extremely rare. They may be characterised by cutaneous lesions, urticaria, oedema or anaphylactoid reactions. Detection of sensitivity by skin testing is of doubtful value.

This product gives rise to methaemoglobinaemia in a dose related fashion. Clinically significant levels of methaemoglobin may occur with cyanosis when doses of prilocaine exceed 600 mg.

Methaemoglobinaemia may occur at lower doses of prilocaine in patients suffering from anaemia, from congenital or acquired haemoglobinopathy (including methaemoglobinaemia), or in patients receiving concomitant therapy e.g. sulphonamides, known to cause such conditions. Infants are particularly susceptible, due to a lower activity of the enzyme which reduces methaemoglobin to haemoglobin.

Methaemoglobinaemia may be treated by the intravenous administration of a 1% solution of methylene blue in a dose of 1 mg/kg, over a period of 5 minutes.

*Use in pregnancy and lactation*: Although there is no evidence of harm to the foetus, as with all drugs Citanest should not be given in early pregnancy unless the benefits are considered to outweigh the risks.

Prilocaine enters the mothers milk but there is generally no risk of effects on the infant at recommended doses.

*Interactions:* Patients receiving concomitant sulphonamide therapy with prilocaine e.g. cotrimoxazole are at increased risk of developing methaemoglobinaemia. Prilocaine should be used with caution in patients receiving other local anaesthetics or agents structurally related to amide-type local anaesthetics since the toxic effects are additive.

*Overdosage*: Treatment of a patient with systemic toxicity consists of arresting convulsions and ensuring adequate ventilation with oxygen, if necessary by assisted or controlled ventilation (respiration). If convulsions occur they must be treated promptly by intravenous injection of thiopentone 100 to 200 mg or diazepam 5 to 10 mg. If cardiac arrest occurs effective cardiopulmonary resuscitation must be instituted. This should include external cardiac compression, artificial ventilation with oxygen, adrenaline and sodium bicarbonate.

**Pharmaceutical precautions** Store below 25°C.

**Legal category** POM

**Package quantities** Polypropylene cartridges of 2.2 ml in boxes of 100.

**Further information** Nil

**Product licence number** 0017/5050R

## CO-BETALOC*

**Presentation** White scored tablets (coded A/MH) containing 100 mg metoprolol tartrate and 12.5 mg hydrochlorothiazide.

*Inactive ingredients:* Lactose, microcrystalline cellulose, sodium starch glycolate, polyvinylpyrrolidone, colloidal silicon dioxide, magnesium stearate.

**Uses** In the management of mild or moderate hypertension. Co-Betaloc may be suitable for use when satisfactory control of arterial blood pressure cannot be obtained with either a diuretic or a β-adrenoreceptor blocking drug used alone.

**Dosage and administration** The dose will depend on patient response. Usually 1–3 tablets per day as a single or divided dose.

*Elderly:* There are no special dosage requirements in otherwise healthy elderly patients.

*Significant hepatic dysfunction:* A reduction in dosage may be necessary.

**Contra-indications, warnings, etc**
*Contra-indications:* AV block. Uncontrolled heart failure. Severe bradycardia. Sick-sinus syndrome. Cardiogenic shock. Severe peripheral arterial disease. Known hypersensitivity to Betaloc or other β-blockers.

Severe kidney and liver failure. Therapy resistant hypokalaemia and hyponatraemia. Hypercalcaemia, symptomatic hyperuricaemia. Anuria. Known hypersensitivity to hydrochlorothiazide or other sulphonamide derivatives.

An anti-diuretic effect has been reported following concomitant treatment with diuretics and lithium. As with all products which contain diuretics, Co-Betaloc is contra-indicated during lithium therapy.

*Warnings:* Metoprolol may aggravate bradycardia, symptoms of peripheral arterial circulatory disorders and anaphylactic shock.

Abrupt interruption of β-blockers is to be avoided. When possible, Co-Betaloc should be withdrawn gradually over a period of 10 days. During its withdrawal patients should be kept under close surveillance, especially those with known ischaemic heart disease.

Co-Betaloc may be administered when heart failure has been controlled. Digitalisation and/or additional diuretic therapy should also be considered for patients with a history of heart failure, or patients known to have a poor cardiac reserve.

Although cardioselective β-blockers may have less effect on lung function than non-selective β-blockers, as with all β-blockers these should be avoided in patients with reversible obstructive airways disease unless there are compelling clinical reasons for their use. When administration is necessary, use of a $\beta_2$-bronchodilator (e.g. terbutaline) may be advisable in some patients.

In labile and insulin-dependent diabetes it may be necessary to adjust the hypoglycaemic therapy.

In patients with a phaeochromocytoma, an α-blocker should be given concomitantly.

In the presence of liver cirrhosis the bioavailability of metoprolol may be increased.

The administration of adrenaline to patients undergoing β-blockade can result in an increase in blood pressure and bradycardia although this is less likely to occur with $\beta_1$-selective drugs.

Co-Betaloc therapy must be reported to the anaesthetist prior to general anaesthesia. If withdrawal of metoprolol is considered desirable, this should if possible be completed at least 48 hours before general anaesthesia.

Co-Betaloc does not interfere with potassium balance. However, at higher doses of hydrochlorothiazide disturbances in the electrolyte and water balance may be experienced. Hyperuricaemia may occur or frank gout may be precipitated in certain patients receiving higher doses of thiazide therapy. Latent diabetes may become manifest during thiazide therapy.

Diuretics in higher doses may precipitate azotemia in patients with renal disease. Cumulative effects of hydrochlorothiazide may develop in patients with impaired renal function. If renal impairment becomes evident metoprolol/hydrochlorothiazide therapy should be discontinued.

*Pregnancy:* Co-Betaloc should not be used in pregnancy or nursing mothers unless the physician considers that the benefit outweighs the possible hazard to the foetus/infant. As with all β-blockers metoprolol may cause side-effects e.g. bradycardia, hypoglycaemia in the foetus, and in the newborn and breastfed infant. Metoprolol has, however, been used in pregnancy associated hypertension under close supervision, after 20 weeks gestation. Although Betaloc crosses the placental barrier and is present in cord blood, no evidence of foetal abnormalities has been reported.

Hydrochlorothiazide can reduce the plasma volume as well as the uteroplacental blood circulation.

*Lactation:* The amount of metoprolol ingested via breast milk should not produce significant β-blocking effects in the neonate if the mother is treated with normal therapeutic doses.

As hydrochlorothiazide passes into breast milk, consideration should be given to withdrawal of Co-Betaloc, replacement by metoprolol in monotherapy or breast-feeding stopped.

*Interactions:* The effects of Co-Betaloc and other antihypertensive drugs on blood pressure are usually additive, and care should be taken to avoid hypotension. However, combinations of antihypertensive drugs may often be used with benefit to improve control of hypertension.

Metoprolol can reduce myocardial contractility and impair intracardiac conduction. Care should be exercised when drugs with similar activity, e.g. antiarrhythmic agents, general anaesthetics, are given concurrently. Like all other β-blockers, metoprolol should not be given in combination with verapamil since this may cause bradycardia, hypotension and asystole. Care should also be exercised when β-blockers are given in combination with sympathetic ganglion blocking agents, other β-blockers (i.e. eye drops) or MAO inhibitors. If combination treatment with clonidine is to be discontinued, metoprolol should be withdrawn several days before clonidine.

As β-blockers may affect the peripheral circulation, care should be exercised when drugs with similar activity e.g. ergotamine are given concurrently.

Metoprolol will antagonise the $\beta_1$-effects of sympathomimetic agents but should have little influence on the bronchodilator effects of $\beta_2$-agonists at normal therapeutic doses. Enzyme inducing agents (e.g. rifampicin) may reduce plasma concentrations of metoprolol, whereas enzyme inhibitors (e.g. cimetidine) may increase plasma concentrations. Metoprolol may impair the elimination of lignocaine.

Indomethacin may reduce the antihypertensive effect of β-blockers.

In general reported interactions have occurred with doses of hydrochlorothiazide higher than those used in this combination. Insulin requirements in diabetic patients may be altered and lithium renal clearance is reduced, increasing the risk of lithium toxicity. Responsiveness to tubocurarine may be increased and arterial responsiveness to noradrenaline may be decreased, but not enough to preclude effectiveness of the pressor agent for therapeutic use. Hypokalaemia may develop during concomitant use of steroids or ACTH, and may sensitise or exaggerate the response of the heart to toxic effects of digitalis.

*Side-effects:* Side-effects to metoprolol are usually mild and infrequent. The most common appear to be lassitude, GI disturbances (nausea, vomiting or abdominal pain) and disturbances of sleep pattern. In many cases these effects have been transient or have disappeared after a reduction in dosage.

Effects related to the CNS which have been reported occasionally are dizziness and headache and rarely paraesthesia, muscle cramps, depression and decreased mental alterness. There have also been isolated reports of personality disorders.

Cardiovascular effects which have been reported occasionally are bradycardia, postural hypotension and rarely, heart failure, palpitations, cardiac arrhythmias, Raynauds phenomenon, peripheral oedema and precordial pain. There have also been isolated reports of cardiac conduction abnormalities, and gangrene in patients with pre-existing severe peripheral circulatory disorders.

Common gastro-intestinal disturbances have been described above but rarely diarrhoea or constipation also occur and there have been isolated cases of dry mouth and abnormal liver function.

Skin rashes (urticaria, psoriasiform, dystrophic skin lesions) and positive anti-nuclear antibodies (not associated with SLE) occur rarely. Isolated cases of photosensitivity, increased sweating and alopecia have been reported. Respiratory effects include occasional reports of dyspnoea on exertion and rare reports of bronchospasm and isolated cases of rhinitis.

Isolated cases of weight gain, thrombocytopenia, disturbances of vision, conjunctivitis, tinnitus and dry or irritated eyes have also been reported.

The reported incidence of skin rashes and/or dry eyes is small and in most cases the symptoms have cleared when treatment was withdrawn. Discontinuation of the drug should be considered if any such reaction is not otherwise explicable.

Hydrochlorothiazide is generally well tolerated at the dose used (12.5 mg) in the combination. However the familiar side-effects of thiazide diuretics may be expected e.g. gastro-intestinal disturbances, metabolic and electrolyte changes, disturbances in sleep patterns, skin rashes and effects relating to the CNS.

*Overdosage:* Poisoning due to an overdose of Co-Betaloc may lead to severe hypotension, sinus bradycardia, atrioventricular block, heart failure, cardiogenic shock, cardiac arrest, bronchospasm, impairment of consciousness, coma, nausea, vomiting, cyanosis, hypoglycaemia and, occasionally, hyperkalaemia. The first manifestations usually appear 20 minutes to 2 hours after drug ingestion.

The most prominent feature of poisoning due to hydrochlorothiazide is acute loss of fluid and electrolytes. The following symptoms may also be observed: dizziness, sedation/impairment of consciousness, hypotension and muscle cramps.

Treatment should include close monitoring of cardiovascular, respiratory and renal function, and blood glucose and electrolytes. Further absorption may be prevented by induction of vomiting, gastric lavage or administration of activated-charcoal if ingestion is recent. Cardiovascular complications should be treated symptomatically, which may require the use of sympathomimetic agents (e.g. noradrenaline, metaraminol), atropine or inotropic agents (e.g. dopamine, dobutamine). Temporary pacing may be required for AV block. Glucagon can reverse the effects of excessive β-blockade, given in a dose of 1–10 mg intravenously. Intravenous $\beta_2$-stimulants e.g. terbutaline may be required to relieve bronchospasm.

Intravenous volume and electrolyte-replacement may be necessary.

Metoprolol cannot be effectively removed by haemodialysis.

**Pharmaceutical precautions** Store below 25°C in a dry place.

**Legal category** POM

**Package quantities** PVC blister strips in an outer carton (7 tablets per strip). Pack size 28.

**Further information** Metoprolol is well absorbed after oral administration, peak plasma concentrations occurring 1.5–2 hours after dosing. The bioavailability of a single dose is approximately 50%, increasing to approximately 70% during repeated administration. The bioavailability also increases if metoprolol is given with food.

Elimination is mainly by hepatic metabolism and the average elimination half-life is 3.5 hours (range 1 to 9 hours). Rates of metabolism vary between individuals, with poor metabolisers (approximately 10%) showing higher plasma concentrations and slower elimination than extensive metabolisers. Within individuals, however, plasma concentrations are stable and reproducible.

Because of variation in rates of metabolism, the dose of metoprolol should always be adjusted to the individual requirements of the patient. As the therapeutic response, adverse effects and relative cardioselectivity are related to plasma concentration, poor metabolisers may require lower than normal doses. Dosage adjustment is not routinely required in the elderly or in patients with renal failure, but dosage may need to be reduced in patients with significant hepatic dysfunction when metoprolol elimination may be impaired.

**Product licence number** 0017/0092

## CO-BETALOC* SA

**Presentation** Yellow, biconvex, film coated tablets engraved A/MC.

Each tablet contains metoprolol tartrate 200 mg embedded in a white tablet layer, from which release takes place slowly, and hydrochlorothiazide 25 mg, in a yellow layer, which is rapidly released.

*Inactive ingredients:* Sodium aluminium silicate, paraffin, ethyl cellulose, magnesium stearate, lactose, microcrystalline cellulose, maize starch, polyvinylpyrrolidone, riboflavin, sodium stearyl fumarate, hydroxypropyl methylcellulose, polyethylene glycol, iron oxide yellow, titanium dioxide.

**Uses** In the management of mild or moderate hypertension. Co-Betaloc SA may be suitable for use when satisfactory control of arterial blood pressure cannot be obtained with either a diuretic or a β-adrenoreceptor blocking drug used alone.

**Dosage and administration** The dose will depend on patient response. Usually one tablet daily, taken whole and swallowed with water.

*Elderly:* There are no special dosage requirements in otherwise healthy elderly patients.

*Significant hepatic dysfunction:* A reduction in dosage may be necessary.

**Contra-indications, warnings, etc**
*Contra-indications:* AV block. Uncontrolled heart failure. Severe bradycardia. Sick-sinus syndrome. Cardiogenic shock. Severe peripheral arterial disease. Known hypersensitivity to metoprolol or other β-blockers.

Severe kidney and liver failure. Therapy resistant hypokalaemia and hyponatraemia. Hypercalcaemia, symptomatic hyperuricaemia. Anuria. Known hypersensitivity to hydrochlorothiazide or other sulphonamide derivatives.

An anti-diuretic effect has been reported following concomitant treatment with diuretics and lithium. As with all products which contain diuretics, Co-Betaloc SA is contra-indicated during lithium therapy.

*Warnings:* Metoprolol may aggravate bradycardia, symptoms of peripheral arterial circulatory disorders and anaphylactic shock.

Abrupt interruption of Co-Betaloc SA is to be avoided. When possible, the drug should be withdrawn gradually over a period of 10 days using Co-Betaloc to help reduce the dose. During withdrawal from treatment patients should be kept under close surveillance, especially those with known ischaemic heart disease.

Co-Betaloc SA may be administered when heart failure has been controlled. Digitalisation and/or diuretic therapy should also be considered for patients with a history of heart failure, or patients known to have a poor cardiac reserve.

Although cardioselective β-blockers may have less effect on lung function than non-selective β-blockers, as with all β-blockers these should be avoided in patients with reversible obstructive airways disease unless there are compelling clinical reasons for their use. When administration is necessary, use of a $\beta_2$-bronchodilator (e.g. terbutaline) may be advisable in some patients.

In labile and insulin dependent diabetes, it may be necessary to adjust the hypoglycaemic therapy.

In patients with phaeochromocytoma, an α-blocker should be given concomitantly.

The bioavailability of metoprolol may be increased in the presence of liver cirrhosis.

The administration of adrenaline to patients undergoing β-blockade can result in an increase in blood pressure and bradycardia although this is less likely to occur with $\beta_1$-selective drugs.

Metoprolol therapy must be reported to the anaesthetist prior to general anaesthetic. If it is desirable to withdraw metoprolol in patients who are to undergo anaesthesia the withdrawal should if possible be completed at least 48 hours before the anaesthesia.

Co-Betaloc SA does not interfere with potassium balance. However, at higher doses of hydrochlorothiazide disturbances in the electrolyte and water balance may be experienced. Hyperuricaemia may occur or frank gout may be precipitated in certain patients receiving higher doses of thiazide therapy. Latent diabetes may manifest itself during thiazide therapy.

Diuretics in higher doses may precipitate azotemia in patients with renal disease. Cumulative effects of hydrochlorothiazide may develop in patients with impaired renal function. If renal impairment becomes evident metoprolol/hydrochlorothiazide therapy should be discontinued.

*Pregnancy:* Co-Betaloc SA should not be used in pregnancy or nursing mothers unless the physician considers that the benefit outweighs the possible hazard to the foetus/infant. As with all β-blockers metoprolol may cause side-effects e.g. bradycardia, hypoglycaemia in the foetus, and in the newborn and breastfed infant. Metoprolol has, however, been used in pregnancy associated hypertension under close supervision, after 20 weeks gestation. Although metoprolol crosses the placental barrier and is present in cord blood, no evidence of foetal abnormalities has been reported.

Hydrochlorothiazide can reduce the plasma volume as well as the uteroplacental blood circulation.

*Lactation:* The amount of metoprolol ingested via breast milk should not produce significant β-blocking effects in the neonate if the mother is treated with normal therapeutic doses.

As hydrochlorothiazide passes into breast milk, consideration should be given to either the withdrawal of Co-Betaloc SA, replacement by metoprolol monotherapy or instructing the patient to stop breast-feeding.

*Interactions:* The effects of metoprolol and other antihypertensive drugs on blood pressure are usually additive, and care should be taken to avoid hypotension. However, combinations of antihypertensive drugs may often be used with benefit to improve control of hypertension.

Metoprolol can reduce myocardial contractility and impair intracardiac conduction. Care should be exercised when drugs with similar activity, e.g. antiarrhythmic agents, general anaesthetics, are given concurrently. Like all other β-blockers, metoprolol should not be given in combination with verapamil since this may cause bradycardia, hypotension and asystole. Care should also be exercised when β-blockers are given in combination with sympathetic ganglion blocking agents, other β-blockers (i.e. eye drops) or MAO inhibitors. If combination treatment with clonidine is to be discontinued, metoprolol should be withdrawn several days before clonidine.

As β-blockers may affect the peripheral circulation, care should be exercised when drugs with similar activity e.g. ergotamine are given concurrently.

Metoprolol will antagonise the $\beta_1$-effects of sympathomimetic agents but should have little influence on the bronchodilator effects of $\beta_2$-agonists at normal therapeutic doses. Enzyme inducing agents (e.g. rifampicin) may reduce plasma concentrations of metoprolol, whereas enzyme inhibitors (e.g. cimetidine) may increase plasma concentrations. Metoprolol may impair the elimination of lignocaine.

Indomethacin may reduce the antihypertensive effect of β-blockers.

In general reported interactions have occurred with doses of hydrochlorothiazide higher than those used in this combination. Insulin requirements in diabetic patients may be altered and lithium renal clearance is reduced, increasing the risk of lithium toxicity. Responsiveness to tubocurarine may be increased and arterial responsiveness to noradrenaline may be decreased, but not enough to preclude effectiveness of the pressor agent for therapeutic use. Hypokalaemia may develop during concomitant use of steroids or ACTH, and may sensitise or exaggerate the response of the heart to toxic effects of digitalis.

*Side-effects:* Side-effects to metoprolol are usually mild and infrequent. The most common appear to be lassitude, GI disturbances (nausea, vomiting or abdominal pain) and disturbances of sleep pattern. In many cases these effects have been transient or have disappeared after a reduction in dosage.

Effects related to the CNS which have been reported occasionally are dizziness and headache and rarely paraesthesia, muscle cramps, depression and decreased mental alertness. There have also been isolated reports of personality disorders.

Cardiovascular effects which have been reported occasionally are bradycardia, postural hypotension and rarely, heart failure, palpitations, cardiac arrhythmias, Raynauds phenomenon, peripheral oedema and precordial pain. There have also been isolated reports of cardiac conduction abnormalities, and gangrene in patients with pre-existing severe peripheral circulatory disorders.

Common gastro-intestinal disturbances have been described above but rarely diarrhoea or constipation also occur and there have been isolated cases of dry mouth and abnormal liver function.

Skin rashes (urticaria, psoriasiform, dystrophic skin lesions) and positive anti-nuclear antibodies (not associated with SLE) occur rarely. Isolated cases of photosensitivity, increased sweating and alopecia have been reported. Respiratory effects include occasional reports of bronchospasm and isolated cases of rhinitis.

Isolated cases of weight gain, thrombocytopenia, disturbances of vision, conjunctivitis, tinnitus and dry or irritated eyes have also been reported.

The reported incidence of skin rashes and/or dry eyes is small and in most cases the symptoms have cleared when treatment was withdrawn. Discontinuation of the drug should be considered if any such reaction is not otherwise explicable.

Hydrochlorothiazide is generally well tolerated at the dose used (25 mg) in the combination. However the familiar side-effects of thiazide diuretics may be expected e.g. gastro-intestinal disturbances, metabolic and electrolyte changes, disturbances in sleep pattern, skin rashes and effects relating to the CNS.

*Overdosage:* Poisoning due to an overdose of metoprolol may lead to severe hypotension, sinus bradycardia, atrioventricular block, heart failure, cardiogenic shock, cardiac arrest, bronchospasm, impairment of consciousness, coma, nausea, vomiting, cyanosis, hypoglycaemia and, occasionally, hyperkalaemia. The first manifestations usually appear 20 minutes to 2 hours after drug ingestion.

The most prominent feature of poisoning due to hydrochlorothiazide is acute loss of fluid and electrolytes. The following symptoms may also be observed: dizziness, sedation/impairment of consciousness, hypotension and muscle cramps.

Treatment should include close monitoring of cardiovascular, respiratory and renal function, and blood glucose and electrolytes. Further absorption may be prevented by induction of vomiting, gastric lavage or administration of activated-charcoal if ingestion is recent. Cardiovascular complications should be treated symptomatically, which may require the use of sympathomimetic agents (e.g. noradrenaline, metaraminol), atropine or inotropic agents (e.g. dopamine, dobutamine). Temporary pacing may be required for AV block. Glucagon can reverse the effects of excessive β-blockade, given in a dose of 1–10 mg intravenously. Intravenous $\beta_2$-stimulants e.g. terbutaline may be required to relieve bronchospasm.

Intravenous volume and electrolyte-replacement may be necessary.

Metoprolol cannot be effectively removed by haemodialysis.

**Pharmaceutical precautions** Store below 25°C in a dry place.

**Legal category** POM

**Package quantities** Calendar packs of 28 tablets.

**Further information** *Metoprolol Tartrate:* Metoprolol is well absorbed after oral administration, peak plasma concentrations occurring 1.5–2 hours after dosing. The bioavailability of a single dose is approximately 50%, increasing to approximately 70% during repeated administration. The bioavailability also increases if metoprolol is given with food.

Elimination is mainly by hepatic metabolism and the average elimination half-life is 3.5 hours (range 1 to 9 hours). Rates of metabolism vary between individuals, with poor metabolisers (approximately 10%) showing higher plasma concentrations and slower elimination than extensive metabolisers. Within individuals, however, plasma concentrations are stable and reproducible.

Because of variation in rates of metabolism, the dose of metoprolol should always be adjusted to the individual requirements of the patient. As the therapeutic response, adverse effects and relative cardioselectivity are related to plasma concentrations, poor metabolisers may require lower than normal doses. Dosage adjustment is not routinely required in the elderly or in patients with renal failure, but dosage may need to be reduced in patients with significant hepatic dysfunction when metoprolol elimination may be impaired.

*Hydrochlorothiazide:* Hydrochlorothiazide is incompletely but rapidly absorbed from the gastrointestinal tract. It is estimated to have a plasma half-life of 3-4 hours with a biological half-life up to 12 hours. It is excreted unchanged in the urine. It crosses the placental barrier and is excreted in breast milk.

**Product licence number** 0017/0202

# COLAZIDE*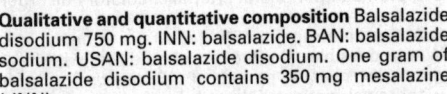

**Qualitative and quantitative composition** Balsalazide disodium 750 mg. INN: balsalazide. BAN: balsalazide sodium. USAN: balsalazide disodium. One gram of balsalazide disodium contains 350 mg mesalazine (rINN).

**Pharmaceutical form** Size 00 hard gelatin capsules with maroon body and red cap.

**Clinical particulars**

*Therapeutic indications:* Colazide is indicated for:
Treatment of mild-to-moderate active ulcerative colitis.

*Posology and method of administration:* To be swallowed whole after food.
*Adults:* 2.25 g (3 capsules) three times daily (6.75 g daily) until remission or for 12 weeks maximum. Rectal or oral steroids can be given concomitantly if necessary.
*Elderly:* As for adults.
*Children:* Colazide is not recommended in children. Treatment with Colazide requires no more supervision than is usual in patients with ulcerative colitis.

*Contra-indications:* Hypersensitivity to any component of the product or its metabolites, including mesalazine. History of hypersensitivity to salicylates. Severe renal impairment (GFR less than 20 ml/minute).

*Special warnings and special precautions for use:* Colazide should be used only with caution in patients with moderate renal impairment or those with established hepatic disease.
Salicylates may worsen asthma.

*Interaction with other medicaments and other forms of interaction:* Plasma levels of digoxin should be monitored in digitalised patients starting Colazide.

*Pregnancy and lactation:* Animal reproduction and fertility studies showed no significant abnormality. Human experience is limited. Colazide should not be given to pregnant or lactating women.

*Effects on ability to drive and use machines:* No evidence of any relevant effect. Presumed to be safe.

*Undesirable effects:* The adverse effects are expected

to be those of mesalazine. In clinical trials of active ulcerative colitis, headache (8.6%), gastrointestinal symptoms such as abdominal pain (7.4%), diarrhoea (5.1%), nausea (4.0%) and vomiting (3.4%) have been reported. Four percent (4%) of patients were withdrawn, usually early in treatment.

With oral mesalazine, rare adverse events such as exacerbation of colitis, nephrotoxicity, pancreatitis, hepatitis, blood dyscrasias and allergic reactions have been reported.

*Overdose:* To date, there are no reports of overdosage with mesalazine-releasing products. Treatment should be symptomatic.

**Pharmacological properties**
*Pharmacodynamic properties:* Balsalazide consists of mesalazine linked to a carrier molecule (4-aminobenzoyl-β-alanine) via an azo bond.

Bacterial azo-reduction releases mesalazine as an active metabolite in the colon. Mesalazine is an intestinal anti-inflammatory agent acting locally on the colonic mucosa. Its precise mechanism of action is unknown. Balsalazide and the carrier do not contribute to the pharmacodynamic action.

*Pharmacokinetic properties:* Balsalazide is only absorbed to a slight degree. After azo-reduction in the colon, up to 20% of the mesalazine and up to 6% of the carrier are absorbed. Both metabolites are rapidly N-acetylated and then highly cleared in urine.

*Preclinical safety data:* No findings have been reported from pre-clinical safety studies which add to the prescribing information given in other sections.

**Pharmaceutical particulars**
*List of excipients:* Inactive ingredients in Colazide capsules are magnesium stearate, colloidal anhydrous silica, gelatin and the colourants E127, E172, E171 and E132.

*Incompatibilities:* None known

*Shelf life:* 3 years.

*Special precautions for storage:* None.

*Nature and contents of container:* High density polyethylene container fitted with tamper-evident, childresistant, high density polyethylene screw caps.
　Pack size of 130 capsules per container.

*Instruction for use/handling:* None.

**Marketing authorisation number** 0017/0394

**Date of approval/revision of the SPC** 14 July 1997.

**Legal category** POM

## DIRYTHMIN* SA

**Presentation** White, film-coated extended release formulation (Durules*), engraved A/DR on one side containing 150 mg disopyramide base as the phosphate.

*Inactive ingredients:* Paraffin, polyvinyl acetate, carboxypolymethylene, magnesium stearate, ethanol 95%, hydroxypropyl methylcellulose, polyethylene glycol 6000, titanium dioxide.

**Uses** Dirythmin SA is a Class IA antiarrhythmic drug, indicated for treatment of a wide range of supraventricular and ventricular arrhythmias including:

　Atrial or ventricular ectopic beats.
　Paroxysmal atrial or ventricular tachycardia.
　Arrhythmias associated with myocardial infarction.
　Wolff-Parkinson-White syndrome.
　Maintenance of sinus rhythm following electroconversion.

Dirythmin SA can be used in both digitalised and nondigitalised patients.

**Dosage and administration** Initiation of treatment, as with other antiarrhythmic agents used to treat lifethreatening ventricular arrhythmias, should be carried out in hospital.

The dosage should be adjusted dependant on the patient response and tolerance. The normal adult dosage is 2 tablets 12 hourly (600 mg daily). Dosage should not normally exceed 750 mg daily.

Patients should be digitalised prior to Dirythmin SA administration for the treatment of atrial flutter/ fibrillation or blocked supraventricular tachycardia.

In patients with moderate renal insufficiency (creatinine clearance >40 ml/min) or hepatic insufficiency, dosage should be limited to 1 Dirythmin SA tablet b.d. In patients with creatinine clearance <40 ml/min Dirythmin SA tablets are not advised.

For patients with cardiomyopathy or compensated cardiac failure, the initial dosage should be limited to 1 tablet b.d. (300 mg daily). Subsequent dosage adjustment should be made with caution.

Patients treated with conventional disopyramide capsules q.i.d. can be transferred to the equivalent dosage of Dirythmin SA e.g. 150 mg disopyramide

q.i.d. is equivalent to 2×150 mg Dirythmin SA tablets b.d.

Transferring to disopyramide from quinidine sulphate or procainamide therapy: Disopyramide may be started 6–12 hours after the last dose of quinidine sulphate or 3–6 hours after the last dose of procainamide.

*Elderly:* The renal function of the patient must be considered in relation to the dose as above.

*Children:* The safety and efficacy of Dirythmin SA in children has not been established.

*Patients with renal or hepatic impairment:* Hepatic impairment causes an increase in the plasma half-life of Dirythmin SA. Dosage should be reduced for such patients. If treatment is warranted, patients should be closely monitored.

Disopyramide is eliminated predominantly by glomerular filtration. The dose administered to patients with significant renal impairment may consequently require adjustment.

Dirythmin SA tablets must not be chewed or crushed. They should be swallowed whole with half a glass of water.

**Contra-indications, warnings, etc**
*Contra-indications:* Dirythmin SA is contra-indicated in patients with second or third degree AV block if no pacemaker is present, cardiomyopathy, cardiogenic shock and hypersensitivity to disopyramide phosphate.

Patients with heart failure or who are susceptible to heart failure should be fully digitalised before Dirythmin SA therapy in order to ensure its mild negative inotropic effect does not contribute to any cardiac insufficiency.

Dirythmin SA should not be administered to patients with hypotension.

*Warnings and precautions:* Disopyramide should not be administered to patients with hypotension, cardiomyopathy or congestive cardiac failure unless cardiac failure is adequately treated.

Severe hypotension has been observed following disopyramide administration primarily in patients with primary cardiomyopathy or inadequately controlled congestive cardiac failure. If hypotension develops, disopyramide should be discontinued. Treatment may later be restarted at a lower dosage and the patient should be closely monitored. In patients with bifascicular bundle branch block, intravenous administration of disopyramide has been reported to induce AV-block in some patients.

If first-degree heart block develops in a patient receiving disopyramide, dosage should be reduced. If the block persists despite reduction of dosage, continuation of the drug must depend upon assessment of benefit vs risk. Development of second or third degree AV-block or significant intraventricular conduction abnormality requires discontinuation of therapy, unless the ventricular rate is adequately controlled by a temporary or permanent ventricular pacemaker.

Like other antiarrhythmic drugs disopyramide may worsen arrhythmias. Disopyramide should be discontinued in the presence of significant (greater than 25%) QRS-widening. QT-prolongation and worsening of the arrhythmia may occur, particularly at high doses. If QT-prolongation of more than 25% appears or the ectopy persists, the patient should be carefully monitored and disopyramide discontinued if necessary.

Disopyramide should not be given simultaneously with other Class I antiarrhythmic agents and/or β-blockers unless life-threatening arrhythmias demonstrably unresponsive to single drug therapy are present. Patients receiving more than one antiarrhythmic agent must be carefully monitored. Caution should be observed during concomitant treatment with other drugs with a negative inotropic action.

There have been reports of hypoglycaemia in association with disopyramide administration, usually in patients with impaired liver function of other conditions predisposing to disturbance of glucoregulatory mechanisms.

Disopyramide may be given to patients with glaucoma if it appears that the overall potential benefits of therapy outweigh the risks of treatment with regard to the glaucoma. Careful monitoring and aggressive therapy of the glaucoma should then be undertaken.

Administration of disopyramide to patients who have or may develop urinary retention is possible, but appropriate corrective measures e.g. catheterisation may be necessary. The potential life-saving effects of disopyramide should be weighed against the disadvantages of treatment in such patients.

Disopyramide should be used with caution in patients with benign prostatic hypertrophy, because its anticholinergic action may precipitate urinary retention.

Disopyramide should be used with extreme caution in the presence of digitalis intoxication. AV-conduction should be monitored carefully in such circumstances.

Antiarrhythmic drugs may be ineffective in patients

with hypokalaemia. Significant potassium deficit should be corrected prior to initiating disopyramide therapy.

Disopyramide should be used with caution in patients with myasthenia gravis.

Administration to children cannot be recommended owing to the lack of clinical studies verifying safety and effect.

*Pregnancy and lactation:* The safety of Dirythmin SA in pregnancy has not been established. Animal teratology and reproduction studies have demonstrated no adverse effects. The benefits of Dirythmin SA therapy must be weighed against the possible hazards to the mother and foetus. Dirythmin SA has been reported to stimulate contractions of the pregnant uterus. However, it is not known whether the use of Dirythmin SA during labour has any effect on either the foetus or the course of labour and delivery.

Disopyramide phosphate is excreted in breast milk, and at the therapeutic doses used, effects on the child are likely.

*Side-effects:* The adverse reactions are mostly doserelated and attributed to the anticholinergic effect or the effect on the cardiovascular system.

Anticholinergic: Occur in about 30% of patients, mainly in the form of dry mouth, urinary retention, constipation and blurred vision.

Cardiovascular: Arrhythmias. In isolated cases hypotension and heart failure.

Gastrointestinal: Nausea, vomiting and diarrhoea.

Metabolic: In isolated cases hypoglycaemia and hypokalaemia.

Miscellaneous: Rarely fatigue, myalgia, muscular weakness and dizziness. In isolated cases acute psychosis and cholestatic jaundice.

*Interactions:* Rifampicin and phenytoin induce the metabolism of disopyramide, leading to reduced plasma concentrations of disopyramide and increased concentrations of the dealkylated metabolite. Atenolol reduces the clearance of disopyramide.

*Overdosage:* Poisoning due to an overdose of Dirythmin SA may lead to widening of the QRS complex and prolongation of the QT interval, atrioventricular block, sinoatrial block or arrest, asystole, paroxysmal ventricular tachycardia, flutter or fibrillation, myocardial depression, severe hypotension and cardiac arrest. Cinchonism, nausea, vomiting, drowsiness and sometimes convulsions also occur. Metabolic acidosis and hypokalaemia may complicate severe poisoning.

Treatment should include close monitoring of cardiovascular, respiratory and renal function, electrolytes and continuous ECG monitoring. Further absorption may be prevented by induction of vomiting or gastric lavage, or administration of activated charcoal if ingestion is recent. Cardiovascular complications should be treated symptomatically, which may require the use of sympathomimetic agents (e.g. noradrenaline, metaraminol), or inotropic agents (e.g. dopamine, dobutamine). Temporary pacing may be required for AV block. Glucagon may be used to treat hypotension, and intravenous sodium bicarbonate to correct acidosis and intravenous diazepam for convulsions.

Disopyramide and its metabolites cannot be removed effectively by peritoneal or haemodialysis, or charcoal column haemoperfusion but repeated oral administration of activated charcoal may enhance elimination. Forced acid diuresis is not recommended.

As Dirythmin SA is an extended release formulation, treatment of overdosage may be required for a longer period.

In case of any impaired renal function, measures to increase the glomerular filtration rate may reduce the toxicity (disopyramide is excreted primarily by the kidney). Altering the urinary pH in humans does not affect the plasma half-life or the amount of disopyramide excreted in the urine.

**Pharmaceutical precautions** Store below 30°C.

**Legal category** POM

**Package quantities** Press-through packages of thermoformed PVC (10 tablets per press-through strip). Pack size 100.

**Further information** Nil

**Product licence number** 0017/0100

## EMLA* CREAM 5%

**Presentation** White cream. Each gramme contains lidocaine base 25 mg and prilocaine base 25 mg in a eutectic mixture as an oil water emulsion also containing arlatone, carboxypolymethylene, sodium hydroxide and purified water.

**Uses** Local anaesthetic for topical use to produce surface anaesthesia of the skin.
　For topical use on the genital mucosa to facilitate the removal of warts in adults.

## Dosage and administration

*Adults (including elderly) and children >1 year:*

| Surface | Procedure | Application |
|---|---|---|
| Skin (apply a thick layer of cream under an occlusive dressing) | Minor dermatological procedures e.g. needle insertion and surgical treatment of localised lesions | Approximately 2 g EMLA applied for a minimum of 60 minutes, maximum 5 hours |
|  | Dermal procedures on larger areas e.g. split skin grafting | Approximately 1.5–3 g/10cm² EMLA applied for a minimum of 2 hours, maximum 5 hours |
| Genital mucosa (Adults) (No occlusive dressing required) | Surgical treatment of localised lesions | Apply up to 10 g EMLA for 5–10 minutes. Commence procedure immediately thereafter |

Analgesic efficacy may decline if the skin application time is more than 5 hours. Procedures on intact skin should begin soon after the occlusive dressing is removed.

On the genital mucosa analgesic efficacy declines after 10–15 minutes and therefore the procedure should be commenced immediately.

Not recommended in infants under one year of age.

### Contra-indications, warnings, etc

*Contra-indications:* Known hypersensitivity to anaesthetics of the amide type.

*Precautions:* Until further clinical experience is available, EMLA Cream should not be applied to wounds, mucous membranes or in areas of atopic dermatitis.

EMLA Cream should not be applied to genital mucosa in children.

EMLA causes corneal irritation and should not be applied to or near the eyes. EMLA, like other local anaesthetics may be ototoxic and should not be instilled in the middle ear nor should it be used for procedures which might allow penetration into the middle ear.

Although the systemic availability of prilocaine by percutaneous absorption of EMLA is low, caution should be exercised in patients with anaemia, congenital or acquired methaemoglobinaemia or patients on concomitant therapy known to produce such conditions.

*Pregnancy and lactation:* Lidocaine and prilocaine cross the placental barrier. However, both drugs have been in widespread clinical use for many years and a large number of women of childbearing age have been exposed to them. No specific effects on the reproductive process have been reported.

Lidocaine and prilocaine are excreted in breast milk in small amounts.

*Adverse events:* Transient paleness, redness and oedema have been reported.

Prilocaine has been known to cause methaemoglobinaemia when given parenterally.

In rare cases local anaesthetics have been associated with allergic reactions including anaphylactic shock.

*Interactions:* Methaemoglobinaemia may be accentuated in patients already taking drugs known to induce the condition, e.g. sulphonamides.

The risk of additional systemic toxicity should be considered when large doses of EMLA are applied to patients already using other local anaesthetics or structurally related drugs e.g. tocainide.

*Overdosage:* Overdosage with EMLA is unlikely but signs of systemic toxicity will be similar in nature to those observed after administration of other local anaesthetics.

**Pharmaceutical precautions**  Store below 30°C.

**Legal category**  POM

**Package quantities**  'Pre-medication pack' containing 10 × 5 g tubes EMLA and 25 occlusive dressings. 30 g tube EMLA. 1 × 5 g tube EMLA without dressing.

**Further information**  Nil

**Product licence number** 0017/0213

## ENTOCORT* CR 3 mg CAPSULES

**Qualitative and quantitative composition**  Each capsule contains budesonide 3 mg.

**Pharmaceutical form**  Entocort CR 3 mg Capsules: Hard gelatin capsules for oral administration with an opaque, light grey body and opaque, pink cap marked $\frac{CIR}{3\,mg}$ in black radial print. Each capsule contains budesonide 3 mg as gastro-resistant, prolonged release granules.

### Clinical particulars

*Therapeutic indications:* Entocort CR Capsules are indicated for the induction of remission in patients with mild to moderate Crohn's disease affecting the ileum and/or the ascending colon.

*Posology and method of administration:*
*Adults: Active Crohn's disease:* The recommended daily dose for induction of remission is 9 mg once daily in the morning, taken before breakfast, for up to eight weeks.

When treatment is to be discontinued, the dose should normally be reduced for the last 2 to 4 weeks of therapy.

*Children:* There is presently no experience with Entocort CR Capsules in children. Entocort is not recommended for use in children.

*Elderly:* No special dose adjustment is recommended. However, experience with Entocort CR Capsules in the elderly is limited.

*Contra-indications:* Bacterial, fungal or viral infections. Known hypersensitivity to any of the ingredients.

*Special warnings and special precautions for use:* Treatment with Entocort CR Capsules results in lower systemic steroid levels than conventional oral steroid therapy. Transfer from other steroid therapy may result in symptoms related to the change in systemic steroid levels. The following warnings apply, in common with other oral steroids.

Use with caution in patients with tuberculosis, hypertension, diabetes mellitus, osteoporosis, peptic ulcer, glaucoma or cataracts or with a family history of diabetes or glaucoma or with any other condition where the use of glucocorticosteroids may have unwanted effects.

Chicken pox and measles may follow a more serious course in patients on oral glucocorticosteroids. Particular care should be taken to avoid exposure in patients who have not previously had these diseases.

Corticosteroids may cause suppression of the HPA axis and reduce the stress response. Where patients are subject to surgery or other stresses, supplementary systemic glucocorticoid treatment is recommended.

In patients with compromised liver function, blood levels of glucocorticosteroid may increase, as with other drugs which are metabolised via the liver.

When treatment is to be discontinued, the dose should normally be reduced for the last 2 to 4 weeks of therapy.

*Interactions with other medicaments and other forms of interaction:* Although not studied, concomitant administration of cholestyramine may reduce Entocort uptake, in common with other drugs.

*Pregnancy and lactation:* Administration during pregnancy should be avoided unless there are compelling reasons for Entocort therapy. In pregnant animals, budesonide, like other glucocorticosteroids, has been shown to cause abnormalities of foetal development. The relevance of this to man has not been established.

There is no information available regarding the passage of budesonide into breast milk.

*Effects on ability to drive and use machines:* No effects are known.

*Undesirable effects:* Undesirable effects characteristic of systemic corticosteroid therapy, such as Cushingoid features, may occur.

In clinical trials other adverse events: dyspepsia, muscle cramps, tremor, palpitations, nervousness, blurred vision, skin reactions (rash, pruritus) and menstrual disorders have been reported. Most of these adverse events were classed as mild to moderate and were not considered serious. In clinical studies, at recommended doses, the incidence of adverse events was comparable to placebo.

Clinical studies showed the frequency of steroid associated side-effects for Entocort CR Capsules to be approximately half that of conventional prednisolone treatment, at equipotent doses. In studies of patients with active disease, receiving Entocort 9 mg daily, the incidence of adverse events was comparable to placebo.

*Overdose:* Acute overdosage with Entocort CR Capsules even at very high doses, is not expected to lead to an acute clinical crisis. Use supportive therapy as required.

Chronic overdosage may lead to systemic corticosteroid effects, such as Cushingoid features. If such changes occur, the dose of Entocort CR Capsules should be gradually reduced until treatment is discontinued, in accordance with normal procedures for the discontinuation of prolonged oral steroid therapy.

### Pharmacological properties

*Pharmacodynamic properties:* The exact mechanism of budesonide in the treatment of Crohn's disease is not fully understood. Data from clinical pharmacology studies and controlled clinical trials strongly indicate that the mode of action of Entocort CR Capsules is based, at least partly, on a local action in the gut. Budesonide is a glucocorticosteroid with a high local anti-inflammatory effect. At doses clinically equivalent to prednisolone, budesonide gives significantly less HPA axis suppression and has a lower impact on inflammatory markers.

At recommended doses, Entocort CR Capsules caused significantly less effect than prednisolone 20-40 mg daily on: morning plasma cortisols; 24 hour plasma cortisol (AUC 0-24h) and 24 hour urine cortisol levels.

ACTH tests have shown Entocort CR Capsules to have significantly less effect than prednisolone on adrenal functions.

*Pharmacokinetic properties:* Budesonide has a high volume of distribution (about 3 litre/kg) and a high systemic clearance (about 1.2 litre/min). Plasma protein binding averages 85-90%. After oral dosing of plain micronized compound, absorption is rapid and seems to be complete. Budesonide then undergoes extensive biotransformation in the liver (approximately 90%) to metabolites of low glucocorticosteroid activity. The glucocorticosteroid activity of the major metabolites, 6β-hydroxybudesonide and 16α-hydroxyprednisolone, is less than 1% of that of budesonide.

In healthy volunteers mean maximal plasma concentrations of 5-10 nmol/litre were seen at 3-5 hours following a single oral dose of Entocort CR Capsules 9 mg, taken before breakfast.

Systemic availability in healthy subjects is approximately 10% for Entocort CR Capsules similar to the systemic availability of plain micronised budesonide, indicating complete absorption.

In patients with active Crohn's disease systemic availability is approximately 20% at the start of treatment, and reduces to around 15% after 8 weeks treatment.

A large proportion of the drug is absorbed from the ileum and ascending colon. Elimination is rate limited by absorption. The average terminal half-life is 4 hours.

*Preclinical safety data:* Results from acute, subacute and chronic toxicity studies show that the systemic effects of budesonide are less severe or similar to those observed after administration of other glucocorticosteroids, e.g. decreased body-weight gain and atrophy of lymphoid tissues and adrenal cortex.

Budesonide, evaluated in six different test systems, did not show any mutagenic or clastogenic effects.

An increased incidence of brain gliomas in male rats in a carcinogenicity study could not be verified in a repeat study, in which the incidence of gliomas did not differ between any of the groups on active treatment (budesonide, prednisolone, triamcinolone acetonide) and the control groups.

Liver changes (primary hepatocellular neoplasms) found in male rats in the original carcinogenicity study were noted again in the repeat study with budesonide as well as the reference glucocorticosteroids. These effects are most probably related to a receptor effect and thus represent a class effect.

Available clinical experience shows that there are no indications that budesonide or other glucocorticosteroids induce brain gliomas or primary hepatocellular neoplasms in man.

The toxicity of Entocort CR Capsules, with focus on the gastro-intestinal tract, has been studied in cynomolgus monkeys in doses up to 5 mg/kg after repeated oral administration for up to 6 months. No effects were observed in the gastrointestinal tract, neither at gross pathology nor in the histopathological examination.

### Pharmaceutical particulars

*List of excipients:* Ethylcellulose, Acetyltributyl citrate, Methacrylic acid copolymer, Triethylcitrate, Antifoam M, Polysorbate 80, Talc, Sucrose, Maize starch, Gelatin, Titanium dioxide (E171), Iron-oxide (E172).

*Incompatibilities:* No known incompatibilities.

*Shelf life:* Entocort CR Capsules have a shelf-life of 2 years when stored below 30°C in the original container.

*Special precautions for storage:* Store in the original container. Replace cap firmly after use. Store out of reach of children.

*Nature and contents of container:* White polyethylene bottles of 100 capsules, having a tamper evident, polypropylene screw cap, with an integral desiccant.

*Instructions for use/handling:* The capsules should be swallowed whole with water. The capsules must not be chewed.

**Marketing authorisation number**  0017/0359

Date of approval/revision of SPC 31 January 1996

Legal category POM

# ENTOCORT* ENEMA

**Qualitative and quantitative composition** 0.02 mg/ml budesonide INN (2 mg budesonide INN/100 ml).

**Pharmaceutical form** Enema.

## Clinical particulars

*Therapeutic indications:* Ulcerative colitis involving rectal and recto-sigmoid disease.

*Posology and method of administration: Adults:* One Entocort Enema nightly for 4 weeks.

*Children:* Not recommended.

*Elderly:* Dosage as for adults.

No dosage reduction is necessary in patients with reduced liver function.

*Contra-indications:* Local bacterial and viral infection. Hypersensitivity to any of the ingredients.

*Special warnings and special precautions for use:* Special care is needed in treatment of patients transferred from systemic steroids to Entocort Enema, as disturbances in the hypothalamic-pituitary-adrenal axis could be expected in these patients.

*Interaction with other medicaments and other forms of interaction:* Information on possible interactions with rectal administration of budesonide is not available presently.

*Pregnancy and lactation:* Administration during pregnancy should be avoided unless there are compelling reasons. In pregnant animals, administration of budesonide has been shown to cause abnormalities of foetal development. The relevance of this to man has not been established.

*Use during lactation:* There is no information available regarding the passage of budesonide into breast milk.

*Effects on ability to drive and use machines:* Entocort Enema does not affect the ability to drive and operate machinery.

*Undesirable effects:* The most common adverse reactions are gastrointestinal disturbances e.g. flatulence, nausea, diarrhoea. Skin reactions (e.g. rash, pruritus) may occur. Less common adverse reactions include agitation and insomnia.

*Overdose:* Acute overdosage with Entocort Enema, even in excessive doses, is not expected to be a clinical problem. The dosage form and route of administration make any prolonged overdosage unlikely.

## Pharmacological properties

*Pharmacodynamic properties:* Budesonide is a glucocorticosteroid with a high local anti-inflammatory effect. Budesonide undergoes an extensive degree (~90%) of biotransformation in the liver to metabolites of low glucocorticosteroid activity. The glucocorticosteroid activity of the major metabolites, 6β-hydroxybudesonide and 16α-hydroxyprednisolone, is less than 1% of that of budesonide.

*Pharmacokinetic properties:* At recommended doses, budesonide causes no or small suppression of plasma cortisol.

The mean maximal plasma concentration after rectal administration of 2 mg budesonide is 3 nmol/litre (range 1–9 nmol/litre), reached within 1.5 hours.

*Preclinical safety data:* Budesonide is a well established active ingredient.

## Pharmaceutical particulars

*List of excipients: Tablet:* Lactose anhydrous PhEur, Riboflavine Sodium Phosphate PhEur, Lactose PhEur, Polyvidone, crosslinked NF, Colloidal Anhydrous Silica PhEur, Magnesium stearate PhEur.

*Vehicle:* Sodium chloride PhEur, Methyl parahydroxybenzoate PhEur, Propyl parahydroxybenzoate PhEur, Water, purified PhEur.

*Incompatibilities:* None stated.

*Shelf-life:* 24 months.

*Special precautions for storage:* Store below 30°C.

*Nature and contents of container:* Entocort Enema 0.02 mg/ml consists of 2 components: A dispersible tablet and a vehicle.

The primary package for the tablets is an aluminium blister package consisting of polyamide 25 micrometre / Aluminium 43 micrometre / polyvinylchloride 60 micrometre / Aluminium 20 micrometre.

The primary package for the vehicle is a polyethylene bottle equipped with a combined seal gasket and non-return valve, a rectal nozzle and a protective cap for the nozzle.

The bottle, the nozzle and the protective cap are made of LD-polyethylene. The combined seal gasket and non-return valve is made of thermoplastic rubber.

*Instructions for use/handling:* None stated.

Marketing authorisation number 0017/0332

Date of approval/revision of SPC October 1996

Legal category POM

# FOSCAVIR*

**Presentation** Solution for intravenous infusion containing foscarnet 24 mg/ml.

1 ml contains 24 mg (80 micromol) foscarnet trisodium hexahydrate for injection, hydrochloric acid for pH adjustment and water for injection. The solution is sterile, clear and isotonic with a pH of 7.4.

**Uses** Therapeutic conditions: Foscavir is indicated for the treatment of cytomegalovirus (CMV) retinitis in patients with AIDS. Induction therapy of mucocutaneous Herpes Simplex Virus (HSV) infections unresponsive to acyclovir in immunocompromised patients.

Following induction therapy over 2–3 weeks Foscavir produced stabilisation of retinal lesions in approximately 80% of cases treated. However, since CMV causes latent infections and since Foscavir exerts a virustatic activity, relapses are likely in the majority of patients with persistent immunodeficiency once treatment is discontinued. Following completion of induction therapy, maintenance therapy should be instituted with a once daily regimen at an initial dose of 60 mg/kg increasing to 90-120 mg/kg if tolerated. A number of patients have received 90 mg/kg over a two hour period as a maintenance therapy starting dose. Maintenance therapy has produced a delay in time to retinitis progression. In patients experiencing progression of retinitis while receiving maintenance therapy or off therapy, reinstitution of induction therapy has shown efficacy equivalent to that of the initial course.

Foscavir is also indicated for the treatment of mucocutaneous HSV infections, clinically unresponsive to acyclovir in immunocompromised patients. The safety and efficacy of Foscavir for the treatment of other HSV infections (e.g. retinitis, encephalitis); congenital or neonatal disease; or HSV in immunocompetent individuals has not been established.

The diagnosis of acyclovir unresponsiveness can be made either clinically by treatment with intravenous acyclovir (5-10 mg/kg t.i.d) for 10 days without response or by *in vitro* testing.

For treatment of acyclovir unresponsive mucocutaneous infections Foscavir was administered at 40 mg/kg every 8 hours over 2–3 weeks or until healing. In a prospective randomised study in patients with AIDS, Foscavir treated patients healed within 11–25 days, had a complete relief of pain within 9 days and stopped shedding HSV virus within 7 days.

Foscavir is not recommended for treatment of CMV infections other than retinitis or HSV or for use in non-AIDS or non-immunocompromised patients.

## Dosage and administration

*Method of administration:* Foscavir should be administered by the intravenous route only, either by a central venous line or in a peripheral vein.

When peripheral veins are used, the solution of foscarnet 24 mg/ml must be diluted. Individually dispensed doses of foscarnet should be aseptically transferred and diluted with equal parts of 0.9% sodium chloride (9 mg/ml) or 5% dextrose (50 mg/ml by the hospital pharmacy. The diluted solutions should be used as soon as possible after preparation but can be stored for up to 24 hours if kept refrigerated.

The solution of foscarnet 24 mg/ml may be given without dilution via a central vein.

*Adults:* Induction therapy for CMV retinitis: Foscavir is administered over 2-3 weeks depending on the clinical response, as intermittent infusions every 8 hours at a dose of 60 mg/kg in patients with normal renal function.

Dosage must be individualised for patients renal function (see dosing chart below). The infusion time should not be shorter than 1 hour.

*Maintenance therapy:* For maintenance therapy, following induction therapy of CMV retinitis, Foscavir is administered seven days a week as long as therapy is considered appropriate. In patients with normal renal function it is a recommended to initiate therapy at 60 mg/kg. Increase to a dose range of 90-120 mg/kg may then be considered in patients tolerating the initial dose level and/or those with progressive retinitis. A number of patients have received 90 mg/kg over a 2 hour period as a starting dose for maintenance therapy. Dosage must be reduced in patients with renal insufficiency (see dosing chart at the end of the dosage section).

Patients who experience progression of retinitis while receiving maintenance therapy may be re-treated with the induction regimen.

*Induction therapy of mucocutaneous HSV infections unresponsive to acyclovir:* Foscavir is administered for 2–3 weeks or until healing of lesions, as intermittent infusions at a dose of 40 mg/kg over one hour every 8 hours in patients with normal renal function. Dosage must be individualised for patients renal function (see dosing chart below). The infusion time should not be shorter than 1 hour.

Efficacy of Foscavir maintenance therapy following induction therapy of acyclovir unresponsive HSV infections has not been established.

Caution – do not administer Foscavir by rapid intravenous injection.

*Foscavir Dosing Chart*
*Induction Therapy*

| Creatinine clearance (ml/kg/min) | CMV every 8 hrs (mg/kg) | HSV every 8 hrs (mg/kg) |
|---|---|---|
| >1.6 | 60 | 40 |
| 1.6-1.4 | 55 | 37 |
| 1.4-1.2 | 49 | 33 |
| 1.2-1.0 | 42 | 28 |
| 1.0-0.8 | 35 | 24 |
| 0.8-0.6 | 28 | 19 |
| 0.6-0.4 | 21 | 14 |
| <0.4 | Treatment not recommended | |

*CMV Maintenance Therapy*

| Creatinine clearance (ml/kg/min) | One infusion dose: mg/kg/day in not less than one hour |
|---|---|
| >1.6 | 60* |
| 1.6-1.4 | 55 |
| 1.4-1.2 | 49 |
| 1.2-1.0 | 42 |
| 1.0-0.8 | 35 |
| 0.8-0.6 | 28 |
| 0.6-0.4 | 21 |
| <0.4 | Treatment not recommended |

* A number of patients have received 90 mg/kg as a starting dose for maintenance therapy

Foscavir is not recommended in patients undergoing haemodialysis since dosage guidelines have not been established.

*Hydration:* Renal toxicity of Foscavir can be reduced by adequate hydration of the patient. It is recommended to establish diuresis by hydration with 0.5-1.0 litre of normal saline at each infusion.

*Elderly:* As for adults.

*Children:* There is very limited experience in treating children.

*Renal or hepatic insufficiency:* The dose must be reduced in patients with renal insufficiency, according to the creatinine clearance level as described in the table above. Dose adjustment is not required in patients with hepatic insufficiency.

*Instructions for use/handling:* Foscarnet contains no preservatives and once the sterility seal of a bottle has been broken the solution should be used within 24 hours

Individually dispensed doses of foscarnet can be aseptically transferred to plastic infusion bags by the hospital pharmacy. The physico-chemical stability of foscarnet and dilutions thereof in equal parts with 0.9% sodium chloride (9 mg/ml) or 5% dextrose (50 mg/ml) in PVC bags is 7 days. However, diluted solutions should be refrigerated and storage restricted to 24 hours.

Accidental skin and eye contact with the foscarnet sodium solution may cause local irritation and burning sensation. If accidental contact occurs the exposed area should be rinsed with water.

Each bottle of Foscavir should only be used to treat one patient with a single infusion. Unused solution should be discarded.

## Contra-indications, warnings, etc

*Contra-indications:* Hypersensitivity to Foscavir, pregnancy and lactation.

*Precautions and warnings:* Foscavir should be used with caution in patients with reduced renal function. Since renal functional impairment may occur at any time during foscarnet administration, serum creatinine should be monitored every second day during induction therapy and once weekly during maintenance therapy and appropriate dose adjustments should be performed according to renal function. Adequate hydration should be maintained in all patients (see *Dosage and Administration*).

Due to Foscavir's propensity to chelate bivalent metal ions, such as calcium, Foscavir administration may be associated with an acute decrease of ionised serum calcium, which may not be reflected in total serum calcium levels. The electrolytes, especially calcium and magnesium, should be assessed prior to and during Foscavir therapy and deficiencies corrected.

Foscavir has local irritating properties and when

excreted in high concentrations in the urine it may induce genital irritation or even ulcerations. Close attention to personal hygiene is recommended after micturition to lessen the potential of local irritation.

When diuretics are indicated, thiazides are recommended.

Following treatment with foscarnet, clinical unresponsiveness can appear which may be due to appearance of virus strains with decreased sensitivity towards foscarnet. Termination of treatment with foscarnet should then be considered.

Mutagenicity studies showed that foscarnet has a genotoxic potential. The possible explanation for the observed effect in the mutagenicity studies is an inhibition of the DNA polymerase in the cell line used. Foscarnet therapeutically acts by inhibition of the herpes virus specific DNA polymerase. The human cellular polymerase $\alpha$ is about 100 times less sensitive to foscarnet. The carcinogenicity studies performed did not disclose any oncogenic potential.

*Side-effects:* In different patient populations Foscavir has been administered to more than 11,500 patients, the majority severely immunocompromised and suffering from serious viral infections.

The patient's physical status, the severity of the underlying disease, other infections and concurrent therapy also contribute to the observed adverse event profile of Foscavir.

Consistent findings associated with Foscavir administration are renal function impairment, impact on serum electrolytes and haemoglobin concentration, convulsions and local genital irritation/ulceration.

The adverse events discussed and tabulated below refer to results for 188 AIDS patients studied in prospective clinical trials and include those events related, unrelated and of unknown relationship to Foscavir. The adverse event profile from marketed use is similar to that reported in clinical studies.

*Renal function impairment:* Twenty-seven percent of the above 188 study patients experienced renal functional impairment recorded as a rise in serum creatinine (19%), decreases in creatinine clearance (6%), abnormal renal function (9%), acute renal failure (2%), uraemia (1%) and polyuria in 2%. Metabolic acidosis was seen in 1%. The overall pattern of these symptoms is consistent with previous experiences although the incidence may vary. Most patients with increased serum creatinine has shown normalisation or a return to pre-treatment levels within 1-10 weeks of treatment discontinuation.

*Electrolytes:* Among the above 188 patients, hypocalcaemia was recorded in 14%. Also, hypomagnesaemia was recorded in 15%. Frequently recorded were also hypokalaemia in 16% and hypophosphataemia and hyperphosphataemia in 8 and 6% respectively. Foscarnet chelates with metal ions ($Ca^{2+}$, $Mg^{2+}$, $Fe^{2+}$, $Zn^{2+}$) and acute hypocalcaemia, sometimes symptomatic, has been a common observation in some 30% of AIDS patients receiving foscarnet. Experimental and clinical data have shown that foscarnet acutely decreases ionised calcium in a dose-related manner. The drop in serum calcium is reversible. It is reasonable to assume that the infusion rate significantly affects the decrease rate of ionised calcium.

*Convulsion:* Among the AIDS patients referred to above, convulsions including grand mal were recorded in 10%. Based on the occurrence of convulsions among immunocompromised patients receiving foscarnet, an association between foscarnet induced hypocalcaemia or a direct action of foscarnet per se and convulsions has been discussed. Although many of the patients experiencing convulsions had pre-existing CNS abnormalities such as cryptococcal meningitis, space occupying lesions or other CNS tumours, an association with foscarnet can not be excluded.

*Haemoglobin concentration:* Decreases of the haemoglobin concentration have been observed in 25-33% of patients. Generally, there has been no consistent pattern of simultaneous decreases in white blood cell and platelet counts. Some 30% of the above study patients were also on concurrent AZT treatment. Many AIDS patients were anaemic already before foscarnet administration.

Local irritation in terms of thrombophlebitis in peripheral veins following infusion of undiluted foscarnet solution and genital irritation/ulcerations have been observed. Since foscarnet is excreted in high concentrations in the urine local irritation/ulceration may ensue especially during induction therapy when high doses of foscarnet are being administered.

*Other adverse events:* Other adverse events that were recorded in the 188 study patients include a variety of symptoms varying in frequency from 1% to approximately 60%, the latter being the incidence for fever. Subgrouped by body system the following adverse events, related, unrelated or of unknown relationship to foscarnet therapy were recorded.

*Body as a whole:* Asthenia, fatigue, malaise and chills were observed in 12, 20, 7 and 13% respectively and sepsis in 7%.

*Gastro-intestinal system disorders:* Nausea and vomiting were observed in 45 and 25% respectively and diarrhoea in 32%. Abdominal pain and occasionally dyspepsia and constipation were observed in 10, 3, and 6% respectively. Isolated cases of pancreatitis have been reported from marketed use.

*Metabolic and nutritional disorders:* Hyponatraemia and oedema in legs were seen in 4 and 1% respectively and increase in LDH and alkaline phosphatases in 2 and 3% respectively. Increased levels of amylase have been reported from marketed use.

*Central/peripheral nervous system disorders:* Paraesthesia was observed in 18%, headache in 25% and dizziness in 12%. Involuntary muscle contractions and tremor were seen in 9 and 5% respectively. Hypoaesthesia, ataxia and neuropathy were observed in 7, 4 and 6% respectively.

*Psychiatric disorders:* Anorexia, anxiety and nervousness were observed in 15 and 5% respectively and depression in 10%, confusion in 7%, psychosis in 1%, agitation in 3% and aggressive reaction in 2%.

*White blood cells:* Adverse events related to white blood cells included leukopenia 9%, granulocytopenia 17%. In these patients over 90% had some degree of leukopenia already before foscarnet administration, in 8% severe or even life-threatening. Moreover in some patients, it is noteworthy that mean WBC counts increased during treatment with foscarnet. Although a few patients worsened in this respect, there is no clear evidence to indicate that foscarnet is myelosuppressive.

*Platelet, bleeding, clotting disorders:* Thrombocytopenia was observed in 4%.

*Skin and appendages:* Rash was observed in 16%.

*Liver and biliary system disorders:* Abnormal liver function was observed in 4% and increase in serum ALAT and ASAT in 3 and 2% respectively and gamma GT in 2%.

*Cardiovascular disorders:* Abnormal ECG, hypertension, and hypotension were observed in 1, 4 and 2% respectively.

*Heart rate and rhythm disorders:* Ventricular arrhythmia has been reported in 2 patients from marketed use.

*Urinary system disorders:* A few cases of diabetes insipidus, usually of the nephrogenic type, have been reported from marketed use.

*Musculo-skeletal disorders:* Muscle weakness has been reported from marketed use.

*Use during pregnancy and lactation:* Foscavir is contra-indicated in pregnancy. Breast feeding should be discontinued before starting Foscavir treatment.

*Interactions:* Since Foscavir can impair renal function, additive toxicity may occur when used in combination with other nephrotoxic drugs such as aminoglycosides and amphotericin B. Moreover, since Foscavir can reduce serum levels of ionised calcium, extreme caution is advised when used concurrently with other drugs known to influence serum calcium levels, like intravenous pentamidine. Renal impairment and symptomatic hypocalcaemia (Trousseau's and Chvostek's signs) have been observed during concurrent treatment with foscarnet and intravenous pentamidine.

The elimination of Foscavir may be impaired by drugs which inhibit renal tubular secretion.

There is no evidence of an increased myelotoxicity when foscarnet is used in combination with zidovudine (AZT). Neither is there any pharmacokinetic interaction between the two drugs.

*Overdose:* Overdose has been reported in 33 patients, the highest dose being about 10 times the prescribed dose. Twenty-eight of the patients experienced adverse events and five patients suffered no ill effects in connection with foscarnet overdosing. Four patients died, one from respiratory/cardiac arrest 3 days after stopping foscarnet, one from progressive AIDS and renal failure approximately 2 months after the last foscarnet dose, one from end stage AIDS and bacteraemia 2 weeks after overdosing and one from multi-organ failure 11 days after stopping foscarnet. The pattern of adverse events reported in connection with overdose was in correspondence with the symptoms previously observed during foscarnet therapy.

Haemodialysis increases foscarnet elimination and may be of benefit in severe overdosage.

*Effects on ability to drive and use machines:* Adverse effects such as dizziness and convulsions may occur during Foscavir therapy. The physician is advised to discuss this issue with the patient, and based upon the condition of the disease and the tolerance of medication, give his recommendation in the individual case.

**Legal category** POM

**Pharmaceutical precautions** Foscavir is not compatible with dextrose 30% solution, amphotericin B, acyclovir sodium, ganciclovir, pentamidine isethionate, trimethoprimsulfamtoxazole and vancomycin hydrochloride. Neither is foscarnet compatible with solutions containing calcium. It is recommended that other drugs should not be infused concomitantly in the same line until further experience is gained.

*Special precautions for storage:* Store below 30°C. Do not refrigerate. If refrigerated or exposed to temperatures below freezing point precipitation may occur. By keeping the bottle at room temperature with repeated shaking the precipitate can be brought into solution again.

**Package quantities** 250 ml or 500 ml glass bottles.

**Further information** Nil

**Product licence number** 0017/0248

## HEMINEVRIN* 0.8% INFUSION

**Presentation** Colourless aqueous solution containing Chlormethiazole Edisylate BP 8 mg/ml.

*Inactive ingredients:* Dextrose anhydrous, sodium hydroxide.

**Uses** Heminevrin is a short acting hypnotic and sedative with anticonvulsant effects used for the treatment of: Pre-eclamptic toxaemia, eclampsia, status epilepticus, acute alcohol withdrawal symptoms where oral administration is not practicable; as a sedative during regional anaesthesia.

**Dosage and administration** When Heminevrin is given by i.v. infusion, the dosage should always be controlled by the desired effect and the patient's response. Exact recommendations on dosage cannot be given because of individual patient variation and the presence or absence of other CNS depressant drugs such as diazepam, paraldehyde or alcohol. The doses given below therefore are guides only and due account must be taken of the patient's age (i.e. children and the very elderly), the general condition and any previous medication.

In general, the infusion should be given as a loading dose to produce the required effect, followed by a maintenance dose. As is the case with intravenous anaesthetics, Heminevrin's brief action is due to redistribution of the drug and not to rapid elimination. Thus stopping the drug, will allow rapid reversal of its sedative effect initially, but after large and prolonged dosage, recovery may be considerably delayed. The patient should be closely and constantly observed.

*Pre-eclamptic toxaemia:* Heminevrin is used to sedate the patient and raise the threshold for eclamptic convulsions.

It is indicated in moderate or severe pre-eclamptic toxaemia under the following circumstances: rapid progression of the disease, symptoms and signs associated with impending eclampsia, when labour is to be induced, during labour and post-partum (a) for up to 12 hours in patients with adequate urine output or (b) until recovery of diuresis in patients with poor urinary output.

During labour most patients will require an average of 0.5 to 0.75 ml/min of Heminevrin 0.8%. As the majority of patients are delivered within 24 hours, prolonged infusion is not necessary. Heminevrin has no analgesic properties and pain relief must be given as necessary. After delivery the intravenous infusion is maintained at 0.5 ml/min for 12 hours. Thereafter oral therapy is continued.

*Eclampsia:* Heminevrin is used to control eclamptic fits or to prevent their recurrence. It is used in conjunction with antihypertensive drugs. If seizures are occurring, Heminevrin 0.8% should be started at an infusion rate of 5–10 ml/min until the fits stop. Once this is achieved the infusion rate is decreased to 0.5–1 ml/min, though this may be varied to suit the individual patient, who should be well sedated but communicative.

If the patient is not having a fit at the start of treatment then Heminevrin is given at 3–5 ml/min until deep sedation occurs. Once the desired level of sedation is achieved this is maintained with an infusion rate of 0.5 to 1 ml/min, though this may be varied to suit the individual patient.

The patient should be lying on one side and adequate oxygenation assured. Loss of the airway, pulmonary aspiration of gastric contents, ventilatory failure and circulatory collapse may occur unless the patient is constantly monitored by experienced staff with oxygen and resuscitation equipment available.

*Status epilepticus:* Adults: 5–15 ml/min should be infused intravenously up to a total of 40–100 ml of Heminevrin 0.8%. This will usually stop convulsions. Thereafter the infusion rate will depend on the patient's response but in most cases 0.5–1 ml/min will be required. The patient should be nursed in the lateral position, to avoid airway obstruction, and turned every 2 hours. The sedation must be maintained until the epileptic convulsions do not recur if the infusion is slowed or stopped. If a prolonged infusion is necessary, fluid and electrolyte balance must be checked.

*Children:* An initial infusion rate of 0.01 ml/kg/min (0.08 mg/kg/min). If seizures continue, the dose is increased every 2 to 4 hours until seizures are abolished or drowsiness occurs. When seizures have ceased for 2 days the rate of infusion may be gradually reduced every 4 to 6 hours. If seizures recur the dose should be increased to the previous level at which they were controlled.

*Acute alcohol withdrawal symptoms; including delirium tremens:* Most patients can be treated with oral Heminevrin but in severe cases an i.v. infusion will give rapid control. The dosing principles mentioned previously, that is, a loading dose for a short period of time followed by maintenance infusion should be used. The initial drip rate should be set in the range of 3 to 7.5 ml/min until shallow sleep is induced from which the patient can easily be awakened. Thereafter, the drip rate should be reduced to a maintenance level, usually 0.5 to 1.0 ml/min, to achieve the lowest possible rate to maintain shallow sleep and adequate spontaneous breathing.

The patients should be nursed on their side to prevent airway obstruction and turned every 2 hours.

For those patients who urgently require deep sedation, an alternative is to give intravenously 40–100 ml of the 0.8% solution over a period of 3–5 minutes. Such treatment should only be given under direct medical supervision. Thereafter maintenance therapy can be established as indicated above.

Because there is a risk of producing unconsciousness with too high a rate of infusion, special attention should be paid to 'Precautions' regarding intravenous administration.

Intravenous administration is usually carried out over a period of 6 to 12 hours during which time usually 500 to 1000 ml of the 0.8% infusion is given. The level of consciousness and the effect of therapy on symptoms should be checked by interrupting the drip flow at intervals. The level of consciousness should lighten rapidly on stopping the drip flow but the longer the administration lasts, the longer the recovery will take. It is desirable to limit the period of intravenous use and to transfer the patient to oral therapy as soon as possible. During prolonged intravenous administration careful attention should be paid to fluid balance and nutrition.

*Sedative during regional anaesthesia:* Pre-medication with atropine or similar antisialogogues will help to prevent nasal congestion and upper airway mucus secretion that otherwise may occur with chlormethiazole. As judged by unresponsiveness to sound and loss of eyelash reflex, unconsciousness should be induced by a fast running intravenous infusion (approx. 25 ml/min) for 1–2 minutes. Thereafter, maintenance must be judged on the patient's reaction but the dose required is of the order of 1–4 ml/min.

If being used as an intravenous sedative in association with regional block anaesthesia e.g. spinal or epidural, the block must be fully effective before surgery begins. Chlormethiazole has no analgesic properties and the patient will respond to painful stimuli by moving.

If the regional block does not fully relieve the pain of operation it is better to give an i.v. opioid analgesic or convert to a volatile inhalation anaesthetic rather than try to increase the dosage of chlormethiazole.

At the end of an operation, stopping the chlormethiazole allows the patient to awaken usually in 1–5 minutes.

*Elderly:* Caution is advised as there may be delayed elimination of chlormethiazole.

**Contra-indications, warnings, etc**
*Contra-indications:* Known sensitivity to chlormethiazole. Acute pulmonary insufficiency.

*Precautions and warnings:* Heminevrin should be used cautiously in patients with chronic pulmonary insufficiency because there is a risk of respiratory depression.

Heminevrin may potentiate or be potentiated by centrally acting depressant drugs, including alcohol and benzodiazepines. Fatal cardiorespiratory collapse has been reported when chlormethiazole was combined with other CNS depressant drugs. When used concomitantly, dosage should be appropriately reduced.

The patient should be kept under close and constant observation by a nurse during the period of continuous infusion. With too high a rate of infusion the sleep induced with Heminevrin can pass unnoticed into deep unconsciousness with the consequent risk of mechanical airway obstruction. With overdosage there is always the possibility of causing centrally induced respiratory depression and circulatory collapse.

Because of the possible danger of mechanical airway obstruction occurring in deep sedation during Heminevrin therapy, the patient's airway may be maintained where necessary by the use of an oral airway tube. In addition, facilities for intubation and

resuscitation equipment should always be close at hand.

Hypoxia resulting from, for example, respiratory insufficiency, can manifest itself as an acute confusional state. Recognition and specific treatment of the cause is essential in such patients and other sedative/hypnotics should be avoided.

Moderate liver disorders associated with alcoholism do not preclude the use of chlormethiazole, but delayed elimination of the drug may require reduced dosage. Great caution should be observed in patients with gross liver damage and decreased liver function, particularly as sedation can mask the onset of liver coma.

Caution should be observed in patients with chronic renal disease.

Paradoxical worsening may occur in the Lennox Gastaut syndrome.

Nasopharyngeal/bronchial secretions may be increased at a time when the heavily sedated patient may be unable to cough or maintain the airway.

There has been a report of thrombophlebitis, fever and headache in young children during prolonged Heminevrin infusion. This may have been due to interaction with plastic i.v. infusion sets and silastic i.v. cannulae. For administration in small children a motor driven glass syringe should be used in preference to a drip set. A teflon intravenous cannula should be used which can be connected to the syringe by a polythene extension tube. If an infusion set is used it should be changed at least every 24 hours.

As Heminevrin is sorbed by PVC giving sets, there may be some loss in concentration before the drug reaches the patient. Dosage must therefore be adjusted to the patient's response and not given on a fixed milligram basis.

When i.v. Heminevrin is given for longer than 24 hours, there is a possibility of electrolyte imbalance due to the water load involved with the glucose vehicle. Electrolytes such as Na, K, Ca and Cl can be added to the infusion bottle to produce physiological concentrations. They will not affect the stability of chlormethiazole over a 24 hour period. Other drugs however, must not be added.

*Interactions:* A combination of chlormethiazole and diazoxide should be avoided as an adverse neonatal reaction suspected to be due to the maternal administration of this combination has been reported.

There is evidence to indicate that the metabolism of chlormethiazole is inhibited by cimetidine, thus the co-administration of these drugs may lead to increased blood/plasma levels of chlormethiazole.

*Pregnancy and lactation:* Do not use in pregnancy, especially during the first trimester, unless there are compelling reasons. There is no evidence of safety in human pregnancy nor is there evidence from animal studies that it is entirely free from hazard.

Chlormethiazole is excreted into breast milk. The effects of even small quantities of sedative/hypnotic and anticonvulsant drugs on the infant brain are not established.

*Adverse effects:* The most common side-effect appears to be a tingling sensation in the nose and sneezing occurring immediately after the start of the intravenous infusion. Conjunctival irritation has also been noted in some cases. Occasionally these symptoms may be severe and may be associated with severe headache. Increased nasopharyngeal/bronchial secretions can occur. Rash and urticaria have also been reported. In rare cases anaphylactic reactions have occurred.

Intravenous administration of Heminevrin solution may be followed by moderate tachycardia and a slight but temporary decrease in blood pressure, which is less pronounced the slower the infusion is given. Rapid infusion may cause transient apnoea and hypotension. Care is needed in patients in whom these events may cause cerebral or cardiac complications e.g. elderly. Thrombophlebitis may occur at the site of injection with intravenous infusion. Neither heparin nor cortisone has been shown to be helpful in preventing such reactions.

*Overdosage:* Overdosage can produce unconsciousness with deep coma accompanied by respiratory and cardiovascular depression similar to that seen with barbiturate overdosage. Treatment consists of securing the airway, giving oxygen (with assisted or controlled ventilation if necessary) and supporting the circulation.

**Legal category** POM

**Pharmaceutical Precautions** Store between 5°C - 8°C.

**Package quantities** Bottles of 500 ml.

**Further information** Nil

**Product licence number** 0017/5007R

# HEMINEVRIN* CAPSULES
# HEMINEVRIN* SYRUP

**Presentation** *Capsules:* Greyish-brown gelatin capsules containing chlormethiazole (base) 192 mg in Miglyol.

*Inactive ingredients:* Miglyol 812.

*Syrup:* Clear, colourless, aqueous solution containing chlormethiazole edisylate 50 mg/ml.

*Inactive ingredients:* Ethanol, sorbitol 70%, cineole, menthol, sodium hydroxide.

**Uses** Heminevrin is a short acting hypnotic and sedative with anticonvulsant effects indicated in the:
Management of restlessness and agitation in the elderly.
Short-term treatment of severe insomnia in the elderly.
Treatment of alcohol withdrawal symptoms where close hospital supervision is also provided.

**Dosage and administration** Doses of capsules and syrup are not strictly equivalent: one capsule contains 192 mg chlormethiazole base; 5 ml of syrup contains the equivalent of 157 mg base.

*Management of restlessness and agitation in the elderly:* One capsule or 5 ml syrup three times daily.

*Severe insomnia in the elderly:* 1–2 capsules or 5–10 ml of the syrup before going to bed. The lower dose should be tried first. As with all psychotropic drugs, treatment should be kept to a minimum, reviewed regularly and discontinued as soon as possible.

*Alcohol withdrawal states:* Heminevrin is not a specific 'cure' for alcoholism. Alcohol withdrawal should be treated in hospital or, in exceptional circumstances, on an outpatient basis by specialist units when the daily dosage of Heminevrin must be monitored closely by community health staff. The dosage should be adjusted to patient response. The patient should be sedated but rousable. A suggested regimen is:
Initial dose: 2 to 4 capsules, if necessary repeated after some hours.
Day 1: first 24 hours: 9 to 12 capsules, divided into 3 or 4 doses.
Day 2: 6 to 8 capsules, divided into 3 or 4 doses.
Day 3: 4 to 6 capsules, divided into 3 or 4 doses.
Days 4 to 6: A gradual reduction in dosage until final dose.
Administration for more than nine (9) days is not recommended. 5 ml of Heminevrin syrup can be substituted for each capsule administered, if desired.

**Contra-indications, warnings, etc**
*Contra-indications:* Known sensitivity to chlormethiazole. Acute pulmonary insufficiency.

*Precautions:* Heminevrin should be used cautiously in patients with chronic pulmonary insufficiency. Heminevrin may potentiate or be potentiated by centrally acting depressant drugs including alcohol and benzodiazepines. Fatal cardiorespiratory collapse has been reported when chlormethiazole was combined with other CNS depressant drugs. When used concomitantly dosage should be appropriately reduced.

Hypoxia, resulting from, for example, cardiac and/or respiratory insufficiency, can manifest itself as an acute confusional state. Recognition and specific treatment of the cause is essential in such patients and in such cases sedative/hypnotics should be avoided.

Moderate liver disorders associated with alcoholism do not preclude the use of chlormethiazole, though an associated increase in systemic availability of oral doses and delayed elimination of the drug may require reduced dosage. Great caution should be observed in patients with gross liver damage and decreased liver function, particularly as sedation can mask the onset of liver coma.

Caution should be observed in patients with chronic renal disease.

Caution must be exercised in prescribing for individuals known to be addiction prone or for those whose histories suggest they may increase the dose on their own initiative since chlormethiazole is not free from the risk of producing psychological and/or physical dependence. After prolonged administration of high doses, physical dependence has been reported with withdrawal symptoms such as convulsions, tremors, and organic psychosis. These reports have mainly been associated with indiscriminate prescribing to outpatient alcoholics and Heminevrin should not be prescribed to patients who continue to abuse alcohol.

As with all centrally acting depressant drugs, the driving of vehicles and the operating of machinery are to be avoided when under treatment.

*Alcoholism:* Alcohol combined with chlormethiazole particularly in alcoholics with cirrhosis can lead to fatal respiratory depression even with short term use. It should not therefore be prescribed for alcoholics who continue to drink alcoholic beverages.

*Elderly:* Caution is advised as there may be increased bioavailability and delayed elimination of chlormethiazole.

*Children:* Oral Heminevrin is not recommended for use in children.

*Interactions:* A combination of chlormethiazole and diazoxide should be avoided as an adverse neonatal reaction suspected to be due to the maternal administration of this combination has been reported.

The combination of propranolol and chlormethiazole has produced profound bradycardia in one patient possibly due to increased bioavailability of propranolol.

There is evidence to indicate that the metabolism of chlormethiazole is inhibited by cimetidine, thus the co-administration of these drugs may lead to increased blood/plasma levels of chlormethiazole.

*Pregnancy:* Do not use in pregnancy, especially during the first and last trimesters, unless there are compelling reasons. There is no evidence of safety in human pregnancy, nor is there evidence from animal studies that it is entirely free from hazard.

*Lactation:* Chlormethiazole is excreted into the breast milk. The effect of even small quantities of sedative/hypnotic and anticonvulsant drugs on the infant brain is not established.

Chlormethiazole should only be used in nursing mothers where the physician considers that the benefit outweighs the possible hazard to the infant.

*Adverse effects:* The most common side-effect is nasal congestion and irritation, which may occur 15 to 20 minutes after drug ingestion. Conjunctival irritation has also been noted in some cases. Occasionally, these symptoms may be severe and may be associated with severe headache. This is commonest with the initial dose following which it decreases in severity with subsequent doses. Increased nasopharyngeal/bronchial secretions can occur.

Rash and urticaria have been reported. In rare cases, bullous skin eruptions have been reported.

Gastrointestinal disturbances have been reported.

Reversible increases of transaminases or bilirubin have been reported.

In rare cases anaphylactic reactions have occurred.

When Heminevrin has been given at higher than recommended doses for other than recommended indications over prolonged periods of time, physical dependence, tolerance and withdrawal reactions have been reported.

Great caution is required in prescribing Heminevrin for patients with a history of chronic alcoholism, drug abuse or marked personality disorder.

When used as a night-time hypnotic, hangover effects in the elderly may occur but are uncommon due to the short half-life.

Excessive sedation may occur, especially with higher doses or when given to the elderly for daytime sedation. Rarely paradoxical excitement or confusion may occur.

*Overdose:* The main effects to be expected with overdose of Heminevrin are: coma, respiratory depression, hypotension and hypothermia.

Hypothermia is thought to be due to a direct central effect as well as a result of lying unconscious for several hours. In addition, patients have increased secretion in the upper airways, which in one series was associated with a high incidence of pneumonia. The effects of overdosage are not usually severe in patients with no evidence of alcoholic liver disease, but they may be exacerbated when chlormethiazole is taken in combination with alcohol and/or CNS depressant drugs, particularly those that are metabolised by the liver. There is no specific antidote to chlormethiazole. Treatment of overdosage should therefore be carried out on a symptomatic basis, applying similar principles to those used in the treatment of barbiturate overdosage.

Charcoal column haemoperfusion is not and cannot be expected to be effective in treating chlormethiazole poisoning.

**Further information** Nil

**Pharmaceutical precautions** Heminevrin Capsules should be stored below 25°C. Heminevrin Syrup should be stored at 2-8°C (refrigerate). Do not freeze.

**Legal category** POM

**Package quantities**

| | |
|---|---|
| Capsules: | Bottles of 60. |
| Syrup: | Bottles of 300 ml. |

**Product licence numbers**

| | |
|---|---|
| Capsules | 0017/5009R |
| Syrup | 0017/0063R |

## IMDUR*

**Presentation** Yellow oval biconvex film coated tablet, scored both sides and coded A/ID. Each tablet contains 60 mg isosorbide mononitrate in an extended release formulation based on Durules*.

**Uses** Prophylactic treatment of angina pectoris.

**Dosage and administration**

*Adults:* Imdur 60 mg (one tablet) once daily to be taken in the morning. The dose may be increased to 120 mg (two tablets) daily, both to be taken once daily in the morning. The dose can be titrated to minimise the possibility of headache, by initiating treatment with 30 mg (half a tablet) for the first 2–4 days.

Imdur tablets must not be chewed or crushed. They should be swallowed whole with half a glass of water.

*Children:* The safety and efficacy of Imdur in children has not been established.

*Elderly:* No evidence of a need for routine dosage adjustment in the elderly has been found, but special care may be needed in those with increased susceptibility to hypotension or marked hepatic or renal insufficiency.

The core of the tablet is insoluble in the digestive juices but disintegrates into small particles when all active substance has been released. Very occasionally the matrix may pass through the gastrointestinal tract without disintegrating and be found visible in the stool, but all active substance has been released.

**Contra-indications, warnings, etc**

*Contra-indications:* Severe cerebrovascular insufficiency or hypotension are relative contra-indications to the use of Imdur.

*Precautions:* Imdur is not indicated for relief of acute angina attacks; in the event of an acute attack, sublingual or buccal glyceryl trinitrate tablets should be used.

*Pregnancy and lactation:* The safety and efficacy of Imdur during pregnancy or lactation has not been established.

*Side-effects:* Most of the adverse reactions are pharmacodynamic mediated and dose dependent. Headache may occur when treatment is initiated but usually disappears after continued treatment. Hypotension with symptoms such as dizziness and nausea has occasionally been reported. These symptoms generally disappear during long-term treatment.

*Overdosage:*

*Symptoms:* Pulsing headache. More serious symptoms are excitation, flushing, cold perspiration, nausea, vomiting, vertigo, syncope, tachycardia and a fall in blood pressure.

*Treatment:* Induction of emesis, activated charcoal. In case of pronounced hypotension the patient should first be placed in the supine position with legs raised. If necessary intravenous administration of fluid.

**Pharmaceutical precautions** Store below 30°C.

**Legal category** POM

**Package quantities** PVC blister strips (7 tablets per strip) 28, 98.

**Further information** Isosorbide mononitrate is an active metabolite of isosorbide dinitrate and exerts qualitatively similar effects. Isosorbide mononitrate is completely absorbed and not metabolised during the first passage through the liver. This reduces the fluctuations in plasma levels and leads to predictable and reliable clinical effects.

Administration of Imdur results in a controlled release of active substance leading to reduced peak plasma levels. Compared to ordinary tablets the absorption phase is prolonged and the duration of effect is extended.

With Imdur 60 mg or 120 mg once daily no development of tolerance with respect to antianginal effects has been detected. The phenomenon of rebound angina between doses as described with intermittent nitrate therapy has not been seen with Imdur.

**Product licence number** 0017/0226

## JECTOFER*

**Presentation** Dark brown liquid for intramuscular injection; Iron Sorbitol Injection BP (contains 50 mg elemental iron per ml).

**Uses** For the treatment of iron-deficiency anaemia and the rapid replenishment of iron stores.

**Dosage and administration** The recommended single dose of Jectofer is 1.5 mg per kg body weight by intramuscular injection to a maximum of 100 mg per injection. A series of daily injections of this single dose should be given to restore haemoglobin levels to normal and replenish iron stores based on the following table.

| Hb gm/100 ml | 5.0 | 6.0 | 7.0 | 8.0 | 9.0 | 10.0 | 11.0 |
|---|---|---|---|---|---|---|---|
| Hb% | 33 | 40 | 46 | 53 | 60 | 66 | 73 |
| No. of injections | 24 | 22 | 20 | 17 | 14 | 12 | 10 |

In elderly or debilitated patients or patients who have a low tolerance threshold to intramuscular iron the injections should be given on alternate days. Not recommended in children under 3 kg (7 lb) body weight.

**Contra-indications, warnings, etc**

*Contra-indications:* Severe liver damage, acute kidney infection, untreated urinary tract infection. Early pregnancy. Intravenous use. Known hypersensitivity to iron or Jectofer.

*Precautions:* Jectofer should not be used to treat anaemias other than iron deficiency anaemia.

Care should be taken when treating patients with iron-storage diseases or haemoglobinopathies.

The importance of using the correct recommended dose in relation to body weight is emphasised, especially in patients who are already markedly underweight.

*Warnings:* Oral iron should be discontinued 24 hours before Jectofer is administered.

Jectofer should not be given intravenously.

*Use in pregnancy and lactation:* Administration is contra-indicated in early pregnancy.

*Side-effects:* Initial local discomfort or temporary discolouration may occur at the site of injection. A transient metallic taste or loss of taste may occur. Nausea, sometimes vomiting, dizziness and flushing may also occur. Occasionally palpitations and pressure sensations in the chest have been reported.

A few cases have been reported of serious reactions of a cardiovascular type with cardiac arrhythmia. Very rarely, anaphylactoid reactions have been reported.

*Interactions:* The concomitant administration of chloramphenicol may delay the response to iron therapy in patients with iron deficiency anaemia.

*Overdosage:* Systemic reactions have been observed when doses higher than recommended are given, especially to patients who are significantly underweight. Similar reactions may rarely occur in debilitated or sensitive patients given recommended doses. See *Side-effects* above.

**Pharmaceutical precautions** Store at 25°C, do not refrigerate.

**Legal category** POM

**Package quantities** 10×2 ml ampoules for intramuscular use.

**Further information** Nil

**Product licence number** 0017/5011R

## KINIDIN* DURULES*

**Presentation** Film-coated white to off-white oval tablets, each containing 250 mg quinidine bisulphate (hydrated) corresponding to Quinidine Sulphate BP 200 mg in an extended release formulation (Durules).

*Inactive ingredients:* Hydroxypropyl methylcellulose, polyethylene glycol, paraffin special, polyvinyl chloride, polyvinyl acetate, magnesium stearate, colour E171.

**Uses** Maintenance of sinus rhythm following cardioversion of atrial fibrillation. Suppression of supraventricular and ventricular tachyarrhythmias.

**Dosage and administration** Initiation of treatment, as with other antiarrhythmic agents used to treat life-threatening ventricular arrhythmias, should be carried out in hospital.

An initial test dose of one tablet should be given to detect hypersensitivity.

Dosage is adjusted according to individual patient requirements. The quinidine dose should preferably be established by determination of the serum concentration after about one week of treatment. The therapeutic plasma concentration range is 1-6 mg/litre (3-18 micromol/litre). The QT-time should be checked before and during treatment. The normal dose is 2–5 tablets (0.4-1.0 g) morning and evening. The normal dose for maintenance treatment after conversion of atrial fibrillation is 3 tablets (0.6 g) morning and evening.

Concomitant food intake may increase the tolerability.

Kinidin Durules must not be chewed or crushed. They should be swallowed whole with half a glass of water.

**Contra-indications, warnings, etc**

*Contra-indications:* Kinidin Durules are contra-indicated in patients with known hypersensitivity to quinidine, a history of quinidine induced thrombocytopenia or complete heart block.

Quinidine should be used with extreme caution in patients with incomplete atrio-ventricular block, uncompensated cardiac failure, digitalis toxicity, myocarditis, severe myocardial damage, or myasthenia gravis.

The use of Kinidin Durules is contra-indicated in pregnancy.

*Precautions:* The patient should be observed after the first dose with special attention to hypersensitivity reactions. Quinidine should be administered with caution to patients with prolonged AV-conduction, sustained decompensation, cardiogenic shock, hypotension, bradycardia or disturbed potassium balance.

Caution is indicated in combined therapy with other class I antiarrhythmic drugs, β-blockers and digitalis glycosides (see further interaction with digoxin and digitoxin). Myocarditis or severe myocardial damage also requires caution.

Heart failure and hypokalaemia should be corrected before quinidine treatment is started. In patients treated with digoxin, the digoxin dosage should be halved if quinidine is given in addition.

Like other antiarrhythmic drugs quinidine may worsen arrhythmias.

At toxic quinidine concentrations, and in some patients even at therapeutic levels, the QT-interval may be considerably prolonged, which increases the risk of ventricular tachycardia, often of the torsades de pointes type and in some cases also ventricular fibrillation.

Kinidin Durules should be used with caution in the presence of obstructive changes in the digestive tract, oesophagus, when there is a potential risk of oesophageal complications.

*Use in pregnancy and lactation:* The use of Kinidin Durules is contra-indicated in pregnancy.

Quinidine is excreted in breast milk but is unlikely to cause effects at therapeutic doses.

*Interactions: Digoxin:* The plasma concentration of digoxin increases (may be doubled) when quinidine is given in addition. This is due to reduced renal clearance and a reduced distribution volume of digoxin. When quinidine is administered, the dose of digoxin should be halved and the plasma concentration of digoxin checked.

This recommendation is based on the assumption that the digoxin concentration is within the therapeutic range when quinidine treatment is started.

*Digitoxin:* The interaction between digitoxin and quinidine is a controversial issue. Several studies indicate, however, that quinidine increases the plasma concentration of digitoxin.

*Cimetidine:* Cimetidine decreases the clearance of quinidine, thereby increasing the plasma level.

*Coumarin derivatives:* Quinidine may enhance the anticoagulant effect of coumarin derivatives.

*Rifampicin, barbituric acid derivatives and phenytoin:* These drugs increase the metabolism of quinidine, thereby reducing the plasma concentration to sub-therapeutic levels if the normal dosage is maintained.

*Verapamil, amiodarone and nifedipine:* Concomitant administration of verapamil or amiodarone can produce clinically important increases in serum quinidine concentrations. Conversely, simultaneous administration of nifedipine has been reported to significantly reduce plasma quinidine levels.

Appropriate quinidine dose changes and ECG monitoring should be carried out when these drugs are added or discontinued. During quinidine therapy 30–50% change in quinidine dosage may be required in order to avoid systemic toxicity or lack of efficacy.

*Desipramine and imipramine:* Quinidine inhibits the metabolism of desipramine and imipramine in the so called rapid hydroxylators resulting in increased plasma concentrations. In addition they have additive antiarrhythmic properties. The combination should be avoided.

*Procainamide:* One case-report indicates that the plasma concentration of procainamide and its main metabolite N-acetyl-procainamide may increase significantly if quinidine is given simultaneously.

*Metoprolol:* In the so called rapid hydroxylators quinidine may inhibit the metabolism of metoprolol resulting in increased plasma concentrations of metoprolol.

*Side-effects:* Gastrointestinal adverse reactions are frequent and occur in approximately 30% of the patients.

*Gastrointestinal:* Diarrhoea, nausea and vomiting.

*Central and peripheral nervous system:* Rarely signs of cinchonism e.g. tinnitus, blurred vision, headache and dizziness.

*Cardiovascular:* Arrhythmias such as ventricular tachycardia, mostly of the torsades de pointes type or ventricular fibrillation. Rarely hypotension and bradycardia, which may lead to cardiac arrest.

*Hypersensitivity reactions:* Rarely urticaria, skin rash and fever. In isolated cases hepatitis, thrombocytopenia, pancytopenia, agranulocytosis, photosensitisation, lupus erythematosus-like syndrome, myalgia and arthralgia.

*Overdosage:* Poisoning due to an overdose of Kinidin Durules may lead to widening of the QRS complex and prolongation of the QT interval, atrioventricular block, sinoatrial block or arrest, asystole, paroxysmal ventricular tachycardia, flutter or fibrillation, myocardial depression, severe hypotension and cardiac arrest. Cinchonism, nausea, vomiting, drowsiness and sometimes convulsions also occur. Metabolic acidosis and hypokalaemia may complicate severe poisoning.

Treatment should include close monitoring of cardiovascular, respiratory and renal function, electrolytes and continuous ECG monitoring. Further absorption may be prevented by induction of vomiting or gastric lavage, or administration of activated charcoal if ingestion is recent. Cardiovascular complications should be treated symptomatically, which may require the use of sympathomimetic agents (e.g. noradrenaline, metaraminol), or inotropic agents (e.g. dopamine, dobutamine). Temporary pacing may be required for AV block. Glucagon may be used to treat hypotension, and intravenous sodium bicarbonate to correct acidosis and intravenous diazepam for convulsions.

Quinidine and its metabolites cannot be removed effectively by peritoneal or haemodialysis, or charcoal column haemoperfusion but repeated oral administration of activated charcoal may enhance elimination. Forced acid diuresis is not recommended.

As Kinidin Durules is an extended release formulation, treatment of overdosage may be required for a longer period.

**Pharmaceutical precautions** Store below 25°C.

**Legal category** POM

**Package quantities** Press-through packages of thermoformed PVC (10 tablets per strip). Pack size 100.

**Further information** The therapeutic plasma concentration is 1 to 6 micrograms per ml (3 to 18 micromol per litre), using modern, more specific, HPLC methodology (Sami, M et al, Am J Cardiol 1981; 48: 147-156, Carliner, NH et al. Am Heart J 1980; 100: 483-9).

**Product licence number** 0017/5015R

## LIGNOSTAB* A

**Presentation** Local anaesthetic injections of lidocaine (lignocaine) 2% with adrenaline 1:80,000. A clear sterile aqueous solution for injection supplied in polypropylene cartridges for use with dental type syringes. Each cartridge contains 2.2 ml of solution.

Each ml of solution contains Lidocaine Hydrochloride PhEur 21.3 mg equivalent to lidocaine hydrochloride anhydrous 20.0 mg and Adrenaline BP 12.5 micrograms.

*Inactive ingredients:* Sodium chloride, disodium edetate, sodium metabisulphite, Water for Injections.

Lidocaine is synonymous with lignocaine.

**Uses** Local anaesthetic solution for use mainly in dental procedures.

Lignostab-A contains adrenaline. The effect of vasoconstrictors is to prolong the local anaesthesia by delaying the diffusion of the anaesthetic into the surrounding tissues. If lidocaine without adrenaline is required, Xylocaine 2% Plain should be used.

**Dosage and administration** The dosage is adjusted according to the response of the patient and the site of administration. The lowest concentration and smallest dose producing the required effect should be given. The maximum single dose of lidocaine hydrochloride is 500 mg or 25 ml when given with a vasoconstrictor. This is equivalent to 11.3 cartridges containing 2.2 ml.

Children and elderly or debilitated patients require smaller doses, commensurate with age and physical status.

### Contra-indications, warnings, etc

*Contra-indications:* Known hypersensitivity to anaesthetics of the amide type or the other constituents.

The use of a vasoconstrictor is contra-indicated for anaesthesia of fingers, toes, tip of nose, ears and penis.

Intravenous use.

*Precautions:* As for other local anaesthetics, use cautiously in patients with epilepsy, impaired cardiac conduction, impaired respiratory function and in patients with impaired hepatic function, if the dose or site of administration is likely to result in high blood levels.

Facilities for resuscitation should be available when local anaesthetics are administered.

The effect of local anaesthetics may be reduced if an injection is made into an inflamed or infected area.

Solutions containing a vasoconstrictor should be used with caution in patients with hypertension, cardiac disease, cerebrovascular insufficiency, thyrotoxicosis, in patients taking tricyclic antidepressants, monoamine oxidase inhibitors, or receiving potent general anaesthetic agents.

Solutions containing adrenaline should be used where possible so as to prolong anaesthesia and reduce systemic absorption. This is particularly important in highly vascular areas.

Use on one patient during one treatment only. Discard unused contents.

*Use in pregnancy:* Although this product crosses the placenta, the low doses used in dental anaesthesia would not be expected to give rise to signs of toxicity in the foetus.

*Side-effects:* In common with other local anaesthetics, adverse reactions are rare and are usually the result of excessively high blood concentrations due to inadvertent intravascular injection, excessive dosage, rapid absorption or diminished tolerance on the part of the patient. In such circumstances systemic effects occur involving the central nervous system and/or the cardiovascular system.

CNS reactions are excitatory and/or depressant, and may be characterised by nervousness, dizziness, blurred vision and tremors, followed by drowsiness, convulsions, unconsciousness and possibly respiratory arrest. The excitatory reactions may be very brief or may not occur at all, in which case the first manifestations of toxicity may be drowsiness, merging into unconsciousness and respiratory arrest.

Cardiovascular reactions are depressant, and may be characterised by hypotension, myocardial depression, bradycardia and possibly cardiac arrest.

Allergic reactions are extremely rare. They may be characterised by cutaneous lesions, urticaria, oedema or anaphylactoid reactions. Detection of sensitivity by skin testing is of doubtful value.

Hypotension may occur as a physiological response to central nerve blocks.

*Symptoms and treatment of overdosage:* The injection of excessive amounts of Lignostab-A may, due to the vasoconstrictor, cause ischaemia. This can be followed by a reactive hyperaemia resulting in post extraction bleeding. Respiratory failure may need assisted ventilation. The circulation can be maintained with electrolyte or plasma infusions. Should convulsions develop these can be controlled with diazepam or a short acting barbiturate.

In cases of overdosage with adrenaline containing solutions, intravenous phentolamine and a β-blocker may be required to control blood pressure.

**Pharmaceutical precautions** Store below 25°C.

**Legal category:** POM

**Package quantities:** Boxes of 500 cartridges (polypropylene).

**Further information** Nil

**Product licence numbers** 0017/0257

## LOSEC* CAPSULES 10 mg 20 mg and 40 mg

**Presentation** Losec Capsules 10 mg: hard gelatin capsules with an opaque pink body, marked 10 and an opaque pink cap marked A/OS in black ink. Each capsule contains omeprazole 10 mg as enteric-coated granules, with an aqueous based coating.

Losec Capsules 20 mg: hard gelatin capsules with an opaque pink body, marked 20 and an opaque reddish-brown cap marked A/OM in black ink. Each capsule contains omeprazole 20 mg as enteric-coated granules, with an aqueous based coating.

Losec Capsules 40 mg: hard gelatin capsules with an opaque reddish-brown body, marked 40 and an opaque reddish-brown cap marked A/OL in black ink. Each capsule contains omeprazole 40 mg as enteric-coated granules, with an aqueous based coating.

**Uses** Treatment of oesophageal reflux disease. In reflux oesophagitis the majority of patients are healed after 4 weeks. Symptom relief is rapid.

Treatment of duodenal and benign gastric ulcers including those complicating NSAID therapy.

Relief of reflux-like symptoms (e.g. heartburn) and/or ulcer-like symptoms (e.g. epigastric pain) associated with acid-related dyspepsia.

Treatment and prophylaxis of NSAID-associated benign gastric ulcers, duodenal ulcers, and gastroduodenal erosions in patients with a previous history of gastroduodenal lesions who require continued NSAID treatment.

Relief of associated dyspeptic symptoms.

*Helicobacter pylori* eradication: Omeprazole should be used in combination with antibiotics for eradication of *Helicobacter pylori (Hp)* in peptic ulcer disease.

Relief of associated dyspeptic symptoms.

Prophylaxis of acid aspiration.

Zollinger-Ellison syndrome.

**Dosage and administration** *Oesophageal reflux disease including reflux oesophagitis:* The usual dosage is 20 mg Losec once daily. The majority of patients are healed after 4 weeks. For those patients not fully healed after the initial course, healing usually occurs during a further 4–8 weeks treatment. Losec has also been used in a dose of 40 mg once daily in patients with reflux oesophagitis refractory to other therapy. Healing usually occurred within 8 weeks. Patients can be continued at a dosage of 20 mg once daily.

*Acid reflux disease:* For long-term management Losec 10 mg once daily is recommended, increasing to 20 mg if symptoms return.

*Duodenal and benign gastric ulcers:* The usual dose is 20 mg Losec once daily. The majority of patients with duodenal ulcer are healed after 4 weeks. The majority of patients with benign gastric ulcer are healed after 8 weeks. In severe or recurrent cases the dose may be increased to 40 mg Losec daily. Long-term therapy for patients with a history of recurrent duodenal ulcer is recommended at a dosage of 20 mg Losec once daily.

For prevention of relapse in patients with duodenal ulcer the recommended dose is Losec 10 mg, once daily, increasing to 20 mg, once daily if symptoms return.

The following groups are at risk from recurrent ulcer relapse; those with *Helicobacter pylori* infections; younger patients (<60 years), those whose symptoms persist for more than one year and smokers. These patients will require initial long-term therapy with Losec 20 mg once daily, reducing to 10 mg once daily, if necessary.

*Acid-related dyspepsia:* The usual dosage is Losec 10 mg or 20 once daily for 2–4 weeks depending on the severity and persistence of symptoms. Patients who do not respond after 4 weeks or who relapse shortly afterwards, should be investigate.

*For the treatment of NSAID-associated gastric ulcers, duodenal ulcers or gastroduodenal erosions:* the recommended dosage of Losec is 20 mg once daily. Symptom resolution is rapid and in most patients healing occurs within 4 weeks. For those patients who may not be fully healed after the initial course, healing usually occurs during a further 4 weeks treatment.

*For the prophylaxis of NSAID-associated gastric ulcers, duodenal ulcers, gastroduodenal erosions and dyspeptic symptoms in patients with a previous history of gastroduodenal lesions who require continued NSAID treatment:* the only recommended dosage of Losec is 20 mg once daily.

*Helicobacter pylori (Hp) eradication regimens in peptic ulcer disease:* Losec is recommended at a dose of 40 mg once daily or 20 mg twice daily in association with antimicrobial agents as detailed below:

*Triple therapy regimens in duodenal ulcer disease:* Losec and the following antimicrobial combinations:

Amoxycillin 500 mg and metronidazole 400 mg both three times a day for one week, **or** Clarithromycin 250 mg and metronidazole 400 mg (or tinidazole 500 mg) both twice a day for one week, **or** Amoxycillin 1 g and clarithromycin 500 mg both twice a day for one week.

*Dual therapy regimens in duodenal ulcer disease:* Losec and amoxycillin 750 mg to 1 g twice daily for two weeks. Alternatively Losec and clarithromycin 500 mg three times a day for two weeks.

*Dual therapy regimens in gastric ulcer disease:* Losec and amoxycillin 750 mg to 1 g twice daily for two weeks.

In each regimen if symptoms return and the patient is *Hp* positive therapy may be repeated or one of the alternative regimens can be used: if the patient is *Hp* negative then see dosage instructions for acid reflux disease.

To ensure healing in patients with active peptic ulcer disease, see further dosage recommendations for duodenal and benign gastric ulcer.

*Prophylaxis of acid aspiration:* For patients considered to be at risk of aspiration of the gastric contents during general anaesthesia, the recommended dosage is Losec 40 mg on the evening before surgery followed by Losec 40 mg 2–6 hours prior to surgery.

*Zollinger-Ellison syndrome:* The recommended initial dosage is 60 mg Losec once daily. The dosage should be adjusted individually and treatment continued as long as clinically indicated. More than 90% of patients with severe disease and inadequate response to other therapies have been effectively controlled on doses of 20–120 mg daily. With doses above 80 mg daily, the dose should be divided and given twice daily.

*Elderly:* Dose adjustment is not required in the elderly.

*Children:* There is no experience of the use of Losec in children.

*Impaired renal function:* Dose adjustment is not required in patients with impaired renal function.

*Impaired hepatic function:* As bioavailability and half-life can increase in patients with impaired hepatic function, the dose requires adjustment with a maximum daily dose of 20 mg.

*Patients with swallowing difficulties:* The capsules may be opened and the contents swallowed alone or suspended in a small amount of fruit juice or yoghurt after gentle mixing. Actual capsules may be sucked and then swallowed. It is important that the contents of the capsules should not be crushed or chewed.

### Contra-indications, warnings, etc.

*Contra-indications:* Known hypersensitivity to omeprazole. When gastric ulcer is suspected, the possibility of malignancy should be excluded before treatment with Losec is instituted, as treatment may alleviate symptoms and delay diagnosis.

*Use in pregnancy and lactation:* There is no evidence on the safety of Losec in human pregnancy. Animal studies have revealed no teratogenic effect, but reproduction studies have revealed reduced litter weights. Avoid in pregnancy unless there is no safer alternative.

There is no information available on the passage of Losec into breast milk or its effects on the neonate. Breast feeding should therefore be discontinued if the use of Losec is considered essential.

*Adverse reactions:* Losec is well tolerated and adverse reactions have generally been mild and reversible. The following have been reported as adverse events in clinical trials or reported from routine use but in many cases a relationship to treatment with omeprazole has not been established.

Skin rash, urticaria and pruritus have been reported, usually resolving after discontinuation of treatment. In addition photosensitivity, bullous eruption, erythema multiforme, angioedema and alopecia have been reported in isolated cases.

Diarrhoea and headache have been reported and may be severe enough to require discontinuation of therapy in a small number of patients. In the majority of cases the symptoms resolved after discontinuation of therapy.

Other gastrointestinal reactions have included constipation, nausea/vomiting, flatulence and abdominal pain. Dry mouth, stomatitis and candidiasis have been reported as isolated cases.

Paraesthesia has been reported. Dizziness, light-headedness and feeling faint have been associated with treatment, but all usually resolve on cessation of therapy. Also reported are somnolence, insomnia and vertigo. Reversible mental confusion, agitation, depression and hallucinations have occurred predominantly in severely ill patients.

Arthritic and myalgic symptoms have been reported and have usually resolved when therapy is stopped.

In isolated cases, the following have been reported: blurred vision, taste disturbance, peripheral oedema, increased sweating, gynaecomastia, leucopenia, thrombocytopenia, agranulocytosis, pancytopenia, anaphylactic shock, malaise, fever, bronchospasm, encephalopathy in patients with pre-existing severe liver disease, hepatitis with or without jaundice, rarely interstitial nephritis and hepatic failure.

Increases in liver enzymes have been observed.

*Interactions:* Due to the decreased intragastic acidity the absorption of ketoconazole may be reduced during omeprazole treatment as it is during treatment with other acid secretion inhibitors. As Losec is metabolised in the liver through cytochrome P450 it can delay the elimination of diazepam, phenytoin and warfarin. Monitoring of patients receiving warfarin or phenytoin is recommended and a reduction of warfarin or phenytoin dose may be necessary. However concomitant treatment with Losec 20 mg daily did not change the blood concentration of phenytoin in patients on continuous treatment with phenytoin. Similarly concomitant treatment with Losec 20 mg daily did not change coagulation time in patients on continuous treatment with warfarin. Plasma concentrations of omeprazole and clarithromycin are increased during concomitant administration. This is considered to be a useful interaction during *H. pylori* eradication. There is no evidence of an interaction with phenacetin, theophylline, caffeine, propranolol, metoprolol, cyclosporin, lidocaine, quinidine, estradiol, amoxycillin or antacids. The absorption of Losec is not affected by alcohol or food.

There is no evidence of an interaction with piroxicam, diclofenac or naproxen. This is considered useful when patients are required to continue these treatments.

Simultaneous treatment with omeprazole and digoxin in healthy subjects lead to a 10% increase in the bioavailability of digoxin as a consequence of the increased intragastric pH.

*Animal toxicology:* Gastric ECL-cell hyperplasia and carcinoids have been observed in life-long studies in rats treated with omeprazole or subjected to partial fundectomy. These changes are the result of sustained hypergastrinaemia secondary to acid inhibition, and not from a direct effect of any individual drug.

*Overdosage:* There is no information available on the effects of overdosage in man and specific recommendations for treatment cannot be given. Single oral doses of up to 400 mg have not resulted in any severe symptoms; elimination remained first order and no specific treatment was needed.

**Pharmaceutical precautions** Store below 30°C.

Bottles: Use within three months of opening. Replace cap firmly after use. Dispense in original container.

**Legal category** POM

**Package quantities** Bottles or blisters of 7, 14 or 28 capsules.

**Further information** Losec is a specific inhibitor of the gastric proton pump (H+,K+ ATPase) in the parietal cell. There it produces dose-dependent inhibition of acid secretion by binding to the enzyme, and effectively reduces gastric acid secretion. Oral dosing with 20 mg Losec once daily produces inhibition of gastric acid secretion within 1–2 hours of the first dose. The maximum effect is achieved within 4 days of starting treatment after which the degree of acid inhibition remains constant. The mean decrease in pentagastrin-stimulated peak acid output twenty-four hours after dosing with Losec is about 70%. The inhibition of acid secretion is directly related to the area under the plasma concentration-time curve (AUC) but not to the plasma concentration at any given time.

Clinical data for omeprazole in the prophylaxis of NSAID induced gastroduodenal lesions are derived from studies of up to 6 months duration.

*Helicobacter pylori (Hp)* is associated with acid peptic disease including duodenal ulcer (DU) and gastric ulcer (GU) in which about 95% and 80% of patients respectively are infected with this bacterium. *Hp* is implicated as a major contributing factor in the development of gastritis and ulcers in such patients. Recent evidence also suggests a causative link between *Hp* and gastric carcinoma.

Omeprazole has been shown to have a bactericidal effect on *Hp* in vitro.

Eradication of *Hp* with omeprazole and antimicrobials is associated with rapid symptom relief, high rates of healing of any mucosal lesions, and long-term remission of peptic ulcer disease, thus reducing complications such as gastrointestinal bleeding as well as the need for prolonged anti-secretory treatment.

In recent clinical data in patients with acute peptic ulcer omeprazole *Hp* eradication therapy improved patients' quality of life.

During long-term treatment an increased frequency of gastric glandular cysts have been reported. These changes are a physiological consequence of pronounced inhibition of acid secretion. The cysts are benign and appear to be reversible. No other treatment related mucosal changes have been observed in patients treated continuously with omeprazole for periods up to 5 years.

**Product licence numbers**

| | |
|---|---|
| Losec Capsules 10 mg | 0017/0337 |
| Losec Capsules 20 mg | 0017/0238 |
| Losec Capsules 40 mg | 0017/0320 |

## MARCAIN* WITH ADRENALINE

**Presentation** Clear, colourless, aqueous, sterile solution 0.25%, 0.5% anhydrous bupivacaine HCl with adrenaline.

0.25% Marcain with adrenaline – 10 ml ampoule containing Bupivacaine Hydrochloride BP 2.5 mg/ml corresponding to bupivacaine hydrochloride monohydrate 2.64 mg/ml. Adrenaline Tartrate PhEur 10.0 micrograms/ml corresponding to adrenaline 5.5 micrograms/ml.

0.5% Marcain with adrenaline – 10 ml ampoule containing Bupivacaine Hydrochloride BP 5.0 mg/ml corresponding to bupivacaine hydrochloride monohydrate 5.28 mg/ml. Adrenaline Tartrate PhEur 10.0 micrograms/ml corresponding to adrenaline 5.5 micrograms/ml.

*Inactive ingredients:* All the above solutions contain sodium chloride to produce isotonic solutions. Those containing adrenaline also contain sodium metabisulphite.

**Uses** Marcain 0.25% and 0.5% solutions are used for the production of local anaesthesia by percutaneous infiltration, peripheral nerve block(s) and central neural block (caudal or epidural), that is, for specialist use in situations where prolonged anaesthesia is required. Because sensory nerve block is more marked than motor block, Marcain is especially useful in the relief of pain, e.g. during labour.

A list of indications and the suggested dose and strength of solution appropriate for each are shown in the table overleaf.

**Dosage and administration** The utmost care should be taken to prevent an accidental intravascular injection, always including careful aspiration. For epidural anaesthesia, a test dose of 3–5 ml of bupivacaine containing adrenaline should be administered, since an intravascular injection of adrenaline will be quickly recognised by an increase in heart rate. Verbal contact and repeated measurement of heart rate should be maintained throughout a period of 5 minutes following the test dose. Aspiration should be repeated prior to administration of the total dose. The main dose should be injected slowly, *25–50 mg/min*, in incremental doses under constant contact with the patient. If mild toxic symptoms occur, the injection should be stopped immediately.

The dosage varies and depends upon the area to be anaesthetised, the vascularity of the tissues, the number of neuronal segments to be blocked, individual tolerance and the technique of anaesthesia used. The lowest dosage needed to provide effective anaesthesia should be administered. For most indications, the duration of anaesthesia with Marcain solutions is such that a single dose is sufficient.

The maximum dosage must be determined by evaluating the size and physical status of the patient and considering the usual rate of systemic absorption from a particular injection site. Experience to date indicates a single dose of up to 150 mg bupivacaine hydrochloride. Doses of up to 50 mg 2-hourly may subsequently be used. The dosages in the following table are recommended as a guide for use in the average adult. For young, elderly or debilitated patients, these doses should be reduced.

**Contra-indications, warnings, etc** Bupivacaine hydrochloride solutions are contra-indicated in patients with a known hypersensitivity to local anaesthetic agents of the amide type or to other components of the injectable formulation.

Solutions of bupivacaine hydrochloride are contra-indicated for intravenous regional anaesthesia (Bier's-block).

Solutions containing adrenaline are contra-indicated in patients with thyrotoxicosis or severe heart disease, particularly when tachycardia is present.

Solutions of bupivacaine hydrochloride with adrenaline should not be used in connection with anaesthesia in areas of the body supplied by end arteries or otherwise having a compromised blood supply such as digits, nose, external ear, penis, etc.

Epidural anaesthesia, regardless of the local anaesthetic used, has its own contra-indications which include: Active disease of the central nervous system such as meningitis, poliomyelitis, intracranial haemorrhage, sub-acute combined degeneration of the cord due to pernicious anaemia and cerebral and spinal tumours. Tuberculosis of the spine. Pyogenic infection of the skin at or adjacent to the site of lumbar puncture. Cardiogenic or hypovolaemic shock. Coagulation disorders or ongoing anticoagulation treatment.

*Precautions:* There have been reports of cardiac arrest with difficult resuscitation or death during use of bupivacaine for epidural anaesthesia in obstetrical patients. In most cases, this has followed use of the 0.75% concentration. Resuscitation has been difficult or impossible despite apparently adequate preparation and appropriate management. Cardiac arrest has occurred after convulsions resulting from systemic toxicity, presumably following unintentional intravascular injection. The 0.75% concentration should be reserved for surgical procedures where a high degree of muscle relaxation and prolonged effect are necessary.

Epidural blockade and large nerve plexus blocks should only be employed by those with the necessary training and experience.

Adequate resuscitation equipment should be available whenever local or general anaesthesia is administered. Overdosage or accidental intravenous injection may give rise to toxic reactions.

Injection of repeated doses of bupivacaine hydrochloride may cause significant increases in blood levels with each repeated dose due to slow accumulation of the drug. Tolerance varies with the status of the patient. Debilitated, elderly or acutely ill patients should be given reduced doses commensurate with their physical status.

Only in rare cases have amide local anaesthetics been associated with allergic reactions (in most severe instances anaphylactic shock).

Patients allergic to ester-type local anaesthetic drugs (procaine, tetracaine, benzocaine, etc.) have not shown cross-sensitivity to agents of the amide type such as bupivacaine.

Local anaesthetics should be used with caution for epidural anaesthesia in patients with impaired cardiovascular function since they may be less able to compensate for functional changes associated with the prolongation of A-V conduction produced by these drugs.

Since bupivacaine is metabolised in the liver, it should be used cautiously in patients with liver disease or with reduced liver blood flow.

Epidural anaesthesia with any local anaesthetic can cause hypotension and bradycardia which should be anticipated and appropriate precautions taken. These may include pre-loading the circulation with crystalloid or colloid solution. If hypotension develops it should be treated with a vasopressor such as ephedrine 10–15 mg intravenously. Severe hypotension may result from hypovolaemia due to haemorrhage or dehydration, or aorto-caval occlusion in patients with massive ascites, large abdominal tumours or late pregnancy. Marked hypotension should be avoided in patients with cardiac decompensation.

Patients with hypovolaemia due to any cause can develop sudden and severe hypotension during epidural anaesthesia.

Epidural anaesthesia can cause intercostal paralysis and patients with pleural effusions may suffer respiratory embarrassment. Septicaemia can increase the risk of intraspinal abscess formation in the postoperative period.

Paracervical block may have a greater adverse effect on the foetus than other nerve blocks used in obstetrics. Due to the systemic toxicity of bupivacaine special care should be taken when using bupivacaine for paracervical block.

Small doses of local anaesthetics injected into the head and neck, including retrobulbar, dental and stellate ganglion blocks, may produce systemic toxicity due to inadvertent intra-arterial injection.

Clinicians who perform retrobulbar blocks should be aware that there have been reports of respiratory arrest following local anaesthetic injection. Prior to retrobulbar block, necessary equipment, drugs and personnel should be immediately available as with all other regional procedures.

Solutions containing adrenaline should be used with caution in patients with hypertension, arteriosclerotic heart disease, cerebrovascular insufficiency or diabetes.

*Drug interactions:* Bupivacaine should be used with care in patients receiving anti-arrhythmic drugs with local anaesthetic activity, e.g. lidocaine, since their toxic effects may be additive.

Solutions containing adrenaline should be used with caution in those patients receiving drugs known to produce blood pressure alterations, i.e. MAO inhibitors, tricyclic antidepressants, phenothiazines, etc., as severe and sustained hypotension or hypertension may occur.

Serious cardiac arrhythmias may occur if preparations containing a vasoconstrictor drug are employed in patients during or following the administration of chloroform, halothane, cyclopropane, trichlorethylene or other related agents.

*Pregnancy and lactation:* Bupivacaine enters the mother's milk, but in such small quantities that there is no risk of affecting the child at therapeutic dose levels.

There is no evidence of untoward effects in human pregnancy. In large doses there is evidence of decreased pup survival in rats and an embryological effect in rabbits if Marcain is administered in pregnancy. Marcain should not therefore be given in early pregnancy unless the benefits are considered to outweigh the risks.

*Side-effects:* Serious systemic adverse reactions are rare, but may occur in connection with overdosage or unintentional intravascular injection.

Bupivacaine causes systemic toxicity similar to that observed with other local anaesthetic agents. It is caused by high plasma concentrations as a result of excessive dosage, rapid absorption or, most commonly, inadvertent intravascular injection. Pronounced acidosis or hypoxia may increase the risk and severity of toxic reactions. Such reactions involve the central nervous system and the cardiovascular system. CNS reactions are characterised by numbness of the tongue, light-headedness, dizziness, blurred vision and muscle twitch, followed by drowsiness, convulsions, unconsciousness and possibly respiratory arrest.

Cardiovascular reactions are related to depression of the conduction system of the heart and myocardium leading to decreased cardiac output, heart block, hypotension, bradycardia and sometimes ventricular arrhythmias, including ventricular tachycardia, ventricular fibrillation and cardiac arrest. Usually these will be preceded or accompanied by major CNS toxicity, i.e. convulsions, but in rare cases cardiac arrest has occurred without prodromal CNS effects.

Epidural anaesthesia itself can cause adverse reactions regardless of the local anaesthetic agent used. These include hypotension and bradycardia due to sympathetic blockade and/or vasovagal fainting.

In severe cases cardiac arrest may occur.

Accidental sub-arachnoid injection can lead to very high spinal anaesthesia possibly with apnoea and severe hypotension.

Neurological damage is a rare but well recognised consequence of regional and particularly epidural and spinal anaesthesia. It may be due to several causes, e.g. direct injury to the spinal cord or spinal nerves, anterior spinal artery syndrome, injection of an irritant substance, or an injection of a non-sterile solution. These may result in localised areas of paraesthesia or anaesthesia, motor weakness, loss of sphincter control and paraplegia. Occasionally these are permanent.

*Treatment of side-effects:* Treatment of a patient with systemic toxicity consists of arresting convulsions and ensuring adequate ventilation with oxygen, if necessary by assisted or controlled ventilation (respiration). If convulsions occur they must be treated promptly by intravenous injection of thiopentone 100 to 200 mg or diazepam 5 to 10 mg. Alternatively succinylcholine 50 mg–100 mg i.v. may be used providing the clinician is capable of performing endotracheal intubation and managing a fully paralysed patient.

Once convulsions have been controlled and adequate ventilation of the lungs ensured, no other treatment is generally required. If hypotension is present, however, a vasopressor, preferably one with inotropic activity, e.g. ephedrine 15 to 30 mg, should be given intravenously.

Cardiac arrest due to bupivacaine can be resistant to electrical defibrillation and resuscitation must be continued energetically for a prolonged period.

High or total spinal blockade causing respiratory paralysis and hypotension during epidural anaesthesia should be treated by ensuring and maintaining a patent airway and giving oxygen by assisted or controlled ventilation.

Hypotension should be treated by the use of vasopressors, e.g. ephedrine 10–15 mg intravenously and repeated until the desired level of arterial pressure is reached. Intravenous fluids, both electrolytes and colloids, given rapidly can also reverse hypotension.

**Pharmaceutical precautions** Store below 25°C.

**Legal category** POM

**Package quantities**

0.25% Marcain with adrenaline 10×10 ml Steripack sterile wrapped ampoules.

0.5% Marcain with adrenaline 10×10 ml Steripack sterile wrapped ampoules.

**Further information** Nil

**Product licence numbers**

0.25% with adrenaline 0017/0118

0.5% with adrenaline 0017/0119

| *Type of block* | % Conc | Each dose ml | Each dose mg | Motor block† |
|---|---|---|---|---|
| *Local infiltration* | 0.25 | up to 60 | up to 150 | – |
| *Lumbar epidural* | | | | |
| Surgical operations | 0.50 | 10 to 20 | 50 to 100 | Moderate to complete |
| | 0.75 | 10 to 20 | 75 to 150 | Complete |
| Analgesia in labour | 0.50 | 6 to 12 | 30 to 60 | Moderate to complete |
| | 0.25 | 6 to 12 | 15 to 30 | Minimal |
| *Caudal epidural* | | | | |
| Surgical operations | 0.50 | 15 to 30 | 75 to 150 | Moderate to complete |
| Children (aged up to 10yrs): | | | | |
| Up to lower thoracic (T10) | 0.25 | 0.3–0.4 ml/kg | 0.75–1.0 mg/kg | |
| Up to mid thoracic (T6) | 0.25 | 0.4–0.6 ml/kg | 1.0–1.5 mg/kg | |
| If total amount greater than 20 ml reduce concentration to 0.2% | | | | |
| Analgesia in labour | 0.50 | 10 to 20 | 50 to 100 | Moderate to complete |
| | 0.25 | 10 to 20 | 25 to 50 | Moderate |
| *Peripheral Nerves* | 0.50 | up to 30 | up to 150 | Moderate to complete |
| | 0.25 | up to 60 | up to 150 | Slight to moderate |
| *Sympathetic blocks* | 0.25 | 20 to 50 | 50 to 125 | |

† With continuous (intermittent) techniques, repeat doses increase the degree of motor block. The first repeat dose of 0.5% may produce complete motor block for intra-abdominal surgery.

# MARCAIN* HEAVY

**Presentation** Clear, colourless solution containing Bupivacaine Hydrochloride BP 5.28 mg/ml equivalent to bupivacaine hydrochloride anhydrous 5 mg per ml, Dextrose Anhydrous PhEur 72.7 mg/ml equivalent to dextrose monohydrate 80 mg/ml. The specific gravity of the solution is 1.026 at 20°C.

*Inactive ingredients:* Sodium hydroxide and water.

**Uses** Spinal anaesthesia for surgery (urological and lower limb surgery lasting 2–3 hours, abdominal surgery lasting 45–60 minutes). Bupivacaine is a long acting local anaesthetic agent of the amide type. Marcain Heavy has rapid onset of action and long duration. The duration of analgesia in the T10–T12 segments is 2–3 hours.

Marcain Heavy produces a moderate muscular relaxation of the lower extremities lasting 2–2.5 hours. The motor blockade of the abdominal muscles makes the solution suitable for performance of abdominal surgery lasting 45–60 minutes. The duration of motor blockade does not exceed the duration of analgesia. The cardiovascular effects of Marcain Heavy are similar or less than those seen with other spinal agents. Bupivacaine 5 mg/ml with glucose 80 mg/ml is exceptionally well tolerated by all tissues with which it comes in contact.

**Dosage and administration** The doses recommended below should be regarded as a guide for use in the average adult.

*Spinal anaesthesia for surgery:* 2–4 ml (10–20 mg bupivacaine hydrochloride).

The spread of anaesthesia obtained with Marcain Heavy depends on several factors, including the volume of solution and the position of the patient during and following the injection. When injected at the L3-L4 intervertebral space with the patient in the sitting position, 3 ml of Marcain Heavy spreads to the T7-T10 spinal segments. With the patient receiving the injection in the horizontal position and then turned supine, the blockade spreads to T4-T7 spinal segments. It should be understood that the level of spinal anaesthesia achieved with any local anaesthetic can be unpredictable in a given patient.

The effects of injections of Marcain Heavy exceeding 4 ml have not yet been studied and such volumes can therefore not be recommended.

**Contra-indications, warnings, etc**
*Contra-indications:* Known hypersensitivity to local anaesthetics of the amide type.

Spinal anaesthesia, regardless of the local anaesthetic used, has its own contra-indications which include: Active disease of the central nervous system such as meningitis, poliomyelitis, intracranial haemorrhage, sub-acute combined degeneration of the cord due to pernicious anaemia and cerebral and spinal tumours. Tuberculosis of the spine. Pyogenic infection of the skin at or adjacent to the site of lumbar puncture. Cardiogenic or hypovolaemic shock. Coagulation disorders or ongoing anticoagulation treatment.

*Precautions:* Spinal anaesthesia should only be undertaken by clinicians with the necessary knowledge and experience. Resuscitative equipment and drugs should be immediately available and the anaesthetist should remain in constant attendance. Spinal anaesthesia with any local anaesthetic can cause hypotension and bradycardia which should be anticipated and appropriate precautions taken. These may include pre-loading the circulation with crystalloid or colloid solution. If hypotension develops it should be treated with a vasopressor such as ephedrine 10–15 mg intravenously. Severe hypotension may result from hypovolaemia due to haemorrhage or dehydration, or aorto-caval occlusion in patients with massive ascites, large abdominal tumours or late pregnancy. Marked hypotension should be avoided in patients with cardiac decompensation.

Patients with hypovolaemia due to any cause can develop sudden and severe hypotension during spinal anaesthesia.

Spinal anaesthesia can cause intercostal paralysis and patients with pleural effusions may suffer respiratory embarrassment. Septicaemia can increase the risk of intraspinal abscess formation in the postoperative period.

*Pregnancy and lactation:* Bupivacaine enters the mother's milk but in such small quantities that there is generally no risk of affecting the child at therapeutic dose levels.

There is no evidence of untoward effects in human pregnancy. In large doses there is evidence of decreased pup survival in rats and an embryological effect in rabbits if Marcain is administered in pregnancy. Marcain should not therefore be given in early pregnancy unless the benefits are considered to outweigh the risks.

*Drug interactions:* Bupivacaine should be used with care in patients receiving antiarrhythmic drugs with local anaesthetic activity, as their toxic effects may be additive.

*Side-effects:* The safety of Marcain Heavy is comparable to that of other local anaesthetics used for spinal anaesthesia.

In rare cases bupivacaine has been associated with allergic reactions and anaphylactic shock.

Spinal anaesthesia itself can cause adverse reactions regardless of the local anaesthetic agent used. These include hypotension and bradycardia due to sympathetic blockade and/or vasovagal fainting.

In severe cases cardiac arrest can occur.

High spinal anaesthesia may result in paralysis of all respiratory muscles.

Postoperatively a post lumbar puncture headache can occur.

Neurological damage is a rare but well recognised consequence of regional and particularly spinal anaesthesia. It may be due to several causes, e.g. direct injury to the spinal cord or spinal nerves, anterior spinal artery syndrome, injection of an irritant substance, or an injection of a non-sterile solution. These may result in localised areas of paraesthesia or anaesthesia, motor weakness, loss of sphincter control and paraplegia. Occasionally these are permanent. Neurological complications of this type have been reported after the use of all local anaesthetics used for spinal anaesthesia.

Systemic toxicity is rarely associated with spinal anaesthesia but might occur after accidental intravascular injection. Systemic adverse reactions are characterised by numbness of the tongue, lightheadedness, dizziness and tremors, followed by convulsions and cardiovascular disorders.

*Treatment of side-effects:* High or total spinal blockade causing respiratory paralysis should be treated by ensuring and maintaining a patent airway and giving oxygen by assisted or controlled ventilation.

Hypotension should be treated by the use of vasopressors, e.g. ephedrine 10–15 mg intravenously and repeated until the desired level of arterial pressure is reached. Intravenous fluids, both electrolytes and colloids, given rapidly can also reverse hypotension.

*Treatment of systemic toxicity:* No treatment is required for milder symptoms of systemic toxicity but if convulsions occur then it is important to ensure adequate oxygenation and to arrest the convulsions if they last more than 15–30 seconds. Oxygen should be given by face mask and the respiration assisted or controlled if necessary. Convulsions can be arrested by injection of thiopentone 100–150 mg intravenously or with diazepam 5–10 mg intravenously. Alternatively, succinylcholine 50–100 mg intravenously may be given but only if the clinician has the ability to perform endotracheal intubation and to manage a totally paralysed patient.

**Pharmaceutical precautions** The solution must not be stored in contact with metals, e.g. needles or metal parts of syringes, as dissolved metal ions may cause swelling at the site of the injection.

The solution should be used immediately after opening of the ampoule. Any remaining solution should be discarded.

Store below 25°C.

**Legal category** POM

**Package quantities** Sterile wrapped ampoules 5×4 ml.

**Further information** Nil

**Product licence number** PL0017/0139

# MARCAIN* POLYAMP* STERIPACK*

**Presentation** Clear, colourless, aqueous, sterile solution 0.25%, 0.375%, 0.5% and 0.75% anhydrous bupivacaine hydrochloride.

0.25% Marcain – 10 ml polyamps containing Bupivacaine Hydrochloride BP 2.64 mg/ml.

0.375% Marcain – 10 ml polyamps containing Bupivacaine Hydrochloride BP 3.96 mg/ml.

0.5% Marcain – 10 ml polyamps containing Bupivacaine Hydrochloride BP 5.28 mg/ml.

0.75% Marcain – 10 ml polyamps containing Bupivacaine Hydrochloride BP 7.92 mg/ml.

**Uses** Marcain 0.25%, 0.375% and 0.5% solutions are used for the production of local anaesthesia by percutaneous infiltration, peripheral nerve block(s) and central neural block (caudal or epidural), that is, for specialist use in situations where prolonged anaesthesia is required. Because sensory nerve block is more marked than motor block, Marcain is especially useful in the relief of pain, e.g. during labour.

A list of indications and the suggested dose and strength of solution appropriate for each are shown in the table overleaf.

Marcain 0.75% solution produces a more prolonged motor block than 0.25%, 0.375% or 0.5% solutions and

is, therefore, recommended for epidural anaesthesia for surgical purposes. Epidural anaesthesia is usually maintained for 3 to 4 hours.

**Dosage and administration** The utmost care should be taken to prevent an accidental intravascular injection, always including careful aspiration. For epidural anaesthesia, a test dose of 3–5 ml of bupivacaine containing adrenaline should be administered, since an intravascular injection of adrenaline will be quickly recognised by an increase in heart rate. Verbal contact and repeated measurement of heart rate should be maintained throughout a period of 5 minutes following the test dose. Aspiration should be repeated prior to administration of the total dose. The main dose should be injected slowly, 25–50 mg/min, in incremental doses under constant contact with the patient. If mild toxic symptoms occur, the injection should be stopped immediately.

The dosage varies and depends upon the area to be anaesthetised, the vascularity of the tissues, the number of neuronal segments to be blocked, individual tolerance and the technique of anaesthesia used. The lowest dosage needed to provide effective anaesthesia should be administered. For most indications, the duration of anaesthesia with Marcain solutions is such that a single dose is sufficient.

The maximum dosage must be determined by evaluating the size and physical status of the patient and considering the usual rate of systemic absorption from a particular injection site. Experience to date indicates a single dose of up to 150 mg bupivacaine hydrochloride. Doses of up to 50 mg 2-hourly may subsequently be used. The dosages in the table below are recommended as a guide for use in the average adult. For young, elderly or debilitated patients, these doses should be reduced.

**Contra-indications, warnings, etc.**
*Contra-indications:* Bupivacaine hydrochloride solutions are contra-indicated in patients with a known hypersensitivity to local anaesthetic agents of the amide type or to other components of the injectable formulation.

Solutions of bupivacaine hydrochloride are contra-indicated for intravenous regional anaesthesia (Bier's-block).

0.75% solution is contra-indicated for epidural use in obstetrics.

Epidural anaesthesia, regardless of the local anaesthetic used, has its own contra-indications which include: Active disease of the central nervous system such as meningitis, poliomyelitis, intracranial haemorrhage, sub-acute combined degeneration of the cord due to pernicious anaemia and cerebral and spinal tumours. Tuberculosis of the spine. Pyogenic infection of the skin at or adjacent to the site of lumbar puncture. Cardiogenic or hypovolaemic shock. Coagulation disorders or ongoing anticoagulation treatment.

*Precautions:* There have been reports of cardiac arrest with difficult resuscitation or death during use of bupivacaine for epidural anaesthesia in obstetrical patients. In most cases, this has followed use of the 0.75% concentration. Resuscitation has been difficult or impossible despite apparently adequate preparation and appropriate management. Cardiac arrest has occurred after convulsions resulting from systemic toxicity, presumably following unintentional intravascular injection. The 0.75% concentration should be reserved for surgical procedures where a high degree of muscle relaxation and prolonged effect are necessary.

Epidural blockade and large nerve plexus blocks should only be employed by those with the necessary training and experience.

Adequate resuscitation equipment should be available whenever local or general anaesthesia is administered. Overdosage or accidental intravenous injection may give rise to toxic reactions.

Injection of repeated doses of bupivacaine hydrochloride may cause significant increases in blood levels with each repeated dose due to slow accumulation of the drug. Tolerance varies with the status of the patient. Debilitated, elderly or acutely ill patients should be given reduced doses commensurate with their physical status.

Only in rare cases have amide local anaesthetics been associated with allergic reactions (in most severe instances anaphylactic shock).

Patients allergic to ester-type local anaesthetic drugs (procaine, tetracaine, benzocaine, etc.) have not shown cross-sensitivity to agents of the amide type such as bupivacaine.

Local anaesthetics should be used with caution for epidural anaesthesia in patients with impaired cardiovascular function since they may be less able to compensate for functional changes associated with the prolongation of A-V conduction produced by these drugs.

Since bupivacaine is metabolised in the liver, it should be used cautiously in patients with liver disease or with reduced liver blood flow.

| Type of block | % Conc | Each dose | | Motor block† |
|---|---|---|---|---|
| | | ml | mg | |
| Local infiltration | 0.25 | up to 60 | up to 150 | – |
| **Lumbar epidural** | | | | |
| Surgical | 0.50 | 10 to 20 | 50 to 100 | Moderate to complete |
| operations | 0.75 | 10 to 20 | 75 to 150 | Complete |
| Analgesia | 0.50 | 6 to 12 | 30 to 60 | Moderate to complete |
| in labour | 0.375 | 6 to 12 | 22.5 to 45 | Moderate to minimal |
| | 0.25 | 6 to 12 | 15 to 30 | Minimal |
| **Caudal epidural** | | | | |
| Surgical operations | 0.50 | 15 to 30 | 75 to 150 | Moderate to complete |
| Children (aged up to 10yrs): | | | | |
| Up to lower thoracic (T10) | 0.25 | 0.3–0.4 ml/kg | 0.75–1.0 mg/kg | |
| Up to mid-thoracic (T6) | 0.25 | 0.4–0.6 ml/kg | 1.0–1.5 mg/kg | |
| If total amount greater than 20 ml reduce concentration to 0.2% | | | | |
| Analgesia | 0.50 | 10 to 20 | 50 to 100 | Moderate to complete |
| in labour | 0.375 | 10 to 20 | 37.5 to 75 | Moderate |
| | 0.25 | 10 to 20 | 25 to 50 | Moderate |
| **Peripheral Nerves** | 0.50 | up to 30 | up to 150 | Moderate to complete |
| | 0.375 | up to 40 | up to 150 | Moderate |
| | 0.25 | up to 60 | up to 150 | Slight to moderate |
| Sympathetic blocks | 0.25 | 20 to 50 | 50 to 125 | – |

† With continuous (intermittent) techniques, repeat doses increase the degree of motor block. The first repeat dose of 0.5% may produce complete motor block for intra-abdominal surgery.

Epidural anaesthesia with any local anaesthetic can cause hypotension and bradycardia which should be anticipated and appropriate precautions taken. These may include pre-loading the circulation with crystalloid or colloid solution. If hypotension develops it should be treated with a vasopressor such as ephedrine 10–15 mg intravenously. Severe hypotension may result from hypovolaemia due to haemorrhage or dehydration, or aorto-caval occlusion in patients with massive ascites, large abdominal tumours or late pregnancy. Marked hypotension should be avoided in patients with cardiac decompensation.

Patients with hypovolaemia due to any cause can develop sudden and severe hypotension during epidural anaesthesia.

Epidural anaesthesia can cause intercostal paralysis and patients with pleural effusions may suffer respiratory embarrassment. Septicaemia can increase the risk of intraspinal abscess formation in the postoperative period.

Paracervical block may have a greater adverse effect on the foetus than other nerve blocks used in obstetrics. Due to the systemic toxicity of bupivacaine special care should be taken when using bupivacaine for paracervical block.

Small doses of local anaesthetics injected into the head and neck, including retrobulbar, dental and stellate ganglion blocks, may produce systemic toxicity due to inadvertent intra-arterial injection.

Clinicians who perform retrobulbar blocks should be aware that there have been reports of respiratory arrest following local anaesthetic injection. Prior to retrobulbar block, necessary equipment, drugs and personnel should be immediately available as with all other regional procedures.

*Drug interactions:* Bupivacaine should be used with care in patients receiving anti-arrhythmic drugs with local anaesthetic activity, e.g. lidocaine, since their toxic effects may be additive.

Serious cardiac arrhythmias may occur if preparations containing a vasoconstrictor drug are employed in patients during or following the administration of chloroform, halothane, cyclopropane, trichlorethylene or other related agents.

*Pregnancy and lactation:* Bupivacaine enters the mother's milk, but in such small quantities that there is no risk of affecting the child at therapeutic dose levels.

There is no evidence of untoward effects in human pregnancy. In large doses there is evidence of decreased pup survival in rats and an embryological effect in rabbits if Marcain is administered in pregnancy. Marcain should not therefore be given in early pregnancy unless the benefits are considered to outweigh the risks.

*Side-effects:* Serious systemic adverse reactions are rare, but may occur in connection with overdosage or unintentional intravascular injection.

Bupivacaine causes systemic toxicity similar to that observed with other local anaesthetic agents. It is caused by high plasma concentrations as a result of excessive dosage, rapid absorption or, most commonly, inadvertent intravascular injection. Pronounced acidosis or hypoxia may increase the risk and severity of toxic reactions. Such reactions involve the central nervous system and the cardiovascular system. CNS reactions are characterised by numbness of the tongue, light-headedness, dizziness, blurred vision and muscle twitch, followed by drowsiness, convulsions, unconsciousness and possibly respiratory arrest.

Cardiovascular reactions are related to depression of the conduction system of the heart and myocardium leading to decreased cardiac output, heart block, hypotension, bradycardia and sometimes ventricular arrhythmias, including ventricular tachycardia, ventricular fibrillation and cardiac arrest. Usually these will be preceded or accompanied by major CNS toxicity, i.e. convulsions, but in rare cases cardiac arrest has occurred without prodromal CNS effects.

Epidural anaesthesia itself can cause adverse reactions regardless of the local anaesthetic agent used. These include hypotension and bradycardia due to sympathetic blockade and/or vasovagal fainting. In severe cases cardiac arrest may occur.

Accidental sub-arachnoid injection can lead to very high spinal anaesthesia possibly with apnoea and severe hypotension.

Neurological damage is a rare but well recognised consequence of regional and particularly epidural and spinal anaesthesia. It may be due to several causes, e.g. direct injury to the spinal cord or spinal nerves, anterior spinal artery syndrome, injection of an irritant substance, or an injection of a non-sterile solution. These may result in localised areas of paraesthesia or anaesthesia, motor weakness, loss of sphincter control and paraplegia. Occasionally these are permanent.

*Treatment of side-effects:* Treatment of a patient with systemic toxicity consists of arresting convulsions and ensuring adequate ventilation with oxygen, if necessary by assisted or controlled ventilation (respiration). If convulsions occur they must be treated promptly by intravenous injection of thiopentone 100 to 200 mg or diazepam 5 to 10 mg. Alternatively succinylcholine 50 mg–100 mg i.v. may be used providing the clinician is capable of performing endotracheal intubation and managing a fully paralysed patient.

Once convulsions have been controlled and adequate ventilation of the lungs ensured, no other treatment is generally required. If hypotension is present, however, a vasopressor, preferably one with inotropic activity, e.g. ephedrine 15 to 30 mg, should be given intravenously.

Cardiac arrest due to bupivacaine can be resistant to electrical defibrillation and resuscitation must be continued energetically for a prolonged period.

High or total spinal blockade causing respiratory paralysis and hypotension during epidural anaesthesia should be treated by ensuring and maintaining a patent airway and giving oxygen by assisted or controlled ventilation.

Hypotension should be treated by the use of vasopressors, e.g. ephedrine 10–15 mg intravenously and repeated until the desired level of arterial pressure is reached. Intravenous fluids, both electrolytes and colloids, given rapidly can also reverse hypotension.

**Pharmaceutical precautions** Store below 30°C. For single use only. Discard any unused solution.

**Legal category** POM

**Package quantities**
0.25% Marcain 10×10 ml Steripack sterile wrapped Polyamps.
0.375% Marcain 10 x 10 ml Steripack sterile wrapped Polyamps.
0.5% Marcain 10×10 ml Steripack sterile wrapped Polyamps.

0.75% Marcain 10×10 ml Steripack sterile wrapped Polyamps.

**Further information** Nil

**Product licence numbers**
| | |
|---|---|
| 0.25% | 0017/0305 |
| 0.375% | 0017/0306 |
| 0.5% | 0017/0307 |
| 0.75% | 0017/0308 |

# NAROPIN* POLYAMP* 2 mg/ml, 7.5 mg/ml and 10 mg/ml ▼
# NAROPIN* INFUSION 2 mg/ml ▼

**Qualitative and quantitative composition** Ropivacaine hydrochloride monohydrate

Molecular formula
$C_{17}H_{26}N_2O*HCl*H_2O$
m.w.:328.9

Naropin 2 mg/ml: 2 mg/ml ropivacaine hydrochloride
Naropin 7.5 mg/ml: 7.5 mg/ml ropivacaine hydrochloride
Naropin 10 mg/ml: 10 mg/ml ropivacaine hydrochloride

**Pharmaceutical form** Solution for injection for perineural and epidural administration (10–20 ml).
Solution for epidural infusion (100 and 200 ml).

**Clinical particulars**
*Therapeutic indications:* Naropin is indicated for:
1. *Surgical anaesthesia:*
   Epidural blocks for surgery, including Caesarean section.
   Field blocks.
2. *Acute pain management:*
   Continuous epidural infusion or intermittent bolus administration during postoperative or labour pain.
   Field blocks.

*Posology and method of administration:* Naropin should only be used by, or under the supervision of, clinicians experienced in regional anaesthesia.
*Posology:* The table below is a guide to dosage for the more commonly used blocks. The smallest dose required to produce an effective block should be used. The clinician's experience and knowledge of the patient's physical status are of importance when deciding the dose.

In general, surgical anaesthesia (e.g. epidural administration) requires the use of the higher concentrations and doses. Naropin 10 mg/ml is recommended for epidural anaesthesia in which a profound motor block is essential for surgery. For analgesia (e.g. epidural administration for acute pain management) the lower concentrations and doses are recommended.

*Method of administration:* Careful aspiration before and during injection is recommended to prevent intravascular injection. When a large dose is to be injected, e.g. in epidural block, a test dose of 3-5 ml lidocaine (lignocaine) with adrenaline (Xylocaine* 2% with Adrenaline 1:200,000) is recommended. An inadvertent intravascular injection may be recognised by a temporary increase in heart rate and an accidental intrathecal injection by signs of a spinal block.

Aspiration should be repeated prior to and during administration of the main dose, which should be injected slowly or in incremental doses, at a rate of 25-50 mg/min, while closely observing the patient's vital functions and maintaining verbal contact. If toxic symptoms occur, the injection should be stopped immediately.

In epidural block for surgery, single doses of up to 250 mg ropivacaine have been used and well tolerated.

When prolonged blocks are used, either through continuous epidural infusion or through repeated bolus administration, the risks of reaching a toxic plasma concentration or inducing local neural injury must be considered. Experience to date indicates that a cumulative dose of up to 675 mg ropivacaine administered over 24 hours is well tolerated in adults. In a limited number of patients higher doses of up to 800 mg/day have been administered with relatively few adverse reactions. However higher doses may be associated with an increased risk of adverse reactions.

For treatment of postoperative pain, the following technique can be recommended: Unless preoperatively instituted, an epidural block with Naropin 7.5 mg/ml is induced via an epidural catheter. Analgesia is maintained with Naropin 2 mg/ml infusion. Infusion rates of 6-10 ml (12-20 mg) per hour provide

| | Conc. mg/ml | Volume ml | Dose mg | Onset minutes | Duration hours |
|---|---|---|---|---|---|
| SURGICAL ANAESTHESIA | | | | | |
| **Lumbar Epidural Administration** | | | | | |
| Surgery | 7.5 | 15–25 | 113–188 | 10–20 | 3–5 |
| | 10 | 15–20 | 150–200 | 10–20 | 4–6 |
| Caesarean Section | 7.5 | 15–20 | 113–150(1) | 10–20 | 3–5 |
| **Thoracic Epidural Administration** | | | | | |
| To establish block for post-operative pain relief | 7.5 | 5–15 (depending on the level of injection) | 38–113 | 10–20 | n/a(2) |
| **Field Block** (e.g. minor nerve blocks and infiltration) | 7.5 | 1–30 | 7.5–225 | 1–15 | 2–6 |
| ACUTE PAIN MANAGEMENT | | | | | |
| **Lumbar Epidural Administration** | | | | | |
| Bolus | 2 | 10–20 | 20–40 | 10–15 | 0.5–1.5 |
| Intermittent injections (top up) (e.g. labour pain management) | 2 | 10–15 (minimum interval 30 mins) | 20–30 | | |
| Continuous infusion (labour pain and postoperative pain management) | 2 | 6–10 ml/h | 12–20 mg/h | n/a(2) | n/a(2) |
| **Thoracic Epidural Administration** | | | | | |
| Continuous infusion (postoperative pain management) | 2 | 4–8 ml/h | 8–16 mg/h | n/a(2) | n/a(2) |
| **Field Block** (e.g. minor nerve blocks and infiltration) | 2 | 1–100 | 2–200 | 1–5 | 2–6 |

The doses in the table are those considered to be necessary to produce a successful block and should be regarded as guidelines for use in adults. Individual variations in onset and duration occur. The figures in the column 'Dose' reflect the expected average dose range needed. For other local anaesthetic techniques standard textbooks should be consulted.

(1) Incremental dosing should be applied, the starting dose of about 100 mg (97.5 mg = 13 ml; 105 mg = 14 ml) to be given over 3–5 minutes. Two additional doses, each of 25 mg, may be administered as needed. The total administered dose should not exceed 150 mg.

(2) n/a = not applicable

adequate analgesia with only slight and non-progressive motor block in most cases of moderate to severe postoperative pain. If some patients do not react adequately, higher doses with an infusion rate of up to 12-14 ml (24-28 mg ropivacaine) per hour may be used.

With this technique a significant reduction in the need for opioids has been observed. Clinical experience supports the use of Naropin epidural infusions for up to 24 hours.

Concentrations above 7.5 mg/ml Naropin have not been documented for Caesarean section.

*Contra-indications:* Naropin solutions are contra-indicated in patients with known hypersensitivity to anaesthetics of the amide type.

General contra-indications related to epidural anaesthesia, regardless of the local anaesthetic used, should be taken into account.

Intravenous regional anaesthesia.

Obstetric paracervical anaesthesia.

Hypovolaemia.

*Special warnings and special precautions for use:* Regional anaesthetic procedures should always be performed in a properly equipped and staffed area. Equipment and drugs necessary for monitoring and emergency resuscitation should be immediately available. For emergency medication, patients receiving major blocks should have an intravenous line inserted before the blocking procedure. The clinician responsible should be appropriately trained and familiar with diagnosis and treatment of side-effects, systemic toxicity and other complications (see *"Overdosage"*).

Certain local anaesthetic procedures, such as injections in the head and neck regions, may be associated with a higher frequency of serious adverse reactions, regardless of the local anaesthetic used. Care should be taken to avoid injections in infected areas.

Naropin cannot be recommended for use in children below the age of 12 years as there is no data with regard to efficacy and safety in this group of patients.

Patients in poor general condition due to ageing or other compromising factors such as partial or complete heart conduction block, advanced liver disease or severe renal dysfunction require special attention, although regional anaesthesia is frequently indicated in these patients.

Patients with hypovolaemia due to any cause can develop sudden and severe hypotension during epidural anaesthesia, regardless of the local anaesthetic used.

Ropivacaine is metabolised in the liver and should therefore be used with caution in patients with severe liver disease. Repeated doses may need to be reduced due to delayed elimination. Normally there is no need to modify the dose in patients with impaired renal function when used for single dose or short term treatment. Acidosis and reduced plasma protein concentration, frequently seen in patients with chronic renal failure, may increase the risk of systemic toxicity.

A possible cross-hypersensitivity with other amide-type local anaesthetics should be taken into account.

*Interaction with other medicaments and other forms of interaction:* Naropin should be used with caution in patients receiving other local anaesthetics or agents structurally related to amide-type local anaesthetics, e.g. certain antiarrhythmics, since the toxic effects are additive. Simultaneous use of Naropin with general anaesthetics or opioids may potentiate each others (adverse) effects.

There is a potential risk for metabolic interaction when Naropin is used in combination with CYP1A-inhibitors, e.g. fluvoxamine and verapamil, which may result in increased plasma levels of Naropin.

*Pregnancy and lactation:*

*Pregnancy:* The safety of ropivacaine for use in human pregnancy has not been established. Evaluation of experimental animal studies does not indicate direct or indirect harmful effects. The use of ropivacaine at recommended doses during child birth has not shown any harmful effects.

*Lactation:* There is no data available concerning the excretion of ropivacaine into human milk.

*Effects on ability to drive and use machines:* No data is available. Depending on the dose, local anaesthetics may have a very mild effect on mental function and co-ordination even in the absence of overt CNS toxicity and may temporarily impair locomotion and alertness.

*Undesirable effects:*

*General:* The adverse reaction profile for Naropin is similar to those for other long acting local anaesthetics of the amide type.

Adverse reactions to local anaesthetics are very rare in the absence of overdose or inadvertent intravascular injection. They should be distinguished from the physiological effects of the nerve block itself e.g. a decrease in blood pressure and bradycardia during epidural anaesthesia. The effects of systemic overdose and unintentional intravascular injections can be serious (see *Overdosage).*

*Allergic reactions:* Allergic reactions (in the most severe instances anaphylactic shock) to local anaesthetics of the amide type are rare.

*Neurological complications:* Neuropathy and spinal cord dysfunction (e.g. anterior spinal artery syndrome, arachnoiditis, cauda equina syndrome) have been associated with regional anaesthesia, regardless of the local anaesthetic drug used.

*Acute systemic toxicity:* Naropin may cause acute toxic effects following high doses or if very rapidly rising blood levels occur due to accidental intravascular injection or overdose. (See *Overdosage* and *Pharmacodynamic properties*).

One case of convulsions has been observed after an unintended intravascular injection during an attempted brachial plexus block with 200 mg.

*Most common adverse reactions:* A large number of adverse reactions have been reported during the clinical development, the great majority of which are related to the expected effects of the block and to the clinical situation rather than reactions to the drug. Thus hypotension and nausea have been reported as the most frequent adverse reactions.

The following other reported adverse reactions are considered to be of clinical importance regardless of causal relationship: Bradycardia, vomiting, paraesthesia, temperature elevation, headache, urinary retention, dizziness, hypertension, rigors (chills), tachycardia, anxiety, hypoesthesia.

*Overdose:*

*Symptoms: Acute systemic toxicity:* Accidental intravascular injections of local anaesthetics may cause immediate toxic effects. In the event of overdose, peak plasma concentrations may not be reached for one to two hours, depending on the site of the injection, and signs of toxicity may thus be delayed. Systemic toxic reactions may involve the central nervous system and the cardiovascular system. Such complications can also occur with accidental sub-arachnoid injection.

*Central nervous system:* Central nervous system toxicity is a graded response with symptoms and signs of escalating severity. Initially symptoms such as visual or hearing disturbances, perioral numbness, dizziness, light-headedness, tingling and paraesthesia are seen. Dysarthria, muscular rigidity and muscular twitching are more serious and may precede the onset of generalised convulsions. These signs must not be mistaken for neurotic behaviour. Unconsciousness and grand mal convulsions may follow, which may last from a few seconds to several minutes. Hypoxia and hypercarbia occur rapidly during convulsions due to the increased muscular activity, together with the interference with respiration. In severe cases even apnoea may occur. The respiratory and metabolic acidosis increases and extends the toxic effects of local anaesthetics.

Recovery follows the redistribution of the local anaesthetic drug from the central nervous system and subsequent metabolism and excretion. Recovery may be rapid unless large amounts of the drug have been injected. However, permanent neurological damage after accidental sub-arachnoid injection can occur.

*Cardiovascular toxicity:* Cardiovascular toxicity indicates a more severe situation. Hypotension, bradycardia, arrhythmia and even cardiac arrest may occur as a result of high systemic concentrations of local anaesthetics. In volunteers the intravenous infusion of ropivacaine resulted in signs of depression of conductivity and contractility.

Cardiovascular toxicity effects are generally preceded by signs of toxicity in the central nervous system, unless the patient is receiving a general anaesthetic or is heavily sedated with drugs such as benzodiazepines or barbiturates.

*Treatment of acute toxicity:* Equipment and drugs necessary for monitoring and emergency resuscitation should be immediately available. If signs of acute systemic toxicity appear, injection of the local anaesthetic should be stopped immediately.

In the event of convulsions, treatment will be required. The objectives of treatment are to maintain oxygenation, stop the convulsions and support the circulation. Oxygen must be given and ventilation assisted, when necessary (mask and bag). An anticonvulsant should be given intravenously if the convulsions do not stop spontaneously in 15–20 seconds. Thiopentone 100–150 mg intravenously will abort the convulsions rapidly. Alternatively diazepam 5–10 mg intravenously may be used, although its action is slower. Suxamethonium will stop the muscle convulsions rapidly, but the patient will require controlled ventilation and tracheal intubation.

If cardiovascular depression is evident (hypotension, bradycardia), ephedrine 5–10 mg intravenously should be given and repeated, if necessary, after 2–3 minutes.

Should circulatory arrest occur, immediate cardiopulmonary resuscitation should be instituted. Optimal oxygenation and ventilation and circulatory support as well as treatment of acidosis are of vital importance.

**Pharmacological properties**

*Pharmacodynamic properties:* Ropivacaine is a long-acting amide-type local anaesthetic developed as a pure enantiomer. It has both anaesthetic and analgesic effects. At high doses it produces surgical anaesthesia, while at lower doses it produces sensory block with limited and non-progressive motor block.

The mechanism is a reversible reduction of the membrane permeability of the nerve fibre to sodium ions. Consequently the depolarisation velocity is decreased and the excitable threshold increased, resulting in a local blockade of nerve impulses.

The most characteristic property of ropivacaine is the long duration of action. Onset and duration of the local anaesthetic efficacy are dependant upon the administration site, but are not influenced by the presence of a vasoconstrictor (e.g. adrenaline). For details concerning the onset and duration of action, see table under *Posology and method of administration.*

Healthy volunteers exposed to intravenous infusions tolerated ropivacaine well. The clinical experience with this drug indicates a good margin of safety.

*Pharmacokinetic properties:* The plasma concentration of ropivacaine depends upon the dose , the route of administration and the vascularity of the injection site. Ropivacaine follows linear pharmacokinetics and the $C_{max}$ is proportional to the dose.

Ropivacaine shows complete and biphasic absorption from the epidural space with half-lives of the two phases of the order of 14 min and 4 h. The slow absorption is the rate-limiting factor in the elimination of ropivacaine, which explains why the apparent elimination half-life is longer after epidural than after intravenous administration.

Ropivacaine has a total plasma clearance in the order of 440 ml/min, a renal clearance of 1 ml/min, a volume of distribution at steady state of 47 litres and a terminal half-life of 1.8 h. Ropivacaine has an intermediate hepatic extraction ratio of about 0.4. It is mainly bound to $\alpha_1$-acid glycoprotein in plasma with an unbound fraction of about 6%.

An increase in total plasma concentrations during continuous epidural infusion has been observed, related to a postoperative increase of $\alpha_1$-acid glycoprotein.

Variations in unbound, i.e. pharmacologically active, concentration have been much less than in total plasma concentration.

Ropivacaine readily crosses the placenta and equilibrium in regard to unbound concentration will be rapidly reached. The degree of plasma protein binding in the foetus is less than in the mother, which results in lower total plasma concentrations in the foetus than in the mother.

Ropivacaine is extensively metabolised, predominantly by aromatic hydroxylation. In total, 86% of the dose is excreted in the urine after intravenous administration, of which only about 1% relates to unchanged drug. The major metabolite is 3-hydroxy-ropivacaine, about 37% of which is excreted in the urine, mainly conjugated. Urinary excretion of 4-hydroxy-ropivacaine, the N-dealkylated metabolite and the 4-hydroxy-dealkylated accounts for 1-3%. Conjugated+unconjugated 3-hydroxy-ropivacaine shows only detectable concentrations in plasma. 3-hydroxy and 4-hydroxy-ropivacaine have a local anaesthetic activity although less than that of ropivacaine.

There is no evidence of *in vivo* racemisation of ropivacaine.

*Preclinical safety data:* Results from mutagenicity studies do not give indications of a relevant mutagenicity potential of ropivacaine.

**Pharmaceutical particulars**

*List of excipients:* All forms: Sodium chloride, hydrochloric acid, sodium hydroxide, water for injections.

*Incompatibilities:* Naropin should not be diluted or mixed with other solutions. In alkaline solutions precipitation may occur as ropivacaine shows poor solubility at pH > 6.0.

*Shelf life: Ampoule (Polyamp*):*
Naropin Polyamp 2 mg/ml: 3 years
Naropin Polyamp 7.5 mg/ml: 3 years
Naropin Polyamp 10 mg/ml: 3 years

The expiry date is shown on the package.

*Infusion bag (Polybag*):*
Naropin Infusion 2 mg/ml – 2 years. The expiry date is shown on the package.

*Special precautions for storage:* Store between 15–30°C. Avoid freezing. Store out of reach of children.

*Nature and contents of containers: Naropin Polyamp 2 mg/ml:*

10 ml polypropylene ampoules (Polyamp) in packs of 5 and 10
**10 ml polypropylene ampoules (Polyamp) in sterile blister packs of** 5 and **10†**
20 ml polypropylene ampoules (Polyamp) in packs of 5 and 10
20 ml polypropylene ampoules (Polyamp) in sterile blister packs of 5 and 10

*Naropin Polyamp 7.5 mg/ml:*
10 ml polypropylene ampoules (Polyamp) in packs of 5 and 10
**10 ml polypropylene ampoules (Polyamp) in sterile blister packs of** 5 and **10†**
20 ml polypropylene ampoules (Polyamp) in packs of 5 and 10
20 ml polypropylene ampoules (Polyamp) in sterile blister packs of 5 and 10

*Naropin Polyamp 10 mg/ml:*
10 ml polypropylene ampoules (Polyamp) in packs of 5 and 10
**10 ml polypropylene ampoules (Polyamp) in sterile blister packs of** 5 and **10†**
20 ml polypropylene ampoules (Polyamp) in packs of 5 and 10
20 ml polypropylene ampoules (Polyamp) in sterile blister packs of 5 and 10

*Naropin Infusion 2 mg/ml:*
**100 ml polypropylene bags (Polybag) in sterile blister packs of 5†**
**200 ml polypropylene bags (Polybag) in sterile blister packs of 5†**

The polypropylene ampoules (Polyamp) are specially designed to fit Luer lock and Luer fit syringes.

† Only those pack sizes highlighted in bold are available in the UK.

*Instructions for use/handling:* Naropin products are preservative free and are intended for single use only. Discard any unused solution.

The intact container must not be re-autoclaved. A blistered container should be chosen when a sterile outside is required.

**Marketing authorisation numbers**

| | |
|---|---|
| Naropin Polyamp 2 mg/ml | 0017/0375 |
| Naropin Polyamp 7.5 mg/ml | 0017/0377 |
| Naropin Polyamp 10 mg/ml | 0017/0378 |
| Naropin Infusion 2 mg/ml | 0017/0376 |

**Date of approval/revision of SPC** 17 May 1996

**Legal category** POM

## OXIS* TURBOHALER* 6 ▼

**Qualitative and quantitative composition** Each delivered dose (i.e. the dose leaving the mouthpiece) from Oxis Turbohaler 6 contains 4.5 micrograms formoterol fumarate dihydrate which is derived from a metered dose of 6 micrograms.

Formoterol INN is also known as eformoterol BAN.

**Pharmaceutical form** Inhalation powder.

**Clinical particulars**

*Therapeutic indications:* Oxis Turbohaler is indicated for the relief of broncho-obstructive symptoms in asthmatics when adequate treatment with corticosteroids is not sufficient.

*Posology and method of administration:*
*Adults:* Normal dosage: 1 or 2 actuations once or twice daily. The dose can be administered in the morning and/or at night. Some patients may need 4 actuations once or twice daily. The maximum daily dose is 8 actuations. In the case of nocturnal asthma symptoms the dosage may be given as a single administration at night. The duration of action has in clinical studies been shown to last for about 12 hours. The treatment should always aim for the lowest effective dose. **NB** A higher strength is available as an alternative for patients requiring 2 or more actuations.

*Children:* The use of Oxis Turbohaler in children has not been documented.

*Special patient groups:* No adjustment of dose should be required in the elderly, or in patients with renal or hepatic impairment at the recommended normal doses. (See Special warnings and special precautions for use.)

*Contra-indications:* Hypersensitivity to formoterol or to inhaled lactose.

*Special warnings and special precautions for use:* Asthmatic patients who require therapy with $\beta_2$-agonists, should also receive optimal anti-inflammatory therapy with corticosteroids. Oxis Turbohaler should only be used in patients requiring long-term regular bronchodilator therapy and not as an alternative to short-acting β-agonists used "on demand" or in the event of an acute attack. Patients must be advised to continue taking their anti-inflammatory therapy after the introduction of Oxis Turbohaler even when symptoms decrease. Should symptoms persist, or treatment with $\beta_2$-agonists need to be increased, this indicates a worsening of the underlying condition and warrants a reassessment of the asthma therapy. Therapy should not be initiated or the dose increased during an exacerbation. In the event of an acute attack, a β-agonist with a short duration of action should be used.

Caution should be observed when treating patients with thyrotoxicosis phaeochromocytoma, hypertrophic obstructive cardiomyopathy, idiopathic subvalvular aortic stenosis, severe hypertension, aneurysm or other severe cardiovascular disorders, such as ischaemic heart disease, tachyarrhythmias or severe heart failure.

Caution should be observed when treating patients with prolongation of the QTc-interval. Formoterol itself may induce prolongation of the QTc-interval.

Due to the hyperglycaemic effects of $\beta_2$-agonists, additional blood glucose monitoring is recommended initially in diabetic patients.

Potentially serious hypokalaemia may result from $\beta_2$-agonist therapy. Particular caution is recommended in acute severe asthma as the associated risk may be augmented by hypoxia. The hypokalaemic effect may be potentiated by concomitant treatment with xanthine-derivatives, steroids and diuretics. The serum potassium levels should therefore be monitored.

As with other inhalation therapy, the potential for paradoxical bronchospasm should be considered.

Oxis Turbohaler contains lactose 450 micrograms per delivered dose (corresponding to 600 micrograms per metered dose). This amount does not normally cause problems in lactose intolerant people.

Children up to the age of 12 years should not be treated with Oxis Turbohaler, as insufficient experience is available for this group.

The effect of decreased liver or kidney function on the pharmacokinetics of formoterol and the pharmacokinetics in the elderly is not known. As formoterol is primarily eliminated via metabolism an increased exposure can be expected in patients with severe liver cirrhosis.

*Interaction with other medicaments and other forms of interaction:* No specific interaction studies have been carried out with Oxis Turbohaler.

Concomitant treatment with other sympathomimetic substances may potentiate the undesirable effects of Oxis Turbohaler.

Concomitant treatment with xanthine derivatives, steroids or diuretics may potentiate a possible hypokalaemic effect of $\beta_2$-agonists. Hypokalaemia may increase the disposition towards arrhythmias in patients who are treated with digitalis glycosides.

Concomitant treatment with quinidine, disopyramide, procainamide, phenothiazines, antihistamines (terfenadine), monoamine oxidase inhibitors and tricyclic antidepressants can prolong the QTc-interval and increase the risk of ventricular arrhythmias.

In addition L-Dopa, L-thyroxine, oxytocin and alcohol can impair cardiac tolerance towards $\beta_2$-sympathomimetics.

Concomitant treatment with monoamine oxidase inhibitors including agents with similar properties such as furazolidone and procarbazine may precipitate hypertensive reactions.

There is an elevated risk of arrhythmias in patients receiving concomitant anaesthesia with halogenated hydrocarbons.

β-adrenergic blockers can weaken or inhibit the effect of Oxis Turbohaler. Oxis Turbohaler should therefore not be given together with β-adrenergic blockers (including eye drops) unless there are compelling reasons.

*Pregnancy and lactation:* Clinical experience in pregnant women is limited. In animal studies formoterol has caused implantation losses as well as decreased early postnatal survival and birth weight. The effects appeared at considerably higher systemic exposures than those reached during clinical use of Oxis Turbohaler. During pregnancy, Oxis Turbohaler should, until further experience is available, only be used after special consideration, especially during the first three months and shortly before delivery.

It is not known whether formoterol passes into human breast milk. Oxis Turbohaler should therefore not be given to mothers who are breast feeding their infants. In rats, small amounts of formoterol have been detected in maternal milk.

*Effects on the ability to drive and use machines:* Oxis Turbohaler does not affect the ability to drive or use machines.

*Undesirable effects:*

| | | |
|---|---|---|
| Common (>1/100) | *Central nervous system:* | Headache |
| | *Cardiovascular system:* | Palpitations |
| | *Musculoskeletal system:* | Tremor |
| Uncommon | *Central nervous system:* | Agitation, restlessness, sleep disturbances |
| | *Musculoskeletal system:* | Muscle cramps |
| | *Cardiovascular system:* | Tachycardia |
| Very rare (<1/1000) | *Skin:* | Exanthema, urticaria, pruritus |
| | *Respiratory tract:* | Bronchospasm |
| | *Metabolic:* | Hypokalaemia/hyperkalaemia |

Tremor and palpitations may occur, but tend to be transient and reduce with regular therapy. As with all inhalation therapy, paradoxical bronchospasm may occur in very rare cases.

In isolated cases the following undesirable effects have been reported: Nausea, taste disturbances, dizziness, angina pectoris, variations in the blood pressure, and hyperglycaemia.

Treatment with $\beta_2$-sympathomimetics may result in an increase in blood levels of insulin, free fatty acids, glycerol and ketone bodies.

*Overdose:* There is no clinical experience on the management of overdose. An overdose would likely lead to effects that are typical of $\beta_2$-agonists: tremor, headache, palpitations, and tachycardia. Hypotension, metabolic acidosis, hypokalaemia and hyperglycaemia may also occur. Supportive and symptomatic treatment is indicated.

Use of cardioselective β-blockers may be considered, but only subject to extreme caution since the use of β-adrenergic blocker medication may provoke bronchospasm. Serum potassium should be monitored.

**Pharmacological properties**

*Pharmacodynamic properties:* Formoterol is a selective $\beta_2$-adrenoceptor agonist that produces relaxation of bronchial smooth muscle. Formoterol thus has a bronchodilating effect in patients with reversible airways obstruction. The bronchodilating effect sets in rapidly, within 1–3 minutes after inhalation and has a mean duration of 12 hours after a single dose.

*Pharmacokinetic properties: Absorption:* Inhaled formoterol is rapidly absorbed. Peak plasma concentration is reached about 15 minutes after inhalation.

In studies the mean lung deposition of formoterol after inhalation via Turbohaler ranged from 28–49% of the delivered dose (corresponding to 21–37% of the metered dose). The total systemic availability for the higher lung deposition was around 61% of the delivered dose (corresponding to 46% of the metered dose).

*Distribution and metabolism:* Plasma protein binding is approximately 50%.

Formoterol is metabolised via direct glucuronidation and O-demethylation. The enzyme responsible for O-demethylation has not been identified. Total plasma clearance and volume of distribution has not been determined.

*Elimination:* The major part of the dose of formoterol is eliminated via metabolism. After inhalation 8–13% of the delivered dose (corresponding to 6–10% of the metered dose) of formoterol is excreted unmetabolised in the urine. About 20% of an intravenous dose is excreted unchanged in the urine. The terminal half-life after inhalation is estimated to be 8 hours.

*Preclinical safety data:* The effects of formoterol seen in toxicity studies in rats and dogs were mainly on the cardiovascular system and consisted of hyperaemia, tachycardia, arrhythmias and myocardial lesions. These effects are known pharmacological manifestations seen after the administration of high doses of $\beta_2$-agonists.

A somewhat reduced fertility in male rats was observed at high systemic exposure to formoterol.

No genotoxic effects of formoterol have been observed in *in-vitro* or *in-vivo* tests. In rats and mice a slight increase in the incidence of benign uterine leiomyomas has been observed. This effect is looked upon as a class-effect observed in rodents after long exposure to high doses of $\beta_2$-agonists.

**Pharmaceutical particulars**

*List of excipients:* Lactose monohydrate.

*Incompatibilities:* None stated.

*Shelf life:* 2 years.

*Special precautions for storage:* Should be stored with cover tightened.

*Nature and contents of container:* Oxis Turbohaler is a multidose, inspiratory flow driven, dry powder inhaler. The inhaler is made of plastic parts.

Each inhaler contains 60 doses.

*Instructions for use/handling:* Oxis Turbohaler is inspiratory flow driven which means that, when the patient inhales through the mouthpiece, the substance will follow the inspired air into the airways.

*Note.* It is important to instruct the patient to breathe in forcefully and deeply through the mouthpiece to ensure that an optimal dose is obtained.

The patient may not taste or feel any medication when using Oxis Turbohaler due to the small amount of drug dispensed.

Detailed instructions for use are packed together with each inhaler.

**Marketing authorisation number** 00017/0386

**Date of approval/revision of SPC** March 1997

**Legal category** POM

## OXIS* TURBOHALER* 12 ▼

**Qualitative and quantitative composition** Each delivered dose (i.e. the dose leaving the mouthpiece) from Oxis Turbohaler 12 contains 9 micrograms formoterol fumarate dihydrate which is derived from a metered dose of 12 micrograms.

Formoterol INN is also known as eformoterol BAN.

**Pharmaceutical form** Inhalation powder.

**Clinical particulars**

*Therapeutic indications:* Oxis Turbohaler is indicated for the relief of broncho-obstructive symptoms in asthmatics when adequate treatment with corticosteroids is not sufficient.

*Posology and method of administration:*

*Adults:* Normal dosage: 1 actuation once or twice daily. The dose can be administered in the morning and/or at night. Some patients may need 2 actuations once or twice daily. The maximum daily dose is 4 actuations. In the case of nocturnal asthma symptoms the dosage may be given as a single administration at night. The duration of action has in clinical studies been shown to last for about 12 hours. The treatment should always aim for the lowest effective dose. **NB** A lower strength is also available.

*Children:* The use of Oxis Turbohaler in children has not been documented.

*Special patient groups:* No adjustment of dose should be required in the elderly, or in patients with renal or hepatic impairment at the recommended normal doses. (See Special warnings and special precautions for use.)

*Contra-indications:* Hypersensitivity to formoterol or to inhaled lactose.

*Special warnings and special precautions for use:* Asthmatic patients who require therapy with $\beta_2$-agonists, should also receive optimal anti-inflammatory therapy with corticosteroids. Oxis Turbohaler should only be used in patients requiring long-term regular bronchodilator therapy and not as an alternative to short-acting β-agonists used "on demand" or in the event of an acute attack. Patients must be advised to continue taking their anti-inflammatory therapy after the introduction of Oxis Turbohaler even when symptoms decrease. Should symptoms persist, or treatment with $\beta_2$-agonists need to be increased, this indicates a worsening of the underlying condition and warrants a reassessment of the asthma therapy. Therapy should not be initiated or the dose increased during an exacerbation. In the event of an acute attack, a β-agonist with a short duration of action should be used.

Caution should be observed when treating patients with thyrotoxicosis phaeochromocytoma, hypertrophic obstructive cardiomyopathy, idiopathic subvalvular aortic stenosis, severe hypertension, aneurysm or other severe cardiovascular disorders, such as ischaemic heart disease, tachyarrhythmias or severe heart failure.

Caution should be observed when treating patients with prolongation of the QTc-interval. Formoterol itself may induce prolongation of the QTc-interval.

Due to the hyperglycaemic effects of $\beta_2$-agonists, additional blood glucose monitoring is recommended initially in diabetic patients.

Potentially serious hypokalaemia may result from $\beta_2$-agonist therapy. Particular caution is recommended in acute severe asthma as the associated risk may be augmented by hypoxia. The hypokalaemic effect may be potentiated by concomitant treatment with xanthine-derivatives, steroids and diuretics. The serum potassium levels should therefore be monitored.

As with other inhalation therapy, the potential for paradoxical bronchospasm should be considered.

Oxis Turbohaler contains lactose 450 micrograms per delivered dose (corresponding to 600 micrograms per metered dose). This amount does not normally cause problems in lactose intolerant people.

Children up to the age of 12 years should not be treated with Oxis Turbohaler, as insufficient experience is available for this group.

The effect of decreased liver or kidney function on the pharmacokinetics of formoterol and the pharmacokinetics in the elderly is not known. As formoterol is primarily eliminated via metabolism an increased exposure can be expected in patients with severe liver cirrhosis.

*Interaction with other medicaments and other forms of interaction:* No specific interaction studies have been carried out with Oxis Turbohaler.

Concomitant treatment with other sympathomimetic substances may potentiate the undesirable effects of Oxis Turbohaler.

Concomitant treatment with xanthine derivatives, steroids or diuretics may potentiate a possible hypokalaemic effect of $\beta_2$-agonists. Hypokalaemia may increase the disposition towards arrhythmias in patients who are treated with digitalis glycosides.

Concomitant treatment with quinidine, disopyramide, procainamide, phenothiazines, antihistamines (terfenadine), monoamine oxidase inhibitors and tricyclic antidepressants can prolong the QTc-interval and increase the risk of ventricular arrhythmias.

In addition L-Dopa, L-thyroxine, oxytocin and alcohol can impair cardiac tolerance towards $\beta_2$-sympathomimetics.

Concomitant treatment with monoamine oxidase inhibitors including agents with similar properties such as furazolidone and procarbazine may precipitate hypertensive reactions.

There is an elevated risk of arrhythmias in patients receiving concomitant anaesthesia with halogenated hydrocarbons.

β-adrenergic blockers can weaken or inhibit the effect of Oxis Turbohaler. Oxis Turbohaler should therefore not be given together with β-adrenergic blockers (including eye drops) unless there are compelling reasons.

*Pregnancy and lactation:* Clinical experience in pregnant women is limited. In animal studies formoterol has caused implantation losses as well as decreased early postnatal survival and birth weight. The effects appeared at considerably higher systemic exposures than those reached during clinical use of Oxis Turbohaler. During pregnancy Oxis Turbohaler should, until further experience is available, only be used after special consideration, especially during the first three months and shortly before delivery.

It is not known whether formoterol passes into human breast milk. Oxis Turbohaler should therefore not be given to mothers who are breast feeding their infants. In rats, small amounts of formoterol have been detected in maternal milk.

*Effects on the ability to drive and use machines:* Oxis Turbohaler does not affect the ability to drive or use machines.

*Undesirable effects:*

| | | |
|---|---|---|
| Common (>1/100) | *Central nervous system:* | Headache |
| | *Cardiovascular system:* | Palpitations |
| | *Musculoskeletal system:* | Tremor |
| Uncommon | *Central nervous system:* | Agitation, restlessness, sleep disturbances |
| | *Musculoskeletal system:* | Muscle cramps |
| | *Cardiovascular system:* | Tachycardia |
| Very rare (<1/1000) | *Skin:* | Exanthema, urticaria, pruritus |
| | *Respiratory tract:* | Bronchospasm |
| | *Metabolic:* | Hypokalaemia/hyperkalaemia |

Tremor and palpitations may occur, but tend to be transient and reduce with regular therapy. As with all inhalation therapy, paradoxical bronchospasm may occur in very rare cases.

In isolated cases the following undesirable effects have been reported: Nausea, taste disturbances, dizziness, angina pectoris, variations in the blood pressure, and hyperglycaemia.

Treatment with $\beta_2$-sympathomimetics may result in an increase in blood levels of insulin, free fatty acids, glycerol and ketone bodies.

*Overdose:* There is no clinical experience on the management of overdose. An overdose would likely lead to effects that are typical of $\beta_2$-agonists: tremor, headache, palpitations, and tachycardia. Hypotension, metabolic acidosis, hypokalaemia and hyperglycaemia may also occur. Supportive and symptomatic treatment is indicated.

Use of cardioselective β-blockers may be considered, but only subject to extreme caution since the use of β-adrenergic blocker medication may provoke bronchospasm. Serum potassium should be monitored.

**Pharmacological properties**

*Pharmacodynamic properties:* Formoterol is a selective $\beta_2$-adrenoceptor agonist that produces relaxation of bronchial smooth muscle. Formoterol thus has a bronchodilating effect in patients with reversible airways obstruction. The bronchodilating effect sets in rapidly, within 1–3 minutes after inhalation and has a mean duration of 12 hours after a single dose.

*Pharmacokinetic properties: Absorption:* Inhaled formoterol is rapidly absorbed. Peak plasma concentration is reached about 15 minutes after inhalation.

In studies the mean lung deposition of formoterol after inhalation via Turbohaler ranged from 28–49% of the delivered dose (corresponding to 21–37% of the metered dose). The total systemic availability for the higher lung deposition was around 61% of the delivered dose (corresponding to 46% of the metered dose).

*Distribution and metabolism:* Plasma protein binding is approximately 50%.

Formoterol is metabolised via direct glucuronidation and O-demethylation. The enzyme responsible for O-demethylation has not been identified. Total plasma clearance and volume of distribution has not been determined.

*Elimination:* The major part of the dose of formoterol is eliminated via metabolism. After inhalation 8–13% of the delivered dose (corresponding to 6–10% of the metered dose) of formoterol is excreted unmetabolised in the urine. About 20% of an intravenous dose is excreted unchanged in the urine. The terminal half-life after inhalation is estimated to be 8 hours.

*Preclinical safety data:* The effects of formoterol seen in toxicity studies in rats and dogs were mainly on the cardiovascular system and consisted of hyperaemia, tachycardia, arrhythmias and myocardial lesions.

These effects are known pharmacological manifestations seen after the administration of high doses of $\beta_2$-agonists.

A somewhat reduced fertility in male rats was observed at high systemic exposure to formoterol.

No genotoxic effects of formoterol have been observed in in-vitro or in-vivo tests. In rats and mice a slight increase in the incidence of benign uterine leiomyomas has been observed. This effect is looked upon as a class-effect observed in rodents after long exposure to high doses of $\beta_2$-agonists.

## Pharmaceutical particulars

List of excipients: Lactose monohydrate.

Incompatibilities: None stated.

Shelf life: 2 years.

Special precautions for storage: Should be stored with cover tightened.

Nature and contents of container: Oxis Turbohaler is a multidose, inspiratory flow driven, dry powder inhaler. The inhaler is made of plastic parts.

Each inhaler contains 60 doses.

Instructions for use/handling: Oxis Turbohaler is inspiratory flow driven which means that, when the patient inhales through the mouthpiece, the substance will follow the inspired air into the airways.

Note. It is important to instruct the patient to breathe in forcefully and deeply through the mouthpiece to ensure that an optimal dose is obtained.

The patient may not taste or feel any medication when using Oxis Turbohaler due to the small amount of drug dispensed.

Detailed instructions for use are packed together with each inhaler.

**Marketing authorisation number** PL00017/0387

**Date of approval/revision** March 1997

**Legal category** POM

# PLENDIL* 2.5 mg, 5 mg and 10 mg

## Qualitative and quantitative composition

Plendil 2.5 mg contains Felodipine PhEur 2.5 mg
Plendil 5 mg contains Felodipine PhEur 5 mg
Plendil 10 mg contains Felodipine PhEur 10 mg

**Pharmaceutical form** Circular bio-convex film coated extended-release tablets.

Plendil 2.5 mg - yellow tablets coded A/FL and 2.5 on the reverse.

Plendil 5 mg - pink tablets coded A/FM and 5 on the reverse.

Plendil 10 mg - red-brown tablets coded A/FE and 10 on the reverse.

## Clinical particulars

Therapeutic indications: In the management of hypertension and prophylaxis of chronic stable angina pectoris.

Posology and method of administration: For oral administration

Hypertension:

Adults (including elderly): The dose should be adjusted to the individual requirements of the patient. The recommended starting dose is 5 mg once daily. If necessary the dose may be further increased or another antihypertensive agent added. The usual maintenance dose is 5–10 mg once daily. Doses higher than 20 mg daily are not usually needed. For dose titration purposes a 2.5 mg tablet is available. In elderly patients an initial treatment with 2.5 mg daily should be considered.

Angina pectoris:

Adults: The dose should be adjusted individually. Treatment should be started with 5 mg once daily and if needed be increased to 10 mg once daily.

Administration: The tablets should be taken in the morning irrespective of food intake. Plendil tablets must not be chewed or crushed. They should be swallowed whole with half a glass of water.

Children: The safety and efficacy of Plendil in children has not been established.

Plendil can be used in combination with β-blockers, ACE inhibitors or diuretics. The effects on blood pressure are likely to be additive and combination therapy will usually enhance the antihypertensive effect. Care should be taken to avoid hypotension. In patients with severely impaired liver function the dose of felodipine should be low. The pharmacokinetics are not significantly affected in patients with impaired renal function.

Contra-indications:
Unstable angina pectoris.
Pregnancy.

Patient with a previous allergic reaction to Plendil or other dihydropyridines because of the theoretical risk of cross-reactivity.

Plendil should not be used in patients with clinically significant aortic stenosis, and during or within one month of a myocardial infarction.

As with other calcium channel blockers, Plendil should be discontinued in patients who develop cardiogenic shock.

Special warnings and special precautions for use: As with other vasodilators, Plendil may, in rare cases, precipitate significant hypotension with tachycardia which in susceptible individuals may result in myocardial ischaemia.

There is no evidence that Plendil is useful for secondary prevention of myocardial infarction.

The efficacy and safety of Plendil in the treatment of malignant hypertension has not been studied.

Plendil should be used with caution in patients with severe left ventricular dysfunction.

Interaction with other medicaments and other forms of interaction: Concomitant administration of substances which interfere with the cytochrome P450 system may affect plasma concentrations of felodipine. Enzyme inhibitors such as cimetidine, erythromycin and itraconazole impair the elimination of felodipine, and Plendil dosage may need to be reduced when drugs are given concomitantly. Conversely, powerful enzyme inducing agents such as some anticonvulsants (phenytoin, carbamazepine, phenobarbitone) can increase felodipine elimination and higher than normal Plendil doses may be required in patients taking the drugs.

No dosage adjustment is required when Plendil is given concomitantly with digoxin.

Felodipine does not appear to affect the unbound fraction of other extensively plasma protein bound drugs such as warfarin.

Grapefruit juice results in increased peak plasma levels and bioavailability possibly due to an interaction with flavonoids in the fruit juice. This interaction has been seen with other dihydropyridine calcium antagonists and represents a class effect. Therefore grapefruit juice should not be taken together with Plendil tablets.

Pregnancy and lactation: Felodipine should not be given during pregnancy.

In a study on fertility and general reproductive performance in rats, a prolongation of parturition resulting in difficult labour, increased foetal deaths and early postnatal deaths were observed in the medium– and high–dose groups. Reproductive studies in rabbits have shown a dose-related reversible enlargement of the mammary glands of the parent animals and dose–related digital abnormalities in the foetuses when felodipine was administered during stages of early foetal development.

Felodipine has been detected in breast milk, but it is unknown whether it has harmful effects on the newborn.

Effects on ability to drive and use machines: None.

Undesirable effects: As with other calcium antagonists, flushing, headache, palpitations, dizziness and fatigue may occur. These reactions are usually transient and are most likely to occur at the start of treatment or after an increase in dosage.

As with other calcium antagonists ankle swelling, resulting from precapillary vasodilation, may occur. The degree of ankle swelling is dose related.

In patients with gingivitis/periodontitis, mild gingival enlargement has been reported with Plendil, as with other calcium antagonists. The enlargement can be avoided or reversed by careful dental hygiene.

As with other dihydropyridines, aggravation of angina has been reported in a small number of individuals especially after starting treatment. This is more likely to happen in patients with symptomatic ischaemic heart disease.

The following adverse events have been reported from clinical trials and from Post Marketing Surveillance. In the great majority of cases a causal relationship between these events and treatment with felodipine has not been established.

Skin: rarely – rash and/or pruritus, and isolated cases of photosensitivity.

Musculoskeletal: in isolated cases arthralgia and myalgia.

Central and peripheral nervous system: headache, dizziness. In isolated cases paraesthesia.

Gastrointestinal: in isolated cases nausea, gum hyperplasia.

Hepatic: in isolated cases increased liver enzymes.

Cardiovascular: rarely – tachycardia, palpitations and syncope.

Vascular (extracardiac): peripheral oedema, flush.

Other: rarely – fatigue, in isolated cases hypersensitivity reactions e.g. urticaria, angiooedema.

Overdose: Symptoms: Overdosage may cause excessive peripheral vasodilatation with marked hypotension which may sometimes be accompanied by bradycardia.

Management: Severe hypotension should be treated symptomatically, with the patient placed supine and the legs elevated. Bradycardia, if present, should be treated with atropine 0.5-1 mg i.v. If this is not

sufficient, plasma volume should be increased by infusion of e.g. glucose, saline or dextran. Sympathomimetic drugs with predominant effect on the $\alpha_1$-adrenoceptor may be given e.g. metaraminol or phenylephrine.

## Pharmacological properties

Pharmacodynamic properties: Felodipine is a vascular selective calcium antagonist, which lowers arterial blood pressure by decreasing peripheral vascular residence. Due to the high degree of selectivity for smooth muscle in the arterioles, felodipine in therapeutic doses has no direct effect on cardiac contractility or conduction.

It can be used as monotherapy or in combination with other antihypertensive drugs, e.g. β-receptor blockers, diuretics or ACE-inhibitors, in order to achieve an increased antihypertensive effect. Felodipine reduces both systolic and diastolic blood pressure and can be used in isolated systolic hypertension. In a study of 12 patients, felodipine maintained its antihypertensive effect during concomitant therapy with indomethacin.

Because there is no effect on venous smooth muscle or adrenergic vasomotor control, felodipine is not associated with orthostatic hypotension.

Felodipine has anti-anginal and anti-ischaemic effects due to improved myocardial oxygen supply/demand balance. Coronary vascular resistance is decreased and coronary blood flow as well as myocardial oxygen supply are increased by felodipine due to dilation of both epicardial arteries and arterioles. Felodipine effectively counteracts coronary vasospasm. The reduction in systemic blood pressure caused by felodipine leads to decreased left ventricular afterload.

Felodipine improves exercise tolerance and reduces anginal attacks in patients with stable effort induced angina pectoris. Both symptomatic and silent myocardial ischaemia are reduced by felodipine in patients with vasospastic angina. Felodipine can be used as monotherapy or in combination with β-receptor blockers in patients with stable angina pectoris.

Felodipine possesses a mild natriuretic/diuretic effect and generalised fluid retention does not occur.

Felodipine is well tolerated in patients with concomitant disease such as congestive heart failure well-controlled on appropriate therapy, asthma and other obstructive pulmonary diseases, diabetes, gout, hyperlipidemia impaired renal function, renal transplant recipients and Raynaud's disease. Felodipine has no significant effect on blood glucose levels or lipid profiles.

Haemodynamic effects: The primary haemodynamic effect of felodipine is a reduction of total peripheral vascular resistance which leads to a decrease in blood pressure. These effects are dose-dependent. In patients with mild to moderate essential hypertension, a reduction in blood pressure usually occurs 2 hours after the first oral dose and lasts for at least 24 hours with a trough/peak ratio usually above 50%.

Plasma concentration of felodipine and decrease in total peripheral resistance and blood pressure are positively correlated.

Electrophysiological and other cardiac effects: Felodipine in therapeutic doses has no effect on cardiac contractility or atrioventricular conduction or refractoriness.

Renal effects: Felodipine has a natriuretic and diuretic effect. Studies have shown that the tubular reabsorption of filtered sodium is reduced. This counteracts the salt and water retention observed for other vasodilators. Felodipine does not affect the daily potassium excretion. The renal vascular resistance is decreased by felodipine. Normal glomerular filtration rate is unchanged. In patients with impaired renal function glomerular filtration rate may increase. Felodipine is well tolerated in renal transplant recipients.

Site and mechanism of action: The predominant pharmacodynamic feature of felodipine is its pronounced vascular versus myocardial selectivity. Myogenically active smooth muscles in arterial resistance vessels are particularly sensitive to felodipine.

Felodipine inhibits electrical and contractile activity of vascular smooth muscle cells via an effect on the calcium channels in the cell membrane.

Pharmacokinetic properties: Absorption and distribution: Felodipine is completely absorbed from the gastrointestinal tract after administration of felodipine extended release tablets.

The systemic availability of felodipine is approximately 15% in man and is independent of dose in the therapeutic dose range.

With the extended-release tablets the absorption phase is prolonged. This results in even felodipine plasma concentrations within the therapeutic range for 24 hours.

The plasma protein binding of felodipine is approximately 99%. It is bound predominantly to the albumin fraction.

*Elimination and metabolism:* The average half-life of felodipine in the terminal phase is 25 hours. There is no significant accumulation during long-term treatment. Felodipine is extensively metabolised by the liver and all identified metabolites are inactive. Elderly patients and patients with reduced liver function have an average higher plasma concentration of felodipine than younger patients.

About 70% of a given dose is excreted as metabolites in the urine; the remaining fraction is excreted in the faeces. Less than 0.5% of a dose is recovered unchanged in the urine.

The kinetics of felodipine are not changed in patients with renal impairment.

*Preclinical safety data:* Felodipine is a calcium antagonist and lowers arterial blood pressure by decreasing vascular resistance. In general a reduction in blood pressure is evident 2 hours after the first oral dose and at steady state lasts for at least 24 hours after dose.

Felodipine exhibits a high degree of selectivity for smooth muscles in the arterioles and in therapeutic doses has no direct effect on cardiac contractility. Felodipine does not affect venous smooth muscle and adrenergic vasomotor control.

Electrophysiological studies have shown that felodipine has no direct effect on conduction in the specialised conducting system of the heart and no effect on the AV nodal refractories.

Plendil possesses a mild natriuretic/diuretic effect and does not produce general fluid retention, nor affect daily potassium excretion. Plendil is well tolerated in patients with congestive heart failure.

**Pharmaceutical particulars**
*List of excipients:* Polyoxyl 40 hydrogenated castor oil, Hydroxypropyl cellulose, Propyl gallate, Hydroxypropyl methylcellulose, Sodium aluminium silicate, Microcrystalline cellulose, Lactose anhydrous, Sodium stearyl fumarate, Polyethylene glycol, Colour Titanium dioxide (E171), Colour Iron oxide yellow (E172) and Carnauba wax.

*Incompatibilities:* None stated.

*Shelf life:* 3 years.

*Special precautions for storage:* Store below 30°C.

*Nature and contents of container: PVC/PVDC Blisters:* Press through blister package of PVC/PVDC form foil with an aluminium foil as enclosure web. Each blister strip contains 7 tablets. A single pack contains 28 tablets as multiples of blisters of 7.

*Instructions for use/handling:* None stated.

**Marketing authorisation numbers**

| | |
|---|---|
| Plendil 2.5 mg | 0017/0349 |
| Plendil 5 mg | 0017/0301 |
| Plendil 10 mg | 0017/0302 |

**Date of approval/revision of SPC** February 1997

**Legal category** POM

## PULMICORT*

**Presentation** Pulmicort Inhaler is a metered dose aerosol delivering 200 micrograms budesonide per actuation via a standard or Spacer adapter. Pulmicort L.S. Inhaler is a metered dose aerosol delivering 50 micrograms budesonide per actuation via a standard or L.S. Spacer adapter.

*Inactive ingredients:* Sorbitan trioleate and chlorofluorocarbons 11, 12 and 114.

**Uses** Pulmicort Inhaler and Pulmicort LS Inhaler contain the potent, non-halogenated corticosteroid budesonide. Inhaled budesonide possesses a local anti-inflammatory action in the lungs without giving rise to systemic corticosteroid effects.

Pulmicort is recommended in patients with bronchial asthma.

The specially designed Spacer adapter permits the aerosol propellants to evaporate and the particle velocity to decrease, resulting in reduced drug deposition in the oral cavity. In addition the Spacer adapter diminishes the need for co-ordination between aerosol actuation and inhalation, making this inhaler suitable for patients who have difficulty using conventional inhalers.

**Dosage and administration** *Adults:* 200 micrograms twice daily, in the morning and in the evening. During periods of severe asthma the daily dosage can be increased to up to 1600 micrograms.

In patients well controlled the daily dose may be reduced below 400 micrograms, but should not go below 200 micrograms.

*Children:* 50 to 400 micrograms to be given twice daily. During periods of severe asthma the daily dosage can be increased up to 800 micrograms.

*Elderly:* Dosage as for adults.

**Contra-indications, warnings, etc**

*Contra-indications:* Hypersensitivity to any of the constituents. No other specific contra-indications are known, but special care is needed in patients with lung tuberculosis, fungal and viral infections in the airways.

*Special warnings and precautions: Pregnancy and breast feeding:* In pregnant animals, administration of budesonide causes abnormalities of foetal development. The relevance of this finding to man has not been established. Administration during pregnancy should be avoided unless there are compelling reasons. As yet there is no information regarding the passage of budesonide into breast milk.

*Patients not dependent on steroids:* Treatment with the recommended doses of Pulmicort usually gives a therapeutic benefit within 7 days. However, certain patients may have an excessive collection of mucous secretion in the bronchi, which reduces penetration of the active substance into the airways. In these cases a short course of oral corticosteroids (usually 1 to 2 weeks) should be given in addition to the aerosol. After the course of the oral drug the inhaler alone should be sufficient therapy. Exacerbations of asthma caused by bacterial infections are usually controlled by appropriate antibiotic treatment and possibly increasing the Pulmicort dosage or if necessary, by giving systemic steroids.

*Steroid dependent patients:* Transfer of patients dependent upon oral steroids to treatment with Pulmicort demands special care mainly due to the slow restitution of the disturbed hypothalamic-pituitary function caused by extended treatment with oral corticosteroids. When the Pulmicort treatment is initiated the patient should be in a relatively stable phase. Pulmicort is then given in combination with the previously used oral steroid dose for about 10 days.

After this period of time the reduction of the oral corticoid dose can be started with a dose reduction corresponding to about 1 mg prednisolone per day every week. The oral dose is thus reduced to the lowest level which in combination with Pulmicort gives a stable respiratory capacity.

In many cases it may eventually be possible to withdraw completely the oral steroid with Pulmicort treatment, but other cases may have to be maintained on a low oral steroid dosage.

Some patients may experience uneasiness during the withdrawal period due to a decreased steroid effect. The physician may have to explain the reason for the Pulmicort treatment in order to encourage the patient to continue. The length of time needed for the body to regain its natural production of corticosteroid in sufficient amounts is often extensive. Thus during physically stressing situations such as severe infections, trauma and surgical operations it will be necessary to give the patient an additional oral steroid dose. Acute exacerbations, accompanied by increased mucous viscosity and mucous plugging, require complementary treatment with a short course of oral corticosteroids.

During transfer from oral therapy to Pulmicort a generally lower systemic steroid action will be experienced which may result in the appearance of allergic or arthritic symptoms such as rhinitis, eczema and muscle and joint pain. Specific treatment should be initiated for these conditions.

*Side-effects:* Occasional cases of mild irritation in the throat and hoarseness have been reported. Due to drug deposition in the oral cavity candidiasis of the mouth and throat occurs in some patients. However, the incidence should be less with the Spacer adapter or Nebuhaler as these reduce oral deposition. Advising the patient to rinse the mouth with water after each dosing occasion is also recommended. In most cases this condition responds to topical anti-fungal therapy without discontinuing treatment with Pulmicort.

*Overdosage:* The only harmful effect that follows inhalation of large amounts of the drug over a short period is suppression of hypothalamic-pituitary-adrenal (HPA) function. No special emergency action needs to be taken. Treatment with Pulmicort inhaler should be continued at the recommended dose to control the asthma.

**Pharmaceutical precautions** Store below 30°C.

**Legal category** POM

**Package quantities** Pulmicort Inhaler (200 micrograms/actuation). Aerosol canister containing 200 metered doses complete with standard and Spacer delivery systems.

Pulmicort L.S. Inhaler (50 micrograms/puff). Aerosol canister containing 200 metered doses complete with standard and Spacer delivery systems.

Pulmicort (200 dose, 200 micrograms/puff) and Pulmicort L.S. (200 dose, 50 micrograms/puff) refill canisters are available.

**Further information** Pulmicort and Pulmicort L.S. may also be administered via the Nebuhaler.

**Product licence numbers**

| | |
|---|---|
| (200 micrograms/puff) | 0017/0128 |
| (50 micrograms/puff) | 0017/0113 |

## PULMICORT* RESPULES*

**Presentation** A white to off-white suspension for nebulisation.

Pulmicort Respules 0.5 mg; 2 ml single dose unit ampoules each containing 0.5 mg budesonide.

Pulmicort Respules 1 mg; 2 ml single dose unit ampoules each containing 1 mg budesonide.

*Inactive ingredients:* Sodium chloride, polysorbate 80, citric acid, sodium citrate and disodium edetate.

**Uses** Pulmicort Respules contain the potent non-halogenated corticosteroid, budesonide for use in bronchial asthma in patients where use of a pressurised inhaler or dry powder formulation is unsatisfactory or inappropriate.

Pulmicort Respules are also recommended for use in infants and children with acute laryngotracheobronchitis – croup.

**Dosage and administration**
*Dosage schedules:* Pulmicort Respules should be administered from suitable nebulisers. The dose delivered to the patient varies depending on the nebulising equipment used. The nebulisation time and the dose delivered is dependent on flow rate, volume of nebuliser chamber and volume fill. An airflow rate of 6–8 litres per minute through the device should be employed. A suitable volume fill for most nebulisers is 2–4 ml. The dosage of Pulmicort Respules should be adjusted to the need of the individual.

*Bronchial Asthma:*

*Initiation of therapy:* When treatment is started, during periods of severe asthma and while reducing or discontinuing oral glucocorticosteroids the recommended dose of Pulmicort Respules is:

*Adults (including elderly):* Usually 1–2 mg twice daily. In very severe cases the dosage may be further increased.

*Children 12 years and older:* Dosage as for adults.

*Children 3 months to 12 years:* 0.5–1 mg twice daily.

*Maintenance:* The maintenance dose should be the lowest dose which keeps the patient symptom-free.

Recommended doses are:

*Adults (including elderly and children 12 years and older):* 0.5–1 mg twice daily.

*Children (3 months–12 years):* 0.25–0.5 mg twice daily.

Recommended dosage table :

| | Pulmicort Respule Presentation | |
|---|---|---|
| | 0.5 mg | 1 mg |
| Dose (mg) | Volume (ml) | Volume (ml) |
| 0.25 | 1 | — |
| 0.5 | 2 | 1 |
| 0.75 | 3 | — |
| 1.0 | 4 | 2 |
| 1.5 | 6 | 3 |
| 2.0 | 8 | 4 |

Where an increased therapeutic effect is desired, especially in those patients without major mucus secretion in the airways, an increased dose of Pulmicort is recommended rather than combined treatment with oral corticosteroids because of the lower risk of systemic effects.

*Acute laryngotracheobronchitis–croup:*

In infants and children with croup the usual dose is 2 mg of nebulised budesonide. This dose is given as a single administration or as two 1 mg doses separated by 30 minutes.

**Contra-indications, warnings, etc**
*Contra-indications:* Hypersensitivity to any of the constituents.

*Special warnings and precautions:* Special care is needed in patients with pulmonary tuberculosis and viral infections in the airways.

*Non-steroid dependent patients:* A therapeutic effect is usually reached within 10 days. In patients with excessive mucus secretion in the bronchi a short (about 2 weeks) additional oral corticosteroid regimen can be given initially. After the course of the oral drug Pulmicort Respules alone should be sufficient therapy.

*Steroid dependent patients:* When transfer from oral corticosteroid to treatment with Pulmicort is initiated the patient should be in a relatively stable phase. Pulmicort is then given in combination with the previously used oral steroid dose for about 10 days.

After that the oral dose should be gradually reduced (by for example 2.5 mg prednisolone or the equivalent each month) to the lowest possible level. In many cases, it is possible to completely substitute Pulmicort for the oral corticosteroid.

During transfer from oral therapy to Pulmicort a generally lower systemic corticosteroid action will be experienced which may result in the appearance of allergic or arthritic symptoms such as rhinitis, eczema and muscle and joint pain. Specific treatment should be initiated for these conditions.

Acute exacerbations of asthma may need additional treatment with a short course of oral corticosteroid. The nebuliser chamber should be cleaned after every administration. Wash the nebuliser chamber and mouthpiece or face-mask in hot water using a mild detergent. Rinse well and dry by connecting the nebuliser chamber to the compressor or air inlet.

Pulmicort does not affect the ability to drive and use machines.

Pulmicort Respules can be mixed with 0.9% saline and with solutions of terbutaline, salbutamol, sodium cromoglycate or ipratropium bromide.

*Side-effects:* Mild irritation in the throat, coughing and hoarseness. Candida infection in the oropharynx has been reported. To minimize oropharyngeal thrush the mouth should be rinsed with water after administration. In rare cases inhaled drugs may provoke bronchoconstriction in hyperreactive patients. Facial skin irritation has occurred in a few cases when a nebuliser with face mask has been used. To prevent irritation facial skin should be washed after use of the face mask. Coughing can usually be prevented by inhaling a $\beta_2$-agonist (e.g. terbutaline) 5–10 minutes before inhalation of Pulmicort Respules.

*Use in pregnancy and lactation:* In pregnant animals administration of budesonide causes abnormalities of foetal development. The relevance of this finding to man has not been established. Administration during pregnancy should be avoided unless there are compelling reasons. As yet there is no information regarding the passage of budesonide into breast milk.

*Overdosage:* Pulmicort Respules contains 0.1 mg/ml disodium edetate which has been shown to cause bronchoconstriction at levels above 1.2 mg/ml. Acute overdosage with Pulmicort should not present a clinical problem.

**Pharmaceutical precautions**   Store below 30°C. Use within 3 months of opening the foil envelope. Protect opened ampoule from light. Use within 12 hours of opening.

**Legal category**   POM

**Package quantities**
Packs of 20 x 2 ml Respules.

**Further information**   Nil

**Product licence numbers**
Pulmicort Respules 0.5 mg            0017/0309
Pulmicort Respules 1 mg              0017/0310

## PULMICORT* TURBOHALER*

**Presentation**   Pulmicort Turbohaler 100 is a breath-actuated metered dose powder inhaler delivering 100 micrograms budesonide per actuation.

Pulmicort Turbohaler 200 is a breath-actuated metered dose powder inhaler delivering 200 micrograms budesonide per actuation.

Pulmicort Turbohaler 400 is a breath-actuated metered dose powder inhaler delivering 400 micrograms budesonide per actuation.

Pulmicort Turbohaler 100, Pulmicort Turbohaler 200 and Pulmicort Turbohaler 400 are free from propellants, lubricants, preservatives, carrier substances or other additives.

**Uses**   Pulmicort Turbohaler 100, Pulmicort Turbohaler 200 and Pulmicort Turbohaler 400 contain the potent, non-halogenated corticosteroid budesonide. Clinical studies have shown inhaled budesonide to possess a local anti-inflammatory action in the lungs without giving rise to systemic corticosteroid effects. Investigations with Pulmicort have documented good therapeutic results in bronchial asthma, whilst being well tolerated during prolonged treatment.

Pulmicort is, therefore, recommended in patients with bronchial asthma.

**Dosage and administration**
*Adults:* The dosage of Pulmicort Turbohaler 100, Pulmicort Turbohaler 200 and Pulmicort Turbohaler 400 should be individualised. When starting treatment, during periods of severe asthma and while reducing or discontinuing oral glucocorticosteroids the dosage in adults should be 200–1600 micrograms daily in divided doses. In less severe cases 200–800 micrograms daily may be used; during periods of severe asthma the daily dosage can be increased to up to 1600 micrograms in divided doses.

*Mild to moderate stable asthmatics: Adults (including elderly and children over 12 years):* A once daily regimen of up to 800 micrograms may be used by patients already controlled on inhaled steroids (e.g. budesonide or beclomethasone dipropionate) administered twice daily. The patient should be transferred to once daily dosing at the same equivalent total daily dose. The dose should subsequently be reduced to the minimum needed to maintain good asthma control.

Patients should be instructed to take the once daily dose in the evening. It is important the dose is taken consistently and at a similar time each evening.

There are insufficient data to make recommendations for the transfer of patients from newer inhaled steroids to once daily Pulmicort Turbohaler.

In keeping with accepted medical practice, when transferring patients to Turbohaler from other devices treatment should be individualised and consideration given to the drug and the method of delivery.

*Children:* 200–800 micrograms daily in divided doses. During periods of severe asthma the daily dose can be increased up to 800 micrograms.

A once daily regimen is not recommended for children under 12 years.

*Elderly:* Dosage as for adults.

The maintenance dose should be individualised and should be the lowest possible, whether once or twice daily dosing is being used.

Patients, in particular those receiving once daily treatment should be advised that if their asthma deteriorates (e.g. increased frequency of bronchodilator use or persistent respiratory symptoms) to double their steroid dose, by administering twice daily and advised to contact their doctor as soon as possible.

In patients where an increased therapeutic effect is desired, an increased dose of Pulmicort is recommended because of the lower risk of systemic effects as compared with a combined treatment with oral glucocorticosteroids.

In order to reduce the risk of oral candidiasis and hoarseness, patients should brush their teeth and rinse their mouths out with water after each administration.

When transferring patients to Turbohaler from other devices, treatment should be individualised. The drug and method of delivery should be considered.

Patients should be reminded of the importance of taking prophylactic therapy regularly even when they are asymptomatic.

**Contra-indications, warnings, etc**
*Contra-indications:* Active pulmonary tuberculosis. Hypersensitivity to budesonide.

*Special warnings and precautions:* Special care is needed in patients with quiescent lung tuberculosis, fungal and viral infections in the airways.

*Precautions:*
*Non-steroid dependent patients:* A therapeutic effect is usually reached within 10 days. In patients with excessive mucus secretion in the bronchi a short (about 2 weeks) additional oral corticosteroid regimen can be given initially.

*Steroid dependent patients:* When transfer from oral steroids to Pulmicort Turbohaler is started, the patient should be in a relatively stable phase. A high dose of Pulmicort Turbohaler is given in combination with the previously used oral steroid for about 10 days. After that the oral dose should be gradually reduced (by for example 2.5 mg prednisolone or the equivalent each month) to the lowest possible level. In many cases, it is possible to completely substitute Pulmicort for the oral steroid.
*Note:* During transfer from oral therapy to Pulmicort a generally lower systemic steroid action will be experienced which may result in the appearance of allergic or arthritic symptoms such as rhinitis, eczema and muscle and joint pain. Specific treatment should be initiated for these conditions.

Acute exacerbations of asthma may need an increase in the dose of Pulmicort or additional treatment with a short course of oral corticosteroids and/or an antibiotic if there is an infection.

Inhaled budesonide will not usually affect adrenocortical function. However, a small proportion of patients may experience some systemic effects after prolonged treatment at the maximum recommended daily dose.

Patients, who have previously been dependant on oral steroids may, as a result of prolonged systemic steroid therapy experience the effects of impaired adrenal function. Recovery may take a considerable amount of time after cessation of oral steroid therapy hence oral steroid dependant patients transferred to budesonide may remain at risk from impaired adrenal function for some considerable time. In such circumstances HPA axis functions should be monitored regularly.

Patients whose adrenocortical function is shown to be impaired or patients who are receiving the maximum dose of inhaled steroids may require supplementary systemic steroids during periods of stress such as chest infections, worsening asthma, surgery or trauma and should be instructed to carry a steroid warning card indicating their needs. Treatment with supplementary systemic steroids or Pulmicort should not be stopped abruptly.

*Pregnancy and breast feeding:* In pregnant animals, administration of budesonide causes abnormalities of foetal development. The relevance of this finding to man has not been established. Administration during pregnancy should be avoided unless there are compelling reasons. If treatment with glucocorticosteroids during pregnancy is unavoidable, inhaled glucocorticosteroids should be preferred because of their lower systemic effect compared with equipotent anti-asthmatic doses of oral glucocorticosteroids. There is no information regarding the passage of budesonide into breast milk.

*Side-effects:* Mild irritation in the throat and hoarseness. Candida infection in the oropharynx has been reported. Advising the patient to rinse the mouth with water after each administration is recommended. In most cases this condition responds to topical antifungal therapy without discontinuing treatment with Pulmicort.

Skin reactions such as a rash may occur in rare cases

As with other inhalation therapy, the potential for paradoxical bronchospasm should be kept in mind. If it occurs treatment should be discontinued immediately and if necessary, alternative treatment initiated. Paradoxical bronchospasm responds to a fast acting inhaled bronchodilator.

*Overdosage:* The only harmful effect that follows inhalation of large amounts of the drug over a short period is suppression of hypothalamic-pituitary-adrenal (HPA) function. No special emergency action needs to be taken. Treatment with Pulmicort Turbohaler should be continued at the recommended dose to control the asthma.

**Pharmaceutical precautions**   Store below 30°C.

**Legal category**   POM

**Package quantities**
Pulmicort Turbohaler 100 :   containing 200 actuations.
Pulmicort Turbohaler 200 :   containing 100 actuations.
Pulmicort Turbohaler 400 :   containing 50 actuations.

**Further information**   Pulmicort Turbohaler is breath-actuated and therefore there is no need to co-ordinate the release of the dose and the inhalation.

Treatment with Pulmicort Turbohaler is effective even at low inspiratory flow rates.

**Product licence numbers**
Pulmicort Turbohaler 100            0017/0319
Pulmicort Turbohaler 200            0017/0272
Pulmicort Turbohaler 400            0017/0271

## RHINOCORT* AQUA

**Presentation**   Rhinocort Aqua is a metered pump spray for nasal application delivering 100 micrograms budesonide per actuation. Also contains disodium edetate, potassium sorbate, glucose, microcrystalline cellulose, carboxymethyl cellulose sodium, polysorbate 80, hydrochloric acid and water.

**Uses**   Seasonal and perennial allergic rhinitis and vasomotor rhinitis. Treatment of nasal polyps.

**Dosage and administration**
*Adults: Rhinitis:* The recommended dose is 400 micrograms. Rhinocort Aqua may be given once daily for nasal inhalation (two applications into each nostril in the morning). When good effect has been achieved the dosage may be reduced to one application into each nostril.

Rhinocort Aqua may also be given twice daily (one application into each nostril morning and evening).

*Nasal polyps:* The recommended dose is 200 micrograms twice daily (one application into each nostril morning and evening). This is the maximum recommended total daily dose. Treatment can be continued for up to 3 months.

*Elderly:* Dosage as for adults.

*Children:* There are insufficient data to recommend the use of Rhinocort Aqua in children. However it is unlikely that the risk/benefit ratio in children is different from that in adults.

Patients should be reminded of the importance of taking this medicine regularly.

**Contra-indications, warnings, etc**
*Contra-indication:* Hypersensitivity to any of the ingredients.

*Precautions and warnings:* Special care is demanded in treatment of patients transferred from oral steroids to Rhinocort where disturbance in the hypothalamic-pituitary-adrenal (HPA) axis could be expected.

Special care is needed in patients with fungal and viral infections in the airways, and in patients with lung tuberculosis.

The patient should be informed that full effect of Rhinocort is not achieved until after a few days treatment. Treatment of seasonal rhinitis should, if possible, start before exposure to the allergens. Concomitant treatment may sometimes be necessary to counteract eye symptoms caused by the allergy. In continuous long-term treatment, the nasal mucosa should be inspected regularly e.g. every 6 months.

Rhinocort Aqua does not affect the ability to drive and operate machinery.

*Pregnancy and lactation:* Administation during pregnancy should be avoided unless there are compelling reasons. In pregnant animals administration of budesonide causes abnormalities of foetal development. The relevance of this to man has not been established. There is no information available regarding the passage of budesonide into breast milk. Use in lactation requires that the therapeutic benefit to the mother be weighed against any potential risk to the neonate.

*Side-effects:* Occasionally sneezing, nasal stinging and dryness may follow immediately after the use of the spray. Slight haemorrhagic secretion/epistaxis may occur.

Contact allergy (rash, urticaria, dermatitis) involving the skin of the face may also occur, but is rare.

Ulceration of mucous membrane and nasal septum perforation have been reported following the use of intranasal aerosol corticosteroids, but these are extremely rare.

Rare cases of raised intraocular pressure or glaucoma have been reported following the use of intranasal steroid formulations.

*Overdose:* Acute overdose with Rhinocort should not present clinical problems.

Inhalation of high doses of corticosteroids may lead to suppression of the hypothalamic – pituitary – adrenal (HPA) axis function.

**Pharmaceutical precautions** Store below 30°C. Use within 2 months of starting treatment.

**Legal category** POM

**Package quantities** Rhinocort Aqua is a nasal spray containing 100×100 microgram actuations budesonide.

**Further information** In pharmacological investigations and investigations in human beings budesonide (a non-halogenated corticosteroid) has shown a favourable relationship between anti-inflammatory effects and systemic effects due to the fact that budesonide is inactivated very rapidly in the liver after systemic absorption. With the recommended dosage of Rhinocort Aqua an effective corticosteroid treatment of the nasal mucous membrane is attained with very little risk of systemic side-effects.

**Product licence number** 0017/0304

## THEO-DUR*

**Presentation** An extended release formulation (Durules) containing Theophylline Anhydrous PhEur, designed to give therapeutic blood levels over 8–12 hours.

200 mg tablet: A white, mottled, biconvex, elliptical tablet with the engraving Theo-Dur/200 on one side and a score in the transverse direction on the opposite side.

300 mg tablet: A white, mottled, biconvex, elliptical tablet with the engraving Theo-Dur/300 on one side and a score in the transverse direction on the opposite side.

**Uses** As a bronchodilator in the symptomatic or prophylactic treatment of bronchospasm associated with chronic obstructive airways disease including asthma and chronic bronchitis.

**Dosage and administration**
*Standard dosing: Adults:* the usual maintenance dose is one 300 mg tablet 12 hourly.

*Children:* <35 kg body weight: 100 mg (half a 200 mg tablet) 12 hourly. >35 kg body weight: 200 mg 12 hourly.

*Elderly and patients with liver disease:* Plasma half-life of theophylline may be prolonged and individual dosing should be adopted (see below).

Theophylline clearance is increased in cigarette smokers and such patients may require increased doses of Theo-Dur to achieve a therapeutic effect.

*Individual dosing:* If sufficient therapeutic effect is not achieved or if side-effects occur, the dose of Theo-Dur may be increased or decreased by 100 mg (half a 200 mg tablet) or 150 mg (half a 300 mg tablet) stages. If doses higher than the usual maintenance doses are to be given, it is recommended that the patient's serum theophylline level is determined and the dose adjusted to maintain this level between 10-20 micrograms/ml (55–110 micromols/litre). The following procedure is recommended.

*Adults:* 150 mg (half a 300 mg tablet) 12 hourly for 4–7 days then 300 mg 12 hourly for 7–10 days.

*Children:* <35 kg body weight: 100 mg (half a 200 mg tablet) 12 hourly for 7–14 days. >35 kg body weight: 100 mg (half a 200 mg tablet) 12 hourly for 4–7 days then 200 mg 12 hourly for 7–10 days.

Blood for theophylline assay should be taken 3–8 hours after a dose when there has been no dosage adjustment for at least 4 days and no doses have been missed for 48 hours. The dose of Theo-Dur may be adjusted as follows:

| *Peak serum theophylline level* | *Dosage adjustment* |
|---|---|
| <7.9 micrograms/ml | Increase dose by 50%.* |
| 8–9.9 micrograms/ml | Increase dose by 20%* to the nearest 50 mg. |
| 10–13.9 micrograms/ml | If the patient's symptoms persist, increase the dose by 10% to the nearest 50 mg. |
| 14–19.9 micrograms/ml | Do not adjust the dose unless side-effects occur in which case a 10% decrease, to the nearest 50 mg may be necessary. |
| 20–24.9 micrograms/ml | Decrease dose by 10% to the nearest 50 mg. |
| 25–29.9 micrograms/ml | Miss next dose and decrease maintenance dose by 25%.* |
| >30 micrograms/ml | Miss next two doses and decrease maintenance dose by 50%*. |

* With patients falling into these categories it is advisable to re-check the serum theophylline concentration 3–5 days after dosage adjustment.

*Nocturnal asthma:* For the control of symptoms of nocturnal asthma the appropriately individualised dosage of Theo-Dur should be administered once daily at approximately 8 p.m.

*Note:*

1. The tablet must not be crushed or chewed but swallowed whole or as a half.
2. Any previous theophylline or aminophylline therapy should be discontinued.
3. If a patient has not previously been treated with theophylline or aminophylline or other theophylline salts, it is advisable to give half the maintenance dose of Theo-Dur (100 mg or 150 mg) for the first 4–7 days of treatment. This procedure should reduce the incidence of side-effects.

It is not possible to ensure bioequivalence between different extended release theophylline products. It should therefore be emphasised that patients once titrated to an effective dose should not be changed from Theo-Dur tablets to other extended release preparations or vice versa without retitration and clinical assessment.

After an effective therapeutic regime is attained it is important that practitioners, pharmacists and patients are aware of the possible dangers of inefficacy or toxicity if an alternative extended release theophylline preparation is substituted. This may be a particular hazard because the products are available without prescription. Likewise there may be a hazard if the doctor prescribes "generically" or if the preparation used in hospital is unknown by the general practitioner.

**Contra-indications, warnings, etc**
*Contra-indications:* None known.

*Precautions:* Theophylline should be given with caution to patients with congestive heart failure, liver disease or viral infections, and in the elderly. Plasma half-life of theophylline is prolonged in most of these patients, and the drug may accumulate to toxic concentrations.

*Use in pregnancy and lactation:* Caution is recommended during pregnancy and lactation. When theophylline is prescribed to pregnant and nursing women, the risk-benefit of the treatment must be taken into account.

Theophylline crosses the placenta, but no influence on foetal development or reproductive capacity has been established. Theophylline should not be used routinely in nursing women even though only very small amounts of theophylline are excreted into breast milk.

Premature children with low birthweight have an extremely prolonged theophylline half-life, which may lead to high theophylline plasma levels causing insomnia, agitation and/or anxiety. Full capacity to eliminate theophylline is not reached until the age of 6–12 months. Caution should be used when theophylline is given to infants who cannot complain of minor adverse reactions.

*Side-effects:* Side-effects of theophylline depend to a great extent on serum concentration and are frequent only at theophylline concentration exceeding 20 micrograms/ml. The Theo-Dur extended release formulation reduces fluctuation in serum levels of theophylline, thereby reducing the incidence of side-effects.

The most common side-effects are gastro-intestinal disturbances (nausea, vomiting and anorexia) which, in most cases, disappear on reducing the dose. Monitoring of the serum concentration of theophylline is recommended.

The CNS stimulating effect of theophylline can cause restlessness, irritability, anxiety and insomnia in some patients. Cardiovascular effects such as palpitations and tachycardia may appear.

Severe side-effects (cramps, convulsions and cardiac arrythmias) may appear at very high serum concentration, in which case the medication should be discontinued.

*Drug interactions:* The serum theophylline concentration may increase in patients receiving cimetidine, quinolone derivatives such as ciprofloxacin or macrolide antibiotics such as erythromycin and troleandomycin, concurrently with theophylline preparations. Increase in the theophylline serum concentration is also seen with oestrogen, allopurinol and propranolol. The serum theophylline concentration may be reduced during concurrent therapy with phenobarbitone, phenytoin and rifampicin as these drugs increase theophylline clearance. Theophylline has been shown to decrease the serum concentration of lithium.

Concurrent administration of ketamine with theophylline may reduce the threshold value for inducing convulsions.

Xanthines may potentiate hypokalaemia resulting from $\beta_2$-agonist therapy, steroids, diuretics and hypoxia. Particular caution is advised in severe asthma. It is recommended that serum potassium levels are monitored in such situations.

The concomitant use of theophylline and fluvoxamine should usually be avoided. Where this is not possible, patients should have their theophylline dose halved and plasma theophylline should be monitored closely.

*Treatment of overdosage:* Gastric lavage and symptomatic treatment to maintain fluid and electrolyte balance and correct hypokalaemia. Give oxygen as necessary. Monitor serum theophylline levels. Oral activated charcoal may reduce serum theophylline concentration. In severe cases charcoal haemoperfusion may be required. Tablets in the intestine may continue to release theophylline for several hours.

Possible signs and symptoms of overdosage are insomnia, anorexia, agitation, anxiety, nausea, vomiting, convulsions, hypotension, palpitations, tachycadia and cardiac arrhythmias. Serious toxicity is not always preceded by less severe adverse effects.

**Pharmaceutical precautions** Store below 30°C.

**Legal category** P

**Package quantities** 100 tablets.

**Further information** Nil

**Product licence numbers**

| | |
|---|---|
| 0017/0098 | 200 mg |
| 0017/0099 | 300 mg |

## XYLOCAINE* VIALS 0.5%, 1% and 2%

**Presentation** A sterile clear aqueous solution of Lidocaine Hydrochloride PhEur. Each ml contains:

| | |
|---|---|
| 0.5% solution: | Lidocaine Hydrochloride PhEur 5.35 mg equivalent to lidocaine hydrochloride anhydrous 5 mg. |
| 1.0% solution: | Lidocaine Hydrochloride PhEur 10.7 mg equivalent to lidocaine hydrochloride anhydrous 10 mg. |
| 2% solution: | Lidocaine Hydrochloride PhEur 21.4 mg equivalent to lidocaine hydrochloride anhydrous 20 mg. |

All the above contain sodium chloride to produce isotonic solutions.

**Uses** Xylocaine is a local anaesthetic solution for use in infiltration anaesthesia, intravenous regional anaesthesia and nerve blocks.

**Dosage and administration** The dosage is adjusted according to the response of the patient and site of administration. The lowest concentration and smallest dose producing the required effect should be given. The maximum dose for healthy adults should not exceed 200 mg.

Children and elderly or debilitated patients require

smaller doses, commensurate with age and physical status.

### Contra-indications, warnings, etc
*Contra-indications:* Known hypersensitivity to anaesthetics of the amide type.

*Precautions:* In common with other local anaesthetics, Xylocaine should be used cautiously in patients with epilepsy, impaired cardiac conduction, bradycardia, impaired respiratory function, and in patients with impaired hepatic function, if the dose or site of administration is likely to result in high blood levels.

Facilities for resuscitation should be available when local anaesthetics are administered.

The effect of local anaesthetics may be reduced if an injection is made into an inflamed or infected area.

*Use in pregnancy:* Although there is no evidence from animal studies of harm to the foetus, as with all drugs, Xylocaine should not be given during early pregnancy unless the benefits are considered to outweigh the risks.

*Side-effects:* In common with other local anaesthetics, adverse reactions to Xylocaine are rare and are usually the result of excessively high blood concentrations due to inadvertent intravascular injection, excessive dosage, rapid absorption or occasionally to hypersensitivity, idiosyncrasy or diminished tolerance on the part of the patient. In such circumstances systemic effects occur involving the central nervous system and/or the cardiovascular system.

CNS reactions are excitatory and/or depressant, and may be characterised by nervousness, dizziness, blurred vision and tremors, followed by drowsiness, convulsions, unconsciousness and possibly respiratory arrest. The excitatory reactions may be very brief or may not occur at all, in which case the first manifestations of toxicity may be drowsiness, merging into unconsciousness and respiratory arrest. Cardiovascular reactions are depressant, and may be characterised by hypotension, myocardial depression, bradycardia and possibly cardiac arrest.

Allergic reactions are extremely rare. They may be characterised by cutaneous lesions, urticaria, oedema or anaphylactoid reactions. Detection of sensitivity by skin testing is of doubtful value.

Hypotension may occur as a physiological response to central nerve blocks.

*Interactions:* Cimetidine can impair the metabolism of lidocaine absorbed into the circulation. Elimination will be delayed and the risk of adverse reactions increased.

*Overdosage:* Treatment of a patient with systemic toxicity consists of arresting convulsions and ensuring adequate ventilation with oxygen, if necessary by assisted or controlled ventilation (respiration). If convulsions occur they must be treated promptly by intravenous injection of thiopentone 100 to 200 mg or diazepam 5 to 10 mg. Alternatively succinylcholine 50 mg–100 mg i.v. may be used providing the clinician is capable of performing endotracheal intubation and managing a fully paralysed patient.

Once convulsions have been controlled and adequate ventilation of the lungs ensured, no other treatment is generally required. If hypotension is present, however, a vasopressor, preferably one with inotropic activity, e.g. ephedrine 15 to 30 mg, should be given intravenously.

### Pharmaceutical precautions  Store below 25˚C.

### Legal category  POM

### Package quantities
0.5% solution – 20 ml. Pack of 5 vials.
1.0% solution – 20 ml. Pack of 5 vials.
2.0% solution – 20 ml. Pack of 5 vials.

### Further information  Multidose vial preparations of Xylocaine contain Methyl Parahydroxybenzoate PhEur 1 mg/ml.

### Product licence numbers
0.5%   0017/5031R
1.0%   0017/5032R
2.0%   0017/5034R

## XYLOCAINE* 2% WITH ADRENALINE 1:80,000

**Presentation**   Sterile, clear aqueous solution. Each ml contains Lidocaine Hydrochloride PhEur 21.4 mg/ml equivalent to lidocaine hydrochloride anhydrous 20 mg/ml and Adrenaline Tartrate PhEur 22.7 micrograms equivalent to adrenaline 12.5 micrograms.

*Inactive ingredients:* sodium chloride to produce an isotonic solution, sodium metabisulphite, hydrochloric acid and water for injection.

**Uses**   Xylocaine 2% with Adrenaline is a local anaesthetic solution for use in dental infiltration anaesthesia and all dental nerve block techniques.

**Dosage and administration**   Infiltration – usual dose is 1 ml. Nerve block – usual dose is 1.5 to 2 ml.

The recommended maximum dose for Xylocaine when given with adrenaline is 500 mg.

Children and elderly or debilitated patients require smaller doses.

### Contra-indications, warnings, etc
*Contra-indications:* Known hypersensitivity to anaesthetics of the amide type.

The use of a vasoconstrictor is contra-indicated for anaesthesia of fingers, toes, tip of nose, ears and penis.

Xylocaine with Adrenaline should not be given intravenously.

*Precautions:* In common with other local anaesthetics, Xylocaine with Adrenaline should be used cautiously in patients with epilepsy, impaired cardiac conduction, impaired respiratory function, and in patients with impaired hepatic function if the dose or site of administration is likely to result in high blood levels.

Facilities for resuscitation should be available when local anaesthetics are administered.

The effect of local anaesthetics may be reduced if an injection is made into an inflamed or infected area. Solutions containing adrenaline should be used with caution in patients with hypertension, cardiac disease, cerebrovascular insufficiency, thyrotoxicosis.

Solutions containing adrenaline should be used where possible so as to prolong anaesthesia and reduce systemic absorption. This is particularly important in highly vascular areas.

Use on one patient during one treatment only.

*Use in pregnancy and lactation:* Although there is no evidence from animal studies of harm to the foetus, as with all drugs lidocaine should not be given in early pregnancy unless the benefits are considered to outweigh the risks.

*Interactions:* Use with caution in patients taking tricyclic antidepressants, MAOI's or receiving potent general anaesthetic agents.

*Adverse reactions:* In common with other local anaesthetics, adverse reactions to Xylocaine with Adrenaline are extremely rare in dental practice and are usually the result of excessively high blood concentrations due to inadvertent intravascular injection, excessive dosage, rapid absorption or occasionally to hypersensitivity, idiosyncrasy or diminished tolerance on the part of the patient. In such circumstances systemic effects occur involving the central nervous system and/or the cardiovascular system.

CNS reactions are excitatory and/or depressant, and may be characterised by nervousness, dizziness, blurred vision and tremors, followed by drowsiness, convulsions, unconsciousness and possibly respiratory arrest. The excitatory reactions may be very brief or may not occur at all, in which case the first manifestations of toxicity may be drowsiness, merging into unconsciousness and respiratory arrest.

Cardiovascular reactions are depressant, and may be characterised by hypotension, myocardial depression, bradycardia and possibly cardiac arrest.

Allergic reactions are extremely rare. They may be characterised by cutaneous lesions, urticaria, oedema or anaphylactoid reactions. Detection of sensitivity by skin testing is of doubtful value.

### Pharmaceutical precautions  Store below 15˚C.

### Legal category  POM

### Package quantities  Glass cartridges of 2 ml standard and 2 ml self-aspirating, in boxes of 100.

### Further information  Dental cartridges of Xylocaine 2% with Adrenaline 1:80,000 do not contain an antimicrobial agent.

### Product licence number 0017/5027R

## XYLOCAINE* WITH ADRENALINE 1:200,000

**Presentation**   A sterile clear aqueous solution of Lidocaine Hydrochloride BP. Each ml contains:
0.5% solution:   Lidocaine Hydrochloride PhEur 5.35 mg equivalent to lidocaine hydrochloride anhydrous 5 mg, Adrenaline Tartrate PhEur 10 micrograms equivalent to adrenaline 5 micrograms.
1% solution:   Lidocaine Hydrochloride PhEur 10.7 mg equivalent to lidocaine hydrochloride anhydrous 10 mg, Adrenaline Tartrate PhEur 10 micrograms equivalent to adrenaline 5 micrograms.

2% solution:   Lidocaine Hydrochloride PhEur 21.4 mg equivalent to lidocaine hydrochloride anhydrous 20 mg, Adrenaline Tartrate PhEur 10 micrograms equivalent to adrenaline 5 micrograms.

*Inactive ingredients:* Sodium chloride, sodium metabisulphite, methylparahydroxybenzoate.

**Uses**   Xylocaine with Adrenaline is a local anaesthetic solution for use in infiltration anaesthesia, and nerve blocks.

**Dosage and administration**   The dosage is adjusted according to the response of the patient and the site of administration. The lowest concentration and smallest dose producing the required effect should be given. The maximum single dose of Xylocaine when given with adrenaline is 500 mg.

Children and elderly or debilitated patients require smaller doses, commensurate with age and physical status.

### Contra-indications, warnings, etc
*Contra-indications:* Known hypersensitivity to anaesthetics of the amide type.

The use of a vasoconstrictor is contra-indicated for anaesthesia of fingers, toes, tip of nose, ears and penis.

Xylocaine with Adrenaline should not be given intravenously.

*Precautions:* In common with other local anaesthetics, Xylocaine with Adrenaline should be used cautiously in patients with epilepsy, impaired cardiac conduction, impaired respiratory function, and in patients with impaired hepatic function, if the dose or site of administration is likely to result in high blood levels.

Facilities for resuscitation should be available when local anaesthetics are administered.

The effect of local anaesthetics may be reduced if an injection is made into an inflamed or infected area.

Solutions containing adrenaline should be used with caution in patients with hypertension, cardiac disease, cerebrovascular insufficiency, thyrotoxicosis, in patients taking tricyclic antidepressants, MAOI's, or receiving potent general anaesthetic agents.

Solutions containing adrenaline should be used where possible so as to prolong anaesthesia and reduce systemic absorption. This is particularly important in highly vascular areas.

*Use in pregnancy:* Although there is no evidence from animal studies of harm to the foetus, as with all drugs, Xylocaine should not be given during early pregnancy unless the benefits are considered to outweigh the risks.

*Side-effects:* In common with other local anaesthetics, adverse reactions to Xylocaine with adrenaline are rare and are usually the result of excessively high blood concentrations due to inadvertent intravascular injection, excessive dosage, rapid absorption or occasionally to hypersensitivity, idiosyncrasy or diminished tolerance on the part of the patient. In such circumstances systemic effects occur involving the central nervous system and/or the cardiovascular system.

CNS reactions are excitatory and/or depressant, and may be characterised by nervousness, dizziness, blurred vision and tremors, followed by drowsiness, convulsions, unconsciousness and possibly respiratory arrest. The excitatory reactions may be very brief or may not occur at all, in which case the first manifestations of toxicity may be drowsiness, merging into unconsciousness and respiratory arrest.

Cardiovascular reactions are depressant, and may be characterised by hypotension, myocardial depression, bradycardia and possibly cardiac arrest.

Allergic reactions are extremely rare. They may be characterised by cutaneous lesions, urticaria, oedema or anaphylactoid reactions. Detection of sensitivity by skin testing is of doubtful value.

Hypotension may occur as a physiological response to central nerve blocks.

### Pharmaceutical precautions  Store below 15˚C.

### Legal category  POM

### Package quantities
0.5% with adrenaline: 20 ml vials. Packs of 5 vials.
1% with adrenaline: 20 ml vials. Packs of 5 vials.
2% with adrenaline: 20 ml vials. Packs of 5 vials.

### Further information  Multidose vial preparations of Xylocaine with Adrenaline 1:200,000 contain methylhydroxybenzoate 1 mg/ml.

### Product licence numbers
0.5%   0017/5028R
1.0%   0017/5029R
2.0%   0017/5030R

## XYLOCAINE* 2% PLAIN

**Presentation** A clear sterile aqueous solution for injection supplied in polypropylene cartridges for use with dental type syringes. Each cartridge contains 2.2 ml of solution.

Each ml of solution contains Lidocaine Hydrochloride PhEur 21.3 mg equivalent to lidocaine hydrochloride anhydrous 20.0 mg.

*Inactive ingredients:* sodium chloride and water for injections.

Lidocaine is synonymous with lignocaine.

**Uses** Local anaesthetic solution for use mainly in dental procedures.

NOTE: If a vasoconstrictor is needed to prolong the local anaesthesia by delaying the diffusion of the anaesthetic in the surrounding tissues a product containing lidocaine and adrenaline such as Lignostab-A should be used.

**Dosage and administration** The dosage is adjusted according to the response of the patient and the site of administration. The lowest concentration and smallest dose producing the required effect should be given. The maximum single dose of lidocaine hydrochloride is 200 mg when given alone. This is equivalent to 4 cartridges containing 2.2 ml.

Children and elderly or debilitated patients require smaller doses, commensurate with age and physical status.

**Contra-indications, warnings, etc**
*Contra-indications:* Known hypersensitivity to anaesthetics of the amide type or the other constituents. Intravenous use.

*Precautions:* As for other local anaesthetics, use cautiously in patients with epilepsy, impaired cardiac conduction, impaired respiratory function, and in patients with impaired hepatic function, if the dose or site of administration is likely to result in high blood levels.

Facilities for resuscitation should be available when local anaesthetics are administered.

The effect of local anaesthetics may be reduced if an injection is made into an inflamed or infected area.

Use on one patient during one treatment only. Discard unused contents.

*Use in pregnancy:* Although this product crosses the placenta, the low doses used in dental anaesthesia would not be expected to give rise to signs of toxicity in the foetus.

*Side-effects:* In common with other local anaesthetics, adverse reactions are rare and are usually the result of excessively high blood concentrations due to inadvertent intravascular injection, excessive dosage, rapid absorption or diminished tolerance on the part of the patient. In such circumstances systemic effects occur involving the central nervous system and/or the cardiovascular system.

CNS reactions are excitatory and/or depressant, and may be characterised by nervousness, dizziness, blurred vision and tremors, followed by drowsiness, convulsions, unconsciousness and possibly respiratory arrest. The excitatory reactions may be very brief or may not occur at all, in which case the first manifestations of toxicity may be drowsiness, merging into unconsciousness and respiratory arrest.

Cardiovascular reactions are depressant, and may be characterised by hypotension, myocardial depression, bradycardia and possibly cardiac arrest. Allergic reactions are extremely rare. They may be characterised by cutaneous lesions, urticaria, oedema or anaphylactoid reactions. Detection of sensitivity by skin testing is of doubtful value. Hypotension may occur as a physiological response to central nerve blocks.

**Pharmaceutical precautions** Store below 25°C.

**Legal category** POM

**Package quantities** Boxes of 100 (polypropylene ) cartridges.

**Further information** Nil

**Product licence number** 0017/0256

## XYLOCAINE* ANTISEPTIC GEL 2%
## XYLOCAINE* ACCORDION ANTISEPTIC GEL 2%

**Presentation** A topical anaesthetic/antiseptic gel.

1 g Xylocaine Antiseptic Gel 2% contains:
*Active constituents:* Lidocaine Hydrochloride PhEur 21.6 mg (equivalent to 20 mg lidocaine hydrochloride anhydrous), Chlorhexidine Gluconate Solution BP 2.7 mg.

*Inactive ingredients:* Hydroxypropyl methylcellulose, sodium hydroxide and water, purified.

1 g Xylocaine Accordion Antiseptic Gel 2% contains:
*Active constituents:* Lidocaine Hydrochloride PhEur 21.6 mg (equivalent to lidocaine hydrochloride anhydrous 20 mg), Chlorhexidine Digluconate BP 2.7 mg.

*Inactive constituents:* Hydroxypropyl methylcellulose, sodium hydroxide q.s., water, purified q.s.

Both Xylocaine Antiseptic Gel 2% and Xylocaine Accordion Antiseptic Gel 2% provide prompt and profound anaesthesia of mucous membranes and lubrication which reduces friction. The water miscible base, characterised by high viscosity and low surface tension, brings the anaesthetic into intimate and prolonged contact with the tissue for effective anaesthesia of long duration (approx. 20–30 mins.). Anaesthesia usually occurs rapidly (within e.g. 5 minutes depending upon area of application).

The anaesthetic ingredient of both Xylocaine Antiseptic Gel 2% and Xylocaine Accordion Antiseptic Gel 2% is lidocaine, which stabilises the neuronal membrane and prevents the initiation and conduction of nerve impulses, thereby effecting local anaesthetic action. Lidocaine is absorbed following application to mucous membranes. The absorption occurs most rapidly after intratracheal administration. Blood concentrations of lidocaine after instillation in urethra of doses up to 800 mg are of low range and below toxic levels. The metabolism of lidocaine takes place in the liver and metabolites and unchanged drug are excreted by the kidney.

**Uses** For anaesthesia of the urethra and topical application on mucous membranes wherever an anaesthetic/antiseptic effect is required.

**Dosage and administration** As with any local anaesthetic, reactions and complications are best averted by employing the minimal effective dosage. Debilitated, elderly patients and children should be given doses commensurate with their age and physical condition.

*Urethral anaesthesia: Surface anaesthesia of the male adult urethra:*
Males: 10 ml injected initially followed by 3–5 ml.
Females: Instil 5–10 ml in small portions to fill the whole urethra.

In order to obtain adequate anaesthesia, several minutes should be allowed prior to performing urological procedures.

**Contra-indications, warnings, etc**
*Contra-indications:* Known history of hypersensitivity to local anaesthesia of the amide type or other components of the gel.

*Precautions and warnings:* Absorption from wound surfaces and mucous membranes is relatively high, especially in the bronchial tree. Xylocaine Antiseptic Gel 2% and Xylocaine Accordion Antiseptic Gel 2% should be used with caution in patients with traumatised mucosa and/or sepsis in the region of the proposed application.

If the dose or site of administration is likely to result in high blood levels, lidocaine, in common with other local anaesthetics, should be used cautiously in patients with epilepsy, impaired cardiac conduction, bradycardia, impaired hepatic function and in severe shock.

The oropharyngeal use of topical anaesthetic agents may interfere with swallowing and thus enhance the danger of aspiration. This is particularly important in children because of their frequency of eating. Numbness of the tongue or buccal mucosa may increase the danger of biting trauma.

Care should be taken to avoid instillation of excessive amounts of Xylocaine Antiseptic Gel 2% or Xylocaine Accordion Antiseptic Gel 2% into the rectum. This is of particular importance in infants and children. Systemic absorption of lidocaine may occur from the rectum, and large doses may result in CNS side-effects. On rare occasions convulsions have occurred in children.

*Use in pregnancy and lactation:* Although there is no evidence from animal studies of harm to the foetus, as with all drugs, Xylocaine should not be given during early pregnancy unless the benefits are considered to outweigh the risks. Lidocaine enters the mother's milk, but in such small quantities that there is generally no risk of the child being affected at therapeutic dose levels.

*Side-effects:* In extremely rare cases local anaesthetic preparations have been associated with allergic reactions (in the most severe instances anaphylactic shock).

Systemic adverse reactions are extremely rare and may result from high plasma levels due to excessive dosage or rapid absorption or from hypersensitivity, idiosyncrasy or reduced tolerance on the part of the patient. Such reactions are systemic in nature and involve the central nervous system and/or the cardiovascular system.

CNS reactions are excitatory and/or depressant and may be characterised by nervousness, dizziness, convulsions, unconsciousness and, possibly, respiratory arrest. The excitatory reactions may be very brief or may not occur at all, in which case the first manifestations of toxicity may be drowsiness, merging into unconsciousness and respiratory arrest.

Cardiovascular reactions are depressant and may be characterised by hypotension, myocardial depression, bradycardia and possibly cardiac arrest.

*Interactions:* Lidocaine should be used with caution in patients receiving antiarrhythmic drugs, such as tocainide, since the toxic effects are additive.

*Overdosage:* Treatment of a patient with systemic toxicity consists of arresting convulsions and ensuring adequate ventilation with oxygen, if necessary by assisted or controlled ventilation (respiration). If convulsions occur they must be treated promptly by intravenous injection of thiopentone 100 to 200 mg or diazepam 5 to 10 mg. Alternatively succinylcholine 50 to 100 mg i.v. may be used providing the clinician is capable of performing endotracheal intubation and managing a fully paralysed patient. If ventricular fibrillation or cardiac arrest occurs, effective cardiovascular resuscitation must be instituted. Adrenaline in repeated doses and sodium bicarbonate should be given as rapidly as possible.

**Pharmaceutical precautions** Store below 25°C. Xylocaine Accordion Antiseptic Gel 2% is sterile and is meant for single use only.

**Legal category** P

**Package quantities** Xylocaine Antiseptic Gel 2%: 10 x 20 g tubes. Xylocaine Accordion Antiseptic Gel 2%: blister packs containing 10 syringes. Each syringe contains 20 g of gel.

**Further information** Nil

**Product licence numbers**

| | |
|---|---|
| Xylocaine Antiseptic Gel 2% | 0017/0244R |
| Xylocaine Accordion Antiseptic Gel 2% | 0017/5035R |

## XYLOCAINE* GEL 2%
## XYLOCAINE* ACCORDION GEL 2%

**Presentation** A topical anaesthetic for urological procedures and lubrication of endotracheal tubes.

1 g Xylocaine Gel 2% contains:
*Active constituent:* Lidocaine Hydrochloride PhEur 21.6 mg (equivalent to 20 mg lidocaine hydrochloride anhydrous).

*Inactive constituents:* Hydroxypropyl methylcellulose, methyl parahydroxybenzoate, propyl parahydroxybenzoate, sodium hydroxide, hydrochloric acid and water, purified.

1 g Xylocaine Accordion Gel 2% contains:
*Active constituent:* Lidocaine Hydrochloride PhEur corresponding to lidocaine hydrochloride anhydrous 20 mg.

*Inactive constituents:* Hydroxypropyl methylcellulose, sodium hydroxide q.s., hydrochloric acid q.s., water, purified q.s.

Both Xylocaine Gel 2% and Xylocaine Accordion Gel 2% provide prompt and profound anaesthesia of mucous membranes and lubrication which reduces friction. The water miscible base, characterised by high viscosity and low surface tension, brings the anaesthetic into intimate and prolonged contact with the tissue for effective anaesthesia of long duration (approx. 20–30 min).

Anaesthesia usually occurs rapidly (within 5 minutes depending upon area of application).

The active ingredient of both Xylocaine Gel 2% and Xylocaine Accordion Gel 2% is lidocaine, which stabilises the neuronal membrane and prevents the initiation and conduction of nerve impulses, thereby affecting local anaesthetic action. Lidocaine is absorbed following application to mucous membranes. The absorption occurs most rapidly after intratracheal administration. Blood concentrations of lidocaine after instillation in urethra of doses up to 800 mg are of low range and below toxic levels. The metabolism of lidocaine takes place in the liver and metabolites and unchanged drug are excreted by the kidneys.

**Uses** Surface anaesthesia and lubrication:
– the male and female urethra during cystoscopy, catheterisation, exploration by sound and other endourethral operations.
– nasal and pharyngeal cavities in endoscopic procedures such as gastroscopy and bronchoscopy.
– during proctoscopy and rectoscopy.
– intubation.

Symptomatic treatment of pain in connection with cystitis and urethritis.

**Dosage and administration** As with any local anaesthetic, reactions and complications are best averted by employing the minimal effective dosage. Debilitated, elderly patients and children should be given doses commensurate with their age and physical condition.

*Urethral anaesthesia:* Surface anaesthesia of the male adult urethra: For adequate analgesia in males 20 ml (=400 mg lidocaine hydrochloride) jelly is required. The jelly is instilled slowly until almost half the syringe (10 ml=200 mg lidocaine hydrochloride) is emptied. A penile clamp is then applied for several minutes at the corona; then the rest of the jelly is instilled.

When anaesthesia is especially important, e.g. during sounding or cystoscopy, a larger quantity of jelly, for example 30–40 ml , may be instilled in 3–4 portions and allowed to work for 10–12 minutes before insertion of the instrument.

Surface anaesthesia of the female adult urethra: Instil 5–10 ml in small portions to fill the whole urethra. In order to obtain adequate anaesthesia, several minutes should be allowed prior to performing urological procedures.

*Endoscopy:* Instillation of 10–20 ml is recommended for adequate analgesia and a small amount should be applied on the instrument for lubrication.

*Lubrication for endotracheal intubation:* About 5 ml applied on the surface of the tube just prior to insertion. Care should be taken to avoid introducing the product into the lumen of the tube.

### Contra-indications, warnings, etc

*Contra-indications:* Known history of hypersensitivity to local anaesthetics of the amide type or other components of the gel.

*Precautions:* Absorption from wound surfaces and mucous membranes is relatively high, especially in the bronchial tree. Xylocaine Gel 2%/Accordion Gel 2% should be used with caution in patients with traumatised mucosa and/or sepsis in the region of the proposed application.

If the dose or site of administration is likely to result in high blood levels, lidocaine, in common with other local anaesthetics, should be used cautiously in patients with epilepsy, impaired cardiac conduction, bradycardia, impaired hepatic function and in severe shock.

The oropharyngeal use of topical anaesthetic agents may interfere with swallowing and thus enhance the danger of aspiration. This is particularly important in children because of their frequency of eating. Numbness of the tongue or buccal mucosa may increase the danger of biting trauma.

When used for endotracheal tube lubrication care should be taken to avoid introduction of the jelly into the lumen of the tube. The jelly may dry on the inner surface leaving residue which tend to clump with flexion, narrowing the lumen. There have been rare reports in which this residue has caused the lumen to occlude.

Care should be taken to avoid instillation of excessive amounts of Xylocaine Gel 2%/Accordion Gel 2% into the rectum. This is of particular importance in infants and children. Systemic absorption of lidocaine may occur from the rectum, and large doses may result in CNS side-effects. On rare occasions convulsions have occurred in children.

*Pregnancy:* Although there is no evidence from animal studies of harm to the foetus, as with all drugs, Xylocaine should not be given during early pregnancy unless the benefits outweigh the risks.

*Lactation:* Lidocaine enters the mother's milk, but in such small quantities that there is generally no risk of affecting the child at therapeutic dose levels.

*Side-effects:* In extremely rare cases local anaesthetic preparations have been associated with allergic reactions (in the most severe instances anaphylactic shock).

Systemic adverse reactions are rare and may result from high plasma levels due to excessive dosage, rapid absorption or may result from hypersensitivity, idiosyncrasy or diminished tolerance on the part of the patient. Such reactions involve the central nervous system and/or the cardiovascular system.

CNS reactions are excitatory and/or depressant and may be characterised by nervousness, dizziness, convulsions, unconsciousness and, possibly, respiratory arrest. The excitatory reactions may be very brief or may not occur at all, in which case the first manifestations of toxicity may be drowsiness, merging into unconsciousness and respiratory arrest.

Cardiovascular reactions are depressant and may be characterised by hypotension, myocardial depression, bradycardia and possibly cardiac arrest.

*Interactions:* Lidocaine should be used with caution in patients receiving antiarrhythmic drugs, such as tocainide, since the toxic effects are additive.

*Overdosage:* Treatment of a patient with systemic toxicity consists of arresting convulsions and ensuring adequate ventilation with oxygen, if necessary by assisted or controlled ventilation (respiration). If convulsions occur, they should be treated rapidly by intravenous injection of thiopentone 100 to 200 mg or diazepam 5 to 10 mg. Alternatively succinylcholine 50

to 100 mg i.v. may be used providing the clinician is capable of performing endotracheal intubation and managing a fully paralysed patient. If ventricular fibrillation or cardiac arrest occurs effective cardiovascular resuscitation must be instituted. Adrenaline in repeated doses and sodium bicarbonate should be given as rapidly as possible.

**Pharmaceutical precautions** Xylocaine Gel 2% contains preservatives (see *Presentation*). Store below 25°C.

Xylocaine Accordion Gel 2% is sterile and is meant for single use only. Store below 25°C.

**Legal category** P

**Package quantities** Xylocaine Gel 2%: Packs of 10 x 20 g tubes. Xylocaine Accordion Gel 2%: Packs of 10 × 20 g Accordion syringes.

**Further information** Nil

**Product licence numbers**

| | |
|---|---|
| Xylocaine Gel 2% | 0017/0242R |
| Xylocaine Accordion Gel 2% | 0017/5037R |

## XYLOCAINE* OINTMENT 5%

**Presentation** A water-soluble topical anaesthetic ointment.

1 g Xylocaine Ointment contains: Lidocaine 50 mg, propylene glycol, polyethylene glycols, water purified q.s.

Xylocaine Ointment contains lidocaine which is dissolved in a vehicle consisting of carbowaxes and propylene glycol. Lidocaine penetrates the tissues and exerts a topical anaesthetic effect. The onset of action is 3–5 minutes on mucous membranes. It is ineffective when applied to intact skin. Propylene glycol in the ointment base has an antibacterial effect against many pathogenic micro-organisms. The carbowax base melts readily at body temperature and spreads evenly. The ointment is easily removed with water.

Lidocaine stabilises the neuronal membrane and prevents the initiation and conduction of nerve impulses effecting local anaesthetic action. Lidocaine is absorbed following the application to mucous membranes. The absorption occurs most rapidly after intratracheal administration. The metabolism of lidocaine takes place in the liver and metabolites and unchanged drug are excreted by the kidneys.

**Uses** Temporary relief of pain associated with minor burns and abrasions of the skin, e.g. sunburn, herpes zoster and labialis, pruritus, sore nipples, insect bites.

Anaesthesia of mucous membranes, e.g. various anal conditions such as haemorrhoids and fissures.

For the alleviation of pain during examination and instrumentation, e.g. proctoscopy, sigmoidoscopy, cystoscopy, endotracheal intubation.

Dentistry: Surface anaesthesia of the gums prior to injection, before deep scaling and in conjunction with the fitting of new dentures.

**Dosage and administration** As with any local anaesthetic, reactions and complications are best averted by employing the minimal effective dosage. Debilitated, elderly patients and children should be given dosage commensurate with their age and physical condition.

The ointment should be applied in a thin layer for adequate control of symptoms. A sterile gauze pad is suggested for application to broken and burned tissue. Apply to tube prior to endotracheal intubation.

In dentistry, apply to previously dried oral mucosa, allow at least 3-5 minutes for anaesthesia to become effective. When inserting new dentures, apply to all denture surfaces contacting mucosa.

For tender nipples, apply on a small piece of gauze; the ointment must be washed away before next feeding.

Not more than 35 g of the ointment should be administered in any 24 hour period.

### Contra-indications, warnings, etc

*Contra-indications:* Known history of hypersensitivity to local anaesthetics of the amide type or to other components of the ointment.

*Precautions:* Absorption from wound surfaces and mucous membranes is relatively high, especially in the bronchial tree. This should be taken into special consideration when the ointment is used in children for treatment of large areas.

Xylocaine Ointment should be used with caution in patients with traumatised mucosa and/or sepsis in the region of the proposed application.

If the dose or site of administration is likely to result in high blood levels, lidocaine, in common with other local anaesthetics should be used cautiously in patients with epilepsy, impaired cardiac conduction, bradycardia, impaired hepatic function and in severe shock.

The use of oral topical anaesthetic agents may interfere with swallowing and thus enhance the

danger of aspiration. This is particularly important in children because of their frequency of eating. Numbness of the tongue or buccal mucosa may increase the danger of biting trauma.

When used for endotracheal tube lubrication care should be taken to avoid introduction of the ointment into the lumen of the tube. The ointment may dry on the inner surface leaving residue which tend to clump with flexion, narrowing the lumen. There have been rare reports in which this residue has caused the lumen to occlude.

*Pregnancy:* There is no or inadequate evidence of safety of the drug in human pregnancy but it has been in wide use for many years without apparent ill consequence, animal studies have shown no hazard. If drug therapy is needed in pregnancy, this drug can be used if there is no safer alternative.

*Lactation:* Lidocaine enters the mother's milk, but in such small quantities that there is generally no risk of affecting the child at therapeutic dose levels.

*Side-effects:* In extremely rare cases local anaesthetic preparations have been associated with allergic reactions (in the most severe instances anaphylactic shock).

Systemic adverse reactions are rare and may result from high plasma levels due to excessive dosage, rapid absorption or may result from hypersensitivity, idiosyncrasy or diminished tolerance on the part of the patient. Such reactions involve the central nervous system and/or the cardiovascular system.

CNS reactions are excitatory and/or depressant, and may be characterised by nervousness, dizziness, convulsions, unconsciousness and possible respiratory arrest. The excitatory reactions may be very brief or may not occur at all, in which case the first manifestations of toxicity may be drowsiness, merging into unconsciousness and respiratory arrest.

Cardiovascular reactions are depressant, and may be characterised by hypotension, myocardial depression, bradycardia and possibly cardiac arrest.

*Interactions:* Lidocaine should be used with caution in patients receiving antiarrhythmic drugs, such as tocainide, since the toxic effects are additive.

*Overdosage:* Treatment of a patient with toxic manifestations consists of ensuring adequate ventilation and arresting convulsions. Ventilation should be maintained with oxygen by assisted or controlled respiration as required. If convulsions occur, they should be treated rapidly by intravenous administration of succinylcholine 50–100 mg and/or 5–15 mg diazepam. As succinylcholine will arrest respiration it should only be used if the clinician has the ability to perform endotracheal intubation and to manage a totally paralysed patient. Thiopentone may also be used to abort convulsions in dosage 100–200 mg. If ventricular fibrillation or cardiac arrest occurs, effective cardiovascular resuscitation must be instituted. Adrenaline in repeated doses and sodium bicarbonate should be given as rapidly as possible.

**Pharmaceutical precautions** Store at room temperature.

**Legal category** P

**Package quantities** 15 g tubes.

**Further information** Nil

**Product licence number** 0017/5038R

## XYLOCAINE* SPRAY

**Presentation** Topical anaesthetic pump spray containing lidocaine 10 mg/dose.

*Inactive ingredients:* Ethanol, polyethylene glycol 400, essence of banana, menthol natural, saccharin and purified water.

**Uses** For the prevention of pain associated with the following procedures:

*Otorhinolaryngology:* Puncture of the maxillary sinus and minor surgical procedures in the nasal cavity, pharynx and epipharynx.

Paracentesis.

*Obstetrics:* During the final stages of delivery and before episiotomy and perineal suturing as supplementary pain control.

*Introduction of instruments and catheters into the respiratory and digestive tract:* Provides surface anaesthesia for the oropharyngeal and tracheal areas to reduce reflex activity, attenuate haemodynamic response and to facilitate insertion of the tube or the passage of instruments during endotracheal intubation, laryngoscopy, bronchoscopy and oesophagoscopy.

*Dental practice:* Before injections, dental impressions, X-ray photography, removal of calculus.

**Dosage and administration** As with any local anaesthetic, reactions and complications are best averted by employing the minimal effective dosage. Debilitated or elderly patients and children should be given doses commensurate with their age and physical condition.

Each activation of the metered dose valve delivers 10 mg lidocaine base. It is unnecessary to dry the site prior to application. No more than 20 spray applications should be used in any adult to produce the desired anaesthetic effect.

The number of sprays depend on the extent of the area to be anaesthetised.

*Dental practice:* 1–5 applications to the mucous membranes.

*Otorhinolaryngology:* 3 applications for puncture of the maxillary sinus.

*During delivery:* Up to 20 applications (200 mg lidocaine base).

*Introduction of instruments and catheters into the respiratory and digestive tract:* Up to 20 applications (200 mg lidocaine base) for procedures in pharynx, larynx, and trachea.

### Contra-indications, warnings, etc

*Contra-indications:* Known history of hypersensitivity to local anaesthetics of the amide type or to other components of the spray solution.

*Precautions:* Absorption from wound surfaces and mucous membranes is relatively high, especially in the bronchial tree. Xylocaine Spray should be used with caution in patients with traumatised mucosa and/or sepsis in the region of the proposed application.

If the dose or site of administration is likely to result in high blood levels, lidocaine, in common with other local anaesthetics, should be used with caution in patients with epilepsy, impaired cardiac conduction, bradycardia, impaired hepatic function and in severe shock.

The oropharyngeal use of topical anaesthetic agents may interfere with swallowing and thus enhance the danger of aspiration. This is particularly important in children because of their frequency of eating. Numbness of the tongue or buccal mucosa may increase the danger of biting trauma.

Avoid contact with the eyes.

*Effect on ability to drive and use machines:* Depending on the dose, local anaesthetics may have a very mild effect on mental function and may temporarily impair locomotion and co-ordination.

*Use in pregnancy and lactation:* There is no or inadequate evidence of safety of the drug in human pregnancy but it has been in wide use for many years without apparent ill consequence, animal studies having shown no hazard. If drug therapy is needed in pregnancy, this drug can be used if there is no safer alternative.

Lidocaine enters the mother's milk, but in such small quantities that there is generally no risk of the child being affected at therapeutic dose levels.

*Side-effects:* In extremely rare cases local anaesthetic preparations have been associated with allergic reactions (in the most severe instances anaphylactic shock).

Systemic adverse reactions are extremely rare and may result from high plasma levels due to excessive dosage or rapid absorption or from hypersensitivity, idiosyncrasy or reduced tolerance on the part of the patient. Such reactions involve the central nervous system and/or the cardiovascular system.

CNS reactions are excitatory and/or depressant and may be characterised by nervousness, dizziness, convulsions, unconsciousness and possibly respiratory arrest. The excitatory reactions may be very brief or may not occur at all, in which case the first manifestations of toxicity may be drowsiness, merging into unconsciousness and respiratory arrest.

Cardiovascular reactions are depressant and may be characterised by hypotension, myocardial depression, bradycardia and possibly cardiac arrest.

*Interactions:* Lidocaine should be used with caution in patients receiving antiarrhythmic drugs, such as tocainide, since the toxic effects are additive.

*Overdosage:* The treatment of a patient with toxic manifestations consists of ensuring adequate ventilation and arresting convulsions. Ventilation should be maintained with oxygen by assisted or controlled respiration as required. If convulsions occur, they should be treated rapidly by the intravenous administration of succinylcholine 50–100 mg and/or 5–15 mg diazepam. As succinylcholine will arrest respiration, it should only be used if the clinician has the ability to perform endotracheal intubation and to manage a totally paralysed patient. Thiopentone may also be used to abort convulsions in the dosage 100–200 mg. If ventricular fibrillation or cardiac arrest occurs, effective cardiovascular resuscitation must be instituted. Adrenaline in repeated doses and sodium bicarbonate should be given as rapidly as possible.

**Pharmaceutical precautions** Each depression of the metered valve delivers 10 mg lidocaine base. The contents of the spray bottle are sufficient to provide approximately 500 sprays.

Store below 25°C. During storage at temperatures below +8°C precipitation may occur. The precipitate dissolves on warming up to room temperature.

**Legal category** P

**Package quantities** 50 ml spray bottles (approx. 500 spray doses) with a metering valve with applicator.

**Further information** The nozzle must not be shortened, as it will affect spray function. To clean the nozzle submerge in boiling water for 5 minutes. The nozzle may also be autoclaved.

**Product licence number** 0017/5039R

## XYLOCAINE* 4% TOPICAL

**Presentation** Topical anaesthetic for use on mucous membranes.

1 ml Xylocaine 4% Topical solution contains Lidocaine Hydrochloride PhEur corresponding to lidocaine hydrochloride anhydrous 40 mg, methylparahydroxybenzoate for injection, sodium hydroxide, water for injection q.s. to 1 ml.

The active agent of Xylocaine 4% Topical solution is lidocaine, which provides prompt and profound anaesthesia of accessible mucous membranes. Anaesthesia usually occurs rapidly (within 1–5 minutes depending upon area of application) and persists for approximately 15–30 minutes.

Lidocaine stabilises the neuronal membrane and prevents the initiation of nerve impulses, thereby effecting local anaesthetic action. Lidocaine may be absorbed following topical administration. Its rate of absorption and percentage of dose absorbed depend upon concentration and total dose administered, the specific site of application and duration of exposure. In general, the rate of absorption of local anaesthetic agents following topical application occurs most rapidly after intratracheal administration. The metabolism of lidocaine takes place in the liver and metabolites and unchanged drug are excreted by the kidneys. The elimination half-life of lidocaine is approximately 1.6 hours.

**Uses** Anaesthesia of mucous membranes of the oropharyngeal, tracheal and bronchial areas e.g. in bronchoscopy, bronchography, laryngoscopy, oesophagoscopy and endotracheal intubation.

Biopsy in the mouth and throat: puncture of the maxillary sinus or polypectomy.

Tonsillectomy: resection of nasal turbinates.

In dentistry.

**Dosage and administration** As with any local anaesthetic, reactions and complications are best averted by employing the minimal effective dosage. Debilitated, elderly patients and children should be given dosage commensurate with their age and physical condition.

The suggested dosage for adults is 1–7.5 ml Xylocaine 4% Topical solution (=40–300 mg lidocaine HCl). For children, smaller amounts and a weaker concentration should be administered depending on their age and weight. Doses exceeding 7.5 ml (=300 mg lidocaine) may result in plasma levels which have been associated with toxic manifestations.

*Biopsy:* 3–4 ml may be sprayed on the area or the solution may be applied for a few minutes with a swab. Adrenaline may be added to this solution in order to produce vasoconstriction (add 1–2 drops, 0.05 ml, 1:1,000 solution to 5 ml Xylocaine 4% solution).

*Puncture of maxillary sinus or polypectomy:* A swab soaked in the solution may be applied for two to three minutes. The addition of adrenaline is advised in these procedures, made up on the lines indicated above.

The Xylocaine 4% Topical solution may be applied from a swab, which should be discarded after use. Surface anaesthesia may also be achieved by instillation into a cavity or on to a surface. When spraying, the solution should be transferred from the original container to an atomiser.

### Contra-indications, warnings, etc

*Contra-indications:* Known history of hypersensitivity to local anaesthetics of the amide type or other components of the solution.

*Precautions:* Absorption from wound surfaces and mucous membranes is relatively high, especially in the bronchial tree. Xylocaine 4% Topical solution should therefore be used with caution in patients with traumatised mucosa and/or sepsis in the region of the proposed application.

If the dose or site of administration is likely to result in high blood levels, lidocaine, in common with other local anaesthetics, should be used with caution in patients with epilepsy, impaired cardiac conduction, bradycardia, impaired hepatic function and in severe shock.

The use of oral topical anaesthetic agents may interfere with swallowing and thus enhance the danger of aspiration. This is particularly important in children because of their frequency of eating. Numbness of the tongue or buccal mucosa may increase the danger of biting trauma.

*Effect on ability to drive and use machines:* Depending on the dose, local anaesthetics may have a very mild effect on mental function and may temporarily impair locomotion and co-ordination.

*Use in pregnancy and lactation:* There is no or inadequate evidence of safety of the drug in human pregnancy but it has been in wide use for many years without apparent ill consequence, animal studies have shown no hazard. If drug therapy is needed in pregnancy, this drug can be used if there is no safer alternative.

Lidocaine enters the mother's milk, but in such small quantities that there is generally no risk of affecting the child at therapeutic dose levels.

*Adverse reactions:* In extremely rare cases amide-type local anaesthetic preparations have been associated with allergic reactions (in the most severe instances anaphylactic shock).

Systemic adverse reactions are rare and may result from high plasma levels due to excessive dosage, rapid absorption or may result from hypersensitivity, idiosyncrasy or diminished tolerance on the part of the patient. Such reactions are systemic in nature and involve the central nervous system and/or the cardiovascular system.

CNS reactions are excitatory and/or depressant and may be characterised by nervousness, dizziness, blurred vision and tremors followed by drowsiness, convulsions, unconsciousness and, possibly, respiratory arrest. The excitatory reactions may be very brief or may not occur at all, in which case the first manifestations of toxicity may be drowsiness, merging into unconsciousness and respiratory arrest.

Cardiovascular reactions are depressant and may be characterised by hypotension, myocardial depression, bradycardia and, possibly, cardiac arrest.

*Interactions:* Lidocaine should be used with caution in patients receiving antiarrhythmic drugs, such as tocainide, since the toxic effects are additive.

*Overdosage:* Treatment of a patient with toxic manifestations consists of ensuring adequate ventilation and arresting convulsions. Ventilation should be maintained with oxygen by assisted or controlled respiration as required. If convulsions occur, they must be treated rapidly by intravenous administration of succinylcholine 50–100 mg and/or 5–15 mg diazepam. As succinycholine will arrest respiration, it should only be used if the clinician has the ability to perform endotracheal intubation and to manage a totally paralysed patient. Thiopentone may also be used to abort convulsions in dosage 100–200 mg. Adrenaline in repeated doses and sodium bicarbonate should be given as rapidly as possible.

**Pharmaceutical precautions** Store below 25°C. Avoid freezing.

**Legal category** P

**Package quantities** Bottles of 30 ml.

**Further information** Nil

**Product licence number** 0017/5040R

## XYLOCARD*

**Presentation** *Xylocard 100 mg intravenous bolus injection:* Clear aqueous sterile solution in pre-loaded 5 ml syringe: lidocaine hydrochloride anhydrous 20 mg/ml, equivalent to 21.2 mg Lidocaine Hydrochloride for Injection PhEur.

**Uses** Prevention of ventricular tachyarrhythmias in patients with suspected or proven acute myocardial infarction. Treatment of ventricular tachyarrhythmias associated with acute myocardial infarction. Ventricular extrasystoles and ventricular tachycardia. As antiarrhythmic cover in cases of ventricular fibrillation being DC converted.

### Dosage and administration

*Adults: Xylocard 100 mg i.v. bolus injection:* 1 mg/kg body weight. Normal doses 50–100 mg (2.5–5 ml) as initial treatment to be injected slowly over a period of two minutes. When necessary injection can be repeated once or twice at 5–10 minute intervals. Effect can be observed within two minutes and usually persists for 15–20 minutes. Not more than 200–300 mg should be administered during one hour.

*Children:* The safety and efficacy of lidocaine in children has not been established.

*Elderly:* In patients with cardiac failure, total plasma

clearance will be reduced and lower dosages may be required.

### Contra-indications, warnings, etc

*Contra-indications:* Known hypersensitivity to lidocaine (extremely rare). Known hypersensitivity to the local anaesthetics of the amide type, such as prilocaine, mepivacaine or bupivacaine.

Atrioventricular block is an absolute or relative contra-indication, according to severity and in the absence of pacemaker. Second or third degree AV-block. Other serious conduction disturbances, and cardiac decompensation not dependent on treatable tachyarrhythmias, are also contra-indicated.

*Precautions:* ECG-monitoring should be instituted when lidocaine is administered as an intravenous infusion.

Caution should be observed in patients with cardiac decompensation and hypotension or posterior diaphragmal infarction with a tendency towards heart block.

Lidocaine should be administered with caution to patients with bradycardia, untreated first-degree AV-block with bifascicular block or hypokalaemia.

Severely impaired liver or kidney function may mean a risk of accumulation and toxic reactions as lidocaine is mainly metabolised in the liver and the metabolites are excreted by the kidneys. Caution should be observed during repeated treatment with lidocaine in patients with these functional disorders.

When high doses are used and the patients myocardial function is impaired, combination with other drugs which reduce the excitability of cardiac muscle requires caution. Lidocaine treatment may aggravate arrhythmias.

The potassium concentration should be normalised before lidocaine treatment is started.

In patients with bradycardia complicated by ventricular tachyarrhythmia, lidocaine may have to be combined with atropine or atropine-like drugs or pacemaker treatment.

*Pregnancy and lactation:* Lidocaine has been used by a large number of pregnant women and women of child-bearing age. No specific disturbances to the reproductive process have so far been reported, e.g. an increased incidence of malformations or direct or indirect harmful effects on the foetus.

It is not known whether lidocaine is excreted in breast milk.

*Side-effects:* Most frequent are adverse reactions from the central and peripheral nervous system. They occur in 5-10% of the patients and are mostly dose-related. *Central and peripheral nervous system:* Dizziness, paraesthesia and drowsiness. Rarely persistent dizziness, tinnitus, confusion, blurred vision, tremor, convulsions, loss of consciousness and respiratory depression. *Cardiovascular:* Rarely hypotension and bradycardia, which may lead to cardiac arrest.

*Interactions:* Propranolol and cimetidine can impair the metabolism of lidocaine. Elimination will be delayed, the duration of action prolonged and the risk of adverse reactions increased.

*Overdosage:* Poisoning due to an overdose of lidocaine may lead to CNS excitation with paraesthesia, muscle twitching and convulsions, atrioventricular block, sinoatrial block or arrest, asystole, myocardial depression, severe hypotension and cardiac arrest.

Treatment should include close monitoring of cardiovascular and respiratory function and electrolytes. If convulsions occur, maintenance of a patent airway is mandatory and assisted or controlled ventilation with oxygen may be required. Convulsions may be controlled with intravenous diazepam or a short-acting barbiturate.

Cardiovascular complications should be treated symptomatically, which may require the use of sympathomimetic agents (e.g. noradrenaline, metaraminol), or inotropic agents (e.g. dopamine, dobutamine). Temporary pacing may be required for AV block.

Lidocaine is usually eliminated rapidly from the body, but elimination may be delayed in severe hypotension, cardiac failure or cardiogenic shock.

**Pharmaceutical precautions**   Store below 25°C.

**Legal category**   POM

**Package quantities**   Xylocard 100 mg 5 ml (20 mg/ml): Pre-loaded syringe for immediate use. Box of 10.

**Further information**   All Xylocard syringes are free of bacteriostat and preservatives.

**Product licence number** 0017/5018R

## XYLOPROCT* OINTMENT

**Presentation**   White water-miscible cream. Each gram contains: Lidocaine 50 mg and Hydrocortisone Acetate PhEur 2.75 mg.

*Inactive ingredients:* Zinc oxide, aluminium acetate,

polyethylene glycol, stearyl alcohol, cetyl alcohol and purified water.

**Uses**   For the relief of symptoms such as anal and peri-anal pruritis, pain and inflammation associated with haemorrhoids, anal fissure, fistulas and proctitis. Pruritis vulva.

**Dosage and administration**   To be applied several times daily according to the severity of the condition.

### Contra-indications, warnings, etc

*Contra-indications:* Known hypersensitivity to local anaesthetics of the amide type or any of the other ingredients. Use on atrophic skin.

*Precautions and warnings:* Xyloproct is intended for use for limited periods.

Appropriate antibacterial, antiviral or antifungal therapy should be given with Xyloproct if infection is present at the site of application.

The possibility of malignancy should be excluded before use.

If irritation or rectal bleeding develops treatment should be discontinued.

When using the special applicator, care should be taken to avoid instillation of excessive amounts of Xyloproct Ointment into the rectum. This is of particular importance in infants and children. Systemic absorption of lidocaine may occur from the rectum and large doses may result in CNS side-effects. On rare occasions convulsions have occurred in children. Xyloproct Suppositories should be used in preference to ointment for treatment of proctitis or internal haemorrhoids.

*Side-effects:* Local reactions such as dermatitis have been reported with the use of Xyloproct Ointment.

*Pregnancy and lactation:* Do not use in pregnancy unless considered essential by the physician.

Lidocaine and hydrocortisone acetate are excreted into breast milk but in such small quantities that adverse effects on the child are unlikely at therapeutic doses.

*Interactions:* Lidocaine should be used with caution in patients receiving antiarrhythmic drugs, such as tocainide, since the toxic effects are additive.

**Pharmaceutical precautions**   Store in a refrigerator. The patient may store the ointment at 25°C for 2 months. The product should be discarded 2 months after opening.

**Legal category**   POM

**Package quantities**   Tubes. 30 g ointment complete with applicator.

**Further information**   Nil

**Product licence number** 0017/5023R

## XYLOPROCT* SUPPOSITORIES

**Presentation**   White cone-shaped suppositories each containing Lidocaine 60 mg, Hydrocortisone Acetate PhEur 5 mg.

*Inactive ingredients:* Zinc oxide, aluminium acetate basic powder, hard fat.

**Uses**   For the treatment of symptoms associated with haemorrhoids and other disorders of the anal canal such as proctitis, anal fissure and anal fistula.

**Dosage and administration**   Removing protective foil, use 1 suppository at night before retiring and repeat the treatment after each bowel action.

### Contra-indications, warnings, etc

*Contra-indications:* Known hypersensitivity to local anaesthetics of the amide type or any of the other ingredients. Use on atrophic skin.

*Precautions and warnings:* Xyloproct is intended for use for limited periods.

Appropriate antibacterial, antiviral or antifungal therapy should be given with Xyloproct if infection is present at the site of application.

The possibility of malignancy should be excluded before use.

If irritation or rectal bleeding develops, treatment should be discontinued.

Xyloproct Suppositories should be used in preference to ointment for the treatment of proctitis or internal haemorrhoids.

*Side-effects:* Local reactions such as dermatitis have been reported with the use of Xyloproct Ointment.

*Pregnancy and lactation:* Do not use in pregnancy unless considered essential by the physician.

Lidocaine and hydrocortisone acetate are excreted into breast milk but in such small quantities that adverse effects on the child are unlikely at therapeutic doses.

*Interactions:* Lidocaine should be used with caution in patients receiving antiarrhythmic drugs, such as tocainide, since the toxic effects are additive.

*Overdosage:* Care should be taken to avoid application of excessive quantities of Xyloproct Suppositories into the rectum. This is of particular importance in infants and children. Systemic absorption of lidocaine may occur from the rectum and large doses may result in CNS side-effects. On rare occasions convulsions have occurred in children.

**Pharmaceutical precautions**   Store in a fridge (below 5°C). The patient may store the product at room temperature (25°C) for 2 months whilst in use. Any remaining suppositories should then be discarded. Avoid freezing.

**Legal category**   POM

**Package quantities**   Packs containing 10 separate foil-protected suppositories.

**Further information**   Nil

**Product licence number** 0017/5024R

## XYLOTOX* 2% E80

**Presentation**   Xylotox 2% E80 is a sterile clear aqueous solution of Lidocaine Hydrochloride PhEur 24.65 mg equivalent to lidocaine base 20 mg and Adrenaline Tartrate PhEur 25.0 micrograms corresponding to adrenaline 12.5 micrograms.

Xylotox 2% E80 is supplied in polypropylene cartridges for use in dental type syringes.

*Inactive ingredients:* Sodium chloride, calcium chloride, potassium chloride and sodium metabisulphite.

**Uses**   Local anaesthetic solution with vasoconstrictor for dental infiltration anaesthesia where a vasoconstrictor is indicated.

**Dosage and administration**   Infiltration – 0.5 to 2 ml. Nerve block – 1.5 to 2 ml. Extensive surgery – 3 to 10 ml. Adult maximum dose 500 mg.

In children the maximum dose is considerably less and should be calculated in relation to the body weight.

### Contra-indications, warnings, etc

*Contra-indications:* Known hypersensitivity to local anaesthetics of the amide type.

Xylotox 2% E80 should not be given intravenously.

The use of a vasoconstrictor is contra-indicated for anaesthesia of the fingers, toes, tip of nose and penis.

*Precautions:* In common with other local anaesthetics, Xylotox 2% E80 should be used cautiously in patients with epilepsy, cardiac disease particularly with arrhythmia or hypertension, impaired respiratory function, thyrotoxicosis, hypovolaemia, acute porphyria and impaired hepatic function.

Adequate resuscitation equipment must be available whenever local or general anaesthesia is administered. Though clinical tolerance is remarkably good, overdosage or accidental intravenous injection may give rise to toxic reactions.

These are best avoided by aspiration before making an injection in order to avoid accidental intravascular injection.

*Use in pregnancy and lactation:* There is no or inadequate evidence of safety of the drug in human pregnancy but it has been in wide use for many years without apparent ill consequence, animal studies have shown no hazard. If drug therapy is needed in pregnancy this drug can be used if there is no safer alternative.

Lidocaine enters the mother's milk but in such small quantities that there is generally no risk of affecting the child at therapeutic dose levels.

*Side-effects:* The type of toxic reaction is unpredictable and depends on dosage, route of administration and state of patient. The reactions are primarily of two types, typified by stimulation and depression of the cerebral cortex and medulla respectively. Slow onset – stimulation leading to nervousness, dizziness, blurred vision, nausea, tremor, convulsions and respiratory arrest. Rapid onset – depression leading primarily to respiratory arrest, cardiovascular collapse and cardiac arrest. Symptoms occur rapidly and with little warning.

*Interactions:* Care should be observed in patients taking tricyclic anti-depressants.

*Overdose:* Toxicity is initially manifested as CNS excitation and may be characterised by nervousness, dizziness, blurred vision and tremors followed by drowsiness, convulsions, unconsciousness and possible respiratory arrest. Toxic cardiovascular reactions to local anaesthetics are usually depressant in nature and are characterised by peripheral vasodilation, hypotension, myocardial depression, bradycardia and possibly cardiac arrest.

Treatment of a patient with toxic symptoms consists of assuring a patent airway and supporting ventilation with oxygen and assisted or controlled respiration as required. This will usually be sufficient in the management of most reactions.

Should a convulsion persist despite ventilation therapy, small increments of a benzodiazepine (e.g. diazepam) or an ultra-short acting barbiturate (e.g. thiopentone) may be given intravenously.

Cardiovascular depression may require circulatory assistance in the form of intravenous fluids and/or vasopressor agents as dictated by the clinical situation.

**Pharmaceutical precautions**    Store below 25°C.

**Legal category**    POM

**Package quantities**    Polypropylene cartridges of 2.2 ml in boxes of 100.

**Further information** Nil

**Product licence number**    0017/0141

*Trade Mark

**Baker Norton Pharmaceuticals**
Gemini House
Flex Meadow
Harlow
Essex CM19 5TJ

BAKER
**NORTON**

## AMIL-CO*

**Presentation** Flat, pale peach, bisected tablets with bevelled edges, 8.5 mm diameter, coded 'AMILCO' around the circumference on one side and bearing a twin triangle logo on the reverse, and containing Amiloride Hydrochloride BP equivalent to 5 mg anhydrous amiloride hydrochloride and 50 mg Hydrochlorothiazide BP.

**Uses** Antihypertensive and diuretic with potassium conserving properties. Indicated in the care of patients with hypertension, congestive heart failure, or hepatic cirrhosis with ascites, or where potassium depletion may occur. The amiloride hydrochloride in Amil-Co reduces the possibility of excessive potassium loss during prolonged and vigorous diuresis. Amil-Co is recommended in those conditions where potassium balance is particularly important, for example in patients with congestive heart failure receiving digitalis.

In hapatic cirrhosis with ascites, Amil-Co is likely to provide satisfactory diuresis with diminished potassium loss, thus lessening the risk of metabolic alkalosis.

**Dosage and administration** The rate of weight loss and the level of serum electrolytes should determine the dosage. The ideal target for weight loss after initiation of diuresis being in the range of 0.5–1.0 kg per day in adults. Amil-Co is not recommended for children.

*Hypertension:* Usually 1 or 2 tablets once a day or in divided doses, which may be increased up to a maximum of 4 tablets per day.

Amil-Co may be used alone or in conjunction with other antihypertensive drugs. Since Amil-Co enhances the actions of such agents, the antihypertensive dosage regimen may have to be altered to obviate any hypotensive reaction.

*Hepatic cirrhosis with ascites:* Starting with 1 tablet per day, dosage may be increased if required until there is effective diuresis provided the dose does not exceed 4 tablets per day. Ideally, a gradual weight loss is preferred in cirrhotic patients to minimise the occurrence of untoward reactions associated with diuretic therapy (your attention is drawn to the precautions section). Maintenance doses are sometimes less than the dosage necessary to initiate diuresis; consequently, attempts should be made to reduce the dosage when the patient's weight is stable.

*Congestive heart failure:* The starting dose is 1 or 2 tablets per day, which may be altered if necessary to a maximum of 4 tablets per day. Serum potassium levels and diuretic response will establish the optimal dosage. On the establishment of initial diuresis, maintenance therapy is possible with a dosage reduction, or by the use of intermittent therapy.

The preparation should be used with care in elderly patients. Dosage should be monitored.

**Contra-indications, warnings, etc**
*Contra-indications:* Hyperkalaemia (serum potassium over 5.5 mmol/litre); other potassium-conserving diuretics e.g. spironolactone or triamterene, and potassium supplements; acute renal failure, severe progressive renal disease, severe hepatic failure, diabetic nephropathy; precoma associated with hepatic cirrhosis, hypercalcaemia or Addison's disease; anuria; patients with blood urea over 60 mg per 100 ml or serum creatinine over 1.5 mg per 100 ml, in whom serum electrolyte and blood urea levels cannot be monitored with satisfaction and frequency; a known sensitivity to amiloride hydrochloride or hydrochlorothiazide and related sulphonamides. In renal impairment, use of potassium-conserving agents may result in rapid development of hyperkalaemia.

The safety of amiloride hydrochloride for use in children has not been established; Amil-Co is therefore not recommended in children. For use in pregnancy and the nursing mother see 'Precautions'.

*Precautions:* Patients who are being treated with this preparation require regular supervision with monitoring of fluid and electrolyte state to avoid inadequate potassium supplementation or excessive loss of fluid.

The preparation should be used with care in elderly patients, or those with potential obstructions of the urinary tract.

*Diabetes mellitus:* Hyperkalaemia has been widely reported in diabetic patients on amiloride; mainly associated with chronic renal disease or pre-renal azotaemia. Renal function status should be established before prescribing Amil-Co to known or suspected diabetics. The taking of Amil-Co should be stopped prior to giving a glucose-tolerance test. Restabilising the insulin requirements of diabetic patients may be necessary. Latent diabetes mellitus may become manifest during thiazide therapy.

*Metabolic or respiratory acidosis:* Severely ill patients likely to experience respiratory or metabolic acidosis on introduction of potassium-conserving therapy, should be treated with caution. Categories such as decompensated diabetics or cardiopulmonary cases should be assessed for shifts in acid-base balance which may alter the balance of extracellular-intracellular potassium; the development of acidosis may be associated with a market rise in serum potassium.

*Blood urea increases and electrolyte imbalance:* Very infrequently, amiloride and hydrochlorothiazide, as combined in Amil-Co, fail to overcome the advent of hypokalaemia. In this instance, the use of potassium supplements should be carefully monitored.

Hyponatraemia and hypochloraemia are possible although the likelihood of hypochloraemic alkalosis is reduced with Amil-Co. Ammonium chloride (except in patients with hepatic complications) may be used to overcome any chloride deficit. Normal salt intake will, in the main, prevent any problem in this area.

*Hyperkalaemia (serum potassium level over 5.5 mmol/litre):* It has been noted that hyperkalaemia may be present in patients receiving amiloride either alone or in combination with other diuretics, especially in such categories as diabetics; the aged; congestive heart failure cases with known renal involvement; patients suffering from hepatic cirrhosis, or those subjected to vigorous diuretic therapy or the seriously ill. Careful observation of such categories of patients for manifestation of hyperkalaemia, using clinical, laboratory and ECG evidence should be undertaken as hyperkalaemia is not always accompanied by an abnormal ECG. In any development of hyperkalaemia, Amil-Co therapy should be stopped forthwith and, should it be desirable, reduction of serum potassium levels to normal values should be actively instituted.

Reversible increases in blood urea have been reported in association with vigorous diuresis, notably in cases of hepatic cirrhosis with ascites and metabolic alkalosis or resistant oedema. In these cases, serum electrolyte and blood urea levels should be carefully monitored. Caution is advised with the use of Amil-Co in patients suffering renal impairment (see 'Contra-indications'). Care should be taken to avoid cumulative or toxic effects due to a reduced excretion of its components. Azotaemia may be precipitated or increased by hydrochlorothiazide. Amil-Co should be discontinued if increased azotaemia and oliguria occur during treatment.

*Effects in cirrhotic patients:* Patients with hepatic cirrhosis and ascites are more likely to experience adverse reactions during oral diuretic therapy owing to the fact that these patients are intolerant of acute shifts in electrolyte balance and because they may be subject to pre-existing hypokalaemia due to associated aldosteronism. Hepatic encephalopathy as characterised by coma, confusion and tremors has been reported with patients receiving amiloride and subjects with liver disease on Amil-Co should be observed for this complication. A tenuous relationship between amiloride and a deepening of jaundice in cirrhotic patients has been postulated.

*Hepatic disease:* Thiazide should be used with caution in patients with impaired hepatic function or progressive liver disease.

*Additional precautions:* Thiazides may produce sensitivity reactions in patients with or without a record of allergy or bronchial asthma. The action of other antihypertensive agents is potentiated by hydrochlorothiazide and a reduced dosage may be necessary at the introduction of Amil-Co. The risk of lithium toxicity with patients combined on lithium and diuretics is very high and lithium should not be administered concurrently with Amil-Co. Reports indicate that there exists a possibility that thiazides may activate or exacerbate systemic lupus erythematosus.

Magnesium excretion is increased and calcium excretion is decreased by hydrochlorothiazide.

Hydrochlorothiazide may reduce arterial responsiveness to noradrenaline, but not to such a degree as to prevent the effectiveness of noradrenaline in therapeutic usage. Thiazides may enhance the responsiveness of tubocurarine. In post-sympathectomy patients, the antihypertensive action of thiazides may be enhanced. Should orthostatic hypotension occur, it may be potentiated by narcotics, barbiturates and alcohol.

Concomitant administration of potassium-sparing agents such as amiloride with ACE inhibitors may increase serum potassium levels and is not recommended. However, if the concomitant use of these agents is deemed appropriate, they should be used with caution and with frequent monitoring of plasma potassium. Non-steroidal anti-inflammatory drugs may attenuate the antihypertensive effect of thiazide diuretics.

Indomethacin (and possibly other NSAIDs), potassium supplements and trilostane may cause hyperkalaemia.

In some patients receiving thiazides, gout may be precipitated or hyperuricaemia may occur.

The concomitant administration of this preparation with cardiac glycosides or hypotensive agents may necessitate adjustment of the dosage of those drugs.

There is an increased risk of hypokalaemia when corticosteroids are given with loop diuretics and thiazides and an increased risk of hyponatraemia when chlorpropamide is given with Amil-Co.

There have been isolated reports of pathological changes in parathyroid glands accompanied by hypophosphataemia and hypercalcaemia following prolonged thiazide therapy. Serum concentrations of plasma bound iodine may increase without signs of thyroid disturbance during thiazide therapy. To establish parathyroid function, first discontinue Amil-Co.

As with any recently introduced preparation, patients should be monitored for possible signs of blood dyscrasias, liver dysfunction and idiosyncratic reactions.

*Administration during pregnancy and for the nursing mother:* The use of Amil-Co is not recommended during pregnancy since the use of diuretics may be associated with hypovolaemia, increased blood viscosity and decreased placental perfusion.

Diuretics do not prevent toxaemia of pregnancy and there is no conclusive evidence that they are useful for its treatment. Hazards to the foetus may include foetal or neonatal jaundice, thrombocytopenia, bone marrow depression and possibly other side-effects known to occur in adults. There is no indication for the use of diuretics on a routine basis in the healthy pregnant woman whether or not mild oedema is present.

Thiazides are excreted in breast milk. If continuation of Amil-Co is thought to be essential then the patient should be instructed to stop breast feeding.

*Side-effects:*
*Related to diuresis:* Orthostatic hypotension, muscle cramps, susceptibility to fatigue, weakness, dizziness, vertigo, salivary gland inflammation, transient blurred vision, paraesthesiae, thirst, dry mouth, minor psychiatric changes, e.g. confusion, depression, insomnia.

*Gastro-intestinal:* Constipation and diarrhoea, pain, cramps, gastric irritation, abdominal fullness, vomiting, nausea, anorexia.

*Additional side-effects:* Side-effects associated with thiazide therapy are hyperuricaemia, glycosuria, hyperglycaemia, yellow vision, pancreatitis, renal dysfunction and interstitial nephritis, jaundice (intra-hepatic cholestatic jaundice), restlessness, headache. Fever, necrotising angiitis (vasculitis, cutaneous vasculitis), photosensitivity, urticaria, rash, purpura, haemolytic anaemia, aplastic anaemia, agranulocytosis, leucopenia, thrombocytopenia, respiratory distress including pneumonitis and anaphylactic reactions have also been reported.

Impotence has been reported in patients taking hydrochlorothiazide.

There have been a few reports of gastro-intestinal bleeding in subjects with a background of gastro-intestinal disease receiving amiloride hydrochloride alone; a casual relationship to amiloride, however, has not been established. Rare reversible abnormalities, possibly relating to amiloride hydrochloride, have been noted in liver function tests.

In the case of moderate or severe side-effects, the dosage of Amil-Co should be reduced or withdrawn altogether.

*Treatment of overdosage:* There is no specific antidote. Dehydration, electrolyte imbalance and hepatic coma are treated by the established procedures. Symptoms of fluid or electrolyte imbalance include dry mouth, weakness, lethargy, drowsiness, restlessness, muscle pain or cramps, hypotension, gastro-intestinal disturbances, low urine output. If ingestion is recent, gastric lavage should be performed or emesis induced. Treatment is symptomatic and supportive. Blood pressure, fluid and electrolyte balance should be monitored. If hyperkalaemia occurs, prompt measures should be taken to lower the serum potassium levels. For respiratory impairment, oxygen or artificial respiration should be administered.

**Pharmaceutical precautions** Keep container tightly closed; store in a cool, dry place below 25°C and protect from light.

**Legal category** POM.

**Package quantities** Containers and blister packs of 7, 14, 21, 28, 30, 50, 56, 60, 84, 90, 100, 112, 120, 250, 500 and 5000 tablets.

**Further information** Oral potassium supplements and potassium conserving diuretics must not be given with Amil-Co.

Onset of diuretic action begins within two to four hours after administration of Amil-Co, and reaches a peak at about the fourth hour; there is detectable activity for about 24 hours.

**Product licence number** 0530/0070

*Product licence holder:* Norton Healthcare Limited, Harlow, Essex CM19 5TJ.

## BECLAZONE* 50 INHALER
## BECLAZONE* 100 INHALER
## BECLAZONE* 250 INHALER

**Qualitative and quantitative composition**
Beclazone 50 Inhaler: 50 μg Beclomethasone Dipropionate per dose.
Beclazone 100 Inhaler: 100 μg Beclomethasone Dipropionate per dose.
Beclazone 250 Inhaler: 250 μg Beclomethasone Dipropionate per dose.

**Pharmaceutical form** Metered-dose aerosol inhaler.

**Clinical particulars**
*Therapeutic indications:*
*BECLAZONE 50 AND 100 INHALERS:*

(i) For the prophylactic treatment of patients with worsening asthma and where there is no satisfactory control of symptoms with bronchodilators.

(ii) For patients inadequately controlled with sodium cromoglycate in addition to bronchodilators.

(iii) For patients with severe chronic asthma and those who are dependant on systemic corticosteroids.

*BECLAZONE 250 INHALER:*

(i) Beclazone 250 Inhaler is indicated for those asthmatic patients who have been shown to require high doses (greater than 800–1000 micrograms daily) of beclomethasone dipropionate BP to control their symptoms.

(ii) It may also be indicated for those patients whose asthma is no longer controlled by maximum maintenance doses of bronchodilators and low doses of beclomethasone dipropionate BP (less than 800 micrograms daily). Some patients with severe asthma require oral corticosteroid therapy in addition to low doses of beclomethasone dipropionate BP (less than 800 micrograms daily) for the adequate control of their symptoms. Many of these patients may, on transfer to Beclazone 250 Inhaler, be able to reduce significantly or eliminate their requirement for additional oral corticosteroids.

*Posology and method of administration:*
*BECLAZONE 50 AND 100 INHALERS:*

*(i) Adults:* The usual starting dose is 200 micrograms twice a day. In more severe cases dosage may be started at, or increased to, 600 to 800 micrograms per day, and subsequently reduced when the patient's asthma has stabilised. The total daily dose may be administered as two, three or four divided doses.

*(ii) Elderly:* There is no need to adjust the dose in elderly patients.

*(iii) Children:* 50–100 micrograms should be given two, three or four times daily according to response. Alternatively, 100 or 200 micrograms twice daily may be administered. The usual starting dose is 100 micrograms twice a day.

*(iv) Patients with hepatic or renal impairment:* There is no need to adjust the dose.

*BECLAXONE 250 INHALER:*

*(i) Adults:* Patients should be given a starting dose of inhaled beclomethasone dipropionate which is appropriate for the severity of their disease. The dose may then be adjusted until control is achieved, or reduced to the minimum effective dose according to individual response.

Patients demonstrating a need for high dose inhaled steroid therapy should start on 1,000 micrograms daily.

The usual maintenance dose is two inhalations (500 micrograms) twice daily, or one inhalation (250 micrograms) four times daily. If necessary, dosage may be increased to two inhalations (500 micrograms) three or four times daily according to response.

*(ii) Elderly:* There is no need to adjust the dose in elderly patients.

*(iii) Children:* Beclazone 250 Inhaler is not indicated for use in children.

*(iv) Patients with hepatic or renal impairment:* There is no need to adjust the dose.

*Method of administration:* Oral inhalation.

*Contra-indications:* Beclazone Inhaler is contra-indicated in patients with a history of hypersensitivity to any of its components. Furthermore, it is contra-indicated in patients with pulmonary tuberculosis (active or quiescent).

Beclazone Inhaler is not indicated in the treatment of acute asthmatic attacks.

*Special warnings and special precautions for use:* Patients should be instructed on the proper use of the inhaler to ensure that the drug reaches the target areas within the lungs. They should also be made aware that Beclazone Inhaler has to be used regularly for optimum benefit. Patients should be made aware of the prophylactic nature of therapy with Beclazone Inhaler and that it should be taken regularly, even when they are asymptomatic.

*BECLAZONE 50 AND 100 INHALERS:* The maximum daily intake of Beclazone 50 or 100 Inhaler in adults should not exceed 1 mg. Significant reduction of plasma cortisol levels has been reported in patients who received twice this amount.

The maximum daily intake of Beclazone 50 or 100 Inhalers in children should not exceed 500 micrograms.

In the majority of patients, no significant adrenal suppression occurs until doses of 1,500 micrograms per day are exceeded. Some patients receiving 2,000 micrograms of beclomethasone dipropionate per day may show a degree of adrenocortical suppression although short term adrenal reserve remains intact. In such patients the risks of developing adrenal suppression should be balanced against the therapeutic advantages and precautions should be taken to provide systemic steroid cover in situations of prolonged stress.

*Patients inadequately controlled by brochodilator therapy:* The use of Beclazone 50 or 100 Inhaler in patients who have never taken steroids, or taken only occasional courses of steroids is straightforward. An improvement in respiratory function is normally obvious within a week. The few patients who do not respond during this period usually have excessive mucus in their bronchi so that the drug is unable to penetrate to its site of action. In such cases, a short course of systemic steroid in relatively high dosage should be given to control secretion of mucus and other inflammatory changes in the lungs. Continuation of treatment with Beclazone 50 Inhaler usually maintains the improvement achieved, the oral steroid being gradually withdrawn. Exacerbations of asthma caused by infections is usually controlled by appropriate antibiotic treatment, by increasing the dose of inhaled beclomethasone dipropionate and, if necessary, by giving a systemic steroid. Use of a $\beta_2$-agonist may also be required.

*Oral steroid-dependent patients:* The transfer of oral steroid-dependent patients to Beclazone 50 or 100 Inhaler and their subsequent management needs special care mainly because recovery from impaired adrenocortical function caused by prolonged systemic steroid therapy is slow. The patient should be in a reasonably stable state before being given Beclazone 50 or 100 Inhaler in addition to his usual maintenance dose of systemic steroid. After about a week, gradual withdrawal of the systemic steroid is started by reducing the daily dose by 1 mg prednisolone, or its equivalent of other corticosteroids, at not less than weekly intervals. Patients treated with systemic steroids for long periods of time, or who have received high doses may have adrenocortical suppression. With these patients adrenocortical function should be monitored regularly and their dose of systemic steroid reduced cautiously. Some patients feel unwell during the withdrawal phase despite maintenance or even improvement of respiratory function. They should be encouraged to persevere with the inhaler and withdrawal of systemic steroid continued unless there are objective signs of adrenal insufficiency. Most patients can be successfully transferred to Beclazone 50 or 100 Inhaler with maintenance of good respiratory function, but special care is necessary for the first months after the transfer until the pituitary-adrenal system has sufficiently recovered to enable the patient to cope with emergencies such as trauma, surgery or infections.

Transferred patients whose adrenocortical function is impaired should carry a warning card indicating that they need supplementary systemic steroids during periods of stress, e.g. surgery, chest infection or worsening asthma attacks, but that this can be reduced again after the stress has been resolved. They should also be given a supply of oral steroid to use in emergency, for example when the asthma worsens as a result of a chest infection. The dose of beclomethasone should be increased at this time and then reduced to the maintenance level after the systemic steroid has been discontinued.

Replacement of systemic steroid treatment with Beclazone 50 Inhaler sometimes unmasks allergies such as allergic rhinitis or eczema previously controlled by the systemic drug. These allergies should be symptomatically treated with antihistamine and/or topical preparations.

*BECLAZONE 250 INHALER:* Patients should be instructed on the proper use of the inhaler to ensure that the drug reaches the target areas within the lungs. They should also be made aware that Beclazone 250 Inhaler has to be used regularly for optimum benefit. Patients should be made aware of the prophylactic nature of therapy with Beclazone 250 Inhaler and that it should be taken regularly, even when they are asymptomatic.

Patients being treated with the low doses of beclomethasone dipropionate BP (less than 800 micrograms daily) may be transferred directly to treatment with Beclazone 250 Inhaler.

Increasing use of bronchodilators, in particular short-acting inhaled $\beta_2$-agonists, to relieve symptoms indicates deterioration of asthma control. If patients find that short-acting relief bronchodilator treatment becomes less effective, or they need more inhalations than usual, medical attention must be sought. In this situation patients should be reassessed and consideration given to the need for increased anti-inflammatory therapy (e.g. higher doses of inhaled corticosteroids or a course of oral corticosteroids). Severe exacerbations of asthma must be treated in the normal way. Exacerbations of asthma caused by infections are usually controlled by appropriate antibiotic treatment, by increasing the dose of inhaled beclomethasone dipropionate and, if necessary, by giving a systemic steroid. Use of a $\beta_2$-agonist may also be required.

In the majority of patients, no significant adrenal suppression occurs until doses of 1,500 micrograms per day are exceeded. Some patients receiving 2,000 micrograms of beclomethasone dipropionate per day may show a degree of adrenocortical suppression although short term adrenal reserve remains intact. In such patients the risks of developing adrenal suppression should be balanced against the therapeutic advantages and precautions should be taken to provide systemic steroid cover in situations of prolonged stress.

Patients being treated with oral corticosteroids should be in a stable state before having Beclazone 250 Inhaler added to their current therapy. After about a week, gradual withdrawal of the systemic steroid is started by reducing the daily dose by 1 mg prednisolone, or its equivalent of other corticosteroids, at not less than weekly intervals. Patients who have been treated with systemic steroids for long periods of time or at a high dose may have adrenocortical suppression. With these patients adrenocortical function should be monitored regularly and their dose of systemic steroid reduced cautiously. Some patients feel unwell during the withdrawal phase despite maintenance or even improvement of respiratory function. They should be encouraged to persevere with the inhaler and withdrawal of systemic steroid continued unless there are objective signs of adrenal insufficiency. Most patients can be successfully transferred to Beclazone 250 Inhaler with maintenance of good respiratory function, but special care is necessary for the first months after the transfer until the pituitary-adrenal system has sufficiently recovered to enable the patient to cope with emergencies such as trauma, surgery or infections. Patients recently transferred from oral steroids to Beclazone 250 Inhaler together with those still receiving oral steroids should carry a warning card indicating that they may need to start or increase the dosage of oral steroids during periods of stress, e.g. surgery, chest infection or worsening asthmatic attacks, but that this can be reduced again after the stress has been resolved. A small supply of oral steroids can be given to them for emergency use.

Treatment with Beclazone 250 Inhaler should not be stopped abruptly.

Replacement of systemic steroid treatment with Beclazone 250 Inhaler sometimes unmasks allergies such as allergic rhinitis or eczema previously controlled by the systemic drugs. These allergies should be symptomatically treated with antihistamine and/or topical preparations.

*Interaction with other medicaments and other forms of interaction:* None reported for inhaled beclomethasone dipropionate.

*Pregnancy and lactation:* Beclazone Inhaler should only be used in pregnancy or lactation if the potential benefit outweighs the risk. There is insufficient data regarding safety in human pregnancy. High doses of systemic corticosteroids in pregnant animals can cause abnormalities in foetal development, including cleft palate and intra-uterine growth retardation.

No data regarding excretion of beclomethasone dipropionate in human breast milk is available.

*Effects on ability to drive and use machines:* On the basis of the pharmacodynamic profile, reported adverse drug reactions (ADR) and/or impairment of performance related to driving, Beclazone Inhaler is presumed to be safe or unlikely to produce an effect.

*Undesirable effects:* In some patients hoarseness or throat irritation may occur. Rinsing the mouth and throat with water after each dose to remove residual medication may be helpful.

Paradoxical bronchospasm may occur, in which case use of the inhaler should cease immediately and medical advice should be sought. Alternative therapy should be introduced.

Candidiasis of the mouth and throat (thrush) occurs in some patients; the incidence of which is increased with doses greater than 400 micrograms beclomethasone dipropionate per day. Patients with high blood levels of *Candida precipitins*, indicating a previous infection, are more likely to develop this complication. Such patients may find it helpful to rinse their mouth with water after using the inhaler. Symptomatic candidiasis can be treated with topical anti-fungal therapy whilst still continuing with Beclazone Inhaler.

*Overdose:* The acute toxicity of beclomethasone dipropionate is low. The only harmful effect that follows inhalation of large amounts of the drug over a short period is suppression of hypothalamic-pituitary-adrenal (HPA) function. No special emergency action need be taken. Treatment with Beclazone Inhaler should be continued at the recommended dose to control asthma; HPA function recovers in a day or two.

Reduction of plasma cortisol levels has been reported in patients who received twice the daily recommended maximum dose of beclomethasone dipropionate. In the unlikely event of excessive intake of beclomethasone dipropionate for weeks or months on end, a degree of adrenocortical atrophy could occur in addition to suppression of HPA function. The patient should be treated as steroid-dependent and transferred to a suitable maintenance dose of a systemic steroid such as prednisolone. Once the patient's condition has stabilised he should be transferred to Beclazone Inhaler by the method described in *Special warnings and precautions for use* above.

To guard against the unexpected event of adrenal suppression, regular tests of adrenal function are advised.

**Pharmacological properties**

*Pharmacodynamic properties:* Beclomethasone dipropionate by inhalation has a potent glucocorticoid anti-inflammatory action within the lungs, but at recommended dosage, is without significant systemic activity.

Beclomethasone dipropionate also has vasoconstrictor effects and it inhibits the late responses to antigen challenge.

*Pharmacokinetic properties:* The pharmacokinetics of beclomethasone dipropionate have not been extensively studied. The current available methods are not of sufficient sensitivity to measure the therapeutically relevant plasma concentrations, particularly those occurring following inhalation.

Beclomethasone dipropionate is readily absorbed after oral administration.

About 25% of an inhaled dose reaches the lungs.

The drug and its metabolites are excreted chiefly in the faeces via biliary elimination and to a lesser extent in the urine.

*Preclinical safety data:* Preclinical data were confined to those associated with over-stimulation of the recognised pharmacological action of corticosteroids, which is the only safety concern for human use derived from animal studies. However, information concerning genotoxicity is lacking. See above for further guidance.

**Pharmaceutical particulars**

*List of excipients:* Oleic Acid BP; Trichlorofluoromethane BP 1988; Dichlorodifluoromethane BP 1988.

*Incompatibilities:* None known.

*Shelf life:* 24 months in the container packaged for sale.

*Special precautions for storage:* Store below 30°C. Protect from frost and direct sunlight. The canister is pressurised, it must not be burnt, punctured or broken even when apparently empty. The therapeutic effect of the medication may decrease when the canister is cold.

*Nature and contents of container:* A pressurised aluminium container with a metered dispensing valve.

*Instructions for use/handling:* The instructions for use/handling that appear in the patient information leaflet are as follows:

1. Remove the cap from the inhaler. Make sure the mouthpiece is clean and clear of fluff and dirt.
2. Hold the inhaler upright, with your thumb on the base and your first finger on the top of the can.

Now shake the inhaler vigorously up and down.

3. Breathe out fully to empty the lungs, then place the mouthpiece firmly between the lips.
4. Now breathe in slowly and deeply. At the same time, press the aerosol can with your first finger to fire the aerosol and release Beclomethasone Dipropionate.
5. Remove the inhaler from your mouth and hold your breath for 10 seconds, or as long as possible. Breathe out slowly.
6. If more than one puff is required, wait at least one minute and repeat the procedure from step 2. Replace the cap.

*Important:* Do not rush steps 3 and 4. It is important that you start to breathe in as slowly as possible just before operating your inhaler. Practice in the mirror for the first few times. If you see 'mist' coming from the top of the inhaler or the sides of your mouth you should start again from step 2.

*Cleaning the inhaler:* Your inhaler should be cleaned reguarly, usually at least once a week. To clean, remove the metal canister from the plastic body and rinse the plastic body and the mouthpiece cover in warm water. Dry thoroughly, then replace the canister and mouthpiece cover. Avoid excessive heat. Do not put the metal canister into water.

*Marketing authorisation holder:* Norton (Waterford) Limited, IDA Estate, Waterford, Eire.

**Marketing authorisation numbers**

| | |
|---|---|
| Beclazone 50 Inhaler | 8142/0003 |
| Beclazone 100 Inhaler | 8142/0004 |
| Beclazone 250 Inhaler | 8142/0005 |

**Date of approval/revision of SPC** June 1997

**Legal category** POM

## CARDILATE MR* 20 mg ANGIOPINE MR* 20 mg TABLETS

**Qualitative and quantitative composition** Active ingredient: Nifedipine (INN) PhEur 20 mg.

**Pharmaceutical form** Modified release tablet for oral administration.

**Clinical particulars**

*Therapeutic indications:* Cardilate MR 20 mg/Angiopine MR 20 mg is indicated for the treatment of hypertension and for prophylaxis of chronic stable angina pectoris.

*Posology and method of administration:* Cardilate MR 20 mg/Angiopine MR 20 mg tablets should be taken with a little water.

Tablets must be swallowed whole and not broken or chewed.

The recommended starting dose of nifedipine is 10 mg every 12 hours swallowed with water, with subsequent titration of dosage according to response. The dose may be adjusted to 40 mg every 12 hours.

The pharmacokinetics of nifedipine are altered in the elderly so that lower maintenance doses of nifedipine may be required compared to younger patients.

Cardilate MR 20 mg/Angiopine MR 20 mg (Nifedipine) is not recommended for treatment of children.

Nifedipine is metabolised primarily by the liver and therefore patients with liver dysfunction should be carefully monitored. Patients with renal impairment should not require adjustment of dosage.

*Route of administration:* Oral.

*Contra-indications:* Cardilate MR 20 mg/Angiopine MR 20 mg should not be given to patients with known hypersensitivity to nifedipine, other tablet constituents, or other dihydropyridines, because of the theoretical risk of cross reactivity.

It is contra-indicated in women of child-bearing potential and those breast-feeding their babies.

Cardilate MR 20 mg/Angiopine MR 20 mg is contra-indicated in patients with clinically significant aortic stenosis, unstable angina, porphyria, or those in cardiogenic shock. It should not be used during or within one month of a myocardial infarction.

Cardilate MR 20 mg/Angiopine MR 20 mg tablets should not be used for the treatment of acute attacks of angina.

The safety of nifedipine in malignant hypertension has not been established.

Cardilate MR 20 mg/Angiopine MR 20 mg tablets should not be used for secondary prevention of myocardial infarction.

Cardilate MR 20 mg/Angiopine MR 20 mg tablets should not be administered concomitantly with rifampicin since effective plasma levels of nifedipine may not be achieved owing to enzyme induction.

*Special warnings and special precautions for use:* Cardilate MR 20 mg/Angiopine MR 20 mg should be administered to patients with low cardiac reserve or with severe hypotension with caution. Patients at risk of hypotensive crisis should begin any therapy under close medical supervision.

*Interaction with other medicaments and other forms of interaction:* As with other dihydropyridines, nifedipine should not be taken with grapefruit juice, because bioavailability is increased.

Cardilate MR 20 mg/Angiopine MR 20 mg can be administered concomitantly with other antihypertensives including beta-receptor blockers. These may have additive antihypertensive effects and postural hypotension may therefore occur. Cardilate MR 20 mg/Angiopine MR 20 mg will not prevent the possibility that there might be a rebound effect when other antihypertensive treatment is stopped. Concomitant therapy with cimetidine may potentiate the antihypertensive action of nifedipine. Nifedipine adminstration may suppress serum levels of quinidine.

The simultaneous administration of nifedipine and digoxin may lead to reduced digoxin clearance, and hence an increase in the plasma digoxin. Digoxin levels should be monitored and if necessary, the digoxin dose reduced.

Cardilate MR 20 mg/Angiopine MR 20 mg may modify insulin and glucose responses, requiring adjustment in therapy of treated diabetics.

Cardilate MR 20 mg/Angiopine MR 20 mg tablets should not be administered concomitantly with rifampicin since effective plasma levels of nifedipine may not be achieved owing to enzyme induction (see *Contra-indications*).

*Pregnancy and lactation:* Cardilate MR 20 mg/Angiopine MR 20 mg is contra-indicated in pregnant women and women of child-bearing potential because fetal risks, observed in animal experiments and during human use, far outweigh the potential benefits.

Nifedipine is secreted into breast milk, so Cardilate MR 20 mg/Angiopine MR 20 mg should not be administered during lactation.

*Effects on ability to drive and use machines:* Infrequently, Cardilate MR 20 mg/Angiopine MR 20 mg may cause headaches, dizziness, nausea and tiredness to such a degree that reaction time is affected. These effects can be aggravated by concurrent alcohol. If this occurs, the patient should not be allowed to drive or operate machines.

*Undesirable effects:* Cardilate MR 20 mg/Angiopine MR 20 mg may cause headaches, facial reddening and dizziness and leg oedema. These effects are secondary to vasodilation. Less common side-effects include rash, nausea, lethargy and urinary frequency. Rarely, gingival hyperplasia may occur; this may resolve when treatment is discontinued. Chest pain due to myocardial ischaemia may occur 1–4 hours after ingestion of Cardilate MR 20 mg/Angiopine MR 20 mg. A 'steal' effect has not been observed up to now with Cardilate MR 20 mg/Angiopine MR 20 mg, but treatment should be discontinued in patients in which this does occur. Cases of hypersensitivity to nifedipine resulting in jaundice have been reported.

Exacerbation of angina pectoris may occur rarely at the start of treatment with sustained release formulations of nifedipine. The occurrence of myocardial infarction has been described, although it is not possible to distinguish such an event from the natural course of ischaemic heart disease.

*Overdose:* Toxic affects arise from the three main actions of nifedipine in overdose: dilatation of vascular smooth muscles (predominant effect); decreased myocardial contractility; and depression of AV nodal conduction. Hypotension and tachycardia or bradycardia are the most likely manifestations of overdose. Other toxic effects include nausea, vomiting, drowsiness, dizziness, confusion, lethargy, flushing, coma and convulsions. Cardiac effects may include heart block, AV dissociation and asystole; metabolic disturbances include hyperglycaemia, acidosis, hypo- or hyperkalaemia and hypocalcaemia; pulmonary oedema has been reported.

Primary treatment involves removal of nifedipine by gastric lavage or ipecac and administration of activated charcoal (50 g adults; 10–15 g children). Cardilate MR 20 mg/Angiopine MR 20 mg is a modified release product, therefore activated charcoal should be repeated at 4-hourly intervals (25 g adults; 10 g children). The patient should be closely monitored and treated according to predominating signs:

- for hypotension: the feet should be raised and plasma expanders given. If this is not effective, 10% calcium gluconate or chloride can be given intravenously (calcium chloride should not be given to acidotic patients). If this fails, dopamine may be tried (large doses may be needed). Glucagon may also be of value.
- for bradycardia: treatment with atropine, isoprenaline and cardiac pacing should be given as required.

The value of extracorporeal methods of removal of nifedipine have not been established.

**Pharmacological properties**

*Pharmacodynamic properties:* Nifedipine inhibits the influx of calcium into myocardial cells, the smooth muscle cells of the coronary arteries and the peripheral capillaries. Nifedipine brings about a substantial improvement in the oxygen supply to the myocardium while reducing oxygen demand. It has been shown to exhibit anti-anginal properties. High blood pressure is normalised due to a reduction in the peripheral resistance (vasodilation).

*Pharmacokinetic properties*

*Absorption:* Nifedipine is absorbed rapidly and almost completely following oral administration. Nifedipine can be detected in plasma 30–60 minutes after administration of Cardilate MR 20 mg/Angiopine MR 20 mg and reaches maximal concentration between 0.75 and 5 hours.

*Distribution:* Nifedipine is more than 90% serum protein bound. Animal studies with labelled nifedipine have shown that distribution of the fraction not protein bound is throughout all organs and tissues, with higher concentrations in myocardium than in skeletal muscle. Neither nifedipine nor its metabolites are stored selectively in any tissue.

*Metabolism:* Nifedipine is converted almost compeltely to inactive metabolites.

*Elimination:* 70 to 80% of administered nifedipine is excreted as metabolites by the kidneys with an elimination half-life of approximately 10 hours.

Elimination may be retarded by renal failure or insufficiency.

*Preclinical safety data:* None stated.

**Pharmaceutical particulars**

*List of excipients:* Microcrystalline cellulose; carboxymethyl sodium starch; mannitol; colloidal anhydrous silica; polyvidone; magnesium stearate; sodium lauryl sulphate; methylhydroxypropyl cellulose; polyoxyethelene glycol 6000; polyoxyethylene glycol 400; red ferric oxide (E172); titanium dioxide (E171); talc. Purified water; alcohol (industrial) – not detected in finished product.

*Incompatibilities:* None known.

*Shelf life:* Three years.

*Special precautions for storage:* Cardilate MR 20 mg/Angiopine MR 20 mg should be stored in the original pack below 25°C, in a dry place and protected from light.

Nifedipine is highly sensitive to light and is therefore protected both by materials in the tablet and in the packaging. Nonetheless tablets should not be exposed to direct sunlight and should only be removed from the blister pack when about to be taken.

*Nature and contents of container:* Thermoformed blister packs of PVC/red transparent PVdC/aluminium in boxes of 7, 14, 20, 21, 28, 30, 56, 60, 84, 90, 100, 112 and 120 tablets.

*Instructions for use/handling:* None.

*Marketing authorisation holder:* Norton Healthcare Ltd, Gemini House, Flex Meadow, Harlow, Essex CM19 5TJ.

**Marketing authorisation number** 0530/0488.

**Date of approval/revision of SPC** 17 January 1997.

**Legal category** POM.

## CORDILOX* IV

**Presentation** Colourless glass 2 ml ampoules with breakline containing 5 mg Verapamil Hydrochloride BP per ampoule.

**Uses** The treatment of supraventricular arrhythmias.

*Mode of action:* Cordilox is a calcium channel blocker which inhibits the inward movement of calcium in smooth muscle cells of the systemic and coronary arteries and in the cells of cardiac muscle and the intracardiac conduction system.

Because of its effect on the movement of calcium in the intracardiac conduction system, it reduces automaticity, decreases conduction velocity and increases the refractory period.

**Dosage and administration**

*Acute (IV injection)*

*Adults:* For the treatment of tachyarrhythmias, 5–10 mg (1–2 ampoules) should be injected intravenously over a period of 30 seconds with continuous observation of the patient and, preferably, with simultaneous ECG monitoring.

In cases of paroxysmal tachyarrhythmias a further 5 mg may, if necessary, be injected 5–10 minutes after the first injection with the same precautions being observed. Higher doses are not usually necessary.

*Children:*

Newborn: 0.75–1 mg (0.3–0.4 ml)
Infants: 0.75–2 mg (0.3–0.8 ml)
1–5 years: 2–3 mg (0.8–1.2 ml)
6–15 years: 2.5–5 mg (1.0–2.0 ml)

In many cases smaller doses than those mentioned above are sufficient. The injection should be stopped at the onset of the desired effect.

For concomitant administration with beta-blockers see 'Precautions'.

*Elderly:* No special dosage recommendations except:

(a) In those patients with impaired liver function, particular attention should be paid to dosage because of reduced drug metabolism.

(b) In cardiac conduction disturbances, the effects of Cordilox and beta-blockers or other cardio-depressive drugs may be additive.

(see 'Precautions')

**Contra-indications, warnings, etc**

*Contra-indications:* Hypotension, marked bradycardia (less than 50 beats/minute), second and third degree atrioventricular block, sick sinus syndrome, uncompensated heart failure. Combination with beta-blockers is contra-indicated in patients with poor ventricular function.

*Precautions:* Cordilox may affect impulse conduction and should be used with caution in patients with first degree atrioventricular block. The effects of Cordilox and beta blockers or other drugs with a cardio-depressive action may be additive both with respect to conduction and contraction, therefore care must be exercised when these are administered concurrently or closely together. This is especially true when either drug is administered intravenously.

Patients with atrial fibrillation/flutter and an accessory pathway (eg W-P-W syndrome) may rarely develop increased conduction across the anomalous pathway and ventricular tachycardia may be precipitated.

If there are signs of tachycardia-induced heart failure (energetic exhaustion of the myocardium) digitalisation is necessary before intravenous administration of Cordilox.

*Drug interactions:* Cordilox may have an additive effect with other antihypertensive drugs. Thus, in many cases, with Cordilox, a reduction in the dose of the other antihypertensive drug may be possible.

There is a possibility of an interaction between verapamil and quinidine, causing hypotension, when Cordilox is administered by the intravenous route.

Verapamil hydrochloride has been shown to increase the serum concentration of digoxin and caution should be exercised with regard to digitalis toxicity. The effects of beta-blockers, anti-arrhythmics and general anaesthetics with verapamil may be additive both with respect to conduction and contraction of cardiac muscle.

There is a risk of nephrotoxicity if lithium is given at the same time as Cordilox due to increased lithium levels. Cordilox has also been reported to decrease lithium serum levels.

An increase in serum verapamil levels is possible if cimetidine is given concurrently. The effect of Cordilox may be reduced if given to patients already taking phenytoin, phenobarbitone or rifampicin, due to an increase in its metabolism. Plasma concentrations of carbamazepine, theophylline and cyclosporin may be increased when these drugs are given concurrently with Cordilox.

Cordilox may affect left ventricular contractility as a result of its mode of action. This effect is small and normally not important but cardiac failure may be precipitated or aggravated if it exists. In cases of poor ventricular function therefore, Cordilox should only be given after appropriate therapy for cardiac failure such as digitalis, etc.

Caution should be observed in the acute phase of myocardial infarction.

In patients with impaired liver function, particular attention should be paid to the dosage because of reduced drug metabolism.

Long term verapamil therapy may give rise to potentiation of neuromuscular blocking agents during anaesthesia.

*Use in pregnancy and lactation:* Verapamil is excreted into the breast milk in small amounts and is unlikely to be harmful. However, hypersensitivity reactions have been reported rarely with verapamil and therefore it should only be used during lactation if in the clinician's judgement it is essential to the welfare of the patient.

Animal studies have not shown any teratogenic effect. Cordilox should not be given during the first trimester of pregnancy unless, in the clinician's judgement, it is essential for the welfare of the patient. The possibility that Cordilox can cause relaxation of the uterine muscle should be considered at term.

*Side-effects:* Cordilox is well tolerated and does not exert a bronchoconstrictor effect.

Due to its mode of action, undesired effects on atrioventricular conduction and blood pressure are possible. This applies particularly to patients with atrioventricular block and/or considerably impaired myocardial function. On rare occasions the intravenous administration of Cordilox may lead to an undesired blocking of conduction and, in extreme cases, to asystole. The asystole is usually of short duration and normally sinus rhythm returns spontaneously after a few seconds. However, if on rare occasions asystole persists, treatment should be carried out as described below.

Intravenous administration of Cordilox may lead to a slight transient fall in blood pressure due to a reduction in peripheral resistance. Rarely this may result in severe hypotension.

*Treatment of acute cardiovascular side-effects:* If acute complications occur after intravenous injection of Cordilox (asystole, atrioventricular block or ventricular fibrillation) the usual emergency measures should be applied, e.g. cardiac massage, mechanical ventilation, the intravenous injection of adrenaline, and the intravenous injection of 10–20 ml of calcium gluconate 10% solution. Hypotension following intravenous injection of Cordilox may, if necessary, be controlled without difficulty by the use of vasoconstrictor substances.

*Overdosage:* Symptoms include hypotension, shock, first and second degree AV block, total AV block, asystole, sinus bradycardia and sinus arrest. Bradycardia may be treated with atropine, isoprenaline or cardiac pacing.

**Pharmaceutical precautions** Cordilox IV is incompatible with alkaline solutions (eg Sodium Bicarbonate Intravenous Infusion BP) as this may lead to a precipitation of the verapamil base.

**Legal category** POM.

**Package quantities** Containers of 5×2 ml ampoules.

**Further information** Metabolisable carbohydrate: Nil.

Sodium content: 0.30 mmol/ampoule (0.15 mmol/ml).

**Product licence number** 0530/0387

*Product licence holder:* Norton Healthcare Limited, Harlow, Essex CM19 5TJ.

## CORDILOX TABLETS 40 mg, 80 mg and 120 mg

**Qualitative and quantitative composition**

*Cordilox Tablets:* Verapamil Hydrochloride BP 40 mg.
*Cordilox Tablets:* Verapamil Hydrochloride BP 80 mg.
*Cordilox Tablets:* Verapamil Hydrochloride BP 120 mg.

**Pharmaceutical form** Tablets.

**Clinical particulars**

*Therapeutic indications:*

1. The treatment of prophylaxis of paroxysmal supraventricular tachycardia and of atrial flutter/fibrillation. Verapamil should not be used when atrial flutter/fibrillation complicates Wolff-Parkinson-White syndrome.
2. The treatment of prophylaxis of angina pectoris.
3. The treatment of mild to moderate hypertension and renal hypertension.

*Posology and method of administration:*

(Note: n40 mg, 80 mg, 120 mg, 160 mg and 240 mg presentations of Cordilox are available.)

*1. Supraventricular tachycardia:*

*Adults:* 40 to 120 mg t.d.s. according to the severity of the condition.

*Children:* Up to 2 years: half of a 40 mg tablet 2 to 3 times a day.

2 years and above: 40 to 120 mg 2 to 3 times a day according to age and effectiveness.

*2. Angina pectoris:*

*Adults:* 120 mg t.d.s. In some patients with angina of effort 80 mg t.d.s. can be completely satisfactory. Less than 120 mg t.d.s. is not likely to be effective in angina at rest and variant angina.

*Children:* No data available.

*3. Hypertension:*

*Adults:* The usual dosage is 160 mg twice a day. However, a minority of patients may be successfully controlled on 120 mg twice a day while others may require up to 480 mg daily given in divided doses.

*Children:* Up to 10 mg/kg/day in divided doses, according to severity of disease.

*Elderly dosages:* No special recommendations except:

(a) In those patients with impaired liver function, particular attention should be paid to dosage because of reduced drug metabolism.

(b) In cardiac conduction disturbances, the effects of Cordilox and beta-blockers or other cardio-depressive drugs may be additive.

*Route of administration:* Oral.

*Contra-indications:* Hypotension associated with cardiogenic shock.

Marked bradycardia (less than 50 beats/minute).

Second or third degree atrioventricular block.

Sick sinus syndrome.

Uncompensated heart failure.

Sino-atrial block.

Concomitant ingestion of grapefruit juice.

*Special warnings and precautions for use:* Cordilox may affect impulse conduction and should be used with caution in patients with first degree atrioventricular block. The effects of Cordilox and beta blockers or other drugs with a cardio-depressive action may be additive both with respect to conduction and contraction, therefore care must be exercised when these are administered concurrently or closely together. This is especially true when either drug is administered intravenously.

Patients with atrial flutter/fibrillation in association with an accessory pathway (e.g. W-P-W syndrome), may rarely develop increased conduction across the anomalous pathway and ventricular tachycardia may be precipitated.

If there are signs of tachycardia-induced heart failure (energetic exhaustion of the myocardium) digitalisation is necessary before intravenous administration of Cordilox.

Cordilox may affect left ventricular contractility as a result of its mode of action. This effect is small and normally not important but cardiac failure may be precipitated or aggravated if it exists. In case of poor ventricular function therefore, Cordilox should only be given after appropriate therapy for cardiac failure such as digitalis, etc.

Caution should be observed in the acute phase of myocardial infarction.

In patients with impaired liver function, particular attention should be paid to the dosage because of reduced drug metabolism. The disposition of verapamil in patients with renal impairment has not been fully established and careful patient monitoring is recommended. Verapamil is not removed during dialysis.

*Interactions with other medicaments and other forms of interaction:* The effects of Cordilox and beta-blockers, anti-arrhythmics, general anaesthetics or other drugs with a cardio-depressive action may be additive with respect to conduction and contraction. Cordilox may have an additive effect with other antihypertensive drugs. Thus, in many cases with Cordilox, a reduction in the dose of other antihypertensive drugs may be possible.

The effect of Cordilox may be reduced when combined with phenytoin, phenobarbitone or rifampicin due to an increase in its metabolism.

There is a possibility of an interaction between verapamil and quinidine, causing hypotension when Cordilox is administered by the intravenous route.

Plasma concentrations of carbamazepine, theophylline and cyclosporin may be increased when these drugs are given concurrently with Cordilox.

Verapamil hydrochloride has been shown to increase the serum concentration of digoxin and caution should be exercised with regard to digitalis toxicity.

There is a risk of neurotoxicity when lithium is given at the same time as Cordilox. Cordilox has also been reported to decrease lithium serum levels.

Long term verapamil therapy may give rise to potentiation of neuromuscular blocking agents during anaesthesia.

An increase in serum Verapamil levels is possible when Cimetidine is given concurrently. Grapefruit juice – an increase in verapamil serum levels has been reported.

*Pregnancy and lactation: Pregnancy:* Although animal studies have not shown any teratogenic effects, Cordilox should not be given during the first trimester of pregnancy unless, in the clinician's judgement, it is essential for the welfare of the patients. The possibility

that Cordilox can cause relaxation of the uterine muscle should be considered at term.

*Lactation:* Verapamil is excreted into the breast milk in small amounts and is unlikely to be harmful. However, hypersensivity reactions have been reported rarely with verapamil and therefore it should only be used during lactation if in the clinician's judgement it is essential to the welfare of the patient.

*Effects on ability to drive and use machines:* None stated.

*Undesirable effects:* Constipation (mild) – not common.

Flushing (mild) – occasional.

Headache (mild), dizziness, fatigue and ankle oedema – rare.

Nausea and vomiting (mild) – seldom.

Allergic reaction (mild) – very rare.

Impairment of liver function (reversible).

Characterised increase in transaminase and/or alkaline phosphatase – very rare.

Rash and pruritus, alopecia and urticaria – a possible side effect.

Rarely, reversible gynaecomastia and gingival hyperplasia.

*Overdose:* Symptoms include hypotension, shock, first and second degree AV block, total AV block, asystole, sinus bradycardia and sinus arrest.

For acute cardio-vascular side-effects, gastric lavage, taking the usual precautionary measures, may be appropriate. The usual emergency measure should be followed, e.g. cardiac massage, mechanical ventilation, the intravenous injection of adrenaline, the intravenous injection of 10–20 ml of calcium gluconate 10% solution.

In the case of second or third degree AV block, atropine, isoprenaline or a temporary pacemaker may be necessary. If myocardial insufficiency occurs, dopamine, dobutamine, cardiac glycosides or calcium gluconate (10–20 ml of a 10% solution) may be required. Appropriate positioning of the patient and vasoconstrictor drugs may be indicated in the case of hypotension.

Bradycardia may be treated with atropine, isoprenaline or cardiac pacing.

**Pharmacological properties**

*Pharmacodynamic properties:* Cordilox is a calcium channel blocker which inhibits the inward movement of calcium in cardiac muscle cells of the systemic and coronary arteries and in the cells of cardiac muscle and the intracardiac conduction system.

Cordilox lowers peripheral vascular resistance with little or no reflex tachycardia. Its efficacy in reducing both raised systolic and diastolic blood pressure is thought to be primarily due to this mode of action.

The decrease in systemic and coronary vascular resistance and the sparing effect on intracellular oxygen consumption appear to explain the anti-anginal properties of the product.

Because of its effect on the movement of calcium in the intracardiac conduction system, it reduces automaticity, decreases conduction velocity and increases the refractory period.

*Pharmacokinetic properties:* More than 90% of the orally administered dose of Cordilox is absorbed. Because of rapid biotransformation of verapamil during its first pass through the portal circulation, absolute bioavailability ranges from 20% to 35%. Peak plasma concentrations are reached between 1 and 2 hours after oral administration.

A close relationship exists between verapamil plasma concentration and prolongation of the PR interval. The mean elimination half-life in single dose studies ranged from 2.8 to 7.4 hours. In these same studies, after repetitive dosing, the half-life increased to a range from 4.5 to 12 hours (after less then 10 consecutive doses given 6 hours apart). Half-life may increase during titration due to saturation of hepatic enzyme systems as plasma verapamil levels rise.

Most of the drug in healthy subjects is eliminated in the urine (about 70% of dose in 5 days) and only about 15% in faeces. 12 different metabolites have been identified. Norverapamil is the major metabolite (25% of recovered products) and is the only metabolite with pharmacological activity (dogs). Approximately 90% is bound to plasma proteins.

*Preclinical safety data:* Not applicable.

**Pharmaceutical particulars**

*List of excipients:* Calcium Phosphate Dibasic Dihydrate USP; Sodium Starch Glycollate BP; Maize Starch BP; Magnesium Stearate PhEur; Water Purified PhEur.

*Coating:* Hydroxypropylmethylcellulose 2910 15CPS USP; Titanium Dioxide (E171) BP; Polyethylene Glycol 8000 NF; Polyethylene Glycol 400; Dye, Yellow D&C No. 110 A1 Lake (E104); Dye, Yellow FD&C No. 6 A1 Lake (E110); Acid Sorbic BP; Alcohol 3A; Water Purified PhEur.

*Incompatibilities:* None stated.

*Shelf life:* 5 years for Securitainer, 'Snap-Secure' Container, Tampertainer or Duma Container.

2 years for PVdC coated PVC/Aluminium blisters.

*Special precautions for use:* None stated.

*Nature and contents of container:* Securitainer, 'Snap-Secure' Container, Tampertainer, Duma Container or PVdC coated PVC/Aluminium blister packs (60 mg/m² PVdC on 250 µ PVC/20 µ A1) in pack sizes of 7, 14, 21, 28, 30, 50, 56, 60, 84, 90, 100, 112, 120 tablets.

*Instructions for use/handling:* None.

*Marketing authorisation holder:* Norton Healthcare Limited, Gemini House, Flex Meadow, Harlow, Essex CM19 5TJ.

**Marketing authorisation numbers**

Cordilox Tablets 40 mg    0503/0382
Cordilox Tablets 80 mg    0503/0383
Cordilox Tablets 120 mg    0503/0384

**Date of approval/revision of SPC**  24 April 1997

**Legal category**  POM

## CORDILOX TABLETS 160 mg

**Qualitative and quantitative composition**  Verapamil Hydrochloride BP 160 mg.

**Pharmaceutical form**  Tablets.

**Clinical particulars**

*Therapeutic indications:* The treatment of mild to moderate hypertension and renal hypertension, used alone or in conjunction with other antihypertensive therapy.

*Posology and method of administration:*
*Hypertension:*

*Adults:* The usual dosage is 160 mg twice a day. However, a minority of patients may be successfully controlled on 120 mg twice a day while others may require up to 480 mg daily given in divided doses.

*Children:* Up to 10 mg/kg/day in divided doses, according to severity of disease.

*Elderly dosages:* No special recommendations except:
– in those patients with impaired liver function, particular attention should be paid to dosage because of reduced drug metabolism.
– in cardiac conduction disturbances, the effects of Cordilox and beta-blockers or other cardio-depressive drugs may be additive.

*Route of administration:* Oral.

*Contra-indications:* Hypotension associated with cardiogenic shock.

Marked bradycardia (less than 50 beats/minute).

Second or third degree atrioventricular block.

Sick sinus syndrome.

Uncompensated heart failure.

Sino-atrial block.

Concomitant ingestion of grapefruit juice.

*Special warnings and precautions for use:* Cordilox may affect impulse conduction and should be used with caution in patients with first degree atrioventricular block. The effects of Cordilox and beta blockers or other drugs with a cardio-depressive action may be additive both with respect to conduction and contraction, therefore care must be exercised when these are administered concurrently or closely together. This is especially true when either drug is administered intravenously.

Patients with atrial flutter/fibrillation in association with an accessory pathway (e.g. W-P-W syndrome), may rarely develop increased conduction across the anomalous pathway and ventricular tachycardia may be precipitated.

If there are signs of tachycardia-induced heart failure (energetic exhaustion of the myocardium) digitalisation is necessary before intravenous administration of Cordilox.

Cordilox may affect left ventricular contractility as a result of its mode of action. This effect is small and normally not important but cardiac failure may be precipitated or aggravated if it exists. In case of poor ventricular function therefore, Cordilox should only be given after appropriate therapy for cardiac failure such as digitalis, etc.

Caution should be observed in the acute phase of myocardial infarction.

In patients with impaired liver function, particular attention should be paid to the dosage because of reduced drug metabolism. The disposition of verapamil in patients with renal impairment has not been fully established and careful patient monitoring is recommended. Verapamil is not removed during dialysis.

*Interactions with other medicaments and other forms of interaction:* The effects of Cordilox and beta-blockers, anti-arrhythmics, general anaesthetics or other drugs with a cardio-depressive action may be additive with respect to conduction and contraction. Cordilox may have an additive effect with other antihypertensive drugs. Thus, in many cases with Cordilox, a reduction in the dose of other antihypertensive drugs may be possible. The effect of Cordilox may be reduced when combined with phenytoin, phenobarbitone or rifampicin due to an increase in its metabolism.

There is a possibility of an interaction between verapamil and quinidine, causing hypotension when Cordilox is administered by the intravenous route.

Plasma concentrations of carbamazepine, theophylline and cyclosporin may be increased when these drugs are given concurrently with Cordilox.

Verapamil hydrochloride has been shown to increase the serum concentration of digoxin and caution should be exercised with regard to digitalis toxicity.

There is a risk of neurotoxicity when lithium is given at the same time as Cordilox. Cordilox has also been reported to decrease lithium serum levels.

Long term verapamil therapy may give rise to potentiation of neuromuscular blocking agents during anaesthesia.

An increase in serum Verapamil levels is possible when Cimetidine is given concurrently.

Grapefruit juice – an increase in verapamil serum levels has been reported.

*Pregnancy and lactation:*

*Pregnancy:* Although animal studies have not shown any teratogenic effects, Cordilox should not be given during the first trimester of pregnancy unless, in the clinician's judgement, it is essential for the welfare of the patients. The possibility that Cordilox can cause relaxation of the uterine muscle should be considered at term.

*Lactation:* Verapamil is excreted into the breast milk in small amounts and is unlikely to be harmful. However, hypersensivity reactions have been reported rarely with verapamil and therefore it should only be used during lactation if in the clinician's judgement it is essential to the welfare of the patient.

*Effects on ability to drive and use machines:* None stated.

*Undesirable effects:* Constipation (mild) – not common.

Flushing (mild) – occasional.

Headache (mild), dizziness, fatigue and ankle oedema – rare.

Nausea and vomiting (mild) – seldom.

Allergic reaction (mild) – very rare.

Impairment of liver function (reversible).

Characterised increase in tramsminase and/or alkaline phosphatase – very rare.

Rash and pruritus, alopecia and urticaria – a possible side effect.

Rarely, reversible gynaecomastia and gingival hyperplasia.

*Overdose:* Symptoms include hypotension, shock, first and second degree AV block, total AV block, asystole, sinus brachycardia and sinus arrest.

For acute cardio-vascular side-effects, gastric lavage, taking the usual precautionary measures, may be appropriate. The usual emergency measure should be followed, e.g. cardiac massage, mechanical ventilation, the intravenous injection of adrenaline, the intravenous injection of 10–20 ml of calcium gluconate 10% solution.

In the case of second or third degree AV block, atropine, isoprenaline or a temporary pacemaker may be necessary. If myocardial insufficiency occurs, dopamine, dobutamine, cardiac glycosides or calcium gluconate (10–20 ml of a 10% solution) may be required. Appropriate positioning of the patient and vasoconstrictor drugs may be indicated in the case of hypotension.

Bradycardia may be treated with atropine, isoprenaline or cardiac pacing.

**Pharmacological properties**

*Pharmacodynamic properties:* Cordilox is a calcium channel blocker which inhibits the inward movement of calcium in cardiac muscle cells of the systemic and coronary arteries and in the cells of cardiac muscle and the intracardiac conduction system.

Cordilox lowers peripheral vascular resistance with little or no reflex tachycardia. Its efficacy in reducing both raised systolic and diastolic blood pressure is thought to be primarily due to this mode of action.

The decrease in systemic and coronary vascular resistance and the sparing effect on intracellular oxygen consumption appear to explain the antianginal properties of the product.

Because of its effect on the movement of calcium in the intracardiac conduction system, it reduces automaticity, decreases conduction velocity and increases the refractory period.

*Pharmacokinetic properties:* More than 90% of the orally administered dose of Cordilox is absorbed. Because of rapid biotransformation of verapamil during its first pass through the portal circulation, absolute bioavailability ranges from 20% to 35%. Peak plasma concentrations are reached between 1 and 2 hours after oral administration.

A close relationship exists between verapamil plasma concentration and prolongation of the PR interval. The mean elimination half-life in single dose studies ranged from 2.8 to 7.4 hours. In these same studies, after repetitive dosing, the half-life increased to a range from 4.5 to 12 hours (after less then 10 consecutive doses given 6 hours apart). Half-life may increase during titration due to saturation of hepatic enzyme systems as plasma verapamil levels rise.

Most of the drug in healthy subjects is eliminated in the urine (about 70% of dose in 5 days) and only about 15% in faeces. 12 different metabolites have been identified. Norverapamil is the major metabolite (25% of recovered products) and is the only metabolite with pharmacological activity (dogs). Approximately 90% is bound to plasma proteins.

*Preclinical safety data:* Not applicable.

**Pharmaceutical particulars**

*List of excipients:* Maize Starch BP; Calcium Hydrogen Phosphage BP; Sodium Starch Glycollate BP; Magnesium Stearate BP.

*Coating:* Hydroxypropylmethylcellulose USP; Polyethylene Glycol 8000 NF; Polyethylene Glycol 400; Titanium Dioxide (E171) BP; Dye, Yellow Lake (E104); Dye, Yellow Lake (E110); Sorbic Acid BP.

*Incompatibilities:* None stated.

*Shelf life:* 5 years.

*Special precautions for use:* None stated.

*Nature and contents of container:* Blister Pack, Securitainer, 'Snap-Secure' Container, Tampertainer, Duma Container containing 7, 14, 21, 28, 30, 50, 56, 60, 84, 90, 100, 112 and 120 tablets.

*Instruction for use/handling:* None.

*Marketing authorisation holder:* Norton Healthcare Limited, Gemini House, Flex Meadow, Harlow, Essex CM19 5TJ.

**Marketing authorisation number**    0503/0385

**Date of approval/revision of SPC**    7 March 1997

**Legal category**    POM

## CROMOGEN* 5 mg INHALER

**Qualitative and quantitative composition**   Sodium cromoglycate 5 mg (INN sodium cromoglicate).

**Pharmaceutical form**   Metered-dose aerosol inhaler.

**Clinical particulars**

*Therapeutic indications:* Cromogen 5 mg Inhaler is indicated for the preventative treatment of mild to moderate bronchial asthma, including the prevention of exercise-induced asthma.

*Posology and method of administration:*

*Adults and children:* Initial dose is two inhalations of the aerosol four times daily. Once adequate control of symptoms has been achieved it may be possible to reduce to a maintenance dose of one inhalation four times daily. However, the dose may be increased to two inhalations six or eight times daily in more severe cases or during periods of severe antigen challenge. Additional doses before exercise may also be taken.

*Elderly patients:* No current evidence for alteration of the recommended adult dose.

*Contra-indications:* Cromogen 5 mg Inhaler is contraindicated in patients with known sensitivity to any of its ingredients.

*Special warnings and special precautions for use:*
*Concomitant bronchodilator therapy:* Where a concomitant aerosol bronchodilator is prescribed, it is recommended that this be administered prior to the Cromogen 5 mg Inhaler.

*Concomitant steroid therapy:* In patients currently treated with steroids the addition of Cromogen 5 mg Inhaler to the regimen may make it possible to reduce the maintenance dose or discontinue steroids completely. The patient must be carefully supervised while the steroid dose is reduced, a rate of reduction of 10% weekly is suggested. If reduction of steroid dosage has been possible Cromogen 5 mg Inhaler should not be withdrawn until cover has been re-instituted.

Since the therapy is prophylactic it is important to continue therapy in those patients who benefit. If it is necessary to withdraw this treatment, it should be done progressively over a period of one week. Symptoms of asthma may recur.

Cromogen 5 mg Inhaler is not indicated for the treatment of acute asthma attack.

*Interaction with other medicaments and other forms of interaction:* No major interactions are anticipated with the proposed usage of the product. See *Special warnings and special precautions for use.*

*Pregnancy and lactation:* As with all medication caution should be exercised especially during the first trimester of pregnancy. Cumulative experience with sodium cromoglycate suggest that it has no adverse effects on foetal development. It should only be used in pregnancy where there is a clear need.

It is not known whether sodium cromoglycate is excreted in breast milk but on the basis of its physicochemical properties this is considered unlikely. There is no evidence to suggest that the use of sodium cromoglycate has any undesirable effects on the baby.

*Effects on ability to drive and use machines:* No known effects.

*Undesirable effects:* Sodium cromoglycate is well-tolerated, mild throat irritation, coughing and transient bronchospasm may occur. Very rarely severe bronchospasm associated with a marked fall in pulmonary function has been reported. In such cases treatment should be stopped and should not be re-introduced. Reactions sometimes occurring after several months treatment include aggravation of existing asthma, gastroestinal symptoms (nausea, vomiting), myositis, dizziness, urticaria, rashes and pulmonary infiltration with eosinophilia.

*Overdose:* No action other than medical observation should be necessary.

**Pharmacological properties**

*Pharmacodynamic properties:* Sodium cromoglycate has no intrinsic bronchodilator, anti-histaminic or anti-inflammatory activity.

In vitro and in vivo studies have consistently suggested that sodium cromoglycate inhibits the release of inflammatory mediators from sensitised mast cells. It appears to inhibit reactions caused by both antigenic and non-antigenic stimuli and prevents both the immediate and late asthmatic responses. Most evidence suggests that the effects of sodium cromoglycate are due to a stabilisation of mast cell membranes, although the precise mechanism of action remains unknown.

*Pharmacokinetic properties:* Sodium cromoglycate is poorly absorbed from the gastrointestinal tract. Following inhalation as a fine powder from sodium cromoglycate capsules, about 8% of the total dose administered is deposited in the lungs from where it is rapidly and completely absorbed and excreted unchanged in the urine and bile. The elimination half-life is 1.5–2 hours and the protein binding is 65%. The majority of an inhaled dose is swallowed and excreted unchanged in the faeces.

*Preclinical safety data:* No relevant information.

**Pharmacological particulars**

*List of excipients:* Sorbitan trioleate, trichlorofluoromethane, dichlorodifluoromethane.

*Incompatibilities:* No incompatibilities are anticipated with the proposed usage of the product.

*Shelf life:* Shelf life of the product as packaged for sale is 24 months.

*Special precautions for storage:* Store below 30°C. The canister is pressurised and should be protected from direct sunlight and frost. It must not be punctured or burnt, even when empty.

*Nature and contents of container:* The container consists of an aluminium can with a metered dispensing valve crimped to it. The can is inserted into a plastic oral inhalation applicator with a dust cap.

Each metered-dose aerosol inhaler contains at least 112 actuations.

*Instructions for use/handling:*

1. Remove the cap from the inhaler. Make sure the mouthpiece is clean and clear of fluff or dirt.

2. Hold the inhaler upright, with your thumb on the base and your first finger on the top of the can.
Now shake vigorously, up and down.

3. Breathe out fully to empty the lungs, then place the mouthpiece firmly between the lips.

4. Now breathe in slowly and deeply. At the same time, press the aerosol can with your first finger to fire the aerosol and release sodium cromoglycate.

5. Remove the inhaler from your mouth and hold your breath for 10 seconds, or as long as possible. Breathe out slowly.

6. If more than one puff is required, wait at least one minute and repeat the procedure from step 2. Replace the cap.

*Cleaning your inhaler:* Your inhaler should be cleaned regularly, usually at least once a week. To clean, remove the metal canister from the plastic body and rinse the plastic body and mouthpiece cover in warm water. Dry thoroughly, then replace the canister and mouthpiece cover. Avoid excessive heat. Do not put the metal canister into water.

*Important:* Do not rush steps 3 and 4. It is important that you start to breathe in as slowly as possible just before operating your inhaler. Practice in front of the mirror for the first few times. If you see 'mist' coming from the top of the inhaler or the sides of your mouth you should start again from step 2.

*Marketing authorisation holder:* Norton Healthcare Limited, Harlow, Essex CM19 5TJ.

**Marketing authorisation number**    0530/0319

**Date of approval/revision of SPC**    March 1997

**Legal category**    POM.

## CROMOGEN* 5 mg EASI-BREATHE INHALER

**Qualitative and quantitative composition** Sodium cromoglycate 5 mg (INN cromoglicate acid).

**Pharmaceutical form** Breath-operated metered dose aerosol inhaler.

### Clinical particulars
*Therapeutic indications:* Cromogen 5 mg Easi-Breathe Inhaler is indicated for the treatment of bronchial asthma, including the prevention of exercise-induced asthma.

*Posology and method of administration:*
*Adults and children:* Initial dose is two inhalations of the aerosol four times daily. Once adequate control of symptoms has been achieved it may be possible to reduce to a maintenance dose of one inhalation four times daily. However, the dose may be increased to two inhalations six or eight times daily in more severe cases or during periods of severe antigen challenge. Additional doses before exercise may also be taken.

*Elderly patients:* No current evidence for alteration of the recommended adult dose.

*Contra-indications:* Cromogen 5 mg Easi-Breathe Inhaler is contra-indicated in patients with known sensitivity to any of its ingredients.

*Special warnings and special precautions for use:*
*Concomitant bronchodilator therapy:* Where a concomitant aerosol bronchodilator is prescribed, it is recommended that this be administered prior to the Cromogen 5 mg Easi-Breathe Inhaler.

*Concomitant steroid therapy:* In patients currently treated with steroids the addition of Cromogen 5 mg Easi-Breathe Inhaler to the regimen may make it possible to reduce the maintenance dose or to discontinue steroids completely. The patient must be carefully supervised while the steroid dose is reduced, a rate of reduction of 10% weekly is suggested. If reduction of steroid dosage has been possible Cromogen 5 mg Easi-Breathe Inhaler should not be withdrawn until steroid cover has been re-instituted.

Since the therapy is prophylactic it is important to continue therapy in those patients who benefit. If it is necessary to withdraw this treatment, it should be done progressively over a period of one week. Symptoms of asthma may recur.

*Interaction with other medicaments and other forms of interaction:* No major interactions are anticipated with the proposed usage of the product. See *Special warnings and special precautions for use.*

*Pregnancy and lactation:* As with all medication, caution should be exercised especially during the first trimester of pregnancy. Cumulative experience with sodium cromoglycate suggests that it has no adverse effects on foetal development. It should only be used in pregnancy where there is a clear need.

It is not known whether sodium cromoglycate is excreted in the breast milk but on the basis of its physico-chemical properties this is considered unlikely. There is no evidence to suggest that the use of sodium cromoglycate has any undesirable effects on the baby.

*Effects on ability to drive and use machines:* No known effects.

*Undesirable effects:* Sodium cromoglycate is well-tolerated, mild throat irritation, coughing and transient bronchospasm may occur. Very rarely severe bronchospasm associated with a marked fall in pulmonary function has been reported. In such cases treatment should be stopped and should not be re-introduced. Reactions sometimes occurring after several months treatment include aggravation of existing asthma, urticaria, rashes and pulmonary infiltration with eosinophilia.

*Overdose:* No action other than medical observation should be necessary.

### Pharmacological properties
*Pharmacodynamic properties:* Sodium Cromoglycate has no intrinsic bronchodilator, anti-histaminic or anti-inflammatory activity.

*In vitro* and *in vivo* studies have consistently suggested that sodium cromoglycate inhibits the release of inflammatory mediators from sensitised mast cells. It appears to inhibit reactions caused by both antigenic and non-antigenic stimuli and prevents both the immediate (Type I) and late (Type II) asthmatic responses. Most evidence suggests that the effects of sodium cromoglycate are due to a stabilisation of mast cell membranes, although the precise mechanism of action remains unknown.

*Pharmacokinetic properties:* Sodium cromoglycate is poorly absorbed from the gastrointestinal tract. Following inhalation as a fine powder from sodium cromoglycate capsules, about 8% of the total dose administered is deposited in the lungs from where it is rapidly absorbed and excreted unchanged in the urine and bile. The majority of an inhaled dose is swallowed and excreted unchanged in the faeces.

*Preclinical safety data:* See *Posology, Contra-indications, Special warnings, Interactions, Pregnancy and lactation, Undesirable effects* and *Overdose* sections above.

### Pharmaceutical particulars
*List of excipients:* Sorbitan trioleate, trichlorofluoromethane, dichlorodifluoromethane.

*Incompatibilities:* No incompatibilities are anticipated with the proposed usage of the product.

*Shelf life:* Shelf life of the product as packaged for sale is 24 months.

*Special precautions for storage:* Store below 30°C. The canister is pressurised and should be protected from direct sunlight and frost. It must not be punctured or burnt, even when empty.

*Nature and contents of container:* Breath operated metered dose aerosol inhaler containing at least 112 actuations.

*Instructions for use/handling:*
1. Before use shake the inhaler vigorously.
2. Then, holding the inhaler upright, open the cap.
3. Breathe out normally. Place the mouthpiece firmly between your lips. Make sure that your hand is not blocking the airholes and that you are still holding the inhaler upright.
4. Breathe in slowly through the mouthpiece. Don't stop breathing when the inhaler puffs the dose into your mouth. Carry on until you have taken a deep breath.
5. Hold your breath for 10 seconds or as long as is comfortable, then breathe out slowly.
6. After use, hold the inhaler upright and immediately close the cap.
7. If you need to take more than one puff, wait at least one minute between doses and repeat from Step 1.
8. It is very important to keep the inhaler clean, especially in the mouthpiece area, to prevent build-up of deposits from the aerosol. Washing once a week is recommended.

*How to clean your inhaler*
A. Unscrew the top of the inhaler. Keep this top dry at all times.
B. Remove metal canister.
C. Rinse inhaler body in warm water and dry. Replace canister.
D. Close cap and screw top of inhaler back onto body. Do not wash the top part of the inhaler.

*Marketing authorisation holder:* Norton Healthcare Limited, Gemin House, Flex Meadow, Harlow, Essex CM19 5TJ.

**Marketing authorisation number** 0530/0404

**Date of approval/revision of SPC** 16 February 1995.

**Legal category** POM.

## CROMOGEN* STERI-NEB*

**Presentation** Cromogen Steri-Neb is a sterile sodium cromoglycate solution for inhalation via a power operated nebuliser. Each polyethylene ampoule contains 20 mg of sodium cromoglycate in 2 ml of water.

**Uses** Cromogen Steri-Neb is indicated for the preventive treatment of bronchial asthma which may be due to allergy, exercise, cold air or chemical and occupational irritants. Sodium cromoglycate has no intrinsic bronchodilator, anti-histaminic or anti-inflammatory activity. Most evidence suggests that the effects of sodium cromoglycate are due to a stabilisation of mast cell membranes, although the precise mechanism of action remains unknown.

**Dosage and administration** Cromogen Steri-Neb must only be administered by a power operated nebuliser, via a face mask or a mouthpiece.

*Dosage:* Since Cromogen Steri-Neb therapy is essentially preventive, it is important to continue therapy in those patients who benefit.

*Adults, children and the elderly:* The normal dose is the contents of 1 ampoule (20 mg), four times a day at intervals of 3–6 hours. In severe cases this may be increased to 5 or 6 times daily but with at least a 3 hour interval between administration of each ampoule.

**Contra-indications, warnings, etc**
*Contra-indications:* Cromogen Steri-Neb should not be administered by injection or administered to those patients with a known hypersensitivity to sodium cromoglycate.

*Concomitant steroid therapy:* In patients currently treated with steroids, the addition of Cromogen Steri-Neb to the regime may make it possible to reduce the maintenance dose or to discontinue steroids completely. The patient must be carefully supervised while the steroid dose is reduced; a rate of reduction of 10% weekly is suggested. An increase in steroid dosage may be necessary if symptoms increase and at times of infection, severe antigen challenge or stress. If reduction in steroid dosage has been possible Cromogen Steri-Neb should not be withdrawn until steroid cover has been reinstituted.

*Concomitant bronchodilator therapy:* If bronchodilators are used concomitantly patients may find that the frequency of bronchodilator usage can be reduced as their asthma is stabilised with Cromogen Steri-Neb.

*Side effects:* Sodium cromoglycate is well tolerated, mild throat irritation, coughing and transient bronchospasm may occur. Very rarely, severe bronchospasm associated with a marked fall in pulmonary function has been reported. In such cases treatment should be stopped and should not be re-introduced. Reactions sometimes occurring after several months treatment include aggravation of existing asthma, urticaria, rashes and pulmonary infiltration with eosinophilia.

*Overdosage:* No action other than medical observation should be necessary.

*Withdrawal of therapy:* Since Cromogen Steri-Neb acts prophylactically, it is important to continue treatment in those patients who benefit. The withdrawal of Cromogen Steri-Neb should be done progressively over a period of one week. Symptoms of asthma may recur.

*Use in pregnancy and lactation:* As with all medication, particular caution must be exercised during the first trimester of pregnancy. Cumulative experience with sodium cromoglycate suggest that it has no adverse effects on foetal development. It should only be used in pregnancy where there is a clear need.

It is not known whether sodium cromoglycate is excreted in the breast-milk but on the basis of its physico-chemical properties this is considered unlikely. There is no evidence to suggest that the use of sodium cromoglycate has any undersirable effects on the baby.

**Pharmaceutical precautions** Store in the box below 25°C protected from light. Cromogen Steri-Neb should not be diluted or mixed with other preparations due to possible incompatibility problems.

**Legal category** POM.

**Package quantities** Packs containing 60 Cromogen Steri-Neb ampoules in strips of 5.

**Further information** Nil.

**Product licence number** 0530/0349.

*Product licence holder:* Norton Healthcare Limited, Harlow, Essex CM19 5TJ.

## FRU-CO*

**Qualitative and quantitative composition** Frusemide BP 40 mg and Amiloride Hydrochloride (anhydrous) BP 5 mg.

**Pharmaceutical form** Tablets for oral administration.

**Clinical particulars**
*Therapeutic indications:* Co-amilofruse is indicated where a prompt diuresis is required. It is of particular value in conditions where potassium conservation is important: congestive cardiac failure, nephrosis, corticosteroid therapy, oestrogen therapy, ascites associated with cirrhosis.

*Posology and method of administration:*
*Adults:* One to two tablets taken in the morning.

*Elderly:* The dosage should be adjusted according to diuretic response: serum electrolytes and urea should be carefully monitored.

*Children:* Not recommended.

*Route of administration:* Oral.

*Contra-indications:* Hyperkalaemia (serum potassium >5.3 mmol/litre), Addison's disease, acute renal failure, anuria, severe progressive renal disease, electrolyte imbalance, precomatose states associated with cirrhosis, concomitant potassium supplements, known sensitivity to frusemide or amiloride.

*Special warnings and precautions for use:* Patients who are being treated with this preparation require regular supervision, with monitoring of fluid and electrolyte states to avoid excessive loss of fluid.

Co-amilofruse should be used with particular caution in elderly patients or those with potential obstruction of the urinary tract or disorders rendering electrolyte balance precarious.

Hyponatraemia, hypochloraemia and raised blood urea nitrogen may occur during vigorous diuresis, especially in seriously ill patients. Careful monitoring of serum electrolytes and urea should therefore be undertaken in these patients.

The dosage of concurrently administered cardiac glycosides or antihypertensive agents may require adjustment.

Co-amilofruse should be discontinued before a glucose tolerance test.

*Interaction with other medicaments and other forms of interaction:* ACE inhibitors should be avoided in patients receiving co-amilofruse as serum potassium levels may be increased. If concomitant use of ACE inhibitors is considered essential, serum electrolytes and clinical condition must be monitored carefully. Concomitant administration of potassium supplements may cause severe hyperkalaemia and is contra-indicated.

Nephrotoxicity caused by cephalosporins may be increased by concomitant administration of co-amilofruse.

In common with other diuretics, serum lithium levels may be increased when lithium is given concomitantly with frusemide, necessitating adjustment of the lithium dosage.

Certain non-steroidal anti-inflammatory agents (e.g. indomethacin) may attenuate the action of frusemide and may cause renal failure in cases of pre-existing hypovolaemia.

The effects of curariform muscle relaxants may be enhanced by frusemide, whilst the effects of antidiabetics may be reduced.

The diuretic effects of frusemide may be reduced by concurrent administraiton of phenytoin.

Interactions have also been reported with ototoxic antibiotics. In cases of concomitant glucocorticoid therapy or abuse of laxatives, the risk of an increased potassium loss should be borne in mind.

*Pregnancy and lactation:* The safety of co-amilofruse has not been established during pregnancy and lactation.

*Effects on ability to drive and use machines:* Reduced mental alertness may impair ability to drive or operate dangerous machinery.

*Undesirable effects:* As with other diuretics, electrolytes and water balance may be disturbed as a result of diuresis after prolonged therapy. This may cause symptoms such as headache, hypotension and muscle cramps.

Hyperkalaemia has been observed in patients receiving amiloride hydrichloride.

Frusemide may cause latent diabetes to become manifest. It may be necessary to increase the dose of hypoglycaemic agents in diabetic patients.

Patients with prostatic hypertrophy or inmpairment of micturition have an increased risk of developing acute urinary retention during diuretic therapy.

Serum uric acid levels may rise during treatment with co-amilofruse and acute attacks of gout may be precipitated.

Malaise, gastric upset, nausea, vomiting, diarrhoea, and constipation may occur.

If skin rashes or pruritus occur, treatment should be withdrawn.

Rare complications may include minor psychiatric disturbances, disturbances in liver function tests and ototoxicity.

Bone marrow depression occasionally complicates treatment, necessitating withdrawal of the product.

The haematopoietic state should be regularly monitored during treatment.

Serum calcium level may be reduced; in very rare cases tetany has been observed.

Serum cholesterol and triglyceride levels may rise during frusemide treatment but usually return to normal within six months during long term therapy.

*Overdose:* Treatment of overdosage should be aimed at reversing dehydration and correcting electrolyte imbalance, particularly hyperkalaemia. Emesis should be induced or gastric lavage performed. Treatment is symptomatic and supportive. If hyperkalaemia is seen, appropriate measures to reduce serum potassium must be instituted.

**Pharmacological properties:**
*Pharmacodynamic properties:*
*Amiloride:* Amiloride is a mild diuretic which appears to act mainly on the distal renal tubules. It is described as potassium-sparing since, like spironolactone, it increases the excretion of sodium and chloride and reduces the excretion of potassium. Unlike spironolactone, however, it does not act by inhibiting aldosterone. Amiloride does not inhibit carbonic anhydrase. It takes effect about 2 hours after administration by mouth and its diuretic action has been reported to persist for about 24 hours. The full effect may be delayed until several days of treatment.

*Frusemide:* Frusemide is a potent diuretic with a rapid action. Its effects are evident within 30 minutes to 1 hour after a dose by mouth and lasts for about 4 to 6 hours. After intravenous injection its effects are evident in about 5 minutes and last for about 2 hours. Frusemide inhibits the reabsorption of electrolytes in the ascending limb of the loop of Henle and also in the distal renal tubules. It may also have a direct effect in the proximal tubules. Excretion of sodium, potassium, and chloride ions is increased and water

excretion enhanced. It has no clinically significant effect on carbonic anhydrase.

*Pharmacokinetic properties:*
*Amiloride:* Amiloride is incompletely absorbed from the gastro-intestinal tract; bioavailability of about 50% is reported and is reduced by food. It is not bound to plasma proteins and has a half-life of 6 to 9 hours. It is excreted unchanged by the kidneys.

*Frusemide:* Frusemide is incompletely but fairly rapidly absorbed from the gastro-intestinal tract; bioavailability has been reported to be about 60 to 70% but is reduced in renal failure. It has a biphasic half-life in the plasma with a terminal elimination phase that has been estimated to range up to about 1½ hours although it is prolonged in renal and hepatic insufficiency. It is up to 99% bound to plasma proteins, and is mainly excreted in the bile, non-renal elimination being considerably increased in renal failure. Frusemide crosses the placental barrier and is excreted in milk.

*Preclinical safety data:* Not applicable.

**Pharmaceutical particulars**
*List of excipients:* Lactose BP, Starch BP, Anstead dispersed orange 11348 (E110), Starch (pre-gelatinised) BP, Croscarmellose sodium USP, Magnesium sterate BP, Talc BP.

*Incompatibilities:* None known.

*Shelf life:* 36 months.

*Special precautions for storage:* Store in a dry place below 25°C and protect from light.

*Nature and contents of container:* Polypropylene tubular container with an open end equipped to accept a polyethylene closure with a tamper-evident tear strip, tampertainers or duma containers. Pack sizes 7, 14, 21, 28, 30, 50, 56, 60, 84, 90, 100, 112, 120, 500 and 1000 tablets, or

250 µm opaque UPVC/20 µm hard temper aluminium foil strip packs or PVdC coated PVC/Aluminium blisters (60 g/m² PVdC on 250 µm PVC/20 µm Al) containing 7, 14, 21, 28, 30, 50, 56, 60, 84, 90, 100, 112 and 120 tablets.

*Instructions for use/handling:* No special instructions.

*Marketing authorisation holder:* Norton Healthcare Ltd, Gemini House, Harlow, Essex CM19 5TJ.

**Marketing authorisation number**    0530/0348

**Date of approval/revision of SPC**    20 February 1997

**Legal category**    POM

# GLAUCOL* 0.25% and 0.5%

**Qualitative and quantitative composition**

| Name of ingredient | Amount (g/litre) | |
|---|---|---|
| | 0.25% w/w | 0.5% w/w |
| Timolol Maleate PhEur | 3.417 | 6.834 |
| equivalent to Timolol | 2.5 | 5.0 |

**Pharmaceutical form**    Opththalmic solution.

**Clinical pariculars**
*Therapeutic indications:* Glaucol opththalmic solution is a beta-adrenergic receptor antagonist used topically for the reduction of elevated intra-ocular pressure in various conditions including patients with ocular hypertension, patients with chronic open-angle glaucoma including patients with aphakia; and some patients with secondary glaucoma.

*Posology and method of administration:*
*Dosage schedule:* Recommended therapy is one drop 0.25% solution in the affected eye(s) twice a day.

If clinical response is not adequate, dosage may be increased to one drop 0.5% solution in the affected eye(s) twice daily. If required, timolol maleate ophthalmic solution may be used with miotics, adrenaline or systemically administered carbonic anhydrous inhibitors.

Intra-ocular pressure should be reassessed approximately four weeks after starting treatment because response to Glaucol may take a few weeks to stabilise.

Provided that the intra-ocular pressure is maintained at satisfactory levels, many patients can then be placed on once-a-day therapy.

*Transfer from other agents:* If transferring from another topical beta-blocking agent, its use should be discontinued after a full day of treatment and treatment with Glaucol 0.25% started the next day with one drop twice daily in the affected eye(s). As above, if the clinical response is not adequate, the dosage may be increased to one drop of the 0.5% solution twice daily.

If transferring from a single anti-glaucoma agent which is not a beta-blocker, the agent should be continued and one drop added of the Glaucol 0.25% in the affected eye(s) twice daily. On the following day the previous agent should be discontinued and Glaucol continued. The dosage may be increased to the 0.5% solution twice daily if the clinical response is inadequate.

*Use in children:* Paediatric use is not currently recommended.

*Use in the elderly:* There has been wide experience with the usage of timolol maleate in elderly patients. The dosage recommendations above reflect the clinical data derived from this experience.

*Contra-indications:* Bronchial asthma, history of bronchial asthma, or severe chronic obstructive pulmonary disease, sinus bradycardia, second and third degree AV block, overt cardiac failure, cardiogenic shock, and hypersensitivity to timolol maleate or other beta-blocking agents.

*Special warnings and precautions for use:* Like other topically applied ophthalmic drugs, Glaucol may be absorbed systemically and adverse reactions seen with systemically administered beta-blockers may occur.

Cardiac failure should be adequately controlled before beginning therapy with Glaucol. Patients with a history of severe cardiac disease should be closely observed for signs of cardiac failure and have their pulse rates checked.

Respiratory and cardiac reactions, including death due to bronchospasm in patients with asthma and, rarely, death associated with cardiac failure, have been reported.

The effect on intra-ocular pressure or the known effects of systemic beta-blockade may be exaggerated when Glaucol is given to patients already receiving an oral beta-blocking agent. The response of these patients should be closely watched.

If Glaucol is used to reduce elevated intra-ocular pressure in angle closure glaucoma it should be used with a miotic and not alone.

There have been reports of skin rashes and/or dry eyes associated with the use of beta-adrenergic receptor blocking drugs. The reported incidence is small and in most cases the symptoms have cleared when treatment was withdrawn. Discontinuation of the drug should be considered if any such reaction is not otherwise explicable. Cessation of therapy involving beta-blockade should be gradual.

Glaucol contains benzalkonium chloride as a preservative which may be deposited in soft contact lenses. Therefore Glaucol should not be used while wearing these lenses. The lenses should be removed before application of the drops and not reinserted earlier than 15 minutes after use.

Glaucol has generally been well tolerated in glaucoma patients wearing conventional hard contact lenses. Glaucol has not been studied in patients wearing lenses made of material other than polymethylmethacrylate (PMMA) which is used to make hard contact lenses.

*Interaction with other medicaments and other forms of interactions:* Although Glaucol alone has little or no effect on pupil size, mydriasis has occasionally been reported when Glaucol is given with adrenaline.

Small amounts of Glaucol may be absorbed systemically and potentially add to the effects of oral calcium antagonists, rauwolfia alkaloids or beta-blockers to induce hypotension and/or marked bradycardia.

*Pregnancy and lactation:* Glaucol has not been studied in human pregnancy. The use of Glaucol requires that the anticipated benefit be weighed against possible hazards.

Glaucol is detectable in human milk. A decision for breast-feeding mothers either to stop taking timolol or stop nursing should be based on the importance of the drug to the mother.

*Effects on ability to drive and use machines:* Installation of Glaucol may cause transient blurring of vision. Patients should be warned not to drive or operate moving machinery until any blurring of vision after installation has totally regressed.

*Undesirable effects:* Glaucol is usually well tolerated.

*Special senses:* Signs and symptoms of ocular irritation, including conjunctivitis, blepharitis, keratitis, and decreased corneal sensitivity, have been reported. Visual disturbances, including refractive changes (due to withdrawal of miotic therapy in some cases), diplopia, and ptosis, can occur.

*Cardiovascular:* Bradycardia, arrhythmia, hypotension, syncope, heart block, cerebrovascular accident, cerebral ischaemia, congestive heart failure, palpitation and cardiac arrest may occur and are probably the result of systemic absorption.

*Respiratory:* Bronchospasm (predominantly in patients with pre-existing bronchospastic disease), respiratory failure, and dyspnoea have been reported.

*Generally:* Headache, asthenia, nausea, dizziness, depression and hypersensitivity reactions including localised and generalised rash and urticaria may occasionally occur.

*Causal relationship unknown:* The following adverse events have been reported, but a causal relationship to Glaucol has not been established: Aphakic cystoid macular oedema, dry mouth, nasal congestion, anorexia, dyspepsia, CNS effects (e.g. behavioural change including confusion, hallucinations anxiety, disorientation, nervousness, somnolence and other psychiatric disturbances), hypertension and retroperitoneal fibrosis.

The adverse reactions seen with oral timolol maleate may occur with Glaucol due to systemic absorption.

*Overdose:* Overdosage reactions are more likely to follow oral ingestion of timolol maleate than by systemic absorption through its topical use. No specific data on overdosage in humans by either route are available.

A study in patients with renal failure suggests that timolol does not readily dialyse.

The most common signs and symptoms to be expected following overdosage with a beta-blocker are symptomatic bradycardia, hypotension, bronchospasm and acute cardiac failure. The standard measures to overcome beta-blockade should be undertaken.

**Pharmacological properties**
*Pharmacodynamic properties:* Glaucol ophthalmic solution is a non-selective beta-adrenergic antagonist used for the topical treatment of increased intra-ocular pressure.

Timolol maleate has no intrinsic sympathomimetic activity nor membrane-stabilising activity.

It is thought that the mode of action is by markedly reducing the production of aqueous humor, probably without any effect on the outflow tract.

Glaucol ophthalmic solution is effective in a range of concentrations but the usual recommendation is for 0.25% and 0.5% solution strengths.

*Pharmacokinetic properties:* Glaucol ophthalmic solution lowers intra-ocular pressure within 30–60 minutes of being administered topically, has a maximum IOP-lowering effect 4–5 hours after administration, and the effect persists for 12–14 hours after a single dose.

Minute amounts are absorbed systemically; plasma concentrations of up to 1 ng/ml can be detected after single eye drop administration.

*Preclinical safety data:* None presented.

**Pharmaceutical particulars**
*List of excipients:* Potassium Dihydrogen Phosphate PhEur; Disodium Hydrogen Phosphate PhEur; Sodium Chloride PhEur; Benzalkonium Chloride PhEur; Purified Water PhEur.

*Incompatibilities:* None known.

*Shelf life:* Shelf life of the product as packaged for sale – Two years.

Shelf life after first opening the container – One month.

*Special precautions for storage:* Store below 30°C. Protect from light.

*Nature and contents of container:* A 5 ml low density polyethylene bottle. The dropper insert is made from low density polyethylene and the bottle is closed by a screw cap manufactured from high density polyethylene. The cap is secured by a tamper evident closure.

*Instructions for use/handling:* Unscrew the cap from the bottle. Pull down the bottom lid of the eye to form a pocket. Place the tip close to the lower eye lid and squeeze the container gently. One drop of solution should fall into the eye.

*Marketing authorisation holder:* Norton Healthcare Ltd, Harlow, Essex CM19 5TJ.

**Marketing authorisation numbers**
Glaucol 0.25% 0530/0490
Glaucol 0.5% 0530/0491

**Date of approval/revision of SPC** March 1996

**Legal category** POM

## HAY-CROM AQUEOUS* EYE DROPS

**Presentation** A clear pale straw coloured solution of Sodium Cromoglycate PhEur 2.0% w/v, with benzalkonium chloride 0.01% w/v. Other constituents: Disodium Edetate BP, Purified Water BP.

**Uses** Hay-Crom Aqueous Eye Drops are indicated for the prophylaxis and treatment of acute and chronic allergic conjunctivitis, including hay fever and seasonal kerato conjunctivitis. Most evidence suggests that the effects of sodium cromoglycate are due to stabilisation of sensitised mast cells, although the precise mechanism of action remains unknown.

**Dosage and administration**
*Adults, children and the elderly:* One or two drops into each affected eye up to four times daily.

**Contra-indications, warnings, etc**
*Contra-indications:* Hypersensitivity to sodium cromoglycate, benzalkonium chloride or disodium edetate.

*Precautions:* Since sodium cromoglycate is essentially prophylactic, patients should be advised not to discontinue using the medication unless advised to do so.

*Side-effects:* Following instillation of the drops, transient blurring of vision, burning, stinging or other transient symptoms may occur. Patients should be advised not to drive or operate machinery until clarity of vision is restored.

*Overdosage or ingestion:* Sodium cromoglycate is poorly absorbed through the gastro-intestinal tract. In case of overdosage, no action other than medical observation should be necessary.

*Use in pregnancy and lactation:* Caution should be exercised with respect to administration during pregnancy, especially during the first trimester. No adverse effects on foetal development have been reported with sodium cromoglycate. Hay-Crom Aqueous Eye Drops should be used in pregnancy only where there is a clear need. No data are available on the excretion of sodium cromoglycate in breast milk, but on the basis of its physico-chemical properties it is considered unlikely.

**Pharmaceutical precautions** Store below 30°C. Protect from light.

**Legal category** POM.

**Package quantities** 13.5 ml.

**Further information** Full instructions for use by patients are provided with each pack. As with other ophthalmic preparations, discard any solution remaining 28 days after opening.

Since the product contains benzalkonium chloride as preservative, the eye drops should not be used whilst wearing soft contact lenses.

**Product licence number** 0530/0356

*Product licence holder:* Norton Healthcare Ltd, Harlow, Essex CM19 5TJ.

## IPRATROPIUM STERI-NEB*

**Presentation** Sterile, unit dose, low density polyethylene vial containing a clear, colourless isotonic solution of ipratropium bromide 0.025% w/v (250 micrograms/ml) for administration by inhalation. Two vial sizes are available:

(i) a Steri-Neb vial containing 250 micrograms ipratropium bromide in 1 ml solution;
(ii) a Steri-Neb vial containing 500 micrograms ipratropium bromide in 2 ml solution.

**Uses**
Ipratropium bromide is an anticholinergic bronchodilator. It is indicated for the treatment of reversible airways obstruction.

**Dosage and administration**
The solution may be administered from an intermittent positive pressure ventilator or from suitable nebulisers using the following recommended doses:

*Adult (including the elderly):* 0.4–2.0 ml solution (100–500 micrograms) up to four times daily.

*Children (3–14 years):* 0.4–2.0 ml solution (100–500 micrograms) up to three times daily.

The dose of nebuliser solution may need to be diluted in order to obtain a final volume suitable for the particular nebuliser being used. If dilution is necessary only sterile Sodium Chloride 0.9% PhEur, such as Saline Steri-Neb (Sodium Chloride 0.9% PhEur) should be used.

*Use in the elderly:* No special precautions are required.

**Contra-indications, warnings, etc**
*Contra-indications:* Known hypersensitivity to atropine. Hypersensitivity to any of the components of Ipratropium Steri-Neb.

*Warnings and precautions:* Occasional reports of paradoxical bronchospasm following administration of nebulised solutions of ipratropium bromide have occurred during early treatment. Therefore, use of Ipratropium Steri-Neb should always be initiated in hospital and be subject to close medical supervision during the first week of treatment. The patient should be advised to seek medical advice should a reduced response to treament become apparent.

Patients must be instructed in the correct administration of the nebuliser solution and be warned not to allow the solution or mist to enter the eyes. Caution is advised in the use of anticholinergic agents in patients with glaucoma.

Anticholinergic agents can precipitate acute urinary retention in patients with prostatic hypertrophy should sufficient plasma concentrations be achieved. However, urinary retention has rarely been reported. Nevertheless, caution is advised in patients with prostatic hypertrophy.

*Use in pregnancy:* Animal teratology and reproduction studies have demonstrated no adverse effects. The safety of ipratropium bromide in human pregnancy has not been established.

As with all medicines, Ipratropium Steri-Neb should not be used in pregnancy, especially during the first trimester, unless the expected benefit is thought to outweigh any possible risk to the foetus.

*Use in breast-feeding.* It is not known to what extent ipratropium bromide passes into breast milk. The product should not be administered to nursing mothers unless considered essential by the physician.

*Side-effects:* Anticholinergic side-effects are unlikely at therapeutic doses, but some patients may complain of a dry mouth. Urinary retention and constipation have rarely been reported.

No adverse effect on bronchial secretion has been shown within the therapeutic dose range.

*Overdosage:* Inhaled doses of 5 mg produced an increase in heart rate with palpitations but single inhaled doses of 2 mg in adults and 1 mg in children did not cause side-effects. Single oral doses of ipratropium bromide 30 mg caused anticholinergic side-effects but these were not severe and did not require treatment.

**Pharmaceutical precautions** The vials should be stored at a temperature not exceeding 25°C. Protect from light. The vial should be opened immediately before use and any solution remaining after use should be discarded.

**Legal category** POM

**Package quantities** Packs containing 20 Steri-Nebs in strips of 5.

**Further information** Ipratropium Steri-Neb is an isotonic, sterile, preservative free solution for single use administration.

**Product licence number** 4544/0018

*Product licence holder:* Steripak Limited, Goddard Road, Runcorn, Cheshire WA7 1QE.

## NASOBEC* AQUEOUS

**Qualitative and quantitative composition** Each 100 milligram spray contains 50 micrograms Beclomethasone Dipropionate BP.

**Pharmaceutical form** Nasal spray.

**Clinical particulars**
*Therapeutic indications:* Beclomethasone Dipropionate Aqueous Nasal Spray is indicated for the prophylaxis and treatment of seasonal and perennial allergic rhinitis and vasomotor rhinitis. Beclomethasone Diproprionate BP has anti-inflammatory glucocorticoid properties without significant systemic activity at recommended doses.

*Posology and method of administration:*
*Adults and children over six years old:* Two sprays twice daily into each nostril (400 micrograms beclomethasone dipropionate per day) is the recommended dosage. It may be preferable for some patients to administer a single spray into each nostril three to four times daily.

It should be made clear to patients that full therapeutic benefit will only be achieved after a few days treatment.

*Elderly:* Dosage as for adults.

*Children less than six years old:* Beclomethasone Dipropionate Aqueous Nasal Spray is not indicated for children under six years old, due to insufficient clinical data.

The total dosage for any 24 hour period should not normally exceed eight sprays, i.e. 400 micrograms of beclomethasone dipropionate.

*Contra-indications:* Patients with a history of hypersensitivity to any of its ingredients.

*Special warnings and precautions for use:* Systemic effects rarely occur. These include hypothalamic-pituitary-adrenal (HPA) suppression and growth retardation in children.

Care must be taken while transferring patients from systemic steroid treatment to Beclomethasone Dipropionate Aqueous Nasal Spray where disturbances in the hypothalamic-pituitary-adrenal (HPA) axis could be expected.

Beclomethasone Dipropionate Aqueous Nasal will control seasonal allergic rhinitis in the majority of cases, concomitant therapy to control eye symptoms may be necessary during a heavy challenge to allergens.

*Interactions with other medicaments and other forms of interaction:* None known.

*Pregnancy and lactation:* There is inadequate evidence of safety in human pregnancy. Early studies in animals have demonstrated an increase in foetal cleft palate and growth retardation following maternal ingestion of high corticosteroid doses. However, direct intranasal application at the recommended doses ensures minimal systemic exposure.

*Use during lactation:* It is probable that beclomethasone dipropionate is excreted in milk. However, given the relatively low dose used by the nasal route, the levels are likely to be low. In mothers breast feeding their baby the therapeutic benefits of the drug should be weighed against the potential hazards to mother and baby.

*Effects on ability to drive and use machines:* Beclomethasone Dipropionate Aqueous Nasal Spray does not affect the ability to operate and drive machines.

*Undesirable effects:* In very rare cases septal perforation can develop during therapy.

Dryness and irritation of the nose and throat as well as blood stained crusts in the nose can occur when taking nasal sprays but these conditions are not progressive and are seldom troublesome. An unpleasant smell and taste are rarely reported.

Rare cases of intraocular pressure or glaucoma in association with intranasal formulations of the beclomethasone dipropionate have been reported.

Widespread use of beclomethasone dipropionate for a decade has shown no serious local damage to mucous membranes.

*Overdose:* Suppression of the HPA function is the only harmful effect that would arise from taking large amounts of beclomethasone dipropionate over a short period of time. No emergency procedure need be undertaken and treatment with Beclomethasone Dipropionate Aqueous Nasal Spray should continue at the recommended dose. The HPA function reverts back to normal within a day or two.

**Pharmacological properties**
*Pharmacodynamic properties:* Beclomethasone dipropionate is the diester of beclomethasone, a synthetic glucocorticoid which demonstrates anti-inflammatory and immunosuppressant properties. This drug is stated to exert a topical effect on the lungs without significant systemic activity at recommended doses, although the mechanisms of action are as yet unknown.

*Pharmacokinetic properties:* The pharmacokinetics of beclomethasone dipropionate have not been extensively studied. The currently available chemical methods are not of sufficient sensitivity to measure therapeutically relevant plasma concentrations, particularly those occurring following inhalation.

(a) *General characteristics of the active substance*

*Absorption:* Beclomethasone dipropionate is readily absorbed from the gastro-intestinal tract. It is also well absorbed from sites of local application. When administered by topical application, as in the case of Beclomethasone Dipropionate Aqueous Nasal Spray, sufficient beclomethasone dipropionate may be absorbed to give systemic effects.

*Distribution:* The drug is rapidly distributed to all body tissues. It crosses the placenta and may be excreted in small amounts in breast milk.

*Elimination:* After metabolism in the liver and kidney, the drug is excreted in the urine.

(b) *Characteristics in patients:* As above.

*Preclinical safety data:* See *Contra-indications, Special warnings, Interactions, Pregnancy and lactation, Undesirable effects* and *Overdose* sections above.

**Pharmaceutical particulars**
*List of excipients:* Benzalkonium Chloride Solution BP, Phenylethylalcohol USP, Polysorbate 80 BP, Dextrose Anhydrous BP, Dispersible Cellulose BP, Hydrochloric Acid BP (if necessary – to adjust pH), Purified Water BP.

*Incompatibilities:* None known.

*Shelf life:* 24 months, unopened.

*Special precautions for storage:* Protect from light. Do not refrigerate. Store below 30°C. Discard three months after first using the spray.

*Nature and contents of container:* Beclomethasone Dipropionate Aqueous Nasal Spray is supplied in polyethylene bottles of 30 ml capacity containing a nominal 200 doses. Each bottle is fitted with a metering pump designed to deliver a nominal 100 milligrams of suspension per spray.

*Instructions for use/handling:* No special instructions.

*Marketing authorisation holder:* Norton Healthcare Limited, Harlow, Essex CM19 5TJ.

**Marketing authorisation number** 00530/0492

**Date of approval/revision of SPC** August 1996.

**Legal category** POM.

## PRO-BANTHINE* TABLETS 15 mg

**Qualitative and quantitative composition** Propantheline Bromide BP 15 mg.

**Pharmaceutical form** Tablets.

**Clinical particulars**
*Therapeutic indications:* Adjunctive in GI disorders characterised by smooth muscle spasm.

Hyperhydrosis.
Adult enuresis.

*Posology and method of administration:*
*Adults:* The recommended initial starting dose is one tablet before each meal, and two tablets at bedtime. Subsequently, dosage should be adjusted according to the patient's individual response and tolerance. Doses up to 120 mg may be required in some patients.

*Elderly:* Elderly patients may be more susceptible to anticholinergic side effects; glaucoma and urinary retention may occur. Consideration should be given to the presence of other disease and concomitant drug therapy (see *Contra-indications, warnings*).

*Children:* Safety and efficacy in children have not been established.

*Caution:* Food has been reported to reduce the bioavailability of Pro-banthine. Tablets should be taken at least one hour before meals.

*Route of administration:* Oral.

*Contra-indications:* Pro-banthine is contraindicated in patients with obstructive diseases of the gastrointestinal or urinary tract, pyloric stenosis, intestinal atony, severe ulcerative colitis or toxic megacolon, hiatus hernia associated with reflux oesophagitis, unstable cardiovascular adjustment in acute haemorrhage, myasthenia gravis, glaucoma and in patients who are hypersensitive to propantheline bromide.

*Special warnings and special precautions for use:* In some patients, especially those with ileostomy or colostomy, diarrhoea may be a symptom of incomplete intestinal obstruction. Pro-banthine therapy should be avoided in such patients.

Patients with severe heart disease in whom an increase in heart rate is undesirable should be observed closely if Pro-banthine is administered.

Patients with prostatic hypertrophy may experience some urinary hesitancy. This may be minimised if such patients are advised to micturate at the time the medication is taken.

Patients with ulcerative colitis should be treated with caution, since Pro-banthine may suppress intestinal motility to the point of producing paralytic ileus, thus precipitating or aggravating toxic megacolon.

Pro-banthine should be used with caution in the elderly and all patients with autonomic neuropathy, hepatic or renal disease, hyperthyroidism, coronary heart disease, congestive heart failure, cardiac arrhythmias or hypertension.

*Interaction with other medicaments and other forms of interactions:* Concurrent use of Pro-banthine with slow-dissolving tablets of digoxin may cause increased serum digoxin levels.

Since anticholinergics tend to delay gastric emptying they may alter the absorption of other medication given concomitantly.

Excessive cholinergic blockade may occur if Pro-banthine is given concomitantly with belladonna alkaloids. Synthetic and semi-synthetic anticholinergic agents or other drugs with anticholinergic activity.

The absorption of nitrofurantoin has been reported to be enhanced and that of paracetamol reduced and retarded.

*Pregnancy and lactation:* Animal reproduction and teratology studies have not been performed. Cohort data on parasympatholytics indicate a possible association with minor malformations. In view of this Pro-banthine should not be administered in pregnancy unless considered essential.

It is unknown whether propantheline bromide is excreted in human breast milk. No animal studies have been conducted. In view of this Pro-banthine should not be administered during breast feeding unless considered essential. Suppression of lactation may occur with parasympatholytics.

*Effects on ability to drive and use machines:* Pro-banthine may produce drowsiness or blurred vision. Patients should not drive or operate machinery if affected this way.

*Undesirable effects:* Side-effects of anticholinergics include dryness of the mouth with difficulty in swallowing and thirst, dilatation of the pupils with loss of accommodation and sensitivity to light, increased intra-ocular pressure, flushing, dryness of the skin, decreased sweating, heat stroke, bradycardia followed by tachycardia, palpitations and arrhythmias, urinary hesitancy and retention and constipation.

*Overdose:* Intensification of the usual side effects may occur. In severe intoxication disturbances of the central nervous system may occur resulting in convulsion, coma, circulatory failure, respiratory depression, delirium, hallucinations and restlessness. Toxic doses of propantheline bromide may produce non-depolarising neuromuscular blocking effects with paralysis of voluntary muscle.

In the event of overdosage, empty the stomach and give activated charcoal. Excitement may be controlled by diazepam. Supportive treatment may require oxygen, assisted ventilation and the administration of fluids. In severe cases (convulsions, hyperpyrexia, respiratory depression) the use of intravenous physostigmine (0.5 to 2 mg) should be considered. Since it has a brief duration of action of about 1 to 2 hours, it may be necessary to repeat injections up to a total dose of 5 mg.

**Pharmacological properties**
*Pharmacodynamic properties:* Pro-banthine inhibits parasymptomatic activity by blocking the action of the neurohormone, acetylcholine, on the neuroeffector cell. This blocking action of Pro-banthine is instrumental in reducing gastric acid secretion and gastrointestinal motor activity.

*Pharmacokinetic properties:* Propantheline bromide is extensively metabolised in man. Some enzymic hydrolysis of the drug may occur in the gastrointestinal tract prior to its absorption.

Studies in healthy men demonstrated that peak plasma levels of unchanged drug were reached within 2 hours of a single, oral dose of Propantheline bromide. Following single oral dosing the plasma elimination half-life was about 2–3 hours and some 1–10% of Propantheline bromide was excreted in urine as unchanged drug.

In healthy men studies have shown onset of anticholinergic effects within 1 hour of oral administration. Effects persisted for up to 6 hours after oral dosing.

*Preclinical safety data:* Not applicable.

**Pharmaceutical particulars**
*List of excipients:* Lactose PhEur, corn starch PhEur, talc PhEur, light liquid paraffin BP, magnesium stearate, magnesium carbonate PhEur, castor oil PhEur.

*Coating:* Sucrose PhEur (powdered), sucrose PhEur (granulated), cosmetic red oxide (E171), cosmetic ochre No. 1624 (E172), calcium carbonate PhEur, saccharin sodium BP, titanium dioxide (E171), talc, purified water PhEur, isopropanol BP, beeswax, Carnauba wax, cardice (solid $CO_2$).

*Incompatibilities:* None reported.

*Shelf life:* 5 years.

*Special precautions for storage:* Store below 30°C.

*Nature and contents of container:* HDPE bottles and foil/PVC–PVdC strips of the appropriate size to accommodate 100, 112, 1000 and 5000 tablets.

*Instructions for use/handling:* No special instructions.

*Marketing authorisation holder:* Norton Healthcare Ltd, Gemini House, Harlow, Essex CM19 5TJ.

**Marketing authorisation number** 0530/0376

**Date of approval/revision of SPC** 4 September 1996

## SALAMOL* STERI-NEB* 2.5 mg and 5 mg

**Presentation** Salamol Steri-Nebs 2.5 mg are unit dose polyethylene ampoules containing a sterile, clear, colourless to light yellow aqueous solution of Salbutamol Sulphate BP. Each Steri-Neb contains 2.5 ml of solution equivalent to 2.5 mg salbutamol, i.e. a concentration of 0.1%. The solution is adjusted to a pH of 4.

Salamol Steri-Nebs 5 mg are unit dose polyethylene ampoules containing a sterile, clear, colourless to light yellow aqueous solution of Salbutamol Sulphate BP. Each Steri-Neb contains 2.5 ml of solution equivalent to 5 mg salbutamol, i.e. a concentration of 0.2%. The solution is adjusted to a pH of 4.

**Uses** For use in the routine management of chronic bronchospasm unresponsive to conventional therapy and the treatment of acute severe asthma.

**Dosage and administration**
*Adults:* The usual dose is 2.5 mg given up to three to four times a day by a nebuliser. This may be increased to 5 mg up to three to four times a day if necessary.

In domiciliary practice, however, the benefits of increasing the dose of nebulised salbutamol sulphate should be weighed against the risk that a deterioration in the patient's underlying condition may be masked. In such circumstances a medical assessment should be considered, since alternative therapy may be indicated.

*Children:* The same dosage as for adults.

*Infants:* The clinical efficacy of nebulised salbutamol sulphate in infants under 18 months is uncertain. As transient hypoxaemia may occur, supplemental oxygen therapy should be considered.

*Elderly:* The same dosage as for other adults.

Delivery of the aerosol may be by face mask or 'T' piece.

Salamol Steri-Nebs should be used undiluted. However, if a delivery time in excess of 10 minutes is required, they should be diluted with Sodium Chloride Injection BP or Saline Steri-Neb.

### Contra-indications, warnings, etc

*Contra-indications:* Hypersensitivity to any of the components of Salamol Steri-Nebs.

Although some forms of salbutamol sulphate have been used for the management of premature labour, Salamol Steri-Nebs should not be used for this purpose.

Salamol Steri-Nebs should not be used in threatened abortion.

*Warnings:* The use of nebulised anti-cholinergic agents and nebulised salbutamol sulphate in combination has been reported to precipitate acute angle closure glaucoma. This combination should be used with caution when giving nebuliser therapy to patients with actual or potential glaucoma.

The patient should be warned not to allow the solution or mist to enter the eyes.

*Precautions:* Salamol Steri-Nebs should be used with caution in patients with thyrotoxicosis or in patients known to have received large doses of other sympathomimetic drugs.

Salamol Steri-Nebs are for use with a nebuliser under the direction of a physician. The solution should not be injected or administered orally. Patients who use Salamol Steri-Nebs at home should be warned that if their usual dose is less effective or its duration of action reduced, they should not increase either the dose or frequency of treatment, but should consult their doctor.

Salbutamol and non-selective beta blocking drugs such as propranolol should not usually be prescribed together.

Potentially serious hypokalaemia may result from beta$_2$ agonist therapy. Particular caution is advised in acute severe asthma as this effect may be potentiated by concomitant treatment with xanthine derivatives, steroids, diuretics and by hypoxia. It is recommended that serum potassium levels are monitored in such situations.

*Pregnancy:* Administration of the drug during pregnancy should only be considered if the expected benefit to the mother is greater than any possible risk to the foetus. Salbutamol has been in widespread use for many years in human beings without apparent ill consequence; this includes its well established use in the management of premature labour. However, as with the majority of drugs, there is little published evidence of its safety in the early stages of human pregnancy, but in animal studies there was evidence of some harmful effects on the foetus at very high dose levels.

*Lactation:* As salbutamol is probably secreted in breast milk, its use in nursing mothers requires careful consideration. It is not known whether salbutamol has a harmful effect on the neonate and so its use should be restricted to situations where it is felt that the expected benefit to the mother is likely to outweigh any potential risk to the neonate.

*Side-effects:* A small increase in heart rate may occur in patients who inhale large doses of salbutamol sulphate. This is not usually accompanied by any other changes in the electrocardiogram.

Solutions which are not of neutral pH may rarely cause paradoxical bronchospasm in some patients. As with other inhalation therapy, the potential for paradoxical bronchospasm should be considered. If it occurs, the preparation should be discontinued immediately and alternative therapy given.

Other side-effects which occur with very high doses of salbutamol sulphate by inhalation are peripheral vasodilation and fine tremor of skeletal muscle.

Headaches have been rarely reported. They usually disappear with continued treatment.

There have been rare reports of transient muscle cramps.

Hypersensitivity reactions including angioedema and urticaria, bronchospasm, hypotension and collapse have been reported very rarely. Potentially serious hypokalaemia may result from beta$_2$ agonist therapy.

As with other beta$_2$ agonists, hyperactivity in children has been reported rarely.

*Overdosage:* The most significant symptom of a large overdosage would be a reflex tachycardia. The recommended antidote to overdosage with salbutamol sulphate is a cardioselective beta blocking agent. However, all beta blocking agents should be used with caution in patients with a history of bronchospasm.

### Pharmaceutical precautions

*Storage:* Salamol Steri-Nebs should be stored at a temperature not exceeding 25°C and protected from light.

*Dilution:* Salamol Steri-Nebs may be diluted if required with Sodium Chloride Injection BP or Saline Steri-Neb. Nebuliser solutions should be replaced daily.

### Legal category POM.

### Package quantities Salamol Steri-Nebs 2.5 mg and

5 mg are available in boxes containing 20 Steri-Nebs in 4 strips of 5.

### Further information Nil.

### Product licence numbers
Salamol Steri-Neb 2.5 mg:  4544/0013
Salamol Steri-Neb 5.0 mg:  4544/0017

*Product licence holder:* Steripak Limited, Goddard Road, Astmoor, Runcorn, Cheshire WA7 1QE.

## SALINE STERI-NEB*

**Presentation** Saline Steri-Nebs are unit dose polyethylene ampoules containing a clear, colourless solution of Sodium Chloride PhEur. Each Steri-Neb contains 2.5 ml of a 0.9% w/v solution of sodium chloride.

**Uses** For the dilution of solutions for nebulisation.

### Dosage and administration

*Adults, children and the elderly:* As directed by the physician.

### Contra-indications, warnings, etc
*Contra-indications:* Not for injection.

*Side-effects:* Substantial oral ingestion may require the use of a diuretic to remove excess sodium.

*Precautions:* Do not use unless the product is clear and the pack intact. Discard any surplus after use.

*Use in pregnancy:* As with all medication, particular caution must be exercised during the first trimester of pregnancy.

### Pharmaceutical precautions

*Storage:* Saline Steri-Nebs should be stored between 5°C and 25°C and protected from light. When diluting nebuliser solutions, make up freshly according to the manufacturer's instructions.

### Legal category POM.

### Package quantities Saline Steri-Nebs are available in boxes containing 20 Steri-Nebs in 4 strips of 5.

### Further information Nil.

### Product licence number 4544/0015

*Product licence holder:* Steripak Limited, Goddard Road, Astmoor, Runcorn, Cheshire, WA7 1QE.

## SERENACE* AMPOULES

### Qualitative and quantitative composition
Serenace 5 mg Ampoules: Haloperidol 5 mg.
Serenace 20 mg Ampoules: Haloperidol 20 mg.

**Pharmaceutical form** Solution for intramuscular or intravenous injection.

### Clinical particulars
*Therapeutic indications:* Psychotic disorders – schizophrenia, mania and hypomania, especially paranoid psychoses.

Mental or behavioural problems such as aggression, hyperactivity and self-mutilation in the mentally retarded.

Moderate to severe psychomotor agitation, excitement, violent or dangerously impulsive behaviour.

Gilles de la Tourette syndrome and severe tics.

Restlessness and agitation in the elderly.

*Serenace 5 mg Ampoules:* Nausea and vomiting. Intractable hiccup.

*Posology and method of administration:* There is considerable variation from patient to patient in the response to treatment and the dosage required. As with all antipsychotics, dosage should be individualised according to the needs and response of each patient.

To determine the initial dosage, consideration should be given to the patient's age, severity of symptoms and previous response to other antipsychotic therapy. Oral dosage may be given in single or divided doses. Administration twice daily is sufficient in most cases.

*Adults:* Psychotic behaviour; Mental or behavioural problems; Moderate to severe psychomotor agitation or impulsive behaviour.

*Initial treatment:* For rapid emergency treatment 5 or 10 mg, or infrequently up to 30 mg by intramuscular injection may be required. Depending on the response of the patient, subsequent doses may be given as frequently as every 30 to 60 minutes although 6–12 hourly intervals may be satisfactory. There is a wide variation among individual patients so that cumulative dosage is not predictable in advance. Some patients may have an optimal early response after as little as 10 mg, whereas others may require up to 40 or 50 mg. Higher doses are not usually necessary. Serenace injection may also be administered intravenously.

*Maintenance treatment:* Once a satisfactory therapeutic response has been achieved, dosage should be reduced gradually to the lowest effective maintenance

level which is often as low as 3 to 10 mg daily dependent on the characteristics and response of each individual patient. If possible, maintenance treatment should be oral.

*Gilles de la Tourette syndrome:* Initial dosage is usually 2 mg daily. During the acute phase of treatment, dosage can be increased gradually to obtain maximum control of symptoms and may range between 6 and 50 mg or, exceptionally up to 180 mg daily.

Once a satisfactory therapeutic response has been achieved, dosage should be reduced gradually to the lowest effective maintenance level which for most patients is 4 mg daily.

*Serenace 5 mg Ampoules:*
Nausea and vomiting: 0.5 to 1 mg I.M. daily.
Intractable hiccup: 3 to 15 mg daily in divided doses parenterally has proved useful.

*Elderly:* Half the recommended adult starting dose may be sufficient for therapeutic response in the elderly. The maximum and maintenance dose will generally be lower for debilitated or geriatric patients who may be more sensitive to serenace.

*Children:* Parenteral administration is not recommended for children.

*Route of administration:* By intramuscular or intravenous injection.

*Contra-indications:* Comatose states, patients with Parkinson's disease or a sensitivity to haloperidol and use during lactation.

*Special warnings and precautions for use:* Liver disease, renal failure, phaeochromocytoma, conditions predisposing to epilepsy (e.g. alcohol withdrawal or brain damage). May be given to epileptics, but usual anticonvulsant therapy should be continued.

Use cautiously in thyrotoxic patients and those with arteriosclerosis who may have occult or manifest lesions of the basal ganglia. Such patients may be more prone to develop extrapyramidal symptoms.

Administer with care to patients with severe cardiovascular disorders, because of the possibility of transient hypotension. Should hypotension occur and a vasopressor be required, adrenaline should not be used since haloperidol may block its vasopressor activity and paradoxical further lowering of the blood pressure may occur.

*Interactions with other medicaments and other forms of interaction:* Serenace may potentiate the central nervous system depression produced by other CNS-depressant drugs including alcohol, hypnotics, sedatives or strong analgesics. Enhanced CNS effects (sedation, mental disturbances) have been reported with the combined use of methyldopa and haloperidol. Severe neuromuscular symptoms with impairment of consciousness and fever have been reported with combined use of lithium and haloperidol. A causal relationship has not been established. However, patients receiving such combined therapy should be carefully observed for early evidence of neurological toxicity and treatment should be discontinued if such signs appear.

Serenace may antagonise the action of adrenaline and other sympathomimetic agents.

Possible interactions have been reported between haloperidol and carbamazepine. Haloperidol levels have been shown to be reduced by approximately 50% when carbamazepine is administered concurrently. The psychotic symptoms in some patients have been exacerbated in association with these lowered haloperidol levels but in some instances increased efficacy was seen, possibly as a result of the central action of carbamazepine itself. The mechanism for this interaction is thought to be enzyme induction and increased hepatic metabolism of haloperidol.

*Pregnancy and lactation:* Pregnancy: The safety of serenace in pregnancy has not been established. Reproduction studies in rodents have shown an increased incidence of resorption, reduced fertility and pup mortality. No specific teratogenic effect has been reported in rats, rabbit or dogs, but cleft palate and open eye syndrome have been observed in mice.

No well-controlled studies of haloperidol use in pregnant women have been conducted. Two cases of foetal limb malformation have been reported following maternal use of haloperidol, combined with other drugs during the first trimester. No causal relationship has been established. Use of haloperidol during pregnancy requires that the anticipated benefit be weighed against the possible hazards to mother and foetus.

Lactation: Haloperidol has been detected in breast milk. If use of haloperidol is considered essential, breast feeding should be discontinued.

*Effects on ability to drive and use machines:* Haloperidol may impair alertness, especially at the start of treatment. These effects may be potentiated by alcohol. Patients should be warned of the risks of sedation and advised not to drive or operate machinery during treatment, until their susceptibility is known.

*Undesirable effects:* Extrapyramidal symptoms such as Parkinson-like symptoms, akinesia, akathisia, dyskinesia, dystonia may develop during haloperidol treatment, very rarely dystonia has been reported to produce laryngeal/pharyngeal spasm associated with gagging, respiratory distress and asphyxia.

In common with other antipsychotics haloperidol has been associated with persistent dyskinesia. Tardive dyskinesia may develop in some patients on long term therapy, possibly in relation to total cumulative dose, or may develop after drug therapy has been discontinued. The risk is reported to be greater in elderly patients on high dose therapy. Characteristic symptoms are rhythmical involuntary movements of the tongue, face, mouth or jaw sometimes accompanied by involuntary movements of the extremities. They may persist for many months or even years and, while they gradually disappear in some patients, they appear to be permanent in others.

At the first signs of tardive dyskinesia which may be orofacial dyskinesia the benefit of continued treatment should be carefully assessed against the risk of the development of persistent dyskinesia. Withdrawal of treatment with careful observation of the dyskinesia and psychotic condition has been suggested in order to assess the need for continued neuroleptic therapy and to reveal persisting dyskinesia. Should it be necessary to reinstate treatment, the antipsychotic agent may mask the syndrome. Anti-Parkinsonian agents have proved of little value in this syndrome. In schizophrenia, the response to antipsychotic drug treatment may be delayed. If drugs are withdrawn, recurrence of symptoms may not become apparent for several weeks or months.

Some degree of sedation may occur, particularly with higher doses and at the start of treatment. The elderly appear more susceptible. At low doses in susceptible (especially non-psychotic) individuals, haloperidol may cause unpleasant subjective feelings of being mentally dulled or slowed down, dizziness, headaches or paradoxical effects of excitement, agitation or insomnia.

Other adverse effects reported include gastrointestinal symptoms, nausea, loss of appetite, dyspepsia, autonomic effects such as blurring of vision and, infrequently, tachycardia. Dose-related hypotension is uncommon, but can occur, particularly in the elderly or after parenteral administration. Impairment of sexual function, including erection and ejaculation, oedema; blood dyscrasias, including agranulocytosis and transient leucopenia; skin reactions including exfoliative dermatitis, erythema multiforme and photosensitisation and jaundice, are rarely reported. Transient abnormalities of liver function tests may occur in the absence of jaundice.

Impairment of body temperature could occur at high doses. In common with other antipsychotics, hormonal effects include hyperprolactinaemia which could cause galactorrhoea, gynaecomastia and oligo-or amenorrhoea. Abrupt discontinuation of high doses of antipsychotics has very rarely resulted in acute withdrawal symptoms, including nausea, vomiting and insomnia. Gradual withdrawal is advisable.

Rare cases of sudden and unexplained death have been reported in psychiatric patients receiving treatment with antipsychotics including haloperidol. The nature of the evidence makes it impossible to determine the contributory role, if any, of the drug.

In common with other antipsychotics haloperidol has been associated with rare cases of neuroleptic malignant syndrome, an idiosyncratic response characterised by hyperthermia, muscle rigidity, autonomic instability, altered consciousness and coma. Signs of autonomic dysfunction such as tachycardia, labile arterial pressure and sweating may precede the onset of hyperthermia, acting as early warning signs. Recovery usually occurs within five to seven days of antipsychotic withdrawal. Affected patients should be carefully monitored.

*Overdose:* Intensification of the known pharmacological and adverse effects may occur. The most prominent would be severe extrapyramidal symptoms, hypotension or sedation. The patient may appear comatose with respiratory depression and hypotension which could be severe enough to produce a shock-like state.

Extrapyramidal reactions may include muscular weakness or rigidity and a generalised or localised tremor. With accidental overdosage hypothermia, bradycardia, sinus arrhythmia and hypertension have been reported in young children. No specific antidote has been identified.

In the event of overdosage the stomach should be emptied by aspiration and lavage. Emetics should not be used. Establishment of patent airway and artificial ventilation may be needed. Hypotension may be counteracted by placing the patient in the head-down position and by the use of a plasma expander and careful use of a vasopressor agent such as noradren-

aline. Adrenaline should not be used. Severe extrapyramidal reactions should be treated with parenteral antihistamines or antiparkinsonian drugs. The relatively long plasma elimination half-life of haloperidol should be considered.

### Pharmacological properties

*Pharmacodynamic properties:* Haloperodol is a butyrophenone. Its pharmacological profile of activity includes a pronounced capacity to induce extrapyramidal reactions and a low incidence of autonomic side-effects, such as hypotension.

*Pharmacokinetic properties:* The pharmacokinetics of haloperidol have been studied in healthy volunteers and patients. In volunteers, following a single intravenous or oral dose, serum elimination half-life ranged from 10–19 hours and 12–38 hours respectively. Similar elimination half-lives were observed in patients after administration of a single oral or intramuscular dose of the drug or after withdrawal of the drug from patients who were in a steady state. Steady state serum levels were usually achieved within 6 days on a fixed oral dosage.

*Preclinical safety data:* Not applicable.

### Pharmaceuticl particulars

*List of excipients:* Lactic Acid BP; Sodium Hydroxide BP; Water for Injections PhEur.

*Incompatibilities:* None.

*Shelf life:* 3 years.

*Special precautions for storage:* Store in a dry place below 30°C. Protect from light.

*Nature and contents of container:*
Serenace 5 mg Ampoules: 1 ml printed clear, neutral glass ampoules with a yellow band around the neck constriction, 6 or 10 packed into cardboard cartons.

Serenace 20 mg Ampoules: 2 ml printed, clear, neutral glass ampoules with a yellow band around the neck constriction; 10 packed in cardboard cartons.

*Instructions for use/handling:* No special instructions.

*Marketing authorisation holder:* Norton Healthcare Limited, Gemini House, Flex Meadow, Harlow, Essex CM19 5TJ.

### Marketing authorisation numbers
Serenace 5 mg Ampoules      0530/0368
Serenace 20 mg Ampoules    0530/0369

**Date of approval/revision of SPC**    30 September 1996

**Legal category**    POM

## SERENACE* TABLETS
## SERENACE* LIQUID
## SERENACE* CAPSULUES

### Qualitative and quantitative composition
*Serenace 1.5 mg Tablets:* Haloperidol BP 1.5 mg.
*Serenace 5 mkg Tablets:* Haloperidol BP 5 mg.
*Serenace 10 mg Tablets:* Haloperidol BP 10 mg.
*Serenace 20 mg Tablets:* Haloperidol BP 20 mg.
*Serenace Liquid:* Haloperidol BP 10 mg/5 ml.
*Serenace Capsules:* Haloperidol BP 0.5 mg.

**Pharmaceutical form**    Tablets, hard gelatin capsules or liquid.

### Clinical particulars
*Therapeutic indications:* Psychotic disorders – schizophrenia, mania and hypomania, especially paranoid psychoses.

Mental or behavioural problems such as aggression, hyperactivity and self-mutilation in the mentally retarded.

Moderate to severe psychomotor agitation, excitement, violent or dangerously impulsive behaviour.

Gilles de la Tourette syndrome and severe tics.

Childhood behaviour disorders, especially when associated with hyperactivity and aggression.

Restlessness and agitation in the elderly.

*Serenace 1.5 mg, 5 mg, and 10 mg Tablets and Serenace Liquid 2 mg/ml:* Intractable hiccup.

*Serenace Liquid 2 mg/ml and Serenace 500 mg Capsules:* Nausea and vomiting.

*Serenace 500 mg Capsules:* Adjunct to short-term management of anxiety.

*Posology and method of administration:* There is considerable variation from patient to patient in the response to treatment and the dosage required. As with all antipsychotics, dosage should be individualised according to the needs and response of each patient.

To determine the initial dosage, consideration should be given to the patient's age, severity of symptoms and previous response to other antipsychotic therapy. Oral dosage may be given in single or divided doses. Administration twice daily is sufficient in most cases.

*Adults:* Psychotic behaviour; Mental or behavioural problems; Moderate to severe psychomotor agitation or impulsive behaviour.

*Initial treatment:* Initial dosage may range from as little as 1.5 mg daily to 20 mg daily, dependent on the characteristics, severity of symptoms and response of each individual patient. It may be necessary to increase the dosage gradually to obtain maximum control of symptoms. Severely disturbed or resistant patients may require up to 100 mg daily, or infrequently, up to 200 mg daily.

*Maintenance treatment:* Once a satisfactory therapeutic response has been achieved, dosage should be reduced gradually to the lowest effective maintenance level which is often as low as 3 to 10 mg daily dependent on the characteristics and response of each individual patient.

*Gilles de la Tourette syndrome:* Initial dosage is usually 2 mg daily. During the acute phase of treatment, dosage can be increased gradually to obtain maximum control of symptoms and may range between 6 and 50 mg or, exceptionally up to 180 mg daily.

Once a satisfactory therapeutic response has been achieved, dosage should be reduced gradually to the lowest effective maintenance level which for most patients is 4 mg daily.

*Serenace 1.5 mg, 5 mg, and 10 mg Tablets and Serenace Liquid 2 mg/ml*
*Intractable hiccup:* 3 to 15 mg daily in divided doses, orally has proven useful.

*Serenace Liquid 2 mg/ml and Serenace 500 mg Capsules*
*Nausea and vomiting:* 1 mg daily orally has proved useful.

*Serenace 500 microgram Capsules*
*Anxiety:* 500 micrograms twice daily.

*Elderly:* Half the recommended adult starting dose may be sufficient for therapeutic response in the elderly. The maximum and maintenance dose will generally be lower for debilitated or geriatric patients who may be more sensitive to serenace.

*Children:* (Oral administration): 25 to 50 micrograms per kg body weight per day to a maximum of 10 mg, although, exceptionally, adolescents may require up to 60 mg daily.

*Route of administration:* Oral.

*Contra-indications:* Comatose states, patients with Parkinson's disease or a sensitivity to haloperidol and use during lactation.

*Special warnings and special precautions for use:* Liver disease, renal failure, phaeochromocytoma, conditions predisposing to epilepsy (e.g. alcohol withdrawal or brain damage). May be given to epileptics, but usual anticonvulsant therapy should be continued.

Use cautiously in thyrotoxic patients and those with arteriosclerosis who may have occult or manifest lesions of the basal ganglia. Such patients may be more prone to develop extrapyramidal symptoms.

Administer with care to patients with severe cardiovascular disorders, because of the possibility of transient hypotension. Should hypotension occur and a vasopressor be required, adrenaline should not be used since haloperidol may block its vasopressor activity and further lowering of the blood pressure may occur.

*Interactions with other medicaments and other forms of interaction:* Serenace may potentiate the central nervous system depression produced by other CNS-depressant drugs including alcohol, hypnotics, sedatives or strong analgesics. Enhanced CNS effects (sedation, mental disturbances) have been reported with the combined use of methyldopa and haloperidol. Severe neuromuscular symptoms with impairment of consciousness and fever have been reported with combined use of lithium and haloperidol. A causal relationship has not been established. However, patients receiving such combined therapy should be carefully observed for early evidence of neurological toxicity and treatment should be discontinued if such signs appear.

Serenace may antagonise the action of adrenaline and other sympathomimetic agents.

Possible interactions have been reported between haloperidol and carbamazepine. Haloperidol levels have been shown to be reduced by approximately 50% when carbamazepine is administered concurrently. The psychotic symptoms in some patients have been exacerbated in association with these lowered haloperidol levels but in some instances increased efficacy was seen, possibly as a result of the central action of carbamazepine itself. The mechanism for this interaction is thought to be enzyme induction and increased hepatic metabolism of haloperidol.

*Pregnancy and lactation:* Pregnancy: The safety of Serenace in pregnancy has not been established. Reproduction studies in rodents have shown an increased incidence of resorption, reduced fertility and pup mortality. No specific teratogenic effect has been reported in rats, rabbit or dogs, but cleft palate and open eye syndrome have been observed in mice.

No well-controlled studies of haloperidol use in pregnant women have been conducted. Two cases of foetal limb malformation have been reported following maternal use of haloperidol, combined with other drugs during the first trimester. No causal relationship has been established. Use of haloperidol during pregnancy requires that the anticipated benefit be weighed against the possible hazards to mother and foetus.

Lactation: Haloperidol has been detected in breast milk. If use of haloperidol is considered essential, breast feeding should be discontinued.

*Effects on ability to drive and use machines:* Haloperidol may impair alertness, especially at the start of treatment. These effects may be potentiated by alcohol. Patients should be warned of the risks of sedation and advised not to drive or operate machinery during treatment, until their susceptibility is known.

*Undesirable effects:* Extrapyramidal symptoms such as Parkinson-like symptoms, akinesia, akathisia, dyskinesia, dystonia may develop during haloperidol treatment, very rarely dystonia has been reported to produce laryngeal/pharyngeal spasm associated with gagging, respiratory distress and asphyxia.

In common with other antipsychotics haloperidol has been associated with persistent dyskinesia. Tardive dyskinesia may develop in some patients on long term therapy, possibly in relation to total cumulative dose, or may develop after drug therapy has been discontinued. The risk is reported to be greater in elderly patients on high dose therapy. Characteristic symptoms are rhythmical involuntary movements of the tongue, face, mouth or jaw sometimes accompanied by involuntary movements of the extremities. They may persist for many months or even years and, while they gradually disappear in some patients, they appear to be permanent in others.

At the first signs of tardive dyskinesia which may be orofacial dyskinesia the benefit of continued treatment should be carefully assessed against the risk of the development of persistent dyskinesia. Withdrawal of treatment with careful observation of the dyskinesia and psychotic condition has been suggested in order to assess the need for continued neuroleptic therapy and to reveal persisting dyskinesia. Should it be necessary to reinstate treatment, the antipsychotic agent may mask the syndrome. Anti-Parkinsonian agents have proved of little value in this syndrome. In schizophrenia, the response to antipsychotic drug treatment may be delayed. If drugs are withdrawn, recurrence of symptoms may not become apparent for several weeks or months.

Some degree of sedation may occur, particularly with higher doses and at the start of treatment. The elderly appear more susceptible. At low doses in susceptible (especially non-psychotic) individuals, haloperidol may cause unpleasant subjective feelings of being mentally dulled or slowed down, dizziness, headaches or paradoxical effects of excitement, agitation or insomnia.

Other adverse effects reported include gastrointestinal symptoms, nausea, loss of appetite, dyspepsia, autonomic effects such as blurring of vision and, infrequently, tachycardia. Dose-related hypotension is uncommon, but can occur, particularly in the elderly or after parenteral administration. Impairment of sexual function, including erection and ejaculation, oedema; blood dyscrasias, including agranulocytosis and transient leucopenia; skin reactions including exfoliative dermatitis, erythema multiforme and photosensitisation and jaundice, are rarely reported. Transient abnormalities of liver function tests may occur in the absence of jaundice.

Impairment of body temperature could occur at high doses. In common with other antipsychotics, hormonal effects include hyperprolactinaemia which could cause galactorrhoea, gynaecomastia and oligo- or amenorrhoea. Abrupt discontinuation of high doses of antipsychotics has very rarely resulted in acute withdrawal symptoms, including nausea, vomiting and insomnia. Gradual withdrawal is advisable.

Rare cases of sudden and unexplained death have been reported in psychiatric patients receiving treatment with antipsychotics including haloperidol. The nature of the evidence makes it impossible to determine the contributory role, if any, of the drug.

In common with other antipsychotics haloperidol has been associated with rare cases of neuroleptic malignant syndrome, an idiosyncratic response characterised by hyperthermia, muscle rigidity, autonomic instability, altered consciousness and coma. Signs of autonomic dysfunction such as tachycardia, labile arterial pressure and sweating may precede the onset of hyperthermia, acting as early warning signs. Recovery usually occurs within five to seven days of antipsychotic withdrawal. Affected patients should be carefully monitored.

*Overdose:* Intensification of the known pharmacological and adverse effects may occur. The most prominent would be severe extrapyramidal symptoms, hypotension or sedation. The patient may appear comatosed with respiratory depression and hypotension which could be severe enough to produce a shock-like state.

Extrapyramidal reactions may include muscular weakness or rigidity and a generalised or localised tremor. With accidental overdosage hypothermia, bradycardia, sinus arrhythmia and hypertension have been reported in young children. No specific antidote has been identified.

In the event of overdosage the stomach should be emptied by aspiration and lavage. Emetics should not be used. Establishment of patent airway and artificial ventilation may be needed. Hypotension may be counteracted by placing the patient in the head-down position and by the use of a plasma expander and careful use of a vasopressor agent such as noradrenaline. Adrenaline should not be used. Severe extrapyramidal reactions should be treated with parenteral antihistamines or antiparkinsonian drugs. The relatively long plasma elimination half-life of haloperidol should be considered.

**Pharmacological properties**

*Pharmacodynamic properties:* Haloperodol is a butyrophenone. Its pharmacological profile of activity includes a pronounced capacity to induce extrapyramidal reactions and a low incidence of autonomic side-effects, such as hypotension.

*Pharmacokinetic properties:* The pharmacokinetics of haloperidol have been studied in healthy volunteers and patients. In volunteers, following a single intravenous or oral dose, serum elimination half-life ranged from 10–19 hours and 12–38 hours respectively. Similar elimination half-lives were observed in patients after administration of a single oral or intramuscular dose of the drug or after withdrawal of the drug from patients who were in a steady state. Steady state serum levels were usually achieved within 6 days on a fixed oral dosage.

*Preclinical safety data:* Not applicable.

**Pharmaceutical particulars**

*List of excipients: Serenace Tablets:* Lactose PhEur; Corn Starch PhEur; Pregelatinised Maize Starch BP; Magnesium Stearate PhEur.

*Serenace 5 mg and 10 mg Tablets Additional Excipient:* FD&C Red No. 3 Lake (E127).

*Serenace 20 mg Tablet Additional Excipient:* Anstead Dispersed Red 11652 (E124).

*Serenace Liquid:* Polypropylene Glycol BP; Methyl Hydroxybenzoate BP; Propyl Hydroxybenzoate BP; Lactic Acid BP; Purified Water BP.

*Serenace Capsule:* Lactose PhEur; Corn Starch PhEur. *Hard Gelatin Shell:* Tartrazine (E102); Patent Blue V (E131); Titanium Dioxide (E171).

*Incompatibilities:* None.

*Shelf life:*
*Serenace 1.5 mg and 5 mg Tablets:* 5 years.

*Serenace 10 mg and 20 mg Tablets:* 5 years. 3 years in blister packs.

*Serenace Liquid:* 3 years.

*Serenace Capsules:* 5 years.

*Special precautions for storage:*
*Serenace Tablets and Capsules:* Store in a dry place below 30°C.

*Serenace Liquid:* Store between 15 and 25°C. Protect from light.

*Nature and contents of container:*
*Serenace Tablets:* High density polyethylene bottles with tamper-evident snap closure, or amber glass bottles with metal screw cap in pack sizes of 7, 14, 21, 28, 30, 50, 56, 60, 84, 90, 100, 112, 120, 250, 1000 and 5000 tablets. PVC/Aluminium blisters, or PVdC coated PVC/Aluminium blisters in pack sizes of 7, 14, 21, 28, 30, 50, 56, 60, 84, 90, 100, 112 and 120 tablets.

*Serenace Liquid:* Amber glass bottles with ROPP closures containing 100 ml or 500 ml.

*Serenace Capsules:* Ward pack sizes of 50.

High density polyethylene bottles with tamper-evident snap closure, or amber glass bottles with metal screw cap in pack sizes of 7, 14, 21, 28, 30, 50, 56, 60, 84, 90, 100, 112, 120, 250, 1000 and 5000.

PVC/Aluminium blisters, or PVdC coated PVC/Aluminium blisters in pack sizes of 7, 14, 21, 28, 30, 50, 56, 60, 84, 90, 100, 112 and 120.

*Instructions for use/handling:* No special instructions.

*Marketing authorisation holder:* Norton Healthcare Limited, Gemini House, Flex Meadow, Harlow, Essex CM19 5TJ.

**Marketing authorisation numbers**

| | |
|---|---|
| Serenace 1.5 mg Tablet | 0530/0370 |
| Serenace 5 mg Tablet | 0530/0371 |
| Serenace 10 mg Tablet | 0530/0372 |
| Serenace 20 mg Tablet | 0530/0373 |
| Serenace Liquid 2 mg/ml | 0530/0374 |
| Serenace 500 micrograms Capsules | 0530/0375 |

**Date of approval/revision of SPC** February 1997

**Legal category** POM

## TEMAZEPAM 10 mg TABLETS TEMAZEPAM 20 mg TABLETS

**Presentation** Temazepam 10 mg and 20 mg tablets are white, flat bevel-edged tablets containing 10 mg and 20 mg temazepam. The 10 mg tablets are embossed 'TMZ 10' with a breakline on one side and a twin triangle logo on the reverse. The 20 mg tablets are embossed 'TMZ 20' with a breakline on one side and a twin triangle logo on the reverse.

**Uses** Temazepam is a benzodiazepine; it has anxiolytic, sedative and hypnotic characteristics as well as possible muscle relaxant and anticonvulsant characteristics.

1. As an hypnotic for the short-term management of insomnia only when it is severe, disabling or subjecting the individual to extreme distress.

2. For pre-medication prior to minor surgery or other related procedures.

**Dosage and administration** Treatment should be as short as possible. Generally the duration of treatment varies from a few days to two weeks with a maximum (including tapering off) of four weeks. The tapering off process should be tailored to the individual. In certain cases, extension beyond the maximum treatment period may be necessary; if so, it should not take place without re-evaluation of the patient's status. The product should be taken on retiring or up to 30 minutes before going to bed.

*Insomnia: Adults:* 10–20 mg. In exceptional circumstances, the dose may be increased to 30–40 mg.

*Elderly:* 10 mg. In exceptional circumstances, the dose may be increased to 20 mg.

*Premedication:* The usual dose is 20–40 mg 30–60 minutes before the procedure.

*Children:* Not recommended for use in children.

Treatment should be started with the lowest recommended dose. The maximum dose should not be exceeded. Patients with impaired liver or kidney function should have a reduced dose.

A lower dose is also recommended for patients with chronic respiratory insufficiency due to the risk of respiratory depression.

**Contra-indications, warnings, etc**

*Contra-indications:* Myasthenia gravis; hypersensitivity to benzodiazepines; severe respiratory insufficiency; sleep apnoea syndrome; children; severe hepatic insufficiency.

*Precautions and warnings:* An underlying cause for insomnia should be sought before deciding on the use of benzodiazepines for symptomatic relief.

Some loss of efficacy to the hypnotic effects of short-acting benzodiazepines may develop after repeated use for a few weeks.

The duration of treatment should be as short as possible. Treatment should not exceed 4 weeks, including the tapering off process. Extension beyond this period should not take place without re-evaluation of the situation. It may be useful to inform the patient when treatment is started that it will be of limited duration and to explain precisely how the dosage will be progressively decreased. Moreover, it is important that the patient should be aware of the possibility of rebound phenomena, thereby minimising anxiety over such symptoms should they occur while the medicinal product is being discontinued. There are indications that, in the case of benzodiazepines with a short duration of action, withdrawal phenomena can become manifest within the dosage interval, especially when the dosage is high.

Benzodiazepines may induce anterograde amnesia. The condition occurs most often several hours after ingesting the product, and therefore to reduce the risk, patients should ensure that they will be able to have an uninterrupted sleep of 7–8 hours.

Benzodiazepines are not indicated to treat patients with severe hepatic insufficiency as it may precipitate encephalopathy. Benzodiazepines are not recommended for the primary treatment of psychotic illness.

Benzodiazepines should not be used alone to treat depression or anxiety associated with depression (suicide may be precipitated in such patients).

Benzodiazepines should also be used with extreme caution in patients with a history of alcohol or drug abuse.

Sedation, amnesia, impaired concentration and impaired muscular function may adversely affect the ability to drive or to use machines. If insufficient sleep duration occurs, the likelihood of impaired alertness may be increased.

After medication with temazepam for surgical or

other procedures, patients should be accompanied home afterwards.

*Special precautions:* Use of benzodiazepines may lead to the development of physical and psychic dependence upon these products. The risk of dependence increases with dose and duration of treatment; it is also greater in patients with a history of alcohol or drug abuse or marked personality disorders.

Once physical dependence has developed, abrupt termination of treatment will be accompanied by withdrawal symptoms. These may consist of headaches, muscle pain, extreme anxiety, tension, restlessness, confusion and irritability. In severe cases the following symptoms may occur: derealisation; depersonalisation; hyperacusis; numbness and tingling of the extremities; hypersensitivity to light, noise and physical contact; hallucinations or epileptic seizures.

'Rebound insomnia' a transient syndrome whereby the symptoms that led to treatment with a benzodiazepine recur in an enhanced form, may occur on withdrawal of hypnotic treatment. It may be accompanied by other reactions, including mood changes, anxiety and restlessness.

Since the risk of withdrawal phenomena/rebound phenomena is greater after abrupt discontinuation of treatment, it is recommended that the dosage is decreased gradually.

*Use in pregnancy and lactation:* Insufficient data are available on temazepam to assess its safety during pregnancy and lactation. Therefore temazepam is not recommended for administration during pregnancy and lactation. If the product is prescribed to a woman of childbearing potential, she should be warned to contact her physician regarding stopping the product if she intends to become or suspects that she is pregnant.

If, for compelling medical reasons, temazepam is administered during the late phase of pregnancy, or during labour, effects on the neonate, such as hypothermia, hypotonia and moderate respiratory depression, can be expected due to the pharmacological action of the product.

Moreover, infants born to mothers who took benzodiazepines chronically during the latter stages of pregnancy may have developed physical dependence and may be at some risk of developing withdrawal symptoms in the postnatal period.

Since benzodiazepines are found in the breast milk, temazepam should not be administered to breast-feeding mothers.

*Effects on ability to drive and use machines:* Sedation, amnesia and impaired muscular function may adversely affect the ability to drive or operate machinery.

*Side-effects:* Side-effects include the following: Drowsiness during the day, numbed emotions, reduced alertness, confusion, fatigue, headache, dizziness, muscle weakness, ataxia, or double vision. These phenomena occur predominantly at the start of the therapy and usually disappear with repeated administration. However, sedation, amnesia and impaired muscular function may adversely affect the ability to drive or use machines. Other side effects like gastrointestinal disturbances, changes in libido, skin reactions, vivid dreams/nightmares, dry mouth, restless sleep and palpitations have been reported occasionally.

Anterograde amnesia may occur using therapeutic dosages, the risk increasing at higher dosages. Amnesia may be associated with inappropriate behaviour.

Pre-existing depression may be unmasked during benzodiazepine use.

Reactions like restlessness, agitation, irritability, aggressiveness, delusion, rages, nightmares, hallucinations, psychoses, inappropriate behaviour and other adverse behavioural effects are known to occur with use of benzodiazepines. These reactions are more likely to occur in the elderly. Should this occur, use of the product should be discontinued.

On rare occasions, visual disturbances, urinary retention, blood dyscrasias, increased liver enzymes and jaundice have been reported with some benzodiazepines. If any of these occur, use of the product should be discontinued.

*Interactions:* Not recommended: Concomitant intake with alcohol. The sedative effect may be enhanced when the product is used in combination with alcohol. This affects the ability to drive or use machines.

Take into account: Combination with CNS depressants. Enhancement of the central depressive effect may occur in cases in concomitant use with antipsychotics (neuroleptics), hypnotics, anxiolytics/sedatives, antidepressant agents, narcotic analgesics, antiepileptic drugs, anaesthetics and sedative antihistamines. In the case of narcotic analgesics, enhancement of euphoria may also occur leading to an increase in dependence.

*Overdosage:* As with other benzodiazepines, overdose should not present a threat to life unless combined with other CNS depressants (including alcohol). In the

management of overdose with any medicinal product, it should be borne in mind that multiple agents may have been taken. Following overdose with oral benzodiazepines, vomiting should be induced (within one hour) if the patient is conscious or gastric lavage undertaken with the airway protected if the patient is unconscious. If there is no advantage in emptying the stomach, activated charcoal should be given to reduce absorption. The value of dialysis has not been determined for temazepam.

3-hydroxy benzodiazepines are, as a rule, not dialysable and their metabolites (glucuronides) only dialysable with difficulty. Special attention should be paid to respiratory and cardiovascular functions in intensive care. Overdose of benzodiazepines is usually manifested by degrees of central nervous system depression ranging from drowsiness to coma. In mild cases, symptoms include drowsiness, mental confusion and lethargy. In more serious cases symptoms may include ataxia, hypotonia, hypotension, respiratory depression, rarely coma and very rarely death. Flumazenil may be useful as an antidote.

**Pharmaceutical precautions**    Store in a dry place below 25°C. Protect from light.

**Legal category**    POM

**Package quantities**    10 mg: Containers of 30, 100, 250, 500 and 1000 tablets and 5000 tablets.
20 mg: Containers of 30, 100, 250, 500 and 1000 tablets and 5000 tablets.

**Further information**    The risk of benzodiazepine related dependence may be minimised by adopting the following guidelines for treatment:

  (1) Select patients carefully taking into account the precautions and warnings stated in this data sheet.

  (2) Adopt short-term or intermittent therapy.

  (3) Use lowest dose possible to achieve effective treatment.

  (4) Review treatment regularly; and especially before repeating prescriptions.

  (5) Discontinue treatment gradually taking into account patient reaction at each stage, i.e. 'titrate downwards'.

**Product licence numbers**
10 mg: 0530/0255
20 mg: 0530/0256

*Product licence holder:* Norton Healthcare Limited, Harlow, Essex CM19 5TR.

# TRIAM-CO* TABLETS

**Qualitative and quantitative composition**    Each tablet contains Triamterene BP 50 mg and Hydrochlorothiazide BP 25 mg.

**Pharmaceutical form**    Peach-yellow FBE tablets.

**Clinical particulars**
*Therapeutic indications:* Anti-hypertensive and diuretic with potassium conserving properties indicated in patients for the control of oedema in cardiac failure, cirrhosis of the liver or the nephrotic syndrome and in drug-induced and premenstrual oedema. Triam-co may be used in the treatment of mild to moderate hypertension, alone or in combination with other anti-hypertensive drugs.

*Posology and method of administration:*
*Adults and elderly:* Triam-co should be administered to adults only. However in the case of elderly patients the normally occurring reduction in glomerular filtration with age should be considered when prescribing Triam-co.

*Hypertension:* Starting with 1 tablet a day following the morning meal and thereafter adjusting to the patient's needs but not exceeding 4 tablets. When Triam-co is used in addition to another anti-hypertensive drug the dosage of the latter should be reduced and adjusted if necessary. However, the addition of another anti-hypertensive drug to Triam-co therapy will not normally require reduction of the Triam-co dosage.

*Oedema:* Starting dose: 1 tablet twice a day after meals. The maximum dosage may be 3 tablets a day, 2 after breakfast and 1 after lunch. Adverse reactions have been reported on a dosage of 4 tablets daily therefore this dosage level should not be exceeded.

  Maintenance dose: Dosage should be reduced to one tablet daily or 2 tablets on alternate days as soon as diuresis has been established.

*Children:* Not recommended.

*Route of administration:* Oral.

*Contra-indications:* Triam-co should not be given to patients with hyperkalaemia. Progressive renal or hepatic dysfunction, hypercalcaemia, Addison's disease, diabetic ketoacidosis, or known hypersensitivity to the product's constituents. The use of potassium supplements or other potassium-conserving drugs with Triam-co is not recommended.

*Special warnings and special precautions for use:* Triam-co should be used with caution in patients with hepatic or renal insufficiency. As both triamterene and hydrochlorothiazide can elevate uric acid levels Triam-co should be used with caution in patients who may suffer from gout.

Thiazides may provoke hyperglycaemia and glycosuria and should be prescribed with caution in diabetic patients. Patients with diabetic nephropathy should be treated with care due to possible hyperkalaemia; concomitant sulphonylurea dosage may need increasing. Pancreatitis may be aggravated by Triam-co.

Serum potassium levels, blood urea and electrolytes should be monitored periodically. This is important in the elderly, or renally impaired patients and those receiving concomitant treatment with NSAIDs.

Triam-co may interfere with laboratory tests for thyroid and parathyroid function, and folic acid biossay.

*Interaction with other medicaments and other forms of interaction:* Care should be taken in patients being treated with lithium as reduction in lithium excretion can occur with resultant toxicity. There have been occasional reports of decreased renal function when triamterene has been administered with indomethacin. Triam-co may reduce arterial responsiveness to noradrenaline and may enhance the responsiveness to tubocurarine.

The action of other anti-hypertensive agents is potentiated and a reduced dosage may be necessary at the introduction of Triam-co. The concurrent use of potassium supplements or potassium conserving drugs may cause hyperkalaemia.

Due to the risk of excess potassium loss, care should be taken when Triam-co is taken in conjunction with corticosteroids; also with cardiac glycosides and antiarrhythmic drugs whose toxicity may be enhanced by hypokalaemia.

Carbenoxolone may antagonise the diuretic action of Triam-co and cholestyramine may delay or reduce its absorption.

Concomitant folate antagonists are inadvisable in pregnant women or patients with hepatic cirrhosis because of the risk of folate deficiency.

*Pregnancy and lactation:* Animal studies have indicated that triamterene crosses the placental barrier and is excreted in breast milk.

In humans, hydrochlorothiazide crosses the placental barrier, and appears in milk.

There are no signifciant reports citing foetal abnormalities when using the combination of triamterene and hydrochlorothiazide; however in isolated instances new-born infants of mothers treated with thiazides have been found to be suffering from thrombocytopenia, pancreatitis or hypoglycaemia. The use of Triam-co in pregnant women or nursing mothers should therefore be avoided unless considered essential.

*Effects on ability to drive and use machines:* Patients should be warned that dizziness may occur and therefore should take care when driving or operating machines.

*Undesirable effects:* Nausea, vomiting, diarrhoea, muscle cramps, weakness, headache, dry mouth, undesirable decreases in blood pressure and rash have been reported. Photosensitivity is rare. Renal failure, reversed on stopping treatment, has been reported very rarely. Anaphylaxis is a possibility.

Consideration should be given to the possibility of minor serum electrolyte changes, metabolic acidosis and fluctuation in serum potassium levels. Large doses may induce electrolyte imbalance although this imbalance could be secondary to the condition being treated. Hyperglycaemia, hyperlipidaemia, raised uric acid levels and hypercalcaemia have been reported. Reduction of glomerular filtration rate causing a temporary increase in blood urea and creatinine levels may occur with Triam-co.

Reports of rare cases of thrombocytopenic purpura and megaloblastic anaemia when using triamterene have appeared in the literature as have reports of thiazides causing jaundice, acute pancreatitis and blood dyscrasias including agranulocytosis, thrombocytopenia and leucopenia. Systemic lupus erythematosus has been very rarely reported with this diuretic combination. Triamterene, under certain light conditions, has been known to cause a blue fluorescence in the urine.

*Overdose:* Symptoms of electrolyte imbalance, especially hyperkalaemia, are likely. These include gastrointestinal disturbance, weakness, lassitude, hypotension and cardiac arrhythmias. Treatment consists of gastric lavage with correction of electrolyte imbalance and fluid depletion. Cardiac monitoring is advised as are appropriate measures to correct hyperkalaemia as necessary. There is no specific antidote; however, if hypotension persists after adequate fluid replacement dopamine may be used. In cases of severe overdosage renal dialysis may be of some benefit.

## Pharmaceutical properties

*Pharmacodynamic properties:* Triam-co is a combination of a thiazide diuretic, hydrochlorothiazide, and a potassium sparing diuretic, triamterene.

Hydrochlorothiazide acts on the distal convuleted tubule of the kidney and diuresis is initiated in about two hours and lasts up to twelve hours.

Triamterene causes potassium retention and is used in this particular combination as an alteranative to giving potassium supplements.

*Pharmacokinetic properties:* Hydrochlorothiazide is incompletely but fairly rapidly absorbed from the gastro-intestinal tract. It has been estimated to have a half-life of about 3 to 4 hours with a subsequent longer terminal phase; its biological half-life is up to about 12 hours. It appears to be preferentially bound to red blood cells. It is excreted unchanged in the urine. Hydrochlorothiazide crosses the placental barrier and is excreted in breast milk.

Triamterene is incompletely but fairly rapidly absorbed from the gastro-intestinal tract. It has been estimated to have half-life of about 2 hours. It is extensively metabolised and is mainly excreted in the urine in the form of metabolites with some unchanged triamterene; variable amounts are also excreted in the bile. Animal studies have indicated that triamterene crosses the placental barrier and is excreted in breast milk.

*Preclinical safety data:* Not applicable.

## Pharmaceutical particulars

*List of excipients:* Avicel PH 101 (E460) NF, Explotab NF, Sodium Lauryl Sulphate NF, Cab-O-Sil NF, Magnesium Stearate NF, F.D. & C. Yellow No. 6 (E110).

*Incompatibilities:* None known.

*Shelf life:* 5 years.

*Special precautions for storage:* Store in a cool dry place.

*Nature and contents of container:* Polypropylene tubular container with an open end equipped to accept a polyethylene closure, with tamper-evident tear strip.

Tampertainers – 250 m opaque UPVC/20 μ, hard temper aluminium foil.

Duma Container – PVdC coated PVC/Aluminium blisters (60 g/m² PVdC on 250 mm PVC/20 mm A1).

Of the appropriate size to accommodate 7, 14, 21, 28, 30, 50, 56, 60, 84, 90, 100, 112, 120, 250, 500 or 1000 tablets.

*Instructions for use/handling:* No special instructions.

*Marketing authorisation holder:* Norton Healthcare Ltd, Gemini House, Harlow, Essex CM19 5TJ.

**Marketing authorisation number** 0530/0177

**Date of approval/revision of SPC** 2 December 1996

*\*Trade Mark*

# Bayer plc
## Pharmaceutical Division
Bayer House
Strawberry Hill
Newbury, Berkshire, RG14 1JA

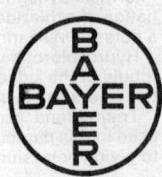

## ADALAT*
## ADALAT* 5

**Presentation** *Adalat capsules:* Orange, soft gelatin ovoid capsules containing a yellow viscous fluid. Each capsule is overprinted with 'ADALAT' and the Bayer cross and contains 10 mg nifedipine.

*Adalat 5 capsules:* Orange, soft gelatin ovoid capsules containing a yellow viscous fluid. Each capsule is overprinted with 'ADALAT 5' and the Bayer cross and contains 5 mg nifedipine.

### Uses

*Mode of action:* As a specific and potent calcium antagonist, the main action of Adalat is to relax arterial smooth muscle both in the coronary and peripheral circulation.

In angina pectoris, Adalat capsules relax peripheral arteries so reducing the load on the left ventricle. Additionally, Adalat dilates submaximally both clear and pre-stenotic, stenotic and post-stenotic coronary arteries, thus protecting the heart against coronary artery spasm and improving perfusion to the ischaemic myocardium.

Adalat capsules reduce the frequency of painful attacks and ischaemic ECG changes, irrespective of the relative contribution from coronary artery spasm or atherosclerosis.

Adalat causes a reduction in blood pressure such that the percentage lowering is directly related to its initial level. In normotensive individuals, Adalat has little or no effect on blood pressure.

*Indications:* For the prophylaxis of chronic stable angina pectoris, the treatment of Raynaud's phenomenon and hypertension.

### Dosage and administration
The capsules should be taken orally with a little water. The recommended starting dose is 5 mg every eight hours with subsequent titration of dose according to response. The dose can be increased to 20 mg every eight hours.

The pharmacokinetics of nifedipine are altered in the elderly so that lower maintenance doses of nifedipine may be required compared to younger patients.

Nifedipine is metabolised primarily by the liver and therefore patients with liver dysfunction should be carefully monitored.

Patients with renal impairment should not require adjustment of dosage.

Treatment may be continued indefinitely.

Nifedipine is not recommended for use in children.

### Contra-indications, warnings, etc
*Contra-indications:* Adalat should not be administered to patients with known hypersensitivity to nifedipine or other dihydropyridines because of the theoretical risk of cross-reactivity.

Adalat should not be administered to women capable of child-bearing or to nursing mothers.

Adalat should not be used in cardiogenic shock, clinically significant aortic stenosis, unstable angina, or during or within one month of a myocardial infarction.

Adalat should not be used for the treatment of acute attacks of angina.

The safety of Adalat in malignant hypertension has not been established.

Adalat should not be used for secondary prevention of myocardial infarction.

Adalat should not be administered concomitantly with rifampicin since effective plasma levels of nifedipine may not be achieved owing to enzyme induction.

*Warnings and precautions:* Adalat may be used in combination with beta-blocking drugs and other antihypertensive agents but the possibility of an additive effect resulting in postural hypotension should be borne in mind. Adalat will not prevent possible rebound effects after cessation of other antihypertensive therapy.

Adalat should be used with caution in patients whose cardiac reserve is poor. Deterioration of heart failure has occasionally been observed with nifedipine.

At doses higher than those recommended, there is some concern about increased mortality and morbid-

ity in the treatment of ischaemic heart disease, in particular after myocardial infarction.

Treatment with short-acting nifedipine may induce an exaggerated fall in blood pressure and reflex tachycardia which can cause cardiovascular complications such as myocardial and cerebrovascular ischaemia.

Caution should be exercised in patients with severe hypotension.

Ischaemic pain has been reported in a small proportion of patients within 30 to 60 minutes of the introduction of Adalat therapy. Although a 'steal' effect has not been demonstrated, patients experiencing this effect should discontinue Adalat.

Diabetic patients taking Adalat may require adjustment of their control.

In dialysis patients with malignant hypertension and hypovolaemia, a marked decrease in blood pressure can occur.

*Interactions:* The antihypertensive effect of Adalat may be potentiated by simultaneous administration of cimetidine.

When used in combination with nifedipine, serum quinidine levels have been shown to be suppressed regardless of dosage of quinidine.

The simultaneous administration of nifedipine and digoxin may lead to reduced digoxin clearance and hence an increase in the plasma digoxin level. Plasma digoxin levels should be monitored and, if necessary, the digoxin dose reduced.

Diltiazem decreases the clearance of nifedipine and hence increases plasma nifedipine levels. Therefore, caution should be taken when both drugs are used in combination and a reduction of the nifedipine dose may be necessary.

Nifedipine may increase the spectrophotometric values of urinary vanillylmandelic acid falsely. However, HPLC measurements are unaffected.

Adalat should not be administered concomitantly with rifampicin since effective plasma levels of nifedipine may not be achieved owing to enzyme induction.

As with other dihydropyridines, nifedipine should not be taken with grapefruit juice because bioavailability is increased.

*Side-effects:* Most side-effects are consequences of the vasodilatory effects of nifedipine. Headache, flushing, tachycardia and palpitations may occur, most commonly in the early stages of treatment with nifedipine. Gravitational oedema, not associated with heart failure or weight gain, may also occur.

Paraesthesia, dizziness, lethargy and gastro-intestinal symptoms such as nausea and altered bowel habit may occur occasionally.

There are reports of skin reactions such as rash, pruritus and urticaria.

Other less frequently reported side-effects include myalgia, tremor and visual disturbances. Impotence may occur rarely.

Increased frequency of micturition may occur.

As with the use of other short-acting dihydropyridines in patients with ischaemic heart disease, exacerbation of angina pectoris may occur frequently at the start of treatment with nifedipine capsules. The occurrence of myocardial infarction has been described although it is not possible to distinguish such an event from the natural course of ischaemic heart disease.

There are reports of gingival hyperplasia and, in older men on long-term therapy, gynaecomastia, which usually regress upon withdrawal of therapy.

Mood changes may occur rarely.

Side-effects which may occur in isolated cases are photosensitivity, exfoliative dermatitis, systemic allergic reactions and purpura. Usually, these regress after discontinuation of the drug.

Rare cases of hypersensitivity-type jaundice have been reported. In addition, disturbances of liver function such as intra-hepatic cholestasis may occur. These regress after discontinuation of therapy.

*Overdosage: Clinical effects:* Reports of nifedipine overdosage are limited and symptoms are not necessarily dose-related. Severe hypotension due to vasodilatation, and tachycardia or bradycardia are the most likely manifestations of overdose.

Metabolic disturbances include hyperglycaemia, metabolic acidosis and hypo- or hyperkalaemia.

Cardiac effects may include heart block, AV dissociation and asystole, and cardiogenic shock with pulmonary oedema.

Other toxic effects include nausea, vomiting, drowsiness, dizziness, confusion, lethargy, flushing, hypoxia and unconsciousness to the point of coma.

*Treatment:* As far as treatment is concerned, elimination of nifedipine and the restoration of stable cardiovascular conditions have priority.

After oral ingestion, gastric lavage is indicated, if necessary in combination with irrigation of the small intestine. Ipecacuanha should be given to children.

Activated charcoal should be given, 50 g for adults, 10–15 g for children.

Blood pressure, ECG, central arterial pressure, pulmonary wedge pressure, urea and electrolytes should be monitored.

Hypotension as a result of cardiogenic shock and arterial vasodilatation should be treated with elevation of the feet and plasma expanders. If these measures are ineffective, hypotension may be treated with 10% calcium gluconate 10–20 ml intravenously over 5–10 minutes. If the effects are inadequate, the treatment can be continued, with ECG monitoring. In addition, beta-sympathomimetics may be given, e.g. isoprenaline 0.2 mg slowly i.v. or as a continuous infusion of 5 µg/min. If an insufficient increase in blood pressure is achieved with calcium and isoprenaline, vasoconstricting sympathomimetics such as dopamine or noradrenaline should be administered. The dosage of these drugs should be determined by the patient's response.

Bradycardia may be treated with atropine, beta-sympathomimetics or a temporary cardiac pacemaker, as required.

Additional fluids should be administered with caution to avoid cardiac overload.

**Pharmaceutical precautions** The capsules should be protected from strong light and stored in the manufacturer's original container.

**Legal category** POM.

**Package quantities** Adalat and Adalat 5 capsules are available in foil strips of 10 in packs of 90. Hospital packs containing 500 Adalat 10 mg capsules are also available.

**Further information** Adalat has no therapeutic anti-arrhythmic effect. Since Adalat does not cause a rise in intraocular pressure, it can be used in patients with glaucoma. Adalat can be used in patients with obstructive airways disease with coexisting hypertension or angina pectoris. Long-term metabolic disturbances have not been observed.

**Product licence numbers**
Adalat      0010/0021
Adalat 5    0010/0079

## ADALAT* LA 30
## ADALAT* LA 60

**Presentation** Pink lacquered tablets each containing 30 mg or 60 mg nifedipine in a modified (extended) release formulation, one side marked Adalat 30 or Adalat 60.

### Uses

*Mode of action:* As a specific and potent calcium antagonist, the main action of nifedipine is to relax arterial smooth muscle both in the coronary and peripheral circulation. The Adalat LA tablet is formulated to achieve controlled delivery of nifedipine in a release profile sufficient to enable once-daily administration to be effective in clinical use.

In hypertension, the main action of nifedipine is to cause peripheral vasodilatation and thus reduce peripheral resistance. Nifedipine administered once-daily provides 24-hour control of raised blood pressure. Nifedipine causes reduction in blood pressure such that the percentage lowering is proportional to its initial level. In normotensive individuals, nifedipine has little or no effect on blood pressure.

In angina, nifedipine reduces peripheral and coronary vascular resistance, leading to an increase in coronary blood flow, cardiac output and stroke volume, whilst decreasing after-load. Additionally, nifedipine dilates submaximally both clear and atherosclerotic coronary arteries, thus protecting the heart against coronary artery spasm and improving perfusion to the ischaemic myocardium. Nifedipine reduces the frequency of painful attacks and the ischaemic ECG changes irrespective of the relative contribution from coronary artery spasm or atherosclerosis.

*Indications:* For the treatment of mild to moderate hypertension.

For the prophylaxis of chronic stable angina pectoris either as monotherapy or in combination with a beta-blocker.

**Dosage and administration** For oral administration, the tablets should be swallowed whole with a glass of water. The tablets should be taken at approximately 24-hour intervals, i.e. at the same time each day, preferably during the morning. Adalat LA tablets must be swallowed whole; under no circumstances should they be bitten, chewed or broken up.

In hypertension and angina pectoris, the recommended initial dose is one 30 mg tablet once-daily. If necessary, the dosage can be increased according to individual requirements up to a maximum of 90 mg once-daily.

Patients in whom hypertension or anginal symptoms are controlled on Adalat capsules or Adalat retard may be switched safely to Adalat LA. Prophylactic anti-anginal efficacy is maintained when patients are switched from other calcium antagonists such as diltiazem or verapamil to Adalat LA. Patients switched from other calcium antagonists should initiate therapy at the recommended initial dose of 30 mg Adalat LA once-daily. Subsequent titration to a higher dose may be initiated as warranted clinically.

The pharmacokinetics of nifedipine are altered in the elderly so that lower maintenance doses of nifedipine may be required compared to younger patients.

Patients with renal impairment should not require adjustment of dosage.

Treatment may be continued indefinitely.

Nifedipine is not recommended for use in children.

**Contra-indications, warnings, etc**

*Contra-indications:* Adalat LA should not be administered to patients with known hypersensitivity to nifedipine or other dihydropyridines because of the theoretical risk of cross-reactivity.

Adalat LA should not be administered to women capable of child-bearing or to nursing mothers.

Adalat LA should not be used in cardiogenic shock, clinically significant aortic stenosis, unstable angina, or during or within one month of a myocardial infarction.

Adalat LA should not be used for the treatment of acute attacks of angina.

The safety of Adalat LA in malignant hypertension has not been established.

Adalat LA should not be used for secondary prevention of myocardial infarction.

Owing to the duration of action of the formulation, Adalat LA should not be administered to patients with hepatic impairment.

Adalat LA should not be administered to patients with a history of gastro-intestinal obstruction, oesophageal obstruction, or any degree of decreased lumen diameter of the gastro-intestinal tract.

Adalat LA is contra-indicated in patients with inflammatory bowel disease or Crohn's disease.

Adalat LA should not be administered concomitantly with rifampicin since effective plasma levels of nifedipine may not be achieved owing to enzyme induction.

*Warnings and precautions:* Adalat LA tablets must be swallowed whole; under no circumstances should they be bitten, chewed or broken up.

The outer membrane of the Adalat LA tablet is not digested and, therefore, what appears to be the complete tablet may be seen in the toilet or associated with the patient's stools.

Caution should be exercised in patients with hypotension as there is a risk of further reduction in blood pressure.

Adalat LA may be used in combination with beta-blocking drugs and other antihypertensive agents but the possibility of an additive effect resulting in postural hypotension should be borne in mind. Adalat LA will not prevent possible rebound effects after cessation of other antihypertensive therapy.

Adalat LA should be used with caution in patients whose cardiac reserve is poor. Deterioration of heart failure has occasionally been observed with nifedipine.

Ischaemic pain has been reported in a small proportion of patients following the introduction of nifedipine therapy. Although a 'steal' effect has not

been demonstrated, patients experiencing this effect should discontinue nifedipine therapy.

Diabetic patients taking Adalat LA may require adjustment of their control.

In dialysis patients with malignant hypertension and hypovolaemia, a marked decrease in blood pressure can occur.

*Interactions:* The antihypertensive effect of Adalat LA may be potentiated by simultaneous administration of cimetidine.

When used in combination with nifedipine, serum quinidine levels have been shown to be suppressed regardless of dosage of quinidine.

The simultaneous administration of nifedipine and digoxin may lead to reduced digoxin clearance and hence an increase in the plasma digoxin level. Plasma digoxin levels should be monitored and, if necessary, the digoxin dose reduced.

Diltiazem decreases the clearance of nifedipine and, hence, increases plasma nifedipine levels. Therefore, caution should be taken when both drugs are used in combination and a reduction of the nifedipine dose may be necessary.

Nifedipine may increase the spectrophotometric values of urinary vanillylmandelic acid falsely. However, HPLC measurements are unaffected.

Adalat LA should not be administered concomitantly with rifampicin since effective plasma levels of nifedipine may not be achieved owing to enzyme induction.

As with other dihydropyridines, nifedipine should not be taken with grapefruit juice because bioavailability is increased.

*Side-effects:* Most side-effects are consequences of the vasodilatory effects of nifedipine. Headache, flushing, tachycardia and palpitations may occur, most commonly in the early stages of treatment with nifedipine. Gravitational oedema, not associated with heart failure or weight gain, may also occur.

Paraesthesia, dizziness, lethargy and gastro-intestinal symptoms such as nausea and altered bowel habit may occur occasionally.

There are reports of skin reactions such as rash, pruritus and urticaria.

Other less frequently reported side-effects include myalgia, tremor and visual disturbances. Impotence may occur rarely.

Increased frequency of micturition may occur.

As with other sustained release dihydropyridines, exacerbation of angina pectoris may occur rarely at the start of treatment with sustained release formulations of nifedipine. The occurrence of myocardial infarction has been described although it is not possible to distinguish such an event from the natural course of ischaemic heart disease.

There are reports of gingival hyperplasia and, in older men on long-term therapy, gynaecomastia, which usually regress upon withdrawal of therapy.

Mood changes may occur rarely.

Side-effects which have been observed in isolated cases are photosensitivity, exfoliative dermatitis, systemic allergic reactions and purpura. Usually, these regress after discontinuation of the drug.

Rare cases of hypersensitivity-type jaundice have been reported. In addition, disturbances of liver function such as intra-hepatic cholestasis may occur. These regress after discontinuation of therapy.

*Overdosage:* There are no reports of overdosage with Adalat LA.

*Clinical effects:* Reports of nifedipine overdosage are limited and symptoms are not necessarily dose-related. Severe hypotension due to vasodilatation, and tachycardia or bradycardia are the most likely manifestations of overdose.

Metabolic disturbances include hyperglycaemia, metabolic acidosis and hypo- or hyperkalaemia.

Cardiac effects may include heart block, AV dissociation and asystole, and cardiogenic shock with pulmonary oedema.

Other toxic effects include nausea, vomiting, drowsiness, dizziness, confusion, lethargy, flushing, hypoxia and unconsciousness to the point of coma.

*Treatment:* As far as treatment is concerned, elimination of nifedipine and the restoration of stable cardiovascular conditions have priority.

After oral ingestion, gastric lavage is indicated, if necessary in combination with irrigation of the small intestine. Ipecacuanha should be given to children.

Elimination must be as complete as possible, including the small intestine, to prevent the otherwise inevitable subsequent absorption of the active substance.

Activated charcoal should be given in 4-hourly doses of 25 g for adults, 10 g for children.

Blood pressure, ECG, central arterial pressure, pulmonary wedge pressure, urea and electrolytes should be monitored.

Hypotension as a result of cardiogenic shock and arterial vasodilatation should be treated with elevation of the feet and plasma expanders. If these measures

are ineffective, hypotension may be treated with 10% calcium gluconate 10–20 ml intravenously over 5–10 minutes. If the effects are inadequate, the treatment can be continued, with ECG monitoring. In addition, beta-sympathomimetics may be given, e.g. isoprenaline 0.2 mg slowly i.v. or as a continuous infusion of 5 µg/min. If an insufficient increase in blood pressure is achieved with calcium and isoprenaline, vasoconstricting sympathomimetics such as dopamine or noradrenaline should be administered. The dosage of these drugs should be determined by the patient's response.

Bradycardia may be treated with atropine, beta-sympathomimetics or a temporary cardiac pacemaker, as required.

Additional fluids should be administered with caution to avoid cardiac overload.

**Pharmaceutical precautions** The tablets should be protected from strong light and stored in the manufacturer's original container.

**Legal category** POM.

**Package quantities** Adalat LA 30 and Adalat LA 60: calendar packs containing 28 tablets.

**Further information** Adalat LA has no therapeutic antiarrhythmic effect. Since Adalat LA does not cause a rise in intraocular pressure, it can be used in patients with glaucoma. Adalat LA can be used in patients with obstructive airways disease with coexisting hypertension or angina. Long-term metabolic disturbances have not been observed.

**Product licence numbers**
Adalat LA 30   0010/0174
Adalat LA 60   0010/0175

## ADALAT* RETARD
## ADALAT* RETARD 10

**Presentation** *Adalat retard:* Pink-grey lacquered tablets each containing 20 mg nifedipine, one side marked 1U and the reverse side with the Bayer cross. *Adalat retard 10:* Pink-grey lacquered tablets each containing 10 mg nifedipine, one side marked A10 and the reverse side with the Bayer cross.

**Uses**
*Mode of action:* Nifedipine is a specific and potent calcium antagonist. In hypertension, the main action of Adalat retard is to cause peripheral vasodilatation and thus reduce peripheral resistance.

In angina, Adalat retard reduces peripheral and coronary vascular resistance, leading to an increase in coronary blood flow, cardiac output and stroke volume, whilst decreasing after-load.

Adalat retard administered twice-daily provides 24-hour control of raised blood pressure. Adalat retard causes reduction in blood pressure such that the percentage lowering is directly related to its initial level. In normotensive individuals, Adalat retard has little or no effect on blood pressure.

*Indications:* For the prophylaxis of chronic stable angina pectoris and the treatment of hypertension.

**Dosage and administration** The recommended starting dose of Adalat retard is 10 mg every 12 hours swallowed with water with subsequent titration of dosage according to response. The dose may be adjusted to 40 mg every 12 hours.

Adalat retard 10 permits titration of initial dosage. The recommended dose is one Adalat retard 10 tablet (10 mg) every 12 hours.

The pharmacokinetics of nifedipine are altered in the elderly so that lower maintenance doses of nifedipine may be required compared to younger patients.

Nifedipine is metabolised primarily by the liver and therefore patients with liver dysfunction should be carefully monitored.

Patients with renal impairment should not require adjustment of dosage.

Treatment may be continued indefinitely.

Nifedipine is not recommended for use in children.

**Contra-indications, warnings, etc**
*Contra-indications:* Adalat retard should not be administered to patients with known hypersensitivity to nifedipine or other dihydropyridines because of the theoretical risk of cross-reactivity.

Adalat retard should not be administered to women capable of child-bearing or to nursing mothers.

Adalat retard should not be used in cardiogenic shock, clinically significant aortic stenosis, unstable angina, or during or within one month of a myocardial infarction.

Adalat retard should not be used for the treatment of acute attacks of angina.

The safety of Adalat retard in malignant hypertension has not been established.

Adalat retard should not be used for secondary prevention of myocardial infarction.

Adalat retard should not be administered concomitantly with rifampicin since effective plasma levels of nifedipine may not be achieved owing to enzyme induction.

*Warnings and precautions:* Adalat retard may be used in combination with beta-blocking drugs and other antihypertensive agents but the possibility of an additive effect resulting in postural hypotension should be borne in mind. Adalat retard will not prevent possible rebound effects after cessation of other antihypertensive therapy.

Adalat retard should be used with caution in patients whose cardiac reserve is poor. Deterioration of heart failure has occasionally been observed with nifedipine.

Caution should be exercised in patients with severe hypotension.

Ischaemic pain has been reported in a small proportion of patients within one to four hours of the introduction of Adalat retard therapy. Although a 'steal' effect has not been demonstrated, patients experiencing this effect should discontinue Adalat retard.

Diabetic patients taking Adalat retard may require adjustment of their control.

In dialysis patients with malignant hypertension and hypovolaemia, a marked decrease in blood pressure can occur.

*Interactions:* The antihypertensive effect of Adalat retard may be potentiated by simultaneous administration of cimetidine.

When used in combination with nifedipine, serum quinidine levels have been shown to be suppressed regardless of dosage of quinidine.

The simultaneous administration of nifedipine and digoxin may lead to reduced digoxin clearance and hence an increase in the plasma digoxin level. Plasma digoxin levels should be monitored and, if necessary, the digoxin dose reduced.

Diltiazem decreases the clearance of nifedipine and hence increases plasma nifedipine levels. Therefore, caution should be taken when both drugs are used in combination and a reduction of the nifedipine dose may be necessary.

Nifedipine may increase the spectrophotometric values of urinary vanillylmandelic acid falsely. However, HPLC measurements are unaffected.

Adalat retard should not be administered concomitantly with rifampicin since effective plasma levels of nifedipine may not be achieved owing to enzyme induction.

As with other dihydropyridines, nifedipine should not be taken with grapefruit juice because bioavailability is increased.

*Side-effects:* Most side-effects are consequences of the vasodilatory effects of nifedipine. Headache, flushing, tachycardia and palpitations may occur, most commonly in the early stages of treatment with nifedipine. Gravitational oedema, not associated with heart failure or weight gain, may also occur.

Paraesthesia, dizziness, lethargy and gastro-intestinal symptoms such as nausea and altered bowel habit may occur occasionally.

There are reports of skin reactions such as rash, pruritus and urticaria.

Other less frequently reported side-effects include myalgia, tremor and visual disturbances. Impotence may occur rarely.

Increased frequency of micturition may occur.

As with other sustained release dihydropyridines, exacerbation of angina pectoris may occur rarely at the start of treatment with sustained release formulations of nifedipine. The occurrence of myocardial infarction has been described although it is not possible to distinguish such an event from the natural course of ischaemic heart disease.

There are reports of gingival hyperplasia and, in older men on long-term therapy, gynaecomastia, which usually regress upon withdrawal of therapy.

Mood changes may occur rarely.

Side-effects which may occur in isolated cases are photosensitivity, exfoliative dermatitis, systemic allergic reactions and purpura. Usually, these regress after discontinuation of the drug.

Rare cases of hypersensitivity-type jaundice have been reported. In addition, disturbances of liver function such as intra-hepatic cholestasis may occur. These regress after discontinuation of therapy.

*Overdosage: Clinical effects:* Reports of nifedipine overdosage are limited and symptoms are not necessarily dose-related. Severe hypotension due to vasodilatation, and tachycardia or bradycardia are the most likely manifestations of overdose.

Metabolic disturbances include hyperglycaemia, metabolic acidosis and hypo- or hyperkalaemia.

Cardiac effects may include heart block, AV dissociation and asystole, and cardiogenic shock with pulmonary oedema.

Other toxic effects include nausea, vomiting, drowsiness, dizziness, confusion, lethargy, flushing, hypoxia and unconsciousness to the point of coma.

*Treatment:* As far as treatment is concerned, elimination of nifedipine and the restoration of stable cardiovascular conditions have priority.

After oral ingestion, gastric lavage is indicated, if necessary in combination with irrigation of the small intestine. Ipecacuanha should be given to children.

Elimination must be as complete as possible, including the small intestine, to prevent the otherwise inevitable subsequent absorption of the active substance.

Activated charcoal should be given in 4-hourly doses of 25 g for adults, 10 g for children.

Blood pressure, ECG, central arterial pressure, pulmonary wedge pressure, urea and electrolytes should be monitored.

Hypotension as a result of cardiogenic shock and arterial vasodilatation should be treated with elevation of the feet and plasma expanders. If these measures are ineffective, hypotension may be treated with 10% calcium gluconate 10–20 ml intravenously over 5–10 minutes. If the effects are inadequate, the treatment can be continued, with ECG monitoring. In addition, beta-sympathomimetics may be given, e.g. isoprenaline 0.2 mg slowly i.v. or as a continuous infusion of 5 μg/min. If an insufficient increase in blood pressure is achieved with calcium and isoprenaline, vasoconstricting sympathomimetics such as dopamine or noradrenaline should be administered. The dosage of these drugs should be determined by the patient's response.

Bradycardia may be treated with atropine, beta-sympathomimetics or a temporary cardiac pacemaker, as required.

Additional fluids should be administered with caution to avoid cardiac overload.

**Pharmaceutical precautions**   The tablets should be protected from strong light and stored in the manufacturer's original container.

**Legal category**   POM.

**Package quantities**   Adalat retard tablets: strips of 14 in packs of 56.

Adalat retard 10 tablets: strips of 14 in packs of 56.

**Further information**   Adalat retard has no therapeutic antiarrhythmic effect. Since Adalat retard does not cause a rise in intraocular pressure, it can be used in patients with glaucoma. Adalat retard can be used in patients with obstructive airways disease with coexisting hypertension or angina pectoris. Long-term metabolic disturbances have not been observed.

**Product licence numbers**
Adalat retard       0010/0078
Adalat retard 10    0010/0151

# BAYCARON*

**Presentation**   A white scored tablet 7 mm × 2 mm, one side scored L/1 and the reverse side with the Bayer cross, containing 25 mg mefruside.

**Uses**   Baycaron is a diuretic agent and is intended for the treatment of hypertension and oedema.

**Dosage and administration**   Baycaron is best taken with a little fluid after meals.

*Hypertension:* 25 mg to 50 mg initially for 10 to 14 days, then maintenance dose of 25 mg each morning. Alternate day dosage may also be used.

*Oedema:* 25 mg to 50 mg every morning increasing if necessary to 75 mg to 100 mg to obtain the desired response. For long-term therapy intermittent dosage is preferable, e.g. 25 mg to 50 mg every second or third day.

Daily doses in excess of 100 mg do not usually increase diuresis further.

Paediatric dosage has not been established.

**Contra-indications, warnings, etc**

*Contra-indications:* Severe renal failure, hepatic coma, Addisons disease, severe hypercalcaemia.

*Warnings and precautions:* It is often necessary to give extra potassium during treatment with diuretics and potassium supplements may be necessary during long-term treatment with Baycaron, especially in patients with impaired liver function or in those also receiving digoxin and other cardiac glycosides.

Particular care is necessary in the elderly because of their susceptibility to electrolyte imbalance.

Although there is no short-term alteration of carbohydrate metabolism in normal subjects on a 50 mg daily dose, the glucose tolerance curve may be prolonged in some diabetics. After Baycaron administration serum uric acid may be raised and therefore it should be used with caution in potential cases of gout.

Baycaron is not suitable for the treatment of acute conditions of fluid excess such as pulmonary and cerebral oedema and glaucoma.

Baycaron should not be administered concurrently with lithium carbonate. Patients with known sulphon-

amide sensitivity may show allergic reactions to Baycaron. Care should be exercised when prescribed with non-steroidal anti-inflammatory drugs. It is always advisable to monitor renal function. Thiazide and thiazide-like diuretics have been implicated in blood dyscrasias and pancreatitis.

*Pregnancy warning:* Baycaron has not been shown to produce teratogenic effects, either after administration to animals, or when used to treat toxaemia of pregnancy. However, the benefits should be carefully weighed against possible risks in the first trimester of pregnancy.

Diuretics are best avoided for the management of oedema of pregnancy or hypertension in pregnancy as their use may be associated with hypovolaemia, increased blood viscosity and reduced placental perfusion.

There is inadequate evidence of safety in human pregnancy and some workers have described foetal bone marrow depression and thrombocytopenia. Foetal and neonatal jaundice have also been described.

*Lactation warning:* As diuretics pass into breast milk they should be avoided in mothers who wish to breast feed.

*Side-effects:* Baycaron is very well tolerated. Occasionally, with daily doses of up to 100 mg, dyspepsia and nausea are encountered initially, but usually subside on continued treatment. There are no reports of postural hypotension nor of any impairment of micturition or bowel habit. Due to its profile of diuretic action, Baycaron does not precipitate acute retention of urine in, for example, cases of prostatic hypertrophy. Impotence is rarely associated with mefruside.

*Overdosage:* There is no special antidote and general supportive measures should be offered together with monitoring of blood pressure, fluid and electrolyte balance, correcting when necessary.

**Pharmaceutical precautions**   There are no special precautions or requirements regarding the storage of Baycaron.

**Legal category**   POM.

**Package quantities**   Bottles of 150 tablets.

**Further information**

*Hypertension:* Baycaron, with its powerful natriuretic effect is particularly suited to the treatment of hypertension, especially in the long term. Baycaron may be administered alone or in combination with other antihypertensive agents.

*Oedema:* By virtue of its prolonged and smooth natriuretic action, Baycaron is suitable for the long-term treatment of oedematous conditions, for example: oedema of cardiac, hepatic, or renal origin, and premenstrual tension. Its profile of action leads to minimum patient inconvenience. Diuresis begins two to four hours following oral administration and is maximal between six and twelve hours after administration.

**Product licence number**   0010/5903R

# BETA-ADALAT*

**Presentation**   Beta-Adalat is presented as reddish brown capsules bearing the name Beta-Adalat with the Bayer cross. Each capsule contains nifedipine retard 20 mg and atenolol 50 mg.

**Uses**

*Mode of action:* Atenolol effects a marked negative inotropic and chronotropic effect thereby reducing cardiac output, myocardial oxygen demand and blood pressure, particularly during exercise. Nifedipine is a powerful coronary and peripheral vasodilator which increases myocardial oxygen supply and reduces blood pressure (afterload) and peripheral resistance. Concomitant use of beta$_1$-blockade, therefore, ameliorates the reflex sympathetic response to nifedipine monotherapy by blocking the rise in heart rate, while atenolol's tendency to increase peripheral resistance is balanced by the vasodilation and increased sympathetic tone induced by the calcium antagonist. Consequently, greater antihypertensive or antianginal efficacy is achieved by the concomitant use of nifedipine and atenolol than either drug alone.

*Indications:* Management of hypertension and of chronic stable angina pectoris where therapy with either a calcium channel blocker or a beta-blocker proves inadequate.

**Dosage and administration**

*Adults: Hypertension:* One capsule daily swallowed with water. If necessary, the dosage may be increased to one capsule dosed every 12 hours. Patients can be transferred to the combination from other antihypertensive treatments with the exception of clonidine (see *Precautions* below).

*Angina:* One capsule every 12 hours swallowed

with water. Where additional efficacy is necessary, prophylactic nitrate therapy or additional nifedipine may be of benefit.

*Children:* There is no paediatric experience with Beta-Adalat and, therefore, this preparation should not be used in children.

*Elderly:* Dosage should not exceed one capsule daily in hypertension or one capsule twice daily in angina.

The pharmacokinetics of nifedipine are altered in the elderly so that lower maintenance doses of nifedipine may be required compared to younger patients.

**Contra-indications, warnings, etc**
*Contra-indications:* Beta-Adalat should not be administered to patients with known hypersensitivity to nifedipine or other dihydropyridines because of the theoretical risk of cross-reactivity.

Beta-Adalat should not be administered to patients with a history of wheezing or asthma.

Beta-Adalat must not be administered to women capable of child-bearing or to nursing mothers.

Beta-Adalat must not be used in the presence of second or third degree heart block, or in patients with evidence of overt heart failure.

Beta-Adalat should not be used in cardiogenic shock, clinically significant aortic stenosis, unstable angina, or during or within one month of a myocardial infarction.

Beta-Adalat should not be used for the treatment of acute attacks of angina.

The safety of Beta-Adalat in malignant hypertension has not been established.

Beta-Adalat should not be used for secondary prevention of myocardial infarction.

Beta-Adalat must not be used in conjunction with other drugs with a cardio-depressant action, e.g. verapamil, as conduction disturbances may ensue.

Beta-Adalat should not be administered concomitantly with rifampicin since effective plasma levels of nifedipine may not be achieved owing to enzyme induction.

*Precautions*
*Cardiac:* Particular care should be taken with patients with conduction defects or whose cardiac reserve is poor. However, in patients already treated with a beta-adrenoceptor antagonist, and/or where signs of cardiac failure have been controlled, Beta-Adalat may be substituted with care if necessary.

Care should be taken in prescribing a beta-adrenoceptor blocking drug with Class 1 antidysrhythmic agents such as disopyramide.

One of the pharmacological actions of beta-adrenoceptor blocking drugs is to reduce heart rate. In the rare instances where symptoms may be attributable to the slow heart rate at a dose of one capsule daily, the drug should be discontinued.

Cessation of therapy with a beta-adrenoceptor blocking drug in patients with ischaemic heart disease should be gradual.

Caution should be exercised when transferring patients from clonidine to beta-adrenoceptor blocking drugs. If beta-adrenoceptor blocking drugs are given concurrently, clonidine should not be discontinued until several days after withdrawal of the beta-adrenoceptor blocking drug.

*Obstructive airways disease:* Although cardioselective (beta$_1$) beta-blockers may have less effect on lung function than non-selective beta-blockers, as with all beta-blockers these should not be administered to patients with reversible obstructive airways disease.

*Renal impairment:* In patients with marked renal impairment (i.e. creatinine clearance below 15 ml/min/1.73 m$^2$, serum creatinine greater than 600 micromol/litre), the use of the combination is considered inappropriate.

*Hepatic impairment:* Care should be taken in patients with marked hepatic impairment. Although no dosage adjustment is suggested from the systemic availability of the monocomponents in patients with cirrhosis, hypertensive patients with clinically significant liver disease have not been studied. Nifedipine is metabolised primarily by the liver and therefore patients with liver dysfunction should be carefully monitored.

*Anaesthesia:* It is not advisable to withdraw beta-adrenoceptor blocking drugs prior to surgery in the majority of patients. However, care should be taken when using anaesthetic agents such as ether, cyclopropane and trichloroethylene. Vagal dominance, if it occurs, may be corrected with atropine (1–2 mg i.v.).

*Diabetes:* The use of nifedipine in diabetic patients may require adjustment of their control.

Beta-Adalat modifies the tachycardia of hypoglycaemia.

*Interactions:* The antihypertensive effect of nifedipine can be potentiated by simultaneous administration of cimetidine.

When used in combination with nifedipine, serum quinidine levels may be suppressed regardless of dosage of quinidine.

The simultaneous administration of nifedipine and digoxin may lead to reduced digoxin clearance and hence an increase in the plasma digoxin level. Plasma digoxin levels should be monitored and, if necessary, the digoxin dose reduced.

Beta-Adalat should not be administered concomitantly with rifampicin since effective plasma levels of nifedipine may not be achieved owing to enzyme induction.

As with other dihydropyridines, nifedipine should not be taken with grapefruit juice because bioavailability is increased.

*Side-effects:* Side-effects which have been reported during treatment with the combination include headache, flushing, fatigue, dizziness and oedema. Side-effects of nifedipine such as flushing and headache may occur at the beginning of the treatment. They are, however, mostly slight and diminish with continuous use.

Impotence may occur rarely as a side-effect of nifedipine.

Rare cases of hypersensitivity-type jaundice have been reported with nifedipine.

There are reports of gingival hyperplasia with nifedipine which may regress on withdrawal of therapy.

There have been reports of skin rashes and/or dry eyes associated with the use of beta-adrenoceptor blocking drugs. The reported incidence is small. Discontinuance of the drug should be considered if any such reaction is not otherwise explicable.

As with other sustained release dihydropyridines, exacerbation of angina pectoris may occur rarely at the start of treatment with sustained release formulations of nifedipine. The occurrence of myocardial infarction has been described although it is not possible to distinguish such an event from the natural course of ischaemic heart disease.

*Overdosage:* Excessive bradycardia can be countered with atropine 1–2 mg intravenously. If necessary, this may be followed by a bolus dose of glucagon 10 mg intravenously. If required, this may be repeated or followed by an intravenous infusion of glucagon 1–10 mg/hour depending on response. If no response to glucagon occurs or if glucagon is unavailable, a beta-adrenoceptor stimulant such as prenalterol 5 mg intravenously, followed if necessary by an intravenous infusion of 5 mg/hour or dobutamine 2.5 to 10 microgram/kg/minute by intravenous infusion may be given.

There is a possibility of hypotension occurring following the use of beta-adrenoceptor agonists but this will be reduced by the more selective agents, prenalterol and dobutamine. In severe cases, cardiac pacing with appropriate cardiorespiratory support may be necessary.

Intravenous calcium gluconate combined with metaraminol may be beneficial for hypotension induced by nifedipine.

**Pharmaceutical precautions** Beta-Adalat should be stored at room temperature, protected from light and moisture.

**Legal category** POM.

**Package quantities** Packs of 28 capsules.

**Further information** When the combined antihypertensive effect or anti-anginal effect of a beta-adrenoceptor antagonist and calcium antagonist is required, Beta-Adalat is a convenient and acceptable therapy. The combination of atenolol and nifedipine retard, given once daily, provides control of raised blood pressure over a 24 hour period and may be expected to improve patient compliance. Given twice daily, the combination provides control of angina.

**Product licence number** 0010/0155

# CANESTEN* GYNAECOLOGICAL PRODUCTS

**Presentation**
*Pessaries:* White convex pessaries measuring 25 mm×6.5 mm×10 mm containing Clotrimazole BP.

Canesten 100 mg Pessary is marked 'Bayer' on one side and 'AD' on the other.

Canesten 200 mg Pessary is marked 'Bayer' on one side and 'F9' on the other.

Canesten 1 Pessary (500 mg) is marked 'Bayer' on one side and 'MU' on the other.

*10% VC:* A white cream containing 10.0% Clotrimazole BP.

*Combi:* A combination pack comprising one Canesten 1 Pessary (500 mg) plus a 20 g tube of Canesten 1% cream (containing 1.0% Clotrimazole BP).

**Uses**
*Pessaries:* The pessaries are indicated for the treatment of candidal vaginitis.

*10% VC:* As for pessaries.

*Combi:* Pessary for candidal vaginitis; cream for associated vulvitis and to treat the sexual partner to prevent re-infection.

**Dosage and administration**
*Adults*
*100 mg Pessaries:* Two pessaries should be inserted daily, preferably at night, for three consecutive days. Alternatively, one pessary daily for six days may be inserted, preferably at night.

*200 mg Pessaries:* One pessary should be inserted daily, preferably at night, for three consecutive days.

*500 mg Pessary:* The single pessary should be inserted, preferably at night.

*10% VC:* Insert the contents of the filled applicator (5 g) intravaginally, preferably at night. A second treatment may be carried out if necessary.

*Combi:* The single pessary should be inserted, preferably at night.

The cream should be applied night and morning to the vulva and surrounding area and/or to the partner's penis to prevent re-infection.

Using the applicator provided, each pessary or dose of vaginal cream should be inserted as deeply as is comfortable into the vagina. This is best achieved when lying back with the legs bent up.

*Children:* As the above products are used with an applicator, paediatric usage is not recommended.

**Contra-indications, warnings, etc**
*Contra-indications:* Hypersensitivity to clotrimazole.

*Warnings and precautions:* Medical advice should be sought if this is the first time the patient has experienced symptoms of candidal vaginitis. Before using the pessaries or cream, medical advice must be sought if any of the following are applicable:
 – More than two infections of candidal vaginitis in the last six months.
 – Previous history of a sexually transmitted disease or exposure to partner with sexually transmitted disease.
 – Pregnancy or suspected pregnancy.
 – Aged under 16 or over 60 years.
 – Known hypersensitivity to imidazoles or other vaginal anti-fungal products.

Canesten pessaries and cream should not be used if the patient has any of the following symptoms, whereupon medical advice should be sought:
 – Irregular vaginal bleeding.
 – Abnormal vaginal bleeding or a blood-stained discharge.
 – Vulval or vaginal ulcers, blisters or sores.
 – Lower abdominal pain or dysuria.
 – Any adverse events such as redness, irritation or swelling associated with the treatment.
 – Fever or chills.
 – Nausea or vomiting.
 – Diarrhoea.
 – Foul smelling vaginal discharge.

If no improvement in symptoms is seen after seven days, the patient should consult their doctor.

*Side-effects:* Rarely patients may experience local mild burning or irritation immediately after applying the cream or inserting the pessaries. Very rarely, the patient may find this irritation intolerable and stop treatment. Hypersensitivity reactions may occur.

*Use in pregnancy:* In animal studies, clotrimazole has not been associated with teratogenic effects but following oral administration of high doses to rats there was evidence of foetotoxicity. The relevance of this effect to topical application in humans is not known. However, clotrimazole has been used in pregnant patients for over a decade without attributable adverse effects. It is therefore recommended that clotrimazole should be used in pregnancy only when considered necessary by the clinician. If used during pregnancy, extra care should be taken when using the applicator to prevent the possibility of mechanical trauma.

*Accidental oral ingestion:* In the event, routine measures such as gastric lavage should be performed as soon as possible after ingestion.

**Pharmaceutical precautions** No special storage precautions are necessary for the pessaries. Canesten 10% VC and Combi should be stored below 25°C.

**Legal category** P.

**Package quantities**
*Pessaries:* 6×100 mg pessaries packed in a blister strip.
 3×200 mg pessaries packed in a blister strip.
 1×500 mg pessary packed in foil.
 An applicator and a patient information leaflet are included.

*Canesten 10% VC:* A prefilled applicator containing 5 g cream. A patient information leaflet is included.

*Combi:* 1×500 mg pessary packed in foil, plus a 20 g tube of Canesten 1% cream. An applicator for the pessary and a patient information leaflet are included.

**Further information** Nil.

**Product licence numbers**

| | |
|---|---|
| 100 mg Pessaries | 0010/0015R |
| 200 mg Pessaries | 0010/0072 |
| 500 mg Pessary | 0010/0083 |
| 10% VC | 0010/0136 |
| Combi: Cream 1% | 0010/0016R |
| 500 mg Pessary | 0010/0083 |

## CANESTEN* TOPICAL PRODUCTS

**Presentation**
*Cream:* A white cream containing 1.0% Clotrimazole BP.

*Atomiser spray:* A clear spray containing 1.0% Clotrimazole BP in 30% isopropanol. The spray is produced by an atomiser and contains no propellant.

*Solution:* A clear solution containing 1.0% Clotrimazole BP in polyethylene glycol 400.

*Powder:* A white powder containing 1.0% Clotrimazole BP.

**Uses** Clotrimazole is a broad spectrum antifungal. It also exhibits activity against *Trichomonas*, staphylococci, streptococci and *Bacteroides*.

Clotrimazole is recommended for the treatment of skin infections due to dermatophytes (e.g. *Trichophyton* species), yeasts (e.g. *Candida* species), moulds and other fungi. These include ringworm (tinea) infections, athlete's foot, paronychia, pityriasis versicolor, erythrasma and intertrigo.

*Cream:* The cream may also be used for the treatment of fungal nappy rash, candidal vulvitis and candidal balanitis.

*Atomiser Spray:* The spray is recommended in particular for infections covering large and/or hairy areas.

*Solution:* The solution is particularly suitable for use on hairy skin and in fungal infections of the outer and middle ear (otitis externa and otomycoses).

*Powder:* The powder is to be used as an adjunct to treatment with cream or atomiser spray and as a prophylactic against re-infection, particularly in infections such as athlete's foot. The powder should be applied to the lesions simultaneously and dusted inside articles of clothing in contact with infected areas.

**Dosage and administration**
*Cream:* Canesten cream should be thinly and evenly applied to the affected area two to three times daily and rubbed in gently.

Treatment should be continued for at least one month for dermatophyte infections, or for at least two weeks for Candidal infections.

If the feet are infected, they should be thoroughly washed and dried, especially between the toes, before applying the cream.

*Atomiser Spray:* Canesten atomiser spray should be applied to the affected area two to three times daily. Treatment should be continued for at least one month for dermatophyte infections, or for at least two weeks for Candidal infections and pityriasis versicolor infections.

*Solution:* Canesten solution should be thinly and evenly applied to the affected area two to three times daily. To prevent relapse treatment should be continued for at least two weeks after the disappearance of all signs of infection.

*Powder:* Sprinkle onto the affected areas two to three times daily after using the cream or atomiser spray. The powder may also be dusted inside articles of clothing and footwear which are in contact with the infected area.

**Contra-indications, warnings, etc**
*Contra-indications:* Hypersensitivity to clotrimazole or, (in the case of the atomiser spray), propylene glycol.

*Warnings and precautions:* Canesten atomiser spray should not be used near a naked flame, should not be allowed to come into contact with the eyes, ears or mucous membranes and should not be inhaled.

*Side-effects:* Rarely patients may experience local mild burning or irritation immediately after applying the cream, solution or atomiser spray. Very rarely, the patient may find this irritation intolerable and stop treatment. Hypersensitivity reactions may occur.

*Use in pregnancy:* In animal studies clotrimazole has not been associated with teratogenic effects but following oral administration of high doses to rats there was evidence of foetotoxicity. The relevance of this effect to topical application in humans is not known. However, clotrimazole has been used in pregnant patients for over a decade without attributable adverse effects. It is therefore recommended that clotrimazole should be used in pregnancy only when considered necessary by the clinician.

*Accidental oral ingestion:* In the event, routine measures such as gastric lavage should be performed as soon as possible after ingestion.

**Pharmaceutical precautions** Cream: Store below 25°C. Atomiser spray, Solution, Powder: No special storage precautions are necessary.

**Legal category** P.

**Package quantities**
Cream: Tubes containing 20 g or 50 g.
Atomiser Spray: Bottles containing 40 ml.
Solution: Dropper bottles containing 20 ml.
Powder: Packs containing 30 g.

**Further information** Nil.

**Product licence numbers**

| | |
|---|---|
| Cream | 0010/0016R |
| Atomiser Spray | 0010/0060R |
| Solution | 0010/0082 |
| Powder | 0010/0067 |

## CANESTEN*HC

**Presentation** A white cream containing 1.0% Clotrimazole BP and 1.0% Hydrocortisone PhEur.

**Uses** Clotrimazole is a broad spectrum antifungal agent. It also exhibits activity against *Trichomonas*, staphylococci, streptococci and *Bacteroides*. It has no effect on lactobacilli.

Hydrocortisone has a vasoconstrictive effect, thus reducing inflammation and oedema and also has an antipruritic effect.

Canesten HC is indicated for the treatment of the following skin infections where co-existing symptoms of inflammation, e.g. itching, require rapid relief:

1. All dermatomycoses due to dermatophytes, (e.g. Trichophyton species), moulds and other fungi.
2. All dermatomycoses due to yeasts (Candida species).
3. Skin diseases showing secondary infection with these fungi.
4. The treatment of nappy rash where infection due to *Candida albicans* is present. Candidal vulvitis, candidal balanitis and candidal intertrigo.

**Dosage and administration** Canesten HC should be thinly and evenly applied to the affected area twice daily and rubbed in gently.

**Contra-indications, warnings, etc**
*Contra-indications:* Hypersensitivity to any of the ingredients.

*Warnings and precautions:* As with all corticosteroids, long term continuous therapy to extensive areas of skin should be avoided, particularly in infants and children. In infants the napkin may act as an occlusive dressing and increase absorption.

Treatment should be for a maximum period of seven days.

*Side-effects:* Rarely patients may experience local mild burning or irritation immediately after applying the cream. Very rarely, the patient may find this irritation intolerable and stop treatment. Hypersensitivity reactions may occur.

*Use in pregnancy:* Topical administration of corticosteroids to pregnant animals can cause abnormalities of foetal development. The relevance of this to humans has not been established.

In animal studies clotrimazole has not been associated with teratogenic effects but following oral administration of high doses to rats there was evidence of foetotoxicity. The relevance of this effect to topical application in humans is not known. However, clotrimazole has been used in pregnant patients for over a decade without attributable adverse effects.

It is therefore recommended that Canesten HC should be used in pregnancy only when considered necessary by the clinician.

*Accidental oral ingestion:* In the event, routine measures such as gastric lavage should be performed as soon as possible after ingestion.

**Pharmaceutical precautions** Store in a cool place.

**Legal category** POM.

**Package quantities** Tubes containing 30 g.

**Further information** Nil.

**Product licence number** 0010/0120

## CANESTEN* HYDROCORTISONE

**Qualitative and quantitative composition** 15 g of cream contains Clotrimazole BP 150 mg (1%) and Hydrocortisone PhEur 150 mg (1%).

**Pharmaceutical form** Cream.

**Clinical particulars**
*Therapeutic Indications:* Canesten Hydrocortisone is indicated for the treatment of the following skin infections where co-existing symptoms of inflammation, e.g. itching, require rapid relief:
(i) Athlete's foot.
(ii) Candidal intertrigo.

*Posology and method of administration:* Canesten Hydrocortisone should be thinly and evenly applied to the affected area twice daily and rubbed in gently. The maximum period of treatment is seven days.

*Contra-indications:* Canesten Hydrocortisone is contra-indicated in the following cases:
- Use on broken skin.
- Use on large areas of skin.
- Use for periods of longer than seven days.
- Hypersensitivity to any of the ingredients.
- To treat cold sores or acne.
- Use on the face, eyes, mouth or mucous membranes.
- Children under 10 years of age, unless prescribed by a doctor.
- Pregnancy and lactation, unless prescribed by a doctor.
- Use on the ano-genital area, unless prescribed by a doctor.
- To treat ringworm, unless prescribed by a doctor.
- To treat secondarily infected skin conditions, unless prescribed by a doctor.

*Special warnings and special precautions for use:* As with all corticosteroids, long-term continuous therapy to extensive areas of skin should be avoided. Therefore, treatment should be for a maximum period of seven days.

Care should be taken not to cover the treated area with a tight bandage or dressing as this may increase absorption of hydrocortisone.

*Interaction with other medicaments and other forms of interaction:* None.

*Pregnancy and lactation:* Topical administration of corticosteroids to pregnant animals can cause abnormalities of foetal development. The relevance of this to humans has not been established. In animal studies, clotrimazole has not been associated with teratogenic effects but following oral administration of high doses to rats, there was evidence of foetotoxicity. The relevance of this effect to topical application in humans is not known. However, clotrimazole has been used in pregnant patients for over a decade without attributable adverse effects. It is therefore recommended that Canesten Hydrocortisone should be used in pregnancy and lactation only when considered necessary by the clinician.

*Effects on ability to drive and use machines:* None applicable.

*Undesirable effects:* Rarely patients may experience local, mild burning or irritation immediately after applying the cream. Very rarely, patients may find this irritation intolerable and stop treatment. Hypersensitivity reactions may occur.

*Overdose:* In the event of accidental oral ingestion, routine measures such as gastric lavage should be performed as soon as possible after ingestion.

**Pharmacological properties**
*Pharmacodynamic properties:* Clotrimazole has a broad spectrum of activity (yeast, dermatophytes, moulds and a number of other fungi). It also exhibits activity against *Trichomonas vaginalis*, staphylococci, streptococci and *Bacteroides*.

Hydrocortisone has a vasoconstrictive effect thus reducing inflammation and oedema. It also has an antipruritic effect.

*Pharmacokinetic properties:* Following application of 1% $^{14}C$-clotrimazole cream (8 mg clotrimazole–200cm$^2$ with occlusive dressing for six hours) to five healthy volunteers, urinary excretion within six days amounted to a maximum of 0.2% of the activity applied. Maximum equivalent concentrations of clotrimazole in the serum remained below 0.0001μg/ml.

A study in 16 healthy volunteers following topical application of 1.5–2.5 g Canesten Hydrocortisone cream (doses of 15–25 mg hydrocortisone) resulted in no measurably effective levels of hydrocortisone in the blood or urine (analytical method used was Amerlex Cortisol $^{125}I$ RIA).

*Preclinical safety data:* The maximum oral dose of Canesten Hydrocortisone that could be administered to mice was not lethal.

Topical administration of the cream to rabbits produced dermatitis. However, the cream is well tolerated in man and the skin irritation seen in rabbits does not apply to human use.

**Pharmaceutical particulars**
*List of excipients:* Canesten Hydrocortisone contains the following excipients: Hostaphosphate KW solid; Cetylstearyl alcohol DAB; Myritol 318 DAB; benzyl alcohol PhEur; purified water PhEur.

*Incompatibilities:* None stated.

*Shelf life:* 30 months.

*Special precautions for storage:* The cream should be stored in a cool place.

*Nature and contents of container:* Aluminium tube with internal lacquer coating and HDPE screw-on cap containing 15 g of cream.

*Instructions for use/handling:* Not applicable.

**Marketing authorisation number** 0010/0216

**Date of approval/revision of SPC** January 1997.

**Legal category** P

# CIPROXIN*

## Presentation

*Infusion:* Clear, almost colourless to pale yellow solution containing 254.4 mg ciprofloxacin lactate (equivalent to 200 mg ciprofloxacin) per 100 ml solution.

*Tablets:* White, round, film-coated tablets marked on one side with the Bayer cross and "CIP 100" on the reverse side. Each tablet contains 116.4 mg ciprofloxacin hydrochloride monohydrate (equivalent to 100 mg ciprofloxacin).

White, scored, round, film-coated tablets, marked on one side with the Bayer cross, and with "CIP 250" on the reverse side. Each tablet contains 291 mg ciprofloxacin hydrochloride monohydrate (equivalent to 250 mg ciprofloxacin).

White, scored, oblong, film-coated tablets marked "BAYER" on one side and "CIP 500" on the reverse side. Each tablet contains 582 mg ciprofloxacin hydrochloride monohydrate (equivalent to 500 mg ciprofloxacin).

White, oblong, film-coated tablets marked "BAYER" on one side and "CIP 750" on the reverse side. Each tablet contains 873 mg ciprofloxacin hydrochloride monohydrate (equivalent to 750 mg ciprofloxacin).

**Uses** Ciprofloxacin is a synthetic, 4-quinolone derivative with bactericidal activity against a wide range of Gram-negative and Gram-positive organisms.

Ciprofloxacin is indicated for the treatment of single infections or mixed infections caused by two or more susceptible organisms. It may be used for infections caused by organisms resistant to other antibiotics, including aminoglycosides, penicillins and cephalosporins.

The extensive tissue penetration of ciprofloxacin combined with its enhanced antibacterial activity (including anti-pseudomonal activity), enables ciprofloxacin to be used alone (pending sensitivity results) or in combination with an aminoglycoside or with beta-lactam antibiotics, for instance when severe neutropenia is present, or with an antibiotic active against anaerobes where the presence of these organisms is suspected.

*Microbiology: In-vitro* studies have shown that the antibacterial action of ciprofloxacin results from the inhibition of bacterial DNA gyrase.

This mode of action differs from that of penicillins, cephalosporins, aminoglycosides and tetracyclines and, therefore, organisms resistant to these antibiotics are generally sensitive to ciprofloxacin.

Ciprofloxacin is active *in-vitro* against the following Gram-negative and Gram-positive organisms: *Citrobacter* spp., *Edwardsiella tarda, Enterobacter* spp., *Escherichia coli, Hafnia alvei, Klebsiella* spp., *Morganella morganii, Proteus* spp. (indole positive and indole negative), *Providencia* spp., *Salmonella* spp., *Serratia* spp., *Shigella* spp., *Yersinia* spp., *Aeromonas* spp., *Campylobacter coli, Campylobacter jejuni, Plesiomonas shigelloides, Pseudomonas aeruginosa, Vibrio* spp., *Haemophilus* spp., *Branhamella catarrhalis, Pasteurella multocida, Moraxella* spp., *Neisseria* spp., *Legionella* spp., *Brucella melitensis, Staphylococcus* spp., *Listeria monocytogenes, Corynebacterium* spp.

Ciprofloxacin is less active against the following organisms. Sensitivity testing should be performed before treatment is commenced: *Acinetobacter* spp., *Alcaligenes* spp., *Flavobacterium* spp., non-*aeruginosa Pseudomonas* spp., *Gardnerella vaginalis, Chlamydia* spp., *Mycoplasma* spp., *Mycobacterium tuberculosis, Mycobacterium fortuitum, Enterococcus faecalis, Streptococcus agalactiae, Streptococcus pneumoniae, Streptococcus pyogenes,* viridans group streptococci.

Anaerobes vary in their susceptibility from being moderately sensitive to resistant. In particular, the *Bacteroides fragilis* group and *Clostridium difficile* are resistant.

In addition, the following organisms are resistant to ciprofloxacin: *Ureaplasma urealyticum, Nocardia asteroides, Enterococcus faecium.*

Ciprofloxacin is not active against *Treponema pallidum.*

*In-vitro* studies have shown that additive activity often results when ciprofloxacin is used concomitantly with other antibacterial agents.

*Indications:* Ciprofloxacin is indicated for the treatment of the following infections caused by sensitive bacteria:

Severe systemic infection: e.g. septicaemia, bacteraemia, peritonitis, infections in immunosuppressed patients with haematological or solid tumours and in patients in intensive care units with specific problems such as infected burns.

Respiratory tract infections: e.g. lobar and bronchopneumonia, acute and chronic bronchitis, acute exacerbation of cystic fibrosis, bronchiectasis, empyema. Ciprofloxacin is not recommended as first-line therapy for the treatment of pneumococcal pneumonia. Ciprofloxacin may be used for treating Gram-negative pneumonia.

Ear, nose and throat infections: e.g. otitis media, sinusitis and mastoiditis, especially if due to Gram-negative bacteria (including *Pseudomonas* spp.). Ciprofloxacin is not recommended for the treatment of acute tonsillitis.

Urinary tract infections: e.g. uncomplicated and complicated urethritis, cystitis, pyelonephritis, prostatitis, epididymitis.

Skin and soft tissue infections: e.g. infected ulcers, wound infections, abscesses, cellulitis, otitis externa, erysipelas, infected burns.

Gastro-intestinal infections: e.g. enteric fever, infective diarrhoea.

Eye infections: e.g. bacterial conjunctivitis.

Infections of the biliary tract: e.g. cholangitis, cholecystitis, empyema of the gall bladder.

Intra-abdominal infections: e.g. peritonitis, intra-abdominal abscesses.

Bone and joint infections: e.g. osteomyelitis, septic arthritis.

Pelvic infections: e.g. salpingitis, endometritis, pelvic inflammatory disease.

Gonorrhoea: including urethral, rectal and pharyngeal gonorrhoea caused by beta-lactamase-producing organisms or organisms moderately sensitive to penicillin.

Ciprofloxacin is also indicated for prophylaxis against infection in elective upper gastro-intestinal surgery and endoscopic procedures where there is an increased risk of infection.

**Dosage and administration** General dosage recommendations: the dosage of ciprofloxacin is determined by the severity and type of infection, the sensitivity of the causative organism(s) and the age, weight and renal function of the patient.

*Adults*

*Ciproxin Infusion:* Ciproxin Infusion in 50 ml (100 mg), 100 ml (200 mg) and 200 ml (400 mg) infusion bottles may be infused directly and should be administered by short-term infusion over periods of 30–60 minutes. The dosage range for adults is 100–400 mg twice daily. The 400 mg dose should be administered over a period of 60 minutes.

In gonorrhoea, a single dose of 100 mg.

Infections of the lower and upper urinary tract, 100 mg twice daily.

For both upper and lower respiratory tract infections, 200–400 mg twice daily depending on the severity of the infection and the sensitivity of the causative organism (see Indications).

Although ciprofloxacin is not recommended as first-line treatment for pneumococcal pneumonia, where it is considered to be appropriate, oral ciprofloxacin may be used (see below).

Cystic fibrosis: In adults with pseudomonal infections of the lower respiratory tract, the dose should be 400 mg twice daily, although as the pharmacokinetics of ciprofloxacin remain unchanged in patients with cystic fibrosis, the low body weight of these patients should be taken into consideration when determining dosage.

In the majority of other infections, 200–400 mg twice daily depending on the severity of the infection.

Initial intravenous administration may be followed by oral treatment.

*Ciproxin Tablets:* Ciproxin Tablets should be swallowed whole with an adequate amount of liquid. The dosage range for adults is 100–750 mg twice daily.

In gonorrhoea, a single dose of 250 mg.

In acute, uncomplicated cystitis in women, 100 mg twice daily. In other infections of the lower and upper urinary tract (depending on severity), 250–500 mg twice daily.

In respiratory tract infections, 250–750 mg twice daily for both upper and lower respiratory tract infections, depending on severity. Although ciprofloxacin is not recommended as first-line treatment for pneumococcal pneumonia, where it is considered to be appropriate, a dosage of 750 mg twice daily should be used.

Cystic fibrosis: In adults with pseudomonal infections of the lower respiratory tract, the normal dose is 750 mg twice daily. As the pharmacokinetics of ciprofloxacin remain unchanged in patients with cystic fibrosis, the low body weight of these patients should be taken into consideration when determining dosage.

In the majority of other infections, 500–750 mg twice daily should be administered. In severe infections, particularly due to *Pseudomonas,* staphylococci and streptococci, the higher dosage of 750 mg twice daily should be used.

For surgical prophylaxis, a single 750 mg dose given 60–90 minutes before the procedure. The tablet may be given with an oral premedicant (but see interactions). In cases of suspected gastro-oesophageal obstructive lesions, ciprofloxacin should be administered in combination with an appropriate antibiotic effective against anaerobes.

*Impaired renal function:* Dosage adjustments are not usually required, except in patients with severe renal impairment (serum creatinine >265 micromole/l or creatinine clearance <20 ml/minute). If adjustment is necessary, this may be achieved by reducing the total daily dose by half, although monitoring of drug serum levels provides the most reliable basis for dose adjustment.

*Impaired hepatic function:* No adjustment of dosage is necessary.

*Elderly:* Although higher ciprofloxacin serum levels are found in the elderly, no adjustment of dosage is necessary.

*Adolescents and children:* As with other drugs in its class, ciprofloxacin has been shown to cause arthropathy in weight-bearing joints of immature animals. Although the relevance of this to man is unknown, its use in children and growing adolescents is not recommended. However, where the benefit of using ciprofloxacin is considered to outweigh this potential risk (e.g. cystic fibrosis), the dosage should be 5-10 mg/kg/day (intravenous) or 7.5–15 mg/kg/day (oral), depending upon the severity of infection, administered in two divided doses.

*Duration of treatment:* The duration of treatment depends upon the severity of infection, clinical response and bacteriological findings.

In acute, uncomplicated cystitis, the treatment period is 3 days.

In other acute infections the usual treatment period is 5 to 7 days with Ciproxin Infusion or 5 to 10 days with Ciproxin Tablets.

Generally, acute and chronic infections (e.g. osteomyelitis and prostatitis, etc), where the causative organism is known to be sensitive to ciprofloxacin, should be treated for at least 3 days after the signs and symptoms of the infection have disappeared.

**Contra-indications, warnings, etc**

*Contra-indications:* Ciprofloxacin is contra-indicated in patients who have shown hypersensitivity to ciprofloxacin or other quinolones.

Ciprofloxacin is also contra-indicated in children and growing adolescents except where the potential benefits of treatment outweigh the risks.

*Warnings and precautions:* Ciprofloxacin should be used with caution in epileptics and patients with a history of CNS disorders and only if the benefits of treatment are considered to outweigh the risk of possible CNS side-effects.

Ciprofloxacin could result in an impairment of the patient's ability to drive or operate machinery, particularly in conjunction with alcohol.

Crystalluria related to the use of ciprofloxacin has been reported. Patients receiving ciprofloxacin should be well hydrated and excessive alkalinity of the urine should be avoided.

Patients with a family history of or actual defects in glucose-6-phosphate dehydrogenase activity are prone to haemolytic reactions with quinolones, and so ciprofloxacin should be used with caution in these patients.

Tendon inflammation and rupture may occur with quinolone antibiotics. Such reactions have been observed particularly in older patients and in those treated concurrently with corticosteroids. At the first sign of pain or inflammation, patients should discontinue Ciproxin and rest the affected limbs.

*Drug interactions:* Ciproxin Tablets should not be administered within 4 hours of medications containing magnesium, aluminium, calcium or iron salts as interference with absorption may occur. When appropriate, patients should be advised not to self-medicate with preparations containing these compounds during therapy with Ciproxin.

Increased plasma levels of theophylline have been observed following concurrent administration with ciprofloxacin. It is recommended that the dose of theophylline should be reduced and plasma levels of theophylline monitored. Where monitoring of plasma levels is not possible, the use of ciprofloxacin should be avoided in patients receiving theophylline. Particular caution is advised in those patients with convulsive disorders.

Prolongation of bleeding time has been reported during concomitant administration of ciprofloxacin and oral anticoagulants.

Animal data have shown that high doses of quinolones in combination with some non-steroidal anti-inflammatory drugs (e.g. fenbufen, but not acetylsalicylic acid) can lead to convulsions.

Transient increases in serum creatinine have been seen following concomitant administration of ciprofloxacin and cyclosporin. Therefore, monitoring of serum creatinine levels is advisable.

The simultaneous administration of quinolones and glibenclamide can on occasion potentiate the effect of glibenclamide, resulting in hypoglycaemia.

Concomitant use with probenecid reduces the renal clearance of ciprofloxacin, resulting in increased quinolone plasma levels.

The use of metoclopramide with ciprofloxacin may accelerate the absorption of ciprofloxacin.

When ciprofloxacin is used for surgical prophylaxis, it is recommended that opiate premedicants (e.g. papaveretum) or opiate premedicants used with anticholinergic premedicants (e.g. atropine or hyoscine) are not used, as the serum levels of ciprofloxacin are reduced and adequate cover may not be obtained during surgery. Co-administration of ciprofloxacin and benzodiazepine premedicants has been shown not to affect ciprofloxacin plasma levels.

*Use in pregnancy and lactation:* Reproduction studies performed in mice, rats and rabbits using parenteral and oral administration did not reveal any evidence of teratogenicity, impairment of fertility or impairment of peri-/post-natal development. However, as with other quinolones, ciprofloxacin has been shown to cause arthropathy in immature animals, and therefore its use during pregnancy is not recommended. Studies have indicated that ciprofloxacin is secreted in breast milk. Administration to nursing mothers is thus not recommended.

*Side-effects:* Ciprofloxacin is generally well tolerated. The most frequently reported adverse reactions are: nausea, diarrhoea, vomiting, dyspepsia, abdominal pain, headache, restlessness, rash, dizziness and pruritus.

The following adverse reactions have been observed:

Gastro-intestinal disturbances, e.g. nausea, diarrhoea, vomiting, dyspepsia, abdominal pain, anorexia, flatulence, dysphagia. Rarely, pseudomembranous colitis.

CNS disturbances, e.g. headache, restlessness, depression, dizziness, tremor, convulsions, confusion, hallucinations, somnolence. Very rarely, sleep disorders and anxiety states. Isolated cases of ciprofloxacin-induced psychoses have been reported. There are isolated reports of intracranial hypertension associated with quinolone therapy.

Hypersensitivity/skin, e.g. rash, pruritus, urticaria, photosensitivity, drug-induced fever, anaphylactic/anaphylactoid reactions. Rarely, erythema nodosum and erythema multiforme. Very rarely, petechiae, haemorrhagic bullae, vasculitis, Stevens-Johnson Syndrome and Lyells Syndrome. Treatment with ciprofloxacin should be discontinued if any of the above occur upon first administration.

Hepatic disturbances, e.g. transient increases in liver enzymes or serum bilirubin (particularly in patients with previous liver damage), hepatitis, jaundice and major liver disorders including hepatic necrosis, which may rarely progress to hepatic failure.

Renal disturbances, e.g. transient increases in blood urea or serum creatinine, renal failure, crystalluria and nephritis.

Musculoskeletal disturbances, e.g. reversible arthralgia, joint swelling and myalgia. Rarely, tenosynovitis. Isolated cases of tendon inflammation have been reported, which may lead to tendon rupture. Treatment should be discontinued immediately if these symptoms occur.

Effects on haematological parameters, e.g. eosinophilia, leucopenia, granulocytopenia, thrombocytopenia, thrombocytosis, altered prothrombin levels and very rarely, haemolytic anaemia.

Special sense disturbances, e.g. very rarely, visual disturbances, impaired taste and smell, tinnitus and transient impairment of hearing, particularly at high frequencies.

Tachycardia has been reported.

In addition with Ciproxin Infusion, local irritation including pain at the site of injection has been reported, accompanied in a small number of patients by phlebitis or thrombophlebitis.

*Overdosage:* Based on the limited information available, in two cases of ingestion of over 18 g of ciprofloxacin, reversible renal toxicity has occurred. Therefore, apart from routine emergency measures, it is recommended to monitor renal function, including urinary pH and acidify, if required, to prevent crystalluria. Patients must be kept well hydrated and in the case of renal damage resulting in prolonged oliguria, dialysis should be initiated.

Calcium or magnesium antacids may be administered as soon as possible after ingestion of Ciproxin Tablets in order to reduce the absorption of ciprofloxacin.

Serum levels of ciprofloxacin are reduced by dialysis.

**Pharmaceutical precautions** Ciproxin Infusion is compatible with sodium chloride 0.9% solution, Ringer's Solution, glucose 5% and 10% solutions, glucose/saline and fructose 10% solution.

Ciproxin Infusion is incompatible with injection solutions (e.g. penicillins, heparin solutions) which are chemically or physically unstable at its pH of 3.9–4.5.

Unless compatibility is proven, the infusion should always be administered separately.

Since Ciproxin Infusion is light-sensitive, the bottles should always be stored in the cardboard outer container. No special precautions are required during the normal 30–60 minute infusion period.

Do not refrigerate Ciproxin Infusion. If the product is inadvertently refrigerated, crystals may form. However, these will redissolve at room temperature and do not affect the product's characteristics.

No special storage precautions are necessary for Ciproxin Tablets.

**Legal category** POM.

**Package quantities** Ciproxin Infusion, bottles of 50 ml, 100 ml or 200 ml.

Ciproxin Tablets 250 mg, 500 mg and 750 mg, blister strips of 10 in packs of 10, 20 and 100 tablets. Ciproxin Tablets 100 mg are available in blister packs of six.

**Further information** Ciproxin Infusion contains 0.01% w/v lactic acid plus 0.9% w/v sodium chloride, equivalent to approximately 154 mmol sodium per litre.

**Product licence numbers**

| | |
|---|---|
| Ciproxin Infusion | 0010/0150 |
| Ciproxin Tablets 100 mg | 0010/0145 |
| Ciproxin Tablets 250 mg | 0010/0146 |
| Ciproxin Tablets 500 mg | 0010/0147 |
| Ciproxin Tablets 750 mg | 0010/0148 |

## CIPROXIN* I.V. FLEXIBAG

**Qualitative and quantitative composition** Ciprofloxacin (INN).

*Quantitative composition per presentation:*

(i) 100 ml: One flexible container with 100 ml infusion solution contains Ciprofloxacin USP 200 mg in the form of ciprofloxacin lactate 254.4 mg, and 5% w/v dextrose.

(ii) 200 ml: One flexible container with 200 ml infusion solution contains Ciprofloxacin USP 400 mg in the form of ciprofloxacin lactate 508.8 mg, and 5% w/v dextrose.

**Pharmaceutical form** Solution for intravenous infusion.

**Clinical particulars**

*Therapeutic indications:* Ciprofloxacin is indicated for the treatment of the following infections caused by sensitive bacteria:

*Severe systemic infections:* e.g. septicaemia, bacteraemia, peritonitis, infections in immunosuppressed patients with haematological or solid tumours and in patients in intensive care units with specific problems such as infected burns.

*Respiratory tract infections:* e.g. lobar and bronchopneumonia, acute and chronic bronchitis, acute exacerbation of cystic fibrosis, bronchiectasis, empyema. Ciprofloxacin is not recommended as first-line therapy for the treatment of pneumococcal pneumonia. Ciprofloxacin may be used for treating Gram-negative pneumonia.

*Ear, nose and throat infections:* e.g. mastoiditis, otitis media and sinusitis, especially if due to Gram-negative bacteria (including *Pseudomonas* spp.). Ciprofloxacin is not recommended for the treatment of acute tonsillitis.

*Eye infections:* e.g. bacterial conjunctivitis.

*Urinary tract infections:* e.g. uncomplicated and complicated urethritis, cystitis, pyelonephritis, prostatitis, epididymitis.

*Skin and soft tissue infections:* e.g. infected ulcers, wound infections, abscesses, cellulitis, otitis externa, erysipelas, infected burns.

*Bone and joint infections:* e.g. osteomyelitis, septic arthritis.

*Intra-abdominal infections:* e.g. peritonitis, intra-abdominal abscesses.

*Infections of the biliary tract:* e.g. cholangitis, cholecystitis, empyema of the gall bladder.

*Gastro-intestinal infections:* e.g. enteric fever, infective diarrhoea.

*Pelvic infections:* e.g. salpingitis, endometritis, pelvic inflammatory disease.

*Gonorrhoea:* including urethral, rectal and pharyngeal gonorrhoea caused by β-lactamase producing organisms or organisms moderately sensitive to penicillin.

*In-vitro* investigations have indicated that ciprofloxacin is active against the following Gram-negative and Gram-positive organisms: *Citrobacter* spp., *Edwardsiella tarda, Enterobacter* spp., *Escherichia coli, Hafnia alvei, Klebsiella* spp., *Morganella morganii, Proteus* spp. (indole positive and indole negative), *Providencia* spp., *Salmonella* spp., *Serratia* spp., *Shigella* spp., *Yersinia* spp., *Aeromonas* spp., *Campylobacter coli, Campylobacter jejuni, Plesiomonas shigelloides, Pseudomonas aeruginosa, Vibrio* spp., *Haemophilus* spp., *Branhamella catarrhalis, Pasteurella multocida, Moraxella* spp., *Neisseria* spp., *Legionella* spp., *Brucella melitensis, Staphylococcus* spp., *Listeria monocytogenes, Corynebacterium* spp.

Ciprofloxacin is less active against the following organisms. Sensitivity testing should be performed before treatment is commenced: *Acinetobacter* spp., *Alcaligenes* spp., *Flavobacterium* spp., non-aeruginosa *Pseudomonas* spp., *Gardnerella vaginalis, Chlamydia* spp., *Mycoplasma* spp., *Mycobacterium tuberculosis, Mycobacterium fortuitum, Enterococcus faecalis, Streptococcus agalactiae, Streptococcus pneumoniae, Streptococcus pyogenes,* viridans group streptococci.

Anaerobes vary in their susceptibility from being moderately sensitive to resistant. In particular, the *Bacteroides fragilis* group and *Clostridium difficile* are resistant.

In addition, the following organisms are resistant to ciprofloxacin: *Ureaplasma urealyticum, Nocardia asteroides, Enterococcus faecium.*

Ciprofloxacin is not active against *Treponema pallidum.*

*In-vitro* studies have shown that additive activity often results when ciprofloxacin is used concomitantly with other antibacterial agents.

*Posology and method of administration:* The dosage of intravenous ciprofloxacin is determined by the severity and type of infection, the sensitivity of the causative organism(s) and the age, weight and renal function of the patient.

The dosage range for adults is 100–400 mg twice daily. The product should be infused directly and administered by short-term infusion over periods of 30–60 minutes. The 400 mg dose should be administered over a period of 60 minutes. Initial intravenous administration may be followed by oral treatment.

*Adults:* The following dosages for specific types of infection are recommended:

Table 1: Recommended adult dosage

| Indication | Dosage i.v. (mg ciprofloxacin) |
|---|---|
| *Treatment* | |
| Gonorrhoea | 100 mg single dose |
| Upper and lower urinary tract infections | 100 mg b.d. |
| Upper and lower respiratory tract infections (depending on severity and sensitivity of causative organism) | 200–400 mg b.d. |
| Pneumococcal pneumonia (second-line PL 0010/0148) | No recommended i.v. dosage, 750 mg p.o. b.d. |
| Cystic fibrosis patients with pseudomonal lower RTI† | 400 mg b.d. |
| Other infections as detailed under *Therapeutic indications* | 200–400 mg b.d. |

† Although the pharmacokinetics of ciprofloxacin remains unchanged in patients with cystic fibrosis, the low bodyweight of these patients should be taken into consideration when determining dosage.

*Impaired renal function:* Dosage adjustments are not usually required, except in patients with severe renal impairment (serum creatinine >265 micromole/l or creatinine clearance <20 ml/minute). If adjustment is necessary, this may be achieved by reducing the total daily dose by half, although monitoring of drug serum levels provides the most reliable basis for dose adjustment.

*Impaired hepatic function:* No adjustment of dosage is necessary.

*Elderly:* Although higher ciprofloxacin serum levels are found in the elderly, no adjustment of dosage is necessary.

*Adolescents and children:* As with other drugs in its class, ciprofloxacin has been shown to cause arthropathy in weight-bearing joints of immature animals. Though the relevance of this to man is unknown, its use in children and growing adolescents is not recommended. However, where the benefit of using ciprofloxacin is considered to outweigh this potential risk (e.g. in cystic fibrosis), the dosage should be 5–10 mg/kg/day, depending upon the severity of infection, administered in two divided doses.

*Duration of treatment:* The duration of treatment depends upon the severity of infection, clinical response and bacteriological findings. The usual treatment period for acute infections is 5–7 days.

Generally, acute and chronic infections (e.g. osteomyelitis and prostatitis, etc), where the causative organism is known to be sensitive to ciprofloxacin, should be treated for at least three days after the signs and symptoms of the infection have disappeared.

*Contra-indications:* Ciprofloxacin is contra-indicated in patients who have shown hypersensitivity to ciprofloxacin or other quinolone anti-infectives.

Ciprofloxacin is also contra-indicated in children and growing adolescents except where the benefits of treatment exceed the risks.

*Special warnings and precautions for use:* Ciprofloxacin should be used with caution in epileptics and patients with a history of CNS disorders and only if the benefits of treatment are considered to outweigh the risk of possible CNS side-effects.

Crystalluria related to the use of ciprofloxacin has been reported. Patients receiving ciprofloxacin should be well hydrated and excessive alkalinity of the urine should be avoided.

Patients with a family history of or actual defects in glucose-6-phosphate dehydrogenase activity are prone to haemolytic reactions with quinolones, and so ciprofloxacin should be used with caution in these patients.

Tendon inflammation and rupture may occur with quinolone antibiotics. Such reactions have been observed particularly in older patients and in those treated concurrently with corticosteroids. At the first sign of pain or inflammation, patients should discontinue ciprofloxacin and rest the affected limbs.

*Interactions with other medicaments and other forms of interaction:* Increased plasma levels of theophylline have been observed following concurrent administration with ciprofloxacin. It is recommended that the dose of theophylline should be reduced and plasma levels of theophylline monitored. Where monitoring of plasma levels is not possible, the use of ciprofloxacin should be avoided in patients receiving theophylline. Particular caution is advised in those patients with convulsive disorders.

Prolongation of bleeding time has been reported during concomitant administration of ciprofloxacin and oral anti-coagulants.

Animal data have shown that high doses of quinolones in combination with some non-steroidal anti-inflammatory drugs (e.g. fenbufen, but not acetylsalicylic acid) can lead to convulsions.

Transient increases in serum creatinine have been seen following concomitant administration of ciprofloxacin and cyclosporin. Therefore, monitoring of serum creatinine levels is advisable.

The simultaneous administration of quinolones and glibenclamide can on occasion potentiate the effect of glibenclamide resulting in hypoglycaemia.

Concomitant use with probenecid reduces the renal clearance of ciprofloxacin, resulting in increased quinolone plasma levels.

*Pregnancy and lactation:* Reproduction studies performed in mice, rats and rabbits using parenteral and oral administration did not reveal any evidence of teratogenicity, impairment of fertility or impairment of peri-/post-natal development. However, as with other quinolones, ciprofloxacin has been shown to cause arthropathy in immature animals, and therefore its use during pregnancy is not recommended. Studies have indicated that ciprofloxacin is secreted in breast milk. Administration to nursing mothers is thus not recommended.

*Effects on ability to drive and use machines:* Ciprofloxacin could result in impairment of the patient's ability to drive or operate machinery, particularly in conjunction with alcohol.

*Undesirable effects:* Ciprofloxacin is generally well tolerated. The most frequently reported adverse reactions are: nausea, diarrhoea, vomiting, dyspepsia, abdominal pain, headache, restlessness, rash, dizziness and pruritus.

The following adverse reactions have been observed:

Local irritation including pain at the site of injection accompanied in a small number of patients by phlebitis or thrombophlebitis.

Gastro-intestinal disturbances, e.g. nausea, diarrhoea, vomiting, dyspepsia, abdominal pain, anorexia, flatulence, dysphagia. Rarely, pseudomembranous colitis.

CNS disturbances, e.g. headache, restlessness, depression, dizziness, tremor, convulsions, confusion, hallucinations, somnolence. Very rarely, sleep disorders and anxiety states. Isolated cases of ciprofloxacin-induced psychoses have been reported. There are isolated reports of intracranial hypertension associated with quinolone therapy.

Hypersensitivity/skin, e.g. rash, pruritus, urticaria, photosensitivity, drug-induced fever, anaphylactic/anaphylactoid reactions. Rarely, erythema nodosum and erythema multiforme. Very rarely, petechiae,

haemorrhagic bullae, vasculitis, Stevens-Johnson Syndrome and Lyells Syndrome. Treatment with ciprofloxacin should be discontinued if any of the above occur upon first administration.

Hepatic disturbances, e.g. transient increases in liver enzymes or serum bilirubin (particularly in patients with previous liver damage), hepatitis, jaundice and major liver disorders including hepatic necrosis, which may rarely progress to hepatic failure.

Renal disturbances, e.g. transient increases in blood urea or serum creatinine, renal failure, crystalluria, nephritis.

Musculoskeletal disturbances, e.g. reversible arthralgia, joint swelling and myalgia. Rarely, tenosynovitis. Isolated cases of tendon inflammation have been reported which may lead to tendon rupture. Treatment should be discontinued immediately if these symptoms occur.

Effects on haematological parameters, e.g. eosinophilia, leucopenia, granulocytopenia, thrombocytopenia, thrombocytosis, altered prothrombin levels, and, very rarely, haemolytic anaemia.

Special sense disturbances, e.g. very rarely, visual disturbances, impaired taste and smell, tinnitus, transient impairment of hearing particularly at high frequencies.

Tachycardia has been reported.

*Overdose:* Based on the limited information available in two cases of ingestion of over 18 g of ciprofloxacin, reversible renal toxicity has occurred. Therefore, apart from routine emergency measures, it is recommended to monitor renal function, including urinary pH and acidify, if required, to prevent crystalluria. Patients must be kept well hydrated, and in the case of renal damage resulting in prolonged oliguria, dialysis should be initiated.

Serum levels of ciprofloxacin are reduced by dialysis.

## Pharmacological properties

*Pharmacodynamic properties:* Ciprofloxacin is a synthetic 4-quinolone derivative, with bactericidal activity. It acts via inhibition of bacterial DNA gyrase, ultimately resulting in interference with DNA function. Ciprofloxacin is highly active against a wide range of Gram-positive and Gram-negative organisms and has shown activity against some anaerobes, *Chlamydia* spp. and *Mycoplasma* spp. Killing curves demonstrate the rapid bactericidal effect against sensitive organisms and it is often found that minimum bactericidal concentrations are in the range of minimum inhibitory concentrations. Ciprofloxacin has been shown to have no activity against *Treponema pallidum* and *Ureaplasma urealyticum*, *Nocardia asteroides*, and *Enterococcus faecium* are resistant.

Plasmid-related transfer of resistance has not been observed with ciprofloxacin and the overall frequency of development of resistance is low ($10^{-9}$–$10^{-7}$). Cross-resistance to penicillins, cephalosporins, aminoglycosides and tetracyclines has not been observed and organisms resistant to these antibiotics are generally sensitive to ciprofloxacin.

Ciprofloxacin is also suitable for use in combination with these antibiotics, and additive behaviour is usually observed.

*Pharmacokinetic properties:* Absorption of oral doses of ciprofloxacin 250 mg, 500 mg and 750 mg tablet formulation occurs rapidly, mainly from the small intestine, the half-life of absorption being 2–15 minutes. Plasma levels are dose-related and peak 0.5–1.5 hours after dosing. The AUC also increases dose proportionately after administration of both single and repeated oral (tablet) and intravenous doses. The pharmacokinetic profile of intravenous ciprofloxacin was shown to be linear over the dose range (100 mg–400 mg). Following intravenous administration of ciprofloxacin, the mean maximum plasma concentrations were achieved at the end of the infusion period. That is, for a 100 mg or 200 mg dose, 30 minutes, and for a 400 mg dose, 60 minutes. Reported plasma levels at this time point were 1.8 mg/l, 3.4 mg/l and 3.9 mg/l, respectively. The absolute bioavailability is reported to be 52–83% and ciprofloxacin is subject to only slight first-pass metabolism.

Distribution of ciprofloxacin within tissues is wide and the volume of distribution high, though slightly lower in the elderly. Protein binding is low (between 19–40%). Ciprofloxacin is present in plasma largely in a non-ionised form.

Only 10–20% of a single oral or intravenous dose is eliminated as metabolites (which exhibit lower activity than the parent drug). Four different antimicrobially active metabolites have been reported, desethylene-ciprofloxacin (M1), sulphociprofloxacin (M2), oxaciprofloxacin (M3) and formylciprofloxacin (M4). M2 and M3 account for one third each of metabolised substance and M1 is found in small amounts (1.3–2.6% of the dose). M4 has been found in very small quantities (<0.1% of the dose). M1–M3 have antimicrobial activity comparable to nalidixic acid and M4 found in the smallest quantity has antimicrobial activity similar to that of norfloxacin.

Elimination of ciprofloxacin and its metabolites occurs rapidly, primarily by the kidney. After single oral and intravenous doses of ciprofloxacin, 55% and 75% respectively are eliminated by the kidney and 39% and 14% in the faeces within 5 days. Renal elimination takes place mainly during the first 12 hours after dosing and renal clearance levels suggest that active secretion by the renal tubules occurs in addition to normal glomerular filtration. Renal clearance is between 0.18–0.3 l/h.kg and total body clearance between 0.48–0.60 l/h.kg. Approximately 1% of a ciprofloxacin dose is excreted via the biliary route. The elimination kinetics are linear and after repeated dosing at 12 hourly intervals, no further accumulation is detected after the distribution equilibrium is attained (at 4–5 half-lives). The elimination half-life of unchanged ciprofloxacin over a period of 24–48 hours post-dose is 3.1–5.1 hours. A total body clearance of approximately 35 l/h was observed after intravenous administration.

Some studies carried out with ciprofloxacin in severely renally impaired patients (serum creatinine >265 micromole/l or creatinine clearance <20 ml/minute) demonstrated either a doubling of the elimination half-life, or fluctuations in half-life in comparison with healthy volunteers, whereas other studies showed no significant correlation between elimination half-life and creatinine clearance. However, it is recommended that in severely renally impaired patients, the total daily dose should be reduced by half, although monitoring of drug serum levels provides the most reliable basis for dose adjustment as necessary.

*Preclinical safety data:* Following extensive oral and intravenous toxicology testing with ciprofloxacin, only two findings which may be considered relevant to the use of ciprofloxacin in man were observed. Crystalluria was noted in those species of animals which had a normally alkaline urine. Kidney damage without the presence of crystalluria was not observed. This effect is considered a secondary inflammatory foreign-body reaction, due to the precipitation of a crystalline complex of ciprofloxacin, magnesium and protein in the distal tubule system of the kidneys. This is considered not to be a problem in man, because the urine is normally acidic. However, to avoid the occurrence of crystalluria, patients should be well hydrated and excessive alkalinity of the urine avoided.

As with other quinolones, damage to the weight-bearing joints of only juvenile rats and dogs treated with ciprofloxacin was noted in repeat dose toxicity testing. This was more noticeable in the dog. Although the relevance of this to man is unknown, the use of ciprofloxacin in children and growing adolescents is not recommended, unless the benefits are considered to outweigh the potential risks. Additionally, because of the potential of arthropathy, the use of ciprofloxacin during pregnancy and lactation is not recommended.

## Pharmaceutical particulars

*List of excipients:* Lactic Acid 20%, prepared from Lactic Acid PhEur and Water for Injections PhEur, Dextrose (hydrous) PhEur, Hydrochloric Acid PhEur and Water for Injections PhEur.

*Incompatibilities:* The Ciproxin I.V. Flexibag should not be mixed with any other drug product or the co-infusion solution 10% Laevulose (D-fructose) since compatibility has not been established with these products. For compatible co-infusion solutions see *Instructions for use/handling.*

*Shelf-life:* For both the 100 ml and 200 ml presentations, the shelf-life is two years.

*Special precautions for storage:* Store between 5–25°C, protected from light; avoid excessive heat and protect from freezing.

*Nature and contents of container:* Clear PVC flexible container, with PVC additive and administration port closures with a rubber sleeve stopper and butadienes-tyrene copolymer cap, containing 100 ml or 200 ml of Ciproxin I.V. Flexibag solution, with an aluminium foil overwrap.

*Instructions for use/handling:* The Ciproxin I.V. Flexibag should be infused directly and be administered by short-term intravenous infusion over a period of 30–60 minutes. The 400 mg/200 ml dose should be administered over 60 minutes. The product should not be mixed with other drug products or the co-infusion solution 10% Laevulose (D-fructose). However, Ciproxin I.V. Flexibag has been shown to be compatible with Ringer's solution, 5% fructose solution, isotonic sodium chloride solution and 10% glucose solution. Unless compatibility is proven, the infusion solution should always be administered separately. In addition, discard any unused portion of product immediately after use.

**Marketing authorisation number**  0010/0220.

**Date of approval/revision of SPC**  June 1996.

**Legal category**  POM.

# DTIC-DOME*

**Presentation** *Active ingredient:* 5-(3,3-dimethyl-1-triazeno) imidazole-4-carboxamide prepared as the citrate salt (dacarbazine).

200 mg vials of sterile dacarbazine.

DTIC-Dome is a colourless to ivory-coloured solid to be reconstituted with Water for Injections BP.

**Uses** *Actions:* Although the exact mechanism of action of dacarbazine is unknown, three hypotheses have been proposed:

1. Inhibition of DNA synthesis by acting as a purine analogue.
2. Action as an alkylating agent.
3. Interaction with sulphydryl groups.

The volume of distribution of dacarbazine exceeds body water content, suggesting localisation in some body tissues. Dacarbazine is only slightly (approximately 5%) protein bound. Its plasma half-life after intravenous administration is approximately 35 minutes. In animal studies, approximately 46% of radiolabelled dose was recovered from the urine after 6 hours. Of this 46%, almost half, was unchanged dacarbazine and a similar quantity was amino-imidazole carboxamide, a metabolite. Dacarbazine is subject to renal tubular secretion rather than glomerular filtration.

*Indications:* Metastatic malignant melanoma.
Sarcoma.
Hodgkin's disease.

In addition, dacarbazine has been shown, when used in combination with other cytotoxic agents, to be of value in treatment of other malignant diseases including: carcinoma of colon, ovary, breast, lung, testicular teratoma, and solid tumours in children.

**Dosage and administration** *Standard dose:* The following dosage schedules are recommended:

1. 2.0–4.5 mg/kg/day for 10 days, which may be repeated at 4 week intervals.
2. 250 mg/m²/day for 5 days, which may be repeated at 3 week intervals.
3. A further alternative is to administer the total schedule dose on the first day.

Other schedules may be used at the discretion of the prescribing physician.

*Children:* The dosage for children is calculated on a mg/kg or mg/m² basis as per the standard dosage.

*Administration:* DTIC-Dome 200 mg vials are reconstituted with 19.7 ml of Water for Injections BP. The resulting solution contains an equivalent of 10 mg/ml of dacarbazine. After the solution has been prepared, the calculated dose is drawn into a syringe and injected intravenously. Injection may be completed in one or two minutes.

If desired, the reconstituted solution may be further diluted with 125–250 ml of Dextrose Injection BP 5% or Sodium Chloride Injection BP 0.9% and administered by intravenous infusion over a period of 15 to 30 minutes.

**Contra-indications, warnings, etc** DTIC-Dome is contra-indicated in patients who have demonstrated a hypersensitivity to it in the past.

This product should not normally be administered to patients who are pregnant or to mothers who are breast feeding.

Studies have demonstrated this agent to have a carcinogenic and teratogenic effect when used on animals.

DTIC-Dome should be administered preferably to patients who are hospitalised and who can be observed carefully and frequently during and after therapy, with particular reference to the haemopoietic system.

Care must be taken to avoid extravasation of the drug subcutaneously during intravenous administration as this may result in tissue damage and severe pain.

Users should avoid contact of DTIC-Dome with the skin and eyes when reconstituting or administering.

It is recommended that DTIC-Dome be administered under the supervision of a physician experienced in the use of cancer chemotherapeutic agents. Since facilities for necessary laboratory studies must be available, hospitalisation is recommended.

Haemopoietic depression is the most common toxic side-effect of dacarbazine and involves primarily the leucocytes and platelets, although mild anaemia may sometimes occur. Leucopenia and thrombocytopenia may be severe enough to cause death. The possible bone marrow depression requires careful monitoring of white blood cell, red blood cell and platelet levels. Haemopoietic toxicity may warrant temporary suspension or cessation of dacarbazine therapy.

Symptoms of anorexia, nausea and vomiting are the most frequently noticed side-effects. Over 90% of patients are affected with the first few doses. The vomiting lasts for 1–12 hours and may be completely but unpredictably palliated by prochlorperazine.

Rarely, dacarbazine causes diarrhoea. Some helpful suggestions include restricting the patient's oral intake of fluids and food for 4–6 hours prior to treatment. The rapid toleration of these symptoms suggests a central nervous system mechanism, and usually these symptoms subside after the first 1 or 2 days.

Infrequently, some patients have experienced an influenza-like syndrome of fever to 39°C, myalgias and malaise. This syndrome occurs usually after large single doses and approximately 7 days after treatment with dacarbazine and lasts 7–21 days, and may recur with successive treatments.

Alopecia has been noted as has facial flushing and facial paraesthesia.

Hepatic toxicity, accompanied by hepatic vein thrombosis and hepatocellular necrosis resulting in death, has been reported. The incidence of such reactions has been low; approximately 0.01% of patients treated. This toxicity has been observed mostly when dacarbazine has been administered concomitantly with other anti-neoplastic drugs; however, it has also been reported in some patients treated with dacarbazine alone.

Anaphylaxis can occur very rarely following administration of dacarbazine.

Erythematous and urticarial rashes have been observed infrequently after administration of dacarbazine.

Rarely photosensitivity reactions may occur.

**Pharmaceutical precautions** Store in a refrigerator between 2°C and 8°C.

Dacarbazine, like all triazenes is sensitive to exposure to light and the reconstituted solution should be protected from light.

After reconstitution in the vial the solution may be stored, suitably protected from light, at 4°C for 72 hours or at normal room temperature for up to 8 hours.

If the reconstituted solution is further diluted in 5% Dextrose Injection BP or Sodium Chloride Injection BP 0.9% the resulting solution may be stored at 4°C for up to 24 hours.

**Legal category** POM.

**Package quantities** Vials containing 200 mg DTIC-Dome as sterile dacarbazine.

**Further information** When reconstituted, the injection contains dacarbazine 10 mg/ml in a solution containing citric acid and mannitol at pH 3.0–4.0.

**Product licence number** 0010/0128

# GLUCOBAY* 50
# GLUCOBAY* 100

**Presentation** *Glucobay 50:* Off-white round tablets of diameter 7 mm, each containing 50 mg acarbose. One side marked G50 and the reverse side marked with the Bayer cross.

*Glucobay 100:* Off-white round tablets of diameter 9 mm, each containing 100 mg acarbose. One side marked G100 with a scoreline and the reverse side marked with the Bayer cross.

**Uses**

*Mode of action:* Glucobay is a competitive inhibitor of intestinal alpha-glucosidases with maximum specific inhibitory activity against sucrase. Under the influence of Glucobay, the digestion of starch and sucrose into absorbable monosaccharides in the small intestine is dose-dependently delayed. In diabetic subjects, this results in a lowering of postprandial hyperglycaemia and a smoothing effect on fluctuations in the daily blood glucose profile.

In contrast to sulphonylureas Glucobay has no stimulatory action on the pancreas.

Treatment with Glucobay also results in a reduction of fasting blood glucose and to modest changes in levels of glycated haemoglobin (HbA₁, HbA₁c). The changes may be a reduction or reduced deterioration in $HbA_1$ or $HbA_{1c}$ levels, depending upon the patient's clinical status and disease progression. These parameters are affected in a dose-dependent manner by Glucobay.

Following oral administration, only 1–2% of the active inhibitor is absorbed.

*Indications:* Glucobay is recommended for the treatment of non-insulin dependent (NIDDM) diabetes mellitus in patients inadequately controlled on diet alone, or on diet and oral hypoglycaemic agents.

**Dosage and administration** Glucobay tablets are taken orally and should be chewed with the first mouthful of food, or swallowed whole with a little liquid directly before the meal. Owing to the great individual variation of glucosidase activity in the intestinal mucosa, there is no fixed dosage regimen, and patients should be treated according to clinical response and tolerance of intestinal side-effects.

*Adults:* The recommended initial dose is 50 mg three

times a day. However, some patients may benefit from more gradual initial dose titration to minimise gastro-intestinal side-effects. This may be achieved by initiating treatment at 50 mg once or twice a day with subsequent titration to a three times a day regimen.

If after six to eight weeks' treatment patients show an inadequate clinical response, the dosage may be increased to 100 mg three times a day. A further increase in dosage to a maximum of 200 mg three times a day may occasionally be necessary. Patients receiving the maximum dose require careful monitoring (see Warnings and Precautions).

Glucobay is intended for continuous long-term treatment.

*Elderly patients:* No modification of the normal adult dosage regimen is necessary.

**Contra-indications, warnings, etc**

*Contra-indications:* Hypersensitivity to acarbose or any of the excipients, use in children aged less than 12 years, pregnancy and in nursing mothers. Glucobay is also contra-indicated in patients with inflammatory bowel disease, colonic ulceration, partial intestinal obstruction or in patients predisposed to intestinal obstruction. In addition, Glucobay should not be used in patients who have chronic intestinal diseases associated with marked disorders of digestion or absorption and in patients who suffer from states which may deteriorate as a result of increased gas formation in the intestine, e.g. larger hernias.

Glucobay is contra-indicated in patients with hepatic impairment.

As Glucobay has not been studied in patients with severe renal impairment, it should not be used in patients with a creatinine clearance of <25 ml/min/ 1.73 m².

*Warnings and precautions*

*Hypoglycaemia:* When administered alone, Glucobay does not cause hypoglycaemia. It may, however, act to potentiate the hypoglycaemic effects of insulin and sulphonylurea drugs, and the dosages of these agents may need to be modified accordingly. Episodes of hypoglycaemia occurring during therapy must, where appropriate, be treated by the administration of glucose, not sucrose. This is because acarbose will delay the digestion and absorption of disaccharides, but not monosaccharides.

*Transaminases:* Glucobay may give rise to transient idiosyncratic elevations of serum hepatic transaminases, especially at higher doses. Patients titrated to the maximum recommended dose of 200 mg three times a day should be closely monitored, preferably at monthly intervals for the first six months. If elevated transaminases are observed, a reduction in dosage or withdrawal of therapy may be warranted, particularly if the elevations persist. In such circumstances, patients should be monitored at weekly intervals until normal values are established.

Intestinal adsorbents (e.g. charcoal) and digestive enzyme preparations containing carbohydrate splitting enzymes (e.g. amylase, pancreatin) may reduce the effect of Glucobay and should not therefore be taken concomitantly.

The concomitant administration of neomycin may lead to enhanced reductions of postprandial blood glucose and to an increase in the frequency and severity of gastro-intestinal side-effects. If the symptoms are severe, a temporary dose reduction of Glucobay may be warranted.

The concomitant administration of cholestyramine may enhance the effects of Glucobay, particularly with respect to reducing postprandial insulin levels. In the rare circumstance that both acarbose and cholestyramine therapy are withdrawn simultaneously, care is needed as a rebound phenomenon has been observed with respect to insulin levels in non-diabetic subjects.

In a pilot study to investigate a possible interaction between Glucobay and nifedipine, no significant or reproducible changes were observed in the plasma nifedipine profiles.

*Side-effects:* Owing to its mode of action, Glucobay results in a greater proportion of dietary carbohydrate being digested in the large bowel. This carbohydrate may also be utilised by the intestinal flora, resulting in the increased formation of intestinal gas. The majority of patients are therefore likely to experience one or more symptoms related to this, particularly flatulence, borborygmi and a feeling of fullness. Abdominal distension, abdominal pain, softer stools and diarrhoea may occur, particularly after sugar or sucrose-containing foods have been ingested. Rarely, these gastrointestinal reactions may be severe and might be confused with paralytic ileus.

The symptoms are both dose and dietary substrate related, and may subside with continued treatment. Symptoms can be reduced by adherence to the prescribed diabetic diet and the avoidance of sucrose or foodstuffs containing sugar. If symptoms are poorly tolerated, a reduction in dosage is recommended.

Should diarrhoea persist, patients should be closely

monitored and the dosage reduced, or therapy withdrawn, if necessary.

The administration of antacid preparations containing magnesium and aluminium salts, e.g. hydrotalcite, has been shown not to ameliorate the acute gastrointestinal symptoms of Glucobay and should therefore not be recommended to patients for this purpose.

Rarely, a transient elevation of serum hepatic transaminases may be observed. Very rarely, jaundice and hepatitis have been reported. Skin reactions may occur rarely.

*Overdosage:* No information on overdosage is available. No specific antidotes to Glucobay are known.

Intake of carbohydrate-containing meals or beverages should be avoided for 4–6 hours.

Diarrhoea should be treated by standard conservative measures.

**Pharmaceutical precautions** The tablets should be stored in the manufacturer's original container in a dry place at temperatures below 25°C.

**Legal category** POM.

**Package quantities** Blister packs in a cardboard outer containing:
Glucobay 50: 90 tablets
Glucobay 100: 90 tablets.

**Product licence numbers**

| | |
|---|---|
| Glucobay 50 | 0010/0171 |
| Glucobay 100 | 0010/0172 |

# KOGENATE* 250
# KOGENATE* 500
# KOGENATE* 1000

**Presentation** Kogenate is a sterile, lyophilised recombinant human Factor VIII preparation for reconstitution with Water for Injections. Kogenate is available as single-dose vials containing 250, 500 or 1000 I.U. Factor VIII. Glycine, sodium chloride, calcium chloride and human albumin are present as excipients.

A vial containing a suitable volume of Water for Injections for reconstitution, a sterile administration set and two alcohol swabs are also provided.

**Uses** Kogenate is indicated in congenital Factor VIII deficiency (haemophilia A) for the treatment and prophylaxis of bleeding in both untreated and previously treated patients without inhibitors. Treatment can be continued in patients who develop Factor VIII inhibitors (neutralising antibodies, less than 10 Bethesda Units (B.U.)) who continue to respond to Kogenate.

Kogenate does not contain von Willebrand Factor and hence is not indicated in von Willebrand's disease.

**Dosage and administration**
*Dosage:* Clinical studies have demonstrated a mean rise of about 2% in Factor VIII activity for each unit of Kogenate administered per kg body weight. The following formulae may be used to estimate (I) the appropriate dose required for a given response, or (II) the response to be expected from a given dose:

I. Required I.U. = body weight (kg) × desired Factor VIII rise (% of normal) × 0.5

II. Expected Factor VIII rise (% of normal) = $\dfrac{2 \times \text{administered I.U.}}{\text{body weight (kg)}}$

The dosage and duration of the substitution therapy should be based upon the patient's body weight, the degree of Factor VIII deficiency, the site and extent of the bleeding, the titre of inhibitors, the Factor VIII level desired and the clinical course. The following provides a guide for Factor VIII minimum blood levels.

*Treatment of haemorrhage:* The required Factor VIII minimum activity (in % of normal) is set out below. These minimal values should be maintained for the specified duration:

*Minor haemorrhage (haemorrhage into joints):* The therapeutically required plasma level of Factor VIII activity is 30% of normal, maintained for at least one day, and is dependent on the severity of haemorrhage.

*Moderate to major haemorrhage (e.g. haemorrhage into muscles or into the oral cavity), surgery (e.g. tooth extraction, operations of medium duration) and mild cranial trauma:* The therapeutically required plasma level of Factor VIII activity is 40–50% of normal maintained for three to four days or until adequate wound healing.

*Major to life-threatening haemorrhage (e.g. intracranial, intra-abdominal or intrathoracic haemorrhages, gastro-intestinal bleeding), major operations (e.g. cardiovascular, orthopaedic surgery) and fractures:* The therapeutically required plasma level of Factor VIII activity is 60–100% of normal, maintained for seven days, then therapy for another seven days to maintain the Factor VIII level at 30–50% of normal.

*Note:* The dose and the frequency of administration should be adapted according to the clinical effectiveness in each individual case. Larger amounts than those calculated may be required, especially at the beginning of treatment.

*Prophylaxis of haemophilia A:* In short or long-term prophylaxis of haemophilia A, doses of 10 to 50 I.U. Kogenate per kg body weight administered at intervals of two to three days have been successful in limiting the number of recurrent bleeding episodes. In some cases, especially in younger patients, shorter dosage intervals or higher doses may be necessary.

*Patients with Factor VIII inhibitors:* Kogenate remains efficacious in patients who have developed Factor VIII inhibitors (neutralising antibodies, less than 10 Bethesda Units (B.U.)), during treatment with Kogenate.

Factor VIII levels and inhibitor titres must be assessed to ensure adequate replacement therapy. The control of bleeding in patients with a high titre of inhibitors (typically above 10 Bethesda Units) may require extensive Factor VIII concentrate infusion therapy but might be impractical because of the very large dose needed to maintain adequate Factor VIII levels. If haemostasis cannot be achieved with Factor VIII concentrate in the presence of high-titre inhibitors, the use of (activated) prothrombin complex concentrate (PCC) should be considered. Such therapy should be undertaken by physicians experienced in the care of patients with haemophilia A.

*Reconstitution and administration:* Sterile conditions are required. Kogenate is intended for intravenous administration only and must be administered within four hours of reconstitution. Do not refrigerate after reconstitution.

Prior to use, clean the rubber stoppers of each vial with the alcohol swabs provided. Ensure that the solvent and the concentrate are warmed to room temperature first (maximum 37°C). To reconstitute the lyophilised powder, add the Water for Injections to the vial containing the lyophilised powder, using the transfer device provided. Use only the solvent provided. Ensure that all the solvent is drawn into the other vial. Remove the solvent vial and transfer device. Swirl continuously until the powder is completely dissolved. **Ensure** that Kogenate is completely dissolved before administration, i.e. a clear liquid is obtained.

Attach the filter needle to the syringe, insert into the rubber stopper of the vial containing the diluted Kogenate after swabbing the stopper, and fill the syringe as required. Remove the filled syringe from the filter needle (which should remain attached to the vial). Attach the venepuncture set to the syringe. Once ready to infuse, transfer Kogenate solution into the venepuncture set by depressing the syringe plunger until the tube is two-thirds full. Puncture vein and secure venepuncture set. Ensure no blood enters the syringe. The reconstituted Kogenate solution should be administered slowly, at not more than 1–2 ml per minute. Discard any unused solution.

If a further dose is required, leave the syringe connected to the venepuncture set until administration of the further dose. Fill a new syringe with reconstituted Kogenate and administer (as above). Remove venepuncture set once all doses have been given, apply pressure to injection site (for approximately two minutes) and apply a small pressure dressing.

**Contra-indications, warnings, etc**
*Contra-indications:* Known hypersensitivity to mouse or hamster protein (see Warnings).

Caution is advised in patients with known allergic reactions to the constituents of Kogenate.

*Warnings:* Kogenate should only be administered intravenously.

If allergic or anaphylactic reactions occur, administration of Kogenate should be stopped immediately and the patient treated for shock.

The required dose can only be calculated approximately. The plasma level of Factor VIII activity should be monitored therefore by appropriate clotting tests. A continuous monitoring of the plasma Factor VIII activity is recommended strongly especially in the case of major surgery or other operations. If bleeding cannot be controlled or the plasma Factor VIII level does not reach calculated values, the presence of Factor VIII inhibitors should be suspected and verified by appropriate tests.

The formation of neutralising antibodies, inhibitors, to Factor VIII is a known complication in the management of haemophilia A (see Side-effects). Therefore, previously untreated patients should be carefully monitored for the development of inhibitory antibodies by appropriate tests.

Animal reproduction studies have not been conducted with Kogenate. Based on the very rare occurrence of haemophilia A in women, experience regarding the use of Kogenate during pregnancy and lactation is not available. Kogenate should only be used during pregnancy and the breast feeding period if clearly necessary.

*Precautions:* No interaction of Factor VIII with other drugs is known.

There are no indications that Factor VIII may impair the ability to drive or to use machines.

Kogenate should not be mixed with other medicinal products or infusion solutions, as this could change its blood clotting activity.

Kogenate should be used promptly and always within four hours of reconstitution. Reconstituted Kogenate should not be refrigerated. Any unused solution must be discarded.

*Side-effects:* Following administration of Kogenate, mild to moderate adverse events have been observed rarely. These include burning, transient erythema and rash at the injection site, chest tightness, dizziness, mild hypotension and nausea.

Development of Factor VIII inhibitors has been observed, predominantly in previously untreated haemophiliacs receiving Kogenate. Thus previously untreated patients should be carefully monitored for the development of inhibitors by appropriate clinical observations and laboratory tests.

No patient in clinical studies with Kogenate developed clinically relevant antibody titres against the trace amounts of mouse and hamster protein present in Kogenate. Caution is advised in patients with known allergic reactions to the constituents of Kogenate.

*Overdosage:* No information on symptoms of overdosage is available.

**Pharmaceutical precautions** For both Kogenate and the solvent Water for Injections, store at +2°C to +8°C.

Do not freeze, since the solvent vial may break.

Do not use after the expiry date.

Do not refrigerate after reconstitution and use within four hours.

In exceptional cases, Kogenate and the solvent Water for Injections may be kept at room temperature (up to 25°C) for a limited period of up to three months. In this case, the expiry date **must** be observed and the date of the end of the three-month period must be noted on the vial and/or the outer packaging.

**Legal category** POM.

**Package quantities** Kogenate 250, Kogenate 500 and Kogenate 1000 are supplied as single dose vials containing 250, 500 or 1000 I.U. Factor VIII together with one vial of Water for Injections for parenteral use containing 2.5, 5.0 or 10.0 ml of solvent, respectively, and two sterile alcohol swabs. A sterile administration set is also provided for single use comprising one transfer device, one filter needle, one venepuncture set and one plastic syringe 5 ml (Kogenate 250 and 500) or 10 ml (Kogenate 1000).

**Further information** Kogenate is a recombinant human antihaemophilic Factor VIII preparation produced from genetically engineered baby hamster kidney cells containing a cloned Human Factor VIII gene.

**Product licence numbers**

| | |
|---|---|
| Kogenate 250, 500, 1000 | 0010/0194–0196 |
| Water for Injections | 0010/0095 |

# LIPOBAY* 100 MICROGRAM TABLETS ▼
# LIPOBAY* 200 MICROGRAM TABLETS ▼
# LIPOBAY* 300 MICROGRAM TABLETS ▼

**Qualitative and quantitative composition**
*Lipobay 100 Microgram Tablets:* Each tablet contains 95.4 micrograms cerivastatin in the form of 100 micrograms cerivastatin sodium.

*Lipobay 200 Microgram Tablets:* Each tablet contains 190.8 micrograms cerivastatin in the form of 200 micrograms cerivastatin sodium.

*Lipobay 300 Microgram Tablets:* Each tablet contains 286.2 micrograms cerivastatin in the form of 300 micrograms cerivastatin sodium.

**Pharmaceutical form** Film-coated tablet for oral administration.

**Clinical particulars**
*Therapeutic indications:* Primary hypercholesterolaemia (Types IIA + II B): The treatment of hypercholesterolaemia in patients who have not responded adequately to an appropriate diet.

*Posology and method of administration:* Prior to initiating Lipobay, secondary causes of hypercholesterolaemia should be excluded. Patients should continue on their standard cholesterol-lowering diet during treatment.

*Adults:* Lipobay should be taken once a day in the evening (at dinner or bed time).

The initial dose is 100 mcg once daily. At intervals of at least 4 weeks, the dosage may be increased by increments of 100 mcg depending on the response. The maximum recommended dose is 300 mcg once daily.

Administration with food does not influence the effect of cerivastatin.

A response to Lipobay is seen within two weeks and the maximum therapeutic response occurs within four weeks. The response is maintained during continuation of therapy.

*Elderly patients:* There is no clinical evidence to suggest the dosage needs to be different in these patients. In common with other agents, treatment should be initiated at the lower end of the dosage range.

*Renal impairment:* Patients with moderate to severe renal disease should initiate treatment at a once daily dose of 100 mcg. Subsequent titration, up to a maximum dose of 200 mcg once daily should be performed with caution.

*Children:* Owing to an absence of clinical experience, use in children is not recommended.

*Concomitant administration:* Whilst Lipobay is effective in lowering total and LDL cholesterol as monotherapy, efficacy may be enhanced when combined with a bile-acid sequestrant (e.g. cholestyramine, see *Interaction with other medicaments and other forms of interaction*).

*Contra-indications:* Known hypersensitivity to any component of Lipobay.

Myopathy, hepatic impairment or unexplained, persistent elevations in serum transaminases.

Pregnancy, lactation or women of childbearing potential unless adequately protected by non-hormonal contraceptive methods.

*Special warnings and precautions for use:*
*Liver function:* As with other statins, increases in liver enzymes have occurred during therapy with Lipobay. In the majority of cases these elevations were minor and asymptomatic. As with other lipid lowering agents, it is recommended that liver function tests be performed before treatment begins and periodically thereafter. Attention should be paid to patients who develop increased transaminase levels and therapy should be discontinued if increases in ALT and AST exceed three times the upper limit of normal (ULN).

Caution should be exercised when Lipobay is administered to patients with a history of heavy alcohol ingestion or a past history of liver disease (active liver disease or unexplained transaminase elevations are contra-indications to the use of Lipobay).

*Muscle:* As with other statins, sporadic elevations of creatine phosphokinase (CPK) have been observed in patients receiving Lipobay. These have usually been of no clinical significance. Rarely, myopathy, associated with marked elevations of CPK ($\geq$ 10 times the ULN) and/or with diffuse myalgias, muscle tenderness or weakness, has been reported with HMG-CoA reductase inhibitors. Patients should be asked to report promptly muscle pain, tenderness or weakness especially if accompanied by malaise or fever. Lipobay should be discontinued if markedly elevated CPK levels occur, or if myopathy is diagnosed or suspected. The risk of myopathy is known to increase in those patients receiving HMG-CoA reductase inhibitors who are concomitantly treated with cyclosporin, fibric acid derivatives, erythromycin, itraconazole and nicotinic acid.

There have been rare cases of renal dysfunction secondary to rhabdomyolysis with drugs of this class. Hence therapy with Lipobay should be temporarily withheld in any patient experiencing a condition predisposing to the development of renal failure secondary to rhabdomyolysis.

*Ophthalmological:* New subcapsular and nuclear opacities have been reported although, as with some other statins, a causal relationship with Lipobay has not been established.

*Interaction with other medicaments and other forms of interaction:* The involvement of cytochrome P450 isozyme CYP 3A4, besides others, in the metabolism of cerivastatin could be demonstrated by in-vitro experiments.

The co-administration of the non-specific cytochrome P450 inhibitor cimetidine did not lead to any significant changes in cerivastatin pharmacokinetics. Interaction studies with cytochrome P450 3A4 inhibitors (i.e. erythromycin, itraconazole, cyclosporin) have not been performed and therefore caution should be exercised when these products are co-prescribed. The effect of cytochrome P450 3A4 inducers (e.g. rifampicin or phenytoin) on cerivastatin pharmacokinetics is unknown.

The possible interaction with other substrates of this isozyme is unknown but should be considered for other drugs with a narrow therapeutic index (e.g. antiarrythmic agents class III including amiodarone).

No clinically significant effects were seen in a range of other interaction studies with drugs commonly prescribed in hypercholesterolaemic patients (e.g. warfarin, digoxin, antacids, cimetidine).

Bile acid sequestering agents: Lipobay should be administered at least four hours after the resin (e.g. cholestyramine) to avoid an interaction due to drug binding to the resin.

*Pregnancy and lactation:* There have been no teratogenic effects observed in animal studies. There are no data available on the use of Lipobay in pregnant women. Both cholesterol and other products of cholesterol biosynthesis are essential components of foetal development. Therefore HMG-CoA reductase inhibitors are contra-indicated during pregnancy and in women of child-bearing potential not taking adequate non-hormonal contraceptive precautions.

Lipobay should not be prescribed to nursing mothers.

*Effects on ability to drive and use machines:* None known.

*Undesirable effects:* In placebo controlled clinical studies of cerivastatin 100 mcg to 300 mcg the following events showed an increase over placebo – sinusitis (placebo subtracted incidence 3.8%), headache (2.2%), rhinitis (1.8%), increased cough (1.8%), insomnia (1.6%), flu syndrome (1.4%), myalgia (1.2%), abdominal pain ( 0.8%), arthralgia (0.7%), back pain (0.5%).

As with other statins, an increase of serum transaminases was observed in patients treated with Lipobay. The majority of the transaminase elevations seen in all treatment groups were mild (less than twice the upper limit of normal). In patients treated with cerivastatin 100 – 300 mcg, 0.46% developed clinically significant elevations of greater than three times the upper limit of normal for aspartate transaminase, and 0.44% similar elevations of alanine transaminase.

Elevated levels of creatine phosphokinase (CPK) greater than three times the upper limit of normal were seen in 1.7% of patients under treatment with cerivastatin for one year, and 2.1% for two years. In patients treated with cerivastatin doses 100 – 300 mcg, 0.18% of patients with normal CPK levels at baseline showed CPK elevations more than ten times the upper limit of normal.

*Overdose:* There is no experience with cerivastatin overdose. No specific antidotes to cerivastatin are known. Should overdose occur, treat symptomatically and institute appropriate supportive measures as required.

## Pharmacological properties

*Pharmacodynamic properties:* Cerivastatin is a synthetic, pure enantiomeric competitive cholesterol synthesis inhibitor which specifically inhibits the enzyme HMG-CoA reductase (hydroxy-methyl-glutaryl coenzyme A). This enzyme catalyses the rate-determining step in the synthesis of cholesterol, the conversion of HMG-CoA to mevalonic acid.

The primary site of action of cerivastatin is the liver.

By reducing intracellular cholesterol content, HMG-CoA reductase inhibitors cause secondary up-regulation of hepatic LDL receptors with increased LDL cholesterol clearance and reduction of both total, and LDL cholesterol in the serum.

*Pharmacokinetic properties:*
*Absorption and bioavailability:* cerivastatin is readily and almost completely absorbed from the gastrointestinal tract reaching maximum plasma concentrations ($C_{max}$) 2 – 3 h after oral administration. Maximum concentration and area under the concentration/time curve (AUC) increase dose-proportionally over the dosing range of 50 to 400 mcg.

The absolute bioavailability of cerivastatin is about 60%. Lipobay tablets show the same bioavailability as a solution (i.e. relative bioavailability is equal to 100%) with similar results for $C_{max}$ and $t_{max}$ The pharmacokinetics of cerivastatin are not influenced by concomitant administration of food.

Distribution: cerivastatin is highly bound to plasma proteins (99.1 – 99.5%). The volume of distribution at steady-state of about 0.3 l/kg body weight indicates that the drug penetrates only moderately into tissues. No accumulation is observed on repeated administration.

*Metabolism:* Two metabolic pathways are equally important in humans: demethylation of the benzylic methyl ether moiety and hydroxylation at one methyl group of the 6-isopropyl substituent. The product from the combined biotransformation reactions is observed as a minor metabolite. All three metabolites are active inhibitors of HMG-CoA reductase at a similar $ED_{50}$ value as the parent drug, contributing to the overall activity of the drug. The involvement of cytochrome P450 isozyme CYP 3A4, besides others, could be demonstrated by in-vitro experiments.

*Elimination:* Cerivastatin is exclusively cleared via cytochrome P450 mediated biotransformation (CYP 3A4 and others) with a plasma elimination half-life of approximately 2 – 3 h. Thirty percent of the dose is excreted as metabolites in urine, and 70% via the faeces. With a clearance of about 13 l/h cerivastatin can be regarded as a low clearance drug.

Cerivastatin intersubject variability for AUC and $C_{max}$ is described by coefficients of variation of approximately 30 to 40 %.

Age and gender have no clinically significant effects on the pharmacokinetics of cerivastatin. Comparable pharmacokinetic data have been found for different ethnic groups investigated.

A single 300 mcg oral dose of cerivastatin was administered to 18 patients with varying degrees of renal impairment (as determined by creatinine clearance ranging from 9 to 84 ml/min) and to 6 healthy young males. For cerivastatin, mean AUC, $C_{max}$, $t_\frac{1}{2}$, and unbound plasma fraction values tended to be higher in the renally impaired patients. The AUC and $t_\frac{1}{2}$ of the main active metabolite also tended to be higher in the renally impaired patients, although $C_{max}$ was lower in those severely impaired.

As cerivastatin is contra-indicated in patients with active liver disease, no pharmacokinetic investigations have been performed in this patient group.

*Preclinical safety data:* Increase in stillbirths and delays in bone development were found in the foetuses of rats treated with an oral dose of 0.3 mg/kg.

In a battery of *in vivo* and *in vitro* tests for the detection of point mutations, chromosomal aberrations and DNA-damage, cerivastatin has not been associated with mutagenic properties.

Liver tumours, known to occur in rodents with other statins, have been observed with cerivastatin in mice at oral doses of 6.75 mg/kg/day (males) and 11.5 mg/kg/day (females). These doses well exceed the therapeutic dose in man. Due to an almost completely different metabolism of cerivastatin in mice, these findings are not considered to be of relevance for man. No tumours have been found in rats.

## Pharmaceutical particulars

*List of excipients:* Lipobay tablets contain the following excipients: Mannitol PhEur, Crospovidone PhEur, Povidone 25 PhEur, Magnesium Stearate PhEur, and Sodium Hydroxide PhEur.

The tablets are film-coated with a mixture comprising Hypromellose PhEur, Macrogol 4000 PhEur, titanium dioxide (E171) and yellow ferric oxide (E172).

*Incompatibilities:* Not applicable.

*Shelf life:* The shelf life of Lipobay is 24 months.

*Special precautions for storage:* The tablets should be stored in the manufacturer's original container, in a dry place at temperatures up to 25°C.

*Nature and contents of container:* Blister strips in hard outers comprising: 300 µm polypropylene foil sealed with a 20 µm aluminium backing foil. Pack sizes: 14, 20, 28, 30, 50, 98, 100 and 160 (10 by 16).

*Instructions for use/handling:* None stated.

**Marketing authorisation numbers**
Lipobay 100 Microgram Tablets    0010/0226
Lipobay 200 Microgram Tablets    0010/0227
Lipobay 300 Microgram Tablets    0010/0228

**Date of approval/revision of SPC** July 1997

**Legal category** POM

## MIGRAVESS*

**Presentation** Round, flat, white tablets, 22 mm diameter marked on one side with a breakline and a letter 'm' in each half of the tablet.

Each dry tablet contains:

| | |
|---|---|
| Metoclopramide Monohydrochloride | 5 mg |
| Aspirin BP | 325 mg |
| Sodium Bicarbonate PhEur | 1180 mg |
| Citric Acid PhEur | 850 mg |

**Uses** Migravess is an analgesic and anti-emetic recommended for the rapid symptomatic relief of headache and nausea associated with migraine.

**Dosage and administration** *Adults:* Two tablets dissolved in water to be taken at the first symptoms of a migraine attack. If the attack persists the dose may be repeated up to a maximum of three doses (six tablets) per day.

*Young adults (12–15 years):* Half the adult dose.

Migravess must be dissolved completely in half a glass of water before taking.

**Contra-indications, warnings, etc**
*Contra-indications:* Migravess is contra-indicated in children under 12 years of age, in patients hypersensitive to aspirin or salicylates and in patients with haemostatic abnormalities or active peptic ulceration.

*Use in pregnancy:* Studies in several animal species have demonstrated no teratogenic effects with metoclopramide. Aspirin may prolong labour and contribute to maternal and neonatal bleeding. Therefore Migravess should only be used when there are compelling reasons. It is not advised during the first trimester and is best avoided at term. Migravess is not recommended during lactation because metoclopramide is excreted in breast milk.

*Warnings and precautions:* Aspirin may induce bronchospasm and asthma attacks in susceptible individuals or may induce gastro-intestinal haemorrhage.

Caution is necessary when patients' renal or hepatic function is impaired.

Care should be taken in patients on other centrally acting drugs, e.g. for epilepsy.

If vomiting persists the patient, especially if under 20 years of age, should be re-assessed in order to avoid masking an underlying disorder, e.g. cerebral irritation.

*Side-effects:* Various extra-pyramidal reactions to metoclopramide have been reported, particularly in the young and the elderly. The incidence may be increased if daily doses in excess of those recommended are administered. The reactions reported include spasm of facial, extraocular or cervical muscles. There may be a generalised increase in muscle tone. Any side-effects normally disappear within 24 hours of withdrawal of the drug. Should treatment be required, an anti-Parkinson drug of the anticholinergic type may be used to counteract these reactions.

Rarely, cases of neuroleptic malignant syndrome, an idiosyncratic response characterised by hyperthermia, muscle rigidity, altered consciousness including coma, and elevated CPK have been reported with metoclopramide.

In common with most anti-emetic drugs, metoclopramide may cause drowsiness but this is less common than with antihistamines. Other reported effects are lethargy, dizziness, insomnia, diarrhoea and flatulence.

Raised serum prolactin levels have been observed during metoclopramide administration. Metoclopramide may induce an acute hypertensive response in patients with phaeochromocytoma.

*Interactions:* Metoclopramide may result in altered absorption of other oral medication, e.g. decrease in digoxin absorption and increase in the absorption of paracetamol and various antibiotics. The effects of sympathomimetic drugs and tricyclic antidepressants may be affected.

Aspirin may enhance the effect of anticoagulants, oral diabetics and methotrexate, and may inhibit the action of diuretics and uricosuric agents.

Aspirin may potentiate the effects and side-effects of other non-steroidal anti-inflammatory drugs and may increase the risk of gastrointestinal bleeding during concomitant therapy with corticosteroids.

Migravess when taken with alcohol may enhance the effects of aspirin on the gastro-intestinal tract.

Migravess should not be administered concomitantly with atropine, any anticholinergic drug or concurrent with the administration of phenothiazines or butyrophenones.

*Overdosage:* If overdosage occurs treat with gastric lavage and supportive therapy. Atropine 2 mg intramuscularly should be given for dystonic reactions in adults.

Forced alkaline diuresis may be used. Restoration of the acid-base balance may be necessary.

**Pharmaceutical precautions**   Store in a dry place below 25°C and do not remove tablets from the foil until required.

**Legal category**   POM.

**Package quantities**   Migravess is available in cartons of 30 tablets (15 strips of 2 tablets). The tablets are packed in moisture-proof aluminium foil laminate.

**Further information**   Each tablet contains 323 mg of elemental sodium.

Migravess presents aspirin and metoclopramide in effervescent form intended to hasten gastric emptying and therefore absorption, with freedom from the side-effects often associated with ergotamine containing preparations.

**Product licence number**   0010/0109

## MIGRAVESS* FORTE

**Presentation**   Round, flat, white tablets, 22 mm diameter marked on one side with a breakline and a letter 'f' in each half of the tablet.

Each dry tablet contains:

| | |
|---|---|
| Metoclopramide Monohydrochloride | 5 mg |
| Aspirin BP | 450 mg |
| Sodium Bicarbonate PhEur | 1230 mg |
| Citric Acid PhEur | 850 mg |

**Uses**   Migravess Forte is an analgesic and anti-emetic recommended for the rapid symptomatic relief of headache and nausea associated with severe migraine.

**Dosage and administration**   *Adults:* Two tablets dissolved in water to be taken at the first symptoms of a migraine attack. If the attack persists the dose may be repeated up to a maximum of three doses (six tablets) per day.

*Young adults (12–15 years):* Half the adult dose.

Migravess Forte must be dissolved completely in half a glass of water before taking.

**Contra-indications, warnings, etc**

*Contra-indications:* Migravess Forte is contra-indicated in children under 12 years of age, in patients hypersensitive to aspirin or salicylates and in patients with haemostatic abnormalities or active peptic ulceration.

*Use in pregnancy:* Studies in several animal species have demonstrated no teratogenic effects with metoclopramide. Aspirin may prolong labour and contribute to maternal and neonatal bleeding. Therefore Migravess Forte should only be used when there are compelling reasons. It is not advised during the first trimester and is best avoided at term. Migravess Forte is not recommended during lactation because metoclopramide is excreted in breast milk.

*Warnings and precautions:* Aspirin may induce bronchospasm and asthma attacks in susceptible individuals or may induce gastro-intestinal haemorrhage.

Caution is necessary when patients' renal or hepatic function is impaired.

Care should be taken in patients on other centrally acting drugs, e.g. for epilepsy.

If vomiting persists the patient, especially if under 20 years of age, should be re-assessed in order to avoid masking an underlying disorder, e.g. cerebral irritation.

*Side-effects:* Various extra-pyramidal reactions to metoclopramide have been reported, particularly in the young and the elderly. The incidence may be increased if daily doses in excess of those recommended are administered. The reactions reported include spasm of facial, extraocular or cervical muscles. There may be a generalised increase in muscle tone. Any side-effects normally disappear within 24 hours of withdrawal of the drug. Should treatment be required, an anti-Parkinson drug of the anticholinergic type may be used to counteract these reactions.

Rarely, cases of neuroleptic malignant syndrome, an idiosyncratic response characterised by hyperthermia, muscle rigidity, altered consciousness including coma, and elevated CPK have been reported with metoclopramide.

In common with most anti-emetic drugs, metoclopramide may cause drowsiness but this is less common than with antihistamines. Other reported effects are lethargy, dizziness, insomnia, diarrhoea and flatulence.

Raised serum prolactin levels have been observed during metoclopramide administration. Metoclopramide may induce an acute hypertensive response in patients with phaeochromocytoma.

*Interactions:* Metoclopramide may result in altered absorption of other oral medication, e.g. decrease in digoxin absorption and increase in the absorption of paracetamol and various antibiotics. The effects of sympathomimetic drugs and tricyclic antidepressants may be affected.

Aspirin may enhance the effect of anticoagulants, oral diabetics and methotrexate, and may inhibit the action of diuretics and uricosuric agents.

Aspirin may potentiate the effects and side-effects of other non-steroidal anti-inflammatory drugs and may increase the risk of gastrointestinal bleeding during concomitant therapy with corticosteroids.

Migravess Forte when taken with alcohol may enhance the effects of aspirin on the gastro-intestinal tract.

Migravess Forte should not be administered concomitantly with atropine, any anticholinergic drug or concurrent with the administration of phenothiazines or butyrophenones.

*Overdosage:* If overdosage occurs treat with gastric lavage and supportive therapy. Atropine 2 mg intramuscularly should be given for dystonic reactions in adults.

Forced alkaline diuresis may be used. Restoration of the acid-base balance may be necessary.

**Pharmaceutical precautions**   Store in a dry place below 25°C and do not remove tablets from the foil until required.

**Legal category**   POM.

**Package quantities**   Migravess Forte is available in cartons of 30 tablets (15 strips of 2 tablets). The tablets are packed in moisture-proof aluminium foil laminate.

**Further information**   Each tablet contains 334 mg of elemental sodium.

Migravess Forte presents aspirin and metoclopramide in effervescent form intended to hasten gastric emptying and therefore absorption, with freedom from the side-effects often associated with ergotamine containing preparations.

**Product licence number**   0010/0108

## MINITRAN*

**Qualitative and quantitative composition**

*Minitran 5* has a surface area of 6.7 sq cm and contains 18 mg of glyceryl trinitrate. The average amount delivered in 24 hours is 5 mg.

*Minitran 10* has a surface area of 13.3 sq cm and contains 36 mg of glyceryl trinitrate. The average amount delivered in 24 hours is 10 mg.

*Minitran 15* has a surface area of 20 sq cm and contains 54 mg of glyceryl trinitrate. The average amount delivered in 24 hours is 15 mg.

**Pharmaceutical form**   Adhesive transdermal patch.

**Clinical particulars**

*Therapeutic indications:* Minitran 5, Minitran 10 and Minitran 15 are indicated for:

1. Prophylaxis of angina pectoris either alone or in combination with other anti-anginal therapy.

Minitran 5 is also indicated for:

2. Maintenance of venous patency at peripheral infusion sites.

*Posology and method of administration:*
*Adults:*

1. *Prophylaxis of angina pectoris:* The response to nitrates differs between individuals, and the minimum effective dose should be prescribed in each case. It is therefore recommended that treatment is started with one Minitran 5 patch per day, with upward dosage titration when necessary. Application can either be for a continuous period of 24 hours or intermittently, incorporating a patch free interval (usually at night). Attenuation of effect has occurred in some patients being treated with sustained release nitrate preparations. On the basis of current clinical studies it is recommended that in such cases Minitran should be applied daily with a patch free interval of 8–12 hours.

Each Minitran patch is contained in a sealed sachet. The adhesive layer is covered by a protective film, which should be removed before application. The Minitran patch should be applied to a clean, dry healthy area of skin on the torso or the arms.

Subsequent patches should not be applied to the same area of skin until several days have elapsed. The Minitran patch adheres easily to the skin, and also stays in place whilst bathing or during physical exercise.

2. *Maintenance of venous patency:* One Minitran 5 patch is applied distal and close to the site of intravenous cannulation at the time of venepuncture. The patch should be changed daily. Treatment with Minitran 5 should be discontinued when intravenous therapy is stopped.

*Elderly:* No specific information on use in the elderly is available, but there is no evidence to suggest that an alteration in dose is required.

*Children:* The safety and efficacy of Minitran in children has yet to be established, and therefore recommendations for its use cannot be made.

*Contra-indications:* The use of glyceryl trinitrate is contra-indicated in cases of known hypersensitivity to nitrates, severe anaemia, increased intra-ocular and intracranial pressure, and marked arterial hypotension. It is also contra-indicated in acute myocardial insufficiency due to obstruction as in aortic or mitral stenosis or of constrictive pericarditis.

*Special warnings and precautions for use:* Minitran is not indicated for the treatment of acute angina attacks requiring rapid relief. Minitran should be used only under strict medical supervision in recent myocardial infarction or acute congestive cardiac insufficiency. Minitran should be used with caution in patients with hypoxaemia, severe anaemia or ventilation perfusion imbalance.

The appearance of cross-tolerance with other nitrates is possible.

The use of products for topical application, especially if prolonged, may give rise to sensitisation phenomena, in which case treatment should be suspended, and suitable therapeutic measures adopted.

Minitran does not contain any metal components, and therefore it is not considered necessary to remove the patch prior to diathermy or cardioversion.

*Interactions with other medicaments and other forms of interaction:* Concomitant use of Minitran and other vasodilatory agents, calcium antagonists, beta-blockers, ACE inhibitors, neuroleptics, diuretics, antihypertensives, tricyclic antidepressants, and alcohol may decrease blood pressure. The effect of Minitran may be weakened by acetylsalicylic acid or other NSAIDs. There is a risk of coronary artery constriction with concurrent administration of dihydroergotamine.

*Pregnancy and lactation:* As with all drugs Minitran should not be prescribed during pregnancy, particularly during the first trimester, unless there are compelling reasons for doing so. It is not known whether the active substance passes into the breast milk. The benefits for the mother must be weighed against the risks for the child.

*Effects on ability to drive and use machines:* The product may give rise to postural hypotension, and it is therefore advisable to warn patients of this possibility, so that they avoid sudden positional changes at the start of treatment. Care should also be exercised when driving vehicles and operating machinery.

*Undesirable effects:*
*Central nervous system:* Glyceryl trinitrate is generally well tolerated. The most frequently encountered side effect is headache, particularly when high doses are used; this usually disappears after a few days, but in particularly intense cases, it may be necessary to reduce the dose or interrupt treatment.
*Cardio-vascular:* Other undesirable effects observed, especially at the start of treatment, are: arterial hypotension (especially postural), tachycardia, fainting, palpitations, hot flushes, dizziness.
*Gastro-intestinal:* Nausea and vomiting are rarely observed.
*Skin:* Reddening of the skin, with or without itching or a slight erythematous reaction is occasionally observed. These effects, however, generally disappear a few hours after removal of the patch without adopting other measures. The site of application should be altered daily to avoid local irritation.

*Overdose:* High doses of glyceryl trinitrate may sometimes induce too rapid a reduction in arterial pressure, causing collapse. Due to the controlled release of glyceryl trinitrate from Minitran, overdosage is likely to be rare. In cases of suspected overdosage the Minitran patch should be removed and any reduction of the arterial blood pressure and symptoms of collapse should be treated by appropriate measures.

**Pharmacological properties**
*Pharmacodynamic properties:* Nitroglycerin, the active constituent of Minitran is a dilator of smooth muscle, producing relaxation by an unknown mechanism. It has no direct effects on the inotropic or chronotropic state of the heart. It affects cardiac output only as a consequence of its effect on venous capacitance and arteriolar resistance vessels. These effects on preload and afterload reduce myocardial oxygen consumption and are primarily responsible for the mechanism by which nitroglycerin relieves the symptoms of angina pectoris. The drug's principal side effects (headache, flushing, dizziness, postural hypotension and tachycardia) are also a result of its smooth muscle relaxing effects.

*Pharmacokinetic properties:* When Minitran is applied to the skin, nitroglycerin is absorbed continuously through the skin into the systemic circulation and thus reaches the target organs (heart, vascular system) before deactivation by the liver. Minitran gives continuous release of nitroglycerin over 24 hours maintaining constant plasma levels. Nitroglycerin is metabolised by hydrolysis to dinitrates and the mononitrate.

*Preclinical safety data:* Not applicable.

**Pharmaceutical particulars**
*List of excipients:* Isooctyl Acrylate/Acrylamide Copolymer (93:7); Ethyl Oleate BP; Glyceryl Monolaurate; Low Density Polyethylene Film; One Side Silicone Coated Polyester Film.

*Incompatibilities:* None known.

*Shelf life:* 3 years.

*Special precautions for storage:* Minitran must be stored at room temperature (below 25 °C) under exclusion of light and moisture.

*Nature and contents of container:* Each patch is individually packed in a heat sealed foil sachet. Cartons contain 30 patches.

*Instructions for use/handling:* The patch is covered by a protective polyester film, which is detached and discarded before use.

**Marketing authorisation numbers**

| | |
|---|---|
| Minitran 5 | 00010/0231 |
| Minitran 10 | 00010/0232 |
| Minitran 15 | 00010/0233 |

**Date of approval/revision of SPC February 1997**

**Legal category** P

## NIMOTOP*
**Presentation**
*Nimotop tablets:* Yellow film-coated tablets marked with the Bayer cross on one side and with the letters SK on the reverse. Each tablet contains 30 mg nimodipine.

*Nimotop solution:* Vials for intravenous infusion, each containing 10 mg nimodipine in 50 ml (0.02%) of sterile aqueous alcoholic solvent.

**Uses**
*Mode of action:* Nimodipine is a calcium channel blocker of the dihydropyridine group with preferential activity on cerebral vessels. Nimodipine increases cerebral perfusion, particularly in poorly perfused areas, by arterial dilatation, an effect which is proportionately greater in smaller than in larger vessels.

*Indications:* Nimotop tablets are recommended for the prevention of ischaemic neurological deficits following aneurysmal or traumatic subarachnoid haemorrhage.
Nimotop solution is recommended for the treatment of ischaemic neurological deficits following aneurysmal or traumatic subarachnoid haemorrhage.

**Dosage and administration**
*Aneurysmal subarachnoid haemorrhage*
*Prophylactic administration:* The recommended dose is two tablets at 4-hourly intervals (total daily dose 360 mg), to be taken with water. Prophylactic administration should commence within four days of onset of subarachnoid haemorrhage and should be continued for 21 days.
In the event of surgical intervention, administration of Nimotop tablets should be continued (dose as above) to complete the 21 days treatment period.

*Therapeutic administration:* For the first two hours of treatment 1 mg of nimodipine, i.e. 5 ml Nimotop solution (about 15 µg/kg bw/h), should be infused each hour via a central catheter.
The dose should be increased after two hours to 2 mg nimodipine, i.e. 10 ml Nimotop solution per hour (about 30 µg/kg bw/h), providing no severe decrease in blood pressure is observed.
Patients of body-weight less than 70 kg or with unstable blood pressure should be started on a dose of 0.5 mg nimodipine per hour (2.5 ml of Nimotop solution), or less if necessary.
Therapeutic administration should commence as soon as cerebral ischaemia occurs, and should continue for at least five days up to a maximum of 14 days.
In the event of surgical intervention during treatment, administration of Nimotop solution should be continued (dose as above) for at least five days.
If cerebral ischaemia occurs during prophylactic administration, tablet treatment may be continued to complete the 21-day treatment period or substituted by Nimotop solution (dosage as above). Nimotop solution may be used with or without pre-treatment with Nimotop tablets. In the event of Nimotop tablets and Nimotop solution being administered sequentially the total duration of treatment should not exceed 21 days. Nimotop solution should not be administered for longer than 14 days. Nimotop solution and tablets should not be used concomitantly.
For administration, Nimotop solution must be drawn up into a 50 ml syringe and connected to a three-way stopcock using the infusion line provided. (The stopcock must allow for concomitant flow of the Nimotop solution and a co-infusion solution.) Nimotop solution must be administered with a co-infusion running at a rate of 40 ml/hr of either sodium chloride 0.9%, glucose 5%, Ringer's lactate solution, dextran 40, human albumin 5% or mannitol 10% which is connected to the second port of the three-way stopcock prior to its connection with the central line catheter.
Nimotop solution must not be added to an infusion bag or bottle and must not be mixed with other drugs.
Nimotop solution may be used during anaesthesia or surgical procedures.

*Traumatic subarachnoid haemorrhage:* Intravenous therapy should be started no later than 12 hours after trauma, as soon as possible after the presence of subarachnoid blood has been diagnosed. Administration of Nimotop solution should be continued for seven to ten days (dosage as for aneurysmal subarachnoid haemorrhage).
On completion of the intravenous therapy, it is recommended that oral administration of Nimotop tablets be continued for eleven to fourteen days, i.e. to complete the 21 day period (dosage as for aneurysmal subarachnoid haemorrhage).
The total duration of treatment with Nimotop should not exceed 21 days.

*Special precautions:* Nimotop solution reacts with polyvinylchloride (PVC). Polyethylene or polypropylene are the recommended plastic materials to be used during nimodipine infusion (see also 'Pharmaceutical precautions').
Polyethylene tubes are supplied with Nimotop solution 50 ml vials.

**Contra-indications, warnings, etc**
*Contra-indications:* Nimodipine should not be administered to patients during or within one month of a myocardial infarction or an episode of unstable angina.

*Warnings:* Nimotop tablets and solution should be used with care when cerebral oedema or severely raised intracranial pressure are present.
Nimotop tablets should not be administered concomitantly with Nimotop solution.
Nimodipine may potentiate the hypotensive effect of anti-hypertensives. Where concomitant administration of other calcium channel blockers (e.g. nifedipine, diltiazem, verapamil), α-methyldopa or beta-blockers is necessary, blood pressure must be monitored, and careful dose titration of nimodipine should be undertaken with possible reduction or discontinuation of the anti-hypertensive agent.
Nimotop solution must be used with caution in hypotensive patients.
Patients with known renal disease and/or receiving nephrotoxic drugs, should have renal function monitored closely during intravenous treatment with Nimotop solution.
Decreased drug clearance may occur in cirrhotic patients receiving Nimotop and therefore close monitoring of blood pressure is recommended in these patients.

*Drug interactions:* Concomitant administration of anti-epileptic drugs (phenobarbitone, phenytoin or carbamazepine) markedly reduces the bioavailability of orally administered nimodipine.
The simultaneous administration of cimetidine or sodium valproate may lead to an increase in the plasma nimodipine concentration.
Nimotop tablets should not be administered concomitantly with rifampicin since the efficacy of nimodipine could be reduced owing to enzyme induction.
The intake of grapefruit juice is not recommended in combination with nimodipine as it can result in increased plasma nimodipine concentrations due to the inhibition of the oxidative metabolism of dihydropyridines.

*Use in pregnancy:* No reproductive toxicology studies following parenteral administration are available. Reproductive toxicology studies in animals after oral administration showed no teratogenic effect. Nimotop tablets and solution should be used with caution in pregnant women, and only when the benefit of treatment is considered to outweigh the risk.

*Side-effects*
*Nimotop solution and tablets:* The following have been reported: decrease in blood pressure, slight increase or decrease in heart rate, flushing, headache, dizziness, gastro-intestinal disorders, nausea, sweating and feeling of warmth. Very rarely thrombocytopenia and ileus have been reported.

*Nimotop solution:* A transient rise in liver enzymes may occur during intravenous administration; this usually reverts to normal on completion of treatment. The infusion contains 20% ethanol and 17% polyethylene glycol-400; this should be taken into account during treatment.

*Overdosage*
*Nimotop Tablets:* If overdosage occurs, gastric lavage should be carried out and activated charcoal administered. If blood pressure is low, a vasopressor should be administered.

*Nimotop Solution:* If overdosage occurs, treatment should be discontinued immediately. If there is a large drop in blood pressure an intravenous injection of dopamine or noradrenaline may be indicated.

**Pharmaceutical precautions** Nimotop tablets should be stored in the manufacturer's original container in a dry place at a temperature not exceeding 25°C.
Nimotop solution is light sensitive and therefore should be stored only in the manufacturer's light-protective container within the cardboard carton at a temperature not exceeding 25°C. The solution when in the syringe must be protected from direct sunlight during administration, but it is stable in diffuse daylight and artificial light for up to 10 hours.
The solution should not be allowed to come into contact with PVC. The only plastic materials suitable for use are polyethylene or polypropylene. Nimotop solution is compatible with glass infusion bottles and infusion packs made of polyethylene (e.g. Polyfusor, Boots).
Nimotop solution 50 ml vials should be infused using a glass or rigid plastic (polyethylene or polypropylene) syringe and giving set (Gillette Sabre syringe; BD plastipak syringe; Monoject disposable syringe, Sherwood Medical Ltd; Combidyn tubes, Braun; Nitrocassette giving set, Imed Ltd.). Nimotop solution is incompatible with infusion bags and any giving sets made of PVC (e.g. Viaflex, Travenol; Steriflex, Boots).

**Legal category** POM.

**Package quantities** *Nimotop tablets:* Each pack contains 100×30 mg tablets in foil strips of 10.

*Nimotop solution:* Each pack contains 5×50 ml (0.02% solution) vials and 5 polyethylene infusion lines.

**Further information** Pharmacokinetic studies have shown the area under the curve to be similar following oral or intravenous administration of Nimotop at the recommended doses.

**Product licence numbers**
Nimotop tablets 0010/0137
Nimotop solution 0010/0138

## NYSTAFORM*-HC OINTMENT
## NYSTAFORM*-HC CREAM

**Presentation** *Nystaform-HC ointment:* Yellow ointment containing Nystatin BP 100,000 Units/g, Chlorhexidine acetate BP 1.0% w/w and Hydrocortisone Ph Eur 1.0% w/w in a water-repellent base.

*Nystaform-HC cream:* Light yellow cream containing Nystatin BP 100,000 Units/g, Chlorhexidine hydrochloride BP 1.0% w/w and Hydrocortisone Ph Eur 0.5% w/w in a water-miscible base.

**Uses** Nystatin is a fungistatic and fungicidal antibiotic primarily effective against *Candida albicans.* Chlorhexidine has activity against a wide range of bacteria. Hydrocortisone exercises a vasoconstrictive effect, thus reducing inflammation and oedema. Hydrocortisone also has an antipruritic effect.

Nystaform-HC preparations are indicated for the treatment of infected dermatoses where fungal (particularly monilial) and/or bacterial infections are present. The choice of cream or ointment depends upon the severity, physical characteristics and site of the condition, and upon the physician's preference.

**Dosage and administration**
*Adults and children:* For topical application only. Apply to the infected areas 2–3 times daily. Treatment should be for a maximum period of 7 days.

**Contra-indications, warnings, etc**
*Contra-indications:* Tuberculous lesions of the skin. Known sensitivity to any of the ingredients.

*Warnings and precautions:* For external use only. Avoid contact with eyes. If sensitivity occurs, or if new infection appears, discontinue use and institute alternative therapy.

In infants, long-term continuous topical steroid therapy should be avoided. Adrenal suppression can occur even without occlusion. As with other topical corticosteroids, systemic absorption may occur when extensive areas are treated, particularly under occlusion.

*Use in pregnancy:* Topical administration of corticosteroids to pregnant animals can cause abnormalities of foetal development including cleft palate and intrauterine growth retardation. The relevance of this finding to humans has not been established. However, topical steroids should not be used extensively in the first trimester of pregnancy and nystatin only with caution. The use of Nystaform-HC products requires that the anticipated benefits outweigh the possible risks.

*Side-effects:* Side-effects are uncommon. Hypersensitivity type reactions including application site reaction and allergic reactions are rarely reported.

*Accidental oral ingestion:* Nystatin is poorly absorbed from the gastro-intestinal tract. In the event, routine measures such as gastric lavage should be performed as soon as possible after ingestion.

**Pharmaceutical precautions** *Storage:* Store in a cool place.

**Legal category** POM.

**Package quantities** Nystaform-HC cream 15 g and 30 g tubes. Nystaform-HC ointment 30 g tubes.

**Further information** The water-miscible base of Nystaform-HC cream is particularly easy to apply to inflamed and tender skin. It is pleasant to use and does not leave the skin feeling greasy. The water-repellent base of Nystaform-HC ointment spreads easily and helps to protect against urine when used in the nappy rash area.

**Product licence numbers**
Nystaform-HC ointment 0010/0124
Nystaform-HC cream 0010/0123

## NYSTAFORM* CREAM

**Presentation** Light yellow cream containing Nystatin BP 100,000 Units/g and Chlorhexidine hydrochloride BP 1.0% w/w in a water-miscible base.

**Uses** Nystatin is a fungistatic and fungicidal antibiotic primarily effective against *Candida albicans.* Chlorhexidine has activity against a wide range of bacteria.

Nystaform preparations are indicated for the treatment of infected skin conditions where fungal (particularly monilial) and/or bacterial infections are present.

**Dosage and administration**
*Adults and children:* For topical application only. Apply to the infected areas 2–3 times daily. Continue application for one week after lesions have healed.

The patient should be advised that if the condition has not improved within seven days, to return to the surgery for further consultation. If the condition does not improve within 14 days of starting treatment, then an alternative treatment should be substituted.

**Contra-indications, warnings, etc**
*Contra-indications:* Known sensitivity to any of the ingredients.

*Warnings and precautions:* For external use only. Avoid contact with eyes. If sensitivity occurs, or if new infection appears, discontinue use and institute alternative therapy.

*Use in pregnancy:* As with all drugs nystatin should be administered with caution during the early months of pregnancy and its use requires that the anticipated benefits outweigh the possible risks.

*Side-effects:* Side-effects are uncommon. Hypersensitivity-type reactions including application site reaction and allergic reactions are rarely reported.

*Accidental oral ingestion:* Nystatin is poorly absorbed from the gastro-intestinal tract. In the event, routine measures such as gastric lavage should be performed as soon as possible after ingestion.

**Pharmaceutical precautions** *Storage:* Store in a cool place.

**Legal category** POM.

**Package quantities** 30 g tubes.

**Further information** The water-miscible base of Nystaform cream is particularly easy to apply to inflamed and tender skin. It is pleasant to use and does not leave the skin feeling greasy.

**Product licence number** 0010/0121

## SECUROPEN*

**Presentation** Vials containing 1.0 g, 2.0 g azlocillin as azlocillin sodium. Infusion vials containing 5.0 g azlocillin as azlocillin sodium. Securopen infusion sets containing 3×5.0 g azlocillin, 3×50 ml Water for Injections, 3 transfer needles and 3 hanging bags.

**Uses** Azlocillin is a broad spectrum antibiotic with especially significant anti-pseudomonal activity. In addition to *Pseudomonas* strains the spectrum of activity of azlocillin includes the following Gram-negative and Gram-positive pathogens: *Escherichia coli, Klebsiella/Enterobacter/Serratia* group, *Proteus* (indole-positive and indole-negative), *Providencia, Citrobacter, Salmonella* and *Shigella,* enterococci, staphylococci (penicillin sensitive), *Haemophilus influenzae,* gonococci, meningococci, pneumococci, streptococci and *Corynebacterium.* The spectrum also includes the anaerobic organisms *Clostridia* and *Bacteroides* species, including *Bacteroides fragilis.*

Azlocillin is indicated for the treatment of systemic and/or local infections due to sensitive organisms, especially infections of the respiratory and urinary tracts, and for septicaemia.

Azlocillin may be administered concomitantly with an aminoglycoside or with beta-lactamase stable isoxazolyl-penicillin, since there is evidence of synergy with these compounds.

**Dosage and administration**
*Adult Dosage:*
*Patients with normal renal function:* Life-threatening infections 5.0 g every 8 hours. In non-life-threatening and urinary tract infections 2.0 g every 8 hours.

*Children's Dosage:*

| *Age* | *Bodyweight (kg)* | *Daily dose (mg/kg bodyweight)* | *(g)* |
|---|---|---|---|
| 6–14 years | 20–40 | 3×75 | 3×1.5–3.0 |
| 2–6 years | 13–20 | 3×75 | 3×1.0–1.5 |
| 1–2 years | 10–13 | 3×75 | 3×0.75–1.0 |
| Infants | | | |
| 7 days–1 year | 3–10 | 3×100 | 3×0.3–1.0 |
| Neonates | | | |
| up to 7 days | 3 | 2×100 | 2×0.3 |
| Premature | 2.5 | 2×50 | 2×0.125 |
| babies | 2.0 | 2×50 | 2×0.100 |
| | 1.5 | 2×50 | 2×0.075 |

*Patients with impaired renal function:* i.e. with serum creatinine above 177 micromol/l (2 mg/dl) or with creatinine clearance less than 30 ml/minute, the unit dose should be as above but at 12-hourly intervals.

In patients presenting with severe impairment of both renal and hepatic functions, a further reduction of the dose may be necessary.

*Patients on haemodialysis:* Azlocillin is dialysable. On non-dialysing days, patients should receive the recommended unit dose of azlocillin twice daily. Before each dialysis an additional unit dose may be given to compensate for the amount of azlocillin removed by dialysis.

*Duration of treatment:* The duration of treatment depends upon the severity of the infection and also the clinical and bacteriological course of the disease. In principle, treatment should be maintained for at least 3 days after fever or clinical symptoms have disappeared. This, on average, requires 7–10 days therapy.

*Administration:* Azlocillin is administered intravenously as a 10% solution in Water for Injections. For doses of 2.0 g or less it is administered as a bolus injection and for higher doses it should be infused over 20–30 minutes.

Supplementary drugs should be injected through the drip tubing and not introduced into the bag or bottle containing azlocillin. In patients already receiving intravenous infusion therapy with other drugs, azlocillin should be infused during the intervening periods or as a parallel infusion. In order to achieve higher initial concentrations in the serum and tissues, up to half of the appropriate dose of azlocillin may be injected slowly through the tubing of the existing infusion.

*Combination therapy:* aminoglycosides, injectable tetracycline derivatives, ciprofloxacin, and metronidazole have proved to be incompatible with azlocillin and must therefore be administered separately. Before administering rarely used solutions or drugs, the compatibility of the individual components must be ascertained; precipitation, cloudiness or discolouration indicate possible incompatibility.

**Contra-indications, warnings, etc**
*Contra-indications:* A history of allergy to other penicillins and cephalosporins. Azlocillin is inactivated by beta-lactamases (penicillinases).

*Use in pregnancy:* Animal studies have shown no evidence of teratogenic or embryotoxic effects of azlocillin. However, as with all drugs, it should be administered with caution during the early months of pregnancy and its use requires that the anticipated benefits outweigh the possible risks.

*Side-effects:* Side-effects are uncommon and typical of other injectable penicillins. These may include: local irritation including pain at the site of injection; gastro-intestinal disturbances e.g. nausea, diarrhoea, vomiting, and occasionally pseudomembranous colitis; hypersensitivity reactions e.g. skin rashes, pruritus. Anaphylactic reactions may also occur.

Since very high serum levels of penicillins may induce seizures, dose adjustment is necessary in patients with severely impaired renal function.

Abnormal clinico-chemical and blood values, may be seen during therapy.

During treatment with high doses of azlocillin a prolongation of bleeding time may occur as a result of a dose-dependent disturbance of thrombocyte function.

*Interactions:* The duration of neuromuscular blockade due to vecuronium may be prolonged if azlocillin is administered at the end of the operation.

Patients being treated with azlocillin and concomitant heparin or other anticoagulants need more frequent control of coagulation parameters.

*Overdosage:* Overdosage should be treated by standard monitoring and supportive measures. Serum levels of azlocillin may be reduced by dialysis.

**Pharmaceutical precautions** *Storage:* Azlocillin should not be stored in temperatures exceeding 25°C. The expiry date is printed on the packaging.

*Dilution and compatibility:* Azlocillin should be freshly prepared immediately before administration by shaking the powder with a suitable volume of Water for Injections until completely dissolved to make a 10% solution – that is, 1.0 g in 10 ml, 2.0 g in 20 ml and 5.0 g in 50 ml. If azlocillin has to be prepared in advance of administration, it may be kept as the 10% solution at room temperature for 6 hours without loss of efficacy. Any unused solution should be discarded.

Azlocillin is compatible and stable in the common infusion fluids provided that the solutions are freshly prepared as above. These include 5% and 10% glucose solutions, fructose 5%, Ringer's solution and sodium chloride 0.9%. Compatibility with rarely used solutions must be ascertained prior to administration; possible incompatibility is indicated by precipitation, cloudiness or discolouration.

**Legal category** POM.

**Package quantities**   1.0 g, 2.0 g vials packed in boxes of 5.
5.0 g vial packed singly.
Infusion pack of 3 × 5.0 g with diluent, transfer needles and hanging bags.

**Further information**
Sodium content:
Each 5.0 g vial contains 10.84 mEq sodium (249.1 mg)
Each 2.0 g vial contains 4.33 mEq sodium (99.6 mg)
Each 1.0 g vial contains 2.17 mEq sodium (49.8 mg)
Displacement value 0.74 ml/g

**Product licence numbers**
Securopen   0010/0075
Water for Injections BP   0010/0095

## SYSCOR* MR

### Qualitative and quantitative composition
Syscor MR 10 1 film-coated tablet contains 10 mg nisoldipine.
Syscor MR 20 1 film-coated tablet contains 20 mg nisoldipine.
Syscor MR 30 1 film-coated tablet contains 30 mg nisoldipine.

**Pharmaceutical form**   Modified (extended) release tablets for oral administration.

### Clinical particulars
*Therapeutic indications:* For the first-line treatment of mild to moderate arterial essential hypertension and the prophylaxis of chronic stable angina pectoris.

*Posology and method of administration:* For oral administration, the tablets should be swallowed whole with a little liquid. The tablets should be taken once-daily at approximately 24-hour intervals, i.e. at the same time each day, preferably during the morning. Syscor MR tablets must be swallowed whole; under no circumstances should they be bitten, chewed or broken up.
A food interaction has been observed with Syscor MR, with an increase in peak plasma concentration and decrease in the area under the plasma concentration/time curve (AUC). It is therefore preferable to administer Syscor MR in the fasting state, i.e. before breakfast.
The recommended initial dose in angina pectoris is 10 mg once-daily. The usual maintenance dose is 20–40 mg once-daily. The maximum recommended dose is 40 mg once-daily.
In hypertension, the recommended initial dose is one 10 mg tablet once-daily. If necessary, the dosage can be increased according to individual requirements up to a maximum of 40 mg once-daily.
Patients should be assessed at least one week after starting on any dosage before titration to a higher dosage.
Patients with renal impairment should not require adjustment of dosage. Nisoldipine is highly protein-bound (>99%) and is not dialysable. Therefore, dose adjustment is not usually required in patients on dialysis.
An alteration of the pharmacokinetics of nisoldipine may be seen in the elderly with peak plasma concentrations and area under the plasma concentration/time curve being increased in some individuals, although there is no alteration of peak:trough fluctuation in plasma levels. Therefore, therapeutic plasma concentrations can be achieved with lower doses without compromising efficacy and safety. Therapy in the elderly with either angina pectoris or hypertension should commence with 10 mg once-daily, titration to higher doses being possible if clinically warranted and according to tolerability.
Treatment may be continued indefinitely.

*Contra-indications:* Syscor MR should not be administered to patients with known hypersensitivity to nisoldipine or other dihydropyridines because of the theoretical risk of cross-reactivity.
Syscor MR should not be administered to pregnant women, to nursing mothers or to children (aged less than 12 years).
Syscor MR should not be used in cardiogenic shock, unstable angina or during or within one month of a myocardial infarction.
Syscor MR should not be used for the treatment of acute attacks of angina.
The safety of Syscor MR in malignant hypertension has not been established.
Syscor MR should not be used for secondary prevention of myocardial infarction.
Syscor MR is contra-indicated in cases where there is a fixed cardiac output obstruction, such as aortic stenosis, as the decrease in peripheral resistance cannot be compensated by an increase in cardiac output, with ensuing risk of severe hypotension.
Owing to the duration of action of the formulation, Syscor MR should not be administered to patients with hepatic impairment.

*Special warnings and special precautions for use:*
Syscor MR tablets must be swallowed whole; under no circumstances should they be bitten, chewed or broken up.
Caution should be exercised in patients with hypotension as there is a risk of further reduction in blood pressure.

*Interactions with other medicaments and other forms of interaction:* Syscor MR may be used in combination with beta-blocking drugs, but the possibility of an additive effect resulting in postural hypotension should be borne in mind. Syscor MR may not prevent possible rebound effects after cessation of other antihypertensive therapy. A study of the interaction of Syscor MR with propranolol did not suggest a significant interaction of either drug on each other's pharmacokinetics, but a possible additive effect of the two drugs must be borne in mind.
The antihypertensive effect of Syscor MR may be potentiated by simultaneous administration of cimetidine. No interaction has been observed with ranitidine.
Decreased plasma levels have been observed with other dihydropyridine calcium antagonists during treatment with rifampicin. As this may also occur with Syscor MR, concomitant administration of rifampicin should be avoided.
Syscor MR does not influence the pharmacokinetics of quinidine, whilst quinidine may cause a small decrease in the AUC of Syscor MR. The clinical relevance of this interaction is probably small but it should be borne in mind that the dose of Syscor MR may need to be increased when using the two drugs concomitantly, to achieve the desired clinical effect.
As interactions have been observed on concomitant administration of phenytoin or carbamazepine with other calcium antagonists, the possibility of an interaction with Syscor MR cannot be excluded.
No interaction has been observed with concomitant administration of Syscor MR and warfarin or digoxin.
The concomitant intake of grapefruit juice may potentiate the effects of Syscor MR during the first 6–8 hours and therefore should be avoided. This effect may be due to a constituent of grapefruit juice which inhibits cytochrome $P_{450}$.

*Pregnancy and lactation:* The use of Syscor MR during pregnancy is contra-indicated.
The safety of Syscor MR for use in human pregnancy has not been established (Category B3). Evaluation of experimental animal studies has shown reproductive toxicity consisting of increased occurrence of phalangeal defects at maternally toxic doses.
Syscor MR is contra-indicated in nursing mothers, as nisoldipine may be present in breast milk.

*Effects on ability to drive and use machines:* None known.

*Undesirable effects:* Gravitational oedema, headache, flushing, tachycardia and palpitation may occur, particularly on commencement of treatment. Gravitational oedema is caused by peripheral dilatation and is not associated with heart failure or weight gain. Most vasodilatory side-effects improve or regress after a few weeks with continuation of therapy. Gravitational oedema may take longer to develop and may remain for longer than other acute vasodilatory side-effects.
Dizziness and gastrointestinal disorders such as nausea and constipation may also occur. Other less frequently reported side-effects include paraesthesia, hypotension, asthenia, dyspnoea and allergic skin reactions (rash, itching).
As with other sustained release dihydropyridines, exacerbation of angina pectoris may rarely occur at the start of treatment with nisoldipine. The occurrence of myocardial infarction has been described although it is not possible to distinguish such an event from the natural course of ischaemic heart disease.
Disturbances of the enzymes AST (SGOT), ALT (SGPT) and CPK may occur on Syscor MR. The abnormalities are usually slight increases in enzyme levels which tend to return to normal with continuation of therapy. If these abnormalities do not regress, or increase, within a few weeks, treatment should be discontinued. Enzyme elevations usually regress on discontinuation of the drug.
Syscor MR has a mild hypouricaemic effect.
Increased diuresis has been observed in isolated cases.

*Overdose:* Overdosage with Syscor MR has not been reported.
Symptoms of nisoldipine overdosage might include a fall in blood pressure, disturbances of cardiac rhythm and shock.
General measures to be taken in the event of nisoldipine overdosage include gastric lavage with the addition of activated charcoal and support of vital functions, with administration of oxygen, possibly mechanical ventilation and volume replacement.
Cardiac rhythm disturbances, especially bradycardia, may be treated symptomatically with beta-sympathomimetics. If these disturbances represent a danger to the patient, a temporary pacemaker may be necessary.
Hypotension due to cardiogenic shock and arterial vasodilatation may be treated with 10–20 ml of a 10% calcium gluconate solution administered slowly intravenously. This can raise the serum calcium level to the high-normal or slightly elevated range. If the effect is insufficient, vasoconstrictive sympathomimetics such as dopamine or noradrenaline must be given in addition. The dosage of these drugs should be determined by the clinical effect observed.

### Pharmacological properties
*Pharmacodynamic properties:* Nisoldipine is a specific and potent calcium antagonist of the dihydropyridine class. Nisoldipine has a selective blocking effect on the slow, voltage-dependent, calcium channels. The anti-anginal and antihypertensive effects of nisoldipine are determined by its high vascular selectivity, its vasodilatory action and consequent reduction of cardiac afterload, and by its natriuretic properties.
Nisoldipine has a coronary-selective action, dilating coronary vessels more potently than peripheral arterial vessels. Consequently, when nisoldipine is used to treat coronary heart disease, there is an improvement in myocardial oxygen supply as a result of coronary dilatation. There is also a reduction in oxygen consumption as a result of the reduction of afterload.
At therapeutic doses, nisoldipine has no negative inotropic effect and does not modify impulse generation or conduction in the heart.
In hypertension, the main effect of nisoldipine is to dilate the peripheral arterial vessels and thus reduce peripheral resistance.
There is no evidence of tolerance developing with Syscor MR during long-term therapy.

*Pharmacokinetic properties:* General characteristics: Orally administered nisoldipine is almost completely absorbed in the gastro-intestinal tract. Nisoldipine undergoes marked first-pass metabolism in the liver and gastro-intestinal tract, giving a systemic availability of approximately 4–8% after oral administration of a solution. Non-metabolised nisoldipine can be detected in the plasma 15–30 minutes after administration of a solution. Nisoldipine is eliminated through metabolism, 70–80% of its metabolites being excreted in the urine. The elimination kinetics are linear within the dosage range proposed. The intrinsic half-lives for nisoldipine are approximately 2 hours (beta-phase) and 10–12 hours (gamma-phase). Over 99% of nisoldipine is bound by plasma proteins.
The Syscor MR tablet is formulated to release nisoldipine in a controlled way to enable once-daily administration.
The pharmacokinetic profile of this formulation is characterised by low peak-trough fluctuation. 0–24 hour plasma-concentration versus time profiles at steady state are plateau-shaped, rendering the MR tablet appropriate for once-daily administration. Bioavailability of the drug in the MR formulation is 5.5%.
*Characteristics in patients:* There are age-related changes in pharmacokinetics of nisoldipine with the AUC of the drug being increased two- to three-fold in the elderly. However, the peak:trough fluctuation is similar to that in the non-elderly, and thus clinical effect may be achieved with lower doses without compromising safety.
There are no significant differences in the pharmacokinetics of nisoldipine between healthy subjects and subjects with renal impairment including anuric patients on haemodialysis. The latter indicates that dosage adjustment is not needed in these patients. Renal dysfunction does not influence the protein binding of nisoldipine.
Nisoldipine is partly metabolised in the liver. In patients with cirrhosis, $C_{max}$ and AUC may be increased approximately four-fold. Owing to the duration of action of the formulation, Syscor MR should not be administered to patients with hepatic impairment.

*Pre-clinical safety data:* In acute oral administration of nisoldipine, the active ingredient is only slightly toxic.
In subacute and subchronic studies in rats, nisoldipine was tolerated without damage at doses of up to 100 mg/kg p.o. Chronic administration to mice (21 months) and rats (2 years) provided no evidence of a drug related carcinogenic effect.
In chronic studies in dogs, with treatment lasting up to one year, the substance was tolerated without damage at doses up to and including 3 mg/kg p.o.
In studies of fertility, embryotoxicity, and perinatal and postnatal development in rats, doses of up to 10 mg/kg were tolerated without damage.
Studies in rabbits have not revealed any general embryotoxic or specific teratogenic effects after doses of up to 10 mg/kg p.o.
In an embryotoxicity study in monkeys, a dose which was maternally toxic (100 mg/kg p.o.) also induced phalangeal defects.
In in-vitro and in-vivo tests, nisoldipine has not been associated with mutagenic properties.

## Pharmaceutical particulars

*List of excipients:* Syscor MR tablets contain the following excipients: Lactose, crospovidone, magnesium stearate, maize starch, microcrystalline cellulose, sodium lauryl sulphate, polyvidone 25, hydroxypropylcellulose (low viscosity), hydroxypropylcellulose (medium viscosity), methylhydroxypropylcellulose, polyethylene glycol 4000, iron oxide yellow (E172), titanium dioxide (E171); 30 mg tablets contain, in addition, iron oxide red (E172).

*Incompatibilities:* Not applicable.

*Shelf life:* Shelf life of the product as packaged for sale:

| Primary packaging material | Shelf life (months) in climatic zones I | II | III | IV |
|---|---|---|---|---|
| 300 µm PP foil, colourless sealed with 20 µm hard aluminium foil with 3.5 g/m² heat-seal coating (PP) | 24 | 24 | 24 | 24 |
| 250 µm transparent PVC foil with 40 g/m² PVDC coating, sealed with 20 µm hard aluminium foil with 7 g/m² heat-seal coating (PVC/PVDC) | 24 | 24 | 24 | 24 |
| Laminated foil, 30 µm soft aluminium with 30 g/m² PE | 24 | 24 | 24 | 24 |
| Brown wide-necked bottles, glass type 3 with PE olive stoppers with tamper evident closure, white opaque | 24 | 24 | 24 | 24 |
| Inner bag: monofoil bag/sack 100 µm PE, colourless, transparent Outer container: fibre drum | 12 | 12 | 12 | 12 |

| | |
|---|---|
| Climatic zone I : | Moderate (20°C/50% r.h.) |
| Climatic zone II : | Warm and humid (Mediterranean, 25°C/60% r.h.) |
| Climatic zone III: | Hot and dry (30°C/50% r.h.) |
| Climatic zone IV: | Hot and humid (30°C/80% r.h.) |

*Special precautions for storage:* The tablets should be protected from strong light and stored in the manufacturer's original container.

*Nature and contents of container:* Calendar packs of PP or PVC, each containing 28 tablets (professional sample pack of 14 tablets also available).

*Instructions for use/handling:* The light-sensitive active ingredient of Syscor MR tablets is protected from light by film-coating the tablets. Nevertheless, it is advisable not to remove the tablets from the manufacturer's original container until immediately before use.

Syscor MR must not be used after the expiry date.

Keep out of the reach of children.

**Marketing authorisation numbers**

| | |
|---|---|
| Syscor MR 10 | 0010/0198 |
| Syscor MR 20 | 0010/0199 |
| Syscor MR 30 | 0010/0200 |

**Date of approval/revision of SPC**  February 1997.

**Legal category** POM.

## TRASYLOL*

**Presentation**  Colourless glass vials containing a solution of aprotinin for injection, each 50 ml vial containing 70 mg aprotinin (=500,000 Kallikrein Inactivator Units, KIU, =277.8 European Pharmacopoeia Units, PhEur units) in 0.9% sodium chloride solution.

**Uses**  Trasylol is an inhibitor of proteolytic enzymes including human trypsin, plasmin, and both plasma and tissue kallikrein.

Trasylol is indicated for the treatment of patients at high risk of major blood loss during and following open heart surgery with extracorporeal circulation. These include:

Patients requiring re-operation through a previous median sternotomy.

Patients with septic endocarditis.

Patients with known blood dyscrasias and coagulopathy, e.g. haemophiliacs, patients with von Willebrand's disease, patients receiving treatment with aspirin.

Trasylol is also indicated for the treatment of patients in whom optimal blood conservation during open heart surgery is an absolute priority. These include:

Jehovah's Witnesses who are to undergo open heart surgery with extracorporeal circulation.

Patients who require open heart surgery and are known carriers of a highly infectious virus, e.g. Hepatitis B, HIV.

Patients with rare blood groups who require open heart surgery.

Since Trasylol can contribute to the re-establishment of haemostasis by inactivating free plasmin, it is indicated for the treatment of life-threatening

haemorrhage due to hyperplasminaemia. Such haemorrhage has occasionally been observed during the mobilisation and dissection of malignant tumours, in acute promyelocytic leukaemia, and following thrombolytic therapy. Trasylol also inhibits the fibrinolytic activity of the plasmin-streptokinase complex formed following thrombolytic therapy with streptokinase.

**Dosage and administration**

*Open heart surgery*

*Adults:* The recommended regimen involves a loading dose, maintenance dose, and a pump prime dose, administered as follows:

*(i) Loading dose:* The loading dose of 200 ml (2 million KIU) should be administered intravenously after induction of anaesthesia and prior to sternotomy. The initial 5 ml (50,000 KIU) should be administered slowly, over several minutes, due to the small risk of allergic or pseudo-allergic reactions. The remainder of the loading dose should then be given as a slow intravenous infusion or injection over a period of 20 minutes.

*(ii) Maintenance dose:* The loading dose should be followed by the administration of a continuous infusion of 50 ml (500,000 KIU) per hour until the end of the operation except in patients with septic endocarditis where it may be continued into the early post-operative period.

*(iii) Pump prime dose:* An additional 200 ml (2 million KIU) should be added to the priming volume of the extracorporeal circuit. In patients with septic endocarditis 300 ml (3 million KIU) should be added to the pump prime.

*Elderly:* No dosage adjustment in the elderly is necessary.

*Children:* The dosage has not been established.

*Hyperplasminaemia*

*Adults:* Initially 50 ml (500,000 KIU) to 100 ml (1 million KIU) should be given by slow intravenous injection or infusion (maximum rate 10 ml/min). If necessary, this should be followed by 20 ml (200,000 KIU) hourly until bleeding stops.

*Children:* The dose should be calculated in proportion to the adult dose on the basis of body weight.

**Contra-indications, warnings, etc**

*Contra-indications:* Known hypersensitivity to aprotinin.

*Side-effects:* Trasylol is generally well tolerated but when given through a peripheral line may occasionally cause local thrombophlebitis.

Hypersensitivity or pseudo-allergic reactions can occur, not only after repeated courses of treatment but also with first administration. These include skin eruptions, tachycardia, pallor or cyanosis, dyspnoea, nausea and anaphylactic shock.

Trasylol should be administered slowly (maximum 10 ml/min) intravenously to the supine patient. If a hypersensitivity reaction occurs during the injection, administration should be stopped immediately and the appropriate therapeutic measures instituted, e.g. adrenaline, antihistamines and intravenous corticosteroids. Intravenous fluids, bronchodilators, and respiratory support may also be needed.

*Warnings:* The addition of Trasylol to heparinised blood will prolong the activated clotting time (ACT). Thus, the ACT should not be taken as a reliable indicator of the need to administer additional heparin during a prolonged period of cardiopulmonary bypass. Furthermore, a prolonged ACT in the presence of Trasylol does not necessarily signify excess heparin requiring additional protamine. It is therefore not necessary to adjust the usual heparin/protamine regimen during treatment with Trasylol.

*Use in pregnancy and lactation:* No evidence of teratogenic or embryotoxic effects has been seen in animals. Experience in human pregnancy and lactation is limited and inadequate to assess safety. As hyperplasminaemia is a life-threatening condition, Trasylol may be used during pregnancy and lactation when the benefit of treatment is considered to outweigh the risk.

*Overdosage:* There is no special antidote or other action to be taken.

**Pharmaceutical precautions**  Any unused solution should be discarded immediately. Trasylol vials are stable at room temperature. However, if the contents are cloudy, the product must not be used. Do not use the contents of the vials after the expiry date shown on the label.

Trasylol has been shown to be incompatible with corticosteroids, heparin, nutrient solutions containing amino acids or fat emulsions, and tetracyclines. Administration of Trasylol in mixed infusions (particularly with beta-lactam antibiotics) should be avoided. Trasylol is compatible with electrolyte and sugar solutions.

**Legal category** POM.

**Package quantities**  Trasylol is supplied as 50 ml vials each containing aprotinin 500,000 KIU (277.8 PhEur units).

**Further information** Nil.

**Product licence number** 0010/5900R

## YOMESAN*

**Presentation**  Yellowish tablets measuring 13 mm × 4 mm, each tablet containing 500 mg Niclosamide BP. One side marked FE, the reverse side with the Bayer cross. The tablets are flavoured with vanilla.

**Uses**  An anthelmintic for treatment of tapeworm infections:

| | |
|---|---|
| *Taenia saginata* | (beef tapeworm) |
| *Taenia solium* | (pork tapeworm) |
| *Diphyllobothrium latum* | (fish tapeworm) |
| *Hymenolepis nana* | (dwarf tapeworm) |

It has no effect in cysticercosis and echinococcosis due to cestode larvae (cysticerci) lodging in extra intestinal tissues.

**Dosage and administration**  *Taenia saginata, Taenia solium, Diphyllobothrium latum.*

| | |
|---|---|
| *Adults and children over 6 years:* | 4 tablets |
| *Children 2 to 6 years:* | 2 tablets |
| *Children under 2 years:* | 1 tablet |

In *Taenia solium* the tablets should be taken as a single dose after a light breakfast but in the case of *Taenia saginata* and *Diphyllobothrium latum* the dose may be divided, half being taken after breakfast and the remainder one hour later.

An aperient should be administered two hours later and in the case of *Taenia solium* a drastic purge should be given.

Infection due to *Hymenolepsis nana* should be treated for 7 days:

First day:

| | |
|---|---|
| *Adults and children over 6 years:* | 4 tablets |
| *Children from 2 to 6 years:* | 2 tablets |
| *Children under 2 years:* | 1 tablet |

The subsequent 6 days:

| | |
|---|---|
| *Adults and children over 6 years:* | 2 tablets |
| *Children from 2 to 6 years:* | 1 tablet |
| *Children under 2 years:* | ½ tablet |

It is important that the tablets are chewed thoroughly before washing down with water. In the case of small children the tablets should be ground up before administration.

**Contra-indications, warnings, etc**

*Contra-indications:* Hypersensitivity to niclosamide.

*Side-effects:* Very rarely the drug may cause mild transient GI disturbances (such as nausea, retching and abdominal pain), light headedness and pruritus.

*Overdosage:* Yomesan is not absorbed and no cases of overdosage have occurred. In the event of overdose a fast acting laxative and enema may be given. Vomiting should not be induced.

*Use in Pregnancy:* In common with most drugs it is wise to avoid treatment in the first trimester of pregnancy. Healthy children have been born to women treated with Yomesan in the first trimester of pregnancy.

Experimental studies in rats showed no embryotoxic or teratogenic effects.

*Warning:* In infections with *Taenia solium* there is always a danger of cysticercosis. A drastic purge is therefore recommended after treatment to eject the lower segment of the tapeworm containing mature eggs.

The hands should be thoroughly scrubbed after defaecation not only on the treatment day but for several days afterwards to avoid reinfection.

The consumption of alcohol during treatment must be avoided.

In the event of constipation it is imperative to restore regular bowel movements before Yomesan treatment.

**Pharmaceutical precautions**  The tablets are light sensitive and should only be stored in the original foil.

**Legal category** P.

**Package quantities**  Packs of 4 tablets of 0.5 g.

**Further information**  Unless the tapeworm is expelled by a drastic purgative, residual parts of it may be eliminated with the stools during the next two or three days. Thereafter, neither tapeworm segments nor ova should be present in the stools. In re-infection with *Taenia saginata* and *Taenia solium* new tapeworm segments or ova should only appear after three months.

In infections with *Hymenolepis nana* the follow-up period is only 14 days as surviving scolices regenerate very rapidly to sexually mature tapeworms and accordingly, after approx. 10 days, ova are eliminated with the stools.

**Product licence number** 0010/5910R

*Trade Mark

## Bayer Bridgend

Bayer House
Strawberry Hill
Newbury
Berkshire RG14 1JA

## GAMIMUNE* N

**Presentation** Gamimune N is a sterile, 5% intra-venous solution (pH 4.25) of unmodified human immunoglobulin stabilised with 10% maltose.

### Uses

*Mode of action:* Gamimune N is a stable preparation of unmodified normal immunoglobulin. It retains the functional activities of the IgG molecule and has a very low level of spontaneous anticomplementary activity.

The precise mode of action in idiopathic thrombocytopenic purpura has yet to be elucidated.

*Indications:* Replacement therapy for congenital agammaglobulinaemia and hypogammaglobulinaemia.

Treatment of idiopathic thrombocytopenic purpura.

Prophylaxis of infection following bone marrow transplantation.

### Dosage and administration

*Dosage:*

*Replacement therapy for congenital agammaglobulinaemia and hypogammaglobulinaemia:* The usual dose of Gamimune N for prophylaxis in immunodeficiency syndromes is 100 mg to 200 mg/kg (2–4 ml/kg) bodyweight, administered once a month by intravenous infusion. The dose may be given more frequently or increased to 400 mg/kg (8 ml/kg) bodyweight if the clinical response is inadequate or the level of IgG achieved in the circulation is felt to be insufficient.

*Idiopathic thrombocytopenic purpura:* The treatment dose is 400 mg/kg bodyweight daily by intravenous infusion for five successive days. A maintenance dose of 400 mg/kg bodyweight may be administered as a single dose every few weeks or as required to maintain the platelet count.

*Bone marrow transplantation:* The prophylactic dose is 500 mg/kg bodyweight and should be administered on both day 7 and day 2 prior to transplant. The same dose should then be administered on day 6 post-operatively and thereafter at weekly intervals until day 90.

*Administration:* Gamimune N should be infused intravenously at an initial rate of 0.01 to 0.02 ml/kg bodyweight per minute for 30 minutes. If well tolerated, the rate may be gradually increased to a maximum of 0.08 ml/kg bodyweight per minute for the remainder of the infusion. If side-effects occur, the rate should be reduced or the infusion interrupted until symptoms subside. The infusion may then be resumed at the rate which is comfortable for the patient.

In patients undergoing bone marrow transplants, Gamimune N can be administered through a central catheter until the patient is discharged. Thereafter infusions may be given via a peripheral vein.

### Contra-indications, warnings, etc

*Contra-indications:* Gamimune N is contra-indicated in individuals who are known to have had an anaphylactic or severe systemic response to Immune Serum Globulin (Human).

Individuals with IgA deficiencies should not receive Gamimune N or any immunoglobulin preparation.

*Warnings:* Gamimune N should be administered only intravenously.

On rare occasions, Gamimune N may cause a precipitous fall in blood pressure and the clinical picture of anaphylaxis, even when the patient has shown no sensitivity to previous administration of immunoglobulin preparations. These reactions appear to be related to the rate of infusion. Accordingly, the infusion rate given under 'Dosage and administration' should be closely followed, at least until the physician has had sufficient experience with a given patient. Patients should be monitored closely and careful observation made for any symptoms throughout the infusion period. Adrenaline should be readily available for treatment of any acute anaphylactoid reaction.

Gamimune N should be administered during pregnancy only if clearly needed. Animal reproduction studies have not been conducted.

The risk of transmission of infection, in particular Non–A, Non–B hepatitis, by intravenous immunoglobulin preparations cannot be entirely excluded.

*Precautions:* Although Gamimune N may be diluted with 5% dextrose no other drug interactions or compatibilities have been evaluated.

Gamimune N should be infused via a separate line and not mixed with other intravenous fluids or medications.

Gamimune N should be used promptly after entering vial. Do not use if turbid.

*Side-effects:* Reported side-effects include chills, headache, nausea, and mild back or hip pain during infusion.

In isolated cases, particularly with high doses of immunoglobulins, symptoms of aseptic meningitis syndrome have been reported. The syndrome is characterised by severe headaches, stiff neck, drowsiness, fever, photophobia, pain on movement of eyes, vertigo and vomiting. The symptoms resolve spontaneously without sequelae.

In rare cases, impairment of renal function and an increase in serum creatinine may occur. This may lead to acute renal failure. The onset may occur after a few days and is reversible on cessation of treatment.

*Overdosage:* Overdosage with Gamimune N has not been reported but any adverse effects would be expected to be similar to those which may occur on rare occasions with normal doses.

**Pharmaceutical precautions** Store at 2°C to 8°C. Do not freeze. Partially used vials must be discarded.

**Legal category** POM.

**Package quantities** Gamimune N is supplied in 0.5 g: 10 ml, 2.5 g: 50 ml or 5.0 g: 100 ml single dose vials.

**Further information** Gamimune N is prepared by cold alcohol fractionation of large pools of human venous plasma. Each individual unit of plasma has been tested and found non-reactive for hepatitis B surface antigen and antibody to human immunodeficiency virus 1 (HIV–1) by approved FDA tests. Each unit used in the manufacture of this product has been found to have an ALT level less than twice the upper limit of normal for the test. The immunoglobulin has not been chemically modified.

Not less than 90% of the gammaglobulin is monomer. The rest is dimer and not more than 5% fragments and 5% aggregates. Also present are traces of IgA and IgM. The distribution of subclasses is similar to that found in normal serum.

Gamimune N has a buffer capacity of 16.5 mEq/l (approximately 0.3 mEq/g of protein). A dose of 150–400 mg/kg (3–8 ml/kg) therefore represents an acid load of 0.0495–0.1320 mEq/kg.

**Product licence number** 0055/0109

*Trade Mark

**Beecham Research**
Welwyn Garden City
Hertfordshire AL7 1EY

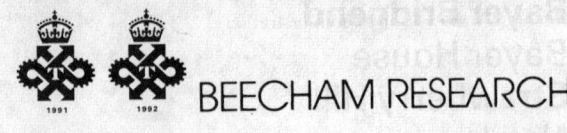

BEECHAM RESEARCH

## AMPICLOX* CAPSULES
## AMPICLOX* SYRUP
## AMPICLOX* NEONATAL SUSPENSION
## AMPICLOX* INJECTION
## AMPICLOX* NEONATAL INJECTION

**Presentation** *Ampiclox Capsules:* Black and amethyst capsules, each containing 250 mg ampicillin as Ampicillin Trihydrate PhEur and 250 mg cloxacillin as Cloxacillin Sodium PhEur.

*Ampiclox Syrup:* Bottles containing powder for the preparation of 100 ml fruit-flavoured syrup. When reconstituted each 5 ml contains 125 mg ampicillin as Ampicillin Trihydrate PhEur and 125 mg cloxacillin as Cloxacillin Sodium PhEur.

*Ampiclox Neonatal Suspension:* Bottles containing powder for the preparation of 10 ml suspension. When reconstituted each 0.6 ml dose contains 60 mg ampicillin as Ampicillin Trihydrate PhEur with 30 mg cloxacillin as Cloxacillin Sodium PhEur. A pipette to measure the 0.6 ml dose is provided.

*Ampiclox Injection:* Vials each containing 250 mg ampicillin as Ampicillin Sodium PhEur with 250 mg cloxacillin as Cloxacillin Sodium PhEur.

*Ampiclox Neonatal Injection:* 75 mg vials each containing 50 mg ampicillin as Ampicillin Sodium PhEur and 25 mg cloxacillin as Cloxacillin Sodium PhEur.

Ampiclox Syrup contains sodium benzoate, disodium edetate and sucrose.

Ampiclox Neonatal Suspension is sugar-free and free from artificial colourings; it contains sodium benzoate.

**Uses** Ampiclox is indicated for the immediate treatment of severe bacterial infections before the infecting organism is identified, and for mixed staphylococcal and Gram-negative infections.

Typical indications include: bronchopneumonia, post-influenzal pneumonia and other severe respiratory infections; post-operative chest and wound infections; septic abortion and infections during the puerperium; septicaemia; infections in patients receiving immunosuppressive drugs; prophylaxis in major surgery.

*Ampiclox Neonatal Suspension and Injection* are indicated for the prophylaxis or treatment of bacterial infections in premature babies or neonates, particularly: suspected or confirmed infections; babies born of mothers with infected liquor or whose membranes ruptured more than 48 hours before delivery; babies requiring certain surgical procedures carrying risk of infection such as exchange transfusions; babies born with respiratory distress necessitating endotracheal procedures, when subsequent infection is a possible hazard; babies following difficult delivery, when inhalation of much liquor, mucus or meconium has occurred.

Parenteral usage is indicated where oral dosage is inappropriate.

**Dosage and administration**

ORAL
*Adult dosage:* one to two capsules or 10–20 ml of syrup every four to six hours.

*Children's dosage: Syrup: one month to two years:* quarter adult dose; *two to 12 years:* half adult dose. *Neonatal Suspension:* 0.6 ml (90 mg) every four hours.

INTRAMUSCULAR/INTRAVENOUS
*Adult dosage (including elderly):* one to two vials (500 mg) every four to six hours.

*Children's dosage: up to two years:* quarter adult dose; *two to 10 years:* half adult dose.

Dosage may be further increased where necessary.

*Premature babies and neonates dosage:* one vial of Neonatal Injection (75 mg) three times a day.

ADMINISTRATION
500 MG VIALS
*Intramuscular:* Dissolve vial contents in 1.5 ml Water for Injections BP.

*Intravenous:* Dissolve vial contents in 10 ml Water for Injections BP and administer slowly (three to four minutes). Ampiclox may also be added to infusion fluids or injected, suitably diluted, into the drip tube over a period of three to four minutes.

*NEONATAL VIALS*
*Intramuscular:* Add 0.5 ml Water for Injections BP to the vial contents.

*Intravenous:* Dissolve the vial contents in 2 ml Water for Injections BP and administer slowly (three to four minutes). Ampiclox Neonatal may also be added to infusion fluids or injected, suitably diluted, into the drip tube over a period of three to four minutes.

**Contra-indications warnings, etc**

*Contra-indications:* Penicillin hypersensitivity; ocular administration. Attention should be paid to possible cross-sensitivity with other β-lactam antibiotics, e.g. cephalosporins.

*Precaution:* Caution should be observed when administering Ampiclox Neonatal Suspension and Injection to babies whose mothers are hypersensitive to penicillin.

*Use in pregnancy and lactation:* Animal studies have shown no teratogenic effects. The product has been in clinical use since 1968 and the limited number of reported cases of use in human pregnancy has shown no evidence of untoward effect. The use of Ampiclox in pregnancy should be reserved for cases considered essential by the clinician. During lactation, trace quantities of penicillins can be detected in breast milk.

*Adverse reactions:* Side-effects, as with other penicillins, are uncommon and mainly of a mild and transitory nature. Gastrointestinal upsets (e.g. nausea, diarrhoea) and skin rashes have been reported infrequently. An urticarial rash suggests penicillin hypersensitivity; an erythematous-type rash may arise in patients receiving ampicillin who have glandular fever. If a skin rash occurs, treatment should be discontinued. Rarely erythema multiforme and Stevens-Johnson syndrome have been reported. In common with other β-lactam antibiotics, angioedema and anaphylaxis have been reported. Pseudomembranous colitis has been reported rarely; cholestatic jaundice has been reported rarely with cloxacillin.

*Incompatibilities:* Ampiclox Injection and Neonatal Injection should not be mixed with blood products or other proteinaceous fluids (e.g. protein hydrolysates) or with intravenous lipid emulsions.

If Ampiclox is prescribed concurrently with an aminoglycoside, the antibiotics should not be mixed in the syringe, intravenous fluid container or giving set because loss of activity of the aminoglycoside and possibly precipitation can occur under these conditions.

*Overdosage:* Problems of overdosage with Ampiclox are unlikely to occur; if encountered they may be treated symptomatically.

**Pharmaceutical precautions** Ampiclox Capsules, Syrup, Injection, Neonatal Suspension and Neonatal Injection should be stored in a cool dry place. The Syrup bottle should be kept tightly closed. Once dispensed, Ampiclox Neonatal Suspension remains stable for five days and Ampiclox Syrup remains stable for seven days, if kept in a cool place. Ampiclox solutions for injection should be used immediately.

Ampiclox 500 mg Injection may be added to most intravenous fluids (e.g. Water for Injections, sodium chloride 0.9%, glucose 5%, sodium chloride 0.18% with glucose 4%). In intravenous solutions containing glucose or other carbohydrates, Ampiclox should be infused within one hour of preparation. Intravenous solutions of Ampiclox in Water for Injections or sodium chloride 0.9% should be infused within 24 hours of preparation. Full particulars are given in the Package Enclosure Leaflet. Preparation of Ampiclox infusion solutions must be carried out under appropriate aseptic conditions if these extended storage periods are required.

**Legal category** POM.

**Package quantities** *Ampiclox Capsules:* Containers of 20 and 100; *Ampiclox Syrup:* Bottles of 100 ml; *Ampiclox Neonatal Suspension:* Packs of 10 ml (OP), with pipette and Patient Information Leaflet; *Ampiclox Neonatal Injection:* Packs of 10 vials; *Ampiclox Injection (500 mg):* Boxes of 10 vials with instructions for use.

**Further information** Ampiclox Neonatal Suspension is sugar-free to minimise the risk of diarrhoea in the newborn. If tube feeding is necessary, the Suspension can easily be passed down a Ryle's tube.

**Product licence numbers**
| | |
|---|---|
| Capsules | 0038/5008R. |
| Syrup | 0038/0115R. |
| Neonatal Suspension | 0038/5009R. |
| Neonatal Injection | 0038/5001R. |
| Injection (500 mg) | 0038/5003R. |

## AUGMENTIN* 375 MG TABLETS
## AUGMENTIN* 625 MG TABLETS
## AUGMENTIN* DISPERSIBLE TABLETS 375 MG
## AUGMENTIN* 250/62 SF SUSPENSION
## AUGMENTIN* 125/31 SF SUSPENSION

**Qualitative and quantitative composition**
*Augmentin 375 mg Tablets:* Each tablet contains co-amoxiclav 250/125.

*Augmentin 625 mg Tablets:* Each tablet contains co-amoxiclav 500/125.

*Augmentin Dispersible Tablets 375 mg:* Each tablet contains co-amoxiclav 250/125.

*Augmentin 250/62 SF Suspension:* When reconstituted each 5 ml contains co-amoxiclav 250/62.

*Augmentin 125/31 SF Suspension:* When reconstituted each 5 ml contains co-amoxiclav 125/31.

In all the above presentations the amoxycillin is present as amoxycillin trihydrate and the clavulanic acid is present as potassium clavulanate.

**Pharmaceutical form**
*Augmentin 375 mg Tablets:* White to off-white oval film-coated tablets engraved Augmentin on one side.

*Augmentin 625 mg Tablets:* White to off-white oval film-coated tablets engraved Augmentin

*Augmentin Dispersible Tablets:* White round tablets engraved Augmentin.

*Augmentin 250/62 SF and 125/31 SF Suspension:* Dry powder for reconstitution in water, at time of dispensing, to form an oral sugar-free suspension.

**Clinical particulars**

*Therapeutic indications:* Augmentin is an antibiotic agent with a notably broad spectrum of activity against the commonly occurring bacterial pathogens in general practice and hospital. The β-lactamase inhibitory action of clavulanate extends the spectrum of amoxycillin to embrace a wider range of organisms, including many resistant to other β-lactam antibiotics.

Augmentin oral preparations are indicated for short-term treatment of bacterial infections at the following sites when amoxycillin-resistant β-lactamase-producing strains are suspected as the cause. In other situations, amoxycillin alone should be considered.

*Upper Respiratory Tract Infections (including ENT)* in particular sinusitis, otitis media, recurrent tonsillitis. These infections are often caused by *Streptococcus pneumoniae, Haemophilus influenzae\*, Moraxella catarrhalis\** and *Streptococcus pyogenes.*

*Lower Respiratory Tract Infections* in particular acute exacerbations of chronic bronchitis (especially if considered severe), bronchopneumonia. These infections are often caused by *Streptococcus pneumoniae, Haemophilus influenzae\** and *Moraxella catarrhalis\*.*

*Genito-urinary Tract and Abdominal Infections* in particular cystitis (especially when recurrent or complicated–excluding prostatitis), septic abortion, pelvic or puerperal sepsis and intra-abdominal sepsis. These infections are often caused by *Enterobacteriaceae\** (mainly *Escherichia coli\**), *Staphylococcus saprophyticus, Enterococcus* species.\*

*Skin and Soft Tissue Infections* in particular cellulitis, animal bites and severe dental abscess with spreading cellulitis. These infections are often caused by *Staphylococcus aureus\*, Streptococcus pyogenes* and *Bacteroides* species\*.

A comprehensive list of sensitive organisms is provided in *Pharmacological properties* section.

\* Some members of these species of bacteria produce β-lactamase, rendering them insensitive to amoxycillin alone.

Mixed infections caused by amoxycillin-susceptible organisms in conjunction with Augmentin-susceptible β-lactamase-producing organisms may be treated with Augmentin. These infections should not require the addition of another antibiotic resistant to β-lactamases.

**Posology and method of administration**

*Usual dosages for the treatment of infection*
*Adults and children over 12 years:* One Augmentin 375 mg Tablet or Dispersible Tablet three times a day. In severe infections one Augmentin 625 mg Tablet three times a day. Therapy can be started parenterally and continued with an oral preparation.

*Children:* The usual recommended daily dosage is 25 mg/kg/day* in divided doses every eight hours. The table below presents guidance for children.

*Augmention Suspension*

| | |
|---|---|
| Under 1 year | 25 mg/kg/day*, for example a 7.5 kg child would require 2 ml Augmentin 125/31 SF Suspension t.d.s. |
| 1–6 years (10–18 kg) | 5 ml Augmentin 125/31 SF Suspension t.d.s. |
| Over 6 years (18–40 kg) | 5 ml Augmentin 250/62 SF Suspension t.d.s. |

In more serious infections the dosage may be increased up to 50 mg/kg/day in divided doses every eight hours.

* Each 25 mg Augmentin provides co-amoxiclav 20/5.

Augmentin 375 mg and 625 mg Tablets are not recommended in children of 12 years and under.

*Dosage in dental infections (e.g. dentoalveolar abscess):*
*Adults and children over 12 years:* One Augmentin Tablet 375 mg three times a day for five days.

*Dosage in renal impairment*
*Adults:*
Mild impairment (Creatinine clearance >30 ml/min): No change in dosage.

Moderate impairment (Creatinine clearance 10–30 ml/min): One 375 mg tablet or one 625 mg tablet 12 hourly

Severe impairment (Creatinine clearance <10 ml/min): Not more than one 375 mg tablet 12 hourly; 625 mg tablets are not recommended.

*Children:* Similar reductions in dosage should be made for children.

*Dosage in hepatic impairment:* Dose with caution; monitor hepatic function at regular intervals.

There are, as yet, insufficient data on which to base a dosage recommendation.

Each 375 mg tablet of Augmentin contains 0.63 mmol (25 mg) of potassium.

*Administration:* Oral: Tablets, dispersible tablets or supsensions. To minimise potential gastrointestinal intolerance, administer at the start of a meal. The absorption of Augmentin is optimised when taken at the start of a meal. Dispersible tablets should be stirred into a little water before taking.

Duration of therapy should be appropriate to the indication and should not exceed 14 days without review.

*Contra-indications:* Penicillin hypersensitivity. Attention should be paid to possible cross-sensitivity with other β-lactam antibiotics, e.g. cephalosporins.

A previous history of Augmentin- or penicillin-associated jaundice/hepatic dysfunction.

*Special warnings and special precautions for use:* Changes in liver function tests have been observed in some patients receiving Augmentin. The clinical significance of these changes is uncertain but Augmentin should be used with caution in patients with evidence of hepatic dysfunction.

Cholestatic jaundice, which may be severe, but is usually reversible, has been reported rarely. Signs and symptoms may not become apparent for several weeks after treatment has ceased.

Serious and occasionally fatal hypersensitivity (anaphylactoid) reactions have been reported in patients on penicillin therapy. These reactions are more likely to occur in individuals with a history of penicillin hypersensitivity (see *Contra-indications* section).

Erythematous rashes have been associated with glandular fever in patients receiving amoxycillin.

Prolonged use may also occasionally result in overgrowth of non-susceptible organisms.

Augmentin Suspensions contain 12.5 mg aspartame per 5 ml dose and therefore care should be taken in phenylketonuria.

*Interaction with other medicaments and other forms of interaction:* Prolongation of bleeding time and prothrombin time have been reported in some patients receiving Augmentin. Augmentin should be used with care in patients on anti-coagulation therapy.

In common with other broad-spectrum antibiotics, Augmentin may reduce the efficacy of oral contraceptives and patients should be warned accordingly.

Concomitant use of allopurinol during treatment with amoxycillin can increase the likelihood of allergic skin reactions. There are no data on the concomitant use of Augmentin and allopurinol.

*Pregnancy and lactation:* Reproduction studies in animals (mice and rats) with orally and parenterally administered Augmentin have shown no teratogenic effects. There is limited experience of the use of Augmentin in human pregnancy. As with all medicines, use should be avoided in pregnancy, especially during the first trimester, unless considered essential by the physician.

Augmentin may be administered during the period of lactation. With the exception of the risk of sensitisation, associated with the excretion of trace quantities in breast milk, there are no known detrimental effects for the breast-fed infant.

*Effects on ability to drive and use machines:* None known.

*Undesirable effects:* Side effects are uncommon and mainly of a mild and transitory nature.

*Gastrointestinal reactions:* Diarrhoea, indigestion, nausea, vomiting, and mucocutaneous candidiasis have been reported. Antibiotic-associated colitis (including pseudomembranous colitis and haemorrhagic colitis) has been reported rarely. Nausea, although uncommon, is more often associated with higher oral dosages. If gastrointestinal side effects occur with oral therapy they may be reduced by taking Augmentin at the start of meals.

As with other antibiotics the incidence of gastrointestinal side effects may be raised in children under two years. In clinical trials, however, only 4% of children under two years were withdrawn from treatment.

Superficial tooth discolouration has been reported rarely, mostly with the suspension. It can usually be removed by brushing.

*Genito-urinary effects:* Vaginal itching, soreness and discharge may occur.

*Hepatic effects:* Moderate and asymptomatic rises in AST and/or ALT and alkaline phosphatases have been reported occasionally. Hepatitis and cholestatic jaundice have been reported rarely. These hepatic reactions have been reported more commonly with Augmentin than with other penicillins.

After Augmentin hepatic reactions have been reported more frequently in males and elderly patients, particularly those over 65 years. The risk increases with duration of treatment longer than 14 days. These reactions have been very rarely reported in children.

Signs and symptoms usually occur during or shortly after treatment but in some cases may not occur until several weeks after treatment has ended. Hepatic reactions are usually reversible but they may be severe and,very rarely, deaths have been reported.

*Hypersensitivity reactions:* Urticarial and erythematous rashes sometimes occur. Rarely erythema multiforme, Stevens-Johnson syndrome, toxic epidermal necrolysis, bullous exfoliative dermatitis, serum sickness-like syndrome and hypersensitivity vasculitis have been reported. Treatment should be discontinued if one of these disorders occurs. In common with other β-lactam antibiotics angioedema and anaphylaxis have been reported. Interstitial nephritis can occur rarely.

*Haematological effects:* As with other β-lactams transient leucopenia, thrombocytopenia and haemolytic anaemia have been reported rarely. Prolongation of bleeding time and prothrombin time has also been reported rarely (see *Interaction with other medicaments and other forms of interaction* section).

*CNS effects:* CNS effects have been seen very rarely. These include reversible hyperactivity, dizziness, headache and convulsions. Convulsions may occur with impaired renal function or in those receiving high doses.

*Overdose:* Problems of overdosage with Augmentin are unlikely to occur; if encountered gastrointestinal symptoms and disturbance of the fluid and electrolyte balances may be evident. They may be treated symptomatically with attention to the water electrolyte balance. Augmentin may be removed from the circulation by haemodialysis.

**Pharmacological properties**

*Pharmacodynamic properties:* Resistance to many antibiotics is caused by bacterial enzymes which destroy the antibiotic before it can act on the pathogen. The clavulanate in Augmentin anticipates this defence mechanism by blocking the β-lactamase enzymes, thus rendering the organisms sensitive to amoxycillin's rapid bactericidal effect at concentrations readily attainable in the body.

Clavulanate by itself has little antibacterial activity; however, in association with amoxycillin as Augmentin, it produces an antibiotic agent of broad spectrum with wide application in hospital and general practice.

Augmentin is bactericidal to a wide range of organisms including:

Gram-positive:

Aerobes: *Enterococcus faecalis**, *Enterococcus faecium**, *Streptococcus pneumoniae, Streptococcus pyogenes, Streptococcus viridans, Staphylococcus aureus**, Coagulase negative staphylococci* (including *Staphylococcus epidermidis**), *Corynebacterium* species, *Bacillus anthracis**, *Listeria monocytogenes.*

Anaerobes: *Clostridium* species, *Peptococcus* species, *Peptostreptococcus.*

Gram-negative:

Aerobes: *Haemophilus influenzae**, *Moraxella catarrhalis** *(Branhamella catarrhalis), Escherichia coli**, *Proteus mirabilis**, *Proteus vulgaris**, *Klebsiella* species*, *Salmonella* species*, *Shigella* species*, *Bordetella pertussis, Brucella* species, *Neisseria gonorrhoeae**, *Neisseria meningitidis**, *Vibrio cholerae, Pasteurella multocida.*

Anaerobes: *Bacteroides* species* including *B. fragilis.*

* Some members of these species of bacteria produce β-lactamase, rendering them insensitive to amoxycillin alone.

*Pharmacokinetic properties:* The pharmacokinetics of the two components of Augmentin are closely matched. Peak serum levels of both occur about one hour after oral administration. Absorption of Augmentin is optimised at the start of a meal. Both clavulanate and amoxycillin have low levels of serum binding; about 70% remains free in the serum.

Doubling the dosage of Augmentin approximately doubles the serum levels achieved.

*Preclinical safety data:* Not relevant

**Pharmaceutical particulars**

*List of excipients:*
*Augmentin 375 mg and 625 mg Tablets:* Each tablet contains magnesium stearate, sodium starch glycollate, colloidal silica, microcrystalline cellulose, titanium dioxide (E171), hydroxypropyl methylcellulose, polyethylene glycol and silicone oil.

*Augmentin Dispersible Tablets 375 mg:* Each tablet contains polyvinylpyrrolidone (cross-linked), silicagel, saccharin sodium, pineapple, strawberry and blood orange dry flavours, magnesium stearate and microcrystalline cellulose.

*Augmentin 250/62 and 125/31 SF Suspensions:* The powder contains xanthan gum, hydroxypropyl methylcellulose, aspartame, silicon dioxide, colloidal silica, succinic acid, raspberry, orange and golden syrup dry flavours.

*Incompatibilities:* None

*Shelf life:*
Augmentin 375 mg Tablets: Blister pack 36 months; glass bottles 48 months.

Augmentin 625 mg Tablets: Blister pack 24 months; glass bottles 36 months.

Augmentin Dispersible Tablets 375 mg : 24 months.

Augmentin 250/62 SF and 125/31 SF Suspension: Dry powder 18 months. Reconstituted suspensions: seven days

*Special precautions for storage:*
*Augmentin 375 mg and 625 mg Tablets* should be stored in a dry place at 25°C or below.

*Augmentin Dispersible Tablets 375 mg* should be stored in a dry place.

*Augmentin 250/62 SF and 125/31 SF Suspensions:* the dry powder should be stored in a dry place. Reconstituted suspensions should be kept in a refrigerator (but not frozen) for up to seven days.

*Nature and contents of container:*
*Augmentin 375 mg Tablets:* Blister packs of 21 in a carton; also amber glass bottles of 50 and 100.

*Augmentin 625 mg Tablets:* Blister packs of 21 in a carton; also amber glass bottles of 50.

*Augmentin Dispersible Tablets 375 mg:* Blister packs of 21 in a carton.

*Augmentin 250/62 SF and 125/31 SF Suspensions:* Clear glass bottles with aluminium screw caps containing powder for reconstitution to 100 ml.

*Instructions for use/handling:*
*Augmentin 375 mg and 625 mg Tablets:* None

*Augmentin Dispersible Tablets 375 mg:* The dispersible tablets should be stirred with a little water before taking.

*Augmentin 250/62 SF and 125/31 SF Suspensions:* At time of dispensing, the dry powder should be reconstituted to form an oral suspension as detailed below:

| *Strength* | *Volume of water to be added to reconstitute* | *Nominal bottle size* | *Final volume of reconstituted oral suspension* |
|---|---|---|---|
| *125/31* | *92 ml* | *150 ml* | *100 ml* |
| *250/62* | *90 ml* | *150 ml* | *100 ml* |

**Marketing authorisation numbers**

| | |
|---|---|
| Augmentin 375 mg Tablets | 0038/0270 |
| Augmentin 625 mg Tablets | 0038/0362 |
| Augmentin Dispersible Tablets 375 mg | 0038/0272 |
| Augmentin 250/62 SF Suspension | 0038/0337 |

Augmentin 125/31 SF Suspension 0038/0298

**Date of approval/revision of SPC** February 1997

**Legal category** POM

## AUGMENTIN* INTRAVENOUS

**Qualitative and quantitative composition** Vials of sterile powder providing co-amoxiclav 500/100 (600 mg Augmentin) or co-amoxiclav 1000/200 (1.2 g Augmentin). For reconstitution as an intravenous injection or infusion.

The amoxycillin is present as amoxycillin sodium and the clavulanic acid is present as potassium clavulanate.

**Pharmaceutical form** Sterile powder for injection.

**Clinical particulars**

*Therapeutic indications:* Augmentin is an antibiotic agent with a notably broad spectrum of activity against the commonly occurring bacterial pathogens in general practice and hospital. The β–lactamase inhibitory action of clavulanate extends the spectrum of amoxycillin to embrace a wider range of organisms, including many resistant to other β–lactam antibiotics.

Augmentin Intravenous is indicated for short-term treatment of bacterial infections at the following sites when amoxycillin resistant beta-lactamase-producing strains are suspected as the cause. In other situations, amoxycillin alone should be considered.

*Upper Respiratory Tract Infections (including ENT)* in particular sinusitis, otitis media, recurrent tonsillitis. These infections are often caused by *Streptococcus pneumoniae, Haemophilus influenzae**, *Moraxella catarrhalis** and *Streptococcus pyogenes.*

*Lower Respiratory Tract Infections* in particular acute exacerbations of chronic bronchitis (especially if considered severe), bronchopneumonia. These infections are often caused by *Streptococcus pneumoniae, Haemophilus influenzae** and *Moraxella catarrhalis**.

*Genito-urinary Tract and Abdominal Infections* in particular cystitis (especially when recurrent or complicated–excluding prostatitis), septic abortion, pelvic or puerperal sepsis and intra-abdominal sepsis. These infections are often caused by *Enterobacteriaceae** (mainly *Escherichia coli**), *Staphylococcus saprophyticus, Enterococcus* species.*

*Skin and Soft Tissue Infections* in particular cellulitis, animal bites and severe dental abscess with spreading cellulitis. These infections are often caused by *Staphylococcus aureus**, *Streptococcus pyogenes* and *Bacteroides* species*.

*Prophylaxis of wound infection associated with surgical procedures* in particular gastrointestinal, pelvic, major head and neck surgery and after limb amputation for infection.

A comprehensive list of sensitive organisms is provided in *Pharmacological properties* section.

* Some members of these species of bacteria produce β-lactamase, rendering them insensitive to amoxycillin alone.

Mixed infections caused by amoxycillin-susceptible organisms in conjunction with Augmentin-susceptible β-lactamase-producing organisms may be treated with Augmentin. These infections should not require the addition of another antibiotic resistant to β-lactamases.

**Posology and method of administration**

*Dosages for the treatment of infection:*

Adults and children over 12 years: Usually 1.2 g eight hourly. In more serious infections, increase frequency to six-hourly intervals.

Children 3 months–12 years: Usually 30 mg/kg * Augmentin eight hourly. In more serious infections, increase frequency to six–hourly intervals.

Children 0–3 months: 30 mg/kg* Augmentin every 12 hours in premature infants and in full term infants during the perinatal period, increasing to eight hours thereafter.

*Each 30 mg Augmentin provides co-amoxiclav 25/5.

*Adult dosage for surgical prophylaxis:* The usual dose is 1.2 g Augmentin Intravenous given at the induction of anaesthesia. Operations where there is a high risk of infection, e.g. colorectal surgery, may require three, and up to four, doses of 1.2 g Augmentin Intravenous in a 24–hour period. These doses are usually given at 0, 8, 16 (and 24) hours. This regimen can be continued for several days if the procedure has a significantly increased risk of infection.

Clear clinical signs of infection at operation will require a normal course of intravenous or oral Augmentin therapy post-operatively.

*Dosage in renal impairment*

*Adults*

| Mild impairment (creatinine clearance >30 ml/min) | Moderate impairment (creatinine clearance 10-30 ml/min) | Severe impairment (creatinine clearance <10 ml/min) |
|---|---|---|
| No change in dosage | 1.2 g IV stat., followed by 600 mg IV 12 hourly | 1.2 g IV stat., followed by 600 mg IV 24 hourly. Dialysis decreases serum concentrations of Augmentin and an additional 600 mg IV dose may need to be given during dialysis and at the end of dialysis |

*Children:* Similar reductions in dosage should be made for children.

*Dosage in hepatic impairment:* Dose with caution; monitor hepatic function at regular intervals.

There are, as yet, insufficient data on which to base a dosage recommendation.

Each 1.2 g vial of Augmentin contains 1.0 mmol of potassium and 3.1 mmol of sodium (approx).

*Administration:* Augmentin Intravenous may be administered either by intravenous injection or by intermittent infusion (see *Instructions for use/handling*). It is not suitable for intramuscular administration.

Duration of therapy should be appropriate to the indication and should not exceed 14 days without review.

*Contra-indications:* Penicillin hypersensitivity. Attention should be paid to possible cross-sensitivity with other β-lactam antibiotics, e.g. cephalosporins.

A previous history of Augmentin- or penicillin-associated jaundice/hepatic dysfunction.

*Special warnings and special precautions for use:* Changes in liver function tests have been observed in some patients receiving Augmentin. The clinical significance of these changes is uncertain but Augmentin should be used with caution in patients with evidence of hepatic dysfunction.

Cholestatic jaundice, which may be severe, but is usually reversible, has been reported rarely. Signs and symptoms may not become apparent for several weeks after treatment has ceased.

Serious and occasionally fatal hypersensitivity (anaphylactoid) reactions have been reported in patients on penicillin therapy. These reactions are more likely to occur in individuals with a history of penicillin hypersensitivity (see *Contra-indications*).

Erythematous rashes have been associated with glandular fever in patients receiving amoxycillin.

Prolonged use may also occasionally result in overgrowth of non-susceptible organisms.

During the administration of high doses of Augmentin adequate fluid intake and urinary output should be maintained to minimise the possibility of crystalluria. When present at high concentrations in urine at room temperature, amoxycillin may precipitate in bladder catheters. A regular check on patency should be maintained.

*Interaction with other medicaments and other forms of interaction:* Prolongation of bleeding time and prothrombin time have been reported in some patients receiving Augmentin. Augmentin should be used with care in patients on anti-coagulation therapy. In common with other broad-spectrum antibiotics, Augmentin may reduce the efficacy of oral contraceptives and patients should be warned accordingly.

Concomitant use of allopurinol during treatment with amoxycillin can increase the likelihood of allergic skin reactions. There are no data on the concomitant use of Augmentin and allopurinol.

*Pregnancy and lactation:* Reproduction studies in animals (mice and rats) with orally and parenterally administered Augmentin have shown no teratogenic effects. There is limited experience of the use of Augmentin in human pregnancy. As with all medicines, use should be avoided in pregnancy, especially during the first trimester, unless considered essential by the physician.

Augmentin may be administered during the period of lactation. With the exception of the risk of sensitisation, associated with the excretion of trace quantities in breast milk, there are no known detrimental effects for the breast-fed infant.

*Effects on ability to drive and use machines:* None known.

*Undesirable effects:* Side effects are uncommon and mainly of a mild and transitory nature.

*Gastrointestinal reactions:* Diarrhoea, indigestion, nausea, vomiting, and mucocutaneous candidiasis have been reported. Antibiotic-associated colitis (including pseudomembranous colitis and haemorrhagic colitis) has been reported rarely. Nausea, although uncommon, is more often associated with higher oral dosages. If gastrointestinal side effects occur with oral therapy they may be reduced by taking Augmentin at the start of meals. Superficial tooth discolouration has been reported rarely, mostly with the suspension. It can usually be removed by brushing.

*Genito-urinary effects:* Vaginal itching, soreness and discharge may occur.

*Hepatic effects:* Moderate and asymptomatic rises in AST and/or ALT and alkaline phosphatases have been reported occasionally. Hepatitis and cholestatic jaundice have been reported rarely. These hepatic reactions have been reported more commonly with Augmentin than with other penicillins.

After Augmentin hepatic reactions have been reported more frequently in males and elderly patients, particularly those over 65 years. The risk increases with duration of treatment longer than 14 days. These reactions have been very rarely reported in children.

Signs and symptoms usually occur during or shortly after treatment but in some cases may not occur until several weeks after treatment has ended. Hepatic reactions are usually reversible but they may be severe and,very rarely, deaths have been reported.

*Hypersensitivity reactions:* Urticarial and erythematous rashes sometimes occur. Rarely erythema multiforme, Stevens-Johnson syndrome, toxic epidermal necrolysis, bullous exfoliative dermatitis, serum sickness-like syndrome and hypersensitivity vasculitis have been reported. Treatment should be discontinued if one of these disorders occurs. In common with other β-lactam antibiotics angioedema and anaphylaxis have been reported. Interstitial nephritis can occur rarely.

*Haematological effects:* As with other β-lactams transient leucopenia, thrombocytopenia and haemolytic anaemia have been reported rarely. Prolongation of bleeding time and prothrombin time has also been reported rarely (see *Interactions with other medicaments and other forms of interaction*).

*CNS effects:* CNS effects have been seen very rarely. These include reversible hyperactivity, dizziness, headache and convulsions. Convulsions may occur with impaired renal function or in those receiving high doses.

*Local:* Thrombophlebitis at the site of injection has been reported occasionally.

*Overdose:* Problems of overdosage with Augmentin are unlikely to occur; if encountered gastrointestinal symptoms and disturbance of the fluid and electrolyte balances may be evident. They may be treated symptomatically with attention to the water electrolyte balance. Augmentin may be removed from the circulation by haemodialysis.

**Pharmacological properties**

*Pharmacodynamic properties:* Resistance to many antibiotics is caused by bacterial enzymes which destroy the antibiotic before it can act on the pathogen. The clavulanate in Augmentin anticipates this defence mechanism by blocking the β-lactamase enzymes, thus rendering the organisms sensitive to amoxycillin's rapid bactericidal effect at concentrations readily attainable in the body.

Clavulanate by itself has little antibacterial activity; however, in association with amoxycillin as Augmentin, it produces an antibiotic agent of broad spectrum with wide application in hospital and general practice.

Augmentin is bactericidal to a wide range of organisms including:

Gram-positive:

Aerobes: *Enterococcus faecalis**, *Enterococcus faecium**, *Streptococcus pneumoniae, Streptococcus pyogenes, Streptococcus viridans, Staphylococcus aureus**, Coagulase negative staphylococci* (including *Staphylococcus epidermidis**), *Corynebacterium* species, *Bacillus anthracis**, *Listeria monocytogenes.*

Anaerobes: *Clostridium* species, *Peptococcus* species, *Peptostreptococcus.*

Gram-negative:

Aerobes: *Haemophilus influenzae**, *Moraxella catarrhalis** *(Branhamella catarrhalis), Escherichia coli**, *Proteus mirabilis**, *Proteus vulgaris**, *Klebsiella* species*, *Salmonella* species*, *Shigella* species*, *Bordetella pertussis, Brucella* species, *Neisseria gonorrhoeae**, *Neisseria meningitidis**, *Vibrio cholerae, Pasteurella multocida.*

Anaerobes: *Bacteroides* species* including *B. fragilis.*

* Some members of these species of bacteria produce β-lactamase, rendering them insensitive to amoxycillin alone.

*Pharmacokinetic properties:* The pharmacokinetics of the two components of Augmentin are closely matched. Both clavulanate and amoxycillin have low levels of serum binding; about 70% remains free in the serum.

Doubling the dosage of Augmentin approximately doubles the serum levels achieved.

*Preclinical safety data:* Not relevant

### Pharmaceutical particulars

*List of excipients:* None

*Incompatibilities:* Augmentin Intravenous should not be mixed with blood products, other proteinaceous fluids such as protein hydrolysates or with intravenous lipid emulsions.

If Augmentin is prescribed concurrently with an aminoglycoside, the antibiotics should not be mixed in the syringe, intravenous fluid container or giving set because loss of activity of the aminoglycoside can occur under these conditions.

*Shelf life:* 2 years

*Special precautions for storage:* Augmentin vials should be stored in a dry place below 25°C.

*Nature and contents of container:* Clear glass vials (PhEur type III) fitted with butyl rubber bungs and aluminium overseals.

*Instructions for use/handling:* 600 mg vial: To reconstitute dissolve in 10 ml Water for Injections BP. (Final volume 10.5 ml.)

1.2 g vial: To reconstitute dissolve in 20 ml Water for Injections BP. (Final volume 20.9 ml.)

Augmentin Intravenous should be given by slow intravenous injection over a period of three to four minutes and used within 20 minutes of reconstitution. It may be injected directly into a vein or via a drip tube.

Alternatively, Augmentin Intravenous may be infused in Water for Injections BP or Sodium Chloride Intravenous Injection BP (0.9% w/v). Add, without delay, 600 mg reconstituted solution to 50 ml infusion fluid or 1.2 g reconstituted solution to 100 ml infusion fluid (e.g. using a minibag or in-line burette). Infuse over 30-40 minutes and complete within four hours of reconstitution. For other appropriate infusion fluids, see Package Enclosure Leaflet.

Any residual antibiotic solutions should be discarded.

Augmentin Intravenous is less stable in infusions containing glucose, dextran or bicarbonate. Reconstituted solution should, therefore, not be added to such infusions but may be injected into the drip tubing over a period of three to four minutes.

**Marketing authorisation number** 0038/0320

**Date of approval/revision of SPC** February 1997

**Legal category** POM

# FLOXAPEN* CAPSULES
# FLOXAPEN* SYRUPS
# FLOXAPEN* INJECTION

**Presentation** *Floxapen Capsules* (Flucloxacillin Capsules BP): Black and caramel capsules overprinted Floxapen, containing 250 mg or 500 mg flucloxacillin as Flucloxacillin Sodium BP.

*Floxapen Vials for Injection* (Flucloxacillin Injection BP): Each vial contains 250 mg, 500 mg or 1 g flucloxacillin as Flucloxacillin Sodium BP as a powder for reconstitution.

*Floxapen Syrups* (Flucloxacillin Oral Suspension BP): Bottles containing powder for the preparation of 100 ml suspension. When reconstituted each 5 ml contains 125 mg or 250 mg flucloxacillin, as Flucloxacillin Magnesium BP.

Floxapen Syrups contain sodium benzoate and sucrose.

**Uses** Floxapen is indicated for the treatment of infections due to Gram-positive organisms, including infections caused by β-lactamase-producing staphylococci. Typical indications include:

*Skin and soft tissue infections:* boils, abscesses, carbuncles, furunculosis, cellulitis; infected skin conditions, e.g. ulcer, eczema and acne; infected wounds, infected burns, protection for skin grafts, otitis media and externa, impetigo.

*Respiratory tract infections:* pneumonia, lung abscess, empyema, sinusitis, pharyngitis, tonsillitis, quinsy.

*Other infections caused by Floxapen-sensitive organisms:* osteomyelitis, enteritis, endocarditis, urinary tract infection, meningitis, septicaemia.

Floxapen is also indicated for use as a prophylactic agent during major surgical procedures where appropriate: for example, cardiothoracic and orthopaedic surgery.

Parenteral usage is indicated where oral dosage is inappropriate.

**Dosage and administration**
*Usual adult dosage (including elderly patients)*

Oral – 250 mg four times a day.
Intramuscular – 250 mg four times a day.
Intravenous – 250 mg to 1 g four times a day.

The above systemic dosages may be doubled where necessary; oral doses should be administered half to one hour before meals.
Osteomyelitis, endocarditis – Up to 8 g daily, in divided doses six to eight hourly.
Surgical prophylaxis – 1 to 2 g IV at induction of anaesthesia followed by 500 mg six hourly IV, IM, or orally for up to 72 hours.

Floxapen may be administered by other routes in conjunction with systemic therapy. (Proportionately lower doses should be given in children.)
Intrapleural – 250 mg once daily.
By nebuliser – 125 to 250 mg four times a day.
Intra-articular – 250 to 500 mg once daily.

*Usual children's dosage*
2–10 years: half adult dose.
Under 2 years: quarter adult dose.

*Abnormal renal function:* In common with other penicillins, Floxapen usage in patients with renal impairment does not usually require dosage reduction. However, in the presence of severe renal failure (creatinine clearance < 10 ml/min) a reduction in dose or an extension of dose interval should be considered.

Floxapen is not significantly removed by dialysis and hence no supplementary dosages need to be administered either during, or at the end of the dialysis period.

*Administration*
*Intramuscular:* Add 1.5 ml Water for Injections BP to 250 mg vial contents or 2 ml Water for Injections BP to 500 mg vial contents.

*Intravenous:* Dissolve 250–500 mg in 5–10 ml Water for Injections BP or 1 g in 15–20 ml Water for Injections BP. Administer by slow intravenous injection (three to four minutes). Floxapen may also be added to infusion fluids or injected, suitably diluted, into the drip tube over a period of three to four minutes.

*Intrapleural:* Dissolve 250 mg in 5–10 ml Water for Injections BP.

*Intra-articular:* Dissolve 250–500 mg in up to 5 ml Water for Injections BP or 0.5% lignocaine hydrochloride solution.

*Nebuliser solution:* Dissolve 125–250 mg of the vial contents in 3 ml sterile water.

**Contra-indications, warnings, etc**

*Contra-indications:* Penicillin hypersensitivity; ocular administration.

*Use in pregnancy and lactation:* Animal studies with Floxapen have shown no teratogenic effects. The product has been in clinical use since 1970 and the limited number of reported cases of use in human pregnancy have shown no evidence of untoward effect. The use of Floxapen in pregnancy should be reserved for cases considered essential by the clinician. During lactation, trace quantities of penicillins can be detected in breast milk.

*Side-effects:* Side-effects, as with other penicillins, are uncommon and mainly of a mild and transitory nature. Gastro-intestinal upsets (e.g. nausea, diarrhoea) and skin rashes have been reported. If a skin rash occurs, treatment should be discontinued. Hepatitis and cholestatic jaundice have been reported. These reactions are related neither to the dose nor to the route of administration. The onset of these effects may be delayed for up to two months post-treatment: in several cases, the course of the reactions has been protracted and lasted for some months. In very rare cases, a fatal outcome has been reported.

Pseudomembranous colitis has been reported rarely and has usually been associated with the use of Floxapen in combination with other antibiotics. In common with other β-lactam antibiotics angioedema and anaphylaxis have been reported.

*Overdosage:* Problems of overdosage with Floxapen are unlikely to occur; if encountered they may be treated symptomatically.

**Pharmaceutical precautions** Floxapen Capsules in Original Packs and Floxapen Syrups should be stored in a dry place. Floxapen Capsules in reclosable containers and Floxapen Vials for Injection should be stored in a cool, dry place.

Once dispensed, Floxapen Syrups (bottles) remain stable for 14 days stored in a refrigerator (5°C). If a dilution of the reconstituted syrup is required, Syrup BP should be used.

Reconstituted solutions for IM or direct IV injection should normally be administered within 30 minutes of preparation. However, aqueous solutions of Floxapen Injection retain their activity for up to 24 hours when stored in a refrigerator (2°–8°C).

Floxapen may be added to most intravenous fluids (e.g. Water for Injections, sodium chloride 0.9%, glucose 5%, sodium chloride 0.18% with glucose 4%).

Once reconstituted, Floxapen solutions should be stored in a refrigerator (2°–8C°) and used within 24 hours of preparation. Full particulars are given in the Package Enclosure Leaflet.

Reconstitution of Floxapen injections and preparation of Floxapen infusion solutions must be carried out under appropriate aseptic conditions if the extended storage periods are required.

N.B. FLOXAPEN VIALS ARE NOT SUITABLE FOR MULTIDOSE USE.

Any residual Floxapen should be discarded.

Floxapen should not be mixed with blood products or other proteinaceous fluids (e.g. protein hydrolysates) or with intravenous lipid emulsions.

If Floxapen is prescribed concurrently with an aminoglycoside, the two antibiotics should not be mixed in the syringe, intravenous fluid container or giving set; precipitation may occur.

**Legal category** POM.

**Package quantities**
*Floxapen Capsules 250 mg:* Original Pack of 28 with Patient Information Leaflet; also containers of 20 and 100.
*Floxapen Capsules 500 mg:* Original Pack of 28 with Patient Information Leaflet; also containers of 100.
*Floxapen Vials 250 mg or 500 mg:* boxes of 10 with instructions for use.
*Floxapen Vials 1 g:* boxes of 5 with instructions for use.
*Floxapen Syrup 125 mg/5 ml:* Original Pack of 100 ml with Patient Information Leaflet.
*Floxapen Syrup 250 mg/5 ml:* Original Pack of 100 ml with Patient Information Leaflet.

**Further information** Floxapen syrups are now formulated using the magnesium salt of flucloxacillin, in preference to the sodium salt, in order to provide two palatable strengths of suspension.

Following oral administration Floxapen gives blood levels comparable to those achieved by intramuscular injection.

**Product licence numbers**

| | |
|---|---|
| Floxapen Capsules 250 mg | 0038/5055R. |
| Floxapen Capsules 500 mg | 0038/5056R. |
| Floxapen Vials for Injection 250 mg | 0038/5051R. |
| Floxapen Vials for Injection 500 mg | 0038/5052R. |
| Floxapen Vials for Injection 1 g | 0038/5053R. |
| Floxapen Syrup 125 mg/5 ml | 0038/0309. |
| Floxapen Syrup 250 mg/5 ml | 0038/0310. |

# MAGNAPEN* CAPSULES
# MAGNAPEN* SYRUP
# MAGNAPEN* INJECTION
*Approved name:* co-fluampicil

**Presentation** *Magnapen Capsules:* Black and turquoise capsules overprinted 'Magnapen', containing 250 mg ampicillin as Ampicillin Trihydrate BP with 250 mg flucloxacillin as Flucloxacillin Sodium BP.

*Magnapen Syrup:* Bottles containing powder for the preparation of 100 ml suspension. When reconstituted each 5 ml contains 125 mg ampicillin as Ampicillin Trihydrate BP with 125 mg flucloxacillin as Flucloxacillin Magnesium BP.

*Magnapen Vials for Injection:* 500 mg Vial: containing 250 mg ampicillin as Ampicillin Sodium BP with 250 mg flucloxacillin as Flucloxacillin Sodium BP.

Magnapen Syrup contains disodium edetate, sodium benzoate and sucrose.

**Uses** Magnapen is indicated for the treatment of severe infections where the causative organism is unknown, and for mixed infections involving β-lactamase-producing staphylococci. Typical indications include:

*In general practice:* chest infections, ENT infections, skin and soft tissue infections, and infections in patients whose underlying pathology places them at special risk.

*In hospital* (prior to laboratory results being available): severe respiratory tract infections, post-operative chest and wound infections; septic abortion, puerperal fever; septicaemia, prophylaxis in major surgery, infections in patients receiving immuno-suppressive therapy.

The spectrum of activity of Magnapen also makes it suitable for the treatment of many mixed infections, particularly those where β-lactamase-producing staphylococci are suspected or confirmed.

Parenteral usage is indicated where oral dosage is inappropriate.

**Dosage and administration**
*Usual adult dosage (including elderly patients):*
Oral: 1 capsule or 10 ml syrup four times a day.
Intramuscular/Intravenous: 500 mg four times a day.

*Usual children's dosage:*
Oral: Under 10 years: 5 ml syrup four times a day.†
Intramuscular/Intravenous: Under 2 years: quarter adult dose.† 2–10 years: half adult dose.

The above dosages for adults and children may be doubled where necessary.

Oral doses should be administered half to one hour before meals.

*Administration:* Intramuscular: 500 mg Vial: add 1.5 ml Water for Injections BP to vial contents.

Intravenous: Dissolve 500 mg in 10 ml Water for Injections BP. Administer by slow intravenous injection (3–4 minutes). Magnapen Injection may be added to infusion fluids or injected, suitably diluted into the drip tube over a period of 3–4 minutes.

### Contra-indications, warnings, etc

*Contra-indications:* Penicillin hypersensitivity; ocular administration.

*Use in pregnancy and lactation:* Animal studies have shown no teratogenic effects. The product has been in clinical use since 1971 and the limited number of reported cases of use in human pregnancy have shown no evidence of untoward effect. The use of Magnapen in pregnancy should be reserved for cases considered essential by the clinician. During lactation, trace quantities of penicillins can be detected in breast milk.

*Side-effects:* Side-effects, as with other penicillins, are uncommon and mainly of a mild and transitory nature. Gastro-intestinal upsets (e.g. nausea, diarrhoea) and skin rashes have been reported. An urticarial rash suggests penicillin hypersensitivity; an erythematous rash may arise in patients receiving ampicillin who have glandular fever. If a skin rash occurs, treatment should be discontinued. Hepatitis and cholestatic jaundice have been reported in association with flucloxacillin. These reactions are related neither to the dose nor to the route of administration. The onset of these effects may be delayed for up to two months post-treatment: in several cases, the course of the reactions has been protracted and lasted for some months. In very rare cases, a fatal outcome has been reported.

Pseudomembranous colitis has been reported rarely. In common with other β-lactam antibiotics angioedema and anaphylaxis have been reported.

*Overdosage:* Problems of overdosage with Magnapen are unlikely to occur; if encountered they may be treated symptomatically.

### Pharmaceutical precautions

Magnapen Capsules and Magnapen Vials for Injection should be stored in a cool, dry place. Magnapen Syrup should be stored in a dry place.

Once dispensed, Magnapen Syrup remains stable for 14 days when kept in a cool place (15°C). If a dilution of the reconstituted suspension is required, Syrup BP should be used.

Magnapen solutions for injection should be used immediately.

Magnapen may be added to most intravenous fluids (e.g. Water for Injections, sodium chloride 0.9%, glucose 5%, sodium chloride 0.18% with glucose 4%). In intravenous solutions containing glucose or other carbohydrates, Magnapen should be infused within two hours of preparation. Intravenous solutions of Magnapen in Water for Injections or sodium chloride 0.9% should be infused within 24 hours of preparation. Full particulars are given in the Package Enclosure Leaflet. Preparation of Magnapen infusion solutions must be carried out under appropriate aseptic conditions if these extended storage periods are required.

Magnapen should not be mixed with blood products, other proteinaceous fluids (e.g. protein hydrolysates) or with intravenous lipid emulsions.

If Magnapen is prescribed concurrently with an aminoglycoside, the antibiotics should not be mixed in the syringe, intravenous fluid container or giving set because loss of activity of the aminoglycoside and possibly precipitation can occur under these conditions.

### Legal category POM.

### Package quantities

*Magnapen Capsules:* Containers of 20 and 100.
*Magnapen Syrup:* Original Pack of 100 ml with Patient Information Leaflet.
*Magnapen Injection:* Box of 10 vials with instructions for use.

### Further information

Infections encountered in medical practice can be of mixed bacteriology, often including β-lactamase-producing strains. Magnapen provides a broad spectrum of activity, which should be considered when dealing with such infections.

Magnapen Syrup is now formulated using the magnesium salt of flucloxacillin in preference to the sodium salt, in order to provide a more palatable suspension with extended stability.

† Ampiclox Neonatal is recommended for the treatment of infections in neonates and premature babies.

### Product licence numbers

| | |
|---|---|
| Magnapen Capsules | 0038/0090R. |
| Magnapen Syrup | 0038/0324. |
| Magnapen Vials 500 mg | 0038/0089R. |

# PENBRITIN* CAPSULES
# PENBRITIN* SYRUPS
# PENBRITIN* PAEDIATRIC SUSPENSION
# PENBRITIN* INJECTION

**Presentation** *Penbritin Capsules* (Ampicillin Capsules BP): black and red capsules overprinted 'Penbritin', containing 250 mg or 500 mg ampicillin as Ampicillin Trihydrate BP.

*Penbritin Syrups* (Ampicillin Oral Suspension BP): Bottles containing powder for the preparation of 100 ml pale cream-coloured suspension. When reconstituted each 5 ml contains 125 mg or 250 mg ampicillin as Ampicillin Trihydrate BP.

*Penbritin Paediatric Suspension:* Bottles containing powder for the preparation of 25 ml off-white suspension. When reconstituted each 1.25 ml contains 125 mg ampicillin as Ampicillin Trihydrate BP. A pipette to measure the 1.25 ml dose is provided.

*Penbritin Vials for Injection* (Ampicillin Sodium BP for Injection): Each vial contains 250 mg or 500 mg ampicillin as Ampicillin Sodium BP.

Penbritin Syrups and Paediatric Suspension contain sodium benzoate and sucrose.

**Uses** Penbritin is a broad-spectrum penicillin, indicated for the treatment of a wide range of bacterial infections caused by ampicillin-sensitive organisms.

Typical indications include: ear, nose and throat infections, bronchitis, pneumonia, urinary tract infections, gonorrhoea, gynaecological infections, septicaemia, peritonitis, endocarditis, meningitis, enteric fever, gastro-intestinal infections.

Extraperitoneal application of Penbritin to wounds can be used to prevent infection following abdominal surgery.

Parenteral usage is indicated where oral dosage is inappropriate.

**Dosage and administration** *Usual adult dosage* (including elderly patients) – oral, except where stated:
*Ear, nose and throat infections:* 250 mg four times a day.
*Bronchitis: Routine therapy:* 250 mg four times a day.
    *High-dosage therapy:* 1 g four times a day.
*Pneumonia:* 500 mg four times a day.
*Urinary tract infections:* 500 mg three times a day.
*Gonorrhoea:* 2 g orally with 1 g probenecid as a single dose. Repeated doses are recommended for the treatment of females.
*Gastro-intestinal infections:* 500–750 mg three to four times daily.
*Enteric: Acute:* 1–2 g four times a day for two weeks.
    *Carriers:* 1–2 g four times a day for four to twelve weeks.
*Septicaemia, endocarditis, osteomyelitis:* 500 mg four to six times a day IM or IV for one to six weeks.
*Peritonitis, intra-abdominal sepsis:* 500 mg four times a day IM or IV.
*Meningitis:* Adult dosage: 2 g six-hourly IV.

*Children's dosage:* 150 mg/kg daily IV in divided doses.

*Usual children's dosage* (under 10 years): half adult routine dosage.

All recommended dosages are a guide only. In severe infections the above dosages may be increased, or Penbritin given by injection. Oral doses of Penbritin should be taken half to one hour before meals.

*Administration:*
*Intramuscular:* Add 1.5 ml Water for Injections BP to 250 mg or 500 mg vial contents.
*Intravenous:* Dissolve 250 mg in 5 ml or 500 mg in 10 ml Water for Injections BP. Administer by slow injection (three to four minutes). Penbritin may also be added to infusion fluids or injected, suitably diluted, into the drip tube over a period of three to four minutes.

Penbritin may also be administered by other routes in conjunction with systemic therapy.
*Intraperitoneal:* 500 mg daily in up to 10 ml Water for Injections BP.
*Intrapleural:* 500 mg daily in 5–10 ml Water for Injections BP.
*Intra-articular:* 500 mg daily, in up to 5 ml Water for Injections BP or sterile 0.5% procaine hydrochloride solution.
*Local use in abdominal surgery:* 1 g sterile powder sprinkled into the wound extraperitoneally or into muscle layers to prevent wound infection post-operatively.

### Contra-indications, warnings, etc

*Contra-indication:* Penicillin hypersensitivity.

*Use in pregnancy and lactation:* Animal studies with Penbritin have shown no teratogenic effects. The product has been in extensive clinical use since 1961 and its use in human pregnancy has been well documented in clinical studies. When antibiotic therapy is required during pregnancy, Penbritin may be considered appropriate.

During lactation, trace quantities of penicillins can be detected in breast milk.

*Side-effects:* Side-effects, as with other penicillins, are uncommon and mainly of a mild and transitory nature. Gastro-intestinal upsets (e.g., nausea, diarrhoea) and skin rashes have been reported infrequently. An urticarial rash suggests penicillin hypersensitivity; an erythematous rash may arise in patients receiving ampicillin who have glandular fever. If a skin rash occurs, treatment should be discontinued. In common with other β-lactam antibiotics angioedema and anaphylaxis have been reported. Pseudomembranous colitis has been reported rarely.

*Overdosage:* Problems of overdosage with Penbritin are unlikely to occur; if encountered they may be treated symptomatically.

### Pharmaceutical precautions

Penbritin Capsules, when packed in blister packs (OP), should be stored in a dry place. All other Penbritin presentations should be stored in a cool dry place.

Once dispensed, Penbritin Syrups and Paediatric Suspension remain stable for seven days if kept in a cool place. If a dilution of the reconstituted syrup is required, Syrup BP should be used.

Penbritin solutions for injection should be used immediately.

Penbritin may be added to most intravenous fluids (e.g. Water for Injections, sodium chloride 0.9%, glucose 5%, sodium chloride 0.18% with glucose 4%). Once reconstituted, Penbritin solutions should be stored in a refrigerator (2–8°C) and used within 24 hours. In intravenous solutions containing glucose or other carbohydrates, Penbritin should be infused within one hour of preparation. Intravenous solutions of Penbritin in Water for Injections or sodium chloride 0.9% should be infused within 24 hours of preparation. Full particulars are given in the Package Enclosure Leaflet. Preparation of Penbritin infusion solutions must be carried out under appropriate aseptic conditions if these extended storage periods are required.

N.B. Penbritin Vials are not suitable for multidose use. Any residual Penbritin solution should be discarded.

Penbritin should not be mixed with blood products or other proteinaceous fluids (e.g. protein hydrolysates) or with intravenous lipid emulsions.

If Penbritin is prescribed concurrently with an aminoglycoside, the antibiotics should not be mixed in the syringe, intravenous fluid container or giving set because loss of activity of the aminoglycoside can occur under these conditions.

### Legal category POM.

### Package quantities

*Penbritin Capsules 250 mg:* Original Pack of 28 with Patient Information Leaflet; also containers of 100.
*Penbritin Capsules 500 mg:* Original Pack of 28 with Patient Information Leaflet; also containers of 100.
*Penbritin Vials for Injection 250 mg, 500 mg:* Boxes of 10 with instructions for use.
*Penbritin Syrups:* Original Packs of 100 ml.
*Penbritin Paediatric Suspension:* Original Pack of 25 ml with pipette and Patient Information Leaflet.

### Further information Nil.

### Product licence numbers

| | |
|---|---|
| Penbritin Capsules 250 mg | 0038/5074R. |
| Penbritin Capsules 500 mg | 0038/5075R. |
| Penbritin Vials for Injection 250 mg | 0038/5060R. |
| Penbritin Vials for Injection 500 mg | 0038/5061R. |
| Penbritin Syrup 125 mg/5 ml | 0038/0265. |
| Penbritin Syrup 250 mg/5 ml | 0038/0266. |
| Penbritin Paediatric Suspension | 0038/5066R. |

# TIMENTIN* 1.6 G, 3.2 G

### Qualitative and quantitative composition

*Timentin 1.6 g:* Contains 100 mg clavulanic acid with 1.5 g ticarcillin.

*Timentin 3.2 g:* Contains 200 mg clavulanic acid with 3.0 g ticarcillin.

The clavulanic acid is present as Potassium Clavulanate BP and the ticarcillin as ticarcillin sodium.

**Pharmaceutical form** Vials containing sterile powder for reconstitution.

### Clinical particulars

*Therapeutic indications:* Timentin is an injectable antibiotic agent with a broad spectrum of bactericidal activity against a wide range of Gram-positive and gram-negative aerobic and anaerobic bacteria. The presence of clavulanate in the formulation extends the spectrum of activity of ticarcillin to include many β-lactamase-producing bacteria normally resistant to ticarcillin and other β–lactam antibiotics.

Timentin is indicated for the treatment of infections in which susceptible organisms have been detected or are suspected.

*Typical indications include:* Severe infections in hospitalised patients and proven or suspected infections in patients with impaired or suppressed host defences including: septicaemia, bacteraemia, peritonitis, intra-abdominal sepsis, post-surgical infections, bone and joint infections, skin and soft tissue infections, respiratory tract infections, serious or complicated renal infections (e.g. pyelonephritis), ear, nose and throat infections.

Timentin is bactericidal to a wide range of organisms including:

Gram-positive:

Aerobes: *Staphylococcus* species including *Staphylococcus aureus* and *Staphylococcus epidermidis, Streptococcus* species including *Enterococcus faecalis.*

Anaerobes: *Peptococcus* species, *Peptostreptococcus* species, *Clostridium* species, *Eubacterium* species.

Gram-negative:

Aerobes: *Escherichia coli, Haemophilus* species including *Haemophilus influenzae, Moraxella catarrhalis, Klebsiella* species including *Klebsiella pneumoniae, Enterobacter* species, *Proteus* species including indole-positive strains, *Providentia stuartii, Pseudomonas* species including *Pseudomonas aeruginosa, Serratia* species including *Serratia marcescens, Citrobacter* species, *Acinetobacter* species, *Yersinia enterocolitica*

Anaerobes: *Bacteroides* species *including Bacteroides fragilis, Fusobacterium* species, *Veillonella* species.

## Posology and method of administration

*Adult dosage (including elderly patients):* The usual dosage is 3.2 g Timentin given six to eight hourly. The maximum recommended dosage is 3.2 g four hourly.

*Children's dosage:* The usual dosage for children is 80 mg Timentin/kg body weight given every six to eight hours.

For premature infants and full-term infants during the perinatal period, the dosage is 80 mg Timentin/kg body weight every 12 hours, increasing to every eight hours thereafter.

*Dosage in renal impairment:*

| Mild impairment (Creatinine Clearance >30 ml/min) | Moderate impairment (Creatinine Clearance 10-30 ml/min) | Severe impairment (Creatinine Clearance <10 ml/min) |
|---|---|---|
| 3.2 g 8 hourly | 1.6 g 8 hourly | 1.6 g 12 hourly |

Similar reductions in dosage should be made for children.

*Administration:* Intravenous infusion

*Contra-indication:* Penicillin hypersensitivity.

*Special warnings and special precautions for use:* Changes in liver function tests have been observed in some patients receiving Timentin. The clinical significance of these changes is uncertain but Timentin should be used with care in patients with evidence of severe hepatic dysfunction.

For patients with abnormal renal function see *Posology and method of administration.* The sodium intake should be monitored in patients with renal impairment. In treating patients on sodium restriction it should be noted that each gram of ticarcillin contains 5.3 mmol of sodium (approx.). Potassium levels should be monitored and supplementation with potassium provided in appropriate cases.

In rare cases bleeding manifestations have been reported following high dosages of ticarcillin. If bleeding manifestations appear with Timentin, treatment should be discontinued and appropriate therapy instituted unless, in the opinion of the physician, no alternative is available.

*Interaction with other medicaments and other forms of interaction:* Timentin acts synergistically with aminoglycosides against a number of organisms including *Pseudomonas.* Timentin prescribed concurrently with an aminoglycoside, may therefore be preferred in the treatment of life-threatening infections, particularly in patients with impaired host defences. In such instances the two products should be administered separately, at the recommended dosages.

*Pregnancy and lactation:* Animal studies with Timentin have shown no teratogenic effects. There is no experience of Timentin in human pregnancy; therefore its use in pregnancy cannot be recommended. During lactation, trace quantities of penicillins can be detected in breast milk.

*Effects on ability to drive and use machines:* None known.

*Undesirable effects:* Side effects (gastrointestinal upsets, rash) are uncommon and typical of other injectable penicillins. If a skin rash occurs, treatment should be discontinued.

Hepatitis and cholestatic jaundice have been reported. Hypokalaemia and eosinophilia have been reported rarely. In common with other β-lactam antibiotics angioedema and anaphylaxis have been reported.

*Overdose:* There is an increased risk of bleeding if ticarcillin is given in excess doses.

Timentin may be removed from the circulation by haemodialysis.

## Pharmacological properties

*Pharmacodynamic properties:* Timentin is an injectable antibiotic, active against a wide range of both Gram-positive and Gram-negative bacteria, including β-lactamase-producing strains.

Resistance to many antibiotics is caused by bacterial enzymes which destroy the antibiotic before it can act on the pathogen. The clavulanate in Timentin anticipates this defence mechanism by blocking the β-lactamase enzymes, thus rendering the organisms sensitive to ticarcillin's rapid bactericidal effect at concentrations readily attainable in the body.

Clavulanate, by itself, has little antibacterial effect; however, in association with ticarcillin, as Timentin it produces an antibiotic agent with a breadth of spectrum suitable for empiric use in a wide range of infections treated parenterally in hospital.

*Pharmacokinetic properties:* The pharmacokinetics of the two components are closely matched and both components are well distributed in body fluids and tissues. Both clavulanate and ticarcillin have low levels of serum binding; about 20% and 45% respectively.

As with other penicillins the major route of elimination for ticarcillin is via the kidney; clavulanate is also excreted by this route.

*Preclinical safety data:* Not applicable.

## Pharmaceutical particulars

*List of excipients:* None.

*Incompatibilities:* Timentin is not compatible with the following:

Proteinaceous fluids (e.g. protein hydrolysates); blood and plasma; intravenous lipids.

If Timentin is prescribed concurrently with an aminoglycoside the antibiotics should not be mixed in the syringe, intravenous fluid container or giving set because loss of activity of the aminoglycoside can occur under these conditions.

*Shelf-life:* 36 months.

*Special precautions for storage:* Timentin should be stored in a dry place at temperatures below 25˚C.

*Nature and contents of container:* Clear glass vials with butyl rubber discs and aluminium seals. Supplied as packs of four vials.

*Instructions for use/handling:* The sterile powder should be dissolved in approximately 10 ml (1.6 g/ 3.2 g vial) prior to dilution into the infusion container (e.g mini-bag) or in-line burette.

The following approximate infusion volumes are suggested:

|  | Water for Injections BP | Glucose Intravenous Infusion BP (5% w/v) |
|---|---|---|
| 3.2 g | 100 ml | 100–150 ml |
| 1.6 g | 50 ml | 100 ml |

Detailed instructions are given in the Package Enclosure Leaflet.

Each dose of Timentin should be infused intravenously over a period of 30–40 minutes; avoid continuous infusion over longer periods as this may result in subtherapeutic concentrations.

800 mg Timentin has a displacement value of 0.55 ml.

Heat is generated when Timentin dissolves. Reconstituted solutions are normally a pale straw colour.

Timentin presentations are not for multi-dose use or for direct IV or IM injection. Any residual antibiotic solution should be discarded if less than the fully made up vial is used.

**Marketing authorisation number** 0038/0329

**Date of approval/revision of SPC** November 1996

**Legal category** POM

*\*Trade Mark*

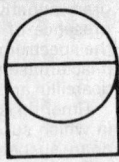

# Bencard
Welwyn Garden City
Hertfordshire AL7 1EY

## AMOXIL* CAPSULES
## AMOXIL* DISPERSIBLE TABLETS
## AMOXIL* SYRUPS SF
## AMOXIL* FIZTAB* TABLETS
## AMOXIL* SACHETS SF
## AMOXIL* PAEDIATRIC SUSPENSION
## AMOXIL* VIALS FOR INJECTION

**Presentation** *Amoxil Capsules:* (Amoxycillin Capsules BP) Maroon and gold capsules overprinted 'Amoxil 250', each providing 250 mg amoxycillin.

Maroon and gold capsules overprinted 'Amoxil 500', each providing 500 mg amoxycillin.

*Amoxil Dispersible Tablets:* Flat, white circular tablets, engraved 'Amoxil 500', each providing 500 mg amoxycillin.

*Amoxil Syrups SF:* (Amoxycillin Oral Suspension BP). Citrus-flavoured sucrose-free syrups providing 125 mg or 250 mg amoxycillin per 5 ml in a sorbitol base. Presented as powder in bottles for preparing 100 ml.

*Amoxil Fiztab Tablets:* Flat, white circular tablets engraved 'Amoxil 125', each providing 125 mg amoxycillin. Flat, white circular tablets, engraved 'Amoxil 250', each providing 250 mg amoxycillin. Flat, white circular tablets, engraved 'Amoxil 500', each providing 500 mg amoxycillin.

*Amoxil Sachets SF:* Sucrose-free sachets providing 750 mg or 3 g amoxycillin in a sorbitol base, for reconstitution in water. Each sachet carries instructions for preparation.

*Amoxil Paediatric Suspension:* Citrus flavoured suspension, providing 125 mg amoxycillin per 1.25 ml (measured by the pipette supplied). Presented as powder in bottles for preparing 20 ml.

*Amoxil Vials for Injection:* Each vial provides 250 mg, 500 mg or 1 g amoxycillin. Presented as sterile powder for reconstitution. Each pack contains instructions for use.

The amoxycillin content per unit dose is present as the trihydrate in Amoxil oral preparations and as the sodium salt in Amoxil injections. Each 1 g vial of Amoxil contains approximately 3.3 mmol of sodium.

Amoxil Syrups SF contain disodium edetate, sodium benzoate (E211) and sorbitol; Amoxil Fiztab Tablets and Sachets SF contain sorbitol; Amoxil Paediatric Suspension contains sodium benzoate (E211) and sucrose; Amoxil Dispersible Tablets contain lactose.

Amoxil Syrups SF, Fiztab Tablets, Sachets SF and Dispersible Tablets are sucrose-free. All Amoxil presentations are free from tartrazine and other azo dyes.

**Uses** *Treatment of Infection:* Amoxil is a broad spectrum antibiotic indicated for the treatment of commonly occurring bacterial infections such as:

Upper respiratory tract infections
Otitis media
Acute and chronic bronchitis
Chronic bronchial sepsis
Lobar and bronchopneumonia
Cystitis, urethritis, pyelonephritis
Bacteriuria in pregnancy
Gynaecological infections including puerperal sepsis and septic abortion
Gonorrhoea
Peritonitis
Intra-abdominal sepsis
Septicaemia
Bacterial endocarditis
Typhoid and paratyphoid fever
Skin and soft tissue infections
Dental abscess (as an adjunct to surgical management)

In children with urinary tract infection the need for investigation should be considered.

*Prophylaxis of endocarditis:* Amoxil may be used for the prevention of bacteraemia, associated with procedures such as dental extraction, in patients at risk of developing bacterial endocarditis.

The wide range of organisms sensitive to the bactericidal action of Amoxil include:

Gram-positive
*Streptococcus faecalis*
*Streptococcus pneumoniae*
*Streptococcus pyogenes*

Gram-negative
*Haemophilus influenzae*
*Escherichia coli*
*Proteus mirabilis*

*Streptococcus viridans*
*Staphylococcus aureus* (penicillin-sensitive)
*Clostridium* species
*Corynebacterium* species
*Bacillus anthracis*
*Listeria monocytogenes*

*Salmonella* species
*Shigella* species
*Bordetella pertussis*
*Brucella* species
*Neisseria gonorrhoeae*
*Neisseria meningitidis*
*Vibrio cholerae*
*Pasteurella septica*

**Dosage and administration** *Treatment of infection:*

*Adult dosage (including elderly patients):*

*Oral:*
*Standard adult dosage:* 250 mg three times daily, increasing to 500 mg three times daily for more severe infections.

*High-dosage therapy* (maximum recommended oral dosage 6 g daily in divided doses): A dosage of 3 g twice daily is recommended in appropriate cases for the treatment of severe or recurrent purulent infection of the respiratory tract.

*Short-course therapy:* Simple acute urinary tract infection: two 3 g doses with 10–12 hours between the doses. Dental abscess: two 3 g doses with 8 hours between the doses. Gonorrhoea: single 3 g dose.

All Fiztab presentations should be chewed thoroughly before swallowing.

*Injectable:*
500 mg IM eight hourly (or more frequently if necessary) in moderate infections. (This dose may be given by slow IV injection if more convenient.)

1 g IV six hourly in severe infections.

*Children's dosage (up to 10 years of age):* Oral: Standard children's dosage: 125 mg three times daily, increasing to 250 mg three times daily for more severe infections.

Amoxil Fiztab Tablets must be chewed and swallowed; therefore this product cannot be recommended in children below three years of age.

Amoxil Paediatric Suspension is recommended for children under six months of age.

In severe or recurrent acute otitis media, especially where compliance may be a problem, 750 mg twice a day for two days may be used as an alternative course of treatment in children aged three to 10 years. The use of Amoxil 750 mg Sachets SF is recommended.

Injectable: 50–100 mg/kg body weight a day, in divided doses.

Parenteral therapy is indicated if the oral route is considered impracticable or unsuitable, and particularly for the urgent treatment of severe infection.

In renal impairment the excretion of the antibiotic will be delayed and, depending on the degree of impairment, it may be necessary to reduce the total daily dosage.

*Prophylaxis of endocarditis:* See table.

*Administration:* Oral: Using capsules, dispersible tablets, syrups, Fiztab tablets, sachets or paediatric suspension.

Intravenous Injection: Dissolve 250 mg in 5.0 ml Water for Injections BP (Final volume = 5.2 ml).

Dissolve 500 mg in 10 ml Water for Injections BP (Final volume = 10.4 ml).

Dissolve 1 g in 20 ml Water for Injections BP (Final volume = 20.8 ml).

Amoxil injection, suitably diluted, may be injected directly into a vein or the infusion line over a period of 3–4 minutes.

Intravenous Infusion: Solutions may be prepared as described for intravenous injections and then added to an intravenous solution in a minibag or in-line burette and administered over a period of half to one hour. Alternatively, using a suitable reconstitution device, the appropriate volume of intravenous fluid may be transferred from the infusion bag into the vial and then drawn back into the bag after dissolution.

Intramuscular: 250 mg: Add 1.5 ml Water for Injections BP † and shake vigorously (Final volume = 1.7 ml).

500 mg: Add 2.5 ml Water for Injections BP † and shake vigorously (Final volume = 2.9 ml).

1 g: Add 2.5 ml Water for Injections†† and shake vigorously (Final volume = 3.3 ml).

† If pain is experienced on intramuscular injection, a sterile 1% solution of lignocaine hydrochloride or 0.5% solution of procaine hydrochloride may be used in place of Water for Injections.

†† The 1 g vial will not dissolve in sterile 1% solution of lignocaine hydrochloride at the required concentration. To minimise pain on injection, 1 g of Amoxil may be given as two separate injections of 500 mg dissolved in a sterile solution of 1% lignocaine hydrochloride (see above).

A transient pink colouration or slight opalescence may appear during reconstitution. Reconstituted solutions are normally a pale straw colour.

**Contra-indications, warnings, etc**
*Contra-indication:* Amoxil is a penicillin and should not be given to penicillin-hypersensitive patients.

*Use in pregnancy and lactation:* Animal studies with Amoxil have shown no teratogenic effects. The product has been in extensive clinical use since 1972 and its suitability in human pregnancy has been well documented in clinical studies. When antibiotic therapy is required during pregnancy, Amoxil may be considered appropriate. During lactation, trace quantities of Amoxil can be detected in breast milk.

*Side-effects:* Side-effects, as with other penicillins, are uncommon and mainly of a mild and transitory nature; they may include diarrhoea, indigestion, or occasionally rash, either urticarial or erythematous. An urticarial rash suggests penicillin hypersensitivity and the erythematous-type rash may arise if Amoxil is administered to patients with glandular fever. In either case treatment should be discontinued. In common with other β-lactam antibiotics angioedema and anaphylaxis have been reported. Pseudomembranous colitis has been reported rarely.

Amoxil Fiztab Tablets and SF formulations contain sorbitol (see *Further Information*).

*Overdosage:* Gross overdosage will produce very high urinary concentrations, more so after parenteral administration. Problems are unlikely if adequate fluid intake and urinary output are maintained; however, crystalluria is a possibility. More specific measures may be necessary in patients with impaired renal function: the antibiotic is removed by haemodialysis.

**Pharmaceutical precautions** Amoxil Fiztab Tablets and Sachets SF should be stored in a dry place below 25°C. Prior to use, other oral presentations of Amoxil should be stored in a dry place. Amoxil injections should be stored in a cool, dry place.

Once dispensed, Amoxil Syrups SF and Amoxil Paediatric Suspension should be stored at 25°C or below and used within 14 days. If dilution of the reconstituted SF product is required, water should be used. Amoxil Paediatric Suspension may be diluted with water or Syrup BP.

When prepared for intramuscular or direct intravenous injection, Amoxil should be administered immediately after reconstitution. The stability of Amoxil in various infusion fluids is dependent upon the concentration and temperature: stability times are given in the package enclosure leaflet.

Amoxil should not be mixed with blood products, other proteinaceous fluids such as protein hydrolysates, or with intravenous lipid emulsions.

If Amoxil is prescribed concurrently with an aminoglycoside, the antibiotics should not be mixed in the syringe, intravenous fluid container or giving set because loss of activity of the aminoglycoside can occur under these conditions.

**Legal category** POM.

**Package quantities** *Amoxil Capsules:* 250 mg: Original Pack of 21 with Patient Information Leaflet; also container of 500. 500 mg: Original Pack of 21 with Patient Information Leaflet; also container of 100.

*Amoxil Dispersible Tablets:* 500 mg: Original Pack of 21 with Patient Information Leaflet.

*Amoxil Syrups SF:* 125 mg and 250 mg per 5 ml: Original Pack of 100 ml with Patient Information Leaflet.

*Amoxil Fiztab Tablets:* 125 mg: Original Pack of 20 with Patient Information Leaflet. 250 mg: Original Pack of 20 with Patient Information Leaflet. 500 mg: Original Pack of 20 with Patient Information Leaflet.

*Amoxil 750 mg Sachet SF:* Original Pack of 4. Each sachet carries instructions for preparation and each pack contains a Patient Information Leaflet.

*Amoxil 3 g Sachet SF:* Original Pack of 2. Each sachet carries instructions for preparation and each pack contains a Patient Information Leaflet.

*Amoxil Paediatric Suspension:* 125 mg per 1.25 ml: Original Pack of 20 ml with pipette and Patient Information Leaflet.

**Prophylaxis of Endocarditis:**

| Condition | | Adults' Dosage (including elderly) | Children's Dosage | Notes |
|---|---|---|---|---|
| Dental Procedures: Prophylaxis for patients undergoing extraction, scaling or surgery involving gingival tissues, and who have not received a penicillin in the previous month. (N.B. Patients with prosthetic heart valves should be referred to hospital – see below.) | Patient not having general anaesthetic. | 3 g Amoxil orally, 1 hour before procedure. A second dose may be given 6 hours later, if considered necessary. | Under 10: Half adult dose. Under 5: Quarter adult dose  The use of Amoxil 500 mg Dispersible Tablets or 750 mg Sachets SF is recommended. | Note 1. If prophylaxis with Amoxil is given twice within one month, emergence of resistant streptococci is unlikely to be a problem. Alternative antibiotics are recommended if more frequent prophylaxis is required, or if the patient has received a course of treatment with a penicillin during the previous month. Note 2. To minimise pain on injection, Amoxil may be given as two injections of 500 mg dissolved in sterile 1% lignocaine solution (see 'Administration'). |
| | Patient having general anaesthetic: if oral antibiotics considered to be appropriate. | Initially 3 g Amoxil orally 4 hours prior to anaesthesia, followed by 3 g orally (or 1 g IV or IM if oral dose not tolerated) as soon as possible after the operation. | | |
| | Patient having general anaesthetic: if oral antibiotics not appropriate. | 1 g Amoxil IV or IM immediately before induction; with 500 mg orally, 6 hours later. | | |
| Dental Procedures: Patients for whom referral to hospital is recommended: (a) patients to be given a general anaesthetic who have been given a penicillin in the previous month. (b) patients to be given a general anaesthetic who have a prosthetic heart valve. (c) patients who have had one or more attacks of endocarditis. | | Initially: 1 g Amoxil IV or IM with 120 mg gentamicin IV or IM, immediately prior to anaesthesia (if given) or 15 minutes prior to dental procedure. Followed by (6 hours later): 500 mg Amoxil orally. | Under 10: The doses of Amoxil should be half the adult dose; the dose of gentamicin should be 2 mg/kg.  Under 5: The doses of Amoxil should be quarter the adult dose: the dose of gentamicin should be 2 mg/kg. | See Note 2. Note 3. Amoxil and gentamicin should not be mixed in the same syringe. Note 4. Please consult the appropriate data sheet for full prescribing information on gentamicin. |
| Genito-urinary Surgery or Instrumentation: Prophylaxis for patients who have no urinary tract infection and who are to have genito-urinary surgery or instrumentation under general anaesthesia. | | Initially: 1 g Amoxil IV or IM with 120 mg gentamicin IV or IM, immediately before induction. Followed by (6 hours later): 500 mg Amoxil orally or IV or IM according to clinical condition. | | See Notes 2, 3 and 4 above. |
| Obstetric and Gynaecological Procedures / Gastro-intestinal Procedures | Routine prophylaxis is recommended only for patients with prosthetic heart valves. | | | |
| Surgery or Instrumentation of the Upper Respiratory Tract | Patients other than those with prosthetic heart valves. | 1 g Amoxil IV or IM immediately before induction; 500 mg Amoxil IV or IM 6 hours later. | Under 10: Half adult dose.  Under 5: Quarter adult dose. | See Note 2 above. Note 5. The second dose of Amoxil may be administered orally as Amoxil Syrup SF. |
| | Patients with prosthetic heart valves. | Initially: 1 g Amoxil IV or IM with 120 mg gentamicin IV or IM, immediately before induction; followed by (6 hours later) 500 mg Amoxil IV or IM. | Under 10: The dose of Amoxil should be half the adult dose; the gentamicin dose should be 2 mg/kg.  Under 5: The dose of Amoxil should be quarter the adult dose; the dose of gentamicim should be 2 mg/kg. | See Notes 2, 3, 4 and 5 above. |

*Amoxil Vials for Injection:* 250 mg, 500 mg and 1 g: packs of 10, 10 and 5 respectively. Each pack carries instructions for use.

**Further information** Amoxil is well absorbed by the oral and parenteral routes. Oral administration, usually at convenient t.d.s. dosage, produces high serum levels independent of the time at which food is taken. Amoxil gives good penetration into bronchial secretions and high urinary concentrations of unchanged antibiotic. It is rapidly bactericidal and possesses the safety profile of a penicillin.
*Sucrose content (approx.):* Amoxil Paediatric Suspension (125 mg) 0.6 g per 1.25 ml.
*Sorbitol content (approx.):* Amoxil Syrups SF (125 mg and 250 mg) 1 g per 5 ml; Amoxil Fiztab Tablets (125 mg) 0.045 g; Amoxil Fiztab Tablets (250 mg) 0.09 g; Amoxil Fiztab Tablets (500 mg) 0.18 g; Amoxil Sachet SF (750 mg) 1.1 g; Amoxil Sachet SF (3 g) 4.2 g.

**Product licence numbers**
| | |
|---|---|
| Amoxil Capsules 250 mg | 0038/0103 |
| Amoxil Capsules 500 mg | 0038/0105 |
| Amoxil Dispersible Tablets 500 mg | 0038/0277 |
| Amoxil Syrup SF 125 mg per 5 ml | 0038/0326 |
| Amoxil Syrup SF 250 mg per 5 ml | 0038/0327 |
| Amoxil Fiztab Tablets 125 mg | 0038/0359 |
| Amoxil Fiztab Tablets 250 mg | 0038/0360 |
| Amoxil Fiztab Tablets 500 mg | 0038/0361 |
| Amoxil 750 mg Sachet SF | 0038/0332 |
| Amoxil 3 g Sachet SF | 0038/0334 |
| Amoxil Paediatric Suspension 125 mg per 1.25 ml | 0038/0107 |
| Amoxil Vials for Injection 250 mg | 0038/0221 |
| Amoxil Vials for Injection 500 mg | 0038/0222 |
| Amoxil Vials for Injection 1 g | 0038/0225 |

## TEMOPEN*

**Presentation** Vial containing 1 g of temocillin as temocillin sodium. Presented as an off-white/pale yellow sterile solid for reconstitution for IM/IV injection or infusion use.

**Uses**
*Action:* Temopen is a bactericidal injectable penicillin which is active against most strains of Enterobacteriaceae (including *E. coli*, *Klebsiella* and *Proteus* species). Other sensitive organisms include *Haemophilus influenzae*. It is stable in the presence of the β-lactamase produced by many Gram-negative organisms and is, therefore, active against many strains of β-lactamase-producing Gram-negative aerobes which are resistant to a number of other antibiotics.
Temocillin is not generally active against *Pseudomonas* species, Gram-positive cocci or anaerobic organisms.

*Indications:* Temopen is indicated for the treatment of septicaemia, urinary tract infection and lower respiratory tract infection in which susceptible Gram-negative bacilli are suspected or confirmed.
In mixed infections where Gram-positive or anaerobic bacteria are also liable to be implicated, co-administration of flucloxacillin and metronidazole may be considered.

**Dosage and administration**
*Adults (including the elderly):* The usual dosage is 1–2 g every 12 hours. In the treatment of acute, uncomplicated urinary tract infections 1 g daily may be used, given as a single dose or in divided dosage.
Temopen may be administered by intravenous injection or infusion or intramuscular injection. High and prolonged serum concentrations are maintained, with an elimination half-life of four to five hours. The main route of excretion is via the kidney. Approximately 75% of a 1 g dose of Temopen is excreted unchanged in the urine within the first 24 hours.

*Children:* Insufficient data are available to recommend an appropriate dosage regime.

*Dosage in patients with impaired renal or hepatic function (adults):* No adjustment to the normal dosage is recommended for patients with a mild degree of renal impairment (creatinine clearance >30 ml/min). In more severe cases adjustment of the interval between doses is recommended (rather than a reduced dosage) as indicated below:

| Degree of renal impairment | Creatinine clearance (ml/min) | Recommended interval between doses |
|---|---|---|
| Moderate | 30–10 | 24 hours |
| Severe (not requiring dialysis) | <10 | 48 hours |

Temopen is removed by haemodialysis. In patients receiving dialysis a further dose of Temopen should be given at the end of each period of dialysis.
Limited experience in patients with impaired hepatic function has not indicated a need for a reduction in dosage.

*Preparation and administration:* Temopen may be administered by intramuscular or intravenous injection, or by intermittent intravenous infusion. Temopen is not intended for multi-dose use; any part-used antibiotic solution should be discarded. Solutions are normally a pale yellow colour.

*Intravenous injection:*

| Dose | Recommended volume of Water for Injections BP to be added for dissolution | Final volume |
|---|---|---|
| 1 g | 20 ml | 20.7 ml |
| 2 g | 20 ml | 21.4 ml |

Temopen solutions should be administered by slow injection into the vein or an infusion line over a period of 3–4 minutes.

*Intravenous infusion:* Solutions should be prepared as described for intravenous injection and then added to an intravenous infusion solution in a mini bag or in-line burette and administered over a period of 30–40 minutes. Alternatively, using a suitable reconstitution device, the appropriate volume of intravenous fluid may be transferred from the infusion bag into the vial and then drawn back into the bag after dissolution.

*Intramuscular injection:*

| Vial strength | Recommended volume of Water for Injections BP to be added for dissolution | Final volume |
|---|---|---|
| 1 g | 2 ml | 2.7 ml |

After addition of water to the vial, shake vigorously.
If pain is experienced at the site of IM injection, a sterile solution of lignocaine hydrochloride 0.5–1% may be used in place of Water for Injections.

## Contra-indications, warnings, etc

*Contra-indication:* Penicillin hypersensitivity.

*Use in pregnancy and lactation:* Animal studies with Temopen have shown no teratogenic effect. There is no experience of Temopen in human pregnancy: therefore its use in pregnancy cannot be recommended. Trace quantities of penicillins can be detected in the milk of lactating mothers.

*Precautions:* In patients with moderate or severe renal impairment, the interval between doses should be increased (see *Dosage and administration* section).

*Side effects:* These are uncommon and typical of the injectable penicillins: they may include diarrhoea; pain at the site of IM injection; occasionally rash, either urticarial or erythematous. If a rash occurs treatment should be discontinued. In common with other β-lactam antibiotics angioedema and anaphylaxis have been reported.

*Overdosage:* There have been no reported cases of overdosage. Dosages of up to 8 g daily have been administered to volunteers without untoward effects.

Temopen may be removed from the circulation by haemodialysis.

**Pharmaceutical precautions**   Vials of Temopen should be stored in a dry place, below 20°C. Temopen is not intended for multi-dose use, and any part-used antibiotic solutions should be discarded.

Temopen solutions for direct injection or IV infusion should normally be administered within 30 minutes of preparation. However, they may be kept for up to 24 hours in a refrigerator (2–8°C). Refrigerated solutions should be restored to ambient temperature before use.

Temopen is compatible with commonly used aqueous intravenous fluids including Water for Injections BP, Sodium Chloride (0.9% w/v) Intravenous Infusion BP, Glucose (5% w/v) Intravenous Infusion BP. Other appropriate infusion fluids are listed in the Package Enclosure Leaflet.

Temopen may be mixed with cloxacillin or flucloxacillin in the same intravenous injection or infusion. Temopen is compatible with intravenous infusion solutions of metronidazole.

If Temopen is prescribed concurrently with an aminoglycoside, the antibiotics should not be mixed in the syringe, intravenous fluid container or giving set because loss of activity of the aminoglycoside can occur under these conditions.

Temopen solutions should not be mixed with blood products or other proteinaceous fluids (e.g. protein hydrolysates) or with intravenous lipid emulsions.

**Legal category**   POM.

**Package quantities**   Temopen vials: 1 g pack of five.
Each pack contains instructions for use.

**Further information**   Temopen offers selective parenteral treatment for appropriate Gram-negative systemic infections, with minimal disturbance of the normal intestinal flora. Each 1 g of Temopen contains approximately 5 mmol of sodium.

Temopen is not a significant inducer of β-lactamase production.

**Product licence number**   0038/0350

*\*Trade Mark*

# Berk Pharmaceuticals Limited
Brampton Road
Hampden Park
Eastbourne
East Sussex
BN22 9AG

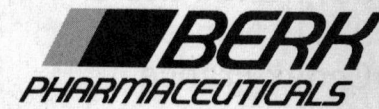

## AlfaD*

**Presentation** AlfaD 0.25 mcg are pink soft gelatin capsules printed '0.25' containing alfacalcidol (1-α hydroxyvitamin D₃) 0.25 micrograms.

AlfaD 1 mcg are orange soft gelatin capsules printed '1.0' containing alfacalcidol (1-α hydroxyvitamin D₃) 1 microgram.

The capsules also contain arachnis (peanut) oil, sodium ethyl hydroxybenzoate (E215) and sodium propyl hydroxybenzoate (E217). The 0.25 mcg capsules contain the colours erythrosine (E127) and black iron oxide (E172). The 1 mcg capsules contain the colours sunset yellow (E110) and black iron oxide (E172).

## Uses

*Action:* Alfacalcidol undergoes rapid hepatic conversion to 1,25-dihydroxyvitamin D₃, the Vitamin D₃ metabolite which acts as a regulator of calcium and phosphate metabolism.

When 1-α hydroxylation by the kidneys is impaired, endogenous 1,25-dihydroxyvitamin D₃ production is reduced. Disorders in which this can occur include renal bone disease, hypoparathyroidism and Vitamin D-dependent rickets. Such conditions require high doses of Vitamin D for their correction but will respond to small doses of AlfaD, which does not depend on the renal 1-α hydroxylation process.

When using parent Vitamin D, the high dose and variable response time can lead to unpredictable hypercalcaemia which may take many weeks, sometimes months, to reverse. With AlfaD, the more rapid onset of response allows better titration of dose and, if hypercalcaemia does occur, it can be reversed within days of stopping treatment.

AlfaD is used for treating conditions in which calcium metabolism is disturbed due to impaired 1-α hydroxylation and other disorders associated with Vitamin D resistance.

The main indications are: Renal osteodystrophy; hypoparathyroidism; hyperparathyroidism (with bone disease); nutritional and malabsorptic rickets and osteomalacia; hypophosphataemic vitamin-D resistant rickets and osteomalacia; pseudo-deficiency (D-dependent Type I) rickets and osteomalacia.

## Dosage and administration

All indications: Starting dose:
*Children 20 kg and over:* 1 microgram/day
*Adults:* 1 microgram/day
*Elderly patients:* 0.5 microgram/day.

The dose should subsequently be adjusted according to the biochemical response. Plasma calcium levels (preferably corrected for protein binding) should initially be measured weekly. The dose of AlfaD can be increased by increments of 0.25 to 0.5 micrograms/day. Most adults respond to doses of 1 to 3 micrograms/day. Once the dose is stabilised, calcium levels may be measured every 2-4 weeks.

Indices of response, in addition to plasma calcium, may include alkaline phosphatase, parathyroid hormone levels, bone radiography and histological investigations. When there is biochemcial or radiographic evidence of bone healing (or in hypoparathyroidism when calcium levels have normalised) the dose required for maintenance generally decreases to around 0.25 to 1 microgram/day. Should hypercalcaemia occur, AlfaD should be stopped until plasma calcium returns to normal (usually about a week) then restarted at one half of the previous dose.

*Renal osteodystrophy:* Patients with already high plasma calcium levels may have autonomous hyperparathyroidism. In this situation they may not respond to alfacalcidol and other therapeutic measures may be indicated.

In patients with chronic renal disease it is particularly important to check the plasma calcium frequently because prolonged hypercalcaemia may further impair renal function.

Before and during AlfaD treatment, the use of phosphate binding agents to prevent hyperphosphataemia may also be considered.

*Hypoparathyroidism:* Low plasma calcium levels can be dangerous and may be restored to normal more quickly with AlfaD than with parent Vitamin D. Severe hypocalcaemia is corrected more rapidly with higher doses of AlfaD (e.g. 3-5 micrograms) together with calcium supplements.

*Hyperparathyroidism:* In patients needing surgery for primary or tertiary hyperparathyroidism, pre-operative treatment with AlfaD for 2-3 weeks can reduce bone pain and myopathy without aggravating hypercalcaemia. To decrease the risk of post-operative hypocalcaemia, AlfaD should be continued until the plasma alkaline phophatase falls to normal or hypercalcaemia occurs.

*Nutritional and malabsorptive rickets and osteomalacia:* Malabsorptive osteomalacia, which responds to large doses of IM or IV parent Vitamin D, will respond to small oral doses of AlfaD. Nutritional rickets and osteomalacia can also be rapidly cured with AlfaD.

*Hypophosphataemic vitamin D-resistant rickets and osteomalacia:* Normal doses of AlfaD rapidly relieve myopathy, when present, and increase calcium and phosphate retention. Phosphate supplements may also be required in some patients. Neither large doses of parent Vitamin D nor phosphate supplements are entirely satisfactory in these conditions.

*Pseudo-deficiency (D-dependent Type I) rickets and osteomalacia:* As with the nutritional conditions, similar oral doses of AlfaD are effective in circumstances which would require high doses of parent Vitamin D.

## Contra-indications, warnings, etc

*Contra-indications:* Alfacalcidol should not be used in patients with evidence of Vitamin D toxicity or known hypersensitivity to the effects of Vitamin D or any of its analogues.

*Precautions:* Alfacalcidol increases the intestinal absorption of calcium and phosphate, serum levels of which should be monitored, particularly in patients with renal failure.

If hypercalcaemia or hypercalciuria occur this can be corrected rapidly by stopping treatment with AlfaD and any calcium supplements until plasma calcium levels return to normal, usually in about a week. AlfaD may then be restarted at half the last dose used.

Response to alfacalcidol may be impaired if the diet is markedly deficient in calcium.

Healing of bone lesions often indicates a decreased requirement for AlfaD in which case appropriate dose adjustments should be made (see Dosage and administration section).

*Use in pregnancy and lactation:* There is insufficient evidence on which to assess the safety of alfacalciol use during pregnancy, although it has been widely used for many years without apparent adverse effects. Animal studies have not revealed any hazard but as with all drugs, AlfaD should only be used during pregnancy if treatment is essential and no better alternative is available.

Although not definitely established, it is likely that increased levels of 1,25-dihydroxyvitamin D₃ will be found in the breast milk of mothers treated with alfacalcidol. This might have an influence on calcium metabolism in a breast-fed infant.

*Use in children:* AlfaD capsules are not indicated in children under 20 kg as the dosage cannot be titrated adequately.

*Use in the elderly:* Initiation of therapy requires a lower dose in elderly patients. The clinical manifestations of hypo- or hypercalcaemia should be considered especially in elderly patients with pre-existing renal or heart conditions.

*Drug interactions:* Hypercalcaemia in patients taking digitalis preparations may precipitate cardiac arrhythmias. Patients taking digitalis concurrently with alfacalcidol must therefore be closely monitored.

Patients on barbiturates or other anticonvulsants may require an increased dose of AlfaD to produce the desired effect.

Absorption of alfacalcidol may be impaired by concurrent use of mineral oil (prolonged use), cholestyramine, colestipol, sucralfate or large amounts of aluminium-based antacids.

Caution should be exercised in the use of magnesium based antacids or laxatives for patients taking alfacalcidol who are on chronic renal dialysis. Hypermagnesaemia may occur.

The risk of hypercalcaemia is increased in patients taking calcium-containing preparations or thiazide diuretics concurrently with alfacalcidol.

Alfacalcidol is a potent derivative of Vitamin D. Pharmacological doses of Vitamin D or its analogues should not be given during alfacalcidol treatment because of the possibility of additive effects and an increased risk of hypercalcaemia.

*Adverse effects:* Adverse effects generally relate to abnormally elevated serum calcium levels and, in the case of renal impairment, elevated serum phosphate levels which may be induced by AlfaD therapy. The dosage should be adjusted to the patient's requirements.

*Overdosage:* Administration of AlfaD should be stopped if hypercalcaemia occurs. Severe hypercalcaemia may require treatment with general supporting measures, with intravenous fluids, with a loop diuretic or with corticosteroids.

In acute overdosage, early treatment with gastric lavage and/or the administration of mineral oil may reduce absorption and promote faecal elimination.

**Pharmaceutical precautions** Store below 25°C.

**Legal category** POM.

**Package quantities**
AlfaD 0.25 mcg: Containers of 100 capsules
AlfaD 1 mcg: Containers of 30 or 100 capsules

**Further information** Nil

**Product licence numbers**
AlfaD 0.25 mcg 6468/0001
AlfaD 1 mcg 6468/0002.

*Product licence holder:* TEVA Pharmaceuticals Industries Limited, PO Box 3190, Petah Tikva, Israel.

*Trade Mark

**Biogen France SA**
55 Avenue des Champs Pierreux
92012 Nanterre
Cedex-France

## AVONEX* ▼

**Qualitative and quantitative composition** Avonex (Interferon beta-1a) is formulated as a white to off-white lyophilised powder, containing a 30 micrograms (6 million IU) dose of Interferon beta-1a per vial.

Using the World Health Organization (WHO) natural interferon beta standard, Second International Standard for Interferon, Human Fibroblast (Gb-23-902-531), 30 micrograms of Avonex contains 6 million IU of antiviral activity. The activity against other standards is not known.

**Pharmaceutical form** Avonex (Interferon beta-1a) is a powder and solvent for solution for injection to be administered intramuscularly after reconstitution.

**Clinical particulars**

*Therapeutic indications:* Avonex (Interferon beta-1a) is indicated for the treatment of ambulatory patients with relapsing multiple sclerosis (MS) characterised by at least 2 recurrent attacks of neurologic dysfunction (relapses) over the preceding 3-year period without evidence of continuous progression between relapses. Avonex slows the progression of disability and decreases the frequency of relapses over a 2-year period.

Avonex has not yet been investigated in patients with progressive multiple sclerosis, and should be discontinued in patients who develop progressive multiple sclerosis.

Not all patients respond to treatment with Avonex. No clinical criteria that would predict the response to treatment have been identified.

*Posology and method of administration:* The recommended dosage of Avonex (Interferon beta-1a) for the treatment of relapsing MS is 30 micrograms injected (1 ml solution) IM once a week (see *Instructions for use*). Treatment should be initiated under supervision of a physician experienced in the treatment of the disease.

The safety and efficacy of doses other than 30 micrograms given IM once weekly in patients with MS have not been evaluated. Therefore, the optimal dose of Interferon beta-1a in MS may not have been established.

The IM injection site should be varied each week (see *Preclinical safety data*).

Prior to injection and for an additional 24 hours after each injection, an antipyretic analgesic is advised to decrease flu-like symptoms associated with Avonex administration. These symptoms are usually present during the first few months of treatment.

There is no experience with Avonex in patients aged 16 years or less. Therefore, Avonex should not be used in children.

At the present time, it is not known for how long patients should be treated. There is currently no clinical experience with Avonex beyond 2 years of treatment. Patients should be clinically evaluated after 2 years of treatment and longer-term treatment should be decided on an individual basis by the treating physician. Treatment should be discontinued if the patient develops chronic progressive multiple sclerosis.

*Contra-indications:* Avonex (Interferon beta-1a) is contra-indicated in patients with a history of hypersensitivity to natural or recombinant interferon beta, human serum albumin, or any other component of the formulation.

Avonex is contra-indicated in pregnant patients (also see *Pregnancy and lactation*), patients with severe depressive disorders and/or suicidal ideation, and in epileptic patients with a history of seizures not adequately controlled by treatment.

*Special warnings and special precautions for use:* There is limited long-term safety experience with Avonex (Interferon beta-1a). To date, a limited number of patients have been followed for up to 2 years.

Patients should be informed of the most common adverse events associated with interferon beta administration, including symptoms of the flu-like syndrome (see *Undesirable effects*). These symptoms tend to be most prominent at the initiation of therapy and decrease in frequency and severity with continued treatment.

Avonex should be used with caution in patients with depression. Depression and suicidal ideation are known to occur in association with interferon use and to occur at an increased frequency in the MS population. Patients treated with Avonex should be advised to immediately report any symptom of depression and/or suicidal ideation to their prescribing physician. Patients exhibiting depression should be monitored closely during therapy with Avonex and treated appropriately. Cessation of therapy with Avonex should be considered.

Caution should be exercised when administering Avonex to patients with pre-existing seizure disorder. For patients without a pre-existing seizure disorder who develop seizures during therapy with Avonex, an aetiologic basis should be established and appropriate anti-convulsant therapy instituted prior to resuming Avonex treatment.

Caution should be used and close monitoring considered when administering Avonex to patients with severe renal and hepatic failure and to patients with severe myelosuppression.

Patients with cardiac disease, such as angina, congestive heart failure or arrhythmia, should be closely monitored for worsening of their clinical condition during initiation of therapy with Avonex. Symptoms of the flu-like syndrome associated with Avonex therapy may prove stressful to patients with cardiac conditions.

Patients should be advised about the abortifacient potential of interferon beta (see *Use during pregnancy and lactation* and *Preclinical safety data*).

Laboratory abnormalities are associated with the use of interferons. Therefore, in addition to those laboratory tests normally required for monitoring patients with multiple sclerosis, complete and differential white blood cell counts, platelet counts, and blood chemistries, including liver function tests, are recommended during Avonex therapy. Patients with myelosuppression may require more intensive monitoring of complete blood cell counts, with differential and platelet counts.

Serum neutralising antibodies against Avonex may develop. The precise incidence rate of antibody formation is as yet uncertain. Initial data suggest that after 12 months of treatment approximately 15% of patients (95% confidence interval, 6–30%) develop serum antibodies to Avonex. This is assumed to represent the plateau for incidence of antibody formation. Data suggest that in some patients the development of antibodies is associated with a reduction of clinical efficacy.

The use of various assays to detect serum antibodies to interferons limits the ability to compare antigenicity among different products.

*Interactions with other medicaments and other forms of interaction:* No formal drug interaction studies have been conducted with Avonex (Interferon beta-1a) in humans.

The interaction of Avonex with corticosteroids or ACTH has not been studied systematically. The clinical studies indicate that multiple sclerosis patients can receive Avonex and corticosteroids or ACTH during relapses.

Interferons have been reported to reduce the activity of hepatic cytochrome P450-dependent enzymes in humans and animals. The effect of high-dose Avonex administration on P450-dependent metabolism in monkeys was evaluated and no changes in liver metabolising capabilities were observed. Caution should be exercised when Avonex is administered in combination with medicinal products that have a narrow therapeutic index and are largely dependent on the hepatic cytochrome P450 system for clearance, e.g. antiepileptics and some classes of antidepressants.

*Use during pregnancy and lactation:* Because of the potential hazards to the foetus, Avonex (Interferon beta-1a) is contra-indicated in pregnancy. There are no studies of Interferon beta-1a in pregnant women. At high doses, in rhesus monkeys, abortifacient effects were observed. It cannot be excluded that such effects will be observed in humans.

Fertile women receiving Avonex should take appropriate contraceptive measures. Patients planning for pregnancy and those becoming pregnant should be informed of the potential hazards and Avonex should be discontinued.

*Nursing mothers:* It is not known whether Avonex is excreted in human milk. Because of the potential for serious advserse reactions in nursing infants, a decision should be made either to discontinue nursing or to discontinue Avonex therapy.

*Effects on the ability to drive and use machines:* Certain less commonly reported undesirable effects on the central nervous system (see *Undesirable effects*) may influence the ability to drive and operate a machine in susceptible patients.

*Undesirable effects:* The highest incidence of adverse events associated with the interferon therapy are related to flu syndrome. The most commonly reported symptoms of the flu syndrome are muscle ache, fever, chills, asthenia, headache, and nausea. Symptoms of the flu syndrome tend to be most prominent at the initiation of therapy and decrease in frequency with continued treatment.

Other less common adverse events include: diarrhoea, anorexia, vomiting, arthralgia, insomnia, dizziness, anxiety, rash, injection site reaction, vasodilation, and palpitations.

Hypersensitivity reactions may occur and appropriate treatment should be initiated.

Seizures and arrhythmia can rarely occur during treatment with Avonex (Interferon beta-1a, see *Special warnings and precautions*).

Depression and suicide have been reported, therefore Avonex should be used with caution in patient with depression (see *Special warnings and precautions*).

Although not usually requiring treatment, certain laboratory abnormalities may occur during treatment with Avonex. Decreases in circulating lymphocytes, white blood cell count, platelet count, neutrophils and hematocrit may occur.

With interferons in general, transient increases in creatinine, potassium, urea nitrogen, alanine transaminase and aspartate transaminase may occur. Transient moderate increases in urinary calcium may also occur.

*Overdose:* There are no reports of overdosage. However, in case of overdosage, patients should be hospitalised for observation and appropriate supportive treatment given.

**Pharmacological properties**

*Pharmacodynamic properties:* Pharmacotherapeutic Group: Cytokines, ATC code L03 AA.

Interferons are a family of naturally occurring proteins that are produced by eukaryotic cells in response to viral infection and other biological inducers. Interferons are cytokines that mediate antiviral, antiproliferative, and immunomodulatory activities. Three major forms of interferons have been distinguished: alpha, beta, and gamma. Interferons alpha and beta are classified as Type I interferons, and interferon gamma is a Type II interferon. These interferons have overlapping but clearly distinguishable biological activities. They can also differ with respect to their cellular sites of synthesis.

Interferon beta is produced by various cell types including fibroblasts and macrophages. Natural interferon beta and Avonex (Interferon beta-1a) are glycosylated and have a single N-linked complex carbohydrate moiety. Glycosylation of other proteins is known to affect their stability, activity, biodistribution, and half-life in blood. However, the effects of interferon beta that are dependent on glycosylation are not fully defined.

Avonex exerts its biological effects by binding to specific receptors on the surface of human cells. This binding initiates a complex cascade of intracellular events that leads to the expression of numerous interferon-induced gene products and markers. These include MHC Class I, Mx protein, 2'/5'-oligoadenylate synthetase, $\beta_2$-microglobulin, and neopterin. Some of these products have been measured in the serum and cellular fractions of blood collected from patients treated with Avonex. After a single IM dose of Avonex, serum levels of these products remain elevated for at least 4 days and up to 1 week.

Whether the mechanism of action of Avonex in multiple sclerosis is mediated by the same pathway as the biological effects described above is not known because the pathophysiology of multiple sclerosis is not well established.

The effects of Avonex in the treatment of multiple sclerosis were demonstrated in a single placebo-controlled study of 301 patients (Avonex, n=158; placebo, n=143) with relapsing MS. Due to the design of the study, patients were followed for variable lengths of time. One hundred and fifty Avonex-treated patients completed 1 year on study and 85 completed 2 years on study. In the study, the cumulative percentage of patients who developed disability progression (by Kaplan-Meier life table analysis) by the end of 2 years was 35% for placebo-treated patients and 22% for Avonex-treated patients. Disability progression was measured as an increase in the Expanded Disability Status Scale (EDSS) of 1.0 point, sustained for at least 6 months. It was also shown that there was a one-third reduction in annual relapse rate. This latter clinical effect was observed after more than one year of treatment.

*Pharmacokinetic properties:* The pharmacokinetic profile of Avonex (Interferon beta-1a) has been investigated indirectly with an assay that measures interferon antiviral activity. This assay is limited in that it is sensitive for interferon but lacks specificity for interferon beta. Alternative assay techniques are not sufficiently sensitive.

Following IM administration of Avonex, serum antiviral activity levels peak between 5 and 15 hours post-dose and decline with a half-life of approximately 10 hours. With appropriate adjustment for the rate of absorption from the injection site, the calculated bioavailability is approximately 40%. The calculated bioavailability is greater without such adjustments. Intramuscular bioavailability is three-fold higher than subcutaneous bioavailability. Subcutaneous administration cannot be substituted for IM administration.

*Preclinical safety data:* Carcinogenesis: No carcinogenicity data for Interferon beta-1a are available in animals or humans.

Chronic toxicity: No chronic toxicity data for Interferon beta-1a is available in animals.

Local tolerance: IM irritation has not been evaluated in animals following repeated administration to the same injection site.

Mutagenesis: Limited but relevant mutagenesis tests have been carried out. The results have been negative.

Impairment of fertility: Fertility and developmental studies in rhesus monkeys have been carried out with a related form of interferon beta-1a. At very high doses, anovulatory and abortifacient effects in test animals were observed. Similar reproductive dose-related effects have also been observed with other forms of alpha and beta interferons.

No teratogenic effects or effects on foetal development have been observed, but the available information on the effects of interferon beta-1a in the peri- and postnatal periods is limited.

No information is available on the effects of the interferon beta-1a on male fertility.

### Pharmaceutical particulars
*List of excipients:* Human serum albumin, di- and monobasic sodium phosphate, sodium chloride.

*Incompatibilities:* None known.

*Shelf life:* The shelf life of Avonex (Interferon beta-1a) is 24 months.

*Special precautions for storage:* Avonex (Interferon beta-1a) can be stored at a temperature up to 25°C. DO NOT FREEZE lyophilised or reconstituted product.

*Nature and contents of container:* Avonex (Interferon beta-1a) is available as a package of four individual doses of: Avonex in a 3 ml clear glass vial with a 13 mm bromobutyl rubber stopper and aluminium seal. It is provided with a 1 ml pre-filled glass syringe of solvent for reconstitution and 2 needles.

*Instructions for use/handling:* Avonex should be administered after reconstitution. However, the reconstituted solution can be stored at 2–8°C for up to 6 hours, prior to injection.

To reconstitute Avonex for injection, the supplied pre-filled syringe of solvent is used. No other solvent should be used. The content of the syringe is injected into the vial of Avonex using the green reconstitution needle. The contents in the vial are gently swirled until all materials are dissolved. DO NOT SHAKE. The reconstituted product is inspected and if it contains particulate matter or is other than colourless to slightly yellow in colour, the vial should be discarded. After reconstitution, 1 ml is drawn from the vial (guidance mark on the pre-filled syringe) for the administration of 30 micrograms Avonex. The needle for IM injection (blue) is provided. The formulation does not contain a preservative. Each vial of Avonex contains a single dose only. The unused portion of any vial should be discarded.

**Marketing authorisation number** EU/1/97/033/001

**Date of approval/revision of SPC** August 1997.

**Legal category** POM.

*\*Trade Mark*

# Bioglan Laboratories Limited
## 5 Hunting Gate
## Hitchin
## Herts SG4 0TJ

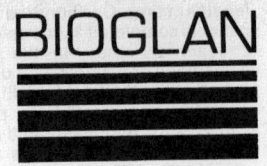

## BARITOP* 100

**Qualitative and quantitative composition** Barium Sulphate PhEur 100% w/v.

**Pharmaceutical form** Barium Sulphate Suspension.

**Clinical particulars**

*Therapeutic indications:* Baritop 100 is an x-ray contrast medium for use in the radiological examination of the gastrointestinal tract.

*Posology and method of administration:* Oral or by enema in accordance with the parts to be examined and examination methods

*Adults and the elderly:*

| Part of GI Tract | Method | Volume (ml) | Concentration (% w/v) |
|---|---|---|---|
| Oesophagus | Oral | 10-150 | 50-100 |
| Stomach and duodenum | Oral, double contrast, distension filling and relief | 10-300 | 30-100 |
| Small intestine | Oral | 100-300 | 30-100 |
| Colon | Enema | 200-2000 | 20-100 |

*Children:* As for adults but in proportion to body weight.

*Infants:* As for adults but in proportion to body weight.

*Contra-indications:*

| Oral use: | Suspected perforation of intestinal organs: Haemorrhage in digestive organs |
|---|---|
| Enema use: | Suspected perforation of intestinal organs: Haemorrhage in digestive organs: Extreme exhaustion |

*Special warnings and precautions for use:* Baritop 100 should be used with great caution in:

| Oral use: | Suspected or known fistula in digestive organs: stricture or signs suggesting obstruction. Suffering from extreme exhaustion. |
|---|---|
| Enema use: | Suspected or known fistula in digestive organs: stricture or signs suggesting obstruction: diseases of internal organs that could lead to perforation (e.g. appendicitis, diverticulitis, ulcerative colitis, invagination tumour, parasitic disease etc). |

*Interaction with other medicaments and other forms of interaction:* None stated.

*Pregnancy and lactation:* At the discretion of the physician.

*Effects on ability to drive and use machines:* None stated.

*Undesirable effects:* May cause constipation, transient diarrhoea, abdominal pain, anal pain and bleeding.

*Overdose:* Treat symptomatically.

**Pharmacological properties**

*Pharmacodynamic properties:* Not applicable.

*Pharmacokinetic properties:* Not applicable.

*Preclinical safety data:* No formal preclinical studies have been undertaken. Barium sulphate is a well established pharmaceutical substance that has been available for many years. It is also the subject of a recognised Pharmacopoeial Monograph.

**Pharmaceutical particulars**

*List of excipients:* In addition to the active ingredient, Baritop 100 contains: Sodium Carboxymethylcellulose BP, Tragacanth HSE, Sodium Saccharin HSE, Glycine BP, Sodium Ascorbate HSE, Silicon Resin Emulsion HSE, Sodium Benzoate BPC, Sodium Dehydroacetate USNF, Cream Soda Essence Flavour HSE, Purified Water BP.

*Incompatabilities:* None known.

*Shelf life:* 24 months.

*Special precautions for storage:* None stated.

*Nature and contents of container:* 300 ml sealed can. Tin free steel coated internally with vinyl resin on epoxy resin.

*Instructions for use/handling:* None stated.

**Marketing authorisation number:** 0041/0024

**Date of approval/revision of SPC** January 1996.

**Legal category** P

## BARITOP* PLUS

**Qualitative and quantitative composition** Barium sulphate JP 94.6% w/w

**Pharmaceutical form** Granules to prepare an aqueous suspension for oral or rectal use as a radiopaque.

**Clinical particulars**
*Therapeutic indications:* Baritop Plus is an x-ray contrast medium for use in the radiological examination of the gastrointestinal tract.

*Posology and method of administration:* After reconstitition with water to make a suspension, Baritop Plus is either taken orally as a barium meal or given rectally as an enema.

*Adult:*

| Part of GI Tract | Method | Volume (ml) | Concentration (% w/v) |
|---|---|---|---|
| Oesophagus | Oral | 10-150 | 50-200 |
| Stomach and duodenum | Oral, double contrast, distension filling and relief | 10-300 | 30-200 |
| Small intestine | Oral | 100-300 | 30-150 |
| Colon | Enema | 200-2000 | 20-130 |

*Children and infants:* As for adults but in proportion to body weight.

*Contra-indications:*

| Oral use: | Suspected perforation of intestinal organs: Haemorrhage in digestive organs |
|---|---|
| Enema use: | Suspected perforation of intestinal organs: Haemorrhage in digestive organs: Extreme exhaustion |

*Special warnings and precautions for use:* Baritop Plus should be used with great caution in:

| Oral use: | Suspected or known fistula in digestive organs: stricture or signs suggesting obstruction. |
|---|---|
| Enema use: | Suspected or known fistula in digestive organs: stricture or signs suggesting obstruction: diseases of internal organs that could lead to perforation (e.g. appendicitis, diverticulitis, ulcerative colitis, invagination tumour, parasitic disease etc). |

*Interaction with other medicaments and other forms of interaction:* None stated.

*Pregnancy and lactation:* At the discretion of the physician.

*Effects on ability to drive and use machines:* None stated.

*Undesirable effects:* May cause constipation.

*Overdose:* Treat symptomatically.

**Pharmacological properties**

*Pharmacodynamic properties:* Not applicable – barium sulphate is not absorbed from the gastrointestinal tract.

*Pharmacokinetic properties:* Not applicable – barium sulphate is not absorbed from the gastro-intestinal tract.

*Preclinical safety data:* No formal preclinical studies have been undertaken. Barium sulphate is a well established pharmaceutical substance that has been available for many years. It is also the subject of a recognised pharmacopoeial monograph.

**Pharmaceutical particulars**

*List of excipients:* In addition to the active ingredient, Baritop Plus contains: Potato Starch (soluble) HSE, Powdered Acacia JP, Silicon Resin Emulsion HSE, Sodium Benzoate JP, Strawberry Oil HSE, Sodium Carboxymethyl Cellulose JSFA, Hydrogenated Maltose Starch Syrup HSE, Purified Water BP.

*Incompatabilities:* None known.

*Shelf life:* 24 months.

*Special precautions for storage:* None stated.

*Nature and contents of container:* Polyethylene – cellulose bags 200 gm pack. Polyethylene – Nylon bags 1000 gm pack.

*Instructions for use/handling:* None stated.

**Marketing authorization number:** 0041/0025

**Date of approval/revision of SPC** January 1996.

**Legal category** P

## BENZAMYCIN* GEL

**Presentation** Benzamycin Gel is presented as a plastic jar containing 20 g of gel and a separate plastic vial (Erythro-pac) containing 0.8 g of erythromycin, which is dissolved in ethanol and added to the gel at the time of dispensing by the pharmacist.

When dispensed Benzamycin Gel is a white gel containing benzoyl peroxide 5% w/w and Erythromycin BP 3% w/w.

**Uses** For the topical treatment of acne vulgaris.

*Pharmacology:* Benzamycin provides an antimicrobial agent with mild keratolytic properties and antibiotic effects. Erythromycin inhibits lipase production whilst benzoyl peroxide reduces the comedone count and has antibacterial action.

**Dosage and administration** Benzamycin should be applied twice daily, morning and evening, to areas usually affected by acne or as directed by the physician. These areas should first be gently washed, rinsed with lukewarm water, and patted dry. Benzamycin should be applied with the fingertips and the hands washed after application.

**Contra-indications, warnings, etc**

*Contra-indications:* Benzamycin is contra-indicated in persons who have shown hypersensitivity to benzoyl peroxide or erythromycin.

*Warnings:* For external use only. Keep away from the eyes, nose, mouth and other mucous membranes. Very fair individuals should begin with a single application at bedtime allowing overnight medication. May bleach hair or dyed fabrics.

*Interactions:* Concomitant topical acne therapy should be used with caution to avoid a possible cumulative irritancy effect. Antagonism has been demonstrated between clindamycin and erythromycin.

*Use in pregnancy and lactation:* The safe use of Benzamycin during pregnancy and lactation has not been established.

*Side effects:* Reported adverse rections have been dryness of the skin and uriticaria.

*Overdose:* Due to the topical administration of this product, overdose is unlikely to occur.

**Pharmaceutical precautions** Prior to reconstitution store at or below 25°C. After reconstitution, store between 2° and 8°C in the refrigerator. Do not freeze.

**Legal category** POM

**Package quantities** 23.3 g as dispensed.

**Further information** Nil.

**Product licence number** 12725/001

*Product licence holder:* Dermik Laboratories Inc, Collegeville, PA, USA.

## BIORPHEN*

**Qualitative and quantitative composition** Orphenadrine Hydrochloride BP 25 mg/5 ml.

**Pharmaceutical form** Aqueous liquid.

*Therapeutic indications:* Parkinsonism, particularly with apathy and depression, and drug induced extrapyramidal syndrome.

*Posology and method of administration:* Oral dose.

*Adults and elderly:* 150 mg daily in divided doses. Maximum dose 400 mg daily. Optimal dose range 150–300 mg and this is usually achieved by raising the dose by 50 mg every two to three days.

*Children:* Not recommended.

*Contra-indications:* Glaucoma, prostatic hypertrophy, urinary retention.

*Special warnings and precautions for use:* Caution in renal and hepatic disease.

*Interaction with other medicaments and other forms of interaction:* Amantidine, antidepressants, antihistamines, disopyramide, phenothiazines, terodiline. May additionally increase anticholinergic activity.

*Pregnancy and lactation:* Caution must be observed.

*Effects on ability to drive and use machines:* None known.

*Undesirable effects:* Dry mouth, blurred vision.

*Overdose:* Gastric lavage, emetic and high enema is recommended. Cholinergics may be useful.

**Pharmacological properties**

*Pharmacodynamic properties:* Orphenadrine is an antimuscarinic agent.

*Pharmacokinetic properties:* No formal pharmacokinetic studies have been performed. The product is an oral solution and the active material is therefore immediately available for absorption.

*Preclinical safety data:* No formal preclinical studies have been undertaken. Orphenadrine hydrochloride is a well-established pharmaceutical substance that has been available for many years. It is also the subject of a recognised pharmacopoeial monograph.

**Pharmaceutical particulars**

*List of excipients:* In addition to the active ingredients Biorphen contains: Sorbitol PhEur, Glycerol PhEur, Anise Water Concentrated BP, Saccharin Sodium BP, Tween 20 PhEur, Benzoic Acid Solution BP, Water Purified PhEur.

*Incompatibilities:* None known.

*Shelf life:* 24 months.

*Special precautions for storage:* None stated.

**Marketing authorization number** 0041/0028

**Date of approval/revision of SPC** January 1996.

**Legal category** POM.

## BROFLEX*

**Qualitative and quantitive composition** Benzhexol Hydrochloride BP 5 mg/5 ml.

**Pharmaceutical form** Syrup.

**Clinical particulars**

*Therapeutic indications:* Parkinsonism and drug induced extrapyramidal syndrome.

*Posology and method of administration:* Oral administration.
*Adults and elderly:* Initial dose 2 mg subsequent doses up to 20 mg as recommended by a physician.
*Children:* Not recommended.

*Contra-indications:* Incipient glaucoma may be precipitated. The following are not absolute contra-indications, nevertheless caution must be observed in patients with: hypertension, cardiac, liver or kidney dysfunction, glaucoma, obstructive diseases of the gastro-intestinal or genito-urinary tracts and in males with prostatic hypertrophy.

*Special warnings and special precautions for use:* None stated.

*Interaction with other medicaments and other forms of interaction:* Monoamine oxidase inhibitors (MAOIs), antihistamines, disopyramide, phenothiazines, tricyclic antidepressants increase the side-effects of blurred vision and dry mouth, constipation, urinary retention, MAOIs and amantadine and some tricyclic antidepressants may also cause excitation, confusion and hallucination.

*Pregnancy and lactation:* At the discretion of the physician.

*Effects on the ability to drive and use machines:* None known.

*Undesirable effects:* Dry mouth, constipation and blurred vision occur and this is more frequent in the elderly but reduces with tolerance.

*Overdose:* There is no specific antidote. Gastric lavage, emetics and high enemas are recommended. Forced fluid intake and general supportive measures are necessary. Atropine antagonists may be helpful.

**Pharmacological properties**

*Pharmacodynamic properties:* None stated.

*Pharmacokinetic properties:* None stated.

*Preclinical safety data:* No formal preclinical studies have been undertaken. Benzhexol Hcl is a well-established pharmaceutical substance that has been available for many years. It is also the subject of a recognised pharmacopoeial monograph.

**Pharmaceutical particulars**

*List of excipients:* In addition to the active ingredients Broflex contains: Anhydrous Citric Acid PhEur, Benzoic Acid PhEur, Propylene Glycol PhEur, Amaranth E123 HSE, Glycerol PhEur, Chloroform Spirit BP, Blackcurrant Flavour A402 HSE, Syrup BP, Purified Water PhEur.

*Incompatibilities:* None known.

*Shelf life:* 24 months.

*Special precautions for storage:* None.

*Nature and contents of container:* 200 ml and 1000 ml pack size in amber glass bottle with polycone lined closure.

*Instructions for use/handling:* None stated.

**Marketing authorization number** 0041/0029

**Date of approval/revision of SPC** December 1996.

**Legal category** POM.

## CITRAMAG*

**Presentation** A sachet containing a white, effervescent powder which produces 17.7 g magnesium citrate in aqueous solution, equivalent in alkalinity to 5 g magnesium oxide.

**Uses** For preparation of the patient for all radiological examinations requiring a completely evacuated bowel. May also be used for colorectal surgery.

**Dosage and administration**

*Dosage:*
*Adults:* The contents of one sachet are to be used as required before the radiological examinations or colorectal surgery. The dose may be reduced for very ill, very thin or elderly patients who may tolerate vigorous purgation poorly.
  *Children (over 10 years):* Reduce the dose to half the adult dose. (5-9 years): Reduce the dose to one third of adult dose

*Administration:* A low residue or a fluid only diet, according to the instructions of the prescribing clinician, is begun thirty six hours before the examination. At 7.30 a.m. on the day before the examination, the aqueous solution is prepared and allowed to dissolve and cool. It is taken orally at 8.00am. Plenty of clear fluids should be drunk between taking Citramag and the examination.

**Contra-indications, warnings etc.** There are no contra-indications. For some patients, particularly those in renal failure, it may be necessary to modify the routine instructions supplied with Citramag.

When any doubts exist about the suitability of the routine instructions, the advice of the treating physician should be obtained. It should be noted that fruit juice, which has a high content of potassium, should be avoided in conditions in which hyperkalaemia can occur, such as Addison's disease, selective hypoaldosteronism, and treatment with spironolactones, triamterene or amiloride.

Similarly, the risk of toxic hypermagnesaemia indicates the need for caution in the administration of magnesium citrate to patients in renal failure.

*Use in pregnancy and lactation:* Use at the discretion of the physician.

**Pharmaceutical precautions** Store in a cool, dry place– below 25C

**Legal category** P

**Package quantities** Sachets containing 29.5 g

**Further information** Nil

**Product licence number** 0041/0030.

## EPADERM*

**Qualitative and quantitative composition** Yellow Soft Paraffin BP, Emulsifying Wax BP.

**Pharmaceutical form** A pale yellow translucent emulsifying ointment.

**Clinical particulars**

*Therapeutic indications:* For general use as an emollient to moisturise and soften dry skin. Epaderm may be used instead of soap.

*Posology and method of administration:* Children, adults and elderly: Epaderm should be massaged into the skin as often as required. Epaderm may also be added to the bath by first producing a dispersion with hot water. When used as a bath additive, care should be taken as it will make the surface slippery.

*Contra-indications:* There are no specific contraindications to the use of Epaderm apart from known sensitivity to any of the components.

*Special warnings and precautions for use:* None stated.

*Interaction with other medicaments and other forms of interaction:* None known.

*Pregnancy and lactation:* The effect of Epaderm during pregnancy and lactation has not been studied. Therefore, there are no recommendations in these conditions.

*Effects on ability to drive and use machines:* None stated.

*Undesirable effects:* None known.

*Overdose:* Overdose is highly unlikely. If necessary, medication should be removed by washing with warm water.

**Pharmacological properties**

*Pharmacodynamic properties:* Epaderm is an emollient preparation for topical application to the skin.

*Pharmacokinetic properties:* Not applicable as this is a topical preparation.

*Preclinical safety data:* The active ingredients are well documented therapeutic agents and therefore preclinical or toxicological data are available from the public domain and not submitted in this instance. Emulsifying wax and yellow soft paraffin are both subjects of pharmacopoeial monographs–both being quoted in the BP.

**Pharmaceutical particulars**

*List of excipients:* In addition to the active ingredients, Epaderm contains: Liquid Paraffin BP.

*Incompatabilities:* None known.

*Shelf life:* 2 years.

*Special precautions for storage:* Store below 25°C in a dry place.

*Nature and contents of container:* 500 g white polypropylene securitub with tamper-evidence closure. 125 g white polypropylene securipot with tamper-evident closure. 50 g white polypropylene securipot with tamper evident closure.

*Instructions for use/handling:* None stated.

**Marketing authorization number** 0041/0049

**Date of approval/revision of the SPC** February 1997.

**Legal category** GSL

## HYDROCAL* CREAM

**Presentation** Hydrocal is a pale pink cream containing Hydrocortisone Acetate BP 1% w/w, in an emollient base containing Calamine BP.

**Uses** Hydrocal is indicated for the relief of the inflammatory manifestations of corticosteroid responsive dermatoses including seborrhoeic dermatitis or eczema with or without associated acne, atopic eczema, photodermatitis, primary irritant and allergic dermatitis, intertrigo, insect bite reactions and napkin rash or urinary dermatitis.

**Dosage and administration** A small quantity should be applied to the affected area two or three times daily.

**Contra-indications, warnings, etc** Primary skin lesions caused by tubercular, fungal, viral and bacterial infections. Known hypersensitivity to Hydrocal or any of its ingredients.

*Precautions and warnings:* Continuous treatment for longer than three weeks should be avoided in patients under the age of three years because of the possibility of adrenocortical suppression.

In infants, the napkin may act as an occlusive dressing and treatment of that area should not exceed seven days.

Prolonged use of uninterrupted occlusion or use with extensive occlusive dressing may suppress adrenocortical function.

Continuous application without interruption may result in local atrophy of the skin, striae, and superficial dilation, particularly on the face.

When treating inflammatory lesions which have become secondarily infected, appropriate antimicrobial therapy should be used.

*Pregnancy and lactation:* Topical administration of corticosteroids to pregnant animals can cause abnormalities of foetal development. The relevance of this finding to man has not been established. Topical steroids should not be administered extensively in pregnancy: ie, in large amounts or for prolonged periods.

*Side-effects:* Preparations containing hydrocortisone are usually well tolerated, but if signs of hypersensitivity appear, application should stop immediately.

Local atrophic changes may occur where skin folds are involved, or in sites such as the nappy area in small children, where constant moist conditions favour the absorption of hydrocortisone. Sufficient systemic absorption may also occur in such sites to produce the features of hypercorticism and suppression of the HPA axis after prolonged treatment. This effect is more likely to occur in infants and children, and if occlusive dressings are used.

**Pharmaceutical precautions**   Store below 25°C.

**Legal category**   POM

**Package quantities**   Hydrocal Cream is supplied in tubes containing 25 g and 100 g.

**Further information**   Ingredients: Hydrocortisone Acetate BP, Calamine BP, emulsifying wax, oleyl alcohol, light mineral oil, Phenonip, Polysorbate 20, Bronopol BP and Purified Water PhEur.

**Product licence number**   0041/0001

## ISOTRATE* 20

**Presentation**   Isotrate 20 tablets are white, round biconvex uncoated tablets engraved 'B20 ISMN' on one side and plain on the reverse. Each tablet contains isosorbide mononitrate 20 mg.

**Uses**   Isotrate is indicated for the prophylaxis of angina pectoris.

Isotrate is not indicated in the management of acute attacks of angina pectoris.

*Mode of action:* Isosorbide-5-mononitrate is an active metabolite of isosorbide dinitrate and from an oral dose exerts qualitatively similar effects. However, unlike the dinitrate which is subject to extensive 'first pass' hepatic metabolism, it has virtually complete systemic availability from an oral dose. Isosorbide mononitrate thus achieves predictable and sustained blood levels. Onset of pharmacological effects occur within 20 minutes of an oral dose and are maintained for more than 8 hours. Isosorbide-5-mononitrate is mainly eliminated via metabolism in the liver. The inactive metabolites are mainly excreted via the kidneys.

**Dosage and administration**

*Adults:* Usually one tablet twice or three times daily. Patients already accustomed to prophylactic nitrate therapy (for example with isosorbide dinitrate) may normally be transferred directly to a therapeutic dose of Isotrate. For patients not receiving prophylactic nitrate therapy, it is recommended that the initial dose should be one Isotrate tablet daily. Maintenance dose in individual patients will be between 20 mg and 120 mg daily.

*Elderly patients:* As for adults, but particular care is required because of susceptibility to hypotension.

The tablets should be swallowed whole with a little fluid.

*Children:* Safety and efficacy in children has not been established.

**Contra-indications, warnings, etc**   A known sensitivity to the drug or to isosorbide dinitrate, acute myocardial infarction with low filling pressures, acute circulatory failure (shock), severe hypotension or cerebral trauma, marked anaemia or hypovolaemia.

*Precautions and warnings:* Side-effects include hypotension, headache, dizziness and nausea. Usually, these respond to temporary reduction in dose on continued therapy.

Nitrates may give rise to symptoms of collapse after the first dose in patients with labile circulation. These symptoms can largely be avoided if the treatment is started with a low dose.

Isosorbide mononitrate should be used with caution in patients who are predisposed to closed angle glaucoma.

Headache may occur at the onset of treatment but will usually subside after a few days; if the headache persists dosage should be temporarily decreased.

Isosorbide mononitrate should be used with caution in patients suffering from hypothyroidism, hypothermia, malnutrition, severe liver or renal disease.

*Pregnancy and lactation:* As with other drugs, nitrates should not be administered to pregnant women and nursing mothers unless essential.

*Overdosage:* Overdosage should be treated symptomatically. The main symptom is likely to be hypotension and this may be treated by elevation of the legs to promote venous return.

**Pharmaceutical precautions**   Store at room temperature. Protect from moisture.

**Legal category**   P

**Package quantities**   Isotrate is blister packed in cartons of 60 sachets.

**Further information**   Isosorbide mononitrate is the British Approved Name for Isosorbide-5-mononitrate.

**Product licence number**   0041/0006.

## METAZEM*

**Qualitative and quantitative composition**   Diltiazem hydrochloride HSE 60 mg per tablet

**Pharmaceutical form**   Tablets intended for internal use.

**Clinical particulars**

*Therapeutic indications:* Prophylaxis and treatment of angina pectoris.

*Posology and method of administration: Adults:* 60 mg three times daily. As patient response may vary, the dose can be increased to a maximum of 360 mg daily in divided doses. Higher doses up to 480 mg/day have been used with benefit in some patients especially in unstable angina.

*Elderly patients with impaired hepatic or renal function:* Initially 60 mg twice daily. Monitoring of the heart rate should be carried out. The dose should not be increased if the rate falls below 50 beats per minute.

*Children:* Not recommended.

*Contra-indications:* Bradycardia, second or third degree heart block, uncontrolled left ventricular failure, sick sinus syndrome. Also contraindicated in pregnancy and in women of childbearing potential.

*Special warnings and precautions for use:* The product should be used with caution in patients with reduced ventricular function. Patients with mild bradycardia, first degree AV block or prolonged PR interval should be observed closely.

*Interaction with other medicaments and other forms of interaction:* The doses of both Metazem and beta-blockers should be reduced when both drugs are used concurrently. Metazem may increase the levels of beta-blockers which have a low bioavailability. Metazem may cause small increases in the plasma levels of digitalis. The blood levels of carbamazipine, cyclosporin and theophylline may be increased when given concurrently with diltiazem hydrochloride. Concurrent administration of $H_2$ antagonists may increase the blood level of Metazem. Concurrent use of Metazem with alpha blockers such as prazosin should be strictly monitored because of the possible synergistic hypotensive effect of this combination.

Metazem treatment has been continued with problem during anaesthesia, but the anaesthetist should be informed that the patient is receiving a calcium antagonist. Metazem, like any calcium antagonist, should not be administered concurrently with dantrolene infusion because of the risk of ventricular fibrillation.

*Pregnancy and lactation:* Metazem is teratogenic in some animal species and therefore should not be used in pregnancy or in women of childbearing potential.

Metazem is excreted in breast milk and therefore should not be used in nursing mothers until an alternative method of infant feeding has been instituted.

*Effects on ability to drive and use machines:* None known.

*Undesirable effects:* Metazem is generally well tolerated. Occasional undesirable effects are nausea, headache, skin rashes, oedema of the legs, flushing, hypotension and fatigue which disappear on cessation of treatment. Metazem may cause depression of atrioventricular nodal conduction and bradycardia. Changes in liver function tests and renal function have been reported in a few cases.

*Overdose:* The clinical syndromes of acute intoxication may include pronounced hypotension or even collapse, and sinus bradycardia with or without atrioventricular conduction defects.

The patient should be closely monitored in hospital to exclude arrhythmias or atrioventricular conduction defects. Gastric lavage and osmotic diuresis should be undertaken when considered appropriate. Symptomatic bradycardia and high grade atrioventricular block may respond to atropine, isoprenaline or occasionally temporary cardiac pacing. Hypotension may require correction with plasma volume expanders, intravenous calcium gluconate and positive inotropic agents.

**Pharmacological properties**

*Pharmacodynamic properties:* Metazem is a calcium antagonist. It restricts the slow channel entry of calcium ions into the cell and so reduces the liberation of calcium from stores in the sarcoplasmic reticulum. This results in a reduction in the amount of available intracellular calcium and consequently a (1) reduction of myocardial oxygen consumption (2) dilation of small and large coronary arteries (3) mild peripheral vasodilation (4) negative dromotropic effects (5) reflex positive chronotrophic and inotropic effects due to reflex sympathetic activity are partially inhibited and result in a slight reduction or no change in heart rate.

The antianginal effect is due to reduction in cardiac oxygen demand with maintenance of coronary blood flow. Cardiac contractility and ventricular ejection fraction are unchanged. Metazem increases exercise capacity and improves indices of myocardial ischaemia in the angina patient. Metazem relieves the spasm of vasospastic (Prinzmetal's) angina.

*Pharmacokinetic properties:* Metazem is rapidly and almost completely absorbed from gastrointestinal tract following oral administration, but undergoes extensive first-pass hepatic metabolism. The bioavailability has been reported to be about 40%, although there is considerable inter-individual variation in plasma concentration. Metazem is about 80% bound to plasma proteins. It is extensively metabolised in the liver; one of the metabolites, desacetyldiltiazem has been reported to have 25 to 50% of the activity of the parent compound. The half-life is reported to be about 3 to 5 hours. Approximately 2 to 4% of a dose is excreted in urine as unchanged diltiazem with the remainder excreted as metabolites in bile and urine.

*Preclinical safety data:* There are no pre-clinical data of relevance to the prescriber which are additional to that already included in other sections of the SPC.

**Pharmaceutical particulars**

*List of excipients:* In addition to the active ingredient, Metazem contains: Lactose Monohydrate PhEur, Hydrogenated Castor Oil USNF, Polyethylene Glycol 6000 USNF, Magnesium Stearate PhEur.

*Incompatibilities:* None known.

*Shelf life:* 3 years.

*Special precautions for storage:* Store below 25°C in a dry place. Keep out of the reach of children.

*Nature and contents of container:* The product is blister packed (10s) in 250µ PVC film faced with 48 g PVDC and sealed with hard tempered aluminium lidding foil. The blister strips are subsequently packed in printed boxboard cartons, in pack sizes of 60, 100 and 500 tablets.

*Instructions for use/handling:* No special precautions.

**Marketing authorization number**   0041/0011

**Date of approval/revision of SPC**   October 1995.

**Legal category** POM

## PRAGMATAR* CREAM

**Presentation**   Pragmatar Cream is a pale, buff-coloured, oil-in-water cream containing 4% w/w cetyl alcohol-coal tar distillate, 3% w/w precipitated sulphur and 3% w/w salicylic acid.

**Uses**   Pragmatar has mild antipruritic, antiseptic and keratolytic properties. It is indicated in the treatment of dandruff, other seborrhoeic conditions, and common scaly skin disorders.

**Dosage and administration**

*Adults and children:* For mild dandruff, apply the cream once a week when the hair is washed. For more severe cases, treat the entire scalp daily at bedtime, applying lightly but thoroughly with the fingertips. The cream can be washed out the next morning or when convenient. For other indicated subacute or chronic skin disorders, apply daily in small quantities to affected areas only.

For use in infants, the cream may be diluted by mixing with a few drops of water in the palm of the hand.

**Contra-indications, warnings, etc**   Do not use in patients who are sensitive to sulphur, or in the presence of acute local infection.

*Warnings (caution):* Use with care near the eyes, mucous membranes, or on acutely inflamed areas. If any cream should accidentally enter the eye, flush with normal saline solution.

*Adverse reactions:* No side effects are to be expected if the cream is used accordingly to directions. Excessive use, however, may cause erythema and irritation.

*Overdosage:* If ingestion occurs, gastro-intestinal disturbances may follow. Treatment consists of rinsing out the mouth together with symptomatic measures if necessary. Even with massive ingestion, salicylate poisoning seems unlikely.

**Pharmaceutical precautions**   Store in a cool place.

**Legal category**   P

**Package quantities**   Tubes containing 25 g and 100 g with applicator.

**Further information** Any queries should be addressed to the Medical Information Department of the Product Licence Holder: Smith Kline & French Laboratories Ltd.

*Ingredients:* Cetyl alcohol-coal tar distillate, Precipitated Sulphur BP, Salicylic Acid BP, Sodium Carboxymethyl cellulose 7MF, Glycerol PhEur, Sodium Lauryl Sulphate BP, Cetyl Alcohol, light Liquid Paraffin BP, Perfume Bouquet 3522, Purified Water PhEur.

**Product licence number** 0002/5044R.

*Product licence holder:* Smith Kline & French Laboratories Ltd, Welwyn Garden City.

*Trade Mark

# Boehringer Ingelheim Limited
Ellesfield Avenue
Bracknell
Berkshire RG12 8YS

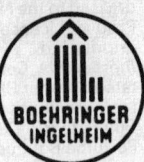

## ALUPENT* METERED AEROSOL

**Presentation** Alupent Metered Aerosol: 15 ml vial (300 metered doses) available as a complete unit with mouthpiece or as a refill vial only. Each metered dose contains orciprenaline sulphate 750 micrograms.

### Uses

*Action:* Alupent is a sympathomimetic amine with bronchodilator properties. The duration of action of a single dose is 3-6 hours.

*Indications:* Alupent is indicated for the relief of reversible airways obstruction.

Alupent metered aerosol is indicated for the relief of acute attacks.

### Dosage and administration By inhalation

*Adults:* The usual starting dose is 1 puff. This may be increased to 2 puffs as necessary. The maximum daily dose should not exceed 12 puffs in 24 hours. Doses should not be repeated within 30 minutes.

*Children 6–12 years:* As for adults. The maximum daily dose should however not exceed 8 puffs in 24 hours. Doses should not be repeated within 30 minutes.

*Children under 6 years:* The usual dose is 1 puff. The maximum daily dose should not exceed 4 puffs in 24 hours. Doses should not be repeated within 30 minutes.

No specific information on the use of this product in the elderly is available. Clinical trials have included patients over 65 years and no adverse reactions specific to this age group have been reported.

### Contra-indications, warnings etc

*Contra-indications:* Hypersensitivity to orciprenaline sulphate or the inactive ingredients of the metered aerosol.

*Precautions:* In patients suffering from bronchial asthma, on demand or symptom-oriented treatment may be preferable to regular use. A chronic requirement for treatment would suggest the need for clinical review of the management of the patient's asthma. The use of inhaled corticosteroids as anti-inflammatory treatment should be considered.

Patients must be instructed in the correct use of a metered aerosol and warned not to exceed the prescribed dose. In the case of acute rapidly worsening dyspnoea a doctor should be consulted immediately. In the event of a previously effective dose of inhaled Alupent failing to give relief lasting at least three hours, the patient should be advised to seek medical advice in order that any necessary additional steps may be taken.

Sympathomimetic agents can cause unwanted effects. The concomitant use of other sympathomimetic drugs should be avoided or only used under strict medical supervision. Alupent and anticholinergic bronchodilators have been administered concurrently in reversible airways obstruction. In some situations, co-administered sympathomimetic agents and anticholinergics have been shown to produce greater bronchodilatation than the use of either agent alone (but see Interactions).

In the following conditions Alupent should only be used after careful risk/benefit assessment, especially when doses higher than those recommended are used: Insufficiently controlled diabetes mellitus, recent myocardial infarction, severe organic heart or vascular disorders, such as hypertrophic obstructive cardiomyopathy and tachyarrhythmias: Hyperthyroidism.

Potentially serious hypokalaemia may result from excessive beta-agonist therapy. This effect may be potentiated by concomitant treatment with xanthine derivatives, glucocorticosteroids and diuretics. Additionally, hypoxia may aggravate the effects of hypokalaemia on cardiac rhythm. It is recommended that serum potassium levels are monitored in such situations.

In view of the possible interaction between beta-adrenergics and monoamine oxidase inhibitors or tricyclic anti-depressants, care should be exercised if it is proposed to administer these compounds concurrently with Alupent.

Beta-adrenergics, anticholinergics and xanthine derivatives may enhance the bronchodilator effect of orciprenaline.

The concurrent administration of the other beta-adrenergics, systemically absorbed anticholinergics and xanthine derivatives may increase the frequency and severity of unwanted effects.

Beta₂-receptor blockers counteract the action of Alupent.

Potentially serious bronchospasm may occur during concurrent administration of beta-blockers to patients with reversible airways obstruction.

*Use in pregnancy:* Although orciprenaline sulphate has been in general use for several years, there is no definite evidence of ill-consequence following administration of the drug during human pregnancy. Only in doses far in excess of the equivalent maximum human dose were effects on foetal development seen in animals.

Alupent should only be used during pregnancy, especially the first trimester, if the potential benefit outweighs the potential risk to the foetus.

The inhibitory effect of orciprenaline sulphate on uterine contraction should be taken into account.

Safety in breast-fed infants has not been established.

*Side-effects:* The most frequently reported undesirable effects observed with Alupent are tremor and nervousness, headache, dizziness, tachycardia, palpitations, gastrointestinal discomfort, nausea and vomiting. Some patients have experienced a feeling of tightness of chest.

In rare cases, local irritation or allergic reactions have been reported.

As with other inhaled bronchodilators, paradoxical broncho-constriction has been reported.

*Overdosage: Symptoms:* The expected symptoms of overdosage with Alupent are those of excessive beta-stimulation such as flushing, tremor, nausea, restlessness, tachycardia, palpitation, dizziness, headache, hypotension, hypertension, a feeling of pressure in the chest, excitation, angina, increased pulse pressure and arrhythmia. Hypokalaemia may occur following overdose with orciprenaline. Serum potassium levels should be monitored.

*Therapy:* Treatment of overdosage should primarily be supportive and symptom-oriented.

If specific therapy is considered necessary, cardio-selective beta-blockers are to be preferred. These should be administered with extreme caution to patients with asthma because of the risk of precipitating severe bronchospasm.

**Pharmaceutical precautions** Alupent preparations should be protected from heat, light and air. Protect aerosol vials from frost. The vials should not be incinerated or opened even when apparently empty.

**Legal category** POM

**Package quantities** Metered aerosol: 15 ml vial (300 metered doses) (OP) complete with mouthpiece. 15 ml refill vial.

**Further information** Alupent is also available as Tablets and Syrup for maintenance therapy.

**Product licence number** 0015/5002

## ALUPENT* SYRUP

**Qualitative and quantitative composition** Clear, colourless syrup with a vanilla-like flavour. Each 5 ml contains orciprenaline sulphate 10 mg.

**Pharmaceutical form** Syrup for oral administration.

### Clinical particulars

*Therapeutic indications:* Alupent is indicated for the relief of reversible airways obstruction.

Alupent Syrup is suggested for maintenance therapy.

*Posology and method of administration:*

*Adults:* The usual dose is 2 x 5 ml four times daily. The maximum recommended daily dosage is 8 x 5 ml spoonfuls.

*Children 3-12 years:* The usual starting dose is 1 x 5 ml four times daily. This may be increased to 2 x 5 ml three times daily as necessary. The maximum recommended daily dosage is 6 x 5 ml spoonfuls.

*Children 1-3 years:* The usual starting dose is ½ x 5 ml four times daily. This may be increased to 1 x 5 ml four times daily as necessary. The maximum recommended daily dosage is 4 x 5 ml spoonfuls.

*Children 0-1 year:* The usual starting dose is ½ x 5 ml three times daily. This may be increased to 1 x 5 ml three times daily as necessary. The maximum recommended daily dosage is 3 x 5 ml spoonfuls.

*Diluents:* Alupent Syrup may be diluted with either Syrup BP or Sorbitol Solution BP

No specific information on the use of this product in the elderly is available. Clinical trials have included patients over 65 years and no adverse reactions specific to this age group have been reported.

*Contra-indications:* Hypersensitivity to any of the ingredients in Alupent Syrup.

*Special warnings and special precautions for use:* A chronic requirement for treatment would suggest the need for clinical review of the management of the patient's asthma. The patient's need for anti-inflammatory therapy (e.g. corticosteroids), or the adequacy of such therapy in patients already receiving it should be assessed.

Patients must be warned not to exceed the prescribed dose. In the case of acute rapidly worsening dyspnoea a doctor should be consulted immediately.

Sympathomimetic agents can cause unwanted effects. The concomitant use of other sympathomimetic drugs should be avoided or only used under strict medical supervision. Alupent and anticholinergic bronchodilators have been administered concurrently in reversible airways obstruction. In some situations, co-administered sympathomimetic agents and anticholinergics have been shows to produce greater bronchodilatation than the use of either agent alone (but see Interactions).

In the following conditions Alupent should only be used after careful risk/benefit assessment, especially when doses higher than those recommended are used: Insufficiently controlled diabetes mellitus, recent myocardial infarction, severe organic heart or vascular disorders, such as hypertrophic obstructive cardiomyopathy and tachyarrhythmia; hyperthyroidism.

Potentially serious hypokalaemia may result from excessive beta-agonist therapy. This effect may be potentiated by concomitant treatment with xanthine derivatives, glucocorticosteroids and diuretics.

Additionally, hypoxia may aggravate the effects of hypokalaemia on cardiac rhythm. It is recommended that serum potassium levels are monitored in such situations.

*Interaction with other medicaments and other forms of interaction:* In view of the possible interaction between beta-adrenergics and monoamine oxidase inhibitors or tricyclic anti-depressants, care should be exercised if it is proposed to administer these compounds concurrently with Alupent.

Beta-adrenergics, anticholinergics and xanthine derivatives may enhance the bronchodilator effect of orciprenaline.

The concurrent administration of the other beta-adrenergics, systemically absorbed anticholinergics and xanthine derivatives may increase the frequency and severity of unwanted effects.

Beta₂-receptor blockers counteract the action of Alupent.

Potentially serious bronchospasm may occur during concurrent administration of beta-blockers to patients with reversible airways obstruction.

*Pregnancy and lactation:* Although orciprenaline sulphate has been in general use for several years, there is no definite evidence of ill-consequence following administration of the drug during human pregnancy. Only in doses far in excess of the equivalent maximum human dose were effects on foetal development seen in animals.

Alupent should only be used during pregnancy, especially the first trimester, if the potential benefit outweighs the potential risk to the foetus.

The inhibitory effect of orciprenaline sulphate on uterine contraction should be taken into account.

Safety in breast-fed infants has not been established.

*Effects on ability to drive and use machines:* None stated.

*Undesirable effects:* The most frequently reported undesirable effects observed with Alupent are tremor and nervousness, headache, dizziness, tachycardia, palpitations, gastro-intestinal discomfort, nausea and vomiting. Some patients have experienced a feeling of tightness of chest.

In rare cases, local irritation or allergic reactions have been reported.

*Overdose: Symptoms:* The expected symptoms of overdosage with Alupent are those of excessive beta-stimulation such as flushing, tremor, nausea, restlessness, tachycardia, palpitation, dizziness, headache, hypotension, hypertension, a feeling of pressure in the chest, excitation, angina, increased pulse pressure and arrhythmia. Hypokalaemia may occur following overdose with orciprenaline. Serum potassium levels should be monitored.

*Therapy:* Treatment of overdosage should primarily be supportive and symptom-oriented.

If specific therapy is considered necessary, cardioselective beta-blockers are to be preferred. These should be administered with extreme caution to patients with asthma because of the risk of precipitating severe bronchospasm.

**Pharmacological properties**

*Pharmacodynamic properties:* Alupent is a sympathomimetic amine with bronchodilator properties. The duration of action of a single dose is 3-6 hours.

*Pharmacokinetic properties:* Following oral administration orciprenaline is absorbed from the GI tract and undergoes extensive first-pass metabolism; about 40% of an oral dose is reported to reach the circulation unchanged. It is excreted in the urine primarily as glucuronide conjugates.

**Pharmaceutical particulars**

*List of excipients:* Sodium metabisulphite; disodium edetate dihydrate; methyl parahydroxybenzoate; propyl parahydroxybenzoate; hydroxyethylcellulose; saccharin; sorbitol solution ; woodruff aroma ; sodium hydroxide; purified water.

*Incompatibilities:* None stated.

*Shelf life:* 5 years.

*Special precautions for storage:* Store below 25°C. Protect from light.

*Nature and contents of container:* 300 ml amber glass bottle (type III glass) with an aluminium roll-on pilfer proof cap.

*Instructions for use/handling:* None stated

**Marketing authorisation number** 0015/0001R

**Date of approval/revision of SPC** October 1996

Legal category POM

## ALUPENT* TABLETS

**Qualitative and quantitative composition** Round, white/off-white compressed tablets scored and impressed with $\frac{20A}{20A}$ on one side and the Boehringer Ingelheim Company logo on the reverse.

Each tablet contains 20 mg of orciprenaline sulphate.

**Pharmaceutical form** Tablets for oral administration.

**Clinical particulars**

*Therapeutic indications:* Alupent is indicated for the relief of reversible airways obstruction. Alupent Tablets are suggested for maintenance therapy.

*Posology and method of administration:*

*Adults:* The usual dose is 1 tablet four times daily. The maximum recommended daily dosage is 4 tablets.

*Children 3–12 years:* The usual starting dose is ½ tablet four times daily. This may be increased to 1 tablet three times daily as necessary. The maximum recommended daily dosage is 3 tablets.

*Children under 3 years:* The syrup is recommended.

*Elderly:* No specific information on the use of this product in the elderly is available. Clinical trials have included patients over 65 years and no adverse reactions specific to this age group have been reported.

*Contra-indications:* Hypersensitivity to any of the ingredients in Alupent Tablets.

*Special warnings and special precautions for use:* A chronic requirement for treatment would suggest the need for clinical review of the management of the patient's asthma. The patient's need for anti-inflammatory therapy (e.g. corticosteroids), or the adequacy of such therapy in patients already receiving it should be assessed.

Patients must be warned not to exceed the prescribed dose. In the case of acute rapidly worsening dyspnoea a doctor should be consulted immediately.

Sympathomimetic agents can cause unwanted effects. The concomitant use of other sympathomimetic drugs should be avoided or only used under strict medical supervision. Alupent and anticholinergic bronchodilators have been administered concurrently in reversible airways obstruction. In some situations, co-administered sympathomimetic agents and anticholinergics have been shown to produce greater bronchodilatation than the use of either agent alone (but see *Interactions*).

In the following conditions Alupent should only be used after careful risk/benefit assessment, especially when doses higher than those recommended are used:

Insufficiently controlled diabetes mellitus, recent myocardial infarction, severe organic heart or vascular disorders, such as hypertrophic obstructive cardiomyopathy and tachyarrhythmia; hyperthyroidism.

Potentially serious hypokalaemia may result from excessive beta-agonist therapy. This effect may be potentiated by concomitant treatment with xanthine derivatives, glucocorticosteroids and diuretics.

Additionally, hypoxia may aggravate the effects of hypokalaemia on cardiac rhythm. It is recommended that serum potassium levels are monitored in such situations.

*Interaction with other medicaments and other forms of interaction:* In view of the possible interaction between beta-adrenergics and monoamine oxidase inhibitors or tricyclic anti-depressants, care should be exercised if it is proposed to administer these compounds concurrently with Alupent.

Beta-adrenergics, anticholinergics and xanthine derivatives may enhance the bronchodilator effect of orciprenaline.

The concurrent administration of the other beta-adrenergics, systemically absorbed anticholinergics and xanthine derivatives may increase the frequency and severity of unwanted effects.

Beta$_2$-receptor blockers counteract the action of Alupent.

Potentially serious bronchospasm may occur during concurrent administration of beta-blockers to patients with reversible airways obstruction.

*Pregnancy and lactation:* Although orciprenaline sulphate has been in general use for several years, there is no definite evidence of ill-consequence following administration of the drug during human pregnancy. Only in doses far in excess of the equivalent maximum human dose were effects on foetal development seen in animals.

Alupent should only be used during pregnancy, especially the first trimester, if the potential benefit outweighs the potential risk to the foetus.

The inhibitory effect of orciprenaline sulphate on uterine contraction should be taken into account.

Safety in breast-fed infants has not been established.

*Effect on ability to drive and use machines:* None stated.

*Undesirable effects:* The most frequently reported undesirable effects observed with Alupent are tremor and nervousness, headache, dizziness, tachycardia, palpitations, gastro-intestinal discomfort, nausea and vomiting. Some patients have experienced a feeling of tightness of chest.

In rare cases, local irritation or allergic reactions have been reported.

*Overdose: Symptoms:* The expected symptoms of overdosage with Alupent are those of excessive beta-stimulation such as flushing, tremor, nausea, restlessness, tachycardia, palpitation, dizziness, headache, hypotension, hypertension, a feeling of pressure in the chest, excitation, angina, increased pulse pressure and arrhythmia. Hypokalaemia may occur following overdose with orciprenaline. Serum potassium levels should be monitored.

*Therapy:* Treatment of overdosage should primarily be supportive and symptom-oriented. If specific therapy is considered necessary, cardioselective beta-blockers are to be preferred. These should be administered with extreme caution to patients with asthma because of the risk of precipitating severe bronchospasm.

**Pharmacological properties**

*Pharmacodynamic properties:* Orciprenaline sulphate is a beta$_2$-adrenergic agonist bronchodilator which decreases reversible bronchospasm. Following oral administration, the effect is usually noted within 30 minutes. The peak effect of bronchodilator activity following orciprenaline sulphate generally occurs within 60–90 minutes, and lasts for 1 to 5 hours.

It is postulated that beta$_2$-adrenergic agonists produce many of their pharmacological effects by activation of adenylcyclase, the enzyme that catalyses the conversion of adenosine triphosphate to adenosine monophosphate.

Orciprenaline sulphate has been shown to inhibit antigen-induced histamine release both *in vitro* in human lung tissue and in isolated mast cells.

Furthermore, an increase in the rate of bronchial ciliary movement has been demonstrated with adrenergic agonists. This enhances mucociliary clearance, a phenomenon that has also been described for orciprenaline sulphate.

*Pharmacokinetic properties:* Oral administration of Alupent Tablets is followed by a rapid absorption with a plasma level maximum between 0.75–3 hours and a half-life of 2.1 hours.

After intravenous administration (1 mg/40 min), the plasma level can be described by a mammalian compartment model; the distribution volume in the steady state is about 60 litres and the total clearance 500 ml. The half-life of the terminal elimination is about 2.7 hours.

The p.o./i.v. quotient of the renally excreted radioactivity of tritium-labelled orciprenaline sulphate is 0.6; from this one can infer an absorption of about 60% of the orally administered dose. The renal excretion of radioactivity after oral administration of tritium-labelled orciprenaline sulphate is 45%.

The active substance is not metabolised by the catechol-0-methyl transferase or monoamine oxidase; it is excreted mainly as the sulphuric acid conjugate.

**Pharmaceutical particulars**

*List of excipients:* Calcium hydrogen phosphate; phosphoric acid 85%; lactose, fine; maize starch, dried; colloidal silica; soluble maize starch; magnesium stearate.

*Incompatibilities:* None stated.

*Shelf life:* The shelf life expiry date for this product is 5 years from the date of its manufacture, when packed in polypropylene securitainers with polythene lids.

The shelf life expiry date for this product is 3 years from the date of its manufacture, when packed in PVC/PVDC blister packs.

*Special precautions for storage:* Store below 25°C. Protect from light. Tablets packed in blister packs should also be stored in a dry place.

*Nature and contents of container:* Polypropylene securitainers with polythene lids containing 28, 50, 112, 250 and 1000 tablets. PVC/PVDC blister packs of 100 tablets.

*Instructions for use/handling:* None stated.

**Marketing authorisation number** 0015/0046R

**Date of approval/revision of SPC** October 1996

**Legal category** POM

## ATROVENT* AEROCAPS*

**Qualitative and quantitative composition** Dark olive/light olive opaque size 3 hard gelatin capsules containing 40 micrograms of ipratropium bromide powder.

**Pharmaceutical form** Capsules containing powder for inhalation.

**Clinical particulars**

*Therapeutic indications:* Atrovent Aerocaps are indicated in the treatment of chronic reversible airways obstruction, particularly in asthma and chronic bronchitis.

*Posology and method of administration:* For inhalation use only. The specially developed Aerohaler* device pierces the capsules making the contents available for inhalation.

*Adults:* 1 capsule three or four times daily. This dose may be doubled safely in patients who are less responsive.

*Children under 12 years:* There is limited experience of the use of Atrovent Aerocaps in children, therefore the product is not recommended for use in children.

*Elderly:* There are no special dosage recommendations in the elderly. Clinical trials have included patients over 65 years and no adverse reactions specific to this age group have been reported.

One Atrovent Aerocap is equivalent to two puffs of Atrovent Inhaler or one puff of Atrovent Forte.

*Contra-indications:* Known hypersensitivity to atropine.

*Special warnings and special precautions for use:* As with other agents, powder-induced bronchoconstriction has been reported occasionally and may occur as wheeze or cough.

The patient should be warned to seek medical advice should a reduced response become apparent.

Patients must be instructed in the correct administration of Atrovent Aerocaps. Generally caution is advocated in the use of anticholinergic agents in patients with glaucoma or prostatic hypertrophy. However, specific studies with Atrovent in patients with glaucoma showed that inhaling cumulative doses of 160 micrograms had no effect on the eye.

*Interaction with other medicaments and other forms of interaction:* There is evidence that the concurrent administration of Atrovent and sympathomimetic drugs produces a greater relief of bronchospasm than either drug given alone.

Atrovent has been shown to produce effective bronchodilation in patients receiving beta-adrenergic blocking agents.

*Pregnancy and lactation:* Atrovent has been in wide general use for many years without apparent ill-consequence during pregnancy: Animal studies have shown no hazard. Nevertheless, medicines should not be used in pregnancy, especially the first trimester, unless the expected benefit is thought to outweigh any possible risk to the foetus.

*Effects on ability to drive and use machines:* None stated.

*Undesirable effects:* Anticholinergic side-effects are unlikely at therapeutic doses, but some patients may complain of a dry mouth. Urinary retention and constipation have only rarely been reported with Atrovent. There is no evidence that in the therapeutic dose range Atrovent has any adverse effect on bronchial secretion.

*Overdose:* Inhaled doses of 5 mg ipratropium bromide have produced an increase in heart rate and palpitation. Single doses of ipratropium bromide 30 mg by mouth caused anticholinergic side effects but these were not severe and did not require specific reversal.

**Pharmacological properties**
*Pharmacodynamic properties:* Ipratropium bromide affects airway function primarily through its neural effect on the para-sympathetic nervous system. Ipratropium bromide blocks the acetylcholine receptors on smooth muscle in the lung. Stimulation of these receptors normally produces contraction and, depending on the degree of activation, bronchoconstriction. Thus, even in normal subjects, ipratropium bromide will cause bronchodilation.

*Pharmacokinetic properties:* Ipratropium bromide is a quaternary ammonium compound which is poorly absorbed from the gastro-intestinal tract and is slow to cross mucous membranes and the blood brain barrier. Following inhalation, uptake into the plasma is minimal; a peak blood concentration is attained $1\frac{1}{2}$ to 3 hours after inhalation (and similarly for oral administration). Excretion is chiefly via the kidneys.

*Preclinical safety data:* There are no pre-clinical data of relevance to the prescriber which are additional to that already included in other sections of the SPC.

**Pharmaceutical particulars**
*List of excipients:* Glucose (ground anhydrous). *Capsule shell:* Titanium dioxide (E171), indigo carmine (E132), iron oxide yellow (E172), iron oxide black (E172), gelatin.

*Incompatibilities:* None stated.

*Shelf life:* 24 months.

*Special precautions for storage:* Store below 25°C. Keep away from heat, including the sun.

*Nature and contents of container:* PVC/Aluminium blister packs containing 30, 50, 60, 90, 100, 120, 180, 240, 300 or 360 Aerocaps (currently only the 100 pack size is marketed: Pack containing 100 Aerocaps and 1 Aerohaler device and refill pack containing 100 Aerocaps).

*Instructions for use/handling:* Full instructions for use are given in the Patient Information Leaflet enclosed in the pack.

**Marketing authorisation number** 0015/0156

**Date of approval/revision of SPC** April 1997

**Legal category** POM

# ATROVENT* METERED DOSE INHALER

**Qualitative and quantitative composition** Atrovent Metered Dose Aerosol is a 10 ml homogeneous cream coloured suspension contained in a 17 ml one-piece aluminium container with a 50 mcl metering valve. Each metered dose delivers 20 micrograms of ipratropium bromide.

**Pharmaceutical form** Metered dose aerosol.

**Clinical particulars**
*Therapeutic indications:* Atrovent Metered Dose Inhaler is indicated in the treatment of chronic reversible airways obstruction, particularly in chronic bronchitis.

*Posology and method of administration:*
*Adults:* Usually 1 or 2 puffs three or four times daily, although some patients may need up to 4 puffs at a time to obtain maximum benefit during early treatment.

*Children:*
6–12 years: Usually 1 or 2 puffs three times daily.
Under 6 years: Usually 1 puff three times daily.
In order to ensure that the inhaler is used correctly, administration should be supervised by an adult.
Some patients may find it beneficial to use the metered dose inhaler with an extension tube.

*Elderly:* No specific information on the use of this product in the elderly is available. Clinical trials have included patients over 65 years and no adverse reactions specific to this age group have been reported.

*Contra-indications:* Known hypersensitivity to atropine.

*Special warnings and special precautions for use:* The patient should be warned to seek medical advice should a reduced response become apparent.

Patients must be instructed in the correct use of a metered dose inhaler and warned against the accidental release of the contents into the eye. Generally, caution is advocated in the use of anticholinergic agents in patients with glaucoma or prostatic hypertrophy. However, specific studies with Atrovent in patients with glaucoma showed that inhaling cumulative doses of 0.16 mg had no effect on the eye. Patients should be informed when starting treatment that onset of action of Atrovent is slower than that of inhaled sympathomimetic bronchodilators.

*Interaction with other medicaments and other forms of interaction:* There is evidence that the concurrent administration of Atrovent and sympathomimetic drugs produces a greater relief of bronchospasm than either drug given alone.

Atrovent has been shown to produce effective bronchodilatation in patients receiving beta adrenergic blocking agents.

There are no serious drug interactions known.

*Pregnancy and lactation:* Atrovent has been in general use for several years and there is no definite evidence of ill-consequence during pregnancy; animal studies have shown no hazard. Nevertheless, medicines should not be used in pregnancy, especially during the first trimester, unless the expected benefit is thought to outweigh any possible risk to the foetus.

*Effect on ability to drive and use machines:* None known.

*Undesirable effects:* Anticholinergic side-effects are unlikely to occur at therapeutic doses although dry mouth has occasionally been reported. Urinary retention and constipation have only rarely been reported with Atrovent.

There is no evidence that in the therapeutic dose range Atrovent has any adverse effect on bronchial secretion.

*Overdose:* Inhaled doses of 5 mg produce an increase in heart rate and palpitation. Single doses of ipratropium bromide 30 mg by mouth caused anticholinergic side-effects but these were not severe and did not require specific reversal.

**Pharmacological properties**
*Pharmacodynamic properties:* Ipratropium bromide affects airway function primarily through its neural effects on the parasympathetic nervous system. Ipratropium bromide blocks the acetylcholine receptors on smooth muscle in the lung. Stimulation of these receptors normally produces contraction and, depending on the degree of activation, bronchoconstriction. Thus, even in normal subjects ipratropium bromide will cause bronchodilatation.

*Pharmacokinetic properties:* Ipratropium bromide is a quaternary ammonium compound which is poorly absorbed from the gastro-intestinal tract, and is slow to cross mucous membranes and the blood-brain barrier. Following inhalation, uptake into the plasma is minimal; a peak blood concentration is attained $1\frac{1}{2}$ to 3 hours after inhalation (and similarly for oral administration). Excretion is chiefly via the kidneys.

**Pharmaceutical particulars**
*List of excipients:* Soya lecithin; monofluorotrichloromethane; difluorotrichloromethane; tetrafluorodichloroethane.

*Incompatibilities:* None known.

*Shelf life:* The shelf life expiry date for this product is 5 years from the date of its manufacture.

*Special precautions for storage:* Protect from heat, including the sun. Protect from frost. The vials should not be opened, punctured or incinerated even when apparently empty.

*Nature and contents of container:* 10 ml of a homogeneous cream coloured suspension in a 17 ml one-piece aluminium container with a 50 mcl metering valve.

*Instructions for use/handling:* To make sure that your inhaler is working, test fire it into the air before using

it for the first time and whenever your inhaler has not been used for a week or more.
1. Remove the dustcap from the mouthpiece and **shake the inhaler vigorously.**
2. Holding the inhaler as shown, breathe out gently and then immediately . . .
3. . . . place the mouthpiece in the mouth and close your lips around it. After starting to breathe in slowly and deeply, through your mouth, press the inhaler firmly as shown to release the Atrovent. *Continue to breathe in as deeply as you can.*
4. Hold your breath for 10 seconds, or as long as is comfortable, before breathing out slowly.
5. If you are to take more than one puff you should wait at least one minute before shaking the inhaler again and repeating steps 2, 3 and 4.
6. After use, replace the dustcap on the mouthpiece.

**Marketing authorisation number** 00015/0043R

**Date of approval/revision of SPC** May 1996

**Legal category** POM

# ATROVENT* AUTOHALER*

**Qualitative and quantitative composition** Each metered dose contains ipratropium bromide 20 micrograms.

**Pharmaceutical form** A breath-actuated pressurised aerosol for inhalation therapy.

**Clinical particulars**
*Therapeutic indications:* Atrovent Autohaler is indicated in the treatment of chronic reversible airways obstruction, particularly in chronic bronchitis.

*Posology and method of administration:* By inhalation.

*Adults:* Usually 1 or 2 puffs three or four times daily, although some patients may need up to 4 puffs at a time to obtain maximum benefit during early treatment.

*Children:* 6–12 years: Usually 1 or 2 puffs three times daily.
Under 6 years: Usually 1 puff three times daily.
In order to ensure that the Autohaler is used correctly, administration should be supervised by an adult.

*Elderly:* No specific information on the use of this product in the elderly is available. Clinical trials have included patients over 65 years and no adverse reactions specific to this age group have been reported.

*Contra-indications:* Known hypersensitivity to atropine.

*Special warnings and special precautions for use:*
*Precautions:* The patient should be warned to seek medical advice should a reduced response become apparent.

Patients must be instructed in the correct use of the Autohaler device. Generally, caution is advocated in the use of anticholinergic agents in patients with glaucoma or prostatic hypertrophy. However, specific studies with Atrovent in patients with glaucoma showed that inhaling cumulative doses of 0.16 mg had no effect on the eye.

Patients should be informed when starting treatment that onset of action of Atrovent is slower than that of inhaled sympathomimetic bronchodilators.

*Interaction with other medicaments and other forms of interaction:* There is evidence that the concurrent administration of Atrovent and sympathomimetic drugs produces a greater relief of bronchospasm than either drug given alone.

Atrovent has been shown to produce effective bronchodilatation in patients receiving beta adrenergic blocking agents. There are no serious drug interactions known.

*Pregnancy and lactation:* Atrovent has been in general use for several years, there is no definite evidence of ill-consequence during pregnancy; animal studies have shown no hazard. Nevertheless, medicines should not be used in pregnancy, especially during the first trimester, unless the expected benefit is thought to outweigh any possible risk to the foetus.

*Effect on ability to drive and use machines:* None known.

*Undesirable effects:* Anticholinergic side-effects are unlikely to occur at therapeutic doses, although dry mouth has occasionally been reported. Urinary retention and constipation have only rarely been reported with Atrovent. There is no evidence that in the therapeutic dose range Atrovent has any adverse effect on bronchial secretion.

*Overdose:* Inhaled doses of 5 mg produce an increase in heart rate and palpitation. Single doses of ipratropium bromide 30 mg by mouth caused anticholinergic side-effects but these were not severe and did not require specific reversal.

**Pharmacological properties**
*Pharmacodynamic properties:* Ipratropium bromide affects airway function primarily through its neural effects on the parasympathetic nervous system. Ipratropium bromide blocks the acetylcholine receptors on smooth muscle in the lung. Stimulation of these receptors normally produces contraction and, depending on the degree of activation, bronchoconstriction. Thus, even in normal subjects ipratropium bromide will cause bronchodilatation.

*Pharmacokinetic properties:* Ipratropium bromide is a quaternary ammonium compound which is poorly absorbed from the gastro-intestinal tract, and is slow to cross mucous membranes and the blood-brain barrier. Following inhalation, uptake into the plasma is minimal; a peak blood concentration is attained 1.5 to 3 hours after inhalation (and similarly for oral administration). Excretion is chiefly via the kidneys.

*Preclinical safety data:* There are no pre-clinical data of relevance to the prescriber which are additional to that already included in other sections of the SPC.

**Pharmaceutical particulars**
*List of excipients:* Soya lecithin, monofluorotrichloromethane, difluorotrichloromethane, tetrafluorodichloroethane.

*Incompatibilities:* None stated.

*Shelf life:* 5 years.

*Special precautions for storage:* Store below 25°C. Protect from direct sunlight. Protect from frost. The vials should not be opened, punctured or incinerated even when apparently empty.

*Nature and contents of container:* 17 ml aluminium aerosol can with metering valve (200 metered doses). Pack size: 10 ml.

Instructions for use/handling:
1. To remove the mouthpiece cover, pull down on the lip at the back.
2. Hold the Authohaler upright as shown. Push the lever up so that it stays up.
3. With the lever still up, shake the Autohaler.
4. Continue to hold the Autohaler device upright, making sure that your hand is not blocking the air vents at the bottom. Breathe out normally and close your lips firmly around the mouthpiece.
5. Breathe in through the mouthpiece. When you hear the slight click, continue to breathe in. This click lets you know you have received your puff of medication. Hold your breath for 10 seconds, or as long as is comfortable, and then breathe out normally.
6. The lever must be lowered after each puff. If your doctor has prescribed more than one puff, wait one minute before repeating steps 2–6. Replace the mouthpiece cover after use.

**Marketing authorisation number** 0015/0160

**Date of approval/revision of SPC** May 1997

**Legal category** POM

## ATROVENT* 250 UDVs*, 1 ml ATROVENT* UDVs*, 2 ml

**Qualitative and quantitative composition** Each single dose unit contains 0.025% w/v ipratropium bromide i.e. 250 micrograms in 1 ml and 500 micrograms in 2 ml.

**Pharmaceutical form** Inhalation solution presented in single dose units of 1 ml and 2 ml.

**Clinical particulars**
*Therapeutic indications:* Atrovent 250 UDVs, 1 ml and Atrovent UDVs, 2 ml, are indicated in the treatment of reversible airways obstruction.

*Posology and method of administration:* By inhalation from an intermittent positive pressure ventilator or from suitable nebulisers.

*Adults:* 0.4–2.0 ml solution (100–500 micrograms) up to 4 times daily.

*Children (3–14 years):* 0.4–2.0 ml solution (100–500 micrograms) up to 3 times daily.

There is no specific information on the use of the isotonic nebuliser solution in the elderly. Clinical trials with the previously available hypotonic formulation included patients over 65 years and no adverse reactions specific to this age group were reported.

The dose of nebuliser solution may need to be diluted in order to obtain a final volume suitable for the particular nebuliser being used; if dilution is necessary use only sterile sodium chloride 0.9% solution.

*Contra-indications:* Known hypersensitivity to atropine.

*Special warnings and precautions for use:* Use of the nebuliser solution should be subject to close medical supervision during initial dosing. There have been rare reports of paradoxical bronchospasm associated with the administration of Atrovent nebuliser solution. The patient should be advised to seek medical advice should a reduced response become apparent.

Patients must be instructed in the correct administration of Atrovent UDVs and warned not to allow the solution or mist to enter the eyes. Acute angle-closure glaucoma has been reported rarely when Atrovent UDVs have been used in conjunction with nebulised $\beta_2$-agonist bronchodilators. Protection of the eyes appears to prevent any increase in intraocular pressure and patients who may be susceptible to glaucoma should be warned specifically on the need for ocular protection. Inhaled doses of Atrovent UDVs up to 1 mg have not been associated with elevation of intraocular pressure.

Caution is advocated in the use of anticholinergic agents in patients with prostatic hypertrophy.

*Interaction with other medicaments and other forms of interaction:* There is evidence to suggest that the concurrent administration of Atrovent and sympathomimetic drugs produces a greater relief of bronchospasm than either drug given alone.

Atrovent has been shown to produce effective bronchodilatation in patients receiving beta-blocking agents.

*Pregnancy and lactation:* Atrovent has been in general use for several years and there is no definite evidence of ill-consequence during pregnancy; animal studies have shown no hazard. Nevertheless, medicines should not be used in pregnancy, especially during the first trimester, unless the expected benefit is thought to outweigh any possible risk to the foetus.

*Effect on ability to drive and use machines:* None stated.

*Undesirable effects:* Anticholinergic side-effects are unlikely at therapeutic doses, but some patients may complain of a dry mouth. Urinary retention and constipation have only rarely been reported with Atrovent.

There is no evidence that in the therapeutic dose range Atrovent has any adverse effect on bronchial secretion.

*Overdose:* Inhaled doses of 5 mg produce an increase in heart rate and palpitation but single doses of 2 mg have been given to adults and 1 mg to children without causing side-effects. Single doses of ipratropium bromide 30 mg by mouth cause anticholinergic side-effects but these are not severe and do not require reversal.

**Pharmacological properties**
*Pharmacodynamic properties:* Ipratropium bromide is an anticholinergic bronchodilator.

*Pharmacokinetic properties:* Ipratropium bromide is poorly absorbed from the gastro-intestinal tract. It has been reported to be partly metabolised following oral administration and to be excreted in the urine and faeces as unchanged drug and metabolites. Little or none is absorbed from the lungs following inhalation.

**Pharmaceutical particulars**
*List of excipients:* Sodium chloride; 1N hydrochloric acid; purified water.

*Incompatibilities:* None stated.

*Shelf life:* The shelf life expiry date for the 2 ml solution shall not exceed 5 years from the date of its manufacture.

The shelf life expiry date for the 1 ml solution shall not exceed 3 years from the date of its manufacture.

*Special precautions for storage:* Store at room temperature. Protect from heat and light.

*Nature and contents of container:* Polyethylene unit dose vials packed in cartons. Each single dose unit contains either 1 ml or 2 ml of solution in pack sizes of 10, 20, 30, 50, 60, 80, 100, 120, 150, 200, 300, 500 and 1000. Pack sizes of 20 and 60 are currently marketed.

*Instructions for use/handling:* Atrovent 250 UDVs, 1 ml and Atrovent UDVs, 2 ml, should only be used in a nebuliser approved by your doctor.
1. Get your nebuliser ready by following the manufacturer's instructions and the advice of your doctor.
2. Carefully separate a new dose unit from the strip. NEVER use one which has been opened already.
3. Open by simply twisting off the top, always taking care to hold it in an upright position.
4. Unless otherwise instructed by your doctor, squeeze all the contents into the nebuliser chamber. If dilution is necessary this should be carried out using ONLY sterile sodium chloride 0.9% solution and as instructed by your doctor.
5. Use your nebuliser as directed by your doctor.
6. After you have finished, throw away any leftover solution.

Follow the manufacturer's instructions for cleaning your nebuliser. It is important that your nebuliser is kept clean.

**Marketing authorisation number** 0015/0108

**Date of approval/revision of SPC** June 1996

Legal category POM

## ATROVENT* FORTE

**Qualitative and quantitative composition** Each metered dose contains ipratropium bromide 40 micrograms.

**Pharmaceutical form** A metered dose inhaler for inhalation therapy.

**Clinical particulars**

*Therapeutic indications:* Atrovent Forte is indicated for the treatment of chronic reversible airways obstruction, particularly in chronic bronchitis.

*Posology and method of administration:* For administration by inhalation only.
*Adults* Usually 1 puff three or four times daily, although some patients may need 2 puffs at a time to obtain maximum benefit during early treatment.

*Children 6-12 years*: usually 1 puff three times daily. In order to ensure that the inhaler is used correctly, administration should be supervised by an adult.

No specific information on the use of this product in the elderly is available. Clinical trials have included patients over 65 years and no adverse reactions specific to this age group have been reported.

*Contra-indications:* Known hypersensitivity to any components of the formulation or atropine.

Since the formulation contains soya lecithin, patients who are hypersensitive to related food products such as soya bean or peanuts are also contra-indicated

*Special warnings and special precautions for use:* The patient should be warned to seek medical advice should a reduced response become apparent.

Patients must be instructed in the correct use of a metered dose inhaler and warned against accidental release of the contents into the eye.

Generally, caution is advocated in the use of anticholinergic agents in patients with glaucoma or prostatic hypertrophy. However, specific studies with Atrovent in patients with glaucoma showed that inhaling cumulative doses of 160 micrograms had no effect on the eye.

*Interaction with other medicaments and other forms of interaction:* There is evidence that the concurrent administration of Atrovent and sympathomimetic drugs produces a greater relief of bronchospasm than either drug given alone. Atrovent has been shown to produce effective bronchodilatation in patients receiving beta-adrenergic blocking agents.

*Pregnancy and lactation:* Atrovent has been in general use for several years, there is no definite evidence of ill-consequence during pregnancy; animal studies have shown no hazard. Nevertheless, medicines should not be used in pregnancy, especially during the first trimester, unless the expected benefit is thought to outweigh any possible risk to the foetus.

*Effects on ability to drive and use machines:* None stated.

*Undesirable effects:* Anticholinergic side-effects are unlikely to occur at therapeutic doses, although dry mouth has occasionally been reported. Urinary retention and constipation have only rarely been reported with Atrovent. There is no evidence that in the therapeutic dose range Atrovent has any adverse effect on bronchial secretion.

*Overdose:* Inhaled doses of 5 mg produce an increase in heart rate and palpitation. Single doses of ipratropium bromide 30 mg by mouth caused anticholinergic side-effects but these were not severe and did not require specific reversal.

**Pharmacological properties**

*Pharmacodynamic properties:* Ipratropium bromide is an anticholinergic bronchodilator which affects airway function primarily through its neural effects on the parasympathetic nervous system. Ipratropium bromide blocks the acetylcholine receptors on smooth muscle in the lung. Stimulation of these receptors normally produces contraction and depending on the degree of activation, bronchconstriction. Thus ipratropium bromide will cause bronchodilatation.

*Pharmacokinetic properties:* Ipratropium bromide is a quaternary ammonium compound which is poorly absorbed from the gastro-intestinal tract, and is slow to cross mucous membranes and the blood brain barrier. Following inhalation, uptake into the plasma is minimal, a peak blood concentration is attained 1½ to 3 hours after inhalation (and similarly for oral administration). Excretion is chiefly via the kidneys.

**Pharmaceutical particulars**

*List of excipients:* Soya lecithin; monofluorotrichloromethane; difluorodichloromethane; tetrafluorodichloroethane

*Incompatibilities:* None stated.

*Shelf life:* Five years

*Special precautions for storage:* Store below 25°C. Protect from heat, including the sun. Protect from frost. The vials should not be opened, punctured or incinerated even when apparently empty.

*Nature and contents of container:* A 17 ml one piece aluminium vial (fill volume 10 ml) with a 50 microlitre metering valve containing 200 metered doses.

*Instructions for use/handling:*
*Correct use of the inhaler:*
1. Remove the dustcap from the mouthpiece and shake the inhaler vigorously.
2. Holding the inhaler as shown, breathe out gently and then immediately. . . . . . .
3. . . . . . . . . place the mouthpiece in the mouth and close your lips around it. After starting to breathe in slowly and deeply, through your mouth, press the inhaler firmly as shown to release the Atrovent Forte. Continue to breathe in as deeply as you can.
4. Hold your breath for 10 seconds, or as long as is comfortable, before breathing out slowly.
5. If you are to take more than one puff you should wait at least one minute before shaking the inhaler again and repeating steps 2,3 and 4.
6. After use, replace the dustcap on the mouthpiece.

*How to clean and care for the inhaler:* Remove the canister and dustcap. Wash and clean the grey mouthpiece in warm soapy water, rinse in warm water, dry.

**Marketing authorisation number** 0015/0107

**Date of approval/revision of SPC** July 1995

**Legal category** POM

## BEROTEC* 100 METERED DOSE INHALER

**Qualitative and quantitative composition** Each actuation delivers 100 micrograms of fenoterol hydrobromide.

**Pharmaceutical form** Pressurised metered aerosol.

**Clinical particulars**
*Therapeutic indications:* For the treatment of reversible airways obstruction in bronchial asthma and chronic obstructive pulmonary disease.

*Posology and method of administration:* By inhalation.

*Adults:* The recommended dose of Berotec 100 is one to two puffs given as a single dose. This may be given 1–3 times daily. Dosing should not exceed two puffs every six hours (i.e. the maximum dose is 800 micrograms daily). Patients with persistent bronchospasm and those who require higher doses may be prescribed Berotec 200.

*Children:* Children aged 6–12 years will normally require one puff. This may be given 1–3 times daily. Dosing should not exceed two puffs every six hours (i.e. the maximum dose is 800 micrograms daily). It is recommended that administration of Berotec 100 to children should be supervised by a responsible adult.

*Elderly:* No specific information on the use of this product in the elderly is available. Clinical trials have included patients over 65 years and no adverse reactions specific to this age group have been reported.

*Contra-indications:* Hypersensitivity to fenoterol hydrobromide or inactive ingredients of the metered aerosol.

*Special warnings and special precautions for use:* In patients suffering from bronchial asthma, on demand or symptom-oriented treatment may be preferable to regular use. A chronic requirement for treatment would suggest the need for clinical review of the management of the patient's asthma. The use of inhaled corticosteroids as anti-inflammatory treatment should be considered.

Patients must be instructed in the correct use of a metered aerosol and warned not to exceed the prescribed dose. In the case of acute rapidly worsening dyspnoea (difficulty in breathing) a doctor should be consulted immediately.

Excessive use of sympathomimetic agents can cause unwanted effects. The concomitant use of other sympathomimetic drugs should be avoided or only used under strict medical supervision. Concurrent administration of Berotec with anticholinergic bronchodilators in reversible airways obstruction has been shown to produce greater bronchodilatation than the use of either agent alone (but see Interactions).

In the following conditions Berotec 100 should only be used after careful risk/benefit assessment, especially when doses higher than those recommended are used:

Insufficiently controlled diabetes mellitus, recent myocardial infarction, severe organic heart or vascular disorders, such as hypertrophic obstructive cardiomyopathy and tachyarrhythmia; hyperthyroidism.

Potentially serious hypokalaemia may result from excessive beta₂-agonist therapy. This effect may be potentiated by concomitant treatment with xanthine derivatives, glucocorticosteroids and diuretics. Additionally, hypoxia may aggravate the effects of hypokalaemia on cardiac rhythm. It is recommended that serum potassium levels are monitored in such situations.

*Interaction with other medicaments and other forms of interaction:* In view of the possible interaction between sympathomimetic amines and monoamine oxidase inhibitors or tricyclic anti-depressants, care should be exercised if it is proposed to administer these compounds concurrently with Berotec.

Beta-adrenergics, anticholinergics, xanthine derivatives and corticosteroids may enhance the bronchodilator effect of fenoterol. The concurrent administration of the other beta-mimetics, systemically absorbed anticholinergics and xanthine derivatives may increase the frequency and severity of unwanted effects.

Potentially serious bronchospasm may occur during concurrent administration of beta-blockers to patients with reversible airways obstruction.

*Pregnancy and lactation:* Although fenoterol hydrobromide has been in general use for several years, there is no definite evidence of ill-consequence following administration of the drug during human pregnancy; animal studies have shown no hazard.

Nonetheless, the usual precautions regarding the use of drug during pregnancy, especially during the first trimester, should be exercised.

The inhibitory effect of fenoterol on uterine contraction should be taken into account.

Preclinical studies have shown that fenoterol is secreted in breast milk.

Safety in breast-fed infants has not been established.

*Effect on ability to drive and use machines:* None stated.

*Undesirable effects:* Frequent undesirable effects observed with Berotec 100 are tremor, nervousness, headache, dizziness, tachycardia, palpitations and oropharyngeal irritation. Allergic reactions have also been reported.

As with other inhaled bronchodilators, cough and paradoxical bronchospasm have been reported.

*Overdose: Symptoms:* Flushing, tremor, nausea, restlessness, tachycardia, palpitation, dizziness, headache, increase in systolic blood pressure, fall in diastolic blood pressure, a feeling of pressure in the chest, excitation and extra systoles may occur following overdose. Hypokalaemia may occur following overdose with fenoterol. Serum potassium levels should be monitored.

*Therapy:* Treatment of overdosage should primarily be supportive and symptom oriented.

If specific therapy is considered necessary, cardioselective beta-blockers are to be preferred. These should be administered with extreme caution to patients with asthma because of the risk of precipitating severe bronchospasm.

**Pharmacological properties**
*Pharmacodynamic properties:* Berotec is highly effective adrenergic exerting a selective effect on the beta₂-receptors of the bronchial tree. The active ingredient, fenoterol hydrobromide, is a sympathomimetic amine where the catechol nucleus of isoprenaline has been replaced by a resorcinol nucleus, and the substituent moiety on the amino group is larger. This substitution has the effect of depressing the affinity of the molecule towards beta₁ (cardiac and lipolytic) adrenergic receptors and enhancing the affinity towards the beta₂ (bronchial vascular and intestinal) adrenergic receptors.

*Pharmacokinetic properties:* Fenoterol hydrobromide is readily absorbed orally in the dog (90%) and maximum blood levels achieved in 30 minutes to one hour. About 78% is excreted in the urine of the dog, with the remainder eliminated by the bile duct or directly through the gastrointestinal tract. No significant enterohepatic circulation was detected in the dog.

The absorbed compound is very rapidly taken up by the tissues and detoxified via the formation of acid conjugates. Excretion of the conjugates is also very rapid. Excretion of the drug by the kidneys is essentially complete after 12 hours.

Renal excretion accounts for 1% after oral administration to rats with 79% in the faeces.

In man fenoterol is very rapidly distributed through the tissues following intravenous administration. The kidneys excrete up to 65% mainly in the form of acidic conjugates. Following oral administration, the plasma levels reach their maximum 2 hours after ingestion and then drop exponentially. The renal excretion is 39% following peroral administration and over 98% of the renal excretory products consist of acidic conjugates. The half life for total excretion is 7.2 hours and absorption was calculated to be 60%.

The duration of action following the use of a metered aerosol is considerably larger and can be explained by the dose independent absorption in the upper bronchial tree. The concentration-independent absorption at this site, from the depot produced by the metered aerosol is maintained for several hours.

**Pharmaceutical particulars**
*List of excipients:* Sorbitan trioleate; monofluorotrichloromethane; difluorodichloromethane; tetrafluorodichloroethane.

*Incompatibilities:* None stated.

*Shelf life:* 5 years.

*Special precautions for storage:* Protect from heat, including the sun. Protect from frost.

The vials should not be opened, punctured or incinerated even when apparently empty.

*Nature and contents of container:* A one piece aluminium vial fitted with a 50 mcl metering valve and containing 10 ml (100 doses) of a white homogeneous suspension, complete with mouthpiece.

*Instructions for use/handling:* The correct administration of the metered aerosol is essential for successful therapy.

To make sure that your inhaler is working, test fire it twice into the air before using it for the first time and whenever your inhaler has not been used for a week or more.

1. Remove the dustcap from the mouthpiece and shake the inhaler vigorously.
2. Holding the inhaler as shown, breathe out gently and then immediately . . .
3. . . . place the mouthpiece in the mouth and close your lips around it. After starting to breathe in slowly and deeply, through your mouth, press the inhaler firmly as shown to release the Berotec. *Continue to breathe in as deeply as you can.*
4. Hold your breath for 10 seconds, or as long as is comfortable, before breathing out slowly.
5. If you are to take more than one puff you should wait at least one minute before shaking the inhaler again and repeating steps 2, 3 and 4.
6. After use, replace the dustcap on the mouthpiece.

**Marketing authorisation number** 0015/0150

**Date of approval/revision of SPC** August 1996

**Legal category** POM

## BEROTEC* 200 METERED DOSE INHALER

**Presentation** Pressurised metered inhaler (10 ml vial) containing 200 metered doses of fenoterol hydrobromide 200 micrograms. Each is available as a complete unit with mouthpiece.

**Uses**
*Action:* Berotec 200 is a potent, rapidly acting, selective beta₂-adrenergic agonist with a duration of action of 6-8 hours.

*Indications:* For the treatment of reversible airways obstruction as in bronchial asthma and chronic obstructive pulmonary disease in patients who are not adequately controlled by Berotec 100.

**Dosage and administration** By inhalation.

*Adults:* The recommended dose of Berotec 200 is two puffs given as a single dose. This may be given 1-3 times daily. Patients who can be controlled with lower doses should be prescribed Berotec 100. Dosing must not exceed two puffs every six hours (i.e. the maximum dose is 1600 micrograms daily).

*Children:* Berotec 200 is not recommended for children under 16 years of age.

*Elderly:* No specific information on the use of this product in the elderly is available. Clinical trials have included patients over 65 years and no adverse reactions specific to this age group have been reported.

**Contra-indications, warnings, etc**
*Contra-indications:* Hypersensitivity to fenoterol hydrobromide or inactive ingredients of the metered aerosol.

*Precautions:* In patients suffering from bronchial asthma, on demand or symptom-oriented treatment may be preferable to regular use. A chronic requirement for treatment would suggest the need for clinical review of the management of the patient's asthma. The use of inhaled corticosteroids as anti-inflammatory treatment should be considered.

Patients must be instructed in the correct use of a metered aerosol and warned not to exceed the prescribed dose. In the case of acute rapidly worsening dyspnoea (difficulty in breathing) a doctor should be consulted immediately.

Excessive use of sympathomimetic agents can cause unwanted effects. The concomitant use of other sympathomimetic drugs should be avoided or only used under strict medical supervision. Concurrent administration of Berotec with anticholinergic bronchodilators in reversible airways obstruction has been shown to produce greater bronchodilatation than the use of either agent alone (but see Interactions).

In the following conditions Berotec 200 should only be used after careful risk/benefit assessment, especially when doses higher than those recommended are used: Insufficiently controlled diabetes mellitus, recent myocardial infarction, severe organic heart or vascular disorders, such as hypertrophic obstructive cardiomyopathy and tachyarrhythmia; hyperthyroidism.

Potentially serious hypokalaemia may result from excessive beta$_2$-agonist therapy. This effect may be potentiated by concomitant treatment with xanthine derivatives, glucocorticosteroids and diuretics. Additionally, hypoxia may aggravate the effects of hypokalaemia on cardiac rhythm. It is recommended that serum potassium levels are monitored in such situations.

*Interactions:* In view of the possible interaction between sympathomimetic amines and monoamine oxidase inhibitors or tricyclic anti-depressants, care should be exercised if it is proposed to administer these compounds concurrently with Berotec.

Beta-adrenergics, anticholinergics, xanthine derivatives and corticosteroids may enhance the bronchodilator effect of fenoterol. The concurrent administration of other beta-mimetics, systemically absorbed anticholinergics and xanthine derivatives may increase the frequency and severity of unwanted effects.

Potentially serious bronchospasm may occur during concurrent administration of beta-blockers to patients with reversible airways obstruction.

*Use in pregnancy and lactation:* Although fenoterol hydrobromide has been in general use for several years, there is no definite evidence of ill-consequence following administration of the drug during human pregnancy; animal studies have shown no hazard.

Nonetheless, the usual precautions regarding the use of drugs during pregnancy, especially during the first trimester, should be exercised.

The inhibitory effect of fenoterol on uterine contraction should be taken into account. Preclinical studies have shown that fenoterol is secreted in breast milk. Safety in breast-fed infants has not been established.

*Side-effects:* Frequent undesirable effects observed with Berotec 200 are tremor, nervousness, headache, dizziness, tachycardia, palpitations and oropharyngeal irritation. Allergic reactions have also been reported.

As with other inhaled bronchodilators, cough and paradoxical bronchospasm have been reported.

*Overdosage: Symptoms:* Flushing, tremor, nausea, restlessness, tachycardia, palpitation, dizziness, headache, increase in systolic blood pressure, fall in diastolic blood pressure, a feeling of pressure in the chest, excitation and extra systoles may occur following overdose. Hypokalaemia may occur following overdose with fenoterol.

Serum potassium levels should be monitored.

*Therapy:* Treatment of overdosage should primarily be supportive and symptom oriented. If specific therapy is considered necessary, cardioselective beta-blockers are to be preferred. These should be administered with extreme caution to patients with asthma because of the risk of precipitating severe bronchospasm.

**Pharmaceutical precautions** Protect from heat, including the sun. Protect from frost.

The vial should not be opened, punctured or incinerated even when apparently empty.

**Legal category** POM

**Package quantities** 10 ml vial (200 metered doses) (OP) complete with mouthpiece.

**Further information** There is evidence to suggest that Berotec may reduce the allergic response of tissues. Animal studies have shown that Berotec also produces an increase in the frequency of movement of the respiratory epithelial cilia and in the rate of mucus transport.

Long-term use has shown Berotec to be free from significant adverse effects, particularly with respect to the blood gases and general biochemistry. Tolerance is not a feature of long-term use.

**Product licence number** 0015/0034

## BUSCOPAN* AMPOULES

**Presentation** Ampoules for intramuscular or intravenous injection, each containing hyoscine-N-butylbromide 20 mg in 1 ml.

### Uses
*Action:* Buscopan is an antispasmodic agent, which relaxes smooth muscle of the organs of the abdominal and pelvic cavities. It is believed to act predominantly on the intramural parasympathetic ganglia of these organs.

*Indications:* Buscopan Ampoules are indicated in acute spasm, as in renal or biliary colic; in radiology for differential diagnosis of obstruction and to reduce spasm and pain in pyelography, and in other diagnostic procedures where spasm may be a problem, e.g. gastro-duodenal endoscopy.

### Dosage and administration
*Children:* Not recommended for children.

*Adults:* By injection: 1 ampoule intramuscularly or intravenously repeated after half-an-hour if necessary. When used in endoscopy this dose may need to be repeated more frequently.

*Diluent:* Buscopan injection solution may be diluted with dextrose or with sodium chloride 0.9% injection solutions. It is also miscible and compatible with most of the commonly used aqueous radiological contrast media such as sodium diatrizoate.

No specific information on the use of this product in the elderly is available. Clinical trials have included patients over 65 years and no adverse reactions specific to this age group have been reported.

### Contra-indications, warnings, etc
*Contra-indications:* Buscopan Ampoules should not be administered to patients with myasthenia gravis, megacolon, glaucoma, tachycardia, benign prostatic hypertrophy with urinary retention and mechanical stenoses in the region of the gastrointestinal tract. In addition, Buscopan should not be used in patients with a known sensitivity to hyoscine-N-butylbromide.

*Precautions:* Buscopan Amoules should be used with caution in conditions characterised by tachycardia such as thyrotoxicosis, cardiac insuffiency or failure and in cardiac surgery where it may further accelerate the heart rate.

Because of the possibility that anticholinergics may reduce sweating, Buscopan should be administered with caution to patients with pyrexia and in situations where the ambient temperature is high. Because of visual accommodation disturbances patients should not drive or operate machinery after parenteral administration of Buscopan until vision has normalised.

*Interactions:* The anticholinergic effect of tricyclic antidepressants, antihistamines, quinidine, amantadine, phenothiazines, butyrophenones and disopyramide may be intensified by Buscopan. The tachycardic effects of beta-adrenergic agents may be enhanced by Buscopan.

*Use in pregnancy and lactation:* Although Buscopan has been in wide general use for many years, there is no definite evidence of ill-consequence during human pregnancy; animal studies have shown no hazard. Nevertheless, medicines should not be used in pregnancy, especially the first trimester, unless the expected benefit is thought to outweigh any possible risk to the foetus. Safety during lactation has not yet been established.

*Side-effects:* Anticholinergic side-effects including dry mouth, visual accommodation disturbances, tachycardia, dizziness, constipation and potentially urinary retention may occur but are generally mild and self-limiting. Allergic reactions including skin reactions, analphylactoid reactions and anaphylactic shock have been reported very rarely. There have been extremely rare reports of dyspnoea in patients with a history of bronchial asthma or allergy. Injection site pain, particularly after intramuscular use, occurs infrequently.

*Overdosage: Symptoms:* Serious signs of poisoning following acute overdosage have not been observed in man. In the case of overdosage, anticholinergic symptoms such as urinary retention, dry mouth, tachycardia, drowsiness, orthostatic hypotension and transient visual disturbances may occur, and Cheynes-Stokes respiration has been reported.

*Therapy:* Symptoms of Buscopan overdosage respond to parasympathomimetics. For patients with glaucoma, pilocarpine should be given locally. Circulation can be supported with sympathomimetics. In the case of orthostatic fall in blood pressure, it is sufficient for the patient to lie flat. Catheterisation may be required for urinary retention. In addition, appropriate supportive measures should be used as required.

**Pharmaceutical precautions** Store below 30°C. Protect from light.

**Legal category** POM

**Package quantities** Pack of 10 x 1 ml ampoules.

**Product licence number** 0015/5055R

## BUSCOPAN* TABLETS

**Presentation** White, sugar-coated tablets containing hyoscine-N-butylbromide 10 mg.

### Uses
*Action:* Buscopan exerts a spasmolytic action on the smooth muscle of the gastrointestinal, biliary and genito-urinary tracts. Peripheral anticholinergic action results from a ganglion-blocking action within the visceral wall as well as from anti-muscarinic activity.

*Indications:* Buscopan Tablets are indicated for the relief of spasm of the genito-urinary tract or gastrointestinal tract, for the symptomatic relief of Irritable Bowel Syndrome, and in the prevention and treatment of spasmodic dysmenorrhoea.

### Dosage and administration
Buscopan Tablets should be swallowed whole with adequate water.

*Adults:* 2 tablets four times daily.

For the symptomatic relief of Irritable Bowel Syndrome, the recommended starting dose is 1 tablet three times daily; this can be increased up to 2 tablets four times daily if necessary. In spasmodic dysmenorrhoea, treatment should commence two days before the expected onset of the period and continue for three days after menstruation has begun.

*Children 6-12 years:* 1 tablet three times daily.

No specific information on the use of this product in the elderly is available. Clinical trials have included patients over 65 years and no adverse reactions specific to this age group have been reported.

### Contra-indications, warnings, etc
*Contra-indications:* Buscopan Tablets should not be administered to patients with myasthenia gravis, megacolon and glaucoma. In addition, Buscopan should not be used in patients with known sensitivity to hyoscine-N-butylbromide.

*Precautions:* Due to the risk of anticholinergic complications, caution should be used in patients susceptible to intestinal or urinary outlet obstructions and in those inclined to tachycardia. Because of the possibility that anticholinergics may reduce sweating, Buscopan should be administered with caution to patients with pyrexia and in situations where the ambient temperature is high.

*Interactions:* The anticholinergic effect of tricyclic antidepressants, antihistamines, quinidine, amantadine, phenothiazines, butyrophenones and disopyramide may be intensified by Buscopan. Concomitant treatment with dopamine antagonists such as metoclopramide may result in diminution of the effects of both drugs on the gastrointestinal tract. The tachycardic effects of beta-adrenergic agents may be enhanced by Buscopan.

*Pregnancy and lactation:* Although Buscopan has been in wide general use for many years, there is no definite evidence of hazard during human pregnancy: animal studies have shown no hazard. Nevertheless, medicines should not be used in pregnancy, especially in the first trimester, unless the expected benefit is thought to outweigh any possible risk to the foetus. Safety during lactation has not yet been established.

*Side-effects:* Anticholinergic side-effects including dry mouth, visual accommodation disturbances, tachycardia, constipation and potentially urinary retention may occur, but are generally mild and self-limiting. Allergic reactions particularly, skin reactions have been reported very rarely. There have been extremely rare reports of dyspnoea in patients with a history of bronchial asthma or allergy. Because of possible visual accommodation disturbances, patients should not drive or operate machinery if affected.

*Overdosage:* Serious signs of poisoning following acute overdosage have not been observed in man. In the case of overdosage, anticholinergic effects such as urinary retention, dry mouth, tachycardia, drowsiness, orthostatic hypotension and transient visual disturbances, may occur, and Cheynes-Stokes respiration has been reported. In the case of oral poisoning, gastric lavage with medicinal charcoal should be followed by magnesium sulphate (15%). Symptoms of Buscopan overdosage respond to parasympathomimetics. For patients with glaucoma, pilocarpine should be given locally. Circulation can be supported with sympathomimetics. In the case of orthostatic fall in blood pressure, it is sufficient for the patient to lie flat. Catheterisation may be required for urinary retention. In addition, appropriate supportive measures should be administered as required.

**Pharmaceutical precautions** Buscopan Tablets should be stored in a dry place below 25°C and protected from light.

**Legal category** POM.

**Package quantities** Blister pack of 56 tablets.

**Further information** Buscopan Tablets are also available in packs of 20 tablets (Pharmacy Only status).

**Product licence number** 0015/0047R.

## CATAPRES* AMPOULES

**Qualitative and quantitative composition** 1 ml colourless glass ampoules containing 0.150 mg clonidine hydrochloride in each 1 ml of solution.

**Pharmaceutical form** Ampoules for injection.

**Clinical particulars**

*Therapeutic indications:* Catapres is indicated for the treatment of hypertensive crises.

*Posology and method of administration:* In hypertensive crises 1 or 2 Catapres Ampoules should be given by slow intravenous injection.

An effect is usually seen within 10 minutes and reaches a maximum about 30 minutes to 1 hour after administration. The duration of effect depends upon the severity of the condition and is commonly of the order of 3-7 hours. Up to 5 ampoules may be given in 24 hours to achieve and maintain the required blood pressure.

Patients undergoing anaesthesia should continue their Catapres treatment before, during and after anaesthesia using oral or intravenous administration according to individual circumstances.

Intravenous injection of Catapres should be given slowly over 10-15 minutes to avoid a possible transient pressor effect.

Catapres injection solution is compatible with 0.9% sodium chloride solution and with 5% Dextrose solution.

No specific information on the use of this product in the elderly is available. Clinical trials have included patients over 65 years and no adverse reactions specific to this age group have been reported.

*Contra-indications:* There are no absolute contra-indications to the use of Catapres.

*Special warnings and special precautions for use:* Sudden withdrawal of Catapres, particularly in those patients receiving high doses may result in rebound hypertension. Termination of long-term therapy with Catapres for any reason should therefore be performed gradually. With Catapres PL this may be achieved by increasing progressively the interval between doses. If a hypertensive episode should nevertheless occur conventional oral or intravenous Catapres should reverse any such effect.

Patients known with a history of depression should be carefully supervised while under long-term treatment with Catapres as there have been occasional reports of further depressive episodes during oral treatment in such patients.

Cautions should be exercised in patients with Raynaud's disease or other peripheral vascular occlusive disease. As with all drugs used in hypertension, Catapres should be used with caution in patients with cerebrovascular, coronary or renal insufficiency.

*Interaction with other medicaments and other forms of interaction:* Concomitant use of diuretics or other antihypertensive agents will usually result in an increased hypotensive effect.

Concomitant administration of tricyclic antidepressants may reduce the hypotensive effect of Catapres.

Alpha-adrenergic blocking drugs antagonise the acute effects of Catapres.

*Pregnancy and lactation:* This product should only be used in pregnancy or lactating women if considered essential by the physician.

*Effects on ability to drive and use machines:* This product may cause drowsiness. Patients who are affected should not drive or operate machinery. Sedation due to the drug may be increased by the concomitant use of other central nervous depressants.

*Undesirable effects:* There are occasional reports of fluid retention during initial stages of oral treatment with clonidine hydrochloride. This is usually transitory and can be corrected by the addition of a diuretic.

A single case of toxic hepatitis has been reported, but the authors commented that the role of clonidine in hepatotoxicity in this patient remains questionable.

Acute administration of clonidine hydrochloride in animals or in man has occasionally induced a transient elevation of blood sugar. This is believed to be due to the initial pharmacological effect of alpha-adrenergic stimulation. Investigators agree that this has no clinical significance. The inclusion of diabetic patients in many clonidine hydrochloride investigations has confirmed its suitability as an antihypertensive agent for such patients.

*Overdose:* Accidental overdosage may cause hypotension, bradycardia, sedation and coma. Transient hypertension may be seen if the total dose is over 10 mg.

Gastric lavage should be performed. In most cases all that is required are general supportive measures. Forced diuresis has been employed. Where bradycardia is severe atropine will increase the heart rate. If hypotension is giving rise to concern the administration of an alpha-adrenergic blocking drug such as phentolamine may help.

**Pharmacological properties**

*Pharmacodynamic properties:* Catapres has been shown to have both central and peripheral sites of action. With long-term treatment Catapres reduces the responsiveness of peripheral vessels to vasoconstrictor and vasodilator substances and to synthetic nerve stimulation. Early in treatment, however, blood pressure reduction is associated with a central reduction of sympathetic outflow and increased vagal tone.

Clinically, there may be reduced venous return and slight bradycardia resulting in reduced cardiac output. Although initially peripheral resistance may be unchanged, it tends to be reduced as treatment continues. There is no interference with myocardial contractility. Studies have shown that cardiovascular reflexes, as shown by the lack of postural hypotension and exercise hypotension, are preserved.

*Pharmacokinetic properties:* Peak plasma concentrations are observed 3-5 hours after administration, declining with a half-life up to about 23 hours. Clonidine is metabolised in the liver. About 65% is excreted in the urine, partly as unchanged clonidine and about 20% is excreted in the faeces.

**Pharmaceutical particulars**

*List of excipients:* Sodium chloride; water for injections.

*Incompatibilities:* None stated.

*Shelf life:* 5 years

*Special precautions for storage:* Store below 30°C. Protect from light.

*Nature and contents of container:* 1 ml colourless glass (PhEur Type I) ampoules, marketed in packs of 5.

*Instructions for use/handling:* None stated.

**Marketing authorisation number** 0015/5008

**Date of approval/revision of SPC** August 1995.

**Legal category** POM

## CATAPRES* TABLETS

**Qualitative and quantitative composition**

*Catapres Tablets 0.1 mg:* white compressed tablets impressed with the motif $\frac{01C}{01C}$ on one side and with the Company symbol on the reverse.

Each tablet contains 100 micrograms of clonidine hydrochloride.

*Catapres Tablets 0.3 mg:* White compressed tablets impressed with the motif $\frac{03C}{03C}$ on one side and with the Company symbol on the reverse.

Each tablet contains 300 micrograms of clonidine hydrochloride.

**Pharmaceutical form** Tablets for oral administration.

**Clinical particulars**

*Therapeutic indications:* Catapres is indicated for the treatment of all grades of essential and secondary hypertension.

*Posology and method of administration:* Oral treatment should commence with 0.05-0.10 mg three times daily. This dose should be increased gradually every second or third day until control is achieved. Most patients will be controlled on divided daily doses of 0.30-1.2 mg. However, some patients may require higher doses, e.g. 1.8 mg or more.

Catapres may be added to an existing antihypertensive regimen where blood pressure control has not been satisfactorily achieved. If side-effects with existing therapy are troublesome the concomitant use of Catapres may allow a lower dose of the established regimen to be employed. Patients changing treatment should have their existing therapy reduced gradually whilst Catapres is added to their regimen.

Patients undergoing anaesthesia should continue their Catapres treatment before, during and after anaesthesia using oral or i.v. administration according to individual circumstances.

No specific information on the use of this product in the elderly is available. Clinical trials have included patients over 65 years and no adverse reactions specific to this age group have been reported.

*Contra-indications:* There are no absolute contra-indications to the use of Catapres.

*Special warnings and special precautions for use:* Initially, sedation or dry mouth are encountered in a few patients. These effects usually subside as treatment continues. Other drug related side-effects which have been mentioned in the literature include dizziness, headache, nocturnal unrest, nausea, euphoria, rash, constipation, impotence (rarely) and agitation on withdrawal of long-term therapy.

There are occasional reports of fluid retention during initial stages of oral treatment. This is usually transitory and can be corrected by the addition of a diuretic.

A single case of toxic hepatitis has been reported, but the authors commented that the role of Catapres in hepatotoxicity in this patient remains questionable.

Acute administration in animals or in man has occasionally induced a transient elevation of blood sugar. This is believed to be due to the initial pharmacological effect of alpha-adrenergic stimulation. Investigators agree that this has no clinical significance. The inclusion of diabetic patients in many Catapres investigations has confirmed its suitability as an antihypertensive agent for such patients.

*Interaction with other medicaments and other forms of interaction:* Concomitant use of diuretics or other antihypertensive agents will usually result in an increased hypotensive effect.

Concomitant administration of tricyclic antidepressants may reduce the hypotensive effect of Catapres.

Alpha-adrenergic blocking drugs antagonise acute effects of Catapres.

*Pregnancy and lactation:* Although clonidine has been in wide general use for many years, there is no definite evidence of hazard during human pregnancy. In animal studies involving doses higher than the equivalent maximum therapeutic dose in man, effects on foetal development were only seen in one species. Foetal malformations did not occur. Medicines should not be used in pregnancy, especially the first trimester, unless the expected benefit is thought to outweigh any possible risk to the foetus.

Catapres should only be given to breast feeding women if considered essential by the physician. There is as yet insufficient experience to enable Catapres to be recommended for children.

*Effects on ability to drive and use machines:* This product may cause drowsiness. Patients who are affected should not drive or operate machinery. Sedation due to the drug may be increased by the concomitant use of other central nervous depressants.

*Undesirable effects:* Sudden withdrawal of Catapres, particularly in those patients receiving high doses, may result in rebound hypertension. As with other antihypertensives, doctors should warn their patients not to stop medication themselves. Termination of long-term therapy with Catapres for any reason should therefore be performed gradually. If a hypertensive episode should nevertheless occur, reintroduction of oral or intravenous Catapres should reverse any such effect. If the use of Catapres is not practical then an alpha-adrenergic blocking drug, such as phentolamine, should be used.

If Catapres is being given concurrently with a beta-blocker, Catapres should not be discontinued until several days after the withdrawal of the beta-blocker.

Patients known with a history of depression should be carefully supervised while under long-term treatment with Catapres as there have been occasional reports of further depressive episodes during oral treatment in such patients.

Caution should be exercised in patients with Raynaud's disease or other peripheral vascular occlusive disease. As with all drugs used in hypertension, Catapres should be used with caution in patients with cerebrovascular, coronary or renal insufficiency.

*Overdose:* Accidental overdosage may cause hypotension, bradycardia, sedation and coma. Transient hypertension may be seen if the total dose is over 10 mg. Gastric lavage should be performed where appropriate. In most cases all that is required are general supportive measures. Forced diuresis has been employed. Where bradycardia is severe atropine will increase the heart rate.

**Pharmacological properties**

*Pharmacodynamic properties:* Catapres has been shown to have both central and peripheral sites of action. With long-term treatment Catapres reduces the responsiveness of peripheral vessels to vasoconstrictor and vasodilator substances and to synthetic nerve stimulation. Early in treatment, however, blood pressure reduction is associated with a central reduction of sympathetic outflow and increased vagal tone.

Clinically, there may be reduced venous return and slight bradycardia resulting in reduced cardiac output. Although initially peripheral resistance may be unchanged, it tends to be reduced as treatment continues. There is no interference with myocardial contractility. Studies have shown that cardiovascular reflexes, as shown by the lack of postural hypotension and exercise hypotension, are preserved.

*Pharmacokinetic properties:* Clonidine is well absorbed from the GI tract. Peak plasma concentrations are observed 3-5 hours after administration, declining with a half life up to about 23 hours. Clonidine is metabolised in the liver. About 65% is excreted in the urine, partly as unchanged clonidine and about 20% is excreted in the faeces.

### Pharmaceutical particulars

*List of excipients:* Lactose; calcium hydrogen phosphate; maize starch; colloidal silica; polyvinylpyrrolidone; starch; stearic acid.

*Incompatibilities:* None stated.

*Shelf life:* 5 years

*Special precautions for storage:* Store in a dry place below 30˚C. Protect from light.

*Nature and contents of container:* Catapres Tablets 0.1 mg and 0.3 mg are currently marketed in PVC blister packs of 100 tablets.

*Instructions for use/handling:* None stated.

### Marketing authorisation numbers
Catapres Tablets 0.1 mg   0015/5009R
Catapres Tablets 0.3 mg   0015/5041R

**Date of approval/revision of SPC**  October 1995

**Legal category** POM

## CATAPRES* PL PERLONGETS

**Qualitative and quantitative composition**  Red/yellow size 2 gelatin capsules. Each Perlonget contains 5 mini tablets constituting 250 micrograms clonidine hydrochloride in a sustained release form.

**Pharmaceutical form** Sustained release capsule for oral administration.

### Clinical particulars

*Therapeutic indications:* All degrees of hypertension excluding hypertensive crisis.

*Posology and method of administration:* Most patients will be satisfactorily controlled on one perlonget daily (usually given in the evening). This dosage can be increased if necessary up to 2 or 3 perlongets daily (one in the morning and one or two at night).

Catapres PL may be added to an existing antihypertensive regimen where blood pressure control has not been satisfactorily achieved. If side effects with existing therapy are troublesome the concomitant use of Catapres PL may allow a lower dose of the established regimen to be employed.

Patients changing treatment should have their existing therapy reduced gradually whilst Catapres is added to their regimen.

*Contra-indications:* There are no absolute contraindications to the use of Catapres PL.

*Special warnings and special precautions for use:* Sudden withdrawal of Catapres PL, particularly in those patients receiving high doses may result in rebound hypertension. Termination of long-term therapy with Catapres PL for any reason should therefore be performed gradually. With Catapres PL this may be achieved by increasing progressively the interval between doses. If a hypertensive episode should nevertheless occur conventional oral or intravenous Catapres should reverse any such effect.

Patients with a known history of depression should be carefully supervised while under long-term treatment with Catapres PL as there have been occasional reports of further depressive episodes during oral treatment in such patients.

Caution should be exercised in patients with Raynaud's disease or other peripheral vascular occlusive disease. As with all drugs used in hypertension, Catapres PL should be used with caution in patients with cerebrovascular, coronary or renal insufficiency.

There is as yet insufficient experience to enable Catapres PL to be recommended in children.

*Interaction with other medicaments and other forms of interaction:* Concomitant use of diuretics or other antihypertensive agents will usually result in an increased hypotensive effect.

Concomitant administration of tricyclic antidepressants may reduce the hypotensive effect of Catapres PL.

Alpha-adrenergic blocking drugs antagonise the acute effects of Catapres PL.

No adverse reaction has been reported following the concurrent administration of clonidine hydrochloride with digoxin, aminophylline, anticonvulsants, or anti-arrhythmic preparations. Monitoring of haematological and hepatic status in large numbers of patients has revealed no drug-related adverse effects. Renal blood flow and glomerular filtration rates are maintained and there is no deterioration in renal

function. There is evidence that plasma renin levels are reduced. Clonidine hydrochloride does not affect the estimation of VMA levels.

*Pregnancy and lactation:* This product should only be used in pregnancy or lactating women if considered essential by the physician.

*Effects on ability to drive and use machines:* This product may cause drowsiness. Patients who are affected should not drive or operate machinery. Sedation due to the drug may be increased by the concomitant use of other central nervous depressants.

*Undesirable effects:* Initially, sedation or dry mouth are encountered in a few patients on treatment with Catapres PL. These effects usually subside as treatment continues. Other drug-related side effects from clonidine hydrochloride which have been mentioned in the literature include: dizziness, headache, nocturnal unrest, nausea, euphoria, constipation, impotence (rarely) and agitation on withdrawal of long-term therapy.

There are occasional reports of fluid retention during initial stages of oral treatment with clonidine hydrochloride. This is usually transitory and can be corrected by the addition of a diuretic.

A single case of toxic hepatitis has been reported, but the authors commented that the role of clonidine in hepatotoxicity in this patient remains questionable.

Acute administration of clonidine hydrochloride in animals or in man has occasionally induced a transient elevation of blood sugar. This is believed to be due to the initial pharmacological effect of alpha-adrenergic stimulation. Investigators agree that this has no clinical significance. The inclusion of diabetic patients in many clonidine hydrochloride investigations has confirmed its suitability as an antihypertensive agent for such patients.

*Overdose:* Accidental overdosage may cause hypotension, bradycardia, sedation and coma. Transient hypertension may be seen if the total dose is over 10 mg.

Gastric lavage should be performed. In most cases all that is required are general supportive measures. Forced diuresis has been employed. Where bradycardia is severe atropine will increase the heart rate. If hypotension is giving rise to concern the administration of an alpha-adrenergic blocking drug such as phentolamine may help.

### Pharmacological properties

*Pharmacodynamic properties:* Catapres PL has been shown to have both central and peripheral sites of action. With long-term treatment Catapres PL reduces the responsiveness of peripheral vessels to vasoconstrictor and vasodilator substances and to synthetic nerve stimulation. Early in treatment, however, blood pressure reduction is associated with a central reduction of sympathetic outflow and increased vagal tone.

Clinically, there may be reduced venous return and slight bradycardia resulting in reduced cardiac output. Although initially peripheral resistance may be unchanged, it tends to be reduced as treatment continues. There is no interference with myocardial contractility. Studies have shown that cardiovascular reflexes, as shown by the lack of postural hypotension and exercise hypotension, are preserved.

*Pharmacokinetic properties:* Catapres PL contains clonidine hydrochloride in a sustained release formulation. Clonidine is well absorbed from the GI tract. Peak plasma concentrations are observed 3-5 hours after administration, declining with a half-life up to about 23 hours. Clonidine is metabolised in the liver. About 65% is excreted in the urine, partly as unchanged clonidine and about 20% is excreted in the faeces.

### Pharmaceutical particulars

*List of excipients:* Lactose; red-brown pigment (E172 and E171); magnesium stearate; povidone; hydroxypropyl methylcellulose; poly (0-ethyl) cellulose; macrogol 6000; titanium dioxide; brown pigment (E172); Lebensmittelblau (E132).

*Incompatibilities:* None stated.

*Shelf life:* 3 years

*Special precautions for storage:* Store below 25˚C. Protect from light.

*Nature and contents of container:* PVC/PVDC blister packs of 56.

*Instructions for use/handling:* None stated.

**Marketing authorisation number**  0015/0072

**Date of approval/revision of SPC**  December 1996.

**Legal category** POM

## COMBIVENT* METERED AEROSOL

**Qualitative and quantitative composition** Combivent Metered Aerosol is a combination of ipratropium

bromide monohydrate and salbutamol sulphate. Each valve activation delivers 21 micrograms of ipratropium bromide monohydrate (corresponds to 20 micrograms ipratropium bromide anhydrous) and 120 micrograms of salbutamol sulphate.

**Pharmaceutical form** Combivent is a metered dose aerosol for inhalation.

### Clinical particulars

*Therapeutic indications:* Combivent is indicated as a bronchodilator for the treatment of bronchospasm associated with chronic obstructive pulmonary disease in patients who require regular treatment with both ipratropium and salbutamol.

*Posology and method of administration:*
*Adults (including elderly patients):* Two inhalations four times a day.

*Children:* There is no experience of the use of Combivent in children below the age of 12 years.

*Contra-indications:* Combivent is contra-indicated in patients with a history of hypersensitivity to any of its components, or to atropine or its derivatives.

*Special warnings and special precautions for use:* Ocular complications

There have been rare reports of ocular complications (i.e. mydriasis, blurring of vision, eye pain) when the contents of metered aerosols containing ipratropium bromide have been sprayed inadvertently into the eye. Care must be taken to prevent Combivent from entering the eye. Should patients develop effects in the eye they should be warned to seek medical advice.

Patients must be instructed in the correct administration of Combivent metered aerosol.

In the following conditions Combivent should only be used after careful risk/benefit assessment: Hypertrophic obstructive cardiomyopathy, tachyarrhythmia, insufficiently controlled diabetes mellitus, recent myocardial infarction and/or severe organic heart or vascular disorders, hyperthyroidism.

The patient should be instructed to consult a doctor immediately in the event of acute, rapidly worsening dyspnoea. In addition, the patient should be warned to seek medical advice should a reduced response become apparent.

Potentially serious hypokalemia may result from beta₂-agonist therapy. Particular caution is advised in severe asthma, as this effect may be potentiated by concomitant treatment with xanthine derivatives, steroids and diuretics. Additionally, hypoxia may aggravate the effects of hypokalemia on cardiac rhythm. It is recommended that serum potassium levels are monitored in such situations.

*Interaction with other medicaments and other forms of interaction:* Beta-adrenergics, xanthine derivatives and corticosteroids may enhance the effect of Combivent. The concurrent administration of other betamimetics, systemically absorbed anticholinergics and xanthine derivatives may increase the side effects.

A potentially serious reduction in effect may occur during concurrent administration of beta-blockers.

Anticholinergic effects of other drugs can be enhanced.

*Pregnancy and lactation:* Ipratropium bromide has been in general use for several years and there is no definite evidence of ill-consequence during pregnancy; animal studies have shown no hazard.

Salbutamol has been in widespread use for many years without apparent ill-consequence during pregnancy. There is inadequate published evidence of safety in the early stages of human pregnancy but in animal studies there has been evidence of some harmful effects on the foetus at very high dose levels.

As with all medicines, Combivent should not be used in pregnancy, especially the first trimester, unless the expected benefit is thought to outweigh any possible risk to the foetus. Similarly, Combivent should not be administered to breast-feeding mothers unless the expected benefit is thought to outweigh any possible risk to the neonate.

*Effects on ability to drive and use machines:* None stated.

*Undesirable effects:* In common with other beta-agonists more frequent undesirable effects of Combivent are fine tremor of skeletal muscles and nervousness, less frequent are tachycardia, dizziness, palpitations or headache, especially in hypersensitive patients.

Potentially serious hypokalemia may result from beta₂-agonist therapy.

In isolated cases there may be local reactions such as dryness of the mouth, throat irritation, or allergic reactions.

As with other bronchodilators, in some cases cough, in very rare instances paradoxical bronchoconstrictions have been observed.

Use of anticholinergic agents (e.g. ipratropium bromide) may precipitate urinary retention, in particular in patients with pre-existing outflow tract obstruction.

*Overdose:* The effects of overdosage are expected to be primarily related to salbutamol because acute overdosage with ipratropium bromide is unlikely as it is not well absorbed systemically after inhalation or oral administration.

Manifestations of overdosage with salbutamol may include anginal pain, hypertension, hypokalaemia and tachycardia. The preferred antidote for overdosage with salbutamol is a cardioselective beta-blocking agent but due care and attention should be used in administering these drugs in patients with a history of bronchospasm.

### Pharmacological properties

*Pharmacodynamic properties:* Ipratropium bromide is an anticholinergic agent which inhibits vagally mediated reflexes by antagonising the action of acetylcholine, the transmitter agent released from the vagus nerve. The bronchodilation following inhalation of ipratropium bromide is primarily local and site specific to the lung and not systemic in nature.

Salbutamol sulphate is a beta$_2$-adrenergic agent which acts on airway smooth muscle resulting in relaxation. Salbutamol relaxes all smooth muscle from the trachea to the terminal bronchioles and protects against all bronchoconstrictor challenges.

Combivent metered aerosol provides the simultaneous release of ipratropium bromide and salbutamol sulphate allowing the synergetic efficacy on the muscarinic and beta$_2$-adrenergic receptors in the lung to cause bronchodilation.

*Pharmacokinetic properties:* Ipratropium bromide is not readily absorbed into the systemic circulation either from the surface of the lung or from the gastrointestinal tract as compared by blood level and renal excretion studies. The half-life elimination is about 3–4 hours after inhalation or intravenous administration. Ipratropium bromide does not penetrate blood brain barrier.

Salbutamol sulphate is rapidly and completely absorbed following oral adminstration either by the inhaled or gastric route. Peak plasma salbutamol concentrations are seen within three hours of administration and the drug is excreted unchanged in the urine after 24 hours. Intravenous salbutamol will cross the blood brain barrier reaching concentrations amounting to about five percent of the plasma concentrations.

From a pharmacokinetic perspective, the additive activity of Combivent is due to the local effect of the fixed dose of the active components (ipratropium bromide and salbutamol sulphate) on the muscarinic and beta$_2$-adrenergic receptors in the lung.

*Preclinical safety data:* The individual active ingredients ipratropium bromide and salbutamol sulphate have been extensively investigated in animal models and the safety concerns are not clinically significant when Combivent is used as metered aerosol at the recommended dosage levels to patients.

### Pharmaceutical particulars

*List of excipients:* Dichlorodifluoromethane; dichlorotetrafluoroethane; trichloromonofluoromethane; soya lecithin.

*Incompatibilities:* None known.

*Shelf life:* 3 years

*Special precautions for storage:* Store below 25°C. Protect from direct sunlight and frost.

*Nature and contents of container:* Combivent Metered Aerosol is a creamy-white suspension of micronised substances in halogenated propellants filled in metal canisters with a metering valve.

*Instructions for use/handling:* The correct operation of the metered aerosol apparatus is essential for successful therapy.

The aerosol should be shaken and the valve depressed once or twice before the apparatus is initially used.

Before each use the following rules should be observed:
1. Remove protective cap.
2. Shake the metered aerosol well before each use.
3. Breathe out deeply.
4. Hold the metered aerosol and close lips over the mouthpiece. The arrow and the base of the container should be pointing upwards.
5. Breathe in as deeply as possible, pressing the base of the container firmly at the same time, this releases one metered dose. Hold the breath for a few seconds, then remove the mouthpiece from the mouth and breathe out.
6. Replace the protective cap after use.

The container is under pressure and should on no account be opened by force or exposed to temperatures exceeding 50°C. As the container is not transparent it is not possible to see when the contents are used up, but if on shaking the container seems to be empty, it probably still contains a further 10 effective inhalations.

The mouthpiece should always be kept clean and can be washed with warm water. If soap or detergent is used, the mouthpiece should be thoroughly rinsed in clear water.

**Marketing authorisation number** 0015/0191

**Date of approval/revision of SPC** September 1996

**Legal category** POM

## COMBIVENT* UDVs*

**Qualitative and quantitative composition** Each 2.5 ml unit-dose vial contains 500 micrograms ipratropium bromide and 3 mg salbutamol sulphate (corresponds to 2.5 mg salbutamol base)

**Pharmaceutical form** Solution for inhalation.

### Clinical particulars

*Therapeutic indications:* Combivent UDVs are indicated for the management of bronchospasm in patients suffering from chronic obstructive pulmonary disease who require regular treatment with both ipratropium and salbutamol.

*Posology and method of administration:* Combivent UDVs may be administered from a suitable nebuliser or an intermittent positive pressure ventilator.

The recommended dose is :
*Adults:* (including elderly patients and children over 12 years): 1 vial three or four times daily.
*Children:* There is no experience of the use of Combivent UDVs in children under 12 years.

*Contra-indications:* Combivent UDVs are contra-indicated in patients with a history of hypersensitivity to ipratropium bromide, salbutamol sulphate or to atropine or its derivatives.

*Special warnings and special precautions for use:* Patients must be instructed in the correct use of Combivent UDVs and warned not to allow the solution or mist to enter the eyes. Acute angle glaucoma has been reported rarely when nebulised solutions of ipratropium bromide have been used in conjunction with beta$_2$-agonist bronchodilators. Protection of the eyes appears to prevent any increase in intra-ocular pressure and patients who may be susceptible to glaucoma should be warned specifically on the need for ocular protection.

In the following conditions Combivent UDVs should only be used after careful risk/benefit assessment : Hypertrophic obstructive cardiomyopathy, tachyarrhythmia, inadequately controlled diabetes mellitus, recent myocardial infarction and/or severe organic heart or vascular disorders, hyperthyroidism.

The patient should be instructed to consult a doctor immediately in the event of acute, rapidly worsening dyspnoea. In addition, the patient should be warned to seek medical advice should a reduced response become apparent.

Potentially serious hypokalaemia may result from beta$_2$-agonist therapy. Particular caution is advised in severe airway obstruction, as this effect may be potentiated by concomitant treatment with xanthine derivatives, steroids and diuretics. Additionally, hypoxia may aggravate the effects of hypokalaemia on cardiac rhythm. It is recommended that serum potassium levels are monitored in such situations.

*Interaction with other medicaments and other forms of interaction:* The use of additional beta-agonists, xanthine derivatives and corticosteroids may enhance the effect of Combivent UDVs. The concurrent administration of other beta-mimetics, systemically absorbed anticholinergics and xanthine derivatives may increase the severity of side effects. A potentially serious reduction in effect may occur during concurrent administration of beta-blockers.

*Pregnancy and lactation:* Ipratropium bromide has been in general use for several years and there is no definite evidence of ill-consequence during pregnancy; animal studies have shown no hazard.

Salbutamol has been in widespread use for many years without apparent ill-consequence during pregnancy. There is inadequate published evidence of safety in the early stages of human pregnancy but in animal studies there has been evidence of some harmful effects on the foetus at very high dose levels.

As with all medicines, Combivent should not be used in pregnancy, especially the first trimester, unless the expected benefit is thought to outweigh any possible risk to the foetus. Similarly, Combivent should not be administered to breast-feeding mothers unless the expected benefit is thought to outweigh any possible risk to the neonate.

*Effects on ability to drive and use machines:* None stated.

*Undesirable effects:* Nebulisation-induced bronchospasm, dyspnoea and cough have been reported infrequently following the use of Combivent UDVs.

In common with other beta-agonist bronchodilators the undesirable effects of Combivent UDVs include fine tremor of skeletal muscles and nervousness and less frequently, tachycardia, dizziness, palpitations or headache, especially in hypersensitive patients.

Potentially serious hypokalaemia may result from beta$_2$-agonist therapy.

Use of anticholinergic agents (e.g. ipratropium bromide) may precipitate urinary retention, in particular in patients with pre-existing obstruction of the urinary tract. Dry mouth has occasionally been reported.

*Overdose:* Acute effects of overdosage with ipratropium bromide are unlikely due to its poor systemic absorption after either inhalation or oral administration. Any effects of overdosage are therefore likely to be related to the salbutamol component.

Manifestations of overdosage with salbutamol may include anginal pain, hypertension, hypokalaemia and tachycardia. The preferred antidote for overdosage with salbutamol is a cardioselective beta-blocking agent but caution should be used in administering these drugs in patients with a history of bronchospasm.

### Pharmacological properties

*Pharmacodynamic properties:* Ipratropium bromide is an anticholinergic agent which inhibits vagally-mediated reflexes by antagonising the action of acetylcholine, the transmitter agent released from the vagus nerve. The bronchodilation following inhalation of ipratropium bromide is primarily local and site specific to the lung and not systemic in nature.

Salbutamol is a beta$_2$-adrenergic agent which acts on airway smooth muscle resulting in relaxation. Salbutamol relaxes all smooth muscle from the trachea to the terminal bronchioles and protects against bronchoconstrictor challenges.

Combivent UDVs provide the simultaneous delivery of ipratropium bromide and salbutamol sulphate allowing effects on both muscarinic and beta$_2$-adrenergic receptors in the lung leading to increased bronchodilation over that provided by each agent singly.

*Pharmacokinetic properties:* Ipratropium bromide is not readily absorbed into the systemic circulation either from the surface of the lung or from the gastrointestinal tract as assessed by blood level and renal excretion studies. The elimination half-life is about 1.5 hours after inhalation or intravenous administration. Ipratropium bromide does not cross the blood-brain barrier.

Salbutamol is rapidly and completely absorbed following oral administration either by the inhaled or the gastric route. Peak plasma salbutamol concentrations are seen within three hours of administration and the drug is excreted unchanged in the urine after 24 hours. The elimination half-life is 4 hours. Salbutamol will cross the blood brain barrier reaching concentrations amounting to about five percent of the plasma concentrations.

It has been shown that co-nebulisation of ipratropium bromide and salbutamol sulphate does not potentiate the systemic absorption of either component and that therefore the additive activity of Combivent UDVs is due to the combined local effect on the lung following inhalation.

*Preclinical safety data:* The individual active ingredients, ipratropium bromide and salbutamol sulphate, have been extensively investigated in animal models and there are no clinically relevant safety issues when Combivent UDVs are used at the recommended doses by patients.

### Pharmaceutical particulars

*List of excipients:* Sodium chloride; hydrochloric acid; purified water.

*Incompatibilities:* None known.

*Shelf life:* 24 months.

*Special precautions for storage:* Store below 25°C. Protect from light. Do not freeze. Do not use if solution is discoloured.

*Nature and contents of container:* Low density polyethylene vials containing 2.5 ml of solution, formed into strips of 10 and packed into cartons containing 60 vials.

*Instructions for use/handling:*
i) Prepare the nebuliser by following the manufacturer's instructions and the advice of your doctor.
ii) Carefully separate a new vial from the strip. NEVER use one that has been opened already.
iii) Open the vial by simply twisting off the top, always taking care to hold it in an upright position.
iv) Unless otherwise instructed by your doctor squeeze all the contents of the plastic vial into the nebuliser chamber.

v) Assemble the nebuliser and use it as directed by your doctor.

vi) After nebulisation clean the nebuliser according to the manufacturer's instructions.

**Marketing authorisation number** 0015/0197

**Date of approval/revision of SPC** June 1995

**Legal category** POM.

## DEXA-RHINASPRAY*

**Presentation** Dexa-Rhinaspray metered nasal spray, complete with nasal applicator. Each 9 g vial contains about 125 metered doses. One metered dose contains: tramazoline hydrochloride 120 micrograms, dexamethasone-21 isonicotinate 20 micrograms, neomycin sulphate 100 micrograms.

### Uses

*Action:* Tramazoline hydrochloride is a sympathomimetic substance with local vasoconstrictor activity. It has a quick-acting, long-lasting decongestant effect on the nasal mucosa. Dexamethasone–21 isonicotinate is a corticosteroid with marked anti-inflammatory and anti-allergic properties. Neomycin sulphate is locally active against a wide range of both Grampositive and Gram-negative bacteria.

*Indication:* Treatment of allergic rhinitis.

### Dosage and administration

*Adults:* 1 metered dose can be applied into each nostril up to six times in 24 hours, although 2 or 3 applications a day are usually sufficient.

*Children 5-12 years:* 1 metered dose into each nostril up to twice daily.

*Children under 5 years:* not recommended.

Each course of treatment should not exceed 14 days.

No specific information on the use of this product in the elderly is available. Clinical trials have included patients over 65 years and no adverse reactions specific to this age group have been reported.

### Contra-indications, warnings, etc

*Contra-indications:* Its use is contra-indicated in infants, patients hypersensitive to neomycin or other aminoglycoside antibiotics, or tramazoline .

*Precautions:* Prolonged use may result in the development of superinfection due to organisms resistant to neomycin. Care should be used to avoid contact with the eyes as conjunctival irritation may occur.

Because of the possibility of adrenocortical suppression Dexa-rhinaspray is not recommended for children under the age of 5 years.

Due to the theoretical risk of foetal ototoxicity from the neomycin component, Dexa-rhinaspray should not be used during pregnancy.

*Side-effects:* A slight burning sensation in the nose, with sneezing, has been reported when using tramazoline hydrochloride alone.

*Overdosage:* There have been no reports of overdosage with Dexa-Rhinaspray, but absorption of tramazoline may produce pallor, sweating, tachycardia and anxiety. These should be treated symptomatically.

**Pharmaceutical precautions** Protect from extremes of temperature. The vials should not be punctured or incinerated even when apparently empty.

**Legal category** POM.

**Package quantities** 9 g vial (125 doses) (OP) complete with nasal applicator.

**Further information** Neomycin sulphate is rarely used systemically. Local use therefore does not prejudice the patient's response to later systemic antibiotic treatment.

**Product licence number** 0015/5010R

## DIXARIT* TABLETS

**Qualitative and quantitative composition** Blue, biconvex, sugar-coated tablets. Each tablet contains clonidine hydrochloride 25 micrograms.

**Pharmaceutical form** Sugar-coated tablets for oral administration.

### Clinical particulars

*Therapeutic indications:*

(a) The prophylactic management of migraine or recurrent vascular headache.

(b) The management of vasomotor conditions commonly associated with the menopause and characterised by flushing.

*Posology and method of administration:*

*Adults:* Initially 2 tablets twice daily. If after two weeks there has been no remission, increase to 3 tablets twice daily.

The duration of treatment depends upon the severity of the condition.

*Children:* Not generally recommended for administration to children under 12 years.

*Elderly:* No specific information on the use of this product in the elderly is available.

Clinical trials have included patients over 65 years and no adverse reactions specific to this age group have been reported.

*Contra-indications:* Dixarit should not be used in patients with sick-sinus syndrome or with known hypersensitivity to the active ingredient, clonidine.

*Special warnings and special precautions for use:* Dixarit should be used with caution in patients with cerebrovascular disease, coronary insufficiency, occlusive peripheral vascular disorders, such as Raynaud's disease, or those with a history of depression.

At doses higher than those recommended above, clonidine is an effective antihypertensive agent. Caution should therefore be observed where antihypertensive agents are being used, as potentiation of the hypotensive effect may occur. Provided the recommended Dixarit dosage regimen is followed, no difficulty with hypotension should arise during the routine management of patients with either migraine or menopausal flushing.

Depending on the dose given, Dixarit can cause bradycardia. In patients with pre-existing cardiac conduction abnormalities, arrhythmias have been observed after high doses of Dixarit.

Patients with renal failure require extreme care.

Clonidine is available for the management of hypertension as Catapres Tablets (100 micrograms and 300 micrograms), Perlongets (250 micrograms) and Ampoules (150 micrograms in 1 ml). Where Catapres is already being used Dixarit therapy is obviously not indicated.

*Interaction with other medicaments and other forms of interaction:* Concurrent administration of antihypertensive agents, vasodilators or diuretics, may lead to an increased hypotensive effect.

Concomitant use of beta-blockers and/or cardiac glycosides can cause bradycardia or dysrhythmia (AV-block) in isolated cases.

If during combined treatment with a beta-blocker there is need to interrupt or discontinue antihypertensive therapy, the beta-blocker must always be discontinued slowly first (reducing the dose gradually to avoid sympathetic hyperactivity) and then the Dixarit, which should also be reduced gradually over several days if previously given in high doses.

As the effects of clonidine can be antagonised by tricyclic anti-depressants, it may be necessary to adjust the dosage of Dixarit, if these agents are administered concurrently. Although there is no experience from clinical trials, the effect of tranquillisers, hypnotics or alcohol could theoretically be potentiated by Dixarit.

*Pregnancy and lactation:* Clonidine has been in wide general use for many years and has shown no evidence of untoward effects when taken during human pregnancy. However, as with all medicines, Dixarit should not be used in pregnancy, especially the first trimester, unless the expected benefit is thought to outweigh any possible risk to the foetus.

In animal studies involving doses higher than the equivalent maximum therapeutic dose in man, effects on foetal development were only seen in one species. Foetal malformations did not occur.

The drug enters breast milk, but is not likely to affect the infant when therapeutic doses are used.

*Effects on ability to drive and use machines:* Because of different individual reactions including drowsiness, the ability to drive or operate machinery may be impaired, particularly in the initial phase of treatment with Dixarit.

*Undesirable effects:* There may be some initial sedation or dry mouth in some patients when Dixarit therapy is started. Dizziness, nausea and nocturnal unrest have been reported. Orthostatic hypotension has been reported, but only following the first administration of high doses.

Rare cases of constipation, impotence and disturbances in peripheral blood flow have been observed.

Very rarely, and only after very high doses of clonidine, have there been reports of hypersensitivity reactions, skin rash, perceptual disorders, nightmares, gynaecomastia, pain in the parotid gland, depressive moods, drying of nasal mucosa and reduced lachrymal flow.

In the management of hypertension a single case of toxic hepatitis has been reported with clonidine. However, the role of clonidine in hepatotoxicity in this patient remains questionable. Monitoring of haematological, renal and hepatic status in large numbers of patients has revealed no drug-related adverse effects.

*Overdose: Symptoms:* Sedation to somnolence, hypotension, orthostatic hypotension, bradycardia, occasionally vomiting, very occasionally hypertension, dryness of the mouth.

*Treatment:* Gastric lavage and/or administration of activated charcoal should be performed where appropriate. In most cases all that is required are general supportive measures.

**Pharmacological properties**

*Pharmacodynamic properties:* Clonidine is an antihypertensive agent which acts centrally by stimulating alpha$_2$-adrenergic receptors and producing a reduction in sympathetic tone, resulting in a fall in diastolic and systolic blood pressure and a reduction in heart rate.

Treatment with Dixarit diminishes the responsiveness of peripheral vessels to constrictor and dilator stimuli, thereby preventing the vascular changes associated with migraine. The same direct action on peripheral vessels moderates the vascular changes associated with menopausal flushing.

*Pharmacokinetic properties:* Clonidine is well absorbed from the gastro-intestinal tract. Peak plasma concentrations are observed 3 to 5 hours post administration, decreasing with a half life of up to approximately 23 hours. Clonidine is metabolised in the liver. About 65% is excreted in the urine, partly as unchanged clonidine and about 20% is excreted in the faeces.

**Pharmaceutical particulars**

*List of excipients: Tablet core:* Calcium hydrogen phosphate; lactose; maize starch; colloidal silica; polyvinylpyrrolidone; soluble starch; colouring E132; magnesium stearate.

*Tablet coating:* Polyvinylpyrrolidone; sucrose; talc; gum arabic; titanium dioxide; colouring E132; polyethylene glycol; carnauba wax; white wax.

*Incompatibilities:* None stated.

*Shelf life:* 5 years.

*Special precautions for storage:* Protect from light.

*Nature and contents of container:* PVC/aluminium blister packs of 84, 100 & 112. Currently the 112 pack is the only marketed pack.

*Instructions for use/handling:* None stated.

**Marketing authorisation number** 0015/5014R

**Date of approval/revision of SPC** July 1996

**Legal category** POM

## DUOVENT* INHALER

**Presentation** Pressurised metered dose inhaler: 10 ml vial (200 metered doses) available as complete unit with mouthpiece. Each metered dose contains fenoterol hydrobromide 100 micrograms and ipratropium bromide 40 micrograms.

### Uses

*Action:* Fenoterol hydrobromide is a highly potent, rapidly acting selective beta$_2$–adrenoceptor stimulant. The degree of selectivity coupled with administration by inhalation allows maximal bronchodilator effect with minimal side-effects.

Ipratropium bromide is an anticholinergic drug with bronchodilator properties.

There is evidence that the concurrent administration of ipratropium bromide and a sympathomimetic drug produces a greater relief of bronchospasm than either drug given alone.

*Indications:* For the treatment of reversible airways obstruction as in bronchial asthma, bronchitis and emphysema.

### Dosage and administration

*Adults:* 1 or 2 puffs three or four times daily.

*Children over 6 years:* 1 puff three times daily. It is recommended that administration of Duovent to children be supervised by an adult.

No specific information on the use of this product in the elderly is available. Clinical trials have included patients over 65 years and no adverse reactions specific to this age group have been reported.

### Contra-indications, warnings, etc

*Contra-indications:* Known sensitivity to atropine.

*Precautions:* Caution should be observed should it be necessary to administer Duovent to patients with thyrotoxicosis, myocardial insufficiency, angina, cardiac dysrhythmias, hypertension or hypertrophic subvalvular aortic stenosis. In view of the possible interaction between sympathomimetic amines and monoamine oxidase inhibitors or tricyclic anti-depressants, care should be exercised if it is proposed to administer these compounds concurrently with Duovent. Duovent should be used with caution in patients already receiving other sympathomimetic agents as cardiovascular effects may be additive.

Potentially serious hypokalaemia may result from beta$_2$–agonist therapy. Particular caution is advised in severe asthma as this effect may be potentiated by concomitant treatment with xanthine derivatives, steroids, diuretics and by hypoxia. It is recommended that serum potassium levels are monitored in such situations.

Generally, caution is advocated in the use of anticholinergic agents in patients with glaucoma and prostatic hypertrophy. However, specific studies with ipratropium bromide in patients with glaucoma showed that inhaling cumulative doses of 160 micrograms had no effect on the eye. Urinary retention and constipation have only rarely been reported.

Patients must be instructed in the correct use of a metered dose inhaler and warned against the accidental release of the contents into the eye. If relief is not obtained after correct use of the inhaler, the dose should not be exceeded and the patient should contact the doctor for advice.

Although both fenoterol hydrobromide and ipratropium bromide have been in general use for several years, there is no definite evidence of ill-consequence during human pregnancy; animal studies have shown no hazard. Beta-adrenergic agents have been shown to prolong pregnancy and inhibit labour although the amount in the prescribed dose of Duovent is probably insufficient to do so.

Medicines should not be used in pregnancy, especially the first trimester, unless the expected benefit is thought to outweigh any possible risk to the foetus.

Beta-adrenergic blocking agents may antagonise fenoterol hydrobromide and reduce its bronchodilator effect if administered concurrently.

*Side-effects:* Potentially serious hypokalaemia may result from beta$_2$–agonist therapy. Transient sympathomimetic side-effects, such as palpitation, tachycardia, headache and tremor may occur, as with other beta–adrenergic agonists, but are uncommon with administration by inhaler.

Anticholinergic side-effects are unlikely to occur at therapeutic doses but some patients may complain of a dry mouth. There is no evidence that in the therapeutic dose range Duovent has any adverse effect on bronchial secretion.

*Overdosage:* Accidental overdosage may give rise to tachycardia, palpitation and tremor. It is suggested that the patient should be treated symptomatically. Should the administration of a beta-adrenergic blocking agent be considered necessary to counteract the effects of over-dosage, its use in a patient liable to bronchospasm should be carefully monitored.

Very high doses (30 mg) of ipratropium bromide by mouth have been reported to cause anticholinergic side-effects but these were not severe and did not require specific reversal.

**Pharmaceutical precautions**  Protect from heat, including the sun. Protect from frost. The canister should not be incinerated or opened even when apparently empty.

**Legal category**  POM.

**Package quantities**  10 ml vial (200 metered doses) (OP) complete with mouthpiece.

**Further information**  There is evidence to suggest that fenoterol may reduce the allergic response of tissues. Animal studies have shown that fenoterol also produces an increase in the frequency of movement of the respiratory epithelial cilia and in the rate of mucus transport.

Long-term use has shown fenoterol and ipratropium to be free from significant adverse effects.

**Product licence number**  0015/0091.


# DUOVENT* AUTOHALER*

**Presentation**  Breath-actuated pressurised aerosol for inhalation therapy. Each actuation delivers fenoterol hydrobromide 100 micrograms and ipratropium bromide 40 micrograms.

**Uses**

*Action:* Fenoterol hydrobromide is a highly potent, rapidly acting selective beta$_2$-adrenoceptor stimulant. The degree of selectivity coupled with administration by inhalation allows maximal bronchodilator effect with minimal side-effects. Ipratropium bromide is an anticholinergic drug with bronchodilator properties. There is evidence that the concurrent administration of ipratropium bromide and a sympathomimetic drug produces a greater relief of bronchospasm than either drug given alone.

*Indications:* For the treatment of reversible airways obstruction as in bronchial asthma, bronchitis and emphysema.

**Dosage and administration**

*Adults:* 1 or 2 puffs three or four times daily.

*Children over 6 years:* 1 puff three times daily. It is recommended that administration of Duovent to children be supervised by an adult.

No specific information on the use of this product in the elderly is available. Clinical trials have included

patients over 65 years and no adverse reactions specific to this age group have been reported.

**Contra-indications, warnings, etc**

*Contra-indications:* Known sensitivity to atropine.

*Precautions :* Caution should be observed should it be necessary to administer Duovent to patients with thyrotoxicosis, myocardial insufficiency, angina, cardiac dysrhythmias, hypertension or hypertrophic subvalvular aortic stenosis. In view of the possible interaction between sympathomimetic amines and monoamine oxidase inhibitors or tricyclic anti-depressants, care should be exercised if it is proposed to administer these compounds concurrently with Duovent. Duovent should be used with caution in patients already receiving other sympathomimetic agents as cardiovascular effects may be additive.

Potentially serious hypokalaemia may result from beta$_2$-agonist therapy. Particular caution is advised in severe asthma as this effect may be potentiated by concomitant treatment with xanthine derivatives, steroids, diuretics and by hypoxia. It is recommended that serum potassium levels are monitored in such situations. Generally, caution is advocated in the use of anti-cholinergic agents in patients with glaucoma and prostatic hypertrophy. However, specific studies with ipratropium bromide in patients with glaucoma showed that inhaling cumulative doses of 160 micrograms had no effect on the eye. Urinary retention and constipation have only rarely been reported.

Patients must be instructed in the correct use of the Autohaler device. If relief is not obtained after correct use of the inhaler, the dose should not be exceeded and the patient should contact the doctor for advice.

Although both fenoterol hydrobromide and ipratropium bromide have been in general use for several years, there is no definite evidence of ill-consequence during human pregnancy; animal studies have shown no hazard. Beta-adrenergic agents have been shown to prolong pregnancy and inhibit labour although the amount in the prescribed dose of Duovent is probably insufficient to do so.

Medicines should not be used in pregnancy, especially the first trimester, unless the expected benefit is thought to outweigh any possible risk to the foetus. Beta-adrenergic blocking agents may antagonise fenoterol hydrobromide and reduce its bronchodilator effect if administered concurrently.

*Side-effects:* Potentially serious hypokalaemia may result from beta$_2$-agonist therapy. Transient sympathomimetic side-effects, such as palpitation, tachycardia, headache and tremor may occur, as with other beta-adrenergic agonists, but are uncommon with administration by inhaler.

Anticholinergic side-effects are unlikely to occur at therapeutic doses but some patients may complain of a dry mouth. There is no evidence that in the therapeutic dose range Duovent has any adverse effect on bronchial secretion.

*Overdosage:* Accidental overdosage may give rise to tachycardia, palpitation and tremor. It is suggested that the patient should be treated symptomatically. Should the administration of a beta-adrenergic blocking agent be considered necessary to counteract the effects of over-dosage, its use in a patient liable to bronchospasm should be carefully monitored. Very high doses (30 mg) of ipratropium bromide by mouth have been reported to cause anticholinergic side-effects but these were not severe and did not require specific reversal.

**Pharmaceutical precautions**  Protect from heat, including the sun. Protect from frost. The canister should not be incinerated or opened even when apparently empty.

**Legal category** POM.

**Package quantities**  10 ml vial (200 metered doses) (OP) complete with mouthpiece.

**Further information**  There is evidence to suggest that fenoterol may reduce the allergic response of tissues. Animal studies have shown that fenoterol also produces an increase in the frequency of movement of the respiratory epithelial cilia and in the rate of mucus transport. Long-term use has shown fenoterol and ipratropium to be free from significant adverse effects.

**Product licence number** 0015/0162.


# DUOVENT* UDVs*

**Qualitative and quantitative composition** Each Unit Dose Vial (UDV) contains fenoterol hydrobromide 1.25 mg and ipratropium bromide, 0.5 mg.

**Pharmaceutical form**  Nebuliser Solution for inhalation.

**Clinical particulars**

*Therapeutic indications:* The management of acute severe asthma or acute exacerbation of chronic

asthma presenting as an emergency requiring treatment by nebuliser.

*Posology and method of administration:* Duovent UDVs may be administered from an intermittent positive pressure ventilator or from a properly maintained and functioning nebuliser.

The recommended dose for adults and children over 14 years is one vial (4 ml) to be nebulised immediately upon presentation. Each dose should be inhaled to dryness from the nebuliser. Repeat dosing may be given at the discretion of the treating physician, up to a maximum of 4 vials in 24 hours.

In acute severe asthma additional doses may be necessary depending on clinical response. Nebuliser treatment of acute severe asthma should be replaced by standard inhaler devices 24-48 hours before discharge unless the patient requires a nebuliser at home.

Clinical trials have included patients over 65 years. No adverse reactions specific to this age group have been reported.

*Contra-indications:* Known hypersensitivity to atropine, ipratropium or fenoterol.

*Special warnings and special precautions for use:* As with other beta-agonists, caution should be observed when using Duovent UDVs in patients with thyrotoxicosis, myocardial insufficiency, angina, cardiac dysrhythmias, hypertension, hypertrophic subvalvular aortic stenosis or hypertrophic obstructive cardiomyopathy.

The administration of nebuliser solutions has occasionally been associated with cases of paradoxical bronchoconstriction.

Patients must be instructed in the correct use of a nebuliser and warned not to exceed the prescribed dose. The patient must be instructed to seek medical advice in the event of Duovent failing to provide relief of bronchospasm.

Care should be taken to prevent the solution or mist from entering the eyes. Acute angle-closure glaucoma has been reported rarely when nebulised ipratropium bromide has been used in conjunction with nebulised beta$_2$-agonist bronchodilators. Protection of the eyes appears to prevent any increase in intra-ocular pressure and patients who may be susceptible to glaucoma should be warned specifically on the need for ocular protection. Inhaled doses of ipratropium bromide nebuliser solution up to 1 mg have not been associated with elevation of intra-ocular pressure.

Caution is advocated in the use of anticholinergic agents in patients with prostatic hypertrophy.

*Interaction with other medicaments and other forms of interaction:* In view of a possible interaction between sympathomimetic amines and monoamine oxidase inhibitors or tricyclic antidepressants, care should be exercised if it is proposed to administer these compounds concurrently with Duovent UDVs.

Duovent UDVs should be used with caution in patients already receiving other sympathomimetic agents as cardiovascular effects may be additive.

Potentially serious hypokalaemia may result from beta$_2$-agonist therapy. Particular caution is advised in severe asthma as this effect may be potentiated by concomitant treatment with xanthine derivatives, steroids, diuretics and by hypoxia. It is recommended that serum potassium levels are monitored on such occasions.

Beta-adrenergic blocking agents may antagonise fenoterol hydrobromide and reduce its bronchodilator effect if administered concurrently.

*Pregnancy and lactation:* Ipratropium bromide and fenoterol hydrobromide have been in wide general use for several years and there is no definite evidence of ill-consequence during pregnancy; animal studies have shown no hazard. Medicines should, however, not be used in pregnancy, especially during the first trimester, unless the expected benefit is thought to outweigh any possible risk to the foetus.

Beta-adrenergic agents have been shown to prolong pregnancy and inhibit labour although the amount in the recommended dose of Duovent UDVs is probably insufficient to do so.

*Effects on ability to drive and use machines:* None stated.

*Undesirable effects:* Anticholinergic side-effects are unlikely at therapeutic doses, but some patients may complain of a dry mouth.

As with other beta-adrenergic agonists transient sympathomimetic side-effects such as tremor, palpitations, tachycardia and headache may occur but are uncommon with administration by inhalation.

Potentially serious hypokalaemia may result from beta$_2$-agonist therapy.

*Overdose:* Inhaled doses of 5 mg ipratropium produce an increase in heart rate and palpitation but single doses of 2 mg have been given to adults and 1 mg to children without causing side effects. Single doses of ipratropium bromide 30 mg by mouth cause anticholinergic side effects but these are not severe and do not require specific reversal.

Accidental overdose with fenoterol may give rise to tachycardia, palpitation, flushing, nausea, restlessness, dizziness, headache and tremor. It is suggested that the patient should be treated symptomatically. Beta$_1$-selective beta-adrenergic blocking agents should be chosen and blood pressure should be monitored. Should the administration of a beta-adrenergic blocking agent be considered necessary to counteract the effects of overdosage, its use in a patient liable to bronchospasm should be carefully monitored.

### Pharmacological properties

*Pharmacodynamic properties:*
*Fenoterol hydrobromide* is a direct acting sympathomimetic agent where the catechol nucleus of isoprenaline has been replaced by a resorcinol nucleus, and the substituent moiety on the amino group is larger. This substitution has the effect of depressing the affinity of the molecule to the beta-1 (cardiac and lipolytic) adrenergic receptors and enhancing the affinity towards the beta-2 (bronchial, vascular and intestinal) adrenergic receptors.

*Ipratropium bromide* affects airway function primarily through its neural effect on the parasympathetic nervous system. Ipratropium bromide blocks the acetylcholine receptors on smooth muscle in the lung. Stimulation of these receptors normally produces contraction and, depending on the degree of actuation, bronchoconstriction. Thus, even in normal subjects, ipratropium bromide will cause bronchodilatation.

*Pharmacokinetic properties:*
*Fenoterol Hydrobromide:* In man fenoterol is very rapidly distributed through the tissues following intravenous administration. The kidneys excrete up to 65% mainly in the form of acidic conjugates. Following oral administration, the plasma levels reach their maximum 2 hours after ingestion and then drop exponentially. Renal excretion is 39% following peroral administration and over 98% of the renal excretory products consist of acidic conjugates. The half life for total excretion is 7.2 hours and absorption was calculated to be 60%.

The duration of action following use of a metered dose aerosol is considerably larger and can be explained by the dose independent absorption in the upper bronchial tree. The concentration-independent absorption at this site, from the depot produced by the metered dose aerosol is maintained for several hours.

*Ipratropium Bromide:* It is a quaternary ammonium compound which is poorly absorbed from the gastro-intestinal tract and is slow to cross mucous membranes and the blood brain barrier. Following inhalation, uptake into the plasma is minimal, a peak blood concentration is attained 1½ to 3 hours after inhalation (and similarly for oral administration). Excretion is chiefly via the kidneys.

### Pharmaceutical particulars

*List of excipients:* Sodium chloride; 1N hydrochloric acid; purified water.

*Incompatibilities:* None stated.

*Shelf life:* 3 years

*Special precautions for storage:* Store below 25°C. Protect from heat and light.

*Nature and contents of container:* Duovent UDVs will be available in low density polyethylene (LDPE) vials formed in strips of 10 packed into cartons containing 20 or 60 vials. Each vial contains 4 ml solution.

**Marketing authorisation number** 0015/0164

**Date of approval/revision of SPC** June 1993

**Legal category** POM.

## MOBIC* TABLETS 7.5 MG ▼

**Qualitative and quantitative composition** Meloxicam 7.5 mg

**Pharmaceutical form** Tablet.

### Clinical particulars

*Therapeutic indications:* Short-term symptomatic treatment of acute exacerbations of osteoarthrosis.
Long-term symptomatic treatment of rheumatoid arthritis (chronic polyarthritis).

*Posology and method of administration:*
Acute exacerbations of osteoarthrosis: 7.5 mg/day (one tablet). If necessary, in the absence of improvement, the dose may be increased to 15 mg/day (two tablets).
Rheumatoid arthritis: 15 mg/day (two tablets).
In elderly patients with rheumatoid arthritis the recommended dose for long term treatment is 7.5 mg per day.

Patients with increased risks for adverse reactions should start treatment with 7.5 mg per day.
DO NOT EXCEED THE DOSE OF 15 mg/day.
The total daily amount should be taken as a single dose, with water or another liquid, during a meal.
In dialysis patients with severe renal failure the dose should not exceed 7.5 mg per day.

*Contra-indications:* Hypersensitivity to meloxicam or to one of the excipients. The possibility exists of crossover sensitivity with aspirin and other non-steroidal anti-inflammatory drugs (NSAIDs). MOBIC should not be given to patients who have developed signs of asthma, nasal polyps, angioneurotic oedema or urticaria following the administration of aspirin or NSAIDs.
Active peptic ulcer during the last six months or a history of recurrent peptic ulcer disease.
Severe hepatic failure.
Non-dialyzed severe renal failure.
Children aged under 15.
Pregnancy (see Pregnancy and lactation).
Lactation.
Gastrointestinal bleeding, cerebrovascular bleeding or other bleeding disorders.

*Special warnings and special precautions for use:*
*Warnings:* As with all NSAIDs, any history of oesophagitis, gastritis and/or peptic ulcer must be sought in order to ensure their total cure before starting treatment with meloxicam.
Attention should routinely be paid to the possible onset of a recurrence in patients treated with meloxicam and with a past history of this type.
As with all NSAIDs, long term administration has been associated with an increased risk of gastrointestinal side effects.
Treatment with meloxicam must be stopped in case of onset of peptic ulcer or of gastrointestinal bleeding.
Withdrawal of treatment with meloxicam must be envisaged in case of onset of cutaneo-mucosal adverse events. The possible occurrence of severe skin reactions and serious life threatening hypersensitivity reactions is known to occur with NSAIDs including oxicams.
In rare instances, NSAIDs may be the cause of interstitial nephritis, glomerulonephritis, renal medullary necrosis or nephrotic syndrome.
As with most NSAIDs, occasional increases in serum transaminase levels, increases in serum bilirubin or other liver function parameters as well as increases in serum creatinine and blood urea nitrogen as well as other laboratory disturbances have been reported. The majority of these instances involved transitory and slight abnormalities. Should any such abnormality prove significant or persistent, the administration of meloxicam should be stopped and appropriate investigations prescribed.
Induction of sodium, potassium and water retention and interference with the natriuretic effects of diuretics and consequently possible exacerbations of the condition of patients with cardiac insufficiency or hypertension may occur with NSAIDs.

*Precautions:* NSAIDs inhibit the synthesis of renal prostaglandins involved in the maintenance of renal perfusion in patients with decreased renal blood flow and blood volume. Administration of NSAIDs in such situations may result in the decompensation of latent renal failure. However renal function returns to its initial status when treatment is withdrawn. This risk concerns all elderly individuals, patients with congestive cardiac failure, cirrhosis of the liver, nephrotic syndrome or renal failure as well as patients on diuretics or having undergone major surgery leading to hypovolaemia. Careful monitoring of urine output and renal function during treatment is necessary in such patients.
Adverse reactions are often less well tolerated in elderly, fragile or weakened individuals, who therefore require careful surveillance. As with other NSAIDs, particular caution is required in the elderly, in whom renal, hepatic and cardiac functions are frequently impaired.
The recommended maximum daily dose should not be exceeded in case of insufficient therapeutic effect nor should an additional NSAID be added to the therapy because this may increase the toxicity while therapeutic advantage has not been proven.

*Interactions with other medicaments and other forms of interaction:*
*Inadvisable combinations:* Other NSAIDs, including high doses of salicylates: administration of several NSAIDs together may increase the risk of ulcers and of gastrointestinal bleeding, via a synergistic effect.
Oral anticoagulants, heparin and ticlopidine: increased risk of bleeding via inhibition of platelet function and damage to the gastroduodenal mucosa. Careful monitoring of the effects of anticoagulants is thus essential if it proves impossible to avoid such combined prescription.
Lithium: NSAIDs increase blood lithium levels, which may then reach toxic values (decreased renal

excretion of lithium). This parameter therefore requires monitoring during the initiation, adjustment and withdrawal of treatment with meloxicam.
Methotrexate: NSAIDs may accentuate the haematologic toxicity of methotrexate. A case of agranulocytosis with meloxicam has been reported in a patient who was also taking methotrexate. The direct causality of meloxicam was not confirmed, but caution is required before prescribing such a combination. Strict monitoring of blood cell count is recommended in this situation.
Intrauterine contraceptive devices: NSAIDs appear to decrease the efficacy of intrauterine contraceptive devices.
*Combinations requiring precautions:* Diuretics: treatment with NSAIDs is associated with a risk of acute renal failure in dehydrated patients (decreased glomerular filtration via decreased renal prostaglandin synthesis). In case of combined prescription of meloxicam and a diuretic, it is essential to ensure that the patient is adequately hydrated and to monitor renal function at the start of treatment.
Nephrotoxicity of cyclosporin may be enhanced by NSAIDs via renal prostaglandin mediated effects. During combined treatment renal function is to be measured.
*Associations needing to be taken into consideration:* Antihypertensive drugs [beta–blockers, angiotensin converting enzyme (ACE) inhibitors, diuretics]: treatment with a NSAID may decrease their antihypertensive effect via inhibition of vasodilator prostaglandin synthesis.
Thrombolytics: increased risk of haemorrhage.
Concomitant administration of antacids, cimetidine, β-acetyl digoxin and frusemide has not given rise to any notable pharmacokinetic interactions with meloxicam. Cholestyramine accelerates the elimination of meloxicam via binding in the digestive tract.
Interactions with oral anti-diabetics cannot be excluded.

*Pregnancy and lactation:*
*Pregnancy:* In animals, lethal effects on the embryo have been reported at doses far higher than those used clinically.
It is advisable to avoid the administration of meloxicam during pregnancy.
During the final three months, all prostaglandin synthesis inhibitors may expose the foetus to cardiopulmonary (pulmonary hypertension with premature closure of the ductus arteriosus) and renal toxicity or inhibit the contraction of the uterus. This effect on the uterus has been associated with an increase in the incidence of dystocia and delayed parturition in animals. Thus all NSAIDs are absolutely contraindicated during the final three months.
*Lactation:* It is unknown whether meloxicam passes into mothers milk. Meloxicam should not be given to nursing mothers.

*Effects on ability to drive and use machines:* There are no specific studies about such effects. However, when adverse effects such as vertigo or drowsiness occur it is advisable to refrain from these activities.

*Undesirable effects:* Digestive system: dyspepsia, nausea, vomiting, abdominal pain, constipation, flatulence, diarrhoea. More rarely, ulcers or occult gastrointestinal bleeding may occur, taking sometimes the form of gastrointestinal blood loss.
Haematologic adverse events: disturbances of blood count, including differential white cell count: anaemia, leukopenia, thrombocytopenia have been described in patients taking meloxicam. Certain cases have been attributed to treatment. Concomitant administration of a potentially myelotoxic drug, in particular methotrexate, appears to be a predisposing factor to the onset of a cytopenia. In particular, a case of agranulocytosis has been described in a patient treated with meloxicam and also taking methotrexate.
Cutaneo-mucosal reactions: stomatitis, oesophagitis, pruritus, skin rash, urticaria, photosensitization have been reported.
Respiratory system: onset of an asthma attack has been reported in certain individuals allergic to aspirin or to other NSAIDs.
Central nervous system: possibility of lightheadedness, headache, vertigo, tinnitus, drowsiness.
Cardiovascular system: oedema, oedema of the lower limbs, palpitations, flushes may occur during treatment.
Genitourinary system: possibility of disturbances of laboratory tests investigating renal function (e.g. raised serum creatinine or urea).
Transitory disturbances of liver function tests (e.g. raised transaminases or bilirubin).

*Overdose:* Appropriate measures are required in case of overdose since there is no known antidote. Evidence was found in one clinical trial of acceleration of the elimination of meloxicam by cholestyramine. Severe gastrointestinal lesions may be treated with antacids and H2 receptor antagonists.

## Pharmacological properties

*Pharmacodynamic properties:* NON-STEROIDAL ANTI-INFLAMMATORY AGENT (M: locomotor system)

Meloxicam is a non-steroidal anti-inflammatory drug (NSAID) of the oxicam family, with anti-inflammatory, analgesic and antipyretic properties.

The anti-inflammatory activity of meloxicam has been proven in classical models of inflammation. As with other NSAIDs, its precise mechanism of action remains unknown. However there is at least one common mode of action shared by all NSAIDs (including meloxicam): inhibition of the biosynthesis of prostaglandins, known inflammation mediators.

*Pharmacokinetic properties:* The bioavailability of meloxicam following oral administration is on the average 89%.

With the doses of 7.5 and 15 mg, plasma concentrations are proportional to dose: 0.4 to 1.0 mg/litre for 7.5 mg and 0.8 to 2.0 mg/litre for 15 mg, on average ($C_{min}$ and $C_{max}$ at steady state).

Meloxicam is very strongly bound to plasma proteins, essentially albumin (99%).

Meloxicam is extensively metabolized, chiefly by oxidation of the methyl radical attached to the thiazolyl ring. Elimination in unchanged form accounts for 3% of the dose. Half of the substance is eliminated in urine and the other half in faeces.

The mean elimination half-life is of the order of 20 hours.

Steady state is reached in 5 days.

In terminal renal failure, the volume of distribution is increased and a daily dose of 7.5 mg must not be exceeded.

Plasma clearance is on average 8 ml/min. Clearance is decreased in the elderly. Volume of distribution is low, on average 11 litres. Interindividual variation is the order of 30-40%.

*Preclinical safety data:* The toxicological profile of meloxicam has been found in preclinical studies to be identical to that of NSAIDs: gastrointestinal ulcers and erosions, renal papillary necrosis at high doses during chronic administration in two animal species. Non toxic doses were 3 to 10 times higher than clinically used doses, according to animal species used.

Reproduction studies have reported lethal effects on the embryo at doses far higher than those used clinically. Fetotoxic effects at the end of gestation, shared by all prostaglandin synthesis inhibitors, have been described. No evidence has been found of any mutagenic effect, either in vitro or in vivo. No carcinogenic risk has been found in the rat and mouse at doses far higher than those used clinically.

## Pharmaceutical particulars

*List of excipients:* Sodium citrate dihydrate; lactose monohydrate; microcrystalline cellulose (AVICEL PH 102); polyvidone (KOLLIDON 25); anhydrous colloidal silica (AEROSIL 200); crospolyvidone (KOLLIDON CL); magnesium stearate.

*Incompatibilities:* None stated.

*Shelf life:* Five years when stored below 25°C for the packaging in blister cards. Five years for packaging in glass bottle and polypropylene tube.

*Special precautions for storage:* Should be stored away from dampness (in the case of blister cards).

*Nature and contents of container:* Glass bottle or polypropylene tube with polyethylene cap. PVC/PVDC-aluminium blister cards.

*Instructions for use/handling:* None stated.

**Marketing authorisation number** 14598/0002

**Date of approval/revision of SPC** November 1996

**Legal category** POM

# MOBIC* TABLETS 15 MG

**Qualitative and quantitative composition** Meloxicam 15 mg

**Pharmaceutical form** Tablet with breakline.

**Clinical particulars**

*Therapeutic indications:* Short-term symptomatic treatment of acute exacerbations of osteoarthrosis

Long-term symptomatic treatment of rheumatoid arthritis (chronic polyarthritis).

*Posology and method of administration:* Acute exacerbations of osteoarthrosis: 7.5 mg/day (half a tablet). If necessary, in the absence of improvement, the dose may be increased to 15 mg/day (one tablet).

Rheumatoid arthritis: 15 mg/day (one tablet).

In elderly patients with rheumatoid arthritis the recommended dose for long term treatment is 7.5 mg per day.

Patients with increased risks for adverse reactions should start treatment with 7.5 mg per day.
DO NOT EXCEED THE DOSE OF 15 mg/day.

The total daily amount should be taken as a single dose, with water or another liquid, during a meal.

In dialysis patients with severe renal failure the dose should not exceed 7.5 mg per day.

*Contra-indications:* Hypersensitivity to meloxicam or to one of the excipients. The possibility exists of crossover sensitivity with aspirin and other non-steroidal anti-inflammatory drugs (NSAIDs). MOBIC should not be given to patients who have developed signs of asthma, nasal polyps, angioneurotic oedema or urticaria following the administration of aspirin or NSAIDs.

Active peptic ulcer during the last six months or a history of recurrent peptic ulcer disease.

Severe hepatic failure.
-Non-dialyzed severe renal failure.
-Children aged under 15.
-Pregnancy (see Pregnancy and lactation).
-Lactation
-Gastrointestinal bleeding, cerebrovascular bleeding or other bleeding disorders.

*Special warnings and special precautions for use:*
*Warnings:* As with all NSAIDs, any history of oesophagitis, gastritis and/or peptic ulcer must be sought in order to ensure their total cure before starting treatment with meloxicam.

Attention should routinely be paid to the possible onset of a recurrence in patients treated with meloxicam and with a past history of this type.

As with all NSAIDs, long term administration has been associated with an increased risk or gastrointestinal side effects.

Treatment with meloxicam must be stopped in case of onset of peptic ulcer or of gastrointestinal bleeding.

Withdrawal of treatment with meloxicam must be envisaged in case of onset of cutaneo-mucosal adverse events. The possible occurrence of severe skin reactions and serious life threatening hypersensitivity reactions is known to occur with NSAIDs including oxicams.

In rare instances. NSAIDs may be the cause of interstitial nephritis, glomerulonephritis, renal medullary necrosis or nephrotic syndrome.

As with most NSAIDs, occasional increases in serum transaminase levels, increases in serum bilirubin or other liver function parameters as well as increases in serum creatinine and blood urea nitrogen as well as other laboratory disturbances have been reported. The majority of these instances involved transitory and slight abnormalities. Should any such abnormality prove significant or persistent, the administration of meloxicam should be stopped and appropriate investigations prescribed.

Induction of sodium, potassium and water retention and interference with the natriuretic effects of diuretics and consequently possible exacerbations of the condition of patients with cardiac insufficiency or hypertension may occur with NSAIDs.

*Precautions:* NSAIDs inhibit the synthesis of renal prostaglandins involved in the maintenance of renal perfusion in patients with decreased renal blood flow and blood volume. Administration of NSAIDs in such situations may result in the decompensation of latent renal failure. However renal function returns to its initial status when treatment is withdrawn. This risk concerns all elderly individuals, patients with congestive cardiac failure, cirrhosis of the liver, nephrotic syndrome or renal failure as well as patients on diuretics or having undergone major surgery leading to hypovolemia. Careful monitoring of urine output and renal function during treatment is necessary in such patients.

Adverse reactions are often less well tolerated in elderly, fragile or weakened individuals, who therefore require careful surveillance. As with other NSAIDs, particular caution is required in the elderly, in whom renal, hepatic and cardiac functions are frequently impaired.

The recommended maximum daily dose should not be exceeded in case of insufficient therapeutic effect nor should an additional NSAID be added to the therapy because this may increase the toxicity while therapeutic advantage has not been proven.

*Interactions with other medicaments and other forms of interaction:*
*Inadvisable combinations:* Other NSAIDs, including high doses of salicylates: administration of several NSAIDs together may increase the risk of ulcers and of gastrointestinal bleeding, via a synergistic effect.

Oral anticoagulants, heparin and ticlopidine: increased risk of bleeding via inhibition of platelet function and damage to the gastroduodenal mucosa. Careful monitoring of the effects of anticoagulants is thus essential if it proves impossible to avoid such combined prescription.

Lithium: NSAIDs increase blood lithium levels, which may then reach toxic values (decreased renal excretion of lithium). This parameter therefore requires monitoring during the initiation, adjustment and withdrawal of treatment with meloxicam.

Methotrexate: NSAIDs may accentuate the haematologic toxicity of methotrexate. A case of agranulocytosis with meloxicam has been reported in a patient who was also taking methotrexate. The direct causality of meloxicam was not confirmed, but caution is required before prescribing such a combination. Strict monitoring of blood cell count is recommended in this situation.

Intrauterine contraceptive devices: NSAIDs appear to decrease the efficacy of intrauterine contraceptive devices.

*Combinations requiring precautions:* Diuretics: treatment with NSAIDs is associated with a risk of acute renal failure in dehydrated patients (decreased glomerular filtration via decreased renal prostaglandin synthesis). In case of combined prescription of meloxicam and a diuretic, it is essential to ensure that the patient is adequately hydrated and to monitor renal function at the start of treatment.

Nephrotoxicity of cyclosporin may be enhanced by NSAIDs via renal prostaglandin mediated effects. During combined treatment renal function is to be measured.

*Associations needing to be taken into consideration:* Antihypertensive drugs [beta–blockers, angiotensin converting enzyme (ACE) inhibitors, diuretics]: treatment with a NSAID may decrease their antihypertensive effect via inhibition of vasodilator prostaglandin synthesis.

Thrombolytics: increased risk of haemorrhage.

Concomitant administration of antacids, cimetidine, β-acetyl digoxin and frusemide has not given rise to any notable pharmacokinetic interactions with meloxicam. Cholestyramine accelerates the elimination of meloxicam via binding in the digestive tract.

Interactions with oral anti-diabetics cannot be excluded.

*Pregnancy and lactation:*
*Pregnancy:* In animals, lethal effects on the embryo have been reported at doses far higher than those used clinically.

It is advisable to avoid the administration of meloxicam during pregnancy.

During the final three months, all prostaglandin synthesis inhibitors may expose the fetus to cardiopulmonary (pulmonary hypertension with premature closure of the ductus arteriosus) and renal toxicity or inhibit the contraction of the uterus. This effect on the uterus has been associated with an increase in the incidence of dystocia and delayed parturition in animals.

Thus all NSAIDs are absolutely contra-indicated during the final three months.

*Lactation:* It is unknown whether meloxicam passes into mothers milk. Meloxicam should not be given to nursing mothers.

*Effects on ability to drive and use machines:* There are no specific studies about such effects. However, when adverse effects such as vertigo or drowsiness occur it is advisable to refrain from these activities.

*Undesirable effects:* Digestive system: dyspepsia, nausea, vomiting, abdominal pain, constipation, flatulence, diarrhoea. More rarely, ulcers or occult gastrointestinal bleeding may occur, taking sometimes the form of gastrointestinal blood loss.

Haematologic adverse events: disturbances of blood count, including differential white cell count: anaemia, leukopenia, thrombocytopenia have been described in patients taking meloxicam. Certain cases have been attributed to treatment. Concomitant administration of a potentially myelotoxic drug, in particular methotrexate, appears to be a predisposing factor to the onset of a cytopenia. In particular, a case of agranulocytosis has been described in a patient treated with meloxicam and also taking methotrexate.

Cutaneo-mucosal reactions: stomatitis, oesophagitis, pruritus, skin rash, urticaria, photosensitization have been reported.

Respiratory system: onset of an asthma attack has been reported in certain individuals allergic to aspirin or to other NSAIDs.

Central nervous system: possibility of lightheadedness, headache, vertigo, tinnitus, drowsiness.

Cardiovascular system: oedema, oedema of the lower limbs, palpitations, flushes may occur during treatment.

Genitourinary system: possibility of disturbances of laboratory tests investigating renal function (e.g. raised serum creatinine or urea).

Transitory disturbances of liver function tests (e.g. raised transaminases or bilirubin).

*Overdose:* Appropriate measures are required in case of overdose since there is no known antidote. Evidence was found in one clinical trial of acceleration of the elimination of meloxicam by cholestyramine. Severe gastrointestinal lesions may be treated with antacids and H2 receptor antagonists.

## Pharmacological properties

*Pharmacodynamic properties:* NON-STEROIDAL ANTI-INFLAMMATORY AGENT (M: locomotor system)

Meloxicam is a non-steroidal anti-inflammatory drug (NSAID) of the oxicam family, with anti-inflammatory, analgesic and antipyretic properties.

The anti-inflammatory activity of meloxicam has been proven in classical models of inflammation. As with other NSAIDs, its precise mechanism of action remains unknown. However there is at least one common mode of action shared by all NSAIDs (including meloxicam): inhibition of the biosynthesis of prostaglandins, known inflammation mediators.

*Pharmacokinetic properties:* The bioavailability of meloxicam following oral administration is on the average 89%.

With the doses of 7.5 and 15 mg, plasma concentrations are proportional to dose:0.4 to 1.0 mg/litre for 7.5 mg and 0.8 to 2.0 mg/litre for 15 mg, on average ($C_{min}$ and $C_{max}$ at steady state).

Meloxicam is very strongly bound to plasma proteins, essentially albumin (99%).

Meloxicam is extensively metabolized, chiefly by oxidation of the methyl radical attached to the thiazolyl ring. Elimination in unchanged form accounts for 3% of the dose. Half of the substance is eliminated in urine and the other half in faeces.

The mean elimination half-life is of the order of 20 hours.

Steady state is reached in 5 days.

In terminal renal failure, the volume of distribution is increased and a daily dose of 7.5 mg must not be exceeded.

Plasma clearance is on average 8 ml/min. Clearance is decreased in the elderly. Volume of distribution is low, on average 11 litres. Interindividual variation is the order of 30-40%.

*Preclinical safety data:* The toxicological profile of meloxicam has been found in preclinical studies to be identical to that of NSAIDs: gastrointestinal ulcers and erosions, renal papillary necrosis at high doses during chronic administration in two animal species. Non toxic doses were 3 to 10 times higher than clinically used doses, according to animal species used.

Reproduction studies have reported lethal effects on the embryo at doses far higher than those used clinically. Fetotoxic effects at the end of gestation, shared by all prostaglandin synthesis inhibitors, have been described. No evidence has been found of any mutagenic effect, either in vitro or in vivo. No carcinogenic risk has been found in the rat and mouse at doses far higher than those used clinically.

## Pharmaceutical particulars

*List of excipients:* Sodium citrate dihydrate; lactose monohydrate; microcrystalline cellulose (AVICEL PH 102); polyvidone (KOLLIDON 25); anhydrous colloidal silica (AEROSIL 200); crospolyvidone (KOLLIDON CL); magnesium stearate.

*Incompatibilities:* None stated.

*Shelf life:* Five years when stored below 25°C for the packaging in blister cards. Five years for packaging in glass bottle and polypropylene tube.

*Special precautions for storage:* Should be stored away from dampness (in the case of blister cards).

*Nature and contents of container:* Glass bottle or polypropylene tube with polyethylene cap. PVC/PVDC-aluminium blister cards.

*Instructions for use/handling:* None stated.

**Marketing authorisation number** 14598/0003

**Date of approval/revision of SPC** November 1996

**Legal category** POM.

## MOBIC* SUPPOSITORIES 15 MG ▼

**Qualitative and quantitative composition** Meloxicam 15 mg

**Pharmaceutical form** Suppository.

### Clinical particulars

*Therapeutic indications:* Long-term symptomatic treatment of rheumatoid arthritis (chronic polyarthritis).

*Posology and method of administration:*
Rheumatoid arthritis : 15 mg/day (one suppository).

In elderly patients with rheumatoid arthritis the recommended dose for long term treatment is 7.5 mg per day.

Patients with increased risks for adverse reactions should start treatment with 7.5 mg per day. MOBIC suppositories are not suitable for the initiation of treatment.

DO NOT EXCEED THE DOSE OF 15 mg/day.

In dialysis patients with severe renal failure the dose should not exceed 7.5 mg per day.

*Contra-indications:* Hypersensitivity to meloxicam or to one of the excipients. The possibility exists of crossover sensitivity with aspirin and other non-steroidal anti-inflammatory drugs (NSAIDs). Meloxicam should not be given to patients who have developed signs of asthma, nasal polyps, angioneurotic oedema or urticaria following the administration of aspirin or NSAIDs.

Active peptic ulcer during the last six months or a history of recurrent peptic ulcer disease.

Severe hepatic failure.

Non-dialyzed severe renal failure.

Children aged under 15.

Past history of proctitis or of rectal bleeding.

Pregnancy (see Pregnancy and lactation).

Lactation.

Gastrointestinal bleeding, cerebrovascular bleeding or other bleeding disorders.

*Special warnings and special precautions for use:*
*Warnings:* As with all NSAIDs, any history of oesophagitis, gastritis and/or peptic ulcer must be sought in order to ensure their total cure before starting treatment with meloxicam.

Attention should routinely be paid to the possible onset of a recurrence in patients treated with meloxicam and with a past history of this type.

As with all NSAIDs, long term administration has been associated with an increased risk of gastrointestinal side effects.

Treatment with meloxicam must be stopped in case of onset of peptic ulcer or of gastrointestinal bleeding.

Withdrawal of treatment with meloxicam must be envisaged in case of onset of cutaneo-mucosal adverse events. The possible occurrence of severe skin reactions and serious life threatening hypersensitivity reactions is known to occur with NSAIDs including oxicams.

In rare instances NSAIDs may be the cause of interstitial nephritis, glomerulonephritis, renal medullary necrosis or nephrotic syndrome.

As with most NSAIDs, occasional increases in serum transaminase levels, increases in serum bilirubin or other liver function parameters as well as increases in serum creatinine and blood urea nitrogen as well as other laboratory disturbances have been reported. The majority of these instances involved transitory and slight abnormalities. Should any such abnormality prove significant or persistent, the administration of meloxicam should be stopped and appropriate investigations prescribed.

Induction of sodium, potassium and water retention and interference with the natriuretic effects of diuretics and consequently possible exacerbations of the condition of patients with cardiac insufficiency or hypertension may occur with NSAIDs.

*Precautions:* NSAIDs inhibit the synthesis of renal prostaglandins involved in the maintenance of renal perfusion in patients with decreased renal blood flow and blood volume. Administration of NSAIDs in such situations may result in the decompensation of latent renal failure. However renal function returns to its initial status when treatment is withdrawn. This risk concerns all elderly individuals, patients with congestive cardiac failure, cirrhosis of the liver, nephrotic syndrome or renal failure as well as patients on diuretics or having undergone major surgery leading to hypovolemia. Careful monitoring of urine output and renal function during treatment is necessary in such patients.

Adverse reactions are often less well tolerated in elderly, fragile or weakened individuals, who therefore require careful surveillance. As with other NSAIDs, particular caution is required in the elderly, in whom renal hepatic and cardiac functions are frequently impaired.

The recommended maximum daily dose should not be exceeded in case of insufficient therapeutic effect nor should an additional NSAID be added to the therapy because this may increase the toxicity while therapeutic advantage has not been proven.

*Interaction with other medicaments and other forms of interaction:*
*Inadvisable combinations:* Other NSAIDs, including high doses of salicylates: administration of several NSAIDs together may increase the risk of ulcers and of gastrointestinal bleeding, via a synergistic effect.

Oral anticoagulants, heparin and ticlopidine: increased risk of bleeding via inhibition of platelet function and damage to the gastroduodenal mucosa. Careful monitoring of the effects of anticoagulants is thus essential if it proves impossible to avoid such combined prescription.

Lithium: NSAIDs increase blood lithium levels, which may then reach toxic values (decreased renal excretion of lithium). This parameter therefore requires monitoring during the initiation, adjustment and withdrawal of treatment with meloxicam.

Methotrexate: NSAIDs may accentuate the haematologic toxicity of methotrexate. A case of agranulocytosis with meloxicam has been reported in a patient

who was also taking methotrexate. The direct causality of meloxicam was not confirmed, but caution is required before prescribing such a combination. Strict monitoring of blood cell count is recommended in this situation.

Intrauterine contraceptive devices: NSAIDs appear to decrease the efficacy of intrauterine contraceptive devices.

*Combinations requiring precautions:* Diuretics: treatment with NSAIDs is associated with a risk of acute renal failure in dehydrated patients (decreased glomerular filtration via decreased renal prostaglandin synthesis). In case of combined prescription of meloxicam and a diuretic, it is essential to ensure that the patient is adequately hydrated and to monitor renal function at the start of treatment.

Nephrotoxicity of cyclosporin may be enhanced by NSAIDs via renal prostaglandin mediated effects. During combined treatment renal function is to be measured.

*Associations needing to be taken into consideration:* Antihypertensive drugs [beta-blockers, angiotensin converting enzyme (ACE) inhibitors, diuretics]: treatment with a NSAID may decrease their antihypertensive effect via inhibition of vasodilator prostaglandin synthesis.

Thrombolytics: increased risk of haemorrhage.

Concomitant administration of antacids, cimetidine, β-acetyl digoxin and frusemide has not given rise to any notable pharmacokinetic interactions with meloxicam. Cholestyramine accelerates the elimination of meloxicam via binding in the digestive tract.

Interactions with oral anti-diabetics cannot be excluded.

*Pregnancy and lactation:*
*Pregnancy:* In animals, lethal effects on the embryo have been reported at doses far higher than those used clinically.

It is advisable to avoid the administration of meloxicam during pregnancy.

During the final three months, all prostaglandin synthesis inhibitors may expose the fetus to cardio-pulmonary (pulmonary hypertension with premature closure of the ductus arteriosus) and renal toxicity or inhibit the contraction of the uterus. This effect on the uterus has been associated with an increase in the incidence of dystocia and delayed parturition in animals.

Thus all NSAIDs are absolutely contra-indicated during the final three months.

*Lactation:* It is unknown whether meloxicam passes into mothers' milk. Meloxicam should not be given to nursing mothers.

*Effects on ability to drive and use machines:* There are no specific studies about such effects. However when adverse effects such as vertigo or drowsiness occur it is advisable to refrain from these activities.

*Undesirable effects:* Digestive system: dyspepsia, nausea, vomiting, abdominal pain, constipation, flatulence, diarrhoea: More rarely, ulcers or occult gastrointestinal bleeding may occur, taking sometimes the form of gastrointestinal blood loss.

Haematologic adverse events: disturbances of blood count, including differential white cell count: anaemia, leukopenia, thrombocytopenia have been described in patients taking meloxicam. Certain cases have been attributed to treatment. Concomitant administration of a potentially myelotoxic drug, in particular methotrexate, appears to be a predisposing factor to the onset of a cytopenia. In particular, a case of agranulocytosis has been described in a patient treated with meloxicam and also taking methotrexate.

Cutaneo-mucosal reactions: stomatitis, oesophagitis, pruritus, skin rash, urticaria, photosensitization have been reported.

Respiratory system: onset of an asthma attack has been reported in certain individuals allergic to aspirin or to other NSAIDs.

Central nervous system: possibility of lightheadedness, headache, vertigo, tinnitus, drowsiness.

Cardiovascular system: oedema, oedema of the lower limbs, palpitations, flushes may occur during treatment.

Genitourinary system: possibility of disturbances of laboratory tests investigating renal function (e.g. raised serum creatinine or urea).

Transitory disturbances of liver function tests (e.g. raised transaminases or bilirubin).

*Overdose:* Appropriate measures are required in case of overdose since there is no known antidote. Evidence was found in one clinical trial of acceleration of the elimination of meloxicam by cholestyramine. Severe gastrointestinal lesions may be treated with antacids and H2 receptor antagonists.

## Pharmacological properties

*Pharmacodynamic properties:* NON-STEROIDAL ANTI-INFLAMMATORY AGENT (M: locomotor system)

Meloxicam is a non-steroidal anti-inflammatory

drug (NSAID) of the oxicam family, with anti-inflammatory, analgesic and antipyretic properties.

The anti-inflammatory activity of meloxicam has been proven in classical models of inflammation. As with other NSAIDs, its precise mechanism of action remains unknown. However there is at least one common mode of action shared by all NSAIDs (including meloxicam): inhibition of the biosynthesis of prostaglandins, known inflammation mediators.

*Pharmacokinetic properties:* Pharmacokinetic studies have involved use of the oral formulation of meloxicam.

Meloxicam suppositories have been shown to be bioequivalent to oral formulations.

The bioavailability of meloxicam following oral administration is on the average 89%.

With the doses of 7.5 and 15 mg plasma concentrations are proportional to dose: 0.4 to 1.0 mg/litre for 7.5 mg and 0.8 to 2.0 mg/litre for 15 mg, on average ($C_{min}$ and $C_{max}$ at steady state).

Meloxicam is very strongly bound to plasma proteins, essentially albumin (99%).

Meloxicam is extensively metabolized, chiefly by oxidation of the methyl radical attached to the thiazolyl ring. Elimination in unchanged form accounts for 3% of the dose. Half of the substance is eliminated in urine and the other half in faeces.

The mean elimination half-life is of the order of 20 hours.

Steady state is reached in 5 days.

In terminal renal failure, the volume of distribution is increased and a daily dose of 7.5 mg must not be exceeded.

Plasma clearance is on average 8 ml/min. Clearance is decreased in the elderly. Volume of distribution is low, on average 11 litres. Interindividual variation is the order of 30-40%.

*Preclinical safety data:* The toxicological profile of meloxicam has been found in preclinical studies to be identical to that of NSAIDs: gastrointestinal ulcers and erosions, renal papillary necrosis at high doses during chronic administration in two animal species. Non toxic doses were 3 to 10 times higher than clinically used doses, according to animal species used.

Reproduction studies have reported lethal effects on the embryo at doses far higher than those used clinically. Fetotoxic effects at the end of gestation, shared by all prostaglandin synthesis inhibitors, have been described. No evidence has been found of any mutagenic effect, either in vitro or in vivo. No carcinogenic risk has been found in the rat and mouse at doses far higher than those used clinically.

**Pharmaceutical particulars**

*List of excipients:* Hard fat (SUPPOCIRE BP); polyoxyethylenated hydrogenated castor oil (CREMOPHOR RH 40)

*Incompatibilities:* None stated.

*Shelf life:* Three years

*Special precautions for storage:* Should be stored at a temperature of below 30°C.

*Nature and contents of container:* Cartons containing 12 suppositories packed in aluminum blister sheets.

*Instructions for use/handling:* None stated.

**Marketing authorisation number** 14598/0001

**Date of approval/revision of SPC** October 1996

**Legal category** POM

## MOTENS*

**Qualitative and quantitative composition** Tablets containing lacidipine 2 mg or 4 mg.

**Pharmaceutical form** Film coated tablets.

**Clinical particulars**

*Therapeutic indications:* Motens is indicated for the treatment of hypertension either alone or in combination with other antihypertensive agents, including β-adrenoceptor antagonists, diuretics, and ACE-inhibitors.

*Posology and method of administration:*

*Adults:* The treatment of hypertension should be adapted to the severity of the condition, and according to the individual response.

The recommended initial dose is 2 mg once daily. The dose may be increased to 4 mg (and then, if necessary, to 6 mg) after adequate time has been allowed for the full pharmacological effect to occur. In practice, this should not be less than 3 to 4 weeks. Daily doses above 6 mg have not been shown to be significantly more effective.

Motens should be taken at the same time each day, preferably in the morning.

Treatment with Motens may be continued indefinitely.

*Patients with kidney disease:* As Motens is not cleared by the kidneys, the dose does not require modification in patients with kidney disease.

*Use in children:* No experience has been gained with Motens in children.

*Contra-indications:* Motens tablets are contra-indicated in patients with known hypersensitivity to any ingredient of the preparation. Motens should only be used with great care in patients with a previous allergic reaction to another dihydropyridine because there is a theoretical risk of cross-reactivity.

In healthy volunteers, patients and pre-clinical studies Motens did not inhibit myocardial contractility. As with other calcium antagonists, Motens should be discontinued in patients who develop cardiogenic shock. In addition, dihydropyridines have been shown to reduce coronary arterial blood-flow in patients with aortic stenosis and in such patients Motens is contra-indicated.

Motens should not be used during or within one month of a myocardial infarction.

*Special warnings and precautions for use:* In specialised studies Motens has been shown neither to affect the spontaneous function of the sinoatrial (SA) node nor to cause prolonged conduction within the atrioventricular (AV) node. However, the theoretical potential for a calcium antagonist to affect the activity of the SA and AV nodes should be noted, and care should be taken in patients with pre-existing abnormalities.

There is no evidence that Motens is useful for secondary prevention of myocardial infarction.

Motens should be used with caution in patients with poor cardiac reserve.

The efficacy and safety of Motens in the treatment of malignant hypertension has not been established.

Caution should be exercised in patients with hepatic impairment because the antihypertensive effect may be increased.

There is no evidence that Motens impairs glucose tolerance or alters diabetic control.

*Interaction with other medicaments and other forms of interaction:* Concomitant administration of Motens with other antihypertensive agents e.g. diuretics, β-adrenoceptor antagonists or ACE-inhibitors may have an additive hypotensive effect.

The plasma concentration of Motens may be increased by simultaneous administration of cimetidine.

As with other dihydropyridines, Motens should not be taken with grapefruit juice as bioavailability may be altered.

Motens is highly protein-bound (>95%) to albumin and alpha$_1$-acid glycoprotein. No specific pharmacodynamic interaction problems have been identified in studies with common antihypertensive agents e.g. β-adrenoceptor antagonists and diuretics, or with digoxin, tolbutamide or warfarin.

*Pregnancy and lactation:* Although some dihydropyridine compounds have been found to be teratogenic in animals, data in the rat and rabbit for Motens provide no evidence of a teratogenic effect. Using doses far above the therapeutic range, in animals Motens shows evidence of maternal toxicity resulting in increased pre- and post-implantation losses and possibly delayed ossification. There is, however, no clinical experience of Motens in pregnancy and lactation. Accordingly, Motens should not be used during pregnancy or lactation.

*Effects on ability to drive and use machines:* None reported.

*Undesirable effects:* Motens is generally well tolerated. Some individuals may experience minor side effects which are related to its known pharmacological action of peripheral vasodilation. The most common of these are headache, flushing, oedema, dizziness and palpitations. Such effects are usually transient and usually disappear with continued administration of Motens at the same dosage.

Asthenia, skin rash (including erythema and itching), gastric upset, nausea, gingival hyperplasia, polyuria muscle cramps and disturbances of mood have also been reported rarely.

As with other dihydropyridines aggravation of underlying angina has been reported in a small number of individuals, especially after the start of treatment. This is more likely to happen in patients with symptomatic ischaemic heart disease. Motens should be discontinued under medical supervision in patients who develop unstable angina.

Transient and reversible increases in alkaline phosphatase have been noted on rare occasions.

*Overdose: Symptoms:* There have been no recorded cases of Motens overdosage. The expected symptoms could comprise prolonged peripheral vasodilation associated with hypotension and tachycardia. Bradycardia or prolonged AV conduction could occur.

*Therapy:* Symptomatic treatment is warranted. There is no specific antidote.

**Pharmacological properties**

*Pharmacodynamic properties:* Motens is a specific and potent calcium antagonist with a predominant selectivity for calcium channels in the vascular smooth muscle. Its main action is to dilate peripheral arterioles, reducing peripheral vascular resistance and lowering blood pressure.

In a study of ten patients with a renal transplant, Motens has been shown to prevent an acute decrease in renal plasma flow and glomerular filtration rate about six hours after administering oral cyclosporin. During the trough phase of cyclosporin treatment, there was no difference in renal plasma flow and glomerular filtration rate between patients with or without Motens.

*Pharmacokinetic properties:* Motens is a highly lipophilic compound; it is rapidly absorbed from the gastrointestinal tract following oral dosing. Absolute bioavailability averages about 10% due to extensive first-pass metabolism in the liver.

Peak plasma concentrations are reached between 30 and 150 minutes. The drug is eliminated primarily by hepatic metabolism. There is no evidence that Motens causes either induction or inhibition of hepatic enzymes.

The principal metabolites possess little, if any, pharmacodynamic activity.

Approximately 70% of the administered dose is eliminated as metabolites in the faeces and the remainder as metabolites in the urine.

The average terminal half-life of Motens ranges from between 13 and 19 hours at steady state.

*Preclinical safety data:* In acute toxicity studies, Motens has shown a wide safety margin.

In repeated dose toxicological studies, findings in animals, related to the safety profile of Motens in man, were reversible and reflected the pharmacodynamic effect of Motens.

No data of clinical relevance have been gained from *in vivo* and *in vitro* studies on reproduction toxicity, genetic toxicity or oncogenicity.

**Pharmaceutical particulars**

*List of excipients:* Lactose (monohydrate); lactose (spray-dried); povidone K30; magnesium stearate.

*Incompatibilities:* None known.

*Shelf life:* 24 months.

*Special precautions for storage:* Store below 30°C. Motens is light sensitive. Motens tablets should, therefore, be protected from light and should not be removed from their foil pack until required for administration. Keep out of the reach of children.

*Nature and contents of container:* Cartons containing 14 and 28 tablets packed in blister strips.

*Instructions for use/handling:* Do not remove from foil pack until required for administration.

**Marketing authorisation numbers**

| | |
|---|---|
| Motens 2 mg | 0015/0188 |
| Motens 4 mg | 0015/0189 |

**Date of approval/revision of SPC** March 1997

**Legal category** POM

## OXIVENT* INHALER

**Qualitative and quantitative composition** Each actuation delivers 100 micrograms of oxitropium bromide.

**Pharmaceutical form** Pressurised metered aerosol.

**Clinical particulars**

*Therapeutic indications:* For the management of airways obstruction in patients suffering from chronic stable asthma and chronic obstructive pulmonary disease.

*Posology and method of administration:* For administration by inhalation only.

*Adults :* Two puffs, two or three times daily.

*Children :* Oxivent has not been evaluated in children.

*Elderly patients :*There are no special dosage requirements for the elderly.

All patients should be instructed in the correct use of a metered dose inhaler.

*Contra-indications:* Oxivent Inhaler is contraindicated in patients with a history of hypersensitivity to soya lecithin or related food products such as soya beans or peanuts.

Oxivent Inhaler should not be taken by patients who have known hypersensitivity to atropine or its derivatives, or to any other component of the product.

*Special warnings and special precautions for use:* Symptoms of aerosol-induced bronchospasm including wheeze, cough and chest tightness, have been reported following the use of Oxivent If patients report respiratory symptoms associated with the use of the inhaler, treatment should be discontinued.

The patient should be warned to seek medical advice should a reduced response become apparent.

Oxivent should be prevented from coming into contact with the eye. Accidental release of Oxivent into the eye should be avoided, as there have been isolated reports of ocular complications (such as mydriasis, increased intraocular pressure, narrow-angle glaucoma and eye pain) following unintended exposure of the eye to anticholinergics. Patients therefore should be instructed in the correct administration of Oxivent Inhaler. Antiglaucoma therapy is also effective in the prevention of acute narrow-angle glaucoma in susceptible individuals.

As patients with cystic fibrosis may be prone to gastrointestinal motility disturbances, Oxivent as with other anticholinergics should be used with caution in these patients.

Caution is advocated in patients with narrow-angle glaucoma or those with prostatic hypertrophy.

*Interaction with other medicaments and other forms of interaction:* Oxivent has been administered in conjunction with sympathomimetic bronchodilators, xanthines, steroids and sodium cromoglycate with no evidence of adverse interaction. There is evidence that the administration of Oxivent with beta$_2$-agonist drugs and xanthine preparations may intensify the bronchodilator effect of Oxivent.

Oxivent has been shown to prevent and reverse propranolol-induced bronchoconstriction in patients with reversible airways obstruction.

*Pregnancy and lactation:* The safety of this product for use in human pregnancy has not been established. Animal studies have shown reproductive toxicity with high doses of Oxitropium. Oxivent should not therefore be used during pregnancy, particularly the first trimester, unless the expected benefit is thought to outweigh any risk to the foetus.

Animal studies have shown that oxitropium bromide can be secreted in mother's milk. It is unlikely that the drug would reach the infant to any great extent, but caution should be exercised by nursing mothers.

*Effects on ability to drive and use machines:* None known.

*Undesirable effects:* The most frequent non-respiratory adverse reactions reported in clinical trials were headache, nausea and dryness of the mouth.

Anticholinergic side effects such as tachycardia, palpitations, visual accommodation disturbances and urinary retention have been reported. The risk of urinary retention may be increased in patients with pre-existing urinary outflow obstruction.

Ocular side effects have been reported (see: *Special warnings and special precautions for use*).

As with other inhaled bronchodilator therapy, cough and paradoxical bronchoconstriction may occur. Cases of unpleasant taste have been reported. Local irritation of the oropharynx may occur.

*Overdose:* No symptoms specific to overdosage have been encountered. The poor absorption of Oxivent, and limited experience of the outcome of overdose with the product in clinical use, suggest that serious anticholinergic symptoms are unlikely. As seen with other anticholinergics, dry mouth, visual accommodation disturbances, tachycardia and urinary retention may occur.

**Pharmacological properties**

*Pharmacodynamic properties:* Oxitropium bromide is an anticholinergic bronchodilator that competitively antagonises the effects of acetylcholine at muscarinic receptors. When administered by inhalation, it produces only local effects on the lung due to its poor absorption through the lungs and gastrointestinal tract.

*Pharmacokinetic properties:* Studies in man have shown that, following oral administration (20 mg), peak plasma levels were not reached for 3 hours (36.5 ng/ml). At 96 hours, 12.6% was excreted by the kidneys and 77% in the faeces. The decline of the plasma level showed a biphasic course. Absorption after oral administration was calculated to be 16.2%. Following inhalation 10.4% was eliminated by the kidneys and 87.9% in the faeces. The absorption after inhalation was 15.4% of the dose.

**Pharmaceutical particulars**

*List of excipients:* Soya lecithin; monofluorotrichloromethane; difluorodichloromethane; tetrafluorodichloroethane.

*Incompatibilities:* None stated.

*Shelf life:* 3 years.

*Special precautions for storage:* Protect from heat, including the sun. The vials should not be punctured or incinerated even when apparently empty. Protect from frost.

*Nature and contents of container:* A one piece aluminium vial fitted with a 50 microlitre metering valve and containing 10 ml (200 doses) of a cream-coloured suspension, complete with mouth piece.

*Instructions for use/handling:*
To make sure that your inhaler is working, test fire it twice into the air before using it for the first time and whenever your inhaler has not been used for a week or more.

1. Remove the dustcap from the mouthpiece and shake the inhaler vigorously.
2. Holding the inhaler as shown, breathe out gently and then immediately. . ..
3. . . .place the mouthpiece in the mouth and close your lips around it. After starting to breathe in slowly and deeply, through your mouth, press the inhaler firmly as shown to release the Oxivent . Continue to breathe in as deeply as you can.
4. Hold your breath for 10 seconds, or as long as is comfortable, before breathing out slowly.
5. If you are to take more than one puff you should wait at least one minute before shaking the inhaler again and repeating steps 2,3 and 4.
6. After use, replace the dustcap on the mouthpiece.

**Marketing authorisation number** 00015/0142

**Date of approval/revision of SPC** August 1996

**Legal category** POM.

## OXIVENT* AUTOHALER*

**Qualitative and quantitative composition** Each actuation delivers 100 micrograms of oxitropium bromide.

**Pharmaceutical form** A breath-actuated pressurised metered aerosol for inhalation therapy.

**Clinical particulars**

*Therapeutic indications:* For the management of airways obstruction in patients suffering from chronic stable asthma and chronic obstructive pulmonary disease.

*Posology and method of administration:* For administration by inhalation only.

*Adults:* Two puffs, two or three times daily.

*Children:* Oxivent has not been evaluated in children.

*Elderly patients:* There are no special dosage requirements for the elderly.

All patients should be instructed in the correct use of the Autohaler device.

*Contra-indications:* Oxivent Autohaler is contraindicated in patients with a history of hypersensitivity to soya lecithin or related food products such as soya beans or peanuts.

Oxivent Autohaler should not be taken by patients who have known hypersensitivity to atropine or its derivatives, or to any other component of the product.

*Special warnings and special precautions for use:* Symptoms of aerosol-induced bronchospasm including wheeze, cough and chest tightness, have been reported following the use of Oxivent. If patients report respiratory symptoms associated with the use of the inhaler, treatment should be discontinued.

The patient should be warned to seek medical advice should a reduced response become apparent.

Oxivent should be prevented from coming into contact with the eye. It is unlikely that correct use of the Oxivent Autohaler would result in accidental release of Oxivent into the eye, however, there have been isolated reports of ocular complications (such as mydriasis, increased intraocular pressure, narrow-angle glaucoma and eye pain) following unintended exposure of the eye to anticholinergics. Patients therefore should be instructed in the correct administration of Oxivent Autohaler. Antiglaucoma therapy is also effective in the prevention of acute narrow-angle glaucoma in susceptible individuals.

As patients with cystic fibrosis may be prone to gastro-intestinal motility disturbances, Oxivent as with other anticholinergics should be used with caution in these patients.

Caution is advocated in patients with narrow-angle glaucoma or those with prostatic hypertrophy.

*Interaction with other medicaments and other forms of interaction:* Oxivent had been administered in conjunction with sympathomimetic bronchodilators, xanthines, steroids and sodium cromoglycate with no evidence of adverse interaction. There is evidence that the administration of Oxivent with beta$_2$-agonist drugs and xanthine preparations may intensify the bronchodilator effect of Oxivent.

Oxivent has been shown to prevent and reverse propranolol-induced bronchoconstriction in patients with reversible airways obstruction.

*Pregnancy and lactation:* The safety of this product for use in human pregnancy has not been established. Animal studies have shown reproductive toxicity with high doses of oxitropium.

Oxivent should not therefore be used during pregnancy, particularly the first trimester, unless the expected benefit is thought to outweigh any risk to the foetus.

Animal studies have shown that oxitropium bromide can be secreted in mother's milk. It is unlikely that the drug would reach the infant to any great extent, but caution should be exercised by nursing mothers.

*Effects on ability to drive and use machines:* None known.

*Undesirable effects:* The most frequent non-respiratory adverse reactions reported in clinical trials were headache, nausea and dryness of the mouth.

Anticholinergic side effects such as tachycardia, palpitations, visual accommodation disturbances and urinary retention have been reported. The risk of urinary retention may be increased in patients with pre-existing urinary outflow obstruction.

Ocular side effects have been reported (see: *Special warnings and special precautions for use*).

As with other inhaled bronchodilator therapy, cough and paradoxical bronchoconstriction may occur. Cases of unpleasant taste have been reported. Local irritation of the oropharynx may occur.

*Overdose:* No symptoms specific to overdosage have been encountered. The poor absorption of Oxivent, and limited experience of the outcome of overdose with the product in clinical use, suggest that serious anticholinergic symptoms are unlikely. As seen with other anticholinergics, dry mouth, visual accommodation disturbances, tachycardia and urinary retention may occur.

**Pharmacological properties**

*Pharmacodynamic properties:* Oxitropium bromide is an anticholinergic bronchodilator that competitively antagonises the effects of acetylcholine at muscarinic receptors. When administered by inhalation, it produces only local effects on the lung due to its poor absorption through the lungs and gastrointestinal tract.

*Pharmacokinetic properties:* Studies in man have shown that, following oral administration (20 mg), peak plasma levels were not reached for 3 hours (36.5 ng/ml). At 96 hours, 12.6% was excreted by the kidneys and 77% in the faeces. The decline of the plasma level showed a biphasic course. Absorption after oral administration was calculated to be 16.2%. Following inhalation 10.4% was eliminated by the kidneys and 87.9% in the faeces. The absorption after inhalation was 15.4% of the dose.

**Pharmaceutical particulars**

*List of excipients:* Soya lecithin; monofluorotrichloromethane; difluorodichloromethane; tetrafluorodichloroethane.

*Incompatibilities:* None stated.

*Shelf life:* 3 years.

*Special precautions for storage:* Protect from heat, including the sun. The vials should not be punctured or incinerated even when apparently empty. Protect from frost.

*Nature and contents of container:* A one piece aluminium vial fitted with a 50 mcl metering valve and containing 10 ml (200 doses) of a cream-coloured suspension, in a breath-actuated device.

*Instructions for use/handling:*

1. To remove the mouthpiece cover, pull down on the lip at the back.
2. Hold the Autohaler device upright as shown. Push the lever up so that it stays up.
3. With the lever still up, shake the Autohaler device.
4. Continue to hold the Autohaler device upright, making sure that your hand is not blocking the air vents at the bottom. Breathe out normally and close your lips firmly around the mouthpiece.
5. Breathe in through the mouthpiece. When you hear the slight click, continue to breathe in. This click lets you know you have received your puff of medication. Hold your breath for 10 seconds, or as long as is comfortable, and then breathe out normally.
6. The lever must be lowered after each puff. If your doctor has prescribed more than one puff, wait one minute before repeating steps 2–6. Replace the mouthpiece cover after use.

**Marketing authorisation number** 0015/0163

**Date of approval/revision of SPC** May 1997

**Legal category** POM

## PAVACOL-D*

**Qualitative and quantitative composition** Dark brown liquid containing 5 mg of Pholcodine BP in each 5 ml.

**Pharmaceutical form** Liquid for oral administration.

## Clinical particulars

*Therepeutic indications:* For the symptomatic treatment of dry troublesome coughs.

*Posology and method of administration:*

*Adults:* One or two 5 ml spoonfuls as required. The dose may be increased to three 5 ml spoonfuls if necessary. No more than 60 ml should be taken in 24 hours.

*Children:*

to 12 years: One 5 ml spoonful four or five times daily.

to 5 years: One 5 ml spoonful three times daily.

to 2 years: Half a 5 ml spoonful three or four times daily.

Pavacol-D may be diluted with Sorbitol Solution BPC.

*Elderly:* No specific information on the use of this product in the elderly is available. Clinical trials have included patients over 65 years and no adverse reactions specific to this age group have been reported.

*Contra-indications:* Hypersensitivity to any of the ingredients, or liver disease.

*Special warnings and special precautions for use:* Cough suppressants may cause sputum retention and this may be harmful in patients with chronic bronchitis and bronchiectasis. If symptoms persist longer than 5 days a physician should be consulted.

*Interaction with other medicaments and other forms of interaction:* Alcohol or other CNS depressants may lead to greater drowsiness and sedation.

*Pregnancy and lactation:* Although Pavacol-D has been in general use for many years, there is no evidence of ill-consequence during human pregnancy.

Medicines should not be used in pregnancy, especially the first trimester, unless the expected benefit is thought to outweigh any possible risk to the foetus.

*Effect on ability to drive and use machines:* Drowsiness occurs occasionally after taking pholcodine.

*Undesirable effects:* Nausea, sputum retention and constipation occur occasionally after taking pholcodine.

*Overdose:* Symptoms of overdosage include nausea, drowsiness, restlessness, excitement, ataxia and respiratory depression.

Treatment consists of emptying the stomach by aspiration and lavage. In case of severe poisoning the specific narcotic antagonist nalaxone may be used. Otherwise, treatment is supportive and symptomatic.

## Pharmacological properties

*Pharmacodynamic properties:* Pholcodine is a specific anti-tussive lacking the unwanted side-effects of opium and its derivatives. The specificity of action suggests that pholcodine acts via a distinct subset of opioid receptors.

*Pharmacokinetic properties:* In a study of male volunteers receiving 15, 30 and 60 mg doses of pholcodine at 7 day intervals, pharmacokinetics were found to be independent of dose. The elimination of pholcodine is described by a two-compartment model with an elimination half-life of 37±4.2 hours. Pholcodine undergoes little conjugation and is not transformed to morphine.

## Pharmaceutical particulars

*List of excipients:* Tolu balsam solution; special flavour; ethanol 96%; anise oil; clove oil; peppermint oil; capsicum tincture; strong ginger tincture; sorbitol solution; saccharin sodium; hydroxyethylcellulose; treacle flavour; caramel; L-menthol; methyl paraben; propyl paraben; deionised water.

*Incompatibilities:* None stated.

*Shelf life:* The shelf life expiry date for Pavacol-D is 3 years from the date of its manufacture.

When Pavacol-D is diluted an in-use shelf life of 14 days is recommended.

*Special precautions for storage:* Store below 25°C. Protect from light.

*Nature and contents of container:* 300 ml round amber glass bottle (Type III glass) with an aluminium roll-on pilfer proof cap.

*Instructions for use/handling:* None stated.

**Marketing authorisation number** 00015/0207

**Date of approval/revision of SPC** February 1996

**Legal category** P

## PERSANTIN*

**Presentation** Persantin Tablets 25 mg: orange sugar-coated tablets containing dipyridamole 25 mg.

Persantin Tablets 100 mg: white sugar-coated tablets containing dipyridamole 100 mg.

**Uses**

*Action:* Dipyridamole has an antithrombotic action based on its ability to modify various aspects of platelet function, such as platelet aggregation, adhesion and survival, which have been shown to be factors associated with the initiation of thrombus formation.

*Indications:* An adjunct to oral anticoagulation for prophylaxis of thromboembolism associated with prosthetic heart valves.

**Dosage and administration**

*Adults:* 300-600 mg daily in three or four doses.

*Children:* The normal total oral daily dose is 5 mg/kg in divided doses.

Persantin should usually be taken before meals.

**Contra-indications, warnings, etc**

*Contra-indications:* There are no absolute contra-indications to the administration of Persantin.

*Precautions:* Persantin is a potent vasodilator and should therefore be used with caution in patients with rapidly worsening angina, subvalvular aortic stenosis or haemodynamic instability associated with a recently sustained myocardial infarction.

There is inadequate evidence of safety in human pregnancy but Persantin has been used for many years without apparent ill-consequence. Animal studies have shown no hazards. Medicines should not be used in pregnancy, especially the first trimester, unless the expected benefit is thought to outweigh any possible risk to the foetus.

The concurrent administration of antacids may reduce the efficacy of Persantin.

It is possible that Persantin may enhance the effects of oral anticoagulants.

Persantin should be used with caution in patients with coagulation disorders.

*Side-effects:* If these occur it is usually during the early part of treatment and they are often dose-related. The vasodilating properties of Persantin may occasionally produce a vascular headache which normally disappears with dosage reduction. Dizziness, faintness, dyspepsia, mild diarrhoea and rash have also been reported occasionally.

*Overdosage:* Overdosage may lead to headache, gastro-intestinal symptoms and hypotension. Coronary vasodilatation may cause chest pain in patients with ischaemic heart disease. General supportive measures should be employed. Coronary vasodilatation may be reversed by administering aminophylline by slow IV injection, whilst monitoring the ECG.

**Pharmaceutical precautions** Protect from heat, light and moisture.

**Legal category** POM.

**Package quantities** Blister packs of 84 (OP)

**Further information** There is evidence that the effects of aspirin and dipyridamole on platelet behaviour are synergistic.

**Product licence numbers**

Persantin Tablets 25 mg　0015/0052R

Persantin Tablets 100 mg　0015/5016R

## PERSANTIN*AMPOULES

**Presentation** Amber glass ampoules containing a yellow solution for intravenous injection. Each ampoule contains dipyridamole 10 mg in 2 ml.

**Uses**

*Action :* Dipyridamole is a powerful coronary vasodilator and produces a marked increase in coronary blood flow.

*Indications:* As an alternative to exercise stress in thallium-201 myocardial imaging, particularly in patients unable to exercise or in those for whom exercise may be contra-indicated.

**Dosage and administration** 0.56 mg/kg injected intravenously over 4 minutes. The injection of thallium-201 should be given from 1-2 minutes after completion of the dipyridamole injection.

The half-life of an intravenous bolus injection of dipyridamole is approximately 30 minutes and therefore repeat imaging to assess redistribution can be performed after 240 minutes.

**Contra-indications, warnings, etc**

*Contra-indications:* Patients with a known hypersensitivity to dipyridamole.

Subvalvular aortic stenosis, aortic disease, hypotension associated with a recently sustained myocardial infarction, significant valvular disease, or uncompensated congestive heart failure. Patients with known cardiac conduction defects or dysrhythmias.

*Precautions:* The product should be administered with care in unstable angina.

As with exercise-induced stress, the use of Persantin ampoules as an adjunct to thallium imaging may occasionally precipitate cardiac arrhythmia in patients with severe heart disease. Dipyridamole-thallium scanning should be performed with continual monitoring of the patient's ECG.

Concurrent administration of a vasodilator may cause a severe hypotensive effect.

There is inadequate evidence of safety in human pregnancy, but dipyridamole has been used for many years without apparent ill-consequence.

*Side-effects:* Some patients may experience chest pain or a worsening of their angina symptoms. These may be reversed, if necessary, with intravenous aminophylline.

Transient headache, dizziness, faintness, facial flushing and nausea are common side effects. A bitter taste has sometimes been experienced after intravenous injection.

**Pharmaceutical precautions** Protect from heat, light and moisture.

**Legal category** POM.

**Package quantities** Ampoules: Packs of 5.

**Further information** Persantin is also available as tablets (100 mg and 25 mg) for use as an adjunct to oral anticoagulation for prophylaxis of thromboembolism associated with prosthetic heart valves.

**Product licence number** 0015/0119.

## PERSANTIN* RETARD 200 mg

**Qualitative and quantitative composition** Each modified release capsule contains dipyridamole 200 mg.

**Pharmaceutical form** Modified release capsule.

**Clinical particulars**

*Therepeutic indications:* Secondary prevention of ischaemic stroke and transient ischaemic attacks either alone or in conjunction with aspirin.

An adjunct to oral anti-coagulation for prophylaxis of thromboembolism associated with prosthetic heart valves.

*Posology and method of administration:* For oral administration.

*Adults, including the elderly:* The recommended dose is one capsule twice daily, usually one in the morning and one in the evening preferably with meals.

The capsules should be swallowed whole without chewing.

*Children:* Persantin Retard 200 mg is not recommended for children.

*Contra-indications:* Hypersensitivity to any component of the product.

*Special warnings and special precautions for use:* Among other properties dipyridamole acts as a potent vasodilator. It should therefore be used in caution in patients with severe coronary artery disease (e.g. unstable angina or recently sustained myocardial infarction), subvalvular aortic stenosis or haemodynamic instability (e.g. decompensated heart failure).

In patients with myasthenia gravis readjustment of therapy may be necessary after changes in dipyridamole dosage (see *Interactions*).

Persantin should be used in caution in patients with coagulation disorders.

*Interaction with other medicaments and other forms of interaction:* Dipyridamole increases the plasma levels and cardiovascular effects of adenosine. Adjustment of adenosine dosage should therefore be considered if use with dipyridamole is unavoidable.

There is evidence that the effects of aspirin and dipyridamole on platelet behaviour are additive.

When dipyridamole is used in combination with anticoagulants and aspirin, the statements on intolerance and risks for these preparations must be observed. Addition of dipyridamole to aspirin does not increase the incidence of bleeding events. When dipyridamole was administered concomitantly with warfarin, bleeding was no greater in frequency or severity than that observed when warfarin was administered alone.

Dipyridamole may increase the hypotensive effect of blood pressure lowering drugs and may counteract the anticholinesterase effect of cholinesterase inhibitors thereby potentially aggravating myasthenia gravis.

*Pregnancy and lactation:* There is inadequate evidence of safety in human pregnancy, but dipyridamole has been used for many years without apparent ill-consequence. Animal studies have shown no hazard. Nevertheless, medicines should not be used in pregnancy, especially the first trimester unless the expected benefit is thought to outweigh the possible risk to the foetus.

Persantin Retard 200 mg should only be used during lactation if considered essential by the physician.

*Effects on ability to drive and use machines:* None stated.

*Undesirable effects:* Adverse reactions at therapeutic doses are usually mild. Vomiting, diarrhoea and symptoms such as dizziness, nausea, dyspepsia, headache and myalgia have been observed. These tend to occur early after initiating treatment and may disappear with continued treatment. As side effects may be dose related dose reduction may need to be considered.

As a result of its vasodilating properties, Persantin Retard 200 mg may cause hypotension, hot flushes and tachycardia. In rare cases, worsening of the symptoms of coronary heart disease has been observed.

Hypersensitivity reactions such as rash and urticaria have been reported. In very rare cases, increased bleeding during or after surgery has been observed.

*Overdose:* Due to the low number of observations, experience with dipyridamole overdose is limited. Symptoms such as feeling warm, flushes, sweating, accelerated pulse, restlessness, feeling of weakness, dizziness, drop in blood pressure and anginal complaints can be expected.

Symptomatic therapy is recommended. Administration of xanthine derivatives (e.g. aminophylline) may reverse the haemodynamic effects of dipyridamole overdose. ECG monitoring is advised in such a situation. Due to its wide distribution to tissues and its predominantly hepatic elimination, dipyridamole is not likely to be accessible to enhanced removal procedures.

### Pharmacological properties

*Pharmacodynamic properties:* The antithrombotic action of dipyridamole is based on its ability to modify various aspects of platelet function such as inhibition of platelet adhesion and aggregation, which have been shown to be factors associated with the initiation of thrombus formation, as well as lengthening shortened platelet survival time.

*Pharmacokinetic properties:* Persantin Retard 200 mg given twice daily has been shown to be bioequivalent to the same total daily dose of Persantin Tablets given in four dividend doses.

Peak plasma concentrations are reached 2–3 hours after administration. Steady state conditions are reached within 3 days.

Metabolism of dipyridamole occurs in the liver predominantly by conjugation with glururonic acid to form a monoglucuronide. In plasma about 70–80% of the total amount is present as parent compound and 20–30% as the monoglucuronide.

Renal excretion is very low (1–5%).

*Preclinical safety data:* Dipyridamole has been extensively investigated in animal models and no clinically significant findings have been observed at doses equivalent to therapeutic doses in humans.

### Pharmaceutical particulars

*List of excipients:* Tartaric acid; povidone; Eudragit S 100; talc; acacia; methylhydroxypropylcellulose phthalate; methylhydroxypropylcellulose; triacetin; dimethicone 300; stearic acid; and in the capsule shells – gelatin; erythrosine (E127); titanium dioxide (E171); red and yellow iron oxides (E172).

*Incompatibilities:* None stated.

*Shelf life:* 3 years.

*Special precautions for storage:* Store below 25°C. Discard any capsules remaining 6 weeks after first opening.

*Nature and contents of container:* White polypropylene tubes with low-density polyethylene Air-sec stoppers filled with dessicating agent (90% white silicon gel/10% molecular sieves).

Packs contain 30, 60 or 100 capsules. Packs of 60 are marketed.

*Instructions for use/handling:* None stated.

**Marketing authorisation number** 0015/0206

**Date of approval/revision of SPC** April 1997

**Legal category** POM

## RINATEC* NASAL SPRAY 0.03%

**Qualitative and quantitative composition** Rinatec Nasal Spray 0.03% is an aqueous formulation (adjusted to pH 4.0–5.0) available as a 15 ml (180 metered doses) and 30 ml (380 metered doses) pump spray. Each valve actuation delivers 70 mcl of solution containing 21 micrograms of ipratropium bromide.

**Pharmaceutical form** Aqueous nasal spray.

**Clinical particulars**

*Therepeutic indications:* Rinatec Nasal Spray 0.03% is indicated for the symptomatic relief of rhinorrhoea in allergic and non-allergic rhinitis.

*Posology and method of administration:*
*Adults:* Two sprays (42 mcg) in each nostril administered 2–3 times a day.

*Children:* The use of Rinatec Nasal Spray 0.03% has not been evaluated in children, and therefore is not recommended for use in patients below the age of 12 years.

*Contra-indications:* Rinatec Nasal Spray 0.03% is contraindicated in patients known to be hypersensitive to atropine-like substances or inactive ingredients of the product.

*Special warnings and special precautions for use:* There have been isolated reports of ocular complications (i.e. mydriasis, increased intraocular pressure, angle-closure glaucoma, eye pain) when nebulised ipratropium bromide either alone or in combination with an adrenergic beta$_2$-agonist, was sprayed into the eyes.

Thus patients must be instructed in the correct administration of Rinatec Nasal Spray 0.03%. Eye pain or discomfort, blurred vision, visual halos or coloured images in association with red eyes from conjunctival and corneal congestion may be signs of acute angle-closure glaucoma. Should any combination of these symptoms develop, treatment with miotic drops should be initiated and specialist advice sought immediately.

*Interaction with other medicaments and other forms of interaction:* The concomitant use of Rinatec Nasal Spray 0.03% with other drugs commonly prescribed for perennial rhinitis i.e. antihistamines, decongestants or nasal steroids does not increase the incidence of nasal or non-nasal side effects.

Anticholinergic adverse events with chronic use of Rinatec Nasal Spray 0.03% are rare, limited to local adverse events of dryness of nose and mouth and are not increased by concomitant use of drugs with anticholinergic properties.

*Pregnancy and lactation:* No adequate or well controlled studies have been conducted in pregnant women. Oral reproduction studies performed in mice, rats and rabbits [at doses approximately 2,000, 200,000 and 25,000 times the maximum recommended human daily dose of Rinatec Nasal Spray 0.03% in perennial rhinitis (252 mcg/day), respectively] and inhalation reproduction studies in rats and rabbits (at doses approximately 305 and 357 times the maximum recommended human daily dose, respectively) have demonstrated no evidence of teratogenic effects as a result of administration of ipratropium bromide. Fertility of male or female rats at oral doses up to approximately 10,000 times the maximum recommended human daily dose was unaffected by ipratropium bromide administration. At doses above 18,000 times the maximum recommended human daily dose, increased resorption and decreased conception rates were observed. Because animal studies are not always predictive of human response, Rinatec Nasal Spray 0.03% should be used during pregnancy only if the potential benefit outweighs the potential risk.

It is not known whether ipratropium bromide is excreted in human milk. Although, lipid-insoluble quaternary bases pass into breast milk, it is unlikely that ipratropium bromide would reach the infant to an important extent, especially when taken intranasally. However, because many drugs are excreted in human milk, caution should be exercised when Rinatec Nasal Spray 0.03% is administered to a nursing woman.

*Effects on ability to drive and use machines:* None known, however see *Overdose*.

*Undesirable effects:* Local reactions can cause nasal drying in 10% of patients and epistaxis in 6% of patients. These effects may necessitate reduced frequency of administration.

Blurring of vision, precipitation or worsening of narrow angle glaucoma or eye pain may result if Rinatec Nasal Spray 0.03% comes into direct contact with the eyes. Patients should read and follow the patient's *Instructions for use* carefully.

*Overdose:* Acute overdosage by intranasal administration is unlikely since ipratropium bromide is not well absorbed systemically after intranasal or oral administration. The oral LD$_{50}$ of ipratropium bromide ranged between 1001 and 2010 mg/kg in mice; between 1667 and more than 4000 mg/kg in rats; and between 400 and 1300 mg/kg in dogs.

**Pharmacological properties**

*Pharmacodynamic properties:* Ipratropium bromide is an anticholinergic drug. As such it directly reduces mucous secretions from the nasal serous and seromucous glands especially in cases where secretion is raised.

*Pharmacokinetic properties:* The active ingredient is adsorbed to the local muscarinic receptor very quickly after both nasal and oral inhalation. Following intranasal administration of an ipratropium bromide solution, plasma ipratropium concentration above 0.1 mgm/ml are not observed. The systemic bioavailability following intranasal administration or after inhalation is estimated to be less than 10.

The basic pharmacokinetic parameters were calculated from the plasma level data after i.v. administration. The active ingredient was eliminated from the plasma with a terminal half-life of 1.6 h. The half-life of the active ingredient and the metabolites was 3.6 h. The three metabolites whose structure has been determined bind poorly to the muscarinic receptor. The total clearance of the active ingredient is 2300 ml/min. Approx. 40% of clearance is renal (872 ml/min) and 60% non-renal i.e. mainly hepato-metabolic. The volume of distribution in the steady state (Vss) is 176 l (corresponding to approx. 2.4 l/kg) and the volume of distribution in the terminal phase (Vz) is 338 l (approx. 4.6 l/kg).

Renal excretion of the active ingredient is given as 46.3% of the dose after intravenous administration, 3.1% of the dose after inhalation, and 3.7% of the dose after intranasal administration.

The plasma protein binding is minimal (0–9%). It was not observed that the blood brain barrier was penetrated consistent with the quaternary amino structure of the molecule.

*Preclinical safety data:* The toxicity of ipratropium bromide has been investigated extensively in the following types of studies: acute, subchronic and chronic toxicity, carcinogenicity, reproductive toxicity and mutagenicity via oral, intravenous, subcutaneous, intranasal and/or inhalation routes. Based on these toxicity studies, the probability of systemic anticholinergic side effects decreases in the following order: intravenous > subcutaneous > oral > inhalation > intranasal.

Pre-clinically, ipratropium bromide was found to be well-tolerated. Two-year carcinogenicity studies in rats and mice have revealed no carcinogenic activity at doses up to approximately 1.200 times the maximum recommended human daily dose for Rinatec Nasal Spray 0.03%. Results of various mutagenicity tests were negative.

**Pharmaceutical particulars**

*List of excipients:* Sodium chloride; benzalkonium chloride; disodium edetate dihydrate; purified water. Hydrochloric acid and sodium hydroxide are used for pH adjustment.

*Incompatibilities:* None known.

*Shelf life:* 2 years.

*Special precautions for storage:* Store between 15°C and 30°C. Avoid excessive heat or freezing.

*Nature and contents of container:* Rinatec Nasal Spray 0.03% is a clear colourless aqueous solution adjusted to the optimum pH 4.0–5.0. The solution is filled into either 15 ml or 30 ml amber glass bottles (Type I glass) fitted with 70 mcl manually activated nasal pump/closures.

*Instructions for use/handling:* To obtain the best results from your nasal spray follow the simple instructions given below. If you are unclear about how to use the nasal spray ask your doctor or pharmacist to explain.

1. Remove the dust cap and safety clip.
2. The nasal spray pump must be primed before Rinatec Nasal Spray is used for the first time. To prime the pump, hold the bottle with your thumb at the base and your index and middle fingers on the white shoulder area. Make sure the bottle points upright and away from your eyes. Press your thumb firmly and quickly against the bottle seven times. The pump is now primed and can be used. Your pump will hold its prime for up to 24 hours. If you have not used your pump for more than 24 hours you will need to prime it again before use. Reprime the pump as before, but this time only two sprays are required. If you have not used your pump for more than 7 days reprime using 7 sprays.
3. Blow your nose to clear your nostrils if necessary.
4. Close one nostril by gently placing your finger against the side of your nose. Tilt your head slightly forward and, keeping the bottle upright, insert the nasal tip into the other nostril. Point the tip toward the back and outer side of the nose.

Press firmly and quickly upwards with the thumb at the base while holding the white shoulder portion of the pump between your index and middle fingers. Following each spray, sniff deeply and breathe out through your mouth.

After spraying the nostril and removing the unit, tilt your head backwards for a few seconds to let the spray spread over the back of the nose.

5. Repeat step 4 in the other nostril.
6. Replace the cap and safety clip.

Avoid spraying Rinatec Nasal Spray in or around your eye. Should this occur, immediately flush your eye with cold tap water for several minutes. If you accidentally spray Rinatec Nasal Spray in your eyes, you may experience a temporary blurring of vision and increased sensitivity to light, which may last a few hours. Follow your doctor's instructions about when and how to take your medicine and always read the label.

If the nasal tip becomes clogged, remove the clear plastic dust cap and safety clip. Hold the nasal tip under running warm tap water for about a minute. Dry the nasal tip, reprime the nasal spray pump and replace the plastic dust cap and safety clip.

**Marketing authorisation number**   0015/0196

**Date of approval/revision of SPC**   March 1997

**Legal category**   POM

## TRANXENE*

**Presentation   Presentation** Tranxene Capsules 15 mg: Pink/grey hard gelatin capsules imprinted with the notation 15 mg and the Company symbol. Each capsule contains dipotassium clorazepate 15 mg.

Tranxene Capsules 7.5 mg: Maroon/grey hard gelatin capsules imprinted with the product name, 7.5 mg and the Company symbol. Each capsule contains dipotassium clorazepate 7.5 mg.

**Uses**   *Action:* Tranxene is a tranquilliser exhibiting many characteristics of the benzodiazepine group of preparations. Particular features which distinguish Tranxene from other members of this group are the rapid appearance in the blood of the anxiolytic compound nordiazepam, the maintenance of satisfactory therapeutic effect in most patients with once daily administration, and little sedation.

*Indications:* For the short-term relief (2–4 weeks) only of anxiety that is severe, disabling or subjecting the individual to unacceptable distress, occurring alone or in association with insomnia or short-term psychosomatic, organic or psychotic illness.

The use of benzodiazepines to treat short-term 'mild' anxiety is considered to be inappropriate and unsuitable.

**Dosage and administration**   Adults only, not generally recommended for children under 16 years. Tranxene 15 mg: one capsule daily, usually administered at night. Tranxene 7.5 mg: one capsule up to three times daily.

Half the normal dose may be sufficient for a therapeutic response in the elderly.

The lowest dose which can control symptoms should be used. It should not be continued beyond 4 weeks.

Long-term chronic use is not recommended.

Treatment should always be tapered off gradually. Patients who have taken benzodiazepines for a long time may require a longer period during which doses are reduced.

**Contra-indications, warnings, etc**

*Contra-indications:* Known hypersensitivity to benzodiazepines; acute pulmonary insufficiency.

*Precautions:* Tranxene is not recommended for acute primary depressive states, chronic major psychoses, phobic or obsessional states. It should not be used alone for the treatment of depression or anxiety associated with depression. The action of Tranxene may potentiate other preparations with central nervous system depressant effects such as barbiturates, narcotics, phenothiazines and alcohol.

Although sedation has not proved to be a problem with Tranxene, in accordance with general principles patients should be advised that their ability to drive or to operate dangerous machinery may be impaired.

Amnesia may occur. In cases of loss or bereavement psychological adjustment may be inhibited by benzodiazepines.

There is no evidence as to drug safety in human pregnancy nor is there evidence from animal work that it is free from hazard. Do not use during pregnancy, especially during the first and last trimesters, unless there are compelling reasons.

Tranxene and its metabolites are excreted in human milk in minimal quantities and therefore use during lactation should be avoided if possible. In labour, high single doses or low repeated doses of benzodiazepines have been reported to produce irregularities of the foetal heart and hypotonia, and poor suckling and hypothermia in the neonate. Caution should be exercised in patients suffering from chronic pulmonary insufficiency, or chronic renal or hepatic disease.

*Side-effects:* Side-effects, which have been reported only rarely, include dizziness, gastro-intestinal upset, nervousness, blurred vision, dry mouth, headache, skin rashes and jaundice. Drowsiness has occasionally been reported but does not constitute a major problem.

Hypotension, urinary retention, changes in libido and blood dyscrasias have also been reported for benzodiazepines in general.

Abnormal psychological reactions to benzodiazepines have been reported. Disinhibiting effects may be manifested in various ways. Suicide may be precipitated in patients who are depressed and aggressive behaviour towards self and others may be precipitated. Extreme caution should therefore be used in prescribing benzodiazepines in patients with personality disorders.

Withdrawal from benzodiazepines may be associated with physiological and psychological symptoms including depression, nervousness, rebound insomnia, irritability, sweating and diarrhoea. Withdrawal symptoms occur with benzodiazepines following normal therapeutic doses given for short periods of time, but particularly on sudden discontinuation of the benzodiazepine, in patients with a history of drug abuse or alcoholism or in patients with marked personality disorders. In such patients treatment should be monitored closely and routine prescriptions avoided, with gradual drug withdrawal when appropriate.

*Overdosage:* An overdose of 900 mg has been reported, causing drowsiness, ataxia, respiratory depression and coma. If vomiting has not occurred spontaneously, it should be induced. Gastric lavage is recommended. General supportive therapy is indicated and specific measures to counteract central nervous system depressant effects may be necessary. Prolonged administration of doses as high as 120 mg daily has not given rise to organ toxicity. Abrupt withdrawal of excessive doses of benzodiazepines has been reported as occasionally producing confusion, toxic psychosis, convulsion or a condition resembling delirium tremens.

**Pharmaceutical precautions**   Tranxene capsules should be protected from heat, light and moisture.

**Legal category**   POM.

**Package quantities**   Blister packs of 20 and 100.

**Further information**   In common with other benzodiazepines, Tranxene has a central muscle-relaxant effect, and synergism with peripherally acting muscle relaxants is a theoretical possibility.

**Product licence numbers**
Tranxene capsules 15 mg     0015/0057R
Tranxene capsules 7.5 mg    0015/0045R

*\*Trade Mark*

# Boehringer Ingelheim Limited–Hospital Division
## Ellesfield Avenue
## Bracknell
## Berkshire RG12 8YS

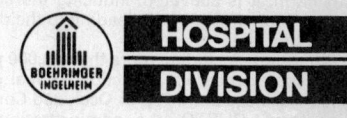

## ACTILYSE*

### Qualitative and quantitative composition
*10 mg/vial:* Actilyse 10 mg contains 10 mg (equivalent to 5.8 million International Units) alteplase (recombinant human tissue-type plasminogen activator) per vial.

*20 mg/vial:* Actilyse 20 mg contains 20 mg (equivalent to 11.6 million International Units) alteplase (recombinant human tissue-type plasminogen activator) per vial.

*50 mg/vial:* Actilyse 50 mg contains 50 mg (equivalent to 29 million International Units) alteplase (recombinant human tissue-type plasminogen activator) per vial.

The specific activity of alteplase in-house reference material is 580,000 International Units/mg. This has been confirmed by comparison with the second international WHO Standard for t-PA. The specification for the specific activity of alteplase batches is 522.000 to 696.000 International Units/mg.

Following reconstitution with the appropriate volume of Water for Injections, the pH of the resulting solution is 7.3±0.5.

**Pharmaceutical form** Vial with freeze–dried product, to be reconstituted with Water for Injection (PhEur), for intravenous administration.

### Clinical particulars
*Therapeutic indications:* Thrombolytic treatment in acute myocardial infarction
- 90 minutes (accelerated) dose regimen (see posology and method of administration): for patients in whom treatment can be started within 6 hours after symptom onset
- 3 hour dose regimen (see posology and method of administration): for patients in whom treatment can be started between 6-12 hours after symptom onset
- provided that the above-mentioned indication is clear
Actilyse has proven to reduce 30-day-mortality in patients with acute myocardial infarction.

Thrombolytic treatment in acute massive pulmonary embolism with haemodynamic instability. The diagnosis should be confirmed whenever possible by objective means such as pulmonary angiography or non-invasive procedures such as lung scanning.

There is no evidence for positive effects on mortality and late morbidity related to pulmonary embolism.

*Posology and method of administration:* Actilyse should be given as soon as possible after symptom onset.

Under aseptic conditions the contents of an injection vial of Actilyse (10 or 20 or 50 mg) dry substance is dissolved with water for injection (10 or 20 or 50 ml depending on the size of the rt–PA vial) to a concentration of 1 mg Actilyse/ml and is then administered intravenously. The reconstituted solution may be diluted further with sterile physiological saline solution (0.9 %) up to a minimal concentration of 0.2 mg/ml.

1) Myocardial infarction
a) 90 minutes (accelerated) dose regimen for patients with myocardial infarction, in whom treatment can be started within 6 hours after symptom onset:
15 mg as an intravenous bolus,
50 mg as an infusion over the first 30 minutes,
followed by an infusion of 35 mg over 60 minutes, up to the maximum dose of 100 mg.
In patients with a body weight below 65 kg the dose should be weight adjusted with 15 mg as an intravenous bolus, and 0.75 mg/kg body weight over 30 minutes (maximum 50 mg), followed by an infusion of 0.5 mg/kg over 60 minutes (maximum 35 mg).
b) 3 hour dose regimen for patients, in whom treatment can be started between 6 and 12 hours after symptom onset:
10 mg as an intravenous bolus,
50 mg as an intravenous infusion over the first hour,
followed by infusions of 10 mg over 30 minutes, up to the maximum dose of 100 mg over 3 hours.
In patients with a body weight below 65 kg the total dose should not exceed 1.5 mg/kg.
The maximum acceptable dose of Actilyse is 100 mg.
*Adjunctive therapy:* Aspirin should be initiated as

soon as possible after symptom onset and continued for several months after myocardial infarction. The recommended dose is 160 - 300 mg/day.

Heparin should be administered concomitantly for at least 24 hours (at least 48 hours with the accelerated dose regimen). An initial intravenous bolus of 5,000 Units prior to thrombolytic therapy is recommended, followed by an infusion of 1,000 Units/hour. The dose of heparin should be adjusted according to repeated measurements of aPTT values of 1.5 to 2.5 fold of the initial value.

*Pulmonary embolism:* A total dose of 100 mg should be administered in 2 hours. The most experience available is with the following dose regimen:
10 mg as an intravenous bolus over 1-2 minutes, 90 mg as an intravenous infusion over 2 hours.
The total dose should not exceed 1.5 mg/kg in patients with a body weight below 65 kg.
*Adjunctive therapy:* After treatment with Actilyse heparin therapy should be initiated (or resumed) when aPTT values are less than twice the upper limit of normal. The infusion should be adjusted according to aPTT values of 1.5 to 2.5 fold of the initial value.

*Contra–indications:* Like all thrombolytic agents, Actilyse should not be used in cases where there is a high risk of haemorrhage such as:
–known haemorrhagic diathesis
–patients receiving oral anticoagulants, e.g. warfarin sodium.
–manifest or recent severe or dangerous bleeding
–any history of stroke or central nervous system damage (i.e. neoplasm, aneurysm, intracranial or spinal surgery)
–haemorrhagic retinopathy, e.g. in diabetes (vision disturbances may indicate haemorrhagic retinopathy)
–recent (less than 10 days) traumatic external heart massage, obstetrical delivery, recent puncture of a non-compressible blood–vessel (e.g. subclavian or jugular vein puncture)
–severe uncontrolled arterial hypertension
–bacterial endocarditis, pericarditis
–acute pancreatitis
–documented ulcerative gastrointestinal disease during the last 3 months, oesophageal varices, arterial aneurismus, arterial/venous malformations
–neoplasm with increased bleeding risk
–severe liver disease, including hepatic failure, cirrhosis, portal hypertension (oesophageal varices) and active hepatitis.
–major surgery or significant trauma in past 3 months

*Special warnings and special precautions for use:* Actilyse should be used by physicians experienced in the use of thrombolytic treatment and with the facilities to monitor that use.
The risk of intracerebral haemorrhage is increased in elderly patients. As the therapeutic benefit is also increased in elderly patients, the risk–benefit–evaluation should be carried out carefully.
As yet, there is only limited experience with the use of Actilyse in children.
As with all thrombolytics, the expected therapeutic benefit should be weighed up particularly carefully against the possible risk, especially in patients with
–smaller recent traumas, such as biopsies, puncture of major vessels, intramuscular injections, cardiac massage for resuscitation
–conditions with an increased risk of haemorrhage which are not mentioned in the *Contra-indications* section.
A dose exceeding 100 mg of alteplase should not be given because it has been associated with an additional increase in intracranial bleeding.
There is limited experience with readministration of Actilyse. Actilyse is not suspected to cause anaphylactic reactions. If an anaphylactoid reaction occurs, the infusion should be discontinued and appropriate treatment initiated.
The use of rigid catheters should be avoided.

*Interaction with other medicaments and other forms of interaction:* The risk of haemorrhage can be increased with the use of coumarine derivatives, platelet aggregation inhibitors, heparin and other agents influencing coagulation.

*Pregnancy and lactation:* There is very limited experience with the use of Actilyse during pregnancy and lactation. In cases of an acute life–threatening disease the benefit has to be evaluated against the potential risk.

In pregnant animals no teratogenic effects were observed after iv. infusion of pharmacologically effective doses. In rabbits embryotoxicity (embryolethality, growth retardation) was induced by more than 3 mg/kg/day. No effects on peri–postnatal development or on fertility parameters were observed in rats with doses up to 10 mg/kg/day.

*Effects on ability to drive and use machines:* Not applicable.

*Undesirable effects:* The most frequent adverse reaction associated with Actilyse is bleeding resulting in a fall in haematocrit and/or haemoglobin values. The type of bleeds associated with thrombolytic therapy can be divided into two broad categories:
-superficial bleeding, normally from punctures or damaged blood vessels,
- internal bleedings into the gastro–intestinal or uro–genital tract, retro–peritoneum or CNS or bleeding of parenchymatous organs.
In clinical studies with Actilyse significant blood–loss was observed occasionally from gastro–intestinal, uro–genital or retro–peritoneal bleeding. Ecchymosis, epistaxis and gingival bleeding are observed rather frequently but usually do not require any specific action. In studies, where patients were treated according to clinical routine, i.e. without acute left–heart catheterisation, a blood transfusion was only occasionally necessary. Intracranial haemorrhage has been reported rarely (less than 1%).
If a potentially dangerous haemorrhage occurs, in particular cerebral haemorrhage, the fibrinolytic therapy must be discontinued. In general, however, it is not necessary to replace the coagulation factors because of the short half–life and the minimal effect on the systemic coagulation factors. Most patients who have bleeding can be managed by interruption of thrombolytic and anticoagulant therapy, volume replacement, and manual pressure applied to an incompetent vessel. Protamine should be considered if heparin has been administered within 4 hours of the onset of bleeding. In the few patients who fail to respond to these conservative measures, judicious use of transfusion products may be indicated. Transfusion of cryoprecipitate, fresh frozen plasma, and platelets should be considered with clinical and laboratory reassessment after each administration. A target fibrinogen level of 1 gram/litre is desirable with cryoprecipitate infusion. Antifibrinolytic agents are available as a last alternative.
Actilyse therapy may lead to cholesterol crystal embolization or thrombotic embolisation in rare cases. The clinical consequences depend on the organ involved (e.g. renal failure in the case of renal involvement).
In patients receiving Actilyse for myocardial infarction successful reperfusion is often accompanied by arrythmias. These may require the use of conventional antiarrhythmic therapies.
In rare cases nausea, vomiting, hypotension and fever have been reported. These reactions can also occur as concomitant symptoms of myocardial infarction.
In rare cases, anaphylactoid reactions (urticaria, bronchospasm, hypotension) have been reported. A causal relationship could not be established. Clinical relevant antibody formation after alteplase administration has not been observed. No definite allergic reactions with Actilyse are known.

*Overdose:* The relative fibrin specificity notwithstanding, a clinically significant reduction in fibrinogen and other blood coagulation components may occur after overdosage. In most cases, it is sufficient to await the physiological regeneration of these factors after the Actilyse therapy has been terminated. If, however, severe bleeding results, the infusion of fresh frozen plasma or fresh blood is recommended and if necessary, synthetic antifibrinolytics may be administered.

### Pharmacological properties
*Pharmacodynamic properties:* The active ingredient of Actilyse (alteplase) is a glycoprotein, which activates plasminogen directly to form plasmin. When

administered intravenously, alteplase remains relatively inactive in the circulatory system. Once bound to fibrin, it is activated, inducing the conversion of plasminogen to plasmin leading to the dissolution of the fibrin clot.

In a study including more than 40,000 patients with an acute myocardial infarction (Global Utilization of Streptokinase and t-PA for Occluded Coronary Arteries Study–GUSTO) the administration of 100 mg alteplase over 90 minutes, with concomitant iv. heparin infusion, led to a lower mortality after 30 days (6.3 %) as compared to the administration of streptokinase, 1.5 million Units over 60 minutes, with sc or iv heparin (7.3%). Actilyse-treated patients showed higher infarct related vessel patency rates at 90 minutes after thrombolysis than the streptokinase-treated patients. No differences in patency rates were noted at 180 minutes or longer.

30-day-mortality is reduced as compared to patients not undergoing thrombolytic therapy (Anglo-Scandinavian Study of Early Thrombolysis–ASSET).

The release of alpha-hydroxybutyrate-dehydrogenase (HBDH) is reduced. Global ventricular function as well as regional wall motion is less impaired as compared to patients receiving no thrombolytic therapy.

A placebo controlled trial with 100 mg Actilyse over 3 hours (Late Assessment of Thrombolytic Efficacy Study–LATE) showed a reduction of 30-day-mortality compared to placebo for patients treated within 6-12 hours after symptom onset. In cases in which clear signs of myocardial infarction are present, treatment initiated up to 24 hours after symptom onset may still be beneficial.

In patients with acute massive pulmonary embolism with haemodynamic instability thrombolytic treatment with Actilyse leads to a fast reduction of the thrombus size and a reduction of pulmonary artery pressure. Mortality data are not available.

Due to its relative fibrin-specificity Actilyse at a dose of 100 mg leads to a modest decrease of the circulating fibrinogen levels to about 60% at 4 hours, which generally reverts to more than 80% after 24 hours. Plasminogen and alpha-2-antiplasmin decrease to about 20% and 35% respectively after 4 hours and increase again to more than 80% at 24 hours. A marked and prolonged decrease of the circulating fibrinogen level is only seen in a few patients.

Actilyse is not suspected to be antigenic.

*Pharmacokinetic properties:* Actilyse is cleared rapidly from the circulating blood and metabolized mainly by the liver (plasma clearance 550 – 680 ml/min.). The relevant plasma half–life $t_{\frac{1}{2}}$alpha is 4-5 minutes. This means that after 20 minutes less than 10% of the initial value is present in the plasma. For the residual amount remaining in a deep compartment, a beta–half–life of about 40 minutes was measured.

*Preclinical safety data:* In subchronic toxicity studies in rats and marmosets no unexpected side effects were found.

No indications of a mutagenic potential were found in mutagenic tests.

**Pharmaceutical particulars**

*List of excipients:* L-Arginine, phosphoric acid and polysorbate 80.

*Incompatibilities:* The reconstituted solution may be diluted further with sterile physiological saline solution (0.9 %) up to 1:5.

It may not, however, be diluted further with water for injection or carbohydrate infusion solutions, e. g. dextrose.

Actilyse must not be mixed with other drugs, neither in the same infusion-vial nor via the same catheter (not even with heparin).

*Shelf life:* 36 months under controlled room temperature storage conditions (not exceeding 25°C, PhEur).

The prepared solution may be stored under refrigeration up to 24 hours and up to 8 hours at a temperature not exceeding 25°C.

*Special precautions for storage:* Protect the lyophilized substance from light.

*Nature and contents of container:* 10, 20 or 50 ml sterilized glass vials, which are stoppered with sterile siliconized grey butyl–lyophilization–type stoppers with aluminium/plastic flip–off caps.

The water for injection is filled into either 10, 20 or 50 ml vials, depending on the size of the rt–PA–vials. The water for injection vials are stoppered with appropriate rubber stoppers and aluminium/plastic flip–off type caps.

*Instructions for use/handling:* Not applicable

**Marketing authorisation number** 0015/0120

**Date of approval/revision of SPC** October 1995.

**Legal category** POM

## BONEFOS* CAPSULES
## BONEFOS* TABLETS

**Presentation**

*Bonefos 400 mg Capsules:* Pale yellow, hard gelatine capsules, each containing the equivalent of 400 mg sodium clodronate.

*Bonefos 800 mg Tablets:* White film-coated, oval-shaped scored tablets, printed with code L 134 on the scored side, each containing the equivalent of 800 mg sodium clodronate.

**Uses**

*Action:* Sodium clodronate is a bisphosphonate which has a high affinity for bone. It suppresses osteoclast-mediated bone resorption producing a decrease in serum calcium and a reduction in urinary excretion of calcium and hydroxyproline, without adversely affecting the normal bone mineralisation process.

*Indication:* Bonefos Capsules/Tablets are indicated for the management of osteolytic lesions, hypercalcaemia and bone pain associated with skeletal metastases in patients with carcinoma of the breast or multiple myeloma.

Bonefos Capsules/Tablets are also indicated for the maintenance of clinically acceptable serum calcium levels in patients with hypercalcaemia of malignancy initially treated with an intravenous infusion of Bonefos concentrate.

**Dosage and administration**

*Adults:* The recommended daily dose of Bonefos is 1600 mg sodium clodronate taken as a single dose or in two divided doses (800 mg bd). The capsules/tablets should be taken with a little fluid, but not milk, at least 1 hour before or 1 hour after food. If necessary, the dose may be increased but should not exceed a maximum of 3200 mg sodium clodronate daily.

*Children:* Bonefos has not been evaluated in children

*Elderly:* There are no special dosage recommendations in the elderly. Clinical trials have included patients over 65 years and no adverse reactions specific to this age group have been reported.

*Renal impairment:* In patients with moderate renal impairment (creatinine clearance between 10 and 30 ml/min), the daily dose should be reduced to half the adult dose, i.e. 800 mg sodium clodronate. Sodium clodronate is contraindicated in patients with creatinine clearance below 10 ml/min.

**Contra-indications, warnings, etc**

*Contra-indications:* Bonefos Capsules/Tablets are contra-indicated in patients with known hypersensitivity to bisphosphonates, in patients with moderate to severe renal failure (serum creatinine greater than 440 micromol/litre or creatinine clearance below 10 ml/min), in children, in pregnant and lactating women, and in patients receiving other bisphosphonates.

*Precautions:* Adequate fluid intake should be maintained during treatment.

Bonefos Capsules/Tablets should be administered with care to patients with renal insufficiency. It is recommended that appropriate monitoring of hydration status and of renal function with serum creatinine measurement be carried out during treatment. Serum calcium should be monitored periodically.

*Use in pregnancy and lactation:* There are insufficient data either from animal or human studies on the effects of sodium clodronate on the foetus and on reproduction. No studies have been conducted on secretion in breast milk. Bonefos Capsules/Tablets are therefore contra-indicated in pregnancy and lactation and should not be given to women of childbearing age unless they are taking adequate contraceptive precautions. Sodium clodronate is likely to adversely affect bone formation both in the foetus and in young children.

*Side-effects:* Gastro-intestinal disturbances, for example, nausea, vomiting and diarrhoea, may occur during oral treatment but these are usually mild. If these symptoms occur, use of the divided dose regimen rather than a single daily dose may improve gastro-intestinal tolerance. Hypersensitivity reactions have been mainly confined to the skin: pruritus, urticaria, exfoliative dermatitis. Bronchospasm has been precipitated rarely in patients with and without a previous history of asthma. Renal dysfunction, including failure, has been reported

Reversible elevations of serum parathyroid hormone, creatinine, lactic acid dehydrogenase, transaminase and alkaline phosphatase have been reported.

Asymptomatic hypocalcaemia has been noted rarely.

*Interactions:* Concomitant use of other bisphosphonates is contra-indicated. Patients receiving NSAIDs in addition to sodium clodronate have developed renal dysfunction. However, a synergistic action has not been established. As aminoglycosides can cause hypocalcaemia, concomitant clodronate should be administered with caution. There is no evidence from clinical experience that sodium clodronate interacts with other medication such as steroids, diuretics, analgesics or chemotherapeutic agents.

Bonefos forms complexes with divalent metal ions and, therefore, simultaneous administration with food, antacids and mineral supplements may impair absorption.

*Overdosage:* No reports of overt poisoning with sodium clodronate have been received. It is theoretically possible that hypocalcaemia may develop up to 2 or 3 days following the overdose. Serum calcium should be monitored and oral or parenteral calcium supplementation may be needed.

**Pharmaceutical precautions** Bonefos Capsules/Tablets should be stored at room temperature, below 25°C.

**Legal category** POM

**Package quantities**

Bonefos 400 mg Capsules: packs of 30, 112 and 120

Bonefos 800 mg Tablets: packs of 10 and 60

**Product licence numbers**

Bonefos Capsules 400 mg 0015/0136

Bonefos Tablets 800 mg 0015/0199

## BONEFOS* CONCENTRATE

**Qualitative and quantitative composition** Colourless 5 ml ampoules containing 60 mg/ml sodium clodronate. One 5 ml ampoule contains 300 mg sodium clodronate.

**Pharmaceutical form** Concentrate for intravenous infusion.

**Clinical particulars**

*Therapeutic indications:* The treatment of hypercalcaemia of malignancy.

*Posology and method of administration:* Patients must be kept adequately hydrated before, during and after the administration of Bonefos Concentrate.

*Adults:* Bonefos Concentrate may be administered to adults as follows:

*Single infusion:* 1500 mg (five 5 ml ampoules) Bonefos Concentrate in 500 ml of either 0.9% w/v saline or 5% glucose solution administered as an intravenous infusion over a period of four hours. Serum calcium levels should start to decrease 24–48 hours after the infusion.

*Multiple infusions:* As an alternative, 300 mg (one 5 ml ampoule) Bonefos Concentrate in 500 ml of either 0.9% w/v saline or 5% glucose solution administered as an intravenous infusion over a period of at least two hours on successive days until normocalcaemia is achieved or to a maximum of 7 days.

*Response:* Whichever method of infusion is employed, most patients will achieve normocalcaemia within 5 days. For those who do not achieve a clinically acceptable serum calcium level, the infusion with Bonefos Concentrate may be repeated.

*Further treatment:* The length of time that a clinically acceptable serum calcium level is maintained after infusion of Bonefos Concentrate varies considerably from patient to patient. The infusion can be repeated as necessary to control the serum calcium level or, alternatively, treatment with oral Bonefos Capsules at a dose of 1600–3200 mg daily may be appropriate.

Renal function and serum calcium levels should be monitored during therapy. Dose reduction is recommended if deterioration in renal function becomes apparent (see below). Treatment should be stopped if hypocalcaemia develops, and serum calcium levels monitored to determine whether further treatment is required.

*Renal impairment:* There are no published data at present on which to base recommendations for dose reduction in renal impairment when considering the option of a single 1500 mg infusion in hypercalcaemia.

The dose of clodronate should be reduced in renal impairment according to creatinine clearance when using divided intravenous doses of 300 mg. Thus in mild renal impairment with creatinine clearance of 50–80 ml/minute a 25% reduction in dose is recommended, in moderate renal impairment (10–50 ml/minute) a 25–50% reduction in dose is recommended. Sodium clodoronate is contra-indicated in patients with creatinine clearance below 10 ml/minute.

*Children:* Bonefos has not been evaluated in children.

*Elderly:* There are no special dosage recommendations in the elderly. Clinical trials have included patients over 65 years and no adverse reactions specific to this age group have been reported.

*Contra-indications:* Bonefos Concentrate is contra-indicated in patients with known hypersensitivity to bisphosphonates, in patients with moderate to severe renal failure (serum creatinine greater than 440 micromol/l or creatinine clearance below 10 ml/minute), in children, in pregnant and lactating women, and in patients receiving other bisphosphonates.

*Special warnings and precautions for use:* Bonefos Concentrate should be administered with care to patients with renal insufficiency. It is recommended that appropriate monitoring of renal function with serum creatinine measurement be carried out during treatment.

*Interaction with other medicaments and other forms of interaction:* Patients receiving NSAIDs in addition to sodium clodronate have developed renal dysfunction. However, a synergistic action has not been established. As aminoglycosides can cause hypocalcaemia concomitant clodronate should be administered with caution. There is no evidence from clinical experience that sodium clodronate interacts with other medication such as steroids, diuretics, analgesics or chemotherapeutic agents.

*Pregnancy and lactation:* There are insufficient data either from animal or human studies on the effects of sodium clodronate on the foetus and on reproduction. No studies have been conducted on secretion in breast milk. Bonefos Concentrate is, therefore, contra-indicated in pregnancy and lactation and should not be given to women of childbearing age unless they are taking adequate contraceptive precautions. Sodium clodronate is likely to adversely affect bone formation both in the foetus and in young children.

*Effects on ability to drive and use machines:* There is no indication to suggest any effects of Bonefos on a patient's ability to drive or use machinery.

*Undesirable effects:* Hypersensitivity reactions have been mainly confined to the skin: pruritus, urticaria, exfoliative dermatitis. Bronchospasm has been precipitated rarely in patients with and without a previous history of asthma. Renal dysfunction, including failure, has been reported.

Transient proteinuria has been noted immediately after intravenous infusion.

Reversible elevations of serum creatinine, parathyroid hormone, lactic acid dehydrogenase and alkaline phosphatase have been reported. Asymptomatic hypocalcaemia has been noted infrequently; symptomatic hypocalcaemia is rare.

*Overdosage:* No reports of overt poisoning with clodronate have been received.

One patient developed fatal renal failure after receiving extremely high doses of intravenous clodronate. Transient increases in serum creatinine have been observed in two studies, suggesting that overdosage of intravenous clodronate may lead to reduced renal function.

It is theoretically possible that hypocalcaemia may develop up to 2 or 3 days following the overdose. Serum calcium should be monitored and oral or parenteral calcium supplementation may be needed.

**Pharmaceutical properties**

*Pharmacodynamic properties:* Clodronate is a bisphosphonate (formerly diphosphonate), a group of analogues of pyrophosphate which have been shown, *in vitro*, to inhibit the formation and dissolution of calcium phosphate (hydroxyapatite). *In vivo*, they have been shown to inhibit bone resorption to a greater or lesser extent, depending on the compound, and clodronate is one of the most effective in this respect.

*Pharmacokinetic properties:* Clodronate is eliminated mainly via the kidneys, and after intravenous doses, 60–80% will be found in urine within 48 hours. Distribution studies in animals suggest that the remainder is retained in bone tissue. Total systemic clearance is, on average, 110 ml/min and the renal clearance 90 ml/min. Clodronate is not metabolised. The half life for elimination from plasma is 2 hours but a second phase with a half life of 13 hours has been identified although less than 10% of total urinary excretion takes place during this phase. The substance which is bound to bone will be excreted more slowly at a rate correspondig to bone turnover. The binding of clodronate to serum proteins is low.

Due to low uptake from gastrointestinal tract, the bioavailability of oral doses is 1–4%. The kinetics of clodronate are linear after both iv and oral doses.

*Preclinical safety data:* No further information relevant to clinical practice is available from preclinical studies.

**Pharmaceutical particulars**

*List of excipients:* Sodium hydroxide, water for injections.

*Incompatibilities:* None stated.

*Shelf life:* The shelf life expiry date for this product shall not exceed 2 years from the date of its manufacture.

*Special precautions for storage:* The ampoules should be stored below 25°C. Diluted solution must be used within 12 hours.

*Nature and contents of container:* Bonefos Concentrate is available in 5 ml colourless ampoules of Type I glass, packed into cartons containing 5 or 10 ampoules.

*Instructions for use/handling:* None stated.

**Marketing authorisation number** 0015/0134

**Date of approval/revision of SPC** June 1997.

**Legal category** POM

## IMMUKIN*

**Presentation** Vials containing an isotonic solution (pH5.0±0.5) for subcutaneous injection. Each vial contains 100 micrograms recombinant human interferon gamma-1b (equivalent to 3 x $10^6$ Units) per 0.5 ml.

When compared with native human interferon gamma which is a mixture of clipped forms of a heterogeneously glycosylated protein with two allelic forms (position 137: arginine or glutamine, respectively) of different polypeptide chain lengths, interferon gamma-1b is a recombinant homogeneous 140 amino acid long non-glycosylated (position 137: arginine) containing a N-terminal methionine.

**Uses**

*Properties:* Interferons are a family of functionally related proteins synthesised by eukaryotic cells in response to viruses and a variety of natural and synthetic stimuli. While alpha, beta and gamma interferons share certain properties, IFN-gamma has potent phagocyte-activating effects not seen with other interferon preparations.

In a placebo-controlled clinical trial in patients with chronic granulomatous disease (CGD), Immukin was shown to reduce the frequency of serious infections during the trial period of 12 months. The overwhelming majority of these patients were also receiving prophylactic antimicrobial therapy.

*Pharmacokinetics:* Immukin is rapidly cleared after intravenous administration and slowly and well absorbed after intramuscular or subcutaneous administration. Clearance is via the liver and kidney.

The mean elimination half-lives were 38 minutes, 2.9 hours and 5.9 hours after administration of a single 100 micrograms/m² injection by intravenous, intramuscular and subcutaneous routes. Peak plasma concentrations occurred approximately 4 hours after i.m. dosing and 7 hours after s.c. dosing. Multiple-dose subcutaneous pharmacokinetic studies were conducted in healthy male subjects. There was no accumulation of Immukin after 12 consecutive daily injections of 100 micrograms/m².

No pharmacokinetic studies have been performed with the recommended dosage regimen.

*Indications:* Immukin is indicated as an adjunct therapy to antibiotics to reduce the frequency of serious infections in patients with chronic granulomatous disease (CGD).

**Dosage and administration** The recommended dose is 50 micrograms/m² or 1.5 micrograms/kg/dose for patients whose body surface area is 0.5 m² or less, to be given by subcutaneous injection three times a week.

The volume withdrawn from the vial should be controlled according to the required dosage before administration. Although the optimum dose of Immukin is not yet known, the recommended dose should not be exceeded. If severe reactions occur, the dosage should be modified (50% reduction) or therapy should be discontinued until the adverse reaction has subsided.

Safety and efficacy in children under the age of 6 months has not been established.

Clinical experience in the elderly is limited.

**Contra-indications, warnings etc**

*Contra-indications:* Immukin is contra-indicated in patients who develop or have known acute hypersensitivity to interferon gamma or known hypersensitivity to closely related interferons.

*Interaction with other medicaments and other forms of interactions:* Immukin does not reduce the efficacy of antibiotics or glucocorticoids in CGD patients.

Immukin can potentially alter the half-lives of simultaneously administered drugs which are metabolised by the cytochrome P-450 system.

It is theoretically possible that hepatotoxic and/or nephrotoxic drugs might have effects on the clearance of Immukin.

Concurrent use of drugs having neurotoxic (including effects on the central nervous system), haemotoxic or cardiotoxic effects may increase the toxicity of interferons in these systems.

The effects of anti-inflammatory drugs, NSAIDs, theophylline, immunosuppressive and cytostatic drugs on the acute cellular effects of Immukin and its therapeutic effects in CGD patients when such drugs are used concomitantly in chronic conditions are not known.

Theoretically, concomitant administration of heterologous serum protein preparations or immunological preparations (e.g. vaccines) might increase the immunogenicity of Immukin.

Immukin should not be mixed with other drugs in the same syringe.

*Effects on ability to drive and use machines:* Immukin may impair the ability to drive or operate machinery. Patients should be warned of this, and that the effect may be enhanced by alcohol.

*Undesirable effects:* The clinical and laboratory toxicity associated with multiple-dose Immukin therapy is dose-, route- and schedule-dependent.

Serious adverse reactions have not been observed in patients receiving the recommended dose of Immukin.

The most common adverse experiences are fever, headache, chills, myalgia or fatigue which may decrease in severity as treatment continues. Vomiting, nausea, arthralgia and injection site tenderness have been reported in some patients.

Acute serious hypersensitivity reactions have not been observed in patients receiving Immukin. However, transient cutaneous rashes, e.g. dermatitis, maculopapular rash, pustular and vesicular eruptions and erythema at injection site have occurred in some patients following injection but have rarely necessitated interruption of treatment.

*Pregnancy and lactation:* There is insufficient information about use during pregnancy in the human to assess possible risk. Immukin should be used during pregnancy only if the potential benefit justifies the potential risk to the foetus. There is no indication of maternal toxicity, embryotoxicity, foetotoxicity or teratogenicity in animal studies.

It is not known whether Immukin is excreted in human milk. Because of unknown risk to the infant breast feeding is inadvisable.

*Other special warnings and precautions:* Patients with serious liver disease and patients with severe renal insufficiency should be treated with caution because of the possibility of interferon gamma-1b accumulation.

Caution should be exercised when treating patients with known seizure disorders and/or compromised central nervous system function.

Although no direct cardiotoxic effects have been demonstrated Immukin should be used with caution in patients with pre-existing cardiac disease, including symptoms of ischaemia, congestive heart failure or arrhythmia.

Simultaneous administration of interferon gamma-1b with other heterologous serum protein preparations or immunological preparations (e.g. vaccines,) should be avoided because of the risk of unexpected amplified immune response.

In addition to tests normally required for monitoring patients with CGD, patients should undergo the following tests before beginning Immukin therapy and at appropriate periods during treatment: haematologic tests, including full blood counts, differential wbc and platelet counts; blood chemistry, including renal and liver function tests; urinalysis.

Although antibodies to interferon gamma-1b have not been detected in several hundred patients, it would be prudent to monitor patients periodically for the presence of antibodies to Immukin.

Parenteral drug products should be inspected visually for particulate matter and discolouration prior to administration.

*Overdose:* Experience of doses in excess of 50 micrograms/m² has been confined to patients with conditions other than CGD.

Central nervous system adverse reactions including decreased mental status, gait disturbance and dizziness have been observed, particularly in cancer patients receiving doses greater than 100 micrograms/m²/day. These abnormalities were reversible within a few days upon dose reduction or discontinuation of therapy.

Reversible neutropenia and elevation of hepatic enzymes have been observed at doses equal to or above 250 micrograms/m²/day. Thrombocytopenia and proteinuria have also been seen rarely.

It is possible that at very high doses (250 micrograms/m²/day or higher), acute, self-limiting constitutional toxicities such as arrhythmia, pulmonary and renal insufficiency, confusion and seizure may exacerbate pre-existing cardiac conditions.

**Pharmaceutical precautions** Store in a refrigerator (2-8°C). Do not freeze. Do not shake vigorously.

The formulation does not contain a preservative. Once opened, the contents of a vial should be used immediately. The unused portion of any vial should be discarded. Immukin is for single use only.

**Legal category** POM.

**Package quantities** Immukin is available in packs containing 6 vials.

**Further information** Immukin also contains mannitol, disodium succinate hexahydrate, succinic acid, polysorbate 20 and water for injection.

**Product licence number** 0015/0154.

## MEXITIL* AMPOULES

**Qualitative and quantitative composition** Colourless, glass, ampoules contains 250 mg mexiletine hydrochloride (equivalnt to 207.7 mg of mexiletine) in 10 ml of solution.

**Pharmaceutical form** Ampoules for intravenous injection.

**Clinical particulars**
*Therapeutic indications:* For the treatment of ventricular arrhythmias which are considered as serious and/or life-threatening by the physician.

i.v. mexiletine has been used successfully in the treatment of ventricular arrhythmias induced by digitalis or other drugs; mexiletine has also been proven to be of some benefit in idiopathic and other arrhythmic states. Mexiletine is often effective in patients with good left ventricular function, in suppressing ventricular arrhythmias refractory to other treatment. Mexiletine is not of proven value in arrhythmias in pre-excitation syndromes.

*Posology and method of administration:*
*Intravenous mexitil:* Mexitil should never be injected in bolus form.

*(a) Loading dose:* i.v. injection of 4–10 ml (100–250 mg) Mexitil given at a suggested rate of 1 ml per minute (25 mg per minute).
THEN
Add 500 mg (2 ampoules) Mexitil to 500 ml of a suitable infusion solution. Administer the first 250 ml by i.v. infusion over 1 hour (4 ml per minute).
THEN
Administer the second 250 ml by i.v. infusion over 2 hours (2 ml per minute).

*(b) Maintenance dose:* Add 250 mg (1 ampoule) Mexitil to 500 ml of a suitable infusion solution. Administer by i.v. infusion at a suggested rate of 1 ml per minute (0.5 mg per minute), according to patient response. Continue for as long as required or until oral maintenance therapy is commenced.

*2. Alternative loading dose regimes:*

(a) Combination i.v. Mexitil and Oral Mexitil Loading Dose: i.v. injection of 8 ml (200 mg) Mexitil given at a suggested rate of 1 ml per minute. On completion of injection or infusion give 400 mg Mexitil orally.
(b) Maintenance dose: As in 1(b) above.

*3. Change over from i.v. to oral Mexitil maintenance:* On discontinuing the i.v. infusion commence the maintenance dose. The first capsule should be taken at, or shortly before, the end of the infusion (an oral loading dose should not be given).

*Notes:*
1. The loading dose regime is designed to compensate for the rapid phase of tissue distribution which occurs especially with i.v. loading.
2. Side effects are more likely to be encountered during the initial tissue loading phase in which case the rate of infusion should be reduced.
3. If the optimum therapeutic effect is not achieved the rate of infusion or oral dosage may be increased, side-effects permitting.
4. When mexiletine therapy is commenced, patients should be monitored closely (ECG and blood pressure, routine laboratory tests) over a period of at least 24 hours, particularly in the following situations: sinus node dysfunction, conduction defects, bradycardia, hypotension or cardiac, renal or hepatic failure. There may be potentiation of tremor in patients with Parkinsonism.

Regular monitoring of cardiac function throughout treatment is advisable.

The duration of treatment required in any patient is of necessity variable, and although no precise guide can be given withdrawal of treatment may be attempted after a suitable period of free arrhythmia. Gradual withdrawal, i.e. over 1–2 weeks, is preferable as arrhythmias which have been satisfactorily controlled may recur.

No specific information on the use of this product in the elderly is available. Clinical trials have included patients over 65 years and no adverse reactions specific to this age group have been reported.

*Instructions for dilution:* Mexitil solution for injection is known to be compatible with the following infusion solutions: sodium chloride 0.9%; sodium chloride 0.9% with potassium chloride 0.3% or 0.6%; dextrose 5%; sodium bicarbonate 1.4%; sodium lactate (M/6). Diluted Mexitil should not be stored for longer than 8 hours.

*Contra-indications:* Hypersensitivity to mexiletine or local anaesthetics, cardiogenic shock and high degree A-V block unless a pacemaker is *in situ*.

Mexitil should not be used in the first three months following myocardial infarction or where cardiac output is limited (left ventricular stroke work <35% except in patients with life-threatening ventricular arrhythmias.

*Warnings:* When using Mexitil, it should be noted that the long-term use of anti-arrhythmic agents has not been shown to prolong life.

*Special warnings and special precautions for use:* Myocardial infarction results in prolonged absorption half-life of mexiletine. Plasma elimination half-life may be prolonged in moderate to severe hepatic disease, and in patients with creatinine clearance of less than 10 ml/min: individual dose titration is advised in these conditions.

*Interaction with other medicaments and other forms of interaction:*
(i) Drugs which delay the rate of absorption (narcotic analgesics, some antacids) may reduce peak plasma concentration of mexiletine.
(ii) Drugs which induce the hepatic mixed function oxidase system (e.g. rifampicin, phenytoin and phenobarbitone) can influence the metabolism and hence lower plasma levels of mexiletine. Conversely, drugs which inhibit hepatic function may increase mexiletine levels in the plasma.
(iii) Drugs which acidify or alkalinise urine will enhance or reduce (respectively) the rate of drug elimination.
(iv) Concurrent administration of mexiletine may increase plasma levels of theophylline and caffeine.
(v) No interactions have been observed with warfarin, diazepam or nitrazepam.
(vi) Mexitil may be used concurrently with the cardiovascular drugs digoxin, amiodarone, quinidine and beta-adrenergic blocking agents. Concomitant i.v. therapy with other local anaesthetic-type agents such as lignocaine or procainamide is not recommended. However, no problems have been encountered when oral mexiletine has been given in conjunction with these drugs.

*Pregnancy and lactation:* Although Mexitil has been in general use for several years, there is no definite evidence of safety during human pregnancy. Mexiletine freely crosses the placenta: however, animal studies have shown no hazard.

As with all medicines, mexiletine should not be used in pregnancy, especially the first trimester, unless the expected benefit is thought to outweigh any possible risk to the foetus.

Mexiletine is secreted in breast milk (at concentrations on average slightly higher than maternal blood), but has not been detected in the plasma of the suckling infant. Nevertheless caution should be exercised, particularly when nursing a premature infant.

*Effect on ability to drive and use machines:* Mexitil may impair the ability to drive or operate machinery, especially when taken in combination with alcohol.

*Indesirable effects:* Side-effects are mainly related to blood concentration and may therefore be seen during the initial phases of both i.v. and oral treatment when fluctuation may occur before the blood and tissue concentrations reach equilibrium. Reducing the rate of injection of infusion or delaying the next oral dose allows the blood concentration to fall and usually reduces side-effects.

Generally side-effects are of the following types:
*Gastrointestinal* – nausea, vomiting, indigestion, constipation, diarrhoea, dry mouth, unpleasant taste, hiccoughs. Oesophageal ulceration may occur if oral Mexitil is swallowed without adequate liquid and is lodged in the oesophagus.
*Central nervous system* – light-headedness, drowsiness, confusion, dizziness, unco-ordination, diplopia, blurred vision, nystagmus, dysarthria, ataxia, tremor, paraesthesiae, convulsion, psychiatric disorders, insomnia. Animals studies using toxic doses have shown that benzodiazepines reduce the CNS effects.
*Cardiovascular* – hypotension, sinus bradycardia, atrial fibrillation, palpitation, conduction defects, exacerbation of arrhythmias and torsade de pointes. When hypotension has occurred this has tended to be in patients with severe illness who have already been given a variety of anti-arrhythmic or other preparations and, if associated with bradycardia, may be reduced by the use of atropine. Pulmonary fibrosis has been observed in isolated cases.
*Haematological* – rash, jaundice, arthralgia, fever, thrombocytopenia and appearance of positive but symptomless antinuclear factor titres. Leucopernia has been observed rarely. Rare cases of Stevens-Johnson Syndrome, some with liver involvement, have been reported in Japan.
*Hepatic* – liver damage has been observed following Mexitil administration.

*Overdose:* The minimum fatal dose is unknown but 4.40 g proved fatal in a healthy young adult.

The clinical features include nausea, vomiting, drowsiness, confusion, ataxia and convulsions. Blurred vision and paraesthesiae have also been reported. Hypotension, sinus bradycardia, atrial fibrillation and cardiac arrest are more specific effects. Arrhythmias should be treated as appropriate and diazepam may be useful to control convulsions.

Acidification of the urine enhances the rate of drug elimiation and so may be useful.

**Pharmacological properties**
*Pharmacodynamic properties:* Mexitil is an anti-arrhythmic agent which depresses the maximum rate of depolarisation with little or no modification of resting potentials or the duration of action potentials.

*Pharmacokinetic properties:* Mexiletine is metabolised in the liver to a number of metabolites. It is excreted in the urine, mainly in the form of its metabolites with a small proportion of unchanged mexiletine; the clearance of mexiletine is increased in acid urine. Mexiletine is widely distributed throughout the body and is about 60–70% bound to plasma proteins. It has a plasma half life of 10 hours in healthy subjects but this may be prolonged in patients with heart disease.

**Pharmaceutal particulars**
*List of excipients:* Sodium chloride; water for injections.

*Incompatibilities:* None stated.

*Shelf life:* The ampoules have a shelf life expiry date of 5 years from date of manufacture. Diluted Mexitil should be discarded after 8 hours.

*Special precautions for storage:* Store below 25°C. Protect from light.

*Nature and contents of container:* Cartons containing 5×10 ml colourless glass ampoules.

*Instructions for use/handling:* None stated.

**Marketing authorisation number** 0015/0065R.

**Date of approval/revision of SPC** January 1996.

**Legal category** POM.

## MEXITIL* CAPSULES

**Qualitative and quantitative composition**
*Mexitil Capsules 50 mg:* Red/purple hard gelatin capsules imprinted with the notation 50 mg and the Company symbol. Each capsule contains mexiletine hydrochloride 50 mg, equivalent to 41.5 mg of mexiletine base.

*Mexitil Capsules 200 mg:* Red/red hard gelatin capsules imprinted with the notation 200 mg and the Company symbol. Each capsule contains mexiletine hydrochloride 200 mg, equivalent to 166.2 mg of mexiletine base.

**Pharmaceutical form** Capsules for oral administration.

**Clinical particulars**
*Therapeutic indications:* For the treatment of ventricular arrhythmias which are considered as serious and/or life-threatening by the physician.

i.v. mexiletine has been used successfully in the treatment of ventricular arrhythmias induced by digitalis or other drugs; mexiletine has also been proven to be of some benefit in idiopathic and other arrhythmic states. Mexiletine is often effective in patients with good left ventricular function, in suppressing ventricular arrhythmias refractory to other treatment. Mexiletine is not of proven value in arrhythmias in pre-excitation syndromes.

*Posology and method of administration:* Capsules should be swallowed whole with ample liquid, preferably with the patient in an upright position. It is advisable to take Mexitil after food.

*(i) Loading dose:* Give 400 mg Mexitil.

*(ii) Maintenance dose:* Give 200–250 mg Mexitil three to four times daily commencing 2 hours after the loading dose. The usual daily dose is between 600–800 mg in divided doses; optimal doses range from 300–1200 mg daily in divided doses.

*Note:* Mexitil is absorbed in the upper part of the small intestine. In acute myocardial infarction and particularly when opiates have been given, *rate* of absorption *but not bioavailability* may be delayed and therefore a larger loading dose e.g. 600 mg may be preferable.

*Alternative loading dose regimes*

(a) *Combination i.v. Mexitil and oral mexitil loading dose:* i.v. injection of 8 ml (200 mg) Mexitil given at a suggested rate of 1 ml per minute. On completion of injection or infusion give 400 mg Mexitil orally. Maintenance dose as in (ii).

(b) *Combination i.v. Lignocaine and oral Mexitil loading dose:* Give i.v. lignocaine according to manufacturer's instructions. On completion of injection give 400 mg Mexitil orally. Maintenance dose as in (ii).

*Change over from i.v. to oral maintenance:* On discontinuing the i.v. infusion commence the maintenance dose. The first capsule should be taken at, or shortly before, the end of the infusion (an oral loading dose should not be given). Give 200–250 mg Mexitil orally three or four times a day.

*Notes:*

1. The loading dose regime is designed to compensate for the rapid phase of tissue distribution which occurs especially with i.v. loading.

2. Side-effects are more likely to be encountered during the initial tissue loading phase in which case the rate of infusion should be reduced.

3. If the optimum therapeutic effect is not achieved the rate of infusion or oral dosage may be increased, side-effects permitting.

4. Gastric emptying time may be delayed in patients with myocardial infarction and/or to whom opiates have been given and thus, it may be necessary to titrate the dose against therapeutic effects and side-effects.

5. The 50 mg capsule is available in order that a more precise dose titration may be undertaken should this be required. Small increments will also reduce the incidence of side effects.

6. When mexiletine therapy is commenced, patients should be monitored closely (ECG and blood pressure, routine laboratory tests) over a period of at least 24 hours, particularly in the following situations: sinus node dysfunction, conduction defect, bradycardia, hypotension or cardiac, renal or hepatic failure. There may be potentiation of tremor in patients with Parkinsonism.

Regular monitoring of cardiac function throughout treatment is advisable.

The duration of treatment required in any patient is of necessity variable, and although no precise guide can be given, withdrawal of treatment may be attempted after a suitable period free of arrhythmia. Gradual withdrawal, i.e. over 1–2 weeks, is preferable as arrhythmias which have been satisfactorily controlled may recur.

No specific information on the use of this product in the elderly is available. Clinical trials have included patients over 65 years and no adverse reactions specific to this age group have been reported.

*Contra-indications:* Hypersensitivity to mexiletine or local anaesthetics, cardiogenic shock and high degree A-V block unless a pacemaker is *in situ*.

Mexitil should not be used in the first three months following myocardial infarction or where cardiac output is limited (left ventricular stoke work <35%) except in patients with life-threatening ventricular arrhythmias.

*Warnings:* When using Mexitil, it should be noted that the long-term use of anti-arrhythmic agents has not been shown to prolong life.

*Special warnings and special precautions for use:* Myocardial infarction results in prolonged absorption half-life of mexiletine. Plasma elimination half-life may be prolonged in moderate to severe hepatic disease, and in patients with creatinine clearance of less than 10 ml/min: individual dose titration is advised in these conditions.

*Interactions with other medicaments and other forms of interaction:*

(i) Drugs which delay the rate of absorption (narcotic analgesics, some antacids) may reduce peak plasma concentration of mexiletine.

(ii) Drugs which induce the hepatic mixed function oxidase system (e.g. rifampicin, phenytoin and phenobarbitone) can influence the metabolism and hence lower plasma levels of mexiletine. Conversely, drugs which inhibit hepatic function may increase mexiletine levels in the plasma.

(iii) Drugs which acidify or alkalinise urine will enhance or reduce (respectively) the rate of drug elimination.

(iv) Concurrent administration of mexiletine may increase plasma levels of theophylline and caffeine.

(v) No interactions have been observed with warfarin, diazepam or nitrazepam.

(vi) Mexitil may be used concurrently with the cardiovascular drugs digoxin, amiodarone, quinidine and beta-adrenergic blocking agents. Concomitant I.V. therapy with other local anaesthetic-type agents such as lignocaine or procainamide is not recommended. However no problems have been encountered when oral mexiletine has been given in conjunction with these drugs.

*Pregnancy and lactation:* Although Mexitil has been in general use for several years, there is no definite evidence of safety during human pregnancy. Mexiletine freely crosses the placenta: however, animal studies have shown no hazard. As with all medicines, mexiletine should not be used in pregnancy, especially the first trimester, unless the expected benefit is thought to outweigh any possible risk to the foetus. Mexiletine is secreted in breast milk (at concentrations on average slightly higher than maternal blood), but has not been detected in the plasma of the suckling infant. Nevertheless caution should be exercised, particularly when nursing a premature infant.

*Effect on ability to drive and use machines:* Mexitil may impair the ability to drive or operate machinery, especially when taken in combination with alcohol.

*Undesirable effects:* Side-effects are mainly related to blood concentration and may, therefore be seen during the initial phases of both i.v. and oral treatment when fluctuation may occur before the blood and tissue concentrations reach equilibrium. Reducing the rate of injection of infusion or delaying the next oral dose allows the blood concentration to fall and usually reduces side-effects.

Generally side-effects are of the following types:

*Gastrointestinal* – nausea, vomiting, indigestion, constipation, diarrhoea, dry mouth, unpleasant taste, hiccoughs. Oesophageal ulceration may occur if oral Mexitil is swallowed without adequate liquid and is lodged in the oesophagus.

*Central nervous system* – light-headedness, drowsiness, confusion, dizziness, unco-ordination, diplopia, blurred vision, nystagmus, dysarthria, ataxia, tremor, paraesthesiae, convulsion, psychiatric disorders, insomnia. Animal studies using toxic doses have shown that benzodiazepines reduce the CNS effects.

*Cardiovascular* – hypotension, sinus bradycardia, atrial fibrillation, palpitation, conduction defects, exacerbation of arrhythmias and torsade de pointes. When hypotension has occurred this has tended to be in patients with severe illness who have already been given a variety of anti-arrhythmic or other preparations and, if associated with bradycardia, may be reduced by the use of atropine. Pulmonary fibrosis has been observed in isolated cases.

*Haematological* – rash, jaundice, arthralgia, fever, thrombocytopenia and appearance of positive but symptomless antinuclear factor titres. Leucopenia has been observed rarely. Rare cases of Stevens-Johnson Syndrome, some with liver involvement, have been reported in Japan.

*Hepatic* – Liver damage has been observed following Mexitil administration.

*Overdose:* The minimum fatal dose is unknown but 4.40 g proved fatal in a healthy young adult.

The clinical features include nausea, vomiting, drowsiness, confusion, ataxia and convulsions. Blurred vision and paraesthesiae have also been reported. Hypotension, sinus bradycardia, atrial fibrillation and cardiac arrest are more specific effects.

Gastric lavage should be performed where appropriate and the patient should be transferred to an intensive/coronary care unit for possible cardiopulmonary support.

Arrhythmias should be treated as appropriate and diazepam may be useful to control convulsions.

Acidification of the urine enhances the rate of drug elimination and so may be useful.

**Pharmacological properties**

*Pharmacodynamic properties:* The basic cellular electrophysiological effect of mexiletine is a slowing of the maximal rate of depolarisation of the action potential. Mexiletine blocks sodium channels with a rapid rate of onset and recovery. Mexiletine may have a vagolytic activity.

In patients, mexiletine increases the functional refractory period of the atrio-ventricular node and atrio-ventricular conduction time, and shifts the Wenckebach point to a lower rate. Mexiletine increases the relative and effective refractory periods of his-purkinje system. (Reference: Campbell, RNF, *NEJ Medicine* 316 29–34 (1987)).

*Pharmacokinetic properties:* Mexiletine is primarily absorbed in the upper portion of the small intestine. Peak plasma levels are reached 1.5 hours after administration to normal subjects; absorption is slower after myocardial infarction. Mexiletine shows a fast distribution phase, a slow distribution phase, and a slow elimination phase. Tissue up-take is substantial. Mexiletine undergoes less than 10% first-pass hepatic metabolism. Bioavailability is about 90%. Renal clearance varies with urine pH but this is unlikely to have clinical significance. In patients the elimination half-life is 10–15 hours. (Reference: Campbell, RNF, *NEJ Medicine* 316 29–34 (1987)).

**Pharmaceutical particulars**

*List of excipients:* Dried maize starch, colloidal silica, magnesium stearate, hard gelatin capsules.

*Incompatibilities:* None stated.

*Shelf life:* The capsules have a shelf life expiry of 5 years from date of manufacture.

*Special precautions for storage:* Store below 25˚C.

*Nature and contents of container:* PVC blister packs (backed with PVC-lacquered aluminium) of 100.

*Instructions for use/handling:* None stated.

**Marketing authorisation numbers**
Mexitil Capsules 50 mg    0015/0062R
Mexitil Capsules 200 mg   0015/0064R

**Date of approval/revision of SPC**   January 1996.

**Legal category**   POM.

## MEXITIL* PL PERLONGETS*

**Qualitative and quantitative composition**   Mexitil PL Perlongets are sustained release hard gelatin capsules consisting of a scarlet opaque cap and a turquoise opaque body and containing five round, biconvex, beige-yellow film-coated tablets wth a dull sheen. Each capsule contains 360 mg of mexiletine hydrochloride (equivalent to 299.1 mg mexiletine).

**Pharmaceutical form**   Sustained release capsules for oral administration.

**Clinical particulars**

*Therapeutic indications:* For the treatment of ventricular arrhythmias which are considered as serious and/or life-threatening by the physician. Mexiletine has also been proven to be of some benefit in idiopathic and other arrhythmic states. Mexiletine is often effective in patients with good left ventricular function, in suppressing ventricular arrhythmias refractory to other treatment. Mexiletine is not of proven value in arrhythmias in pre-excitation syndromes.

*Posology and method of administration:* Capsules should be swallowed whole with ample liquid, preferably with the patient in an upright position. It is advisable to take Mexitil after food.

One Mexitil PL capsule twice daily (twelve hourly) will maintain therapeutic blood levels of mexiletine. If this regimen is used initially in new patients, therapeutic blood levels of mexiletine will be achieved after about 36 hours. If a more rapid effect is required, one of the following loading doses may be used:

(a) Two Mexitil PL capsules. This will give therapeutic blood levels of mexiletine within 6 hours.

(b) One Mexitil PL Capsule together with 250 mg Mexitil as conventional capsules. This will give therapeutic blood levels of mexiletine within $2\frac{1}{2}$ hours.

(c) Intravenous loading dose. See Mexitil Capsules and Ampoules SPCs for details. This will give therapeutic blood levels of mexiletine within 5 minutes.

*Change over from i.v. to Mexitil PL Capsules:* Commence oral maintenance therapy 1–2 hours before the end of the infusion (an oral loading dose should not be given).

*Change over from Mexitil Capsules to Mexitil PL Capsules:* The first Perlonget should be given in the evening, in place of the capsule. Alternatively, the first Perlonget may be given in the morning together with the last capsule.

Where individually adjusted dosage is necessary, titration of dosage may be accomplished with lower-dosed Mexitil capsules, where appropriate.

*Notes:* Gastric emptying time may be delayed in patients with myocardial infarction and/or to whom opiates have been given and thus it may be necessary to titrate the dose against therapeutic effects and side-effects. When mexiletine therapy is commenced, patients should be monitored closely (ECG and blood pressure, routine laboratory tests) over a period of at least 24 hours, particularly in the following situations: Sinus node dysfunction, conduction defect, bradycardia, hypotension or cardiac, renal or hepatic failure. There may be potentiation of tremor in patients with Parkinsonism.

Regular monitoring of cardiac function throughout treatment is advisable.

The duration of treatment required in any patient is of necessity variable, and although no precise guide can be given, withdrawal of treatment may be attempted after a suitable period free of arrhythmia. Gradual withdrawal, i.e. over 1–2 weeks, is preferable as arrhythmias which have been satisfactorily controlled may recur.

No specific information on the use of this product in the elderly is available. Clinical trials have included patients over 65 years and no adverse reactions specific to this age group have been reported.

*Contra-indications:* Hypersensitivity to mexiletine or local anaesthetics, cardiogenic shock and high degree A-V block unless a pacemaker is *in situ*.

Mexitil should not be used in the first three months following myocardial infarction or where cardiac output is limited (left ventricular stroke work <35%)

except in patients with life-threatening ventricular arrhythmias.

When using Mexitil, it should be noted that the long-term use of antiarrhythmic agents has not been shown to prolong life.

*Special warnings and special precautions for use:* Myocardial infarction results in prolonged absorption half-life of mexiletine. Plasma elimination half-life may be prolonged in moderate to severe hepatic disease, and in patients with creatinine clearance of less than 10 ml/min: individual dose titration is advised in these conditions.

*Interactions with other medicaments and other forms of interaction:*

(i) Drugs which delay the rate of absorption (narcotic analgesics, some antacids) may reduce peak plasma concentration of mexiletine.

(ii) Drugs which induce the hepatic mixed function oxidase system (e.g. rifampicin, phenytoin and phenobarbitone) can influence the metabolism and hence lower plasma levels of mexiletine. Conversely, drugs which inhibit hepatic function may increase mexiletine levels in the plasma.

(iii) Drugs which acidify or alkalinise urine will enhance or reduce (respectively) the rate of drug elimination.

(iv) Concurrent administration of mexiletine may increase plasma levels of theophylline and caffeine.

(v) No interactions have been observed with warfarin, diazepam or nitrazepam.

(vi) Mexitil may be used concurrently with the cardiovascular drugs digoxin, amiodarone, quinidine and beta-adrenergic blocking agents. Concomitant i.v. therapy with other local anaesthetic-type agents such as lignocaine or procainamide is not recommended. However no problems have been encountered when oral mexiletine has been given in conjunction with these drugs.

*Pregnancy and lactation:* Although Mexitil has been in general use for several years, there is no definite evidence of safety during human pregnancy. Mexiletine freely crosses the placenta; however animal studies have shown no hazard. As with all medicines, mexiletine should not be used in pregnancy, especially the first trimester, unless the expected benefit is thought to outweigh any possible risk to the foetus. Mexiletine is secreted in breast milk (at concentrations on average slightly higher than maternal blood), but has not been detected in the plasma of the suckling infant. Neverthelss caution should be exercised, particularly when nursing a premature infant.

*Effect on ability to drive and use machines:* Mexitil may impair the ability to drive or operate machines, especially when taken in combination with alcohol.

*Undesirable effects:* Side-effects are mainly related to blood concentration and may therefore be seen during the initial phases of both i.v. and oral treatment when fluctuation may occur before the blood and tissue concentrations reach equilibrium. Reducing the rate of injection or infusion or delaying the next oral dose allows the blood concentration to fall and usually reduces side-effects. Generally side-effects are of five types:

*Gastro-intestinal* – Nausea, vomiting, indigestion, constipation, diarrhoea, dry mouth, unpleasant taste, hiccoughs. Oesophageal ulceration may occur if oral Mexitil is swallowed without adequate liquid and is lodged in the oesophagus.

*Central nervous system* – Light headedness, drowsiness, confusion, dizziness, unco-ordination, diplopia, blurred vision, nystagmus, dysarthria, ataxia, tremor, paraesthesiae, convulsion, psychiatric disorders, insomnia. Animal studies using toxic doses have shown that benzodiazepines reduce the CNS effects.

*Cardiovascular* – Hypotension, sinus bradycardia, atrial fibrillation, palpitation, conduction defects, exacerbation of arrhythmias and torsade de pointes.

When hypotension has occurred this has tended to be in patients with severe illness who have already been given a variety of anti-arrhythmic or other preparations and, if associated with bradycardia, may be reduced by the use of atropine. Pulmonary fibrosis has occurred in isolated cases.

*Haematological* – rash, jaundice, arthralgia, fever, thrombocytopenia and appearance of positive but symptomless antinuclear factor titres. Leucopenia has been observed rarely. Rare cases of Stevens-Johnson syndrome, some with liver involvement, have been reported in Japan.

*Hepatic* – Liver damage has been observed following Mexitil administration.

*Overdose:* The minimum fatal dose is unknown but 4.40 g proved fatal in a healthy young adult. The clinical features include: nausea, vomiting, drowsiness, confusion, ataxia and convulsions. Blurred vision and paraesthesiae have also been reported. Hypotension, sinus bradycardia, atrial fibrillation and cardiac arrest are more specific effects.

Gastric lavage should be performed where appro-priate and the patient should be transferred to an intensive/coronary care unit for possible cardio-pulmonary support. Arrhythmias should be treated as appropriate and diazepam may be useful to control convulsions. Acidification of the urine enhances the rate of drug elimination and so may be useful.

**Pharmacological properties**

*Pharmacodynamic properties:* Mexitil is an anti-arrhythmic agent which depresses the maximum rate of depolarisation with little or no modification of resting potentials or the duration of action potentials.

*Pharmacokinetic properties:* Mexiletine is readily and almost completely absorbed from the gastrointestinal tract, peak plasma concentrations being obtained 2–4 hours after oral administration.

**Pharmaceutical particulars**

*List of excipients: Tablet core:* Lactose; povidone; yellow iron oxide; magnesium stearate. *Tablet coating:* Ethylcellulose; polyethylene glycol 6000. *Capsule shell:* Gelatin; erythrosine; indigo carmine; titanium dioxide; yellow iron oxide; black iron oxide.

*Incompatibilities:* None stated.

*Shelf Life:* 5 years.

*Special precautions for storage:* Store below 25°C.

*Nature and content of container:* Mexitil PL Perlongets are packed into blister packs of 56 and 60 consisting of aluminium foil coated with a heat seal lacquer (PVC/PVDC combination) and a PVC/PVDC film is used as the sealing surface.

*Instructions for use/handling:* None stated.

**Marketing authorisation number** 0015/0084.

**Date of approval/revision of SPC** November 1996.

**Legal category** POM.

# MYDRILATE*

**Presentation** Isotonic, sterile aqueous solutions of Cyclopentolate Hydrochloride BP 0.5% and 1.0% w/v buffered to pH 5 and containing 0.01% w/v benzalkonium chloride.

*Uses:* Cyclopentolate is an anti-muscarinic agent used topically in the eye as a mydriatic and cycloplegic. The effects are similar to those of atropine but with a more rapid onset and shorter duration of action. It is indicated for:

(i) Diagnostic purposes for fundoscopy and cycloplegic refraction.

(ii) Dilating the pupil in inflammatory conditions of the iris and uveal tract.

**Dosage and administration**

*(i) Refraction/Fundoscopy*
*Adults (and the elderly):* One drop of 0.5% solution instilled into the eye, repeated after 15 minutes if necessary, approximately 40 minutes before examination. Deeply pigmented eyes may require the use of a 1% solution.

N.B. : Maximum effect is reached after 30-60 minutes.

*Children 6-16 years:* One drop of 1% solution instilled into the eye, repeated after 15 minutes if necessary, approximately 40 minutes before examination.

*Children under 6 years:* One or two drops of 1% solution instilled into the eye, repeated after 15 minutes if necessary, approximately 40 minutes before examination.

*(ii) For Uveitis, Iritis and Iridocyclitis*
*Adults (and the elderly):* One or two drops of 0.5% solution instilled into the eye up to 4 times daily or as required. Deeply pigmented eyes may require the use of a 1% solution.

*Children:* At the discretion of the physician.

Do not use during the first three months of life due to possible association between the cycloplegia produced and the development of amblyopia and also the increased risks of systemic toxicity in neonates.

Cycloplegia following administration is quick in onset and short-lived. Maximal cycloplegia is achieved within 15-45 minutes of instillation and lasts on average about 20 minutes. Recovery normally takes place in about 4 hours, but very occasionally some effect persists for up to 24 hours.

Mydriasis is produced very rapidly and an average pupil diameter of 7 mm is usually reached 15-30 minutes after instillation of one drop of 0.5% solution. Complete recovery from the mydriatic effect generally occurs spontaneously in not more than 20 hours.

No specific information on the use of this product in the elderly is available. Clinical trials have included patients over 65 years and no adverse reactions specific to this group have been reported.

**Contra-indications, warnings etc**

*Contra-indications:* Mydrilate is contra-indicated for use in patients with narrow-angle glaucoma or those with a tendency towards glaucoma e.g. patients with a shallow anterior chamber; known hypersensitivity to cyclopentolate hydrochloride, benzalkonium chloride or any other components of the formulation; paralytic ileus and use in children with organic brain syndromes, including congenital or neuro-developmental abnormalities, particularly those predisposing to epileptic seizures.

This preparation contains benzalkonium chloride and should not be used whilst soft contact lenses are being worn.

*Precautions and warnings:* Because of the risk of precipitating angle-closure glaucoma in the elderly and others prone to raised intraocular pressure, an estimate of the depth of the anterior chamber should be made before use, particularly if therapy is likely to be intense or protracted.

Caution should be observed when drugs of this group are administered to patients with prostatic enlargement, coronary insufficiency or cardiac failure, or ataxia. Atropine-like effects have been reported as side-effects.

Extreme caution is advised for use in children and individuals susceptible to belladonna alkaloids because of the increased risk of systemic toxicity.

Patients should be warned of the oral toxicity of this preparation, and advised to wash their hands after use. If accidentally swallowed, patients should be advised to seek medical attention.

Use with caution in an inflamed eye as the hyperaemia greatly increases the rate of systemic absorption through the conjunctiva.

To reduce systemic absorption the lacrimal sac should be compressed at the medial canthus by digital pressure for at least two minutes after instillation of the drops.

May cause blurred vision, difficulty in focussing and sensitivity to light. Patients should be warned not to drive or engage in other hazardous activities (e.g. climbing ladders and scaffolding) unless vision is clear. Complete recovery from the effects of Mydrilate Eye Drops may take up to 24 hours.

*Drug interactions:* The effects of anti-muscarinic agents may be enhanced by the concomitant administration of other drugs with anti-muscarinic properties such as some antihistamines, butyrophenones, phenothiazines, tricyclic antidepressants and amantadine.

*Use in pregnancy and lactation:* There is insufficient evidence as to drug safety in pregnancy and lactation. This product should not be used during pregnancy unless it is considered essential by a physician.

*Side-effects:* Increased intraocular pressure, transient stinging, and sensitivity to light secondary to pupillary dilation. Prolonged administration may lead to local irritation, hyperaemia, oedema and conjunctivitis.

Systemic anticholinergic toxicity is manifested by dryness of the mouth, flushing, dryness of the skin, bradycardia followed by tachycardia with palpitations and arrhythmias, urinary urgency, difficulty and retention, reduction in the tone and motility of the gastro-intestinal tract leading to constipation.

Vomiting, giddiness and staggering may occur, a rash may be present in children, abdominal distension in infants. Psychotic reactions, behavioural disturbances and cardio-respiratory collapse may occur in children.

*Overdosage:* Systemic toxicity may occur following topical use, particularly in children. It is manifested by flushing and dryness of the skin, (a rash may be present in children,) blurred vision, a rapid and irregular pulse, fever, abdominal distension in infants, convulsions and hallucinations and the loss of neuro-muscular co-ordination.

Treatment is supportive (there is no evidence that physostigmine is superior to supportive management). In infants and small children the body surface must be kept moist. If accidentally ingested, induce emesis or perform gastric lavage.

**Pharmaceutical precautions:** Do not dilute or dispense from any container other than the original bottle. Discard one month after opening.

Store at 2-8°C (refrigerate; do not freeze), protect from light.

**Legal category** POM

**Package quantities** 5 ml dropper bottles of 0.5% and 1.0% solutions.

When using the product for the first time, remove both the cap and collar. Replace the cap and screw down firmly to pierce the seal at the tip of the plastic nozzle.

**Further information** Mydrilate is non-irritant and sensitivity reactions are uncommon. The onset of cycloplegia is at least as fast as that obtained by any other preparation used for the purpose. In the normal eye it has little or no effect on intra-ocular tension.

Mydrilate Eye Drops also contain boric acid, potassium chloride, benzalkonium chloride and purified water.

### Product licence numbers
Mydrilate 0.5% Eye Drops   1416/5030R
Mydrilate 1.0% Eye Drops   1416/5031R

## ORAMORPH* ORAL SOLUTION
## ORAMORPH* CONCENTRATED ORAL SOLUTION

### Presentation
*Oramorph Oral Solution:* A clear, colourless solution of Morphine Sulphate BP, 10 mg/5 ml.

*Oramorph Concentrated Oral Solution:* A clear, red solution of Morphine Sulphate BP 20 mg/ml.

### Uses For the relief of severe pain.

### Dosage and administration
*Adults:* Usual dose 10-20 mg every 4 hours.

*Children 6-12 years:* Maximum dose 5–10 mg every 4 hours.

*Children 1-5 years:* Maximum dose 5 mg every 4 hours.

*Children under 1 year:* Not recommended.

Dosage can be increased under medical supervision according to the severity of the pain and the patient's previous history of analgesic requirement. Reductions in dosage may be appropriate in the elderly and in debilitated patients.

When patients are transferred from other morphine preparations to Oramorph Oral preparations dosage titration may be appropriate.

Morphine Sulphate BP is readily absorbed from the gastro-intestinal tract following oral administration. However, when oral Oramorph preparations are used in place of parenteral morphine, a 50% to 100% increase in dosage is usually required in order to achieve the same level of analgesia.

*Oramorph Concentrated Oral Solution:* A calibrated dropper is supplied with this dosage form for accurate and convenient dose adjustment. The required dose may be added to a soft drink immediately prior to administration.

### Contra-indications, warnings, etc
*Contra-indications:* Respiratory depression, obstructive airways disease, known morphine sensitivity, acute hepatic disease, acute alcoholism, head injuries, coma, convulsive disorders and where intracranial pressure is raised. Concurrent administration of monoamine oxidase inhibitors or within two weeks of discontinuation of their use.

*Warnings and precautions:* Care should be exercised if morphine sulphate is given in the first 24 hours post-operatively, in hyperthyroidism or hypothyroidism, and where there is reduced respiratory reserve, such as kyphoscoliosis, emphysema and severe obesity. Morphine sulphate should not be given if paralytic ileus is likely to occur. It is wise to reduce dosage in chronic hepatic and renal disease, myxoedema, adrenocortical insufficiency, prostatic hypertrophy or shock. Tolerance and dependence may occur.

*Interactions:* The depressant effects of morphine are enhanced by depressants of the central and peripheral nervous system such as alcohol, anaesthetics, muscle relaxants, hypnotics and sedatives, tricyclic antidepressants and phenothiazines.

*Side-effects:* In normal doses, the commonest side effects of morphine sulphate are nausea, vomiting, constipation, drowsiness and confusion. If constipation occurs, this may be treated with appropriate laxatives. Micturition may be difficult and there may be ureteric or biliary spasm. There is also an antidiuretic effect. Dry mouth, sweating, facial flushing, vertigo, bradycardia, palpitations, orthostatic hypotension, hypothermia, restlessness, changes of mood and miosis can also occur. These effects are more common in ambulant patients than in those who are bedridden. Raised intracranial pressure occurs in some patients. As a consequence of histamine release, urticaria and/or pruritis may occur in some individuals.

*Use in pregnancy and lactation:* Although morphine sulphate has been in general use for many years, there is inadequate evidence of safety in human pregnancy and lactation. Morphine is known to cross the placenta and is excreted in breast milk, and may thus cause respiratory depression in the newborn infant.

Medicines should not be used in pregnancy, especially the first trimester, unless the expected benefit outweighs any possible risk to the foetus.

*Effects on ability to drive and use machinery:* Patients

should be warned not to drive or operate dangerous machinery after taking Oramorph.

*Overdosage:* Signs of morphine toxicity and overdosage: These are likely to consist of pin-point pupils, respiratory depression and hypotension. Circulatory failure and deepening coma may occur in more severe cases. Convulsions may occur in infants and children. Death may occur from respiratory failure.

Treatment of morphine overdosage: Managed with intravenous naloxone therapy at an initial dose of 400 micrograms (10 micrograms per kilogram body weight in children). If the desired degree of counteraction and improvement is not observed within 2-3 minutes repeat dosing or establish an infusion of 2 mg in 500 ml of normal saline or 5 % dextrose to provide a concentration of 4 micrograms/ml. Empty the stomach. A 0.02% aqueous solution of potassium permanganate may be used for lavage. Assist respiration if necessary. Maintain fluid and electrolyte levels.

### Pharmaceutical precautions Store at below 25°C. Protect from light.
*Oramorph Oral Solution:* Discard 90 days after opening.

*Oramorph Concentrated Oral Solution:* Discard 120 days after opening.

### Legal category
Oramorph Oral Solution POM, CD(Sch 5)
Oramorph Concentrated Oral Solution POM, CD(Sch 2)

### Further information
*Oramorph Oral Solution:* Formulated to have a bland flavour to make it acceptable to the patient regardless of taste perception. It contains sugar, alcohol and preservatives.

*Oramorph Concentrated Oral Solution:* Contains preservatives.

### Package quantities
*Oramorph Oral Solution:* Bottles of 100 ml, 300 ml and 500 ml

*Oramorph Concentrated Oral Solution:* Bottles of 30 ml and 120 ml with calibrated dropper.

### Product licence numbers
Oramorph Concentrated Oral Solution 0015/0125
Oramorph Oral Solution 0015/0122

## ORAMORPH SR TABLETS

### Qualititative and quantitative composition
*Oramorph SR Tablets 10 mg:* each tablet contains 10 mg Morphine Sulphate BP, equivalent to 7.5 mg anhydrous morphine.

*Oramorph SR Tablets 30 mg:* each tablet contains 30 mg Morphine Sulphate BP, equivalent to 22.5 mg anhydrous morphine.

*Oramorph SR Tablets 60 mg:* each tablet contains 60 mg Morphine Sulphate BP, equivalent to 45.0 mg anhydrous morphine.

*Oramorph SR Tablets 100 mg:* each tablet contains 100 mg Morphine Sulphate BP, equivalent to 75.0 mg anhydrous morphine.

### Pharmaceutical form Slow release morphine tablet.

### Clinical particulars
*Therapeutic indication:* For the prolonged relief of severe pain.

*Posology and method of administration:* Oramorph SR tablets must be swallowed whole and not chewed.

The dosage of Oramorph SR tablets is dependent upon the severity of the pain and the patient's previous history of analgesic requirements. Oramorph SR should normally be administered twice daily at 12 hourly intervals.

One Oramorph SR 30 mg tablet twice daily is the recommended starting dose if Oramorph is taken to replace a weaker opioid analgesic (such as co-proxamol).

One or two Oramorph SR 10 mg tablets twice daily is the recommended starting dosage for a patient presenting with severe pain who has not been previously treated with a weaker opioid analgesic. With increasing severity of pain it is recommended that the dosage of morphine be increased to achieve the desired relief. The dosage may be varied by choosing combinations of the available strengths (10, 30, 60 and 100 mg) or by using higher strength tablets alone.

Alternatively, the effective dose of Oramorph SR Tablets can be found by giving Oramorph liquid every 4 hours in increasing doses until the pain has been controlled and then transferring the patient to the same total 24 hour dose of Oramorph SR, divided into 2 portions taken 12-hourly. The first dose of Oramorph SR should be given 4 hours after the last dose of the oral solution.

It is recommended that a patient transferred from

another oral morphine preparation, having similar bioavailability to oral morphine liquid, should receive the same total morphine dose in one twenty-four hour period, divided between the morning and evening dose.

If it is necessary to transfer a patient from another modified release preparation to Oramorph SR it is recommended that the patient receive the same total dose in one 24 hour period, divided into two portions for 12-hourly administration. The first dose of Oramorph SR should not be administered before the dosing interval of the previous morphine preparation has been completed. The patient should be monitored initially and the dose of Oramorph SR adjusted if necessary.

Where a patient had previously received parenteral morphine prior to being transferred to Oramorph SR tablets, a higher total dosage of Oramorph SR may be required. Individual dosage adjustment will be necessary to compensate for any reduction in analgesic effect associated with oral administration.

Oramorph SR tablets should be used with caution post-operatively (as with all morphine preparations) but especially in cases of 'acute abdomen' and following abdominal surgery. Gastric motility should have returned and be maintained.

When Oramorph SR is to be given for the relief of post-operative pain, it is not advisable to administer it during the first 24 hours. Following this initial period, the dosage should be at the physician's discretion.

As with all modified release morphine preparations, breakthrough pain may occur. An immediate release form of morphine should, therefore, be available to the patient as rescue medication. Careful attention should be paid to the total daily morphine dosage. The prolonged effects of morphine in the Oramorph SR formulation should also be borne in mind.

Oramorph SR is not recommended for use in children.

*Contra-indications:* Respiratory depression, obstructive airways disease, known morphine sensitivity, acute hepatic disease, acute abdomen, paralytic ileus, acute alcoholism, head injuries and where the intracranial pressure is raised. Concurrent administration of monoamine oxidase inhibitors or within two weeks of discontinuation of their use. Oramorph SR Tablets should not be given during an attack of bronchial asthma nor in heart failure secondary to chronic lung disease.

*Special warnings and special precautions for use:*
*Precautions:* Nausea, vomiting and confusion may be troublesome. Care should be exercised in hypothyroidism, and where there is reduced respiratory reserve, such as kyphoscoliosis, emphysema and severe obesity. If constipation occurs, this may be treated with appropriate laxatives.

It is wise to reduce dosage in chronic hepatic and renal disease, myxoedema, adrenocortical insufficiency, prostatic hypertrophy or shock. It should be used with caution in patients with either obstructive bowel disorders, convulsive disorders or myasthenia gravis. Tolerance and dependence may occur.

*Interaction with other medicaments and other forms of interaction:* Phenothiazine anti-emetics may be given with morphine, but it should be noted that morphine potentiates the effects of tranquillisers, anaesthetics, hypnotics, sedatives and alcohol. Morphine's gastrointestinal effects may also delay the absorption of certain drugs, e.g. mexiletine, or be counteractive, as with metoclopramide.

*Pregnancy and lactation:* Although morphine sulphate has been in general use for many years, there is inadequate evidence of safety in human pregnancy and lactation. Morphine is known to cross the placenta and is excreted in breast milk, and may thus cause respiratory depression in the newborn infant.

Medicines should not be used in pregnancy, especially the first trimester, unless the expected benefit outweighs any possible risk to the foetus.

*Effects on ability to drive and use machines:* Patients taking Oramorph SR tablets should not operate dangerous machinery. Patients should be warned that Oramorph may affect their ability to drive.

*Undesirable effects:* Morphine may cause dry mouth, sweating, facial flushing, vertigo, bradycardia, palpitations, orthostatic hypotension, hypothermia, restlessness, changes of mood and miosis. Micturition may be difficult and there may be ureteric or biliary spasm. There is also an antidiuretic effect. These effects are more common in ambulant patients than in those who are bedridden. Raised intracranial pressure occurs in some patients.

*Overdose:*
*Signs of morphine toxicity and overdosage:* These are likely to consist of pin-point pupils, respiratory depression and hypotension. Circulatory failure and deepening coma may occur in more severe cases. Convulsions may occur in infants and children. Death may occur from respiratory failure.

*Treatment of morphine overdosage:* Administer

naloxone 400 micrograms intravenously. Repeat at 2–3 minute intervals as necessary, or by an infusion of 2 mg in 500 ml of normal saline or 5% dextrose (4 micrograms/ml). Empty the stomach. A 0.02% aqueous solution of potassium permanganate may be used for lavage. Assist respiration if necessary. Maintain fluid and electrolyte levels.

### Pharmacological properties

*Pharmacodynamic properties:* Morphine is an opioid analgesic. It acts mainly on the central nervous system and thus on smooth muscle. Although morphine is predominantly a central nervous system depressant it has some central stimulant actions which result in nausea and vomiting and miosis. Morphine generally increases smooth muscle tone, especially the sphincters of the gastro-intestinal tract.

Morphine and related analgesics may produce both physical and psychological dependence and should therefore be used with discrimination. Tolerance may also develop.

Morphine is an alagesic used for the symptomatic relief of moderate to severe pain, especially that associated with neoplastic disease, myocardial infarction and surgery. When pain is likely to be of short duration, a short-acting analgesic is usually preferred. In addition to relieving pain, morphine also alleviates the anxiety associated with severe pain. It is useful as a hypnotic where sleeplessness is due to pain and may also relieve the pain of biliary or renal colic, although an antispasmodic may also be required since morphine may increase smooth muscle tone.

Morphine reduces motility and is used in the symptomatic treatment of diarrhoea. It also relieves the dyspnoea of left ventricular failure and of pulmonary oedema. It is effective for the suppression of cough, but codeine is usually preferred as there is less risk of dependence. Morphine has been used pre-operatively as an adjunct to anaesthesia for pain relief and to allay anxiety. It has also been used in high doses as a general anaesthetic in specialised procedures. Morphine is usually administered as the sulphate, although the hydrochloride and the tartrate are used in simular doses; the acetate has also been used. Routes of administration include the oral, subcutaneous, intramuscular, intravenous, intraspinal and rectal routes. Parenteral doses may be intermittent injections or continuous or intermittent infusions adjusted according to individual analgesic requirements.

*Pharmacokinetic properties:* Morphine has a plasma half-life of about 2 to 3 hours and if given I.V. must be administered frequently. Oramorph SR on the other hand, being a sustained release preparation of morphine, has the advantage that it is only administered twice daily.

A summary of the morphine pharmacokinetic parameters is given below:

(a) Half-life; Plasma half-life; about 2–3 hours
(b) volume of Distribution; about 3–5 litres/kg
(c) Clearance; Plasma clearance; about 15 to 20 ml/min/kg
(d) Protein Binding; in plasma 20–35%

Pharmacokinetic parameters pertinent to Oramorph SR are summarised in the following table:

| Parameters | Oramorph SR Fasting (A) | Oramorph SR Food (B) |
|---|---|---|
| AUC$_{0-t}$ (NG.HR/ML) | 46.02±18.85 | 59.88±20.52 |
| C$_{max}$ (NG/ML) | 9.2±3.6 | 13.6±4.6 |
| T$_{max}$ (Hours) | 2.5±1.7 | 3.9±1.6 |

*Preclinical safety data:* No preclinical safety data are available which are additional to the experience gained in man over many years.

### Pharmaceutical particulars

*List of excipients:* Lactose, hydroxyethylcellulose, hypromellose, polyvinylpyrrolidone, talc, magnesium stearate, Opadry buff OY-3607 (10 mg tablet), Opadry violet OY-6708 (30 mg tablet), Opadry orange OY-3533 (60 mg tablet), and Opadry grey OY-8238 (100 mg tablet). The coating agents contain the following constituents:

*Opadry Buff OY-3607:* Hypromellose; polyethylene glycol 400; titanium dioxide (E171); iron oxide yellow (E172); iron oxide red (E172).

*Opadry Orange OY-3533:* Hypromellose; polyethylene glycol 400; titanium dioxide (E171); sunset yellow FCF aluminium lake (E110).

*Opadry Violet OY-6708:* Hypromellose; polyethylene glycol 400; titanium dioxide (E171); erythrosine aluminium lake (E121); indigo carmine aluminium lake (E132); sunset yellow FCF aluminium lake (E110).

*Opadry Grey OY-8238:* Hypromellose; polyethylene glycol 400; titanium dioxide (E171); iron oxide black (E172).

*Incompatibilities:* None known.

*Shelf life:* 3 years below 25°C.

*Special precautions for storage:* Store below 25°C in a dry place and protect from light.

*Nature and contents of container:* Polypropylene securitainers with low density polyethylene caps, containing 10 or 60 tablets; or blister packs of a hard-tempered aluminium foil (20 microns), coated outside with nitrocellulose lacquer and inside with a heat-seal lacquer bonded to clear PVC (250 microns) containing 10 or 60 tablets.

*Instructions for use/handling:* No special handling instructions are required.

**Marketing authorisation numbers**
Oramorph SR Tablets 10 mg　　　　0015/0208
Oramorph SR Tablets 30 mg　　　　0015/0209
Oramorph SR Tablets 60 mg　　　　0015/0210
Oramorph SR Tablets 100 mg　　　　0015/0211

**Date of approval/revision of SPC**　October 1995.

**Legal category**　CD (Sch 2), POM.

## ORAMORPH* UNIT DOSE VIALS

**Presentation**　Clear, colourless solution in 5 ml polyethylene Unit Dose Vials containing 10 mg/5 ml, 30 mg/5 ml, 100 mg/5 ml Morphine Sulphate.

**Uses**　Oramorph Unit Dose Vials are indicated for the relief of severe pain.

**Dosage and administration**　For oral use only.

*Adults:* The usual starting dose is 10-20 mg (5-10 ml) or Oramorph 10 mg/5 ml Unit Dose Vials every 4 hours.

The dosage can be increased under medical supervision according to the severity of the pain and the patients previous history of analgesic requirements, using Oramorph 30 mg/5 ml Unit Dose Vials or Oramorph 100 mg/5 ml Unit Dose Vials.

*Children under 5 years:* Not recommended.

*6-12 years:* Maximum dose 10 mg (5 ml of Oramorph 10 mg/5 ml Unit Dose Vial) every 4 hours.

Reductions in dosage may be appropriate in the elderly or in debilitated patients or where sedation is undesirable.

The required dose may be added to a soft drink immediately prior to administration.

When patients are transferred from other morphine preparations to Oramorph Unit Dose Vials, dosage titration may be appropriate. Morphine sulphate BP is readily absorbed from the gastro-intestinal tract following oral administration. However, when Oramorph Unit Dose Vials are used in place of parenteral morphine, a 50% to 100% increase in dosage is usually required to achieve the same level of analgesia.

*Contra-indications, warnings, etc:* Respiratory depression, obstructive airways disease, known morphine sensitivity, acute hepatic disease, acute alcoholism, head injuries, coma, convulsive disorders and where the intracranial pressure is raised. Concurrent administration of monoamine oxidase inhibitors or within 10 days of discontinuation of their use.

*Precautions:* Nausea, vomiting and constipation may be troublesome. Phenothiazine anti-emetics may be given with morphine, but it should be noted that morphine potentiates the effects of tranquillisers, anaesthetics, hypnotics, sedatives and alcohol.

Care should be exercised if morphine sulphate is given in the first 24 hours post-operatively, in hyperthyroidism, and where there is reduced respiratory reserve, such as kyphoscoliosis, emphysema and severe obesity. Morphine sulphate should not be given if paralytic ileus is likely to occur. If constipation occurs, this may be treated with appropriate laxatives.

It is wise to reduce dosage in chronic hepatic and renal disease, myxoedema, adrenocortical insufficiency, prostatic hypertrophy or shock. Tolerance and dependence may occur.

*Side effects:* In routine clinical practice, the commonest side effects of morphine sulphate are nausea, vomiting, constipation, drowsiness and confusion. If constipation occurs, this may be treated with appropriate laxatives. Micturition may be difficult and there may be ureteric or biliary spasm. There is also an antidiuretic effect. Dry mouth, sweating, facial flushing, vertigo, bradycardia, palpitations, orthostatic hypotension, hypothermia, restlessness, changes of moods and miosis can also occur. These effects are more common in ambulant patients than in those who are bedridden. Raised intracranial pressure occurs in some patients. As a consequence of histamine release, urticaria and/or pruritus may occur in some individuals.

*Use in pregnancy and lactation:* Although morphine sulphate has been in general use for many years, there is inadequate evidence of safety in human pregnancy and lactation. Morphine is known to cross the placenta and is excreted in breast milk, and may thus cause respiratory depression in the new born infant.

Medicines should not be used in pregnancy, especially the first trimester, unless the expected benefit outweighs any possible risk to the foetus.

*Effects on ability to drive and use machinery:* Morphine may cause drowsiness and confusion. Patients should be warned not to drive or operate dangerous machinery after taking Oramorph.

*Overdosage: Signs of morphine toxicity and overdosage:* These are likely to consist of pin-point pupils, respiratory depression and hypotension. Circulatory failure and deepening coma may occur in more severe cases. Convulsions may occur in infants and children. Death may occur from respiratory failure.

*Treatment of morphine overdosage:* Administer 400 micrograms naloxone intravenously.

Thereafter repeat at 2-3 minute intervals as necessary, or by an infusion of 2 mg in 500 ml of normal saline or 5% dextrose (4 micrograms/ml). Empty the stomach. A 0.02% aqueous solution of potassium permanganate may be used for lavage. Assist respiration if necessary. Maintain fluid and electrolyte levels.

**Pharmaceutical precautions**　Store below 25°C. Protect from light. Discard unused solution after administration.

**Legal category**
10 mg/5 ml UDV POM
30 mg/5 ml UDV POM, CD
100 mg/5 ml UDV POM, CD

**Package quantities**　Packs containing 25 vials.

**Further information**　Oramorph UDVs do not contain preservatives

Oramorph is also available as Oramorph Oral Solution (10 mg/5 ml), Oramorph Concentrated Oral Solution (20 mg/5 ml) and Oramorph SR Tablets.

**Product licence numbers**
10 mg/5 ml UDV　0015/0157
30 mg/5 ml UDV　0015/0158
100 mg/5 ml UDV　0015/0159

## POSIJECT*

**Presentation**　Posiject (dobutamine hydrochloride for injection): ampoules containing 5 ml of a colourless to pale yellow sterile solution for intravenous use only. Each ml contains 50 mg dobutamine, 1 mg ascorbic acid and water for injections.

**Uses**

*Actions:* The primary action of dobutamine is to augment cardiac contractility by stimulating the β1 receptors of the heart. It is a direct-acting agent.

*Indications:* Posiject is indicated for adults who require inotropic support in the treatment of low output cardiac failure associated with myocardial infarction, open heart surgery, cardiomyopathies, septic shock and cardiogenic shock. Posiject can also increase or maintain cardiac output during positive end expiratory pressure (PEEP) ventilation.

Posiject may also be used for cardiac stress testing as an alternative to exercise in patients for whom routine exercise testing cannot be satisfactorily performed. This use of dobutamine should only be undertaken in units which already perform exercise stress testing and all normal care and precautions required for such testing are also required when using dobutamine for this purpose.

**Dosage and administration**　For intravenous administration only.

Posiject Solution must be diluted to at least 50 ml with either: Sodium Chloride Intravenous Infusion BP or 5% Dextrose Intravenous Infusion BP.

Dilution to 250 ml or 500 ml, will give the following concentrations:

250 ml contains 1,000 micrograms/ml of dobutamine.

500 ml contains 500 micrograms/ml of dobutamine.

The final volume administered should be determined by the fluid requirements of the patient. Concentrations as high as 5,000 micrograms/ml have been used in patients on a restricted fluid intake. High concentrations of dobutamine should only be given with an infusion pump, to ensure accurate dosage.

The diluted solution may be stored for up to 24 hours in a refrigerator.

*Administration:* Due to its short half life, Posiject must be administered as a continuous intravenous infusion. After dilution, Posiject should be administered intravenously through an intravenous needle or catheter. An i.v. drip chamber or other suitable metering device is essential for controlling the rate of flow in drops per minute.

*Recommended dosage for adults and the elderly:*
*Cardiac stress testing:* When used as an alternative to exercise for cardiac stress testing the content of one

ampoule (250 mg) should be diluted to 250 ml with Sodium Chloride Intravenous Infusion BP or 5% Dextrose Intravenous Infusion BP to give a final concentration of 1,000 micrograms/ml. The diluted solution should be administered with an infusion pump to ensure accurate delivery. The recommended dose is an incremental increase of 5 micrograms/kg/minute from 5 up to 20 micrograms/kg/minute, each dose being infused for 8 minutes. Continuous ECG monitoring is essential and the infusion should be terminated in the event of >3 mm ST segment depression or any ventricular arrhythmia. The infusion should also be terminated if heart rate reaches the age/sex maximum, systolic blood pressure rises above 220 mm Hg or any side-effects occur – see 'Side-effects'.

*Other uses:* Most patients will respond satisfactorily to doses ranging from 2.5 to 10 micrograms/kg/minute. Occasionally, however, a dose as low as 0.5 micrograms/kg/minute will elicit a response.

The rate of administration and the duration of therapy should be adjusted according to the individual patient's response.

Rather than abruptly discontinuing therapy with Posiject, it is advisable to decrease the dosage gradually.

Side-effects, which are dose-related, are infrequent when Posiject is administered at rates below 10 micrograms/kg/minute. Rates as high as 40 micrograms/kg/minute have been used occasionally without significant adverse effects.

*Paediatric use:* The safety and efficacy of dobutamine for use in children have not been established.

### Contra-indications, warnings, etc
*Contra-indications:* Previous hypersensitivity to dobutamine. Patients with hypovolaemia.

*Warnings:* If an undue increase in heart rate or systolic blood pressure occurs or if an arrythmia is precipitated the dose of dobutamine should be reduced or the drug should be discontinued temporarily.

Dobutamine may precipitate or exacerbate ventricular ectopic activity: rarely it has caused ventricular tachycardia or fibrillation. Because dobutamine facilitates atrioventricular conduction, patients with atrial flutter or fibrillation may develop rapid ventricular responses.

Particular care should be exercised when dobutamine is used in patients with acute myocardial infarction because any significant increase in heart rate or excessive increases in arterial pressure that occur may intensify ischaemia and cause anginal pain and ST segment elevation.

Inotropic agents, including dobutamine, do not improve haemodynamics in most patients with mechanical obstruction that hinders either ventricular filling or outflow, or both. Inotropic response may be inadequate in patients with markedly reduced ventricular compliance. Such conditions are present in cardiac tamponade, valvular aortic stenosis, and idiopathic hypertrophic subaortic stenosis.

Minimal vasoconstriction has occasionally been observed, most notably in patients recently treated with a β-blocking drug. As the inotropic effect of dobutamine stems from stimulation of cardiac $\beta_1$ receptors, this effect is prevented by β-blocking drugs. However, dobutamine has been shown to counteract the cardiodepressive effects of β-blocking drugs. Conversely, α-adrenergic blockade may make the $\beta_1$ and $\beta_2$ effects apparent, resulting in tachycardia and vasodilatation.

The use of dobutamine as an alternative to exercise for cardiac stress testing is not recommended for patients with unstable angina, bundle branch block, valvular heart disease, aortic outflow obstruction or any cardiac condition that could make them unsuitable for exercise stress testing.

*Usage in pregnancy:* Reproduction studies performed in rats and rabbits have revealed no evidence of impaired fertility, harm to the fetus, or teratogenic effects due to dobutamine. As there are no adequate and well-controlled studies in pregnant women, and as animal reproduction studies are not always predictive of human response, dobutamine should not be used during pregnancy unless the potential benefits outweigh the potential risks to the fetus.

*Precautions:* During the administration of dobutamine, as with any parenteral catecholamine, heart rate and rhythm, arterial blood pressure, and infusion rate should be monitored closely. When initiating therapy, electrocardiographic monitoring is advisable until a stable response is achieved. Dobutamine should only be used in specialist units in which adequate facilities are available for patient surveillance and the monitoring of responses.

Precipitous decreases in blood pressure have occasionally been described in association with dobutamine therapy. Decreasing the dose or discontinuing the infusion typically results in rapid return of blood pressure to base line values, but rarely intervention may be required and reversibility may not be immediate. Dobutamine should be used with caution in the presence of severe hypotension complicating cardiogenic shock (mean arterial pressure less than 70 mm Hg).

Hypovolaemia should be corrected when necessary with whole blood or plasma before dobutamine is administered.

If arterial blood pressure remains low or decreases progressively during administration of dobutamine despite adequate ventricular filling pressure and cardiac output, consideration may be given to the concomitant use of a peripheral vasoconstrictor agent, such as dopamine or noradrenaline.

*Side-effects:* For cardiovascular effects, see *Warnings* and *Precautions.*

The following side-effects have been reported rarely: nausea, headache, anginal pain, non-specific chest pain, palpitations, shortness of breath, and reactions suggestive of hypersensitivity, including rash, fever, eosinophilia and bronchospasm.

As with other catecholamines, decreases in serum potassium concentrations have occurred, rarely to hypokalaemic values.

*Reactions at site of intravenous infusion:* Phlebitis has occasionally been reported. Local inflammatory changes have been described following inadvertent infiltration.

*Long-term safety:* Infusions for up to 72 hours have revealed no adverse effects other than those seen with shorter infusions. There is evidence that partial tolerance develops with continuous infusions of dobutamine for 72 hours or more; therefore, higher doses may be required to maintain the same effects.

*Overdosage:* Overdoses of dobutamine have been reported rarely. The symptoms of toxicity may include anorexia, nausea, vomiting, tremor, anxiety, palpitations, headache, shortness of breath and anginal and non-specific chest pain. The positive inotropic and chronotropic effects of dobutamine may cause hypertension, tachyarrhythmias, myocardial ischaemia and ventricular fibrillation. Hypotension may result from vasodilatation.

The duration of action of dobutamine hydrochloride is generally short (half-life approximately 2 minutes).

Temporarily discontinue dobutamine until the patient's condition stabilises. The patient should be monitored and any appropriate resuscitative measures initiated promptly.

Forced diuresis, peritoneal dialysis, or charcoal haemoperfusion have not been established as beneficial.

If the product is ingested, unpredictable absorption may occur from the mouth and gastrointestinal tract.

**Pharmaceutical precautions** Store undiluted ampoules of Posiject below 25°C and protect from light. If solid particles are evident, do not use.

Prior to administration, Posiject Concentrate must be further diluted to at least 50 ml with either: Sodium Chloride Intravenous Infusion BP or 5% Dextrose Intravenous Infusion BP.

The diluted solution may be stored for up to 24 hours in a refrigerator.

No other intravenous preparation should be administered in the same solution as Posiject.

Posiject should not be mixed with alkaline solutions.

Discard any unused contents of the ampoule.

**Legal category** POM.

**Package quantities** Packs containing 5×5 ml ampoules.

**Further information** Nil.

**Product licence number** 0015/0180.

*Trade Mark

# Boehringer Mannheim UK Limited
## Simpson Parkway
## Kirkton Campus
## Livingston, West Lothian
## EH54 7BH

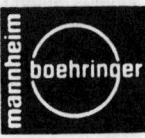

## BEZALIP*

**Presentation** Bezalip is presented as white, round film-coated tablets bearing the identification code BM/G6. Each tablet contains 200 mg bezafibrate.

The product contains lactose. No synthetic colouring substances are present in the formulation.

**Uses** Bezalip is indicated for use in hyperlipidaemias of Type IIa, IIb, III, IV and V (Fredrickson classification).

Bezalip should be employed only in patients with a fully defined and diagnosed lipid abnormality which is inadequately controlled by dietary means, or by other changes in life-style such as physical exercise and weight reduction, and in whom the long-term risks associated with the condition warrant treatment.

The rationale for the use of Bezalip is to control abnormalities of serum lipids and lipoproteins to reduce or prevent the long term adverse effects which have been shown by many epidemiological studies to be positively and strongly correlated with such hyperlipidaemias.

## Dosage and administration

*Adults:* The recommended dosage for Bezalip tablets is three tablets daily, equivalent to 600 mg bezafibrate. The tablets should be swallowed whole with a little fluid after each meal.

*Elderly:* No specific dosage reduction is necessary in elderly patients.

*Children:* At present there is inadequate information regarding an appropriate dosage in children.

*Renal impairment:* In patients with renal insufficiency the dose should be adjusted according to serum creatinine levels or creatinine clearance as shown in the following table.

| Serum creatinine (micromol/l) | Creatinine clearance (ml/min) | Dosage (tablets/day) |
|---|---|---|
| Up to 135 | Over 60 | 3 |
| 136–225 | 60–40 | 2 |
| 226–530 | 40–15 | 1 every 1 or 2 days |
| Over 530 | Less than 15 | 1 every 3rd day |
| Dialysis Patients | | 1 every 3rd day |

The response to therapy is normally rapid, although a progressive improvement may occur over a number of weeks. Treatment should be withdrawn if an adequate response has not been achieved within 3 to 4 months.

## Contra-indications, warnings, etc

*Contra-indications:* Significant hepatic disease (other than fatty infiltration of the liver associated with raised triglyceride values), gall bladder disease with or without cholelithiasis, nephrotic syndrome. Hypersensitivity to bezafibrate.

*Pregnancy and lactation:* Although the drug substance has not been shown in animal studies to have any adverse effects on the foetus, it is recommended that Bezalip should not be administered to either pregnant women or to those who are breast feeding.

*Warnings:* The chronic administration of a high dose of bezafibrate to rats was associated with hepatic tumour formation in females. This dosage was in the order of 30 to 40 times the human dosage. No such effect was apparent at reduced intake levels approximating more closely to the lipid-lowering dosage in humans.

*Interactions:* Care is required in administering Bezalip to patients taking coumarin-type anti-coagulants, the action of which may be potentiated. The dosage of anti-coagulant should be reduced by up to 50% and readjusted by monitoring blood coagulation.

As bezafibrate improves glucose utilisation the action of antidiabetic medication, including insulin, may be potentiated. Hypoglycaemia has not been observed although increased monitoring of the glycaemic status may be warranted for a brief period after introduction of Bezalip.

Should combined therapy with an ion-exchange resin be considered necessary, there should be an interval of 2 hours between the intake of the resin and Bezalip as the absorption of bezafibrate otherwise may be impaired.

Combination therapy with HMG CoA reductase inhibitors and fibric acid derivatives has been reported to increase the risk of myopathy and should therefore be used with caution. Patients should be monitored for signs of myopathy and increased creatine kinase activity. This combination therapy should not be used in patients with predisposing factors for myopathy (impaired renal function, severe infection, trauma, surgery, disturbances of hormone or electrolyte balance).

MAO-inhibitors (with hepatotoxic potential) should not be administered together with bezafibrate.

Since oestrogens may lead to a rise in lipid levels, the necessity for treatment with Bezalip in patients receiving oestrogens or oestrogen containing preparations should be considered on an individual basis.

*Adverse effects:* Adverse effects during treatment with Bezalip most frequently are gastro-intestinal in nature, such as loss of appetite, nausea or gastric discomfort. These symptoms generally are transient and do not require withdrawal of therapy. In susceptible patients a slowly increasing dosage over 5 to 7 days may help to avoid such symptoms. More rarely there may be allergic skin reactions such as pruritus or urticaria or general hypersensitivity reactions. Increased hair loss and disturbances of potency have been reported. There have also been reports of marked elevations of creatinine kinase, myositis, myopathy and rarely rhabdomyolysis. Patients who develop signs of myotoxicity should be monitored closely and serum creatine kinase levels checked. Treatment with Bezalip should be stopped if myopathy is suspected or if creatine kinase increases to ≥10 times the upper limit of normal. All of these adverse effects generally resolve rapidly following withdrawal of therapy. Rarely headache, dizziness, decreases of haemoglobin, leucocytes, platelets and single cases of increases in transaminases have been reported. Slight increases in serum creatinine may occur. Special care is needed in patients with renal disease as progressive increases in the serum creatinine level and/or failure to follow the dosage guidelines may result in myotoxicity (rhabdomyolysis).

Bezafibrate may increase the lithogenic index in some patients although studies have shown inconsistent results. There have been isolated reports of the occurrence of gallstones. However, there is no evidence that the administration of Bezalip is associated with an increased frequency of gallstones.

*Overdosage:* The effects of acute overdosage are unknown although no serious biochemical or clinical effects are likely. Treatment, if necessary, should be symptomatic.

**Pharmaceutical precautions** Bezalip requires no special storage conditions. As with most medicines, however, and in accordance with normal pharmaceutical practice, the tablets should be stored in a cool, dry place.

**Legal category** POM.

**Package quantities** Packs of 100 tablets.

**Further information** The protein-binding of bezafibrate in serum is approximately 95%. The elimination half-life is in the order of 2.1 hours although elimination is markedly slowed in the presence of limited renal function. Elimination may be increased in forced diuresis. The drug substance is non-dialysable (cuprophane filter).

Studies have shown bezafibrate to be effective in treating hyperlipidaemia in patients with diabetes mellitus. Some cases showed a beneficial reduction in fasting blood glucose.

Significant reductions in serum fibrinogen levels have been observed in hyperfibrinogenaemic patients treated with bezafibrate.

**Product licence number** 15722/0006.

## BEZALIP MONO*

**Presentation** Bezalip Mono is a white, round, film-coated tablet with a white core and is imprinted BM/D9. Each modified release tablet contains 400 mg bezafibrate. Lactose is present in the formulation.

**Uses** Bezalip Mono is indicated for use in hyperlipidaemias of Type IIa, IIb, III, IV and V (Fredrickson classification).

Bezalip Mono should be employed only in patients with a fully defined and diagnosed lipid abnormality which is inadequately controlled by dietary means, or by other changes in life-style such as physical exercise and weight reduction, and in whom the long-term risks associated with the condition warrant treatment.

The rationale for the use of Bezalip Mono is to control abnormalities of serum lipids and lipoproteins to reduce or prevent the long term adverse effects which have been shown by many epidemiological studies to be positively and strongly correlated with such hyperlipidaemias.

## Dosage and administration

*Adults:* The dosage for Bezalip Mono is one tablet daily, equivalent to 400 mg bezafibrate. The tablets should be swallowed whole with a little fluid after a meal either at night or in the morning.

*Elderly:* No specific dosage reduction is necessary in elderly patients.

*Children:* At present there is inadequate information regarding an appropriate dosage in children.

*Renal impairment:* Bezalip Mono is contraindicated in patients with renal impairment with serum creatinine greater than 135 micromol/l or creatinine clearance less than 60 ml/min. Such patients may be treated with conventional Bezalip tablets (200 mg bezafibrate) using an appropriately reduced daily dosage.

The response to therapy is normally rapid, although a progressive improvement may occur over a number of weeks. Treatment should be withdrawn if an adequate response has not been achieved within 3 to 4 months.

## Contra-indications, warnings, etc

*Contra-indications:* Significant hepatic disease (other than fatty infiltration of the liver associated with raised triglyceride values), gall bladder disease with or without cholelithiasis, nephrotic syndrome or renal impairment (serum creatinine greater than 135 micromol/l or creatinine clearance less than 60 ml/min). Patients undergoing dialysis. Hypersensitivity to bezafibrate.

*Pregnancy and lactation:* Although the drug substance has not been shown in animal studies to have any adverse effects on the foetus, it is recommended that Bezalip Mono should not be administered to either pregnant women or to those who are breast feeding.

*Warnings:* The chronic administration of a high dose of bezafibrate to rats was associated with hepatic tumour formation in females. This dosage was in the order of 30 to 40 times the human dosage. No such effect was apparent at reduced intake levels approximating more closely to the lipid-lowering dosage in humans.

*Interactions:* Care is required in administering Bezalip Mono to patients taking coumarin-type anti-coagulants, the action of which may be potentiated. The dosage of anti-coagulant should be reduced by up to 50% and readjusted by monitoring blood coagulation.

As bezafibrate improves glucose utilisation the action of antidiabetic medication, including insulin, may be potentiated. Hypoglycaemia has not been observed although increased monitoring of the glycaemic status may be warranted for a brief period after introduction of Bezalip Mono.

Should combined therapy with an ion-exchange resin be considered necessary, there should be an interval of 2 hours between the intake of the resin and Bezalip Mono as the absorption of bezafibrate otherwise may be impaired.

Combination therapy with HMG CoA reductase inhibitors and fibric acid derivatives has been reported to increase the risk of myopathy and should therefore be used with caution. Patients should be monitored for signs of myopathy and increased creatine kinase activity. This combination therapy should not be used in patients with predisposing factors for myopathy (impaired renal function, severe infection, trauma, surgery, disturbances of hormone or electrolyte balance).

MAO-inhibitors (with hepatotoxic potential) should not be administered together with bezafibrate.

Since oestrogens may lead to a rise in lipid levels, the necessity for treatment with Bezalip Mono in patients receiving oestrogens or oestrogen containing preparations should be considered on an individual basis.

*Adverse effects:* Adverse effects during treatment with Bezalip Mono most frequently are gastro-intestinal in nature, such as loss of appetite, nausea or gastric discomfort. These symptoms generally are transient and do not require withdrawal of therapy. In susceptible patients a slowly increasing dosage over 5 to 7 days with Bezalip Mono tablets may help to avoid such symptoms. More rarely there may be allergic skin reactions such as pruritus or urticaria or general hypersensitivity reactions. Increased hair loss and disturbances of potency have been reported. There have also been reports of marked elevations of creatine kinase, myositis, myopathy and rarely rhabdomyolysis. Patients who develop signs of myotoxicity should be monitored closely and serum creatine kinase levels checked. Treatment with Bezalip Mono should be stopped if myopathy is suspected or if creatine kinase increases to ≥10 times the upper limit of normal. All of these adverse effects generally resolve rapidly following withdrawal of therapy. Rarely headache, dizziness, decreases of haemoglobin, leucocytes, platelets and single cases of increases in transaminases have been reported. Slight increases in serum creatinine may occur. Special care is needed in patients with renal disease as progressive increases in the serum creatinine level and/or failure to follow the dosage guidelines may result in myotoxicity (rhabdomyolysis).

Bezafibrate may increase the lithogenic index in some patients although studies have shown inconsistent results. There have been isolated reports of the occurrence of gallstones. However, there is no evidence that the administration of Bezalip Mono is associated with an increased frequency of gallstones.

*Overdosage:* The effects of acute overdosage are unknown although no serious biochemical or clinical effects are likely. Treatment, if necessary, should be symptomatic.

**Pharmaceutical precautions** Bezalip Mono requires no special storage conditions. As with most medicines, however, and in accordance with normal pharmaceutical practice, the tablets should be stored in a cool, dry place.

**Legal category** POM.

**Package quantities** Calendar packs of 28 tablets.

**Further information** The protein-binding of bezafibrate in serum is approximately 95%. The elimination half-life is in the order of 2.1 hours although elimination is markedly slowed in the presence of limited renal function. Elimination may be increased in forced diuresis. The drug substance is non-dialysable (cuprophane filter).

Studies have shown bezafibrate to be effective in treating hyperlipidaemia in patients with diabetes mellitus. Some cases showed a beneficial reduction in fasting blood glucose.

Significant reductions in serum fibrinogen levels have been observed in hyperfibrinogenaemic patients treated with bezafibrate.

**Product licence number** 15722/0013.

## CORO-NITRO* PUMP SPRAY (CFC FREE)

**Qualitative and quantitative composition** In terms of the active ingredients: Glyceryl trinitrate 0.4 mg per shot.

**Pharmaceutical form** Oromucosal spray.

**Clinical particulars**

*Therapeutic indications:* Treatment and prophylaxis of angina pectoris.

*Posology and method of administration*

*Adults:* The normal dosage is one or two spray puffs (0.4 to 0.8 mg glyceryl trinitrate) as required for relief of anginal pain or for short term prophylaxis before physical or emotional stress or other factors known to precipitate anginal attacks. Occasionally up to 3 spray puffs (1.2 mg glyceryl trinitrate) may be needed at a single time in severe cases. In no circumstances should this be exceeded.

*Elderly:* As for adults. No special dosage requirements.

*Children:* Not recommended.

*Contra-indications:* Coro-Nitro Pump Spray is contra-indicated in hypotensive disorders including shock, in cases of significant cerebral trauma, acute myocardial infarction with low left ventricular filling pressure and in patients hypersensitive to glyceryl trinitrate.

*Special warnings and precautions for use:* None.

*Interactions with other medicaments and other forms of interactions:* The hypotensive effects of other drugs may be potentiated. Concomitant alcohol intake may enhance side effects and should be avoided.

*Pregnancy and lactation:* There is inadequate evidence of safety of glyceryl trinitrate in human pregnancy although nitrates have been in wide use for many years without apparent ill consequence, animal studies having shown no adverse effects on the foetus. Use in pregnancy and lactation is not recommended unless considered essential by the patient's physician.

*Effects on ability to drive and use machines:* The ability to drive or operate machinery may be impaired especially if the patient has been consuming alcohol or is taking other hypotensive medication.

*Undesirable effects:* A number of nitrate related adverse effects may occur including headache, facial flushing, dizziness, nausea, vomiting, feelings of weakness, postural hypotension and reflex tachycardia.

An initial burning or stinging sensation in the oral mucosa may occur. This is more likely if the patient has oral ulcers, cuts or other oral inflammation. Alternative therapy may be necessary.

*Overdose*

*Symptoms and signs:* Excessive dosage may promote severe headache, facial flushing, hypotension and fainting and, rarely, cyanosis and methaemoglobinaemia. In some cases the effect of overdose will closely resemble shock.

*Treatment:* Recovery normally occurs spontaneously. The patient should lie in a supine position with the legs elevated to promote venous return. Symptomatic treatment may be needed if there is severe circulatory or respiratory collapse. Methaemoglobinaemia will respond to methylene blue infusion.

**Pharmacological properties**

*Pharmacodynamic properties:* Glyceryl trinitrate reduces cardiac workload by venous dilation and may also have a beneficial action through dilation of coronary arteries. These actions bring about a reduction in the requirement for oxygenated blood and may also increase the amount of oxygenated blood reaching the ischaemic heart.

*Pharmacokinetic properties:* Glyceryl trinitrate enters the blood stream very quickly over the mucous membrane of the mouth.

Following buccal administration of 0.8 mg glyceryl trinitrate in the form of 2 spray puffs of Coro-Nitro Pump Spray, peripheral vascular effects (measured by finger plethysmography) are evident within 2 minutes. The maximum effect is achieved within 10 minutes of application and this returns to the 2 minute level after 30 minutes. A residual dilation remains 60 minutes after application.

*Preclinical safety data:* Glyceryl trinitrate is a well established medicinal drug. No special preclinical studies were conducted for Coro-Nitro Pump Spray.

**Pharmaceutical particulars**

*List of excipients:* Alcohol (ethanol), medium chain triglycerides.

*Incompatibilities:* Not applicable.

*Shelf-life:* 24 months at room temperature.

*Special precautions for storage:* Coro-Nitro Pump Spray should be stored below 25°C and not close to direct sources of heat. The spray should not be used near naked flames.

*Nature and contents of container:* Glass bottles encased in red transparent PVC with metering valve and spray nozzle covered with a polypropylene cap.

Each Coro-Nitro Pump Spray will deliver 200 metered doses of 0.4 mg glyceryl trinitrate.

*Instructions for use/handling:* Coro-Nitro Pump Spray is for buccal administration and patients must be warned not to inhale the spray. During use the Pump Spray should be held upright, near to the open mouth. Pressure on the valve will release a single dose of 0.4 mg glyceryl trinitrate. The spray should be directed into the mouth preferably onto or under the tongue.

The valve of the Coro-Nitro Pump Spray must be pressed down three times prior to initial use. This fills the pumping chamber and ensures complete spray capacity. Subsequently the spray can be used immediately unless it has not been used for several days, in which case the valve should be pressed 1–2 times prior to use.

**Marketing authorisation number** 15722/0032.

**Date of approval/revision of SPC** March 1997.

**Legal category** P.

## EUCARDIC*

**Qualitative and quantitative composition** Eucardic 12.5 tablets each contain 12.5 mg carvedilol. Eucardic 25 tablets each contain 25.0 mg carvedilol.

**Pharmaceutical form** Tablets for oral administration.

**Clinical particulars**

*Therapeutic indications:* Treatment of hypertension.

*Posology and method of administration:*

*Adults:* The recommended dose for initiation of therapy is 12.5 mg once a day for the first two days. Thereafter the recommended dosage is 25 mg once a day. Although this is an adequate dose in most patients, if necessary the dose may be titrated up to a recommended daily maximum dose of 50 mg given once a day or in divided doses.

Dose titration should occur at intervals of at least two weeks.

*Elderly:* An initial dose of 12.5 mg daily is recommended. This has provided satisfactory control in some cases. If the response is inadequate the dose may be titrated up to the recommended daily maximum dose of 50 mg given once a day or in divided doses.

*Children:* Safety and efficacy in children has not yet been established.

*Contra-indications:* Second or third degree heart block, severe bradycardia, cardiogenic shock, uncontrolled heart failure, obstructive airways disease, hepatic impairment, hypersensitivity to carvedilol.

*Special warnings and precautions for use:* Special care should be taken in patients whose cardiac reserve is poor. Heart failure should be satisfactorily controlled with appropriate therapy before carvedilol is started.

Although angina has not been reported on stopping treatment, withdrawal should be gradual in patients with ischaemic heart disease as carvedilol has beta-blocking activity.

As with other beta-blocking drugs carvedilol may mask the symptoms of hyperthyroidism and early signs of acute hypoglycaemia may be masked in patients with diabetes mellitus. Alternatives to beta-blocking agents are generally preferred in insulin-dependent diabetic patients.

As for other drugs which produce changes in blood pressure, patients taking carvedilol should be warned not to drive or operate machinery if they experience dizziness or related symptoms. This may be most relevant when starting or changing treatment and when alcohol is taken.

The following warnings will be included on the outer packaging and leaflet:

*Packaging:* Do not take this medicine if you have a history of wheezing or asthma.

*Leaflet:* Do not take this medicine if you have a history of wheezing or asthma, Consult your doctor or pharmacist first.

*Interactions:* As with other anti-hypertensives, there is a potential for pronounced hypotension during general anaesthesia.

As with other agents with beta-blocking activity, carvedilol may potentiate the effect of other concomitantly administered drugs that are anti-hypertensive in action or have hypotension as part of their adverse effect profile.

As with other drugs with beta-blocking activity, caution should be exercised when administering Class I antiarrhythmic drugs or calcium antagonists such as verapamil. These drugs should not be administered intravenously.

Trough plasma digoxin levels may be increased in patients co-administered carvedilol and digoxin. Increased monitoring of digoxin levels is recommended when initiating, adjusting or discontinuing carvedilol.

Care may be required in those receiving inducers of mixed function oxidases e.g. rifampicin, as serum levels of carvedilol may be reduced.

*Use during pregnancy and lactation:* There is no evidence from animal studies that carvedilol has any teratogenic effects. Embryotoxicity was observed only after large doses in rabbits. The relevance of these findings for humans is uncertain. Animal studies have shown that carvedilol crosses the placental barrier and is excreted in breast milk and therefore the possible consequences of alpha and beta blockade in the human foetus and neonate should be borne in mind. With other alpha and beta blocking agents, effects have included perinatal and neonatal distress (bradycardia, hypotension, respiratory depression, hypoglycaemia, hypothermia). Carvedilol is therefore not recommended for use in pregnancy or in breast feeding mothers.

*Effects on ability to drive and use machines:* As for other drugs which produce changes in blood pressure, patients taking carvedilol should be warned not to drive or operate machinery if they experience dizziness or related symptoms.

*Undesirable effects:* Eucardic is usually well tolerated.

Symptomatic postural hypotension, mainly on the initiation of therapy or when increasing the dose, may occur but the incidence is minimised when the drug is used as recommended. Dizziness, headache, fatigue, gastrointestinal upset and bradycardia have been observed. These are usually mild, transient and occur early in the course of treatment.

Diminished peripheral circulation, dry eyes and flu-like symptoms have occurred occasionally.

Rarely angina pectoris, A-V block or exacerbation of symptoms in intermittent claudication may occur.

Skin reactions (e.g. allergic exanthema, urticaria, pruritus and lichen planus-like reactions) have been reported rarely. Psoriatic skin lesions may occur or existing lesions be exacerbated.

Stuffy nose, wheezing, depressed mood, sleep disturbance, paraesthesiae and progression of heart failure have been reported in isolated cases.

There have been isolated reports of changes in serum transaminases, thrombocytopaenia and leucopaenia.

*Overdosage:*
*Symptoms and signs:* Profound cardiovascular effects such as hypotension and bradycardia would be expected after massive overdose. Heart failure, cardiogenic shock and cardiac arrest may follow. Gastric lavage or induced emesis may be useful in the first few hours after ingestion.

Patients should be placed in the supine position. Atropine, 0.3 mg to 3 mg i.v. and/or glucagon 10 mg i.v. (followed by a slow i.v. infusion of 1 to 10 mg/hour if necessary) may be given when bradycardia is present. For excessive hypotension, intravenous fluids may be administered. In addition, noradrenaline may be given, either 5 to 10 micrograms i.v., repeated according to blood pressure response, or 5 micrograms per minute by infusion titrated to blood pressure. Bronchospasm may be treated using salbutamol or other beta$_2$-agonists.

**Pharmacological properties**
*Pharmacodynamics:* Carvedilol is a dual action cardiovascular agent with beta blocking and vasodilating properties. The beta blockage is non-cardioselective and is devoid of intrinsic sympathomimetic activity. Vasodilation is predominantly mediated through alpha$_1$ receptor antagonism.

*Pharmacokinetics:* The absolute bioavailability of carvedilol capsules (bioequivalent to the tablet formulation intended for marketing) was 22% in humans (range 10 to 49%).

Carvedilol exhibits a considerable first pass effect. The metabolite pattern reveals intensive metabolism with glucuronidation as one of the major steps.

Serum levels peak 1 to 3 hours after an oral dose. There is a linear relationship between the dose and serum concentrations. The average elimination half-life is 6 hours. The primary route of excretion is via the faeces.

Food does not affect bioavailability, residence time or the maximum serum concentration although the time to reach maximum serum concentration is delayed.

The pharmacokinetics of carvedilol are not affected by age. In a study in patients with cirrhotic liver disease, the bioavailability of carvedilol was four times greater and the peak plasma level five times higher than in healthy subjects. Since carvedilol is primarily excreted via the faeces, significant accumulation in patients with renal impairment is unlikely.

*Preclinical safety data*
*Acute toxicity:*

| Species | Test | I.V. | I.P. | P.O. |
|---|---|---|---|---|
| Mouse, female | LD$_{50}$ | 36 mg/kg | 364 mg/kg | >8000 mg/kg |
| Mouse, male | LD$_{50}$ | 27 mg/kg | 568 mg/kg | >8000 mg/kg |
| Rat, female | LD$_{50}$ | 25 mg/kg | 769 mg/kg | >8000 mg/kg |
| Rat, male | LD$_{50}$ | 27 mg/kg | 1244 mg/kg | >8000 mg/kg |

*Chronic toxicity:* No substance-related toxic effects were observed in animal studies.

*Oncogenicity and mutagenicity:* In two-year studies conducted in rats and mice employing dosages up to 75 mg/kg/day and 200 mg/kg/day, respectively (150 to 400 times the human dose), carvedilol had no carcinogenic effect.

Carvedilol was not mutagenic in *in vitro* or in *in vivo* non-mammalian and mammalian tests.

*Reproduction toxicity:* Carvedilol at dosages ≥200 mg/kg/day (≥400 times the human dose) was toxic to adult rats (sedation, reduced weight gain) and was associated with a reduced number of successful matings, prolonged mating time, significantly fewer corpora lutea and implants per dam and complete resorption of 18% of the litter. The no observed effect level for overt toxicity and impairment of fertility was 60 mg/kg/day (120 times the human dose).

**Pharmaceutical particulars**
*List of excipients:* All tablet strengths (12.5 mg, 25 mg and 50 mg) contain Sucrose Ph.Eur, Lactose Ph.Eur, Povidone USP, Colloidal Silicon Dioxide Ph.Eur, Cros-

povidone USNF and Magnesium Stearate Ph.Eur as inactive ingredients. The 12.5 mg tablet also contains yellow iron oxide and red iron oxide.

*Incompatibilities:* Not applicable.

*Shelf life:* 4 years in blister packs for 12.5 mg tablets. 5 years for 25 mg tablets in blister packs. 4 years in standard polypropylene tube packs for 25 mg tablets. 3 years in standard polypropylene tube packs for 12.5 mg tablets.

*Special precautions for storage:* Store in a dry place below 25°C. Protect from light (special labelling not required as protection given by carton).

*Nature and contents of containers:* Blister packs, opaque PVC/aluminium, containing 14, 28, 30, 56 or 100 tablets. Standard polypropylene tube packs of 100 tablets.

**Marketing authorisation numbers**
Eucardic 12.5     15722/0020
Eucardic 25     15722/0021.

**Date of approval/revision of SPC**   May 1997.

**Legal category**   POM.

## ISMO*

**Presentation**   Ismo tablets are white, circular, uncoated and contain isosorbide mononitrate. Lactose is present in the formulation.

The presentations available are:

*Ismo 10:* 10 mg isosorbide mononitrate. Each tablet is marked Ismo on one face and 10 on the reverse.

*Ismo 20:* 20 mg isosorbide mononitrate. Each tablet is marked with a score line and BMB3 on both faces.

*Ismo 40:* 40 mg isosorbide mononitrate. Each tablet is marked Ismo on one face and 40 on the reverse.

The Ismo Starter Pack contains both Ismo 10 and Ismo 20 tablets for initiation of therapy in new patients.

**Uses**   Ismo products are indicated for use in the treatment and prophylaxis of angina pectoris and as adjunctive therapy in congestive heart failure which does not respond adequately to cardiac glycosides and/or diuretics.

**Dosage and administration**
*Adults:* The recommended dosage is from 20 to 120 mg isosorbide mononitrate daily in divided doses. The majority of patients will require a dosage in the range of 40 to 60 mg daily in divided doses. The tablets should be taken with fluid and swallowed whole without chewing.

For patients who have not previously received prophylactic nitrate therapy it is recommended that the Ismo Starter Pack be employed. This provides an initial dosage of 10 mg isosorbide mononitrate (1 tablet) daily for 2 days followed by a dosage of 20 mg daily (1 tablet morning and evening) for a further 3 days. Subsequently the daily dosage may be increased to the normal prophylactic level using the Ismo 20 tablets also included in the Starter Pack. Patients already accustomed to chronic nitrate therapy normally may be transferred directly to a therapeutic dose of Ismo. For those previously treated with isosorbide dinitrate in conventional form the dosage of Ismo should be the same initially. Ismo is effectively twice as potent as sustained release forms of isosorbide dinitrate and patients transferred from such treatment initially should receive Ismo at half the previous dosage.

*Elderly:* There is no evidence to suggest an adjustment of dose is necessary. However, caution may be required in elderly patients who are known to be susceptible to the effects of hypotensive medication.

*Children:* The safety and efficacy of Ismo in children has not been established.

*Renal and hepatic impairment:* No dosage reduction is necessary.

**Contra-indications, warnings, etc**
*Contra-indications:* Ismo tablets are contra-indicated in patients with a known hypersensitivity to isosorbide mononitrate or isosorbide dinitrate and in cases of marked low blood pressure, shock and acute myocardial infarction with low left ventricular filling pressure.

*Precautions:* Ismo is not indicated for relief of an acute attack, sublingual or buccal glyceryl trinitrate tablets or spray should be used. In the case of acute myocardial infarction, Ismo tablets should be continued only under strict medical supervision. Since a rebound phenomenon cannot be excluded, therapy with isosorbide mononitrate should be terminated gradually rather than stopping abruptly.

*Use in pregnancy and lactation:* There is inadequate evidence of safety of isosorbide mononitrate in human pregnancy although nitrates have been in wide use for many years without ill consequence, animal studies having shown no adverse effects on the foetus. There is no information on excretion of

isosorbide mononitrate in breast milk. Use in pregnancy and lactation is not recommended unless considered essential by the patient's physician.

*Adverse effects:* A number of nitrate-related adverse effects may occur during treatment including headache and feelings of dizziness. The incidence of such effects is normally highest at the commencement of treatment and tends to decline with time. The Ismo Starter Pack is provided to assist in minimising such effects initially. In highly sensitive patients hypotension may occur, especially after a high dose. Other reactions, including feelings of weakness, nausea or vomiting may occur occasionally. Side-effects which have been associated with isosorbide dinitrate (e.g. flushing, postural hypotension, dry rash, exfoliative dermatitis) may also occur.

In theory, the ability to drive or to operate machinery may be impaired in patients experiencing hypotensive side effects.

*Interactions:* The hypotensive effects of other drugs may be potentiated.

*Overdosage:* In the event of overdosage the main sign is liable to be hypotension. The stomach should be aspirated to remove any remaining tablets. The patient should be placed in a supine position with the legs elevated to promote venous return. Symptomatic and supportive treatment e.g. plasma expanders and, if necessary, the careful use of vasopressor agents to counterbalance the hypotensive effects may be necessary. Methaemoglobinaemia will normally respond to methylene blue infusion.

**Pharmaceutical precautions**   No special storage or handling precautions apply although it is recommended that Ismo products be kept in a cool, dry place in accordance with good pharmaceutical practice.

**Legal category**   P.

**Package quantities**   Ismo Starter Pack: 8 tablets of Ismo 10 and 60 tablets of Ismo 20 in blister strips (OP).
Ismo 10: Packs of 100 tablets and packs of 60 tablets in blister strips (OP).
Ismo 20: Packs of 100 tablets and packs of 60 tablets in blister strips (OP).
Ismo 40: Packs of 100 tablets and packs of 60 tablets in blister strips (OP).

**Further information**   Ismo provides long term nitrate treatment of angina pectoris and heart failure in a form with complete biological availability due to lack of any significant hepatic first-pass metabolism. This provides consistently uniform blood levels of drug substance and a predictable clinical response. The onset of activity occurs within 20 minutes and, depending on dosage, is maintained for up to 10 hours.

Beta-blocking drugs have a different pharmacological action in angina and may have a complementary effect when co-administered with Ismo.

**Product licence numbers**   15722/0014, 15722/0011, 15722/0012.

## ISMO* RETARD

**Presentation**   Circular, white, sugar coated tablets containing 40 mg isosorbide mononitrate in a sustained release form. Lactose is present in the formulation.

**Uses**   Ismo Retard is indicated for the prophylaxis of angina pectoris.

**Dosage and administration**   Ismo Retard has been developed to provide a convenient, once daily dosage form of isosorbide mononitrate. It is designed to achieve therapeutic blood concentrations within 30 minutes which persist up to 17 hours. A nitrate free interval of up to 7 hours makes the development of anti-anginal tolerance during chronic therapy unlikely.

The tablets should be taken with fluid and swallowed whole without chewing.

*Adults:* One tablet daily, to be taken in the morning.

*Elderly:* There is no evidence to suggest an adjustment of dose is necessary. However, caution may be required in elderly patients who are known to be susceptible to the effects of hypotensive medication.

*Children:* The safety and efficacy of Ismo Retard in children has not been established.

*Renal and hepatic impairment:* No dosage reduction is necessary.

**Contra-indications, warnings, etc**
*Contra-indications:* Ismo Retard is contra-indicated in patients with a known hypersensitivity to isosorbide mononitrate or isosorbide dinitrate and in cases of marked low blood pressure, shock and acute myocardial infarction with low left ventricular filling pressure.

*Precautions:* Ismo Retard is not indicated for relief of acute anginal attacks. In the event of an acute attack, sublingual or buccal glyceryl trinitrate tablets or sprays should be used.

Patients who have not previously received nitrates may be started with a low dose, which should be increased gradually, before introducing Ismo Retard.

In the case of acute myocardial infarction, Ismo Retard should be continued only under strict medical supervision. Since a rebound phenomenon cannot be excluded, therapy with isosorbide mononitrate should be terminated gradually rather than stopping abruptly.

*Use in pregnancy and lactation:* There is inadequate evidence of safety of the drug in human pregnancy although nitrates have been in wide use for many years without ill consequence, animal studies having shown no adverse effects on the foetus.

There is no information on excretion of isosorbide mononitrate in breast milk. Use in pregnancy and lactation is not recommended unless considered essential by the patient's physician.

*Adverse effects:* A number of nitrate-related adverse effects may occur during treatment, including headache and feelings of dizziness. The incidence of such effects is normally highest at the commencement of treatment and tends to decline with time. Other reactions, including feelings of weakness, nausea or vomiting may occur occasionally. Side effects which have been associated with isosorbide dinitrate (e.g. flushing, postural hypotension, dry rash, exfoliative dermatitis) may also occur.

*Interactions:* The hypotensive effects of other drugs may be potentiated.

*Overdosage:* In the event of overdosage with Ismo Retard the main sign is likely to be hypotension. The stomach should be aspirated to remove any remaining tablets. The patient should be placed in a supine position with the legs elevated to promote venous return. Symptomatic and supportive treatment e.g. plasma expanders and, if necessary, the careful use of vasopressor agents to counterbalance the hypotensive effects may be necessary. Methaemoglobinaemia will normally respond to methylene blue infusion.

**Pharmaceutical precautions** No special handling or storage precautions apply. As with all medicines, however, it is recommended that Ismo Retard be stored in a cool, dry place.

**Legal category** P.

**Package quantities** Packs of 28 tablets (OP).

**Further information** Beta-blocking drugs have a different pharmacological action in angina and may have a complementary effect when co-administered with Ismo Retard.

**Product licence number** 15722/0015.

## LORON* 520

**Presentation** Loron 520 tablets are white, oblong, film-coated tablets with bilateral score lines, containing 520 mg sodium clodronate for oral administration. Each tablet is marked BM E9. Lactose is included in the film coating.

**Uses**

*Indication:* Loron 520 is indicated for the management of osteolytic bone lesions, hypercalcaemia and bone pain associated with skeletal metastases in patients with carcinoma of the breast or multiple myeloma. Loron 520 is also indicated for the maintenance of clinically acceptable serum calcium levels in patients with hypercalcaemia of malignancy initially treated with an intravenous infusion of sodium clodronate.

*Properties:* Sodium clodronate is a bisphosphonate which has a high affinity to bone. It is mainly the portion of the dose adsorbed to bone which is pharmacologically active. The pharmacological effect of sodium clodronate is to suppress osteoclast-mediated bone resorption as judged by bone histology and decreases in serum calcium, urine calcium and urinary excretion of hydroxyproline, without adversely affecting mineralisation.

**Dosage and administration**

*Adults:* The recommended dose is two tablets daily (1040 mg). If necessary, the dosage may be increased, but should not exceed a maximum of four tablets daily (2080 mg).

The tablets may be taken as a single dose or in two equally divided doses if necessary to improve gastro-intestinal tolerance. Loron 520 tablets should be swallowed with a little fluid, but not milk, at least one hour before or one hour after food.

When changing therapy from Loron capsules (400 mg) to Loron 520 tablets (520 mg), it should be noted that two Loron capsules are equivalent to one Loron 520 tablet. This is due to greater bioavailability of the tablet formulation.

*Elderly:* No specific dosage recommendations.

*Children:* Safety and efficacy in children has not been established.

*Use in renal impairment:* In patients with renal insufficiency, with creatinine clearance between 10 and 30 ml/min, the daily dose should be reduced to one half the recommended adult dose. Serum creatinine should be monitored during therapy. Sodium clodronate is contra-indicated in patients with creatinine clearance below 10 ml/min.

**Contra-indications, warnings, etc**

*Contra-indications:* Hypersensitivity to sodium clodronate. Acute, severe inflammatory conditions of the gastro-intestinal tract. Pregnancy and lactation. Renal failure with creatinine clearance below 10 ml/min, except for short term use in the presence of purely functional renal insufficiency caused by elevated serum calcium levels. Concomitant use of other bisphosphonates.

*Precautions and warnings:* No information is available on the potential carcinogenicity of sodium clodronate, but patients have been treated in clinical trials for up to 2 years. The duration of treatment, therefore is at the discretion of the physician, according to the status of the underlying malignancy.

It is recommended that appropriate monitoring of renal function with serum creatinine be carried out during treatment. Serum calcium and phosphate should be monitored periodically. Monitoring of liver enzymes and white cell counts is advised (see side effects).

*Use in pregnancy and lactation:* There are insufficient data either from animal studies or from experience in humans of the effects of sodium clodronate on the embryo and foetus. No studies have been conducted on excretion in breast milk. Consequently, sodium clodronate is contra-indicated in pregnancy and lactation.

*Side-effects:* Patients may experience a mild gastro-intestinal upset, usually in the form of nausea or mild diarrhoea. The symptoms may respond to the use of a twice daily dosage regime, rather than a single dose. It is not normally required to withdraw therapy or to provide medication to control these effects. Asymptomatic hypocalcaemia has been noted rarely. A reversible elevation of serum parathyroid hormone may occur. In a small proportion of patients a mild, reversible increase in serum lactate dehydrogenase and a modest transient leucopenia have been reported although these may have been associated with concurrent chemotherapy. Renal dysfunction, including renal failure has been reported. Hypersensitivity reactions have been mainly confined to the skin: pruritus, urticaria and rarely exfoliative dermatitis. However, bronchospasm has been precipitated in patients with or without a previous history of asthma.

*Interactions:* No other bisphosphonate drugs should be given with Loron tablets. The calcium-lowering action of clodronate can be potentiated by the administration of aminoglycosides either concomitantly or one to several weeks apart. Severe hypocalcaemia has been observed in some cases. Hypomagnesaemia may also occur simultaneously. Patients receiving NSAIDs in addition to sodium clodronate have developed renal dysfunction. However, a synergistic action has not been established. There is no evidence from clinical experience that sodium clodronate interacts with other medication such as steroids, diuretics, calcitonin, non NSAID analgesics or chemotherapeutic agents. Calcium rich foods, mineral supplements and antacids may impair absorption.

*Overdosage:* There is no experience of acute overdosage in humans. The development of hypocalcaemia is possible for up to two or three days following the overdosage. Serum calcium should be monitored and oral or parenteral calcium supplementation may be required. Acute overdosage may be associated with gastro-intestinal symptoms such as nausea and vomiting. Treatment should be symptomatic.

**Pharmaceutical precautions** No special handling or storage precautions apply. It is recommended however, that Loron 520 be stored in a cool, dry place in accordance with normal pharmaceutical practice.

**Legal category** POM.

**Package quantities** Packs of 10 and original pack of 60 tablets.

**Further information** Nil.

**Product licence number** 15722/0029.

## LORON* CAPSULES

**Qualitative and quantitative composition** Each Loron capsule contains 400 mg disodium clodronate.

**Pharmaceutical form** Capsules for oral administration.

**Clinical particulars**

*Therapeutic indications:* Loron is indicated for the management of osteolytic lesions, hypercalcaemia and bone pain associated with skeletal metastases in patients with carcinoma of the breast or multiple myeloma. Loron capsules are also indicated for the maintenance of clinically acceptable serum calcium levels in patients with hypercalcaemia of malignancy initially treated with an intravenous infusion of disodium clodronate.

*Posology and method of administration*

*Adults:* The recommended dose is 4 capsules (1600 mg disodium clodronate) daily. If necessary, the dosage may be increased but should not exceed a maximum of 8 capsules (3200 mg disodium clodronate) daily.

The capsules may be taken as a single dose or in two equally divided doses if necessary to improve gastro-intestinal tolerance. Loron capsules should be swallowed with a little fluid, but not milk, at least one hour before or one hour after food.

*Elderly:* No special dosage recommendations.

*Children:* Safety and efficacy in children has not been established.

*Use in renal impairment:* In patients with renal insufficiency with creatinine clearance between 10 and 30 ml/min., the daily dose should be reduced to half the recommended adult dose. Serum creatinine should be monitored during therapy. Disodium clodronate is contra-indicated in patients with creatinine clearance below 10 ml/min.

*Contra-indications:* Hypersensitivity to disodium clodronate. Acute, severe inflammatory conditions of the gastro-intestinal tract. Pregnancy and lactation. Renal failure with creatinine clearance below 10 ml/min, except for short term use in the presence of purely functional renal insufficiency caused by elevated serum calcium levels. Concomitant use of other bisphosphonates.

*Special warnings and precautions for use:* No information is available on the potential carcinogenicity of disodium clodronate, but patients have been treated in clinical trials for up to 2 years. The duration of the treatment is therefore at the discretion of the physician, according to the status of the underlying malignancy.

*Interactions with other medicaments and other forms of interaction:* No other bisphosphonate drugs should be given with Loron capsules.

The calcium-lowering action of clodronate can be potentiated by the administration of aminoglycosides either concomitantly or one to several weeks apart. Severe hypocalcaemia has been observed in some cases. Hypomagnesaemia may also occur simultaneously. Patients receiving NSAIDs in addition to disodium clodronate have developed renal dysfunction. However, a synergistic action has not been established. There is no evidence from clinical experience that disodium clodronate interacts with other medication such as steroids, diuretics, calcitonin, non-NSAID analgesics or chemotherapeutic agents. Calcium rich foods, mineral supplements and antacids may impair absorption.

*Pregnancy and lactation:* There are insufficient data either from animal studies or from experience in humans of the effects of disodium clodronate on the embryo and foetus. No studies have been conducted on excretion in breast milk. Consequently, disodium clodronate is contra-indicated in pregnancy and lactation.

*Effects on ability to drive and use machines:* No effects.

*Undesirable effects:* Patients may experience a mild gastro-intestinal upset, usually in the form of nausea or mild diarrhoea. The symptoms may respond to the use of a twice daily dosage regime, rather than a single dose. It is not normally required to withdraw therapy or to provide medication to control these effects. Asymptomatic hypocalcaemia has been noted rarely. A reversible elevation of serum parathyroid hormone may occur. In a small proportion of patients a mild, reversible increase in serum lactate dehydrogenase and a modest transient leucopenia have been reported although these may have been associated with concurrent chemotherapy. Renal dysfunction, including renal failure, has been reported. Hypersensitivity reactions have been mainly confined to the skin: pruritus, urticaria and rarely exfoliative dermatitis. However, bronchospasm has been precipitated in patients with or without a previous history of asthma.

*Overdosage:* There is no experience of acute overdosage in humans. The development of hypocalcaemia is possible for up to 2 or 3 days following the overdosage. Serum calcium should be monitored and oral or parenteral calcium supplementation may be required. Acute overdosage may be associated with gastro-intestinal symptoms such as nausea and vomiting. Treatment should be symptomatic.

## Pharmacological properties

*Pharmacodynamic properties:* Disodium clodronate is a bisphosphonate which has a high affinity to bone. It is mainly the portion of the dose adsorbed to bone which is pharmacologically active. The pharmacological effect of disodium clodronate is to suppress osteoclast mediated bone resorption as judged by bone histology and decreases in serum calcium, urine calcium and urinary excretion of hydroxyproline, without adversely affecting mineralisation.

*Pharmacokinetic properties:* Oral bioavailability is in the order of 2%.

Disodium clodronate is not metabolised. The volume of distribution is approximately 0.3 L/kg. Elimination from serum is rapid, 75% of the dose is recovered unchanged in urine within 24 hours.

The elimination kinetics best fit a 3 compartment model. The first two compartments have relatively short half-lives. The third compartment is probably the skeleton. Elimination half-life is approximately 12–13 hours.

*Preclinical safety data:* Disodium clodronate shows relatively little toxicity either on single oral administration or after daily oral administration for a period of up to 6 months. In rats, a dose of 200 mg/kg/day in the chronic toxicity test is at the limit of tolerability. In dogs, 40 mg/kg/day chronically is within the tolerated range.

On daily administration of 500 mg/kg for 6 weeks to rats, signs of renal failure with a clear rise in BUN, and initial liver parenchymal reaction with rises of SGOT, SGPT and AP occurred. No significant haematological changes were found in the toxicological investigations.

Investigations for mutagenic properties did not show any indication of mutagenic potency.

Reproduction toxicology investigations did not provide any indication of peri- and post-natal disorders, teratogenic damage or disorders of fertility.

It is not known if disodium clodronate passes into the mother's milk or through the placenta.

## Pharmaceutical particulars

*List of excipients:* Loron capsules also contain talc, maize starch, magnesium stearate and sodium starch glycollate. The capsule shell is made of gelatin.

*Incompatibilities:* Not applicable.

*Shelf-life:* HDPE container: 3 years. PVC/aluminium blister packs: 5 years.

*Special precautions for storage:* None.

*Nature and contents of container:* HDPE tubes, containing 30, 112 or 120 capsules, PVC/aluminium foil blister packs containing 20, 60 or 120 capsules.

*Instructions for use/handling:* None.

**Marketing authorisation number** 15722/0016.

**Date of approval/revision of SPC** January 1997.

**Legal category** POM.

## LORON* FOR INFUSION

**Qualitative and quantitative composition** Each ampoule contains 300 mg disodium clodronate.

**Pharmaceutical form** Clear colourless sterile liquid for use by intravenous infusion after dilution.

### Clinical particulars

*Therapeutic indications:* Loron for Infusion is indicated for the normalisation of serum calcium levels in patients with hypercalcaemia of malignancy in conjunction with full rehydration of patients as appropriate.

*Posology and method of administration:* Loron for Infusion is a concentrated presentation which must be diluted before use. The only recommended diluent is 0.9% w/v sodium chloride intravenous infusion. No other drugs or nutrients may be added.

Loron for Infusion may be administered either as a single infusion or as multiple infusions. Slow infusion is important for safety. It is recommended that oral or intravenous fluids be administered to establish or maintain full hydration.

*Adults: Single infusion:* Five ampoules of Loron for Infusion (1500 mg disodium clodronate) should be added aseptically to 500 ml of sodium chloride intravenous infusion (0.9%). The diluted infusion solution should be administered by slow intravenous infusion over a period of not less than 4 hours.

*Multiple infusions:* One ampoule of Loron for Infusion (300 mg disodium clodronate) should be added aseptically to 500 ml of sodium chloride intravenous infusion (0.9%). The diluted infusion solution should be administered by slow intravenous infusion over a period of not less than 2 hours on successive days. The duration of treatment by multiple infusion depends on patient response but should not exceed 10 days.

*Response:* In most cases, an elevated serum calcium level can be lowered to within the normal range after 3–5 days, whichever method of infusion is used. Normocalcaemia may be maintained thereafter with oral administration of Loron 520 or Loron capsules. If hypercalcaemia recurs, the intravenous infusion may be reintroduced.

*Elderly:* No special dosage recommendations.

*Children:* Safety and efficacy in children has not been established.

*Use in renal impairment:* The effect of disodium clodronate in patients with moderate to severe renal impairment (serum creatinine greater than 440 micromol/l) has not been systematically examined in clinical trials. Since disodium clodronate is excreted unchanged by the kidney its use is contra-indicated in these patients. In patients with normal renal function or mild renal impairment (serum creatinine less than 440 micromol/l) serum creatinine should be monitored during therapy.

*Contra-indications:* Hypersensitivity to disodium clodronate. Pregnancy and lactation. Moderate to severe renal failure (serum creatinine greater than 440 micromol/l). Concomitant use of other bisphosphonates.

*Special warnings and precautions for use:* Intravenous infusion of disodium clodronate may be associated with a transient proteinuria immediately after infusion even when the correct dosage and administration recommendations are followed (see Undesirable effects). Hypercalcaemia may promote or worsen renal dysfunction and the use of disodium clodronate has normally been demonstrated to improve renal function as the serum calcium concentration is lowered. Nevertheless, care is required with the intravenous route of administration and the recommended dosage must not be exceeded.

It is recommended that appropriate monitoring of renal function with serum creatinine be carried out during treatment with Loron for Infusion. Serum calcium and phosphate should also be monitored periodically. Monitoring of liver enzymes and white cell counts is advised (see Undesirable effects).

*Interactions with other medicaments and other forms of interaction:* No other bisphosphonate drugs should be given with Loron for Infusion. The calcium-lowering action of clodronate can be potentiated by the administration of aminoglycosides either concomitantly or one to several weeks apart. Severe hypocalcaemia has been observed in some cases. Hypomagnesaemia may also occur simultaneously. Patients receiving NSAIDs in addition to disodium clodronate have developed renal dysfunction. However, a synergistic action has not been established. There is no evidence from clinical experience that disodium clodronate interacts with other medication, such as steroids, diuretics, calcitonin, non-NSAID analgesics or chemotherapeutic agents.

*Pregnancy and lactation:* There are insufficient data either from animal studies or from experience in humans of the effects of disodium clodronate on the embryo and foetus. No studies have been conducted on excretion in breast milk. Consequently, disodium clodronate is contra-indicated in pregnancy and lactation.

*Effects on ability to drive and use machines:* No effects.

*Undesirable effects:* Asymptomatic hypocalcaemia has been noted rarely. A reversible elevation of serum parathyroid hormone may occur. In a small proportion of patients, a mild reversible increase in serum lactate dehydrogenase and a modest transient leucopenia have been reported although these may have been associated with concurrent chemotherapy. Renal dysfunction, including renal failure, has been reported. Transient proteinuria has been reported immediately after intravenous infusion (see Special warnings and precautions). The clinical significance is uncertain. However, chronic proteinuria following infusion has not been observed. Hypersensitivity reactions have been mainly confined to the skin: pruritus, urticaria and rarely exfoliative dermatitis. However, bronchospasm has been precipitated in patients with or without a previous history of asthma.

*Overdose:* There is no experience of acute overdosage in humans. An overdosage by intravenous infusion, or injection of undiluted infusion concentrate, could provoke renal damage and renal function should be monitored. The development of hypocalcaemia is possible for up to 2 or 3 days following the overdosage. Serum calcium should be monitored and oral or parenteral calcium supplementation may be required. Acute overdosage may be associated with gastro-intestinal symptoms such as nausea and vomiting. Treatment should be symptomatic.

### Pharmacological properties

*Pharmacodynamic properties:* Disodium clodronate is a bisphosphonate which has a high affinity to bone. It is mainly the portion of a dose adsorbed to bone which is pharmacologically active. The pharmacological effect of disodium clodronate is to suppress osteoclast-mediated bone resorption as judged by bone histology and decreases in serum calcium, urine calcium and urinary excretion of hydroxyproline, without adversely affecting mineralisation.

*Pharmacokinetic properties:* Disodium clodronate is not metabolised. The volume of distribution is approximately 0.3 L/kg. Elimination from serum is rapid, 75% of the dose is recovered unchanged in urine within 24 hours.

The elimination kinetics best fit a 3 compartment model. The first two compartments have relatively short half-lives. The third compartment is probably the skeleton. Elimination half-life is approximately 12–13 hours.

*Preclinical safety data:* Disodium clodronate shows relatively little toxicity either on single oral administration or after daily oral administration for a period of up to 6 months. In rats, a dose of 200 mg/kg/day in the chronic toxicity test is at the limit of tolerability. In dogs, 40 mg/kg/day chronically is within the tolerated range.

On daily administration of 500 mg/kg for 6 weeks to rats, signs of renal failure with a clear rise in BUN, and initial liver parenchymal reaction with rises of SGOT, SGPT and AP occurred. No significant haematological changes were found in the toxicological investigations.

Investigations for mutagenic properties did not show any indication of mutagenic potency.

Reproduction toxicology investigations did not provide any indication of peri- and post-natal disorders, teratogenic damage or disorders of fertility.

It is not known if disodium clodronate passes into the mother's milk or through the placenta.

### Pharmaceutical particulars

*List of excipients:* Loron for Infusion also contains sodium bicarbonate, water for injections and hydrochloric acid.

*Incompatibilities:* None known.

*Shelf-life:* Unopened ampoule – 2 years. Diluted solution – 12 hours.

*Special precautions for storage:* None.

*Nature and contents of container:* Clear glass ampoules, each containing 10 ml solution. 5 ampoules to a carton.

*Instruction for use/handling:* None.

**Marketing authorisation number** 15722/0017.

**Date of approval/revision of SPC** January 1997.

**Legal category** POM.

## PALFIUM*

**Presentation** Palfium products contain Dextromoramide Tartrate BP, and the dose and strength are expressed as dextromoramide base. The presentations available cover the oral and rectal routes of administration:

*Palfium tablets, 5 mg:* white, scored tablets for oral use (Dextromoramide Tablets BP, 5 mg).

*Palfium tablets, 10 mg:* peach, scored tablets for oral use (Dextromoramide Tablets BP, 10 mg).

*Palfium suppositories, 10 mg:* light cream coloured suppositories for rectal administration.

Lactose is present in Palfium tablets and suppositories. Palfium tablets 10 mg contain colouring agent E110.

**Uses** Palfium is a potent analgesic for relief of the severe pain of inoperable carcinoma and for the relief of other forms of severe and intractable pain.

**Dosage and administration** *Adult dosage: First dose:* Not more than 5 mg by mouth or 10 mg rectally.

*Subsequent doses:* The size of subsequent doses depends upon the needs of the patient, that is, upon the severity of the pain. In cases of severe pain 10 mg Palfium may be required, repeated as necessary in order to maintain analgesia. The dose required may also be influenced by the patient's body weight. Regardless of body weight, however, not more than 20 mg should be given as a single dose. The dose frequency and the total daily dosage may vary significantly and should be titrated according to the needs of the individual patient.

In postoperative pain the initial dose of Palfium in the immediate postoperative period should be restricted, for example, to 2.5 mg, as the patient may still be under the influence of circulating anaesthetic agents and premedications. For subsequent postoperative care, 5 mg three times daily as required is usually sufficient.

*Administration:* Palfium tablets should be given before meals, if possible. Palfium is also fully effective rectally and a 10 mg dose may be administered by suppository, particularly at night.

*Child dosage:* A paediatric dosage regime has not yet been established. Should the need arise to administer

Palfium to a child, the initial dosage should be not more than 0.08 mg per kg of body weight.

**Contra-indications, warnings, etc** Palfium is contra-indicated in patients with respiratory depression or obstructive airways disease, and in female patients during child-birth. It is also contra-indicated in patients receiving monoamine oxidase inhibitors and two to three weeks should be allowed to elapse before Palfium is administered to patients who have been treated with these agents.

The use of Palfium in pregnant patients is not recommended, although there is no evidence from animal studies to suggest that it is potentially harmful. In cases where the rate of metabolism of dextromoramide may be reduced, such as in the elderly and in patients with hypothyroidism or chronic hepatic insufficiency, it may be advisable to employ a reduced dosage regime.

Palfium may give rise to dizziness and sweating, especially in the ambulant patient. These effects may be minimised by advising the patient to rest, preferably supine, for a short period after administration of the first few doses. Nausea and vomiting may be troublesome but tend to occur only rarely. As with other potent analgesics tolerance and addiction may occur with continued use of Palfium. Concurrent administration of CNS depressants, including alcohol, must be carefully considered as such agents may enhance the central effects of Palfium and consequently the risk of respiratory depression.

Respiratory depression is unlikely to occur when Palfium is employed on its own in a normal therapeutic dosage. In the event of oral overdosage gastric lavage may be useful in the first few hours after ingestion. If consciousness is impaired and respiration depressed a suitable antagonist such as naloxone may be administered using the appropriate dosage. The circulation should be maintained with intravenous infusion of plasma or suitable electrolyte solutions and assisted respiration may be necessary until spontaneous breathing is restored.

**Pharmaceutical precautions** Store Palfium tablets below 25°C and protect from moisture. Palfium suppositories must be stored in a cool location well away from radiators and other sources of heat.

**Legal category** CD (Sch 2) POM.

**Package quantities** Palfium tablets 5 mg and 10 mg, blister packs of 60.

Palfium suppositories, packs of 10.

**Further information** The analgesic effect is rapid by both routes of administration (typically 20–30 minutes).

Palfium provides pain relief normally without clouding consciousness or mental activity, and does not cause constipation. It may be advantageous in some cases to provide simultaneous administration of a sedative, hypnotic or tranquilliser, such as chlorpromazine, with Palfium. A cautious approach should be made to establish the most satisfactory dosage regime. In most cases only half the normal dose of the ancillary drug will be required.

**Product licence numbers**

| | |
|---|---|
| Palfium Tablets 5 mg | 15722/0004. |
| Palfium Tablets 10 mg | 15722/0005. |
| Palfium Suppositories | 15722/0003. |

## RAPILYSIN* 10 U ▼

**Qualitative and quantitative composition** 1 vial contains 1.16 g powder for injection with 10 U reteplase (rINN). 1 prefilled syringe contains 10 ml water for injections. Potency of reteplase is expressed in units (U) by using a reference standard which is specific for reteplase and is not comparable with units used for other thrombolytic agents.

**Pharmaceutical form** Powder for intravenous injection following reconstitution.

**Clinical particulars**

*Therapeutic indications:* Thrombolytic therapy of acute myocardial infarction (AMI) (within 12 hours after the onset of AMI symptoms).

*Posology and method of administration:* Reteplase is supplied as a freeze-dried substance in vials. The lyophilizate is reconstituted with the contents of the accompanying syringe (see *Instructions for use and handling*). The reconstituted solution should be used immediately.

Treatment with reteplase should be initiated as soon as possible after the onset of AMI symptoms.

Reteplase is administered as a 10+10 U double bolus injection. Each bolus is administered as a slow intravenous injection over not more than 2 minutes. The second bolus is given 30 minutes after initiation of the first bolus injection.

The bolus injection is given via an intravenous line. It should be ensured that the injection is not mistakenly

given paravenously. Only clear, colourless solutions should be injected. No other medication should be added to the injection solution.

Heparin and acetylsalicylic acid should be administered concomitantly with and following the administration of reteplase to reduce the risk of rethrombosis. The recommended heparin dose is 5000 I.U. given as a bolus injection prior to reteplase therapy followed by an infusion of 1000 I.U. per hour starting after the second reteplase bolus. Heparin should be administered for at least 24 hours, preferably for 48 (–72) hours, aiming to keep aPTT values 1.5 to 2 times normal.

The initial dose of acetylsalicylic acid prior to thrombolysis should be at least 250 mg (250–350 mg) followed by 75–150 mg/day at least until discharge.

*Contra-indications:* Because thrombolytic therapy increases the risk of bleeding, reteplase is contra-indicated in the following situations:

– known haemorrhagic diathesis
– patients with current concomitant therapy with oral anticoagulants (e.g. warfarin sodium)
– intracranial neoplasm, arteriovenous malformation or aneurysm
– neoplasm with increased bleeding risk
– history of cerebrovascular accident
– recent (<10 days) prolonged and vigorous external heart massage
– severe uncontrolled hypertension
– active peptic ulceration
– portal hypertension (oesophageal varices)
– severe liver or renal dysfunction
– acute pancreatitis, pericarditis, bacterial endocarditis
– diabetic haemorrhagic retinopathy or other haemorrhagic ophthalmic conditions
– within 3 months of severe bleeding, major trauma or major surgery (e.g. coronary artery bypass graft, intracranial or intraspinal surgery or trauma), obstetric delivery, organ biopsy, previous puncture of noncompressible vessels.

*Special warnings and special precautions for use:* Reteplase should be used by physicians experienced in the use of thrombolytic treatment and with the facilities to monitor that use.

Each patient being considered for therapy with reteplase should be carefully evaluated.

*Bleeding:* The most common complication encountered during reteplase therapy is bleeding. The concomitant use of heparin anticoagulation may contribute to bleeding. As fibrin is lysed during reteplase therapy, bleeding from recent puncture sites may occur. Therefore, thrombolytic therapy requires careful attention to all possible bleeding sites (including catheter insertion sites, arterial and venous puncture sites, cutdown sites and needle puncture sites). The use of rigid catheter as well as intramuscular injections and nonessential handling of the patient should be avoided during treatment with reteplase.

Should serious bleeding, in particular cerebral haemorrhage, occur any concomitant heparin should be terminated immediately. In addition, the second bolus of reteplase should not be given if the serious bleeding occurs before it is administered. In general, however, it is not necessary to replace the coagulation factors because of the relatively short half-life of reteplase. Most patients who have bleeding can be managed by interruption of thrombolytic and anticoagulant therapy, volume replacement and manual pressure applied to an incompetent vessel. Protamine should be considered if heparin has been administered within 4 hours of the onset of bleeding. In the patients who fail to respond to these conservative measures, judicious use of transfusion products may be indicated. Transfusions of cryoprecipitate, fibrinogen, fresh frozen plasma and platelets should be considered with clinical and laboratory reassessment after each administration. A target fibrinogen level of 1 g/l is desirable with cryoprecipitate or fibrinogen infusion.

In the following conditions, the risks of reteplase therapy may be increased and should be weighed against the anticipated benefits:

– cerebrovascular disease
– systolic blood pressure at entry >160 mmHg
– recent gastrointestinal or genitourinary bleeding (within 10 days)
– high likelihood of left heart thrombus e.g. mitral stenosis with atrial fibrillation
– septic thrombophlebitis or occluded arteriovenous cannula at seriously infected site
– advanced age i.e. over 75 years old
– any other conditions in which bleeding constitutes a significant hazard or would be particularly difficult because of its location.

At present, insufficient data in patients with diastolic blood pressure >100 mgHg prior to thrombolytic therapy are available for reteplase.

*Arrhythmias:* Coronary thrombolysis may result in arrhythmias associated with reperfusion. It is strongly

recommended that antiarrhythmic therapy for bradycardia and/or ventricular tachyarrhythmias (e.g. ventricular tachycardia or fibrillation) is available when reteplase is administered.

*Readministration:* Since at present there is no experience with readministration of reteplase, readministration is not recommended. However, no antibody formation to the reteplase molecule has been observed.

If an anaphylactoid reaction occurs, the injection should be discontinued immediately and appropriate therapy should be initiated.

*Use in children:* Safety and effectiveness of reteplase in children have not been established. At present the administration of reteplase in children is not recommended.

*Interactions with other medicaments and other forms of interaction:* No formal interaction studies with reteplase and drugs commonly administered in patients with AMI have been performed. Retrospective analyses of clinical studies did not reveal any clinical relevant interactions with drugs used concomitantly with reteplase in patients with acute myocardial infarction. Heparin, vitamin K antagonists and drugs that alter platelet function (such as acetylsalicylic acid, dipyridamole) may increase the risk of bleeding if administered prior to, during or after reteplase therapy.

Attention should be paid to this effect especially during periods of low plasma fibrinogen (up to about 2 days after fibrinolytic therapy of AMI).

*Use during pregnancy and lactation:* No experience in pregnant women is available for reteplase. Except in life-saving situations the use in pregnancy is contraindicated because animal studies have shown a risk of pregnancy loss; foetal effects have not been studied in animals and there are insufficient data on effects on postnatal development.

It is not known whether reteplase is excreted into breast milk. Breast milk should be discarded within the first 24 hours after thrombolytic therapy.

*Effects on ability to drive and use machines:* Not applicable.

*Undesirable effects:*

*Haemorrhage:* The most frequent adverse drug reaction associated with reteplase treatment is haemorrhage, predominantly at the injection site, occasionally as gastrointestinal, gingival or genitourinary bleeding; haemopericardium, retroperitoneal bleeding, cerebral haemorrhage and epistaxis were observed rarely (each in less than 1%). Systolic blood pressure over 160 mmHg before thrombolysis with reteplase was associated with greater risk for cerebral bleeding. Blood transfusions were required rarely.

*Cardiovascular:* As with other thrombolytic agents in the context of acute myocardial infarction, arrhythmias (e.g. complete AV-block, ventricular tachycardia and fibrillation) and hypotension have been observed occasionally.

*Hypersensitivity:* Rarely, allergic reactions have been reported. One anaphylactoid/anaphylactic reaction has been observed in a clinical trial.

*Overdose:* In the event of overdosage one might expect depletion of fibrinogen and other blood coagulation components (e.g. coagulation factor V) with a consequent risk of bleeding.

Should serious bleeding occur, in particular cerebral haemorrhage, any concomitant heparin should be terminated immediately. In addition, the second bolus of reteplase should not be given if serious bleeding occurs before it is administered. In general, however, it is not necessary to replace coagulation factors because of the relatively short half-life of reteplase. Most patients who have bleeding can be managed by interruption of thrombolytic and anticoagulant therapy, volume replacement and manual pressure applied to an incompetent vessel. Protamine should be considered if heparin has been administered within 4 hours of the onset of bleeding. In patients who fail to respond to these conservative measures, judicious use of transfusion products may be indicated. Transfusions of cryoprecipitate, fibrinogen, fresh frozen plasma and platelets should be considered with clinical and laboratory reassessment after each administration. A target fibrinogen level of 1 g/l is desirable with cryoprecipitate or fibrinogen infusion.

**Pharmacological properties**

*Pharmacodynamic properties:* Pharmaco-therapeutic group: antithrombotic agent.

Reteplase is a recombinant plasminogen activator which catalyses the cleavage of endogenous plasminogen to generate plasmin. This plasminogenolysis occurs preferentially by interaction with fibrin. Plasmin in turn degrades fibrinogen and fibrin, which is a component of the matrix of thrombi, thereby exerting its thrombolytic action.

Reteplase (10+10 U) dose dependently reduces plasma fibrinogen levels by about 60 to 80%. The fibrinogen level normalises within 2 days. As with other plasminogen activators a rebound phenomenon then occurs during which fibrinogen levels reach a maximum within 9 days and remain elevated for up to 18 days.

Reductions of plasma levels of plasminogen and $\alpha_2$-antiplasmin normalise within 1 to 3 days. Coagulation factor V, clotting factor VIII, $\alpha_2$-macroglobulin and C1-esterase inhibitor are only slightly reduced and normalise within 1 to 2 days. Plasminogen activator inhibitor (PAI-1) activity can be reduced to around zero but rapidly normalises within 2 hours showing a rebound phenomenon. Prothrombin activation fragment 1 levels and thrombin-antithrombin III-complexes increase during thrombolysis indicating thrombin production of which the clinical relevance is unknown.

A large comparative mortality trial (INJECT) in approx. 6000 patients showed that reteplase reduced the incidence of heart failure (secondary efficacy criterion) in a significant manner and was at least equally effective in terms of reducing mortality (primary efficacy criterion) when compared to streptokinase. In two clinical trials aiming primarily at patency (RAPID I and II) reteplase was associated with higher early patency rates (primary efficacy criterion), as well as with a lower incidence of heart failure (secondary efficacy criterion) than alteplase (3 hour and 'accelerated' dosage regimes).

*Pharmacokinetic properties:* Following intravenous bolus injection of 10+10 U in patients with acute myocardial infarction reteplase antigen is distributed in plasma with a dominant half-life ($t_{1/2}\alpha$) of 18±5 min and eliminated with a terminal half-life ($t_{1/2}\beta$) of 5.5 hours ±12.5 min at a clearance rate of 121±25 ml/min. Reteplase activity is cleared from the plasma at a rate of 283±101 ml/min, resulting in a dominant half-life ($t_{1/2}\alpha$) of 14.6±6.7 min and a terminal half-life ($t_{1/2}\beta$) of 1.6 hours ±39 min. Only minor amounts of reteplase were immunologically detected in the urine. Exact data of the main elimination routes for reteplase in humans are not available and the consequences of hepatic or renal insufficiency are not known. Experiments in rats indicate that the liver and the kidneys are the main organs of active uptake and lysosomal degradation.

Additional studies in human plasma samples *in vitro* suggest that complexation with C1-inactivator, $\alpha_2$-antiplasmin and $\alpha_2$-antitrypsin contributes to the inactivation of reteplase in plasma. The relative contribution of the inhibitors to inactivation of reteplase decreases as follows: C1-inactivator $>\alpha_2$-antiplasmin$>\alpha_2$-antitrypsin.

The half-life of reteplase was increased in patients with AMI as compared to healthy volunteers. An additional increase of half-life of activity in patients with myocardial infarction and severely impaired liver and renal function cannot be excluded, but no clinical data of pharmacokinetics of reteplase in these patients are available. Animal data show that, in cases of severely impaired renal function with a pronounced increase in serum creatinine and serum urea, an increase in half-life of reteplase has to be expected. Mild impairment of renal function did not significantly affect the pharmacokinetic properties of reteplase.

*Preclinical safety data:* Acute toxicity studies have been performed in rats, rabbits and monkeys and subacute toxicity studies were performed in rats, dogs and monkeys. The predominant acute symptom after single high doses of reteplase in rats and rabbits was transient apathy shortly after injection. In cynomolgus monkeys, the sedative effect ranged from slight apathy to unconsciousness, caused by a reversible dose-related drop in blood pressure. There was increased local haemorrhage at the injection site.

Sub acute toxicity studies did not reveal any unexpected adverse events. In dogs, repeated dosing of the human peptide reteplase led to immunologic-allergic reactions. Genotoxicity of reteplase was excluded by a complete battery of tests at different genetic end points *in vitro* and *in vivo*.

**Pharmaceutical particulars**

*List of excipients:* Arginine, phosphoric acid, polysorbate 20.

*Incompatibilities:* None known to date.

*Shelf life:* Reteplase 10 U vials have a shelf-life of 2 years at temperatures of 2°C to 25°C when stored in the original pack. When reconstituted as directed, the solution should be used immediately. Chemical stability has been proven for 4 hours.

*Special precautions for storage:* Protect the lyophilizate during extended storage from excessive exposure to light.

*Nature and content of container:* 2 vials with powder for injection. 2 syringes with diluent. 2 reconstitution devices and 2 needles 19G1.

*Instructions for use and handling:*
1. Use aseptic technique throughout.
2. Remove the protective flip-cap from the vial of

reteplase and clean the rubber closure with an alcohol wipe.
3. Open the package containing the reconstitution spike, remove the protective cap from the Luer lock port of the reconstitution spike.
4. Open the package containing the 10 ml syringe with Luer tip. Remove the tip cap from the syringe and connect the syringe to the reconstitution spike.
5. Remove the protective cap from the spike end of the reconstitution spike and insert the spike through the rubber closure into the vial of reteplase. Transfer the 10 ml of diluent into the vial of reteplase.
6. With the reconstitution spike and syringe still attached to the vial, swirl the vial gently to dissolve the reteplase powder. DO NOT SHAKE. The reconstituted preparation results in a clear colourless solution.
7. Withdraw 10 ml of reteplase solution back into the syringe. A small amount of solution may remain in the vial due to overfill.
8. Disconnect the syringe from the reconstitution spike and attach the sterile needle provided. The dose is now ready for intravenous administration.

**Marketing authorisation holder:** Boehringer Mannheim GmbH, Sandhofer Strasse 116, D-68298 Mannheim, Germany.

**Marketing authorisation number** EU/1/96/018/001.

**Date of approval/revision of SPC** August 1996.

**Legal category** POM.

# RECORMON*

**Qualitative and quantitative composition** In terms of the active ingredients:

*Recormon 1000:* 1000 international units (IU) (corresponding to 8.3 micrograms epoetin beta) with 1 ml Water for Injections.

*Recormon 2000:* 2000 international units (IU) (corresponding to 16.6 micrograms epoetin beta) with 1 ml Water for Injections.

*Recormon 5000:* 5000 international units (IU) (corresponding to 41.5 micrograms epoetin beta) with 1 ml Water for Injections.

*Recormon 10,000:* 10,000 international units (IU) (corresponding to 83 micrograms epoetin beta) with 1 ml Water for Injections.

*Recormon S:* Recormon S packs contain Recormon with 1 ml Water (Recormon diluent) in a syringe. (Recormon packs contain Water in ampoules).

**Pharmaceutical form** Recormon contains epoetin beta (a recombinant human erythropoietin) as a freeze-dried powder for injection. Provided with each vial is either an ampoule or syringe containing Water for reconstitution of the powder.

**Clinical particulars**

*Therapeutic indications:* Recormon is indicated for use in the treatment of anaemia associated with chronic renal failure (renal anaemia) in patients on dialysis.

Recormon is also indicated for use in the treatment of symptomatic renal anaemia in patients not yet undergoing dialysis.

Recormon is also indicated for use in the prevention of anaemias of prematurity in infants with a birth weight of 750 to 1500 g and a gestational age of less than 34 weeks.

Recormon is indicated for the treatment of anaemia in adult patients with ovarian carcinoma and treated with platinum-based chemotherapy prone to induce anaemia (cisplatin: 75 mg/m²/cycle or more; carboplatin 350 mg/m²/cycle or more).

Recormon can be used to increase the yield of autologous blood from patients in a predonation programme initiated to avoid the use of homologous blood. Treatment is only indicated in patients with moderate, non-iron deficient anaemia (haemoglobin approximately 11 g to 13 g per 100 ml) when blood conserving procedures are insufficient or unavailable (i.e. a large volume of blood is required or when there is only a short time period for collection of blood).

*Posology and method of administration*

*Administration:* For administration the freeze-dried powder should be dissolved in the Water supplied. The dissolved substance which must be used immediately, i.e. within 2 hours, can be administered either subcutaneously or by the intravenous route or by short term intravenous infusion.

For subcutaneous administration the contents of the vial of freeze-dried powder should be dissolved in the Water provided.

Recormon S packs are provided with syringes for subcutaneous administration.

For intravenous injection, e.g. via the A-V fistula at the end of dialysis, administration should take place over approximately 2 minutes.

Alternatively, for administration by short term infusion, each dose of Recormon can be dissolved in at least 100 ml of sodium chloride solution 0.9%.

*Dosage in anaemia associated with renal failure:* Adults, including the elderly, and children: Treatment with Recormon is divided into two stages:

1. *Correction phase:* The usual target haemoglobin level is 10 to 12 g per 100 ml by increasing the level by at least 1 g per 100 ml per month. A haemoglobin level of 12 g per 100 ml should not be exceeded.

With subcutaneous administration the initial dosage for the first 4 weeks of treatment is 60 IU per kg of bodyweight per week. The total weekly dose can be administered in one dose or divided in up to 7 individual daily doses. If necessary, increases of 60 IU per kg of bodyweight per week may be made at 4 week intervals in order to achieve the target haemoglobin level (if the response is less than 1 g per 100 ml per month).

The initial dosage for intravenous administration for the first four weeks of treatment is 40 IU per kg of bodyweight three times per week. This may be increased after 4 weeks to 80 IU per kg of bodyweight three times per week. If necessary further increases of 20 IU per kg of bodyweight three times a week may be made at monthly intervals in order to achieve the target haemoglobin level.

For both routes of administration, the maximum correction dosage should not exceed 720 IU per kg of bodyweight per week.

2. *Maintenance phase:* To maintain a haemoglobin in the range 10 to 12 g per 100 ml (haematocrit 30 to 35%), the previous correction dose should be reduced by half initially. Subsequent doses are dependent upon the patient's response with further adjustments made at one or two week intervals to maintain a haemoglobin level not exceeding 12 g per 100 ml.

Although the dosage recommendations should be followed for children, clinical trial results showed that on average the required dosage of epoetin, per kg bodyweight, tended to be higher, the younger the child. However the individual response cannot be predicted.

Whilst treatment with Recormon is normally a lifelong therapy it may be interrupted or terminated, if necessary, at any time at the discretion of the physician.

*Dosage in prevention of anaemias of prematurity:* Recormon may be administered subcutaneously at a dose of 250 IU per kg of bodyweight three times per week. Recormon treatment should be started as early as possible, preferably by day 3 of life and continued for 6 weeks. Premature infants who have already received a blood transfusion before the start of Recormon treatment are unlikely to benefit as much as untransfused infants.

*Dosage in anaemic patients with ovarian cancer:* The dose should be administered subcutaneously. The weekly dose can be divided into 3 to 7 single doses.

Recormon treatment is indicated in patients receiving platinum-based chemotherapy if the haemoglobin value ≤11 g per 100 ml (6.9 mmol/l) at the start of chemotherapy. The recommended initial dose is 450 IU/kg/week. If after 4 weeks, a patient does not show a satisfactory response to in terms of haemoglobin values and transfusion rate, then the dose should be doubled. The therapy should be continued up to 3 weeks after the end of chemotherapy.

If the haemoglobin level falls by more than 1 g per 100 ml (0.6 mmol/l) in the first cycle of chemotherapy, despite concomitant Recormon therapy, further therapy may not be effective.

An increase in haemoglobin >2 g per 100 ml (1.25 mmol/l) per month or to above 14 g per 100 ml should be avoided. If haemoglobin increases by more than 2 g per 100 ml (1.25 mmol/l) per month, the Recormon dose should first be reduced by 50%. If values exceed 14 g per 100 ml (8.8 mmol/l), Recormon therapy should be interrupted until a value ≤12 g per 100 ml (7.5 mmol/l) is achieved and then restarted with 50% of the previous weekly dose.

*Dosage in donation of autologous blood:* Recormon may be administered twice weekly for 4 weeks either by intravenous injection or by short term infusion.

The required amount of predonated blood is expressed in units (one unit contains 450 ml whole blood with a haematrocit of 40%).

The dose of Recormon required should be calculated once prior to the first donation of blood. This dose should then be administered twice weekly throughout the period of donation.

The ability of a patient to donate blood depends predominantly on the patient's whole blood volume and the pre-donation haematocrit. The minimum haematocrit for donation is 33% (haemoglobin 11 g per 100 ml).

The variables of whole blood volume and haematocrit (before Recormon treatment) determine the surplus volume (if any) of whole blood cells which is available for donation. This can be regarded as the *endogenous red cell reserve.*

The capacity to donate blood is represented by:

endogenous red cell reserve (ml) =

$$\frac{\text{whole blood volume (ml)} \times (\text{haematocrit} - 33)}{100}$$

whole blood volume = 44 [ml/kg] × bodyweight [kg] + 1600 [ml] (men)

whole blood volume = 41 [ml/kg] × bodyweight [kg] + 1200 [ml] (women)

By using the nomogram provided, the dosage of Recormon required per administration can be identified by the point of interception of the anticipated volume of blood to be replaced (units) and the patient's endogenous red cell reserve (ml).

Recormon administration may be timed to follow the donation of blood if appropriate.

The maximum weekly dose should not exceed 1600 IU per kg of bodyweight. During the treatment period the haematocrit should not exceed 48% (haemoglobin 16 g per 100 ml).

*Contra-indications:* Recormon should not be used in patients with hypertension which is poorly controlled or in patients with known hypersensitivity to the product.

*Special warnings and precautions for use:* Recormon should be used with caution in the presence of refractory anaemia with excess blasts in transformation, in those with epilepsy, in patients with a raised platelet count (thrombocytosis) or chronic hepatic failure.

Deficiencies of folic acid and vitamin $B_{12}$ reduce the effectiveness of Recormon and should be excluded or corrected. In most cases, the increase in haemoglobin is accompanied by reduced serum ferritin values. Iron therapy, e.g. 200 to 300 mg/day orally (and additional intravenous iron, if indicated), is recommended during Recormon treatment for those donating autologous blood and also in renal anaemia and anaemia associated with ovarian cancer for all patients with serum ferritin values below 100 micrograms per litre or whose transferrin saturation is below 20%. In most premature infants a fall in serum ferritin values is observed and iron supplementation is recommended (at least 2 mg/day $Fe^{2+}$ orally). This should be started as soon as possible (by day 14 of life at the latest), dosing modified according to the serum ferritin level (e.g. if serum ferritin <100 ng/ml or there are other laboratory signs of iron deficiency, iron supplementation should be increased to 5 to 10 mg/day $Fe^{2+}$) and continued until laboratory signs of iron deficiency disappear.

Female

Anticipated volume of blood to be replaced (units)

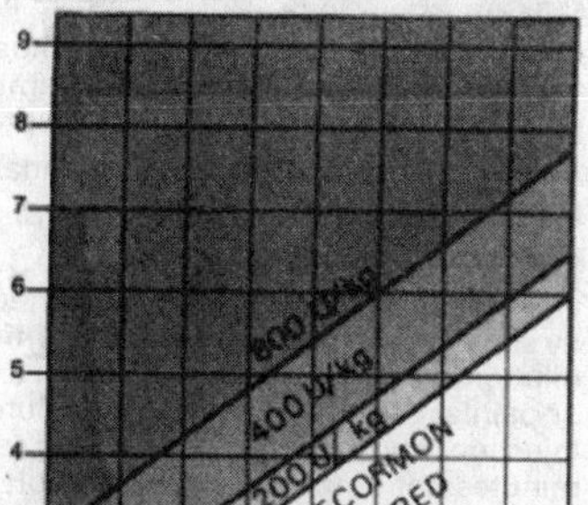


Male

Anticipated volume of blood to be replaced (units)

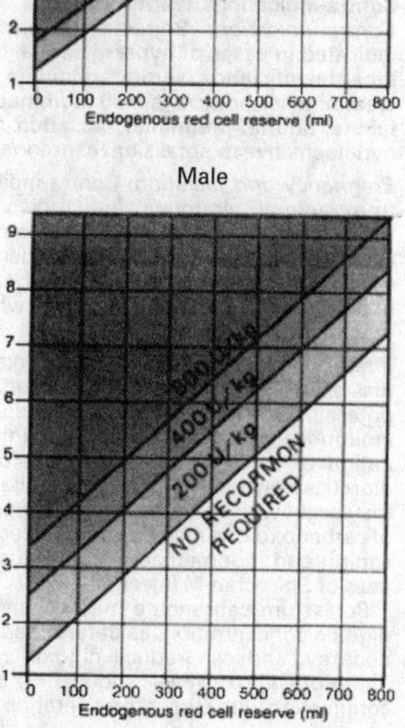


Severe aluminium toxicity in chronic renal failure patients may compromise the effectiveness of Recormon.

Serum potassium levels should be monitored regularly. Potassium elevation has been reported in a few uraemic patients receiving Recormon although causality has not been established. If an elevated or rising potassium level is observed consideration should be given to stopping Recormon administration until the level has been corrected.

In hypertensive patients or those with existing cardiovascular, cerebrovascular, or peripheral vascular disease, the target haemoglobin level may have to be lower than in other patient groups. In some patients the optimum haemoglobin level may be below 10 g per 100 ml.

The need for Recormon in anaemic nephrosclerotic renal disease patients not yet requiring dialysis should be carefully considered as the possible acceleration of the progression of renal failure has not been discounted.

In an autologous predonation programme, only patients with a haemoglobin ≥11 g per 100 ml should donate; special care is required in patients whose bodyweight is less than 50 kg; a single donation of blood should not exceed approximately 12% of the patient's estimated blood volume. Treatment should be reserved for those patients in whom it is important to avoid homologous blood transfusion taking into consideration the risk/benefit.

Use of Recormon where not medically indicated may lead to excessive increases in haemoglobin associated with life-threatening cardiovascular complications.

*Interactions with other medicaments and other forms of interaction:* There is no evidence from clinical usage so far to indicate that Recormon interacts with any other drug therapy.

Animal experiments revealed that Recormon does not increase the myelotoxicity of mitosis-inhibiting cytostatic drugs like etoposide, cisplatin, cyclophosphamide and fluorouracil.

*Pregnancy and lactation:* Animal studies showed no embryotoxic, foetotoxic or teratogenic effects. As experience in human pregnancy is inadequate, Recormon is not recommended for use during pregnancy. Similarly there is little experience of the use of Recormon in patients who are breast-feeding.

*Effects on ability to drive and use machines:* No special instructions are required.

*Undesirable effects:* In renal anaemia patients the most frequent adverse effect during treatment with Recormon is a dose-dependent increase in blood pressure or a worsening of existing hypertension especially in cases of rapid haematocrit increase. These increases in blood pressure may be treated with appropriate medication. If blood pressure remains uncontrolled a transient interruption of Recormon therapy may be appropriate. Monitoring of blood pressure is recommended between dialysis sessions and especially at the commencement of therapy. In patients with otherwise normal or low blood pressure there have been isolated cases of hypertensive crisis with encephalopathy-like symptoms (e.g. headache and confusional state, sensorimotor disorders such as speech disturbance, impaired gait or generalised tonic/clonic seizures requiring immediate medical attention). Particular attention should be paid to sudden stabbing migraine-like headaches as a possible warning sign.

Occasionally in patients with ovarian cancer there may be an increase in blood pressure which can be treated with drugs. It is therefore recommended that blood pressure is monitored, in particular in the initial treatment phase. Headache may also occur occasionally.

There may be a moderate dose-dependent increase in the platelet count within the normal range during treatment with Recormon, especially following intravenous administration and in patients in a predonation programme, the effect regressing as treatment continues. Development of thrombocytosis is extremely rare. It is recommended that the platelet count is monitored regularly during the first 8 weeks of therapy in renal anaemia. In anaemias of prematurity, particularly before day 12 to 14 of life, there may be a slight rise in platelet counts and therefore regular monitoring of platelets is recommended. Although no increase in the incidence of thromboembolic events has been observed in clinical trials in anaemia patients with ovarian cancer, regular monitoring of platelet counts is advised. In patients donating autologous blood the platelet count should be monitored at least once a week and if the increase is greater than $150 \times 10^9$/l or if the platelet count rises above the normal range, Recormon therapy should be discontinued.

Due to the increase in haematocrit and haemoglobin during therapy the viscosity of the blood increases. An increase in the dose of heparin during haemodialysis frequently may be necessary, therefore, as occlusion of the dialysis system is possible if heparinisation is not optimised.

In dialysis patients shunt thromboses may also occur, especially in patients with a tendency to hypotension or who have had previous arteriovenous fistula complications, for example, as a result of stenosis, aneurysms, etc. Early shunt revision or prophylaxis against thrombosis is recommended.

As isolated cases of transient increases in serum potassium and phosphate levels have been observed, regular monitoring is recommended.

Anaphylactoid reactions have been observed in isolated cases.

*Overdose:* No serious adverse effects are likely to occur in cases of acute overdosage. If necessary, treatment in such cases should be symptomatic.

**Pharmacological properties**

*Pharmacodynamic properties:* Epoetin beta is identical in its amino acid and carbohydrate composition to erythropoietin isolated from the urine of anaemic patients.

Erythropoietin is a glycoprotein that stimulates the formation of erythrocytes from precursors of the stem cell compartment. It acts as a mitosis stimulating factor and differentiating hormone.

There is no evidence of the development of neutralising antibodies to epoetin beta in humans.

*Pharmacokinetic properties:* The half-life of intravenously administered Recormon is between 4 and 12 hours in both healthy volunteers and uraemic patients. Following subcutaneous administration absorption is protracted and serum concentrations reach a plateau with a maximum concentration 12 to 28 hours after administration. The terminal half-life following subcutaneous administration is approximately 13 to 28 hours and absolute bioavailability is between 23 and 42%.

*Preclinical safety data:* No adverse findings were observed in a 3 month toxicity studies in rats with doses up to 10,000 IU per kg bodyweight, or in dogs with doses of up to 3000 IU per kg bodyweight administered daily either s.c. or i.v., with the exception of fibrotic changes of the bone marrow. These effects occurred if the haematocrit values exceeded 80% (Hb >30 g per 100 ml). A further study in dogs revealed that the myelofibrosis does not occur if the haematocrit is kept below 60% (Hb <22 g per 100 ml). The observation of myelofibrosis in preclinical studies is therefore irrelevant to the clinical situation in man.

**Pharmaceutical particulars**

*List of excipients:* Urea, sodium chloride, polysorbate 20, sodium dihydrogen phosphate, sodium monohydrogen phosphate, calcium chloride, glycine, L-leucine, L-isoleucine, L-threonine, L-glutamic acid, L-phenylalanine.

*Incompatibilities:* To avoid incompatibility or loss of activity it is important to:

- Use only plastic materials for injection or short term infusion. Avoid the use of glass.
- Do not use any solvent other than those specified.
- Do not mix the solution with other drugs.

*Shelf-life:* Recormon 1000, 2000, 5000 and 10000 vials are stable for 24 months when stored between +2°C and +8°C.

Following reconstitution, the solution must be used immediately, i.e. within 2 hours.

*Special precautions for storage:* Recormon must be stored at a temperature of +2°C to +8°C, that is, in a refrigerator.

To enable transportation, the cooling chain may be interrupted for a period of up to 5 days at room temperature (25°C).

Once reconstituted, any material which is not used immediately should be discarded.

*Nature and contents of container:* The freeze-dried powder is contained in glass vials (hydrolytic class I) with burgundy red, freeze-drying stoppers made of chlorobutyl rubber without plasticizer. The diluent (water) is contained either in clear, colourless glass ampoules (hydrolytic class I) or prefilled colourless glass syringes (borosilicate type I) with chlorobutyl rubber stopper, stainless steel needle cannula and rubber needle shield.

| | |
|---|---|
| Recormon 1000: | 10 vials + 10 ampoules |
| Recormon S 1000: | 10 vials + 10 syringes |
| Recormon 2000: | 10 vials + 10 ampoules |
| Recormon S 2000: | 10 vials + 10 syringes |
| Recormon 5000: | 5 vials + 5 ampoules |
| Recormon S 5000: | 5 vials + 5 syringes |
| Recormon 10000: | 5 vials + 5 ampoules |
| Recormon S 10000: | 5 vials + 5 syringes |

*Instructions for use/handling:* Before administration the Recormon solution should be inspected for visible particles. Only solutions which are colourless, clear or slightly opalescent should be injected.

**Marketing authorisation numbers**
Recormon 1000, 2000:        0075/0065
Recormon 5000:              0075/0083
Recormon 10000:             0075/0084
Water for Injections:       0075/0066

**Date of approval/revision of SPC**  June 1997.

**Legal category**  POM.

## SPIROCTAN*

### Qualitative and quantitative composition
Spiroctan 25 contains 25 mg Spironolactone BP.
Spiroctan 50 contains 50 mg Spironolactone BP.
Spiroctan 100 contains 100 mg Spironolactone BP.

### Pharmaceutical form
*Spiroctan 25:* Light blue coated tablets marked BM B2 and containing 25 mg Spironolactone BP.
*Spiroctan 50:* Green coated tablets marked BM A8 and containing 50 mg Spironolactone BP.
*Spiroctan 100:* Light green hard gelatin capsules marked BM A7 and containing 100 mg Spironolactone BP.

### Clinical particulars
*Therapeutic indications:* Spiroctan is recommended for the treatment of congestive cardiac failure, cirrhosis with ascites and oedema, malignant ascites, nephrotic syndrome and also for diagnosis and treatment of primary hyperaldosteronism.

*Posology and method of administration:*
*Adults:* Adequate maintenance dosage is usually between 50 and 200 mg daily, depending on the patient's response. This may be increased to 300 to 400 mg daily when necessary. A single dose of 100 mg should not be exceeded.

*Elderly:* In elderly patients, caution is advised. It is suggested that treatment should begin at the lowest dose, increasing gradually up to the normal adult dose, until the desired response is achieved.

*Children:* The daily dosage for children is based on an intake of 1.5 to 3.0 mg per kg body weight as shown in the following guidelines.
Age 1–3 years (up to approximately 15 kg): One tablet Spiroctan 25 every other day.
Age 4–7 years (up to approximately 23 kg): One tablet Spiroctan 25 each day.
Age 8–12 years (up to approximately 37 kg): One tablet Spiroctan 25 twice daily.
Children should be treated for more than 30 days only if deemed essential.
Spiroctan tablets and capsules should be taken with fluid. For children who cannot swallow solid dosage forms, the tablets may be crushed and taken with food or drink.

*Contra-indications:* Spiroctan is contra-indicated in cases of renal insufficiency (serum creatinine >180 μmol/litre or creatinine clearance <30 ml/min), acute renal insufficiency, anuria, where hyperkalaemia or hyponatraemia is present, pregnancy, lactation and in patients hypersensitive to spironolactone.

*Special warnings and precautions for use:* Although the dose of Spiroctan does not generally need to be reduced in hepatic dysfunction, such patients should be monitored carefully as hepatic coma may be precipitated in susceptible subjects.
Periodic estimation of serum electrolytes is recommended.

*Interactions:* Potassium supplements should not be administered with Spiroctan except initially in cases of hypokalaemia, and the use of Spiroctan with other potassium-sparing diuretics or ACE inhibitors should be avoided. Combination of spironolactone, ACE inhibitors and loop diuretics may lead to acute renal failure.
The effect of carbenoxolone may be decreased. Acetylsalicylic acid, indomethacin and other inhibitors of prostaglandin synthesis may reduce the inhibiting effects of Spiroctan on aldosterone.
The action of other diuretics may be potentiated. The initial dose should be half that normally administered and the dosage should be adjusted to the patient's needs. Spiroctan may enhance the effect of antihypertensive agents.
Spironolactone may falsely elevate serum digoxin concentration, as determined by radioimmunoassay and can reduce digoxin and renal clearance. Therefore digoxin levels should only be interpreted in conjunction with clinical presentation.

*Pregnancy and lactation:* Use of Spiroctan during pregnancy is contraindicated. Animal teratogenicity studies have shown evidence of feminisation of the male foetus. As metabolites of spironolactone may be excreted in breast milk, the use of Spiroctan in patients who are breast feeding is not recommended.

*Effects on ability to drive and operate machines:* Alertness may be impaired.

*Undesirable effects:* These are infrequent and normally mild. Occasionally central nervous system side effects such as headaches, drowsiness, lethargy or ataxia may occur, and the ability to drive or operate machinery may be impaired. Gastrointestinal effects are possible.
Hyperkalaemia may occur occasionally, especially in patients with renal dysfunction, and a reversible increase in BUN and creatinine may occur even when kidney function is normal. Hyponatraemia and reversible induction or aggravation of hyperchloraemic metabolic acidosis is possible. Occasionally a rise in serum uric acid may occur.
It is theoretically possible that in chronic therapy there may be antiandrogenic effects such as nipple sensitivity and gynaecomastia in men and mastodynia in women. Hirsutism and occasional disorders of menstruation – in rare cases amenorrhoea – have been observed in women. In men there may be occasional disorders of potency. In rare cases there may be irreversible changes in voice pitch. This risk should be considered carefully in patients for whom voice control is important, for example in actors and teachers. There have been isolated cases of skin rashes, alopecia, osteomalacia, hepatotoxicity, hepatitis and agranulocytosis. Rarely eosinophilia (in patients with liver cirrhosis) and thrombocytopenia may occur.

*Overdose:* Toxic effects in overdosage are due to hyperkalaemia. Clinical symptoms include irregular pulse, lassitude and muscular weakness, and it may be difficult to differentiate clinically from hypokalaemia. Treatment is by cessation of therapy, administration of potassium-excreting diuretics, use of ion-exchange resins etc.

### Pharmacological properties
*Pharmacodynamic properties:* Spiroctan promotes diuresis by competitive inhibition of aldosterone, a sodium-retaining, potassium-excreting hormone. It acts on the distal portion of the renal tubule, and may be used in conjunction with more proximally acting diuretics.
After initiation of therapy, the diuretic response develops slowly over 2–3 days.

*Pharmacokinetic properties:* Absorption of spironolactone is proportional to dose up to 100 mg. Thereafter an assumed saturation mechanism is apparent. Spironolactone is rapidly and completely metabolised following administration, and unchanged spironolactone cannot be detected in the urine. The main active metabolites of spironolactone are canrenone, 7α thiomethylspironolactone and sulphur containing metabolites. 10% of a single dose of spironolactone shows antimineralocorticoid activity. This increases to 25% during steady state administration.
The metabolites have a long plasma half-life. Following a single administration of spironolactone, the plasma half-life of canrenone is in the order of 18.5 to 20 hours, and that of the other metabolites 15 to 16 hours.
Following oral administration, within 6 days approximately 53% of the dose is excreted in the urine, and approximately 36% in the faeces.
The renal excretion half life is approximately 22 hours.

*Preclinical safety data:* Spironolactone has been shown to produce tumours in rats when administered at high doses over a long period of time. The significance of these findings with respect to clinical use is not certain. However, the long-term use of spironolactone in young patients requires careful consideration of the benefits and the potential hazard involved. No mutagenic potential was demonstrated in in-vivo experiments.
Spironolactone crosses the placental barrier. In animal experiments (rats and dogs) spironolactone shows a feminising effect on male foetuses due to its antiandrogenic properties at doses much higher than those recommended for humans.

### Pharmaceutical particulars
*List of excipients:* Spiroctan tablets also contain lactose, talc, sodium carboxymethylamylopectin, maize starch, magnesium stearate, sodium lauryl sulphate, agar, colloidal silicon dioxide. The sugar coating contains sucrose, kaolin, polyethylene glycol, glucose, titanium dioxide, povidone and montanic acid/ethanediol ester. Both Spiroctan 25 and 50 contain the colouring agents E102 and E132. Spiroctan 50 also contains E110 . (The sugar content of each tablet is less than 0.125 g).
Spiroctan 100 capsules contain lactose, maize starch, colloidal silicon dioxide, microcrystalline cellulose, sodium carboxymethylamylopectin, sodium lauryl sulphate, polyoxyethylene stearate, magnesium stearate, talc, titanium dioxide, gelatin and the colouring agents E104 and E132.

*Incompatibilities:* Not applicable.

*Shelf life:*
Spiroctan 25: 5 years.
Spiroctan 50: 5 years.
Spiroctan 100: 5 years.

*Special precautions for storage:* No special storage precautions are necessary. As with all medicines, however, it is recommended that Spiroctan be stored in a cool dry place.

*Nature and contents of containers:*
Spiroctan 25: Polypropylene tube packs with low density polyethylene caps containing 100 tablets.
Spiroctan 50: Polypropylene tube packs with low density polyethylene caps containing 100 tablets.
Spiroctan 100: PVC/Al blister strips containing 28 capsules.

*Instruction for use/handling:* None.

**Marketing authorisation numbers**
Spiroctan 25                 15722/0007.
Spiroctan 50                 15722/0008.
Spiroctan 100                15722/0009.

**Date of approval/revision of SPC**  January 1997.

**Legal category**  POM.

## SPIROCTAN-M* INJECTION

**Presentation**  A clear, yellow, aqueous solution containing 200 mg potassium canrenoate in each 10 ml ampoule. The formulation also contains sodium carbonate and sodium chloride.

### Uses
*Pharmacology:* Potassium canrenoate is rapidly metabolised to canrenone, a known metabolite of spironolactone, with further intensive metabolism thereafter. Like spironolactone, potassium canrenoate promotes diuresis by competitive antagonism of aldosterone.

*Indications for use:* Spiroctan-M Injection is indicated for use in patients with oedema associated with secondary aldosteronism in cases such as ascites, oedema associated with liver disease and oedema associated with chronic, decompensated heart disease.
Spiroctan-M Injection is also indicated for use in the diagnosis and treatment of primary hyperaldosteronism.
Use of Spiroctan-M Injection is recommended only when treatment with other diuretic agents is inadequate and when oral aldosterone antagonists cannot be administered.

### Dosage and administration
*Adult patients only:* The dosage of Spiroctan-M Injection should be adjusted to the needs and response of the individual patient. Depending on the severity of the aldosterone excess, 1 to 2 ampoules (200 to 400 mg potassium canrenoate) should be administered daily increasing to 4 ampoules (800 mg potassium canrenoate) daily in exceptional cases.

*Elderly:* No special dose recommendation (see adults above).

*Children:* Not recommended.

Administration is by the intravenous route, either by slow intravenous injection or by infusion following dilution in a suitable vehicle. In order to avoid irritation or pain at the site of injection undiluted Spiroctan-M Injection should be administered slowly, 2 to 3 minutes per ampoule, and preferably not into a thin vein.

### Contra-indications, warnings, etc
*Contra-indications:* Spiroctan-M Injection is contra-indicated in cases of hyperkalaemia, hyponatraemia, renal insufficiency (serum creatinine >180 μmol/l or creatinine clearance is <30 ml/minute) acute renal failure, anuria, pregnancy, lactation and in patients hypersensitive to potassium canrenoate.

*Pregnancy and lactation:* Contra-indicated. No data from animal teratogenicity studies are available. However studies with spironolactone (also metabolised to canrenone) have shown evidence of feminisation of the male foetus. Traces of canrenone have been detected in human breast milk where the mother was taking oral spironolactone.

*Interactions:* It is possible that hyperkalaemia may be provoked if Spiroctan-M Injection is administered with potassium or potassium sparing diuretics such as amiloride, triamterene or with ACE inhibitors. Combination of spironolactone, ACE inhibitors and loop diuretics may lead to acute renal failure. Potentiation may occur with antihypertensive drugs and the action of carbenoxolone may be antagonised. Drugs such as aspirin and indomethacin may reduce the effectiveness of Spiroctan-M Injection.
Potassium canrenoate may falsely elevate serum digoxin concentration, as determined by radioimmunoassay, and can reduce digoxin renal clearance. Therefore digoxin levels should only be interpreted in conjunction with clinical presentation.

*Precautions:* Electrolyte balance should be monitored regularly during long term therapy.

*Adverse effects:* Adverse effects may include irritation or pain at the site of injection if undiluted Spiroctan-M Injection is not administered slowly. A transient confusion syndrome has been observed during therapy with high doses (1000 mg/day or more). Occasionally central nervous system side effects such as headaches, drowsiness, lethargy or ataxia may occur and the ability to drive or operate machinery may be impaired. Gastrointestinal effects are possible.

Hyperkalaemia may occur occasionally, especially in patients with renal dysfunction, and a reversible increase in BUN may occur even when kidney function is normal. Hyponatraemia and reversible induction or aggravation of hyperchloraemic metabolic acidosis is possible. Occasionally a rise in serum uric acid may occur.

It is theoretically possible that in chronic therapy there may be antiandrogenic effects such as nipple sensitivity and gynaecomastia in men and mastodynia in women.

Hirsutism and occasional disorders of menstruation—in rare cases amenorrhoea—have been observed in women. In men there may be occasional disorders of potency. In rare cases there may be irreversible changes in voice pitch. This risk should be carefully considered in patients for whom voice control is important for example in actors and teachers. There have been isolated cases of skin rashes, alopecia, osteomalacia, hepatotoxicity, hepatitis and agranulocytosis. Rarely eosinophilia (in patients with liver cirrhosis) and thrombocytopenia may occur.

Normally treatment with Spiroctan-M is of short duration. Treatment may be continued, if appropriate, using oral spironolactone capsules or tablets. The potency ratio of 0.7 should be considered in converting from Spiroctan-M Injection to oral spironolactone (spironolactone ÷0.7=potassium canrenoate).

*Carcinogenicity:* In long term studies of potassium canrenoate administered to rats for 2 years by the oral route myelocytic leukaemia and other neoplastic changes were observed. Use of Spiroctan-M Injection thus should be limited to as short a time as possible and the necessity for its use should be monitored continuously. Use in young patients particularly requires careful consideration of the benefits and potential hazards involved.

*Overdosage:* In overdosage, effects noted may include nausea, vomiting, transient confusion and possibly hyperkalaemia. Treatment is by cessation of therapy, anti-emetic medication and use of a potassium-eliminating drug if hyperkalaemia is present.

**Pharmaceutical precautions** Spiroctan-M Injection should be stored away from light. For slow intravenous infusion Spiroctan-M Injection may be diluted with 250 ml of either dextrose solution 5% or sodium chloride solution 0.9%. No other drugs or nutrients may be added. Use the diluted preparation within 12 hours and check visually for the absence of precipitation before use.

**Legal category** POM.

**Package quantities** The ampoules are supplied in packs of 5.

**Further information** Diuresis normally commences within the first 24 hours although long latent periods have been reported in refractory cases. Spiroctan-M Injection does not adversely affect glucose metabolism or the management of diabetes mellitus.

**Product licence number** 15722/0010.

# TOREM 5 mg/ml INJECTION*

**Qualitative and quantitative composition** Torem Injection 2 ml ampoules each contain 10 mg torasemide in 2 ml aqueous solution.

Torem Injection 4 ml ampoules each contain 20 mg torasemide in 4 ml aqueous solution.

**Pharmaceutical form** Ampoules containing aqueous solution for intravenous administration.

**Clinical particulars**
*Therapeutic indications:* Oedema due to congestive heart failure. Oedema of hepatic, pulmonary and renal origin.

*Posology and method of administration:* Torem injection solution must be administered by slow intravenous infusion.

*Adults:* Oedema due to congestive heart failure; oedema of hepatic origin. Therapy should be started with one intravenous administration of 10 mg torasemide daily. If this is not sufficient, the dose may be increased up to 20 mg daily. A maximum dose of 40 mg torasemide should not be exceeded.

In acute situations e.g. pulmonary oedema, 20 mg is recommended as an initial dose. If necessary, the dose can be repeated after 30 minutes, and may be increased stepwise to a maximum of 200 mg daily.

*Oedema of renal origin:* Therapy is started with 20 mg torasemide daily, and may be increased stepwise according to individual needs up to a maximum of 200 mg torasemide daily.

For long-term treatment, oral administration of Torem tablets is recommended. Clinical experience of intravenous administration is limited to one week's therapy.

*Elderly:* No special dosage adjustments are necessary.

*Children:* There is no experience of torasemide in children.

*Contra-indications:* Renal failure with anuria; hepatic coma and precoma; hypotension; pregnancy and lactation; hypersensitivity to torasemide and sulphonylureas.

*Special warnings and precautions for use:* Hypokalaemia, hyponatraemia, hypovolaemia and disorders of micturition must be corrected before treatment.

On long term treatment with torasemide, regular monitoring of the electrolyte balance, glucose, uric acid, creatinine and lipids in the blood, is recommended.

Careful monitoring of patients with a tendency to hyperuricaemia and gout is recommended. Carbohydrate metabolism in latent or manifest diabetes mellitus should be monitored.

As for other drugs which produce changes in blood pressure, patients taking torasemide should be warned not to drive or operate machinery if they experience dizziness or related symptoms.

*Interactions:* When used simultaneously with cardiac glycosides, a potassium and/or magnesium deficiency may increase sensitivity of the cardiac muscle to such drugs. The kaliuretic effect of mineralo- and glucocorticoids and laxatives may be increased.

As with other diuretics, the effect of antihypertensive drugs given concomitantly may be potentiated.

Torasemide, especially at high doses, may potentiate the toxicity of aminoglycoside antibiotics, cisplatin preparations, the nephrotoxic effects of cephalosporins, and the cardio- and neurotoxic effect of lithium. The action of curare-containing muscle relaxants and of theophylline can be potentiated. In patients receiving high doses of salicylates, salicylate toxicity may be increased. The action of anti-diabetic drugs may be reduced.

Sequential or combined treatment, or starting a new co-medication with an ACE inhibitor may result in transient hypotension. This may be minimised by lowering the starting dose of the ACE inhibitor and/or reducing or stopping temporarily the dose of torasemide. Torasemide may decrease arterial responsiveness to pressor agents e.g. adrenaline, noradenaline.

*Pregnancy and lactation:* There are no data from experience in humans of the effect of torasemide on the embryo and foetus. Whilst studies in the rat have shown no teratogenic effect, malformed foetuses have been observed after high doses in pregnant rabbits. No studies have been conducted on excretion in breast milk. Consequently, torasemide is contraindicated in pregnancy and lactation.

*Effects on ability to drive and use machines:* As for other drugs which produce changes in blood pressure, patients taking torasemide should be warned not to drive or operate machinery if they experience dizziness or related symptoms.

*Undesirable effects:*
*Related to diuretic action:* As with other diuretics, depending on the dosage and duration of treatment, there may be disturbances of water and electrolyte balance, especially with markedly limited salt intake.

Hypokalaemia (especially if a low potassium diet is being taken, or if vomiting, diarrhoea or excessive use of laxatives takes place, or in cases of hepatic failure); raised serum uric acid, gamma GT, glucose or lipids; aggravation of metabolic acidosis. Raised serum urea and creatinine; dryness of the mouth.

Symptoms and signs of electrolyte and volume depletion, such as headache, dizziness, weakness, loss of appetite and cramps may occur if diuresis is marked, especially at the start of treatment, and in elderly patients. Dose adjustment may be necessary. In patients with urinary outflow obstruction, retention of urine may be precipitated.

*Occasional:* Gastrointestinal symptoms.
*Rare:* Paraesthesia in the limbs.
*Isolated cases:* Thromboembolic complications and circulatory disturbances due to haemoconcentration; decreases in red and white blood cells, and platelets; allergic reactions such as pruritus, rash and photosensitivity; visual disturbance.

*Overdosage*
*Symptoms and signs:* No typical picture of intoxication is known. If overdosage occurs, then there may be a marked diuresis with the danger of loss of fluid and electrolytes which may lead to somnolence and confusion, hypotension, circulatory collapse. Gastrointestinal disturbances may occur.
*Treatment:* No specific antidote is known. Symptoms and signs of overdosage require the reduction

of the dose or withdrawal of torasemide, and simultaneous replacement of fluid and electrolytes.

**Pharmacological properties**
*Pharmacodynamic properties:* Torasemide is a loop diuretic. However, at low doses its pharmacodynamic profile resembles that of the thiazide class regarding the level and duration of diuresis. At higher doses, torasemide induces a brisk diuresis in a dose dependant manner with a high ceiling of effect.

*Pharmacokinetic properties*
*Absorption:* Torasemide is absorbed rapidly and almost completely after oral administration, and peak serum levels are reached after 1–2 hours.

*Serum protein binding:* More than 99% of torasemide is bound to plasma proteins.

*Distribution:* The apparent distribution volume is 16 litres.

*Metabolism:* Torasemide is metabolised to three metabolites, M1, M3 and M5 by stepwise oxidation, hydroxylation or ring hydroxylation.

*Elimination:* The terminal half-life of torasemide and its metabolites is 3–4 hours in healthy subjects. Total clearance of torasemide is 40 ml/min and renal clearance about 10 ml/min. About 80% of the dose administered is excreted as torasemide and metabolites into the renal tubule – torasemide 24%, M1 12%, M3 3%, M5 41%. In the presence of renal failure, elimination half-life of torasemide is unchanged.

*Preclinical safety data:*
*Toxicity: Acute toxicity* – Very low toxicity.
*Chronic toxicity* – The changes observed in toxicity studies in dogs and rats at high doses are attributable to an excess pharmacodynamic action (diuresis). Changes observed were weight reduction, increases in creatinine and urea and renal alterations such as tubular dilatation and interstitial nephritis. All drug induced changes were shown to be reversible.
*Teratogenicity* – Reproduction toxicology studies in the rat have shown no teratogenic effect, but malformed foetuses have been observed after high doses in pregnant rabbits. No effects on fertility have been seen.

Torasemide showed no mutagenic potential. Carcinogenicity studies in rats and mice showed no tumorigenic potential.

**Pharmaceutical particulars**
*List of excipients:* The injection solution also contains sodium hydroxide, trometamol, macrogol 400, water for injection.

*Incompatibilities:* Not applicable.

*Shelf life:* 4 years.

*Special precautions for storage:* Store in a cool dry place below 25°C.

*Nature and contents of containers:* Colourless clear glass ampoules (2 ml or 4 ml).

**Marketing authorisation number** 15722/0027.

**Date of approval/revision of SPC** March 1997.

**Legal category** POM.

# TOREM TABLETS*

**Qualitative and quantitative composition**
Torem 2.5 each contain 2.5 mg torasemide.
Torem 5 each contain 5.0 mg torasemide.
Torem 10 each contain 10.0 mg torasemide.

**Pharmaceutical form** Tablets for oral administration.
Torem 2.5: Round, white, marked BM/B4.
Torem 5: Round, white, marked BM/C9, with scoreline.
Torem 10: Round, white, marked BM/D7, with scoreline.

**Clinical particulars**
*Therapeutic indications:*
Torem 2.5: Essential hypertension.
Torem 5: Essential hypertension; oedema due to congestive heart failure; hepatic, pulmonary or renal oedema.
Torem 10: Oedema due to congestive heart failure; hepatic, pulmonary or renal oedema.

*Posology and method of administration:*
*Adults: Essential hypertension:* A dose of 2.5 mg torasemide p.o. once daily is recommended. If necessary, the dose may be increased to 5 mg once daily. Studies suggest that doses above 5 mg daily will not lead to further reduction in blood pressure. The maximum effect is exhibited after approximately 12 weeks of continuous treatment.
*Oedema:* The usual dose is 5 mg p.o. once daily. If necessary, the dose can be increased stepwise up to 20 mg once daily. In individual cases, as much as 40 mg torasemide/day has been administered.
*Elderly:* No special dosage adjustments are necessary.
*Children:* There is no experience of torasemide in children.

*Contra-indications:* Renal failure with anuria; hepatic

coma and pre-coma; hypotension; pregnancy and lactation; hypersensitivity to torasemide and sulphonylureas.

*Special precautions for use:* Hypokalaemia, hyponatraemia, hypovolaemia and disorders of micturition must be corrected before treatment.

On long term treatment with torasemide, regular monitoring of the electrolyte balance, glucose, uric acid, creatinine and lipids in the blood, is recommended.

Careful monitoring of patients with a tendency to hyperuricaemia and gout is recommended. Carbohydrate metabolism in latent or manifest diabetes mellitus should be monitored.

As for other drugs which produce changes in blood pressure, patients taking torasemide should be warned not to drive or operate machinery if they experience dizziness or related symptoms.

*Interactions:* When used simultaneously with cardiac glycosides, a potassium and/or magnesium deficiency may increase sensitivity of the cardiac muscle to such drugs. The kaliuretic effect of mineralo- and glucocorticoids and laxatives may be increased.

As with other diuretics, the effect of antihypertensive drugs given concomitantly may be potentiated.

Torasemide, especially at high doses, may potentiate the toxicity of aminoglycoside antibiotics, cisplatin preparations, the nephrotoxic effects of cephalosporins, and the cardio- and neurotoxic effect of lithium. The action of curare-containing muscle relaxants and of theophylline can be potentiated. In patients receiving high doses of salicylates, salicylate toxicity may be increased. The action of anti-diabetic drugs may be reduced.

Sequential or combined treatment, or starting a new co-medication with an ACE inhibitor may result in transient hypotension. This may be minimised by lowering the starting dose of the ACE inhibitor and/or reducing or stopping temporarily the dose of torasemide. Torasemide may decrease arterial responsiveness to pressor agents e.g. adrenaline, noradrenaline.

*Pregnancy and lactation:* There are no data from experience in humans of the effect of torasemide on the embryo and foetus. Whilst studies in the rat have shown no teratogenic effect, malformed foetuses have been observed after high doses in pregnant rabbits. No studies have been conducted on excretion in breast milk. Consequently, torasemide is contraindicated in pregnancy and lactation.

*Effects on ability to drive and use machines:* As for other drugs which produce changes in blood pressure,

patients taking torasemide should be warned not to drive or operate machinery if they experience dizziness or related symptoms.

*Undesirable effects:*
*Related to diuretic action:* As with other diuretics, depending on the dosage and duration of treatment, there may be disturbances of water and electrolyte balance, especially with markedly limited salt intake.

Hypokalaemia (especially if a low potassium diet is being taken, or if vomiting, diarrhoea or excessive use of laxatives takes place, or in cases of hepatic failure); raised serum uric acid, gamma GT, glucose or lipids; aggravation of metabolic acidosis. Raised serum urea and creatinine; dryness of the mouth.

Symptoms and signs of electrolyte and volume depletion, such as headache, dizziness, weakness, loss of appetite and cramps may occur if diuresis is marked, especially at the start of treatment, and in elderly patients. Dose adjustment may be necessary. In patients with urinary outflow obstruction, retention of urine may be precipated.

*Occasional:* Gastrointestinal symptoms.
*Rare:* Paraesthesia in the limbs.
*Isolated cases:* Thromboembolic complications and circulatory disturbances due to haemoconcentration; decreases in red and white blood cells, and platelets; allergic reactions such as pruritus, rash and photosensitivity; visual disturbance.

*Overdosage:*
*Symptoms and signs:* No typical picture of intoxication is known. If overdosage occurs, then there may be marked diuresis with the danger of loss of fluid and electrolytes which may lead to somnolence and confusion, hypotension, circulatory collapse. Gastrointestinal disturbances may occur.

*Treatment:* No specific antidote is known. Symptoms and signs of overdosage require the reduction of the dose or withdrawal of torasemide, and simultaneous replacement of fluid and electrolytes.

*Pharmacological properties*
*Pharmacodynamic properties:* Torasemide is a loop diuretic. However, at low doses its pharmacodynamic profile resembles that of the thiazide class regarding the level and duration of diuresis. At higher doses, torasemide induces a brisk diuresis in a dose dependant manner with a high ceiling of effect.

*Pharmacokinetic properties:*
*Absorption:* Torasemide is absorbed rapidly and almost completely after oral administration, and peak serum levels are reached after 1–2 hours.

*Serum protein binding:* More than 99% of torasemide is bound to plasma proteins.
*Distribution:* The apparent distribution volume is 16 litres.
*Metabolism:* Torasemide is metabolised to three metabolites, M1, M3 and M5 by stepwise oxidation, hydroxylation or ring hydroxylation.
*Elimination:* The terminal half-life of torasemide and its metabolites is 3–4 hours in healthy subjects. Total clearance of torasemide is 40 ml/min and renal clearance about 10 ml/min. About 80% of the dose administered is excreted as torasemide and metabolites into the renal tubule – torasemide 24%, M1 12%, M3 3%, M5 41%.

In the presence of renal failure, elimination half-life of torasemide is unchanged.

*Preclinical safety data*
*Toxicity: Acute toxicity* – Very low toxicity.
*Chronic toxicity* – The changes observed in toxicity studies in dogs and rats at high doses are attributable to an excess pharmacodynamic action (diuresis). Changes observed were weight reduction, increases in creatinine and urea and renal alterations such as tubular dilatation and interstitial nephritis. All drug induced changes were shown to be reversible.
*Teratogenicity* – Reproduction toxicology studies in the rat have shown no teratogenic effect, but malformed foetuses have been observed after high doses in pregnant rabbits. No effects on fertility have been seen.

Torasemide showed no mutagenic potential. Carcinogenicity studies in rats and mice showed no tumorigenic potential.

**Pharmaceutical particulars**
*List of excipients:* All strengths of tablet contain lactose, maize starch, colloidal silicon dioxide, magnesium stearate.
*Incompatibilities:* Not applicable.
*Shelf life:* Torem 2.5 and Torem 10: 4 years. Torem 5: 5 years.
*Special precautions for storage:* Not applicable.
*Nature and contents of container:* Blister packs, PVC/aluminium, containing 14, 28, 100 or 112 tablets.

**Marketing authorisation numbers**
Torem 2.5 Tablets      15722/0023
Torem 5 Tablets        15722/0024
Torem 10 Tablets       15722/0025.

**Date of approval/revision of SPC** March 1997.

**Legal category** POM.

*\*Trade Mark*

# Bristol-Myers Pharmaceuticals
Bristol-Myers Squibb House
Staines Road
Hounslow TW3 3JA

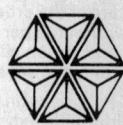

## ALPHA KERI* BATH OIL

**Presentation** Alpha Keri Bath Oil is a clear colourless water dispersible anti-pruritic bath additive.

The product contains the following active ingredients: mineral oil (91.7%) and lanolin oil (3.0%).

Other ingredients: Oxybenzone, perfume, PEG-4-dilaurate.

**Uses** Alpha Keri effectively deposits a thin uniform emulsified film of oil over the skin, and thus retards evaporation of moisture, helps to relieve itching, lubricates and softens the skin.

Alpha Keri is valuable as an aid in the management of dry pruritic skin, especially in senile pruritus, ichthyosis and other dermatoses where dermal hydration is an important part of the therapy (as in the prevention of decubitus ulcer).

Alpha Keri Bath Oil is particularly suitable for infant bathing. The preparation also overcomes the problem of cleansing the skin in conditions where the use of soaps, soap substitutes and colloid or oat-meal baths prove irritating.

**Dosage and administration** Alpha Keri should always be either added to water or rubbed onto wet skin.

Because of its inherent cleansing properties soap should not be used with Alpha Keri.

*Bath:* Add 10–20 ml to the bath water. Soak for 10–20 minutes.

*Sponge bath:* Add 10–20 ml to a basin of warm water. Apply over entire body with a sponge or flannel.

*Infant bath:* Add 5 ml to bath water.

*Skin cleansing:* Rub a small amount onto wet skin, rinse and pat dry.

*Shower:* Pour a small amount onto a wet sponge or flannel and rub onto wet skin, rinse and pat dry.

**Contra-indications, warnings, etc** As Alpha Keri deposits a film of oil over the skin, special care should be taken to guard against slipping, especially in the bath or shower.

Alpha Keri contains lanolin oil and is therefore contra-indicated in those patients allergic to this ingredient.

**Pharmaceutical precautions** Store at room temperature.

**Legal category** P.

**Package quantities** Alpha Keri Bath Oil is available in bottles containing 240 ml and 480 ml (original packs).

**Further information** Nil.

**Product licence number** 0125/0141.

## AMIKIN* INJECTION

**Qualitative and quantitative composition** Each vial contains in 2 ml amikacin sulphate equivalent to amikacin activity 100 mg (100,000 international units).

Each vial contains in 2 ml amikacin sulphate equivalent to amikacin activity 500 mg (500,000 international units)

**Pharmaceutical form** Solution for administration to human beings by injection.

**Clinical particulars**

*Therapeutic indications:* Amikacin sulphate is an aminoglycoside antibiotic which is active against a broad spectrum of gram-negative organisms, including *Pseudomonas* spp., *Escherichia coli*, indole-positive and indole-negative *Proteus* spp. *Klebsiella-Enterobacter-Serratia* spp, *Salmonella, Shigella, Minea-Herellae, Citrobacter freundii* and *Providencia* spp.

Many strains of these gram-negative organisms resistant to gentamicin and tobramycin may show sensitivity to amikacin *in vitro*. The principal gram-positive organism sensitive to amikacin is *Staphylococcus aureus*, including methicillin-resistant strains. Amikacin has some activity against other gram-positive organisms including certain strains of *Streptococcus pyogenes*, Enterococci and *Diplococcus pneumoniae*.

Amikin is indicated in the short-term treatment of serious infections due to susceptible strains of gram-negative bacteria. It may also be indicated for the treatment of known or suspected staphylococcal disease.

*Posology and method of administration:* For most infections the intramsucular route is preferred, but in life-threatening infections, or in patients in whom intramuscular injection is not feasible the intravenous route may be used.

*Intramuscular and intravenous administration:* At the recommended dosage level, uncomplicated infections due to sensitive organisms should respond to therapy within 24 to 48 hours.

If clinical response does not occur within three to five days consideration should be given to alternative therapy.

*Adults and children:* 15 mg/kg/day in two equally divided doses (equivalent to 500 mg b.i.d. in adults): use of the 100 mg/2 ml strength is recommended for children for the accurate measurement of the appropriate dose.

*Neonates and premature infants:* An initial loading dose of 10 mg/kg followed by 15 mg/kg/day in two equally divided doses.

*Elderly:* Amikacin is excreted by the renal route, renal function should be assessed whenever possible and dosage adjusted as described under impaired renal function.

*Life-threatening infections and/or those caused by pseudomonas:* The adult dose may be increased to 500 mg every eight hours but should neither exceed 1.5 g/day nor be administered for a period longer than 10 days. A maximum total adult dose of 15 g should not be exceeded.

*Urinary tract infections: (other than pseudomonal infections):* 7.5 mg/kg/day in two equally divided doses (equivalent to 250 mg b.i.d. in adults). As the activity of amikacin is enhanced by increasing the pH, a urinary alkalising agent may be administered concurrently.

*Impaired renal function:* In patients with impaired renal function, the daily dose should be reduced and/or the intervals between doses increased to avoid accumulation of the drug. A suggested method for estimating dosage in patients with known or suspected diminished renal function is to multiply the serum creatinine concentration (in mg/100 ml) by 9 and use the resulting figure as the interval in hours between doses.

| Serum Creatinine Concentration (mg/100 ml) | | Interval between AMIKACIN doses of 7.5 mg/kg/IM (hours) |
|---|---|---|
| 1.5 | | 13.5 |
| 2.0 | | 18 |
| 2.5 | | 22.5 |
| 3.0 | | 27 |
| 3.5 | | 31.5 |
| 4.0 | X9 = | 36 |
| 4.5 | | 40.5 |
| 5.0 | | 45 |
| 5.5 | | 49.5 |
| 6.0 | | 54 |

As renal function may alter appreciably during therapy, the serum creatinine should be checked frequently and the dosage regimen modified as necessary.

*Intraperitoneal use:* Following exploration for established peritonitis, or after peritoneal contamination due to faecal spill during surgery, Amikin may be used as an irrigant after recovery from anaesthesia in concentrations of 0.25% (2.5 mg/ml). If instillation is desired in adults, a single dose of 500 mg is diluted in 20 ml of sterile distilled water and may be instilled through a polyethylene catheter sutured into the wound at closure. If possible, instillation should be postponed until the patient has fully recovered from the effects of anaesthesia and muscle-relaxing drugs.

*Other routes of administration:* Amikin in concentrations of 0.25% may be used satisfactorily as an irrigating solution in abscess cavities, the pleural space, the peritoneum and the cerebral ventricles

*Contra-indications:* None.

*Special warnings and special precautions for use:*

Patients should be well hydrated during amikacin therapy.

In patients with impaired renal function or diminished glomerular filtration, amikacin should be used cautiously. In such patients, renal function should be assessed by the usual methods prior to therapy and periodically during therapy. Daily doses should be reduced and/or the interval between doses lengthened in accordance with serum creatinine concentrations to avoid accumulation of abnormally high blood levels and to minimise the risk of ototoxicity.

As with other aminoglycosides, ototoxicity and/or nephrotoxicity can result from the use of amikacin; precautions on dosage and adequate hydration should be observed.

If signs of renal irritation appear (such as albumin, casts, red or white blood cells), hydration should be increased and a reduction in dosage may be desirable. These findings usually disappear when treatment is completed. However, if azotaemia or a progressive decrease in urine output occurs, treatment should be stopped.

The use of amikacin in patients with a history of allergy to aminoglycosides or in patients who may have subclinical renal or eighth nerve damage induced by prior administration of nephrotoxic and/or ototoxic agents such as streptomycin, dihydrostreptomycin, gentamicin, tobramycin, kanamycin, bekanamycin, neomycin, polymyxin B, colistin, cephaloridine, or viomycin should be considered with caution, as toxicity may be additive.

In these patients amikacin should be used only if, in the opinion of the physician, therapeutic advantages outweigh the potential risks.

The intraperitoneal use of amikacin is not recommend in young children.

*Interactions with other medicaments and other forms of interaction:* The risk of ototoxicity is increased when amikacin is used in conjunction with rapidly acting diuretic drugs, particularly when the diuretic is administered intravenously. Such agents include frusemide and ethacrynic acid. Irreversible deafness may result.

The intraperitoneal use of amikacin is not recommended in patients under the influence of anaesthetics or muscle-relaxing drugs (including ether, halothane, d-tubocurarine, succinylcholine and decamethonium) as neuromuscular blockade and consequent respiratory depression may occur.

*Pregnancy and lactation:* The safety of Amikin in pregnancy has not yet been established.

*Effects on ability to drive and use machines:* None stated.

*Undesirable effects:* When the recommended precautions and dosages are followed the incidence of toxic reactions, such as tinnitus, vertigo, and partial reversible or irreversible deafness, skin rash, drug fever, headache, paraesthesia, nausea and vomiting is low. Urinary signs of renal irritation (albumin, casts, and red or white blood cells), azotaemia and oliguria have been reported.

*Overdose:* In the event of overdosage or toxic reaction, peritoneal dialysis or haemodialysis will aid in the removal of amikacin from the blood.

**Pharmacological properties**

*Pharmacodynamic properties:* Amikacin sulphate is an aminoglycoside antibiotic which is active against a broad spectrum of gram-negative organisms, including *Pseudomonas* spp, *Escherichia coli*, indole-positive and indole-negative *Proteus* spp. *Klebsiella-Enterobacter-Serratia* spp, *Salmonella, Shigella, Minea-Herellae, Citrobacter Freundii* and *Providencia* spp.

Many strains of these gram-negative organisms resistant to gentamicin and tobramycin may show sensitivity to amikacin *in vitro*. The principal gram-positive organism sensitive to amikacin is *Staphylococcus aureus*, including methicillin-resistant strains. Amikacin has some activity against other gram-positive organisms including certain strains of *Streptococcus pyogenes*, Enterococci and *Diplococcus pneumoniae*.

*Pharmacokinetic properties:* Amikin is rapidly absorbed after intramuscular injection. Peak serum levels of approximately 11 mg/l and 23 mg/l are reached one hour after i.m. doses of 250 mg and 500 mg respectively. Levels 10 hours after injection are of the order of 0.3 mg/l and 2.1 mg/l respectively.

Twenty per cent or less is bound to serum protein and serum concentrations remain in the bactericidal range for sensitive organisms for 10 to 12 hours.

*Pharmacokinetic properties:* Amikin diffuses readily through extracellular fluids and is excreted in the urine unchanged, primarily by glomerular filtration. Half-life in individuals with normal renal functions is two to three hours.

Following intramuscular administration of a 250 mg dose, about 65% is excreted in six hours and 91% within 24 hours. The urinary concentrations average 563 mg/l in the first 6 hours and 163 mg/l over 6 to 12 hours. Mean urine concentrations after a 500 mg i.m. dose average 832 mg/l in the first six hours.

Single doses of 500 mg administered to normal adults as an intravenous infusion over a period of 30 minutes produce a mean peak serum concentration of 38 mg/l at the end of the infusion. Repeated infusions do not produce drug accumulation.

Amikin has been found in cerebrospinal fluid, pleural fluid, amniotic fluid and in the peritoneal cavity following parenteral administration.

*Preclinical safety data:* No further relevant information.

### Pharmaceutical particulars

*List of excipients:* Sodium Citrate, Sodium Bisulphite, Sulphuric Acid, Water for Injection.

*Incompatibilities:* None.

*Shelf life:* 36 months.

*Special precautions for storage:* Store below 25°C.

*Nature and contents of container:* 2 ml flint glass Type 1 vial with butyl rubber stopper and aluminium seal.

*Instructions for use/handling:* None stated.

**Marketing authorisation numbers**
100 mg/2 ml     0125/0090R
500 mg/2 ml     0215/0092R

**Date of approval/revision of SPC**  October 1995

**Legal category**  POM

## ANGETTES 75*

**Presentation**  White circular tablets embossed 'AJA' on one side, each tablet containing Aspirin BP 75 mg.
Other ingredients: Lactose, maize starch, sodium saccharin.

**Uses**  As a platelet antiaggregatory agent for the prevention of secondary myocardial infarction and in patients suffering from unstable angina.

### Dosage and administration

*Adults:* Following myocardial infarction; two tablets to be taken once daily. Treatment should commence as soon as possible. Patients suffering from unstable angina; four tablets once daily.

*Elderly patients:* The risk/benefit ratios in the elderly have not been fully established.

*Children:* WARNING: Not recommended for children under 12 years old.

### Contra-indications, warnings, etc

*Contra-indications:* Active peptic ulceration, haemophilia and other bleeding disorders, hypersensitivity to aspirin.

*Use in pregnancy:* There is clinical and epidemiological evidence of safety in human pregnancy.

Aspirin may prolong labour and contribute to maternal and neonatal bleeding, and should be avoided at term.

*Precautions:* Aspirin may enhance the effects of anticoagulants and may inhibit the action of uricosurics. Aspirins may precipitate bronchospasm and may induce attacks of asthma in susceptible subjects.

*Warnings and adverse effects:* Aspirin may induce gastro-intestinal haemorrhage, occasionally major. Patients with hypertension should be carefully monitored.

*Overdose:* Overdosage is unlikely due to the low level of aspirin in Angettes. If necessary gastric lavage, forced alkaline diuresis and supportive therapy may be employed. Restoration of acid/base balance may be required.

**Pharmaceutical precautions**  Store at room temperature.

**Legal category**  P.

**Package quantities**  Original packs of 56 tablets.

**Further information**  Nil.

**Product licence number**  0125/5020R.

## BAXAN*

**Presentation**  *Baxan Capsules:* white capsules imprinted with the number 7244 containing cefadroxil monohydrate equivalent to 500 mg cefadroxil activity.

Other ingredients: Colloidal silicon dioxide, lactose, magnesium stearate; gelatin capsules contain titanium dioxide.

*Baxan Suspension:* supplied as a bottle containing powder for reconstitution to provide 125 mg, 250 mg or 500 mg per 5 ml.

Other ingredients: Flavours, polysorbate 40, sodium benzoate, sucrose, titanium dioxide, xanthan gum.

**Uses**  Baxan is a cephalosporin antibiotic bactericidal *in vitro* against a wide range of Gram-positive and Gram-negative micro-organisms. Sensitive Gram-positive organisms include: penicillinase and non-penicillinase-producing *staphylococci*, beta-haemolytic *streptococci*, *Streptococcus pneumoniae* and *Streptococcus pyogenes*. Sensitive Gram-negative organisms include *Escherichia coli*, Klebsiella species, *Proteus mirabilis, Moraxella [Branhamella] catarrhalis* and *Bacteroides spp.* (excluding *Bacteroides fragilis*) and some strains of *Haemophilus influenzae*.

Baxan is indicated in the treatment of the following infections when due to susceptible micro-organisms.

*Respiratory tract infections:* Tonsillitis, pharyngitis, lobar and bronchopneumonia, acute and chronic bronchitis, pulmonary abscess, empyema, pleurisy, sinusitis, laryngitis, otitis media.

*Skin and soft-tissue infections:* Lymphadenitis, abscesses, cellulitis, decubitus ulcers, mastitis, furunculosis, erysipelas.

*Genitourinary tract infections:* Pyelonephritis, cystitis, urethritis, gynaecological infections.

*Other infections:* Osteomyelitis, septic arthritis.

### Dosage and administration

*Adults and children weighing more than 40 kg (88 lbs):* 500 mg to 1 g twice a day, depending upon the severity of infection.

Alternatively, in skin and soft tissue and uncomplicated urinary tract infections, 1 g once a day.

In the treatment of beta-haemolytic streptococcal infections, Baxan should be administered for at least 10 days.

*Children weighing less than 40 kg (88 lbs):*
Under 1 year: 25 mg/kg daily in divided doses, e.g. 2.5 ml of the 125 mg per 5 ml suspension twice a day for a 6 month old infant weighing 5 kg, or 5 ml of the 125 mg per 5 ml suspension twice a day for a 1 year old infant weighing 10 kg.
1–6 years: 250 mg twice a day
Over 6 years: 500 mg twice a day.

*Elderly:* No specific dosage recommendations or precautions for use in the elderly except to monitor those patients with impaired renal function.

The bioavailability and consequent chemotherapeutic effects of cefadroxil are unaffected by food. It may, therefore, be taken with meals or on an empty stomach.

*Renal Impairment Dosage:* In patients with renal impairment, the dosage should be adjusted according to creatinine clearance rates to prevent drug accumulation and serum levels should be monitored. A modified dosage schedule is unnecessary in patients with creatinine clearance rates of greater than 50 ml/min. In those patients with creatinine clearance rates of 50 ml/min or less, the following reduced dosage schedule is recommended as a guideline, based upon the creatinine clearance rate (ml/min/1.73m²).

Patients with renal insufficiency may be treated with an initial dose of 500 mg to 1000 mg of Baxan. Subsequent doses may be administered according to the following table:

| Creatinine clearance | Dose | Dose Interval |
|---|---|---|
| 0–10 ml/min/1.73m² | 500–1000 mg | 36 hrs |
| 11–25 ml/min/1.73m² | 500–1000 mg | 24 hrs |
| 26–50 ml/min/1.73m² | 500–1000 mg | 12 hrs |

Baxan can be removed from the body by haemodialysis.

**Contra-indications, warnings, etc**  Baxan is contra-indicated in patients with a history of hypersensitivity to any of the ingredients.

*Use in pregnancy and lactation:* Although animal studies and clinical experience have not shown any evidence of teratogenicity the safe use of Baxan during pregnancy has not been established. Baxan is excreted in breast milk and should be used with caution in lactating mothers.

*Precautions:* In patients with a history of penicillin allergy, Baxan should be used with caution. There is evidence of partial cross-allergenicity between the penicillins and the cephalosporins. Should an allergic reaction to Baxan occur, the drug should be discontinued and the patient treated with the usual agents (pressor amines, corticosteroids and/or antihistamines), depending on the severity of the reaction.

As experience in premature infants and neonates is limited, the use of Baxan in these patients should only be undertaken with caution.

As with all antibiotics, prolonged use may result in over-growth of non-susceptible organisms.

As with other broad spectrum antibiotics, pseudo-membranous colitis has been reported. It is important to consider its diagnosis in patients who develop diarrhoea in association with Baxan therapy.

*Adverse reactions:* The most commonly reported side-effects are gastrointestinal disturbances and hypersensitivity phenomena. Rash, pruritus, urticaria, angioneurotic oedema have been observed infrequently. Serum sickness, erythema multiforme and anaphylaxis have been reported rarely. Side effects, including nausea, vomiting, diarrhoea, dyspepsia, abdominal discomfort, fever, dizziness, headache, arthralgia and genital candidiasis may also occur. Reversible neutropenia may occur rarely, as may leucopenia, thrombocytopenia, agranulocytosis and minor elevations in serum transaminase and Stevens-Johnson Syndrome. Colitis, including rare instances of pseudo-membraneous colitis, has been reported.

*Overdosage:* Ingestion of <250 mg/kg in children under six years of age was not associated with significant outcomes. The patient should be observed and treated symptomatically. For amounts >250 mg/kg gastric lavage or stimulation of vomiting is appropriate.

*Drug interactions:* There are not sufficient data available to indicate whether the concurrent use of Baxan and potential nephrotoxic agents such as aminoglycosides causes any alteration in their nephrotoxic effects.

A false-positive Coombs' reaction may occur in some patients receiving Baxan.

Urine from patients treated with Baxan may give a false-positive glycosuria reaction when tested with Benedict's or Fehling's solutions. This does not occur with enzyme based tests.

**Pharmaceutical precautions**  Store below 30°C in a dry place.

**Legal category**  POM.

**Package quantities**  Capsules – Containers of 100.
Suspension – Bottles containing 60 ml

**Further information**  Nil.

**Product licence numbers**
Baxan 500 mg capsules          0125/0107
Baxan 125 mg/5 ml suspension    0125/0110
Baxan 250 mg/5 ml suspension    0125/0111
Baxan 500 mg/5 ml suspension    0125/0112

## BiCNU*

**Presentation**  *BiCNU Injection:* each package contains a 30 ml vial containing 100 mg carmustine and a 5 ml vial containing 3 ml sterile ethanol diluent.

**Uses**  BiCNU is indicated as palliative therapy as a single agent or in established combination therapy with other approved chemotherapeutic agents in the following:

1. Brain tumours – Glioblastoma, brainstem glioma, medulloblastoma, astrocytoma, ependymoma, and metastatic brain tumours.
2. Multiple myeloma – In combination with prednisone.
3. Hodgkin's Disease – As secondary therapy in combination with other approved drugs in patients who relapse while being treated with primary therapy, or who fail to respond to primary therapy.
4. Non-Hodgkin's lymphomas – As secondary therapy in combination with other approved drugs in patients who relapse while being treated with primary therapy, or who fail to respond to primary therapy.

### Dosage and administration

*Intravenous administration:* The recommended dose of BiCNU as single agent in previously untreated patients is 200 mg/m² intravenously every six weeks. This may be given as a single dose or divided into daily injections such as 100 mg/m² on two successive days.

When BiCNU is used in combination with other myelosuppressive drugs or in patients in whom bone marrow reserve is depleted the doses should be adjusted accordingly.

A repeat course of BiCNU should not be given until circulating blood elements have returned to acceptable levels (platelets above 100,000/mm³; leucocytes above 4,000/mm³) and this is usually in six weeks. Blood counts should be monitored frequently and repeat courses should not be given before six weeks because of delayed toxicity.

Doses subsequent to the initial dose should be adjusted according to the haematological response of the patient to the preceding dose. The following schedule is suggested as a guide to dosage adjustment.

| Nadir after Prior Dose | | Percentage of prior dose to be given |
|---|---|---|
| Leucocytes (/mm³) | Platelets (/mm³) | |
| > 4000 | > 100,000 | 100 |
| 3000–3999 | 75,000–99,999 | 100 |
| 2000–2999 | 25,000–74,999 | 70 |
| < 2000 | < 25,000 | 50 |

*Children:* BiCNU should be used with extreme caution in children due to the high risk of pulmonary toxicity (see *Warnings*).

*Elderly:* No dosage adjustment is required on the grounds of age.

**Contra-indications, warnings, etc** *Contra indications:* BiCNU should not be given to individuals who have demonstrated a previous hypersensitivity to it.

BiCNU should not be given to individuals with decreased circulating platelets, leucocytes, or erythrocytes either from previous chemotherapy or other causes.

*Warnings and precautions:* Pulmonary toxicity characterised by pulmonary infiltrates and/or fibrosis has been reported to occur with a frequency ranging up to 30%. This may occur within 3 years of therapy and appears to be dose related with total cumulative doses of 1200–1500 mg/m² being associated with increased likelihood of lung fibrosis. Risk factors include smoking, the presence of a respiratory condition, pre-existing radiographic abnormalities, sequential or concomitant thoracic irradiation and association with other agents that cause lung damage.

Cases of late pulmonary fibrosis, occurring up to 17 years after treatment, have also been reported. In a long-term follow-up of 17 patients who survived childhood brain tumours eight (47%) died of lung fibrosis. Of these eight deaths, two occurred within 3 years of treatment and 6 occurred 8–13 years after treatment. Of the patients who died, the median age at treatment was 2.5 years (range 1–12); the median age of the long-term survivors was 10 years (5–16 years at treatment). All five patients treated under the age of 5 years have died of pulmonary fibrosis. In this study, the dose of BiCNU did not influence fatal outcome nor did co-administration of vincristine or spinal irradiation. Of the remaining survivors available for follow-up, evidence of lung fibrosis was detected in all patients. The risks and benefits of BiCNU therapy must be carefully considered especially in young patients, due to extremely high risk of pulmonary toxicity.

BiCNU should be administered by individuals experienced in antineoplastic therapy. Bone marrow toxicity is a common and severe toxic effect of BiCNU. Complete blood counts should be monitored frequently for at least six weeks after a dose. Repeat doses of BiCNU should not be given more frequently than every six weeks. The bone marrow toxicity of BiCNU is cumulative and therefore dosage adjustment must be considered on the basis of nadir blood counts from prior dose (see Dosage Adjustment Table under Dosage).

It is recommended that liver function, kidney function and pulmonary function also be monitored.

*Pregnancy and lactation:* BiCNU should not normally be administered to patients who are pregnant or mothers who are breast-feeding. Male patients should be advised to use adequate contraceptive measures.

Safe use in pregnancy has not been established and therefore the benefit to risk of toxicity must be carefully weighed. BiCNU is embryotoxic and teratogenic in rats and embryotoxic in rabbits at dose levels equivalent to the human dose. BiCNU also affects fertility in male rats at doses somewhat higher than the human dose.

BiCNU is carcinogenic in rats and mice, producing a marked increase in tumour incidence in doses approximating those employed clinically.

*Adverse reactions:* Haematological: Delayed myelosuppression is a frequent and serious adverse event associated with BiCNU administration. It usually occurs four to six weeks after drug administration and is dose-related. Platelet nadirs occur at four to five weeks; leucocyte nadirs occur at five to six weeks post therapy. Thrombocytopenia is generally more severe than leucopenia. However both may be dose limiting toxicities. Anaemia also occurs, but is generally less severe. The occurrence of acute leukaemia and bone marrow dysplasias have been reported in patients following long term nitrosourea therapy.

*Gastro-intestinal:* Nausea and vomiting after i.v. administration of BiCNU are noted frequently. This reaction appears within two hours of dosing, usually lasting four to six hours and is dose-related. Prior

administration of anti-emetics is effective in diminishing and sometimes preventing this side-effect.

*Hepatic:* When high doses of BiCNU have been employed, a reversible type of hepatic toxicity, manifested by increased transaminase, alkaline phosphatase and bilirubin levels, has been reported in a small percentage of patients.

*Pulmonary:* See *Warnings and Precautions.*

*Renal:* Renal abnormalities consisting of decrease in kidney size, progressive azotaemia and renal failure have been reported in patients who receive large cumulative doses after prolonged therapy with BiCNU and related nitrosoureas. Kidney damage has also been reported in patients receiving lower total doses.

*Cardiovascular:* Hypotension, tachycardia have been reported.

*Local:* Burning at the site of injection is common but true thrombosis is rare.

*Other:* Rapid i.v. infusion of BiCNU may produce intense flushing of the skin and suffusion of the conjunctiva within two hours, lasting about four hours. Neuroretinitis, chest pain, headache, allergic reactions have been reported.

**Pharmaceutical precautions IMPORTANT NOTE:** The lyophilised dosage formulation contains no preservatives and is not intended as multiple dose vial. Reconstitutions and further dilutions should be carried out under aseptic conditions.

Unopened vials of the dry powder must be stored in a refrigerator (2–8°C).

Once reconstituted as recommended, resulting solutions, undiluted or further diluted (with 500 ml of sodium chloride for injection or 500 ml of 5% glucose for injection) may be stored up to a total of 24 hours when stored at 2–8°C and protected from light.

*Compatibility/incompatibility with containers:* The intravenous solution is suitable for infusion in polythene or glass containers. Studies have shown carmustine to be incompatible with PVC containers as it is readily absorbed on plastic.

*Preparation of intravenous solution:* Dissolve BiCNU with 3 ml of the supplied sterile diluent (absolute ethanol) and then aseptically add 27 ml of sterile water for injection to the alcohol solution. Each ml of the resulting solution will contain 3.3 mg of BiCNU in 10% ethanol and has a pH of 5.6 to 6.0.

Reconstitution as recommended results in a clear colourless solution which may be further diluted with sodium chloride for injection, or 5% glucose for injection.

The reconstituted solution must be given intravenously and should be administered by i.v. drip over a one- to two-hour period. Injection of BiCNU over shorter periods of time may produce intense pain and burning at the site of injection.

**IMPORTANT NOTE:** BiCNU has a low melting point (approximately 30·5–32·0°C or 86·9–89·6°F). Exposure of the drug to this temperature or above will cause the drug to liquefy and appear as an oil film in the bottom of the vials. This is a sign of decomposition and vials should be discarded.

*Guidelines for the safe handling of antineoplastic agents:*

1. Trained personnel should reconstitute the drug.
2. This should be performed in a designated area.
3. Adequate protective gloves should be worn.
4. Precautions should be taken to avoid the drug accidentally coming into contact with the eyes. In the event of contact with the eyes, flush with copious amounts of water and/or saline.
5. The cytotoxic preparation should not be handled by pregnant staff.
6. Adequate care and precaution should be taken in the disposal of items (syringes, needles etc) used to reconstitute cytotoxic drugs. Excess material and body waste may be disposed of by placing in double sealed polythene bags and incinerating at a temperature of 1,000°C. Liquid waste may be flushed with copious amounts of water.
7. The work surface should be covered with disposable plastic-backed absorbent paper.
8. Use Luer-Lock fittings on all syringes and sets. Large bore needles are recommended to minimise pressure and the possible formation of aerosols. The latter may also be reduced by the use of a venting needle.

**Legal category** POM.

**Package quantities** BiCNU Injection packed in cartons of 10 units, each unit consisting of one vial of carmustine 100 mg and one vial of sterile absolute alcohol 3 ml.

**Further information** BiCNU alkylates DNA and RNA and has also been shown to inhibit several enzymes by carbamoylation of amino acids in proteins.

Intravenously administered BiCNU is rapidly degraded, with no intact drug detectable after 15 minutes. However, in studies with $C_{14}$ labelled drug,

prolonged levels of the isotope were observed in the plasma and tissue, probably representing radioactive fragments of the parent compound.

It is thought that the antineoplastic and toxic activities of BiCNU may be due to metabolites. Approximately 60 to 70% of a total dose is excreted in the urine in 96 hours and about 10% as respiratory $CO_2$. The fate of the remainder is undetermined.

Because of the high lipid solubility and the relative lack of ionisation at a physiological pH, BiCNU crosses the blood brain barrier.

Levels of radioactivity in the CSF are at least 50% higher than those measured concurrently in plasma.

**Product licence number** 0125/0108.

## BUSPAR*

**Presentation** Buspar 5 mg tablets: white, pillow-shaped biconvex tablet engraved '5' on one face. Each tablet contains buspirone hydrochloride 5 mg.

Buspar 10 mg tablets: white, pillow-shaped biconvex tablet, engraved '10' and a scoreline on one face. Each tablet contains buspirone hydrochloride 10 mg.

Other ingredients: Colloidal silicon dioxide, lactose anhydrous, magnesium stearate, microcrystalline cellulose, sodium starch glycollate.

**Uses** Buspar is indicated for the short-term management of anxiety disorders and the relief of symptoms of anxiety with or without accompanying depression.

**Dosage and administration** Dosage should be adjusted according to response for maximum effect. The recommended initial dose is 5 mg two to three times daily and this may be increased every two to three days. The usual therapeutic dose is 15 to 30 mg daily in divided doses with a maximum recommended dose of 45 mg daily in divided doses.

*Elderly:* Dosage should be adjusted according to response for maximum effect. The recommended initial dose is 5 mg two to three times daily and this may be increased as required. The usual therapeutic dose is 15 to 30 mg daily in divided doses with a maximum recommended dose of 45 mg daily in divided doses.

*Children:* Use in children has not been established.

**Contra-indications, warnings, etc**

*Contra-indications:* Buspar should not be used in patients hypersensitive to buspirone hydrochloride. Buspar should not be used in patients with epilepsy. In patients with a history of renal or hepatic impairment buspirone should be used with caution. Buspar should not be used in patients with severe renal impairment, defined as a creatinine clearance of 20 ml/minute or below, or a plasma creatinine above 200 micromoles/litre. Buspar should not be used in patients with severe hepatic disease.

*Use in pregnancy and lactation:* In some studies, administration of high doses of buspirone to pregnant animals produced effects on survival, birth and weanling weights, although there was no effect on foetal development. Since the relevance of this finding in humans has not been established, Buspar is contra-indicated in pregnancy and in lactation.

*Precautions:* In controlled studies in healthy volunteers Buspar in single doses up to 20 mg caused no significant impairment of cognitive or psychomotor functions, unlike the benzodiazepines, diazepam or lorazepam. In studies in healthy volunteers, Buspar did not potentiate the psychomotor impairment produced by alcohol, in contrast to a comparative benzodiazepine. However no data is available on concomitant use of alcohol and Buspar at single doses greater than 20 mg. It is prudent therefore to avoid alcohol while taking Buspar.

As Buspar does not exhibit cross-tolerance with benzodiazepines and other common sedative/hypnotic agents, it will not block the withdrawal syndrome often seen with cessation of therapy with these compounds. Before starting therapy with Buspar, it is advisable to withdraw patients gradually from prior chronic treatment with these agents.

*Drug interactions:* The occurrence of elevated blood pressure in patients receiving both buspirone and monoamine oxidase inhibitors (phenelzine and tranylcypromine) has been reported. It is therefore recommended that Buspar should not be used concomitantly with a monoamine oxidase inhibitor.

*In vitro* studies have shown that buspirone does not displace warfarin, digoxin, phenytoin or propranolol from plasma proteins.

In a study in normal volunteers, no interaction with amitriptyline was seen. A similar study with diazepam showed a slight increase in metabolite (nordiazepam) levels.

*Side-effects:* Buspar is generally well tolerated. If side-effects occur they are normally observed at the beginning of treatment and usually subside with continued use and/or decreased dosage.

In controlled trials, the only side-effects that occurred with significantly greater frequency with buspirone treatment than with placebo were dizziness, headache, nervousness, light-headedness, excitement and nausea. Tachycardia, palpitations, chest pain, drowsiness, confusion, dry mouth, fatigue and sweating/clamminess have also been reported rarely.

*Overdose:* There is no specific antidote to Buspar. Buspar is not removed by haemodialysis. The stomach should be emptied as quickly as possible. Treatment should be symptomatic and supportive. The ingestion of multiple agents should be suspected.

Death by deliberate or accidental overdose has not been observed. A dose of 375 mg per day in healthy volunteers produced no significant adverse effects. As maximum dose levels are reached symptoms most commonly observed are: nausea, vomiting, dizziness, drowsiness and miosis.

**Pharmaceutical precautions** Buspirone tablets should be stored at room temperature.

**Legal category** POM.

**Package quantities** 5 mg: 100 tablet bottle; 6 × 21 tablet calendar pack. 10 mg: 100 tablet bottle.

**Further information** Buspar is an azaspirodecanedione. The exact mechanism of Buspar anxioselective action is not fully known. It does not act on benzodiazepine receptor sites and lacks sedative, anticonvulsant and muscle relaxant properties. From animal studies it is known to interact with serotonin, noradrenaline, acetylcholine and dopamine systems of the brain. Buspar enhances the activity of specific noradrenergic and dopaminergic pathways, whereas the activity of serotonin and acetylcholine are reduced.

Buspar is rapidly absorbed when given orally. It is then subject to considerable first-pass metabolism. Peak plasma levels occur 60–90 minutes after dosing. Plasma concentration is linearly related to dose. Following multiple dosing steady state plasma concentrations are achieved within 2 days. Buspar is 95% protein bound. Buspar is eliminated primarily by liver metabolism. In pharmacokinetic studies mean plasma half-lives have varied from 2 to 11 hours.

**Product licence numbers**
5 mg tablets      0125/0162.
10 mg tablets     0125/0163

## KERI* THERAPEUTIC LOTION

**Presentation** Keri Therapeutic Lotion is a white lotion containing mineral oil, 16%.

Other ingredients: Carbomer 934, glyceryl monostearate, lanolin oil, laureth 4, methyl hydroxybenzoate, perfume, PEG-4 dilaurate, polyethylene glycol 40 stearate, propyl hydroxybenzoate, propylene glycol, quaternium 15, sodium dioctyl sulphosuccinate, triethanolamine, water.

**Uses** Keri Therapeutic Lotion has emollient properties. It is indicated for the symptomatic treatment of dermatitis, eczema, ichthyosis, ammoniacal dermatitis (nappy rash), protection of raw and abraded skin areas, pruritus and related conditions where dry scaly skin is a problem. It is also indicated as an emollient before bathing for dry/eczematous skin, to alleviate drying effects.

**Dosage and administration** Keri Therapeutic Lotion should be gently massaged into the skin three times daily or as often as required.

*Elderly:* No dosage adjustment is necessary.

**Contra-indications, warnings, etc** Keri Therapeutic Lotion contains lanolin oil and is therefore contra-indicated in those patients allergic to this ingredient.

**Pharmaceutical precautions** Store at room temperature.

**Legal category** P.

**Package quantities** Bottles containing 190 ml & 380 ml.

**Further information** Nil.

**Product licence number** 0125/0152

## MEGACE* TABLETS

**Qualitative and quantitative composition** Each tablet contains Megestrol Acetate BP 40 or 160 mg.

**Pharmaceutical form** Oral tablets.

**Clinical particulars**
*Therapeutic indications:* Megace is a progestational agent, indicated for the treatment of certain hormone dependent neoplasms, such as a endometrial or breast cancer.

*Posology and method of administration:*
*Breast cancer:* 160 mg/day (40 mg qid or 160 mg taken once daily).

*Endometrial cancer:* 40–320 mg/day in divided doses (40–80 mg one to four times daily or one to two 160 mg tablets daily).

At least two months of continuous treatment is considered an adequate period for determining the efficacy of Megace.

*Children:* Megace is not recommended for use in children.

*Elderly:* No dosage adjustments is necessary.

*Contra-indications:* Megace is contra-indicated in patients who have demonstrated hypersensitivity to the drug.

*Special warnings and special precautions for use:*
*Precautions:* Megace should be used with caution in patients with a history of thrombophlebitis.

*Interactions with other medicaments and other forms of interaction:* None stated.

*Pregnancy and lactation:* Megace should not normally be administered to women who are pregnant or to mothers who are breast feeding.

Fertility and reproduction studies with high doses of megestrol acetate have shown a reversible feminising effect on some male rat foetuses.

Several reports suggest an association between intrauterine exposure to progestational drugs in the first trimester of pregnancy and genital abnormalities in male and female foetuses. The risk of hypospadias in male foetuses may be approximately doubled with the exposure to progestational drugs.

If a patient is exposed to Megace during the first four months of pregnancy or if she becomes pregnant whilst taking Megace, she should be apprised of the potential risks to the foetus.

Women of child bearing potential should be advised to avoid becoming pregnant.

Because of the potential for adverse effects, nursing should be discontinued during treatment with Megace.

*Effects on the ability to drive and use machines:* None stated.

*Undesirable effects:* The major side-effect experienced by patients while taking megestrol acetate, particularly at high doses, is weight gain, which is usually not associated with water retention, but which is secondary to an increased appetite and food intake. Other occasionally noted side effects are nausea, vomiting, oedema and breakthrough uterine bleeding. Rare reports have been received of patients developing dyspnoea, heart failure, hypertension, hot flushes, mood changes, cushingoid faces, tumour flare (with or without hypercalcaemia), hyperglycaemia, alopecia and carpal tunnel syndrome while taking megestrol acetate. Thromboembolic phenomena including thrombophlebitis and pulmonary embolism (in some cases fatal) have been reported. A rarely encountered side effect of prolonged administration of megestrol acetate is urticaria, presumably an idiosyncratic reaction to the drug. The drug is devoid of the myelosuppressive activity characteristic of many cytotoxic drugs and it causes no significant changes in haematology, blood chemistry or urinalysis.

Clinical and laboratory evidence of mild adrenal suppression has been observed in patients receiving Megace.

*Overdose:* No serious side-effects have resulted from studies involving Megace (megestrol acetate) administered in dosages as high as 1600 mg/day.

There is no specific antidote to overdosage and treatment should therefore be symptomatic.

**Pharmacological properties**
*Pharmacodynamic properties:* Megace (megestrol acetate) possesses pharmacological properties similar to those of natural progesterone. Its progestational activity is slightly greater than that of medroxyprogesterone acetate, norethindrone, norethindrone acetate and norethynodrel; slightly less than that of chlormadinone acetate; and substantially less than that of norgestrel.

Megestrol acetate is a potent progestogen that exerts significant anti-oestrogenic effects. It has no androgenic or oestrogenic properties. It has antigonadotropic, anti-uterotropic and anti-androgenic/anti-myotropic actions. It has a slight but significant glucocorticoid effect and a very slight mineralocorticoid effect.

The progestational activity of megestrol acetate has been assessed in a number of standard tests, including clauberg-mcphail, mcginty, uterotropic and carbonic anhydrase tests in rabbits; pregnancy maintenance and delay-of-implantation tests in rats; endometrial response in rhesus monkeys; conversion of an oestrogen-primed endometrium to a secretory one in normal women and in those with secondary amenorrhea with resultant withdrawal bleeding; induction of pseudopregnancy for treatment of endometriosis; and the delay-of-menses and thermogenic tests. In all these tests, progestational activity was high.

It has been demonstrated that megestrol acetate blocks oestrogen effects in the uteri of rats and mice

in human cervical mucus and vaginal mucosa. Anti-gondotropic activity has been demonstrated in rats of both sexes.

*Pharmacokinetic properties:*
*Animal:* Peak plasma levels occur four to six hours after oral administration of radioactively labelled megestrol acetate to female rats. High concentrations are found in the liver, fat, adrenal glands, ovaries and kidneys. Radioactivity is almost wholly cleared within a week, chiefly by biliary excretion to the faeces.

In dogs, megestrol acetate metabolite are excreted primarily in the faeces. In rabbits, the principal route of metabolic excretion is urinary and the major metabolites are the 2-alpha-hydroxy-6-hydroxymethyl and 6-hydroxymethyl derivatives.

*Human:* Peak plasma levels of tritiated megestrol acetate and metabolites occur one to three hours after oral administration. When 60 to 91 mg doses of c-labelled megestrol acetate were administered to women, urinary excretion of radioactivity accounted for 57% to 78% of the dose within 10 days, while 8% to 30% was excreted in the faeces. There is no unchanged drug in the urine and no apparent a-ring aromatisation to oestrogenic substances. Three major metabolites excreted in urine as glucuronide conjugates have been identified as 17-alpha-acetoxy-2-alpha hydroxy-6-methylpregna-4,6-diene-3,20-dione; 17-alpha-acetoxy-6-hydroxymethylpregna-4,6-diene-3,20-dione,; and 17-alpha-acetoxy-2-alpha-hydroxy-6-hydromethylpregna-4,6-diene-3,20-dione.

Serum concentrations were measured after the administration of single and multiple oral doses of megestrol acetate. Both men and women participated in the study. All were healthy volunteer adults not more than 65 years of age and the women were postmenopausal.

Megestrol acetate is readily absorbed following oral administration of 20, 40, 80 and 200 mg doses. Megestrol serum concentrations increase with increasing doses, the relationship between increasing dosage and increasing serum levels not being arithmetically proportional. Average peak serum concentrations for the four doses tested were 89, 190, 209 and 465 ng/ml.

Mean peak serum concentrations are found three hours after single-dose administration for all dosage levels studied. The serum concentration curve appears biphasic, and the beta-phase half-life is 15 to 20 hours longer.

After multiple doses over a three-day period, serum levels increase each day and are estimated to reach 80% to 90% predicted steady-state levels on the third day.

*Preclinical safety data:* No further relevant data.

**Pharmaceutical particulars**
*List of excipients: 40 mg Tablets:* Acacia, calcium hydrogen phosphate, lactose, magnesium stearate, maize starch, silicon dioxide. *160 mg Tablets:* Colloidal silicon dioxide, lactose monohydrate, magnesium stearate, microcrystalline cellulose, povidone, sodium starch glycollate.

*Incompatibilities:* None stated.

*Shelf life:* 36 months.

*Special precautions for storage:* Megace tablets should be stored below 25°C.

*Nature and contents of container:*
40 mg tablet – blister packs of 100 tablets.
160 mg tablet – blister packs of 30 tablets.

*Instructions for use handling:* None.

**Marketing authorisation numbers**
Megace 40 mg    0125/0144
Megace 160 mg   0125/0173

**Date of approval/revison of SPC** 24 January 1996.

**Legal Category** POM.

## PARAPLATIN* SOLUTION

**Qualitative and quantitative composition** Paraplatin Solution contains carboplatin (cis-diammine (1,1-cyclobutane-dicarboxylato) platinum) as a 10 mg/ml solution in water for injection.

**Pharmaceutical form** Solution for intravenous injection.

**Clinical particulars**
*Therapeutic indications:* Paraplatin is indicated for the treatment of:

1. advanced ovarian carcinoma of epithelial origin in:
   a. first line therapy
   b. second line therapy, after other treatments have failed.
2. small cell carcinoma of the lung.

*Posology and method of administration:* Paraplatin should be used by the intravenous route only. The recommended dosage of Paraplatin in previously untreated adult patients with normal kidney function is 400 mg/m² as a single i.v. dose administered by a 15 to 60 minutes infusion. Alternatively, see Calvert formula below. Therapy should not be repeated until four weeks after the previous Paraplatin course and/or until the neutrophil count is at least 2,000 cells/mm³ and the platelet count is at least 100,000 cells/mm³.

Reduction of the initial dosage by 20-25% is recommended for those patients who present with risk factors such as prior myelosuppressive treatment and low performance status (ECOG-Zubrod 2-4 or Karnofsky below 80).

Determination of the haematological nadir by weekly blood counts during the initial courses of treatment with Paraplatin is recommended for future dosage adjustment.

*Impaired Renal Function:* The optimal use of Paraplatin in patients presenting with impaired renal function requires adequate dosage adjustments and frequent monitoring of both haematological nadirs and renal function.

Dosage (mg) = target AUC (mg/ml x min) x [GFR ml/min + 25]

Note: With the Calvert formula, the total dose of carboplatin is calculated in mg, not mg/m².

| Target AUC | Planned Chemotherapy | Patient treatment status |
|---|---|---|
| 5-7 mg/ml.min | single agent carboplatin | Previously untreated |
| 4-6 mg/ml.min | single agent carboplatin | Previously treated |
| 4-6 mg/ml.min | carboplatin plus cyclophosphamide | Previously untreated |

*Combination therapy:* The optimal use of Paraplatin in combination with other myelosuppressive agents requires dosage adjustments according to the regimen and schedule to be adopted.

*Paediatrics:* Sufficient usage of Paraplatin in paediatrics has not occurred to allow specific dosage recommendations to be made.

*Elderly:* Dosage adjustment, initially or subsequently, may be necessary, dependent on the physical condition of the patient.

*Dilution and reconstitution:* See *Instructions for use/handling.*

*Contra-indications:* Paraplatin should not be used in patients with severe pre-existing renal impairment (creatinine clearance at or below 20 ml/minute).

It should not be employed in severely myelosuppressed patients. It is also contra-indicated in patients with a history of several allergic reactions to Paraplatin or other platinum containing compounds.

*Special warnings and special precautions for use Warnings:* Paraplatin should be administered by individuals experienced in the use of anti-neoplastic therapy.

Paraplatin myelosuppression is closely related to its renal clearance. Patients with abnormal kidney function or receiving concomitant therapy with other drugs with nephrotoxic potential are likely to experience more severe and prolonged myelotoxicity. Renal function parameters should therefore be carefully assessed before and during therapy. Paraplatin courses should not be repeated more frequently than monthly under normal circumstances. Thrombocytopenia, leukopenia and anaemia occur after administration of Paraplatin. Frequent monitoring of peripheral blood counts is recommended throughout and following therapy with Paraplatin. Paraplatin combination therapy with other myelosuppressive compounds must be planned very carefully with respect to dosages and timing in order to minimise additive effects. Supportive transfusional therapy may be required in patients who suffer severe myelosuppression.

Paraplatin can cause nausea and vomiting. Premedication with anti-emetics has been reported to be useful in reducing the incidence and intensity of these effects.

Renal and hepatic function impairment may be encountered with Paraplatin. Very high doses of Paraplatin (>5 times single agent recommended dose) have resulted in severe abnormalities in hepatic and renal function. Although no clinical evidence on compounding nephrotoxicity has been accumulated, it is recommended not to combine Paraplatin with aminoglycosides or other nephrotoxic compounds.

Infrequent allergic reactions to Paraplatin have been reported, i.e. skin reactions usually designated as a rash. Rarely anaphylaxis, angio-oedema and anaphylactoid reactions including bronchospasm, urticaria and facial oedema have occurred. These reactions are similar to those observed after administration of other platinum containing compounds and may occur within minutes. Patients should be observed carefully for possible allergic reactions and managed with appropriate supportive therapy.

The carcinogenic potential of Paraplatin has not been studied but compounds with similar mechanisms of action and mutagenicity have been reported to be carcinogenic.

*Precautions:* Peripheral blood counts and renal and hepatic function tests should be monitored closely. Blood counts at the beginning of the therapy and weekly to assess haematological nadir for subsequent dose adjustment are recommended. Neurological evaluations should also be performed on a regular basis.

*Interactions with other medicaments and other forms of interaction:* The use of Paraplatin with nephrotoxic compounds is not recommended.

*Pregnancy and lactation:* The safe use of Paraplatin during pregnancy has not been established: Paraplatin has been shown to be an embryotoxin and teratogen in rats. If Paraplatin is used during pregnancy the patient should be apprised of the potential hazard to the foetus. Women of child-bearing potential should be advised to avoid becoming pregnant.

Carboplatin has been shown to be mutagenic *in vivo* and *in vitro.*

*Nursing mothers:* It is not known whether Paraplatin is excreted in human milk.

*Effects on ability to drive and use machines:* None reported.

*Undesirable effects:* Incidences of adverse reactions reported hereunder are based on cumulative data obtained in a large group of patients with various pretreatment prognostic features.

*Haematological toxicity:* Myelosuppression is the dose-limiting toxicity of Paraplatin. At maximum tolerated dosages of Paraplatin administered as a single agent, thrombocytopenia, with nadir platelet counts of less than 50 x 10⁹/L, occurs in about a quarter of the patients.

The nadir usually occurs between days 14 and 21, with recovery within 35 days from the start of therapy. Leukopenia has also occurred in approximately 14% of patients but its recovery from the day of nadir (day 14-28) may be slower and usually occurs within 42 days from the start of therapy. Neutropenia with granulocyte counts below 1 x 10⁹/L occurs in approximately one fifth of patients. Anaemia with haemoglobin values below 11 g/dL has been observed in more than two-thirds of patients with normal baseline values.

Myelosuppression may be more severe and prolonged in patients with impaired renal function, extensive prior treatment, poor performance status and age above 65. Myelosuppression is also worsened by therapy combining Paraplatin with other compounds that are myelosuppressive.

Myelosuppression is usually reversible and not cumulative when Paraplatin is used as a single agent and at the recommended dosages and frequencies of administration.

Infectious complications have occasionally been reported. Haemorrhagic compli-cations, usually minor, have also been reported.

*Nephrotoxicity:* Renal toxicity is usually not dose-limiting in patients receiving Paraplatin, nor does it require preventive measures such as high volume fluid hydration or forced diuresis. Nevertheless, increasing blood urea or serum creatinine levels can occur. Renal function impairment, as defined by a decrease in the creatinine clearance below 60 ml/min, may also be observed. The incidence and severity of nephrotoxicity may increase in patients who have impaired kidney function before Paraplatin treatment. It is not clear whether an appropriate hydration programme might overcome such an effect, but dosage reduction or discontinuation of therapy is required in the presence of severe alteration of renal function tests.

Decreases in serum electrolytes (sodium, magnesium, potassium and calcium) have been reported after treatment with Paraplatin but have not been reported to be severe enough to cause the appearance of clinical signs or symptoms.

Cases of hyponatraemia have been reported. Haemolytic uraemic syndrome has been reported rarely.

*Gastrointestinal toxicity:* Nausea without vomiting occurs in about 15% of patients receiving Paraplatin; vomiting has been reported in over half of the patients and about one-fifth of these suffer severe emesis. Nausea and vomiting usually disappear within 24 hours after treatment and are usually responsive to (and may be prevented by) anti-emetic medication. A fifth of patients experience no nausea or vomiting.

Cases of anorexia have been reported.

*Allergic reactions:* Infrequent allergic reactions to Paraplatin have been reported. These reactions are similar to those observed after administration of other platinum-containing compounds, i.e. erythematous rash, fever with no apparent cause and pruritus.

*Ototoxicity:* Subclinical decrease in hearing acuity, consisting of high-frequency (4000-8000 Hz) hearing loss determined by audiogram, has been reported in 15% of the patients treated with Paraplatin. However, only 1% of patients present with clinical symptoms, manifested in the majority of cases by tinnitus. In patients who have been previously treated with cisplatin and have developed hearing loss related to such treatment, the hearing impairment may persist or worsen.

*Neurotoxicity:* The incidence of peripheral neuropathies after treatment with Paraplatin is 4%. In the majority of the patients neurotoxicity is limited to paraesthesia and decreased deep tendon reflexes. The frequency and intensity of this side effect increases in elderly patients and those previously treated with cisplatin.

Paraesthesia present before commencing Paraplatin therapy, particularly if related to prior cisplatin treatment, may persist or worsen during treatment with Paraplatin.

*Ocular toxicity:* Transient visual disturbances, sometimes including transient sight loss, have been reported rarely with platinum therapy. This is usually associated with high dose therapy in renally impaired patients.

*Other:* Abnormalities of liver function tests (usually mild to moderate) have been reported with Paraplatin in about one-third of the patients with normal baseline values. The alkaline phosphatase level is increased more frequently than SGOT, SGPT or total bilirubin. The majority of these abnormalities regress spontaneously during the course of treatment.

Infrequent events consisting of taste alteration, asthenia, alopecia, fever and chills without evidence of infection have occurred.

*Overdose:* There is no known antidote for Paraplatin overdosage. The anticipated complications of overdosage would be related to myelosuppression as well as impairment of hepatic and renal function.

**Pharmacological properties**

*Pharmacodynamic properties:* Carboplatin is an anti-neoplastic agent. Its activity has been demonstrated against several murine and human cell lines.

Carboplatin exhibited comparable activity to cisplatin against a wide range of tumours regardless of implant site.

Alkaline elution techniques and DNA binding studies have demonstrated the qualitatively similar modes of action of carboplatin and cisplatin. Carboplatin, like cisplatin, induces changes in the superhelical conformation of DNA which is consistent with a "DNA shortening effect".

*Pharmacokinetic properties:* Paraplatin has biochemical properties similar to that of cisplatin, thus producing predominantly interstrand and intrastrand DNA crosslinks. Following administration of Paraplatin in man, linear relationships exist between dose and plasma concentrations of total and free ultrafilterable platinum. The area under the plasma concentration versus time curve for total platinum also shows a linear relationship with the dose.

Repeated dosing during four consecutive days did not produce an accumulation of platinum in plasma. Following the administration of Paraplatin reported values for the terminal elimination of half-lives of free ultrafilterable platinum and Paraplatin in man are approximately 6 hours and 1.5 hours respectively. During the initial phase, most of the free ultrafilterable platinum is present as Paraplatin. The terminal half-life for total plasma platinum is 24 hours. Approximately 87% of plasma platinum is protein bound within 24 hours following administration. Paraplatin is excreted primarily in the urine, with recovery of approximately 70% of the administered platinum within 24 hours. Most of the drug is excreted in the first 6 hours. Total body and renal clearances of free ultrafilterable platinum correlate with the rate of glomerular filtration but not tubular secretion.

*Preclinical safety data:* Paraplatin has been shown to be embryotoxic and teratogenic in rats. (See *Pregnancy and lactation.*) It is mutagenic in vivo and in vitro and although the carcinogenic potential of Paraplatin has not been studied, compounds with similar mechanisms of action and mutagenicity have been reported to be carcinogenic.

**Pharmaceutical particulars**

*List of excipients:* Water for Injections.

*Incompatibilities:* Needles or intravenous sets containing aluminium parts that may come into contact with Paraplatin should not be used for preparation or administration of Paraplatin.

*Shelf life:* Unopened product: 18 months. After dilution: 8 hours at room temperature (15–25°C), or 24 hours under refrigeration (2–8°C)

*Special precautions for storage:* Paraplatin should be stored at room temperature (15–25°C) and protected from light. When diluted as directed, it is recommended that any Paraplatin Solution be discarded after 8 hours from dilution if stored at room temperature (15–25°C) or after 24 hours if stored refrigerated (2–8°C).

*Nature and contents of container:* Cardboard carton

containing a flint glass vial with a rubber or Daikyo compound Teflon coated stopper and aluminium closure with polypropylene top, containing either 50 mg, 150 mg or 450 mg carboplatin as a 10 mg/ml solution.

*Instructions for use/handling:* This product is for single dose use only.

*Reconstitution:* The product may be diluted with 5% Glucose for Injection BP, or 0.9% Sodium Chloride for Injection BP, to concentrations as low as 0.5 mg/ml (500 micrograms / ml).

When diluted as directed, Paraplatin solutions are stable for eight hours stored at room temperature or 24 hours stored under refrigeration. Since no antibacterial preservatives are contained in the formulation, it is recommended that any Paraplatin solution be discarded after eight hours from dilution if stored at room temperature or after 24 hours if stored refrigerated. This product is for single dose use only.

*Guidelines for the safe handling of anti-neoplastic agents:*

1. Trained personnel should reconstitute the drug.
2. This should be performed in a designated area.
3. Adequate protective gloves should be worn.
4. Precautions should be taken to avoid the drug accidentally coming into contact with the eyes. In the event of contact with the eyes, wash with water and/or saline.
5. The cytotoxic preparation should not be handled by pregnant staff.
6. Adequate care and precautions should be taken in the disposal of items (syringes, needles, etc.) used to reconstitute cytotoxic drugs. Excess material and body waste may be disposed of by placing in double sealed polythene bags and incinerating at a temperature of 1,000 degrees C. Liquid waste may be flushed with copious amounts of water.

*Reconstitution:*

7. The work surface should be covered with disposable plastic-backed absorbent paper.
8. Use Luer-Lock fittings on all syringes and sets. Large bore needles are recommended to minimise pressure and the possible formation of aerosols. The latter may also be reduced by the use of a venting needle.

**Marketing authorisation number** 0125/0201

**Date of approval/revision of SPC** January 1997

**Legal category** POM

## QUESTRAN* QUESTRAN LIGHT*

**Presentation** Questran sachets containing 9 g of orange-flavoured powder which produces a pale orange-coloured suspension when reconstituted with water. Each sachet supplies 4 g of anhydrous cholestyramine (a basic anion-exchange resin).

Other ingredients: Acacia, citric acid anhydrous, flavours, polysorbate 80, propylene glycol alginate, sucrose, sunset yellow.

Questran Light sachets containing 5 g of orange-flavoured powder which produces a pale orange-coloured suspension when reconstituted with water. Each sachet supplies 4 g of anhydrous cholestyramine. Questran Light sachets contain aspartame.

Other ingredients: Aspartame, citric acid anhydrous, colloidal silicon dioxide, flavours, propylene glycol alginate, quinoline yellow, sucrose, xanthan gum.

**Uses** Questran is used for:

1. Primary prevention of coronary heart disease in men between 35 and 59 years of age and with primary hypercholesterolaemia who have not responded to diet and other appropriate measures.

2. Reduction of plasma cholesterol in hypercholesterolaemia, particularly in those patients who have been diagnosed as Fredrickson's Type II (high plasma cholesterol with normal or slightly elevated triglycerides).

3. Relief of pruritus associated with partial biliary obstruction and primary biliary cirrhosis.

4. Relief of diarrhoea associated with ileal resection, Crohn's disease, vagotomy and diabetic vagal neuropathy.

5. Management of radiation-induced diarrhoea.

**Dosage and administration** *Adults:* As a precautionary measure, where concurrent drug therapy exists then such drugs should be administered at least one hour before or 4–6 hours after Questran.

1. For primary prevention of coronary heart disease and to reduce cholesterol: After initial introduction over a three to four week period, 3 to 6 Questran sachets per day, administered either as a single daily dose or in divided doses up to four times daily according to dosage requirements and patient acceptability. Dosage may be modified according to response and can be increased to 9 sachets per day if necessary.

Occasional slight gastro-intestinal upsets e.g. constipation, may occur when starting Questran. These usually pass with continued usage of Questran and are minimised by starting therapy gradually.

| *Final dose required* | *Sachets per day* | | | |
|---|---|---|---|---|
| | *Week 1* | *Week 2* | *Week 3* | *Week 4* |
| 3 | 1 | 2 | 3 | 3 |
| 4 | 1 | 2 | 3 | 4 |
| 6 | 1 | 2 | 3 | 6 |

2. To relieve pruritus: One or two sachets daily are usually sufficient.

3. To relieve diarrhoea: As for reduction of cholesterol but it may be possible to reduce this dosage.

Questran should not be taken in its dry form.

Questran should be administered mixed with water or a suitable liquid, such as fruit juice, and stirred to a uniform consistency.

Questran may also be mixed with skimmed milk, thin soups, pulpy fruits with high moisture content, e.g. apple sauce etc.

*Children 6–12 years:* The initial dose is determined by the following formula:

$$\frac{\text{child's weight in kg} \times \text{adult dose}}{70}$$

Subsequent dosage adjustment may be necessary where clinically indicated.

The dose has not been established in infants and children under 6 years.

*Elderly:* No dosage adjustment is necessary.

**Contra-indications, warnings, etc**

*Contra-indications:* Questran is likely to be ineffective in patients with complete biliary obstruction, since Questran cannot be effective where bile is not secreted into the intestine.

*Side-effects:* Since Questran may interfere with the absorption of fat soluble vitamins the diet may require supplementation with vitamins A, D and K during prolonged high dose administration.

Chronic use of Questran may be associated with increased bleeding tendency due to hypoprothrombinemia associated with Vitamin K deficiency. This will usually respond promptly to parenteral Vitamin K administration. Recurrences can be prevented by oral administration of Vitamin K.

Hyperchloraemic acidosis has occasionally been reported following the prolonged use of anion exchange resins.

Gastro-intestinal side effects are those most frequently reported. The principal complaint is constipation which may be controlled with the usual remedies, and frequently disappears on continued usage of Questran. Large doses of Questran can cause diarrhoea.

*Use in pregnancy and lactation:* As with other drugs, Questran should not be given in pregnancy or lactation unless considered essential.

*Interactions:* Questran may delay or reduce the absorption of certain drugs (such as digitalis and its alkaloids, tetracycline, chlorothiazide, warfarin and thyroxine). The response to concomitant medication should be closely monitored and appropriate adjustments made if necessary.

Patients should take other drugs at least one hour before or 4–6 hours after Questran to minimise possible interference with their absorption.

*Overdose:* Overdosage with Questran has not been reported. The potential problem in overdosage would be obstruction of the gastro-intestinal tract.

**Pharmaceutical precautions** Questran should not be taken in its dry form. The powder should be prepared immediately prior to administration. Store in a dry place.

**Legal category** POM.

**Package quantities** Questran and Questran Light are available in original packs containing 180 sachets.

**Further information** The correlation between high blood cholesterol levels and ischaemic heart conditions has prompted the dietary control of patients who have shown signs or symptoms of coronary artery disease. With Questran it is possible to reduce cholesterol levels without recourse to excessively stringent dietary measures or systemically absorbed drugs.

Questran (cholestyramine) is a basic anion exchange resin. It is not absorbed in the gut and its affinity for bile acids in the intestinal tract prevents their reabsorption. To compensate for the faecal loss of bile acids, their major precursor, cholesterol, is oxidised at an increased rate in the liver and plasma cholesterol levels are thus lowered.

**Product licence numbers**

Questran 0125/5009R.
Questran Light 0125/0192.

## SOTACOR*

**Qualitative and quantitative composition**

*Sotacor tablets:* White, circular tablets engraved 'SOTACOR 80' or 'SOTACOR 160' on one face, each tablet containing 80 mg or 160 mg sotalol hydrochloride.

*Sotacor injection:* Ampoules containing sotalol hydrochloride 40 mg in each 4 ml of solution.

**Pharmaceutical forms** Oral tablets. Intravenous injection.

**Clinical particulars**

*Therapeutic indications: Sotacor tablets* are indicated for: Ventricular arrhythmias: treatment of life-threatening ventricular tachyarrhythmias; treatment of symptomatic non-sustained ventricular tachyarrhythmias.

Supraventricular arrhythmias: prophylaxis of paroxysmal atrial tachycardia, paroxysmal atrial fibrillation, paroxysmal A-V nodal re-entrant tachycardia, paroxysmal A-V re-entrant tachycardia using accessory pathways, and paroxysmal supraventricular tachycardia after cardiac surgery; maintenance of normal sinus rhythm following conversion of atrial fibrillation or atrial flutter.

*Sotacor injection* is indicated for: termination of acute and life-threatening arrhythmias, including life-threatening ventricular tachyarrhythmias, symptomatic non-sustained ventricular tachyarrhythmias; testing of drug efficacy during programmed electrical stimulation in patients with inducible ventricular and supraventricular tachyarrhythmias; transitory substitution for oral Sotacor in patients temporarily unable to take oral medications.

*Posology and method of administration:* The initiation of treatment or changes in dosage with Sotacor should follow an appropriate medical evaluation including ECG control with measurement of the corrected QT interval, and assessment of renal function, electrolyte balance, and concomitant medication (see Warnings and precautions).

As with other antiarrhythmic agents, it is recommended that Sotacor be initiated and doses increased in a facility capable of monotoring and assessing cardiac rhythm. The dosage must be individualised and based on the patient's response. Proarrhythmic events can occur not only at initiation of therapy, but also with each upward dosage adjustment.

In view of its β-adrenergic blocking properties, treatment with Sotacor should not be discontinued suddenly, especially in patients with ischaemic heart disease (angina pectoris, prior acute myocardial infarction) or hypertension, to prevent exacerbation of the disease (see Warnings).

The following dosing schedule can be recommended:

*Sotacor tablets:* The initial dose is 80 mg, administered either singly or as two divided doses. Oral dosage of Sotacor should be adjusted gradually allowing 2–3 days between dosing increments in order to attain steady-state, and to allow monitoring of QT intervals. Most patients respond to a daily dose of 160 to 320 mg administered in two divided doses at appoximately 12 hour intervals. Some patients with life-threatening refractory ventricular arrhythmias may require doses as high as 480–640 mg/day. These doses should be used under specialist supervision and should only be prescribed when the potential benefit outweighs the increased risk of adverse events, particularly proarrhythmias (see Warnings).

*Sotacor injection:* For the management of acute arrhythmias, dosage range is from 20–120 mg intravenously (0.5 mg to 1.5 mg/kg). The total calculated dose has been safely administered over a 10-minute period and can be repeated at 6-hour intervals if necessary. For high risk patients with acute myocardial infarction and/or congestive heart failure, careful monitoring for hemodynamic or electrocardiographic changes is recommended.

For programmed electrical stimulation, an initial bolus of 1.5 mg/kg should be given over 10 to 20 minutes, followed by maintenance infusion at a rate of between 0.2 and 0.5 mg/kg/hour.

For substitution in place oral therapy, infusion of between 0.2 and 0.5 mg/kg/hour should be used with the total daily dose not exceeding 640 mg.

*Children:* Sotacor is not intended for administration to children.

*Dosage in renally impaired patients:* Because Sotacor is excreted mainly in urine, the dosage should be reduced when the creatinine clearance is less than 60 ml/min according to the following table:

| *Creatinine clearance (ml/min)* | *Adjusted doses* |
|---|---|
| >10 | Recommended Sotacor Dose |
| 30–60 | $\frac{1}{2}$ recommended Sotacor Dose |
| 10–30 | $\frac{1}{4}$ recommended Sotacor Dose |
| <10 | Avoid |

The creatinine clearance can be estimated from serum creatinine by the Cockcroft and Gault formula:

Men:

$$\frac{(140-\text{age})\times\text{weight (kg)}}{72\times\text{serum creatinine (mg/dl)}}$$

Women: idem×0.85

When serum creatinine is given in μmol/l, divide the value by 88.4 (1 mg/dl = 88.4 μmol/l).

*Dosage in hepatically impaired patients:* No dosage adjustment is required in hepatically impaired patients.

*Contra-indications:* Sotacor should not be used where there is evidence of sick sinus syndrome; second and third degree AV heart block unless a functioning pacemaker is present; congenital or acquired long QT syndromes; torsades de pointes; symptomatic sinus bradycardia; uncontrolled congestive heart failure; cardiogenic shock; anaesthesia that produces myocardial depression; untreated phaeochromocytoma; hypotension (except due to arrhythmia); Raynaud's phenomenon and severe peripheral circulatory disturbances; history of chronic obstructive airway disease or bronchial asthma; hypersensitivity to any of the components of the formulation; metabolic acidosis; renal failure (creatinine clearance <10 ml/min).

*Special warnings and special precautions for use:*

*Abrupt withdrawal:* Hypersensitivity to catecholamines is observed in patients withdrawn from beta-blocker therapy. Occasional cases of exacerbation of angina pectoris, arrhythmias, and in some cases, myocardial infarction have been reported after abrupt discontinuation of therapy. Patients should be carefully monitored when discontinuing chronically administered Sotacor, particularly those with ischaemic heart disease. If possible the dosage should be gradually reduced over a period of one or two weeks, if necessary at the same time initiating replacement therapy. Abrupt discontinuation may unmask latent coronary insufficiency. In addition, hypertension may develop.

*Proarrhythmias:* The most dangerous adverse effect of Class I and Class III antiarrhythmic drugs (such as sotalol) is the aggravation of pre-existing arrhythmias or the provocation of new arrhythmias. Drugs that prolong the QT-interval may cause torsades de pointes, a polymorphic ventricular tachycardia associated with prolongation of the QT-interval. Experience to date indicates that the risk of torsades de pointes is associated with the prolongationof the QT-interval, reduction of the heart rate, reduction in serum potassium and magnesium, high plasma sotalol concentrations and with the concomitant use of solatol and other medications which have been associated with torsades de pointes (see Interactions). Females may be at increased risk of developing torsades de pointes.

The incidence of torsades de pointes is dose dependent. Torsades de pointes usually occurs early after initiating therapy or escalation of the dose and can progress to ventricular fibrillation.

In clinical trials of patients with sustained VT/VF the incidence of severe proarrhythmia (torsades de pointes or new sustained VT/VF) was <2% at doses up to 320 mg. The incidence more than doubled at higher doses.

Other risk factors for torsades de pointes were excessive prolongation of the $QT_c$ and history of cardiomegaly or congestive heart failure. Patients with sustained ventricular tachycardia and a history of congestive heart failure have the highest risk of serious proarrhythmia (7%). Proarrhythmic events must be anticipated not only on initiating therapy but with every upward dose adjustment. Initiating therapy at 80 mg with gradual upward dose titration thereafter reduces the risk of proarrhythmia. In patients already receiving Sotacor caution should be used if the $QT_c$ exceeds 500 msec whilst on therapy, and serious consideration should be given to reducing the dose or discontinuing therapy when the $QT_c$-interval exceeds 550 msec. Due to the multiple risk factors associated with torsades de pointes, however, caution should be exercised regardless of the $QT_c$-interval.

*Electrolyte disturbances:* Sotacor should not be used in patients with hypokalaemia or hypomagnesaemia prior to correction of imbalance; these conditions can exaggerate the degree of QT prolongation, and increase the potential for torsades de pointes. Special attention should be given to electrolyte and acid-base balance in patients experiencing severe or prolonged diarrhoea or patients receiving concomitant magnesium- and/or potassium-depleting drugs.

*Congestive heart failure:* Beta-blockade may further depress myocardial contractility and precipitate more severe heart failure. Caution is advised when initiating therapy in patients with left ventricular dysfunction controlled by therapy (i.e. ACE Inhibitors, diuretics, digitalis, etc); a low initial dose and careful dose titration is appropriate.

*Recent MI:* In post-infarction patients with impaired left ventricular function, the risk versus benefit of sotalol administration must be considered. Careful monitoring and dose titration are critical during initiation and follow-up of therapy. Sotacor should be avoided in patients with left ventricular ejection fractions ≤40% without serious ventricular arrhythmias.

*Electrocardiographic changes:* Excessive prolongation of the QT-interval can be a sign of toxicity and should be avoided (see *Proarrhythmias* above). Bradycardia increases the risk of torsades de pointes.

*Anaphylaxis:* Patients with a history of anaphylactic reaction to a variety of allergens may have a more severe reaction on repeated challenge while taking beta-blockers. Such patients may be unresponsive to the usual doses of adrenaline used to treat the allergic reaction.

*Anaesthesia:* As with other beta-blocking agents, Sotacor should be used with caution in patients undergoing surgery and in association with anaesthetics that cause myocardial depression, such as cyclopropane or trichloroethylene.

*Diabetes mellitus:* Sotacor should be used with caution in patients with diabetes (especially labile diabetes) or with a history of episodes of spontaneous hypoglycaemia, since beta-blockade may mask some important signs of the onset of acute hypoglycaemia, e.g. tachycardia.

*Thyrotoxicosis:* Beta-blockade may mask certain clinical signs of hyperthyroidism (e.g., tachycardia). Patients suspected of developing thyrotoxicosis should be managed carefully to avoid abrupt withdrawal of beta-blockade which might be followed by an exacerbation of symptoms of hyperthyroidism, including thyroid storm.

*Renal impairment:* As sotalol is mainly eliminated via the kidneys the dose should be adjusted in patients with renal impairment (see dosage).

*Psoriasis:* Beta-blocking drugs have been reported rarely to exacerbate the symptoms of psoriasis vulgaris.

*Interactions with other medicaments and other forms of interaction:*

*Antiarrhythmias:* Class 1a antiarrhythmic drugs, such as disopyramide, quinidine and procainamide and other antiarrhythmic drugs such as amiodarone and bepridil are not recommended as concomitant therapy with Sotacor, because of their potential to prolong refractoriness (see Special Warnings and Precautions). The concomitant use of other beta-blocking agents with Sotacor may result in additive Class II defects.

*Other drugs prolonging the QT-interval:* Sotacor should be given with extreme caution in conjugation with other drugs known to prolong the QT-interval such as phenothiazines, tricyclic antidepressants, terfenadine and astemizole. Other drugs that have been associated with an increased risk for torsades de pointes include vincamine, fénoxedil, erythromycin IV, halofantrine, pentamidine, sultopride.

*Floctafenine:* Beta-adrenergic blocking agents may impede the compensatory cardiovascular reactions associated with hypotension or shock that may be induced by Floctafenine.

*Calcium channel blocking drugs:* Concurrent administration of beta-blocking agents and calcium channel blockers has resulted in hypotension, bradycardia, conduction defects, and cardiac failure. Beta-blockers should be avoided in combination with cardiodepressant calcium-channel blockers such as verapamil and diltiazem because of the additive effects on atrioventricular conduction, and ventricular function.

*Potassium-depleting diuretics:* Hypokalaemia or hypomagnesaemia may occur, increasing the potential for torsade de pointes (see Special Warnings and Precautions for Use).

*Other potassium-depleting drugs:* Amphotericin B (IV route), corticosteroids (systemic administration), and some laxatives may also be associated with hypokalaemia; Potassium levels should be monitored and corrected appropriately during concomitant administration with Sotacor.

*Clonidine:* Beta-blocking drugs may potentiate the rebound hypertension sometimes observed after discontinuation of clonidine; therefore, the beta-blocker should be discontinued slowly several days before the gradual withdrawal of clonidine.

*Digitalis glycosides:* Single and multiple doses of Sotacor do not significantly affect serum digoxin levels. Proarrhythmic events were more common in sotalol treated patients also receiving digitalis glycosides; however, this may be related to the presence of CHF, a known risk factor for proarrhythmia, in patients receiving digitalis glycosides. Association of digitalis glycosides with beta-blockers may increase auriculo-ventricular conduction time.

*Catecholamine-depleting agents:* Concomitant use of catecholamine-depleting drugs, such as reserpine, guanethidine, or alpha methyldopa, with a beta-blocker may produce an excessive reduction of resting sympathetic nervous tone. Patients should be closely monitored for evidence of hypotension and/or marked bradycardia which may produce syncope.

*Insulin and oral hypoglycaemics:* Hypoglycaemia may occur, and the dosage of antidiabetic drugs may require adjustment. Symptoms of hypoglycaemia (tachycardia) may be masked by beta-blocking agents.

*Neuromuscular blocking agents like Tubocurarine:* The neuromuscular blockade is prolonged by beta-blocking agents.

*Beta-2-receptor stimulants:* Patients in need of beta-agonists should not normally receive Sotacor. However, if concomitant therapy is necessary beta-agonists may have to be administered in increased dosages.

*Drug/laboratory interaction:* The presence of sotalol in the urine may result in falsely elevated levels of urinary metanephrine when measured by photometric methods. Patients suspected of having phaeochromocytoma and who are treated with sotalol should have their urine screened utilising the HPLC assay with solid phase extraction.

*Pregnancy and lactation:*

*Pregnancy:* Animal studies with sotalol hydrochloride have shown no evidence of teratogenicity or other harmful effects on the foetus. Although there are no adequate and well-controlled studies in pregnant women, sotalol hydrochloride has been shown to cross the placenta and is found in amniotic fluid. Beta-blockers reduce placental perfusion, which may result in intrauterine foetal death, immature and premature deliveries. In addition, adverse effects (especially hypoglycaemia and bradycardia) may occur in foetus and neonate. There is an increased risk of cardiac and pulmonary complications in the neonate in the postnatal period. Therefore, Sotacor should be used in pregnancy only if the potential benefits outweigh the possible risk to the foetus. The neonate should be monitored very carefully for 48–72 hours after delivery if it was not possible to interrupt maternal therapy with Sotacor 2–3 days before the birthdate.

Most beta-blockers, particularly lipophilic compounds, will pass into breast milk although to a variable extent. Breast feeding is therefore not recommended during administration of these compounds.

*Effect on ability to drive and use machines:* There are no data available, but the occasional occurrence of side-effects such as dizziness and fatigue should be taken into account (see Undesirable effects).

*Undesirable effects:* The most frequent adverse effects of sotalol arise from its beta-blockade properties. Adverse effects are usually transient in nature and rarely necessitate interruption of, or withdrawal from treatment. If they do occur, they usually disappear when the dosage is reduced. The most significant adverse effects, however, are those due to proarrhythmia, including torsades de pointes (see Warnings).

The following are adverse events considered related to therapy, occurring in 1% or more of patients treated with Sotacor.

*Cardiovascular:* Bradycardia, dyspnoea, chest pain, palpitations, oedema, ECG abnormalities, hypotension, proarrhythmia, syncope, heart failure, presyncope.

*Dermatologic:* Rash.

*Gastro-intestinal:* Nausea/vomiting, diarrhoea, dyspepsia, abdominal pain, flatulence.

*Musculoskeletal:* Cramps.

*Nervous/psychiatric:* Fatigue, dizziness, asthenia, lightheadedness, headache, sleep disturbances, depression, paresthesia, mood changes, anxiety.

*Urogenital:* Sexual dysfunction.

*Special senses:* Visual disturbances, taste abnormalities, hearing disturbances.

*Body as a whole:* Fever.

In trials of patients with cardiac arrhythmia, the most common adverse events leading to discontinuation of Sotacor were fatigue 4%, bradycardia (<50 bpm) 3%, dyspnoea 3%, protarrhythmia 2%, asthenia 2%, and dizziness 2%.

*Overdose:* Intentional or accidental overdosage with Sotacor has rarely resulted in death. Haemodialysis results in a large reduction of plasma levels of sotalol.

Symptoms and treatment of overdosage: The most common signs to be expected are bradycardia, congestive heart failure, hypotension, bronchospasm and hypoglycaemia. In cases of massive intentional overdosage (2–16 g) of Sotacor the following clinical findings were seen: hypotension, bradycardia, prolongation of QT-interval, premature ventricular complexes, ventricular tachycardia, torsades de pointes.

If overdosage occurs, therapy with Sotacor should

be discontinued and the patient observed closely. In addition if required, the following therapeutic measures are suggested:

*Bradycardia:* Atropine (0.5 to 2 mg IV), another anticholinergic drug, a beta-adrenergic agonist (isoprenaline, 5 microgram per minute, up to 25 microgram, by slow IV injection) or transvenous cardiac pacing.

*Heart block (second and third degree):* Transvenous cardiac pacing.

*Hypotension:* Adrenaline rather than isoprenaline or noradrenaline may be useful, depending on associated factors.

*Bronchospasm:* Aminophylline or aerosol beta-2-receptor stimulant.

*Torsades de pointes:* DC cardioversion, transvenous cardiac pacing, adrenaline, and/or magnesium sulphate.

**Pharmacological properties**

*Pharmacodynamic properties:* D,l-sotalol is a non-selective hydrophilic β-adrenergic receptor blocking agent, devoid of intrinsic sympathomimetic activity or membrane stabilising activity.

Sotacor has both beta-adrenoreceptor blocking (Vaughan Williams Class II) and cardiac action potential duration prolongation (Vaughan Williams Class III) antiarrhythmic properties. Sotalol has no known effect on that upstroke velocity and therefore no effect on the depolarisation phase.

Sotalol uniformly prolongs the action potential duration in cardiac tissues by delaying the repolarisation phase. Its major effects are prolongation of the atrial, ventricular and accessory pathway effective refractory periods.

The Class II and III properties may be reflected on the surface electrocardiogram by a lengthening of the PR, QT and QT$_c$ (QT corrected for heart rate) intervals with no significant alteration in the QRS duration.

The d- and l-isomers of sotalol have similar Class III antiarrhythmic effects while the l-isomer is responsible for virtually all of the beta-blocking activity. Although significant beta-blockade may occur at oral doses as low as 25 mg, Class III effects are usually seen at daily doses of greater than 160 mg.

Its β-adrenergic blocking activity causes a reduction in heart rate (negative chronotropic effect) and a limited reduction in the force of contraction (negative inotropic effect). These cardiac changes reduce myocardial oxygen consumption and cardiac work. Like other β-blockers, sotalol inhibits renin release. The renin-suppressive effect of sotalol is significant both at rest and during exercise. Like other beta adrenergic blocking agents, Sotacor produces a gradual but significant reduction in both systolic and diastolic blood pressures in hypertensive patients. Twenty-four-hour control of blood pressure is maintained both in the supine and upright positions with a single daily dose.

*Pharmacokinetic properties:* The bioavailability of oral sotalol is essentially complete (greater than 90%). After oral administration, peak levels are reached in 2.5 to 4 hours, and steady-state plasma levels are attained within 2–3 days. The absorption is reduced by approximately 20% when administered with a standard meal, in comparison to fasting conditions. Over the dosage range 40–640 mg/day Sotacor displays dose proportionality with respect to plasma levels. Distribution occurs to a central (plasma) and a peripheral compartment, with an elimination half-life of 10–20 hours. Sotalol does not bind to plasma proteins and is not metabolised. There is very little inter-subject variability in plasma levels. Sotalol crosses the blood brain barrier poorly, with cerebrospinal fluid concentrations only 10% of those in plasma. The primary route of elimination is renal excretion. Approximately 80 to 90% of a dose is excreted unchanged in the urine, while the remainder is excreted in the faeces. Lower doses are necessary in conditions of renal impairment (see Dosage and Administration in patients with renal dysfunction). Age does not significantly alter the pharmacokinetics, although impaired renal function in geriatric patients can decrease the excretion rate, resulting in increased drug accumulation.

*Preclinical safety data:* No further particulars.

**Pharmaceutical particulars**

*List of excipients:*

Sotacor tablets: Sotacor 80 mg: lactose, magnesium stearate, maize starch, talc.

Sotacor 160 mg: magnesium stearate, maize starch, microcrystalline cellulose, pregelatinised starch.

Sotacor injection: Glacial acetic acid, sodium chloride, sodium hydroxide, water.

*Incompatibilities:* There are no known incompatibilities.

*Shelf life:* Three years.

*Special precautions for storage:* Store below 30°C in a dry place, protect from light.

*Nature and contents of container:*

Sotacor 80 mg and 160 mg tablets: Original packs of 28 – blister strips of 14 tablets with 2 strips to a carton.

Sotacor injection: is supplied as 40 mg sotalol hydrochloride in 4 ml ampoules, with 5 ampoules per box.

*Instructions for use handling:* Sotacor injection fluid can be administered as an intravenous infusion with 5% glucose intravenous infusion or 0.9% sodium chloride intravenous infusion. The final concentration should be between 0.01–2 mg/ml.

In concentrations of 0.01–2 mg/ml, dilution of Sotacor injection fluid with 5% glucose intravenous infusion or 0.9% sodium chloride intravenous infusion, is chemically and physically stable during at least 4 days at room temperature (15–25°C) and 3 weeks under refrigeration (2–8°C).

As the formulation does not contain a preservative, the solutions of Sotacor should be prepared in an aseptic manner. Prompt use of the solution is recommended.

**Marketing authorisation numbers**

Sotacor 80 mg tablets          0125/0076
Sotacor 160 mg tablets         0125/0093
Sotacor Injection 40 mg/4 ml   0125/0123

**Date of approval/revision of SPC** March 1996.

**Legal category** POM.

## VEPESID* CAPSULES
## VEPESID* INJECTION

**Presentation** Vepesid Injection-vials containing 100 mg etoposide in 5 ml.

Other ingredients: Benzyl alcohol, citric acid anhydrous, dehydrated ethanol, polyethylene glycol, polysorbate 80.

Vepesid Capsules-soft gelatin, pale pink capsules containing 50 mg and 100 mg etoposide.

Other ingredients: citric acid, glycerol, polyethylene glycol 400, water; gelatin capsules containing glycerol, iron oxide, sodium hydroxybenzoic acid, ethyl ester, sodium propyl hydroxybenzoate, titanium dioxide, water.

**Uses** Vepesid is an anti-neoplastic drug for intravenous or oral use, which can be used alone or in combination with other oncolytic drugs.

Present data indicate that Vepesid is applicable in the therapy of: small cell lung cancer, resistant non-seminomatous testicular carcinoma.

**Dosage and administration** The recommended course of Vepesid Injection is 60–120 mg/m², i.v., daily for five consecutive days. As Vepesid produces myelosuppression, courses may not be repeated more frequently than at 21 day intervals. In any case, repeat courses of Vepesid should not be given until the blood picture has been checked for evidence of myelosuppression and found to be satisfactory

Immediately before administration, the required dose of Vepesid Injection must be diluted with 0.9% saline solution for injection to give a solution concentration of not more than 0.25 mg/ml of etoposide; it should then be given by intravenous infusion over a period of not less than 30 minutes.

Care should be taken to avoid extravasation.

If oral dosing is preferred, 120–240 mg/m² should be given daily, for five consecutive days. The dose of Vepesid capsules is based on the recommended i.v. dose with consideration given to the bioavailability of Vepesid capsules appearing to be dependent upon the dose administered. The bioavailability also varies from patient to patient following any oral dose. This should be taken into consideration when prescribing this medication. In view of significant intra-patient variability, dose adjustments may be required in order to achieve the desired therapeutic effect. As Vepesid produces myelosuppression, courses may not be repeated more frequently than at 21 day intervals. In any case, a repeat course of Vepesid should not be given until the blood picture has been checked for evidence of myelosuppression and found to be satisfactory.

The capsules should be taken on an empty stomach.

*Elderly:* No dosage adjustment is necessary.

*Paediatric use:* Safety and effectiveness in children have not been established.

**Contra-indications, warnings, etc** Vepesid is contra-indicated in patients with severe hepatic dysfunction or in those patients who have demonstrated hypersensitivity to the drug.

Vepesid must not be given by intra-cavitary injection.

*Warnings*

*Use in pregnancy:* Vepesid is teratogenic in rats and mice at dose levels equivalent to those employed clinically. There are no adequate and well-controlled studies in pregnant women.

Vepesid should not normally be administered to patients who are pregnant or to mothers who are breast feeding. Women of childbearing potential should be advised to avoid becoming pregnant.

The influence of Vepesid on human reproduction has not been determined.

In-vitro tests indicate that Vepesid is mutagenic.

*Precautions:* Vepesid should be administered by individuals experienced in the use of antineoplastic therapy.

When Vepesid is administered intravenously care should be taken to avoid extravasation.

If radiotherapy and/or chemotherapy has been given prior to starting Vepesid treatment, an adequate interval should be allowed to enable the bone marrow to recover. If the leucocyte count falls below 2,000/mm³, treatment should be suspended until the circulating blood elements have returned to acceptable levels (platelets above 100,000mm³, leucocytes above 4,000/mm³), this is usually within 10 days.

Peripheral blood counts and liver function should be monitored. (See Adverse Reactions.)

Bacterial infections should be brought under control before treatment with Vepesid commences.

The occurrence of acute leukaemia, which can occur with or without a preleukaemic phase has been reported rarely in patients treated with etoposide in association with other anti-neoplastic drugs.

*Adverse reactions: Haematological:* The dose limiting toxicity of Vepesid is myelosuppression, predominantly leucopenia and thrombocytopenia. Anaemia occurs infrequently.

The leucocyte count nadir occurs approximately 21 days after treatment.

*Alopecia:* Alopecia occurs in approximately two-thirds of patients and is reversible on cessation of therapy.

*Gastrointestinal:* Nausea and vomiting are the major gastrointestinal toxicities and occur in over one-third of patients. Anti-emetics are useful in controlling these side effects. Abdominal pain, anorexia, diarrhoea, oesophagitis and stomatitis occur infrequently.

*Other Toxicities:* Hypotension may occur following an excessively rapid infusion and may be reversed by slowing the infusion rate.

Anaphylactoid reactions have been reported following administration of Vepesid. Higher rates of anaphylactoid reactions have been reported in children who received infusions at concentrations higher than those recommended. The role that concentration of infusion (or rate of infusion) plays in the development of anaphylactoid reactions is uncertain. These reactions have usually responded to cessation of therapy and administration of pressor agents, corticosteroids, antihistamines or volume expanders as appropriate.

Apnoea with spontaneous resumption of breathing following discontinuation of etoposide injection has been reported. Sudden fatal reactions associated with bronchospasm have been reported. Hypertension and/or flushing have also been reported. Blood pressure usually returns to normal within a few hours after cessation of the infusion.

The use of etoposide has been reported infrequently to cause peripheral neuropathy.

Vepesid has been shown to reach high concentrations in the liver and kidney, thus presenting a potential for accumulation in cases of functional impairment.

Somnolence, fatigue, aftertaste, fever, rash, pigmentation, pruritus, urticaria, dysphagia, transient cortical blindness and a single case of radiation recall dermatitis have also been reported following the administration of Vepesid.

*Overdosage:* No proven antidotes have been established for Vepesid overdosage. Treatment should be symptomatic and supportive.

Total doses of 2.4 to 3.5 g/m² administered i.v. over three days have resulted in severe mucositis and myelotoxicity. Metabolic acidosis and cases of severe hepatic toxicity have been reported in patients receiving higher than recommended doses of etoposide.

**Pharmaceutical precautions** Vepesid injection should be stored at room temperature. The injection should be protected from light. Vepesid capsules should be stored between 10–25°C. Do not open any blister in which there is evidence of capsule leakage.

*Preparation of intravenous solution:* Immediately before administration the required dose of Vepesid Injection must be diluted with 0.9% sodium chloride for injection to give a solution concentration of not more than 0.25 mg/ml of etoposide; it should then be given by intravenous infusion over a period of not less than 30 minutes. The infusion solution should be kept at room temperature and should be used within six hours of preparation. Solutions of concentration greater than 0.25 mg/ml may show signs of precipitation, and are therefore not recommended. Any solutions showing signs of precipitation should be discarded.

The intravenous solution is suitable for infusion in glass or PVC containers.

Hard plastic devices made of acrylic or ABS (a polymer composed of acrylonitrile, butadiene and styrene) have been reported to crack and leak when used with undiluted Vepesid Injection. This effect has not been reported with diluted Vepesid Injection.

*Vepesid should not be physically mixed with any other drug.*

*Guidelines for the safe handling of antineoplastic agents:*

1. Trained personnel should reconstitute the drug.
2. This should be performed in a designated area.
3. Adequate protective gloves should be worn.
4. Precautions should be taken to avoid the drug accidentally coming into contact with the eyes. In the event of contact with the eyes, irrigate with large amounts of water and/or saline.
5. The cytotoxic preparation should not be handled by pregnant staff.
6. Adequate care and precautions should be taken in the disposal of items (syringes, needles etc) used to reconstitute cytotoxic drugs. Excess material and body waste may be disposed of by placing in double sealed polythene bags and incinerating at a temperature of 1,000°C. Liquid waste may be flushed with copious amounts of water.

7. The work surface should be covered with disposable plastic-backed absorbent paper.

8. Use Luer-Lock fittings on all syringes and sets. Large bore needles are recommended to minimise pressure and the possible formation of aerosols. The latter may also be reduced by the use of a venting needle.

**Legal category** POM.

**Package quantities** Vepesid injection is packed in cartons of 10 vials, each vial containing 100 mg etoposide in 5 ml of solution.

Vepesid 100 mg capsules are packed in blister packs of 10 capsules, each capsule containing 100 mg etoposide.

Vepesid 50 mg capsules are packed in blister packs of 20 capsules, each capsule containing 50 mg etoposide.

**Further information** Etoposide is a semisynthetic derivative of podophyllotoxin.

Experimental data indicate that etoposide arrests the cell cycle in the $G_2$ phase. Etoposide differs from the vinca alkaloids in that it does not cause an accumulation of cells in metaphase, but prevents cells from entering mitosis or destroys cells in the $G_2$ phase. The incorporation of thymidine into DNA is inhibited in-vitro by etoposide. Etoposide does not interfere with microtubule assembly. Etoposide is approximately 94% protein-bound in human serum. Plasma decay kinetics follow a bi-exponential curve and correspond to a two compartmental model. The mean volume of distribution is approximately 32% of body weight. Etoposide demonstrates relatively poor penetration into the cerebrospinal fluid. Urinary excretion is approximately 45% of an administered dose, 29% being excreted unchanged in 72 hours.

An information sheet on the storage, preparation and handling of the product is available

**Product licence numbers**

| | |
|---|---|
| Vepesid 50 mg Capsules | 0125/0153 |
| Vepesid 100 mg Capsules | 0125/0124 |
| Vepesid Injection | 0125/0184 |

*Trade Mark

# Bristol-Myers Squibb Pharmaceuticals Ltd
Bristol-Myers Squibb House
Staines Road
Hounslow TW3 3JA

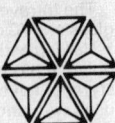

## DUTONIN*

**Qualitative and quantitative composition** Nefazodone is a phenylpiperazine antidepressant, available as tablets containing 50, 100 and 200 mg of nefazodone HCl.

Nefazodone tablets contain the following inactive ingredients: microcrystalline cellulose, povidone, sodium starch glycollate, colloidal silicon dioxide, magnesium stearate and iron oxides.

**Pharmaceutical form** Nefazodone is supplied as flat faced, bevelled edged, hexagonal shaped tablets containing 50 mg, 100 mg or 200 mg of nefazodone HCl. Tablets are imprinted with the product strength on one side. The 100 and 200 mg tablets are bisect scored. Tablet colours are pink (50 mg), white (100 mg) and light yellow (200 mg).

### Clinical particulars

*Therapeutic indications:* Nefazodone is indicated for the symptomatic treatment of all types of depressive illness, including depressive syndromes accompanied by anxiety or sleep disturbances.

*Posology and method of administration:*
*Adults:* The usual therapeutic dose is 200 mg twice daily. The recommended starting dose is 50-100 mg twice daily which should be increased to 200 mg twice daily after 5-7 days. Depending on the clinical response, the daily dose can be increased gradually to a maximum of 300 mg twice daily.

In patients being transferred from another CNS medication, treatment should be initiated at a dose of 50 mg twice daily before being titrated at weekly intervals to the usual therapeutic dose.

While benefit is seen during the first week of treatment, as with all antidepressants, up to 4 weeks' treatment may be required to obtain the full antidepressant effect in some patients. It is recommended that treatment should continue for a sufficient period which may be several months. Patients treated with nefazodone for up to one year have shown continued beneficial response.

*Elderly:* The effects of the starting dose (50 mg twice daily) and the rate of subsequent dose titration should be carefully assessed, since increased plasma concentrations have been seen to occur in the elderly, especially females. Maximum therapeutic benefit is usually achieved at doses of 100-200 mg twice daily.

*Renal impairment:* No significant relationship between pharmacokinetic parameters and degree of renal impairment has been observed. However, with chronic administration, accumulation of nefazodone or its metabolites may occur in patients with severely impaired renal function, and use of the lower end of the dose range is advised.

*Hepatic impairment:* The elimination half-life of nefazodone in patients with cirrhosis was significantly prolonged. This suggests that if nefazodone is administered to patients with liver disease, dosage should be restricted to the lower end of the dose range.

*Children:* The use of nefazodone in children is not recommended, as safety and effectiveness in children below the age of 18 years have not yet been established.

*Contra-indications:* Nefazodone is contra-indicated in patients with known hypersensitivity to nefazodone hydrochloride, any of the inactive ingredients, or other phenylpiperazine antidepressants.

*Special warnings and special precautions for use:*
*Hepatic or renal impairment:* see section *Posology and method of administration.*
*Electro-convulsive therapy:* There are no clinical studies involving the combined use of ECT and nefazodone.
*Epilepsy:* As with other antidepressants, nefazodone should be used with caution in patients with epilepsy.
*History of mania/hypomania:* Nefazodone should be used with caution in these patients as rare occurrences of activation of mania / hypomania have been reported.
*Cardiovascular:* Patients with a recent history of myocardial infarction or unstable heart disease should be treated with caution.
*Sexual function:* Unlike other antidepressants, nefazodone has not been associated with impotence and abnormal ejaculation in men or inability to achieve orgasm in women. Priapism has been reported with another phenylpiperazine compound and, should this occur during nefazodone treatment, the patient should be advised to discontinue therapy immediately and seek medical attention.

*Suicide:* The possibility of suicide attempt in seriously depressed patients is inherent to the illness and may persist even during apparent improvement of symptoms. Close supervision of high risk patients is advised.

*Interactions with other medicaments and other forms of interaction:*
*Centrally active medication:* As with all centrally acting drugs, caution is advised when drugs are used in combination. Concurrent or immediate pretreatment with fluoxetine increases the AUC of the nefazodone metabolite m-chlorophenylpiperazine (mCPP). Such patients may experience transient increased side effects which can be minimised by reducing the dose of nefazodone or allowing an adequate washout period.
*Benzodiazepines:* In healthy volunteers, the half-life of triazolam, a short-acting sedative hypnotic, was significantly increased (from 2.3 to 7 h) when co-administered with nefazodone. The pharmacokinetics of nefazodone were not altered. When alprazolam and nefazodone were co-administered the half life of alprazolam was doubled and, although the nefazodone concentration was unaffected, the concentration of its metabolite, mCPP, was increased. A reduction in the alprazolam dosage is recommended. The co-administration of lorazepam and nefazodone resulted in minimal changes in the pharmacokinetic parameters of either drug. No dosage adjustment is required. Caution should be exercised when using nefazodone and other benzodiazepines concomitantly.
*Protein binding:* Nefazodone is extensively (>99%) bound to plasma proteins in man. The effect of nefazodone on the plasma protein binding of co-administered drugs should be considered. The protein binding of chlorpromazine, desipramine, diazepam, phenytoin, lidocaine, prazosin, propranolol, verapamil or warfarin was not affected by nefazodone *in vitro.*
*Warfarin:* No significant clinical or pharmacokinetic interactions between nefazodone and warfarin were observed in a multidose study using healthy male subjects.
*Terfenadine/astemizole/cisapride:* Nefazodone has been shown *in vitro* to be an inhibitor of cytochrome $P_{450}$ III A4. Therefore, the concomitant use of nefazodone with terfenadine, astemizole or cisapride, which are all metabolised by this isoenzyme, is not recommended.
*Other drugs metabolised by cytochrome $P_{450}III_{A4}$:* As their clearance may be affected, caution is indicated in the combined use of nefazodone with other drugs metabolised by this isoenzyme.
*Lithium:* Co-administration of nefazodone with lithium did not cause any untoward effects (e.g. tremor, hyperthermia) associated with serotonin syndrome. However, caution should be exercised when using nefazodone and lithium concomitantly.
*Carbamazepine:* Monitoring of carbamazepine plasma concentrations is recommended when coadministered with nefazodone as a 23% increase of both $C_{max}$ and AUC for carbamazepine was observed in a multidose volunteer study. No adjustment in the initial dose of nefazodone is necessary when administered with carbamazepine but, based on clinical effect, subsequent dose adjustments may be required due to marked decreases in nefazodone plasma concentrations.
*Haloperidol:* In a multi-dose study involving healthy volunteers, the AUC of haloperidol was increased by 35% with no significant increase in the $C_{max}$ or $T_{max}$ when co-administered with nefazodone. Slight protein binding displacement of haloperidol was also noted. Caution should be exercised when using nefazodone and haloperidol concomitantly.
*Monoamine oxidase inhibitors:* As with other antidepressants, nefazodone should not be used in combination with an MAOI or within two weeks of discontinuing treatment with an MAOI. Conversely, at least one week should be allowed after stopping nefazodone before starting an MAOI.
*Cimetidine:* No significant clinical or pharmacokinetic interactions between nefazodone and cimetidine were observed in a multiple dose clinical trial involving healthy volunteers.
*Cardiovascular:* Although nefazodone is not a potent alpha-adrenergic blocking agent, there have been reports of orthostatic hypotension and syncope occurring in nefazodone-treated patients. Concomitant administration of antihypertensive therapy, e.g. propranolol, and nefazodone may require an adjustment in the dose of the antihypertensive drug. Caution is advised with co-administration of nefazodone and digoxin as serum concentrations of digoxin have been shown to increase by as much as 30%. Other cardiovascular agents have not been formally studied but the potential for interaction exists.
*Theophylline:* There was no effect on $FEV_1$ values, nor any change in the pharmacokinetics of either nefazodone or theophylline when co-administered to patients with chronic obstructive pulmonary disease.
*General anaesthetics:* Concomitant use of nefazodone with general anaesthetics has not been formally evaluated but the potential for interaction exists; therefore, prior to elective surgery, nefazodone should be discontinued for as long as clinically feasible.
*Alcohol:* Whilst in a controlled trial with young normal volunteers, nefazodone did not alter the psychomotor or cognitive impairment caused by alcohol, it is prudent to avoid concomitant use of alcohol and nefazodone.

*Pregnancy and lactation:* The safety of nefazodone for use in human pregnancy has not been established. An evaluation of experimental animal studies does not indicate direct or indirect harmful effects with respect to development of the embryo: however, both maternal and foetal / neonatal toxicities occurred. Findings consisted of non-specific delay in foetal development and increased mortality and decreased body weight in the neonates. Because animal reproductive studies are not always predictive of human response, this drug should be used during pregnancy only if clearly needed.

It is not known whether nefazodone or its metabolites are excreted in human milk. Hence use in nursing mothers is not recommended.

*Effects on ability to drive and use machines:* In healthy volunteers nefazodone caused a modest decrease in some psychomotor function tests but no impairment of cognitive function. However, any psychoactive drug may impair judgement, cognitive or motor skills, and patients should be cautioned about operating hazardous machinery, including automobiles.

*Undesirable effects:* Nefazodone is generally well tolerated. If side effects occur, they are normally observed at the beginning of treatment and usually subside with decreased dosage. In controlled clinical trials, certain side effects occurred with significantly greater frequency than placebo: the most frequent were asthenia, dry mouth, nausea, constipation, somnolence, dizziness and lightheadedness; side effects which sometimes occurred were chills, fever, postural hypotension, vasodilation, abnormal dreams, paraesthesia, arthralgia, memory impairment, confusion, ataxia, amblyopia and other minor visual disturbances; a side effect which rarely occurred was syncope.

Over a six week trial period, there was evidence of progressive adaptation with continued therapy to the following adverse experiences: asthenia, visual disturbances, constipation, dizziness, dry mouth, lightheadedness, nausea and somnolence.

*Overdose:* There have been rare reported cases of overdose with nefazodone (up to 11.2 g). No death has occurred. The reactions most frequently reported from overdose have been drowsiness and vomiting. Overdosage may cause an increase in incidence or severity of any of the reported adverse reactions (see *Undesirable effects*).

Any patient suspected of having taken an overdose should have the stomach emptied by gastric lavage. Treatment should be symptomatic and supportive in the case of hypotension or excessive sedation. There is no specific antidote for nefazodone.

### Pharmacological properties
*Pharmacodynamic properties:* Nefazodone blocks serotonin type 2 ($5HT_2$) receptors and inhibits serotonin uptake. It lacks anticholinergic and antihistamine effects, has little alpha$_1$-adrenergic blocking activity

and does not potentiate the sedative effects of alcohol in man or pentobarbital in animal studies.

In elderly volunteers, nefazodone caused a small fall in mean supine blood pressure and pulse rate; however, no significant orthostatic blood pressure or ECG changes were observed.

Nefazodone has positive effects on sleep architecture. It slightly decreased (20%) the time between sleep initiation and the first REM episode, increased total REM sleep time, and did not affect the number or timing of REM episodes through the night. There were no changes in detumescence time for nocturnal erections associated with REM episodes. Additionally, Dutonin decreased the number of arousals and wakefulness during sleep in patients with major depression.

*Pharmacokinetic properties:* Nefazodone is rapidly and completely absorbed with peak plasma concentrations 1-3 hours after oral administration. It undergoes extensive presystemic metabolism and is highly protein bound (>99%). The estimated systemic bioavailability of nefazodone is 15-23%. The plasma elimination half-life is 2-4 hours for nefazodone, with elimination primarily by liver metabolism. Steady state is reached within 3-4 days after initiating treatment or making a dose adjustment. Pharmacokinetic parameters are non-linear with relatively higher peak serum levels and greater AUCs occurring as doses are increased through the recommended dosage range. Nefazodone is eliminated within 24 hours of discontinuing treatment.

*Effect of age, gender and phenotype:* In repeat dose studies, plasma levels of nefazodone and its major metabolite were higher in elderly than in young females. In male subjects, no significant effect of age was observed. The pharmacokinetics of nefazodone and its metabolites were unchanged in slow metabolisers of dextromethorphan, except that the clearance of the metabolite, m-chloro-phenylpiperazine (mCPP), is reduced in this phenotype.

*Effect of food:* Food delays the absorption of nefazodone and decreases the systemic exposure to nefazodone (AUC) on average by approximately 20%. These effects are not considered to be clinically significant.

*Preclinical safety data:* There is no evidence of carcinogenic, mutagenic or genotoxic effects with nefazodone. There were no specific organ toxicities noted in animal studies.

## Pharmaceutical particulars

*List of excipients:* Microcrystalline Cellulose; Povidone; Sodium Starch Glycollate; Colloidal Silicon Dioxide; Magnesium Stearate; Red Ferric Oxide; Yellow Ferric Oxide.

*Incompatibilities:* Not applicable.

*Shelf life:* PVC, PVDC blisters on foil flexible packaging: 24 months

*Special precautions for storage:* Storage should be below 30°C, in a dry place.

*Nature and contents of container:* Polyvinyl chloride (PVC) or polyvinylidene chloride (PVDC) blister packs on foil flexible packaging, containing 14 or 56 tablets per carton. Treatment initiation pack containing blisters of 14 pink 50 mg, 14 white 100 mg and 28 light yellow 200 mg tablets.

*Instructions for use/handling:* No special handling instructions.

## Marketing authorisation numbers

Dutonin Tablets 50 mg       11184/0027
Dutonin Tablets 100 mg      11184/0028
Dutonin Tablets 200 mg      11184/0029

Date of approval/revision of SPC January 1997

**Legal category** POM

## LIPOSTAT* TABLETS

### Qualitative and quantitative composition

*Lipostat tablets 10 mg:* Yellow capsule shaped biconvex tablet each containing pravastatin sodium 10 mg. Each tablet is engraved '10' on one side, with a breakline.

*Lipostat tablets 20 mg:* Yellow capsule shaped biconvex tablet each containing pravastatin sodium 20 mg. Each tablet is engraved '20' on one side, with a breakline.

*Lipostat tablets 40 mg:* Yellow capsule shaped biconvex tablet each containing pravastatin sodium 40 mg. Each tablet is engraved '40' on one side.

**Pharmaceutical form** Uncoated tablet

### Clinical particulars

*Therapeutic indications:*
*Hypercholesterolaemia:* The reduction of elevated total and LDL cholesterol levels in patients with primary hypercholesterolaemia who have not responded adequately to dietary measures.

*Coronary heart disease:* As an adjunct to diet to slow the progressive course of coronary atherosclerosis and reduce the incidence of clinical cardiac events in patients with hypercholesterolaemia and documented atherosclerotic coronary artery disease.

*Prevention of coronary heart disease:* As an adjunct to diet in hypercholesterolaemic patients without clinically evident coronary heart disease to:

- reduce the risk of fatal and non-fatal myocardial infarction;
- reduce the need to undergo myocardial revascularisation procedures;
- improve survival by reducing cardiovascular deaths.

*Posology and method of administration:* Prior to initiating Lipostat, secondary causes of hypercholesterolaemia should be excluded and patients should be placed on a standard cholesterol-lowering diet which should be continued during treatment. In addition, physicians are recommended to consult guidelines issued by consensus groups such as the European Atherosclerosis Society.

*Adults:* The usual dosage range is 10-40 mg administered once a day at bedtime.

The maximal effect of a given dose occurs within four weeks, therefore periodic lipid determinations should be performed and the dosage adjusted accordingly.

*Elderly patients and patients with hepatic or renal impairment:* There is no clinical evidence to suggest the dose range needs to be different in these patients. In common with other treatments, treatment should be initiated at the lower end of the dosage range.

*Children:* There are insufficient clinical data to recommend use in individuals less than 18 years old.

*Concomitant therapy:* The effects of Lipostat on lowering total and LDL cholesterol are enhanced when combined with a bile acid-binding resin. When administering a bile acid-binding resin (e.g. cholestyramine, colestipol) Lipostat should be given either one hour or more before or at least four hours after the resin. The bioavailability of pravastatin is not altered by concurrent administration with nicotinic acid, probucol and gemfibrozil (see *Precautions, Skeletal Muscle*).

Patients taking immunosuppressive drugs such as cyclosporin (see *Precautions, Skeletal Muscle*) concomitantly with pravastatin, should begin treatment with 10 mg of pravastatin once daily and be titrated to higher doses with caution.

*Contra-indications:* Hypersensitivity to any component of this medication.

Active liver disease or unexplained persistent elevations in liver function tests.

Pregnancy and Lactation (see *Pregnancy and lactation* section).

*Special warnings and special precautions for use:* Lipostat should not be used when hypercholesterolaemia is due to elevated HDL-C or in patients with homozygotic familial hypercholesterolaemia.

*Liver function:* As with other lipid-lowering agents, liver function tests should be performed periodically. Special attention should be given to patients who develop increased transaminase levels and therapy should be discontinued if increases in alanine aminotransferase (ALT) and aspartate aminotransferase (AST) exceed three times the upper limit of normal and persist.

In clinical trials 0.5% of patients treated with pravastatin had marked persistent increases (greater than 3 times the upper limit of normal) in serum transaminases. These elevations were not associated with clinical signs and symptoms of liver disease and usually declined to pre-treatment levels upon discontinuation of therapy.

Caution should be exercised when pravastatin is administered to patients with a history of liver disease or heavy alcohol ingestion.

*Skeletal muscle:* As with other HMG-CoA reductase inhibitors, sporadic elevations of creatine phosphokinase levels (CPK [MM fraction]) have been observed. If a markedly elevated (greater than 10 times upper limit of normal) serum CPK develops, or if myopathy is suspected, discontinuation of pravastatin therapy is recommended. There have been rare reports of rhabdomyolysis with renal dysfunction secondary to myoglobinuria. An increase in the incidence of myositis and myopathy has been seen in patients receiving HMG-CoA reductase inhibitors, especially those being treated concomitantly with cyclosporin (see Drug Interactions), fibric acid derivatives and nicotinic acid.

In clinical trials involving small numbers of patients who were treated concurrently with pravastatin and nicotinic acid, there were no reports of myopathy. However, such combinations should continue to be used with caution.

The combined use of pravastatin and fibric acid derivatives may be useful in selected patients requiring further lipid level reductions. However, since the occurrence of myopathy cannot be excluded, concom-

itant use of pravastatin and fibric acid derivatives should generally be avoided.

*Interactions with other medicaments and other forms of interaction:* No clinically significant effects were seen in a range of interaction studies.

*Cholestyramine/Colestipol:* There was no clinically significant decrease in bioavailability or therapeutic effect when pravastatin was administered one hour before or four hours after cholestyramine or one hour before colestipol and a standard meal. Concomitant administration resulted in approximately 40 to 50% decrease in the bioavailability of pravastatin.

*Cyclosporin:* Some investigators have measured cyclosporin plasma levels in patients receiving pravastatin and cyclosporin concomitantly and to date these results indicate no clinically meaningful elevations in cyclosporin levels. In one single-dose study, pravastatin plasma levels were found to be increased in cardiac transplant patients receiving cyclosporin.

*Warfarin:* Bioavailability parameters at steady state for pravastatin were not altered following administration with warfarin. Chronic dosing of the two drugs did not produce any changes in the anticoagulant action of warfarin.

In interaction studies with aspirin, antacids (one hour prior to Lipostat) cimetidine, gemfibrozil, nicotinic acid or probucol, no statistically significant differences in bioavailability were seen.

*Other drugs:* During clinical trials, no noticeable drug interactions were reported when Lipostat was added to: diuretics, antihypertensives, digitalis, converting-enzyme inhibitors, calcium channel blocker, beta-blockers, or nitroglycerins.

*Pregnancy and lactation:* There have been no teratogenic effects seen in animal studies. The safety of pravastatin therapy during pregnancy has not been established. Lipostat should only be used in women of child-bearing potential who are protected by effective contraception. As cholesterol and other products of cholesterol synthesis are essential components for foetal development, HMG-CoA reductase inhibitors are contra-indicated during pregnancy.

A small amount of pravastatin is excreted in human milk. Breastfeeding should be discontinued during pravastatin therapy.

*Effects on ability to drive and use machines:* None.

*Undesirable effects:* Lipostat is generally well tolerated. Adverse events, both clinical and laboratory are usually mild and transient. Pravastatin was not associated with cataract formation in patients treated for up to a year or more in clinical studies nor in long-term animal studies.

In placebo controlled studies, the following events showed a small increase in incidence over placebo: those occurring with a frequency >1% were rash, myalgia, headache, non-cardiac chest pain; those occurring with a frequency >0.1% were nausea/vomiting, diarrhoea, fatigue.

Pravastatin has been administered concurrently with cholestyramine, colestipol, nicotinic acid and probucol. No adverse reactions unique to the combination or in addition to those previously reported for each drug alone have been reported.

*Overdose:* To date there have been only two reported cases of overdose, both of which were asymptomatic and did not give rise to abnormal laboratory tests. In the event of accidental overdose patients should be treated symptomatically.

### Pharmacological properties

*Pharmacodynamic properties:* Pravastatin sodium is a competitive inhibitor of 3-hydroxy-3-methylglutaryl-coenzyme A (HMG-CoA) reductase, the enzyme catalysing the early rate-limiting step in cholesterol biosynthesis, and produces its lipid-lowering effect in two ways. First, it effects modest reductions in intracellular pools of cholesterol which results in an increased number of LDL-receptors on cell surfaces, enhanced receptor-mediated catabolism and clearance of circulating low density lipoprotein cholesterol (LDL-C). Second, pravastatin inhibits LDL-C production by inhibiting hepatic synthesis of very low density lipoprotein (VLDL-C), the LDL-C precursor. These effects result in a reduction of total cholesterol (Total-C), LDL-C, VLDL-C, apolipoprotein B and triglycerides, whilst increasing high density, lipoprotein cholesterol (HDL-C) and apolipoprotein A. Unlike other HMG-CoA reductase inhibitors, Lipostat has little effect on cholesterol synthesis in other tissues (e.g. lens, adrenal glands). *In vitro* studies demonstrated that pravastatin is transported into hepatocytes with substantially less uptake into other cells.

In controlled clinical trials, pravastatin was shown to reduce the progression of atherosclerosis and cardiovascular events (e.g. fatal and non-fatal M.I.) or death, in patients with moderate hypercholesterolaemia with or without atherosclerotic cardiovascular disease.

*Pharmacokinetic properties:* Pravastatin is administered orally in the active form and is rapidly absorbed, with peak plasma levels occurring 1 to 1.5 hours after dosing. Whilst the presence of food reduces the systemic biovailability, the lipid-lowering effect is unaffected. Pravastatin undergoes extensive first-pass extraction in the liver which is its primary site of action and the primary site of cholesterol synthesis and of LDL-C clearance. Plasma levels are of limited value in predicting lipid-lowering efficacy. Approximately 50% of the circulating drug is bound to plasma proteins. The plasma elimination half life of pravastatin is between 1.5 and 2 hours. After oral dosing approximately 20% of the dose is excreted in the urine and 70% in the faeces. Although there are dual routes of elimination, and the potential exists for compensatory excretion by the alternate route, accumulation of drug and/or metabolites may occur in patients with renal or hepatic insufficiency. The major metabolite of pravastatin has one-tenth to one-fortieth of the activity of the parent compound.

*Preclinical safety data:* Pravastatin has not demonstrated any carcinogenic potential in mice. However, in a 2 year study in male rats given 125 times the maximum human dose of pravastatin, a statistically significant increase in the incidence of hepatocellular carcinomas was observed. This change was not seen in male rats given less than or equal to 50 times the recommended human dose, or in female rats at any dose level.
*In vitro* toxicology studies have shown no evidence of mutagenic potential.

**Pharmaceutical particulars**

*List of excipients:* Croscarmellose sodium, lactose, magnesium stearate, magnesium oxide, microcrystalline cellulose, polyvidone, yellow ferric oxide E172.

*Incompatibilities:* Not applicable.

*Shelf life:* 36 months

*Special precautions for storage:* Store below 30°C. Protect from light and moisture.

*Nature and contents of container:* PVC blister or aluminium foil packs of 28 tablets.

*Instructions for use/handling:* Not applicable.

**Marketing authorisation numbers**

| | |
|---|---|
| Lipostat 10 mg | 11184/0055 |
| Lipostat 20 mg | 11184/0056 |
| Lipostat 40 mg | 11184/0057 |

**Date of approval/revision of SPC** 10 January 1997

**Legal category** POM

## SULPAREX* TABLETS 200 MG

**Presentation** Plain white round tablets with BMS 1510 on one side and a break bar on the other, each containing 200 mg sulpiride.
Other ingredients: magnesium stearate, maize starch, microcrystalline cellulose and polyvidone.

**Uses** For the treatment of acute and chronic schizophrenia.
Sulparex is a highly selective dopamine antagonist with bi-modal dose-dependant antidepressant and antipsychotic activity. Florid schizophrenic symptoms respond to high doses of Sulparex, whereas administration of lower doses results in mood elevation and alerting effect. Schizophrenia characterised by lack of social contact can benefit strikingly from treatment. Improvement of both florid and negative symptoms occurs, often within the first few days of treatment. The sedation and blunted effect characteristically associated with classical neuroleptics of the phenothiazine or butyrophenone type are not features of Sulparex therapy.

**Dosage and administration** *Adults:* The initial dose depends on the nature of the symptoms.
Predominantly positive symptoms (formal thought disorder, hallucinations, delusions, incongruity of effect) respond to higher doses, and a starting dose of at least 400 mg twice daily is recommended, increasing if necessary up to a suggested maximum of 1200 mg twice daily. Increasing the dose beyond this level has not been shown to produce further improvement.
Predominantly negative symptoms (flattening of effect, poverty of speech, anergia, apathy), as well as depression, usually respond best to a total of 200 mg to 400 mg daily, given in divided doses.
Patients with mixed positive and negative symptoms, with neither predominating, will normally respond to dosage of 200 mg to 600 mg twice daily.
*Elderly:* The same dose ranges may be required in the elderly but, as a general rule with the use of psychotropics in elderly patients, starting doses should be lower and increased gradually, particularly in those with renal impairment.
*Children:* Clinical experience in children under 14 years of age is insufficient to permit specific recommendations.

**Contra-indications, warnings, etc**
*Contra-indications:* Hypersensitivity to any of the ingredients of Sulparex. Phaeochromocytoma. Severe hepatic, renal or haematological disease. Alcoholic intoxication or other disorders which depress CNS function.
*Warnings:* Increased motor agitation has been reported at low dosage in a small number of patients. Low doses of Sulparex may aggravate symptoms in aggressive, agitated, or excited phases of the disease process. Consequently, low doses are not recommended when hypomania is present. Insomnia may occur in a small percentage of patients.
Extra-pyramidal reactions, including akathisia, have been reported in a small number of cases. If warranted, reduction in dosage or anti-parkinsonian medication may be necessary.
Tardive dyskinesia has occurred rarely.
As with all neuroleptic drugs, the presence of unexplained hyperthermia could indicate the neuroleptic malignant syndrome (NMS). In this event Sulparex and any associated neuroleptic treatment should be discontinued until the origin of the fever has been determined.
Hormonal effects of neuroleptic drugs include hyperprolactinaemia, which may cause galactorrhoea, gynaecomastia and oligomenorrhoea/amenorrhoea. Sexual function may be increased or decreased. These side-effects are reversible on cessation of treatment. In long term animal studies with neuroleptic compounds, including sulpiride, an increase of various endocrine tumours (a small proportion of which were malignant) have been seen in some but not all strains of rats and mice studied. The significance of these findings to man is not known; there is no evidence of an association between Sulparex use and tumour risk in man. However, when prescribing neuroleptics to patients with existing mammary neoplasia or a personal history of this disease, possible risk should be weighed against benefits of therapy.
*Precautions:* As with all drugs for which the kidney is the major elimination pathway, caution should be exercised when administering Sulparex to patients with impairment of renal function. Dose levels and/or the frequency of administration may need to be amended.
Although Sulparex is less prone to produce drowsiness than conventional neuroleptic compounds, patients receiving high doses of medication should be warned about the hazards of driving or operating machinery until the compound has been shown not to interfere with their physical or mental ability.
Patients should be warned against taking alcohol with sulpiride as reaction capacity may be impaired.
*Patients with epilepsy:* Although Sulparex produces only slight modifications to the EEG, anti-convulsant medication should be continued unchanged in epileptics. Patients with unstable epilepsy should be monitored frequently.
*Drug interactions:* As with other psychotropic compounds, sulpiride may increase the effect of antihypertensives and CNS depressants (including alcohol) or stimulants.
*Use in pregnancy and lactation:* Despite the negative results of teratogenicity studies in animals and the lack of teratogenic effects during widespread clinical use, Sulparex should not be considered an exception to the general principle of avoiding drug treatment during pregnancy, particularly during the first 16 weeks, with potential benefits being weighed against possible hazards.
Passage of sulpiride into breast milk has been reported.
*Side-effects:* Hepatic reactions, including jaundice and hepatitis, have been reported.
Cases of convulsions, sometimes in patients with no previous history, have been reported.
*Toxicity and treatment of overdose:* Overdoses have been reported ranging from 1 g to 16 g but no death has occurred even at the 16 g dose. Doses of 1 g to 3 g have been reported to produce restlessness and clouding of consciousness and (rarely) extrapyramidal symptoms. Doses of 3 g to 7 g may produce a degree of agitation, confusion, low blood pressure and extrapyramidal symptoms. In cases where coma has occurred, Sulparex has been administered in conjunction with other psychotropic medication. The duration of intoxication is generally short, the symptoms disappearing within a few hours. There are no specific complications from overdose. In particular no haematological or hepatic toxicity has been reported.
Overdose may be treated with alkaline osmotic diuresis and, if necessary, anti-parkinsonian drugs. Emetic drugs are unlikely to be effective. Coma needs appropriate nursing.

**Pharmaceutical precautions** Store below 30°C.

**Legal category** POM.

**Package quantities** Cardboard cartons containing blister strips of 100 tablets.

**Further information** Sulparex is a member of the group of substituted benzamides, which are structurally distinct from the phenothiazines, butyrophenones and thioxanthenes. Current evidence suggests that the actions of Sulparex hint at an important distinction between different types of dopamine receptors or receptor mechanisms in the brain. Behaviourally and biochemically, Sulparex shares with these conventional neuroleptics a number of properties indicative of cerebral dopamine receptor antagonism. Essential and intriguing differences include lack of catalepsy at doses active in other behavioural tests, lack of effect in the dopamine sensitive adenylate cyclase systems, lack of effect upon noradrenaline or 5HT turnover, negligible anticholinesterase activity, no effect on muscarinic or GABA receptor binding, and a radical difference in the binding of tritiated sulpiride to striatal preparations *in-vitro*, compared to $^3$H-spiperone or $^3$H-haloperidol. These findings indicate a major differentiation between Sulparex and conventional neuroleptics which lack such specificity.
Sulparex is slowly absorbed after oral dosing.
Peak sulpiride serum levels are reached 2–6 hours after an oral dose. The majority of studies have shown that the elimination half-life in plasma is 6–8 hours. Approximately 40% sulpiride is bound to plasma proteins. The mean concentration of sulpiride in the cerebrospinal fluid is 13% of its serum concentration. 95% of the compound is excreted in the urine and faeces as unchanged sulpiride.
Sulparex has no significant cardiovascular or anticholinergic activity.

**Product licence number** 11184/0032.

## TAXOL*
## TAXOL*-100

**Qualitative and quantitative composition** Taxol vials contain 30 mg or 100 mg paclitaxel per vial as a 6 mg/ml solution.

**Pharmaceutical form** Concentrate for solution for infusion.

**Clinical particulars**

*Therapeutic indications:*
*Ovarian carcinoma*: The primary treatment of carcinoma of the ovary, in combination with cisplatin, in patients with advanced disease or residual disease (>1cm) after initial laparotomy.
The secondary treatment of metastatic carcinoma of the ovary after failure of standard platinum containing therapy.
*Breast carcinoma*: The treatment of metastatic carcinoma of the breast in patients who have failed, or are not candidates for, standard anthracycline containing therapy.
*Posology and method of administration:*
*Primary treatment of ovarian carcinoma:* although other dosage regimens are under investigation, a combination regimen is recommended consisting of Taxol 135 mg/m² administered over 24 hours, followed by cisplatin 75 mg/m², with a 3 week interval between courses (see Interactions).
Secondary treatment of ovarian and breast carcinoma: the recommended dose of Taxol is 175 mg/m² administered over a period of 3 hours, with a 3 week interval between courses.
Subsequent doses of Taxol should be administered according to individual patient tolerance.
Taxol should not be readministered until the neutrophil count is $\geq 1.5\times 10^9$/L and the platelet count is $\geq 100\times 10^9$/L. Patients who experience severe neutropenia (neutrophil count $<0.5\times 10^9$/L for ≥7 days) or severe peripheral neuropathy should receive a dose reduction of 20% for subsequent courses (see Special warnings).
All patients must be premedicated with corticosteroids, antihistamines, and $H_2$ antagonists prior to Taxol, eg.

| *Drug* | *Dose* | *Administration prior to Taxol* |
|---|---|---|
| dexamethasone | 20 mg oral | approximately 12 and 6 hours |
| diphenhydramine *or* | 50 mg IV | 30 to 60 minutes |
| chlorpheniramine | 10 mg IV | |
| cimetidine *or* | 300 mg IV | 30 to 60 minutes |
| ranitidine | 50 mg IV | |

Taxol should be administered through an in-line filter with a microporous membrane ≤0.22μ m (see *Instructions for use/handling*).
*Contra-indications:* Taxol is contra-indicated in patients with severe hypersensitivity reactions to

paclitaxel or any other component of the formulation, especially polyethoxylated castor oil.

Taxol is contra-indicated during pregnancy and lactation.

Taxol should not be used in patients with baseline neutrophils <1.5x10⁹/L.

*Special warnings and special precautions for use:* Taxol should be administered under the supervision of a physician experienced in the use of cancer chemotherapeutic agents. Since significant hypersensitivity reactions may occur, appropriate supportive equipment should be available.

Patients must be pretreated with corticosteroids, antihistamines and $H_2$ antagonists (see *Posology and method of administration*).

Taxol should be given *before* cisplatin when used in combination (see *Interactions*).

Significant hypersensitivity reactions characterized by dyspnea and hypotension requiring treatment, angioedema and generalized urticaria have occurred in < 1% of patients receiving Taxol after adequate premedication. These reactions are probably histamine-mediated. In the case of severe hypersensitivity reactions, Taxol infusion should be discontinued immediately, symptomatic therapy should be initiated and the patient should not be rechallenged with the drug.

Bone marrow suppression (primarily neutropenia) is the dose-limiting toxicity. Frequent monitoring of blood counts should be instituted. Patients should not be retreated until neutrophils recover to a level ≥1.5x10⁹/L and platelets recover to a level ≥100x10⁹/L.

Severe cardiac conduction abnormalities have been reported rarely. If patients develop significant conduction abnormalities during Taxol administration, appropriate therapy should be administered and continuous cardiac monitoring should be performed during subsequent therapy with Taxol. Hypotension, hypertension, and bradycardia have been observed during Taxol administration; patients are usually asymptomatic and generally do not require treatment. Frequent vital sign monitoring, particularly during the first hour of Taxol infusion, is recommended.

Although the occurrence of peripheral neuropathy is frequent, the development of severe symptoms is unusual. In severe cases, a dose reduction of 20% is recommended for all subsequent courses of Taxol.

There is no evidence that the toxicity of Taxol is increased when given as a 3-hour infusion to patients with mildly abnormal liver function. No data are available for patients with severe baseline cholestasis. When Taxol is given as a longer infusion, increased myelosuppression may be seen in patients with moderate to severe hepatic impairment.

Taxol is not recommended in patients with severely impaired hepatic function.

Since Taxol contains dehydrated alcohol (396 mg/mL), consideration should be given to possible CNS and other effects.

Special care should be taken to avoid intra-arterial administration of Taxol. In animal studies investigating local tolerance, severe tissue reactions occurred following intra-arterial administration.

*Interactions with other medicaments and other forms of interaction:* Paclitaxel clearance is not affected by cimetidine premedication.

The recommended regimen of Taxol administration for the primary treatment of ovarian carcinoma is for Taxol to be given *before* cisplatin. When Taxol is given *before* cisplatin, the safety profile of Taxol is consistent with that reported for single-agent use. When Taxol was given *after* cisplatin, patients showed a more profound myelosuppression and an approximately 20% decrease in paclitaxel clearance.

There is possible inhibition of paclitaxel metabolism in patients treated with ketoconazole. As a result, caution should be exercised when treating patients with Taxol if they are receiving concomitant therapy with ketoconazole.

*Pregnancy and lactation:* Taxol has been shown to be embryotoxic and fetotoxic in rabbits, and to decrease fertility in rats.

There is no information on the use of Taxol in pregnant women. As with other cytotoxic drugs, Taxol may cause fetal harm, and is therefore contraindicated during pregnancy. Women should be advised to avoid becoming pregnant during therapy with Taxol, and to inform the treating physician immediately should this occur.

It is not known whether paclitaxel is excreted in human milk. Taxol is contraindicated during lactation. Breastfeeding should be discontinued for the duration of Taxol therapy.

*Effect on ability to drive and use machines:* Taxol has not been demonstrated to interfere with this ability. However, it should be noted that the formulation contains alcohol (see *Special warnings* and *List of excipients*).

*Undesirable effects:* Unless otherwise stated, the following safety data relate to 95 patients with ovarian

cancer and 289 patients with breast cancer treated with 175 mg/m² over a 3 hour infusion in three phase III clinical trials. Data from these clinical trials demonstrate that Taxol given at the recommended dose and schedule is well tolerated and none of the observed toxicities was clearly influenced by age.

Safety has also been evaluated in a large randomised trial (GOG-111) which compared Taxol (135 mg/m² over 24 hours)/cisplatin (75 mg/m²) with cyclophosphamide/cisplatin in 410 patients (196 receiving Taxol). Unless otherwise mentioned, the combination of Taxol with platinum agents or the infusion of Taxol over 24 hours did not result in any clinically relevant changes to the safety profile of Taxol.

The most frequent significant undesirable effect of Taxol was bone marrow suppression. Severe neutropenia (<0.5x10⁹/L) occurred in 28% of patients, but was not associated with febrile episodes. Only 1% of patients experienced severe neutropenia for 7 days or more.

Twenty-four percent of patients had an infectious episode. In the phase III clinical trials, 2 fatal infections were seen at the recommended dose and infusion schedule.

Thrombocytopenia was reported in 11% of patients. Three percent of patients had a platelet count nadir <50x10⁹/L at least once while on study.

Anemia was observed in 64% of patients, but was severe (Hb<8 g/dL) in only 6% of patients. Incidence and severity of anemia is related to baseline hemoglobin status.

One case each of acute myeloid leukemia and myelodysplastic syndrome has been reported outside the phase III trials.

Myelosuppression is less frequent and less severe with a 3-hour infusion than with a 24-hour infusion schedule. The recommended Taxol/cisplatin regimen for the primary treatment of ovarian cancer caused more severe myelosuppression than single dose Taxol using the recommended schedule of 175 mg/m² over 3 hour infusion. However, there was no increase in clinical sequelae.

A significant hypersensitivity reaction with possible fatal outcome (defined as hypotension requiring therapy, angioedema, respiratory distress requiring bronchodilator therapy, or generalized urticaria) occurred in 2 (<1%) patients. Thirty-four percent of patients (17% of all courses) experienced minor hypersensitivity reactions. These minor reactions, mainly flushing and rash, did not require therapeutic intervention nor did they prevent continuation of Taxol therapy.

Hypotension and bradycardia were experienced by 22% and 5% of patients, respectively. The degree of change was usually mild and did not require therapeutic intervention.

Seventeen percent of patients had an abnormal ECG during clinical trials. In most cases, no clear relationship between Taxol and ECG alterations could be defined and these alterations were of little or no clinical relevance.

One (<1%) patient experienced hypertension during Taxol therapy. In addition, 2 (<1%) patients presented severe thrombotic events (upper extremity thrombosis and thrombophlebitis). One patient each (<1%) experienced the following significant cardiovascular events: hypotension associated with septic shock, cardiomyopathy and tachycardia associated with fever. In early clinical studies, conducted with varying dosages and infusion schedules, 2% patients experienced severe cardiovascular events possibly related to Taxol which included asymptomatic ventricular tachycardia, tachycardia with bigeminy, AV block and syncope.

Cases of myocardial infarction have been reported rarely. Congestive heart failure has been reported typically in patients who have received other chemotherapy, notably anthracyclines.

Peripheral neuropathy, mainly manifested by paresthesia, affected 66% of patients, but was severe in only 5% of patients. Peripheral neuropathy can occur following the first course and can worsen with increasing exposure to Taxol. Peripheral neuropathy was the cause of Taxol discontinuation in 3 cases. Sensory symptoms have usually improved or resolved within several months of Taxol discontinuation. Pre-existing neuropathies resulting from prior therapies are not a contraindication for Taxol therapy. Among patients treated with Taxol outside these randomized trials, grand mal seizures, encephalopathy, motor neuropathy with resultant minor distal weakness, autonomic neuropathy resulting in paralytic ileus, and orthostatic hypotension have been reported. Optic nerve and/or visual disturbances (scintillating scotomata) have also been reported, particularly in patients who have received higher doses than recommended. These effects generally have been reversible.

Arthralgia or myalgia affected 60% of patients and was severe in 13% of patients.

Alopecia was observed in almost all patients.

Transient and mild nail and skin changes have been observed. Rare reports of skin abnormalities related to radiation recall have been received outside the phase III trials.

Gastrointestinal side effects were usually mild to moderate: nausea/vomiting, diarrhea and mucositis were reported by 43%, 28% and 18% of patients, respectively. Other gastrointestinal events reported outside these randomized trials included bowel obstruction/perforation, and (mesenteric thrombosis including ischemic) colitis.

Severe elevations (> 5 x normal values) in AST (SGOT), alkaline phosphatase or bilirubin were seen in 5%, 4%, and <1% of patients, respectively. Hepatic necrosis and hepatic encephalopathy have been reported in patients treated with Taxol outside the phase III trials.

Injection site reactions during intravenous administration may lead to localized edema, pain, erythema, and induration; on occasion, extravasation can result in cellulitis. Skin discoloration may also occur. Recurrence of skin reactions at a site of previous extravasation following administration of Taxol at a different site, ie. "recall", has been reported rarely. A specific treatment for extravasation reactions is unknown at this time.

Radiation pneumonitis has been reported in patients receiving concurrent radiotherapy.

*Overdose:* There is no known antidote for Taxol overdosage. The primary anticipated complications of overdosage would consist of bone marrow suppression, peripheral neurotoxicity and mucositis.

**Pharmacological properties**

*Pharmacodynamic properties:* Pharmacotherapeutic group/ATC code: cystostatic agent, L01C D01.

Paclitaxel is a novel antimicrotubule agent that promotes the assembly of microtubules from tubulin dimers and stabilizes microtubules by preventing depolymerization. This stability results in the inhibition of the normal dynamic reorganization of the microtubule network that is essential for vital interphase and mitotic cellular functions. In addition, paclitaxel induces abnormal arrays or bundles of microtubules throughout the cell cycle and multiple asters of microtubules during mitosis.

The safety and efficacy of Taxol (135 mg/m² over 24 hr) immediately followed by cisplatin (75 mg/m²) was evaluated in a major randomized, double-blind, controlled clinical trial (GOG-111). Patients in the control group received cyclophosphamide 750 mg/m² + cisplatin 75 mg/m². The trial involved over 400 patients with stage III/IV primary ovarian cancer with a >1cm residual disease after staging laparotomy or with distant metastases. There were statistically significant gains in median time to progression (> 3.5 months) and overall median survival (>11 months) for the Taxol arm. The level of serious toxicity was comparable between the two groups.

*Pharmacokinetic properties:* Following intravenous administration, paclitaxel exhibits a biphasic decline in plasma concentrations.

The pharmacokinetics of paclitaxel were determined following 3 and 24 hour infusions at doses of 135 and 175 mg/m². Mean terminal half-life estimates ranged from 3.0 to 52.7 hours, and mean, noncompartmentally derived, values for total body clearance ranged from 11.6 to 24.0 L/hr/m²; total body clearance appeared to decrease with higher plasma concentrations of paclitaxel. Mean steady-state volume of distribution ranged from 198 to 688 L/m², indicating extensive extravascular distribution and/or tissue binding. With the 3-hour infusion, increasing doses result in non-linear pharmacokinetics. For the 30% increase in dose from 135 mg/m² to 175 mg/m², the $C_{MAX}$ and $AUC_{0-\infty}$ values increased 75% and 81%, respectively.

Intrapatient variability in systemic paclitaxel exposure was minimal. There was no evidence of accumulation of paclitaxel with multiple treatment courses.

*In vitro* studies of binding to human serum proteins indicate that 89-98% of drug is bound. The presence of cimetidine, ranitidine, dexamethasone or diphenhydramine did not affect protein binding of paclitaxel.

The disposition of paclitaxel has not been fully elucidated in humans. Mean values for cumulative urinary recovery of unchanged drug have ranged from 1.3 to 12.6% of the dose, indicating extensive non-renal clearance. Hydroxylated metabolites have been demonstrated to be the principal metabolites. Hepatic metabolism and biliary clearance may be the principal mechanism for disposition of paclitaxel. The effect of renal or hepatic dysfunction on the disposition of paclitaxel following a 3-hour infusion has not been investigated formally. Pharmacokinetic parameters obtained from one patient undergoing hemodialysis who received a 3-hour infusion of Taxol 135 mg/m² were within the range of those defined in non-dialysis patients.

*Preclinical safety data:* The carcinogenic potential of Taxol has not been studied. However, paclitaxel is a potential carcinogenic and genotoxic agent, based upon its pharmacodynamic mechanism of action. Taxol has been shown to be mutagenic in both *in vitro* and *in vivo* mammalian test systems.

### Pharmaceutical particulars

*List of excipients:* Dehydrated alcohol (396 mg/mL), cleaned polyethoxylated castor oil.

*Incompatibilities:* Polyethoxylated castor oil can result in DEHP [di-(2-ethylhexyl)phthalate] leaching from plasticized polyvinyl chloride (PVC) containers, at levels which increase with time and concentration. Consequently, the preparation, storage and administration of diluted Taxol should be carried out using non-PVC-containing equipment.

*Shelf life:* Unopened vials are stable until the date indicated on the package (24 months), when stored between 15-25°C in the original carton.

If unopened vials are refrigerated, a precipitate may form that redissolves with little or no agitation upon reaching room temperature. Product quality is not affected. If the solution remains cloudy or if an insoluble precipitate is noted, the vial should be discarded. Freezing does not adversely affect the product.

*Special precautions for storage:* Store the unopened vials between 15-25°C in the original cartons to protect from light.

*Nature and contents of container:* Glass vials with butyl rubber stoppers containing 30 mg or 100 mg of paclitaxel as a 6 mg/ml solution. The vials are available individually packed in a carton or in a shelf pack of 10 cartons.

*Instructions for use/handling:* Handling: as with all antineoplastic agents, caution should be exercised when handling Taxol. Dilution should be carried out under aseptic conditions by trained personnel in a designated area. Adequate protective gloves should be worn. Precautions should be taken to avoid contact with the skin and mucous membranes. In the event of contact with the skin, the area should be washed with soap and water. Following topical exposure, tingling, burning and redness have been observed. In the event of contact with the mucous membranes, these should be flushed thoroughly with water. Upon inhalation, dyspnea, chest pain, burning throat and nausea have been reported.

The Chemo-Dispensing Pin device or similar devices with spikes should not be used since they can cause the vial stopper to collapse, resulting in loss of sterile integrity.

*Preparation for IV administration:* Prior to infusion, Taxol must be diluted, using aseptic techniques, in 0.9% Sodium Chloride Injection, or 5% Dextrose Injection, or 5% Dextrose and 0.9% Sodium Chloride Injection, or 5% Dextrose in Ringer's Injection, to a final concentration of 0.3 to 1.2 mg/mL. The prepared solutions are physically and chemically stable for up to 27 hours (including preparation and administration) at ambient temperature (approximately 25°C) and room lighting conditions. Diluted solutions should not be refrigerated.

Upon preparation, solutions may show haziness, which is attributed to the formulation vehicle, and is not removed by filtration. Taxol should be administered through an in-line filter with a microporous membrane ≤0.22µ m. No significant losses in potency have been noted following simulated delivery of the solution through IV tubing containing an in-line filter.

To minimize patient exposure to DEHP, which may be leached from plasticized PVC infusion bags, sets, or other medical instruments, diluted Taxol solutions should be stored in non-PVC bottles (glass, polypropylene) or plastic bags (polypropylene, polyolefin) and administered through polyethylene-lined administration sets. Use of filter devices (eg. IVEX-2*) which incorporate short inlet and/or outlet plasticized PVC tubing has not resulted in significant leaching of DEHP.

There have been rare reports of precipitation during Taxol infusions, usually towards the end of a 24 hour infusion period. Although the cause of this precipitation has not been elucidated, it is probably linked to the supersaturation of the diluted solution. To reduce the precipitation risk, Taxol should be used as soon as possible after dilution and excessive agitation, vibration or shaking should be avoided. The infusion sets should be flushed thoroughly before use. During infusion the appearance of the solution should be inspected regularly and the infusion should be stopped if precipitation is present.

*Disposal:* All items used for preparation, administration or otherwise coming into contact with Taxol should undergo disposal according to local guidelines for the handling of cytotoxic compounds.

### Marketing authorisation numbers

| | |
|---|---|
| Taxol | 11184/0026 |
| Taxol-100 | 11184/0058 |

**Date of approval/revision of SPC** March 1997

**Legal category** POM

## VIDEX* TABLETS

**Qualitative and quantitative composition** Chewable/dispersible buffered tablets containing didanosine 25 mg and 100 mg.

**Pharmaceutical form** Tablets.

**Clinical particulars**

*Therapeutic indications:* Videx is indicated, preferably in combination with other antiretroviral agents, for the treatment of HIV-infected adults and children with progressive or advanced immunodeficiency.

Clinical benefit of Videx was demonstrated in several important clinical trials (see *Pharmacodynamic properties*).

*Posology and method of administration:* Because of reduced absorption in the presence of food, it is recommended that Videx be administered at least 30 minutes before a meal. (see *Pharmacokinetic properties*). Although the optimal dose of Videx has not been finally established, the following recommendations can be made:

*Dosage:*

*Adults:* The recommended starting dose is dependent on weight; the dosing interval should be approximately 12 hours (BID). Doses up to 750 mg/day (sachet) or 600 mg/day (tablet) have been used in clinical trials. The recommended average starting doses are outlined in the table below.

*Adult dosing guidelines*

| Patient Baseline Weight | Videx tablets (†) |
|---|---|
| ≥60 kg | 200 mg BID |
| <60 kg | 125 mg BID |

(†) To ensure that patients taking Videx tablets receive a sufficient amount of antacid, each dose must be given as 2 tablets.

*Children:* The recommended starting dose, based on body surface area, is 240 mg/m²/day (180 mg/m²/day in combination with ZDV). The recommended dosing interval is 12 hours.

Insufficient clinical experience exists to recommend a dosing regimen in infants under 3 months of age.

*Dose adjustment:* Significant elevations of serum amylase should prompt discontinuation of therapy and careful evaluation of the possibility of pancreatitis, even in the absence of symptoms of pancreatitis. Fractionation of amylase may help distinguish amylase of salivary origin. Only after pancreatitis has been ruled out or after clinical and biological parameters have returned to normal, should dosing be resumed, and then only if treatment is considered essential. Treatment should be re-initiated with low doses and increased slowly, if appropriate.

Many patients who present with symptoms of neuropathy and who experience resolution of symptoms upon drug discontinuation will tolerate a reduced dose of Videx.

*Renal impairment:* Although there are insufficient data to recommend a specific dose adjustment of Videx in patients with mild or moderate renal impairment, a dose reduction should be considered. In anuric patients requiring dialysis, half of the recommended total daily dose of Videx should be administered once a day. The dose should be administered after dialysis (see *Special warnings*).

*Hepatic impairment:* There are insufficient data to recommend a specific dose adjustment of Videx in patients with hepatic impairment, but an adjustment in the dose in these patients should also be considered (see *Special warnings*).

*Contra-indications:* Videx is contra-indicated in patients with hypersensitivity to any of the components of the formulations.

*Special warnings and special precautions for use:* *Pancreatitis* is a known serious complication among HIV-infected patients. It has also been associated with Videx therapy and has been fatal in some cases. Videx should be used only with extreme caution in patients with a history of pancreatitis. Positive relationships have been found between the risk of pancreatitis and daily dose.

Whenever warranted by clinical conditions, Videx dosing should be suspended until the diagnosis of pancreatitis is excluded by appropriate laboratory and imaging techniques. Similarly, when treatment with other drugs known to cause pancreatic toxicity is required (e.g. i.v. pentamidine), didanosine should be suspended during therapy wherever possible. If concomitant therapy is unavoidable there should be close observation. Dose suspension should also be considered when biochemical markers of pancreatitis have increased to a clinically significant degree above the upper limit of normal, even in the absence of symp-

toms. Significant elevations of triglycerides are a known cause of pancreatitis and warrant close observation.

*Peripheral neuropathy:* Patients on Videx may develop toxic peripheral neuropathy, usually characterized by bilateral symmetrical distal numbness, tingling, and pain in feet and, less frequently, hands. Whenever warranted by clinical conditions, Videx therapy should be suspended until resolution of symptoms. Many patients tolerate a reduced dose after resolution of symptoms.

*Hyperuricaemia:* Videx has been associated with hyperuricaemia. Treatment should be suspended if significant elevations in uric acid levels occur during treatment.

*Liver failure of unknown etiology* has occurred rarely in patients on Videx. Patients should be observed for liver enzyme elevations and Videx should be suspended if enzymes rise to a clinically significant level above the upper limit of normal. Rechallenge should be considered only if the potential benefits of Videx treatment clearly outweigh the potential risks for the individual patient

Paediatric patients on Videx therapy have demonstrated **retinal or optic nerve changes** on rare occasions, particularly at doses above those recommended. There have been reports of retinal depigmentation in adult patients. Especially for children, periodic dilated retinal examinations (every 6 months), or if a change in vision occurs, should be considered.

Insufficient clinical experience exists to recommend a dosing regimen in infants under 3 months of age.

Patients receiving Videx or any antiretroviral therapy may continue to develop opportunistic infections and other complications of HIV infection or therapy. They therefore should remain under close clinical observation by physicians experienced in the treatment of patients with HIV associated diseases. To carry out the treatment in an appropriate way, one needs access to appropriate equipment, e.g., the possibility to carry out special laboratory tests including the necessary controls of T4-lymphocytes and biochemical markers of pancreatitis.

*Renal impairment:* Although there are insufficient data to recommend a specific dose adjustment of Videx in patients with mild or moderate renal impairment, a dose reduction should be considered as these patients may be at greater risk of toxicity from Videx. Further, the magnesium content of each Videx tablet is 8.7 mEq which may represent an excessive load of magnesium to patients with significant renal impairment. In anuric patients requiring dialysis, half the recommended total daily dose of Videx should be administered once a day. The dose should be administered after dialysis (see *Posology and method of administration*).

*Hepatic impairment:* There are insufficient data to recommend a specific dose adjustment of Videx in patients with hepatic impairment, but an adjustment of the dose in these patients should also be considered (see *Posology and method of administration*).

*Phenylketonurics:* Videx tablets contain 36.5 mg phenylalanine (from the aspartame). Therefore, the use of Videx in phenylketonuria patients should be considered only if clearly indicated.

*Interaction with other medicaments and other forms of interaction:* Combination studies of Videx (up to 500 mg/day) and zidovudine (ZDV) (up to 600 mg/day) have not revealed any unexpected toxicities.

Specific drug interaction studies have been conducted with ZDV, ranitidine, loperamide, metoclopramide and rifabutin without evidence of interaction. Based upon the results from a study with ketoconazole, it is recommended that drugs which can be affected by stomach acidity (eg. oral azoles such as ketoconazole and itraconazole), be given at least 2 hours prior to dosing with Videx.

Concomitant administration of ganciclovir and Videx (200 mg BID) was associated with an increase in the steady state AUC for didanosine and a minor change in this parameter for ganciclovir. It is not known whether these changes are associated with alterations in either the safety of Videx or the efficacy of ganciclovir. Significant but clinically tolerable myelosuppression with haemoglobin levels < 8.0 g/dL was observed in a few patients receiving the combination of Videx and ganciclovir.

Coadministration of Videx with drugs that are known to cause peripheral neuropathy or pancreatitis may increase the risk of these toxicities. Patients who receive these drugs should be carefully observed.

As with other products containing aluminum and/or magnesium antacid components, Videx tablets should not be taken with any tetracycline antibiotic. Likewise, plasma concentrations of some quinolone antibiotics (eg. ciprofloxacin) are decreased by administration with antacids contained in or adminstered with Videx. It is recommended that drugs that may interact with antacids be administered at least 2 hours prior or 4 hours after a dose of Videx.

As experience of drug interactions with Videx is still limited, care should be taken in combining other drug regimens with Videx.

Ingestion of Videx with food reduces the amount of didanosine absorbed by approximately 50% (see 5.2)

*Pregnancy and lactation: Pregnancy:* There are no adequate and well-controlled studies in pregnant women and it is not known whether didanosine can cause foetal harm or affect reproductive capacity when administered during pregnancy. Therefore, the use of Videx during pregnancy should be considered only if clearly indicated, and only when the potential benefit outweighs the possible risk.

Teratology studies in rats and rabbits did not produce evidence of embryotoxic, foetotoxic, or teratogenic effects. A study in rats showed that didanosine and/or its metabolites are transferred to the foetus through the placenta.

*Lactation:* It is not known whether didanosine is excreted in human milk. It is recommended that women taking Videx do not breast-feed because of the potential for serious adverse reactions from didanosine in nursing infants.

At the 1000 mg/kg/day dose levels in rats, didanosine was slightly toxic to females and pups during mid and late lactation (reduced food intake and body weight gains), but the physical and functional development of the subsequent offsprings were not impaired. A further study showed that, following oral administration, didanosine and/or its metabolites were excreted into the milk of lactating rats.

*Reproduction:* In rats, didanosine did not impair the reproduction ability of male or female parents following treatment prior to and during mating, gestation and lactation at daily didanosine doses up to 1000 mg/kg/day. In a perinatal and postnatal reproduction study in rats, didanosine did not induce toxic effects.

*Effects on ability to drive and use machines:* At present, no data are known regarding these effects.

*Undesirable effects:*
*Adults:* Most of the serious adverse events observed have generally reflected the recognized clinical course of AIDS and HIV infection. Concurrent dosing with a variety of drugs was allowed in the studies. Therefore, it is difficult to distinguish which events are related to Videx, to the disease itself, or to other therapy-related events.Clinically significant undesirable effects reported in controlled clinical studies which may be possibly related to treatment with Videx at the recommended dose include pancreatitis and elevations in serum amylase and lipase levels. Pancreatitis, which may be fatal in some cases, was more frequent in patients who were treated with doses above those recommended; patients with advanced HIV disease or a history of pancreatitis may also be at increased risk of developing pancreatitis. Peripheral neuropathy has been associated with Videx therapy. Abnormal liver function tests, with rare reports of liver failure and death have also been reported. Events of less clinical importance which may possibly be associated with Videx treatment include diarrhoea, nausea/vomiting, allergic reactions, diabetes mellitus, dry mouth and elevated uric acid levels. Retinal or optic nerve changes have been reported rarely.

*Children:* Undesirable effects were generally similar to those seen in adults. A higher incidence of haematotoxicity has been reported in patients treated with the combination with ZDV compared with Videx monotherapy. Retinal or optic nerve changes have been reported in a small number of paediatric patients usually at doses above those recommended. It is recommended that children on Videx treatment undergo dilated retinal examination every 6 months or if a change in vision occurs.

*Overdose:* There is no known antidote for didanosine overdosage. Experience in early studies, in which didanosine was initially administered at doses ten times the recommended doses indicates that the anticipated complications of overdosage would be secondary to hyperuricaemia or, possibly, to hepatic dysfunction.

Didanosine is not dialyzable by peritoneal dialysis, although there is some clearance by hemodialysis. (The fractional removal of didanosine during an average hemodialysis session of 3 to 4 hours was approximately 20-35% of the dose present in the body at the start of dialysis.)

**Pharmacological properties**

*Pharmacodynamic properties:* Didanosine (2',3'-dideoxyinosine) is an inhibitor of the *in vitro* replication of HIV in cultured human cells and cell lines. After didanosine enters the cell, it is enzymatically converted to dideoxyadenosine-triphosphate (ddATP), its active metabolite. In viral nucleic acid replication, incorporation of this 2'-3'-dideoxynucleoside prevents chain extension, and thereby inhibits viral replication.

In addition, ddATP inhibits HIV-reverse transcriptase by competing with dATP for binding to the enzyme's active site, preventing proviral DNA synthesis.

The relationship between *in vitro* susceptibility of HIV to didanosine, and clinical response to therapy has not been established. Likewise, *in vitro* sensitivity results vary greatly and methods to establish virologic responses have not been proven.

The effect of Videx, alone or in combination with ZDV (zidovudine), was evaluated in several major randomized, controlled clinical trials (ACTG 175, ACTG 152, DELTA, CPCRA 007). These trials confirmed the reduced risk of HIV disease progression or death with Videx therapy, alone or in combination with ZDV, as compared with ZDV monotherapy in HIV-infected individuals, including symptomatic and asymptomatic adults with CD4 counts < 500 cells/mm$^3$ and children with evidence of immunosuppression. The clinical benefits of initial Videx therapy were demonstrated in adults with CD4 counts 200-500 cells/mm$^3$, as well as in children. The ACTG 175 trial showed that eight weeks of treatment with ZDV,Videx, or Videx plus ZDV decreased mean plasma HIV RNA by 0.26, 0.65 and 0.93 $\log_{10}$ copies /mL, respectively.

*Pharmacokinetic properties:*
*Adults:* Didanosine is rapidly degraded at an acidic pH. Therefore, all oral formulations must contain buffering agents designed to increase gastric pH. The administration of didanosine with a meal results in a significant decrease in bioavailability. This decrease is about 50 % with the tablet. All Videx formulations should be administered at least 30 minutes before a meal. A study in 10 asymptomatic HIV seropositive patients demonstrated that administration of Videx tablets 30 min to 1 hr before a meal did not result in any significant changes in the bioavailability of didanosine compared to administration under fasting conditions. Administration of the tablets 1 to 2 hr after a meal was associated with a 55% decrease in CMAX and AUC values, which was comparable to the decrease observed when the formulation was given immediately after a meal.

The volume of distribution at steady state averages 54 L, suggesting that there is some uptake of didanosine by body tissues.

The level of didanosine in the cerebrospinal fluid (CSF), one hour after infusion, averages 21% of that of the simultaneous plasma level.

The average elimination half-life after intravenous administration of didanosine is approximately 1.4 hours. Renal clearance represents 50% of total body clearance (800 mL/min), indicating that active tubular secretion, in addition to glomerular filtration, is responsible for the renal elimination of didanosine.

Urinary recovery of didanosine is approximately 20% of the dose after oral treatment. There is no evidence of didanosine accumulation after the administration of oral doses for 4 weeks.

*Children:* Variability in the amount of didanosine (non-buffered Videx powder reconstituted with water and antacid) absorbed in children is greater than in adults. The absolute bioavailability of didanosine administered orally was approximately 36% after the first dose and 47% at steady state.

The CSF didanosine level averages 46% of that of the simultaneous plasma level after intravenous administration of doses of 60 or 90 mg/m$^2$ and equivalent oral doses of 120 or 180 mg/m$^2$. Measurable concentrations of didanosine in the CSF were detectable for up to 3.5 hours after dosing.

The average elimination half-life after intravenous didanosine administration is approximately 0.8 hours. Renal clearance represents approximately 59% of the total body clearance (315 mL/min/m$^2$), indicating that both renal and nonrenal pathways are involved in the elimination.

Urinary recovery of didanosine is approximately 17% of dose after oral treatment.

There is no evidence of didanosine accumulation after oral administration for an average of 26 days.

The metabolism of didanosine in man has not been evaluated. However, based on animal studies, it is presumed that it follows the same pathways responsible for the elimination of endogenous purines.

*In vitro* human plasma protein binding is less than 5% with didanosine, indicating that drug interactions involving binding site displacement are not anticipated.

There are currently incomplete data concerning the effect of impaired renal or hepatic function on the pharmacokinetics of didanosine.

*Preclinical safety data:* The lowest dose to cause death in acute toxicity studies in the mouse, rat and dog was greater than 2000 mg/kg which is equivalent to approximately 300 times the maximum recommended human dose of the tablet formulation. Repeat-dose oral toxicity studies revealed evidence of a dose-limiting skeletal muscle toxicity in rodents (but not in dogs) following long-term (> 90 days) dosing with didanosine at doses that were approximately 1.2–12 times the estimated human dose. Additionally, in repeat dose studies, leucopenia was observed in dogs and rats, and gastrointestinal disturbances (soft stool, diarrhoea) were seen in dogs at doses approximately 5–14 times the maximum human dose. In the carcinogenicity studies, non-neoplastic alterations have been observed including skeletal muscle myopathy, hepatic alterations and an exacerbation of spontaneous age-related cardiomyopathy. Results from the genotoxicity studies suggest that didanosine is not mutagenic at biologically and pharmacologically relevant doses. At significantly elevated concentrations in vitro, the genotoxic effects of didanosine are similar in magnitude to those seen with natural DNA nucleosides. Lifetime dietary carcinogenicity studies were conducted in mice and rats for 22 or 24 months, respectively. No drug-related neoplasms were observed in any didanosine-treated groups of mice during, or at the end of, the dosing period. In rats, statistically significant increased incidences of granulosa cell tumors in females receiving the high dose, of subcutaneous fibrosarcomas and histiocytic sarcomas in males receiving the high dose and of hemangiomas in males receiving the high and intermediate dose of didanosine were noted. The drug-relationship and clinical relevance of these statistical findings were not clear.

**Pharmaceutical particulars**

*List of excipients:* Aspartame, calcium carbonate, crospovidone, magnesium hydroxide, magnesium stearate, mandarin orange flavour, microcrystalline cellulose, sorbitol.

*Incompatibilities:* None.

*Shelf life:* 24 months at room temperature (15-30°C). If dispersed in water, the dose may be held for up to 1 hour at ambient temperature.

*Special precautions for storage:* Store in tightly closed bottles at room temperature.

*Nature and contents of container:* High-density polyethylene bottle with child-resistant cap (60 tablets per bottle).

*Instructions for use/handling:*
*Method of preparation:*
*Adults:* Patients should take two tablets in each dose, to provide sufficient antacid against acid degradation of didanosine. The tablets should be thoroughly chewed, or crushed, or dispersed in at least 30 mL of water prior to consumption. To disperse tablets, stir until a uniform dispersion forms, and drink the entire dispersion immediately. If additional flavouring is desired, the dispersion may be diluted with 30 mL of clear apple juice.

Stir the further dispersion just prior to consumption. The dispersion with clear apple juice is stable at room temperature for up to one hour.

*Children:* Children older than 1 year of age should receive a 2-tablet dose, children under 1 year should receive a 1-tablet dose. Tablets should be chewed, or crushed, or dispersed in water prior to consumption, as described in the preceding Adult Dosing Method of Preparation. When a one tablet dose is required, the volume of water for dispersion should be 15 mL. Fifteen mL of clear apple juice may be added to the dispersion as a flavouring.

**Marketing authorisation numbers**

| | |
|---|---|
| 25 mg: | 11184/0008 |
| 100 mg: | 11184/0010 |

**Date of approval/revision of SPC** 18 July 1996

**Legal category** POM

**Trade Mark*

# Britannia Pharmaceuticals Limited
## 41–51 Brighton Road
## Redhill
## Surrey RH1 6YS

## ALEC*

**Presentation** ALEC is presented as a vial of white, sterile, freeze-dried powder stored under nitrogen together with a 5 ml syringe, catheter, and 2 ml ampoule of sterile sodium chloride 0.9% w/v.

Each vial of ALEC contains 100 mg pumactant for reconstitution with 1.2 ml of cold, sterile sodium chloride solution 0.9% w/v. ALEC is for intratracheal administration.

When reconstituted the product appears as a white, creamy suspension. The reconstituted product contains 0.18 mmol (10.8 mg) of sodium.

**Uses** ALEC treatment reduces neonatal mortality in newborn babies of an estimated gestational age of 25–29 weeks, and who are intubated and undergoing mechanical ventilation because they are at risk of developing, or have developed Respiratory Distress Syndrome (RDS).

**Dosage and administration** ALEC must be reconstituted with 1.2 ml of cold, sterile sodium chloride solution 0.9% w/v before administration.

*Dosage: Adults and older children*—Not applicable.

*Neonates:* The reconstituted contents of one vial (i.e. 100 mg pumactant) should be given via the endotracheal tube as soon as possible after the baby is intubated. If the baby remains intubated, a second dose should be given 1 hour later. A third dose should be given at 24 hours from the time of intubation, but only if the baby is still undergoing mechanical ventilation.

Infants should not be intubated solely for the purpose of administering ALEC.

*Reconstitution:* ALEC should be reconstituted immediately before use as it contains no antimicrobial preservatives. The reconstituted product should be used within 8 hours.

The phospholipids in reconstituted ALEC will undergo a physical transition when warmed to body temperature to give molecular lamellar structures. This change involves a rapid spreading of the phospholipids, and it is essential that this occurs only after ALEC has been instilled into the endotracheal tube. Therefore, care should be taken to ensure that ALEC is kept cool up to the time of administration. ALEC (powder, syringe, catheter and the sterile sodium chloride solution 0.9% w/v) must be stored in the refrigerator (below 8°C) before use, BOTH as the packaged product AND as the reconstituted suspension ready for use. Do not freeze.

ONLY preservative-free sodium chloride solution 0.9% w/v for injection should be used for reconstitution, which should be performed as follows:

1. Remove the centre of the metal cover on the pumactant vial. Tap the vial to loosen the powder which may have settled on storage.

2. Draw 1.2 ml of cold, sterile sodium chloride solution 0.9% w/v into the 5 ml syringe. Push the syringe needle through the stopper of the pumactant vial and inject the sodium chloride solution. Withdraw the syringe with needle still attached.

3. Shake the vial gently, just enough to ensure dispersal of the pumactant; the contents of the vial should appear as a creamy suspension with a few lumps. (Any lumps of pumactant remaining in the vial will be disrupted in drawing up the reconstituted ALEC or will melt on warming to body temperature after administration).

Vigorous shaking will cause the suspension to form a foam, and should be avoided.

4. Draw 2 ml of air into the syringe and push the syringe needle through the rubber stopper of the pumactant vial. Inject the air to create a positive pressure.

5. Invert the vial and carefully draw as much of the suspension as possible into the syringe, followed by about 1 ml of air. Withdraw the syringe with needle still attached.

6. Hold the syringe with the needle pointing upwards and expel air so that the final volume reading on the syringe is 1.2 ml. Remove the needle from the syringe.

7. Attach the catheter supplied in the pack of ALEC to the syringe.

*Administration:* ALEC should be administered only by those trained and experienced in the care and resuscitation of preterm infants.

ALEC is administered rapidly from the syringe through the catheter which has been passed to the end of the endotracheal tube. It is necessary to disconnect the ventilator from the neonate temporarily during administration, although the time taken to deliver a whole single dose of ALEC should not generally be more than a few seconds.

The administration of ALEC should be performed as follows:

1. Prepare the ALEC as described under *Reconstitution* above, and have it ready to use before proceeding to the following steps.

2. Disconnect the ventilator (or the resuscitation bag in the event of the baby being hand-ventilated) from the endotracheal tube. Proceed quickly through the next five steps.

3. Suction the baby's airway to clear any mucous immediately before ALEC is administered. This will not be appropriate if the dose is being given immediately after the baby has been intubated and it is known that the endotracheal tube is essentially clear from any obstruction.

4. Having noted the length of the endotracheal tube, pass the catheter on the syringe containing ALEC down it so that the lower end is just at the end of the endotracheal tube.

5. Instill ALEC by quickly injecting the suspension and air from the syringe into the trachea; it should not take more than two seconds.

6. With the catheter still in the endotracheal tube, quickly disconnect the syringe from the catheter. Draw 3 ml of air into the syringe and reconnect to the catheter. Rapidly inject all the air down the endotracheal tube into the neonate; this empties the syringe and catheter of any residual ALEC suspension.

7. Withdraw the catheter from the endotracheal tube and reconnect the ventilator (or the resuscitation bag) to the endotracheal tube.

Some 'milky' surfactant suspension will be seen in the endotracheal tube. This should NOT be aspirated; it will melt on warming from body heat and spread slowly into the baby's lungs.

8. Ensure that satisfactory ventilation has been re-established. Arterial oxygen monitors may record a more than transitory depression of arterial oxygen suggestive of a blockage of the endotracheal tube. If there is any concern that the airways have been obstructed by surfactant the first action should be hand ventilation with oxygen and resuscitation bag. If this is unsuccessful the endotracheal tube should be aspirated. If this does not remedy the problem, the baby should be re-intubated.

Care should be taken to avoid prolonged disconnection from the ventilator.

**Contra-indications, warnings, etc**

*Contra-indications:* There are no known contra-indications to the use of ALEC.

*Precautions:* ALEC should only be administered where there are adequate facilities for ventilation and monitoring of neonates with, or at risk from, RDS.

Preterm birth is hazardous. Surfactant administration can be expected to diminish the severity of RDS and hence to diminish the complications of intensive care, especially the ventilatory support required for the treatment of RDS, but cannot be expected to eliminate entirely the mortality and morbidity associated with preterm delivery. Infants who, but for the administration of surfactant, might have died from RDS may be exposed to other complications of their immaturity.

As a consequence of the surfactant properties of ALEC, chest expansion may improve rapidly after dosing, necessitating rapid reduction in peak ventilator inspiratory pressure.

The improvement in lung mechanics resulting from ALEC administration may result in rapid improvement in arterial oxygen concentration. After any appropriate reduction in ventilator pressure, rapid reduction in inspired oxygen concentration may be needed to avoid hyperoxia.

ALEC was non-mutagenic in Chinese Hamster Ovaries cells. No long-term studies have been performed in animals to determine whether ALEC has carcinogenic potential. The only constituents of pumactant are synthetic phospholipids which are also naturally occurring in human lung surfactant. These are not known to be carcinogenic.

The effects of ALEC on fertility have not been studied.

*Side-effects:* In rare instances (less than 1% of cases) ALEC administration has been associated with obstruction of the endotracheal tube. In infants in whom endotracheal tube obstruction is suspected this should be treated, according to normal practice, by hand-ventilation with oxygen and a resuscitation bag, followed by suction of the tube, or by replacement of the tube if this is unsuccessful.

*Pregnancy and lactation:* Not applicable.

*Interactions:* No drug interactions have been reported with ALEC.

*Treatment of overdosage:* ALEC contains only phospholipids which are naturally occurring in human lung surfactant. There have been no reports of overdosage with ALEC.

In case of a severe accidental overdosage, as much as possible of the surfactant should be aspirated and the baby should then be managed with supportive treatment.

**Pharmaceutical precautions** ALEC (powder, syringe, catheter and 2 ml ampoule of sterile sodium chloride 0.9% w/v) must be stored in the refrigerator (below 8°C) before use, BOTH as the packaged product AND as the reconstituted product ready for use.

Do not freeze packs of ALEC or the reconstituted product.

ALEC should be used within 8 hours from reconstitution.

**Legal category** POM.

**Package quantities** ALEC contains one vial of pumactant, packaged with a 5 ml syringe, catheter and 2 ml ampoule of sterile sodium chloride 0.9% w/v.

**Further information** ALEC contains pumactant which is a 7:3 mixture (by weight) of dipalmitoylphosphatidylcholine (DPPC) and unsaturated phosphatidylglycerol (PG). Both of these phospholipids are naturally occurring in human lung surfactant. ALEC contains no protein, alcohol or other artificial surface-active agents.

Neonates with RDS have a deficiency in lung surfactant, and what surfactant is present has an abnormal composition compared to that of healthy full-term babies. ALEC mimics closely the properties of natural lung surfactant and can improve lung compliance. In a multicentre clinical trial, ALEC was able to reduce neonatal mortality from 27% to 14% in babies of less than 30 weeks gestation.

**Product licence number** 04483/0040.

## BRITAJECT*

**Presentation** Britaject Pen 10 mg/ml is a disposable multiple dose pen injector system incorporating a clear glass cartridge containing apomorphine hydrochloride 10 mg/ml in aqueous solution for subcutaneous injection. It contains sodium bisulphite 0.093% w/v as an antioxidant.

Britaject Injection 10 mg/ml is presented as ampoules each containing apomorphine hydrochloride 10 mg/ml in aqueous solution for subcutaneous injection. It contains sodium metabisulphite 0.1% w/v as an antioxidant.

Britaject Pen 10 mg/ml contains 3 ml of solution and Britaject Injection 10 mg/ml is available in ampoules of 2 ml and 5 ml.

**Uses**

*Indication:* Britaject is indicated for the management of refractory motor fluctuations in Parkinson's disease; i.e. patients with disabling fluctuations in motor performance ('off' episodes) which are inadequately controlled by levodopa or other dopamine agonists (e.g. bromocriptine, lisuride, pergolide, etc.).

*Properties:* Apomorphine HCl is a potent dopamine agonist with antiparkinsonian activity. Other pharmacological effects include induction of emesis, nausea, retching, sedation, and yawning.

Apomorphine HCl is recommended for use in parkinsonian patients who have reached a stage of the disease at which they are exhibiting frequent 'on-off' disabling fluctuations in motor performance which are inadequately controlled by conventional antiparkinsonian medication.

Benefits are best seen in those Parkinson's disease patients who have good quality motor performance with levodopa, but in whom the duration of 'on' time is frequently unsatisfactory and is associated with unpredictable, disabling motor fluctuations.

Apomorphine HCl has an onset of action of between 5–10 minutes with a duration of action of about one hour, and, when administered by subcutaneous injection, may prevent an 'off' episode.

**Dosage and administration** The following general guidance applies to initiation and maintenance of apomorphine HCl therapy. It is administered as a subcutaneous injection. The optimal dosage of apomorphine HCl has to be determined on an individual patient basis. Hospital admission under appropriate specialist supervision is advised when establishing a patient's therapeutic regime.

It is essential that the patient is established on the antiemetic domperidone for at least 3 days prior to initiation of therapy.

*Patient selection:* Apomorphine HCl injections are only considered to be suitable for Parkinson's disease patients capable of recognising and anticipating 'off' episodes in motor performance. Patients must be capable and motivated for apomorphine HCl to be used effectively. Adult patients through all age ranges have been successfully managed with apomorphine HCl injections. Apomorphine HCl is contra-indicated in children and adolescents up to 18 years of age.

Elderly patients, in appropriate circumstances, can be successfully managed with apomorphine HCl.

The practical steps described below should be followed when commencing a patient on treatment;
- Pre-treat with domperidone.
- Discontinue all existing antiparkinsonian medication to provoke an 'off' episode in motor performance.
- Determine the threshold dose response to apomorphine HCl that produces an unequivocal motor response.
- Re-establish other antiparkinsonian agents.
- Determine effective treatment regimen for apomorphine HCl.
- Teach patient and/or carer how and when to administer.
- Discharge from hospital.
- Monitor frequently and adjust dosage regimen as appropriate.

Full details are given below:

*Pre-treatment:* Patient admission to hospital at least 3 days before initiation of apomorphine HCl treatment is recommended. On admission treatment with domperidone should be commenced (see *Use of domperidone with apomorphine HCl*, below). Over the following 3 days a clinical assessment must be made of the fluctuations in the patient's motor performance and response to conventional antiparkinsonian drug therapy.

*Provoking and assessing an 'off' state:* After at least 3 days of hospitalisation all anti-parkinsonian therapy is withheld overnight to provoke an 'off'-state in motor performance and to undertake a baseline motor assessment as follows:
(a) Alternate, unilateral hand-tapping for 30 seconds on mounted digital counters (preferably 20 cm apart) (Ref. Hughes, AJ et al., Lancet, 1990; *336*: 32–34).
(b) Time taken to walk 12 metres.
(c) Clinical assessment of tremor and dyskinesia according to a four point scale (0=nil, 1=mild, 2=moderate, 3=severe).
(d) Scoring on a modified Webster disability scale to assess 12 features of parkinsonism (maximum disability score of 36) (Ref. Kempster, PA et al., J Neurol Neurosurg Psychiatry, 1989; *52*: 718–23).

*Determination of the threshold dose:* Following baseline motor assessment the patient is challenged for apomorphine responsiveness according to the following schedule;
- 1.5 mg apomorphine HCl (0.15 ml) is injected subcutaneously and the patient is observed over 30 minutes for motor responsiveness.
- if no or poor response is obtained, a second dose of 3 mg apomorphine HCl (0.3 ml) is given 40 minutes after the first dose, and the patient observed for a further 30 minutes.
- The dosage is increased in an incremental fashion every 40 minutes and the patient observed carefully for an unequivocal motor response. The third dose is 5 mg s.c., and the fourth dose is 7 mg s.c. If the patient shows no response to the 7 mg dose then the patient must be classified as a non-responder to apomorphine HCl and no further attempts to provoke a motor response should be made. If the patient shows only a mild response to the 7 mg dose, a maximum dose of 10 mg can be used to see if an unequivocal motor response is possible.
- The lowest dose producing an unequivocal motor response is called the 'threshold dose'. For the majority of patients the threshold dose is less than 7 mg apomorphine HCl (0.7 ml), although very occasionally it can be up to 10 mg apomorphine HCl (1.0 ml).

Since Britaject Pen 10 mg/ml can only be administered in unit increments of 1 mg of apomorphine hydrochloride, it is recommended that the determination of the threshold dose is carried out with Britaject Injection 10 mg/ml.

Motor responsiveness is judged to be positive if 2 or more of the following are seen:
(a) More than 15% increase in tapping score.
(b) More than 25% improvement in walking time.
(c) An improvement of at least 2 points of tremor score.
(d) An improvement of Webster's score of 3 or more.

*Initiation of treatment:* Following establishment of an acceptable threshold dose of apomorphine HCl injection, the patient should be restarted on conventional antiparkinsonian therapy.

A subcutaneous injection of the established threshold dose may then be given into the lower abdomen or outer thigh at the first signs of an 'off' episode. The patient should then be observed over the following hour and the quality of their 'on' period noted. It may be appropriate to modify the dose of apomorphine HCl according to the patient's response.

Close monitoring of therapeutic benefits and side-effects under specialist supervision is required after initiation of treatment. The daily dose can vary between patients and will typically be in the range of 3 mg up to 30 mg per day in divided doses. The frequency of injection will also vary between patients and may be between 1 to 10 per day but in rare cases may be up to 12 times per day.

Patients who have shown a good 'on' period response during the initiation stage, but whose overall control remains unsatisfactory using intermittent injections, or who require many and frequent injections (more than 10 per day), may be commenced on or transferred to continuous subcutaneous infusion by minipump as follows;

Continuous infusion is started at a rate of 1 mg apomorphine HCl (0.1 ml) per hour then increased according to the individual response. Increases in the infusion rate should not exceed 0.5 mg per hour at intervals of not less than 4 hours. Hourly infusion rates may range between 1 mg and 4 mg (0.1 ml and 0.4 ml), equivalent to 0.015–0.06 mg/kg/hour. Infusions should run for waking hours only. Unless the patient is experiencing severe night-time problems, 24-hour infusions are not advised. In any event, the infusion site should be changed every 12 hours.

Patients normally need to supplement their continuous infusion with intermittent bolus boosts via the pump system as necessary. Patients who experience severe dyskinesias should only use bolus doses when absolutely necessary.

It is recommended that the total daily dose of apomorphine HCl should not exceed 100 mg and that individual bolus injections should not exceed 10 mg.

*Transferring patients established on intermittent apomorphine injections using standard syringes to Britaject Pen 10 mg/ml:* Britaject Pen 10 mg/ml is a convenient delivery system for administering frequent intermitttent injections. Patients already receiving apomorphine injections may be transferred to Britaject Pen 10 mg/ml but should be given a clear explanation by suitably trained medical staff on the use of the new delivery system. Some patients may require re-training in the administration technique. Full instructions for use are given in the leaflet enclosed with each pack.

Patients who are injecting apomorphine HCl in mg doses corresponding to whole digits may transfer directly to the corresponding mg dose on Britaject Pen 10 mg/ml.

However, since the dose dial increments on Britaject Pen 10 mg/ml are in single whole digits, patients who receive doses in between (e.g. 3.5 mg) will need to retitrate their dose on transferring to the Pen.

The appropriate dose (either up or down to the single, whole digit) should be selected according to the requirements of the individual patient. This can be established by instructing the patient to use the lower dose at the first sign of an off-episode. If the response is considered to be sub-optimal, a higher dose may be used for subsequent off-episodes.

In cases where over or under-dosing is achieved with Britaject Pen 10 mg/ml, it may be necessary to revert back to the original dose using their previous delivery system, or alternatively, the patient may be referred to their hospital specialist physician to determine whether he or she may be successfully transferred to Britaject Pen 10 mg/ml.

*Monitoring treatment:* Long-term specialist supervision of patients is advised.

There is a high probability of adverse effects to apomorphine HCl therapy (see *Side-effects*, below).

The frequency and severity of adverse events should be monitored carefully at regular intervals and a reassessment of the patient carried out if appropriate. Adjustments to the dosage or discontinuation may be necessary.

*Use of domperidone with apomorphine HCl:* Domperidone maleate is a peripherally acting dopamine receptor antagonist and is recommended for the treatment of drug-induced nausea and vomiting in Parkinson's disease. Pre-treatment with domperidone is necessary during the initiation of therapy to control apomorphine's emetic actions.

The typical pre-treatment dose of domperidone used in specialist centres during the clinical development of Britaject, was 20 mg three times a day. However, the appropriate pre-treatment and maintenance doses of domperidone should be established on an individual patient basis. Domperidone treatment can normally be withdrawn gradually over several weeks to 6 months, according to the degree of nausea being experienced by the patient, although occasionally it has to be continued indefinitely. Where nausea and vomiting occur during treatment it is usually as a result of omission or sub-therapeutic dosing of domperidone.

**Contra-indications, warnings, etc**

*Contra-indications:* Apomorphine HCl is contra-indicated in patients with respiratory or central nervous system depression. Apomorphine HCl should not be administered to patients who are sensitive to morphine or its derivatives.

Apomorphine HCl can lead to neuropsychiatric disturbances and should not be administered to patients with pre-existing neuropsychiatric problems or dementias due to other pathological processes, e.g. dementia of the Alzheimer's type or multiinfarct dementia.

Apomorphine HCl treatment is not suitable for patients who have an 'on' response to levodopa which is marred by severe dyskinesia, hypotonia or psychotoxicity.

*Use in pregnancy and lactation:* Animal reproduction studies have not been conducted with apomorphine HCl. It is not known whether apomorphine can damage the foetus or affect the mother's reproductive capacity. Therefore, apomorphine HCl is not recommended for use in women of child bearing potential.

It is not known whether apomorphine is excreted in breast milk. However, breast-feeding is not recommended where a nursing mother is on apomorphine HCl therapy.

*Precautions:* Apomorphine HCl should be given with caution to patients with endocrine, renal, pulmonary or cardiovascular disease and persons prone to nausea and vomiting.

Extra caution is recommended during initiation of therapy in elderly and/or debilitated patients. Periodic evaluation of hepatic, haemopoietic, renal and cardiovascular functions is advised.

If the patient has a history of postural hypotension, particularly if associated with other dopamine agonists, extra caution is recommended during the initiation stages of therapy with lying and standing blood pressure monitored before and after apomorphine test doses.

Patients selected for treatment with apomorphine HCl are almost certain to be taking concomitant medications for their Parkinson's disease. In the initial stages of apomorphine HCl therapy the patient should be monitored for unusual side-effects or signs of potentiation of effect.

Drugs which interfere with central amine mechanisms such as reserpine, tetrabenazine, metoclopramide, antipsychotic dopamine-blocking agents (such as phenothiazines, thioxanthines, and butyrophenones), amphetamines and papaverine should be avoided if possible. If, however, their administration is considered essential, extreme care should be taken and the patient monitored for signs of potentiation, antagonism or other interactions and for any unusual side-effects.

*Side-effects:* Local induration and nodules often develop at subcutaneous sites of injection. In patients on high doses of apomorphine HCl these may persist and give rise to areas of erythema, tenderness and induration. Panniculitis has been reported from those patients where a skin biopsy has been undertaken. These local subcutaneous effects can sometimes be reduced by rotation of injection sites, dilution of the solution with Sodium Chloride 0.9% injection, and possibly the use of ultrasound to areas of nodularity and induration. Care should be taken to ensure that areas of ulceration do not become infected. Rarely, cutaneous ulceration has led to cessation of apomorphine HCl therapy.

Drug-induced dyskinesias during 'on' periods can be severe, and in a few patients may result in cessation of therapy. Postural instability, falls, increasing cognitive impairment, personality change and disabling dyskinesias during the 'on' phase can mar the therapeutic response in some patients. Motor deficits in skilled tasks can still be detectable during 'on' periods, and impaired speech and balance may not improve with apomorphine HCl therapy.

Nausea and vomiting may occur, usually as a result of the omission of domperidone (*see Use of Domperidone*, above).

Neuropsychiatric disturbances are common in parkinsonian patients. Apomorphine HCl can lead to neuropsychiatric disturbances and should not be given to patients with pre-existing neuropsychiatric problems or dementias due to other pathological processes, e.g. dementia of the Alzheimer's type or multiinfarct dementia. Transient mild confusion and visual hallucinations have occurred during apomorphine HCl therapy, most commonly in patients reporting previous levodopa-induced neuropsychiatric complications. In the event of the continued development of confusion or hallucinations during treatment with apomorphine HCl an attempt should be made to identify the contributing factor under the direct supervision of a hospital specialist. The dose of apomorphine HCl should be reduced gradually and the effects on the patient's motor and psychiatric states closely observed.

Transient sedation with each dose of apomorphine HCl at the start of therapy is common; this usually resolves over the first few weeks. Postural hypotension is seen infrequently and is usually transient.

Euphoria, light-headedness, restlessness and tremors have also been reported.

The use of apomorphine HCl in conjunction with levodopa treatment may cause Coombs' positive haemolytic anaemia. An initial screen prior to commencement of treatment and at 6 monthly intervals is recommended. In the event of the development of a haemolytic anaemia, a haematological specialist should be consulted. The dose of apomorphine HCl and/or levodopa should be reduced, with careful monitoring of the patient's motor state. It may be necessary to discontinue treatment with levodopa and/or apomorphine HCl in the event that it is not possible to control the anaemia satisfactorily.

Eosinophilia has occurred in only a few patients during treatment with apomorphine HCl.

*Treatment of overdosage:* In a few cases hypotension and bradycardic episodes have occurred during test doses with apomorphine HCl. These are usually transient. If necessary, measures should be taken to increase the blood pressure, e.g. raising the foot of the bed. There is no clearly established pharmacological antidote to excessive doses of apomorphine HCl. However, treatment with an opioid antagonist such as naloxone has been reported to reduce yawning, sleepiness, nausea, retching, and vomiting when administered prior to a dose of apomorphine HCl. (Ref. Bonuccelli, U et al., Clin Neuropharmacol 1991, *14*: 442–449) and may be considered in severe cases where excessive doses of apomorphine HCl have been given.

Domperidone maleate is a recognised peripherally acting dopamine antagonist and is used to counter the emetic actions of apomorphine. Its use may be considered in cases of overdose.

Antipsychotic (neuroleptic) drugs, which interfere with dopaminergic transmission in the brain by blocking dopamine receptors, may be considered in the treatment of overdosage with apomorphine HCl.

### Pharmaceutical precautions
*Britaject Pen 10 mg/ml:* Store in a cool dry place (below 25°C) but not in a refrigerator. Do not store in direct heat or sunlight. Do not use if the solution turns green. Discard each pen no later than 48 hours from first use.

*Britaject Injection 10 mg/ml ampoules:* Protect from light and store at a temperature not exceeding 25°C. Do not use if the solution turns green. Britaject ampoules do not contain an antimicrobial preservative, so solutions should be used within 24 hours of opening.

### Legal category POM.

### Package quantities
*Britaject Pen 10 mg/ml:* Each pen contains apomorphine hydrochloride 10 mg/ml in 3 ml solution. The pens are supplied in cartons of 5.

*Britaject Injection 10 mg/ml* is presented as ampoules containing apomorphine hydrochloride 10 mg/ml:
   20 mg apomorphine hydrochloride in 2 ml of solution.
   50 mg apomorphine hydrochloride in 5 ml of solution.
The ampoules are supplied in cartons of 5.

### Further information Nil.

### Product licence numbers
Britaject Pen 10 mg/ml 4483/0042.
Britaject Injection 10 mg/ml 2 ml and 5 ml ampoules 4483/0038.

## BRITLOFEX* TABLETS 0.2 mg

**Presentation** Round, peach, film coated tablets; 6.5 mm diameter containing 0.2 mg lofexidine hydrochloride.

**Uses** To relieve symptoms in patients undergoing opiate detoxification.

**Dosage and administration** Initial dosage should be one 0.2 mg tablet twice daily. The dose may be increased by increments of 0.2–0.4 mg per day up to a maximum of 2.4 mg (12 tablets) per day, according to the patient's response. In cases where no opiate use occurs during detoxification a duration of treatment of 7–10 days is recommended. In some cases a longer treatment period may be warranted.

At the end of treatment dosage should be reduced gradually over a period of at least 2–4 days (see under Precautions).

**Contra-indications, warnings, etc**
*Contra-indications:* Lofexidine is contra-indicated in cases of sensitivity to other Imidazoline derivatives.

*Interactions:* Lofexidine may enhance the CNS depressive effects of alcohol, barbiturates and other sedatives, although concurrent medication to aid sleeping has frequently been used in withdrawal studies. Concomitant use of tricyclic antidepressants may reduce the efficacy of lofexidine.

*Pregnancy:* The safety of lofexidine in pregnant women has not been established and it should only be administered during pregnancy if the benefit outweighs the potential risk to mother and foetus. It is not known whether lofexidine is excreted in human milk and caution should be exercised when it is administered to nursing mothers.

*Precautions:* Lofexidine may have a mild sedative effect. If affected, patients should be advised not to drive or operate machinery.

Lofexidine does not normally produce any clinically significant effects on blood pressure, but since lofexidine possesses mild hypotensive properties it should be used with caution in patients with severe coronary insufficiency, recent myocardial infarction, cerebrovascular disease or chronic renal failure. Lofexidine should not be discontinued abruptly, but withdrawn gradually over 2–4 days, or longer, to minimise any risk of blood pressure elevation and associated signs and symptoms. It should also be used with caution in patients with marked bradycardia (55 beats per minute); pulse rate should be assessed frequently. Patients with a history of depression should be carefully observed during long term therapy with lofexidine.

*Side-effects:* The side-effects of lofexidine are primarily related to its central alpha-adrenergic effects and comprise drowsiness and related symptoms and dryness of mucous membranes especially mouth, throat and nose. Hypotension and bradycardia may occur.

*Treatment of overdosage:* Overdosage may cause hypotension, bradycardia, sedation and coma. Gastric lavage should be carried out where appropriate. In most cases all that is required are general supportive measures.

**Pharmaceutical precautions** Protect from heat, moisture and light.

**Legal category** POM.

**Package quantities** 60 tablets.

**Further information** Nil.

**Product licence number** 4483/0036.

## CRYSTAPEN* INJECTION

**Presentation** Vials containing 600 mg (1 mega unit) sodium benzylpenicillin (penicillin G) as a white crystalline water-soluble powder for the preparation of Benzylpenicillin Injection BP. Each vial contains a single dose for use on one occasion only.

**Uses** Crystapen has bactericidal activity in infections due to penicillin-sensitive organisms, particularly streptococci, pneumococci (*Streptococcus pneumoniae*), meningococci, gonococci and staphylococci (excluding penicillinase-producing strains). Crystapen is indicated for most wound infections, pyogenic infections of the skin, soft tissue infections and infections of the nose, throat, nasal sinuses, respiratory tract and middle ear, etc. Generalised infections, septicaemia and pyaemia from susceptible bacteria. Acute and chronic osteomyelitis, subacute bacterial endocarditis and meningitis caused by susceptible organisms. Gonorrhoea. Suspected meningococcal disease.

**Dosage and administration** The following dosages apply to both intramuscular and intravenous injection.
*Adults:* Usually 600 to 1,200 mg (1 to 2 mega units)

daily, divided into 2 to 4 doses. Higher doses (up to 14.4 g/day (24 mega units) in divided doses) may be given in adult meningitis. In bacterial endocarditis, 4.8 g (8 mega units) or more may be given daily in divided doses by the intravenous route, often by infusion. Intravenous doses in excess of 1.2 g (2 mega units) should be given slowly, taking at least one minute for each 300 mg (0.5 mega unit) to avoid high levels causing irritation of the central nervous system. High dosage of sodium benzylpenicillin may result in hypernatraemia and hypokalaemia unless the sodium content is taken into account.
*Children aged 1 month to 12 years:* 100 mg/kg/day in four divided doses.
*Infants:* 75 mg/kg/day in three divided doses.
*Newborn infants:* 50 mg/kg/day in two divided doses.

**Meningitis in infants and children:**
*Newborn infants:* 100 mg/kg/day in two divided doses.
*Infants 1–4 weeks:* 150 mg/kg/day in three divided doses.
*Children 1 month to 12 years:* 180–300 mg/kg/day in four to six divided doses.

**Suspected meningococcal disease:**
*Adults and children over 10 years:* 1,200 mg i.v. (or i.m.).
*Children 1–9 years:* 600 mg i.v. (or i.m.).
*Children under 1 year:* 300 mg i.v. (or i.m.).
*PREPARATION OF SOLUTIONS*
*Intramuscular injection:* A 600 mg (1 mega unit) dose is usually dissolved in 1.6 to 2.0 ml of Water for Injections BP.
*Intravenous injection:* A suitable concentration is 600 mg (1 mega unit) dissolved in 4 to 10 ml of Water for Injections BP.
*Intravenous infusion:* It is recommended that 600 mg (1 mega unit) should be dissolved in at least 10 ml of Sodium Chloride Injection BP or other transfusion solution.
*OTHER ROUTES OF ADMINISTRATION* – These usually supplement systemic dosage.
*Subconjunctival injection:* 300 to 600 mg dissolved in 0.5 to 1 ml of Water for Injections BP.
*Intrathecal injection:* Must be diluted by hospital pharmacy. Only freshly prepared solutions should be used. For adults, 6 mg (10,000 units) dissolved in 10 ml of Sodium Chloride Injection BP. Maximum dose, 12 mg (20,000 units).
For infants and children, 0.1 mg/kg (170 units/kg) is suitable.
The concentration of penicillin in the injection should not exceed 0.6 mg/ml (1,000 units/ml).
*Overdosage can cause convulsions, paralysis and may be fatal.* Use of a disposable membrane filter of 0.45 micron pore size is convenient for ensuring clarity of the solution.

**Contra-indications, warnings, etc**
*Contra-indications:* Allergy to penicillins. Hypersensitivity to any ingredient of the preparation.
*Precautions:* Massive doses of sodium penicillin can cause hypokalaemia and sometimes hypernatraemia. Use of a potassium-sparing diuretic may be helpful.

In the presence of impaired renal function large doses of penicillin (e.g. more than 8 grams/day in an adult) can cause cerebral irritation, convulsions and coma.

Overdosage by the intrathecal route can cause convulsions, paralysis and may be fatal (see Preparation of Solutions).

Skin sensitisation may occur in persons handling the antibiotic, and care should be taken to avoid contact with the substance. It should be recognised that any patient with a history of allergy, especially to drugs, is more likely to develop a hypersensitivity reaction to penicillin.

*Pregnancy:* Crystapen has been taken by a large number of pregnant women and women of childbearing age without an increase in malformations or other direct or indirect harmful effects on the foetus having been observed.

*Side-effects:* Anaphylactic reactions and immediate and delayed hypersensitivity reactions have been reported.

There have been rare reports of paraesthesia following long term administration.

Haemolytic anaemia and granulocytopenia, agranulocytosis, thrombocytopenia and coagulation disorders have been reported in patients receiving prolonged high dosage of parenteral benzylpenicillin sodium (e.g. in subacute bacterial endocarditis).

*Overdosage:* Excessive blood levels of penicillin G can be corrected by haemodialysis.

In the event of overdosage by the intrathecal route, CSF lavage to reduce the toxic concentration of penicillin G may be considered.

**Pharmaceutical precautions** Store below 25°C. Reconstituted solutions of penicillin are intended for immediate administration but may be stored for up to 24 hours at 2–8°C if necessary. For intrathecal injection only freshly prepared solutions should be used.

**Legal category** POM.

**Package quantities** 600 mg (1,000,000 units) unbuffered, box of 25 vials and 'GP pack' containing 2 vials.

**Further information** 600 mg Crystapen in solution displaces 0.4 ml. Each mega unit of unbuffered Crystapen represents 1.68 mmol of sodium.

**Product licence number** 4483/0039.

## RIMSO-50*

**Presentation** Sterile aqueous solution containing dimethyl sulphoxide 50% w/w in water.

**Uses** Indicated only for the symptomatic relief of patients with interstitial cystitis (Hunner's Ulcer).
For bladder instillation only.
Not for IM or IV injection.

**Dosage and administration** Instillation of 50 ml of Rimso-50 (dimethyl sulphoxide) directly into the bladder may be accomplished by catheter or bladder syringe and allowed to remain for 15 minutes. Application of an analgesic lubricant gel such as lignocaine jelly to the urethra is suggested prior to the insertion of the catheter to avoid spasm. The medication is expelled by spontaneous voiding. It is recommended that treatment be repeated every two weeks until maximum symptomatic relief is obtained. Thereafter, time intervals between therapy may be in-

creased appropriately. In selected cases where symptomatic relief is not complete, the bladder may be gently distended by gravity instillation with up to 500 ml of a solution prepared immediately prior to instillation in a glass bottle, with one part Rimso-50 and one part sterile water prior to the instillation of the standard dose of 50 ml of Rimso-50. After retention of Rimso-50 for 15 minutes the medication is again expelled by spontaneous voiding. Administration of oral analgesic medication prior to instillation of Rimso-50 can reduce bladder spasm in particularly sensitive patients.

In patients with very sensitive bladders, the treatment should be done under anaesthesia (preferably saddle block type).

Rimso-50 is recommended for bladder instillation only.

A garlic-like taste may be noted by the patient within a few minutes after instillation of RIMSO-50 (dimethyl sulphoxide). This taste may last several hours and because of the presence of metabolites, an odour on the breath and skin may remain for 72 hours.

**Contra-indications, warnings, etc**
*Contra-indications:* Nursing mothers and children.

*Precautions:* Changes in the refractive index and lens opacities have been seen in monkeys, dogs and rats given dimethyl sulphoxide chronically. No ophthalmic changes attributable to intravesical instillation of dimethyl sulphoxide have been reported in patients carefully followed for up to 17 months; nevertheless, full eye evaluations, including slit lamp examinations, are recommended prior to and at six month intervals during treatment.

Along with the ophthalmological examinations, patients should be investigated with respect to biochemical parameters, particularly renal and hepatic function, at six month intervals.

Intravesical instillation of Rimso-50 may be harmful to patients with urinary tract malignancy because of dimethyl sulphoxide-induced vasodilation.

*Warnings:* Dimethyl sulphoxide can initiate the liberation of histamine and there has been an occasional hypersensitivity reaction with topical administration of dimethyl sulphoxide. This hypersensitivity has not occurred in patients receiving intravesical Rimso-50; however, the physician should be cognizant of this possibility in prescribing Rimso-50. If anaphylactoid symptoms develop, appropriate therapy should be instituted. Some data indicates that dimethyl sulphoxide potentiates other concomitantly administered medications.

*Use in pregnancy:* The safety of dimethyl sulphoxide for the human foetus has not been established, hence it should be given to pregnant women only when the potential benefits to the mother have been weighed against possible hazards to the child.

**Pharmaceutical precautions** Store in a cool place protected from light.

**Legal category** POM.

**Package quantities** Bottles of 50 ml.

**Further information** Nil.

**Product licence number** 4047/0001.

*\*Trade Mark*

# Cambridge Laboratories
Richmond House
Old Brewery Court
Sandyford Road
Newcastle upon Tyne NE2 1XG

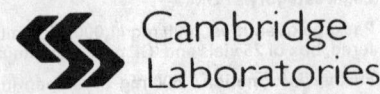

## ACTIDOSE-AQUA*

**Qualitative and quantitative composition** Actidose-Aqua contains 1.040 g of activated charcoal/5 ml.

**Pharmaceutical form** Suspension for oral administration.

### Clinical particulars

*Therapeutic indications:* For the emergency treatment of acute poisoning and drug overdosage where substances such as those listed below have been ingested. The list is not exhaustive and Actidose-Aqua may be of benefit following ingestion of many other toxins.

Also indicated for a limited number of systemic poisonings resulting from parenteral overdosage or when the ingested toxin has been totally absorbed. This usually involves repeated doses of Actidose-Aqua to remove compounds which undergo enterohepatic recycling or which can diffuse into the gastrointestinal tract along a concentration gradient. Under these circumstances, multiple doses of Actidose-Aqua adsorb the toxin, thereby preventing its reabsorbtion and increasing the concentration gradient in favour of further diffusion of the toxin into the gastrointestinal tract. Compounds most effectively transferred by this mechanism are lipophilic, uncharged and not excessively protein-bound. Examples of compounds which can be eliminated more rapidly by 'gastrointestinal dialysis' in this way are phenobarbitone and theophylline.

*Posology and method of administration:* The container should be shaken thoroughly prior to administration. If the dose of poison that has been ingested is known, a ratio of 10:1 (activated charcoal:toxin) may be used to determine the optimal dose of activated charcoal, subject to the limits of practicality. In the absence of any information regarding the amount of poison ingested, the following doses are recommended:

*Adults (including the elderly) and children over 12 years of age:* For single dose therapy, 50–100 grams of activated charcoal (240–480 ml) taken as soon as possible after ingestion of the poison.

For multiple dose therapy, 25–50 grams of activated charcoal (120–240 ml) every 4–6 hours.

*Children aged 1–12 years:* For single dose therapy, 25–50 grams of activated charcoal (120–240 ml) taken as soon as possible after ingestion of the poison. For multiple dose therapy, the dose may be repeated every 4–6 hours.

*Children under 1 year:* For single dose therapy, 1 g or 5 ml per kg bodyweight taken as soon as possible after ingestion of the poison. For multiple dose therapy, the dose may be repeated every 4–6 hours.

When syrup of ipecac is used to produce emesis, administration of Actidose-Aqua should be delayed until 30–60 minutes after vomiting has ceased. If gastric lavage is being used to facilitate stomach evacuation, a single dose of Actidose-Aqua may be administered early in the procedure. This has the advantage of prompt administration of activated charcoal, but the gastric lavage returns will be black which may make it difficult to evaluate what the patient ingested by visual examination.

Actidose-Aqua may be effective even when several hours have elapsed after ingestion of the poison if gastrointestinal motility is reduced by the toxin or if the drug is subject to enterohepatic or enteroenteric recycling.

*Contra-indications:* Use of Actidose-Aqua is contra-indicated in persons who are not fully conscious.

*Special warnings and precautions for use:* Actidose-Aqua is not recommended for patients who have ingested corrosive agents such as strong acids or alkalis since the activated charcoal may obscure endoscopic visualisation of oesophageal and gastric lesions produced by the toxin. Actidose-Aqua is of little or no value in the treatment of poisoning with cyanides, alcohols, iron salts, malathion and DDT.

Actidose-Aqua is an adjunct in the management of poisoning emergencies. Prior to its use, proper basic life support measures must be implemented where required, as well as the appropriate gastric emptying technique if indicated.

Actidose-Aqua should be used with caution in patients who have been exposed to toxins which interfere with gastrointestinal motility (e.g. anticholinergics, opioids). Bowel sounds should be monitored frequently to assess peristaltic action, especially in patients undergoing multiple dose activated charcoal therapy.

*Interactions with other medicaments and other forms of interaction:* Actidose-Aqua will adsorb most medicaments and many other chemical substances. If a specific antidote is to be administered, the likelihood of its adsorption by activated charcoal should be borne in mind and a parenteral route of administration used if possible. Thus, in the case of paracetamol, Actidose-Aqua should not be given as well as oral methionine but may be used alone or in conjunction with intravenous N-acetylcysteine.

Other concurrent medications to counteract shock or associated infection should also be given parenterally since orally administered drugs may be bound to the activated charcoal in the gut.

*Pregnancy and lactation:* The safety of this medicinal product for use in human pregnancy has not been established. Experimental animal studies are insufficient to assess the safety with respect to the development of the embryo or foetus, the course of gestation and peri- and postnatal development.

Activated charcoal is, however, essentially inert pharmacologically and is not absorbed from the gastrointestinal tract. No hazard is therefore anticipated from its use during pregnancy or lactation.

*Effects on ability to drive and use machines:* None known.

*Undesirable effects:* Both the patient and health care professionals should be aware that Actidose-Aqua will produce black stools. A laxative may be given concurrently to accelerate the removal of the activated charcoal-toxin complex, but should be used with caution and only intermittently during multiple dose activated charcoal therapy since profuse and protracted diarrhoea may lead to fluid and electrolyte imbalance.

Aspiration of activated charcoal has been reported to produce airways obstruction and appropriate precautions should be taken. Gastrointestinal obstruction associated with the use of multiple dose activated charcoal therapy has been reported rarely.

*Overdose:* Actidose-Aqua is well tolerated and due to its lack of toxicity, overdosage requiring treatment is unlikely. A laxative may be administered to enhance elimination of the product.

### Pharmacological properties

*Pharmacodynamic properties:* Activated charcoal has a high adsorptive capacity for a wide range of compounds, including many of those which are most commonly encountered in deliberate and accidental poisoning. Substances adsorbed include the following:

Aspirin and other salicylates
Barbiturates
Benzodiazepines
Chlormethiazole
Chloroquine
Chlorpromazine and related phenothiazines
Clonidine
Cocaine and other stimulants
Digoxin and digitoxin
Ibuprofen
Mefenamic Acid
Mianserin
Nicotine
Paracetamol
Paraquat
Phenelzine and other monoamine oxidase inhibitors
Phenytoin
Propranolol and other beta-blockers
Quinine
Theophylline
Zidovudine

*Pharmacokinetic properties:* Activated charcoal is not absorbed from the gastrointestinal tract or subject to any metabolic processes. It is eliminated in the faeces.

*Preclinical safety data:* Activated charcoal is essentially inert pharmacologically and it would therefore be expected to be virtually devoid of toxicity, other than any ill-effects arising from mechanical obstruction of the gut or, if inhaled, the lungs.

The excipients in the product are all well known and widely used in medicinal products and should not give rise to any toxicological problems.

### Pharmaceutical particulars

*List of excipients:* Methylparaben, propylparaben, butylparaben, potassium sorbate, sucrose, propylene glycol, glycerine, citric acid, purified water.

*Incompatibilities:* None known.

*Shelf life:* Two years.

*Special precautions for storage:* Store at 15–30°C. Do not refrigerate.

*Nature and contents of container:*
1. Low density polyethylene bottles containing 120 ml
2. Low density polyethylene bottles containing 240 ml
3. Low density polyethylene tubes containing 120 ml.

*Instructions for use/handling:* Shake well before use.

**Marketing authorisation number** 12070/0011.

**Date of approval/revision of SPC** March 1996.

**Legal category** P.

## DEBRISOQUINE TABLETS

**Presentation** Round, white tablets with 'ROCHE 10' imprinted on one face and a single break bar on the other, containing 12.8 mg debrisoquine sulphate (equivalent to 10 mg base).

### Uses

*Properties:* Debrisoquine lowers blood pressure markedly and promptly in the hypertensive patient. It does this by blocking the transmission of sympathetic nerve impulses at the nerve terminals, thereby decreasing peripheral vascular resistance. Reduction in post-ganglionic sympathetic transmission is achieved by interfering with the physiological release of noradrenaline, without depleting major catecholamine stores in cardiovascular tissues and without impairing the cardiac contractile mechanism. The action, as with other alpha-adrenergic blocking agents, is most marked in the standing position. Debrisoquine normally acts within 4–10 hours and its effects usually last for 9–24 hours, although an occasional patient may show a longer response. There is no accumulation on maintenance dosage.

*Indications:* Debrisoquine is indicated for the treatment of all grades of hypertension. It can be given either alone or together with other antihypertensive drugs or diuretics.

### Dosage and administration

*Adults: Mild to moderate hypertension:* 10 mg once or twice daily. This dose can be increased by 10 mg at 3-day intervals. The total dose usually falls within the range 20–60 mg daily.

*Adults: Severe hypertension:* 20 mg once or twice daily. This dose can be increased, depending on response, by 10–20 mg every 3 or 4 days provided a close check is kept on the blood pressure. When initially treating severe hypertension with Debrisoquine, the diastolic pressure should not be reduced below 110 mmHg as impaired autoregulatory mechanisms may lead to impaired perfusion of vital organs. The total dose usually falls within the range 40–120 mg but in cases of severe hypertension 300 mg or more daily may be given. Although some tolerance to the drug may occur during long-term therapy, requiring increased dosage, this has usually been moderate and has not posed special problems.

Should postural hypotension occur with a dosage that controls the blood pressure, the total daily dose should be adjusted to give a small dose in the morning, a relatively large dose at midday and a moderate evening dose. Adequate control of blood pressure is frequently obtained with Debrisoquine alone but, if necessary, its effects can be enhanced by the addition of therapy with a diuretic or another antihypertensive drug (e.g. a beta-adrenergic blocking agent).

*Elderly:* There is inadequate evidence of the safety of Debrisoquine in the elderly, although it has been in wide use for many years without apparent ill-consequence specifically relating to elderly populations. However, as with other potent hypotensive agents, including α-adrenergic blockers, the possibility of postural hypotension occurring should be borne in mind.

*Children:* There is inadequate evidence of the safety of Debrisoquine in children, although it has been in wide use for many years without apparent ill-consequence specifically relating to childhood.

Debrisoquine Tablets are for oral administration.

**Contra-indications, warnings, etc**
*Contra-indications:* Debrisoquine should not be given to patients with a phaechromocytoma or with a recent history of cerebral or myocardial infarction. It is contra-indicated in patients who have shown hypersensitivity to the drug.

*Use in pregnancy:* There is inadequate evidence of safety of Debrisoquine in human pregnancy but it has been in wide use for many years without apparent ill-consequence, animal studies having shown no hazard.

*Precautions:* Debrisoquine should be used with caution in patients with renal or hepatic insufficiency; smaller or more widely spread doses may be appropriate. Debrisoquine may give rise to exertional and postural hypotension (see Side-effects). Caution should therefore be exercised in patients with coronary or cerebral insufficiency.

The possibility of an enhanced hypotensive effect should be borne in mind when any drug with a tendency to lower blood pressure is given concomitantly with Debrisoquine.

As with other potent hypotensive agents, including α-adrenergic blockers, the possibility of postural hypotension occurring in the elderly should be borne in mind. Patients on antihypertensive drugs often have a lower blood pressure in warm weather, therefore in hot climates their dose of Debrisoquine may need to be reduced. Evidence from both animal experiments and clinical observation suggests that the hypotensive action of adrenergic neurone-blocking drugs such as debrisoquine may be inhibited by simultaneous treatment with tricyclic antidepressants, monoamine oxidase inhibitors and fenfluramine. Extra care should be taken when prescribing antihypertensive drugs in patients being treated with levodopa. Patients taking Debrisoquine are sensitive to sympathomimetic drugs.

If anaesthesia for surgery or dentistry is necessary, the anaesthetist should be informed that the patient is being treated with Debrisoquine.

Abrupt cessation of Debrisoquine should be avoided as this may lead to rebound hypertension.

*Side-effects:* Debrisoquine is well tolerated. Overdosage causes postural hypotension, most noticeable in the early morning or with long standing and associated with weakness, giddiness, fatigue and very rarely syncope. The patient should be warned of the possibility of these symptoms occurring. This can be minimised by reducing the dose. Other reported side-effects include malaise, nausea, headache, sweating, oedema, muscle weakness, failure of ejaculation in the male, and sometimes disturbances of micturition and nocturia. Diarrhoea, common with some other anti-hypertensive agents, is seen only very rarely. Aggravation of angina pectoris has been reported in a few cases.

*Effects of overdose and their treatment:* Excessive fall in blood pressure will be shown by orthostatic collapse. This will usually respond rapidly to placing the patient in a recumbent position. Patients receiving Debrisoquine are particularly sensitive to the effects of catecholamines. Sympathomimetic agents should therefore be administered only with great caution.

**Pharmaceutical precautions**
*Storage:* No special storage precautions required.

**Legal category** POM.

**Package quantities** Debrisoquine Tablets 10 mg in packings of 100 and 500.

**Further information** The metabolism of Debrisoquine is subject to genetic polymorphism such that non-metabolisers may show a marked response (e.g. orthostatic hypotension) to doses that have little effect in metabolisers.

New patients should be carefully monitored during the initial treatment to determine possible non-metabolisers (approximately 8 per cent of Caucasian populations).

**Product licence number** 14576/0001.

*Product licence holder:* Lifehealth Limited, Richmond House, Old Brewery Court, Sandyford Road, Newcastle upon Tyne NE2 1XG.

## DICOBALT EDETATE INJECTION 300 mg

**Presentation** Clear 20 ml ampoules filled with a rose-coloured solution and each containing 300 mg Dicobalt Edetate INN (15 mg/ml).

*Excipients:* Dextrose, water for injections.

**Uses**
*Indications:* Dicobalt edetate is a specific antidote for acute cyanide poisoning. In view of the difficulty of certain diagnosis in emergency situations, it is recommended that Dicobalt edetate only be given when the patient is tending to lose, or has lost, consciousness. The product should not be used as a precautionary measure (see *Warnings* section).

*Pharmacology:* Cyanide blocks intracellular respiration by binding to cytochrome oxidase. Dicobalt edetate forms a stable complex with the cyanide thereby acting as an antidote.

**Dosage and administration**
*Adults:* One 300 mg ampoule intravenously over approximately one minute. If the patient shows inadequate response, a second ampoule may be given. If there is no response after a further five minutes, a third ampoule may be administered.

Each ampoule of Dicobalt edetate may be followed immediately by 50 ml Dextrose Intravenous Infusion BP 500 g/l.

When the patient's condition is less severe but, in the physician's judgement, still warrants the use of Dicobalt edetate, the period over which the injection is given should be extended to 5 minutes.

*Children:* There is no clincial experience of the use of Dicobalt edetate in children. As with adults, the dose required will be related to the quantity of cyanide ingested.

*Elderly:* There is no clinical experience of the use of Dicobalt edetate in the elderly, but there is no reason to believe that the dosage schedule should be different from that for adults.

Cyanide poisoning must be treated as quickly as possible and intensive supportive measures must be instituted: clear airways and adequate ventilation are essential. 100% oxygen should be administered concurrently with Dicobalt edetate.

Expert advice on the treatment of poisoning is available from the local Poisons Centre.

**Contra-indications, warnings, etc**
*Warnings:* There is a reciprocal antidote action between cyanide and cobalt. Thus in the absence of cyanide, Dicobalt edetate is itself toxic. It is therefore essential that the product only be used in cases of cyanide poisoning. When the patient is fully conscious, it is unlikely that the extent of poisoning warrants the use of Dicobalt edetate.

*Adverse reactions:* The initial effects of Dicobalt edetate are vomiting, a fall in blood pressure, and compensatory tachycardia. After this the patient should recover.

*Overdosage:*
*Signs and symptoms:* These may be due to cobalt toxicity or to an anaphylactic type reaction, which may be dramatic. Oedema (particularly of the face and neck), vomiting, chest pain, sweating, hypotension, cardiac irregularities and rashes may occur.

*Treatment:* Intensive supportive therapy is required.

**Pharmaceutical precautions** Store below 25°C away from light. The shelf-life is 3 years.

**Legal category** POM.

**Package quantities** 6 ampoules.

**Further information** Nil.

**Product licence number** 14945/0001.

*Product licence holder:* L'Arguenon Limited, 82 Kings Ride, Camberley, Surrey GU15 5LN.

## EDROPHONIUM INJECTION BP 10 mg/1 ml

**Presentation** Ampoules containing 10 mg edrophonium chloride in 1 ml. The ampoule solution is almost colourless. Excipients: Sodium sulphite, sodium citrate, citric acid and water for injections.

**Uses**
*Properties:* Edrophonium is an antagonist to cholinesterase, the enzyme which normally destroys acetylcholine. The action of edrophonium can briefly be described, therefore, as the potentiation of naturally occurring acetylcholine. It differs from neostigmine and pyridostigmine in the rapidity and brevity of its action.

*Pharmacokinetics:* Following intravenous injection of edrophonium an initial rapid phase of elimination (0.5–2 minutes) precedes a much slower decline (24–45 minutes). It is suggested that the rapid fall in plasma concentration of edrophonium is not primarily due to metabolism and excretion but to the rapid uptake of the drug by other tissues.

*Indications:* Myasthenia gravis, as a diagnostic test; to distinguish between overdosage and underdosage of cholinergic drugs in myasthenic patients; diagnosis of suspected 'dual block'; antagonist to non-depolarising neuromuscular blockade.

**Dosage and administration**
*Adults: Test for myasthenia gravis*
A syringe is filled with the contents of 1 ampoule edrophonium (10 mg) and 2 mg is given intravenously, the needle and syringe being left *in situ*. If no response occurs within 30 seconds, the remaining 8 mg is injected. In adults with unsuitable veins, 10 mg is given by intramuscular injection.

*To differentiate between 'myasthenic' and 'cholinergic' crisis:* In a myasthenic patient who is suffering from marked muscle weakness, in spite of taking large doses of pyridostigmine or neostigmine, a test dose of 2 mg edrophonium is given intravenously one hour after the last dose of the cholinergic compound. If therapy has been inadequate, there is a rapid transient increase of muscle strength; if the patient has been overtreated, edrophonium causes a transient increase of muscle weakness.

*Diagnosis of suspected 'dual block':* Edrophonium 10 mg intravenously. If the block is due to depolarisation, it is briefly potentiated, whereas in a 'dual block' it is reversed.

*Children: Diagnostic tests:* A total dose of 100 micrograms/kg body-weight may be given intravenously. One-fifth of this dose should be injected initially; if no reaction occurs, the remainder of the dose is administered 30 seconds later.

*Antagonist to non-depolarising neuromuscular blockade:* Generally, reversal of neuromuscular block with edrophonium should not be attempted until there is evidence of spontaneous recovery from paralysis. It is recommended that the patient be well ventilated and a patent airway maintained until complete recovery of normal respiration is assured.

*Adults and children:* Edrophonium 500–700 micrograms/kg body-weight and atropine 7 micrograms/kg body-weight, by slow intravenous injection over several minutes, is usually adequate for reversal of non-depolarising muscle relaxants within 5–15 minutes. The two drugs are usually given simultaneously, but in patients who show bradycardia the pulse rate should be increased to about 80/minute with atropine before administering edrophonium.

The speed of recovery from neuromuscular blockade is primarily determined by the intensity of the block at the time of antagonism but it is also subject to other factors, including the presence of drugs (e.g. anaesthetic agents, antibiotics, antiarrhythmic drugs) and physiological changes (electrolyte and acid-base imbalance, renal impairment). These factors may prevent successful reversal with edrophonium or lead to recurarisation after apparently successful reversal. Therefore it is imperative that patients should not be left unattended until these possibilities have been excluded.

*Elderly:* There are no specific dosage recommendations for edrophonium in elderly patients.

Edrophonium ampoules are for intramuscular or intravenous injection.

In view of the possibility of provoking a cholinergic crisis it is recommended that facilities for resuscitation should be available whenever edrophonium is administered.

Edrophonium ampoules may be diluted with Water for Injections. However, maintenance of stability cannot be guaranteed when edrophonium ampoule solution is diluted.

**Contra-indications, warnings, etc**
*Contra-indications:* Edrophonium should not be given to patients with mechanical intestinal or urinary obstruction.

Edrophonium is contra-indicated in patients with known hypersensitivity to the drug.

With doses above 10 mg, especially the higher dosage employed to antagonise neuromuscular blockade, edrophonium should not be used in conjunction with depolarising muscle relaxants such as suxamenthonium as neuromuscular blockade may be potentiated and prolonged apnoea may result.

*Use in pregnancy and lactation:* The safety of edrophonium during pregnancy or lactation has not been established. Although the possible hazards to mother and child must be weighed against the potential benefits in every case, experience with edrophonium in pregnant patients with myasthenia gravis has revealed no untoward effect of the drug on the course of pregnancy.

There is no information on the excretion of edrophonium into breast milk. Although only negligible amounts would be expected to be present, due regard should be paid to possible effects on the breast-feeding infant.

*Precautions:* Extreme caution is required when administering edrophonium to patients with bronchial asthma.

Care should also be taken in patients with bradycardia, recent coronary occlusion, vagotonia, hypotension, peptic ulcer, epilepsy or Parkinsonism.

In diagnostic uses of edrophonium, a syringe containing 1 mg of atropine should be kept at hand to counteract severe cholinergic reactions, should they occur. In view of the possibility of provoking a cholinergic crisis it is recommended that facilities for resuscitation should always be available.

When edrophonium is used as an antagonist to neuromuscular blockade bradycardia may occur, to a possibly dangerous level, unless atropine is given simultaneously. In this indication, edrophonium should not be given during cyclopropane or halothane anaesthesia; however it may be used after withdrawal of these agents.

There is no evidence to suggest that edrophonium has any special effects in elderly. However, elderly patients may be more susceptible to dysrhythmias than younger adults.

*Side-effects and adverse reactions:* These may include nausea and vomiting, increased salivation, diarrhoea and abdominal cramps.

*Treatment of overdosage:* Edrophonium overdosage may give rise to bradycardia, arrhythmias, hypotension and bronchiolar spasm. Perspiration, gastro-intestinal hypermotility and visual disturbances may also occur.

Artificial ventilation should be instituted if respiration is severely depressed. Atropine sulphate 1–2 mg intravenously is an antidote to the muscarinic effects.

**Pharmaceutical precautions**   *Storage:* Edrophonium ampoule solution should be protected from light.

**Legal category**   POM.

**Package quantities**   Edrophonium ampoules in packs of 10.

**Further information**   Nil.

**Product licence number**   12070/0008.

# FLUOROURACIL

**Presentation**   Ampoules containing 250 mg of fluorouracil in the form of the sodium salt in 10 ml Water for Injections BP. The ampoule solution is colourless to slightly yellow.

Capsules with powder opaque cap and orange opaque body with ROCHE printed in black along both cap and body, containing 250 mg fluorouracil.

**Uses**

*Properties:* Fluorouracil, a cytostatic agent, is a fluorinated pyrimidine belonging to the category of anti-metabolites. It inhibits cell division by interfering with the synthesis of deoxyribonucleic acid (DNA) and to a lesser extent of ribonucleic acid (RNA).

*Indications:* The palliative treatment of carcinoma.

**Dosage and administration**   Various techniques are employed when using Fluorouracil in the treatment of carcinoma. The following examples are given for guidance.

*Adults by the intravenous route:* Fluorouracil may be administered by intravenous infusion or by intravenous injection. Dosages are generally based on the patient's body weight. If the patient is obese or there has been a spurious gain due to oedema, ascites or other forms of fluid retention, the patient's ideal weight should be used in calculating the dosage. The initial dose given below should be reduced by one-third to a half if the following conditions are present: poor nutritional state; after major surgery (within the previous 30 days); poor bone-marrow function (anaemia, leucopenia, thrombocytopenia); impaired hepatic or renal function.

*Initial treatment:* This may be in the form of an infusion or injection, the former usually being preferred because of lesser toxicity.

*Infusion:* A daily dose of 15 mg/kg, but not more than 1 g per infusion, is diluted in 500 ml 5% dextrose solution or 500 ml 0.9% sodium chloride solution and given by intravenous infusion at the rate of 40 drops per minute over 4 hours. Alternatively, the daily dose may be infused over 30–60 minutes, or given as a continuous infusion over 24 hours. This daily dose is given on successive days until toxicity occurs or until 12 to 15 g has been given. This sequence of injections constitutes a 'course' of therapy. Some patients have

received up to 30 g at a maximum rate of 1 g daily. The daily dose should never exceed 1 g. An interval of four to six weeks should be allowed between any two 'courses' of Fluorouracil.

*Injection:* A dose of 12 mg/kg i.v. daily on three consecutive days. If there are no signs of toxicity the patient receives 6 mg/kg on the 5th, 7th and 9th days. If toxicity occurs the signs should be allowed to regress before further doses are administered.

Maintenance therapy consists of 5 to 15 mg/kg i.v. once weekly.

A more recent alternative method is to give 15 mg/kg i.v. once a week throughout the course of treatment. This obviates the need for an initial period of daily administration.

*Regional perfusion intra-arterially:* Continuous infusion of Fluorouracil into an artery supplying a localised growth has been shown to produce a better result in some tumours than would have been expected from systemic administration by the intravenous route, together with a decrease in toxicity. The usual dose is 5 to 7.5 mg/kg daily.

*In combination with radiotherapy:* Irradiation combined with Fluorouracil has been found to be useful in the treatment of certain types of metastatic lesions in the lungs and for relief of pain caused by recurrent, inoperable growth. The standard dose of Fluorouracil is used.

*By the oral route:* Fluorouracil may be administered orally using either the capsule or the ampoule solution. Oral administration is not recommended when Fluorouracil is being used initially as the sole agent in palliative treatment of carcinoma.

Oral administration may be useful in: palliative therapy employing a combination of drugs; long-term maintenance or post-operative prophylactic therapy in weekly doses; and where therapy with Fluorouracil is indicated, but it is impractical to administer the drug parenterally.

The usual dosage for maintenance treatment is 15 mg/kg once weekly. For palliative therapy a more rapid onset of therapeutic effect may be obtained by giving a daily dose of 15 mg/kg on six successive days. This is followed by maintenance therapy of 15 mg/kg once weekly. The daily dose should not exceed 1 g. The capsules should be taken with water after a meal.

The solution may be mixed with fruit juice or other similar beverages immediately before oral ingestion to mask its rather bitter taste. Multi-dose preparations must not be made up.

*Elderly:* Fluorouracil should be used in the elderly with similar consideration as in younger adults, notwithstanding that incidence of concomitant medical illness is higher in the former group.

*Children:* No dosage recommendations are made for the administration of Fluorouracil to children.

Fluorouracil Ampoules are for intra-arterial, intravenous or oral administration.

Fluorouracil Capsules are for oral administration.

**Contra-indications, warnings, etc**

*Contra-indication:* Fluorouracil should not be used in the management of non-malignant disease.

*Use in pregnancy:* Fluorouracil has been shown to be teratogenic. It therefore should not normally be administered to patients who are pregnant. Fluorouracil should also be regarded as contra-indicated in mothers who are breast-feeding.

*Precautions:* It is recommended that Fluorouracil be given only by or under the supervision of a physician who is experienced in cancer chemotherapy and who is well versed in the use of potent antimetabolites. Because of the possibility of severe toxic reactions, all patients should be admitted to hospital for initial treatment. Fluorouracil should be used with great care in debilitated patients.

The margin between the effective and toxic doses of Fluorouracil is narrow and a therapeutic response is unlikely without some evidence of toxicity. Even with meticulous selection of patients and careful adjustment of dosage, there may be severe haematological toxicity and gastro-intestinal haemorrhage. Severe toxicity is more likely in poor-risk patients.

Treatment should be discontinued promptly whenever one of the following signs of toxicity appears: Leucopenia (WBC under 3,500 per mm³). Thrombocytopenia (platelets under 100,000 per mm³). Stomatitis (the first small ulceration at the inner margin of the lips is a signal for stopping treatment. Severe diarrhoea (frequent bowel movements and watery stools). Gastro-intestinal ulceration and bleeding. Haemorrhage at any site.

Isolated cases of angina, ECG abnormalities and, rarely, myocardial infarction have been reported following Fluorouracil administration. Caution should therefore be exercised in treating patients who experience chest pain during courses of therapy, or patients with a history of heart disease.

The carcinogenic potential of Fluorouracil has not

been evaluated but, as with all cytostatic drugs, this possibility should be borne in mind when designing long-term management of patients.

*Side-effects:* During treatment, diarrhoea, nausea and vomiting commonly occur, but may be controlled by the use of appropriate drugs.

Leucopenia usually follows an adequate course of treatment with Fluorouracil. The lowest white cell count commonly occurs between the seventh and fourteenth days after the first dose, but it may be delayed for as long as the twentieth day. By the thirtieth day, the count has usually returned to the normal range. Because of the importance of leucopenia, the white cell count should be checked frequently throughout the course. If it falls, it is advisable to obtain differential counts. If the total is less than 2,000 per mm³, and especially if there is granulocytopenia, it is recommended that the patient be placed in protective isolation in the hospital and treated with appropriate measures for the prevention of systemic infection.

Alopecia and dermatitis may occur in a substantial proportion of cases. Female patients particularly should be warned as to the possibility of alopecia. Since the alopecia appears to be reversible, special measures do not seem to be indicated.

*Treatment of overdosage:* Signs and symptoms are qualitatively similar to the side-effects, and similar measures should be taken to treat them.

*Handling precautions:* Fluorouracil is irritant, contact with skin and mucous membranes should be avoided.

*Handling guidelines:*

*Ampoules:* Fluorouracil Ampoules should only be opened by trained staff and as with all cytotoxic agents, precautions should be taken to avoid exposing staff during pregnancy. Preparation of solution for administration should be carried out in a designated handling area and working over a washable tray or disposable plastic-backed absorbent paper.

Suitable eye protection, disposable gloves, face mask and disposable apron should be worn. Syringes and infusion sets should be assembled carefully to avoid leakage (use of Luer lock fittings is recommended).

On completion, any exposed surface should be thoroughly cleaned and hands and face washed.

*Capsules:* Undamaged capsules present minimal risk of contamination but in accordance with good hygiene requirements, direct handling should be avoided. As with all cytotoxic agents, precautions should be taken to avoid exposing staff during pregnancy.

*Disposal guidelines:* All sharps should be placed in an appropriate container and all other disposable items in a sealed plastic bag which should be incinerated with other clinical waste.

Waste material may be disposed of by incineration. Waste ampoule solution may first be absorbed on to cotton wool and double wrapped in sealed polythene bags.

*First aid:* Eye contact: Irrigate immediately with water and seek medical advice.

Skin contact: Wash thoroughly with soap and water and remove contaminated clothing.

Inhalation, ingestion: Seek immediate medical attention.

**Pharmaceutical precautions**

*Storage:* Fluorouracil Ampoule solution should be stored between 15°C and 25°C. Fluorouracil Capsules in blister packings should be stored in a dry place; the recommended maximum storage temperature is 25°C.

*Additives:* Fluorouracil Ampoule solution may be diluted with dextrose injection, sodium chloride injection or Water for Injections BP immediately before parenteral use.

Fluorouracil Ampoule solution may be diluted with fruit juice or other similar beverages immediately before use to facilitate ingestion by the oral route. Fluorouracil Ampoule solution must not be made up into multidose preparations.

**Legal category**   POM

**Package quantities**   Fluorouracil Ampoules in packings of 10.

Fluorouracil Capsules in blister packings of 30.

**Further information**   *Availability:* Fluorouracil Ampoules are available through hospital pharmacies for use in hospitals and hospital clinics and can be supplied to retail chemists for dispensing prescriptions for patients whose treatment has been initiated in hospital practice.

**Product licence numbers**
Ampoules     14576/0002
Capsules     14576/0003

# GESTRONOL HEXANOATE AMPOULES

**Qualitative and quantitative composition** 1 ml of solution contains 100 mg of gestronol hexanoate.

**Pharmaceutical form** Solution for injection.

## Clinical particulars

*Therapeutic indications:* For the treatment of endometrial carcinoma and benign prostatic hyperplasia in adults.

*Posology and method of administration:* To be administered by slow intramuscular injection.

*Endometrial carcinoma, before hysterectomy and for advanced disease:* Gestronol hexanoate is a well-tolerated adjunct to other therapy. To inhibit metastatic spread before and after operation, 200–400 mg intramuscularly every 5–7 days, starting immediately following diagnosis and continuing for a minimum of 12 weeks.

For treating existing metastases: 200–400 mg can be administered intramuscularly every 5–7 days. If the metastases are hormone-responsive, improvement will be observed within 8–12 weeks of therapy. Treatment should than be continued for as long as it appears beneficial.

*Benign prostatic hyperplasia:* Where (a) the patient is an operation risk; (b) symptoms are mild; (c) there is a waiting list for operation, the following standard dosage applies: 200 mg weekly by intramuscular injection. In view of Gestronol hexanoate's good tolerance, this dosage can confidently be increased. In trials, 300 mg and 400 mg weekly have been used. The full benefit of treatment is unlikely to be established in a shorter period than three months, and trial results suggest that improvement can continue during substantially longer periods.

*Contra-indications:* Pregnancy. History of herpes gestationis. Previous or existing liver tumours (in progressive endometrial carcinoma only if these are not due to metastases).

*Special warnings and precautions for use:* Patients suffering from bronchial asthma, diabetes, epilepsy or migraine should be supervised closely.

In patients with chronic liver damage it is advisable to check liver function at intervals during long-term treatment or repeated courses of Gestronol hexanoate. Transient moderate rises in bromsulphthalein retention and serum transaminases have occasionally been observed but have always proved harmless.

In rare cases benign and, in even rarer cases malignant liver tumours leading in isolated cases to life-threatening intra-abdominal haemorrhage, have been observed after the use of hormonal substances such as Gestronol hexanoate. If severe upper abdominal complaints, liver enlargement or signs of intra-abdominal haemorrhage occur, a liver tumour should be considered in the differential diagnosis.

During treatment of prostatic adenoma, supervision of bladder and renal function is necessary.

*Interactions with other medicaments and other forms of interaction:* The requirement for oral antidiabetic agents or insulin can change.

*Pregnancy and lactation:* Gestronol hexanoate is contra-indicated in pregnancy.

*Effects on ability to drive and use machines:* None stated.

*Undesirable effects:* Rarely, local reactions may occur at the site of injection. Exacerbation of bronchial asthma, diabetes, epilepsy and migraine may sometimes occur. Side-effects are infrequent.

In males, a reversible depression of libido and gynaecomastia with discomfort have been reported by a few patients. Spermatogenesis is temporarily inhibited.

In rare cases, coughing, dyspnoea and circulatory irregularities may develop during, or immediately after, the injection.

Experience has shown that these reactions can be avoided by injecting very slowly.

Should severe or repeated symptomatology occur despite this injection technique, withdrawal of therapy will have to be considered.

*Overdose:* Overdose with injectable drugs is unlikely to occur, but if it does arise, treatment should be symptomatic.

## Pharmacological properties

*Pharmacodynamic properties:* Gestronol hexanoate is 25 times more potent than its parent substance progesterone. In the female, the action of Gestronol hexanoate is concentrated on the endometrium. This action is direct and does not involve suppression via the pituitary. Except in some highly anaplastic tumours, Gestronol hexanoate has a strong antimitotic effect, with regression or arrest of primary endometrial carcinoma and of soft-tissue metastases.

In the male, Gestronol hexanoate has been shown to reduce prostatic weight significantly. It may effect an objective improvement in peak urine flow rates

and residual urine and in subjective symptoms such as nocturia.

*Pharmacokinetic properties:* Gestronol hexanoate is administered intramuscularly as an oily solution. Therapeutic effects are dependent upon the release of gestronol hexanoate from its intramuscular depot which is retarded but complete. Liberation of active ingredient from the depot, however, is slower than its elimination from the plasma. This is why the disposition half-lives from plasma reflect the liberation process from the oily depot. About 3 days after administration, peak plasma levels reach about 420 ng/ml. Plasma levels decrease with a half-life of about 7.5 days.

The unchanged drug substance is probably responsible for the therapeutic effects observed. Its fraction of the whole sum of metabolites in plasma may not exceed 5%, however. The predominant part of the main metabolite is rapidly conjugated. There is virtually no free gestronol hexanoate.

Gestronol hexanoate is excreted mainly in the faeces (72%) and also in the urine (25%). The recovery was 48% of the administered dose within 14 days and 85% within 37 days. The observed half-lives of renal (3.2 days; with urine) and biliary (3.7 days; with faeces) excretion reflect the release of drug substance from its oily depot.

Gestronol hexanoate is completely bioavailable.

*Preclinical safety data:* There are no preclinical safety data which could be of relevance to the prescriber and which are not already included in other relevant sections of the SPC.

## Pharmaceutical particulars

*List of excipients:* Benzyl benzoate; castor oil for injection.

*Imcompatibilities:* None known.

*Shelf life:* 5 years.

*Special precautions for storage:* Store below 25˚C. Protect from light.

*Nature and contents of container:* 2 ml amber glass ampoules in packs of 5 ampoules.

*Instruction for use/handling:* Keep out of the reach of children.

*Marketing authorisation holder:* Cambridge Selfcare Diagnostics Limited, Newcastle upon Tyne NE2 1XG.

**Marketing authorisation number** 12070/0014.

**Date of approval/revision of SPC** March 1996.

**Legal category** POM.

# ISOCARBOXAZID

**Presentation** Round, pink tablets with CL 3M3 imprinted across one face and a single break bar on the other, containing 10 mg isocarboxazid. Also contains lactose and other ingredients.

## Uses

*Properties:* Isocarboxazid is a monoamine oxidase inhibitor, effective in small doses. Its antidepressant action is thought to be related to its effect on physiological amines such as serotonin and noradrenaline, and this effect is cumulative and persistent.

*Pharmacokinetics:* Isocarboxazid is readily absorbed after oral administration. Most of the drug-related material is excreted as metabolites in the urine.

*Indications:* Treatment of the symptoms of depressive illness.

## Dosage and administration

*Adults:* A daily dose of 30 mg, in single or divided doses, should be given until improvement is obtained. The maximal effect is only observed after a period varying from 1–4 weeks. If no improvement has been seen by 4 weeks, doses up to 60 mg may be tried, according to the patient's tolerance, for no longer than 4–6 weeks, provided the patient is closely monitored because of the increased risk of adverse reactions occurring. Once the optimal effect is achieved, the dose should be reduced to the lowest possible amount sufficient to maintain the improvement. Clinical experience has shown this to be usually 10–20 mg daily but up to 40 mg daily may be required in some cases.

*Elderly:* The elderly are more likely to experience adverse reactions such as agitation, confusion and postural hypotension. Half the normal maintenance dose may be sufficient to produce a satisfactory clinical response.

*Children:* Isocarboxazid is not indicated for paediatric use. Isocarboxazid tablets are for oral administration.

## Contra-indications, warnings, etc

*Contra-indications:* Isocarboxazid is contra-indicated in patients with any impairment of hepatic function, cerebrovascular disorders or severe cardiovascular disease, and in those with actual or suspected phaeochromocytoma.

*Use in pregnancy and lactation:* Do not use in pregnancy, especially during the first and last trimesters, unless there are compelling reasons. There is no evidence as to drug safety in human pregnancy, nor is there evidence from animal work that it is free from hazard. In addition, the effect of psychotropic drugs on the fine brain structure of the foetus is unknown. Since there is no information on the secretion of the drug into breast milk, Isocarboxazid is contra-indicated during lactation.

*Warnings:* Like other monoamine oxidase inhibitors, Isocarboxazid potentiates the action of a number of drugs and foods. Patients being treated with a monoamine oxidase inhibitor should not receive indirectly-acting sympathomimetic agents such as amphetamines, metaraminol, fenfluramine or similar anorectic agents, ephedrine or phenylpropanolamine (contained in many proprietary 'cold-cure' medications), dopamine or levodopa. Patients should also be warned to avoid foodstuffs and beverages with a high tyramine content: mature cheeses (including processed cheeses), hydrolysed yeast or meat extracts, alcoholic beverages, particularly heavy red wines such as Chianti, non-alcoholic beers, lagers and wines and other foods which are not fresh and are fermented, pickled, 'hung', 'matured' or otherwise subject to protein degradation before consumption. Broad bean pods (which contain levodopa) and banana skins may also present a hazard.

In extreme cases interactions may result in severe hypertensive episodes. Isocarboxazid should therefore be discontinued immediately upon the occurrence of palpitations or frequent headaches.

Pethidine should not be given to patients receiving monoamine oxidase inhibitors as serious, potentially fatal reactions, including central excitation, muscle rigidity, hyperpyrexia, circulatory collapse, respiratory depression and coma, can result. Such reactions are less likely with morphine, but experience of the interaction of Isocarboxazid with narcotic analgesics other than pethidine is limited and extreme caution is therefore necessary when administering morphine to patients undergoing therapy with Isocarboxazid.

Isocarboxazid should not be administered together with other monoamine oxidase inhibitors or most tricyclic antidepressants (clomipramine, desipramine, imipramine, butriptyline, nortriptyline or protriptyline). Although there is no proof that combined therapy will be effective, refractory cases of depression may be treated with Isocarboxazid in combination with amitriptyline or trimipramine, provided appropriate care is taken.

Hypotensive and other adverse reactions are likely to be increased.

An interval of 1–2 weeks should be allowed after treatment with Isocarboxazid before the administration of anti-depressants with a different mode of action or any other drug which may interact. A similar interval is recommended before administration of Isocarboxazid when another antidepressant has been used; in the case of drugs with a very long half-life (such as Fluoxetine), it may be advisable to extend this interval.

Isocarboxazid should be discontinued for at least 2 weeks prior to elective surgery requiring general anaesthesia. The anaesthetist should be warned that a patient is being treated with Isocarboxazid, in the event of emergency surgery being necessary.

*Precautions:* Concurrent administration of Isocarboxazid with other central nervous system depressants (especially barbituates and phenothiazines), stimulants, local anaesthetics, ganglion-blocking agents and other hypotensives (including methyldopa and reserpine), diuretics, vasopressors, anticholinergic drugs and hypoglycaemic agents may lead to potentiation of their effects. This should be borne in mind if dentistry, surgery or a change in treatment of a patient becomes necessary during treatment with Isocarboxazid.

All patients taking Isocarboxazid should be warned against self-medication with proprietary 'cold-cure' preparations and nasal decongestants and advised of the dietary restrictions listed under 'Warnings'.

With Isocarboxazid, as with other drugs acting on the central nervous system, patients should be instructed to avoid alcohol while under treatment, since the individual response cannot be foreseen. Like all medicaments of this type, Isocarboxazid may modify patients' reactions (driving ability, operation of machinery, etc.) to a varying extent, depending on dosage and individual susceptibility.

Some monoamine oxidase inhibitors have occasionally caused hepatic complications and jaundice in patients, therefore regular monitoring of liver function should be carried out during Isocarboxazid therapy. If there is any evidence of a hepatotoxic reaction, the drug should be withdrawn immediately.

The drug should be used cautiously in patients with impaired renal function, to prevent accumulation taking place, and also in the elderly or debilitated and those with cardiovascular disease, diabetes or blood dyscrasias.

In restless or agitated patients, Isocarboxazid may precipitate states of excessive excitement. Isocarboxazid appears to have varying effects in epileptic patients; while some have a decrease in frequency of seizures, others have more seizures.

*Side-effects and adverse reactions:* In general, Isocarboxazid is well tolerated by the majority of patients. Side-effects, if they occur, are those common to the group of monoamine oxidase inhibitors. The most frequently reported have been orthostatic hypotension, associated in some patients with disturbances in cardiac rhythm, peripheral oedema, complaints of dizziness, dryness of the mouth, nausea and vomiting, constipation, blurred vision, insomnia, drowsiness, weakness and fatigue. These side-effects can usually be controlled by dosage reduction.

There have been infrequent reports of mild headaches, sweating, paraesthesiae, peripheral neuritis, hyperreflexia, agitation, overactivity, muscle tremor, confusion and other behavioural changes, difficulty in micturition, impairment of erection and ejaculation, and skin rashes. Although rare, blood dyscrasias (purpura, granulocytopenia) have been reported. Response to Isocarboxazid may be accompanied by increased appetite and weight gain.

*Treatment of overdosage:* The primary symptoms of overdosage include dizziness, ataxia and irritability. In acute cases, hypotension or hypertension, tachycardia, pyrexia, psychotic manifestations, convulsions, respiratory depression and coma may occur and continue for 8–14 days before recovery.

Gastric lavage should be performed soon after ingestion and intensive supportive therapy carried out.

Sympathomimetic agents should not be given to treat hypotension but plasma expanders may be used in severe cases. Hypertensive crises may be treated by pentolinium or phentolamine, severe shock with hydrocortisone. Diazepam may be used to control convulsions or severe excitement. Dialysis is of value in eliminating the drug in severe cases.

### Pharmaceutical precautions
*Storage:* Isocarboxazid tablets should be stored in well-closed containers. The recommended maximum storage temperature is 25°C.

**Legal category** POM.

**Package quantities** Isocarboxazid tablets in packs of 56.

**Further information** Nil.

**Product licence number** 12070/0003.

## ISONIAZID AMPOULES

**Presentation** Ampoules containing 50 mg isoniazid in 2 ml. The ampoule solution is almost colourless. Excipients: Hydrochloric acid and water for injections.

### Uses
*Properties:* Isoniazid is a highly active tuberculostatic drug. It is easily absorbed and has a high rate of diffusion so that the tuberculostatic action affects intracellular as well as extracellular bacilli.

*Indications:* All forms of pulmonary and extra-pulmonary tuberculosis.

**Dosage and administration** Isoniazid ampoules are for intramuscular, intravenous, intrapleural, or intrathecal injection.

*Adults and children:* The usual intramuscular or intravenous dose for adults is 200 to 300 mg as a single daily dose, for children 100 to 300 mg daily (10–20 mg/kg), but doses much larger than these are sometimes given, especially in conditions such as tuberculous meningitis. It is recommended to give an intravenous dose slowly as an undiluted bolus injection, although other methods may be employed.

*Neonates:* The recommended intravenous or intramuscular dose for neonates is 3–5 mg/kg with a maximum of 10 mg/kg daily. Isoniazid may be present in the milk of lactating mothers (see 'Use in pregnancy').

*Elderly:* No dosage reduction is necessary in the elderly.

*Intrapleural use:* 50 to 250 mg may be instilled intrapleurally after aspiration of pus, the dosage or oral isoniazid on that day being correspondingly reduced. The ampoule solution is also used for the local treatment of tuberculous ulcers, for irrigation of fistulae, etc.

*Intrathecal use:* It should be noted that CSF concentrations of isoniazid are approximately 90% of plasma concentrations. Where intrathecal use is required 25–50 mg daily has been given to adults and 10–20 mg daily for children, according to age.

It is usual to give Isoniazid together with other

antituberculous therapy, as determined by current practice and/or sensitivity testing. It is recommended that pyridoxine 10–50 mg daily be given during Isoniazid therapy to minimise adverse reactions, especially in malnourished patients and those predisposed to neuropathy (e.g. diabetics and alcoholics).

*Use in renal and hepatic impairment:* No dosage reduction of Isoniazid is necessary when given to patients with mild renal failure. Patients with severe renal failure (glomerular filtration rate of less than 10 ml/minute) and slow acetylator status might require a dose reduction of about 100 mg to maintain trough plasma levels at less than 1 microgram/ml.

The possible risks of administration of Isoniazid to patients with pre-existing non-tuberculous hepatic disease should be balanced against the benefits expected from treating tuberculosis.

### Contra-indications, warnings, etc
*Contra-indications:* Isoniazid should not be given to patients with a history of sensitivity to isoniazid.

*Use in pregnancy:* While Isoniazid is generally regarded to be safe in pregnancy, there is a possibility of an increased risk of foetal malformations occurring when isoniazid is given in early pregnancy. If pregnancy cannot be excluded possible risks should be balanced against therapeutic benefits.

Isoniazid is excreted in breast milk at concentrations equivalent to those found in maternal plasma, i.e. 6–12 micrograms/ml. This could result in an infant ingesting up to 2 mg/kg/day.

*Precautions:* For use in renal and hepatic impairment. See '*Dosage and administration*'. Care is also required in chronic alcoholism and when prescribing isoniazid for patients with pre-existing hepatitis.

Convulsions and psychotic reactions have occurred, especially in patients with a previous history of these conditions. These manifestations usually subside rapidly when the drug is withdrawn. Isoniazid should therefore be given with caution to patients with convulsive disorders and should be avoided in those with manic or hypomanic psychoses.

Isoniazid may inhibit the metabolism of phenytoin, primidone and carbamazepine. Plasma levels of these drugs should be monitored if concurrent therapy with Isoniazid is necessary.

*Side-effects and adverse reactions:* Isoniazid is generally well tolerated. Side-effects have been reported mainly in association with high doses or in slow acetylators who develop higher blood levels of the drug. Fever, peripheral neuropathy (preventable with pyridoxine), optic neuritis and atrophy, allergic skin conditions (including erythema multiforme) and rarely lupoid syndrome, pellagra, purpura and haematological reactions have occurred during isoniazid therapy. Hyperglycaemia and gynaecomastia have been reported with isoniazid treatment.

Isoniazid, especially if given with rifampicin, may induce abnormalities in liver function, particularly in patients with pre-existing liver disorders, in the elderly, the very young and the malnourished. Monthly review is suggested to detect and limit the severity of this side-effect by stopping treatment if plasma transaminases exceed three times the upper limit of normal. There is conflicting opinion as to the relationship of this side-effect to acetylator status.

*Treatment of overdosage:* In severe poisoning the main risk is of epileptiform convulsions. In addition any of the side-effects listed above may occur together with metabolic acidosis and hyperglycaemia. Treatment should be directed to the control of convulsions and large doses of pyridoxine may limit the occurrence of other adverse effects. Metabolic acidosis may require sodium bicarbonate infusion. The drug is removed by dialysis.

### Pharmaceutical precautions
*Storage:* The recommended maximum storage temperature for Isoniazid ampoules is 25°C. The ampoules should be protected from light.

*Dilution:* Isoniazid ampoule solution may be diluted with Water for Injections. Maintenance of stability cannot be guaranteed when Isoniazid ampoule solution is diluted.

**Legal category** POM.

**Package quantities** Isoniazid ampoules in packs of 10.

**Further information** Isoniazid is metabolised by acetylation, which is subject to genetic variation. The 'slow acetylators' may be more susceptible to drug-induced peripheral neuropathy. However, dose adjustment is not normally required.

**Product licence number** 12070/0005.

## LEVODOPA

**Presentation** Round, white tablets with CL3L3 imprinted on one face and two break bars on the other, containing 500 mg levodopa.

### Uses
*Properties:* Levodopa is an anti-Parkinsonian agent. Levodopa is the metabolic precursor of dopamine. The latter is severely depleted in the striatum, pallidum and substantia nigra of Parkinsonian patients and it is considered that administration of Levodopa raises the level of available dopamine in these centres.

Treatment with Levodopa gives worthwhile sustained relief in about two-thirds of these patients. Akinesia usually responds first, then rigidity, and then tremor. Amelioration may be seen in other symptoms, including oculogyric crises. It may take six months or more before maximal improvement in achieved.

*Indication:* Parkinsonism-idiopathic, post-encephalitic, arteriosclerotic. Previous neurosurgery is not a contra-indication to Levodopa.

**Dosage and administration** Dosage and administration are variable and no more than a guide can be given.

*Adults: Hospitalised patients:* Initially 0.25 to 1 g daily in up to five divided doses immediately after food. Dosage should be increased by 0.5 to 1 g every three to four days until adequate improvement results or intolerable side-effects appear. If severe side-effects appear, the dosage should be gradually decreased to the maximum tolerated. The majority of patients will tolerate the rapid dose increase outlined above, but occasionally intolerance may prevent patients from reaching effective dosage levels. When patients discontinue therapy due to intolerance they should be restarted on 0.25 to 0.5 g daily in small divided doses, increasing by 0.125 to 0.5 g at weekly intervals.

*Adults: General practice patients and out-patients:* Initially 0.125 g twice daily immediately after food. After one week, the dose may be increased to 0.125 g four or five times daily. Thereafter dosage should be increased at weekly intervals by 0.375 g daily, the total daily dose being given in four or five divided doses. The response of individual patients varies and some patients may tolerate a more rapid rate of increase, e.g. by 0.25 to 0.5 g daily at intervals of three to four days.

Improvement is usually seen in two to three weeks with the normal dosage range being 2.5 to 8 g daily, but further improvement may occur up to six months or even longer.

When the optimum daily dosage for any particular patient has been reached, it may need to be redistributed throughout the day to meet fluctuations in the individual's requirements. Most patients find a four or five times daily dosage scheme satisfactory; some obtain a smoother effect with two-hourly administration; others, who develop akinetic crises at particular times of the day, learn by experience the daily dosage scheme most suited to their needs.

After a period at the maximum tolerated dosage level, side-effects may slowly develop, usually in the form of involuntary movements. These generally regress without loss of therapeutic effect if the dosage is slightly reduced.

Anticholinergic drugs should be continued during Levodopa therapy. As treatment with Levodopa proceeds and the therapeutic effect is found, the dosage of the anticholinergic drugs may need to be changed.

*Elderly:* Elderly patients with Parkinson's disease have been treated with Levodopa. However, Levodopa tolerance is less in the elderly and produces more severe hypotensive side effects in older patients with Parkinson's disease especially those with a history of myocardial infarction.

*Children:* No dosage recommendations are made for the administration of Levodopa to children.

Levodopa tablets are for oral administration.

### Contra-indications, warnings, etc
*Contra-indications:* Levodopa is contra-indicated in narrow-angle glaucoma (it may be used in wide-angle glaucoma provided that the intra-ocular pressure remains under control); severe psychoneuroses or psychoses; severe endocrine, renal, hepatic or cardiac disorders.

It should not be given in conjunction with monoamine oxidase inhibitors (except selective MAO-B inhibitors) or within two weeks of their withdrawal.

It should not be given to patients under 25 years of age.

Suspicion has arisen that levodopa may activate a malignant melanoma. Therefore, Levodopa should not be used in persons who have a history of, or who may be suffering from, a malignant melanoma.

*Use in pregnancy:* There is no, or inadequate evidence of safety of the drug in human pregnancy; it has been in wide use for many years without apparent ill-consequence; there is evidence of harmful effects in pregnancy in animals.

Levodopa therapy may interfere with lactation; this should be borne in mind if treatment is required in breast-feeding mothers.

*Precautions:* Pyridoxine (vitamin B₆), which is often

included in multivitamin preparations, is known to block the effects of levodopa.

When other drugs must be given in conjunction with Levodopa, the patient should be carefully observed for unusual side-effects or potentiating effects.

Drugs which interfere with central amine mechanisms, such as rauwolfia alkaloids (reserpine), tetrabenazine, metoclopramide, phenothiazines, thioxanthenes, butyrophenones, amphetamines and papaverine, should be avoided where possible. If, however, their administration is considered essential, extreme care should be exercised and a close watch kept for any signs of potentiation, antagonism or other interactions and for unusual side-effects.

In the event of general anaesthesia being required, Levodopa therapy may be continued as long as the patient is able to take fluids and medication by mouth. If therapy is temporarily interrupted, the usual daily dosage may be administered as soon as the patient is able to take oral medication. Whenever therapy has been interrupted for longer periods, dosage should again be adjusted gradually; however, in many cases the patient can rapidly be returned to his previous therapeutic dosage.

There have been occasional reports of a neuroleptic malignant-like syndrome, involving hyperthermia, on abrupt withdrawal of levodopa preparations. Sudden discontinuation of Levodopa without close supervision, or 'drug holidays' should therefore be avoided.

Care should be taken when using Levodopa in the following circumstances: in endocrine, renal, pulmonary or cardiovascular disease, particularly where there is a history of myocardial infarction or arrhythmia; psychiatric disturbances; hepatic disorder; peptic ulcer; osteomalacia; where sympathomimetic drugs may be required (e.g. bronchial asthma), due to possible potentiation of the cardiovascular effects of levodopa; where antihypertensive drugs are being used, due to possible increased hypotensive action.

Periodic evaluation of hepatic, haemopoietic, renal and cardiovascular functions is advised.

Patients who improve on Levodopa therapy should be advised to resume normal activities gradually as rapid mobilization may increase the risk of injury.

*Side-effects and adverse reactions:* Tolerance to Levodopa varies widely between patients and is often related to the rate of dosage increase. Post-encephalitic Parkinsonian patients tolerate the drug less well. Side-effects, usually dose-related, occur at some time in most patients. During the initiation of therapy nausea and vomiting, anorexia, weakness and hypotension, which is usually postural (but a labile hypertension may rarely be seen), are most frequent. Nausea and vomiting may be minimised by administering Levodopa immediately after food; an antiemetic, e.g. cyclizine hydrochloride 50 mg three times daily, may also be helpful.

Psychiatric disturbances are common in Parkinsonian patients, including those being treated with levodopa. They include mild elation, anxiety, agitation, insomnia, depression, aggression, delusions, hallucinations and 'unmasking' of psychoses. Although there have been rare reports of possible antagonism of levodopa by diazepam, in general diazepam and nitrazepam have been found to be useful in the treatment of anxiety and insomnia, respectively, occurring in Parkinsonism. Depression may be treated with tricyclic antidepressants although isolated cases of hypertensive crisis have been reported with the concomitant use of tricyclic drugs. ECT may be administered if appropriate. MAO inhibitors, except selective MAO-B inhibitors, must not be used.

Involuntary movements, commonly in the form of oral dyskinesias, often accompanied by 'paddling' foot movements, or of the choreo-athetoid type, are common, particularly on long-term administration. These are usually dose-dependent and may disappear or become tolerable after dose adjustment.

With long-term administration, fluctuations in the therapeutic response may be encountered. They include 'freezing' episodes, end-of-dose deterioration and the so-called 'on-off' effect. Patients may be helped by dosage reduction or by giving smaller and more frequent doses.

Other side-effects which have occasionally been reported with levodopa therapy include gastrointestinal bleeding, flushing, sweating and drowsiness.

On some occasions the urine passed during Levodopa treatment may be altered in colour; usually red-tinged, this will turn dark on standing. These changes are due to metabolites and are no cause for concern.

Transient rises in SGOT, SGPT and alkaline phosphatase values have been noted: serum uric acid and blood urea nitrogen levels are occasionally increased. In rare instances, haemolytic anaemia, mild transient leucopenia and thrombocytopenia have been reported.

Also, in rare instances, headache and peripheral neuropathy have been reported.

Levodopa may interfere chemically with several diagnostic laboratory tests including those for glucose, ketone bodies or catecholamines in urine and for glucose or uric acid in blood. Levodopa therapy has been reported to inhibit the response to protirelin in tests of thyroid function.

*Treatment of overdosage:* Symptoms of overdosage are qualitatively similar to the side-effects but may be of greater magnitude.

Treatment should include gastric lavage, general supportive measures, intravenous fluids and the maintenance of an adequate airway.

Electrocardiographic monitoring should be instituted and the patient carefully observed for the possible development of arrhythmias. If necessary, anti-arrhythmic therapy should be given and other symptoms treated as they arise.

**Pharmaceutical precautions**
*Storage:* Levodopa tablets should be stored in well-closed containers, protected from light.

**Legal category** POM.

**Package quantities** Levodopa tablets in packs of 200.

**Further information** Nil.

**Product licence number** 12070/0002.

## MENADIOL SODIUM DIPHOSPHATE

**Presentation** Round, white to pale pink tablets with CL 1L3 imprinted on one face and a single break bar on the other, containing 12.63 mg of tetra-sodium salt of 2-methyl-1, 4-naphthahydroquinone diphosphate (equivalent to 10 mg of the free ester).

Menadiol sodium diphosphate is a vitamin K analogue. It contains the substance chemically described as the sodium salt of 2-methyl-1, 4-naphthahydroquinone diphosphate. Also contains lactose and other ingredients.

**Uses**
*Properties:* Menadiol sodium diphosphate is a water-soluble vitamin K analogue. The presence of vitamin K is essential for the formation within the body of prothrombin, factor VII, factor IX and factor X. Lack of vitamin K leads to increased tendency to haemorrhage.

*Indications:* Menadiol sodium diphosphate is indicated in the treatment of haemorrhage or threatened haemorrhage associated with a low blood level of prothrombin or factor VII. The main indication is obstructive jaundice (before and after surgery).

**Dosage and administration**
*Adults:* Usual therapeutic dose: 10 to 40 mg daily.

*Children:* If, on the recommendation of a physician, a children's dosage is required, it is suggested that 5 to 20 mg daily be given.

*Use in the elderly:* Recommendations for use in the elderly do not differ from those for other adults.

Menadiol sodium diphosphate tablets are for oral administration.

**Contra-indications, warnings, etc**
*Contra-indications:* The administration of Menadiol sodium diphosphate to neonates, infants or to mothers in the pre- and post-natal periods is contra-indicated. Moderate doses of Menadiol sodium diphosphate have produced haemolytic anaemia, hyperbilirubinaemia and kernicterus, especially in premature infants, even when administered prior to delivery. In the treatment of haemorrhagic disease of the newborn, vitamin K₁ (Konakion*) is the preferred drug of choice.

*Use in pregnancy:* There is evidence of hazard if Menadiol sodium diphosphate is used in human pregnancy. It is known to be associated with a small risk of haemolytic anaemia, hyperbilirubinaemia and kernicterus in the infant if administered to the mother in late pregnancy or during labour. Menadiol sodium diphosphate is therefore contra-indicated during late pregnancy.

*Precautions:* Large doses of Menadiol sodium diphosphate may decrease patient sensitivity to anticoagulants.

*Side-effects and adverse reactions:* Menadiol sodium diphosphate may induce haemolysis (especially in the newborn infant) in the presence of erythrocyte glucose-6-phosphate dehydrogenase deficiency or low concentrations of alpha-tocopherol in the blood.

**Pharmaceutical precautions**
*Storage:* The recommended maximum storage temperature for Menadiol sodium diphosphate tablets is 30°C. Menadiol sodium diphosphate tablets should be protected from light.

**Legal category** P.

**Package quantities** Menadiol sodium diphosphate tablets in packs of 100.

**Further information** In almost all circumstances Menadiol sodium diphosphate is as effective as the natural vitamin (Vitamin K₁). However, for cases of severe drug-induced hypoprothrombinaemia or bleeding as produced in association with coumarin or indandione anticoagulants or salicylates. Konakion (vitamin K₁) should be used.

**Product licence number** 12070/0007.

## NABILONE

**Presentation** Capsules (blue and white, coded Lilly 3101) containing 1 mg nabilone.

**Uses** Nabilone is indicated for the control of nausea and vomiting, caused by chemotherapeutic agents used in the treatment of cancer, in patients who have failed to respond adequately to conventional anti-emetic treatments.

**Dosage and administration** Nabilone is for oral administration to adults only. It is not recommended for use in children younger than 18 years of age as safety and efficacy have not been established.

The usual adult dosage is 1 mg or 2 mg twice a day. To minimise side-effects, it is recommended that the lower starting dose is used and that the dose is increased as necessary. The first dose should be administered the night before initiation of chemotherapy, and the second dose should be given one to three hours before the first dose of the oncolytic agent is administered. The maximum daily dose should not exceed 6 mg, given in three divided doses.

Nabilone may be administered throughout each cycle of chemotherapy and, if necessary, for 48 hours after the last dose of each cycle. Data on the chronic use of nabilone are not available.

*The elderly:* As for adults (see 'Precautions').

**Contra-indications, warnings, etc**
*Contra-indications:* Nabilone is contra-indicated in patients with a known allergy to cannabinoid agents and when the nausea and vomiting arises from any cause other than cancer chemotherapy.

*Warnings:* As nabilone is excreted primarily by the biliary route, the drug is not recommended for use in patients with severe liver dysfunction.

Nabilone may impair the mental and/or physical abilities required for the performance of potentially hazardous tasks such as operating machinery or driving a car; therefore the patient should be advised accordingly. The effects of nabilone may persist for a variable and unpredictable period of time following its oral administration. Adverse psychiatric reactions can persist for 48 to 72 hours following cessation of treatment.

Patients receiving nabilone should be closely observed, if possible, within an in-patient setting. This is especially important during the treatment of naive patients. However, even patients experienced with cannabinoid agents may have serious untoward responses not predicted by prior uneventful exposures.

Patients should be made aware of possible changes of mood and other adverse behavioural effects of the drug.

*Use in pregnancy:* Laboratory studies have so far shown no evidence of teratogenicity. There are no adequate and well controlled studies in pregnant women. Nabilone should be used during pregnancy only if clearly needed.

Reproduction studies performed in rats at 150 times the human dose and rabbits at 40 times the human dose revealed a dose-related reduction in litter size, an increase in the incidence of foetal resorptions, and an increase in the incidence of stillborn pups. The number of implantations was unaffected by treatment. These effects appear related to the dose-dependent reduction in maternal food intake and gain in body weight induced by nabilone. At 150 times the maximum recommended human dose, nabilone produced a reduction in neonatal survival that may be related to reduced milk production by mothers. Nabilone is known to have an inhibitory effect on prolactin release, which could contribute to the observed reduction in milk production. Hypothermia was also reported in the offspring of high-dose groups of female rats, which may have also contributed to reduced neonatal survival.

*Nursing mothers:* It is not known whether this drug is excreted in breast milk. It is not recommended that nabilone be given to nursing mothers.

*Precautions:* Since nabilone can elevate supine and standing heart rates and cause postural hypotension, it should be used with caution in the elderly and in patients with hypertension and heart disease.

Nabilone should be administered with caution to patients who are taking other psychoactive drugs or CNS depressants, including alcohol, barbiturates and narcotic analgesics, or to those with a history of psychiatric disorder (including manic-depressive illness and schizophrenia). Nabilone has been shown to have an additive CNS depressant effect when given with either diazepam, secobarbitone sodium, alcohol or codeine.

*Side-effects:* During controlled clinical trials of nabilone, virtually all patients experienced at least one adverse reaction. These included psychotomimetic reactions.

In these trials, the commonest statistically significant adverse events (in decreasing order of incidence) were: drowsiness, vertigo/dizziness, euphoria (high), dry mouth, ataxia, visual disturbance, concentration difficulties, sleep disturbance, dysphoria, hypotension, headache and nausea.

Other reported events include confusion, disorientation, hallucinations, psychosis, depression, decreased co-ordination, tremors, tachycardia, decreased appetite and abdominal pain.

Tolerance to such CNS effects as relaxation, drowsiness and euphoria develops rapidly and is readily reversible.

*Drug abuse and dependence:* Nabilone is an abusable substance, capable of producing subjective side-effects, such as euphoria or 'high', at therapeutic doses. Prescriptions should be limited to the amount necessary for a single cycle of chemotherapy (i.e., a few days). The physical dependence capability of Nabilone is unknown. Patients who participated in clinical trials, up to 5 days duration, showed no withdrawal symptoms on cessation of dosing.

*Overdosage:* Signs and symptoms are an extension of the psychotomimetic and physiological effects of nabilone. Overdosage may be considered to have occurred, even at prescribed dosages, if disturbing psychiatric symptoms are present. Subsequent doses should be withheld until patients have returned to their baseline mental status; routine dosing, possibly at a lower dose, may then be resumed if clinically indicated. In controlled clinical trials, alterations in mental status, related to the use of nabilone, resolved within 72 hours without specific medical therapy. Vital signs should be monitored, since hypertension, hypotension and tachycardia have occurred.

No cases of overdosage with more than 10 mg/day of nabilone have been reported during clinical trials. Signs and symptoms to be anticipated in large overdose situations are psychotic episodes, including hallucinations and anxiety reactions, respiratory depression and coma.

*Treatment:* Conservative management, if possible (i.e. verbal support and comfort). In more severe cases, antipsychotic drugs may be useful, although they have not been systematically evaluated. Such patients should be closely monitored because of the potential for drug interactions (e.g., additive CNS depressant effects due to nabilone and chlorpromazine).

General supportive care is recommended. Consider giving activated charcoal to decrease absorption from the gastrointestinal tract. The use of forced diuresis, peritoneal dialysis, haemodialysis, charcoal haemoperfusion, or cholestyramine, has not been reported. Most of a dose of nabilone is eliminated through the biliary system.

Treatment for respiratory depression and comatose state consists of symptomatic and supportive therapy. Attention should be paid to the occurrence of hypothermia. Consider fluids, inotropes and/or vasopressors for hypotension.

**Pharmaceutical precautions**   Keep containers tightly closed. Store at room temperature (15°C–25°C).

**Legal category**   POM.

**Package quantities**   Bottles and blister packs of 20.

**Further information**   For supply to hospitals only.

**Product licence number**   12070/0013.

## NEOSTIGMINE BROMIDE TABLETS

**Presentation**   Round, white tablets with 'PROSTIGMIN' imprinted on one face with a single break bar on the other, containing 15 mg neostigmine bromide.

**Uses**

*Properties:* Neostigmine Bromide is an antagonist to cholinesterase, the enzyme which normally destroys acetylcholine. The action of Neostigmine Bromide can briefly be described, therefore, as the potentiation of naturally occurring acetylcholine.

*Indications:* Myasthenia gravis, antagonist to non-depolarising neuromuscular blockade; paralytic ileus; post-operative urinary retention.

**Dosage and administration**   Neostigmine Bromide has a slower onset of effect when given orally than when given parenterally, but the duration of action is longer and the intensity of action more uniform.

To facilitate change of treatment from one route of administration to another, the following doses are approximately equivalent in effect:

0.5 mg intravenously = 1–1.5 mg intramuscularly or subcutaneously = 15 mg orally.

*Myasthenia gravis*
*Adults:* Doses of 15 to 30 mg by mouth are given at intervals throughout the day when maximum strength is needed (for example, on rising and before mealtimes). The usual duration of action of a dose is two to four hours. The total daily dose is usually in the range of 5–20 tablets but doses higher than these may be needed by some patients.

*Newborn infants:* Neostigmine Bromide (Prostigmin) ampoules are recommended.

*Other children:* Children under 6 years old should receive an initial dose of half a tablet (7.5 mg) of Neostigmine Bromide; children 6–12 years old should receive one tablet (15 mg). Dosage requirements should be adjusted according to the response but are usually in the range of 15–90 mg orally per day. The requirement for Neostigmine Bromide is usually markedly decreased after thymectomy, or when additional therapy (steroids, immunosuppressant drugs) is given.

When relatively large doses of Neostigmine Bromide are taken by myasthenic patients, it may be necessary to give atropine or other anticholinergic drugs to counteract the muscarinic effects. It should be noted that the slower gastro-intestinal motility caused by these drugs may affect the absorption of oral Neostigmine Bromide.

In all patients the possibility of 'cholinergic crisis', due to overdosage of Neostigmine Bromide, and its differentiation from 'myasthenic crisis', due to increased severity of disease, must be borne in mind. Both types of crisis are manifested by increased muscle weakness, but whereas myasthenic crisis may require more intensive anticholinesterase treatment, cholinergic crisis calls for immediate discontinuation of this treatment and institution of appropriate supportive measures, including respiratory assistance.

*Antagonist to non-depolarising neuromuscular blockade:* Neostigmine Bromide (Prostigmin) ampoules are recommended.

*Other indications: Adults:* The usual dose is 1 to 2 tablets orally.
*Children:* 2.5–15 mg orally.
The frequency of these doses may be varied according to the needs of the patient.

*The elderly:* There are no specific dosage recommendations for Neostigmine Bromide in elderly patients.

Neostigmine Bromide Tablets are for oral administration.

**Contra-indications, warnings, etc**

*Contra-indication:* Neostigmine Bromide should not be given to patients with mechanical gastro-intestinal or urinary obstruction.

Neostigmine Bromide is contra-indicated in patients with known hypersensitivity to the drug and to bromides.

Neostigmine Bromide should not be used in conjunction with depolarising muscle relaxants such as suxamethonium as neuromuscular blockade may be potentiated and prolonged apnoea may result.

*Use in pregnancy:* The safety of Neostigmine Bromide during pregnancy or lactation has not been established. Although the possible hazards to mother and child must therefore be weighed against the potential benefits in every case, experience with Neostigmine Bromide in pregnant patients with myasthenia gravis has revealed no untoward effect of the drug on the course of pregnancy. As the severity of myasthenia gravis often fluctuates considerably, particular care is required to avoid cholinergic crisis, due to overdosage of the drug, but otherwise management is no different from that in non-pregnant patients. Observations indicate that only negligible amounts of Neostigmine Bromide are excreted in breast milk; nevertheless due regard should be paid to possible effects on the breast-feeding infant.

*Precautions:* Extreme caution is required when administering Neostigmine Bromide to patients with bronchial asthma.

Care should also be taken in patients with bradycardia, recent corony occlusion, hypotension, peptic ulcer, vagotonia, epilepsy or Parkinsonism. There is no evidence to suggest that Neostigmine Bromide has any special effects in the elderly. However, elderly patients may be more susceptible to dysrhythmias than the younger adult.

Neostigmine Bromide should not be given during cyclopropane or halothane anaesthesia; however, it may be used after withdrawal of these agents.

*Side-effects:* These may include nausea and vomiting, increased salivation, diarrhoea and abdominal cramps.

*Treatment of overdosage:* Signs of overdose due to muscarinic effects may include abdominal cramps, increased peristalsis, diarrhoea, nausea and vomiting, increased bronchial secretions, salivation, diaphoresis

and miosis. Nicotinic effects consist of muscular cramps, fasciculations and general weakness. Bradycardia and hypotension may also occur.

Artificial ventilation should be instituted if respiration is severely depressed. Atropine sulphate 1 to 2 mg intravenously is an antidote to the muscarinic effects.

**Pharmaceutical precautions**

*Storage:* The recommended maximum storage temperature is 30°C. The tablets should be protected from light.

**Legal category**   POM.

**Package quantities**   Neostigmine Bromide Tablets in packs of 140.

**Further information**   Nil.

**Product licence number**   14576/0004.

*Product licence holder:* Lifehealth Limited, Richmond House, Old Brewery Court, Sandyford Road, Newcastle upon Tyne NE2 1XG.

## PROCARBAZINE CAPSULES 50 mg

**Presentation**   Capsules with opaque ivory cap and body, containing 58.3 mg procarbazine hydrochloride (equivalent to 50 mg of procarbazine).

**Uses**

*Properties:* Procarbazine is a cytostatic agent with weak MAO inhibitor properties. Its exact mode of action on tumour cells is unknown. It may be effective in patients who have become resistant to radiation therapy and other cytostatic agents.

Procarbazine is readily absorbed from the gastrointestinal tract. It is rapidly metabolized, the primary circulating metabolite is the azo-derivative while the major urinary metabolite has been shown to be N-isopropylterephthalamic acid.

*Indications:* The main indication is Hodgkin's disease (lymphoma).

Procarbazine may also be useful in other advanced lymphomata and a variety of solid tumours which have proved resistant to other forms of therapy.

**Dosage and administration**

*In combination chemotherapeutic regimens:* Procarbazine is usually administered concomitantly with other appropriate cytostatic drugs in repeated four-to-six-weekly cycles. In most such combination chemotherapy regimens currently in use (e.g. the so-called MOPP schedule with mustine, vincristine and prednisone) procarbazine is given daily on the first 10–14 days of each cycle in a dosage of 100 mg per m² of body surface (to nearest 50 mg).

*As sole therapeutic agent:*

*Adults:* Treatment should begin with small doses which are increased gradually up to a maximum daily dose of 250 to 300 mg, divided as evenly as possible throughout the day.

Initial dosage scheme:

| | |
|---|---|
| 1st day: | 50 mg |
| 2nd day: | 100 mg |
| 3rd day: | 150 mg |
| 4th day: | 200 mg |
| 5th day: | 250 mg |
| 6th day: | et seq.: 250–300 mg |

*Further procedure:* Treatment should be continued with 250 or 300 mg daily until the greatest possible remission has been obtained, after which a maintenance dose is given.

*Maintenance dose:* 50 to 150 mg daily. Treatment should be continued until a total dose of at least 6 g has been given; otherwise, a negative result is not significant.

*Elderly:* Procarbazine should be used with caution in the elderly. Patients in this group should be observed very closely for signs of early failure or intolerance of treatment.

*Children:* If, on the recommendation of a physician, a children's dosage is required, 50 mg daily should be given for the first week. Daily dosage should then be maintained at 100 mg per m² of body surface (to nearest 50 mg) until leucopenia or thrombocytopenia occurs or maximum response is obtained.

Procarbazine capsules are for oral administration.

**Contra-indications, warnings, etc**

*Contra-indications:* Pre-existing severe leucopenia or thrombocytopenia from any cause; severe hepatic or renal damage.

Procarbazine should not be used in the management of non-malignant disease.

*Use in pregnancy and lactation:* Procarbazine is teratogenic in animals. Isolated human foetal malformations have been reported following MOPP combination therapy. Therefore procarbazine should not be administered to patients who are pregnant unless considered absolutely essential by the physician.

Procarbazine should not be given to breast feeding mothers.

*Precautions:* Procarbazine should be given only under the supervision of a physician who is experienced in cancer chemotherapy and having facilities for regular monitoring of clinical and haematological effects during and after administration. Introduction of therapy should only be effected under hospital conditions.

Caution is advisable in patients with hepatic or renal dysfunction, cardiovascular or cerebrovascular disease, phaeochromocytoma, or epilepsy.

Regular blood counts are of great importance. If, during the initial treatment, the total white-cell count falls to 3,000 per mm³ or the platelet count to 80,000 per mm³, treatment should be suspended temporarily until the leucocyte and/or platelet levels recover, when therapy with the maintenance dose may be resumed.

Treatment should be interrupted on the appearance of allergic skin reactions.

Procarbazine is a weak MAO inhibitor and therefore interactions with certain foodstuffs and drugs, although very rare, must be borne in mind. Thus, owing to possible potentiation of the effect of barbiturates, narcotic analgesics (especially pethidine), drugs with anticholinergic effects (including phenothiazine derivatives and tricyclic antidepressants), other central nervous system depressants (including anaesthetic agents) and antihypertensive agents, these drugs should be given concurrently with caution and in low doses. Intolerance to alcohol (disulfiram-like reaction) may occur.

Procarbazine has been shown to be carcinogenic in animals. The increased risk of carcinogenicity in man should be borne in mind when long-term management of patients is proposed.

*Side-effects and adverse reactions:* Loss of appetite and nausea occur in most cases, sometimes with vomiting. These symptoms are usually confined to the first few days of treatment and then tend to disappear.

Procarbazine causes leucopenia and thrombocytopenia. These haematological changes are almost always reversible and seldom require complete cessation of therapy.

*Treatment of overdosage:* Signs of overdosage include severe nausea and vomiting, dizziness, hallucinations, depression and convulsions; hypotension or tachycardia may occur.

Gastric lavage and general supportive treatment should be performed, with prophylactic treatment against possible infection, and frequent blood counts.

*Handling guidelines:* Undamaged capsules present minimal risk of contamination, but in accordance with good hygiene requirements, direct handling should be avoided. As with all cytotoxics, precautions should be taken to avoid exposing staff during pregnancy.

Waste material may be disposed of by incineration.

**Pharmaceutical precautions**
*Storage:* Procarbazine capsules should be stored in a dry place; the recommended maximum storage temperature is 25°C.

**Legal category** POM.

**Package quantities** Procarbazine capsules in packs of 50.

**Further information** Nil.

**Product licence number** 12070/0004.

## RAZOXANE

**Presentation** Razoxane Tablets, each containing 125 mg razoxane, are white to pale cream, and marked on one side CL5 and a bisection line on the other. Inactive ingredients are alginic acid, magnesium stearate, microcrystalline cellulose and povidone.

**Uses** In contrast to most anti-cancer agents Razoxane interferes with cell division at the $G_2M$ phase of the cycle.

Razoxane in combination with radiotherapy may be used for all forms of soft-tissue, chondro- and osteosarcomas. In comparison with radiotherapy alone, this combination may increase the response rate and reduce recurrence. Razoxane can produce remissions in previous radio-resistant lesions.

Razoxane may be useful alone or in combination with other antimitotic agents in the treatment of malignant lymphomas, including mycosis fungoides, acute leukaemias, especially the acute blast cell-crisis of chronic myeloid leukaemia, and Kaposi's sarcoma. Experience to date has been in open studies which indicate that the product is of value in patients in whom previous therapies have been unsuccessful.

**Dosage and administration**
*Note:* Because of an association between administration of Razoxane and the development of acute myeloid leukaemia or skin epitheliomata, the drug should only be used in the above malignant conditions and then when its administration is essential such as when other treatments have failed.

*Adults and children:* Razoxane is administered orally. The following guidelines are based on the regimens with which responses have been obtained. In all regimens, if unacceptable degrees of leucopenia, thrombocytopenia or gastrointestinal disturbance occur, the dosage of Razoxane should be reduced or temporarily withdrawn to allow recovery.

*Soft-tissue, osteo- and chondro-sarcomata:* 125 mg (1 tablet) twice daily 3 days before the start of radiotherapy, continued throughout that therapy. On days when radiation is given, 1 tablet of Razoxane should be taken 1–4 hours before radiotherapy; the other tablet in the evening. The dosage of radiation should be selected and administered using normal criteria.

*Malignant lymphomas (including mycosis fungoides):* 0.5–1.5 g/m²/week should be administered orally as long as a remission is maintained. For example the dosage can be given as:

(a) 125 mg (1 tablet) twice daily on 3–5 days/week or

(b) three doses of 375 mg (3 tablets) given eight hours apart and repeated weekly.

If an inadequate response is obtained the dosage may be increased, provided that the white cell count permits.

*Acute leukaemias (including blast cell crisis of chronic myeloid leukaemia):* 150–500 mg/m²/day for 3–5 days. Treatment should be repeated at 14–28 day intervals, depending on the peripheral blood count. Allopurinol may also be given to prevent uric acid deposition.

*Kaposi's sarcoma:* 333 mg/m² three times daily for 3 days every 3 weeks, and adjusted as necessary according to peripheral blood count.

*Elderly patients:* There are no special dosage recommendations for the elderly, but it may be advisable to monitor elderly patients so that optimum dosage can be individually determined.

**Contra-indications, warnings, etc** Razoxane is contra-indicated in the treatment of non-malignant conditions such as psoriasis.

Razoxane is contra-indicated in pregnancy because of its action on cell division. Animal studies have revealed abnormalities of foetal development. It should not normally be administered to mothers who are breast feeding.

Mice and rats developed tumours following long term intraperitoneal administration of Razoxane. There is an association between the development of acute myeloid leukaemia or skin epitheliomata and the administration of Razoxane in man.

The peripheral blood count should be monitored throughout Razoxane therapy. Unacceptable degrees of leucopenia or thrombocytopenia are quickly reversed on cessation of treatment. Unacceptable degrees of myelosuppression are more likely to occur in patients who have received extensive chemotherapy previously.

*Side-effects:* The principal reported side-effects include leucopenia, thrombocytopenia, nausea, vomiting, diarrhoea, skin reactions and alopecia. Early skin reactions in patients receiving Razoxane plus radiotherapy may be more marked than those expected from radiotherapy alone. Severe late subcutaneous fibrosis has been reported in some patients receiving the combined therapy. There appears to be an increased likelihood of oesophagitis and pneumonitis in patients who require radiotherapy for thoracic lesions.

*Overdosage:* In cases of overdosage, signs and symptoms are likely to be qualitatively similar to side-effects; there is no specific antidote and treatment must be symptomatic.

**Pharmaceutical precautions** Store below 25°C, protected from light and moisture.

It is recommended that adequate protective gloves be worn when handling Razoxane Tablets and that Razoxane Tablets should not be handled by pregnant staff.

**Legal category** POM.

**Package quantities** Containers of 30 tablets.

**Further information** In contrast to most anti-cancer agents, Razoxane interferes with cell division at the $G_2M$ phase of the cell cycle and in multiple-drug chemotherapy regimens, it is logical to combine Razoxane with agents acting at the other phases of the cell cycle.

**Product licence number** 12070/0012.

## RHEOMACRODEX* IN DEXTROSE

**Qualitative and quantitative composition** Dextran 40 – 10 g in 100 mls.

**Pharmaceutical form** Colourless, clear, slightly viscous sterile solution 500 ml.

**Clinical particulars**
*Therapeutic indications:* Rheomacrodex is used for the early fluid replacement or for plasma volume expansion in the adjunctive treatment of certain types of shock or in impending shock including those resulting from burns, surgery, haemorrhage or trauma in which circulatory volume deficit is present.

Rheomacrodex is not a substitute for whole blood or blood products where these are clearly indicated.

Rheomacrodex may be used in embolic episodes and for prophylaxis of venous thrombosis and pulmonary embolism in patients at moderate or high risk of thromboembolism.

Rheomacrodex is also used as a priming fluid during extracorporeal circulation.

Rheomacrodex is used in conditions where improvement of microcirculatory flow is required.

*Posology and method of administration:* Rheomacrodex is for intravenous administration only.

The recommended dosage is dependent upon the age, weight and clinical condition of the patient.

The solution is hyperoncotic and draws extravascular fluid into the vascular space such that 500 ml infused rapidly into a normally hydrated patient may produce an expansion of almost one litre. This expansion is short lived due to excretion of smaller molecules, and by 3 hours expansion will have declined to about 520 ml, by 6 hours 430 ml and 12 hours 360 ml. Such expansion rapidly fills circulation deficit, reduces haematocrit and concentration of clotting factors, and may produce oozing from recent surgical incisions due to increase in capillary flow.

Dehydration must be corrected before giving the drug.

*In shock:* The suggested total adult dose for the first 24 hours should not exceed 20 ml per kg body weight. The first 10 ml per kg may be infused as rapidly as necessary to effect improvement. Monitoring central venous pressure; strongly recommended as guide to infusion. Daily doses after the first 24 hours should not exceed 10 ml per kg and therapy should not be continued beyond 5 days.

*For the treatment of thromboembolism:* Initially 500–1000 ml over 4–6 hours on the first day followed by 500 ml over 4–6 hours the next day. Then, the treatment may be continued with 500 ml over 4–6 hours on alternate days for a maximum of 10 days.

*For the prophylaxis of thromboembolism:* Infuse 500 ml over 4–6 hours during or at the end of surgery followed by 500 ml over 4–6 hours the next day. In high-risk patients, the treatment may be continued with 500 ml over 4–6 hours on alternate days for a maximum of 10 days.

*In extracorporeal perfusion:* The dose of Rheomacrodex will depend upon the volume needed to prime the pump oxygenator. Usually, a total dose of 10–20 ml per kg of body weight is added to the perfusion circuit. The total dose should not exceed 2 g per kg of body weight and this can be limited and controlled by adding other priming fluids.

*In improvement of microcirculatory flow:* Infuse 500–1000 ml in the first 24 hours. 500 ml is given the next day and then alternate days to a maximum of two weeks.

*Infants:* up to 5 ml per kg of body weight.

*Children:* up to 10 ml per kg of body weight.

*Elderly:* as per adults, but take extra care regarding dehydration, overloading and renal function.

*Contra-indications:* Rheomacrodex is contra-indicated in the presence of thrombocytopenia, hypofibrinogenaemia, severe congestive heart failure, renal disease with severe oliguria or anuria and where there is known intolerance to dextran.

Rheomacrodex in sodium chloride should not be administered to patients in whom sodium restriction is indicated. Rheomacrodex in 5% dextrose is available.

*Special warnings and special precautions for use:*
*Warnings:* Because Rheomacrodex is a colloidal solution it withdraws water from the extravascular space and the resultant fluid shifts may become critical in poorly hydrated patients. The renal excretion of dextran is associated with elevations of the specific gravity of the urine and these may become significant in patients with reduced renal function. It is therefore, essential that the patient's state of hydration is assessed before Rheomacrodex is administered. If signs of dehydration are present, appropriate parenteral fluids should be administered and the infusion of Rheomacrodex limited to 500 ml per hour. An osmotic diuretic like mannitol may be used to maintain urine excretion following adequate hydration. Urine flow should be kept above 250 ml/6 hours and the s.g. below 1.065.

Recommended dosage of Rheomacrodex effects only minor and transient changes in the coagulation of the blood. Excessive dosage may induce a prolonged bleeding time. Therefore, the physician should be aware of the possibility of a slight increase in blood loss.

It is strongly recommended that central venous pressure is frequently monitored during the initial infusion of Rheomacrodex. With monitoring, the first 500 ml may be administered rapidly, but should be immediately discontinued if there is a steep rise in central venous pressure. Without monitoring, the intravenous infusion should be slower and the patient carefully observed for signs of circulatory overloading.

Following the administration of Rheomacrodex, an increase in urinary output usually occurs in oliguric patients. If no increase is observed after the administration of 500 ml, the infusion should be discontinued until adequate diuresis develops spontaneously or can be provoked by other means.

The amount of Rheomacrodex given should not cause a depression of the haemoglobin concentration below 9 g% for more than a short time. Care should be taken to prevent a depression of the haematocrit below 30% volume.

*Precautions:* Although dextrans of higher molecular weight produce erythrocyte aggregation which may interfere with blood-typing and cross-matching, no such interference occurs with Rheomacrodex. Blood sugar determinations that employ high concentrations of acid may result in hydrolysis of dextran, yielding falsely elevated glucose assay results. This has been observed both with sulphuric acid and with acetic acid. In other laboratory tests, the presence of dextran in the blood may result in the development of turbidity, which can interfere with the assay. This has been observed in bilirubin assays in which alcohol is employed and in total protein assays employing biuret reagent. Thus consideration should be given to withdrawal of blood for chemical laboratory tests prior to initiation of therapy.

Patients should be closely observed for signs of anaphylaxis during the first few minutes and resuscitative measures should be readily available. Large doses may result in pulmonary oedema. Caution is advised in patients with poor cardiac function.

In patients in whom restriction of sodium is indicated Rheomacrodex in glucose should be used, and conversely, in patients in whom dextrose restriction is indicated, Rheomacrodex in saline should be used.

*Interaction with other medicaments and other forms of interaction:* Rheomacrodex crystallises occasionally due to swings of temperature causing expansion changes of meniscus level. Seed crystals form on the meniscus line which may grow into full crystals. Storage should therefore, be at a constant temperature not exceeding 25˚C. If flakes of dextran appear, these can be redissolved by heating for a short time at a low temperature not to exceed 100˚C. The solution should then be cooled to 37˚C before infusion.

As with all parenterals, compatibilities should be checked when additives are used.

Thorough and careful mixing of any additives is mandatory.

Avoid storage of solution so prepared.

*Pregnancy and lactation:* Although anaphylactic reactions to Rheomacrodex are rare, the product should only be used during pregnancy when strictly indicated, since anaphylactic reactions in the mother have been reported to cause anoxic brain damage which has resulted in death of the foetus in a number of cases.

*Effects on ability to drive and use machines:* Not applicable.

*Undesirable effects:* Mild urticarial reactions, rarely severe anaphylactoid reactions, increase in viscosity and specific gravity of urine, reversible tubular vacuolisation, and occasionally transient acidosis due to improved tissue perfusion. Rarely renal failure has been reported.

*Overdose:* In the event of an accidental over infusion, treatment should temporarily be either discontinued or rate of infusion decreased significantly, depending on extent of over infusion. The patient should be observed for symptoms and signs of cardiorespiratory decompensation and hepatic and renal functions, and fluid and electrolyte balance should be carefully monitored together with any evidence of bleeding diathesis, other symptomatic and supportive measures should be provided.

**Pharmacological properties**

*Pharmacodynamic properties:* Dextran 40 has a mean molecular weight of 40,000. Dextran of this weight binds about 20 ml of water per gram of dextran when in the circulation and the dextran 40 is known to have disaggregative effects on erythrocytes. This effect combined with the volume expansion and haemodilution produced by the infusion serves to improve microcirculatory flow. Inhibition of platelet adhesiveness combined with haemodilution, improved flow due to reduced viscosity and dilution of clotting factors serve to inhibit post surgical thrombo embolic

disease without altering normal haemostasis. Thrombi formed in the presence of dextran have a structure more readily attacked by body lytic processes.

The solution is hyperoncotic and draws extravascular fluid into the vascular space such that 500 ml infused rapidly into a normal hydrated patient may produce an expansion of almost one litre. This expansion is short lived due to excretion of smaller molecules and by 3 hours expansion will have declined to about 520 ml, by 6 hours 430 ml and 12 hours 360 ml. Such expansion rapidly fills circulatory deficit, reduces haematocrit and concentration of clotting factors and may produce oozing from recent surgical incisions due to increase in capillary flow.

Dehydration must be corrected before giving the drug.

*Pharmacokinetic properties:* Following intravenous infusion the dextran 40 remains largely in the vasculature, producing the volume changes outlined above. Molecules below a mw of about 50,000 are rapidly excreted through the kidneys, about 60% of the dextran in the first 6 hours. The large molecules are metabolised at about 70–100 mg/kg/body weight/day by the reticulo endothelial system (mainly the liver) to glucose, which joins the body pool. This slower mode of elimination means that by 24 hours only 70% of the dextran has gone.

*Preclinical safety data:* None stated.

**Pharmaceutical particulars**

*List of excipients:* Dextrose Monohydrate PhEur; water for injections.

*Incompatibilities:* The slight acid pH of Rheomacrodex despite negligible buffering capacity (<2mEq/L) may precipitate salts of weak acids such as the various penicillins, unless they are buffered. Aminocaproic acid, dihydrallazine mesylate, warfarin sodium (dextrose vehicle only). 95% ethanol, dexamethasone sodium phosphate, isoxaprin hydrochloride and propantheline bromide have been reported incompatible.

*Shelf life:* 5 years.

*Special precautions for storage:* Store at steady temperature not exceeding 30˚C. Do not freeze.

*Nature and contents of container:* Type II. Glass infusion bottle complying with EP and DIN 58363, bromo chlorbutyl rubber stoppers to DIN 58363 and EP. Aluminium seal.

*Instructions for use/handling:* None stated.

*Marketing authorisation holder:* Medisan Pharmaceuticals AB, AR4, S-741 74 Uppsala, Sweden.

**Marketing authorisation number**  15135/0001.

**Date of approval/revision of SPC**  15 March 1996.

**Legal category**  POM.

## RHEOMACRODEX* IN NORMAL SALINE

**Qualitative and quantitative composition**  Dextran 40 – 10 g in 100 mls.

**Pharmaceutical form**  Colourless, clear, slightly viscous sterile solution 500 ml.

**Clinical particulars**

*Therapeutic indications:* Rheomacrodex is used for the early fluid replacement or for plasma volume expansion in the adjunctive treatment of certain types of shock or in impending shock including those resulting from burns, surgery, haemorrhage or trauma in which circulatory volume deficit is present.

Rheomacrodex is not a substitute for whole blood or blood products where these are clearly indicated.

Rheomacrodex may be used in embolic episodes and for prophylaxis of venous thrombosis and pulmonary embolism in patients at moderate or high risk of thromboembolism.

Rheomacrodex is also used as a priming fluid during extracorporeal circulation.

Rheomacrodex is used in conditions where improvement of microcirculatory flow is required.

*Posology and method of administration:* Rheomacrodex is for intravenous administration only.

The recommended dosage is dependent upon the age, weight and clinical condition of the patient.

The solution is hyperoncotic and draws extravascular fluid into the vascular space such that 500 ml infused rapidly into a normal hydrated patient may hydrated patients. The renal excretion of dextran is associated with elevations of the specific gravity of the urine and these may become significant in patients with reduced renal function. It is therefore, essential that the patient's state of hydration is assessed before Rheomacrodex is administered. If signs of dehydration are present, appropriate parenteral fluids should be administered and the infusion of Rheomacrodex limited to 500 ml per hour. An osmotic diuretic like mannitol may be used to maintain urine excretion

following adquate hydration. Urine flow should be kept above 250 ml/6 hours and the s.g. below 1.065.

Recommended dosage of Rheomacrodex effects only minor and transient changes in the coagulation of the blood. Excessive dosage may induce a prolonged bleeding time. Therefore, the physician should be aware of the possibility of a slight increase in blood loss.

It is strongly recommended that central venous pressure is frequently monitored during the initial infusion of Rheomacrodex. With monitoring, the first 500 ml may be administered rapidly, but should be immediately discontinued if there is a steep rise in central venous pressure. Without monitoring, the intravenous infusion should be slower and the patient carefully observed for signs of circulatory overloading.

Following the administration of Rheomacrodex, an increase in urinary output usually occurs in oliguric patients. If no increase is observed after the administration of 500 ml, the infusion should be discontinued until adequate diuresis develops spontaneously or can be provoked by other means.

The amount of Rheomacrodex given should not cause a depression of the haemoglobin concentration below 9 g% for more than a short time. Care should be taken to prevent a depression of the haematocrit below 30% volume.

*Precautions:* Although dextrans of higher molecular weight produce erythrocyte aggregation which may interfere with blood-typing and cross-matching, no such interference occurs with Rheomacrodex. Blood sugar determinations that employ high concentration of acid may result in hydrolysis of dextran, yielding falsely elevated glucose assay results. This has been observed both with sulphuric acid and with acetic acid. In other laboratory tests, the presence of dextran in the blood may result in the development of turbidity, which can interfere with the assay. This has been observed in bilirubin assays in which alcohol is employed and in total protein assays employing biuret reagent. Thus consideration should be given to withdrawal of blood for chemical laboratory tests prior to initiation of therapy.

Patients should be closely observed for signs of anaphylaxis during the first few minutes and resuscitative measures should be readily available. Large doses may result in pulmonary oedema. Caution is advised in patients with poor cardiac function.

In patients in whom restriction of sodium is indicated Rheomacrodex in glucose should be used, and conversely, in patients in whom dextrose restriction is indicated, Rheomacrodex in saline should be used.

*Interaction with other medicaments and other forms of interaction:* Rheomacrodex crystallises occasionally due to swings of temperature causing expansion changes of meniscus level. Seed crystals form on the meniscus line which may grow into full crystals. Storage should therefore, be at a constant temperature not exceeding 25˚C. If flakes of dextran appear, these can be redissolved by heating for a short time at a low temperature not to exceed 100˚C. The solution should then be cooled to 37˚C before infusion.

As with all parenterals, compatibilities should be checked when additives are used.

Thorough and careful mixing of any additives is mandatory.

Avoid storage of solution so prepared.

*Pregnancy and lactation:* Although anaphylactic reactions to Rheomacrodex are rare, the product should only be used during pregnancy when strictly indicated, since anaphylactic reactions in the mother have been reported to cause anoxic brain damage which has resulted in death of the foetus in a number of cases.

*Effects on ability to drive and use machines:* Not applicable.

*Undesirable effects:* Mild urticarial reactions, rarely severe anaphylactoid reactions, increase in viscosity and specific gravity of urine, reversible tubular vacuolisation and occasionally transient acidosis due to improved tissue perfusion. Rarely renal failure has been reported.

*Overdose:* In the event of an accidental over infusion, treatment should temporarily be either discontinued or rate of infusion decreased significantly, depending on extent of over infusion. The patient should be observed for symptoms and signs of cardiorespiratory decompensation and hepatic and renal functions, and fluid and electrolyte balance should be carefully monitored together with any evidence of bleeding diathesis, other symptomatic and supportive measures should be provided.

**Pharmacological properties**

*Pharmacodynamic properties:* Dextran 40 has a mean molecular weight of 40,000. Dextran of this weight binds about 20 ml of water per gram of dextran when in the circulation and the dextran 40 is known to have disaggregative effects on erythrocytes. This effect combined with the volume expansion and haemodilution produced by the infusion serve to improve microcirculatory flow. Inhibition of platelet adhesiveness combined with haemodilution, improved flow due to reduced viscosity and dilution of clotting factors serves to inhibit post surgical thrombo embolic disease without altering normal haemostasis. Thrombi formed in the presence of dextran have a structure more readily attacked by body lytic processes.

The solution is hyperoncotic and draws extravascular fluid into the vascular space such that 500 ml infused rapidly into a normal hydrated patient may produce an expansion of almost one litre. This expansion is short lived due to excretion of smaller molecules and by 3 hours expansion will have declined to about 520 ml, by 6 hours 430 ml and 12 hours 360 ml. Such expansion rapidly fills circulatory deficit, reduces haematocrit and concentration of clotting factors and may produce oozing from recent surgical incisions due to increase in capillary flow.

Dehydration must be corrected before giving the drug.

*Pharmacokinetic properties:* Following intravenous infusion the dextran 40 remains largely in the vasculature, producing the volume changes outlined above. Molecules below a mw of about 50,000 are rapidly excreted through the kidneys, about 60% of the dextran in the first 6 hours. The large molecules are metabolised at about 70–100 mg/kg/body weight/day by the reticulo endothelial system (mainly the liver) to glucose, which joins the body pool. This slower mode of elimination means that by 24 hours only 70% of the dextran has gone.

*Preclinical safety data:* None stated.

**Pharmaceutical particulars**

*List of excipients:* Sodium chloride; water for injections.

*Incompatibilities:* The slight acid pH of Rheomacrodex despite negligible buffering capacity (<2mEq/L) may precipitate salts of weak acids such as the various penicillins, unless they are buffered. Aminocaproic acid, dihydrallazine mesylate, warfarin sodium (dextrose vehicle only), 95% ethanol, dexamethasone sodium phosphate, isoxaprin hydrochloride and propantheline bromide have been reported incompatible.

*Shelf life:* 5 years.

*Special precautions for storage:* Store at steady temperature not exceeding 25°C. Do not freeze.

*Nature and contents of container:* Type II. Glass infusion bottle complying with EP and DIN 58363, bromo or chlorbutyl rubber stoppers to DIN 58363 and EP. Aluminium seal.

*Instructions for use/handling:* None stated.

*Marketing authorisation holder:* Medisan Pharmaceuticals AB, AR4, S-741 74 Uppsala, Sweden.

**Marketing authorisation number** 15135/0002.

**Date of approval/revision of SPC** 24 May 1996.

**Legal cateogry** POM.

## TESTOSTERONE ENANTHATE AMPOULES

**Qualitative and quantitative composition** Each ampoule contains 250 mg Testosterone Enanthate PhEur in oily solution.

**Pharmaceutical form** Solution for injection.

**Clinical particulars**

*Therapeutic indications:* Mammary carcinoma in the female. Androgen deficiency in the male.

*Posology and method of administration:*

*Females – mammary carcinoma:* 250 mg every two weeks by intramuscular injection.

*Males – Hypogonadism:* To stimulate development of underdeveloped androgen-dependent organs and for initial treatment of deficiency symptoms, 250 mg Testosterone Enanthate intramuscularly every two to three weeks.

*For maintenance treatment:* 250 mg Testosterone Enanthate intramuscularly every three to six weeks, according to individual requirement.

*Contra-indications:* Prostatic carcinoma, mammary carcinoma in males and pregnancy. Previous or existing liver tumours (in advanced mammary carcinoma in females only) if these are not due to metastases.

*Special warnings and precautions for use:* Androgens should not be used for enhancing muscular development in healthy individuals or for increasing physical ability.

High dose or long-term administration of testosterone occasionally increases the tendency to water retention and oedema. Caution should therefore be exercised in patients predisposed to oedema.

In rare cases benign and in even rarer cases malignant liver tumours leading in isolated cases to life-threatening intra-abdominal haemorrhage have been observed after the use of hormonal substances such as testosterone enanthate. If severe upper abdominal complaints, liver enlargement or signs of intra-abdominal haemorrhage occur, a liver tumour should be included in the differential diagnosis and, if necessary, the preparation should be withdrawn. Regular examination of the prostate is advisable for men receiving androgen therapy.

If, in individual cases, frequent or persistent erections occur, the dose should be reduced or the treatment discontinued in order to avoid injury to the penis.

In women: If hypercalcaemia develops, therapy must be discontinued.

*Interactions with other medicaments and other forms of interaction:* Phenobarbitone increases the breakdown of steroid hormones in the liver (possible impairment of efficacy).

The clotting status should be monitored particularly closely when testosterone enanthate is administered together with coumarin derivatives.

*Pregnancy and lactation:* Contra-indicated in pregnancy.

*Effects on ability to drive and use machines:* None known.

*Undesirable effects:* Women treated with Testosterone Enanthate may develop signs of virilisation, (e.g. acne, hirsutism, voice changes). Particular care is therefore necessary in women whose occupations involve singing or speaking.

Spermatogenesis is inhibited by long-term and high-dose treatment with testosterone enanthate.

In rare cases, coughing, dyspnoea and circulatory irregularities may occur during or immediately after the injection. Experience has shown that these reactions can be avoided by injecting very slowly.

*Overdose:* Acute toxicity data show that Testosterone Enanthate can be classified as non-toxic following a single intake. Even in the case of an inadvertent administration of a multiple of the dose required for therapy, no acute toxicity risk is expected.

**Pharmacological properties**

*Pharmacodynamic properties:* Testosterone enanthate is an ester of the natural male sex hormone testosterone and exhibits all the pharmacological effects of the natural hormone. It differs in that it has a depot effect, due to the fact that testosterone enanthate is only slowly degraded to testosterone in the body.

*Pharmacokinetic properties:* Following intramuscular administration of 200 mg of testosterone enanthate to 6 hypogonadal males:

– Peak serum testosterone levels of 1233±484 ng/ml were achieved at 24 hours.

– Physiological levels of testosterone (approx. 500 ng/ml) were maintained for 11 days.

Half-life in blood was 2–3 days (healthy male volunteers).

*Preclinical safety data:* Studies in animals showed that the formulation has minimal potential for causing sensitisation or local irritation following intramuscular injection. Long-term systemic studies showed no evidence of testicular toxicity although a temporary inhibition of spermatogenesis may occur. No fertility studies with testosterone enanthate have been carried out. Administration of Testosterone Enanthate is contraindicated during pregnancy due to the possibility of virilisation of the female foetus. However, investigations into embryotoxic, in particular teratogenic, effects gave no indication that further impairment of organ development may occur.

*In vitro* investigations of mutagenicity gave negative results.

**Pharmaceutical particulars**

*List of excipients:* Benzyl benzoate; castor oil for injection.

*Incompatibilities:* None so far known.

*Shelf life:* 5 years.

*Special precautions for storage:* Protect from light.

*Nature and contents of container:* Clear glass ampoules of 1 ml in packs of 3.

*Instruction for use/handling:* Not applicable.

*Marketing authorisation holder:* Cambridge Selfcare Diagnostics Limited, Newcastle upon Tyne NE2 1XG.

**Marketing authorisation number** 12070/0015.

**Date of approval/revision of SPC** April 1996.

**Legal category** POM.

## TETRABENAZINE TABLETS

**Presentation** Round, yellowish-buff tablets with 'Roche' imprinted across one face and a single break bar on the other, containing 25 mg tetrabenazine.

**Uses**

*Properties:* The central effects of Tetrabenazine closely resemble those of reserpine, but it differs from the latter in having less peripheral activity and being much shorter-acting.

It is known from animal experiments that Tetrabenazine intervenes in the metabolism of biogenic amines, such as serotonin and noradrenaline, and that this activity is mainly limited to the brain. It is thought that the effect of Tetrabenazine on brain amines explains its clinical effects in man.

*Pharmacokinetics:* Tetrabenazine has a low and erratic bioavailability. It appears to be extensively metabolised by first-pass metabolism. The major metabolite, hydroxytetrabenazine, is formed by reduction. Little unchanged tetrabenazine can be detected in the urine. Since hydroxybenazine is reported to be as active as tetrabenazine in depleting brain amines, it is likely that this is the major therapeutic agent.

*Indications:* Movement disorders associated with organic central nervous system conditions, e.g. Huntington's chorea, hemiballismus and senile chorea.

**Dosage and administration**

*Adults:* Dosage and administration are variable and only a guide is given. An initial starting dose of 25 mg three times a day is recommended. This can be increased by 25 mg a day every three or four days until 200 mg is being given or the limit of tolerance, as dictated by unwanted effects, is reached, whichever is the lowest dose. If there is no improvement at the maximum dose in seven days, it is unlikely that the compound will be of benefit to the patient, either by increasing the dose or by extending the duration of treatment.

*Elderly:* No specific studies have been performed in the elderly, but Tetrabenazine has been administered to elderly patients in standard dosage without apparent ill effect.

*Children:* No specific dosage recommendations are made for the administration of Tetrabenazine to children, although it has been used without ill effect. Tetrabenazine tablets are for oral administration.

**Contra-indications, warnings, etc**

*Contra-indications:* Tetrabenazine blocks the action of reserpine.

*Use in pregnancy:* There is inadequate evidence of safety of the drug in human pregnancy and no evidence from animal work, but it has been in wide use for many years without apparent ill consequence.

Tetrabenazine should be avoided in breast-feeding mothers.

*Precautions:* Levodopa should be administered with caution in the presence of Tetrabenazine.

Patients should be advised that Tetrabenazine may cause drowsiness and therefore may modify their performance at skilled tasks (driving ability, operation of machinery, etc.) to a varying degree, depending on dose and individual susceptibility.

*Side-effects:* Side-effects are usually mild with little hypotensive action and few digestive disorders. The main unwanted effect reported to date has been drowsiness, which occurs with higher doses. If depression occurs, it can be controlled by reducing the dose or by giving antidepressant drugs such as the monoamine oxidase inhibitors. However, Tetrabenazine should not be given immediately after a course of any of the monoamine oxidase inhibitors as such treatment may lead to a state of restlessness, disorientation and confusion. In man, a Parkinsonian-like syndrome has been reported on rare occasions, usually in doses above 200 mg per day, but this disappears on reducing the dose.

*Effects of overdosage and their treatment:* Signs and symptoms of overdose may include drowsiness, sweating, hypotension and hypothermia. Treatment is symptomatic.

**Pharmaceutical precautions**

*Storage:* Tetrabenazine tablets should be stored in well-closed containers. The recommended maximum storage temperature is 30°C.

**Legal category** POM.

**Package quantities** Tetrabenazine tablets in packings of 120.

**Further information** Nil.

**Product licence number** 14576/0005.

*Product licence holder:* Lifehealth Limited, Richmond House, Old Brewery Court, Sandyford Road, Newcastle upon Tyne NE2 1XG.

## TRH-CAMBRIDGE*

**Presentation** Plain glass ampoules containing 200 micrograms TRH-Cambridge in 2 ml. The ampoule solution is almost colourless to faintly yellow. TRH-Cambridge contains the substance known as thyrotrophin releasing hormone and has the approved name protirelin. It is chemically described as L-pyro-gluta-myl-L-histidyl-L-proline-amide. Excipients: Mannitol, acetic acid, sodium hydroxide, hydrochloric acid and water for injections.

## Uses
*Properties:* TRH-Cambridge stimulates the secretion of thyroid stimulating hormone (TSH). Intravenous injection results in a prompt rise in serum TSH levels in normal subjects, peak levels being observed about 20 minutes after administration. There is a concomitant rise in serum levels of prolactin.

TRH rapidly disappears from the plasma after intravenous injection. Over 90% is removed within 20 minutes with a half-life of about 5.3 minutes. About 5.5% of the dose is excreted in the urine, mostly within 30 minutes.

*Indications:* The administration of TRH-Cambridge provides a means of assessing thyroid function and the reserve of TSH in the pituitary gland and is recommended as a test procedure where such assessment is indicated.

It is particularly useful as a diagnostic test for:
1. Mild hyperthyroidism.
2. Ophthalmic Graves' disease.
3. Mild or preclinical hypothyroidism.
4. Hypopituitarism.
5. Hypothalamic disease.
It may also be used in place of the $T_3$ suppression test.

## Dosage and administration
*Adults*
*Intravenous injection:* Tests employing intravenous TRH-Cambridge are based on the serum TSH response to a standard dose. They provide a means of both quantitative and qualitative assessment of thyroid function. It is essential for each laboratory to establish its own normal range of values for serum TSH before attempting quantitative assessment of TRH-Cambridge responses by this means.

*Intravenous TRH-Cambridge test*
(a) Blood sample taken for control TSH assay.
(b) TRH-Cambridge 200 micrograms given as a single bolus injection.
(c) Blood sample taken 20 minutes after injection for peak TSH assay.
(d) If necessary, a further blood sample may be taken 60 minutes after injection to detect a delayed TSH response.
The ampoule solution should not be diluted.

*Use in the elderly:* The use of TRH-Cambridge in the elderly has been well documented. Dosage requirements and the side-effects are similar to those of younger adults. The response may be altered in sick elderly subjects.

*Children:* The procedures for administering TRH-Cambridge to children are identical with those outlined above. An intravenous dose of 1 microgram/kg body weight may be used.

*Interpretation of results:* Interpretation of the responses of TRH-Cambridge is based on the increase in TSH and/or PBI, $T_3$ or $T_4$ levels from the basal values. In normal subjects, there is a prompt rise in serum levels of TSH. The changes observed in various conditions are briefly outlined below:
1. Hyperthyroidism – no rise in serum TSH or thyroid hormone levels.
2. Ophthalmic Graves' disease – often no rise in serum TSH or thyroid hormone levels.
3. Primary hypothyroidism – exaggerated and prolonged rise in serum TSH but no change in thyroid hormone levels.
4. Hypopituitarism – absent or impaired TSH or thyroid hormone response implies diminished TSH reserve.
5. Hypothalamic disease – a rise in serum TSH or thyroid hormone levels can occur in the presence of hypothyroidism; delayed responses are common.
The TRH-Cambridge test provides, in most instances, information similar to that obtained from a $T_3$ suppression test in that an absent or impaired response usually correlates with an absent or impaired response to $T_3$ suppression.
The response to TRH-Cambridge may be modified in subjects taking $T_3$, $T_4$, antithyroid drugs, corticosteroids, oestrogens, theophylline, levodopa, phenothiazines, metoclopramide, bromocriptine, salicylates, benzodiazepines, amiodarone, carbamazepine, lithium or spironolactone.

## Contra-indications, warnings, etc
*Precautions:* There are no absolute contra-indications to TRH-Cambridge. In view of the postulated effect of bolus injections of TRH-Cambridge on smooth muscle, patients with bronchial asthma or other types of obstructive airways disease should be closely monitored. Caution should also be observed in patients with myocardial ischaemia and severe hypopituitarism.

*Use in pregnancy:* There is some clinical evidence of safety in human pregnancy, animal studies having shown no hazard. Nevertheless, the established medical principle of not administering drugs during early pregnancy should be observed.

*Side-effects and adverse reactions:* TRH-Cambridge is well tolerated. No impairment of respiratory, hepatic, renal or haematological function has been reported. Following rapid intravenous injection, side-effects of a mild and transient nature may be experienced. They comprise nausea, a desire to micturate, a feeling of flushing, slight dizziness and a peculiar taste, and have been attributed to a local action of the bolus of TRH-Cambridge on the plain muscle of the gastrointestinal and genito-urinary tracts. A transient increase in pulse rate and blood pressure may also be noted.

*Effects of overdosage:* No symptoms of overdosage have been noted in patients receiving up to 1 mg intravenously.

## Pharmaceutical precautions
*Storage:* The recommended maximum storage temperature for TRH-Cambridge ampoules is 30˚C.

*Additives:* TRH-Cambridge ampoule solution should not be diluted.

**Legal category** POM.

**Package quantities** TRH-Cambridge ampoules containing 200 micrograms TRH-Cambridge in 2 ml in packs of 10.

## Further information
*Availability:* TRH-Cambridge is available through hospitals, pharmacies and clinics.

**Product licence number** 12070/0009.

# TRIMETAPHAN CAMSYLATE

**Presentation** Ampoules containing 250 mg trimetaphan camsylate in 5 ml. The ampoule solution is colourless to pale yellow. Excipients: Sodium acetate, hydrochloric acid and water for injections.

## Uses
*Properties:* Trimetaphan is a ganglion-blocking agent which also has a direct dilator effect on peripheral vessels. It has a rapid, short and readily reversible action, which permits minute-to-minute control of the blood pressure.

*Pharmacokinetics:* Trimetaphan crosses the placenta. Further pharmacokinetic data are unavailable as there is no acceptable assay procedure for the determination of trimetaphan in biological specimens, however most of a parenteral dose is excreted unchanged by the kidney.

*Indications:* Trimetaphan is used to induce controlled hypotension during certain surgical procedures. These may include: neurosurgery; vascular surgery; prostatectomy; chest surgery; thyroidectomy; bone and joint surgery.

## Dosage and administration
*Adults and children*
(a) Dilution to 250 ml with normal saline or dextrose-saline gives a 0.1 per cent solution (1 mg per ml) which is the strength usually used for an intravenous drip. The Trimetaphan drip is started at an average of 60 drops (approximately 3 to 4 mg) per minute and, having ascertained the patient's response, the rate of administration is then adjusted to maintain the desired level of hypotension. Since there is marked variation in individual response, continuous blood pressure monitoring is essential to maintain proper control.
(b) If a weaker solution is preferred, a 0.05 per cent solution can be prepared by diluting the 5 per cent ampoule solution to 500 ml.
(c) It may be necessary to use a more concentrated solution in operations in which intravenous fluid should be restricted. For such patients a solution containing 0.25 per cent Trimetaphan should be prepared by diluting the original 5 per cent solution to 100 ml with normal saline or dextrose-saline. The rate at which the drip is given should be correspondingly reduced.
(d) The undiluted solution has also been used by intermittent intravenous injection.
As with other hypotensive drugs, Trimetaphan should be stopped before wound closure to allow the blood pressure to rise.
Trimetaphan ampoules are for administration by intravenous drip and intermittent intravenous injection.
Trimetaphan ampoule solution may be diluted with Water for Injections, normal saline or dextrose-saline immediately before use.

## Contra-indications, warnings, etc
*Contra-indications:* Trimetaphan should not be used for hypotensive surgery in patients with severe arteriosclerosis, severe cardiac disease, or pyloric stenosis.

*Precautions:* Trimetaphan should be used with caution in the elderly, in patients with cerebral or coronary vascular insufficiency, diabetes mellitus, hepatic or renal insufficiency and in adrenal insufficiency. Care should also be taken in patients receiving neuromuscular blocking agents (especially suxamethonium), other anti-hypertensive agents, myocardial depressants or systemic corticosteroids.

Since the effect of Trimetaphan is neutralised by vasopressor drugs such as adrenaline, noradrenaline and ephedrine, local adrenaline infiltration at the site of incision is contra-indicated. Trimetaphan may sensitise patients to the cardiovascular effects of sympathomimetic agents.

*Use in pregnancy:* Use of Trimetaphan in pregnancy should be avoided due to the risk of producing paralytic ileus or meconium ileus in the newborn.

*Use in the elderly:* No specific data are available on the use of Trimetaphan in the elderly. Whilst there is no indication that this is accompanied by particular problems, it is known that the elderly may be more sensitive to hypotensive drugs.

Trimetaphan should be used with particular caution in patients with coronary artery disease, prostatic hypertrophy or glaucoma (cf. pupillary dilatation effect).

*Use in other special groups:* Extreme caution should also be exercised when using Trimetaphan in patients with degenerative disease of the central nervous system, Addison's disease and diabetes. Owing to its histamine-releasing effects, Trimetaphan should be used with caution in subjects with a history of allergy.

*Side-effects and adverse reactions:* Ganglionic blockade due to Trimetaphan may reduce gastro-intestinal motility and bladder function and affect visual accommodation. Constipation, mydriasis, increased intra-ocular pressure, decreased oral and nasal secretion, respiratory arrest (on rapid infusion of greater than 5 mg/minute), hypoglycaemia and hypokalaemia may also rarely occur.

*Treatment of overdosage:* The major effect will be a marked fall in blood pressure below the desired level of hypotension. Tachycardia and respiratory depression may result, particularly if Trimetaphan is used concomitantly with a muscle relaxant.

Vasopressor agents such as phenylephrine, ephedrine or noradrenaline are antidotes and may be used to effect a rapid return to normotensive level.

## Pharmaceutical precautions
*Storage:* The recommended maximum storage temperature is 6˚C; avoid freezing.

*Additives:* It is inadvisable to use the Trimetaphan drip as a vehicle for administering other drugs. Trimetaphan is known to be incompatible with thiopentone, gallamine triethiodide, strongly alkaline solutions, iodides and bromides.

**Legal category** POM.

**Package quantities** Trimetaphan ampoules in packs of 10.

**Further information** Nil.

**Product licence number** 12070/0001.

# VITAMIN A PALMITATE
# AMPOULES 100,000 IU/2 ml

**Presentation** Ampoules containing 100,000 international units (IU) vitamin A as the palmitate (30 mg retinol equivalent) in 2 ml colloidal aqueous solution.

The ampoule solution, which is strongly opalescent greenish-yellow to yellow-brown in colour, contains a polyethoxylated castor oil as solubilising agent. Other excipients: DL-alpha-tocopherol, sodium benzoate, hydrochloric acid and purified water.

## Uses
*Properties:* Vitamin A Palmitate is a synthetic vitamin A preparation. Vitamin A may be considered to act chiefly as a regulator of the growth and activity of epithelial tissues. It plays an essential role in the visual cycle through its participation in the synthesis of rhodopsin by the retina.

The cardinal signs and symptoms of Vitamin A deficiency are those affecting the eyes, such as xerosis, swelling and destruction of the cornea and night-blindness. Hyperkeratosis of the skin and keratinising and metaplastic changes in the mucous membranes of the respiratory, digestive and urinary tracts have been reported.

*Pharmacokinetics:* After a single injection of 100,000 IU of vitamin A palmitate in a water miscible preparation the following results were obtained.

Plasma levels of vitamin A palmitate of up to 6,000 mcg/l were obtained at 10 to 20 hours after administration.

Baseline levels of 10 to 50 mcg/l were reached after approximately 150 hours. Elimination from plasma appears to be governed by non-linear kinetics.

The bioavailability of this water miscible preparation is approximately 50%.

*Indications:* Prevention and treatment of vitamin A deficiency symptoms.

Vitamin A Palmitate ampoules are indicated when oral therapy is inappropriate (e.g. in malabsorption syndrome).

### Dosage and administration

*Adults:* A maintenance dose of 100,000 IU by deep intramuscular injection once monthly is usually sufficient.

In acute deficiency states 100,000 IU may be given once weekly. However, if patients are receiving high doses continuously for a prolonged period, it is recommended that Vitamin A Palmitate be given in courses of no longer than six weeks separated by treatment-free intervals of two weeks in order to minimise the risk of hypervitaminosis A.

In patients with liver disease, a dose of 100,000 IU once every two to four months by deep intramuscular injection is recommended subject to a regular check of vitamin A status.

*Children:* For children, and infants under one year of age, a dose of 50,000 IU by deep intramuscular injection once monthly is recommended.

*Elderly:* No specific studies of vitamin A have been performed in elderly patients but Vitamin A Palmitate has been widely used for many years in the dosages recommended for younger adults without apparent ill consequence.

Vitamin A Palmitate ampoule solution should not be diluted or mixed with other agents before injection. In particular mixing of the water miscible Vitamin A Palmitate ampoule solution with oil-based formulations (e.g. Calciferol Injection BP) may be expected to result in emulsification.

Vitamin A Palmitate ampoule solution is only suitable for deep intramuscular injection.

### Contra-indications, warnings, etc

*Contra-indications:* Use in patients with a known hypersensitivity to any of the constituents (see 'Precautions').

*Use in pregnancy:* High doses of vitamin A can be teratogenic. Vitamin A Palmitate is therefore contra-indicated during pregnancy.

*Precautions:* Small children are sometimes sensitive to single doses of 100,000 IU vitamin A. While children are taking Vitamin A Palmitate no other vitamin supplement containing vitamin A should be taken, unless under medical supervision.

Massive doses of vitamin A are required to produce toxicity and therefore it is extremely unlikely that even exceptionally large single doses would cause hypervitaminosis A, except possibly in children, and in patients with underlying liver disease where enhanced susceptibility to vitamin A toxicity should be anticipated.

Vitamin A Palmitate ampoules contain a polyethoxylated castor oil as solubiliser. In animal studies, polyethoxylated castor oil can produce severe anaphylactoid reactions associated with histamine release. There is strong circumstantial evidence that

similar reactions occurring in patients may have been caused by polyethoxylated castor oil. If such a reaction should occur the usual measures should be taken (e.g. administration of glucocorticoids and/or antihistamines).

Local injection site reactions have been reported following co-administration of Vitamin A Palmitate ampoules with oil based formulations.

Vitamin A Palmitate should not, therefore, be mixed with oil-based formulations.

*Side-effects and adverse reactions:* Yellowing of skin is one of the signs of toxicity associated with high doses.

*Overdose:* Manifestations of acute overdosage in children include severe headache, nausea or vomiting, drowsiness, irritability and pruritus. In chronic overdosage in children the following have been noted after periods of 2.5 to 15 months: hydrocephaly, alopecia, painful swelling over the long bones, with bone and joint pains, hyperostosis, and deep, hard, tender swellings in the extremities. Adults are likely to complain of bone and joint pains.

In the event of overdosage the vitamin should be discontinued. Symptoms of acute overdosage subside within 72 hours and of chronic overdosage over a period of several months, without further treatment.

### Pharmaceutical precautions

*Storage:* Vitamin A Palmitate ampoules should be protected from light and stored below 15°C.

If ampoules show signs of flocculation (as may be the case after unsuitable storage) they must not be used.

### Legal category  POM.

**Package quantities**  Vitamin A Palmitate ampoules in packs of 10.

**Further information**  Nil.

**Product licence number**  12070/0006.

# VITAMIN E SUSPENSION

**Presentation**  A water miscible suspension of tocopheryl acetate, 500 mg/5 ml. Also contains benzoic acid, castor oil polyethylene glycol ether, sorbic acid, sucrose and other ingredients.

### Uses

*Properties:* Vitamin E Suspension contains a synthetic vitamin E preparation. The exact role of vitamin E in the animal organism has not yet been established. Vitamin E is known to exert an important physiological function as an antioxidant for fats, with a sparing action on vitamin A, carotenoids and on unsaturated fatty acids. Other work has demonstrated that vitamin E is connected with the maintenance of certain factors essential for the normal metabolic cycle.

Vitamin E is absorbed from the gastro-intestinal tract. Most of the vitamin appears in the lymph and is then widely distributed to all tissues. Most of the dose is slowly excreted in the bile and the remainder is eliminated in the urine as glucuronides of tocopheronic acid or other metabolites.

*Indications:* Vitamin E Suspension is indicated for the correction of vitamin E deficiency occurring in malabsorption disorders, i.e. cystic fibrosis, chronic cholestasis and abetalipoproteinaemia.

### Dosage and administration

*Adults and the elderly:* For the treatment of malabsorption disorders the following doses should be administered:

cystic fibrosis                 100–200 mg/day
abetalipoproteinaemia   50–100 mg/kg/day

*Children:* For the treatment of cystic fibrosis a dose of 50 mg/day should be given to children less than 1 year of age and 100 mg/day to children 1 year and over.

The adult dosage should be used for the treatment of abetalipoproteinaemia (50–100 mg/kg/day).

Infants with vitamin E deficiency which is secondary to chronic cholestasis may be treated with doses of 150–200 mg/kg/day.

Vitamin E Suspension may be diluted with Syrup BP but should then be used immediately and not stored.

Vitamin E Suspension is for oral administration.

### Contra-indications, warnings, etc

*Contra-indications:* Known hypersensitivity to vitamin E.

*Use in pregnancy and lactation:* There is no evidence of the safety of high doses of vitamin E in pregnancy nor is there evidence from animal work that it is free from hazard, therefore do not use in pregnancy especially in the first trimester.

No information is available on excretion into breast milk, therefore it is advisable not to use Vitamin E Suspension during lactation.

*Precautions:* Vitamin E has been reported to increase the risk of thrombosis in patients who are predisposed to this condition, including patients taking oestrogens. This finding has not been confirmed but should be borne in mind when selecting patients for treatment with Vitamin E Suspension, in particular women taking oral contraceptives containing oestrogens.

A higher incidence of necrotising enterocolitis has been noted in lower weight premature infants (less than 1.5 kg) treated with vitamin E.

*Side-effects and adverse reactions:* Diarrhoea and abdominal pain may occur with doses greater than 1 g daily.

*Treatment of overdosage:* Transient gastro-intestinal disturbances have been reported with doses greater than 1 g daily and, where necessary, general supportive measures should be employed.

**Pharmaceutical precautions**  Vitamin E Suspension may be diluted with Syrup BP but the diluted suspension should be used immediately and not stored.

*Storage:* Vitamin E Suspension should be stored at or below 25°C and should be used within 1 month after opening the bottle.

**Legal category**  GSL.

**Package quantities**  Bottles of 100 ml.

**Further information**  Nil.

**Product licence number**  12070/0010.

*Trade Mark

# Centeon Limited
RPR House
52 St. Leonards Road
Eastbourne
East Sussex BN21 3YG

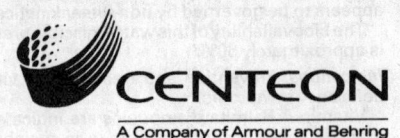

**CENTEON**
A Company of Armour and Behring

## ALBUMINAR*-5

**Presentation** Albuminar-5 is a sterile aqueous solution of Human Albumin 5% obtained from large pools of adult human venous plasma. Each 100 ml of Albuminar-5 contains 5 g of human albumin which is osmotically equivalent to normal human plasma.

The product conforms to the monograph for Human Albumin Solution PhEur.

Other ingredients are: Sodium acetyltryptophanate, sodium caprylate, sodium chloride, sodium bicarbonate, sodium hydroxide, glacial acetic acid, water for injection.

**Indications** Albuminar-5 is indicated in: The emergency treatment of shock and in other conditions where the restoration of blood volume is urgent.

Serious burns to prevent haemoconcentration and to combat fluid and sodium losses.

Clinical situations associated with low plasma protein (hypoproteinaemia) with or without oedema, provided that sodium restriction is not imperative.

Therapeutic Plasma Exchange as a replacement fluid for apheresed plasma.

**Dosage and administration** (a) *Administration:* Albuminar-5 is for intravenous infusion.

Albuminar-5 may be given intravenously without further dilution; 5% solution is approximately isotonic and isosmotic with citrated plasma.

When albumin solution is administered to patients with normal blood volume, particular attention should be given to the rate of infusion so that the plasma volume is not expanded too rapidly.

(b) *Standard dose: Urgent restoration of blood volume:* In the emergency treatment of shock, the amount of albumin and duration of therapy must be based on the responsiveness of the patient as indicated by blood pressure, central venous pressure, degree of pulmonary congestion and haematocrit. The initial dose may be followed by additional albumin within 15–30 minutes if the response is deemed inadequate. If there has been considerable loss of blood, transfusion with whole blood is indicated, or if there is continued loss of protein, blood or plasma it may also be desirable to give whole blood and/or other blood fractions.

*Burns:* Albuminar-5 may be used to prevent marked haemoconcentration and to maintain appropriate electrolyte balance. An optimal regimen involving the use of albumin, crystalloids and water has not been established. Suggested therapy in the treatment of burns includes administration of large volumes of crystalloid solution during the first 24 hours to maintain an adequate plasma volume, even when albumin is infused. Continuation of therapy beyond 24 hours usually requires more albumin and less crystalloid solution. Duration of treatment varies depending on the extent of protein loss through renal excretion, denuded areas of skin and decreased albumin synthesis. Attempts to raise the albumin level above 40 g/litre may only result in an increased rate of catabolism.

*Conditions associated with hypoproteinaemia:* In these conditions, 1,000 to 1,500 ml of Albuminar-5 may be required to reduce oedema and to bring serum protein values to normal. Since such patients usually have approximately normal blood volume, doses of more than 500 ml of Albuminar-5 should not be given faster than 500 ml in 30–45 minutes for acute replacement of protein lost in hypoproteinaemic conditions, with careful monitoring of cardiovascular status. Further therapy should be guided by clinical response, blood pressure and assessments of serum protein levels and degree of anaemia. If slower administration is desired, e.g. in patients with hypertension or cardiac insufficiency, 1,000 ml of Albuminar-5 may be administered by continuous drip at a rate of 100 ml of this solution per hour. Unless the pathological condition responsible for the hypoproteinaemia can be corrected, albumin in any form can afford only symptomatic or supportive relief. The 5% solution should not be administered in situations where sodium restriction is imperative.

*Therapeutic plasma exchange:* In plasma exchange procedures the volume of plasma removed may be replaced with an equivalent volume of Albuminar-5.

(c) *Children:* The amount of albumin given and the duration of therapy must be determined by the child's condition, response and other parameters, as stated under 'Standard Dose'. However, when treating children, their body weight should also be taken into account.

*Pharmacology: Action:* Albuminar-5 is active osmotically and is therefore important in regulating the volume of circulating blood. When the circulating blood volume has been depleted, the haemodilution following albumin administration persists for many hours. In individuals with normal blood volumes, it usually lasts only a few hours.

**Contra-indications, warnings, etc** *Contra-indications:* Albuminar-5 may be contra-indicated in patients with severe anaemia or cardiac failure or with known hypersensitivity to human albumin.

*Precautions:* If dehydration is present additional fluids must accompany or follow the administration of Albuminar-5.

The rise in blood pressure which may follow rapid administration of albumin necessitates careful observation of the injured patient to detect bleeding points which failed to bleed at the lower blood pressure; otherwise new haemorrhage and shock may occur.

Albuminar-5 should be administered with caution to patients with low cardiac reserve or with no albumin deficiency, because a rapid increase in plasma volume may cause circulatory embarrassment or pulmonary oedema. In cases of hypertension or cardiac insufficiency, a slower rate of administration is desirable, at a rate of 5 g of albumin (100 ml) per hour. A careful watch must be kept for the possible development of pulmonary oedema. Should pulmonary oedema occur, the infusion must be stopped immediately.

*Use in pregnancy:* There is some experience of albumin being used in the treatment of pre-eclampsia and eclampsia. However, there is very little experience of the use of albumin in the early stages of pregnancy. There is no evidence either in human pregnancy or in animal work that administration of albumin is free from hazard.

*Warnings and adverse effects:* Do not use if the solution is turbid or contains a deposit. Since the solution contains no preservative, it should be used within 3 hours after entering the vial.

The incidence of adverse reactions to human albumin 5% is low, although nausea, vomiting, increased salivation, urticaria and febrile reactions may occasionally occur. Anaphylactic reactions may rarely occur, in which cases the infusion should be stopped and appropriate treatment initiated.

When medical products prepared from human blood or plasma are administered, infectious diseases due to the transmission of infective agents cannot be totally excluded. This applies also to pathogens of hitherto unknown nature. See also 'Further information'.

*Toxicity and treatment of overdosage:* Administration of large quantities of albumin should be supplemented with red cell concentrates or replaced by whole blood to combat the relative anaemia which would follow such use. If circulatory embarrassment or pulmonary oedema should develop, the infusion must be stopped immediately and specific treatment given.

**Pharmaceutical precautions**
(a) *Presentation and Composition:* Albuminar-5 is a sterile, clear, yellowish, slightly viscous aqueous solution of human serum albumin. It is stabilised with 0.004 M sodium acetyltryptophanate and 0.004 M sodium caprylate and the pH of the solution is adjusted with sodium bicarbonate or acetic acid. The solution contains approximately 145 mmol/l of sodium and not more than 200 micrograms/l of aluminium. The solution contains no preservative.

(b) *Incompatibilities:* Albuminar-5 should not be mixed with protein hydrolysates, amino acid mixtures or solutions containing alcohol.

(c) *Storage:* Albuminar-5 should be stored at a temperature between 2° and 25°C. Freezing will not harm the solution, but might damage the container and allow contamination of the contents.

Protect solution from light.

When stored as directed Albuminar-5 has a shelf-life of 3 years.

**Legal category** POM.

**Package quantities**
Albuminar-5 is supplied as a 5% solution in:
250 ml glass vials containing 12.5 grams of albumin
500 ml glass vials containing 25.0 grams of albumin
1,000 ml glass vials containing 50.0 grams of albumin.

**Further information** The source plasma or blood from which Albuminar-5 is prepared has been tested and found non-reactive for hepatitis B surface antigen (HBsAg), negative for antibody to hepatitis C and negative for antibody to human immunodeficiency viruses (Anti-HIV-1-and Anti-HIV-2). In addition, Albuminar-5 is pasteurized at 60°C for 10 hours, a procedure designed to reduce the risks of viral transmission. So prepared, Albuminar-5, unlike whole blood or plasma, has not been associated with homologous serum hepatitis or AIDS transmission.

Albuminar-5 may be given in conjunction with other parenteral fluids, such as whole blood, plasma, saline, dextrose, or sodium lactate. It is convenient to use, since no cross-matching is required and the absence of cellular elements removes the danger of sensitisation with repeated infusions.

Albuminar-5 contains none of the recognised components of the clotting mechanism of normal blood or plasma. It does not interfere with the normal clotting of blood.

**Product licence number** 0231/0056.

## ALBUMINAR-20

**Presentation** Albuminar-20 is a sterile aqueous solution of Human Albumin 20% obtained from large pools of adult human venous plasma. Each 100 ml of Albuminar-20 contains 20 g of human serum albumin which is osmotically equivalent to 400 ml of normal human plasma.

Other ingredients are: Sodium acetyltryptophanate, sodium caprylate, sodium chloride, sodium bicarbonate, sodium hydroxide, glacial acetic acid, water for injection.

The product conforms to the monograph for Human Albumin Solution Ph Eur.

**Indications** Albuminar-20 is indicated in: The emergency treatment of shock and in other conditions where the restoration of blood volume is urgent.

Serious burns to prevent haemoconcentration and to combat fluid and sodium losses.

Clinical situations associated with low plasma protein (hypoproteinaemia) with or without oedema.

As an adjunct to exchange transfusion for the treatment of hyperbilirubinaemia in haemolytic disease of the newborn.

In priming heart lung machines for cardiopulmonary by-pass surgery.

**Dosage and administration**
(a) *Administration:* Albuminar-20 is for intravenous infusion.

Albuminar-20 may be given intravenously without dilution or it may be diluted with normal saline or 5% dextrose before administration, 250 ml per litre gives a solution which is approximately isotonic and isosmotic with citrated plasma.

When undiluted albumin solution is administered to patients with normal blood volume, particular attention should be given to the rate of infusion so that the plasma volume is not expanded too rapidly.

(b) *Standard dose: Urgent restoration of blood volume:* In these conditions the effectiveness of Albuminar-20 depends on its ability to draw tissue fluid into the blood stream, when such fluid is available. Therefore, if dehydration is present, other fluids must be administered by any available route, either with albumin or following it. In the emergency treatment of shock, the amount of albumin and duration of therapy must be based on the responsiveness of the patient as indicated by blood pressure, central venous pressure, degree of pulmonary congestion and haematocrit. The initial dose may be followed by additional albumin within 15–30 minutes if the response is deemed inadequate. If there has been considerable loss of blood, transfusion with whole blood is indicated, or if there is continued loss of protein, blood or plasma it may also be desirable to give whole blood and/or other blood fractions.

*Burns:* Albuminar-20 may be used in conjunction with normal saline or dextrose to prevent marked haemoconcentration and to maintain appropriate electrolyte balance. An optimal regimen involving the use of albumin, crystalloids and water has not been established. Suggested therapy in the treatment of burns includes administration of large volumes of crystalloid solution during the first 24 hours to maintain an adequate plasma volume, even when albumin is infused. Continuation of therapy beyond 24 hours usually requires more albumin and less crystalloid solution. Duration of treatment varies depending on the extent of protein loss through renal excretion, denuded areas of skin and decreased albumin synthesis. Attempts to raise the albumin level above 40 g/litre may only result in an increased rate of catabolism.

*Conditions associated with hypoproteinaemia:* In these conditions, 200 to 300 ml of Albuminar-20 may be required to reduce oedema and to bring serum protein values to normal. Since such patients usually have approximately normal blood volume, doses of more than 100 ml of Albuminar-20 should not be given faster than 100 ml in 30–45 minutes for acute replacement of protein lost in hypoproteinaemic conditions, with careful monitoring of cardiovascular status. Further therapy should be guided by clinical response, blood pressure and assessments of serum protein levels and degree of anaemia. If slower administration is desired, e.g. in patients with hypertension or cardiac insufficiency, 250 ml of Albuminar-20 may be mixed with 250 ml of 10% dextrose solution and administered by continuous drip at a rate of 100 ml of this dextrose solution per hour. Unless the pathological condition responsible for the hypoproteinaemia can be corrected, albumin in any form can afford only symptomatic or supportive relief.

*Hyperbilirubinaemia in haemolytic disease of the newborn:* In neonates, with serum bilirubin levels above 20 mg per 100 ml severe cerebral damage can develop due to kernicterus. In hypoalbuminaemia the reserve binding capacity for bilirubin is decreased and consequently bilirubin toxicity increases and with it the risk of cerebral damage. The risk of cerebral damage can be reduced by correction of the bilirubin binding capacity with Albuminar-20.

If immediate protection of the patient is required an intravenous injection of 1.0–1.5 g/kg albumin (5–7 ml Albuminar-20/kg bodyweight) can be given. Following this injection the exchange transfusion procedure should be instituted within 6 hours.

If albumin is intended for increasing the removal of bilirubin during exchange transfusion, it is suggested that 1.5–2.5 g albumin (7–12 ml Albuminar-20) is added to each 100 ml donor blood during exchange transfusion.

*In Priming Heart Lung Machines for Cardiopulmonary By-Pass Surgery:* Pre-operative dilution of the blood by use of a pump prime consisting of only albumin and crystalloid has been shown to be well tolerated during clinical studies. An albumin concentration of 5 g per cent has been widely used. A commonly employed programme is an albumin and crystalloid pump prime adjusted so as to achieve a haematocrit reading of 20 per cent and a plasma albumin level of 2.5 g/100 ml in the patient.

(c) *Children:* The amount of albumin given and the duration of therapy must be determined by the child's condition, response and other parameters, as stated under 'Standard Dose'. However, when treating children, their body weight should also be taken into account.

*Pharmacology: Action:* Albuminar-20 is active osmotically and is therefore important in regulating the volume of circulating blood. When injected intravenously, 50 ml of Albuminar-20 draws approximately 3 volumes of additional fluid into the circulation within 15 minutes, except in the presence of marked dehydration. This extra fluid reduces haematocrit and blood viscosity. The degree of volume expansion is dependent on the initial blood volume. When circulating blood volume has been depleted, the haemodilution following albumin administration persists for many hours. In individuals with normal blood volume, it usually lasts only a few hours.

### Contra-indications, warnings, etc

*Contra-indications:* Albuminar-20 may be contra-indicated in patients with severe anaemia or cardiac failure or with known hypersensitivity to human albumin.

*Precautions:* If dehydration is present additional fluids must accompany or follow the administration of Albuminar-20.

The rise in blood pressure which may follow rapid administration of albumin necessitates careful observation of the injured patient to detect bleeding points which failed to bleed at the lower blood pressure; otherwise new haemorrhage and shock may occur.

Albuminar-20 should be administered with caution to patients with low cardiac reserve or with no albumin deficiency, because a rapid increase in plasma volume may cause circulatory embarrassment or pulmonary oedema. In cases of hypertension or cardiac insufficiency, a slower rate of administration is desirable: 250 ml of Albuminar-20 may be mixed with 250 ml of 10% dextrose solution and administered at a rate of 10 g of albumin (100 ml) per hour. A careful watch must be kept for the possible development of pulmonary oedema. Should pulmonary oedema occur, the infusion must be stopped immediately.

*Use in pregnancy:* There is some experience of albumin being used in the treatment of pre-eclampsia and eclampsia. However, there is very little experience of the use of albumin in the early stages of pregnancy. There is no evidence either in human pregnancy or in animal work that administration of albumin is free from hazard.

*Warnings and adverse effects:* Do not use if the solution is turbid or contains a deposit. Since the solution contains no preservative, it should be used within 3 hours after entering the vial.

The incidence of adverse reactions to human albumin 20% is low, although nausea, vomiting, increased salivation, urticaria and febrile reactions may occasionally occur. Anaphylactic reactions may rarely occur, in which cases the infusion should be stopped and appropriate treatment initiated.

When medical products prepared from human blood or plasma are administered, infectious diseases due to the transmission of infective agents cannot be totally excluded. This applies also to pathogens of hitherto unknown nature. See also 'Further information'.

*Toxicity and treatment of overdosage:* Administration of large quantities of albumin should be supplemented with red cell concentrates or replaced by whole blood to combat the relative anaemia which would follow such use.

If circulatory embarrassment or pulmonary oedema should develop, the infusion must be stopped immediately and specific treatment given.

### Pharmaceutical precautions

(a) *Presentation and composition:* Albuminar-20 is a sterile, clear, brownish, slightly viscous aqueous solution of human albumin. It is stabilised with 0.016 M sodium acetyltryptophanate and 0.016 M sodium caprylate and the pH of the solution is adjusted with sodium bicarbonate or acetic acid. The solution contains approximately 145 mmol/l of sodium and not more than 200 micrograms/l of aluminium. The solution contains no preservative.

(b) *Incompatibilities:* Albuminar-20 should not be mixed with protein hydrolysates, amino acid mixtures or solutions containing alcohol.

(c) *Storage:* Albuminar-20 should be stored at a temperature between 2° and 25°C. Freezing will not harm the solution, but might damage the container and allow contamination of the contents. Protect solution from light.

When stored as directed, Albuminar-20 has a shelf-life of 3 years.

### Legal category POM.

### Package quantities Albuminar-20 is supplied as a 20% solution in:

50 ml vials containing 10.0 grams of albumin;
100 ml vials containing 20.0 grams of albumin.

### Further information

The source plasma or blood from which Albuminar-20 is prepared has been tested with licensed reagents and found non-reactive for hepatitis B surface antigen (HBsAg), negative for antibody to hepatitis C and negative for antibody to human immunodeficiency viruses (Anti-HIV-1 and Anti-HIV-2). In addition, Albuminar-20 is pasteurized at 60°C for 10 hours, a procedure designed to reduce the risks of viral transmission. So prepared, Albuminar-20, unlike whole blood or plasma, has not been associated with homologous serum hepatitis of AIDS transmission.

Albuminar-20 may be given in conjunction with other parenteral fluids, such as whole blood, plasma, saline, dextrose, or sodium lactate. It is convenient to use, since no cross-matching is required and the absence of cellular elements removes the danger of sensitisation with repeated infusions.

Albuminar-20 contains none of the recognised components of the clotting mechanism of normal blood or plasma. It does not interfere with the normal clotting of blood.

### Product licence number 0231/0057

## ALBUMINAR-25

### Presentation
Albuminar-25 is a sterile aqueous solution of Human Albumin 25% obtained from large pools of adult human venous plasma. Each 100 ml of Albuminar-25 contains 25 g of human serum albumin which is osmotically equivalent to 500 ml of normal human plasma.

Other ingredients are: Sodium acetyltryptophanate, sodium caprylate, sodium chloride, sodium bicarbonate, sodium hydroxide, glacial acetic acid, water for injection.

The product conforms to the monograph for Human Albumin Solution PhEur.

### Indications
Albuminar-25 is indicated in: The emergency treatment of shock and in other conditions where the restoration of blood volume is urgent.

Serious burns to prevent haemoconcentration and to combat fluid and sodium losses.

Clinical situations associated with low plasma protein (hypoproteinaemia) with or without oedema.

As an adjunct to exchange transfusion for the treatment of hyperbilirubinaemia in haemolytic disease of the newborn.

In priming heart-lung machines for cardiopulmonary by-pass surgery.

### Dosage and administration

(a) *Administration:* Albuminar-25 is for intravenous infusion.

Albuminar-25 may be given intravenously without dilution or it may be diluted with normal saline or 5% dextrose before administration; 200 ml per litre gives a solution which is approximately isotonic and isosmotic with citrated plasma.

When undiluted albumin solution is administered to patients with normal blood volume, particular attention should be given to the rate of infusion so that it is slow enough to prevent too rapid expansion of plasma volume.

(b) *Standard dose: Urgent restoration of blood volume:* In these conditions the effectiveness of Albuminar-25 depends on its ability to draw tissue fluid into the blood stream, when such fluid is available. Therefore, if dehydration is present, other fluids must be administered by any available route, either with albumin or following it. In the emergency treatment of shock, the amount of albumin and duration of therapy must be based on the responsiveness of the patient as indicated by blood pressure, central venous pressure, degree of pulmonary congestion and haematocrit. The initial dose may be followed by additional albumin within 15–30 minutes if the response is deemed inadequate. If there has been considerable loss of blood, transfusion with whole blood is indicated, or if there is continued loss of protein, blood or plasma it may also be desirable to give whole blood and/or other blood fractions.

*Burns:* Albuminar-25 may be used in conjunction with normal saline or dextrose to prevent marked haemoconcentration and to maintain appropriate electrolyte balance. An optimal regimen involving the use of albumin, crystalloids and water has not been established. Suggested therapy in the treatment of burns includes administration of large volumes of crystalloid solution during the first 24 hours to maintain an adequate plasma volume, even when albumin is infused. Continuation of therapy beyond 24 hours usually requires more albumin and less crystalloid solution. Duration of treatment varies depending on the extent of protein loss through renal excretion, denuded areas of skin and decreased albumin synthesis. Attempts to raise the albumin level above 40 g/litre may only result in an increased rate of catabolism.

*Conditions associated with hypoproteinaemia:* In these conditions, 200 to 300 ml of Albuminar-25 may be required to reduce oedema and to bring serum protein values to normal. Since such patients usually have approximately normal blood volume, doses of more than 100 ml of Albuminar-25 should not be given faster than 100 ml in 30–45 minutes for acute replacement of protein lost in hypoproteinaemic conditions, with careful monitoring of cardiovascular status. Further therapy should be guided by clinical response, blood pressure and assessments of serum protein levels and degree of anaemia. If slower administration is desired, e.g. in patients with hypertension or cardiac insufficiency, 200 ml of Albuminar-25 may be mixed with 300 ml of 10% dextrose solution and administered by continuous drip at a rate of 100 ml of this dextrose solution per hour. Unless the pathological condition responsible for the hypoproteinaemia can be corrected, albumin in any form can afford only symptomatic or supportive relief.

*Hyperbilirubinaemia in haemolytic disease of the newborn:* In neonates with serum bilirubin levels above 20 mg per 100 ml severe cerebral damage can develop due to kernicterus. In hypoalbuminaemia the reserve binding capacity for bilirubin is decreased and consequently bilirubin toxicity increases and with it the risk of cerebral damage. The risk of cerebral damage can be reduced by correction of the bilirubin binding capacity with Albuminar-25.

If immediate protection of the patient is required an intravenous injection of 1.0–1.5 g/kg albumin (4–6 ml Albuminar-25/kg bodyweight) can be given. Following this injection the exchange transfusion procedure should be instituted within 6 hours.

If albumin is intended for increasing the removal of bilirubin during exchange transfusion, it is suggested that 1.5–2.5 g albumin (6–10 ml Albuminar-25) is added to each 100 ml donor blood during exchange transfusion.

*In Priming Heart Lung Machines for Cardiopulmonary By-Pass Surgery:* Pre-operative dilution of the blood by use of a pump prime consisting of only albumin and crystalloid has been shown to be well tolerated during clinical studies. An albumin concentration of 5 g per cent has been widely used. A commonly employed programme is an albumin and crystalloid pump prime adjusted so as to achieve a haematocrit reading of 20 per cent and a plasma albumin level of 2.5 g/100 ml in the patient.

(c) *Children*: The amount of albumin given and the duration of therapy must be determined by the child's condition, response and other parameters, as stated under 'Standard Dose'. However, when treating children, their body weight should also be taken into account.

*Pharmacology: Action:* Albuminar-25 is active osmotically and is therefore important in regulating the volume of circulating blood. When injected intravenously, 50 ml of Albuminar-25 draws approximately 175 ml of additional fluid into the circulation within 15 minutes, except in the presence of marked dehydration. This extra fluid reduces haematocrit and blood viscosity. The degree of volume expansion is dependent on the initial blood volume. When circulating blood volume has been depleted, the haemodilution following albumin administration persists for many hours. In individuals with normal blood volume, it usually lasts only a few hours.

**Contra-indications, warnings, etc**
*Contra-indications:* Albuminar-25 may be contra-indicated in patients with severe anaemia or cardiac failure or with known hypersensitivity to human albumin.

*Precautions:* If dehydration is present additional fluids must accompany or follow the administration of Albuminar-25.

The rise in blood pressure which may follow rapid administration of albumin necessitates careful observation of the injured patient to detect bleeding points which failed to bleed at the lower blood pressure; otherwise new haemorrhage and shock may occur.

Albuminar-25 should be administered with caution to patients with low cardiac reserve or with no albumin deficiency, because a rapid increase in plasma volume may cause circulatory embarrassment or pulmonary oedema. In cases of hypertension or cardiac insufficiency, a slower rate of administration is desirable: 200 ml of Albuminar-25 may be mixed with 300 ml of 10% dextrose solution and administered at a rate of 10 g of albumin (100 ml) per hour. A careful watch must be kept for the possible development of pulmonary oedema. Should pulmonary oedema occur, the infusion must be stopped immediately.

*Use in pregnancy:* There is some experience of albumin being used in the treatment of pre-eclampsia and eclampsia. However, there is very little experience of the use of albumin in the early stages of pregnancy. There is no evidence either in human pregnancy or in animal work that administration of albumin is free from hazard.

*Warnings and adverse effects:* Do not use if the solution is turbid or contains a deposit. Since the solution contains no preservative, it should be used within 3 hours after entering the vial.

The incidence of adverse reactions to human albumin 25% is low, although nausea, vomiting, increased salivation, urticaria and febrile reactions may occasionally occur. Anaphylactic reactions may rarely occur, in which case the infusion should be stopped and appropriate treatment initiated.

When medicinal products prepared from human blood or plasma are administered, infectious diseases due to the transmission of infective agents cannot be totally excluded. This applies also to pathogens of hitherto unknown nature.

*Toxicity and treatment of overdosage:* Administration of large quantities of albumin should be supplemented with red cell concentrates or replaced by whole blood to combat the relative anaemia which would follow such use.

If circulatory embarrassment or pulmonary oedema should develop, the infusion must be stopped immediately and specific treatment given.

**Pharmaceutical precautions**
(a) *Presentation and composition:* Albuminar-25 is a sterile, clear, brownish, slightly viscous aqueous solution of human albumin. It is stabilised with 0.02 M sodium acetyltryptophanate and 0.02 M sodium caprylate and the pH of the solution is adjusted with sodium bicarbonate or acetic acid. The solution contains approximately 145 mmol/l of sodium and not more than 200 micrograms/l of aluminium. The solution contains no preservative.

(b) *Incompatibilities:* Albuminar-25 should not be mixed with protein hydrolysates, amino acid mixtures or solutions containing alcohol.

(c) *Storage:* Albuminar-25 should be stored at a temperature between 2° and 25°C. Freezing will not harm the solution, but might damage the container and allow contamination of the contents. Protect solution from light.

When stored as directed, Albuminar-25 has a shelf-life of 3 years.

**Legal category** POM

**Package quantities** Albuminar-25 is supplied as a 25% solution in:
 50 ml vials containing 12.5 grams of albumin;
 100 ml vials containing 25.0 grams of albumin.

**Further information** The source plasma or blood from which Albuminar-25 is prepared has been tested with licensed reagents and found non-reactive for hepatitis B surface antigen (HBsAg), negative for antibody to hepatitis C and negative for antibody to human immunodeficiency viruses (Anti-HIV-1 and Anti-HIV-2). In addition, Albuminar-25 is pasteurized at 60°C for 10 hours, a procedure designed to reduce the risks of viral transmission. So prepared, Albuminar-25, unlike whole blood or plasma, has not been associated with homologous serum hepatitis or AIDS transmission.

Albuminar-25 may be given in conjunction with other parenteral fluids, such as whole blood, plasma, saline, dextrose, or sodium lactate. It is convenient to use, since no cross-matching is required and the absence of cellular elements removes the danger of sensitisation with repeated infusions.

Albuminar-25 contains none of the recognised components of the clotting mechanism of normal blood or plasma. It does not interfere with the normal clotting of blood.

**Product licence number** 0231/0045.

# HAEMATE P* ▼

**Presentation** Haemate P (Factor VIII HS, heat treated) is presented in clear glass vials containing 250 or 500 units of Factor VIII as a lyophilised concentrate. When reconstituted with the vial of solvent provided, the solution will contain 25 IU Factor VIII per ml.

**Uses** Prophylaxis and therapy of haemorrhages in Hemophilia A and other diseases with Factor VIII deficiency.

**Dosage and administration** Unless prescribed otherwise the dosage should depend on the degree of Factor VIII deficiency and the extent and location of the bleeding. The amount of Factor VIII required can be estimated as follows: On administration of 1 IU/kg body-weight a rise in Factor VIII activity by about 1% of the normal is to be expected.

In the case of the following haemorrhagic events, the Factor VIII activity should not fall below the given level (in per cent of normal) in the corresponding period:

| Haemorrhagic event | Therapeutically necessary blood level of Factor VIII | Period during which it is necessary to maintain the therapeutic blood level |
| --- | --- | --- |
| 1. Haemorrhages into joints; Gastro-intestinal haemorrhages; Bite injuries in the oral cavity; Slighter injuries (where local therapy is unsuccessful) | 10–20% | 2–3 days |
| 2. Haemorrhages into muscles; Larger injuries; Minor operations; (Teeth extractions) | 20–30% | 3–4 days |
| 3. Intracranial, intra-abdominal or intrathoracic haemorrhages; Medium operations; Fractures | 30–50% | 4–14 days or until wound completely healed. |
| 4. Major operations | over 50% | 14–21 days or until wound completely healed |

The amount to be administered should always be oriented to the clinical effectiveness in the individual case. Under certain circumstances larger amounts than those calculated can be required, especially in the case of the initial dose.

In the case of major surgical interventions in particular, a precise monitoring of the substitution therapy by means of coagulation analyses is indispensable.

*Administration:* The contents of one vial should be dissolved, by slow swirling of the vial, in the appropriate amount of water for injection previously brought to 20°-37°C. The material will dissolve in less than 10 minutes to give a clear to slightly opalescent solution.

*Injection:* Using a filter needle, withdraw solution from the vial into a syringe. Inject the solution slowly (maximum 4 ml per minute) intravenously. Administration may be effected with the infusion set or with a suitable injection needle. Do not use the filter needle for injection.

*Infusion:* Dissolve the preparation as described and infuse slowly by means of a disposable transfusion set (with filter inset).

**Contra-indications, warnings, etc**
*Contra-indications:* None known.

*Warnings:* In the case of patients with known allergic diathesis, antihistamines and corticosteroids should be administered as prophylaxis. Caution should be observed in cases of impaired liver or kidney function.

In the case of massive therapy, symptoms of hypervolaemia and–in rare cases–haemolytic reactions through blood-group isoagglutinins should be watched for.

The therapeutic effect may not be achieved if the blood of the patient contains a high level of inhibitors for Factor VIII ('inhibitor hemophilia'). In such cases an attempt must be made to override the inhibitors by administration of large amounts of Factor VIII.

This concentrate has been prepared from large pools of human plasma non-reactive for hepatitis B surface antigen (HbsAg). However, such plasma may contain one or more causative agents of viral hepatitis. Haemate P is heated to 60°C for 10 hours in solution form. However, no procedure has been shown to be totally effective in removing hepatitis infectivity from Antihemophilic Factor (Human).

*Side-effects:* Haemate P is usually tolerated without reaction. Rare cases of allergic reactions and rise in temperature have been observed. Therapeutic countermeasures depend on nature and severity of the side-effect. In the case of slight reactions, corticosteroids and antihistamines may be used.

In the case of severe reactions (anaphylactic shock), immediate discontinuation of the preparation and injection of adrenalin slowly iv supplemented by high doses of corticosteroids slowly iv.

**Pharmaceutical precautions** Haemate P should be stored in a refrigerator at +2°C to +8°C and used on or before the expiry date given on the pack. The dissolved preparation should be used within 3 hours of reconstitution.

**Legal category** POM.

**Package quantities** The product is supplied as a single vial with an ampoule containing Water for Injections.

**Further information** Haemate P is a specific hemostatic agent for intravenous application in hemophilia A. The lyophilised preparation is sterile and pyrogen-free and does not contain any preservative. No fibrinogen can be detected by the Clauss method.

Haemate P is obtained from HBsAg-negative and anti HIV-negative plasma of healthy donors. In addition the ALT in the plasma is determined and donations with pathological values are rejected. The pasteurisation process, heating to 60°C for 10 hours in solution form, has been shown to inactivate several DNA viruses (Epstein Barr, cytomegalovirus, herpes simplex and hepatitis B) and RNA viruses (rubella, mumps, measles, poliomyelitis and HIV), and the pathogens of hepatitis non-A/non-B (Hutchison Pool).

Haemate P prepared from cryoprecipitate experimentally infected with Hepatitis B virus was given to chimpanzees. After 6 and 9 months follow-up the test animals remained serologically negative.

**Product licence number** 15036/0001.

*Product licence holder:* Centeon Pharma GmbH, PO Box 1230, 35002 Marburg, Germany.

# MONOCLATE-P*

**Presentation** Sterile vials containing nominally 250, 500 or 1000iu Freeze Dried Human Coagulation Factor VIII Ph Eur, highly purified by affinity chromatography using a murine antibody to von Willebrand's Factor.

Supplied with Water for Injection for reconstitution prior to intravenous administration.

The concentrate as formulated contains pasteurised Human Albumin Solution as a stabiliser, resulting in a concentrate with a specific activity between 5 and 10 units/mg of total protein. In the absence of this pasteurised Human Albumin stabiliser, specific activity has been determined to exceed 3000 units/mg of protein.

The lyophilised vials also contain sodium chloride, histidine, calcium chloride and mannitol.

The product has been pasteurised in aqueous solution at 60°C for 10 hours during manufacture to further reduce the risk of viral transmission.

**Uses** Monoclate-P is indicated for the treatment of classical haemophilia (Haemophilia A). Affected individuals frequently require therapy following minor accidents. Surgery, when required in such individuals, must be preceded by temporary correction of the clotting abnormality. Pre-surgical correction of severe Factor VIII (AHF) deficiency can be accomplished with a small volume of Monoclate-P.

Monoclate-P is not effective in controlling the bleeding of patients with von Willebrand's disease.

**Dosage and administration** Freeze-Dried Human Coagulation Factor VIII, Monoclate-P, Factor VIII: C Pasteurised is for intravenous administration only. As a general rule one unit of Factor VIII activity per kg will increase the circulating Factor VIII by 2%. The following formula provides a guide for dosage calculations:

$$\text{Number of Factor VIII IU Required} = \frac{\text{Body weight}}{\text{(in kg)}} \times \frac{\text{desired Factor VIII}}{\text{increase (\% normal)}} \times 0.5$$

Although dosage must be individualised according to the needs of the patient (weight, severity of haemorrhage, presence of inhibitors), the following general dosages are suggested.

*Mild haemorrhages:* Minor haemorrhagic episodes will generally subside with a single infusion if a level of 30% of normal or more is attained.

*Moderate haemorrhage and minor surgery:* For more serious haemorrhages and minor surgical procedures, the patient's Factor VIII level should be raised to 30–50% of normal, which usually requires an initial dose of 15–25 IU per kg. If further therapy is required a maintenance dose is 10–15 IU per kg every 8–12 hours.

*Severe haemorrhage:* In haemorrhages near vital organs (neck, throat, subperitoneal) it may be desirable to raise the Factor VIII level to 80–100% of normal which can be achieved with an initial dose of 40–50 IU per kg and a maintenance dose of 20–25 IU per kg every 8–12 hours.

*Major surgery:* For surgical procedures a dose of Factor VIII sufficient to achieve a level 80–100% of normal should be given an hour prior to surgery. A second dose, half the size of the priming dose, should be given five hours after the first dose. Factor VIII levels should be maintained at a daily minimum of at least 30% of normal for a period of 10–14 days post-operatively. Close laboratory control to maintain Factor VIII plasma levels deemed appropriate to maintain haemostasis is recommended.

*Reconstitution and administration:* Specific instructions for reconstitution and administration are included on the package insert and patient instruction leaflet.

Monoclate-P is for intravenous injection only. Plastic disposable syringes are recommended with Monoclate-P solution. The ground glass surfaces of all-glass syringes tend to stick with solutions of this type.

A winged infusion needle with microbore tubing is supplied with each pack. Use of other winged needles without microbore tubing, although compatible with the concentrate, will result in a larger retention of solution within the infusion set.

**Contra-indications, warnings, etc**
*Contra-indications:* None known.

*Warnings:* Monoclate-P is prepared from pooled units of human plasma which may contain the causative agents of hepatitis B, non-A non-B hepatitis (hepatitis C), acquired immune deficiency syndrome (AIDS) and other viral diseases. Each unit of plasma used in the production of Monoclate-P has been tested and found nonreactive for hepatitis B surface antigen ($HB_sAg$), negative for antibody to human immunodeficiency viruses (Anti-HIV-1 and Anti-HIV-2) and negative for antibody to hepatitis C virus by FDA approved tests, and has been shown to have ALT levels not exceeding two times the upper limit of normal. Additional screening procedures used to eliminate high risk plasma donors, and the purification techniques and pasteurisation step used in the manufacturing process, are all designed to reduce the risk of transmitting viral infection. However, testing methods presently available are not sensitive enough to detect all units of potentially infectious plasma, and treatment methods have not been shown to be totally effective in eliminating any of the aforementioned viral diseases from this concentrate. Accordingly, the benefits and risks of treatment with this concentrate should be carefully assessed prior to use.

Individuals who have not received multiple infusions of blood or plasma products are likely to develop signs and/or symptoms of some viral infections, especially non-A non-B hepatitis as shown by recent data, when treated with coagulant factor concentrates. However, a group of such patients treated with Monoclate, Heat-Treated, did not demonstrate signs or symptoms of a non-A, non-B hepatitis over observation periods ranging from 6 months to 36 months.

*Precautions:* Patients should be informed of the early signs of hypersensitivity reactions including hives, generalised urticaria, tightness of the chest, wheezing, hypotension and anaphylaxis, and should be advised to discontinue use of the concentrate and contact their physician if these symptoms occur.

*Adverse reactions:* Products of this type are known to cause allergic reactions, mild chills, nausea or stinging at the infusion site.

**Pharmaceutical precautions** Monoclate-P should not be mixed with other drugs before injection.

*Storage:* When stored at refrigerator temperature, 2°–8°C (36°–46°F), Monoclate-P, is stable for the period indicated by the expiration date on its label. Within this period, Monoclate-P may be stored at room temperature not to exceed 30°C (86°F), for up to six months. Avoid freezing which may damage the container for the diluent.

**Legal category** POM.

**Package quantities** Monoclate-P is supplied in a single dose vial. IU activity is stated on the label of each vial. Nominal strengths available are 250, 500 and 1000 IU. A patient user kit is supplied with each vial of Monoclate-P. The kit includes a vial of sterile Water for Injections, sterile 10 ml plastic syringe, sterile vented filter spike, sterile winged infusion set, sterile double ended transfer needle, sterile plaster dressing, disposable alcohol swabs and plastic disposal bag.

**Further information** Upon reconstitution, a clear, colourless solution is obtained, containing 50 to 150 times as much Factor VIII: C as does an equivalent volume of plasma.

Each vial contains the labelled amount of Factor VIII: C activity as expressed in terms of International Units of Factor VIII: C activity. One unit of antihaemophilic activity is equivalent to that quantity of Factor VIII: C present in one ml of normal human plasma. When reconstituted as recommended, the resulting solution contains approximately 300 to 450 millimoles of sodium ions per litre and has 2–3 times the tonicity of saline. It contains approximately 2–5 millimoles of calcium per litre, contributed as calcium chloride, approximately 1–2% pasteurised Human Albumin Solution, 0.8% mannitol, and 1.2 mM histidine. The pH is adjusted with hydrochloric acid and/or sodium hydroxide. Monoclate-P also contains trace amounts (less than 50 ng per 100 IU Factor VIII) of mouse protein.

The half-life of the second elimination phase in haemophiliacs is 17.5±4.8 hours and recovery 1.9 units/dl increase per unit per kg BW (95%) which is comparable to other commercially available Factor VIII products.

The pasteurisation process used in the manufacture of this concentrate has demonstrated in vitro inactivation of 10.5 logs of Human Immunodeficiency Virus (HIV-1) and 7.8 logs of murine encephalomyocarditis (EMC), a non-lipid encapsulated model virus were inactivated to undetectable levels.

The purification and preparative steps used in the production of Monoclate-P are capable of providing a non-specific viral reduction of approximately 5–6 logs independent of the pasteurisation process.

**Product licence numbers**

| | |
|---|---|
| 250 IU/vial | 0231/0090 |
| 500 IU/vial | 0231/0091 |
| 1,000 IU/vial | 0231/0092 |
| Diluent | 0231/0107 |

## MONONINE*

**Presentation** Mononine (Freeze Dried Human Coagulation Factor IX PhEur) is supplied as a sterile freeze dried concentrate in single dose vials of nominally 250, 500 or 1000 International Units (iu) with diluent for intravenous administration. Other ingredients include histidine (approximately) 10 mM), sodium chloride (approximately 66 mM) and mannitol (approximately 165 mM).

Unlike lower purity concentrates of Factor IX which are typically complexes of Factor IX with other vitamin K-dependent clotting factors, this product is further purified by a process which includes affinity chromatography using a murine antibody.

**Uses** Mononine is indicated for the prevention and control of bleeding in Factor IX deficiency, also known as Haemophilia B or Christmas disease.

Mononine is not indicated in the treatment or prophylaxis of Haemophilia A patients with inhibitors to Factor VIII. It contains non-detectable levels of Factors II, VII and X and is, therefore, not indicated for replacement therapy of these clotting factors. Mononine is also not indicated in the treatment or reversal of coumarin-induced anticoagulation or in a haemorrhagic state caused by hepatitis-induced lack of production of liver dependent coagulation factors.

**Dosage and administration** Mononine is intended for intravenous administration only. It should be reconstituted with the volume of Water for Injections PhEur supplied with the batch, and administered within three hours of reconstitution. Do not refrigerate after reconstitution. After administration, any unused solution and the administration equipment should be discarded.

As a general rule, one unit of Factor IX activity per kg can be expected to increase the circulating level of Factor IX by 1% of normal. The following formula provides a guide for dosage calculations:

$$\begin{matrix}\text{Number of} \\ \text{Factor IX iu} \\ \text{required}\end{matrix} = \begin{matrix}\text{Body} \\ \text{weight} \\ \text{(in kg)}\end{matrix} \times \begin{matrix}\text{Desired Factor} \\ \text{IX increase} \\ \text{(\% normal)}\end{matrix} \times 1.0\,\text{iu/kg}$$

The amount of Mononine to be infused, as well as the frequency of infusions, will vary with each patient and with the clinical situation.

As a general rule, the level of Factor IX required for treatment of different conditions is as follows:

| | *Minor spontaneous haemorrhage, prophylaxis* | *Major trauma or surgery* |
|---|---|---|
| Desired levels of Factor IX for haemostasis | 15–25% | 25–50% |
| Initial loading dose to achieve desired level | up to 20–30 iu/kg | up to 75 iu/kg |
| Frequency of dosing | once; repeated in 24 hours if necessary | every 18–30 hours, depending on $T_{1/2}$ and measured Factor IX levels |
| Duration of treatment | once; repeated if necessary | up to 10 days, depending upon nature of insult |

Recovery of the loading dose varies from patient to patient. Doses administered should be titrated to the patient's response.

In the presence of an inhibitor to Factor IX, higher doses of Mononine might be necessary to overcome the inhibitor. No data on the treatment of patients with inhibitors to Factor IX with Mononine are available.

*Reconstitution and administration:* Specific instructions for reconstitution and administration are included on the package insert and patient instruction leaflet.

Plastic disposable syringes are recommended with Mononine solution. The ground glass surfaces of all-glass syringes tend to stick with solutions of this type.

A winged infusion needle with microbore tubing is supplied with each pack. Use of other winged needles without microbore tubing, although compatible with the concentrate, will result in a larger retention of solution within the winged infusion set.

*Rate of administration:* The rate of administration should be determined by the response and comfort of the patient; intravenous dosage administration rates of up to 225 units/minute have been regularly tolerated without incident. When reconstituted as directed, i.e. to approximately 100 units/ml, Mononine should be administered at a rate of approximately 2.0 ml per minute.

**Contra-indications, warnings, etc**
*Contra-indications:* Known hypersensitivity to mouse protein.

*Warnings:* This product is prepared from pooled human plasma which may contain the causative agents of hepatitis, AIDS and other viral diseases. Prescribed manufacturing procedures utilised at the plasma collection centres, plasma testing laboratories, and the fractionation facilities are designed to reduce the risk of transmitting viral infection. However, the risk of viral infectivity from this product cannot be totally eliminated. Accordingly, the benefits and risks of treatment with this concentrate should be carefully assessed prior to use.

Individuals who receive infusions of blood or plasma products may develop signs and/or symptoms of some viral infections, particularly nonA nonB hepatitis.

Since the use of Factor IX Complex concentrates has historically been associated with the development of thromboembolic complications, the use of Factor IX containing products may be potentially hazardous in patients with signs of fibrinolysis and in patients with disseminated intravascular coagulation (DIC).

*Precautions:* The administration of Factor IX Complex concentrates, containing Factors II, VII, IX and X, has been associated with the development of thromboembolic complications. Although Mononine contains highly purified Factor IX, the potential risk of thrombosis or disseminated intravascular coagulation observed with the use of other products containing Factor IX should be recognised. Patients should be given Mononine under specialist direction with appropriate facilities for clinical and laboratory monitoring and observed closely for signs or symptoms of intravascular coagulation or thrombosis. Because of the potential risk of thromboembolic complications, caution should be exercised when administering this concentrate to patients with liver disease, to patients post-operatively, to neonates, or to patients at risk of thromboembolic phenomena or disseminated intravascular coagulation. In each of these situations, the potential benefit of treatment with Mononine should be weighed against the risk of these complications.

The product should be administered intravenously at a rate that wil permit observation of the patient for any immediate reaction. Rates of infusion of up to 225 units per minute have been regularly tolerated with no adverse reactions. If any reaction takes place that is thought to be related to the administration of Mononine, the rate of infusion should be decreased or the infusion stopped, as dictated by the response of the patient.

During the course of treatment, determination of daily Factor IX levels is advised to guide the dose to be administered and the frequency of repeated infusions. Individual patients may vary in their response to Mononine, achieving different levels of in vivo recovery and demonstrating different half-lives.

The use of high doses of Factor IX Complex concentrates has been reported to be associated with instances of myocardial infarction, disseminated intravascular coagulation, venous thrombosis and pulmonary embolism. Generally a Factor IX level of 25% to 50% is considered adequate for haemostasis, including major haemorrhages and surgery. Attempting to maintain Factor IX levels of >75% to 100% during treatment is not recommended. To achieve Factor IX

levels that will remain above 25% between once-a-day administrations, each daily dose should attempt to raise the level to 50–60% (see 'Dosage and administration').

No data are available regarding the use of ε-amino caproic acid following an initial infusion of Mononine for the prevention or treatment of oral bleeding following trauma or dental procedures such as extractions.

*Formation of antibodies to mouse protein:* Although no hypersensitivity reactions have been observed, because Mononine contains trace amounts of mouse protein (<50 ng per 100 Factor IX activity units), the possibility exists that patients treated with Mononine may develop hypersensitivity to the mouse protein.

*Information for patients:* Patients shouuld be informed of the early signs of hypersensitivity reactions including hives, generalised urticaria, tightness of the chest, wheezing, hypotension and anaphylaxis, and should be advised to discontinue use of the concentrate and contact their physician if these symptoms occur.

*Use in pregnancy:* Animal reproduction studies have not been conducted with Mononine. It is also not known whether it can cause foetal harm when administered to a pregnant woman or can affect reproduction capacity. Mononine should therefore be given to a pregnant woman only if clearly needed.

*Adverse reactions:* In clinical trials there were occasional reports of sinusitis, pruritus, rash, fatigue and bitter taste. As with the administration of any product intravenously, the following reactions may be observed following administration: headache, fever, chills, flushing, nausea, vomiting, tingling, lethargy, hives; stinging or burning at the infusion site or other manifestations of allergic reactions.

There is a potential risk of thromboembolic episodes following the administration of Mononine (see *Warnings and Precautions*).

*Overdosage:* See *Precautions.*

**Pharmaceutical precautions**  Mononine should be administered by a separate infusion line without mixing with other drugs or medication.

*Storage:* Mononine should be stored at 2°–8°C. Mononine does not contain a preservative. Upon reconstitution, it is advisable that Mononine be administered immediately; in any case it should be administered within three hours in order to assure sterility.

Stability data for Mononine stored under room

temperature conditions support the stability of the product for a period of up to one month at a temperature of ≤30°C. These data would suooort a one-time-only storage of Mononine at room temperature in cases where refrigeration is not available and such storage is unavoidable. Precautions should be followed to monitor the time and temperature conditions to assure that they do not exceed one month and 30°C, respectively.

Avoid freezing which may damage the diluent container.

**Legal category**  POM

**Package quantities**  Mononine is supplied in a single dose vial with diluent, double-end needle for reconstitution, vented filter spike for withdrawal, winged infusion set, sterile 10 ml plastic syringe, alcohol swabs, sterile plaster dressing and plastic disposal bag. Factor IX activity in International Units (iu) is stated on the label of each vial which contains nominally 250, 500 or 1000 iu.

One iu represents the activity of Factor IX present in 1 ml of normal, pooled plasma.

**Further information**  Infusion of Freeze-Dried Human Coagulation Factor IX, Mononine into ten patients with severe or moderate Haemophilia B has shown a mean recovery of 67% and a mean half-life of 22.6 hours. Determinations of half-life and recovery six months later in nine of the same ten patients showed a mean recovery of 68% and a mean half-life of 25.3 hours. This pharmacokinetic profile compares favourably to published results for prothrombin complex concentrates.

This concentrate has been processed by monoclonal antibody immunoaffinity chromatography during its manufacture which has been shown to be capable of reducing the risk of viral transmission. Additionally, a chemical treatment protocol and two ultrafiltration steps used in its manufacture have been shown to be capable of significant viral reductions. However, no procedure has been shown to be totally effective in removing viral infectivity from coagulation factor concentrates.

**Product licence numbers**

| 250 iu/vial | 0231/0097 |
| 500 iu/vial | 0231/0098 |
| 1,000 iu/vial | 0231/0099 |
| Diluent | 0231/0100 |

*\*Trade Mark*

# Chauvin Pharmaceuticals Ltd
## Ashton Road
## Harold Hill
## Romford
## Essex RM3 8SL

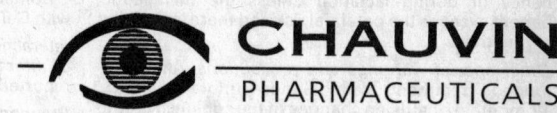

## EPPY*

**Presentation** L-adrenaline base 1% in a buffered ophthalmic solution containing benzalkonium chloride 0.01% w/v as the preservative. The other ingredients are purified water, ammonium lactate, N-acetyl-L-cysteine and ammonium hydroxide.

**Uses** Indicated for the treatment of elevated intraocular pressure in open-angle (chronic simple) glaucoma.

It may be used in combination with miotics, beta-adrenergic blocking agents or carbonic anhydrase inhibitors where indicated.

### Dosage and administration
*Adults (including the elderly):* One or two drops to each eye, usually once or twice daily. (May be given as infrequently as once every three days.) Determine the frequency of instillation by tonometry.

When used in conjunction with miotics, instil this drug five or ten minutes after the miotic drops.

*Children:* As directed by a physician. Safety and efficacy of use in children has not been established.

### Contra-indications, warnings, etc
*Contra-indications:* Closed-angle glaucoma (unless previously treated with iridectomy).

Patients with a narrow angle prone to angle block precipitated by mydriatics.

Hypersensitivity to adrenaline or any other component of the preparation.

This product contains benzalkonium chloride and should not be used when soft contact lenses are worn.

*Interactions:*
*Monoamine oxidase inhibitors:* There is an increased risk of adrenergic reactions when used simultaneously with or up to three weeks after the administration of MAOIs.

*Tricyclic antidepressants:* The pressor response to adrenergic agents and the risk of cardiac arrhythmia may be potentiated in patients receiving tricyclic antidepressants (or within several days of their discontinuation).

*Halothane:* Because of the increased risk of ventricular fibrillation, adrenaline should not be given during general anaesthesia with anaesthetic agents which sensitise the myocardium to sympathomimetics.

*Effects on the ability to drive and use machines:* May cause temporarily blurred vision. Warn patients not to drive or operate hazardous machinery unless vision is clear.

*Other undesirable effects:*
*Local:* Severe smarting on instillation, blurred vision, photophobia, eye pain, conjunctival hyperaemia (resulting in a red eye as a frequent response). Conjunctival sensitisation and allergy and local skin reactions occur occasionally. Pigmentary deposits in the conjunctiva, cornea or eyelids may occur after prolonged use.

*CNS:* Headache or browache are also common but usually diminish as treatment is continued.

*Systemic:* Systemic adverse reactions are rare following topical use at normal dosage. However, palpitations, tachycardia, raised blood pressure, extrasystoles, cardiac arrhythmias, faintness, sweating, pallor, trembling and perspiration may occur.

*Use in pregnancy and lactation:* Safety for use in pregnancy and lactation has not been established. This product should not be used during pregnancy unless it is considered essential by a physician.

*Other special warnings and precautions:* Do not use until the diagnosis of glaucoma has been verified and the nature of the glaucoma has been confirmed (as the use of adrenaline is contra-indicated in narrow-angle glaucoma).

To reduce the risk of precipitating an attack of narrow-angle glaucoma, evaluate the anterior chamber angle by gonioscopy before initiating therapy.

Adrenaline eye drops should be used with caution by patients with hypertension, cardiac disease, aneurysms, arrhythmia or tachycardia, hyperthyroidism, cerebral arteriosclerosis and diabetes mellitus.

Maculopathy with a central scotoma may occur following use in aphakic patients. Discontinue use in such patients if visual acuity deteriorates.

Systemic absorption of adrenaline from eye drops may be reduced by compressing the lacrimal sac at the medial canthus for a minute during and following the instillation of the drops. (This blocks the passage of the drops via the naso-lacrimal duct to the wide absorptive area of the nasal and pharyngeal mucosa. It is especially advisable in children.)

*Overdose:* Systemic reactions to topical adrenaline are unlikely at normal doses. Greater caution is necessary in children and the elderly and those patients predisposed to such reactions e.g. hypertensive cardiac disease or thyrotoxicosis. A severe reaction to adrenaline is of rapid onset and short duration. The treatment of a severe toxic reaction is an immediate intravenous injection of a quick-acting alpha-adrenoceptor blocking agent such as 2 mg to 5 mg of phentolamine. This is followed by intravenous administration of a beta-adrenoceptor blocking agent (such as 1 mg of propranolol injected over 1 minute and repeated, if necessary, at 2 minute intervals up to a maximum of 10 mg (5 mg in anaesthesia)). Adrenaline is almost totally inactive when given by mouth as a result of enzymic degradation in the gut and first pass metabolism in the liver.

*Incompatibilities:* None known.

**Pharmaceutical precautions** Eppy should not be diluted or dispensed from any container other than the original bottle. It should be stored below 25°C in its carton away from strong light. Do not freeze. Eppy should not be used if the solution has become dark amber. Eppy should be discarded one month after opening.

**Legal category** POM

**Package quantities** 7.5 ml of Eppy is supplied as a sterile ophthalmic solution in a plastic dropper bottle. Each bottle is enclosed in a nitrogen-filled nylon/aluminium pouch inside a carton. OP.

**Further information** In common with other sympathomimetic agents, Eppy does not affect accommodation.

There has been work that suggests that as adrenaline probably exerts its effect on increasing outflow via Beta-2 receptors, additive effect on reducing I.O.P. may be expected if a Beta-1 selective beta-blocker is used in conjunction with adrenaline, but not if a non-selective beta-blocker is used.

**Product licence number** 0033/5022R

## FLUORETS*

**Presentation** Sterile, individually wrapped paper strips each impregnated with approximately 1 mg Fluorescein Sodium BP. There are no other ingredients.

**Uses** Fluorescein is a corneal stain and can be used in diagnostic examinations including Goldmann tonometry and the fitting of hard contact lenses.

### Dosage and administration
*Adults and children:* One Fluoret moistened with tear fluid, sterile water or sterile ophthalmic solution should be sufficient to provide adequate corneal staining. Pull tabs apart at right-hand end of envelope and withdraw Fluoret. Moisten tip as above, then gently stroke the Fluoret across the conjunctiva. For the best results the patient should blink several times.

**Contra-indications, warnings, etc** Not to be used with soft contact lenses. The applicator should be used once and then discarded. Care should be taken to handle the strip by the non-impregnated end only.

May cause transient blurring of vision on instillation. Warn patients not to drive or operate hazardous machinery unless vision is clear.

Safety for use in pregnancy and lactation has not been established. Therefore, use only when considered essential by the physician.

**Pharmaceutical precautions** No special precautions.

**Legal category** P

**Package quantities** Gravity-delivered cartons of 100 individually wrapped Fluorets. OP.

**Further information** Fluorescein does not stain a normal cornea but conjunctival abrasions are stained yellow or orange, corneal abrasions or ulcers are stained a bright green and foreign bodies are surrounded by a green ring.

**Product licence number** 0033/5095R

## GANDA*

**Presentation** Ganda is a clear, viscous, colourless to almost colourless liquid, available in two strengths: Ganda 1+0.2 (Guanethidine Monosulphate PhEur 1% w/v + Adrenaline BP 0.2% w/v); Ganda 3+0.5 (Guanethidine Monosulphate PhEur 3% w/v + Adrenaline BP 0.5% w/v), in a buffered solution containing benzalkonium chloride 0.01% w/v as the preservative. The other ingredients are purified water, N-acetyl-L-cysteine, ammonium dihydrogen phosphate, hydroxyethylcellulose and ammonium hydroxide. Ganda is supplied in a plastic dropper bottle packed in a nitrogen-filled pouch.

**Uses** For the treatment of primary open-angle or secondary glaucoma. It may be used in conjunction with miotics or carbonic anhydrase inhibitor therapy.

### Dosage and administration
*Adults (including the elderly):* One drop to be instilled into the eye once or twice daily, or at the discretion of the physician.

*Children:* At the discretion of the physician.

Light pressure may be applied for a few minutes to the inner canthus to reduce systemic absorption via the naso-lacrimal duct.

When used in conjunction with miotics, Ganda should follow the miotic after an interval of 5-10 minutes.

### Contra-indications, warnings, etc
*Contra-indications:* Ganda should not be used in the case of a narrow angle between the iris and cornea as pupillary dilation may precipitate angle closure.

*Interactions:*
*Miotics* and other forms of glaucoma treatment produce an enhancement of the therapeutic effect of Ganda.

*Monoamine oxidase inhibitors:* There is an increased risk of adrenergic reactions when used simultaneously with or up to three weeks after the administration of MAOIs.

*Tricyclic antidepressants:* The pressor response to adrenergic agents and the risk of cardiac arrhythmia may be potentiated in patients receiving tricyclic antidepressants (or within several days of their discontinuation).

*Halothane:* Because of the increased risk of ventricular fibrillation, adrenaline should not be given during general anaesthesia with halothane or other anaesthetic agents which sensitise the myocardium to sympathomimetics.

*Effects on the ability to drive and use machines:* May cause stinging and temporarily blurred vision. Warn patients not to drive or operate hazardous machinery until vision is clear.

*Other undesirable effects:*
*Local:* Occasionally a patient may complain of orbital discomfort or red eye. Rarely, headache, irritation and local skin reactions may occur. As with other adrenaline preparations, melanosis may occasionally occur, but this has no pathological significance. Topical adrenaline has been shown to occasionally cause macular oedema in aphakic eyes and thus the use of adrenaline-containing eye drops in aphakic patients is not recommended.

*Systemic:* Systemic effects are rare but can include tachycardia, extrasystoles, and elevation of blood pressure. Although no reports of such reactions to Ganda have been received, caution is recommended in patients with thyrotoxicosis, hypertension or cardiovascular problems including tachycardia and arrhythmias.

Systemic absorption may be reduced by compressing the lacrimal sac at the medial canthus for a minute during and following the instillation of the drops. (This blocks the passage of the drops via the naso-lacrimal duct to the wide absorptive area of the nasal and pharyngeal mucosa. It is especially advisable in children.)

*Use in pregnancy and lactation:* No data are available on the use of Ganda in pregnancy and lactation, therefore, Ganda cannot be recommended in pregnancy or during lactation unless the therapeutic benefit exceeds the potential risk and there is no safer alternative.

*Other special warnings and precautions:* After prolonged treatment with Ganda (more than 9-12 months) cicatrising changes of the conjunctiva and cornea leading to corneal ulceration and scarring have been reported in some patients. If the initial changes are detected on slit lamp examination, treatment with Ganda should be stopped. These cicatrising changes develop slowly and six-monthly examination of the conjunctiva and cornea will enable Ganda to be withdrawn in any patients who are starting to show conjunctival damage.

One clinical investigator has reported that in two cases out of 21, a paradoxical increase of intraocular pressure occurred for which no explanation was offered.

Some degree of ptosis may represent an adverse effect in glaucoma, but will usually respond to a reduction in dosage or in the frequency of administration.

At prolonged high dosage a tendency to superficial punctate keratitis has been reported, responding either to a reduction in dosage or termination of treatment.

*Overdose:* Overdose is unlikely to occur at normal doses, however, caution is necessary in children, the elderly and patients with predisposing conditions e.g. hypertensive cardiac disease or thyrotoxicosis. A severe reaction to adrenaline is of rapid onset and short duration. The treatment of a severe toxic reaction is an immediate intravenous injection of a quick-acting alpha-adrenoceptor blocking agent such as 2 mg to 5 mg of phentolamine. This is followed by intravenous administration of a beta-adrenoceptor blocking agent (such as 1 mg of propranolol injected over 1 minute and repeated, if necessary, at 2 minute intervals up to a maximum of 10 mg (5 mg in anaesthesia)). Adrenaline is almost totally inactive when given by mouth as a result of enzymic degradation in the gut and first pass metabolism in the liver.

**Pharmaceutical precautions** Ganda is supplied in a plastic dropper bottle in a nitrogen-filled pouch, inside a carton. It should be stored in its carton in a cool place away from strong light. The carton only should be removed before supplying to the patient. Ganda should not be diluted, nor should it be dispensed from any container other than the original bottle. Ganda should not be used if the solution has become dark amber. The contents of the bottle should be discarded one month after removal from the pouch.

**Legal category** POM

**Package quantities** 7.5 ml of Ganda is supplied as a sterile ophthalmic solution in a plastic dropper bottle. Each bottle is enclosed in a nitrogen-filled, nylon/aluminium foil pouch inside a carton. OP.

**Further information** The use of the nitrogen-filled overwrap ensures the long shelf-life of Ganda.

Ganda is a unique combination of Adrenaline BP and Guanethidine Monosulphate PhEur in a plastic dropper bottle which has been specially designed for patient convenience. Its special formulation gives improved stability and includes a viscoliser to enhance comfort and effectiveness.

In common with other sympathomimetic agents Ganda does not affect accommodation.

**Product licence numbers**
Ganda 1+0.2    0033/0075
Ganda 3+0.5    0033/0071

## GELTEARS

**Qualitative and quantitative composition** Clear, colourless gel containing 0.2% w/w Carbomer 940.

**Pharmaceutical form**  Sterile eye gel.

**Clinical particulars**

*Therapeutic indications:* Substitution of tear fluid in the management of dry eye conditions, including keratoconjunctivitis sicca and unstable tear film.

*Posology and method of administration:*
*Adults (including the elderly) and children:* One drop to be instilled into the conjunctival fold of each affected eye 3–4 times daily or as required, depending on the degree of discomfort.

*Contra-indications:* Use in patients with a known hypersensitivity to any component of the preparation.

*Special warnings and precautions for use:* Blurred vision can occur if too much gel is instilled at one time, or if the gel is used too frequently. This effect can last for up to an hour. Recovery can be aided by blinking vigorously for a few seconds. If this fails, the lower eyelid should be manipulated until the gel returns to the lower fornix and normal vision is restored.

Contact lenses should be removed during treatment with GelTears.

*Interaction with other medicaments and other forms of interaction:* No significant interactions have been reported.

*Pregnancy and lactation:* Safety for use in pregnancy and lactation has not been established, therefore, GelTears should not be used in these circumstances.

*Effects on ability to drive and use machines:* As with other ophthalmic preparations, transient blurring of vision may occur on instillation. If affected, the patient should be advised not to drive or operate hazardous machinery until normal vision is restored.

*Undesirable effects:* Corneal irritation due to benzalkonium chloride could possibly occur with prolonged use.

*Overdose:* Not applicable.

**Pharmacological properties**

*Pharmacodynamic properties:* GelTears contains Carbomer 940, a hydrophilic, high molecular weight polymer of carboxyvinylic acid. The gel forms a transparent lubricating and moistening film on the surface of the eye. The preparation has a pH similar to that found in the normal tear film and is slightly hypotonic with respect to tears. GelTears relieves the symptoms of irritation linked with dry eye syndromes and protects the cornea against drying out.

The use of vital stains has provided objective evidence that the corneal and conjunctival epithelial lesions associated with dry eye syndromes show improvement on treatment with GelTears. The gel remains on the surface of the eye for longer than low viscosity artificial tears and hence, less frequent application is required.

*Pharmacokinetic properties:* No human pharmacokinetic studies are available, however, absorption or accumulation in ocular tissues is likely to be negligible due to the high molecular weight of the active ingredient.

*Preclinical safety data:* No adverse safety issues were detected during the development of this formulation. The ingredients are well established in clinical ophthalmology.

**Pharmaceutical particulars**

*List of excipients:* Benzalkonium chloride 0.01% w/w (as a preservative); purified water; sorbitol; sodium hydroxide.

*Incompatibilities:* None known.

*Shelf life:* The shelf life expiry date shall not exceed 3 years from the date of its manufacture when stored below 25°C. Any remaining gel should be discarded 28 days after first opening the tube.

*Special precautions for storage:* The product should be transported in the original packaging. It should be stored below 25°C.

*Nature and contents of container:* Sterile ophthalmic gel presented in 5 g and 10 g plasticised, lacquered aluminium tubes, closed with a tamper evident polyethylene cap. Each tube is individually cartonned with a patient information leaflet.

**Marketing authorisation number** 0033/0149

**Date of approval/revision of SPC**    January 1996

**Legal category**    P

## MINIMS* AMETHOCAINE HYDROCHLORIDE 0.5%

**Presentation** Single-use, clear, colourless, sterile eye drops containing a 0.5% w/v solution of Amethocaine (Tetracaine) Hydrochloride PhEur. The other ingredients are purified water and hydrochloric acid. There are no preservatives in the formulation.

**Uses** As a topical anaesthetic.

**Dosage and administration** One drop, or as required.
Each Minims unit should be discarded after a single use.

**Contra-indications, warnings, etc** Amethocaine is hydrolysed in the body to p-amino-benzoic acid and should not, therefore, be used in patients being treated with sulphonamides.
In view of the immaturity in premature babies of the enzyme system which metabolises ester-type local anaesthetics, amethocaine should be avoided in these patients.
Amethocaine may give rise to dermatitis in hypersensitive patients.
On instillation an initial burning sensation may be complained of, but this passes off in less than half a minute.

The anaesthetised eye should be protected from dust and bacterial contamination.

The cornea may be damaged by prolonged application of anaesthetic drops.

May cause transient blurring of vision on instillation. Warn patients not to drive or operate hazardous machinery unless vision is clear.

Safety for use in pregnancy and lactation has not been established. Therefore, use only when considered essential by the physician.

Systemic absorption may be reduced by compressing the lacrimal sac at the medial canthus for a minute during and following the instillation of the drops. (This blocks the passage of the drops via the naso-lacrimal duct to the wide absorptive area of the nasal and pharyngeal mucosa. It is especially advisable in children.)

**Pharmaceutical precautions** Minims Amethocaine Hydrochloride should be stored below 25°C and should not be exposed to strong light. Do not freeze.

**Legal category** POM

**Package quantities** Cartons of 20 units, each containing approximately 0.5 ml. OP.

**Further information** Nil.

**Product licence number** 0033/5000R

## MINIMS* AMETHOCAINE HYDROCHLORIDE 1%

**Quantitative and qualitative composition** Single-use, clear, colourless, sterile eye drops Amethocaine (Tetracaine) Hydrochloride PhEur 1% w/v solution.

**Pharmaceutical form** Single-use, sterile eye drops.

**Clinical particulars**

*Therapeutic indications:* Ocular anaesthetic for topical instillation into the conjunctival sac.

*Posology and method of administration:*
*Adults (including the elderly) and children:* One drop or as required.

*Contra-indications:* Not to be used in patients with a known hypersensitivity to the product.
Amethocaine is hydrolysed in the body to p-aminobenzoic acid and should not therefore be used in patients being treated with sulphonamides.
In view of the immaturity of the enzyme system which metabolises the ester-type local anaesthetics in premature babies, amethocaine should be avoided in these patients.

*Special warnings and precautions for use:* The anaesthetised eye should be protected from dust and bacterial contamination.
Amethocaine may give rise to dermatitis in hypersensitive patients.
On instillation an initial burning sensation may be experienced. This may last for up to 30 seconds.
The cornea may be damaged by prolonged application of anaesthetic eye drops.
Systemic absorption may be reduced by compressing the lacrimal sac at the medial canthus for a minute during and following the instillation of the drops. (This blocks the passage of the drops via the naso lacrimal duct to the wide absorptive area of the nasal and pharyngeal mucosa. It is especially advisable in children.)

*Interaction with other medicaments and other forms of interaction:* Amethocaine should not be used in patients being treated with sulphonamides (see *Contra-indications* above).

*Pregnancy and lactation:* Safety for use in pregnancy and lactation has not been established, therefore, use only when considered essential by the physician.

*Effects on ability to drive and use machines:* May cause transient blurring of vision on instillation. Warn patients not to drive or operate hazardous machinery unless vision is clear.

*Undesirable effects:* Not applicable.

*Overdose:* Not expected.

**Pharmacological properties**

*Pharmacodynamic properties:* Amethocaine hydrochloride is used as a local anaesthetic which acts by reversibly blocking the propagation and conduction of nerve impulses along nerve axons. Amethocaine stabilises the nerve membrane, preventing the increase in sodium permeability necessary for the production of an action potential.

*Pharmacokinetic properties:* Amethocaine is a weak base (pK$_a$ 8.5), therefore, significant changes in the rate of ionised lipid soluble drug uptake may occur with changes in the acid base balance.
In vitro studies have shown that amethocaine has a high affinity for melanin, therefore, differences in duration of action may be expected between deeply pigmented eyes and less pigmented eyes.

The primary site of metabolism for amethocaine is the plasma. Pseudocholinesterases in the plasma hydrolyse amethocaine to 4-aminobenzoic acid. Unmetabolised drug is excreted in the urine.

*Preclinical safety data:* No adverse safety issues were detected during the development of this formulation. The active ingredient is well established in clinical ophthalmology.

**Pharmaceutical particulars**

*List of excipients:* Hydrochloric acid; purified water.

*Incompatibilities:* None known.

*Shelf life:* 15 months.

*Special precautions for storage:* Store below 25°C. Do not freeze. Protect from light.

*Nature and contents of container:* A sealed conical shaped polypropylene container fitted with a twist and pull off cap. Overwrapped in an individual polypropylene/paper pouch. Each container holds approximately 0.5 ml of solution.

*Instructions for use/handling:* Each Minims unit should be discarded after a single use.

**Marketing authorisation number**  0033/5001R

**Date of approval/revision of the SPC** April 1997

**Legal category**  POM

## MINIMS* ARTIFICIAL TEARS

**Qualitative and quantitative composition**  Clear, colourless, sterile eye drops containing Hydroxyethylcellulose 0.44% w/w BP and Sodium Chloride PhEur 0.35% w/w.

**Pharmaceutical form** Sterile single-use eye drop.

**Clinical particulars**

*Therapeutic indications:* For the relief of dry eye syndromes associated with deficient tear secretion.

*Posology and method of administration:* One or two drops instilled into the affected eye three or four times daily, or as often as is required.

*Contra-indications:* None known.

*Special warnings and precautions for use:* If irritation persists or worsens or continued redness occurs, discontinue use and consult a physician or ophthalmologist.

*Interaction with other medicaments and other forms of interaction:* None known.

*Pregnancy and lactation:* There is no evidence of safety of the drug in human pregnancy but it has been in wide use for many years without apparent ill consequence. If drug therapy is needed in pregnancy this preparation can be used if recommended by a physician and it is considered that the benefits outweigh the possible risks.

*Effects on ability to drive and use machines:* May cause transient blurring of vision on instillation. Do not drive or operate hazardous machinery unless vision is clear.

*Undesirable effects:* May cause transient mild stinging or temporarily blurred vision.

*Overdose:* Overdose would not be expected to produce symptoms.

**Pharmacological properties**

*Pharmacodynamic properties:* The viscolising properties of hydroxyethylcellulose combined with sodium chloride have been shown to increase the tear break-up time in animal models, whilst also acting as a lubricating agent for dry eyes.

*Pharmacokinetic properties:* Not applicable.

*Preclinical safety data:* No adverse safety issues were detected during the development of this formulation. The active ingredients are well-established in clinical ophthalmology.

**Pharmaceutical particulars**

*List of excipients:* Purified water; borax; boric acid.

*Incompatibilities:* None known.

*Shelf life:* 15 months.

*Special precautions for storage:* Store below 25°C. Do not freeze. Protect from light.

*Nature and contents of container:* A sealed conical shaped polypropylene container fitted with a twist and pull off cap. Each Minims unit is overwrapped in an individual polypropylene/paper pouch.

*Instructions for use/handling:* Do not use if solution is more than pale yellow in colour. Each Minims unit should be discarded after a single use.

**Marketing authorisation number**  0033/0137

**Date of approval/revision of SPC** December 1996

**Legal category**  P

## MINIMS* ATROPINE SULPHATE

**Presentation** Single-use, clear, colourless, sterile eye drops available as a 1% w/v solution of Atropine Sulphate PhEur. The other ingredients are purified water and hydrochloric acid. No preservatives are included in the formulation.

**Uses** As a mydriatic and cycloplegic.

**Dosage and administration** One drop, or as required.
Each Minims unit should be discarded after a single use.

**Contra-indications, warnings, etc** The protracted mydriasis which is difficult to reverse, may be a disadvantage. All mydriatics and cycloplegics are contra-indicated in eyes where the filtration angle is narrow, as an acute attack of angle closure glaucoma may be precipitated. If in doubt it is recommended that homatropine is used, since its action can be reversed by eserine (physostigmine).
May cause transient blurring of vision on instillation. Warn patients not to drive or operate hazardous machinery unless vision is clear.
Safety for use in pregnancy and lactation has not been established. Therefore, use only when considered essential by the physician.
Systemic absorption may be reduced by compressing the lacrimal sac at the medial canthus for a minute during and following the instillation of the drops. (This blocks the passage of the drops via the naso-lacrimal duct to the wide absorptive area of the nasal and pharyngeal mucosa. It is especially advisable in children.)

**Pharmaceutical precautions** Minims Atropine Sulphate should be stored below 25°C and should not be exposed to strong light. Do not freeze.

**Legal category**  POM.

**Package quantities** Cartons of 20 units, each unit containing approximately 0.5 ml. OP.

**Further information** Dilation of the pupil occurs within half an hour after application.

**Product licence number**  0033/5002R

## MINIMS* BENOXINATE (OXYBUPROCAINE) HYDROCHLORIDE

**Presentation** Single-use, clear, colourless, sterile eye drops, available as a 0.4% w/v solution of Benoxinate (Oxybuprocaine) Hydrochloride USP. The other ingredients are purified water and hydrochloric acid. No preservatives are included in the formulation.

**Uses** As a topical anaesthetic.

**Dosage and administration** One drop of benoxinate 0.4% is sufficient when dropped into the conjunctival sac to anaesthetise the surface of the eye to allow tonometry after one minute. A further drop after 90 seconds provides adequate anaesthesia for the fitting of contact lenses.
Three drops at 90 second intervals provides sufficient anaesthesia after five minutes for a foreign body to be removed from the corneal epithelium, or for incision of a Meibomian cyst through the conjunctiva.
Corneal sensitivity is normal again after about one hour.
Each Minims unit should be discarded after a single use.

**Contra-indications, warnings etc** The anaesthetised eye should be protected from dust and bacterial contamination. The cornea may be damaged by prolonged application of anaesthetic eye drops.
May cause transient blurring of vision on instillation. Warn patient not to drive or operate hazardous machinery unless vision is clear.
Safety for use in pregnancy and lactation has not been established. Therefore, use only when considered essential by the physician.
Systemic absorption may be reduced by compressing the lacrimal sac at the medial canthus for a minute during and following the instillation of the drops. (This blocks the passage of the drops via the naso-lacrimal duct to the wide absorptive area of the nasal and pharyngeal mucosa. It is especially advisable in children.)

**Pharmaceutical precautions** Minims Benoxinate (Oxybuprocaine) Hydrochloride should be stored below 25°C and should not be exposed to strong light. Do not freeze.

**Legal category**  POM.

**Package quantities** Cartons of 20 units, each unit containing approximately 0.5 ml. OP.

**Further information** When applied to the conjunctiva, benoxinate is less irritant than amethocaine in normal concentrations.

**Product licence number** 0033/5004R

## MINIMS* CHLORAMPHENICOL

**Presentation** Single-use, clear, colourless, sterile eye drops, available as a 0.5% w/v solution of Chloramphenicol PhEur. The other ingredients are purified water, borax and boric acid. No preservatives are included in the formulation.

**Uses** Chloramphenicol is a broad-spectrum bacteriostatic antibiotic. It is active against a wide variety of Gram-negative and Gram-positive organisms as well as rickettsiae and spirochaetes. It is indicated for use as a topical antibacterial in the treatment of superficial ocular infections caused by sensitive organisms.

**Dosage and administration**

*Adults (including the elderly) and Children:* One to two drops applied to each affected eye up to six times daily or more frequently if required. (Severe infections may require one to two drops every fifteen to twenty minutes initially, reducing the frequency of instillation gradually as the infection is controlled.)
Each Minims unit should be discarded after a single use.

**Contra-indications, warnings, etc**
*Contra-indications:* Hypersensitivity to chloramphenicol or to any component of the preparation.

*Interactions:* Chymotrypsin will be inhibited if given simultaneously with chloramphenicol.

*Effects on ability to drive and use machines:* May cause transient blurring of vision on instillation. Warn patients not to drive or operate hazardous machinery unless vision is clear.

*Other undesirable effects:*
*Local:* Sensitivity reactions such as transient irritation, burning, stinging, itching and dermatitis.
*Systemic:* Several cases of major adverse haematological events (bone marrow depression, aplastic anaemia and death) have been reported following ocular use of chloramphenicol.

*Use in pregnancy and lactation:* Safety for use in pregnancy and lactation has not been established. Therefore, use only when considered essential by the physician.

*Other special warnings and precautions:* In severe infections, topical use of chloramphenicol should be supplemented with appropriate systemic treatment.
Aplastic anaemia has followed topical use of chloramphenicol eye drops and, whilst this hazard is a rare one, it should be considered when the benefits of the use of chloramphenicol are assessed.
Prolonged use should be avoided as it may increase the likelihood of sensitisation and the emergence of resistant organisms.
Contact lenses should be removed during the period of treatment.
Systemic absorption may be reduced by compressing the lacrimal sac at the medial canthus for a minute during and following the instillation of the drops. (This blocks the passage of the drops via the naso-lacrimal duct to the wide absorptive area of the nasal and pharyngeal mucosa. It is especially advisable in children.)

*Overdose:* Not applicable.

*Incompatibilities:* None known.

**Pharmaceutical precautions** Minims Chloramphenicol should be stored between 2°C and 8°C. Do not freeze.

**Legal category** POM

**Package quantities** Cartons of 20 units, each unit containing approximately 0.5 ml. OP.

**Further information** Nil.

**Product licence number** 0033/0055R

## MINIMS* CYCLOPENTOLATE HYDROCHLORIDE

**Presentation** Single-use, clear, colourless, sterile eye drops. Two strengths are available: Cyclopentolate Hydrochloride BP 0.5% and 1% w/v solutions. The other ingredients are purified water and hydrochloric acid. No preservatives are included in the formulation.

**Uses** As a mydriatic and cycloplegic.

**Dosage and administration**
*Adults:* One or two drops as required. Maximum effect is induced 30-60 minutes after instillation. In iritis or iridocyclitis 1 or 2 drops of a 0.5% w/v solution are instilled every six to eight hours. One or two drops of a 0.5% w/v solution are also used for breaking down adhesions of the iris to the lens. For refraction the

instillation of 1 drop of a 0.5% w/v solution, repeated after 5 minutes is usually sufficient. Deeply pigmented eyes may require a 1% solution.

*Children:* At the discretion of the physician.

Each Minims unit should be discarded after a single use.

**Contra-indications, warnings, etc** Should not be used in neonates except where, on expert evaluation, the need is considered to be compelling.

All mydriatics and cycloplegics are contra-indicated in eyes where the filtration angle is narrow, as an acute attack of angle closure glaucoma may be precipitated.

There have been reports of allergic reactions, manifesting as cutaneous sensitivity, following use of Minims Cyclopentolate.

May cause transient blurring of vision on instillation. Warn patients not to drive or operate hazardous machinery unless vision is clear.

Safety for use in pregnancy and lactation has not been established. Therefore, use only when considered essential by the physician.

Systemic absorption may be reduced by compressing the lacrimal sac at the medial canthus for a minute during and following the instillation of the drops. (This blocks the passage of the drops via the naso-lacrimal duct to the wide absorptive area of the nasal and pharyngeal mucosa. It is especially advisable in children.)

**Pharmaceutical precautions** Minims Cyclopentolate Hydrochloride should be stored below 25°C and should not be exposed to strong light. Do not freeze.

**Legal category** POM

**Package quantities** Cartons of 20 units, each unit containing approximately 0.5 ml. OP.

**Further information** Recovery of accommodation occurs within 24 hours.

**Product licence numbers**
Cyclopentolate Hydrochloride 0.5%    0033/5005R
Cyclopentolate Hydrochloride 1%      0033/5006R

## MINIMS* FLUORESCEIN SODIUM

**Presentation** Single-use, clear, orange-red, sterile eye drops. Two strengths are available: Fluorescein Sodium BP 1% and 2% w/v solutions. Purified water is the only other ingredient. No preservatives are included in the formulation.

**Uses** Fluorescein is a corneal stain and can be used in diagnostic examinations including Goldmann tonometry. It is also used in the fitting of hard contact lenses.

**Dosage and administration** Sufficient solution should be applied to stain the damaged areas. Excess may be washed away with sterile saline solution.

Each Minims unit should be discarded after a single use.

**Contra-indications, warnings, etc** Not to be used with soft contact lenses.

Special care should be taken to avoid microbial contamination. *Pseudomonas aeruginosa* grows well in fluorescein solutions, therefore, a unit-dose preparation is preferred.

May cause transient blurring of vision on instillation. Warn patient not to drive or operate hazardous machinery unless vision is clear.

Safety for use in pregnancy and lactation has not been established. Therefore, use only when considered essential by the physician.

**Pharmaceutical precautions** Minims Fluorescein should be stored below 25°C and should not be exposed to strong light. Do not freeze.

**Legal category** P

**Package quantities** Cartons of 20 units, each unit containing approximately 0.5 ml. OP.

**Further information** Fluorescein does not stain a normal cornea but conjunctival abrasions are stained yellow or orange, corneal abrasions or ulcers are stained a bright green and foreign bodies are surrounded by a green ring.

**Product licence numbers**
Fluorescein Sodium 1%    0033/0079
Fluorescein Sodium 2%    0033/5008R

## MINIMS* GENTAMICIN SULPHATE

**Presentation** Single-use, clear, colourless sterile eye drops containing Gentamicin Sulphate BP equivalent to 0.3% w/v gentamicin base. The other ingredients are purified water, sodium chloride, borax and sodium hydroxide. No preservatives are included in the formulation.

**Uses** As a broad-spectrum bactericidal antibiotic, for the treatment of ocular infections caused by both Gram-positive and Gram-negative organisms.

**Dosage and administration**
*Adults (including the elderly):* One drop as required.

*Children:* At the discretion of the physician.

Each Minims unit should be discarded after a single use.

**Contra-indications, warnings, etc** Gentamicin should not be used in patients with hypersensitivity to gentamicin and/or other aminoglycosides.

Gentamicin has been used topically without any evidence of significant absorption of the drug causing systemic reactions. Gentamicin is well tolerated when applied topically to the eye.

The use of sulphacetamide with gentamicin in the treatment of eye infections is not recommended. Concomitant administration of frusemide and gentamicin may reduce the renal clearance of gentamicin but this is unlikely to be of significance with topical use.

Gentamicin is incompatible with amphotericin, cephalosporins, erythromycin, heparin, penicillins, sodium bicarbonate and sulphadiazine sodium. This is unlikely to be relevant regarding topical use.

The use of gentamicin during pregnancy is not recommended.

Gentamicin should not be the first choice antibiotic for minor infections, in order to minimise the possibility of bacterial resistance.

Systemic absorption may be reduced by compressing the lacrimal sac at the medial canthus for a minute during and following the instillation of the drops. (This blocks the passage of the drops via the naso-lacrimal duct to the wide absorptive area of the nasal and pharyngeal mucosa. It is especially advisable in children.)

**Pharmaceutical precautions** Minims Gentamicin Sulphate should be stored below 25°C and should not be exposed to strong light. Do not freeze.

**Legal category** POM

**Package quantities** Cartons of 20 units, each unit containing approximately 0.5 ml. OP.

**Further information** Nil.
**Product licence number** 0033/0094

## MINIMS* HOMATROPINE HYDROBROMIDE

**Presentation** Single-use, clear, colourless sterile eye drops, available as a 2% w/v solution of Homatropine Hydrobromide PhEur. The other ingredients are purified water and hydrochloric acid. No preservatives are included in the formulation.

**Uses** As a mydriatic and cycloplegic.

**Dosage and administration** One drop as required.

Each Minims unit should be discarded after a single use.

**Contra-indications, warnings, etc**
*Contra-indications:* All mydriatics and cycloplegics are contra-indicated in eyes where the filtration angle is narrow, as an acute attack of angle closure glaucoma may be precipitated.

Minims Homatropine should not be used in patients who are hypersensitive to atropine, patients with myasthenia gravis or patients with tachycardia secondary to cardiac insufficiency or thyrotoxicosis.

*Warnings:* Use with caution in patients with fever or in those who may be exposed to elevated environmental temperatures, as there is a risk of heat prostration and hyperthermia.

Minims Homatropine should not be used during the first three months of life. The safety and effectiveness of homatropine in children has not been established. Children with blond hair and blue eyes are more susceptible to the effects of homatropine.

Systemic absorption may be reduced by compressing the lacrimal sac at the medial canthus for a minute during and following the instillation of the drops. (This blocks the passage of the drops via the naso-lacrimal duct to the wide absorptive area of the nasal and pharyngeal mucosa. It is especially advisable in children.)

Safety for use in pregnancy and lactation has not been established, therefore, use only when considered essential by the physician.

May cause transient blurring of vision on instillation. Warn patients not to drive or operate hazardous machinery unless vision is clear.

**Pharmaceutical precautions** Minims Homatropine Hydrobromide should be stored below 25°C and should not be exposed to strong light. Do not freeze.

**Legal category** POM

**Package quantities** Cartons of 20 units, each unit containing approximately 0.5 ml. OP.

**Further information** Nil.

**Product licence number** 0033/5010R

## MINIMS* LIGNOCAINE AND FLUORESCEIN

**Presentation** Single-use, clear, yellow, sterile eye drops containing Lignocaine (Lidocaine) Hydrochloride PhEur 4.0% w/v and Fluorescein Sodium BP 0.25% w/v. The other ingredients are purified water, polyvinyl pyrrolidone and hydrochloric acid. No preservatives are included in the formulation.

**Uses** As a diagnostic stain and topical anaesthetic combined. Minims Lignocaine and Fluorescein units are used in the measurement of intraocular pressure by Goldmann tonometry.

**Dosage and administration**
*Adults:* One or more drops as required.

*Children:* At the discretion of the physician.

Each Minims unit should be discarded after a single use.

**Contra-indications, warnings etc** Known hypersensitivity to lignocaine and other local anaesthetics.

Special care should be taken to protect the anaesthetised eye from foreign body contamination, particularly in elderly patients in whom the duration of anaesthesia may exceed 30 minutes.

This combination has been in use during pregnancy and lactation for a number of years without apparent ill consequence.

Overdose is not expected to cause adverse effects. However, overuse of local anaesthetics can cause keratitis, with loss of corneal epithelium and stromal opacity.

**Pharmaceutical precautions** Minims Lignocaine and Fluorescein should be stored below 25°C and should not be exposed to strong light. Do not freeze.

**Legal category** POM

**Package quantities** Cartons of 20 units, each unit containing approximately 0.5 ml. OP.

**Further information** Nil.

**Product licence number** 0033/0073

## MINIMS* METIPRANOLOL

**Presentation** Single-use, clear, colourless, sterile eye drops. Two strengths are available: 0.1% w/v and 0.3% w/v Metipranolol. The other ingredients are purified water, sodium chloride, hydrochloric acid and sodium hydroxide. No preservatives are included in the formulation.

**Uses** Metipranolol is a non-selective beta-adrenoceptor blocking agent.

Minims Metipranolol is indicated for the treatment of raised intraocular pressure. It is particularly suitable for the control of post-operative intraocular pressure and for the treatment of chronic open-angle glaucoma in patients who are allergic to preservatives.

The use of Minims Metipranolol in patients with chronic glaucoma should be restricted only to those patients who are allergic to the preservatives commonly used in multidose preparations, or those patients wearing soft contact lenses in whom benzalkonium chloride should be avoided.

**Dosage and administration**
*Adults (including the elderly):* The recommended dose is one drop instilled into the affected eye twice daily. Newly diagnosed patients should be treated in the first instance with the 0.1% w/v strength, changing to a higher strength if adequate control is not achieved or maintained.

In the treatment of post-operative rises in intraocular pressure, the dosage and frequency should be at the discretion of the physician.

*Children:* At the discretion of the physician. No clinical trials in children have been carried out.

Each Minims unit should be discarded after a single use.

**Contra-indications, warnings, etc**
*Contra-indications:* Bronchial asthma, history of bronchial asthma, chronic obstructive airways disease, sinus bradycardia, second or third degree atrioventricular block, cardiac failure, cardiogenic shock, hypersensitivity to any of the components of the preparation.

*Precautions and warnings:* As with other topically applied beta-blockers, systemic absorption may occur giving adverse reactions similar to those of orally administered beta-blockers.

Cardiac and respiratory reactions have been reported with topically applied beta-blockers including, rarely, death due to bronchospasm or cardiac failure.

Congestive cardiac failure should be adequately controlled before starting therapy with Minims Metipranolol. If the patient has a history of cardiac disease, pulse rate should be monitored.

Diabetic control should be monitored during Minims Metipranolol therapy in patients with labile diabetes.

Granulomatous anterior uveitis has been reported in association with the use of the multidose preparation of metipranolol in patients with chronic glaucoma. In any case where a patient shows symptoms or signs suggestive of anterior uveitis, Minims Metipranolol should be withdrawn and an alternative ocular hypotensive agent substituted.

Systemic absorption may be reduced by compressing the lacrimal sac at the medial canthus for a minute during and following the instillation of the drops. (This blocks the passage of the drops via the naso-lacrimal duct to the wide absorptive area of the nasal and pharyngeal mucosa. It is especially advisable in children.)

*Use in pregnancy:* Although there is no evidence to suggest that metipranolol has teratogenic properties, its use during pregnancy should be avoided unless the potential benefits are considered to outweigh the possible hazards.

*Use in lactation:* As beta-blockers can pass into breast milk, consideration should be given to stopping breast-feeding if Minims Metipranolol is considered necessary.

*Side-effects:*
*Ocular:* Transient burning or stinging on instillation, blurred vision, superficial punctate keratitis, blepharoconjunctivitis and anterior uveitis have been reported.

*Cardiovascular:* Bradycardia and hypotension can occasionally occur following the systemic absorption of topically applied beta-blockers.

*Respiratory:* Bronchospasm can occur, predominantly in patients with a history of reversible obstructive airways disease. Dyspnoea and respiratory failure have also been reported with topically applied beta-blockers.

*CNS:* Headache, ataxia, weakness and lethargy can occur.

*Dermatological:* Local manifestations of contact sensitivity. Reactions around the eyes can involve skin rashes on the lower lids and cheeks and periorbital oedema.

*Drug interactions:* Caution should be exercised if used in conjunction with oral beta-blockers as additive effects on systemic beta-blockade may occur. In particular, care should be taken in patients with sinus bradycardia and greater than first-degree heart block.

Beta-blockers should not be given with verapamil and neither drug should be administered within several days of discontinuing the other.

**Pharmaceutical precautions** Minims should be stored below 25°C and should not be exposed to strong light. Do not freeze.

**Legal category** POM

**Package quantities** Cartons of 20 units, each unit containing approximately 0.5 ml solution. OP.

**Further information** Metipranolol has little or no effect on pupil size or accommodation. Metipranolol is generally well tolerated but some patients may experience slight transient stinging. Transient headaches have been reported.

**Product licence numbers**
Metipranolol 0.1%     0033/0121
Metipranolol 0.3%     0033/0122

# MINIMS* NEOMYCIN SULPHATE

**Qualitative and quantitative composition** Clear, colourless, sterile eye drops, available as a 0.5% w/v solution of Neomycin Sulphate PhEur.

**Pharmaceutical form** Sterile single-use eye drop.

**Clinical particulars**

*Therapeutic indications:* For the topical treatment of superficial ocular infections caused by sensitive pathogens.

*Posology and method of administration:* One or two drops applied to each affected eye up to six times daily or more frequently if required. (Severe infections may require one or two drops every fifteen to twenty minutes initially, reducing the frequency of instillation gradually as the infection is controlled.)

*Contra-indications:* Hypersensitivity to neomycin or to any component of the preparation. (Cross-sensitivity with other aminoglycoside antibiotics may occur.)

*Special warnings and special precautions for use:*
(a) In severe infections topical use of neomycin should be supplemented with appropriate systemic treatment.

(b) Prolonged use should be avoided as it may lead to skin sensitisation and the emergence of resistant organisms.

(c) Neomycin may cause irreversible, partial or total deafness when given systemically or when applied topically to open wounds or damaged skin. This effect is dose-related and is enhanced by renal or hepatic impairment. Although this effect has not been reported following topical ocular use, the possibility should be considered when high dose topical treatment is given to small children or infants.

(d) Contact lenses should be removed during the period of treatment.

(e) Systemic absorption may be reduced by compressing the lacrimal sac at the medial canthus for a minute during and following the instillation of the drops. (This blocks the passage of the drops via the naso lacrimal duct to the wide absorptive area of the nasal and pharyngeal mucosa. It is especially advisable in children.)

*Interaction with other medicaments and other forms of interaction:* None relevant to topical use.

*Pregnancy and lactation:* Safety for use in pregnancy and lactation has not been established therefore use only when considered essential by the physician.

*Effects on ability to drive and use machines:* May cause transient blurring of vision on instillation. Warn patients not to drive or operate hazardous machinery until vision is clear.

*Undesirable effects:* Hypersensitivity reactions, usually of the delayed type, occur frequently with local treatment with neomycin. Irritation, burning, stinging, itching and dermatitis may occur.

*Overdose:* Please see 'Special warnings and special precautions for use' above.

**Pharmacological properties**

*Pharmacodynamic properties:* Neomycin is a broad spectrum antibiotic effective against a wide range of Gram-positive and Gram-negative micro-organisms. It has no activity against viruses or fungi.

*Pharmacokinetic properties:* No specific human topical ocular pharmacokinetic data are available.

*Preclinical safety data:* No unexpected safety issues were identified during the development of this product.

**Pharmaceutical particulars**

*List of excipients:* Purified water; sodium dihydrogen phosphate; disodium edetate.

*Incompatibilities:* None applicable.

*Shelf life:* 15 months.

*Special precautions for storage:* Store below 25°C. Do not freeze. Protect from light.

*Nature and contents of container:* A sealed conical shaped polypropylene container fitted with a twist and pull off cap. Each Minims unit is overwrapped in an individual polypropylene/paper pouch.

*Instructions for use/handling:* Each Minims unit should be discarded after a single use.

**Marketing authorisation number** 0033/5012R

**Date of approval/revision of SPC** July 1996

**Legal category** POM

# MINIMS* PHENYLEPHRINE HYDROCHLORIDE

**Quantitative and qualitative composition**

**Pharmaceutical form** Single-use, clear, colourless, sterile eye drops. Two strengths are available: Phenylephrine Hydrochloride BP 2.5% and 10% w/v solutions. No preservatives are included in the formulation.

**Clinical particulars**

*Therapeutic indications:* Phenylephrine is a directly acting sympathomimetic agent used topically in the eye as a mydriatic. It may be indicated to dilate the pupil in diagnostic or therapeutic procedures.

*Posology and method of administration:*
*Adults:* Apply one drop to each eye. If necessary, this dose may be repeated once only, at least one hour after the first drop.
N.B. The use of a drop of topical anaesthetic a few minutes before instillation of phenylephrine is recommended to prevent stinging.
*Children and the elderly:* The use of phenylephrine 10% solution is contra-indicated in these groups because of the increased risks of systemic toxicity.

*Contra-indications:* Patients with cardiac disease, hypertension, aneurysms, thyrotoxicosis, long-standing insulin dependent diabetes mellitus and tachycardia. Patients on monoamine oxidase inhibitors, tricyclic

antidepressants and anti-hypertensive agents (including beta-blockers).

Patients with closed angle glaucoma (unless previously treated with iridectomy) and patients with a narrow angle prone to glaucoma precipitated by mydriatics.

Hypersensitivity to phenylephrine or any component of the preparation.

*Special warnings and precautions for use:* Use with caution in the presence of diabetes, cerebral arteriosclerosis or long standing bronchial asthma.

To reduce the risk of precipitating an attack of narrow angle glaucoma evaluate the anterior chamber angle before use.

Corneal clouding may occur if phenylephrine 10% is instilled when the corneal epithelium has been denuded or damaged.

Systemic absorption may be minimised by compressing the lacrimal sac at the medial canthus for one minute during and after the instillation of the drops. This blocks the passage of the drops via the naso-lacrimal duct to the wide absorptive area of the nasal and pharyngeal mucosa.

*Interaction with other medicaments and other forms of interaction:*
*Anti-hypertensive agents:* Topical phenylephrine should not be used as it may reverse the action of many anti-hypertensive agents with possibly fatal consequences.
*Monoamine oxidase inhibitors:* There is an increased risk of adrenergic reactions when used simultaneously with, or up to three weeks after, the administration of MAOIs.
*Tricyclic Antidepressants:* The pressor response to adrenergic agents and the risk of cardiac arrhythmia may be potentiated in patients receiving tricyclic antidepressants (or within several days of their discontinuation).
*Halothane:* Because of the increased risk of ventricular fibrillation, phenylephrine should be used with caution during general anaesthesia with anaesthetic agents which sensitise the myocardium to sympathomimetics.
*Cardiac glycosides or quinidine:* There is an increased risk of arrhythmias.

*Pregnancy and lactation:* Safety for use in pregnancy and lactation has not been established. This product should only be used during pregnancy if it is considered by the physician to be essential.

*Effects on ability to drive and use machines:* May cause stinging and temporarily blurred vision. Warn patients not to drive or operate hazardous machinery until vision is clear.

*Undesirable effects:*
*Local:* Eye pain and stinging on instillation (use of a drop of topical anaesthetic a few minutes before the instillation of phenylephrine is recommended), temporarily blurred vision and photophobia, conjunctival sensitisation and allergy may occur.
*Systemic:* Palpitations, tachycardia, extrasystoles, cardiac arrhythmias and hypertension.
Serious cardiovascular reactions including coronary artery spasm, ventricular arrhythmias and myocardial infarctions have occurred following topical use of 10% phenylephrine. These sometimes fatal reactions have usually occurred in patients with pre-existing cardiovascular disease.

*Overdose:* Because a severe toxic reactions to phenylephrine is of rapid onset and short duration, treatment is primarily supportive. Prompt injection of a rapidly acting alpha-adrenergic blocking agent such as phentolamine (dose 2 to 5 mg iv) has been recommended.

**Pharmacological properties**

*Pharmacodynamic properties:* Phenylephrine is a direct acting sympathomimetic agent. It causes mydriasis via the stimulation of alpha receptors. There is almost no cycloplegic effect.

Maximal mydriasis occurs in 60- 90 minutes with recovery after 5–7 hours.

The mydriatic effects of phenylephrine can be reversed with thymoxamine.

*Pharmacokinetic properties:* Phenylephrine is a weak base at physiological pH. The extent of ocular penetration is determined by the condition of the cornea. A healthy cornea presents a physical barrier, in addition to which, some metabolic activity may occur. Where the corneal epithelium is damaged, the effect of the barrier and the extent of metabolism are reduced, leading to greater absorption.

*Preclinical safety data:* The use of phenylephrine in ophthalmology has been well-established for many years. No unexpected adverse safety issues were identified during the development of the Minims format.

**Pharmaceutical particulars**

*List of excipients:* Purified water; sodium metabisulphite; disodium edetate.

*Incompatibilities:* None relevant.

*Shelf life:* 15 months.

*Special precautions for storage:* Store below 25°C. Do not freeze. Protect from light.

*Nature and contents of container:* A sealed conical shaped polypropylene container fitted with a twist and pull off cap. Overwrapped in an individual polypropylene/paper pouch. Each container holds approximately 0.5 ml of solution.

*Instructions for use/handling:* Each Minims unit should be discarded after a single use.

### Marketing authorisation numbers
Minims Phenylephrine 2.5%     0033/0117
Minims Phenylephrine 10%      0033/5021R

### Date of approval/revision of SPC
Minims Phenylephrine 2.5%     September 1996
Minims Phenylephrine 10%      January 1997

### Legal category   P

## MINIMS* PILOCARPINE NITRATE

**Quantitative and qualitative composition** Three strengths are available: Pilocarpine Nitrate PhEur 1%, 2% and 4% w/v solutions. No preservatives are included in the formulation.

**Pharmaceutical form** Single-use, clear, colourless, sterile eye drops.

### Clinical particulars

*Therapeutic indications:* Pilocarpine is used as a miotic for reversing the action of weaker mydriatics and in the emergency treatment of glaucoma.

*Posology and method of administration:*

*Adults (including the elderly) and children:* Instil dropwise into the eye according to the recommended dosage.

To induce miosis, one or two drops should be used.

In cases of emergency treatment of acute narrow-angle glaucoma, one drop should be used every five minutes until miosis is achieved.

*Contra-indications:* Conditions where pupillary constriction is undesirable e.g. acute iritis, anterior uveitis and some forms of secondary glaucoma.

Hypersensitivity to any component of the preparation.

Patients with soft contact lenses should not use this preparation.

*Special warnings and precautions for use:* Systemic reactions rarely occur when treating chronic simple glaucoma at normal doses. However, in the treatment of acute closed-angle glaucoma the possibility of systemic reactions must be considered because of the higher doses given. Caution is particularly advised in patients with acute heart failure, bronchial asthma, peptic ulceration, hypertension, urinary tract obstruction, Parkinson's disease and corneal abrasions.

Retinal detachments have been caused in susceptible individuals and those with pre-existing retinal disease, therefore, fundus examination is advised in all patients prior to the initiation of therapy.

Patients with chronic glaucoma on long-term pilocarpine therapy should have regular monitoring of intraocular pressure and visual fields.

Systemic absorption may be minimised by compressing the lacrimal sac at the medial canthus for one minute during and after the instillation of the drops. This blocks the passage of the drops via the naso-lacrimal duct to the wide absorptive area of the nasal and pharyngeal mucosa.

*Interaction with other medicaments and other forms of interaction:* Although clinically not proven, the miotic effects of pilocarpine may be antagonised by long-term topical or systemic corticosteroid therapy, systemic anticholinergics, antihistamines, pethidine, sympathomimetics or tricyclic antidepressants.

Concomitant administration of two miotics is not recommended because of inter-drug antagonism and the risk that unresponsiveness may develop to both drugs.

*Pregnancy and lactation:* Safety for use in pregnancy and lactation has not been established. This product should only be used during pregnancy if it is considered by the physician to be essential.

*Effects on ability to drive and use machines:* Causes difficulty with dark adaptation, therefore, caution is necessary when night driving and when hazardous tasks are undertaken in poor illumination. May cause accommodation spasm. Patients should be advised not to drive or use machinery if vision is not clear.

*Undesirable effects:*

*Local:* Burning, itching, smarting, blurring of vision, ciliary spasm, conjunctival vascular congestion, induced myopia, sensitisation of the lids and conjunctiva, reduced visual acuity in poor illumination, lens changes with chronic use, increased pupillary block, retinal detachments and vitreous haemorrhages.

*CNS:* Browache and headache (especially in younger patients who have recently started therapy).

*Systemic:* Systemic reactions rarely occur in the treatment of chronic simple glaucoma but they may include hypertension, tachycardia, bronchial spasm, pulmonary oedema, salivation, sweating, nausea, vomiting, diarrhoea and lacrimation.

*Overdose:* If accidentally ingested, induce emesis or perform gastric lavage. Observe for signs of toxicity (salivation, lacrimation, sweating, bronchial spasm, cyanosis, nausea, vomiting and diarrhoea).

### Pharmacological properties

*Pharmacodynamic properties:* Pilocarpine is a direct acting parasympathomimetic drug. It duplicates the muscarinic effect of acetyl choline, but not its nicotinic effects. Consequently, pilocarpine stimulates the smooth muscle and secretary glands but does not affect the striated muscle.

*Pharmacokinetic properties:* Pilocarpine has a low ocular bioavailability when topically applied and this has been attributed to extensive pre-corneal drug loss in conjunction with the resistance to normal corneal penetration. Further, pilocarpine appears to bind to the eye pigments from which it is gradually released to the muscles.

Inactivation of pilocarpine in the eye is thought to occur by a hydrolysing enzyme. The amount of this enzyme is not changed by the prolonged use of pilocarpine by glaucoma patients, nor is it changed in patients poorly controlled by glaucoma therapy.

*Preclinical safety data:* There are no preclinical data of relevance to the prescriber which are additional to that already included in other sections of the SPC.

### Pharmaceutical particulars

*List of excipients:* Purified water.

*Incompatibilities:* None known.

*Shelf life:* 15 months.

*Special precautions for storage:* Store below 25°C. Do not freeze. Protect from light.

*Nature and contents of container:* A sealed conical shaped polypropylene container fitted with a twist and pull off cap. Overwrapped in an individual polypropylene/paper pouch. Each container holds approximately 0.5 ml of solution.

*Instructions for use/handling:* Each Minims unit should be discarded after a single use.

### Marketing authorisation numbers
Minims Pilocarpine 1%     0033/5013R
Minims Pilocarpine 2%     0033/5014R
Minims Pilocarpine 4%     0033/5016R

### Date of approval/revision of SPC   February 1997

### Legal category   POM

## MINIMS* PREDNISOLONE SODIUM PHOSPHATE

**Quantitative and qualitative composition** Clear, colourless, sterile eye drops containing Prednisolone Sodium Phosphate BP 0.5% w/v.

**Pharmaceutical form** Single-use, sterile eye drops.

### Clinical particulars

*Therapeutic indications:* Non-infected inflammatory conditions of the eye.

*Posology and method of administration:*
*Adults (including the elderly):* One or two drops applied topically to the eye as required.
*Children:* At the discretion of the physician.

*Contra-indications:* Use is contra-indicated in viral, fungal, tuberculous and other bacterial infections.

Prolonged application to the eye of preparations containing corticosteroids has caused increased intraocular pressure and therefore the drops should not be used in patients with glaucoma.

In children, long-term, continuous topical corticosteroid therapy should be avoided due to possible adrenal suppression.

*Special warnings and precautions for use:* Care should be taken to ensure that the eye is not infected before Minims Prednisolone is used.

Systemic absorption may be reduced by compressing the lacrimal sac at the medial canthus for a minute during and following the instillation of the drops. (This blocks the passage of drops via the naso-lacrimal duct to the wide absorptive area of the nasal and pharyngeal mucosa. It is especially advisable in children.)

*Interaction with other medicaments and other forms of interaction:* Corticosteroids are known to increase the effects of barbiturates, sedative hypnotics and tricyclic antidepressants.

They will, however, decrease the effects of anticholinesterases, antiviral eye preparations and salicylates.

*Pregnancy and lactation:* Topical administration of corticosteroids to pregnant animals can cause abnormalities of foetal development and although the relevance of this finding to human beings has not been established, the use of Minims Prednisolone during pregnancy should be avoided.

*Effects on ability to drive and use machines:* None known.

*Undesirable effects:* Prolonged treatment with corticosteroids in high dosage is occasionally associated with cataract.

The systemic effects of steroids are possible following the use of Minims Prednisolone, but are, however, unlikely due to the reduced absorption of topical eye drops.

*Overdose:* As Minims are single dose units, overdose is unlikely to occur.

### Pharmacological properties

*Pharmacodynamic properties:* The actions of corticosteroids are mediated by the binding of the corticosteroid molecules to receptor molecules located within sensitive cells. Corticosteroid receptors are present in human trabecular meshwork cells and in rabbit iris ciliary body tissue.

Prednisolone, in common with other corticosteroids, will inhibit phospholipase A2 and thus decrease prostaglandin formation.

The activation and migration of leucocytes will be affected by prednisolone. A 1% solution of prednisolone has been demonstrated to cause a 5.1% reduction in polymorphonuclear leucocyte mobilisation to an inflamed cornea. Corticosteroids will also lyse and destroy lymphocytes. These actions of prednisolone all contribute to its anti-inflammatory effect.

*Pharmacokinetic properties:* The oral availability, distribution and excretion of prednisolone is well documented. A figure of $82 \pm 13\%$ has been quoted as the oral availability and $1.4 \pm 0.3$ ml/min/kg as the clearance rate. A half life of 2.1–4.0 hours has been calculated.

With regard to ocular pharmacokinetics, prednisolone sodium phosphate is a highly water soluble compound and is almost lipid insoluble. Therefore, theoretically it should not penetrate the intact corneal epithelium. Nevertheless, 30 minutes after instillation of a drop of 1% drug, corneal concentrations of 10μg/g and aqueous levels of 0.5μg/g have been attained. When a 0.5% solution was instilled in rabbit eyes every 15 minutes for an hour, an aqueous concentration of 2.5μg/ml was measured. Considerable variance exists in the intraocular penetration of prednisolone depending on whether the cornea is normal or abraded.

It can be seen that only low levels of prednisolone will be absorbed systemically, particularly where the cornea is intact.

Any prednisolone which is absorbed will be highly protein-bound in common with other corticosteroids.

*Preclinical safety data:* The use of prednisolone in ophthalmology is well-established. Little specific toxicology work has been reported, however, the breadth of clinical experience confirms its suitability as a topical ophthalmic agent.

### Pharmaceutical particulars

*List of excipients:* Disodium edetate; disodium dihydrogen phosphate; sodium chloride; sodium hydroxide for pH adjustment; purified water.

*Incompatibilities:* None known.

*Shelf life* 15 months.

*Special precautions for storage:* Store below 25°C. Do not freeze. Protect from light.

*Nature and contents of container:* A sealed conical shaped polypropylene container fitted with a twist and pull off cap. Overwrapped in an individual polypropylene/paper pouch. Each container holds approximately 0.5 ml of solution.

*Instructions for use/handling:* Each Minims unit should be discarded after a single use.

**Marketing authorisation number**   0033/0091

**Date of approval/revision of SPC** December 1996

**Legal category**   POM

## MINIMS* PROXYMETACAINE

**Quantitative and qualitative composition** Clear, colourless to pale yellow 0.5% w/v solution of Proxymetacaine Hydrochloride BP.

**Pharmaceutical form** Single-use, sterile eye drops.

**Clinical particulars**

*Therapeutic indications:* To be used as a topical ocular anaesthetic.

*Posology and method of administration:*
*Adults (including the elderly) and children:*
Deep anaesthesia: Instil 1 drop every 5–10 minutes for 5–7 applications.
Removal of sutures: Instil 1 or 2 drops 2–3 minutes before removal of sutures.
Removal of foreign bodies: Instil 1 or 2 drops prior to operating.
Tonometry: Instil 1 or 2 drops immediately before measurement.

*Contra-indications:* Use in patients with a known hypersensitivity to proxymetacaine.

In view of the immaturity of the enzyme system which metabolises the ester-type local anaesthetics in premature babies, this product should be avoided in these patients.

*Special warnings and precautions for use:* This product should be used cautiously and sparingly in patients with known allergies, cardiac disease or hyperthyroidism because of the increased risk of sensitivity reactions.

Minims Proxymetacaine is not miscible with fluorescein, however, fluorescein can be added to the eye after it has been anaesthetised with Minims Proxymetacaine.

This product is not intended for long term use. Regular and prolonged use of topical ocular anaesthetics e.g. in conjunction with contact lens insertion, may cause softening and erosion of the corneal epithelium, which could produce corneal opacification with accompanying loss of vision.

Protection of the eye from rubbing, irritating chemicals and foreign bodies during the period of anaesthesia is very important. Patients should be advised to avoid touching the eye until the anaesthesia has worn off.

Tonometers soaked in sterilising or detergent solutions should be thoroughly rinsed with sterile distilled water prior to use.

Systemic absorption may be reduced by compressing the lacrimal sac at the medial canthus for a minute during and following the instillation of the drops. (This blocks the passage of the drops via the naso lacrimal duct to the wide absorptive area of the nasal and pharyngeal mucosa. It is especially advisable in children.)

*Interaction with other medicaments and other forms of interaction:* None stated.

*Pregnancy and lactation:* Safety for use in pregnancy and lactation has not been established, therefore, use only when considered essential by the physician.

*Effects on ability to drive and use machines:* May cause transient blurring of vision on instillation. Warn patients not to drive or operate hazardous machinery unless vision is clear.

*Undesirable effects:* Pupillary dilatation or cycloplegic effects have rarely been observed with proxymetacaine preparations. Irritation of the conjunctiva or other toxic reactions have occurred only rarely. A severe, immediate-type apparently hyperallergic corneal reaction may rarely occur. This includes acute, intense and diffuse epithelial keratitis, a grey ground-glass appearance, sloughing of large areas of necrotic epithelium, corneal filaments and sometimes, iritis with descemetitis.

*Overdose:* Not applicable.

**Pharmacological properties**

*Pharmacodynamic properties:* Proxymetacaine, in common with other local anaesthetics, reversibly blocks the initiation and conduction of nerve impulses by decreasing the permeability of the neuronal membrane to sodium ions.

The delay to onset of effect, duration of effect and potency of proxymetacaine are similar to those of amethocaine.

*Pharmacokinetic properties:* Proxymetacaine is readily absorbed into the systemic circulation where, in common with other ester-type local anaesthetics, it is hydrolysed by plasma esterases. Proxymetacaine is also subject to hepatic metabolism.

*Preclinical safety data:* No adverse safety issues were identified during the development of this formulation. The ingredients are well established in clinical ophthalmology.

**Pharmaceutical particulars**

*List of excipients:* Purified water; hydrochloric acid; sodium hydroxide

*Incompatibilities:* None known.

*Shelf life:* 2 years.

*Special precautions for storage:* The product should be transported in the original packaging. It should be stored at 2–8°C. Do not freeze.

*Nature and contents of container:* A sealed conical shaped polypropylene container fitted with a twist and pull off cap. Each Minims unit contains approximately 0.5 ml of solution. Each unit is overwrapped in a polyethylene sachet. 20 units are packed into a suitable carton.

*Instructions for use/handling:* Do not use if solution is more than pale yellow in colour.

Each Minims unit should be discarded after a single use.

**Marketing authorisation number**   0033/0151

**Date of approval/revision of SPC**   March 1996

**Legal category**   POM

## MINIMS* PROXYMETACAINE AND FLUORESCEIN

**Quantitative and qualitative composition**   Clear, yellow solution containing 0.5% w/v Proxymetacaine Hydrochloride BP and 0.25% w/v Fluorescein Sodium BP.

**Pharmaceutical form**   Single-use, sterile eye drops.

**Clinical particulars**

*Therapeutic indications:* As a combined topical ocular anaesthetic and diagnostic stain. Uses include tonometry, removal of corneal foreign bodies and other corneal or conjunctival procedures of short duration.

*Posology and method of administration:*
*Adults (including the elderly) and children:* Instil one or two drops into the conjunctival sac prior to the procedure.

Each Minims unit should be discarded after a single use to avoid risk of cross infection.

*Contra-indications:* Do not use in patients with a known hypersensitivity to any component of the preparation. In view of the immaturity of the enzyme system which metabolises the ester type local anaesthetics in premature babies, this product should be avoided in these patients.

*Special warnings and precautions for use:* This product should be used cautiously and sparingly in patients with known allergies, cardiac disease or hyperthyroidism because of the increased risk of sensitivity reactions.

This product is not intended for long term use. Regular and prolonged use of topical ocular anaesthetics e.g. in conjunction with contact lens insertion, may cause softening and erosion of the corneal epithelium, which could produce corneal opacification with accompanying loss of vision.

Protection of the eye from rubbing, irritating chemicals and foreign bodies during the period of anaesthesia is very important. Patients should be advised to avoid touching the eye until the anaesthesia has worn off.

Tonometers soaked in sterilising or detergent solutions should be thoroughly rinsed with sterile distilled water prior to use.

Systemic absorption may be reduced by compressing the lacrimal sac at the medial canthus for a minute during and following instillation of the drops. (This blocks the passage of the drops via the naso-lacrimal duct to the wide absorptive area of the nasal and pharyngeal mucosa. It is especially advisable in children.)

*Interaction with other medicaments and other forms of interaction:* None stated.

*Pregnancy and lactation:* Safety for use in pregnancy and lactation has not been established, therefore, use only when considered essential by the doctor or eye specialist.

*Effects on ability to drive and use machines:* May cause transient blurring of vision on instillation. Warn patients not to drive or operate hazardous machinery unless vision is clear.

*Undesirable effects:* Transient mild stinging or blurring of vision may occur immediately following the use of this product.

Pupillary dilatation or cycloplegic effects have been observed infrequently with proxymetacaine preparations. Irritation of the conjunctiva or other toxic reactions have occurred only rarely. A severe, immediate-type apparently hyperallergic corneal reaction may rarely occur. This includes acute, intense and diffuse epithelial keratitis; a grey ground-glass appearance; sloughing of large areas of necrotic epithelium; corneal filaments and sometimes, iritis with descemetitis.

*Overdose:* Not applicable.

**Pharmacological properties**

*Pharmacodynamic properties:* Proxymetacaine, in common with other local anaesthetics, reversibly blocks the initiation and conduction of nerve impulses by decreasing the permeability of the neuronal membrane to sodium ions.

The time to onset of effect, duration of effect and potency of proxymetacaine are similar to those of amethocaine.

Fluorescein does not stain a normal cornea but conjunctival abrasions are stained yellow or orange, corneal abrasions are stained a bright green and foreign bodies are surrounded by a green ring.

*Pharmacokinetic properties:* Proxymetacaine is readily absorbed into the systemic circulation where, in common with other ester-type local anaesthetics, it is hydrolysed by plasma esterases. Proxymetacaine is also subject to hepatic metabolism.

Fluorescein will resist penetration of a normal cornea and most will therefore be carried with the tear film away from the conjunctival sac. The majority will be lost through the naso-lacrimal ducts and absorbed via the gastro-intestinal tract from where it is converted rapidly to glucuronide and excreted via the urine.

If fluorescein crosses the cornea it will enter the Bowman's membrane, stroma and possibly the anterior chamber. Aqueous flow and diffusion into the blood in the anterior area finally remove fluorescein from the eye and it is excreted unchanged in the urine.

*Preclinical safety data:* No adverse safety issues were identified during the development of this formulation. The ingredients are well established in clinical ophthalmology.

**Pharmaceutical particulars**

*List of excipients:* Purified water; Povidone K30; hydrochloric acid; sodium hydroxide.

*Incompatibilities:* None known.

*Shelf life:* 18 months.

*Special precautions for storage:* The product should be transported in the original packaging. It should be stored at 2–8°C and prevented from freezing.

*Nature and contents of container:* A sealed conical shaped polypropylene container fitted with a twist and pull off cap. Each Minims unit contains approximately 0.5 ml of solution. Each unit is overwrapped in a polyethylene sachet. 20 units are packed into a suitable carton.

*Instructions for use/handling:* Each Minims unit should be discarded after a single use. Excess solution may be washed away with sterile saline solution.

**Marketing authorisation number**   0033/0152

**Date of approval/revision of SPC**   February 1997

**Legal category**   POM

## MINIMS* ROSE BENGAL

**Presentation**   Single-use, clear, dark-red, sterile eye drops, available as a 1% w/v solution of Rose Bengal. The other ingredients are purified water and sodium hydroxide. No preservatives are included in the formulation.

**Uses**   As a diagnostic stain. Rose Bengal solution stains degenerated conjunctival and corneal epithelial cells. It is particularly useful in demonstrating these changes in Sjögren's syndrome, where lack of tears has caused damage. Pressure marks from contact lenses are shown by Rose Bengal, indicating that alteration of the lens may be necessary.

**Dosage and administration**   One or two drops as required.

Each Minims unit should be discarded after a single use.

**Contra-indications, warnings, etc**   Rose Bengal can produce severe stinging in dry eyes, where it should be used with care. The solution should not be instilled into the eye when the patient is wearing contact lenses. Rose Bengal may discolour the eyelids and/or conjunctiva.

May cause transient blurring of vision on instillation. Warn patients not to drive or operate hazardous machinery unless vision is clear.

The use of Rose Bengal in pregnancy and lactation over many years has not shown any adverse effects. In the absence of any teratology studies, however, Rose Bengal is not recommended in pregnancy unless the therapeutic benefit exceeds the potential risk.

**Pharmaceutical precautions**   Minims Rose Bengal should be stored below 25°C and should not be exposed to strong light. Do not freeze.

**Legal category** P

**Package quantities**   Cartons of 20 units, each unit containing approximately 0.5 ml. OP.

**Further information** Nil.

**Product licence number** 0033/0048R

# MINIMS* SODIUM CHLORIDE

**Presentation** Single-use, clear, colourless, sterile eye drops, available as a 0.9% w/v solution of Sodium Chloride PhEur. Purified water is the only other ingredient. No preservatives are included in the formulation.

**Uses** As an irrigating solution.

**Dosage and administration** Adequate solution should be used to irrigate the eye.

Each Minims unit should be discarded after a single use.

**Contra-indications, warnings, etc** None.

**Pharmaceutical precautions** Minims Sodium Chloride should be stored below 25°C and should not be exposed to strong light. Do not freeze.

**Legal category** P

**Package quantities** Cartons of 20 units, each unit containing approximately 0.5 ml. OP.

**Further information** Nil.

**Product licence number** 0033/5017R

# MINIMS* TROPICAMIDE

**Presentation** Single-use, clear, colourless, sterile eye drops. Two strengths are available: Tropicamide BP 0.5% and 1% w/v solutions. The other ingredients are purified water, hydrochloric acid and sodium hydroxide. No preservatives are included in the formulation.

**Uses** As a mydriatic and cycloplegic.

**Dosage and administration**

*Adults:* 2 drops at five minute intervals, with a further 1 or 2 drops after 30 minutes if required.

*Children:* At the discretion of the physician.

Each Minims unit should be discarded after a single use.

**Contra-indications, warnings, etc** All mydriatics and cycloplegics are contra-indicated in eyes where the filtration angle is narrow, as an acute attack of angle closure glaucoma may be precipitated.

Patients who receive a mydriatic may suffer from photophobia and this may impair their ability to drive under certain circumstances.

There is no evidence as to the drug's safety in human pregnancy nor is there evidence from animal work that it is free from hazard. This product should only be used during pregnancy if considered essential by the physician.

Systemic effects from Minims Tropicamide are not expected. Absorption, however, may be reduced by compressing the lacrimal sac at the medial canthus for a minute during and following the instillation of the drops. (This blocks the passage of the drops via the naso-lacrimal duct to the wide absorptive area of the nasal and pharyngeal mucosa. It is especially advisable in children.)

Should an overdosage occur causing local effects eg. sustained mydriasis, physostigmine 0.25% w/v should be applied.

**Pharmaceutical precautions** Minims Tropicamide should be stored below 25°C and should not be exposed to strong light. Do not freeze.

**Legal category** POM

**Package quantities** Cartons of 20 units, each unit containing approximately 0.5 ml. OP.

**Further information** The 0.5% solution in particular may be expected to cause little or no cycloplegia.

**Product licence numbers**
Minims Tropicamide 0.5%    0033/0077
Minims Tropicamide 1%      0033/0078

# SIMPLENE*

**Qualitative and quantitative composition** Clear, viscous, colourless to almost colourless liquid containing Adrenaline BP. Two strengths are available: 0.5% and 1.0% w/v Adrenaline BP in a buffered solution preserved with benzalkonium chloride 0.01% w/v.

**Pharmaceutical form** Multidose eye drops.

**Clinical particulars**

*Therapeutic indications:* Indicated for the treatment of elevated intraocular pressure in open-angle (chronic simple) glaucoma. It may be used in combination with miotics, beta-adrenergic blocking agents or carbonic anhydrase inhibitors where indicated.

*Posology and method of administration:*
*Adults (including the elderly):* One or two drops to each eye, usually once or twice daily. (May be given as infrequently as every three days.) Determine the frequency of instillation by tonometry.

When used in conjunction with miotics, instil this drug 5 to 10 minutes after the miotic drops.

*Children:* As directed by a physician. Safety and efficacy of use in children has not been established.

*Contra-indications:* Closed-angle glaucoma (unless previously treated with iridectomy). Patients with a narrow angle prone to angle block precipitated by mydriatics. Hypersensitivity to adrenaline or any other component of the preparation. This product contains benzalkonium chloride and should not be used when soft contact lenses are worn.

*Special warnings and special precautions for use:* Do not use until the diagnosis of glaucoma has been verified and the nature of the glaucoma has been confirmed (as the use of adrenaline is contra-indicated in narrow-angle glaucoma).

To reduce the risk of precipitating an attack of narrow-angle glaucoma, evaluate the anterior chamber angle by gonioscopy before initiating therapy.

Adrenaline eye drops should be used with caution by patients with hypertension, cardiac disease, aneurysms, arrhythmia or tachycardia, hyperthyroidism, cerebral arteriosclerosis and diabetes mellitus.

Maculopathy with a central scotoma may occur following use in aphakic patients. Discontinue use in such patients if visual acuity deteriorates.

Systemic absorption of adrenaline from eye drops may be minimised by compressing the lacrimal sac at the medial canthus for a minute during and following the instillation of the drops. (This blocks the passage of the drops via the naso-lacrimal duct to the wide absorptive area of the nasal and pharyngeal mucosa. It is especially advisable in children.)

*Interaction with other medicaments and other forms of interaction:*
*Monoamine oxidase inhibitors:* There is an increased risk of adrenergic reactions when used simultaneously with or up to three weeks after the administration of MAOIs.

*Tricyclic antidepressants:* The pressor response to adrenergic agents and the risk of cardiac arrhythmia may be potentiated in patients receiving tricyclic antidepressants (or within several days of their discontinuation).

*Halothane:* Because of the increased risk of ventricular fibrillation, adrenaline should not be given during general anaesthesia with anaesthetic agents which sensitise the myocardium to sympathomimetics.

*Pregnancy and lactation:* Safety for use in pregnancy and lactation has not been established. This product should not be used during pregnancy unless it is considered essential by the physician.

*Effects on ability to drive and use machines:* May cause temporarily blurred vision. Warn patients not to drive or operate hazardous machinery unless vision is clear.

*Undesirable effects:*
*Local:* Severe smarting on instillation, blurred vision, photophobia, eye pain, conjunctival hyperaemia (resulting in a red eye as a frequent response). Conjunctival sensitisation and allergy and local skin reactions occur occasionally. Pigmentary deposits in the conjunctiva, cornea or eyelids may occur after prolonged use.

*CNS:* Headache or browache are also common but usually diminish as treatment is continued.

*Systemic:* Systemic adverse reactions are rare following topical use at normal dosage. However, palpitations, tachycardia, raised blood pressure, extrasystoles, cardiac arrhythmias, faintness, sweating, pallor, trembling and perspiration may occur.

*Overdose:* Systemic reactions to topical adrenaline are unlikely at normal doses. Greater caution is necessary in children and the elderly and those patients predisposed to such reactions e.g. hypertensive cardiac disease or thyrotoxicosis. A severe reaction to adrenaline is of rapid onset and short duration. The treatment of severe toxic reaction is an immediate intravenous injection of a quick-acting alpha-adrenoceptor blocking agent (such as 2 mg to 5 mg of phentolamine) followed by a beta-adrenoceptor blocking agent (such as 1 mg of propranolol injected over 1 minute and repeated, if necessary at 2 minute intervals up to a maximum of 10 mg (5 mg in anaesthesia)). Adrenaline is almost totally inactive when given by mouth as a result of enzymic degradation in the gut and first pass metabolism in the liver.

**Pharmacological properties**

*Pharmacodynamic properties:* Adrenaline is a sympathomimetic drug which acts as an agonist on both alpha and beta type receptors. In the eye, this sympathomimetic action initiates a contraction of the radial muscle of the iris, which leads to a mydriatic effect on the pupil. Adrenaline is also capable of causing local vasoconstriction in the conjunctiva and increased uveal vascular resistance. Except where angle block is produced in eyes with a narrow angle,

the intraocular pressure is reduced via actions on both the production and drainage of aqueous humour.

*Pharmacokinetic properties:* There are no data on the pharmacokinetics of topical Simplene.

Caution should be exercised when treating patients with cardiovascular disease and thyrotoxicosis.

No reports have been received which would indicate that clinically significant systemic reactions have occurred following the use of Simplene.

*Preclinical safety data:* Adrenaline is a naturally occurring molecule; its use in ophthalmology is well established. Little specific toxicology work has been carried out, however, the breadth of clinical experience confirms its suitability as a topical ophthalmic agent.

**Pharmaceutical particulars**

*List of excipients:* Benzalkonium chloride 50% solution (as preservative); purified water; ammonium lactate (as 60% syrup); N-acetyl-L-cysteine; hydroxyethylcellulose; 0.880 ammonium hydroxide.

*Incompatibilities:* Not known.

*Shelf life:* Unopened: 24 months. Opened: 28 days.

*Special precautions for storage:* Store below 25°C. Protect from light.

*Nature and contents of container:* 7.5 ml of Simplene is supplied in a dropper bottle fitted with a polystyrene or polyethylene pilfer proof cap. Each bottle is enclosed in a nitrogen filled sealed pouch inside a carton. Simplene has a shelf life of 2 years provided the pouch remains unopened.

*Instructions for use/handling:* Contact between the dropper nozzle and other surfaces should be avoided.

Discard any remaining solution 28 days after first opening the container.

**Marketing authorisation numbers**
Simplene 0.5%    0033/0072
Simplene 1%      0033/0057R

**Date of approval/revision of SPC**
Simplene 0.5%    May 1992
Simplene 1%      October 1995

**Legal category** POM

# SNO* PHENICOL

**Qualitative and quantitative composition** Multidose, colourless to pale straw coloured eye drops containing Chloramphenicol BP 0.5% w/v.

**Pharmaceutical form** Multidose sterile eye drops.

**Clinical particulars**

*Therapeutic indications:* Chloramphenicol is a broad spectrum bacteriostatic antibiotic. It is active against a wide variety of gram-negative and gram-positive organisms as well as *rickettsiae* and *spirochaetes*. It is indicated for use as a topical antibacterial in the treatment of superficial ocular infections caused by sensitive organisms.

*Posology and method of administration:*

*Adults (including the elderly):* One to two drops applied to each affected eye up to six times daily or more frequently if required. (Severe infections may require one to two drops every fifteen to twenty minutes initially, reducing the frequency of instillation gradually, as the infection is controlled.)

*Children:* One drop as required.

*Contra-indications:* This product is not intended as a long term treatment for dry eye syndromes. Hypersensitivity to chloramphenicol or to any component of the formulation.

*Special warnings and special precautions for use:* In severe infections topical use of chloramphenicol should be supplemented with appropriate systemic treatment.

Aplastic anaemia has followed topical use of chloramphenicol eye drops and, whilst this hazard is a rare one, it should be considered when the benefits of the use of chloramphenicol are assessed.

Prolonged use should be avoided as it may increase the likelihood of sensitisation and the emergence of resistant organisms.

Contact lenses should be removed during the period of treatment.

Systemic absorption may be reduced by compressing the lacrimal sac at the medial canthus for a minute during and following instillation of the drops. (This blocks the passage of the drops via the naso-lacrimal duct to the wide absorptive area of the nasal and pharyngeal mucosa. This procedure is especially advisable in children).

*Interaction with other medicaments and other forms of interaction:* Chymotrypsin will be inhibited if given simultaneously with chloramphenicol.

*Pregnancy and lactation:* Safety for use in pregnancy

and lactation has not been established. Therefore, use only when considered essential by the physician.

*Effects on ability to drive and use machines:* May cause transient blurring of vision on instillation. Warn patients not to drive or operate hazardous machinery unless vision is clear.

*Undesirable effects:*
*Local:* Sensitivity reactions such as transient irritation, burning, stinging, itching and dermatitis.

*Systemic:* Several cases of major adverse haematological events (bone marrow depression, aplastic anaemia and death) have been reported following ocular use of chloramphenicol.

*Overdose:* Not applicable.

## Pharmacological properties

*Pharmacodynamic properties:* Chloramphenicol binds to the 50S subunit of 70S ribosomes. This prevents the translation of mRNA into protein by inhibiting peptide bond synthesis.

*Pharmacokinetic properties:* Systemically absorbed chloramphenicol is widely distributed throughout the body. Approximately 53% of the absorbed dose is bound to plasma protein. Plasma half life has a mean of around 5 hours. Excretion is mainly in the form of the glucuronide.

*Preclinical safety data:* There are no preclinical data of relevance to the prescriber which are additional to that already included in other sections of the SPC.

## Pharmaceutical particulars

*List of excipients:* Chlorhexidine acetate 0.01% w/v as a preservative; purified water; polyvinyl alcohol; disodium citrate; citric acid.

*Incompatibilities:* None known.

*Shelf life:* Unopened: 18 months. After opening: 28 days.

*Special precautions for storage:* Store between 2°C and 8°C. Do not freeze.

*Nature and contents of container:* Sno phenicol is supplied as a sterile ophthalmic solution in a 10 ml polyethylene bottle with a polyethylene dropper and a polyethylene or polystyrene cap.

*Instructions for use/handling:* Contact between the dropper nozzle and other surfaces should be avoided.
Discard any remaining solution 28 days after first opening the container.

**Marketing authorisation number** 0033/0076

**Date of approval/revision of SPC** April 1996

**Legal category** POM

## SNO* PILO

**Presentation** Multi-dose, clear, colourless to pale yellow eye drops, supplied in a plastic dropper bottle. Three strengths are available 1%, 2% and 4% w/v Pilocarpine Hydrochloride BP preserved with 0.01% benzalkonium chloride. The other ingredients are purified water, polyvinyl alcohol, sodium acetate and acetic acid.

**Uses** Sno pilo is a directly-acting miotic used for the treatment of glaucoma. Indicated for chronic simple glaucoma, acute (closed-angle) glaucoma and as a miotic to counter the effects of mydriasis produced by sympathomimetic agents. Pilocarpine may be used alone or in conjunction with other agents to decrease intraocular pressure prior to surgical treatment.

## Dosage and administration
*Adults (including the elderly):* One or two drops up to four times daily or as prescribed.
The frequency of instillation and concentration of

drops used are determined by the severity of the glaucoma and the response to treatment.

*Children:* At the discretion of the physician. Safety and efficacy of use in children has not been established.

## Contra-indications, warnings etc
*Contra-indications:* Conditions where pupillary constriction is undesirable eg. acute iritis, anterior uveitis and some forms of secondary glaucoma.
Hypersensitivity to any component of the preparation.
Patients with soft contact lenses should not use this preparation.

*Interactions:* Although clinically not proven, the miotic effects of pilocarpine may be antagonised by longterm topical or systemic corticosteroid therapy, systemic anticholinergics, antihistamines, pethidine, sympathomimetics or tricyclic antidepressants. Concomitant administration of two miotics is not recommended because of interdrug antagonism, and unresponsiveness may develop to both drugs.

*Effects on ability to drive and use machines:* Causes difficulty with dark adaptation, therefore, caution is necessary with night driving and when hazardous tasks are undertaken in poor illumination. May cause accommodation spasm. Patients should be advised not to drive or use machinery if vision is not clear.

*Other undesirable effects:*
*Local:* Burning, itching, smarting, blurring of vision, ciliary spasm, conjunctival vascular congestion, induced myopia, sensitisation of the lids and conjunctiva, reduced visual acuity in poor illumination, lens changes with chronic use, increased pupillary block, retinal detachments and vitreous haemorrhages.
*CNS:* Browache and headache (especially in younger patients who have recently started therapy).
*Systemic:* Systemic reactions rarely occur in the treatment of chronic simple glaucoma but they may include hypertension, tachycardia, bronchial spasm, pulmonary oedema, salivation, sweating, nausea, vomiting, diarrhoea and lacrimation.

*Use in pregnancy and lactation:* Safety for use in pregnancy and lactation has not been established, therefore, use only when clearly indicated.

*Other special warnings and precautions:* Systemic reactions rarely occur when treating chronic simple glaucoma at normal doses. However, in the treatment of acute closed-angle glaucoma the possibility of systemic reactions must be considered because of the higher doses given. Caution is particularly advised in patients with acute heart failure, bronchial asthma, peptic ulceration, hypertension, urinary tract obstruction, Parkinson's disease and corneal abrasions.
Retinal detachments have been caused in susceptible individuals and those with pre-existing retinal disease, therefore, fundus examination is advised in all patients prior to the initiation of therapy.
Patients with chronic simple glaucoma on longterm pilocarpine therapy should have regular monitoring of intraocular pressure and visual fields.
Systemic absorption may be reduced by compressing the lacrimal sac at the medial canthus for a minute during and following the instillation of the drops. (This blocks the passage of the drops via the naso-lacrimal duct to the wide absorptive area of the nasal and pharyngeal mucosa. It is especially advisable in children.)

*Overdose:* If accidentally ingested, induce emesis or perform gastric lavage. Observe for signs of toxicity (salivation, lacrimation, sweating, bronchial spasm, cyanosis, nausea, vomiting and diarrhoea).

*Incompatibilities:* None known.

**Pharmaceutical precautions** Sno pilo should not be diluted or dispensed from any container other than

the original bottle and should be stored in a cool place. Sno pilo, like other eye drops, should be discarded one month after opening.

**Legal category** POM

**Package quantities** Sno pilo is supplied as a sterile ophthalmic solution in a 10 ml plastic dropper bottle. OP.

**Further information** The solution is formulated with a viscoliser for patient comfort.

**Product licence numbers**
Sno pilo 1%          0033/0065R
Sno pilo 2%          0033/0066R
Sno pilo 4%          0033/0068R.

## SNO* TEARS

**Presentation** Sno tears is a clear, colourless, slightly viscous solution in a plastic dropper bottle containing polyvinyl alcohol 1.4% w/v preserved with benzalkonium chloride 0.004% w/v. The other ingredients are purified water, sodium chloride, disodium edetate, hydroxyethylcellulose and sodium hydroxide.

**Uses** Sno tears is used topically to provide tear-like lubrication for the symptomatic relief of dry eyes and eye irritation associated with deficient tear production (usually in cases of keratoconjunctivitis sicca and xerophthalmia). Also used as an ocular lubricant for artificial eyes.

## Dosage and administration
*Adults, children and the elderly:* The dose depends on the need for lubrication. Usually one or more drops as required or as prescribed.

## Contra-indications, warnings, etc
*Contra-indications:* Hypersensitivity to any component of the preparation.
Contains benzalkonium chloride and should not be used when soft contact lenses are worn.

*Interactions:* None known.

*Effects on ability to drive and use machines:* May cause transient blurring of vision on instillation. Do not drive or operate hazardous machinery unless vision is clear.

*Other undesirable effects:* May cause transient, mild stinging or temporarily blurred vision.

*Use in pregnancy and lactation:* There is no, or inadequate, evidence of safety of the drug in human pregnancy, but it has been in wide use for many years without apparent ill-consequence. If drug therapy is needed in pregnancy this preparation can be used if recommended by a physician.

*Other special warnings and precautions:* If irritation persists or worsens, or headache, eye pain, vision changes or continued redness occur, discontinue use and consult a physician or ophthalmologist.
To preserve sterility, do not allow the dropper to touch the eye or any other surface.

*Incompatibilities:* None known.

**Pharmaceutical precautions** Sno tears should be stored below 25°C. Sno tears, as with other eye drops, should be discarded one month after opening.

**Legal category** P

**Package quantities** Sno tears is supplied as a sterile ophthalmic solution in a 10 ml plastic dropper bottle. OP.

**Further information** Nil.

**Product licence number** 0033/0097

*Trade Mark

# Chugai Pharma UK Limited
Mulliner House,
Flanders Road,
Turnham Green,
London W4 1NN

## GRANOCYTE* ▼

**Qualitative and quantitative composition** Granocyte contains lenograstim, a recombinant glycoprotein (rHuG-CSF) equivalent to the Human Granulocyte Colony-Stimulating Factor isolated from CHU-2, a human cell line. Lenograstim is expressed and glycosylated in a mammalian host cell system, Chinese hamster ovary (CHO) cells.

*Composition of the lyophilisate*

|  | Granocyte-34 | Granocyte-13 |
| --- | --- | --- |
| Lenograstim (rHuG-CSF) | 33.6 MIU‡ | 13.4 MIU‡ |
|  | 263.0 µg | 105.0 µg |
| Human Albumin | 1.0 mg | 1.0 mg |
| Mannitol | 50.0 mg | 50.0 mg |
| Polysorbate 20 | 0.1 mg | 0.1 mg |
| Disodium phosphate | qs pH 6.5 | qs pH 6.5 |
| Sodium dihydrogen phosphate | qs pH 6.5 | qs pH 6.5 |

*Composition of the solvent*

| Water for Injections | 1.05 ml | 1.05 ml |
| --- | --- | --- |

‡ as measured by the GNFS-60 bioassay in comparison with the WHO International Standard.

Both vials and solvent are over-filled by 5%. The extractable volume of the solvent is 1.05 ml to be used for reconstitution of the lyophilisate in order to be able to extract 1 ml of reconstituted Granocyte for use.

When reconstituted, Granocyte-13 contains 13.4 MIU (105 µg) in 1 ml.

When reconstituted, Granocyte-34 contains 33.6 MIU (263 µg) in 1 ml.

The reconstituted product is formulated in an aqueous buffer at pH 6.5 and contains Mannitol 5%, Human Albumin 0.1%, and Polysorbate 20 0.01%.

**Pharmaceutical form** Granocyte is presented as a single-use vial of freeze-dried product with an ampoule of solvent containing Water for Injections BP.

*Presentations:*
1 pack of 1 13.4 MIU (105 µg) vial + 1 ampoule
1.05 ml solvent (WFI)
1 pack of 5 33.6 MIU (263 µg) vials + 5 ampoules
1.05 ml solvent (WFI)

**Clinical particulars**
*Therapeutic indications:* Reduction in the duration of neutropenia and the associated complications in patients with non-myeloid malignancy who have undergone autologous or allogeneic bone marrow transplantation, or treatment with established cytotoxic chemotherapy regimens associated with a significant incidence of febrile neutropenia.

Mobilisation of autologous peripheral blood progenitor cells (PBPCs).

*Posology and method of administration:* For reduction in the duration of neutropenia and the associated complications in patients who have undergone bone marrow transplantation, or treatment with cytotoxic chemotherapy, the recommended dose of Granocyte is 150 micrograms (19.2 MIU) per m² daily.

For mobilisation of PBPCs with Granocyte after cytotoxic chemotherapy, the recommended dose of Granocyte is 150 micrograms (19.2 MIU) per m² daily.

This recommended dose of Granocyte 150 micrograms (19.2 MIU) per m² daily, is therapeutically equivalent to 5 micrograms per kg daily, as used in clinical studies.

In these indications, Granocyte-13 is used in patients with a body surface area up to 0.7 m² and Granocyte-34 is used in patients with a body surface area up to 1.8 m².

For mobilisation of PBPCs with Granocyte alone, the recommended dose of Granocyte is 10 micrograms per kg daily.

*Adults:*
*In bone marrow transplantation:* Granocyte should be diluted in Sodium Chloride Injection BP and administered daily as a 30-minute intravenous infusion, starting the day after transplantation. Daily dosing should continue until the expected nadir has passed and the neutrophil count returns to within the normal range, with a maximum of 28 consecutive days of treatment if necessary.

It is anticipated that by day 14 after bone marrow transplantation, 50% of patients will achieve neutrophil recovery.

*In established cytotoxic chemotherapy:* Granocyte should be administered as a subcutaneous injection starting 24 hours after chemotherapy administration ends. Daily dosing should continue until the expected nadir has passed and the neutrophil count returns to within the normal range, usually within 8 to 14 days after starting treatment, with a maximum of 28 consecutive days of treatment if necessary. A transient increase in neutrophil count may occur within the first two days of treatment. Granocyte treatment should not be stopped, since the subsequent nadir usually occurs earlier and recovers more quickly if treatment continues.

*In peripheral blood progenitor cell mobilisation:* After cytotoxic chemotherapy, Granocyte should be administered daily as a subcutaneous injection starting on the day following completion of chemotherapy. Daily dosing should continue until the expected nadir has passed and the neutrophil count returns to a stable level compatible with treatment discontinuation.

Leucapheresis should be performed when the post-nadir leucocyte count is rising, or after assessment of CD34+ cell count by a validated method. For patients who have not received extensive chemotherapy, one leucapheresis is often sufficient to obtain the acceptable minimum yield (≥2 × 10⁶ CD34+ cells per kg bodyweight) for adequate haematologic reconstitution.

In peripheral blood progenitor cell mobilisation with Granocyte alone, Granocyte should be administered as a subcutaneous injection daily for 4 to 6 days, with leucapheresis between days 5 and 7. For patients who have not received extensive chemotherapy, one leucapheresis is often sufficient to obtain the acceptable minimum yield (≥2 × 10⁶ CD34+ cells per kg bodyweight) for adequate haematologic reconstitution.

Granocyte therapy should only be given in collaboration with an experienced oncology and/or haematology centre.

*Elderly:* Clinical trials with Granocyte have included a small number of patients up to the age of 70 years, but special studies have not been performed in the elderly. Specific dose recommendations cannot be made.

*Children:* The safety and efficacy of Granocyte have been established in children older than 2 years in bone marrow transplantation.

*Contra-indications:* Granocyte should not be administered to patients with known hypersensitivity to the product or its constituents.

Granocyte should not be used to increase the dose-intensity of cytotoxic chemotherapy beyond established dose regimens, since it does not affect the non-haematological toxicity of cytotoxic drugs.

Granocyte should not be administered concurrently with cytotoxic chemotherapy.

Granocyte should not be administered to patients with myeloid malignancy.

*Special precautions and special warnings for use:*
*Malignant cell growth:* Granulocyte colony stimulating factors can promote the growth of myeloid cell lines in vitro. The safety and efficacy of Granocyte administration to patients with acute myelogenous leukaemia, or chronic myelogenous leukaemia have not been established, and because of the possibility of tumour growth, Granocyte should not be used in any myeloid malignancy.

Clinical trials have not established whether or not Granocyte influences the progression of myelodysplastic syndrome to acute myelogenous leukaemia. Caution should be exercised in using Granocyte in any pre-malignant myeloid condition.

Some tumour cell lines with non-specific characteristics can, exceptionally, express a G-CSF receptor. This should be considered if unexpected tumour regrowth is observed concomitantly with Granocyte therapy.

*Leucocytosis:* In view of the potential risks associated with severe leucocytosis, white blood cell count should be monitored regularly during Granocyte therapy. A leucocyte count greater than 50 × 10⁹/L has not been observed in any of the clinical trial patients treated with 5 micrograms per kg daily following bone marrow transplantation. White blood cell counts of ≥70 × 10⁹/L have been observed in less than 5% of

patients who received cytotoxic chemotherapy and were treated with Granocyte at 5 micrograms per kg daily. No adverse events attributable to this degree of leucocytosis have been reported.

After bone marrow transplantation, or cytotoxic chemotherapy, if the leucocyte count exceeds 50 × 10⁹/L after the expected nadir, Granocyte should be discontinued immediately.

For PBPC mobilisation, Granocyte should be discontinued if the leucocyte count exceeds 70 × 10⁹/L.

*Risks associated with increased doses of chemotherapy:* The safety and efficacy of Granocyte have yet to be established in the context of dose-intensified chemotherapy. Due to non-haematological toxicity of the cytotoxic chemotherapy, Granocyte should not be used to decrease the intervals between chemotherapy courses beyond established limits, and/or to increase the doses of chemotherapy agents beyond established limits. Non-haematological toxicities were the limiting factors in a chemotherapy intensification trial with Granocyte.

*Peripheral blood progenitor cell mobilisation:*
*Choice of mobilisation method:* Trials have shown that the PBPC yield is higher when Granocyte is given after cytotoxic chemotherapy than when Granocyte is administered alone. For each patient, the choice of mobilisation should be considered in relation to the overall treatment objectives.

*Prior exposure to radiotherapy and/or cytotoxic chemotherapy agents:* Patients who have previously undergone extensive cytotoxic chemotherapy and/or radiotherapy treatment may not mobilise sufficient PBPCs to achieve the minimum acceptable yield for haematologic reconstitution (≥2 × 10⁶ CD34+ cells per kg bodyweight). PBPC transplantation should be defined early in the patient's treatment program. Before proceeding to myelosuppressive, or myeloablative cytotoxic chemotherapy, the yield of PBPC should be considered carefully, and if yields are low, an alternative to PBPC transplantation implemented.

*Assessment of PBPC yield:* Results of flow cytometric analysis of CD34+ cells vary between laboratories. Particular attention should be paid to the method of progenitor cell quantification.

*Minimum PBPC yield:* The minimum number of PBPCs required for haematological reconstitution is not well defined and the recommendation of ≥2 × 10⁶ CD34+ cells per kg bodyweight is based on available published experience. The time to haematological recovery is related to the dose of CD34+ cells reinfused. Infusion of ≥2 × 10⁶ CD34+ cells per kg bodyweight is associated with a relatively more rapid recovery compared to reinfusion of <2 × 10⁶ CD34+ cells per kg bodyweight.

*Other special precautions:* The safety and efficacy of Granocyte have not been defined in patients with severe impairment of hepatic or renal function.

In patients with substantially reduced myeloid progenitor cells (e.g. due to prior intensive radiotherapy or chemotherapy), neutrophil response is sometimes diminished and the safety of Granocyte has not been established.

*Interactions with other medicaments and other forms of interaction:* Rapidly dividing myeloid cells are sensitive to cytotoxic chemotherapy. The use of Granocyte is not recommended from 24 hours before cytotoxic chemotherapy administration until 24 hours after administration ends.

Possible interactions with other haematopoietic growth factors and cytokines have yet to be investigated in clinical trials.

*Pregnancy and lactation:* The safety of Granocyte has not been established in pregnant women.

There is no evidence from studies in rats and rabbits that Granocyte is teratogenic. An increased frequency of embryo loss has been observed in rabbits, but no malformation has been seen. In pregnancy, the possible risk to the foetus of Granocyte use must be weighed against the expected therapeutic benefits.

Granocyte is not recommended for use in nursing women, as it is not known whether Granocyte is excreted in human breast milk.

*Effects on ability to drive or use machines:* None.

*Undesirable effects:*

*In bone marrow transplantation:* Special attention must be paid to platelet recovery, since in trials the mean platelet count was lower in patients treated with Granocyte than in patients treated with placebo. This did not result in an increased frequency of adverse events related to blood loss, and the median number of days following bone marrow transplantation to last platelet infusion was similar in treated and untreated groups.

In trials, the most frequently reported adverse events occurred with equal frequency in patients treated with Granocyte or placebo. Events were those usually encountered with conditioning regimens and were apparently unrelated to Granocyte, which did not prevent them. They were infection/inflammatory disorder of the buccal cavity, fever, diarrhoea, rash, abdominal pain, vomiting, alopecia, sepsis and infection.

The effect of Granocyte on the incidence and severity of acute and chronic graft versus host disease has not been defined.

*In Chemotherapy-Induced Neutropenia:* The safety of Granocyte use with cytotoxic chemotherapy agents that have cumulative bone marrow toxicity, or predominant toxicity to the platelet lineage, e.g. nitrosourea, mitomycin, has not been established. The use of Granocyte with such agents may result in increased platelet toxicity.

In trials, the overall incidence of reported adverse events was the same in patients treated with either Granocyte or placebo. The most commonly reported adverse events were alopecia, nausea, vomiting, fever, and headache, similar to those observed in cancer patients treated with chemotherapy. In patients treated with Granocyte, bone pain and injection site reaction were reported with slightly higher frequency (10% and 5% higher respectively) compared to patients treated with placebo.

*Overdose:* The effects of Granocyte overdose have not been fully established. Discontinuation of Granocyte therapy usually results in a 50% decrease in circulating neutrophils within 1 to 2 days, with a return to normal levels within 1 to 7 days. In humans, doses up to 40 micrograms per kg daily were not associated with toxic side effects, except for musculoskeletal pain.

In animals, acute toxicity studies (up to 1000 micrograms per kg daily in mice) and subacute toxicity studies (up to 100 micrograms per kg daily in monkeys) showed that the effects of overdose were restricted to an exaggerated and reversible pharmacological effect. See *Special precautions and special warnings for use: Leucocytosis.*

## Pharmacological properties

*Pharmacodynamic properties:* Granocyte (lenograstim, rHuG-CSF) belongs to the cytokine group of biologically active proteins which regulate cell differentiation and growth. rHuG-CSF stimulates neutrophil precursor cells, increasing CFU-S and CFU-GM cell counts in peripheral blood. Granocyte induces a marked increase in peripheral blood neutrophil counts within 24 hours of administration.

Elevations in neutrophil counts are dose-dependent over the range 1–10 micrograms per kg daily. At the recommended dose, repeated doses induce an enhancement of the neutrophil reponse. Neutrophils produced in response to Granocyte show normal chemotactic and phagocytic functions.

Use of Granocyte in patients who have undergone bone marrow transplantation, or treatment with cytotoxic chemotherapy, leads to significant reductions in the duration of neutropenia and the associated complications.

Use of Granocyte alone, or after cytotoxic chemotherapy mobilises haematopoietic progenitor cells into peripheral blood. These autologous cells can be harvested and reinfused after high-dose chemotherapy, either in place of, or in addition to bone marrow transplantation.

Reinfused PBPCs, obtained following mobilisation with Granocyte, have been shown to reconstitute haematopoiesis. This reduces time to engraftment compared to autologous bone marrow transplantation, leading to a marked reduction in the number of days to independence from platelet transfusions.

*Pharmacokinetic properties:* The pharmacokinetics of Granocyte are dose and time dependent. During repeated subcutaneous or intravenous dosing, peak serum concentrations are proportional to the injected dose. Repeated dosing with Granocyte by these routes showed no evidence of drug accumulation.

At the recommended dose, the absolute bioavailability of Granocyte is 30%. The apparent distribution volume ($V_d$ area) is approximately 1L per kg body-weight and the mean residence time after subcutaneous dosing approaches 7 hours.

The apparent serum half-life of Granocyte at steady state (repeated dosing) is approximately 3–4 hours, and is shorter, 1–1.5 hours, following repeated intravenous infusion.

Plasma clearance of rHuG-CSF increased 3-fold, from 50 to 150 ml/min, during repeated subcutaneous dosing. Less than 1% of the dose is excreted unchanged in urine, and Granocyte is considered to be metabolised to peptides. During multiple subcutaneous dosing at the recommended dose, peak serum concentrations are close to 100 picograms per ml. There is a positive correlation between the dose and the serum concentration of Granocyte, and between the neutrophil response and the total amount of Granocyte recovered in serum.

## Pharmaceutical particulars

*List of excipients:* Human albumin, mannitol, polysorbate 20, disodium phosphate, sodium dihydrogen phosphate, sodium chloride.

*Incompatibilities:* Dilution of Granocyte-13 to a final concentration of less than 0.26 MIU/ml (2 micro-grams/ml), i.e. approximately 1 vial into 50 ml of infusion fluid, is not recommended.

Dilution of Granocyte-34 to a final concentration of less than 0.32 MIU/ml (2.5 micrograms/ml), i.e. approximately 1 vial into 100 ml of infusion fluid, is not recommended.

*Shelf life:* Two years when stored in a refrigerator between 2°C and 8°C.

*Special precautions for storage:* Granocyte should be stored in a refrigerator between 2°C and 8°C.

A single, short exposure (up to two weeks) of the vials to temperatures up to 30°C does not affect the product stability.

Granocyte should not be reconstituted and diluted more than 24 hours before administration. Solutions should be stored in a refrigerator between 2°C and 8°C.

Granocyte vials are for single use only.

After reconstitution in Water for Injections as recommended, the product is stable for 24 hours at 25°C.

When diluted for infusion in Sodium Chloride Injection BP to a final concentration of not less than 0.26 MIU/ml (2 micrograms/ml) for Granocyte-13, or 0.32 MIU/ml (2.5 micrograms/ml) for Granocyte-34, the product is stable for 24 hours when stored at 5°C or 25°C.

*Nature and contents of container:*

*Granocyte-13, Granocyte-34:* A PhEur Type 1 borosilicate glass vial, with isobutylene-isoprepene rubber seal, held by an aluminium cap and polypropylene lid.

*Water for Injections Ampoule:* A PhEur Type 1 borosilicate glass ampoule.

*Instructions for use:* Immediately prior to administration, aseptically add the extractable contents (1.05 ml) of one ampoule of solvent (Water for Injections) to the Granocyte-13, or Granocyte-34 vial.

Mix gently until completely dissolved (about 5 seconds). **Do not shake vigorously.**

Withdraw the required volume from the vial.

For intravenous infusion, Granocyte should be diluted with Sodium Chloride Injection BP. After reconstitution, the maximum dilution volume should not exceed 50 ml for 1 vial of Granocyte-13, or 100 ml for 1 vial of Granocyte-34.

Granocyte should be used within 24 hours of reconstitution.

Diluted solutions should be stored in a refrigerator between 2°C and 8°C.

When diluted in Sodium Chloride Injection BP, Granocyte is compatible with the commonly used giving sets for injection, e.g. polyvinyl chloride.

Granocyte vials are for single use only.

**Marketing authorisation number** 12185/0002.

**Date of approval/revision of SPC** January 1997.

**Legal category** POM.

*\*Trade Mark*

# CIBA Vision Ophthalmics
Flanders Road
Hedge End
Southampton
Hampshire SO30 2LG

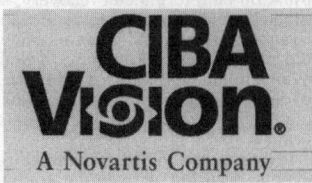

## HYPOTEARS*

**Presentation** A sterile colourless, hypotonic aqueous solution, containing 1.0% w/v polyvinyl alcohol. It also contains disodium edetate, benzalkonium chloride (preservative), polyethylene glycol and purified water.

**Uses** An ocular lubricant for the treatment and symptomatic relief of physiological dry eye conditions and associated irritation.

**Dosage and administration**

*Adults:* One or two drops in the affected eye(s) as required.

*Elderly and children:* No dosage amendment is necessary in the elderly or in children.

**Contra-indications, warnings, etc**

*Contra-indications:* Patients with known hypersensitivity to benzalkonium chloride.

Due to the presence of benzalkonium chloride this product should not be prescribed for patients who wear soft contact lenses.

*Precautions:* Discontinue use if allergy develops to any component of the preparation. To avoid contamination of the solution, do not touch dropper tip to any surface, particularly the eyelids or surrounding area. For topical use only. Discard any remainder 28 days after opening. If eye irritation persists discontinue use and seek medical advice.

*Pregnancy:* There is no experience regarding the safety of Hypotears in human pregnancy or lactation.

*Side-effects:* As with other lubricating artificial tear solutions, transient stinging and/or burning has been reported.

*Overdosage:* Not applicable.

*Effect on ability to drive or use machines:* Hypotears does not have any sedative effect and so will not affect ability to drive and to use machines.

**Pharmaceutical precautions** Store below 30°C

**Legal category** P

**Package quantities** 15 ml

**Further information** Hypotears is an ocular lubricant which relieves irritation or dryness of eyes due to physiological dry eye conditions. Hypotears normalises the pre-corneal tear film by balancing tear film osmolarity and stabilises the mucin and aqueous tear layers. The polyvinyl alcohol contained in Hypotears has mucomimetic properties to soothe and lubricate the dry eye and enhance tear film stability. Polyvinyl alcohol also reduces the surface tension of the tears to increase the wetting of the cornea by the tear film.

There are no pharmacologically active constituents in Hypotears. The action of polyvinyl alcohol in the eye is based on its demulcent and lubricating properties rather than chemical or pharmacological actions.

**Product licence number** 8685/0012

## IOCARE* BALANCED SALT SOLUTION

**Presentation** A sterile, colourless, isotonic solution, each 1 ml contains: sodium chloride 0.64% w/v, potassium chloride 0.075% w/v, calcium chloride 0.048% w/v, magnesium chloride 0.03% w/v, sodium acetate 0.39% w/v and sodium citrate 0.17% w/v.

**Uses** For intraocular or topical irrigation of the eye during surgical procedures.

**Dosage and administration**

*Dosage:* Adults, elderly and children: To be used according to the ophthalmic surgeon during surgical procedures.

*Administration:*

*15 ml bottle:* Ensure that the blister and paper backing are intact. If the blister package is damaged sterility cannot be assured.

Open under aseptic conditions.

The adapter plug is designed to accept an irrigating needle. Tissues may be irrigated by attaching the needle to the bottle as explained below. External irrigation may be done without an irrigating needle.

Aseptically remove from the blister pack.

Snap on irrigator needle. Push firmly into place. Test assembly for proper function before use.

Squeeze out several drops of solution before inserting into the anterior chamber of the eye. The needle should be removed from the anterior chamber prior to releasing pressure to prevent suction.

*500 ml bag:* If the fluid bag is damaged, sterility cannot be assured.

Follow directions of the particular administration set to be used. Insert the administration set spike aseptically into the fluid bag. Allow the fluid to flow and remove air from the tubing before irrigation begins.

**Contra-indications, warnings, etc**

*Contra-indications:* There are no specific contra-indications to the use of Balanced Salt Solution for tissue irrigation.

*Precautions:* The solution contains no preservative and should not be reused. Any remainder should be discarded. The product may not be resterilised.

Not for injection or IV infusion.

*Pregnancy and lactation:* There is no pharmacologically active ingredient in Balanced Salt Solution. Reproductive studies have not been conducted to assess the safety of this product for use during pregnancy and lactation. As with all medicines, however, careful consideration should be given to the treatment of pregnant and lactating patients.

*Drug interactions:* Not known.

*Side-effects:* When the corneal endothelium is abnormal, irrigation, or any other trauma, may result in bullous keratopathy.

*Overdosage:* Not applicable.

*Effects on ability to drive or use machinery:* Not applicable.

**Pharmaceutical precautions** Store below 25°C. Discard any remainder, do not resterilise.

**Legal category** P

**Package quantities** 15 ml bottle x 12; 500 ml bag.

**Further information** Iocare is a physiological irrigating solution containing essential ions for normal cell metabolism.

**Product licence numbers**
15 ml 8685/0011
500 ml 8685/0010

## LIVOSTIN* EYE DROPS ▼

**Presentation** White sterile ophthalmic microsuspension (pH6-8) containing levocabastine hydrochloride equivalent to 0.5 mg/ml levocabastine. Livostin eye drops also contain benzalkonium chloride, disodium edetate, propylene glycol, polysorbate 80, disodium phosphate, monosodium phosphate, hypromellose and water.

**Uses** Levocabastine is a selective histamine $H_1$ antagonist.

Livostin eye drops are indicated for the symptomatic treatment of seasonal allergic conjunctivitis.

**Dosage and administration** As Livostin eye drops are a microsuspension, the bottle should be shaken before each application.

*Adults, the elderly and children 9 years and over:* The usual dose is 1 drop of Livostin eye drops per eye, twice a day. The dose may be increased to 1 drop per eye 3 to 4 times daily, if necessary. Treatment should not be continued beyond 4 weeks. Exposure to the product is limited to a total of 4 weeks in any one year.

It is not useful to continue treatment for more than 3 days if no improvement is seen.

*Use in children:* Livostin eye drops are not recommended for use in children less than 9 years.

**Contra-indications, warnings, etc**

*Contra-indications:* Hypersensitivity to any of the ingredients.

*Precautions:* As with all ophthalmic preparations containing benzalkonium chloride patients are ad-

vised not to wear soft (hydrophilic) contact lenses whilst being treated with Livostin eye drops.

*Use in pregnancy and lactation:* In mice, rats and rabbits, Livostin, at oral doses up to 8,300 times the recommended ocular clinical dose, did not reveal any embryotoxic or teratogenic effect. In rodents, at 16,500 times this dose and higher, teratogenicity and/or increased embryonal resorption were observed.

There are no adequate data on the use of Livostin eye drops in pregnant women, therefore Livostin eye drops should not be used during pregnancy, unless the potential benefit justifies the potential risk to the foetus.

Based on determinations of levocabastine concentrations in saliva and breast milk in a nursing woman, it was calculated that the daily dose of levocabastine in the infant would not exceed 0.5μg after ophthalmic treatment of the mother. Therefore levocabastine eye drops can be given to nursing mothers.

*Effects on ability to drive or use machines:* Sedation has rarely been reported during concomitant use of the eye drops and nasal spray. This should be borne in mind when special alertness is necessary eg in connection with driving or in performance of skilled tasks.

*Side-effects:* Effects such as local irritation, blurring of vision, eye oedema, urticaria, dyspnoea and headache have been reported after instillation of Livostin Eye Drops. If effects are severe it may be necessary to discontinue treatment.

*Overdosage:* Overdosage is unlikely following topical use. In the event of accidental oral ingestion, supportive measures should be taken.

**Pharmaceutical precautions** Store below 25°C. Use within one month of opening the bottle. Shake well before use

**Legal category** POM

**Package quantities** White plastic bottles containing 4 ml microsuspension.

**Further information** Nil

**Product licence number** 0242/0151

## LIVOSTIN* NASAL SPRAY ▼

**Presentation** White sterile microsuspension (pH6-8) containing levocabastine hydrochloride equivalent to 0.5 mg/ml levocabastine. Livostin nasal spray also contains benzalkonium chloride, disodium edetate, propylene glycol, polysorbate 80, disodium phosphate, monosodium phosphate, hypromellose and water.

**Uses** Levocabastine is a selective histamine $H_1$ antagonist.

Livostin nasal spray is indicated for the symptomatic treatment of seasonal allergic rhinitis.

**Dosage and administration** As Livostin nasal spray is a microsuspension, the bottle should be shaken before each application.

*Adults and children 9 years and over:* The usual dose is 2 sprays per nostril of Livostin nasal spray, twice daily. The dose may be increased to 2 sprays per nostril 3 to 4 times daily, if necessary. Treatment should not be continued for more than 4 weeks.

Patients should be instructed to clean the nasal passages prior to administering the spray and to inhale gently through the nose during spraying. Before using the pump delivery system for the first time the pump reservoir should be filled up by squeezing the bottle once or twice until a fine spray is delivered.

*Use in the elderly:* As for adults

*Use in children:* Livostin nasal spray is not recommended for use in children less than 9 years of age.

**Contra-indications, warnings, etc**

*Contra-indications:* Hypersensitivity to any of the ingredients.

The main route of excretion of levocabastine is via the kidneys. In patients with renal impairment elimination of levocabastine was found to be prolonged.

Use of Livostin nasal spray in patients with significant renal impairment is therefore contraindicated.

*Use in pregnancy and lactation*: In mice, rats and rabbits, levocabastine, at oral doses up to 1,250 times the recommended nasal clinical dose, did not reveal any embryotoxic or teratogenic effect. In rodents, at 2,500 times this dose and higher, teratogenicity and/or increased embryonal resorption were observed.

There are no adequate data on the use of Livostin nasal spray in pregnant women. Livostin nasal spray should therefore not be used during pregnancy, unless the potential benefit justifies the potential risk to the foetus.

Based on determination of levocabastine concentrations in saliva and the breast milk in a nursing woman, it was calculated that the daily dose of levocabastine in the infant would not exceed 3.5µg after nasal treatment of the mother. Livostin nasal spray can therefore be given to nursing mothers.

*Interactions*: No interaction with alcohol or with any other drugs was reported during clinical trials. In specially designed psychoperformance studies, no interaction with diazepam or alcohol was observed.

Treatment with Livostin nasal spray may cause sedation in some patients. This should be borne in mind when special alertness is necessary, eg in connection with driving or the performance of skilled tasks. Excess alcohol should be avoided.

*Side-effects*: Symptoms of local irritation (eg nasal stinging and burning), have been reported following the application of Livostin nasal spray.

Headache, fatigue and somnolence have also been reported. Conclusive evidence of the causation of these effects has not been demonstrated.

*Overdosage*: Overdosing with Livostin nasal spray is unlikely. In the event of accidental oral ingestion, supportive measures should be taken.

**Pharmaceutical precautions** Store at room temperature, not greater than 30°C. Shake well before use.

**Legal category** POM

**Package quantities** White plastic bottles with a spray pump containing 10 ml microsuspension.

**Further information** Nil

**Product licence number** 0242/0152
*Product licence holder:* Janssen-Cilag Ltd

## MIOCHOL*

**Presentation** A vial of two compartments containing, acetylcholine chloride 20 mg and mannitol 60 mg in the lower chamber and water for injection 2 ml in the upper chamber. On reconstitution 2 ml of a 1:100 solution of acetylcholine chloride in 3% mannitol is obtained. Mannitol renders the reconstituted solution isotonic with blood and serum. It is not considered an active ingredient

**Uses** To obtain rapid and complete miosis after delivery of the lens in cataract surgery as well as in penetrating keratoplasty, iridectomy and other anterior segment surgery where rapid complete miosis is required.

**Dosage and administration**
*Adults and elderly:* In most cases a satisfactory miosis, which will last for approximately 20 minutes, is produced in seconds by 0.5–2.0 ml. A second application may be made at the discretion of the surgeon if prolonged miosis is required.

*Children:* Safety and effectiveness in children have not been established.

Miochol is for intraocular irrigation only. A freshly prepared 1% solution should be used in the anterior chamber of the eye during surgery.

**Contra-indications, warnings,etc**
*Contra-indications:* There are no known contraindications to the use of Miochol in cataract or anterior segment surgery.

*Precautions*: In cataract surgery, Miochol should be used only after delivery of the lens. If miosis is to be obtained quickly and completely, obstructions to miosis such as anterior or posterior synechiae may require surgery prior to administration of Miochol.

If blister or paper backing is damaged or broken, sterility of the Miochol vial cannot be assured. The solvent should be in the upper chamber before use. If the centre rubber plug in the univial does not go down when the plunger-stopper is pressed or is already down, the vial should not be used.

*Pregnancy and lactation*: The safety and efficacy of Miochol in pregnancy and lactation have not been established. Miochol should not be used in pregnant or lactating patients.

*Drug interactions:* Although clinical studies with acetylcholine chloride and animal studies with acetylcholine or carbachol revealed no interference, and there is no known pharmacological basis for an interaction, there have been reports that acetylcholine chloride and carbachol have been ineffective when used in patients treated with topical non-steroidal anti-inflammatory agents.

*Side-effects:* Adverse reactions which are indicative of systemic absorption have been reported rarely in the literature. Symptoms include bradycardia, hypotension, flushing, breathing difficulties and sweating. Isolated cases of corneal oedema, corneal clouding and corneal decompensation have been reported with the use of Miochol, although a causal relationship has not been established.

*Overdosage:* The symptoms of overdosage are likely to be effects resulting from systemic absorption, ie bradycardia, hypotension, flushing, breathing difficulties and sweating. Atropine sulphate (0.5–1 mg) should be given intramuscularly or intravenously and should be readily available to counteract possible overdosage. Adrenaline (0.1–1.0 mg subcutaneously) is also of value in overcoming severe cardiovascular or bronchoconstrictor responses.

*Effects on ability to drive or use machines:* Not applicable

**Pharmaceutical precautions** Store below 25°C. Protect from freezing. Aqueous solutions of Miochol are unstable. The solution should therefore be prepared immediately before use. Any remainder should be discarded.

Acetylcholine is incompatible with solutions of acidic or alkaline pH but this is unlikely to be relevant during clinical use.

Sterile unless pack is open or broken. Do not resterilise.

**Legal category** POM

**Package quantities** 2 ml x 12 vials

**Further information** Nil

**Product licence number** 8685/0014

## OTRIVINE-ANTISTIN* STERILE EYE DROPS

**Presentation** A clear colourless odourless solution containing Xylometazoline Hydrochloride BP 0.05% w/v and antazoline sulphate 0.5% w/v with Benzalkonium Chloride Ph Eur 0.01% w/v as a preservative.

Also contains: boric acid, disodium edetate, sodium tetraborate and water.

**Uses** Otrivine-Antistin is a combination of a long acting vasoconstrictor and an antihistamine. The eye drops are for temporary relief of redness and itching of the eye due to seasonal and perennial allergies such as hay fever, or allergy due to house dust.

**Dosage and administration** Otrivine-Antistin Eye Drops are intended for local administration to the eye.

*Adults:* 1 or 2 drops instilled 2-3 times per day into the conjunctival sac.

*Children 5–12 years and the elderly:* No specific studies have been performed in these patients. Due to possible systemic effects caution must be exercised and the dosage reduced to 1 drop instilled 2-3 times per day.

The eye drops should not be used in children under the age of 5 years.

When necessary, mydriatics or miotics may be administered simultaneously with Otrivine-Antistin Eye Drops.

**Contra-indications, warnings, etc**
*Contra-indications:* Hypersensitivity to any of the components of the formulation. Presence of narrow angle glaucoma. The use of monoamine oxidase inhibitors within the last 14 days. Otrivine-Antistin is not recommended in patients who wear contact lenses of any type.

*Precautions:* In patients who are receiving medication for hypertension, cardiac irregularities, hyperthyroidism or diabetes mellitus particular caution should be exercised. Caution should be observed in patients with relevant previous eye disease or surgery. Otrivine-Antistin is not suitable for patients suffering from dry eyes without first seeking medical advice. Rebound congestion may follow continued use. Inflammation arising from infection should receive appropriate antibacterial therapy.

*Use in pregnancy and lactation:* In line with common practice, the use of medication during pregnancy is not recommended unless considered essential.

*Drug interactions:* No interactions with other drugs have been reported. There is a theoretical potential for interaction with clonidine.

*Side-effects:* Otrivine-Antistin Eye Drops are well tolerated in the eye and for the majority of the patients will be non-irritant, but in a few cases, slight transient local stinging may occur. Other side effects which have been reported very occasionally are blurred vision, headache and drowsiness.

*Overdosage:* There is no experience of overdosage.

**Pharmaceutical precautions** Protect from heat. The drops should not be used later than one month after first breaking the seal.

**Legal category** P

**Package quantities** Otrivine-Antistin Sterile Eye drops 10 ml (OP)

**Further information** Nil

**Product licence number** 8685/0002

## TEOPTIC* EYE-DROPS

**Presentation** A clear colourless odourless sterile solution containing carteolol hydrochloride 1% or 2% w/v with Benzalkonium Chloride PhEur 0.005% w/v as a preservative.

Also contains: sodium chloride, dibasic sodium phosphate, monobasic sodium phosphate and water.

**Uses** Teoptic is a beta-adrenergic-receptor-blocking agent possessing intrinsic sympathomimetic activity. Teoptic Eye-Drops are a topical treatment for the reduction of intra-ocular pressure, eg in ocular hypertension, chronic open angle glaucoma, some secondary glaucomas.

**Dosage and administration** Teoptic Eye-Drops are for local administration to the eye. Initially, the recommended adult dose is one drop of Teoptic 1% Eye-Drops instilled twice daily in each affected eye. If the clinical response is not adequate, the dosage may be altered to one drop of Teoptic 2% Eye-Drops instilled twice daily in each affected eye.

Teoptic Eye-Drops may, if necessary, be used in association with pilocarpine, adrenaline, carbachol and carbonic anhydrase inhibitors.

*Children:* Teoptic Eye-Drops have not been studied in children. Their use in these patients is, therefore, not recommended.

*Use in the elderly:* In clinical trials, the efficacy and tolerability profiles of Teoptic Eye-Drops were similar in elderly patients and in the general adult patient population. The usual recommended adult dose may, therefore, be considered suitable for elderly patients.

**Contra-indications, warnings, etc**
*Contra-indications:* Unsatisfactorily controlled cardiac insufficiency; bronchospasm, including bronchial asthma, or chronic obstructive pulmonary disease; pregnancy; hypersensitivity to any of the components of the formulation.

*Precautions:* As with other topically applied ophthalmic preparations, Teoptic may be absorbed systemically. Teoptic Eye-Drops should, therefore, be used with caution in patients receiving systemic beta-adrenergic-receptor-blocking therapy and in patients with known contra-indications to systemic beta-blockers, eg sinus bradycardia, second and third degree atrioventricular block, cardiogenic shock, right ventricular insufficiency due to pulmonary hypertension and congestive heart failure, unsatisfactorily controlled diabetes mellitus.

As with all ophthalmic preparations containing benzalkonium chloride, soft contact lenses (hydrophilic lenses) should not be worn during treatment with Teoptic Eye-Drops.

*Side-effects:* Local ocular reactions such as irritation, burning, itching and pain, blurred vision, photophobia, xerosis, conjunctival hyperaemia, conjunctival discharge and corneal disorders such as diffuse superficial keratitis may occasionally develop. As with all beta-blocking agents, bradycardia, bronchospasm, rashes, dyspnoea, headache, lassitude and vertigo have occasionally been reported.

*Use in pregnancy and lactation:* Teoptic Eye-Drops have not been studied in human pregnancy and lactation. Use during pregnancy is, therefore, contra-indicated. In animal studies, orally administered carteolol has been shown to penetrate the breast milk and the use of Teoptic Eye-Drops in lactating mothers should, therefore, be at the discretion of the physician.

*Overdosage:* There is no experience of overdosage with Teoptic Eye-Drops. However, potential symptoms (typical of beta-blocking agents) which may occur after accidental oral ingestion include bradycardia, severe hypotension, acute cardiac failure, bronchospasm, hypoglycaemia, delirium and unconsciousness. Initially, treatment should be by removal of any unabsorbed drug (eg gastric lavage) and general supportive measures, ie marked bradycardia should be treated in the first instance by intravenous atropine sulphate at a dose of 500 micrograms-2.0 mg depending on severity; intravenous glucagon and cardiac pacemakers may be required in more severe cases; bronchospasm should be treated with appropriate bronchodilators, including B₂-agonists and aminophylline where necessary. Patients should be monitored for several days as the beta-blocking effects of Teoptic may exceed its plasma half life.

**Pharmaceutical precautions**  Protect from heat. Teoptic Eye-Drops are sterile until the seal is broken.The container should not be accepted for initial use if the seal is damaged. The drops should not be used later than one month after first breaking the seal.

**Legal category**  POM

**Package quantities**  1%: 1 X 5 ml dropper-bottle, 3 X 5 ml dropper-bottle; 2%: 1 X 5 ml dropper-bottle; 3 X 5 ml dropper-bottle

**Further information**  Unlike miotics, Teoptic Eye-Drops reduce intra-ocular pressure without altering accommodation or pupil diameter. A slight increase in pupil diameter may be noted, however, if patients are transferred from miotic therapy to Teoptic Eye-Drops.

**Product licence numbers**
1% Eye-Drops: 8685/0005
2% Eye-Drops: 8685/0006

## VISCOTEARS* LIQUID GEL

**Presentation**  Sterile, colourless and translucent liquid gel, containing 2.0 mg/g Carbomer 940 (polyacrylic acid). It also contains cetrimide (0.1 mg/g), sorbitol, disodium edetate, sodium hydroxide and water.

**Uses**  Substitute of tear fluid for management of dry eye conditions including keratoconjunctivitis sicca, and for unstable tear film.

**Dosage and administration**
*Adults:* 1 drop 3–4 times daily or as required, depending upon the severity of the disease

*Elderly:* No dosage amendment is necessary in the elderly

*Children:* No specific studies with Viscotears have been performed in children. Use in these patients, is therefore, at the responsibility of the physician.

Hold the tube vertically. This results in the formation of a small drop which readily becomes detached from the tube opening. This drop is instilled into the conjunctival sac.

**Contra-indications,warnings,etc**
*Contra-indications:* Patients with known hypersensitivity to one of the components of the gel.

*Precautions:* Contact lenses should not be worn during instillation of the drug. After instillation there should be an interval of at least 30 minutes before reinsertion.

*Pregnancy and lactation:* There is no experience regarding the safety of Viscotears Liquid Gel in human pregnancy or lactation. Administration during pregnancy and lactation is therefore not recommended, except for compelling reasons.

*Drug interactions:* In case of any additional local ocular treatment (eg glaucoma therapy) there should be an application interval of at least 5 minutes between the two medications, Viscotears Liquid Gel always should be the last medication instilled.

*Side-effects:* In clinical studies with Viscotears Liquid Gel the following adverse events have been occasionally reported: mild, transient burning sensation; sticky eyelid; blurred vision after instillation of the gel.

*Overdosage:* Not applicable

*Effects on ability to drive or use machines:* Viscotears Liquid Gel may temporarily influence the visual acuity. Patients with blurred vision driving a vehicle or operating machines should be alerted to the possibility of impaired reactions.

**Pharmaceutical precautions**  Store below 30°C.

**Legal category**  P

**Package quantities**  Viscotears Liquid Gel 10 g (OP)

**Further information**  Viscotears Liquid Gel is a stable, well preserved liquid gel containing Carbomer 940. After local instillation it spreads rapidly over the conjunctiva and cornea and forms a lubricating film with prolonged contact time.

The retention times of Viscotears Liquid Gel and a conventional tear substitute based on polyvinylalcohol were studied in 30 healthy volunteers with fluorescein staining. The retention time of Viscotears Liquid Gel was approximately 16 minutes compared with approximately 2 minutes for the conventional artificial tears eye drops.

Tear film stability was maintained for a period of up to 6 hours. Data of clinical studies on healthy volunteers, patients with dry eye and patients in intensive care or during operation suggest evidence that Viscotears Liquid Gel improves tear film stability and prolongs tear break-up time (BUT).

There are no controlled animal or human pharmacokinetic studies available. However, absorption or accumulation in eye tissues can presumably be excluded due to the high molecular weight of polyacrylic acid (4 mio D).

**Product licence number**  8685/0009

## VOLTAROL* OPHTHA

**Presentation**  A clear, slightly yellow, sterile eye drop solution presented in single dose units, containing 0.1% (w/v) diclofenac sodium in a preservative free formulation.

Also contains boric acid, polyoxyl 35 castor oil, tromethamine and water.

**Uses**  Inhibition of peroperative miosis during cataract surgery. Voltarol Ophtha does not have intrinsic mydriatic properties and does not replace standard mydriatic agents. Voltarol Ophtha is also indicated for the treatment of post-operative inflammation in cataract surgery, and the control of ocular pain and discomfort associated with corneal epithelial defects after excimer PRK (photorefractive keratectomy) surgery.

**Dosage and administration**
*Adults:* For the prophylaxis of peroperative miosis: apply 1 drop four times during the 2 hours prior to surgery.

For the control of post-operative inflammation: apply 1 drop four times daily for up to 28 days.

For the control of post-PRK pain and discomfort: apply 1 drop 2 times in the hour prior to surgery, one drop 2 times five minutes apart immediately after PRK surgery and then post-operatively 1 drop every 2–5 hours while awake for up to 24 hours.

*Elderly patients:* No dosage amendment is necessary in the elderly.

*Children:* Safety and efficacy in children have not been established.

*Note:* Each Voltarol Ophtha single dose unit should be used for a single dose only. Discard the single dose unit immediately after use. Do not save unused contents.

**Contra-indications, warnings,etc**
*Contra-indications:* Patients with known hypersensitivity to any of the ingredients of the formulation.

Like other non-steroidal anti-inflammatory agents, Voltarol Ophtha is also contraindicated in patients in whom attacks of asthma, urticaria, or acute rhinitis are precipitated by acetylsalicylic acid or by other drugs with prostaglandin synthetase inhibiting activity. Intraocular use during surgical procedure is also contraindicated

*Special precautions and warnings:* In the presence of infection, or if there is a risk of infection, appropriate therapy (eg antibiotic) should be given concurrently with Voltarol Ophtha.

Although there have been no reported adverse events, there is a theoretical possibility that patients receiving other medications which may prolong bleeding time, or with known haemostatic defects may experience exacerbation with Voltarol Ophtha.

*Adverse reactions:* In clinical studies with Voltarol Ophtha, the following adverse events have been reported:
Frequent: a mild to moderate burning sensation
Rare: blurred vision immediately after instillation of the eye drops, hypersensitivity reactions with itching and reddening, photosensitivity, keratitis punctata.

*Use during pregnancy and lactation:* There is no experience concerning the safety of Voltarol Ophtha in human pregnancy. Administration during pregnancy and lactation is therefore not recommended except for compelling reasons.

*Overdosage:* There is practically no risk of adverse effects due to accidental oral ingestion, since the eye drop solution in a block of ten units contains only 3 mg of diclofenac sodium, corresponding to about 1.8% of the recommended maximum daily adult dose of Voltarol after oral administration. By way of comparison, the maximum oral daily dose for diclofenac sodium recommended in children is 2 mg/kg body weight.

*Drug interactions:* None reported to date. Clinical findings have shown that Voltarol Ophtha can, if necessary, be combined with steroid containing eye drops.

To prevent the active substances from being washed out when additional ophthalmic medication is used, an interval of at least 5 minutes between each application should be adhered to.

*Ability to drive and operate machinery:* Patients with blurred vision should refrain from driving a vehicle or operating machinery.

**Pharmaceutical precautions**  Store below 15°C until the pack is dispensed. The pack is then stable for 28 days when stored below 25°C. The single dose units should not be used more than 28 days after dispensing. Discard each single dose unit after single dose use.

**Legal category**  POM

**Package quantities**  Voltarol Ophtha is available in packs of 5 and 40 single dose units.

**Further information**  Voltarol Ophtha solution contains diclofenac sodium, a non-steroidal compound with pronounced anti-inflammatory and analgesic properties. Inhibition of prostaglandin biosynthesis, which has been demonstrated experimentally, is regarded as having an important bearing on its mechanism of action.

Prostaglandins play a major role in miosis which occurs during ocular surgery through the constriction of the iris sphincter and in the causation of inflammation and pain.

In clinical trials Voltarol Ophtha has been found to inhibit miosis during cataract surgery, to reduce inflammation following surgical interventions and to reduce ocular pain and discomfort associated with corneal epithelial defects after excimer PRK surgery.

Penetration of diclofenac into the anterior chamber has been confirmed in humans. No measurable plasma levels of diclofenac could be found in humans after ocular application of diclofenac eye drops.

**Product licence number**  0001/0172

*Trade Mark

# Cox Pharmaceuticals
## A. H. Cox & Co. Limited
Whiddon Valley
Barnstaple
North Devon EX32 8NS

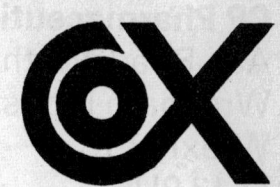

## COBADEX*

**Presentation** Cobadex Cream is a white cream available in two strengths containing Hydrocortisone BP 1.0% w/w and Dimethicone 350 BP 20% w/w.

**Uses** Cobadex Cream is formulated to include volatile and skin-penetrating solvents. This enables the hydrocortisone to be carried into the skin by the organic solvent vehicle, and at the same time evaporation of water will take place from the external surface of the cream, leaving a water-repellent silicone film in contact with the air. Cobadex is indicated, therefore, in all steroid responsive dermatoses wherever water, soap, chemicals, etc. cause irritation, e.g. contact dermatitis (especially of hands and body).

**Dosage and administration** A thin layer of cream should be applied to the affected area two or three times daily.

**Contra-indications, warnings, etc**
*Contra-indications:* Bacterial (impetigo), viral (herpes simplex) or fungal (candida or dermatophyte) infections. The cream should not be used on raw, weeping surfaces because it tends to hold back any exudate. The area of skin around the eye should be avoided.

*Use in pregnancy and lactation:* There is inadequate evidence of safety in human pregnancy. Topical administration of corticosteroids to pregnant animals can cause abnormalities of foetal development including cleft palate and intra-uterine growth retardation. There may therefore be a very small risk of such effects in the human foetus.

*Other undesirable effects:* Discontinue treatment should sensitisation occur.

*Other special warnings and precautions:* Steroid therapy in infants should not exceed seven days, since adrenal suppression may occur, even without occlusion.

**Pharmaceutical precautions** Cobadex should be stored in a cool place; avoid freezing.

**Legal category** POM.

**Package quantities** Cobadex is available in 20 g tubes.

**Further information** Cobadex Cream also contains propylene glycol, cetostearyl alcohol, paraffin, isopropyl myristate, cetomacrogol, polysorbate, methyl and propyl hydroxy benzoates, isobornyl acetate and disodium edetate.

**Product licence number** 0142/0201.


## KLOREF*

**Presentation** White, effervescent, lemon and lime flavoured tablets impressed 'Kloref' on one face; each tablet contains Potassium Bicarbonate BPC, Potassium Chloride BP, potassium benzoate and Betaine Hydrochloride BPC 1949, which provides 6.7 mmol potassium (K+) and 6.7 mmol chloride (Cl-) (equivalent to 500 mg potassium chloride) when dissolved in water.

**Uses** Kloref is indicated in all cases of potassium depletion resulting from prolonged or intensive diuretic therapy, an inadequate dietary potassium intake, and those receiving digitalis – here the elderly population are a special risk. A lack of cellular potassium in the latter can increase the toxic effect of digitalis.

Other indications are corticosteroid therapy, use of carbenoxolone sodium, advanced hepatic cirrhosis, chronic renal disease, Cushing's syndrome, diabetic ketosis, patients on a low-salt diet and in conditions requiring potassium supplementation due to prolonged or chronic diarrhoea or vomiting.

**Dosage and administration** Each tablet should be fully dissolved in at least 100 ml of cold or refrigerated water before drinking. The tablets themselves should not be swallowed.

*Adults:* In most cases 1–2 tablets three times daily (20–40 mmol K+ and Cl-). A few patients may need considerably bigger doses.

*Children and pregnant women:* Treatment should only be initiated under close medical supervision in hospital, with frequent monitoring of serum electrolytes.

*Elderly:* The elderly also require monitoring of serum electrolytes.

**Contra-indications, warnings, etc**
*Contra-indications:* Hyperchloraemia; renal tubular or metabolic acidosis.

*Use in pregnancy and lactation:* Potassium may be indicated as replacement therapy for pregnant women with low potassium levels such as those receiving diuretics. Serum levels should be closely monitored.

Administration of potassium during lactation is considered to be safe providing that maternal serum levels are maintained in the physiological range.

*Other special warnings and precautions:* Cautious administration is required in cases of chronic renal disease.

*Overdosage:* Hyperkalaemia. Poisoning is usually minimal below 6.5 mmol/l, moderate between 6.5 and 8 mmol/l and severe above that level. The absolute toxicity is governed by both pH and associated sodium levels.

Hyperkalaemic symptoms and particularly the ECG effects, may be transiently controlled by calcium gluconate, administration of glucose or glucose and insulin, sodium bicarbonate or hypertonic sodium infusions, cation exchange resins or by haemodialysis and peritoneal dialysis. Caution should be exercised in patients who are digitalised and who may experience acute digitalis intoxication in the course of potassium removal.

**Pharmaceutical precautions** Kloref Tablets should be stored in a tightly closed container in a cool dry place. Avoid storing at temperatures in excess of 25°C.

**Legal category** P.

**Package quantities** Kloref is available in packs of 50 tablets.

**Further information** The addition of each tablet to water brings about a reaction between the betaine hydrochloride and potassium bicarbonate; effervescence results from the liberation of carbon dioxide.

Betaine is a naturally occurring substance found in beet, and is metabolised by the body.

Kloref also contains citric acid, povidone, macrogol, saccharin calcium and dioctyl sodium sulphosuccinate.

**Product licence number** 0142/0275.


## KLOREF-S*

**Presentation** Lemon and lime flavoured effervescent granules in individual sachets; each sachet contains Potassium Bicarbonate BPC, Potassium Chloride BP and Betaine Hydrochloride BPC 1949, which provide 20 mmol potassium (K+) and 20 mmol chloride (Cl-) (equivalent to 1.5 g potassium chloride) when dissolved in water.

**Uses** Kloref-S is indicated in all cases of potassium depletion resulting from intensive or prolonged diuretic therapy, an inadequate potassium dietary intake, and those receiving digitalis – here the elderly popu-lation are a special risk. A lack of cellular potassium in the latter can increase the toxic effect of digitalis.

Other indications are corticosteroid therapy, use of carbenoxolone sodium, advanced hepatic cirrhosis, chronic renal disease, Cushing's syndrome, diabetic ketosis, patients on a low-salt diet and in conditions requiring potassium supplementation due to prolonged or chronic diarrhoea or vomiting.

**Dosage and administration** *Adults:* In most cases 1 or 2 sachets daily (20–40 mmol K+ and Cl-) preferably after meals. A few patients may need considerably bigger doses. Each sachet should be dissolved in at least 200 ml of cold water.

*Children and pregnant women:* Treatment should only be initiated under close medical observation in hospital, with frequent monitoring of serum electrolytes.

*Elderly:* The elderly also require monitoring of serum electrolytes.

**Contra-indications, warnings, etc**
*Contra-indications:* Contra-indicated in hyperchloraemia, renal tubular or metabolic acidosis.

*Use in pregnancy and lactation:* Potassium may be indicated as replacement therapy for pregnant women with low potassium levels such as those receiving diuretics. Serum levels should be closely monitored.

Administration of potassium during lactation is considered to be safe providing that maternal serum levels are maintained in the physiological range.

*Other special warnings and precautions:* Cautious administration is required in cases of chronic renal disease.

Periodic evaluation of the patient's clinical status, serum electrolytes and the ECG should be carried out when replacement therapy is undertaken. This is particularly important in patients with cardiac disease and in those receiving digitalis.

The following warnings appear on the product labelling: 'To be taken only under medical supervision. Keep out of the reach of children'.

*Overdosage:* Hyperkalaemia. Poisoning is usually minimal below 6.5 mmol/l, moderate between 6.5 and 8 mmol/l and severe above that level. The absolute toxicity is governed by both pH and associated sodium levels.

Hyperkalaemic symptoms and particularly the ECG effects, may be transiently controlled by calcium gluconate, administration of glucose or glucose and insulin, sodium bicarbonate or hypertonic sodium infusions, cation exchange resins or by haemodialysis and peritoneal dialysis. Caution should be exercised in patients who are digitalised and who may experience acute digitalis intoxication in the course of potassium removal.

**Pharmaceutical precautions** Kloref-S should be stored in a cool dry place. Avoid storing at temperatures in excess of 25°C.

**Legal category** P.

**Package quantities** Kloref-S is available in boxes of 30 sachets.

**Further information** The addition of each sachet to water brings about a reaction between the betaine hydrochloride and potassium bicarbonate; effervescence results from the liberation of carbon dioxide.

Betaine is a naturally occurring substance found in beet, and is metabolised by the body.

Kloref-S also contains citric acid and saccharin calcium.

**Product licence number** 0142/0367.


*Trade Mark

# CP Pharmaceuticals Limited
Ash Road North
Wrexham Industrial Estate
Wrexham
LL13 9UF

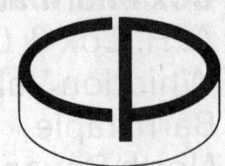

## CANUSAL*

**Presentation** A sterile, pyrogen-free, clear, colourless solution of porcine mucosal Heparin Sodium BP in Sodium Chloride Injection BP adjusted to pH 5 to 8. The solution is preservative free. Each 2 ml ampoule contains 200 iu heparin sodium (100 iu per ml).

**Uses** Heparin is an anticoagulant. It acts by potentiating the naturally occurring inhibitors of thrombin and factor X (Xa).

Canusal is indicated in any clinical circumstances in which it is desired to maintain the patency of indwelling intravascular catheters/cannulae, attendant lines or heparin locks.

Canusal is not recommended for systemic use.

### Dosage and administration
*Adults:* Flush with 2 ml (200 iu) every 4 hours or as required.

*Children/elderly:* As for adults.

### Contra-indications, warnings, etc
*Contra-indications:* Established hypersensitivity to heparin which occurs only rarely.

*Precautions:* When used as directed, it is extremely unlikely that the low levels of heparin reaching the blood will have any systemic effect.

Rigorous aseptic technique should be observed at all times in its use.

*Use in pregnancy:* The safety of Canusal in pregnancy is not established but the dose of heparin involved would not be expected to constitute a hazard.

Heparin does not appear in breast milk.

**Pharmaceutical precautions** Heparin may be incompatible with solutions of certain other drugs, e.g. some antibiotics, opioid analgesics and antihistamines. Canusal should be stored below 25°C. It should not be frozen and should be stored protected from light.

**Legal category** POM.

**Package quantities** Box of 10 ampoules.

**Further information** Nil.

**Product licence number** 4543/0322.

## CHENDOL* CAPSULES 125 mg
## CHENDOL* TABLETS 250 mg
## COMBIDOL* TABLETS
## URDOX* TABLETS 300 mg

### Qualitative and quantitative composition
*Chendol Capsules 125 mg* contain chenodeoxycholic acid 125 mg.

*Chendol Tablets 250 mg* contain chenodeoxycholic acid 250 mg.

*Combidol Tablets* contain chenodeoxycholic acid 125 mg and ursodeoxycholic acid 125 mg.

*Urdox Tablets 300 mg* contain ursodeoxycholic acid 300 mg.

### Pharmaceutical form
*Chendol Capsules 125 mg:* Capsule for oral use.
*Chendol Tables 250 mg:* Tablet for oral use.
*Combidol Tablets:* Tablet for oral use.
*Urdox Tablets 300 mg:* Tablet for oral use.

### Clinical particulars
*Therapeutic indications*
*Gall-stone dissolution:* Chendol Capsules 125 mg, Chendol Tablets 250 mg, Combidol Tablets and Urdox Tablets 300 mg are indicated for the dissolution of small to medium sized radiolucent, cholesterol-rich gall-stones in functioning gall bladders.

Cholesterol stones coated with calcium or stones composed of bile pigments are not dissolved by chenodeoxycholic acid and ursodeoxycholic acid. Chendol Capsules 125 mg, Chendol Tablets 250 mg, Combidol Tablets and Urdox Tablets 300 mg have a particular place in the treatment of patients in whom surgery is contraindicated or who are anxious to avoid surgery.

*Lithotripsy support:* Combidol Tablets are used for therapy beginning two to three weeks prior to litho-tripsy and continuing for two to three months following apparent complete dissolution of the fragments.

*Posology and method of administration:*
*Chendol Capsules 125 mg, Chendol Tablets 250 and Combidol Tablets*
*Adults and elderly:* The usual dose is 10–15 mg/kg/day either as a single night time dose or in divided doses.

The dose of Chendol (capsules or tablets) may be increased to 18–20 mg/kg/day in obese patients, if necessary.

The duration of treatment may be up to two years, depending on the size of the stone(s), and should be continued for two to three months after the apparent dissolution of the stone(s).

*Children:* Not recommended.

*Urdox Tablets 300 mg*
*Adults and elderly:* The usual dose is 6–12 mg/kg/day either as a single night time dose or in divided doses. This may be increased to 15 mg/kg/day in obese patients, if necessary. The duration of treatment may be up to two years, depending on the size of the stone(s), and should be continued for three months after the apparent dissolution of the stone(s).

*Children:* Not recommended.

*Contra-indications:* Use in patients with radio-opaque calcified gall-stones, or in those with non-functioning gall bladders.

Use in women who may become pregnant.

Use in patients with chronic liver disease, peptic ulcers or in those with inflammatory diseases of the small intestine and colon.

*Special warnings and special precautions for use:* None known.

*Interactions with other medicaments and other forms of interaction:* Chendol Capsules 125 mg, Chendol Tablets 250 mg, Combidol Tablets and Urdox Tablets 300 mg should not be administered with oral contraceptives, oestrogenic hormones and other drugs which reduce the blood cholesterol level and increase the bile cholesterol level. Antacids bind bile acids in the gut. Drugs such as charcoal, colestipol and cholestyramine bind bile acids *in vitro.* All the above should be avoided during bile acid therapy as they may limit the effectiveness of therapy.

*Pregnancy and lactation:* These products should not be used during pregnancy or lactation. Measures should be taken to prevent pregnancy if given to women of childbearing age. A non-hormonal contraceptive should be used. Treatment should be discontinued immediately if pregnancy occurs and medical advice sought.

*Effects on ability to drive and to use machines:* None known.

*Undesirable effects*
*Chendol Capsules 125 mg, Chendol Tablets 250 mg, Combidol Tablets:* Chendol and Combidol may give rise to mild transient diarrhoea, which has been found to respond to a reduction in dose for several days. Subsequent treatment should be gradually increased to the previous level. Mild pruritus may occur. Serum transaminase levels may be elevated and hypercholesterolaemia has been reported.

Because of the reduced levels of both drugs in Combidol, side-effects are less frequent than with single agent therapy.

*Urdox Tablets 300 mg:* Urdox may give rise to nausea, vomiting, diarrhoea and pruritus. A calcified layer may develop on the surface of the stone making it unable to be dissolved by bile acid therapy, resulting in surgery for some patients.

*Overdose:* Bile acids are removed in the faeces either unchanged or as bacterial metabolites. It is unlikely therefore that serious toxicity would occur following overdose. The most likely result is diarrhoea which should be treated symptomatically and supportively.

*Pharmacological properties*
*Pharmacodynamic properties:* When given by mouth, chenodeoxycholic acid and ursodeoxycholic acid reduce the ratio of cholesterol to bile salts plus phospholipids in bile, causing desaturation of cholesterol saturated bile. The exact mechanism of action has not been fully elucidated.

*Pharmacokinetic properties:* Chenodeoxycholic acid and ursodeoxycholic acid are absorbed from the gastro-intestinal tract and undergo first pass metabolism and enterohepatic recycling. Both chenodeoxycholic acid and ursodeoxycholic acid are partially conjugated in the liver before being excreted into bile and undergoing 7-∝-dehydroxylation to lithocholic acid some of which is excreted directly in the faeces. The rest is absorbed and mainly conjugated and sulphated by the liver before excretion in the faeces.

*Preclinical safety data:*
*Chendol Capsules 125 mg, Chendol Tablets 250 and Combidol Tablets:* Chenodeoxycholic acid given in long term studies in doses of 600 mg/kg/day to rats and 1000 mg/kg/day to mice induced malignant liver cell tumours in female rats and benign liver cell tumours in female rats and mice. The clinical significance of these findings is not known.

*Urdox Tablets 300 mg:* There are no pre-clinical data of relevance to the prescriber which are additional to those already included in other sections.

**Pharmaceutical particulars**
*List of excipients*
*Chendol Capsules 125 mg:* Lactose PhEur; Maize Starch PhEur; Sodium Starch Glycollate PhEur; Talc PhEur; Colloidal Silicon Dioxide USP; Magnesium Stearate PhEur.

Capsule shell: Gelatin PhEur; E104; E127; E171.

*Chendol Tablets 250 mg:* Maize Starch PhEur; Povidone PhEur; Polyethylene Glycol 4000 PhEur; Sodium Starch Glycollate PhEur; Magnesium Stearate PhEur.

Tablet coating: Hydroxypropylmethylcellulose (E464) USP; Opaspray M-1-3460 (E110, E171) HSE; Polyethylene Glycol 400 USP.

*Combidol Tablets and Urdox Tablets:* Lactose PhEur; Maize Starch PhEur; Povidone PhEur; Sodium Starch Glycollate PhEur; Magnesium Stearate PhEur.

Tablet coating: Hydroxypropylmethylcellulose (E464) PhEur; Titanium Dioxide (E171) PhEur; Polyethylene Glycol 400 PhEur.

*Incompatibilities:* None known.

*Shelf life:* Three years.

*Special precautions for storage:*
*Chendol Capsules 125 mg, Chendol Tablets 250 mg and Combidol Tablets:* Store below 25°C.

*Urdox Tablets 300 mg:* Store below 25°C. Protect from light.

*Nature and contents of container:*
*Chendol Capsules 125 mg:* Polypropylene or polyethylene container of 100 or 224 capsules.

*Chendol Tablets 250 mg:* Polypropylene or polyethylene tablet container with tamper evident closure containing 50 or 112 tablets.

*Combidol Tablets:* Polypropylene or polyethylene tablet containers with polyethylene closures. Strips of UPVC and hard tempered aluminium foil.

*Urdox Tablets 300 mg:* Polypropylene or polyethylene tablet container with tamper evident closure. Strips of white opaque 250 micron UPVC with 20 micron hard tempered foil.

*Instructions for use/handling:* None.

**Marketing authorisation numbers**
Chendol Capsules 125 mg 4543/0229
Chendol Tablets 250 mg 4543/0215
Combidol Tablets 4543/0321
Urdox Tablets 300 mg 4543/0318

**Date of approval/revision of SPC** May 1997.

**Legal category** POM.

## DIAMORPHINE INJECTION BP

**Qualitative and quantitative composition** Each ampoule contains 5 mg, 10 mg, 30 mg, 100 mg, 250 mg or 500 mg of Diamorphine Hydrochloride BP.

**Pharmaceutical form** A white to off-white, sterile, freeze dried powder of Diamorphine Hydrochloride BP for reconstitution for injection.

**Clinical particulars**
*Therapeutic indications:* Diamorphine may be used in

the treatment of severe pain associated with surgical procedures, myocardial infarction or pain in the terminally ill and for the relief of dyspnoea in acute pulmonary oedema.

*Posology and method of administration:* Diamorphine may be given by the intramuscular, intravenous or subcutaneous routes. Glucose intravenous infusion is the preferred diluent, particularly when the drug is administered by a continuous infusion pump over 24 to 48 hours, although it is also compatible with sodium chloride intravenous infusion.

The dose should be suited to the individual patient.

*Adults:*

*Acute pain,* 5 mg repeated every four hours if necessary (up to 10 mg for heavier, well muscled patients) by subcutaneous or intramuscular injection. By slow intravenous injection, one quarter to one half the corresponding intramuscular dose.

*Chronic pain,* 5–10 mg regularly every four hours by subcutaneous or intramuscular injection. The dose may be increased according to individual needs.

*Myocardial infarction,* 5 mg by slow intravenous injection (1 mg/minute) followed by a further 2.5 mg to 5 mg if necessary.

*Acute pulmonary oedema,* 2.5 mg to 5 mg by slow intravenous injection (1 mg/minute).

*Children and elderly:* As diamorphine has a respiratory depressant effect, care should be taken when giving the drug to the very young and the elderly and a lower starting dose than normal is recommended.

*Contra-indications:* Respiratory depression and obstructive airways disease.

Phaeochromocytoma (endogenous release of histamine may stimulate catecholamine release).

Raised intracranial pressure.

Concurrent use of monoamine oxidase inhibitors or within two weeks of their discontinuation.

*Special warnings and special precautions for use:* Diamorphine should be administered with care to patients with head injuries as there is an increased risk of respiratory depression which may lead to elevation of CSF pressure. The sedation and pupillary changes produced may interfere with accurate monitoring of the patient.

Repeated administration of diamorphine may lead to dependence and tolerance developing. Abrupt withdrawal in patients who have developed dependence may precipitate a withdrawal syndrome. Great caution should be exercised in patients with a known tendency or history of drug abuse.

Use with caution in patients with toxic psychosis, CNS depression, myxoedema, prostatic hypertrophy or urethral stricture, kyphoscoliosis, actue alcoholism, delirium tremens, severe inflammatory or obstructive bowel disorders, adrenal insufficiency or severe diarrhoea. Care should be exercised in treating the elderly or debilitated patients and those with hepatic or renal impairment.

*Interaction with other medicaments and other forms of interaction:* The depressant effects of diamorphine may be exaggerated and prolonged by phenothiazines, monoamine oxidase inhibitors, tricyclic antidepressants, anxiolytics and hypnotics. There may be antagonism of the gastrointestinal effects of cisapride, domperidone and metoclopramide. The risk of severe constipation and/or urinary retention is increased by administration of antimuscarinic drugs (e.g. atropine). There may be increased risk of toxicity with 4-quinolone antibacterials.

Alcohol may enhance the sedative and hypotensive effects of diamorphine.

Cimetidine inhibits metabolism of opioid analgesics.

Hyperpyrexia and CNS toxicity have been reported when opioid analgesics are used with selegiline.

*Pregnancy and lactation:* Safety has not been established in pregnancy.

Administration during labour may cause respiratory depression in the neonate and gastric stasis during labour, increasing the risk of inhalation pneumonia.

Diamorphine should not be given to women who are breast-feeding as there is limited information available on diamorphine in breast milk.

*Effects on ability to drive and to use machines:* Diamorphine causes drowsiness and mental clouding. If affected patients should not drive or use machines.

*Undesirable effects:* The most serious hazard of therapy is respiratory depression although circulatory depression is also possible. The most common side effects are sedation, nausea and vomiting, constipation and sweating. Other side effects include dizziness, miosis, confusion, urinary retention, biliary spasm, orthostatic hypotension, facial flushing, vertigo, palpitations, mood changes, dry mouth, dependence, urticaria, pruritus and raised intracranial pressure.

*Overdose: Symptoms:* Respiratory depression, pulmonary oedema, muscle flaccidity, coma or stupor, constricted pupils, cold, clammy skin and occasionally bradycardia and hypotension.

*Treatment:* Respiration and circulation should be maintained and naloxone is indicated if coma or bradypnoea are present. A dose of 0.4 to 2 mg repeated at intervals of two to three minutes (up to 10 mg) may be given by subcutaneous, intramuscular or intravenous injection. The usual initial dosage for children is 10 micrograms per kg body weight. Naloxone may also be given by continuous intravenous infusion, 2 mg diluted in 500 ml, at a rate adjusted to the patient's response. Oxygen and assisted ventilation should be administered if necessary.

**Pharmacological properties**

*Pharmacodynamic properties:* Diamorphine is a narcotic analgesic which acts primarily on the central nervous system and smooth muscle. It is predominantly a central nervous system depressant but it has stimulant actions resulting in nausea, vomiting and miosis.

*Pharmacokinetic properties:* Diamorphine is a potent opiate analgesic which has a more rapid onset of activity than morphine as the first metabolite, monoacetylmorphine, more readily crosses the blood brain barrier. In man, diamorphine has a half life of two to three minutes. Its first metabolite, monoacetylmorphine, is more slowly hydrolysed in the blood to be concentrated mainly in skeletal muscle, kidney, lung, liver and spleen. Monoacetylmorphine is metabolised to morphine. Morphine forms conjugates with glucuronic acid. The majority of the drug is excreted via the kidney as glucuronides and to a much lesser extent as morphine. About 7–10% is eliminated via the biliary sytem into the faeces.

Diamorphine does not bind to protein. However, morphine is about 35% bound to human plasma proteins, mainly to albumin. The analgesic effect lasts approximately three to four hours.

*Preclinical safety data:* There are no additional preclinical data of relevance to the prescriber.

**Pharmaceutical particulars**

*List of excipients:* Water for Injections BP removed during the freeze drying process.

*Incompatibilities:* Physical incompatibility has been reported with mineral acids and alkalis.

*Shelf life:* Three years from date of manufacture.

*Special precautions for storage:* Store below 25°C. Protect from light.

*Nature and contents of container:* Neutral glass ampoules containing a plug of white sterile freeze dried powder packed in cartons of 5, 10 or 50 ampoules.

*Instruction for use/handling:* The solution should be used immediately after preparation.

**Marketing authorisation numbers**

Diamorphine Injection BP 5 mg    4543/0303
Diamorphine Injection BP 10 mg   4543/0304
Diamorphine Injection BP 30 mg   4543/0305
Diamorphine Injection BP 100 mg 4543/0306
Diamorphine Injection BP 250 mg 4543/0307
Diamorphine Injection BP 500 mg 4543/0308

**Date of approval/revision of SPC**   July 1997.

**Legal category**   CD(Sch 2), POM.

# DIAZEPAM INJECTION BP

**Qualitative and quantitative composition**  Diazepam BP 5.0 mg/ml.

**Pharmaceutical form**   Solution for Injection.

**Clinical particulars**

*Therapeutic indications:* Diazepam injection may be used in severe or disabling anxiety and agitation; for the control of status epilepticus, epileptic and febrile convulsions; to relieve muscle spasm; as a sedative in minor surgical and dental procedures; or other circumstances in which a rapid effect is required.

*Posology and method of administration:* Dosage depends on individual response, age and weight.

*Adults:*

In *severe anxiety or acute muscle spasm,* diazepam 10 mg may be given intravenously or intramuscularly and repeated after 4 hours.

In *tetanus,* 0.1 to 0.3 mg per kg body weight may be given intravenously and repeated every 1–4 hours; alternatively, a continuous infusion of 3 to 10 mg per kg every 24 hours may be used or similar doses may be given by nasoduodenal tube.

In *status epilepticus or epileptic convulsions,* 0.15– 0.25 mg per kg (usually 10–20 mg) is given by intravenous injection. If no effect is seen after 5 minutes, the dose can be repeated, up to a maximum of 30 mg. One the patient is controlled, recurrence of seizures may be prevented by a slow infusion (maximum total dose 3 mg per kg over 24 hours).

In *minor surgical procedures and dentistry,* 0.1– 0.2 mg per kg by injection (usually 10–20 mg) adjusted to the patient's requirements.

*Elderly:* Elderly or debilitated patients should be given not more than half of the usual dose.

*Hepatic/renal impairment:* Dosage reduction may also be required in patients with liver or kidney dysfunction.

*Children:*

In *status epilepticus, epileptic or febrile convulsions:* 0.2–0.3 mg per kg (or 1 mg per year of life) is given by intravenous injection. If no effect is seen after 5 minutes, the dose can be repeated.

*Sedation or muscle relaxation:* up to 0.2 mg per kg may be given parenterally.

*Neonates:* Not recommended; dosage has not been established.

**IMPORTANT: In order to reduce the likelihood of adverse effects during intravenous administration the injection should be given slowly (1.0 ml solution per minute). It is advisable to keep the patient supine for at least an hour after administration. Except in emergencies, a second person should always be present during intravenous use and facilities for resuscitation should always be available.**

It is recommended that patients should remain under medical supervision until at least one hour has elapsed from the time of injection. They should always be accompanied home by a responsible adult, with a warning not to drive or operate machinery for 24 hours.

Intravenous injection may be associated with local reactions and thrombophlebitis and venous thrombosis may occur. In order to minimise the likelihood of these effects, intravenous injections of diazepam should be given into a large vein of the antecubital fossa.

Where continuous intravenous infusion is necessary it is suggested that 2 ml Diazepam Injection is mixed with at least 200 ml of infusion fluid such as Sodium Chloride Injection or Dextrose Injection and that such solutions should be used immediately. There is evidence that diazepam is adsorbed onto plastic infusion bags and giving sets. It is therefore recommended that glass bottles should be used for the administration of diazepam by intravenous infusion.

*Contra-indications:* Known sensitivity to benzodiazepines or any of the ingredients. Myasthenia gravis. Severe respiratory insufficiency.

Diazepam Injection should not be used in phobic or obsessional states nor be used alone in the treatment of depression or anxiety associated with depression due to the risk of suicide being precipitated in this patient group. Diazepam Injection should not be used in the treatment of chronic psychosis. In common with other benzodiazepines the use of diazepam may be associated with amnesia and Diazepam Injection should not be used in cases of loss or bereavement as psychological adjustment may be inhibited.

*Special warnings and precautions for use:* Diazepam injection should be used with caution in patients with renal or hepatic dysfunction, chronic pulmonary insufficiency, closed angle glaucoma or organic brain changes, particularly arteriosclerosis.

Diazepam may enhance the effects of other CNS depressants; their concurrent use should be avoided.

The dependence potential of diazepam is low when limited to short term use. Withdrawal symptoms may occur with benzodiazepines following normal use of therapeutic doses for only short periods and may be associated with physiological and psychological sequelae, including depression. This should be considered when treating patients for more than a few days.

As with other benzodiazepines extreme caution should be used if prescribing diazepam for patients with personality disorders. The disinhibiting effects of benzodiazepines may be manifested as the precipitation of suicide in patients who are depressed or show aggressive behaviour towards self and others.

*Interactions with other medicaments and other forms of interaction:* Enhanced sedation or respiratory and cardiovascular depression may occur if diazepam is given with other drugs that have CNS depressant properties (e.g. antipsychotics, anxiolytics, sedatives, antidepressants, hypnotics, narcotic analgesics, anaesthetics, antiepileptics).

If such centrally acting depressant drugs are given parenterally in conjunction with intravenous diazepam, severe respiratory and cardiovascular depression may occur. When intravenous diazepam is to be administered concurrently with a narcotic analgesic agent (e.g. in dentistry) it is recommended that diazepam be given after the analgesic and that the dose be carefully titrated to meet the patient's needs.

Agents that interfere with metabolism by hepatic enzymes (e.g. isoniazid, disulfiram, cimetidine, omeprazole, oral contraceptives) have been shown to reduce the clearance of benzodiazepines and may potentiate their actions, whilst known inducers of hepatic enzymes, for example, rifampicin, may increase the clearance of benzodiazepines.

Diazepam metabolism is accelerated by theophylline and smoking.

Diazepam may interact with other hepatically metabolised drugs, causing inhibition (levodopa) or potentiation (phenytoin, muscle relaxants).

*Pregnancy and lactation:* There is no evidence regarding the safety of diazepam in pregnancy. It should not be used, especially in the first and third trimesters, unless the benefit is considered to outweigh the risk.

In labour, high single doses or repeated low doses have been reported to produce hypothermia, hypotonia, respiratory depression and poor suckling (floppy infant syndrome) in the neonate and irregularities in the foetal heart.

Diazepam is excreted in the breast milk and therefore its use during lactation should be avoided.

*Effects on ability to drive and use machines:* Patients treated with Diazepam Injection should not drive or use machinery.

*Undesirable effects:* High dosage or parenteral administration can produce respiratory depression and hypotension.

The side effects of diazepam are usually mild and infrequent. The most common side effects are sedation, drowsiness, headaches, muscle weakness, dizziness (with risk of falls in the elderly), ataxia, confusion, slurred speech, tremor, numbed emotions, reduced alertness, fatigue, double vision, anterograde amnesia and a hangover effect. Elderly or debilitated patients are particularly susceptible to side effects and may require lower doses. Other effects which may occur rarely are dry mouth, increased appetite, gastrointestinal and visual disturbances, jaundice, urinary retention, hypotension, bradycardia, changes in libido, menstrual disturbances, skin reactions, blood dyscrasias, laryngeal spasm, chest pain, respiratory depression and apnoea.

In susceptible patients, an unnoticed depression may become evident. Paradoxical reactions (restlessness, agitation, instability, rages, hallucinations) are known to occur with benzodiazepines and are more likely in children and the elderly.

*Overdose: Symptoms:* The symptoms of mild overdose may include confusion, somnolence, ataxia, dysarthria, hypotension, muscular weakness. In severe overdose, depression of vital functions may occur, particularly the respiratory centre. As drug levels fall severe agitation may develop.

*Treatment:* Treatment is symptomatic. Respiration, heart rate, blood pressure and body termperature should be monitored and supportive measures taken to maintain cardiovascular and respiratory function. Flumazenil is indicated to counteract the central depressive effect of benzodiazepines.

**Pharmacological properties**

*Pharmacodynamic properties:* Diazepam is a psychotropic substance from the class of 1,4-benzodiazepines with marked properties of suppression of tension, agitation and anxiety as well as sedative and hypnotic effects. In addition, diazepam demonstrates muscle relaxant and anticonvulsive properties. It is used in the short-term treatment of anxiety and tension states, as a sedative and premedicant, in the control of muscle spasm and in the management of alcohol withdrawal symptoms.

Diazepam binds to specific receptors in the central nervous system and particular peripheral organs. The benzodiazepine receptors in the CNS have a close functional connection with receptors of the GABA-ergic transmitter system. After binding to the benzodiazepine receptor, diazepam augments the inhibitory effect of GABA-ergic transmission.

*Pharmacokinetic properties:* Diazepam is highly lipid soluble and crosses the blood brain barrier. These properties qualify it for intravenous use in short term anaesthetic procedures since it acts promptly on the brain, and its initial effects decrease rapidly as it is distributed into fat deposits and tissues. Following the administration of an adequate intravenous dose of diazepam, effective plasma concentrations are usually reached within 5 minutes (ca. 150–400 ng/ml).

Absorption is erratic following intramuscular administration and lower peak plasma concentrations may be obtained than those following oral administration.

Diazepam is extensively protein bound (95–99%). The volume of distribution is between 0.95 and 2 l/kg depending on age. Diazepam and its main metabolite, N-desmethyldiazepam, cross the placenta and are secreted in breast milk.

Diazepam is metabolised predominantly in the liver. Its metabolites, N-desmethyldiazepam (nordiazepam), temazepam and oxazepam, which appear in the urine as glucuronides, are also pharmacologically active substances. Only 20% of the metabolites are detected in the urine in the first 72 hours.

Diazepam has a biphasic half life with an initial rapid distribution phase followed by a prolonged terminal elimination phase of 1–2 days. For the active metabolites N-desmethyldiazepam, temazepam and oxazepam, the half lives are 30–100 hours, 10–20 hours and 5–15 hours, respectively.

Excretion is mainly renal and also partly biliary. It is dependent on age as well as hepatic and renal function.

Metabolism and elimination in the neonate are markedly slower than in children and adults. In the elderly, elimination is prolonged by a factor of 2 to 4. In patients with impaired renal function, elimination is also prolonged. In patients with hepatic disorders (liver cirrhosis, hepatitis), elimination is prolonged by a factor of 2.

*Preclinical safety:* Chronic toxicity studies have demonstrated no evidence of drug induced changes. There are no long term animal studies to investigate the carcinogenic potential of diazepam. Severel investigations pointed to a weakly mutagenic potential at doses far above the human therapeutic dose.

Local tolerability has been studied following single and repeat dose applications into the conjunctival sac of rabbits and the rectum of dogs. Only minimal irritation was observed. There were no systemic changes.

In humans it would appear that the risk of congenital abnormalities from the ingestion of therapeutic doses of benzodiazepines is slight, although a few epidemiological studies have pointed to an increased risk of cleft palate. There are case reports of congenital abnormalities and mental retardation in prenatally exposed children following overdosage and intoxication with benzodiazepines.

**Pharmaceutical particulars**

*List of excipients:* Benzoic acid; ethanol; propylene glycol; sodium benzoate; benzyl alcohol; water for injections.

*Incompatibilities:* Diazepam Injection should not be mixed with other drugs in the same infusion solution or the same syringe.

*Shelf life:* Three years.

*Special precautions for storage:* Store protected from light. Store below 25°C.

*Nature and contents of container:* Amber glass ampoules (2 ml or 4 ml) packed in 10s in an outer printed carton.

*Instructions for use/handling:* None.

**Marketing authorisation number**   4543/0179

**Date of approval/revision of SPC**   May 1996.

**Legal category**   CD(Sch 4), POM.

# DIAZEPAM RECTUBES*

**Qualitative and quantitative composition**
Diazepam PhEur 2.5 mg in 1.25 ml (2 mg/ml).
Diazepam PhEur 5 mg in 2.5 ml (2 mg/ml).
Diazepam PhEur 10 mg in 2.5 ml (4 mg/ml).
Diazepam PhEur 20 mg in 5.0 ml (4 mg/ml).

**Pharmaceutical form**   Solution in rectal tube – rectal use.

**Clinical particulars**

*Therapeutic indications:* Diazepam rectal tubes may be used in severe or disabling anxiety and agitation; epileptic and febrile convulsions; to relieve muscle spasm caused by tetanus; as a sedative in minor surgical and dental procedures, or other circumstances in which a rapid effect is required but where intravenous injection is impracticable or undesirable.

Diazepam rectal tubes may be of particular value for the immediate treatment of convulsions in children.

*Posology and method of administration:* Dosage depends on age and weight.

*Children:* 0.5 mg/kg (not recommended in infants under 10 kg).

*Adults:* 0.5 mg/kg.

If convulsions are not controlled other anticonvulsive measures should be instituted. The dose can be repeated every 12 hours.

Elderly and debilitated patients should be given not more than one half the appropriate adult dose.

Dosage reduction may also be required in patients with liver or kidney dysfunction.

*Contra-indications:* Known hypersensitivity to benzodiazepines or any of the ingredients. Myasthenia gravis. Severe respiratory insufficiency.

Diazepam should not be used in phobic or obsessional states, nor be used alone in the treatment of depression or anxiety associated with depression due to the risk of suicide being precipitated in this patient group. Diazepam should not be used in the treatment of chronic psychosis. In common with other benzodiazepines the use of diazepam may be associated with amnesia and diazepam should not be used in cases of loss or bereavement as psychological adjustments may be inhibited.

*Special warnings and special precautions for use:* Diazepam should be used with caution in patients with renal or hepatic dysfunction, chronic pulmonary insufficiency, closed angle glaucoma or organic brain changes, particularly arteriosclerosis.

Diazepam may enhance the effects of other CNS depressants, their concurrent use should be avoided.

The dependence potential of diazepam is low when limited to short-term use. Withdrawal symptoms may occur with benzodiazepines following normal use of therapeutic doses for only short periods and may be associated with physiological and psychological sequelae, including depression. This should be considered when treating patients for more than a few days.

As with other benzodiazepines extreme caution should be used if prescribing diazepam for patients with personality disorders. The disinhibiting effects of benzodiazepines may be manifested as the precipitation of suicide in patients who are depressed or show aggressive behaviour towards self and others.

*Interaction with other medicaments and other forms of interactions:* Enhanced sedation or respiratory and cardiovascular depression may occur if diazepam is given with other drugs that have CNS depressant properties (e.g. antipsychotics, anxiolytics, sedatives, antidepressants, hypnotics, narcotic analgesics, anaesthetics, antiepileptics) or with agents that interfere with its metabolism by hepatic enzymes (e.g. isoniazid, disulfiram. cimetidine, omeprazole, oral contraceptives). Cimetidine and omeprazole have been shown to reduce the clearance of benzodiazepines and may potentiate their action whilst known inducers of hepatic enzymes e.g. rifampicin may increase the clearance of benzodiazepines.

Diazepam metabolism is accelerated by theophylline and smoking.

Diazepam may interact with other hepatically metabolised drugs, causing inhibition (levodopa) or potentiation (phenytoin, muscle relaxants).

*Pregnancy and lactation:* There is no evidence regarding the safety of diazepam in pregnancy. It should not be used especially in the first and third trimesters, unless the benefit is considered to outweight the risk.

In labour, high single doses or repeated low doses have been reported to produce hypothermia, hypotonia, respiratory depression and poor suckling (floppy infant syndrome) in the neonate and irregularities in the foetal heart.

Diazepam is excreted in the breast milk and therefore its use during lactation should be avoided.

*Effects on ability to drive and use machines:* Patients treated with Diazepam Rectal Tubes should not drive or operate machines.

*Undesirable effects:* The side effects of diazepam are usually mild and infrequent. The most common side effects are sedation, drowsiness, headaches, muscle weakness, dizziness (with risk of falls in the elderly), ataxia, confusion, slurred speech, tremor, numbed emotions, reduced alertness, fatigue, double vision, anterograde amnesia and a hangover effect. Elderly or debilitated patients are particularly susceptible to side effects and may require lower doses. Other effects which may occur rarely are dry mouth, increased appetite, gastrointestinal and visual disturbances, jaundice, urinary retention, hypotension, bradycardia, changes in libido, menstrual disturbances, skin reactions, blood dyscrasias, laryngeal spasm, chest pain, respiratory depression and apnoea.

In susceptible patients, an unnoticed depression may become evident. Paradoxical reactions (restlessness, agitation, instability, rages, hallucinations) are known to occur with benzodiazepines and are more likely in children and the elderly.

*Overdose*

*Symptoms:* The symptoms of mild overdose may include confusion, somnolence, ataxia, dysarthria, hypotension, muscular weakness. In severe overdose, depression of vital functions may occur, particularly the respiratory centre. As drug levels fall severe agitation may develop.

*Treatment:* Treatment is symptomatic. Respiration, heart rate, blood pressure and body temperature should be monitored and supportive measures taken to maintain cardiovascular and respiratory function. Flumazenil is indicated to counteract the central depressive effect of benzodiazepines.

**Pharmacological properties**

*Pharmacodynamic properties:* Diazepam is a psychotropic substance from the class of 1,4-benzodiazepines with marked properties of suppression of tension, agitation and anxiety as well as sedative and hypnotic effects. In addition, diazepam demonstrates muscle relaxant and anticonvulsive properties. It is used in the short-term treatment of anxiety and tension states, as a sedative and premedicant, in the control of muscle spasm and in the management of alcohol withdrawal symptoms.

Diazepam binds to specific receptors in the central nervous system and particular peripheral organs. The benzodiazepine receptors in the CNS have a close functional connection with receptors of the GABA-ergic transmitter system. After binding to the benzodiazepine receptor, diazepam augments the inhibitory effect of GABA-ergic transmission.

*Pharmacokinetic properties:* After rectal administration of the solution, diazepam is absorbed rapidly and almost completely from the rectum.

The onset of the therapeutic effect occurs within a few minutes of rectal administration. The rapidity of the rise in the serum level following rectal administration corresponds approximately to that following an intravenous dose but peak plasma concentrations are lower after rectal tubes than after intravenous administration. In adults maximal plasma concentrations following the administration of 10 mg diazepam in rectal solution are reached after about 10–30 minutes (ca. 150–400 ng/ml).

Diazepam is extensively protein bound (95–99%). The volume of distribution is between 0.95 and 2 l/kg depending on age. Diazepam is lipophilic and rapidly enters the cerebrospinal fluid. Diazepam and its main metabolite, N-desmethyldiazepam, cross the placenta and are secreted in breast milk.

Diazepam is metabolised predominantly in the liver. Its metabolites, N-desmethyldiazepam (nordiazepam), temazepam and oxazepam, which appear in the urine as glucuronides, are also pharmacologically active substances. Only 20% of the metabolites are detected in the urine in the first 72 hours.

Diazepam has a biphasic half life with an initial rapid distribution phase followed by a prolonged terminal elimination phase of 1–2 days. For the active metabolites N-desmethyldiazepam, temazepam and oxazepam, the half lives are 30–100 hours, 10–20 hours and 5–15 hours, respectively.

Excretion is mainly renal and also partly biliary. It is dependent on age as well as hepatic and renal function.

Metabolism and elimination in the neonate are markedly slower than in children and adults. In the elderly, elimination is prolonged by a factor of 2 to 4. In patients with impaired renal function, elimination is also prolonged. In patients with hepatic disorders (liver cirrhosis, hepatitis), elimination is prolonged by a factor of 2.

*Preclinical safety data:* Chronic toxicity studies in animals have demonstrated no evidence of drug-induced changes. There are no long-term animal studies to investigate the carcinogenic potential of diazepam. Several investigations pointed to a weakly mutagenic potential at doses far above the human therapeutic dose.

Local tolerability has been studied following single and repeat dose applications into the conjunctival sac of rabbits and the rectum of dogs. Only minimal irritation was observed. There were no systemic changes.

In humans it would appear that the risk of congenital abnormalities from the ingestion of therapeutic doses of benzodiazepines is slight, although a few epidemiological studies have pointed to an increased risk of cleft palate. There are case reports of congenital abnormalities and mental retardation in prenatally exposed children following overdosage and intoxication with benzodiazepines.

**Pharmaceutical particulars**
*List of excipients:* Benzyl alcohol, alcohol, propylene glycol, benzoic acid, sodium benzoate, purified water.

*Incompatabilities:* None known.

*Shelf life:* Three years in alufoil pack.

*Special precautions for storage:* Store below 25°C. Short-term exposure to higher temperatures (e.g. in emergencies), is of no consequence.

*Nature and contents of container:*
2.5 mg: Packs of 5 rectal tubes each containing 1.25 ml of solution.
5 mg: Packs of 5 rectal tubes each containing 2.5 ml of solution.
10 mg: Packs of 5 rectal tubes each containing 2.5 ml of solution.
20 mg: Packs of 5 rectal tubes each containing 5 ml of solution.

The tubes are made of low desnity polyethylene.

*Instructions for use/handling:* The solution is administered rectally. Adults should be in the lateral position; children should be in the prone or lateral position.

(a) Tear open the foil pack. Remove the cap.
(b) Insert the tube nozzle completely into the rectum. For children under 15 kg, insert only half way. Hold the tube with the spout downwards. The contents of the tube should be completely emptied by using firm pressure with the index finger and thumb.
(c) To avoid suction, maintain pressure on the tube until it is withdrawn from the rectum. Press together the patient's buttocks for a short time.

**Marketing authorisation numbers**

| | |
|---|---|
| 2.5 mg | 4543/0364 |
| 5 mg | 4543/0340 |
| 10 mg | 4543/0341 |
| 20 mg | 4543/0363 |

**Date of approval/revision of SPC** August 1996

**Legal category** CD (Sch 4), POM.

## HEPSAL* 10 iu/ml

**Qualitative and quantitative composition** Heparin Sodium (Mucous) BP 10 iu per ml.

**Pharmaceutical form** Injection.

**Clinical particulars**
*Therapeutic indications:* Heparin is an anticoagulant and acts by potentiating the naturally occurring inhibitors of thrombin and factor X (Xa).

Hepsal is indicated in any clinical circumstances in which it is desired to maintain the patency of indwelling catheters/cannulae, attendant lines or heparin locks. Hepsal is not recommended for systemic use.

*Posology and method of administration:* Route of administration – For cleaning indwelling cannulae. Material to be used as a cannula flush (5 ml; 50 units) every 4 hours or as required.

*Contra-indications:* The very rare occurrence of established hypersensitivity to heparin is the only contra-indication to Hepsal.

*Special warnings and special precautions for use:* Rigorous aseptic technique should be observed at all times in its use.

*Interaction with other medicaments:* None stated.

*Pregnancy and lactation:* None stated.

*Effects on ability to drive and to use machinery:* None stated.

*Undesirable effects:* Used as directed, it is extremely unlikely that the low levels of heparin reaching the blood will have any systemic effect.

*Overdose:* None stated.

**Pharmacological properties**
*Pharmacodynamic properties:* Hepsal, containing only 50 iu of sodium heparin per ampoule (5 ml), is to be used as directed for flushing indwelling cannulae. This is unlikely to produce blood levels of heparin having any systemic effect.

*Pharmacokinetic properties:* None stated.

*Preclinical safety data:* Heparin has not been the subject of toxicity tests now required for newer compounds.

**Pharmaceutical particulars**
*List of excipients:* Sodium Chloride BP; Water for Injection BP; Hydrochloric Acid 3M; Sodium Hydroxide 3M.

*Incompatibilities:* None stated.

*Shelf life:* 36 months in glass ampoules. 24 months in polypropylene ampoules.

*Special precautions for storage:* Store below 25°C. Do not freeze.

*Nature and contents of container:* 5 ml clear glass ampoules: carton contains 10 ampoules. 5 ml polypropylene ampoules: carton contains 30 ampoules.

*Instructions for use/handling:* Not applicable.

**Marketing authorisation numbers**
Glass ampoules 4543/0228
Polypropylene ampoules 4543/0358

**Date of approval/revision of SPC** July 1996.

**Legal category** POM.

## HYALASE*
## Hyaluronidase Injection BP

**Qualitative and quantitative composition** Each ampoule contains 1,500 international units of Hyaluronidase for Injection BP (ovine).

**Pharmaceutical form** 1 ml neutral glass ampoule containing a white, sterile, freeze dried powder of the enzyme hyaluronidase for subcutaneous and intramuscular injection.

**Clinical particulars**
*Therapeutic indications:* Hyalase can be used to enhance permeation of subcutaneous or intramuscular injections, local anaesthetics and subcutaneous infusions and to promote resorption of excess fluids and blood in the tissues.

*Posology and method of administration*
*Adults, children and the elderly:*

*With subcutaneous infusion (hypodermoclysis):* 1500 IU of Hyalase dissolved in 1 ml of water for injections or normal saline injected into the site, before the infusion is set up, or injected into the tubing of the infusion set, about 2 cm back from the needle, at the start of the infusion. 1500 IU is sufficient for administration of 500–1000 ml of most fluids. Care should be taken in young children and the elderly to control the speed and total volume of fluid administered and to avoid over-hydration, especially in renal impairment.

*With subcutaneous or intramuscular injections:* 1500 IU of Hyalase dissolved directly in solution to be injected.

*With local anaesthetics:* 1500 IU Hyalase is mixed with the quantity of local anaesthetic solution to be used. In ophthalmology 15 IU of Hyalase per ml is recommended.

*Extravasation:* Where dispersal rather than localisation is indicated, 1500 IU of Hyalase in 1 ml water for injections or normal saline infiltrated into the affected area as soon as possible after the extravasation is noted.

*Haematoma:* 1500 IU of Hyalase dissolved in 1 ml water for injections or normal saline infiltrated into the affected area.

Immediately before use dissolve the freeze-dried powder in approx 1 ml of water for injections or directly in the solution with which Hyalase is to be combined.

Solutions for subcutaneous administration should be isotonic with extracellular fluid. Hyalase is physically compatible with the commonly used infusion fluids. Use in hypodermoclysis has been reported with 0.9% sodium chloride, 0.18% sodium chloride with 4% glucose, 0.45% sodium chloride with 2.5% glucose and 5% glucose.

Potassium 34 mmol/litre has been administered in isotonic glucose or saline. Electrolyte-free fluids are less preferable than those containing electrolytes and should not be given too rapidly. Hyalase has also been mixed with morphine, diamorphine, hydromorphone, chlorpromazine, metoclopramide, promazine, dexamethasone, local anaesthetics and adrenaline (see *Incompatibilities*).

*Contra-indications: Hypersensitivity to hyaluronidase.* Not to be used to reduce the swelling of bites or stings or at sites where infection or malignancy is present. Not to be used in cases of unexplained premature labour.

*Special warnings and precautions for use:* Do not apply direct to the cornea. Not to be used for intravenous injections.

*Interactions with other medicaments and other forms of interaction:* None stated.

*Pregnancy and lactation:* It is not known whether the drug enters breast milk although it is unlikely to harm the breast fed infant. Caution should be exercised in administering it to nursing mothers.

There is no evidence on the drug's safety in human pregnancy nor is there evidence from animal work that it is free from hazard. Avoid use in pregnancy unless there is no safer alternative.

*Effects on ability to drive and to use machines:* None known.

*Undesirable effects:* Oedema has been reported in association with hypodermoclysis. Severe allergic reactions have been reported rarely. Local irritation, infection, bleeding and bruising also occur rarely.

*Overdose:* No cases of overdose appear to have been reported.

**Pharmacological properties** *Pharmacodynamic properties:* Hyaluronidase is an enzyme which has a temporary and reversible depolymerising effect on the polysaccharide hyaluronic acid which is present in the intercellular matrix of connective tissue.

*Pharmacokinetic properties:* Not applicable.

*Preclinical safety data:* There are no additional preclinical data of relevance to the prescriber.

**Pharmaceutical particulars**
*List of excipients:* Water for Injections BP removed during the freeze drying process.

*Incompatibilities:* Physical incompatibility has been reported with heparin and adrenaline, although in clinical practice very low concentrations of adrenaline are combined with hyaluronidase without problems. Frusemide, the benzodiazepines and phenytoin have been found to be incompatible with hyaluronidase.

*Shelf life:* Three years from date of manufacture.

*Special precautions for storage:* Store below 25°C.

*Nature and contents of container:* 1 ml neutral glass ampoule containing a plug of white freeze dried powder.

*Instructions for use/handling:* The solution should be used immediately after preparation.

**Marketing authorisation number** 4543/0337

**Date of approval/revision of SPC** September 1996.

**Legal category** POM.

# HYPURIN* BOVINE NEUTRAL CARTRIDGES
# HYPURIN* BOVINE ISOPHANE CARTRIDGES

**Qualitative and quantitative composition** Highly Purified Crystalline Bovine Insulin PhEur 100 international units/ml.

## Pharmaceutical form
*Neutral:* Sterile injection for subcutaneous, intramuscular or intravenous injection.

*Isophane:* Sterile injection for subcutaneous or intramuscular injection.

## Clinical particulars
*Therapeutic indications:* The treatment of insulin dependent diabetes mellitus.

*Hypurin Bovine Neutral:* May be used for diabetics who require an insulin of prompt onset and short duration. It is a suitable preparation for admixture with longer acting insulins. It is particularly useful where intermittent, short term or emergency therapy is required, during initial stabilisation and in the treatment of labile diabetes.

*Hypurin Bovine Isophane:* May be used for diabetics requiring a depot insulin of medium duration. Where a more rapid, intense onset is desirable it may be mixed with Hypurin Neutral.

*Posology and method of administration:* To be determined by the physician according to the needs of the patient.

*Hypurin Bovine Neutral:* Usually administered subcutaneously but where necessary it may be given intramuscularly or intravenously. After subcutaneous injection onset of action occurs within 30–60 minutes with an overall duration of 6–8 hours. Maximum effect is exerted over the mid-range.

*Hypurin Bovine Isophane:* Usually administered subcutaneously but where necessary it may be given intramuscularly in which case onset is more rapid and overall duration shorter. It should not be given intravenously. Onset of action occurs within 2 hours after subcutaneous injection with an overall duration of 18–24 hours. Maximum effect is exerted between 6–12 hours.

*Contra-indications:* Hypoglycaemia.

*Special warnings and special precautions for use:* In no circumstances must Hypurin Bovine Isophane be given intravenously.

Blood or urinary glucose concentrations should be monitored and the urine tested for ketones by patients on insulin therapy.

Patients transferred to Hypurin Bovine insulins from other commercially available preparations may require dosage adjustments. Patients whose blood glucose control is greatly improved, e.g. by intensified insulin therapy, may lose some or all of the warning symptoms of hypoglycaemia and should be advised accordingly.

*Interactions with other medicaments and other forms of interaction:* Insulin requirements may increase during illness, puberty or emotional upset or during concurrent administration of drugs associated with hyperglycaemic activity e.g. oral contraceptives, chlorpromazine, thyroid hormone replacement therapy, thiazide diuretics and sympathomimetic agents.

Insulin requirements may decrease with liver or kidney disease, disease of the adrenal, pituitary or thyroid glands or during concomitant use of drugs with hypoglycaemic activity, e.g. salicylates, anabolic steroids, monoamine oxidase inhibitors, NSAIDS. Drugs which may decrease or increase insulin requirements include alcohol, cyclophosphamide, isoniazid and beta blockers (which may also mask some of the warning signs of insulin-induced hypoglycaemia).

Insulin requirements are usually reduced but occasionally increased during periods of increased activity.

*Pregnancy and lactation:* A decreased requirement for insulin may be observed in the early stages of pregnancy. However, in the second and third trimesters, insulin requirements may increase. Diabetic patients who are breast feeding may require adjustments in their insulin dose.

*Effects on ability to drive and to use machines:* The product itself should not affect the ability to drive but patients whose condition is not adequately stabilised with respect to insulin dosage may not be in a fit condition to drive or operate machinery.

*Undesirable effects:* Lipodystrophy (atrophy or hypertrophy of the fat tissue) or oedema may occur at the injection site. Insulin hypersensitivity can occur with animal insulins, but appears less likely with purified

insulins and there is minimal evidence that such effects occur with Hypurin Bovine insulins.

Intolerability reactions to phenol and m-cresol contained as preservative may occur.

*Overdose: Symptoms:* Overdosage causes hypoglycaemia. Symptoms include weakness, sweating, trembling, nervousness, excitement and irritability which, if untreated, will lead to collapse and coma.

*Treatment:* Mild hypoglycaemia will respond to oral administration of glucose or sugar and rest.

Moderately severe hypoglycaemia can be treated by intramuscular or subcutaneous injection of glucagon followed by oral carbohydrate when the patient is sufficiently recovered.

For patients who are comatose or who have failed to respond to glucagon injection an intravenous injection of Strong Dextrose Injection BP should be given.

## Pharmacological properties
*Pharmacodynamic properties:* Insulin output from the pancreas of a healthy person is about 50 units per day, which is sufficient to maintain the fasting blood sugar concentration in the range 0.8±0.2 mg/ml. In diabetes mellitus, the blood sugar rises in an uncontrolled manner. Parenterally administered insulin causes a fall in blood sugar concentration and increased storage of glycogen in the liver. In the diabetic it raises the respiratory quotient after a carbohydrate meal and prevents the formation of ketone bodies. The rise in blood sugar concentration caused by adrenaline and corticosteroids, glucagon and posterior pituitary extract is reversed by insulin.

*Pharmacokinetic properties:* Insulin is rapidly absorbed from subcutaneous tissue or muscle following injection. Insulin is metabolised mainly in the liver and a small amount is excreted in the urine. The plasma half life is 4 to 5 minutes. The half life after subcutaneous injection is about 4 hours and after intramuscular injection about 2 hours.

*Preclinical safety data:* There are no preclinical data of relevance to the prescriber which are additional to those already included in other sections.

## Pharmaceutical particulars
*List of excipients:*
*Neutral:* m-cresol, Phenol PhEur, Sodium Phosphate PhEur, Glycerol PhEur, Water for Injections PhEur.

*Isophane:* Protamine Sulphate PhEur, Zinc Chloride PhEur, m-cresol, Phenol PhEur, Sodium Phosphate PhEur, Glycerol PhEur, Water for Injections PhEur.

*Incompatibilities:* None.

*Shelf life:* 24 months. Following injection of the first dose the product should be used within 28 days. Discard any unused material after this time.

*Special precautions for storage:* Store between 2°C and 8°C. Do not freeze.

*Nature and contents of container:* 1.5 ml neutral glass cartridge sealed with a rubber bung and metal closure.

*Instructions for use/handling:* Prior to use the cartridge of Hypurin Bovine Isophane should be inverted at least ten times. The Injection should then be made immediately.

The cartridge must not be used if the contents have been frozen or it contains lumps that do not disperse on mixing.

**Marketing authorisation numbers**
Hypurin Bovine Neutral cartridge     4543/0366
Hypurin Bovine Isophane cartridge    4543/0367

**Date of approval/revision of SPC** July 1997.

**Legal category** P.

# HYPURIN* BOVINE NEUTRAL VIALS
# HYPURIN* BOVINE ISOPHANE VIALS
# HYPURIN* BOVINE LENTE VIALS
# HYPURIN* BOVINE PROTAMINE ZINC VIALS

**Qualitative and quantitative composition** Highly Purified Crystalline Bovine Insulin PhEur 100 international units/ml.

## Pharmaceutical form
*Neutral:* Sterile injection for subcutaneous, intramuscular or intravenous injection.

*Isophane:* Sterile injection for subcutaneous or intramuscular injection.

*Lente:* Sterile suspension for subcutaneous injection.

*Protamine Zinc:* Sterile suspension for subcutaneous injection.

## Clinical particulars
*Therapeutic indications:* The treatment of insulin dependent diabetes mellitus.

*Hypurin Bovine Neutral:* May be used for diabetics who require an insulin of prompt onset and short duration. It is a suitable preparation for admixture

with longer acting insulins. It is particularly useful where intermittent, short term or emergency therapy is required, during initial stabilisation and in the treatment of labile diabetes.

*Hypurin Bovine Isophane:* May be used for diabetics requiring a depot insulin of medium duration. Where a more rapid, intense onset is desirable it may be mixed with Hypurin Neutral.

*Hypurin Bovine Lente:* May be used for diabetics requiring a depot insulin of medium to extended duration.

*Hypurin Bovine Protamine Zinc:* May be used for diabetics requiring a depot insulin of extended duration. It is characteristically slow in onset and is commonly used in conjunction with Hypurin Neutral.

*Posology and method of administration:* To be determined by the physician according to the needs of the patient.

*Hypurin Bovine Neutral:* Usually administered subcutaneously but where necessary it may be given intramuscularly or intravenously. After subcutaneous injection onset of action occurs within 30–60 minutes with an overall duration of 6–8 hours. Maximum effect is exerted over the mid-range.

*Hypurin Bovine Isophane:* Usually administered subcutaneously but where necessary it may be given intramuscularly in which case onset is more rapid and overall duration shorter. It should not be given intravenously. Onset of action occurs within 2 hours after subcutaneous injection with an overall duration of 18–24 hours. Maximum effect is exerted between 6–12 hours.

*Hypurin Bovine Lente:* Administered subcutaneously. It is not recommended for intramuscular use and should not be given intravenously. Onset of action occurs approximately 2 hours after subcutaneous injection with an overall duration extending up to 30 hours. Maximum effect is exerted between 8–12 hours.

*Hypurin Bovine Protamine Zinc:* Administered subcutaneously. It is not recommended for intramuscular use and should not be given intravenously. Onset of action occurs after 4–6 hours with an overall duration of 24–36 hours. Maximum effect is exerted between 10–20 hours.

*Contra-indications:* Hypoglycaemia.

*Special warnings and special precautions for use:* In no circumstances must Hypurin Bovine Isophane, Hypurin Bovine Lente or Hypurin Bovine Protamine Zinc be given intravenously.

Blood or urinary glucose concentrations should be monitored and the urine tested for ketones by patients on insulin therapy.

Patients transferred to Hypurin Bovine insulins from other commercially available preparations may require dosage adjustments. Patients whose blood glucose control is greatly improved, e.g. by intensified insulin therapy, may lose some or all of the warning symptoms of hypoglycaemia and should be advised accordingly.

*Interactions with other medicaments and other forms of interaction:* Insulin requirements may increase during illness, puberty or emotional upset or during concurrent administration of drugs associated with hyperglycaemic activity e.g. oral contraceptives, chlorpromazine, thyroid hormone replacement therapy, thiazide diuretics and sympathomimetic agents.

Insulin requirements may decrease with liver or kidney disease, disease of the adrenal, pituitary or thyroid glands or during concomitant use of drugs with hypoglycaemic activity, e.g. salicylates, anabolic steroids, monoamine oxidase inhibitors, NSAIDs. Drugs which may decrease or increase insulin requirements include alcohol, cyclophosphamide, isoniazid and beta blockers (which may also mask some of the warning signs of insulin-induced hypoglycaemia).

Insulin requirements are usually reduced but occasionally increased during periods of increased activity.

*Pregnancy and lactation:* A decreased requirement for insulin may be observed in the early stages of pregnancy. However, in the second and third trimesters, insulin requirements may increase. Diabetic patients who are breast feeding may require adjustments in their insulin dose.

*Effects on ability to drive and to use machines:* The product itself should not affect the ability to drive but patients whose condition is not adequately stabilised with respect to insulin dosage may not be in a fit condition to drive or operate machinery.

*Undesirable effects:* Lipodystrophy (atrophy or hypertrophy of the fat tissue) or oedema may occur at the injection site. Insulin hypersensitivity can occur with animal insulins, but appears less likely with purified insulins and there is minimal evidence that such effects occur with Hypurin Bovine insulins.

Intolerability reactions to phenol and m-cresol contained as preservative may occur.

*Overdose: Symptoms:* Overdosage causes hypoglycaemia. Symptoms include weakness, sweating, trembling, nervousness, excitement and irritability which, if untreated, will lead to collapse and coma.

*Treatment:* Mild hypoglycaemia will respond to oral administration of glucose or sugar and rest.

Moderately severe hypoglycaemia can be treated by intramuscular or subcutaneous injection of glucagon followed by oral carbohydrate when the patient is sufficiently recovered.

For patients who are comatose or who have failed to respond to glucagon injection an intravenous injection of Strong Dextrose Injection BP should be given.

### Pharmacological properties

*Pharmacodynamic properties:* Insulin output from the pancreas of a healthy person is about 50 units per day, which is sufficient to maintain the fasting blood sugar concentration in the range 0.8±0.2 mg/ml. In diabetes mellitus, the blood sugar rises in an uncontrolled manner. Parenterally administered insulin causes a fall in blood sugar concentration and increased storage of glycogen in the liver. In the diabetic it raises the respiratory quotient after a carbohydrate meal and prevents the formation of ketone bodies. The rise in blood sugar concentration caused by adrenaline and corticosteroids, glucagon and posterior pituitary extract is reversed by insulin.

*Pharmacokinetic properties:* Insulin is rapidly absorbed from subcutaneous tissue or muscle following injection. Insulin is metabolised mainly in the liver and a small amount is excreted in the urine. The plasma half life is 4 to 5 minutes. The half life after subcutaneous injection is about 4 hours and after intramuscular injection about 2 hours.

*Preclinical safety data:* There are no preclinical data of relevance to the prescriber which are additional to those already included in other sections.

### Pharmaceutical particulars
*List of excipients:*

*Neutral:* m-cresol, Phenol PhEur, Sodium Phosphate PhEur, Glycerol PhEur, Water for Injections PhEur.

*Isophane:* Protamine Sulphate PhEur, Zinc Chloride PhEur, m-cresol, Phenol PhEur, Sodium Phosphate PhEur, Glycerol PhEur, Water for Injections PhEur.

*Lente:* Sodium Chloride PhEur, Sodium Acetate PhEur, Methylparahydroxybenzoate PhEur, Zinc Chloride PhEur, Water for Injections PhEur.

*Protamine Zinc:* Protamine Sulphate PhEur, Zinc Chloride PhEur, Glycerol PhEur, Sodium Phosphate PhEur, Phenol PhEur, Water for Injections PhEur.

*Incompatibilities:* None.

*Shelf life:* 24 months.

Following injection of the first dose the product should be used within 28 days. Discard any unused material after this time.

*Special precautions for storage:* Store between 2°C and 8°C. Do not freeze.

*Nature and contents of container:* 10 ml neutral glass vial sealed with a rubber bung and metal closure.

*Instructions for use/handling:* The vial must not be used if the contents have been frozen or it contains lumps that do not disperse on mixing. Prior to use the vial of Hypurin Bovine Isophane or Hypurin Bovine Lente or Hypurin Bovine Protamine Zinc should be rolled gently between the palms or inverted several times.

Hypurin Bovine Isophane and Hypurin Bovine Lente may be mixed with Hypurin Bovine Neutral in the syringe, in which case Hypurin Bovine Neutral should be the first dose to be withdrawn.

Hypurin Bovine Neutral and Hypurin Bovine Protamine Zinc should not be mixed together in the syringe. The injection should then be made immediately upon withdrawal of the contents.

### Marketing authorisation numbers
Hypurin Bovine Neutral    4543/0203
Hypurin Bovine Isophane    4543/0196
Hypurin Bovine Lente    4543/0214
Hypurin Bovine Protamine Zinc    4543/0199

**Date of approval/revision of SPC**  July 1997.

**Legal category**  P.

# HYPURIN* PORCINE NEUTRAL CARTRIDGES
# HYPURIN* PORCINE ISOPHANE CARTRIDGES
# HYPURIN* PORCINE BIPHASIC ISOPHANE 30/70 MIX CARTRIDGES

**Qualitative and quantitative composition**  Highly Purified Crystalline Porcine Insulin PhEur 100 international units/ml.

### Pharmaceutical form
*Neutral:* Sterile injection for subcutaneous, intramuscular or intravenous injection.

*Isophane and Biphasic Isophane:* Sterile injection for subcutaneous or intramuscular injection.

### Clinical particulars
*Therapeutic indications:* The treatment of insulin dependent diabetes mellitus.

*Hypurin Porcine Neutral:* May be used for diabetics who require an insulin of prompt onset and short duration. It is a suitable preparation for admixture with longer acting insulins. It is particularly useful where intermittent, short term or emergency therapy is required, during initial stabilisation and in the treatment of labile diabetes.

*Hypurin Porcine Isophane:* May be used for diabetics requiring a depot insulin of medium duration. Where a more rapid, intense onset is desirable it may be mixed with Hypurin Porcine Neutral.

*Hypurin Porcine Biphasic Isophane 30/70 Mix:* May be used for diabetics requiring a depot insulin of intermediate duration.

*Posology and method of administration:* To be determined by the physician according to the needs of the patient.

*Hypurin Porcine Neutral:* Usually administered subcutaneously but where necessary it may be given intramuscularly or intravenously. After subcutaneous injection onset of action occurs within 30–60 minutes with an overall duration of 6–8 hours. Maximum effect is exerted over the mid-range.

*Hypurin Porcine Isophane:* Usually administered subcutaneously but where necessary it may be given intramuscularly in which case onset is more rapid and overall duration shorter. It should not be given intravenously. Onset of action occurs within 2 hours after subcutaneous injection with an overall duration of 18–24 hours. Maximum effect is exerted between 6–12 hours.

*Hypurin Porcine Biphasic Isophane 30/70 Mix:* Usually administered subcutaneously but where necessary it may be given intramuscularly in which case onset is more rapid and overall duration shorter. It should not be given intravenously. Onset of action occurs within 2 hours after subcutaneous injection with an overall duration up to 24 hours. Maximum effect is exerted between 4–12 hours.

*Contra-indications:* Hypoglycaemia.

*Special warnings and special precautions for use:* In no circumstances must Hypurin Porcine Isophane or Hypurin Porcine Biphasic Isophane 30/70 be given intravenously.

Blood or urinary glucose concentrations should be monitored and the urine tested for ketones by patients on insulin therapy.

Patients transferred to Hypurin Porcine insulins from other commercially available preparations may require dosage adjustments. Patients whose blood glucose control is greatly improved, e.g. by intensified insulin therapy, may lose some or all of the warning symptoms of hypoglycaemia and should be advised accordingly.

*Interactions with other medicaments and other forms of interaction:* Insulin requirements may increase during illness, puberty or emotional upset or during concurrent administration of drugs associated with hyperglycaemic activity e.g. oral contraceptives, chlorpromazine, thyroid hormone replacement therapy, thiazide diuretics and sympathomimetic agents.

Insulin requirements may decrease with liver or kidney disease, disease of the adrenal, pituitary or thyroid glands or during concomitant use of drugs with hypoglycaemic activity, e.g. salicylates, anabolic steroids, monoamine oxidase inhibitors, NSAIDs. Drugs which may decrease or increase insulin requirements include alcohol, cyclophosphamide, isoniazid and beta blockers (which may also mask some of the warning signs of insulin-induced hypoglycaemia).

Insulin requirements are usually reduced but occasionally increased during periods of increased activity.

*Pregnancy and lactation:* A decreased requirement for insulin may be observed in the early stages of pregnancy. However, in the second and third trimesters, insulin requirements may increase. Diabetic patients who are breast feeding may require adjustments in their insulin dose.

*Effects on ability to drive and to use machines:* The product itself should not affect the ability to drive but patients whose condition is not adequately stabilised with respect to insulin dosage may not be in a fit condition to drive or operate machinery.

*Undesirable effects:* Lipodystrophy (atrophy or hypertrophy of the fat tissue) or oedema may occur at the injection site. Insulin hypersensitivity can occur with animal insulins, but appears less likely with purified insulins.

Intolerability reactions to phenol and m-cresol contained as preservative may occur.

*Overdose: Symptoms:* Overdosage causes hypoglycaemia. Symptoms include weakness, sweating, trembling, nervousness, excitement and irritability which, if untreated, will lead to collapse and coma.

*Treatment:* Mild hypoglycaemia will respond to oral administration of glucose or sugar and rest.

Moderately severe hypoglycaemia can be treated by intramuscular or subcutaneous injection of glucagon followed by oral carbohydrate when the patient is sufficiently recovered.

For patients who are comatose or who have failed to respond to glucagon injection an intravenous injection of strong Dextrose Injection BP should be given.

### Pharmacological properties

*Pharmacodynamic properties:* Insulin output from the pancreas of a healthy person is about 50 units per day, which is sufficient to maintain the fasting blood sugar concentration in the range 0.8±0.2 mg/ml. In diabetes mellitus, the blood sugar rises in an uncontrolled manner. Parenterally administered insulin causes a fall in blood sugar concentration and increased storage of glycogen in the liver. In the diabetic it raises the respiratory quotient after a carbohydrate meal and prevents the formation of ketone bodies. The rise in blood sugar concentration caused by adrenaline and corticosteroids, glucagon and posterior pituitary extract is reversed by insulin.

*Pharmacokinetic properties:* Insulin is rapidly absorbed from subcutaneous tissue or muscle following injection. Insulin is metabolised mainly in the liver and a small amount is excreted in the urine. The plasma half life is 4 to 5 minutes. The half life after subcutaneous injection is about 4 hours and after intramuscular injection about 2 hours.

*Preclinical safety data:* There are no preclinical data of relevance to the prescriber which are additional to that already included in other sections.

### Pharmaceutical particulars
*List of excipients*

*Neutral:* m-cresol, Phenol PhEur, Sodium Phosphate PhEur, Glycerol PhEur, Water for Injections PhEur.

*Isophane:* Protamine Sulphate PhEur, Zinc Chloride PhEur, m-cresol, Phenol PhEur, Sodium Phosphate PhEur, Glycerol PhEur, Water for Injections PhEur.

*Biphasic Isophane:* Protamine Sulphate PhEur, Zinc Chloride PhEur, m-cresol, Phenol PhEur, Sodium Phosphate PhEur, Glycerol PhEur, Water for Injections PhEur.

*Incompatibilities:* None.

*Shelf life:* 24 months. Following injection of the first dose the product should be used within 28 days. Discard any unused material after this time.

*Special precautions for storage:* Store between 2°C and 8°C. Do not freeze.

*Nature and contents of container:* 1.5 ml neutral glass cartridge sealed with a rubber bung and metal closure.

*Instructions for use/handling:* Prior to use the cartridge of Hypurin Porcine Isophane or Hypurin Porcine Biphasic Isophane 30/70 Mix should be inverted at least ten times. The injection should then be made immediately.

The cartridge must not be used if the contents have been frozen or it contains lumps that do not disperse on mixing.

### Marketing authorisation numbers
Hypurin Porcine Neutral cartridge    4543/0373
Hypurin Porcine Isophane cartridge    4543/0374
Hypurin Porcine Biphasic Isophane 30/70 cartridge    4543/0375

**Date of approval/revision of SPC**  April 1997.

**Legal category**  P.

# HYPURIN* PORCINE NEUTRAL VIALS
# HYPURIN* PORCINE ISOPHANE VIALS
# HYPURIN* PORCINE BIPHASIC ISOPHANE 30/70 MIX VIALS

**Qualitative and quantitative composition**  Highly Purified Crystalline Porcine Insulin PhEur 100 international units/ml.

### Pharmaceutical form
*Neutral:* Sterile injection for subcutaneous, intramuscular or intravenous injection.

*Isophane and Biphasic Isophane:* Sterile injection for subcutaneous or intramuscular injection.

### Clinical particulars
*Therapeutic indications:* The treatment of insulin dependent diabetes mellitus.

*Hypurin Porcine Neutral:* May be used for diabetics who require an insulin of prompt onset and short duration. It is a suitable preparation for admixture with longer acting insulins. It is particularly useful where intermittent, short term or emergency therapy is required, during initial stabilisation and in the treatment of labile diabetes.

*Hypurin Porcine Isophane:* May be used for diabetics requiring a depot insulin of medium duration. Where a more rapid, intense onset is desirable it may be mixed with Hypurin Neutral.

*Hypurin Porcine Biphasic Isophane 30/70 Mix:* May be used for diabetics requiring a depot insulin of intermediate duration.

*Posology and method of administration:* To be determined by the physician according to the needs of the patient.

*Hypurin Porcine Neutral:* Usually administered subcutaneously but where necessary it may be given intramuscularly or intravenously. After subcutaneous injection onset of action occurs within 30–60 minutes with an overall duration of 6–8 hours. Maximum effect is exerted over the mid-range.

*Hypurin Porcine Isophane:* Usually administered subcutaneously but where necessary it may be given intramuscularly in which case onset is more rapid and overall duration shorter. It should not be given intravenously. Onset of action occurs within 2 hours after subcutaneous injection with an overall duration of 18–24 hours. Maximum effect is exerted between 6–12 hours.

*Hypurin Porcine Biphasic Isophane 30/70 Mix:* Usually administered subcutaneously but where necessary it may be given intramuscularly in which case onset is more rapid and overall duration shorter. It should not be given intravenously. Onset of action occurs within 2 hours after subcutaneous injection with an overall duration up to 24 hours. Maximum effect is exerted between 4–12 hours.

*Contra-indications:* Hypoglycaemia.

*Special warnings and special precautions for use:* In no circumstances must Hypurin Porcine Isophane or Hypurin Porcine Biphasic Isophane 30/70 Mix be given intravenously.

Blood or urinary glucose concentrations should be monitored and the urine tested for ketones by patients on insulin therapy.

Patients transferred to Hypurin Porcine insulins from other commercially available preparations may require dosage adjustments. Patients whose blood glucose control is greatly improved, e.g. by intensified insulin therapy, may lose some or all of the warning symptoms of hypoglycaemia and should be advised accordingly.

*Interactions with other medicaments and other forms of interaction:* Insulin requirements may increase during illness, puberty or emotional upset or during concurrent administration of drugs associated with hyperglycaemic activity e.g. oral contraceptives, chlorpromazine, thyroid hormone replacement therapy, thiazide diuretics and sympathomimetic agents.

Insulin requirements may decrease with liver or kidney disease, disease of the adrenal, pituitary or thyroid glands or during concomitant use of drugs with hypoglycaemic activity, e.g. salicylates, anabolic steroids, monoamine oxidase inhibitors, NSAIDs. Drugs which may decrease or increase insulin requirements include alcohol, cyclophosphamide, isoniazid and beta blockers (which may also mask some of the warning signs of insulin-induced hypoglycaemia).

Insulin requirements are usually reduced but occasionally increased during periods of increased activity.

*Pregnancy and lactation:* A decreased requirement for insulin may be observed in the early stages of pregnancy. However, in the second and third trimesters, insulin requirements may increase. Diabetic patients who are breast feeding may require adjustments in their insulin dose.

*Effects on ability to drive and use machines:* The product itself should not affect the ability to drive but patients whose condition is not adequately stabilised with respect to insulin dosage may not be in a fit condition to drive or operate machinery.

*Undesirable effects:* Lipodystrophy (atrophy or hypertrophy of the fat tissue) or oedema may occur at the injection site. Insulin hypersensitivity can occur with animal insulins, but appears less likely with purified insulins and there is minimal evidence that such effects occur with Hypurin insulins.

Intolerability reactions to phenol and m-cresol contained as preservative may occur.

*Overdose: Symptoms:* Overdosage causes hypoglycaemia. Symptoms include weakness, sweating, trembling, nervousness, excitement and irritability which, if untreated, will lead to collapse and coma.

*Treatment:* Mild hypoglycaemia will respond to oral administration of glucose or sugar and rest.

Moderately severe hypoglycaemia can be treated by intramuscular or subcutaneous injection of glucagon followed by oral carbohydrate when the patient is sufficiently recovered.

For patients who are comatose or who have failed to respond to glucagon injection an intravenous injection of strong Dextrose Injection BP should be given.

**Pharmacological properties**

*Pharmacodynamic properties:* Insulin output from the pancreas of a healthy person is about 50 units per day, which is sufficient to maintain the fasting blood sugar concentration in the range 0.8±0.2 mg/ml. In diabetes mellitus, the blood sugar rises in an uncontrolled manner. Parenterally administered insulin causes a fall in blood sugar concentration and increased storage of glycogen in the liver. In the diabetic it raises the respiratory quotient after a carbohydrate meal and prevents the formation of ketone bodies. The rise in blood sugar concentration caused by adrenaline and corticosteroids, glucagon and posterior pituitary extract is reversed by insulin.

*Pharmacokinetic properties:* Insulin is rapidly absorbed from subcutaneous tissue or muscle following injection. Insulin is metabolised mainly in the liver and a small amount is excreted in the urine. The plasma half life is 4 to 5 minutes. The half life after subcutaneous injection is about 4 hours and after intramuscular injection about 2 hours.

*Preclinical safety data:* There are no preclinical data of relevance to the prescriber which are additional to those already included in other sections.

**Pharmaceutical particulars**

*List of excipients:*

*Neutral:* m-cresol, Phenol PhEur, Sodium Phosphate PhEur, Glycerol PhEur, Water for Injections BP.

*Isophane:* Protamine Sulphate PhEur, Zinc Chloride PhEur, m-cresol, Phenol PhEur, Sodium Phosphate PhEur, Glycerol PhEur, Water for Injections BP.

*Biphasic Isophane:* Protamine Sulphate PhEur, Zinc Chloride PhEur, m-cresol, Phenol PhEur, Sodium Phosphate PhEur, Glycerol PhEur, Water for Injections BP.

*Incompatibilities:* None.

*Shelf life:* 24 months. Following withdrawal of the first dose the product should be used within 28 days. Discard any unused material.

*Special precautions for storage:* Store between 2°C and 8°C. Do not freeze.

*Nature and contents of container:* 10 ml neutral glass vial sealed with a rubber bung and metal closure.

*Instruction for use/handling:* Prior to use the vial of Hypurin Porcine Isophane or Hypurin Porcine Biphasic Isophane 30/70 Mix should be gently rolled between the palms or inverted several times.

The vial must not be used if the contents have been frozen or it contains lumps that do not disperse on mixing.

The injections should be made immediately upon withdrawal of the contents.

**Marketing authorisation numbers**

Hypurin Porcine Neutral vials 4543/0370
Hypurin Porcine Isophane vials 4543/0371
Hypurin Porcine Biphasic Isophane 30/70 Mix vials 4543/0372

**Date of approval/revision of SPC** April 1997.

**Legal category** P.

## MONOPARIN*

**Qualitative and quantitative composition**

Monoparin 1,000 iu/ml: Heparin Sodium (Mucous) BP 1,000 iu/ml.
Monoparin 5,000 iu/ml: Heparin Sodium (Mucous) BP 5,000 iu/ml.
Monoparin 10,000 iu/ml: Heparin Sodium (Mucous) BP 10,000 iu/ml.
Monoparin 25,000 iu/ml: Heparin Sodium (Mucous) BP 25,000 iu/ml.

**Pharmaceutical form**

*Monoparin 1,000 iu/ml:* Intravenous injection.

*Monoparin 5,000 iu/ml, Monoparin 10,000 iu/ml and Monoparin 25,000 iu/ml:* Intravenous and subcutaneous injection.

**Clinical particulars**

*Therapeutic indications:*

*Monoparin 1,000 iu/ml, 5,000 iu/ml, 10,000 iu/ml, 25,000 iu/ml:* Treatment of deep vein thrombosis, pulmonary embolism, unstable angina pectoris and acute peripheral arterial occlusion.

In extracorporeal circulation and haemodialysis.

*Monoparin 5,000 iu/ml, 10,000 iu/ml, 25,000 iu/ml:* Prophylaxis of deep vein thrombosis and pulmonary embolism.

Prophylaxis of mural thrombosis following myocardial infarction.

*Posology and method of administration:* By continuous intravenous infusion in 5% glucose or 0.9% sodium chloride or by intermittent intravenous injection or (exept Monoparin 1,000 iu/ml) by subcutaneous injection.

As the effects of heparin are short-lived, administration by intravenous infusion is preferable to intermittent intravenous injections.

*Recommended dosage:*

*Treatment of deep vein thrombosis, pulmonary embolism, unstable angina pectoris, acute peripheral arterial occlusion (Monoparin 1,000 iu/ml, 5,000 iu/ml, 10,000 iu/ml, 25,000 iu/ml):*

*Adults:*

*Loading dose:* 5,000 units intravenously (10,000 units may be required in severe pulmonary embolism).

*Maintenance:* 1,000–2,000 units/hour by intravenous infusion,

*or* 5,000–10,000 units 4-hourly by intravenous injection,

*or* (except Monoparin 1,000 iu/ml) 10,000–20,000 units 12 hourly subcutaneously.

*Elderly:* Dosage reduction may be advisable.

*Children and small adults:*

*Loading dose:* 50 units/kg intravenously.

*Maintenance:* 15–25 units/kg/hour by intravenous infusion,

*or* 100 units/kg 4-hourly by intravenous injection,

*or* (except Monoparin 1,000 iu/ml) 250 units/kg 12 hourly subcutaneously.

**Daily laboratory monitoring (ideally at the same time each day, starting 4–6 hours after initiation of treatment) is essential during full-dose heparin treatment, with adjustment of dosage to maintain an APTT value 1.5–2.5 x midpoint of normal range or control value.**

*In extracorporeal circulation and haemodialysis (Monoparin 1,000 iu/ml, 5,000 iu/ml, 10,000 iu/ml, 25,000 iu/ml):*

*Adults:*

*Cardiopulmonary bypass:* Initially 300 units/kg intravenously, adjusted thereafter to maintain the activated clotting time (ACT) in the range 400–500 seconds.

*Haemodialysis and haemofiltration:* Initially 1–5,000 units. Maintenance: 1–2,000 units/hour, adjusted to maintain clotting time >40 minutes.

*Route of administration*

*Prophylaxis of deep vein thrombosis and pulmonary embolism (Monoparin 5,000 iu/ml, 10,000 iu/ml, 25,000 iu/ml only):*

*Adults:*

2 hours pre-operatively: 5,000 units subcutaneously followed by: 5,000 units subcutaneously every 8–12 hours, for 7–10 days or until the patient is fully ambulant.

No laboratory monitoring should be necessary during low dose heparin prophylaxis. If monitoring is considered desirable, anti-Xa assays should be used as the activated partial thromboplastin time (APTT) is not significantly prolonged.

*During pregnancy:* 5,000–10,000 units every 12 hours, subcutaneously, adjusted according to APTT or anti-Xa assay.

*Elderly:* Dosage reduction and monitoring of APTT may be advisable.

*Children:* No dosage recommendations.

*Prophylaxis of mural thrombosis following myocardial infarction (Monoparin 5,000 iu/ml, 10,000 iu/ml, 25,000 iu/ml only):*

*Adults:* 12,500 units 12 hourly subcutaneously for at least 10 days.

*Elderly:* Dosage reduction may be advisable.

*Contra-indications:* Patients who consume large amounts of alcohol, who are sensitive to the drug, who are actively bleeding or who have haemophilia, purpura, severe hypertension, active tuberculosis or increased capillary permeability.

Patients with present or previous thrombocytopenia. The rare occurrence of skin necrosis in patients receiving heparin contra-indicates the further use of heparin either by subcutaneous or intravenous routes because of the risk of thrombocytopenia. Because of the special hazard of post-operative haemorrhage heparin is contra-indicated during surgery of the brain, spinal cord and eye, and in patients undergoing lumbar puncture or regional anaesthetic block.

The relative risks and benefits of heparin should be carefully assessed in patients with a bleeding tendency or those patients with an actual or potential bleeding site e.g. hiatus hernia, peptic ulcer, neoplasm, bacterial endocarditis, retinopathy, bleeding haemorrhoids, suspected intracranial haemorrhage, cerebral thrombosis or threatened abortion.

Menstruation is not a contra-indication.

*Special warnings and special precautions for use:* Platelet counts should be measured in patients receiving heparin treatment for longer than 5 days and the treatment should be stopped immediately in those who develop thrombocytopenia.

In patients with advanced renal or hepatic disease, a reduction in dosage may be necessary.

Although heparin hypersensitivity is rare, it is advisable to give a trial dose of 1,000 iu in patients with a history of allergy.

In most patients, the recommended low-dose regimen produces no alteration in clotting time. However, patients show an individual response to heparin, and it is therefore essential that the effect of therapy on coagulation time should be monitored in patients undergoing major surgery.

*Interactions with other medicaments and other forms of interaction:* Drugs that interfere with platelet aggregation e.g. aspirin, dextran solutions, dipyridamole or any other drug which may interfere with coagulation, should be used with care.

*Pregnancy and lactation:* Heparin is not contra-indicated in pregnancy. Heparin does not cross the placenta or appear in breast milk. The decision to use heparin in pregnancy should be taken after evaluation of the risk/benefit in any particular circumstances.

*Effects on ability to drive and to use machines:* None stated.

*Undesirable effects:* Haemorrhage (see *Overdose*).

Thrombocytopenia has been observed occasionally (see *Warnings*). There is some evidence that prolonged dosing with heparin (i.e. over many months) may cause alopecia and osteoporosis. Significant bone demineralisation has been reported in women taking more than 10,000 iu per day of heparin for at least 6 months.

Hypersensitivity reactions, local irritation and skin necrosis may occur but are rare.

*Overdose:* A potential hazard of heparin therapy is haemorrhage, but this is usually due to overdosage and the risk is minimised by strict laboratory control. Slight haemorrhage can usually be treated by withdrawing the drug. If bleeding is more severe, clotting time and platelet count should be determined. Prolonged clotting time will indicate the presence of an excessive anticoagulant effect requiring neutralisation by intravenous protamine sulphate, at a dosage of 1 mg for every 100 iu of heparin to be neutralised. The bolus dose of protamine sulphate should be given slowly over about 10 minutes and not exceed 50 mg. If more than 15 minutes have elapsed since the injection of heparin, lower doses of protamine will be necessary.

**Pharmacological properties**
*Pharmacodynamic properties:* Heparin is an anticoagulant and acts by inhibiting thrombin and by potentiating the naturally occurring inhibitors of activated Factor X (Xa).

*Pharmacokinetic particulars:* As heparin is not absorbed from the gastrointestinal tract and sublingual sites it is administered by injection. After injection heparin extensively binds to plasma proteins.

Heparin is metabolised in the liver and the inactive metabolic products are excreted in the urine.

The half life of heparin is dependent on the dose.

*Preclinical safety data:* There are no pre-clinical data of relevance to the prescriber which are additional to those already included in other sections.

**Pharmaceutical particulars**
*List of excipients:* Water for Injections BP; Sodium Hydroxide Solution 3M; Hydrochloric Acid 3M.

*Incompatibilities:* Heparin is incompatible with many injectable preparations e.g. some antibiotics, opioid analgesics and antihistamines.

*Shelf life:* 36 months.

*Special precautions for storage:* Monoparin should be stored below 25°C.

*Nature and contents of container:* Monoparin 1,000 iu/ml: Neutral glass ampoules (Type I PhEur) of 1 ml, 5 ml, 10 ml and 20 ml capacity containing 1 ml, 5 ml, 10 ml and 20 ml of solution respectively. Cartons contain 10 ampoules.

*Monoparin 5,000 iu/ml:* Neutral glass ampoules (Type I PhEur) of 1 ml and 5 ml capacity containing 1 ml and 5 ml of solution respectively. Cartons contain 10 ampoules.

*Monoparin 10,000 iu/ml:* Neutral glass ampoules (Type I PhEur) of 1 ml capacity containing 1 ml of solution. Cartons contain 10 ampoules.

*Monoparin 25,000 iu/ml:* Neutral glass ampoules (Type I PhEur) of 1 ml capacity containing 0.2 ml, 0.5 ml and 1 ml of solution respectively and 5 ml ampoules containing 5 ml of solution. Cartons contain 10, 15 or 50 ampoules.

*Instructions for use/handling:* Not applicable.

**Marketing authorisation numbers**
Monoparin 1,000 iu/ml 4543/0221
Monoparin 5,000 iu/ml 4543/0208
Monoparin 10,000 iu/ml 4543/0209
Monoparin 25,000 iu/ml 4543/0210

**Date of approval/revision of SPC** April 1997.

**Legal category** POM.

## MONOPARIN-CA*

**Qualitative and quantitative composition**
Monoparin Ca 1,000 iu/ml: Heparin Calcium (Mucous) BP 1,000 iu/ml.
Monoparin Ca 5,000 iu/ml: Heparin Calcium (Mucous) BP 5,000 iu/ml.
Monoparin Ca 25,000 iu/ml: Heparin Calcium (Mucous) BP 25,000 iu/ml.

**Pharmaceutical form**
*Monoparin-Ca 1,000 iu/ml:* Intravenous injection.

*Monoparin-Ca 5,000 iu/ml and Monoparin-Ca 25,000 iu/ml:* Intravenous or subcutaneous injection.

**Clinical particulars**
*Therapeutic indications:*
*Monoparin-Ca 1,000 iu/ml, 5,000 iu/ml, 25,000 iu/ml:* Treatment of deep vein thrombosis, pulmonary embolism, unstable angina pectoris and acute peripheral arterial occlusion.

In extracorporeal circulation and haemodialysis.

*Monoparin-Ca 5,000 iu/ml and Monoparin-Ca 25,000 iu/ml:* Prophylaxis of deep vein thrombosis and pulmonary embolism. Prophylaxis of mural thrombosis following myocardial infarction.

*Posology and method of administration:*
*Route of administration:* By continuous intravenous infusion in 5% glucose or 0.9% sodium chloride or by intermittent intravenous injection or (except Monoparin-Ca 1,000 iu/ml) by subcutaneous injection.

As the effects of heparin are short-lived, administration by intravenous infusion is preferable to intermittent intravenous injections.

*Recommended dosage:*
*Treatment of deep vein thrombosis, pulmonary embolism, unstable angina pectoris, acute peripheral arterial occulation (Monoparin-Ca 1,000 iu/ml, 5,000 iu/ml, 25,000 iu/ml):*
*Adults:*
 Loading dose: 5,000 units intravenously (10,000 units may be required in severe pulmonary embolism)
 Maintenance: 1,000–2,000 units/hour by intravenous infusion.
 or 5,000–10,000 units 4-hourly by intravenous injection.
 or (except Monoparin-Ca 1,000 iu/ml) 10,000–20,000 units 12 hourly subcutaneously.
*Elderly:* Dosage reduction may be advisable.

*Children and small adults:*
 Loading dose: 50 units/kg intravenously.
 Maintenance: 15–25 units/kg/hour by intravenous infusion,
 or 100 units/kg 4-hourly by intravenous injection
 or (except Monoparin-Ca 1,000 iu/ml) 250 units/kg 12 hourly subcutaneously.

**Daily laboratory monitoring (ideally at the same time each day, starting 4–6 hours after initiation of treatment) is essential during full-dose heparin treatment, with adjustment of dosage to maintain an APTT value 1.5–2.5 x midpoint of normal range or control value.**

*In extracorporeal circulation and haemodialysis (Monoparin-Ca 1,000 iu/ml, 5,000 iu/ml, 25,000 iu/ml):*
*Adults:*
*Cardiopulmonary bypass:* Initially 300 units/kg intravenously, adjusted thereafter to maintain the activated clotting time (ACT) in the range 400–500 seconds.

*Haemodialysis and haemofiltration:* Initially 1–5,000 units. Maintenance: 1–2,000 units/hour, adjusted to maintain clotting time >40 minutes.

*Route of administration:* By continuous intravenous infusion in 5% glucose or 0.9% sodium chloride or by intermittent intravenous injection, or by subcutaneous injection.

As the effects of heparin are short-lived, administration by intravenous infusion or subcutaneous injection is preferable to intermittent intravenous injections.

*Prophylaxis of deep vein thrombosis and pulmonary embolism (Monoparin-Ca 5,000 iu/ml, 25,000 iu/ml only):*
*Adults:*
2 hours pre-operatively: 5,000 units subcutaneously followed by: 5,000 units subcutaneously every 8–12 hours, for 7–10 days or until the patient is fully ambulant.

No laboratory monitoring should be necessary during low dose heparin prophylaxis.

If monitoring is considered desirable, anti-Xa assays should be used as the activated partial thromboplastin time (APTT) is not significantly prolonged.

*During pregnancy:* 5,000–10,000 units every 12 hours, subcutaneously, adjusted according to APTT or anti-Xa assay.

*Elderly:* Dosage reduction and monitoring of APTT may be advisable.

*Children:* No dosage recommendations.

*Prophylaxis of mural thrombosis following myocardial infarction (Monoparin 5,000 iu/ml, 25,000 iu/ml only):*
*Adults:* 12,500 units 12 hourly subcutaneously for at least 10 days.

*Elderly:* Dosage reduction may be advisable.

*Contra-indications:* Patients who consume large amounts of alcohol, who are sensitive to the drug, who are actively bleeding or who have haemophilia, purpura, severe hypertension, active tuberculosis or increased capillary permeability.

Patients with present or previous thrombocytopenia. The rare occurrence of skin necrosis in patients receiving heparin contra-indicates the further use of heparin either by subcutaneous or intravenous routes because of the risk of thrombocytopenia. Because of the special hazard of post-operative haemorrhage heparin is conta-indicated during surgery of the brain, spinal cord and eye, and in patients undergoing lumbar puncture or regional anaesthetic block.

The relative risks and benefits of heparin should be carefully assessed in patients with a bleeding tendency or those patients with an actual or potential bleeding site e.g. hiatus hernia, peptic ulcer, neoplasm, bacterial endocarditis, retinopathy, bleeding haemorrhoids, suspected intracranial haemorrhage, cerebral thrombosis or threatened abortion.

Menstruation is not a contra-indication.

*Special warnings and special precautions for use:* Platelet counts should be measured in patients receiving heparin treatment for longer than 5 days and the treatment should be stopped immediately in those who develop thrombocytopenia.

In patients with advanced renal or hepatic disease, a reduction in dosage may be necessary.

Although heparin hypersensitivity is rare, it is advisable to give a trial dose of 1,000 iu in patients with a history of allergy.

In most patients, the recommended low-dose regimen produces no alteration in clotting time. However, patients show an individual response to heparin, and it is therefore essential that the effect of therapy on coagulation time should be monitored in patients undergoing major surgery.

*Interactions with other medicaments and other forms of interaction:* Drugs that interfere with platelet aggregation e.g. aspirin, dextran solutions, dipyridamole or any other drug which may interfere with coagulation, should be used with care.

*Pregnancy and lactation:* Heparin is not contra-indicated in pregnancy. Heparin does not cross the placenta or appear in breast milk. The decision to use heparin in pregnancy should be taken after evaluation of the risk/benefit in any particular circumstances.

*Effects on ability to drive and use machines:* None stated.

*Undesirable effects:* Haemorrhage (see *Overdosage*).

Thrombocytopenia has been observed occasionally (see *Warnings*).

There is some evidence that prolonged dosing with heparin (i.e. over many months) may cause alopecia and osteoporosis. Significant bone demineralisation has been reported in women taking more than 10,000 iu per day of heparin for at least 6 months.

Hypersensitivity reactions, local irritation and skin necrosis may occur but are rare.

*Overdose:* A potential hazard of heparin therapy is haemorrhage, but this is usually due to overdosage and the risk is minimised by strict laboratory control. Slight haemorrhage can usually be treated by withdrawing the drug. If bleeding is more severe, clotting time and platelet count should be determined. Prolonged clotting time will indicate the presence of an excessive anticoagulant effect requiring neutralisation by intravenous protamine sulphate, at a dosage of 1 mg for every 100 iu of heparin to be neutralised. The bolus dose of protamine sulphate should be given slowly over about 10 minutes and not exceed 50 mg. If more than 15 minutes have elapsed since the injection of heparin, lower doses of protamine will be necessary.

**Pharmacological properties**
*Pharmacodynamic properties:* Heparin is an anticoagulant and acts by inhibiting thrombin and by potentiating the naturally occurring inhibitors of activated Factor X (Xa).

*Pharmacokinetic properties:* As heparin is not absorbed from the gastrointestinal tract and sublingual sites it is administered by injection. After injection heparin extensively binds to plasma proteins.

Heparin is metabolised in the liver and the inactive metabolic products are excreted in the urine.

The half life of heparin is dependent on the dose.

*Preclinical safety data:* There are no pre-clinical data

of relevance to the prescriber which are additional to those already included in other sections.

**Pharmaceutical particulars**
*List of excipients:* Water for Injections BP, Calcium Hydroxide Solution 3M, Hydrochloric Acid 3M.

*Incompatibilities:* Heparin is incompatible with many injectable preparations e.g. some antibiotics, opioid analgesics and antihistamines.

*Shelf life:* 36 months.

*Special precautions for storage:* Monoparin-Ca should be stored below 25°C.

*Nature and contents of container:*
Monoparin-Ca 1,000 iu/ml: Neutral glass ampoules (Type I PhEur) of 1 ml and 5 ml capacity containing 1 ml and 5 ml of solution respectively. Cartons contain 10 ampoules.

Monoparin-Ca 5,000 iu/ml: Neutral glass ampoule (Type I PhEur) of 1 ml and 5 ml capacity containing 1 ml and 5 ml of solution respectively. Cartons contain 10 ampoules.

Monoparin-Ca 25,000 iu/ml: Neutral glass ampoules (Type I PhEur) of 1 ml capacity containing 0.2 ml of solution. Cartons contain 10 ampoules.

*Instructions for use/handling:* Not applicable.

**Marketing authorisation numbers**
Monoparin-Ca 1,000 iu/ml  4543/0211
Monoparin-Ca 5,000 iu/ml  4543/0212
Monoparin-Ca 25,000 iu/ml 4543/0213

**Date of approval/revision of SPC**  April 1997.

**Legal category**  POM.


# MULTIPARIN*

**Qualitative and quantitative composition**
Multiparin 1,000 iu/ml: Heparin Sodium (Mucous) BP 1,000 iu/ml.
Multiparin 5,000 iu/ml: Heparin Sodium (Mucous) BP 5,000 iu/ml.
Multiparin 25,000 iu/ml: Heparin Sodium (Mucous) BP 25,000 iu/ml.

**Pharmaceutical form**
*Multiparin 1,000 iu/ml:* Intravenous injection.

*Multiparin 5,000 iu/ml and Multiparin 25,000 iu/ml:* Intravenous or subcutaneous injection.

**Clinical particulars**
*Therapeutic indications:*
*Multiparin 1,000 iu/ml, 5,000 iu/ml, 25,000 iu/ml:* Treatment of deep vein thrombosis, pulmonary embolism, unstable angina pectoris and acute peripheral arterial occlusion.

In extracorporeal circulation and haemodialysis.

*Multiparin 5,000 iu/ml and Multiparin 25,000 iu/ml:* Prophylaxis of deep vein thrombosis and pulmonary embolism. Prophylaxis of mural thrombosis following myocardial infarction.

*Posology and method of administration*
*Route of administration:* By continuous intravenous infusion in 5% glucose or 0.9% sodium chloride or by intermittent intravenous injection or (except Multiparin 1,000 iu/ml) by subcutaneous injection.

The intravenous injection volume of Multiparin should not exceed 15 ml.

As the effects of heparin are short-lived, administration by intravenous infusion is preferable to intermittent intravenous injections.

*Recommended dosage:*
Treatment of deep vein thrombosis, pulmonary embolism, unstable angina pectoris, acute peripheral arterial occlusion (Multiparin 1,000 iu/ml, 5,000 iu/ml, 25,000 iu/ml):
*Adults:*
Loading dose: 5,000 units intravenously (10,000 units may be required in severe pulmonary embolism)
    Maintenance: 1,000–2,000 units/hour by intravenous infusion,
        or 5,000–10,000 units 4-hourly by intravenous injection,
        or (except Multiparin 1,000 iu/ml) 10,000–20,000 units 12 hourly subcutaneously.
*Elderly:* Dosage reduction may be advisable.

*Children and small adults:*
Loading dose: 50 units/kg intravenously.
    Maintenance: 15–25 units/kg/hour by intravenous infusion,
        or 100 units/kg 4-hourly by intravenous injection,
        or (except Multiparin 1,000 iu/ml) 250 units/kg 12 hourly subcutaneously.

**Daily laboratory monitoring (ideally at the same time each day, starting 4–6 hours after initiation of treatment) is essential during full-dose heparin treatment, with adjustment of dosage to maintain an APTT value 1.5–2.5 x midpoint of normal range or control value.**

*In extracorporeal circulation and haemodialysis (Multiparin 1,000 iu/ml, 5,000 iu/ml, 25,000 iu/ml):*
*Adults:*
*Cardiopulmonary bypass:* Initially 300 units/kg intravenously, adjusted thereafter to maintain the activated clotting time (ACT) in the range 400–500 seconds.
*Haemodialysis and haemofiltration:* Initially 1–5,000 units. Maintenance: 1–2,000 units/hour, adjusted to maintain clotting time >40 minutes.
*Prophylaxis of deep vein thrombosis and pulmonary embolism (Multiparin 5,000 iu/ml, 25,000 iu/ml only):*
*Adults:*
2 hours pre-operatively: 5,000 units subcutaneously, followed by: 5,000 units subcutaneously every 8–12 hours, for 7–10 days or until the patient is fully ambulant.
    No laboratory monitoring should be necessary during low dose heparin prophylaxis. If monitoring is considered desirable, anti-Xa assays should be used as the activated partial thromboplastin time (APTT) is not significantly prolonged:
*During pregnancy:* 5,000–10,000 units every 12 hours, subcutaneously, adjusted according to APTT or anti-Xa assay.
*Elderly:*
Dosage reduction and monitoring of APTT may be advisable.
*Children:* No dosage recommendations.

*Prophylaxis of mural thrombosis following myocardial infarction (Multiparin 5,000 iu/ml, 25,000 iu/ml only):*
*Adults:* 12,500 units 12 hourly subcutaneously for at least 10 days.
*Elderly:* Dosage reduction may be advisable.

*Contra-indications:* Patients who consume large amounts of alcohol, who are sensitive to the drug, who are actively bleeding or who have haemophilia, purpura, severe hypertension, active tuberculosis or increased capillary permeability.
    Patients with present or previous thrombocytopenia. The rare occurrence of skin necrosis in patients receiving heparin contra-indicates the further use of heparin either by subcutaneous or intravenous routes because of the risk of thrombocytopenia. Because of the special hazard of post-operative haemorrhage heparin is contra-indicated during surgery of the brain, spinal cord and eye, and in patients undergoing lumbar puncture or regional anaesthetic block.
    The relative risks and benefits of heparin should be carefully assessed in patients with a bleeding tendency or those patients with an actual or potential bleeding site e.g. hiatus hernia, peptic ulcer, neoplasm, bacterial endocarditis, retinopathy, bleeding haemorrhoids, suspected intracranial haemorrhage, cerebral thrombosis or threatened abortion.
    Menstruation is not a contra-indication.

*Special warnings and special precautions for use:* Platelet counts should be measured in patients receiving heparin treatment for longer than 5 days and the treatment should be stopped immediately in those who develop thrombocytopenia.
    In patients with advanced renal or hepatic disease, a reduction in dosage may be necessary.
    Although heparin hypersensitivity is rare, it is advisable to give a trial dose of 1,000 iu in patients with a history of allergy.
    In most patients, the recommended low-dose regimen produces no alteration in clotting time. However, patients show an individual response to heparin, and it is therefore essential that the effect of therapy on coagulation time should be monitored in patients undergoing major surgery.

*Interactions with other medicaments and other forms of interaction:* Drugs that interfere with platelet aggregation e.g. aspirin, dextran solutions, dipyridamole or any other drug which may interfere with coagulation, should be used with care.

*Pregnancy and lactation:* Heparin is not contra-indicated in pregnancy. Heparin does not cross the placenta or appear in breast milk. The decision to use heparin in pregnancy should be taken after evaluation of the risk/benefit in any particular circumstances.

*Effects on ability to drive and use machines:* None stated.

*Undesirable effects:* Haemorrhage (see *Overdose*). Thrombocytopenia has been observed occasionally (see *Warnings*). There is some evidence that prolonged dosing with heparin (i.e. over many months) may cause alopecia and osteoporosis. Significant bone demineralisation has been reported in women taking more than 10,000 iu per day of heparin for at least 6 months.
    Hypersensitivity reactions, local irritations and skin necrosis may occur but are rare.

*Overdose:* A potential hazard of heparin therapy is haemorrhage, but this is usually due to overdosage and the risk is minimised by strict laboratory control. Slight haemorrhage can usually be treated by with-

drawing the drug. If bleeding is more severe, clotting time and platelet count should be determined. Prolonged clotting time will indicate the presence of an excessive anticoagulant effect requiring neutralisation by intravenous protamine sulphate, at a dosage of 1 mg for every 100 iu of heparin to be neutralised. The bolus dose of protamine sulphate should be given slowly over about 10 minutes and not exceed 50 mg. If more than 15 minutes have elapsed since the injection of heparin, lower doses of protamine will be necessary.

**Pharmacological properties**
*Pharmacodynamic properties:* Heparin is an anticoagulant and acts by inhibiting thrombin and by potentiating the naturally occurring inhibitors of activated Factor X (Xa).

*Pharmacokinetic properties:* As heparin is not absorbed from the gastrointestinal tract and sublingual sites it is administered by injection. After injection heparin extensively binds to plasma proteins.
    Heparin is metabolised in the liver and the inactive metabolic products are excreted in the urine.
    The half life of heparin is dependent on the dose.

*Preclinical safety data:* There are no pre-clinical data of relevance to the prescriber which are additional to those already included in other sections.

**Pharmaceutical particulars**
*List of excipients:* Chlorocresol 0.15%, Water for Injections BP, Sodium Hydroxide Solution 3M, Hydrochloric Acid 3M.

*Incompatibilities:* Heparin is incompatible with many injectable preparations e.g. some antibiotics, opioid analgesics and antihistamines.

*Shelf life:* 36 months.

*Special precautions for storage:* Multiparin should be stored below 25°C.

*Nature and contents of container:* 5 ml multidose neutral glass (Type I, PhEur) vial. Carton containing 10 vials.

*Instructions for use/handling:* Not applicable.

**Marketing authorisation numbers**
Multiparin 1,000 iu/ml  4543/0218
Multiparin 5,000 iu/ml  4543/0219
Multiparin 25,000 iu/ml 4543/0220

**Date of approval/revision of SPC**  April 1997.

**Legal category**  POM.


# ORLEPT* TABLETS
# ORLEPT* (SF) LIQUID

**Qualitative and quantitative composition**
*Orlept Tablets:* Sodium Valproate BP 200 mg or 500 mg.

*Orlept Liquid:* Sodium Valproate PhEur 200 mg in 5 ml.

**Pharmaceutical form**
*Orlept Tablets:* Enteric coated tablet for oral administration.

*Orlept Liquid:* Oral liquid.

**Clinical particulars**
*Therapeutic indications:* Sodium valproate is used in the treatment of all forms of epilepsy.

*Posology and method of administration:* Dosage requirements vary according to age and body weight and should be adjusted individually to achieve adequate seizure control. The tablets or liquid may be given in divided doses.

*Monotherapy:* Usual requirements are as follows:
*Adults:* Dosage should start at 600 mg daily increasing by 200 mg at three day intervals until control is achieved. This is generally within the dosage range 1,000 mg to 2,000 mg per day i.e. 20–30 mg/kg body weight daily. Where adequate control is not achieved within this range the dose may be further increased to a maximum of 2,500 mg per day.

*Children over 20 kg:* Initial dosage should be 400 mg/day increasing until control is achieved. This is usually within the range 20–30 mg/kg body weight per day.

*Children under 20 kg:* 20 mg/kg of body weight per day; in severe cases this may be increased up to 40 mg/kg/day.

*Use in the elderly:* Care should be taken when adjusting dosage in the elderly since the pharmacokinetics of sodium valproate are modified. Dosage should be determined by seizure control.

*Combined therapy:* In certain cases it may be necessary to raise the dose by 5 to 10 mg/kg/day when used in combination with liver enzyme inducing drugs such as phenytoin, phenobarbitone and carbamazepine.

*Contra-indications:* Liver disease. Hypersensitivity to valproate.

*Special warnings and special precautions for use:* Clinical symptoms are a more sensitive indicator in the early stages of hepatic failure than laboratory investigations. The onset of an acute illness, especially within the first six months, which may include symptoms of vomiting, lethargy or weakness, drowsiness, anorexia, jaundice or loss of seizure control is an indication for immediate withdrawal of the drug.

Patients should be instructed to report any such signs to the clinician should they occur.

Routine measurement of liver function should be undertaken in those at risk before and during the first six months of therapy including children under three years, especially those with mental retardation, organic brain damage or metabolic disorder. The drug should be discontinued if signs of liver damage occur or if serum amylase levels are elevated.

Valproic acid inhibits the second stage of platelet aggregation. If spontaneous bruising or bleeding occurs medication should be withdrawn. It is recommended that patients receiving sodium valproate be monitored for platelet function and clotting time before major surgery.

Withdrawal of sodium valproate or transition to another antiepileptic should be made gradually to avoid precipitation of an increase in seizure frequency.

Sodium valproate may give false positives for ketone bodies in the urine testing of diabetics.

*Interactions with other medicaments and other forms of interaction:* Concomitant use of hepatic enzyme inducers (e.g. barbiturates, carbamazepine, phenytoin) may enhance metabolism of valproic acid, while cimetidine has been reported to decrease clearance. Valproic acid has been reported to have variable effects on blood levels of other hepatically metabolised or highly protein bound agents. Caution is recommended when administering with other drugs affecting clotting (e.g. warfarin, aspirin). Other hepatotoxic drugs should be avoided. Antidepressants and antipsychotics may lower the threshold for convulsions and higher doses of sodium valproate may be needed.

*Pregnancy and lactation:* There is an increased incidence of congenital abnormalities in offspring born to mothers with epilepsy, both untreated and treated.

The benefits of anti-epileptic therapy in pregnancy should be evaluated against the possible risks. There have been reports of foetal abnormalities including neural tube defects in women receiving valproate during the first trimester. This incidence has been estimated to be in the region of 1%. Women should be informed of the possible risk and carefully screened by alpha foetoprotein measurement and ultra sound, and if indicated, amniocentesis.

The concentration of valproate in breast milk is very low, between 1% and 10% of total maternal plasma levels, and at this level appears not to have harmful effects on the nursing child.

*Effects on ability to drive and use machines:* Sodium valproate in appropriate doses may not impair driving skills but driving should be restricted to patients whose seizures are adequately controlled. Administration of the drug may occasionally induce drowsiness.

*Undesirable effects:* Most frequently, gastrointestinal disturbances, particularly on initiation of therapy. Less commonly, increased appetite and weight gain, tremor, drowsiness, ataxia, confusion, headache, reversible prolongation of bleeding time, thrombocytopenia, leucopenia and bone marrow depression have been reported. Occasionally rashes, transient alopecia with regrowth of curly hair. Transient elevation of liver enzyme levels is common and dose related. Liver dysplasia and hepatic failure (rarely fatal) occurs occasionally, usually in the first few months, necessitating withdrawal. Hyperammonaemia without liver failure, hyperglycinaemia and pancreatitis have been reported.

Congenital malformations have been reported in women receiving anti-epileptic agents including sodium valproate during pregnancy.

*Overdose:* Treatment includes induced vomiting, gastric lavage, assisted ventilation and forced diuresis.

**Pharmacological properties**
*Pharmacodynamic properties:* The mode of action of valproic acid in epilepsy is not fully understood but may involve an elevation of gamma-amino butyric acid levels in the brain.

*Pharmacokinetic properties:* Sodium valproate is rapidly and completely absorbed after oral administration; the rate of absorption is delayed by administration as enteric coated tablets.

Sodium valproate is extensively metabolised in the liver, it is excreted in the urine almost entirely in the form of its metabolites.

Sodium valproate is extensively bound to plasma protein. Peak plasma levels are attained 1–4 hours after oral dosing and the half life is of the order of 8–22 hours. Sodium valproate crosses the blood brain barrier and small amounts are excreted in milk. Data

from animal studies indicate that sodium valproate crosses the placenta.

*Preclinical safety data:* There are no additional preclinical data of relevance to the prescriber which have not been included in the main body of the text.

**Pharmaceutical particulars**
*List of excipients:*
*200 mg and 500 mg Tablets:* Microcrystalline Cellulose Anhydrous PhEur, Methylated Colloidal Anhydrous Silica HSE, Enzymatically Hydrolysed Gelatin HSE, Calcium Behenate DAB, Talc PhEur. *Coating:* Methacrylic Acid Copolymer USP, Talc PhEur, Triacetin USP, Titanium Dioxide PhEur, Polyethylene Glycol 6000 PhEur.

*Oral liquid:* Maltilol Solution (Syrup), Nipasept, Cherry Flavour Blank NA D3923, 3M hydrochloride acid, 3M sodium hydroxide, purified water.

*Incompatibilities:* None known.

*Shelf life:*
*Tablets:* 24 months in polypropylene or polyethylene container or glass bottles. 24 months in blister strips of PVC/PVDC and aluminium foil.
*Oral liquid:* 24 months.

*Special precautions for storage:*
*Tablets:* Store below 25°C in a dry place.
*Oral liquid:* Store below 25°C and protect from light.

*Nature and contents of container:*
*Tablets:* Polypropylene or polyethylene containers or glass bottles containing 100 tablets. Blister strips of rigid PVC/PVDC film and aluminium foil of 10 tablets used in multiples of 5, 6 or 10 giving pack sizes of 10, 50, 60 or 100 tablets.
*Oral liquid:* 100 ml opaque HDPE bottles with polypropylene caps. 300 ml, 500 ml and 2,000 ml amber glass bottles with black bakelite screw-on caps.

*Instructions for use/handling:* None.

**Marketing authorisation numbers**
Orlept Tablets 200 mg 4543/0283
Orlept Tablets 500 mg 4543/0284
Orlept (SF) Liquid     4543/0323

**Date of approval/revision of SPC** April 1997.

**Legal category** POM.

# PROSULF*

**Qualitative and quantitative composition** Protamine Sulphate PhEur 50 mg.

**Pharmaceutical form** Solution for injections.

**Clinical particulars**
*Therapeutic indications:* Protamine sulphate is used to counteract the anticoagulant effect of heparin: before surgery; after renal dialysis; after open-heart surgery; if excessive bleeding occurs and when an overdose has inadvertently been given.

*Posology and method of administration:*
*Adults:* Prosulf should be administered by slow intravenous injection over a period of about 10 minutes. No more than 50 mg of protamine sulphate should be given in any one dose.

The dose is dependent on the amount and type of heparin to be neutralised, its route of administration and the time elapsed since it was last given, since heparin is continuously being excreted. Ideally, the dose required to neutralise the action of heparin should be guided by blood coagulation studies or calculated from a protamine neutralisation test.

Patients should be carefully monitored using either the activated partial thromboplastin time or the activated coagulation time, carried out 5–15 minutes after protamine sulphate administration. Further doses may be needed because protamine is cleared from the blood more rapidly than heparin, especially low molecular weight heparin.

In gross excess, protamine itself acts as an anticoagulant.

*Neutralisation of unfractionated (UF) heparins:* 1 mg of protamine sulphate will usually neutralise at least 100 international units of mucous heparin or 80 units of lung heparin. The dose of protamine sulphate should be reduced if more than 15 minutes have elapsed since intravenous injection.

For example, if 30–60 minutes have elapsed since heparin was injected intravenously, 0.5–0.75 mg protamine sulphate per 100 units of mucous heparin is recommended. If two hours or more have elapsed, 0.25–0.375 mg per 100 units of mucous heparin should be administered.

If the patient is receiving an intravenous infusion of heparin, the infusion should be stopped and 25–50 mg of protamine sulphate given by slow intravenous injection.

If heparin was administered subcutaneously, 1 mg protamine sulphate should be given per 100 units of mucous heparin – 25–50 mg by slow intravenous injection and the balance by intravenous infusion over 8–16 hours.

In the reversal of UF heparin following cardiopulmonary bypass, either a standard dose of protamine may be given, as above, or the dose may be titrated according to the activated clotting time.

*Neutralisation of low molecular weight (LMW) heparins:* A dose of 1 mg per 100 units is usually recommended but the manufacturer's own guidelines should be consulted.

The anti-Xa activity of LMW heparins may not be completely reversible with protamine sulphate and may persist for up to 24 hours after administration.

The longer half-life of LMW heparins (approximately twice that of UF heparin) should also be borne in mind when estimating the dose of protamine sulphate required in relation to the time which has elapsed since the last heparin dose.

Theoretically, the dose of protamine sulphate should be halved when one half-life has elapsed since the last LMW heparin dose. Intermittent injections or continuous infusion of protamine sulphate have been recommended for the neutralisation of LMW heparin following subcutaneous administration, as there may be continuing absorption from the subcutaneous depot.

*Elderly:* There is no current evidence for alteration of the recommended dose.

*Children:* Safety and efficacy in children have not been established. Not recommended.

*Contra-indications:* None known.

*Special warnings and special precautions for use:* Too rapid administration of protamine sulphate may cause severe hypotension and anaphylactoid reactions. Facilities for resuscitation and treatment of shock should be available.

Protamine sulphate is not suitable for reversing the effects of oral anticoagulants. Caution should be observed when administering protamine sulphate to patients who may be at increased risk of allergic reaction to protamine. These patients include those who have previously undergone procedures such as coronary angioplasty or cardio-pulmonary by-pass which may include use of protamine, diabetics who have been treated with protamine insulin, patients allergic to fish and men who have had a vasectomy or are infertile and may have antibodies to protamine.

Patients undergoing prolonged procedures involving repeated doses of protamine should be subject to careful monitoring of clotting parameters. A rebound bleeding effect may occur up to 18 hours postoperatively which responds to further doses of protamine.

*Interaction with other medicaments and other forms of interaction:* None known.

*Pregnancy and lactation:* As with most drugs, to be used only if clearly indicated in pregnancy and with caution during lactation.

*Effects on ability to drive and use machines:* None.

*Undesirable effects:* When used at doses in excess of that required to neutralise the anticoagulant effect of heparin, protamine sulphate exerts its own anticoagulant effect. Following injection of protamine sulphate the following effects have been observed; a sudden fall in blood pressure, bradycardia, pulmonary and systemic hypertension, dyspnoea, transitory flushing and a feeling of warmth, back pain, nausea and vomiting, lassitude. Hypersensitivity reactions and fatal anaphylaxis have been reported.

*Overdose: Symptoms:* Overdosage may cause hypotension, bradycardia and dyspnoea with a sensation of warmth, nausea, vomiting, lassitude and transitory flushing.

*Treatment:* Includes monitoring of coagulation tests, respiratory ventilation and symptomatic treatment. If bleeding is a problem, fresh frozen plasma or fresh whole blood should be given.

**Pharmacological properties**
*Pharmacodynamic properties:* Although protamine is a potent antidote for heparin, its precise mechanism of action is unknown. However, when the strongly basic protamine combines with the strongly acid heparin, a stable salt is formed lacking in anticoagulant activity. One mg of protamine sulphate neutralises between 80 and 120 units of heparin. However, methods of standardisation and the use of heparin from different sources (mucosal, lung) may produce different responses to protamine.

*Pharmacokinetic properties:* The onset of action of protamine occurs within five minutes following intravenous administration. The fate of the protamine-heparin complex is unknown, but it may be partially degraded, thus freeing heparin.

*Preclinical safety data:* No data are available.

**Pharmaceutical particulars**
*List of excipients:* sodium chloride, hydrochloric acid 3M, sodium hydroxide 3M, water for injections.

*Incompatibilities:* Protamine sulphate is incompatible

with certain antibiotics, including several cephalosporins and penicillin.

*Shelf life:* 48 months in glass ampoules. 24 months in polypropylene ampoules.

*Special precautions for storage:* Store between 15˚C and 25˚C.

*Nature and contents of container:* 5 ml and 10 ml neutral type I hydrolytic glass ampoules in pack sizes of 10 ampoules in cartons. 5 ml polypropylene ampoules.

*Instructions for use/handling:* Not applicable.

### Marketing authorisation numbers
Glass ampoules                4543/0234
Polypropylene ampoules        4543/0359

**Date of approval/revision of SPC**   July 1997.

**Legal category**  POM.

## UNIPARIN-Ca*

**Qualitative and quantitative composition**  Heparin Calcium (Mucous) BP 25,000 iu/ml.

**Pharmaceutical form**  Subcutaneous injection.

### Clinical particulars
*Therapeutic indications:* Prophylaxis of deep vein thrombosis and pulmonary embolism. Prophylaxis of mural thrombosis following myocardial infarction.

*Posology and method of administration:*
*Route of administration:* By subcutaneous injection.

*Recommended dosage:*
*Prophylaxis of deep vein thrombosis and pulmonary embolism:*
*Adults:*
2 hours pre-operatively: 5,000 units subcutaneously followed by: 5,000 units subcutaneously every 8–12 hours, for 7–10 days or until the patient is fully ambulant.

No laboratory monitoring should be necessary during low dose heparin prophylaxis. If monitoring is considered desirable, anti-Xa assays should be used as the activated partial thromboplastin time (APTT) is not significantly prolonged.

*During pregnancy:* 5,000–10,000 units every 12 hours, subcutaneously, adjusted according to APTT or anti-Xa assay.

*Elderly:* Dosage reduction and monitoring of APTT may be advisable.

*Children:* No dosage recommendations.

*Prophylaxis of mural thrombosis following myocardial infarction:*
*Adults:* 12,500 units 12 hourly subcutaneously for at least 10 days.

*Elderly:* Dosage reduction may be advised.

*Contra-indications:* Patients who consume large amounts of alcohol, who are sensitive to the drug, who are actively bleeding or who have haemophilia, purpura, severe hypertension, active tuberculosis or increased capillary permeability.

Patients with present or previous thrombocytopenia. The rare occurrence of skin necrosis in patients receiving heparin contra-indicates the further use of heparin either by subcutaneous or intravenous routes because of the risk of thrombocytopenia. Because of the special hazard of post-operative haemorrhage heparin is contra-indicated during surgery of the brain, spinal cord and eye, and in patients undergoing lumbar puncture or regional anaesthetic block.

The relative risks and benefits of heparin should be carefully assessed in patients with a bleeding tendency or those patients with an actual or potential bleeding site, e.g. hiatus hernia, peptic ulcer, neoplasm, bacterial endocarditis, retinopathy, bleeding haemorrhoids, suspected intracranial haemorrhage, cerebral thrombosis or threatened abortion.

Menstruation is not a contra-indication.

*Special warnings and special precautions for use:* Platelet counts should be measured in patients receiving heparin treatment for longer than 5 days and the treatment should be stopped immediately in those who develop thrombocytopenia.

In patients with advanced renal or hepatic disease, a reduction in dosage may be necessary.

Although heparin hypersensitivity is rare, it is advisable to give a trial dose of 1,000 iu in patients with a history of allergy.

In most patients, the recommended low-dose regimen produces no alteration in clotting time. However, patients show an individual response to heparin, and it is therefore essential that the effect of therapy on coagulation time should be monitored in patients undergoing major surgery.

*Interactions with other medicaments and other forms of interaction:* Drugs that interfere with platelet aggregation e.g. aspirin, dextran solutions, dipyridamole or any other drug which may interfere with coagulation, should be used with care.

*Pregnancy and lactation:* Heparin is not contra-indicated in pregnancy. Heparin does not cross the placenta or appear in breast milk. The decision to use heparin in pregnancy should be taken after evaluation of the risk/benefit in any particular circumstances.

*Effects on ability to drive and use machines:* None stated.

*Undesirable effects:* Haemorrhage (see *Overdose*). Thrombocytopenia has been observed occasionally (see *Warnings*). There is some evidence that prolonged dosing with heparin (i.e. over many months) may cause alopecia and osteoporosis. Significant bone demineralisation has been reported in women taking more than 10,000 iu per day of heparin for at least 6 months.

Hypersensitivity reactions, local irritations and skin necrosis may occur but are rare.

*Overdose:* A potential hazard of heparin therapy is haemorrhage, but this is usually due to overdosage and the risk is minimised by strict laboratory control. Slight haemorrhage can usually be treated by withdrawing the drug. If bleeding is more severe, clotting time and platelet count should be determined. Prolonged clotting time will indicate the presence of an excessive anticoagulant effect requiring neutralisation by intravenous protamine sulphate, at a dosage of 1 mg for every 100 iu of heparin to be neutralised. The bolus dose of protamine sulphate should be given slowly over about 10 minutes and not exceed 50 mg. If more than 15 minutes have elapsed since the injection of heparin, lower doses of protamine will be necessary.

### Pharmacological properties
*Pharmacodynamic properties:* Heparin is an anticoagulant and acts by inhibiting thrombin and by potentiating the naturally occurring inhibitors of activated Factor X (Xa).

*Pharmacokinetic properties:* As heparin is not absorbed from the gastrointestinal tract and sublingual sites it is administered by injection. After injection heparin extensively binds to plasma proteins.

Heparin is metabolised in the liver and the inactive metabolic products are excreted in the urine.

The half life of heparin is dependent on the dose.

*Preclinical safety data:* There are no pre-clinical data of relevance to the prescriber which are additional to those already included in other sections.

### Pharmaceutical particulars
*List of excipients:* Water for Injections BP, Calcium Hydroxide Solution 3M, Hydrochloric Acid 3M.

*Incompatibilities:* Heparin is incompatible with many injectable preparations e.g. some antibiotics, opioid analgesics and antihistamines.

*Shelf life:* 36 months.

*Special precautions for storage:* Uniparin-Ca should be stored below 25˚C and protected from light.

Other preparations should not be mixed with Uniparin-Ca in the disposable syringe.

*Nature and contents of container:* 0.5 ml Becton Dickenson Hypak disposable syringes containing 0.2 ml or 0.5 ml of solution. Cartons contain 10, 15 or 50 syringes.

*Instructions for use/handling:* Not applicable.

**Marketing authorisation number**  4543/0207

**Date of approval/revision of SPC**   July 1996.

**Legal category**  POM.

## UNIPARIN FORTE*

**Qualitative and quantitative composition**  Heparin Sodium (Mucous) 10,000 iu 0.4 ml.

**Pharmaceutical form**  Subcutaneous injection.

### Clinical particulars
*Therapeutic indications:* Prophylaxis of deep vein thrombosis and pulmonary embolism. Prophylaxis of mural thrombosis following myocardial infarction.

*Posology and method of administration:*
*Route of administration:* By subcutaneous injection.

*Recommended dosage:*
*Prophylaxis of deep vein thrombosis and pulmonary embolism:*
*Adults:*
2 hours pre-operatively: 5,000 units subcutaneously followed by: 5,000 units subcutaneously every 8–12 hours, for 7–10 days or until the patient is fully ambulant.

No laboratory monitoring should be necessary during low dose heparin prophylaxis. If monitoring is considered desirable, anti-Xa assays should be used as the activated partial thromboplastin time (APTT) is not significantly prolonged.

*During pregnancy:* 5,000–10,000 units every 12 hours, subcutaneously, adjusted according to APTT or anti-Xa assay.

*Elderly:* Dosage reduction and monitoring of APTT may be advisable.

*Children:* No dosage recommendations.

*Prophylaxis of mural thrombosis following myocardial infarction:*
*Adults:* 12,500 units 12 hourly subcutaneously for at least 10 days.

*Elderly:* Dosage reduction may be advised.

*Contra-indications:* Patients who consume large amounts of alcohol, who are sensitive to heparin, who are actively bleeding or who have haemophilia, purpura, severe hypertension, active tuberculosis or increased capillary permeability.

Patients with present or previous thrombocytopenia. The rare occurrence of skin necrosis in patients receiving heparin contra-indicates the further use of heparin either by subcutaneous or systemic routes because of the risk of thrombocytopenia.

The relative risks and benefits of heparin should be carefully assessed in patients with a bleeding tendency or those patients with an actual or potential bleeding site e.g. hiatus hernia, ulcerative lesions of the gastrointestinal tract, neoplasm, bacterial endocarditis, retinopathy, bleeding haemorrhoids, suspected intracranial haemorrhage, cerebral thrombosis or threatened abortion.

Heparin should be withheld during surgery of the brain, spinal cord and eye, and should not be administered to patients undergoing lumbar puncture or regional anaesthetic block.

*Special warnings and special precautions for use:* In patients with advanced renal or hepatic disease, a reduction in dosage may be necessary.

Although heparin hypersensitivity is rare, it is advisable to give a trial dose of 1,000 iu in patients with a history of allergy.

In most patients, the recommended low-dose regimen produces no alteration in clotting time. However, patients show an individual response to heparin, and it is therefore essential that the effect of therapy on coagulation time should be monitored in patients undergoing major surgery. Drugs that interfere with platelet aggregation e.g. aspirin, dextran solutions, should be used with care.

*Interactions with other medicaments and other forms of interaction:* Drugs that interfere with platelet aggregation e.g. aspirin, dextran solutions, dipyridamole, should be used with care.

*Pregnancy and lactation:* Neither pregnancy nor menstruation is contra-indicated. Heparin does not cross the placenta or appear in breast milk.

*Effects on ability to drive and use machines:* None stated.

*Undesirable effects:* Haemorrhage (see *Overdose*). Thrombocytopenia has been observed occasionally.

There is some evidence that prolonged dosing with heparin (i.e. over many months) may cause alopecia and osteoporosis. Significant bone demineralisation has been reported in women taking more than 10,000 iu per day of heparin for at least 6 months.

Hypersensitivity reactions may occur but are rare.

*Overdose:* Symptoms: A potential hazard of heparin therapy especially associated with overdose is haemorrhage, though the risk is minimised by strict laboratory control.

Treatment: Slight haemorrhage can usually be treated by withdrawing the drug. If bleeding is more severe, clotting time and platelet count should be determined. Prolonged clotting time will indicate the presence of an overly anticoagulant effect requiring neutralisation by intravenous protamine sulphate, at a dosage of 1 mg for every 100 iu of heparin to be neutralised. The bolus dose of protamine sulphate should be given slowly over about 10 minutes and not exceed 50 mg. If more than 15 minutes have elapsed since the injection of heparin, lower doses of protamine will be necessary.

### Pharmacological properties
*Pharmacodynamic properties:* Heparin is an anticoagulant and acts by inhibiting thrombin and by potentiating the naturally occurring inhibitors of activated Factor X (Xa).

*Pharmacokinetic properties:* As heparin is not absorbed from the gastrointestinal tract and sublingual sites it is administered by injection. After injection heparin extensively binds to plasma proteins.

Heparin is metabolised in the liver and the inactive metabolic products are excreted in the urine.

The half life of heparin is dependent on the dose.

*Preclinical safety data:* There are no pre-clinical data of relevance to the prescriber which are additional to those already included in other sections.

### Pharmaceutical particulars
*List of excipients:* Water for Injections PhEur, Sodium Hydroxide Solution 3M, Hydrochloric Acid 3M.

*Incompatibilities:* Heparin is incompatible with many injectable preparations.

*Shelf life:* 36 months.

*Special precautions for storage:* Store in a cool place (below 25°C). Do not freeze. Protect from light.

*Nature and contents of container:* 0.5 ml Becton Dickenson Hypak disposable syringes containing 0.4 ml of solution. Cartons contain 10 or 50 syringes.

*Instructions for use/handling:* Not applicable.

**Marketing authorisation number** 4543/0230

**Date of approval/revision of SPC** July 1997.

**Legal category** POM.

*Trade Mark

# Delandale Laboratories Limited
Foundation Park
Roxborough Way
Maidenhead, Berkshire, SL6 3UD

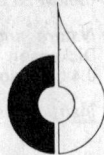

## DOLMATIL* 200 mg TABLETS
## DOLMATIL* 400 mg TABLETS

### Qualitative and quantitative composition
*Dolmatil 200 mg Tablets:* Active ingredient is sulpiride 200 mg. Sulpiride is a benzamide derivative.

*Dolmatil 400 mg Tablets:* Active ingredient is sulpiride 400 mg. Sulpiride is a benzamide derivative.

### Pharmaceutical form
*Dolmatil 200 mg Tablets:* Plain white round tablet with a transverse breakline on one side and D200 on the other.

*Dolmatil 400 mg Tablets:* White film coated stick shaped tablet with break bar engraved SLP 400 on one side.

### Clinical particulars
*Therapeutic indications:* Acute and chronic schizophrenia.

*Posology and method of administration:*

*Adults:* A starting dose of 400 mg to 800 mg daily, given in two divided doses (morning and early evening) is recommended.

Predominantly positive symptoms (formal thought disorder, hallucinations, delusions, incongruity of affect) respond to higher doses, and a starting dose of at least 400 mg twice daily is recommended, increasing if necessary up to a suggested maximum of 1200 mg twice daily. Increasing the dose beyond this level has not been shown to produce further improvement. Predominantly negative symptoms (flattening of affect, poverty of speech, anergia, apathy), as well as depression, respond to doses below 800 mg daily; therefore, a starting dose of 400 mg twice daily is recommended. Reducing this dose towards 200 mg twice daily will normally increase the alerting effect of Dolmatil.

Patients with mixed positive and negative symptoms, with neither predominating, will normally respond to dosage of 400–600 mg twice daily.

*Children:* Clinical experience in children under 14 years of age is insufficient to permit specific recommendations.

*Elderly:* The same dose ranges may be required in the elderly, but should be reduced if there is evidence of renal impairment.

*Contra-indications:* Phaeochromocytoma and acute porphyria. There are no cardiovascular contra-indications.

*Special warnings and special precautions for use:* Increased motor agitation has been reported at high dosage in a small number of patients: in aggressive, agitated or excited phases of the disease process, low doses of Dolmatil may aggravate symptoms. Care should be exercised where hypomania is present.

Extrapyramidal reactions, principally akathisia have been reported in a small number of cases. If warranted, reduction in dosage of anti-parkinsonian medication may be necessary.

As with all neuroleptic drugs, the presence of unexplained hyperthermia could indicate the neuroleptic malignant syndrome (NMS). In this event Dolmatil and any associated neuroleptic treatment should be discontinued until the origin of the fever has been determined.

Hepatic reactions have been reported. Although Dolmatil only induces slight EEG modifications, caution is advised in prescribing it for patients with unstable epilepsy. Patients requiring Dolmatil who are receiving anti-convulsant therapy should continue unchanged on the latter medication. Cases of convulsions, sometimes in patients with no previous history, have been reported. Dolmatil has no significant anticholinergic or cardiovascular activity. As with all drugs for which the kidney is the major elimination pathway, the usual precautions should be taken in cases of renal failure.

*Interaction with other medicaments and other forms of interaction:* While no drug interactions are known, unnecessary polypharmacy should be avoided. As with other psychotropic compounds, sulpiride may increase the effect of antihypertensives and CNS depressants or stimulants.

*Pregnancy and lactation:* Despite the negative results of teratogenicity studies in animals and the lack of teratogenic effects during widespread clinical use in other countries, Dolmatil should not be considered an exception to the general principle of avoiding drug treatment during pregnancy, particularly during the first 16 weeks, with potential benefits being weighed against possible hazards.

*Effects on ability to drive and operate machines:* None stated.

*Undesirable effects:* Dolmatil is very well tolerated and usually only minor side-effects occur, if at all, at the recommended doses.

After over a decade of widespread use in many countries, tardive dyskinesia has occurred rarely. Insomnia has been reported.

Many medicines, including neuroleptics, raise serum prolactin levels, which may be associated with galactorrhoea and amenorrhoea, and less frequently with gynaecomastia. In long-term animal studies with neuroleptic drugs, including sulpiride, an increased incidence of various endocrine tumours (some of which have occasionally been malignant) has been seen in some but not all strains of rats and mice studied. The significance of these findings to man is not known; there is no current evidence of any association between neuroleptic use and tumour risk in man. However, when prescribing neuroleptics to patients with existing mammary neoplasia or a history of this disease, possible risks should be weighed against benefits of therapy.

*Overdose:* The range of single toxic doses is 1 to 16 g but no death has occurred even at the 16 g dose.

The clinical manifestations of poisoning vary depending upon the size of the dose taken. After single doses of 1 to 3 g restlessness and clouding of consciousness have been reported and (rarely) extrapyramidal symptoms. Doses of 3 to 7 g may produce a degree of agitation, confusion and extrapyramidal symptoms; more than 7g can cause, in addition, coma and low blood pressure.

The duration of intoxication is generally short, the symptoms disappearing within a few hours. Comas which have occurred after large doses have lasted up to four days. There are no specific complications from overdose. In particular no haematological or hepatic toxicity has been reported.

Overdose may be treated with alkaline osmotic diuresis and, if necessary, anti-parkinsonian drugs. Coma needs appropriate nursing. Emetic drugs are unlikely to be effective in Dolmatil overdosage.

### Pharmacological properties
*Pharmacodynamic properties:* One of the characteristics of Dolmatil is its bimodal activity, as it has both antidepressant and neuroleptic properties. Schizophrenia characterised by a lack of social contact can benefit strikingly. Mood elevation is observed after a few days treatment, followed by disappearance of the florid schizophrenic symptoms. The sedation and lack of effect characteristically associated with classical neuroleptics of the phenothiazine or butyrophenone type are not features of Dolmatil therapy.

Dolmatil is a member of the group of substituted benzamides, which are structurally distinct from the phenothiazines, butyrophenones and thioxanthenes. Current evidence suggests that the actions of Dolmatil hint at an important distinction between different types of dopamine receptors or receptor mechanisms in the brain.

Behaviourally and biochemically, Dolmatil shares with these classical neuroleptics a number of properties indicative of cerebral dopamine receptor antagonism. Essential and intriguing differences include lack of catalepsy at doses active in other behavioural tests, lack of effect in the dopamine sensitive adenylate cyclase systems, lack of effect upon noradrenaline or 5HT turnover, negligible anticholinesterase activity, no effect on muscarinic or GABA receptor binding, and a radical difference in the binding of tritiated sulpiride to striatal preparations in-vitro, compared to $^3$H-spiperone or $^3$H-haloperidol. These findings indicate a major differentiation between Dolmatil and classical neuroleptics which lack such specificity.

*Pharmacokinetic properties:* Peak sulpiride serum levels are reached 3–6 hours after an oral dose. The plasma half-life in man is approximately 8 hours. Approximately 40% sulpiride is bound to plasma proteins. 95% of the compound is excreted in the urine and faeces as unchanged sulpiride.

*Preclinical safety data:* No further information is available.

### Pharmaceutical particulars
*List of excipients:* Starch, lactose, methylcellulose, magnesium stearate, talc, silica.

*Incompatibilities:* None known.

*Shelf life:* 5 years.

*Special precautions for storage:* Store at or below 25°C.

*Nature and contents of container:* Cartons containing 100 tablets in blister strips.

*Product licence holder:* Delagrange Ltd, Foundation Park, Roxborough Way, Maidenhead SL6 3UD.

**Marketing authorisation number** 5299/0006.

**Date of approval/revision of SPC** 15 January 1997.

**Legal category** POM.

## PRIADEL*
## PRIADEL* 200

**Qualitative and quantitative composition** Priadel tablets contain 400 mg lithium carbonate. Priadel 200 tablets contain 200 mg lithium carbonate.

### Pharmaceutical form
*Priadel:* White, circular, bi-convex tablets engraved PRIADEL on one side, scored on the other side, in a controlled release formulation.

*Priadel 200:* White, scored, capsule-shaped tablets engraved P200 on one side, in a controlled release formulation.

### Clinical particulars
*Therapeutic indications:*
1. In the management of acute mania or hypomanic episodes.
2. In the management of episodes of recurrent depressive disorders where treatment with other antidepressants has been unsuccessful.
3. In the prophylaxis against bipolar affective disorders.
4. Control of aggressive behaviour or intentional self harm.

*Posology and method of administration:* A simple treatment schedule has been evolved which except for some minor variations should be followed whether using Priadel therapeutically or prophylactically. The minor variations to this schedule depend on the elements of the illness being treated and these are described later.

1. In patients of average weight (70 kg) an initial dose of 400–1,200 mg of Priadel may be given as a single daily dose in the morning or on retiring. Alternatively, the dose may be divided and given morning and evening. The tablets should not be crushed or chewed. When changing between lithium preparations serum lithium levels should first be checked, then Priadel therapy commenced at a daily dose as close as possible to the dose of the other form of lithium. As bioavailability varies from product to product (particularly with regard to retard or slow release preparations) a change of product should be regarded as initiation of new treatment.

2. Four to five days after starting treatment (and never longer than one week) a blood sample should be taken for the estimation of serum lithium level.

3. The objective is to adjust the Priadel dose so as to maintain the serum lithium level permanently within the diurnal range of 0.5–1.5 mmol/l. In practice, the blood sample should be taken between 12 and 24 hours after the previous dose of Priadel. 'Target' serum lithium concentrations at 12 and 24 hours are shown in the table below.

|  | 'Target' serum lithium concentrations (mmol/l) | |
| --- | --- | --- |
|  | At 12 hours | At 24 hours |
| Once daily dosage | 0.7–1.0 | 0.5–0.8 |
| Twice daily dosage | 0.5–0.8 |  |

Both strengths have breaklines, therefore they can be divided accurately to provide dosage requirements as small as 100 mg. Serum lithium levels should be monitored weekly until stabilisation is achieved.

4. Lithium therapy should not be initiated unless adequate facilities for routine monitoring of serum concentrations are available. Following stabilisation of serum lithium levels, the period between subsequent estimations can be increased gradually but should not normally exceed three months. Additional measurements should be made following alteration of dosage, on development of intercurrent disease, signs of manic or depressive relapse, following significant change in sodium or fluid intake, or if signs of lithium toxicity occur.

5. Whilst a high proportion of acutely ill patients may respond within three to seven days of the commencement of Priadel therapy, Priadel should be continued through any recurrence of the affective disturbance. This is important as the full prophylactic effect may not occur for 6 to 12 months after the initiation of therapy.

6. In patients who show a positive response to Priadel therapy, treatment is likely to be long term. Careful clinical appraisal of the patient should be exercised throughout medication (see *Precautions*).

*Prophylactic treatment of bipolar affective disorders and control of aggressive behaviour or intentional self harm:* It is recommended that the described treatment schedule is followed.

*Treatment of acute manic or hypomanic episodes and recurrent depressive disorders:* It is likely that a higher than normal Priadel intake may be necessary during an acute phase and divided doses would be required here. Therefore as soon as control of mania or depression is achieved, the serum lithium level should be determined and it may be necessary, dependent on the results, to lower the dose of Priadel and re-stabilise serum lithium levels. In all other details the described treatment schedule is recommended.

*Elderly:* In elderly patients or those below 50 kg in weight, it is recommended that the starting dose is 400 mg. Elderly patients may be more sensitive to undesirable effects of lithium and also may require lower doses in order to maintain therapeutic serum lithium levels. It follows therefore that long-term patients often require a reduction in dosage over a period of years.

*Children and adolescents:* Not recommended.

*Contra-indications:* Cardiac failure. Clinically significant renal impairment. Addison's disease. Untreated hypothyroidism.

*Special warnings and precautions for use:* When considering Priadel therapy, it is necessary to ascertain whether patients are receiving lithium in any other form. If so, check serum levels before proceeding. It is important to ensure that renal function is normal – if necessary a creatinine clearance test or other renal function test should be performed. Cardiac and thyroid function should be assessed before commencing lithium treatment. Patients should be euthyroid before the initiation of lithium therapy. Renal function, cardiac function and thyroid function should be re-assessed periodically.

Clear instructions regarding the symptoms of impending toxicity should be given by the doctor to all patients receiving long term lithium therapy (see toxic effects). Patients should also be warned to report if polyuria or polydipsia develop. Episodes of nausea and vomiting or other conditions leading to salt/water depletion (including severe dieting) should also be reported.

Elderly patients are particularly liable to lithium toxicity.

Caution should be exercised to ensure that diet and fluid intake are normal thus maintaining a stable electrolyte balance. This may be of special importance in very hot weather or work environment. Infectious diseases including colds, influenza, gastroenteritis and urinary infections may also alter fluid balance and thus affect serum lithium levels. Treatment should be discontinued during any intercurrent infection and should only be reinstituted after the patient's physical health has returned to normal.

*Interactions with other medicaments and other forms of interaction:* Concurrent use of lithium and diuretics may cause reduced lithium clearance, leading to intoxication. If a diuretic has to be prescribed for a lithium patient, the lithium dosage should first be lowered and the patient re-stabilised with frequent monitoring. Similar precautions should be exercised on diuretic withdrawal. Other drugs affecting electrolyte balance, e.g. steroids, may alter lithium excretion and should be avoided in patients on lithium. If other psychotropic drugs are used they should be initiated at a lower dosage than usual, as their side effects may be potentiated by the use of lithium. This has been shown to be of particular importance for the concurrent use of lithium and haloperidol or flupenthixol.

Concomitant use with NSAIDs can increase serum lithium concentrations, possibly resulting in lithium toxicity. Serum lithium concentrations should be monitored more frequently if NSAID therapy is initiated or discontinued.

There have been isolated reports of possible interactions between lithium and diazepam (resulting in hypothermia), methyldopa, tetracyclines, phenytoin, carbamazepine, indomethacin and other prostaglandin-synthetase inhibitors.

*Pregnancy and lactation:* Lithium should not be used during pregnancy since there is evidence that the drug may harm the foetus. Because lithium is secreted into breast milk, it is recommended that breast-feeding be discontinued during use.

Should the use of lithium be unavoidable, close monitoring of serum concentrations should be made during pregnancy and parturition.

Babies may show signs of lithium toxicity necessitating fluid therapy in the neonatal period. Babies born with low serum lithium concentrations may have a flaccid appearance which returns to normal without any treatment. Lithium is secreted in breast milk, therefore bottle feeding is recommended.

*Effects on ability to drive and use machines:* None.

*Undesirable effects:* Side-effects are less common in patients with plasma lithium concentrations below 1.0 mmol/l. Mild gastrointestinal effects, nausea, vertigo, muscle weakness and a dazed feeling may occur initially, but frequently disappear after stabilisation. Fine hand tremors, polyuria and mild thirst may persist. Weight gain or oedema may present in some patients but should not be treated with diuretics.

Hypercalcaemia, hypermagnesaemia and hyperparathyroidism have been reported. Skin conditions including acne, psoriasis, generalised pustular psoriasis, rashes and leg ulcers have occasionally been reported as being aggravated by lithium treatment.

Long term treatment with lithium may be associated with disturbances of thyroid function, including goitre, hypothyroidism and thyrotoxicosis. Lithium-induced hypothyroidism may be managed successfully with concurrent thyroxine.

Memory impairment may occur during long term use.

*Nephrotoxicity:* Up to one third of patients on lithium may develop polyuria with a urinary output of up to three litres per day. This is usually due to lithium blocking the effect of ADH and is reversible on lithium withdrawal. However, long term treatment with lithium may also result in permanent changes in kidney histology and impairment of renal function. High serum concentrations of lithium including episodes of acute lithium toxicity may aggravate these changes. The minimum clinically effective dose of lithium should always be used. In patients who develop polyuria or polydipsia, renal function should be monitored, e.g. with measurement of blood urea, serum creatinine and urinary protein levels in addition to the routine serum lithium estimations.

After a period lasting 3–5 years, patients should be carefully assessed to ensure that benefit persists.

*Toxic effects:* Such effects are indicative of impending lithium intoxication and fall into two groups:

1. Gastro-intestinal: increasing anorexia, diarrhoea and vomiting.

2. Central nervous system: muscle weakness, lack of co-ordination, drowsiness or lethargy progressing to giddiness with ataxia, tinnitus, blurred vision, dysarthria, coarse tremor and muscle twitching.

At blood levels above 2–3 mmol/l there may be a large output of dilute urine, with increasing disorientation, seizures, coma and death.

Patients should be instructed to stop taking their tablets if toxic symptoms appear and to report immediately for a serum lithium estimation.

*Overdose:* There is no specific antidote to lithium poisoning. In the event of accumulation, lithium should be stopped and serum estimation should be carried out every 6 hours.

Under no circumstances should a diuretic be used. Osmotic diuresis (mannitol or urea infusion) or alkalinisation of the urine (sodium lactate or sodium bicarbonate infusion) should be initiated. If the serum lithium level is over 4.0 mmol/l, if there is a deterioration in the patient's condition, or if the serum lithium concentration is not falling at a rate corresponding to a half-life of under 30 hours, peritoneal or haemodialysis should be instituted promptly. This should be continued until there is no lithium in the serum or dialysis fluid. Serum lithium levels should be monitored for at least a further week to take account of any possible rebound in serum lithium levels as a result of delayed diffusion from body tissues.

**Pharmacological properties** The mode of action of lithium is still not fully understood. However, lithium modifies the production and turnover of certain neurotransmitters, particularly serotonin, and it may also block dopamine receptors.

It modifies concentrations of some electrolytes, particularly calcium and magnesium, and it may reduce thyroid activity.

*Pharmacokinetic properties:* Lithium has a half life of about 24 hours although this increases to about 36 hours in the elderly due to a progressive decrease in renal lithium clearance with age. Lithium is 95% eliminated in the urine. Time to peak serum level for controlled release Priadel tablets is about 2 hours and approximately 90% bioavailability would be expected.

*Preclinical safety data:* Nothing of therapeutic relevance.

**Pharmaceutical particulars**

*List of excipients:* Priadel and Priadel 200 contain precirol, mannitol, acacia powder, sodium lauryl sulphate, magnesium stearate, maize starch and primojel. In addition Priadel 200 may contain imwitor.

*Incompatibilities:* None stated.

*Shelf life:* Three years.

*Special precautions for storage:* Store in a cool, dry place.

*Nature and contents of container:* Pack sizes:

*Priadel:* Securitainers 1,000, 100 and 50. Blister packs 100. Hospital packs 100.

*Priadel 200:* Securitainers 500, 100. Blister packs 100.

*Instructions for use/handling:* Not applicable.

**Marketing authorisation numbers**
Priadel          0357/5000R
Priadel 200      0357/0028

**Date of approval/revision of SPC** March 1996.

**Legal category** POM.

## PRIADEL* LIQUID

**Presentation** A clear, colourless pineapple flavoured sugar free syrup containing 520 mg lithium citrate (equivalent to 200 mg lithium carbonate) per 5 ml.

**Uses**
1. Treatment of mania and hypomania.
2. Lithium may also be tried in the treatment of some patients with recurrent bipolar depression, where treatment with other antidepressants has been unsuccessful.
3. Prophylactic treatment of recurrent affective disorders.
4. Control of aggressive or self-mutilating behaviour.

**Dosage and administration** A simple treatment schedule has been evolved which except for some minor variations should be followed whether using Priadel Liquid therapeutically or prophylactically. The minor variations to this schedule depend on the elements of the illness being treated and these are described later.

1. In patients of average weight (70 kg) an initial total daily dose of 10–30 ml of Priadel Liquid (equivalent to 400–1200 mg lithium carbonate) should be given in divided doses, ideally twice a day.

When changing between lithium preparations serum lithium levels should first be checked, then Priadel Liquid therapy commenced at a daily dose as close as possible to that of the other form of lithium. As bioavailability varies from product to product (particularly with regard to slow release preparations) a change of product should be regarded as initiation of new treatment.

2. Four to five days after starting treatment (and never longer than one week) a blood sample should be taken for the estimation of serum lithium level.

3. The objective is to adjust the Priadel Liquid dose so as to maintain the serum lithium level permanently within the diurnal range of 0.5–1.5 mmol/l. In practice, the blood sample should be taken 12 hours after the previous dose of Priadel Liquid. 'Target' serum lithium concentration at 12 hours should be 0.5–0.8 mmol/l.

Priadel Liquid is supplied with a 2.5/5 ml double ended spoon to provide dosage adjustments equivalent to 100 mg and 200 mg lithium carbonate respectively. Serum lithium levels should be monitored weekly until stabilisation is achieved.

4. Lithium therapy should not be initiated unless adequate facilities for routine monitoring of serum concentrations are available. Following stabilisation of serum lithium levels, the period between subsequent estimations can be increased gradually but should not normally exceed three months. Additional measurements should be made following alteration of dosage, on development of intercurrent disease, signs of manic or depressive relapse, following significant change in sodium or fluid intake, or if signs of lithium toxicity occur.

5. Whilst a high proportion of acutely ill patients may respond within three to seven days of the commencement of therapy with Priadel Liquid, it should be continued through any recurrence of the

affective disturbance. This is important as the full prophylactic effect may not occur for 6 to 12 months after the initiation of therapy.

6. In patients who show a positive response to therapy with Priadel Liquid, treatment is likely to be long term. Careful clinical appraisal of the patient should be exercised throughout medication (see Precautions).

*Prophylactic treatment of recurrent affective disorders:* It is recommended that the described treatment schedule is followed.

*Treatment of acute mania, hypomania and recurrent bipolar depression:* It is likely that a higher than normal intake of Priadel Liquid may be necessary during an acute phase. As soon as control of mania or depression is achieved, the serum lithium level should be determined and it may be necessary, dependent on the results, to lower the dose of Priadel Liquid and to restabilise serum lithium levels.

*Use in elderly:* In elderly patients or those below 50 kg in weight, it is recommended that a starting dose of 5 ml (equivalent to 200 mg lithium carbonate) taken twice daily. Elderly patients may be more sensitive to undesirable effects of lithium and also may require lower doses in order to maintain normal serum lithium levels. It follows therefore that long term patients often require a reduction in dosage over a period of years.

*Use in children and adolescents:* Not recommended.

### Contra-indications, warnings, etc

*Contra-indications.* Renal insufficiency, cardiovascular insufficiency, Addison's disease and untreated hypothyroidism are all contra-indications to lithium therapy.

*Use in pregnancy:* There is epidemiological evidence that lithium may be harmful to the foetus in human pregnancy.

| Total no. 'lithium babies' reported | Malformed infants | Ebstein's anomaly and other major cardiovascular malformations |
|---|---|---|
| 225 | 25 (11%) | 18 (8%) |

It is strongly recommended that lithium be discontinued before a planned pregnancy. If it is considered essential to maintain treatment with Priadel Liquid during pregnancy, serum lithium levels should be monitored closely since renal function changes gradually during pregnancy and suddenly at parturition, requiring dosage adjustments. It is recommended that administration of Priadel Liquid be discontinued shortly before delivery and recommenced a few days postpartum.

Babies may show signs of lithium toxicity necessitating fluid therapy in the neonatal period. Babies born with low serum lithium concentrations may have a flaccid appearance which returns to normal without any treatment. Lithium is secreted in breast milk, therefore bottle feeding is recommended.

*Precautions:* When considering therapy with Priadel Liquid, it is necessary to ascertain whether patients are receiving lithium in any other form. If so, check serum levels before proceeding. It is important to ensure that renal function is normal – if necessary a creatinine clearance test or other renal function test should be performed. Cardiac and thyroid function should be assessed before commencing lithium treatment. Patients should be euthyroid before the initiation of lithium therapy. Renal function, cardiac function and thyroid function should be reassessed periodically.

Clear instructions regarding the symptoms of impending toxicity should be given by the doctor to all patients receiving long term lithium therapy (see Toxic effects). Patients should also be warned to report if polyuria or polydipsia develop. Episodes of nausea and vomiting or other conditions leading to salt/water depletion (including severe dieting) should also be reported. Elderly patients are particularly liable to lithium toxicity.

Caution should be exercised to ensure that diet and fluid intake are normal thus maintaining a stable electrolyte balance. This may be of special importance in very hot weather or work environment. Infectious diseases including colds, influenza, gastroenteritis and urinary infections may alter fluid balance and thus affect serum lithium levels. Treatment should be discontinued during any intercurrent infection and should only be reinstituted after the patient's physical health has returned to normal.

*Drug interactions:* Concurrent use of lithium and diuretics may result in reduced lithium clearance, leading to intoxication. If a diuretic has to be prescribed for a lithium patient, the lithium dosage should first be lowered and the patient restabilised with frequent monitoring. Similar precautions should be exercised on diuretic withdrawal. Other drugs affecting electrolyte balance e.g. steroids, may alter lithium excretion and should be avoided in patients on lithium. If other psychotropic drugs are used they should be initiated at a lower dosage than usual, as their side effects may be potentiated by the use of lithium. This has been shown to be of particular importance for the concurrent use of lithium and haloperidol or flupenthixol.

Concomitant use with NSAIDs can increase serum lithium concentrations, possibly resulting in lithium toxicity. Serum lithium concentrations should be monitored more frequently if NSAID therapy is initiated or discontinued.

There have been isolated reports of possible interactions between lithium and diazepam (resulting in hypothermia), methyldopa, tetracyclines, phenytoin, carbamazepine, indomethacin and other prostaglandinsynthetase inhibitors.

### Warnings and adverse effects

*Side effects:* Side effects are usually related to serum lithium concentrations and are infrequent at levels below 1.0 mmol/l.

Mild gastrointestinal effects, nausea, vertigo, muscle weakness and a dazed feeling may occur initially, but frequently disappear after stabilisation. Fine hand tremors, polyuria and mild thirst may persist. Weight gain or oedema may present in some patients but should not be treated with diuretics.

Hypercalcaemia, hypermagnesaemia and hyperparathyroidism have been reported. Skin conditions including acne, psoriasis, generalised pustular psoriasis, rashes and leg ulcers have occasionally been reported as being aggravated by lithium treatment.

Long term treatment with lithium may be associated with disturbances of thyroid function, including goitre, hypothyroidism and thyrotoxicosis. Lithium-induced hypothyroidism may be managed successfully with concurrent thyroxine.

Memory impairment may occur during long term use.

*Nephrotoxicity:* Up to one third of patients on lithium may develop polyuria with a urinary output of up to three litres per day. This is usually due to lithium blocking the effect of ADH and is reversible on lithium withdrawal. However, long term treatment with lithium may also result in permanent changes in kidney histology and impairment of renal function. High serum concentrations of lithium including episodes of acute lithium toxicity may aggravate these changes. The minimum clinically effective dose of lithium should always be used. In patients who develop polyuria or polydipsia, renal function should be monitored, e.g. with measurement of blood urea, serum creatinine and urinary protein levels in addition to the routine serum lithium estimations.

After a period lasting 3–5 years, patients should be carefully assessed to ensure that benefit persists.

*Toxic effects:* Such effects are indicative of impending lithium intoxication and fall into two groups:

(a) Gastrointestinal: increasing anorexia, diarrhoea and vomiting.

(b) Central nervous system: muscle weakness, lack of coordination, drowsiness or lethargy progressing to giddiness with ataxia, tinnitus, blurred vision, dysarthria, coarse tremor and muscle twitching.

At blood levels above 2–3 mmol/l there may be a large output of dilute urine, with increasing disorientation, seizures, coma and death.

Patients should be instructed to stop taking their Priadel Liquid if toxic symptoms appear and to report immediately for a serum lithium estimation.

*Lithium intoxication:* There is no specific antidote to lithium poisoning. In the event of accumulation, lithium should be stopped and serum estimations should be carried out every six hours.

Under no circumstances should a diuretic be used. Osmotic diuresis (mannitol or urea infusion) or alkalinisation of the urine (sodium lactate or sodium bicarbonate infusion) should be initiated.

If the serum lithium level is over 4.0 mmol/l, if there is a deterioration in the patient's condition, or if the serum lithium concentration is not falling at a rate corresponding to a half-life of under 30 hours, peritoneal or haemodialysis should be instituted promptly. This should be continued until there is no lithium in the serum or dialysis fluid. Serum lithium levels should be monitored for at least a further week to take account of any possible rebound in serum lithium levels as a result of delayed diffusion from body tissues.

**Pharmaceutical precautions** Store at or below 25°C. Protect from direct sunlight. Dilution of Priadel Liquid is not recommended.

**Legal category** POM.

**Package quantities** Priadel Liquid is available in bottles of 150 ml.

**Further information** Nil.

**Product licence number** 0357/0032.

*\*Trade Mark*

# Dermal Laboratories Limited
Tatmore Place
Gosmore, Hitchin
Herts, SG4 7QR

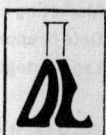

## ANHYDROL* FORTE

**Qualitative and quantitative composition** Aluminium Chloride Hexahydrate 20.0% w/v.

**Pharmaceutical form** Clear, colourless evaporative topical solution.

**Clinical particulars**

*Therapeutic indications:* For the topical treatment of hyperhidrosis specifically involving axillae, hands or feet.

*Posology and method of administration:* For adults, children and the elderly. Apply to the affected sites at night, as required, and allow to dry. Wash off in the morning.

*Contra-indications:* Not to be used in cases of sensitivity to any of the ingredients.

*Special warnings and special precautions in use:* Care should be taken to restrict the application to the affected sites only. Keep away from the eyes and mucous membranes. Care should be taken to avoid Anhydrol Forte coming into direct contact with clothing, polished surfaces, jewellery or metal. Replace cap tightly after use. For external use only.

*Interaction with other medicaments and other forms of interaction:* Do not bathe immediately before use and, if the axillae are treated, do not shave or use depilatories on this area within 12 hours before or after use.

*Pregnancy and lactation:* No special precautions.

*Effects on ability to drive and use machines:* None known.

*Undesirable effects:* If applied too frequently, Anhydrol Forte may cause irritation which should be treated with a mild topical hydrocortisone cream.

*Overdose:* See section above (*Undesirable effects*).

**Pharmacological properties**

*Pharmacodynamic properties:* Aluminium chloride is believed to denature the protein content of sweat issuing from eccrine glands, and to combine with the intraductal keratin fibrils, producing a functional closure. The antibacterial action of the aluminium ion also precludes the development of miliaria. Accordingly, there is no secondary inflammation. The intraluminal pressure rises to the point where it acts as a feedback system, shutting off acinar secretion.

The formulation of Anhydrol Forte has been tested in widespread clinical practice, and has been shown to be effective when used in accordance with the recommended instructions.

*Pharmacokinetic properties:* As the active ingredient is applied in an alcoholic solution of low surface tension, it therefore penetrates into the terminal pores of the sweat ducts, when applied, as recommended, to dry skin. The alcohol then evaporates off, leaving the salt deposited in close contact with the lining of the duct. The use of the preparation is restricted to small areas of skin, namely the axillae, hands or feet, to ensure that there are no detrimental effects from widespread obstruction of sweating.

*Preclinical safety data:* No special information.

**Pharmaceutical particulars**

*List of excipients:* IMS BP.

*Incompatibilities:* None known.

*Shelf life:* 36 months.

*Special precautions for storage:* Highly flammable. Store at room temperature (not exceeding 25°C). Store upright and away from flames.

*Nature and contents of container:* 60 ml plastic bottle with roll on applicator and screwcap. This is supplied as an original pack (OP).

*Instructions for use/handling:* Not applicable.

**Marketing authorisation number** 0173/0030.

**Date of approval/revision of SPC** February 1995.

**Legal category** P.

## BETACAP* SCALP APPLICATION

**Presentation** Transparent, slightly gelled emollient scalp application containing 0.1% w/w betamethasone as valerate. The vehicle also contains isopropyl alcohol, which has antiseptic activity.

*Ingredients:* Betamethasone Valerate BP; PEG-7 Glyceryl Cocoate (a water-dispersible derivative of coconut oil); Isopropyl Alcohol BP; Carbomer; Sodium Hydroxide BP; Purified Water BP.

**Uses** For the treatment of dermatoses of the scalp, such as psoriasis and seborrhoeic dermatitis unresponsive to less potent corticosteroids.

**Dosage and administration**
*For adults, including the elderly, and children over the age of six:* Betacap Scalp Application should be applied sparingly to the scalp night and morning until improvement is noticeable. It may then be possible to sustain improvement by applying once a day, or less frequently. For the treatment of seborrhoeic dermatitis in children, this product should not be used for longer than 5 to 7 days.

**Contra-indications, warnings, etc**
*Contra-indications:* Do not use in cases of bacterial, fungal and/or viral infection of the scalp or where there is a known sensitivity to any of the ingredients. Do not use on children under six years old.

*Precautions:* Care must be taken to keep the preparation away from the eyes. As it is highly flammable, do not use the product near a fire or naked flame. Allow treated scalp to dry naturally.

Continuous long-term treatment should be avoided, particularly in children, as systemic side-effects can occur even without occlusion.

Complications sometimes associated with topical corticosteroids in psoriasis include the possibility of rebound relapses, development of tolerance, risk of generalised pustular psoriasis and development of local or systemic toxicity due to impaired barrier function of the skin. If used in psoriasis careful patient supervision is therefore important.

Development of secondary infection requires withdrawal of topical corticosteroid therapy and commencement of appropriate systemic antimicrobial treatment.

*Use in pregnancy and lactation:* There is inadequate evidence of safety in human pregnancy. Topical administration of corticosteroids to pregnant animals can cause abnormalities of foetal development, including cleft palate and intra-uterine growth retardation. There may therefore be a very small risk of such effects in the human foetus. The risk/benefit needs to be carefully assessed, therefore, before prescribing this medicine.

*Side-effects:* Betamethasone preparations are usually well tolerated, but if signs of hypersensitivity appear, application should be stopped immediately.

As with other topical corticosteroids, prolonged use of large amounts, or treatment of extensive areas, can result in sufficient systemic absorption to produce the features of hypercorticism and suppression of the HPA axis. These effects are more likely to occur in infants and children, and if occlusive dressings are used. Local atrophy may occur after prolonged treatment, particularly under occlusion.

In rare instances, treatment of psoriasis with corticosteroids (or its withdrawal) is thought to have provoked the pustular form of the disease.

*Overdosage:* Acute overdosage is very unlikely to occur. In the case of chronic overdosage or misuse, the features of hypercorticism may appear and in this situation treatment with Betacap Scalp Application should be discontinued.

**Pharmaceutical precautions** Store upright at room temperature (not exceeding 25°C), with the cap replaced. Return bottle to carton between use. Protect from light. Avoid spillage.

**Legal category** POM.

**Package quantity** Betacap Scalp Application is supplied in a plastic squeeze bottle with integral nozzle applicator, containing 100 ml. This is supplied as an original pack (OP).

**Further information** Betacap Scalp Application is

specially formulated to include a coconut-oil related emollient ingredient designed to reduce the drying effect that a standard alcoholic vehicle may otherwise have on the scalp. The viscosity of the preparation has been adjusted so that it spreads easily without being too fluid. The squeeze bottle and nozzle also allow easy application direct to the scalp through the hair.

**Product licence number** 0173/0149.

## CAPASAL* THERAPEUTIC SHAMPOO

**Qualitative and quantitative composition** Salicylic Acid BP 0.5% w/w; Coconut Oil BP 1.0% w/w; Distilled Coal Tar 1.0% w/w.

**Pharmaceutical form** Golden brown therapeutic shampoo.

**Clinical particulars**

*Therapeutic indications:* For use as a shampoo in the treatment of dry, scaly scalp conditions such as seborrhoeic eczema, seborrhoeic dermatitis, pityriasis capitis, psoriasis, and cradle cap in children. It may also be used to remove previous scalp applications.

*Posology and method of administration:* For adults, children and the elderly. Use as a shampoo, daily if necessary. Wet the hair thoroughly. Massage a small amount of the shampoo into the scalp, leaving on for a few minutes before washing out. Repeat, producing a rich lather. Rinse hair well and dry.

*Contra-indications:* Not to be used in cases of sensitivity to any of the ingredients.

*Special warnings and special precautions for use:* Keep away from the eyes. Keep out of the reach of children. In case of irritation, discontinue treatment. For external use only.

*Interaction with other medicaments and other forms of interaction:* None known.

*Pregnancy and lactation:* No known side-effects.

*Effects on ability to drive and use machines:* None known.

*Undesirable effects:* None known.

*Overdose:* There are no known toxic effects resulting from excessive use of Capasal Therapeutic Shampoo.

**Pharmacological properties**

*Pharmacodynamic properties:* The preparation has been designed for use in the treatment of dry, scaly scalp conditions by incorporating into a convenient shampoo formulation three well known ingredients which have been established as safe and effective, for example, in Coconut Oil Compound Ointment (Ung Cocois Co), for use in these indications. They are as follows:

0.5% salicylic acid – mild keratolytic
1.0% coconut oil – emollient, softening agent and lubricant
1.0% distilled coal tar – anti-pruritic, keratoplastic
The preparation may also be used conveniently to remove any previous topical application.

*Pharmacokinetic properties:* The active ingredients of the formulation are readily available for intimate contact with the skin, as the shampoo is massaged into the scalp and left on for a few minutes before washing out. This is then repeated in order to produce a rich lather. The detergent effect of the shampoo will also remove any previous application to the scalp.

*Preclinical safety data:* No special information.

**Pharmaceutical particulars**

*List of excipients:* Lauric Acid Diethanolamide; Coco Amido Propyl Dimethyl Betaine; Triethanolamine Lauryl Sulphate; Phenoxyethanol BP; Water.

*Incompatibilities:* None known.

*Shelf life:* 36 months.

*Special precautions for storage:* Store at room temperature (not exceeding 25°C) and away from direct sunlight.

*Nature and contents of container:* Polyethylene bottle containing 250 ml. This is supplied as an original pack (OP).

*Instructions for use/handling:* Not applicable.

**Marketing authorisation number** 0173/0048.

**Date of approval/revision of SPC** January 1996.

**Legal category** P.

## DERMOL* 500 LOTION

**Qualitative and quantitative composition** Benzalkonium Chloride BP 0.1% w/w; Chlorhexidine Hydrochloride BP 0.1% w/w; Liquid Paraffin BP 2.5% w/w; Isopropyl Myristate BP 2.5% w/w.

**Pharmaceutical form** White, non-greasy aqueous lotion.

**Clinical particulars**

*Therapeutic indications:* An antimicrobial emollient for the management of dry and pruritic skin conditions, especially eczema and dermatitis. The lotion is suitable for direct application, and for use as a soap substitute.

*Posology and method of administration:* For adults, children and the elderly. For application to the skin: apply the lotion to the affected areas as required. Massage well into the skin, until absorbed. For periodic use as a soap substitute: as required, use the lotion in the bath or shower, or for other toiletry purposes, instead of ordinary soap or shower gel.

*Contra-indications:* Do not use in cases of known sensitivity to any of the ingredients.

*Special warnings and special precautions for use:* Avoid contact with the eyes.

*Interaction with other medicaments and other forms of interaction:* None known.

*Pregnancy and lactation:* No special precautions.

*Effects on ability to drive and use machines:* None known.

*Undesirable effects:* Although the lotion has been specially formulated for use on dry or problem skin, in the unlikely event of a reaction discontinue treatment.

*Overdose:* Not applicable.

**Pharmacological properties**

*Pharmacodynamic properties:* Bacteria (especially *Staphylococcus aureus*) are implicated in the pathogenesis of inflammatory dry skin conditions such as atopic eczema or dermatitis. Dermol 500 Lotion contains 5% of emollient oils in a non-greasy aqueous lotion which also contains the well-known and effective antiseptics benzalkonium chloride and chlorhexidine hydrochloride. Its antimicrobial properties assist in overcoming infection, whether from *Staph. aureus*, the pathogen which often complicates eczema and associated pruritus, or secondary infection caused by scratching.

Massaged into the skin, the emollients, liquid paraffin and isopropyl myristate, permit rehydration of dry skin by forming an occlusive barrier within the skin surface, thus reducing drying from evaporation of water that diffuses from the underlying layers.

*Pharmacokinetic properties:* The active ingredients are presented in an aqueous lotion and so are readily absorbed into the stratum corneum when the product is gently massaged over the areas of dry skin. The antiseptic ingredients are in intimate contact with the skin, and as they are in solution, their availability is optimal.

*Preclinical safety data:* No special information.

**Pharmaceutical particulars**

*List of excipients:* Cetostearyl Alcohol BP; Cetomacrogol 1000 BP; Phenoxyethanol BP; Purified Water BP.

*Incompatibilities:* None known.

*Shelf life:* 30 months in unopened container. Use within 18 months of first opening.

*Special precautions for storage:* Store at room temperature (not exceeding 25°C).

*Nature and contents of container:* High density polyethylene 500 ml bottle with a white polypropylene pump dispenser. Supplied as an original pack (OP).

*Instructions for use/handling:* Not applicable.

**Marketing authorisation number** 0173/0051.

**Date of approval/revision of SPC** October 1996.

**Legal category** P.

## DIODERM*

**Presentation** White aqueous cream containing Hydrocortisone BP 0.1% w/w.

*Ingredients:* Hydrocortisone BP; Citric Acid BP; Emul-

sifying Ointment BP; Propylene Glycol BP; Purified Water BP.

**Uses** Topical treatment of eczema and dermatitis.

**Dosage and administration**

*Adults, children and the elderly:* Apply to the affected areas twice daily.

**Contra-indications, warnings, etc** As with all topical steroids, Dioderm is contra-indicated where there is a bacterial, viral or fungal infection. It should not be applied to open wounds, ulcers or broken skin. It may also be hazardous in psoriasis for a number of reasons including rebound relapses following development of tolerance, risk of generalised pustular psoriasis and local and systemic toxicity due to impaired barrier function of the skin. In such patients, careful patient supervision is important. Dioderm should not normally be used under occlusion. Keep away from the eyes. Do not use if sensitive to any of the ingredients.

*Use in pregnancy:* There is inadequate evidence of safety in human pregnancy. Topical administration of corticosteroids to pregnant animals can cause abnormalities of foetal development including cleft palate and intra-uterine growth retardation. There may therefore be a very small risk of such effects in the human foetus.

*Use in infants:* Although generally regarded as safe, even for long-term administration in adults, there is a potential for overdosage in infancy. Extreme caution is required in dermatoses of infancy, including napkin eruption. In such patients, courses of treatment should not normally exceed 7 days.

*Overdosage:* Under exceptional circumstances, if Dioderm is used excessively, particularly in young children, it is theoretically possible that adrenal suppression and skin thinning may occur. The symptoms are normally reversible on cessation of treatment.

**Pharmaceutical precautions** Store at room temperature (not exceeding 25°C). Replace cap tightly after use.

**Legal category** POM.

**Package quantity** Dioderm is supplied in a collapsible tube containing 30 g. This is supplied as an original pack (OP).

**Further information** Although Dioderm contains the relatively low concentration of 0.1% hydrocortisone, the formulation is designed to provide clinical activity at least equivalent to the usual strength of 1.0% Hydrocortisone Cream BP.

**Product licence number** 0173/0047.

## DITHROCREAM*

**Presentation** Pale yellow aqueous creams containing Dithranol BP 0.1%, 0.25%, 0.5%, 1.0% or 2.0% w/w.

*Ingredients:* Dithranol BP; White Soft Paraffin BP; Salicylic Acid BP; Cetostearyl Alcohol BP; Chlorocresol BP; Ascorbic Acid BP; Sodium Lauryl Sulphate BP; Purified Water BP.

Dithrocream 2.0% also contains Liquid Paraffin BP. The packs are colour coded as follows:

| | |
|---|---|
| 0.1% | pale blue |
| 0.25% | red |
| 0.5% | purple |
| 1.0% | brown |
| 2.0% | yellow |

**Uses** Dithrocream is recommended for the topical treatment of sub-acute and chronic psoriasis, including psoriasis of the scalp. Dithrocream 0.5%, Dithrocream 1.0% and Dithrocream 2.0% should only be used for those patients who have failed to respond to lower strengths of dithranol. Dithrocream 1.0% and 2.0% should normally only be applied for 'short contact' periods.

**Dosage and administration**

*Adults, children and the elderly:* It is important to determine each patient's optimal treatment strength, as too high a strength may induce a burning sensation. Where the response to Dithrocream has not previously been established, always commence treatment with Dithrocream 0.1%, continuing for at least one week and then, if necessary, increase to the 0.25% followed by the 0.5%, the 1.0%, and finally the 2.0% strength. The aim should be to build up gradually over approximately 4 weeks to the highest tolerated strength to produce the optimum therapeutic effect. This optimum concentration will depend upon such factors as the thickness and location of the psoriatic plaques, as well as the variation between individual patients in their reaction to dithranol. Dithrocream 0.5%, Dithrocream 1.0% and Dithrocream 2.0% should always be used under medical supervision.

Dithrocream should be applied once every 24 hours, at any convenient time of the day or evening, and

then removed by washing off, usually no more than one hour after application. Alternatively, it may be applied at night before retiring and washed off in the morning.

Dithrocream should be applied sparingly, only to the affected areas. Rub the cream gently and carefully into the skin until completely absorbed. It is most important to avoid applying an excessive amount of the cream, which may cause unnecessary soiling and staining of clothing and/or bed linen. After each period of treatment, a bath/shower should be taken to remove any residual cream. To prevent the possibility of discolouration, particularly where Dithrocream 1.0% or 2.0% has been used, always rinse the bath/shower with hot water immediately after washing/showering and then use a suitable cleanser to remove any deposit on the surface of the bath or shower.

For use on the scalp, first comb the hair to remove scalar debris and, after suitably parting, rub the cream well into the affected areas. After use on the scalp, a shampoo may be used to remove the Dithrocream residue. Great care must be taken when washing out the shampoo (which may contain some Dithrocream residue), to ensure that it does not get into the eyes or on the face. This is particularly important when the higher strengths of Dithrocream have been used.

Treatment should be continued until the skin is entirely clear, i.e. when there is nothing to feel with the fingers and the texture is normal.

By gradually increasing the strength of cream applied, it should be possible to clear psoriasis patches within 4 to 6 weeks.

**Contra-indications, warnings, etc** Not to be used on the face, or for acute or pustular psoriasis. Not to be used in cases of sensitivity to any of the ingredients.

Although a feeling of warmth at the application site is normal, if this amounts to a burning sensation, or if the lesions spread, treatment should be stopped at once, and the dosage re-evaluated by a doctor. Dithrocream is not normally recommended for use on areas of folded skin such as in the groin and beneath the breasts. Do not use high strengths on these sites. Keep away from the eyes and mucous membranes. Always wash the hands after use.

As long term use of topical corticosteroids is known to destabilise psoriasis, and withdrawal may give rise to a rebound phenomenon, an interval of at least one week should be allowed between the discontinuance of such steroids and the commencement of Dithrocream therapy. A suitably bland emollient may usefully be applied in the intervening period.

Contact with fabrics, plastics and other materials may cause permanent staining and should be avoided.

Dithrocream may cause temporary staining of the skin and/or hair.

*Use in pregnancy:* Although there is no experimental evidence to support the safety of the drug in pregnancy, no adverse effects have been reported.

*Use in children:* No additional special precautions necessary. However, use cautiously with regular supervision.

*Accidental oral ingestion:* Dithranol is a cathartic (laxative) and, if accidentally swallowed, should be removed by gastric lavage.

**Pharmaceutical precautions** Store at room temperature (not exceeding 25°C). Replace cap tightly after use.

**Legal category** P except for Dithrocream 2.0% (POM).

**Package quantities** All strengths of Dithrocream are supplied in collapsible tubes containing 50 g. These are supplied as original packs (OP).

**Further information** Dithrocream has been developed as a cream formulation of dithranol for particular convenience for home treatment, and is especially suitable for the exposed surfaces and hairy regions of the body, including psoriasis of the scalp.

**Product licence numbers**

| | |
|---|---|
| Dithrocream 0.1% | 0173/0029 |
| Dithrocream 0.25% | 0173/0028 |
| Dithrocream 0.5% | 0173/0027 |
| Dithrocream 1.0% | 0173/0039 |
| Dithrocream 2.0% | 0173/0045 |

## EMULSIDERM* EMOLLIENT

**Presentation** Pale blue/green liquid emulsion containing Benzalkonium Chloride BP 0.5% w/w, Liquid Paraffin BP 25% w/w and Isopropyl Myristate BP 25% w/w.

*Ingredients:* Benzalkonium Chloride BP; Liquid Paraffin BP; Isopropyl Myristate BP; Sorbitan Monostearate BP; Polysorbate 60 BP; Methylene Blue; IMS BP; Purified Water BP.

**Uses** For the treatment of dry skin conditions, including those associated with dermatitis and psoriasis. It permits re-hydration of the keratin by replacing lost lipids, and its antibacterial properties assist in overcoming *Staph. aureus*, the pathogen which often complicates atopic eczema and associated pruritus.

**Dosage and administration**

*Adults, children and the elderly:* Shake bottle before use.

Add 7 to 30 ml to a bath of warm water (more or less according to the size of the bath and individual patient requirements). Soak for 5 to 10 minutes. Pat dry.

For application to the skin: rub a small amount of undiluted emollient into the dry areas of skin until absorbed.

**Contra-indications, warnings, etc** Keep away from the eyes. Take care to avoid slipping in the bath.

Do not use if sensitive to any of the ingredients.

**Pharmaceutical precautions** Store at room temperature (not exceeding 25˚C). Replace cap after use.

**Legal category** P.

**Package quantities** Emulsiderm is supplied in polythene bottles; a 300 ml with a measuring cap, and a 1 litre with a measuring cup. These are supplied as original packs (OP).

**Further information** Bacteria (especially *Staph. aureus*) have been implicated in the pathogenesis of inflammatory dry skin conditions such as atopic eczema or dermatitis. Dual action bactericidal and emollient Emulsiderm is specially formulated in a unique emulsion system optimised for convenient application to the skin, either directly or via the patient's bath water.

**Product licence number** 0173/0036.

# EXTEROL*

**Qualitative and quantitative composition** Urea Hydrogen Peroxide 5.0% w/w.

**Pharmaceutical form** Clear, straw-coloured, viscous ear drops.

**Clinical particulars**

*Therapeutic indications:* As an aid in the removal of hardened ear wax.

*Posology and method of administration:* For adults, children and the elderly. Instil up to 5 drops into the ear. Retain drops in ear for several minutes by keeping the head tilted and then wipe away any surplus. Repeat once or twice daily for at least 3 to 4 days, or as required.

*Contra-indications:* Do not use if the eardrum is known or suspected to be damaged, in cases of dizziness, or if there is, or has been, any other ear disorder (such as pain, discharge, inflammation, infection or tinnitus). Do not use after ill-advised attempts to dislodge wax using fingernails, cotton buds or similar implements, as such mechanical efforts can cause the ear's delicate inner lining to become damaged, inflamed or infected, whereupon the use of ear drops can be painful. For similar reasons, it is inadvisable to use Exterol within 2 to 3 days of syringing. Do not use where there is a history of ear problems, unless under close medical supervision. Do not use if sensitive to any of the ingredients.

*Special warnings and special precautions for use:* Keep Exterol away from the eyes. For external use only.

*Interaction with other medicaments and other forms of interaction:* Exterol should not be used at the same time as anything else in the ear.

*Pregnancy and lactation:* No known side-effects.

*Effects on ability to drive and use machines:* None known.

*Undesirable effects:* Due to the release of oxygen, patients may experience a mild, temporary effervescence in the ear. Stop usage if irritation or pain occurs. Instillation of ear drops can aggravate the painful symptoms of excessive ear wax, including some loss of hearing, dizziness and tinnitus. Very rarely, unpleasant taste has been reported. If patients encounter any of these problems, or if their symptoms persist or worsen, they should discontinue treatment and consult a doctor.

*Overdose:* No adverse effects.

**Pharmacological properties**

*Pharmacodynamic properties:* After insertion of the drops into the ear, the urea hydrogen peroxide complex liberates oxygen which acts to break up the hardened wax. The hydrogen peroxide component is also an antiseptic, especially in sites with relative anaerobiosis. The glycerol assists in softening the wax, so that it may more easily be removed from the ear, either with or without syringing. The urea acts as a mild keratolytic, helping to reduce the keratin-load

in the wax debris, thereby assisting penetration of the other components.

*Pharmacokinetic properties:* Exterol is intended only for the treatment of impacted wax in the *external* auditory canal. The ingredients of the formulation are therefore readily available for intimate contact with the affected area, as the drops are instilled into the ear and retained therein for several minutes by tilting the head.

*Preclinical safety:* No special information.

**Pharmaceutical particulars**

*List of excipients:* 8-Hydroxyquinoline; Glycerol BP.

*Incompatibilities:* None known.

*Shelf life:* 30 months.

*Special precautions for storage:* Store at room temperature (not exceeding 25˚C). Replace cap after use, and return bottle to carton.

*Nature and contents of container:* 8 ml easy squeeze plastic dropper bottle. This is supplied as an original pack (OP).

*Instructions for use/handling:* Not applicable.

**Marketing authorisation number** 0173/0037.

**Date of approval/revision of SPC** January 1997.

**Legal category** P.

# GLUTAROL*

**Qualitative and quantitative composition** Glutaraldehyde 10.0% w/v.

**Pharmaceutical form** Colourless, evaporative wart paint.

**Clinical particulars**

*Therapeutic indications:* For the topical treatment of warts, especially plantar warts.

*Posology and method of administration:* For adults, children and the elderly.

1. Gently rub the surface of the wart with a piece of pumice stone or manicure emery board, or pare down any hard skin.
2. Using the applicator provided, carefully apply a few drops of the paint to the wart, taking care to localise the application to the affected area. Allow each drop to dry before the next is applied.
3. Repeat twice daily.
4. On subsequent days, repeat steps 1 to 3.

It is not necessary to cover the treated wart(s) with an adhesive plaster.

*Contra-indications:* Not to be used in cases of sensitivity to any of the ingredients. Not to be used on the face, anal or perineal region. Not to be used on moles or on any other skin lesion for which it is not indicated.

*Special warnings and special precautions for use:* Keep away from the eyes and mucous membranes. Avoid spreading onto surrounding uninvolved skin. Avoid spillage. Avoid inhaling vapour. Replace cap tightly after use. For external use only.

*Interaction with other medicaments and other forms of interaction:* None known.

*Pregnancy and lactation:* No special precautions.

*Effects on ability to drive and use machines:* None known.

*Undesirable effects:* Undesirable effects occur very occasionally and mostly involve mild local skin rashes and irritation. Very rarely, a severe reaction may occur particularly on the hands or when the product is used excessively and allowed to spread onto surrounding normal skin. If mild irritation should occur, apply a reduced amount (taking special care to avoid spreading beyond the wart or verruca) and apply less often. If the irritation is severe, patients should stop treatment immediately and seek medical advice.

*Overdose:* Accidental oral ingestion should be treated immediately by gastric lavage with 2 to 5% aqueous sodium bicarbonate solution. Fluid and electrolyte balance should be monitored and appropriate supportive measures should be provided. Symptoms include headache, nausea, vomiting, diarrhoea and respiratory depression.

**Pharmacological properties**

*Pharmacodynamic properties:* Glutaraldehyde is virucidal and thus inactivates the wart virus. On the skin, it also acts as an anhidrotic, drying the warts and surrounding skin, thus reducing the spread of lesions and simplifying the removal of persistent warts by curettage.

As glutaraldehyde stains the outer layer of the skin brown, treatment can be seen to be carried out. This stain soon disappears after cessation of treatment.

*Pharmacokinetic properties:* Addition of ethanol to the formulation stabilises the glutaraldehyde against

irreversible polymerisation during storage but at the same time diminishes its activity. However, when the aqueous ethanolic solution is applied to the skin, the alcohol rapidly evaporates leaving a concentrated aqueous solution of glutaraldehyde which is highly reactive and attacks the wart before it has time to polymerise. Thus, the ethanolic formulation is stable in storage, as confirmed by stability tests, but is immediately activated when applied to the skin and the alcohol is allowed to evaporate.

*Preclinical safety data:* No special information.

**Pharmaceutical particulars**

*List of excipients:* Bitrex; IMS BP; Purified Water BP.

*Incompatibilities:* None known.

*Shelf life:* 36 months.

*Special precautions for storage:* Flammable. Keep away from flames. Store upright at room temperature (not exceeding 25˚C).

*Nature and contents of container:* 10 ml amber glass bottle incorporating a specially designed spatula for ease of application. This is supplied as an original pack (OP).

*Instructions for use/handling:* Not applicable.

**Marketing authorisation number** 0173/0022.

**Date of approval/revision of SPC** April 1996.

**Legal category** P.

# IBUGEL*

**Qualitative and quantitative composition** Ibuprofen BP 5.0% w/w.

**Pharmaceutical form** Non-greasy, fragrance-free, clear, colourless aqueous-alcoholic gel.

**Clinical particulars**

*Therapeutic indications:* For the topical treatment of backache, rheumatic and muscular pain, sprains, strains and neuralgia. Ibugel is also indicated for symptomatic relief of pain due to non-serious arthritic conditions.

*Posology and method of administration:* Apply the gel to the affected areas, up to three times daily, or as directed by the physician. On each occasion apply only enough gel to thinly cover the affected area, and gently massage well into the skin, until completely absorbed. Do not use excessively. Therapy should be reviewed after a few weeks, particularly if symptoms worsen or persist.

The same dosage and dosage schedule applies to all age groups, although Ibugel is not normally recommended for use on children under the age of 14 years, unless instructed by their doctor.

*Contra-indications:* Not to be used in cases of sensitivity to any of the ingredients, particularly if asthmatic and have previously shown hypersensitivity to aspirin or ibuprofen. Not to be used on broken skin.

*Special warnings and special precautions for use:* Seek medical advice if symptoms worsen or persist. Oral NSAIDs, including ibuprofen, can sometimes be associated with renal impairment, aggravation of active peptic ulcers, and can induce allergic bronchial reactions in susceptible asthmatic patients. Although the systemic absorption of topically applied ibuprofen is less than for oral dosage forms, these complications can occur in rare cases. For these reasons, patients with an active peptic ulcer, a history of kidney problems, asthma or intolerance to aspirin or ibuprofen taken orally should seek medical advice before using Ibugel. Keep Ibugel away from the eyes and mucous membranes. For external use only.

*Interaction with other medicaments and other forms of interaction:* Non-steroidal anti-inflammatory drugs may interact with blood pressure lowering drugs, although the chance of this occurring with a topically administered preparation is extremely remote.

*Pregnancy and lactation:* Do not use during pregnancy or lactation.

*Effects on ability to drive and use machines:* None known.

*Undesirable effects:* Local side-effects do not normally occur. In rare instances, skin rashes may occur, in which case the application of Ibugel should be stopped.

*Overdose:* Not applicable. Any overdose with a topical presentation of ibuprofen is extremely unlikely.

**Pharmacological properties**

*Pharmacodynamic properties:* Ibugel is a topical preparation which has anti-inflammatory and analgesic properties. It contains the active ingredient, ibuprofen, which exerts its effects directly in inflamed tissues underlying the site of application, mainly by inhibiting prostaglandin biosynthesis.

Because it is formulated in an aqueous/alcoholic gel, Ibugel also exerts a soothing and cooling effect when applied to the affected area.

*Pharmacokinetic properties:* Specially formulated for external application, the active ingredient penetrates through the skin rapidly and extensively, achieving high, therapeutically relevant local concentrations in underlying soft tissues, joints and synovial fluid, whilst producing plasma levels that are unlikely to be sufficient to cause any systemic side-effects, other than in rare individuals who are hypersensitive to ibuprofen.

Furthermore, there do not appear to be any appreciable differences between the oral and topical routes of administration regarding metabolism or excretion of ibuprofen.

*Preclinical safety data:* Published information on subchronic toxicity studies confirms that topically applied ibuprofen is well tolerated both locally and by the gastro-intestinal tract. Any local erythema is only mild and no signs of mucosal lesions or ulcerogenic effects have been determined in the gastro-intestinal tract.

In the course of assessing mucosal tolerance, topical ibuprofen has been found to cause acute, but reversible, irritant reactions in the eyes and mucous membranes.

**Pharmaceutical particulars**

*List of excipients:* IMS BP; Carbomer; Propylene Glycol BP; Diethylamine; Purified Water BP.

*Incompatibilities:* None known.

*Shelf life:* 36 months.

*Special precautions for storage:* Store at room temperature (not exceeding 25°C).

*Nature and contents of container:* 100 g membrane sealed, epoxy resin coated, tamper-evident collapsible aluminium tube, fitted with a screw cap. This is supplied as an original pack (OP).

*Instructions for use/handling:* Not applicable.

**Marketing authorisation number** 0173/0050.

**Date of approval/revision of SPC** November 1996.

**Legal category** P.

## IBUSPRAY*

**Qualitative and quantitative composition** Ibuprofen BP 5.0% w/w.

**Pharmaceutical form** Clear, colourless, fragrance-free, aqueous-alcoholic topical spray.

**Clinical particulars**

*Therapeutic indications:* For the topical treatment of backache, rheumatic and muscular pain, sprains, strains and neuralgia. Ibuspray is also indicated for symptomatic relief of pain due to non-serious arthritic conditions.

*Posology and method of administration:* Holding the bottle upright or upside down, spray approximately 4 inches to 6 inches away from the skin. After every 2 to 3 sprays, gently massage the preparation into the skin, spreading the product over a wide area around the affected site. The exact amount to be applied will vary, depending on the extent and severity of the condition, but it should normally be sufficient to apply 5 to 10 sprays (1 to 2 ml). This amount may be repeated three to four times daily, or more often if required.

Therapy should be reviewed after a few weeks, particularly if symptoms worsen or persist.

The same dosage and dosage schedule applies to all age groups, although Ibuspray is not normally recommended for use on children under the age of 14 years, unless instructed by their doctor.

*Contra-indications:* Not to be used in cases of sensitivity to any of the ingredients, particularly if asthmatic and have previously shown hypersensitivity to aspirin or ibuprofen. Not to be used on broken skin.

*Special warnings and special precautions for use:* This product is flammable. Do not spray near flames, electric heaters or similar objects. Patients should seek medical advice if symptoms worsen or persist. Oral NSAIDs, including ibuprofen, can sometimes be associated with renal impairment, aggravation of active peptic ulcers, and can induce allergic bronchial reactions in susceptible asthmatic patients. Although the systemic absorption of topically applied ibuprofen is less than for oral dosage forms, these complications can occur in rare cases. For these reasons, patients with an active peptic ulcer, a history of kidney problems, asthma or intolerance to aspirin or ibuprofen taken orally should seek medical advice before

using Ibuspray. Keep away from the eyes and mucous membranes. For external use only.

*Interaction with other medicaments and other forms of interaction:* Non-steroidal anti-inflammatory drugs may interact with blood pressure lowering drugs, although the chance of this occurring with a topically administered preparation is extremely remote.

*Pregnancy and lactation:* Do not use during pregnancy or lactation.

*Effects on ability to drive and use machines:* None known.

*Undesirable effects:* The side-effects known to occur with oral ibuprofen are theoretically possible, although much less likely with topical application. In rare instances, skin rashes may occur, in which case the application of Ibuspray should be stopped.

*Overdose:* Not applicable. Any overdose with a topical presentation of ibuprofen is extremely unlikely.

**Pharmacological properties**

*Pharmacodynamic properties:* Ibuspray is a topical preparation which has anti-inflammatory and analgesic properties. It contains the active ingredient, ibuprofen, which exerts its effects directly in inflamed tissues underlying the site of application, mainly by inhibiting prostaglandin biosynthesis. Because it is formulated in an evaporative aqueous/alcoholic solution, Ibuspray also exerts a soothing and cooling effect when applied to the affected area.

*Pharmacokinetic properties:* Specially formulated for external application, the active ingredient penetrates through the skin rapidly and extensively, achieving high, therapeutically relevant local concentrations in underlying soft tissues, joints and synovial fluid, whilst producing plasma levels that are unlikely to be sufficient to cause any systemic side effects, other than in rare individuals who are hypersensitive to ibuprofen. Furthermore, there do not appear to be any appreciable differences between the oral and topical routes of administration regarding metabolism or excretion of ibuprofen.

*Preclinical safety data:* Published information on subchronic toxicity studies confirms that topically applied ibuprofen is well tolerated both locally and by the gastro-intestinal tract. Any local erythema is only mild and no signs of mucosal lesions or ulcerogenic effects have been determined in the gastro-intestinal tract.

In the course of assessing mucosal tolerance, topical ibuprofen has been found to cause acute, but reversible, irritant reactions in the eyes and mucous membranes.

**Pharmaceutical particulars**

*List of excipients:* IMS BP; Polyethylene Glycol 300 BP; Cetomacrogol 1000 BP; Purified Water BP.

*Incompatibilities:* None known.

*Shelf life:* 30 months.

*Special precautions for storage:* Store at room temperature (not exceeding 25°C).

*Nature and contents of container:* 100 ml plastic bottle incorporating a controlled metered-dose spray pump dispenser and overcap. This is supplied as an original pack (OP). Ibuspray is not an aerosol, does not contain potentially irritant propellants and is ozone-friendly.

*Instructions for use/handling:* Not applicable.

**Marketing authorisation number** 0173/0150.

**Date of approval/revision of SPC** November 1996.

**Legal category** P.

## PERINAL* SPRAY

**Presentation** Colourless, aqueous spray solution containing Hydrocortisone BP 0.2% w/w and Lignocaine Hydrochloride BP 1.0% w/w.

*Ingredients:* Hydrocortisone BP; Lignocaine Hydrochloride BP; Cetomacrogol 1000 BP; Citric Acid BP; Phenoxyethanol BP; Purified Water BP.

**Uses** For use as a spray for the symptomatic relief of anal and perianal itch, irritation and pain such as associated with haemorrhoids.

**Dosage and administration**

*Adults and the elderly:* Spray twice over the affected area up to three times daily, depending on the severity of the condition.

**Contra-indications, warnings, etc** Not to be used if sensitive to lignocaine or any other of the ingredients. Not to be used on broken or infected skin. Not to be used internally (inside the anus). Perinal Spray is intended for use for limited periods and so should not be used continuously for longer than seven days without medical advice. Patients should be instructed to seek medical advice if they experience persistent

pain or bleeding from the anus, especially where associated with a change in bowel habit, if the stomach is distended or if they are losing weight. Prompt medical treatment may be very important under such circumstances. A temporary tingling sensation may be experienced locally after initial application. Hypersensitivity to lignocaine has rarely been reported, and the incidence in no way approaches the known reactions to benzocaine, cinchocaine or amethocaine. Keep away from the eyes, nose and mouth.

*Use in pregnancy:* There is inadequate evidence of safety in human pregnancy. Topical administration of corticosteroids to pregnant animals can cause abnormalities of foetal development including cleft palate and intra-uterine growth retardation. There may therefore be a very small risk of such effects in the human foetus. The risk/benefit needs to be carefully assessed, therefore, before prescribing this medicine.

*Use in children:* Not normally recommended for children under the age of 14 years, unless on medical advice.

*Overdosage:* Under exceptional circumstances, if Perinal Spray is used excessively, particularly in young children, it is theoretically possible that adrenal suppression and skin thinning may occur. The symptoms are normally reversible on cessation of treatment.

**Pharmaceutical precautions** Store at room temperature (not exceeding 21°C).

**Legal category** P.

**Package quantity** Perinal Spray is supplied in 30 ml quantities in a collapsible laminate tube fitted with a metered-dose pump spray which is ozone friendly. For added convenience, the spray device will operate when held in any orientation. This is supplied as an original pack (OP).

Perinal Spray is *not* an aerosol and does *not* contain potentially irritant propellants.

**Further information** The preparation combines the well-known local anti-inflammatory and anti-pruritic properties of hydrocortisone and the analgesic effect of lignocaine in an aqueous spray formulation. On application, finger contact with the affected area can be avoided which makes for improved hygiene, and lessens the risk of infection. The active ingredients are readily available for intimate contact with the skin and mucous membranes, as the preparation is sprayed in small droplets which dry after application to leave the active ingredients in close contact with the affected area. Because the preparation is a clear solution, it is entirely homogeneous, and the availability of the active ingredients is optimal.

**Product licence number** 0173/0049.

## PSORIDERM* BATH EMULSION

**Qualitative and quantitative composition** Distilled Coal Tar 40.0% w/v.

**Pharmaceutical form** Buff coloured liquid emulsion.

**Clinical particulars** The use of coal tar has long been advocated as a therapeutic agent in the management of psoriasis. Psoriderm Bath Emulsion conveniently provides a coal tar bath which may be used alone, or as part of a more extensive treatment regime.

*Therapeutic indications:* For use topically as an aid in the treatment of sub-acute and chronic psoriasis.

*Posology and method of administration:* For adults, children and the elderly. Add 30 ml of the emulsion to a standard bath of warm water. Soak for 5 minutes, pat dry.

*Contra-indications:* Not to be used in cases of sensitivity to any of the ingredients.

*Special warnings and special precautions for use:* Do not use product undiluted. Keep away from the eyes and broken or inflamed skin. Replace cap after use. Avoid spillage. For external use only.

*Interaction with other medicaments and other forms of interaction:* None known.

*Pregnancy and lactation:* No special precautions.

*Effects on ability to drive and use machines:* None known.

*Undesirable effects:* Local side-effects do not normally occur. In rare cases of skin irritation, discontinue treatment.

*Overdose:* There are no known toxic effects resulting from excessive use of Psoriderm Bath Emulsion. In case of accidental ingestion, patients should contact a doctor or hospital immediately.

**Pharmacological properties**

*Pharmacodynamic properties:* Coal tar has been used dermatologically for hundreds of years and has been shown to be safe and effective in the treatment of scaly skin conditions such as psoriasis. The British Pharmacopoeia contains monographs on coal tar and coal tar solution, and many formulations of coal tar are used in hospitals throughout the country. The coal tar used in Psoriderm Bath Emulsion has been specially distilled and is based on a neutral fraction which has been shown to be effective in the treatment of psoriasis.

The precise mechanism of action of coal tar is not understood, largely as a result of it comprising up to 10 000 components. There is evidence that topical application of coal tar improves psoriasis by reducing the excessive rate of mitotic epidermal cell division.

*Pharmacokinetic properties:* Dry scales, which are a common feature of psoriasis, generally reduce the effectiveness of topically applied treatments by reducing absorption of the active ingredient. An established means of overcoming this problem is to add a mild softening agent such as lecithin. In the case of Psoriderm Bath Emulsion, however, no such softening agent is included because the dosage and administration regime involves prolonged soaking (5 minutes) in a warm water emulsion which achieves a similar effect.

*Preclinical safety data:* No special information.

**Pharmaceutical particulars**

*List of excipients:* Polysorbate 20 BP; Triethanolamine BP; Phenoxyethanol BP; Water.

*Incompatibilities:* None known.

*Shelf life:* 36 months.

*Special precautions for storage:* Store at room temperature (not exceeding 25°C).

*Nature and contents of container:* Amber glass bottle containing 200 ml. This is supplied as an original pack (OP).

*Instructions for use/handling:* Not applicable.

**Marketing authorisation number** 0173/5003R.

**Date of approval/revision of SPC** March 1995.

**Legal category** P.

## PSORIDERM* CREAM

**Qualitative and quantitative composition** Distilled Coal Tar 6.0% w/w; Lecithin 0.4% w/w.

**Pharmaceutical form** Buff coloured cream.

**Clinical particulars** The use of coal tar has long been advocated as a therapeutic agent in the management of psoriasis. Psoriderm Cream may be used alone, or as part of a more extensive treatment regime, and is particularly suitable for treating the hair bearing parts of the body and the flexures.

*Therapeutic indications:* For the topical treatment of sub-acute and chronic psoriasis, including psoriasis of the scalp and flexures.

*Posology and method of administration:* For adults, children and the elderly. Apply to the affected area once or twice daily, or as recommended by the physician. Wash hands after use.

*Contra-indications:* Not to be used for acute psoriasis. Not to be used in cases of sensitivity to any of the ingredients.

*Special warnings and special precautions for use:* Keep away from the eyes and mucous membranes. Replace cap after use. Avoid spillage. For external use only.

*Interaction with other medicaments and other forms of interaction:* None known.

*Pregnancy and lactation:* No special precautions.

*Effects on ability to drive and use machines:* None known.

*Undesirable effects:* Local side-effects do not normally occur. In rare cases of skin irritation, discontinue treatment.

*Overdose:* There are no known toxic effects resulting from excessive use of Psoriderm Cream.

**Pharmacological properties**

*Pharmacodynamic properties:* Coal tar has been used dermatologically for hundreds of years and has been shown to be safe and effective in the treatment of scaly scalp conditions such as psoriasis. The British Pharmacopoeia contains monographs on coal tar and coal tar solution, and many formulations of coal tar are used in hospitals throughout the country. The coal tar used in Psoriderm Cream has been specially distilled and is based on a neutral fraction which has been shown to be effective in the treatment of psoriasis.

The precise mechanism of action of coal tar is not understood, largely as a result of it comprising up to 10 000 components. There is evidence that topical application of coal tar improves psoriasis by reducing the excessive rate of mitotic epidermal cell division.

Lecithin is a well known phospholipid which is present in foodstuffs. It is added to Psoriderm Cream to soften psoriasis scales and thereby enhance the absorption of the coal tar.

*Pharmacokinetic properties:* Not applicable.

*Preclinical safety data:* No special information.

**Pharmaceutical particulars**

*List of excipients:* Stearic Acid BP; Isopropyl Palmitate; Propylene Glycol BP; Triethanolamine BP; Phenoxyethanol BP; Purified Water BP.

*Incompatibilities:* None known.

*Shelf life:* 36 months.

*Special precautions for storage:* Store in a cool, dark place.

*Nature and contents of container:* Amber glass jar containing 225 ml. This is supplied as an original pack (OP).

*Instructions for use/handling:* Not applicable.

**Marketing authorisation number** 0173/5000R.

**Date of approval/revision of SPC** September 1995.

**Legal category** P.

## PSORIDERM* SCALP LOTION

**Qualitative and quantitative composition** Distilled Coal Tar 2.5% w/v; Lecithin 0.3% w/v.

**Pharmaceutical form** Golden brown coloured foaming therapeutic shampoo.

**Clinical particulars** The use of coal tar has long been advocated as a therapeutic agent in the management of psoriasis. Psoriderm Scalp Lotion may be used alone as a coal tar shampoo, or as part of a more extensive treatment regime.

*Therapeutic indications:* For the topical treatment of psoriasis of the scalp.

*Posology and method of administration:* For adults, children and the elderly. Wet the hair thoroughly. Apply a small amount of the shampoo to the scalp, and massage gently until a rich lather has been generated. Retain on the scalp for a few minutes. Remove excess lather with the hands before rinsing with warm water. Repeat the above procedure.

*Contra-indications:* Not to be used for acute psoriasis. Not to be used in cases of sensitivity to any of the ingredients.

*Special warnings and special precautions for use:* Keep away from the eyes and mucous membranes. Replace cap after use. Avoid spillage. For external use only.

*Interaction with other medicaments and other forms of interaction:* None known.

*Pregnancy and lactation:* No special precautions.

*Effects on ability to drive and use machines:* None known.

*Undesirable effects:* Local side-effects do not normally occur. In rare cases of skin irritation, discontinue treatment.

*Overdose:* There are no known toxic effects resulting from excessive use of Psoriderm Scalp Lotion.

**Pharmacological properties**

*Pharmacodynamic properties:* Coal tar has been used dermatologically for hundreds of years and has been shown to be safe and effective in the treatment of scaly scalp conditions such as psoriasis. The British Pharmacopoeia contains monographs on coal tar and coal tar solution, and many formulations of coal tar are used in hospitals throughout the country. The coal tar used in Psoriderm Scalp Lotion has been specially distilled and is based on a neutral fraction which has been shown to be effective in the treatment of psoriasis.

The precise mechanism of action of coal tar is not understood, largely as a result of it comprising up to 10 000 components. There is evidence that topical application of coal tar improves psoriasis by reducing the excessive rate of mitotic epidermal cell division.

Lecithin is a well known phospholipid which is present in foodstuffs. It is added to Psoriderm Scalp Lotion to soften psoriasis scales and thereby enhance the absorption of the coal tar.

*Pharmacokinetic properties:* Not applicable.

*Preclinical safety data:* No special information.

**Pharmaceutical particulars**

*List of excipients:* Triethanolamine Lauryl Sulphate; Lauric Acid Diethanolamide; Disodium Edetate BP; Sodium Chloride BP; Phenoxyethanol BP; Purified Water BP.

*Incompatibilities:* None known.

*Shelf life:* 36 months.

*Special precautions for storage:* Store in a cool, dark place.

*Nature and contents of container:* Polyethylene bottle containing 250 ml. This is supplied as an original pack (OP).

*Instructions for use/handling:* Not applicable.

**Marketing authorisation number** 0173/5001R.

**Date of approval/revision of SPC** April 1995.

**Legal category** P.

## SALACTOL*

**Qualitative and quantitative composition** Salicylic Acid BP 16.7% w/w; Lactic Acid BP 16.7% w/w.

**Pharmaceutical form** Colourless or pale yellow/brown evaporative wart paint.

**Clinical particulars**

*Therapeutic indications:* For the topical treatment of warts, verrucas, corns and calluses.

*Posology and method of administration:* For adults, children and the elderly. Soak the affected site in warm water and pat dry. Gently rub the surface of the wart, verruca, corn or callus with a pumice stone or manicure emery board to remove any hard skin. Using the applicator provided, carefully apply a few drops of Salactol to the lesion, taking care to localise the application to the affected area. Plantar warts should be covered with an adhesive plaster. Leave for 24 hours. Repeat the procedure daily, removing old collodion on each occasion.

*Contra-indications:* Not to be used on or near the face, intertriginous or anogenital regions. Not to be used by diabetics or individuals with impaired peripheral blood circulation. Not to be used in cases of sensitivity to any of the ingredients. Not to be used on moles, birthmarks, hairy warts or on any other skin lesions for which Salactol is not indicated.

*Special warnings and special precautions for use:* Keep away from the eyes and mucous membranes. Avoid spreading onto surrounding normal skin. If the treated area becomes inflamed or painful, treatment should be suspended until the inflammation resolves. Extremely flammable. Avoid spillage. Avoid inhaling vapour. Replace cap tightly after use. For external use only.

*Interaction with other medicaments and other forms of interaction:* None known.

*Pregnancy and lactation:* No special precautions.

*Effects on ability to drive and use machines:* None known.

*Undesirable effects:* Salactol may be irritant on the skin in certain patients.

*Overdose:* Any excessive use of Salactol could cause irritation of the skin. If this occurs, Salactol should be used more sparingly or applied less frequently. Accidental oral ingestion should be treated immediately by gastric lavage with a 2 to 5% aqueous sodium bicarbonate solution. Fluid and electrolyte balance should be monitored and appropriate supportive measures should be provided. Symptoms include headache, nausea, vomiting, diarrhoea and respiratory depression.

**Pharmacological properties**

*Pharmacodynamic properties:* The combination of salicylic acid and lactic acid in flexible collodion has been shown to be particularly efficacious in treating warts, verrucas, corns and calluses.

Salicylic acid has bacteriostatic and fungicidal actions as well as keratolytic properties. Its effectiveness for topical treatment of hyperkeratotic skin lesions is based on mild keratolytic action which produces slow and painless destruction of the epithelium. In the treatment of warts, a mild irritant reaction, which may render the virus more prone to immunologic stimulation or response, may add to the mechanical removal of infected cells. Apart from its antiseptic and caustic properties, lactic acid enhances the availability of salicylic acid from the dried collodion.

*Pharmacokinetic properties:* Salactol contains 16.7% salicylic acid and 16.7% lactic acid in flexible collodion. The bioavailability of salicylic acid is reduced as the collodion film dries on the skin due to entrapment of the drug which inhibits release. The addition of lactic acid to salicylic acid collodion provides more efficient release of the salicylic acid, since the non-volatile lactic acid remains in the film, thus permitting continued release of the keratolytic which may otherwise be entrapped within the dried collodion film. Systemic absorption of salicylic acid or lactic acid after application to small circumscribed areas is exceedingly unlikely.

*Preclinical safety data:* No special information.

**Pharmaceutical particulars**

*List of excipients:* Pyroxylin BP; Colophony BP; Castor Oil BP; IMS BP; Solvent Ether BP.

*Incompatibilities:* None known.

*Shelf life:* 36 months in unopened container. 3 months in opened container.

*Special precautions for storage:* Store at room temperature (not exceeding 25°C).

*Nature and contents of container:* Amber glass bottle containing 10 ml, incorporating a specially designed spatula for ease of application. This is supplied as an original pack (OP).

*Instructions for use/handling:* Not applicable.

**Marketing authorisation number**  0173/5006R.

**Date of approval/revision of SPC**  February 1996.

**Legal category**  P.

## SALATAC* GEL

**Qualitative and quantitative composition**  Salicylic Acid BP 12.0% w/w; Lactic Acid BP 4.0% w/w.

**Pharmaceutical form**  Clear, colourless, collodion-like wart gel.

**Clinical particulars**

*Therapeutic indications:* For the topical treatment of warts, verrucas, corns and calluses.

*Posology and method of administration:* For adults, children and the elderly. Salatac Gel should be applied once daily. The gel should be applied once every night. Treatment can take up to twelve (12) weeks for resistant lesions to disappear, and it is necessary to persevere with treatment.

1. Every night, soak the affected site in warm water for 2 to 3 minutes.
2. Dry thoroughly with the patient's own towel.
3. Carefully apply one or two drops of the gel to the lesion and allow to dry over its surface. Take care to avoid spreading on to surrounding normal skin. No adhesive plaster is necessary.
4. The following evening, carefully peel off and discard the elastic film formed from the previous application, and apply fresh gel again.

5. Once a week, gently rub away the treated surface using an emery board, as provided, or pumice stone used only for this purpose, before re-applying the gel.
6. The wart, verruca, corn or callus may take up to twelve (12) weeks to disappear and it is important to persevere with the treatment.

*Contra-indications:* Not to be used on or near the face, intertriginous or anogenital regions, or by diabetics or individuals with impaired peripheral blood circulation. Not to be used on moles or on any other skin lesions for which the gel is not indicated. Not to be used in cases of sensitivity to any of the ingredients.

*Special warnings and special precautions for use:* Keep away from the eyes, mucous membranes and from cuts and grazes. Apply only to warts, verrucas, corns and calluses, avoiding surrounding normal skin. Do not use excessively. Some mild, transient irritation may be expected, but in cases of more severe inflammation, treatment should be suspended. Avoid inhaling vapour, and keep cap firmly closed when not in use. Contact with clothing, fabrics, plastics and other materials may cause damage, and should be avoided. For external use only.

*Interaction with other medicaments and other forms of interaction:* None known.

*Pregnancy and lactation:* No special precautions.

*Effects on ability to drive and use machines:* None known.

*Undesirable effects:* Salatac Gel may be irritant on the skin in certain patients.

*Overdose:* Any excessive use of Salatac Gel could cause irritation of the skin. If this occurs, Salatac Gel should be used more sparingly or applied less frequently.

**Pharmacological properties**

*Pharmacodynamic properties:* The active ingredients, salicylic acid and lactic acid, are well-established pharmacopoeial substances. In combination, they are routinely used in the treatment of verrucas, warts, corns and calluses for their keratolytic properties.

When applied topically, and in high enough concentrations, salicylic acid acts by achieving a slow, painless destruction of the thickened stratum corneum. It softens and destroys the stratum corneum of the affected tissue by reducing the adhesiveness of the corneocytes while causing the cornified epithelium to swell, soften, macerate and finally desquamate. In the treatment of warts, a mild irritant reaction,

which may render the virus more prone to immunologic stimulation or response, may add to the mechanical removal of infected cells. The other active ingredient, lactic acid, enhances the availability of the salicylic acid from the dried collodion, in addition to having antiseptic and caustic properties.

*Pharmacokinetic properties:* Salatac Gel contains 12% salicylic acid and 4% lactic acid in an evaporative collodion-like gel which forms a cohesive and adhesive film on the skin.

The formulation is presented in a collapsible aluminium tube fitted with a special applicator nozzle allowing the formulation to be dispensed precisely to the affected areas only. This minimises the spread of the preparation onto the surrounding healthy skin.

The gel quickly forms a surface film, well before it dries completely, thereby prolonging the period during which the keratolytic solution can properly infiltrate and achieve intimate contact with the surface layers of the thickened stratum corneum.

Furthermore, even when the film appears to have dried completely, the inclusion of the non-evaporative lactic acid ensures that a proportion of the salicylic acid remains in solution within the vehicle, thus permitting continued release of the keratolytic, which may otherwise be entrapped within the collodion-like film.

Systemic absorption of salicylic acid or lactic acid after application of the recommended daily dose of one or two drops of the preparation to small, circumscribed areas is exceedingly unlikely.

*Pre-clinical safety data:* No special information.

**Pharmaceutical particulars**

*List of excipients:* Camphor BP; Pyroxylin BP; Ethanol (96%) BP; Ethyl Acetate.

*Incompatibilities:* None known.

*Shelf life:* 36 months.

*Special precautions for storage:* Highly flammable – keep away from flames. Store at room temperature, not exceeding 25°C.

*Nature and contents of container:* Collapsible tube containing 8 g, complete with special applicator, emery board and instructions. This is supplied as an original pack (OP).

*Instructions for use/handling:* Not applicable.

**Marketing authorisation number**  0173/0046.

**Date of approval/revision of SPC**  February 1996.

**Legal category** P.

*Trade Mark

# E. C. De Witt & Company Limited
## Tudor Road, Manor Park
## Runcorn, Cheshire WA7 1SZ

## FLEET* MICRO-ENEMA

**Presentation** A ready-to-use, disposable micro-enema contained in a 5 ml tube, with an integral finger guard and a soft pre-lubricated Comfortip* with a protective sheath. Fleet Micro-enema delivers 5 ml of a smooth white, opaque solution rectally, and contains 450 mg Sodium Citrate BP and 45 mg Sodium Lauryl Sulphoacetate. Excipients: Glycerin BP/PhEur, Sorbitol BP/PhEur, Propylene Glycol BP, Carbomer BP.

**Uses** For the treatment of occasional constipation in bedridden patients, geriatrics, paediatrics and obstetrics.

**Dosage and administration**
*Dosage: Adults and children aged 3 years and over:* Administer the contents of one Fleet Micro-enema rectally 15 minutes before effect is wanted. Do not administer to children under 3 years of age.
For rectal use only.
*Directions for use:* Lie on left side with both knees bent and arms at rest.

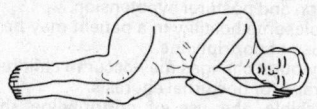

*Remove orange protective shield.* Pull shield gently while grasping grooved cap underneath finger guard.

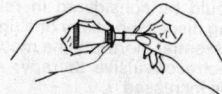

With steady pressure, gently insert pre-lubricated nozzle full length into the rectum with tip pointing towards navel. Squeeze tube until contents are expelled.
Discontinue use if resistance is encountered – forcing an enema can result in injury.

**Contra-indications, warnings, etc**
*Contra-indications:* It is advisable to avoid the use of Fleet Micro-enema in cases of haemorrhoid eruptions and in patients with inflammatory bowel disease.
*Warnings:* Excessive use may cause diarrhoea and fluid loss, which should be treated symptomatically. Propylene Glycol can cause local irritancy and hypersensitivity. Frequent or prolonged use of a laxative for more than one week may result in dependence.
Rectal bleeding or failure to have a bowel movement after use of a laxative may indicate a serious condition. Discontinue use and consult a doctor.
In case of accidental ingestion, seek medical advice.
*Use in pregnancy and lactation:* Use only under medical supervision.
Keep out of reach of children.

**Pharmaceutical precautions** Store below 25°C.

**Legal category** P.

**Package quantities** 5 ml ready-to-use, disposable tubes, packed in 12s.

**Further information** The laxative action is due to the combined action of sodium citrate and sodium lauryl sulphoacetate. Sodium citrate acts by retaining fluid in the bowel by osmosis and by changing the pattern of water distribution in the faeces, while sodium lauryl sulphoacetate is a wetting agent.

**Product licence number** 0083/0045.


## FLEET* PHOSPHO-SODA*

**Presentation** Two polyethylene bottles, each containing 45 ml of a clear, colourless, ginger-lemon flavoured solution for oral use, with the equivalent of 24.4 g (54.3% w/v) Sodium Dihydrogen Phosphate Dihydrate PhEur and 10.8 g (24.0% w/v) Disodium Phosphate Dodecahydrate PhEur per 45 ml. Sodium content is 5.0 g per 45 ml. Excipients: Glycerol, Sodium Saccharin, Sodium Benzoate (E211), Ginger-lemon flavouring, Purified water. The product is sugar free.

**Uses** For use as a purgative for bowel cleansing in preparation for surgery or preparing the colon for x-ray or endoscopic examination.

**Dosage and administration**
*Dosage: Adults only:* Unless directed by a physician, Fleet Phospho-soda should be taken in the morning and in the evening on the day before examination or surgery.
Note: No solid foods may be taken for breakfast, lunch or evening meal on the day of taking this medicine. The liquid 'diet' indicated should be strictly adhered to.
*1st dose – At 7 a.m. (morning) on the day before examination or surgery:* Dilute total contents of one bottle (45 ml) in half a glass (120 ml) of cool water. Drink this solution, followed by one full glass (240 ml) of cool water. At mid-day, follow with at least three full glasses (720 ml) of water or 'clear liquid', more if desired.
'Clear liquids' include water, clear soup, strained fruit juices without pulp, black tea or black coffee, clear carbonated and non-carbonated soft drinks.
*2nd dose – At 7 p.m. (evening) on the day before examination or surgery:* Dilute total contents of the second bottle (45 ml) in half a glass (120 ml) of cool water. Drink this solution followed by one full glass (240 ml) of cool water. Additional 'clear liquid' may be taken up until midnight if necessary.
Not to be given to children.
This product normally produces a bowel movement in ½–6 hours.

**Contra-indications, warnings, etc**
*Contra-indications:* Fleet Phospho-soda is contra-indicated in patients with known or suspected gastro-intestinal obstruction or ileus. Do not use in patients with congestive heart failure, Hirschsprung's Disease or congenital megacolon. Do not use when nausea, vomiting or abdominal pain are present, unless directed by a physician.
*Warnings:* Use with caution in patients with impaired renal function, heart disease, colostomy or on a low salt diet as hyperphosphataemia, hypocalcaemia, hypernatraemic dehydration and acidosis may occur.
Patients should be warned to expect frequent, liquid stools.
*Interactions:* Use with caution in patients taking calcium channel blockers, diuretics, lithium treatment or other medication that might affect electrolyte levels as hyperphosphataemia, hypocalcaemia, hypernatraemic dehydration and acidosis may occur.
*Use in pregnancy and lactation:* Use under medical supervision only.
Keep out of reach of children.
*Overdose:* Recovery from the toxic effects of accidental excess ingestion can normally be achieved by rehydration, though the intravenous administration of 10% calcium gluconate may be necessary.

**Pharmaceutical precautions** Store below 25°C. Do not refrigerate.

**Legal category** P.

**Package quantities** Two single-dose disposable bottles, each containing 45 ml of solution in a single carton.

**Further information** Fleet Phospho-soda is a saline laxative which acts by osmotic processes to increase fluid retention in the lumen of the small intestine. Fluid accumulation in the ileum produces distension, in turn promoting peristalsis and evacuation.

**Product licence number** 0083/0044.


## FLEET* READY-TO-USE ENEMA

**Presentation** A ready-to-use, self-contained, disposable enema. Each 118 ml (delivered dose) contains the equivalent of Sodium Acid Phosphate 21.4 g (18.1% w/v) and Sodium Phosphate 9.4 g (8.0% w/v). Sodium content: 4.4 g per delivered dose. Excipients: Benzalkonium Chloride, Disodium Edetate, Purified Water.

**Uses** For use in the relief of occasional constipation. For pre- and post-operative bowel cleansing, in obstetrics and prior to proctoscopy, sigmoidoscopy or X-ray examination.

**Dosage and administration**
*Adults and children 12 years and over:* One enema (118 ml delivered dose), no more than once daily or as directed by a physician.
*Children 3 years to under 12:* As directed by physician.
Do not administer to children under 3 years of age.
For rectal use only.
*Directions for use:* Remove protective orange shield before use. *Positioning:* Lie on left side, with both knees bent, arms at rest.

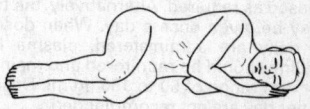

The enema should be gently inserted into the anus with steady pressure, bottle tip pointing towards the navel. The bottle should then be squeezed until nearly all the liquid is expelled. The bottle contains more than the amount of liquid needed for effective use.
Maintain patient position until the urge to evacuate is strong – usually within 2 to 5 minutes.
Application should be discontinued if resistance is encountered, as injury may otherwise occur.

**Contra-indications, warnings, etc**
*Contra-indications:* Do not use in patients with congenital megacolon, Hirschsprung's Disease, imperforate anus or congestive heart failure. Use with caution in patients with impaired renal function, heart disease, colostomy, or pre-existing electrolyte disturbances such as dehydration or those secondary to the use of diuretics as hyperphosphataemia, hypocalcaemia, hypernatraemia and acidosis may occur.
*Warnings, precautions:* Rectal bleeding or failure to have a bowel movement after use of a laxative may indicate a serious condition. Use should be discontinued and medical advice sought.
*Special precautions:* Fleet Ready-to-use enema should be administered according to the directions for use to be found above and on the carton.
*Use in pregnancy and lactation:* For use only under medical supervision.
*Interactions:* Use with caution in patients on calcium channel blockers, diuretics or other medications which may affect electrolyte levels as hypocalcaemia, hyperphosphataemia, hypernatraemia and acidosis may occur.
*Special warnings:* Do not use when nausea, vomiting or abdominal pain is present unless directed by a physician. Do not use for more than two weeks without advice from a physician.
As with all laxatives, prolonged, repeated use is not recommended, as dependence may result.
Keep out of reach of children.
In case of accidental ingestion or overdose seek medical advice.

**Pharmaceutical precautions** Store below 25°C. Do not refrigerate.

**Legal category** P.

**Further information** Phosphates act as a mild saline laxative when administered by the rectal route as enemas. They stimulate peristalsis, leading to an approximately normal bowel movement, in that only the rectum, sigmoid colon and part of the descending colon are involved.

**Product licence number** 0083/0043.

*Trade Mark

**Dista Products Limited**
Kingsclere Road,
Basingstoke,
Hants. RG21 6XA

1996
THE QUEEN'S AWARD FOR EXPORT ACHIEVEMENT

DISTA

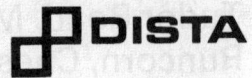

## ALLEGRON*

**Presentation** Tablets each containing Nortriptyline Hydrochloride BP equivalent to 25 mg nortriptyline. The tablets are orange, scored and have a diameter of 8 mm. They are marked 'DISTA'.

Tablets each containing Nortriptyline Hydrochloride BP equivalent to 10 mg nortriptyline. The tablets are white, unscored and have a diameter of 5.5 mm. They are marked 'DISTA'.

**Uses** Allegron is indicated for the relief of symptoms of depression. It may also be used for the treatment of some cases of nocturnal enuresis.

**Dosage and administration** For oral administration.

*Adults:* The usual adult dose is 25 mg three or four times daily. Dosage should begin at a low level and be increased as required. Alternatively, the total daily dose may be given once a day. When doses above 100 mg daily are administered, plasma levels of nortriptyline should be monitored and maintained in the optimum range of 50 to 150 ng/ml. Doses above 150 mg per day are not recommended.

Lower than usual dosages are recommended for elderly patients and adolescents. Lower dosages are also recommended for outpatients than for hospitalised patients who will be under close supervision. The physician should initiate dosage at a low level and increase it gradually, noting carefully the clinical response and any evidence of intolerance. Following remission, maintenance medication may be required for a longer period of time at the lowest dose that will maintain remission.

If a patient develops minor side-effects, the dosage should be reduced. The drug should be discontinued promptly if adverse effects of a serious nature or allergic manifestations occur.

*The elderly:* 30 to 50 mg/day in divided doses.

*Adolescent patients:* 30 to 50 mg/day in divided doses.

*Plasma levels:* Optimal responses to nortriptyline have been associated with plasma concentrations of 50 to 150 ng/ml. Higher concentrations may be associated with more adverse experiences. Plasma concentrations are difficult to measure, and physicians should consult the laboratory professional staff.

Many antidepressants (tricyclic antidepressants, including nortriptyline, selective serotonin re-uptake inhibitors and others) are metabolised by the hepatic cytochrome P450 isoenzyme P450IID6. Three to ten per cent of the population have reduced isoenzyme activity ('poor metabolisers') and may have higher than expected plasma concentrations at usual doses. The percentage of 'poor metabolisers' in a population is also affected by its ethnic origin.

Older patients have been reported to have higher plasma concentrations of the active nortriptyline metabolite 10-hydroxynortriptyline. In one case, this was associated with apparent cardiotoxicity, despite the fact that nortriptyline concentrations were within the 'therapeutic range'. Clinical findings should predominate over plasma concentrations as primary determinants of dosage changes.

*Children:* (for nocturnal enuresis only).

| Age (years) | Weight kg | Weight lb | Dose (mg) |
|---|---|---|---|
| 6-7 | 20-25 | 44-55 | 10 |
| 8-11 | 25-35 | 55-77 | 10-20 |
| >11 | 35-54 | 77-119 | 25-35 |

The dose should be administered thirty minutes before bedtime.

The maximum period of treatment should not exceed three months. A further course of treatment should not be started until a full physical examination, including an ECG, has been made.

**Contra-indications, warnings, etc**

*Contra-indications:* Hypersensitivity to nortriptyline.

Recent myocardial infarction, any degree of heart block or other cardiac arrhythmias.

Severe liver disease. Mania.

Nortriptyline is contra-indicated for the nursing mother and for children under the age of six years.

Please also refer to 'Drug interactions' section.

*Warnings:* As improvement may not occur during the initial weeks of therapy, patients, especially those posing a high suicidal risk, should be closely monitored during this period.

Withdrawal symptoms, including insomnia, irritability and excessive perspiration, may occur on abrupt cessation of therapy.

The use of nortriptyline in schizophrenic patients may result in an exacerbation of the psychosis or may activate latent schizophrenic symptoms. If administered to overactive or agitated patients, increased anxiety and agitation may occur. In manic-depressive patients, nortriptyline may cause symptoms of the manic phase to emerge.

Cross sensitivity between nortriptyline and other tricyclic antidepressants is a possibility.

Patients with cardiovascular disease should be given nortriptyline only under close supervision because of the tendency of the drug to produce sinus tachycardia and to prolong the conduction time. Myocardial infarction, arrhythmia and strokes have occurred. Great care is necessary if nortriptyline is administered to hyperthyroid patients or to those receiving thyroid medication, since cardiac arrhythmias may develop.

The use of nortriptyline should be avoided, if possible, in patients with a history of epilepsy. If it is used, however, the patients should be observed carefully at the beginning of treatment, for nortriptyline is known to lower the convulsive threshold.

Nortriptyline may impair the mental and/or physical abilities required for the performance of hazardous tasks, such as operating machinery or driving a car; therefore the patient should be warned accordingly.

*Drug interactions:* Under no circumstances should nortriptyline be given concurrently with, or within two weeks of cessation of, therapy with monoamine oxidase inhibitors. Hyperpyretic crises, severe convulsions and fatalities have occurred when similar tricyclic antidepressants were used in such combinations.

Nortriptyline should not be given with sympathomimetic agents such as adrenaline, ephedrine, isoprenaline, noradrenaline, phenylephrine and phenylpropanolamine.

Nortriptyline may decrease the antihypertensive effect of guanethidine, debrisoquine, bethanidine and possibly clonidine. Concurrent administration of reserpine has been shown to produce a 'stimulating' effect in some depressed patients. It would be advisable to review all antihypertensive therapy during treatment with tricyclic antidepressants.

Barbiturates may increase the rate of metabolism of nortriptyline.

Anaesthetics given during tricyclic antidepressant therapy may increase the risk of arrhythmias and hypotension. If surgery is necessary, the drug should be discontinued, if possible, for several days prior to the procedure, or the anaesthetist should be informed if the patient is still receiving therapy.

Tricyclic antidepressants may potentiate the CNS depressant effect of alcohol.

The potentiating effect of excessive consumption of alcohol may lead to increased suicidal attempts or overdosage, especially in patients with histories of emotional disturbances or suicidal ideation.

Steady-state serum concentrations of the tricyclic antidepressants are reported to fluctuate significantly as cimetidine is either added to or deleted from the drug regimen. Higher than expected steady-state serum concentrations of the tricyclic antidepressant have been observed when therapy is initiated in patients already taking cimetidine. A decrease may occur when cimetidine therapy is discontinued.

Because nortriptyline's metabolism (like other tricyclic and SSRI antidepressants) involves the hepatic cytochrome P450IID6 isoenzyme system, concomitant therapy with drugs also metabolised by this system may lead to drug interactions. Lower doses than are usually prescribed for either the tricyclic antidepressant or the other drug may therefore be required.

Greater than two-fold increases in previously stable plasma levels of nortriptyline have occurred when fluoxetine was administered concomitantly. Fluoxetine and its active metabolite, norfluoxetine, have long half-lives (4–16 days for norfluoxetine).

Concomitant therapy with other drugs that are metabolised by this isoenzyme, including other antidepressants, phenothiazines, carbamazepine, propafenone, flecainide and encainide, or that inhibit this enzyme (e.g. quinidine), should be approached with caution.

Supervision and adjustment of dosage may be required when nortriptyline is used with other anticholinergic drugs.

*Usage in pregnancy:* The safety of nortriptyline for use during pregnancy has not been established, nor is there evidence from animal studies that it is free from hazard; therefore the drug should not be administered to pregnant patients or women of childbearing age unless the potential benefits clearly outweigh any potential risk.

*Usage in nursing mothers:* See *Contra-indications.*

*Precautions:* The elderly are particularly liable to experience adverse reactions, especially agitation, confusion and postural hypotension.

Troublesome hostility in a patient may be aroused by the use of nortriptyline.

Behavioural changes may occur in children receiving therapy for nocturnal enuresis.

If possible, the use of nortriptyline should be avoided in patients with narrow angle glaucoma or symptoms suggestive of prostatic hypertrophy.

The possibility of a suicide attempt by a depressed patient remains after the initiation of treatment. This possibility should be considered in relation to the quantity of drug dispensed at any one time.

When it is essential, nortriptyline may be administered with electroconvulsive therapy, although the hazards may be increased.

Both elevation and lowering of blood sugar levels have been reported. Significant hypoglycaemia was reported in a Type II diabetic patient maintained on chlorpropamide (250 mg/day), after the addition of nortriptyline (125 mg/day).

*Side-effects:* Included in the following list are a few adverse reactions that have not been reported with this specific drug. However, the pharmacological similarities among the tricyclic antidepressant drugs require that each of the reactions be considered when nortriptyline is administered.

*Cardiovascular:* Hypotension, hypertension, tachycardia, palpitation, myocardial infarction, arrhythmias, heart block, stroke.

*Psychiatric:* Confusional states (especially in the elderly) with hallucinations, disorientation, delusions; anxiety, restlessness, agitation; insomnia, panic, nightmares; hypomania; exacerbation of psychosis.

*Neurological:* Numbness, tingling, paraesthesia of extremities; inco-ordination, ataxia, tremors; peripheral neuropathy; extrapyramidal symptoms; seizures, alteration of EEG patterns; tinnitus.

*Anticholinergic:* Dry mouth and, rarely, associated sublingual adenitis or gingivitis; blurred vision, disturbance of accommodation, mydriasis; constipation, paralytic ileus; urinary retention, delayed micturition, dilation of the urinary tract.

*Allergic:* Rash, petechiae, urticaria, itching, photosensitisation (avoid excessive exposure to sunlight); oedema (general or of face and tongue), drug fever, cross-sensitivity with other tricyclic drugs.

*Haematological:* Bone-marrow depression, including agranulocytosis; aplastic anaemia; eosinophilia; purpura; thrombocytopenia.

*Gastro-intestinal:* Nausea and vomiting, anorexia, epigastric distress, diarrhoea; peculiar taste, stomatitis, abdominal cramps, black tongue, constipation, paralytic ileus.

*Endocrine:* Gynaecomastia in the male; breast enlargement and galactorrhoea in the female; increased or decreased libido, impotence; testicular swelling; elevation or depression of blood sugar levels; syndrome of inappropriate secretion of antidiuretic hormone.

*Other:* Jaundice (simulating obstructive); altered liver function, hepatitis and liver necrosis; weight gain or loss; sweating; flushing; urinary frequency, nocturia; drowsiness, dizziness, weakness, fatigue; headache; parotid swelling; alopecia.

*Withdrawal symptoms:* Though these are not indicative of addiction, abrupt cessation of treatment after prolonged therapy may produce nausea, headache and malaise.

*Overdosage*

*Signs and symptoms:* 50 mg of a tricyclic antidepressant can be an overdose in a child. Of patients who are alive at presentation, mortality of 0-15% has been reported. Symptoms may begin within several hours and may include blurred vision, confusion, restlessness, dizziness, hypothermia, hyperthermia, agitation, vomiting, hyperactive reflexes, dilated pupils, fever, rapid heart rate, decreased bowel sounds, dry mouth, inability to void, myoclonic jerks, seizures, respiratory depression, myoglobinuric renal failure, nystagmus, ataxia, dysarthria, choreoathetosis, coma, hypotension and cardiac arrhythmias. Cardiac conduction may be slowed, with prolongation of QRS complex and QT intervals, right bundle branch and AV block, ventricular tachyarrhythmias (including Torsade de pointes and fibrillation) and death. Prolongation of QRS duration to more than 100 msec is predictive of more severe toxicity. The absence of sinus tachycardia does not ensure a benign course. Hypotension may be caused by vasodilatation, central and peripheral alpha-adrenergic blockade and cardiac depression. In a healthy young person, prolonged resuscitation may be effective; one patient survived 5 hours of cardiac massage.

*Treatment:* Symptomatic and supportive therapy is recommended. Activated charcoal may be more effective than emesis or lavage to reduce absorption.

Ventricular arrhythmias, especially when accompanied by lengthened QRS intervals, may respond to alkalinisation by hyperventilation or administration of sodium bicarbonate. Serum electrolytes should be monitored and managed. Refractory arrhythmias may respond to propranolol, bretylium or lignocaine. Quinidine and procainamide usually should not be used because they may exacerbate arrhythmias and conduction already slowed by the overdose.

Seizures may respond to diazepam. Phenytoin may treat seizures and cardiac rhythm disturbances. Physostigmine may antagonise atrial tachycardia, gut immotility, myoclonic jerks and somnolence. The effects of physostigmine may be short-lived.

Diuresis and dialysis have little effect. Haemoperfusion is unproven. Monitoring should continue, at least until the QRS duration is normal.

**Pharmaceutical precautions** Store below 25°C.

**Legal category** POM.

**Package quantities**
Tablets 25 mg: Bottles of 100
Tablets 10 mg: Bottles of 100

**Further information** Nil.

**Product licence numbers**
Tablets 25 mg: 0006/5003
Tablets 10 mg: 0006/5002

## CAPASTAT*

**Presentation** Capreomycin sulphate as sterile white powder for intramuscular injection only, in sealed vials each containing 1,000,000 units (approximately equivalent to 1 g capreomycin base).

**Uses**

*Actions:* Capreomycin is active against human strains of *Mycobacterium tuberculosis.*

Frequent cross-resistance occurs between capreomycin and viomycin. Varying degrees of cross-resistance between capreomycin and kanamycin and neomycin have been reported. No cross-resistance has been observed between capreomycin and isoniazid, aminosalicylic acid, cycloserine, streptomycin, ethionamide or ethambutol.

*Indications:* Capastat should be used concomitantly with other appropriate antituberculous agents for the treatment of pulmonary infections caused by capreomycin-susceptible strains of *Mycobacterium tuberculosis* when the primary agents (isoniazid, rifampicin, streptomycin and ethambutol) have been ineffective or cannot be used because of toxicity or the presence of resistant tubercle bacilli.

**Dosage and administration** The usual dose is 1 g daily (but 20 mg/kg/day should not be exceeded) given by deep intramuscular injection only for 60 to 120 days, followed by 1 g intramuscularly two or three times a week. Capastat is always administered in combination with at least one other antituberculous agent to which the patient's strain of tubercle bacillus is susceptible.

Capastat should be dissolved in 2 ml of 0.9% Sodium Chloride Intravenous Infusion BP or Water for Injections PhEur. Two to three minutes should be allowed for complete solution.

For administration of a 1 g dose, the entire contents of the vial should be given. For dosages of less than 1 g the following dilution table may be used:

| *Diluent to be added (ml)* | *Approximate volume of Capastat solution (ml)* | *Approximate average concentration (mg/ml) in terms of mg of capreomycin activity* |
|---|---|---|
| 2.15 | 2.85 | 350 |
| 2.63 | 3.33 | 300 |
| 3.3 | 4.0 | 250 |
| 4.3 | 5.0 | 200 |

*The elderly:* As for adults. Reduce dosage if renal function is impaired.

*Patients with reduced renal function:* A reduced dosage should be given based on creatinine clearance using the guidance given in the following table. These dosages are designed to achieve a mean steady-state capreomycin level of 10 micrograms/ml, at various levels of renal function:

| *Creatinine clearance (ml/min)* | *Capreomycin clearance (l/kg/h X $10^{-2}$)* | *Half-life (hours)* | *Dose for these dosing intervals (mg/kg)* | | |
|---|---|---|---|---|---|
| | | | *24 h* | *48 h* | *72 h* |
| 0 | 0.54 | 55.5 | 1.29 | 2.58 | 3.87 |
| 10 | 1.01 | 29.4 | 2.43 | 4.87 | 7.30 |
| 20 | 1.49 | 20.0 | 3.58 | 7.16 | 10.70 |
| 30 | 1.97 | 15.1 | 4.72 | 9.45 | 14.20 |
| 40 | 2.45 | 12.2 | 5.87 | 11.70 | |
| 50 | 2.92 | 10.2 | 7.01 | 14.00 | |
| 60 | 3.40 | 8.8 | 8.16 | | |
| 80 | 4.35 | 6.8 | 10.40 | | |
| 100 | 5.31 | 5.6 | 12.70 | | |
| 110 | 5.78 | 5.2 | 13.90 | | |

*Infants and children:* Not for paediatric use, since the safety of capreomycin for use in infants and children has not been established.

**Contra-indications, warnings, etc**

*Contra-indication:* Hypersensitivity to capreomycin.

*Warnings:* The use of capreomycin in patients with renal insufficiency or pre-existing auditory impairment must be undertaken with great caution, and the risk of additional eighth cranial nerve impairment or renal injury should be weighed against the benefits to be derived from treatment.

Simultaneous administration of other antituberculous drugs which also have ototoxic and nephrotoxic potential (e.g. streptomycin, viomycin) is not recommended. Also, use with other drugs that are not given for the treatment of tuberculosis but have ototoxic or nephrotoxic potential (e.g. polymyxin, colistin sulphate, amikacin, gentamicin, tobramycin, vancomycin, kanamycin and neomycin) should also be undertaken only with great caution.

*Pregnancy:* The safety of capreomycin for use during pregnancy has not been established. Capreomycin has been shown to be teratogenic in rats when given at 3.5 times the human dose. There are no adequate and well controlled studies in pregnant women. Capastat should be used during pregnancy only if the potential benefit justifies the potential risk to the foetus.

Studies have not been performed to determine potential for carcinogenicity, mutagenicity, or impairment of fertility.

*Nursing mothers:* It is not known whether capreomycin is excreted in human milk. Caution should be exercised when administering to a nursing woman.

*Precautions:* As capreomycin is potentially ototoxic, audiometry and assessment of vestibular function should be performed before starting treatment and at regular intervals during treatment.

Regular tests of renal function should be made throughout the period of treatment, and reduced dosage should be used in patients with known, or suspected, renal impairment (see 'Dosage and administration').

Since hypokalaemia may occur during capreomycin therapy, serum potassium levels should be determined frequently.

A partial neuromuscular block can occur after large doses of capreomycin.

Capreomycin should be administered cautiously to patients with a history of allergy, particularly to drugs.

*Side-effects*

*Renal:* Elevation of serum creatinine or blood urea and abnormal urine sediment have been observed. Toxic nephritis was reported in one patient with tuberculosis and portal cirrhosis who was treated with capreomycin (1 g) and aminosalicylic acid daily for one month. This patient developed renal insufficiency and oliguria and died. The post-mortem showed subsiding acute tubular necrosis.

Electrolyte disturbances resembling Bartter's syndrome have been reported in one patient.

*Hepatic:* A decrease in bromsulphthalein excretion without change in serum enzymes has been noted in the presence of pre-existing liver disease. Abnormal results in liver function tests have occurred in many patients receiving capreomycin in combination with other antituberculous agents which are also known to cause changes in hepatic function. Periodic determinations of liver function are recommended.

*Haematological:* Leucocytosis and leucopenia have been observed. Rare cases of thrombocytopenia have been reported. Most patients receiving daily capreomycin have had eosinophilia exceeding 5%, but this has subsided with the reduction of capreomycin dosage to two or three times weekly.

*Hypersensitivity:* Urticaria and maculopapular rashes associated in some cases with febrile reactions have been reported when capreomycin and other antituberculous drugs were given concomitantly.

*Otic:* Clinical and subclinical auditory loss has been noted. Some audiometric changes have proved reversible and others with permanent loss have not been progressive following withdrawal of capreomycin. Tinnitus and vertigo have occurred.

*Injection site reactions:* Pain and induration at injection sites have been observed. Excessive bleeding and sterile abscesses have also been reported at these sites.

*Overdosage*

*Signs and symptoms:* Hypokalaemia, hypocalcaemia, hypomagnesaemia and an electrolyte disturbance resembling Bartter's syndrome have been reported to occur in patients with capreomycin toxicity. Nephrotoxicity, including acute tubular necrosis; and ototoxicity, including dizziness, tinnitus, vertigo and loss of high-tone acuity (see 'Warnings' and 'Precautions'). Neuromuscular blockage or respiratory paralysis may occur following rapid intravenous administration.

If capreomycin is ingested, toxicity is unlikely because less than 1% is absorbed from an intact gastro-intestinal system.

*Treatment:* Symptomatic and supportive therapy is recommended. Activated charcoal may be more effective than emesis or lavage in reducing absorption.

Patients who have received an overdose of capreomycin and have normal renal function should be hydrated to maintain a urine output of 3-5 ml/kg/hr. Fluid balance electrolytes and creatinine clearance should be monitored.

Haemodialysis is effective in patients with significant renal disease.

**Pharmaceutical precautions** Store below 25°C. The reconstituted product should be used within 24 hours.

The solution may acquire a pale straw colour and darken with time, but this is not associated with loss of potency or the development of toxicity.

**Legal category** POM.

**Package quantities** Vials of 1,000,000 units (1 g base approximately): Pack of 5 vials.

**Further information** Capastat must be used only in conjunction with adequate doses of other antituberculous drugs. The use of Capastat alone allows the rapid development of strains resistant to it.

**Product licence number** 0006/5005.

## DISTACLOR*

**Presentation** Capsules (violet and grey, printed Lilly 3062) containing 500 mg cefaclor.

Granules (pink) for suspension containing 125 mg cefaclor/5 ml.

Granules (pink) for suspension containing 250 mg cefaclor/5 ml.

**Uses** Distaclor is indicated for the treatment of the following infections due to susceptible micro-organisms:

Respiratory tract infections, including pneumonia, bronchitis, exacerbations of chronic bronchitis, pharyngitis and tonsillitis, and as part of the management of sinusitis
Otitis media
Skin and soft tissue infections
Urinary tract infections, including pyelonephritis and cystitis
Distaclor has been found to be effective in both acute and chronic urinary tract infections.

Cefaclor is active against the following organisms *in vitro:*
Alpha- and beta-haemolytic streptococci
Staphylococci; including coagulase-positive, coagulase-negative and penicillinase-producing strains
*Streptococcus pneumoniae*
*Streptococcus pyogenes* (group A beta-haemolytic streptococci)
*Branhamella catarrhalis*
*Escherichia coli*
*Proteus mirabilis*
*Klebsiella* species
*Haemophilus influenzae,* including ampicillin-resistant strains.

Cefaclor has no activity against *Pseudomonas* species or *Acinetobacter* species. Methicillin-resistant staphylococci and most strains of enterococci (e.g. *Str. faecalis*) are resistant to cefaclor. Cefaclor is not active against most strains of *Enterobacter* spp, *Serratia* spp, *Morganella morganii*, *Proteus vulgaris* and *Providencia rettgeri*.

Cefaclor is generally effective in the eradication of streptococci from the nasopharynx, however, data establishing efficacy in the subsequent prevention of either rheumatic fever or bacterial endocarditis are not available.

**Dosage and administration** Distaclor is administered orally.

*Adults:* The usual adult dosage is 250 mg every eight hours. For more severe infections or those caused by less susceptible organisms, doses may be doubled. Doses of 4 g per day have been administered safely to normal subjects for 28 days, but the total daily dosage should not exceed this amount.

Please see the separate Distaclor MR data sheet for extended release tablets of cefaclor, equivalent to 375 mg cefaclor.

Distaclor may be administered in the presence of impaired renal function. Under such conditions dosage is usually unchanged (see *Precautions*).

*Patients undergoing haemodialysis:* Haemodialysis shortens serum half-life by 25–30%. In patients undergoing regular haemodialysis, a loading dose of 250 mg–1 g administered prior to dialysis and a therapeutic dose of 250–500 mg every six to eight hours maintained during interdialytic periods is recommended.

*The elderly:* As for adults.

*Children:* The usual recommended daily dosage for children is 20 mg/kg/day in divided doses every eight hours, as indicated. For bronchitis and pneumonia, the dosage is 20 mg/kg/day in divided doses administered 3 times daily. For otitis media and pharyngitis, the total daily dosage may be divided and administered every 12 hours. Safety and efficacy have not been established for use in infants aged less than one month.

*Distaclor Suspension*

|  | 125 mg/5 ml | 250 mg/5 ml |
|---|---|---|
| <1 year (9 kg) | 2.5 ml t.i.d. | |
| 1–5 years (9–18 kg) | 5.0 ml t.i.d. | |
| Over 5 years | | 5.0 ml t.i.d. |

In more serious infections, otitis media, sinusitis and infections caused by less susceptible organisms, 40 mg/kg/day in divided doses is recommended, up to a daily maximum of 1 g.

In the treatment of beta-haemolytic streptococcal infections, therapy should be continued for at least 10 days.

**Contra-indications, warnings, etc**
*Contra-indication:* Hypersensitivity to cephalosporins.

*Warnings:* Before instituting therapy with cefaclor, every effort should be made to determine whether the patient has had previous hypersensitivity reactions to cefaclor, cephalosporins, penicillins or other drugs. Cefaclor should be given cautiously to penicillin-sensitive patients, because cross-hypersensitivity, including anaphylaxis, among beta-lactam antibiotics has been clearly documented.

If an allergic reaction to cefaclor occurs, the drug should be discontinued and the patient treated with the appropriate agents.

Pseudomembranous colitis has been reported with virtually all broad-spectrum antibiotics, including macrolides, semi-synthetic penicillins and cephalosporins. It is important, therefore, to consider its diagnosis in patients who develop diarrhoea in association with the use of antibiotics. Such colitis may range in severity from mild to life-threatening. Mild cases usually respond to drug discontinuance alone. In moderate to severe cases, appropriate measures should be taken.

*Usage in pregnancy:* Animal studies have shown no evidence of impaired fertility or teratogenicity. However, since there are no adequate or well-controlled studies in pregnant women, caution should be exercised when prescribing for the pregnant patient.

*Usage in nursing mothers:* Small amounts of cefaclor have been detected in breast milk following administration of single 500 mg doses. Average levels of about 0.2 micrograms/ml or less were detected up to 5 hours later. Trace amounts were detected at one hour. As the effect on nursing infants is not known, caution should be exercised when cefaclor is administered to a nursing woman.

*Precautions:* Cefaclor should be administered with caution in the presence of markedly impaired renal function. Since the half-life of cefaclor in anuric patients is 2.3 to 2.8 hours (compared to 0.6–0.9 hours

in normal subjects), dosage adjustments for patients with moderate or severe renal impairment are not usually required. Clinical experience with cefaclor under such conditions is limited; therefore, careful clinical observation and laboratory studies should be made.

Broad-spectrum antibiotics should be prescribed with caution in individuals with a history of gastro-intestinal disease, particularly colitis.

Prolonged use of cefaclor may result in the overgrowth of non-susceptible organisms. If superinfection occurs during therapy, appropriate measures should be taken.

Positive direct Coombs' tests have been reported during treatment with the cephalosporin antibiotics. In haematological studies or in transfusion cross-matching procedures, when anti-globulin tests are performed on the minor side, or in Coombs' testing of newborns whose mothers have received cephalosporin antibiotics before parturition, it should be recognised that a positive Coombs' test may be due to the drug.

A false-positive reaction for glucose in the urine may occur with Benedict's or Fehling's solutions or with copper sulphate test tablets.

*Drug interactions:* There have been rare reports of increased prothrombin time, with or without clinical bleeding, in patients receiving cefaclor and warfarin concomitantly. It is recommended that in such patients, regular monitoring of prothrombin time should be considered, with adjustment of dosage if necessary.

The renal excretion of cefaclor is inhibited by probenecid.

*Side-effects*
*Gastro-intestinal:* The most frequent side-effect has been diarrhoea. It is rarely severe enough to warrant cessation of therapy. Colitis, including rare instances of pseudomembranous colitis, has been reported. Nausea and vomiting have also occurred.

*Hypersensitivity:* Allergic reactions such as morbilliform eruptions, pruritus and urticaria have been observed. These reactions usually subside upon discontinuation of therapy. Serum sickness-like reactions (erythema multiforme minor, rashes or other skin manifestations accompanied by arthritis/arthralgia, with or without fever) have been reported. Lymphadenopathy and proteinuria are infrequent, there are no circulating immune complexes and no evidence of sequelae. Occasionally, solitary symptoms may occur, but do not represent a serum sickness-like reaction. Serum sickness-like reactions are apparently due to hypersensitivity and have usually occurred during or following a second (or subsequent) course of therapy with cefaclor. Such reactions have been reported more frequently in children than in adults. Signs and symptoms usually occur a few days after initiation of therapy and usually subside within a few days of cessation of therapy. Antihistamines and corticosteroids appear to enhance resolution of the syndrome. No serious sequelae have been reported.

There are rare reports of erythema multiforme major (Stevens-Johnson syndrome), toxic epidermal necrolysis, and anaphylaxis. Anaphylaxis may be more common in patients with a history of penicillin allergy. Anaphylactoid events may present as solitary symptoms, including angioedema, asthenia, oedema (including face and limbs), dyspnoea, paraesthesias, syncope, or vasodilatation.

Rarely, hypersensitivity symptoms may persist for several months.

*Haematological:* Eosinophilia, positive Coombs' tests and, rarely, thrombocytopenia. Transient lymphocytosis, leucopenia and, rarely, haemolytic anaemia, aplastic anaemia, agranulocytosis and reversible neutropenia of possible clinical significance. See 'Drug interactions'.

*Hepatic:* Transient hepatitis and cholestatic jaundice have been reported rarely, slight elevations in AST, ALT or alkaline phosphatase values.

*Renal:* Reversible interstitial nephritis has occurred rarely, also slight elevations in blood urea or serum creatinine or abnormal urinalysis.

*Central Nervous System:* Reversible hyperactivity, agitation, nervousness, insomnia, confusion, hypertonia, dizziness, hallucinations and somnolence have been reported rarely.

*Miscellaneous:* Genital pruritus, vaginitis and vaginal moniliasis.

*Overdosage:* Symptoms of nausea, vomiting, epigastric distress and diarrhoea would be anticipated.
*Treatment:* Unless 5 times the normal total daily dose has been ingested, gastro-intestinal decontamination will not be necessary.

General management may consist of supportive therapy.

**Pharmaceutical precautions** Store below 25°C. Keep containers tightly closed and protect from light.

After reconstitution, the 125 mg/5 ml and 250 mg/

5 ml suspensions should be stored in a refrigerator (2°-8°C) and be used within 14 days. When dilution is unavoidable, Syrup BP should be used after the suspension has been prepared according to the manufacturer's instructions.

**Legal category** POM.

**Package quantities**
Capsules 500 mg: Bottles of 50
Suspension 125 mg/5 ml: Bottles of 100 ml
Suspension 250 mg/5 ml: Bottles of 100 ml

**Further information** Nil.

**Product licence numbers**
Capsules 500 mg: 0006/0119
Suspension 125 mg/5 ml: 0006/0120
Suspension 250 mg/5 ml: 0006/0121

## DISTACLOR MR*

**Presentation** Extended release tablets of cefaclor 'Modified Release' (blue, printed Distaclor MR 375), equivalent to 375 mg cefaclor.

Cefaclor 'Modified Release' differs from cefaclor in its rate of dissolution, producing a lower peak serum concentration, but retaining sustained measurable serum concentrations, which provides the advantage of twice daily dosing.

**Uses** Distaclor MR is indicated in the treatment of the following infections when caused by susceptible strains of the designated organisms:

*Acute bronchitis and acute exacerbations of chronic bronchitis* caused by *Streptococcus pneumoniae, Haemophilus influenzae* (including beta-lactamase producing strains), *Haemophilus parainfluenzae, Moraxella catarrhalis* (including beta-lactamase producing strains) and *Staphylococcus aureus.*

*Pharyngitis and tonsillitis* caused by *Streptococcus pyogenes* (group A streptococci).

*Pneumonia* caused by *S. pneumoniae, H. influenzae* (including beta-lactamase producing strains) and *M. catarrhalis* (including beta-lactamase producing strains).

*Uncomplicated lower urinary tract infections,* including cystitis and asymptomatic bacteriuria, caused by *Escherichia coli, Klebsiella pneumoniae, Proteus mirabilis* and *Staphylococcus saprophyticus.*

*Skin and skin structure infections* caused by *S. pyogenes* (group A streptococci), *S. aureus* (including beta-lactamase producing strains) and *Staphylococcus epidermidis* (including beta-lactamase producing strains).

Bacteriological studies, to determine the causative organism and its susceptibility to cefaclor, should be performed. Therapy may be started while awaiting the results of these studies. Once these results become available, antimicrobial therapy should be adjusted accordingly.

Note: Distaclor MR is generally effective in the eradication of streptococci from the oropharynx. However, data establishing the efficacy of this antibiotic in the subsequent prevention of rheumatic fever are not available.

Distaclor MR has been shown to be active *in vitro* against most strains of the following organisms, although clinical efficacy has not been established:

**Gram-negative organisms:**
  *Citrobacter diversus*
  *Neisseria gonorrhoeae*

**Anaerobic organisms:**
  *Propionibacterium acnes*
  *Bacteroides* species (excluding *Bacteroides fragilis*)
  Peptococci
  Peptostreptococci
Note: *Pseudomonas* sp, *Acinetobacter calcoaceticus*, most strains of enterococci, *Enterobacter* sp, indole-positive *Proteus* and *Serratia* sp are resistant to cefaclor. Cefaclor is inactive against methicillin-resistant staphylococci.

Cefaclor is a semi-synthetic cephalosporin antibiotic.

**Dosage and administration** Distaclor MR is administered orally.

*Adults and the elderly: Pharyngitis, bronchitis, tonsillitis, skin and skin structure infections:* 375 mg twice daily.
*Lower urinary tract infections:* 375 mg twice daily.
*Pneumonia:* 750 mg twice daily.

In clinical trials, doses of 1.5 g/day of Distaclor MR have been administered safely for 14 days. Doses of 4 g/day of cefaclor have been administered safely, to normal subjects, for 28 days.

Elderly subjects with normal renal function do not require dosage adjustment.

*Children:* The safety and effectiveness of Distaclor MR have not been established. Cefaclor suspensions are available (see Distaclor data sheet for dosages).

In the treatment of infections caused by *S. pyogenes* (group A streptococci), a therapeutic dosage should be administered for at least 10 days.

Distaclor MR is well absorbed from the gastro-intestinal tract. Since absorption is enhanced by administration with food, Distaclor MR should be taken with meals.

The tablets should not be cut, crushed or chewed.

There is no evidence of metabolism in humans.

### Contra-indications, warnings, etc

*Contra-indication:* Hypersensitivity to cefaclor and other cephalosporins.

*Warnings:* Before instituting therapy with cefaclor, every effort should be made to determine whether the patient has had previous hypersensitivity reactions to the cephalosporins, penicillins or other drugs. Cefaclor should be given cautiously to penicillin-sensitive patients and to any patient who has demonstrated some form of allergy, particularly to drugs.

If an allergic reaction to cefaclor occurs, the drug should be discontinued and the patient treated with the appropriate agents.

Pseudomembranous colitis has been reported with virtually all broad-spectrum antibiotics, including macrolides, semi-synthetic penicillins and cephalosporins. It is important, therefore, to consider its diagnosis in patients who develop diarrhoea in association with the use of antibiotics. Such colitis may range in severity from mild to life-threatening. Mild cases usually respond to drug discontinuance alone. In moderate to severe cases, appropriate measures should be taken.

*Usage in pregnancy:* Although animal studies have shown no evidence of impaired fertility or harm to the foetus due to cefaclor, there are no adequate and well-controlled studies in pregnant women. Distaclor MR should be used during pregnancy only if clearly needed.

*Usage in nursing mothers:* Small amounts of cefaclor have been detected in breast milk following administration of single 500 mg doses. Average levels of about 0.2 micrograms/ml or less were detected up to 5 hours later. Trace amounts were detected at one hour. As the effect on nursing infants is not known, caution should be exercised when cefaclor is administered to a nursing woman. No studies have been done with Distaclor MR.

*Usage during labour and delivery:* Treatment should be given only if clearly needed.

*Precautions:* Prolonged use of cefaclor may result in the overgrowth of non-susceptible organisms. If superinfection occurs during therapy, appropriate measures should be taken.

A false-positive reaction for glucose in the urine may occur with Benedict's or Fehling's solutions or with copper sulphate test tablets.

*Drug interactions:* The extent of absorption of Distaclor MR is diminished if magnesium hydroxide or aluminium hydroxide containing antacids are taken within 1 hour of administration. $H_2$ blockers do not alter either the rate or extent of absorption.

The renal excretion of cefaclor is inhibited by probenecid.

*Adverse reactions:* The majority of adverse reactions observed in clinical trials of Distaclor MR were mild and transient. Drug-related adverse reactions requiring discontinuation of therapy occurred in 1.7% of patients. The following adverse reactions were reported in clinical trials. Incidence rates were less than 1 in 100 (less than 1%), except as stated:

*Gastro-intestinal:* Diarrhoea (3.4%), nausea (2.5%), vomiting and dyspepsia.

*Hypersensitivity:* Rash, urticaria or pruritus occurred in approximately 1.7% of patients. One serum sickness-like reaction (0.03%) was reported among the 3,272 patients treated with Distaclor MR during the controlled clinical trials.

Serum sickness-like reactions (erythema multiforme minor, rashes or other skin manifestations accompanied by arthritis/arthralgia, with or without fever) have been reported with cefaclor. Lymphadenopathy and proteinuria are infrequent, there are no circulating immune complexes and no evidence of sequelae. Occasionally, solitary symptoms may occur, but do not represent a serum sickness-like reaction. Serum sickness-like reactions are apparently due to hypersensitivity and have usually occurred during or following a second (or subsequent) course of therapy with cefaclor. Such reactions have been reported more frequently in children than in adults. Signs and symptoms usually occur a few days after initiation of therapy and usually subside within a few days of cessation of therapy. Antihistamines and corticosteroids appear to enhance resolution of the syndrome. No serious sequelae have been reported.

*Haematological and lymphatic systems:* Eosinophilia.

*Genitourinary:* Vaginal moniliasis (2.5%) and vaginitis (1.7%).

The following adverse effects have been reported, but causal relationship is uncertain:

*Central nervous system:* Headache, dizziness and somnolence.

*Hepatic:* Transient elevations in AST, ALT and alkaline phosphatase.

*Renal:* Transient increase in BUN or creatinine.

*Laboratory tests:* Transient thrombocytopenia, leucopenia, lymphocytosis, neutropenia and abnormal urinalysis.

In addition to the adverse reactions listed above that have been observed in patients taking Distaclor MR, the following have been reported in patients treated with cefaclor:

Erythema multiforme, fever, anaphylaxis (may be more common in patients with a history of penicillin allergy), Stevens–Johnson syndrome, positive direct Coombs' test and genital pruritus. Symptoms of pseudomembranous colitis may appear either during or after antibiotic treatment. Anaphylactoid events may present as solitary symptoms, including angioedema, asthenia, oedema (including face and limbs), dyspnoea, paraesthesias, syncope, or vasodilatation.

Rarely, hypersensitivity symptoms may persist for several months.

The following reactions have been reported rarely in patients treated with cefaclor:

Toxic epidermal necrolysis, reversible interstitial nephritis, hepatic dysfunction, including cholestasis, increased prothrombin time in patients receiving cefaclor and warfarin concomitantly, reversible hyperactivity, agitation, nervousness, insomnia, confusion, hallucinations, hypertonia, aplastic anaemia, agranulocytosis and haemolytic anaemia.

The following adverse reactions have been reported in patients treated with other beta-lactam antibiotics:

Colitis, renal dysfunction and toxic nephropathy.

Several beta-lactam antibiotics have been implicated in triggering seizures, particularly in patients with renal impairment when the dosage was not reduced. If seizures associated with drug therapy should occur, the drug should be discontinued. Anticonvulsant therapy can be given if clinically indicated.

*Overdosage:* Symptoms of nausea, vomiting, epigastric distress and diarrhoea would be anticipated.

General management consists of supportive therapy. Consider activated charcoal instead of, or in addition to, gastric emptying.

Forced diuresis, peritoneal dialysis, haemodialysis or charcoal haemoperfusion have not been established as beneficial.

**Pharmaceutical precautions** Store at room temperature (15°–25°C). Protect from light.

**Legal category** POM

**Package quantity** Blister packs of 14 tablets

**Product licence number** 0006/0274

# DISTALGESIC*
## Approved name: Co-proxamol

**Qualitative and quantitative composition** Each tablet contains 32.5 mg Dextropropoxyphene Hydrochloride BP (equivalent to approximately 30 mg dextropropoxyphene base) with 325 mg Paracetamol PhEur.

**Pharmaceutical form** White, pillow-shaped, film coated tablets, 14 mm in length and marked 'DG'.

### Clinical particulars

*Therapeutic indications:*

*Actions:* Dextropropoxyphene is a mild narcotic analgesic structurally related to methadone.

*Indication:* For the management of mild to moderate pain.

*Posology and method of administration:* For oral administration to adults only. The usual dose is 2 tablets three or four times daily and should not normally be exceeded.

Consideration should be given to a reduced total daily dosage in patients with hepatic or renal impairment.

*The elderly:* There is evidence of prolonged half-life in the elderly, so reduction in dosage should be considered.

*Children:* Distalgesic is not recommended for use in children.

*Contra-indications:* Hypersensitivity to dextropropoxyphene or paracetamol.

Use in patients who are suicidal or addiction-prone.

*Special warnings and special precautions for use:*

*Warnings:* PATIENTS SHOULD BE ADVISED NOT TO EXCEED THE RECOMMENDED DOSE AND TO AVOID ALCOHOL.

Dextropropoxyphene products in excessive doses, either alone or in combination with other CNS depressants, including alcohol, are a major cause of drug-related deaths. Fatalities within the first hour of overdosage are not uncommon and can occur within 15 minutes. Some deaths have occurred as a consequence of the accidental ingestion of excessive quantities of Distalgesic alone, or in combination with other drugs.

Overdosage may damage the liver, due predominantly to the accumulation of intermediate metabolites of paracetamol which cause hepatic necrosis.

Distalgesic should be prescribed with caution for those patients whose medical condition requires the concomitant administration of sedatives, tranquillisers, muscle relaxants, antidepressants or other CNS-depressant drugs; patients should be advised of the additive depressant effects of these combinations. Distalgesic should also be prescribed with caution in patients who use alcohol in excess.

*Drug dependence:* Dextropropoxyphene, when taken in higher than recommended doses over long periods of time, can produce drug dependence.

*Precautions:* Distalgesic should be administered with caution to patients with hepatic or renal impairment since higher serum concentrations or delayed elimination may occur.

*Interaction with other medicaments and other forms of interaction:*

*Drug interactions:* The CNS-depressant effect of dextropropoxyphene is additive with that of other CNS depressants, including alcohol.

Dextropropoxyphene may interfere with the metabolism of antidepressants, anticonvulsants and warfarin-like drugs. Severe neurological signs, including coma, have occurred with concomitant use of carbamazepine.

*Pregnancy and lactation:*

*Pregnancy:* Safety in pregnancy has not been established relative to possible adverse effects on fetal development. Withdrawal symptoms in neonates have been reported following use during pregnancy. Therefore, Distalgesic should not be used in pregnant women unless, in the judgment of the physician, the potential benefits outweigh the possible hazards.

*Nursing mothers:* Low levels of dextropropoxyphene have been detected in human milk. In postpartum studies involving nursing mothers who were given dextropropoxyphene, no adverse effects were noted in the infants.

*Effects on ability to drive and use machines:*

*Ambulatory patients:* Dextropropoxyphene may impair abilities required for tasks such as driving a car or operating machinery. The patient should be cautioned accordingly.

*Undesirable effects:* The most frequently reported have been dizziness, sedation, nausea and vomiting. Some of these side-effects may be alleviated if the patient lies down.

Other side-effects include constipation, abdominal pain, rashes, light-headedness, headache, weakness, euphoria, dysphoria, hallucinations and minor visual disturbances.

Dextropropoxyphene therapy has been associated with abnormal liver function tests and, more rarely, with instances of reversible jaundice (including cholestatic jaundice).

Hepatic necrosis may result from acute overdose of paracetamol. In chronic alcohol abusers, this has been reported rarely with short-term use of paracetamol dosages of 2.5 to 10 g/day. Fatalities have occurred.

Renal papillary necrosis may result from chronic paracetamol use, particularly when the dosage is greater than recommended and when combined with aspirin.

Subacute painful myopathy has occurred following chronic dextropropoxyphene overdosage.

Chronic ingestion of dextropropoxyphene in doses exceeding 720 mg per day has caused toxic psychoses and convulsions.

*Overdose:* Initial consideration should be given to the management of the CNS effects of dextropropoxyphene overdosage. Resuscitative measures should be initiated promptly.

*Dextropropoxyphene:* In the acute phase dextropropoxyphene produces symptoms typical of narcosis, with somnolence or coma and respiratory depression, sometimes with convulsions. Blood pressure falls and cardiac performance deteriorates. Cardiac arrhythmias and conduction delay may be present. A combined respiratory-metabolic acidosis occurs, which may be severe if large amounts of salicylates have also been ingested. Death may occur.

Naloxone will reduce the respiratory depression and 0.4-2 mg IV should be administered promptly. (This may be repeated at 2-3 minute intervals, but if there is no response after 10 mg of naloxone the diagnosis should be questioned.) The duration of antagonism may be brief and need repeating for up to 24 hours. Mechanical ventilation, with oxygen may be required, and PEEP ventilation is desirable if pulmonary oedema is present.

Blood gases, pH and electrolytes should be monitored and electrocardiographic monitoring is essential. Ventricular fibrillation or cardiac arrest may occur. Respiratory acidosis rapidly subsides as ventilation is restored and hypercapnoea eliminated, but lactic acidosis may require IV bicarbonate for prompt correction. In addition to the use of a narcotic antagonist, the patient may require titration with an anti-convulsant to control convulsions. Gastric lavage may be useful and activated charcoal can absorb a significant amount of ingested dextropropoxyphene.

*Treatment of dextropropoxyphene overdose in children:* See general comments above. Naloxone at 0.01 mg/kg body weight IV should be administered promptly. If there is no response a dose of 0.1 mg/kg IV may be used.

*Paracetamol:* Overdose symptoms may not become apparent until later but early measurement of paracetamol levels is essential. N-acetylcysteine given as early as possible is effective in reducing the toxic effects of paracetamol. Treatment should be instituted within 16 hours of ingestion. Initial symptoms may be anorexia, nausea, vomiting, profuse sweating, malaise and abdominal pain, but the patient may have no symptoms. Subsequent evidence of liver dysfunction may be apparent up to 72 hours after ingestion, and if severe lead to irreversible hepatic necrosis and death within 3-7 days.

In adults, hepatic toxicity has rarely been reported with acute overdoses of less than 10 g and fatalities with less than 15 g.

Acute renal failure may accompany the hepatic dysfunction and can occur without signs of fulminant hepatic failure. Typically renal impairment is more apparent 6-9 days after overdose.

### Pharmacological properties

*Pharmacodynamic properties:* The product is a compound analgesic containing the non-narcotic drug (paracetamol) for the relief of pain of musculoskeletal conditions and a narcotic drug (dextropropoxyphene) for the relief of pain of visceral origin.

*Pharmacokinetic properties:* Single dose studies have shown peak plasma levels of 0.06 mg/l two hours after administration of 65 mg of dextropropoxyphene HCl. Variation of plasma levels between subjects may be due to individual differences in drug absorption and metabolism.

Multiple dose studies have shown that differences in plasma levels obtained with the hydrochloride salt or the napsylate salt have little therapeutic significance and that a 65 mg dextropropoxyphene HCl dose administered six hourly will achieve steady state plasma levels in the 0.13-0.19 mg/l range after 48 hours. The minimum lethal dose of dextropropoxyphene has been reported to be 500-800 mg and could result in blood concentrations of 0.45-0.74 mg/l. Mean half lives of 11.8 hours for dextropropoxyphene and 36.6 hours for norpropoxyphene have been demonstrated.

*Preclinical safety data:* There are no preclinical data of relevance to the prescriber in addition to that summarised in other sections of the summary of product characteristics.

### Pharmaceutical particulars

*List of excipients:* Maize Starch; Pregelatinised Maize Starch; Magnesium Stearate; Methylhydroxypropylcellulose 15; Glycerol; Titanium Dioxide.

*Incompatibilities:* Not applicable.

*Shelf life:* 3 years.

*Special precautions for storage:* None.

*Nature and contents of container:* Blister packs containing 100 white, pillow-shaped, film coated tablets, 14 mm in length and marked 'DG' (10 strips of 10 tablets).

*Instructions for use/handling:* None.

**Marketing authorisation number**   PL 0006/5000

**Date of approval/revision of SPC**   April 1996

**Legal category**   CD (Sch 5), POM

## DISTAMINE*

**Presentation**   Tablets each containing 125 mg or 250 mg D-penicillamine base. The 125 mg tablets are white, coated and have a diameter of 8 mm. They are marked 'DS' on one face and '125' on the other. The 250 mg tablets are white, coated and have a diameter of 10 mm. They are marked 'DM' on one face and '250' on the other.

**Uses**

(a) Severe active rheumatoid arthritis, including juvenile forms.

(b) Wilson's disease (hepatolenticular degeneration).

(c) Cystinuria—dissolution and prevention of cystine stones.

(d) Lead poisoning.

(e) Chronic active hepatitis.

**Dosage and administration**   For oral administration.

*(a) Rheumatoid arthritis: Adults:* 125–250 mg daily for the first month. Increase by the same amount every 4 to 12 weeks until remission occurs. The minimum maintenance dose to achieve suppression of symptoms should be used and treatment should be discontinued if no benefit is obtained within twelve months. Improvement may not occur for some months.

The usual maintenance dose is 500–750 mg daily. Up to 1.5 g daily may be required. If possible, penicillamine should be taken at least half an hour before meals, or on retiring.

If remission is established and has been sustained for six months, gradual reduction by 125–250 mg amounts every 12 weeks may be attempted.

*The elderly:* Increased toxicity has been observed in this patient population regardless of renal function. Initial dose should not exceed 125 mg daily for the first month, increasing by a similar increment every 4 to 12 weeks until the minimum maintenance dose to suppress symptoms is reached. Daily dosage should not exceed 1 g.

*Children:* 15-20 mg/kg/day is considered appropriate in the majority of cases. The initial dose should be 2.5–5.0 mg/kg/day and increased at four-weekly intervals over a period of three to six months. Please note that as the smallest available tablet is 125 mg, this may not be suitable for children under 8 years.

*(b) Wilson's disease: Adults:* 1.5-2 g daily in divided doses 30 minutes before food. Dose may be reduced to 750 mg-1 g daily when control of the disease is achieved. Patients must be maintained in negative copper balance and the minimum dosage of penicillamine required to achieve this should be given.

It is advisable that a dose of 2 g/day should not be continued for more than a year.

*The elderly:* 20 mg/kg/day in divided doses. Adjust dosage to control disease and maintain negative copper balance.

*Children:* Up to 20 mg/kg/day in divided doses before food. Minimum dose 500 mg/day.

*(c) Cystinuria:* Ideally, establish the lowest effective dose by quantitative amino acid chromatography of urine.

(i) *Dissolution of cystine stones: Adults:* 1-3 g daily in divided doses 30 minutes before food, where possible.

Urine cystine levels of not more than 200 mg/l should be maintained.

(ii) *Prevention of cystine stones: Adults:* 500 mg-1 g on retiring. Fluid intake should be not less than 3 litres/day.

Urine cystine levels of not more than 300 mg/l should be maintained.

*The elderly:* Use the minimum dose to maintain urinary cystine levels below 200 mg/l.

*Children:* No dose range established, but urinary cystine levels must be kept below 200 mg/l. The minimum dose of penicillamine required to achieve this should be given.

*(d) Lead poisoning: Adults:* 1-1.5 g daily in divided doses before food until urinary lead is stabilised at less than 0.5 mg/day.

*The elderly:* 20 mg/kg/day in divided doses until urinary lead is stabilised at less than 0.5 mg/day.

*Children:* 20 mg/kg/day.

*(e) Chronic active hepatitis: Adults:* For maintenance treatment after the disease process has been brought under control with corticosteroids. The initial dosage of 500 mg daily, in divided doses, should be increased gradually over three months to a maintenance dose of 1.25 g daily. During this period, the dosage of corticosteroids should be phased out. Throughout therapy, liver function tests should be carried out periodically to assess the disease status.

*The elderly:* Not recommended.

*(f) Desensitisation:* No fixed dose regimen. An initial dose of 25 mg daily is suggested, this to be gradually increased in accordance with the response of the patient. Higher initial doses have been employed in cystinuric patients.

**Contra-indications, warnings, etc**

*Contra-indications:* Hypersensitivity to penicillamine, except in a life-threatening situation, when desensitisation should be attempted (see 'Dosage and Administration').

Agranulocytosis or severe thrombocytopenia due to penicillamine.

Lupus erythematosus.

*Warnings*

*Usage in pregnancy:* The safety of penicillamine for use during pregnancy has not been established. It has been shown to be teratogenic in rats when given in doses several times higher than those recommended for human use.

*Wilson's disease:* There has been one case reported of reversible cutis laxa in an infant born to a mother taking 1.5 g penicillamine daily throughout pregnancy. Although there have been no controlled studies on the use of penicillamine during pregnancy, two retrospective studies have reported the successful delivery of 43 normal infants to 28 women receiving between 0.5 g and 2 g of penicillamine daily.

*Cystinuria:* There have been reports of patients delivered of normal infants, and one report of a severe connective tissue abnormality in the infant of a mother who received 2 g penicillamine daily throughout pregnancy. Whenever possible, penicillamine should be withheld during pregnancy, but if stones continue to form, the benefit of resuming treatment must be weighed against the possible risk to the foetus.

*Rheumatoid arthritis or chronic active hepatitis:* Penicillamine should not be administered to patients who are pregnant, and therapy should be stopped when pregnancy is diagnosed or suspected, unless considered to be absolutely essential by the physician.

*Precautions:* Full blood and platelet counts should be performed and renal function should be assessed prior to treatment with penicillamine. Monitoring of blood and platelet counts should be carried out at appropriate intervals, together with urinalysis for detection of haematuria and proteinuria.

If concomitant oral iron therapy is indicated, this should not be given within two hours of taking penicillamine.

Caution should be observed when anti-inflammatory or other drugs with known propensity for causing marrow injury are taken concurrently with penicillamine.

Care should be exercised in patients with renal insufficiency; modification of dosage may be necessary.

*Side-effects:* NB: The incidence and severity of some of the adverse reactions, noted below, varies according to the dosage and nature of the disease under treatment.

Nausea, anorexia, fever and rash may occur early in therapy, especially when full doses are given from the start. Antihistamines, steroid cover, or temporary reduction of dose will control urticarial reactions.

Reversible loss of taste may occur. Mineral supplements to overcome this are not recommended. Rarely, mouth ulceration stomatitis has occurred.

Thrombocytopenia occurs commonly and neutropenia less often. These reactions may occur at any time during treatment and are usually reversible. Deaths from agranulocytosis and aplastic anaemia have occurred. Full blood counts should be carried out weekly or fortnightly during the first eight weeks of therapy, in the week after any increase in dose, and otherwise monthly thereafter. In cystinuria or Wilson's disease, longer intervals may be adequate.

Withdrawal of treatment should be considered if platelets fall below 120,000 or white blood cells below 2,500/mm³, or if three successive falls are noted within the normal range. Treatment may be restarted at a reduced dosage when counts return to normal, but should be permanently withdrawn on recurrence of neutropenia or thrombocytopenia.

Proteinuria occurs in up to 30 per cent of patients and is partially dose-related. Urine should be tested weekly at first and after each increase in dose, then monthly, though again longer intervals may be adequate with cystinuria and Wilson's disease. Increasing proteinuria may necessitate withdrawal of treatment.

Haematuria is rare, but if it occurs in the absence of renal stones or other known cause, treatment should be stopped immediately.

Other rare adverse reactions are as follows: alopecia and inflammatory conditions of the respiratory system, such as bronchiolitis and pneumonitis.

Other complications have included haemolytic anaemia, nephrotic syndrome, drug induced lupus erythematosus, and conditions closely resembling myasthenia gravis, polymyositis (with rare cardiac involvement), dermatomyositis, pemphigus, Goodpasture's syndrome, Stevens-Johnson syndrome and rheumatoid arthritis.

A late rash, described as acquired epidermolysis bullosa and penicillamine dermopathy, may occur after several months or years of therapy. This may necessitate a reduction in dosage. Pseudoxanthoma elasticum and skin laxity have been reported rarely.

*Overdosage:* No instances of adverse reactions to an overdose of penicillamine have been recorded and no specific measures are indicated.

**Further information** Nil.

**Pharmaceutical precautions** Store in a dry place below 25°C. Keep containers tightly closed.

**Legal category** POM.

**Package quantities**
Tablets 125 mg: Bottles of 100
Tablets 250 mg: Bottles of 100

**Product licence numbers**
Tablets 125 mg: 0006/0090
Tablets 250 mg: 0006/5008

# ILOSONE*

**Qualitative and quantitative composition** Erythromycin Estolate.

Equivalent to base 250 mg (pulvules) or base 500 mg (tablets).

**Pharmaceutical form** The capsules are ivory/red, marked DISTA, and are 2.1cm long.

The tablets are pink, para-capsule shaped, 1.9cm long and coded DISTA DI.

**Clinical particulars**

*Therapeutic indications:* Antibiotic. Erythromycin is indicated in the treatment of the following infections when due to susceptible organisms:

Upper and lower respiratory tract infections

Otitis media

Skin and soft-issue infections, including erythrasma and acne

Dental infections

Genito-urinary infections, including gonorrhoea, syphilis, and chlamydial infections

Intestinal amoebiasis (extra-enteric amoebiasis requires treatment with other agents)

Erythromycin is also indicated for the following:

*Endocarditis:* Continuous or short-term prophylaxis against bacterial endocarditis, especially prior to dental or other operative procedures, in patients with a history of rheumatic fever or congenital heart disease and who are hypersensitive to penicillin. Erythromycin is not suitable for prophylaxis prior to genito-urinary or gastro-intestinal tract surgery.

*Diphtheria:* As an adjunct to antitoxin, to prevent establishment of carriers, and to eradicate the organism in carriers.

*Whooping cough:* When given early after exposure, erythromycin may reduce the risk of development of classical symptoms.

*Legionnaires' disease:* Limited clinical experience would suggest that erythromycin may be effective in treating Legionnaires' disease.

Erythromycin is active against the following organisms *in vitro: Streptococcus pyogenes; Str. pneumoniae;* Alpha-haemolytic streptococci (viridans group); *Staphylococcus aureus; Haemophilus influenzae; Mycoplasma pneumoniae; Corynebacterium* spp.; *Listeria monocytogenes; Bordetella pertussis; Legionella pneumophila; Helicobacter* spp.; *Neisseria gonorrhoeae; Treponema pallidum; Chlamydia trachomatis;* Anaerobic bacteria, including *Bacteroides* spp., *Clostridium* spp. and *Propionibacterium acnes; Entamoeba histolytica.*

*Posology and method of administration:* For oral administration.

*Adults:* The usual dose is 250 mg every six hours. This may be increased up to 4 g per day according to the severity of the infection. Dosage should be limited to a maximum of 1.5 g daily in patients with severe renal impairment.

*The elderly:* As for adults.

*Children:* Age, weight and severity of the infection are important factors in determining the correct dosage. The usual range is 20-50 mg/kg/day in divided doses.

If administration on a twice daily schedule is desirable, one-half of the total daily dose may be given every 12 hours. Twice daily dosing is not recommended when doses larger than 1 g daily are administered.

*Streptococcal infections:* For streptococcal pharyngitis and tonsillitis, the usual dosage range is 20-50 mg/kg/day in divided doses. In the treatment of group A beta-haemolytic streptococcal infections, a therapeutic dosage of erythromycin should be administered for at least 10 days. In continuous prophylaxis of streptococcal infections in persons with a history of rheumatic heart disease, the dosage is 250 mg twice daily.

When Ilosone is used prior to surgery to prevent endocarditis caused by alpha-haemolytic streptococci (viridans group), a recommended schedule for adults is 1 g pre-operatively (20 mg/kg for children) and 500 mg (10 mg/kg for children) 6 hours later.

*Pertussis:* Doses of erythromycin estolate utilised in reported clinical studies were 40-50 mg/kg/day, given in divided doses for five to 14 days.

*Gonorrhoea:* For disseminated infection, 500 mg four times daily for 7 days.

*Syphilis:* A regimen of 20 g of erythromycin estolate in divided doses over a period of 10 days has been shown to be effective.

*Amoebic dysentery:* Dosage for adults is 250 mg four times daily for 10 to 14 days: for children, 30-50 mg/kg/day in divided doses for 10 to 14 days.

*Legionnaires' disease:* Although optimum regimens have not been established, 1-4 g daily in divided doses has been utilised in reported clinical studies.

*Urogenital infections during pregnancy due to C. trachomatis:* 500 mg four times a day for at least seven days. For women who cannot tolerate this regimen, a decreased dose of 250 mg four times a day should be used for at least fourteen days.

For adults with uncomplicated urethral, endocervical, or rectal infections caused by *C. trachomatis in whom tetracyclines are contra-indicated or not tolerated:* 500 mg four times a day for at least seven days.

*Contra-indications:* Hypersensitivity to erythromycin.

Patients who have previously developed jaundice or who have pre-existing liver disease or dysfunction.

Patients taking terfenadine or astemizole.

*Special warnings and special precautions for use:* The administration of erythromycin estolate has been associated with the infrequent occurrence of reversible cholestatic hepatitis. Hepatic dysfunction with or without jaundice has occurred, chiefly in adults. It may be accompanied by malaise, nausea, vomiting, abdominal colic and fever. In some instances severe abdominal pain may simulate the pain of biliary colic, pancreatitis, perforated ulcer, or an acute abdominal surgical problem. In other instances, clinical symptoms and results of liver function tests have resembled findings in extrahepatic obstructive jaundice. Laboratory findings have been characterised by abnormal hepatic function test values, peripheral eosinophilia and leucocytosis. If the above findings occur, discontinue Ilosone promptly.

Initial symptoms have developed in some cases after a few days of treatment, but generally have followed one or two weeks of continuous therapy. Symptoms re-appear promptly, usually within 48 hours, after the drug is re-administered to sensitive patients. The syndrome seems to result from a form of sensitisation, occurs chiefly in adults, and has been reversible when medication is discontinued.

The diagnosis of pseudomembranous colitis should be considered should diarrhoea develop. Mild cases usually respond to drug discontinuation alone. Additional measures will be required in more severe cases, which may be life-threatening.

The antibacterial activity of erythromycin is markedly greater in alkaline than in neutral or acid media. Urinary alkalinisation should be considered when treating urinary infections.

*Laboratory tests:* Erythromycin interferes with some clinical laboratory tests, for example, high SGOT values may be artefacts and may not necessarily reflect changes in liver function.

During prolonged or repeated therapy, there is a possibility of overgrowth of non-susceptible bacteria or fungi. If such infections arise, the drug should be discontinued and appropriate therapy instituted.

*Interaction with other medicaments and other forms of interaction:*

*Drug interactions:* Erythromycin significantly alters the metabolism of terfenadine or astemizole when taken concomitantly. Rare cases of serious cardiovascular events, including death, cardiac arrest, torsade de pointes and other ventricular arrhythmias, have been observed (see *Contra-indications*).

Since probenecid inhibits tubular re-absorption of erythromycin in animals, it prolongs maintenance of plasma levels.

Erythromycin and lincomycin or clindamycin may, under some conditions, be antagonistic. Lincomycin or clindamycin therapy should be avoided in treatment of infections due to erythromycin-resistant organisms.

The use of erythromycin in patients who are receiving concomitant high doses of theophylline may be associated with an increase in serum theophylline levels and potential theophylline toxicity. If symptoms of toxicity or elevated serum theophylline levels develop, the dose of theophylline should be reduced.

Concomitant administration of erythromycin and digoxin has been reported to result in elevated digoxin serum levels.

There have been reports of increased anticoagulant effects when erythromycin and oral anticoagulants were used concomitantly. Increased anticoagulation effects due to this drug interaction may be more pronounced in the elderly.

Concurrent use of erythromycin and ergotamine or dihydroergotamine has been associated in some patients with acute ergot toxicity characterised by severe peripheral vasospasm and dysaesthesia.

Erythromycin has been reported to decrease the clearance of triazolam and midazolam, and thus may increase the pharmacological effect of these benzodiazepines.

The use of erythromycin in patients concurrently taking drugs metabolised by the cytochrome P450 system may be associated with elevation in serum levels of these other drugs. Elevated serum concentrations of the following drugs have been reported when administered concurrently with erythromycin: carbamazepine, cyclosporin, hexobarbitone, phenytoin, alfentanil, disopyramide, lovastatin and bromocriptine. Serum concentrations of such drugs should be monitored closely in patients concurrently receiving erythromycin.

*Pregnancy and lactation:*

*Usage in pregnancy:* Reproduction studies in rats, mice and rabbits, with doses several times the usual human dose, have revealed no evidence of impaired fertility or foetal harm related to erythromycin. There are no adequate studies in pregnant women. Because animal reproductive studies are not always predictive of human response, this drug should be used during pregnancy only if clearly needed.

*Usage in nursing mothers:* Erythromycin is excreted in breast milk. Caution should be exercised when it is administered to a nursing woman.

*Effects on ability to drive and use machines:* Not applicable.

*Undesirable effects:* The most frequent side-effects of erythromycin preparations are gastro-intestinal (eg, abdominal cramping and discomfort) and are dose-related. Nausea, vomiting and diarrhoea occur infrequently with usual oral doses.

Mild allergic reactions, such as urticaria and other skin rashes, have occurred. Serious allergic reactions, including anaphylaxis, have been reported.

There have been isolated reports of hearing loss and/or tinnitus occurring chiefly in patients with renal or hepatic insufficiency and in patients receiving high doses of erythromycin. Ototoxic effects are usually reversible upon discontinuation, but in rare instances, involving intravenous administration, the ototoxic effect has been irreversible.

Rarely, erythromycin has been associated with ventricular arrhythmias, including ventricular tachycardia and torsade de pointes, in individuals with prolonged QT intervals.

*Overdose:*

*Symptoms:* Nausea, vomiting and dose-related epigastric distress and diarrhoea. Reversible mild acute pancreatitis has been reported. Hearing loss, with or without tinnitus and vertigo, may occur (see *Undesirable effects*).

*Treatment:* Unless 5 times the normal single dose has been ingested, gastro-intestinal decontamination should not be necessary. Consider activated charcoal instead of, or in addition to, gastric emptying.

Forced diuresis, peritoneal dialysis, haemodialysis, or charcoal haemoperfusion have not been established as beneficial.

**Pharmacological properties**

*Pharmacodynamic properties:* Erythromycin acts by interfering with bacterial protein synthesis and is bacteriostatic or bactericidal, depending on the concentration of the drugs and the type of organism.

*Pharmacokinetic properties:* Erythromycin estolate is stable to acid, and is not affected by food to the same extent as other erythromycins. It is rapidly absorbed, with peak serum levels being achieved within 4 hours in adults. Serum concentrations are significantly higher than those obtained with the base or other esters.

*Preclinical safety data:* Reproduction studies in rats, mice and rabbits, with doses several times the usual human dose, have revealed no evidence of impaired fertility or foetal harm related to erythromycin.

**Pharmaceutical particulars**

*List of excipients:*
*Capsules:* Talc; Silica Gel Powder; Magnesium Stearate; Liquid Paraffin; Erythrosine (E127); Titanium Dioxide (E171); Quinoline Yellow (E104); Red Iron Oxide (E172); Yellow Iron Oxide (E172); Gelatin.

*Tablets:* Magnesium Stearate; Starch; Amaranth Aluminium Lake (E123); Erythrosine Aluminium Lake (E127); Sunset Yellow Aluminium Lake (E110).

*Incompatibilities:* Not applicable.

*Shelf life:* 5 years.

*Special precautions for storage:*
*Capsules:* Store below 25°C.
*Tablets:* Store in a cool, dry place (6-15°C).
Keep tightly closed.

*Nature and contents of container:* High density polyethylene bottle.

*Package quantities*
Capsules 250 mg: Bottles of 100.
Tablets 500 mg: Bottles of 12.

*Instructions for use/handling:* Not applicable.

**Marketing authorisation numbers**
Capsules: PL 0006/5022R
Tablets: PL 0006/5015R

**Date of approval/revision of SPC** September 1996

**Legal category** POM

## KEFADOL*

**Presentation** 10 ml vials containing cefamandole nafate for injection equivalent to 1 g cefamandole.

The vials also contain 63 mg Sodium Carbonate USP per gram of cefamandole. The total sodium content is approximately 77 mg per gram of cefamandole activity.

**Uses** Cefamandole is indicated in the treatment of infections of the lower respiratory tract, genito-urinary tract, bones and joints, bloodstream (septicaemia), skin and soft tissue, gall bladder and peritoneum, and pelvic inflammatory disease in women, when due to susceptible micro-organisms.

*Prophylactic use:* Perioperative administration of cefamandole may reduce the incidence of postoperative infections in patients undergoing contaminated or potentially contaminated surgical procedures associated with a high risk of infection, or where the occurrence of a postoperative infection could be especially serious.

Cefamandole is usually active against the following organisms *in vitro* and in clinical infections:

Gram-positive:

Staphylococci, including coagulase-positive, coagulase-negative (e.g. *Staphylococcus epidermidis*) and penicillinase-producing strains

Beta-haemolytic and other streptococci (most strains of enterococci, e.g. *Enterococcus faecalis*, are resistant)

*Streptococcus pneumoniae*

Gram-negative:

*Escherichia coli*

*Klebsiella* spp.

*Enterobacter* spp. (initially susceptible organisms occasionally may become resistant during therapy)

*Haemophilus influenzae*

*Proteus mirabilis*

*Providencia rettgeri*

*Morganella morganii*

*Proteus vulgaris* (some strains of *P. vulgaris* have been shown by *in vitro* tests to be resistant to cefamandole and certain other cephalosporins)

Anaerobic organisms:

Gram-positive and gram-negative cocci (including *Peptococcus* and *Peptostreptococcus* spp.)

Gram-positive bacilli (including *Clostridium* spp.)

Gram-negative bacilli (including *Bacteroides*)

Most strains of *Bacteroides fragilis* are resistant.

*Pseudomonas, Acinetobacter calcoaceticus* and most *Serratia* strains are resistant to cefamandole and certain other cephalosporins. Cefamandole is resistant to degradation by β–lactamases from certain members of the *Enterobacteriaceae*.

**Dosage and administration** Cefamandole nafate may be given intravenously or by deep intramuscular injection into a large muscle mass to minimise pain.

*Adults and the elderly:* The dosage range for cefamandole is 500 mg to 2 g every four to eight hours, depending on the severity and site of infection.

*Impaired renal function:* When renal function is impaired, a reduced dosage must be employed and serum concentrations should be monitored when feasible. After an initial dose of 1 to 2 g (depending on the severity of infection), a maintenance dosage schedule should be followed (see table). Continued dosage should be determined by degree of renal impairment, severity of infection and susceptibility of the causative organism.

*Maintenance dosage of cefamandole in patients with impaired renal function*

| *Creatinine clearance ml/min/1.73 m²* | *Life-threatening infections* | *Severe infections* | *Less severe infections* |
|---|---|---|---|
| 80-50 | 2 g q 6 h | 1.5 g q 6 h | 0.75 g q 6 h |
| 50-25 | 2 g q 8 h | 1.5 g q 8 h | 0.75 g q 8 h |
| 25-10 | 1.25 g q 8 h | 1.0 g q 8 h | 0.5 g q 8 h |
| 10-2 | 1 g q 12 h | 0.75 g q 12 h | 0.5 g q 12 h |
| <2 | 0.75 g q 12 h | 0.5 g q 12 h | 0.25 g q 12 h |

*Intramuscular administration:* Each gram of cefamandole should be reconstituted with 3 ml of Water for Injections PhEur or Sodium Chloride Intravenous Infusion BP. Shake well until dissolved.

*Intravenous administration:* Intravenous route may be preferable for bacterial septicaemia, localised parenchymal abscesses, peritonitis, or other severe or life-threatening infections.

1. *For direct intermittent intravenous administration*, each gram of cefamandole should be reconstituted with 10 ml of Water for Injections PhEur, 5% Dextrose Intravenous Infusion BP, or Sodium Chloride Intravenous Infusion BP. Slowly inject directly into the vein over a period of three to five minutes or give through the tubing of an administration set while the patient is also receiving one of the following intravenous fluids:

Sodium Chloride Intravenous Infusion BP
5% Dextrose Intravenous Infusion BP
10% Dextrose Intravenous Infusion BP
5% Dextrose and 0.9% Sodium Chloride Intravenous Infusion BP
5% Dextrose and 0.45% Sodium Chloride Intravenous Infusion BP
Sodium Lactate Intravenous Infusion BP

2. *Intermittent intravenous infusion with a Y-type administration set or volume control set* can also be accomplished while any of the above mentioned intravenous fluids are being infused. However, during infusion of the solution containing cefamandole, it is desirable to discontinue the other solution. When this technique is employed, careful attention should be paid to the volume of the solution containing cefamandole so that the calculated dose will be infused. When a Y-tube connection is used, 100 ml of an appropriate diluent should be added to 2 g cefamandole. If Water for Injections PhEur is used as the diluent, reconstitute with approximately 20 ml per g to avoid a hypotonic solution.

3. *For continuous intravenous infusion*, each gram of cefamandole should be diluted with 10 ml of Water for Injections PhEur. An appropriate quantity of the resulting solution may be added to an i.v. bottle containing one of the previously mentioned intravenous fluids.

If combination therapy with cefamandole and an aminoglycoside is indicated, each of these should be administered at separate sites.

*Infants and children:* Administration of 50 to 100 mg/kg/day in equally divided doses every four to eight hours has been effective for most infections susceptible to cefamandole. This may be increased to a total daily dose of 150 mg/kg (not to exceed the maximum adult dose) for serious infections.

*Infants:* Cefamandole has been effectively used in this age group, but all laboratory parameters have not been extensively studied in infants between 1 and 6 months of age. Safety of this product has not been established in prematures and infants under 1 month of age; therefore, if cefamandole is to be administered to infants, the physician should determine whether the potential benefits outweigh the possible risks involved. Accumulation of cephalosporins (with resulting prolongation of drug half-life) has been reported in neonates.

*Prophylactic use:* The following schedules are recommended for perioperative use:

*Adults and the elderly:* 1 or 2 g intravenously or intramuscularly one-half to one hour prior to surgical incision, followed by 1 or 2 g every six hours for 24 to 48 hours.

For patients undergoing procedures involving implantation of prosthetic devices, administration for up to 72 hours is recommended.

*Children (more than three months of age):* 50–100 mg/kg/day in equally divided doses by the same routes and schedule designated for adults.

If signs of infection occur, cultures should be obtained and appropriate therapy instituted.

Kefadol should be continued for a minimum of 48 to 72 hours after the patient becomes asymptomatic or bacterial eradication has occurred. A minimum of 10 days treatment is recommended in infections caused by group A beta-haemolytic streptococci. In chronic urinary tract infection, frequent bacteriological and clinical appraisal is necessary during therapy and possibly for several months after completion. Persistent infections may require treatment for several weeks.

**Contra-indications, warnings, etc**

*Contra-indication:* Cefamandole is contra-indicated in patients with known allergy to the cephalosporin group of antibiotics.

*Warnings:* Before cefamandole therapy is instituted, careful enquiry should be made concerning previous hypersensitivity reactions to cephalosporins, penicillins or other drugs. Kefadol should be given cautiously to penicillin-sensitive patients.

There is some clinical and laboratory evidence of partial cross-allergenicity of the penicillins and the cephalosporins. Patients have been reported to have had severe reactions (including anaphylaxis) to both drugs.

Antibiotics should be administered with caution to any patient who has demonstrated some form of allergy, particularly to drugs.

Pseudomembranous colitis has been reported with most broad-spectrum antibiotics. Its diagnosis should be considered in patients who develop diarrhoea with antibiotics. Such colitis may range from mild to life-threatening.

*Usage in pregnancy:* Reproduction studies in rats given doses of 500 or 1000 mg/kg/day (approximately 5 times the maximum clinical dose) revealed no evidence of impaired fertility or harm to the foetus due to cefamandole nafate. There are, however, no adequate and well-controlled studies in pregnant women. Because animal studies are not always predictive of human response, this drug should be used during pregnancy only if clearly needed.

*Nursing mothers:* Caution should be exercised.

*Precautions:* Although cefamandole rarely produces alteration in kidney function, evaluation of renal status is recommended, especially in seriously ill patients receiving maximum doses. Patients with impaired renal function should be placed on the dosage schedule recommended under 'Dosage and administration'. Usual doses in such individuals may result in excessive serum concentrations.

Nephrotoxicity has been reported following concomitant administration of aminoglycoside antibiotics and cephalosporins.

The results of experimental studies in animals suggest that the concurrent use of potent diuretics such as frusemide or ethacrynic acid may also increase the risk of renal toxicity with cephalosporin antibiotics.

As with other broad-spectrum antibiotics, hypoprothrombinaemia with or without bleeding has been reported rarely, but it has been promptly reversed by administration of vitamin K. Such episodes have usually occurred in elderly, debilitated or otherwise compromised patients with deficient stores of vitamin K. Prophylactic administration of vitamin K may be indicated in such patients, especially when intestinal sterilisation and surgical procedures are performed.

In a few patients receiving cefamandole, nausea, vomiting and vasomotor instability with hypotension and peripheral vasodilatation, has occurred following the ingestion of alcohol. Cefamandole inhibits the enzyme acetaldehyde dehydrogenase in laboratory animals. This causes accumulation of acetaldehyde when ethanol is administered concurrently.

Broad-spectrum antibiotics should be prescribed with caution in individuals with a history of gastro-intestinal disease, particularly colitis.

Prolonged use of cefamandole may result in the overgrowth of non-susceptible organisms. Careful observation of the patient is essential. If superinfection occurs during therapy, appropriate measures should be taken.

A false positive reaction for glucose in the urine may occur with Benedict's or Fehling's solutions or with Clinitest tablets. A false positive test for proteinuria may occur with acid and denaturisation precipitation tests.

*Impairment of fertility:* Very high doses of cefamandole (equivalent to approximately 5 times the maximum clinical dose) have been found to delay maturation of the testicular germinal epithelium in rats. This effect was seen only when cefamandole was given to neonatal rats during initial spermatogenic development. The clinical significance of this finding is unknown due to differences in the time of initiation of spermatogenesis, rate of spermatogenic development and duration of puberty.

*Side-effects*

*Hypersensitivity:* Anaphylaxis, maculopapular rash, urticaria, eosinophilia and drug fever have been reported. These reactions are more likely to occur in patients with a history of allergy, particularly to penicillin.

*Haematological:* Thrombocytopenia has been reported rarely. Neutropenia has been reported, especially in long courses of treatment. Some individuals have developed positive direct Coombs' tests during treatment with the cephalosporin antibiotics.

*Gastro-intestinal:* Nausea and vomiting occur rarely. Colitis, including rare instances of pseudomembranous colitis, has been reported.

*Liver:* Transient rise in AST, ALT and ALP levels have been noted. Transient hepatitis and cholestatic jaundice have been reported rarely.

*Kidney:* Decreased creatinine clearance has been reported in patients with prior renal impairment. As with some other cephalosporins, transitory elevations of blood urea have occasionally been observed; their frequency increases in patients over 50 years of age. In some of these cases, there was also a mild increase in serum creatinine.

*Local reactions:* Pain on intramuscular injection is infrequent. Thrombophlebitis occurs rarely.

*Overdosage:* The administration of inappropriately large doses of parenteral cephalosporins may cause seizures, particularly in patients with renal impairment. Dosage reduction is necessary when renal function is impaired (see 'Dosage and administration'). If seizures occur, the drug should be promptly discontinued; anticonvulsant therapy may be administered if clinically indicated.

In the event of serious overdosage, general supportive care is recommended, with monitoring of haematological, renal and hepatic functions, and coagulation status, until the patient is stable. Haemodialysis may be considered in cases of overwhelming overdosage.

**Pharmaceutical precautions**  *Unreconstituted vials:* Store below 25°C. Protect from light.

It is good practice to reconstitute immediately before use. If this is not feasible, reconstituted solutions may be stored in a refrigerator (2°-8°C) and used within 96 hours. If kept below 25°C, use within 24 hours. During storage at room temperature, carbon dioxide develops inside the vial after reconstitution. This pressure may be dissipated prior to withdrawal of the vial contents, or it may be used to aid withdrawal if the vial is inverted over the syringe needle and the contents are allowed to flow into the syringe.

The pH of freshly reconstituted solutions usually ranges from 6.0 to 8.5.

Do not mix an aminoglycoside with cefamandole in the same intravenous fluid container.

**Legal category**  POM.

**Package quantities**  Vials 1 g: Individual vials in packs of 10.

**Further information**  Solutions of cefamandole range from light yellow to amber, depending upon a variety of factors, including concentration and the diluent used.

**Product licence number** 0006/0111.

# PROZAC*

**Presentation**  Capsules (green and yellow, coded 3105) each containing 20 mg fluoxetine, as the hydrochloride.

Capsules (yellow, coded 3109) each containing 60 mg fluoxetine, as the hydrochloride.

Liquid (clear, colourless, mint odoured) containing 20 mg fluoxetine, as the hydrochloride, per 5 ml syrup.

**Uses**

*Depression:* Prozac is indicated for the treatment of the symptoms of depressive illness, with or without associated anxiety symptoms, especially where sedation is not required.

*Obsessive-compulsive disorder.*

*Bulimia nervosa:* Prozac is indicated for the reduction of binge-eating and purging activity.

**Dosage and administration**  For oral administration to adults only.

*Depression, with or without associated anxiety symptoms – adults and the elderly:* A dose of 20 mg/day is recommended.

*Obsessive-compulsive disorder:* 20 mg/day to 60 mg/day. A dose of 20 mg/day is recommended as the initial dose. Although there may be an increased potential for side-effects at higher doses, a dose increase may be considered after several weeks if there is no response.

*Bulimia nervosa – adults and the elderly:* A dose of 60 mg/day is recommended.

Fluoxetine has a half-life of 1 to 3 days after acute administration. The half-life may be prolonged to 4 to 6 days after chronic administration. The active metabolite, norfluoxetine, has a mean half-life of 9.3 days after multiple dosing (range 4 to 16 days). Steady state plasma concentrations are only achieved after continuous dosing for weeks.

When dosing is stopped, active drug substances will persist in the body for weeks. This should be borne in mind when starting or stopping treatment.

Plasma concentrations do not appear to increase without limit because, in addition to metabolism by the hepatic cytochrome P450IID6 isoenzyme system, there are non-saturable pathways. Patients receiving fluoxetine for as long as 3 years exhibited average plasma concentrations, similar to those seen among patients treated for 4 or 5 weeks.

The capsule and liquid dosage forms are bioequivalent.

*Children:* The use of Prozac in children is not recommended, as safety and efficacy have not been established.

*Patients with renal and/or hepatic dysfunction:* See 'Contra-indications' and 'Precautions' sections.

**Contra-indications, warnings, etc**

*Contra-indications:* Hypersensitivity to fluoxetine.

Fluoxetine should not be administered to patients with severe renal failure (GFR <10 ml/min) because accumulation may occur in these patients during chronic treatment.

*Usage in nursing mothers:* Prozac should not be prescribed to nursing mothers. In one breast milk sample the concentration of fluoxetine, plus norfluoxetine, was 70.4 ng/ml, compared to 295.0 ng/ml in the mother's plasma. No adverse effects on the infant were noted. In another infant the plasma level of fluoxetine was 340 ng/ml and 208 ng/ml of norfluoxetine on the second day of breast feeding from a mother on Prozac. This infant developed crying, sleep disturbance, vomiting and watery stools.

*Monoamine oxidase inhibitors:* At least 14 days should elapse between discontinuation of an MAOI and initiation of treatment with Prozac. At least five weeks (longest if fluoxetine has been prescribed chronically and/or at higher doses) should elapse between discontinuation of Prozac and initiation of therapy with an MAOI.

Serious, sometimes fatal reactions (including hyperthermia, rigidity, myoclonus, autonomic instability with possible rapid fluctuations of vital signs, and mental status changes that include extreme agitation progressing to delirium and coma) have been reported with concomitant use or when fluoxetine had been recently discontinued and an MAOI started. Some cases presented with features resembling neuroleptic malignant syndrome. Cyproheptadine or dantrolene may benefit patients experiencing such reactions.

*Warnings*

*Rash and allergic reactions:* Angioneurotic oedema, urticaria and other allergic reactions have been reported. Upon the appearance of rash or of other allergic phenomena for which an alternative aetiology cannot be identified, Prozac should be discontinued.

*Pregnancy:* The safety of fluoxetine in human pregnancy has not been established; accordingly, the drug should be avoided in pregnancy unless there is no safer alternative. There was no evidence of teratogenicity from animal studies but full testing was limited by maternal toxicity.

*Lactation:* See 'Contra-indications'.

*Precautions:* Prozac should be discontinued in any patient who develops seizures. Prozac should be avoided in patients with unstable epilepsy; patients with controlled epilepsy should be carefully monitored. There have been rare reports of prolonged seizures in patients on fluoxetine receiving ECT treatment.

Fluoxetine is extensively metabolised by the liver and excreted by the kidneys. A lower dose, e.g., alternate day dosing, is recommended in patients with significant hepatic dysfunction or mild to moderate renal failure (GFR 10–50 ml/min).

Clinical experience in acute cardiac disease is limited, therefore caution is advisable. However, the ECG of 312 patients who received fluoxetine in double-blind trials were retrospectively evaluated; no conduction abnormalities that resulted in heart block were observed.

Prozac may cause weight loss which may be undesirable in underweight depressed patients. Only rarely have depressed or bulimic patients been discontinued for weight loss when treated with fluoxetine.

In patients with diabetes, fluoxetine may alter glycaemic control. Hypoglycaemia has occurred during therapy with fluoxetine and hyperglycaemia has developed following discontinuation. Insulin and/or oral hypoglycaemic dosage may need to be adjusted.

There have been reports of abnormal bleeding in several patients, but causal relationship to fluoxetine and clinical importance are unclear.

Although fluoxetine has been shown not to affect psychomotor performance in healthy volunteers, any psychoactive drug may impair judgement or skills. Therefore, patients should be cautioned that their ability to perform potentially hazardous tasks (e.g., driving, operating machinery) may be impaired.

As improvement may not occur during the first two or more weeks of treatment, patients should be closely monitored during this period. The possibility of a suicide attempt is inherent in depression and may persist until significant remission occurs.

*Drug interactions:* Monoamine oxidase inhibitors: (see 'Contra-indications').

Caution is advised if the concomitant administration of Prozac and CNS active drugs, including lithium, is required. There have been reports of both increased and decreased lithium levels when used concomitantly with fluoxetine. Cases of lithium toxicity have been reported. Lithium levels should be monitored.

Because fluoxetine's metabolism (like tricyclic antidepressants and other selective serotonin antidepressants) involves the hepatic cytochrome P450IID6 isoenzyme system, concomitant therapy with drugs also metabolised by this enzyme system may lead to drug interactions.

Concomitant therapy with drugs predominantly metabolised by this isoenzyme, and which have a narrow therapeutic index (such as flecainide, encainide, vinblastine, carbamazepine and tricyclic antidepressants), should be initiated at or adjusted to the low end of their dose range. This will also apply if fluoxetine has been taken in the previous 5 weeks.

Greater than two-fold increases of previously stable plasma levels of cyclic antidepressants have been observed when Prozac has been administered in combination.

Agitation, restlessness and gastro-intestinal symptoms have been reported in a small number of patients receiving fluoxetine in combination with tryptophan.

Patients on stable doses of phenytoin have developed elevated plasma phenytoin concentrations and clinical phenytoin toxicity following initiation of concomitant fluoxetine treatment.

The long elimination half-lives should be borne in mind (see 'Dosage and administration') when considering pharmacodynamic or pharmacokinetic drug interactions.

Fluoxetine is bound to plasma protein and concurrent administration may alter plasma concentrations of other plasma protein bound drugs or conversely fluoxetine. In formal testing, no drug interaction of clinical significance has been observed between fluoxetine and chlorothiazide, ethanol, secobarbital and tolbutamide.

In formal testing, no drug interaction of clinical significance has been observed between fluoxetine and warfarin. Possible interactions have been reported rarely.

Fluoxetine does not appear to potentiate the effects of alcohol.

*Adverse effects*

*Body as a whole:* Asthenia, fever.

*Digestive system:* Nausea, diarrhoea, dry mouth, appetite loss, dyspepsia, vomiting. Abnormal liver function tests have been reported rarely.

*Nervous system:* Headache, nervousness, insomnia, drowsiness, anxiety, tremor, dizziness, fatigue, decreased libido, seizures (see 'Precautions'). Hypomania or mania occurred in approximately one per cent of fluoxetine treated trial patients. Dyskinesia (including, for example, a case of buccal-lingual-masticatory syndrome, which resolved following drug discontinuation), movement disorders developing in patients with risk factors (including drugs associated with such events) and worsening of pre-existing movement disorders, and neuroleptic malignant syndrome-like events have been reported.

*Respiratory system:* Pharyngitis, dyspnoea. Pulmonary events (including inflammatory processes of varying histopathology and/or fibrosis) have been reported rarely. Dyspnoea may be the only preceding symptom.

*Skin and appendages:* A small percentage of patients developed rash and/or urticaria (see 'Warnings'). Serious systemic reactions, possibly related to vasculitis, have developed in patients with rash, and rarely death has been reported. Excessive sweating, arthralgia, myalgia, serum sickness and anaphylactoid reactions have also been reported. Hair loss, usually reversible, has been reported.

*Urinogenital system:* Sexual dysfunction (delayed or inhibited orgasm).

Hyponatraemia (including serum sodium below 110 mmol/l) has been rarely reported and appeared to be reversible when Prozac was discontinued. Some cases were possibly due to the syndrome of inappropriate antidiuretic hormone secretion. The majority of reports were associated with older patients, and patients taking diuretics or otherwise volume depleted.

The following have been reported in association with fluoxetine but no causal relationship has been established: aplastic anaemia, cerebral vascular accident, confusion, ecchymoses, eosinophilic pneumonia, gastro-intestinal haemorrhage, hyperprolactinaemia, immune-related haemolytic anaemia, pancreatitis, pancytopenia, suicidal ideation, thrombocytopenia, thrombocytopenic purpura, vaginal bleeding after drug withdrawal and violent behaviour.

*Overdosage:* On the evidence available, fluoxetine has a wide margin of safety in overdose. Since introduction, reports of death attributed to overdosage of fluoxetine alone have been extremely rare.

One patient who reportedly took 3000 mg of fluoxetine experienced 2 grand mal seizures that remitted spontaneously. Nausea and vomiting were prominent in overdoses involving higher fluoxetine doses. Agitation, restlessness, hypomania and other signs of CNS excitation were also observed.

*Management:* No specific antidote is known.

An airway should be established. Cardiac and vital

signs monitoring is recommended, along with general symptomatic and supportive measures.

An extended time for close medical observation may be needed in patients who have taken excessive quantities of a tricyclic antidepressant if they are also taking, or have recently taken, fluoxetine. Accumulation of the parent tricyclic or an active metabolite may increase the possibility of clinically relevant sequelae.

Based on experience with animals, fluoxetine-induced seizures which fail to remit spontaneously may respond to diazepam. Due to the large volume of distribution of fluoxetine, forced diuresis, dialysis, haemoperfusion and exchange transfusion are unlikely to be of benefit. Activated charcoal, which may be used with sorbitol, may be as or more effective than emesis or lavage.

**Pharmaceutical precautions**   Store at room temperature (15°–25°C).

**Legal category**   POM.

**Package quantities**
20 mg: Calendar packs of 30 capsules (2 strips of 15 capsules).
20 mg: Packs of 98 capsules (14 strips of 7 capsules).
60 mg: Packs of 30 capsules (3 strips of 10 capsules).
Bottles of 70 ml liquid.

**Further information**   Fluoxetine is chemically unrelated to tricyclic and tetracyclic antidepressant agents. It is a specific serotonin (5-hydroxytryptamine, 5-HT) reuptake inhibitor, whose specificity is unaltered by its major metabolite. Fluoxetine is a 50:50 mixture of

two isomers which have equivalent pharmacological activity in animals. Individuals with reduced P450IID6 isoenzyme activity (3–10% of the normal human population – 'poor metabolisers') were compared to normal metabolisers. The total sum at steady state of the two isomers and their active norfluoxetine metabolites was similar. Thus, net pharmacodynamic activities were essentially the same.

**Product licence numbers**
20 mg capsules:      0006/0195
60 mg capsules:      0006/0198
Liquid:               0006/0272

*Trade Mark

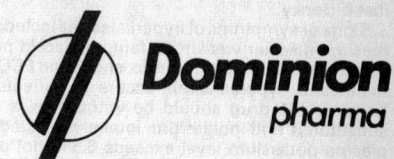

## CLOBURATE* EYE DROPS

**Presentation** Cloburate Eye Drops contain clobetasone 17-butyrate 0.1% w/v as an off-white suspension that is sterile until the bottle is opened. Also contains: benzalkonium chloride 0.01% w/v (preservative), polyethylene glycol 300, sodium citrate and citric acid.

**Uses** For short-term treatment of steroid responsive inflammatory conditions of the eye after clinical exclusion of bacterial, viral and fungal infections. In these conditions it has been shown to have comparable anti-inflammatory activity to Betamethasone Sodium Phosphate Eye Drops.

Cloburate Eye Drops have less adverse effect on intraocular pressure than hydrocortisone (1%), betamethasone sodium phosphate (0.1%), prednisolone sodium phosphate (0.5%), or dexamethasone (0.1%) eye drops.

**Dosage and administration**
*Adults (and the elderly) and children:* The usual dosage is one or two drops four times a day; for severe inflammatory conditions one or two drops should be instilled into the eye every one or two hours until signs of improvement are apparent, when the frequency may be reduced.

**Contra-indications, warnings, etc**
*Contra-indications:* Bacterial, viral, fungal, tuberculous or purulent conditions of the eye.

Use is contra-indicated if glaucoma is present, or where herpetic keratitis (e.g.: dendritic ulcer) is considered a possibility. Inadvertent use of topical steroids in the latter condition can lead to enlargement of the ulcer and marked visual deterioration.

Hypersensitivity to the preparation.

Cloburate Eye Drops contain benzalkonium chloride as a preservative and therefore should not be used to treat patients who wear soft contact lenses.

*Precautions:* Topical corticosteroids should never be given for an undiagnosed red eye as inappropriate use is potentially blinding.

Prolonged use may lead to the risk of adrenal suppression in infants.

Although Cloburate Eye Drops have been shown to have little adverse effect on intra-ocular pressure in most patients, ophthalmological treatment with corticosteroid preparations should not be repeated or prolonged without regular review to exclude raised intra-ocular pressure, cataract formation or unsuspected infections.

Cataract is reported to have occurred after unduly prolonged treatment with some topical corticosteroids and in those diseases which cause thinning of the cornea, perforation has been known to occur.

May cause transient blurring of vision on instillation. Warn patients not to drive or operate hazardous machinery unless vision is clear.

*Pregnancy:* Safety for use in pregnancy and lactation has not been established. There is inadequate evidence of safety in human pregnancy. Administration of topical corticosteroids to pregnant animals can cause abnormalities of foetal development including cleft palate and intra-uterine growth retardation. There may therefore be a very small risk of such effects in the human foetus.

*Side-effects:* Hypersensitivity reactions, usually of the delayed type, may occur leading to irritation, burning, stinging, itching and dermatitis. Topical steroid use may result in increased intra-ocular pressure leading to optic nerve damage, reduced visual acuity and visual field defects.

Rises in intra-ocular pressure have been reported in susceptible patients but these are generally much less than with other corticosteroid eye preparations, including hydrocortisone.

Intensive or prolonged use of topical corticosteroids may lead to formation of posterior subcapsular cataracts.

In those diseases causing thinning of the cornea or sclera, corticosteroid therapy may result in thinning of the globe leading to perforation.

*Overdosage:* Long-term intensive topical use may lead to systemic effects. Oral ingestion of the contents of one bottle (up to 10 ml) is unlikely to lead to any serious adverse effects.

**Pharmaceutical precautions** The contents should not be used more than four weeks after first opening the bottle.

**Legal category** POM

**Package quantities** Plastic dropper bottles containing 10 ml

**Further information** Nil

**Product licence number** 10622/0014

## CLOBURATE-N* EYE DROPS

**Presentation** Cloburate-N Eye Drops contain clobetasone 17-butyrate 0.1% and neomycin sulphate 0.5% w/v as an off-white suspension that is sterile until the bottle is opened. Also contains: benzalkonium chloride 0.01% w/v (preservative), polyethylene glycol 300, disodium hydrogen orthophosphate and citric acid.

**Uses** For short-term treatment of steroid responsive conditions of the eye when prophylactic antibiotic treatment is also required, after excluding the presence of fungal and viral disease. In these conditions it has been shown to have comparable anti-inflammatory activity to Betamethasone Sodium Phosphate with Neomycin Eye Drops.

**Dosage and administration**
*Adults (and the elderly) and children:* The usual dosage is one or two drops four times a day; for severe inflammatory conditions one or two drops should be applied to each affected eye up to six times daily or more frequently if required.

**Contra-indications, warnings, etc**
*Contra-indications:* Viral, fungal, tuberculous or purulent conditions of the eye. Use is contra-indicated if glaucoma is present or herpetic keratitis (e.g.: dendritic ulcer) is considered a possibility. Use of topical steroids in the latter condition can lead to extension of the ulcer and marked visual deterioration.

Hypersensitivity to the preparation.

Cloburate-N Eye Drops contain benzalkonium chloride as a preservative and therefore should not be used to treat patients who wear soft contact lenses.

*Precautions:* Topical corticosteroids should never be given for an undiagnosed red eye as inappropriate use is potentially blinding.

Treatment with corticosteroid/antibiotic combinations should not be continued for more than 7 days in the absence of any clinical improvement, since prolonged use may lead to occult extension of infection due to the masking effect of the steroid. Prolonged use may also lead to skin sensitisation and the emergence of resistant organisms.

Prolonged use may lead to the risk of adrenal suppression in infants.

Treatment with corticosteroid preparations should not be repeated or prolonged without regular review to exclude raised intra-ocular pressure, cataract formation or unsuspected infections.

Aminoglycoside antibiotics may cause irreversible, partial or total deafness when given systemically or when applied topically to open wounds or damaged skin. This effect is dose related and is enhanced by renal or hepatic impairment. Although this effect has not been reported following topical ocular use, the possibility should be considered when high dose topical treatment is given to small children or infants.

May cause transient blurring of vision on instillation. Warn patients not to drive or operate hazardous machinery unless vision is clear.

*Pregnancy and lactation:* Safety for use in pregnancy and lactation has not been established. There is inadequate evidence of safety in human pregnancy. Topical administration of corticosteroids to pregnant animals can cause abnormalities of foetal development including cleft palate and intra-uterine growth retardation. There may, therefore, be a very small risk of such effects in the human foetus. There is a risk of foetal ototoxicity if aminoglycoside antibiotic preparations are administered during pregnancy.

*Side-effects:* Hypersensitivity reactions, usually of the delayed type, may occur leading to irritation, burning, stinging, itching and dermatitis.

Topical steroid use may result in increased intra-ocular pressure leading to optic nerve damage, reduced visual acuity and visual field defects.

Rises in intra-ocular pressure have been reported in susceptible patients, but these are generally much less than with other corticosteroid eye preparations, including hydrocortisone.

Intensive or prolonged use of topical corticosteroids may lead to formation of posterior subcapsular cataracts.

In those diseases causing thinning of the cornea or sclera, corticosteroid therapy may result in thinning of the globe leading to perforation.

*Overdosage:* Long-term intensive topical use may lead to systemic effects. Oral ingestion of the contents of one bottle (up to 10 ml) is unlikely to lead to any serious adverse effects.

**Pharmaceutical precautions** The contents should not be used more than four weeks after first opening the bottle.

**Legal category** POM

**Package quantities** Plastic dropper bottles containing 10 ml

**Further information** Nil

**Product licence number** 10622/0015

## KALSPARE*

**Qualitative and quantitative composition** Chlorthalidone BP 50 mg, Triamterene BP 50 mg

**Pharmaceutical form** Coated tablets

**Clinical particulars**

*Therapeutic indications:* Management of mild to moderate hypertension. Oedema associated with congestive cardiac failure, nephrosis, corticosteroid or oestrogen therapy. Ascites associated with hepatic cirrhosis.

*Posology and method of administration:* Hypertension: Usually one tablet daily taken after breakfast. If necessary the dose may be increased to two tablets taken once daily. Oedema: The usual dose is one tablet daily taken after breakfast. If oedema persists after seven to ten days the dose may be increased to two tablets daily.

Dosage in children has not been established and Kalspare is recommended for the treatment of adults only.

The elderly may require a lower dosage schedule.

*Contra-indications:* Hypersensitivity to the individual components or to other sulphonamide-derived drugs. Progressive renal failure. Concomitant lithium therapy. Kalspare should not be used in the presence of hyperkalaemia (plasma potassium above 5.0 mmol/litre) or in patients receiving other potassium-sparing agents such as spironolactone or amiloride.

*Special warnings and precautions:* Caution should be exercised in patients with severe kidney disease, impaired liver function or progressive liver disease.

As with thiazide diuretics and chlorthalidone, treatment with Kalspare may result in hyperuricaemia or the precipitation of acute gout in certain patients.

Potassium supplements should not be given with Kalspare except in the presence of hypokalaemia.

Chlorthalidone has, in common with other sulphonamide diuretics, occasionally aggravated or precipitated diabetes mellitus. The effect is usually reversible on cessation of therapy.

Chlorthalidone and related drugs may decrease serum protein bound iodine levels without signs of thyroid disturbance.

Triamterene may cause a decreasing alkali reserve, with the possibility of metabolic acidosis.

Although no clinically significant hyperkalaemia has occurred in studies with Kalspare, all potassium conserving diuretic combinations can cause an abnormal elevation of plasma potassium. It is recommended that measurements of potassium are made at the time of dosage adjustments and at appropriate intervals during therapy, particularly in elderly or diabetic patients with confirmed or suspected renal insufficiency.

Signs or symptoms of hyperkalaemia include paresthesia, muscular weakness, fatigue, flaccid paralysis of the extremities, bradycardia, shock and ECG abnormalities. If hyperkalaemia occurs in patients taking Kalspare the drug should be withdrawn, a diuretic substituted and potassium intake restricted. If the plasma potassium level exceeds 6.5 mmol per litre, active measures should be taken to reduce it. Such measures include the intravenous administration of sodium bicarbonate solution or oral or parenteral glucose with a rapid-acting insulin preparation.

If progressive renal impairment becomes evident, Kalspare therapy should be withdrawn and alternative therapy instituted if necessary.

*Interactions with other medicaments and other forms of interaction:* Kalspare may add to or potentiate the action of other antihypertensive drugs. Any tendency to orthostatic hypotension on Kalspare treatment may be aggravated by concomitant alcohol, barbiturates or narcotics. Chlorthalidone and related drugs may increase the responsiveness to tubocurarine.

*Pregnancy and lactation:* Thiazide diuretics have been shown to cross the placenta and also to appear in breast milk. In rare instances, thrombocytopenia, pancreatitis or hypokalaemia have been reported in newborn infants of mothers treated with thiazide diuretics. The use of Kalspare in pregnant or nursing mothers should therefore be avoided unless essential.

*Effects on ability to drive and use machines:* None

*Undesirable effects:* Side effects are similar to those that have been associated with thiazide therapy and include nausea, dry mouth, constipation, leg cramp, headaches, dizziness and fatigue. Rare cases of megaloblastic anaemia have been reported in association with triamterene.

*Overdosage:* The stomach contents should be emptied immediately. Treatment should be symptomatic and supportive with correction of electrolyte imbalance and fluid depletion. No specific antidote exists for Kalspare.

**Pharmacological properties**

*Pharmacodynamic properties:* Kalspare is a long acting potassium sparing diuretic and antihypertensive of particular value in conditions where potassium conservation is important.

Chlorthalidone blocks the reabsorption of sodium and chloride in the cortical diluting segment of the nephron thereby increasing both the quantity of sodium delivered to the distal tubule and the volume of water excreted. However, a portion of the additional sodium reaching the distal tubule is exchanged at this site for potassium and hydrogen.

Triamterene is a weak diuretic found to spare potassium. It acts on the membrane of the lumen in the collecting duct of the kidney to inhibit the reabsorption of sodium and decrease the passive forces influencing the secretion of potassium and hydrogen.

*Pharmacokinetic properties:* Triamterene is incompletely but fairly rapidly absorbed from the gastrointestinal tract. It is extensively metabolised and mainly excreted in the urine as metabolites with some unchanged triamterene.

Chlorthalidone is also incompletely absorbed from the gastro-intestinal tract and is mainly excreted unchanged in the urine.

From a bioequivalence single dose study
*Serum triamterene levels*:
C max (ng/ml) mean: 67.05
T max (h) median: 1
Auc to 24 hours mean: 257.75
*Urinary chlorthalidone levels:*
Peak urinary excretion rate (mg/h) mean: 0.804
Time to peak urinary excretion rate (h) median: 3
Total amount excreted by 120 hours (mg) mean: 15.856
Auc to 120 hours mean: 15.85

*Preclinical safety data:* There are no pre-clinical data of relevance to the prescriber which are additional to that in other sections of the SPC.

**Pharmaceutical particulars**

*List of excipients*: Lactose BP, Starch BP, STA RX 1500 starch, Microcrystalline cellulose BP, Sodium starch glycollate BP, Magnesium stearate BP, Hypromellose, Polyethylene glycol 4000, Polyethylene glycol 400, Antifoam, Sodium propyl hydroxybenzoate BP, Carnauba wax BP, Titanium dioxide E171, Sunset Yellow E110.

*Incompatibilities:* None known

*Shelf life*: 36 months

*Special precautions for storage:* Store in a dry place, below 25°C.

*Nature and contents of container:* PVC/aluminium blister strips containing 4 or 14 tablets.

4 or 28 tablets (2 strips) are packed into cardboard cartons.

*Instructions for use/handling:* None stated.

**Marketing authorisation number** 10622/0019

**Date of approval/revision of SPC** January 1997

**Legal category** POM

## LOMEXIN* PESSARY ▼

**Qualitative and quantitative composition** Fenticonazole nitrate 200 mg or 600 mg

**Pharmaceutical form** Pessary

**Clinical particulars**

*Therapeutic indications:* Vulvovaginal candidiasis

*Contra-indications:* Ascertained hypersensitivity to the product and other imidazole derivatives.

*Side-effects:* After intravaginal administration slight transient burning–which usually disappears rapidly–may occasionally occur.

*Precautions:* In the event of hypersensitivity reactions or development of resistant organisms, treatment should be discontinued and the physician consulted.

*Use during pregnancy and lactation:* Oral administration of fenticonazole in rats has been reported to produce prolonged gestation and embryotoxic effects after doses above 40 mg/kg/day. Fenticonazole does not interfere with the function of male and female gonads and does not modify the first phases of reproduction.

Fenticonazole has shown no teratogenic effects in rats and rabbits.

Fenticonazole or its metabolites cross the placental barrier in pregnant rats and rabbits after vaginal application and are excreted in milk of lactating rats.

Since there is no experience of use during pregnancy and lactation Lomexin should not be used unless the physician considers it essential to the welfare of the patient.

*Interactions with other medicaments:* Not yet investigated. Since fenticonazole systemic absorption after vaginal application is low, interactions with other drugs are unlikely to occur.

*Dosage and administration:* Adults: One 200 mg pessary at bedtime for 3 days, or one 600 mg pessary once only, at bedtime. The pessary must be introduced deep into the vagina.

Children: The use of Lomexin in children is not recommended.

Lomexin is not greasy, does not soil and can easily be removed with water.

*Overdosage:* Because of the low systemic absorption after vaginal application, overdosage is unlikely. In case of a suspected oral accidental ingestion emesis should be induced or gastric lavage may be attempted. Irrespective of success in inducing emesis make patient drink water or lemonade with active charcoal and a laxative. Symptomatic therapy may be administered if indicated.

*Special warnings:* Prolonged topical application may cause sensitisation reactions. The product should not be used in conjunction with barrier contraceptives.

*Effects on driving ability and control of machinery:* None

**Pharmacological properties**

*Pharmacodynamic properties:* Lomexin is a broad-spectrum antimycotic agent.

In vitro: high fungistatic and fungicidal activity against *Candida albicans*.

In vivo: healing of vaginal mycoses due to candida within 5 days in mice.

*Pharmacokinetic properties:* Pharmacokinetic studies in humans have shown that systemic absorption of fenticonazole nitrate after vaginal administration is minimal.

*Preclinical safety data:* In mice, rats and dogs, the oral $LD_{50}$ values were 3000 mg/kg, 3000 mg/kg and 1000 mg/kg, respectively.

Long term oral administration to rats and dogs at and above 60 mg/kg/day has been reported to produce morphological and functional modifications of the liver, while cutaneous and ocular reactions were noticed in dogs only.

Fenticonazole has no mutagenic potential.

Satisfactory results were obtained in tolerability tests performed in rabbit, dog, guinea pig and mini-pig.

Fenticonazole has shown no evidence of phototoxicity and photoallergy.

**Pharmaceutical particulars**

*List of excipients:* Lomexin 200 mg: Triglycerides of saturated fatty acids, colloidal silicon dioxide, gelatin, glycerin, titanium dioxide, sodium ethyl hydroxybenzoate, sodium propyl hydroxybenzoate.

Lomexin 600 mg: Liquid paraffin, white soft paraffin, soya lecithin, gelatin, titanium dioxide, sodium ethyl hydroxybenzoate, sodium propyl hydroxybenzoate.

*Incompatibilities:* None

*Shelf life:* in integral package: 36 months.

*Special precautions for storage:* No special storage conditions are required.

*Nature and contents of container:*

200 mg Pessary: PVC/PVDC/aluminium foil blisters in packs of 3 pessaries

600 mg Pessary: PVC/PVDC/aluminium foil blisters in packs of 1 pessary

**Marketing authorisation numbers**
200 mg Pessary 10622/0024
600 mg Pessary 10622/0025

**Date of approval/revision of SPC** 9 March 1995

**Legal category** POM

## LOTRIDERM* CREAM

**Presentation** Smooth uniform white to off-white cream free of foreign matter, containing 0.05% betamethasone as the dipropionate ester and 1% clotrimazole.

**Uses** Lotriderm Cream combines the broad spectrum antifungal activity of clotrimazole with the sustained anti-inflammatory, antipruritic and vasoconstrictive actions of betamethasone dipropionate and is indicated for short-term topical treatment of the following dermal infections: *Trichophyton rubrum, T. mentagrophytes, Epidermophyton floccosum* and *Microsporum canis*; candidiasis due to *Candida albicans*.

**Dosage and administration** Gently massage sufficient Lotriderm Cream into the affected and surrounding skin areas twice daily, in the morning and evening for two weeks in tinea cruris, tinea corporis and candidiasis and four weeks in tinea pedis.

Clinical improvement, with relief of erythema and pruritus, usually occurs within the first 3 to 5 days of treatment. If a patient with tinea cruris, tinea corporis or candidiasis shows no clinical improvement after one week of treatment with Lotriderm, the diagnosis should be reviewed. Similarly in tinea pedis diagnosis should be reviewed if no improvement is shown after two weeks of treatment.

**Contra-indications, warnings, etc** Lotriderm is contra-indicated in those patients with history of sensitivity to any of its components or to other corticosteroids or imidazoles.

If irritation or sensitisation develops with the use of Lotriderm Cream, treatment should be discontinued and appropriate therapy instituted.

Lotriderm is contra-indicated in facial rosacea, acne vulgaris, perioral dermatitis, perianal and genital pruritus, napkin eruptions and bacterial or viral infections.

In the presence of bacterial or viral infections appropriate concomitant therapy should be administered. If a favourable response does not occur promptly, treatment with Lotriderm should be discontinued until the infection has been controlled adequately.

Any of the side-effects that are reported following systemic use of corticosteroids, including adrenal suppression, may also occur with topical steroids, especially in infants and children.

Local and systemic toxicity is common especially following long continued use on large areas of damaged skin, and in flexures. If used in children or on the face courses should be limited to 5 days. Long term continuous therapy should be avoided in all patients irrespective of age.

Lotriderm Cream should not be used with occlusive dressing.

The safety and effectiveness of Lotriderm Cream has not been established in children below the age of 12.

Lotriderm Cream is not intended for ophthalmic use.

Topical corticosteroids may be hazardous in psoriasis for a number of reasons including rebound relapses following the development of tolerance, risk of generalised pustular psoriasis and local and systemic toxicity due to impaired barrier function of the skin.

There is inadequate evidence of safety in pregnancy. Clotrimazole has shown no teratogenic effect in animals but is foetotoxic at high oral doses. Topical administration of corticosteroids to pregnant animals can cause abnormalities of foetal development including cleft palate and intra-uterine growth retardation. There may therefore be a very small risk of such effects in the human foetus. Hence Lotriderm Cream should only be used in pregnancy if the benefit justifies the potential risk to the foetus and such use should not be extensive, i.e. in large amounts or for long periods.

It is not known whether the components of Lotriderm are excreted in human milk and therefore caution should be exercised when treating nursing mothers.

Adverse reactions reported for Lotriderm include: burning and stinging, maculopapular rash, oedema and secondary infection.

Reported reactions to clotrimazole include erythema, stinging, blistering, peeling, oedema, pruritus, urticaria and general irritation of the skin.

Reactions to betamethasone dipropionate include: burning, itching, irritation, dryness, folliculitis, hypertrichosis, acneiform eruptions, hyperpigmentation, perioral dermatitis, allergic contact dermatitis, maceration of the skin, secondary infection, skin atrophy, striae and miliaria.

**Pharmaceutical precautions**  Store at or below 25°C.

**Legal category**  POM

**Package quantities**  Tubes of 15 g.

**Further information**  Nil.

**Product licence number** 0201/0081

*Product licence holder:* Schering-Plough Ltd., Welwyn Garden City

## MASNODERM* CREAM

**Presentation**  A white cream containing 1.0% Clotrimazole BP in a dispersible base. Also contains: 2-octyldodecanol, stearyl alcohol, cetyl alcohol, cetyl esters wax, sorbitan monostearate, polysorbate 60, benzyl alcohol and water.

**Uses**  Clotrimazole is a broad spectrum antifungal agent, which also exhibits activity against Trichomonas spp., Staphylococcus spp., Streptococcus spp. and Bacteroides spp.

Clotrimazole is indicated for the treatment of skin infections due to dermatophytes (e.g. Trichophyton spp.), yeasts (e.g. Candida spp.), moulds and other fungi. These include ringworm (tinea) infections, athlete's foot, paronychia, pityriasis versicolor, erythrasma and intertrigo as well as fungal nappy rash, candidal vaginitis and candidal balanitis.

**Dosage and administration**  Two or three times daily. Masnoderm cream should be thinly and evenly applied to the affected area and rubbed in gently.

Treat dermatophyte infections for at least one month and candida infections for at least two weeks.

If used to treat infections of the feet, wash and dry thoroughly before applying the cream. In the treatment of the intertriginous areas, thorough drying of the lesion after washing is essential.

### Contra-indications, warnings, etc

*Contra-indications:* Known hypersensitivity to any of the components.

*Warnings and precautions:* No special precautions necessary.

*Side-effects:* Rarely patients may experience local mild burning or irritation immediately after applying the cream. Rarely hypersensitivity reactions have occurred.

*Use in pregnancy:* Not recommended.

*Overdosage:* Accidental ingestion: in cases of accidental oral ingestion routine supporting measures such as gastric lavage should be performed as soon as possible.

**Pharmaceutical precautions**  No special storage precautions are necessary.

**Legal category**  P

**Package quantities**  Tubes containing 20 g

**Further information**  Nil

**Product licence number** 10622/0004

## MODRASONE* CREAM
## MODRASONE* OINTMENT

**Qualitative and quantitative composition**  Alclometasone dipropionate 0.05% w/w.

**Pharmaceutical form**  Cream/ointment for topical use.

**Clinical particulars**

*Therapeutic indications:* Alclometasone dipropionate is a non-fluorinated topically active synthetic corticosteroid. Modrasone is indicated for the treatment of inflammatory and pruritic manifestations of corticosteroid responsive dermatoses.

*Posology and method of administration:*

*Adult and children:* A thin film of Modrasone should be applied to the affected area two or three times daily or as directed by the physician. Massage gently into the skin until the medication disappears.

*Contra-indications:* Hypersensitivity to any of the ingredients; rosacea; acne and perioral dermatitis; tuberculous and viral lesions of the skin, particularly Herpes Simplex; vaccinia; varicella.

Modrasone should not be used in fungal or bacterial skin infections.

*Special warnings and precautions:* As with all topical steroids, long term continuous therapy should be avoided where possible, particularly in infants and children as adrenal suppression may occur even without occlusion. In infants the napkin may act as an occlusive dressing and thus increase absorption.

*Interactions with other medicaments and other forms of interaction:* None known.

*Pregnancy and lactation:* Topical administration of corticosteroids to pregnant animals can cause abnormalities in foetal development. The relevance of this finding to human beings has not been established; however, topical steroids should not be used extensively in pregnancy i.e. in large amounts or for long periods.

It is not known whether topical administration of corticosteroids could result in sufficient systemic absorption to produce detectable quantities in breast milk. Modrasone should be administered to nursing mothers only after careful consideration of the benefit/risk relationship.

*Effects on ability to drive and use machines:* Not applicable.

*Undesirable effects:* Excessive prolonged use may result in local atrophy of the skin, striae and superficial vascular dilation, particularly on the face.

*Overdosage:* Excessive prolonged use of topical corticosteroids can suppress pituitary-adrenal function resulting in secondary adrenal insufficiency which is usually reversible. In such cases appropriate symptomatic treatment is indicated. In cases of chronic toxicity, corticosteroids should be withdrawn.

The steroid content is so low as to have little or no effect in the unlikely event of accidental oral ingestion.

**Pharmacological properties**

*Pharmacodynamic properties:* Alclometasone dipropionate is a non-fluorinated, topically active synthetic corticosteroid. Alclometasone dipropionate suppresses local inflammation at doses producing minimal systemic effects. Studies have shown alclometasone dipropionate to be approximately 2/3 as potent as betamethasone valerate and 60 x as potent as hydrocortisone.

*Pharmacokinetic properties:* Not applicable in view of topical action and application.

*Preclinical safety data:* Modrasone appears to be a relatively non-toxic and non-irritating drug product that produces no unusual or unexpected teratologic effects in laboratory animals. A wide margin of safety was demonstrated in all species studied. Acute oral and intraperitoneal doses more than 3,000 times the proposed topical human dose were without any toxicologically significant effects.

**Pharmaceutical particulars**

*List of excipients:* Cream: Propylene Glycol PhEur, White Soft Paraffin BP, Cetostearyl Alcohol BP, Glyceryl stearate PEG 100 stearate, Polyoxyethylene (20) cetyl ether, Sodium dihydrogenium phosphate dihydrate, 4-Chloro-M-Cresol BP, Phosphoric Acid Ph Eur, Purified Water PhEur.

Ointment: Hexylene glycol, Propylene glycol monostearate, White Beeswax BP, White Soft Paraffin BP.

*Incompatibilities:* None known

*Shelf life:* Cream and ointment: 60 months

*Special precautions for storage:* Store below 25°C.

*Nature and contents of container:* Cream and Ointment: Aluminium tubes with white LDPE caps. Pack size: 50 g

*Instructions for use/handling:* Not applicable

*Marketing authorisation holder:* Schering-Plough Ltd., Welwyn Garden City.

**Marketing authorisation numbers**
Cream: 0201/0060
Ointment: 0201/0061

**Date of approval/revision of SPC**  March 1996

**Legal category** POM

## NEO-CORTEF* EYE/EAR DROPS
## NEO-CORTEF* EYE/EAR OINTMENT

**Qualitative and quantitative composition**
Eye/Ear Drops: Hydrocortisone acetate 15 mg and neomycin sulphate 5 mg (equivalent to neomycin 3.5 mg) per ml.
Eye/Ear Ointment: Hydrocortisone acetate 15 mg and neomycin sulphate 5 mg (equivalent to neomycin 3.5 mg) per g.

**Pharmaceutical form**
Eye/Ear Drops
Eye/Ear Ointment

**Clinical particulars**

*Therapeutic indications:*
Eye: Short-term treatment of steroid responsive conditions of the eye when prophylactic antibiotic treatment is also required, after excluding the presence of fungal and viral disease.
Eyelid: Blepharitis
Ear: Otitis externa caused by susceptible organisms

*Posology and method of administration:*
*Adults and children:*
DROPS:
Eye: One or two drops to be applied to each eye up to six times daily or more frequently if required.
Ear: Two or three drops to be instilled into the ear three to four times daily.
OINTMENT:
Eye: Apply sparingly two or three times daily, or at night if drop treatment is given during the day.
Ear: Apply once or twice daily.
*Elderly patients:* There is no information to suggest that a change in dosage is warranted in the elderly, however care should be taken when the drops/ointment are administered in this group (see Special warnings and special precautions for use).
Do not exceed the recommended dose.

*Contra-indications:* Viral, fungal, tuberculous or purulent conditions of the eye. Use is contra-indicated if glaucoma is present or herpetic keratitis (eg dendritic ulcer) is considered a possibility.
Use of topical steroids in the latter condition can lead to extension of the ulcer and marked visual deterioration.
Otitis externa should not be treated when the eardrum is perforated because of the risk of ototoxicity.
Hypersensitivity to any of the ingredients of the preparation.

*Special warnings and precautions:* Topical corticosteroids should never be given for an undiagnosed red eye as inappropriate use is potentially blinding.
Treatment with corticosteroid/antibiotic combinations should not be continued for more than 7 days in the absence of any clinical improvement, since prolonged use may lead to occult extension of infection due to the masking effect of the steroid. Prolonged use may also lead to skin sensitisation and the emergence of resistant organisms.
Prolonged use may lead to the risk of adrenal suppression in infants.
Treatment with corticosteroid preparations should not be repeated or prolonged without regular review to exclude raised intra-ocular pressure, cataract formation or unsuspected infections.
Aminoglycoside antibiotics may cause irreversible, partial or total deafness when given systemically or when applied topically to open wounds or damaged skin. This effect is dose related and is enhanced by renal or hepatic impairment. Although this effect has not been reported following topical ocular use, the possibility should be considered when high dose topical treatment is given to small children or infants and patients suffering from renal impairment.
Care should also be taken when the drops/ointment are administered to the elderly and those with existing hearing loss.

*Interactions with other medicaments and other forms of interaction:* None relevant to ocular/aural use.

*Pregnancy and lactation:* Safety for use in pregnancy and lactation has not been established. There is inadequate evidence of safety in human pregnancy. Topical administration of corticosteroids to pregnant animals can cause abnormalities of foetal development including cleft palate and intra-uterine growth retardation. There may therefore be a very small risk of such effects in the human foetus. There is a risk of foetal ototoxicity if aminoglycoside antibiotic preparations are administered during pregnancy.

*Effects on ability to drive and use machines:* Transient blurring of vision on instillation or application. Warn patients not to drive or operate hazardous machinery unless vision is clear.

*Undesirable effects:* Hypersensitivity reactions, usually of the delayed type, may occur leading to irritation, burning, stinging, itching and dermatitis.

Topical steroid use may result in increased intra-ocular pressure leading to optic nerve damage, reduced visual acuity, and visual field defects.

In those diseases causing thinning of the cornea or sclera, corticosteroid therapy may result in thinning of the globe leading to perforation.

*Overdosage:* Long-term intensive topical use may lead to systemic effects.

Oral ingestion of the contents of one bottle is unlikely to lead to any serious adverse effects.

### Pharmacological properties

*Pharmacodynamic properties:* Neomycin is an aminoglycoside antibiotic. It has activity against many Gram-negative bacteria (not *Pseudomonas* spp), and *Staphylococcus aureus.*

Hydrocortisone is a mild corticosteroid.

*Pharmacokinetic properties:* Activity is intended to be restricted locally to the eye/ear.

*Preclinical safety data:* There are no pre-clinical data of relevance to the prescriber which are additional to that in other sections of the SPC.

### Pharmaceutical particulars

*List of excipients:*
Eye/Ear Drops: Sodium citrate, polyethylene glycol, myristyl gamma-picolinium chloride, povidone, water.

Eye/Ear Ointment: White soft paraffin, wool fat, liquid paraffin.

*Incompatibilities:* None known

*Shelf life:*
Eye/Ear Drops: 36 months
Eye/Ear Ointment: 48 months

*Special precautions for storage:*
Eye/Ear Drops: Store at room temperature below 25°C. Protect from freezing.
Eye/Ear Ointment: Store at room temperature below 25°C.

*Nature and contents of container:*
Eye/Ear Drops: Polyethylene squeeze bottle with applicator tip, containing 10 ml of sterile suspension.
Eye/Ear Ointment: Collapsible, internally lacquered tubes, containing 3.9 g ointment.

*Instructions for use/handling:*
Eye/Ear Drops: The contents are sterile whilst the bottle seal is intact. Discard one month after opening.
Eye/Ear Ointment: Discard one month after opening.

*Marketing authorisation holder:* Pharmacia & Upjohn Limited, Milton Keynes

**Marketing authorisation numbers**
Eye/Ear Drops: 0032/5026
Eye/Ear Ointment: 0032/5027

**Date of approval/revision of SPC** December 1996

**Legal category** POM

## NEOSPORIN* EYE DROPS

**Presentation** A colourless to very pale yellow, slightly hazy solution. Each ml contains:

| | |
|---|---|
| Polymyxin B Sulphate BP | 5,000 units |
| Neomycin Sulphate BP | 1,700 units |
| Gramicidin USP | 25 units |

Also contains Thiomersal BP (0.001%) as a preservative.

**Uses** Topical antibacterial agent. For the prophylaxis and treatment of external bacterial infections of the eye. Prophylactically, it is useful following removal of foreign bodies, and before and after ophthalmic surgery, to help provide and maintain a sterile field.

**Dosage and administration** *Adults and children:* 1 or 2 drops in the affected eye, two to four times daily or more frequently as required. In severe infections, therapy should be started with 1 or 2 drops every 15 to 30 minutes, reducing the frequency of instillation gradually as the infection is controlled.

*Use in the elderly:* No special comment.

### Contra-indications, warnings, etc

*Contra-indications:* Hypersensitivity to polymyxins, gramicidin or neomycin group of antibiotics.

*Precautions:* Neomycin is ototoxic and nephrotoxic if absorbed from open surfaces. Polymyxin B and gramicidin are also nephrotoxic. However, these effects are unlikely with ocular administration.

Neosporin Eye Drops should not be used during surgical procedures nor before surgery in circumstances where access of the product to intra-ocular fluids could occur.

*Side- and adverse effects:* Allergic reactions following the topical application of neomycin have been reported in the literature, but such reactions following the application of polymyxin B and gramicidin are rare events.

As with all antibacterial preparations prolonged use

may result in the overgrowth of non-susceptible organisms including fungi.

*Use in pregnancy and lactation:* Neosporin Eye Drops have been in use for many years. There has been no evidence of untoward effects in pregnancy. However, caution should be exercised by balancing the potential benefits of treatment against any possible hazard.

No information is available regarding the excretion of the active ingredients or their metabolites in human breast milk.

*Toxicity and treatment of overdosage:* Not applicable.

**Pharmaceutical precautions** Store below 15°C. Keep dry. Protect from light. Not suitable for injection. Discard four weeks after opening.

**Legal category** POM

**Package quantities** Special dropper bottle of 5 ml (OP).

**Further information** Neosporin is a non-irritating isotonic solution and is well tolerated by the sensitive structures of the eye.

**Product licence number** 0003/5108R

*Product licence holder:* The Wellcome Foundation Limited, Greenford, Middlesex.

## NITROMIN* SPRAY

**Qualitative and quantitative composition** Glyceryl trinitrate 400 micrograms/dose

**Pharmaceutical form** Oromucosal spray

### Clinical particulars

*Therapeutic indications:* For the treatment and prophylaxis of angina pectoris.

*Posology and method of administration:*
*Adult:* At the onset of an attack: 1 or 2 sprays (400-800 micrograms). Dose should not exceed more than 3 sprays at any one time.

For prophylaxis: 1-2 sprays (400-800 micrograms) immediately prior to an angina inducing event.

The patient should be in the sitting position. The spray should be held upright and should not be inhaled. After spraying under the tongue the mouth should be closed immediately after each dose.

*Elderly:* As adult.

*Children:* Not recommended.

*Contra-indications:* Hypersensitivity to nitrates. Hypotensive shock. Severe anaemia. Cerebral haemorrhage and brain trauma. Mitral stenosis. Angina caused by hypertrophic obstructive cardiomyopathy.

*Special warnings and precautions:* Tolerance and cross-tolerance to other nitrates may occur.

*Interactions with other medicaments and other forms of interaction:* Alcohol may potentiate the hypotensive effects.

Nitromin may be employed in conjunction with other nitrate containing products, but care should be taken to avoid excessive total intake. In practical terms this means that sublingual GTN tablets should not be taken in addition to Nitromin for the same anginal attack unless under close medical supervision (this does not apply to long acting nitrate preparations used for attack prevention).

*Pregnancy and lactation:* There are no specific data available on the use of Nitromin in human pregnancy. Since angina is uncommon in pregnancy it is unlikely that the need for Nitromin would arise. In all cases, the benefit of treatment to the patient must be balanced against any possible hazard to the foetus. There is no information regarding excretion of glyceryl trinitrate in breast milk.

*Effects on ability to drive and use machines:* Nitromin should not impair ability to drive or use machines, however, patients should be advised not to drive etc. if they feel unwell or faint after using the spray.

*Undesirable effects:* The following side effects occur in approximately 30-40% of patients: taste disturbance (metallic taste), headache, postural hypotension, flushing, and palpitations. These are usually mild and disappear within a few minutes.

*Overdosage:* Symptoms—flushing, severe headache, a feeling of suffocation, hypotension, fainting. Rarely cyanosis and methaemoglobinaemia. In a few patients a reaction comparable to shock with nausea, vomiting, weakness, sweating and syncope.

Emergency procedures—recovery often occurs without special treatment. Elevate legs to promote venous return.

Antidote—treat methaemoglobinaemia with intravenous methylene blue. Treat symptomatically for serious respiratory and circulatory effects.

### Pharmacological properties

*Pharmacodynamic properties:* Glyceryl trinitrate relaxes smooth muscle and reduces blood pressure. Its

anti-anginal effects are believed to depend on reducing myocardial oxygen demand by means of peripheral vasodilation.

*Pharmacokinetic properties:* The onset of action following sublingual administration is within 2 minutes. Duration of action is about 30 minutes.

*Preclinical safety data:* No animal toxicological studies have been performed using Nitromin. Animal studies using inorganic nitrates have shown toxic effects due to excessive pharmacodynamic action (e.g. hypovolaemia, shock, and circulatory collapse) or due to the effects of methaemoglobinaemia. These effects have always occurred at doses proportional to doses in the toxic range in humans.

Studies in pregnant animals have shown similar toxic effects but no evidence of a direct teratogenic effect.

### Pharmaceutical particulars

*List of excipients:* Propylene glycol BP, Ethanol (96%) v/v BP

*Incompatibilities:* None known

*Shelf life:* Opened and unopened: 36 months.

*Special precautions for storage:* Store in a cool place below 25°C. Protect from sunlight and do not expose to temperatures above 50°C. Do not pierce or burn after use. Do not spray on to a naked flame or any incandescent material.

*Nature and contents of container:* Aluminium canister with metered dosing valve and nozzle. Plastic protective cap. Each canister contains 10 grams (180 doses).

*Instructions for use/handling:* None stated.

**Marketing authorisation number** 10622/0011

**Date of approval/revision of SPC** July 1996

**Legal category** P

## OCUSERT*

**Qualitative and quantitative composition**
Ocusert Pilo 20: Pilocarpine USP 5.0 mg per unit
Ocusert Pilo 40: Pilocarpine USP 11.0 mg per unit.

**Pharmaceutical form** Ocular inserts. Elliptically shaped units designed to release pilocarpine continuously following placement into the upper or lower conjunctival sac.

The systems consist of a core reservoir of pilocarpine surrounded by a membrane which controls the drug's diffusion from the system into the tear fluid. Two systems are available, Ocusert Pilo 20 and Ocusert Pilo 40, which release 20 and 40 micrograms per hour, respectively, for one week. The Ocusert Pilo 20 system is 5.7 x 13.4 mm across its axis, 0.3 mm thick and contains 5 mg pilocarpine: the Ocusert Pilo 40 system is 5.5 x 13 mm across its axis, 0.5 mm thick, and contains 11 mg pilocarpine. Except for the opaque white margin, the systems are clear.

### Clinical particulars

*Therapeutic indications:* The Ocusert pilocarpine system is indicated for control of elevated intra-ocular pressure in glaucoma, in pilocarpine-responsive patients.

*Posology and method of administration:*
Route of administration: Placement in the conjunctival sac. Suitable for use with contact lenses.
Recommended doses and dosage schedules:
*Adults and elderly. Initiation of therapy:* The Ocusert Pilo 20 system will usually control a patient previously controlled by 1 per cent or 2 per cent pilocarpine eye drops; a patient who has used higher strengths of pilocarpine eye drops may require the Ocusert Pilo 40. However, there is no direct correlation between the two strengths of Ocusert and the strength of pilocarpine eye drops necessary to achieve the required reduction of pressure. The Ocusert systems reduce the amount of pilocarpine necessary to achieve adequate reduction of intra-ocular pressure; therapy may be started therefore with the Ocusert Pilo 20 system irrespective of the strength of pilocarpine eye drops used previously by the patient. If the pressure is satisfactorily reduced with the Ocusert Pilo 20 system the patient should continue with its use, replacing each unit every 7 days; if greater reduction of intra-ocular pressure is required, the patient should be transferred to the Ocusert Pilo 40 system. Depending on the patient's age, family history, and disease status, the ophthalmologist may elect to begin therapy with the Ocusert Pilo 40 system.

*Concomitant therapy:* Where necessary, adrenaline or timolol eye drops or a diuretic of the carbonic anhydrase inhibitor type may be used concurrently with Ocusert systems. The release rate of pilocarpine from the Ocusert system is not influenced by the beta adrenoceptor antagonists, carbonic anhydrase inhibitors, adrenaline eye drops, fluorescein or local anaesthetics, antibiotics or anti-inflammatory steroid eye drops.

*Placement and removal of the Ocusert systems:* Patient instructions for the replacement of the Ocusert systems in the eye and their removal are included in each package. It is strongly recommended that the patient's ability to manage the placement and removal of the system be reviewed at the first patient visit after initiation of therapy.

Since pilocarpine-induced myopia from the Ocusert system may occur during the first few hours of therapy, the patient should be advised to place the system into the conjunctival sac at bedtime. By morning the induced myopia is at a stable level.

*Handling precautions:* Patients should be instructed to wash their hands thoroughly with soap and water before touching or manipulating the Ocusert systems. If a displaced unit contacts unclean surfaces, rinsing with cool tap water before replacing is advisable. Bacteriologically contaminated units should be discarded and replaced with fresh ones.

*Retention in the eye:* During the initial adaptation period, the Ocusert unit may slip out of the conjunctival sac to the cheek. The patient is usually aware of such movement and can replace the unit without difficulty. In those patients in whom retention of the Ocusert is a problem, placement in the upper conjunctival sac maybe more acceptable. The Ocusert unit can be manipulated from the lower to the upper conjunctival sac by a gentle digital massage through the lid, a technique readily learned by the patient. For best retention, the unit should be moved before sleep to the upper conjunctival sac. Should the unit slip out of the conjunctival sac during sleep, its ocular hypotensive effect continues for a period of time comparable to that following instillation of eye drops. The patient should be instructed to check for the presence of the Ocusert unit before sleep and on rising.

*Children:* Not recommended.

*Contra-indications:* Ocusert systems are contra-indicated where pupillary constriction is undesirable, such as glaucomas associated with acute inflammatory disease of the anterior segment of the eye, and glaucomas occurring or persisting after extra-capsular cataract extraction where posterior synechiae may occur.

*Special warnings and precautions:* Ocusert systems should not be used in patients with acute infectious conjunctivitis or keratitis except on specialist advice. Damaged or deformed systems should not be placed or retained in the eye. Systems believed to be associated with an unexpected increase in drug action should be removed and replaced with new systems.

The safety of Ocusert systems in patients with retinal detachment or with filtration blebs has not been established.

Although withdrawal of the peripheral iris from the anterior chamber angle by miosis may reduce the tendency for narrow angle closure, miotics can occasionally precipitate angle closure by increasing the resistance to aqueous flow from posterior to anterior chamber. Miotic agents may also cause retinal detachment; thus, care should be exercised with all miotic therapy especially in young myopic patients.

The use of pilocarpine eye drops should be considered when intense miosis is desired in certain ocular conditions.

*Interaction with other medicaments and other forms of interaction:* Although eye drops have been used effectively in conjunction with the Ocusert systems, systemic reactions consistent with an increased rate of absorption from the eye of an automotive drug, such as adrenaline, have been observed. In rare instances, reactions of this type can be severe. The conjunctival erythema and oedema associated with adrenaline eye drops are not substantially altered by concomitant use of an Ocusert system.

*Pregnancy and lactation:* Pilocarpine has no known effect on pregnancy and lactation.

*Effect on the ability to drive and use machines:* The effect of Pilocarpine on visual accommodation may affect the patient's ability to drive and use machinery.

*Undesirable effects:* Ciliary spasm is encountered with Pilocarpine usage but is not a contra-indication to continued therapy unless the induced myopia is debilitating to the patient. Irritation from Pilocarpine has been infrequently encountered and may require cessation of therapy depending on judgement of the doctor. True allergic reactions are uncommon, but require discontinuation of therapy if they occur.

Some patients may notice signs of conjunctival irritation including mild erythema with or without a slight increase in mucous secretion when they first use Ocusert systems. These signs tend to lessen or disappear after the first week of therapy. In rare instances a sudden increase in pilocarpine effect has been reported.

*Overdose:* Patients are unlikely to experience pilocarpine overdosage with the use of the Ocusert system.

**Pharmacological properties**

*Pharmacodynamic properties:* Pilocarpine is released from the Ocusert system as soon as it is placed in contact with the conjunctival surfaces. Pilocarpine is a direct acting parasympathomimetic drug which produces pupillary constriction, stimulates the ciliary muscle and increased aqueous humour outflow facility.

*Pharmacokinetic properties:* The ocular hypotensive effect of both the Ocusert Pilo 20 and Ocusert Pilo 40 systems is fully developed within 1½ to 2 hours after placement in the conjunctival sac and is maintained for 24 hours a day for seven days.

*Pre clinical safety data:* Not applicable

**Pharmaceutical particulars**

*List of excipients:* Alginic acid, Ethylene vinyl acetate, Titanium dioxide. Ocusert Pilo 40 also contains Di (2-Ethylhexyl) phthalate.

*Incompatibilities:* None known

*Shelf life:* 36 months

*Special precautions for storage:* Ocusert Pilo 20/40 should be stored in a refrigerator at 2-8°C.

*Nature and contents of container:* Containers of 1, 2, 4 or 8 inserts (sterile units)

*Instructions for use/handling:* None

**Marketing authorisation numbers**
Ocusert Pilo 20 10622/0012
Ocusert Pilo 40 10622/0013

**Date of approval/revision of SPC** October 1996

**Legal category** POM

## PERCUTOL*

**Qualitative and quantitative composition** The active ingredient of Percutol is glyceryl trinitrate 2 %w/w.

**Pharmaceutical form** A homogeneous cream coloured ointment.

**Clinical particulars**

*Therapeutic indications:* Prophylaxis of angina pectoris.

*Posology and method of administration:* Topical application.

*Adults (including elderly):* The usual dose is 1 to 2 inches squeezed from the tube, although some patients may require more. This dose may be repeated every 3 to 4 hours as required.

The dose may be titrated to individual patients' needs by finding the dose that causes headache and then reducing this dose by half an inch. Half an inch of ointment should be applied on the first day, one inch on the second, etc. increasing by half an inch per day until headache occurs and then reducing by half an inch. If several applications per day are required the dose may need to be reduced.

The ointment may be conveniently measured and applied using the paper "Applirules" enclosed in the carton. After squeezing the required length of ointment onto the "Applirule" it should be pressed on to any convenient area of skin (e.g. chest, thigh, or arm) until the ointment is spread in a thin layer under the paper. The ointment should not be rubbed in. The "Applirule" may be secured in place with surgical tape.

*Children:* The safety and efficacy of Percutol in children has not been established.

*Contra-indications:* May be contra-indicated in patients with marked anaemia, or raised intra cranial pressure. Should not be employed in patients with known idiosyncrasies to nitrates.

*Special warnings and precautions:* In the elderly the development of postural hypotension may be more pronounced especially on sudden rising. Caution should be exercised in patients with cerebrovascular disease. As with other vasodilators chronic therapy should not be discontinued abruptly. The frequency of application and the dosage should gradually be reduced (over a period of 4 to 6 weeks).

*Interactions with other medicaments and other forms of interaction:* Some effects of glyceryl trinitrate are enhanced by alcohol.

*Pregnancy and lactation:* The safety of Percutol in pregnancy is not established. The product should therefore be given during pregnancy, only if clearly needed. It is not known whether glyceryl trinitrate is excreted in human milk, therefore caution should be exercised when administered to a nursing mother.

*Effects on ability to drive and use machines:* Glyceryl trinitrate may cause dizziness. In consequence until the effect of treatment is known, patients should be warned not to take charge of vehicles or machinery.

*Undesirable effects:* Headache, flushing, dizziness or postural hypotension.

*Overdosage:* A hypotensive headache is a sign of overdosage. High doses of glyceryl trinitrate may cause marked hypotension and collapse, however topical application reduces the likelihood of overdosage and the effect can be quickly terminated by washing the ointment off the skin.

**Pharmacological properties**

*Pharmacodynamic properties:* The active ingredient relaxes smooth muscle and reduces blood pressure. Its use as a vasodilator in the prophylaxis and treatment of angina pectoris is well established.

*Pharmacokinetic properties:* In human volunteers the mean absorption of glyceryl trinitrate from 1 inch of ointment was 0.8 mg/hour.

*Preclinical safety data:* There are no preclinical data of relevance to the prescriber which are additional to that already included in other sections of the SPC.

**Pharmaceutical particulars**

*List of excipients:* Percutol also contains lanolin anhydrous USP, purified water USP, white petroleum USP, and lactose anhydrous USP.

*Incompatibilities:* None stated.

*Shelf life:* 36 months.

*Special precautions for storage:* Store below 25°C.

*Nature and contents of container:* Collapsible aluminium tube containing 60 g.

*Instructions for use/handling:* None stated.

*Marketing authorisation holder:* Rorer Pharmaceuticals, West Malling.

**Marketing authorisation number** 5272/0001

**Date of approval/revision of SPC** February 1997

**Legal category** P

## POLYFAX* OINTMENT

**Presentation** Polyfax Ointment contains 10,000 units of Polymyxin B Sulphate BP and 500 units of Zinc Bacitracin BP per gram, in a stable petrolatum base. The translucent ointment is off-white in colour.

**Uses** Topical antibacterial agent. Polyfax Ointment is indicated for the treatment of infected wounds, burns, skin grafts, ulcers, pyoderma, sycosis barbae, impetigo, and in secondarily infected skin lesions of scabies, pediculosis, tinea pedis and contact and allergic dermatitis.

**Dosage and administration**

*Adults:* Polyfax Ointment should be applied thinly over the affected area, which is best left exposed. Two or more applications a day may be necessary, depending on the severity of the condition.

*Children:* As for adults.

*Use in the elderly:* No specific studies have been carried out in the elderly, however it may be advisable to monitor renal function in these patients and if there is any impairment then caution should be exercised.

**Contra-indications, warnings, etc**

*Contra-indications:* Hypersensitivity to bacitracin, polymyxins or cross-sensitising substances.

*Precautions:* The following statements take into account the possibility that the constituent drugs of Polyfax Ointment may be absorbed to a significant degree after topical application. However, the normal use of Polyfax is unlikely to present any risk of systemic toxicity unless the application were excessive eg more than 200 g per day in adults or proportionately less in children and in patients with compromised renal function.

Nephrotoxicity may result from the absorption of bacitracin, and nephrotoxicity and neurotoxicity from polymyxin B.

As with all antibacterial preparations prolonged use may result in the overgrowth of non-susceptible organisms including fungi.

*Side- and adverse effects:* Allergic reactions following topical application of polymyxin B and zinc bacitracin have rarely been reported.

Anaphylactic reactions have been reported, as rare events, following topical application of zinc bacitracin. Following significant systemic absorption, polymyxin B can intensify and prolong the respiratory depressant effects of neuromuscular blocking agents.

*Use in pregnancy and lactation:* Due to a lack of detailed information, the use of Polyfax Ointment during pregnancy and lactation cannot be recommended in circumstances where significant systemic absorption of the active ingredients may occur.

No information is available regarding the excretion of the active ingredients or their metabolites in human milk.

*Toxicity and treatment of overdosage:* In the unlikely event of significant systemic absorption of the active ingredients of Polyfax Ointment occurring, signs of neurotoxicity and nephrotoxicity may be noted. In such an event, the patient's general status and renal function should be monitored and blood levels of polymyxin B and zinc bacitracin determined.

**Pharmaceutical precautions**   Store below 25°C.

**Legal category**   POM

**Package quantities**   Tube of 20 g (OP)

**Further information**   Nil

**Product licence number** 0003/5230

*Product licence holder:* The Wellcome Foundation Limited, Greenford, Middlesex.

## POLYFAX* OPHTHALMIC OINTMENT

**Qualitative and quantitative compositions** 10K IU Polymyxin B Sulphate EP, 500 IU Bacitracin Zinc EP

**Pharmaceutical form** Ointment

**Clinical particulars**

*Therapeutic indications:* Polyfax Ophthalmic Ointment is indicated for the treatment of bacterial infections of the eye and its adnexa, including conjunctivitis, keratitis, corneal ulceration and ulcerative blepharitis.

Polyfax Ophthalmic Ointment may be applied both pre- and post-operatively to prevent ocular infection following surgical procedures, including the removal of foreign bodies from the eye.

The use of Polyfax does not exclude concomitant systemic therapy or other forms of local therapy where appropriate.

*Posology and method of administration:*
*Adults:* A thin film of ointment should be applied to the affected part or inside of the lower eyelid two or more times a day depending on the severity of the condition.

Treatment should be continued until at least two days after the eye has apparently recovered.
*Children:* As for adults.
*Use in the elderly:* No special comment.

*Contra-indications:* Hypersensitivity to bacitracin, polymixin B sulphate or cross-sensitising substances.

*Special warnings and special precautions for use:* Ocular administration of Polyfax Ophthalmic Ointment is extremely unlikely to lead to significant absorption of the constituents and therefore present no risk of systemic toxicity.

*Interaction with other medicaments and other forms of interaction:* None known.

*Pregnancy and lactation:* Polyfax has been used for several years without any untoward effect in pregnancy. The clinical benefit of the treatment to the patient must be balanced against any possible but unknown hazards to the developing foetus. No information is available regarding the excretion of the active ingredients or their metabolites in human milk.

*Undesirable effects:* Allergic reactions following topical (dermatological) application of polymyxin B and bacitracin zinc is rare but has been reported.

As with other antibacterial preparations, prolonged use may result in the overgrowth of non-susceptible organisms, including fungi.

*Overdose:* Not applicable

**Pharmacological properties**

*Pharmacodynamic properties:* Polymyxin B sulphate and bacitracin zinc are both bactericidal antibiotics. The former exerts its action by binding with the cellular membrane and the latter by inhibiting bacterial cell wall development.

It has been shown in animal studies that both polymyxin B sulphate and bacitracin zinc may be absorbed into the aqueous humour following topical application to the eye, especially in circumstances where the cornea is either abraded or inflamed.

In vitro activity: Gram positive: Species of staphylococcus; streptococcus, including
*S. Pyogenes* (B haemolytic streptococcus) and *S. Pneumoniae* (Pneumococcus); and corynebacterium.

Gram negative: Species of pseudomonas (including *P. Aeruginosa*), haemophilus, klebsiella. enterobacter, escherichia and neisseria.

**Pharmaceutical particulars**

*List of excipients:* White Petrolatum USP.

*Incompatibilities:* None known.

*Shelf life:* 5 years.

*Special precautions for storage:* Store below 25°C.

*Nature and contents of container:* Pack size 4 g. Laminate ophthalmic ointment tubes with polyolefin screw caps.

*Instructions for use/handling:* No special instructions.

*Marketing authorisation holder:* The Wellcome Foundation Limited, Greenford, Middlesex.

**Marketing authorisation number** 0003/5229R

**Date of approval/revision of SPC**   April 1996

**Legal category** POM

## POLYTRIM* EYE DROPS

**Presentation**   A clear, colourless, sterile, aqueous solution containing in each ml Trimethoprim BP 1 mg and Polymyxin B Sulphate BP 10,000 units. Thiomersal BP (0.05 mg per ml) is included as a preservative.

**Uses**   Antibacterial agent. For the treatment and prophylaxis of external bacterial infections of the eye including conjunctivitis, keratitis, corneal ulceration, ulcerative blepharitis with associated conjunctivitis, and chronic dacryocystitis. Prophylactically, it is useful following removal of foreign bodies, and before and after ophthalmic surgery to help provide and maintain a sterile field. Use of Polytrim does not exclude concomitant systemic therapy or other forms of local therapy, where appropriate.

**Dosage and administration**
*Adults and children:* 1 drop in affected eye four times daily. More frequent administration may be required, depending on the severity of the condition. Treatment should normally be continued for at least forty-eight hours after the eye has apparently returned to normal.

*Use in the elderly:* No special precautions.

**Contra-indications, warnings, etc**
*Contra-indications:* Contra-indicated in individuals who have a history of hypersensitivity to trimethoprim, polymyxins, or cross-sensitising substances, such as the polypeptide group of antibiotics.

*Precautions:* As with all antibacterial preparations, prolonged use may result in the overgrowth of non-susceptible organisms including fungi.

*Side- and adverse effects:* Polytrim is isotonic with tear fluid and is well tolerated in the eye. No local adverse effects are to be expected except, rarely, a hypersensitivity reaction. If one is suspected during treatment, administration should be discontinued.

*Use in pregnancy and lactation:* The active ingredients of Polytrim Eye Drops have been used for several years without any evidence of untoward effect in pregnancy, however the clinical benefit of treatment to the patient must be balanced against any possible hazard to the developing foetus.

No information is available regarding the excretion of polymyxin B sulphate or its metabolites in human breast milk.

Trimethoprim is excreted in breast milk following *systemic* administration but this presents a negligible risk to the suckling infant. No information, however, is available on the excretion of trimethoprim or its metabolites in human breast milk following topical application.

*Toxicity and treatment of overdosage:* Not applicable.

**Pharmaceutical precautions**   Do not use if the container seal has been broken. Use within one month of opening container. Store below 25°C, and protect from light. Not suitable for injection.

**Legal category**   POM

**Package quantities**   Screw-capped plastic dropper bottle containing 5 ml (OP).

**Further information**   The combination is effective

against a wide variety of Gram-positive and Gram-negative bacterial ocular pathogens, including *Pseudomonas aeruginosa*.

**Product licence number** 0003/0153

*Product licence holder:* The Wellcome Foundation Limited, Greenford, Middlesex.

## POLYTRIM* OPHTHALMIC OINTMENT

**Presentation**   A white to off-white sterile ointment containing Trimethoprim BP 0.5% w/w and Polymyxin B Sulphate BP 10,000 units per gram in a sterile, anhydrous, soft paraffin base.

**Uses**   An antibacterial agent for the treatment and prophylaxis of external bacterial infections of the eye and surrounding tissues including conjunctivitis, keratitis, corneal ulceration, ulcerative blepharitis with associated conjunctivitis, and chronic dacryocystitis. Prophylactically, it can be used following removal of foreign bodies, and before and after ophthalmic surgery to help provide and maintain a sterile field.

**Dosage and administration**
*Dosage in adults:* Apply a thin film of ointment either directly to the affected part or inside the lower conjunctival sac 3 to 4 times a day depending on the severity of the condition.

*Dosage in children:* As for adults. Suitable for use in subjects of all ages including infants.

Treatment should normally be continued until at least forty-eight hours after the eye has apparently returned to normal. Debris such as crusts or pus should be removed prior to application of the ointment.

*Use in the elderly:* No special studies have been carried out in the elderly, although no special precautions are expected to be applied to this group.

**Contra-indications, warnings, etc**
*Contra-indications:* Contra-indicated in individuals who have a history of hypersensitivity to trimethoprim or to polymyxins.

*Precautions:* As with all antibacterial preparations prolonged use may result in the overgrowth of non-susceptible organisms including fungi.

*Side- and adverse effects:* Rarely, hypersensitivity reactions may occur. If one is suspected during treatment, administration should be discontinued.

*Use in pregnancy and lactation:* There is no evidence of safety of Polytrim Ophthalmic Ointment in human pregnancy, however the active ingredients have been in use for many years without apparent ill consequence. In high systemic dosage (40 times the human systemic dose), trimethoprim had been shown to be teratogenic in rats. Although topical application is unlikely to be associated with risk, the clinical benefit of treatment to the patient must be balanced against any possible but unknown hazards to the developing foetus.

No information is available on the excretion of polymyxin in breast milk.

Excretion of trimethoprim into breast milk has been noted after oral administration to lactating women, but this represents a negligible risk to the suckling infant.

*Toxicity and treatment of overdosage:* Not applicable.

**Pharmaceutical precautions**   Do not use if the container seal has been broken. Use within one month of opening container. Store below 25°C.

**Legal category**   POM

**Package quantities**   Tubes of 4 g (OP).

**Further information**   The combination is effective against a wide variety of Gram-positive and Gram-negative bacterial ocular pathogens, including *Pseudomonas aeruginosa*, but not *Neisseria gonorrhoeae*.

**Product licence number** 0003/0223

*Product licence holder:* The Wellcome Foundation Limited, Greenford, Middlesex.

*\*Trade Mark*

# Dumex Limited
Tring Business Centre
Upper Icknield Way
Tring
Herts HP23 4JX

# DUMEX

## ANTABUSE*

**Presentation** White scored tablet marked DUMEX 110L. Each tablet contains 200 mg Disulfiram BP. Inactive ingredients include lactose.

**Uses** Alcoholic deterrent compound. Antabuse is indicated as an adjuvant in the treatment of carefully selected and co-operative patients with drinking problems. Its use should be supported by appropriate supportive treatment.

### Dosage and administration

*Adults and the elderly:* It is recommended that treatment with Antabuse should be initiated only in a hospital or specialised clinic and by physicians experienced in its use.

On the first day of treatment: 4 tablets as a single dose. The second day: 3 tablets, followed on the third day by 2 tablets and on each of the fourth and fifth days by 1 tablet. Subsequently, 1 or half a tablet daily for the duration of the treatment. Treatment should not be continued for longer than six months without review.

In the routine management of the alcoholic an alcoholic challenge test is not recommended. If it is considered that this test is necessary for the success of the therapy, this should be carried out in a specialised unit by physicians acquainted with the procedure since severe reactions can occur. Full resuscitation facilities should be immediately available.

*Children:* Not applicable.

### Contra-indications, warnings, etc

*Contra-indications:* Antabuse is contra-indicated in the presence of cardiac failure, coronary artery disease, previous history of CVA, hypertension, severe personality disorder, suicidal risk or psychosis.

*Warnings/precautions:* Caution should be exercised in the presence of renal failure, hepatic or respiratory disease, diabetes mellitus and epilepsy.

Before initiating treatment it is advised that appropriate examinations should be carried out to establish the suitability of the patient for treatment. Patients must not have taken alcohol for at least 24 hours prior to initiation of Antabuse therapy, during treatment or for 1 week after cessation of treatment with Antabuse. Patients should be warned of the unpredictable and potentially severe nature of an Antabuse-alcohol reaction as in rare cases deaths have been reported following the drinking of alcohol by patients receiving Antabuse. Personnel involved in administration of therapy should be made aware that disulfiram should not be given during a drinking episode. Adequate social and family support to avoid ingestion of alcohol should be available.

Liquid medicines, remedies, tonics and foods may contain sufficient alcohol to elicit an Antabuse-alcohol reaction and patients should be made aware of this.

*Use in pregnancy and lactation:* The use of disulfiram in the first trimester of pregnancy is not advised. The risk/benefit ratio in assessing adverse effects of alcoholism in pregnancy should be taken into account when considering the use of disulfiram in pregnancy.

There have been rare reports of congenital abnormalities in infants whose mothers have received disulfiram in conjunction with other medicines.

No information is available on whether disulfiram is excreted in breastmilk. Its use during breast feeding is not advised.

*Drug interactions:* Antabuse may potentiate the toxic effects of warfarin, antipyrine, phenytoin, chlordiazepoxide and diazepam by inhibiting their metabolism. The intensity of the Antabuse-alcohol reaction may be increased by amitriptyline and decreased by diazepam. Chlorpromazine, while decreasing certain components of the Antabuse-alcohol reaction, may increase the overall Lintensity. Disulfiram inhibits the oxidation and renal excretion of rifampicin. Animal studies have indicated similar inhibition of metabolism of pethidine, morphine and amphetamines. A few case reports of increased confusion and changes in affective behaviour have been noted with the concurrent administration of metronidazole, isoniazid or paraldehyde. Potentiation of organic brain syndrome with amitriptyline and choreoathetosis following pimozide have occurred very rarely.

*Side-effects:* During initial treatment, drowsiness and fatigue may occur. Nausea, vomiting, halitosis and reduction in libido have been reported. If side-effects are marked the dosage may be reduced. Psychotic reactions, including depression, paranoia, schizophrenia and mania occur rarely in patients receiving Antabuse. There are occasional reports of allergic dermatitis, peripheral neuritis and hepatic cell damage.

*Treatment of Antabuse-alcohol reaction:* Antabuse interferes with the metabolism of alcohol and leads to an accumulation of acetaldehyde in the bloodstream. The Antabuse-alcohol reaction can occur within 10 minutes of ingestion of alcohol and may last several hours. It is characterised by violent flushing, dyspnoea, headache, palpitations, tachycardia, nausea and vomiting.

Intensive supportive therapy should be available in the event of severe reaction to alcohol. Oxygen should be available and supportive measures may be necessary to counteract hypotension.

Severe vomiting may occur which may require administration of intravenous fluids.

*Overdosage and treatment of overdose:* Antabuse has low toxicity. Ingestion of quantities of up to 25 g have resulted in central and peripheral neurological symptoms which have resolved without sequelae. Treatment should be symptomatic; gastric lavage and observation are recommended.

**Pharmaceutical precautions** Keep tightly closed, protect from light.

**Legal category** POM.

**Package quantities** Pack of 50 tablets.

**Further information** Antabuse is rapidly absorbed from the gastro-intestinal tract but is very slowly eliminated and may be detected in body fluids up to seven days after cessation of administration.

**Product licence number** 4938/0011.

## DIAZEMULS*

**Presentation** Ampoules of a white, opaque emulsion containing Diazepam BP 10 mg in 2 ml.

**Uses** *Action:* Diazepam is a potent anxiolytic, anticonvulsant and central muscle relaxant mediating its effects mainly via the limbic system as well as the polysynaptic spinal reflexes. The formulation of diazepam in an oil-in-water emulsion similar to Intralipid reduces the incidence of local pain and thrombophlebitis after injection.

*Indications:*

1. Sedation prior to procedures such as endoscopy, dentistry, cardiac catheterisation and cardioversion.
2. Premedication prior to anaesthesia.
3. Control of acute muscle spasm due to tetanus or poisoning.
4. Control of convulsions; status epilepticus.
5. Management of severe acute anxiety or agitation including delirium tremens.

**Dosage and administration** Diazemuls may be administered by slow intravenous injection (1 ml per min), or by continuous infusion. Diazemuls should be drawn up into the syringe immediately prior to administration.

1. *Sedation:* 0.1–0.2 mg diazepam/kg body weight by iv injection. The normal adult dose is 10–20 mg, but dosage should be titrated to the patient's response.
2. *Premedication:* 0.1–0.2 mg diazepam/kg body weight by iv injection. Dosage should be titrated to the patient's response. In this indication, prior treatment with diazepam leads to a reduction in fasciculations and postoperative myalgia associated with the use of suxamethonium.
3. *Tetanus:* 0.1–0.3 mg diazepam/kg body weight by iv injection repeated every 1–4 hours as required. Alternatively, a continuous infusion (see below) of 3–10 mg/kg body weight every 24 hours may be used.
4. *Status epilepticus:* An initial dose of 0.15–0.25 mg/kg body weight by iv injection repeated in 30 to 60 minutes if required, and followed if necessary by infusion (see below) of up to 3 mg/kg body weight over 24 hours.
5. *Anxiety and tension, acute muscle spasm, acute states of excitation, delirium tremens:* The usual dose is 10 mg repeated at intervals of 4 hours, or as required.

*Elderly or debilitated patients:* Elderly or debilitated patients are particularly sensitive to benzodiazepines. Dosage should initially be reduced to one half of the normal recommendations.

If a continuous infusion is required Diazemuls may be added to 5% or 10% dextrose solution to achieve a final diazepam concentration within the range 0.1–0.4 mg/ml (i.e. 2–8 ml Diazemuls per 100 ml dextrose solution). A dextrose solution containing added Diazemuls should be used within 6 hours of the admixture. Diazemuls can be mixed in all proportions with Intralipid 10% or 20% but not with saline solutions. It can be injected into the infusion tube during an ongoing infusion of isotonic saline or dextrose solution 5% or 10%. As with other diazepam injections, adsorption may occur to plastic infusion equipment. This adsorption occurs at a lesser degree with Diazemuls than with aqueous diazepam injection preparations when mixed with dextrose solutions.

**Contra-indications, warnings, etc** As with other benzodiazepine preparations:

1. Should not be used in phobic or obsessional states since there is inadequate evidence of efficacy and safety.
2. Should not be used in the treatment of chronic psychosis.

*Warnings and precautions:*

1. Treatment with diazepam may cause drowsiness and increase the patient's reaction time. This should be considered in situations where alertness is required, e.g. driving a car.
2. Use with caution in patients with impairment of renal or hepatic function and in patients with pulmonary insufficiency or myasthenia gravis.
3. Should not be used alone to treat depression or anxiety associated with depression.
4. Amnesia may occur. In cases of loss or bereavement psychological adjustment may be inhibited by benzodiazepines.
5. Disinhibiting effects may be manifested in various ways. Suicide may be precipitated in patients who are depressed and aggressive behaviour toward self and others may be precipitated. Extreme caution should therefore be used in prescribing benzodiazepines in patients with personality disorders.
6. Physiological and psychological symptoms of withdrawal including depression may be associated with discontinuation of benzodiazepines even after normal therapeutic doses for short periods of time.

*Interactions with other medicaments:* Concomitant use of central nervous system depressants, e.g. alcohol, general anaesthetics, narcotic analgesics, or antidepressants, including MAOI's will result in accentuation of their sedative effects. When Diazemuls is combined with centrally depressant drugs administered parenterally, severe respiratory and cardiovascular depression may occur. It is recommended that Diazemuls is administered following the analgesic, and that the dose should be carefully titrated to the patient's response. Diazepam clearance is increased by concomitant administration of phenobarbitone, and is decreased by administration of cimetidine.

*Use in pregnancy:* Diazepam crosses the placenta and should not be used during pregnancy. Maternal doses administered during delivery may produce clinical effects in the newborn, for example hypotonia and hypothermia.

*Lactation:* Diazepam can be transmitted in breast milk and clinical effects may occur in the breast-fed infant. Diazemuls should be administered during lactation only if considered essential.

*Side-effects:* This formulation may rarely cause local pain or thrombophlebitis in the vein used for administration.

Rare instances have been reported of a local

painless erythematous rash around the site of injection, which has resolved in 1–2 days. Urticaria and, rarely, anaphylaxis have been reported following the injection of Diazemuls.

*Overdosage:* CNS depression and coma. Treatment symptomatic.

**Pharmaceutical precautions** For full information on admixture see dosage and administration. Diazemuls should only be mixed in the same container or syringe with dextrose solution 5% or 10% or Intralipid 10% or 20%. The contents of the ampoule should not be mixed with any drugs other than the infusion solutions mentioned above. Store at room temperature. Do not freeze.

**Legal category** CD (Sch 4), POM.

**Package quantities** Boxes of 10×2 ml ampoules.

**Further information** During prolonged administration, for example in the treatment of tetanus, the plasma concentration of desmethyldiazepam, the main (and similarly potent) active metabolite of diazepam, may exceed that of the parent compound. Accordingly, there is a risk of accumulation and prolonged CNS depression if the dosage is not reduced following continuous administration for 5–7 days.

The clinician should be aware that intravenous sedation is associated with a significant incidence of anterograde and retrograde amnesia.

**Product licence number** 10183/0001.

## DUMICOAT* DENTURE LACQUER

**Presentation** Dumicoat denture lacquer contains miconazole 50 mg/g. Each bottle contains 1 g of denture lacquer. After application to the upper surface of the upper denture, the lacquer forms a film, which slowly releases miconazole during the course of a week.

**Uses** Dumicoat denture lacquer is to be used in the treatment of Candida-associated denture stomatitis. Miconazole is an imidazole antifungal active against Candida spp., e.g. C. albicans, dermatophytes, Aspergillus spp., and Pityrosporon spp.

*Kinetics:* Miconazole is incompletely absorbed from the gastrointestinal tract after oral ingestion, the bioavailability being about 25–30%.

The apparent volume of distribution is about 1400 L. More than 90% of the drug is bound to plasma proteins. Miconazole is metabolised in the liver to inactive metabolites, with less than 1% excreted unchanged in the urine. About 50% of an oral dose may be recovered, mainly unchanged in the faeces. The elimination half-life is 20–25 hours.

**Dosage and administration**

*Adults:* One gram of denture lacquer (content of one bottle) is applied to the upper surface of the upper denture 3 times with weekly intervals. It may be necessary to repeat the treatment after a time.

Before each application, the denture must be cleaned thoroughly, as described in the directions for use. The lacquer is applied with a brush to the upper surface of the denture down to the rim of the teeth. When the lacquer is dry, the denture may be replaced in the mouth. It should be noted that the lacquer is not suitable for use with soft linings, nor to be used with poorly fitting dentures.

*Use in the elderly:* As for adults.

**Contra-indications, warnings, etc**

*Contra-indications:* There are no known contra-indications to the use of miconazole denture lacquer.

*Warnings and precautions:* Miconazole may potentiate the effect of oral anticoagulants, anti-epileptics, and hypoglycaemic drugs.

*Side-effects:* Transient smarting has been reported in a few cases immediately after the lacquered denture was placed in the mouth.

*Use in pregnancy:* Miconazole has shown no teratogenic effects in animals. No information is available regarding secretion into human breast milk. Dumicoat denture lacquer is considered to be safe for use during pregnancy, owing to the small amount of miconazole administered.

**Pharmaceutical precautions** Nil.

**Legal category** POM.

**Package quantities** Three glass bottles, each containing 1 g of Dumicoat denture lacquer, 3 brushes, and 4 cleaning tissues to a carton.

**Further information** Nil.

**Product licence number** 10183/0007.

## ELYZOL* 25% DENTAL GEL

**Presentation** Elyzol dental gel is an off-white semi-solid suspension containing metronidazole benzoate corresponding to 250 mg metronidazole per g.

The dental gel is designed for application into gingival pockets. After application the gel assumes greater flowability and fills the pockets. On contact with the gingival fluid it forms a highly viscous gel. This is slowly broken down and metronidazole is released gradually from the gel.

**Uses** Elyzol dental gel is to be used in the treatment of chronic periodontal disease as an adjunct to conventional therapy.

Metronidazole is an antibiotic active against most of the organisms that are predominant in the subgingival flora in adult periodontitis. Metronidazole has a bactericidal effect against *Bacteroides spp., Fusobacterium, Selemonas, Wolinella, Spirochetes* and other obligate anaerobic organisms, but does not affect aerobic bacteria. Also some facultatively anaerobic bacteria, such as *Actinobacillus actinomycetemcomitans* are sensitive to the concentrations of metronidazole obtained after local application of Elyzol 25% dental gel. Development of resistance against metronidazole is seldom reported, and only with high doses after long-term use. Metronidazole does not affect the commensal flora.

*Kinetics:* After application of Elyzol 25% dental gel, metronidazole concentrations of above 100 µg/ml are measurable locally in the crevicular fluid for at least 8 hours. At 36 hours, concentrations above 1 µg/ml are still measurable. Metronidazole is released slowly from the dental gel with a bioavailability of about 70%. The maximal plasma concentration is found after about four hours. Systemic concentrations above 1.3 µg/ml have not been found.

Metronidazole is metabolised by means of hydroxylation and oxidation, and it conjugates with glucuronic acid. Metronidazole is mainly excreted with urine, in which 15–20% is found unchanged, and the rest as metabolites. A certain amount is excreted in the bile.

**Dosage and administration** Elyzol 25% dental gel is administered into the periodontal pocket twice with a one week interval. Dosage is individual, dependent upon the number of teeth to be treated.

Treatment should not normally be repeated within six months of initial therapy.

**Contra-indications, warnings, etc**

*Contra-indications:* Known hypersensitivity to metronidazole.

*Precautions:* In some patients metronidazole may have an effect similar to that of disulfiram on the metabolism of alcohol, resulting in intolerance symptoms.

*Side-effects:* Because of the low plasma concentrations after local application of the dental gel, the risk of systemic side-effects is low. The most frequent side-effects are local and occur directly in connection with the application, such as bitter taste and temporary local tenderness. Headache has been reported.

*Interactions:* Some potentiation of anticoagulant therapy has been reported when metronidazole has been used with warfarin type oral anticoagulants. Metronidazole and disulfiram taken concurrently may cause a confusional condition.

*Use in pregnancy:* Metronidazole should not be given during the first trimester of pregnancy unless it is considered essential.

*Lactation:* Metronidazole is excreted in milk but the risk of affecting the child seems unlikely with therapeutic doses.

**Pharmaceutical precautions** Use each applicator on one patient during one session of treatment only. If only part is used the remainder should be discarded.

**Legal category** POM.

**Package quantities** Disposable applicator containing 1 g dental gel. Cartons of 2×1 g.

**Further information** Nil.

**Product licence number** 4938/0007.

## LITAREX*

**Presentation** Oval, white, biconvex, scored, controlled release tablets marked 160I on one side. Each tablet contains lithium citrate 564 mg equivalent to 6 mmol lithium.

**Uses** Litarex is a source of lithium ions in a controlled release dosage form. Lithium may act by competing with sodium ions at various sites in the body. It changes the electrolyte composition of body fluids and increases the intracellular and total body water volume. The mechanism of action in affective disorders is not known. For the prophylaxis and treatment of mania. For the prophylaxis of manic depression and depression.

**Dosage and administration** Tablets should be swallowed whole and not chewed and taken in single or divided doses as necessary.

*Adults – Prophylactic long term treatment:* Start with a low dosage and then increase step-wise over a period of several weeks. Treatment is managed by monitoring clinical symptoms and by measuring plasma lithium concentration. Plasma concentrations should initially be taken after 48 hours then, following any required adjustments to the dosage, at weekly intervals for a period of one month and thereafter at monthly intervals for the duration of treatment.

The initial dose is one tablet (6 mmol $Li^+$) each morning and evening. The dosage should be adjusted to produce a concentration of about 0.80 mmol/litre. In some patients effective plasma lithium may be within the range 0.4 to 1.0 mmol/litre. Toxic symptoms are usually associated with plasma lithium exceeding 1.2 mmol/litre. During prophylactic treatment, blood samples for estimation of lithium should be taken 12 hours after the evening dose.

*Adults – Treatment of acute mania:* Initiate in hospital. There is considerable biological variation in renal lithium clearance and thus the number of Litarex tablets required by individual patients to reach their particular effective plasma concentration is variable. The initial dose required for the acute treatment of mania may be high, for example 48 mmol lithium daily. Close monitoring of plasma lithium is necessary to maintain the plasma lithium concentration within the optimum range. The dose of Litarex may need to be reduced as soon as the acute phase has passed and restabilisation of plasma lithium levels may be required. Lithium concentrations should not exceed 1.2 mmol/litre.

*Use in elderly:* Elderly patients, or patients below 50 kg in weight, may require smaller doses of Litarex. Elderly patients may be more sensitive to the undesirable effects of lithium. Plasma lithium levels should be adjusted to the lower end of the recommended range and not exceeding 1.0 mmol/litre.

**Contra-indications, warnings, etc**

*Use in children:* Not recommended.

*Contra-indications:* Renal disease, sodium depletion, cardiovascular disease or Addison's disease and in women who are breast feeding.

*Precautions:* Lithium therapy should not be initiated unless adequate facilities for monitoring serum concentrations are available.

The use of lithium for long-term prophylactic treatment requires careful supervision. Plasma lithium concentration should be monitored regularly and determined from a blood sample drawn 12 hours after the last dose. More frequent monitoring is advisable after a change in dose; during an intercurrent illness provoking fluid loss; after starting a slimming diet; in the treatment of elderly patients; if signs of lithium toxicity on mania or depressive relapse occur.

As bioavailability varies from product to product, a change of product should be regarded as initiation of new treatment. Blood levels should therefore be monitored weekly until restabilisation is achieved.

ECG, renal function and thyroid function should be determined prior to treatment. Patients should be euthyroid before starting treatment.

Renal function should be routinely monitored in patients with polyuria and polydypsia. Clear instructions regarding the symptoms of impending toxicity should be given by the doctor to all patients receiving long-term lithium therapy. Patients should also be warned to report the development of polyuria or polydypsia. Episodes of nausea and vomiting or other conditions leading to salt/water depletion should also be reported. Patients should be advised to maintain their usual salt and fluid intake.

*Use in pregnancy:* The lithium ion crosses the placenta. It is therefore, advisable that a pregnancy test should be carried out prior to treatment, that women treated with lithium should adopt adequate contraceptive methods, and that treatment should be withdrawn for the first trimester of pregnancy. Treatment with lithium throughout pregnancy is associated with an incidence of congenital abnormality greater than that for the general population. Lithium dosage requirements may vary during pregnancy and after delivery; serum lithium concentrations should be monitored closely. Lithium is excreted in breast milk, and therefore lithium-treated patients should not breast feed.

*Drug interactions: ACE inhibitors and NSAIDs* reduce excretion of lithium, possibility of toxicity. Antacids and adsorbents, e.g. sodium bicarbonate increases excretion of lithium (reduced plasma lithium concentration). Lithium toxicity has been reported with metronidazole and spectinomycin. Serum lithium concentrations may increase during concomitant therapy with tetracycline.

*Antidepressants,* e.g. fluoxetine, fluvoxamine, paroxetine and sertraline increases the risk of CNS toxicity. Symptoms of nephrogenic diabetes are particularly prevalent in patients receiving concurrent treatment with tri/tetracyclic anti-depressants.

*Antidiabetics:* Lithium may occasionally impair glucose tolerance.

*Antiepileptics:* Neurotoxicity may occur with carbamazepine and phenytoin without increase in plasma-lithium concentration.

*Antihypertensives:* Neurotoxicity may occur with methyldopa without increased plasma-lithium concentration.

*Antipsychotics:* Increased risk of extrapyramidal effects and possibility of neurotoxicity (notably with haloperidol). Symptoms of nephrogenic diabetes insipidus are particularly prevalent in patients receiving concurrent treatment with tri/tetracyclic antidepressants.

*Calcium-channel blockers:* Neurotoxicity may occur with diltiazem and verapamil without increased plasma-lithium concentration.

*Cholinergics:* Lithium antagonises the effect of neostigmine and pyridostigmine.

*Diuretics:* Lithium excretion is reduced by loop diuretics and thiazide (increased plasma-lithium concentration and risk of toxicity; loop diuretics are safer than thiazides); lithium excretion is increased by acetazolamide.

*Domperidone and metoclopramide:* Increased risk of extrapyramidal effects and possibility of neurotoxicity with metoclopramide.

*Muscle relaxants:* Muscle relaxant effect enhanced by lithium; baclofen possibly aggravates hyperkinesis.

*Sumatriptan:* Risk of CNS toxicity.

*Theophylline:* Lithium excretion increased (reduced plasma lithium concentration).

*Other interactions:* Lithium treatment may lead to aggravation of myasthenia gravis. Lithium intake should be stopped 2 days before major surgery. A low sodium intake facilitates lithium re-absorption in the renal tubule and may lead to lithium accumulation. Raised plasma levels of ADH may occur during treatment.

*Side-effects:* Thirst and polyuria, fine tremor of the hands, muscular weakness, nausea and loose stools are the commonest side-effects during the first days or weeks of treatment. These often subside as treatment progresses.

During maintenance therapy fine hand tremor, weight gain, oedema, polyuria, hypothyroidism and goitre may occur.

More serious side-effects which may signal imminent lithium toxicity include loss of appetite, slurred speech, drowsiness, coarse hand tremor, vomiting, diarrhoea, fasciculation, vertigo and confusion. Mild cognitive impairment may occur during long-term use.

Hypercalcaemia, hypermagnesaemia, hyperparathyroidism and an increase in antinuclear antibodies have also been reported. Exacerbation of psoriasis may occur.

Long-term treatment with lithium may result in permanent changes in the kidney and impairment of renal function. High serum concentrations of lithium, including episodes of acute lithium toxicity may enhance these changes. The minimum clinically effective dose of lithium should always be used. Patients should be maintained on lithium after 3–5 years only if benefit persists.

*Overdosage:* Early signs of toxicity (see side effects) may respond to a reduction in, or cessation of, lithium therapy.

Symptoms of severe lithium poisoning include hyper-reflexia, attacks of hyper-extension of the limbs, epileptic seizures, toxic psychosis, syncope, oliguria, circulatory failure and coma. Deaths have been reported.

Treatment consists of the induction of vomiting and/or gastric lavage together with appropriate supportive and symptomatic measures. It is essential that fluid and electrolyte balance and adequate renal function are maintained. In cases of gross overdosage (plasma concentrations greater than 3 mmol per litre) lithium clearance can be enhanced by haemodialysis or peritoneal dialysis.

Since Litarex is a controlled-release preparation, clinicians should be aware of the possibility of lithium release continuing over a period of time. Following overdose, plasma lithium levels should be monitored for at least 24 hours and subsequently as considered necessary.

**Pharmaceutical precautions** No special requirements.

**Legal category** POM.

**Package quantities** Containers of 100.

**Further information** The lithium citrate in Litarex tablets is distributed in a plastic/lipid matrix from which the lithium salt is released over a period of four to five hours during passage through the gastro-intestinal tract. The tablets are formulated in such a way as to give absorption which is slow and even, so that rapid increases and high peak levels in serum lithium concentrations are avoided.

**Product licence number** 4938/0012.

## METRONIDAZOLE TABLETS 500 mg

**Qualitative and quantitative composition** Each tablet contains metronidazole 500 mg.

**Pharmaceutical form** Tablets.

**Clinical particulars**

*Therapeutic indications:* Metronidazole is active against infections caused by *Trichomonas vaginalis, Gardnerella vaginalis, Giardia lamblia,* and *Entamoeba histolytica.* It is also active against a broad spectrum of obligate anaerobic bacteria, including Bacteroides, Fusobacterium, Clostridium and various anaerobic cocci. The action is trichomonacidal, amoebacidal and bactericidal.

Metronidazole tablets may be used in the treatment of *Trichomonas vaginalis* infestations in men and women; *Gardnerella vaginalis*; giardiasis (lambliasis); amoebiasis; and infections in which anaerobic bacteria have been identified or are suspected as pathogens.

Metronidazole tablets may be used in combination with other recommended agents in the treatment of *Helicobacter pylori* infection associated with peptic ulcer.

Metronidazole tablets may be used in the prevention of postoperative infections caused by anaerobic bacteria, particularly following gynaecological and gastrointestinal surgery.

Metronidazole tablets may be used in acute ulcerative gingivitis (Vincent's Infection).

*Posology and method of administration:* As given below under the specific indications.

The dose should be reduced in the presence of severe liver insufficiency.

*Trichomoniasis:* 2 g (4 tablets) in a single dose or 250 mg (½ tablet) each morning and evening for 6 days. In severe cases 500 mg each morning and evening for 6 days. Both the patient and partner should be treated simultaneously.

*Gardnerella vaginalis:* 500 mg (1 tablet) each morning and evening for 7 days.

*Amoebiasis – acute intestinal amoebiasis:* 2 to 2.5 g (4 to 5 tablets) in a single dose for 2 to 3 days or 750 mg three times daily for 5 to 10 days.

*Hepatic amoebiasis:* 1.5 to 2.5 g (3 to 5 tablets) in a single dose for 2 to 3 days or 500 mg three times daily for 5 days.

*Eradication of cysts in symptomless carriers: Adults:* 500 to 750 mg three times daily for 5 to 10 days.

*Children:* Half the adult dose.

*Infants:* 50 mg/kg body weight daily.

*Giardiasis: Adults:* 2 g (4 tablets) in 3 single dose for 3 days or 500 mg (1 tablet) twice daily for 1 to 10 days.

*Children:* 250 mg (½ tablet) once daily for 10 days.

*Infants:* 25 mg/kg body weight for 10 days.

*Eradication of Helicobacter pylori in infected patients:* Generally, metronidazole treatment should be given for at least 7 days in triple combination with other agents recommended for use in the treatment of Helicobacter pylori infection.

*Adults:* 500 mg two to three daily for 7–14 days.

There are no specific recommendations for use in children.

*Acute ulcerative gingivitis: Adults:* 250 mg (½ tablet) three times daily for 3 days.

*Treatment of anaerobic infections:* Generally metronidazole treatment should be given for at least 7 days.

*Adults and children over 12 years of age:* 500 mg every 8 hours.

*Children under 12 years:* 7 mg/kg body weight every 8 hours.

*Prevention of anaerobic infections:* Generally metronidazole prophylaxis should be given for 3 to 7 days.

*Elective surgery:* e.g. hysterectomy and colonic surgery.

*Preoperatively: Adults and children over 12 years of age:* 24 hours before surgery 1 g (2 tablets) followed by 500 mg by mouth every 8 hours until preoperative starvation.

*Children under 12 years:* 7 mg/kg body weight every 8 hours.

*Postoperative periods: Adults and children over 12 years of age:* 500 mg (1 tablet) every 8 hours once oral medication is possible.

*Children under 12 years:* 7 mg/kg body weight every 8 hours once oral medication is possible.

*Acute surgery:* e.g. appendectomy, gastrointestinal perforation.

*Adults and children over 12 years of age:* 500 mg (1 tablet) every 8 hours postoperatively, once oral medication is possible.

*Children under 12 years:* 7 mg/kg body weight every 8 hours postoperatively, once oral medication is possible.

*Contra-indications:* A history of known allergy to metronidazole.

*Special warnings and precautions for use:* Metronidazole tablets should not be used in patients with blood dyscrasias or with active non-infectious disease of the central nervous system. High doses of metronidazole may mask the presence of syphilis.

The dose should be prescribed with caution in patients with renal or hepatic impairment.

Regular clinical and biological surveillance are advised if administration of metronidazole tablets for more than 10 days is considered necessary.

*Interaction with other medicaments and other forms of interaction:* Metronidazole may provoke a disulfiram-like reaction with alcohol. Concurrent ingestion of disulfiram may cause conditions of acute confusion.

Metronidazole enhances the activity of warfarin. Anticoagulant therapy should be closely monitored in patients receiving metronidazole concurrently.

Cimetidine decreases the plasma clearance of metronidazole by 30%. This is not thought to have major clinical significance.

Metronidazole has exhibited synergism with several agents active against anaerobes, for instance clindamycin, erythromycin, nifampicin and nalidixic acid. Phenobarbitone increases the metabolism of metronidazole, reducing the half-life to about three hours.

*Pregnancy and lactation:* Should not be used unless the physician considers it essential.

*Effect on ability to drive and use machines:* None.

*Undesirable effects:* Serious adverse reactions occur rarely. Side effects of metronidazole are usually mild and may include gastrointestinal disturbances, nausea, unpleasant taste in the mouth, coated tongue, headache and skin rashes. There have been occasional reports of erythema multiforme, urticaria and angioedema, which may be reversed on drug withdrawal. Anaphylaxis may occur rarely. Drowsiness, dizziness, depression and darkening of the urine have been reported.

Abnormal liver function tests, cholestatic hepatitis and jaundice, which may be reversed upon drug withdrawal have been reported. During intensive and/or prolonged metronidazole therapy, peripheral neuropathy, transient epileptiform seizures and paraesthesia i.e. tingling, have been reported.

There have been reports of bone marrow depression disorders, such as agranulocytosis, neutropenia, thrombocytopenia and pancytopenia, which may be reversed on drug withdrawal, although fatalities have been reported.

*Overdose:* There is no specific treatment for gross overdosage of metronidazole.

**Pharmacological properties**

*Pharmacodynamic properties:* Metronidazole is active against obligate anaerobic bacteria, *Gardnerella vaginalis, Trichomonas vaginalis, Giardia lamblia* and *Entamoeba histolytica.*

*Pharmacokinetic properties:* Metronidazole is absorbed readily and almost completely from the gastrointestinal tract. Maximum concentrations occur after about 1 hour. Metronidazole penetrates well into body tissues and fluids. About 10% of the drug is bound to plasma proteins.

At least half the dose is excreted in the urine as metronidazole and its metabolites, including an acid oxidation product, a hydroxy derivative and a glucuronide. The elimination half-life of metronidazole is about 8.5 hours.

*Preclinical data:* None.

**Pharmacological particulars**

*List of excipients:* Lactose, maize starch, povidone, magnesium stearate ac-di-sol, microcrystalline cellulose, purified water, ethanol, methocel E5, propylene glycol, dimethicone, titanium dioxide (E-171).

*Incompatibilities:* None.

*Shelf life:* 3 years.

*Special precautions for storage:* Store below 25°C. Protect from light.

*Nature and contents of container:* Amber glass bottle (500 tablets). Blister packs (21 tablets).

*Instruction for use/handling:* Not applicable.

**Marketing authorisation holder:** A/S Dumex (Dumex Ltd), Prags Boulevard 37, DK-2300 Copenhagen S.

**Marketing authorisation number** 4938/0014.

**Date of approval/revision of SPC** 16 July 1996.

**Legal category** POM.

## STESOLID* RECTAL TUBES

**Presentation** Transparent, yellow, polyethylene Rectal Tubes containing a clear, colourless to slightly yellowish solution of 2 mg/ml or 4 mg/ml diazepam. The formulation also includes the following inactive ingredients: benzoic acid, benzyl alcohol, ethanol, propylene glycol and sodium benzoate. Approximately 2.5 ml can be squeezed from each tube, giving an individual dose of 5 mg or 10 mg diazepam. The small amount left in the tube will not affect the correct dose.

**Uses** Diazepam has anti-convulsant, sedative and muscle relaxant properties. It is used in the treatment of severe anxiety and tension states, as a sedative and premedicant in the control of muscle spasm and in the management of alcohol withdrawal symptoms.

Stesolid Rectal Tubes may be used in acute severe anxiety and agitation, epileptic and febrile convulsions, tetanus, as a sedative in minor surgical and dental procedures or other circumstances in which a rapid effect is required but where intravenous injection is impracticable or undesirable. Stesolid Rectal Tubes may be of particular value for the immediate treatment of convulsions in children. (1 year and over).

**Dosage and administration** Sensitivity to diazepam varies with age.

*Children:* 1 to 3 years of age – one 5 mg tube. Insert tube half way to mark on nozzle. Over 3 years of age – one 10 mg tube. Note: these recommendations assume normal frame size for age. In particularly small children the depth of insertion should be reduced accordingly.

*Adults:* One 10 mg tube.

*Elderly patients:* One 5 mg tube.

If no effect is seen after five minutes, one further tube (5 mg or 10 mg) diazepam respectively can be administered. Further doses of Stesolid Rectal Tubes should be administered only after consultation with a physician. If convulsions are still not controlled, then other anti-convulsive measures should be instituted.

**Contra-indications, warnings, etc**

*Contra-indications:* Known sensitivity to any of the ingredients. Acute pulmonary insufficiency, respiratory depression.

*Use in pregnancy and lactation:* There is no evidence as to the safety of diazepam in human pregnancy. It should not be used, especially during the first and last trimesters, unless the benefit is considered to outweigh the potential risk.

In labour, high single doses or repeated low doses have been reported to produce hypotonia, poor suckling and hypothermia in the neonate and irregularities in the foetal heart.

Diazepam is excreted in breast milk and therefore its use during lactation should be avoided.

*Warnings:* Stesolid Rectal Tubes should not be used in phobic or obsessional states as there is insufficient evidence of efficacy and safety in this situation, nor should they be used alone in the treatment of depression or anxiety associated with depression due to the risk of suicide being precipitated in this patient group. Stesolid Rectal Tubes should not be used in the treatment of chronic psychosis. In common with other benzodiazepines the use of diazepam may be associated with amnesia and Stesolid Rectal Tubes should not be used in cases of loss or bereavement as psychological adjustment may be inhibited.

As with other benzodiazepines extreme caution should be used if prescribing Stesolid Rectal Tubes for patients with personality disorders. The disinhibiting effects of benzodiazepines may be manifested as the precipitation of suicide in patients who are depressed and aggressive behaviour towards self and others.

Withdrawal symptoms occur with benzodiazepines following normal therapeutic doses given for short periods of time and may be associated with physiological and psychological sequelae including depression.

*Precautions:* Stesolid Rectal Tubes should be used with caution in patients with renal or hepatic dysfunction, chronic pulmonary insufficiency or close-angle glaucoma.

Elderly or debilitated patients are particularly susceptible to side-effects and may require lower doses.

Alertness and performance at skilled tasks may be impaired. Patients should be warned not to drive or operate machinery. Alcohol may potentiate these effects.

*Drug interactions:* Diazepam may enhance the effects of other CNS depressants. Their concurrent use should be avoided. Diazepam may potentiate the effect of phenytoin when taken concurrently. Sodium valproate displaces protein bound diazepam and inhibits its metabolism. Occasionally, diazepam has been reported to antagonise the effect of levodopa.

Cimetidine may potentiate the effect of diazepam because of decreased hepatic metabolism.

Alcohol may alter the response to diazepam.

*Side-effects:* The side-effects of diazepam are usually mild and infrequent. The most common side-effects are drowsiness, light-headedness, unsteadiness and ataxia.

Elderly and debilitated patients are particularly susceptible to these effects and may require lower doses. Other rare side-effects include hypotension, apnoea, respiratory depression, gastro-intestinal and visual disturbances, skin rashes, urinary retention, headache, confusion, vertigo, changes in libido, blood dyscrasias and jaundice.

Paradoxical reactions to benzodiazepines have been reported, provoking excitement instead of sedation.

*Treatment of overdosage:* The symptoms of overdose are hypnosis, hypotension, respiratory depression and coma. Treatment is symptomatic, with airway maintenance. Intravenous fluids may be administered. Flumazenil is a specific I.V. antidote for use in emergency situations. Patients requiring such intervention should be monitored closely in hospital.

**Pharmaceutical precautions** Stesolid Rectal Tubes should be stored at a temperature below 25°C. Do not open the foil before use.

**Legal category** CD (Sch 4), POM.

**Package quantities** Single-packed Rectal Tubes, 5 tubes to a carton.

**Further information** Shelf life of two and a half years from date of manufacture.

**Product licence numbers**

| | |
|---|---|
| 5 mg Rectal Tube | 10183/0003 |
| 10 mg Rectal Tube | 10183/0004 |

## VANCOMYCIN CAPSULES

**Qualitative and quantitative composition** Vancomycin 125 mg (125,000 IU) per capsule and 250 mg (250,000 IU) per capsule as vancomycin hydrochloride.

**Pharmaceutical form** Capsules.

**Clinical particulars**

*Therapeutic indications:* Staphylococcal enterocolitis and pseudomembraneous colitis due to *Clostridium difficile*.

Vancomycin is not significantly absorbed from the normal gastro-intestinal tract and is therefore not effective by the oral route for other types of infection.

*Posology and method of administration:*

*Adults and the elderly:* The usual daily dose is 500 mg in 4 divided doses for 7 to 10 days. In severe cases up to 2 g daily in 3 or 4 divided doses. The total daily dose should not exceed 2 g.

*Children:* 40 mg/kg daily in 3 or 4 divided doses for 7 to 10 days. The total daily dosage should not exceed 2 g.

*Contra-indications:* Hypersensitivity to vancomycin.

*Special warnings and precautions for use:* Although in general very little vancomycin is absorbed from the gastro-intestinal tract following oral administration, absorption may be enhanced in patients with inflammatory disorders of the intestinal mucosa. These patients may be at risk for the development of adverse reactions. The risk is greater in patients with renal impairment. The greater the renal impairment, the greater the risk of developing the adverse reactions associated with the parental administration of vancomycin.

Monitoring of serum concentrations of these patients should therefore be performed. It should be noted that the total systemic and renal clearances of vancomycin are reduced in the elderly.

*Nephrotoxicity:* Nephrotoxicity has occurred in patients receiving vancomycin. It has been reported mostly in patients who have been given excessive intravenous doses, have a pre-existing kidney dysfunction, or are receiving concomitant treatment with aminoglycoside.

In order to minimise the risk of nephrotoxicity when treating patients with underlying renal dysfunction or patients receiving concomitant therapy with an aminoglycoside, serial monitoring at renal function should be performed.

*Ototoxicity:* Ototoxicity has occurred in patients receiving vancomycin. It may be transient or permanent. It has been reported mostly in patients who have been given excessive intravenous doses, have a pre-existing hearing loss, or are receiving concomitant treatment with an ototoxic drug. Serial tests of auditory function may be helpful in order to minimise the risk of ototoxicity.

*Haematological:* Haematological problems have occurred in patients receiving vancomycin. Most of the conditions are reversible.

*Interaction with other medicaments and other forms of interaction:* None known.

*Pregnancy and lactation:* Teratology studies have been performed at 5 times the human dose in rats and 3 times the human dose in rabbits, and have revealed no evidence of harm to the foetus due to vancomycin. In a controlled clinical study, the potential ototoxic and nephrotoxic effects of vancomycin hydrochloride on infants were evaluated when the drug was administered to pregnant women for serious staphylococcal infections complicating intravenous drug abuse. Vancomycin hydrochloride was found in cord blood. No sensorineural hearing loss or nephrotoxocity attributable to vancomycin was noted. One infant, whose mother received vancomycin in the third trimester, experienced conductive hearing loss that was not attributable to vancomycin. Because vancomycin was administered only in the second and third trimesters. It is not known whether it causes foetal harm, Vancomycin should therefore, only be given to pregnant women if clearly needed.

Vancomycin hydrochloride is excreted in human milk. Caution should be exercised when vancomycin is administered to a nursing woman.

*Effect on ability to drive and use machines:* Not applicable.

*Undesirable effects:* Since vancomycin is not usually significantly absorbed from the gastro-intestinal tract, the adverse reactions encountered with parental therapy is unlikely to occur after oral administration.

*Nephrotoxicity:* Rarely, renal failure, principally manifested by increased serum creatinine or blood urea concentrations, have been observed, especially in patients given large doses of intravenously administered vancomycin. Rare cases of interstitial nephritis have been reported. Most occurred in patients who were given aminoglycosides concomitantly or who had pre-existing kidney dysfunction.

*Ototoxicity:* Hearing loss associated with intravenously administered vancomycin has been reported. Most of those patients had kidney dysfunction, pre-existing hearing loss, or concomitant treatment with an ototoxic drug. Vertigo, dizziness, and tinnitus have been reported rarely.

*Haematological:* Reversible neutropenia, usually starting one week or more after onset of intravenous therapy or after a total dose of more than 25 g. Neutropenia appears to be promptly reversible when vancomycin is discontinued. Thrombocytopenia and reversible agranulocytosis (granulo-cyte count less than 500/mm³) have been reported rarely.

*Miscellaneous:* Anaphylaxis, chills, drug fever, eosinophilia, hypotension, wheezing, dyspnoea, urticaria, pruritus, flushing of the upper body, pain, muscle spasm of the chest and back, nausea and rashes, including exfoliative dematitis, Stevens-Johnson syndrome and rare cases of vasculitis.

*Overdose: Symptoms:* See *Undesirable effects.*

*Treatment:* Supportive care is advised, with maintenance of glomeruler filtration. Vancomycin is poorly removed by dialysis. Haemofiltration and haemoperfusion with Amberlite resin XAD-4 have been reported to be of limited benefit.

**Pharmacological properties**

*Pharmacodynamic properties:* Vancomycin is a narrow spectrum antibiotic. The mechanism of action is an inhibition of the enzyme glycopeptide synthetase which is reponsible for condensation of the glycopeptide backbone of the cell wall.

Vancomycin has a bactericidal effect against gram-positive bacteria, especially Staphylococcus aureus. Staphylococcus epidermis, streptococcus faecalis, and Clostridium difficile. All gram negative organisms are resistant.

Resistance is not readily acquired *in vitro* and it has not been observed during the use of vancomycin *in vivo*. There is no cross resistance with other known antibiotics.

*Pharmacokinetic properties:* Vancomycin is not normally absorbed from the gastro-intestinal tract, but in patients with inflammatory disorders of the intestinal mucosa some systemic absorption may occur. The orally administered drug is active only locally within the gut lumen, making it useful in enterocolitis. An oral dose is excreted exclusively in the faeces.

*Preclinical safety data:* None.

**Pharmacological particulars**

*List of excipients:* Polyethylene glycol 6000.

Capsule 125 mg: Black iron oxide E-172, titanium-dioxide E-171, yellow iron oxide E-172, gelatin.

Capsule 250 mg: Black iron oxide E-172, titanium-dioxide E-171, yellow iron oxide E-172, indigo carmine E-132, gelatin.

*Incompatibilities:* Not applicable.

*Shelf life:* 2 years.

*Special precautions for storage:* Room temperature (15–25°C). Protect from moisture.

*Nature and contents of container:* Unit dose blister

packs of PVC/PVdC (250/35 µm) on aluminium foil (20 µm). Pack sizes: 28 capsules.

*Instructions for use/handling:* Not applicable.

*Marketing authorisation holder:* Dumex-Alphama A/S, Dalslandsgrade 11, DK-23000 Copenhagen S, Denmark.

### Marketing authorisation numbers
125 mg Capsules     4938/0015
250 mg Capsules     4938/0016

**Date of approval/revision of SPC**    28 May 1996

**Legal category**    POM

# VANCOMYCIN POWDER for INFUSION

**Qualitative and quantitative composition** *Vancomycin Powder for Infusion 1 g:* Vancomycin 1 g (equivalent to 1,000,000 IU) as vancomycin hydrochloride.

*Vancomycin Powder for Infusion 500 mg:* Vancomycin 500 mg (equivalent to 500,000 IU) as vancomycin hydrochloride.

**Pharmaceutical form**    Powder for infusion.

### Clinical particulars
*Therapeutic indications:* Severe infections caused by bacteria that are susceptible to vancomycin and resistant to other antibiotics; when therapy fails; and in the presence of allergy to penicillin. For instance, sepsis and/or endocarditis, peritonitis in dialysis patients which is caused by Staphlococcus aureus or Staphylococcus epidermidis.

*Posology and method of administration:*
*Adults:* 500 mg every six hours or 1 g every twelve hours by slow intravenous infusion.

*Children:* 40 mg/kg body weight every 24 hours divided into 2 doses given by slow intravenous infusion.

The rate of infusion should not exceed 10 mg/min, corresponding to a rate of 2 ml/min with a concentration of vancomycin of 5 mg/ml.

The dose must be reduced in the presence of decreased renal function. The initial dose is at least 15 mg/kg. The following tables give a guideline for use in patients with decreased renal function.

| Creatinine clearance<br>ml/min | Dose Vancomycin<br>mg/24 hours |
|---|---|
| >100 | 2000–1500 |
| 100–70 | 1500–1000 |
| 70–30 | 1000–50 |
| 20 | 300 |
| 10 | 150 |

*Contra-indications:* None.

*Special warnings and precautions for use:* The serum concentation must be determined daily and the dose regulated accordingly. Two hours after completion of infusion serum concentrations are in the region of 18–26 mg/litre. Serum concentrations measured immediately prior to the next dose should be in the 5–10 mg/litre range.

Care must be exercised in administration to patients with decreased kidney function and in elderly patients.

Concomitant treatment with potentially ototoxic or nephrotoxic medication should be avoided.

*Interactions with other medicaments and other forms of interaction:* None.

*Pregnancy and lactation:*
*Pregnancy:* Reproduction studies of animals have been faulty or non-existent. The data available gives no reason to suspect an increased frequency in foetal damage or other serious effects on the reproductive process. Should not be given in pregnancy, except when the clinical suituation is sufficiently serious to outweigh potential foetal risks.

*Lactation:* Vancomycin is secreted into breast milk. Information on the levels of vancomycin in breast milk is insufficient to judge the risk to the infant. During lactation avoid breast feeding.

*Effects on ability to drive and use machines:* None.

*Undesirable effects:* Commonest are phlebitis and pseudo-allergic reactions occurring when the information is given too quickly.

*Frequent (> 1/100):*
    *General:* Anaphylactoid reactions including hypotension, wheezing, dyspnoea, urticaria, pruritus, and flushing of the upper body (red man effect), pain and muscle spasm of the chest and back.
    *Circulation:* Thrombophlebitis.
    *Urogenital:* Elevated serum creatinine and serum urea, indicating nephrotoxicity.

*Less frequent:*
    *Skin:* Rash.
    *Ears:* Reduced hearing.

*Rare:*
    *Miscellaneous:* Anaphylaxis, fever, chills, dizziness.
    *Haematological:* Thrombocytopenia, neutropenia.
    *Skin:* Exfoliative dermatitis.
    *Ears:* Tinnitus.

Reversible agranulocystosis and pseudomembranous colitis have been reported in a few cases. Ototoxicity may be reversible or permanent, and has been reported mainly in patients given an overdose, in patients with a history of reduced hearing, and with concomitant therapy with other ototoxoc drugs, such as aminoglycosides.

*Overdose:* Symptoms: see *Undesirble effects.*
    Treatment: Symptomatic. Cannot be removed by haemodialysis.

### Pharmacological properties
*Pharmacodynamic properties:* Vancomycin inhibits the construction of the cellular wall of gram-positive bacteria. It has a rapid bacterial action on bacteria in the growth phase. Vancomycin is active against gram-positive cocci, especially Staphylococcus aureus, Staph. epidermidis, Streptococcus faecalis, and gram-positive rods, particularly Clostridium difficile. Other micro-organisms are resistant.

*Pharmacokinetic properties:* Intravenous administration of 2 g over 24 hours produces a mean serum concentration of 10–20 micg/ml. Protein binding is 55%. Vancomycin is distributed rapidly to most tissue and body fluids after intravenous infusion. It penetrates the intact blood-brain barrier only to a low degree. Elimination occurs via kidneys and more than 95% of the dose administered is recovered in the urine. The plasma half-life in adults is 4–6 hours, in children 2–3 hours, and 6–10 hours in the newborn.

*Preclinical safety data:* $LD_{50}$ values after intravenous administration: 489 mg/kg (mice), 319 mg/kg (rats). Teratogenic and mutagenic effects have not been demonstrated in animal studies.

### Pharmaceutical particulars
*List of excipients:* Nitrogen, Water for Injections.

*Incompatibilities:* After reconstitution in sterile water, the pH value is 2.8–4.5. Should only be dissolved in or mixed with the infusion fluids described under *Instruction for use/handling.* The prepared infusion fluid should not be mixed with other drugs.

*Shelf life:* Powder for infusion: 2 years at a temperature below 25˚C.
    Dissolved powder for infusion: 24 hours in a refrigerator at 2–8˚C.

*Special precautions for storage:* Temperature below 25˚C.

*Nature and contents of container:*
*Nature:* Vials, closed with stoppers of chlorobutyl type 1 coated with silicone, sealed with a grey flip-off capsule of aluminium with polypropylene tops, and packaged into a carton.

*Contents of container:*
*Vancomycin Powder for Infusion 1 g:* 1 vial containing 1 g vancomycin packaged into a carton.

*Vancomycin Powder for Infusion 500 mg:* 1 vial containing 500 mg vancomycin packaged into a carton.

*Instruction for use/handling:*
*Vancomycin Powder for Infusion 1 g:* Dissolve the powder for infusion in and dilute to a strength of 50 mg/ml with 20 ml of sterile water. Dilute this stock solution with at least 200 ml of sodium chloride infusion fluid 9 mg/ml or glucose infusion fluid 50 mg/ml.

*Vancomycin Powder for Infusion 500 mg:* Dissolve the powder for infusion in and dilute to a strength of 50 mg/ml with 10 ml of sterile water. Dilute this stock solution with at least 100 ml of sodium chloride infusion fluid 9 mg/ml or glucose infusion fluid 50 mg/ml.

*Marketing authorisation holder:* Dumex-Alpharma A/S, Dalslandsgade 11, DK-2300 Copenhagen S.

**Marketing authorisation number**    0438/0018

**Date of approval/revision of SPC**    2 April 1997

**Date of (partial) revision of the text**    22 January 1997

*Trade Mark

## Du Pont Pharmaceuticals Limited

Avenue One
Letchworth Garden City
Hertfordshire SG6 2HU


DU PONT PHARMA

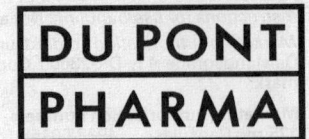

### CARACE

**Presentation** Blue, half scored, oval tablets, marked 'MSD 15', containing 2.5 mg lisinopril.

White, half-scored, oval tablets, marked 'CARACE' and '5', containing 5 mg lisinopril.

Yellow, half-scored, oval tablets, marked 'CARACE' and '10', containing 10 mg lisinopril.

Orange, half-scored, oval tablets, marked 'CARACE' and '20', containing 20 mg lisinopril.

**Uses**

*Indications*

*Hypertension:* All grades of essential hypertension and renovascular hypertension. Carace may be used alone or with other antihypertensive agents.

*Heart failure:* In heart failure, Carace should be used as an adjunctive therapy with non-potassium-sparing diuretics and, where appropriate, digitalis.

*Severe heart failure:* Treatment with Carace should always be initiated in hospital under close medical supervision.

*Mild to moderate heart failure:* Treatment with Carace should always be initiated under close medical supervision.

*Acute myocardial infarction:* Carace is indicated for the treatment of haemodynamically stable patients, defined as patients not in cardiogenic shock and who have a systolic blood pressure greater than 100 mmHg. Carace may be initiated within 24 hours of acute myocardial infarction to prevent the subsequent development of left ventricular dysfunction or heart failure and to improve survival. Patients should receive, as appropriate, the standard recommended treatments such as thrombolytics, aspirin and beta-blocker.

*Action:* Lisinopril is a peptidyl dipeptidase inhibitor. It inhibits the angiotensin converting enzyme (ACE) that catalyses the conversion of Angiotensin I to the vasoconstrictor peptide, Angiotensin II. Angiotensin II also stimulates aldosterone secretion by the adrenal cortex. Inhibition of ACE results in decreased concentrations of Angiotensin II which results in decreased vasopressor activity and reduced aldosterone secretion. The latter decrease may result in a small increase in serum potassium concentration.

While the mechanism through which lisinopril lowers blood pressure is believed to be primarily suppression of the renin-angiotensin-aldosteronesystem, lisinopril is antihypertensive even in patients with low-renin hypertension. ACE is identical to kinanase II, an enzyme that degrades bradykinin. Whether increased levels of bradykinin, a potent vasodilatory peptide, play a role in the therapeutic effects of lisinopril remains to be elucidated.

The disposition of lisinopril in patients with renal insufficiency was similar to that in patients with normal renal function until the glomerular filtration rate reached 30 ml/min or less. Older patients have higher blood levels and higher values for the area under the plasma concentration time curve than younger patients. Lisinopril can be removed by dialysis.

Following oral administration of lisinopril, peak serum concentrations occur within about 7 hours. On multiple dosing lisinopril has an effective half life of accumulation of 12.6 hours.

Declining serum concentrations exhibited a prolonged terminal phase which did not contribute to drug accumulation. This terminal phase probably represents saturable binding to ACE and was not proportional to dose. Lisinopril did not appear to be bound to other plasma proteins.

Based on urinary recovery, the mean extent of absorption of lisinopril is approximately 25%, with interpatient variability (6–60%) at all doses tested (5–80 mg).

Lisinopril does not undergo metabolism and absorbed drug is excreted unchanged entirely in the urine. Lisinopril absorption is not affected by the presence of food in the gastrointestinal tract.

Studies in rats indicate that lisinopril crosses the blood-brain barrier poorly.

**Dosage and administration** The absorption of Carace is not affected by food.

*Hypertension:* The need for dosage titration should be determined by measurement of the blood pressure just before the next dose.

*Essential and renovascular hypertension:* Treatment should be started with 2.5 mg once daily, and titrated upwards to achieve optimal blood pressure control. A 2.5 mg dose seldom achieves a therapeutic response.

The usual effective dose range is 10–20 mg once daily.

The maximum recommended dose is 40 mg daily.

*Diuretic-treated patients:* If possible, the diuretic should be discontinued or the dose reduced, two to three days before beginning therapy with Carace (see 'Precautions') and may be resumed later if required.

*Use in the elderly:* Age alone does not appear to affect the efficacy or safety profile of Carace. Thus, elderly patients should start treatment with Carace as directed above.

*Congestive heart failure:* Carace may be used as adjunctive therapy with non-potassium-sparing diuretics with or without digitalis.

*Initial dosage:* Therapy with Carace should be initiated under close medical supervision (in hospital for severe heart failure) with a recommended starting dose of 2.5 mg once daily. If possible, the dose of diuretic should be reduced before beginning treatment.

Blood pressure and renal function should be monitored closely both before and during treatment because severe hypotension and, more rarely, consequent renal failure have been reported with angiotensin-converting enzyme (ACE) inhibitors (see 'Precautions').

The appearance of hypotension after the initial dose of Carace does not preclude subsequent careful dose adjustment with the drug, following effective treatment of the hypotension.

Some patients, other than those with severe heart failure, are considered to be at higher risk when started on an ACE inhibitor and are recommended for initiation of therapy in hospital. Research data have shown such patients to be: those on multiple or high-dose diuretics (e.g., >80 mg frusemide); patients with hypovolaemia; hyponatraemia (serum sodium <130 mEq/1); pre-existing hypotension (systolic blood pressure <90 mm HG); patients with unstable cardiac failure; renal impairment (serum creatinine >150 micromol/l); those on high-dose vasodilator therapy; patients aged 70 years or over.

*Maintenance dosage:* The dose should be gradually increased, depending on the patient's response, to the usual maintenance dose (5–20 mg). This dose adjustment may be performed over a two- to four-week period, or more rapidly if clinically indicated.

*Acute myocardial infarction:* Treatment with Carace may be started within 24 hours of the onset of symptoms. The first dose of Carace is 5 mg given orally, followed by 5 mg after 24 hours, 10 mg after 48 hours and then 10 mg once daily thereafter. Patients with a low systolic blood pressure (120 mmHg or less) should be given a lower dose – 2.5 mg orally (see precautions). If hypotension occurs (systolic blood pressure less than or equal to 100 mmHg) a daily maintenance dose of 5 mg may be given with temporary reductions to 2.5 mg if needed. If prolonged hypotension occurs (systolic blood pressure less than 90 mmHg for more than 1 hour) Carace should be withdrawn.

Dosing for patients with acute myocardial infarction should continue for six weeks. The benefit appears to be greatest in patients with large myocardial infarctions and evidence of impaired left ventricular function. For patients who develop symptoms of heart failure, see Dosage and administration, Congestive heart failure.

Carace is compatible with intravenous or transdermal glyceryl trinitrate.

*Impaired renal function:* Carace is excreted by the kidney, and should be used with caution in patients with renal insufficiency.

Carace is dialysable. Dialysis patients may be given the usual dose of 'Carace' on dialysis days. On the days when patients are not on dialysis the dosage should be tailored to the blood pressure response.

*Paediatric use:* Carace has not been studied for use in children.

**Contra-indications, warnings, etc**

*Contra-indications*

*Pregnancy:* The use of Carace during pregnancy is not recommended. When pregnancy is determined Carace should be discontinued as soon as possible unless it is considered life-saving for the mother (see Precautions).

*Hypersensitivity* to Carace, and in patients with a history of angioneurotic oedema relating to previous treatment with an ACE inhibitor.

*Precautions*

*Assessment of renal function:* Evaluation of the patient should include assessment of renal function prior to initiation of therapy, and during treatment.

*Impaired renal function:* Carace should be used with caution in patients with renal insufficiency, as they may require reduced or less frequent doses (see 'Dosage'). Close monitoring of renal function during therapy should be performed as deemed appropriate in those with renal insufficiency. In the majority, renal function will not alter, or may improve.

Renal failure has been reported in association with ACE inhibitors and has been mainly in patients with severe congestive heart failure or underlying renal disease, including renal artery stenosis. If recognised promptly and treated appropriately, renal failure is usually reversible.

Some hypertensive patients, with no apparent pre-existing renal disease, have developed increases in blood urea and creatinine when Carace has been given concurrently with a diuretic. Dosage reduction of Carace and/or discontinuation of the diuretic may be required. This situation should raise the possibility of underlying renal artery stenosis (see 'Renovascular hypertension').

*Symptomatic hypotension* was seen rarely in uncomplicated hypertensive patients. It is more likely to occur in patients who have been volume-depleted by diuretic therapy, dietary salt restriction, dialysis, diarrhoea, or vomiting. In these patients, by discontinuing diuretic therapy or significantly reducing the diuretic dose for two to three days prior to initiating Carace, the possibility of this occurrence is reduced.

Similar caution and close supervision may apply also to patients with ischaemic heart or cerebrovascular disease in whom severe hypotension could result in a myocardial infarct or cerebrovascular accident.

Severe hypotension has been reported with ACE inhibitors, mainly in patients with severe heart failure. Many of these patients were on high doses of loop diuretics, and some had hyponatraemia or functional renal impairment. If hypotension develops, the patient should be placed in a supine position. Volume repletion with oral fluids or intravenous normal saline may be required. Intravenous atropine may be necessary if there is associated bradycardia. Treatment with Carace may be restarted with careful dose titration following restoration of effective blood volume and pressure.

In some patients with congestive heart failure who have normal or low blood pressure, additional lowering of systemic blood pressure may occur with Carace. If such hypotension becomes symptomatic, a reduction of dose or discontinuation of Carace may become necessary.

The appearance of hypotension after the initial dose of Carace does not preclude subsequent careful dose titration with the drug after effective management of hypotension.

*Hypotension in acute myocardial infarction:* Treatment with lisinopril must not be initiated in acute myocardial infarction patients who are at risk of further serious haemodynamic deterioration after treatment with a vasodilator. These are patients with systolic blood pressure of 100 mmHg or lower or cardiogenic shock. During the first 3 days following the infarction, the dose should be reduced if the systolic blood pressure is 120 mmHg or lower. Maintenance doses should be reduced to 5 mg or temporarily to 2.5 mg if systolic blood pressure is 100 mmHg or lower. If hypotension persists (systolic blood pressure less than 90 mmHg for more than 1 hour) then Carace should be withdrawn.

*Renovascular hypertension:* Carace can be used when surgery is not indicated, or prior to surgery. In some patients with bilateral renal artery stenosis or stenosis of the artery to a solitary kidney, increases of blood urea and creatinine, reversible upon discontinuation of therapy, have been seen. This is especially likely in patients treated with diuretics and/or those with renal insufficiency.

In acute myocardial infarction, treatment with lisinopril should not be initiated in patients with evidence of renal dysfunction, defined as serum creatinine concentration exceeding 177 micromol/l and/or proteinuria exceeding 500 mg/24 h. If renal dysfunction develops during treatment with Carace (serum creatinine concentration exceeding 265 micromol/l or a doubling from the pre-treatment value) then the physician should consider withdrawal of Carace.

*Angioneurotic oedema:* It has been reported with angiotensin-converting enzyme inhibitors, including Carace. This may occur at any time during treatment. In such cases, Carace should be discontinued promptly and appropriate monitoring should be instituted to ensure complete resolution of symptoms prior to dismissing the patient. Where swelling is confined to the face, lips and mouth, the condition will usually resolve without further treatment although antihistamines may be useful in relieving symptoms. These patients should be followed carefully until the swelling has resolved. However, where there is involvement of the tongue, glottis or larynx likely to cause airways obstruction, appropriate therapy such as subcutaneous adrenaline (0.5 ml 1:1,000) should be administered promptly.

Patients with a history of angioedema unrelated to ACE-inhibitor therapy may be at an increased risk of angioedema while receiving an ACE inhibitor (see also 'Contra-indications').

Other hypersensitivity reactions have been reported.

*Haemodialysis patients:* Anaphylactoid reactions have been reported in patients dialysed with high-flux membrances (e.g. AN 69®) and treated concomitantly with an ACE inhibitor. In these patients consideration should be given to using a different type of dialysis membrane or a different class of antihypertensive agent.

*Cough:* Cough has been reported with the use of ACE-inhibitors. Characteristically, the cough is non-productive, persistent, and resolves after discontinuation of therapy. ACE-inhibitor-induced cough should be considered as part of the differential diagnosis of cough.

*Surgery/anaesthesia:* In patients undergoing major surgery or during anaesthesia with agents that produce hypotension, Carace blocks angiotensin II formation secondary to compensatory renin release. This may lead to hypotension which can be corrected by volume expansion.

*General:* Carace should not be used in patients with aortic stenosis, cor pulmonale or outflow tract obstruction.

Where Carace is used as a single agent in hypertension, Afro-Caribbean patients may show a reduced therapeutic response.

*Drug interactions:* When Carace is combined with other antihypertensive agents such as beta-blockers and diuretics the antihypertensive effect is usually additive.

Carace minimises the development of thiazide-induced hypokalaemia and hyperuricaemia.

Carace has been used with nitrates without significant clinical interaction.

Indomethacin may reduce the antihypertensive efficacy of Carace.

As Carace may reduce the elimination of lithium, serum levels of lithium should be monitored if lithium salts are administered.

*Plasma potassium* usually remains within normal limits, although a few cases of hyperkalaemia have occurred. If Carace is given with a diuretic, the likelihood of diuretic-induced hypokalaemia may be lessened. Carace may elevate plasma potassium levels in patients with renal failure. Potassium supplements, potassium-sparing diuretics and potassium-containing salt substitutes are not recommended.

*Use in pregnancy and lactation:* The use of Carace during pregnancy is not recommended. When pregnancy is detected Carace should be discontinued as soon as possible, unless it is considered life-saving for the mother.

ACE inhibitors can cause foetal and neonatal morbidity and mortality when administered to pregnant women during the second and third trimesters. Use of ACE inhibitors during this period has been associated with foetal and neonatal injury including hypotension, renal failure, hyperkalaemia, and/or skull hypoplasia in the newborn. Maternal oligohydramnios, presumably representing decreased foetal renal function, has occurred and may result in limb contractures, craniofacial deformations and hypoplastic lung development. If Carace is used, the patient should be appraised of the potential hazard to the foetus.

These adverse effects to the embryo and foetus do not appear to have resulted from intrauterine ACE-inhibitor exposure limited to the first trimester.

In those rare cases where ACE inhibitor use during pregnancy is deemed essential, serial ultrasound examinations should be performed to assess the intraamniotic environment. If oligohydramnios is detected, Carace should be discontinued unless it is considered life-saving to the mother. Patients and physicians should be aware, however, that oligohydramnios may not appear until after the foetus has sustained irreversible injury.

Infants whose mothers have taken Carace should be closely observed for hypertension, oliguria and hyperkalaemia. Lisinopril, which crossed the placenta, has been removed from the neonatal circulation by peritoneal dialysis with some clinical benefit, and theoretically may be removed by exchange transfusion.

*Nursing mothers:* It is not known whether Carace is excreted in human milk. Because many drugs are secreted in human milk, caution should be exercised if Carace is given to a nursing mother.

*Side-effects:* Hypotension has occurred in association with therapy with Carace. This appears to occur in certain specific sub-groups (see 'Precautions').

*Hypersensitivity/angioneurotic oedema:* Angioneurotic oedema of the face, extremities, lips, tongue, glottis and/or larynx has been reported rarely (see 'Precautions').

*Other adverse reactions:* Dizziness, headache, diarrhoea, fatigue, cough, and nausea are the most frequent. Other less frequent side effects include: orthostatic effects (including hypotension), rash, and asthenia.

Rare side-effects include myocardial infarction or cerebrovascular accident possibly secondary to excessive hypotension in high-risk patients (see 'Precautions'), palpitation, tachycardia, pancreatitis, abdominal pain, dry mouth, hepatitis (hepatocellular or cholestatic), mood alterations, mental confusion, urticaria, diaphoresis, uraemia, oliguria/anuria, renal dysfunction, acute renal failure, impotence.

There have been reports of haemolytic anaemia in patients taking lisinopril, although no causal relationship has been established.

A symptom complex has been reported which may include fever, vasculitis, myalgia arthralgia/arthritis, a positive ANA, elevated erythrocyte sedimentation rate, eosinophilia, and leucocytosis. Rash, photosensitivity, or other dermatological manifestation may occur.

*Laboratory test findings:* Increases in blood urea and creatinine, reversible on discontinuation of Carace, are most likely in the presence of bilateral renal artery stenosis, especially in patients with renal insufficiency (see 'Precautions'). However, increases in blood urea and creatinine may occur without evidence of pre-existing renal impairment, especially in patients taking diuretics. In this event, undiagnosed renal artery stenosis should be suspected. Dosage reduction of Carace and/or discontinuation of the diuretic should be considered. Rare cases of neutropenia have been reported, although no causal relationship has been established.

Increases in liver enzymes and serum bilirubin have occurred which are usually reversible on discontinuation of Carace.

Decreases in haemoglobin and haematocrit have been reported in a few patients but were rarely of clinical importance unless another cause of anaemia was present.

Hyperkalaemia and hyponatraemia have occurred occasionally (see also 'Plasma potassium').

Thrombocytopenia and leukopenia have been reported: a causal relationship to therapy with Carace cannot be excluded.

*Overdosage:* There are no data on overdosage in humans. The most likely manifestation of overdosage would be hypotension, which can be treated, if necessary, by intravenous infusion of normal saline solution. Carace can be removed by haemodialysis.

**Pharmaceutical precautions** Store in a dry place below 25°C.

**Legal category** POM.

**Package quantities**
Tablets 20 mg: Calendar packs of 28 tablets.
Tablets 10 mg: Calendar packs of 28 tablets.
Tablets 5 mg: Calendar packs of 28 tablets.
Tablets 2.5 mg: Calendar packs of 28 tablets.

**Further information** Nil.

**Product licence numbers**

| | |
|---|---|
| 2.5 mg tablet | 11173/0027 |
| 5 mg tablet | 11173/0028 |
| 10 mg tablet | 11173/0029 |
| 20 mg tablet | 11173/0030 |

## CARACE * 10 PLUS and CARACE 20 PLUS

**Presentation** Carace 10 Plus: Blue, hexagonal, biconvex tablet with the product code 145 on one side. Each tablet contains 10 mg lisinopril and 12.5 mg hydrochlorothiazide.

Carace 20 Plus: Hexagonal, yellow tablets marked MSD 140 on one side and scored. Each tablet contains 20 mg lisinopril and 12.5 mg hydrochlorothiazide.

**Uses** For the management of mild to moderate hypertension in patients who have been stabilised on the individual components given in the same proportions.

*Action:* Carace 10 Plus and Carace 20 Plus are fixed combinations of an angiotensin-converting enzyme inhibitor (lisinopril) and a diuretic (hydrochlorothiazide). Carace 10 Plus and Carace 20 Plus are highly effective in the treatment of hypertension. Hydrochlorothiazide stimulates the renin-angiotensin-aldosterone system which produces an additive effect with lisinopril.

Lisinopril is an inhibitor of the angiotensin-converting enzyme (ACE). Inhibition of the formation of angiotensin II results in vasodilation and a fall in blood pressure.

Hydrochlorothiazide is a diuretic and antihypertensive agent. Use of this agent alone results in increased renin secretion. Although lisinopril alone is antihypertensive, even in patients with low renin hypertension, concomitant administration with hydrochlorothiazide results in a greater reduction in blood pressure. Lisinopril attenuates the potassium loss associated with hydrochlorothiazide.

**Dosage and administration**
*Adults*

*Essential hypertension:* The usual dosage of Carace 10 Plus or Carace 20 Plus is 1 tablet, administered once daily. If necessary, the dosage may be increased to 2 tablets, administered once daily.

*Dosage in renal insufficiency:* Thiazides may not be appropriate diuretics for use in patients with renal impairment and are ineffective at creatinine clearance values of 30 ml/min or below (i.e. moderate or severe renal insufficiency).

Carace 10 Plus or Carace 20 Plus are not to be used as initial therapy in any patient with renal insufficiency.

In patients with creatinine clearance of >30 and <80 ml/min, Carace 10 Plus or Carace 20 Plus may be used, but only after titration of the individual components.

*Prior diuretic therapy:* Symptomatic hypotension may occur following the initial dose of Carace 10 Plus or Carace 20 Plus: this is more likely in patients who are volume and/or salt depleted as a result of prior diuretic therapy. If possible, the diuretic therapy should be discontinued for 2–3 days prior to initiation of therapy with lisinopril alone, in a 2.5 mg dose.

*Use in the elderly:* Lisinopril was equally effective in elderly (65 years or older) and non-elderly hypertensive patients. In elderly hypertensive patients, monotherapy with lisinopril was as effective in reducing diastolic blood pressure as monotherapy with either hydrochlorothiazide or atenolol. In clinical studies, age did not affect the tolerability of lisinopril.

In clinical studies the efficacy and tolerability of lisinopril and hydrochlorothiazide, administered concomitantly, were similar in both elderly and younger hypertensive patients.

*Paediatric use:* Safety and effectiveness in children have not been established.

**Contra-indications, warnings, etc**
*Contra-indications:* Carace 10 Plus or Carace 20 Plus are contra-indicated in patients with anuria or aortic stenosis or hyperkalaemia.

Carace 10 Plus or Carace 20 Plus are contra-indicated in patients who are hypersensitive to any component of the product and in patients with a history of angioneurotic oedema relating to previous treatment with an angiotensin-converting-enzyme inhibitor.

Carace 10 Plus and Carace 20 Plus are contra-indicated in patients who are hypersensitive to other sulphonamide-derived drugs.

The use of Carace 10 Plus or Carace 20 Plus during pregnancy is not recommended. When pregnancy is detected Carace 10 Plus or Carace 20 Plus should be discontinued as soon as possible, unless it is considered life-saving for the mother.

ACE inhibitors can cause foetal and neonatal morbidity and mortality when administered to pregnant women during the second and third trimesters. Use of ACE inhibitors during this period has been associated with foetal and neonatal injury including hypotension, renal failure, hyperkalaemia, and/or skull hypoplasia in the newborn. Maternal oligohydramnios, presumably representing decreased foetal renal function, has occurred and may result in limb contractures, craniofacial deformations and hypoplastic lung development.

These adverse effects to the embryo and foetus do not appear to have resulted from intrauterine ACE inhibitor exposure limited to the first trimester.

The routine use of diuretics in otherwise healthy pregnant women is not recommended and exposes mother and foetus to unnecessary hazard including foetal or neonatal jaundice, thrombocytopenia and possibly other adverse reactions which have occurred in the adult.

If Carace 10 Plus or Carace 20 Plus are used during pregnancy, the patient should be apprised of the potential hazard to the foetus. In those rare cases where use during pregnancy is deemed essential, serial ultrasound examinations should be performed to assess the intraamniotic environment. If oligohydramnios is detected, Carace 10 Plus or Carace 20 Plus should be discontinued unless it is considered life-saving for the mother. Patients and physicians should be aware, however, that oligohydramnios may not appear until after the foetus has sustained irreversible injury.

Infants whose mothers have taken Carace 10 Plus or Carace 20 Plus should be closely observed for hypotension, oliguria and hyperkalaemia. Lisinopril, which crosses the placenta, has been removed from the neonatal circulation by peritoneal dialysis with some clinical benefit, and theoretically may be removed by exchange transfusion. There is no experience with the removal of hydrochlorothiazide, which also crosses the placenta, from the neonatal circulation.

Carace 10 Plus or Carace 20 Plus are contra-indicated in lactating women who are breast-feeding infants. It is not known whether lisinopril is excreted in human milk. Thiazides do appear in human milk.

See also 'Breast-feeding mothers' under 'Precautions'.

*Precautions*

*Hypotension and electrolyte/fluid imbalance:* As with all antihypertensive therapy, symptomatic hypotension may occur in some patients. This was rarely seen in uncomplicated hypertensive patients but is more likely in the presence of fluid or electrolyte imbalance, e.g. volume depletion, hyponatraemia, hypochloraemic alkalosis, hypomagnesaemia or hypokalaemia which may occur from prior diuretic therapy, dietary salt restriction, dialysis, or during intercurrent diarrhoea or vomiting. Periodic determination of serum electrolytes should be performed at appropriate intervals in such patients.

Particular consideration should be given when therapy is administered to patients with ischaemic heart or cerebrovascular disease, because an excessive fall in blood pressure could result in myocardial infarction or cerebrovascular accident.

If hypotension occurs, the patient should be placed in the supine position and, if necessary, should receive an intravenous infusion of normal saline. A transient hypotensive response is not a contra-indication to further doses. Following restoration of effective blood volume and pressure, reinstitution of therapy at reduced dosage may be possible; or either of the components may be used appropriately alone.

*Renal function impairment:* Thiazides may not be appropriate diuretics for use in patients with renal impairment and are ineffective at creatinine clearance values of 30 ml/min or below (i.e. moderate or severe renal insufficiency). Carace 10 Plus or Carace 20 Plus should not be administered to patients with renal insufficiency (creatinine clearance <80 ml/min) until titration of the individual components has shown the need for the doses present in the combination tablet.

Some hypertensive patients, with no apparent pre-existing renal disease, have developed usually minor and transient increases in blood urea and serum creatinine when lisinopril has been given concomitantly with a diuretic. If this occurs during therapy with Carace 10 Plus or Carace 20 Plus the combination should be discontinued. Reinstitution of therapy at reduced dosage may be possible, or either of the components may be used appropriately alone.

In some patients, with bilateral renal artery stenosis or stenosis of the single artery to a solitary kidney, increases in blood urea and serum creatinine, reversible upon discontinuation of therapy, have been seen with angiotensin-converting enzyme (ACE) inhibitors.

*Haemodialysis patients:* The use of Carace 10 Plus or Carace 20 Plus are not indicated in patients requiring dialysis for renal failure. A high incidence of anaphylactoid reactions have been reported in patients dialysed with high-flux membrances (e.g. AN 69®) and treated concomitantly with an ACE inhibitor. These combinations should therefore be avoided.

*Hepatic disease:* Thiazides should be used with caution in patients with impaired hepatic function or progressive liver disease, since minor alterations of fluid and electrolyte balance may precipitate hepatic coma.

*Surgery/anaesthesia:* In patients undergoing major surgery or during anaesthesia with agents that produce hypotension, lisinopril may block angiotensin II formation secondary to compensatory renin release. If hypotension occurs and is considered to be due to this mechanism, it can be corrected by volume expansion.

*Metabolic and endocrine effects:* Thiazide therapy may impair glucose tolerance. Dosage adjustment of antidiabetic agents, including insulin, may be required.

Thiazides may decrease urinary calcium excretion and may cause intermittent and slight elevation of serum calcium. Marked hypercalcaemia may be evidence of hidden hyperparathyroidism. Thiazides should be discontinued before carrying out tests for parathyroid function.

Increases in cholesterol and triglyceride levels may be associated with thiazide diuretic therapy.

Thiazide therapy may precipitate hyperuricaemia and/or gout in certain patients. However, lisinopril may increase urinary uric acid and thus may attenuate the hyperuricaemic effect of hydrochlorothiazide.

*Hypersensitivity/angioneurotic oedema:* Angioneurotic oedema of the face, extremities, lips, tongue, glottis, and/or larynx has been reported rarely in patients treated with angiotensin-converting enzyme inhibitors, including lisinopril. This may occur at anytime during treatment. In such cases, Carace 10 Plus or Carace 20 Plus should be discontinued promptly, and appropriate monitoring should be instituted to ensure complete resolution of symptoms prior to dismissing the patient.

In those instances where swelling has been confined to the face and lips, the condition generally resolved without treatment, although antihistamines have been useful in relieving symptoms. Angioneurotic oedema associated with laryngeal oedema may be fatal. Where there is involvement of the tongue, glottis or larynx, likely to cause airway obstruction, appropriate therapy such as subcutaneous adrenaline solution 1:1,000 (0.3 ml to 0.5 ml) should be administered promptly. Patients with a history of angioedema unrelated to ACE-inhibitor therapy may be at increased risk of angioedema while receiving an ACE inhibitor. (See also 'Contra-indications').

In patients receiving thiazides, sensitivity reactions may occur with or without a history of allergy or bronchial asthma. Exacerbation or activation of systemic lupus erythematosus has been reported with the use of thiazides.

*Anaphylactoid reactions during hymenoptera desensitization:* Rarely, patients receiving ACE inhibitors during desensitization with hymenoptera venom have experienced life-threatening anaphylactoid reactions. These reactions were avoided by temporarily withholding ACE inhibitor therapy prior to each desensitisation.

*Cough:* Cough has been reported with the use of ACE inhibitors. Characteristically, the cough is non-productive, persistent, and resolves after discontinuation of therapy. ACE inhibitor-induced cough should be considered as part of the differential diagnosis of cough.

*Breast-feeding mothers:* It is not known whether lisinopril is secreted in human milk; however, thiazides do appear in human milk. Because of the potential for serious reactions in nursing infants, a decision should be made whether to discontinue breast-feeding or to discontinue Carace 10 Plus or Carace 20 Plus, taking into account the importance of the drug to the mother.

*Drug interactions:*

*Serum potassium:* The potassium-losing effect of thiazide diuretics is usually attenuated by the potassium-conserving effect of lisinopril.

The use of potassium supplements, potassium-sparing agents or potassium-containing salt substitutes, particularly in patients with impaired renal function, may lead to a significant increase in serum potassium. If concomitant use of Carace 10 Plus or Carace 20 Plus and any of these agents is deemed appropriate, they should be used with caution and with frequent monitoring of serum potassium.

*Lithium:* Lithium generally should not be given with diuretics or ACE inhibitors. Diuretic agents and ACE inhibitors reduce the renal clearance of lithium and add a high risk of lithium toxicity. Refer to prescribing information for lithium preparations before use of such preparations.

*Other agents:* Indomethacin may diminish the hypertensive effect of concomitantly administered Carace 10 Plus or Carace 20 Plus. The antihypertensive effect of Carace 10 Plus or Carace 20 Plus may be potentiated when given concomitantly with other agents likely to cause postural hypotension.

Thiazides may increase the responsiveness to tubocurarine.

*Side-effects:* Carace 10 Plus or Carace 20 Plus are usually well tolerated. In clinical studies, side effects have usually been mild and transient, and in most instances have not required interruption of therapy. The side-effects that have been observed have been limited to those reported previously with lisinopril or hydrochlorothiazide.

One of the most common clinical side-effects was dizziness, which generally responded to dosage reduction and seldom required discontinuation of therapy.

Other, less frequent side-effects were headache, dry cough, fatigue, and hypotension including orthostatic hypotension.

Still less common were diarrhoea, nausea, vomiting, dry mouth, rash, gout, palpitation, chest discomfort, muscle cramps and weakness, paraesthesia, asthenia, and impotence.

Pancreatitis has been reported rarely with lisinopril and with hydrochlorothiazide and therefore is a potential side-effect of Carace 10 Plus and Carace 20 Plus.

*Hypersensitivity/angioneurotic oedema:* Angioneurotic oedema of the face, extremities, lips, tongue, glottis and/or larynx has been reported rarely (see 'Precautions').

A symptom complex has been reported which may include fever, vasculitis, myalgia, arthralgia/arthritis, a positive ANA, elevated ESR, eosinophilia, and leucocytosis. Rash photosensitivity, or other dermatological manifestations may occur.

*Laboratory test findings:* Laboratory side-effects have rarely been of clinical importance. Occasional hyperglycaemia, hyperuricaemia and hyperkalaemia or hypokalaemia have been noted. Usually minor and transient increases in blood urea nitrogen and serum creatinine have been seen in patients without evidence of pre-existing renal impairment. If such increases persist, they are usually reversible upon discontinuation of Carace 10 Plus or Carace 20 Plus. Small decreases in haemoglobin and haematocrit have been reported frequently in hypertensive patients treated with Carace 10 Plus or Carace 20 Plus but were rarely of clinical importance unless another cause of anaemia co-existed. Rarely, elevation of liver enzymes and/or serum bilirubin have occurred, but a causal relationship to Carace 10 Plus or Carace 20 Plus has not been established.

Other side-effects reported with the individual components alone, and which may be potential side-effects with Carace 10 Plus or Carace 20 Plus, are:

*Lisinopril:* Myocardial infarction or cerebrovascular accident possibly secondary to excessive hypotension in high-risk patients (see 'Precautions'), tachycardia, abdominal pain, hepatitis – either hepatocellular or cholestatic jaundice, mood alterations, mental confusion, bronchospasm, urticaria, pruritis, diaphoresis, alopecia, uraemia, oliguria/anuria, renal dysfunction, acute renal failure, thrombocytopenia, leukopenia, hyponatraemia. Rare cases of neutropenia have been reported, although no causal relationship has been established. There have been reports of haemolytic anaemia in patients taking lisinopril, although no causal relationship has been established.

*Hydrochlorothiazide:* Anorexia, gastric irritation, constipation, jaundice (intrahepatic cholestatic jaundice), sialoadenitis, vertigo, xanthopsia, leucopenia, agranulocytosis, thrombocytopenia, aplastic anaemia, haemolytic anaemia, purpura, photosensitivity, urticaria, necrotising angiitis (vasculitis, cutaneous vasculitis), fever, respiratory distress including pneumonitis and pulmonary oedema, anaphylactic reactions, hyperglycaemia, glycosuria, hyperuricaemia, electrolyte imbalance including hyponatraemia, muscle spasm, restlessness, transient blurred vision, renal failure, renal dysfunction, and interstitial nephritis.

*Overdosage:* No specific information is available on the treatment of overdosage with Carace 10 Plus or Carace 20 Plus. Treatment is symptomatic and supportive. Therapy with Carace 10 Plus or Carace 20 Plus should be discontinued and the patient observed closely. Suggested measures include induction of emesis and/or gastric lavage, if ingestion is recent, and correction of dehydration, electrolyte imbalance and hypotension by established procedures.

*Lisinopril:* The most likely features of overdosage would be hypotension, for which the usual treatment would be intravenous infusion of normal saline solution.

Lisinopril may be removed from the general circulation by haemodialysis.

*Hydrochlorothiazide:* The most common signs and symptoms observed are those caused by electrolyte depletion (hypokalaemia, hypochloraemia, hyponatraemia) and dehydration resulting from excessive diuresis. If digitalis has also been administered, hypokalaemia may accentuate cardiac arrhythmias.

**Pharmaceutical precautions** Store in a dry place below 25°C.

**Legal category** POM.

**Package quantities** Calendar packs of 28 tablets.

**Further information** Nil.

**Product licence numbers**

Carace 10 Plus        11173/0036.
Carace 20 Plus        11173/0033

# MODURET 25*

**Presentation** Moduret 25 is available as off-white, diamond-shaped tablets, with a break line and marked '923', containing Amiloride Hydrochloride BP equivalent to 2.5 mg anhydrous amiloride hydrochloride and 25 mg Hydrochlorothiazide BP.

**Uses** Potassium-conserving diuretic and antihypertensive.

Moduret 25 is indicated alone or as an adjunct to other antihypertensive agents in: hypertension, congestive heart failure, hepatic cirrhosis with ascites and oedema.

Moduret 25 is intended for the treatment of patients in whom potassium depletion might be suspected or anticipated. The presence of amiloride hydrochloride minimises the likelihood of potassium loss during vigorous diuresis for long term maintenance therapy. The combination is thus indicated especially in conditions where potassium balance is particularly important.

**Dosage and administration**

*Hypertension:* Usually two or four Moduret 25 tablets given once a day or in divided doses. Some patients may require only one Moduret 25 Tablet a day. The dosage may be increased if necessary, but must not exceed eight Moduret 25 tablets a day.

*Congestive heart failure:* Initially two or four tablets of Moduret 25 a day, subsequently adjusted if required, but not exceeding eight Moduret 25 tablets a day. Optimal dosage is determined by the diuretic response and the plasma potassium level. Once an initial diuresis has been achieved, reduction in dosage may be attempted for maintenance therapy. Maintenance therapy may be on an intermittent basis.

*Hepatic cirrhosis with ascites:* Initiate therapy with a low dose. A single daily dose of two Moduret 25 tablets may be increased gradually until there is an effective diuresis. Dosage should not exceed eight Moduret 25 tablets a day. Maintenance dosages may be lower than those required to initiate diuresis; dosage reduction should therefore be attempted when the patient's weight is stabilised. A gradual weight reduction is especially desirable in cirrhotic patients to reduce the likelihood of untoward reactions associated with diuretic therapy.

*Paediatric use:* Moduret 25 is not recommended for children (see 'Contra-indications').

*Use in the elderly:* Particular caution is needed in the elderly because of their susceptibility to electrolyte imbalance; the dosage should be carefully adjusted to renal function and clinical response.

**Contra-indications, warnings, etc**

*Contra-indications:* Hyperkalaemia (plasma potassium over 5.5 mmol/l); other potassium-conserving diuretics. Potassium supplements or potassium-rich food (except in severe and/or refractory cases of hypokalaemia under careful monitoring); concomitant use with spironolactone or triamterene; anuria; acute renal failure, severe progressive renal disease, severe hepatic failure, precoma associated with hepatic cirrhosis, Addison's disease, hypercalcaemia, concurrent lithium therapy, diabetic nephropathy; patients with blood urea over 10 mmol/l, patients with diabetes mellitus, or those with serum creatinine over 130 umol/l in whom serum electrolyte and blood urea levels cannot be monitored carefully and frequently. Prior hypersensitivity to amiloride hydrochloride, hydrochlorothiazide or other sulphonamide derived drugs. Because the safety of amiloride hydrochloride for use in children has not been established, Moduret 25 is not recommended for children. For 'Use in pregnancy' and 'Use in breast-feeding mothers', see 'Precautions'.

*Precautions:* Hyperkalaemia has been observed in patients receiving amiloride hydrochloride, either alone or with other diuretics, particularly in the aged or in hospital patients with hepatic cirrhosis or congestive heart failure with renal involvement, who were seriously ill, or were undergoing vigorous diuretic therapy. Such patients should be carefully observed for clinical, laboratory, and ECG evidence of hyperkalaemia (not always associated with an abnormal ECG).

Neither potassium supplements nor a potassium-rich diet should be used with Moduret 25 except under careful monitoring in severe and/or refractory cases of hypokalaemia.

Some deaths have been reported in this group of patients.

*Treatment of hyperkalaemia:* Should hyperkalaemia develop, discontinue treatment immediately and, if necessary, take active measures to reduce the plasma potassium to normal.

*Impaired renal function:* Renal function should be monitored because the use of Moduret 25 in impaired renal function may result in the rapid development of hyperkalaemia. Thiazide diuretics become ineffective when creatinine levels fall below 30 ml/min.

*Electrolyte imbalance:* Although the likelihood of electrolyte imbalance is reduced by Moduret 25, careful check should be kept for such signs of fluid and electrolyte imbalance as hyponatraemia, hypochloraemic alkalosis, hypokalaemia and hypomagnesaemia. It is particularly important to make serum and urine electrolyte determinations when the patient is vomiting excessively or receiving parenteral fluids. Warning signs or symptoms of fluid or electrolyte imbalance include: dryness of the mouth, weakness, lethargy, drowsiness, restlessness, seizures, muscle pains or cramps, muscular fatigue, hypotension, oliguria, tachycardia, and gastro-intestinal disturbances such as nausea and vomiting.

Hypokalaemia may develop, especially as a result of brisk diuresis, after prolonged therapy or when severe cirrhosis is present. Hypokalaemia can sensitise or exaggerate the response of the heart to the toxic effects of digitalis (e.g. increased ventricular irritability).

Diuretic-induced hyponatraemia is usually mild and asymptomatic. It may become severe and symptomatic in a few patients who will then require immediate attention and appropriate treatment.

Thiazides may decrease urinary calcium excretion. Thiazides may cause intermittent and slight elevation of serum calcium in the absence of known disorders of calcium metabolism. Therapy should be discontinued before carrying out tests for parathyroid function.

Azotaemia may be precipitated or increased by hydrochlorothiazide. Cumulative effects of the drug may develop in patients with impaired renal function. If increasing azotaemia and oliguria develop during treatment of renal disease, Moduret 25 should be discontinued.

*Hepatic disease:* Thiazides should be used with caution in patients with impaired hepatic function or progressive liver disease (see 'Contra-indications'), since minor alterations of fluid and electrolyte balance may precipitate hepatic coma.

*Metabolic:* Hyperuricaemia may occur, or gout may be precipitated or aggravated, in certain patients receiving thiazides. Thiazides may impair glucose tolerance. Diabetes mellitus may be precipitated or aggravated by therapy with Moduret 25 (see 'Contra-indications'). Dosage adjustment of antidiabetic agents, including insulin, may be required.

Increases in cholesterol and triglyceride levels may be associated with thiazide diuretic therapy.

To minimise the risk of hyperkalaemia in diabetic or suspected diabetic patients, the status of renal function should be determined before initiating therapy with Moduret 25. Therapy should be discontinued at least three days before giving a glucose tolerance test. Potassium-conserving therapy should be initiated only with caution in severely ill patients in whom metabolic or respiratory acidosis may occur, e.g. patients with cardiopulmonary disease or patients with inadequately controlled diabetes.

Shifts in acid-base balance alter the balance of extracellular/intracellular potassium, and the development of acidosis may be associated with rapid increases in plasma potassium.

*Sensitivity reactions:* The possibility that thiazides may activate or exacerbate systemic lupus erythematosus has been reported.

*Ability to drive and to use machines:* Infrequently, patients may experience weakness, fatigue, dizziness, stupor and vertigo. Should any of these occur, the patient should be cautioned not to drive or operate machinery.

*Use in pregnancy:* The routine use of diuretics in otherwise healthy pregnant women with or without mild oedema is not indicated, because they may be associated with hypovolaemia, increased blood viscosity, and decreased placental perfusion. Diuretics do not prevent the development of toxaemia of pregnancy and there is no satisfactory evidence that they are useful for its treatment.

Since thiazides cross the placental barrier and appear in cord blood, use where pregnancy is present or suspected requires that the benefits of the drug be weighed against possible hazards to the fetus. These hazards include fetal or neonatal jaundice, thrombocytopenia, bone marrow depression and possibly other side effects that have occurred in the adult.

*Use in breast-feeding mothers:* Although it is not known whether amiloride hydrochloride is excreted in human milk, it is known that thiazides do appear in breast milk. If use of the drug combination is deemed essential, the patient should stop breast-feeding.

*Drug interactions:* When amiloride hydrochloride is administered concomitantly with an ACE inhibitor, the risk of hyperkalaemia may be increased. Therefore,

if concomitant use of these agents is indicated because of demonstrated hypokalaemia, they should be used with caution and with frequent monitoring of serum potassium.

When given concurrently, the following drugs may interact with thiazide diuretics:

Alcohol, barbiturates or narcotics: Co-administration may potentiate orthostatic hypotension. Oral and parenteral antidiabetic drugs may require adjustment of dosage with concurrent use. Other antihypertensive drugs may have an additive effect. Therefore the dosage of these agents, especially adrenergic-blockers, may need to be reduced when Moduret 25 is added to the regimen. Diuretic therapy should be discontinued for 2–3 days prior to initiation of therapy with an ACE inhibitor to reduce the likelihood of first dose hypotension. Corticosteroids or ACTH may intensify any thiazide-induced electrolyte depletion, particularly hypokalaemia. Pressor amines such as adrenaline may show decreased arterial responsiveness when used with Moduret 25 but this reaction is not enough to preclude their therapeutic usefulness. Non-depolarising muscle relaxants such as tubocurarine may possibly interact with Moduret 25 to increase muscle relaxation. Lithium may accumulate as a result of reduced renal clearance. Non-steroidal anti-inflammatory drugs may attenuate the diuretic, natriuretic and antihypertensive effects of diuretics. Chlorpropamide: Moduret 25 can act synergistically with chlorpropramide to increase the risk of hyponatraemia. Drug/laboratory tests: Because thiazides may affect calcium metabolism, Moduret 25 may interfere with tests for parathyroid function.

*Side-effects:* Although minor side effects are relatively common, significant side effects are infrequent.

Reported side effects are generally associated with diuresis, thiazide therapy, or with the underlying disease.

No increase in the risk of adverse reactions has been seen over those of the individual components.

The reported adverse reactions of the combination:

Body as a whole: headache, weakness, fatigue, malaise, chest pain, back pain, syncope.

Cardiovascular: arrhythmias, tachycardia, digitalis toxicity, orthostatic hypotension, angina pectoris.

Digestive: anorexia, nausea, vomiting, diarrhoea, constipation, abdominal pain, GI bleeding, appetite changes, abdominal fullness, flatulence, thirst, hiccups.

Metabolic: elevated plasma potassium levels (above 5.5 mmol/l), electrolyte imbalance, hyponatraemia, gout, dehydration, symptomatic hyponatraemia.

Integumentary: rash, pruritis, flushing, diaphoresis.

Musculoskeletal: leg ache, muscle cramps, joint pain.

Nervous: dizziness, vertigo, paraesthesiae, stupor.

Psychiatric: insomnia, nervousness, mental confusion, depression, sleepiness.

Respiratory: dyspnoea.

Special senses: bad taste, visual disturbance, nasal congestion.

Urogenital: impotence, dysuria, nocturia, incontinence, renal dysfunction including renal failure.

The reported adverse reactions of amiloride:

Body as a whole: neck/shoulder ache, pain in extremities.

Digestive: abnormal liver function, activation of probable pre-existing peptic ulcer, dyspepsia, jaundice.

Integumentary: dry mouth, alopecia, diaphoresis.

Nervous: tremors, encephalopathy.

Haematological: aplastic anaemia, neutropenia.

Cardiovascular: one patient with partial heart block developed complete heart block, palpitation.

Psychiatric: decreased libido, somnolence.

Respiratory: cough.

Special senses: tinnitus, increased intra-ocular pressure.

Urogenital: polyuria, urinary frequency, bladder spasm.

The reported adverse reactions of hydrochlorothiazide:

Body as a whole: anaphylactic reaction, fever.

Cardiovascular: necrotising angiitis (vasculitis, cutaneous vasculitis).

Digestive: jaundice (intrahepatic cholestatic jaundice), pancreatitis, cramping, gastric irritation.

Endocrine/Metabolic: glycosuria, hyperglycaemia, hyperuricaemia.

Integumentary: photosensitivity, sialadenitis, urticaria.

Haematological: agranulocytosis, aplastic anaemia, haemolytic anaemia, leucopenia, purpura, thrombocytopenia.

Psychiatric: restlessness.

Renal: interstitial nephritis.

Respiratory: respiratory distress, including pneumonitis, pulmonary oedema.

Special senses: transient blurred vision, xanthopsia.

*Overdosage:* No specific data are available on overdosage with Moduret 25. No specific antidote is available, and it is not known whether the drug is dialysable.

Treatment should be symptomatic and supportive. Therapy should be discontinued and the patient watched closely. Emesis should be induced and/or gastric lavage performed. The most common signs and symptoms of overdosage with amiloride hydrochloride are dehydration and electrolyte imbalance. Blood pressure should be monitored and corrected where necessary. If hyperkalaemia occurs, active measures should be taken to reduce the plasma potassium levels.

Electrolyte depletion (hypokalaemia, hypochloraemia, hyponatraemia) and dehydration are the most common signs and symptoms of hydrochlorothiazide overdosage. If digitalis has been administered, hypokalaemia may accentuate cardiac arrhythmias.

The plasma half-life of hydrochlorothiazide is 5.6 hours with a subsequent longer terminal half-life: the plasma half-life of amiloride is about six hours.

**Pharmaceutical precautions** Store in a dry place below 25°C, protected from light.

**Legal category** POM.

**Package quantities** Calendar packs of 28 tablets.

**Further information** The combination of amiloride with hydrochlorothiazide has been shown to cause less magnesium excretion than either the thiazides or the loop diuretics when used alone.

Onset of diuretic action begins within two hours after administration, and reaches a peak at about the fourth hour; there is detectable activity for about 24 hours.

**Product licence number** 0025/0178.

*Product licence holder:* Merck Sharp & Dohme Limited, Hertford Road, Hoddesdon, Hertfordshire, EN11 9BU.

## MODURETIC*

**Presentation** Moduretic is available as peach-coloured, half-scored, diamond shaped tablets, marked 'MSD 917', containing amiloride hydrochloride BP, equivalent to 5 mg anhydrous amiloride hydrochloride and 50 mg hydrochlorothiazide BP.

Moduretic is also available as aniseed/peppermint-flavoured solution containing amiloride hydrochloride BP, equivalent to 5 mg anhydrous amiloride hydrochloride, and 50 mg hydrochlorothiazide BP in each 5 ml.

**Uses** Potassium-conserving diuretic and antihypertensive.

Moduretic is indicated in patients with: hypertension, congestive heart failure, hepatic cirrhosis with ascites and oedema. In hypertension, Moduretic may be used alone or in conjunction with other antihypertensive agents.

Moduretic is intended for the treatment of patients in whom potassium depletion might be suspected or anticipated. The presence of amiloride hydrochloride minimises the likelihood of potassium loss during vigorous diuresis for long term maintenance therapy. The combination is thus indicated especially in conditions where potassium balance is particularly important.

**Dosage and administration**

*Hypertension:* Usually one or two Moduretic tablets given once a day or in divided doses. Some patients may require only half a Moduretic tablet a day. The dosage may be increased if necessary, but must not exceed four Moduretic tablets (or equivalent) a day.

*Congestive heart failure:* Initially one or two tablets of Moduretic a day, subsequently adjusted if required, but not exceeding four Moduretic tablets (or equivalent) a day. Optimal dosage is determined by the diuretic response and the plasma potassium level. Once an initial diuresis has been achieved, reduction in dosage may be attempted for maintenance therapy. Maintenance therapy may be on an intermittent basis.

*Hepatic cirrhosis with ascites:* Initiate therapy with a low dose. A single daily dose of one Moduretic tablet or equivalent may be increased gradually until there is an effective diuresis. Dosage should not exceed four Moduretic tablets (or equivalent) a day. Maintenance dosages may be lower than those required to initiate diuresis; dosage reduction should therefore be attempted when the patient's weight is stabilised. A gradual weight reduction is especially desirable in cirrhotic patients to reduce the likelihood of untoward reactions associated with diuretic therapy.

*Paediatric use:* Moduretic is not recommended for children (see 'Contra-indications').

*Use in the elderly:* Particular caution is needed in the elderly because of their susceptibility to electrolyte imbalance; the dosage should be carefully adjusted to renal function and clinical response.

**Contra-indications, warnings, etc**

*Contra-indications:* Hyperkalaemia (plasma potassium over 5.5 mmol/l); other potassium-conserving diuretics. Potassium supplements or potassium-rich food (except in severe and/or refractory cases of hypokalaemia under careful monitoring); concomitant use with spironolactone or triamterene; anuria; acute renal failure, severe progressive renal disease, severe hepatic failure, precoma associated with hepatic cirrhosis, Addison's disease, hypercalcaemia, concurrent lithium therapy, diabetic nephropathy; patients with blood urea over 10 mmol/l, patients with diabetes mellitus, or those with serum creatinine over 130 umol/l in whom serum electrolyte and blood urea levels cannot be monitored carefully and frequently. Prior hypersensitivity to amiloride hydrochloride, hydrochlorothiazide or other sulphonamide derived drugs. Because the safety of amiloride hydrochloride for use in children has not been established, Moduretic is not recommended for children. For 'Use in pregnancy' and 'Use in breast-feeding mothers', see 'Precautions'.

*Precautions:* Hyperkalaemia has been observed in patients receiving amiloride hydrochloride, either alone or with other diuretics, particularly in the aged or in hospital patients with hepatic cirrhosis or congestive heart failure with renal involvement, who were seriously ill, or were undergoing vigorous diuretic therapy. Such patients should be carefully observed for clinical, laboratory, and ECG evidence of hyperkalaemia (not always associated with an abnormal ECG).

Neither potassium supplements nor a potassium-rich diet should be used with Moduretic except under careful monitoring in severe and/or refractory cases of hypokalaemia.

Some deaths have been reported in this group of patients.

*Treatment of hyperkalaemia:* Should hyperkalaemia develop, discontinue treatment immediately and, if necessary, take active measures to reduce the plasma potassium to normal.

*Impaired renal function:* Renal function should be monitored because the use of Moduretic in impaired renal function may result in the rapid development of hyperkalaemia. Thiazide diuretics become ineffective when creatinine levels fall below 30 ml/min.

*Electrolyte imbalance:* Although the likelihood of electrolyte imbalance is reduced by Moduretic, careful check should be kept for such signs of fluid and electrolyte imbalance as hyponatraemia, hypochloraemic alkalosis, hypokalaemia and hypomagnesaemia. It is particularly important to make serum and urine electrolyte determinations when the patient is vomiting excessively or receiving parenteral fluids. Warning signs or symptoms of fluid or electrolyte imbalance include: dryness of the mouth, weakness, lethargy, drowsiness, restlessness, seizures, muscle pains or cramps, muscular fatigue, hypotension, oliguria, tachycardia, and gastro-intestinal disturbances such as nausea and vomiting.

Hypokalaemia may develop, especially as a result of brisk diuresis, after prolonged therapy or when severe cirrhosis is present. Hypokalaemia can sensitise or exaggerate the response of the heart to the toxic effects of digitalis (e.g. increased ventricular irritability).

Diuretic-induced hyponatraemia is usually mild and asymptomatic. It may become severe and symptomatic in a few patients who will then require immediate attention and appropriate treatment.

Thiazides may decrease urinary calcium excretion. Thiazides may cause intermittent and slight elevation of serum calcium in the absence of known disorders of calcium metabolism. Therapy should be discontinued before carrying out tests for parathyroid function.

Azotaemia may be precipitated or increased by hydrochlorothiazide. Cumulative effects of the drug may develop in patients with impaired renal function. If increasing azotaemia and oliguria develop during treatment of renal disease, Moduretic should be discontinued.

*Hepatic disease:* Thiazides should be used with caution in patients with impaired hepatic function or progressive liver disease (see 'Contra-indications'), since minor alterations of fluid and electrolyte balance may precipitate hepatic coma.

*Metabolic:* Hyperuricaemia may occur, or gout may be precipitated or aggravated, in certain patients receiving thiazides. Thiazides may impair glucose tolerance. Diabetes mellitus may be precipitated or aggravated by therapy with Moduretic (see 'Contra-indications'). Dosage adjustment of antidiabetic agents, including insulin, may be required.

Increases in cholesterol and triglyceride levels may be associated with thiazide diuretic therapy.

To minimise the risk of hyperkalaemia in diabetic or suspected diabetic patients, the status of renal function should be determined before initiating therapy with Moduretic. Therapy should be discontinued at least three days before giving a glucose tolerance test. Potassium-conserving therapy should be initiated only with caution in severely ill patients in whom metabolic or respiratory acidosis may occur, e.g. patients with cardiopulmonary disease or patients with inadequately controlled diabetes.

Shifts in acid-base balance alter the balance of extracellular/intracellular potassium, and the development of acidosis may be associated with rapid increases in plasma potassium.

*Sensitivity reactions:* The possibility that thiazides may activate or exacerbate systemic lupus erythematosus has been reported.

*Ability to drive and to use machines:* Infrequently, patients may experience weakness, fatigue, dizziness, stupor and vertigo. Should any of these occur, the patient should be cautioned not to drive or operate machinery.

*Use in pregnancy:* The routine use of diuretics in otherwise healthy pregnant women with or without mild oedema is not indicated, because they may be associated with hypovolaemia, increased blood viscosity, and decreased placental perfusion. Diuretics do not prevent the development of toxaemia of pregnancy and there is no satisfactory evidence that they are useful for its treatment.

Since thiazides cross the placental barrier and appear in cord blood, use where pregnancy is present or suspected requires that the benefits of the drug be weighed against possible hazards to the foetus. These hazards include foetal or neonatal jaundice, thrombocytopenia, bone marrow depression and possibly other side effects that have occurred in the adult.

*Use in breast-feeding mothers:* Although it is not known whether amiloride hydrochloride is excreted in human milk, it is known that thiazides do appear in breast milk. If use of the drug combination is deemed essential, the patient should stop breast-feeding.

*Drug interactions:* When amiloride hydrochloride is administered concomitantly with an ACE inhibitor, the risk of hyperkalaemia may be increased. Therefore, if concomitant use of these agents is indicated because of demonstrated hypokalaemia, they should be used with caution and with frequent monitoring of serum potassium.

When given concurrently, the following drugs may interact with thiazide diuretics:

Alcohol, barbiturates or narcotics: Co-administration may potentiate orthostatic hypotension. Oral and parenteral antidiabetic drugs may require adjustment of dosage with concurrent use. Other antihypertensive drugs may have an additive effect. Therefore the dosage of these agents, especially adrenergic-blockers, may need to be reduced when Moduretic is added to the regimen. Diuretic therapy should be discontinued for 2–3 days prior to initiation of therapy with an ACE inhibitor to reduce the likelihood of first dose hypotension. Corticosteroids or ACTH may intensify any thiazide-induced electrolyte depletion, particularly hypokalaemia. Pressor amines such as adrenaline may show decresed arterial responsiveness when used with Moduretic but this reaction is not enough to preclude their therapeutic usefulness. Non-depolarising muscle relaxants such as tubocurarine may possibly interact with Moduretic to increase muscle relaxation. Lithium may accumulate as a result of reduced renal clearance. Non-steroidal anti-inflammatory drugs may attenuate the diuretic, natriuretic and antihypertensive effects of diuretics. Chlorpropamide: Moduretic can act synergistically with chlorpropramide to increase the risk of hyponatraemia. Drug/laboratory tests: Because thiazides may affect calcium metabolism, Moduretic may interfere with tests for parathyroid function.

*Side-effects:* Although minor side effects are relatively common, significant side effects are infrequent.

Reported side effects are generally associated with diuresis, thiazide therapy, or with the underlying disease.

No increase in the risk of adverse reactions has been seen over those of the individual components.

The reported adverse reactions of the combination:

Body as a whole: headache, weakness, fatigue, malaise, chest pain, back pain, syncope.

Cardiovascular: arrhythmias, tachycardia, digitalis toxicity, orthostatic hypotension, angina pectoris.

Digestive: anorexia, nausea, vomiting, diarrhoea, constipation, abdominal pain, GI bleeding, appetite changes, abdominal fullness, flatulence, thirst, hiccups.

Metabolic: elevated plasma potassium levels (above 5.5 mmol/l), electrolyte imbalance, hyponatraemia, gout, dehydration, symptomatic hyponatraemia.

Integumentary: rash, pruritis, flushing, diaphoresis.

Musculoskeletal: leg ache, muscle cramps, joint pain.

Nervous: dizziness, vertigo, paraesthesiae, stupor.

Psychiatric: insomnia, nervousness, mental confusion, depression, sleepiness.

Respiratory: dyspnoea.

Special senses: bad taste, visual disturbance, nasal congestion.

Urogenital: impotence, dysuria, nocturia, incontinence, renal dysfunction including renal failure.

The reported adverse reactions of amiloride:

Body as a whole: neck/shoulder ache, pain in extremities.

Digestive: abnormal liver function, activation of probable pre-existing peptic ulcer, dyspepsia, jaundice.

Integumentary: dry mouth, alopecia, diaphoresis.

Nervous: tremors, encephalopathy.

Haematological: aplastic anaemia, neutropenia.

Cardiovascular: one patient with partial heart block developed complete heart block, palpitation.

Psychiatric: decreased libido, somnolence.

Respiratory: cough.

Special senses: tinnitus, increased intra-ocular pressure.

Urogenital: polyuria, urinary frequency, bladder spasm.

The reported adverse reactions of hydrochlorothiazide:

Body as a whole: anaphylactic reaction, fever.

Cardiovascular: necrotising angiitis (vasculitis, cutaneous vasculitis).

Digestive: jaundice (intrahepatic cholestatic jaundice), pancreatitis, cramping, gastric irritation.

Endocrine/Metabolic: glycosuria, hyperglycaemia, hyperuricaemia.

Integumentary: photosensitivity, sialadenitis, urticaria.

Haematological: agranulocytosis, aplastic anaemia, haemolytic anaemia, leucopenia, purpura, thrombocytopenia.

Psychiatric: restlessness.

Renal: interstitial nephritis.

Respiratory: respiratory distress, including pneumonitis, pulmonary oedema.

Special senses: transient blurred vision, xanthopsia.

*Overdosage:* No specific data are available on overdosage with Moduretic. No specific antidote is available, and it is not known whether the drug is dialysable.

Treatment should be symptomatic and supportive. Therapy should be discontinued and the patient watched closely. Emesis should be induced and/or gastric lavage performed. The most common signs and symptoms of overdosage with amiloride hydrochloride are dehydration and electrolyte imbalance. Blood pressure should be monitored and corrected where necessary. If hyperkalaemia occurs, active measures should be taken to reduce the plasma potassium levels.

Electrolyte depletion (hypokalaemia, hypochloraemia, hyponatraemia) and dehydration are the most common signs and symptoms of hydrochlorothiazide overdosage. If digitalis has been administered, hypokalaemia may accentuate cardiac arrhythmias.

The plasma half-life of hydrochlorothiazide is 5.6 hours with a subsequent longer terminal half-life: the plasma half-life of amiloride is about six hours.

**Pharmaceutical precautions** Keep container tightly closed. Store in a dry place below 25°C, protected from light. Moduretic Solution should not be diluted.

**Legal category** POM.

**Package quantities** Calendar packs of 28 tablets. Moduretic Tablets: Bottles of 100 and 500 tablets. Moduretic Solution: Bottles of 200 ml solution.

**Further information** The combination of amiloride with hydrochlorothiazide has been shown to cause less magnesium excretion than either the thiazides or the loop diuretics when used alone.

Onset of diuretic action begins within two hours after administration, and reaches a peak at about the fourth hour; there is detectable activity for about 24 hours.

**Product licence numbers**
Moduretic Tablets          0025/5016.
Moduretic Solution         0025/0165.

*Product licence holder:* Merck Sharp & Dohme Limited, Hertford Road, Hoddesdon, Hertfordshire, EN11 9BU.

# NALOREX*

**Presentation** Pale yellow, film coated capsule-shaped tablet, debossed on one side with 'Du Pont' and scored and debossed with '11' on the other side, containing naltrexone hydrochloride 50 mg.

**Uses** Nalorex is indicated as an adjunctive therapy in the maintenance of detoxified, formerly opioid-dependent patients.

**Dosage and administration** Nalorex treatment

should be initiated in a drug addiction centre and supervised by suitably qualified physicians.

Nalorex is an opioid antagonist with only minimal agonist activity under ordinary conditions. It is extensively metabolised in the liver. One of its metabolites, 6-Beta-Naltrexol, may also have activity as an opioid antagonist. It is excreted mainly in urine.

The initial dose of Nalorex should be 25 mg (half a tablet) followed by 50 mg (one tablet) daily.

A three-times a week dosing schedule may be considered if it is likely to result in better compliance, e.g. 100 mg on Monday, 100 mg on Wednesday and 150 mg on Friday.

Treatment with Nalorex should be considered only in patients who have remained opioid-free for a minimum of 7–10 days.

Narcan* (Naloxone hydrochloride) challenge is recommended to minimise the chance of a prolonged withdrawal syndrome precipitated by Nalorex (see also 'Warnings').

As Nalorex is a prophylactic agent and full recovery from opioid dependence is variable, no standard duration of therapy can be recommended; an initial period of three months should be considered. However, prolonged administration may be necessary.

**Contra-indications, warnings, etc**

*Contra-indications:* Nalorex should not be given to patients currently dependent on opioids since an acute withdrawal syndrome may ensue.

Nalorex should not be used in conjunction with an opioid-containing medication.

Nalorex should not be given to patients who are hypersensitive to it.

Nalorex should not be given to patients with acute hepatitis or liver failure.

*Warnings:* It is not uncommon for opioid abusing individuals to have impaired liver functions. Liver function test abnormalities have been reported in obese and elderly patients taking naltrexone who have no history of drug abuse. Liver function tests should be carried out both before and during treatment.

A withdrawal syndrome may be precipitated by Nalorex* in opioid dependent patients; signs and symptoms may develop within 5 minutes and last up to 48 hours.

Treatment should be symptomatic and may include opioid administration.

Narcan (Naloxone hydrochloride) challenge is recommended to screen for presence of opioid use; a withdrawal syndrome precipitated by Narcan* will be of shorter duration than one precipitated by Nalorex*. The recommended procedure is as follows:

– i.v. injection of 0.2 mg Narcan
– if after 30 seconds no adverse reactions occur, a further i.v. injection of 0.6 mg Narcan may be administered.
– continue to observe the patient for withdrawal effects for a further 30 minutes.

If doubt exists that the patient is opioid-free, the challenge may be repeated with a Narcan dose of 1.6 mg.

If there is no evidence of a reaction, Nalorex administration may be initiated with 25 mg by mouth (half a tablet).

*Drug interactions:* Concomitant administration of Nalorex with an opioid containing medication should be avoided. Patients should be warned that attempts to overcome the blockade may result in acute opioid intoxication which may be life threatening. In an emergency requiring opioid analgesia an increased dose of opioid may be required to control pain. The patient should be closely monitored for evidence of respiratory depression or other adverse symptoms and signs.

*Use in pregnancy:* Animal studies do not suggest a teratogenic effect.

Because of absence of documented clinical experience Nalorex should only be given to pregnant or breast-feeding women when, in the judgement of the attending physician, the potential benefits outweigh the possible risks.

*Use in children:* Safe use in children has not been established.

*Use in elderly:* There is no experience of use in the elderly.

*Precautions:* Since Nalorex* is extensively metabolised by the liver and excreted predominantly in the urine, caution should be observed in administering the drug to patients with impaired hepatic or renal function.

*Adverse effects:* The following adverse reactions have been reported before and during naltrexone medication: an incidence of more than 10% in detoxified opioid abusers; difficulty in sleeping, anxiety, nervousness, abdominal pain/cramps, nausea and/or vomiting, low energy, joint and muscle pain, and headache: an incidence of less than 10%; loss of appetite, diarrhoea, constipation, increased thirst,

increased energy, feeling down, irritability, dizziness, skin rash, delayed ejaculation, decreased potency, chills, chest pain, increased sweating, and increased lacrimation. Occasional liver function abnormalities have also been reported. One case of reversible idiopathic thrombocytopenic purpura has occurred in a patient taking Nalorex*.

*Overdose:* There is no clinical experience with Nalorex* overdose in patients. There was no evidence of toxicity in volunteers receiving 800 mg/day for seven days, however, in case of overdose, patients should be monitored and treated symptomatically in a closely supervised environment.

**Pharmaceutical precautions** Store below 30°C. Protect from light.

**Legal category** POM.

**Package quantities** Bottles of 50 tablets.

**Further information** The development of tolerance and dependence have not been observed with Nalorex.

**Product licence number** 11173/0026.

*Product licence holder:* Du Pont Pharmaceuticals Limited, Avenue One, Letchworth Garden City, Herts SG6 2HU.

# NARCAN*
# NARCAN* NEONATAL

**Presentation** A sterile, clear, colourless solution of naloxone hydrochloride in clear, colourless ampoules.

*Narcan (1 ml ampoules):* each 1 ml of solution contains 400 micrograms naloxone hydrochloride.

*Narcan Neonatal (2 ml ampoules):* each 1 ml of solution contains 20 micrograms naloxone hydrochloride.

**Uses** Narcan may be used for the complete or partial reversal of opioid depression, including mild to severe respiratory depression induced by natural and synthetic opioids, the agonist/antagonists nalbuphine and pentazocine, or dextropropoxyphene. It may also be used for the diagnosis of suspected acute opioid overdosage. Narcan Neonatal may be used to counteract respiratory and other CNS depression in the new-born resulting from the administration of analgesics to the mother during childbirth.

Narcan usually acts within two minutes of intravenous administration and the onset of action is only slightly less rapid following intramuscular or subcutaneous injection. The duration of action is dependent upon the dose, route of administration; intramuscular injection producing a more prolonged effect than intravenous doses. However, the need for repeat doses of Narcan also depends on the amount, type and route of administration of the opioid being antagonised.

**Dosage and administration** Narcan is for intravenous, intramuscular or subcutaneous injection or intravenous infusion.

*Intravenous infusion:* Narcan may be diluted for intravenous infusion in normal saline (0.9%) or 5% dextrose in water or saline: the addition of 2 mg of Narcan in 500 ml of either solution provides a concentration of 4 micrograms/ml. Mixtures should be used within 12 hours. After 12 hours, the remaining unused solution must be discarded. The rate of administration should be titrated in accordance with the patient's response to both the Narcan infusion and to any previous bolus doses administered.

Parenteral drug products should be inspected visually for particulate matter and discoloration prior to administration whenever solution and container permit. Narcan should not be mixed with preparations containing bisulphite, metabisulphite, long-chain or high molecular weight anions or any solution having an alkaline pH. No drug or chemical agent should be added to Narcan unless its effect on the chemical and physical stability of the solution has first been established.

*Adults:*

*Opioid overdosage (known or suspected):* An initial dose of 400 to 2000 micrograms of Narcan may be administered intravenously. If the desired degree of counteraction and improvement in respiratory function is not obtained it may be repeated at 2 to 3 minute intervals. If no response is observed after 10 mg of Narcan have been administered the diagnosis of opioid-induced or partial opioid-induced toxicity should be questioned. Intramuscular or subcutaneous administration may be necessary if dosing by the intravenous route is not feasible.

N.B. The duration of action of certain opioids can outlast that of an IV bolus of Narcan, e.g. dextropropoxyphene (present in commonly prescribed analgesics which in over-dosage have been associated with suicide), dihydrocodeine and methadone. In situations where one of these opioids is known or suspected it is recommended that an infusion of Narcan (see above) be used to produce sustained antagonism to the opioid without repeated injection.

*Post-operative use:* When Narcan is used post-operatively, the dose should be titrated for each patient in order to obtain optimum respiratory response while maintaining adequate analgesia. Intravenous doses of 100–200 micrograms (1.5–3 micrograms/kg body weight) are usually sufficient, but a full two minutes should be allowed between each 100 micrograms increment of Narcan administered. Further intramuscular doses may be needed within one to two hours, depending on the interval since the last opioid administration and the amount and type (i.e. long or short-acting) of drug used. Alternatively Narcan may be administered as an intravenous infusion (see above).

*Children:* The usual initial dose in children is 10 micrograms per kg body weight given IV. If this dose does not result in the desired degree of clinical improvement, a subsequent dose of 100 micrograms per kg of body weight may be administered. Narcan may be required by infusion as described above. If an IV route of administration is not feasible, Narcan may be administered IM or SC in divided doses.

*Neonatal use:* An adequate airway should be established in the apnoeic infant before Narcan is administered. The usual dose for opioid-induced depression is 10 micrograms/kg body weight administered IV, IM or SC. If the desired degree of counteraction and improvement in respiratory function is not obtained it may be repeated at 2 to 3 minute intervals. Alternatively, a single dose of 200 micrograms (approximately 60 micrograms/kg body weight) may be given intramuscularly at birth. It should, however, be noted that onset of action is slower following IM injection. In neonates needing infusion of Narcan in saline care should be taken to avoid excessive sodium intake.

### Contra-indications, warnings, etc

*Contra-indication:* Narcan should not be given to patients who are known to be hypersensitive to it.

*Warnings:* It should be administered cautiously to patients who have received large doses of opioids or to those physically dependent on opioids since too rapid reversal of opioid effects by Narcan may precipitate an acute withdrawal syndrome in such patients. The same caution is needed when giving Narcan to neonates delivered of such patients.

Patients who have responded satisfactorily to Narcan should be kept under observation. Repeated doses of Narcan may be necessary since the duration of action of some opioids may exceed that of Narcan.

Narcan is not effective against respiratory depression caused by non-opioid drugs. Reversal of buprenorphine-induced respiratory depression may be incomplete. If an incomplete response occurs, respirations should be mechanically assisted.

*Use in elderly:* There have been no specific studies of use in the elderly.

*Precautions:* Several instances of hypotension, hypertension, ventricular tachycardia and fibrillation, and pulmonary oedema have been reported. These have occurred in postoperative patients, most of whom had pre-existing cardiovascular disorders or received other drugs which may have similar adverse cardiovascular effects. Although a direct cause and effect relationship has not been established, Narcan should be used with caution in patients with pre-existing cardiac disease or patients who have received potentially cardiotoxic drugs.

In addition to Narcan, other resuscitative measures such as maintenance of a free airway, artificial ventilation, cardiac massage and vasopressor agents should be available and employed when necessary to counteract acute poisoning.

*Use in pregnancy and lactation:* The safety of this medicinal product for use in human pregnancy has not been established. Evaluation of experimental animal studies does not indicate direct or indirect harmful effects with respect to the development of the embryo or foetus, the course of gestation and peri- and postnatal development. Narcan should, like all drugs, be used with caution during pregnancy. Narcan may be administered to mothers during the second stage of labour to correct respiratory depression caused by opioids used to provide obstetrical analgesia.

It is not known whether Narcan is excreted in human milk, caution should be exercised when Narcan is administered to a nursing mother.

*Adverse effects:* Abrupt reversal of narcotic depression may result in nausea, vomiting, sweating, tachycardia, increased blood pressure, tremulousness, seizures and cardiac arrest. In postoperative patients, larger than necessary dosage of Narcan may result in significant reversal of analgesia and excitement. Hypotension, hypertension, ventricular tachycardia

and fibrillation, and pulmonary oedema have been associated with the use of Narcan postoperatively.

*Overdosage:* There have been no reports of acute overdosage with Narcan. Single doses of 10 mg intravenously and subcutaneous doses of 15 mg every four hours for two weeks have been administered without producing either respiratory depression or psychotomimetic effects.

**Pharmaceutical precautions**   Protect from light.

**Legal category**   POM.

**Package quantities**   Narcan ampoules each containing 1 ml (equivalent to 400 micrograms naloxone hydrochloride) are supplied in boxes of 3 or 10 ampoules.

Narcan Neonatal ampoules each containing 2 ml (equivalent to 40 micrograms naloxone hydrochloride) are supplied in boxes of 10 ampoules.

**Further information**   Narcan has not been shown to produce tolerance nor to cause physical or psychological dependence.

**Product Licence Numbers**

Narcan (400 micrograms/ml)
    1 ml Ampoule             11173/0009
Narcan Neonatal (20 micrograms/ml)
    2 ml Ampoule             11173/0012

*Product licence holder:* Du Pont Pharmaceuticals Ltd, Avenue One, Letchworth Garden City, Herts SG6 2HU.

## NUBAIN*

**Presentation**   Ampoules containing a clear colourless sterile aqueous solution of 20 mg nalbuphine hydrochloride in 2 ml or 10 mg nalbuphine hydrochloride in 1 ml.

**Uses**   Nubain injection is indicated for the relief of moderate to severe pain. It can also be used as a premedication, for pre- and post-operative analgesia, and as a component of balanced anaesthesia. It can also be used in the management of pain due to suspected myocardial infarction.

**Dosage and administration**   Nubain injection may be administered subcutaneously, intramuscularly or intravenously. It may also be administered by patient-controlled on demand intravenous infusion, using a delivery system which is appropriately calibrated and does not interact with the drug.

*Adults:* The usual recommended dosage is 10 mg–20 mg for a 70 kg individual. The dosage should be adjusted according to the severity of pain, physical status of the patient and other medications the patient may be receiving.

*Balanced anaesthesia*

    Induction: 0.3 mg/kg to 1 mg/kg I.V. over a 10–15 minute period.

      Maintenance: 0.25–0.5 mg/kg at 30 minute intervals.

      Premedication: 0.1–0.2 mg/kg.

*Suspected myocardial infarction:* Usual dose 20 mg by slow intravenous injection. Some patients may be successfully managed on 10 mg while others may need to have the dose increased to 30 mg. In the absence of pain relief a repeat dose of 20 mg may be given within 30 minutes.

*Children:* An initial dose of up to 0.3 mg/kg IV, IM or SC which may be repeated once or twice as necessary.

**Contra-indications, warnings, etc**

*Contra-indications:* Nubain should not be administered to patients who are hypersensitive to it.

*Warnings:* Drug dependence: Nubain has low abuse potential. However, caution should be observed in prescribing it for emotionally unstable patients or for patients with a history of opioid abuse.

When Nubain is selected for the control of chronic pain, its suggested prolonged activity may delay the need for larger or more frequent doses.

Abrupt discontinuation of Nubain following prolonged use has been followed by symptoms of opioid withdrawal.

Nubain should only be used if considered essential and then with extreme caution to provide analgesia in patients with head injury and increased intracranial pressure.

*Use in ambulatory patients:* Nubain may impair the mental or physical abilities required for the performance of potentially dangerous tasks such as driving a car or operating machinery. Therefore, Nubain should be administered with caution to ambulatory patients who should be warned to avoid such hazards.

*Use in pregnancy and lactation:* Safe use of Nubain in pregnancy (including labour) has not been established. A few cases of severe foetal respiratory depression and bradycardia have been reported when Nubain has been used during labour.

Although animal studies have not revealed teratogenic or embryotoxic effects, nalbuphine should only

be administered to pregnant women when, in the judgement of the physician, the potential benefits outweigh the possible hazards.

It is not known whether Nubain is excreted in human milk. Because many drugs are excreted in human milk, caution should be exercised when Nubain is administered to a nursing woman.

*Precautions:* Nubain used as a premedication causes some respiratory depression. Caution should therefore be observed in administering the drug to patients with impaired respiration, or with other medications which produce respiratory depression.

During evaluation of Nubain in anaesthesia, a higher incidence of bradycardia has been reported in patients not administered pre-operative atropine.

In the presence of bronchial asthma, uraemia, severe infection, cyanosis or respiratory obstruction, Nubain should be administered with caution and in reduced doses.

Nubain should be used with caution and administered in reduced amounts in patients with impaired renal or hepatic function.

*Drug interactions:* Patients receiving an opioid analgesic, general anaesthetic, phenothiazine or other tranquillizer, sedative, hypnotic or other CNS depressant (including alcohol) concomitantly with Nubain may exhibit an additive effect. When such combined therapy is contemplated, the dose of one or both agents should be reduced.

*Adverse effects:* The most frequently seen reaction to Nubain is sedation. Less frequent are sweating, nausea, vomiting, dizziness, dry mouth, vertigo and headache. Rarely seen are CNS effects such as nervousness, depression, confusion and dysphoria. Also reported have been hyper- and hypotension, bradycardia, tachycardia, urticaria, speech difficulty, blurred vision and flushing.

*Overdosage:* The immediate intravenous administration of Narcan* (naloxone hydrochloride) is a specific antidote. Oxygen, intravenous fluids, vasopressors and other supportive measures should be used as indicated.

**Pharmaceutical precautions**   Protect from light. Store at room temperature.

**Legal category**   POM.

**Package quantities**

Nubain 2 ml ampoules are supplied in boxes of 10.
Nubain 1 ml ampoules are supplied in boxes of 10.

**Further information**   Nubain is compatible with 0.9% sodium chloride, 5% dextrose, 4.3% dextrose/0.18% saline and Hartmann's solution used in glass, PVC and polyethylene infusion containers.

**Product licence number**   11173/0013.

*Product licence holder:* Du Pont Pharmaceuticals Ltd, Avenue One, Letchworth Garden City, Herts SG6 2HU.

## SINEMET*

**Presentation**

*Sinemet-LS* is available as yellow, half-scored, oval tablets, marked 'SINEMET LS', containing 12.5 mg carbidopa (as carbidopa monohydrate) and 50 mg levodopa.

*Sinemet-110* is available as dapple-blue, half-scored, oval tablets, marked 'MSD 647' containing 10 mg carbidopa (as carbidopa monohydrate) and 100 mg levodopa.

*Sinemet-Plus* is available as yellow, half-scored, oval tablets, marked 'SINEMET PLUS', containing 25 mg carbidopa (as carbidopa monohydrate) and 100 mg levodopa.

*Sinemet-275* is available as dapple-blue, half-scored, oval tablets, marked 'MSD 654', containing 25 mg carbidopa (as carbidopa monohydrate) and 250 mg levodopa.

**Uses**   Antiparkinsonian agent.

For treatment of Parkinson's disease and syndrome. Sinemet is useful in relieving many of the symptoms of parkinsonism, particularly rigidity and bradykinesia. It is frequently helpful in the management of tremor, dysphagia, sialorrhoea, and postural instability associated with Parkinson's disease and syndrome.

When response to levodopa alone is irregular, and signs and symptoms of Parkinson's disease are not controlled evenly throughout the day, substitution of Sinemet usually reduces fluctuations in response. By reducing some of the adverse reactions produced by levodopa alone, Sinemet permits more patients to obtain adequate relief of the symptoms of Parkinson's disease.

Sinemet may be given to patients with Parkinson's disease and syndrome who are taking vitamin preparations that contain pyridoxine hydrochloride (Vitamin B6).

**Dosage and administration**   The optimum daily

dosage of Sinemet must be determined by careful titration for each patient.

Sinemet Tablets are available in a ratio of 1:4 or 1:10 of carbidopa to levodopa to provide facility for fine dosage titration for each patient.

*General considerations:* Studies show that the peripheral enzyme dopa-decarboxylase is fully inhibited (saturated) by carbidopa at doses between 70 and 100 mg a day. Patients receiving less than this amount of carbidopa are more likely to experience nausea and vomiting.

Standard anti-parkinsonism drugs other than levodopa alone, may be continued while 'Sinemet' is being administered, although their dosage may have to be adjusted.

Because both therapeutic and adverse effects are seen more rapidly with Sinemet than with levodopa, patients should be carefully monitored during the dosage adjustment period. Involuntary movements, particularly blepharospasm, are a useful early sign of excess dosage in some patients.

If general anaesthesia is required, therapy with Sinemet may be continued for as long as the patient is permitted to take fluids and medicines by mouth. If therapy has to be stopped temporarily, Sinemet may be restarted as soon as oral medication can be taken at the same daily dosage as before.

*Patients not receiving levodopa:* Dosage may be best initiated with one tablet of Sinemet-Plus three times a day. This dosage schedule provides 75 mg of carbidopa per day. Dosage may be increased by one tablet of Sinemet-LS or Sinemet-Plus every day or every other day, as necessary, until a dosage equivalent of eight tablets of Sinemet-Plus a day is reached.

If Sinemet-110 or Sinemet-LS is used, dosage may be initiated with one tablet three or four times a day. Titration upward may be required in some patients to achieve optimum dosage of carbidopa. The dosage may be increased by one tablet every day or every other day until a total of eight tablets (two tablets q.d.s.) is reached. For patients starting with Sinemet-275, the initial dose is one-half tablet taken once or twice daily. However, this may not provide the optimal amount of carbidopa needed by many patients. If necessary, add one-half tablet every day or every other day until optimal response is reached.

Response has been observed in one day, and sometimes after one dose. Fully effective doses usually are reached within seven days as compared to weeks or months with levodopa alone.

Sinemet-LS or Sinemet-110 may be used to facilitate dosage titration according to the needs of the individual patient.

*Patients receiving levodopa:* Discontinue levodopa at least 12 hours (24 hours for slow-release preparations) before starting therapy with Sinemet. The easiest way to do this is to give Sinemet as the first morning dose after a night without any levodopa. The dose of Sinemet should be approximately 20% of the previous daily dosage of levodopa.

Patients taking less than 1,500 mg levodopa a day should be started on one tablet of Sinemet-Plus three or four times a day dependent on patient need. The suggested starting dose for most patients taking more than 1,500 mg levodopa a day is one tablet of Sinemet-275 three or four times a day.

*Maintenance:* Therapy with Sinemet should be individualised and adjusted gradually according to response. When a greater proportion of carbidopa is required, each tablet of Sinemet-110 may be replaced with a tablet of Sinemet-Plus or Sinemet-LS.

When more levodopa is required, Sinemet-275 should be substituted at a dosage of one tablet three or four times a day. If necessary, the dosage of Sinemet-275 may be increased by half to one tablet every other day to a maximum of eight tablets a day. Experience with a total daily dosage greater than 200 mg carbidopa is limited.

*Patients receiving other antiparkinsonian agents:* The combination of Sinemet with MAO-B inhibitors (e.g. selegiline) has been reported to improve the efficacy of Sinemet in controlling episodes of akinesia and/or dyskinesia.

*Use in children:* The safety of Sinemet in patients under 18 years of age has not been established.

*Use in the elderly:* There is wide experience in the use of this product in elderly patients. The recommendations set out above reflect the clinical data derived from this experience.

### Contra-indications, warnings, etc

*Contra-indications:* MAO-inhibitors (except low doses of selective MAO-B inhibitors) and Sinemet should not be given concomitantly (these must be discontinued at least two weeks before starting Sinemet); narrow-angle glaucoma; known hypersensitivity to any component of this medication. Because levodopa may activate a malignant melanoma, it should not be used in patients with suspicious undiagnosed skin

lesions or a history of melanoma. See also 'Pregnancy and lactation', under 'Precautions'.

*Precautions:* Sinemet is not recommended for the treatment of drug-induced extrapyramidal reactions.

Sinemet should be administered cautiously to patients with severe cardiovascular or pulmonary disease, bronchial asthma, renal, hepatic or endocrine disease; or a history of peptic ulcer disease (because of the possibility of upper gastrointestinal haemorrhage).

Care should be exercised when Sinemet is administered to patients with a history of myocardial infarction who have atrial, nodal, or ventricular arrhythmias. Cardiac function should be monitored with particular care in such patients during the period of initial dosage adjustment.

All patients should be monitored carefully for the development of mental changes, depression with suicidal tendencies, and other serious antisocial behaviour. Patients with current psychoses should be treated with caution.

Dyskinesias may occur in patients previously treated with levodopa alone, because carbidopa permits more levodopa to reach the brain and, thus, more dopamine to be formed. The occurence of dyskinesias may require dosage reduction.

As with levodopa, Sinemet may cause involuntary movements and mental disturbances. Patients with a history of severe involuntary movements or psychotic episodes when treated with levodopa alone should be observed carefully when Sinemet is substituted. These reactions are thought to be due to increased brain dopamine following administration of levodopa, and use of Sinemet may cause a recurrence. A syndrome resembling the neuroleptic malignant syndrome including muscular rigidity, elevated body temperature, mental changes and increased serum creatine phosphokinase has been reported with the abrupt withdrawal of antiparkinsonian agents. Therefore, any abrupt dosage reduction or withdrawal of Sinemet should be carefully observed, particularly in patients who are also receiving neuroleptics.

Concomitant administration of psycho-active drugs such as phenothiazines or butyrophenones should be carried out with caution, and the patients carefully observed for loss of antiparkinsonian effect. Patients with a history of convulsions should be treated with caution.

As with levodopa, periodic evaluations of hepatic haemoptopoietic, cardiovascular and renal functions are recommended during extended therapy.

Patients with chronic wide-angle glaucoma may be treated cautiously with Sinemet, provided the intraocular pressure is well controlled and the patient monitored carefully for changes in intra-ocular pressure during therapy.

*Laboratory tests:* Commonly, levels of blood urea, creatinine and uric acid are lower during administration of Sinemet than with levodopa. Transient abnormalities include elevated levels of blood urea, AST (SGOT), ALT (SGPT), LDH, bilirubin, alkaline phosphatase, and protein-bound iodine.

Decreased haemoglobin, haematocrit, elevated serum glucose, and white blood cells, bacteria and blood in the urine have been reported.

Positive Coombs tests have been reported, both with Sinemet and levodopa alone, but haemolytic anaemia is extremely rare.

Sinemet may cause a false positive result when a dipstick is used to test for urinary ketone; and this reaction is not altered by boiling the urine. The use of glucose oxidase methods may give false negative results for glycosuria.

*Drug interactions:* Caution should be exercised when the following drugs are administered concomitantly with Sinemet:

*Antihypertensive agents:* Postural hypotension can occur when Sinemet is added to the treatment of patients already receiving antihypertensive drugs. Dosage adjustments of the antihypertensive agent may be required.

*Antidepressants:* Rarely, reactions including hypertension and dyskinesia have been reported with the concomitant use of tricyclic antidepressants. (See the Contra-indications for patients receiving MAOIs.)

*Other drugs:* Phenothiazines, butyrophenones, phenytoin and papaverine may reduce the therapeutic effect of levodopa. Patients taking these drugs with Sinemet should be carefully observed for loss of therapeutic response.

Since levodopa competes with certain amino acids, the absorption of Sinemet may be impaired in some patients on a high protein diet.

*Pregnancy:* Although the effects of Sinemet on human pregnancy are unknown, both levodopa and combinations of carbidopa and levodopa have caused visceral and skeletal malformations in rabbits. Therefore, use of Sinemet in women of childbearing potential requires that the anticipated benefits of the

drug be weighed against possible hazards should pregnancy occur.

*Breast-feeding mothers:* It is not known whether carbidopa or levodopa is excreted in human milk. Because many drugs are excreted in human milk and because of the potential for serious adverse reactions in infants, a decision should be made whether to discontinue breast-feeding or to discontinue the use of Sinemet taking into account the importance of the drug to the mother.

*Side-effects:* Side-effects that occur frequently with Sinemet are those due to the central neuropharmacological activity of dopamine. These reactions can usually be diminished by dosage reduction. The most common are dyskinesias including choreiform, dystonic, and other involuntary movements. Muscle twitching and blepharospasm may be taken as early signs to consider dosage reduction.

Other serious side-effects are mental changes, including paranoid ideation and psychotic episodes; depression, with or without development of suicidal tendencies; and dementia. A common but less serious side effect is nausea.

Less frequent side-effects are cardiac irregularities and/or palpitations, orthostatic hypotensive episodes, bradykinetic episodes (the 'on-off' phenomenon), anorexia, vomiting, dizziness, and somnolence.

Gastro-intestinal bleeding, development of duodenal ulcer, hypertension, phlebitis, leucopenia, haemolytic and non-haemolytic anaemia, thrombocytopenia, agranulocytosis, chest pain, dyspnoea and paraesthesia have occurred rarely.

Other side-effects that have been reported with levodopa and may be potential side effects with Sinemet include:

Neurological: ataxia, numbness, increased hand tremor, muscle twitching, muscle cramp, trismus, activation of latent Horner's syndrome.

Psychiatric: confusion, insomnia, nightmares, hallucinations, delusions, agitation, anxiety, euphoria.

Gastro-intestinal: dry mouth, bitter taste, sialorrhoea, dysphagia, bruxism, hiccups, abdominal pain and distress, constipation, diarrhoea, flatulence, burning sensation of the tongue.

Metabolic: weight gain or loss, oedema.

Integumentary: flushing, increased sweating, dark sweat, rash, hair loss.

Genito-urinary: urinary retention, urinary incontinence, dark urine, priapism.

Special senses: diplopia, blurred vision, dilated pupils, oculogyric crises.

Miscellaneous: weakness, faintness, fatigue, headache, hoarseness, malaise, hot flushes, sense of stimulation, bizarre breathing patterns, neuroleptic malignant syndrome, malignant melanoma (see 'Contra-indications').

Other side-effects that have been reported with Sinemet CR and may be potential side-effects with Sinemet include:

Neurological: Falling, gait abnormalities.

*Overdosage:* Management of acute overdosage with Sinemet is basically the same as management of acute overdosage with levodopa; however, pyridoxine is not effective in reversing the actions of Sinemet. ECG monitoring should be instituted, and the patient carefully observed for the possible development of arrhythmias; if required, appropriate anti-arrhythmic therapy should be given.

The possibility that the patient may have taken other drugs as well as Sinemet should be taken into consideration. To date, no experience has been reported with dialysis, and hence its value in the treatment of overdosage is not known.

The terminal half-life of levodopa is about two hours in the presence of carbidopa.

**Pharmaceutical precautions** Keep container tightly closed; store in a cool place, protected from light.

**Legal category** POM.

**Package quantities**
Sinemet-LS in bottles of 84.
Sinemet-110 in bottles of 100.
Sinemet-Plus in bottles of 100.
Sinemet-275 in bottles of 100.

**Further information** Levodopa relieves the symptoms of Parkinson's disease presumably by being decarboxylated to dopamine in the brain. Carbidopa, which does not cross the blood-brain barrier, inhibits only the extra-cerebral decarboxylation of levodopa, making more levodopa available for transport to the brain and subsequent conversion to dopamine. This obviates the need for large doses of levodopa at frequent intervals. The lower dosage reduces or eliminates many adverse reactions, some of which are attributed to dopamine being formed in extra-cerebral tissues.

**Product licence numbers**

| | |
|---|---|
| Sinemet-LS | 0025/0226 |
| Sinemet-110 | 0025/0084 |
| Sinemet-Plus | 0025/0150 |
| Sinemet-275 | 0025/0085 |

*Product licence holder:* Merck, Sharp & Dohme Limited, Hertford Road, Hoddesdon, Hertfordshire EN11 9BU.

## SINEMET* CR HALF SINEMET CR

**Presentation** Sinemet CR is available as peach coloured, oval tablets marked 'DPP' and '521' containing carbidopa monohydrate equivalent to 50 mg anhydrous carbidopa and 200 mg levodopa. Half Sinemet CR is available as pink coloured, oval tablets marked 'DPP' and '601' containing carbidopa monohydrate equivalent to 25 mg anhydrous carbidopa and 100 mg kevodopa.

**Uses** Antiparkinson agent.

Idiopathic Parkinson's disease, in particular to reduce off-period in patients who previously have been treated with levodopa/decarboxylase inhibitors, or with levodopa alone and who have experienced motor fluctuations. The experience is limited with Sinemet CR and Half Sinemet CR in patients who have not been treated with levodopa before.

*Action:* Sinemet CR and Half Sinemet CR are a combination of carbidopa, an aromatic amino acid decarboxylase inhibitor, and levodopa, the metabolic precursor of dopamine, in a polymer-based controlled-release tablet formulation, for use in the treatment of Parkinson's disease. Sinemet CR and Half Sinemet CR are particularly useful to reduce 'off' time in patients treated previously with a conventional levodopa/decarboxylase inhibitor combination who have had dyskinesias and motor fluctuations.

Patients with Parkinson's disease treated with preparations containing levodopa may develop motor fluctuations characterised by end-of-dose failure, peak dose dyskinesia, and akinesia. The advanced form of motor fluctuations ('on-off' phenomenon) is characterised by unpredictable swings from mobility to immobility. Although the causes of the motor fluctuations are not completely understood, it has been demonstrated that they can be attenuated by treatment regimens that produce steady plasma levels of levodopa.

Levodopa relieves the symptoms of Parkinson's disease by being decarboxylated to dopamine in the brain. Carbidopa, which does not cross the blood-brain barrier, inhibits only the extracerebral decarboxylation of levodopa, making more levodopa available for transport to the brain and subsequent conversion to dopamine. This normally obviates the necessity for large doses of levodopa at frequent intervals. The lower dosage reduces or may help eliminate gastrointestinal and cardiovascular side-effects, especially those which are attributed to dopamine being formed in extracerebral tissues.

Sinemet CR and Half Sinemet CR are designed to release their active ingredients over a four-six hour period. With this formulation there is less variation in plasma levodopa levels and the peak plasma levodopa level is 60% lower than with conventional Sinemet, as established in healthy volunteers.

In clinical trials, patients with motor fluctuations experienced reduced 'off'-time with Sinemet CR when compared with Sinemet. The reduction of the 'off'-time is rather small (about 10%) and the incidence of dyskinesias increases slightly after administration of Sinemet CR compared to standard Sinemet.

Global ratings of improvement and activities of daily living in the 'on' and 'off' state, as assessed by both patient and physician, were better during therapy with Sinemet CR than with Sinemet. Patients considered Sinemet CR to be more helpful for their clinical fluctuations, and preferred it over Sinemet. In patients without motor fluctuations, Sinemet CR under controlled conditions, provided the same therapeutic benefit with less frequent dosing than with Sinemet. Generally, there was no further improvement of other symptoms of Parkinson's disease.

**Dosage and administration** Sinemet CR and Half Sinemet CR tablets contain a 1:4 ratio of carbidopa to levodopa (Sinemet CR: carbidopa 50 mg levodopa 200 mg per tablet; Half Sinemet CR 25 mg/100 mg per tablet). The daily dosage of Sinemet CR must be determined by careful titration. Patients should be monitored closely during the dose adjustment period, particularly with regard to appearance or worsening of nausea or abnormal involuntary movements, including dyskinesias, chorea and dystonia.

Sinemet CR and Half Sinemet CR may only be administered as whole tablets. So that the controlled release properties of the tablet can be maintained, tablets should not be chewed, crushed, or halved.

Standard antiparkinson drugs, other than levodopa alone, may be continued while Sinemet CR or Half Sinemet CR are being administered, although their dosage may have to be adjusted.

Since carbidopa prevents the reversal of levodopa effects caused by pyridoxine, Sinemet CR or Half Sinemet CR can be given to patients receiving supplemental pyridoxine (vitamin $B_6$).

*Initial dose*

*Patients currently treated with conventional levodopa/decarboxylase inhibitor combinations:* Dosage with Sinemet CR should be substituted initially at an amount that provides no more than approximately 10% more levodopa per day when higher dosages are given (more than 900 mg per day). The dosing interval between doses should be prolonged by 30 to 50% at intervals ranging from 4 to 12 hours. It is recommended to give the smaller dose, if divided doses are not equal, at the end of the day. The dose needs to be titrated further depending on clinical response, as indicated below under 'Titration'. Dosages that provide up to 30% more levodopa per day may be necessary.

A guide for substitution of Sinemet CR treatment for conventional levodopa/decarboxylase inhibitor combinations is shown in the table.

*Guidelines for conversion from Sinemet to Sinemet CR*

| *Sinemet* | *Sinemet CR* | |
|---|---|---|
| *Daily dosage Levodopa (mg)* | *Daily dosage Levodopa (mg)* | *Dosage regimen* |
| 300– 400 | 400 | 1 2×daily |
| 500– 600 | 600 | 1 3×daily |
| 700– 800 | 800 | 4 Tablets in 3 or more divided doses |
| 900–1000 | 1000 | 5 Tablets in 3 or more divided doses |
| 1100–1200 | 1200 | 6 Tablets in 3 or more divided doses |
| 1300–1400 | 1400 | 7 Tablets in 3 or more divided doses |
| 1500–1600 | 1600 | 8 Tablets in 3 or more divided doses |

Half Sinemet CR is available to facilitate titration when 100 mg steps are required.

*Patients currently treated with levodopa alone:* Levodopa must be discontinued at least eight hours before therapy with Sinemet CR is started. In patients with mild to moderate disease, the initial recommended dose is one tablet of Sinemet CR twice daily.

*Patients not receiving levodopa:* In patients with mild to moderate disease, the initial recommended dose is one tablet of Sinemet CR twice daily. Initial dosages should not exceed 600 mg per day of levodopa, nor be given at intervals of less than six hours.

*Titration:* Following initiation of therapy, doses and dosing intervals may be increased or decreased, depending upon therapeutic response. Most patients have been adequately treated with two to eight tablets per day, administered as divided doses at intervals ranging from four to twelve hours during the waking day. Higher doses (up to 12 tablets) and shorter intervals (less than 4 hours) have been used, but are not usually recommended.

When doses of Sinemet CR are given at intervals of less than 4 hours, or if the divided doses are not equal, it is recommended that the smaller doses be given at the end of the day. In some patients the onset of effect of the first morning dose may be delayed for up to one hour compared with the response usually obtained from the first morning dose of Sinemet.

An interval of at least three days between dosage adjustments is recommended.

*Maintenance:* Because Parkinson's disease is progressive, periodic clinical evaluations are recommended and adjustment of the dosage regimen of Sinemet CR or Half Sinemet CR may be required.

*Addition of other antiparkinson medication:* Anticholinergic agents, dopamine agonists and amantadine can be given with Sinemet CR or Half Sinemet CR. Dosage adjustment of Sinemet CR or Half Sinemet CR may be necessary when these agents are added to an existing treatment for Sinemet CR or Half Sinemet CR.

*Interruption of therapy:* Patients should be observed carefully if abrupt reduction or discontinuation of Sinemet CR or Half Sinemet CR is required, especially if the patient is receiving antipsychotics (see Warnings and Precautions).

If general anesthesia is required, Sinemet CR or Half Sinemet CR may be continued as long as the patient is permitted to take oral medication. If therapy is interrupted temporarily, the usual dosage should be administered as soon as the patient is able to take oral medicine.

**Contra-indications, warnings, etc**

*Contra-indications:* Sinemet CR or Half Sinemet CR should not be given when administration of a sympathomimetic amine is contraindicated.

Monoamine oxidase inhibitors (except low doses of selective MAO-B inhibitors) and Sinemet CR or Half Sinemet CR should not be given concomitantly. These inhibitors must be discontinued at least two weeks prior to initiating therapy with Sinemet CR or Half Sinemet CR.

Sinemet CR or Half Sinemet CR is contraindicated in patients with known hypersensitivity to any component of this medication, and in patients with narrow-angle glaucoma.

Because levodopa may activate a malignant melanoma, Sinemet CR or Half Sinemet CR should not be used in patients with suspicious undiagnosed skin lesions or a history of melanoma.

*Warnings:* When patients are receiving levodopa monotherapy, levodopa must be discontinued at least eight hours before therapy with Sinemet CR or Half Sinemet CR is started (at least 12 hours if slow-release levodopa has been administered).

Sinemet CR and Half Sinemet CR are not recommended for the treatment of drug-induced extra-pyramidal reactions or for the treatment of Huntington's chorea.

*Use in children:* Safety and effectiveness of Sinemet CR or Half Sinemet CR in infants and children have not been established, and its use in patients below the age of 18 is not recommended.

*Pregnancy and lactation:* There are insufficient data to evaluate the possible harmfulness of this substance when used in human pregnancy. The medicine has appeared harmful in animal trials (visceral and skeletal malformations in rabbits). It is not known whether carbidopa or levodopa is excreted in human milk. Sinemet CR or Half Sinemet CR should not be given during pregnancy and to nursing mothers.

*Effects on ability to drive and to use machines:* No data are known about the effect on this product on the ability to drive. If they occur, side-effects such as dizziness or somnolence may affect the ability to drive or to operate machinery.

*Precautions:* Based on the pharmacokinetic profile of Sinemet CR the onset of effect in patients with early morning dyskinesias may be slower than with conventional Sinemet. The incidence of dyskinesias is slightly higher during treatment with Sinemet CR than with conventional Sinemet (16.5% vs 12.2%) in advanced patients with motor fluctuations.

Dyskinesias may occur in patients previously treated with levodopa alone because carbidopa permits more levodopa to reach the brain and, thus, more dopamine to be formed. The occurrence of dyskinesias may require dosage reduction.

Sinemet CR should be administered cautiously to patients with severe cardiovascular or pulmonary disease, bronchial asthma, renal, hepatic or endocrine disease, or with a history of peptic ulcer disease or of convulsions.

Care should be exercised in administering Sinemet CR or Half Sinemet CR to patients with a history of recent myocardial infarction who have residual atrial, nodal, or ventricular arrhythmia. In such patients, cardiac function should be monitored with particular care during the period of initial dosage administration and titration.

As with levodopa, Sinemet CR or Half Sinemet CR may cause involuntary movements and mental disturbances. Patients with a history of severe involuntary movements or psychotic episodes when treated with levodopa alone or levodopa/decarboxylase inhibitor combination should be observed carefully when Sinemet CR or Half Sinemet CR is substituted. These reactions are thought to be due to increased brain dopamine following administration of levodopa and use of Sinemet CR or Half Sinemet CR may cause recurrence. Dosage reduction may be required. All patients should be observed carefully for the development of depression with concomitant suicidal tendencies. Patients with past or current psychoses should be treated with caution.

A symptom complex resembling the neuroleptic malignant syndrome including muscular rigidity, elevated body temperature, mental changes, and increased serum creatinine phosphokinase has been reported when antiparkinsonian agents were withdrawn abruptly. Therefore, patients should be observed carefully when the dosage of carbidopa-levodopa combinations is reduced abruptly or discontinued, especially if the patient is receiving anti-psychotics.

Patients with chronic wide-angle glaucoma may be treated cautiously with Sinemet CR or Half Sinemet CR, provided the intraocular pressure is well controlled and the patient monitored carefully for changes in intraocular pressure during therapy.

Periodic evaluations of hepatic, haematopoietic, cardiovascular and renal function are recommended during extended therapy.

*Laboratory tests:* Abnormalities in various laboratory

tests have occurred with carbidopa-levodopa preparations and may occur with Sinemet CR or Half Sinemet CR. These include elevations of liver function tests such as alkaline phosphatase, SGOT (AST), SGPT (ALT), LDH, bilirubin, blood urea and positive Coombs' test.

Carbidopa-levodopa preparations may cause a false-positive reaction for urinary ketone bodies when a test tape is used for determination of ketonuria. This reaction will not be altered by boiling the urine specimen. False-negative tests may result with the use of glucose-oxidase methods of testing for glycosuria.

*Drug interactions:* Caution should be exercised when the following drugs are administered concomitantly with Sinemet CR or Half Sinemet CR.

*Antihypertensive agents:* Symptomatic postural hypotension has occurred when levodopa/decarboxylase inhibitor combinations were added to the treatment of patients receiving some antihypertensive drugs. Therefore when therapy with Sinemet CR or Half Sinemet CR is started, dosage adjustment of the antihypertensive drug may be required.

*Antidepressants:* There have been rare reports of adverse reactions, including hypertension and dyskinesia, resulting from the concomitant use of tricyclic antidepressants and carbidopa-levodopa preparations. (For patients receiving monomine oxidase inhibitors, see contraindications).

*Anticholinergics:* Anticholinergics may affect the absorption and thus the patient's response.

*Other drugs:* Antipsychotics may reduce the therapeutic effects of levodopa. The beneficial effects of levodopa in Parkinson's disease have been reported to be reversed by phenytoin and papaverine. Patients taking these drugs with Sinemet CR or Half Sinemet CR should be observed carefully for loss of therapeutic response.

Since levodopa competes with certain amino acids, the absorption of levodopa may be impaired in some patients on a high protein diet.

The effect of simultaneous administration of antacids with Sinemet CR on the bioavailability of levodopa has not been studied.

*Adverse effects:* In controlled clinical trials in patients with moderate to severe motor fluctuations Sinemet CR did not produce side-effects which were unique to the controlled-release formulation.

The side-effect reported most frequently was dysksinesia (a form of abnormal involuntary movements). A greater incidence of dyskinesias was seen with Sinemet CR than with Sinemet.

Other side-effects that also were reported frequently (above 2%) were: nausea, hallucinations, confusion, dizziness, chorea and dry mouth.

Side-effects occurring less frequently (1–2%) were: dream abnormalities, dystonia, somnolence, insomnia, depression, asthenia, vomiting and anorexia.

Side-effects observed rarely (0.5%–1%) were: headache, on-off phenomenon, constipation, disorientation, parasthesia, dyspnea, fatigue, orthostatic effects, palpitation, dyspepsia, intestinal pain, muscle cramps, decreased mental acuity, chest pain, diarrhoea, weight loss, agitation, anxiety, falling, gait abnormalities and blurred vision.

Other side-effects that have been reported with levodopa or levodopa-carbidopa combinations and may be potential side-effects with Sinemet CR are listed below:

Nervous system: Ataxia, numbness, increased hand tremor, muscle twitching, blepharospasm, trismus, activation of latent Horner's syndrome.

Psychiatric: Euphoria, paranoid ideation and psychotic episodes, and dementia.

Gastrointestinal: Bitter taste, sialorrhoea, dysphagia, bruxism, hiccups, gastrointestinal bleeding, flatulence, burning sensation of tongue, development of duodenal ulcer.

Cardiovascular: Cardiac irregularities, hypertension, phlebitis.

Integumentary: Flushing, increased sweating, dark sweat, rash, hair loss.

Genitourinary: Urinary retention, urinary incontinence, dark urine, priapism.

Special senses: Diplopia, dilated pupils, oculogyric crises.

Haematological: Leukopenia, haemolytic and non-haemolytic anaemia, thrombocytopenia, agranulocytosis.

Miscellaneous: Weakness, faintness, hoarseness, malaise, hot flushes, sense of stimulation, bizarre breathing patterns, hypertension, phlebitis, neuroleptic malignant syndrome, malignant melanoma (see contra-indications). Convulsions have occured; however, a causal relationship with levodopa or levodopa-carbidopa combinations has not been established.

*Laboratory tests:* Laboratory tests which have been reported to be abnormal are alkaline phosphatase, SGOT (AST), SGPT (ALT), LDH, bilirubin, blood urea nitrogen and Coomb's test.

Decreased haemoglobin and haematocrit, elevated serum glucose and white blood cells, bacteria and blood in the urine have been reported with standard Sinemet.

*Overdosage:* Management of acute overdosage with Sinemet CR or Half Sinemet CR is basically the same as management of acute overdosage with levodopa; however, pyridoxine is not effective in reversing the actions of Sinemet CR or Half Sinemet CR.

Electrocardiographic monitoring should be instituted and the patient observed carefully for the development of arrhythmias; if required, appropriate antiarrhythmic therapy should be given. The possibility that the patient may have taken other drugs as well as Sinemet CR or Half Sinemet CR should be taken into consideration. To date, no experience has been reported with dialysis; hence, its value in overdosage is not known.

**Pharmaceutical precautions** Keep container tightly closed; avoid storage above 30°C. The expiration date is mentioned on the package.

**Legal category** POM

**Package quantities** Bottles of 56.

**Further information** The pharmacokinetics of levodopa following administration of Sinemet CR were studied in young and elderly healthy volunteers. The mean time to peak plasma levodopa level after Sinemet CR was approximately two hours compared to 0.75 hours with Sinemet. The mean peak plasma levodopa levels were 60 per cent lower with Sinemet CR than with Sinemet. The in vivo absorption of levodopa following administration of Sinemet CR was continuous for 4 to 6 hours. In these studies, as with patients, plasma levodopa concentrations fluctuated in a narrower range than with Sinemet. Because the bioavailability of levodopa from Sinemet CR relative to Sinemet is approximately 70 percent, the daily dosage of levodopa in the controlled release formulation will usually be higher than that with conventional formulations. There was no evidence that Sinemet CR released its ingredients in a rapid or uncontrolled fashion.

The pharmacokinetics of levodopa following administration of Half Sinemet CR were studied in patients with Parkinson's disease. Chronic three month, open-label, twice daily dosing with Half Sinemet CR (range: 50 mg carbidopa, 200 mg levodopa up to 150 mg carbidopa, 600 mg levodopa per day) did not result in accumulation of plasma levodopa. The dose-adjusted bioavailability for one Half Sinemet CR tablet was equivalent to that for one Sinemet CR tablet. The mean peak concentration of levodopa following administration of one Half Sinemet CR tablet was greater than 50% of that following one Sinemet CR tablet. Mean time-to-peak plasma levels may be slightly less for Half Sinemet CR than for Sinemet CR.

It is not known whether or not to what extent the absorption is influenced by a protein rich diet. The bioavailability may be influenced by drugs which affect the gastrointestinal propulsion.

**Product licence numbers**
Sinemet CR 0025/0269
Half Sinemet CR 0025/0287

*Product licence holder:* Merck Sharp & Dohme Limited, Hertford Road, Hoddesdon, Hertfordshire EN11 9BU

## VIAZEM XL*

**Qualitative and quantitative composition** Diltiazem hydrochloride : 120-180-240-300-360 mg per capsule. Each capsule of Viazem XL is composed of coated pellets.

**Pharmaceutical form** Prolonged release capsule. For oral administration.

**Clinical particulars**

*Therapeutic indications:* Mild to moderate hypertension.

*Posology and method of administration:*

*Adults:* One capsule per day, before or during a meal. The dose should be taken at approximately the same time each day. The usual daily dose is 300 mg, to be adapted according to the patient's response. This range of capsule strengths facilitates titration to the optimal dose.

*Elderly and patients with impaired hepatic or renal function:* Plasma levels of diltiazem can be increased in the elderly, and in patients with impaired renal or hepatic function. In these cases, the starting dose should be one 120 mg Viazem XL capsule once daily. Dose adjustment may be required to obtain a satisfactory clinical response.

*Children:* Safety and efficacy in children have not been established.

The capsule should not be chewed but swallowed whole.

*Contra-indications:* Diltiazem is contra-indicated in pregnancy and in women of child-bearing potential. Diltiazem is excreted in breast milk in concentrations similar to those in serum. If use of diltiazem is considered essential during lactation, an alternative method of infant feeding should be instituted.

Diltiazem depresses atrioventricular node conduction and is therefore contra-indicated in patients with marked bradycardia, sick sinus syndrome, left ventricular failure with stasis, or second or third degree AV block except in the presence of a functioning pacemaker.

*Special warnings and precautions for use:* Diltiazem should be used with caution in patients with reduced left ventricular function. Patients with mild bradycardia, first degree AV block or prolonged PR interval should be observed closely.

No special precautions are necessary in cases of isolated branch block. In cases of general anaesthesia, the anaesthetist should be informed that the drug is being taken.

Diltiazem may be used without risk in patients with chronic respiratory diseases.

*Interaction with other medicaments and other forms of interaction:* Combinations contra-indicated as a safety measure:

In animals, fatal ventricular fibrillations are constantly seen during administration of verapamil and dantrolene via the i.v. route. The combination of a calcium antagonist and dantrolene is therefore potentially dangerous.

Combinations requiring safety precautions:

In common with other calcium antagonists, when diltiazem is used with drugs which may induce bradycardia or with antiarrhythmic or other antihypertensive drugs the possibility of an additive effect should be borne in mind.

Diltiazem has been used safely in combination with beta-blockers, diuretics, ACE-inhibitors and other antihypertensive agents. It is recommended that patients receiving these combinations should be regularly monitored. Concomitant use of diltiazem with alpha-blockers such as prazosin should be strictly monitored because of the possible synergistic hypotensive effect of this combination.

Case reports have suggested that blood levels of carbamazepine, cyclosporin and theophylline may be increased when given concurrently with diltiazem. Care should be exercised in patients taking these drugs. In common with other calcium antagonists diltiazem may cause small increases in plasma levels of digoxin.

In patients taking $H_2$-antagonists concurrently with diltiazem there may be increased levels of diltiazem.

Magnification of the hypotensive and lipothymic effects (summation of vasodilator properties) of nitrate derivatives can occur. In patients on calcium inhibitors, prescription of nitrate derivatives should be made at progressively increasing doses. Diltiazem treatment has been continued without problem during anaesthesia, but the anaesthetist should be informed that the patient is receiving a calcium antagonist.

*Pregnancy and lactation:*

*Pregnancy:* Diltiazem is teratogenic in some animal species. In the absence of adequate evidence of safety in human pregnancy, Viazem XL should not be used in pregnancy or in women of childbearing potential.

*Lactation:* Diltiazem is excreted in breast milk in concentrations similar to those in serum. If the use of diltiazem is considered essential, an alternative method of infant feeding should be instituted.

*Effects on ability to drive and use machines:* None of note at the recommended dosage.

*Undesirable effects:* Certain undesirable effects may lead to suspension of treatment : sinus bradycardia, sinoatrial heart block, 2nd and 3rd degree atrioventricular heart block, skin rash, oedema of the lower limbs.

In hypertensive patients, adverse effects are generally mild and transient and are most commonly vasodilatory related events

The following have been described in decreasing order of frequency : lower limb oedema, headache, hot flushes/flushing, asthenia/fatigue, palpitations, malaise, minor gastro-intestinal disorders (dyspepsia, abdominal pain, dry mouth) and skin rash. Vasodilatory related events (in particular, oedema) are dose-dependent and appear to be more frequent in elderly subjects.

Rare cases of symptomatic bradycardia and exceptionally sino-atrial block and atrioventricular block were also recorded.

Experience with use in other indications and with other formulations, has shown that skin rashes are usually localised and are limited to cases of erythema, urticaria or occasionally desquamative erythema, with or without fever, which regress when treatment is discontinued.

Isolated cases of moderate and transient elevation of liver transaminases have been observed at the start of treatment. Isolated cases of clinical hepatitis have been reported which resolved on cessation of therapy.

*Overdose:* The clinical consequences of overdose can be severe hypotension leading to collapse, and sinus bradycardia which may be accompanied by isorhythmic dissociation and atrioventricular conduction disturbances. Observation in a coronary care unit is advisable. Vasopressors such as adrenaline may be indicated in patients exhibiting profound hypotension. Calcium gluconate may help reverse the effects of calcium entry blockade. Atropine administration and temporary cardiac pacing may be required to manage bradycardia and/or conduction disturbances.

Glucagon can be used in cases of established hypoglycaemia.

Diltiazem and its metabolites are very poorly dialysable.

## Pharmacological properties

*Pharmacodynamic properties:* Diltiazem hydrochloride is a calcium antagonist. It selectively reduces calcium entry through voltage-dependent calcium-n channels into vascular smooth muscle cells and myocardial cells. This lowers the concentration of intracellular calcium which is available to activate contractile proteins. This action of diltiazem results in dilation of coronary arteries causing an increase in myocardial oxygen supply. It reduces cardiac work by moderating the heart rate and by reducing systemic vascular resistance thus reducing oxygen demand.

*Pharmacokinetic properties:* The kinetics of diltiazem are linear and non-saturable. In the healthy volunteer, following a single oral administration, diltiazem is well absorbed (90%).

Viazem XL formulations allow a prolonged absorption of the active element. In most cases, the 300 mg capsule translates into therapeutic levels (50-200 ng/ml) over 24 hours following chronic administration. In other cases the therapeutic level is obtained with lower or higher dosages.

Diltiazem is bound to plasma proteins in proportions of 80 to 85%. It is metabolised by the liver.

After chronic administration, the unchanged substance is found in the urine at levels of 1 to 3%.

Deacetyldiltiazem, the active metabolite, represents 15% of circulating levels of diltiazem. Food does not significantly alter the kinetics of diltiazem when administered as the Viazem XL formulation.

Diltiazem and its metabolites are very poorly dialysable.

The apparent half-life of elimination is from 5 to 7 hours.

*Preclinical safety data:*
*Toxicity: Toxicity by single ingestion:* The LD$_{50}$ for rats

and mice are 560 mg/kg/day and 508 mg/kg/day respectively by the oral route. By the intravenous route, the LD$_{50}$ are 38 mg/kg/day (males) and 39 mg/kg/day (females) in rats, and 61 mg/kg/day (males) and 58 mg/kg/day (females) in mice. It has been estimated that the smallest lethal dose in dogs is 40 mg/kg/day.

*Subacute toxicity:* In rats, 500 mg/kg/day for 30 days via the oral route or 25 mg/kg/day via the intraperitoneal route constitute lethal doses. In dogs, the lethal dose is 50 mg/kg/day.

*Chronic toxicity:* In studies carried out in rats for 6 months, a 60% mortality rate was noted at a dose of 125 mg/kg/day. In dogs after the same period, a sole death took place with a dose of 40 mg/kg/day.

*Fertility and general capacity for reproduction:* The effects of diltiazem on fertility and reproductive function were studied in rats. Toxic effects were revealed at an oral dose of 100 mg/kg/day and via the intraperitoneal route at a dose of 80 mg/kg/day. Via the intravenous route, a dose of 18 mg/kg/day produced toxic effects.

*Embryotoxicity–Teratogenicity:* In mice, a teratogenic effect is evidenced via the oral route from doses of 50 mg/kg/day. In rats, oral administration of diltiazem from the 9th to the 14th days of gestation at high doses (200 to 400 mg/kg/day) induce toxic effects.

In rabbits, doses from 18 to 70 mg/kg/day exert a teratogenic effect, which becomes lethal to the embryo at doses of 35 mg/kg/day.

*Peri- and post natal toxicity:* In rats, oral doses (from 100 mg/kg/day) produce maternal toxicity. A teratogenic effect has been observed in the retina and in the tongue upwards of 30 mg/kg/day. Toxic effects become evident at a dose of 130 mg/kg/day via the intravenous route on the neonatal survival rate and on the average growth rate.

*Mutagenesis–Carcinogenesis:* Diltiazem has no known carcinogenic potential.

*Toxicity in man:* The lethal dose in man is not known.

## Pharmaceutical particulars

*List of excipients:* Saccharose stearate; Microcrystalline cellulose; Polyvidone; Magnesium stearate; Talc; Titanium; Methylhydroxypropylcellulose; Polysorbate 80; Polyacrylate dispersion 30% (dry); Simethicone emulsion.

| | Capsule body | Capsule cap |
|---|---|---|
| 120 mg | Lavender opaque (1) | Lavender opaque (1) |
| 180 mg | White opaque (2) | Blue green opaque (3) |
| 240 mg | Blue green opaque (3) | Lavender opaque (1) |
| 300 mg | White opaque (2) | Lavender opaque (1) |
| 360 mg | Blue green opaque (3) | Blue green opaque (3) |

(1) Colour is composed of Erythrosine E127, Indigotine E132, and Titanium Dioxide E171.
(2) Colour is composed of Titanium Dioxide.
(3) Colour is composed of Quinoline Yellow E104, Indigotine E132 and Titanium Dioxide E171.

*Gelatin capsule markings (printed radially):*

| | Capsule body | Capsule cap |
|---|---|---|
| 120 mg | Viazem XL 120 (white ink EEC approved) | Viazem XL 120 (white ink EEC approved) |
| 180 mg | Viazem XL 180 (black ink EEC approved) | Viazem XL 180 (black ink EEC approved) |
| 240 mg | Viazem XL 240 (white ink EEC approved) | Viazem XL 240 (white ink EEC approved) |
| 300 mg | Viazem XL 300 (black ink EEC approved) | Viazem XL 300 (black ink EEC approved) |
| 360 mg | Viazem XL 360 (white ink EEC approved) | Viazem XL 360 (white ink EEC approved) |

*Incompatibilities:* Not applicable.

*Shelf life:* 3 years.

*Special precautions for storage:* At room temperature (at or below 25˚C), avoiding excessive humidity.

*Nature and contents of container:* The capsules are packed in PVC/aluminium blisters.

*Instructions for use/handling:* Swallow capsules whole, do not chew.

*Marketing authorisation holder:* Biovail (UK) Ltd, Thames House, Wellington Street, London SE18 6NZ.

**Marketing authorisation numbers**
Viazem XL 120 mg　　15136/0006
Viazem XL 180 mg　　15136/0007
Viazem XL 240 mg　　15136/0008
Viazem XL 300 mg　　15136/0009
Viazem XL 360 mg　　15136/0010

**Date of approval/revision of SPC** April 1997

**Legal category POM.**

*Trade Mark

# Eastern Pharmaceuticals Ltd
Coomb House
St John's Road
Isleworth
Middlesex TW7 6NA

## AMORAM*

**Presentation** Red/white opaque capsules each containing 250 mg amoxycillin. The Red shell has a white band with a reversed radial print Amoram. The white body has a red band with a reversed radial print 250.

Red/white opaque capsules each containing 500 mg amoxycillin. The Red shell has a white band with a reversed radial print Amoram. The white body has a red band with a reversed radial print 500.

Amoram suspensions (Amoxycillin Mixture BP). Sugar free. Amoram suspension is prepared by adding water to the powder, containing 125 mg and 250 mg In each 5 ml.

**Uses** Amoram is a broad spectrum antibiotic for the treatment of commonly-occurring bacterial infections such as: Upper respiratory infections; otitis media; acute and chronic bronchitis; chronic bronchial sepsis; lobar and bronchopneumonia; cystitis, urethritis pyelonephritis; bacteriuria in pregnancy: gynaecological infections including puerperal sepsis abortion; gonorrhoea; peritonitis; intra-abdominal sepsis; septicemia; bacterial endocarditis; typhoid and paratyphoid fever; skin and soft tissue infections; osteomyelitis; dental abscess (as an adjunct to surgical management).

In children with urinary tract infection the need for investigation should be considered.

**Dosage and administration**

*Adult (including elderly patients):*
*Standard adult* dosage: 250 mg three times a day. In severe infections doses should be doubled.

*High dosage therapy* (maximum recommended oral dosage 6 g daily in divided doses): a dosage of 3 g twice daily is recommended in appropriate cases for the treatment of severe or recurrent purulent infection of the respiratory tract.

*Short course therapy:* Simple acute urinary tract infection, two 3 g doses with 10-12 hours between the doses. Dental abscess: two 3 g doses with 8 hours between the doses. Gonorrhoea: single 3 g dose.

Amoram suspension is recommended for children under 10 years of age. Children's dosage: Standard children dosage: 125 mg three times a day. In severe infections doses should be doubled. Amoram suspension is not recommended for Paediatric use. In renal impairment the excretion of the antibiotic will be delayed and depending on the degree of impairment it may be necessary to reduce the total daily dosage.

**Contra-indications warnings, etc** Amoram is a penicillin and should not be given to penicillin hypersensitive patients.

*Use in pregnancy and lactation.* When antibiotic therapy is required during pregnancy Amoram may be considered appropriate. During lactation, trace quantities of Amoram can be detected in breast milk.

*Side-effects:* Side-effects as with other penicillins are usually of a mild and transitory nature they may include diarrhoea, indigestion or occasionally rash, either urticarial or erythematous. An urticaral rash suggests penicillin hypersensitivity and the erythematous type rash may arise if Amoram is administered to patients with glandular fever. In either case treatment should be discontinued.

*Overdosage:* Gross overdose will produce very high urinary concentrations, problems are likely if adequate fluid intake and urinary output are maintained, however, crystalluria is a possibility. More specific measures may be necessary in patients with impaired renal function; the antibiotic is removed by Haemodialysis.

**Pharmaceutical precautions** Store in a cool place. Amoram suspension should be used within two weeks of preparation.

**Legal category** POM.

**Package quantities** Amoram 250 mg and 500 mg: Packs of 100 capsules. Amoram 125 mg/5 ml, 250 mg/ 5 ml suspension: Bottles of 100 ml.

**Further information** Nil.

**Product licence numbers**
Amoram 250 mg Capsules 11382/0001
Amoram 500 mg Capsules 11382/0002
Amoram 125 mg/5 ml Suspension 11382/0003
Amoram 250 mg/5 ml Suspension 11382/0004

## DALIVIT* DROPS

**Presentation** Deep yellow liquid with a characteristic taste and odour in a 25 ml amber glass bottle with integral dropper. Each 0.6 ml contains:

| | |
|---|---|
| Vitamin A Palmitate | 5,000 Units |
| Ergocalciferol (Vitamin D₂) | 400 Units |
| Thiamine Hydrochloride | 1 mg |
| Riboflavine | 400 micrograms |
| Pyridoxine Hydrochloride | 500 micrograms |
| Ascorbic Acid | 50 mg |
| Nicotinamide | 5 mg |

**Uses** As a supplement for the prevention of vitamin deficiency states and as an aid to the maintenance of normal health and growth in infants and young children.

**Dosage and administration** Dalivit Drops are administered orally.

*Infants from 6 weeks up to one year:* 0.3 ml daily (7 drops).

*Older children, adults:* 0.6 ml daily (14 drops) or as directed by the physician.

**Contra-indications, warnings, etc**
*Contra-indications:* Hypersensitivity to any of the ingredients. Hypercalcaemia.

*Interactions:* None known.

*Effects on ability to drive and to use machines:* None known.

*Other undesirable effects:* Excessive doses of Vitamin A and D can lead to hypervitaminosis.

*Use in pregnancy and lactation:* During first trimester of pregnancy large doses of Vitamin A may be teratogenic. Patients should be warned not to take Vitamin A supplements if pregnant or likely to become pregnant, except on the advice of a doctor or ante-natal clinic. Vitamin D is secreted in breast milk and may cause hypercalcaemia in infants.

*Other special warnings and precautions:* When multivitamin preparations are prescribed allowance must be made for vitamins from other sources.

*Overdose:* Symptoms of vitamin overdosage may include anorexia, nausea, vomiting, rough dry skin, polyuria, thirst, loss of hair, painful bones and joints as well as raised plasma and urine calcium and phosphate concentration.

*Incompatibilities:* None known.

**Pharmaceutical precautions** Store in a cool place protected from light.

**Legal category** GSL.

**Package quantities** 1 x 25 ml and 2 x 25 ml dropper bottles.

**Further information** Dalivit Drops are prescribable on the NHS. A daily dose of 14 drops is useful for preventing vitamin deficiency in the elderly who may find drops easier to take than other forms of vitamin supplementation.

**Product licence number** 11382/0015

## ELECTROLADE*

**Presentation** Paper/aluminium foil sachet containing white free flowing powder, flavoured with banana, melon, blackcurrant, oange, lemon and lime or plain. Each sachet contains:

| | |
|---|---|
| Sodium Chloride PhEur | 0.236 g |
| Potassium Chloride PhEur | 0.309 g |
| Sodium Bicarbonate PhEur | 0 500 9 |
| Anhydrous Dextrose PhEur | 4.000 9 |
| Saccharin Sodium | 0.003 9 |
| Also contains flavourings | |

**Uses** Oral replacement therapy of electrolyte and fluid loss in children and adults arising from dehydration associated with diarrhoea of various origins (including viral). Also a corrective treatment of dehydration associated with other feverish illnesses.

**Dosage and administration**
*Reconstitution:* Only with water and at the volume stated.

*Adults and children:* The contents of each sachet should be dissolved in approximately 200 ml of cool, fresh, clean drinking water. The resulting solution is both clear and colourless.

*Infants:* The water should be boiled then cooled before reconstitution as above.

The reconstituted cooled solution should be used immediately and the unused remainder discarded, or stored in a refrigerator for no longer than 24 hours. Do not boil after reconstitution. The product must only be used at the recommended dilution.

*Dosage:* Oral fluid replacement and maintenance therapy must be tailored by the physician to individual patients needs. The volume of solution used will depend on the weight and age of the patient, using the basic principle of firstly rehydrating the patient by replacing lost fluid and thereafter maintaining fluid replacement in line with the volume of fluid lost from stools or vomiting plus normal daily requirements. As a basic guide, a daily intake of 150 ml/kg bodyweight for infants (under 2 years of age) or 100-120 ml/kg for adults and children is needed.

*Replacement of fluid losses with Electrolade solution:* Infants (under 2 years of age): Reconstitute sachets according to directions and administer at 1-1.5 times usual feed volume. No milk (other than breast milk) or solids should be given during the first 24 hours. In breast-fed infants, Electrolade should be given before the feed. The re-introduction of normal feeding should only take place when symptoms of diarrhoea are abating and should be added gradually to make up the total daily fluid requirements.

*Children:* One sachet after every loose motion, up to 12 sachets in 24 hours.

*Adults:* 1-2 sachets after every loose motion, up to 16 sachets in 24 hours.

*Elderly persons:* As for adults but care must be taken not to over-hydrate.

In adults and children Electrolade can be given in amounts necessary to satisfy thirst. As with infants, solids should be avoided during the first day, but may be gradually resumed as necessary during day 2.

It is extremely difficult to over-hydrate by mouth, thus when there is normal renal function, it is better to give more Electrolade than less.

*Pregnancy and lactation:* The dose is the above adult dose. Breast feeding can be continued as normal. If vomiting is a problem then Electrolade solution should be taken in frequent small volumes.

**Contra-indications, warnings, etc** There are no absolute contra-indications to using Electrolade. However, it would be unwise to give the solution where there is renal failure with oliguria, in acute abdominal patients prior to surgery or where parenteral therapy should be given.

The solution must be made up without adding extra sugar or salt. In treating diabetics with gastro-enteritis, the sugar content must be noted.

Solution of greater concentration may result in hypernatraemia. Those of greater dilution may result in inadequate replacement.

*Overdosage:* In oral electrolyte replacement therapy, toxicity is rare in previously healthy people. In subjects with renal impairment, hypernatraemia and hyperkalaemia might occur. If these conditions occur full biochemical profile under hospital conditions will be needed and the physician should take the appropriate measures.

**Pharmaceutical precautions** Electrolade should be stored in a dry place below 25 C.

**Legal category** P.

**Package quantities** Box of 6 or 20 sachets containing a patient information leaflet.

**Further information** A reconstituted solution of Electrolade (1 sachet/200 ml) has the following composition:

| | |
|---|---|
| Sodium | 50 |
| Potassium | 20 |
| Chloride | 40 |
| Bicarbonate | 30 |
| Dextrose | 111 |

The sodium and dextrose concentration should give optimum water replacement; solutions with higher concentrations reverse this process.

Potassium and bicarbonate included in the formula will replace the large amounts lost in diarrhoea and will combat metabolic acidosis.

**Product licence numbers**

| | |
|---|---|
| Electrolade Melon | 11382/0018 |
| Electrolade Banana | 11382/0019 |
| Electrolade Blackcurrant | 11382/0020 |
| Electrolade Orange | 11382/0022 |
| Electrolade Plain | 11382/0024 |
| Electrolade Lemon and Lime | 11382/0025 |

## ISOCARD* TRANSDERMAL SPRAY

**Presentation** Active ingredient: Isosorbide dinitrate. Each metered dose contains 30 mg isosorbide dinitrate. Metered dose aerosol for application to skin.

**Uses** For the long-term treatment of angina pectoris and prevention of anginal attacks including the postinfarction phase.

**Dosage and administration**
*Adults:* 1-2 actuations sprayed on the skin in the morning after washing and if necessary in the evening before going to bed. For patients receiving nitrates for the first time a dosage titration is recommended e.g one actuation daily for three days, then if necessary two actuations daily for the next three days, followed by two actuations twice daily.

*Children:* Not recommended.

*The elderly:* There are no specific dosage recommendations for elderly patients but as with all drug treatment the lowest effective dose should be used.

**Contra-indication, warnings, etc**
*Contra-indications:* Shock. acute myocardial infarction with low filling pressure, orthostatic hypotension, hypersensitivity to organic nitrates, anaemia cerebral haemorrhage.

Use with caution in patients who are predisposed to closed angle glaucoma. Avoid contact with the eyes. Do not spray into mouth or inhale the spray. Do not use near a naked flame.

*Interaction:* Antihypertensive drugs, other vasodilators, calcium antagonists, tricyclic antidepressants and alcohol can potentiate the hypotensive effect of Isocard Transdennal spray.

*Use in pregnancy and lactation:* There is no evidence of the safety of the drug in human pregnancy. It should therefore not be used in pregnancy or lactation unless the physician considers it essential.

*Effects on ability to drive and use machinery:* No specific effects.

*Other undesirable effects:* At the start of therapy, postural hypotension and an increase in heart rate may occur. The most frequent side-effects are headaches, vertigo, dizziness, transient flushing, tachycardia rashes, mild skin burning and nausea

*Overdosage:* The main symptom of overdose is hypotension, in such event the drug should be withheld and the patient carefully monitored, passive exercise and elevation of the legs of the recumbent patient will promote venous return. In life threatening situations, administration of vasopressors should be considered.

*Pharmacodynamic properties:* Isosorbide dinitrate is an organic nitrate which has been widely used as a coronary vasodilator. Its mode of action at the cellular level is not yet fully understood but its pharmacological properties are very similar to those of glyceryl trinitrate. Cardiac workload is reduced by venodilation with peripheral pooling of blood and by a mild reduction in arterial tone. Increased blood flow to ischaemic areas of the myocardium occurs.

*Pharmacokinetic properties:* Absorption following oral administration is variable and subject to a substantial first-pass metabolism. This results in the formation of mononitrates which also have vasodilator activity. The half-life of the dinitrate and of the 2- and 5- mononitrate metabolites are 0.5, 1.5, and 4.5 hours respectivelyAdministration via the buccal and transdermal routes avoids the first pass effect and in the fomer case provides very rapid absorption whilst the latter route gives a slow absorption enabling twice daily dosage to be employed

*Preclinical properties:* No further information available.

**Pharmaceutical precautions**
*List of excipients:* diisopropyl adipate, polyethylene glycol DAB, citric acid PhEur, ethanol.

*Incompatibilities:* None stated.

*Shelf life:* 3 years.

*Precautions for storage:* Store below 25°C.

**Legal category** P

**Package quantities** 25 g metered dose aerosol delivers 65 metered doses of 30 mg.

**Further information** *Instructions for use:* The spray should be applied to the chest from a distance of about 20cm and then spread and rubbed gently over the skin with the finger tips. The can should be kept vertical. After drying, the skin can be covered with clothes. The skin may be washed 20 minutes after the application.

**Product licence number** 11382/0026

## KONSYL*

**Presentation** Konsyl is a micronised preparation of Ispaghula husk which is supplied in the form of fine powder. In addition to Konsyl Sugar Free, the product is also available in a flavoured version, Konsyl Orange, and one with a sweetening agent, Konsyl Dex.

**Uses** Konsyl functions as a bulk laxative by absorbing water in the gastro-intestinal tract which increases faecal volume and stimulates peristalsis. It has no purgative effects but results can usually be expected within 24 hours of administration. In some cases 2 or 3 days of medication may be required for the full effect to be obtained.

Because it has no purgative action Konsyl may also be used in treating the irritable bowel syndrome, diarrhoea and for the management of patients with colostomies, where its use results in well formed stools which are easily evacuated, which contributes to the establishment of regular control.

**Dosage and administration**
*Adults:* One sachet to be taken one to three times daily, before or after meals.

*Children (6 years or older):* Half the adult dose or less.

*Elderly:* As for adults.

*Diarrhoea treatment:* The standard dose should be administered three times daily until symptoms subside.

The measured dose of Konsyl should be stirred vigorously into half a glass of water and swallowed immediately. It may be necessary to adjust the dose to suit individual patients.

**Contra-indications, warnings, etc**
*Contra-indications:* Known hypersensitivity to ispaghula.

*Precautions:* Konsyl should not be given to patient with intestinal obstruction or conditions likely to lead to this. Since Konsyl decreases intestinal transit time there is a theoretical possibility of interference the absorption of other drugs. Flatulence and abdominal distension can occur and intestinal obstruction has been rarely reported and it is essential that an adequate fluid intake be maintained in order to avoid such events. Konsyl Dex should not be use in diabetics. Konsyl should be swallowed immediately after mixing and it is advisable that administration to debilitated or very elderly patients should be supervised by a carer in order to avoid any possibility of inadvertent inhalation.

*Pregnancy:* There are no known contra-indications to use during pregnancy or lactation but the usual practice of avoiding the unnecessary use during first trimester should be observed.

*Side effects:* Nil.

*Overdosage:* Overdosage with Konsyl may cause intestinal obstruction, which should be treated appropriately.

**Pharmaceutical precautions** Store in a cool dry place below 25°C.

**Legal category** GSL.

**Package quantities** 6 g Konsyl Sugar Free (6 g Ispaghula Husk BP/sachet) packed in 30 sachets. 6.5 9 Konsyl Dex (3.4 g Ispaghula Husk BP/sachet) packed in 60 sachets. 12 g Konsyl Orange (3.4 g Ispaghula Husk BP/sachet) packed in 60 sachets.

**Further information** Nil.

**Product licence numbers**

| | |
|---|---|
| Konsyl Sugar Free | 11170/0001 |
| Konsyl Dex | 11170/0002 |
| Konsyl Orange | 11170/0003 |

## VOLRAMAN*

**Presentation** Orange enteric coated tablets, coded V on one side and 25 on other, each containing 25 mg diclofenac sodium.

Orange enteric coated tablets, coded V on one and 50 on other, each containing 50 mg diclofenac sodium.

**Uses**
*Adults:* Rheumatoid arthritis, osteoarthrosis, low back pain and other acute musculo-skeletal disorders, acute gout, control of pain and inflammation in orthopaedic, dental and other minor surgery.

*Children:* Juvenile chronic arthritis.

**Dosage and administration**
*Adults:* A total of 75-150 mg daily given in two or three divided doses.

*Children:* 1-3 mg/kg per day in divided doses.

*Elderly:* The standard adult dose may be used.

**Contra-indications, warnings, etc**
*Contra-indications:* Active or suspected ulcer or gastro-intestinal bleeding, previous sensitivity to diclofenac, pregnancy, asthmatic patients in whom attacks of asthma, urticaria or acute rhinitis are precipitated by aspirin or other non-steroidal anti-inflammatory agents.

*Precautions:* History of gastro-intestinal ulceration, haematemesis or melaena, ulcerative colitis, Crohn's disease, bleeding diathesis or haematological abnormalities.

Patients with severe hepatic, cardiac, or renal insufficiency or the elderly should be kept under close surveillance.

Volraman should not be prescribed during pregnancy or lactation.

Volraman should be given with care to those who are receiving coumarin anti-coagulants.

Diclofenac may increase plasma concentrations of lithium and digoxin.

Side-effects reported include epigastric pain, eructation, nausea and diarrhoea, headache or slight dizziness. These side-effects are usually of a mild nature. Central nervous side-effects, such as tiredness, insomnia or irritability, have occurred in rare stances.

Occasionally skin reactions, fluid retention and abnormalities of serum transaminases have been reported.

There have been reports of gastro-intestinal ulceration, haematemesis and melaena. Jaundice, hepatitis, renal failure and nephrotic syndrome have also been reported. If these occur Volraman should withdrawn.

*Overdosage:* No known antidote, treatment is symptomatic. Immediate treatment is forced emesis.

**Pharmaceutical precautions** Store in a cool dry place.

**Legal category** POM.

**Package quantities** Packs of 100 tablets.

**Further information** Diclofenac sodium has been reported to depress salicylate levels and vice versa. There have been isolated reports of anaphylactoid reactions and blood dyscrasias.

**Product licence numbers**
25 mg Tablets 11382/0007
50 mg Tablets 11382/0008.

## ZITA*

**Presentation** Green film-coated tablets engraved EASTERN on one side and ZITA 200, ZITA 400 and ZITA 800 on the other, depending on the cimetidine content in milligrammes. The 200 mg tablet is round, the 400 mg capsule shape and the 800 mg elliptical shape.

**Uses** Zita is an H2 receptor antagonist which reduces pepsin production and inhibits both basal and stimulated gastric acid secretion. It is indicated for conditions where a reduction of gastric acid is beneficial (see table).

Antacids can be given until symptoms cease.

*Adults:*

| Condition | Dose | Duration |
|---|---|---|
| Duodenal & gastric ulcers Short bowel syndrome Pancreatic insufficiency Stomach ulceration | 800 mg at night or 400 mg twice daily or 400 mg qid if above adequate | Minimum 4 Optimum 8 weeks |
| Oesophageal reflux Zollinger-Ellison syndrome | 400 mg tid and 400 mg at night | Minimum 4 Optimum 8 weeks |

| Condition | Dose | Duration |
|---|---|---|
| Haemorrhage prophylaxis in stress ulcers | Between 200 mg and 400 mg 6 hourly | As long as risk exists |
| Prevention of gastric acid aspiration during anaesthesia | 400 mg, 90 to 120 minutes prior to induction or at start of labour | Repeat 400 mg at 4-hourly intervals up to 2.5 G max per 24 hours |

*Elderly:* The normal adult dose may be employed unless renal function is impaired.

*Chilldren:*Over one year of age a daily close of between 25 and 30 mg/kilo body-weight may be given, in divided doses.

**Contra-indications, warnings, etc**
*Contra-indications:* Hypersensitivity to cimetidine. Pregnancy and lactation.

*Precautions:* Reduce dosage in patients with impaired renal function. Exclude malignant disease before and during treatment.
   Monitor patients on long-term treatment especially with NSAIDs.

*Interactions:* Oral anticoagulants, theophylline, phenytoin, lidocaine, diazepam, chlordiazepoxide, propranolol, imipramine and morphine. Restrict alcohol intake during treatment.

*Adverse reactions:* Diarrhoea, dizziness, rash, tiredness and headache. Gynaecomastia, mental contusion in the elderly or very ill and effects on liver function. Very rarely interstitial nephritis,

acutepancreatitis, thrombocytopaenia, agranulocytosis, myalgia, arthralgia, tachycardia, bradycardia, and heart block all of which were reversible on treatment withdrawal.

**Pharmaceutical precautions** Store below 25 degrees centigrade in a dry place. Protect from direct light.

**Legal category** POM.

**Package quantities** Blister packs of 200 mg (120), 400 mg (60), 800 mg (30).

**Further information** Nil.

**Product licence numbers**
Zita 200   11382/0012
Zita 400   11382/0013
Zita 800   11382/0014

*Trade Mark

# Eisai Ltd
## Hammersmith International Centre
## 3 Shortlands
## London W6 8EE

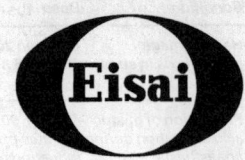

## ARICEPT* 5 mg, 10 mg ▼

**Qualitative and quantitative composition** 5 mg donepezil hydrochloride tablets each containing 4.56 mg donepezil free base. 10 mg donepezil hydrochloride tablets each containing 9.12 mg free base.

**Pharmaceutical form** Coated tablets.

**Clinical particulars**
*Therapeutic indications:* Aricept tablets are indicated for the symptomatic treatment of mild or moderate dementia in Alzheimer's disease.

*Posology and method of administration:*
*Adults/elderly:* Treatment is initiated at 5 mg/day (once-a-day dosing). Aricept should be taken orally, in the evening, just prior to retiring. The 5 mg/day dose should be maintained for at least one month in order to allow the earliest clinical responses to treatment to be assessed and to allow steady-state concentrations of donepezil hydrochloride to be achieved. Following a one month clinical assessment of treatment at 5 mg/day, the dose of Aricept can be increased to 10 mg/day (once-a-day dosing). The maximum recommended daily dose is 10 mg. Doses greater than 10 mg/day have not been studied in clinical trials.

Upon discontinuation of treatment, a gradual abatement of the of the beneficial effects of Aricept is seen. There is no evidence of a rebound effect after abrupt discontinuation of therapy.

*Renal and hepatic impairment:* A similar dose schedule can be followed for patients with renal or mild to moderate hepatic impairment as clearance of donepezil hydrochloride is not affected by these conditions.

*Children:* Aricept is not recommended for use in children

*Contra-indications:* Aricept is contra-indicated in patients with a known hypersensitivity to donepezil hydrochloride, piperidine derivatives, or to any excipients used in the formulation.

*Special warnings and precautions for use:*
*Anaesthesia:* Aricept, as a cholinesterase inhibitor is likely to exaggerate succinylcholine-type muscle relaxation during anaesthesia.

*Cardiovascular conditions:* Because of their pharmacological action, cholinesterase inhibitors may have vagotonic effects on heart rate (e.g. bradycardia). The potential for this action may be particularly important to patients with "sick sinus syndrome" or other supraventricular cardiac conduction conditions.

*Gastro-intestinal conditions:* Patients at increased risk for developing ulcers, e.g. those with a history of ulcer disease or those receiving concurrent nonsteroidal anti-inflammatory drugs (NSAIDs), should be monitored for symptoms. However, the clinical studies with Aricept showed no increase, relative to placebo, in the incidence of either peptic ulcer disease or gastrointestinal bleeding.

*Genito-urinary:* Although not observed in clinical trials of Aricept, cholinomimetics may cause bladder outflow obstruction.

*Neurological conditions:* Seizures: Cholinomimetics are believed to have some potential to cause generalised convulsions. However, seizure activity may also be a manifestation of Alzheimer's disease.

*Pulmonary conditions:* Because of their cholinomimetic actions, cholinesterase inhibitors should be prescribed with care to patients with a history of asthma or obstructive pulmonary disease.

*Interaction with other medicaments and other forms of interaction:* The metabolism of donepezil hydrochloride is slow and does not appear to be saturable following therapeutic doses, consistent with the observation that donepezil hydrochloride and/or any of its metabolites does not inhibit the metabolism of theophylline, warfarin, cimetidine or digoxin in humans. The metabolism of donepezil hydrochloride is not affected by the concurrent administration of digoxin or cimetidine. However, donepezil hydrochloride has the potential to interfere with medications having anticholinergic activity. There is also the potential to for synergistic activity with concomitant treatment involving medications such as succinylcholine, other neuro-muscular blocking agents or cholinergic agonists.

In long-term open-label studies, no adverse effects related to drug interactions were reported when patients were concomitantly administered Aricept and selective serotonin reuptake inhibitors, neuroleptics or (in a small number of cases) anti-Parkinsonian treatment.

*Pregnancy and lactation:*
*Pregnancy:* Teratology studies conducted in pregnant rats at doses up to approximately 80 times the human dose and in pregnant rabbits at doses up to approximately 50 times the human dose did not disclose any evidence for a teratogenic potential. However, in a study in which pregnant rats were given approximately 50 time the human dose from day 17 of gestation through day 20 postpartum, there was a slight increase in stillbirths and a slight increase in stillbirths and a slight decrease in pup survival through day 4 postpartum. No effect was observed at the next lower dose tested, approximately 15 times the human dose. Aricept should only be used during pregnancy if the potential benefit justifies the potential risk to the foetus.

*Lactation:* It is not known whether donepezil hydrochloride is excreted in human breast milk and there are no studies in lactating women. Aricept should only be used by a woman who is breast feeding if the potential benefit outweighs the potential risk to the infant.

*Effects on ability to drive and use machines:* Based on the pharmacodynamic properties and the adverse event profile, it is unlikely that Aricept would cause an impairment of driving performance or compromise the ability to use machinery. However, Alzheimer's Dementia may cause impairment of driving performance or compromised the ability to use machinery.

*Undesirable effects:* Most adverse events are mild in severity and transient in nature.

The most common (incidence ≥ 5% and twice the frequency of placebo) were diarrhoea and muscle cramps.

Other side effects (incidence ≥ 5%) were fatigue, nausea, vomiting, insomnia and dizziness.

No notable abnormalities in laboratory values were observed. Treatment can be associated with minor increases in muscle creatine kinase blood concentrations.

*Overdose:* The estimated median lethal dose of donepezil hydrochloride following administration of a single oral dose in mice and rats is 45 and 32 mg/kg, respectively, or approximately 225 and 160 times the maximum recommended human dose of 10 mg per day. Dose-related signs of cholinergic stimulation were observed in animals and included reduced spontaneous movement, prone position, staggering gait, lacrimation, clonic convulsions, depressed respiration, salivation, miosis, fasciculation and lower body surface temperature.

Overdosage with cholinesterase inhibitors can result in cholinergic crisis characterized by severe nausea, vomiting, salivation, sweating, bradycardia, hypotension, respiratory depression, collapse and convulsions. Increasing muscle weakness is a possibility and may result in death if respiratory muscles are involved.

As in any case of overdose, general supportive measures should be utilised. Tertiary anticholinergics such as atropine may be used as an antidote for Aricept overdosage. Intravenous atropine sulphate titrated to effect is recommended: an initial dose of 1.0 to 2.0 mg IV with subsequent doses based upon clinical response. Atypical responses in blood pressure and heart rate have been reported with other cholinomimetics when co-administered with quaternary anticholinergics such as glycopyrrolate. It is not known whether donepezil hydrochloride and/or its metabolites can be removed by dialysis (haemodialysis peritoneal dialysis, or haemofiltration).

**Pharmacological properties**
*Pharmacodynamic properties:* Donepezil hydrochloride is a specific and reversible inhibitor of acetylcholinesterase, the predominant cholinesterase in the brain. Donepezil hydrochloride is over 1000 times more potent an inhibitor of this enzyme than of butyrylcholinesterase, an enzyme which is present mainly outside the central nervous system.

In patients with Alzheimer's Dementia participating in clinical trials, administration of single daily doses of 5 mg or 10 mg of Aricept produced steady-state inhibition of acetylcholinesterase activity (measured in erythrocyte membranes) of 63.3% and 77.3% respectively when measured post dose. The inhibition of acetylcholinesterase (AChE) in red blood cells by donepezil hydrochloride has been shown to correspond closely to the effects in the cerebral cortex. In addition, significant correlation was demonstrated between plasma levels of donepezil hydrochloride, AChE inhibition and change in ADAS-cog, a sensitive scale which examines memory.

*Pharmacokinetic properties–General characteristics:*
*Absorption:* Oral administration of Aricept produces predictable plasma concentrations with maximal values achieved approximately 3 to 4 hours after dose administration. Plasma concentrations and area under the curve rise in proportion to the dose. The terminal disposition half-life is approximately 70 hours, thus, administration of multiple single-daily doses results in gradual approach to steady-state. Approximate steady-state is achieved within 3 weeks after initiation of therapy. Once at steady-state, plasma donepezil hydrochloride concentrations and the related pharmacodynamic activity show little variability over the course of the day.

Food did not affect the absorption of donepezil hydrochloride.

*Distribution:* Donepezil hydrochloride is approximately 95% bound to human plasma proteins. The distribution of donepezil hydrochloride in various body tissues has not been definitively studied. However, in a mass balance study conducted in healthy male volunteers, 240 hours after the administration of a single 5 mg dose of $^{14}$C-labelled donepezil hydrochloride, approximately 28% of the label remained unrecovered. This suggests that donepezil hydrochloride and/or its metabolites may persist in the body for more than 10 days.

*Metabolism/excretion:* Donepezil hydrochloride is both excreted in the urine intact and metabolised by the cytochrome P450 system to multiple metabolites, not all of which have been identified. Following administration of a single 5 mg dose of $^{14}$C-labelled donepezil hydrochloride, plasma radioactivity, expressed as a percent of the administered dose, was present primarily as intact donepezil hydrochloride (30%), 6-O-desmethyl donepezil (11%–only metabolite that exhibits activity similar to donepezil hydrochloride), donepezil-cis-N-oxide (9%), 5-O-desmethyl donepezil (7%) and the glucuronide conjugate of 5-O-desmethyl donepezil (3%).

Approximately 57% of the total administered radioactivity was recovered from the urine and 14.5% was recovered from the faeces, suggesting biotransformation and urinary excretion as the primary routes of elimination. There is no evidence to suggest enterohepatic recirculation of donepezil hydrochloride and/ or any of its metabolites.

Plasma donepezil concentrations decline with a half-life of approximately 70 hours.

Sex, race and smoking history have no clinically significant influence on plasma concentrations of donepezil hydrochloride.

*Pharmacokinetic/dynamic properties–Characteristics in patients:* As an inhibitor of AChE, donepezil hydrochloride is postulated to augment cholinergic function in the central nervous system, thereby providing its therapeutic benefit. The enzyme AChE occurs peripherally in red blood cells; therefore, measurement of AChE activity in erythrocyte membranes provides an index for donepezil hydrochloride pharmacodynamics, This surrogate marker has been evaluated in several human pharmacokinetic/pharmacodynamic trials and in controlled clinical trials.

The population plasma donepezil hydrochloride concentrations and AChE inhibition measurements verified that patients in clinical trials experienced exposure to donepezil hydrochloride and its pharmacodynamic actions as predicted.

The results from therapeutic drug monitoring showed no apparent relationship between plasma concentration and adverse drug reactions.

In two double-blind randomized trials, statistically significant drug placebo differences were present for each of the two primary outcome measures (ADAS-cog/CIBIC plus).

*Preclinical safety data:* Extensive testing in experimental animals has demonstrated that this compound causes few effects other than the intended pharmacological effects consistent with its action as a cholinergic stimulator (See *Overdose* section above).

Donepezil hydrochloride was not mutagenic in the Ames reverse mutation assay in bacteria or in the mouse lymphoma forward mutation assay *in vitro*. Donepezil hydrochloride did not induce unscheduled DNA synthesis in rat primary hepatocyte cultures following oral dosing of the animals.

Some clastogenic effects were observed in Chinese Hamster Lung cells *in vitro*, but only at concentrations approaching those overtly toxic to the cells and more than 3000 times the steady-state plasma concentrations observed in patients during clinical trials. Donepezil hydrochloride was not clastogenic in the mouse micronucleus model *in vivo*.

Donepezil hydrochloride had no effect on fertility in rats, and was not teratogenic in rats or rabbits, but had a slight effect on still births and early pup survival when administered to pregnant rats at 50 times the human dose (see *Pregnancy and lactation* section above).

**Pharmaceutical particulars**

*List of excipients:* Inactive ingredients are lactose monohydrate, maize starch, microcrystalline cellulose, hydroxypropyl cellulose, and magnesium stearate. The film coating contains talc, polyethylene glycol, hydroxypropyl methylcellulose and titanium dioxide. Additionally, the 10 mg tablet contains yellow iron oxide (synthetic) as a colouring agent.

*Incompatibilities:* None.

*Shelf life:* 36 months.

*Special precautions for storage:* Store below 30°C.

*Nature and contents of container:* 5 mg tablets: Bottles (HDPE) of 28,30 and 100. Unit Dose blister strips (PVC/foil) of 7, 14 and 15.

10 mg tablets: Bottles (HDPE) of 28,30 and 100. Unit Dose blister strips (PVC/foil) of 7, 14 and 15.

*Instructions for use/handling:* No special instructions.

**Marketing authorisation numbers**
5 mg          10555/0006
10 mg         10555/0007

**Date of approval/revision of SPC** February 1997

**Legal category** POM

*\*Trade Mark*

# Elan Pharma Ltd
Lambert Court
Chestnut Avenue
Eastleigh
Hants SO53 3ZQ

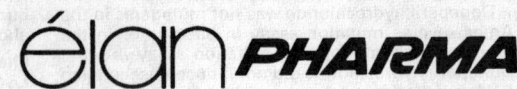

## DILZEM* SR

### Presentation
*Dilzem SR 60:* Contains 60 mg Diltiazem hydrochloride USP. Size 3, beige, hard gelatin capsule, containing sustained release beads. Each capsule is overprinted with the product strength.

*Dilzem SR 90:* Contains 90 mg Diltiazem hydrochloride USP. Size 2, beige, hard gelatin capsule, containing sustained release beads. Each capsule is overprinted with the product strength.

*Dilzem SR 120:* Contains 120 mg Diltiazem hydrochloride USP. Size 1, beige, hard gelatin capsule, containing sustained release beads. Each capsule is overprinted with the product strength.

### Uses
*Action:* Diltiazem has pharmacologic actions similar to those of other calcium channel blocking agents such as nifedipine or verapamil. The principal physiologic action of diltiazem is to inhibit the transmembrane influx of extracellular calcium ions across the membranes of myocardial cells and vasular smooth muscle cells.

Calcium plays important roles in the excitation-contraction coupling processes of the heart and vascular smooth muscle cells and in the electrical discharge of the specialised conduction cells of the heart. The membranes of these cells contain numerous channels that carry a slow inward current and that are selective for calcium.

By inhibiting calcium influx, diltiazem inhibits the contractile processes of cardiac and vascular smooth muscle, thereby dilating the main coronary and systemic arteries. Dilation of systemic arteries by diltiazem results in a decrease in total peripheral resistance, a decrease in systemic blood pressure and a decrease in the afterload of the heart. The reduction in afterload, seen at rest and with exercise and its resultant decrease in myocardial oxygen consumption are though to be responsible for the beneficial effects of diltiazem in patients with chronic stable angina pectoris. In patients with Prinzmetal variant angina, inhibition of spontaneous and ergometrine-induced coronary artery spasm by diltiazem results in increased myocardial oxygen delivery.

*Indications:* Treatment of angina pectoris including Prinzmetal's angina. Treatment of mild to moderate hypertension.

### Dosage and administration
*Route of administration:* Oral.

*Adults: Hypertension:* The usual initial dose is 90 mg twice daily (corresponding to 180 mg of diltiazem hydrochloride daily). Depending upon clinical response the patient's dosage may be increased stepwise to 180 mg twice daily if required.
*Angina pectoris:* The usual initial dose is 90 mg twice daily (corresponding to 180 mg of diltiazem hydrochloride daily). Depending upon clinical response the patient's dosage may be increased stepwise to 180 mg twice daily if required.

*Elderly patients and those with renal or hepatic impairment:* Dosage should commence at the lower level of 60 mg twice daily and be increased slowly. Do not increase the dose if the heart rate falls below 50 beats per minute.

*Children:* Not recommended.

### Contra-indications, warnings, etc
*Contra-indications:* (1) Use in women of child-bearing potential. (2) Concomitant administration of dantrolene infusion due to the risk of ventricular fibrillation. (3) Shock. (4) Acute cardiac infarct with complications (bradycardia, severe hypotension, left heart insufficiency). (5) Bradycardia (pulse rate, at rest, of less than 50 beats per minute), hypotension (less than 90 mm Hg systole), second or third degree heart block or sick sinus syndrome except in the presence of a functioning ventricular pacemaker. (6) Atrial fibrillation / flutter and simultaneous presence of a WPW (Wolff-Parkinson-White) syndrome (increased risk of triggering a ventricular tachycardia). (7) Manifest myocardial insufficiency. (8) Left ventricular failure with stasis. (9) Hypersensitivity to diltiazem or any of the excipients.

*Use in pregnancy and lactation:* Diltiazem must not be taken during pregnancy as experimental studies have shown indications of teratogenicity. There is no experience of its effects in humans. As diltiazem is known to enter the breast milk and there is no experience of possible effects in infants, infants should be weaned if treatment of the mother with diltiazem is necessary.

*Adverse effects:* In studies carried out to date, serious adverse reactions with diltiazem have been rare; however, it should be recognised that patients with impaired ventricular function and cardiac conduction abnormalities have usually been excluded from these studies.

In 900 patients with hypertension, the most common adverse effects were oedema (9%), headache (8%), dizziness (6%), asthenia (5%), sinus bradycardia (3%), flushing (3%) and first degree AV block (3%). Only oedema and perhaps bradycardia were dose related. The most common adverse events (>1%) observed in clinical studies of over 2100 angina and hypertensive patients receiving diltiazem were oedema (5.4%), headache (4.5%), dizziness (3.4%), asthenia (2.8%), first degree AV block (1.8%), flushing (1.7%), nausea (1.6%), bradycardia (1.5%) and rash (1.5%). Less common adverse events have included the following: *Cardiovascular:* angina, arrhythmia, AV block (second or third degree), congestive heart failure, hypotension, palpitations, syncope. *Nervous system:* amnesia, depression, gait abnormality, hallucinations, insomnia, nervousness, paraesthesia, personality change, somnolence, tinnitus, tremor. *Gastro-intestinal:* anorexia, constipation, diarrhoea, dyspepsia, mild elevations of alkaline phosphatase, SGOT, SGPT and LDH (see *Precautions and warnings*), vomiting, weight increase, gingivitis. *Dermatologic:* Petechiae, pruritus, photosensitivity, urticaria. Allergic skin reactions including erythema multiforme, vasculitis, lymphadenopathy and eosinophilia have been observed in isolated cases. Dermatological events may be transient and may disappear despite continued use of diltiazem. Should a dermatologic reaction persist, the drug should be discontinued. *Other:* amblyopia, CK elevation, dyspnoea, epistaxis, eye irritation, hyperglycaemia, nasal congestion, nocturia, osteoarticular pain, polyuria, sexual difficulties.

*Precautions and warnings:* Capsules should not be sucked or chewed.

The use of diltiazem hydrochloride in diabetic patients may require adjustment of their control.

The product should be used with caution in patients with hepatic dysfunction. Abnormalities of liver function may occur during therapy. Very occasional reports of abnormal liver function have been received, these reactions have been reversible upon discontinuation of therapy.

First degree AV block or prolonged PR interval. Dilzem prolongs AV node refractory periods without significantly prolonging sinus node recovery time, except in patients with sick sinus syndrome. This effect may rarely result in abnormally slow heart rates (particularly in patients with sick sinus syndrome) or second- or third- degree AV block (see Interactions section for information concerning beta-blockers and digitalis).

Mild bradycardia.
Patients with reduced left ventricular function.
Renally impaired patients.

As with any drug given over prolonged periods, laboratory parameters should be monitored at regular intervals.

*Interactions:* Diltiazem undergoes biotransformation by cytochrome P-450 mixed function oxidase. Coadministration with other agents which follow the same route of biotransformation may result in competitive inhibition of metabolism.

Diltiazem hydrochloride should only be administered with great care to patients receiving concurrent treatment with antihypertensives or other hypotensive agents including halogenated anaesthetics or drugs with moderate protein binding.

Diltiazem hydrochloride will not protect against the effects of withdrawal of beta-adrenoceptor blocking agents, nor the rebound effects seen with various antihypertensives. Combination with beta-adrenoceptor blockers having a significant 'first pass' loss, eg. propanolol may require a decrease in their dose and may lead to bradycardia. There may be an additive effect when used with drugs which may induce bradycardia or with other antihypertensives.

Concomitant $H_2$ antagonist therapy may increase diltiazem blood levels.

Diltiazem may affect the blood levels of concomitant carbamazepine, theophylline, cyclosporin and digoxin. Careful attention should therefore be given to signs of overdosage. If necessary, the levels should be determined and the dose of carbamazepine, theophylline, cyclosporin or digoxin reduced if necessary. Patients receiving beta-blockers, diuretics, ACE inhibitors or other antihypertensive agents should be regularly monitored. Use with alpha blockers should be strictly monitored.

The simultaneous administration of diltiazem with drugs such as beta-blockers, antiarrythmics or heart glycosides may cause a greater degree of AV blocking, reduce the heart rate or induce a hypotensive effect.

Intravenous administration of beta-blockers should be discontinued during therapy with diltiazem.

Anaesthetists should be warned that a patient is on a calcium antagonist. The depression of cardiac contractility, conductivity and automaticity as well as the vascular dilation associated with anaesthetics may be potentiated by calcium channel blockers. When used concomitantly, anaesthetics and calcium channel blockers should be titrated carefully.

There have been reports in the literature of diltiazem interactions with warfarin, rifampicin and lithium.

*Overdosage:* Experience of overdosage in man is limited but cases of spontaneous recovery have been reported. However, it is recommended that patients with suspected overdose, should be placed under observation in a coronary care unit with facilities available for treatment of any possible hypotension and conduction disturbances that may occur.

Most patients suffering from overdosage of diltiazem become hypotensive within 8 hours of ingestion. With bradycardia and first to third degree atrioventricular block also developing cardiac arrest may ensue. Hyperglycaemia is also a recognised complication. The elimination half-life of diltiazem after overdosage is estimated to be about 5.5-10.2 hours. If a patient presents early after overdose, gastric lavage should be performed and activated charcoal administered to reduce diltiazem absorption.

Hypotension should be corrected with plasma expanders, intravenous calcium gluconate and inotropic agents (dopamine, dobutamine or isoprenaline), symptomatic bradycardia and high grade AV block may respond to atropine, isoprenaline or occasionally cardiac pacing which may be useful if cardiac standstill occurs.

**Pharmaceutical precautions** Store in a dry place at a temperature not exceeding 25°C.

**Legal category** POM.

**Package quantities**
*Dilzem SR 60:* Blister pack containing 100 capsules
*Dilzem SR 90:* Blister pack containing 60 capsules
*Dilzem SR 120:* Blister pack containing 60 capsules

**Further information** None

**Product licence numbers**
Dilzem SR 60    0018/0205
Dilzem SR 90    0018/0206
Dilzem SR 120   0018/0207

*Product licence holder:* Parke Davis & Company, Usk Road, Pontypool, NP4 0YH

## DILZEM* XL

**Presentation** Dilzem XL 120, 180, 240 (Sustained release capsules). Each capsule contains Diltiazem hydrochloride USP 120 mg, 180 mg and 240 mg respectively. The capsules are off-white in colour and overprinted with the product strength and the Elan Company logo.

### Uses
*Action:* Diltiazem has pharmacologic actions similar to those of other calcium channel blocking agents

such as nifedipine or verapamil. The principal physiologic action of diltiazem is to inhibit the transmembrane influx of extracellular calcium ions across the membranes of myocardial cells and vasular smooth muscle cells.

Calcium plays important roles in the excitation-contraction coupling processes of the heart and vascular smooth muscle cells and in the electrical discharge of the specialised conduction cells of the heart. The membranes of these cells contain numerous channels that carry a slow inward current and that are selective for calcium.

By inhibiting calcium influx, diltiazem inhibits the contractile processes of cardiac and vascular smooth muscle, thereby dilating the main coronary and systemic arteries. Dilation of systemic arteries by diltiazem results in a decrease in total peripheral resistance, a decrease in systemic blood pressure and a decrease in the afterload of the heart. The reduction in afterload, seen at rest and with exercise and its resultant decrease in myocardial oxygen consumption are though to be responsible for the beneficial effects of diltiazem in patients with chronic stable angina pectoris. In patients with Prinzmetal variant angina, inhibition of spontaneous and ergometrine-induced coronary artery spasm by diltiazem results in increased myocardial oxygen delivery.

*Indications:* Prophylaxis and treatment of angina pectoris. For the treatment of mild to moderate hypertension.

**Dosage and administration**
*Route of administration:* Oral.

*Adults: Hypertension:* The usual initial dose is one 180 mg capsule per day (corresponding to 180 mg of diltiazem hydrochloride once daily). Depending upon clinical response the dosage may be increased stepwise to 360 mg/day if required as a single daily dose.

*Angina pectoris:* The usual initial dose is one 180 mg capsule per day (corresponding to 180 mg of diltiazem hydrochloride once daily). Depending upon clinical response, the dosage may be increased stepwise to 360 mg/day if required, as a single daily dose.

*Elderly patients and those with renal or hepatic impairment:* Dosage should commence at the lower level of 120 mg once daily and be increased slowly. Do not increase the dose if the heart rate falls below 50 beats per minute.

*Children:* This product is not recommended for use in children.

**Contra-indications, warnings, etc** *Contra-indications:* (1) Use in women of child-bearing potential. (2) Concomitant administration of dantrolene infusion due to the risk of ventricular fibrillation. (3) Shock. (4) Acute cardiac infarct with complications (bradycardia, severe hypotension, left heart insufficiency). (5) Bradycardia (pulse rate, at rest, of less than 50 beats per minute), hypotension (less than 90 mm Hg systole), second or third degree heart block or sick sinus syndrome except in the presence of a functioning ventricular pacemaker. (6) Atrial fibrillation / flutter and simultaneous presence of a WPW (Wolff-Parkinson-White) syndrome (increased risk of triggering a ventricular tachycardia). (7) Manifest myocardial insufficiency. (8) Left ventricular failure with stasis. (9) Hypersensitivity to diltiazem or any of the excipients.

*Use in pregnancy and lactation:* Diltiazem must not be taken during pregnancy as experimental studies have shown indications of teratogenicity. There is no experience of its effects in humans. As diltiazem is known to enter the breast milk and there is no experience of possible effects in infants, infants should be weaned if treatment of the mother with diltiazem is necessary.

*Adverse effects:* In studies carried out to date, serious adverse reactions with diltiazem have been rare; however, it should be recognised that patients with impaired ventricular function and cardiac conduction abnormalities have usually been excluded from these studies.

In 900 patients with hypertension, the most common adverse effects were oedema (9%), headache (8%), dizziness (6%), asthenia (5%), sinus bradycardia (3%), flushing (3%) and first degree AV block (3%). Only oedema and perhaps bradycardia were dose related. The most common adverse events (>1%) observed in clinical studies of over 2100 angina and hypertensive patients receiving diltiazem were oedema (5.4%), headache (4.5%), dizziness (3.4%), asthenia (2.8%), first degree AV block (1.8%), flushing (1.7%), nausea (1.6%), bradycardia (1.5%) and rash (1.5%). Less common adverse events have included the following: *Cardiovascular:* angina, arrhythmia, AV block (second or third degree), congestive heart failure, hypotension, palpitations, syncope. *Nervous system:* amnesia, depression, gait abnormality, hallucinations, insomnia, nervousness, paraesthesia, personality change, somnolence, tinnitus, tremor. *Gastro-intestinal:* anorexia, constipation, diarrhoea, dyspepsia, mild elevations of alkaline phosphatase, SGOT, SGPT and LDH (see *Precautions and warnings*), vomiting, weight increase, gingivitis. *Dermatologic:* Petechiae, pruritus, photosensitivity, urticaria. Allergic skin reactions including erythema multiforme, vasculitis, lymphadenopathy and eosinophilia have been observed in isolated cases. Dermatological events may be transient and may disappear despite continued use of diltiazem. Should a dermatologic reaction persist, the drug should be discontinued. *Other:* amblyopia, CK elevation, dyspnoea, epistaxis, eye irritation, hyperglycaemia, nasal congestion, nocturia, osteoarticular pain, polyuria, sexual difficulties.

*Precautions and warnings:* Capsules should not be sucked or chewed.

The use of diltiazem hydrochloride in diabetic patients may require adjustment of their control.

The product should be used with caution in patients with hepatic dysfunction. Abnormalities of liver function may occur during therapy. Very occasional reports of abnormal liver function have been received, these reactions have been reversible upon discontinuation of therapy.

First degree AV block or prolonged PR interval. Dilzem prolongs AV node refractory periods without significantly prolonging sinus node recovery time, except in patients with sick sinus syndrome. This effect may rarely result in abnormally slow heart rates (particularly in patients with sick sinus syndrome) or second- or third- degree AV block (see Interactions section for information concerning beta-blockers and digitalis).

Mild bradycardia.

Patients with reduced left ventricular function.

Renally impaired patients.

As with any drug given over prolonged periods, laboratory parameters should be monitored at regular intervals.

*Interactions:* Diltiazem undergoes biotransformation by cytochrome P-450 mixed function oxidase. Coadministration with other agents which follow the same route of biotransformation may result in competitive inhibition of metabolism.

Diltiazem hydrochloride should only be administered with great care to patients receiving concurrent treatment with antihypertensives or other hypotensive agents including halogenated anaesthetics or drugs with moderate protein binding.

Diltiazem hydrochloride will not protect against the effects of withdrawal of beta-adrenoceptor blocking agents, nor the rebound effects seen with various antihypertensives. Combination with beta-adrenoceptor blockers having a significant 'first pass' loss, eg. propanolol may require a decrease in their dose and may lead to bradycardia. There may be an additive effect when used with drugs which may induce bradycardia or with other antihypertensives.

Concomitant $H_2$ antagonist therapy may increase diltiazem blood levels.

Diltiazem may affect the blood levels of concomitant carbamazepine, theophylline, cyclosporin and digoxin. Careful attention should therefore be given to signs of overdosage. If necessary, the levels should be determined and the dose of carbamazepine, theophylline, cyclosporin or digoxin reduced if necessary. Patients receiving beta-blockers, diuretics, ACE inhibitors or other antihypertensive agents should be regularly monitored. Use with alpha blockers should be strictly monitored.

The simultaneous administration of diltiazem with drugs such as beta-blockers, antiarrythmics or heart glycosides may cause a greater degree of AV blocking, reduce the heart rate or induce a hypotensive effect.

Intravenous administration of beta-blockers should be discontinued during therapy with diltiazem.

Anaesthetists should be warned that a patient is on a calcium antagonist. The depression of cardiac contractility, conductivity and automaticity as well as the vascular dilation associated with anaesthetics may be potentiated by calcium channel blockers. When used concomitantly, anaesthetics and calcium channel blockers should be titrated carefully.

There have been reports in the literature of diltiazem interactions with warfarin, rifampicin and lithium.

*Overdosage:* Experience of overdosage in man is limited but cases of spontaneous recovery have been reported. However, it is recommended that patients with suspected overdose, should be placed under observation in a coronary care unit with facilities available for treatment of any possible hypotension and conduction disturbances that may occur.

Most patients suffering from overdosage of diltiazem become hypotensive within 8 hours of ingestion. With bradycardia and first to third degree atrioventricular block also developing cardiac arrest may ensue. Hyperglycaemia is also a recognised complication. The elimination half-life of diltiazem after overdosage is estimated to be about 5.5-10.2 hours. If a patient presents early after overdose, gastric lavage should be performed and activated charcoal administered to reduce diltiazem absorption.

Hypotension should be corrected with plasma expanders, intravenous calcium gluconate and inotropic agents (dopamine, dobutamine or isoprenaline), symptomatic bradycardia and high grade AV block may respond to atropine, isoprenaline or occasionally cardiac pacing which may be useful if cardiac standstill occurs.

**Pharmaceutical precautions** Store in a dry place at a temperature not exceeding 25°C.

**Legal category** POM.

**Package quantities** Securitainer containing 30 Dilzem XL 120 mg, 180 mg or 240 mg capsules

**Further information** None

**Product licence numbers**

| | |
|---|---|
| Dilzem XL 120 | 0018/0216 |
| Dilzem XL 180 | 0018/0217 |
| Dilzem XL 240 | 0018/0218 |

*Product licence holder:* Parke Davis & Company, Usk Road, Pontypool, NP4 0YH

## ERYMAX*

**Presentation** Each capsule contains 250 mg Erythromycin PhEur orange and white enteric coated pellets in a size 0 capsule with an opaque orange cap and a clear orange body, radially imprinted Erymax 250 mg on each capsule half.

**Uses** Erythromycin is an antibiotic effective in the treatment of bacterial disease caused by susceptible organisms.

Examples of its use are in the treatment of upper and lower respiratory tract infections of mild to moderate severity; skin and soft tissue infections including pustular acne.

Erythromycin is usually active against the following organisms *in vitro* and in clinical infection: *Streptococcus pyogenes; Alpha haemolytic streptococci; Staphylococcus aureus; Streptococcus pneumoniae; Mycoplasma pneumoniae; Treponema pallidum; Corynebacterium diphtheriae; Corynebacterium minutissimum; Entamoeba histolytica; Listeria monocytogenes; Neisseria gonorrhoeae; Bordetella pertussis; Legionella pneumophila; Haemophilus influenzae; Chlamydia trachomatis, Propionibacterium acnes.*

**Dosage and administration** Oral

*Adults:* 250 mg every six hours – before or with meals. 500 mg every twelve hours may be given if desired; b.i.d. dosage should not be used if dosage exceeds one gram.

See below for dosage recommendations for specific indications.

*Elderly (over 65 years):* As for adults.

*Children:* 30-50 mg/kg/day in divided doses given every six hours or twice daily. For the treatment of more severe infections, this dose may be doubled; elevated doses should be given every six hours. The drug should be given before or with meals. This product may be given to children of any age group who can swallow the intact capsules.

*Streptococcal Infections: For active infection*–a full therapeutic dose is given for at least ten days.

*For continuous prophylaxis* against recurrences of streptococcal infections in patients with evidence of rheumatic heart disease, the dose is 250 mg b.i.d.

*For the prevention of bacterial endocarditis* in patients with valvular disease scheduled for dental or surgical procedures of the upper respiratory tract, adult dose is 1.0 gram (children 20 mg/kg) 2 hours before surgery. Following surgery, 500 mg for adults (children 10 mg/kg) orally every six hours for 8 doses.

*Primary syphilis* 30-40 grams given in divided doses over a period of 10-15 days.

*Intestinal amoebiasis* 250 mg four times daily for 10 to 14 days for adults: 30 to 50 mg/kg/day in divided doses for 10 to 14 days for children.

*Legionnaires' disease* 1–4 g daily until clinical signs and symptoms indicate a clinical cure. Treatment may be prolonged.

*Pertussis* 30-50 mg/kg/day given in divided doses for 5–14 days, depending upon eradication of a positive culture.

*Acne* Initially, 250 mg twice daily, which may be reduced to a maintenance dose of 250 mg once daily after one month according to response.

**Contra-indications, warnings, etc**
*Contra-indications:* Erymax is contraindicated in patients with known hypersensitivity to erythromycin. Erythromycin is contraindicated with either astemizole or terfenadine.

*Precautions and warnings:* In patients with impaired hepatic function, liver function should be monitored, since a few reports of hepatic dysfunction have been received in patients taking erythromycin as the estolate, base, or stearate. Extended administration requires regular evaluation, particularly of liver function. Therapy should be discontinued if significant hepatic dysfunction occurs.

Prolonged use of erythromycin has caused overgrowth of nonsusceptible bacteria or fungi; this is a rare occurrence.

*Use in pregnancy:* Like all drugs, erythromycin should be used in pregnancy only when clearly indicated. Erythromycin crosses the placental barrier.

Nursing mothers – erythromycin is excreted in human milk and should be used in lactating women only if clearly needed.

*Drug interactions:* Concomitant administration of erythromycin and digoxin has been reported to result in elevated digoxin serum levels.

The use of erythromycin in patients taking concurrent drugs which are metabolised by the cytochrome P450 system may be associated with elevated serum levels of these other drugs.

Concomitant use of erythromycin with terfenadine or astemizole is likely to result in an enhanced risk of cardiotoxicity with these drugs. The concomitant use of erythromycin with either astemizole or terfenadine is therefore contraindicated.

There have been reports of interactions of erythromycin with cyclosporin, hexobarbital and phenytoin.

In a few patients receiving high doses of theophylline, concomitant use of erythromycin has caused increase of serum theophylline levels and signs of toxicity.

Erythromycin administration in patients receiving carbamazepine has been reported to cause increased serum levels of carbamazepine with subsequent development of signs of carbamazepine toxicity.

There have been reports of increased anticoagulant effects when erythromycin and oral anticoagulants were used concomitantly.

There are reports that ischaemic reactions may occur when erythromycin is given concurrently with ergotamine containing drugs.

Erythromycin should be used with caution if administered concomitantly with lincomycin, clindamycin or chloramphenicol, as competitive inhibition may occur.

The concomitant use of erythromycin with alfentanil can significantly inhibit the clearance of alfentanil and may increase the risk of prolonged or delayed respiratory depression.

Patients receiving concomitant lovastatin and erythromycin should be carefully monitored as cases of rhabdomyolysis have been reported in seriously ill patients.

*Side-effects:* Serious allergic reaction, including anaphylaxis, has been reported. Nausea and abdominal discomfort can occur at elevated doses; diarrhoea and vomiting are less common. Hepatotoxicity: There have been reports of hepatic dysfunction, with or without jaundice, occurring in patients receiving erythromycin products due to combined cholestatic and hepatocellular injury although less commonly than with erythromycin estolate.

Superinfections including pseudomembranous colitis have been occasionally reported to occur in association with erythromycin therapy.

Transient hearing disturbances and deafness have been reported with doses of erythromycin usually greater than 4 g daily, and usually given intravenously.

There have been isolated reports of transient central nervous system side effects including confusion, hallucinations, seizures, and vertigo; however, a cause and effect relationship has not been established.

*Overdosage:* Nausea, vomiting and diarrhoea have been reported.

*Treatment:* Gastric lavage and general supportive therapy. Erythromycin is not removed by peritoneal dialysis or haemodialysis.

**Pharmaceutical precautions** Store below 25°C. Protect from moisture and light.

**Legal category** POM.

**Package quantities** Blister packs of 30 or 100 capsules

**Further information** Nil

**Product licence number** 0018/0133

*Product licence holder:* Parke Davis & Company, Usk Road, Pontypool, NP4 0YH

## ERYMIN* SUSPENSION

**Qualitative and quantitative composition** Erythromycin 250 mg/5 ml as erythromycin ethylsuccinate.

**Pharmaceutical form** Oral suspension.

**Clinical particulars**
*Therapeutic indications:* Erythromycin is an antibiotic effective in the treatment of bacterial disease caused by susceptible organisms.

Examples of its use are in the treatment of upper and lower respiratory tract infections of mild to moderate severity; skin and soft tissue infections including pustular acne. Erythromycin is usually active against the following organisms in vitro and in clinical infection: *Streptoccus pyogenes;* Alpha haemolytic streptococci; *Staphylococcus aureus; Streptococcus pneumoniae; Mycoplasma pneumoniae; Treponema pallidum; Corynebacterium diphtheriae; Corynebacterium minutissimum; Entamoeba histolytica; Listeria monocytogenes; Neisseria gonorrhoeae; Bordetella pertussis; Legionella pneumophila; Haemophilus influenzae; Chlamydia trachomatis, Propionibacterium acnes.*

*Posology and method of administration:* The suspension is administered orally. The normal recommended dosage range is:

Children up to 2 years: 125 mg (2.5 ml) twice daily.
Children 2 to 8 years: 250 mg (5 ml) twice daily.
Adults and children over 8 years: 625 mg (12.5 ml) twice daily.

For severe infections doses may be doubled.

Erymin should be taken fasted or more than one hour before or after eating.

*Contra-indications:* Erymin is contra-indicated in patients with known hypersensitivity to erythromycin. Erythromycin is contra-indicated with either astemizole or terfenadine.

*Special warnings and special precautions for use:* In patients with impaired hepatic function, liver function should be monitored, since a few reports of hepatic dysfunction have been received in patients taking erythromycin as the estolate, base or stearate. Extended administration requires regular evaluation, particularly of liver function. Therapy should be discontinued if significant hepatic dysfunction occurs. Prolonged use of erythromycin has caused overgrowth of nonsusceptible bacteria or fungi; this is a rare occurrence.

*Interactions:* Concomitant administration of erythromycin and digoxin has been reported to result in elevated digoxin serum levels. The use of erythromycin in patients taking concurrent drugs which are metabolised by the cytochrome P450 system may be associated with elevated serum levels of these other drugs.

Concomitant use of erythromycin with terfenadine or astemizole is likely to result in an enhanced risk of cardiotoxicity with these drugs. The concomitant use of erythromycin with either astemizole or terfenadine is therefore contra-indicated.

There have been reports of interactions of erythromycin with cyclosporin, hexobarbital and phenytoin.

In a few patients receiving high doses of theophylline, concomitant use of erythromycin has caused increase of serum theophylline levels and signs of toxicity.

Erythromycin administration in patients receiving carbamazepine has been reported to cause increased serum levels of carbamazepine with subsequent development of signs of carbamazepine toxicity.

There have been reports of increased anticoagulant effects when erythromycin and oral anticoagulants were used concomitantly.

There are reports that ischaemic reactions may occur when erythromycin is given concurrently with ergotamine containing drugs.

Erythromycin should be used with caution if administered concomitantly with lincomycin, clindamycin or chloramphenicol as competitive inhibition may occur.

The concomitant use of erythromycin with alfentanil can significantly inhibit the clearance of alfentanil and may increase the risk of prolonged or delayed respiratory depression.

Patients receiving concomitant lovastatin and erythromycin should be carefully monitored as cases of rhabdomyolysis have been reported in seriously ill patients.

*Pregnancy and lactation:* Like all drugs, erythromycin should be used in pregnancy only when clearly indicated. Erythromycin crosses the placental barrier. Erythromycin is excreted in human milk and should be used in lactating women only if clearly needed.

*Effects on ability to drive and use machinery:* Not applicable.

*Undesirable effects:* Serious allergic reactions, including anaphylaxis, have been reported. Nausea and abdominal discomfort can occur at elevated doses; diarrhoea and vomiting are less common. Hepatotoxicity: There have been reports of hepatic dysfunction with or without jaundice, occurring in patients receiving erythromycin products due to combined cholestatic and hepatocellular injury although less commonly than with erythromycin estolate.

Superinfections including pseudomembranous colitis have been occasionally reported to occur in association with erythromycin therapy. Transient hearing disturbances and deafness have been reported with doses of erythromycin usually greater than 4 g daily, and usually given intravenously. There have been isolated reports of transient central nervous system side effects including confusion, hallucinations, seizures and vertigo; however, a cause and effect relationship has not been established.

*Overdose:* Nausea, vomiting, loss of hearing and diarrhoea have been reported.

*Treatment:* Gastric lavage and general supportive therapy. Erythromycin is not removed by peritoneal dialysis or haemodialysis.

**Pharmacological properties**
*Pharmacodynamic properties:* Erythromycin is a macrolide antibiotic with a macrocyclic lactone nucleus containing 14 atoms substituted by sugars via glycoside bonds. Its mechanism of actions involves inhibition of microsomal protein synthesis in susceptible organisms by inhibiting the translocation process. Specific binding to the 50S subunit or 70S ribosome occurs in these organisms, but there is no binding to the stable 80S mammalian ribosome.

Erythromycin is effective against many gram positive bacteria, some gram negative bacteria and mycoplasmas and chlamydia. It is particularly effective against streptococci. Its action is bacteriostatic or bactericidal depending on the organism and the concentrations achieved. Recommended dose range is from 1 to 4 g daily, depending on the severity of infection. Erythromycin resistance due to mutation is uncommon and unstable. In staphylococci continuously exposed to sub-inhibitory concentrations it may be extended to other macrolides as well. Constitutive resistance may also be generalised to include lincosamides. The effects of erythromycin in combination with other antibiotics are unpredictable. The synthesis of penicillinase is variably affected, resulting in synergy or antagonism with susceptible β-lactams. The listericidal effects of penicillins, rifampicin and gentamicin are antagonised. Erythromycin is synergistic with sulphonamides against *Haemophilus influenzae.*

*Pharmacokinetic properties:* Erythromycin is incompletely, but adequately absorbed in the upper part of the small intestine. Peak concentrations occur 1 to 4 hours after ingestion and vary from 0.3 to 0.5 mcg/ml after 250 mg erythromycin base, and 0.3 to 1.9 mcg/ml after 500 mg. Various factors improve absorption. Peak concentrations after 500 mg are approximately 1.5 mcg/ml. The ester is a pro-drug for the active base, levels of which will be at 0.5 mcg/ml after 500 mg, 1 to 2 hours post dosing.

Erythromycin readily diffuses into intercellular fluids, but does not cross the blood/brain barrier into the brain and CSF. Tissue levels may be high, and it is difficult to correlate tissue levels with plasma levels, given the difficulty measuring the latter. Erythromycin base is 70–75% protein bound in plasma. Erythromycin is concentrated in the liver and excreted in active form in the bile. Only 2–5% of orally dosed erythromycin is excreted in the urine, in active form. The plasma half life is short, approximately 1.6 hours. This can be prolonged in patients with anuria, but dose reduction in such circumstances has not been recommended. It is not removed significantly by haemodialysis or peritoneal dialysis.

In Erymin, erythromycin as the ethylsuccinate ester is coated with a polymer prior to suspension in an oil-based vehicle. These formulation factors are believed to enhance the stability of the active ingredient, particularly in the acid environment of the stomach. In pharmacokinetic analyses, blood levels of erythromycin free base and the ethylsuccinate ester were measured. Free base was measured by differential extraction, with total erythromycin activity measured by the traditional microbiological assays. In these measurements, ethylsuccinate levels were estimated by the difference of free base from total erythromycin activity. A corroborative HPLC assay was also used to measure base and ester levels simultaneously. Both the free base and ethylsuccinate moieties showed good evidence of linearity of dose.

Steady state comparisons of Erymin 250 mg/5 ml against a standard erythromycin reference product 500 mg/5 ml demonstrated Erymin to be superbioavailable with respect to the comparator at a ratio of 1.6 to 1 respectively. As expected for the higher dose of erythromycin in the reference product the $C_{max}$ values are higher ($0.53 \pm 0.22$ for the reference versus Erymin $0.40 \pm 0.25$) with correspondingly faster $T_{max}$ values for the reference ($1.14 \pm 0.66$) versus Erymin ($1.72 \pm 0.67$). This data was consistently demonstrated for erythromycin free base, as described above, and the ethylsuccinate ester. ($C_{max}$ of $1.86 \pm 0.95$ versus $1.53 \pm 0.47$ and $T_{max}$ of $0.86 \pm 0.59$ versus $1.50 \pm 0.57$).

These pharmacokinetic parameters clearly demonstrate the sustained delivery characteristic for the formulation.

Dosing with high fat meals was found to decrease the rate and extent of absorption of Erymin whereas no effect on bioavailability was found when dosing with a standard meal.

## Pharmaceutical particulars

*List of excipients:* Ethylcellulose; citric acid; soya oil; aspartame; colloidal silicon dioxide; mixed tocopherols (Tenox GT-1); banana flavour; Hexane; Cyclohexane*.

* These ingredients are used in the method of manufacture but are not present in the final presentation.

*Incompatibilities:* Not applicable.

*Shelf life:* The proposed shelf life of the product is 2 years.

*Special precautions for storage:* Store below 25°C. Protect from moisture and light.

*Nature and contents of the container:* Erymin is packaged in 70 ml round amber soda glass bottles. Starter packs of 15 ml are also available.

*Instructions for use/handling:* Erymin should be taken fasting (on an empty stomach), or more than one hour before or one hour after eating. Shake well before use.

**Marketing authorisation number** PL 10038/0019.

**Date of approval/revision of SPC** July 1996.

**Legal category** POM.

# PONSTAN * CAPSULES
# PONSTAN* PAEDIATRIC SUSPENSION

**Presentation** *Capsules:* An off-white powder in a No 1 hard gelatin capsule with an ivory opaque body and an aqua-blue opaque cap, radially printed 'PONSTAN 250'.
*Composition:* Each capsule contains mefenamic acid BP 250 mg.
*Paediatric Suspension:* An off-white suspension with typical aroma and taste.
*Composition:* Each 5 ml suspension contains mefenamic acid BP 50 mg.

## Uses

*Action:* Mefenamic acid is a non-steroidal anti-inflammatory agent with analgesic properties, and a demonstrable antipyretic effect. It has been shown to inhibit prostaglandin activity.

*Indications:* 1. As an anti-inflammatory analgesic for the symptomatic relief of rheumatoid arthritis (including Still's Disease), osteoarthritis and pain including muscular, traumatic and dental pain, headaches of most aetiology, post-operative and post-partum pain; pyrexia in children.
2. Primary dysmenorrhoea.
3. Menorrhagia due to dysfunctional causes and presence of an IUD when other pelvic pathology has been ruled out.

## Dosage and administration Oral

*Adults:* 2 capsules (500 mg) three times daily.
In dysmenorrhoea to be administered at the onset of menstrual pain and continued according to the judgement of the physician.
In menorrhagia to be administered on the first day of excessive bleeding and continued according to the judgement of the physician.

*Elderly (over 65 years):* As for adults. Whilst no pharmacokinetic or clinical studies specific to the elderly have been undertaken with Ponstan, it has been used at normal dosage in trials which included many elderly patients.
Ponstan should be used with caution in elderly patients suffering from dehydration and renal disease.
Non-oliguric renal failure and proctocolitis have been reported mainly in elderly patients who have not discontinued Ponstan after the development of diarrhoea.

*Children:* It is recommended that children under 12 years of age should be given PONSTAN Paediatric Suspension (50 mg/5 ml) in the following dosage regime:
Infants over 6 months: 25 mg/kg of bodyweight daily in divided doses, or,
6 months to 1 year: one 5 ml spoonful
2 years to 4 years: two 5 ml spoonfuls
5 years to 8 years: three 5 ml spoonfuls
9 years to 12 years: four 5 ml spoonfuls

Dose may be repeated as necessary, up to three times daily.
Apart from the treatment of Still's Disease, therapy should not be continued for longer than 7 days in children.
Do not exceed the stated dose.

## Contra-indications, warnings, etc

*Contra-indications:* Patients hypersensitive to mefenamic acid. Mefenamic acid is contra-indicated in inflammatory bowel disease and in patients suffering from peptic and/or intestinal ulceration and in patients with renal or hepatic impairment.
Because the potential exists for cross-sensitivity to aspirin or other non-steroidal anti-inflammatory drugs, mefenamic acid should not be given to patients in whom these drugs induce symptoms of bronchospasm, allergic rhinitis, or urticaria.

*Precautions and warnings:* Safety in pregnancy has not been established and because of the effects of drugs in this class on the foetal cardiovascular system, the use of mefenamic acid in pregnant women is not recommended.
Trace amounts of mefenamic acid may be present in breast milk and transmitted to the nursing infant. Therefore, mefenamic acid should not be taken by nursing mothers.
Patients suffering from dehydration and renal disease, particularly the elderly.
Concurrent therapy with other plasma protein binding drugs may necessitate a modification in dosage. In the case of anticoagulants the dose of the anticoagulant may need to be reduced.
Concurrent administration of mefenamic acid with oral anticoagulant drugs requires careful prothrombin time monitoring.
The following interactions have been reported with NSAIDs but have not necessarily been associated with Ponstan Capsules or Suspension.
*Antihypertensives and diuretics:* a reduction in antihypertensive and diuretic effect have been observed.
*Cardiac glycosides:* NSAIDs may exacerbate cardiac failure and increase in plasma cardiac glycoside levels may occur when renal function is affected.
*Lithium and methotrexate:* Elimination of these drugs can be reduced.
*Cyclosporin:* The risk of nephrotoxicity of cyclosporin may be increased with NSAIDs.
*Mifepristone:* NSAIDs should not be taken for 8-12 days after mifepristone administraion, NSAIDs can reduce the effects of mifepristone.
*Corticosteroids:* Concomitant use may increase the risk of gastrointestinal bleeding.
*Quinolone antibiotics:* Animal data indicates that NSAIDs can increase the risk of convulsions associated with quinolone antibiotics. Patients taking NSAIDs and quinolones may have an increased risk of developing convulsions.
*Other analgesics:* Concomitant use of two or more NSAIDs should be avoided.
In dysmenorrhoea and menorrhagia lack of response should alert the physician to investigate other causes.
Caution should be exercised when treating patients suffering from epilepsy.

*Side-effects:* Diarrhoea occasionally occurs following the use of mefenamic acid. Although this may occur soon after starting treatment, it may also occur after several months of continuous use. The diarrhoea has been investigated in some patients who have continued this drug in spite of its continued presence. These patients were found to have associated proctocolitis. If diarrhoea does develop the drug should be withdrawn immediately and this patient should not receive mefenamic acid again.
Skin rashes have been observed following the administration of mefenamic acid and the occurrence of a rash is a definite indication to withdraw medication. There have been rare reports of Stevens-Johnson syndrome, Lyell's syndrome (toxic epidermal necrolysis) and erythema multiforme.
Serious gastrointestinal toxicity such as bleeding, ulceration and perforation can occur at any time with or without warning symptoms, in patients treated chronically with NSAID therapy. GI bleeding has been associated with a previous history of peptic ulcer, smoking and alcohol use.
Elderly or debilitated patients seem to tolerate ulceration or bleeding less well than other individuals and most spontaneous reports of fatal GI events are in this population.
As with other prostaglandin inhibitors allergic glomerulonephritis has occurred occasionally. There have also been reports of acute interstitial nephritis with haematuria and proteinuria and occasionally nephrotic syndrome. Non-oliguric renal failure has been reported on a few occasions in elderly patients with dehydration usually from diarrhoea. Toxicity has been seen in patients with pre-renal conditions leading to a reduction in renal blood flow or blood volume. Patients at greatest risk of this reaction are those with impaired renal function, heart failure, liver dysfunction, those taking diuretics and the elderly. The drug should not be administered to patients with significantly impaired renal function. It has been suggested that the recovery is more rapid and complete than with other forms of analgesic induced renal impairment, with discontinuation of NSAID therapy being typically followed by recovery to the pre-treatment state.
Thrombocytopenic purpura has been reported with mefenamic acid. In some cases reversible haemolytic anaemia has occurred. Temporary lowering of the white blood cell count which may have been due to mefenamic acid has been reported. Rarely eosinophilia, agranulocytosis, pancytopenia and aplastic anaemia have been reported. Blood studies should therefore be carried out during long term administration and the appearance of any dyscrasia is an indication to discontinue therapy..
Bronchospasm and/or urticaria may be precipitated in patients suffering from, or with a previous history of, bronchial asthma or allergic disease.
Borderline elevations of one or more liver function tests may occur in some patients receiving mefenamic acid therapy. A patient with symptoms and/or signs suggesting liver dysfunction, or in whom an abnormal liver test has occurred, should have their therapy discontinued. Patients on prolonged therapy should be kept under surveillance with particular attention to liver dysfunction. Pancreatitis and cholestatic jaundice have also been reported.

*Other adverse reactions:* Nausea, vomiting, abdominal pain, headache, facial oedema, laryngeal oedema and anaphylaxis. Drowsiness, dizziness, abnormal vision, palpitations, glucose intolerance in diabetic patients and hypotension have rarely been reported.
*Note:* A positive reaction in certain tests for bile in the urine of patients receiving mefenamic acid has been demonstrated to be due to the presence of the drug and its metabolites and not to the presence of bile.

*Overdosage (including treatment):* Gastric lavage in the conscious patient and intensive supportive therapy where necessary. Vital functions should be monitored and supported. Activated charcoal has been shown to be a powerful adsorbent for mefenamic acid and its metabolites. Studies in experimental animals and human volunteers have shown that a 5 to 1 ratio of charcoal to mefenamic acid results in considerable suppression of absorption of the drug. Haemodialysis is of little value since mefenamic acid and its metabolites are firmly bound to plasma proteins. Overdose has led to fatalities.
Mefenamic acid has a tendency to induce tonic-clonic (grand mal) convulsions in overdose. Acute renal failure and coma have been reported with mefenamic acid overdose. It is important that the recommended dose is not exceeded and the regime adhered to since some reports have involved daily dosages under 3 g.

**Pharmaceutical precautions** Capsules and Suspension: Store at a temperature not exceeding 30°C.

**Legal category** POM.

**Package quantities** Capsules: available in packs of 6, 10, 42, 100.
Suspension: available in bottles of 125 ml.

**Further information** Nil

**Product licence numbers**
Ponstan Capsules 0018/0094R
Ponstan Paediatric Suspension 0018/5025R

*Product licence holder:* Parke Davis & Company, Usk Road, Pontypool, NP4 0YH.

# PONSTAN* FORTE

**Qualitative and quantitative composition** Mefenamic Acid BP 500 mg

**Pharmaceutical form** Yellow film coated tablet, inscribed 'Ponstan Forte' on one side.

## Clinical particulars

*Therapeutic indications:* Mefenamic acid is a nonsteroidal anti-inflammatory agent with analgesic properties, and a demonstrable antipyretic effect. It has been shown to inhibit prostaglandin activity.
*Indications:* 1. As an anti-inflammatory analgesic for the symptomatic relief of rheumatoid arthritis (including Still's Disease), osteoarthritis and pain including muscular, traumatic and dental pain, headaches of most aetiology, post-operative and post-partum pain.
2. Primary dysmenorrhoea.
3. Menorrhagia due to dysfunctional causes and presence of an IUD when other pelvic pathology has been ruled out.

*Posology and method of administration:* Oral

*Adults:* 1 tablet (500 mg) three times daily.
In menorrhagia to be administered on the first day of excessive bleeding and continued according to the judgement of the physician.
In dysmenorrhoea to be administered at the onset of menstrual pain and continued according to the judgement of the physician.

*Elderly (over 65 years):* As for adults. Whilst no pharmacokinetic or clinical studies specific to the elderly have been undertaken with Ponstan Forte tablets, it has been used at normal dosage in trials which included many elderly patients.
Ponstan Forte tablets should be used with caution in elderly patients suffering from dehydration and renal disease. Non-oliguric renal failure and proctocolitis have been reported mainly in elderly patients

who have not discontinued Ponstan Forte tablets after the development of diarrhoea.

*Children:* It is recommended that children under 12 years of age should be given mefenamic acid paediatric suspension.

Do not exceed the stated dose.

*Contra-indications:* Patients hypersensitive to mefenamic acid.

Mefenamic acid is conta-indicated in inflammatory bowel disease and in patients suffering from peptic and/or intestinal ulceration and in patients with renal or hepatic impairment.

Because the potential exists for cross-sensitivity to aspirin or other nonsteroidal anti-inflammatory drugs, mefenamic acid should not be given to patients in whom these drugs induce symptoms of bronchospasm, allergic rhinitis or urticaria.

*Special warnings and special precautions for use:* Precaution should be taken in patients suffering from dehydration and renal disease, particularly the elderly.

In dysmenorrhoea and menorrhagia, lack of response should alert the physician to investigate other causes.

Caution should be exercised when treating patients suffering from epilepsy

*Interactions with other medicaments and other forms of interaction:* Concurrent therapy with other plasma protein binding drugs may necessitate a modification in dosage. In the case of anticoagulants the dose of the anticoagulant may need to be reduced.

Concurrent administration of mefenamic acid with oral anticoagulant drugs requires careful prothrombin time monitoring.

The following interactions have been reported with NSAIDs but have not necessarily been associated with Ponstan Forte Tablets.

*Antihypertensives and diuretics:* a reduction in antihypertensive and diuretic effect have been observed.

*Cardiac glycosides:* NSAIDs may exacerbate cardiac failure and increase in plasma cardiac glycoside levels may occur when renal function is affected.

*Lithium and methotrexate:* Elimination of these drugs can be reduced.

*Cyclosporin:* The risk of nephrotoxicity of cyclosporin may be increased with NSAIDs.

*Mifepristone:* NSAIDs should not be taken for 8-12 days after mifepristone administraion, NSAIDs can reduce the effects of mifepristone.

*Corticosteroids:* Concomitant use may increase the risk of gastrointestinal bleeding.

*Quinolone antibiotics:* Animal data indicates that NSAIDs can increase the risk of convulsions associated with quinolone antibiotics. Patients taking NSAIDs and quinolones may have an increased risk of developing convulsions.

*Other analgesics:* Concomitant use of two or more NSAIDs should be avoided.

*Use in pregnancy and lactation:* Safety in pregnancy has not been established, and because of the effects of drugs in this class on the foetal cardiovascular system, the use of mefenamic acid in pregnant women is not recommended.

Trace amounts of mefenamic acid may be present in breast milk and transmitted to the nursing infant. Therefore, mefenamic acid should not be taken by nursing mothers.

*Effects on ability to drive and use machines:* Drowsiness and dizziness have rarely been reported.

*Undesirable effects:* Diarrhoea occasionally occurs following the use of mefenamic acid. Although this may occur soon after starting treatment, it may also occur after several months of continuous use. The diarrhoea has been investigated in some patients who have continued this drug in spite of its continued presence. These patients were found to have associated proctocolitis. If diarrhoea does develop the drug should be withdrawn immediately and this patient should not receive mefenamic acid again.

Skin rashes have been observed following the administration of mefenamic acid and the occurrence of a rash is a definite indication to withdraw medication. There have been rare reports of Stevens-Johnson syndrome, Lyell's syndrome (toxic epidermal necrolysis) and erythema multiforme.

Serious gastrointestinal toxicity such as bleeding, ulceration, and perforation can occur at any time with or without warning symptoms, in patients treated chronically with NSAID therapy. GI bleeding has been associated with a previous history of peptic ulcer, smoking and alcohol use.

Elderly or debilitated patients seem to tolerate ulceration or bleeding less well than other individuals and most spontaneous reports of fatal GI events are in this population.

As with other prostaglandin inhibitors allergic glomerulonephritis has occurred occasionally. There have also been reports of acute interstitial nephritis with haematuria and proteinuria and ocassionally nephrotic syndrome. Non-oliguric renal failure has been reported on a few occasions in elderly patients with dehydration usually from diarrhoea. Toxicity has been seen in patients with pre-renal conditions leading to a reduction in renal blood flow or blood volume. Patients at greatest risk of this reaction are those with impaired renal function, heart failure, liver dysfunction, those taking diuretics and the elderly. The drug should not be administered to patients with significantly impaired renal function. It has been suggested that the recovery is more rapid and complete than with other forms of analgesic induced renal impairment, with discontinuation of NSAID therapy being typically followed by recovery to the pre-treatment state.

Thrombocytopenic purpura has been reported with mefenamic acid. In some cases reversible haemolytic anaemia has occurred. Temporary lowering of the white blood cell count which may have been due to mefenamic acid has been reported. Rarely eosinophilia, agranulocytosis, pancytopenia and aplastic anaemia have been reported. Blood studies should therefore be carried out during long term administration and the appearance of any dyscrasia is an indication to discontinue therapy.

Bronchospasm and/or urticaria may be precipitated in patients suffering from, or with a previous history of, bronchial asthma or allergic disease.

Borderline elevations of one or more liver function tests may occur in some patients receiving mefenamic acid therapy. A patient with symptoms and/or signs suggesting liver dysfunction, or in whom an abnormal liver test has occurred, should have their therapy discontinued. Patients on prolonged therapy should be kept under surveillance with particular attention to liver dysfunction. Pancreatitis and cholestatic jaundice have also been reported.

*Other adverse reactions:* nausea, vomiting, abdominal pain, headache, facial oedema, laryngeal oedema and anaphylaxis. Drowsiness, dizziness, abnormal vision, palpitations, glucose intolerance in diabetic patients and hypotension have rarely been reported.

*Note:* A positive reaction in certain tests for bile in the urine of patients receiving mefenamic acid has been demonstrated to be due to the presence of the drug and its metabolites and not to the presence of bile.

*Overdose:* Gastric lavage in the conscious patient and intensive supportive therapy where necessary. Vital functions should be monitored and supported. Activated charcoal has shown to be a powerful adsorbant for mefenamic acid and its metabolites. Studies in experimental animals and human volunteers have shown that a 5 to 1 ratio of charcoal to mefenamic acid results in considerable suppression of absorption of the drug. Haemodialysis is of little value since mefenamic acid and its metabolites are firmly bound to plasma proteins. Overdose has led to fatalities.

Mefenamic acid has a tendency to induce tonic-clonic (grand mal) convusions in overdose. Acute renal failure and coma have been reported with mefenamic acid overdose. It is important that the recommended dose is not exceeded and the regime adhered to since some reports have involved daily dosages under 3 g.

**Pharmacological properties**

*Pharmacodynamic properties:*
*Animal models:* Mefenamic acid is a non-steroidal anti-inflammatory drug (NSAID) with anti-inflammatory, analgesic and antipyretic properties.

Its anti-inflammatory effect was first established in the UV erythema model of inflammation. Further studies included inhibition of granulation tissue growth into subcutaneous cotton pellets in rats and carrageenin induced rat paw oedema tests.

Antipyretic activity was demonstrated in yeast-induced pyresis in rats. In this model its antipyretic activity was roughly equal to that of phenylbutazone and flufenamic acid, but less than that of indomethacin.

Analgesic activity was demonstrated in tests involving pain sensitivity of rats paws inflamed by brewers yeast. Mefenamic acid was less potent than flufenamic acid in this model.

Prostaglandins are implicated in a number of disease processes including inflammation, modulation of the pain response, dysmenorrhoea, menorrhagia and pyrexia.

In common with most NSAID's mefenamic acid inhibits the action of prostaglandin synthetase (cyclo-oxygenase). This results in a reduction in the rate of prostaglandin synthesis and reduced prostaglandin levels.

The anti-inflammatory activity of NSAID's in the rat paw oedema test has been correlated with their ability to inhibit prostaglandin synthetase. When mefenamic acid is ranked in both these tests it falls between indomethacin and phenylbutazone and it is probable that inhibition of prostaglandin synthesis contributes to the pharmacological activity and clinical efficacy of mefenamic acid.

There is also considerable evidence that the fenamates inhibit the action of prostaglandins after they have been formed. They therefore both inhibit the synthesis and response to prostaglandins. This double blockade may well be important in their mode of action

*Pharmacokinetic properties:*
*Absorption and distribution:* Mefenamic acid is absorbed from the gastro-intestinal tract. Peak levels of 10 mg/l occur two hours after the administration of a 1 g oral dose to adults.

*Metabolism:* Mefenamic acid is extensively metabolised, first to A3 hydroxymethyl derivative (metabolite I) and then A3 carboxyl derivative (metabolite II). Both metabolites undergo secondary conjugation to form glucuronides.

*Elimination:* Fifty two percent of a dose is recovered from the urine, 6% as mefenamic acid, 25% as metabolite I and 21% as metabolite II. Assay of stools over a 3 day period accounted for 10-20% of the dose chiefly as unconjugated metabolite II.

The plasma levels of unconjugated mefenamic acid decline with a half life of approximately two hours.

*Preclinical safety data:* Preclinical safety data does not add anything of further significance to the prescriber.

**Pharmaceutical particulars**

*List of excipients:* Each tablet contains: Lactose, pregelatinised starch, maize starch, polyvidone, silicon dioxide, talc, magnesium stearate, croscarmellose sodium type A, sodium lauryl sulphate, purified water*, Opadry OY-LS-22808 (H.P.M.C. 2910 15cP, lactose, polyethylene glycol 4000, vanillin, E104, E110, E171), Opaglos AG7350 (purified water, beeswax white, carnauba wax yellow, polysorbate 20, sorbic acid).

* not detectable

*Incompatibilities:* None known.

*Shelf life:* 48 months.

*Special precautions for storage:* Store below 30°C.

*Nature and contents of container:* Amber polystyrene bottle with a high density polyethene anti-arthritic closure containing 100 capsules

*Instructions for use/handling:* Not applicable.

*Marketing authorisation holder:* Parke Davis & Company, Usk Road, Pontypool, NP4 0YH

**Marketing authorisation number**  0018/0234

**Date of approval/revision of SPC**  October 1996

**Legal category**  POM

*\*Trade Mark*

# Ethical Generics Ltd
West Point
46–48 West Street
Newbury
Berkshire RG14 1BD

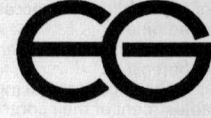

ethical
generics

## DIGENAC* XL 100

**Qualitative and quantitative composition** Each tablet contains Diclofenac Sodium BP 100 mg.

**Pharmaceutical form** White, circular, biconvex tablets embossed with DSR on one side and plain on reverse.

### Clinical particulars
*Therapeutic indications:* In the management of rheumatoid arthritis, osteoarthrosis, low back pain, acute musculo-skeletal disorders such as periarthritis (especially frozen shoulder), tendinitis, tenosynovitis, bursitis, sprains, strains and dislocations, relief of pain in fractures, ankylosing spondylitis, acute gout, psoriatic arthropathy, dysmenorrhoea, including associated menorrhagia.

In the management of post operative pain and inflammation in orthopaedic, dental and other minor surgery.

*Posology and method of administration*
*Adults:* The usual dosage is 100 mg (one tablet) daily.

*Elderly:* The pharmacokinetics of diclofenac sodium sustained release tablets are not impaired in elderly patients and the standard adult dose may be used. Non-steroidal anti-inflammatory drugs (NSAIDs) should be used with caution in older patients who generally are more prone to adverse reactions.

*Children:* Diclofenac sodium sustained release tablets are not recommended for use in children.

*Contra-indications:* Diclofenac is contra-indicated in patients with known hypersensitivity to the drug and in patients in whom asthma, rhinitis or urticaria is precipitated by aspirin or other NSAIDs. Diclofenac may precipitate allergic symptoms in aspirin-sensitive individuals who have no previous exposure to the drug. NSAIDs generally are contra-indicated in patients in whom urticaria, angioedema, bronchospasm, severe rhinitis or shock is precipitated by aspirin or other NSAIDs, although the drugs have occasionally been used in NSAID-sensitive patients who have undergone desensitisation.

*Special warnings and precautions for use:* Caution should be exercised in treating patients with a history of gastro-intestinal ulceration, haematemesis or melaena, ulcerative colitis, Crohn's disease, bleeding diathesis or haematological abnormalities.

Patients with severe hepatic, cardiac or renal insufficiency should be kept under close surveillance. All patients who are receiving long-term treatment with NSAIDs should be monitored as a precautionary measure (e.g. renal, hepatic function and blood counts).

The importance of prostaglandins in maintaining renal blood flow should be taken into account in patients with impaired cardiac or renal function, those being treated with diuretics or recovering from major surgery.

Patients who experience dizziness or other central nervous system disturbances while taking NSAIDs should refrain from driving or operating machinery. Diclofenac sodium, in common with other NSAIDs, can reversibly inhibit platelet aggregation.

*Interactions with other medicaments and other forms of interaction:* Diclofenac is bound practically completely to plasma albumin (99.7%) and consequently displacement reactions with high protein binding affinity must be borne in mind.

Diclofenac sodium may cause increased plasma concentrations of concurrently administered lithium and digoxin.

Pharmacodynamic studies have shown no potentiation of oral hypoglycaemic and anticoagulant drugs, but caution and adequate monitoring are nevertheless advised.

Caution should be exercised if NSAIDs and methotrexate are administered within 24 hours of each other, since NSAIDs may increase methotrexate plasma levels, resulting in increased toxicity.

Concomitant therapy with other systemic NSAIDs may increase the frequency of side-effects.

Various NSAIDs are liable to inhibit the activity of some diuretics. Concomitant treatment with potassium-sparing diuretics may be associated with increased serum potassium levels, hence serum potassium should be monitored.

*Pregnancy and lactation:* Diclofenac sodium should not be prescribed during pregnancy and lactation unless considered essential by the physician. Use of prostaglandin synthetase inhibitors may result in premature closure of the ductus arteriosus or uterine inertia; such drugs are therefore not recommended during the last trimester of pregnancy. Traces of the drug are detectable in breast milk but are not clinically significant.

*Effects on ability to drive and use machines:* None.

*Undesirable effects:* Side-effects include gastro-intestinal disturbances and bleeding, irritability, fluid retention, rash, hepatitis, renal dysfunction, anaphylaxis and rarely blood dyscrasias, bronchospasm and erythema multiforme.

*Overdose:* Management of acute poisoning with NSAIDs essentially consists of supportive and symptomatic measures. There is no typical clinical picture resulting from diclofenac sodium overdosage. The therapeutic measures to be taken are: absorption should be prevented as soon as possible after overdosage by means of gastric lavage and treatment with activated charcoal, supportive and symptomatic treatment should be given for complications such as hypotension, renal failure, convulsions, gastro-intestinal irritation and respiratory depression; specific therapies such as forced diuresis, dialysis or haemoperfusion are probably of no help in eliminating NSAIDs due to their high rate of protein binding and extensive metabolism.

### Pharmacological properties
*Pharmacodynamic properties:* Diclofenac sodium possesses analgesic, antipyretic and anti-inflammatory activities. It is an inhibitor of cyclo-oxygenase and its potency is substantially greater than that of indomethacin, naproxen or several other agents. In addition, diclofenac sodium appears to reduce intracellular concentrations of free arachidonate in leukocytes, perhaps by altering the release or uptake of the fatty acid.

*Pharmacokinetic properties:* Diclofenac sodium is rapidly absorbed from the gastro-intestinal tract but is subject to first-pass metabolism. Peak plasma concentrations occur about 6–8 hours after administration of the sustained release tablets when taken with a meal. Food and antacids decrease the rate but not the extent of absorption of diclofenac. The active substance is 99.7% bound to plasma proteins, mainly albumin. Diclofenac enters the synovial fluid and synovial fluid concentrations at steady state exceed plasma concentrations. Furthermore, elimination from synovial fluid is slower than from plasma. Diclofenac and its metabolites cross the placenta and traces of diclofenac have been found in the milk of lactating women. The half-life for the terminal elimination phase is 1–2 hours. Approximately 60% of the administered dose is excreted via the kidneys in the form of metabolites and less than 1% in unchanged form. About 30% of the dose is excreted via the bile in metabolised form. In patients with impaired renal function accumulation of diclofenac sodium has not been reported. However, the half-life of diclofenac may be prolonged in patients with severe renal impairment.

*Pre-clinical safety data:* No information submitted.

### Pharmaceutical particulars
*List of excipients:* Ethanol 96% BP*, Hydrogenated Vegetable Oil Type 1 USNF, Lactose BP, Magnesium Stearate BP, Povidone K30 PhEur, Talc BP.
* Not detected in the finished product.

*Incompatibilities:* No incompatibilities stated.

*Shelf life:* 3 years.

*Special precautions for storage:* Store below 25°C in a dry place.

*Nature and contents of container:*
(i) Blister packs consisting of PVC and aluminium foil. Pack sizes: 28 and 30 tablets.
(ii) Polypropylene tubes with low density polyethylene caps. Pack sizes: 56, 100, 250 and 500 tablets.
(iii) Scanstar containers: High density polyethylene containers with low density polyethylene screw caps. Pack sizes: 56, 100, 250 and 500 tablets.

*Instructions for use/handling:* No instructions stated for use/handling.

*Marketing authorisation holder:* Clonmel Healthcare Limited, Waterford Road, Clonmel, Co. Tipperary, Ireland.

**Marketing authorisation number** 0790/0109

**Date of approval/revision of SPC** June 1994.

**Legal category** POM.

## TENSIPINE* MR 10 and 20

**Qualitative and quantitative composition**
*Tensipine MR 20 tablets:* Pink-grey lacquered modified release tablets each containing 20 mg nifedipine, one side marked TMR and the reverse side marked 20.

*Tensipine MR 10 tablets:* Pink-grey lacquered modified release tablets each containing 10 mg nifedipine, one side marked TMR and the reverse side marked 10.

**Pharmaceutical form** Modified release tablets for oral administration.

### Clinical particulars
*Therapeutic indications:* For the prophylaxis of chronic stable angina pectoris and the treatment of hypertension.

*Posology and method of administration:*
*Adults:* The recommended starting dose of Tensipine MR is 10 mg every 12 hours swallowed with water with subsequent titration of dosage according to response. The dose may be adjusted to 40 mg every 12 hours.

Tensipine MR 10 permits titration of initial dosage. The recommended dose is one Tensipine MR 10 tablet (10 mg) every 12 hours.

Nifedipine is metabolised primarily by the liver therefore patients with liver dysfunction should be carefully monitored.

Patients with renal impairment should not require adjustment of dosage.

*Elderly patients:* The pharmacokinetics of nifedipine are altered in the elderly so that lower maintenance doses of nifedipine may be required compared to younger patients.

*Children:* Nifedipine is not recommended for use in children.

Treatment may be continued indefinitely.

*Contra-indications:* Tensipine MR should not be administered to patients with known hypersensitivity to nifedipine or other dihydropyridines because of the theoretical risk of cross-reaction, to women capable of child-bearing or to nursing mothers.

Tensipine MR should not be used in cardiogenic shock, clinically significant aortic stenosis, unstable angina, or during or within one month of a myocardial infarction.

Tensipine MR should not be used for the treatment of acute attacks of angina.

The safety of Tensipine MR in malignant hypertension has not been established.

Tensipine MR should not be used for secondary prevention of myocardial infarction.

Tensipine MR should not be administered concomitantly with rifampicin since effective plasma levels of nifedipine may not be achieved owing to enzyme induction.

*Special warnings and precautions for use:* Tensipine MR is not a beta-blocker and therefore gives no protection against the dangers of abrupt beta-blocker withdrawal; any such withdrawal should be by gradual reduction of the dose of beta-blocker preferably over 8–10 days.

Tensipine MR may be used in combination with beta-blocking drugs and other antihypertensive agents but the possibility of an additive effect resulting in postural hypotension should be borne in mind. Tensipine MR will not prevent possible rebound effects after cessation of other antihypertensive therapy.

Tensipine MR should be used with caution in

patients whose cardiac reserve is poor. Deterioration of heart failure has occasionally been observed with nifedipine.

Caution should be exercised in patients with severe hypotension.

Diabetic patients taking Tensipine MR may require adjustment of their control.

In dialysis patients with malignant hypertension and hypovolaemia, a marked decrease in blood pressure can occur.

*Interactions with other medicaments and other forms of interaction:* The antihypertensive effect of Tensipine MR may be potentiated by simultaneous administration of cimetidine.

When used in combination with nifedipine, serum quinidine levels have been shown to be suppressed regardless of dosage of quinidine.

The simultaneous administration of nifedipine and digoxin may lead to reduced digoxin clearance and hence an increase in the plasma digoxin level. Plasma digoxin levels should be monitored and, if necessary, the digoxin dose reduced.

Diltiazem decreases the clearance of nifedipine and hence increases plasma nifedipine levels. Therefore, caution should be taken when both drugs are used in combination and a reduction of the nifedipine dose may be necessary.

Nifedipine may increase the spectrophotometric values of urinary vanillylmandelic acid falsely. However, HPLC measurements are unaffected.

Rifampicin interacts with nifedipine (see Contra-indications).

As with other dihydropyridines, nifedipine should not be taken with grapefruit juice because bioavailability is increased.

*Pregnancy and lactation:* Tensipine MR is contraindicated in women capable of child-bearing and nursing mothers.

*Effects on ability to drive and use machines:* None known.

*Undesirable effects:* Ischaemic pain has been reported in a small proportion of patients within one to four hours of the introduction of Tensipine MR therapy. Although a 'steal' effect has not been demonstrated, patients experiencing this effect should discontinue Tensipine MR.

Most side-effects are consequences of the vasodilatory effects of nifedipine. Headache, flushing, tachycardia and palpitations may occur, most commonly in the early stages of treatment with nifedipine. Gravitational oedema not associated with heart failure or weight gain may also occur.

Paraesthesia, dizziness, lethargy and gastro-intestinal symptoms such as nausea and altered bowel habit occur occasionally.

There are reports of skin reactions such as rash, pruritus and urticaria.

Other less frequently reported side-effects include myalgia, tremor and visual disturbances.

Impotence may occur rarely.

Increased frequency of micturition may occur.

There are reports of gingival hyperplasia and, in older men on long-term therapy, gynaecomastia, which usually regress upon withdrawl of therapy.

Mood changes may occur rarely.

Side-effects which may occur in isolated cases are photosensitivity, exfoliative dermatitis, systemic allergic reactions and purpura. Usually, these regress after discontinuation of the drug.

Rare cases of hypersensitivity-type jaundice have been reported. In addition, disturbances of liver function such as intra-hepatic cholestasis may occur. These regress after discontinuation of therapy.

As with other sustained release dihydropyridines, exacerbation of angina pectoris may occur rarely at the start of treatment. The occurrence of myocardial infarction has been described although it is not possible to distinguish such as an event from the natural course of ischaemic heart disease.

*Overdose:*
*Clincial effects:* Reports of nifedipine overdosage are limited and symptoms are not necessarily dose-related.

Severe hypotension due to vasodilatation, and tachycardia or bradycardia are the most likely manifestations of overdose.

Metabolic disturbances include hyperglycaemia, metabolic acidosis and hypo- or hyperkalaemia.

Cardiac effects may include heart block, AV dissociation and asystole, and cardiogenic shock with pulmonary oedema.

Other toxic effects include nausea, vomiting, drowsiness, dizziness, confusion, lethargy, flushing, hypoxia and unconsciousness to the point of coma.

*Treatment:* As far as treatment is concerned, elimination of nifedipine and the restoration of stable cardiovascular conditions have priority.

After oral ingestion, gastric lavage is indicated, if necessary in combination with irrigation of the small intestine. Ipecacuanha should be given to children.

Elimination must be as complete as possible, including the small intestine, to prevent the otherwise inevitable subsequent absorption of the active substance. Activated charcoal should be given in 4-hourly doses of 25 g for adults, 10 g for children.

Blood pressure, ECG, central arterial pressure, pulmonary wedge pressure, urea and electrolytes should be monitored.

Hypotension as a result of cardiogenic shock and arterial vasodilatation should be treated with elevation of the feet and plasma expanders. If these measures are ineffective, hypotension may be treated with 10% calcium gluconate 10–20 ml intravenously over 5–10 minutes. If the effects are inadequate, the treatment can be continued, with ECG monitoring. In addition, beta-sympathomimetics may be given, e.g. isoprenaline 0.2 mg slowly i.v. or as a continuous infusion of 5 mcg/min. If an insufficient increase in blood pressure is achieved with calcium and isoprenaline, vasoconstricting sympathomimetics such as dopamine or noradrenaline should be administered. The dosage of these drugs should be determined by the patient's response.

Bradycardia may be treated with atropine, beta-sympathomimetics or a temporary cardiac pacemaker, as required.

Additional fluids should be administered with caution to avoid cardiac overload.

**Pharmacological properties**
*Pharmacodynamic properties*
*Mode of action:* Nifedipine is a specific and potent calcium antagonist. In hypertension, the main action of Tensipine MR is to cause peripheral vasodilatation and thus reduce peripheral resistance.

In angina, Tensipine MR reduces peripheral and coronary vascular resistance, leading to an increase in coronary blood flow, cardiac output and stroke volume, whilst decreasing after-load.

Additionally, nifedipine dilates submaximally both clear and atherosclerotic coronary arteries, thus protecting the heart against coronary artery spasm and improving perfusion to the ischaemic myocardium.

Nifedipine reduces the frequency of painful attacks and the ischaemic ECG changes irrespective of the relative contribution from coronary artery spasm or atherosclerosis.

Tensipine MR administered twice-daily provides 24-hour control of raised blood pressure. Tensipine MR causes reduction in blood pressure such that the percentage lowering is directly related to its initial level. In normotensive individuals, Tensipine MR has little or no effect on blood pressure.

*Pharmacokinetic properties:* Nifedipine is absorbed almost completely from the gastro-intestinal tract regardless of the oral formulation used and undergoes extensive metabolism in the liver to inactive metabolites, with less than 1% of the parent drug appearing unchanged in the urine. The rate of absorption determines the drug's apparent elimination. The terminal elimination half-life of the modified release formulation is 6–11 hours.

After enteral or intravenous doses, 70–80% of activity is eliminated (primarily as metabolites) via the urine. Remaining excretion is via the faeces.

After 24 hours, 90% of the administered dose is eliminated.

Protein binding of nifedipine exceeds 90% in human serum.

*Pre-clinical safety data*
*Reproduction toxicology:* Nifedipine administration has been associated with a variety of embryotoxic, placentotoxic and fetotoxic effects in rats, mice and rabbits. All of the doses associated with the teratogenic, embryotoxic or fetotoxic effects in animals were maternally toxic and several times the recommended maximum dose for humans.

**Pharmaceutical particulars**
*List of excipients:* Tensipine MR tablets contain the following excipients:

Microcrystalline cellulose, maize starch, lactose, polysorbate 80, magnesium stearate, hydroxypropyl methylcellulose, polyethylene glycol 4000, iron oxide red and titanium dioxide.

*Incompatibilities:* Not applicable.

*Shelf life:* PVC blister strips: 48 months. PP blister strips: 30 months.

*Special precautions for storage:* The tablets should be protected from strong light and stored in the manufacturer's original container.

*Nature and contents of container:* Tensipine MR 10 tablets: blister strips of 14 tablets in a cardboard outer container, packs of 56 tablets.

Tensipine MR 20 tablets: blister strips of 14 tablets in a cardboard outer container, packs of 56 tablets.

Blister strips are composed of red polypropylene foil (0.3 mm) with aluminium backing foil (0.02 mm) or red PVC foil (0.3 mm) with aluminium backing foil (0.02 mm).

*Instructions for use/handling:* No additional information.

**Marketing authorisation numbers**
Tensipine MR 10 tablets 6831/0048
Tensipine MR 20 tablets 6831/0049

**Date of approval/revision of SPC** November 1996.

**Legal category** POM.

## UNIPINE* XL

**Qualitative and quantitative composition** Circular, biconvex, red, film-coated tablets marked 'UXL 30' on one side and blank on the other side containing 30 mg Nifedipine PhEur.

**Pharmaceutical form** Nifedipine (30 mg) in tablet form for oral administration. It is a sustained release preparation.

**Clinical particulars**
*Therapeutic indications:* Unipine XL is indicated for the treatment of hypertension.

*Posology and method of administration: Adults and elderly:* The recommended starting dose of nifedipine is 30 mg every 24 hours swallowed with water with subsequent titration of dosage according to response. The dose may be adjusted to 60 mg every 24 hours.

Nifedipine should be taken with a little water. Tablets should be swallowed whole. Do not chew. *Not* to be taken with or immediately after food.

The pharmacokinetics of nifedipine are altered in the elderly so that lower maintenance doses of nifedipine may be required compared to younger patients.

Nifedipine is metabolised primarily by the liver and therefore patients with liver dysfunction should be carefully monitored. Patients with renal impairment should not require adjustment of dosage.

*Children:* Nifedipine is not recommended for use in children.

*Contra-indications:* Hypersensitivity to nifedipine or other dihydropyridines because of the theoretical risk of cross reactivity.

Nifedipine should not be used in clinically significant aortic stenosis, unstable angina, or during or within one month of a myocardial infarction.

Nifedipine should not be used for the treatment of acute attacks of angina.

The safety of nifedipine in malignant hypertension has not been established.

Nifedipine should not be used for secondary prevention of myocardial infarction.

Nifedipine should not be administered concomitantly with rifampicin since effective plasma levels of nifedipine may not be achieved owing to enzyme induction.

*Special warnings and precautions for use:* Unipine XL should be used with caution in patients whose cardiac reserve is poor and in patients with hepatic impairment. A marked decrease in blood pressure may occur in dialysis patients with malignant hypertension and hypovolaemia.

Unipine XL should be discontinued in patients who experience ischaemic pain following its administration.

*Interactions with other medicaments and other forms of interaction:* When Unipine XL is used in combination with beta-blocking drugs and other antihypertensive drugs, there is the possibility of an additive effect resulting in postural hypotension.

Decreased plasma quinidine and increased plasma phenytoin and theophylline concentrations have been reported when nifedipine is administered concomitantly.

Adjustment of hypoglycaemic medication may be required in diabetic patients.

There may be potentiation of the antihypertensive action of nifedipine when administered simultaneously with cimetidine.

Unipine XL is not a beta-blocker and therefore gives no protection against the dangers of abrupt beta-blocker withdrawal. Any such withdrawal should be by gradual reduction of the dose of beta-blocker preferably over 8 to 10 days. Unipine XL will not prevent possible rebound effects after cessation of antihypertensive therapy.

The simultaneous administration of nifedipine and digoxin may lead to reduced digoxin clearance and hence an increase in the plasma digoxin. Digoxin levels should be monitored and, if necessary the digoxin dose reduced.

Nifedipine should not be administered concomitantly with rifampicin since effective plasma levels of nifedipine may not be achieved owing to enzyme induction (see *Contra-indications*).

As with other dihydropyridines, nifedipine should not be taken with grapefruit juice because bioavailability is increased.

*Pregnancy and lactation:* Unipine XL should not be

administered to women who are pregnant, women of child-bearing potential or to nursing mothers.

*Effects on ability to drive and use machines:* Not applicable.

*Undesirable effects:* Side-effects, mainly associated with the vasodilatory action of nifedipine include headache, dizziness, flushing and gravitational oedema. These effects usually disappear with continued treatment. Common side-effects include rash, nausea, lethargy, increased frequency of micturition, hypersensitivity type jaundice and gingival hyperplasia.

As with other sustained release dihydropyridines, exacerbation of angina pectoris may occur rarely at the start of treatment with sustained release formulations of nifedipine. The occurrence of myocardial infarction has been described although it is not possible to distinguish such an event from the natural course of ischaemic heart disease.

*Overdose:* Following overdosage, the stomach should be emptied by aspiration and lavage and charcoal instillation. Standard measures such as atropine and noradrenaline may be used for resultant bradycardia and hypotension. Intravenous calcium gluconate may be of benefit combined with metaraminol.

## Pharmacological properties

*Pharmacodynamic properties:* Nifedipine is a potent and specific Class II calcium antagonist. The main action is to reduce contraction of vascular smooth muscle in both the coronary and peripheral circulation resulting in a reduction in blood pressure.

*Pharmacokinetic properties:* Nifedipine is absorbed over the whole length of the gastrointestinal tract the majority of an oral dose being absorbed in the jejunum. There is however considerable inter-individual variation in the rate and extent to which nifedipine is absorbed. It undergoes extensive yet variable first pass metabolism. The absorption of nifedipine from Nifedipine (30 mg) SR Tablets occurs over several hours which is typical of a sustained release preparation. At steady state $C_{max}$ was approximately 20 ng/ml with $T_{max}$ of 7 hours. At 24 hours the mean plasma concentration was approximately 8 ng/ml supporting once daily administration. In a single dose study the mean elimination half life was shown to be 10 hours (range 3.5–16.5 hours) in the fasting state.

*Pre-clinical safety data:* The $LD_{50}$ of oral nifedipine has been found to be 494 mg/kg in mice and 1022 mg/kg in rats. Reproductive studies have shown reduced fertility in male and female rats dosed 100 mg/kg/day nifedipine for 10 weeks. Pregnant rats and rabbits receiving 30 mg/kg/day nifedipine showed increased rates of resorption and abortion. In pregnant mice dosed at 24 mg/kg/day nifedipine caused a low incidence of embryo lethality and a dosage-related reduction in foetal weight.

Nifedipine showed no mutagenic activity in the dominant lethal or micronucleus tests in mice, or in an *in vivo* cytogenic study in hamsters. Nor was it carcinogenic in rats.

The widespread clinical usage of nifedipine in accordance with the data sheet has established its safety and efficacy in man in the treatment of hypertension.

## Pharmaceutical particulars

*List of excipients:* Povidone, Ammoniomethacrylate copolymer, Lactose, Hydrogentated castor oil, Talc, Colours E110, E171, E120, E132.

*Incompatibilities:* Unipine XL should not be taken with cimetidine as this causes potentiation of the antihypertensive action of nifedipine.

*Shelf life:* 2 years.

*Special precautions for storage:* Unipine XL should be protected from light and stored below 25°C, in a dry place in the manufacturer's original container.

*Nature and contents of container:* Unipine XL is available in blister packs each containing 28 tablets.

*Instructions for use/handling:* No special instructions.

**Marketing authorisation number** 6831/0047.

**Date of approval/revision of SPC** February 1997.

**Legal category** POM.

*Trade Mark

# Euroderma Limited
The Old Coach House
34 Elm Road
Chessington
Surrey KT9 1AW

**EURODERMA LIMITED**

## ACNISAL*

**Presentation** Acnisal is an off-white solution containing 2% w/w Salicylic Acid BP in a surfactant blend for topical application. Other ingredients include benzyl alcohol.

**Uses** For the management of acne. Helps prevent new comedones, papules and pustules.

**Dosage and administration** Acnisal is for topical application.
Wash the affected area 2–3 times daily. Lather with warm water, massage into skin, rinse and dry.

**Contra-indications, warnings, etc** Patients with a known sensitivity to salicylic acid should not use Acnisal.
For external use only. Take care to keep the product away from contact with the mouth, the eyes and other mucous membranes to avoid irritation.
Skin irritation may develop. If undue skin irritation develops or increases, the patient should adjust the usage schedule or consult their physician. With topical preparations containing salicylic acid, excessive prolonged use may result in symptoms of salicylism.

**Legal category** P.

**Package quantities** Acnisal is available in a 6 oz (177 ml) plastic bottle.

**Further information** The base of Acnisal is a blend of surfactants with an emollient designed to assist in cleansing and removal of excess sebum whilst not being too drying or irritating and being non-comedogenic.

**Product licence number** 10670/0004.

## AXSAIN* CREAM

**Presentation** A smooth white cream containing 0.075% capsaicin in an emollient base. Other ingredients include benzyl alcohol.

**Uses** For the symptomatic relief of neuralgia associated with and following herpes zoster infections (post herpetic neuralgia), after open skin lesions have healed or the symptomatic management of painful diabetic neuropathy.

**Dosage and administration** Axsain is for topical application on unbroken skin.
*Adults and the elderly:* Apply sparingly to affected area 3 or 4 times daily.

**Contra-indications, warnings, etc** Axsain should only be used in diabetic patients under the direct supervision of a hospital consultant.
Axsain may cause burning on application. This burning is observed more frequently when application schedules of less than 3 or 4 times daily are used.
Axsain is contra-indicated for use on broken or irritated skin and should not come into contact with the eyes. If it does, wash thoroughly with copious water.
Do not bandage tightly over Axsain cream. If the condition worsens the patient should seek medical advice.
Keep the product away from the eyes. After applying Axsain cream with the fingers, hands should be washed immediately.
Other side effects are erythema, dry skin at the application site, coughing or sneezing.
Not suitable for use in children.
*Pregnancy and lactation:* The safety of Axsain during pregnancy or lactation has not been established in either humans or animals. However, in the small amounts absorbed transdermally from Axsain Cream, it is considered unlikely that capsaicin will cause any adverse effects in humans.

**Legal category** POM.

**Package quantities** Axsain cream 0.075% is available in 45 g tubes.

**Further information** Evidence suggests that Axsain exerts its topical analgesic effect by depleting Substance P in peripheral sensory neurons (C fibres);

Substance P is held to be the principal pain neurotransmitter.

**Product licence number** 10670/0003.

## METED* SHAMPOO

**Presentation** A viscous, yellow shampoo containing salicylic acid 3.0% w/w and colloidal sulphur equivalent to 5% w/w in the following excipients: magnesium aluminium silicate, hydroxypropyl methyl cellulose, panthenol, sodium laureth sulphate, sodium cocoyl sarcosinate, cocamido propyl betaine, fragrance and purified water.

**Uses** Meted shampoo is used for the relief of itching, irritation, redness, flaking and scaling due to dandruff, seborrhoeic dermatitis or psoriasis of the scalp.

**Dosage and administration** For topical application. The hair should be thoroughly wetted and sufficient Meted shampoo applied to produce an abundant lather. The hair should be rinsed and the procedure repeated. Use at least twice weekly or as otherwise directed by a physician.

**Contra-indications, warnings, etc** Meted shampoo should not be used on patients sensitive to any of the ingredients. Salicylic acid is a mild irritant and may cause dermatitis. Contact of Meted shampoo with the eyes should be avoided. If this occurs rinse thoroughly with water. If the condition of the scalp worsens or does not improve after regular use of the shampoo as directed, the patient should consult a physician.
*Overdosage:* There is no evidence of systemic absorption following the use of Meted shampoo. There are no reports of its ingestion.

**Pharmaceutical precautions** Shake the bottle thoroughly before use.

**Legal category** P.

**Package quantities** Meted shampoo is available in bottles of 120 ml.

**Further information** Meted contains panthenol to condition the hair and counteract the drying effect of the salicylic acid and sulphur.

**Product licence number** 10670/0001.

## OCCLUSAL*

**Presentation** Occlusal is a clear solution for topical application containing 26% w/w Salicylic Acid BP in a polyacrylic vehicle made up by polyvinyl butyral, dibutyl phthalate, isopropyl alcohol, butyl acetate and acrylates co-polymer.

**Uses** Occlusal is indicated for the treatment and removal of common warts and plantar warts.

**Dosage and administration** Occlusal is for topical application. There are no differences in dosage for children, adults or the elderly. Prior to application soak wart in warm water for five minutes. Remove loose tissue with a brush, pumice stone or emery board. Dry thoroughly with a towel not used by others to avoid contagion. Carefully apply Occusal twice to the wart using the brush applicator allowing the first application to dry before applying the second. Thereafter repeat treatment once daily or as directed by physician. Do not apply to surrounding healthy skin. Clinically visible improvement should occur in one to two weeks but maximum effect may be expected after four to six weeks.

**Contra-indications, warnings, etc**
*Contra-indications:* Occlusal should not be used by diabetics or patients with impaired blood circulation. Do not use on moles, birthmarks, unusual warts with hair growth, on facial warts, or in the anal or perineal region.
*Warnings:* Occlusal is for external use only. Do not permit contact with eyes or mucous membranes. If contact occurs flush with water for 15 minutes. Do not allow contact with normal skin around wart. Avoid using in areas of broken or damaged skin. Discontinue treatment if excessive irritation occurs.

*Pregnancy and lactation:* The chronic use of this product during pregnancy and lactation, particularly when large areas of skin are involved, should be avoided.
*Side-effects:* A localised irritant reaction may occur if Occlusal is applied to normal skin surrounding the wart. This may normally be controlled by temporarily discontinuing the use of Occlusal and by being careful to apply the solution only to the wart itself when treatment is resumed.
*Overdosage:* Salicylism can occur following large doses of salicylic acid or prolonged use of topical salicylic acid preparations, or in the unlikely event of accidental consumption.

**Pharmaceutical precautions** Occlusal should be stored at room temperature. Occlusal is flammable and should be kept away from flame or fire. Keep the bottle tightly capped when not in use. Do not allow the solution to drip from the brush onto the bottle neck thread, otherwise subsequent opening of the bottle may be difficult.

**Legal category** P.

**Package quantities** Occlusal is available in 10 ml amber glass bottles with an applicator brush in the cap.

**Further information** The vehicle of Occlusal when dry forms a self-occluding barrier over the wart, maximising the keratolytic action of the salicylic acid and requires no bandage or plasters.

**Product licence number** 10670/0006.

## PAPULEX* GEL

**Presentation** Translucent topical gel containing 4% w/w nicotinamide.

**Uses** Papulex is indicated for use in the topical treatment of mild to moderate inflammatory acne vulgaris.

**Dosage and administration** Cleanse the affected and surrounding area with soap and warm water. Dry and apply a thin film of Papulex Gel, sufficient to cover the affected area, twice daily.

**Contra-indications, warnings, etc**
*Contra-indications:* Papulex is contraindicated in persons with known hypersensitivity to any of its components.
*Warnings and precautions:* Papulex is for external use only and should be kept away from the eyes and mucous membranes, including those of the nose and mouth. If excessive dryness, irritation or peeling occurs reduce the dosage to one application per day or every other day.
*Pregnancy and lactation:* Vitamin $B_3$ derivative requirements, such as nicotinamide, are increased during pregnancy and infancy. Nicotinamide is excreted in breast milk. As with all medicines, care should be exercised during the first trimester of pregnancy.
*Side-effects:* The most frequently encountered adverse effect reported with Papulex is dryness of the skin. Other less frequent adverse effects include pruritus, erythema, burning sensation and irritation.

**Pharmaceutical precautions** Store below 25°C.

**Legal category** P.

**Package quantities** 60 g tubes.

**Further information** Nicotinamide is not an antibiotic and has not been associated with the emergence of resistant bacterial strains.

**Product licence number** 10670/0009.

## PENTRAX* SHAMPOO

**Presentation** Pentrax is a clear, burgundy-brown coloured shampoo containing Fractar 5, an extract of coal tar equivalent to coal tar 4.3% with the following excipients: sodium laureth sulphate, laureth 23, co-camide DEA, lauramine oxide, PEG 8, dioctyl sodium sulphosuccinate.

**Uses** Pentrax shampoo is used for the relief of itching, irritation, redness, flaking and scaling associated with dandruff, seborrhoeic dermatitis and psoriasis.

**Dosage and administration** For topical application. The hair should be wetted and the shampoo massaged into the wet hair and scalp to produce a lather. The hair should be rinsed and the shampoo reapplied liberally allowing the lather to remain on the hair for up to ten minutes. The hair should be thoroughly rinsed.

Pentrax shampoo should be used at least twice weekly or as otherwise directed by a physician.

**Contra-indications, warnings, etc** Pentrax shampoo should not be used in patients sensitive to any of the ingredients. Coal tar may cause irritation to the skin and hypersensitivity to coal tar has been reported.

Contact of Pentrax shampoo with the eyes should be avoided. If this occurs the eyes should be rinsed thoroughly with water.

If the scalp condition does not improve or worsens after regular use with Pentrax shampoo as directed, consult a physician.

*Overdosage:* There is no evidence of systemic absorption following the use of Pentrax shampoo nor are there any reports of its ingestion.

**Pharmaceutical precautions** Nil.

**Legal category** P.

**Package quantities** Pentrax shampoo is available in plastic bottles of 120 ml.

**Further information** Fractar-5 is an extract of crude coal tar with improved cosmetic acceptability, being combined in Pentrax with surfactants and conditioners.

**Product licence number** 10670/0002.

*Trade Mark

# Evans Medical Limited

Evans House
Regent Park
Kingston Road
Leatherhead
Surrey KT22 7PQ

# EVANS

## ARILVAX* YELLOW FEVER VACCINE, LIVE BP

**Qualitative and quantitative composition** The composition in terms of active ingredients is as follows:

Each 0.5 ml dose of reconstituted vaccine contains the equivalent of not less than 1000 mouse $LD_{50}$ units as defined by the World Health Organisation requirements

**Pharmaceutical form** Stabilised freeze-dried preparation, reconstituted with Water for Injections, BP prior to subcutaneous injection in humans

### Clinical particulars

*Therapeutic indications:* For active immunisation of residents in yellow fever endemic areas. Yellow fever endemic areas are limited to the African and South American continents and Central America.

For active immunisation of travellers to and from such areas.

For the issue of an International Certificate of Vaccination, as required by the national health authorities of certain countries which consider these zones as infected areas (although the 'yellow fever endemic zones' are in fact no longer included in the International Health Regulations). The International Health Regulations define the form of certificate of vaccination to be used which, in the case of primary vaccination, is valid for a period of 10 years from the 10th day after vaccination. In the case of revaccination within 10 years, the certificate is valid at once.

*Posology and method of administration:*
Children aged 9 months and over, adults and elderly: The dose is 0.5 ml of reconstituted vaccine, given subcutaneously. This dose is the same for persons of all ages.

Children under 9 months of age: Not recommended.

It is good practice to record the title, dose and lot numbers of all vaccines and the dates of administration.

*Contra-indications:* The vaccine should not be administered to a subject who has experienced a serious reaction (e.g. anaphylaxis) to a previous dose of this vaccine or who is known to be hypersensitive to any component thereof. It is advisable to avoid vaccination during an acute infection. Since the vaccine is prepared in chick embryos and contains small quantities of neomycin and polymyxin, it should not be administered to individuals who are hypersensitive to egg or chick protein or to these antibiotics.

The vaccine should not be given to those with impaired immune responsiveness, whether congenital, idiopathic or as a result of treatment with steroids (with the exception of standard doses of locally-acting, e.g. topical or inhaled, steroids), radiotherapy, cytotoxic drugs or other agents.

The vaccine should not be given to either symptomatic or asymptomatic HIV positive individuals since there is insufficient evidence as to the safety of its use.

*Special warnings and precautions for use:* The vaccine is not recommended for use in children under the age of 9 months. The decision to vaccinate infants under this age must depend on the anticipated risk of exposure to the disease, since the small number of cases of encephalitis that have been reported, have nearly all occurred in infants under this age.

It is advisable to avoid administration of the vaccine within 6 weeks following the administration of immune globulin on general principles. Similarly, on theoretical grounds it is advisable to avoid the administration of immune globulin within 2 weeks following vaccination. An interval of not less than 3 weeks should normally be allowed to lapse between the administration of any two live vaccines. If time does not permit then they might be given simultaneously at separate sites.

Although anaphylaxis is rare, facilities for its management should always be available during vaccination

*Interaction with other medicaments and other forms of interaction:* None stated.

*Pregnancy and lactation:* On theoretical grounds the vaccine should not be administered during pregnancy and lactation.

*Effects on ability to drive and use machines:* None stated.

*Undesirable effects:* Severe reactions to the vaccine are extremely rare and include encephalitis and allergic reactions. Occasionally some redness, soreness and swelling may occur at the site of injection, and headache has been reported. Myalgia and low-grade fever may occur a few days after immunisation.

Rare cases of urticaria, bursitis, jaundice and neuritis have been reported in a temporal relationship to vaccination.

Any untoward reactions should be reported to the regulatory authorities and to the manufacturer.

*Overdose:* Not applicable

**Pharmacological particulars** Not applicable

*Pharmacodynamic properties:* Not applicable

*Pharmacokinetic properties:* Not applicable

*Preclinical safety data:* Not applicable

**Pharmaceutical particulars**

*List of excipients:* The excipients contained in the preparation are as follows: Polymyxin B sulphate BP, Neomycin sulphate BP, Sorbitol BP, Hydrolysed gelatin HSE*, Sodium chloride PhEur, Disodium hydrogen orthophosphate HSE*, Potassium chloride HSE*, Potassium dihydrogen orthophosphate HSE*, Water for Injections PhEur

Prior to use the vaccine is diluted with Water for Injections BP.

*HSE House specification

*Incompatibilities:* None stated.

*Shelf life:*
Vaccine: In filled containers:- 3 years at 2-8°C. After reconstitution:- 1 hour kept cool
Diluent: In filled containers: 3 years at below 25°C

*Special precautions for storage:* The freeze-dried vaccine should be stored between 2-8°C. Protect from light. Diluent should not be frozen but should be stored below 25°C. After reconstitution the vaccine should be kept cool, protected from light and used within one hour.

*Nature and contents of container:*
Vaccine: Single Dose: PhEur Type I clear neutral glass vials, 3 ml capacity with grey butyl rubber stopper, aluminium seal and a blue polypropylene flip-off top.

Multi-dose: PhEur Type I clear neutral glass vials, 8 ml capacity with either grey butyl rubber stopper, aluminium seal and a blue polypropylene flip-off top, or red chlorbutyl rubber stopper, aluminium seal and a yellow polypropylene flip-off top.

Diluent : PhEur type I clear neutral glass ampoules, 1 ml or 5 ml.

*Instructions for use and handling:* Only the Water for Injections BP supplied should be used for reconstitution using a sterile syringe and needle. The entire contents of the appropriate diluent container are injected into the vaccine vial and gently agitated to ensure reconstitution. The vacuum in the vaccine vial may be broken to facilitate withdrawal of the vaccine solution. After reconstitution, the vaccine should be kept cool and used within one hour.

Contamination with bactericides is to be avoided. Use a fresh sterile disposal syringe and needle free from traces of spirit and disinfectant for each injection.

Disposal should be by incineration at a temperature of not less than 1100°C at a registered waste disposal contractor.

No attempt should be made to obtain more than the stated number of doses from the vial.

**Marketing authorisation numbers**
Yellow Fever Vaccine, Live BP     0039/0476
Water for Injections BP     0039/5704

**Date of approval/revision of SPC** November 1994

**Legal category** POM

## ASMABEC* SPACEHALER*

**Qualitative and quantitative composition**
Asmabec Spacehaler 50 micrograms: Each actuation contains 50 micrograms Beclomethasone Dipropionate BP.

Asmabec Spacehaler 100 micrograms: Each actuation contains 100 micrograms Beclomethasone Dipropionate BP.

Asmabec Spacehaler 250 micrograms: Each actuation contains 250 micrograms Beclomethasone Dipropionate BP.

**Pharmaceutical form** Metered-dose inhaler with Spacehaler actuator.

The Spacehaler is a vortex generating actuator which acts to reduce the velocity of the emitted dose. Compared with a standard actuator it decreases the proportion of non-respirable drug particles within the emitted dose cloud whilst achieving a similar respirable fraction.

### Clinical particulars

*Therapeutic indications:*
Asmabec Spacehaler 50 and 100 micrograms:

(i) Treatment of patients whose asthma is becoming worse, and the relief provided by bronchodilators is less effective.

(ii) Treatment of patients with severe asthma who are dependent on systemic corticosteroids or adrenocorticotrophic hormone (ACTH) or its synthetic equivalent.

(iii) Treatment of patients who are inadequately controlled by sodium cromoglycate in addition to bronchodilators.

(iv) Particularly important for managing severe asthma in children because good control can be achieved without retardation of growth.

Asmabec Spacehaler 250 micrograms:

(i) Asmabec Spacehaler 250 micrograms is indicated for those asthmatic patients who have been shown to require high doses (greater than 800-1000 micrograms daily) of Beclomethasone Dipropionate BP to control their symptoms.

(ii) It may also be indicated for those patients whose asthma is no longer controlled by maximum maintenance doses of bronchodilators and Asmabec Spacehaler 50 micrograms or Asmabec Spacehaler 100 micrograms. Some patients with severe asthma require oral corticosteroid therapy in addition to Asmabec Spacehaler 50 micrograms or Asmabec Spacehaler 100 micrograms for the adequate control of their symptoms. Many of these patients may, on transfer to Asmabec Spacehaler 250 micrograms, be able to reduce significantly or eliminate their requirement for additional oral corticosteroids .

*Posology and method of administration:*

Asmabec Spacehaler 50 and 100 micrograms:

Adults: The usual starting dose is 200 micrograms twice a day. In more severe cases dosage may be started at, or increased to 600-800 micrograms per day, and subsequiently reduced when the patient's asthma has stabilised. The total daily dose may be administered as two, three or four divided doses.

Elderly: There is no need to adjust the dose in elderly patients or in those with hepatic or renal impairment.

Children: 50-100 micrograms should be given two, three or four times daily according to response. Alternatively, 100 or 200 micrograms twice daily may be administered. The usual starting dose is 100 micrograms twice a day.

Asmabec Spacehaler 250 micrograms:

Adults: Patients should be given a starting dose of inhaled beclomethasone dipropionate which is appropriate for the severity of their disease. The dose may then be adjusted until control is achieved, or reduced to the minimum effective dose according to individual response.

Patients demonstrating a need for high dose inhaled steroid therapy should start on 1,000 micrograms daily.

The usual maintenance dose is two inhalations (500 micrograms) twice daily, or one inhalation (250 micrograms) four times daily. If necessary, dosage may be increased to two inhalations (500 micrograms) three or four times daily according to response.

Elderly: There is no need to adjust the dose in elderly patients or in those with hepatic or renal impairment.

Children: Asmabec Spacehaler 250 micrograms is not indicated for use in children.

*Contra-indications:* Patients with a history of hypersensitivity to any of its components. Special care is necessary in patients with active or quiescent pulmonary tuberculosis.

*Special warnings and precautions for use:* Patients should be instructed on the proper use of the inhaler to ensure that the drug reaches the target areas within the lungs. They should also be made aware that Asmabec Spacehaler has to be used regularly for optimum benefit. Patients should be made aware of the prophylactic nature of therapy with Asmabec Spacehaler and that it should be taken regularly, even when they are asymptomatic.

Patients being treated with Asmabec Spacehaler 50 micrograms or Asmabec Spacehaler 100 micrograms may be transferred directly to treatment with Asmabec Spacehaler 250 micrograms.

The maximum daily intake of Asmabec Spacehaler 50 micrograms and 100 micrograms should not exceed 1,000 micrograms. The maximum daily dose of Asmabec Spacehaler 250 micrograms should not exceed 2,000 micrograms. Significant reduction of plasma cortisol levels has been reported in patients who received in excess of 2,000 micrograms.

In the majority of patients, no significant adrenal suppression occurs until doses of 1,500 micrograms per day are exceeded. Some patients receiving 2,000 micrograms of beclomethasone dipropionate per day may show a degree of adrenocortical suppression although short term adrenal reserve remains intact. In such patients the risks of developing adrenal suppression should be balanced against the therapeutic advantages and precautions should be taken to provide systemic steroid cover in situations of prolonged stress.

Patients inadequately controlled by bronchodilator therapy: The use of Asmabec Spacehaler in patients who have never taken steroids or taken only occasional courses of steroids is straightforward. An improvement in respiratory function is normally obvious within a week. The few patients who do not respond during this period usually have excessive mucus in their bronchi so that the drug is unable to penetrate to its site of action. In such cases, a short course of systemic steroid in relatively high dosage should be given to control secretion of mucus and other inflammatory changes in the lungs. Continuation of treatment with Asmabec Spacehaler usually maintains the improvement achieved, the oral steroid being gradually withdrawn. Exacerbation of asthma caused by infections is usually controlled by appropriate antibiotic treatment, by increasing the dose of inhaled beclomethasone dipropionate and, if necessary, by giving a systemic steroid. Use of a β2-agonist may also be required.

Oral steroid-dependent patients: The transfer of oral steroid-dependent patients to Asmabec Spacehaler and their subsequent management needs special care mainly because recovery from impaired adrenocortical function caused by prolonged systemic steroid therapy is slow. The patient should be in a reasonably stable state before being given Asmabec Spacehaler in addition to his usual maintenance dose of systemic steroid. After about a week, gradual withdrawal of the systemic steroid is started by reducing the daily dose by 1 mg prednisolone, or its equivalent of other corticosteroids, at not less than weekly intervals. Patients treated with systemic steroids for long periods of time or who have received high doses may have adrenocortical suppression. With these patients adrenocortical function should be monitored regularly and their dose of systemic steroid reduced cautiously. Some patients feel unwell during the withdrawal phase despite maintenance or even improvement of respiratory function. They should be encouraged to persevere with the inhaler and withdrawal of systemic steroid continued unless there are objective signs of adrenal insufficiency. Most patients can be successfully transferred to Asmabec Spacehaler with maintenance of good respiratory function, but special care is necessary for the first months after the transfer until the pituitary-adrenal system has sufficiently recovered to enable the patient to cope with emergencies such as trauma, surgery or infections.

Transferred patients whose adrenocortical function is impaired should carry a warning card indicating that they need supplementary systemic steroids during periods of stress, e.g. surgery, chest infection or worsening asthma attacks, but that this can be reduced again after the stress has been resolved. They should also be given a supply of oral steroid to use in emergency, for example when the asthma worsens as a result of a chest infection. The dose of beclomethasone should be increased at this time and then reduced to the maintenance level after the systemic steroid has been discontinued. Replacement of systemic steroid treatment with Asmabec Spacehaler sometimes unmasks allergies such as allergic rhinitis or eczema previously controlled by the systemic drug. These allergies should be symptomatically treated with antihistamine and/or topical preparations.

Asmabec Spacehaler 250 micrograms: Increasing use of bronchodilators, in particular short-acting inhaled β2-agonists, to relieve symptoms indicates deterioration of asthma control. If patients find that short-acting relief bronchodilator treatment becomes less effective, or they need more inhalations than usual, medical attention must be sought. In this situation patients should be reassessed and consideration given to the need for increased anti-inflammatory therapy (e.g. higher doses of inhaled corticosteroids or a course of oral corticosteroids). Severe exacerbations of asthma must be treated in the normal way.

Treatment with Asmabec Spacehaler 250 micrograms should not be stopped abruptly.

*Interactions with other medicaments and other forms of interaction:* None known

*Pregnancy and lactation:* Beclomethasone dipropionate should only be used in pregnancy or lactation if the potential benefit outweighs the risk. There is insufficient data regarding safety in human pregnancy. High doses of systemic corticosteroids in pregnant animals can cause abnormalities in foetal development, including cleft palate and intra-uterine growth retardation.

No data regarding excretion of beclomethasone dipropionate in human breast milk is available. However, the dosages recommended for Asmabec Spacehalers suggest a lower potential for transfer to the foetus or infant than with systemic corticosteroids.

*Effects on ability to drive and use machines:* On the basis of the pharmacodynamic profile, reported adverse drug reactions (ADR) and/or impairment of driving performance related to driving, the medicine is presumed to be safe or unlikely to produce an effect.

*Undesirable effects:* In some patients hoarseness or throat irritation may occur. Rinsing the mouth and throat with water after each dose to remove residual medication may be helpful.

Paradoxical bronchospasm may occur, in which case use of the inhaler should cease immediately and medical advice should be sought. Alternative therapy should be introduced.

Candidiasis of the mouth and throat (thrush) occurs in some patients; the incidence of which is increased with doses greater than 400 micrograms beclomethasone dipropionate per day. Patients with high blood levels of Candida precipitins, indicating a previous infection, are more likely to develop this complication. Such patients may find it helpful to rinse their mouth with water after using the inhaler. Symptomatic candidiasis can be treated with topical anti-fungal therapy whilst still continuing with Asmabec Spacehaler.

*Overdose:* The acute toxicity of beclomethasone dipropionate is low. The only harmful effect that follows inhalation of large amounts of the drug over a short period is suppression of hypothalamic-pituitary-adrenal (HPA) function. No special emergency action need be taken. Treatment with Asmabec Spacehaler should be continued at the recommended dose to control the asthma; HPA function recovers in a day or two.

Reduction of plasma cortisol levels has been reported in patients who received twice the daily recommended maximum dose of beclomethasone dipropionate. In the unlikely event of excessive intake of beclomethasone dipropionate for weeks or months on end, a degree of adrenocortical atrophy could occur in addition to suppression of HPA function. The patient should be treated as steroid-dependent and transferred to a suitable maintenance dose of a systemic steroid such as prednisolone. Once the patient's condition has stabilised they should be transferred to Asmabec Spacehaler.

To guard against the unexpected event of adrenal suppression, regular tests of adrenal function are advised.

## Pharmacological properties

*Pharmacodynamic properties:* Beclomethasone dipropionate by inhalation has a potent glucocorticoid anti-inflammatory action within the lungs, but at recommended dosage, is without significant systemic activity.

Beclomethasone dipropionate also has vasoconstrictor effects and it inhibits the late responses to antigen challenge.

*Pharmacokinetic properties:* The pharmacokinetics of beclomethasone dipropionate have not been extensively studied. The currently available chemical methods are not of sufficient sensitivity to measure therapeutically relevant plasma concentrations, particularly those occurring following inhalation.

*a) general characteristics of the active substance*

| | |
|---|---|
| absorption | Beclomethasone dipropionate is readily absorbed from the gastro-intestinal tract. It is also well absorbed from sites of local application. |
| distribution | About 25% of an inhaled dose reaches the lungs. The drug is rapidly distributed to all body tissues. It crosses the placenta and may be excreted in small amounts in breast milk. |
| elimination | The drug and its metabolites are excreted chiefly in the faeces via biliary elimination and to a lesser extent in the urine. |

*b) characteristics in patients*
As above

*Preclinical safety data:* See Clinical Particulars sections above.

## Pharmaceutical particulars

*List of excipients:* Oleic Acid BP, Trichlorofluoromethane (1988) BP, Dichlorodifluoromethane (1988) BP

*Incompatibilities:* None known

*Shelf life:* Shelf-life in the product as packaged for sale: 24 months.

*Special precautions for storage:* Store below 30°C. Protect from frost and direct sunlight. The canister is pressurised, it must not be burnt, punctured or broken even when apparently empty. The therapeutic effect of the medication may decrease when the canister is cold.

*Nature and contents of container:* The container consists of a seamless aluminium can with a metering dispensing valve crimped to it. The can is inserted into a plastic oral inhalation actuator with a dust cap.

The can is a 19 ml nominal capacity aerosol can of deep drawn NS4 aluminium with either a debossed or plain base.

The metering aerosol valves used are 20 mm types, with a nominal 63 microlitre dosing capacity. The valve is composed of metal and rubber components and is assembled into a metal ferrule.

The actuator supports the container during actuation and directs the sprayed aerosol particles into the mouth. The actuator is injection moulded polypropylene which may be plain, printed or embossed with the name of the product. A mouthpiece cover is fitted over the actuator mouthpiece to prevent the ingress of particulates into the mouthpiece cavity between uses.

*Instructions for use/handling:* Instructions as shown in the leaflet:

1. Remove the cap from the inhaler mouthpiece. Make sure the mouthpiece is clean and clear of fluff and dirt.
2. Hold the inhaler upright, with your thumb on the base and your first finger on the top of the can. Now shake the inhaler gently up and down.
3. Breathe out fully to empty the lungs and then place the mouthpiece firmly between the lips.
4. Now breathe in slowly and deeply. At the same time press the aerosol can with your first finger to fire the aerosol and release the drug.
5. Remove the inhaler from your mouth and hold breath for 10 seconds or as long as is comfortable. Breathe out slowly.
6. If more than one puff is required, wait at least one minute and repeat procedure from step 2. Replace the cap.
7. Your inhaler should be cleaned regularly usually at least once a week. To clean, remove the metal canister from the plastic body and remove the plastic cover from the mouthpiece. Rinse the plastic body and the mouthpiece cover in warm water. Dry thoroughly then replace the canister and mouthpiece cover. Avoid excessive heat. Do not put the metal canister into water.

Important: Do not rush steps 3 and 4. It is important that you start to breathe in as slowly as possible just before operating your inhaler. Practice in the mirror for the first few times. If you see a 'mist' coming from the top of your inhaler or the sides of your mouth, you should start again from step 2.

## Marketing authorisation numbers
Asmabec Spacehaler 50 micrograms     0039/0480
Asmabec Spacehaler 100 micrograms    0039/0481
Asmabec Spacehaler 250 micrograms    0039/0482

**Date of approval/revision of SPC**    May 1997

**Legal category**    POM

# ASMASAL* CLICKHALER*

**Qualitative and quantitative composition** The inhaler contains a powder blend of Salbutamol Sulphate PhEur with Lactose PhEur. Each metered actuation contains the equivalent of 95 micrograms Salbutamol base.

**Pharmaceutical form** An inhaler which delivers the drug as an inhalation powder by means of a specially designed actuator.

## Clinical particulars

*Therapeutic indications:* Asmasal Clickhaler is indicated both for the treatment and prophylaxis of bronchospasm in bronchial asthma and other conditions with associated reversible airways obstruction.

Salbutamol acts rapidly and Asmasal Clickhaler may be used when necessary to relieve attacks of acute dyspnoea. It may also be used before exertion to prevent exercise-induced bronchospasm or before exposure to a known unavoidable allergen challenge.

*Posology and method of administration:*
*Adults:* For the relief of acute bronchospasm and for managing intermittent episodes of asthma, one inhalation may be administered as a single dose; this may be increased to two inhalations if necessary. The recommended dose for prophylactic therapy is two inhalations three or four times a day.

To prevent exercise-induced bronchospasm, two inhalations should be taken before exertion.

*Elderly:* As for adults.

*Children:* One inhalation is the recommended dose for the relief of acute bronchospasm, in the management of episodic asthma or before exercise. One inhalation should be administered three or four times a day for prophylactic therapy. These doses may be increased to two inhalations if necessary.

On demand use should not exceed four times daily. The bronchodilator effect of each administration of inhaled salbutamol lasts for at least four hours except in patients whose asthma is becoming worse. Such patients should be warned not to increase their usage of the inhaler, but should seek medical advice in case treatment with an inhaled and/or systemic glucocorticosteroid is indicated.

As there may be adverse effects associated with excessive dosing, the dosage or frequency of administration should only be increased on medical advice.

*Contra-indications:* Inhaled salbutamol preparations are not appropriate for managing premature labour. Salbutamol presentations should not be used for threatened abortion.

Asmasal Clickhaler is contra-indicated in patients with a history of hypersensitivity to any of the components.

*Special warnings and precautions for use:* Bronchodilators should not be the only or main treatment in patients with severe or unstable asthma. Severe asthma requires regular medical assessment including lung function testing as patients are at risk of severe attacks and even death. Physicians should consider using oral corticosteroid therapy and/or the maximum recommended dose of inhaled corticosteroid in these patients. Increasing use of bronchodilators, in particular short-acting inhaled beta-2-agonists to relieve symptoms, indicates deterioration of asthma control. If patients find that short-acting bronchodilator treatment becomes less effective or they need more inhalations than usual, medical attention must be sought. In this situation, patients should be reassessed and consideration given to the need for increased anti-inflammatory therapy (e.g. higher doses of inhaled corticosteroids or a course of oral corticosteroids).

Severe exacerbations of asthma must be treated in the normal way. In the event of a previously effective dose of inhaled salbutamol failing to give relief lasting at least three hours, the patient should be warned to seek medical advice in order that any necessary additional steps may be taken.

The dosage or frequency of administration should only be increased on medical advice.

Salbutamol should be administered cautiously to patients suffering from thyrotoxicosis.

Salbutamol and non-selective beta-blocking drugs such as propranolol, should not usually be prescribed together.

Potentially serious hypokalaemia may result from beta-2-agonist therapy. Particular caution is advised in acute severe asthma as this effect may be potentiated by concomitant treatment with xanthine derivatives, steroids, diuretics and by hypoxia. It is recommended that serum potassium levels are monitored in such situations.

*Interaction with other medicaments and other forms of interaction:* Only those mentioned under *Special warnings and precautions for use* are known.

*Pregnancy and lactation:*
*Pregnancy* Administration of salbutamol during pregnancy should only be considered if the expected benefit to the mother is greater than any possible risk to the foetus. As with the majority of drugs there is little published evidence of its safety in the early stages of pregnancy, but in animal studies, there was evidence of some harmful effects in the foetus at very high dose levels.

*Lactation* Salbutamol may be secreted in breast milk. It is not known whether salbutamol has a harmful effect on the neonate and so its use should be restricted to situations where it is felt that the expected benefit to the mother is likely to outweigh any potential risk to the neonate.

*Effects on ability to drive and use machines:* None known.

*Undesirable effects:* Salbutamol may cause mild tremor, headache, slight tachycardia and a feeling of tenseness. These usually disappear with continued treatment.

There have been rare reports of transient muscle cramps.

Hypersensitivity reactions including angioedema and urticaria, bronchospasm, hypotension and collapse have been reported very rarely.

Potentially serious hypokalaemia may result in beta-2-agonist therapy.

As with other inhalation therapy, the potential for paradoxical bronchospasm should be kept in mind. If it occurs, the preparation should be discontinued immediately and alternative therapy instituted. As with other beta-2-agonists, hyperactivity in children has been reported rarely.

*Overdose:* The preferred antidote for overdosage with salbutamol is a cardioselective beta-blocking agent but beta-blocking drugs should be used with caution in patients with a history of bronchospasm.

## Pharmacological particulars

*Pharmacodynamic properties:* Salbutamol is a beta-adrenergic stimulant which has a highly selective action on bronchial beta-2-adrenoceptors and little or no effect on cardiac beta-1-receptors at therapeutic doses.

Salbutamol is also highly active in preventing antigen-induced release of histamine and slow reacting substance of anaphylaxis, SRS(A), from mast cells in human lung sensitised by IgE antibody. Such Type 1 hypersensitivity reactions are generally considered to be the primary triggers of the allergic asthma syndrome.

Salbutamol causes bronchodilation in normal subjects and in patients with asthma or chronic obstructive airways disease. Other actions on the respiratory system include enhanced mucociliary clearance and an anti-allergic effect due to inhibition of mediator release. The clinical relevance of these latter actions is not established.

The drug also causes vasodilation leading to a reflex chronotropic effect and widespread metabolic effects, including hypokalaemia.

*Pharmacokinetic properties:* Pre-systemic metabolism of salbutamol is considerable and occurs primarily in the gastrointestinal tract and by conjugation to form an inactive sulphate ester.

Following treatment with salbutamol by inhalation, only approximately 10% or less of the drug is deposited in the airways and the remainder is swallowed. Plasma concentrations are of no relevance to the effects of drug inhalation; the therapeutic effect is seen much sooner after inhalation than the time of peak plasma levels which suggests a local action; little therapeutic effect may be detectable at the time of peak plasma levels. Salbutamol is well absorbed from the gastrointestinal tract.

Following treatment with conventional tablets (4 mg), peak plasma levels of 10-16.9 micrograms/litre are recorded after 2-3 hours at which time the ratio of free drug to metabolite is about 1:5. The plasma half life is 2.7-5 hours and the major route of excretion is renal.

*Preclinical safety data:* Acute toxicity studies on salbutamol have indicated low toxicity. Selective beta-2-agonists, including salbutamol, have been shown to induce benign mesovarian leiomyomas in certain strains of rat susceptible to this type of tumour. There is no evidence of carcinogenicity, teratogenicity or mutagenicity.

## Pharmaceutical particulars

*List of excipients:* Lactose PhEur.

*Incompatibilities:* None known.

*Shelf life:* 2 years in unopened foil pouch. 6 months when removed from foil pouch.

*Special precautions for storage:* Store at up to 30°C in a dry place.

*Nature and contents of container:* A plastic inhaler device incorporating a specially designed actuator enclosed within an aluminium foil heat sealed bag. Each device contains a nominal 200 actuations.

*Instructions for use and handling:*
1. Remove mouthpiece cover from the inhaler.
2. Shake the inhaler well.
3. Hold the inhaler upright with thumb on the base and finger on the push button. Press the dosing button down firmly–once only.
4. Breathe out as far as is comfortable. Note: do not blow into the device at any time.
5. Place mouthpiece in your mouth. Close lips firmly around it (do not bite it).
6. Breathe in through your mouth steadily and deeply, to draw the medicine into your lungs.
7. Hold your breath, take the inhaler from your mouth and continue holding your breath for about 5 seconds.
8. For the second puff, keep the inhaler upright and repeat steps 2-7.
9. Replace the mouthpiece cover.

**Marketing authorisation number** 0039/0497.

**Date of approval/revision of SPC** April 1997

**Legal category** POM

# ASMASAL* SPACEHALER*

**Qualitative and quantitative composition** Each metered-dose contains 100 micrograms Salbutamol BP.

**Pharmaceutical form** Metered-dose inhaler with Spacehaler actuator.

The Spacehaler is a vortex generating actuator which acts to reduce the velocity of the emitted dose. Compared with a standard actuator it decreases the proportion of non-respirable drug particles within the emitted dose cloud whilst achieving a similar respirable fraction.

## Clinical particulars

*Therapeutic indications:*
(i) Treatment and prophylaxis of bronchial asthma.
(ii) Treatment of bronchitis and emphysema and conditions associated with reversible airways obstruction.
(iii) Relief of acute dyspnoea associated with reversible airways obstruction.
(iv) Particularly suitable for treatment of bronchospasm and in patients with co-existing heart disease or hypertension.

*Posology and method of administration:* Each inhalation, as delivered by the metering valve, contains 100 micrograms Salbutamol BP.
*Adults:*

| | |
|---|---|
| acute bronchospasm and intermittent episodes of asthma | one or two inhalations as a single dose |
| chronic maintenance or prophylactic therapy | two inhalations three or four times a day |
| to prevent exercise–induced bronchospasm | two inhalations should be taken before exercise |

*Children:*

| | |
|---|---|
| acute bronchospasm, episodic asthma or before exercise | one inhalation |
| routine maintenance or prophylactic therapy | one inhalation three or four times daily |

*Elderly:*
The dosage is the same as for other adults.

*Contra-indications:* In spite of the fact that salbutamol has been used intravenously and orally in the management of uncomplicated premature labour, Asmasal Spacehaler is not appropriate for such use.

Salbutamol is contra-indicated in patients with a history of hypersensitivity to any of its components.

*Special warnings and precautions for use:* Patients with hyperthyroidism or who are especially susceptible to salbutamol should use Asmasal Spacehaler with caution as should those patients suffering from diabetes mellitus, serious cardiovascular disorders or hypertension.

Asthmatic patients whose condition deteriorates despite salbutamol therapy or where a previously effective dose fails to give relief for at least three hours should seek medical advice. Alternative or additional therapy including corticosteroids should be instituted promptly.

*Interactions with other medicaments and other forms of interaction:* Adverse metabolic effects of high doses of salbutamol may be exacerbated by concomitant administration of high dose of corticosteroids.

Potentially serious hypokalaemia may result from β2-agonist therapy. Particular caution is advised in severe asthma as this effect may be potentiated by concomitant treatment with xanthine derivatives, steroids, diuretics and by hypoxia. It is recommended that serum potassium levels are monitored in such situations.

There is no evidence that adverse interactions occur between cardio-selective betablockers and sympathomimetic bronchodilators. Propranolol and other non-cardioselective beta-adrenoceptor blocking agents antagonise the effects of salbutamol.

*Pregnancy and lactation:* In spite of the fact that salbutamol has been used intravenously and orally in the management of uncomplicated premature labour, Asmasal Spacehaler is not appropriate for such use.

The existing data regarding the use of inhaled salbutamol during human pregnancy is insufficient to be able to assess possible harmful effects. Similarly little data is known regarding the possible harmful effects for breast-fed babies during lactation. It is therefore advised that salbutamol should be used in pregnancy only after careful consideration by the medical practitioner.

Use during lactation: Salbutamol should be used in lactation only after careful consideration by the medical practitioner.

*Effects on ability to drive and use machines:* On the basis of the pharmacodynamic profile, reported ADR and/or impairment of driving performance or performance related to driving, the medicine is presumed to be safe or unlikely to produce an effect.

*Undesirable effects:* Potentially serious hypokalaemia may result from β2-agonist therapy.

Salbutamol in large dosage may cause fine tremor of skeletal muscle (particularly the hands), palpitations and muscle cramps. Slight tachycardia, tenseness, headaches and peripheral vasodilatation have also been reported after large doses but these are less usually associated with the inhalation dosage form.

*Overdose:* Overdosage may result in skeletal muscle tremor, tachycardia, tenseness, headache and peripheral vasodilatation. Preferred treatment is with cautious use of cardioselective beta-adrenoceptor blocking agents.

### Pharmacological properties

*Pharmacodynamic properties:* Salbutamol is a direct acting sympathomimetic bronchodilator agent with a predominantly beta-adrenergic activity and a selective action on β2-receptors.

*Pharmacokinetic properties:* Salbutamol is readily absorbed from the gastro-intestinal tract. It is subject to first pass metabolism in the liver; about half is excreted in the urine as an inactive sulphate conjugate following oral administration (the rest being unchanged salbutamol). Salbutamol does not appear to be metabolised in the lung, therefore its behaviour following inhalation depends upon the delivery method used which determines the proportion of inhaled salbutamol relative to the proportion inadvertently swallowed. Spacehaler is considered to reduce buccal deposition and therefore the proportion of drug swallowed, compared with a standard metered dose inhaler.

The plasma half-life has been estimated to range from about two to seven hours.

*Preclinical safety data:* No preclinical data are available since salbutamol has been used clinically for over 20 years. The safety and efficacy of salbutamol have been proven.

Please see *Clinical Particulars* sections above for further guidance.

### Pharmaceutical particulars

*List of excipients:* Oleic Acid BP, Dichlorodifluoromethane BP 1988, Trichlorofluoromethane BP 1988

*Incompatibilities:* None known

*Shelf life:* Thirty-six months

*Special precautions for storage:* Store below 30°C. Keep away from direct sunlight or heat. Protect from frost. Do not puncture or burn the canister even when it seems empty.

*Nature and contents of container:* Aerosol for inhalation supplied in a pressurised aluminium container with metering valve crimped in place, containing 80, 200 or 300 metered actuations of Salbutamol BP.

*Instructions for use/handling:* Instructions as shown in the leaflet:

1. Remove the cap from the inhaler mouthpiece. Make sure the mouthpiece is clean and clear of fluff and dirt.
2. Hold the inhaler upright, with your thumb on the base and your first finger on the top of the can. Now shake the inhaler gently up and down.
3. Breathe out fully to empty the lungs and then place the mouthpiece firmly between the lips.
4. Now breathe in slowly and deeply. At the same time press the aerosol can with your first finger to fire the aerosol and release the drug.
5. Remove the inhaler from your mouth and hold breath for 10 seconds or as long as is comfortable. Breathe out slowly.
6. If more than one puff is required, wait at least one minute and repeat procedure from step 2. Replace the cap.
7. Your inhaler should be cleaned regularly usually at least once a week. To clean, remove the metal canister from the plastic body and remove the plastic cover from the mouthpiece. Rinse the plastic body and the mouthpiece cover in warm water. Dry thoroughly then replace the canister and mouthpiece cover. Avoid excessive heat. Do not put the metal canister into water.

Important: Do not rush steps 3 and 4. It is important that you start to breathe in as slowly as possible just before operating your inhaler. Practice in the mirror for the first few times. If you see a 'mist' coming from the top of your inhaler or the sides of your mouth, you should start again from step 2.

**Marketing authorisation number**   0039/0479

**Date of approval/revision of SPC**   May 1997

**Legal category**   POM

## BETA-CARDONE* TABLETS

### Presentation

*Beta-Cardone Tablets 200 mg:* White, circular, scored tablets engraved Evans/BC20, each containing sotalol hydrochloride 200 mg.

*Beta-Cardone Tablets 80 mg:* Pink, circular, scored tablets engraved Evans/BC8, each containing sotalol hydrochloride 80 mg.

*Beta-Cardone Tablets 40 mg:* Green, circular, scored tablets engraved Evans/BC4, each containing sotalol hydrochloride 40 mg.

### Uses

*Ventricular arrhythmias:* Treatment of life-threatening ventricular tachyarrhythmias and symptomatic non-sustained ventricular tachyarrhythmias.

*Supraventricular arrhythmias:* Prophylaxis of paroxysmal atrial tachycardia, paroxysmal atrial fibrillation, paroxysmal A-V nodal re-entrant tachycardia, paroxysmal A-V re-entrant tachycardia using accessory pathways, and paroxysmal supraventricular tachycardia after cardiac surgery. Maintenance of normal sinus rhythm following conversion of atrial fibrillation or atrial flutter.

Beta-Cardone has both β-adrenoceptor blocking (Vaughan Williams Class II) and cardiac action potential duration prolongation (Vaughan Williams Class III) antiarrhythmic properties. Its action is devoid of intrinsic sympathomimetic and local anaesthetic activity. Its major therapeutic effect is to protect the heart from undesirable sympathetic activity. Beta-Cardone reduces the rate and force of contraction of the heart; cardiac work and oxygen consumption are diminished.

### Dosage and administration

*Oral administration in adults:*
*General instructions:* When administering Beta-Cardone to a patient for the first time, it is desirable to start with a low dose and gradually increase the dose until the desired response is obtained; as a general rule the heart rate should not be reduced to less than 55 beats per minute.

Before starting treatment or increasing the dose the corrected QT interval should be measured and renal function, electrolyte balance, and concomitant medications assessed. Treatment with Beta-Cardone should be initiated and doses increased in a facility capable of monitoring and assessing cardiac rhythm. The dosage must be individualised and based on the patient's response. Proarrhythmic events can occur not only at initiation of therapy, but also with each upward dosage adjustment.

Treatment with Beta-Cardone should not be discontinued suddenly, especially in patients with ischaemic heart disease (angina pectoris, prior acute myocardial infarction) or hypertension, to prevent exacerbation of the disease (see section 'Abrupt withdrawal' under 'Special warnings').

The following are guidelines for oral administration. The initial dose is 80 mg, as one or two divided doses. Oral dosage should be adjusted gradually allowing 2–3 days between dosing increments in order to attain steady-state, and to allow monitoring of QT intervals. Most patients respond to 160 to 320 mg per day, in two divided doses.

The dosage should be reduced in renal impairment. Creatinine clearance: 60–30 ml/min: ½ recommended dose. Creatinine clearance 30–10 ml/min: ¼ recommended dose.

*Administration in children:* Beta-Cardone is not intended for administration to children.

### Contra-indications, warnings, etc

*Contra-indications:* Beta-Cardone should not be given to patients with sick sinus syndrome; long QT syndromes, torsades de pointes; symptomatic sinus bradycardia; uncontrolled congestive heart failure; cardiogenic shock; anaesthesia that produces myocardial depression; untreated phaeochromocytoma; hypotension (except due to arrhythmia); Raynaud's phenomenon and severe peripheral circulatory disturbances; chronic obstructive airway disease or bronchial asthma; renal failure (creatinine clearance < 10 ml/min).

Beta-Cardone should not be given to patients suffering from heart block or who may have a history of bronchospasm. In patients with poor cardiac reserve β-blockade can precipitate heart failure; in such cases, Beta-Cardone therapy should not be commenced until the patient has been controlled by therapy (ACE inhibitors, cardiac glycosides or, if necessary, diuretic therapy – see *Interactions*).

Beta-Cardone should not be given to patients suffering from diabetic keto-acidosis or metabolic acidosis; therapy with Beta-Cardone can be commenced or resumed when the metabolic condition has been corrected.

*Interactions:* In combined therapy, clonidine should not be discontinued until several days after withdrawal of Beta-Cardone. Use with great caution with drugs that also prolong QT interval, e.g. disopyramide, amiodarone, Class I antiarrhythmic agents, calcium antagonists of the verapamil type or tricyclic antidepressants.

Concomitant potassium-depleting diuretics may increase the potential for torsade de pointes.

Proarrhythmic events are more common in patients also receiving digitalis glycosides.

Interactions also occur with phenothiazines, terfenadine, astemizole and diltiazem.

Concomitant use of reserpine, guanethidine, or alpha methyldopa requires close monitoring for evidence of hypotension and/or marked bradycardia, syncope.

Tubocurarin: Neuromuscular blockade is prolonged by beta-blocking agents.

*Effects on ability to drive and use machines:* Side-effects such as dizziness and fatigue should be taken into account.

*Side-effects:* The most significant adverse effects are those due to proarrhythmia, including torsades de pointes.

Bradycardia, dyspnoea, chest pain, palpitations, oedema, ECG abnormalities, hypotension, proarrhythmia, syncope, heart failure and presyncope can occur. Nausea/vomiting, diarrhoea, dyspepsia, abdominal pain, flatulence, cramps, fatigue, dizziness, asthenia, lightheadedness, headache, sleep disturbances, depression, paraesthesia, mood changes, anxiety, sexual dysfunction, visual disturbances, taste abnormalities, hearing disturbances and fever have also been reported.

Beta-blockers, even those with apparent cardioselectivity should not be used in patients with asthma or a history of obstructive airways disease unless no alternative treatment is available. In such cases, the risk of inducing bronchospasm should be appreciated and appropriate precautions taken. If bronchospasm should occur after the use of Beta-Cardone it can be treated with beta₂-agonist by inhalation e.g. salbutamol (the dose of which may need to be greater than the usual dose in asthma) and, if necessary, intravenous atropine 1 mg.

There have been reports of skin rashes and/or dry eyes associated with the use of β-adrenoceptor-blocking drugs. The reported incidence is small and in most cases the symptoms have cleared when the treatment was withdrawn. Discontinuance of the drug should be considered if any such reaction is not otherwise explicable. Cessation of therapy with a β-blocker should be gradual.

*Use in pregnancy and lactation:*
*Pregnancy:* Animal studies with sotalol hydrochloride have shown no evidence of teratogenicity or other harmful effects on the foetus. Nevertheless its use throughout pregnancy should be avoided unless it is absolutely necessary as it crosses the placenta and may cause foetal bradycardia.
*Lactation:* Infants should not be fed with breast milk from mothers being treated with Beta-Cardone.

*Other special warnings and precautions:*
*Abrupt withdrawal:* Patients should be carefully monitored when discontinuing chronically administered sotalol, particularly those with ischaemic heart disease. If possible the dosage should be gradually reduced over a period of 1 to 2 weeks, if necessary at the same time initiating replacement therapy. Hypersensitivity to catecholamines is observed in patients withdrawn from β-blocker therapy. Occasional cases of exacerbation of angina pectoris, arrhythmias and in some cases myocardial infarction have been reported after abrupt discontinuation of therapy. Abrupt discontinuation may unmask latent coronary insufficiency. In addition, hypertension may develop.

*Proarrhythmias:* Rarely, Beta-Cardone causes aggravation of pre-existing arrhythmias or the provocation of new arrhythmias.

Risk factors for torsades de pointes include prolongation of the QT interval, bradycardia, reduction in serum potassium and magnesium, and history of cardiomegaly or congestive heart failure, sustained ventricular tachycardia.

Proarrhythmic events can occur on initiating therapy and with every upward dose adjustment, The incidence of torsades de pointes is dose dependent.

Caution should be used if the $QT_c$ exceeds 500 msec whilst on therapy. It is advisable to reduce dose or discontinue therapy when the $QT_c$ interval exceeds 550 msec.

*Electrolyte disturbances:* Beta-Cardone should not be used in patients with hypokalaemia or hypomagnesaemia. Potassium levels should be monitored. In conditions likely to provoke hypokalaemia/hypomagnesaemia, such as persistent diarrhoea, appropriate corrective clinical measures should be taken.

*Heart failure:* Beta-blockade may precipitate heart failure.

Following myocardial infarction careful monitoring and dose titration are critical during initiation and follow-up of therapy. Sotalol should be avoided in patients with left ventricular ejection fractions ≤ 40% without serious ventricular arrhythmias.

*Thyrotoxicosis:* Beta-blockade may mask certain clinical signs of hyperthyroidism.

*Treated diabetes:* Beta-Cardone, like other β-blocking agents, may reduce or mask the usual pre-hypoglycaemic warning signs. It may be necessary to adjust the dose of anti-diabetic therapy.

*General anaesthesia:* If desired, Beta-Cardone may be stopped four days prior to surgery under specialist supervision. However, where sudden withdrawal might expose the patient to severe angina or arrhythmias, anaesthesia can proceed provided that the following precautions are taken.

1. Vagal dominance is counteracted by premedication with atropine sulphate (0.25 to 2.0 mg) administered intravenously.
2. Anaesthetic agents such as ether, chloroform, cyclopropane, trichlorethylene, methoxyflurane and enflurane, are not used.

*Alcoholism:* β-adrenoceptor blocking drugs may precipitate cardiac failure in alcoholic patients.

*Upper respiratory infections:* In these conditions, patients without a history of airways obstruction may suffer bronchospasm from β-blockade.

The product labelling will bear a statement warning against use in patients with a history of wheezing or asthma.

*Overdosage:* Overdosage causes excessive bradycardia and hypotension; to counteract this atropine sulphate (0.25 to 2.0 mg) should be administered intravenously and, if need be, isoprenaline (about 5 micrograms per minute) by slow intravenous injection. In severe overdose, intravenous glucagon may be preferred: an initial bolus dose of 5 to 10 mg in dextrose or saline should be followed by an intravenous infusion of 4 mg/hour or as sufficient to maintain cardiac output. Prolongation of the Q-Tc interval has been reported. Transvenous pacing may be required.

**Pharmaceutical precautions** Beta-Cardone Tablets should be protected from light.

**Legal category** POM.

**Package quantities**
*Beta-Cardone 200 mg* are available in containers of 30 tablets (OP).
*Beta-Cardone 80 mg* are available in containers of 100 tablets (OP).
*Beta-Cardone 40 mg* are available in containers of 100 tablets (OP).

**Further information** Beta-Cardone is not metabolised and, in the main, is excreted in the urine. After oral administration the plasma half life has been shown to be 17 hours; the lipid solubility is very low.

**Product licence numbers**
Beta-Cardone Tablets 200 mg    0039/0416
Beta-Cardone Tablets 80 mg    0039/0415
Beta-Cardone Tablets 40 mg    0039/0414

## BETNELAN* TABLETS

**Qualitative and quantitative composition** Each tablet contains 500 micrograms (0.5 mg) betamethasone.

**Pharmaceutical form** Small white tablets engraved 'Betnelan Evans' on one side and scored on the reverse. The product complies with the specification for Betamethasone Tablets BP.

**Clinical particulars**

*Therapeutic indications:* Betamethasone is a glucocorticosteroid which is about eight to ten times as active as prednisolone on a weight-for-weight basis.

A wide variety of diseases may sometimes require corticosteroid therapy. Some of the principal indications are:

Bronchial asthma, severe hypersensitivity reactions, anaphylaxis; rheumatoid arthritis, systemic lupus erythematosis, dermatomyositis, mixed connective tissue disease (excluding systemic sclerosis), polyarteritis nodosa; inflammatory skin disorders, including pemphigus vulgaris, bullous pemphigoid and pyoderma gangrenosum; minimal change nephrotic syndrome, acute interstitial nephritis; ulcerative colitis, Crohn's disease; sarcoidosis; rheumatic carditis; haemolytic anaemia (auto-immune), acute and lymphatic leukaemia, malignant lymphoma, multiple myeloma, idiopathic thrombocytopenia purpura; immuno-suppression in transplantation.

*Posology and method of administration:* The lowest dosage that will produce an acceptable result should be used; when it is possible to reduce the dosage, this must be accomplished in stages. During prolonged therapy, dosage may need to be increased temporarily during periods of stress or in exacerbation of illness (see *Special warnings and precautions for use*).

Adults: The dose used will depend upon the disease, its severity, and the clinical response obtained. The following regimens are for guidance only.

Short-term treatment: 2 to 3 mg daily for the first few days, subsequently reducing the daily dosage by 250 or 500 micrograms (0.25 or 0.5 mg) every two to five days, depending upon the response.

Rheumatoid arthritis: 500 micrograms (0.5 mg) to 2 mg daily. For maintenance therapy the lowest effective dosage is used.

Most other conditions: 1.5 to 5 mg daily for one to three weeks, then reducing to the minimum effective dosage.

Larger doses may be needed for mixed connective tissue diseases and ulcerative colitis.

Children: A proportion of the adult dosage may be used (e.g. 75% at twelve years, 50% at seven years and 25% at one year) but clinical factors must be given due consideration (see *Special warnings and precautions for use*).

*Contra-indications:* Systemic infections, unless specific anti-infective therapy is employed. Hypersensitivity to any component of the tablets.

*Special warnings and precautions for use:* A Patient Information Leaflet should be supplied with this product.

Undesirable effects may be minimised by using the lowest effective dose for the minimum period, administering the daily requirement as a single morning dose, or as a single morning dose on alternate days whenever possible. Frequent patient review is required to appropriately titrate the dose against disease activity (see *Posology and method of administration*).

Suppression of the inflammatory response and immune function increases the susceptibility to infections and their severity. The clinical presentation may often be atypical and serious infections such as septicaemia and tuberculosis may be masked and may reach an advanced stage before being recognised.

Chickenpox is of particular concern since this normally minor illness may be fatal in immunosuppressed patients. Patients (or parents of children) without a definite history of chickenpox should be advised to avoid close personal contact with chickenpox or herpes zoster and if exposed they should seek urgent medical attention. Passive immunisation with varicella/zoster immunoglobulin (VZIG) is needed by exposed non-immune patients who are receiving systemic corticosteroids or who have used them within the previous 3 months; this should be given within 10 days of exposure to chickenpox. If a diagnosis of chickenpox is confirmed, the illness warrants specialist care and urgent treatment. Corticosteroids should not be stopped and the dose may need to be increased.

Live vaccines should not be given to individuals with impaired immune responsiveness. The antibody response to other vaccines may be diminished.

Adrenal suppression: Adrenal cortical atrophy develops during prolonged therapy and may persist for years after stopping treatment. Withdrawal of corticosteroids after prolonged therapy must therefore always be gradual to avoid acute adrenal insufficiency, being tapered off over weeks or months according to the dose and duration of treatment. During prolonged therapy any intercurrent illness, trauma or surgical procedure will require a temporary increase in dosage; if corticosteroids have been stopped following prolonged therapy they may need to be temporarily re-introduced.

Special precautions: Particular care is required when considering the use of systemic corticosteroids in patients with the following conditions and frequent patient monitoring is necessary.

A. Osteoporosis (post-menopausal females are particularly at risk).
B. Hypertension or congestive heart failure.
C. Existing or previous history of severe affective disorders (especially previous steroid psychosis).
D. Diabetes mellitus (or a family history of diabetes).
E. History of tuberculosis.
F. Glaucoma (or a family history of glaucoma).
G. Previous corticosteroid-induced myopathy.
H. Liver failure – blood levels of corticosteroid may be increased, (as with other drugs which are metabolised in the liver).
I. Renal insufficiency.
J. Epilepsy.
K. Peptic ulceration.

Patients should carry 'steroid treatment' cards which give clear guidance on the precautions to be taken to minimise risk and which provide details of prescriber, drug, dosage and the duration of treatment.

Use in children: Corticosteroids cause dose-related growth retardation in infancy, childhood and adolescence, which may be irreversible. Treatment should be limited to the minimum dosage for the shortest possible time. In order to minimise suppression of the HPA axis and growth retardation, consideration should be given to administration of a single dose on alternate days.

Use in the elderly: The common adverse effects of systemic corticosteroids may be associated with more serious consequences in old age, especially osteoporosis, hypertension, hypokalaemia, diabetes, susceptibility to infection and thinning of the skin. Close clinical supervision is required to avoid life-threatening reactions.

*Interactions with other medicaments and other forms of interaction* Steroids may reduce the effects of anticholinesterases in myasthenia gravis, cholecystographic X-ray media and non-steroidal anti-inflammatory agents.

Rifampicin, rifabutin, carbamazepine, phenobarbitone, phenytoin, primidone, aminoglutethimide and ephedrine enhance the metabolism of corticosteroids; thus the corticosteroid therapeutic effect may be reduced.

The desired effects of hypoglycaemic agents (including insulin), anti-hypertensives and diuretics are antagonised by corticosteroids, and the hypokalaemic effects of acetazolamide, loop diuretics, thiazide diuretics and carbenoxolone are enhanced.

The efficacy of coumarin anticoagulants may be enhanced by concurrent corticosteroid therapy and close monitoring of the INR or prothrombin time is required to avoid spontaneous bleeding.

The renal clearance of salicylates is increased by corticosteroids and steroid withdrawal may result in salicylate intoxication.

*Pregnancy and lactation:* Intrauterine growth retardation in the foetus and a small increased risk of cleft palate have been reported. Hypoadrenalism may occur in the neonate. When corticosteroids are essential, however, patients with normal pregnancies may be treated as if they were in the non-gravid state. Patients with pre-eclampsia or fluid retention require close monitoring.

Corticosteroids are excreted in small amounts in breast milk and infants of mothers taking pharmacological doses of steroids should be monitored carefully for signs of adrenal suppression.

*Effects on ability to drive and use machine:s* None known

*Undesirable effects:* The incidence of predictable undesirable effects, including hypothalamic-pituitary-adrenal (HPA) axis suppression correlates with the relative potency of the drug, dosage, timing of administration and the duration of treatment (see *Special warnings and precautions for use*).

Endocrine/metabolic: Suppression of the hypothalamic-pituitary-adrenal axis, growth suppression in infancy, childhood and adolescence, menstrual irregularity and amenorrhoea. Cushingoid facies, hirsutism, weight gain, impaired carbohydrate tolerance with increased requirement for antidiabetic therapy. Negative protein and calcium balance. Increased appetite.

Anti-inflammatory and immunosuppressive effects: Increased susceptibility to and severity of infections with suppression of clinical symptoms and signs, opportunistic infections, recurrence of dormant tuberculosis (see *Special warnings and precautions for use*).

Musculoskeletal: Osteoporosis, vertebral and long bone fractures, avascular osteonecrosis, tendon rupture, proximal myopathy.

Fluid and electrolyte disturbance: Sodium and water retention, hypertension, potassium loss, hypokalaemic alkalosis.

Neuropsychiatric: Euphoria, psychological dependence, depression, psychosis, insomnia, and aggravation of schizophrenia. Increased intra-cranial pressure with papilloedema in children (pseudotumour cerebri), usually after treatment withdrawal. Aggravation of epilepsy.

Ophthalmic: Increased intra-ocular pressure, glaucoma, papilloedema, posterior subcapsular cataracts, corneal or scleral thinning, exacerbation of ophthalmic viral or fungal diseases.

Gastrointestinal: Dyspepsia, peptic ulceration with perforation and haemorrhage, acute pancreatitis, candidiasis.

Dermatological: Impaired healing, skin atrophy, bruising, telangiectasia, striae, acne.

General: Hypersensitivity including anaphylaxis, has been reported. Leucocytosis. Thrombo-embolism.

Withdrawal symptoms and signs: Too rapid a reduction of corticosteroid dosage following prolonged treatment can lead to acute adrenal insufficiency, hypotension and death (see Special warnings and precautions for use).

A 'withdrawal syndrome' may also occur including; fever, myalgia, arthralgia, rhinitis, conjunctivitis, painful itchy skin nodules and loss of weight.

Overdose: Treatment is unlikely to be needed in cases of acute overdosage.

## Pharmacological properties

Pharmacodynamic properties: Betamethasone is a glucocorticoid which is about eight to ten times as active as prednisolone on a weight-for-weight basis.

Pharmacokinetic properties: Corticosteroids are bound to plasma proteins in varying degrees. Corticosteroids are metabolised primarily in the liver and are then excreted by the kidneys.

## Pharmaceutical particulars

List of excipients: Lactose, Starch Maize , Gelatin, Magnesium Stearate, Purified Water

Incompatibilities: None known

Shelf life: 3 years

Special precautions for storage: Store below 30°C and protect from light.

Nature and contents of container: Tubular glass vial with a polyurethane snap-plug closure containing 100 tablets

Tamper evident polypropylene container with a polyurethane foam wad and a low density polyethylene lid.

**Marketing authorisation number** 0039/0392

**Date of approval/revision of SPC** July 1997

**Legal category** POM

# BETNESOL* EYE, EAR AND NOSE PREPARATIONS

**Presentation** Betnesol Drops contains betamethasone sodium phosphate 0.1% w/v, and benzalkonium chloride 0.02% w/v in a clear, colourless to pale yellow aqueous solution that is sterile until the bottle is opened. This product complies with the BPC specification for Betamethasone Eye Drops.

Betnesol Eye Ointment contains betamethasone sodium phosphate 0.1 % w/w in a bland, soft paraffin base of white, translucent appearance. Sterile until opened.

**Uses**

Ointment: Short-term treatment of steroid responsive inflammatory conditions of the eye after clinical exclusion of bacterial, viral and fungal infections.

Drops: In addition to the above: Non-infected inflammatory conditions of the ear or nose.

**Dosage and administration** The frequency of dosing depends on the clinical response. If there is no clinical response within 7 days of treatment, the treatment should be discontinued. Treatment should be the lowest effective dose for the shortest possible time. After more prolonged treatment (over 6 to 8 weeks), the drops or ointment should be withdrawn slowly to avoid relapse.

Ointment:

Adults (and the Elderly) and Children: An extrusion of the ointment about 1/4 inch long may be introduced beneath the lower lid two or three times daily and/or at night or as directed by physician.

Drops:

Eyes: I or 2 drops instilled into the eye every one or two hours until control is achieved, when the frequency may be reduced.

Ears: 2 or 3 drops instilled into the ear every two or three hours until control is achieved, when the frequency may be reduced.

Nose: 2 or 3 drops instilled into each nostril two or three times daily.

**Contra-indications, warnings, etc.**

Contra-indications:

Drops and Ointment: Bacterial, viral, fungal, tuberculous or purulent conditions of the eye. Use is contra-

indicated if glaucoma is present, or herpetic keratitis (e.g. dendritic ulcer) is considered a possibility.

Use of topical steroids in the latter condition can lead to the extension of the ulcer and marked visual deterioration.

Cortisoteroids should not be used in patients with a perforated tympanic membrane.

Hypersensitivity to any component of the preparation.

Topical corticosteroids should never be given for an undiagnosed "red eye" as inappropriate use is potentially blinding.

Drops: In addition to the above: Betnesol Drops contain benzalkonium chloride as a preservative and therefore should not be used as eye drops to treat patients who wear soft contact lenses.

Precautions: Topical corticosteroids should not be used in the eye for longer than one week except under the direction and supervision of an opthalmologist in the management of certain specific eye disorders, to exclude raised intra-ocular pressure, cataract formation, or unsuspected infections. Prolonged continuous use should be avoided.

Prolonged use may lead to the risk of adrenal suppression in infants.

Pregnancy and lactation: Safety for use in pregnancy and lactation has not been established. There is inadequate evidence of safety in human pregnancy. Topical administration of corticosteroids to pregnant animals can cause abnormalities of fetal development including cleft palate and intra-uterine growth retardation. There may, therefore, be a very small risk of such effects in the human foetus.

Side-effects: Hypersensitivity reactions, usually of the delayed type, may occur leading to irritation, burning, stinging, itching and dermatitis.

Topical steroid use may increase intra-ocular pressure leading to optic nerve damage, reduced visual acuity and visual field defects.

Intensive or prolonged use of topical corticosteroids may lead to formation of posterior subcapsular cataracts.

In those diseases causing thinning of the cornea or sclera, corticosteroid therapy may result in thinning of the globe leading to perforation.

Mydriasis, ptosis and epithelial punctate keratitis have also been reported following ophthalmic use of corticosteroids.

Following nasal administration, the most common effects are nasal irritation and dryness, although sneezing, headache, lightheadedness, urticaria, nausea, epistaxis, rebound congestion, bronchial asthma, perforation of the nasal septum and anosmia have also been reported.

Excessive and prolonged intranasal usage above the recommended dose may induce systemic side effects.

May cause transient blurring of vision on instillation. Warn patients not to drive or operate hazardous machinery unless vision is clear.

Overdosage: Oral ingestion of the contents of one bottle (up to 10 ml) of drops, or one tube (up to 3 g) of ointment is unlikely to lead to any serious adverse effects.

Long term intensive topical use may lead to systemic effects.

**Pharmaceutical precautions** Store at a temperature not exceeding 25°C. The product should not be used later than 28 days from the date of breaking its protective seal and any contents remaining after this date should be discarded.

**Legal category** POM.

**Package quantities**

Betnesol Drops Plastic dropper bottles containing 10 ml

Betnesol Eye Ointment Narrow-nozzle tubes containing 3 g.

**Further information** Nil

**Product licence numbers**
Betnesol Drops          0039/0387
Betnesol Eye Ointment   0039/0388

# BETNESOL* INJECTION

**Qualitative and quantitative composition** Each ampoule of ready-prepared Betnesol Injection contains 4 mg betamethasone as the sodium phosphate ester in 1 ml of sterile aqueous solution.

**Pharmaceutical form** 1 ml ampoules containing a clear colourless to pale yellow solution.

**Clinical particulars**

Therapeutic indications: Betamethasone is a glucocorticosteroid which is about eight to ten times as active as prednisolone on a weight-for-weight basis. It may be indicated in the following conditions:

Status asthmaticus and acute allergic reactions, including anaphylactic reactions to drugs. Betnesol Injection supplements the action of adrenaline.

Severe shock arising from surgical or accidental trauma or overwhelming infection.

Acute adrenal crisis caused by abnormal stress in Addison's disease, Simmonds' disease, hypopituitarism following adrenalectomy, and when adrenocortical function has been suppressed by prolonged corticosteroid therapy.

Soft tissue lesions such as tennis elbow, tenosynovitis and bursitis.

N.B. Betnesol Injection does not replace other forms of therapy for the treatment of shock and status asthmaticus.

Posology and method of administration: The incidence of predictable undesirable effects, including hypothalamic-pituitary-adrenal (HPA) axis suppression correlates with the relative potency of the drug, dosage, timing of administration and the duration of treatment (see Special warnings and precautions for use). Betnesol Injection is not intended for long-term use.

Systemic therapy in adults: 4 to 20 mg betamethasone (1 to 5 ml) administered by slow intravenous injection over half to one minute. Alternatively, Betnesol Injection may be given by intravenous infusion. The same dose can be given by deep intramuscular injection but the response is likely to be less rapid, especially in shock.

This dose can be repeated three or four times in 24 hours depending upon the condition being treated and the clinical response.

Systemic therapy in children: Infants up to 1 year may be given 1 mg betamethasone intravenously; children aged 1 to 5 years, 2 mg; 6 to 12 years, 4 mg (1 ml). This dose can be repeated three or four times in 24 hours, depending upon the condition being treated and the clinical response.

Other routes: Local injections of 4 to 8 mg Betnesol may be used when treating soft tissue lesions in adults; children may require smaller doses. This dose can be repeated on two or three occasions depending upon the clinical response.

Betnesol Injection has also been administered subconjunctivally as a single injection of 0.5 to 1 ml. Intrathecal use is not recommended.

Contra-indications: Systemic infections, unless specific anti-infective therapy is employed.

Betnesol Injection contains sodium metabisulphite (0.1% w/v) as a preservative and therefore should not be used to treat patients with known hypersensitivity to bisulphite, metabisulphite or any other component of the injection.

Betnesol Injection should not be injected directly into tendons.

Special warnings and precautions for use: A patient information leaflet should be supplied with this product.

Undesirable effects may be minimised by using the lowest effective dose for the minimum period, and by administering the daily requirement as a single morning dose, or whenever possible as a single morning dose on alternate days. Frequent patient review is required to appropriately titrate the dose against disease activity (see Posology and method of administration).

Suppression of the inflammatory response and immune function increases the susceptibility to infections and their severity. The clinical presentation may often be atypical and serious infections such as septicaemia and tuberculosis may be masked and may reach an advanced stage before being recognised.

Chickenpox is of particular concern since this normally minor illness may be fatal in immunosuppressed patients. Patients (or parents of children) without a definite history of chickenpox should be advised to avoid close personal contact with chickenpox or herpes zoster and if exposed they should seek urgent medical attention. Passive immunisation with varicella zoster immunoglobulin (VZIG) is needed by exposed non-immune patients who are receiving systemic corticosteroids or who have used them within the previous 3 months; this should be given within 10 days of exposure to chickenpox. If a diagnosis of chickenpox is confirmed, the illness warrants specialist care and urgent treatment. Corticosteroids should not be stopped and the dose may need to be increased.

Live vaccines should not be given to individuals with impaired immune responsiveness. The antibody response to other vaccines may be diminished.

In the treatment of cerebral oedema due to brain trauma, gastrointestinal bleeding may occur and stool examination may be helpful in diagnosis.

Adrenal suppression: Adrenal cortical atrophy develops during prolonged therapy and may persist for years after stopping treatment. Withdrawal of corticosteroids after prolonged therapy must therefore always be gradual to avoid acute adrenal insufficiency, it should be tapered off over weeks or months according to the dose and duration of treatment. During prolonged therapy any intercurrent illness, trauma or surgical procedure will require a temporary increase in dosage; if corticosteroids have been stopped following prolonged therapy they may need to be temporarily re-introduced.

Special precautions: Particular care is required when considering the use of systemic corticosteroids in patients with the following conditions and frequent patient monitoring is necessary.

A. Osteoporosis (post-menopausal females are particularly at risk).
B. Hypertension or congestive heart failure.
C. Existing or previous history of severe affective disorders (especially previous steroid psychosis).
D. Diabetes mellitus (or a family history of diabetes).
E. History of, or active, tuberculosis.
F. Glaucoma (or a family history of glaucoma).
G. Previous corticosteroid-induced myopathy.
H. Liver failure – blood levels of corticosteroid may be increased, as with other drugs which are metabolised in the liver.
I. Renal insufficiency.
J. Epilepsy.
K. History of, or active, peptic ulceration.
L. Herpes simplex keratitis.
M. Diverticulitis.
N. Thromboembolic tendencies.

Patients should carry 'steroid treatment' cards which give clear guidance on the precautions to be taken to minimise risk and which provide details of prescriber, drug, dosage and the duration of treatment.

Use in children: Corticosteroids cause dose-related growth retardation in infancy, childhood and adolescence, which may be irreversible. Treatment should be limited to the minimum dosage for the shortest possible time. In order to minimise suppression of the HPA axis and growth retardation, consideration should be given to administration of a single dose on alternate days.

Use in the elderly: The common adverse effects of systemic corticosteroids may be associated with more serious consequences in old age, especially osteoporosis, hypertension, hypokalaemia, diabetes, susceptibility to infection and thinning of the skin. Close clinical supervision is required to avoid life-threatening reactions.

Interactions with other medicaments and other forms of interaction: Steroids may reduce the effects of anticholinesterases in myasthenia gravis cholecystographic x-ray media and non-steroidal anti-inflammatory agents.

Rifampicin, rifabutin, carbamazepine, phenobarbitone, phenytoin, primidone, aminoglutethimide and ephedrine enhance the metabolism of corticosteroids and their therapeutic effects may be reduced.

The desired effects of hypoglycaemic agents (including insulin), anti-hypertensives and diuretics are antagonised by corticosteroids, and the hypokalaemic effects of acetazolamide, loop diuretics, thiazide diuretics and carbenoxolone are enhanced.

The efficacy of coumarin anticoagulants may be enhanced by concurrent corticosteroid therapy and close monitoring of the INR or prothrombin time is required to avoid spontaneous bleeding.

The renal clearance of salicylates is increased by corticosteroids and steroid withdrawal may result in salicylate intoxication.

There have been rare reports of convulsions in patients on high dose corticosteroids and cyclosporin.

Pregnancy and lactation: Intra-uterine growth retardation in the foetus and a small increased risk of cleft palate have been reported. Hypoadrenalism may occur in the neonate. When corticosteroids are essential however, patients with normal pregnancies may be treated as though they were in the non-gravid state. Patients with pre-eclampsia or fluid retention require close monitoring.

Corticosteroids are excreted in small amounts in breast milk and infants of mothers taking pharmacological doses of steroids should be monitored carefully for signs of adrenal suppression.

Effects on ability to drive and use machines: None known

Undesirable effects: The incidence of predictable undesirable effects, including hypothalamic-pituitary-adrenal (HPA) axis suppression correlates with the relative potency of the drug, dosage, timing of administration and the duration of treatment (see Special warnings and precautions for use).

Endocrine/metabolic: Suppression of the hypothalamic-pituitary-adrenal (HPA) axis, growth suppression in infancy, childhood and adolescence, menstrual irregularity and amenorrhoea. Cushingoid facies, hirsutism, weight gain, impaired carbohydrate tolerance with increased requirement for antidiabetic

therapy. Negative protein and calcium balance. Increased appetite.

Anti-inflammatory and immunosuppressive effects: Increased susceptibility and severity of infections with suppression of clinical symptoms and signs, opportunistic infections, recurrence of dormant tuberculosis (see Special warnings and precautions for use).

Musculoskeletal: Osteoporosis, vertebral and long bone fractures, avascular osteonecrosis, tendon rupture, proximal myopathy.

Fluid and electrolyte disturbance: Sodium and water retention, hypertension, potassium loss, hypokalaemic alkalosis.

Neuropsychiatric: Euphoria, psychological dependence, depression, psychosis, insomnia, and aggravation of schizophrenia. Increased intra-cranial pressure with papilloedema in children (pseudotumour cerebri), usually after treatment withdrawal. Aggravation of epilepsy.

Ophthalmic: Increased intra-ocular pressure, glaucoma, papilloedema, posterior subcapsular cataracts, corneal or scleral thinning, exacerbation of ophthalmic viral or fungal diseases.

Gastrointestinal: Dyspepsia, peptic ulceration with perforation and haemorrhage, acute pancreatitis, candidiasis.

Dermatological: Impaired healing, skin atrophy, bruising, telangiectasia, striae, acne.

General: Hypersensitivity including anaphylaxis, has been reported. Leucocytosis. Thrombo-embolism.

Withdrawal symptoms and signs: Too rapid a reduction of corticosteroid dosage following prolonged treatment can lead to acute adrenal insufficiency, hypotension and death (see Special warnings and precautions for use).

A 'withdrawal syndrome' may also occur including; fever, myalgia, arthralgia, rhinitis, conjunctivitis, painful itchy skin nodules and loss of weight.

Overdose: Should overdosage occur, the possibility of adrenal suppression should be minimised by a gradual reduction of dosage over a period of time. The patient may need support during any further trauma.

### Pharmacological properties

Pharmacodynamic properties: Betamethasone is a glucocorticoid which is about eight to ten times as active as prednisolone on a weight-for-weight basis.

Pharmacokinetic properties: Corticosteroids are bound to plasma proteins in varying degrees. Corticosteroids are metabolised primarily by the liver and then excreted by the kidneys.

### Pharmaceutical particulars

List of excipients Disodium edetate, Sodium metabisulphite, Sodium chloride, Sodium hydroxide/hydrochloric acid, Water for injection.

Incompatibilities: None known

Shelf life: 2 years

Special precautions for storage: Store below 30°C and protect from light.

Nature and contents of container: 1 ml clear neutral glass ampoules in packs of five.

**Marketing authorisation number** 0039/0391

**Date of approval/revision of SPC** July 1997

**Legal category** POM

## BETNESOL* TABLETS

**Qualitative and quantitative composition** Each tablet contains 500 micrograms (0.5 mg) betamethasone as the sodium phosphate ester.

**Pharmaceutical form** Small, soluble, pink tablets engraved "Betnesol Evans" on one side and scored on the reverse.

The tablets comply with the specification for Betamethasone Sodium Phosphate Tablets BP.

### Clinical particulars

Therapeutic indications: A wide variety of diseases may sometimes require corticosteroid therapy. Some of the principal indications are as follows.

Bronchial asthma, severe hypersensitivity reactions, anaphylaxis, rheumatoid arthritis, systemic lupus erythematosus, dermatomyositis, mixed connective tissue disease (excluding systemic sclerosis), polyarteritis nodosa; inflammatory skin disorders, including pemphigus vulgaris, bullous pemphigoid and pyoderma gangrenosum; minimal change nephrotic syndrome, acute interstitial nephritis; ulcerative colitis, Crohn's disease; sarcoidosis; rheumatic carditis; haemolytic anaemia (auto-immune), acute and lymphatic leukaemia, malignant lymphoma, multiple myeloma, idiopathic thrombocytopenic purpura; immunosuppression in transplantation.

Posology and method of administration: Betnesol

Tablets are best taken dissolved in water, but they can be swallowed whole without difficulty. The lowest dosage that will produce an acceptable result should be used; when it is possible to reduce the dosage, this must be accomplished by stages. During prolonged therapy, dosage may need to be increased temporarily during periods of stress or in exacerbations of illness (see Special warnings and precautions for use).

Adults: Short term treatment: 2000-3000 micrograms (4-6 tablets) daily for the first few days, then reducing the daily dose by 250-500 micrograms ($\frac{1}{2}$ or 1 tablet) every two to five days, depending upon the response.

Rheumatoid arthritis: 500-2000 micrograms (1-4 tablets) daily. For long-term treatment the lowest effective dosage is used.

Most other conditions: 1500-5000 micrograms (3-10 tablets) daily for one to three weeks, then gradually reducing to the minimum effective dosage. Larger doses may be needed for mixed connective tissue diseases and ulcerative colitis.

Children: A proportion of the adult dosage may be used (e.g. 75% at 12 years, 50% at 7 years and 25% at 1 year).

Contra-indications: Systemic infections, unless specific anti-infective therapy is employed. Hypersensitivity to any component of the tablets.

Special warnings and precautions for use: A patient information leaflet should be supplied with this product.

Undesirable effects may be minimised by using the lowest effective dose for the minimum period, and by administering the daily requirement as a single morning dose, or whenever possible as a single morning dose on alternate days. Frequent patient review is required to appropriately titrate the dose against disease activity (see Posology and method of administration).

Suppression of the inflammatory response and immune function increases the susceptibility to infections and their severity. The clinical presentation may often be atypical and serious infections such as septicaemia and tuberculosis may be masked and may reach an advanced stage before being recognised.

Chickenpox is of particular concern since this normally minor illness may be fatal in immunosuppressed patients. Patients (or parents of children) without a definite history of chickenpox should be advised to avoid close personal contact with chickenpox or herpes zoster and if exposed they should seek urgent medical attention. Passive immunisation with varicella zoster immunoglobulin (VZIG) is needed by exposed non-immune patients who are receiving systemic corticosteroids or who have used them within the previous 3 months; this should be given within 10 days of exposure to chickenpox. If a diagnosis of chickenpox is confirmed, the illness warrants specialist care and urgent treatment. Corticosteroids should not be stopped and the dose may need to be increased.

Live vaccines should not be given to individuals with impaired immune responsiveness. The antibody response to other vaccines may be diminished.

Adrenal suppression: Adrenal cortical atrophy develops during prolonged therapy and may persist for years after stopping treatment. Withdrawal of corticosteroids after prolonged therapy must therefore always be gradual to avoid acute adrenal insufficiency; and thus should be tapered off over weeks or months according to the dose and duration of treatment. During prolonged therapy any intercurrent illness, trauma or surgical procedure will require a temporary increase in dosage; if corticosteroids have been stopped following prolonged therapy they may need to be temporarily re-introduced.

Special precautions: Particular care is required when considering the use of systemic corticosteroids in patients with the following conditions and frequent patient monitoring is necessary.

A. Osteoporosis (post-menopausal females are particularly at risk).
B. Hypertension or congestive heart failure.
C. Existing or previous history of severe affective disorders (especially previous steroid psychosis).
D. Diabetes mellitus (or a family history of diabetes).
E. History of tuberculosis.
F. Glaucoma (or a family history of glaucoma).
G. Previous corticosteroid-induced myopathy.
H. Liver failure – blood levels of corticosteroid may be increased, (as with other drugs which are metabolised in the liver).
I. Renal insufficiency.
J. Epilepsy.
K. Peptic ulceration.

Patients should carry 'steroid treatment' cards which give clear guidance on the precautions to be taken to minimise risk and which provide details of prescriber, drug, dosage and the duration of treatment.

Use in children: Corticosteroids cause dose-related

growth retardation in infancy, childhood and adolescence, which may be irreversible. Treatment should be limited to the minimum dosage for the shortest possible time. In order to minimise suppression of the HPA axis and growth retardation, consideration should be given to administration of a single dose on alternate days.

Use in the elderly: The common adverse effects of systemic corticosteroids may be associated with more serious consequences in old age, especially osteoporosis, hypertension, hypokalaemia, diabetes, susceptibility to infection and thinning of the skin. Close clinical supervision is required to avoid life-threatening reactions.

*Interactions with other medicaments and other forms of interaction:* Steroids may reduce the effects of anticholinesterases in myasthenia gravis cholecystographic x-ray media and non-steroidal anti-inflammatory agents.

Rifampicin, rifabutin, carbamazepine, phenobarbitone, phenytoin, primidone, aminoglutethimide and ephedrine enhance the metabolism of corticosteroids; thus the corticosteroid therapeutic effect may be reduced.

The desired effects of hypoglycaemic agents (including insulin), anti-hypertensives and diuretics are antagonised by corticosteroids, and the hypokalaemic effects of acetazolamide, loop diuretics, thiazide diuretics and carbenoxolone are enhanced.

The efficacy of coumarin anticoagulants may be enhanced by concurrent corticosteroid therapy and close monitoring of the INR or prothrombin time is required to avoid spontaneous bleeding.

The renal clearance of salicylates is increased by corticosteroids and steroid withdrawal may result in salicylate intoxication.

*Pregnancy and lactation:* Intra-uterine growth retardation in the foetus and a small increased risk of cleft palate have been reported. Hypoadrenalism may occur in the neonate. When corticosteroids are essential however, patients with normal pregnancies may be treated as though they were in the non-gravid state. Patients with pre-eclampsia or fluid retention require close monitoring.

Corticosteroids are excreted in small amounts in breast milk and infants of mothers taking pharmacological doses of steroids should be monitored carefully for signs of adrenal suppression.

*Effects on ability to drive and use machines:* None known

*Undesirable effects:* The incidence of predictable undesirable effects, including hypothalamic-pituitary-adrenal (HPA) axis suppression correlates with the relative potency of the drug, dosage, timing of administration and the duration of treatment (see *Special warnings and precautions for use*).

Endocrine/metabolic: Suppression of the hypothalamic-pituitary-adrenal axis, growth suppression in infancy, childhood and adolescence, menstrual irregularity and amenorrhoea. Cushingoid facies, hirsutism, weight gain, impaired carbohydrate tolerance with increased requirement for antidiabetic therapy. Negative protein and calcium balance. Increased appetite.

Anti-inflammatory and immunosuppressive effects: Increased susceptibility to and severity of infections with suppression of clinical symptoms and signs, opportunistic infections, recurrence of dormant tuberculosis (see *Special warnings and precautions for use*).

Musculoskeletal: Osteoporosis, vertebral and long bone fractures, avascular osteonecrosis, tendon rupture, proximal myopathy.

Fluid and electrolyte disturbance: Sodium and water retention, hypertension, potassium loss, hypokalaemic alkalosis.

Neuropsychiatric: Euphoria, psychological dependence, depression, psychosis, insomnia, and aggravation of schizophrenia. Increased intra-cranial pressure with papilloedema in children (pseudotumour cerebri), usually after treatment withdrawal. Aggravation of epilepsy.

Ophthalmic: Increased intra-ocular pressure, glaucoma, papilloedema, posterior subcapsular cataracts, corneal or scleral thinning, exacerbation of ophthalmic viral or fungal diseases.

Gastrointestinal: Dyspepsia, peptic ulceration with perforation and haemorrhage, acute pancreatitis, candidiasis.

Dermatological: Impaired healing, skin atrophy, bruising, telangiectasia, striae, acne.

General: Hypersensitivity, including anaphylaxis, has been reported. Leucocytosis. Thrombo-embolism.

Withdrawal symptoms and signs: Too rapid a reduction of corticosteroid dosage following prolonged treatment can lead to acute adrenal insufficiency, hypotension and death (see *Special warnings and precautions for use*).

A 'withdrawal syndrome' may also occur including; fever, myalgia, arthralgia, rhinitis, conjunctivitis, painful itchy skin nodules and loss of weight.

*Overdose* Treatment is unlikely to be needed in cases of acute overdosage.

## Pharmacological properties

*Pharmacodynamic properties:* Betamethasone is a glucocorticosteroid (which is about eight to ten times as active as prednisolone on a weight-for-weight basis) with topical anti-inflammatory activity.

*Pharmacokinetic properties:* The vast majority of corticosteroids, including betamethasone, are absorbed from the gastrointestinal tract.

Corticosteroids are metabolised mainly in the liver but also in the kidney, and are excreted in the urine.

Synthetic corticosteroids, such as prednisolone, have increased potency when compared to the natural corticosteroids, due to their slower metabolism and lower protein-binding affinity.

## Pharmaceutical particulars

*List of excipients:* Sodium Bicarbonate, Sodium Acid Citrate, Saccharin Sodium, Povidone, Erythrosine (E127), Sodium Benzoate.

*Incompatibilities:* None known

*Shelf life:* 3 years

*Special precautions for storage:* Store at a temperature not exceeding 25°C.

*Nature and contents of container:* The tablets are sealed into individual pockets in an aluminium/polyethylene laminate (30 micron and 38 micron respectively). The tablets are strip packed in cartons of 100.

**Marketing authorisation number**  0039/0386

**Date of approval/revision of SPC**  July 1997

**Legal category**  POM

# BETNESOL-N* EYE, EAR AND NOSE PREPARATIONS

**Presentation**  Betnesol-N Drops contain betamethasone sodium phosphate 0.1% w/v, neomycin sulphate 0.5% w/v and benzalkonium chloride 0.01 % w/v in a clear, colourless to pale yellow aqueous solution. Sterile until opened.

Betnesol-N Eye Ointment contains betamethasone sodium phosphate 0.1 % w/w and neomycin sulphate 0.5% w/w in a bland, soft paraffin base of white translucent appearance. Sterile until opened.

**Uses**  Betamethasone has topical corticosteroid activity. The presence of neomycin should prevent the development of bacterial infection.

*Drops and ointment*
*Eye:* For the short-term treatment of steroid responsive conditions of the eye when prophylactic antibiotic treatment is also required, after excluding the presence of fungal and viral disease.

*Drops only*
*Ear:* Otitis externa or other steroid responsive conditions where prophylactic antibiotic treatment is also required.
*Nose:* Steroid responsive inflammatory conditions where prophylactic antibiotic treatment is also required.

**Dosage and administration**
*Adults: (and the Elderly) and Children:* The frequency of dosing depends on the clinical response. If there is no clinical response within 7 days of treatment, the treatment should be discontinued.

Treatment should be the lowest effective dose for the shortest possible time. Normally Betnesol-N Drops or Ointment should not be given for more than 7 days, unless under expert supervision. After more prolonged treatment (over 6 to 8 weeks), the drops or ointment should be withdrawn slowly to avoid relapse.

*Drops:*
*Eyes:* 1 or 2 drops applied to each affected eye up to six times daily or more frequently if required.
*Ears:* 2 or 3 drops instilled into the ear three or four times daily.
*Nose:* 2 or 3 drops instilled into each nostril two or three times daily.

*Ointment:* An extrusion of the ointment about 5 mm long may be introduced beneath the lower lid two or three times daily and/or at night.

**Contra-indications, warnings, etc.**
*Contra-indications:* Viral, fungal, tuberculous or purulent conditions of the eye. Use is contra-indicated if glaucoma is present or herpetic keratitis (e.g. dendritic ulcer) is considered a possibility. Use of topical steroids in the latter condition can lead to extension of the ulcer and marked visual deterioration.

Otitis externa should not be treated when the eardrum is perforated because of the risk of ototoxicity.

Corticosteroids should not be used in patients with a perforated tympanic membrane.

Hypersensitivity to any component of the preparation.

Betnesol-N Drops contain benzalkonium chloride as a preservative and should not be used as eye drops to treat patients who wear soft contact lenses.

Topical corticosteroids should never be given for an undiagnosed "red eye" as inappropriate use is potentially blinding.

*Precautions:* Treatment with corticosteroid/antibiotic combinations should not be continued for more than 7 days in the absence of any clinical improvement, since prolonged use may lead to occult extension of infection due to the masking effect of the steroid. Prolonged use may also lead to skin sensitisation and the emergence of resistant organisms.

Prolonged use may lead to the risk of adrenal suppression in infants.

Treatment with corticosteroid preparations should not be repeated or prolonged without regular review to exclude raised intra-ocular pressure, cataract formation or unsuspected infections.

Aminoglycoside antibiotics may cause irreversible, partial or total deafness when given systemically or when applied topically to open wounds or damaged skin. This effect is dose related and is enhanced by renal or hepatic impairment. Although this effect has not been reported following topical ocular use, the possibility should be considered when high dose topical treatment is given to small children or infants.

Excessive or prolonged use intranasally may lead to the appearance of systemic corticosteroid effects.

May cause transient blurring of vision on instillation.

Warn patients not to drive or operate hazardous machinery unless vision is clear.

Acute sensitisation to neomycin is a rare event.

*Pregnancy and lactation:* Safety for use in pregnancy and lactation has not been established. There is inadequate evidence of safety in human pregnancy. Topical administration of corticosteroids to pregnant animals can cause abnormalities of foetal development including cleft palate and intra-uterine growth retardation. There may therefore be a very small risk of such effects in the human foetus. There is a risk of foetal ototoxicity if aminoglycoside antibiotic preparations are administered during pregnancy.

*Side-effects:* Hypersensitivity reactions, usually of the delayed type, may occur leading to irritation, burning, stinging, itching and dermatitis.

Topical steroid use may result in increased intraocular pressure leading to optic nerve damage, reduced visual acuity and visual field defects.

Intensive or prolonged use of topical corticosteroids may lead to formation of posterior subcapsular cataracts.

In those diseases causing thinning of the cornea or sclera, corticosteroid therapy may result in thinning of the globe leading to perforation.

Mydriasis, ptosis and epithelial punctate keratitis have also been reported following ophthalmic use of corticosteroids.

Following nasal administration, the most common effects are nasal irritation and dryness, although sneezing, headache, lightheadedness, urticaria, nausea, epistaxis, rebound congestion, bronchial asthma, perforation of the nasal septum and anosmia have also been reported.

*Overdosage:* Long-term intensive topical use may lead to systemic effects.

Oral ingestion of the contents of one bottle (up to 10 ml) of drops, or one tube (3 g) is unlikely to lead to any serious adverse effects.

**Pharmaceutical precautions**  Store below 25°C. The product should not be used later than 28 days from the date of breaking its protective seal and any contents remaining after this date should be discarded.

**Legal category**  POM.

**Package quantities**
*Betnesol-N Drops:* Plastic dropper bottles containing 10 ml.
*Betnesol-N Eye Ointment:* Tubes containing 3 g.

**Further information**  Nil.

**Product licence numbers**
Betnesol-N Drops          0039/0389
Betnesol-N Eye Ointment   0039/0390

# BETTAMOUSSE*

**Qualitative and quantitative composition**  Betamethasone Valerate BP 0.12% w/w

**Pharmaceutical form**  Hydroalcoholic foam mousse

## Clinical particulars

*Therapeutic indications:* Steroid responsive dermatoses of the scalp, such as psoriasis.

*Posology and method of administration:* Adults, the elderly and children (over the age of six years): No more than a 'golf-ball' sized amount of mousse (containing approximately 3.5 mg betamethasone), or proportionately less for children, to be massaged into the affected areas of the scalp twice daily (in the morning and evening) until the condition improves. If there is no improvement after 7 days, treatment should be discontinued. Once the condition has cleared, it may be possible to maintain improvement by applying only once a day, or even less frequently. For the treatment of seborrhoeic dermatitis in children, this product should not be used for longer than 5 to 7 days.

Patients should be advised to use the product sparingly.

As with other topical corticosteroids, at least monthly clinical review is recommended if treatment is prolonged. Allow the treated scalp to dry naturally.

*Contra-indications:* Bacterial, fungal or viral infections of the scalp, for example ringworm. Hypersensitivity to any component of the preparation. Dermatoses in children under six years of age.

*Special warnings and precautions for use:* Care must be taken to keep the preparation away from the eyes. Do not use near a naked flame. The least amount of mousse required to control the disease should be used for the shortest possible time. This should minimise the potential for long term side effects. This is particularly the case in children, as adrenal suppression can occur even without its use with an occlusive dressing. The use of topical corticosteroids in psoriasis requires careful supervision. There is a risk of the development of generalised, pustular psoriasis or local or systemic toxicity due to impaired barrier function of the skin. Tolerance may develop and rebound relapse may occur on withdrawal of treatment. Development of secondary infection requires withdrawal of topical corticosteroid therapy and commencement of appropriate systemic antimicrobial therapy.

*Interactions with other medicaments and other forms of interaction:* Not relevant to topical use.

*Pregnancy and lactation:* There is inadequate evidence of safety in human pregnancy. Topical administration of corticosteroids to pregnant animals can cause abnormalities of foetal development including cleft palate and intra-uterine growth retardation. There may, therefore, be a very small risk of such effects in the human foetus.

*Effects on ability to drive and use machines:* None known

*Undesirable effects:* Betamethasone preparations are usually well tolerated, but if signs of hypersensitivity appear, application should be stopped immediately.

As with other topical corticosteroids, prolonged use of large amounts, or treatment of extensive areas can result in sufficient systemic absorption to produce the features of hypercorticism and suppression of the hypothalamic-pituitary-adrenal axis. These effects are more likely to occur in infants and children, and if occlusive dressings are used. Local atrophy may occur after prolonged treatment.

In rare instances, treatment of psoriasis with corticosteroids (or their withdrawal) is thought to have provoked the pustular form of the disease (see Precautions).

*Overdose:* Acute overdosage is very unlikely to occur. However, in the case of chronic overdosage or misuse, the features of hypercorticism may appear and in this situation topical steroids should be discontinued under careful clinical supervision, with supportive therapy if appropriate.

## Pharmacological properties

*Pharmacodynamic properties:* Betamethasone is a glucocorticosteroid which has topical anti-inflammatory activity.

*Pharmacokinetic properties:* Under conditions of normal use, topical administration of betamethasone is not associated with clinically significant systemic absorption.

*Preclinical safety data:* Topical administration of corticosteroids to pregnant animals has been associated with abnormalities of foetal development and growth retardation. It is, therefore, considered that there may be a very small risk of such effects in the human foetus.

## Pharmaceutical particulars

*List of excipients:* Cetyl alcohol, Stearyl alcohol, Polysorbate 60, Ethanol, Purified Water, Propylene glycol, Citric acid anhydrous, Potassium Citrate, Butane/Propane.

*Incompatibilities:* None known

*Shelf life:* 2 years

*Special precautions for storage:* Store at a temperature not exceeding 25°C.

*Nature and contents of container:* Aluminium EP-lined Cebal can with Precision valve and clear cover cap, with a net weight of 100 g.

**Marketing authorisation number** 0039/0488

**Date of approval/revision of SPC** April 1996

**Legal category** POM

# ADSORBED TETANUS VACCINE, BP (CLOSTET*)

**Qualitative and quantitative composition** Each 0.5 ml dose contains: Not less than 40IU tetanus toxoid adsorbed onto aluminium hydroxide.

**Pharmaceutical form** Adsorbed Tetanus Vaccine is a suspension of purified tetanus toxoid, prepared by chemical detoxification of *Clostridium tetani* exotoxin, adsorbed on aluminium hydroxide.

## Clinical particulars

*Therapeutic indications:* For active immunisation against tetanus and for reinforcement of immunity to tetanus.

Primary immunisation against tetanus in infancy is usually carried out by the administration of combined Adsorbed Diphtheria, Tetanus and Pertussis Vaccine (DTPer/Vac/Ads) or Adsorbed Diphtheria and Tetanus Vaccine (CHILD) (DT/Vac/Ads(Child)).

*Posology and method of administration:* Each dose is 0.5 ml given by intramuscular or deep subcutaneous injection. The intervals between immunisations may be exceeded without the need to repeat the full course of immunisation. A five dose course of injections (3 primary doses and 2 reinforcing doses) should give lifelong protection. Further injections should not usually be given except in the event of a tetanus-prone wound occurring more than 10 years after the last dose.

Shake well before each dose is withdrawn.

Children under 10 years of age: Primary course; one 0.5 ml dose at 2, 3 and 4 months of age. Reinforcing dose; one 0.5 ml dose at least 3 years after the last dose of the primary course (usually pre-school booster). Final reinforcing dose; one 0.5 ml dose at 15-19 years of age or on leaving school.

Children aged 10 years and over, adults and elderly: Primary course; three 0.5 ml doses with an interval of one month between each dose. Reinforcing doses; one 0.5 ml dose 10 years after completion of the primary course and a further dose 10 years after that should give lifelong protection.

Tetanus-prone wounds: For the majority of fully immunised subjects, reinforcement on wounding should only be required if more than 10 years has elapsed since the previous vaccination. Tetanus vaccination should not be given to any patient who has received a reinforcing dose in the preceding year because of the risk of considerable local reactions.

Specific anti-tetanus prophylaxis
(1992 Edition of Immunisation Against Infectious Disease)

| Immunisation Status | Type of Wound Clean | Type of Wound Tetanus prone |
|---|---|---|
| Last of 3 dose course, or reinforcing dose within last 10 years. | Nil. | Nil–(A dose of adsorbed vaccine may be given if risk of infection is considered especially high, e.g. contamination with stable manure). |
| Last of 3 dose course or reinforcing dose more than 10 years previously. | A reinforcing dose of adsorbed vaccine. | A reinforcing dose of adsorbed vaccine plus a dose of human tetanus immunoglobulin. |
| Not immunised or immunisation status not known with certainty. | A full 3 dose course of adsorbed vaccine. | A full 3 dose course of vaccine, plus a dose of tetanus immunoglobulin in a different site. |

Persons of all ages are susceptible to tetanus unless they have received appropriate immunisation. Rarely, if ever, is natural immunity developed even in persons who have recovered from severe tetanus. Since most tetanus cases follow trivial wounds, all persons should, if possible, be actively immunised against the disease.

Adsorbed Tetanus Vaccine may be administered simultaneously with human tetanus immunoglobulin or tetanus antitoxin but must be given at separate sites. The antibody response of subjects to subsequent doses of vaccine is not significantly impaired by this procedure.

Oral Poliomyelitis Vaccine, BP may be given at the same time as Adsorbed Tetanus Vaccine.

It is good practice to record the title, dose and lot numbers of all vaccines and dates of administration.

*Contra-indications:* Adsorbed Tetanus Vaccine must not be given intradermally since it may give rise to a persistent skin nodule.

The vaccine should not be administered to a subject who has experienced a serious reaction (e.g. anaphylaxis) to a previous dose of this vaccine or who is known to be hypersensitive to any component thereof.

Adsorbed Tetanus Vaccine should not be given to an individual suffering from an acute febrile illness except in the presence of a tetanus-prone wound.

Tetanus vaccine should not be given to any patient who has received a booster dose in the preceding year.

*Special warnings and precautions for use:* Although anaphylaxis is rare, facilities for its management should always be available during vaccination.

*Interactions with other medicaments and other forms of interaction:* None known.

*Pregnancy and lactation:* In countries where the risks of neonatal tetanus are high, tetanus vaccines are widely administered during pregnancy without any apparent significant adverse effect on pregnancy or foetal development.

No relevant information on the immunisation of lactating women is available.

*Effects on ability to drive and use machines:* None known.

*Undesirable effects:* Local reactions of swelling, redness and pain may develop at the injection site and persist for several days. Delays of up to 10 days before symptoms develop are reported. Occasionally these local reactions may be quite marked, with tenderness and swelling of a large area. Local reactions are rare in children, the incidence increases with age and according to the number of previously administered doses of tetanus toxoid containing vaccine. However, reactions may occur after the first dose. Subjects who develop reactions frequently have high titres of circulating antitoxin. Women develop reactions more frequently than men.

General reactions are uncommon but may include arthralgia, lymphadenopathy, faintness, nausea, headache, lethargy, malaise, myalgia and pyrexia. They do not usually persist for more than a few hours. Urticaria, angioneurotic oedema and acute anaphylactic reactions are sometimes seen.

Serum sickness and peripheral neuropathy have been described. Calcifying dermatomyositis has been observed in temporal association with tetanus vaccination.

Persistent nodules at the site of injection may occasionally follow administration of adsorbed vaccines especially if the inoculation is into the superficial layers of subcutaneous tissue.

Any untoward reactions should be reported to the regulatory authorities and to the manufacturer.

*Overdose:* Not applicable.

**Pharmacological properties** Immunisation with Adsorbed Tetanus vaccine protects by stimulating the production of antitoxin which provides immunity against the effects of tetanus toxin. The immunogen is prepared by treating a cell-free preparation of toxin with formaldehyde and thereby converting it into the inoculous tetanus toxoid. Tetanus toxoid alone is a relatively poor immunogen, and for vaccine use it is adsorbed onto an adjuvant such as aluminium hydroxide.

## Pharmaceutical particulars

*List of excipients* Each 0.5 ml dose contains:
Aluminium hydroxide 1.5 mg
Sodium thimerfonate 0.025 mg
Sodium chloride 4.25 mg
Water for Injections to 0.5 ml

*Incompatibilities (Major):* None known.

*Shelf life:* Ampoules: 36 months when stored at 2-8°C unopened. Pre-filled syringes: 24 months when stored at 2-8°C unopened.

*Special precautions for storage:* Store between 2 and 8°C. Protect from light. Do not freeze. Vaccine which has been frozen should not be used.

*Nature and contents of container:* Ampoules: Single dose (0.5 ml) 1 ml clear neutral type 1 glass complying with the PhEur requirements for containers for injectables. Pre-filled syringes: Single dose 1 ml Hypack SCF pre-filled syringe containing 0.5 ml vaccine.

*Instructions for use/handling* Disposal should be by incineration at a temperature of not less than 1100°C at a registered waste disposal contractor.

**Marketing authorisation number**  0039/0444

**Date of approval/revision of SPC**  February 1996

**Legal category**  POM

## COCOIS* COCONUT OIL COMPOUND

**Presentation**  Cocois is a presentation of coconut oil compound ointment. It is a buff coloured ointment containing Coal Tar Solution BP 12% w/w, Precipitated Sulphur BP 4% w/w and Salicylic Acid PhEur 2% w/w in a coconut oil emollient base.

**Uses**  Cocois is indicated as a adjunctive treatment of common scaly scalp disorders such as psoriasis, eczema, seborrhoeic dermatitis and dandruff. It has a mild antipruritic and keratolytic action.

**Dosage and administration**  Part the hair and squeeze a thin ribbon of Cocois onto the affected area(s) of the scalp using the applicator provided. Gently rub in the ointment and leave in contact for approximately 1 hour. Wash out using warm water and a mild shampoo.

For severe scaly scalp conditions, use daily for 3-7 days until improvement has been obtained and then intermittently as necessary.

For less severe conditions such as dandruff, use intermittently as necessary, e.g. once a week.

If symptoms persist after four weeks, consult your doctor.

For children between 6-12 years use under medical supervision only.

Cocois is not recommended for use in children below the age of six years.

**Contra-indications, warnings, etc**
*Contra-indications:* Do not use in the presence of acute skin infections of the scalp, acute pustular psoriasis or known sensitivity to any of the ingredients including sulphur and salicylates.

*Adverse effects:* It has been reported that coal tar may cause skin irritation, folliculitis and rarely, photosensitivity. In the event of such a reaction, discontinue use.

*Warnings and precautions:* Avoid contact with the eyes and wash the hands immediately after application.

Coal tar may stain bed linen and jewellery. Care should be taken to protect these items during treatment.

*Use in pregnancy:* There are no data on the use of Cocois in pregnancy.

**Pharmaceutical precautions**  Store between 10°C and 25°C.

**Legal category**  GSL.

**Package quantities**  Tubes of 40 g and 100 g and applicator.

**Further information**  Cocois is based upon a formulation developed at St John's Hospital for Diseases of the Skin, London.

*Ingredients:* Coal Tar Solution BP 12% w/w, Salicylic Acid PhEur 2% w/w, Precipitated Sulphur BP 4% w/w, Coconut Oil BP, White Soft Paraffin BP, Glycerol PhEur, Cetostearyl Alcohol BP, Liquid Paraffin PhEur, Polyoxyethylene Glycerol Monostearate (Tagat S2), Paraffin Hard BP.

**Product licence number**  0039/0499

## CO-DANTHRUSATE

**Presentation**
*Capsules:* Co-danthrusate (Normax) capsules, containing 50 mg danthron and 60 mg docusate sodium. Dark brown capsules, overprinted with the product name 'Normax'.

*Suspension:* Co-danthrusate (Normax) suspension, containing 50 mg danthron and 60 mg docusate sodium per 5 ml. An orange-yellow suspension with an odour of peppermint.

**Uses**
*Principal action:* Danthron is a mild peristaltic stimulant acting on the lower bowel to encourage normal bowel movement without causing irritation. Docusate sodium is a softening agent which prevents excessive colonic dehydration and hardening of stools.

*Indications:* Constipation in geriatric practice. Analgesic-induced constipation in terminally ill patients over 6 years old. Constipation in cardiac failure and coronary thrombosis (conditions in which defaecation must be free of strain).

**Dosage and administration**  For oral administration only.
*Adults (including elderly patients):* 1-3 capsules or 5-15 ml suspension at bedtime.

*Children (6-12 years):* 1 capsule or 5 ml suspension at bedtime.

Prolonged use is not recommended.

**Contra-indications, warnings, etc.**
*Contra-indications:* In common with all laxatives, Co-danthrusate is contra-indicated in cases of non-specific abdominal pain and when intestinal obstruction is suspected.

*Caution:* Danthron is excreted in the urine and metabolised danthron in the faeces. There is evidence that these may cause erythema in patients with urinary and or faecal incontinence. It is recommended therefore that co-danthrusate should be used with caution in all incontinent patients.

*Use in pregnancy and lactation:* Co-danthrusate should not be used during pregnancy or lactation.

*Other special warnings:* In experimental animals, danthron has been associated with adenocarcinomas in the bowel and tumours in the liver.

*Adverse reactions:* The griping often found with other types of laxative is not an appreciable problem with Co-danthrusate. Occasionally, an orange tint in the urine may be observed due to the danthron component.

*Overdosage:* The patient should be encouraged to drink fluids. An anticholinergic preparation may be used to ease excessive intestinal motility if necessary.

**Pharmaceutical precautions**
*Capsules:* Store in a dry place.

*Suspension:* Store at a temperature not exceeding 25°C and protect from light.

**Legal category**  POM.

**Package quantities**
*Capsules:* Capsules in blister packs of 63.
*Suspension:* 200 ml bottle.

**Further information**  Nil.

**Product licence numbers**
Co-danthrusate capsules       0039/0380
Co-danthrusate suspension     0039/0381

## CORACTEN* CAPSULES

**Qualitative and quantitative composition**  Each capsule contains 10 mg or 20 mg Nifedipine USP in sustained release form.

**Pharmaceutical form**

*10 mg:* Sustained release capsules with opaque grey body and opaque brownish-pink cap, overprinted in white with 'Coracten' on the body and '10 mg' on the cap, and filled with yellow pellets.

*20 mg:* Sustained release capsules with opaque brownish-pink body and opaque reddish-brown cap, overprinted in white with 'Coracten' on the body and '20 mg' on the cap, and filled with yellow pellets.

**Clinical particulars**

*Therapeutic indications:* Coracten Capsules are indicated for the prophylaxis of chronic stable angina pectoris and the treatment of hypertension.

They are also indicated for the treatment of Prinzmetal (variant) angina when diagnosed by a cardiologist.

*Posology and method of administration:*
*Adults only:* The recommended starting dose of Coracten Capsules is 10 mg every 12 hours swallowed with water with subsequent titration of dosage according to response. The dose may be adjusted to 40 mg every 12 hours.
*Children:* Coracten Capsules are not recommended for use in children.
*Elderly:* The pharmacokinetics of nifedipine are altered in the elderly so that lower maintenance doses of nifedipine may be required compared to younger patients.
*Hepatic impairment:* Caution should be exercised in treating patients with hepatic impairment. In these patients the use of one 10 mg Coracten Capsule every 12 hours, together with careful monitoring, is suggested when commencing therapy.
*Renal impairment:* Dosage adjustments are not usually required in patients with renal impairment.

*Contra-indications:* Coracten Capsules are contra-indicated in patients with known hypersensitivity to nifedipine or other dihydropyridines because of the theoretical risk of cross reactivity. They should not be used in women who are or who may become pregnant (see section *Pregnancy and Lactation*).

Coracten Capsules should not be used in clinically significant aortic stenosis, unstable angina, or during

or within one month of a myocardial infarction. They should not be used in patients in cardiogenic shock.

Coracten Capsules should not be used for the treatment of acute attacks of angina, or in patients who have had ischaemic pain following its administration previously.

The safety of Coracten Capsules in malignant hypertension has not been established.

Coracten Capsules should not be used for secondary prevention of myocardial infarction.

Coracten Capsules are contra-indicated in patients with acute porphyria.

Coracten Capsules should not be administered concomitantly with rifampicin since effective plasma levels of nifedipine may not be achieved owing to enzyme induction.

*Special warnings and precautions for use:* Nifedipine should be used with caution in patients who are hypotensive; in patients with poor cardiac reserve; in patients with heart failure or significantly impaired left ventricular function as their condition may deteriorate; in diabetic patients as they may require adjustment of their diabetic therapy; and in dialysis patients with malignant hypertension and irreversible renal failure with hypovolaemia, since a significant drop in blood pressure may occur due to the vasodilator effects of nifedipine.

Since nifedipine has no beta-blocking activity, it gives no protection against the dangers of abrupt withdrawal of beta-blocking drugs. Withdrawal of any previously prescribed beta-blockers should be gradual, preferably over 8 to 10 days.

Nifedipine may be used in combination with beta-blockers and other antihypertensive agents, but the possibility of an additive effect resulting in postural hypotension and/or cardiac failure must be borne in mind.

Cardiac ischaemic pain has been reported in a minority of patients within 30 minutes of starting nifedipine treatment; such patients should stop treatment.

*Interaction with other medicaments and other forms of interaction:* As with other dihydropyridines, nifedipine should not be taken with grapefruit juice because bioavailability is increased.

The simultaneous administration of nifedipine and digoxin may lead to reduced digoxin clearance and hence an increase in the plasma digoxin. Digoxin levels should be monitored and, if necessary, the digoxin dose reduced.

Nifedipine may increase the spectrophotometric values of urinary vanillylmandelic acid falsely. However, HPLC measurements are unaffected.

Coracten Capsules should not be administered concomitantly with rifampicin since effective plasma levels of nifedipine may not be achieved owing to enzyme induction (see section 4.3. Contra-indications).

Increased plasma levels of nifedipine have been reported during concomitant use of $H_2$-receptor antagonists (specifically cimetidine), other calcium channel blockers (specifically diltiazem), alcohol and cyclosporin.

**Plasma levels of nifedipine are possibly decreased by the concomitant use of antiepileptics.**

**When used in combination with nifedipine, plasma concentrations of quinidine have been shown to be suppressed regardless of quinidine dosage.** The plasma concentrations of phenytoin, theophylline and non-depolarising muscle relaxants (e.g. tubocurarine) are increased when used in combination with nifedipine.

Profound hypotension has been reported with nifedipine and intravenous magnesium sulphate in the treatment of pre-eclampsia.

*Pregnancy and lactation:*
*Pregnancy:* Because animal studies show embryotoxicity and teratogenicity, Coracten Capsules are contra-indicated during pregnancy (see also section 4.3. Contra-indications). Embryotoxicity was noted at 6 to 20 times the maximum recommended dose for Coracten Capsules given to rats, mice and rabbits, and teratogenicity was noted in rabbits given 20 times the maximum recommended dose for Coracten Capsules.

*Lactation:* Nifedipine is excreted in breast milk, therefore Coracten Capsules are not recommended during lactation.

*Effects on ability to drive and use machines:* None known.

*Undesirable effects:* Side-effects are generally transient and mild, and usually occur at the start of treatment only. They include headache, flushing and, usually at higher dosages, nausea, dyspepsia, heartburn, dizziness, lethargy, skin reactions (such as rash, pruritus and urticaria), paraesthesia, hypotension, palpitation, tachycardia, dependent oedema, increased frequency of micturition, eye pain, depression, fever, gingival hyperplasia and telangiectasia. Other less frequently reported side-effects include myalgia, tremor and visual disturbances. Impotence may occur rarely.

As with other sustained release dihydropyridines, exacerbation of angina pectoris may occur rarely at the start of treatment with sustained release formulations of nifedipine. The occurrence of myocardial infarction has been described although it is not possible to distinguish such an event from the natural course of ischaemic heart disease.

There are reports in older men on long-term therapy of gynaecomastia which usually regresses upon withdrawal of therapy.

Side-effects which may occur in isolated cases are photosensitivity, exfoliative dermatitis, systemic allergic reactions and purpura. Usually, these regress after discontinuation of the drug.

Rare cases of hypersensitivity-type jaundice have been reported. In addition, disturbances of liver function such as intra-hepatic cholestasis may occur. These regress after discontinuation of therapy.

*Overdose:*
*Human experience:* Reports of nifedipine overdosage are limited and symptoms are not necessarily dose-related. Severe hypotension due to vasodilation, and tachycardia or bradycardia are the most likely manifestations of overdose.

Metabolic disturbances include hyperglycaemia, metabolic acidosis and hypo- or hyperkalaemia.

Cardiac effects may include heart block, AV dissociation and asystole, and cardiogenic shock with pulmonary oedema.

Other toxic effects include nausea, vomiting, drowsiness, dizziness, confusion, lethargy, flushing, hypoxia, unconsciousness and coma.

*Management of overdose in man:* Treatment consists of gastric lavage followed by oral activated charcoal together with supportive and symptomatic measures, principally intravenous fluids to maintain circulating blood volume. If the latter is not sufficient, dopamine or dobutamine may be given. Intravenous calcium gluconate may be considered as an antidote.

**Pharmacological particulars**

*Pharmacodynamic properties:* Nifedipine is a potent calcium-channel blocker which, by dilating peripheral arterial smooth muscle, decreases cardiac work and myocardial oxygen requirement. It also dilates coronary arteries, thereby improving myocardial perfusion and reducing coronary artery spasm. In hypertension, it reduces blood pressure but has little or no effect in normotensive subjects. It has no therapeutic antiarrhythmic effect.

*Pharmacokinetic properties:* Coracten Capsules are a sustained release formulation of nifedipine designed to provide less fluctuation and more prolonged nifedipine blood concentrations than standard immediate release preparations.

Nifedipine is highly protein bound. It undergoes hepatic oxidation to inactive metabolites which are excreted in the urine (80%) and faeces (20%).

*Preclinical safety data:* There are no pre-clinical data of relevance to the prescriber which are additional to that already included in other sections of the SPC.

**Pharmaceutical particulars**

*List of excipients:*
*Capsule contents:* Sucrose PhEur, Maize Starch PhEur, Lactose PhEur, Povidone K30 PhEur, Methacrylic acid copolymer type A (Eudragit L100) NF, Talc PhEur, Purified Water PhEur.

*Capsule shells:* Gelatin BP, Red iron oxide (E172), Yellow iron oxide (E172), Titanium dioxide (E171) and in Coracten 10 mg tablets only black iron oxide (E172).

*Incompatibilities:* None known.

*Shelf life:* 36 months.

*Special precautions for storage:* Store in original pack at a temperature not exceeding 30°C and protect from light.

*Nature and contents of container:* Coracten Capsules are presented in blister strips packed in cartons containing 60 capsules. The blister strips are formed from PVC with a coating of PVdC backed with aluminium foil.

(Cartons of 10, 15, 30, 56, 100, 150, 250, 500 and 600 capsules are licensed but not marketed.)

*Instructions for use and handling:* None.

**Marketing authorisation numbers**
10 mg    0039/0365
20 mg    0039/0367

**Date of approval/revision of SPC**  October 1996

**Legal category**  POM

## CORLAN* PELLETS

**Presentation**  Small white pellets engraved 'Corlan Evans' on one side. Each pellet contains 2.5 mg hydrocortisone in the form of the water soluble ester

hydrocortisone sodium succinate. They also contain lactose, acacia, magnesium stearate, industrial methylated spirit and purified water. The pellets comply with the specification for Hydrocortisone Lozenges BPC.

**Uses**  Local use in previously diagnosed aphthous ulceration of the mouth, whether simple or occurring as a complication in diseases such as sprue, idiopathic steatorrhoea or ulcerative colitis.

**Dosage and administration**
*Adults and elderly:* Corlan Pellets should not be sucked, but kept in the mouth and allowed to dissolve slowly in close proximity to the ulcers. One pellet should be used in this way four times a day. If the ulcers have not healed after 5 days of treatment (completion of one pack), or if they recur quickly after healing, a doctor should be consulted.

Children under 12 years of age: Children under 12 years old must see a doctor before starting each course of Corlan Pellets.

**Contra-indications, warnings, etc.**
*Contra-indications:* Corlan Pellets should not be used in the presence of oral infection unless effective appropriate anti-infective therapy is also employed. Hypersensitivity to any component of the product.

*Precautions:* If aphthous ulceration is severe or recurring, serious underlying disease should be excluded.

There is inadequate evidence of safety in human pregnancy. Topical administration of corticosteroids to pregnant animals can cause abnormalities of foetal development including cleft palate and intra-uterine growth retardation. There may, therefore, be a very small risk of such effects in the human foetus.

*Side effects:* Corticosteroids may worsen diabetes.

Occasionally, topical steroid therapy may result in an exacerbation of local infection.

*Overdosage:* Treatment is unlikely to be needed in cases of acute overdosage.

**Pharmaceutical precautions**  Store below 25°C. Replace cap firmly after use.

**Legal category**  P.

**Package quantities**  Container of 20 pellets (OP).

**Further information**  Nil.

**Product licence number**  0039/0397

## CRYSTACIDE* CREAM 1%

**Qualitative and quantitative composition**  Hydrogen peroxide 1.0% (w/w)

**Pharmaceutical form**  Crystacide cream is a smooth, white cream with iridescent crystals.

The cream vehicle consists of water and lipid crystals of glyceryl monolaurate, and glyceryl monomyristate. Stabilisers are added in order to obtain a satisfactory stability of hydrogen peroxide.

**Clinical particulars**
*Therapeutic indications:* Crystacide cream is intended for topical administration for the treatment of primary and secondary superficial skin infections.

*Posology and method of administration:*
*Adults, elderly and children:* Crystacide cream is applied 2-3 times a day, or when needed, on the lesions. If an occlusive dressing is used, one application a day is sufficient. A dry film will appear on the skin after application, this can be washed off with water.

*Contra-indications:* Known hypersensitivity to hydrogen peroxide.

*Special warnings and precautions for use:* Contact with the eyes should be avoided.

*Interaction with other medicaments and other forms of interaction:* Crystacide cream is incompatible with iodine, permanganates and other stronger oxidising agents.

*Pregnancy and lactation:* Not applicable.

*Effects on ability to drive and use machines:* Not applicable.

*Undesirable effects:* Crystacide is generally well tolerated and not associated with any serious side effects. However, a mild sensation of burning may be experienced for a short time after application.

*Overdose:* Not applicable.

**Pharmacological particulars**

*Pharmacodynamic properties:* Hydrogen peroxide is a well-known antiseptic agent, and is effective against a majority of pathogenic micro-organisms.
*In vitro* pharmacology studies have shown that hydrogen peroxide has both activity against a wide variety of micro-organisms, and is a potent antibacterial agent with effect against Gram-positive as well as Gram-negative bacteria.

*In vitro* studies have shown that the bactericidal activity of Crystacide cream 1% is equal in effect compared with a 1% aqueous solution of hydrogen peroxide, and the duration of action is longer for the cream.

There are no known pathogenic bacteria or fungi that develop resistance to hydrogen peroxide.

*Pharmacokinetic properties:* Reports on the rate of absorption, distribution and excretion of hydrogen peroxide after oral administration are sparse. In the absence of stabilising agent, hydrogen peroxide gradually decomposes to oxygen and water. The decomposition is rapid in the presence of the endogenous enzyme catalase or peroxidase.

*Preclinical safety data:* There are no pre-clinical data of relevance to the prescriber which are additional to that already included in other sections of the SPC.

**Pharmaceutical particulars**

*List of excipients:* Glyceryl monolaurate, Glyceryl monomyristate, Polyoxyethylene (100) stearate, Propylene glycol, Citric acid anhydrous, Sodium hydroxide, Sulphuric acid, 1M, Sodium oxalate, Salicylic acid, Disodium edetate, Sodium pyrophosphate, Sodium stannate, Purified water.

*Incompatibilities:* Iodine, permanganates and other stronger oxidising agents.

*Shelf life:* The shelf life for Crystacide cream is 2 years from the date of manufacture.

*Special precautions for storage:* Store below 25°C, in a dry place.

*Nature and contents of container:* Crystacide cream is filled into polyethylene tubes pigmented with titanium dioxide, and fitted with polypropylene caps. Each tube is subsequently packed in a unit, printed boxboard carton, in pack sizes of 10 g and 25 g. 5 g and 40 g tubes are licensed but not marketed.

*Instructions for use and handling:* Not applicable.

*Product licence holder:* Bioglan Laboratories Limited, 5 Hunting Gate, Hitchin, Hertfordshire, SG4 0TJ

**Marketing authorisation number**  0041/0043

**Date of approval/revision of SPC**  January 1996

**Legal category**  P

## CYTAMEN*

**Presentation**  Cytamen '1000' is a clear, red solution containing 1,000 micrograms cyanocobalamin per ml.

Cytamen complies with the specification of Cyanocobalamin Injection BP.

**Uses**  Addisonian pernicious anaemia. Prophylaxis and treatment of other macrocytic anaemias associated with vitamin $B_{12}$ deficiency. Schilling test.

**Dosage and administration**  The following dosage schemes are suitable for adults and children.

*Addisonian pernicious anaemia and other macrocytic anaemias without neurological involvement:* Initially: 250 to 1,000 micrograms intramuscularly on alternate days for one to two weeks then 250 micrograms weekly until blood count is normal.

Maintenance: 1,000 micrograms monthly.

*Addisonian pernicious anaemia and other macrocytic anaemias with neurological involvement:* Initially: 1,000 micrograms intramuscularly on alternate days as long as improvement is occurring.

Maintenance: 1,000 micrograms monthly.

*Prophylaxis of macrocytic anaemia associated with vitamin $B_{12}$ deficiency resulting from gastrectomy, some malabsorption syndromes and strict vegetarianism:* 250 to 1,000 micrograms monthly.

*Schilling Test:* An intramuscular injection of 1,000 micrograms cyanocobalamin is an essential part of this test.

**Contra-indications, warnings, etc.**
*Contra-indications:* Hypersensitivity to cyanocobalamin.

Not indicated for treatment of toxic amblyopias–use Neo-Cytamen.

*Precautions:* The dosage schemes given above are usually satisfactory, but regular examination of the blood is advisable. If megaloblastic anaemia fails to respond to Cytamen, folate metabolism should be investigated.

Doses in excess of 10 micrograms daily may produce a haematological response in patients with folate deficiency. Indiscriminate administration may mask the true diagnosis. Cardiac arrhythmias secondary to hypokalaemia during initial therapy have been reported. Plasma potassium should therefore be monitored during this period.

*Pregnancy:* Cytamen should not be used for the treatment of megaloblastic anaemia of pregnancy unless vitamin $B_{12}$ deficiency has been demonstrated.

Cytamen is secreted into breast milk but this is unlikely to harm the infant, and may be beneficial if the mother and infant are vitamin $B_{12}$ deficient.

*Side-effects:* Hypersensitivity reactions have been reported including skin reactions (e.g. rash, itching) and exceptionally anaphylaxis. Other symptoms reported include fever, chills, hot flushing, dizziness, malaise, nausea, acneiform and bullous eruptions.

*Effects on ability to drive and use machines:* None.

*Interactions:* Chloramphenicol-treated patients may respond poorly to Cytamen.

Chloramphenicol-treated patients may respond poorly to Cytamen. Serum concentrations of hydroxocobalamin may be lowered by oral contraceptives but this interaction is unlikely to have clinical significance.

Antimetabolites and most antibiotics invalidate vitamin $B_{12}$ assays by microbiological techniques.

*Overdosage:* Treatment is unlikely to be needed in cases of overdosage.

**Pharmaceutical precautions**  Protect from light.

**Legal category**  POM.

**Package quantities**  Ampoules of 1 ml in boxes of 5.

**Further information**  Nil.

**Product licence number**  0039/0403

## DEXEDRINE* TABLETS

**Presentation**  Half-scored, white tablets (marked Evans above breakline and DB5 below) each containing 5 mg dexamphetamine sulphate.

**Uses**  Dexedrine is a sympathomimetic amine with central stimulant and anorectic activity. It is indicated in narcolepsy. It is also indicated for children with refractory hyperkinetic states under the supervision of a physician specialising in child psychiatry.

### Dosage and administration
*Adults:* In narcolepsy, the usual starting dose is 10 mg Dexedrine a day, given in divided doses. Dosage may be increased if necessary by 10 mg a day at weekly intervals to a suggested maximum of 60 mg a day.

*Elderly:* Start with 5 mg a day, and increase by increments of 5 mg at weekly intervals.

*Children:* In hyperkinetic states, the usual starting dosage for children aged 3-5 years is 2.5 mg a day, increased if necessary by 2.5 mg a day, at weekly intervals; for children aged 6 years and over, the usual starting dose is 5-10 mg a day increasing if necessary by 5 mg at weekly intervals.

The usual upper limit is 20 mg a day though some older children have needed 40 mg or more for optimal response.

### Contra-indications, warnings, etc.
*Contra-indications:* Do not use in patients known to be intolerant of sympathomimetic amines, during, or for 14 days after, treatment with an MAO inhibitor, in those with a history of drug abuse, with symptomatic cardiovascular disease and/or moderate or severe hypertensive disease, in those suffering from hyperthyroidism or hyperexcitability or in those with glaucoma; Gilles de la Tourette Syndrome or similar dystonias; porphyria.

*Precautions and warnings:* Use with caution in patients with mild hypertension or a family history of dystonias. If tics develop, discontinue treatment with Dexedrine. Dexamphetamine is likely to reduce the convulsant threshold therefore caution is advised in patients with epilepsy. Height and weight should be carefully monitored in children as growth retardation may occur.

Adrenoceptor blocking drugs (e.g. propanolol), Lithium and α-methyltyrosine may antagonise the effects of Dexamphetamine. Disulfiram may inhibit metabolism and excretion. Guanethidine may be antagonised by Dexamphetamine.

The concurrent use of tricyclic antidepressants may increase the risk of cardiovascular side effects.

In common with other drugs acting on the CNS, Dexedrine may affect ability to drive or operate machinery.

*Use in pregnancy and lactation:* Dexamphetamine has been thought to produce embryotoxic effects in rodents, and retrospective evidence of uncertain significance in man has suggested a similar possibility. Dexedrine should therefore be avoided in pregnancy, especially during the first trimester. Dexedrine passes into breast milk, therefore, it should be avoided in breast-feeding mothers.

*Adverse reactions:* Insomnia (especially with dosage later in the day), restlessness, irritability, euphoria, tremor, dizziness, headache and other symptoms of over-stimulation have been reported. Also dry mouth, anorexia and other gastro-intestinal symptoms, sweating, and cardiovascular effects such as tachy-

cardia, palpitation and minor increases in blood pressure. Rhabdomolysis and renal damage.

There have been isolated reports of cardiomyopathy associated with chronic amphetamine use.

Drug dependence, with consumption of increasing doses to levels many times those recommended, may occur as tolerance develops. At such levels, a psychosis which may be clinically indistinguishable from schizophrenia can occur.

Treatment should be stopped gradually since abrupt cessation may produce extreme fatigue and mental depression.

Intracranial haemorrhages have been reported, presumably precipitated by the hypertensive effect and possibly associated with pre-existing vascular malformation.

A toxic hypermetabolic state, characterised by transient hyperactivity, hyperpyrexia, acidosis and death due to cardiovascular collapse have been reported.

*Overdosage:* Symptoms of overdosage include excitement, hallucinations, convulsions leading to coma; tachycardia and cardiac arrhythmias, and respiratory depression.

Treatment consists of the induction of vomiting and/or gastric lavage together with supportive and symptomatic measures. Excessive stimulation or convulsions may be treated with diazepam. Excretion of dexamphetamine may be increased by forced acid diuresis.

**Pharmaceutical precautions**  No special storage precautions are necessary.

**Legal category**  CD (Sch 2), POM.

**Package quantities**  Blister pack of 28 tablets.

**Further information**  Inactive ingredients include lactose and sucrose.

**Product licence number**  0039/0385

## DIAMORPHINE HYDROCHLORIDE BP FOR INJECTION

**Presentation**  Ampoules containing 5, 10, 30, 100 and 500 mg of preservative-free Diamorphine Hydrochloride BP as a white freeze-dried plug. The colour of the plugs in the larger strength ampoules is off-white, and occasionally the integral plug may break up to produce a crystalline powder.

**Uses**  Diamorphine is a powerful narcotic analgesic which is more potent than morphine and more likely to produce euphoria and addiction, but relatively less nausea, constipation and hypotension.

It is readily absorbed after injection and rapidly hydrolysed to 6-monoacetylmorphine in the blood, and then more slowly metabolised to morphine the major active metabolite. Up to 80% of a dose is excreted in the urine in 24 hours, mainly as morphine-3-glucuronide together with about 5 to 7% of the dose as free morphine.

Diamorphine is used to control severe pain, such as that associated with cancer, acute myocardial infarction and in the treatment of acute pulmonary oedema.

### Dosage and administration
*Administration:* The drug may be given by the intramuscular, subcutaneous or intravenous routes, the latter two routes using either bolus injection or infusion.

Its solubility in water is 1 in 1.6, and the small volume of diluent required is of obvious benefit in treating an emaciated patient. Presentations up to 100 mg will readily dissolve in 1 ml of diluent. Because of the bulk of material in the 500 mg ampoule, a minimum of 2 ml of diluent is required to effect solution and it is recommended that the plug be tapped down, thoroughly wetted and the ampoule gently shaken until the plug dissolves.

*Dosage:* It is important that the dosage be suited to the individual patient, taking into account the properties of the drug, the nature of the pain, the total condition of the patient and previous or concurrent medication.

*5, 10, 30, 100 and 500 mg are recommended for:*

*Cancer:* Use of Diamorphine or other narcotic analgesics although very important, should be only one part of the comprehensive approach to total pain control, which ideally should include non-drug measures and psychosocial support. Diamorphine may be used parenterally when oral administration of narcotic analgesics is no longer possible because of the dosage required, impaired absorption, intestinal disorders, nausea and vomiting or difficulty in swallowing.

An initial dosage of 5 to 10 mg every 4 hours may be suitable, but higher doses are reported in the literature (Dover SB. BMJ 1987;294:553-555.). The initial dosage will usually depend on the doses and drugs given previously. Persistent pain is controlled by titrating the dose against the degree of pain, until

the smallest dose required to remove the pain is reached. This dose is maintained and the patient's condition continually reassessed, the dose being increased or decreased as necessary. The therapeutic objective must be to control the pain by regular administration of the correct dose when this is determined, and continuous infusion may be preferred to intermittent therapy.

*5 mg and 10 mg ampoules are recommended for:*

*Acute myocardial infarction:* A dose of 5 mg may be given by slow intravenous injection (1 mg per minute), followed by 2.5 to 5 mg if necessary.

*Acute pulmonary oedema:* A dose of 2.5 to 5 mg may be given by slow intravenous injection (1 mg per minute).

**Equivalent Doses of Morphine Sulphate by mouth (as oral solution or standard tablets or as modified-release tablets) or of Diamorphine Hydrochloride by Intramuscular Injection or by Subcutaneous Infusion:**

These equivalences are approximate only and may need to be adjusted according to response:

| ORAL MORPHINE | | PARENTERAL MORPHINE | |
|---|---|---|---|
| Morphine sulphate oral solution or standard tablets | Morphine sulphate modified-release tablets | Diamorphine hydrochloride by intramuscular injection | Diamorphine hydrochloride by subcutaneous infusion |
| every 4 hours | every 12 hours | every 4 hours | every 24 hours |
| 5 mg | 20 mg | 2.5 mg | 15 mg |
| 10 mg | 30 mg | 5 mg | 20 mg |
| 15 mg | 50 mg | 5 mg | 30 mg |
| 20 mg | 60 mg | 7.5 mg | 45 mg |
| 30 mg | 90 mg | 10 mg | 60 mg |
| 40 mg | 120 mg | 15 mg | 90 mg |
| 60 mg | 180 mg | 20 mg | 120 mg |
| 80 mg | 240 mg | 30 mg | 180 mg |
| 100 mg | 300 mg | 40 mg | 240 mg |
| 130 mg | 400 mg | 50 mg | 300 mg |
| 160 mg | 500 mg | 60 mg | 360 mg |
| 200 mg | 600 mg | 70 mg | 400 mg |

*Use in children and the elderly:* Mainly because of its respiratory depressant effect, caution should be exercised when giving the drug to the elderly and a reduced dose should be used.

Diamorphine has been used in the treatment of terminally ill children. Diamorphine has been administered in reduced doses to children with neoplastic disease when it becomes difficult to give treatment orally. The starting dose should be selected according to age, size, symptoms and previous analgesic requirements and administered 4 hourly; the dose being titrated according to the degree of pain. If treatment continues for more than 24 hours it may be appropriate to use a syringe driver (Burne R, Hunt A. Palliative Medicine 1987;11:27-30.).

### Contra-indications, warnings, etc.
*Contra-indications:* Respiratory depression, obstructive airways disease and concurrent administration of monoamine oxidase inhibitors or within two weeks of their discontinuation. Biliary colic. Phaeochromocytoma.

*Warnings:* Administration to patients with head injuries or raised intracranial pressure increases the risk of respiratory depression and further elevation of CSF pressure. The sedation and pupillary changes produced may interfere with accurate monitoring of the patient.

The drug can cause hypotension in patients who already have conditions or drug therapy that interfere with the ability to maintain normal blood pressure.

Concurrent administration of other CNS sedative/hypnotic drugs may have an additive effect necessitating their dosage reduction. Administration of drugs having anti-muscarinic activity (atropine and synthetic anticholinergics) may increase the risk of severe constipation and/or urinary retention.

*Precautions:* Tolerance and physical dependence on the drug is likely to develop in most patients after a few weeks of treatment, but this does not prevent reduction of dosage or discontinuation when considered necessary, and drug abuse is not normally a problem in patients with severe pain. Great caution should be exercised however, in using the drug in patients with a known tendency to, or history of, drug abuse.

Care should be exercised in treating the elderly, debilitated patients, and those with hepatic or renal impairment. It is recommended that a lower than normal initial dose is given to these patients.

Careful consideration should be given before treating patients with myxoedema or hypothyroidism, adrenocortical insufficiency, toxic psychoses, CNS depression, prostatic hypertrophy or urethral stricture, kyphoscoliosis, acute alcoholism and delirium tremens, severe inflammatory bowel disease and severe diarrhoea.

*Use in pregnancy:* There is inadequate evidence of safety in human pregnancy, therefore, as with all drugs it is not advisable to administer diamorphine during pregnancy. Use during labour is not advisable due to the risk of respiratory depression in the newborn.

There is limited information on diamorphine levels in breast milk and it is, therefore, not advisable for patients on high doses of diamorphine to breast feed.

*Side-effects:* The most serious hazards of therapy are respiratory depression and arrest, although circulatory depression, shock and cardiac arrest can occur.

The most common side-effects are sedation, nausea and vomiting, constipation and sweating.

Other side-effects include tachycardia, postural hypotension, palpitations, faintness and syncope; euphoria, dysphoria, weakness, insomnia, dizziness, confusional symptoms and occasionally hallucinations; dry mouth, anorexia, cramps, taste alterations; urinary retention, reduced libido or potency; pruritus, urticaria and other skin rashes.

*Overdosage:* The symptoms of serious overdosage are respiratory depression, stupor or coma, muscle flaccidity, cold clammy skin, constricted pupils and occasionally bradycardia and hypotension.

The specific antidote naloxone is indicated if coma or bradypnoea are present. A dose of 0.4 to 2 mg may be given by SC, IM or IV injection repeated at intervals of 2-3 minutes up to a maximum of 10 mg if respiratory function does not improve. The dosage for children is 10 micrograms per kg body weight. Alternatively naloxone may be given by continuous IV infusion, 2 mg diluted in 500 ml intravenous solution, at a rate adjusted to the patient's response.

**Pharmaceutical precautions** Diamorphine is incompatible with mineral acids and alkalis. Store below 25°C. Protect from light.

Refer to 'Further information' for pharmaceutical compatibility of diamorphine with continuous infusions or co-administered anti-emetics.

**Legal category**　CD(Sch2), POM.

**Package quantities**　Ampoules of 5, 10, 30 mg in cartons of 5 boxes of 100. Ampoules of 100 mg and 500 mg in cartons of 5.

**Further information**　Diamorphine hydrochloride is compatible with Dextrose and Sodium Chloride intravenous infusions, and an aqueous solution has maximum stability of several days at pH 3.8 to 4.4, the stability reducing as the pH rises. For this reason Dextrose Intravenous Infusion is the preferred diluent, particularly when the drug is administered by a continuous infusion pump over 24 to 48 hours.

The occurrence of nausea and vomiting may require the concurrent administration of an anti-emetic. If given together with diamorphine as a bolus injection, normal infusion or in a continuous infusion pump, hyoscine hydrobromide, metoclopramide and methotrimeprazine are compatible with diamorphine concentrations of up to 50 mg/ml, for at least 24 hours. Haloperidol and cyclizine have also been co-administered with diamorphine hydrochloride, but precipitation may occur when using high concentrations of diamorphine hydrochloride and these antiemetics (data on file). Chlorpromazine and prochlorperazine are also compatible with diamorphine hydrochloride, but are not appropriate for administration via the subcutaneous route.

**Product licence numbers**
| | |
|---|---|
| 5 mg | 0039/5662 |
| 10 mg | 0039/5663 |
| 30 mg | 0039/5665 |
| 100 mg | 0039/0154 |
| 500 mg | 0039/0163 |

## ADSORBED DIPHTHERIA AND TETANUS VACCINE, BP (CHILD)

**Qualitative and quantitative composition**　The composition in terms of active ingredients is as follows:
| | |
|---|---|
| Diphtheria toxoid | not less than 30IU (HSE) |
| Tetanus toxoid | not less than 40IU (HSE) |

Quantities expressed per 0.5 ml dose.

**Pharmaceutical form**　Sterile suspension for deep subcutaneous or intramuscular injection to humans.

**Clinical particulars**

*Therapeutic indications:* For active immunisation against diphtheria and tetanus in children under 10 years of age.

Adsorbed Diphtheria and Tetanus Vaccine (CHILD) is used for the primary immunisation of infants and children under 10 years of age against tetanus and diphtheria where the use of Adsorbed Diphtheria, Tetanus and Pertussis Vaccine (DTPer/Vac/Ads) is contra-indicated or not required. It is also given to reinforce immunity in children under 10 years of age immunised in infancy with Adsorbed Diphtheria and Tetanus Vaccine (CHILD), or Adsorbed Diphtheria, Tetanus and Pertussis Vaccine (DT/Vac/Ads (Child), DTPer/Vac/Ads).

*Posology and method of administration:* Children under 10 years of age: Each dose is 0.5 ml, given by intramuscular or deep subcutaneous injection. The primary course of immunisation consists of three doses with an interval of at least one month between each dose.

The intervals between immunisations may be exceeded without need to repeat the full course of immunisation.

The primary course should start at 2 months of age with an interval of at least one month between each dose.

Primary course in children: Primary immunisation against diphtheria and tetanus may be carried out by the administration of combined Adsorbed Diphtheria, Tetanus and Pertussis Vaccine (DTPer/Vac/Ads) or Adsorbed Diphtheria and Tetanus Vaccine (CHILD) (DT/Vac/Ads (Child)) in infancy. One 0.5 ml dose is given at 2, 3 and 4 months of age.

Reinforcing doses in children: Children who have received the primary course of immunisation in infancy require reinforcement of immunity against diphtheria and tetanus. This can be achieved by giving one dose (0.5 ml) Adsorbed Diphtheria and Tetanus Vaccine (CHILD) (DT/Vac/Ads (Child)), at least three years after the last dose of the primary course. The reinforcing dose is commonly given prior to school entry.

A reinforcing dose (0.5 ml) of either Adsorbed Diphtheria and Tetanus Vaccine for Adults and Adolescents or Adsorbed Tetanus Vaccine may be given at 15-19 years of age or on leaving school.

Oral Poliomyelitis Vaccine, BP may be given at the same time as Adsorbed Diphtheria and Tetanus Vaccine (CHILD).

Children aged 10 years and over, adults and elderly: NOT RECOMMENDED. In adults and elderly, reinforcement of immunity to diphtheria and/or tetanus can be achieved by administering one dose (0.5 ml) of either Adsorbed Diphtheria Vaccine for Adults and Adolescents, Adsorbed Diphtheria and Tetanus Vaccine for Adults and Adolescents or Adsorbed Tetanus Vaccine. For children aged 10 years and over, see Reinforcing doses in children.

Shake well before each dose is withdrawn. It is good practice to record the title, dose and lot numbers of all vaccines and the dates of administration.

*Contra-indications:* Adsorbed Diphtheria and Tetanus Vaccine (CHILD) must not be given intradermally since it may give rise to a persistent skin nodule.

ADSORBED DIPHTHERIA AND TETANUS VACCINE (CHILD) SHOULD NOT BE ADMINISTERED TO CHILDREN AGED 10 YEARS AND OVER, ADULTS AND ELDERLY.

The vaccine should not be administered to a subject who has experienced a serious reaction (e.g. anaphylaxis) to a previous dose of this vaccine or who is known to be hypersensitive to any component thereof.

It is advisable to avoid vaccination during an acute infection.

*Special warnings and precautions for use* Although anaphylaxis is rare, facilities for its management should always be available during vaccination.

*Interactions with other medicaments and other forms of interaction:* None stated.

*Pregnancy and lactation:* Accurate information is not available on the safety of Adsorbed Diphtheria and Tetanus Vaccine (CHILD) in pregnancy or on the immunisation of lactating women. The vaccine should not be used in pregnancy or lactation.

*Effects on ability to drive and use machines:* None stated.

*Undesirable effects:* Local reactions to diphtheria and tetanus vaccines are uncommon in young children. Local reactions consist of swelling, redness and tenderness at the injection-site and may occasionally be severe.

General reactions consisting of transient fever, malaise and headache occur infrequently. Acute allergic reaction-anaphylaxis, urticaria, pallor, cyanosis and polyradiculoneuritis have been reported very rarely after diphtheria/tetanus vaccines.

Angioneurotic oedema, dyspnoea, serum sickness, peripheral neuropathy, neuropathy and polyneuritis have followed the administration of tetanus vaccine.

Calcifying dermatomyositis has been observed in temporal association with tetanus vaccination.

A small painless nodule may form at the injection-site, but usually disappears without sequelae. Occasionally these nodules persist, especially if the inoculation is introduced into the superficial layers of subcutaneous tissue. Very rarely, circumscribed hypertrichosis and eczema are associated with such nodules.

Transverse myelitis has been reported after simultaneous administration of diphtheria and tetanus vaccine and oral polio vaccine, but a cause and effect relationship has not been established.

Any untoward reactions should be reported to the regulatory authorities and to the manufacturer.

*Overdose:* Not applicable.

**Pharmacological properties**　Not applicable.

**Pharmaceutical particulars**

*List of excipients:* The excipients contained in the preparation are as follows:-
| | |
|---|---|
| Aluminium hydroxide | HSE |
| Disodium tetraborate (Sodium borate) | BP |
| Succinic acid | HSE |
| Sodium chloride | PhEur |
| Thiomersal | BP |
| Water for injections | PhEur |

HSE house specification

*Incompatibilities:* None stated.

*Shelf life:* In filled containers: 2 years.

*Special precautions for storage:* Store between 2-8°C. Protect from light. Vials should be stored upright. Do not freeze.

*Nature and contents of container:* PhEur type 1 clear neutral glass ampoules, 1 ml capacity (0.5 ml fill). Multidose PhEur type 1 clear neutral glass vials, 8 ml capacity (5 ml fill) with butyl rubber plug with an aluminium collar and pigmented polypropylene flip-off top.

*Instructions for use/handling:* Vaccine which has been frozen should not be used.

Discard any partly used vaccine vials at the end of the vaccination session.

Disposal should be by incineration at a temperature not less than 1100°C at a registered waste disposal contractor.

**Marketing authorisation number**　0039/0467

**Date of approval/revision of SPC**　May 1996.

**Legal category**　POM

## ADSORBED DIPHTHERIA VACCINE, BP (CHILD)

**Qualitative and quantitative composition**　The composition in terms of active ingredients is as follows:- Diphtheria toxoid–not less than 30 IU. Quantities expressed per 0.5 ml dose.

**Pharmaceutical form**　Sterile suspension for deep subcutaneous or intramuscular injection to humans.

**Clinical particulars**

*Therapeutic indications:* For active immunisation against diphtheria in children under 10 years of age.

Primary immunisation against diphtheria in infancy is usually carried out by the administration of combined Adsorbed Diphtheria, Tetanus and Pertussis Vaccine (DTPer/Vac/Ads) or Adsorbed Diphtheria and Tetanus Vaccine (CHILD) (DT/Vac/Ads (Child)). Primary immunisation against diphtheria alone for children under 10 years of age may be carried out with Adsorbed Diphtheria Vaccine (CHILD) (Dip/Vac/Ads (Child)).

*Posology and method of administration:* Children under 10 years of age: Each dose is 0.5 ml, given by intramuscular or deep subcutaneous injection. The primary course of immunisation consists of three doses with an interval of at least one month between each dose.

The intervals between immunisations may be exceeded without the need to repeat the full course of immunisation.

Primary course in children: Primary immunisation against diphtheria may be carried out by the administration of combined Adsorbed Diphtheria, Tetanus and Pertussis Vaccine (DTPer/Vac/Ads), Adsorbed Diphtheria and Tetanus Vaccine (CHILD) (DT/Vac/Ads (Child)) or Adsorbed Diphtheria Vaccine (CHILD) (Dip/Vac/Ads (Child)) in infancy. One 0.5 ml dose is given at 2, 3 and 4 months of age.

Reinforcing doses in children: Children who have received the primary course of immunisation in infancy require reinforcement of immunity against diphtheria. This can be achieved by giving one dose (0.5 ml) Adsorbed Diphtheria and Tetanus Vaccine (CHILD) (DT/Vac/Ads (Child)) or Adsorbed Diphtheria Vaccine (CHILD) (Dip/Vac/Ads (Child)), at least three years after the last dose of the primary course. The reinforcing dose is commonly given prior to school entry.

A reinforcing dose (0.5 ml) of either Adsorbed Diphtheria and Tetanus Vaccine for Adults and Adolescents or Adsorbed Tetanus Vaccine may be given at 15-19 years of age or on leaving school.

Oral Poliomyelitis Vaccine, BP may be given at the same time as Adsorbed Diphtheria Vaccine (CHILD).

Children aged 10 years and over, adults and elderly: NOT RECOMMENDED. In adults and elderly, reinforcement of immunity can be achieved by administering one dose (0.5 ml) of Adsorbed Diphtheria Vaccine for Adults and Adolescents. Adsorbed Diphtheria and Tetanus Vaccine for Adults and Adolescents may be used if simultaneous reinforcement of immunity against diphtheria and tetanus is required. For children aged 10 years and over, see "Reinforcing doses in children".

Shake well before each dose is withdrawn. It is good practice to record the title, dose and lot numbers of all vaccines and dates of administration.

*Contra-indications:* Adsorbed Diphtheria Vaccine (CHILD) should not be administered intradermally since it may give rise to a persistent skin nodule.

ADSORBED DIPHTHERIA VACCINE (CHILD) SHOULD NOT BE ADMINISTERED TO CHILDREN AGED 10 YEARS AND OVER, ADULTS OR ELDERLY.

The vaccine should not be administered to a subject who has experienced a serious reaction (e.g. anaphylaxis) to a previous dose of this vaccine or who is known to be hypersensitive to any component thereof.

It is advisable to avoid vaccination during an acute infection.

*Special warnings and precautions for use:* Although anaphylaxis is rare, facilities for its management should always be available during vaccination.

*Interactions with other medicaments and other forms of interaction:* None known

*Pregnancy and lactation:* Accurate information is not available on the safety of Adsorbed Diphtheria Vaccine (CHILD) in pregnancy or on the immunisation of lactating women. The vaccine should not be used in pregnancy or lactation.

*Effects on ability to drive and use machines:* None stated

*Undesirable effects:* Reactions may be local or general and they may be more frequent and severe after the second injection. Local reactions are uncommon in children under two years of age. Local reactions consisting of swelling, redness and tenderness at the injection-site may occur and may occasionally be severe.

The incidence and severity of local reactions increases rapidly after the age of 10 years, occurring frequently in adults.

General reactions consisting of transient fever, malaise and headache may occur.

Allergic reactions, urticaria, pallor and dyspnoea have been reported following injection of Adsorbed Diphtheria Vaccine (CHILD).

A small painless nodule may form at the injection-site but usually disappears without sequelae. Occasionally these nodules persist, especially if the inoculation is introduced into the superficial layers of subcutaneous tissue. Very rarely, circumscribed hypertrichosis and eczema are associated with such nodules.

Any untoward reactions should be reported to the regulatory authorities and to the manufacturer.

*Overdose:* Not applicable

**Pharmacological properties** Not applicable

**Pharmaceutical particulars**

*List of excipients:* The excipients contained in the preparation are as follows:-

| | |
|---|---|
| Aluminium phosphate | HSE |
| Sodium succinate | HSE |
| Sodium chloride | PhEur |
| Thiomersal | BP |
| Water for injections | PhEur |

HSE House specification

*Incompatibilities:* None stated

*Shelf life:* In filled containers: 2 years

*Special precautions for storage:* Store between 2 and 8°C. Protect from light. Do not freeze.

*Nature and contents of container:* PhEur type 1 clear neutral glass ampoules of 1 ml capacity (0.5 ml fill).

*Instructions for use/handling:* Vaccine which has been frozen should not be used. Disposal should be by incineration at a temperature not less than 1100°C at a registered waste disposal contractor.

**Marketing authorisation number** 0039/0466

**Date of approval/revision of SPC** February 1996.

**Legal category** POM

## EUDEMINE* TABLETS 50MG

**Presentation** White sugar-coated tablets each containing Diazoxide BP 50 mg.

**Uses** Eudemine tablets are used orally in the treatment of intractable hypoglycaemia. Diazoxide also causes salt and water retention.

*Hypoglycaemia:* Eudemine administered orally is indicated for the treatment of intractable hypoglycaemia with severe symptoms from a variety of causes including: idiopathic hypoglycaemia in infancy, leucine-sensitive or unclassified; functional islet-cell tumours both malignant and benign if inoperable; extra-pancreatic neoplasms producing hypoglycaemia; glycogen storage disease; hypoglycaemia of unknown origin.

**Dosage and administration**
*Hypoglycaemia:* In hypoglycaemia the dosage schedule of Eudemine Tablets is determined according to the clinical needs and the response of the individual patient. For both adults and children a starting oral dose of 5 mg/kg body weight divided into 2 or 3 equal doses per 24 hours will establish the patient's response and thereafter the dose can be increased until the symptoms and blood glucose level respond satisfactorily. Regular determinations of the blood in the initial days of treatment are essential. The usual maintenance dose is 3–8 mg/kg/day given in two or three divided doses. Reduced doses may be required in patients with impaired renal function. In children with leucine-sensitive hypoglycaemia, a dosage range of 15 to 20 mg/kg/day is suggested.

In adults with benign or malignant islet-cell tumours producing large quantities of insulin, high dosages of up to 1,000 mg per day have been used.

**Contra-indications, warnings, etc.**
*Contra-indications:* In the treatment of hypoglycaemia, Eudemine is contra-indicated in all cases which are amenable to surgery or other specific therapy.

Hypersensitivity to any component of the preparation or to other thiazides.

*Precautions:* In the treatment of hypoglycaemia it is necessary that the blood pressure be monitored regularly.

Retention of sodium and water is likely to necessitate therapy with oral diuretic such as frusemide or ethacrynic acid. The dosage of either of the diuretics mentioned may be up to 1 g daily. It must be appreciated that if diuretics are employed then both the hypotensive and the hyperglycaemic activities of diazoxide will be potentiated and it is likely that the dosage of diazoxide will require adjustment downwards. In patients with severe renal failure it is desirable to maintain, with diuretic therapy, urinary volumes in excess of 1 litre daily. Hypokalaemia should be avoided by adequate potassium replacement.

Diazoxide should be used with caution in patients with impaired cardiac reserve, in whom sodium and water retention may precipitate congestive heart failure (see *side effects*). Diazoxide should be administered with caution to patients with hyperuricaemia or a history of gout, and it is advisable to monitor serum uric acid concentration.

Whenever Eudemine is given over a prolonged period regular haematological examinations are indicated to exclude changes in white blood cell and platelet counts. Also in children there should be regular assessment of growth, bone and psychological maturation.

The very rapid almost complete protein binding of diazoxide requires cautious dosage to be used in patients whose plasma proteins may be lower than normal.

*Interactions:* Drugs potentiated by diazoxide therapy include: oral diuretics, anti-hypertensive agents and anticoagulants.

Phenytoin levels should be monitored as increased dosage may be needed if administered concurrently with diazoxide.

The risk of hyperglycaemia may be increased by concurrent administration of corticosteroids of oestrogen-progestogen combinations.

*Use in pregnancy:* Eudemine Tablets are only to be used in pregnant women when the indicated condition is deemed to put the mother's life at risk.

Eudemine should not be given to nursing mothers as the safety of diazoxide during lactation has not been established.

*Side-effects:* Prolonged oral therapy of Eudemine during pregnancy has been reported to cause alopecia in the new-born.

With oral therapy nausea is common in the first two or three weeks and may require relief with an antinauseant. Prolonged therapy has given rise to reports of hypertrichosis lanuginosa, anorexia and hyperuricaemia.

Extra-pyramidal side-effects have been reported with oral diazoxide. It was found that extra-pyramidal effects such as Parkinsonian tremor, cogwheel rigidity and oculogyric crisis could be easily suppressed by intravenous injection of an anti-Parkinson drug such as procyclidine and that they could be prevented by maintenance therapy with such a drug given orally.

Other adverse effects of Eudemine which have been reported are hyperosmolar non-ketotic coma, cardiomegaly, leucopenia, thrombocytopenia and hirsutism.

Sodium and water retention occur frequently in patients receiving multiple doses of diazoxide, and may precipitate cardiac failure in susceptible patients (e.g. those with impaired cardiac reserve). Symptoms of disturbed cardiac function (tachycardia arrhythmias), inappropriate hypotension or hyperglycaemia (including ketoacidosis) have also been reported.

Diazoxide may cause gastrointestinal disturbances including nausea, vomiting, abdominal pain, anorexia, diarrhoea, ileus and constipation. Changes in hepatic and renal function have been observed occasionally, including increased AST, alkaline phosphatase, azotemia, decreased creatinine clearance, reversible nephrotic syndrome, haematuria and albuminuria.

Disorders of blood components (decreased haemoglobin and/or haematocrit, eosinophilia, bleeding) have been reported. Hypogamma-globulinaemia may also occur. Other reported side effects of diazoxide treatment include: headache, dyspnoea, musculo-skeletal pain, hypersensitivity reactions (rash, fever, leucopenia), blurred vision, transient cataracts. Voice changes in children and abnormal facial features in children on long term treatment have also been reported.

*Overdosage:* Excessive dosage of Eudemine can result in hyperglycaemia which will respond to insulin, and/or hypotension which will necessitate maintenance of blood volume with intravenous fluids.

**Pharmaceutical precautions** None.

**Legal category** POM.

**Package quantities** Eudemine Tablets 50 mg are packed in containers of 100 (OP).

**Further information** Nil.

**Product licence number** 0039/0412

## FLUVIRIN*

**Qualitative and quantitative composition** Each 0.5 ml dose contains haemagglutinin and neuraminidase proteins of the following strains of influenza virus, as recommended by the WHO:

| | | |
|---|---|---|
| A/Singapore/6/86 (H1N1)–Like strain [A/Texas/36/91 (H1N1) is the actual strain] | 15µg haemagglutinin | |
| A/Wuhan/359/95 (H3N2)–Like strain [A/Nanchang/933/95 is the actual strain] | 15µg haemagglutinin | |
| B/Beijing/184/93–Like strain [B/Harbin/7/94 is the actual strain] | 15µg haemagglutinin | |

**Pharmaceutical form** An aqueous suspension intended for deep subcutaneous or intramuscular injection.

**Clinical particulars**

*Therapeutic indications:* To induce active immunity to influenza in those groups regarded as being at special risk, especially the elderly, which include those suffering from the following conditions:

Chronic pulmonary disease, e.g. chronic bronchitis and emphysema, asthma, bronchiectasis, pulmonary tuberculosis and pulmonary fibrosis.

Chronic heart disease, e.g. valvular and hypertensive heart disease.

Chronic renal disease, e.g. chronic nephritis; patients with renal disease on immunosuppressive drugs.

Diabetes and possibly other less common endocrine disorders.

Patients who are being actively considered for immunosuppressive therapy.

Immunisation also recommended in:

Persons living in residential establishments, especially the elderly, in which rapid spread is likely to follow the introduction of infection.

Doctors, nurses, ambulance crew and others at special risk of infection by reason of their contacts with persons suffering from influenza.

*Posology and method of administration:* Adults and children aged 4 years and over: One dose of 0.5 ml vaccine. Young children under the age of thirteen not previously infected or not having received trivalent influenza vaccine in last 4 years may require two doses at intervals of 4 to 6 weeks.

Route of administration: For human medicinal use by deep subcutaneous or intramuscular injection.

Adults and children are normally immunised in the deltoid muscle; young children in the anterolateral aspect of the thigh.

*Contra-indications:* Fluvirin [Inactivated Influenza Vaccine (Surface Antigen) PhEur] should not be given to persons sensitive to eggs, chicken protein, chicken feathers or influenzal viral protein.

The occurrence of any neurological symptoms or

signs following administration of any vaccine is a contraindication to further use. Immunisation should be deferred in a patient with any active neurological disorder.

Immunisation should be delayed if there is active or suspected infection.

*Special warnings and special precautions for use:* Because the vaccine contains purified haemagglutinin and neuraminidase antigens, the total viral protein content of the vaccine has been reduced to about one tenth of that of whole virus vaccines. In the event of an allergic reaction, adrenaline by injection should be available for use.

If spirit is used to swab the injection site, it should be allowed to dry completely before vaccination, and should not come in contact with the vaccine.

Very small quantities of neomycin and polymyxin are used during manufacture. Theoretically the vaccine purification process removes these antibiotics, and no adverse effects have been reported. Nevertheless caution should be exercised with very hypersensitive patients.

*Interactions with other medicaments and other forms of interaction:* None known. It is not known if Fluvirin interacts with warfarin or theophylline although it has been reported that influenza vaccination can inhibit their clearance. Studies have failed to establish any adverse clinical effects attributable to these drugs in patients receiving influenza vaccine.

*Use during pregnancy and lactation:* Animal studies have not been conducted, therefore the effects of vaccination during pregnancy or lactation are unknown. Use in pregnancy or lactation should be avoided unless directed by the patient's doctor and then restricted to patients where there is an indication for its use.

*Effects on ability to drive and use machines:* None.

*Undesirable effects:* Systemic effects such as headache, pyrexia, and a feeling of malaise, beginning 6 to 12 hours after injection and lasting for up to 48 hours, may occur. Local effects such as redness and soreness at the site of injection may occur. Rarely neurological disorders such as encephalomyelitis, neuritis and Guillain Barre Syndrome have been reported but without any clear causal relationship with the vaccine.

*Overdose:* No research has been conducted in relation to overdosage and, in view of the nature of this product and the mode of administration of the drug, the likelihood of overdosage is negligible.

**Pharmacological particulars** This vaccine is used for active immunisation against influenza, principally for the vaccination of those groups regarded as being at special risk, especially the elderly and children.

The vaccine stimulates production of antibodies with a specific protective capacity against influenza.

**Pharmaceutical particulars**

*List of excipients:*

| | |
|---|---|
| Disodium Hydrogen Phosphate | 0.1278% w/v |
| Potassium Dihydrogen Phosphate | 0.01362% w/v |
| Sodium Chloride | 0.87% w/v |
| Water for Injection | to 100.0% v/v |

*Incompatibilities:* Spirit should not be allowed to come into contact with the vaccine.

*Shelf life:* 12 months as presented for sale. Syringes should be used immediately after opening.

*Special precautions for storage:* Store between 2 and 8°C. Do not freeze. Protect from light.

*Nature and contents of container:* Pre-filled syringe: Neutral (type 1) clear glass syringe with siliconised rubber stoppers, containing 0.5 ml vaccine.

*Instructions for use/handling:* If the vaccine has been stored in a refrigerator it should be allowed to reach room temperature before use.

The syringe should be well shaken immediately before making the injection.

**Marketing authorisation number**    00039/0490

**Date of approval/revision of SPC**    May 1996

## INTRADERMAL BCG VACCINE, BP

**Qualitative and quantitative composition** Each 0.1 ml dose contains:

*10 dose vaccine:* Bacillus Calmette Guerin (Copenhagen sub-strain 1077) 1.0 to 2.6 x 10⁶ viable units.

*20 and 50 dose vaccine:* Bacillus Calmette Guerin (Copenhagen sub-strain 1077) 0.8 to 2.6 x 10⁶ viable units.

**Pharmaceutical form** Freeze-dried standardised preparation of a sub-strain of Bacillus Calmette-Guerin to be reconstituted with Water for Injections, BP or Sodium Chloride Injection, BP prior to intradermal administration.

**Clinical particulars**

*Therapeutic indications:* For active immunisation against tuberculosis. Vaccinated persons normally become Mantoux-positive after eight weeks, but sometimes up to 14 weeks are needed.

*Posology and method of administration:* The INTRADERMAL inoculation should be given in the arm, over the insertion of the deltoid muscle onto the humerus. Administration in the leg has been associated with more severe reactions in neonates and should be avoided. The administration of INTRADERMAL BCG Vaccine should preferably be carried out with a syringe fitted with a short bevel gauge 25 needle. The use of jet injectors to administer the vaccine is not recommended.

*Children aged 3 months and over, adults and elderly:* 0.1 ml strictly by **INTRADERMAL** injection (subcutaneous injection must be avoided). A tuberculin skin test must be conducted before BCG immunisation.

*Infants under 3 months of age:* 0.05 ml strictly by **INTRADERMAL** injection (subcutaneous injection must be avoided).

*Reconstitution:* The vaccine must not be contaminated with any antiseptic or detergent. Avoid contamination with bactericides. If alcohol is used to swab the rubber stopper of the vial, it must be allowed to evaporate before the stopper is penetrated with the syringe needle.

The vaccine suspension is prepared by adding 1 ml of Water for Injections, BP or Sodium Chloride Injection, BP to the 10 dose vial. When using the 50 dose vial, 5 ml of Sodium Chloride Injection, BP (not Water for Injections, BP) should be added. DO NOT shake as this causes frothing. Allow to stand for one minute, then draw into the syringe twice to ensure homogeneity.

*Intradermal injection technique:* The vaccine must not be contaminated with any antiseptic or detergent. Avoid contamination with bactericides. If alcohol is used to swab the skin, it must be allowed to evaporate before the vaccine is injected.

The upper arm must be approximately 45° to the body. After cleaning and allowing to dry, the skin should be stretched between thumb and forefinger. The needle should be inserted (bevel upwards) slowly for about 2 mm into the superficial layers of dermis. The needle is almost parallel with the skin surface and should be visible through the epidermis during insertion. A raised, blanched bleb showing tips of hair follicles is a sign of correct injection. If considerable resistance is not felt, the needle should be removed and reinserted.

The injection site is best left uncovered to facilitate healing.

It is good practice to record the title, dose and lot numbers of all vaccines and dates of administration.

*Contra-indications:* INTRADERMAL BCG VACCINE MUST NOT BE ADMINISTERED USING THE MULTIPLE PUNCTURE TECHNIQUE.

INTRADERMAL BCG Vaccine should NOT be given to persons receiving systemic corticosteroids or immunosuppressive treatment including radiotherapy, those suffering from malignant conditions (e.g. lymphoma, leukaemia, Hodgkin's Disease or other tumours of the reticuloendothelial system), those in whom normal immunological mechanism is impaired (e.g. hypogammaglobulinaemia), those known or suspected to be HIV-positive, including infants born to HIV-positive mothers and persons with pyrexia or generalised infected skin conditions. The effect of INTRADERMAL BCG Vaccine may be exaggerated in these patients and a more generalised infection is possible. Eczema is not a contra-indication, but the vaccine site must be lesion free.

INTRADERMAL BCG Vaccine should not be given to patients who are receiving prophylactic doses of anti-tuberculous drugs.

Tuberculin-positive persons, i.e. those with induration of 5 mm or greater in diameter in the Mantoux test, or those in Heaf grades 2 to 4, do not require the vaccine. Its administration to these persons may result in an accelerated local reaction of larger size than normal.

The vaccine should not be administered to a subject who is known to be hypersensitive to any component of the vaccine.

*Special warnings and precautions for use:* INTRADERMAL BCG Vaccine may be given concurrently with another live vaccine, including Oral Poliomyelitis Vaccine, BP. An interval of not less than three weeks should normally be allowed to lapse between the administration of any two live vaccines, if they are not given at the same time. However, when INTRADERMAL BCG Vaccine is given to infants, there is no need to delay the primary childhood immunisations which includes polio vaccine.

No further vaccination should be given for at least three months in the arm used for BCG vaccination, because of the risk of regional lymphadenitis.

Although anaphylaxis is rare, facilities for its management should always be available during vaccination.

Infectious mononucleosis, viral infections in general, including those of the upper respiratory tract, live viral vaccines, Hodgkin's disease, sarcoidosis, corticosteroid therapy and immunosuppressing treatment or diseases, including HIV, may suppress the reaction to the tuberculin skin test.

*Interaction with other medicaments and other forms of interaction:* None known.

*Pregnancy and lactation:* No reproductive studies have been conducted in animals. There are no data on the use of this vaccine in pregnancy or lactation. Vaccination should be avoided in early pregnancy and if possible delayed until after delivery. The vaccine should not normally be used during lactation unless the benefit outweighs the risk.

*Effects on ability to drive and use machines:* None known.

*Undesirable effects:* Normally following intradermal administration of BCG, a local reaction develops at the injection site within two to six weeks. This begins as a small papule which increases in size for a few weeks widening into a circular area up to 7 mm in diameter with scaling, crusting and occasional bruising. The lesion slowly subsides over several months and eventually heals leaving only a small, flat scar. Occasionally an ulcer up to 10 mm in diameter develops.

Rash, fever, local induration, pain and lymphadenopathy may occur.

Occasionally an excessive response to INTRADERMAL BCG Vaccine results in a discharging ulcer. This may be attributable to inadvertent subcutaneous injection or to excessive dosage. The ulcer should be encouraged to dry and abrasion avoided, e.g. by tight clothes. Waterproof dressings should not be used. If the ulcer persists, it can be treated by application of a mild corticosteroid cream and/or a topical antibiotic.

In rare cases of severe local reaction with abscess formation, aspiration may be carried out and anti-tuberculous therapy considered. Enlargement of axillary lymph glands is unlikely except occasionally in young infants.

Anaphylactic reactions have been reported on rare occasions.

Any untoward reactions should be reported to the Regulatory Authorities and to the Marketing Authorisation Holder.

*Overdose:* If gross overdosage occurs and there is reason to suspect the development of a more generalised infection with BCG, systemic treatment with isoniazid or any other suitable anti-tuberculous drug should be given.

**Pharmacological particulars** This vaccine is used for active immunisation against tuberculosis, principally for the vaccination of selected groups of the population and of persons likely to be exposed to infection.

The vaccine stimulates production of cell mediated immunity with a specific protective capacity against tuberculosis.

In British schoolchildren efficacy (protection against tuberculosis) is 70-80% with protection lasting at least 15 years.

**Pharmaceutical particulars**

*List of excipients:* Before freeze-drying, each vial contains 0.5 to 1.0 ml* (±10%) of freeze-drying medium of the following composition: Dextran 8.3%, Glucose 7.5%, Triton WR 1339 0.025%, Water for Injections, BP 100.0%.

* the amount of freeze-drying medium used is such that the depth of suspension in the vial is suitable for freeze-drying.

Water for Injections, BP (PL00039/5704) and Sodium Chloride Injection, BP (PL00039/5699) are provided as diluents with the vaccine.

*Incompatibilities:* None known.

*Shelf life:*

10 dose vaccine: 36 months when stored at 2-8°C unopened. 4 hours after reconstitution.

20 and 50 dose vaccine: 24 months when stored at 2-8°C unopened. 4 hours after reconstitution.

*Special precautions for storage:* The freeze-dried vaccine should be stored between 2-8°C. Protect from light. Diluent should not be frozen but should be stored below 25°C.

*Nature and contents of container:*

Size: 3 ml vials (10 and 20 dose), 5 ml vials (50 dose).

Type: Neutral (type 1) amber glass vials complying with the PhEur requirements for containers for injectables.

Seals: Siliconised rubber peg bungs with aluminium overseals and polypropylene flip top caps.

*Instructions for use and handling:* The vaccine suspension is prepared by adding 1 ml of Water for Injections BP or Sodium Chloride Injection BP to the 10 dose vial. When using the 50 dose vial, 5 ml of Sodium

Chloride Injection BP (not Water for Injections BP) should be added. DO NOT shake as this causes frothing. Allow to stand for one minute, then draw into the syringe twice to ensure homogeneity.

After reconstitution the vaccine should be kept cool, protected from light and used in the same session, i.e. within 4 hours. Any reconstituted vaccine remaining at the end of the session (maximum 4 hours) should be discarded.

Disposal should be by incineration at a temperature not less than 1100°C at a registered waste disposal contractor.

**Marketing authorisation number** 0039/0435

**Date of approval/revision of SPC** March 1997

**Legal category** POM

## INTRADERMAL BCG VACCINE, BP ISONIAZID RESISTANT

**Qualitative and quantitative composition** Each 0.1 ml dose contains: Bacillus Calmette-Guerin (Isoniazid resistant sub-strain) 0.8 to 2.6 x $10^6$ viable units.

**Pharmaceutical form** Freeze-dried standardised preparation of an isoniazid resistant sub-strain of Bacillus Calmette-Guerin to be reconstituted with Water for Injections, BP or Sodium Chloride Injection, BP prior to intradermal administration.

**Clinical particulars**

*Therapeutic indications:* For active immunisation against tuberculosis in tuberculous contacts while they are receiving prophylactic treatment with isoniazid.

It is well established that BCG vaccination of contacts confers protection against tuberculosis and it is especially useful in this respect for new-born infants of tuberculous mothers or infants born into tuberculous households. However, under such circumstances segregation is necessary until Mantoux testing has shown conversion. This undesirable segregation period of a few weeks can be abolished by giving isoniazid to the infant from birth, but the adoption of this procedure suffers from the disadvantage that concurrent administration of isoniazid interferes with the response to normal BCG vaccine. This can be avoided by the use of an isoniazid resistant BCG vaccine, when administration of isoniazid need only continue until the post-BCG tuberculin test becomes positive.

*Posology and method of administration:* The **INTRADERMAL** inoculation should be given in the arm, over the insertion of the deltoid muscle onto the humerus. The administration of INTRADERMAL BCG Vaccine, BP Isoniazid Resistant should preferably be carried out with a syringe fitted with a short bevel gauge 25 needle. The use of jet injectors to administer the vaccine is not recommended.

*Children aged 3 months and over, adults and elderly:* 0.1 ml strictly by **INTRADERMAL** injection (subcutaneous injection must be avoided). A tuberculin skin test must be conducted before BCG immunisation.

*Infants under 3 months of age:* 0.05 ml strictly by **INTRADERMAL** injection (subcutaneous injection must be avoided).

*Reconstitution:* The vaccine must not be contaminated with any antiseptic or detergent. Avoid contamination with bactericides. If alcohol is used to swab the rubber stopper of the vial, it must be allowed to evaporate before the stopper is penetrated with the syringe needle.

The vaccine suspension is prepared by adding 1 ml of Water for Injections, BP or Sodium Chloride Injection, BP to the vial. Do NOT shake as this causes frothing. Allow to stand for one minute, then draw into the syringe twice to ensure homogeneity.

*Intradermal injection technique:* The vaccine must not be contaminated with any antiseptic or detergent. Avoid contamination with bactericides. If alcohol is used to swab the skin, it must be allowed to evaporate before the vaccine is injected.

The upper arm must be approximately 45° to the body. After cleaning and allowing to dry, the skin should be stretched between thumb and forefinger. The needle should be inserted (bevel upwards) slowly for about 2 mm into the superficial layers of dermis. The needle is almost parallel with the skin surface and should be visible through the epidermis during insertion. A raised, blanched bleb showing tips of hair follicles is a sign of correct injection. If considerable resistance is not felt, the needle should be removed and reinserted.

The injection site is best left uncovered to facilitate healing.

It is good practice to record the title, dose and lot numbers of all vaccines and dates of administration.

*Contra-indications:* INTRADERMAL BCG VACCINE, BP ISONIAZID RESISTANT MUST NOT BE ADMINISTERED BY THE MULTIPLE PUNCTURE TECHNIQUE.

INTRADERMAL BCG Vaccine, BP Isoniazid Resistant should NOT be given to persons receiving systemic corticosteroids or immunosuppressive treatment including radiotherapy, those suffering from malignant conditions (e.g. lymphoma, leukaemia, Hodgkin's Disease or other tumours of the reticuloendothelial system), those in whom normal immunological mechanism is impaired (e.g. hypogammaglobulinaemia), those known or suspected to be HIV-positive, including infants born to HIV positive mothers, and persons with pyrexia or generalised infected skin conditions. The effect of INTRADERMAL BCG Vaccine, BP Isoniazid Resistant may be exaggerated in these patients and a more generalised infection is possible. Eczema is not a contra-indication, but the vaccine site must be lesion free.

Tuberculin-positive persons, i.e. those with induration of 5 mm or greater in diameter in the Mantoux test, or those in Heaf grades 2 to 4, do not require the vaccine. Its administration to these persons may result in an accelerated local reaction of larger size than normal.

The vaccine should not be administered to a subject who is known to be hypersensitive to any component of the vaccine.

*Special warnings and precautions for use:* INTRADERMAL BCG Vaccine, Isoniazid Resistant, may be given concurrently with another live vaccine, including Oral Poliomyelitis Vaccine, BP.. An interval of not less than three weeks should normally be allowed to lapse between the administration of any two live vaccines, if they are not given at the same time. However, when INTRADERMAL BCG Vaccine, Isoniazid Resistant is given to infants, there is no need to delay primary childhood immunisations which include polio vaccine.

No further vaccination should be given for at least three months in the arm used for BCG vaccination, because of the risk of regional lymphadenitis.

Although anaphylaxis is rare, facilities for its management should always be available during vaccination.

Infectious mononucleosis, viral infections in general, including those of the upper respiratory tract, live viral vaccines, Hodgkin's disease, sarcoidosis, corticosteroid therapy and immunosuppressing treatment or diseases, including HIV, may suppress the reaction to the tuberculin skin test.

*Interaction with other medicaments and other forms of interaction:* None known.

*Pregnancy and lactation:* No reproductive studies have been conducted in animals. There are no data on the use of this vaccine in pregnancy or lactation. Vaccination should be avoided in early pregnancy and if possible delayed until after delivery. The vaccine should not normally be used during lactation unless the benefit outweighs the risk.

*Effects on ability to drive and use machines:* None known.

*Undesirable effects:* Normally following intradermal administration of BCG, a local reaction develops at the injection site within two to six weeks. This begins as a small papule which increases in size for a few weeks widening into a circular area up to 7 mm in diameter with scaling, crusting and occasional bruising. The lesion slowly subsides over several months and eventually heals leaving only a small, flat scar. Occasionally an ulcer up to 10 mm in diameter develops.

Rash, fever, local induration, pain and lymphadenopathy may occur. Occasionally an excessive response to INTRADERMAL BCG Vaccine, BP Isoniazid Resistant results in a discharging ulcer. This may be attributable to inadvertent subcutaneous injection or to excessive dosage. The ulcer should be encouraged to dry and abrasion avoided, e.g. by tight clothes. Waterproof dressings should not be used. If the ulcer persists, it can be treated by application of a mild corticosteroid cream and/or a topical antibiotic.

In rare cases of severe local reaction with abscess formation, aspiration may be carried out and antituberculous therapy considered. Enlargement of axillary lymph glands is unlikely except occasionally in young infants.

Anaphylactic reactions have been reported on rare occasions with INTRADERMAL BCG Vaccine, BP and PERCUTANEOUS BCG Vaccine, BP.

Any untoward reactions should be reported to the regulatory authorities and to the Marketing Authorisation Holder.

*Overdose:* Not applicable.

**Pharmacological particulars** This vaccine is suitable for vaccinating tuberculous contacts while they are receiving prophylactic treatment with isoniazid. The vaccine contains an isoniazid resistant sub-strain of Bacillus Calmette-Guerin prepared by repeated subcultivation in the presence of isoniazid.

The vaccine stimulates production of cell mediated immunity with a specific protective capacity against tuberculosis.

**Pharmaceutical particulars**

*List of excipients:* Before freeze-drying, each vial contains 0.5 ml ± (10%)* of freeze-drying medium of the following composition: Dextran 8.3%, Glucose 7.5%, Triton WR 1339 0.025%, Water for Injections, BP 100.0%.

* the amount of freeze-drying medium used is such that the depth of suspension in the vial is suitable for freeze-drying.

*Incompatibilities:* None known.

*Shelf life:* 24 months when stored at 2-8°C unopened. 4 hours after reconstitution.

*Special precautions for storage:* Store between 2 and 8°C. Protect from light.

*Nature and contents of container:*

Size: 3 ml vial (10 dose).

Type: Neutral (type 1) amber glass vials complying with the PhEur requirements for containers for injectables.

Seals: Siliconised rubber peg bungs with aluminium overseals and polypropylene flip top caps.

*Instructions for use and handling:* The vaccine suspension is prepared by adding 1 ml of Water for Injections BP or Sodium Chloride Injection BP to the 10 dose vial. Do NOT shake as this causes frothing. Allow to stand for one minute, then draw into the syringe twice to ensure homogeneity.

After reconstitution the vaccine should be kept cool, protected from light and used in the same session, i.e. within 4 hours. Any reconstituted vaccine remaining at the end of the session (maximum 4 hours) should be discarded.

Disposal should be by incineration at a temperature not less than 1100°C at a registered waste disposal contractor.

**Marketing authorisation number** 0039/0437

**Date of approval/revision of SPC** January 1997

**Legal category** POM

INTRADERMAL BCG Vaccine, BP Isoniazid Resistant is not marketed, and is available to the profession on request only.

## MICANOL* CREAM 1%
## MICANOL* CREAM 3%

**Qualitative and quantitative composition** Dithranol BP 1.0% or 3.0% w/w

**Pharmaceutical form** Cream

**Clinical particulars**

*Therapeutic indications:* Treatment of sub-acute and chronic psoriasis, including psoriasis of the scalp, by the short contact therapy method.

*Posology and method of administration:*

*Adults including the elderly:* Apply Micanol cream only to the affected areas being careful to avoid contact with normal skin. Use only a small amount, rubbing it in gently and thoroughly until it no longer smears.

Micanol cream should be applied once every 24 hours and removed by washing off usually no more than 30 minutes after application. The cream must be washed off using plenty of lukewarm water only. This may be easiest in a bath or shower, particularly if the treated area is extensive.

When removing the cream, it is important that the water is not too hot and soap is not used, as these can damage the Micanol cream base and cause increased staining of the skin. Soap may be used for washing after the Micanol cream has been rinsed off.

The treatment should start with 1% cream on a limited surface. Where the response to dithranol has not been previously established, contact with 1% cream should initially be not greater than 10 minutes. This may gradually be increased to 30 minutes over a period of about seven days depending on the individual response.

After 1-2 weeks patients may progress to Micanol 3% if necessary provided they do not show any sign of skin irritation.

If the skin is irritated, patients should revert to 1% cream. Treatment should be continued until the skin is clear of psoriasis.

For use on the scalp, first wash the hair with shampoo, rinse and then apply Micanol cream while the hair is still damp. Leave in contact for up to 30 minutes and then rinse off using plenty of lukewarm water only. Further shampoo may be used after the cream has been removed.

Micanol 3% cream should always be used under medical supervision.

Micanol cream may cause staining of clothing and bed linen. To remove staining on clothing or bed linen rinse in lukewarm water only (not more than 30°C). To prevent the possibility of discolouration to the bath or shower always rinse with lukewarm water. Should any deposit be left on the surface a suitable cleanser may be used.

*Children:* There is no evidence of adverse effects in children. However, caution should be exercised and the treatment supervised regularly.

Micanol is not suitable for the treatment of infants and young children.

*Contra-indications:* Acute pustular psoriasis or presence of inflammation of skin, including folliculitis; erythroderma; hypersensitivity to Dithranol or any other component of Micanol*.

*Special warnings and precautions for use:* Use with caution if potent steroids have been administered recently. Do not apply to the face and keep away from eyes; if accidentally applied to the eyes, severe conjunctivitis, keratinitis, or corneal opacity may result. If accidental contact occurs, wash with plenty of lukewarm water.

Do not apply to mucous membrane, genitalia or intertriginous skin, do not apply to blistered, raw or oozing area of the skin.

When excessive redness or burning is observed, reduce frequency or concentration, or discontinue application. Such irritation is more likely with higher concentrations.

If sensitivity reactions occur, especially on the normal skin surrounding the plaque site, discontinue use.

Wash hands thoroughly after use.

*Interaction with other medicaments and other forms of interaction:* Photosensitising medications (concurrent use of these medications with Dithranol may enhance their photosensitising effects).

Propylene glycol containing drugs (Dithranol would be oxidised and inactivated).

Withdrawal of long term steroids in psoriasis may cause a rebound phenomenon. An interval of one or two weeks should therefore be left between stopping long term steroids and starting Micanol treatment. A bland emollient may be used in the intervening period.

*Pregnancy and lactation:* There is no experimental evidence to support the safety of dithranol in pregnancy. Micanol cream should be given to pregnant women only if clearly needed.

Nursing mothers should not apply Micanol on the breast area, and avoid accidental contamination of the skin or mouth of the baby.

*Effects on ability to drive and use machines:* None reported and none expected.

*Undesirable effects:*
*Frequent:* Perilesional erythema and burning, lesional burning (usually mild or moderate). These reactions usually lessen after one or two weeks of treatment.

*Rarely:* Allergic reaction (skin rash).

Staining of the treated and surrounding skin may appear. It will disappear within 1 to 2 weeks after the end of treatment.

May temporarily discolour fingernails or grey or white hair, may stain fabrics.

*Overdose:* Excessive application of the cream and prolonged usage causes burning and deep staining of the skin.

The skin should be rinsed firstly with water only and then washed, never wash at a temperature exceeding 30°C.

Dithranol is a cathartic (laxative) and if accidentally swallowed, should be removed by gastric lavage.

**Pharmacological particulars**

*Pharmacodynamic properties:* Dithranol belongs to the family of Hydroxyanthrones, which have been used in the treatment of psoriasis for more than a century.

The therapeutic action of dithranol has been linked to its ability to generate free radicals.

Dithranol has been shown to accumulate in the mitochondria where it induces morphological and functional changes. This affects the cellular energy supply which, in turn, results in inhibition of energy dependent processes such as DNA replication which slows down excessive cell division as seen in psoriasis plaque. Cyclic nucleosides are important in the regulation of epidermal cell division.

The psoriatic hyperproliferative epidermis contains elevated levels of cyclic guanosine monophosphate. As dithranol has been shown to reduce the elevated level of cGMP back to normal, this could represent an additional mechanism of action.

*Pharmacokinetic properties:*
*Absorption and distribution:* In vitro studies with human skin showed that more dithranol penetrates into skin with impaired stratum corneum barrier in 30 minutes than into intact skin during 16 hours. The concentration reaches its maximum after 30-60 minutes contact time and remains rather constant thereafter. In intact skin, however, the concentration continues to increase with time.

The highest concentration of unchanged dithranol is found in the horny layer where it can be detected

for 24-48 hours, even after the skin has been washed. In deeper dermal layers relatively small amounts of unoxidised dithranol are detected whereas higher concentrations of the dithranol dimer are found.

*Metabolism:* The unstable dithranol is oxidised to danthron, to dithranol dimer and to further insoluble polymerisation products.

*Elimination:* There are no studies which indicate that unchanged dithranol is absorbed through the human skin. However, small quantities of oxidation products have been detected in the urine of patients after topical application.

*Preclinical safety data:* There are no pre-clinical data of relevance to the prescriber which are additional to that already included in other sections of the SPC.

**Pharmaceutical particulars**

*List of excipients:* Glyceryl Monolaurate, Glyceryl Monomyristate, Anhydrous Citric Acid PhEur, Sodium Hydroxide PhEur, Purified Water PhEur.

*Incompatibilities:* Oxidants (like Propylene glycol).

*Shelf life:* 2 years.

*Special precautions for storage:* Store below 25°C, in a dry place.

*Nature and contents of container:* Micanol cream is packed in aluminium tubes lined internally with a protective lacquer and sealed at the nozzle end with an aluminium membrane, and fitted with polypropylene caps.

The tubes are subsequently packed, together with the patient information leaflet, in unit, printed boxboard cartons in a pack size of 50 g. A 5 g tube is licensed but not marketed.

*Instructions for use and handling:* Micanol may stain fabrics and contact should be avoided if possible. It is especially formulated so that it is easily washed off using lukewarm water only. Do not use very hot water or soap as these may increase the staining of Micanol.

*Product licence holder:* Bioglan Laboratories Limited, 5 Hunting Gate, Hitchin, Hertfordshire, SG4 0TJ

**Marketing authorisation numbers**
1%    0041/0041
3%    0041/0042

**Date of approval/revision of SPC** January 1996

**Legal category** 1%-P, 3%-POM

## MICRALAX* MICRO-ENEMA

**Presentation** A disposable plastic tube with 2 inch pliable plastic nozzle, which contains 5 ml of a colourless viscous liquid incorporating 450 mg sodium citrate, 45 mg sodium alkylsulphoacetate and 5 mg sorbic acid, together with glycerin, sorbitol and purified water.

**Uses** Micralax combines the action of sodium citrate, a 'peptizing' agent which can displace bound water present in the faeces; sorbitol, which enhances this action; and sodium alkylsulphoacetate, a wetting agent. Micralax is indicated whenever an enema is necessary to relieve constipation: in dyschezia, especially in bedridden patients; in geriatrics, paediatrics and obstetrics; and in preparation for X-ray examination, proctoscopy and sigmoidoscopy.

**Dosage and administration**
*Adults and children aged 3 years and over:* Administer the contents of one micro-enema rectally, inserting the full length of the nozzle. No lubricant is needed as a drop of the mixture is sufficient.

**Contra-indications, warnings, etc.**
*Contra-indications:* Do not use in patients with inflammatory bowel disease.

*Adverse reactions:* Excessive use may cause diarrhoea and fluid loss, which should be treated symptomatically.

**Pharmaceutical precautions** Store below 25°C.

**Legal category** P

**Package quantities** Packs of 12.

**Further information** Inactive ingredients include sorbic acid.

**Product licence number** 0039/0368

## NEO-CYTAMEN*

**Presentation** Ampoules containing a clear, red solution which provides 1,000 micrograms (Neo-Cytamen '1000') of hydroxocobalamin per ml. Neo-Cytamen Injection complies with the specification of Hydroxocobalamin Injection BP.

**Uses** Addisonian pernicious anaemia. Prophylaxis and treatment of other macrocytic anaemias associated with vitamin B12 deficiency. Tobacco amblyopia and Leber's optic atrophy.

**Dosage and administration** The following dosage schemes are suitable for adults and children.

*Addisonian pernicious anaemia and other macrocytic anaemias without neurological involvement:* Initially: 250 to 1,000 micrograms intramuscularly on alternate days for one or two weeks, then 250 micrograms weekly until the blood count is normal. Maintenance: 1,000 micrograms every two to three months.

*Addisonian pernicious anaemia and other macrocytic anaemias with neurological involvement.:* Initially: 1,000 micrograms on alternate days as long as improvement is occurring. Maintenance: 1,000 micrograms every two months.

*Prophylaxis of macrocytic anaemia associated with vitamin B12 deficiency resulting from gastrectomy, some malabsorption syndromes and strict vegetarianism:* 1,000 micrograms every two or three months.

*Tobacco amblyopia and Lober's optic atrophy:* Initially: 1,000 micrograms or more daily by intramuscular injection for two weeks then twice weekly as long as improvement is occurring. Maintenance: 1,000 micrograms monthly.

**Contra-indications, warnings, etc.**
*Contra-indications:* Hypersensitivity to any ingredient in the preparation.

*Precautions:* The dosage schemes given above are usually satisfactory, but regular examination of the blood is advisable. If megaloblastic anaemia fails to respond to Neo-Cytamen, folate metabolism should be investigated. Doses in excess of 10 micrograms daily may produce a haematological response in patients with folate deficiency. Indiscriminate administration may mask the true diagnosis.

Cardiac arrhythmias secondary to hypokalaemia during initial therapy have been reported- Plasma potassium should therefore be monitored during this period.

*Interactions:* Chloramphenicol-treated patients may respond poorly to Neo-Cytamen. Serum concentrations of hydroxocobalamin may be lowered by oral contraceptives but this interaction is unlikely to have clinical significance. Antimetabolites and most antibiotics invalidate Vitamin $B_{12}$ assays by microbiological techniques.

*Side-effects:* Hypersensitivity reactions have been reported including skin reactions (e.g. rash, itching) and exceptionally anaphylaxis. Other symptoms reported include fever, chills, hot flushing, dizziness, malaise, nausea, vomiting, diarrhoea, acneiform and bullous eruptions.

*Pregnancy and lactation:* Neo-Cytamen should not be used for the treatment of megaloblastic anaemia of pregnancy unless Vitamin $B_{12}$ deficiency has been demonstrated. Neo-Cytamen is secreted into breast milk but this is unlikely to harm the infant, and may be beneficial if the mother and infant are vitamin $B_{12}$ deficient.

*Overdosage:* Treatment is unlikely to be needed in cases of overdosage

**Pharmaceutical precautions** Protect from light.

**Legal category** POM.

**Package quantities** Ampoules of 1 ml in boxes of 5.

**Further information** An intramuscular injection of hydroxocobalamin produces higher serum levels than the same dose of cyanocobalamin, and these levels are well maintained.

**Product licence numbers** 0039/0405

## O.P.V. POLIOMYELITIS VACCINE, LIVE (ORAL) BP TRIVALENT (SABIN TYPE)

**Qualitative and quantitative composition** The vaccine contains live attenuated strains of poliomyelitis virus, types I, II and III at the following levels per dose:

Type I    $10^6$ $TCID_{50}$
Type II   $10^5$ $TCID_{50}$
Type III  $10^{5.5}$ $TCID_{50}$

$TCID_{50}$–Tissue Culture Infective Dose required to infect 50% of a specific cell culture population.

**Pharmaceutical form** The attenuated vaccine strain of each type of poliovirus has antibody-inducing characteristics similar to its virulent counterpart. Extensive studies have shown that there is little risk of Sabin attenuated virus reverting to a virulent condition.

The vaccine is a clear pale yellow liquid.

Each dose of OPV, Poliomyelitis Vaccine, Live (Oral) contains up to 6IU polymyxin B sulphate and up to 0.5IU neomycin sulphate. In common with all vaccine derived from Sabin seed it may also contain traces of penicillin and streptomycin.

**Clinical particulars**

*Therapeutic indications:* For active immunisation against poliomyelitis.

*Posology and method of administration:* For oral use only.

*Adults and children:* The contents of one single dose polythene tube constitutes one dose. The primary course consists of three doses of poliomyelitis vaccine at intervals of not less than four weeks. If there is a known risk of exposure to poliomyelitis in those who have completed a primary course, a single reinforcing dose of OPV, Poliomyelitis Vaccine Live (Oral) is recommended.

*Elderly:* As for adults.

*Administration of the vaccine:* Separate a single-dose tube from the strip. The tube should be held by the large tab and shaken down, as with a thermometer, to propel the entire contents to the corrugated end. The tube should be held upright without applying pressure to the tube, and the narrow end removed by twisting the top. Incline tube and shake gently to move the vaccine to the open end.

The contents are then expelled by exerting gentle pressure to the tube just above the surface of the liquid (a small residue of vaccine may remain).

A course of Poliomyelitis Vaccine, Live (Oral) is usually administered simultaneously with Trivax-AD* (DTPer/Vac/Ads)) or Adsorbed Diphtheria and Tetanus Vaccine (CHILD) (DT/Vac/Ads (Child)). Thereafter, it is recommended that all immunised children are given a single reinforcing dose of OPV, Poliomyelitis Vaccine, Live (Oral) at school entry when they receive their reinforcing dose of Diphtheria and Tetanus Vaccine and again at 15-19 years of age or on leaving school.

Adults may be given a single reinforcing dose of OPV, Poliomyelitis Vaccine, Live (Oral) if already immunised or a primary immunisation course if their immunisation histories are uncertain or absent.

OPV, Poliomyelitis Vaccine, Live (Oral) may be administered as early as six weeks of age and the response has been shown to be unaffected by breast-feeding from this age onwards.

If parents or siblings of an infant due for immunisation have never been immunised then, provided there is no contra-indication, it is preferable to immunise them with OPV, Poliomyelitis Vaccine, Live (Oral) at the same time in order to reduce the remote risk of contact paralysis.

Alternatively, two doses of Inactivated Poliomyelitis Vaccine (IPV), one month apart, may be given to the adults before administration of OPV, Poliomyelitis Vaccine, Live (Oral) to the infant.

Administration of oral poliomyelitis vaccine induces circulating antibodies and local antibody responses in the intestine. However, one type of poliovirus in the vaccine may inhibit another from establishing immunity. Thus, when only a single dose of trivalent oral polio vaccine is given successful immunisation against all three types of poliovirus may not occur. Therefore in the primary course the vaccine is administered on at least three occasions to ensure that each type of vaccine poliovirus is given an opportunity of establishing immunity.

It is good practice to record title, dose and lot numbers of all vaccines and the dates of administration.

*Contra-indications:* The antibiotic content of the vaccine does not normally contra-indicate use except in cases of extreme hypersensitivity, e.g. anaphylaxis following its administration.

No data are available on the co-administration of OPV, Poliomyelitis Vaccine, Live (Oral) and live attenuated Typhoid Vaccine (Ty21a). Concurrent vaccination with OPV, Poliomyelitis Vaccine, live (Oral) and Oral Ty21a is therefore contra-indicated.

The efficacy of the vaccine may be impaired if given while the subject has diarrhoea or vomiting. The vaccine should not be given to those with acute febrile illness or severe chronic illness.

Any patient who has previously experienced a serious reaction to the vaccine or any component thereof should not be re-vaccinated.

Persons residing in the household of susceptible immuno-compromised individuals should not be vaccinated because viable poliomyelitis vaccine virus may be excreted in the faeces of the recipient and be communicated to susceptible persons within the household; IPV should be given.

The vaccine should not be given to those with impaired immune responsiveness, whether congenital, idiopathic or as a result of treatment with steroids (with the exception of locally acting eg topical or inhaled steroids), radiotherapy, cytotoxic drugs or other agents.

The vaccine should not be given either to symptomatic or asymptomatic HIV-positive individuals, since there is insufficient evidence as to the safety of its use.

*Special warnings and precautions for use:* Although anaphylaxis is rare, facilities for its management should always be available during vaccination.

The vaccine should not be administered on foods containing preservatives, as they may inactivate OPV, Poliomyelitis Vaccine, Live (Oral).

Vaccinees, parents and other household contacts should be made aware of the possible risk of recipient and contact paralysis prior to vaccination.

Any untoward reactions should be reported to the regulatory authorities and to the manufacturer.

*Interaction with other medicaments and other forms of interaction:* None known.

*Pregnancy and lactation:* The safety of OPV, Poliomyelitis Vaccine Live (Oral), for use in human pregnancy and breast-feeding has not been established. Therefore, routine vaccination during pregnancy and breast-feeding should be avoided. The benefits of using OPV, a live attenuated poliomyelitis vaccine, during pregnancy and breast-feeding should be weighed against any possible risks.

*Effects on ability to drive and use machines:* None known.

*Undesirable effects:* Vaccine-related paralysis in recipients or contacts may occur on very rare occasions.

*Overdose:* Not applicable.

**Pharmacological particulars** Not applicable.

**Pharmaceutical particulars**

*List of excipients:* The excipients contained in the preparation are as follows: Polymyxin B sulphate PhEur, Neomycin sulphate PhEur, Sucrose PhEur, L-glutamic acid HSE, Human albumin solution (20% w/v) PhEur, Potassium dihydrogen orthophosphate anhydrous HSE, Dipotassium hydrogen orthophosphate anhydrous HSE, Water for Injections PhEur.

*Incompatibilities:* None known.

*Shelf life:* 2-8°C: 6 months

*Special precautions for storage:* The vaccine should be stored between 2 and 8°C until its expiry date.

*Nature and contents of container:* 2 strips of 5 polyethylene dropper tubes with twist-off ends, each containing one dose.

*Instructions for use and handling:* Since the vaccine contains live attenuated poliomyelitis virus, care should be taken to avoid transfer of virus to immuno-deficient subjects.

When the vaccine tubes are opened the vaccine should be administered immediately to reduce the risk of contamination with bacteria and moulds which may result in a reduction of vaccine potency.

Caution should be exercised to avoid spillage. All parts of the containers should be subject to disposal by incineration at a temperature not less than 1100°C. If a spoon was used, it should either be incinerated or sterilised in a 0.1% aqueous hypochlorite solution yielding 1000 ppm available chlorine (e.g. 1:10 Milton 1%) and then rinsed thoroughly in water.

**Marketing authorisation number**  0039/0468

**Date of approval/revision of SPC**  May 1996

**Legal category**  POM

# PARVOLEX*

**Presentation**  Parvolex is a clear, colourless, sterile, aqueous solution of 20%w/v Acetylcysteine BP (N-acetyl-3-mercapto-alanine) adjusted to pH 7.0 with sodium hydroxide. Each ampoule of Parvolex contains 2 grams of N-acetylcysteine in 10 ml of solution.

**Uses**  N-acetylcysteine is a derivative of the naturally occurring amino acid L-cysteine.

In paracetamol overdosage the observed hepatotoxicity is due to the formation of a toxic metabolite which is thought to cause liver cell damage and necrosis. Hepatic-reduced glutathione inactivates the toxic metabolite by conjugation but glutathione stores are rapidly depleted with hepatotoxic doses of paracetamol. Acetylcysteine, being a sulphydryl (SH) group donor, protects the liver possibly by restoring depleted hepatic-reduced glutathione or by acting as an alternative substrate for the toxic paracetamol metabolite.

*Indications:* Parvolex (N-acetylcysteine) is indicated for the treatment of paracetamol overdosage.

**Dosage and administration**

*Adults:* An initial dose of 150 mg/kg body weight of N-acetylcysteine is infused in 200 ml 5% dextrose intravenously over 15 minutes, followed by an intravenous infusion of 50 mg/kg in 500 ml 5% dextrose over the next 4 hours, then 100 mg/kg in 1 litre of 5% dextrose over the next 16 hours. (This gives a total dose of 300 mg/kg in 20 hours.)

*Children:* Children should be treated with the same doses and regimen as adults; however, the quantity of intravenous fluid used should be modified to take into account age and weight, as fluid overload is a potential danger. The National Poisons Centres in the UK and Ireland have provided the following guidance:

*Children weighing 20 kg or more:* 150 mg/kg intravenous infusion in 100 ml 5% dextrose over 15 minutes; then 50 mg/kg intravenous infusion in 250 ml 5% dextrose over 4 hours; then 100 mg/kg intravenous infusion in 500 ml 5% dextrose over 16 hours.

*Children under 20 kg:* Volumes for infusion of the above doses are the responsibility of the prescriber and should be based on the daily maintenance requirements of the child by weight.

*Critical times:* N-acetylcysteine (Parvolex) is very effective in preventing paracetamol-induced hepatoxicity when administered during the first 8 hours after a paracetamol overdose. When administered after the first 8 hours, the protective effect diminishes progressively as the overdose-treatment interval increases. However, clinical experience indicates that N-acetylcysteine can still be of benefit when administered up to 24 hours after paracetamol overdose, without any change in its safety profile. It may also be administered after 24 hours in patients at risk of severe liver damage. In general, for patients presenting later than 24 hours after a paracetamol overdose, guidance should be sought from a National Poisons Centre.

*Treatment 'nomogram':* Plasma paracetamol concentration in relation to time after the overdose is commonly used to determine whether a patient is at risk of hepatotoxicity and should therefore receive treatment with an antidote such as N-acetylcysteine.

For the majority of otherwise healthy patients, a line joining points of 200 mg/l at 4 hours and 30 mg/l at 15 hours on a semilogarithmic plot is used (Treatment Line A – see graph). This line can be extended to 24 hours after overdose, based on a paracetamol half-life of 4 hours. It is recommended that patients whose plasma paracetamol concentrations fall on or above this line receive N-acetylcysteine. If there is doubt about the timing of the overdose, consideration should be given to treatment with N-acetylcysteine.

Patients with induced hepatic microsomal oxidase enzymes (such as chronic alcoholics and patients taking anticonvulsant drugs) are susceptible to paracetamol-induced hepatotoxicity at lower plasma paracetamol concentrations (see below under 'Contra-indications, warnings, etc') and should be assessed against Treatment Line B (see graph).

In patients who have taken staggered overdoses, blood levels are meaningless in relation to the treatment graph. These patients should all be considered for treatment with N-acetylcysteine.

NB: Blood samples taken less than 4 hours after a paracetamol overdose give unreliable estimates of the serum paracetamol concentration.

**Contra-indications, warnings, etc**

*Contra-indications:* Hypersensitivity to any ingredient in the preparation.

*Precautions:* Administer with caution in patients with asthma or a history of bronchospasm.

*Pregnancy:* The safety of N-acetylcysteine in pregnancy has not been investigated in formal prospective clinical trials. However, clinical experience indicates that use of N-acetylcysteine in pregnancy for the treatment of paracetamol overdose is effective. Prior to use in pregnancy, the potential risks should be balanced against the potential benefits.

*Liver enzyme-inducing drugs; Chronic alcohol abuse:* Patients taking drugs that induce liver enzymes, such as some anticonvulsant drugs (e.g. phenytoin, phenobarbitone, primidone and carbamazepam) and rifampicin, and patients who routinely consume alcohol above recommended levels are believed to be at risk of hepatotoxity from paracetamol poisoning at lower plasma paracetamol concentrations than other patients. It is recommended that such patients whose plasma paracetamol concentrations fall on or above a treatment line joining 100 mg/l at 4 hours after overdose and 15 mg/l at 15 hours after overdose on a semilogarithmic plot, (i.e. Treatment Line B – see graph) be given N-acetylcysteine.

*Other patients predisposed to toxicity:* Patients suffering from malnutrition, for example, patients with anorexia or AIDS, may have depleted glutathione reserves. It has been recommended that paracetamol overdose in such patients be treated as for chronic alcohol consumers or patients taking anticonvulsant drugs (Treatment Line B – see graph).

*Side-effects:* 'Anaphylactoid' or 'hypersensitivity-like' reactions have been reported. They include nausea/vomiting, injection-site reactions, flushing, itching, rashes/urticaria, angioedema, bronchospasm/respiratory distress, hypotension, and rarely, tachycardia or hypertension, These have usually occurred between 15 and 60 minutes after the start of infusion.

In many cases, symptoms have been relieved by stopping the infusion. Occasionally, an antihistamine drug may be necessary. Corticosteroids may occasionally be required. Once an anaphylactoid reaction

## TREATMENT LINES

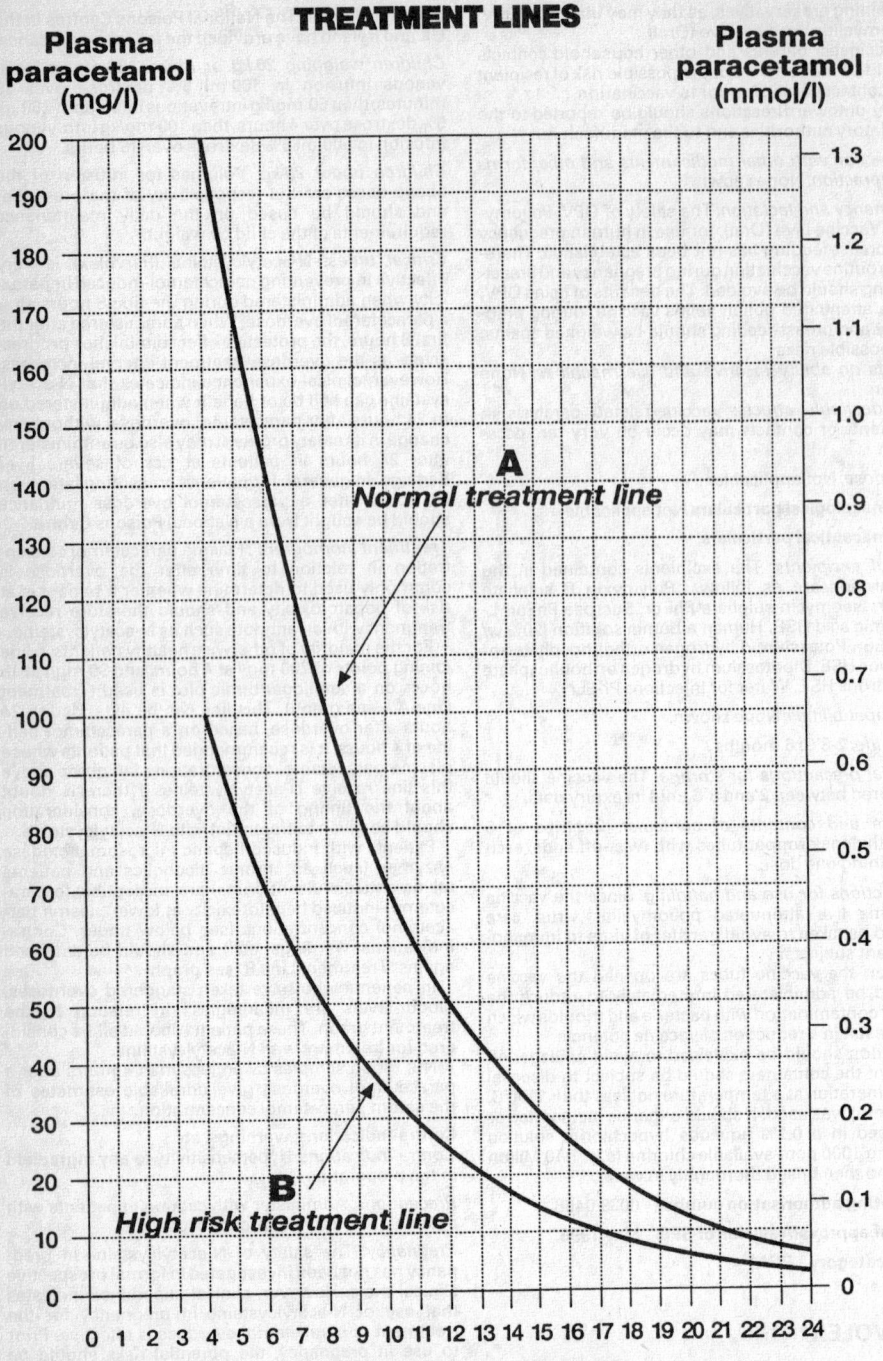

**Plasma paracetamol (mg/l)**

**Plasma paracetamol (mmol/l)**

A — *Normal treatment line*

B — *High risk treatment line*

**Hours after ingestion**

Plasma paracetamol concentrations in relation to time after overdosage as a guide to prognosis.
From Guidelines agreed by National Poisons Centres – June 1995
Parvolex is indicated in patients with values on or above the appropriate treatment line.

is under control, the infusion can normally be restarted at the lowest infusion rate (100 mg/kg in 1 litre over 16 hours).

In rare instances, the following side-effects have occurred: coughing, chest tightness or pain, puffy eyes, sweating, malaise, raised temperature, vasodilation, blurred vision, bradycardia, facial or eye pain, syncope, acidosis, thrombocytopenia, respiratory or cardiac arrest, stridor, anxiety, extravasation, arthropathy, arthralgia, deterioration of liver function, generalised seizure, cyanosis, lowered blood urea. Rare instances of fatality have also occurred.

Hypokalaemia and ECG changes have been noted in patients with paracetamol poisoning irrespective of the treatment given. Monitoring of plasma potassium concentration is therefore recommended.

If any side-effects to Parvolex (N-acetylcysteine) develop, advice should be sought from a National Poisons Centre to ensure that the patient receives adequate treatment of the paracetamol overdose.

*Overdosage:* There is a theoretical risk of hepatic encephalopathy. Overdosage of N-acetylcysteine has been reported to be associated with effects similar to the 'anaphylactoid' reactions noted above, but they may be more severe. General supportive measures should be carried out. Such reactions are managed with antihistamines and steroids in the usual way. There is no specific antidote.

**Pharmaceutical precautions**   Store below 25°C. N-acetylcysteine is not compatible with rubber or metals, particularly iron, copper and nickel. Silicone rubber and plastic are satisfactory for use with Parvolex.

A change in the colour of the solution to light purple has sometimes been noted and is not thought to indicate significant impairment of safety or efficacy.

**Legal category**   POM

**Package quantities**   Parvolex is supplied in ampoules of 10 ml and packed in printed cartons of 10 ampoules per carton.

**Further information**   Guidelines on the management of acute paracetamol overdose are available from the National Poisons Centre.

**Product licence number**   0039/0410

## PERCUTANEOUS BCG VACCINE, BP

**Qualitative and quantitative composition**   Each vial contains :Bacillus Calmette-Guerin (Copenhagen sub-strain 1077) 50 to 250 x 10⁶ viable units

**Pharmaceutical form**   Freeze-dried standardised preparation of a sub-strain of Bacillus Calmette-Guerin to be reconstituted with Water for Injections, BP or

Sodium Chloride Injection, BP prior to percutaneous administration.

**Clinical particulars**

*Therapeutic indications:* For active immunisation against tuberculosis in neonates, infants and very young children only. Vaccinated persons normally become Mantoux-positive after eight weeks, but sometimes up to 14 weeks are needed.

*Posology and method of administration:* PERCUTANEOUS BCG Vaccine is used with a **MULTIPLE PUNCTURE APPARATUS** equipped with 18–20 needles giving reliable penetration of the skin to a depth of 2 mm. The inoculation should be given in the arm, over the insertion of the deltoid muscle onto the humerus. A tuberculin skin test must be conducted before BCG immunisation in children aged 3 months and over.

The multiple puncture apparatus must be properly sterilised each time after use according to the manufacturer's instructions. Alternatively a disposable head may be used each time. Any alcohol should be burnt off before the apparatus is used, which must be allowed to cool before use. Detergents or antiseptics should not be used.

The vaccine must not be contaminated with any antiseptic or detergent. Avoid contamination with bactericides. If alcohol is used to swab the rubber stopper of the vial, it must be allowed to evaporate before the stopper is penetrated with the syringe needle.

The vaccine suspension is prepared by adding 0.3 ml of Water for Injections, BP or 0.3 ml Sodium Chloride Injection, BP to the 10 dose vial. DO NOT shake as this causes frothing. Allow to stand for one minute, then draw into the syringe twice to ensure homogeneity.

The vaccine must not be contaminated with any antiseptic or detergent. Avoid contamination with bactericides. If alcohol is used to swab the skin, it must be allowed to evaporate before the vaccine is injected. Transfer a small amount (about 0.03 ml) of reconstituted vaccine onto the skin using a glass rod, platinum loop or spatula. The treated area of skin is then immediately punctured with the multiple puncture apparatus.

The injection site is best left uncovered to facilitate healing.

It is good practice to record the title, dose and lot numbers of all vaccines and dates of administration.

*Contra-indications:* PERCUTANEOUS BCG VACCINE MUST NOT BE ADMINISTERED BY INTRADERMAL INJECTION.

PERCUTANEOUS BCG Vaccine should NOT be given to persons receiving systemic corticosteroids or immunosuppressive treatment including radiotherapy, those suffering from malignant conditions (e.g. lymphoma, leukaemia, Hodgkin's Disease or other tumours of the reticuloendothelial system), those in whom normal immunological mechanism is impaired (e.g. hypogammaglobulinaemia), those known or suspected to be HIV-positive, including infants born to HIV-positive mothers and persons with pyrexia or generalised infected skin conditions. The effect of PERCUTANEOUS BCG Vaccine may be exaggerated in these patients and a more generalised infection is possible. Eczema is not a contra-indication, but the vaccination site must be lesion free.

PERCUTANEOUS BCG Vaccine should not be given to patients who are receiving prophylactic doses of anti-tuberculous drugs.

Tuberculin-positive persons, i.e. those with induration of 5 mm or greater in diameter in the Mantoux test, or those in Heaf grades 2 to 4, do not require the vaccine. Its administration to these persons may result in an accelerated local reaction of larger size than normal.

The vaccine should not be administered to a subject who is known to be hypersensitive to any component of the vaccine.

*Special warnings and precautions for use:* PERCUTANEOUS BCG Vaccine may be given concurrently with another live vaccine, including Oral Poliomyelitis Vaccine, BP. An interval of not less than three weeks should normally be allowed to lapse between the administration of any two live vaccines, if they are not given at the same time. However, when PERCUTANEOUS BCG Vaccine is given to infants, there is no need to delay the primary childhood immunisations which include polio vaccine.

No further vaccination should be given for at least three months in the arm used for BCG vaccination, because of the risk of regional lymphadenitis.

Although anaphylaxis is rare, facilities for its management should always be available during vaccination.

Infectious mononucleosis, viral infections in general, including those of the upper respiratory tract, live viral vaccines, Hodgkin's disease, sarcoidosis, corticosteroid therapy and immunosuppressing treatment or diseases, including HIV, may suppress the reaction to the tuberculin skin test.

*Interaction with other medicaments and other forms of interaction:* None known.

*Pregnancy and lactation* PERCUTANEOUS BCG Vaccine is for use in neonates, infants and very young children only.

*Effect on ability to drive and use machinery:* None known.

*Undesirable effects:* Normally following PERCUTANEOUS BCG Vaccine administration, a small amount of erythema occurs. The erythema and 18–20 point marks fade quickly. After about eight weeks there is little to see at the injection site; this may take longer in pigmented skin. A visible long term scar is unlikely.

Rash, fever, local induration, pain and lymphadenopathy may occur. Occasionally an excessive response to PERCUTANEOUS BCG Vaccine results in a discharging ulcer. The ulcer should be encouraged to dry and abrasion avoided, e.g. by tight clothes. Waterproof dressings should not be used. If the ulcer persists, it can be treated by application of a mild corticosteroid cream and/or a topical antibiotic.

In rare cases of severe local reaction with abscess formation, aspiration may be carried out and antituberculous therapy considered. Enlargement of axillary lymph glands is unlikely except occasionally in young infants.

Anaphylactic reactions have been reported on rare occasions.

Any untoward reactions should be reported to the regulatory authorities and to the Marketing Authorisation Holder.

*Overdose:* If gross overdosage occurs and there is reason to suspect the development of a more generalised infection with BCG, systemic treatment with isoniazid or any other suitable anti-tuberculous drug should be given.

**Pharmacological properties**

*Pharmacodynamic properties:* This vaccine is used for active immunisation against tuberculosis; principally for the vaccination of selected groups of the population and of persons likely to be exposed to infection.

The vaccine stimulates production of cell mediated immunity with a specific protective capacity against tuberculosis.

**Pharmaceutical particulars**

*List of excipients:* Before freeze-drying, each vial contains 0.5 ml ± 10%* of freeze-drying medium of the following composition : Dextran 8.3%, Glucose 7.5%, Triton WR 1339 0.025%, Water for Injections, BP 100.0%

* the amount of freeze-drying medium used is such that the depth of suspension in the vial is suitable for freeze-drying.

*Incompatibilities:* None known.

*Shelf life:* 24 months when stored at 2–8°C unopened. 4 hours after reconstitution.

*Special precautions for storage:* Store between 2 and 8°C. Protect from light.

*Nature and contents of container:* Size: 3 ml vial (10 dose), Type: Neutral (type 1) amber glass vials complying with the PhEur requirements for containers for injectables, Seals: Siliconised rubber peg bungs with aluminium overseals and polypropylene flip top caps.

*Instructions for use/handling:* The vaccine suspension is prepared by adding 0.3 ml of Water for Injections BP or 0.3 ml Sodium Chloride Injection BP to the 10 dose vial. DO NOT shake as this causes frothing. Allow to stand for one minute, then draw into the syringe twice to ensure homogeneity.

After reconstitution the vaccine should be kept cool, protected from light and used in the same session, i.e. within 4 hours. Any reconstituted vaccine remaining at the end of the session (maximum 4 hours) should be discarded.

Disposal should be by incineration at a temperature not less than 1100°C at a registered waste disposal contractor.

**Marketing authorisation number** 0039/0436

**Date of approval/revision of SPC** January 1997

**Legal category** POM

## PREDSOL* DROPS FOR EYE AND EAR

**Presentation** Predsol Drops contain prednisolone sodium phosphate 0.5% w/v and benzalkonium chloride 0.02% w/v in a sterilised clear and colourless aqueous solution.

**Uses** Short-term treatment of corticosteroid responsive inflammatory conditions of the eye after clinical exclusion of bacterial, viral and fungal infections.

Non-infected inflammatory conditions of the ear.

**Dosage and administration**

*Eyes:* 1 or 2 drops instilled into the eyes every one or two hours until control is achieved, when the frequency may be reduced.

*Ears:* 2 or 3 drops instilled into the ear every two or three hours until control is achieved, when the frequency can be reduced.

Frequency of dosing depends on clinical response. If there is no clinical response within 7 days treatment, the drops should be discontinued. Treatment should be the lowest effective dose for the shortest possible time. After more prolonged treatment (over 6–8 weeks), the drops should be withdrawn slowly to avoid relapse.

**Contra-indications, warnings, etc.**

*Contra-indications:* Bacterial, viral, fungal, tuberculous or purulent conditions of the eye. Use in the eye is contra-indicated if glaucoma is present or where herpetic keratitis (e.g. dendritic ulcer) is considered a possibility. Inadvertent use of topical steroids in the latter condition can lead to the extension of the ulcer and marked visual deterioration.

Hypersensitivity to any component of the preparation.

In the ear topical corticosteroids in patients with fungal diseases of the auricular structure and in those with a perforated tympanic membrane.

Predsol Eye Drops contain benzalkonium chloride as a preservative and therefore should not be used to treat patients who wear soft contact lenses.

*Precautions:* Topical corticosteroids should never be given for an undiagnosed red eye as inappropriate use is potentially blinding. Prolonged use may lead to the risk of adrenal suppression in infants. Ophthalmological treatment with steroid preparations should not be repeated or prolonged without regular review to exclude raised intraocular pressure, cataract formation or unsuspected infections.

The use of corticosteroids may reduce resistance to or mask the signs of infection. Appropriate anti-infective agents should be used if infection is present.

May cause transient blurring of vision on instillation. Warn patients not to drive or operate hazardous machinery until vision is clear.

*Use in pregnancy and lactation:* Safety for use in pregnancy and lactation has not been established. There is inadequate evidence of safety in human pregnancy. Topical administration of corticosteroids to pregnant animals can cause abnormalities of foetal development including cleft palate and intrauterine growth retardation. There may, therefore, be a very small risk of such effects in the human foetus.

*Side-effects:* Hypersensitivity reactions, usually of the delayed type, may occur leading to irritation, burning, stinging, itching and dermatitis.

Topical corticosteroid use may result in increased intra-ocular pressure leading to optic nerve damage, reduced visual acuity and visual field defects.

Other side effects include mydriasis, ptosis, epithelial punctate keratitis and possible corneal or scleral malacia. Within a few days after discontinuing topical ophthalmic corticosteroid therapy, acute anterior uveitis has occured in patients (mainly blacks) without pre-existing ocular inflammation or infection.

Intensive or prolonged use of topical corticosteroids may lead to formation of posterior subcapsular cataracts.

In those diseases causing thinning of the cornea or sclera, corticosteroid therapy may result in thinning of the globe leading to perforation.

*Overdose:* Long-term intensive topical use may lead to systemic effects. Oral ingestion of the contents of one bottle (up to 10 ml) is unlikely to lead to any serious adverse effects.

**Pharmaceutical precautions** Store below 25°C. Avoid freezing. Always replace bottle in carton to protect contents from light. Sterility of the drops is assured until cap seal is broken.

The bottle contents should not be used more than four weeks after first opening it.

**Legal category** POM

**Package quantities** Plastic dropper bottles containing 10 ml.

**Further information** Nil.

**Product licence number** 0039/0393

## PREDSOL* RETENTION ENEMA

**Qualitative and quantitative composition** 20 mg prednisolone as the sodium phosphate ester

**Pharmaceutical form** 100 ml disposable plastic bags, each containing 20 mg prednisolone as the sodium phosphate ester in a buffered solution. The product complies with the specification for Prednisolone Enema BP.

**Clinical particulars**

*Therapeutic indications:* Predsol Retention Enema provides local corticosteroid treatment for rectal and rectosigmoidal disease in ulcerative colitis and Crohn's disease.

*Posology and method of administration:* Adults: 1 enema used nightly, for 2 to 4 weeks. Treatment may be continued in patients showing progressive improvement, but it should not be continued if the response has been inadequate. Some patients may relapse after an interval but are likely to respond equally well to a repeated course of treatment.

The enema is used each night on retiring. It may be warmed before administration by placing the bag in a vessel of warm water for a few minutes. Before use lie in bed on the left side with knees drawn up. Hold the bag with tube upwards and squeeze the base of the tube where it joins the bag. Remove the stopper from the bag, lubricate the nozzle with petroleum jelly and gently insert about half the length of the nozzle into the rectum. The bag should then be squeezed gently until it is emptied, taking a minute or two to do so. The nozzle should then be removed and the whole unit discarded. The patient should then roll over to lie face down for 3 to 5 minutes but may sleep in any comfortable position.

Although Predsol Retention Enema is applied locally, it should be borne in mind that there is likely to be substantial systemic absorption, especially when the bowel is inflamed.

The volume of the enema is considered to be the optimum to ensure maximum coverage of the affected area. However, undesirable effects may be minimised by using for the minimum period.

Frequent patient review is required to monitor therapeutic effect against disease activity.

Children: Predsol Retention Enema is not suitable for use in children.

*Contra-indications:* Systemic or local infection unless specific anti-infective therapy is employed. Hypersensitivity to any ingredient of the preparation.

*Special warnings and precautions for use:* Although Predsol Retention Enema is applied locally, it should be borne in mind that there is likely to be substantial systemic absorption, especially when the bowel is inflamed.

The volume of the enema is considered to be the optimum to ensure maximum coverage of the affected area. However, undesirable effects may be minimised by using for the minimum period.

Frequent patient review is required to monitor therapeutic effect against disease activity (see *Posology and method of administration*).

Suppression of the inflammatory response and immune function increases the susceptibility to infections and their severity. The clinical presentation may often be atypical and serious infections such as septicaemia and tuberculosis may be masked and may reach an advanced stage before being recognised.

Chickenpox is of particular concern since this normally minor illness may be fatal in immunosuppressed patients. Patients without a definite history of chickenpox should be advised to avoid close personal contact with chickenpox or herpes zoster and if exposed they should seek urgent medical attention. Passive immunisation with varicella zoster immunoglobulin (VZIG) is needed by exposed non-immune patients who are receiving systemic corticosteroids or who have used them within the previous 3 months; this should be given within 10 days of exposure to chickenpox. If a diagnosis of chickenpox is confirmed, the illness warrants specialist care and urgent treatment. Corticosteroids should not be stopped and the dose may need to be increased.

Live vaccines should not be given to individuals with impaired immune responsiveness. The antibody response to other vaccines may be diminished.

Corticosteroid treatment may reduce the response of the pituitary adrenal axis to stress, and relative insufficiency can persist for up to a year after withdrawal of prolonged therapy. Withdrawal of corticosteroids after prolonged therapy must therefore always be gradual to avoid acute adrenal insufficiency, being tapered off over weeks or months depending on the duration of treatment. During prolonged therapy any intercurrent illness, trauma or surgical procedure will require a temporary increase in dosage. If corticosteroids have been stopped following prolonged therapy they may need to be temporarily re-introduced.

Special precautions: Particular care is required when considering the use of systemic corticosteroids in patients with the following conditions and frequent patient monitoring is necessary.

A. Osteoporosis (post-menopausal females are particularly at risk).
B. Hypertension or congestive heart failure.
C. Existing or previous history of severe affective disorders (especially previous steroid psychosis).
D. Diabetes mellitus (or a family history of diabetes).
E. History of tuberculosis.
F. Glaucoma (or a family history of glaucoma).
G. Previous corticosteroid-induced myopathy.
H. Liver failure – blood levels of corticosteroid may be increased, (as with other drugs which are metabolised in the liver).
I. Renal insufficiency.
J. Epilepsy.
K. Peptic ulceration.

Patients should carry 'steroid treatment' cards which give clear guidance on the precautions to be taken to minimise risk and which provide details of prescriber, drug, dosage and the duration of treatment.

Use in the elderly: The common adverse effects of systemic corticosteroids may be associated with more serious consequences in old age, especially osteoporosis, hypertension, hypokalaemia, diabetes, susceptibility to infection and thinning of the skin. Close clinical supervision is required to avoid life-threatening reactions.

*Interactions with other medicaments and other forms of interaction:* Systemic absorption of prednisolone should be borne in mind, especially when there is local inflammation. Thus the following interactions are possible.

Rifampicin, rifabutin, carbamazepine, phenobarbitone, phenytoin, primidone, aminoglutethimide enhance the metabolism of corticosteroids and its therapeutic effects may be reduced.

The desired effects of hypoglycaemic agents (including insulin), anti-hypertensives and diuretics are antagonised by corticosteroids, and the hypokalaemic effects of acetazolamide, loop diuretics, thiazide diuretics and carbenoxolone are enhanced.

The efficacy of coumarin anticoagulants may be enhanced by concurrent corticosteroid therapy and close monitoring of the INR or prothrombin time is required to avoid spontaneous bleeding.

The renal clearance of salicylates is increased by corticosteroids and steroid withdrawal may result in salicylate intoxication.

*Pregnancy and lactation:* Topical administration of corticosteroids to pregnant animals can cause abnormalities of foetal development including cleft palate and intrauterine growth retardation. There may therefore be a very small risk of such effects in the human foetus. Also, hypoadrenalism may occur in the neonate. When corticosteroids are essential however, patients with normal pregnancies may be treated as though they were in the non-gravid state. Patients with pre-eclampsia or fluid retention require close monitoring.

Corticosteroids are excreted in small amounts in breast milk and infants of mothers taking pharmacological doses of steroids should be monitored carefully for signs of adrenal suppression.

*Effects on ability to drive and use machines:* None known

*Undesirable effects:* The incidence of predictable undesirable effects, including hypothalamic-pituitary-adrenal (HPA) axis suppression correlates with the relative systemic potency of the drug, dosage, timing of administration and the duration of treatment. (see *Special warnings and precautions for use*).

Endocrine/metabolic: Suppression of the hypothalamic-pituitary-adrenal axis, growth suppression in infancy, childhood and adolescence, menstrual irregularity and amenorrhoea. Cushingoid facies, hirsutism, weight gain, impaired carbohydrate tolerance with increased requirement for antidiabetic therapy. Negative protein and calcium balance. Increased appetite.

Anti-inflammatory and immunosuppressive effects: Increased susceptibility and severity of infections with suppression of clinical symptoms and signs, opportunistic infections, recurrence of dormant tuberculosis (see 'Other Special Warnings and Precautions').

Musculoskeletal: Osteoporosis, vertebral and long bone fractures, avascular osteonecrosis, tendon rupture, proximal myopathy.

Fluid and electrolyte disturbance: Sodium and water retention, hypertension, potassium loss, hypokalaemic alkalosis.

Neuropsychiatric: Euphoria, psychological dependence, depression, insomnia, and aggravation of schizophrenia. Increased intra-cranial pressure with papilloedema in children (pseudotumour cerebri), usually after treatment withdrawal. Aggravation of epilepsy.

Ophthalmic: Increased intra-ocular pressure, glaucoma, papilloedema, posterior subcapsular cataracts, corneal or scleral thinning, exacerbation of ophthalmic viral or fungal diseases.

Gastrointestinal: Dyspepsia, peptic ulceration with perforation and haemorrhage, acute pancreatitis, candidiasis.

Dermatological: Impaired healing, skin atrophy, bruising, telangiectasia, striae, acne.

General: Hypersensitivity including anaphylaxis, has been reported. Leucocytosis. Thrombo-embolism.

Withdrawal symptoms and signs: Too rapid a reduction of corticosteroid dosage following prolonged treatment can lead to acute adrenal insufficiency, hypotension and in severe cases this could be fatal.

A 'withdrawal syndrome' may also occur including; fever, myalgia, arthralgia, rhinitis, conjunctivitis, painful itchy skin nodules and loss of weight.

*Overdose* Treatment is unlikely to be needed in cases of acute overdosage.

**Pharmacological properties**  Not applicable

**Pharmaceutical particulars**

*List of excipients:* E214, E216, E218, Butyl 4-hydroxybenzoate, Disodium Edetate, Sodium Acid Phosphate, Disodium Hydrogen Phosphate Anhydrous, Sodium Hydroxide, Purified Water.

*Incompatibilities:* None known.

*Shelf life:* 2 years

*Special precautions for storage:* Store below 25°C and protect from light.

*Nature and contents of container:* Boxes of seven 100 ml disposable bags (instructions to patients enclosed).

**Marketing authorisation number**  0039/0396

**Date of approval/revision of SPC**  June 1997

**Legal category**  POM

## PREDSOL SUPPOSITORIES

**Qualitative and quantitative composition**  5 mg prednisolone as the sodium phosphate ester.

**Pharmaceutical form**  White, opaque suppositories.

**Clinical particulars**

*Therapeutic indications:* Prednisolone is a glucocorticosteroid which is about four times as potent as hydrocortisone on a weight for weight basis.

Predsol Suppositories are indicated for the treatment of haemorrhagic and granular proctitis and the anal complications of Crohn's disease.

*Posology and method of administration:*
Adults and children: 1 suppository inserted at night and one in the morning after defaecation. When the response is good, treatment is usually continued for some months. If symptoms recur later, treatment should be resumed.

*Contra-indications:* Systemic or local infection unless specific anti-infective therapy is employed. Hypersensitivity to any ingredient.

*Special warnings and precautions for use:* Although Predsol Suppositories are applied locally, it should be borne in mind that substantial systemic absorption is a possibility, especially when the bowel is inflamed.

Undesirable effects may be minimised by using the minimum period.

Frequent patient review is required to monitor therapeutic effect against disease activity.

Suppression of the inflammatory response and immune function increases the susceptibility of infections and their severity. The clinical presentation may often be atypical and serious infections such as septicaemia and tuberculosis may be masked and may reach an advanced stage before being recognised.

Chickenpox is of particular concern since this normally minor illness may be fatal in immunosuppressed patients. Patients without a definite history of chickenpox should be advised to avoid close personal contact with chickenpox or herpes zoster and if exposed they should seek urgent medical attention. Passive immunisation with varicella zoster immunoglobulin (VZIG) is needed by exposed non-immune patients who are receiving systemic corticosteroids or who have used them within the previous 3 months; this should be given within 10 days of exposure to chickenpox. If a diagnosis of chickenpox is confirmed, the illness warrants specialist care and urgent treatment. Corticosteroids should not be stopped and the dose may need to be increased.

Live vaccines should not be given to individuals with impaired immune responsiveness. The antibody response to other vaccines may be diminished.

Corticosteroid treatment may reduce the response of the pituitary adrenal axis to stress, and relative insufficiency can persist for up to a year after withdrawal of prolonged therapy. Withdrawal of corticosteroids after prolonged therapy must there-

fore always be gradual to avoid acute adrenal insufficiency, being tapered off over weeks or months according to the dose and duration of treatment. During prolonged therapy any intercurrent illness, trauma or surgical procedure will require a temporary increase in dosage; if corticosteroids have been stopped following prolonged therapy they may need to be temporarily re-introduced.

Special precautions: Particular care is required when considering the use of systemic corticosteroids in patients with the following conditions and frequent patient monitoring is necessary.

A. Osteoporosis (post-menopausal females are particularly at risk).
B. Hypertension or congestive heart failure.
C. Existing or previous history of severe affective disorders (especially previous steroid psychosis).
D. Diabetes mellitus (or a family history of diabetes).
E. History of tuberculosis.
F. Glaucoma (or a family history of glaucoma).
G. Previous corticosteroid-induced myopathy.
H. Liver failure–blood levels of corticosteroid may be increased (as with other drugs which are metabolised in the liver).
I. Renal insufficiency.
J. Epilepsy.
K. Peptic ulceration.

Patients should carry 'steroid treatment' cards which give clear guidance on the precautions to be taken to minimise risk and which provide details of prescriber, drug, dosage and the duration of treatment.

Use in the elderly: The common adverse effects of systemic corticosteroids may be associated with more serious consequences in old age, especially osteoporosis, hypertension, hypokalaemia, diabetes, susceptibility to infection and thinning of the skin. Close clinical supervision is required to avoid life-threatening reactions.

*Interaction with other medicaments and other forms of interaction:* Systemic absorption of prednisolone should be borne in mind, especially when there is local inflammation. Thus the following interactions are possible.

Rifampicin, rifabutin carbamazepine, phenobarbitone, phenytoin, primidone, aminoglutethimide enhance the metabolism of corticosteroids and its therapeutic effects may be reduced.

The desired effects of hypoglycaemic agents (including insulin), anti-hypertensives and diuretics are antagonised by corticosteroids, and the hypokalaemic effects are acetazolamide, loop diuretics, thiazide diuretics and carbenoxolone are enhanced.

The efficacy of coumarin anticoagulants may be enhanced by concurrent corticosteroid therapy and close monitoring of the INR or prothrombin time is required to avoid spontaneous bleeding.

The renal clearance of salicylates is increased by corticosteroids and steroid withdrawal may result in salicylate intoxication.

*Pregnancy and lactation:* Topical administration of corticosteroids to pregnant animals can cause abnormalities of foetal development including cleft palate and intrauterine growth retardation. There may therefore be a very small risk of such effects in the human foetus. Also, hypoadrenalism may occur in the neonate. When corticosteroids are essential however, patients with normal pregnancies may be treated as though they were in the non-gravid state. Patients with pre-eclampsia or fluid retention require close monitoring.

Corticosteroids are excreted in small amounts in breast milk and infants of mothers taking pharmacological doses of steroids should be monitored carefully for signs of adrenal suppression.

*Effects on ability to drive and use machines:* None known.

*Undesirable effects:* The incidence of predictable undesirable effects, including hypothalamic-pituitary-adrenal (HPA) axis suppression correlates with the relative systemic potency of the drug, dosage, timing of administration and the duration of treatment. (See *Special warnings and precautions for use.*)

Endocrine/metabolic: Suppression o f the hypothalamic-pituitary-adrenal axis, growth suppression in infancy, childhood and adolescence, menstrual irregularity and amenorrhoea. Cushingoid facies, hirsutism, weight gain, impaired carbohydrate tolerance with increased requirement for antidiabetic therapy. Negative protein and calcium balance. Increased appetite.

Anti-inflammatory and immunosuppressive effects: Increased susceptibility and severity of infections with suppression of clinical symptoms and signs, opportunistic infections, recurrence of dormant tuberculosis (see *Special warnings and precautions for use*).

Musculoskeletal: Osteoporosis, vertebral and long bone fractures, avascular osteonecrosis, tendon rupture, proximal myopathy.

Fluid and electrolyte disturbance: Sodium and water

retention, hypertension, potassium loss, hypokalaemic alkalosis.

Neuropsychiatric: Euphoria, psychological dependence, depression, insomnia, and aggravation of schizophrenia. Increased intra-cranial pressure with papilloedema in children (pseudotumour cerebri), usually after treatment withdrawal. Aggravation of epilepsy.

Ophthalmic: Increased intra-ocular pressure, glaucoma, papilloedema, posterior subcapsular cataracts, corneal or scleral thinning, exacerbation of ophthalmic viral or fungal diseases.

Gastrointestinal: Dyspepsia, peptic ulceration with perforation and haemorrhage, acute pancreatitis, candidiasis.

Dermatological: Impaired healing, skin atrophy, bruising, telangiectasia, striae, acne.

General: Hypersensitivity including anaphylaxis, has been reported. Leucocytosis. Thrombo-embolism.

Withdrawal symptoms and signs: Too rapid a reduction of corticosteroid dosage following prolonged treatment can lead to acute adrenal insufficiency, hypotension and in severe cases this could be fatal (see *Other Special Warnings and Precautions*).

A 'withdrawal syndrome' may also occur including fever, myalgia, arthralgia, rhinitis, conjunctivitis, painful itchy skin nodules and loss of weight.

*Overdose:* Treatment is unlikely to be needed in cases of acute overdosage.

### Pharmacological particulars

*Pharmacodynamic properties:* Prednisolone sodium phosphate is an active corticosteroid with topical anti-inflammatory activity.

*Pharmacokinetic properties:* Corticosteroids are metabolised mainly in the liver but also in the kidney and are excreted in the urine.

Synthetic corticosteroids such as prednisolone have increased potency when compared with the natural corticosteroids, due to their slower metabolism and lower protein-binding affinity.

*Preclinical safety data:* There are no pre-clinical data of relevance to the prescriber which are additional to that already included in other sections of the SPC.

### Pharmaceutical particulars

*List of excipients:* Witepsol H15.

*Incompatibilities:* None known.

*Shelf life:* 2 years.

*Special precautions for storage:* Store below 25˚C.

*Nature and contents of container:* Fin sealed plastic cavities moulded from 100 micron non-toxic PVC. Each cartoned plastic mould contains 10 suppositories (2 strips of 5 suppositories).

**Marketing authorisation number** 0039/0395

**Date of approval/revision of SPC** May 1997

**Legal category** POM

## PREDSOL-N* DROPS FOR EYE AND EAR

**Presentation** Predsol-N Drops contain prednisolone sodium phosphate 0.5% w/v, neomycin sulphate 0.5% w/v and benzalkonium chloride 0.01% w/v in a clear, colourless, aqueous solution. Also contains: disodium edetate, polyethylene glycol, sodium formate, anhydrous sodium sulphate, disodium hydrogen phosphate anhydrous, sodium acid phosphate and sodium hydroxide/phosphoric acid buffer. Sodium content not more than 0.2 g per bottle. Sterile until opened.

### Uses

*Eye:* For the short-term treatment of steroid responsive conditions of the eye when prophylactic antibiotic treatment is also required, after excluding the presence of fungal and viral disease.

*Ear:* Otitis externa or other steroid responsive conditions where prophylactic antibiotic treatment is also required.

### Dosage and administration

*Adults (and the Elderly) and Children:* Frequency of dosing depends on clinical response. If there is no clinical response within 7 days treatment, the drops should be discontinued.

Treatment should be the lowest effective dose for the shortest possible time. Normally, do not give for more than 7 days, unless under expert supervision. After more prolonged treatment (over 6–8 weeks), the drops should be withdrawn slowly to avoid relapse.

*Eyes:* 1 or 2 drops applied to each affected eye up to six times daily or more frequently if required.

*Ears:* 2 or 3 drops instilled into the ear three to four times daily.

### Contra-indications, warnings, etc.

*Contra-indications:* Viral, fungal, tuberculous or purulent conditions of the eye. Use is contra-indicated if glaucoma is present, or herpetic keratitis (e.g. dendritic ulcer) is considered a possibility. Use of topical steroids in the latter condition can lead to extension of the ulcer and marked visual deterioration.

Otitis externa should not be treated when the eardrum is perforated because of the risk of ototoxicity.

Hypersensitivity to the preparation.

Predsol-N Eye Drops contain benzalkonium chloride as a preservative and, therefore, should not be used to treat patients who wear soft contact lenses.

*Precautions:* Topical corticosteroids should never be given for undiagnosed red-eye as inappropriate use is potentially blinding. Topical corticosteroid/antibiotic combinations should not be continued for more than 7 days in the absence of any clinical improvement, since prolonged use may lead to occult extension of infection due to the masking effect of the steroid, and the emergence of resistant organisms. Prolonged use may also lead to skin sensitisation and the emergence of resistant organisms.

In infants prolonged use may lead to the risk of adrenal suppression.

Treatment with corticosteroid preparations should not be repeated or prolonged without regular review to exclude raised intra-ocular pressure, cataract formation or unsuspected infections.

Aminoglycoside antibiotics may cause irreversible, partial or total deafness when given systemically or when applied topically to open wounds or damaged skin. This effect is dose related and is enhanced by renal or hepatic impairment. Although this effect has not been reported following topical ocular use, the possibility should be considered when high dose topical treatment is given to small children or infants.

*Effects on ability to drive and use machines:* May cause transient blurring of vision on instillation. Warn patients not to drive or operate machinery unless vision is clear.

*Pregnancy and lactation:* Safety for use in pregnancy and lactation has not been established. There is inadequate evidence of safety in human pregnancy. Topical administration of corticosteroids to pregnant animals can cause abnormalities of foetal development including cleft palate and intra-uterine growth retardation. There may therefore be a very small risk of such effects in the human foetus. There is a risk of foetal ototoxicity if aminoglycoside antibiotic preparations are administered during pregnancy.

*Side-effects:* Hypersensitivity reactions, usually of the delayed type, may occur leading to irritation, burning, stinging, itching and dermatitis.

Topical corticosteroid use may result in increased intraocular pressure leading to optic nerve damage, reduced visual acuity and visual field defects.

Intensive or prolonged use of topical corticosteroids may lead to formation of posterior subcapsular cataracts.

In those diseases causing thinning of the cornea or sclera, corticosteroid therapy may result in thinning of the globe leading to perforation.

Other side effects include mydriasis, ptosis, epithelial punctate keratitis and possible corneal or scleral malacia. Within a few days after discontinuing topical ophthalmic corticosteroid therapy and occasionally during therapy, acute anterior uveitis has occurred in patients (mainly blacks) without pre-existing ocular inflammation or infection.

*Overdosage:* Long-term intensive topical use may lead to systemic effects.

Oral ingestion of the contents of one bottle (up to 10 ml) is unlikely to lead to any serious adverse effects.

**Pharmaceutical precautions** The contents should not be used more than four weeks after first opening the bottle. Store at a temperature not exceeding 25˚C.

**Legal category** POM

**Package quantities** Plastic dropper bottles containing 10 ml.

**Further information** Nil.

**Product licence number** 0039/0394

## PREGADAY* TABLETS

**Presentation** Pregaday Tablets are brownish pink, film-coated tablets engraved 'Pregaday' on one face. Each tablet contains Ferrous Fumarate BP equivalent to 100 mg ferrous iron and 350 micrograms (0.35 mg) anhydrous folic acid.

**Uses** There is evidence that a daily intake of 100 mg of elemental iron in the ferrous form is adequate to prevent development of iron deficiency in expectant mothers. If a mild iron deficiency is present when Pregaday administration is started, this will be corrected by increased absorption of iron. The daily folate requirement rises steeply during the final trimester of pregnancy, and evidence of maternal depletion may be found. To ensure normal tissue folate levels in the mother after delivery, a daily supplement of about 300 micrograms is required during the second and third trimester of pregnancy. This dose does not obscure the blood picture of Addisonian pernicious anaemia. Pregaday is indicated during the second and third trimester of pregnancy for prophylaxis against iron deficiency and megaloblastic anaemia of pregnancy. Pregaday is not intended as a treatment for established megaloblastic anaemia of pregnancy.

**Dosage and administration** It is usual to begin therapy with Pregaday about the thirteenth week of pregnancy (see 'Precautions') either as routine prophylaxis or selectively if the haemoglobin concentration is less than 11 g/100 ml (less than 75% of normal).

One tablet daily by mouth (the foil enclosing the tablets is printed with the days of the week in sequence).

### Contra-indications, warnings, etc.

*Contra-indications:* Vitamin $B_{12}$ deficiency.

Known hypersensitivity to the product, Paroxysmal nocturnal haemoglobinuria, haemosiderosis, haemochromatosis, active peptic ulcer, repeated blood transfusion, regional enteritis and ulcerative colitis.

Pregaday must not be used in the treatment of anaemias other than those due to iron deficiency.

*Pregnancy:* Administration of Pregaday during the first trimester of pregnancy may be undesirable.

A minority of pregnant women are not protected by physiological doses of folic acid, The development of anaemia despite prophylaxis with Pregaday calls for investigation.

*Other special warnings and precautions:* Some post-gastrectomy patients show poor absorption of iron. Care is needed when treating iron deficiency anaemia in patients with treated or controlled peptic ulceration.

Caution should be exercised when administering folic acid to patients who may have folate dependant tumours.

Since anaemia due to combined iron and Vitamin $B_{12}$ or folate deficiencies may be microcytic in type, patients with microcytic anaemia resistant to therapy with iron alone should be screened for Vitamin $B_{12}$ or folate deficiency.

*Side-effects:* Gastrointestinal disorders have been reported including gastrointestinal discomfort, anorexia, nausea, vomiting, constipation and diarrhoea. Darkening of the stools may occur.

Rarely, allergic reactions may occur.

*Interactions:* Iron reduces the absorption of penicillamine. Absorption of both iron and antibiotic may be reduced if Pregaday is given with a tetracycline.

Concurrent administration of antacids may reduce absorption of iron.

Co-trimoxazole, chloramphenicol or sulphasalazine may interfere with folate metabolism. Serum levels of anticonvulsant drugs may be reduced by administration of folate. Oral chloramphenicol delays plasma iron clearance, incorporation of iron into red blood cells and interferes with erythropoiesis.

Some inhibition of iron absorption may occur if it is taken with cholestyramine, tea, eggs or milk.

*Overdosage:* Acute overdosage of oral iron requires emergency treatment. In young children 200 to 250 mg/kg ferrous fumarate is considered to be extremely dangerous.

Symptoms and signs of abdominal pain, vomiting and diarrhoea appear within 60 minutes. Cardiovascular collapse with coma may follow. Some improvement may occur after this phase which in some patients is followed by recovery, in others after about sixteen hours deterioration may occur involving diffuse vascular congestion, pulmonary oedema, convulsions, anuria, hypothermia, severe shock, metabolic acidosis, coagulation abnormalities or hypoglycaemia.

Vomiting should be induced immediately, followed as soon as possible by parenteral injection of desferrioxamine mesylate and then gastric lavage. In the meantime, it is helpful to give milk and/or 5% sodium bicarbonate solution by mouth.

Dissolve 2 g desferrioxamine mesylate in 2 to 3 ml Water for Injections and give intramuscularly. A solution of 5 g desferrioxamine in 50 to 100 ml of fluid may be left in the stomach. If desferrioxamine is not available, leave 300 ml of 1% to 5% sodium bicarbonate solution in the stomach. Fluid replacement is essential.

Recovery may be complicated by long-term sequelae such as hepatic necrosis, pyloric stenosis or acute toxic encephalitis which may lead to CNS damage.

**Pharmaceutical precautions** Protect from light. Pregaday tablets should be kept out of the reach of children.

**Legal category** P.

**Package quantities** Cartons of two calendar blister packs of 14 tablets (OP).

**Further information** Nil.

**Product licence numbers** 0039/0398

# RUBILIN* RUBELLA VACCINE, LIVE BP

**Qualitative and quantitative composition:** The composition in terms of active ingredient is as follows:

Each 0.5 ml dose of reconstituted vaccine contains not less than 1000 $CCID_{50}$ live attenuated virus (Wistar RA 27/3).

**Pharmaceutical form** Freeze-dried preparation, reconstituted with Water for Injections BP prior to intramuscular or deep subcutaneous injection to humans.

The reconstituted vaccine may vary in colour from pale straw to pink.

## Clinical particulars

*Therapeutic indications:* For active immunisation against rubella.

It is recommended that all girls between the ages of 10 and 14 and seronegative non-pregnant women of child-bearing age, should be vaccinated. The latter group should be advised not to become pregnant within 1 month of vaccination. Because clinical diagnosis without laboratory tests is unreliable a past history of rubella is not a reliable guide to immune status.

One dose of vaccine will produce a seroconversion rate of over 95% in vaccinees.

*Posology and method of administration:*
*Children, adults and elderly:* One 0.5 ml dose of reconstituted vaccine is given by intramuscular or deep subcutaneous injection. The freeze-dried plug should be reconstituted by slowly adding the 0.5 ml Water for Injections BP provided, immediately prior to use.

*Contra-indications:* The vaccine must not be given to pregnant women and pregnancy should be avoided for one month after vaccination.

The vaccine should not be administered to a subject who has experienced a serious reaction (e.g. anaphylaxis) to a previous dose of this vaccine or who is known to be hypersensitive to any component thereof. The vaccine contains a small amount of neomycin and polymyxin and should not be given to individuals known to be hypersensitive to either of them.

The vaccine should not be given to subjects suffering from a febrile illness.

The vaccine should not be given to those suffering from malignant conditions (e.g. lymphoma, leukaemia, Hodgkin's Disease), impaired immunological mechanism (e.g. hypogammaglobulinaemia) or impaired immune responsiveness, whether congenital, idiopathic or as a result of treatment with steroids (with the exception of standard doses of locally acting, e.g. topical or inhaled, steroids), radiotherapy, cytotoxic drugs or other agents.

*Special warnings and precautions for use:* Although anaphylaxis is rare, facilities for its management should always be available during vaccination.

The vaccine may depress tuberculin skin sensitivity for 4 weeks or longer.

The vaccine virus is not transmitted and there is no risk to pregnant women from contact with vaccinees.

An interval of not less than 3 weeks should normally be allowed to lapse between the administration of any two live vaccines. If time does not permit they may be given simultaneously at separate sites. A 3 week interval should be allowed between the administration of Rubella Vaccine and BCG.

Rubella Vaccine should not be given within three months of an injection of immunoglobulin. The vaccine should not normally be given within 3 months of a transfusion of blood or plasma. If these have been used near the time of vaccination, the presence of antibodies should be checked at a later date.

Do not attempt to obtain more than the stated number of doses from the vial. It is good practice to record the title, dose and lot numbers of all vaccines and dates of administration

*Interaction with other medicaments and other forms of interaction:* The vaccine is inactivated by alcohol and if this is used to clean the skin prior to vaccination, it must be allowed to evaporate before the vaccine is given. Avoid contamination with bactericides. Use only sterile disposable syringes and needles which are free from traces of disinfectants or spirits. Use a fresh needle and syringe for each injection.

*Pregnancy and lactation:* There is a possibility that live attenuated virus administered during pregnancy could infect and damage the foetus, producing congenital abnormalities. Therefore, pregnant women must not be vaccinated. After vaccination women must ensure they do not conceive in the following one month until the theoretical risk of congenital abnormality returns to baseline.

*Effects on ability to drive and use machines:* Not applicable.

*Undesirable effects:* Fever, malaise, headache, sore throat, lymphadenopathy, rash, arthralgia and arthritis may occur. Such symptoms commence between one and three weeks after vaccination, and are usually mild and self limiting. Induration, pain and erythema at the injection site may occur. Joint symptoms are more common in adult females than in children and adolescents. Neurological symptoms have been reported on rare occasions. Thrombocytopenia has occasionally been reported after vaccination.

Any untoward reactions should be reported to the regulatory authorities and to the manufacturer

*Overdose:* Not applicable.

**Pharmacological particulars** Not applicable

**Pharmaceutical particulars**

*List of excipients:* The excipients contained in the preparation are as follows: Polymyxin BP, Neomycin BP, 199 Medium HSE, Sucrose BP, Sorbitol BP, Glutamic Acid (L) sodium salt HSE, Potassium dihydrogen phosphate HSE, Dipotassium hydrogen phosphate HSE, Peptone (Proteose) HSE, Water for Injections HSE.

*Incompatibilities:* None stated.

*Shelf life:*
2 to 8°C: 12 months
37°C: 1 week

*Special precautions for storage:* Store between 2 and 8°C. Do not freeze. Protect from light. Use the reconstituted vaccine within one hour after which time any remaining vaccine should be discarded.

*Nature and contents of container:* The vaccine is supplied as single dose vials in packs of 1 and 10 with siliconised rubber bungs, aluminium overseals and polypropylene flip off tops. Each vial contains freeze-dried powder for reconstitution of one dose of vaccine with 0.5 ml of Water for Injections. Each 0.5 ml Water for Injections is supplied in a glass ampoule.

*Instructions for use and handling:* After reconstitution with supplied Water for Injections, the vaccine should be administered immediately to reduce the risk of contamination with bacteria and moulds which may result in a reduction of vaccine potency.

Disposal should be by incineration at a temperature of not less than 1100°C at a registered waste disposal contractor.

**Marketing authorisation number** 0039/0349

**Date of approval/revision of SPC** February 1996

**Legal category** POM

# STREPTOMYCIN SULPHATE BP STERILE POWDER

**Qualitative and quantitative composition** Each vial contains 1.342 g Streptomycin Sulphate Sterile BP (equivalent to 1 g Streptomycin base).

**Pharmaceutical form** A white sterile powder for preparation of Streptomycin Sulphate Injection BP, intended for intramuscular injection.

## Clinical particulars

*Therapeutic indications:* Streptomycin may be used in the treatment of tuberculosis and other serious infections resistant to alternative antibiotics.

*Posology and method of administration:*

*Monitoring advice:* Serum levels should be monitored, especially if there is renal impairment. Dosages may need to be adjusted to avoid toxicity. In general, peak levels should not exceed 40 mcg/ml and trough levels 3 mcg/ml. In the elderly, the trough may need to be even lower (1 mcg/ml).

*Route of administration:* By deep intramuscular injection.

The injection should be given deeply into muscle and the site changed for each injection.

A 1 g dose is usually dissolved in 2 or 3 ml of Water for Injections. (The displacement volume of 1 g is approximately 0.75 ml). Use of a sterile disposable membrane filter of 0.45 micron pore size is convenient to ensure clarity of the solution.

*Tuberculosis:* Streptomycin is always given together with other antituberculosis drugs. It can be given on a daily basis or three times a week if intermittent treatment is more appropriate.

*Adults under 40 years of age AND bodyweight greater than 50 kg:* 1 g daily or intermittently.

*Elderly and adults over 40 years of age OR bodyweight less than 50 kg:* 0.5-0.75 g per day if given daily; 0.75 g per day if given intermittently. (See also monitoring advice).

*Children:* 15-20 mg/kg bodyweight (up to 1 g maximum) daily or intermittently.

*Renal impairment:* Dosages may need to be adjusted (see monitoring advice).

Streptomycin treatment should usually continue for the initial 2 month treatment phase and may be included in the subsequent continuation phase. Treatment should be supervised by a specialist physician.

*Non-tuberculous infections:*
*Adults:* Usually 1 g per day for 3-7 days.
*Elderly:* The adult dosage may require some adjustment (see monitoring advice).
*Children:* Up to 40 mg/kg bodyweight (up to 1 g maximum) daily for 3-7 days. Divided doses are often used.

*Note:* in urinary-tract infections the urine should be kept alkaline as aminoglycosides are inhibited by acidic environments.

*Maximum tolerated daily dose and maximum dose for an entire course of therapy:* Side-effects increase after a cumulative dose of 100 g, which should only be exceeded in exceptional circumstances.

*In tuberculosis treatment:* Intramuscular dosages of 2 g daily (divided) for 6 weeks and 1 g twice daily for up to 8 weeks have been administered.

*In non-tuberculous treatment:* Intramuscular dosage of 2.4 g daily (divided) for up to 14 days has been administered.

*Contra-indications:* Streptomycin is contra-indicated in patients with known hypersensitivity to the drug; in patients with diseases of the ear, particularly suppurative otitis media and labyrinthine disturbances; in pregnancy; in patients with myasthenia gravis and in patients with impaired renal function, unless the dosage is adjusted (see *Posology and method of administration*).

*Special warnings and precautions for use:* Intrathecal administration of streptomycin is not recommended.

Renally impaired and elderly patients should have dosages adjusted and plasma concentrations monitored as indicated under *Posology and method of administration.*

Skin sensitisation may occur in persons handling the antibiotic and care should be taken to avoid contact with the substance. Use of rubber gloves is recommended.

*Interactions with other medicaments and other forms of interaction:* Streptomycin should not be given with potentially ototoxic diuretics (e.g. frusemide and ethacrynic acid); if concurrent use is unavoidable administration of the aminoglycoside and of the diuretic should be separated by as long a period as practicable.

Concurrent use with other nephrotoxic drugs, including other aminoglycosides, vancomycin and some of the cephalosporins, should be avoided as they increase the risk of toxicity.

Streptomycin and benzylpenicillin act synergistically against *Streptococcus faecalis*. They should not be given together unless the preparation is freshly made because the combination rapidly becomes less active on storage.

*Pregnancy and lactation:*
*Pregnancy:* Streptomycin is contra-indicated during pregnancy as it crosses the placenta and can cause foetal eighth nerve damage.
*Lactation:* The drug enters breast milk but the exact significance is unknown. However, the risk of possible sensitisation should be borne in mind.

*Effects on ability to drive and use machines:* None known.

*Undesirable effects:* The main adverse effect is ototoxicity: some impairment of vestibular function (less often of auditory function) can occur, particularly with prolonged or intensive therapy, in the presence of renal dysfunction and in the elderly and neonate. Reported symptoms include giddiness, vertigo, tinnitus, ataxia and deafness, which is sometimes irreversible.

Paraesthesia in and around the mouth is not uncommon after intramuscular injection and other neurological symptoms, including peripheral neuropathies, optic neuritis and scotoma have occasionally occurred.

Nephrotoxicity can also occur; evidence of minor renal tubular dysfunction, such as urinary casts and minor degrees of albuminuria are common, but severe renal damage (proximal tubular necrosis) is rare.

Cutaneous and generalised hypersensitivity reactions, such as rash and fever, are common. (Note precautions (*Special warnings and precautions for use*) for persons handling the drug.) Occasional allergic-type reactions, rarely severe and often responding to antihistamine treatment. Severe exfoliative dermatitis and anaphylactic shock have been reported.

Aplastic anaemia and agranulocytosis have also been rarely reported.

*Overdose*
*Human experience:* Acute haemolytic anaemia and renal failure have been reported following repeated injection of streptomycin for 15 years.

*Management of overdose in man:* Streptomycin can be removed from the body by haemodialysis.

**Pharmacological particulars**

*Pharmacodynamic properties:* Streptomycin is an aminoglycoside antibiotic which is active against *Mycobacterium tuberculosis*. It is not active against *Pseudomonas aeruginosa*. Resistance develops fairly rapidly in many organisms, limiting its use.

*Pharmacokinetic properties:* Oral absorption of streptomycin is poor (0-40%) and it is thus administered parenterally. Following parenteral administration, approximately 50-60% of the dose is excreted unchanged in the urine within 24 hours. The plasma half life is approximately 2.5 hours, increasing to approximately 100 hours when blood urea nitrogen concentrations are in the range of 100-150 mg per 100 ml. A small proportion of the dose (about 1%) is excreted in the bile, this proportion falling when there is chronic hepatic dysfunction. Approximately 20% of the dose cannot be accounted for by urinary excretion but no metabolites have yet been identified.

*Preclinical safety data:* There are no pre-clinical data of relevance to the prescriber which are additional to that already included in other sections of the Summary of Product Characteristics.

**Pharmaceutical particulars**

*List of excipients:* None.

*Incompatibilities:* Streptomycin is incompatible with acids and alkalis.

*Shelf life:* Dry powder: 4 years.

*Special precautions for storage:* Dry powder: Store at a temperature not exceeding 25°C.

*Nature and contents of container:* Streptomycin Sulphate BP Sterile Powder is presented in glass vials which are packaged in cartons containing 10 vials.

*Instructions for use/handling:* Sterile solutions of streptomycin should be used as soon as possible after reconstitution.
*Note:* skin sensitisation can occur in persons handling the drug and care should be taken to avoid contact with the substance. Use of rubber gloves is recommended.

**Marketing authorisation number**  0039/6002R

**Date of approval/revision of SPC**  April 1996

**Legal category**  POM.

## ADSORBED TETANUS VACCINE, BP

**Qualitative and quantitative composition**  The composition in terms of active ingredient is as follows:-
Tetanus toxoid not less than 40IU. Quantities expressed per 0.5 ml dose.

**Pharmaceutical form**  Sterile suspension for deep subcutaneous or intramuscular injection to humans.

**Clinical particulars**

*Therapeutic indications:* For active immunisation against tetanus. Primary immunisation against tetanus in infancy is usually carried out by administration of combined Adsorbed Diphtheria, Tetanus and Pertussis Vaccine (DTPer/Vac/Ads) or Adsorbed Diphtheria and Tetanus Vaccine (CHILD) (DT/Vac/Ads (Child)).

*Posology and method of administration:* Children, adults and elderly: Each dose is 0.5 ml given by intramuscular or deep subcutaneous injection.

The primary course of immunisation against tetanus consists of three doses with an interval of one month between each dose. The intervals between immunisations may be exceeded without the need to repeat the full course of immunisation. Reinforcing doses are given to maintain immunity against tetanus.

Primary course in children: Primary immunisation against tetanus may be carried out by the administration of combined Adsorbed Diphtheria, Tetanus and Pertussis Vaccine (DTPer/Vac/Ads), Adsorbed Diphtheria and Tetanus Vaccine (CHILD) (DT/Vac/Ads (Child)) or Adsorbed Tetanus Vaccine (Tet/Vac/Ads) in infancy. Three 0.5 ml doses are given, with a dose at 2, 3 and 4 months of age.

Reinforcing doses in children: Children who have received the primary course of immunisation in infancy require reinforcement of immunity against tetanus. This can be achieved by giving one dose (0.5 ml) Adsorbed Diphtheria and Tetanus Vaccine (CHILD) (DT/Vac/Ads (Child)) or Adsorbed Tetanus Vaccine (Tet/Vac/Ads), after at least three years from the last dose of the primary course. The reinforcing dose is commonly given prior to school entry.

A reinforcing dose (0.5 ml) of either Adsorbed Diphtheria and Tetanus Vaccine for Adults and Adolescents or Adsorbed Tetanus Vaccine (Tet/Vac/Ads) may be given at 15 to 19 years of age or on leaving school.

Primary course in adults: Primary immunisation against tetanus consists of three doses separated by intervals of not less than four weeks.

Reinforcing doses in adults: A single dose of vaccine given at any time after completion of the primary course of three injections can be expected to provide an effective reinforcement of immunity.

The administration of a reinforcing dose approximately 10 years after the completion of a primary immunisation course is recommended. Thereafter, a further vaccination at 10 years is thought to provide the potential for lifelong protection. However, this does not preclude the need to consider administration of additional doses in the event of injuries which may give rise to tetanus. Such prophylaxis requires consideration on a patient to patient basis e.g. immunisation history, immune status etc. For the majority of fully immunised subjects, reinforcement of immunity on wounding should only be required if >10 years have elapsed since the previous vaccination. Reinforcing doses of tetanus vaccine at frequent intervals may provoke hypersensitivity reactions and tetanus vaccine should not be given to any patient who has received a booster dose in the preceding year.

Persons of all ages are susceptible to tetanus unless they have received appropriate immunisation. Rarely, if ever, is natural immunity developed even in persons who have recovered from severe tetanus. Since most tetanus cases follow trivial wounds, all persons should, if possible, be actively immunised against the disease.

Adsorbed Tetanus Vaccine may be administered simultaneously with human tetanus immunoglobulin or tetanus antitoxin but must be given at separate sites. The antibody response of subjects to subsequent doses of vaccine is not significantly impaired by this procedure.

Oral Poliomyelitis Vaccine BP may be given at the same time as Adsorbed Tetanus Vaccine.

Shake well before each dose is withdrawn. It is good practice to record the title, dose and lot numbers of all vaccines and dates of administration.

*Contra-indications:* Adsorbed Tetanus Vaccine must not be given intradermally since it may give rise to a persistent skin nodule.

The vaccine should not be administered to a subject who has experienced a serious reaction (e.g. anaphylaxis) to a previous dose of this vaccine or who is known to be hypersensitive to any component thereof.

Adsorbed Tetanus Vaccine should not be given to an individual suffering from an acute febrile illness except in the presence of a tetanus-prone wound.

Tetanus vaccine should not be given to any patient who has received a booster dose in the preceding year.

*Special warnings and precautions for use:* Although anaphylaxis is rare, facilities for its management should always be available during vaccination.

*Interactions with other medicaments and other forms of interaction:* None known.

*Pregnancy and lactation:* In countries where the risks of neonatal tetanus are high, tetanus vaccines are widely administered during pregnancy without any apparent significant adverse effect on pregnancy or foetal development. No information on the immunisation of lactating women is available.

*Effects on ability to drive and use machines:* None stated.

*Undesirable effects:* Local reactions consisting of swelling, redness and pain may develop at the injection site and persist for several days. Delays of up to 10 days before symptoms develop are reported. Occasionally these local reactions may be quite marked, with tenderness and swelling of a large area. Local reactions are rare in children, the incidence increases with age and according to the number of previously administered doses of tetanus toxoid containing vaccine. However, reactions may occur after the first dose. Subjects who develop reactions frequently have high titres of circulating antitoxin. Women develop reactions more frequently than men.

General reactions are uncommon but may include arthralgia, lymphadenopathy, faintness, nausea, headache, lethargy, malaise, myalgia and pyrexia. They do not usually persist for more than a few hours. Urticaria, angioneurotic oedema and acute anaphylactic reactions are sometimes seen.

Serum sickness and peripheral neuropathy have been described. Calcifying dermatomyositis has been observed in temporal association with tetanus vaccination.

Persistent nodules at the site of injection may occasionally follow administration of adsorbed vaccines especially if the inoculation is into the superficial layers of subcutaneous tissue.

Any untoward reactions should be reported to the regulatory authorities and to the manufacturer.

*Overdose:* Not applicable.

**Pharmacological properties**  Not applicable.

**Pharmaceutical particulars**

*List of excipients:* The excipients contained in the preparation are as follows:-

| | |
|---|---|
| Aluminium hydroxide | HSE* |
| Disodium Tetraborate (Sodium borate) | BP |
| Succinic acid | HSE* |
| Sodium chloride | PhEur |
| Thiomersal | BP |
| Water for injections | PhEur |

* HSE house specification

*Incompatibilities:* None stated.

*Shelf life:* In filled containers: 2 years.

*Special precautions for storage:* Store between 2-8°C. Protect from light. Do not freeze. Vials should be stored upright.

*Nature and contents of container:* PhEur type 1 clear neutral glass ampoules, 1 ml capacity (0.5 ml fill). Multidose PhEur type 1 clear neutral glass vials, 8 ml capacity (5 ml fill), with red butyl rubber plug with an aluminium collar and blue polypropylene flip-off top.

*Instructions for use/handling:* Vaccine which has been frozen should not be used.

Discard partly used vials at the end of the vaccination session.

Disposal should be by incineration at a temperature of not less than 1100°C at a registered waste disposal contractor.

**Marketing authorisation number**  0039/0473

**Date of approval/revision of SPC**  May 1996

**Legal category**  POM

## TRANDATE* INJECTION

**Presentation**  Trandate Injection: 20 ml ampoules each containing 100 mg (5 mg/ml) labetalol hydrochloride in an aqueous colourless solution. Labetalol hydrochloride is 2-hydroxy-5-[1-hydroxy-2-(1-methyl-3-phenyl-propylamino) ethyl] benzamide hydrochloride.

**Uses**
*Indications:* Trandate Injection is indicated when rapid control of blood pressure is essential in severely hypertensive patients including severe hypertension of pregnancy and for use in anaesthesia where a hypotensive technique is indicated.

It is also indicated in hypertensive episodes following acute myocardial infarction.

*Mode of action:* Trandate lowers the blood pressure primarily by blocking alpha-adrenoceptors in peripheral arterioles and thereby reducing the peripheral resistance.

Concurrent beta-blockade protects the heart from reflex sympathetic drive normally induced by peripheral vasodilatation. Cardiac output is not significantly reduced at rest or after moderate exercise. Increases in systolic pressure during exercise are, however, reduced after Trandate, corresponding changes in diastolic pressure are essentially normal. All these effects would be expected to benefit hypertensive patients.

**Dosage and administration**
*Adults:* Trandate Injection is intended for intravenous use in hospitalised patients. The plasma concentrations achieved after intravenous doses of Trandate in severe hypertension are substantially greater than those following oral administration of the drug and provide the greater degree of blockade of alpha-adrenoceptors necessary to control the more severe disease. Patients should, therefore, always receive the drug whilst in the supine or left lateral position. Raising the patient into the upright position, within three hours of intravenous Trandate administration, should be avoided since excessive postural hypotension may occur.

*Bolus Injection:* If it is essential to reduce the blood pressure quickly, as for example, in hypertensive encephalopathy, a dose of 50 mg of Trandate should be given by intravenous injection over a period of at least one minute. If necessary, doses of 50 mg may be repeated at five minute intervals until a satisfactory response occurs. The total dose should not exceed 200 mg. After bolus injection, the maximum effect usually occurs within five minutes and the effective duration of action is usually about six hours but may be as long as eighteen hours.

*Intravenous Infusion:* An alternative method of administering Trandate is intravenous infusion of a solution made by diluting the contents of two ampoules (200 mg) to 200 ml with Sodium Chloride and Dextrose Injection BP or 5% Dextrose Intravenous Infusion BP. The resultant infusion solution contains 1 mg/ml of Trandate. It should be administered using a paediatric giving set fitted with a 50 ml graduated burette to facilitate dosage.

*In the hypertensions of pregnancy:* The infusion can be started at the rate of 20 mg per hour and this dose may be doubled every thirty minutes until a satisfactory reduction in blood pressure has been obtained or a dosage of 160 mg per hour is reached. Occasionally, higher doses may be necessary.

*In hypertensive episodes following acute myocardial infarction:* Infusion should be commenced at 15 mg per hour and gradually increased to a maximum of 120 mg per hour depending on the control of blood pressure.

*In hypertension due to other causes:* The rate of infusion of Trandate should be about 2 mg (2 ml of infusion solution) per minute, until a satisfactory response is obtained; the infusion should then be stopped. The effective dose is usually in the range of 50-200 mg, depending on the severity of the hypertension. For most patients it is unnecessary to administer more than 200 mg but larger doses may be required especially in patients with phaeochromocytoma. The rate of infusion may be adjusted according to the response, at the discretion of the physician. The blood pressure and pulse rate should be monitored throughout the infusion.

It is desirable to monitor the heart rate after injection and during infusion. In most patients, there is a small decrease in the heart rate; severe bradycardia is unusual but may be controlled by injecting atropine 1-2 mg intravenously. Respiratory function should be observed particularly in patients with any known impairment.

Once the blood pressure has been adequately reduced, maintenance therapy with Trandate Tablets should be instituted with a starting dose of one 100 mg tablet twice daily. (See Trandate Tablets Data Sheet for further details). Trandate Injection has been administered to patients with uncontrolled hypertension already receiving other hypotensive agents, including beta-blocking drugs, without adverse effects.

*In hypotensive anaesthesia:* Induction should be with standard agents (e.g. sodium thiopentone) and anaesthesia maintained with nitrous oxide and oxygen with or without halothane. The recommended starting dose of Trandate Injection is 10-20 mg intravenously depending on the age and condition of the patient. Patients for whom halothane is contra-indicated usually require a higher initial dose of Trandate (25-30 mg). If satisfactory hypotension is not achieved after five minutes, increments of 5-10 mg should be given until the desired level of blood pressure is attained.

Halothane and Trandate act synergistically therefore the halothane concentration should not exceed 1 to 1.5% as profound falls in blood pressure may be precipitated.

Following Trandate Injection the blood pressure can be quickly and easily adjusted by altering the halothane concentration and/or adjusting table tilt. The mean duration of hypotension following 20-25 mg of Trandate is fifty minutes.

Hypotension induced by Trandate Injection is readily reversed by atropine 0.6 mg and discontinuation of halothane.

Tubocurarine and pancuronium may be used when assisted or controlled ventilation is required. IPPV may further increase the hypotension resulting from Trandate Injection and/or halothane.

*Children:* Safety and efficacy have not been established.

### Contra-indications, warnings, etc

*Contra-indications:* History of wheezing or asthma, hypersensitivity to labetalol, second or third degree heart block, cardiogenic shock and other conditions associated with severe and prolonged hypotension or severe bradycardia. Uncontrolled, incipient or digitalis-refractory heart failure.

Where peripheral vasoconstriction suggests low cardiac output, the use of Trandate Injection to control hypertensive episodes following acute myocardial infarction is contra-indicated.

*Precautions:* There have been rare reports of severe hepatocellular injury with labetalol therapy. The hepatic injury is usually reversible and has occurred after both short and long term treatment. Appropriate laboratory testing should be done at the first sign or symptom of liver dysfunction.

If there is laboratory evidence of liver injury or the patient is jaundiced, labetalol therapy should be stopped and not re-started.

Where cardiac reserve is poor, control with a cardiac

glycoside and a diuretic should be obtained prior to the cautious use of Trandate Injection.

Beta-blockers, even those with apparent cardioselectivity, should not be used in patients with a history of obstructive airways disease unless no alternative treatment is available. In such cases, the risk of inducing bronchospasm should be appreciated and appropriate precautions taken. If bronchospasm should occur after the use of Trandate, it can be treated with a $\beta_2$–agonist by inhalation e.g. salbutamol (the dose of which may need to be greater than the usual dose in asthma) and if necessary intravenous atropine 1 mg. It is not necessary to discontinue Trandate therapy in patients requiring anaesthesia but they should be given intravenous atropine prior to induction; the effect of halothane on blood pressure may be enhanced by Trandate. During anaesthesia Trandate may mask the compensatory physiological responses to sudden haemorrhage (tachycardia and vasoconstriction). Close attention must therefore be paid to blood loss and the blood volume maintained.

Care should be taken in the concomitant use of labetalol and either Class I antiarrhythmic agents or calcium antagonists of the verapamil type.

*Risk of anaphylactic reaction:* While taking beta-blockers, patients with a history of severe anaphylactic reaction to a variety of allergens may be more reactive to repeated challenge, either accidental, diagnostic or therapeutic. Such patients may be unresponsive to the usual doses of adrenaline used to treat allergic reaction.

*Pregnancy:* Although no teratogenic effects have been demonstrated in animals, Trandate should only be used during the first trimester of pregnancy if the potential benefit outweighs the potential risk. Trandate crosses the placental barrier and the possibility of the consequences of alpha- and beta-adrenoceptor blockade in the fetus and neonate should be borne in mind.

Perinatal and neonatal distress (bradycardia, hypotension, respiratory depression, hypoglycaemia, hypothermia) has been rarely reported. Sometimes these symptoms developed a day or two after birth. Response to supportive measures (e.g. intravenous fluids and glucose) is usually prompt but with severe pre-eclampsia, particularly after prolonged intravenous labetalol, recovery may be slower. This may be related to diminished liver metabolism in premature babies. Intra-uterine and neonatal deaths have been reported but other drugs (e.g. vasodilators, respiratory depressants) and the effects of pre-eclampsia, intra-uterine growth retardation and prematurity were implicated.

Such clinical experience warns against unduly prolonging high dose labetalol and delaying delivery and against co-administration of hydralazine.

Trandate is excreted in breast milk. No adverse effects in breast feeding infants have been reported.

*Side-effects:* Trandate Injection is usually well tolerated. Excessive postural hypotension may occur if patients are allowed to assume the upright position within three hours of receiving Trandate Injection.

There have been a few reports of nasal congestion and rare reports of hypersensitivity: rash, pruritus, angioedema and dyspnoea.

There are rare reports of raised liver function tests, jaundice (both hepatocellular and cholestatic), hepatitis and hepatic necrosis. The signs and symptoms are usually reversible on withdrawal of the drug. There are reports of bradycardia and heart block.

*Overdosage:* Profound cardiovascular effects are to be expected e.g. excessive, posture-sensitive hypotension and sometimes bradycardia. Patients should be laid supine with legs raised. Use a cardiac glycoside and a diuretic in cardiac failure; for bronchospasm, administer a $\beta_2$-agonist per aerosol. Intravenous atropine 0.25 to 3 mg should be given to relieve bradycardia. Intravenous noradrenaline 5 to 10 micrograms initially, repeated according to response, may be preferable to isoprenaline to improve the circulation. Alternatively, noradrenaline may be infused at a rate of 5 micrograms per minute until the response is satisfactory.

In severe overdose, intravenous glucagon may be preferred: an initial bolus dose of 5 to 10 mg in dextrose or saline should be followed by an intravenous infusion of 5 mg/hour or as sufficient to maintain cardiac output. Transvenous pacing may be required.

Oliguric renal failure has been reported after massive overdosage of labetalol orally. In one case, the use of dopamine to increase the blood pressure may have aggravated the renal failure.

Haemodialysis removes less than 1% labetalol hydrochloride from the circulation.

**Pharmaceutical precautions** Protect from light.

Trandate Injection has been shown to be incompatible with Sodium Bicarbonate Injection BP 4.2% w/v.

**Legal category** POM.

**Package quantities** Trandate Injection 20 ml ampoules: Boxes of 5.

**Further information** Trandate does not adversely affect renal function and is a particularly suitable drug for use in hypertensive patients with renal disease. The metabolites of Trandate are excreted in the faeces as well as in the urine and so the drug is unlikely to accumulate in the body even in renal failure.

The plasma half-life of Trandate is about 4 hours. Only about 50% of Trandate in blood is protein bound.

Trandate fluoresces in alkaline solution at an excitation wavelength of 334nm and a fluorescence wavelength of 412nm and may therefore interfere with the assays of certain fluorescent substances.

The presence of labetalol metabolites in the urine may result in falsely elevated levels of urinary catecholamines, metanephrine, normetanephrine, and vanillylmandelic acid (VMA) when measured by fluorimetric or photometric methods. In screening patients suspected of having a phaeochromocytoma and being treated with Trandate a specific method, such as a high performance liquid chromatographic assay with solid phase extraction (e.g. J. Chromatogr. 385, 241, 1987) should be employed in determining levels of catecholamines.

**Product licence number** 0039/0492

## TRANDATE* TABLETS

**Presentation** Trandate Tablets: Circular, orange-coloured, film-coated, biconvex tablets marked TRANDATE and the strength in milligrams on one face.

Trandate Tablets 50 mg: each containing labetalol hydrochloride 50 mg.

Trandate Tablets 100 mg: each containing labetalol hydrochloride 100 mg.

Trandate Tablets 200 mg: each containing labetalol hydrochloride 200 mg.

Trandate Tablets 400 mg: each containing labetalol hydrochloride 400 mg.

Labetalol hydrochloride is 2 hydroxy-5[1-hydroxy-2(1-methyl-3-phenyl-propylamino) ethyl] benzamide hydrochloride.

### Uses

*Indications:* Trandate Tablets are indicated in mild, moderate and severe hypertension including the hypertensions of pregnancy, when oral therapy is desirable. Trandate Tablets are also indicated in angina pectoris with existing hypertension.

*Mode of action:* Trandate lowers blood pressure by blocking peripheral arteriolar alpha-adrenoceptors, thus reducing peripheral resistance and by concurrent beta-blockade, protects the heart from reflex sympathetic drive that would otherwise occur. Cardiac output is not significantly reduced at rest or after moderate exercise. Increases in systolic blood pressure during exercise are reduced but corresponding changes in diastolic pressure are essentially normal.

In patients with anginal pectoris coexisting with hypertension, the reduced peripheral resistance decreases myocardial afterload and oxygen demand. All these effects would be expected to benefit hypertensive patients and those with coexisting angina.

**Dosage and administration** Trandate Tablets should be taken with food.

*Adults:* Hypertension: Treatment should start with 100 mg twice daily. In patients already being treated with antihypertensives and in those of low body weight this may be sufficient to control blood pressure. In others, increase in dosage of 100 mg twice daily should be made at fortnightly intervals. Many patients' blood pressure is controlled by 200 mg twice daily and up to 800 mg daily may be given as a twice daily regimen. In severe, refractory hypertension, daily doses up to 2400 mg have been given. Such doses should be divided into a three or four times a day regimen.

*Elderly:* In elderly patients, an initial dose of 50 mg twice daily is recommended. This has provided satisfactory control in some cases.

*In hypertensions of pregnancy:* The initial dosage of 100 mg twice daily may be increased if necessary, at weekly intervals by 100 mg twice daily. During the second and third trimesters, the severity of the hypertension may require further dose titration to a three times daily regimen, ranging from 100 mg tds to 400 mg tds. A total daily dose of 2400 mg should not be exceeded.

Hospital in-patients with severe hypertension, particularly of pregnancy, may have daily increases in dosage.

*General:* If rapid reduction of blood pressure is necessary, see the data sheet for Trandate Injection. If long-term control of hypertension following the use of Trandate Injection is required, oral therapy with Trandate Tablets should start with 100 mg twice daily.

Additive hypotensive effects may be expected if

Trandate Tablets are administered together with other antihypertensives, e.g. diuretics, methyldopa etc. When transferring patients from such agents. Trandate Tablets should be introduced with a dosage of 100 mg twice daily and the previous therapy gradually decreased. Abrupt withdrawal of clonidine or beta-blocking agents is undesirable.

*Angina coexisting with hypertension:* In patients with angina pectoris coexisting with hypertension, the dose of Trandate will be that required to control the hypertension.

*Children:* Safety and efficacy in children have not been established.

**Contra-indications, warnings, etc**
*Contra-indications:* Trandate Tablets are contra-indicated in history of wheezing or asthma, second or third degree heart block, cardiogenic shock, other conditions associated with severe and prolonged hypotension or severe bradycardia and uncontrolled, incipient or digitalis-refractory heart failure.

Labetalol is contra-indicated for patients known to have a hypersensitivity to the drug.

*Warnings:* There have been reports of skin rashes and/or dry eyes associated with the use of beta-adrenoceptor blocking drugs. The reported incidence is small and in most cases the symptoms have cleared when the treatment was withdrawn. Gradual discontinuance of the drug should be considered if any such reaction is not otherwise explicable.

There have been rare reports of severe hepatocellular injury with labetalol therapy. The hepatic injury is usually reversible and has occurred after both short-term and long-term treatment. Appropriate laboratory testing should be done at the first sign or symptom of liver dysfunction. If there is laboratory evidence of liver injury or the patient is jaundiced, labetalol should be stopped and not re-started.

*Precautions:* Special care should be taken with patients whose cardiac reserve is poor and heart failure should be controlled with a cardiac glycoside and a diuretic before starting Trandate therapy.

Beta-blockers, even those with apparent cardioselectivity, should not be used in patients with a history of obstructive airways disease unless no alternative treatment is available. In such cases, the risk of inducing bronchospasm should be appreciated and appropriate precautions taken. If bronchospasm should occur after the use of Trandate, it can be treated with a $\beta_2$-agonist by inhalation e.g. salbutamol (the dose of which may need to be greater than the usual dose in asthma) and, if necessary, intravenous atropine 1 mg.

Trandate Tablets need not be discontinued prior to anaesthesia but patients should receive intravenous atropine prior to induction. Trandate may enhance the hypotensive effect of halothane. Care should be taken if labetalol is used concomitantly with either Class I anti-arrhythmic agents or calcium antagonists of the verapamil type.

Patients, particularly those with ischaemic heart disease, should not interrupt/discontinue abruptly Trandate therapy.

*Risk of anaphylactic reaction:* While taking beta-blockers, patients with a history of severe anaphylactic reaction to a variety of allergens may be more reactive to repeated challenge, either accidental, diagnostic or therapeutic. Such patients may be unresponsive to the usual doses of adrenaline used to treat allergic reaction.

*Pregnancy:* Although not teratogenic effects have been demonstrated in animals, Trandate should only be used during the first trimester of pregnancy if the potential benefit outweighs the potential risk. Trandate crosses the placental barrier and the possibility of the consequences of alpha- and beta-adrenoceptor blockade in the fetus and neonate should be borne in mind.

Perinatal and neonatal distress (bradycardia, hypotension, respiratory depression, hypoglycaemia, hypothermia) has been rarely reported. Sometimes these symptoms developed a day or two after birth. Response to supportive measures (e.g. intravenous fluids and glucose) is usually prompt but with severe pre-eclampsia, particularly after prolonged intravenous labetalol, recovery may be slower. This may be related to diminished liver metabolism in premature babies. Intra-uterine and neonatal deaths have been reported but other drugs (e.g. vasodilators, respiratory depressants) and the effects of pre-eclampsia, intra-uterine growth retardation and prematurity were implicated. Such clinical experience warns against unduly prolonging high dose labetalol and delaying delivery and against co-administration of hydralazine.

Trandate is excreted in breast milk. No adverse effects in breast feeding infants have been reported.

*Side-effects:* Most side-effects are transient and occur during the first few weeks of treatment. They include headache, tiredness, dizziness, depressed mood, lethargy, nasal congestion, sweating, and rarely, ankle oedema. Postural hypotension is uncommon except at very high doses or if the initial dose is too high or doses are increased too rapidly. A tingling sensation in the scalp, usually transient, also may occur in a few patients early in treatment. Tremor has been reported in the treatment of hypertensions of pregnancy. Acute retention of urine, difficulty in micturition, ejaculatory failure, epigastric pain, nausea and vomiting have been reported. There have been rare reports of positive anti-nuclear antibodies unassociated with disease as well as rare cases of systemic lupus erythematosus and very rarely drug fever.

There have been very rare reports of toxic myopathy. Rare reports of hypersensitivity: rash, pruritus, angioedema and dyspnoea. A reversible lichenoid rash has occurred rarely. Blurred vision, eye irritation and cramps have been reported but were not necessarily related to Trandate. There are rare reports of raised liver function tests, jaundice (both hepatocellular and cholestatic), hepatitis and hepatic necrosis. The signs and symptoms are usually reversible on withdrawal of the drug. There are rare reports of bradycardia and heart block.

*Drug interactions:* Concomitant use of tricyclic antidepressants may increase the incidence of tremor. Cimetidine may increase the bioavailability of labetalol and care is required in the oral dosing of the latter.

*Overdosage:* Profound cardiovascular effects are to be expected e.g. excessive, posture-sensitive hypotension and sometimes bradycardia. Patients should be laid supine with the legs raised. Gastric lavage or induced emesis is warranted for a few hours after ingestion; use a cardiac glycoside and a diuretic in cardiac failure; for bronchospasm, administer a $\beta_2$-agonist per aerosol. Intravenous atropine 0.25 to 3 mg should be given to relieve bradycardia. Intravenous noradrenaline 5 to 10 micrograms initially, repeated according to response, may be preferable to isoprenaline to improve the circulation. Alternatively, noradrenaline may be infused at a rate of 5 micrograms per minute until the response is satisfactory.

In severe overdose, intravenous glucagon may be preferred: an initial bolus dose of 5 to 10 mg in dextrose or saline should be followed by an intravenous infusion of 5 mg/hour or as sufficient to maintain cardiac output. Transvenous pacing may be required.

Oliguric renal failure has been reported after massive overdosage of labetalol orally. In one case, the use of dopamine to increase the blood pressure may have aggravated the renal failure.

Haemodialysis removes less than 1% labetalol hydrochloride from the circulation.

**Pharmaceutical precautions** No special storage precautions are required.

**Legal category** POM.

**Package quantities** Trandate Tablets 100 mg and 200 mg are available in containers of 250; Trandate Tablets 400 mg in containers of 56 (OP) and 250; Trandate Tablets 50 mg, 100 mg and 200 mg are also available in calendar blister packs of 56 tablets (OP).

**Further information** Trandate does not adversely affect renal function and is particularly suitable for use in hypertensive patients with renal disease. Its metabolites are excreted in faeces as well as urine and the drug is unlikely to accumulate in the body even in renal failure.

The plasma half-life of Trandate is about 4 hours. Only 50% of labetalol in the blood is protein bound. It fluoresces in alkaline solution at an excitation wavelength of 334nm and a fluorescence wavelength of 412nm and may therefore interfere with the assays of certain fluorescent substances including catecholamines.

The presence of labetalol metabolites in the urine may result in falsely elevated levels of urinary catecholamines, metanephrine, normetanephrine, and vanillylmandelic acid (VMA) when measured by fluorimetric or photometric methods. In screening patients suspected of having a phaeochromocytoma and being treated with Trandate a specific method, such as a high performance liquid chromatographic assay with solid phase extraction (e.g. J. Chromatrogr. 385, 241, 1987) should be employed in determining levels of catecholamines.

**Product licence numbers**

| | |
|---|---|
| Trandate Tablets 50 mg | 0039/0493 |
| Trandate Tablets 100 mg | 0039/0494 |
| Trandate Tablets 200 mg | 0039/0495 |
| Trandate Tablets 400 mg | 0039/0496 |

## TRIVAX-AD*. Adsorbed Diphtheria, Tetanus and Pertussis Vaccine, BP

**Qualitative and quantitative composition** The composition in terms of active ingredients is as follows:

| | |
|---|---|
| Diphtheria toxoid | not less than 30IU |
| Tetanus toxoid | not less than 60IU |
| Bordetella pertussis | not more than 20,000 million chemically killed organisms with a potency of not less than 4IU |

Quantities expressed per 0.5 ml dose.

**Pharmaceutical form** Sterile suspension for deep subcutaneous or intramuscular injection to humans.

**Clinical particulars**

*Therapeutic indications:* For active immunisation against diphtheria, tetanus and whooping cough in infants and children under 10 years of age.

*Posology and method of administration:* Children aged 10 years and over, adults and elderly: NOT RECOMMENDED.

Children under 10 years of age: Each dose is 0.5 ml, given by intramuscular or deep subcutaneous injection. The primary course of immunisation consists of three doses with an interval of at least one month between each dose. The intervals between immunisations may be exceeded without the need to repeat the full course of immunisation.

The primary course should start at 2 months of age, with an interval of at least one month between each dose.

When Adsorbed Diphtheria and Tetanus Vaccine (CHILD) has been administered at the start of a primary course, Adsorbed Diphtheria, Tetanus and Pertussis Vaccine may be administered for subsequent doses. Once three doses of Adsorbed Diphtheria and Tetanus Vaccine (CHILD) have been administered, monovalent pertussis vaccine may be given at monthly intervals to complete the course.

A single dose of Adsorbed Diphtheria, Tetanus and Pertussis Vaccine is recommended as the initial dose of a primary pertussis vaccination course for children who require simultaneous reinforcement of immunity to diphtheria and tetanus. Vaccination against pertussis should be completed using monovalent pertussis vaccine.

Reinforcing doses: Children who have received the primary course of Adsorbed Diphtheria, Tetanus and Pertussis Vaccine do not require further immunisation against pertussis. Reinforcement of immunity against diphtheria and tetanus is necessary. This can be achieved by giving one dose (0.5 ml) Adsorbed Diphtheria and Tetanus Vaccine (CHILD) after at least three years from the last dose of the primary course. The reinforcing dose is commonly given prior to school entry. A reinforcing dose (0.5 ml) of either Adsorbed Diphtheria and Tetanus Vaccine for Adults and Adolescents or Adsorbed Tetanus Vaccine may be given at 15 to 19 years of age or on leaving school.

Shake well before withdrawing a dose. It is good practice to record title, dose and lot numbers of all vaccines and dates of administration.

*Contra-indications:* Current acute febrile illness (e.g. temperature above 39.5°C).

Progressive degenerative neurological disorder.

Severe local reaction to previous dose of the vaccine or one of its components–an area of erythema, swelling and induration involving most of the antero-lateral thigh or a major part of the circumference of the upper arm.

Severe general reaction to a previous dose of the vaccine or one of its components–for example:

(a) Prolonged inconsolable crying or screaming for over 3 hours.
(b) A convulsion or temperature >40.5°C occurring within 72 hours, for which no other cause was found.
(c) Hypotonia–hyporesponsive episode occurring within 72 hours.
(d) Severe, acute neurological illness occurring within 72 hours.
(e) Immediate allergic reaction (severe or anaphylactic) to a previous dose of Diphtheria, Tetanus or Pertussis Vaccine.

Any child exhibiting a severe local or significant general reaction to a previous dose of a pertussis-containing vaccine should not be given a further dose of pertussis-containing vaccine. However, protection against diphtheria and tetanus is advisable and can be accomplished by giving Adsorbed Diphtheria and Tetanus Vaccine (CHILD).

The vaccine should not be injected intradermally.

ADSORBED DIPHTHERIA, TETANUS AND PERTUSSIS VACCINE SHOULD NOT BE ADMINISTERED TO CHILDREN AGED 10 YEARS AND OVER, ADULTS AND ELDERLY.

*Special warnings and precautions for use:* When there is a family or personal history of febrile convulsions, there is an increased risk of these occurring after pertussis immunisation. In such children, immunisation is recommended but advice on prevention of fever should be given at the time of immunisation.

In a recent British study, children with a personal or

family history of epilepsy were immunised with pertussis vaccine without any significant adverse events. These childrens' developmental progress has been normal. In children with a close family history (first degree relatives) of idiopathic epilepsy there may be a risk of developing this condition irrespective of vaccination. Immunisation is recommended for these children. Children whose epilepsy is well controlled may receive pertussis vaccine.

**Advice on the prevention of fever should be given.** When there is still an evolving neurological problem, immunisation should be deferred until the condition is stable. When there has been a documented history of cerebral damage in the neonatal period, immunisation should be carried out unless there is evidence of an evolving neurological abnormality. A personal or family history of allergy is not a contraindication to immunisation with pertussis nor are stable neurological conditions such as cerebral palsy or spina bifida. Where there is doubt, appropriate advice should be sought from a consultant peadiatrician, district (Health Board) Immunisation coordinator or a consultant in communicable disease control rather than withholding the vaccine. HIV positive individuals may receive pertussis vaccine in the absence of contraindications.

Although anaphylaxis is rare, facilities for its management should always be available during vaccination.

Antipyretic measurs may be indicated in those who experience a febrile convulsion following vaccination.

Use of Adsorbed Diphtheria, Tetanus and Pertussis Vaccine in individuals aged 10 years and over may be associated with severe hypersensitivity reactions.

*Interactions with other medicaments and other forms of interaction:* None stated.

*Pregnancy and lactation:* No reproductive studies have been conducted in animals since simultaneous vaccination against diphtheria, tetanus and pertussis in adults is uncommon. There is no accurate information on the safety of this vaccine in pregnancy therefore this vaccine should not be used in pregnancy or during lactation.

*Effects on ability to drive and use machines:* Not applicable

*Undesirable effects:* Local reactions, particularly erythema at the site of injection, are commonly seen during the 24 hours following vaccination. They normally subside without treatment. A nodule may be found at the site of injection, especially if the inoculation is introduced into the superficial layers of subcutaneous tissue.

A transient rise in temperature, restlessness, irritability, crying or loss of appetite may sometimes occur a few hours after vaccination, but does not generally call for treatment. Systemic reactions such as headache, malaise and somnolence have been reported. Allergic manifestations including pallor, dyspnoea and collapse have been observed rarely.

Neurological events have occasionally been observed following the administration of pertussis-containing vaccines. The events reported do not appear to constitute a single, identifiable clinical syndrome but include isolated febrile convulsions, infantile spasms, episodes of persistent screaming and severe encephalopathy resulting in permanent brain damage or death. These events cannot be distinguished from those occurring in unvaccinated children of similar age. In the absence of a common, identifiable pathological mechanism, it is not possible to produce a reliable estimate of the incidence of neurological events attributable to pertussis vaccination *per se*.

An increased incidence of reactions may occur due to failure to shake the container and re-suspend the vaccine before withdrawing a dose, to inadvertent intravenous administration, or to an over-rapid injection.

Since combined diphtheria, tetanus and pertussis vaccines are widely used in a population in which sudden illnesses of undefined origin are not uncommon, intercurrent illness bearing a temporal but not a causal relationship to vaccination may be expected.

Any untoward reactions should be reported to the regulatory authorities and to the manufacturer.

*Overdose:* Not applicable

**Pharmacological properties** Not applicable

**Pharmaceutical particulars**

*List of excipients:* The excipients contained in the preparation are as follows:-

| | |
|---|---|
| Aluminium hydroxide | HSE |
| Disodium tetraborate (Sodium borate) | BP |
| Succinic acid | HSE |
| Sodium chloride | PhEur |
| Thiomersal | BP |
| Water for injections | PhEur |

HSE House specification

*Incompatibilities:* None stated

---

*Shelf life:* In filled containers: 2 years

*Special precautions for storage* Store between 2 and 8°C. Protect from light. Do not freeze.

*Nature and contents of container:* PhEur type 1 clear neutral glass ampoules, 1 ml capacity (0.5 ml fill).

*Instructions for use/handling:* Vaccine which has been frozen should not be used.

Disposal should be by incineration at a temperature not less than 1100°C at a registered waste disposal contractor.

**Marketing authorisation number** 0039/0474

**Date of approval/revision of SPC** June 1997

**Legal category** POM

## TUBERCULIN PURIFIED PROTEIN DERIVATIVE (PPD) BP

**Qualitative and quantitative composition**
Tuberculin PPD 1000 u/ml.
Tuberculin PPD 100 u/ml.
Tuberculin PPD 10 u/ml.
Control solution for Mantoux test contains no active ingredient.

**Pharmaceutical form** Sterile aqueous solutions for intradermal injection containing Tuberculin PPD BP are prepared from human strains of *Mycobacterium tuberculosis* or sterile aqueous solutions containing Tuberculin PPD BP intended for parenteral administration to human beings.

Control solution for Mantoux Test is a sterile aqueous solution intended for parenteral administration to human beings.

**Clinical particulars**

*Therapeutic indications:* As an intradermal diagnostic test for hypersensitivity to Tubercle bacilli. For use with Mantoux Test only.

*Posology and method of administration:*
*Mantoux Test:* Dose: 0.1 ml by INTRADERMAL INJECTION. The inoculation should preferably be carried out with a syringe fitted with a short bevel gauge 25 or 26 needle.

The skin of the volar surface of the left forearm is cleaned with alcohol and allowed to dry. Using a disposable syringe and needle the dose is administered intradermally so that a bleb is produced, typically of 7 mm diameter.

Routinely one dose (0.1 ml) of 100 units per ml Tuberculin PPD (equivalent to 10 units) is given. If there is any doubt about interpretation of the area of induration produced, a second dose (0.1 ml) of 1000 units per ml Tuberculin PPD (equivalent to 100 units) may be given 3 days later. If that reading is negative, the patient is normally assessed as tuberculin negative.

If there is concern that a person may be hypersensitive to tuberculin or in whom tuberculosis is suspected, a dose (0.1 ml) of 10 units per ml Tuberculin PPD (equivalent to 1 unit) or even less should be given.

A positive reaction is characterised by an area of 5 mm or greater of palpable induration, which may sometimes be surrounded by erythema. The results should be read after 72 hours, but usually a valid reading can be obtained up to 96 hours. Tuberculin positive subjects should not be given BCG vaccine.

Control Solution for Mantoux Test may be used at the same time but at a different site, to assess an individual patient's response to the vehicle used.

A tuberculin skin test must be conducted prior to BCG vaccination in all subjects with the exception of infants aged under three months of age.

*Contra-indications:* Caution should be exercised in giving tuberculin to patients who have, or are suspected of having active tuberculosis. The reaction to the tuberculin skin test may be suppressed by the following factors: ultra-violet light treatment, corticosteroid therapy, immunosuppressive diseases, including HIV, sarcoidosis, Hodgkin's disease, live viral vaccines, glandular fever and viral infections in general, including those of the upper respiratory tract.

Subjects who have a negative test but who may have had a upper respiratory tract or other viral infection at the time of testing should be retested 2–3 weeks after clinical recovery before being given BCG. Tuberculin testing should not be carried out within three weeks of receiving a live viral vaccine.

*Special warnings and precautions for use:* The potency of the Tuberculin PPD may be affected if it is diluted with diluents which differ in composition from the vehicle used in its preparation. Where it is necessary to dilute, Control Solution for Mantoux Test should be used.

Use contents of ampoule as soon as possible and within 1 hour of opening provided adequate aseptic

---

precautions are taken. Care should be taken to avoid contamination of the ampoule contents.

*Interaction with other medicaments and other forms of interaction:* None stated.

*Pregnancy and lactation:* Vaccination with BCG vaccines (INTRADERMAL, INTRADERMAL Isoniazid Resistant and PERCUTANEOUS) should be avoided during early pregnancy and if possible delayed until after delivery. Similarly, use of the tuberculin skin test should be avoided during pregnancy unless subsequent immunisation with BCG vaccine is considered appropriate should the skin test reading be negative.

*Effects on ability to drive and use machines:* No specific warning.

*Undesirable effects:* Nausea, headache, malaise and rash have occasionally been reported after tuberculin skin testing.

Immediate local reactions have been reported following tuberculin testing and these reactions were more common in atopic subjects. Rarely vesicular or ulcerating local reactions, regional adenopathy and fever may occur. Use of a dry dressing may be appropriate with local reactions of this severity.

Lymphangitis and anaphylactic reactions have been reported very rarely.

Tuberculin PPD can cause a severe local reaction in some individuals if the solution is allowed to come into contact with open cuts, the eyes or the mouth. The affected area should be washed with copious quantities of water followed, if necessary, by a topical corticosteroid.

*Overdose:* Not applicable

**Pharmacological particulars** When the Tuberculin protein is injected into the skin a delayed hypersensitivity reaction is induced in persons previously sensitised by micro-organisms of the same species. The active fraction which is predominantly protein is isolated by precipitation.

**Pharmaceutical particulars**

*List of excipients:*
*Tween/Phosphate Buffered Diluent*

| | |
|---|---|
| Polysorbate 80 (Tween 80) | 0.005% v/v |
| Potassium dihydrogen phosphate | 0.138% w/v |
| Disodium hydrogen phosphate | 0.724% w/v |
| Sodium chloride | 0.457% w/v |
| Water for injection | 100.000% v |

*Incompatibilities:* Control solution for Mantoux Test should not be used with tuberculins other than those manufactured by Evans Medical Ltd.

*Shelf life:* Tuberculin PPD 1000 u/ml, 100 u/ml and 10 u/ml shelf life is 12 months when stored unopened. Use contents of ampoule at once and within one hour provided adequate aseptic precautions are taken.

Control solution for Mantoux Test shelf life is 36 months when stored unopened. Use contents of ampoule at once and within one hour provided adequate aseptic precautions are taken.

*Special precautions for storage:* Store between 2°C and 8°C. Do not freeze. Protect from light. Disposal should be by incineration at a temperature not less than 1100°C at a registered waste disposal contractor.

*Nature and contents of container:* Sealed labelled neutral glass ampoules contained within printed cardboard carton and held in position by divided plastic tray.

*Instructions for use and handling:* Use contents of ampoule as soon as possible and within 1 hour of opening provided adequate aseptic precautions are taken. Care should be taken to avoid contamination of the ampoule contents.

**Marketing authorisation numbers**

| | |
|---|---|
| Tuberculin PPD 1000 u/ml | 0039/0440 |
| Tuberculin PPD 100 u/ml | 0039/0441 |
| Tuberculin PPD 10 u/ml | 0039/0442 |
| Control solution for Mantoux Test | 0039/0443 |

**Date of approval/revision of SPC** May 1996

**Legal category** POM

## TUBERCULIN PURIFIED PROTEIN DERIVATIVE (PPD) BP 100 000 U/ML

**Qualitative and quantitative composition** Tuberculin PPD BP 10 x 10⁴ u/ml.

**Pharmaceutical form** Sterile aqueous solutions for intradermal injection containing Tuberculin PPD BP are prepared from human strains of *Mycobacterium tuberculosis* or Sterile aqueous solutions containing Tuberculin PPD BP intended for parenteral administration to human beings.

**Clinical particulars**

*Therapeutic indications:* As an intradermal diagnostic test for hypersensitivity to Tubercle bacilli. For use with the Heaf multiple puncture apparatus only.

*Posology and method of administration:* ***Heaf Test:*** The following preparation is used: **100,000 UNITS PER ML.**

The skin of the volar surface of the left forearm is cleaned with alcohol and allowed to dry. A small amount of the undiluted tuberculin is transferred to the cleaned skin using a syringe needle or loop. The solution is then dispersed over a circular area of skin just larger than the diameter of the perforated head of the Heaf apparatus. The puncture depth of the needles of the Heaf multiple puncture apparatus should be adjusted to give 1 mm for children under two years of age or 2 mm for children aged two years and over and adults.

Holding the apparatus at right angles to the skin, place the end plate firmly and evenly in the centre of the film of tuberculin and press the handle to release the needles. Withdraw the apparatus, wipe off any excess tuberculin solution and observe the presence of six puncture marks (if these are not present the test has not been adequately applied). No dressing need be applied however perfumes and cosmetics should be avoided.

It is very important that the gun is properly sterilised after each application, or sterile disposable end plates may be used.

The test should read between 3 and 10 days. The reaction is graded 0–4 according to the degree of induration produced.

| | |
|---|---|
| Grade 0– | no induration at the puncture sites. |
| Grade 1– | discrete induration at 4 or more needle sites. |
| Grade 2– | induration around each needle site merging with the next, forming a ring of induration but with a clear centre. |
| Grade 3– | the centre of the reaction becomes filled with induration to form one uniform circle of induration 5–10 mm wide. |
| Grade 4– | solid induration over 10 mm wide. Vesiculation or ulceration may also occur. |

Grades 0 and 1 are regarded as negative. Grades 2 to 4 are regarded as positive. Tuberculin positive subjects should not be given BCG vaccine.

A tuberculin skin test must be conducted prior to BCG vaccination in all subjects with the exception of infants aged under three months of age.

*Contra-indications:* Caution should be exercised in giving tuberculin to persons who have, or are suspected of having active tuberculosis. The reaction to the tuberculin skin test may be suppressed by the following factors: ultra-violet light treatment, corticosteroid therapy, immunosuppressive diseases, including HIV, sarcoidosis, Hodgkin's disease, live viral vaccines, glandular fever and viral infections in general, including those of the upper respiratory tract.

Subjects who have a negative test but who may have had an upper respiratory tract or other viral infection at the time of testing should be retested 2–3 weeks after clinical recovery before being given BCG. Tuberculin testing should not be carried out within three weeks of receiving a live viral vaccine.

*Special warnings and precautions for use:* The potency of the Tuberculin PPD may be affected if it is diluted with diluents which differ in composition from the vehicle used in its preparation. Where it is necessary to dilute, Control Solution for Mantoux Test should be used. The Heaf multiple puncture apparatus should be checked at regular intervals to ensure the needles are sufficiently sharp to penetrate the skin.

Use contents of ampoule as soon as possible and within 1 hour of opening provided adequate aseptic precautions are taken. Care should be taken to avoid contamination of the ampoule contents.

*Interaction with other medicaments and other forms of interaction:* None stated.

*Pregnancy and lactation* Vaccination with BCG vaccines (INTRADERMAL, INTRADERMAL Isoniazid Resistant and PERCUTANEOUS) should be avoided during early pregnancy and if possible delayed until after delivery. Similarly, use of the tuberculin skin test should be avoided during pregnancy unless subsequent immunisation with BCG vaccine is considered appropriate should the skin test reading be negative.

*Effect on ability to drive and use machinery:* No specific warning.

*Undesirable effects:* Nausea, headache, malaise and rash have occasionally been reported after tuberculin skin testing.

Immediate local reactions have been reported following tuberculin testing and these reactions were more common in atopic subjects. rarely vesicular of ulcerating local reactions, regional adenopathy and fever may occur. Use of a dry dressing may be appropriate with local reactions of this severity.

Lymphangitis and anaphylactic reactions have been reported very rarely.

Tuberculin PPD can cause a severe local reaction in some individuals if the solution is allowed to come into contact with open cuts, the eyes or the mouth. the affected area should be washed with copious quantities of water followed, if necessary, by a topical corticosteroid.

*Overdose:* Not applicable.

**Pharmacological properties** When the Tuberculin protein is injected into the skin a delayed hypersensitivity reaction is induced in persons previously sensitised by micro-organisms of the same species. The active fraction which is predominantly protein is isolated by precipitation.

**Pharmaceutical particulars**

*List of excipients:*

*Tween/Phosphate Buffered Diluent*

| | |
|---|---|
| Glycerol | 20.00% v/v |
| Phenol | 0.25% w/v |
| Polysorbate 80 (Tween 80) | 0.005% w/v |
| Potassium dihydrogen phosphate | 0.138% w/v |
| Disodium hydrogen phosphate | 0.724% w/v |
| Sodium chloride | 0.457% w/v |
| Water for injection | 100.000% v |

*Incompatibilities:* None stated.

*Shelf life:* Tuberculin PPD 100,000 u/ml shelf life is 24 months when stored unopened. Use contents of ampoule at once and within one hour provided adequate aseptic precautions are taken.

*Special precautions for storage:* Store between 2 and 8°C. Do not freeze. Protect from light. Disposal should be by incineration at a temperature not less than 1100°C at a registered waste disposal contractor.

*Nature and contents of container:* Sealed labelled neutral glass ampoules contained within printed cardboard carton and held in position by divided plastic tray.

*Instructions for use/handling:* Use contents of ampoule as soon as possible and within 1 hour of opening provided adequate aseptic precautions are taken. Care should be taken to avoid contamination of the ampoule contents.

**Marketing authorisation number** 0039/0439

**Date of approval/revision of SPC** October 1995

**Legal category** POM

## VIVOTIF*

**Qualitative and quantitative composition** The composition in terms of active ingredients is as follows:- *Salmonella typhi* Ty21a not less than 2 x $10^9$ viable cells. Quantities expressed per capsule.

**Pharmaceutical form** Enteric coated capsule, for oral administration to humans.

**Clinical particulars**

*Therapeutic indications:* For active oral immunisation against typhoid fever, in children aged 6 years and over, adults and elderly.

*Posology and method of administration:* The blister containing the vaccine capsules should be inspected to ensure that the foil seal and capsules are intact.

*Children aged 6 years and over, adults and elderly:* One capsule is to be swallowed approximately one hour before a meal with a cold or lukewarm (temperature not to exceed body temperature, e.g. 37°C (98.6°F)) drink on alternate days, e.g. days 1, 3 and 5. The vaccine capsule should not be chewed and should be swallowed as soon as possible after placing in the mouth.

A complete immunisation schedule is the ingestion of 3 vaccine capsules as described above. Unless a complete immunisation schedule is followed, an optimum immune response may not be achieved. Not all recipients of Vivotif will be fully protected against typhoid fever. Travellers should take all necessary precautions to avoid contact or ingestion of potentially contaminated food or water.

Protection against typhoid fever commences approximately 7–10 days after ingesting the last dose of vaccine. Under conditions of repeated or continuous exposure to *S.typhi* protection persists for at least 3 years. In the case of travel from a non-endemic to an area where typhoid fever is endemic an annual booster consisting of three doses is to be taken.

*Children:* Safety and efficacy have not been established in children under 6 years of age.

*Use in the elderly:* No special comment.

*Contra-indications:* The vaccine should not be administered to any subject who is known to be hypersensitive to any component of the vaccine or the enteric-coated capsule. Patients with congenital or acquired immune deficiency, including treatment with immunosuppressive or antimitotic drugs, should not be treated.

Vivotif is not to be taken during an acute febrile illness or in the face of acute gastrointestinal illness. Postpone taking the vaccine if persistent diarrhoea or vomiting is occurring.

*Special warnings and precautions for use:* None.

*Interaction with other medicaments and other forms of interaction:* The vaccine should not be administered to individuals receiving sulphonamides or antibiotics since these agents may be active against the vaccine strain and prevent a sufficient degree of multiplication to occur in order to induce a protective immune response.

In the case of simultaneous malaria prophylaxis with mefloquine it is not recommended to take Vivotif and mefloquine on the same day. If they must be taken on the same day, their ingestion should be separated by at least 12 hours. Simultaneous administration of live or inactivated parenterally administered vaccines and of human gamma globulin preparations is not contraindicated.

*Pregnancy and lactation* Animal reproduction studies have not been conducted with Vivotif®. It is not known whether Vivotif can cause foetal harm when administered to pregnant women or can affect reproduction capacity. Vivotif should be given to a pregnant woman only if clearly needed.

There are not data to warrant the use of the product in nursing mothers. It is not known if Vivotif is excreted in human milk.

*Effect on ability to drive and use machinery:* None.

*Undesirable effects:* Transient mild nausea, vomiting, abdominal cramps, diarrhoea, headache, fever, influenza-like illness and urticarial exanthema may occur in less than 1% of all cases.

Although rarely reported, occasional allergic reactions, including anaphylaxis, may occur.

*Overdose:* Doses five-fold higher than the recommended dose do not produce vomiting, acute abdominal distress or fever. However overdosing can increase the possibility of shedding the *S. typhi* Ty21a vaccine in the faeces.

**Pharmacological properties**

*Pharmacodynamic properties:* As a result of irreversible changes in cell wall biosynthesis, the patented Ty21a strain is devoid of pathogenicity but retains its full immunogenic capacity. *S. typhi* is the etiological agent of typhoid fever, an acute febrile enteric disease. This vaccine will not afford protection against species of *Salmonella* other than *S. typhi,* or other bacteria that cause enteric disease.

*Pharmacokinetic properties:* Pharmacokinetic parameters using doses approximately 50 times greater than those in the present vaccine were assessed by taking stool or rectal swabs daily for a period extending 7 days beyond the last dose of vaccine. Sera for determination of antibodies to O, H and Vi antigens were obtained prior to vaccination and biweekly for 8 weeks. The rate of excretion of the vaccine strain in the stools was low, and the vaccine strain could not be recovered from small bowel aspirates one or more days after vaccination. Fourfold or greater responses in titre of 0 antibody only was observed.

There was no correlation between faecal excretion of the strain Ty21a organisms and seroconversion with respect to titre of any of the antibodies tested.

**Pharmaceutical particulars**

*List of excipients:* The excipients contained in the preparation are as follows: Sucrose PhEur, Ascorbic acid PhEur, Casein hydrolysate (Hy-Case Sf Sheffield) HSE, Lactose–fast flow dried USP, Lactose–dried PhEur, Magnesium stearate PhEur, Inactivated *S.typhi* Ty21a Berna cells HSE.

*Capsule:* Gelatin, Titanium dioxide (white), Titanium dioxide (red), Erythosine red No. 3, Ferric oxide (yellow), Ferric oxide (red).

*Capsule coating:* Hydroxypropyl methyl cellulose–phthalate (HP-MCP)–50, Ethylene glycol, Dibutyl phthalate, Diethyl phthalate.

*Incompatibilities:* None known.

*Shelf life: In filled containers:* 15 months from date of packing unopened, at 2-8°C. *After opening container:* Not applicable.

*Special precautions for storage:* Store at 2–8°C.

*Nature and contents of container:* Blister packs (PVC/PVDC 200/40). Each blister pack contains 3 capsules.

*Instructions for use/handling:* No special instructions.

*Product licence holder:* Instituto Sieroterapico Berna s.r.l., Via Bellinzona 39, I-22100 Como, Italy

**Marketing authorisation number** 15747/0001

**Date of approval/revision of SPC** December 1996

**Legal category** POM

*Trade Mark

# Faulding Pharmaceuticals Plc
Spartan Close
Tachbrook Park
Warwick CV34 6RS

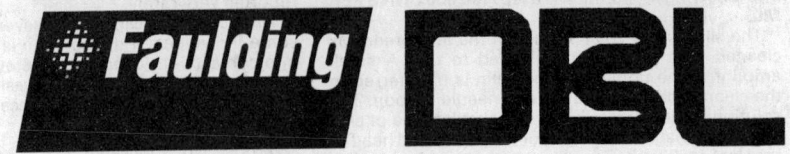

## ACICLOVIR I.V. FOR INTRAVENOUS INFUSION

### Qualitative and quantitative composition

|  | 250 mg/ 10 mL | 500 mg/ 20 mL | 1 g/40 mL |
|---|---|---|---|
| *Active constituent* Aciclovir PhEur | 250 mg | 500 mg | 1 gram |
| *Other constituents* Sodium hydroxide PhEur | 46.45 mg | 92.9 mg | 185.8 mg |
| Water for injections PhEur | to10 ml | to 20 ml | to 40 ml |

**Pharmaceutical form** Aciclovir iv is a clear colourless or almost colourless sterile solution containing the equivalent of 25 mg/ml aciclovir in water for injections b.p; the aciclovir is present as aciclovir sodium. It is available in the following concentrations 250 mg/ 10 ml, 500 mg/20 ml, 1 g/40 ml.

### Clinical particulars

*Therapeutic indications:* Aciclovir i.v. is indicated for the treatment of *Herpes simplex* infections in immunocompromised patients and severe initial genital herpes in the non-immunocompromised.

Aciclovir i.v. is indicated for the prophylaxis of *Herpes simplex* infections in Immunocompromised patients.

Aciclovir i.v. is indicated for the treatment of *Varicella zoster* infections.

Aciclovir i.v. is indicated for the treatment of herpes encephalitis.

Aciclovir i.v. is indicated for the treatment of *Herpes simplex* infections in the Neonate and infant up to 3 months of age.

*Posology and method of administration:* A course of treatment with aciclovir i.v. usually lasts 5 days, but this may be adjusted according to the patient's condition and response to therapy. Treatment for herpes encephalitis and neonatal *Herpes simplex* infections usually lasts 10 days.

The duration of prophylactic administration of aciclovir i.v. is determined by the duration of the period at risk.

*Dosage in adults:* Patients with *Herpes simplex* (except herpes encephalitis) or *Varicella zoster* infectionsshould be given aciclovir i.v in doses of 5 mg/kg bodyweight every 8 hours.

Immunocompromised patients with *Varicella zoster* infections or patients with herpes encephalitis should be given aciclovir i.v in doses of 10 mg/kg bodyweight every 8 hours provided renal function is not impaired. (see dosage in renal impairment).

*Dosage in children:* the dose of aciclovir i.v. for children aged between 3 months and 12 years is calculated on the basis of body surface area.

Children with *Herpes simplex* (except herpes encephalitis) or *Varicella zoster* infections should be given aciclovir i.v in doses of 250 mg per square metre of body surface area every 8 hours.

In immunocompromised children with *Varicella zoster* infections or children with herpes encephalitis, aciclovir i.v. should be given in doses of 500 mg per square metre body surface area every 8 hours if renal function is not impaired.

Children with impaired renal function require an appropriately modified dose, according to the degree of impairment.

The dosage of aciclovir i.v. in neonates and infants up to 3 months of age is calculated on the basis of bodyweight.

Neonates and infants up to 3 months of age with *Herpes simplex* infections should be given aciclovir i.v. in doses of 10 mg/kg bodyweight every 8 hours. Treatment for neonatal *Herpes simplex* infections usually lasts 10 days.

*Dosage in the elderly:* in the elderly, total aciclovir body clearance declines in parallel with creatinine clearance. Special attention should be given to dosage reduction in elderly patients with impaired creatinine clearance. It is recommended that the state of hydration and the creatinine clearance should be evaluated before the administration of high dosages of aciclovir, especially in elderly patients, who may have reduced renal function despite a normal serum creatinine concentration.

Dosage in renal impairment: caution is advised when administering aciclovir i.v. to patients with impaired renal function since the drug is excreted through the kidneys. The following adjustments in dosage are suggested:

| Creatinine clearance | Dosage |
|---|---|
| 25 to 50 ml/min | the dose recommended above (5 or 10 mg/kg bodyweight or 500 mg/m²) should be given every 12 hours. |
| 10 to 25 ml/min | the dose recommended above (5 or 10 mg/kg bodyweight or 500 mg/m²) should be given every 24 hours. |
| 0(anuric) to 10 ml/min | in patients receiving continuous ambulatory peritoneal dialysis (capd) the dose recommended above (5 or 10 mg/kg bodyweight or 500 mg/m²) should be halved and administered every 24 hours. In patients receiving haemodialysis the dose recommended above (5 or 10 mg/kg bodyweight or 500 mg/m²) should be halved and administered every 24 hours and after dialysis. |

*Administration:* the required dose of aciclovir i.v. should be administered by slow intravenous infusion over a one-hour period.

Aciclovir i.v. may be administered by a controlled-rate infusion pump.

For adults, it is recommended that infusion bags containing 100 ml of infusion fluid are used, even when this would give an aciclovir concentration substantially below 0.5% w/v. Thus one 100 ml infusion bag may be used for any dose between 250 mg and 500 mg aciclovir but a second bag must be used for doses between 500 and 1000 mg. Aciclovir injection should not be diluted to a concentration greater than 5 mg/ml (0.5%w/v) for administration by infusion. After addition of aciclovir iv to an infusion solution the mixture should be shaken to ensure through mixing.

For children and neonates, where it is advisable to keep the volume of infusion fluid to a minimum, it is recommended that dilution is on the basis of 4 ml of solution, (100 mg aciclovir), added to 20 ml of infusion fluid.

When diluted in accordance with the recommended schedules, aciclovir i.v. is known to be compatible with the following infusion fluids and stable for up to 24 hours at room temperature, below 25 c:

Sodium chloride intravenous infusion BP 0.9% w/v;
Sodium chloride (0.18% w/v) and glucose (4% w/v) intravenous infusion BP;
Sodium chloride (0.9% w/v) and glucose (5% w/v) intravenous infusion BP;
Compound sodium lactate intravenous infusion BP (hartmann's solution).

Aciclovir i.v. when diluted in accordance with the above schedule will give an aciclovir concentration not greater that 0.5% w/v.

Aciclovir iv contains no preservative. Dilution should therefore be carried out immediately before use and any unused solution should be discarded.

Should any visible turbidity or crystallisation appear in the solution before or during infusion, the preparation should be discarded.

The solution should not be refrigerated as this causes precipitation of crystals.

*Contra-indications:* Aciclovir i.v. is contra-indicated in patients known to be previously hypersensitive to aciclovir.

*Special warnings and special precautions for use:* Aciclovir i.v. is intended for intravenous infusion only and should not be used by any other route.

*Special warnings and special precautions for use*: The dose of aciclovir i.v. must be adjusted in patients with impaired renal function in order to avoid accumulation of aciclovir in the body. Infusions of aciclovir must be given over a period of at least one hour in order to avoid renal tubular damage. (see dosage in renal impairment).

Although the aqueous solubility of aciclovir exceeds 100 mg/ml, precipitation of aciclovir crystals in renal tubules and the consequent renal tubular damage can occur if the maximum solubility of free aciclovir (2.5 mg/ml at 37°C in water) is exceeded. Aciclovir infusions must be accompanied by adequate hydration. Since maximum urine concentration occurs within the first few hours following infusion particular attention should be given to establish sufficient urine flow during that period. Concomitant use of other nephrotoxic drugs, pre-existing renal disease and dehydration increase the risk of further renal impairment by aciclovir.

In patients receiving aciclovir i.v. at higher doses (e.g. For herpes encephalitis), specific care regarding renal function should be taken, particularly when patients are dehydrated or have any renal impairment.

Aciclovir i.v. has a ph of approximately 11.0 and should not be administered by mouth.

*Interaction with other medicaments and other forms of interaction:* Probenecid increases the aciclovir mean half-life and area under the plasma concentration-time curve. Other drugs affecting renal physiology could potentially influence the pharmacokinetics of aciclovir. However, clinical experience has not identified other drug interactions with aciclovir.

*Pregnancy and lactation:* Limited data are available on the use of aciclovir during pregnancy. Aciclovir should not be used during pregnancy unless the potential benefits to the patient outweigh the potential risk to the foetus.

Limited human data show that aciclovir is excreted in human breast milk. Aciclovir should only be administered to nursing mothers if the benefits to the mother outweigh the potential risks to the baby.

*Effects on ability to drive and use machines:* Not applicable.

*Undesirable effects: Renal:* Rapid increases in blood urea and creatinine levels may occasionally occur in patients given aciclovir i.v. these are usually reversible but progression to acute renal failure can occur in rare cases. The rapid increases in blood urea and creatinine levels are believed to be related to peak plasma levels and the state of hydration of the patient. To avoid this effect the drug should not be given as an intravenous bolus injection but by slow infusion over a one hour period. Adequate hydration of the patient should be maintained.

The risk of renal damage is increased by concomitant use of other nephrotoxic drugs and pre-existing renal disease.

Renal impairment developing during treatment with aciclovir i.v. usually responds rapidly to rehydration of the patient and/or dosage reduction or withdrawal of the drug. Progression to acute renal failure, however, can occur in exceptional cases.

*Skin:* Severe local inflammatory reactions or phlebitis have occurred at the injection site sometimes leading to breakdown of the skin. Rashes and hives may occur.

Local necrosis and inflammation have occurred when aciclovir i.v. has been inadvertently infused into extravascular tissues.

*Neurological:* Reversible neurological reactions such as confusion, lethargy, hallucinations, agitation, tremors, somnolence, psychosis, convulsions and coma have been associated with aciclovir i.v. therapy, usually in medically complicated cases.

Therefore aciclovir should be used with caution in patients with underlying neurological abnormalities. It should also be used with caution in patients who have manifested neurological reactions to cytotoxic drugs or are receiving concomitantly interferon or intrethecal methotrexate.

*Other:* Other events reported in patients receiving aciclovir i.v. include increases in liver-related enzymes, fever and decreases in haematological indices (anaemia, thrombocytopenia, leucopoenia).

Aciclovir should be used with caution in patients with significant hypoxia or serious hepatic or electrolyte abnormalities.

Other less frequent adverse effects reported in patients receiving therapy with aciclovir i.v include, diaphoresis, haematuria, hypotension, reversible psychiatric effects and headache, nausea and vomiting.

*Overdose:* Toxicity and treatment of overdosage: There is little experience concerning overdosage with aciclovir however single doses of aciclovir i.v. up to 80 mg/kg bodyweight have been inadvertently administered without adverse effects. Effects of overdosage may be expected to be similar in nature to those described under adverse reactions. Adequate hydration is essential to reduce the possibility of crystal formation in the urine. Aciclovir can be removed from the circulation by haemodialysis.

**Pharmacological properties**

*Pharmacodynamic properties: Mode of action:* aciclovir is a synthetic acyclic purine nucleoside analogue with in vitro and in vivo inhibitory activity against human herpes viruses, including herpes simplex virus types 1 and 2 and varicella zoster virus (vzv), epstein barr virus (ebv) and cytomegalovirus (cmv). In cell culture aciclovir has the greatest antiviral activity against hsv-1, followed (in decreasing order of potency) by hsv-2, vzv, ebv, and cmv.

The inhibitory activity of aciclovir for hsv-1, hsv-2, vzv and ebv is highly selective. The enzyme thymidine kinase (tk) of normal, uninfected cells does not use aciclovir effectively as a substrate, hence toxicity to mammalian host cells is low; however, tk encoded by hsv,vzv and ebv converts aciclovir to aciclovir monophosphate, a nucleoside analogue, which is further converted to the diphosphate and finally to the triphosphate by cellular enzymes. Aciclovir needs to be phosphorylated to the active compound aciclovir triphosphate, in order to become active against the virus. Aciclovir triphosphate acts as an inhibitor of, and a substrate for, the herpes specified dna polymerase preventing further viral dna synthesis.

Animal studies indicate that at high does aciclovir is cytotoxic.

*Pharmacokinetic properties: Pharmacokinetics:* in adults, the terminal plasma half-life of aciclovir after the administration of aciclovir i.v. is about 2.9 hours. Approximately 60% of the drug is excreted unchanged by the kidney. Renal clearance aciclovir is substantially greater than creatinine clearance, indicating that tubular secretion, in addition to glomerular filtration, contributes to the renal elimination of the drug.

When aciclovir is given one hour after 1 gram of probenecid the terminal half-life and the area under the plasma concentration time curve, are extended by 18% and 40% respectively. 9-carboxymethoxymethylguanine is the major significant metabolite of aciclovir and accounts for 10 to 15% of the dose excreted in the urine.

In adults, mean steady state peak plasma concentrations ($c^{ss}max$) following a one-hour infusion of 2.5 mg/kg, 5 mg/kg, 10 mg/kg and 15 mg/kg were 22.7 micromolar (5.1 microgram/ml), 43.6 micromolar (9.8 microgram/ml), 92 micromolar (20.7 microgram/ml) and 105 micromolar (23.6 microgram/ml); respectively. The corresponding trough levels ($c^{ss}min$) 7 hours later were 2.2 micromolar (0.5 microgram/ml), 3.1 micromolar (0.7 microgram/ml) 10.2 micromolar (2.3 microgram/ml), and 8.8 micromolar (2.0 microgram/ml), respectively. In children over 1 year of age similar mean peak ($c^{ss}max$) and trough ($c^{ss}min$) levels were observed when a dose of 250 mg/m$^2$ was substituted for 5 mg/kg and a dose of 500 mg/m$^2$ was substituted for 10 mg/kg. Ir. Neonates (0 to 3 months of age) treated with doses of 10 mg/kg administered by infusion over a one-hour period every 8 hours the $c^{ss}max$ was found to be 61.2 micromolar (13.8 microgram/ml) and the $c^{ss}min$. To be 10.1 micromolar (2.3 microgram/ml).

The terminal plasma half-life in these patients was 3.8 hours. In the elderly, total body clearance falls with increasing age and is associated with decreases in creatinine clearance although there is little change in the terminal plasma half-life.

In patients with chronic renal failure the mean terminal half-life was found to be 19.5 hours. The mean aciclovir half-life during haemodialysis was 5.7 hours. Plasma aciclovir levels dropped approximately 60% during dialysis.

Cerebrospinal fluid levels are approximately 50% of corresponding plasma levels.

Plasma protein binding is relatively low (9 to 33%) and drug interactions involving binding site displacement are not anticipated.

*Preclinical safety data:* The results of a wide range of mutagenicity test in vitro and in vivo indicate that aciclovir is unlikely to pose a genetic risk to man.

Aciclovir was not found to be carcinogenic in long-term studies in the rat and the mouse.

Systemic administration of aciclovir in internationally accepted standard tests did not produce embryotoxic or teratogenic effects in rabbits, rats or mice.

In a non-standard test in rats, foetal abnormalities were observed but only following such high subcutaneous doses that maternal toxicity was produced. The clinical relevance of these findings is uncertain.

Largely reversible adverse effects on spermatogenesis in association with overall toxicity in rats and dogs have been reported only at doses of aciclovir greatly in excess of those employed therapeutically. Two-generation studies in mice did not reveal any effect of (orally administered) aciclovir on fertility.

There is no experience of the effect of aciclovir i.v. on human fertility. Aciclovir tablets have shown to have no definitive effect upon sperm count, morphology or motility in man.

**Pharmaceutical particulars**

*List of excipients:*

| | *250 mg/ 10 mL* | *500 mg/ 20 mL* | *1 g/40 mL* |
|---|---|---|---|
| Sodium hydroxide PhEur | 46.45 mg | 92.9 mg | 185.8 mg |
| Water for injections PhEur | to10 ml | to 20 ml | to 40 ml |

*Incompatibilities:* Aciclovir sodium is reported to be incompatible with solutions of dobutamine hydrochloride, dopamine hydrochloride, amsacrine, fludarabine phosphate, foscarnet sodium, idarubicin hydrochloride, ondansetron hydrochloride, and piperacillin sodium–tazobactam sodium. Diltiazem hydrochloride 5 mg/ml, pethidine hydrochloride 10 mg/ml and morphine sulphate 1 mg/ml cause precipitation, although solutions containing lower concentrations of these drugs are compatible with aciclovir.

Biologic or colloidal fluids (e.g. Blood products, protein containing solutions) are incompatible with aciclovir sodium.

*Shelf life:* 24 months.

*Special precautions for storage:* Store below 25°C.

*Instructions for use/handling:* Aciclovir i.v. contains no preservative. Dilution should therefore be carried out immediately before use and any unused solution should be discarded.

Diluted solutions should not be refrigerated.

**Marketing authorisation number** 4515/0098.

**Date of approval/revision of SPC** May 1997

**Legal category** POM

## AMIKACIN SULPHATE INJECTION

**Qualitative and quantitative composition**

| | |
|---|---|
| Amikacin (as Amikacin Sulphate USP) | 500.0 mg |
| Sodium Citrate BP | 50.0 mg |
| Sodium metabisulphite BP | 4.8 mg |
| Water for Injections BP | 2.0 ml |

**Pharmaceutical form** Each vial contains in 2 ml, amikacin sulphate equivalent to amikacin activity 500 mg.

**Clinical particulars**

*Therapeutic indications:* Amikacin Sulphate Injection is a semi-synthetic, aminoglycoside antibiotic which is active against a broad spectrum of Gram-negative organisms, including pseudomonas and some Gram-positive organisms.

Sensitive Gram-negative organisms include; *Pseudomonas aeruginosa, Escherichia coli*, indole-positive and indole-negative Proteus spp, Klebsiella, Enterobacter and Serratia spp, *Citrobacter freundii*, Salmonella, Shigella, Acinetobacter and Providencia spp.

Many strains of these Gram-negative organisms resistant to gentamicin and tobramycin show sensitivity to amikacin in vitro.

The principal Gram-positive organism sensitive to amikacin is *Staphylococcus aureus*, including some methicillin-resistant strains.

Amikacin is indicated in the short-term treatment of serious infections due to susceptible strains of Gram-negative bacteria, including Pseudomonas species. Although amikacin is not the drug of choice for infections due to staphylococci, at times it may be indicated for the treatment of known or suspected staphylococcal disease. These situations include: the initiation of therapy for severe infections when the organisms suspected are either Gram-negative or staphylococci, patients allergic to other antibiotics, and mixed staphylococcal/Gram-negative infections.

Therapy with amikacin may be instituted prior to obtaining the results of sensitivity testing. Surgical procedures should be performed where indicated.

*Posology and method of administration:* At the recommended dosage level, uncomplicated infections due to sensitive organisms should respond to therapy within 24 to 48 hours.

If clinical response does not occur within two to three days, consideration should be given to alternative therapy.

Amikacin Sulphate Injection can be administered by intramuscular injection or the intravenous route, when either a slow bolus (two to three minutes) or an infusion (0.25% over 30 minutes) maybe used. The dosage is identical for either route of administration and should be used on an estimate of ideal body weight.

If required, suitable diluents for intravenous use are: Normal saline, 5% dextrose in water. Once the product has been diluted the solution must be used as soon as possible and NOT STORED.

*Adults and children*: 15 mg/kg/day in two equally divided doses (equivalent to 500 mg b.i.d.in adults).

*Neonates and premature infants*: In neonates an initial loading dose of 10 mg/kg followed by 15 mg/kg/day in two equally divided doses.

Sufficient extensive clinical use has not been achieved to enable firm dosage guidelines to be given in premature infants.

*Use in elderly*: Amikacin is excreted by the renal route, renal function should be assessed whenever possible and dosage adjusted as described under impaired renal function.

*Life-threatening infections and/or those caused by pseudomonas:* The adult dose may be increased to 500 mg every eight hours but should never exceed 1.5 g/day nor be administered for a period longer than 10 days. A maxium total adult dose of 15 g should not be exceeded.

*Urinary tract infections: (other than pseudomonas infections):* 7.5 mg/kg/day in two equally divided doses (equivalent to 250 mg b.i.d. in adults). As the activity of amikacin is enhanced by increasing the pH, a urinary alkalinising agent may be administered concurrently.

*Impaired renal function:* In patients with impaired renal function, the daily dose should be reduced and/or the intervals between doses increased to avoid accumulation of the drug. A suggested method for estimating dosage in patients with known or suspected diminished renal function is to multiply the serum creatinine concentration (in mg/100 ml) by 9 and use the resulting figure as the interval in hours between doses.

| *Serum creatinine concentration (mg/100 ml)* | | *Interval between Amikacin doses of 7.5 mg/kg/IM (hours)* |
|---|---|---|
| 1.5 | | 13.5 |
| 2.0 | | 18.0 |
| 2.5 | | 22.5 |
| 3.0 | | 27.0 |
| 3.5 | x 9 = | 31.5 |
| 4.0 | | 36.0 |
| 4.5 | | 40.5 |
| 5.0 | | 45.0 |
| 5.5 | | 49.5 |
| 6.0 | | 54.0 |

As renal function may alter appreciably during therapy, the serum creatinine should be checked frequently and the dosage regimen modified as necessary.

*Intraperitoneal use*: Following exploration for established peritonitis, or after peritoneal contamination due to faecal spill during surgery, amikacin may be used as an irrigant after recovery from anaesthesia in concentrations of 0.25% (2.5 mg/ml).

*Other routes of administration*: Amikacin in concentrations 0.25% (2.5 mg/ml) may be used satisfactorily as an irrigating solution in abscess cavities, the pleural space, the peritoneum and the cerebral ventricles.

*Contra-indications:* Patients should be well hydrated during amikacin therapy. In patients with impaired renal function or diminished glomerular filtration amikacin should be used with caution.

If therapy is expected to last seven days or more in patients with renal impairment, or 10 days in other patients, a pre-treatment audiogram should be obtained and repeated during therapy. Amikacin therapy should be stopped if tinnitus or subjective hearing loss develops, or if follow-up audiograms show significant loss of high frequency response.

As with other aminoglycosides, ototoxicity and/or nephrotoxicity can result from the use of amikacin; precautions on dosage and adequate hydration should be observed.

If signs of renal irritation appear (such as albumin, casts, red or white blood cells), hydration should be increased and a reduction in dosage may be desirable. These findings usually disappear when treatment is completed. However, if azotaemia or a progressive decrease in urine output occurs, treatment should be stopped.

The use of amikacin in patients with a history of allergy to aminoglycosides or in patients who may have subclinical renal or eighth nerve damage induced by prior administration of nephrotoxic and/or ototoxic agents such as streptomycin, gentamicin, tobramycin, kanamycin, neomycin, polymyxin B, colistin, cephaloridine, should be considered with caution, as toxicity may be additive. In these patients amikacin should be used only if, in the opinion of the physician, therapeutic advantages outweigh the potential risks.

The risk of ototoxicity is increased when amikacin is used in conjunction with rapidly acting diuretic drugs, particularly when the diuretic is administered intravenously. Such agents include frusemide and ethacrynic acid. Irreversible deafness may result.

The intraperitoneal use of amikacin is not recommended in young children or in patients under the influence of anaesthetics or muscle-relaxing drugs (including ether, halothane, d-tubocurarine, succinylcholine and deca methonium) as neuromuscular blockade and consequent respiratory depression may occur.

*Special warnings and special precautions for use:* In such patients, renal function should be assessed by the usual methods prior to therapy and periodically during therapy. Daily doses should be reduced and/or the interval between doses lengthened in accordance with serum creatinine concentrations to avoid accumulation of abnormally high blood levels and tominimise the risk of ototoxicity. Regular monitoring of serum drug concentration and of renal function is particularly important in elderly patients, who may have reduced renal function that may not be evident in the results of routine screening tests ie. blood urea and serum creatinine.

If signs of renal irritation appear (such as albumin, casts, red or white blood cells), hydration should be increased and a reduction in dosage may be desirable. These findings usually disappear when treatment is completed. However, if azotaemia or a progressive decrease in urine output occurs, treatment should be stopped.

*Interaction with other medicaments and other forms of interaction:* Amikacin sulphate is incompatible with some penicillins and cephalosporins, amphotericin chlorothiazide sodium, erythromycin gluceptate, heparin, nitrofurantoin sodium, phenytoin sodium, thiopentone sodium and warfarin sodium, and depending on the composition and strength of the vehicle, tetracyclines, vitamins of the B group with vitamin C, and potassium chloride.

*Pregnancy and lactation:* The safety of amikacin in pregnancy has not yet been established

*Effects on ability to drive and use machines:* Not applicable.

*Undesirable effects:* When the recommended precautions and dosages are followed the incidence of toxic reactions, such as tinnitis, vertigo, and partial reversible deafness, skin rash, drug fever, headache, paraesthesia, nausea and vomiting is low. Urinary signs of renal irritation (albumen, casts, and red or white cells), azotaemia and oliguria have been reported.

*Overdose:* In the event of overdosage or toxic reaction, peritoneal dialysis or haemodialysis will aid in the removal of amikacin from the blood.

**Pharmacological properties**

*Pharmacodynamic properties:* Amikacin is a semi-synthetic aminoglycoside antibiotic derived from Kanamycin A. It is active against a broad spectrum of Gram-negative organisms, including pseudomonas, Escherichia coli and some Gram-positive organisms, e.g. *Staphylococcus aureus.*

Aminoglycoside antibiotics are bactericidal in action. Although the exact mechanism of action has not been fully elucidated, the drugs appear to inhibit protein synthesis in susceptible bacteria by irreversibly binding to 30S ribosomal subunits.

*Pharmacokinetic properties:* Amikacin is rapidly absorbed after intramuscular injection. Peak plasma concentrations equivalent to about 20 mg/mL are achieved one hour after I.M. doses of 500 mg, reducing to about 2ug/mL 10 hours after injections.

Single doses of 500 mg administered as an intravenous infusion over a period of 30 minutes produce a mean peak serum concentration of 38ug/ml. Repeated infusions do not produce drug accumulation in adults with normal renal function. However, decreased renal function will lead to accumulation

In adults with normal renal function the plasma elimination half-life of amikacin is usually 2-3 hours. 94-98% of a single I.M. or I.V. dose of amikacin is excreted unchanged by glomerular filtration within 24 hours. Urine concentrations of amikacin average 563ug/mL for 6 hours following a single 250-mg I.M. dose and 832ug/mL following a single 500-mg I.M. dose in adults with normal renal function.

Amikacin diffuses readily through extracellular fluids. It has been found in pleural fluid, amniotic fluid and in the peritoneal cavity following parenteral administration.

*Preclinical safety data:* There are no pre-clinical data of relevance to the prescriber which are additional to that already included in other sections of the SPC.

**Pharmaceutical particulars**

*List of excipients:*

| | |
|---|---|
| Sodium Citrate BP | 50.0 mg |
| Sodium metabisulphite BP | 4.8 mg |
| Water for Injections BP | 2.0 ml |

*Incompatibilities:* Amikacin sulphate is incompatible with some penicillins and cephalosporins, amphotericin chlorothiazide sodium, erythromycin gluceptate, heparin, nitrofurantoin sodium, phenytoin sodium, thiopentone sodium and warfarin sodium, and depending on the composition and strength of the vehicle, tetracyclines, vitamins of the B group with vitamin C, and potassium chloride.

*Shelf life:* 36 months shelf life in the medicinal product as packaged for sale.

*Special precautions for storage:* At times, amikacin may be indicated as concurrent therapy with other antibacterial agents in mixed or superinfections. In such instances, amikacin should not be physically mixed with other antibacterial agents in syringes, infusion bottles or any other equipment. Each agent should be administered separately.

Store below 25°C. The solution may darken from colourless to a pale yellow but this does not indicate a loss of potency

**Marketing authorisation number** 4515/0075

**Date of approval/revision of SPC** December 1995

**Legal category** POM

## ATRACURIUM BESILATE INJECTION

**Qualitative and quantitative composition** Atracurium besilate 10 mg/ml

**Pharmaceutical form** Solution for injection

**Clinical particulars**

*Therapeutic indications:* Atracurium Besilate Injection is indicated as an adjunct to general anaesthesia, to facilitate endotracheal intubation and to relax skeletal muscles during surgery or controlled ventilation.

*Posology and method of administration:* Atracurium Besilate Injection should only be administered by intravenous injection. Do not give Atracurium Besilate Injection intramuscularly since this may result in tissue irritation and there are no clinical data to support this route of administration.

To avoid distress to the patient, Atracurium Besilate Injection should not be administered before unconsciousness has been induced. Atracurium Besilate Injection should not be mixed in the same syringe, or administered simultaneously through the same needle, with alkaline solutions (e.g. barbiturate solutions).

In common with all neuromuscular blocking agents, monitoring of neuromuscular function is recommended during the use of Atracurium Besilate Injection in order to individualise dosage requirements.

*Initial bolus doses for intubation:* An initial atracurium besilate dose of 0.3 to 0.6 mg/kg (depending on the duration of full block required), given as an intravenous bolus injection, is recommended. This will provide adequate relaxation for about 15 to 35 minutes.

Endotracheal intubation can usually be accomplished within 90 seconds of the intravenous injection of 0.5 to 0.6 mg/kg. Maximum neuromuscular blockade is generally achieved approximately 3 to 5 minutes after administration. Spontaneous recovery from the end of full block occurs in about 35 minutes as measured by the restoration of the tetanic response to 95% of normal neuromuscular function.

Although atracurium is potentiated by isoflurane or enflurane anaesthesia, the same initial atracurium besilate dose (0.3 to 0.6 mg/kg) may be used for intubation if given prior to the administration of these inhalation agents. However if the initial atracurium dose is administered after steady state anaesthesia with isoflurane or enflurane has been achieved, the dose of atracurium should be reduced by approximately one-third. Smaller dosage reductions may be considered with concomitant halothane anaesthesia since it has only a marginal (approximately 20%) potentiating effect on atracurium.

*Maintenance doses–intermittent IV injection:* During prolonged surgical procedures neuromuscular blockade may be maintained with atracurium besilate maintenance doses of 0.1 to 0.2 mg/kg. The need for maintenance doses should be determined by the individual patient's requirements and response. Successive supplementary dosing does not give rise to accumulation of neuromuscular blocking effect.

*Reversal of neuromuscular blockade:* The neuromuscular blockade induced by atracurium can be reversed with an anticholinesterase agent such as neostigmine or pyridostigmine, usually in conjunction with an anticholinergic agent such as atropine to prevent the adverse muscarinic effects of the anticholinesterase. Under balanced anaesthesia, reversal can be usually be attempted approximately 20 to 35 minutes after the initial atracurium dose, or approximately 10 to 30 minutes after the last atracurium maintenance dose, when recovery of muscle twitch has started. Complete reversal of neuromuscular blockade is usually achieved within 8 to 10 minutes after administration of the reversing agents.

Rare instances of breathing difficulties, possibly related to incomplete reversal, have been reported following attempted pharmacological antagonism of atracurium induced neuromuscular blockade. As with other agents in this class, the tendency for residual neuromuscular block is increased if reversal is attempted at deep levels of blockade or if inadequate doses of reversal agents are employed.

*Use as an infusion:* After the initial atracurium bolus dose, neuromuscular blockade may be maintained during prolonged surgical procedures by administering atracurium besilate as a continuous intravenous infusion at a rate of 0.3 to 0.6 mg/kg/hour. The infusion should not be commenced until early spontaneous recovery from the initial atracurium bolus dose is evident.

Atracurium besilate infusion solutions may be prepared by admixing Atracurium Besilate Injection with an appropriate diluent (see below) to give an atracurium besilate concentration of 0.5 mg/ml to 5 mg/ml.

Atracurium Besilate Injection can be administered by infusion during cardiopulmonary bypass surgery at the recommended infusion rates. Induced hypothermia to a body temperature of 25 to 26°C reduces the rate of inactivation of atracurium, and therefore full neuromuscular block may be maintained with approxyimately half the original infusion rate at these temperatures.

*Compatibility with infusion solutions:*

Atracurium Besilate Injection diluted to 0.5 mg/ml with the following infusion solutions, and stored at 30°C protected from light, was shown to be stable for the times stated below.

| *Infusion Solution* | *Period of stability* |
|---|---|
| Sodium Chloride 0.9% Intravenous Infusion | 24 hours |
| Glucose 5% Intravenous Infusion | 24 hours |
| Glucose 4% and Sodium Chloride 0.18% Intravenous Infusion | 24 hours |
| Ringer's Injection USP | |
| Compound Sodium Lactate Intravenous Infusion | 24 hours |
| (Hartmann's Solution for Injection) | 4 hours |

Atracurium Besilate Injection diluted to 5 mg/ml with the following infusion solutions, and stored at 30°C in 50 ml plastic syringes, was shown to be stable for the times stated below.

| *Infusion Solution* | *Period of stability* |
|---|---|
| Sodium Chloride 0.9% Intravenous Infusion | 24 hours |
| Glucose 5% Intravenous Infusion | 24 hours |
| Glucose 4% and Sodium Chloride 0.18% Intravenous Infusion | 24 hours |
| Ringer's Injection USP | |
| Compound Sodium Lactate Intravenous Infusion | 24 hours |
| (Hartmann's Solution for Injection) | 8 hours |

*Dosage considerations*

*Use in children:* The dosage in children over the age of one month is similar to that in adults on a body weight basis.

*Use in the elderly:* The standard dose of atracurium may be used in elderly patients, however, it is recommended that the initial dose be at the lower end of the range and that it be administered slowly.

*Use in patients with reduced renal and/or hepatic function:* Standard dosages may be used at all levels of renal or hepatic function, including endstage failure.

*Use in patients with cardiovascular disease:* In patients with significant cardiovascular disease the initial dose of atracurium should be administered over a period of 60 seconds.

See also "Special warnings and special precautions for use".

*Contra-indications:* Known or suspected hypersensitivity to the product.

*Special warnings and special precautions for use:* Atracurium Besilate Injection should be used only by those skilled in the management of artificial respiration and only when facilities are immediately available for endotracheal intubation and for providing adequate ventilation support, including the administration of oxygen under positive pressure and the elimination of carbon dioxide. The clinician must be prepared to assist or control ventilation, and anticholinesterase agents should be immediately available for reversal of neuromuscular blockade.

Atracurium has no known effect on consciousness, pain threshold, or cerebration. It should be used only with adequate anaesthesia.

In common with other neuromuscular blocking agents, the potential for histamine release exists in susceptible patients during administration of atracurium besilate. Caution should be exercised in patients with a history suggestive of an increased sensitivity to the effects of histamine.

Do not give Atracurium Besilate Injection by intramuscular administration.

Atracurium Besilate Injection has an acid pH and therefore should not be mixed with alkaline solutions (e.g. barbiturate solutions) in the same syringe or administered simultaneously during intravenous infusion through the same needle. Depending on the resultant pH of such mixtures, Atracurium Besilate Injection may be inactivated and a free acid may be precipitated.

When a small vein is selected as the injection site, Atracurium Besilate Injection should be flushed through the vein with physiological saline after injection. When other anaesthetic drugs are administered through the same indwelling needle or cannula as Atracurium Besilate Injection, it is important that each drug is flushed through with an adequate volume of physiological saline.

Atracurium may have profound effects in patients with myasthenia gravis, Eaton-Lambert syndrome, or other neuromuscular diseases in which potentiation of non-depolarising agents has been noted. A reduced dosage of atracurium and the use of a peripheral nerve stimulator for assessing neuromuscular blockade is especially important in these patients. Similar precautions should be taken in patients with severe electrolyte disorders or carcinomatosis.

Atracurium does not have significant vagal or ganglion blocking properties in the recommended dosage range. Consequently, atracurium will not counteract the bradycardia produced by many anaesthetic agents or by vagal stimulation during surgery. Therefore, bradycardia during anaesthesia may be more common with atracurium than with other muscle relaxants.

As with other non-depolarising neuromuscular blocking agents, resistance to atracurium may develop in patients suffering from burns. Such patients may require increased doses of atracurium depending on the time elapsed since the burn injury and the extent of the burn.

Atracurium Besilate Injection should be administered over a period of 60 seconds to patients who may be unusually sensitive to falls in arterial blood pressure, for example those who are hypovolaemic.

Atracurium Besilate Injection is not suitable for long term use (continuous use over a period of days) for maintenance intubation and muscle paralysis in tetanus, chest trauma, etc. as serum laudanosine levels may accumulate in these situations and thereby may increase the potential for causing CNS excitation.

*Interaction with other medicaments and other forms of interaction:* As with other non-depolarising neuromuscular blocking agents, the magnitude and/or duration of atracurium's effects may be increased as a result of an interaction with the following agents.

*Inhalation anaesthetics:* atracurium is potentiated by isoflurane and enflurane anaesthesia, and only marginally potentiated by halothane anaesthesia.

*Antibiotics:* including the aminoglycosides, polymyxins, spectinomycin, tetracyclines, lincomycin, clindamycin and vancomycin.

*Antiarrhythmic drugs:* lignocaine, procainamide, quinidine

*Beta-blockers:* propranolol.

*Calcium channel blockers:* verapamil

*Diuretics:* frusemide, thiazides, acetazolamide and possibly mannitol.

*Ganglion blocking agents:* trimetaphan, hexamethonium.

*Others:* magnesium sulphate, ketamine, lithium salts and quinine.

The administration of combinations of non-depolarising neuromuscular blocking agents in conjunction with atracurium may produce a degree of neuromuscular blockade in excess of that which might be expected were an equipotent total dose of atracurium administered. Any synergistic effect may vary between different drug combinations.

A depolarising muscle relaxant such as suxamethonium chloride should not be administered to prolong the neuromuscular blocking effects of non-depolarising blocking agents such as atracurium, as this may result in a prolonged and complex block which can be difficult to reverse with anticholinesterase drugs.

Rarely, certain drugs may aggravate or unmask latent myasthenia gravis or actually induce a myasthenic syndrome. Such drugs include various antibiotics, beta-blockers (propranolol, oxprenolol), antiarrhythmic drugs (procainamide, quinidine), antirheumatic drugs (chloroquine, d-penicillamine), trimetaphan, chlorpromazine, steroids, phenytoin and lithium. In these situations a consequent increased sensitivity to atracurium would be expected.

The onset of neuromuscular blockade is likely to be lengthened and the duration of blockade shortened in patients receiving chronic anticonvulsant therapy (e.g. carbamazepine, phenytoin).

*Pregnancy and lactation:* Atracurium crosses the placenta but there have been no demonstrated adverse effects in the foetus or newborn infant. Animal studies have indicated that atracurium has no adverse effects on foetal development. Nevertheless, as with all neuromuscular blocking agents, atracurium should be used during pregnancy only if the potential benefit to the mother outweighs any potential risk to the foetus.

It is not known whether muscle relaxants administered during vaginal delivery have immediate or delayed effects on the foetus or increase the likelihood that resuscitation of the newborn infant will be necessary. The possibility that a forceps delivery will be necessary may increase.

In an open study, atracurium besilate (0.3 mg/kg) was administered to 26 pregnant women during delivery by caesarean section. No harmful effects were attributable to atracurium in any of the newborn infants, although small amounts of atracurium were shown to cross the placental barrier. The possibility of respiratory depression in the newborn infant should always be considered following caesarean section during which a neuromuscular blocking agent has been administered. In patients receiving magnesium sulphate, the reversal of neuromuscular blockade may be unsatisfactory and the atracurium dose should be lowered as indicated.

It is not known whether atracurium is excreted in human milk. Caution should be exercised when Atracurium Besilate Injection is administered to a nursing mother.

*Effects on ability to drive and use machines:* As atracurium is indicated for use with general anaesthetics consideration of the effects of atracurium on the ability to drive and use machines is irrelevant.

*Undesirable effects:*

*Adverse reactions:* During extensive clinical trials atracurium was well tolerated and produced few adverse reactions. As with most neuromuscular blocking agents, the potential exists for adverse reactions suggestive of histamine release in susceptible patients. In clinical trials involving 875 patients, reports of skin flushing ranged from 1% at doses up to 0.3 mg/kg, to 29% at doses of 0.6 mg/kg or greater. The incidence of transient hypotension ranged from 1 to 14% respectively for the corresponding dosages. Other reactions reported included bronchospasm, tachycardia and rarely anaphylactoid reactions.

In large scale atracurium surveillance studies, adverse reactions considered possibly or probably related to atracurium were observed in approximately 10% of patients. Localised skin reactions, generalised flushing and hypotension each occurred in approximately 2 to 3% of patients. Hypertension, tachycardia and bradycardia were observed in approximately 1% of patients. Bronchospasm was reported in approximately 0.2% of patients.

The following adverse reactions have been reported for atracurium:

General: Allergic reactions (i.e. anaphylactic or anaphylactoid responses) which in rare instances were severe (e.g. cardiac arrest), angioneurotic oedema.

Musculoskeletal: Inadequate block, prolonged block.

Cardiovascular: Hypotension, hypertension, vasodilatation (flushing), tachycardia, bradycardia, hypoxaemia.

Respiratory: Dyspnoea, bronchospasm, laryngospasm, wheezing.

Dermatological: Rash, urticaria, generalised erythema, skin flushing, reaction at injection site.

There have been rare reports of seizures in ICU patients following long-term infusion of atracurium to support mechanical ventilation. There are insufficient data to define the contribution, if any, of atracurium and/or its metabolite laudanosine.

*Overdose:* There is limited experience with atracurium overdosage following parenteral administration. The possibility of iatrogenic overdosage can be minimised by carefully monitoring muscle twitch response to peripheral nerve stimulation. Excessive doses of atracurium are likely to produce symptoms consistent with extensions of the usual pharmacological effects. Overdosage may increase the risk of histamine release and adverse cardiovascular effects, especially hypotension. If cardiovascular support is necessary, this should include proper positioning, fluid administration, and the use of vasopressor agents if necessary. It is essential to maintain a patent airway with assisted positive pressure ventilation until spontaneous respiration is adequate. Full sedation will be required since consciousness is not impaired. The duration of neuromuscular blockade may be prolonged and a peripheral nerve stimulator should be used to monitor recovery. Recovery may be hastened by the administration of an anticholinesterase agent such as neostigmine or pyridostigmine in conjunction with an anticholinergic agent such as atropine, once evidence of spontaneous recovery is present.

**Pharmacological properties**

*Pharmacodynamic properties:* Atracurium besilate is a non-depolarising neuromuscular blocking agent with an intermediate duration of action, administered intravenously to produce skeletal muscle relaxation.

Non-depolarising neuromuscular blocking agents antagonise the action of the neurotransmitter acetylcholine by competitively binding with cholinergic receptor sites on the motor endplate of the myoneural junction. These effects may be inhibited or reversed by the administration of anticholinesterases such as neostigmine or pyridostigmine.

The duration of neuromuscular blockade produced by equipotent doses of atracurium is approximately one-third to one-half that induced by tubocurarine and pancuronium, but similar or slightly longer than that induced by vecuronium. As with other non-depolarising neuromuscular blocking agents, the time to onset or paralysis is reduced, and the duration of maximum effect prolonged, with increasing atracurium doses.

The neuromuscular blocking effects of atracurium is enhanced in the presence of potent inhalation anaesthetics. For example, isoflurane and enflurane increase the potency of atracurium and prolong neuromuscular blockade by approximately 35%. However, halothane has only a marginal potentiating effect (approximately 20%) on the action of atracurium.

Repeated administration of atracurium maintenance doses has no cumulative effect on the duration of neuromuscular blockade. Therefore, doses can be administered at relatively regular intervals with predictable results. After an initial atracurium besilate dose of 0.4 to 0.5 mg/kg under balanced anaesthesia, the first maintenance dose (0.08 to 0.10 mg/kg) is generally required within 20 to 45 minutes, and subsequent maintenance doses are usually required at approximately 15 to 25 minute intervals.

Once recovery from atracurium's neuromuscular blocking effects begins, it proceeds more rapidly than recovery from tubocurarine, alcuronium, and pancuronium. Regardless of the atracurium dose, the time from start of recovery (from complete block) to complete recovery (as measured by restoration of the tetanic response to 95% of normal) is approximately 30 minutes under balanced anaesthesia, and approximately 40 minutes under halothane, enflurane or isoflurane anaesthesia. Repeated doses have no cumulative effect on recovery rate.

Reversal of the neuromuscular blocking effects produced by atracurium can be achieved with an anticholinesterase agent such as neostigmine or pyridostigmine, in conjunction with an anticholinergic agent such as atropine. Under balanced anaesthesia, reversal can usually be attempted approximately 20 to 35 minutes after an initial atracurium besilate dose of 0.4 to 0.5 mg/kg, or approximately 10 to 30 minutes after a maintenance dose of 0.08 to 0.10 mg/kg, when recovery of muscle twitch has started. Complete reversal is usually accomplished within 8 to 10 minutes after administration of the reversing agents.

Rare cases of breathing difficulties, possibly related to incomplete reversal, have been reported following attempted pharmacological antagonism of atracurium induced neuromuscular blockade. As with other agents in this class, the tendency for residual neuromuscular block is increased if reversal is attempted at deep levels of blockade or if inadequate doses of reversal agents are employed.

*Pharmacokinetic properties:* The pharmacokinetics of atracurium besilate in humans are essentially linear within the dose range of 0.3 to 0.6 mg/kg. The elimination half-life is approximately 20 minutes. *The duration of neuromuscular blockade produced by atracurium does not correlate with plasma pseudocholinesterase levels and is not altered by the absence of renal function.* This is consistent with the results of *in vitro* studies which have shown that atracurium is inactivated in plasma via two non-oxidative pathways: ester hydrolysis, catalysed by non-specific esterases; and Hofmann elimination, a non-enzymatic chemical process which occurs at physiological pH and body temperature. The rate of Hofmann elimination, which is the principal route of elimination for atracurium, is increased at a higher pH or at higher temperatures, and reduced at a lower pH or lower temperatures. Some placental transfer occurs in humans.

Radiolabel studies demonstrated that atracurium undergoes extensive degradation in cats, and that neither the renal nor hepatic routes play a major role in its elimination. Biliary and urinary excretion were the major routes of excretion of radioactivity (totalling >90% of the labelled dose within 7 hours of dosing), of which atracurium represented only a minor fraction. The metabolites in bile and urine were similar, including products of Hofmann elimination and ester hydrolysis. A major metabolite is laudanosine which accumulates during long-term use (i.e. over a period of days) and has CNS activating properties. In normal use, the levels of laudanosine obtained do not produce any significant pharmacological effects.

The effects of haemodialysis, haemoperfusion and haemofiltration on plasma levels of atracurium and its metabolites are unknown.

With initial atracurium besilate doses up to 0.5 mg/kg, plasma histamine levels were shown to increase by 15% in a dose dependant way, but haemodynamic changes were minor within this dose range. Following the administration of 0.6 mg/kg of atracurium besilate, histamine levels were shown to increase by 92%, and were shown to correlate with a transient (5 minutes) decrease in blood pressure and a brief (2 to 3 minutes) episode of skin flushing. While these effects are of little clinical significance in most patients, the possibility of substantial histamine release at recommended doses must be considered in sensitive individuals, or in patients in whom substantial histamine release would be especially hazardous (e.g. patients with significant respiratory or cardiovascular disease).

It is not known whether the prior use of other non-depolarising neuromuscular blocking agents has any effect on the activity of atracurium. The prior use of suxamethonium reduces the onset (to maximum blockade) by approximately 2 to 3 minutes, and may increase the depth of neuromuscular blockade by atracurium.

*Preclinical safety data:*
*Carcinogenicity/Mutagenicity:* Carcinogenesis and fertility studies have not been performed. However, mutagenicity tests showed that atracurium was non-mutagenic in both the Ames Salmonella assay (at concentrations up to 1000 μg/plate) and in a rat bone marrow cytogenicity assay (at up to paralysing doses). A positive response was observed in the mouse lymphoma assay under conditions (80 and 100 μg/ml, in the absence of metabolic activation) which killed over 80% of the treated cells. There was no mutagenicity at 60 μg/ml and lower, concentrations which killed up to half of the treated cells. A far weaker response was observed in the presence of metabolic activation at concentrations (1200 μg/ml and higher) which also killed over 80% of the treated cells.

Mutagenicity testing is intended to simulate chronic (years to lifetime) exposure in an effort to determine potential carcinogenicity. Thus, a single positive mutagenicity response for a drug used infrequently and/or briefly is of questionable clinical relevance.

**Pharmaceutical particulars**

*List of excipients:* Benzenesulphonic acid and water for injections.

*Incompatibilities:* Atracurium Besilate Injection has an acid pH and therefore should not be mixed with alkaline solutions (e.g. barbiturate solutions) in the same syringe or administered simultaneously during intravenous infusion through the same needle.

*Shelf life:* 18 months

*Special precautions for storage:* Store at 2 to 8°C. Protect from light. Do not freeze.

*Instructions for use/handling:* There are no relevant data additional to the information already included under the section *Posology and method of administration.*

**Marketing authorisation number** 4515/0099

**Date of approval/revision of SPC** 16 January 1997

**Legal category** POM

# CALCIUM LEUCOVORIN INJECTION

**Qualitative and quantitative composition**

| | *3 mg/mL* | *15 mg/2 mL* | *10 mg/mL presentations* |
|---|---|---|---|
| *Active Constituent* | | | |
| Leucovorin Calcium USP | 3.24 mg | 8.1 mg | 10.8 mg |
| Equivalent to Leucovorin USP | 3.0 mg | 7.5 mg | 10.0 mg |
| *Other Constituents* | | | |
| Sodium Chloride BP | 8.6 mg | 8.1 mg | 8.5 mg |
| Water for Injections BP | to 1.0 ml | to 1.0 ml | to 1.0 ml |

There is no overage included in the formulation.

**Pharmaceutical form** Sterile solution for injection.

**Clinical particulars**
*Therapeutic indications:* Calcium Leucovorin is indicated in:

a. Neutralising the immediate toxic effects of folic acid antagonists, e.g. Methotrexate.
b. Calcium Leucovorin Rescue–a treatment technique using Calcium Leucovorin in conjunction with folic acid antagonists, e.g. methotrexate, to minimise systemic toxicity.
c. The treatment of megaloblastic anaemias due to sprue, nutritional deficiency, pregnancy, infancy, liver disease and malabsorption syndrome.
d. Enhancement of 5-Fluorouracil cytotoxicity in the treatment of advanced colorectal cancer.

*Posology and method of administration:*
*Adults and children:* Calcium Leucovorin may be given parenterally by intramuscular injection, intravenous injection or intravenous infusion. When required for intravenous infusion, it may be diluted with 5% glucose injection of 0.9% sodium chloide injection. Such solutions are stable for 24 hours when stored below 25°C.

Treatment of Overdosage of Folic Acid Antagonists: In cases of overdosage of folic acid antagonists, Calcium Leucovorin maybe administered by intravenous infusion in doses of up to 75 mg within 12 hours, followed by 12 mg intramuscularly every 6 hours for 4 doses.

In general, where overdosage is suspected, the dose of Calcium Leucovorin should be equal to or greater than the offending dose of the folic acid antagonist administered, and should be given as soon as possible; preferably within the first hour and certainly within 4 hours after which it may not be effective.

Calcium Leucovorin Rescue: Calcium Leucovorin may be used in conjunction with folic acid antagonists, e.g. methotrexate, to reduce their systemic toxicity. It is given 12 to 24 hours after the antineoplastic drug. Doses of up to 120 mg may be given over 12 to 24 hours by intramuscular injection or intravenous injection or infusion, followed by 12 to 15 mg intramuscularly, or 15 mg orally, every 6 hours for the next 48 hours. With lower doses of methotrexate, leucovorin 15 mg orally every 6 hours for 48 to 72 hours may be sufficient.

Treatment of Megaloblastic Anaemia: The dose should not exceed 1 mg daily given intramuscularly. When given orally, the recommended dosage is one Calcium Leucovorin Tablet (15 mg) daily. Children up to 12 years: 0.25 mg/kg/day. Normal adult dosage: 10-20 mg daily.

Enhancement of 5-Fluorouracil cytotoxicity in advanced colorectal cancer. Adults and the Elderly: Administration: Calcium Leucovorin Injection should be used to administer the high doses of calcium leucovorin required in combination regimens.

When used in combination regimens with 5-FU, calcium leucovorin should only be given by the intravenous route. The agents should not be mixed together.

*Dosage:* Various combination regimens have been studied and based on the available clinical evidence the following regimen has been found to be effective in advanced colorectal carcinoma:

Calcium leucovorin given at a dose of 200 mg/m² by slow intravenous injection, followed immediately by 5-FU at an initial dose of 370 mg/m² by intravenous injection. The injection of leucovorin should not be given more rapidly than over 3-5 minutes because of the calcium content of the solution. This treatment is repeated daily for 5 consecutive days. Subsequent courses may be given after a treatment-free interval of 21-28 days.

For the above regimen, modification of the 5-FU dosage and the treatment-free interval may be necessary depending on patient condition, clinical response and dose limiting toxicity. A reduction of Calcium leucovorin dosage is not required. The number of repeat cycles used is at the discretion of the clinician.

On the basis of the available data, no specific dosage modifications are recommended in the use of the combination regimen with 5-FU in the elderly. However, particular care should be taken when treating elderly or debilitated patients as these patients are at increased risk of severe toxicity with this therapy.

Children: There are no data available on the use of this combination in children.

*Contra-indications:* Calcium Leucovorin Injection is contra-indicated in the treatment of pernicious anaemia or other megaloblastic anaemias where vitamin $B_{12}$ is deficient. Its use can lead to an apparent response of the haematopoietic system, but neurological damage may occur or progress if already present.

*Special warnings and special precautions for use:*
*Warnings:* In the treatment of inadvertent overdosage of a folic acid antagonist, leucovorin should be administered as soon as possible; if a period exceeding 4 hours intervenes, the treatment may not be effective.

In the combination regimen with 5-FU, the toxicity profile of 5-FU is enhanced by calcium leucovorin. The commonest manifestations are leucopenia, mucositis, stomatitis and/or diarrhoea which may be dose limiting. When calcium leucovorin and 5-FU are used in the treatment of colorectal cancer, the 5-FU dosage must be reduced more in cases of toxicity than when 5-FU is used alone. Toxicities observed in patients treated with the combination are qualitatively similar to those observed in patients treated with 5-FU alone. Gastrointestinal toxicities are observed more commonly and may be more severe or even life threatening. In severe cases, treatment is withdrawal of 5-FU and calcium leucovorin, and supportive intravenous therapy. Elderly or debilitated patients are at a greater risk of severe toxicity with this therapy.

*Precautions:* In general, Calcium Leucovorin should not be given simultaneously with folicacid antagonists, e.g. methotrexate, to abort clinical toxicity as the therapeutic effect of the antagonist may be nullified. However, Calcium Leucovorin given concurrently with folate antagonists, such as pyrimethamine and trimethoprim does not inhibit their antibacterial activity.

Parenteral administration of leucovorin is preferable to oral dosing following chemotherapy with folic acid antagonists if there is a possibility that the patient may vomit and not absorb the leucovorin.

Calcium Leucovorin Injection should be given with haematological control.

*Interaction with other medicaments and other forms of interaction:* Not applicable.

*Pregnancy and lactation:* Animal reproduction studies have not been performed with Leucovorin. It is also not known whether Leucovorin can cause foetal harm, when administered to pregnant women. Leucovorin should be used during pregnancy only when clearly needed.

Since it is not known if Leucovorin is distributed into milk, the drug should be used with caution in nursing women.

*Effects on ability to drive and use machines:* Not applicable.

*Undesirable effects:* Adverse reactions are rare but occasional allergic reactions have been reported; pyrexia has occurred after parenteral administration.

*Overdose:* Not applicable.

**Pharmacological properties**
*Pharmacodynamic properties:* Leucovorin is a derivative of tetrahydrofolic acid, the reduced form of folic acid, which is involved as a cofactor for 1-carbon transfer reactions in the biosynthesis of purine and pyrimidines of nucleic acids.

Impairment of thymidylate synthesis in patients with folic acid deficiency is thought to account for the defective DNA synthesis that leads to megaloblast formation and megaloblastic and macrocytic anaemias. Because of its ready conversion to other tetrahydrofolic acid derivatives, Leucovorin is a potent antidote for both hematopoietic and reticuloendothelial toxic effects of folic acid antagonists, (e.g. Methotrexate, Pyrimethamine, Trimethoprim). It is postulated that in some cancers, Leucovorin enters and 'rescues' normal cells from the toxic effects of folic acid antagonists, in preference to tumour cells, because of a difference in membrane transport mechanisms; this principle is the basis of high-dose Methotrexate therapy with 'Leucovorin rescue'.

*Pharmacokinetic properties:* Absorption and distribution: In vivo, Leucovorin Calcium is rapidly and extensively converted to other tetrahydrofolic acid derivatives including 5-methyl tetrahydrofolate, which is the major transport and storage form of folate in the body.

Normal total serum folate concentrations have been reported to range from 0.005-0.015 mcg/mL. Folate is actively concentrated in CSF, and normal CSF concentrations are reported to be about 0.016-0.021 mcg/mL. Normal erythrocyte folate concentrations range from 0.175-0.316 mcg/mL.

In general, serum folate concentrations less than 0.005 mcg/mL indicate folate deficiency and concentrations less than 0.002 mcg/mL usually result in megaloblastic anaemia. Following i.m. administration of a 15 mg (7.5 mg/m²) dose in healthy men, mean peak serum folate concentrations of 0.241 mcg/mL occur within about 40 minutes. Following oral administration of a 15 mg (7.5 mg/m²) dose in healthy men, mean peak serum folate concentrations of 0.268 mcg/mL occur within about 1.72 hours. Areas under the serum folate concentration-time curves (AUCs) are reported to be about 8% less following i.m. injection in the gluteal region than in the deltoid region and about 12% less following i.m. injection in the gluteal region than following i.v. or oral administration.

Tetrahydrofolic acid and its derivatives are distributed to all body tissues; the liver contains about one-half of total body folate stores. In a small number of patients, biliary concentration of folates was about 4.5 times the plasma folate concentration after oral administration of a 2 mg dose of Leucovorin; this is believed to represent the hepatic folate pool rather than excretion of the administered dose.

Elimination: Leucovorin is excreted in urine, mainly as 10-formyl tetrahydrofolate and 5, 10-methenyl tetrahydrofolate. There is some evidence that 5-methyltetrahydrofolate may be conserved by the kidneys in preference to 5-formyltetrahydrofolate (Leucovorin). Loss of folate in the urine becomes approximately logarithmic as the amount of Leucovorin administered exceeds 1 mg.

**Pharmaceutical particulars**

*List of excipients:*

| | 3 mg/mL | 7.5 mg/mL | 10 mg/mL |
|---|---|---|---|
| Sodium Chloride BP | 8.6 mg | 8.1 mg | 8.5 mg |
| Water for Injections BP | to 1.0 mL | to 1.0 mL | to 1.0 mL |

There is no overage included in the formulation.

*Incompatibilities:* Immediate precipitation results when combined with Droperidol in syringe.

*Shelf life:* 24 months.

*Special precautions for storage:* Store 2°C-8°C. Protect from light.

Ampoules and Vials of Calcium Leucovorin do not contain a preservative. They should be used once and discarded.

*Instructions for use/handling:* Not applicable.

**Marketing authorisation number** 4515/0032.

**Date of approval/revision of SPC** February 1997

**Legal category** POM

## CARBOPLATIN INJECTION SOLUTION 10MG PER ML

**Qualitative and quantitative composition**

| | per unit dose | | per vial | |
|---|---|---|---|---|
| Carboplatin | 10 mL | 50 mg | 150 mg | 450 mg |
| Water for Injection BP | 1.0 mL | 5.0 mL | 15.0mL | 45.0mL |

**Pharmaceutical form** Aqueous solution for injection.

**Clinical particulars**

*Therapeutic indications:* Antineoplastic agent indicated in the treatment of ovarian carcinoma of epithelial origin or in the treatment of small cell lung carcinoma.

*Posology and method of administration:* The recommended dose of Carboplatin in previously untreated adults with normal renal function is 400 mg/m2 given as a single short term intravenous infusion over 15 to 60 minutes. Therapy should not be repeated until 4 weeks after the previous Carboplatin course.

Initial dosage should be reduced by 20-25% in patients with risk factors such as previous myelosuppressive therapy and/or poor performance status.

Determination of haematologic nadir by weekly blood counts during initial courses is recommended for future dosage adjustment and scheduling of Carboplatin.

*Impaired renal function:* In patients with impaired renal function dosage of Carboplatin should be reduced and haematological nadirs and renal function monitored.

A suggested dosage schedule based on creatinine clearance is as follows:

| *Creatinine Clearance (ml/min)* | *Dosage of Carboplatin* |
|---|---|
| 40 ml per minute | 400 mg per square metre |
| 20–39 ml per minute | 250 mg per square metre |

*Elderly:* Dosage adjustment may be necessary in elderly patients and also in patients receiving combination chemotherapy.

*Children:* Specific dosage recommendations for use in children and infants cannot be made due to insufficient use in paediatrics at this time.

*Contra-indications:* Carboplatin is contra-indicated in patients with severe myelosuppressions, preexisting severe renal impairment (with creatinine clearance of less than 20 ml per minute) and a history of severe allergic reaction to Carboplatin, other platinum containing compounds or Mannitol. Dosage adjustment may allow use in the presence of mild renal impairment (See *Posology and method of administration*).

*Special warnings and special precautions for use:*

*Warnings:* Myelosuppression as a result of Carboplatin treatment is closely related to the renal clearance of the drug. Therefore, in patients with abnormal renal function, or who are receiving concomitant therapy with nephrotoxic drugs, myelosuppression, especially thrombocytopenia, may be more severe and prolonged.

The occurrence, severity and protraction of toxicity is likely to be greater in patients who have received extensive prior treatment for their disease, have poor performance status and are advanced in years. Renal function parameters should be assessed prior to, during, and after Carboplatin therapy. Peripheral blood counts (including platelets, white blood cells and haemoglobin) should be followed during and after therapy. Combination therapy with other myelosuppressive drugs may require modification of dosage/timing of schedules in order to minimize additive effects.

Carboplatin courses should not, in general, be repeated more frequently than every 4 weeks in order to ensure that the nadir in blood counts has occurred and there has been recovery to a satisfactory level.

Precautions:

Carboplatin should only be administered under the supervision of a qualified physician who is experienced in the use of chemotherapeutic agents. Diagnostic and treatment facilities should be readily available for management of therapy and possible complications.

Peripheral blood counts and renal function tests should be monitored closely. Blood counts should be performed prior to commencement of Carboplatin therapy, and at weekly intervals thereafter. This will monitor toxicity and help determine the nadir and recovery of haematological parameters, and assist in subsequent dosage adjustments. Lowest levels of platelets are generally seen between days 14 and 21 of initial therapy. A greater reduction is seen in patients who previously received extensive myelosuppressive chemotherapy. Lowest Levels of white cells occur generally between days 14 and 28 of initial therapy. If levels fall below 2000 cells/mm3 or platelets less than 50,000 cells/mm3 then postponement of Carboplatin therapy until bone marrow recovery is evident, should be considered. This recovery usually takes 5 to 6 weeks. Transfusions may be necessary and dosage reductions recommended for subsequent treatment.

Renal toxicity is not usually dose limiting. Pretreatment and post-treatment hydration is not necessary. However, about 25% of patients show a decrease in creatinine clearance and, less frequently, a rise in serum creatinine and blood urea nitrogen. Impairment of renal function is more likely in patients who have previously experienced nephrotoxicity as a result of Cisplatin therapy.

Neurological evaluation and an assessment of hearing should be performed on a regular basis. Neurotoxicity, such as parasthesia, decreased deep tendon reflexes, and ototoxicity are more likely seen in patients previously treated with Cisplatin.

Aluminium containing equipment should not be used during preparation and administration of Carboplatin (see *Interactions*).

*Interaction with other medicaments and other forms of interaction:* Carboplatin may interact with aluminium to form a black precipitate. Needles, syringes, catheters or IV administration sets that contain aluminium parts which may come into contact with Carboplatin should not be used for the preparation or administration of the drug.

Concurrent therapy with nephrotoxic drugs may increase or exacerbate toxicity due to Carboplatin induced changes in renal clearance.

Combination therapy with other myelosuppressive agents may require dose changes or rescheduling of doses in order to minimise the additive myelosuppressive effects.

*Pregnancy and lactation:* Safe use of Carboplatin in pregnancy has not been established and its use is not recommended during pregnancy. It is not known whether Carboplatin is excreted in breast milk. To avoid possible harmful effects in the infant, breast feeding is not advised during Carboplatin therapy.

*Effects on ability to drive and use machines:* None known.

*Undesirable effects:*

*Adverse reactions:* Myelosuppression is the dose limiting toxic reaction of Carboplatin. It is generally reversible and not cumulative when Carboplatin is used as a single agent at recommended frequencies of administration. Adverse reactions which have occurred in studies to date can be grouped under the following systems:

Haemopoietic System: Leucopenia (55%), thrombocytopenia (32%) and anaemia (59%) of patients. Transfusion support has been required in about 20% of patients.

Gastrointestinal System: Nausea and vomiting (53%), nausea only in 25%. Nausea and vomiting are generally delayed until 6 to 12 hours after administration of Carboplatin, are readily controlled or prevented with antiemetics and disappear within 24 hours. Diarrhoea occurred in 6% and constipation in 3% of patients.

Renal System: Creatinine clearance decreased in 25% of patients. Increases in uric acid (25%), blood urea nitrogen (16%) and serum creatinine (7%).

Biochemistry: Decreased serum levels of Magnesium (37% patients), potassium (16% patients) and calcium (5% patients) have occurred although not severe enough to cause clinical symptoms.

Neurotoxicity: Mild peripheral neuropathy occurred in 6% of patients and dysgeusia in less than 1% of patients. Parasthesias present prior to treatment, especially if caused by Cisplatin, may persist or worsen during Carboplatin therapy. (See Precautions).

Ototoxicity: A subclinical decrease in hearing acuity in the high frequency range (4000-8000 Hz), determined by audiogram, occurred in 15% of patients. Clinical ototoxicity also manifested itself as tinnitus (1% of patients). Hearing loss as a result of Cisplatin therapy may give rise to persistent or worsening symptoms.

Hepatic System: Transient increases in liver enzymes have been reported in some patients. Alkaline phosphatase was increased in 30% of patients, with aspartate aminotransferase (15% patients) and elevated serum bilirubin (4% patients) occurring less frequently.

Allergic Reactions: Erythematous rash, fever and pruritis have been observed in less than 2% of patients treated. These were reactions similar to those seen after Cisplatin therapy but in a few cases no cross-reactivity was present.

Other Reactions: Rare events have included alopecia (2%), a flu-like syndrome (1%) and reaction at the injection site (<1%).

*Overdose:* No overdosage occurred during clinical trials. If necessary, however, the patient may need supportive treatment relating to myelosuppression, renal and hepatic impairment. Reports of doses up to 1600 mg/m2 indicate patients feeling extremely ill with diarrhoea and alopecia developing.

**Pharmacological properties**

*Pharmacodynamic properties:* Carboplatin, like Cisplatin, interferes with DNA intrastrand and interstrand crosslinks in cells exposed to the drug. DNA reactivity has been correlated with cytotoxicity.

*Pharmacokinetic properties:* After a 1 hour infusion (20-520 mg/m²) plasma levels of total platinum and free (ultrafilterable) platinum decay biphasically following first order kinetics. For free platinum the initial phase (t alpha) half life is approximately 90 minutes, and the later phase (t beta) half life approximately 6 hours. All free platinum is in the form of Carboplatin in the first 4 hours after administration.

Carboplatin is excreted primarily by glomerular filtration in urine, with recovery of 65% of a dose within 24 hours. Most of the drug is excreted within the first 6 hours. Approximately 32% of a given dose of Carboplatin is excreted unchanged.

Protein binding of Carboplatin reaches 85-89% within 24 hours of administration although during the first 4 hours only up to 29% of the dose is protein bound. Patients with poor renal function may require dosage adjustments due to altered pharmacokinetics of Carboplatin.

**Pharmaceutical particulars**

*List of excipients:* Water for Injection BP

*Incompatibilities:* Aluminium-containing equipment should not be used (see *Interactions*).

*Shelf life:* A shelf life of 24 months when stored below 25˚C and protected from light.

*Special precautions for storage:* Store below 25˚C. Protect from light.

Carboplatin Injection Solution may be further diluted in Glucose 5% or Sodium Chloride 0.9% BP and administered as an intravenous infusion. This infusion solution is chemically stable for 24 hours when stored at room temperature.

The reconstituted solution should be prepared immediately before use and is stable for 24 hours at room temperature. The solution contains no preservative and any unused portion should be discarded immediately.

*Instructions for use/handling:*
*Handling:* Carboplatin should be prepared for administration only by professionals who have been trained in the safe use of chemotherapeutic agents.

Reconstitution of the powder and transfer to syringes and infusion containers should be carried out only in the designated area. Personnel carrying out these procedures should be adequately protected with clothing, gloves, and an eye shield.

Pregnant personnel are advised not to handle chemotherapeutic agents.

*Contamination:* In the event of contact of Carboplatin with eyes or skin, wash the affected area with copious amounts of water or Normal Saline. A bland cream may be used to treat transient stinging of skin. Medical advice should be sought if the eyes are affected.

In the event of spillage, two operators should put on gloves and mop up the spilled material with a sponge kept for that purpose. In the event of powder spillage, cover with a cloth and moisten with water before mopping up. Rinse the area twice with water. Put all solutions and sponges in a plastic bag, seal and label with the words 'CYTOTOXIC WASTE' and incinerate.

*Disposal:* Syringes, containers, absorbent materials, solutions and any other material which has come into contact with Carboplatin should be placed in a thick plastic bag or other impervious container and incinerated at 1000˚C.

**Marketing authorisation number**   4515/0050

**Date of approval/revision of SPC**   June 1995

**Legal category**   POM

# CISPLATIN INJECTION SOLUTION

## Qualitative and quantitative composition

|  | 10 mg | 50 mg | 100 mg |
|---|---|---|---|
| *Active Constituent* Cis-Diammine Dicloroplatinum (II) HSE | 10.0 mg | 50.0 mg | 100.0 mg |
| *Other Constituents* Mannitol BP | 10.0 mg | 50.0 mg | 100.0 mg |
| Sodium Chloride BP | 90.0 mg | 450.0 mg | 900.0 mg |
| Dilute Hydrochloric Acid BP | QS | QS | QS |
| Water for Injections BP to: | 10.0 ml | 50.0 ml | 100.0 ml |

There is no overage included in the above formulations.

**Pharmaceutical form** A sterile, clear, colourless to pale yellow preservative-free solution free from visible particulates.

## Clinical particulars
*Therapeutic indications:* Cisplatin is indicated in metastatic, non-seminomatous germ cell carcinoma, advanced stage and refractory ovarian carcinoma, advanced stages and refractory bladder carcinoma and squamous cell carcinoma of head and neck.

Cisplatin is indicated in combination with other antineoplastic agents for the treatment of metastatic testicular tumours. The combination of Cisplatin, Vinblastine and Bleomycin is reported to be highly effective.

*Posology and method of administration:*
*Adults and children:* Cisplatin should be administered by I.V. infusion over a 6-8 hour period. The recommended dose of Cisplatin in adults and children is 50 to 100 mg/m² as a single I.V. dose every 3 to 4 weeks, or 15 to 20 mg/m² intravenously daily for 5 days every 3 to 4 weeks.

Interaction with aluminium:
Cisplatin may interact with metal aluminium to form a black precipitate of platinum. All aluminium-containing I.V. sets, needles, catheters and syringes should be avoided.

1. Pretreatment Hydration: Pretreatment hydration is required to induce diuresis during (and after) Cisplatin administration. This hydration is achieved by giving 2 litres of either 0.9% Sodium Chloride or Dextrose 4% in one-fifth Normal Saline (0.18%) over a 2-hour period. During the last 30 minutes of the pre-treatment hydration or after the hydration, administer by side arm drip 37.5 g of Mannitol (i.e., 375 ml of Mannitol 10% Injection).
2. Preparation of Cisplatin Infusion: Cisplatin Injection Solution 1 mg/mL may be diluted in 2 litres of 0.9% Sodium Chloride Injection. Do not refrigerate solutions.
3. Treatment: Following prehydration, administer the Cisplatin infusion over 1 to 2 hours. It has been proposed that a longer infusion time of 6 to 8 hours may decrease the gastrointestinal and renal toxicities. The container should be covered to exclude light. Discard remaining contents after use.
4. Post Treatment Hydration: Continue I.V. hydration with the aim of administering another 2 litres of Sodium Chloride 0.9% Injection, or Dextrose 4% in Sodium Chloride 0.18% Injection, over a period of 6 to 12 hours.

*Contra-indications:* Cisplatin may give allergic reactions in some patients. Use is contraindicated in those patients with a history of allergic reaction to Cisplatin or other platinum containing compounds. Cisplatin induces nephrotoxicity which is cumulative. It is therefore contraindicated in patients with renal impairment. The serum creatinine BUN and creatinine clearance should be measured prior to initiating therapy and monitored throughout treatment with Cisplatin. To reduce nephrotoxicity of Cisplatin treatment pretreatment hydration prcedures, together with maintenance of hydration and urinary output during the 24 hours following administration are necessary.

Cisplatin has been shown to be cumulatively ototoxic and should not be given to patients with hearing impairment. It is recommended that hearing function should be monitored prior to and during treatment with Cisplatin. Cisplatin is also contraindicated in myelosuppressed patients.

*Special warnings and precautions for use:*
*Warnings and precautions:* Cisplatin must only be used by physicians experienced in cytotoxic chemotherapy.

Cisplatin reacts with metallic aluminium to form a black precipitate of platinum. All aluminium containing I.V. sets, needles, catheters and syringes should be avoided.

The solution for infusion should not be mixed with other drugs or additives.

*Interactions with other medicaments and other forms of interaction:* Cisplatin and antihypertensive therapy with Frusemide, Hydralazine Diazoxide and Propanolol have been reported to cause nephrotoxicity.

Cisplatin may interact with aluminium. See *Dosage and Administration.*

*Pregnancy and lactation:*
*Use in pregnancy:* The safe use of Cisplatin in human pregnancy has not been established. Cisplatin has been shown to be mutagenic in bacteria. It produces chromosome aberrations in tissue-cultures of animal cells and is teratogenic and embryotoxic in mice.
*Use in lactation:* Cisplatin should not normally be administered to mothers who are breastfeeding.

*Effects on ability to drive and use machines:* Not applicable.

*Undesirable effects:*
1. Nephrotoxicity: Renal toxicity has been shown in 28-38% of patientstreated with a single dose of Cisplatin 50 mg/m². Renal toxicity becomes more prolonged and severe with repeated courses of the drug. Renal function must be restored before additional Cisplatin therapy is used.
2. Ototoxicity: Ototoxicity has occurred in up to 31% of patients treated with a single dose of Cisplatin 50 mg/m². Ototoxicity may be more severe in children and more frequent and severe with repeated doses.
3. Haemotoxicity: Myelosuppression is observed in about 30% of patients treated with Cisplatin. Leucopenia and thrombocytopenia are more pronounced at higher doses.
4. Myelosuppression: This may occur in patients treated with Cisplatin. The nadirs in circulating platelets and leucocytes generally occur between days 18-32 (range 7.3 to 45) with most patients recovering by day 39 (range 13 to 62). Leucopenia and thrombocytopenia are more pronounced at doses greater than 50 mg/m². Anaemia (decreases of greater than 2 g% haemoglobin) occurs at approximately the same frequency, but generally with a later onset than leucopenia and thrombocytopenia. Subsequent courses of Cisplatin should not be instituted until platelets are present at levels greater than 100.000/mm² and white cells greater than 4.000/mm². A high incidence of severe anaemia requiring transfusion of packed red cells has been observed in patients receiving combination chemotherapy including Cisplatin.
5. Anaphylaxis: Reactions possibly secondary to Cisplatin therapy have been occasionally reported in patients who were previously exposed to Cisplatin. Patients who are particularly at risk are those with a prior history or family history of atopy. Facial oedema, wheezing, tachycardia, hypotension and skin rashes of urticarial non-specific maculopapular type can occur within a few minutes of administration. Serious reactions seem to be controlled by I.V. adrenaline, corticosteroids or antihistamines.
6. Hypomagnesaemia and Hypocalcaemia: Hypomagnesaemia occurs quite frequently with Cisplatin administration, while hypocalcaemia occurs less frequently. The loss of magnesium seems to be associated with renal tubular damage which prevents resorption of this cation. Where both electrolytes are deficient, tetany may result. It does not appear to be dose related. Monitoring of electolytes is necessary.
7. Neurotoxicity and Seizures: Peripheral neuropathy, postural hypotension and seizures may occur with Cisplatin administration. This appears to be common after Cisplatin administration. The development of clinically significant symptoms should generally contra-indicate further Cisplatin usage.

*Overdose:* Overdosage can be expected to cause the toxic effects described above, but to an exaggerated degree. Adequate hydration and osmotic diuresis may help reduce the toxicity of Cisplatin if administered promptly following overdosage.

Convulsions may be treated with appropriate anticonvulsants. Renal function, cardiovascular function and blood counts should be monitored daily in order to assess the potential toxicity to these systems. Serum magnesium and calcium levels should be carefully monitored as should symptoms and signs of voluntary muscle irritability. If symptomatic tetany develops, electrolyte supplements should be administered. Serum liver enzymes and uric acid should also be monitored daily after an acute overdose.

If fever develops during prolonged myelosuppression, appropriate presumptive antibiotic coverage should be instilled after cultures have been obtained.

**Pharmacological properties**
*Pharmacodynamic properties:* Cisplatin has biochemical properties similar to those of bifunctional alkylating agents. The drug inhibits DNA synthesis by producing intrastrand and interstrand cross links in DNA. Protein and RNA synthesis are also inhibited to a lesser extent.

Although the principal mechanism of action of Cisplatin appears to be inhibition of DNA synthesis, other mechanisms, including enhancement of tumour immunogenicity, may be involved in its antineoplastic activity. Cisplatin also has immunosuppressive, radiosensitising, and antimicrobial properties.

Cisplatin dose not appear to be cell cycle specific.

*Pharmacokinetic properties:* There is good uptake of Cisplatin by the kidneys, liver and intestine. More than 90% of platinum containing species remaining in the blood are bound (possibly irreversibly) to plasma proteins.

Penetration into the CSF is poor although significant amounts of Cisplatin can be detected in intracerebral tumours.

The clearance of total platinum from plasma is rapid during the first four hours after intravenous administration, but then proceeds more slowly because of covalent binding to serum proteins. Levels of unbound platinum fall with a half-life of 20 minutes to 1 hour depending on the rate of drug infusion.

The elimination of intact drug and various platinum-containing biotransformation products is via the urine. About 15-25% of administered platinum is rapidly excreted in the first 2-4 hours after administration of Cisplatin. This early excretion is mostly of intact Cisplatin. In the first 24 hours after administration, 20-80% is excreted, the remainder representing drug bound to tissues or plasma protein.

*Preclinical safety data:* There are no pre-clinical data of relevance to the prescriber which are additional to that already included in other sections of the SPC.

**Pharmaceutical particulars**
*List of excipients:*

|  | 10 mg | 50 mg | 100 mg |
|---|---|---|---|
| Mannitol BP | 10.0 mg | 50.0 mg | 100.0 mg |
| Sodium Chloride BP | 90.0 mg | 450.0 mg | 900.0 mg |
| Dilute Hydrochloric Acid BP | QS | QS | QS |
| Water for Injections BP to: | 10.0 ml | 50.0 ml | 100.0 ml |

There is no overage included in the above formulations.

*Incompatibilities:* There is a total loss of Cisplatin in 30 minutes at room temperature when mixed with Metoclopramide and Sodium Metabisulphite in concentrations equivalent to those that would be found on mixing with a commercial formulation of Metoclopramide.

Cisplatin and Sodium Bisulphite have been known to react chemically. Such antioxidants might inactivate Cisplatin before administration if they are present in intravenous fluids.

*Shelf life:* 48 months.

*Special precautions for storage:* All preparations and reconstituted solutions must be stored between 15°C and 25°C. Do not store in refrigerator. Protect from light.

*Instruction for use/handling:* Not applicable.

**Marketing authorisation number** 4515/0026

**Date of approval/revision of SPC** 12 March 1996

**Legal category** POM

## STERILE CO-TRIMOXAZOLE CONCENTRATE BP

### Qualitative and quantitative composition

| | 480 mg/ 5 ml | 960 mg/ 10 ml | 1920 mg/ 20 ml |
|---|---|---|---|
| *Active Constituent* | | | |
| Trimethoprim BP | 80 mg | 160 mg | 320 mg |
| Sulphamethoxazole BP | 400 mg | 800 mg | 1600 mg |
| *Other Constituents* | | | |
| Diethanolamine HSE | 0.015 mL | 0.030 mL | 0.06 mL |
| Propylene Glycol BP | 2.0 mL | 4.0 mL | 8.0 mL |
| Ethanol BP | 0.5 mL | 1.0 mL | 2.0 mL |
| Sodium Metabisulphite BP | 5.0 mL | 10 mg | 20 mg |
| Sodium Hydroxide BP | 62.5 mg | 125 mg | 250 mg |
| Water for Injections BP to: | 5.0 mL | 10 mL | 20 mL |

There is no overage included in the above formulations.

**Pharmaceutical form** Strong sterile solution.

### Clinical particulars

*Therapeutic indications:* Co-trimoxazole is an antibacterial combination product. It is bactericidal at concentrations at which the components are usually bacteriostatic, and is frequently active against organisms which are resistant to one of the components.

Treatment and prophylaxis (primary and secondary) of Pneumocystis carinii pneumonitis in adults and children.

Treatment and prophylaxis of toxoplasmosis, treatment of nocardia.

Treatment of urinary tract infections and acute exacerbations of chronic bronchitis, where there is bacterial evidence of sensitivity to Cotrimoxazole and good reason to prefer this combination to a single antibiotic.

Treatment of acute otitis media in children, where there is a good reason to prefer cotrimoxazole to a single antibiotic.

Parenteral administration of Co-trimoxazole is indicated where oral dosage is not desirable or practical, e.g. pre- and post-operative infections associated with surgery, trauma and gynaecology.

*Posology and method of administration:* Sterile Cotrimoxazole Concentrate BP MUST BE DILUTED prior to administration.

It should be administered intravenously only in the form of an infusion solution, and may not be injected undiluted either intravenously or directly into infusion tube.

The prepared infusion should be shaken well to ensure thorough mixing. Should visible turbidity or crystallisation appear in the solution at any time before or during infusion, the mixture should be discarded and replaced by a freshly prepared solution.

It is recommended that infusion of co-trimoxazole be commenced within half an hour of preparation and the duration of infusion should not exceed one and a half hours. However, this should be balanced against the fluid requirements of the patient.

Sterile Co-trimoxazole Concentrate BP may be mixed only with the following infusion solutions:

Glucose Injection BP 5% or 10%
Laevulose Injection BP 5%
Sodium Chloride Injection BP 0.45% or 0.9%
Sodium Chloride Injection BP 0.45% in Glucose 2.5%
Sodium Chloride Injection BP 0.18% in Glucose 4%
Dextran 40 Injection BP
Dextran 70 Injection BP
Dextran Injection BP 6% or 10% in Glucose 5%
Dextran Injection BP 6% or 10% in normal saline
Ringer's Injection USP

No other agent should be added to or mixed with the infusion.

It is important to adhere to the following dilution scheme:

Add 5 mL Sterile Co-trimoxazole Concentrate BP to 125 mL infusion solution

10 mL Sterile Co-trimoxazole Concentrate BP to 250 mL infusion solution 15 mL to 500 mL infusion solution or an equivalent dilution

In addition, dilutions of the following for the treatment of patients with PCP can be used:

2 x 5 mL amps in 125 mL of 5% dextrose, normal saline or saline/dextrose.

or

4 x 5 mL amps in 125 mL of normal saline injection solution

*Dosage for adults and children over 12 years:* Standard dose: 10 ml diluted and infused twice daily.

For severe infections: 15 ml diluted and infused twice daily.

*Dosage for children up to 12 years:* The recommended dosage is approximately 6 mg trimethoprim and 30 mg sulphamethoxazole per kg bodyweight per day, divided into two equal doses, morning and evening.

As a guide, the following doses of Sterile Cotrimoxazole Concentrate BP may be used:

6 weeks to 5 months: 1.25 mL diluted to 30 mL and infused twice daily.

6 months to 5 years: 2.5 mL diluted to 60 mL and infused twice daily.

6 years to 12 years: 5 mL diluted to 120 mL and infused twice daily.

In severe infections the paediatric dosage may be increased by 50%.

*Table 1: Co-trimoxazole dosages in impaired renal function*

| Criteria of kidney function | | Recommended dosage regimens |
|---|---|---|
| Creatinine Clearance (ml/min.) | Serum Creatinine (µmol/l) (a) | One standard dose for adults. 160 mg trimethoprim and 800 mg sulphamethoxazole. |
| Above 30 | Men <260 Women < 170 | Dosage as for patients with normal kidney function. |
| 30-15 | Men 260-600 Women 170-400 | One standard dose every 12 hours for 3 days; thereafter one standard dose every 24 hours as long as allowed by control analyses (b). |
| Below 15 | Men >600 Women >400 | Until further experience is gained, the combination should be given only if patients can undergo haemodialysis when necessary (c); under this condition one standard dose may be administered every 24 hours as long as allowed by control analyses (b). |

a. Serum creatinine levels can be used as the basis of dosing only in cases of stable chronic renal impairment, but not acute or subacute kidney failure.

b. The concentration of total sulphamethoxazole should be measured in plasma samples obtained 12 hours after every third day of treatment.

Treatment must be interrupted if at any time the determined plasma level of total sulphamethoxazole exceeds 150 microgram/ml. As soon as the value of total sulphamethoxazole drops again below 120 microgram/ml (e.g. in patients undergoing haemodialysis), treatment can be continued as recommended.

c. Both trimethoprim and sulphamethoxazole are readily dialysable, leading to a significantly shortened half-life for each drug during dialysis. It is suggested that patients undergoing haemodialysis receive a dose just before and at the end of the procedure.

No data are available relating to dosage in children with renal failure.

The recommended dosage for patients with documented Pneumocystis carinii pneumonitis is 20 mg/kg trimethoprim and 100mg/kg sulphamethoxazole per 24 hours given in equally divided doses every 6 hours for 14 days.

*Duration of treatment:* Sterile Co-trimoxazole Concentrate BP should be used ONLY during such periods as the patient is unable to accept oral therapy. In general, administration is unlikely to be required for more than a few days.

*Dosage in impaired renal function:* In patients with impaired renal function, the dosage and/or frequency of administration of co-trimoxazole needs to be modified. Dosages are suggested in Table 1.

*Contra-indications:* Co-trimoxazole should not be given to patients with known hypersensitivity or with documented megaloblastic anaemia secondary to folate deficiency.

It is contraindicated in patients showing marked liver parenchymal damage, blood dyscrasias and severe renal insufficiency where repeated measurements of the plasma concentrations cannot be performed.

Infants under 6 weeks of age except in the management of PCP where this may be from 4 weeks of age should not be given co-trimoxazole because sulphamethoxazole may interfere with the serum albumin binding of bilirubin and produce kernicterus.

*Special warnings and special precautions for use:*
*Warnings:* Prolonged parenteral administration of preparations containing propylene glycol can lead to lactic acidosis.

A number of serious side effects; aplastic anaemia, pancytopenia and thrombocytopenia are reported as occurring more frequently in the elderly. Accordingly, co-trimoxazole should not be prescribed in elderly patients unless the benefits are felt to exceed the increased risk of these serious side effects.

Fatalities may occur in severe skin, hepatic and blood disorders and pulmonary hypersensitivity; discontinue immediately with skin rashes; haemolysis in patients with G6PD deficiency; avoid in patients at risk of acute porphyria; do not use in Group A beta-haemolytic streptococci; can be used in patients with phenylketonuria on special diet.

*Precautions:* Care should be taken when giving Co-trimoxazole, to patients with liver damage, renal damage, urinary obstruction, blood dyscrasias, allergies or bronchial asthma.

In renal impairment reduced or less frequent dosage is recommended in order to avoid accumulation of trimethoprim in the blood. For such patients serum assays are necessary and adequate fluid intake must be maintained in order to avoid crystalluria and stone formation (see Table 1).

Because of the possible interference with folate metabolism, regular blood counts are advisable in patients on long-term therapy; in those who are predisposed to folate deficiency (i.e. the elderly, chronic alcoholics and rheumatoid arthritics), in malabsorption syndromes, malnutrition states or during the treatment of epilepsy with anticonvulsant drugs such as phenytoin, primidone and barbiturates.

Finally, the possibility of super-infection with a non-sensitive organism should be born in mind.

*Interaction with other medicaments and other forms of interaction:* Sulphamethoxazole may displace methotrexate from protein binding sites.

PABA or its derivatives may antagonise the antibacterial effects of sulphamethoxazole, while rifampicin may decrease trimethoprim concentrations. Increased sulphamethoxazole blood levels may occur in patients who are also receiving urinary acidifiers, oral anticoagulants, phenylbutazone, oxyphenbutazone and indomethacin.

As co-trimoxazole possesses anti-folate properties, the drug increases the incidence of folate deficiencies induced by other drugs such as phenytoin and pyrimethamine when used concomitantly.

Cross sensitisation may exist between Co-trimoxazole and some antithyroid agents, diuretics (acetazolamide), cyclosporin and oral hypoglycaemic drugs.

Care should be taken in patients receiving warfarin and sulphonylurea hypoglycaemic agents and cations at physiological pH, e.g. procainamide, amantadine and digoxin since their action could be increased.

*Pregnancy and lactation*
*Use in pregnancy:* Since trimethoprim is a folate antagonist, it might be expected to cause teratogenic effects. Foetal malformations commonly associated with lack of folic acid have occurred in several animal species when trimethoprim was administered to the pregnant female. The teratogenic effects were prevented concurrent administration of dietary folates. No teratogenic effects have yet been reported in women. Nevertheless, since folate levels are probably marginal in pregnant women, the combination of trimethoprim and sulphamethoxazole is generally

contraindicated, or should only be used with the full knowledge of the potential danger during pregnancy.

Furthermore, sulphamethoxazole should not be administered in late pregnancy because of the risk of kernicterus.

*Use in lactation:* Both trimethoprim and sulphamethoxazole are excreted in breast milk at concentrations comparable or somewhat lower than that in the blood. Although the quantity of Co-trimoxazole ingested by a breast-feeding infant is small, it is recommended that the possible risks be balanced against the therapeutic benefits.

*Effects on ability to drive and use machines:* Not applicable.

*Undesirable effects:* At the recommended dose Co-trimoxazole is well tolerated, but may occasionally give rise to local side effects in the form of mild to moderate venous pain and phlebitis.

In general, the adverse reactions (5-7%) correspond to those of a sulphonamide of moderately low toxicity.

During the administration of Co-trimoxazole, the possibility of blood dyscrasias should be taken into account.

Nausea and vomiting are the most frequent gastro-intestinal reactions to Cotrimoxazole, but glossitis, stomatitis, abdominal pain, pancreatitis, diarrhoea, anorexia, raised hepatic transaminases, rarely cholestatic jaundice and hepatic necrosis have been reported.

Haematological changes have been observed in some patients, particularly the elderly. The great majority of these changes were mild, asymptomatic and proved reversible on withdrawal of the drug. The reported changes consist primarily of neutropenia and thrombocytopenia. Leucopenia, aplastic and haemolytic anaemia, purpura, agranulocytosis and bone marrow depression rare. Reports have also been noted of megaloblastic anaemia, methaemoglobinaemia, haemolysis in patients with G6PD deficiency; reactions may be worse in patients with poor hepatic or renal function and poor folate status.

A number of serious side effects; aplastic anaemia, pancytopenia and thrombocytopenia are reported as occurring more frequently in the elderly. Accordingly, Co-trimoxazole should not be prescribed in elderly patients the benefits are felt to exceed the increased risk of these serious side effects.

Pseudomembranous colitis has been reported as well as several cases of Stevens-Johnson and Lyell's syndrome. Jaundice rarely occurs and has usually been mild and transient, frequently occurring in patients with a past history of infectious hepatitis.

Skin reactions which have been noted include rashes, photosensitivity, exfoliative dermatitis and erythema multiforme.

Allergic reactions which have been noted include serum sickness, anaphylaxis, allergic myocarditis, angiodema, drug fever, peri-arteritis nodosa and SLE.

Neurological reactions which have been noted include aseptic meningitis (reversible on withdrawal), convulsions, peripheral neuritis, ataxia, vertigo, tinnitus, headache, depression, dizziness and hallucinations.

Genitourinary reactions include impaired renal function and rarely interstitial nephritis.

Reported respiratory reactions include cough, dyspnoea, pulmonary infiltration and indicative of hypersensitivity.

Reported metabolic reactions include hyperkalaemia and hyponatraemia, which may be worse in the elderly and with high doses.

Musculoskeletal reactions which have been noted include arthralgia and myalgia.

It should be noted that adverse reactions may be more severe in the management of PCP.

*Overdose:* Stop therapy. Force fluids orally or parenterally if renal function is normal.

In excessive overdosage in patients with impaired renal function, consider dialysis, since both drugs are readily dialysable.

Calcium leucovorin may be used as an effective antidote for adverse effects in the haemopoietic system caused by trimethoprim.

**Pharmacological properties**

*Pharmacodynamic properties:* Co-trimoxazole usually is bactericidal. Of its components, sulphamethoxazole is bacteriostatic and trimethoprim usually is bactericidal. Co-trimoxazole acts by sequentially inhibiting enzymes of the folic acid pathway; sulphamethoxazole inhibits the formation of dihydrofolic acid from p-aminobenzoic acid and, by inhibiting dihydrofolate reductase, trimethoprim inhibits the formation of tetrahydrofolic acid from dihydrofolic acid.

By inhibiting synthesis of tetrahydrofolic acid, the metabolically active form of folic acid, co-trimoxazole inhibits bacterial thymidine synthesis.

Sequential inhibition by co-trimoxazole of two steps in the folic acid pathway appears to be responsible for the antibacterial synergism of the trimethoprim-sulphamethoxazole combination. For most organisms optimum synergistic antibacterial action occurs in vitro at a trimethoprim : sulphamethoxazole ratio about 1 : 20, which is also the approximate peak serum concentration ratio of 2 drugs achieved following oral or I.V. administration of co-trimoxazole. Synergistic activity also has been observed in vitro at trimethoprim : sulphamethoxazole ratios of 1:1 - 1:40.

Susceptibility of organisms to trimethoprim usually is more critical to the efficacy of co-trimoxazole than is susceptibility to sulphamethoxazole.

Many organisms that are resistant to sulphamethoxazole but susceptible to trimethoprim will show synergistic antibacterial response to co-trimoxazole. However, for Neisseria gonorrhoeae, susceptibility to sulphamethoxazole is required for antibacterial response to co-trimoxazole.

*Pharmacokinetic properties:* Co-trimoxazole is rapidly and well absorbed from the G.I. tract. Peak serum concentrations of 1-2 mg/ml of trimethoprim and 40-60 mg/ml of unbound sulphamethoxazole are reached 1-4 hours after a single oral dose of co-trimoxazole containing 160 mg trimethoprim and 800 mg of sulphamethoxazole.

Co-trimoxazole is widely distributed into body tissues and fluids including sputum, aqueous humour, middle ear fluid, prostatic fluid, vaginal fluid, bile and CSF. Trimethoprim is approximately 44% and sulphamethoxazole is approximately 70% bound to plasma proteins. Co-trimoxazole readily crosses the placenta and is distributed into breast milk. High concentrations of co-trimoxazole are achieved in the urine.

Sulphamethoxazole and trimethoprim are both excreted unchanged and as metabolites mainly by the kidneys. Both compounds have elimination half-lives of approximately 12 hours.

Renal Impairment: Because both compounds are cleared largely via the kidneys, their half-lives are significantly increased in patients with creatinine clearance less than 30 ml per minute. This reduction of dosage is required when patients with renal impairment are treated with co-trimoxazole.

**Pharmaceutical particulars**

*List of excipients:*

| | *480 mg/ 5 ml* | *960 mg/ 10 ml* | *1920 mg/ 20 ml* |
|---|---|---|---|
| Diethanolamine HSE | 0.015 mL | 0.030 mL | 0.06 mL |
| Propylene Glycol BP | 2.0 mL | 4.0 mL | 8.0 mL |
| Ethanol BP | 0.5 mL | 1.0 mL | 2.0 mL |
| Sodium Metabisulphite BP | 5.0 mL | 10 mg | 20 mg |
| Sodium Hydroxide BP | 62.5 mg | 125 mg | 250 mg |
| Water for Injections BP to: | 5.0 mL | 10 mL | 20 mL |

There is no overage included in the above formulations.

*Incompatibilities:* No other agent should be added to or mixed with the infusion.

*Shelf life:* 36 months.

*Special precautions for storage:* Store below 30°C. Do not refrigerate. Protect from light. If stored at low temperatures, precipitation may occur, and solutions in which precipitation has occurred could be discarded.

*Instructions for use/handling:* Not applicable.

**Marketing authorisation number** 4515/0023.

**Date of approval/revision of SPC** 5 February 1996

**Legal category** POM

## CYTARABINE INJECTION SOLUTION 20MG/ML

**Qualitative and quantitative composition**

*Active Constituent*

Cytarabine BP 2.0% w/v

*Other Constituents*

Sodium Chloride BP 6.8 mg

Water for Injections BP to 1.0 mL

There is no overage in the formulation.

**Pharmaceutical form** Aqueous, sterile isotonic solution for injection.

**Clinical particulars**

*Therapeutic indications:* Cytarabine may be used alone or in combination with other antineoplastic agents. It is indicated alone or in combination for induction of remission and/or maintainance in patients with acute myeloid leukaemia, acute non-lymphoblastic leukaemias, acute lymphoblastic leukaemias, acute lymphocytic leukaemia, erythroleukaemia, blast crises of chronic myeloid leukaemia, diffuse histiocytic lymphomas (non-hodgkin's lymphomas of high malignancy), meningeal leukaemia and meningeal neoplasms. Clinicians should refer to the current literature on combination therapy before initiating treatment.

*Posology and method of administration:* Cytarabine Injection Solution is a ready to use solution with a concentration of 20 mg/mL. The 20 mg/mL presentation is suitable for intravenous, subcutaneous and intrathecal use.

Cytarabine Injection Solution can be diluted with Sterile Water for Injection BP, Glucose 5% Injection BP or Sodium Chloride 0.9% Injection BP Prepared infusions, in the recommended diluents should be used immediately. Alternatively, the diluted infusion fluids may be stored at 2-8°C, protected from light, but portions remaining unused after 24 hours must be discarded.

Remission induction: Adults

Continuous dosing: The usual dose in leukaemia, is 2 mg/kg by rapid intravenous injection daily for ten days. If after ten days neither therapeutic response not toxicity has been observed, the dose may be increased to 4 mg per kg until a therapeutic response or toxicity is evident. Daily blood counts should be taken. Almost all patients can be carried to toxicity with these doses.

Alternatively, 0.5 to 1 mg/kg may be infused daily in 1-24 hours for ten days, and then at a rate of 2 mg/kg/day until toxicity is observed. Continue to toxicity or until remission occurs. Results from one hour infusions have been satisfactory in the majority of patients.

Intermittent dosing: Cytarabine may be given as intermittent IV doses of 3-5 mg/kg daily, for five consecutive days This course of treatment can be repeated after an interval of 2 to 9 days, and repeated until the therapeutic response or toxicity is exhibited.

Evidence of bone marrow inprovement has been reported to occur 7-64 days days after the beginning of therapy.

In general, if a patient shows neither remission or toxicity after a trial period, then cautiously administered higher doses can be administered. Generally patients tolerate higher doses given by rapid intravenous injection rather than slow infusion.

As a single agent for induction of remissions in patients with acute leukaemia, Cytarabine has been given in doses of 200 mg/m² by continuous IV Infusion for five days at approximately 2 week intervals.

Maintainance therapy: To maintain remission, doses of 1-1.5 mg/kg may be given intravenously or subcutaneously, once or twice weekly.

Leukaemic meningitis: Therapy for established meningitis employs a wide variety of dose regimens but a recommended total daily dose not exceeding 100 mg, alternating with Methotrexate (given either systemically or intrathecally) is recommended. Cytarabine Injection has been given intrathecally at doses of 10-30 mg per m2 three times a week until CSF findings return to normal.

Myelosuppression, anaemia and thrombocytopenia occur almost to all patients given daily infusions or injections. Myelosuppression is biphasic and nadirs at 7-9 and 15-24 days. Evidence of bone marrow improvement may be expected 7-64 (mean 28) days after the beginning of treatment.

Children: Children appear to tolerate higher doses of Cytarabine than adults, and where the range of doses is given, children should receive the higher dose.

Elderly: No data is available to suggest that a change in dose is necessary in the elderly. However, the elderly patient is more susceptable to toxic reactions and therefore particular attention should be paid to drug induced leucopenia, thrombocytopenia and anaemia.

*Contra-indications:* Cytarabine is contra-indicated in patients with known hypersensitivity to the drug. Therapy with Cytarabine should not be considered in patients with pre-existing drug-induced bone marrow suppression, unless in the opinion of the physician the potential benefits outweigh the hazards. Cytarabine should not be used in the management of non-malignant disease, except for immunosuppression.

*Special warnings and special precautions for use:* Cytarabine is a potent bone marrow suppressant. Patients receiving the drug should be kept under close medical supervision. Leucocyte and platelet counts should be performed frequently and daily during induction. One case of anaphylaxis that resulted in cardiopulmonary arrest and necessitated resusitiation has been reported. This occurred immediately after intravenous Cytarabine was administered.

Severe and at times fatal CNS, GI and pulmonary toxicity (different from that seen with conventional therapy regimens of dosage schedules). These reactions include reversible corneal toxicity; cerebral and cerebellar dysfunction, usually reversible; severe gastrointestinal ulceration including pneumatosis cysteroides intestinalis, leading to peritonitis; sepsis and liver abscess; and pulmonary oedema.

Cytarabine has been shown to be mutagenic and carcinogenic in animals.

Cytarabine should only be used under the constant supervision by physicians experienced in therapy with cytotoxic agents. Hyperuricaemia secondary to lysis of neoplastic cells may occur in patients receiving Cytarabine; serum uric acid concentrations should be monitored.

Periodic determinations of renal and hepatic functions and bone marrow should also be performed and the drug should be used with caution in patients with impaired hepatic function.

However, dosage reduction does not appear to be necessary in patients with impaired renal function. The human liver apparently detoxifies a substantial fraction of the administered dose. The drug should be used with caution and at a reduced dose when liver function is poor. Frequent platelet and leucocyte counts are manditory. Therapy should be suspended or modified when drug-induced bone marrow depression results in a platelet count of less than 50,000 or a polymorphonuclear count of under 1000 per cubic mm. Counts may continue to fall after the therapy has been discontinued and may reach lowest values after five to seven days. Therapy may be restarted when the bone marrow appears to be recovering on successive bone marrow studies. Therapy should not wait until the normal blood values are obtained to be re-initiated.

When intravenous doses are given quickly, patients may become nauseated and may vomit for several hours afterwards. The problem tends to be less severe when infused.

When given intrathecally, as with any other intrathecal drug, care must be taken with radiotherapy given either during or after treatment; it is well recognised that this can exacerbate the toxicity of radiotherapy.

The safety of the drug has not been established in infants.

*Interaction with other medicaments and other forms of interaction*

(i) *Cardiac glycosides:* G.I. absorption of oral digoxin tablets may be substantially reduced in patients receiving combination chemotherapy regimens (including regimens containing cytarabine), possibly as a result of temporary damage to intestinal mucosa caused by the cytotoxic agents. Limited data suggest that the extent of G.I. absorption of digitoxin is not substantially affected by concomitant administration of combination chemotherapy regimens known to decrease absorption of digoxin.

(ii) *Anti-infective agents:* One in vitro study indicates that cytarabine may antagonise the activity of gentamicin against *Klebsiella pneumoniae*. Limited data may suggest that cytarabine may antagonise the anti-infective activity of flucytosine, possibly by competitive inhibition of the anti-infective uptake by fungi.

*Pregnancy and lactation:* Cytarabine is teratogenic in some animal species. It should not be used in pregnant women (especially during the first trimester) or in those who may become pregnant, unless the possible benefits outweigh the potential risks. Women who are, or become, pregnant during treatment with Cytarabine should be informed of the risks.

It is not known if Cytarabine or its metabolite is distributed into breast milk, and it should not be used.

*Effects on ability to drive and use machines:* No documented effect on ability to drive or operate machinery.

*Undesirable effects:*

*Haematological effects:* The major adverse effect of Cytarabine is the haematological toxicity. Myelosuppression is manifested by megaloblastosis, reticulocytopenia, thrombocytopenia and anaemia.

These appear to be more evident after high doses and continuous infusions; the severity depends on the dose of the drug and schedule of administration.

*GI effects:* Nausea and vomiting occur and are generally more frequent following rapid IV administration than with continuous IV infusion of the drug.

Diarrhoea, anorexia, oral and anal inflammation or ulceration and less frequently abdominal pain, sore throat, oesphagitis, oesophageal ulceration and gastrointestinal haemorrhage may also occur.

Other reported adverse effects of Cytarabine include fever, rash, alopecia, skin ulceration, conjunctivitis, chest pain, urinary retention, dizziness, neuritis or neural toxicity and pain, cellulitis or thrombophlebitis at the site of injection. Cytarabine has also been associated with renal dysfunction, hepatic dysfunction and jaundice in some patients. It has also been associated with sepsis, irritation or sepsis at the injection site, neuritis or neurotoxicity rash, freckling, skin and mucosal bleeding, chest pain, joint pain and reduction in reticulocytes.

A Cytarabine reaction is characterised by fever, myalgia, bone pain, occasionally chest pain, maculopapular rash, conjunctivitis and malaise. It usually occurs 6-12 hours after administration. Corticosteroids have been shown to be beneficial in treating or preventing this syndrome. If the symptoms of the syndrome are serious enough to warrant treatment, corticosteroids should be contemplated as well as continuation of Cytarabine therapy.

*Overdose:* Cessation of therapy followed by management of ensuing bone marrow depression including whole blood or platelet transfusion and antibiotics as required.

**Pharmacological properties**

*Pharmacodynamic properties:* Cytarabine (ARA-C) is metabolised in vivo to ARA-CTP phosphorylated compound. This competitively inhibits DNA polymerase and may also inhibit certain acid kinase enzymes. Primarily the drug acts as a false nucleoside and competes for enzymes involved in the conversion of Cytidine nucleotide to deoxycytidine nucleotide and also incorporation into the DNA.

Cytarabine has no effect on non proliferating cells nor on proliferating cells unless in the S phase. It is a cell cycle specific antineoplastic drug.

*Pharmacokinetic properties:* Oral administration is ineffective due to rapid deamination in the gut. Cytidine deaminase is concentrated in the liver and intravenous doses show biphasic elimination with half lifes of approximately 10 minutes and 1-3 hours.

After 24 hours 80% of a dose has been eliminated either as the inactive metabolite or as the unchanged Cytarabine, mostly in urine but some in bile.

CSF levels of 50% of plasma levels are achieved with IV infusion. Intrathecal dosing results in slower elimination (T1/2 2-11 hours).

Cytarabine is rapidly and widely distributed into tissues, crosses the blood brain barrier and also the placenta.

*Preclinical safety data:* Not applicable.

**Pharmaceutical particulars**

*List of excipients:*

| | |
|---|---|
| Sodium Chloride BP | 6.8 mg |
| Water for Injections BP | to 1.0 mL |

There is no overage in the formulation.

*Incompatibilities:* Solutions of Cytarabine have been reported to be incompatible with various drugs, i.e. Carbenicillin Sodium, Cephalothin Sodium, Fluorouracil, Gentamicin Sulphate, Heparin Sodium, Hydrocortisone Sodium Succinate, Insulin-regular, Methylprednisolone Sodium Succinate, Nafacillin Sodium, Oxacillin Sodium, Penicillin G Sodium. However, the incompatibility depends on several factors (e.g. concentrations of the drug, specific diluents used, resulting pH, temperature). Specialised references should be consulted for specific compatibility information.

*Shelf life:* 36 months.

*Special precautions for storage:* Store below 25°C. Protect from light.

In diluted infusion fluids store at 2-8°C and protect from light for a maximum of 24 hours.

*Instructions for use/handling:* Not applicable.

**Marketing authorisation number** 4515/0040.

**Date of approval/revision of SPC** March 1996

**Legal category** POM

## CYTARABINE INJECTION SOLUTION 100MG/ML

**Qualitative and quantitative composition**

*Active constituent*

| | |
|---|---|
| Cytarabine BP | 10.0 % w/v |

*Other constituents*

| | |
|---|---|
| Water for Injections BP to | 1.0 mL |

There is no overage in the formulation

**Pharmaceutical form** Aqueous, sterile hypertonic solution for injection.

**Clinical particulars**

*Therapeutic indications:* Cytarabine may be used alone or in combination with other antineoplastic agents. It is indicated alone or in combination for induction of remission and/or maintainance in patients with acute myeloid leukaemia, acute non-lymphoblastic leukaemias, acute lymphoblastic leukaemias, acute lymphocytic leukaemia, erythroleukaemia, blast crises of chronic myeloid leukaemia, diffuse histiocytic lymphomas (non-hodgkin's lymphomas of high malignancy), meningeal leukaemia and meningeal neoplasms. Clinicians should refer to the current literature on combination therapy before initiating treatment.

*Posology and method of administration:* Cytarabine Injection Solution is a ready to use solution with a concentration of 100 mg/mL.

Cytarabine Injection Solution 100 mg/mL can be administered by the intravenous and subcutaneous routes. Cytarabine Injection Solution 100 mg/mL should not be administered by the intrathecal route due to the slight hypertonicity of this formulation.

Cytarabine Injection Solution can be diluted with Sterile Water for Injection BP, Glucose Injection BP or Sodium Chloride 0.9% Injection BP Prepared infusions, in the recommended diluents should be used immediately. Alternatively, the diluted infusion fluids may be stored at 2-8°C, protected from light, but portions remaining unused after 24 hours must be discarded.

*Remission induction:* Adults

*Continuous dosing:* The usual dose in leukaemia, is 2 mg/kg by rapid intravenous injection daily for ten days. If after ten days neither therapeutic response not toxicity has been observed, the dose may be increased to 4 mg per kg until a therapeutic response or toxicity is evident. Daily blood counts should be taken. Almost all patients can be carried to toxicity with these doses.

Alternatively, 0.5 to 1 mg/kg may be infused daily in 1-24 hours for ten days, and then at a rate of 2 mg/kg/day until toxicity is observed. Continue to toxicity or until remission occurs. Results from one hour infusions have been satisfactory in the majority of patients.

Intermittent dosing: Cytarabine may be given as intermittent IV doses of 3-5 mg/kg daily, for five consecutive days This course of treatment can be repeated after an interval of 2 to 9 days, and repeated until the therapeutic response or toxicity is exhibited.

Evidence of bone marrow inprovement has been reported to occur 7-64 days after the beginning of therapy.

In general, if a patient shows neither remission or toxicity after a trial period, then cautiously administered higher doses can be administered. Generally patients tolerate higher doses given by rapid intravenous injection rather than slow infusion.

As a single agent for induction of remissions in patients with acute leukaemia, Cytarabine has been given in doses of 200 mg/m2 by continuous IV Infusion for five days at approximately 2 week intervals.

Maintainance therapy: To maintain remission, doses of 1-1.5 mg/kg may be given intravenously or subcutaneously, once or twice weekly.

*Leukaemic meningitis:* Therapy for established meningitis employs a wide variety of dose regimens but a recommended total daily dose not exceeding 100 mg, alternating with Methotrexate (given either systemically or intrathecally) is recommended. Cytarabine Injection has been given intrathecally at doses of 10-30 mg per m2 three times a week until CSF findings return to normal. Cytarabine Injection Solution 100 mg/mL should not be administered by the intrathecal route due to the slight hypertonicity of this formulation.

Myelosuppression, anaemia and thrombocytopenia occur almost to all patients given daily infusions or injections. Myelosuppression is biphasic and nadirs at 7-9 and 15-24 days. Evidence of bone marrow improvement may be expected 7-64 (mean 28) days after the beginning of treatment.

*Children:* Children appear to tolerate higher doses of Cytarabine than adults, and where the range of doses is given, children should receive the higher dose.

*Elderly:* No data is available to suggest that a change in dose is necessary in the elderly. However, the elderly patient is more susceptable to toxic reactions and therefore particular attention should be paid to drug induced leucopenia, thrombocytopenia and anaemia.

*Contra-indications:* Cytarabine is contra-indicated in patients with known hypersensitivity to the drug. Therapy with Cytarabine should not be considered in patients with pre-existing drug-induced bone marrow suppression, unless in the opinion of the physician the potential benefits outweigh the hazards. Cytarabine should not be used in the management of non-malignant disease, except for immunosuppression.

*Special warnings and special precautions for use:* Cytarabine is a potent bone marrow suppressant. Patients receiving the drug should be kept under close medical supervision. Leucocyte and platelet counts should be performed frequently and daily during induction. One case of anaphylaxis that resulted in cardiopulmonary arrest and necessitated resusitiation has been reported. This occurred immediately after intravenous Cytarabine was administered.

Severe and at times fatal CNS, GI and pulmonary toxicity (different from that seen with conventional therapy regimens of dosage schedules). These reactions include reversible corneal toxicity; cerebral and cerebellar dysfunction, usually reversible; severe gastrointestinal ulceration including pneumatosis cysteroides intestinalis, leading to peritonitis; sepsis and liver abscess; and pulmonary oedema.

Cytarabine has been shown to be mutagenic and carcinogenic in animals.

Cytarabine should only be used under the constant supervision by physicians experienced in therapy with cytotoxic agents. Hyperuricaemia secondary to lysis of neoplastic cells may occur in patients receiving Cytarabine; serum uric acid concentrations should be monitored.

Periodic determinations of renal and hepatic functions and bone marrow should also be performed and the drug should be used with caution in patients with impaired hepatic function.

However, dosage reduction does not appear to be necessary in patients with impaired renal function. The human liver apparently detoxifies a substantial fraction of the administered dose. The drug should be used with caution and at a reduced dose when liver function is poor. Frequent platelet and leucocyte counts are manditory. Therapy should be suspended or modified when drug-induced bone marrow depression results in a platelet count of less than 50,000 or a polymorphonuclear count of under 1000 per cubic mm. Counts may continue to fall after the therapy has been discontinued and may reach lowest values after five to seven days. Therapy may be restarted when the bone marrow appears to be recovering on successive bone marrow studies. Therapy should not wait until the normal blood values are obtained to be re-initiated.

When intravenous doses are given quickly, patients may become nauseated and may vomit for several hours afterwards. The problem tends to be less severe when infused.

The safety of the drug has not been established in infants.

*Interaction with other medicaments and other forms of interaction:*

(I) Cardiac glycosides: G.I. absorption of oral digoxin tablets may be substantially reduced in patients receiving combination chemotherapy regimens (including regimens containing cytarabine), possibly as a result of temporary damage to intestinal mucosa caused by the cytotoxic agents. Limited data suggest that the extent of G.I. absorption of digitoxin is not substantially affected by concomitant administration of combination chemotherapy regimens known to decrease absorption of digoxin.

(ii) Anti-infective agents: One in vitro study indicates that cytarabine may antagonise the activity of gentamicin against Klebsiella pneumoniae. Limited data may suggest that cytarabine may antagonise the anti-infective activity of flucytosine, possibly by competitive inhibition of the anti-infective uptake by fungi.

*Pregnancy and lactation:* Cytarabine is teratogenic in some animal species. It should not be used in pregnant women (especially during the first trimester) or in those who may become pregnant, unless the possible benefits outweigh the potential risks. Women who are, or become, pregnant during treatment with Cytarabine should be informed of the risks.

It is not known if Cytarabine or its metabolite is distributed into breast milk, and it should not be used.

*Effects on ability to drive and use machines:* No documented effect on ability to drive or operate machinery.

*Undesirable effects:*
*Haematological effects:* The major adverse effect of Cytarabine is the haematological toxicity. Myelosuppression is manifested by megaloblastosis, reticulocytopenia, thrombocytopenia and anaemia.

These appear to be more evident after high doses and continuous infusions; the severity depends on the dose of the drug and schedule of administration.

*GI effects:* Nausea and vomiting occur and are generally more frequent following rapid IV administration than with continuous IV infusion of the drug.

Diarrhoea, anorexia, oral and anal inflammation or ulceration and less frequently abdominal pain, sore throat, oesphagitis, oesophageal ulceration and gastrointestinal haemorrhage may also occur.

Other reported adverse effects of Cytarabine include fever, rash, alopecia, skin ulceration, conjunctivitis, chest pain, urinary retention, dizziness, neuritis or neural toxicity and pain, cellulitis or thrombophlebitis at the site of injection. Cytarabine has also been associated with renal dysfunction, hepatic dysfunction and jaundice in some patients. It has also been associated with sepsis, irritation or sepsis at the injection site, neuritis or neurotoxicity rash, freckling, skin and mucosal bleeding, chest pain, joint pain and reduction in reticulocytes.

A Cytarabine reaction is characterised by fever, myalgia, bone pain, occasionally chest pain, maculopapular rash, conjunctivitis and malaise. It usually occurs 6-12 hours after administration. Corticosteroids have been shown to be beneficial in treating or preventing this syndrome. If the symptoms of the syndrome are serious enough to warrant treatment, corticosteroids should be contemplated as well as continuation of Cytarabine therapy.

*Overdose:* Cessation of therapy followed by management of ensuing bone marrow depression including whole blood or platelet transfusion and antibiotics as required.

**Pharmacological properties**

*Pharmacodynamic properties:* Cytarabine (ARA-C) is metabolised in vivo to ARA-CTP phosphorylated compound. This competitively inhibits DNA polymerase and may also inhibit certain acid kinase enzymes. Primarily the drug acts as a false nucleoside and competes for enzymes involved in the conversion of Cytidine nucleotide to deoxycytidine nucleotide and also incorporation into the DNA.

Cytarabine has no effect on non proliferating cells nor on proliferating cells unless in the S phase. It is a cell cycle specific antineoplastic drug.

*Pharmacokinetic properties:* Oral administration is ineffective due to rapid deamination in the gut. Cytidine deaminase is concentrated in the liver and intravenous doses show biphasic elimination with half lifes of approximately 10 minutes and 1-3 hours.

After 24 hours 80% of a dose has been eliminated either as the inactive metabolite or as the unchanged Cytarabine, mostly in urine but some in bile.

CSF levels of 50% of plasma levels are achieved with IV infusion. Intrathecal dosing results in slower elimination (T1/2 2-11 hours).

Cytarabine is rapidly and widely distributed into tissues, crosses the blood brain barrier and also the placenta.

*Preclinical safety data:* Not applicable.

**Pharmaceutical particulars**

*List of excipients:* Water for Injections BP to 1.0 mL. There is no overage in the formulation.

*Incompatibilities:* Solutions of Cytarabine have been reported to be incompatible with various drugs, i.e. Carbenicillin Sodium, Cephalothin Sodium, Fluorouracil, Gentamicin Sulphate, Heparin Sodium, Hydrocortisone Sodium Succinate, Insulin-regular, Methylprednisolone Sodium Succinate, Nafacillin Sodium, Oxacillin Sodium, Penicillin G Sodium. However, the incompatibility depends on several factors (e.g. concentrations of the drug, specific diluents used, resulting pH, temperature). Specialised references should be consulted for specific compatibility information.

*Shelf life:* Conventional Glass Vials and Onco-Tain* Vials: 36 months. Shell Glass Vials: 24 months

*Special precautions for storage:*
Conventional Glass Vials and Onco-Tain* Vials: Store below 25°C. Protect from light.

In diluted infusion fluids store at 2-8°C and protect from light for a maximum of 24 hours.

Shell Glass Vials: Store below 25°C. Protect from light.

Unused portions of opened vials or prepared infusions if not used immediately must be stored at 2-8°C for no longer than 24 hours from the time of opening or preparation.

*Instructions for use/handling:* Not applicable.

**Marketing authorisation number** 4515/0057

**Date of approval/revision of SPC** April 1995

**Legal category** POM

## DACARBAZINE FOR INJECTION

**Qualitative and quantitative composition** Dacarbazine for Injection BP is a cytotoxic agent presented as vials containing 100 mg and 200 mg of sterile dacarbazine as a white/pale yellow powder or plug which is to be reconstituted with Water for Injections BP.

When reconstituted as directed each ml of the solution of the 100 mg vial contains dacarbazine 10 mg, citric acid 10 mg, mannitol 5 mg, and sodium hydroxide 1N has been used to adjust the pH. Each ml of the 200 mg vial contains dacarbazine 20 mg, citric acid 20 mg, mannitol 7.5 mg, and sodium hydroxide 1N has been used to adjust the pH.

**Pharmaceutical form** Freeze dried powder for injection.

**Clinical particulars**

*Therapeutic indications:*

1. Metastatic malignant melanoma
2. Sarcoma
3. Hodgkin's disease.

In addition, dacarbazine has been shown, when used in combination with other cytotoxic agents, to be of use in the treatment of other malignant diseases including: carcinoma of the colon, ovary, breast, lung, testicular teratoma, and solid tumours in children.

*Posology and method of administration:*
*Dosage:* Standard dose. The following dosage schedules are recommended:

1. 2.0-4.5 mg/kg/day for 10 days, which may be repeated at 4 week intervals.
2. 250 mg/m²/day for five days, which may be repeated at 3 week intervals.
3. A further alternative is to administer the total schedule dose on the first day.

Other schedules may be used at the discretion of the prescribing physician.

*Children:* The dosage for children is calculated on a mg/kg or mg/m² basis as per the standard dosage. There is no indication that children require a different dosage range or metabolise or react differently to the drug.

*Geriatric:* As for paediatric use.

*With impaired hepatic function:* As the drug partly undergoes metabolism in the liver, impairment of liver function is likely to necessitate a variation in dosage.

*With impaired renal function:* As the drug is excreted 50% unchanged in the urine by tubular secretion, impairment of renal function is likely to necessitate a change in dosage.

*Administration:* Administration is by the IV route only.

Dacarbazine 100 mg and 200 mg vials should be reconstituted with 9.9 ml and 19.7 ml respectively, with Water for Injections BP. The resulting solutions contain the equivalent of 10 mg/ml of dacarbazine and have a pH of 3 to 4. The resultant solution should be injected intravenously over one to two minutes.

If desired the reconstituted solution can be further diluted with 125-250 ml of Dextrose Injection BP 5% or Sodium Chloride Injection BP 0.9% and administered by intravenous infusion over 15-30 minutes.

*Contra-indications:* Dacarbazine is contra-indicated in patients who have demonstrated a hypersensitivity to Dacarbazine in the past.

Dacarbazine should not be administered to patients who are pregnant or may become pregnant or breast feeding mothers.

Patients who have previously had severe myelosuppression.

*Special warnings and special precautions for use:*
*Warnings:* Haemopoietic depression is the most common toxic side-effect of dacarbazine and involves primarily the leucocytes and platelets, although mild anaemia may sometimes occur. Leucopenia and thrombocytopenia may be severe enough to cause death. Possible bone marrow depression requires careful monitoring of white blood cells, red blood cells and platelet levels. Such toxicity may necessitate temporary suspension or cessation of therapy.

Hepatic toxicity, accompanied by hepatic vein thrombosis and hepatocellular necrosis resulting in death, have been reported. The incidence of such reactions has been low. This toxicity has been observed mostly when dacarbazine has been administered concommitantly with other anti-neoplastic drugs; however, it has also been reported in some patients treated with dacarbazine alone.

*Precautions:* The drug can produce severe and possibly fatal, haematologic or hepatic toxicity and severe GI reactions and should be administered to patients preferably within the hospital setting, where they can be observed frequently during and after therapy, particularly with regards to the haemopoietic toxicity.

It is recommended that dacarbazine be administered by physicians experienced in the use of cytotoxic therapy. Laboratory facilities should be available for blood monitoring.

Restriction of food intake for 4-6 hours prior to treatment may reduce the severity of the nausea and vomiting which occurs in most patients particularly during the first two days of treatment. Administration of an anti-emetic may also reduce the severity of these effects.

Impairment of renal and liver function: See dosage in impaired renal and liver function

Care must be taken to avoid extravasation during intravenous administration as this may cause tissue damage and severe pain.

Care should be taken to avoid contact with the skin and eyes when reconstituting or administering dacarbazine.

*Interaction with other medicaments and other forms of interaction:* Microsomal liver enzyme inducers eg barbiturates, rifampicin, phenytoin may theoretically hasten the activation of dacarbazine to aminoimidazole-carboxamide.

Mercaptopurine, azathioprine, allopurinol: dacarbazine inhibits xanthine oxidase and may theoretically potentiate the activity of these drugs.

Patients receiving Dacarbazine should not receive immunisation with live vaccines. Dacarbazine may impair the immunological response to the vaccine with the development of a generalised vaccinia.

*Pregnancy and lactation:* Studies have demonstrated that this agent is carcinogenic and teratogenic when administered to animals. Dacarbazine therefore should not be administered to pregnant or lactating women unless the benefit clearly justifies the potential risk to the foetus.

*Effects on ability to drive and use machines:* Dacarbazine in appropriate doses should not impair the ability to drive. However, rare adverse reactions affecting the nervous system may cause blurred vision, seizures, headache, confusion, malaise and lethargy. Patients affected by these adverse effects should not drive or operate machinery.

*Undesirable effects:*
*Common reactions:* Symptoms of anorexia, nausea, and vomiting are the most frequent side-effects. Vomiting may last for 1-12 hours and is incompletely and unpredictably palliated with prochlorperazine. Diarrhoea is a rarer side-effect of Dacarbazine therapy. Rarely have intractable nausea and vomiting have necessitated discontinuation of therapy.

It is suggested that restriction fo the patients oral fluid intake and food 4-6 hours prior to treatment may be helpful. The rapid toleration of these symptoms suggests a central nervous system mechanism, and usually these symptoms subside after the first 1-2 days.

Haematological:Bone marrow depression, leucocytopenia, thrombocytopenia.

Haemopoietic toxicity may warrant temporary suspension or cessation of Dacarbazine therapy.

*Less common reactions:*
Cardiovascular: Facial flushing
Dermatological: Transient rash, alopecia

General : Infrequently some patients have experienced an influenza type syndrome of fever, myalgias and malaise. This syndrome usually occurs after large single doses and approximately seven days after treatment with dacarbazine and lasts 7-21 days, and may reoccur with successive treatments.

Hepatic: Increases in transaminases (AST, ALT), alkaline phosphatase, LDH. Levels usually return to normal within two weeks; hepatic toxicity accompanied by hepatic vein thrombosis and hepatocellular necrosis,(Budd-Chiari Syndrome) resulting in death.

Nervous System: Blurred vision, seizures, headache, facial paraesthesia, confusion, malaise, lethargy.

Anaphylaxis can occur very rarely following administration of Dacarbazine.

Photosensitivity reactions may occur rarely.

*Overdose:* Signs and Symptoms: Severe bone marrow depression and gastrointestinal effects such as nausea, vomiting and diarrhoea may be expected.

Treatment: Cease dacarbazine administration and institute supportive measures, eg appropriate transfusions for bone marrow suppression.

**Pharmacological properties**

*Pharmacodynamic properties:* Dacarbazine is an imidazole dimethyltriazene with reproducible activity in patients with metastatic melanoma. The structure of Dacarbazine bears a striking resemblance to the metabolite 5-aminoimidazole-4-carboxamide (AIC) which is converted to inosinic acid by enzymes involved in purine synthesis.

It was therefore initially thought to act as an antimetabolite, by inhibiting purine metabolism and nucleic acid synthesis. However the similarity of structure is of little relevance since Dacarbazine is extensively metabolised by the cytochrome P450 system in the liver by N-demethylation reaction. The monomethyl derivative then spontaneously cleaves to yield AIC and an intermediate compound, probably diazomethane, which decomposes to produce the methyl carbonium ion. This ion attached to nucleophilic groups on nucleic acids and other macromolecules, thus acting as an alkylating agent. The 7-position of guanine on DNA is especially susceptible to alkylation.

Dacarbazine is thought to act as an alkylating agent in man. It interferes with the synthesis of DNA, RNA and proteins but its cytotoxicity is not specific for any phase of the cell cycle. In general, it is most effective in inhibiting synthesis of RNA. Dacarbazine kills cells slowly and no immunosuppressive action has been shown in man. There are no systemic studies of dose-response effects but one anecdotal report has suggested that there may be an increased chance of response as the dose increases.

Dacarbazine undergoes spontaneous photodegradation in light, decomposing into 5-diazoimidazole-4-carboxamide and dimethylamine. 5-Diazoimidazole-4-carboxamide can attack nucleophilic groups of DNA and also undergoes structural rearrangement to form 2-azahypoxanthine. However, the products of photodegradation of dacarbazine probably do not contribute greatly to its cytotoxicity, although they may be implicated in the local burning pain on intravenous injection and systemic problems associated with the drug.

*Pharmacokinetic properties:* The volume of distribution of dacarbazine exceeds body water content, suggesting localisation in some body tissues, probably the liver. Dacarbazine is only slightly (approximately 5%) bound to plasma proteins. Its plasma half-life after intravenous administration is approximately 35 minutes. In animal studies, approximately 46% of radio-labelled dose was recovered from the urine after 6 hours. Of this 46%, almost half, was unchanged dacarbazine and a similar quantity was amino-imidazole carboxamide, a metabolite. Dacarbazine is subject to renal tubular secretion rather than glomerular filtration.

Dacarbazine crosses the blood-brain barrier to a limited extent; CSF concentrations are reported to be about 14% of plasma concentrations. It is not known if dacarbazine crosses the placenta or distributes into milk.

*Preclinical safety data:* Not applicable.

**Pharmaceutical particulars**

*List of excipients:* Citric Acid BP; Mannitol BP; Sodium Hydroxide 1.0N.

*Incompatibilities:* Dacarbazine is incompatible with hydrocortisone sodium succinate in solution, forming an inmediate precipitate.

It has been reported to be incompatible with heparin, although only with concentrated solutions (25 mg/ml).

*Shelf life:* 3 years.

*Special precautions for storage:* Store between 2-8°C. Protect from light.

After reconstitution the vial should be stored, protected from light, at 2-8°C and the contents used within 24 hours. If the reconstituted solution is further diluted in 5% Dextrose Injection BP or Sodium Chloride 0.9% BP the resulting solution should be stored protected from light, at 2-8°C and used within 24 hours.

*Instructions for use/handling:* Dacarbazine for Injection should only be prepared for administration by professionals who have been trained in the safe use of the preparation. In the event of spillage, operators should put on gloves and mop up the spilled material with a sponge kept in the area for that purpose, and transfer the sponge to a plastic bag. The procedure should be repeated and the area rinsed with water and absorbed solution placed in the plastic bag, which is then sealed. Repeat if necessary. The plastic container should then be incinerated and the gloves destroyed.

**Marketing authorisation numbers**
100 mg 4515/0091
200 mg 4515/0092

**Date of approval/revision of SPC** November 1995

**Legal category** POM

# DEXAMETHASONE SODIUM PHOSPHATE INJECTION.

**Qualitative and quantitative composition** 4 mg/1 mL, 8 mg/2 mL, 120 mg/5 mL.

**Pharmaceutical form** Sterile solution for injection.

**Clinical particulars**

*Therapeutic indications:* Dexamethasone Injection is indicated in acute conditions in which oral glucocorticoid therapy is not feasible such as:

Shock: of haemorrhagic, traumatic, surgical or septic origin; Cerebral oedema associated with cerebral neoplasm; Inflammatory diseases of joints and soft tissue such as rheumatoid arthritis

Short term management of acute self-limited allergic conditions such as angioneurotic oedema or acute exacerbations of chronic allergic disorders such as bronchial asthma or serum sickness.

High doses of Dexamethasone are intended for the adjunctive treatment of shock where massive doses of corticosteroids are needed. There is a lack of evidence that use of corticosteriods in septic shock affects mortality in the long term. Use must be accompanied by the appropriate concomitant systemic antibiotic treatment and supportive measures which the patient's condition may require.

*Posology and method of administration:* Dosage of Dexamethasone Sodium Phosphate is usually expressed in terms of Dexamethasone Phosphate.

The lowest effective dose should be used for the minimum period and this should be reviewed frequently to appropriately titrate the dose against disease activity. (See Warnings Section).

Dexamethasone Sodium Phosphate Injection 4 mg/ml may be administered by intramuscular, intra-articular or direct intravenous injection, intravenous infusion or soft tissue infiltration.

Dexamethasone Sodium Phosphate Injection 24 mg/ml is for intravenous administration only.

*Intravenous and intramuscular administration:* I.M. or I.V. dosage of Dexamethasone Phosphate is variable, depending on the condition being treated. It usually ranges from 0.5-24 mg daily. The duration of therapy is dependent on the clinical response of the patient and as soon as improvement is indicated, the dosage should be adjusted to the minimum required to maintain the desired clinical response. Withdrawal of the drug on completion of therapy should be gradual.

*Shock:* A single I.V. injection of 2 to 6 mg/kg bodyweight which may be repeated in 2-6 hours if shock persists. High-dose therapy should be continued only until the patient's condition has stabilised and usually for no longer than 48-72 hours. This bolus injection can then be followed by continuous I.V. infusion of 3 mg/kg bodyweight per 24 hours. Dexamethasone Sodium Phosphate Injection can be diluted with Sodium Chloride Injection BP or Glucose Injection BP

*Cerebral oedema associated with neoplasm:* An initial dose of 10 mg I.V. followed by 4 mg I.M. every 6 hours until the symptoms of oedema subside (usually after 12 to 24 hours). After 2 to 4 days the dosage should be reduced and gradually stopped over a period of 5 to 7 days. In patients with recurrent or inoperable neoplasms, maintenance therapy may be effective at doses of 2 mg I.M. or I.V. 2-3 times daily.

*Life-Threatening Cerebral Oedema:*

*High Dose Schedule:*

| | *Adults* | *Children > 35 kg* | *Children <35 kg* |
|---|---|---|---|
| Initial dose | 50 mg IV | 25 mg IV | 20 mg IV |
| 1st day | 8 mg IV every 2 hrs | 4 mg IV every 2 hrs | 4 mg IV every 3 hrs |
| 2nd day | 8 mg IV every 2 hrs | 4 mg IV every 2 hrs | 4 mg IV every 3 hrs |
| 3rd day | 8 mg IV every 2 hrs | 4 mg IV every 2 hrs | 4 mg IV every 3 hrs |
| 4th day | 4 mg IV every 2 hrs | 4 mg IV every 4 hrs | 4 mg IV every 6 hrs |
| 5th-8th day | 4 mg IV every 4 hrs | 4 mg IV every 6 hrs | 4 mg IV every 6 hrs |
| After 8 days | decrease by 4 mg daily | decrease by 2 mg daily | decrease by 1 mg daily |

Note: The intravenous and intramuscular routes of administration of Dexamethasone Sodium Phosphate should only be used where acute illness or life-threatening situations exist. Oral therapy should be substituted as soon as possible.

*Intra-articular and soft tissue injections:* Dosage varies with the degree of inflammation and the size and location of the affected area. Injections may be repeated from once every 3-5 days (e.g. for bursae) to once every 2-3 weeks (for joints).

| *Site of injection* | *Dosage* |
|---|---|
| Large Joint | 2 mg to 4 mg |
| Small Joints | 800 microgram to 1 mg |
| Bursae | 2 mg to 3 mg |
| Tendon Sheaths | 400 microgram to 1 mg |
| Soft Tissue Infiltration | 2 mg to 6 mg |
| Ganglia | 1 mg to 2 mg |

*Children:* Dosage requirements are variable and may have to be changed according to individual need. Usually 200 micrograms/kg to 400 micrograms/kg of body weight daily.

Corticosteroids cause growth retardation in infancy, childhood and adolescence, which may be irreversible. Treatment should be limited to the minimum dosage for the shortest possible time. In order to minimise suppression of the hypothalamopituitary-adrenal axis and growth retardation, treatment should be limited, where possible, to a single dose on alternative days.

Growth and development of infants and children on prolonged corticosteriod therapy should be carefully monitored.

*Elderly:* Treatment of elderly patients, particularly long-term, should be planned, bearing in mind the more serious consequences in old age. Such effects include osteoporosis, hypertension, hypokalaemia, diabetes, susceptibility to infection, thinning and fragility of the skin. Close clinical supervision is required to avoid life-threatening reactions.

*Contra-indications:* Unless considered to be life-saving systemic administration of corticosteroids are generally contraindicated in patients with systemic infections, (unless specific anti-infective therapy is employed). Hypersensitivity to any components of the injection.

*Special warnings and special precautions for use:*
*Warnings:* A Patient Information Leaflet should be supplied with this product.

The lowest effective dose of corticosteroid should be used to control the condition under treatment for the minimum period. Frequent patient review is required to appropriately titrate the dose against disease activity (see dosage section). When dose reduction is possible, it should occur gradually. Too rapid a reduction of dexamethasone dosage following prolonged treatment can lead to acute adrenal insufficiency, hypotension and death.

A 'withdrawal syndrome' may also occur including fever, myalgia, arthralgia, rhinitis, conjunctivitis, painful itchy skin nodules and loss of weight.

Adrenal suppression: Adrenal cortical atrophy develops during prolonged therapy and may persist for years after stopping treatment. Withdrawal of corticosteroids after prolonged therapy must, therefore, be gradual to avoid acute adrenal insufficiency, being tapered off over weeks or months according to the dose and duration of treatment. During prolonged therapy any intercurrent illness, trauma or surgical procedure will require a temporary increase in dosage; if corticosteroids have been stopped following prolonged therapy they may need to be temporarily reintroduced.

Patients should carry 'steroid treatment' cards which give clear guidance on the precautions to be taken to minimise risk and which provide details of prescriber, drug, dosage and the duration of treatment.

There is lack of evidence to support the prolonged use of corticosteroids in septic shock. Although they may be of value in the early treatment, the overall survival may not be influenced.

Severe anaphylactoid reactions have occurred after administration of parenteral corticosteroids, particularly in patients with history of allergy. Appropriate precautions should be taken prior to administration.

The slower rate of absorption after intramuscular injection should be noted.

Intra-articular corticosteroids are associated with a substantially increased risk of an inflammatory response in the joint, particularly a bacterial infection introduced with the injection. Great care is required and all intra-articular corticosteroid injections should be undertaken in an aseptic environment. Charcot like arthropathies have been reported particularly after repeated injections.

Prior to intra-articular injection the joint fluid should be examined to exclude a septic process. A marked increase in pain, accompanied by local swelling, further restriction of joint motion, fever and malaise are suggestive of septic arthritis. If this complication occurs and sepsis is confirmed, appropriate antimicrobial therapy should be commenced.

Patients should be impressed strongly with the importance of not overusing joints in which symptomatic benefit has been obtained, but the inflammatory process remains active.

Suppression of the inflammatory response and the immune function increases the susceptibility to infections and their severity. The clinical presentation may be atypical and serious infections, such as septicaemia and tuberculosis, may be masked and may reach an advanced stage before being recognised.

Chickenpox is of particular concern since this normally minor illness may be fatal in immunosuppressed patients. Patients (or parents of children) without a definite history of chickenpox should be advised to avoid close personal contact with chickenpox or herpes zoster and if exposed they should seek urgent medical attention. Passive immunisation with varicella/zoster immunoglobulin (VZIG) is needed by exposed non-immune patients who are receiving systemic dexamethasone or who have received it during the previous 3 months; this should be given within 10 days of exposure to chicken pox. If a diagnosis of chickenpox is confirmed, the illness warrants specialist care and urgent treatment. Dexamethasone should not be stopped and the dose may need to be increased.

Live vaccines should not be given to individuals with impaired immune responsiveness. The antibody response to other vaccines may be diminished.

False negative results may occur with the nitroblue tetrazolium test for bacterial infection.

Extreme caution should be exercised in the treatment of patients with the following conditions and frequent patient monitoring is necessary:

Liver failure, chronic renal failure, congestive heart failure, hypertension, epilepsy, migraine.

Osteoporosis, since corticosteroids increase calcium excretion. Post-menopausal women are at particular risk.

Latent tuberculosis, as corticosteroids can cause reactivation.

Hypothyroidism or cirrhosis, because such patients often show an exaggerated response to corticosteroids.

Latent amoebiasis, as corticosteroids may cause reactivation. Prior to treatment, amoebiasis should be ruled out in any patient with unexplained diarrhoea or who has recently spent time in the tropics.

Ocular herpes simplex, because corticosteroids may cause corneal perforation.

Corticosteroids should also be used with caution in patients with diabetes mellitus (or a family history of diabetes), affective disorders (especially previous steroid psychosis), glaucoma (or a family history of glaucoma), peptic ulceration or previous corticosteroid-induced myopathy.

*Interaction with other medicaments and other forms of interaction:* Liver enzyme inducing drugs such as barbiturates, ephedrine, rifampicin, rifabutin, carbamazepine, phenytoin, primidone and aminoglutethimide may enhance the metabolism of corticosteroids, resulting in a decrease in pharmacological action, and a need for dosage adjustment.

The efficacy of coumarin anticoagulants may be enhanced by concurrent corticosteroid therapy and close monitoring of prothombin time or INR is required to avoid spontaneous bleeding. Corticosterioids may affect glucose tolerance and increase the dosage requirement for hypoglycaemic drugs (including insulin).

The incidence of gastro-intestinal ulceration is increased in patients receiving concomitant nonsteroidal anti-inflammatory drugs and corticosteroids.

The renal clearance of salicylates is increased by corticosteroids and steroid withdrawal may result in salicylate intoxication.

Diuretics are antagonised by corticosteroids and the hypokalaemic effects of acetozolamide, loop diuretics, thiazide diuretics and carbenoxolone are enhanced. Patients receiving corticosteroids and potassium depleting diuretics and/or cardiac glycosides, should be monitored for hypokalaemia. This is of particular importance in patients receiving cardiac glycosides, since hypokalamia increases the toxicity of these drugs. The effects of anti-hypertensive drugs are also antagonised by corticosteroids.

*Pregnancy and lactation:*

*Use in pregnancy:* There may be a very small risk of cleft palate and intrauterine growth retardation in the foetus. There is evidence of harmful effects on pregnancy in animals. Infants born to mothers who have received substantial doses of corticosteroids during the pregnancy should be carefully observed, for signs of adrenal insufficiency.

When corticosteroids are essential however, patients with normal pregnancies may be treated as though they were in the non-gravid state. Patients with pre-eclampsia or fluid retention require close monitoring.

*Use in lactation:* Corticosteroids are excreted in small amounts in breast milk. Suppression of growth or other adverse effects may occur. Infants of mothers taking pharmacological doses of steroids should be monitored carefully for signs of adrenal suppression.

*Effects on ability to drive and use machines:* Not applicable.

*Undesirable effects:*

*Adverse reactions:* The incidence of predictable undesirable effects, including hypothalamic-pituitary-adrenal suppression correlates with the relative potency of the drug, dosage, timing of administration and the duration of treatment (see *Other Special Warnings and Precautions*).

High doses of Dexamethasone Sodium Phosphate are intended for short term therapy and therefore adverse reactions are uncommon. However, peptic ulceration and bronchospasm may occur.

Except for hypersensitivity, the following adverse effects have been associated with prolonged systemic corticosteroid therapy.

Endocrine and metabolic disturbances: Suppression of the hypothalamic-pituitary adrenal axis; Cushing-like syndrome, hirsuitism and weight gain; suppression of growth in infants, children and adolescents; secondary adrenocortical unresponsiveness, particularly in times of stress, as in surgery or trauma; menstrual irregularities and amenorrhoea; impaired glucose tolerance with increased requirement for anti-diabetic therapy; hyperglycaemia; negative protein/nitrogen and calcium balance; increased appetite.

Metabolic: Electrolyte imbalance (retention of sodium and water with oedema and hypertension); nitrogen depletion; hyperglycaemia; hypokalaemic alkalosis; increased calcium and potassium excretion and hypertension.

Anti-inflammatory and Immunosupressive effects: Increased susceptibility to and severity of infection with supression of clinical symptoms and signs; opportunistic infections; recurrence of dormant tuberculosis. (See Warnings Section).

Musculoskeletal: Muscular atrophy, proximal myopathy, premature epiphyseal closure, osteoporosis, avascular osteonecrosis, muscle weakness, tendon rupture, vertebral compression and long bone fractures.

Gastro-intestinal: Dyspepsia, peptic ulceration with perforation and haemorrhage, oesophageal ulcerations, acute pancreatitis and candidiasis.

Dermatological: Impaired wound healing; skin atrophy; bruising; telangiectasia and striae; petechiae and ecchymoses; erythema; increased sweating; possible suppression of skin tests; burning or tingling; bruising; allergic dermatitis; urticaria, candidiasis, acne.

Neurological: Mental disturbances, psychological dependence, euphoria, depression, insomnia, headache, convulsions, vertigo. Aggravation of epilepsy and schizoprenia. Increased intra-cranial pressure with papilloedema in children (pseudotumour cerebri), usually after treatment withdrawal.

Ophthalmic: Posterior sub-capsular cataracts or increased intraocular pressure may result in glaucoma or occasionally damage to the optic nerve; exophthalmos papilloedema; corneal or scleral thinning; exacerbation of ophthalmic viral or fungal diseases.

Other: Hypersensitivity including anaphylaxis, has been reported; blindness associated with intralesional therapy around the face and neck; hyperpigmentation; hypopigmentation; subcutaneous and cutaneous atrophy; sterile abscess; post injection flare (following intra-articular injection): Charcot-like arthropathy. Leucocytosis. Thromboembolism.

Withdrawal symptoms and signs: Too rapid a reduction of corticosteroid dosage following prolonged treatment can lead to acute adrenal insufficiency, hypotension and death. (See Warnings Section).

A 'withdrawal syndrome' may also occur including fever, myalgia, arthralgia, rhinitis, conjunctivitis, painful itchy skin nodules and loss of weight.

*Overdose:* Treat anaphylaxis with adrenaline and positive pressure ventilation. Other supportive measures aimed to maintain the patient unstressed.

**Pharmacological properties**

*Pharmacodynamic properties:* Pharmacology of the corticosteroids is complex and the drugs affect almost all body systems. Maximum pharmacologic activity lags behind peak blood concentrations, suggesting that most effects of the drugs result from modification of enzyme activity rather than from direct actions by the drugs.

*Pharmacokinetic properties:* Intramuscular injections of Dexamethasone Phosphate gives maximum plasma concentrations of Dexamethasone at 1 hour. Dexamethasone is readily absorbed from the gastro-intestinal tract. Its biological half-life in plasma is about 190 minutes. Binding of Dexamethasone to plasma proteins is less than for most other corticosteroids. Dexamethasone penetrates into tissue fluids and cerebrospinal fluids. Metabolism of the drug takes place in the kidneys and liver and excretion is via the urine.

*Preclinical safety data:* Not applicable.

**Pharmaceutical particulars**

*List of excipients:*

| | *4 mg* | *8 mg* | *120 mg* |
|---|---|---|---|
| Dexamethasone Sodium Phosphate BP, equivalent to Dexamethasone Phosphate: | 4.0 mg | 8.0 mg | 120.0 mg |
| Creatinine | 8.0 mg | 16.0 mg | 40.0 mg |
| Disodium Edetate BP | | | 2.5 mg |
| Sodium Citrate BP | 10.0 mg | 20.0 mg | 50.0 mg |
| Water for Injection BP to | 1.0 mL | 2.0 mL | 5.0 mL |

*Incompatibilities:* Dexamethasone Sodium Phosphate is physically incompatible with Daunorubicin, Doxorubicin and Vancomycin and should not be admixed with solutions containing these drugs. Also incompatible with Doxapram HCl and glycopyrrolate in syringe.

*Shelf life:* 3 years.

*Special precautions for storage:* Store below 25°C and protect from freezing and from light. Do not use heat to sterilise the exterior of vials. Any unused portion should be discarded immediately after use.

When Dexamethasone Sodium Phosphate is given by intravenous infusion, only Sodium Chloride Injection BP or Glucose Injection BP should be used as diluents. The exact concentration of Dexamethasone Sodium Phosphate per infusion container should be determined by the desired dose, patient fluid intake and drip rate required. Dilutions should be used within 24 hours and discarded after use.

*Instructions for use/handling:* Not applicable.

**Marketing authorisation numbers**

| | |
|---|---|
| 120 mg/5 ml | 4515/0018 |
| 4 mg/1 ml | 4515/0019 |
| 8 mg/2 ml | 4515/0020 |

**Date of approval/revision of SPC** July 1995

**Legal category** POM

## STERILE DOBUTAMINE HYDROCHLORIDE CONCENTRATE.

**Qualitative and quantitative composition**

| | per vial | per mL |
|---|---|---|
| Dobutamine Hydrochloride USP | 280.2 mg* | 14.01 mg |
| (equivalent to Dobutamine) | (250.0 mg) | (12.50 mg) |
| Sodium Metabisulphite BP | 4.4 mg | 0.22 mg |
| Water for Injections BP to | 20.0 mL | 1.0 mL |

* No overage is required in the formulation.

**Pharmaceutical form** Aqueous solution for injection.

**Clinical particulars**

*Therapeutic indications:* Dobutamine Hydrochloride is a sympathomimetic agent which acts by stimulating the ß1 adrenergic receptors of the heart promoting a prominent inotropic action on the heart, increasing cardiac contractility and stroke volume It is a direct acting agent.

Dobutamine is indicated for adults who require inotropic support in the treatment of low output cardiac failure associated with organic heart disease, myocardial infarction, open heart surgery, cardiomyopathies, septic shock and cardiogenic shock. Dobutamine can increase or maintain cardiac output during positive end expiratory pressure (PEEP) ventilation. The drug should not be used in patients with marked mechanical obstruction, ie. severe valvular aortic stenosis.

*Posology and method of administration:* Dobutamine Hydrochloride should be administered by IV infusion only using an infusion pump or other apparatus to control the flow rate.

Dobutamine Hydrochloride must be diluted to a final volume of at least 50 mL with the following IV infusion solutions:

Sodium Chloride Intravenous Infusion BP
5% Dextrose Intravenous Infusion BP

If diluting to 250 mL or 500 mL, dilution will give a concentration for administration as follows:

250 mL contains 1,000 micrograms/ml of Dobutamine

500 mL contains 500 micrograms/ml of Dobutamine
1000 mL contains 250 micrograms/ml of Dobutamine

Diluted solution should be used within 24 hours, when aseptically prepared and stored in the refrigerator.

*Administration:* The concentration of Dobutamine administered depends upon the dosage and fluid requirements of the individual patient. Concentrations of 5000 microgram/ml have been used in fluid restricted patients but this concentration should not be exceeded. High concentrations of Dobutamine should only be given with an infusion pump to ensure accurate dosage. Due to it's short half-life Dobutamine should be administered as a continuous intravenous infusion. Dobutamine should be administered intravenously through an intravenous needle or catheter. An intravenous pump or other suitable apparatus should be used to control the flow rate in drops per minute.

*Dosage:*
*Adults:* The usual rate is 2.5 to 10 mcg per kg bodyweight per minute,which should be adjusted according to the patients heart rate, blood pressure, cardiac output and urine output. Up to 40 micrograms per kg per minute may occasionally be required but this is rare. Dobutamine infusions have been given for up to 72 hours without a decrease in effectiveness. It is recommended that treatment with Dobutamine should be discontinued gradually.

Side-effects which are dose related, are infrequent when Dobutamine is administered at rates below 10 microgram/kg/min. Rates as high as 40 microgram/kg/min have been used occasionally without significant adverse effects.

*Children:* The safety and efficacy of Dobutamine has not been established in children.

*Contra-indications:* Dobutamine is contra-indicated in patients with idiopathic hypertrophic subaortic stenosis or with known hypersensitivity to Dobutamine.

*Special warnings and special precautions for use:*
*Warnings:* If an undue increase in heart rate or systolic blood pressure occurs or if an arrythmia is precipitated the dose of Dobutamine should be reduced or the drug should be discontinued temporarily.

Dobutamine may precipitate or exacerbate ventricular ectopic activity, rarely has it caused ventricular tachycardia or fibrillation. Because Dobutamine increases atrioventricular conduction, patients with atrial flutter or fibrillation may develop a rapid ventricular response, and therefore should be digitalised prior to administration of Dobutamine.

Experience with the use of Dobutamine following acute myocardial infarction is limited. However there is a possibility that Dobutamine can cause a significant increase in heart rate or excessive increase in arterial pressure which may intensify or extend myocardial ischaemia, cause anginal pain and elevate ST segment, therefore care should be exercised following myocardial infarction.

Dobutamine will not improve haemodynamics in most patients with mechanical obstruction affecting ventricular filling or outflow, or both. Inotropic response may be inadequate in patients with markedly reduced ventricular compliance, eg. with cardiac tamponade, valvular aortic stenosis, and idiopathic hypertrophic subaortic stenosis.

Minor vasoconstriction has been observed in patients treated with beta blocking drugs. This may occur due to the inotropic effect of Dobutamine which stimulates cardiac ß1 receptors and which is blocked by ß blockers. Conversely alpha adrenergic blockade may make the ß1 and ß2 effects apparent, resulting in tachycardia and vasodilatation.

*Precautions:* Before administration of Dobutamine, hypovolaemia should be corrected with an appropriate plasma volume expander. The ECG, blood pressure and when possible, cardiac output and pulmonary wedge pressure should be monitored.

Like other drugs with ß2 agonist activity, Dobutamine may produce slight reductions in serum potassium concentrations and hypokalaemia may occur occasionally. Consideration should be given to monitoring serum potassium during Dobutamine therapy.

During administration of Dobutamine heart rate and rhythm, arterial blood pressure, and infusion rate should be monitored closely. When starting therapy, electrocardiographic monitoring is recommended until a stable response is obtained.

*Interaction with other medicaments and other forms of interaction:* ß-Adrenergic blocking agents: In animals the cardiac effects of Dobutamine are antagonised by ß-adrenergic blocking agents such as propranolol and metoprolol, resulting in predominance of alpha-adrenergic blocking agents and increased peripheral resistance.

General anaesthetics: Ventricular arrythymias have been reported in animals receiving usual doses of Dobutamine during Halothane or Cyclopropane anaesthesia; therefore, caution should be exercised when administering Dobutamine to patients receiving these anaesthetics.

*Pregnancy and lactation:* Safe use of Dobutamine during pregnancy has not been established. Reproductive studies in rats and rabbits have not revealed any evidence of impaired fertility, evidence of harm to the foetus or teratogenic effects. Dobutamine should not be used in pregnant women unless the possible benefits outweigh the potential risks.

It is not known if Dobutamine crosses the placenta or is distributed into milk.

*Effects on ability to drive and use machines:* Not applicable.

*Undesirable effects:*
*Adverse effects:* Principal adverse effects are ectopic heart beats, increased heart rate, angina, chest pain, palpitation and elevations in blood pressure. All of these cardiovascular effects are usually dose related, and dosage should be reduced or temporarily discontinued if they occur. Rarely Dobutamine has caused ventricular tachycardia.

Other less frequent adverse effects include nausea, vomiting, tingling sensation, parasthesia, dyspnoea, headache and mild leg cramps; pruritis of the scalp during IV infusion of Dobutamine has been reported as with other reactions indicative of hypersensitivity, including rash, fever, eosinophilia and bronchospasm.

Phlebitis at the site of the IV infusion has been reported occasionally. Inadvertant subcutaneous infiltration of Dobutamine has caused local inflammatory changes and local pain without local ischaemia, however rarely dermal necrosis has been reported.

As with other catecholamines, decreases in serum potassium concentrations have occurred, rarely to hypokalaemic values.

Infusions for up to 72 hours have revealed no adverse effects other than those seen with shorter infusions. There is evidence that partial tolerance develops with continuous infusions of Dobutamine for 72 hours or more; therefore higher doses may be required to maintain the same effects.

*Overdose:* Overdosage have been reported rarely. The symptoms of toxicity may include anorexia, nausea, vomiting, tremor, anxiety, palpitations, headache, shortness of breath, fatigue and anginal and specific chest pain. The positive inotropic and chronotropic effects of Dobutamine may cause hypertension, tachyarrythmias, myocardial ischaemia and ventricular fibrillation. Hypotension may result from vasodilatation. The duration of action of Dobutamine Hydrochloride is generally short (half-life, approximately 2 minutes).

Temporarily discontinue Dobutamine until the patient's condition stabilises. The patient should be monitored and any appropriate resusitative measures started immediately.

Forced diuresis, peritoneal dialysis, haemodialysis or charcoal haemoperfusion have not been established as beneficial.

If the product is ingested, unpredictable absorption may occur from the mouth and gastrointestinal tract.

Dobutamine should be used with caution in severe hypotension complicating cardiogenic shock (mean arterial pressure less than 70 mm Hg). If the blood pressure drops quickly decreasing the dose or stopping the infusion typically results in a return to baseline blood pressure values. Occasionally intervention may be required and reversibility may not be immediate.

If arterial blood pressure remains low or decreases progressively during administration of Dobutamine despite adequate ventricular filling pressure and cardiac output consideration may be given to the use of a peripheral vasoconstrictor agent eg Noradrenaline or Dopamine.

DBL Dobutamine Hydrochloride contains sodium metabisulphite in the formulation. This may cause allergic type reactions including anaphylaxis and life-threatening or less severe asthmatic episodes, in certain susceptable individuals. The overall prevalence of sulphite sensitivity in the general population is unknown but probably low; such sensitivity seems to occur more frequently in asthmatic patients.

**Pharmacological properties**

*Pharmacodynamic properties:* Dobutamine is a selective ß-adrenergic agonist whose mechanism of action is complex.

It is believed that the ß-adrenergic effects result from stimulation of adenyl cyclase activity. In therapeutic doses, Dobutamine also has mild ß2- and a1-adrenergic receptor agonist effects, which are relatively balanced and result in minimal net direct effect on systemic vasculature. Dobutamine does not cause release of endogenous norepinephrine. The main effect of therapeutic doses of Dobutamine is cardiac stimulation. While the positive inotropic effect of the drug on the myocardium appears to be mediated principally via ß1-adrenergic stimulation, experimental evidence suggests that a1-adrenergic stimulation may also be involved and that the a1-adrenergic activity results mainly from the (-)-stereoisomer of the drug.

The ß1-adrenergic effects of Dobutamine exert a positive inotropic effect on the myocardium and result in an increase in cardiac output due to increased myocardial contractility and stroke volume. Increased left ventricular filling pressure decreases in patients with congestive heart failure. In therapeutic doses, Dobutamine causes a decrease in peripheral resistance; however, systolic blood pressure and pulse pressure may remain unchanged or be increased because of augmented cardiac output. With usual doses, heart rate is usually not substantially changed. Coronary blood flow and myocardial oxygen consumption are usually increased because of increased myocardial contractility.

Dobutamine facilitates atrioventricular conduction and shortens or causes no important change in intraventricular conduction. The tendency of Dobutamine to induce cardiac arrhythmias may be slightly less than that of dopamine and is considerably less than that of isoproterenol or other catecholamines. Pulmonary vascular resistance may decrease if it is elevated initially and mean pulmonary artery pressure may decrease or remain unchanged. Dobutamine does not seem to affect dopaminergic receptors and causes no renal or mesenteric vasodilation; however, urine flow may increase because of increased cardiac output.

*Pharmacokinetic properties:*
*Absorption:* Orally administered Dobutamine is rapidly metabolized in the GI tract. Following IV administration, the onset of action of Dobutamine occurs within 2 minutes. Peak plasma concentrations of the drug and peak effects occur within 10 minutes after initiation of an IV infusion. The effects of the drug cease shortly after discontinuing an infusion.

*Distribution:* It is not known if Dobutamine crosses the placenta or is distributed into milk.

*Elimination:* The plasma half-life of Dobutamine is about 2 minutes. Dobutamine is metabolized in the liver and other tissues by catechol-O-methyltransferase to an inactive compound, 3-O-methyldobutamine, and by conjugation with glucuronic acid. Conjugates of Dobutamine and 3-O-methyldobutamine are excreted mainly in urine and to a minor extent in faeces.

**Pharmaceutical particulars**

*List of excipients:*

| | |
|---|---|
| Sodium Metabisulphite BP | 0.22 mg |
| Water for Injections BP | to 1.0 mL. |

*Incompatibilities:* Dobutamine Hydrochloride has been reported to be incompatible with alkaline solutions and should not be mixed with sodium bicarbonate 5%, or other strong alkaline solutions ie. aminophylline, frusemide. Precipitation has occured with bumetanide, calcium gluconate, insulin, diazepam and phenytoin Because of the potential physical incompatibilities, it is recommended that Dobutamine Hydrochloride not be mixed with other drugs in the same solution.

Dobutamine should not be used with drugs or diluents containing bisulphites or ethanol.

*Shelf life:* 24 months

*Special precautions for storage:* Undiluted vials of Dobutamine Hydrochloride should be stored below 25°C.

Prepared intravenous solutions are stable for 24 hours, when aseptically prepared and stored in the refrigerator.

Solutions of Dobutamine Hydrochloride may have a pink discolouration. This discolouration, which will increase with time, results from a slight oxidation of the drug. However, there is no significant loss of drug potency within the recommended storage times for solutions of the drug.

*Instructions for use/handling:* Not applicable.

**Marketing authorisation number** 4515/0077.

**Date of approval/revision of SPC** September 1995

**Legal category** POM

# STERILE DOPAMINE CONCENTRATE

## Qualitative and quantitative composition
*Active constituent*
Dopamine Hydrochloride HSE    800.0 mg   200.0 mg
*Other constituents*
Sodium Metabisulphite BP    50.0 mg   50.0 mg
Water for Injections BP    5.0 mL   5.0 mL

There is no overage included in the formulation.

**Pharmaceutical form** Concentrated solution for intravenous infusion.

## Clinical particulars

*Therapeutic indications:* Dopamine is indicated for the correction of haemodynamic imbalance present in:

a. Acute hypotension or shock associated with myocardial infarction, endotoxic septicaemia, trauma and renal failure.

b. As an adjunct after open heart surgery, where there is persistent hypotension after correction of hypovolaemia.

c. In chronic cardiac decompensation as in congestive failure.

*Posology and method of administration:* Dopamine is a potent drug; it must be diluted before administration. *Adults:* Where appropriate, the circulating blood volume must be restored with a suitable plasma expander or whole blood, prior to administration of dopamine hydrochloride.

Begin infusion of dopamine hydrochloride solution at doses of 2.5 mcg/kg/min in patients who are likely to respond to modest increments of heart force and renal perfusion.

In more severe cases, administration may be initiated at a rate of 5 mcg/kg/min and increased gradually in 5 to 10 mcg/kg/min increments up to 20 to 50 mcg/kg/min as needed. If doses in excess of 50 mcg/kg/min are required, it is advisable to check urine output frequently.

Should urinary flow begin to decrease in the absence of hypotension, reduction of dopamine dosage should be considered. It has been found that more than 50% of patients have been satisfactorily maintained on doses less than 20 mcg/kg/min.

In patients who do not respond to these doses, additional increments of dopamine may be given in an effort to achieve adequate blood pressure, urine flow and perfusion generally.

Treatment of all patients requires constant evaluation of therapy in terms of blood volume, augmentation of cardiac contractility, and distribution of peripheral perfusion and urinary output.

Dosage of dopamine should be adjusted according to the patient's response, with particular attention to diminution of established urine flow rate, increasing tachycardia or development of new dysrhythmias as indications for decreasing or temporarily suspending the dosage.

*Preparation of infusion solutions:*
*Suggested dilution:* Aseptically transfer Sterile Dopamine Concentrate into the I.V. solution as shown in the following table :

| Strength | Volume (mL) | I.V. solution volume (mL) | Final concentration (microgram/ mL) |
|---|---|---|---|
| 200 mg/5 ml | 5 | 500 | 400 |
| 200 mg/5 ml | 5 | 250 | 800 |
| 200 mg/5 ml | 10 | 250 | 1600 |
| 200 mg/5 ml | 20 | 500 | 1600 |
| 800 mg/5 ml | 5 | 500 | 1600 |
| 800 mg/5 ml | 5 | 250 | 3200 |

Dopamine Hydrochloride can be diluted with:
   0.9% Sodium Chloride Injection
   5% Dextrose / 0.45% Sodium Chloride Solution
   Compound Sodium Lactate (Hartmann's) Solution
Dilution in these fluids retain at least 95% of the original potency for 48 hours at room temperature under normal fluorescent light. Dilutions should be discarded immediately after use.
   Children: The safety and efficacy of Dopamine in paediatric patients has not been established.
   Geriatric: No variation in dosage is suggested for geriatric patients. However, close monitoring is suggested for blood pressure, urine flow and peripheral tissue perfusion.

*Contra-indications:* Dopamine should not be used in patients with phaeochromocytoma or hyperthyroidism.

Dopamine should not be used in the presence of uncorrected arterial or ventricular tachyarrhythmias or ventricular fibrillation.

Cyclopropane and halogenated hydrocarbon anaesthetics should be avoided.

*Special warnings and special precautions for use:*
*Warnings:* Dopamine should not be used in the presence of uncorrected tachyarrhythmias or ventricular fibrillation. Nor should it be used in patients with phaeochromocytoma or hyperthyroidism. Cyclopropane and halogenated hydrocarbon anaesthetics should be avoided.

Patients who have been treated with MAO inhibitors prior to Dopamine should be given reduced doses; the starting dose should be one tenth (1/10th) of the usual dose.

Excess administration of potassium-free solutions may result in significant hypokalaemia. The intravenous administration of these solutions can cause fluid and/or solute overloading resulting in dilution of serum electrolyte concentrations, overhydration, congested states or pulmonary oedema.

*Precautions:* Hypovolaemia should be corrected where necessary prior to Dopamine infusion. Low doses should be used in shock due to acute myocardial infarction.

If a disproportionate rise in diastolic pressure (i.e. a marked decrease in pulse pressure) is observed, the infusion rate should be decreased and the patients observed carefully for further evidence of predominant vasoconstriction activity, unless such an effect is desired.

Patients with a history of peripheral vascular disease should be closely monitored for any changes in colour or temperature of the skin of the extremities. If a change of skin colour or temperature occurs and is thought to be the result of compromised circulation to the extremities, the benefits of continued dopamine infusion should be weighed against the risk of possible necrosis. These changes may be reversed by decreasing the rate or discontinuing the infusion.

Dopamine hydrochloride in 5% dextrose injection should be infused into a large vein whenever possible to prevent the possibility of infiltration of perivascular tissue adjacent to the infusion site. Extravasation may cause necrosis and sloughing of the surrounding tissue. Ischaemia can be reversed by infiltration of the affected area with 10-15 ml of saline containing 5 to 10 mg phentolamine mesylate. A syringe with a fine hypodermic needle should be used to liberally infiltrate the ischaemic area as soon as extravasation is noted.

Dopamine should be used with extreme caution in patients inhaling cyclopropane or halogenated hydrocarbon anaesthetics due to the arterial arrhythmogenic potential.

Dextrose solutions should be used with caution in patients with known subclinical or overt diabetes mellitus.

*Interaction with other medicaments and other forms of interaction:*
   Anaesthetics: The myocardium is sensitised by the effect of Dopamine, Cyclopropane or halogenated hydrocarbon anaesthetics, and these should be avoided. This interaction applies both to pressor activity and cardiac beta adrenergic stimulation.
   Alpha and beta blockers: The cardiac effects of Dopamine are antagonised by β-adrenergic blocking agents such as Propanolol and Metoprolol, and the peripheral vasoconstriction caused by high doses of

Dopamine is antagonised by a-adrenergic blocking agents. Dopamine-induced renal and mesenteric vasodilation is not antagonised by either a or β-adrenergic blocking agents but, in animals, is antagonised by Haloperidol or other butyrophenones, phenothiazines, and opiates.

   Monoamine Oxidase (MAO) Inhibitors: MAO inhibitors potentiate the effect of Dopamine and its duration of action. Patients who have been treated with monoamine oxidase (MAO) inhibitors prior to dopamine should be given reduced doses; the starting dose should be one tenth (1/10th) of the usual dose.

   Phenytoin: Administration of I.V. Phenytoin to patients receiving Dopamine has resulted in hypotension and bradycardia; some clinicians recommend that Phenytoin be used with extreme caution, if at all, in patients receiving Dopamine.

*Pregnancy and lactation:*
Use in pregnancy: Animal studies have shown no evidence of teratogenic effects with dopamine. However, the effect of Dopamine on the human foetus is unknown therefore the drug should be used in pregnant women only when the expected benefits outweight the potential risk to the foetus.

Use in lactation: It is not known if Dopamine is excreted in breast milk nor if there is any effect of the infant.

*Effects on ability to drive and use machines:* Not applicable.

*Undesirable effects:* Adverse reactions to dopamine are related to its pharmacological action.
*More common reactions:*
   Cardiovascular: Ectopic beats, tachycardia, anginal pain, palpitation, hypotension, vasoconstriction.
   Gastrointestinal. Nausea, vomiting.
   Nervous System. Headache.
   Respiratory. Dyspnoea.
*Less common reactions:*
   Biochemical Abnormalities. Azotaemia.
   Cardiovasular. Aberrant conduction, bradycardia, widened QRS complex, hypertension, gangrene.
   Nervous system. Piloerection.
*Serious or life-threatening reactions:* Gangrene of the feet has occurred following doses of 10-14 mcg/kg/min and higher in a few patients with pre-existing vascular disease.

*Overdose:* Excessive elevation of blood pressure and vasoconstriction can occur due to the alpha adrenergic actions of dopamine, especially in patients with a history of occlusive vascular disease. If desired, this condition can be rapidly reversed by dose reduction or discontinuing the infusion, since dopamine has a half-life of less than 2 minutes in the body. Should these measures fail, an infusion of an alpha adrenergic blocking agent eg., phentolamine mesylate should be considered. Dopamine at the infusion site can cause local vasoconstriction, hence the desirability of infusing into a large vein. The resulting ischaemia can be reversed by infiltration of the effected area with 10-15 ml of saline containing 5 to 10 mg phentolamine mesylate. A syringe with a fine hypodermic needle should be used to liberally infiltrate the ischaemic area as soon as extravasation is noted.

*Accidental overdosage:* Accidental overdosage as evidenced by excessive blood pressure elevation can be controlled by dose reduction or discontinuing the dopamine infusion for a short period, since the duration of action of dopamine is short.

Should these measures fail, an infusion of phentolamine mesylate should be considered.

### Pharmacological properties

*Pharmacodynamic properties:* Dopamine stimulates adrenergic receptors of the sympathetic nervous system. The drug has principally a direct stimulatory effect on β1-adrenergic receptors, but also appears to have an indirect effect by releasing norepinephrine from its storage sites. Dopamine also appears to act on specific dopaminergic receptors in the renal, mesenteric, coronary, and intracerebral vascular beds to cause vasodilation. The drug has little or no effect on β2-adrenergic receptors.

In I.V. doses of 0.5-2 mcg/kg per minute, the drug acts predominantly on dopaminergic receptors; in I.V. doses of 2-10 mcg/kg per minute, the drug also stimulates β1-adrenergic receptors. In higher therapeutic doses, a-adrenergic receptors are stimulated and the net effect of the drug is the result of a-adrenergic, β1-adrenergic, and dopaminergic stimulation. The main effects of Dopamine depend on the dose administered. In low doses, cardiac stimulation and renal vascular dilation occur and in larger doses vasoconstriction occurs. It is believed that a-adrenergic effects result from inhibition of the production of cyclic adenosine -31, 51-monophosphate (cAMP) by inhibition of the enzyme adenyl cyclase, whereas β-adrenergic effects result from stimulation of adenyl cyclase activity.

*Pharmacokinetic properties:*
Absorption: Orally administered Dopamine is rapidly

metabolised in the G.I. tract. Following I.V. administration, the onset of action of Dopamine occurs within 5 minutes, and the drug has a duration of action of less than 10 minutes.

*Distribution:* The drug is widely distributed in the body but does not cross the blood-brain barrier to a substantial extent. It is not known if Dopamine crosses the placenta.

*Elimination:* Dopamine has a plasma half-life of about 2 minutes. Dopamine is metabolised in the liver, kidneys, and plasma by monoamine oxidase (MAO) and catechol-0-methyltransferase to the inactive compounds homovanillic acid (HVA) and 3,4-dihydroxyphenylacetic acid. In patients receiving MAO inhibitors, the duration of action of Dopamine may be as long as 1 hour. About 25% of a dose of Dopamine is metabolised to norepinephrine within the adrenergic nerve terminals.

Dopamine is excreted in urine principally as HVA and its sulphate and glucuronide conjugates and as 3,4-dihydroxyphenylacetic acid. A very small fraction of a dose is excreted unchanged. Following administration of radio labelled Dopamine, approximately 80% of the radioactivity reportedly is excreted in urine within 24 hours.

**Pharmaceutical particulars**

*List of excipients:*

| | |
|---|---|
| Sodium Metabisulphite BP | 50.0 mg |
| Water for Injections BP | 5.0 mL. |

There is no overage included in the formulation.

*Incompatibilities:* Sterile Dopamine Concentrate should not be added to any alkaline intravenous solutions, i.e. Sodium Bicarbonate. Any solution which exhibits physical or chemical incompatibility through a colour change or precipitate should not be administered.

It is suggested that admixtures containing Gentamicin Sulphate, Cephalothin Sodium, Cephalothin Sodium Neutral or Oxacillin Sodium should be avoided unless all other viable alternatives have been exhausted.

Admixtures of Ampicillin and Dopamine in 5% Glucose Solution are alkaline and incompatible and result in decomposition of both drugs. They should not be admixed.

Admixtures of Dopamine, Amphotericin B in 5% Glucose Solution are incompatible as a precipitate forms immediately on mixing.

*Shelf life:* 36 months.

*Special precautions for storage*: Store below 30°C. Protect from light.

Do not add dopamine to 5% sodium bicarbonate or other alkaline solutions, since the drug is inactivated. Store below 30°C, protect from light, do not use if discoloured. Any solution which exhibits physical or chemical incompatibility through a colour change or precipitate should not be administered.

*Instructions for use/handling*: Not applicable.

**Marketing authorisation numbers**

| | |
|---|---|
| 800 mg/5 mL | 4515/0022 |
| 200 mg/5 mL | 4515/0011 |

**Date of approval/revision of SPC** November 1993

**Legal category** POM

## DOXORUBICIN HYDROCHLORIDE FOR INJECTION

**Qualitative and quantitative composition**

| *Active constituent* | *10 mg* | *50 mg* |
|---|---|---|
| Doxorubicin USP | 10.0 mg | 50.0 mg |

**Pharmaceutical form** Sterile freeze dried powder for injection.

**Clinical particulars**

*Therapeutic indications:* Doxorubicin has been used successfully in the treatment of neoplastic conditions such as acute leukaemia, soft tissue and osteogenic sarcomas, breast carcinoma, lymphomas , bronchogenic (lung) carcinoma. It has also been used in the treatment of paediatric malignancy. Doxorubicin is frequently used in combination chemotherapy regimen involving other cytotoxic drugs. Doxorubicin can be used in the treatment of non-metastatic transitional cell carcinoma, carcinoma in situ and papillary tumours of the bladder, by intravesical administration.

*Posology and method of administration:* When used as a single agent, the recommended dosage schedule is 60- 75 mg/m² body surface area, as a single intravenous injection administered at 21 day intervals. If using body weight to calculate the dose, then dosages of 1.2–2.4 mg/kg are recommended.

It has been shown that giving doxorubicin as a single dose every three weeks greatly reduces the distressing toxic effect, mucositis. However, there are some regimens which divide the dose over three successive days (20-25 mg/m² or 0.4-0.8 mg/kg). It is thought that this regimen has greater effectiveness although at a cost of higher toxicity

Administration of doxorubicin in a weekly regimen has been shown to be as effective as the three weekly regimen. The recommended dosage is 20 mg/m² once a week although objective responses have been seen at 6-12 mg/m². This regimen of weekly dosing also reduces the incidence of cardiotoxicity.

It is particularly important to reduce the dose of doxorubicin if it is used in combination with other drugs with a similar toxicity profile. The recommended lifetime cumulative dose limit is 450-550 mg doxorubicin hydrochloride/m² body surface area.

It is recommended that doxorubicin be slowly administered into the tubing of a freely running intravenous infusion of Sodium Chloride Injection 0.9% or 5% Dextrose Injection. The tubing should be attached to a Butterfly needle inserted preferably into a large vein. The rate of administration is dependent on the size of the vein and the dosage. However the dose should be administered in not less than 3 to 5 minutes. This technique minimises the risk of thrombosis or perivenous extravasation which can lead to severe cellulitis and vesication.

Intravenous infusion is not advised due to the tissue damage that may occur if the infusion infiltrates the tissues. If a central vein catheter is used then infusion of Doxorubicin in Sodium Chloride 0.9% Injection is advised.

Local erythematous streaking along the vein as well as facial flushing may be indicative of too rapid administration. A burning or stinging sensation may be indicative of perivenous infiltration and the infusion should be immediately terminated and restarted in another vein. Doxorubicin should not be mixed with heparin since it has been reported that these drugs are incompatible to the extent that a precipitate may form. Until specific compatibility data are available, it is not recommended that doxorubicin be mixed with other drugs.

*Intravesical administration:* This technique may be used for the treatment of transitional cell carcinoma, papillary bladder tumours and carcinoma in situ. It should not be used for invasive tumours of the bladder which have penetrated the bladder wall.

Many regimens are in use, making interpretation difficult, but the following procedure may be a helpful guide:

1. Patient should be instructed not to drink fluids for 12 hours prior to the examination.
2. Dissolve 50 mg of doxorubicin in 50 mL of normal saline and instil via the catheter into the bladder.
3. The catheter should be removed and the patient instructed to be on one side. At 15 minute intervals the patient should make a quarter turn over a 1 hour period. At the end of this period, the patient may void.
4. The procedure may be repeated at monthly intervals.

*Intra-arterial administration:* Doxorubicin Hydrochloride has been administered as an intra-arterial infusion in an attempt to produce local intense activity and reduce systemic toxicity. However it must be recognised that this route of administration is potentially extremely hazardous and can lead to widespread necrosis of perfused tissue unless careful precautions are taken. Intraarterial administration should be undertaken only by experienced professionals.

*Paediatric:* Adult dosage regimens may be suitable for paediatric cases, but may need to be reduced.

*Geriatric:* It is recommended that the total cumulative dose of doxorubicin for adults aged 70 or older be restricted to 450 mg/m² body surface area. Adult doses may be suitable for geriatric patients, but may need to be reduced.

*Impaired hepatic function:* Doxorubicin is metabolised by the liver and excreted in bile. Impairment of liver function results in slower excretion of the drug and consequently increased retention and accumulation in the plasma and tissues, resulting in enhanced clinical toxicity.

Doxorubicin dosage must be reduced if hepatic function is impaired according to the following table:

| *Serum bilirubin levels* | *BSP retention* | *Recommended dose* |
|---|---|---|
| 1.2–3.0 mg/100 mL | 9–15% | 50% normal dose |
| over 3.0 mg/100 mL | over 15% | 25% normal dose |

*Impaired renal function:* Doxorubicin and metabolites are excreted in the urine to a minor degree and there are no clear indications that the pharmacokinetics or toxicity of doxorubicin are altered in patients with impaired renal function.

*Contra-indications:* Dosage should not be repeated in cases of bone marrow depression or buccal ulceration or buccal burning sensation, which can precede ulceration.

Experienced Physician: Doxorubicin should be administered only under the supervision of a physician who is experienced in the use of cancer chemotherapeutic agents.

*Special warnings and special precautions for use:*

*Warnings:* Cardiac toxicity: Special attention must be given to the cardiac toxicity exhibited by doxorubicin. This may present as tachycardia or ECG changes including supraventricular tachycardia. Severe cardiac failure may occur suddenly, without premonitory ECG changes.

It is recommended that the cumulative total lifetime dose of doxorubicin (including related drugs such as daunorubicin) should not exceed 450–550 mg/sq m body surface area. Above this dosage, the risk of irreversible congestive cardiac failure increases greatly. Total dose should also take account of any previous or concomitant mediastinal irradiation, other anthracycline chemotherapy or concurrent high dose cyclophosphamide, which may also exhibit cardiotoxic effects.

Congestive heart failure and/or cardiomyopathy may be encountered several weeks after discontinuation of doxorubicin therapy and for this reason extreme care should be taken in patients with existing associated heart disease.

Cardiac failure is often not favourably affected by presently known medical or physical therapy for cardiac support. Early clinical diagnosis of drug induced heart failure appears to be essential for successful treatment with digitalis, diuretics, low salt diet and bed rest. Severe cardiac toxicity may occur precipitously without antecedent ECG changes. Base line ECG and periodic follow up ECG during and immediately after active drug therapy is an advisable precaution. Transient ECG changes, such as T-wave flattening, S-T depression and arrhythmias are not considered indications for suspension of doxorubicin therapy. A persistent reduction in the voltage of the QRS wave is presently considered more specifically predictive for cardiac toxicity. If this occurs, the benefit of continued therapy must be carefully evaluated against the risk of producing irreversible cardiac damage.

Bone marrow depression: There is a high incidence of bone marrow depression, primarily of leucocytes, requiring careful haematological monitoring. With the recommended dosage schedule, leucopenia is usually transient, reaching its nadir at 10–14 days after treatment, with recovery usually occurring by the 21st day. White blood cell counts as low as 1000/cubic mm are to be expected during treatment with appropriate doses of doxorubicin. Red blood cell and platelet levels should also be monitored, since they may also be depressed.

Haematologic toxicity may require dose reduction or suspension or delay of doxorubicin therapy.

Immunosuppression: Doxorubicin is a powerful but temporary immunosuppressant agent. Appropriate measures should be taken to prevent secondary infection.

Severe myelosuppression: Persistent severe myelosuppression may result in superinfection or haemorrhage.

Enhanced toxicity: It has been reported that doxorubicin may enhance the severity of the toxicity of anticancer therapies, such as cyclophosphamide induced haemorrhagic cystitis, mucositis induced by radiotherapy and hepatotoxicity of 6-mercaptopurine.

Infertility: Doxorubicin may cause infertility during the time of drug administration. Although ovulation and menstruation appear to return after termination of therapy, there is no information about the restoration of male fertility.

Hepatic impairment: Toxicity to recommended doses of doxorubicin is enhanced by hepatic impairment. It is recommended that an evaluation of hepatic function be carried out prior to individual dosing, using conventional clinical laboratory tests such as AST, ALT, alkaline phosphatase, bilirubin and BSP. If required, dosage schedules should be reduced accordingly (see Dosage and administration).

Extravasation: On intravenous administration of doxorubicin, a stinging or burning sensation signifies extravasation and, even if blood return from aspiration of the infusion needle is good, the injection or infusion should be immediately terminated and restarted in another vein.

Should extravasation occur, stop the infusion immediately and apply ice packs to the injection site. Local injection of dexamethasone or hydrocortisone may be used to minimise local tissue necrosis. Hydrocortisone cream 1% may also be applied locally.

*Precautions:* Initial treatment with doxorubicin requires close observation of the patient and extensive laboratory monitoring.

It is strongly recommended therefore, that patients be hospitalised at least during the first phase of treatment. Blood count and liver function tests should be carried out prior to each doxorubicin treatment.

*Interaction with other medicaments and other forms of interaction:* Not applicable.

*Pregnancy and lactation:*
Use In pregnancy*:* The drug is embryotoxic and teratogenic in rats and embryotoxic and abortifacient in rabbits, and trace amounts of the drug have been found in mouse foetuses and in one aborted human foetus. Although there is no conclusive evidence, there is data which suggests that doxorubicin may harm the foetus. It is therefore recommended that doxorubicin is not administered to women who are pregnant.
Use In lactation: Doxorubicin is distributed into milk. Experimental data suggests that doxorubicin may harm the infant and should therefore not be administered to mothers who are breast feeding.

*Use In intravesical administration:* Urine cytologies and blood counts should be monitored monthly, and cytoscopic examinations should be performed at regular intervals.

*Effects on ability to drive and use machines:* Not known.

*Undesirable effects:*
*Adverse reactions–more common reactions:*
Cardiovascular: Cardiotoxicity i.e. cardiomyopathy, congestive heart failure, supraventricular tachycardia.
Dermatological: Doxorubicin extravasation, skin necrosis, cellulitis, vesication, phlebitis, reversible alopecia, erythematous streaking along the vein proximal to the site of injection, phlebosclerosis. Hair growth returns to normal after cessation of treatment.
Gastrointestinal: Nausea and vomiting, mucositis (stomatitis and oesophagitis), diarrhoea. Mucositis is a frequent and painful complication of doxorubicin treatment. Mucositis most commonly develops 5 to 10 days after treatment, and typically begins as a burning sensation in the mouth and pharynx. It may involve the vagina, rectum and oesophagus, and progress to ulceration with risk of secondary infection and usually subsides in 10 days. Retrospective comparison of the incidence of mucositis suggests that it is less frequent as the intervals between doses increase. Mucositis may be severe in patients who have had previous irradiation to the mucosae.
General: Dehydration, facial flushing (if an injection has been given too rapidly). Administration of Doxorubicin may cause red colouration of the urine. Patients should be advised that this is no cause for alarm.
Haematological: Myelosuppression, leucopenia.
*Less common reactions:*
Dermatological: Urticarial rash, hyperpigmentation of nailbeds and dermal increases (primarily in children in a few cases), recall of skin reaction due to prior radiotherapy.
General: Chills and fever, anorexia, anaphylaxis.
Haematological: Leucopenia, thrombocytopenia, anaemia. Myelosuppression is more common in patients who have had extensive radiotherapy, bone infiltration by tumour, impaired liver function (when appropriate dosage reduction has not been adopted. See DOSAGE: WITH IMPAIRED HEPATIC FUNCTION) and simultaneous treatment with other myelosuppressive agents. The nadir (time from treatment to peripheral blood evidence of maximal myelosuppression) of leucopenia and thrombocytopenia is 10 to 15 days after treatment, and counts return to normal before day 21.
Nervous System: Drowsiness.
Ocular: Conjunctivitis.
Renal: Renal damage.

*Overdose:* Clinical features: The symptoms of overdosage are likely to be an extension of doxorubicin's pharmacological action. Single doses of 250 mg and 500 mg of doxorubicin have proved fatal. Such doses may cause acute myocardial degeneration within 24 hours, and severe myelosuppression, the greatest effects of which are seen between 10 and 15 days after administration.
Delayed cardiac failure may occur up to six months after the overdose. Patients should be monitored carefully and if symptoms appear, conventional treatment started.
Management: Symptomatic supportive measures should be instituted. Particular attention should be given to prevention and treatment of possible severe haemorrhage or infections secondary to severe, persistent bone marrow depression. Blood transfusion and reverse barrier nursing may be considered.

**Pharmacological properties**
*Pharmacodynamic properties:* Doxorubicin hydrochloride is a cytotoxic anthracycline antibiotic.
Although not completely elucidated, the mechanism of action of doxorubicin is related to its ability to bind to DNA and inhibit nucleic acid synthesis. Cell culture studies have demonstrated rapid cell penetration and perinucleolar chromatin binding, rapid inhibition of mitotic activity and nucleic acid synthesis, mutagenesis and chromosomal aberrations.
The specificity of doxorubicin toxicity appears to be related primarily to proliferative activity of normal tissue. Thus, bone marrow, gastro-intestinal tract and gonads are the main normal tissues damaged.
Doxorubicin is not suitable for oral administration as less than 5% of the drug is absorbed.

*Pharmacokinetic properties:* Pharmacokinetic studies show the intravenous administration of normal or radiolabelled doxorubicin for injection is followed by rapid plasma clearance and significant tissue binding. No information on plasma-protein binding of doxorubicin is available.
The metabolism and disposition of doxorubicin is still to be defined. The drug is metabolised predominantly by the liver to doxorubicinol and several aglycone metabolites. It should be noted that several of the metabolites are cytotoxic. However, it is not certain whether any are more cytotoxic than the parent compound. High levels of metabolites appear rapidly in plasma and undergo a distribution phase with a measurable short initial half-life. Metabolism may be impaired in patients with abnormal liver function.
The disappearance of doxorubicin and its metabolites from the plasma follows a triphasic pharmacokinetic pattern with a mean half-life of the first phase of 12 minutes, of a second phase of 3.3 hours and a prolonged third phase of 29.6 hours.
Urinary excretion of doxorubicin hydrochloride and its metabolites is prolonged and accounts for only 5% of the drug excreted during the first 5 days. Approximately 50% of an administered dose is excreted in bile.
Impairment of liver function results in slower excretion, and consequently, increased retention and accumulation in plasma and tissues. Doxorubicin does not cross the blood brain barrier. However it is known to cross the placenta barrier.

**Pharmaceutical particulars**

*List of excipients:*

| | | |
|---|---|---|
| Doxorubicin content | *10 mg* | *50 mg* |
| Lactose monohydrate BP | 52.6 mg | 263.1 mg |

There is no overage included in the above formulations.

*Incompatibilities:* Doxorubicin should not be mixed with heparin since it has been reported that these drugs are incompatible to the extent that a precipitate may form. Until specific compatibility data are available, it is not recommended that doxorubicin be mixed with other drugs.

*Shelf life*: 36 months.

*Special precautions for storage:* Store below 25°C and protect from light.

*Instructions for use/handling*: Doxorubicin is a potent cytotoxic agent which should only be prescribed, prepared and administered by professionals who have been trained in the safe use of the preparation. The following guidelines should be followed when handling, preparing and disposing of Doxorubicin.
*Preparation:*
1. Reconstitution of powder, transfer to syringes or infusion bags should be carried out in designated areas, preferably a laminar flow station.
2. Personnel must be adequately protected with suitable clothing, gloves, mask and eye shield.
3. Pregnant women should be excluded from handling cytotoxic agents.
*Contamination:*
1. In the event of contact with the skin or eyes, the affected area should be washed with copious amounts of water or Normal saline. A bland cream may be used to treat transient stinging of skin. Medical advice should be sought if the eyes are affected.
2. In the event of spillage treat with 1% Sodium Hypochlorite solution using a cloth/sponge kept in the designate area. Rinse twice with water. Put all cloths into a plastic bag and seal for incineration.
*Disposal:* All items used during preparation or administration including syringes,containers, absorbent materials, residual solutions should all be placed in a thick plastic bag and incinerated at 700oC.
*Preparation of the injection:* The contents of the vial should be reconstituted with Water for Injection BP, Sodium Chloride 0.9%, or Dextrose 5% Injection to a solution concentration of 2 mg per ml.
The reconstituted solution is stable at room temperature, in the vial or in a polypropylene (Terumo) syringe, in the presence or absence of light, for a period of 48 hours. However, it is recommended that the solution be stored at 2-8°C in a refrigerator, and used within 24 hours, in line with good pharmaceutical practice.

**Marketing authorisation number** 4515/0072-73

**Date of approval/revision of SPC** May 1996

**Legal category** POM

# ERYTHROMYCIN LACTOBIONATE FOR I.V. INJECTION.

**Qualitative and quantitative composition**

| | |
|---|---|
| Erythromycin BP | 1000.0 mg |
| Lactobionic Acid H.S.E. | 448.0 mg |

**Pharmaceutical form** Freeze dried powder for injection in a vial.

**Clinical particulars**

*Therapeutic indications:*

1. Upper respiratory tract infections (tonsillitis, pharyngitis, sinusitis, secondary bacterial infections).
2. Lower respiratory tract infections (pneumonia, bronchitis, primary atypical pneumonia, Legionnaire's disease).
3. Skin and soft tissue infections (furunculosis, erysipelas).
4. Other infections–diphtheria carriers and cases as an adjunct to antitoxin, syphilis and gonorrhoea (in cases of penicillin allergy), subacute bacterial endocarditis, otitis media.

*Posology and method of administration:* Intravenous injection by:

1. Continuous I.V. infusion.
2. Intermittent I.V infusion. (Small volume I.V. infusion, minimum volume 100 ml, is the preferred method so as to minimise venous irritation).
3. Slow intravenous injection should be made over a period of 3-5 minutes.

Intravenous administration of erythromycin is suitable to patients who are unable to tolerate oral medication or when it is necessary to produce a high blood concentration to control severe infections. Oral administration should replace parenteral administration as soon as practicable.
Due to the local irritant effects of erythromycin as well as reports of QT interval prolongation and ventricular arrhythmias (some of which have been fatal) being associated with elevated serum concentrations of erythromycin, the drug must not be administered rapidly by direct intravenous injection (IV push).
Erythromycin lactobionate vials labelled as containing 1 gram of Erythromycin should be initially reconstituted by adding 20 ml of Sterile Water for Injections BP without preservative, to provide a solution containing 50 mg per ml. No other diluent should be used to prepare this initial solution. It is important to ensure that the product is completely dissolved by vigorous shaking before transferring to infusion containers. Prior to administration the concentrated solution should be further diluted in glass or flexible plastic containers of 0.9% Sodium Chloride Injection. If, for clinical reasons, 0.9% saline is not suitable, then neutralised Glucose Intravenous Infusion BP 5% w/v may be used. Neutralised glucose solution is prepared by the addition of 5 ml of sterile 8.4% w/v sodium bicarbonate solution to each litre of Glucose Intravenous Injection BP 5% w/v.
It is necessary to buffer the glucose solution in this way because the stability of Erythromycin Lactobionate is adversely affected below pH 5.5.
To ensure potency, all solutions for administration should be used within 8 hours of preparation.
It is recommended that a clarifying filter is used to minimise the particulate levels in resultant infusions.
For continuous I.V. infusion the concentrated solution should be diluted to a concentration of 1 mg per ml. If required, solution strengths up to 5 mg/ml (0.5% solution) may be used, but should not be exceeded. Higher concentrations may result in pain along the vein. Bolus injection is not recommended.
For intermittent I.V. infusion the appropriate daily dose can be given as 4 doses once every 6 hours. The erythromycin concentration should not exceed 5 mg per ml and the infusion should be administered over 60 minutes, as a rapid infusion is more likely to be associated with arrhythmias or hypotension. A longer period of infusion should be used in patients with risk factors or previous evidence of arrhythmias. Not less than 100 ml of diluent should be used for preparing intermittent I.V. solutions.
Intravenous therapy should be replaced by oral administration at the appropriate time.
*Adults*: The usual adult dose is the equivalent of 25-50 mg/kg per day in divided doses of erythromycin, by intravenous infusion every 6 hours, or the equivalent of 1 to 2 g of erythromycin daily by intermittent intravenous infusion over 20 to 60 minutes every 6 hours or by infusion over 24 hours. The equivalent of 4 gram daily has been recommended for severe infections.
Small volume I.V. infusion, minimum volume 100 ml, is the preferred method so as to minimise venous irritation.
*Children*: 25-50 mg per kg by intravenous injection, daily in divided doses.
*Elderly*: Use adult dosage with care, taking into

consideration any impairments in liver or biliary functions.

*Patients with impaired hepatic function*: In the presence of normal hepatic function, erythromycin is concentrated in the liver and excreted in the bile. Although the effect of hepatic dysfunction on the excretion of erythromycin and its half-life in such patients is not known, caution should be exercised in administering the antibiotic in such cases.

*Patients with impaired renal function*: The low proportion of renal excretion would suggest that dosage modification in patients with impaired renal function may not be necessary. In severely impaired patients however, toxicity has been reported and dosage adjustment in these cases may be warranted.

*Contra-indications:* Patients with known hypersensitivity to erythromycin.

Erythromycin is contraindicated with either astemizole or terfenadine.

Prolongation of the QT interval and development of ventricular arrhythmias (some of which have been fatal), including atypical ventricular tachycardia (torsades de pointes) have been reported with the intravenous administration of erythromycin. Limited data suggest that these adverse effects may be associated with abnormally elevated serum erythromycin concentrations following rapid administration. Erythromycin therefore must not be administered rapidly by direct intravenous injection (IV push).

*Special warnings and precautions for use:* Allergic reactions ranging from urticaria to anaphylaxis have been reported with intravenous erythromycin.

Superinfection may occur with prolonged use, giving rise to overgrowth of non susceptible organisms.

Erythromycin is excreted principally via the liver and caution should be exercised when using erythromycin in patients with a degree of hepatic impairment.

In severe renal impairment the half life may be prolonged to 4-7 hours requiring a dose modification.

*Interactions with other medicaments and other forms of interaction:* Penicillin: Erythromycin, in low bacteriostatic concentrations, may inhibit the actions of bactericidal drugs. In high concentrations, erythromycin may act synergistically with penicillin.

Use of erythromycin in patients receiving digoxin, warfarin, carbemazepine or high doses of theophylline may result in potentiation of the effects due to impairment of excretion. A possible interaction between Erythromycin and Vinblastine has been reported in which patients receiving the two agents concurrently may experience myalgia, neutropenia and fever. It is recommended that patients should avoid receiving erythromycin and vinblastine at the same time.

Increased plasma levels of cyclosporin may occur in patients on erythromycin.

Ergotism has been reported in patients receiving erythromycin in combination with ergot derivatives.

Concomitant use of erythromycin with terfenadine or astemizole is likely to result in an enhanced risk of cardiotoxicity with these drugs. The concomitant use of erythromycin with either astemizole or terfenadine is therefore contraindicated.

Laboratory tests used for measurement of urinary catecholamines, SGOT and 17-hydroxycorticosteroids, may be affected if a colorimetric test is used. This interference may complicate interpretation of liver function tests. Suppression of growth of Lactobacillus casei by erythromycin, may interfere with serum folate measurements.

*Pregnancy and lactation:* Erythromycin crosses the placenta and gives rise to foetal plasma levels which are approximately 5-20% of maternal levels. However the risks associated with this phenomenon have not been clearly established. Erythromycin should not be administered to pregnant women unless the benefits outweigh the potential risks.

In lactating women, erythromycin is secreted into breast milk in quantities of between 0.5 and 6.2 micrograms/ml. These quantities are not known to be harmful. Erythromycin is not recommended for nursing mothers unless the expected benefits outweigh the potential risks.

*Effects on ability to drive and use machines:* Not applicable.

*Undesirable effects:*

Hepatic: Administration may be followed, in up to 10% of cases, by increases in AST and ALT enzymes, which sometimes recur on challenge.

Cardiovascular: Thrombophlebitis, venous irritation. Irritation can be reduced by either slow I.V. injection, or preferably a small volume I.V. infusion.

Prolongation of the QT interval and development of ventricular arrhythmias (some of which have been fatal), including atypical ventricular tachycardia (torsades de pointes), have been reported with the intravenous administration of erythromycin. Limited data suggest that these adverse effects may be associated with abnormally elevated serum erythromycin concentrations following rapid administration.

Auditory/Vestibular: In very high doses, erythromycin may cause transient perceptive deafness.

Dermatological: Mild allergic reactions, urticaria, skin eruptions, rashes with fever, and reports of erythema multiforme reaction have been noted.

*Overdose:* The toxicity is low. Overdosage may be associated with ototoxicity. No specific treatment has been proposed other than general supportive measures.

**Pharmacological properties** Erythromycin binds to the ribosomes of bacteria and affects protein synthesis without affecting nucleic acid synthesis. Erythromycin does not bind to cytoplasmic membranes of the host cells. This is a possible explanation of its low toxicity and safety record.

Erythromycin is bacteriostatic and bactericidal depending on its concentration and the type of organism. It inhibits protein synthesis by binding to ribosmal subunits, inhibiting translocation of aminocyl transfer RNA and inhibiting polypeptide synthesis without causing any alteration in the nucleic acid cycle.

*Distribution:* The apparent volume of distribution of erythromycin is around 45% of body weight in normal subjects. This large distribution volume is consistent with the extensive tissue penetration of erythromycin.

Erythromycin diffuses readily into most body fluids, except the cerebrospinal fluid. However, in cases of meningeal inflammation, higher concentrations are apparent.

*Metabolism:* In studies using rabbit microsomes it has been shown that erythromycin is demethylated to des-N-methyl erythromycin and formaldehyde.

*Excretion:* In the presence of normal hepatic function, erythromycin is concentrated in the liver and excreted in the bile; the effect of hepatic dysfunction on excretion of erythromycin by the liver is not known.

From 12% to 15% of intravenously administered erythromycin is excreted in active form in the urine.

The drug is also excreted in the faeces.

*Half-life:* The plasma elimination half-life in patients with normal renal function is about 2 hours. In severe renal impairment the half-life may be prolonged to between 4 and 7 hours.

*Preclinical safety data:* There are no preclinical data of relevance to the prescriber which are additional to that already included in other sections of the SPC.

**Pharmaceutical particulars**

*List of excipients:* None.

*Incompatibilities:* Erythromycin should not be reconstituted with inorganic salt solutions. Use only Water for Injections.

Subsequent dilution into infusion fluids should be made prior to administration. Recommended fluids are Sodium Chloride Injection BP 0.9%, or Dextrose 5% Injection BP

The stability of solutions of Erythromycin Lactobionate is adversely affected below pH 5.5. 5 ml of sterile 8.4% sodium bicarbonate solution will neutralise 1 litre of Glucose Injection BP 5% and should be added to the bag prior to addition of Erythromycin Lactobionate.

*Shelf life:* 24 months.

*Special precautions for storage:* Store below 25°C. Diluted solutions should be used within 8 hours of preparation.

*Instruction for use/handling:* Not applicable.

**Marketing authorisation number** 4515/0054

**Date of approval/revision of SPC** July 1996

**Legal category** POM

# FENTANYL CITRATE INJECTION

**Qualitative and quantitative composition**

*Fentanyl Citrate Injection 100 micrograms in 2 mL:*

| | *per unit dose* | *per mL* |
|---|---|---|
| Fentanyl (as Fentanyl Citrate BP) | 100 micrograms (157 micrograms) | 50 micrograms (78.5 micrograms/mL) |
| Water for Injections BP to | 2 mL | 1 mL |

*Fentanyl Citrate Injection 500 micrograms in 10 mL:*

| | *per unit dose* | *per mL* |
|---|---|---|
| Fentanyl (as Fentanyl Citrate BP) | 500 micrograms (785 micrograms) | 50 micrograms (78.5 micrograms/mL) |
| Water for Injections BP to | 10 mL | 1 mL |

**Pharmaceutical form** Aqueous injection solution.

**Clinical particulars**

*Therapeutic indications:* Fentanyl is a narcotic analgesic indicated for short term analgesia during short surgical procedures. Alternatively, in higher doses, it may be used in ventilated patients as an analgesic and respiratory depressant. In combination with a neuroleptic agent, Fentanyl may be used in the technique of neuroleptanalgesia.

*Posology and method of administration:* Fentanyl Citrate Injection is for administration by the intravenous or intramuscular routes. When administered as an analgesic to patients with spontaneous respiration, adult doses should be as follows:

Initial dose: 50–200 micrograms. Supplemental: 50 micrograms

Doses in excess of 200 micrograms are for general anaesthesia only. Patients on assisted ventilation may be given the following intravenous doses of Fentanyl Citrate:

Initial dose: 300–3500 micrograms. Supplemental: 100-200 micrograms

Fentanyl may also be given intramuscularly, 30–60 minutes before induction of anaesthesia, in doses of 50–100 micrograms.

*Dosage in children:* In children, Fentanyl Citrate is given on a bodyweight basis according to the following schedule:

Spontaneous respiration: Initially 3–5 micrograms per kg, followed by 1 microgram per kg.

Assisted ventilation: Initially 15 micrograms per kg, followed by 1–3 micrograms per kg.

Safe use of Fentanyl has not been established in children under 2 years of age, and it should not be administered to such patients.

*Dosage in the elderly:* Because of the adverse reactions associated with Fentanyl, particularly those affecting the respiratory and cardiovascular systems, it is wise to use reduced doses in treatment of the elderly.

Fentanyl Citrate has a short duration of action and a single dose may be expected to provide analgesia for 10–20 minutes in an unpremedicated adult patient. Larger doses provide analgesia for up to 4 hours when doses of 50 micrograms per kg are used. It is important to assess the degree of stimulation, effect of other drugs and the duration of the surgical procedure when calculating the dosage.

*Contra-indications:* Fentanyl citrate is contraindicated in patients with a known hypersensitivity to the drug, or in patients who have received monoamine oxidase inhibitor (MAOI) drugs within the previous 2 weeks. In addition, patients with obstructive airway disease or respiratory depression should not be treated with Fentanyl Citrate.

*Special warnings and special precautions for use:*
*Warnings:* At high doses (more than 200 micrograms), respiratory depression occurs, which can be reversed by administration of Naloxone 100–200 micrograms in adult patients, or 10–20 micrograms in children.

A transient fall in blood pressure may occur after intravenous administration. Bradycardia, which can be reversed by atropine, may also occur.

Muscular rigidity may occur which can affect respiration, particularly in myasthenia gravis patients. The effects can be minimised by a slow intravenous injection, or alternatively muscle relaxants can be used to treat the rigidity.

In combination with other narcotic analgesics, Fentanyl may cause additive effects on CNS depression and respiration. Resuscitative measures should be available at all times, and the patient kept under close medical supervision. As Fentanyl is a narcotic drug, tolerance and dependence may occur. Nausea and vomiting may also be a problem although the incidence is lower than with other opiates.

As with all potent opioids, profound analgesia is accompanied by marked respiratory depression, which may persist into or recur in the early postoperative period. Care should be taken after large doses or infusions of fentanyl to ensure that adequate spontaneous breathing has been established and maintained before disharging the patient from the recovery area. Hyperventilation during anaesthesia may alter the patient's response to $CO_2$, thus affecting respiration postoperatively. Use of opioid premedication may enhance or prolong the respiratory depressant effects of fentanyl.

Where early discharge is envisaged patients should be advised not to drive or operate machinery. Fentanyl is for single use only. Use once and any unused product must be discarded.

*Precautions:* Fentanyl should only be administered by experienced clinicians to patients under close medical supervision. It should be administered with caution to patients in the following cases:

(a) Severe, chronic liver or renal impairment
(b) Severe impairment of pulmonary function
(c) Myasthenia gravis
(d) Hypothyroidism

When used in conjunction with neuroleptics, the different duration of action should be taken into account.

*Interaction with other medicaments and other forms of interaction:* Used in combination with CNS depressants, Fentanyl may have additive or potentiating effects. MAO inhibitors are known to interact with narcotic analgesics, and the safe use of Fentanyl Citrate has not been established in this situation.

*Pregnancy and lactation:*
Use in pregnancy: Administration in labour may induce respiratory depression in the newborn. Safe use has not been established during pregnancy and it should not be used unless the benefits to the mother outweigh the potential risks to mother and child.

Use in lactation: Safe use of Fentanyl Citrate has not been established in mothers who are breast feeding their children. However, because of the nature of the drug and its indications it is unlikely that Fentanyl would be administered to a lactating mother.

*Effects on ability to drive and use machines:* Where early discharge is envisaged patients should be advised not to drive or operate machinery.

*Undesirable effects:* As with all opiates, profound analgesia is accompanied by respiratory depression which may persist longer than the analgesic effect, through into the immediate post-operative period.

Respiratory depression can be immediately reversed with a narcotic agonist and is more likely to occur following too rapid intravenous administration.

Muscular rigidity can be reversed by intravenous administration of a relaxant such as suxamethonium, in combination with assisted ventilation.

Bradycardia may occur, but is less likely if atropine is included in the premedication regimen.

Other reported adverse effects include hypertension, hypotension, blurred vision, dizziness, nausea, vomiting, laryngospasm, sweating, itching and spasm of the sphincter of Oddi.

*Overdose:* The symptoms of overdosage are extensions of the pharmacological effects. Respiratory depression may be reversed using naloxone in combination with other supportive measures.

If respiratory depression is associated with muscular rigidity, then use of suxamethonium has been successful in reversing the effects. Bradycardia may be treated with atropine sulphate.

### Pharmacological properties

*Pharmacodynamic properties:* Fentanyl is a potent narcotic analgesic, chemically related to pethidine and estimated to be about 80 times as potent as morphine as an analgesic. Fentanyl is a centrally acting opiate analgesic which produces profound analgesia of short duration, which is reversed by narcotic antagonists such as naloxone. Its primary indication is for analgesia during short term surgical procedures, or at higher doses, for analgesia in ventilated patients.

*Pharmacokinetic properties:* Following IV administration, the onset of action is within a few minutes, with analgesia lasting for 30-60 minutes following one dose of 100 micrograms. Following IM administration, onset of action occurs with 7-15 minutes, and duration is 1-2 hours.

Fentanyl is rapidly metabolised and excreted in the urine. The short duration of action is primarily due to redistribution. Up to 70% of a dose may be protein bound. The drug also crosses the placental barrier.

### Pharmaceutical particulars

*List of excipients:* Water for Injections BP qs.

*Incompatibilities:* Fentanyl is stated to be chemically incompatible with Thiopentone Sodium, Methohexitone and Phenobarbitone.

*Shelf life:* The medicinal product as packaged for sale has a 2 year shelf life.

*Special precautions for storage:* Storage is recommended below 25°C. Protect from light. Store as specified in Misuse of Drugs Act in respect of Schedule 2 drugs.

*Instructions for use/handling:* Not applicable.

### Marketing authorisation numbers

| | |
|---|---|
| 100 micrograms in 2 ml | 4515/0046 |
| 500 micrograms in 10 ml | 4515/0046 |

**Date of approval/revision of SPC**    26 July 1995

**Legal category**    CD(Sch 2), POM

## FLUOROURACIL INJECTION BP 25MG/ML

### Qualitative and quantitative composition

| | 250mg in 10ml | 500mg in 20ml | 2.5gm in 100ml |
|---|---|---|---|
| *Active Ingredient* | | | |
| Fluorouracil BP | 250mg | 500mg | 2.5gram |
| *Other Ingredients* | | | |
| Sodium Hydroxide BP | 69.7mg | 139.4mg | 697mg |
| Water for Injections BP | to 10ml | to 20ml | to 100ml |

No overage is required in the formulation.

**Pharmaceutical form** Aqueous solution for injection.

### Clinical particulars

*Therapeutic indications:* Fluorouracil may be used alone or in combination, for its palliative action in the management of common malignancies particularly cancer of the colon and breast.

*Posology and method of administration:*
*Routes of administration:* Fluorouracil Injection BP can be given by intravenous injection or intravenous or intra-arterial infusion.

*Adults:* Selection of an appropriate dose and treatment regime depends upon the condition of the patient, the type of carcinoma being treated and whether fluorouracil is to be administered alone or in combination with other therapy. Initial treatment should be given in hospital and the *total daily dose should not exceed 0.8–1 gram.* It is customary to calculate the dose in accordance with the patient's actual bodyweight unless there is obesity, oedema or some form of abnormal fluid retention such as ascites. Ideal weight is used as the basis for calculation in such cases.

The initial dose should be reduced by one-third to one half in patients with any of the following:

1. Cachexia.
2. Major surgery within preceding 30 days.
3. Reduced bone marrow function.
4. Impaired hepatic or renal function.

The following regimen have been recommended for use as a single agent:

Initial Treatment: This may be in the form of an infusion or an injection, the former usually being preferred because of lesser toxicity.

*Intravenous infusion:* 15 mg/kg bodyweight but not more than 1 g per infusion, diluted in 300–500 ml of 5% glucose or 9% NaCl injection and given over 4 hours. Alternatively the daily dose may be infused over 30–60 minutes or may be given as a continuous infusion over 24 hours. The infusion may be repeated daily until there is evidence of toxicity or a total dose of 12–15 g has been reached.

Intravenous Injection: 12 mg/kg bodyweight may be given daily for 3 days and then, if there is no evidence of toxicity, 6 mg/kg on alternate days for 3 further doses.

An alternative regimen is 15 mg/kg as a single intravenous injection once a week throughout the course.

*Intra-arterial infusion:* 5/7.5 mg/kg bodyweight daily may be given by 24 hour continuous intra-arterial infusion.

*Maintenance therapy:* An initial intensive course may be followed by maintenance therapy providing there are no significant toxic effects.

In all instances, toxic side effects must disappear before maintenance therapy is started.

The initial course of fluorouracil can be repeated after an interval of 4 to 6 weeks from the last dose or, alternatively, treatment can be continued with intravenous injections of 5-15 mg/kg bodyweight at weekly intervals. This sequence constitutes a course of therapy. Some patients have received up to 30 g at a maximum rate of 1 g daily.

A more recent alternative method is to give 15 mg/kg IV once a week throughout the course of treatment. This obviates the need for an initial period of daily administration.

In combination with Irradiation

Irradiation combined with 5-FU has been found to be useful in the treatment of certain types of metastatic lesions in the lungs and for the relief of pain caused by recurrent, inoperable growth. The standard dose of 5FU should be used.

*Children:* No recommendations are made regarding the use of fluorouracil in children.

*Elderly:* Fluorouracil should be used in the elderly with similar considerations as in younger adults, notwithstanding that incidence of concomitant medical illness is higher in the former group.

*Contra-indications:* Fluorouracil is contra-indicated in seriously debilitated patients or those with bone marrow depression after radiotherapy or treatment with other antineoplastic agents.

Fluorouracil is strictly contra-indicated in pregnant or breast feeding women.

Fluorouracil should not be used in the management of non-malignant disease.

Special warnings and special precautions for use Precautions

It is recommended that fluorouracil be given only by, or under the strict supervision of, a qualified physician who is conversant with the use of potent antimetabolites.

All patients should be admitted to hospital for initial treatment.

Adequate treatment with fluorouracil is usually followed by leucopoenia, the lowest white blood cell (W.B.C.) count commonly being observed between

the 7th and 14th day of the first course, but occasionally being delayed for as long as 20 days.

The count usually returns to normal by the 30th day. Daily monitoring of platelet and W.B.C. count is recommended and treatment should be stopped if platelets fall below 100,000 per mm³ or the W.B.C. count falls below 3,500 per mm³. If the total count is less than 2000 per mm³, and especially if there is granulocytopenia, it is recommended that the patient be placed in protective isolation in the hospital and treated with appropriate measures to prevent systemic infection.

Treatment should also be stopped at the first sign of oral ulceration or if there is evidence of gastrointestinal side effects such as stomatitis, diarrhoea, bleeding from the G.I. tract or haemorrage at any site. The ratio between effective and toxic dose is small and therapeutic response is unlikely without some degree of toxicity. Care must be taken, therefore, in the selection of patients and adjustment of dosage.

Fluorouracil should be used with caution in patients with reduced renal or liver function or jaundice. Isolated cases of angina, ECG abnormalities and rarely, myocardial infarction have been reported following administration of Fluorouracil. Caution should therefore be exercised in treating patients who experience chest pain during courses of treatment, or patients with a history of heart disease.

*Interaction with other medicaments and other forms of interaction:* Various agents have been reported to biochemically modulate the antitumour efficacy or toxicity of Fluorouracil, common drugs include Methotrexate, Metronidazole, Leucovorin as well as Allopurinol and Cimetidine which can affect the availability of the active drug.

*Pregnancy and lactation:* Fluorouracil is strictly contra-indicated in pregnant or breast feeding women.

*Effects on ability to drive and use machines:* Not applicable.

*Undesirable effects:* Diarrhoea, nausea and vomiting are observed quite commonly during therapy and may be treated symptomatically. An antiemetic may be given for nausea and vomiting. Alopecia may be seen in a substantial number of cases, particularly in females, but is reversible. Other side effects include dermatitis, pigmentation, changes in the nails, ataxia and fever.

There have been reports of chest pain, tachycardia, breathlessness and ECG changes after administration of fluorouracil. Special attention is therefore advisable in treating patients with a history of heart disease or those who develop chest pain during treatment.

Leucopoenia is common and the precautions described above should be followed.

Systemic fluorouracil treatment has been associated with various types of ocular toxicity.

Additionally several other reports have been noted including:

Incidences of excessive lacrimation, dacryostenosis, visual changes and photophobia.

A transient reversible cerebellar syndrome can occur after the use of 5-fluorouracil. Rarely, a reversible confusional state may occur. Both neurological conditions usually respond to withdrawal of 5-fluorouracil.

Palmar-Plantar Erythrodysesthesia Syndrome has been reported as an unusual complication of high dose bolus or protracted continuous therapy with fluorouracil.

Thrombophlebitis/vein tracking.

*Overdose:* The symptoms and signs of overdosage are qualitatively similar to the adverse reactions and should be managed as indicated under *Precautions* and *Adverse Reactions.*

### Pharmacological properties

*Pharmacodynamic properties:* Fluorouracil is an analogue of uracil, a component of ribonucleic acid. The drug is believed to function as an antimetabolite. After intracellular conversion to the active deoxynucleotide, it interferes with the synthesis of DNA by blocking the conversion of deoxyuridylic acid to thymidylic acid by the cellular enzyme thymidylate synthetase. Fluorouracil may also interfere with RNA synthesis.

*Pharmacokinetic properties:* After intravenous administration, Fluorouracil is distributed through the body water and disappears from the blood within 3 hours. It is preferentially taken up by actively dividing tissues and tumours after conversion to its nucleotide. Fluorouracil ready enters the C.S.F and brain tissue.

Following IV administration, the plasma elimination half-life averages about 16 minutes and is dose dependant. Following a single IV dose of Fluorouracil approximately 15% of the dose is excreted unchanged in the urine within 6 hours; over 90% of this is excreted in the first hour. The remainder is mostly metabolised in the liver by the usual body mechanisms for uracil.

## Pharmaceutical particulars

*List of excipients:*

| | 250 mg in 10 ml | 500 mg in 20 ml | 2.5 gm in 100 ml |
|---|---|---|---|
| Sodium Hydroxide BP | 69.7 mg | 139.4 mg | 697 mg |
| Water for Injections BP | to 10 ml | to 20 ml | to 100 ml |

No overage is required in the formulation.

*Incompatibilities:* 5-Fluorouracil is incompatible with Carboplatin, Cisplatin, Cytarabine, Diazepam, Doxorubicin, other Anthracyclines and possibly Methotrexate.

Formulated solutions are alkaline and it is recommended that admixture with acidic drugs or preparations should be avoided.

*Shelf life:* 24 months.

*Special precautions for storage:* Fluorouracil Injection BP should be stored between 15°C and 25°C and should be protected from light. The pH of Fluorouracil Injection BP is 8.9 and the drug has maximal stability over the pH range 8.6 to 9.0.

If a precipitate has formed as a result of exposure to low temperatures, redissolve by heating to 60°C accompanied by vigorous shaking. Allow to cool to body temperature prior to use.

*Instructions for use/handling:* Fluorouracil is an irritant, contact with skin and mucous membranes should be avoided. Please refer to company for COSHH hazard datasheets.

*Diluents:* Fluorouracil Injection BP may be diluted with Glucose or Sodium Chloride Injection BP or Water for Injections BP immediately before parenteral use. The remainder of solutions should be discarded after use: do not make up into multidose preparations. Fluorouracil Injection should only be prepared for administration by professionals who have been trained in the safe use of the preparation. Preparation should only be carried out in a designated area.

*First aid:* Eye contact: Irrigate immediately with water and seek medical advice.

Skin contact: Wash thorughly with soap and water and remove contaminated clothing.

Inhalation, Ingestion: Seek medical advice.

**Marketing authorisation number** 4515/0024.

**Date of approval/revision of SPC** 22 July 1996

# FLUOROURACIL INJECTION BP 50MG/ML

**Qualitative and quantitative composition** Fluorouracil Injection BP 50 mg/ml is available in the following presentations:- 250 mg/5 ml, 500 mg/10 ml and 2.5 g/50 ml conventional glass vials and Onco-Tain* vials

**Pharmaceutical form** Sterile solution for injection.

## Clinical particulars

*Therapeutic indications:* Fluorouracil may be used alone, or in combination for its palliative action in the management of common malignancies particularly cancer of the colon and breast, either as a single agent or in combination with other cytotoxic agents.

*Posology and method of administration:* Selection of an appropriate dose and treatment regime will depend upon the condition of the patient, the type of carcinoma being treated and whether Fluorouracil is to be administered alone or in combination with other therapy. Initial treatment should be given in hospital and the total daily dose should not exceed 1 gram. It is customary to calculate the dose in accordance with the patient's actual weight unless there is obesity, oedema or some other form of abnormal fluid retention such as ascites. In this case, ideal weight should be used as the basis for the calculation. Reduction of the dose is advisable in patients with any of the following:

(1) Cachexia
(2) Major surgery within preceding 30 days
(3) Reduced bone marrow function
(4) Impaired hepatic or renal function

Fluorouracil injection can be given by intravenous injection or, intravenous or intra-arterial infusion.

*Adult dose:* The following regimes have been recommended for use as a single agent:

Initial treatment: This may be in the form of an infusion or an injection, the former usually being preferred because of lesser toxicity.

*Intravenous infusion:* 15 mg/kg bodyweight but not more than 1 g per infusion, diluted in 500 ml of 5% glucose or 0.9% NaCl injection and given by intravenous infusion at a rate of 40 drops per minute over 4 hours. Alternatively the daily dose may be infused over 30–60 minutes or may be given as a continuous infusion over 24 hours. The infusion may be repeated

daily until there is evidence of toxicity or a total dose of 12–15 g has been reached.

*Intravenous injection:* 12 mg/kg bodyweight may be given daily for 3 days and then if there is no evidence of toxicity 6 mg/kg on alternate days for 3 further doses. An alternative regime is 15 mg/kg as a single intravenous injection once a week throughout the course.

*Intra-arterial infusion:* 5-7.5 mg/kg may be given by 24 hour continuous intra-arterial infusion.

*Maintenance therapy:* An initial intensive course may be followed by maintenance therapy providing there are no significant toxic effects. In all instances, toxic side effects must disappear before maintainance therapy is started.

The initial course of Fluorouracil can be repeated after an interval of 4 to 6 weeks from the last dose, or alternatively, treatment can be continued with intravenous injections of 5-15 mg/kg at weekly intervals. This sequence constitutes a course of therapy. Some patients have received up to 30 g at a maximum rate of 1 g daily. A more recent alternative method is to give 15 mg/kg IV Once a week throughout the course of treatment. This obviates the need for an initial period of daily administration.

In combination with irradiation: Irradiation combined with 5-FU has been found to be useful in the treatment of certain types of metastatic lesions in the lungs and for the relief of pain caused by recurrent, inoperable growth. The standard dose of 5-FU should be used.

*Children:* No recommendations are made regarding the use of Fluorouracil in children.

*Elderly:* Fluorouracil should be used in the elderly with similar considerations as with normal adult dosages.

*Contra-indications:* Fluorouracil is contra-indicated in seriously debilitated patients or those with bone marrow depression after radiotherapy or treatment with other antineoplastic agents.

Fluorouracil is strictly contra-indicated in pregnant or breast feeding women.

Fluorouracil should not be used in the management of non-malignant disease.

*Special warnings and special precautions for use:* It is recommended that Fluorouracil be given only by, or under the strict supervision of, a qualified physician who is conversant with the use of potent antimetabolites.

All patients should be admitted to hospital for initial treatment.

Adequate treatment with Fluorouracil is usually followed by leucopenia, the lowest white blood cell (W.B.C.) count comonly being observed between the 7th and 14th day of the first course, but occasionally being delayed for as long as 20 days.

The count usually returns to normal by the 30th day. Daily monitoring of platelet and W.B.C. count is recommended and treatment should be stopped if platelets fall below 100,000 per mm3 or the W.B.C. count falls below 3,500 per mm³. If the total count is less than 2000 mm³, and especially if there is granulocytopenia, it is recommended that the patient be placed in protective isolation in the hospital and treated with appropriate measures to prevent systemic infection.

Treatment should also be stopped at the first sign of oral ulceration or if there is evidence of gastrointestnal side effects such as stomatitis, diarrhoea, bleeding from the G.I. tract ot haemorrage at any site. The ratio between effective and toxic dose is small and therapeutic response is unlikely without some degree of toxicity. Care must be taken therefore, in the selection of patients and adjustment of dosage.

Fluorouracil should be used with caution in patients with reduced renal or liver function or jaundice. Isolated cases of angina, ECG abnormalities and rarely, myocardial infarction have been reported following administration of Fluorouracil. Care should therefore be exercised in treating patients who experience chest pain during courses of treatment, or patients with a history of heart disease.

Interaction with other medicaments and other forms of interaction

*Drug interactions:* Various agents have been reported to biochemically modulate the antitumour efficacy or toxicity of Fluorouracil, common drugs include Methotrexate, Metronidazole, Leucovorin as well as Allopurinol and Cimetidine which can affect the availability of the active drug.

*Pregnancy and lactation:* Fluorouracil is strictly contra-indicated in pregnant and breast feeding women.

*Effects on ability to drive and use machines:* Not applicable.

*Undesirable effects:* Diarrhoea, nausea and vomiting are observed quite commonly during therapy and may be treated symptomatically. An anti-emetic may be given for nausea and vomiting.

Alopecia may be seen in a substantial number of

cases, partcularly females, but is reversible. Other side effects include dermatitis, pigmentation, changes in the nails, ataxia and fever.

There have been reports of chest pain, tachycardia, breathlessness and E.C.G. changes after administration of Fluorouracil. Special attention is advisable in treating patients with a history of heart disease or those who develop chest pain during treatment.

Leucopenia is common and the precautions described above should be followed.

Systemic Fluorouracil treatment has been associated with various types of ocular toxicity.

A transient reversible cerebellar syndrome can occur after the use of 5-fluorouracil. Rarely, a reversible confusional state may occur. Both neurological conditions usually respond to withdrawal of 5-fluorouracil.

Additionally several other reports have been noted including:

Incidences of excessive lacrimation, dacryostenosis, visual changes and photophobia.

Palmar-Plantar Erythrodysesthesia Syndrome has been reported as an unusual complication of high dose bolus or protracted continuous therapy with fluorouracil.

Thrombophlebitis/Vein Tracking

*Overdose:* The symptoms and signs of overdosage are qualitatively similar to the adverse reactions and should be managed as indicated under *Other Undesirable Effects* and *Special Warnings and Precautions.*

## Pharmacological properties

*Pharmacodynamic properties:* Fluorouracil is an analogue of uracil, a component of ribonucleic acid. The drug is believed to function as an antimetabolite. After intracellular conversion to the active deoxynucleotide, it interferes with the synthesis of DNA by blocking the conversion of deoxyuridylic acid to thymidylic acid by the cellular enzyme thymidylate synthetase. Fluorouracil may also interfere with RNA synthesis.

*Pharmacokinetic properties:* After intravenous administration, Fluorouracil is distributed through the body water and disappears from the blood within 3 hours. It is preferentially taken up by actively dividing tissues and tumours after conversion to its nucleotide. Fluorouracil ready enters the C.S.F and brain tissue.

Following IV administration, the plasma elimination half-life averages about 16 minutes and is dose dependant. Following a single IV dose of Fluorouracil approximately 15% of the dose is excreted unchanged in the urine within 6 hours; over 90% of this is excreted in the first hour. The remainder is mostly metabolised in the liver by the usual body mechanisms for uracil.

*Preclinical safety data:* Not applicable.

## Pharmaceutical particulars

*List of excipients:* Sodium Hydroxide BP; Water for Injections BP.

*Incompatibilities:* Fluorouracil is incompatible with Carboplatin, Cisplatin, Cytarabine, Diazepam, Doxorubicin, other Anthracyclines and possibly Methotrexate.

Formulated solutions are alkaline and it is recommended that admixture with acidic drugs or preparations should be avoided.

*Shelf life:* 24 months.

*Special precautions for storage:* Storage: Fluorouracil Injection BP should be stored between 15°C and 25°C and should be protected from light. Do not refrigerate. Unused portions of opened vials or prepared infusions if not used immediately must be stored at 2-8°C for no longer than 24 hours from the time of opening or preparation.

The pH of Fluorouracil Injection BP is 8.9 and the drug has maximal stability over the pH range 8.6 to 9.0.

If a precipitate has formed as a result of exposure to low temperatures, redissolve by heating to 60°C accompanied by vigorous shaking. Allow to cool to body temperature prior to use.

The product should be discarded if it appears brown or dark yellow in solution.

*Instructions for use/handling:* Cytotoxic Handling Guidelines: Should be administered only by or under the direct supervision of a qualified physician who is experienced in the use of cancer chemotherapeutic agents.

Fluorouracil Injection should only be prepared for administration by professionals who have been trained in the safe use of the preparation. Preparation should only be carried out in a designated area.

In the event of spillage, operators should put on gloves, face mask, eye protection and disposible apron and mop up the spilled material with a absorbant material kept in the area for that purpose. The area should then be cleaned and all contaminated material transferred to a cytotoxic spillage bag or bin and sealed for incineration.

Contamination: Fluorouracil is an irritant, contact with skin and mucous membranes should be avoided.

In the event of contact with the skin or eyes, the affected area should be washed with copious amounts of water or normal saline. A bland cream may be used to treat the transient stinging of the skin. Medical advice should be sought if the eyes are affected or if the preparation is inhaled or ingested.

Please refer to company for COSHH hazard datasheets.

*Preparation guidelines:*

a. Chemotherapeutic agents should be prepared for administration only by professionals who have been trained in the safe use of the preparation.
b. Operations such as reconstitution of powder and transfer to syringes should be carried out only in the designated area.
c. The personnel carrying out these procedures should be adequately protected with clothing, gloves and eye shield.
d. Pregnant personnel are advised not to handle chemotherapeutic agents.

Disposal: Syringes containing remaining solution, absorbent materials, and any other contaminated material should be placed in a thick plastic bag or other impervious container and incinerated at 700°C.

Diluents: Fluorouracil Injection BP may be diluted with Glucose or Sodium Chloride Injection BP or Water for Injections BP immediately before parenteral use.

**Marketing authorisation number** 4515/0088

**Date of approval/revision of SPC** 22 July 1996

**Legal category** POM

## FLUPHENAZINE DECANOATE INJECTION BP 25 mg/mL

**Qualitative and quantitative composition**

*Fluphenazine Decanoate Injection BP*

| | *per ml* | *per unit dose* | *per unit dose* | *per unit dose* |
|---|---|---|---|---|
| Fluphenazine Decanoate | 25 mg | 12.5mg | 25 mg | 50 mg |
| Sesame Oil | to 1mL | to 0.5mL | to 1 ml | in 2 ml |

**Pharmaceutical form** Oily injection solution.

**Clinical particulars**

*Therapeutic indications:* The management of schizophrenic patients and those with paranoid psychoses. Fluphenazine is also particularly useful in the managment of patients who are unreliable at taking oral medication and of those who do not absorb their oral phenothiazines in adequate amounts.

*Posology and method of administration:* Fluphenazine Decanoate is given by deep intramuscular injection into the gluteal muscle region, using a needle of at least 21 gauge size. Dosage will depend on any previous exposure to Fluphenazine or other phenothiazines prior to treatment.

*Adults*: In patients with no previous treatment, initially 12.5 mg to 25 mg should be given. Onset of action will normally occur between 24 and 72 hours after injection with an antipsychotic effect being noticed within 2 to 4 days. Subsequent dosages schedules must be determined with the individual patient response. Maintenance therapy can be effected using a single injection for as long as four to six weeks, although most patients symptoms can be contolled on 12.5–100 mg given at two to five week intervals.

Dosage would not normally exceed 100 mg. If doses in excess of 50 mg are required then increments of 12.5 mg should be implemented.

Fluphenazine Decanoate Injection 100 mg per ml is indicated for those patients requiring high doses as part of maintenance therapy and where a small injection volume is required. When transferring from Fluphenazine Decanoate 25 mg/ml to Fluphenazine Decanoate 100 mg/ml Injection the dose volume should be divided by four to obtain equivalent milligram dosage.

*Children:* Fluphenazine Decanoate and Fluphenazine Decanoate 100 mg/ml Injection are not recommended for use in children under the age of twelve.

*Elderly:* Reduced maintenance doses may be needed in patients showing extra-pyramidal symptoms, following initial dosing as above.

Initial dose–0.25 ml (25 mg)

Patients not previously treated with a depot fluphenazine formulation, and over sixty years of age, should receive a lower initial dose.

*Contra-indications:* Fluphenazine Decanoate is contraindicated in comatose patients or those under the influence of central nervous system depressants. The presence of liver damage, history of jaundice and renal insufficiency preclude use of Fluphenazine Decanoate. Cerebral atherosclerosis, phaeochromocytoma, severely depressed states and severe cardiac insufficiency are also contra-indications for Fluphenazine Decanoate therapy.

*Special warnings and special precautions for use:*
*Warnings:* Sudden, unexplained deaths have been reported in hospitalised psychotic patients receiving phenothiazines. Autopsy findings have revealed acute, fulminating pneumonia, aspiration of gastric contents or intramyocardial lesions. Some patients exhibited acute exacerbations of psychotic behaviour shortly prior to their death.

Fluphenazine Decanoate may impair the mental and physical abilities required for driving or operating machinery. Potentiation of the central nervous system depressant effects of alcohol may occur.

The drug should be administered under the direction of a physician experienced in the use of psychotropic drugs. Hepatic and renal function should be monitored periodically as well as haemotological monitoring.

*Precautions:* Fluphenazine Decanoate should be used with caution in patients with cardiovascular or respiratory disease.

The drug may cause cross sensitivity with other phenothiazines, so caution is necessary in patients with a known history of hypersensitivity to phenothiazines.

On prolonged therapy patients may show symptoms of liver damage, pigmentary retinopathy, corneal deposits and irreversible dyskinesia.

The preparation should be used with caution in patients with a history of convulsive disorders, and grand mal seizures have been reported in patients on Fluphenazine.

Psychotic patients on high doses who will be undergoing surgery may be at risk to hypotension, and may additionally require reduced amounts of anaesthetic agents or central nervous system depressants. Body temperature control mechanisms may be affected giving rise to hypothermia or hyperpyrexia in patients on high doses of Fluphenazine Decanoate. In addition elderly patients or those subjected to extremes of temperature and humidity may be affected.

The anticholinergic effects of atropine may be potentiated. Antiparkinsonian drug effects may be diminished in patients on Fluphenazine therapy.

*Interaction with other medicaments and other forms of interaction:* Fluphenazine Decanoate may interact additionally with CNS depressants (alcohol, barbiturates, hypnotics, sedatives and strong analgesics) to enhance their depressant effects. Guanethidine and levodopa efficacy may be impaired. Plasma levels of Fluphenazine may be increased by high doses of tricyclic antidepressants, and lowered by barbiturates.

Adrenaline action may be reversed and the antihypertensive properties of adrenergic blocking drugs may be antagonised. The antiparkinsonian effect of Levodopa may be impaired as well as the effects of anticonvulsants.

*Pregnancy and lactation:*
*Use in pregnancy:* The safety of this drug during pregnancy has not been established. The possible hazards should be weighed against the benefits when administering the drug to pregnant patients.

*Use in lactation:* Fluphenazine Decanoate may possibly be excreted in breast milk, as other phenothiazines are. Breast feeding is therefore not recommended during treatment.

*Effects on ability to drive and use machines:* Use may impair mental and physical abilities to drive or operate heavy machinery.

*Undesirable effects:*
*Adverse reactions:* Extrapyramidal disturbances: Extrapyramidal side effects occur with Fluphenazine Decanoate including pseudo-parkinsonism, dystonia, dyskinesia, akathisia, oculogyric crises, opisthotonos and hyperreflexia.

Dystonic reactions such as acute spasm of facial, neck and back muscles may occur within 24 hours of an injection and require immediate administration of an anticholinergic such as benztropine, benzhexol oir procyclidine. This may need to be continued orally for a few days to prevent recurrence. Young male patients seem most at risk from dystonic reactions.

Parkinsonism effects occur frequently, particularly in elderly patients, usually within 2-5 days after an injection. Early detection is important so that the patients neurological system can be examined regularly. Extrapyramidal symptoms are persistent but usually reversible.

Tardive dyskinesia: As with all antipsychotic agents, tardive dyskinesia may occur in patients on long-term therapy or after drug treatment has been discontinued. The risk seems greatest in elderly female patients on high doses. Symptoms are persistent and may be irreversible. The disorder consists of repetitive involuntary movements of the tongue, face, and muscles of mastication. The trunk and limbs are less frequently involved. Fine vermicular movements of the tongue may be an early sign of the syndrome, and if medication is stopped at this stage, the syndrome may not develop.

There is no known effective treatment for tardive dyskinesia. Increasing the dose of medication may result in temporary suppression but with subsequent deterioration. Anticholinergic drugs may exacerbate the problem. All antipsychotic agents may be withdrawn if these symptoms appear. Subsequently symptoms of dyskinesia may be masked if a different antipsychotic agent is used, or if the dose of Fluphenazine Decanoate is increased.

Other central nervous system effects: Drowsiness, lethargy may necessitate a reduction in dosage. Phenothiazine derivatives have been known to cause restlessness, excitement or bizarre dreams.

Autonomic nervous system: Hypotension is infrequently found except in patients with pre-existing cerebrovascular disease or cardiac insufficiency such as mitral valve disease. Such patients should be closely monitored when the drug is administered. In acute hypotension, supportive measures including the use of intravenous vasopressor drugs is recommended, but excluding the use of adrenaline which has been found to further lower blood pressure through drug interaction with Fluphenazine Decanoate.

Nausea, and loss of appetite, salivation, polyuria, perspiration, dry mouth, headache and constipation may occur. These can usually be controlled by a dosage reduction or temporary discontinuation of treatment. Blurred vision, glaucoma, constipation, urinary incontinence and epileptiform attacks are also occasionally seen.

Allergic reactions: Skin disorders such as itching, erythema, urticaria, and dermatitis have been reported occasionally. SLE and skin pigmentation have rarely been reported.

Haemopoietic system: Blood dyscrasias including transient leucopenia, thrombocytopenia and agranulocytosis have been reported. Accordingly, if patients show signs of sore throat, gums or mouth, then regular blood counts should be instituted and if symptoms persist, the treatment be discontinued until the haemotological system has recovered.

Hepatic system: Cholestatic jaundice may occur during the first three months of treatment, and if so therapy should be stopped. Alterations in liver function tests have been reported in the absence of jaundice.

Metabolic and endocrine system: Weight changes, peripheral oedema, gynacomastia, alterations in lactation, menstrual irregularities and impotence have been reported. Blood glucose levels may also be erratic causing problems in diabetic patients.

Cardiovascular system: Phenothiazines may cause changes in ECG patterns which are dose related. Moderate to high dosages can cause prolongation of QT interval and alteration in T waves. Rarely these effects precede serious arrhythmias including ventricular tachycardia and fibrillation.

*Overdose:* Supportive and symptomatic treatment should be used. Oral or parenteral procyclidine or benztropine will control extrapyramidal symptoms. In severe hypotension, management of circulatory failure should be instituted including vasoconstrictors and intravenous fluids.

N.B. Avoid the use of adrenaline as this may exacerbate the hypotension due to interaction with Fluphenazine.

**Pharmacological properties**

*Pharmacodynamic properties:* Fluphenazine is a piperazine phenothiazine used widely in the treatment of schizophrenia. The action is thought to be through dopamine receptor blockade in the mesolimbic system. Fluphenazine has weak anticholinergic effects, sedative effects, antiadrenal effects and neuroendocrine effects. Side effects from extrapyramidal symptoms are common.

In an oil vehicle as the decanoate, fluphenazine ester slowly diffuses into the circulation. After hydrolysis, the drug passes the blood brain barrier as free drug.

*Pharmacokinetic properties:* Esterification of fluphenazine slows the rate of release from fat and thus prolongs the duration of action. Further delay is achieved by formulation in an oily solvent. Onset of action is within 48-72 hours, duration may be 1-6 weeks with an average of 2 weeks.

Distribution and metabolism are not fully described. Plasma half life has been shown to be 6-9 days following intramuscular administration of the decanoate.

**Pharmaceutical particulars**

*List of excipients:*

*Fluphenazine Decanoate Injection BP 25 mg in 1 mL*

| | per unit dose | per mL |
|---|---|---|
| Sesame Oil | to 1 mL | to 1 mL |

*Incompatibilities:* Not applicable. An oily injection for intramuscular use only.

*Shelf life:* The medicinal product as packaged for sale has a 24 month shelf life.

*Special precautions for storage:* Storage: store between 15°C–25°C. Protect from light. Do not refrigerate.

*Instructions for use/handling:* Not applicable.

**Marketing authorisation number**  4515/0048

**Date of approval/revision of SPC**  21 July 1997

**Legal category**  POM

# FLUPHENAZINE DECANOATE INJECTION BP 100 mg/mL

## Qualitative and quantitative composition

*Fluphenazine Decanoate Injection BP*

| | per ml | per unit dose | per unit dose |
|---|---|---|---|
| Fluphenazine Decanoate | 100mg | 50mg | 100mg |
| Sesame Oil | to 1 mL | to 0.5mL | to 1 ml |

**Pharmaceutical form** Oily injection solution.

## Clinical particulars

*Therapeutic indications:* The management of schizophrenic patients and those with paranoid psychoses. Fluphenazine is also particularly useful in the management of patients who are unreliable at taking oral medication and of those who do not absorb their oral phenothiazines in adequate amounts.

*Posology and method of administration:*
*Adults:* Suitable where a reduced injection volume is desirable and therefore most suitable for patients on high dose maintenance therapy.

Not previously treated: Initially 0.5 ml by deep intramuscular injection into the gluteal region given at 2-5 week intervals, depending on patient response. Most patients are maintained on dose range of 0.5–4 ml.

If doses in excess of 100 mg are needed, increments of 12.5 mg (0.125 ml) should be implemented.
Previously treated:
(i) Oral: Dosage must be titrated as for new patients.
(ii) Depot: Restart on same dose as previously, possibly required at shorter dose intervals in the early weeks of treatment.

*Children:* Not recommended for patients under 12 years of age.
*Elderly:* Reduced maintenance doses may be needed in patients showing extrapyramidal symptoms, following initial dosing as above.
Initial dose–0.25 ml (25 mg).
N.B. Dose should not be increased without close supervision. Patients will respond in varying degrees to the drug. The response may be delayed. Symptoms may not recur for several weeks after discontinuation of treatment.

*Contra-indications:* Comatose patients, hepatic damage, jaundice, renal insufficiency, marked cerebral atherosclerosis, phaeochromocytoma, cardiac insufficiency and severely depressed states.

Special warnings and special precautions for use
Sudden, unexplained death has been reported in patients on phenothiazines, revealing at autopsy an acute, fulminating pneumonia with aspiration.

The drug should be administered under the direction of an experienced clinician. Renal and hepatic function should be monitored periodically during treatment.

Use with caution in patients with cardiovascular disease, known hypersensitivity to other phenothiazines, convulsive disorders. Patients undergoing surgery may be at risk to hypotension. Body temperature controls may become altered particularly at high doses. Atropinic effects may be potentiated.

*Interaction with other medicaments and other forms of interaction:*

CNS depressants: (alcohol, barbiturates, hypnotics, sedatives, strong analgesics all may show increased depressant effects).
May impair:
Antiparkinson effect of levodopa
Effect of anticonvulsants
Metabolism of tricyclic antidepressants
Control of diabetes
Action of adrenalin and other sympathomimetics.
May interact with lithium.

May enhance:
Cardiac depressant effect of quinidine
Absorption of corticosteroids
Absorption of digoxin
Absorption of neuromuscular blocking agents
Effect of anticoagulants.

*Pregnancy and lactation:*
*Use in pregnancy:* The safety of this drug during pregnancy has not been established. The possible hazards should be weighed against the benefits when administering the drug to pregnant patients.
*Use in Lactation:* Fluphenazine Decanoate may possibly be excreted in breast milk, as other phenothiazines are. Breast feeding is therefore not recommended during treatment.

*Effects on ability to drive and use machines*
Use may impair mental and physical abilities to drive or operate heavy machinery.

*Undesirable effects:*
*Adverse reactions:* Acute dystonic reactions occur frequently, usually within 24-48 hours. In susceptible individuals they may occur after small doses. Reaction may include oculogyric crises and opisthotonos. Rapidly relived by intravenous antiparkinsonian agent such as procyclidine.

Parkinsonian-like state may occur particularly between second and fifth day after injection. Can be reduced by using smaller doses more frequently or concomitant use of benzhexol, benztropine or procyclidine. Antiparkinson drugs should not be prescribed routinely because of the risk of aggravating antiucholinergic side effects or precipitating toxic confusion states or impairing therapeutic response. Careful monitoring will minimise use of antiparkinsonian drugs.

Tardive dyskinesia may appear on long term therapy or after drug has been discontinued. Elderly female patients on high doses seem to be most at risk. Symptoms are persistent and in some cases irreversible. The syndrome is characterised by rhythmical, involuntary movement of the tongue, face, mouth or jaw. Sometimes accompanied by involuntary movements of limbs. There is no known effective treatment. Antiparkinson drugs do not usually alleviate symptoms. It is suggested that antipsychotic agents be discontinued if such symptoms occur. It is reported that fine vermicular movements of the tongue may be an early sign of the syndrome, and cessation of treatment at this stage may prevent development of the full syndrome.

Drowsiness, lethargy, blurred vision, dryness of the mouth, constipation, urinary hesitancy or incontinence, mild hypotension, impairment of judgement and mental skills, epileptic form attacks are all occasionally seen.

Blood dyscrasias are rarely reported. Blood counts should be performed if persistent infection develops. Transient leucopenia and thrombocytopenia have been reported. Antinuclear antibodies and SLE are very rarely reported.

Jaundice and transient abnormalities of liver function are rarely reported.

Long term high dose phenothiazine use may result occasionally in abnormal skin pigmentation and lens opacity.

Skin rashes have been rarely reported.

Elderly patients may be more susceptible to sedative or hypertensive effects.

Cardiovascular effects of phenothiazines are dose related. ECG changes, including prolongation of QT interval and T wave changes have been reported commonly in patients treated with moderate to high dose therapy. The effects are reversible on reducing the dose. Rarely the effects may precipitate arrhythmias including ventricular tachycardia and fibrillation. These effects may also occur on overdosage.

Sudden, unexplained death has also been reported in hospitalised psychotic patients receiving phenothiazines.

Phenothiazines may impair body temperature regulation. Severe hypothermia or hyperpyrexia have been reported in association with moderate or high doses. Elderly patients may be particularly susceptible to hypothermia. Hyperpyrexia may be increased by hot or humid weather or by antiparkinsonian drugs which impair sweating.

Neuroleptic malignant syndrome (NMS) is rarely reported. The syndrome is characterised by hyperthermia, together with some or all of the following: muscular rigidity, autonomic instability, akinesia, altered consciousness, sometimes progressing to coma or stupor. Leucocytoses, elevated CPK, liver function abnormalities and acute renal failure. Neuroleptic drug therapy should be discontinued immediately. The syndrome is potentially fatal, and must be treated with vigorous symptomatic treatment.

Hormonal effects of phenothiazines include hyperprolactinaemia, which may cause galactorrhoea, gynacomastia and oligo or ammenorrhoea. Sexual function may be impaired.

*Overdose:* Supportive measures and symptomatic treatment. Extrapyramidal symptoms can be controlled with procyclidine or benztropine. Hypotension can be treated with vasoconstrictors and fluid replacement–but avoid using adrenalin.

## Pharmacological properties

*Pharmacodynamic properties:* Fluphenazine is a piperazine phenothiazine used widely in the treatment of schizophrenia. The action is thought to be through dopamine receptor blockade in the mesolimbic system. Fluphenazine has weak anticholinergic effects, sedative effects, antiadrenal effects and neuroendocrine effects. Side effects from extrapyramidal symptoms are common.

In an oil vehicle as the decanoate, fluphenazine ester slowly diffuses into the circulation. After hydrolysis, the drug passes the blood brain barrier as free drug.

*Pharmacokinetic properties:* Esterification of fluphenazine slows the rate of release from fat and thus prolongs the duration of action. Further delay is achieved by formulation in an oily solvent. Onset of action is within 48-72 hours, duration may be 1-6 weeks with an average of 2 weeks.

Distribution and metabolism are not fully described. Plasma half life has been shown to be 6-9 days following intramuscular administration of the decanoate.

## Pharmaceutical particulars

*List of excipients:*

*Fluphenazine Decanoate Injection BP 50 mg in 0.5 mL*

| | per unit dose | per mL |
|---|---|---|
| Sesame Oil BP | to 0.5 mL | to 1 mL |

*Fluphenazine Decanoate Injection BP 100 mg in 1 mL*

| | per unit dose | per mL |
|---|---|---|
| Sesame Oil | to 1 mL | to 1 mL |

*Incompatibilities:* Not applicable. An oily injection for intramuscular use only.

*Shelf life:* The medicinal product as packaged for sale has an 24 month shelf life.

*Special precautions for storage:* Store between 15°C–25°C. Protect from light.

*Instructions for use/handling:* Not applicable.

**Marketing authorization numbers**

| | |
|---|---|
| 50 mg in 0.5 ml | 4515/0056. |
| 100 mg in 1 ml | 4515/0056. |

**Date of approval/revision of SPC**  20 February 1996

**Legal category**  POM

# GENTAMICIN INJECTION BP

**Qualitative and quantitative composition** Active constituent: Gentamicin Sulphate BP, equivalent to Gentamicin Base: 40 mg/mL solutions, presented as 1 mL and 2 mL ampoules and 2 mL vials. 3.5% overage included in formulation.

**Pharmaceutical form** Sterile solution of Gentamicin Sulphate BP in Water for Injections BP

## Clinical particulars

*Therapeutic indications:* Gentamicin is bactericidal and is active against many strains of Gram-positive and Gram-negative pathogens including species of *Escherichia, Enterobacter, Klebsiella, Salmonella, Serratia, Shigella, Staphylococcus aureus*, some *Proteus* and against *Pseudomonas aeruginosa*. Gentamicin is often effective against strains of these organisms which are resistant to other antibiotics such as streptomycin, kanamycin and neomycin. Gentamicin is effective against penicillin-resistant *Staphylococci*, but rarely effective against *Streptococci*.

Gentamicin is indicated in the treatment of the following infections when caused by susceptible organisms:
Severe Gram-negative Infections
Upper and lower urinary tract infections
Burn and wound infections
Septicaemia, bacteraemia
Abscesses
Subacute bacterial endocarditis
Respiratory tract infections (bronchopneumonia)
Neonatal infections
Gynaecological infections
Gram-positive Infections:
Bacteraemia
Abscesses
Accidental and operative trauma
Burns and serious skin lesions

*Posology and method of administration:* Gentamicin is normally given by the intramuscular route, but can be given intravenously when intramuscular administration is not feasible.

Gentamicin is normally given by the intramuscular route, but can be given intravenously when intramuscular administration is not feasible, e.g. in shocked or severely burned patients. When given intravenously, the prescribed dose should be administered slowly over 2 to 3 minutes directly into a vein or into the rubber tubing of a giving set. Rapid, direct intravenous administration may give rise, initially, to potentially neurotoxic concentrations and it is essential that the prescribed dose is administered over the recommended period of time. Alternatively the prescribed dose should be dissolved in up to 100 ml of normal saline or 5% glucose in water, but not solutions containing bicarbonate (see *Incompatibilities*), and the solution infused over a period of 20 to 30 minutes.

The same dosage schedule is recommended for intramuscular and intravenous dosing. Dosage is related to the severity of infection, the age of the patient and the patient's renal function.

Dosage in Patients with Normal Renal Function:

*Adult dosage:*

| Type of infection | Dosage | Time interval between doses | Duration of therapy |
|---|---|---|---|
| Systemic and urinary tract infections | 3 mg/kg/day up to 80 mg | 8 hours | 7-10 days |
| Life threatening infections | 5 mg/kg/day initially then 3 mg/kg/day as soon as improvement is indicated | 6-8 hours | 7-10 days (Longer therapy may be required. If so, auditory renal and vestibular functions should be monitored). |

*Paediatric dosage:*

| Infection | Age | Dose/Route | Frequency |
|---|---|---|---|
| Systemic | 0–7 days | 5 mg/kg/day IM | 12 hours |
| | 1 week–1 yr | 6 mg/kg/day IM | 12 hours |
| | 1 yr–12 yrs | 4.5 mg/kg/day IM | 8 hours |
| Urinary tract infections | - | 3 mg/kg/day IM | 8 hours–12 hours |
| Life threatening infections | 0–7 days | 5 mg/kg/day | 12 hours |
| | 1 week–1 yr | 7.5 mg/kg/day | 8 hours |
| | 1 yr–12 yrs | 6 mg/kg/day | 8 hours |

*Doses in patients with impaired renal function:* Dosage is adjusted for patients with renal impairment to minimise the risk of toxicity. The first dose should be as normal–after this, doses should be given less frequently, the interval being determined by results of renal function tests as below:

*Renal function tests:*

| Dose | Creatinine clearance (ml/mn) | Serum creatinine (mmol/l) | BUN (mmol/l) | Interval between doses |
|---|---|---|---|---|
| 80 mg | over 70 | less than 0.12 | less than 6.5 | 8 hours |
| | 35-70 | 0.12-0.17 | 6.5-10 | 12 hours |
| | 24-34 | 0.18-0.25 | 11-14 | 18 hours |
| | 16-23 | 0.26-0.33 | 15-18 | 24 hours |
| | 10-15 | 0.34-0.47 | 19-26 | 36 hours |
| | 5-9 | 0.48-0.64 | 27-36 | 48 hours |

Serum levels should be monitored daily.

Peak levels in infants and young children: Peak serum levels are reached in 1 hour and dosage should be adjusted to achieve levels of more than 4 micrograms/ml, but not exceed 10 micrograms/ml.

*Contra-indications:* Patients being treated with Gentamicin should be under close clinical observation because of its potential toxicity. There are no absolute contraindications other than a history of hypersensitivity to Gentamicin. Gentamicin should be used with caution in premature infants because of their renal immaturity, in elderly people and generally in patients with impaired renal function. Diabetes, auditory vestibular dysfunctions, otitis media, a history of otitis media, previous use of ototoxic drugs and a geneti-

cally determined high sensitivity to aminoglycoside induced ototoxicity, are other main factors which may pre-dispose the patient to toxicity.

*Special warnings and precautions for use:* As with other aminoglycosides toxicity is related to serum concentration. At serum levels more than 10 micrograms/ml the vestibular mechanism may be affected. Toxicity can be minimised by monitoring serum concentrations and it is advisable to check serum levels to confirm that peak levels (one hour) do not exceed 10 micrograms/ml and that trough levels (one hour before next injection) do not exceed 2 micrograms/ml. Evidence of toxicity requires adjustment of dosage or withdrawal of the drug.

Concurrent use of other neurotoxic and/or nephrotoxic drugs can increase the possibility of Gentamicin toxicity. Co-administration with the following agents should be avoided:

Neuromuscular blocking agents such as succinylcholine and tubocurarine.

Other potentially nephrotoxic or ototoxic drugs such as cephalosporins and methicillin.

Potent diuretics such as ethacrynic acid and frusemide.

Other aminoglycosides.

*Interactions with other Medicaments and other forms of Interaction:*

(i) Antibacterials: increased risk of nephrotoxicity with *cephalosporins notably cephalothin*.

(ii) Gentamicin has been known to potentiate anticoagulants such as warfarin and phenindione.

(iii) Antifungals: increased risk of nephrotoxicity with *amphotericin*.

(iv) Cholinergics: antagonism of effect of *neostigmine and pyridostigmine*.

(v) Cyclosporin: increased risk of nephrotoxicity.

(vi) Cytotoxics: increased risk of nephrotoxicity and possible risk of ototoxicity with *cisplatin*.

(vii) Diuretics: increased risk of ototoxicity with *loop diuretics*.

(viii) Muscle relaxants: effect of non-depolarising muscle relaxants such as *tubocurarine* enhanced.

*Pregnancy and lactation:*

Use in pregnancy: Although no teratogenic effects have been observed, Gentamicin is known to cross the placenta. Ototoxicity in the foetus is also a potential hazard. The benefits should, therefore, be weighed against such hazards to the foetus before using Gentamicin during pregnancy.

Use in lactation: Small amounts of Gentamicin have been reported in breast milk. Because of the potential for serious adverse reactions to an aminoglycoside in nursing infants, a decision should be made whether to discontinue nursing or the drug, taking into account the importance of the drug to the woman.

*Effects on ability to drive and use machines:* Not applicable.

*Undesirable effects:* Ototoxicity and nephrotoxicity are the most common side effects associated with Gentamicin therapy. Both effects are related to renal impairment and hence the dosage in such patients should be altered as suggested.

Other adverse reactions associated with Gentamicin therapy include nausea, vomiting, urticaria, reversible granulocytopenia, allergic contact sensitization and neuromuscular blockade.

*Overdose:* As in the case of other aminoglycosides, toxicity is associated with serum levels above a critical value. In patients with normal renal function it is unlikely that toxic serum levels (in excess of 10 micrograms/ml) will be reached after administration of recommended doses. Where higher levels occur because of renal impairment, dosage should be reduced. In the event of an overdose or toxic reaction, peritoneal dialysis or haemodialysis will lower serum Gentamicin levels.

## Pharmacological properties

*Pharmacodynamic properties:* Gentamicin is usually bactericidal in action. Although the exact mechanism of action has not been fully elucidated, the drug appears to inhibit protein synthesis in susceptible bacteria by irreversibly binding to 30S ribosomal subunits.

In general, Gentamicin is active against many aerobic gram-negative bacteria and some aerobic gram-positive bacteria. Gentamicin is inactive against fungi, viruses, and most anaerobic bacteria.

In vitro, Gentamicin concentrations of 1-8μg/mL inhibit most susceptible strains of *Escherichia coli*, *Haemophilus influenzae*, *Moraxella lacunata*, *Neisseria*, indole positive and indole negative *Proteus*, *Pseudomonas* (including most strains of *Ps. aeruginosa*), *Staphylococcus aureus*, *S. epidermidis*, and *Serratia*. However, different species and different strains of the same species may exhibit wide variations in susceptibility *in vitro*. In addition, *in vitro* susceptibility does not always correlate with *in vivo*

activity. Gentamicin is only minimally active against *Streptococci*.

Natural and acquired resistance to Gentamicin has been demonstrated in both gram-negative and gram-positive bacteria. Gentamicin resistance may be due to decreased permeability of the bacterial cell wall, alteration in the ribosomal binding site, or the presence of a plasmid-mediated resistance factor which is acquired by conjugation. Plasmid-mediated resistance enables the resistant bacteria to enzymatically modify the drug by acetylation, phosphorylation, or adenylylation and can be transferred between organisms of the same or different species. Resistance to other aminoglycosides and several other anti-infectives (e.g. chloramphenicol, sulphonamides, tetracycline) may be transferred on the same plasmid.

There is partial cross-resistance between Gentamicin and other aminoglycosides.

*Pharmacokinetic properties:* Gentamicin and other aminoglycosides are poorly absorbed from the gastrointestinal tract but are rapidly absorbed after intramuscular injection. Average peak plasma concentrations of about 4μg per mL have been obtained 30 to 60 minutes after intramuscular administration of a dose equivalent to 1 mg of Gentamicin per kg body-weight although there may be considerable individual variation and higher concentrations in patients with renal failure. Similar concentrations are obtained after intravenous administration. Several doses are required before equilibrium concentrations are obtained in the plasma and this may represent the saturation of binding sites in body tissues such as the kidney. Binding of Gentamicin to plasma proteins is usually low.

Following parenteral administration Gentamicin and other aminoglycosides diffuse mainly into extracellular fluids and factors which affect the volume of distribution will also affect plasma concentrations. However, there is little diffusion into the cerebrospinal fluid and even when the meninges are inflamed effective concentrations may not be achieved; diffusion into the eye is also poor. Aminoglycosides diffuse readily into the perilymph of the inner ear. Gentamicin crosses the placenta but only small amounts have been reported in breast milk.

Systemic absorption of Gentamicin and other aminoglycosides has been reported after topical use on denuded skin and burns and following instillation into and irrigation of wounds, body-cavities, and joints.

*Preclinical safety data:* There are no preclinical data of relevance to the prescriber which are additional to that already included in other sections of the SPC.

## Pharmaceutical particulars

List of excipient:

| | |
|---|---|
| Sodium Metabisulphite BP | 6.4 mg |
| Disodium Edetate BP | 0.2 mg |
| Water for Injections BP | 2.0 ml |
| Sulphuric Acid (2.5N) BP | Q.S. |
| Sodium Hydroxide (2.5N) BP | Q.S. |
| (In presentations with bactericide only): | |
| Methyl Hydroxybenzoate BP | 3.6 mg |
| Propyl Hydroxybenzoate BP | 0.4 mg |

*Incompatibilities:* Gentamicin Injection should not be mixed with other drugs before injection and where co-administration of penicillins, cephalosporins, erythromycin, sulphadiazine, frusemide and betalactam antibiotics and heparin is necessary, the drugs should be administered separately, either as bolus injections into the tubing of the giving set or at separate sites. Addition of Gentamicin to solutions containing bicarbonate may lead to the release of carbon dioxide.

*Shelf life:* 36 months.

*Special precautions for storage:* Store below 25˚C.

*Instruction for use/handling:* Not applicable.

**Marketing authorisation numbers**

| | |
|---|---|
| Ampoules | 4515/0028 |
| 80 mg/2 mL vial | 4515/0037 |

**Date of approval/revision of SPC** 24 January 1997

**Legal category** POM

## GLYCERYL TRINITRATE FOR INJECTION 5MG/1ML.

**Qualitative and quantitative composition**

*Active Constituent*

| | |
|---|---|
| Glyceryl Trinitrate HSE | 5.0 mg. |

*Other Constituents*

| | |
|---|---|
| Ethanol BP | 30.0% v/v |
| Propylene Glycol BP | 30.0% v/v |
| Water for Injections BP | to 1.0 mL. |

There is no overage included in the formulation.

**Pharmaceutical form** A sterile, non-pyrogenic, clear, practically colourless solution.

**Clinical particulars**

*Therapeutic indications:* Surgery: Glyceryl Trinitrate is indicated for the prompt control of hypertension during cardiac surgery.

It may also be used for the production and maintenance of controlled hypotension during surgical procedures.

Glyceryl Trinitrate may be given for the control of myocardial ischaemia both during and following cardiovascular surgery.

Unresponsive congestive cardiac failure secondary to acute myocardial infarction: Glyceryl Trinitrate may be used in patients presenting with unresponsive congestive heart failure secondary to acute myocardial infarction.

Unstable angina: Glyceryl Trinitrate Infusion may be used to reduce myocardial oxygen demand in proportion to the reduction in pre- and after-load. It may be indicated for the control of anginal episodes in patients with unstable angina who do not respond to standard treatment and/or beta-blockers.

It is recommended that blood pressure and pulse rate are regularly monitored during infusion of Glyceryl Trinitrate.

*Posology and method of administration:* Glyceryl Trinitrate for Injection is a concentrated, potent drug which must be diluted in Dextrose (5%) Injection BP or Sodium Chloride (0.9%) Injection BP prior to its infusion.

The dosage range for most patients is 10-20mcg/min. However, doses up to 400 mcg/min may be required during surgical procedures.

*Compatibility:* Glyceryl Trinitrate for Injection is compatible with glass infusion bottles and some rigid infusion packs made of polyethylene. Examples of such suitable infusion packs are: Boots polyfusor and the bottle pack distributed by Dylade, Cheshire UK (bottlepak, flatpak) or Antigen Ltd. Roscrea, Eire (Braun).

Glyceryl Trinitrate for Injection may also be administered using a syringe pump or rigid plastic syringe (Gillette Sabre syringe, Brunswick Disposable, Plastipak syringe or Monojet disposable syringe).

Suitable giving sets are Types A261 or A2001 available from David Bull Laboratories or Avon Medicals. Lectrocath tubing (Vygon UK Ltd) is also known to be compatible with the preparation.

The method of choice of administration should ensure that the drug is given at a constant infusion rate.

*Incompatibility:* Glyceryl Trinitrate for Injection is incompatible with polyvinyl chloride (PVC) since 40-80% of the total amount thereof in the final diluted solution for infusion is absorbed by the PVC tubing of the intravenous administration sets.

*Dosage:* The recommended dose range is 10-200 mcg/min, although larger doses than this have been used. During some surgical procedures, doses of up to 400 mcg/min may be required. In order to maintain the appropriate infusion rate, clinical assessment and regular blood pressure monitoring are necessary. Measurement of pulmonary capillary wedge pressure and cardiac out-put may also be used to titrate dosage to response.

*Surgery:* For the control of hypertensive episodes the recommended starting dose is 25 mcg/min increasing in steps to 25 mcg/min at 5 minute intervals until the desired drop in blood pressure is achieved. Although most patients respond to doses between 10-200 mcg/min, doses up to 400 mcg/min have been required during some surgical procedures. In the treatment of perioperative myocardial ischaemia, the recommended starting dose is 15-20 mcg/min increasing in steps of 10-15 mcg/min until the desired effect is achieved.

*Unresponsive congestive cardiac failure secondary to acute myocardial infarction:* The recommended starting dose is 20-25 mcg/min which can be decreased to 10 mcg/min or increased in steps of 20-25 mcg/min at 15-30 minute intervals until the desired effect is achieved.

*Unstable angina:* The recommended starting dose is 10 mcg/min increasing in steps of 5-10 mcg/min at approximately 30 minute intervals.

*Children and the elderly:* The use of Glyceryl Trinitrate in children and elderly patients is not recommended, as the safety and effectiveness of Glyceryl Trinitrate in children and elderly patients have not been established.

*Contra-indications:* To those who have or are:

1. Hypersensitive to Glyceryl Trinitrate
2. Hypotensive or hypovolaemic
3. Increased intracranial pressure
4. Constrictive pericarditis and pericardial tamponade
5. Severe anaemia and arterial hypoxaemia.

*Special warnings and special precautions for use:*
*Warnings:* DBL Glyceryl Trinitrate for Injection contains propylene glycol which can lead to lactic acidosis. It is recommended that the use of this preparation be restricted to not more than three successive days.

*Precautions:* Glyceryl Trinitrate for Injection should not be administered to patients known to be hypersensitive to organic nitrates, nor should it be given to patients with uncorrected hypovolaemia, severe anaemia or cerebral haemorrhage or hypotension.

Glyceryl Trinitrate should be used with caution in patients presenting with malnutrition, hypothyroidism, severe hypothermia, or severe impairment of hepatic and/or renal function.

Evidence is not available to demonstrate the safety of Glyceryl Trinitrate for intracoronary injection.

Glyceryl Trinitrate for Injection should be used with caution in patients predisposed to closed angle glaucoma.

*Interaction with other medicaments and other forms of interaction:*

Anti-arrhythmics: disopyramide may reduce effect of sublingual nitrates (owing to dry mouth)

Anti-depressants: tricyclics may reduce effects of sublingual nitrates (owing to dry mouth)

Antimuscarinics: antimuscarinics such as atropine and propantheline may reduce effect of sublingual nitrates (owing to dry mouth).

*Pregnancy and lactation:* The safety of Glyceryl Trinitrate during pregnancy and lactation has not been demonstrated and therefore it should not be used in these situations unless considered essential by the physician.

*Effects on ability to drive and use machines:* Not applicable.

*Undesirable effects:* Adverse reactions to organic nitrates which have been reported include hypotension, tachycardia, nausea, retching, diaphoresis, apprehension, headache, restlessness, muscle twitching, retrosternal discomfort, palpitations, dizziness, and abdominal pain, paradoxical bradycardia has rarely been observed.

*Overdose:* Overdosage usually results in hypotension and tachycardia and can be reversed by elevating the legs or decreasing or terminating the infusion. In severe cases of overdosage, intravenous administration of methoxamine or phenylephrine is recommended.

**Pharmacological properties**

*Pharmacodynamic properties:* Glyceryl Trinitrate, an organic nitrate, is a vasodilator. The principal pharmacological action of Glyceryl Trinitrate is the relaxation of vascular smooth muscle. Glyceryl Trinitrate produces, in a dose-related manner, dilation of both arterial and venous beds. Dilatation of the post-capillary vessels, including large veins, promotes peripheral pooling of blood and decreases venous return to the heart, reducing left ventricular end-diastolic pressure (pre-load).

Arteriolar relaxation reduces systemic vascular resistance and arterial pressure (after-load). Myocardial oxygen consumption or demand (as measured by the pressure-rate product, tension time index and stroke work index) is decreased by both arterial and venous effects of Glyceryl Trinitrate, and a more favourable supply demand ratio can be achieved.

Therapeutic doses of intravenous Glyceryl Trinitrate reduce systolic, diastolic and mean arterial blood pressure. Effective coronary perfusion pressure is usually maintained, but can be compromised if blood pressure falls excessively or increased heart rate decreases diastolic filling time.

Glyceryl Trinitrate reduces elevated central venous and pulmonary capillary wedge pressures, pulmonary vascular resistance and systemic vascular resistance. Heart rate is usually slightly increased, presumably a reflex response to the fall in blood pressure. Cardiac index may be increased, decreased or unchanged.

Patients with elevated left ventricular filling pressure and systemic vascular resistance values in conjunction with a depressed cardiac index are likely to experience an improvement in cardiac index. Alternatively, when filling pressures and cardiac index are normal, cardiac index may be slightly reduced by intravenous Glyceryl Trinitrate.

*Pharmacokinetic properties:* Glyceryl Trinitrate is widely distributed in the body with an apparent volume of distribution of 200 L in adult male subjects, and is rapidly metabolised to dinitrates and mononitrates, with a short half-life estimated at 1-4 minutes. This results in a low plasma concentration after intravenous infusion. Glyceryl Trinitrate is also well absorbed from the gastro-intestinal tract, but it is not known if it is distributed into milk.

At plasma concentrations of between 50 and 500ng/ml, the binding of Glyceryl Trinitrate to plasma proteins is approximately 60% and 30% respectively. The plasma half-life of Glyceryl Trinitrate is about 1-4 minutes. Glyceryl mononitrate which is inactive, is the principal metabolite.

*Preclinical safety data:* Not applicable.

**Pharmaceutical particulars**

*List of excipients:*

| | |
|---|---|
| Ethanol BP | 30.0% v/v |
| Propylene Glycol BP | 30.0% v/v |
| Water for Injections BP | to 1.0 mL. |

There is no overage included in the formulation.

*Incompatibilities:* The manufacturers of Glyceryl Trinitrate for Injection recommend that this concentrated and potent drug must be diluted in Dextrose (5%) Injection BP or Sodium Chloride (0.9%) Injection BP prior to its infusion. They also state that no other drug should be admixed with it.

*Shelf life:* 36 months.

*Special precautions for storage:* Store below 25°C. Protect from light.

Open ampoules of Glyceryl Trinitrate should be used immediately and any unused portion discarded.

Dilutions of Glyceryl Trinitrate for Injection in Sodium Chloride Injection or Dextrose Injection are stable for 40 hours at room temperature when stored in glass containers or recommended plastic containers. Similar dilutions are stable for 7 days at 2°C-8°C.

Solutions containing 1 mg or 4 mg per Glyceryl Trinitrate, diluted in Dextrose 5% Injection BP are stable for up to 72 hours, at room temperature protected from light, using either polycarbonate (Plastipak) or polypropylene syringes.

Glyceryl Trinitrate is rapidly lost from solutions stored in polyvinylchloride (PVC) containers, and the use of such infusion packs should therefore be avoided.

Glyceryl Trinitrate should be administered in the recommended plastic containers (see under compatibility).

Glyceryl Trinitrate should be protected from strong light.

Do not use if the solution is discoloured.

*Instructions for use/handling:* Not applicable.

**Marketing authorisation number** 4515/0006

**Date of approval/revision of SPC** August 1995

**Legal category** POM

# METHOTREXATE INJECTION

**Qualitative and quantitative composition**

*2.5 mg/mL presentations*

| *Presentation* | *5 mg/2 mL* | |
|---|---|---|
| *Active Constituent* | *per unit dose* | *per mL* |
| Methotrexate BP | 5.0 mg* | 2.5 mg |

*There is a 5% manufacturing overage included in the formulation.

*25 mg/mL presentations*

| *Presentation* | *50 mg/2 mL* | | *500 mg/20 mL* | |
|---|---|---|---|---|
| *Active Constituent* | *per unit dose* | *per mL* | *per unit dose* | *per mL* |
| Methotrexate BP | 50.0 mg* | 25.0 mg | 500.0 mg* | 25.0 mg. |

*There is a 5% manufacturing overage included in the formulation.

*100 mg/mL presentations*

| *Presentation* | *1 g/10 mL* | | *5 g/50 mL* | |
|---|---|---|---|---|
| *Active Constituent* | *per unit dose* | *per mL* | *per unit dose* | *per mL* |
| Methotrexate BP | 1000.0 mg* | 100.0 mg | 5000.0 mg* | 100.0 mg. |

*There is a 5% manufacturing overage included in the formulation.

**Pharmaceutical form** Sterile solution of Methotrexate in Water for Injections.

**Clinical particulars**

*Therapeutic indications:* Methotrexate is indicated in the treatment of neoplastic disease, such as trophoblastic neoplasms and leukaemia, and the symptomatic treatment of severe recalcitrant disabling psoriasis which is not adequately responsive to other forms of treatment.

Methotrexate Injection BP may be given by the intramuscular, intravenous, intra-arterial, intrathecal routes.

NOTE: Methotrexate Injection BP 1 g in 10 ml and 5 g in 50 ml are hypertonic and therefore are not suitable for intrathecal use. The 500 mg in 20 ml should not be administered by the intrathecal route.

*Posology and method of administration:*
*Adults and children: Antineoplastic chemotherapy:* Methotrexate is active orally and parenterally. Methotrexate Injection BP may be given by the intramuscular, intravenous, intra-arterial or intrathecal routes. Dosage is related to the patient's body weight or surface area. Methotrexate has been used with beneficial effect in a wide variety of neoplastic diseases, alone and in combination with other cytotoxic agents. Note: Methotrexate Injection BP 1 g in 10 ml and 5 g in 50 ml are hypertonic and thus are not recommended for intrathecal use.

*Choriocarcinoma and Similar Trophoblastic Dis-*

*eases:* Methotrexate is administered orally or intramuscularly in doses of 15-30 mg daily for a 5 day course. Such courses may be repeated for 3-5 times as required, with rest periods of one or more weeks interposed between courses until any manifesting toxic symptoms subside.

The effectiveness of therapy can be evaluated by 24 hours quantitative analysis of urinary chorionic gonadotrophin hormone (HCG). Alternation of Methotrexate, and combination therapy with other cytotoxic drugs, has also been reported as useful.

Hydatidiform mole may precede or be followed by choriocarcinoma, and Methotrexate has been used in similar doses for the treatment of hydatidiform mole and chorioadenoma destruens.

*Breast Carcinoma:* Prolonged cyclic combination with Cyclophosphamide, Methotrexate and Fluorouracil has given good results when used as adjuvant treatment to radical mastectomy in primary breast cancer with positive axillary lymph nodes. Methotrexate dosage was 40 mg/m2 intravenously on the first and eight days.

*Leukaemia:* Acute granulocytic leukaemia is rare in children but common in adults and this form of leukaemia responds poorly to chemotherapy.

Methotrexate is not generally a drug of choice for induction of remission of lymphoblastic leukaemia. Oral Methotrexate dosage of 3.3 mg/m2 daily, and Prednisolone 40-60 mg/m2 daily for 4-6 weeks has been used. After a remission is attained, Methotrexate in a maintenance dosage of 20-30 mg/m2 orally or by I.M. injection has been administered twice weekly. Twice weekly doses appear to be more effective than daily drug administration. Alternatively, 2.5 mg/kg has been administered I.V. every 14 days.

*Meningeal Leukaemia:* Some patients with leukaemia are subject to leukaemic invasions of the central nervous system and the CSF should be examined in all leukaemia patients.

Passage of Methotrexate from blood to the cerebrospinal fluid is minimal and for adequate therapy the drug should be administered intrathecally. Methotrexate may be given in a prophylactic regimen in all cases of lymphocytic leukaemia. Methotrexate is administered by intrathecal injection in doses of 200-500 micrograms/kg body weight. The administration is at intervals of 2 to 5 days and is usually repeated until the cell count of cerebrospinal fluid returns to normal. At this point one additional dose is advised. Alternatively, Methotrexate 12 mg/m2 can be given once weekly for 2 weeks, and then once monthly. Large doses may cause convulsions and untoward side effects may occur as with any intrathecal injection, and are commonly neurological in character.

NOTE: Methotrexate Injection BP 1 g in 10 ml, 5 g in 50 ml and 500 mg in 20 ml are not recommended for intrathecal use.

*Lymphomas:* In Burkitt's Tumour, stages 1-2, Methotrexate has prolonged remissions in some cases. Recommended dosage is 10-25 mg per day orally for 4 to 8 days. In stage 3, Methotrexate is commonly given concomitantly with other antitumour agents. Treatment in all stages usually consists of several courses of the drug interposed with 7 to 10 day rest periods, and in stage 3 they respond to combined drug therapy with Methotrexate given in doses of 0.625 mg to 2.5 mg/kg daily. Hodgkin's Disease responds poorly to Methotrexate and to most types of chemotherapy.

*Mycosis Fungoides:* Therapy with Methotrexate appears to produce clinical remissions in one half of the cases treated. Recommended dosage is usually 2.5 to 10 mg daily by mouth for weeks or months and dosage should be adjusted according to the patient's response and haematological monitoring. Methotrexate has also been given intramuscularly in doses of 50 mg once weekly or 25 mg twice weekly.

*Psoriasis Chemotherapy:* Cases of severe uncontrolled psoriasis, unresponsive to conventional therapy, have responded to weekly single, oral, I.M. or I.V. doses of 10-25 mg per week, and adjusted according to the patient's response. An initial test dose one week prior to initiation of therapy is recommended to detect any idiosyncrasy. A suggested dose range is 5-10 mg parenterally.

An alternative dosage schedule consists of 2.5 to 5 mg of Methotrexate administered orally at 12 hour intervals for 3 doses each week or at 8-hour intervals for 4 doses each week; weekly dosages should not exceed 30 mg.

A daily oral dosage schedule of 2 to 5 mg administered orally for 5 days followed by a rest period of at least 2 days may also be used. The daily dose should not exceed 6.25 mg.

The patient should be fully informed of the risks involved and the clinician should pay particular attention to the appearance of the liver toxicity by carrying out liver function tests before starting Methotrexate treatment, and repeating these at 2 to 4 month intervals during therapy. The aim of therapy should be to reduce the dose to the lowest possible level with the longest possible rest period. The use of Methotrexate may permit the return to conventional topical therapy which should be encouraged.

*Contra-indications:* Impaired renal or hepatic function. Pre-existing blood dyscrasias, such as marrow hypoplasia, leukopenia, thromocytopenia or anaemia.

Pregnancy and lactation: Methotrexate is contraindicated in pregnancy. Because of the potential for serious adverse reactions from methotrexate in breast fed infants, breast feeding is contra-indicated in women taking methotrexate. Patients with a known allergic hypersensitivity to methotrexate should not receive methotrexate.

*Special warnings and special precautions for use:*
*Warnings:* Methotrexate must be used only by physicians experienced in antimetabolic chemotherapy.

Because of the possibility of fatal or severe toxic reactions, the patient should be fully informed by the physician of the risks involved and be under his constant supervision.

Deaths have been reported with the use of Methotrexate in the treatment of psoriasis.

In the treatment of psoriasis, Methotrexate should be restricted to severe recalcitrant, disabling psoriasis which is not adequately responsive to other forms of therapy, but only when the diagnosis has been established as by biopsy and/or after dermatological consultation.

1. Methotrexate may produce marked depression of bone marrow, anaemia, leukopenia, thrombocytopenia and bleeding.

2. Methotrexate may be hepatotoxic, particularly at high dosage or with prolonged therapy. Liver atrophy, necrosis, cirrhosis, fatty changes, and periportal fibrosis have been reported. Since changes may occur without previous signs of gastrointestinal or haematological toxicity, it is imperative that hepatic function be determined prior to initiation of treatment and monitored regularly throughout therapy. Special caution is indicated in the presence of pre-existing liver damage of impaired hepatic function. Concomitant use of other drugs with hepatotoxic potential (including alcohol) should be avoided.

3. Methotrexate has been shown to be teratogenic; it has caused foetal death and/or congenital anomalies. Therefore it is not recommended in women of childbearing potential unless there is appropriate medical evidence that the benefits can be expected to outweigh the considered risks. Pregnant psoriatic patients should not receive Methotrexate.

4. Impaired renal function is usually a contraindication.

5. Diarrhoea and ulcerative stomatitis are frequent toxic effects and require interruption of therapy, otherwise haemorrhagic enteritis and death from intestinal perforation may occur.

6. Methotrexate affects gametogenesis during the period of its administration and may result in decreased fertility which is thought to be reversible on discontinuation of therapy. Conception should be avoided during the period of Methotrexate administration and for at least 6 months thereafter. Patients and their partners should be advised to this effect.

7. Methotrexate has some immunosuppressive activity and immunological responses to concurrent vaccination may be decreased. The immunosuppressive effect of Methotrexate should be taken into account when immune responses of patients are important or essential.

8. Patients with pleural effusions or ascites should have these drained if appropriate before treatment or treatment should be withdrawn.

9. Deaths have been reported with the use of methotrexate. Serious adverse reactions including deaths have been reported with concomitant administration of methotrexate (usually in high doses) along with some non-steroidal anti-inflammatory drugs (NSAIDs).

10. Concomitant administration of folate antagonists such as trimethoprim/sulphamethoxazole has been reported to cause an acute megaloblastic pancytopenia in rare instances.

*Precautions:* Methotrexate has a high potential toxicity, usually dose related, and should be used only by physicians experienced in antimetabolite chemotherapy, in patients under their constant supervision. The physician should be familiar with the various characteristics of the drug and its established clinical usage.

Before beginning methotrexate therapy or reinstituting methotrexate after a rest period, assessment of renal function, liver function and blood elements should be made by history, physical examination and laboratory tests.

It should be noted that intrathecal doses are transported into the cardiovascular system and may give rise to systemic toxicity. Systemic toxicity of methotrexate may also be enhanced in patients with renal dysfunction, ascites, or other effusions due to prolongation of serum half-life.

High doses may cause the precipitation of methotrexate or its metabolites in the renal tubules. A high fluid throughout and alkalinisation of the urine to pH 6.5-7.0 by oral or intravenous administration of sodium bicarbonate (5 x 625 mg tablets every three hours) or acetazolamide (500 mg orally four times a day) is recommended as a preventative measure.

Carcinogenesis, mutagenesis, and impairment of fertility: Animal carcinogencity studies have demonstrated methotrexate to be free of carcinogenic potential. Although methotrexate has been reported to cause chromosomal damage to animal somatic cells and bone marrow cells in humans, these effects are transient and reversible. In patients treated with methotrexate, evidence is insufficient to permit conclusive evaluation of any increased risk of neoplasia.

Methotrexate has been reported to cause impairment of fertility, oligospermia, menstrual dysfunction and amenorrhoea in humans, during and for a short period after cessation of therapy. In addition, methotrexate causes, embryotoxicity, abortion and foetal defects in humans. Therefore the possible risks of effects on reproduction should be discussed with patients of childbearing potential (see 'Warnings').

Patients undergoing therapy should be subject to appropriate supervision so that signs or symptoms of possible toxic effects or adverse reactions may be detected and evaluated with minimal delay. Pretreatment and periodic haematological studies are essential to the use of Methotrexate in chemotherapy because of its common effect of haematopoietic suppression. This may occur abruptly and on apparent safe dosage, and any profound drop in blood cell count indicates immediate stopping of the drug and appropriate therapy. In patients with malignant disease who have pre-existing bone marrow aplasia, leukopenia, thrombocytopenia or anaemia, the drug should be used with caution, if at all.

Methotrexate is excreted primarily by the kidneys. Its use in the presence of impaired renal function may result in accumulation of toxic amounts or even additional renal damage. The patient's renal status should be determined prior to or during Methotrexate therapy and proper caution exercised, should significant renal impairment be disclosed.

Drug dosage should be reduced or discontinued until renal function is improved or restored.

In general, the following laboratory tests are recommended as part of essential clinical evaluation and appropriate monitoring of patients chosen for or receiving Methotrexate therapy: complete haemogram; haematocrit; urinalysis; renal function tests; and liver function tests.

A chest X-ray is also recommended. The purpose is to determine any existing organ dysfunction or system impairment. The tests should be performed prior to therapy, at appropriate periods during therapy and after termination of therapy. It may be useful or important to perform liver biopsy or bone marrow aspiration studies where high dose or long term therapy is being followed.

Methotrexate is bound in part to serum albumin after absorption, and toxicity may be increased because of displacement by certain drugs such as salicylates, sulphonamides, phenytoin, and some antibacterials such as tetracycline, chloramphenicol and para-aminobenzoic acid. These drugs, especially salicylates and sulphonamides, whether antibacterial, hypoglycaemic or diuretic, should not be given concurrently until the significance of these findings is established.

Vitamin preparations containing folic acid or its derivatives may alter response to Methotrexate.

Methotrexate should be used with extreme caution in the presence of infection, peptic ulcer, ulcerative colitis, debility, and in extreme youth and old age. If profound leukopenia occurs during therapy, bacterial infection may occur or become a threat. Cessation of the drug and appropriate antibiotic therapy is usually indicated. In severe bone marrow depression, blood or platelet transfusions may be necessary.

Since it is reported that Methotrexate may have an immunosuppressive action, this factor must be taken into consideration in evaluating the use of the drug where immune responses in a patient may be important or essential.

In all instances where the use of Methotrexate is considered for chemotherapy, the physician must evaluate the need and usefulness of the drug against the risks of toxic effects or adverse reactions. Most such adverse reactions are reversible if detected early. When such effects or reactions do occur, the drug should be reduced in dosage or discontinued and appropriate corrective measures should be taken according to the clinical judgement of the physician. Reinstitution of Methotrexate therapy should be carried out with caution, with adequate consideration of further need for the drug and alertness as to the possible recurrence of toxicity.

*Interaction with other medicaments and other forms of interaction:* Methotrexate is extensively protein bound and may be displaced by certain drugs such as salicylates, hypoglycaemics, diuretics, sulphonamides, diphenylhydantoins, tetracyclines, chloramphenicol and p-aminobenzoic acid, and the acidic anti-inflammatory agents, so causing a potential for increased toxicity when used concurrently. Concomitant use of other drugs with nephrotoxic or hepatotoxic potential (including alcohol) should be avoided. Vitamin preparations containing folic acid or its derivatives may decrease the effectiveness of methotrexate.

Caution should be used when NSAIDs and salicylates are administered concomitantly with methotrexate. These drugs have been reported to reduce the tubular secretion of methotrexate in an animal model and thereby may enhance its toxicity. Renal tubular transport is also diminished by probenecid; use of methotrexate with this drug should be carefully monitored.

Patients using constant dosage regimens of NSAIDs have received concurrent doses of methotrexate problems. Therefore, until more is known about the NSAIDs/methotrexate interaction, it is recommended that methotrexate dosage be carefully controlled during treatment with NSAIDs.

Methotrexate should be used with caution in patients taking drugs known to have an antifolate potential.

*Pregnancy and lactation:* Abortion, foetal death, and/ or congenital anomalies have occurred in pregnant women receiving Methotrexate, especially during the first trimester of pregnancy. Methotrexate is contraindicated in the management of psoriasis or rheumatoid arthritis in pregnant women. Women of childbearing potential should not receive Methotrexate until pregnancy is excluded. For the management of psoriasis or rheumatoid arthritis, Methotrexate therapy in women should be started immediately following a menstrual period and appropriate measures should be taken in men or women to avoid conception during and for at least 12 weeks following Methotrexate therapy.

Both men and women receiving Methotrexate should be informed of the potential risk of adverse effects on reproduction. Women of childbearing potential should be fully informed of the potential hazard to the foetus should they become pregnant during Methotrexate therapy. In cancer chemotherapy, Methotrexate should not be used in pregnant women or women of childbearing potential who might become pregnant unless the potential benefits to the mother outweigh the possible risks to the foetus.

Defective oogenesis or spermatogenesis, transient oligospermia, menstrual dysfunction, and infertility have been reported in patients receiving Methotrexate.

Methotrexate is distributed into breast milk. Because of the potential for serious adverse reactions to Methotrexate in nursing infants, a decision should be made whether to discontinue nursing or the drug, taking into account the importance of the drug to the woman.

*Effects on ability to drive and use machines:* Not applicable.

*Undesirable effects:* The most common adverse reactions include ulcerative stomatitis, leukopenia, nausea and abdominal distress. Although very rare, anaphylactic reactions to methotrexate have occurred. Others reported are malaise, undue fatigue, chills and fever, dizziness and decreased resistance to infection. In general, the incidence and severity of side effects are considered to be dose-related. Adverse reactions as reported for the various systems are as follows:

Skin: Erythematous rashes, pruritus, urticaria, photosensitivity, depigmentation, alopecia, ecchymosis, telangiectasia, acne, furunculosis. Lesions of psoriasis may be aggravated by concomitant exposure to ultraviolet radiation. Skin ulceration has been reported in psoriatic patients. The recall phenomenon has been reported in both radiation and solar damaged skin.

Blood: Bone marrow depression, leukopenia, thrombocytopenia, anaemia, hypogammaglobulinaemia, haemorrhage from various sites, septicaemia.

Alimentary System: Gingivitis, pharyngitis, stomatitis, anorexia, vomiting, diarrhoea, haematemesis, melena, gastrointestinal ulceration and bleeding, enteritis, hepatic toxicity resulting in active liver atrophy, necrosis, fatty metamorphosis, periportal fibrosis, or hepatic cirrhosis. In rare cases the effect of methotrexate on the intestinal mucosa has led to malabsorption or toxic megacolon.

Hepatic: Hepatic toxicity resulting in significant elevations of liver enzymes, acute liver atrophy, necrosis, fatty metamorphosis, periportal fibrosis or cirrhosis or death may occur, usually following chronic administration.

Urogenital System: Renal failure, azotaemia, cystitis, haematuria, defective oogenesis or spermatogenesis, transient oligospermia, menstrual dysfunction, infertility, abortion, foetal defects, severe nephropathy. Vaginitis, vaginal ulcers, cystitis, haematuria and nephropathy have also been reported.

Pulmonary System: Infrequently an acute or chronic interstitial pneumonitis, often associated with blood eosinophilia, may occur and deaths have been reported. Acute pulmonary oedema has also been reported after oral and intrathecal use. Pulmonary fibrosis is rare. A syndrome consisting of pleuritic pain and pleural thickening has been reported following high doses.

Central Nervous System: Headaches, drowsiness, blurred vision, aphasia, hemiparesis and convulsions have occurred possibly related to haemorrhage or to complications from intra-arterial catheterization. Convulsion, paresis, Guillain-Barre syndrome and increased cerebrospinal fluid pressure have followed intrathecal administration.

Other reactions related to, or attributed to the use of Methotrexate such as pneumonitis, metabolic changes, precipitation of diabetes, osteoporotic effects, abdominal changes in tissue cells and even sudden death have been reported.

There have been reports of leukoencephalopathy following intravenous methotrexate in high doses, or low doses following cranial-spinal radiation.

Adverse reactions following intrathecal methotrexate are generally classified into three groups, acute, subacute, and chronic. The acute form is a chemical arachnoiditis manifested by headache, back or shoulder pain, nuchal rigidity, and fever. The subacute form may include paresis, usually transient, paraplegia, nerve palsies, and cerebellar dysfunction. The chronic form is a leukoencephalopathy manifested by irritability, confusion, ataxia, spasticity, occasionally convulsions, dementia, somnolence, coma, and rarely, death. There is evidence that the combined use of cranial radiation and intrathecal methotrexate increases the incidence of leukoencephalopathy.

Additional reactions related to or attributed to the use of methotrexate such as osteoporosis, abnormal (usually 'megaloblastic') red cell morphology, precipitation of diabetes, other metabolic changes, and sudden death have been reported.

*Overdose:* Calcium Folinate (Calcium Leucovorin) is a potent agent for neutralizing the immediate toxic effects of Methotrexate on the haematopoietic system. Where large doses or overdoses are given, Calcium Folinate may be administered by intravenous infusion in doses up to 75 mg within 12 hours, followed by 12 mg intramuscularly every 6 hours for 4 doses. Where average doses of Methotrexate appear to have an adverse effect 6-12 mg of Calcium Folinate may be given intramuscularly every 6 hours for 4 doses. In general, where overdosage is suspected, the dose of Calcium Folinate should be equal to or higher than, the offending dose of Methotrexate and should be administered as soon as possible; preferably within the first hour and certainly within 4 hours after which it may not be effective. Other supporting therapy such as blood transfusion and renal dialysis may be required.

**Pharmacological properties**

*Pharmacodynamic properties*

Methotrexate is an antimetabolite which acts principally by competitively inhibiting the enzyme, dihydrofolate reductase. In the process of DNA synthesis and cellular replication, folic acid must be reduced to tetrahydrofolic acid by thisenzyme, and inhibition by Methotrexate interfers with tissue cell reproductions. Actively proliferating tissues such as malignant cells are generally more sensitive to this effect of Methotrexate. It also inhibits antibody synthesis.

Methotrexate also has immunosuppressive activity, in part possibly as a result of inhibition of lymphocyte multiplication. The mechanism(s) of action in the management of rheumatoid arthritis of the drug is not known, although suggested mechanisms have included immunosuppressive and/or anti-inflammatory effect.

*Pharmacokinetic properties*

In doses of 0.1 mg (of Methotrexate) per kg, Methotrexate is completely absorbed from the G.I. tract; larger oral doses may be incompletely absorbed. Peak serum concentrations are achieved with 0.5–2 hours following I.V., I.M. or intra-arterial administration. Serum concentrations following oral administration of Methotrexate may be slightly lower than those following I.V. injection.

Methotrexate is actively transported across cell membranes. The drug is widely distributed into body tissues with highest concentrations in the kidneys, gall bladder, spleen, liver and skin. Methotrexate is retained for several weeks in the kidneys and for months in the liver. Sustained serum concentrations and tissue accumulation may result from repeated daily doses. Methotrexate crosses the placental barrier and is distributed into breast milk. Approximately 50% of the drug in the blood is bound to serum proteins.

In one study, Methotrexate had a serum half-life of 2-4 hours following I.M. administration. Following oral doses of 0.06 mg/kg or more, the drug had a serum half-life of 2-4 hours, but the serum half-life was reported to be increased to 8-10 hours when oral doses of 0.037 mg/kg were given.

Methotrexate does not appear to be appreciably metabolised. The drug is excreted primarily by the kidneys via glomerular filtration and active transport. Small amounts are excreted in the faeces, probably via the bile. Methotrexate has a biphasic excretion pattern. If Methotrexate excretion is impaired accumulation will occur more rapidly in patients with impaired renal function. In addition, simultaneous administration of other weak organic acids such as salicylates may suppress Methotrexate clearance.

**Pharmaceutical particulars**

*List of excipients:*

*2.5 mg/mL presentations*

| *Presentation* | *5 mg/2 mL per unit dose* | *per mL* |
|---|---|---|
| Sodium Chloride BP | 17.2 mg | 8.6 mg |
| Sodium Hydroxide BP | qs | qs |
| Water for Injections BP | to 2.0 mL | to 1.0 mL |

*25 mg/mL presentations*

| *Presentation* | *50 mg/2 mL per unit dose* | *per mL* | *500 mg/20 mL per unit dose* | *per mL* |
|---|---|---|---|---|
| Sodium Chloride BP | 9.8 mg | 4.90 mg | 98 mg | 4.90 mg |
| Sodium Hydroxide BP | qs | qs | qs | qs |
| Water for Injections BP | to 2.0 mL | to 1.0 mL | to 20 mL | to 1.0 mL |

There is a 5% manufacturing overage included in the formulation.

*100 mg/mL presentations*

| *Presentation* | *1 g/10 mL per unit dose* | *per mL* | *5 g/50 mL per unit dose* | *per mL* |
|---|---|---|---|---|
| Sodium Hydroxide BP | qs | qs | qs | qs |
| Water for Injections BP | to 10.0 mL | to 1.0 mL | to 50.0 mL | to 1.0 mL |

*Incompatibilities:* Immediate precipitation or turbidity results when combined with certain concentrations of Droperidol, Heparin Sodium, Metoclopramide Hydrochloride, Ranitidine Hydrochloride in syringe.

*Shelf life:* 24 months.

*Special precautions for storage:* Store below 25°C. Protect from light and freezing.

Unused portions of opened vials or prepared infusions if not used immediately must be stored at 2-8°C for no longer than 24 hours from the time of opening or preparation.

*Instructions for use/handling:* Not applicable.

**Marketing authorisation numbers**

| | |
|---|---|
| 2.5 mg/mL | 4515/0013 |
| 25 mg/mL | 4515/0015 |
| 100 mg/mL | 4515/0038 |

**Date of approval/revision of SPC** June 1994

**Legal category** POM

## METHOTREXATE TABLETS BP

**Qualitative and quantitative composition** *Active constituent:* Methotrexate PhEur 2.5 mg and 10.0 mg. There is no overage included in the formulation.

**Pharmaceutical form** Tablet for oral administration.

**Clinical particulars**

*Therapeutic indications:* Methotrexate is indicated in the treatment of neoplastic disease, such as trophoblastic neoplasms and leukaemia and in the control of severe recalcitrant psoriasis which is not responsive to other forms of therapy.

*Posology and method of administration:*
*Adults and children:*

*Antineoplastic chemotherapy:* Methotrexate is active orally and parenterally. Methotrexate Injection BP may be given by the intramuscular, intravenous, intra-arterial or intrathecal routes. Dosage is related to the patient's body weight or surface area. Methotrexate has been used with beneficial effect in a wide variety of neoplastic *diseases, alone and in combination with other cytotoxic agents.*

*Choriocarcinoma and similar trophoblastic diseases:* Methotrexate is administered orally or intramuscularly in doses of 15-30 mg daily for a 5 day course. Such courses may be repeated for 3-5 times as required, with rest periods of one or more weeks interposed between courses until any manifesting toxic symptoms subside.

The effectiveness of therapy can be evaluated by 24 hours quantitative analysis of urinary chorionic gonadotrophin hormone (HCG). Alternation of Methotrexate, and combination therapy with other cytotoxic drugs, has also been reported as useful.

Hydatidiform mole may precede or be followed by choriocarcinoma, and Methotrexate has been used in similar doses for the treatment of hydatidiform mole and chorioadenoma destruens.

*Breast Carcinoma:* Prolonged cyclic combination with Cyclophosphamide, Methotrexate and Fluorouracil has given good results when used as adjuvant treatment to radical mastectomy in primary breast cancer with positive axillary lymph nodes. Methotrexate dosage was 40 mg/m2 intravenously on the first and eight days.

*Leukaemia:* Acute granulocytic leukaemia is rare in children but common in adults and this form of leukaemia responds poorly to chemotherapy.

Methotrexate is not generally a drug of choice for induction of remission of lymphoblastic leukaemia. Oral Methotrexate dosage of 3.3 mg/m2 daily, and Prednisolone 40-60 mg/m2 daily for 4-6 weeks has been used. After a remission is attained, Methotrexate in a maintenance dosage of 20-30 mg/m2 orally or by I.M. injection has been administered twice weekly. Twice weekly doses appear to be more effective than daily drug administration. Alternatively, 2.5 mg/kg has been administered I.V. every 14 days.

*Meningeal Leukaemia:* Some patients with leukaemia are subject to leukaemic invasions of the central nervous system and the CSF should be examined in all leukaemia patients.

Passage of Methotrexate from blood to the cerebrospinal fluid is minimal and for adequate therapy the drug should be administered intrathecally. Methotrexate may be given in a prophylactic regimen in all cases of lymphocytic leukaemia. Methotrexate is administered by intrathecal injection in doses of 200-500 micrograms/kg body weight. The administration is at intervals of 2 to 5 days and is usually repeated until the cell count of cerebrospinal fluid returns to normal. At this point one additional dose is advised. Alternatively, Methotrexate 12 mg/m2 can be given once weekly for 2 weeks, and then once monthly. Large doses may cause convulsions and untoward side effects may occur as with any intrathecal injection, and are commonly neurological in character.

*Lymphomas:* In Burkitt's Tumour, stages 1-2, Methotrexate has prolonged remissions in some cases. Recommended dosage is 10-25 mg per day orally for 4 to 8 days. In stage 3, Methotrexate is commonly given concomitantly with other antitumour agents. Treatment in all stages usually consists of several courses of the drug interposed with 7 to 10 day rest periods, and in stage 3 they respond to combined drug therapy with Methotrexate given in doses of 0.625 mg to 2.5 mg/kg daily. Hodgkin's Disease responds poorly to Methotrexate and to most types of chemotherapy.

*Mycosis Fungoides:* Therapy with Methotrexate appears to produce clinical remissions in one half of the cases treated. Recommended dosage is usually 2.5 to 10 mg daily by mouth for weeks or months and dosage should be adjusted according to the patient's response and haematological monitoring. Methotrexate has also been given intramuscularly in doses of 50 mg once weekly or 25 mg twice weekly.

Psoriasis Chemotherapy: Cases of severe uncontrolled psoriasis, unresponsive to conventional therapy, have responded to weekly single, oral, I.M. or I.V. doses of 10-25 mg per week, and adjusted according to the patient's response. An initial test dose one week prior to initiation of therapy is recommended to detect any idiosyncrasy. A suggested dose range is 5-10 mg parenterally.

An alternative dosage schedule consists of 2.5 to 5 mg of Methotrexate administered orally at 12 hour intervals for 3 doses each week or at 8-hour intervals for 4 doses each week; weekly dosages should not exceed 30 mg.

A daily oral dosage schedule of 2 to 5 mg administered orally for 5 days followed by a rest period of at least 2 days may also be used. The daily dose should not exceed 6.25 mg.

The patient should be fully informed of the risks involved and the clinician should pay particular attention to the appearance of the liver toxicity by carrying out liver function tests before starting Methotrexate treatment, and repeating these at 2 to 4 month intervals during therapy. The aim of therapy should be to reduce the dose to the lowest possible level with the longest possible rest period. The use of Methotrexate may permit the return to conventional topical therapy which should be encouraged.

*Contra-indications:* Impaired renal or hepatic function.

Pre-existing blood dyscrasias, such as marrow hypoplasia, leukopenia, thromocytopenia or anaemia. Methotrexate is contraindicated in pregnancy.

Methotrexate is contra-indicated in pregnant patients. Because of the potential for serious adverse reactions from methotrexate in breast fed infants, breast feeding is contra-indicated in women taking methotrexate. Patients with a known allergic hypersensitivity to methotrexate should not receive methotrexate.

*Special warnings and special precautions for use:*
*Warnings:* Methotrexate must be used only by physicians experienced in antimetabolic chemotherapy.

Because of the possibility of fatal or severe toxic reactions, the patient should be fully informed by the physician of the risks involved and be under his constant supervision.

Deaths have been reported with the use of Methotrexate in the treatment of psoriasis.

In the treatment of psoriasis, Methotrexate should be restricted to severe recalcitrant, disabling psoriasis which is not adequately responsive to other forms of therapy, but only when the diagnosis has been established as by biopsy and/or after dermatological consultation.

1. Methotrexate may produce marked depression of bone marrow, anaemia, leukopenia, thrombocytopenia and bleeding.

2. Methotrexate may be hepatotoxic, particularly at high dosage or with prolonged therapy. Liver atrophy, necrosis, cirrhosis, fatty changes, and periportal fibrosis have been reported. Since changes may occur without previous signs of gastrointestinal or haematological toxicity, it is imperative that hepatic function be determined prior to initiation of treatment and monitored regularly throughout therapy. Special caution is indicated in the presence of pre-existing liver damage of impaired hepatic function. Concomitant use of other drugs with hepatotoxic potential (including alcohol) should be avoided.

3. Methotrexate has been shown to be teratogenic; it has caused foetal death and/or congenital anomalies. Therefore it is not recommended in women of childbearing potential unless there is appropriate medical evidence that the benefits can be expected to outweigh the considered risks. Pregnant psoriatic patients should not receive Methotrexate.

4. Impaired renal function is usually a contraindication.

5. Diarrhoea and ulcerative stomatitis are frequent toxic effects and require interruption of therapy, otherwise haemorrhagic enteritis and death from intestinal perforation may occur.

6. Methotrexate affects gametogenesis during the period of its administration and may result in decreased fertility which is thought to be reversible on discontinuation of therapy. Conception should be avoided during the period of Methotrexate administration and for at least 6 months thereafter. Patients and their partners should be advised to this effect.

7. Methotrexate has some immunosuppressive activity and immunological responses to concurrent vaccination may be decreased. The immunosuppressive effect of Methotrexate should be taken into account when immune responses of patients are important or essential.

8. Patients with pleural effusions or ascites should have these drained if appropriate before treatment or treatment should be withdrawn.

9. Deaths have been reported with the use of methotrexate. Serious adverse reactions including deaths have been reported with concomitant administration of methotrexate (usually in high doses) along with some non-steroidal anti-inflammatory drugs (NSAIDs).

10. Concomitant administration of folate antagonists such as trimethoprim/sulphamethoxazole has been reported to cause an acute megaloblastic pancytopenia in rare instances.

*Precautions:* Methotrexate has a high potential toxicity, usually dose related, and should be used only by physicians experienced in antimetabolite chemotherapy, in patients under their constant supervision. The physician should be familiar with the various characteristics of the drug and its established clinical usage.

Before beginning methotrexate therapy or reinstituting methotrexate after a rest period, assessment of renal function, liver function and blood elements should be made by history, physical examination and laboratory tests.

It should be noted that intrathecal doses are transported into the cardiovascular system and may give rise to systemic toxicity. Systemic toxicity of methotrexate may also be enhanced in patients with renal dysfunction, ascites, or other effusions due to prolongation of serum half-life.

High doses may cause the precipitation of methotrexate or its metabolites in the renal tubules. A high fluid throughout and alkalinisation of the urine to pH 6.5-7.0 by oral or intravenous administration of sodium bicarbonate (5 x 625 mg tablets every three hours) or acetazolamide (500 mg orally four times a day) is recommended as a preventative measure.

Carcinogenesis, mutagenesis, and impairment of fertility: Animal carcinogencity studies have demonstrated methotrexate to be free of carcinogenic potential. Although methotrexate has been reported to cause chromosomal damage to animal somatic cells and bone marrow cells in humans, these effects are transient and reversible. In patients treated with methotrexate, evidence is insufficient to permit conclusive evaluation of any increased risk of neoplasia.

Methotrexate has been reported to cause impairment of fertility, oligospermia, menstrual dysfunction and amenorrhoea in humans, during and for a short period after cessation of therapy. In addition, methotrexate causes, embryotoxicity, abortion and foetal defects in humans. Therefore the possible risks of effects on reproduction should be discussed with patients of childbearing potential (see 'Warnings').

Patients undergoing therapy should be subject to appropriate supervision so that signs or symptoms of possible toxic effects or adverse reactions may be detected and evaluated with minimal delay. Pretreatment and periodic haematological studies are essential to the use of Methotrexate in chemotherapy because of its common effect of haematopoietic suppression. This may occur abruptly and on apparent safe dosage, and any profound drop in blood cell count indicates immediate stopping of the drug and appropriate therapy. In patients with malignant disease who have pre-existing bone marrow aplasia, leukopenia, thrombocytopenia or anaemia, the drug should be used with caution, if at all.

Methotrexate is excreted primarily by the kidneys. Its use in the presence of impaired renal function may result in accumulation of toxic amounts or even additional renal damage. The patient's renal status should be determined prior to or during Methotrexate therapy and proper caution exercised, should significant renal impairment be disclosed.

Drug dosage should be reduced or discontinued until renal function is improved or restored.

In general, the following laboratory tests are recommended as part of essential clinical evaluation and appropriate monitoring of patients chosen for or receiving Methotrexate therapy: complete haemogram; haematocrit; urinalysis; renal function tests; and liver function tests.

A chest X-ray is also recommended. The purpose is to determine any existing organ dysfunction or system impairment. The tests should be performed prior to therapy, at appropriate periods during therapy and after termination of therapy. It may be useful or important to perform liver biopsy or bone marrow aspiration studies where high dose or long term therapy is being followed.

Methotrexate is bound in part to serum albumin after absorption, and toxicity may be increased because of displacement by certain drugs such as salicylates, sulphonamides, phenytoin, and some antibacterials such as tetracycline, chloramphenicol and para-aminobenzoic acid. These drugs, especially salicylates and sulphonamides, whether antibacterial, hypoglycaemic or diuretic, should not be given concurrently until the significance of these findings is established.

Vitamin preparations containing folic acid or its derivatives may alter response to Methotrexate.

Methotrexate should be used with extreme caution in the presence of infection, peptic ulcer, ulcerative colitis, debility, and in extreme youth and old age. If profound leukopenia occurs during therapy, bacterial infection may occur or become a threat. Cessation of the drug and appropriate antibiotic therapy is usually indicated. In severe bone marrow depression, blood or platelet transfusions may be necessary.

Since it is reported that Methotrexate may have an immunosuppressive action, this factor must be taken into consideration in evaluating the use of the drug where immune responses in a patient may be important or essential.

In all instances where the use of Methotrexate is considered for chemotherapy, the physician must evaluate the need and usefulness of the drug against the risks of toxic effects or adverse reactions. Most such adverse reactions are reversible if detected early. When such effects or reactions do occur, the drug should be reduced in dosage or discontinued and appropriate corrective measures should be taken according to the clinical judgement of the physician. Reinstitution of Methotrexate therapy should be carried out with caution, with adequate consideration of further need for the drug and alertness as to the possible recurrence of toxicity.

*Interaction with other medicaments and other forms of interaction:* Methotrexate is extensively protein bound and may be displaced by certain drugs such as salicylates, hypoglycaemics, diuretics, sulphonamides, diphenylhydantoins, tetracyclines, chloramphenicol and p-aminobenzoic acid, and the acidic anti-inflammatory agents, so causing a potential for increased toxicity when used concurrently. Concomitant use of other drugs with nephrotoxic or hepatotoxic potential (including alcohol) should be avoided. Vitamin preparations containing folic acid or its derivatives may decrease the effectiveness of methotrexate.

Caution should be used when NSAIDs and salicylates are administered concomitantly with methotrexate. These drugs have been reported to reduce the tubular secretion of methotrexate in an animal model and thereby may enhance its toxicity. Renal tubular transport is also diminished by probenecid; use of methotrexate with this drug should be carefully monitored.

Patients using constant dosage regimens of NSAIDs have received concurrent doses of methotrexate problems. Therefore, until more is known about the NSAIDs/methotrexate interaction, it is recommended that methotrexate dosage be carefully controlled during treatment with NSAIDs.

Methotrexate should be used with caution in patients taking drugs known to have an antifolate potential.

*Pregnancy and lactation:* Abortion, foetal death, and/or congenital anomalies have occurred in pregnant women receiving Methotrexate, especially during the first trimester of pregnancy. Methotrexate is contraindicated in the management of psoriasis or rheumatoid arthritis in pregnant women. Women of childbearing potential should not receive Methotrexate until pregnancy is excluded. For the management of psoriasis or rheumatoid arthritis, Methotrexate therapy in women should be started immediately following a menstrual period and appropriate measures should be taken in men or women to avoid conception during and for at least 12 weeks following Methotrexate therapy.

Both men and women receiving Methotrexate should be informed of the potential risk of adverse effects on reproduction. Women of childbearing potential should be fully informed of the potential hazard to the foetus should they become pregnant during Methotrexate therapy. In cancer chemotherapy, Methotrexate should not be used in pregnant women or women of childbearing potential who might become pregnant unless the potential benefits to the mother outweigh the possible risks to the foetus.

Defective oogenesis or spermatogenesis, transient oligospermia, menstrual dysfunction, and infertility have been reported in patients receiving Methotrexate.

Methotrexate is distributed into breast milk. Because of the potential for serious adverse reactions to Methotrexate in nursing infants, a decision should be made whether to discontinue nursing or the drug, taking into account the importance of the drug to the woman.

*Effects on ability to drive and use machines:* Not applicable.

*Undesirable effects:* The most common adverse reactions include ulcerative stomatitis, leukopenia, nausea and abdominal distress. Although very rare, anaphylactic reactions to methotrexate have occurred. Others reported are malaise, undue fatigue, chills and fever, dizziness and decreased resistance to infection. In general, the incidence and severity of side effects are considered to be dose-related. Adverse reactions as reported for the various systems are as follows:

Skin: Erythematous rashes, pruritus, urticaria, photosensitivity, depigmentation, alopecia, ecchymosis, telangiectasia, acne, furunculosis. Lesions of psoriasis may be aggravated by concomitant exposure to ultraviolet radiation. Skin ulceration has been reported in psoriatic patients. The recall phenomenon has been reported in both radiation and solar damaged skin.

Blood: Bone marrow depression, leukopenia, thrombocytopenia, anaemia, hypogammaglobulinaemia, haemorrhage from various sites, septicaemia.

Alimentary System: Gingivitis, pharyngitis, stomatitis, anorexia, vomiting, diarrhoea, haematemesis, melena, gastrointestinal ulceration and bleeding, enteritis, hepatic toxicity resulting in active liver atrophy, necrosis, fatty metamorphosis, periportal fibrosis, or hepatic cirrhosis. In rare cases the effect of methotrexate on the intestinal mucosa has led to malabsorption or toxic megacolon.

Hepatic: Hepatic toxicity resulting in significant elevations of liver enzymes, acute liver atrophy, necrosis, fatty metamorphosis, periportal fibrosis or cirrhosis or death may occur, usually following chronic administration.

Urogenital System: Renal failure, azotaemia, cystitis, haematuria, defective oogenesis or spermatogenesis, transient oligospermia, menstrual dysfunction, infertility, abortion, foetal defects, severe nephropathy. Vaginitis, vaginal ulcers, cystitis, haematuria and nephropathy have also been reported.

Pulmonary System: Infrequently an acute or chronic interstitial pneumonitis, often associated with blood eosinophilia, may occur and deaths have been reported. Acute pulmonary oedema has also been reported after oral and intrathecal use. Pulmonary fibrosis is rare. A syndrome consisting of pleuritic pain and pleural thickening has been reported following high doses.

Central Nervous System: Headaches, drowsiness, blurred vision, aphasia, hemiparesis and convulsions have occurred possibly related to haemorrhage or to complications from intra-arterial catheterization. Convulsion, paresis, Guillain-Barre syndrome and increased cerebrospinal fluid pressure have followed intrathecal administration.

Other reactions related to, or attributed to the use of Methotrexate such as pneumonitis, metabolic changes, precipitation of diabetes, osteoporotic effects, abdominal changes in tissue cells and even sudden death have been reported.

There have been reports of leukoencephalopathy following intravenous methotrexate in high doses, or low doses following cranial-spinal radiation.

Adverse reactions following intrathecal methotrexate are generally classified into three groups, acute, subacute, and chronic. The acute form is a chemical arachnoiditis manifested by headache, back or shoulder pain, nuchal rigidity, and fever. The subacute form may include paresis, usually transient, paraplegia, nerve palsies, and cerebellar dysfunction. The chronic form is a leukoencephalopathy manifested by irritability, confusion, ataxia, spasticity, occasionally convulsions, dementia, somnolence, coma, and rarely, death. There is evidence that the combined use of cranial radiation and intrathecal methotrexate increases the incidence of leukoencephalopathy.

Additional reactions related to or attributed to the use of methotrexate such as osteoporosis, abnormal (usually 'megaloblastic') red cell morphology, precipitation of diabetes, other metabolic changes, and sudden death have been reported.

*Overdose:* Calcium Folinate (Calcium Leucovorin) is a potent agent for neutralizing the immediate toxic effects of Methotrexate on the haematopoietic system. Where large doses or overdoses are given, Calcium Folinate may be administered by intravenous infusion in doses up to 75 mg within 12 hours, followed by 12 mg intramuscularly every 6 hours for 4 doses. Where average doses of Methotrexate appear to have an adverse effect 6-12 mg of Calcium Folinate may be given intramuscularly every 6 hours for 4 doses. In general, where overdosage is suspected, the dose of Calcium Folinate should be equal to or higher than, the offending dose of Methotrexate and should be administered as soon as possible; preferably within the first hour and certainly within 4 hours after which it may not be effective.

Other supporting therapy such as blood transfusion and renal dialysis may be required.

**Pharmacological properties**

*Pharmacodynamic properties:* Methotrexate is an antimetabolite which acts principally by competitively inhibiting the enzyme, dihydrofolate reductase. In the process of DNA synthesis and cellular replication, folic acid must be reduced to tetrahydrofolic acid by this enzyme, and inhibition by Methotrexate interfers with tissue cell reproductions. Actively proliferating tissues such as malignant cells are generally more sensitive to this effect of Methotrexate. It also inhibits antibody synthesis.

Methotrexate also has immunosuppressive activity, in part possibly as a result of inhibition of lymphocyte multiplication. The mechanism(s) of action in the management of rheumatoid arthritis of the drug is not known, although suggested mechanisms have included immunosuppressive and/or anti-inflammatory effect.

*Pharmacokinetic properties:* In doses of 0.1 mg (of Methotrexate) per kg, Methotrexate is completely absorbed from the G.I. tract; larger oral doses may be incompletely absorbed. Peak serum concentrations are achieved with 0.5–2 hours following I.V., I.M. or intra-arterial administration. Serum concentrations following oral administration of Methotrexate may be slightly lower than those following I.V. injection.

Methotrexate is actively transported across cell membranes. The drug is widely distributed into body tissues with highest concentrations in the kidneys, gall bladder, spleen, liver and skin. Methotrexate is retained for several weeks in the kidneys and for months in the liver. Sustained serum concentrations and tissue accumulation may result from repeated daily doses. Methotrexate crosses the placental barrier and is distributed into breast milk. Approximately 50% of the drug in the blood is bound to serum proteins.

In one study, Methotrexate had a serum half-life of 2-4 hours following I.M. administration. Following oral doses of 0.06 mg/kg or more, the drug had a serum half-life of 2-4 hours, but the serum half-life was reported to be increased to 8-10 hours when oral doses of 0.037 mg/kg were given.

Methotrexate does not appear to be appreciably metabolised. The drug is excreted primarily by the kidneys via glomerular filtration and active transport.

Small amounts are excreted in the faeces, probably via the bile. Methotrexate has a biphasic excretion pattern. If Methotrexate excretion is impaired accumulation will occur more rapidly in patients with impaired renal function. In addition, simultaneous administration of other weak organic acids such as salicylates may suppress Methotrexate clearance.

**Pharmaceutical particulars**

*List of excipients:*

| | 2.5 mg tablets | 10 mg tablets |
| --- | --- | --- |
| Maize Starch PhEur | 30.0 mg | 27.6 mg |
| Lactose PhEur | 41.8 mg | 38.5 mg |
| Pre gelatinized Starch (Prejel PA5) USNF | 2.5 mg | 2.5 mg |
| Polysorbate 80 PhEur | 0.2 mg | 0.2 mg |
| Microcrystalline Cellulose (AVICEL 101) USNF | 20.0 mg | 18.2 mg |
| Magnesium Stearate PhEur | 3.0 mg | 3.0 mg |

There is no overage included in the formulation.

*Incompatibilities:* Immediate precipitation or turbidity results when combined with certain concentrations of Droperidol, Heparin Sodium, Metaclopramide Hydrochloride, Ranitidine Hydrochloride in syringe.

*Shelf life:* 60 months.

*Special precautions for storage:* There are no specific storage requirements.

*Instructions for use/handling:* Not applicable.

**Marketing authorisation numbers**
10 mg tabs      4515/0005
2.5 mg tabs     4515/0004

**Date of approval/revision of SPC**   May 1996

**Legal category**   POM

# METHYLENE BLUE INJECTION USP

**Presentation** Methylene Blue Injection USP is presented as a clear, blue coloured sterile solution containing in each 5.0 mL ampoule; Methylene Blue Trihydrate USP 50.0 mg, approximately a 1% solution. The pH of the solution ranges between 3.0 and 4.5.

**Uses** Methylene blue is primarily used in the treatment of drug-induced and genetic methaemoglobinaemia that are not due to a structural abnormality of haemoglobin.

**Dosage and administration** Methylene blue may be administered orally or by intravenous (IV) injection. In the treatment of acute methaemoglobinaemia, the IV route of administration is usually preferred because it provides a more rapid onset of effect. However, in large doses, methylene blue can itself produce methaemoglobinaemia and the methaemoglobin concentration should therefore be closely monitored during treatment. The usual IV dose of methylene blue for adults and children is as a 1% solution in doses of 1 to 2 mg/kg body weight injected over a period of several minutes. A repeat dose may be given after one hour if required.

When treatment is less urgent, and for chronic dosing of genetic methaemoglobinaemias, methylene blue 3-6 mg/kg (generally 300 mg daily in adults) is given orally in divided doses over 24 hours with ascorbic acid 500 mg daily. A suitable dilution for oral dosing would be 5-10 mL of the 1% solution diluted to 100-200 mL with water for injection. The high volume is suggested to reduce the degree of gastrointestinal disturbance and dysuria.

The dosage of methylene blue should be calculated on the basis of lean body weight.

**Contra-indications, warnings, etc**
*Contra-indications:* Use of methylene blue in pregnancy and lactation is contraindicated as its safe use during pregnancy has not yet been established

Methylene blue is contra-indicated in patients with severe renal impairment or a known hypersensitivity to the drug.

Methylene blue should not be used for the treatment of methaemoglobinaemia due to chlorate poisoning as it may convert the chlorate to hypochlorite which is an even more toxic compound.

Methylene blue may cause haemolytic anaemia in patients with glucose-6-phosphate dehydrogenase deficiency.

Intrathecal injection of methylene blue can result in neural damage and is therefore contraindicated.

*Warnings/precautions:* Long-term administration of methylene blue may result in marked anaemia due to accelerated destruction of erythrocytes; haemoglobin concentrations should be checked frequently. If methylene blue is injected subcutaneously or if extravasation occurs, necrotic abscesses may result.

*Use in pregnancy:* Safe use of methylene blue during pregnancy has not been established. Therefore, the drug should be used in pregnant women only if clearly indicated.

Although intra-amniotic injection of methylene blue has been used to diagnose premature rupture of foetal membranes or to identify separate amniotic sacs in twin pregnancies, there have been several reports of haemolytic anaemia and hyperbilirubinaemia in neonates exposed to methylene blue in the amniotic activity.

*Use in lactation:* There is no information on whether or not the drug passes into the breast milk. Consequently, the potential hazard to the infant must be considered prior to administration of the drug to nursing mothers.

*Drug interactions:* No information available.

*Adverse reactions:* After intravenous administration, methylene blue may cause nausea, vomiting, abdominal and chest pain, headache, dizziness, mental confusion, profuse sweating and hypotension; with very high doses methaemoglobinaemia and haemolysis may occur. Infants and patients with glucose-6-phosphate dehydrogenase deficiency are particularly susceptible to haemolysis from treatment with methylene blue.

Oral administration may cause gastrointestinal disturbances (nausea, vomiting and diarrhoea) and dysuria.

High doses, if not adequately diluted, could cause thrombophlebitis. Not more than 350 mg of methylene blue should be diluted in each 500 mL of infusion fluid.

Methylene blue imparts a blue colour to the saliva, urine and faeces.

*Overdosage:* No specific information is available. However, in high concentrations, methylene blue can oxidize haemoglobin to methaemoglobinemia, thus increasing methaemoglobinemia. Nonspecific side effects seen with high doses included precordial pain, dyspnea, restlessness, apprehension, tremors, and a sense of oppression. Large doses are irritant to the urinary tract. In addition, it can produce a mild haemolysis with moderate hyper bilrubinemia, reticulosis and slight anaemia. Rarely, however, a severe haemolytic anaemia with Heinz body formation has resulted. Methylene blue in large doses could cause a blue discolouration to the skin after methaemoglobin levels had returned to normal.

*Treatment of overdosage:* General supportive care and removal of the toxin should be carried out. Depending on the severity of the poisoning and the etiologic agent, this may include removal of contaminated clothing, rinsing the skin with water, ipecac-induced emesis or gastric lavage, charcoal, cathartics, and even haemodialysis.

There is no specific antidotal therapy. Although in severe and refractory cases of methaemoglobinemia, blood transfusions and even exchange transfusions, and (possibly) hyperbaric oxygen therapy maybe the only alternative available. Ascorbic acid works slowly and is probably no benefit in the acute situation. Removal of the toxic compound and supportive therapy are essential.

**Pharmaceutical precautions**

*Incompatibilities:* Methylene blue is reported to be incompatible with caustic alkalis, iodides and dichromates and oxidising and reducing substances.

*Storage:* Methylene Blue Injection USP is to be stored below 25°C and protected from light.

**Legal category** POM

**Package quantities** 1% solution: 5×5 ml ampoules.

**Further information** Nil

**Product licence number** 4515/0079

## METHYLPREDNISOLONE SODIUM SUCCINATE FOR INJECTION

**Qualitative and quantitative composition**

| | | |
|---|---|---|
| Active Constituents | 500 mg | 1 gram |
| Methylprednisolone HSE (as Sodium Succinate) | 500.0 mg | 1.0 gm |
| Prepared in situ from: | | |
| Methylprednisolone Hemisuccinate USP | 633.6 mg | 1.267 gm |
| Other Constituents | | |
| Sodium Hydroxide BP | 53.4 mg | 106.8 mg |
| Disodium Hydrogen Phosphate HSE | 69.8 mg | 139.6 mg |
| Sodium Dihydrogen Phosphate HSE | 6.4 mg | 12.8 mg |
| Sodium Hydroxide BP | QS | QS |
| Hydrochloric Acid BP | QS | QS |
| Water for Injections BP | removed on lyophilisation | removed on lyophilisation |

There is no overage in these formulations.

**Pharmaceutical form** Sterile freeze dried powder for injection.

**Clinical particulars**

*Therapeutic indications:* Parenteral, short term treatment of:

1. Acute anaphylactic and severe allergic reactions such as bronchial asthma, severe seasonal and perennial allergic rhinitis or angioneurotic oedema.
2. Gastrointestinal disease such as Crohns disease or ulcerative colitis.
3. Severe dermatological disease such as erythema multiforme.
4. Aspiration of gastric contents, with appropriate supportive treatment.
5. Tuberculosis, in combination with appropriate anti tubercular chemotherapy, for example TB meningitis or fulminating disseminated tuberculosis.
6. Cerebral oedema secondary to neoplasm.
7. Organ transplant rejection as part of a treatment regimen.

*Posology and method of administration:* Intravenous injection.

Intravenous infusion in the recommended diluents. Injection.

High doses should be administered as an intermittent infusion over at least 30 minutes.

The product should be reconstituted with Water for Injections BP.

The drug may be safely diluted in either Sodium Chloride 0.9% or Dextrose 5% Infusion fluids before administration.

The normal adult dose is 10-500 mg repeated up to 4 hourly. In severe shock, doses of 100 mg-250 mg four hourly may be used or up to 30 mg/kg every four hours have been used for limited periods.

Intramuscular doses are the same as for intravenous administration.

Intravenous infusion of Methylprednisolone Sodium Succinate may be administered by diluting the reconstituted solution in either Dextrose 5%, Sodium Chloride 0.9% or Dextrose 5% in Sodium Chloride 0.9%.

In the treatment of organ transplant rejection and also in autoimmune disorders, intermittent infusion of 1 gram in 100 ml Sodium Chloride 0.9% has been used. This regimen may be given daily or on alternate days, depending on the indication.

In an acute situation or medical crisis, direct intravenous injection should be administered over at least five minutes.

When treating patients with organ transplant rejection, three daily doses of Methylprednisolone Sodium Succinate 1 gram diluted in 100 ml infusion fluid is given over 30 minutes for maximum period of 72 hours.

In the management of autoimmune disorders a number of different regimens have been used including three doses of 1 gram diluted in 100 ml infusion fluid, given on alternate days. This course may be repeated at intervals where necessary.

In anaphylactic reactions, adrenaline or noradrenaline should be administered before methylprednisolone, in order to acheive the required haemodynamic effect.

In allergic reactions, the effect can commence within 1 -2 hours. Status asthmaticus patients are given 40 mg IV repeated as necessary.

Cerebral oedema treated with corticosteroids must have a tapering dosage programme to avoid rebound increases in intracranial pressure. The following are recommended schedules:

| *A:* | *Dose* | *Route* | *Interval* | *Duration* |
|---|---|---|---|---|
| Preoperative | 20 mg | IM | 3-6 hours | |
| During surgery | 20-40mg | IV | hourly | |
| Post operative | 20 mg | IM | 3 hourly | Day 1 |
| | 16 mg | IM | 3 hourly | Day 2 |
| | 12 mg | IM | 3 hourly | Day 3 |
| | 8 mg | IM | 3 hourly | Day 4 |
| | 4 mg | IM | 3 hourly | Day 5 |
| | 4 mg | IM | 6 hourly | Day 6 |
| | 4 mg | IM | 12 hourly | Day 7 |
| *B:* | | | | |
| Preoperative | 40 mg | IM | 6 hourly | 2-3 days |
| Post operative | 40 mg | IM | 6 hourly | 3-5 days |
| | 20 mg | oral | 6 hourly | 24 hours |
| | 12 mg | oral | 6 hourly | 24 hours |
| | 8 mg | oral | 8 hourly | 24 hours |
| | 4 mg | oral | 12hourly | 24 hours |
| | 4 mg | oral | 24 hours | 24 hours |

*Children:* Dosage may be determined by disease state and response but should be not more than 1 gram per day. Normal doses are 30 mg/kg/day for the treatment of haemotological, rheumatic, renal or dermatological conditions. Doses may be repeated either daily or on alternate days, for three days.

10-20 mg/kg/day for organ transplant rejection reactions. Repeated for up to three days, to a maximum of 1 gram per day.

1-4 mg/kg/day for treatment of status asthmaticus, repeated for up; to three days.

N.B. Corticosteroids cause dose-related growth retardation in infancy, childhood and adolescence which may be irreversible (see *Warnings* section).

*Elderly:* There is no indication that dosage adjustment is necessary in elderly patients although the detailed warnings and precautions should be considered when treatment is considered.

*Contra-indications:* Severe infections and septic shock do not appear to respond to Methylprednisolone and this drug should preferably not be used in this situation.

Methylprednisolone is contraindicated when there is hypersensitivity to the drug or its excipients.

Various local or systemic infections are contraindications for use of corticosteroid therapy unless specific anti-infective therapy is employed.

*Special warnings and precautions for use:*

*Warnings:* A patient information leaflet should be supplied with this product.

Short term administration of corticosteroids and short courses of high dose intermittent Methylprednisolone are unlikely to produce harmful effects provided the drug is given at the recommended rate of administration. However if used for longer than 48-72 hours continuously, severe endocrinological and cardiovascular side effects can occur. Secondary adrenocortical insufficiency leading to adrenal atrophy and generalised protein depletion have been reported. Antibiotic therapy should be initiated in patients treated for long periods of time.

Adrenal cortical atrophy develops during prolonged therapy and may persist for years after treatment has ceased. Withdrawal of corticosteroids after prolonged therapy must therefore be gradual to avoid acute adrenal insufficiency, being tapered off over weeks or months according to the dose and duration of treatment, (see *Dosage and Administration* section). During prolonged therapy any intercurrent illness, trauma or surgical procedure will require a temporary increase in dosage, if corticosteroids have been stopped following prolonged therapy they may need to be temporarily re-introduced.

Undesirable effects may be minimised by using the lowest effective dose for the minimum period. Frequent patient review is required to appropriately titrate the dose against disease activity (see *Dosage and Administration* section).

Patients should carry 'steroid treatment' cards which give clear guidance on the precautions to be taken to minimise the risk and which provide details of prescriber, drug, dosage and duration of treatment.

If used to treat adrenal insufficiency a mineralocorticoid drug will also be necessary as Methylprednisolone has only minimal mineralocorticoid action.

Intramuscular injection repeated at the same site may cause subcutaneous atrophy and should be avoided. Deep injection into the gluteal muscle is recommended.

Use in children may cause growth retardation in infancy, childhood and adolescence. Minimise the suppression of hypothalamic-pituitary-adrenal axis by administering the drug as a single dose on alternate days, where possible (see *Dosage* section).

*Use in the elderly:* The common adverse effects of systemic corticosteroids may be associated with more serious consequences in old age, especially osteoporosis, hypertension, hypokalaemia, diabetes, susceptibility to infection and thinning of the skin. Close clinical supervision is required to avoid life-threatening reactions.

High dose intravenous injection must be administered in diluted form and given slowly over at least 30 minutes to avoid the possibility of cardiovascular toxicity. Occasional reports of cardiac arrhythmia, congestive heart failure, circulatory collapse or cardiac arrest have been reported following high doses given over a very short period of time. Monitoring facilities should be available at all times when high dose intravenous therapy is used.

Suppression of the anti-inflammatory response increases the susceptibility to infections and their severity. The clinical presentation may often be atypical and serious infections such as septicaemia and tuberculosis may be masked and may reach an advanced stage before being recognised.

Use in the treatment of tuberculosis should be confined to fulminating disseminated tuberculosis, or TB meningitis. If use in latent disease, a reactivation of the disease may occur. During prolonged treatment these patients should receive chemotherapy prophylactically.

Chickenpox is of particular concern since this normally minor illness may be fatal in immunosuppressed patients. Patients (or parents of children) without a definite history of chickenpox should be advised to avoid close personal contact with chickenpox of herpes zoster and if exposed they should seek urgent medical attention. Passive immunisation with varicella/zoster immunoglobulin (VZIG) is needed by exposed non-immune patients who are receiving systemic corticosteroids or who have had them within the previous 3 months; this should be given within 10 days of exposure of chickenpox. If a diagnosis of chickenpox is confirmed, the illness warrants specialist care and urgent treatement. Corticosteroids should not be stopped and the dose may need to be increased.

Live vaccines should not be given to individuals with impaired immune responsiveness. The antibody response to other vaccines may be diminished.

*Precautions:* Gastric irritation may occur in patients with cerebral oedema induced by trauma, and prophylactic antacids may be advisable.

*Special precautions:* Particular care is required when considering the use of systemic corticosteroids in patients with the following conditions and frequent patient monitoring is necessary.

a. Osteoporosis (post-menopausal females are particularly at risk).
b. Hypertension or congestive heart failure.
c. Existing or previous history of severe affective disorders (especially previous steroid psychosis).
d. Diabetes mellitus (or a family history of diabetes).
e. History of tuberculosis.
f. Glaucoma (or a family history of glaucoma).
g. Previous corticosteroid-induced myopathy.
h. Liver failure.
i. Renal insufficiency.
j. Epilepsy.
k. Peptic ulceration.
l. Myasthenia gravis.
m. Ulcerative colitis, if there is a probability of impending perforation, abscess or other infection.
n. Fresh anastomoses.
o. Diverticulosis.
p. Herpes simplex keratitis.
q. Cushing's syndrome.
r. Cerebral oedema in malaria.

*Interactions with other medicaments and other forms of interaction:* Non steroidal anti-inflammatory drugs may increase the risk of gastrointestinal ulceration.

Vaccinations are not recommended during treatment due to the inhibitory effect on antibody responses.

Concurrent use of non-steroidal anti-inflammatory drugs may increase the risk of gastrointestinal ulceration.

Rifampicin, rifabutin, carbamazepine, phenobarbitone, phenytoin, primidone and aminoglutethimide enhance the metabolism of corticosteroids and its therapeutic effects may be reduced.

The desired effects of hypoglycaemic agents (including insulin), anti-hypertensives and diuretics are antagonised by corticosteroids, and the hypokalaemic effects of acetazolamide, loop diuretics, thiazide diuretics and carbenoxolone are enhanced. Potassium depleting diuretics may enhance the potassium wasting effects of glucocorticoids. Serum potassium levels should be closely monitored during treatment.

The efficacy of coumarin anticoagulants may be enhanced by concurrent corticosteroid therapy and close monitoring of the INR or prothrombin time is required to avoid spontaneous bleeding.

The renal clearance of salicylates is increased by corticosteroids and steroid withdrawal may result in salicylate intoxication.

*Pregnancy and lactation:*

Use in pregnancy: There may be a small risk of cleft palate and intrauterine growth retardation. There is evidence of harmful effects on pregnancy in animals. Hypoadrenalism may also occur in the neonate. When corticosteroids are essential however, patients with normal pregnancies may be treated as though they were in a non-gravid state. Patients with pre-eclampsia or fluid retention require close monitoring.

Use in lactation: Corticosteroids may be distributed into breast milk and could suppress growth or cause adverse effects in nursing infants. Infants or mother taking pharmacological doses of steroids should be monitored carefully for signs of adrenal suppression.

*Effects on ability to drive and use machines:* Not applicable.

*Undesirable effects:*

*Side effects:* The incidence of predictable undesirable effects, including hypothalamic-pituatary-adrenal suppression correlates with the relative potency of the drug, dosage, timing and administration and duration of treatment (see *Warnings* section).

Gastrointestinal: Dyspepsia, peptic ulceration with perforation and haemorrhage. Abdominal distention, oesophageal ulceration or candidiasis, acute pancreatitis, liver failure. Nausea, vomiting and bad taste may occur with repeated administration.

Musculoskeletal: Proximal myopathy, osteoporosis, long bone or vertebral fracture, avascular osteonecrosis, tendon rupture.

Sodium and water retention, hypertension, potassium loss, hypokalaemic alkalosis.

Dermatological: Impaired wound healing, skin atrophy, bruising, striae, telangiectasia, acne.

Endocrine: Suppression of the hypothalamic-pituitary-adrenal axis, growth suppression in infancy, childhood and adolescence, menstrual irregularity and amenorrhoea, Cushinoid face, hirsutism, weight gain, diabetes mellitus, a family history of diabetes or impaired carbohydrate tolerance with increased requirement for antidiabetic therapy, negative protein and calcium balance and increased appetite.

Neuropsychiatric: Existing or previous history of severe affective disorders, euphoria, psychological dependence, depression, insomnia, intracranial hypertension with papilloema in children (pseudotumour cerebri), usually after treatment, withdrawal, aggravation of schizophrenia and epilepsy.

Ophthalmic: Increased intraocular pressure, glaucoma or family history of glaucoma, papiolloedema, posterior subcapsular cataracts, corneal or scleral thinning, exacerbation of opthalmic viral or fungal disease.

Anti-inflammatory and Immunosuppresive effects: Increased susceptibility and severity of infections with suppression of clinical symptoms and signs, opportunistic infections, recurrence of dormant tuberculosis (see *Warnings* and *Precautions*).

General: Hypersensitivity including anaphylaxis, has been reported. Leucocytosis, thromboembolism.

Withdrawal symptoms and signs: Too rapid a reduction of corticosteroid dosage following prolonged treatment can lead to acute adrenal insufficiency, hypotension and death. (See Warnings and Precautions).

A 'withdrawal syndrome' may also occur including, fever, myalgia, arthralgia, rhinitis, conjunctivitis, painful itchy skin nodules and loss of weight.

*Overdose:* Adrenal suppression may occur and appropriate measures should be taken during the withdrawal period. There is no known antidote to Methylprednisolone sodium succinate.

**Pharmacological properties**

*Pharmacodynamic properties:* A potent anti-inflammatory corticosteriod with predominantly glucocorticoid activity.

Methylprednisolone Sodium Succinate is primarily used in the acute treatment of shock, as part of post transplant rejection regimens, in severe rheumatoid arthritis, collagen vascular disease and in severe anaphylaxis or allergic reactions.

Methylprednisolone may cause profound metabolic effects and modify the body's immune response. Use of the parenteral form should therefore be confined to short term treatment.

Methylprednisolone stabilises leucocyte lysosomal membranes, preventing release of destructive acid hydrolases, inhibiting macrophage accumulation, reducing leucocyte adhesion, reducing capilliary wall permeability and antagonising histamine activity.

The immune system is suppressed by reducing the activity and volume of the lymphatic system, decreasing immunoglobulin and complement and decreasing the passage of immune complexes through membranes.

*Pharmacokinetic properties:* Methylprednisolone is rapidly removed from the plasma and widely distributed. The drug is extensively bound to plasma proteins. The drug may also cross the placenta and be distributed into milk.

Metabolism is primarily by reduction in the liver to biologically inactive compounds and subsequent excretion through the kidney.

*Preclinical safety data:* There are no pre-clinical data of relevance to the prescriber which are additional to that already included in other sections of the SPC.

**Pharmaceutical particulars**

*List of excipients:*

| | *500 mg* | *1 gram* |
|---|---|---|
| Disodium Hydrogen Phosphate HSE | 69.8 mg | 139.6 mg |
| Sodium Dihydrogen Phosphate HSE | 6.4 mg | 12.8 mg |
| Sodium Hydroxide BP | QS | QS |
| Hydrochloric Acid BP | QS | QS |
| Water for Injections BP | removed on lyophilisation | removed on lyophilisation |

There is no overage in these formulations.

*Incompatibilities:* Infusion solutions of methylprednisolone sodium succinate in the recommended diluents are stable for 24 hours at room temperature exposed to light. Only clear solutions should be used and any solutions developing a haze after preparation should be discarded. Methylprednisolone has approximately five times the glucocorticoid potency of hydrocortisone. Each gram of Methylprednisolone Sodium Succinate contains 2 mmol of Sodium.

*Shelf life:* 24 months.

*Special precautions for storage:* Methylprednisolone sodium succinate for Injection should be stored below 25°C and protected from light. Do not freeze, reconstituted solutions using the recommended diluent should be stored at 2-8°C and used within 24 hours of preparation.

*Instruction for use/handling:* Not applicable.

**Marketing authorisation number** 4515/0042

**Date of approval/revision of SPC** July 1995

**Legal category** POM

## MITOMYCIN FOR INJECTION

**Qualitative and quantitative composition**

| | | |
|---|---|---|
| Active Constituent | 10 mg/vial | 20 mg/vial |
| Mitomycin USP | 10.0 mg | 20.0 mg |

**Pharmaceutical form** Mitomycin for Injection is a sterile, lyophilised product intended for intravenous administration upon reconstitution with Water for Injections.

**Clinical particulars**

*Therapeutic indications:* Antimitotic and Cytotoxic: Mitomycin for Injection is recommended for certain types of cancer, either in combination with other drugs or after primary therapy has failed. In particular, Mitomycin for Injection has been successfully used to improve subjective and objective symptoms in a wide range of neoplastic conditions:

It has been used as a single agent in the treatment of superficial bladder cancer. In addition it has been shown that post-operative instillations of Mitomycin for Injection can reduce recurrence rates in newly diagnosed patients with superficial bladder cancer.

As a single agent and in combination with other drugs in metastatic breast cancer.

In combination with other agents in advanced squamous cell carcinoma of the uterine cervix.

It shows a degree of activity as part of combination therapy in carcinoma of the stomach, pancreas and lung (particularly non-small cell).

It shows a degree of activity as a single agent and in combination in liver cancer when given by the intra-arterial route.

It has a possible role in combination with other cytotoxic drugs in colorectal cancer.

It shows a degree of activity as a single agent or part of combination therapy in cancer of the head and neck.

It shows a degree of activity as a single agent in cancer of the prostate.

It has a possible role in skin cancer.

It has a degree of activity in leukaemia and non solid tumours.

It has a possible role in sarcomas.

It has been successfully used in combination with surgery, preoperatively (oesophageal, squamous cell carcinoma) and post-operatively (gastric cancer).

It has been shown to be effective when used in combination with radiotherapy.

*Posology and method of administration:* Reconstitution and Administration: Mitomycin for Injection is administered via a functioning I.V. catheter, ***care should be taken to avoid extravasation of the drug,*** and it is recommended that the reconstituted solution be administered through the tubing of an I.V. infusion. (If extravasation occurs, cellulitis, ulceration, and tissue sloughing may result).

Mitomycin for Injection is reconstituted by adding 10 or 20 mL of sterile water for injection to a vial labelled as containing 10 or 20 mg of mitomycin respectively, to provide a solution containing approximately 1 mg/ml. The vial should be shaken to enhance dissolution; if the powder for injection does not dissolve immediately, allow to stand at room temperature until complete dissolution occurs.

Dosage: For systemic administration, Mitomycin for Injection should be given intravenously using great care to avoid extravasation. The usual initial dosage is in the range 10-20 mg per m² body-surface given as a single dose through a running intravenous infusion and repeated every 6-8 weeks. Alternatively it may be given intravenously in divided doses of 2 mg per m² daily for 5 days, repeated after 2 days. Subsequent doses are adjusted according to the effect on bone marrow and treatment should not be repeated until leucocyte count is above 3000/mm³, and the platelet count above at least 75,000/mm³.

Dosage of Mitomycin subsequent to the initial dose maybe adjusted according to the following suggested schedule:

| Nadir after prior dose (cells/mm³) | | Percentage of prior dose to be given |
|---|---|---|
| Leucocytes | Platelets | |
| >4000 | >100,000 | 100% |
| 3000-3999 | 75,000-99,999 | 100% |
| 2000-2999 | 25,000-74,999 | 70% |
| <2000 | <25,000 | Nil |

Dosage may be reduced when used in combination with other antineoplastics. However, when disease continues to progress after 2 courses of Mitomycin therapy, the drug should be discontinued since the likelihood of response is minimal.

For administration to specific tissues, Mitomycin for Injection can be given by the intra-arterial route in the treatment of liver tumours.

Because of cumulative myelosuppression and/or thrombocytopenia patients should be fully re-evaluated after each course of Mitomycin for Injection and the dose reduced if the patient has experienced any toxic effects. Doses greater than 20 mg/m² increase the risk of toxicity and have not been shown to be more effective than lower doses.

Treatment of superficial urinary bladder tumours: In the prevention of recurrent bladder tumours the usual dose is the equivalent of 4-10 mg potency of Mitomycin for Injection instilled into the bladder through a urethral catheter once or three times a week. In the treatment of bladder tumours, the usual dose is the equivalent of 10-40 mg potency of Mitomycin for Injection instilled into the bladder either weekly or three times a week for a total of 20 doses. In either case, it should be dissolved in 10 ml–40 ml of water for injections before use. The dose should be adjusted in accordance with the age and condition of the patient.

*Contra-indications:* Mitomycin is contra-indicated in patients with platelet counts of less than 75,000/mm³, white cell counts of less than 2,500/mm³ or ⁸ serum creatinine concentration greater than 1.7 mg/dL.

Mitomycin is contraindicated in patients who have substantial prolongation of prothrombin time or bleed time, coagulation disorders, increased bleeding due to other causes, or potentially serious infections.

Mitomycin is contraindicated in patients who have demonstrated a hypersensitive or idiosyncratic reaction to it in the past.

*Special warnings and special precautions for use:* Mitomycin for Injection should not be administered orally, intrathecally, into tissues (such as intramuscularly or subcutaneously). Mitomycin is a highly toxic drug with a low therapeutic index. The drug should be used only under the supervision of a physician experienced in cytotoxic cancer chemotherapy. Patients should be monitored closely during each course of treatment, paying particular attention to peripheral blood count including platelet count.

The principal toxicity of Mitomycin for Injection is bone marrow suppression, particularly thrombocytopenia and leucopenia. The nadir is usually around four weeks after treatment and toxicity is cumulative, with increasing risk after each course of treatment.

No repeat dosage should be given until the bone marrow nadir has passed. If disease progression continues after two courses of treatment, the drug should be stopped since the chances of response are then minimal.

Severe renal toxicity has occasionally been reported after treatment and renal function should be monitored before starting treatment and again after each course. The incidence of this is reduced considerably if the total cumulative dose does not exceed 120 mg; this may of course temporize the therapeutic response. Nausea and vomiting are sometimes experienced immediately after treatment but these are usually mild and of short duration. Local ulceration and cellulitis may be caused by tissue extravasation during intravenous injection and utmost care should be taken in administration. In the event of extravasation following an intravenous injection of Mitomycin for Injection, it is recommended that 5 ml of Sodium Bicarbonate 8.4% solution is immediately infiltrated into the area where extravasation has occurred followed by an injection of 4 mg of Dexamethasone. In addition, a systemic injection of 200 mg Vitamin B6 may be of some value in promoting the regrowth of tissues that have been damaged.

The person administering the injection of Mitomycin for Injection should not allow the solution to come into contact with his or her skin.

Treatment of skin or eye contact: Any Mitomycin for Injection substance or solution in contact with the skin should be washed several times with 8.4% sodium bicarbonate solution, followed by washing with soap and water. Use of handcreams or other emollient preparations is inappropriate as this may assist the penetration of any traces of Mitomycin for Injection into the epidermal tissue.

Contact with the eye: The eye should be rinsed several times with sodium bicarbonate eye lotion and the eye examined for several days after contact for evidence of corneal damage. If this occurs, appropriate treatment should be instituted.

*Interaction with other medicaments and other forms of interaction:*
*Potentially hazardous interactions::* As free radical generation is noted with this drug, there may be some synergistic cardiotoxicity with adriamycin. The possible enhancement of lung damage by nitrosoureas and doxorubicin has been reported.

Microsomal enzyme inducers such as barbiturates or liver enzyme inhibitors such as cimetidine may alter activity by an effect on host and tumour metabolism.

*Potentially useful interactions:* Mitomycin may show synergy with 5-Fluorouracil.

Mitomycin may enhance cell kill induced by radiation therapy, particularly under hypoxic conditions.

*Pregnancy and lactation:* Mitomycin for Injection should not normally be administered to patients who are pregnant or to mothers who are breast feeding. Teratological changes have been noted in animal studies. The effect of Mitomycin for Injection on fertility is unknown.

*Effects on ability to drive and use machines:* None known.

*Undesirable effects:*
*Adverse reactions: Potentially life-threatening effects:* A microangiopathic haemolytic anaemia (renal failure syndrome with anaemia, thrombocytopenia, haematuria, proteinuria. hypertension and neurological abnormalities) has been reported and is frequently fatal. It usually occurs after 6 months treatment, but has been reported earlier. In small series where renal histopathology has been studied, fibrin deposition in the glomeruli has been noted, but the precise mechanism is not known. Hepatic veno-occlusive disease has been reported in one high-dose study.
*Severe or irreversible adverse effects:* The dose-limiting toxicity is myelosuppression, which may be delayed with a nadir at 4-8 weeks. The effect is cumulative and affects both leucocytes and platelets. Diffuse pulmonary infiltration has also been recorded and exposure to oxygen in high concentration may be contributory. This side effect is thought to be related to generation of free radicals following activation of the drug.
*Symptomatic adverse effects:* Nausea and vomiting of moderate severity are seen in about 25% of patients and alopecia, stomatitis and diarrhoea are also observed. Local tissue necrosis is observed if the solution is extravasated from a vein or artery.

*Overdose:* No specific antidote for mitomycin is known. Management of overdose should include general supportive measures to sustain the patient through any period of oxicity that might occur.

## Pharmacological properties

*Pharmacodynamic properties:* Mitomycin for Injection is an antitumour antibiotic that is activated in the tissues to an alkylating agent which disrupts deoxyribonucleic acid (DNA) in cancer cells by forming a complex with DNA and also acts by inhibiting division of cancer cells by interfering with the biosynthesis of DNA. In high concentrations, the drug may also inhibit RNA and protein synthesis.

*Pharmacokinetic properties: In vivo,* Mitomycin for Injection is rapidly cleared from the serum after intravenous administration. The time required to reduce the serum concentration by 50% after a 30 mg bolus injection is 17 minutes. After injection of 30 mg, 20 mg, or 10 mg intravenously, the maximal serum concentrations were 2.4 mcg/ml, 1.7 mcg/ml and 0.52 mcg/ml respectively. Clearance is effected primarily by metabolism in the liver but metabolism occurs in other tissues as well. The rate of clearance is inversely proportional to the maximal serum concentration because, it is thought, of saturation of the degradative pathways. Approximately 10% of a dose of Mitomycin for Injection is excreted unchanged in the urine. Since metabolic pathways are saturated at relatively low doses, the percentage dose excreted in the urine increases with increasing dose. In children, excretion of intravenously administered Mitomycin for Injection is similar to that in adults.

In animals, highest mitomycin concentration are found in the kidneys followed by muscles, eyes, lungs, intestines and stomach. The drug is not detectable in the liver, spleen or brain which rapidly inactivate mitomycin. Higher concentrations of the drug are generally present in cancer tissues than in normal tissues.

## Pharmaceutical particulars

*List of excipients:*

| | per 10mg vial | per 20mg vial | per mL | Function | Reference to Standards |
|---|---|---|---|---|---|
| Mannitol | 20mg | 40mg | 2.0mg | Bulking agent | BP |
| Water for Injections* | qs 10ml | qs 20ml | qs 1.00ml | Solvent* | BP/USP |

*Removed during the lyophilisation process.

*Incompatibilities:* Concentrations of Mitomycin for Injection of 10 mg and 50 mg/L in sodium chloride 0.9% resulted in a 20% and 54% loss respectively in bleomycin activity when added to a 20-30 units/L solution of bleomycin.

*Shelf life:*
(1) 3 years shelf life in the medicinal product as packaged for sale.
(2) The reconstituted product should be used immediately and any unused portion discarded.

*Special precautions for storage:* Unreconstituted Mitomycin for Injection remains stable for three years from the date of manufacture when stored below 25°C. Reconstitution, as directed, should be accomplished using aseptic technique and the resulting solutions should be used immediately. Any unused portion should be discarded. When reconstituted solution is added to infusion fluids, especially where these contain dextrose, the resulting solution should be used immediately, and any unused portion discarded.

*Instructions for use/handling:* There is limited but increasing concern that personnel involved in preparation and administration of parenteral antineoplastics may be at some risk because of the potential mutagenicity, teratogenicity, and/or carcinogenicity of these agents, although the actual risk is unknown. Cautious handling both in preparation and disposal of antineoplastic agents is recommended.

Precautions that have been suggested include:
Use of a biological containment cabinet during reconstitution and dilution of parenteral medications and wearing of disposable surgical gloves and masks.

Use of proper technique to prevent contamination of the medication, work area, and operator during transfer between containers (including proper training of personnel in this technique).

Cautious and proper disposal of needles, syringes, vials, ampoules and unused medication.

## Marketing authorisation numbers
Mitomycin for Injection 10 mg Vial          4515/0093
Mitomycin for Injection 20 mg Vial          4515/0094

**Date of approval/revision of SPC**  26 June 1996

**Legal category**  POM

# NALOXONE HYDROCHLORIDE INJECTION

## Qualitative and quantitative composition
*Active Constituents*
Naloxone Hydrochloride USP          400 mcg
*Other Constituents*
Sodium Chloride BP          9.0 mg
Water for Injections BP to          1.0 mL

There is no overage in this formulation.

**Pharmaceutical form** Aqueous solution for injection.

## Clinical particulars

*Therapeutic indications:*

1. Treatment of respiratory depression induced by synthetic and natural opiates.
2. Treatment of respiratory depression induced by partial opiate agonists.
3. Diagnosis of suspected acute opiate overdosage.

*Posology and method of administration:* Intravenous, intramuscular and subcutaneous injection.
*Adults:* Overdosage of narcotics–known or suspected: 400-2000 micrograms intravenously repeated at 2-3 minute intervals up to 10 mg. Dosage is similar if intramuscular or subcutaneous routes are used.
Postoperative Respiratory Depression: 100-200 micrograms intravenously at 2-3 minute intervals, to the required degree of reversal.
*Children:* This presentation of Naloxone is not recommended for use in children.
*Elderly:* No dosage adjustment is necessary for use in elderly patients.
Naloxone Hydrochloride is compatible with either Sodium Chloride 0.9% Infusion BP or Dextrose 5% Infusion BP for a period of 24 hours when stored at room temperature in fluorescent light.

*Contra-indications:* Naloxone is contra-indicated in patients with known hypersensitivity to the drug.

*Special warnings and precautions for use:* Naloxone should be given with caution to patients known or suspected to be physically dependent on opiates (including neonates born to women who are opiate dependent), because the drug may precipitate severe withdrawal symptoms.

Patients who have satisfactorily responded to naloxone should be carefully monitored since the duration of action of some opiates may exceed that of naloxone. Repeated doses of naloxone should be administered when necessary.

Naloxone is not effective against respiratory depression not due to opioid drugs.

When naloxone is used in the management of acute opioid overdosage, other resuscitative measures such as maintenance of a free airway, artificial ventilation, cardiac massage and vasopressor agents should be readily available and used when necessary.

Naloxone should be used with caution in patients with pre-existing cardi-vascular disease or in those receiving potentially cardiotoxic drugs, since serious adverse cardiovascular effects (e.g. ventricular tachycardia and fibrillation) have occurred in postoperative patients following naloxone administration.

Excessive dosage of naloxone following the use of opiates in surgery should be avoided because it may result in excitement, increased blood pressure and clinically important reversal of analgesia. Too rapid reversal of opiate effects may induce nausea, vomiting, sweating or tachycardia.

*Interactions with other medicaments and other forms of interaction* Not known.

*Pregnancy and lactation:* Reproduction studies in mice and rats using naloxone hydrochloride in doses up to 1000 times the usual human dosage revealed no evidence of impaired fertility or harm to the foetus. There are no adequate and controlled studies to date in pregnant women. Naloxone should be administered to pregnant patients only when, in the judgement of the physician, the potential benefits outweigh the possible hazards.

It is not known whether naloxone is excreted in human milk. Therefore, naloxone should be used with caution in nursing women.

*Effects on ability to drive and use machines:* Not applicable.

*Undesirable effects:* Abrupt reversal of narcotic depression has been reported to result in nausea, vomiting, sweating, tachycardia, tremor and hyperventilation. In postoperative patients excessive dosage of naloxone may result in excitement, increased blood pressure and significant reversal of analgesia.

Hypertension, pulmonary oedema, atrial and ventricular arrhythmias and cardiac-arrest have been reported in certain patients, particularly those with pre-existing cardiac abnormalities.

Seizures have occurred rarely following administration of naloxone, however, a causal relationship has not been established.

*Overdose:* No documented reports of acute overdosage are available.

**Pharmacological properties**

*Pharmacodynamic properties:* Naloxone hydrochloride is essentially a pure opiate antagonist, it has little or no agonistic activity. Naloxone is thought to act as a competitive antagonist at μ-, k- and σ- opioid receptors in the CNS. Small doses (0.4 mg to 0.8 mg) of naloxone given intramuscularly or intravenously prevent or promptly reverse the effects of opioids. In patients with respiratory depression, there is an increase in respiratory rate within 1 or 2 minutes. Sedative effects are reversed and blood pressure, if depressed, returns to normal. Naloxone also reverses the psychotomimetic and dysphoric effects of agonist-antagonists such as pentazocine, but higher doses (10-15 mg) are required. One milligram of naloxone intravenously completely blocks the effects of 25 mg of diacetylmorphine.

When administered in usual doses to patients who have not recently received opiates, naloxone exerts little or no pharmacological effect. Even extremely high doses (10 times the usual therapeutic dose) produce insignificant analgesia, only slight drowsiness, and no respiratory depression, psychotomimetic effects, circulatory changes, or miosis.

Naloxone does not produce tolerance or physical or psychological dependence.

Parenteral administration (S.C., I.M. or I.V.) of naloxone will produce withdrawal symptoms in patients physically dependent on opiates or pentazocine.

*Pharmacokinetic properties:* Naloxone has an onset of action within 1-2 minutes following I.V. administration and within 2-5 minutes following subcutaneous or intramuscular administration. The duration of action depends on the dose and route of administration and is more prolonged following I.M. administration than after I.V. administration. Duration of action is reported up to several hours but practical duration probably 1 hour or less.

Following parenteral administration, naloxone is rapidly distributed into body tissues and fluids. It is rapidly metabolised in the liver, principally by conjugation with glucuronic acid, and is excreted in the urine. The plasma half-life of naloxone has been reported to be 60-90 minutes in adults and about 3 hours in neonates.

*Preclinical safety data:* There are no pre-clinical data of relevance to the prescriber which are additional to that already included in other sections of the SPC.

**Pharmaceutical particulars**

*List of excipients:*

| | |
|---|---|
| Sodium Chloride BP | 9.0 mg |
| Water for Injections BP | to 1.0 mL |

There is no overage in this formulation.

*Incompatibilities:* None known.

*Shelf life:* 24 months.

*Special precautions for storage:* Store below 25°C. Protect from light.

*Instruction for use/handling:* Not applicable.

**Marketing authorisation number** 4515/0052

**Date of approval/revision of SPC** 12 March 1996

**Legal category** POM

## PANCURONIUM BROMIDE INJECTION BP

**Qualitative and quantitative composition** *Active constituent:* Pancuronium Bromide BP 2 mg per mL. There is no overage in this formulation.

**Pharmaceutical form** Aqueous solution for injection.

**Clinical particulars**

*Therapeutic indications:* The active substance of Pancuronium Bromide is an amino steroid which effectively blocks transmission of motor nerve impulses to the striated muscle receptors. It is a non-depolarising neuromuscular blocking agent with a medium duration of action and is used in the following indications:

1. As an adjuvant in surgical anaesthesia to obtain relaxation of skeletal muscles in a wide range of surgical procedures.
2. Use in intensive care as a non-depolarising neuromuscular blocker for the treatment of various pathologies eg intractable status asthmaticus and tetanus.

*Posology and method of administration:* Pancuronium should be administered intravenously.

It is not recommended to be given by infusion.

The dosage should be individualised as there is a wide variation in individual response to muscle relaxants. When determining the dose, the method of anaesthesia, expected duration of surgery, potential interaction with other drugs that are administered before and during anaesthesia and the condition of the patient should be taken into account.

The use of a peripheral nerve stimulator is recommended for monitoring the neuromuscular block and recovery.

*Adult:* Initial dosage range 80-100 micrograms/kg body weight depending on the surgical procedure and for intubation. Incremental doses10-20 micrograms/kg.

For endotracheal intubation when Pancuronium is given in the dosage range of 80-100 microgram/kg conditions satisfactory for intubation are usually present within 1-2 minutes.

*Paediatric:* 60-80 micrograms/kg initially I/V by increments increased by increments of 10-20 micrograms/kg thereafter.

*Neonates:* Doses of Pancuronium in neonates up to one month of age must be carefully individualised since neonates are particularly sensitive to non-depolarising neuromuscular blocking agents.

Dosage 30-40 micrograms/kg initially I/V followed by 10-20 micrograms/kg thereafter.

*Elderly:* The neuromuscular blocing activity of Pancuronium is prolonged in the elderly and lower doses may be necessary.

*Obesity:* In heavy obese patients doses of Pancuronium based on a mg/kg basis may lead to overdosage. Dosage must be adjusted according to response.

*Intensive care:* Pancuronium is longer acting in the intensive care patient, and an intravenous dose of 60 micrograms/kg every one to one and a half hours, or even less frequently is usually adequate.

*Impaired liver and renal function:* Care must be exercised in patients with impaired liver or renal function as mentioned in the special warnings and precautions section.

Hyperdiuresis may result in a decreased neuromuscular blocking effect.

In the control of tetanus, duration of Pancuronium relaxation probably depends upon the severity of the spasm, therefore duration of effect can be variable.

The duration of action depends upon the clinical condition of the patient and the dose administered, but in normal subjects receiving perioperative muscle relaxant doses the duration of action is usually 45-60 minutes.

Pancuronium should not be mixed with other agents in the same syringe, or with solutions for intravenous infusions as a change in pH may cause precipitation.

Discard any unused solution.

*Contra-indications:* Patients with a known hypersensitivity to Pancuronium or the Bromide ion Concurrent use of a depolarising neuromuscular blocking agent eg Suxamethonium.

*Special warnings and precautions for use:*
*Renal failure:* As Pancuronium Bromide is excreted mainly in the renal system, the elimination half-life is prolonged in renal failure, resulting in a reduction in plasma clearance and prolonged duration of action.

*Impaired hepatic/biliary tract disease:* The duration of action may be prolonged in these conditions and resistance to neuromuscular blocking action of Pancuronium Bromide may occur because of the increased volume of distribution of the drug.

In such conditions, the drug has a slower onset and coupled with the increased total dosage requirements, there may be a prolongation of blockade and recovering time in these patients.

As with other non-depolarising muscle relaxants Pancuronium should be used with care in patients with pre-existing pulmonary, hepatic or renal disease and with particular care in patients with muscular dystrophies, myasthenia gravis and myasthenic syndrome unless it is intended to administer prolonged post-operative respiratory assistance. Before administration of Pancuronium conditions such as electrolyte disturbance, altered pH, and dehydration should be corrected if possible. Pancuronium should be used cautiously in patients with a tendancy to hypertension.

Pancuronium can cause a reduction in the partial prothromboplastin time and prothrombin time. Conditions associated with slower circulation times eg cardiovascular disease, oedema, old age result in an increased volume of distribution which may lead to an increased onset time.

Pancuronium should be used with particular care in neo-nates, in ill or cachetic patients, in the presence of liver disease or obstructive jaundice (resistant to the effects of drugs) in states with altered plasma protein levels or when there is diminished renal blood flow or renal disease. In operations employing the hypothermic techniques the neuromuscular blocking effect of non-depolarising drugs is decreased and increased by warming the patient.

Pancuronium should be administered in carefully adjusted dosage or under the supervision of a qualified anaesthetist and only when facilities for controlled ventilation, insufflation with oxygen and endotracheal intubation are available for immediate use.

*Interactions with other medicaments and other forms of interaction:*

1. Suxamethonium. Used prior to Pancuronium (for endotracheal intubation) enhances the relaxation effect of the Pancuronium and the duration of action. Therefore administration of Pancuronium should be delayed until Suxamethonium shows signs of wearing off.
2. Anaesthetics. The following anaesthetics may potentiate the neuromuscular blocking activity of Pancuronium, Halothane, Ether, Enflurane, Isoflurane, Methoxyflurane, Cyclopropane, Thiopentone, Methohexitone.
3. The following drugs may influence the duration of action of Pancuronium and the intensity of neuromuscular block.

Potentiation: Other muscle relaxants, antibiotics of the polypeptide and aminoglycoside groups, diazepam, propranolol, thiamine (high dose), MAO inhibiting agents, quinidine, magnesium sulphate, protamine, nitroglycerin, narcotic analgesics, diuretics, phenytoin, alpha adrenergic blocking agents, imidazoles, metronidazole, noradrenaline and adrenaline.

Decreased effect: Neostigmine, edrophonium, corticosteriods (high dose), adrenaline, potassium chloride, calcium chloride, sodium chloride, heparin (temporary decrease), azathioprine, theophylline, pyridostigmine.

Pancuronium should be given with caution to patients receiving chronic tricyclic antidepressant therapy who are anaesthetised with Halothane or any inhalation anaesthetic since this enhances the predisposition to the development of cardiac arrythmias associated with tricyclic antidepressants.

*Pregnancy and lactation:* The use of Pancuronium in pregnant or breast feeding women with respect to safety has not been established. Therefore the drug should only be administered to pregnant women when the attending physician decides that the potential benefits outweigh the risks.

Pancuronium may be used for caesarian section but the reversal of Pancuronium may be unsatisfactory in patients receiving Magnesium sulphate for toxaemia of pregnancy because magnesium salts enhance neuromuscular blockade.

*Effects on ability to drive and use machines:* Not applicable.

*Undesirable effects:* High doses of a depolarising drug may cause end-plate desensitisation and prolong post-operative apnoea.

Cardiovascular: Increased pulse rate and cardiac output. Blood pressure may rise. Arrhythmias may occur occasionally.

Gastrointestinal: Salivation is sometimes noted during anaesthesia.

Hypersensitivity: Occasional transient rash has been noted.

Injection Site Reactions: Pain or local skin reactions noted at the site of injection.

Respiratory: Bronchospasm has rarely been reported. Patients with carcinomatosis especially associated with bronchial carcinoma may exhibit a marked sensitivity to this agent, and the neuromuscular block produced may respond poorly to Neostigmine.

Serious or life threatening reactions: Severe anaphylactoid reactions have been reported uncommonly.

*Overdose:* Clinical features: The symptoms are those of prolonged apnoea, respiratory depression and/or muscle weakness. Death may follow acute respiratory failure.

Management: Neostigmine at a dose of 2.5 mg and Atropine at a dose of 1.2 mg can be administered to reverse the neuromuscular block whilst ventilation is continued. When administration of the cholinesterase inhibiting agent fails to reverse the neuromuscular blocking effects of Pancuronium ventilation must continue until spontaneous breathing is restored.

**Pharmacological properties**

*Pharmacodynamic properties:* Pancuronium bromide produces pharmacologic effects similar to those other non-depolarising neuromuscular blocking agents. The drug may produce an increase in heart rate which appears to result from a direct blocking effect on the acetylcholine receptors of the heart. The increase in heart rate appears to be dose related and is minimal with usual doses. Pancuronium causes little or no histamine release and no ganglionic blockade and therefore does not cause hypotension or bronchospasm. Despite its steroidal structure, the drug exhibits no hormonal activity.

*Pharmacokinetic properties:* Following I/V administration of Pancuronium Bromide 0.06 mg/kg, muscle relaxation reaches a level suitable for endotracheal intubation within 2-3 minutes, slightly more rapidly than with tubocurarine. The onset and duration of paralysis are dose related. After a dose of 0.06 mg/kg, the effects of the drug begin to subside in about 35-45 minutes. Supplemental doses may increase the magnitude and duration of the neuromuscular blockade. The duration of action depends upon the clinical condition of the patient and the dose administered, but in normal subjects receiving perioperative muscle relaxant doses the duration of action is usually 45-60 minutes.

Protein binding of Pancuronium does not appear to be substantial. The activity of the drug is not greatly affected by plasma carbon dioxide concentrations or pH. Redistribution is responsible for the termination of activity following single doses. Pancuronium crosses the placenta in small amounts.

Plasma concentrations appear to decline in a triphasic manner. In adults with normal renal and hepatic function, the half-life in the terminal phase is about 2 hours. The elimination half-life may be prolonged in patients with impaired renal and/or hepatic function. The drug is eliminated mainly unchanged by the kidneys, although small amounts may be metabolised and some of the drug may be eliminated in the bile.

*Preclinical safety data:* There are no pre-clinical data of relevance to the prescriber which are additional to that already included in other sections of the SPC.

**Pharmaceutical particulars**

*List of excipients*

| | |
|---|---|
| Sodium Chloride BP | 8.0 mg |
| Sodium Acetate BP | 2.0 mg |
| Acetic Acid 6N BP | Q.S. |
| Sodium Hydroxide 1N BP | Q.S. |
| Nitrogen BP | Q.S. |
| Water for Injections BP | to 1.0 ml |

There is no overage in this formulation.

*Incompatibilities:* Do not mix other solutions in the same syringe as a change in pH can cause precipitation.

Pancuronium should be stored at 2-8˚C.

*Shelf life:* 24 months.

*Special precautions for storage:* Store between 2-8˚C. Protect from light. Do not freeze.

*Instruction for use/handling:* Not applicable.

**Marketing authorisation number**    4515/0062

**Date of approval/revision of SPC**    June 1997

**Legal category**    POM

# PHENYTOIN INJECTION BP

**Qualitative and quantitative composition** Phenytoin Sodium BP 250 mg in 5 mL

**Pharmaceutical form** Sterile Solution for Injection

**Clinical particulars**

*Therapeutic indications:* Control of status epilepticus and the prevention of seizures occurring during or following neurosurgery. Treatment of certain cardiac dysrhythmias, particularly those unresponsive to conventional antidysrhythmic agents or to cardioversion.

*Posology and method of administration:* Phenytoin Injection BP solution is suitable for use as long as it remains free of haziness and precipitate. A precipitate might form if the product has been kept in a refrigerator or freezer. This precipitate will dissolve if allowed to stand at room temperature. The product will then be suitable for use.

Phenytoin Injection BP should be injected slowly and directly into a large vein through a large-gauge needle or intravenous catheter. It must be administered slowly. Intravenous administration should not exceed 50 mg/minute in adults. In neonates the drug should be administered at a rate not exceeding 1 to 3 mg/kg/min. Each injection should be followed by an injection of 0.9% sodium chloride through the same needle or catheter to avoid local venous irritation due to the alkalinity of the solution.

For infusion administration the parenteral phenytoin should be diluted in 50–100 ml of normal saline, with the final concentration of phenytoin in the solution not exceeding 10 mg/ml. Administration should commence immediately after the mixture has been prepared and must be completed within one hour (the infusion mixture should not be refrigerated). An in-line filter (0.22–0.50 microns) should be used. The diluted form is suitable for use as long as it remains free of haziness and precipitate.

Continuous monitoring of the electrocardiogram and blood pressure is essential. Cardiac resuscitative equipment should be available. The patient should be observed for signs of respiratory depression. If administration of intravenous Phenytoin Injection does not terminate seizures, the use of other measures, including general anaesthesia, should be considered.

For the control of status epilepticus, 150 to 250 mg should be given by slow intravenous injection at a rate not exceeding 50 mg/minute to avoid hypotension. This dose can be repeated if necessary after 30 minutes. A previously untreated adult may require 10-15 mg/kg. The loading dose is then followed by a maintenance dose of 100 mg given orally or intravenously every 6-8h. In geriatric patients with heart disease, it has been recommended that the drug be given at a rate of 50 mg over 2-3 minutes. Dosage for children is usually determined according to weight. Paediatric dosage may also be calculated on the basis of 250 mg/m² of body surface area or 15-20 mg/kg administered in 2 or 3 equally divided doses. Subsequent dosage should be adjusted carefully and slowly according to the patients requirements. Maintenance dosage for children usually ranges from 4-8 mg/kg daily.

Determination of phenytoin serum levels is advised when using Phenytoin Injection BP in the management of status epilepticus and in the subsequent establishing of maintenance dosage. The clinically effective level is usually 10-20 mg/l although some cases of tonic-clonic seizures may be controlled with lower serum levels of phenytoin.

In a patient who has not previously received the drug, Phenytoin Injection, 100 mg-200 mg (2-4 ml), maybe given intramuscularly at approximately 4 hourly intervals prophylactically during neurosurgery and continued during the postoperative period for 48-72 hours. The dosage should then be reduced to a maintenance dose of 300 mg and adjusted according to serum level estimations.

When given by intramuscular injection, phenytoin precipitates out at the injection site and is absorbed slowly and erratically. This route is not, therefore, recommended for treating status epilepticus. If phenytoin is administered by intramuscular injection to patients unable to take the drug orally, the dose should be increased by 50% over the previously

established oral dose. To avoid drug accumulation resulting from eventual absorption from intramuscular injection sites, it is recommended that for the first week back on oral therapy the dose is reduced to one-half the original dose. Monitoring of serum concentrations is also recommended. Intramuscular therapy should generally be limited to I week.

Phenytoin sodium can be useful in ventricular arrhythmias, particularly those due to digitalis. The recommended dosage is one intravenous injection of Phenytoin Injection BP of 3 to 5 mg/kg bodyweight initially, repeating if necessary.

*Contra-indications:* In patients with a known hypersensitivity to phenytoin or other hydantoins.

In patients with sinus bradycardia, sino-atrial block, second and third degree AV block or Adams-Stokes syndrome.

Intra-arterial administration must be avoided in view of the high pH of the preparation.

*Special warnings and special precautions for use:* Warnings: This drug must be administered slowly, at a rate not exceeding 50 mg/minute in adults. In neonates, the drug should be administered at a rate not exceeding 1-3 mg/kg/min. The response to phenytoin may be significantly altered by the concomitant use of other drugs (see Interactions with other Drugs).

Rapid administration may result in hypotension. In patients with cardiovascular disease, parenteral administration may result in atrial and ventricular conduction depression, ventricular fibrillation or reduced cardiac output. Severe complications are most commonly encountered in elderly or gravely ill patients. In these patients, the drug should be administered at a rate not exceeding 25 mg/minute, and if necessary, at a slow rate of 5 to 10 mg/minute.

Serum levels of phenytoin sustained above the optimal range may produce encephalopathy, or confusional states (delirium psychosis), or rarely irreversible cerebellar dysfunction. Plasma level determinations are recommended at the first signs of acute toxicity. If plasma levels are excessive, then dosage reduction is indicated. Termination is recommended if symptoms persist.

Abrupt withdrawal of phenytoin in epileptic patients may precipitate status epilepticus. When it is necessary to reduce the dose of phenytoin, this should be done gradually. In hypersensitivity reactions, where rapid substitution of therapy is warranted, the alternative drug should be one not belonging to the hydantoin class of compounds.

Subcutaneous or perivascular injection should be avoided because of the highly alkaline nature of the solution. Such injection may cause irritation of the tissues varying from slight tenderness to extensive necrosis, sloughing and in rare instances has led to amputation.

The intramuscular route is not recommended for the treatment of status epilepticus because of slow absorption. Serum levels of phenytoin in the therapeutic range cannot be rapidly achieved by this method.

Precautions: The liver is the principal site of biotransformation of phenytoin; patients with impaired liver function, elderly patients, or those who are gravely ill may show early signs of toxicity.

Patients with renal function impairment should also be carefully observed when prescribing phenytoin, as excretion and protein binding may be altered.

A small percentage of individuals who have been treated with phenytoin have been shown to metabolize the drug slowly. Slow metabolism appears to be due to limited enzyme availability and lack of induction, which may be genetically determined.

Phenytoin should be used with caution in diabetic patients as hyperglycaemia may be potentiated.

Measurement of serum phenytoin levels is recommended when using phenytoin in the management of status epilepticus and in establishing a maintenance dose. The usually accepted therapeutic level is 10-20 mg/L, although some patients with tonic-clonic seizures can be controlled with lower serum levels.

Phenytoin is not effective for petit mal seizures. Therefore, combined therapy is required if both grand mal and petit mal seizures are present.

*Interaction with other medicaments and other forms of interaction:* Drugs which may increase serum levels of phenytoin include: chloramphenicol, coumarin anticoagulants, disulfiram, phenylbutazone, isoniazid, salicylates, chlordiazepoxide, phenothiazines, diazepam, oestrogens, ethosuximide, sulthiame, halothane, methylphenidate, trimethadione, mephenytoin, sulphonamides, cimetidine, trazodone, ranitidine, fluconazole, ketoconazole, miconazole.

Drugs which may decrease serum levels of phenytoin include: carbamazepine, reserpine, bleomycin, carboplatin, carmustine, cisplatin, methotrexate, vinblastine, folic acid, calcium folinate, rifampicin.

Drugs which may either increase or decrease serum levels of phenytoin and vice versa include: barbiturates, valproic acid and sodium valproate, primidone.

Acute alcoholic intake may increase serum levels of phenytoin while chronic alcoholic use may decrease them.

Tricyclic antidepressants, haloperidol, monoamine oxidase inhibitors and thioxanthenes may precipitate seizures in susceptible patients and phenytoin dosage may need to be adjusted.

Phenytoin impairs the efficacy of several drugs, including:

anticonvulsants, corticosteroids, coumarin anticoagulants, cyclosporine, dacarbazine, vitamin D, digoxin, disopyramide, doxycycline, frusemide, L-dopa, mexiletine, oestrogens, oral contraceptives, quinidine, succinimide and xanthines.

Caution is advised when nifedipine or verapamil are used concurrently with phenytoin. All are highly protein bound medications and therefore changes in serum concentrations of the free, unbound medications may occur.

Phenytoin may increase serum glucose levels and therefore dosage adjustments for Insulin or oral antidiabetic agents may be necessary.

Concurrent use of phenytoin and oral diazoxide may decrease the efficacy of phenytoin and the hyperglycaemic effect of diazoxide and is not recommended.

Use of intravenous phenytoin in patients maintained on dopamine may produce sudden hypotension and bradycardia. This appears to be dose-dependent. If anticonvulsant therapy is necessary during administration of dopamine, an alternative to phenytoin should be considered.

Concurrent use of intravenous phenytoin with lignocaine or beta-blockers may produce additive cardiac depressant effects. Phenytoin may also increase the metabolism of lignocaine.

*Pregnancy and lactation:*

Use in pregnancy: Adverse effects on the foetus of status epilepticus, specifically hypoxia, make it imperative to control the condition. However, Phenytoin readily crosses the placenta about 10% of exposed fetuses have been noted to show minor craniofacial and digital abnormalities–the so-called fetal hydrantoin syndrome. Common features include broad lower nasal bridge, epicanthic folds, hypertelorism, malformed ears, wide mouth and hypoplasia of the distal phalanges and nails. A few of these babies have microencephaly and are retarded. Facial clefts and congenital heart disease are also seen more commonly than might be expected. Overall, however, the risk of having an abnormal child as a result of medication is far outweighed by the dangers to the mother and foetus of uncontrolled epilepsy.

The adverse effects on the foetus of status epilepticus, specifically hypoxia, make it imperative to control the condition in the shortest possible time.

The pharmacokinetics of phenytoin are altered in pregnancy. A fall in plasma albumin together with more efficient hepatic metabolism act to a reduce total and unbound plasma phenytoin concentrations. Neonatal coagulation defects have been reported within the first 24 hours in babies born to epileptic mothers receiving phenytoin. Vitamin K has been shown to prevent or correct this defect and may be given to the mother before delivery and to the neonate after birth.

Use in lactation: Phenytoin concentrations in breast milk are 20 to 25% of simultaneous maternal plasma levels. If maternal plasma levels are within the therapeutic range, and considering the daily volume of milk taken by the infant, it is unlikely that the infant will be exposed to clinically significant phenytoin concentrations. Breast feeding is not, therefore, contraindicated.

*Effects on ability to drive and use machines:* Phenytoin in appropriate doses may as such impair driving skills but epilepsy itself dictates the practice of driving. Patients affected by drowsiness should not drive or operate machinery.

*Undesirable effects:* The most notable signs of toxicity are cardiovascular collapse and/or depression of the central nervous system. Hypotension can occur when the drug is administered rapidly by intravenous injection. Toxicity should be minimised by following the appropriate directions (see *Dosage and Administration*).

Cardiovascular: Severe cardiotoxic reactions and fatalities have been reported, most commonly in gravely ill patients or the elderly (see *Warnings*).

Central Nervous System: There are the most common reactions encountered with phenytoin and include nystagmus, ataxia, slurred speech, decreased coordination and mental confusion. Cases of dizziness, insomnia, transient nervousness, motor twitchings and headaches have also been reported. These side effects are usually dose related.

There have also been rare reports of phenytoin induced dyskinesias, including chorea, dystonia, tremor and asterixis, similar to those induced by phenothiazine and other neuroleptic drugs. These may be due to sudden intravenous administration for status epilepticus. The effect usually lasts 24-48h after discontinuation.

A predominantly sensory peripheral polyneuropathy has been reported for patients on long-term phenytoin therapy.

Gastrointestinal: Nausea, vomiting and constipation.

Dermatological: A measle-like rash is the most common dermatological manifestation. Rashes are sometimes accompanied by fever, and are generally more common in children and young adults. Other types of rashes are more rare, and more serious forms which may be fatal include bullous, exfoliative or purpuric dermatitis, lupus erythematosus, Stevens-Johnson syndrome and toxic epidermal necrolysis. Phenytoin should be discontinued if a skin rash appears. If the rash is exfoliative, purpuric, or bullous or if lupus erythematosus, Stevens-Johnson syndrome or toxic epidermal necrolysis is suspected, phenytoin should not be resumed. If the rash is mild (measles-like or scarlatiniform), therapy may be resumed when the rash has completely disappeared. However, in the case of the rash recurring upon reinstitution of therapy, further phenytoin medication is contraindicated.

Haemopoietic: Some fatal haemopoietic complications have occasionally been reported in association with the use of phenytoin. These have included thrombocytopenia, leukopaenia, granulocytopaenia, agranulocytosis, and pancytopaenia with or without bone marrow suppression. Although macrocytosis and megaloblastic anaemia have occurred, these conditions usually respond to folic acid therapy. There have been a number of reports suggesting a relationship between phenytoin and the development of local or generalised lymphadenopathy, including benign lymph node hyperplasia, lymphoma, pseudolymphoma and Hodgkin's Disease. Although a cause and effect relationship has not been established, the occurrence of lymphadenopathy indicates the need to differentiate such a condition from other types of lymph node pathology. Lymph node involvement may occur with or without symptoms resembling serum sickness e.g. rash, fever and liver involvement. In all cases of lymphadenopathy, seizure control should be sought using alternative antiepileptic drugs and observation of patients for an extended period is recommended.

Injection Site: Local irritation, inflammation and tenderness. Necrosis and sloughing have been reported after subcutaneous or perivascular injection. Subcutaneous or perivascular injection should be avoided. Soft tissue irritation and inflammation have occurred at the site of injection with or without extravasation of intravenous phenytoin.

Others: Gingival hyperplasia is common with long-term therapy. Its incidence may be reduced by maintaining good oral hygiene such as frequent brushing, gum massage and appropriate dental care.

Coarsening of the facial features, enlargement of the lips, hypertrichosis, Peyronies Disease, systemic lupus erythematosus, periarteritis nodosa, toxic hepatitis, liver damage, and immunoglobulin abnormalities may occur.

Rare reports of pulmonary infiltrates or fibrosis, with symptoms including fever, troubled or quick, shallow breathing, unusual tiredness or weakness, loss of appetite and weight and chest discomfort, have also occurred.

*Overdose:*

Symptoms: The lethal dose in adults is considered to be 2 to 5 grams. The lethal dose in children is not known. The initial symptoms are nystagmus, ataxia, and dysarthria. Other signs are tremor, hyperflexia, lethargy, slurred speech, nausea and vomiting. The patient may become comatose and hypotensive. Death is due to respiratory and circulatory depression.

Treatment: Treatment is nonspecific since there is no known antidote. (If ingestion has taken place, the stomach should be emptied). If the gag reflex is absent, the airway should be supported. Oxygen and assisted ventilation may be necessary for central nervous system, respiratory and cardiovascular depression. Haemodialysis can be considered since phenytoin is not completely bound to plasma proteins. Total exchange transfusion has been utilised in the treatment of severe intoxication in children.

**Pharmacological properties**

*Pharmacodynamic properties:* Phenytoin sodium inhibits the spread of seizure activity in the motor cortex. It appears that by promoting sodium efflux from neurons, phenytoin sodium tends to stabilise the threshold against hyperexcitability caused by environmental changes or excessive stimulation capable of reducing membrane sodium gradient. This includes the reduction of post tetanic potentiation of synapses. Loss of post tetanic potentiation prevents cortical seizure foci from detonating adjacent cortical areas. Phenytoin thereby reduces the over-activity of brain stem centres responsible for the tonic phase of grand mal seizures.

Phenytoin sodium antiarrhythmic action may be attributed to the normalization of influx of sodium and calcium to cardiac Purkinje fibres. Abnormal ventricular automaticity and membrane responsiveness are decreased. It also shortens the refractory period, and therefore shortens the QT interval and the duration of the action potential.

Hydantoins induce production of liver microsomal enzymes, thereby accelerating the metabolism of concomitantly administered drugs.

*Pharmacokinetic properties:* The onset of action after an intravenous dose is 30 to 60 minutes and the effect persists up to 24 hours. Phenytoin is about 90% protein bound. Protein binding may be lower in neonates and hyperbilirubinemic infants; also altered in patients with hypoalbuminaemia, uraemia or acute trauma, and in pregnancy. Optimum control without clinical signs of toxicity occurs most often with serum levels between 10 and 20μg/mL. In renal failure or hypoalbuminaemia, 5 to 12μg/mL or even less may be therapeutic.

Phenytoin is metabolised in the liver, the major inactive metabolite is 5-(p-hydroxyphenyl)-5-phenylhydantoin (HPPH). The rate of metabolism is increased in younger children, pregnant women, in women during menses and in patients with acute trauma. The rate decreases with advancing age. Phenytoin may be metabolised slowly in a small number of individuals due to genetic factors, which may cause limited enzyme availability and lack of induction.

The plasma half-life is normally from 10 to 15 hours. Because phenytoin exhibits saturable or dose-dependent pharmacokinetics, the apparent half-life of phenytoin changes with dose and serum concentration. At therapeutic concentrations of the drug, the enzyme system responsible for metabolising phenytoin becomes saturated. Thus a constant amount of drug is metabolised, and small increases in dose may cause disproportionately large increases in serum concentrations and apparent half-life, possibly causing unexpected toxicity.

**Pharmaceutical particulars**

*List of excipients*

| | |
|---|---|
| Propylene Glycol BP | 2.0 ml |
| Absolute Alcohol BP | 0.5 ml |
| Water for Injection BP | to 5.0 ml |

*Incompatibilities:* Incompatible with amikacin sulphate, cephapirin sodium clindamycin phosphate, and many other drugs. It is recommended that phenytoin sodium not be mixed with other drugs or with any infusion solution other than sodium chloride 0.9%.

*Shelf life:* 24 months.

*Special precautions for storage:* Phenytoin Injection BP should be stored below 25°C and protected from light. The product should be visually inspected for particulate matter and discolouration prior to administration.

*Instructions for use/handling:* See under *Posology and Method of Administration.*

**Marketing authorisation number** 4515/0083

**Date of approval/revision of SPC** May 1996

**Legal category** POM

## SODIUM NITROPRUSSIDE FOR INJECTION BP 50MG

**Qualitative and quantitative composition** Active constituent: Sodium Nitroprusside Dihydrate BP 50.0 mg. There is no overage included in the formulation.

**Pharmaceutical form** Lyophilised powder for reconstitution with Glucose Injection BP

**Clinical particulars**

*Therapeutic indications:* Sodium Nitroprusside is indicated for the immediate reduction of blood pressure in patients in hypertensive crises.

The drug is effective in the management of hypertensive emergencies, irrespective of aetiology, and may be useful when other drugs have failed.

Sodium nitroprusside may also be used to produce controlled hypotension during anaesthesia in order to reduce bleeding in surgical procedures when surgeon and anaesthetist deem it appropriate.

Nitroprusside has also been used in the treatment of heart failure and other cardiac disorders where it is necessary to quickly reduce left ventricular outflow (afterload) and lower raised ventricular pressure (preload).

*Posology and method of administration:* Sodium Nitroprusside is to be administered only by intravenous infusion using a controlled infusion device, infusion pump, drip regulator, micro-drip regulator or similar device that will allow precise measurements of flow rate. Care should be taken to avoid extravasation.

Reconstitution of Sodium Nitroprusside for Injection BP to produce the Intravenous Infusion

Reconstitution can only be carried out using Glucose Injection BP A concentrated solution of sodium nitroprusside may be prepared by dissolving 50 mg of the drug in 2-3 ml of glucose Injection BP The concentrated solution should be further diluted in 250, 500, or 1000 ml of Glucose Injection BP to provide solutions containing 200, 100 or 50 micrograms per ml respectively. Nitroprusside solutions should be protected from light by promptly wrapping the containers in aluminium foil or other opaque material. Both the concentrated solution and the infusion solution should be freshly prepared and any unused portion discarded after 24 hours. The freshly prepared infusion solution has a very faint brownish tint; if it is highly coloured it should be discarded.

Administration should be carried out at all times under close supervision. No other drug should be added to the infusion fluid for simultaneous administration with sodium nitroprusside and in hypotensive patients receiving concomitant antihypertensive medication, smaller doses of sodium nitroprusside might be required.

It is recommended that the blood pressure should not be allowed to drop rapidly and that systolic pressure should not be lowered below 60 mmHg. This can be achieved by increasing the dose slowly which should also prevent any physiological compensatory reactions resulting from the release of catecholamines and renins into the blood, which would lead to tachycardia.

The rate of administration should be adjusted to maintain the desired hypotensive effect, as determined by continous blood pressure monitoring.

In order to avoid excessive levels of cyanide and thiocyanate and lessen the possibility of a precipitous drop in blood pressure, infusion rates greater than 10 micrograms per kilogram per minute should not be used. If, at this rate, an adequate reduction of blood pressure is not obtained within 10 minutes, the administration of sodium nitroprusside should be stopped.

The intravenous infusion should not be stopped suddenly as this might lead to an excessive rebound rise in blood pressure, but rather over a period of 15 to 30 minutes. In hypertensive emergencies sodium nitroprusside infusion may be continued until an alternative oral therapy can be safely introduced.

Intravenous infusion of sodium nitroprusside may be continued for several days but care must be taken to ensure that the blood cyanide concentration does not exceed 100 micrograms per 100 ml and that the serum cyanide concentration does not exceed 8 micrograms per 100 ml. If infusion is carried out for a period in excess of three days then the blood thiocyanate concentration should be checked and not exceed 100 micrograms per ml.

*Dosage in adults:*

Hypertensive crisis: Dosage varies considerably between patients, hence the need for individual titration. In adults not receiving other hypotensive agents, the average dosage of sodium nitroprusside is 3 micrograms per kilogram per minute.The initial dose is normally within the range of 0.5-1.5 micrograms per kilogram per minute, but can then be adjusted in a stepwise fashion, e.g. in increments of 0.5 micrograms per kilogram per minute every 5 minutes, to fall between 0.5–8 micrograms per kilogram per minute.To maintain the blood pressure at 30 to 40 % lower than the pretreatment diastolic blood pressure levels an average of 200 micrograms/minute (range of 20 to 400 micrograms/minute) is usually sufficient. In hypertensive patients receiving concomitant antihypertensive medication, smaller doses might be required.

Heart failure: The initial dose should be between 10-15 micrograms per minute increased every 5-10 minutes in increments of 10 to 15 micrograms per minute as necessary to the normal range of 10-200 microgram per minute to obtain the desired response.In some patients the additive effects of a vasodilator and a potent inotropic agent may be used to advantage. If a vasodilator is used haemodynamic monitoring should be used to guide its administration.If during treatment signs of hypotension, hypoperfusion or any other adverse effects are observed the infusion rate should be reduced or administration stopped.The infusion may be continued until an alternative oral therapy can be safely introduced. The infusion therapy should not normally exceed 3 days.

In controlled hypotension during general anaesthesia: For the induction of hypotension during anaesthesia a maximum dose of 1.5 microgram per kilogram bodyweight per minute is recommended. The intrinsic hypotensive effect of many anaesthetic agents must be remembered and all normal procedures for hypotensive techniques should be carried out.

Geriatric Patients: Commence therapy with low doses since geriatric patients appear to be more sensitive to the hypotensive effects of the drug. Therefore the drug should be administered with caution in this age group.

Children: Dosage recommendations have not been established.

*Contra-indications:*

1. Treatment of compensatory hypertension, e.g. arteriovenous shunt or coarctation of the aorta.
2. Inadequate cerebral circulation
3. Cyanide and thiocyanate are metabolites of nitroprusside and may interfere with the metabolism of cyanocobalamin. Nitroprusside is therefore contraindicated in patients suffering from severe vitamin B12 deficiency, hepatic failure and Leber's optic atrophy.

*Special warnings and special precautions for use:*
*Precautions:* Thiocyanate may accumulate in the blood of patients receiving sodium nitroprusside therapy, especially those with impaired renal function or hyponatraemia. Since thiocyanate inhibits both uptake and binding of iodine, symptoms of hypothyroidism may occur.

Sodium nitroprusside should be administered only when adequate facilities are available to frequently monitor blood pressure, since the hypotensive effect is rapid. When I.V. infusion of sodium nitroprusside is decreased or discontinued, blood pressure usually begins to increase immediately and returns to pretreatment levels within 1-10 minutes.

Because sodium nitroprusside may interfere with vitamin B12 distribution and metabolism, the drug should be used with caution in patients with low plasma vitamin B12 concentrations.

The drug should be used with extreme caution if the patient is hypothermic.

*Interaction with other medicaments and other forms of interaction:* e hypotensive effects of Sodium Nitroprusside are additive when used concomitantly with ganglionic blocking agents, general anaesthetics (e.g. halothane, enflurane), and with most other circulatory depressants.

*Pregnancy and lactation:*
Use in pegnancy: Adequate reproduction studies have not been performed with sodium nitroprusside, and its its use in pregnancy or women of child bearing potential requires that the potential benefits be weighed against possible hazards to the mother and child or foetus.

Use in lctation: It is not known if sodium nitroprusside is distributed into milk, therefore the drug should be used with caution in nursing mothers.

*Effects on ability to drive and use machines:* Not applicable.

*Undesirable effects:* Nausea, retching, diaphoresis, apprehension, headache, restlessness, muscle twitching, retrosternal discomfort, palpitations, drowsiness, dizziness, paraesthesial warmth and abdominal pain have been noted when the reduction in blood pressure is too rapid, but these symptoms quickly disappear when the rate of infusion is decreased or the infusion is temporarily discontinued and do not reappear with continued slower rate of administration.

Tachycardia and postural hypotension have also been reported. Irritation and reddening of the skin may occur at the injection site.

*Overdose:* Overdosage will result in a fall in blood pressure below the desired level. Discontinuation of administration or a reduction in the rate of administration are usually sufficient measures for managing an overdose of sodium nitroprusside.

Infusion rates exceeding 10 micrograms per kilogram per minute may result in cyanide intoxication. This is best managed by the intravenous injection of sodium nitrate in conjunction with sodium thiosulphate.

**Pharmacological properties**

*Pharmacodynamic properties:* When Sodium Nitroprusside is administered by IV infusion to hypertensive or normotensive patients, a marked lowering of arterial blood pressure is produced. Venous pressure is also lowered and a moderate reduction in total peripheral resistance occurs. The effects of the drug on blood pressure are more pronounced in hypertensive than in normotensive patients.

The hypotensive action of Sodium Nitroprusside results from peripheral vasodilation caused by a direct action on vascular smooth muscle. Animal tests performed in situ have demonstrated no relaxation of other smooth muscle tissue, such as the uterus or duodenum, by Sodium Nitroprusside. The drug has no direct effect on vasomotor centres, sympathetic nerves, or adrenergic receptors. The hypotensive effect of Sodium Nitroprusside is augmented by concomitant use of other hypotensive agents and is not blocked by adrenergic blocking agents or vagotomy. Pressor agents such as epinephrine which

stimulate the myocardium directly are the only drugs that cause an increase in blood pressure during Sodium Nitroprusside therapy. Resistance to the drug's hypotensive effects and tachyphylaxis are very rare.

The effects of Sodium Nitroprusside on cardiac performance appear to depend on preexisting performance. Changes in cardiac performance are attributed mainly to a reduction in left ventricular afterload resulting from vasodilation but may also be related to reduction in venous return to the heart resulting from peripheral vascular pooling of blood, decreased arteriolar resistance, and increased diastolic compliance. The drug has no direct effect on the myocardium, but it may exert a direct coronary vasodilator effect. When Sodium Nitroprusside is administered to hypertensive patients, a slight increase in heart rate usually occurs and cardiac output is usually decreased slightly. Decreases in cardiac index and stroke index are common; however, these decreases do not occur consistently and increases have occurred in some patients. When Sodium Nitroprusside is administered to patients with refractory heart failure and/or acute myocardial infarction, substantial improvement in left ventricular performance results with cardiac output, cardiac index, and stroke volume being increased and left ventricular filling pressure being decreased. In patients with congestive heart failure, a slight but clinically important slowing of the heart rate results, as well as reduction or cessation of arrhythmias.

A reduction in myocardial oxygen consumption during Sodium Nitroprusside use has been noted which could prove beneficial when infarcted areas of the heart are already short of oxygen. In patients with congestive heart failure, improvement in cardiac performance is accompanied by prompt diuresis, with urine volume and sodium excretion both being increased.

Moderate doses of Sodium Nitroprusside in hypertensive patients produce renal vasodilation without an appreciable increase in renal blood flow or a decrease in glomerular filtration. Mean renal arterial pressure and renal vascular resistance are slightly decreased. The acute reduction in mean arterial pressure is accompanied by an increase in renin activity of renal venous plasma.

*Pharmacokinetic properties:*
Absorption: IV infusion of Sodium Nitroprusside produces an almost immediate reduction in blood pressure. Blood pressure begins to rise immediately when the infusion is slowed or stopped and returns to pretreatment levels within 1-10 minutes.

Distribution: Distribution of Nitroprusside in the body as well as passage across the placenta into milk, or across the blood-brain barrier has not been studied.

Elimination: Sodium Nitroprusside is rapidly metabolised, probably by interaction with sulphhydryl groups in the erythrocytes and tissues. Cyanogen (cyanide radical) is produced which is converted to thiocyanate in the liver by the enzyme rhodanase. A thiocyanate oxidase present in the erythrocytes may oxidise small quantities of thiocyanate back to cyanogen. Toxic symptoms begin to appear at plasma thiocyanate concentrations of 50-100µg/ml; fatalities have been reported at concentrations of 200µg/ml.

Sodium Nitroprusside is excreted entirely as metabolites, principally thiocyanate. In animals, Sodium Nitroprusside metabolites are excreted mainly in urine, exhaled air, and probably in faeces. The elimination half-life of thiocyanate is 2.7-7 days when renal function is normal but is longer in patients with impaired renal function or hyponatraemia.

**Pharmaceutical particulars**

*List of excipients:* Not applicable. There is no overage included in the formulation.

*Incompatibilities:* Nitroprusside forms highly coloured reaction products with a wide variety of therapeutic agents, and admixture should be avoided.

*Shelf life:* 36 months.

*Special precautions for storage:* Sodium nitroprusside vials and infusion solution should be protected from light; heat and moisture. Reconstituted intravenous infusion should be protected from light by covering with aluminium foil or other opaque material as quickly as possible.

Sodium Nitroprusside when reconstituted should be discarded after 24 hours. If the reconstituted solution is highly coloured, the solution should be discarded.

No preparation other than Glucose Injection BP should be added to the sodium nitroprusside vial or mixed with the infusion solution.

*Instructions for use/handling:* Not applicable.

**Marketing authoristion number** 4515/0016

**Date of approval/revision of SPC** 31 January 1997

**Legal category** POM

## TOBRAMYCIN INJECTION BP

**Presentation** Tobramycin Injection BP is a sterile, colourless solution. It contains tobramycin 40 mg per ml or 10 mg per ml (paediatric formulation only). The solution also contains in each ml; 0.1 mg disodium edetate BP, and 2.4 mg metabisulphite presented in clear glass vials.

**Uses** Tobramycin is an aminoglycoside antibiotic obtained from cultures of Streptomyces tenebrarius. Tobramycin Injection BP is indicated in the treatment of the following serious infections caused by susceptible micro-organisms:

1. central nervous system infections including meningitis, septicaemia and neonatalsepsis;
2. gastro-intestinal infections including peritonitis;
3. complicated and recurrent urinary tract infections such as pyelonephritis and cystitis;
4. lower respiratory tract infections, including pneumonia, bronchopneumonia and acutebronchitis;
5. skin, bone and soft tissue infections including burns.

Tobramycin may be considered in serious staphylococcal infections for which penicillin or other less potentially toxic drugs are contra-indicated and when bacterial susceptibility testing and clinical judgement indicate its use.

Tobramycin is usually active against most strains of the following organisms:

Pseudomonas aeruginosa

Proteus species (indole-positive and indole-negative), including *Pr. mirabilis*, *Pr. rettgeri* and *Pr. vulgaris*; *Morganella morganii*, *Escherichia coli*, Klebsiella-Enterobacter-Serratia species, Citrobacter species, Providencia species, Staphylococci including *Staphylococcus aureus* (coagulase-positive and coagulase-negative).

Most strains of enterococci demonstrate resistance although some strains of group D streptococci are susceptible in vivo. The combination of tobramycin and carbenicillin is synergistic in vitro against most strains of *Ps. aeruginosa.* Other Gram-negative organisms may be affected synergistically by the combination of tobramycin and a cephalosporin.

Prior to initiation of tobramycin therapy, appropriate specimens should be collected for identification of the causative organism and in vitro susceptibility tests. Tobramycin may be started pending results of susceptibility tests but should be discontinued if the causative organism is shown to be resistant to the drug. The decision to continue tobramycin therapy should be based upon the results of susceptibility studies, severity of the infection, and the important additional concepts discussed under 'Warnings'.

**Dosage and administration** Tobramycin may be given intramuscularly or intravenously and the dosage is the same for either route of administration. To calculate the correct dosage, the patients pretreatment bodyweight should be obtained.

*Patients with normal renal funtion:*

*Adults:* For adults with serious infections the usual recommended dosage is 3 mg/kg/day, administered in three equal doses every eight hours (see Table 1)

Patients with life-threatening infections, dosages up to 5 mg/kg/day may be administered in three or four equal dosages. The dosage should be reduced to 3 mg/kg/day as soon as clinically indicated. Dosage should not exceed 5 mg/kg/day, unless serum levels are monitored in order to prevent increased toxicity due to excessive blood levels (See *Warnings and Precautions*).

It may be necessary to administer up to 8 to 10 mg/kg/day in equally divided doses, to achieve therapeutic serum levels for patients with cystic fibrosis. Serum levels should be monitored because serum concentrations of tobramycin vary from patient to patient.

In adults with normal renal function, mild to moderate infections of the urinary tract have responded to a dosage of 2-3 mg/kg/day administered as a single intramuscular injection.

*Table 1: Dosage schedule for adults with normal renal function*

*(Dosage at 8-hour intervals)*

| *Patient Weight* | *Usual dose for Serious Infections 1 mg/kg q 8h. (Total 3 mg/kg/day)* | | *Maximum dose for Life-threatening Infections (Reduce as soon as possible) 1.66 mg/kg q 8h (Total 5 mg/kg/day- unless monitored)* | |
|---|---|---|---|---|
| *kg* | *mg/dose* | *ml/dose** | *mg/dose* | *ml/dose** |
| 120 | 120 | 3.0 | 200 | 5.0 |
| 100 | 100 | 2.5 | 166 | 4.0 |
| 80 | 80 | 2.0 | 133 | 3.0 |
| 60 | 60 | 1.5 | 100 | 2.5 |
| 40 | 40 | 1.0 | 66 | 1.6 |

* Applicable to 40 mg/ml product forms.

*Elderly:* As for adults, but see recommendations for patients with impaired renal function.

*Children:* The recommended dosage is 6-7.5 mg/kg/day, administered in 3 or 4 equally divided doses. It may be necessary to administer higher doses in some patients.

*Premature or full-term neonates:* Dosages of up to 4 mg/kg/day may be administered in two equal doses every 12 hours, for children between 1.5 and 2.5 kg body weight.

The usual length of treatment is seven to ten days. However, in difficult and complicated infections, a longer course of therapy may be necessary. In such cases monitoring of renal, auditory and vestibular functions is advised because neurotoxicity is more likely to occur when treatment is extended longer than ten days.

To ensure the correct dosage is given, it is recommended that blood levels should be determined whenever possible. Blood levels should always be determined in patients with chronic infections such as cystic fibrosis, or where longer duration of treatment may be necessary, or in patients with decreased renal function.

*Patients with impaired renal function:* Following a loading dose of 1 mg/kg, subsequent dosage must be adjusted, either with lower doses administered at 8hr intervals or with normal doses at prolonged intervals, (see Table 2). Both these regimens are suggested as guides to be used when serum levels of tobramycin can not be measured directly. They are based on either the creatinine clearance or the serum creatinine of the patient, because these values correlate with the half-life of tobramycin. Neither regimen should be used when dialysis is being performed.

*Regimen I*–Reduced dosage at 8-hour intervals: An appropriate reduced dosage range can be found in the accompanying table, (Table 2) for any patient for whom the creatinine clearance or serum creatinine values are known. The choice of dose within the indicated range should be based on the severity of the infection, the sensitivity of the pathogen, and individual patient considerations, especially renal function. Another rough guide for determining reduced dosage at 8-hour intervals, e.g. for patients whose steady-state serum creatinine values are known is to divide the normally recommended dose by the patient's serum creatinine value (mg/100 ml).

*Regimen II* - Normal dosage at prolonged intervals: Table 2 illustrates the recommended intervals between doses. As a general rule, the dosage frequency in hours can be determined by multiplying the patient's serum creatinine level (expressed as mg/100 ml) by six.

The dosage schedules derived from either method should be used in conjunction with careful clinical and laboratory observations of the patient and should be modified as necessary (see *Warnings*).

*Intramuscular administration:* Tobramycin may be administered by withdrawing the appropriate dose directly from the vial.

*Intravenous administration*: Tobramycin Injection BP may be given by intravenous infusion or by direct intravenous injection. When given by infusion, tobramycin may be diluted (with 0.9% Sodium Chloride Intravenous Infusion BP or 5% Dextrose Intravenous Infusion BP) to volumes of 50-100 ml for adult doses. For children, the volume of diluent should be proportionately less than for adults. The diluted solution should be infused over a period of 20-60 minutes avoiding admixture with any other drug. Tobramycin may be administered by direct intravenous injection or into the tubing of a drip set. When given in this way, serum levels may exceed 12 mg/L for a short time (See *Contra-indications, warnings, etc*).

It is recommended that both peak and trough serum levels should be determined whenever possible to ensure the correct dosage is given.

Following IM administration of a single dose of tobramycin of 1 mg/kg in adults with normal renal function, peak plasma tobramycin concentrations averaging 4-6μg/mL are attained within 30-90 minutes; plasma concentrations of the drug are 1μg/mL or less at 8 hours. Following intravenous infusion of the same dose over 30-60 minutes, similar plasma concentrations of the drug are obtained. In neonates, average peak plasma tobramycin concentrations of about 5μg/mL are attained 30-60 minutes after a single IM dose of 2 mg/kg; plasma concentrations average 1-2μg/mL at 12 hours.

**Contra-indications, warnings, etc**

*Contra-indications*: Intrathecal administration. Because of the known cross-allergenicity of drugs in this class, hypersensitivity to any aminoglycoside is a contraindication to the use of tobramycin.

*Warnings:* Tobramycin contains sodium metabisulphite which may cause allergic-type reactions, including anaphylactic symptoms and life-threatening or less severe asthmatic episodes, in certain susceptible people. The overall prevalence of sulphite sensitivity in the general population is unknown and probably low, but it occurs more frequently in asthmatic patients.

Cross-allergenicity among aminoglycosides has been known to occur. Patients treated with aminoglycoside antibiotics such as tobramycin should be under close clinical observation because these drugs have an inherent potential for causing nephrotoxicity and ototoxicity.

Both vestibular and auditory ototoxicity can occur. Eighth nerve impairment may develop in patients with pre-existing renal damage, and if tobramycin is administered for longer periods or in higher doses than those recommended. Other manifestations of neurotoxicity may include numbness, skin tingling, muscle twitching and convulsions. The risk of aminoglycoside-induced hearing loss increases with the degree of exposure to either high peak or high trough serum concentrations. Patients who develop cochlear damage may not have symptoms during therapy to warn of eighth-nerve toxicity, and partial or total irreversible bilateral deafness may continue to develop after the drug has been discontinued. Rarely, nephrotoxicity may not become manifest until the first few days after cessation of therapy. Aminoglycoside-induced nephrotoxicity is usually reversible. Therefore, renal and eighth cranial nerve function should be closely monitored in patients with known or suspected renal impairment and also in those whose renal function is initially normal but who develop signs of renal dysfunction during therapy. Evidence of impairment in renal, vestibular and/or auditory function requires discontinuation of the drug or dosage adjustment.

In elderly patients, it is particularly important to monitor renal function, when reduced renal function may not be evident in the results of routine screening tests, such as blood urea or serum creatinine. A creatinine clearance determination may be more useful.

Serum concentrations should be monitored when possible, and prolonged concentrations above 12 mg/L should be avoided. A useful guideline would be to perform serum level assays after 2 or 3 doses and also at 3 or 4 day intervals during therapy, so that the dosage could be adjusted if necessary. In the event of changing renal function, more frequent serum levels should be obtained and the dosage or dosage intervals adjusted according to the guidelines provided in the

*Table 2: Two maintenance regimens based on renal function and body weight following a loading dose of 1 mg/kg**

| *Renal Function°* | | | *Regimen I* | | *or Regimen II* |
|---|---|---|---|---|---|
| | | | *Adjusted doses at 8-hour intervals* | | *Normal dosage at prolonged intervals* |
| *Serum Creatinine* | | *Creatinine Clearance* | *Weight* | | *Weight/Dose* |
| *mg/100 ml* | *mmol/L* | *ml/min* | *50-60 kg* | *60-80 kg* | *50-60 kg : 60 mg*<br>*60-80 kg : 80 mg* |
| < 1.3 | < 114.9 | > 70 | 60 mg | 80 mg | q. 8h |
| 1.4–1.9 | 123.8–168 | 69–40 | 30–60 mg | 50–80 mg | q. 12h |
| 2.0–3.3 | 176.8–291.7 | 39–20 | 20–25 mg | 30–45 mg | q. 18h |
| 3.4–5.3 | 300.6–468.5 | 19–10 | 10–18 mg | 15–24 mg | q. 24h |
| 5.3–7.5 | 477.4–663 | 9–5 | 5–9 mg | 7–12 mg | q. 36h |
| > 7.6 | > 671.8 | < 4 | 2.5–4.5 mg | 3.5–6 mg | q. 48h† |

* For life-threatening infections, dosages 50% above those normally recommended may be used. The dosages should be reduced as soon as possible when improvement is noted.

° If used to estimate degree of renal impairment, serum creatinine concentrations should reflect a steady state of renal azotaemia.

† When dialysis is not being performed.

'Dosage and Administration' section. In order to measure the peak level, a serum sample should be drawn about 30 minutes following intravenous infusion or at one hour after intramuscular injection. Trough levels are measured by obtaining serum samples at 8 hours or just prior to the next dose of tobramycin.

Urine should be examined for increased excretion of protein, cells and casts. Serum creatinine or creatinine clearance (preferred over blood urea) should be measured periodically. When possible, it is recommended that serial audiograms be obtained in patients old enough to be tested, particularly high-risk patients.

In patients with normal renal function who do not receive tobramycin in higher doses or for longer periods of time than those recommended, the risk of toxic reactions is low. However, patients with reduced renal function are prone to the potential ototoxic and nephrotoxic effects of this drug, so dosage should be adjusted carefully on the basis of regular monitoring of serum drug concentrations and of renal function.

Concurrent and sequential use of other nephrotic, neurotoxic or ototoxic drugs, particularly streptomycin, neomycin, kanamycin, gentamicin, cephaloridine, paromomycin, viomycin, polymyxin B, colistin, cisplatin, vancomycin and amikacin, should be avoided. Advanced age and dehydration may also increase patient risk.

Tobramycin should not be given concurrently with potent diuretics. Some diuretics themselves cause ototoxicity, and diuretics administered intravenously enhance aminoglycoside toxicity by altering antibiotic concentrations in serum and tissue.

*Use in pregnancy and lactation:*

*Use in pregnancy:* Aminoglycosides can cause foetal harm when administered to a pregnant woman. Aminoglycosides such as tobramycin cross the placenta. Serious side-effects to mother, foetus, or newborn have not been reported in the treatment of pregnant women with other aminoglycosides, but tobramycin should not be administered to the pregnant patient unless the potential benefits clearly outweigh any potential risk. If tobramycin is used during pregnancy or if the patient becomes pregnant whilst taking tobramycin, she should be informed of the potential hazard to the foetus.

*Use in lactation:* Tobramycin is excreted in the breast milk and should be avoided in nursing women.

*Precautions:*

*Use in neonates:* Tobramycin should be used with caution and in reduced dosage in premature and full term neonate infants younger than 6 weeks of age because of their renal immaturity and the resulting prolongation of serum half-life of the drug.

*General:* It is desirable to measure both peak and trough serum concentrations as high doses of drug may be associated with a greater risk of toxicity.

Serum calcium, magnesium and sodium should be monitored. It is particularly important to monitor serum levels closely in patients with known renal impairment.

In patients with extensive burns, altered pharmacokinetics may result in reduced serum drug levels. Dosage must be based on measured serum levels in these patients.

Aminoglycosides may be absorbed in significant quantities from body surfaces for local irrigation or application and may cause neurotoxicity and nephrotoxicity.

Aminoglycosides should be used with caution in patients with muscular disorders, such as myasthenia gravis or parkinsonism, since these drugs may aggravate muscle weakness because of their potential curare-like effect on neuromuscular function.

The possibility of prolonged secondary apnoea should be considered if tobramycin is administered to anaesthetised patients who are also receiving neuromuscular blocking agents such as succinylcholine, tubocurarine or decamethonium, or to patients receiving massive transfusions of citrated blood. If neuromuscular blockade occurs, it may be reversed by the administration of calcium salts.

The inactivation of tobramycin by beta-lactam-type antibiotics (penicillins or cephalosporins) has been demonstrated in vitro and in patients with severe renal impairment. Such inactiviation has not been found in patients with normal renal function if the drugs are administered by separate routes.

If overgrowth of non-susceptible organisms occurs appropriate therapy should be initiated.

*Side-effects:* Renal function changes such as rising blood urea and serum creatinine and by oliguria, cylindruria and increased proteinuria, have been reported, especially in patients with a history of renal impairment who are treated for longer periods or with higher doses than these recommended. These changes can occur in patients with initially normal renal function.

In patients receiving high doses or prolonged therapy, side effects on both vestibular and auditory branches of the eighth cranial nerve have been reported. Similar effects have been noted in those given previous courses of therapy with an ototoxin, and in cases of dehydration. Symptoms include dizziness, vertigo, tinnitus, roaring in the ears and hearing loss. Hearing loss is usually irreversible and is manifested initially by diminution of high tone acuity.

Other side effects attributed to tobramycin have been reported such as increased AST, ALT, and serum bilirubin; decreased serum calcium, magnesium, sodium, potassium; anaemia, granulocytopenia, thrombocytopenia, leucopenia, leucocytosis and eosinophilia; and fever, rash, itching, urticaria, nausea, vomiting, headache, lethargy, pain at injection site, mental confusion and disorientation.

*Overdose:* Severity of the manifestations of a tobramycin overdose depend on the dose, the patient's renal function, state of hydration, age and whether concurrent medication with similar toxicities is being given.

Nephrotoxicity following the parenteral administration of an aminoglycoside is most closely related to the AUC of serum concentrations versus time. Nephrotoxicity is more likely if trough levels fail to fall below 2μg/mL and is also proportional to the average blood concentration. Patients who are elderly, have renal impairment, are receiving other nephrotoxic or ototoxic drugs, or are volume depleted, are at greater risk for developing acute tubular necrosis or auditory and vestibular toxicity. These patients often experience dizziness, tinnitus, vertigo and a loss of high-tone acuity. Neuromuscular blockade or respiratory failure may occur following rapid intravenous administration of many aminoglycosides. These reactions and prolonged respiratory paralysis may occur more commonly in patients with myasthenia gravis or Parkinson's disease, or those receiving decamethonium, tubocurarine or succinylcholine.

Toxicity from ingested tobramycin is unlikely because aminoglycosides are poorly absorbed from an intact gastro-intestinal tract.

*Treatment of overdose:* Haemodialysis or peritoneal dialysis will help remove tobramycin from the blood in the event of overdosage or toxic reactions. Depending on the duration and type of dialysis employed, approximately 25-70% of the administered dose may be removed. Haemodialysis is the more effective method. Calcium salts given intravenously have been used to counter neuromuscular blockade, the effectiveness of neostigmine has been variable.

**Pharmaceutical precautions**

*Incompatibilities:* Incompatibility or loss of activity has been reported between tobramycin sulphate and some cephalosporins and penicillins and also heparin sodium. Solutions with clindamycin phosphate in glucose injection are reported to be unstable.

Tobramycin Injection BP should not be physically premixed with other drugs but should be administered separately according to the recommended dose and route.

*Storage:* Store below 25°C and protect from light.

**Legal category** POM

**Package quantities** All presentations are available in packs of 5.

**Further information** Nil.

**Product licence numbers**

| | |
|---|---|
| 40 mg/ml | 4515/0066 |
| 80 mg/2 ml | 4515/0066 |
| 20 mg/2 ml | 4515/0067 |

## VANCOMYCIN HYDROCHLORIDE FOR INJECTION BP

**Qualitative and quantitative composition** Vancomycin BP 500 mg and 1 gram.

**Pharmaceutical form** Freeze dried powder in clear glass vial for reconstitution before injection.

**Clinical particulars**

*Therapeutic indications:* Vancomycin is an amphoteric glycopeptide antimicrobial substance produced by the growth of certain strains of *Nocardia orientalis* (formerly known as *Streptomyces orientalis*). It is bactericidal against many gram-positive organisms. Vancomycin is not chemically related to any of the presently used antimicrobial agents.

Vancomycin is indicated in potentially life-threatening infections due to susceptible gram-positive organisms which cannot be treated by other effective, less toxic antimicrobial drugs, such as the penicillins and cephalosporins. As Vancomycin is the only currently available antibiotic to which nearly all strains of Staphylococcus remain susceptible, it should be reserved for those cases where there is a specific indication, to minimise the chance of resistance emerging. Vancomycin is one of the agents of choice in treating methicillin resistant Staphylococcal infection.

*Staphylococcal infections:* Vancomycin is useful in therapy of severe Staphylococcal infections in patients who cannot receive or who have failed to respond to the penicillins and cephalosporins or who have infections with Staphylococci that are resistant to other antibiotics, including methicillin. Vancomycin has been used successfully alone in the treatment of staphylococcal endocarditis. Its efficacy has been documented in other infections due to staphylococci, including osteomyelitis, pneumonia, septicaemia and soft tissue infections.

Pseudomembranous colitis:

Oral Vancomycin is indicated for severe cases of antibiotic-associated pseudomembranous colitis (usually involving *Clostridium difficile*). Vancomycin is not absorbed from the gastrointestinal tract and faecal levels are many times higher than the M.I.C.'s needed. The incidence of relapse is approximately 14% and usually occurs 4 to 21 days after Vancomycin is discontinued. Patients appear to respond to a second course of oral Vancomycin. (Note: Intravenous Vancomycin is ineffective in treating pseudomembranous colitis.)

*Posology and method of administration:* The usual adult intravenous dose is 500 mg every six hours or 1 g every twelve hours. Staphylococcal infections normally respond within 48 to 72 hours. Duration of therapy depends on type and severity of infections and patient response. For bacterial endocarditis, the generally accepted regimen is 500 mg Vancomycin intravenously every six hours for a minimum of three weeks either alone or in combination with other antibiotics.

*Therapeutic range of serum levels:* During chronic therapy peak concentration should be kept within the range 10-20 micrograms/ml.

Pseudomembranous colitis: The recommended dose is 250 mg taken orally every six hours for 5 to 10 days. Even doses of 125 mg six hourly, produce faecal levels of Vancomycin well above those needed to kill most strains of C. difficile. Relapse rate is about 14% and may appear within 1 to 3 weeks of stopping therapy but responds to a further course of Vancomycin.

*Preparation of solution:* At the time of use, add 10 ml of sterile Water for Injections BP to a 500 mg vial of Vancomycin powder for Injection. Similarly, add 20 ml of sterile Water for Injections BP to a 1 gram vial of Vancomycin powder for Injection. Vials reconstituted in this manner will give a solution of 50 mg/ml. Further dilution is required depending on method of administration.

*Intravenous:* Intermittent infusion (the preferred method of administration): Reconstituted solutions containing 500 mg Vancomycin must be diluted with at least 100 ml diluent. Reconstituted solutions containing 1 g vancomycin must be diluted with at least 200 ml diluent. Sodium Chloride Intravenous infusion BP or 5% Dextrose Intravenous Infusion BP are suitable diluents. The desired dose should be given by intravenous infusion over a period of at least 60 minutes. If administered over a shorter period of time or in higher concentrations there is the possibility of inducing marked hypotension in addition to thrombophlebitis. Rapid administration may also produce flushing and a transient rash over the neck and shoulders.

Continuous infusion (should only be used when intermittent infusion not feasible): 1 g or 2 g of Vancomycin may be added to a sufficiently large volume of Sodium Chloride 0.9% Injection or Glucose 5% in Water for Injection to permit the desired dose to be infused over twenty-four hours.

Oral: After initial reconstitution of the vial, the selected dose 250 mg (5 ml) or 125 mg (2.5 ml) may be diluted in 30 ml of water and given to the patient to drink or the diluted material may be given down a nasogastric tube. Vancomycin is not effective orally for conditions other than pseudomembranous colitis.

*Paediatric: Intravenous:* The usual intravenous dosage is 10 mg/kg per dose given every 6 hours (total daily dosage 40 mg/kg of body weight). Each dose should be administered over a period of at least 60 minutes. In neonates and young infants, the total daily dosage may be lower. An initial dose of 15 mg/kg is suggested, followed by 10 mg/kg every 12 hours in the first week of life and every 8 hours thereafter until one month of age. Each dose should be administered over 60 minutes. Close monitoring of serum vancomycin concentrations may be warranted in these patients.

*Oral:* Can be administered using 40 mg per kg body weight in three or four divided doses for 7–10 days. The total daily dose of Vancomycin is normally 125 mg every six hours for a period of 7-14 days for the treatment of antibiotic associated diarrhoea caused by *Clostridium difficile*.

*Geriatric:* Because of its ototoxicity and nephrotoxicity, Vancomycin should be used with caution in patients with renal insufficiency or previous hearing loss. The elderly are particularly at risk. Doses should be titrated on the basis of serum levels. The elderly are particularly susceptible to auditory damage and should be given serial tests for auditory function if over the age of 60. Concurrent or sequential use of other neurotoxic substances should be avoided.

With impaired renal function: In patients with impaired renal function, dosage regimen of Vancomycin must be modified in response to degree of renal impairment, severity of infection, susceptibility of causative organism and serum concentrations of the drug. A suggested starting dose in patients with impaired renal function is 15 mg/kg with subsequent doses based mainly on renal function and serum concentrations of the drug.

In patients on haemodialysis, the drug is not significantly removed by haemodialysis. A dose of 1 g of Vancomycin every seven days produces effective blood levels. Serum levels should be monitored to avoid drug accumulation and resultant toxicity. The serum half-life ranges from 120 to 216 hours.

In patients undergoing peritoneal dialysis, the half-life of Vancomycin has been reported at around 18 hours. To prevent undue lowering of serum levels during peritoneal dialysis, an additional amount of Vancomycin could be added to the dialysate in a concentration of 25 microgram per ml.

*Contra-indications:* Vancomycin is contra-indicated in patients with known hypersensitivity to this drug.

*Special warnings and special precautions for use:* *Warnings:* Because of its toxicity and nephrotoxicity, Vancomycin should be used with care in patients with renal impairment. The risk of toxicity is increased by high blood concentrations or prolonged therapy. Therefore, blood levels should be monitored and dosage adjusted if it is necessary to use Vancomycin in such patients.

The concurrent or sequential use of other nephrotoxic drugs requires careful monitoring and should be avoided if possible.

Vancomycin should, if possible, be avoided in patients with previous hearing loss. If used it is very important that the dose be adjusted by monitoring the blood concentrations of the drug. Deafness may be preceded by tinnitus. The elderly are more susceptible to auditory damage. Experience with other antibiotics suggests that deafness may be progressive despite cessation of treatment.

*Precautions:* Vancomycin is very irritating to tissue and causes necrosis if injected intramuscularly. Pain and thrombophlebitis occur in many patients receiving Vancomycin and are occasionally severe. The frequency and severity of thrombophlebitis can be minimised if the drug is administered in a volume of at least 200 ml of glucose or saline solution and if the sites of injection are changed regularly. Complications of occasional severe hypotension, histamine like responses and maculopapular or erythematous rash ('red man's syndrome' or 'red neck syndrome') are thought to be related to the rate of the infusion and can be avoided by administration of the recommended dilute solutions over at least 20 to 30 minutes. One gram doses should be given over at least one hour and slow infusions over one hour are recommended for infants and children.

All patients receiving Vancomycin should have periodic haematological studies, urine analysis, liver and renal function tests.

Anaesthetic induced myocardial depression may be enhanced by Vancomycin. During anaesthesia, doses must be well diluted and administered slowly with close cardiac monitoring. Position changes should be delayed until the infusion is completed to allow for postural adjustment.

Patients taking oral Vancomycin should be warned of its offensive taste.

*Interaction with other medicaments and other forms of interaction:* Concurrent administration with other neurotoxic or nephrotoxic antibiotics, e.g. streptomycin, neomycin, gentamicin, kanamycin, amikacin, tobramycin, polymyxin B and colistin requires careful monitoring.

Diuretics such as ethacrynic acid and frusemide may aggravate ototoxicity.

Cholestyramine has been shown to bind Vancomycin in-vitro. Therefore, if oral Vancomycin is used with cholestyramine, the two drugs should be administered several hours apart.

*Pregnancy and lactation:*

Use in pregnancy: As there is little information on the use of Vancomycin in pregnancy, the drug should not be used in pregnant women or those likely to become pregnant unless the expected benefits outweigh any potential risk.

Use in lactation: Vancomycin is excreted in breast milk but it is not known whether it is harmful to the newborn. Therefore, it is not recommended for nursing mothers unless the expected benefits outweigh any potential risk.

*Effects on ability to drive and use machines:* Not applicable.

*Undesirable effects:*

*Adverse reactions: Auditory and vestibular:* Sensorineural deafness which may be accompanied by tinnitus has occurred but the incidence is low. Permanent deafness is more likely to occur in patients with compromised auditory or renal function but reversible deafness has been reported in normal patients.

*Cardiovascular:* Hypotension, palpitations, substernal pressure, tachycardia. (All effects due to excessively rapid infusion or insufficient dilution of drug.)

*Dermatological:* Pruritus at injection site, generalised flushing, erythematous macular rash with intense pruritus over face, neck and upper body have occurred after too rapid injection of the drug. Tissue irritation and necrosis occurs after I.M. injection or extravasation from I.V. site.

*Gastrointestinal:* Oral doses are extremely unpalatable. In leukaemic patients, oral dosing regimens are associated with frequent nausea, diarrhoea and occasional vomiting.

*General:* The use of Vancomycin may result in overgrowth of non-susceptible organisms resulting in new bacterial or fungal infections.

*Genitourinary:* Transient elevations of urea and granular casts in the urine occasionally occur. Nephrotoxicity in the presence of normal renal function at therapeutic serum levels is rare.

*Haematological:* Eosinophilia and neutropenia have been reported.

*Immunological:* Histamine release with chills, nausea, urticaria, macular rash, fever and rigors, even at normal doses but usually following rapid drug administration. Anaphylactoid reactions have been reported.

*Ocular:* Subconjunctival injections have infrequently been used in the treatment of bacterial corneal ulcers but may cause severe inflammation or sloughing.

*Overdose:* No information available except for that given under *Adverse Reactions* above.

**Pharmacological properties**

*Pharmacodynamic properties:* Vancomycin is a biological material, described as a tricyclic glycopeptide obtained from cultures of *Nocardia orientalis (Streptomyces orientalis)*. It is structurally unrelated to other antibiotics and is presented as the hydrochloride salt for parenteral administration. The drug is not absorbed from the gastrointestinal tract, and an aqueous solution of the product can be administered orally in the treatment of Pseudomembranous colitis.

Vancomycin is a bactericidal antibiotic and appears to bind to the bacterial cell wall causing blocckage of glycopeptide polymerisation. This effect produces immediate inhibition of cell wall synthesis and secondary damage to the cytoplasmic membrane. It is active against may gram positive organisms including staphylococci, group A beta haemolytic streptococci, streptococcus pneumoniae, enterococci, corynebacterium and clostridium species. It does not demonstrate clinical efficacy against gram negative bacteria, fungi or yewasts, and hence the product literature only indicates use in severe infections caused by gram positive organisms.

*Pharmacokinetic properties:* Vancomycin is poorly absorbed by mouth. An intravenous dose of 1 g produces serum levels averaging 25 microgram per ml after two hours in patients with normal renal function. Serum levels are higher in patients with renal impairment and toxicity may result. Vancomycin is excreted unchanged in the urine, at least 80% is excreted in the first 24 hours. It has a half-life of about 6 hours in patients with normal renal function.

Vancomycin readily diffuses into pleural, pericardial, ascitic and synovial fluids. It does not diffuse into cerebrospinal fluid with normal meninges, but therapeutic concentrations may be reached in patients with acute meningitis. Vancomycin is active against many gram-positive organisms including staphylococci, streptococci, corynebacterium and clostridium, including Clostridium difficile. Gram-negative bacteria, mycobacteria and fungi are highly resistant. Many strains of gram-positive bacteria are sensitive in-vitro toVancomycin concentrations of 0.5 to 5 microgram/ml, but a few Staph. aureus strains require 10-20 microgram/ml for inhibition.

Using the Bauer-Kirby method of disc susceptibility testing, a 30 microgram Vancomycin disc should produce a zone of more than 11 mm when tested against a Vancomycin sensitive strain.

Vancomycin appears to act by inhibiting the production of bacterial cell wall mucopeptide. This effect occurs at a site different from that affected by penicillins and produces immediate inhibition of cell wall synthesis and secondary damage to the cytoplasmic membrane.

*Preclinical safety data:* Not applicable.

**Pharmaceutical particulars**

*List of excipients:* Water for Injections BP removed during lyophilisation.

*Incompatibilities:* Chemically incompatible with Dexamethasone sodium phosphate, Heparin sodium, Methicillin sodium, phenobarbitone sodium, sodium bicarbonate.

*Shelf life:* 18 months.

*Special precautions for storage:* Store below 25°C and protect from light.

When aseptically prepared, the product may be stored for up to 24 hours at 2°C to 8°C. The product does not contain an antimicrobial preservative. Therefore if aseptic preparation cannot be ensured, the product should be prepared immediately before use and any unused portion discarded.

*Instructions for use/handling:* Vancomycin is very irritating to tissue and causes necrosis if injected intramuscularly. Pain and thrombophlebitis occur in many patients receiving vancomycin and are occasionally severe. The frequency and severity of thrombophlebitis can be minimised if the drug is administered in a volume of at least 200 ml of glucose or saline solution and if the sites of injection are changed regularly.

Complications of occasional severe hypotension, histamine like responses and maculopapular or erythematous rash ('red man's syndrome' or 'red neck syndrome') are thought to be related to the rate of the infusion and can be avoided by administration of the recommended dilute solutions over at least 20 to 30 minutes. One gram doses should be given over at least one hour and slow infusions over one hour are recommended for infants and children.

All patients receiving vancomycin should have periodic haematological studies, urine analysis, liver and renal function tests.

Anaesthetic induced myocardial depression may be enhanced by vancomycin. During anaesthesia, doses must be well diluted and administered slowly with close cardiac monitoring. Position changes should be delayed until the infusion is completed to allow for postural adjustment.

Patients taking oral vancomycin should be warned of its offensive taste.

**Marketing authorisation number** 4515/0053

**Date of approval/revision of SPC** 12 February 1997

**Legal category** POM

## VINBLASTINE SULPHATE INJECTION SOLUTION 10MG/10ML

**Qualitative and quantitative composition**

| | *per unit dose* | *per mL* |
|---|---|---|
| Vinblastine Sulphate | 10 mg | 1 mg |
| Sodium Chloride | 90 mg | 9 mg |
| Water for Injection | to 10 mL | to 1 mL |

1N Sodium Hydroxide or 1N Sulphuric Acid is added to adjust the pH to be approximately 4.5

**Pharmaceutical form** Vinblastine Sulphate Injection Solution is a clear, colourless, sterile solution of Vinblastine Sulphate BP in Water for Injection BP It is presented in conventional glass vials and Onco-Tain* vials containing 10 ml of a 1 mg/ml solution of Vinblastine Sulphate BP and 9 mg/ml Sodium Chloride BP The solution does not contain any preservatives.

**Clinical particulars**

*Therapeutic indications:* Vinblastine Sulphate is a cytotoxic drug that arrests cell growth at the metaphase. Its actions are more pronounced on the rapidly dividing cell than on the normal cell. It appears to act, like Vincristine, by binding to the microtubular proteins of the mitotic spindle, preventing polymerisation.

Vinblastine Sulphate is effective as a single agent, but its therapeutic effect is enhanced when used in combination with other antineoplastic drugs. Vinblastine Sulphate has been used in the treatment of Hodgkin's Disease (Stages III and IV); lymphocytic lymphoma (nodular and diffuse, poorly and well differentiated); histiocytic lymphoma; advanced stages of mycosis fungoides; advanced carcinoma of the testis; Kaposi's sarcoma and Letterer-Siwe disease (histocytosis X). Vinblastine Sulphate may be used in the treatment of choriocarcinoma resistant to other chemotherapeutic agents; carcinoma of the breast, unresponsive to appropriate endocrine surgery and hormonal therapy.

*Posology and method of administration:* The solution may be injected either directly into the vein or into the injection site of a running intravenous infusion. Injection of Vinblastine Sulphate may be completed in about one minute.

This preparation is for intravenous use only. Intrathecal administration usually results in death. (See warnings).

Syringes containing this product should be overlabelled with the intrathecal warning label provided –'NOT FOR INTRATHECAL USE'.

Dosage: Vinblastine Sulphate is given intravenously at weekly intervals according to the needs of the patient. Therapy is initiated by a single intravenous dose in accordance with the following dosage table, and white blood cell counts should be made to determine the sensitivity of the patient to Vinblastine. Dosage should not be increased after that dose which reduces the white cell count to approximately 3000 cells/mm³.

|  | Adults mg/m² bsa | Children mg/m² bsa |
|---|---|---|
| First Dose | 3.7 | 2.5 |
| Second Dose | 5.5 | 3.75 |
| Third Dose | 7.4 | 5.0 |
| Fourth Dose | 9.25 | 6.25 |
| Fifth Dose | 11.1 | 7.5 |

Dosage increase may be continued but must not exceed 18.5 mg/m² for adults or 12.5 mg/m² for children.

Patients should be maintained on the maximum weekly dose that does not cause the above degree of leucopenia.

For most adult patients this dosage will be 5.5 mg/m²–7.4 mg/m², however, leucopenia can be produced at 3.7 mg/m², other patients may require 11.1 mg/m² and, very rarely, 18.5 mg/m².

A FURTHER DOSE OF VINBLASTINE SHOULD NOT BE GIVEN UNTIL THE WHITE CELL COUNT HAS RETURNED TO AT LEAST 4000/mm³, EVEN THOUGH 7 DAYS MAY HAVE ELAPSED.

In some cases, oncolytic activity may be encountered before the leucopenic effect and, when this occurs, there is no necessity to increase subsequent doses.

Duration of maintenance therapy is dependent upon the disease state and the antineoplastic agent combination.

Differing clinical opinions are held for the appropriate duration of maintenance therapy in Hodgkin's Disease. Prolonged chemotherapy for maintaining remissions involves several risks such as life-threatening infections, sterility and possibly the appearance of other cancers through suppression of immune response.

Vinblastine should not be given intramuscularly, subcutaneously or intrathecally.

*Contra-indications:* This preparation is for intravenous use only. Intrathecal administration usually results in death (see *Warnings*).

Vinblastine Sulphate is contra-indicated in patients who are leucopenic. It should not be used in the presence of bacterial infection. Such infections should be brought under control with antiseptics or antibiotics before the initiation of therapy with Vinblastine Sulphate.

*Special warnings and special precautions for use: Warnings:* Vinblastine Sulphate must be used only by physicians experienced in cytotoxic chemotherapy.

Syringes containing this product should be overlabelled with the intrathecal warning label provided –'NOT FOR INTRATHECAL USE'.

The following treatment successfully arrested progresive paralysis in a single patient mistakenly given the related vincristine sulphate, intrathecally. This treatment should be initiated immediately:

1. Removal of as much CSF as is safely possible.
2. Flushing with Lactated Ringer's solution by continuous infusion at 150 ml/h, through a catheter in a cerebral lateral ventricle and removed through lumbar access, until fresh plasma became available.
3. Fresh frozen plasma, 25 ml, diluted with 1 L of Lactated Ringer's was then infused similarly at 75 ml/h. The rate of infusion should be adjusted to maintain a spinal fluid protein level of 150 mg/dl.
4. Glutamic acid, 10 gm, was given iv over 24 hours, followed by 500 mg tds by mouth for 1 month. Glutamic acid may not be essential.

Vinblastine SHOULD NOT BE GIVEN intramuscularly, subcutaneously or intrathecally.

Caution is necessary with the use of Vinblastine Sulphate during pregnancy. There is insufficient information to assess Vinblastine Sulphate's effect on fertility in men and women. However, aspermia has been reported in man.

Animal studies suggest that teratogenic effects may occur. The drug should not be used in pregnant women unless the expected benefit outweighs the potential risk.

As with other antineoplastic agents, vinblastine may cause a severe local reaction on extravasation. If leakage into the surrounding tissue should occur during intravenous administration of Vinblastine Sulphate, the injection should be discontinued immediately and any remaining portion of the dose should

be introduced into another vein. Local injection of hyaluronidase with the application of heat has been used to disperse the drug in order to minimise discomfort and the possibility of tissue damage.

Liver disease may alter the elimination of vinblastine in the bile, markedly increasing toxicity to peripheral nerves and necessitating a dosage modification in affected patients.

*Precautions:* Patients should be carefully monitored for infection until the white cell count has returned to normal levels, if leucopenia with less than 2000 white blood cells per mm3 occurs following a dose of Vinblastine Sulphate.

When cachexia or ulcerated areas of the skin are present, a more profound leucopenic response may be produced by vinblastine. Therefore, its use should be avoided in older persons suffering from either of these conditions.

Leucocyte and platelet counts have sometimes fallen precipitously after moderate doses of Vinblastine Sulphate in patients with malignant cell infiltration of the bone marrow.

Further use of the drug in such patients is inadvisable. Avoid contamination of the eye with Vinblastine Sulphate injection. If accidental contamination occurs, severe irritation or corneal ulceration may result. The affected eye should be thoroughly irrigated with water immediately.

*Interaction with other medicaments and other forms of interaction:*

(i)  Vinblastine used as part of a combination regimen with mitomycin may result in acute respiratory distress and pulmonary infiltration.
(ii)  Cases of respiratory distress with interstitial pulmonary infiltrates have been reported in patients given a regimen comprising vinblastine, mitomycin, and progesterone (MVP).

*Pregnancy and lactation:* Although information on the use of vinblastine during pregnancy is limited, the drug may cause foetal toxicity when administered to pregnant women. The drug causes resorption of foetuses in animals and produces gross foetal abnormalities in surviving offspring. There are no adequate and controlled studies to date using vinblastine in pregnant women, and the drug should be used during pregnancy only in life-threatening situations or severe disease for which safer drugs cannot be used or are ineffective. Women of childbearing potential should be advised to avoid becoming pregnant while receiving the drug. When vinblastine is administered during pregnancy or the patient becomes pregnant while receiving the drug, the patient should be informed of the potential hazard to the foetus.

The effect of vinblastine on fertility in humans is not fully known. Aspermia has occurred in some individuals during vinblastine therapy.

It is not known whether vinblastine is excreted in human milk. Because of the potential for serious adverse reactions due to vinblastine in nursing infants, a decision should be made whether to discontinue nursing or the drug, taking into account the importance of the drug to the mother.

*Effects on ability to drive and use machines:* Not applicable.

*Undesirable effects:* The incidence of side effects with Vinblastine Sulphate appears to be dose related and most do not persist longer than 24 hours. Neurological effects are uncommon but can occur and may last longer than 24 hours.

Leucopenia is the most common side effect and dose limiting factor.

The following side effects have been reported:

Gastrointestinal: nausea, vomiting, constipation, vesiculation of the mouth, diarrhoea, anorexia, abdominal pain, rectal bleeding, pharyngitis, haemorrhagic enterocolitis, bleeding for an old peptic ulcer.

Neurological: numbness, paraesthesias, peripheral neuritis, mental depression, loss of deep tendon reflexes, headache, convulsions.

Miscellaneous: malaise, weakness, dizziness, pain in tumour site, vesiculation of the skin, alopecia.

Antiemetics may be used to control nausea and vomiting. Alopecia is usually not total and in some cases the hair regrows during maintenance therapy.

Extravasation during intravenous injection may result in cellulitis and phlebitis. In extreme instances sloughing may occur.

*Overdose:* Side-effects following the use of vinblastine are dose related. Therefore, following administration of more than the recommended dose, patients can be expected to experience these effects in an exaggerated fashion.

In addition, neurotoxicity similar to that seen with vincristine sulphate may be observed.

Treatment: Supportive care should include: (1) prevention of the side effects that result from the syndrome of inappropriate secretion of antidiuretic hormone. This includes restriction of fluid intake and perhaps the use of a diuretic acting on the loop of

Henle and distal tubule function; (2) administration of an anticonvulsant; (3) prevention and treatment of ileus; (4) monitoring the patient's cardiovascular system; and (5) daily blood counts for guidance in transfusion requirement.

The major effect of excessive doses of vinblastine will be on granulocytopoeisis, and this may be life-threatening.

**Pharmacological properties**

*Pharmacodynamic properties:* Although the mechanism of action has not been definitely established, vinblastine appears to bind to or crystallize critical microtubular proteins of the mitotic spindle, thus preventing their proper polymerization and causing metaphase arrest. In high concentrations, vinblastine also exerts complex effects on nucleic acid and protein synthesis. Vinblastine reportedly also interferes with amino acid metabolism by blocking cellular utilization of glutamic acid and thus inhibits purine synthesis, the citric acid cycle, and the formation of urea. Vinblastine exerts some immunosuppressive activity.

*Pharmacokinetic properties:* Vinblastine sulphate is unpredictably absorbed from the GI tract. Following intravenous administration, the drug is rapidly cleared from the blood and distributed into body tissues.

Vinblastine crosses the blood-brain barrier poorly and does not appear in the CSF in therapeutic concentrations. Vinblastine is reported to be extensively metabolized, primarily in the liver, to desacetyl-vinblastine, which is more active than the parent compound on a weight basis. The drug is excreted slowly in urine and in faeces via the bile.

**Pharmaceutical particulars**

*List of excipients:*
| | |
|---|---|
| Sodium Chloride BP | 9.0 mg |
| Water for Injection BP | to 10.0 mL. |

*Incompatibilities:* Vinblastine Sulphate is incompatible with furosemide, when injected sequentially into Y-site with no flush between or when mixed in syringe. Immediate precipitation results.

*Shelf life:* 24 months.

*Special precautions for storage:* The product must be stored between 2°C and 8°C and protected from light.

*Instructions for use/handling: Cytotoxic Handling Guidelines:*
Administration: Should be administered only by or under the direct supervision of a qualified physician who is experienced in the use of cancer chemotherapeutic agents.

*Preparation (Guidelines)*
(a) Chemotherapeutic agents should be prepared for administration only by professionals who have been trained in the safe use of the preparation.
(b) Operations such as reconstitution of powder and transfer to syringes should be carried out only in the designated area.
(c) The personnel carrying out these procedures should be adequately protected with clothing, gloves and eye shield.
(d) Pregnant personnel are advised not to handle chemotherapeutic agents.

*Contamination*
(a) In the event of contact with the skin or eyes, the affected area should be washed with copious amounts of water or normal saline. A bland cream may be used to treat the transient stinging of skin. Medical advice should be sought if the eyes are affected.
(b) In the event of spillage, operators should put on gloves and mop up the spilled material with a sponge kept in the area for that purpose. Rinse the area twice with water. Put all solutions and sponges into a plastic bag and seal it.

*Disposal:* Syringes, containers, absorbent materials, solution and any other contaminated material should be placed in a thick plastic bag or other impervious container and incinerated.

**Marketing authorisation number**    4515/0051

**Date of approval/revision of SPC**    9 August 1996

**Legal category**    POM

# VINCRISTINE SULPHATE INJECTION SOLUTION

**Qualitative and quantitative composition**
*Active Constituent*
| | |
|---|---|
| Vincristine Sulphate BP | 1.0 mg. |

*Other Constituents*
| | |
|---|---|
| Mannitol BP | 100.0 mg |
| Water for Injections BP | to 1.0 mL. |

There is no overage in this formulation.

**Pharmaceutical form** A sterile, colourless solution.

**Clinical particulars**

*Therapeutic indications:* Vincristine Sulphate is used primarily as a component of various chemotherapeutic regimens for the treatment of acute leukaemias. It has also been used in conjunction with other oncolytic drugs in the treatment of Hodgkin's Disease, all forms of lymphoma, Wilm's tumour, sarcomas and tumours of the breast, brain and lung.

*Posology and method of administration:* This preparation is for intravenous use only. Intrathecal administration usually results in death (see *Warnings* for treatment).

Vincristine Sulphate is administered by intravenous injection at weekly intervals, the precise dose being determined by body weight.

Great care should be exercised in calculating the dose as overdosage may be extremely serious or even fatal. The dose should not be increased beyond the level which produces therapeutic benefit. In general, individual doses should not exceed 2 mg; and white cell counts should be carried out before and after giving each dose.

Vincristine Sulphate for Injection BP after reconstitution as directed (see below) or Vincristine Sulphate Injection Solution may be injected into the tubing or side arm of a free-flowing I.V. infusion or directly into a vein over a one-minute period. For safety reasons when administering Vincristine Injection into a side arm of a fast running infusion, please ensure that pressure is maintained on the syringe plunger during administration, to avoid back pressure from the infusion forcing the plunger out of the syringe barrel. Care should be taken to avoid extravasation as this may cause local ulceration.

Because of the narrow range between therapeutic and toxic levels and variations in response, the dosage must always be adjusted to the individual.

The following dosage regimens have been used:

*Acute leukaemia:*
*Adults:* The suggested dose is 25-75 micrograms/kg body weight (1.4 mg/m2 body surface area) by weekly intravenous injection.

*Children:* Weekly intravenous injections starting with 50 micrograms/kg body weight (1.5-2 mg/m2 body surface area) increasing by weekly increments of 25 micrograms/kg body weight to a maximum of 150 micrograms/kg body weight. The dose should not be increased after a response has been obtained and it may be possible to maintain remission with a reduced dose.

*Elderly:* The normal adult dose is still appropriate in the elderly.

*Other tumours:* 25 micrograms/kg body weight by weekly intravenous injection until a response is observed and 5-10 micrograms/kg body weight thereafter for maintenance.

*Contra-indications:* Intrathecal administration of Vincristine Sulphate is usually fatal. Although there are no other known contraindications to the use of Vincristine Sulphate, careful notice should be given to those conditions listed under *Warnings* and *Precautions*.

Breast feeding during treatment.

*Special warnings and special precautions for use:*
*Warnings:* Syringes containing this product should be labelled 'VINCRISTINE FOR INTRAVENOUS USE ONLY'.

After intrathecal administration, removal of cerebrospinal fluid, and flushing with Lactated Ringer's and other solutions, has not prevented ascending paralysis leading to death. In one adult paralysis was arrested, with some recovery, by the following treatment initiated immediately:-

1. Removal of as much CSF as is safely possible.
2. Flushing with Lactated Ringer's solution by continuous infusion at 150 ml/h, through a catheter in a cerebral lateral ventricle and removed through lumbar access, until fresh frozen plasma became available.
3. Fresh frozen plasma, 25 ml, diluted with 1l of Lactated Ringer's was then infused similarly at 75 ml/h. The rate of infusion was adjusted to maintain a spinal fluid protein level of 150 mg/dl.
4. Glutamic acid, 10 gm, was given iv over 24 hours, followed by 500 mg tds by mouth for 1 month. Glutamic acid may not be essential.

Vincristine Sulphate should only be administered by physicians experienced in cytotoxic chemotherapy.

Vincristine Sulphate should not be given by intrathecal, intramuscular or subcutaneous injection.

Vincristine Sulphate is a vesicant and may cause a severe local reaction or extravasation. If leakage into the surrounding tissue should occur during I.V. administration of Vincristine Sulphate, the injection should be discontinued immediately and any remaining portion of the dose should be introduced into another vein. Local injection of hyaluronidase with the application of heat has been used to disperse the drug in order to minimise discomfort and the possibility of tissue damage.

Precautions: Leucopenia is less likely following therapy with Vincristine Sulphate than is the case with other oncolytic agents. However, because of its possibility both physician and patient should remain alert for signs of any complicating infection. If leucopenia or a complicating infection is present, then administration of the next dose of Vincristine Sulphate warrants careful consideration.

Acute uric acid nephropathy, which may occur after administration of oncolytic agents, has also been reported with Vincristine Sulphate.

As Vincristine Sulphate penetrates the blood-brain barrier poorly, additional agents and routes of administration may be required for central nervous system leukaemias.

The neurotoxic effect of Vincristine Sulphate may be additive with other neurotoxic agents or increased by spinal cord irradiation and neurological disease. Elderly patients may be more susceptible to the neurotoxic effects of Vincristine Sulphate.

The elimination of Vincristine Sulphate may be reduced in the presence of impaired hepatic or biliary function and the dose must be decreased accordingly.

Care should be exercised to avoid accidental contamination of the eyes as Vincristine Sulphate is highly irritant and can cause corneal ulceration.

*Interaction with other medicaments and other forms of interaction:* Allopurinol, pyridoxine and isoniazid may increase the incidence of cytotoxic induced bone marrow depression. The mechanism for this potentiation has not been fully classified.

The neurotoxicity of Vincristine Sulphate may be additive with that of other drugs acting on the peripheral nervous system.

Vincristine Sulphate appears to increase the cellular uptake of Methotrexate by malignant cells and this principle has been applied in high-dose Methotrexate therapy.

*Pregnancy and lactation:* Safe use of Vincristine Sulphate during pregnancy has not been established. The drug should not be used in women who are or who may become pregnant, unless the expected benefit outweighs the potential risk. Women being treated with Vincristine should take appropriate contraceptive measures during therapy. Vinca alkaloids may effect fertility and have been shown to be embryocidal.

Vincristine Sulphate should not be used in women who are breastfeeding, unless the expected benefit outweighs the potential risk.

*Effects on ability to drive and use machines:* Not applicable.

*Undesirable effects:* Vincristine is a vesicant and may cause a severe local reaction on extravasation. It should only be administered by physicians experienced in cytotoxic chemotherapy.

Vincristine may cause granulocytopenia and users should be alert to signs of infection. Preexisting granulocytopenia does not preclude treatment, but care should be taken in such patients.

Daily administration of small doses of Vincristine Sulphate may result in the prolongation of side-effects which would otherwise be of short duration.

Side-effects of Vincristine Sulphate appear to be dose-related and, particularly in the case of neurotoxicity, related to the total accumulated dose given.

Neuropathies are the most common side effect in all age groups and are often dose-limiting. The neuropathy may occur as neuritic pain, paraesthesia, sensory loss and peroneal weakness resulting in foot drop and impaired gait. Headache and jaw pain are associated with cranial nerve involvement. No reversal agent for the neuromuscular effects has been reported as yet.

Gastrointestinal side-effects such as constipation, abdominal cramps, paralytic ileus, vomiting and diarrhoea may be encountered. The prophylactic use of stool softeners and mild cathartics is recommended to avoid impaction as a result of constipation.

Bladder neuropathies are uncommon but have been reported.

Reversible alopecia occurs in approximately 20% of all cases treated with Vincristine Sulphate and patients should be warned of this possibility. Other side effects reported in a small number of patients are weight loss, polyuria, dysuria and fever.

*Overdose:* Symptoms are those associated with acute neurotoxicity, seizures, fluid retention, paralytic ileus.

Side effects of Vincristine Sulphate are dose related and are exaggerated by overdosage. There is, as yet, no antidote for Vincristine Sulphate.

Support therapy should be directed to the prevention of the side effects resulting from hypersecretion of antidiuretic hormone by restriction of fluid intake and possibly the use of an appropriate diuretic. Anticonvulsants, e.g. phenobarbitone may be necessary for control of seizure and cathartics administered to prevent ileus.

Routine cardiovascular monitoring is recommended together with daily haematology as an indicator for transfusion requirements.

Folinic Acid has been used for the treatment of overdosage. An intravenous injection of 15 mg Folinic Acid may be given every 3 hours for 24 hours, then every 6 hours for at least 48 hours.

**Pharmacological properties**

*Pharmacodynamic properties:* Although the mechanism of action has not been definitely established, Vincristine appears to bind to or crystallize critical microtubular proteins of the mitotic spindle, thus preventing their proper polymerization and causing metaphase arrest. In high concentrations, the drug also exerts complex effects on nucleic acid and protein synthesis. Vincristine exerts some immuno-suppressive activity.

*Pharmacokinetic properties:* Vincristine is not reliably absorbed from the gastro-intestinal tract. After intravenous injection it disappears rapidly from the blood. It is extensively protein bound and it is reported to be concentrated in blood platelets. It is metabolised in the liver and excreted primarily in the bile–about 70% of a dose is found in faeces, as unchanged drug and metabolites, over 72 hours. Some also appears in the urine. Vincristine does not appear to cross the blood-brain barrier in significant amounts.

Following rapid I.V. injection of Vincristine, serum concentrations of the drug appear to decline in a triphasic manner. The terminal elimination half-life of Vincristine has ranged from 10.5-15.5 hours.

**Pharmaceutical particulars**

*List of excipients:*

| | |
|---|---|
| Mannitol BP | 100.0 mg |
| Water for Injections BP | to 1.0 mL. |

There is no overage in this formulation.

*Incompatibilities:* It is not recommended that Vincristine Sulphate should be mixed with any other drug and should not be diluted in solutions that raise or lower the pH outside the range 3.5 to 5.5. Frusemide both in syringe and injected sequentially into Y-site with no flush between, results in immediate precipitation.

*Shelf life:* 24 months.

*Special precautions for storage:* Store between 2°C and 8°C. Protect from light.

**Marketing authorisation number** 4515/0008

**Date of approval/revision of SPC** August 1996

**Legal category** POM

*Trade Mark

# Ferring Pharmaceuticals Ltd
Greville House
Hatton Road
Feltham
Middlesex TW14 9PX

**FERRING**
PHARMACEUTICALS

## APROTININ INJECTION BP

**Presentation** A sterile, pyrogen-free, clear, colourless solution of Aprotinin 5.56 BP/EP Units per ml/ 10,000 KIU (Kallikrein Inactivator Units) per ml in 0.9% sodium chloride solution presented in 50 ml vials containing 70 mg aprotinin (500,000 KIU) and 5 ml ampoules containing 7 mg aprotinin (50,000 KIU).

**Uses** Aprotinin is a polyvalent protease inhibitor, isolated from animal tissue. It is active against certain proteolytic enzymes such as kallikrein, kinin, trypsin, chymotrypsin, plasmin, plasmin-activator, fibrin enzymes and tissue proteases. Aprotinin may be used therapeutically or prophylactically when these enzyme systems fail.

Aprotinin is a haemostatic. High doses offer major reductions in peri-operative blood loss and the need for donor blood transfusions. It is indicated for the treatment of life-threatening haemorrhage due to hyperplasminaemia.

**Dosage and administration** Intravenously by slow injection or infusion.

*Dosage in adults:* 500,000 to 1,000,000 KIU (277.8–555.6 EP Units) given by slow IV infusion (maximum rate 5 ml/min), followed by 200,000 KIU (111.1 EP Units) hourly until bleeding stops.

*Dosage in the elderly:* The dosage given above applies to persons of average bodyweight. Reductions of these doses should be considered in patients of below average weight.

*Dosage in children:* It is recommended that a dose proportional to the adult dose is calculated.

**Contra-indications, warnings, etc**
*Contra-indications:* Known hypersensitivity to aprotinin.

*Interactions:* None known.

*Effects on ability to drive/use machines:* None known; unlikely to be applicable as indications are for hospitalised patients.

*Side-effects:* Aprotinin is usually well tolerated but local thrombophlebitis, nausea and vomiting, diarrhoea, muscle pains, and blood-pressure changes can occur.

Allergic reactions such as erythema, urticaria, and bronchospasm have occasionally been reported and can occur on first administration. On repeated dosage, a reddening may occur at the point of injection, but this disappears after 1 or 2 hours. Anaphylaxis, tachycardia, pallor or cyanosis and dyspnoea have also occurred.

*Use in pregnancy/lactation:* There is no evidence that aprotinin has teratogenic or embryotoxic effects in animals. Experience in human pregnancy and lactation is limited and inadequate to assess safety. As the use of aprotinin is in life-threatening situations it may be used in pregnancy and lactation when the benefit is considered to outweigh the risk.

*Warnings/precautions:* Rapid IV injection of large doses should be avoided for the high basicity of aprotinin may cause liberation of histamine and lead to an anaphylactic reaction. Aprotinin should be administered slowly (maximum 5 ml/min) with the patient lying down. Care should be taken in treating patients intermittently and in those who have received Aprotinin previously. If hypersensitivity reactions are observed, the injection/infusion must be stopped immediately and the appropriate therapeutic measures initiated (administration of adrenaline, antihistamines, intravenous corticosteroids). Intra-ocular or intra-dermal testing may be useful for detecting allergic patients.

*Overdose:* There is no specific antidote and symptomatic treatment is advised. The use of more than $6{\times}10^6$ KIU (equivalent to 12×50 ml vials) per day is not recommended.

*Incompatibilities:* Antibiotics which react with proteins, corticosteroid and nutrient solutions containing amino-acids or fat emulsions.

**Pharmaceutical precautions** Store at a temperature not exceeding 25°C and protect from light. Both 5 ml ampoules and 50 ml vials should be considered as single dose containers and any contents not used in a single administration should be discarded.

**Legal category** POM.

**Package quantities** 5 ml ampoules each containing 50,000 KIU in boxes of 10 ampoules; 50 ml vials containing 500,000 KIU.

**Further information** Nil.

**Product licence numbers**
5 ml ampoule     0051/0027
50 ml vial          0051/0028
*Product licence holder:* Paines and Byrne Ltd, West Byfleet, Surrey KT14 6RA.

## DDAVP* TABLETS

**Presentation** Uncoated, white, flat, round tablets of 8 mm diameter, scored on one side and marked '0.1' on the other side, each containing desmopressin acetate 0.1 mg.

Uncoated, white, flat, round tablets of 8 mm diameter, scored one side and marked "0.2" on the other side, each containing desmopressin acetate 0.2 mg.

**Uses** DDAVP Tablets are indicated for the treatment of vasopressin-sensitive cranial diabetes insipidus or in the treatment of post-hypophysectomy polyuria/polydipsia.

DDAVP Tablets are also indicated for the treatment of primary nocturnal enuresis.

**Dosage and administration**
*Treatment of diabetes insipidus:* Dosage is individual but clinical experience has shown that the total daily dose normally lies in the range of 0.2 to 1.2 mg. A suitable starting dose in adults and children is 0.1 mg three times daily. This dosage regimen should then be adjusted in accordance with the patient's response. For the majority of patients, the maintenance dose is 0.1 mg to 0.2 mg three times daily.

*Post-hypophysectomy polyuria/polydipsia:* The dose of DDAVP Tablets should be controlled by measurement of urine osmolality.

*Primary nocturnal enuresis:* Children (from 5 years of age) and adults (up to 65 years of age) with normal urine concentrating ability who have primary nocturnal enuresis should take 0.2 mg at bedtime and only if needed should the dose be increased to 0.4 mg.

The need for continued treatment should be reassessed after 3 months by means of a period of at least 1 week without DDAVP Tablets.

During the treatment of enuresis the fluid intake should be limited to a minimum and only to satisfy thirst for 8 hours following administration.

**Contra-indications, warnings, etc**
*Contra-indications:* DDAVP Tablets are contraindicated in cases of cardiac insufficiency and other conditions requiring treatment with diuretic agents. When used to control primary nocturnal enuresis DDAVP Tablets should only be used in patients with normal blood pressure.

Before prescribing DDAVP Tablets the diagnoses of psychogenic polydipsia and alcohol abuse should be excluded.

Desmopressin should not be prescribed to patients over the age of 65 for the treatment of primary nocturnal enuresis.

*Use in pregnancy:* DDAVP Tablets should be given with caution to pregnant patients, although the oxytocic effect of desmopressin is very low.

Reproduction studies performed in rats and rabbits with doses of more than 100 times the human dose have revealed no evidence of a harmful action of desmopressin on the fetus. There have been rare reports of malformations in children born to mothers treated for diabetes insipidus during pregnancy. However, a review of available data suggests no increase in the rate of malformations in children exposed to desmopressin throughout pregnancy.

*Use in lactation:* Results from analyses of milk from nursing mothers receiving high dose desmopressin (300 micrograms intranasally) indicate that the amounts of desmopressin that may be transferred to the child are considerably less than the amounts required to influence diuresis.

*Precautions:* Care should be taken with patients who have reduced renal function and/or cardiovascular disease or cystic fibrosis. In chronic renal disease the antidiuretic effect of DDAVP Tablets would be less than normal.

Patients being treated for primary nocturnal enuresis should be warned to avoid ingesting water while swimming and to discontinue DDAVP Tablets during an episode of vomiting and/or diarrhoea until their fluid balance is once again normal.

*Special precautions for use:* Precautions to prevent fluid overload must be taken in:
– conditions characterised by fluid and/or electrolyte imbalance
– patients at risk for increased intracranial pressure

*Side-effects:* Occasional side-effects include headache, stomach pain and nausea. Treatment with desmopressin without concomitant reduction of fluid intake may lead to fluid retention, hyponatraemia and in more serious cases, convulsions.

*Interactions:* Indomethacin may augment the magnitude but not the duration of response to desmopressin.

Substances which are known to release antidiuretic hormone e.g. tricyclic antidepressants, chlorpromazine and carbamazepine, may cause an additive antidiuretic effect and increase the risk of water retention.

*Overdose:* An overdose of DDAVP Tablets can lead to hyponatraemia and convulsions.

*Treatment of overdose:* Overdosage increases the risk of fluid retention and hyponatraemia. If hyponatraemia occurs desmopressin treatment should immediately be discontinued and fluid intake restricted until serum sodium is normalised.

**Pharmaceutical precautions** DDAVP Tablets should be stored at room temperature.

**Legal category** POM.

**Package quantities** Cartons containing 90 tablets in blister strip packing.

**Further information** Oral administration of desmopressin acetate results in an antidiuretic effect lasting about eight hours.

The antidiuretic effect of DDAVP Tablets is not influenced by concomitant food intake.

**Product licence numbers**
DDAVP Tablets 0.1 mg 3194/0040
DDAVP Tablets 0.2 mg 3194/0041.

## DDAVP*/DESMOPRESSIN INJECTION

**Presentation** Ampoules containing a clear colourless solution of 4 micrograms desmopressin acetate in 1 ml normal saline.

**Uses** DDAVP/Desmopressin Injection is indicated as follows:
1. Diagnosis and treatment of cranial diabetes insipidus.
2. To increase Factor VIII:C and Factor VIII:Ag in patients with mild to moderate haemophilia or von Willebrand's disease undergoing surgery or following trauma.
3. To establish renal concentration capacity.
4. To treat headache resulting from a lumbar puncture.
5. To test for fibrinolytic response.

**Dosage and administration**
*Diabetes insipidus:* By subcutaneous, intramuscular or intravenous injection.

*Adults:* The usual dose is 1 to 4 micrograms given once daily.

*Children and infants:* Doses from 0.4 micrograms (0.1 ml) may be used.

The diagnostic dose in adults and children is 2 micrograms given by subcutaneous or intramuscular injection. Failure to elaborate a concentrated urine after water deprivation, followed by the ability to do so after the administration of Desmopressin confirms a diagnosis of cranial diabetes insipidus. Failure to concentrate after the administration suggests nephrogenic diabetes insipidus.

When used for diagnostic purposes the fluid intake must be limited and not exceed 0.5 litres from 1 hour before until 8 hours after administration.

*Mild to moderate haemophilia and von Willebrand's Disease:* By intravenous administration.

The dose for adults, children and infants is 0.4 micrograms per kilogram body weight.

The dose should be diluted in 50 ml of 0.9% sodium chloride for injection and given over 20 minutes immediately prior to surgery. During administration of intravenous desmopressin, vasodilation may occur resulting in decreased blood pressure and tachycardia with facial flushing in some patients.

Increase of Factor VIII levels are dependent on basal levels and are normally between 2 and 5 times the pre-treatment levels. If results from a previous administration of desmopressin are not available then blood should be taken pre-dose and 20 minutes post-dose for assay of Factor VIII levels in order to monitor response.

Further doses may be administered at 12 hourly intervals so long as cover is required. As some patients have shown a diminishing response to successive doses, Factor VIII levels should continue to be monitored.

Unless contra-indicated, when surgery is undertaken tranexamic acid may be given orally at the recommended dose from 24 hours beforehand until healing is complete.

*Renal function testing:* By subcutaneous or intramuscular injection.

Adults and children can be expected to achieve urine concentrations above 700 mOsm/kg in the period of 5 to 9 hours following a dose of 2 micrograms DDAVP/Desmopressin injection. It is recommended that the bladder should be emptied at the time of administration.

When used for diagnostic purposes the fluid intake must be limited and not exceed 0.5 litres from 1 hour before until 8 hours after administration.

In normal infants, a urine concentration of 600 mOsm/kg should be achieved in the five hour period following a dose of 0.4 micrograms DDAVP/Desmopressin Injection. The fluid intake at the two meals following the administration should be restricted to 50% of the ordinary intake to avoid water overload.

*Post lumbar puncture headache:* By subcutaneous or intramuscular injection.

Where a headache is thought to be due to a lumbar puncture, an adult patient can be given a dose of 4 micrograms desmopressin which may be repeated 24 hours later if necessary.

Alternatively, a prophylactic dose of 4 micrograms can be given immediately prior to the lumbar puncture and repeated 24 hours later.

*Fibrinolytic response testing:* By intravenous administration.

The dose for adults and children is 0.4 micrograms per kilogram body weight. The dose should be diluted in 50 ml of 0.9% sodium chloride for injection and given over 20 minutes.

A sample of venous blood should be taken 20 minutes after the infusion. In patients with a normal response the sample should show fibrinolytic activity of euglobulin clot precipitate on fibrin plates of at least 240 mm$^2$.

**Contra-indications, warnings, etc**
*Contra-indications:* DDAVP/Desmopressin Injection is contra-indicated in cases of:

*General:* habitual and psychogenic polydipsia.

*Renal function testing, treatment of lumbar puncture headache or fibrinolytic response testing:* Should not be carried out in patients with hypertension, heart disease, cardiac insufficiency and other conditions requiring treatment with diuretic agents.

*For haemostatic use:*
- unstable angina pectoris
- decompensated cardiac insufficiency
- von Willebrand's Disease Type IIB where the administration of desmopressin may result in pseudothrombocytopenia due to the release of clotting factors which cause platelet aggregation.

*Use in pregnancy:* DDAVP/Desmopressin Injection should be given with caution to pregnant patients, although the oxytocic effect of desmopressin is very low.

Reproduction studies performed in rats and rabbits with doses of more than 100 times the human dose have revealed no evidence of a harmful action of desmopressin on the fetus. There have been rare reports of malformations in children born to mothers treated for diabetes insipidus during pregnancy. However, a review of available data suggests no increase in the rate of malformations in children exposed to desmopressin throughout pregnancy.

*Use in lactation:* Results from analyses of milk from nursing mothers receiving high dose desmopressin (300 micrograms intranasally) indicate that the amounts of desmopressin that may be transferred to the child are considerably less than the amounts required to influence diuresis or haemostasis.

*Precautions:*

*General:* Precautions to prevent fluid overload must be taken in:
- conditions characterised by fluid and/or electrolyte imbalance
- patients at risk for increased intracranial pressure.

Care should be taken with patients who have reduced renal function and/or cardiovascular disease or cystic fibrosis.

*For renal concentration capacity testing:* Testing in children below the age of 1 year should only be performed under carefully supervised conditions in hospital.

*For haemostatic use:* When repeated doses are used to control bleeding in haemophilia or von Willebrand's disease, care should be taken to prevent fluid overload. Fluid should not be forced, orally or parenterally, and patients should only take as much fluid as they require to satisfy thirst. Intravenous infusions should not be left up as a routine after surgery. Fluid accumulation can be readily monitored by weighing the patient or by determining plasma sodium or osmolality.

Measures to prevent fluid overload must be taken in patients with conditions requiring treatment with diuretic agents.

*Special warnings:* Special attention must be paid to the risk of water retention. The fluid intake should be restricted to the least possible and the body weight should be checked regularly.

If there is a gradual increase of the body weight, decrease of serum sodium to below 130 mmol/l or plasma osmolality to below 270 mOsm/kg, the fluid intake must be reduced drastically and the administration of DDAVP/Desmopressin Injection interrupted.

During infusion of DDAVP/Desmopressin Injection for haemostatic use, it is recommended that the patient's blood pressure is monitored continuously.

DDAVP/Desmopressin Injection does not reduce prolonged bleeding time in thrombocytopenia.

*Side-effects:* Occasional side-effects include headache, stomach pain, and nausea. Treatment with desmopressin without concomitant reduction of fluid intake may lead to fluid retention, hyponatraemia and in more severe cases, convulsions.

During infusion of DDAVP/Desmopressin Injection for haemostatic indications, vasodilation may occur, resulting in decreased blood pressure and tachycardia with facial flushing. This side effect is normally avoided by infusing the product over 20 minutes.

*Interactions:* Indomethacin may augment the magnitude but not the duration of the antidiuretic response to desmopressin.

Substances which are known to release antidiuretic hormone e.g. tricyclic antidepressants, chlorpromazine and carbamazepine, may cause an additive antidiuretic effect and increase the risk of water retention.

*Overdose:* An overdose of DDAVP/Desmopressin Injection can lead to hyponatraemia and convulsions.

*Treatment of overdose:* Overdosage increases the risk of fluid retention and hyponatraemia. If hyponatraemia occurs, desmopressin treatment should immediately be discontinued and fluid intake restricted until serum sodium is normalised.

**Pharmaceutical precautions** DDAVP/Desmopressin injection should be stored in the refrigerator at 4 to 8°C and must be protected from light. Doses of less than 4 micrograms (1 ml) should be measured using a suitable syringe because dilution may result in the loss of desmopressin by adsorption onto glass or plastic surfaces.

**Legal category** POM.

**Package quantities** Cartons containing 10 × 1 ml ampoules.

**Further information** Desmopressin is a structural analogue of vasopressin in which the antidiuretic activity has been increased and the duration of action prolonged. Desmopressin also retains the ability of vasopressin to increase the levels of clotting factors, Factor VIII:C, Factor VIIIR:Ag, Factor VIII:Rcof and Plasminogen Activator. Pressor activity is reduced to less than 0.01% of vasopressin as a result of which side-effects are rarely seen.

**Product licence number** 3194/0002.

## DDAVP*/DESMOPRESSIN INTRANASAL SOLUTION

**Presentation** 2.5 ml dropper bottle containing a clear solution of desmopressin acetate 100 micrograms per ml. DDAVP/Desmopressin Intranasal contains chlorbutol 0.5% as a preservative.

**Uses** DDAVP/Desmopressin Intranasal is indicated for:
1. The diagnosis and treatment of vasopressin-sensitive cranial diabetes insipidus.
2. The treatment of primary nocturnal enuresis.
3. The treatment of nocturia associated with multiple sclerosis where other treatments have failed.
4. Establishing renal concentration capacity.

**Dosage and administration**
*Treatment of diabetes insipidus:* Dosage is individual but clinical experience has shown that the average maintenance doses are as follows:

*Adults:* 10 to 20 micrograms once or twice daily.

*Children:* 5 to 20 micrograms daily, (a lower dose may be required for infants).

*Diagnosis of diabetes insipidus:* The diagnostic dose in adults and children is 20 micrograms. Failure to elaborate a concentrated urine after water deprivation, followed by the ability to do so after the administration of desmopressin confirms the diagnosis of cranial diabetes insipidus. Failure to concentrate after the administration suggests nephrogenic diabetes insipidus.

When used for diagnostic purposes the fluid intake must be limited and not exceed 0.5 litres from 1 hour before until 8 hours after administration.

*Primary nocturnal enuresis:* The starting dose for children (from 5 years of age) and adults (up to 65 years of age) with normal urine concentrating ability who have primary nocturnal enuresis is 20 micrograms at bedtime and only if needed should the dose be increased up to 40 micrograms.

The need for continued treatment should be reassessed after 3 months by means of a period of at least one week without DDAVP/Desmopressin Intranasal.

During the treatment of enuresis the fluid intake should be limited to a minimum and only to satisfy thirst for 8 hours following administration.

*Treatment of nocturia:* For multiple sclerosis patients up to 65 years of age with normal renal function suffering from nocturia the dose is 10 to 20 micrograms at bedtime. Not more than one dose should be used in any 24 hour period.

During the treatment of nocturia the fluid intake should be limited to a minimum and only to satisfy thirst for 8 hours following adminstration.

*Renal function testing:* Recommended doses for the renal concentration capacity test:
Adults: 40 micrograms.
Children (1–15 years): 20 micrograms.
Infants (to 1 year): 10 micrograms.

Adults and children with normal renal function can be expected to achieve concentrations above 700 mOsm/kg in the period of 5–9 hours following administration of DDAVP/Desmopressin Intranasal. It is recommended that the bladder should be emptied at the time of administration.

When used for diagnostic purposes the fluid intake must be limited and not exceed 0.5 litres from 1 hour before until 8 hours after administration.

In normal infants a urine concentration of 600 mOsm/kg should be achieved in the 5 hour period following the administration of DDAVP/Desmopressin Intranasal. The fluid intake at the two meals following the administration should be restricted to 50% of the ordinary intake in order to avoid water overload.

**Contra-indications, warnings, etc**
*Contra-indications:* DDAVP/Desmopressin Intranasal is contra-indicated in cases of:
- cardiac insufficiency and other conditions requiring treatment with diuretic agents
- hypersensitivity to the preservative

When used to control primary nocturnal enuresis DDAVP/Desmopressin Intranasal should only be used in patients with normal blood pressure.

Before prescribing DDAVP/Desmopressin Intranasal the diagnoses of psychogenic polydipsia and alcohol abuse should be excluded.

When used to control nocturia in patients with multiple sclerosis, desmopressin should not be used in patients with hypertension or cardiovascular disease.

Desmopressin should not be prescribed to patients over the age of 65 for the treatment of primary nocturnal enuresis or nocturia associated with multiple sclerosis.

*Use in pregnancy:* DDAVP/Desmopressin Intranasal should be given with caution to pregnant patients, although the oxytocic effect of desmopressin is very low.

Reproduction studies performed in rats and rabbits

with doses of more than 100 times the human dose have revealed no evidence of a harmful action of desmopressin on the fetus. There have been rare reports of malformations in children born to mothers treated for diabetes insipidus during pregnancy. However, a review of available data suggests no increase in the rate of malformations in children exposed to desmopressin throughout pregnancy.

*Use in lactation:* Results from analyses of milk from nursing mothers receiving high dose desmopressin (300 micrograms intranasally) indicate that the amounts of desmopressin that may be transferred to the child are considerably less than the amounts required to influence diuresis.

*Precautions:* Care should be taken with patients who have reduced renal function and/or cardiovascular disease or cystic fibrosis.

Patients being treated for primary nocturnal enuresis should be warned to avoid ingesting water while swimming and to discontinue DDAVP/Desmopressin Intranasal during an episode of vomiting and/or diarrhoea until their fluid balance is once again normal.

When DDAVP/Desmopressin Intranasal is used in the treatment of nocturia, periodic assessments should be made of blood pressure and weight to monitor the possibility of fluid overload.

Following diagnostic testing for diabetes insipidus or renal concentration capacity, care should be taken to prevent fluid overload. Fluid should not be forced, orally or parenterally, and patients should only take as much fluid as they require to satisfy thirst.

*Special precautions for use:* Precautions to prevent fluid overload must be taken in:
– conditions characterised by fluid and/or electrolyte imbalance
– patients at risk for increased intracranial pressure
  Additional precautions for using the renal concentration capacity test: Renal concentration capacity test in children below the age of 1 year should only be performed under carefully supervised conditions in hospital.

*Side-effects:* Occasional side-effects include headache, stomach pain, nausea, nasal congestion, rhinitis and epistaxis. Allergic reactions to the preservative have been reported rarely. Treatment with desmopressin without concomitant reduction of fluid intake may lead to fluid retention, hyponatraemia and in more serious cases, convulsions.

*Interactions:* Indomethacin may augment the magnitude but not the duration of response to desmopressin.
  Substances which are known to release antidiuretic hormone e.g. tricyclic antidepressants, chlorpromazine and carbamazepine, may cause an additive antidiuretic effect and increase the risk of water retention.

*Overdose:* An overdose of DDAVP/Desmopressin Intranasal can lead to hyponatraemia and convulsions.

*Treatment of overdose:* Overdosage increases the risk of fluid retention and hyponatraemia. If hyponatraemia occurs, desmopressin treatment should immediately be discontinued and fluid intake restricted until serum sodium is normalised.

**Pharmaceutical precautions** DDAVP/Desmopressin Intranasal should be stored in the refrigerator at 2 to 8˚C and must be protected from light.

**Legal category** POM.

**Package quantities** 2.5 ml bottle.

**Further information** Patients sensitive to chlorbutol should use DDAVP* Tablets or Desmotabs*.

**Product licence number** 3194/0001.

## DESMOSPRAY*

**Presentation** Metered-dose, pre-compression atomiser delivering 60 doses of 10 micrograms desmopressin acetate per spray.
  Desmospray contains benzalkonium chloride preservative.

**Uses** Desmospray is indicated for:
1. The treatment of primary nocturnal enuresis.
2. The treatment of nocturia associated with multiple sclerosis where other treatments have failed.
3. The diagnosis and treatment of vasopressin-sensitive cranial diabetes insipidus.
4. Establishing renal concentration capacity.

**Dosage and administration**
*Primary nocturnal enuresis:* The starting dose for children (from 5 years of age) and adults (up to 65 years of age) with normal urine concentrating ability who have primary nocturnal enuresis is one spray (10 micrograms) into each nostril (a total of 20 micrograms) at bedtime and only if needed should the dose be increased up to two sprays (20 micrograms) into each nostril (a total of 40 micrograms).
  The need for continued treatment should be reassessed after 3 months by means of a period of at least 1 week without Desmospray.
  During the treatment of enuresis the fluid intake should be limited to a minimum and only to satisfy thirst for 8 hours following administration.

*Treatment of nocturia:* For multiple sclerosis patients up to 65 years of age with normal renal function suffering from nocturia the dose is one or two sprays intranasally (10 to 20 micrograms) at bedtime. Not more than one dose should be used in any 24 hour period. If a dose of two sprays is required, this should be as one spray into each nostril.
  During the treatment of nocturia the fluid intake should be limited to a minimum and only to satisfy thirst for 8 hours following administration.

*Treatment of diabetes insipidus:* Dosage is individual but clinical experience has shown that the average maintenance dose in adults and children is one or two sprays (10 to 20 micrograms) once or twice daily. If a dose of two sprays is required, this should be as one spray into each nostril.

*Diagnosis of diabetes insipidus:* The diagnostic dose in adults and children is two sprays (20 micrograms).
  Failure to elaborate a concentrated urine after water deprivation, followed by the ability to do so after the administration of Desmospray confirms the diagnosis of cranial diabetes insipidus. Failure to concentrate after the administration suggests nephrogenic diabetes insipidus.
  When used for diagnostic purposes the fluid intake must be limited and not exceed 0.5 litres from 1 hour before until 8 hours after administration.

*Renal function testing:* Recommended doses for the renal concentration capacity test:
Adults: Two sprays into each nostril (a total of 40 micrograms).
Children (1–15 years): One spray into each nostril (a total of 20 micrograms).
Infants (to 1 year): One spray (10 micrograms).
  Adults and children with normal renal function can be expected to achieve concentrations above 700 mOsm/kg in the period of 5 to 9 hours following administration of Desmospray. It is recommended that the bladder should be emptied at the time of administration.
  When used for diagnostic purposes the fluid intake must be limited and not exceed 0.5 litres from 1 hour before until 8 hours after administration.
  In normal infants a urine concentration of 600 mOsm/kg should be achieved in the 5 hour period following administration of Desmospray. The fluid intake at the two meals following the administration should be restricted to 50% of the ordinary intake in order to avoid water overload.

**Contra-indications, warnings, etc**
*Contra-indications:* Desmospray is contraindicated in cases of:
– cardiac insufficiency and other conditions requiring treatment with diuretic agents
– hypersensitivity to the preservative
  When used to control primary nocturnal enuresis Desmospray should only be used in patients with normal blood pressure.
  Before prescribing Desmospray the diagnoses of psychogenic polydipsia and alcohol abuse should be excluded.
  When used to control nocturia in patients with multiple sclerosis, desmopressin should not be used in patients with hypertension or cardiovascular disease.
  Desmopressin should not be prescribed to patients over the age of 65 for the treatment of primary nocturnal enuresis or nocturia associated with multiple sclerosis.

*Use in pregnancy:* Desmospray should be given with caution to pregnant patients, although the oxytocic effect of desmopressin is very low.
  Reproduction studies performed in rats and rabbits with doses of more than 100 times the human dose have revealed no evidence of a harmful action of desmopressin on the fetus. There have been rare reports of malformations in children born to mothers treated for diabetes insipidus during pregnancy. However, a review of available data suggests no increase in the rate of malformations in children exposed to desmopressin throughout pregnancy.

*Use in lactation:* Results from analyses of milk from nursing mothers receiving high dose desmopressin (300 micrograms intranasally) indicate that the amounts of desmopressin that may be transferred to the child are considerably less than the amounts required to influence diuresis.

*Precautions:* Care should be taken with patients who have reduced renal function and/or cardiovascular disease or cystic fibrosis.

Patients being treated for primary nocturnal enuresis should be warned to avoid ingesting water while swimming and to discontinue Desmospray during an episode of vomiting and/or diarrhoea until their fluid balance is once again normal.

When Desmospray is used in the treatment of nocturia, periodic assessments should be made of blood pressure and weight to monitor the possibility of fluid overload.

Following diagnostic testing for diabetes insipidus or renal concentration capacity, care should be taken to prevent fluid overload. Fluid should not be forced, orally or parenterally, and patients should only take as much fluid as they require to satisfy thirst.

*Special precautions for use:* Precautions to prevent fluid overload must be taken in:
– conditions characterised by fluid and/or electrolyte imbalance
– patients at risk for increased intracranial pressure
  Additional precautions for using the renal concentration capacity test: Renal concentration capacity test in children below the age of 1 year should only be performed under carefully supervised conditions in hospital.

*Side-effects:* Occasional side-effects include headache, stomach pain, nausea, nasal congestion, rhinitis and epistaxis. Allergic reactions to the preservative have been reported rarely. Treatment with desmopressin without concomitant reduction of fluid intake may lead to fluid retention, hyponatraemia and in more serious cases, convulsions.

*Interactions:* Indomethacin may augment the magnitude but not the duration of response to desmopressin.
  Substances which are known to release antidiuretic hormone e.g. tricyclic antidepressants, chlorpromazine and carbamazepine, may cause an additive antidiuretic effect and increase the risk of water retention.

*Overdose:* An overdose of Desmospray can lead to hyponatraemia and convulsions.

*Treatment of overdose:* Overdosage increases the risk of fluid retention and hyponatraemia. If hyponatraemia occurs, desmopressin treatment should immediately be discontinued and fluid intake restricted until serum sodium is normalised.

**Pharmaceutical precautions** Desmospray should be stored at room temperature (up to 25˚C) and must be protected from light.

**Legal category** POM.

**Package quantities** 6 ml bottle (60 doses of 10 micrograms desmopressin acetate per spray).

**Further information** Children requiring doses of less than 10 micrograms should use DDAVP Tablets, Desmotabs 0.2 mg or DDAVP/Desmopressin Intranasal solution which employs a small plastic calibrated catheter to administer doses of 5 to 20 micrograms. Patients sensitive to benzalkonium chloride should use DDAVP* Tablets or Desmotabs* 0.2 mg.

**Product licence number** 3194/0024.

## DESMOTABS* 0.2 mg

**Presentation** Uncoated, white, flat, round tablets of 8 mm diameter, scored one side and marked '0.2' on the other side, each containing desmopressin acetate 0.2 mg.

**Uses** Desmotabs are indicated for the treatment of primary nocturnal enuresis.

**Dosage and administration**
*Primary nocturnal enuresis:* Children (from 5 years of age) and adults (up to 65 years of age) with normal urine concentrating ability who have primary nocturnal enuresis should take 0.2 mg at bedtime and only if needed should the dose be increased to 0.4 mg.
  The need for continued treatment should be reassessed after 3 months by means of a period of at least 1 week without Desmotabs.
  During the treatment of enuresis the fluid intake should be limited to a minimum and only to satisfy thirst for 8 hours following administration.

**Contra-indications, warnings, etc**
*Contra-indications:* Desmotabs are contra-indicated in cases of cardiac insufficiency and other conditions requiring treatment with diuretic agents. Desmotabs should only be used in patients with normal blood pressure.
  Before prescribing Desmotabs the diagnoses of

psychogenic polydipsia and alcohol abuse should be excluded.

Desmopressin should not be prescribed to patients over the age of 65 for the treatment of primary nocturnal enuresis.

*Use in pregnancy:* Desmotabs should be given with caution to pregnant patients, although the oxytocic effect of desmopressin is very low.

Reproduction studies performed in rats and rabbits with doses of more than 100 times the human dose have revealed no evidence of a harmful action of desmopressin on the fetus. There have been rare reports of malformations in children born to mothers treated for diabetes insipidus during pregnancy. However, a review of available data suggests no increase in the rate of malformations in children exposed to desmopressin throughout pregnancy.

*Use in lactation:* Results from analyses of milk from nursing mothers receiving high dose desmopressin (300 micrograms intranasally) indicate that the amounts of desmopressin that may be transferred to the child are considerably less than the amounts required to influence diuresis.

*Precautions:* Care should be taken with patients who have cystic fibrosis.

Patients being treated for primary nocturnal enuresis should be warned to avoid ingesting water while swimming and to discontinue Desmotabs during an episode of vomiting and/or diarrhoea until their fluid balance is once again normal.

*Special precautions for use:* Precautions to prevent fluid overload must be taken in:
– conditions characterised by fluid and/or electrolyte imbalance;
– patients at risk for increased intracranial pressure.

*Side-effects:* Occasional side-effects include headache, stomach pain and nausea. Treatment with desmopressin without concomitant reduction of fluid intake may lead to fluid retention, hyponatraemia and in more serious cases, convulsions.

*Interactions:* Indomethacin may augment the magnitude but not the duration of response to desmopressin.

Substances which are known to release antidiuretic hormone e.g. tricyclic antidepressants, chlorpromazine and carbamazepine, may cause an additive antidiuretic effect and increase the risk of water retention.

*Overdose:* An overdose of Desmotabs can lead to hyponatraemia and convulsions.

*Treatment of overdose:* Overdosage increases the risk of fluid retention and hyponatraemia. If hyponatraemia occurs, desmopressin treatment should immediately be discontinued and fluid intake restricted until serum sodium is normalised.

**Pharmaceutical precautions**  Desmotabs should be stored at room temperature.

**Legal category**  POM.

**Package quantities**  Cartons containing 28 tablets in blister strip packing.

**Further information**  Oral administration of Desmopressin acetate results in an antidiuretic effect lasting about eight hours.

The antidiuretic effect of Desmotabs is not influenced by concomitant food intake.

**Product licence number**  3194/0046.

## GESTONE*

**Presentation**  Ampoules of a sterile straw-coloured solution of Progesterone BP 25 or 50 mg per ml in ethyl oleate for injection containing 10% v/v benzyl alcohol.

**Uses**  Gestone is indicated for the treatment of dysfunctional uterine bleeding.

It is also indicated for the maintenance of early pregnancy in cases of documented history of repeated miscarriages due to luteal phase defect and in selected cases as an adjunct to successful treatment of infertility with techniques such as in-vitro fertilisation (IVF) or gamete intra-fallopian transfer (GIFT) in order to facilitate uterine implantation of the fertilised ovum.

**Dosage and administration**  Gestone is given by intramuscular injection. It should be injected deep into the buttock, rather than the thigh or deltoid, using a 1.5 inch (3.8 cm) needle. This site has ample fat cells where a depot of progesterone can be formed for slow release.

*Dysfunctional uterine bleeding:* 5–10 mg daily for 5–10 days until 2 days before anticipated onset of menstruation.

*Maintenance of pregnancy:* Twice weekly or more frequent (maximum: daily) injections of 25–100 mg from approximately day 15, or day of transfer of embryo or gametes usually until 8–16 weeks of pregnancy when secretion of progesterone from the placenta should be established.

Daily dosage can be increased to 200 mg at the discretion of the physician.

As the indications for Gestone are restricted to women of child-bearing age, dosage recommendations for children and the elderly are not appropriate.

**Contra-indications, warnings, etc**
*Contra-indications:* Hypersensitivity to progestins, undiagnosed vaginal bleeding, missed or incomplete abortion, mammary or genital tract carcinoma, thrombophlebitis, cerebral haemorrhage, marked hepatic dysfunction. Contraindicated as a diagnostic test for pregnancy.

*Interactions:* Gestone may interfere with the effects of bromocriptine. Gestone may affect the results of laboratory tests of hepatic and/or endocrine functions. Gestone may raise the plasma concentration of cyclosporin.

*Effects on ability to drive and use machinery:* No known effect.

*Other undesirable effects:* Breakthrough bleeding, change in menstrual flow, amenorrhoea, changes in cervical erosion and secretions, breast changes, oedema, weight gain, catabolism, cholestatic jaundice, allergic reactions and rashes, acne, chloasma, mental depression, pyrexia, insomnia, somnolence, nausea, alopecia, hirsutism, local reactions at site of injection.

*Use in pregnancy and lactation:* Gestone may be used to maintain pregnancy where there is deficient production of endogenous progesterone from the corpus luteum. It should not be necessary to administer Gestone once there is adequate secretion of placental progesterone. Gestone contains progesterone itself, the same as the naturally secreted hormone, and is not associated with masculinization of a female foetus as are synthetic progestins.

Detectable amounts of progesterone enter the breast milk. As the effect on the suckling infant has not been determined, the use of Gestone during lactation is not recommended.

*Other special warnings and precautions:* Gestone should be used cautiously in patients with conditions that might be aggravated by fluid retention (e.g. hypertension, cardiac disease, renal disease, epilepsy), with a history of mental depression, diabetes, mild to moderate hepatic dysfunction, acute intermittent porphyria, migraine or photosensitivity.

If unexplained, sudden or gradual, partial or complete loss of vision, proptosis or diplopia, papilloedema, retinal vascular lesions or migraine occur during therapy, the drug should be discontinued and appropriate diagnostic and therapeutic measures instituted.

*Overdosage:* This is unlikely and is not expected to produce any adverse effects. Treatment is observation and, if necessary, symptomatic and supportive measures should be provided.

**Pharmaceutical precautions**  Protect from light. On storage, solid matter may separate and this should be redissolved by warming before use.

**Legal category**  POM.

**Package quantities**  Ampoules containing: 25 mg in 1 ml; 50 mg in 1 ml; 100 mg in 2 ml. Boxes of 10.

**Further information**  Nil.

**Product licence numbers**
25 mg   3194/0061
50 mg   3194/0062
100 mg  3194/0063.

## GLYPRESSIN*

**Presentation**  Glypressin 1 mg. Freeze-dried powder for injection. Supplied with 5 ml ampoule of sterile diluent.

**Uses**  Glypressin (triglycyl-lysine-vasopressin) is a hormonogen. When injected into the blood the glycyl residues of the molecule are slowly cleaved off by enzymatic action generating the release of vasopressin. Glypressin may thus be regarded as a circulating depot, releasing vasopressin at a constant rate.

The beneficial effect of injection of vasopressin in patients with bleeding oesophageal varices is established. However, the side-effects of vasopressin given in the doses necessary to obtain a satisfactory haemostatic effect have induced a cautious attitude in many clinicians. These side-effects are primarily the pressor response of vasopressin of the blood pressure and the release into the circulation of plasminogen activator which leads to increased fibrinolytic activity in the blood. Smooth muscle constriction in the g.i. tract also occurs with unmodified vasopressin leading to abdominal colic while coronary vasoconstriction may lead to cardiac ischaemia.

Extensive tests in animals and humans have shown that Glypressin in itself is without hormonal activity. Appropriate doses of glypressin however, lead to a reduction of portal vein pressure, but arterial blood pressure changes are far less marked than after vasopressin and further Glypressin does not increase the fibrinolytic activity of the blood.

Glypressin is indicated in the treatment of bleeding oesophageal varices.

**Dosage and administration**  In acute variceal bleeding, 2 mg Glypressin should be administered by intravenous bolus injection followed by 1 or 2 mg every 4 to 6 hours until bleeding is controlled, up to a maximum of 72 hours.

**Contra-indications, warnings, etc**
*Contra-indications:* Due to its effect on smooth muscle Glypressin is contra-indicated in pregnancy.

*Warnings and precautions:* The pressor and antidiuretic effects of Glypressin are reduced (compared with lysine or arginine vasopressin) but the product should still be used with great caution in patients with hypertension, advanced atherosclerosis, cardiac dysrhythmias or coronary insufficiency. Constant monitoring of blood pressure, serum sodium and potassium fluid balance are essential. The possibility of immunological sensitisation cannot be excluded.

*Side-effects:* Because the severity of pressor and antidiuretic activities are reduced, few side-effects have been recorded. Infrequent effects include: abdominal cramps, headache, transient blanching, increase in arterial blood pressure.

*Drug interactions:* Glypressin is intended for the short term treatment of acute bleeding oesophageal varices. No interactions are known with other products likely to be used concurrently.

*Treatment of overdose:* Increase in blood pressure following the use of Glypressin in patients with known hypertension has been controlled with clonidine 150 micrograms intravenously.

**Pharmaceutical precautions**  Freeze-dried powder and the diluent may be stored at room temperature, protected from direct sunlight. Each 1 mg vial of Glypressin should be reconstituted with 5 ml diluent supplied and used immediately.

**Legal category**  POM.

**Package quantity**  Glypressin Terlipressin 1 mg freeze dried powder: Single use vial. Diluent 5 ml ampoule supplied with each vial. Cartons of five vials and ampoules.

**Product licence number**  3194/0018.

## CHORAGON 5000 U and CHORAGON SOLVENT*

**Presentation**  Choragon 5000 U is presented in ampoules containing a white, sterile, freeze-dried plug of 5000 Units of Chorionic Gonadotrophin PhEur (HCG) in the inactive carrier mannitol, for injection. It is supplied with a 1 ml ampoule of solvent for reconstitution of the powder.

**Uses**  Human chorionic gonadotrophin (HCG) is obtained from the urine of pregnant women. The action of HCG is predominantly that of the pituitary luteinising hormone.

*In the female:* In the management of anovulatory infertility, Choragon can be given to induce ovulation after follicular development has been stimulated with follicle stimulating hormone.

*In the male:* HCG stimulates the interstitial cells to secrete testosterone. Choragon can therefore be used in the management of delayed puberty, undescended testes and oligospermia.

**Dosage and administration**  Choragon is given by intramuscular injection. Treatment should only commence after expert assessment.

*In the female: Induction of ovulation:* 10,000 units mid-cycle if plasma oestrogen levels are favourable following follicular stimulation.

*In the male: Delayed puberty:* Dose should be titrated against plasma testosterone, starting with 500 units twice weekly. Treatment should be continued for 4–6 weeks.

*Undescended testes:* Treatment should begin before puberty, the optimum age range being 7–10 years. 500 units three times weekly is a suitable starting dose, but this may be increased up to 4000 units thrice weekly if necessary. Treatment should continue for 6–10 weeks. In males over 17 years of age a commencing dose of 1000 units twice weekly can be given. Treatment should be continued for one or two months after testicular descent.

*Oligospermia:* Dose should be titrated against seminal analysis starting with 500 units two or three times weekly. Treatment should be continued for 16 weeks.

**Contra-indications, warnings, etc**
*Contra-indications:* HCG should not be given to patients with disorders that might be exacerbated by androgen release.

*Warnings:* HCG should be given with care to patients in whom fluid retention might be a hazard, as in asthma, epilepsy, migraine, or cardiac or renal disorders.

Allergic reactions may occur and patients thought to be susceptible should be given skin tests before treatment.

HCG preparations should only be used under the supervision of a specialist having available adequate facilities for appropriate laboratory monitoring.

*In the female:* Use in induction of ovulation may result in ovarian enlargement or cysts, acute abdominal pain, superovulation, or multiple pregnancies, particularly if endocrine monitoring is inadequate.

*In the male:* Treatment for undescended testes may produce precocious puberty; use should cease immediately. Gynaecomastia has been reported. A growth spurt may also be associated with use and this should be kept in mind particularly where epiphyseal growth is still potentially active.

*Side-effects:* Headache, tiredness and mood changes have been described.

**Pharmaceutical precautions** Choragon in the dry state, in sealed ampoules, will remain stable if protected from light and stored at a temperature not exceeding 20°C. Solutions are unstable and should be freshly prepared.

**Legal category** POM.

**Package quantities** Cartons containing 3 ampoules of Choragon 5000 U and solvent for reconstitution of the powder.

**Further information** The solvent contains 0.9% Sodium Chloride in Water for Injection PhEur.

**Product licence number** 03194/0065

## PENTASA* MESALAZINE ENEMA

**Presentation** Individually foil-wrapped unit dose plastic enema bottles with protective sleeve. Each bottle contains 100 ml aqueous suspension containing 1 g mesalazine.

**Uses** Treatment of ulcerative colitis affecting the distal colon and rectum.

**Dosage and administration** *Adults:* The recommended dosage is one enema at bedtime.
*Children:* Not recommended.

**Contra-indications, warnings, etc** *Contra indications:* Known sensitivity to salicylates.

*Special precautions and warnings:* Serious blood dyscrasias have been reported very rarely with mesalazine. Haematological investigations should be performed if the patient develops unexplained bleeding, bruising, purpura, anaemia, fever or sore throat. Treatment should be stopped if there is suspicion or evidence of blood dyscrasia.

*Use during pregnancy and lactation:* Pentasa should be used with caution during pregnancy and lactation and only if the potential benefit outweighs the possible hazards in the opinion of the physician. No data are available on teratogenicity but negligible quantities of mesalazine cross the placenta and none can be detected in breast milk during sulphasalazine therapy.

*Use in the Elderly:* Pentasa should be used with caution in the elderly and should only be used in those patients with normal renal function.

*Adverse reactions:* Minor side effects which may occasionally occur include headache, nausea, diarrhoea and abdominal pain. Mesalazine may be associated with an exacerbation of the symptoms of colitis in those patients who have previously had such problems with sulphasalazine. There have been rare reports of leucopenia, neutropenia, agranulocytosis, aplastic anaemia and thrombocytopenia, pancreatitis, hepatitis, allergic lung reactions, lupus-erythematosus-like reactions and rash (including urticaria), interstitial nephritis and nephrotic syndrome with oral mesalazine treatment, usually reversible on withdrawal. Renal failure has been reported. Mesalazine-induced nephrotoxocity should be suspected in patients developing renal dysfunction during treatment. Pentasa is not recommended in patients with renal impairment. Patients with raised blood urea or proteinuria should be treated with caution.

*Treatment of overdosage:* There is no specific antidote; intravenous infusion of electrolytes may be used to promote diuresis.

**Pharmaceutical precautions** Store at room temperature. Protect from light. Use immediately after opening the individual foil pack.

**Legal category** POM.

**Package quantities** Cartons containing seven individually foil-wrapped 100 ml enemas.

**Further information** A plastic sleeve bearing administration instructions is provided for each enema bottle. The sleeve also facilitates hygienic application of the enema and disposal after use.

**Product licence number** 3194/0027.

*Product licence holder:* Ferring Pharmaceuticals Ltd, Feltham, Middx.

## PENTASA* SLOW RELEASE TABLETS

**Presentation** Pentasa Slow Release Tablets 250 mg: Round, white to light grey mottled tablets with a break line on the front face. The tablets are marked '250' on the front face, and 'PENTASA' on the reverse. Each tablet contains 250 mg mesalazine in a slow release presentation.

Pentasa Slow Release Tablets 500 mg: Round, white to light grey mottled tablets with a break line on the front face. The tablets are marked '500' on the front face, and 'PENTASA' on the reverse. Each tablet contains 500 mg mesalazine in a slow release presentation.

**Uses** For the treatment of mild to moderate acute exacerbations of ulcerative colitis.

For the maintenance of remission of ulcerative colitis.

**Dosage and administration** The tablets may be dispersed in water to facilitate swallowing but they should not be chewed.
*Adults:*
*Acute treatment:* Individual dosage up tp 4 g mesalazine daily in 2 or 3 divided doses.
*Maintenance treatment:* Individual dosage. Recommended starting dose is 1500 mg of mesalazine daily in 2 or 3 divided doses.
*Children:* Not recommended.
*Elderly patients:* Pentasa is not recommended in patients with renal impairment. Otherwise, the usual adult dose applies.

**Contra-indications, warnings, etc**
*Contra-indications:* Children under the age of 15 years. Known sensitivity to salicylates.

*Special precautions and warnings:* Serious blood dyscrasias have been reported very rarely with mesalazine. Haematological investigations should be performed if the patient develops unexplained bleeding, bruising, purpura, anaemia, fever or sore throat. Treatment should be stopped if there is suspicion or evidence of blood dyscrasia.

*Use during pregnancy and lactation:* Pentasa should be used with caution during pregnancy and lactation and only if the potential benefit outweighs the possible hazards in the opinion of the physician. No data are available on teratogenicity but negligible quantities of mesalazine cross the placenta and none can be detected in breast milk.

*Adverse reactions:* Minor side effects which may occasionally occur include headache, nausea, diarrhoea and abdominal pain. Mesalazine may be associated with an exacerbation of the symptoms of colitis in those patients who have previously had such problems with sulphasalazine. There have been rare reports of leucopenia, neutropenia, agranulocytosis, aplastic anaemia and thrombocytopenia, pancreatitis, hepatitis, allergic lung reactions, lupus-erythematosus-like reactions and rash (including urticaria), interstitial nephritis and nephrotic syndrome with oral mesalazine treatment, usually reversible on withdrawal. Renal failure has been reported. Mesalazine-induced nephrotoxocity should be suspected in patients developing renal dysfunction during treatment. Pentasa is not recommended in patients with renal impairment. Patients with raised blood urea or proteinuria should be treated with caution.

*Treatment of overdose:* There is no specific antidote; intravenous infusion of electrolytes may be used to promote diuresis.

**Pharmaceutical precautions** Store at room temperature. Protect from light.

**Legal category** POM.

**Package quantities** Amber glass screw-top bottles each containing 200×250 mg tablets. Double aluminium foil blister packages in cartons containing 100×500 mg tablets.

**Further information** Pentasa Slow Release Tablets disintegrate in the stomach to yield coated slow release granules which are conveyed into the intestinal tract. The release of mesalazine from the granulation takes place at all physiological pH values but is slower in the acidic conditions found in the upper gastrointestinal tract. This approach ensures that mesalazine is available in the lumen of the intestine for topical activity in ulcerative colitis. Plasma levels of mesalazine and its metabolites are similar to those observed during therapy with sulphasalazine.

**Product licence numbers**
Pentasa Slow Release Tablets 250 mg 3194/0043.
Pentasa Slow Release Tablets 500 mg 3194/0044.

*Product licence holder:* Ferring Pharmaceuticals Ltd, Feltham, Middlesex.

## PENTASA* SUPPOSITORY 1 g

**Presentation** Oval, compressed grey to pale brown, specked suppositories each containing 1 g mesalazine in a macrogol 6000 base.

**Uses** For the treatment of ulcerative proctitis.

**Dosage and administration**
*Adults:*
*Acute treatment:* Recommended dosage: 1 suppository daily for 2–4 weeks.
*Maintenance Treatment:* 1 suppository daily.
*Children:* Not recommended.
*Elderly patients:* Pentasa is not recommended in patients with renal impairment. Otherwise, the usual adult dose applies.

**Contra-indications, warnings, etc**
*Contra-indications:* Children under the age of 15 years. Known sensitivity to salicylates.

*Precautions and warnings:* Serious blood dyscrasias have been reported very rarely with mesalazine. Haematological investigations should be performed if the patient develops unexplained bleeding, bruising, purpura, anaemia, fever or sore throat. Treatment should be stopped if there is suspicion or evidence of blood dyscrasia.

*Use during pregnancy and lactation:* Pentasa should be used with caution during pregnancy and lactation and only if the potential benefit outweighs the possible hazards in the opinion of the physician. No data are available on teratogenicity but negligible quantities of mesalazine cross the placenta and none can be detected in breast milk.

*Adverse reactions:* Minor side effects which may occasionally occur include headache, nausea, diarrhoea and abdominal pain. Mesalazine may be associated with an exacerbation of the symptoms of colitis in those patients who have previously had such problems with sulphasalazine. There have been rare reports of leucopenia, neutropenia, agranulocytosis, aplastic anaemia and thrombocytopenia, pancreatitis, hepatitis, allergic lung reactions, lupus-erythematosus-like reactions and rash (including urticaria), interstitial nephritis and nephrotic syndrome with oral mesalazine treatment, usually reversible on withdrawal. Renal failure has been reported. Mesalazine-induced nephrotoxocity should be suspected in patients developing renal dysfunction during treatment. Pentasa is not recommended in patients with renal impairment. Patients with raised blood urea or proteinuria should be treated with caution.

*Treatment of overdose:* There is no specific antidote; intravenous infusion of electrolytes may be used to promote diuresis.

**Pharmaceutical precautions** Store at room temperature. Protect from light. Use immediately after opening the individual foil pack.

**Legal category** POM.

**Package quantities** Each suppository is individually packed in double aluminium foil and is available in cartons of 28 suppositories.

**Further information** Each pack contains administration instructions for patients and rubber finger-protectors to facilitate hygenic insertion. The release profile for the Pentasa Suppositories is comparable to Pentasa Enemas.

**Product licence number** 3194/0045.

*Product licence holder:* Ferring Pharmaceuticals Ltd, Feltham, Middlesex.

## PICOLAX*

**Presentation** Sachets each containing 16.1 g of powder for oral administration. Active ingredients: Sodium picosulphate 10 mg with magnesium citrate formed in solution. Packed in complete treatment packs of 2 sachets in outers of 25×2 sachets.

**Uses** For clearance of the bowel prior to examination by radiography, endoscopy or surgery.

**Dosage and administration**
*Adults:* The contents of one sachet are dissolved in a cup of water. Stir for 2–3 minutes and drink the

mixture. If the solution becomes hot, wait until it cools sufficiently to drink.

1st dose – 1 sachet before 8 am on the day prior to examination.

2nd dose – 1 sachet between 2 and 4 pm on the day prior to examination.

*Children:* Timings as above.

1–2 years: ¼ sachet morning, ¼ sachet afternoon.

2–4 years: ½ sachet morning, ½ sachet afternoon.

4–9 years: 1 sachet morning, ½ sachet afternoon.

9 and above: adult dose.

*Elderly patients:* As for adults.

A low residue diet is recommended for 2 days prior to examination, and a liberal intake of clear fluids. Patients should drink as much as is required to satisfy thirst. A suggested diet plan is given in the Patient Information Leaflet. Patients should be warned to expect frequent, loose bowel movements starting within 3 hours of the first dose. Some authorities recommend a high fluid intake but no food at all during the 24 hours prior to examination.

**Contra-indications, warnings, etc** The usual general contraindications to purgatives apply. In patients with severely reduced renal function, accumulation of magnesium in plasma may occur. Another preparation should be used in such cases.

Picolax should not be used in suspected toxic dilatation of the colon. Picolax is also contraindicated in patients with clinical evidence of bowel obstruction.

*Use in pregnancy and lactation:* Reproduction studies with sodium picosulphate performed in animals have revealed no evidence of a harmful action on the fetus. However, clinical experience of the use of Picolax during pregnancy is limited and caution should be observed, particularly during the first trimester.

Neither sodium picosulphate nor magnesium citrate have been shown to be excreted in breast milk.

*Warnings and precautions:* Picolax should not be used in patients with undiagnosed abdominal symptoms. Care should also be taken in patients with inflammatory bowel disease and in patients with suspected bowel obstruction.

A suboptimal oral intake of water and electrolytes could create clinically significant deficiencies in less fit patients. In this regard, elderly, debilitated and patients at risk of hypokalaemia may need particular attention.

The period of bowel cleansing should not exceed 24 hours because longer preparation may increase the risk of water and electrolyte imbalance.

*Side effects:* As with other bowel cleansing regimens, treatment with Picolax may cause headache, tiredness, nausea, griping and anal pain. Isolated cases have been reported of allergic reactions including anaphylaxis or of vomiting and severe diarrhoea leading to hyponatraemia and convulsions in the absence of adequate salt replacement.

*Interactions:* As a purgative, Picolax increases gastro-intestinal transit rate. Absorption of other orally administered medicines may therefore be modified during the treatment period. The efficacy of Picolax is lowered by bulk-forming laxatives.

Care should be taken with patients already receiving drugs which may be associated with hypokalaemia (such as diuretics or corticosteroids, or drugs where hypokalaemia is a particular risk i.e. cardiac glycosides).

*Treatment of overdose:* Overdosage would lead to profuse diarrhoea. Treatment is by general supportive measures and maintenance of fluid intake.

**Pharmaceutical precautions** Store at room temperature, in a cool dry place.

**Legal category** P.

**Package quantity** Treatment units of two sachets in cartons of 25×2 sachets.

**Product licence number** 3194/0014

## PROPESS*-RS ▼

**Presentation** Propess-RS is presented as a thin, flat, semi-opaque polymeric pessary which is rectangular in shape with radiused corners contained within a knitted polyester retrieval system.

Each pessary consists of a non-biodegradable polymeric drug delivery device containing dinoprostone ($PGE_2$) dispersed throughout its matrix, and releasing approximately 5 mg $PGE_2$ over 12 hours. The reservoir of 10 mg dinoprostone serves to maintain constant release.

The retrieval system, within which each pessary is supplied, consists of a one-piece knitted polyester pouch and withdrawal tape. This ensures easy and reliable removal of the pessary when the patient's requirement for $PGE_2$ has been fulfilled or an obstetric event makes it necessary to stop further drug administration.

**Uses** Propess-RS is indicated for the initiation and/or continuation of cervical ripening in patients at term (from 38 weeks gestation) when there is a singleton cephalic presentation. The ripeness of the cervix should be assessed by a Bishop's Score or modification thereof. Propess-RS is indicated for induction of labour when the score is 6 or less by the original Bishop's Score (Bishop, E.H., (1964) Obstetrics & Gynecology, *24* (2), 266–268). There should be no fetal or maternal contra-indications.

**Dosage and administration**

*Dosage:* One pessary. This is usually sufficient to achieve cervical ripening.

If there has been insufficient cervical ripening in 8–12 hours, the pessary should be removed. It may be replaced by a second pessary. This should also be removed not more than 12 hours later. Not more than 2 consecutive pessaries should be used in the course of therapy.

*Administration:* Do not remove the pessary from the retrieval system in which it is supplied.

The pessary should be inserted high into the posterior vaginal fornix using only small amounts of water soluble lubricants to aid insertion. After the pessary has been inserted, the withdrawal tape may be cut with scissors always ensuring there is sufficient tape outside the vagina to allow removal. No attempt should be made to tuck the end of the tape into the vagina as this may make retrieval more difficult.

The patient should be recumbent for 20 mins–30 mins after insertion. As $PGE_2$ will be released continuously over a period of 12 hours, it is important to monitor uterine contractions and fetal condition at frequent regular intervals.

*Retrieval:* It is necessary to remove the pessary to terminate drug administration when cervical ripening is judged to be complete or for any of the reasons listed below.

The pessary can be removed quickly and easily by gentle traction on the retrieval tape.

The pessary should be removed immediately under any of the following circumstances:

1. Onset of labour. For the purpose of induction of labour with Propess-RS, the onset of labour is defined as the presence of regular painful uterine contractions occurring every 3 minutes irrespective of any cervical change. There are two important points to note:

(i) Once regular, painful contractions have been established with Propess-RS they will not reduce in frequency or intensity as long as Propess-RS remains *in situ* because $PGE_2$ is still being administered.

(ii) Patients, particularly multigravidae, may develop regular painful contractions without any apparent cervical change. Effacement and dilatation of the cervix may not occur until uterine activity is established. Because of this, once regular painful uterine activity is established with Propess-RS *in situ*, the pessary should be removed irrespective of cervical state to avoid the possibility of uterine hyperstimulation.

2. Spontaneous rupture of the membranes and at artificial rupture of membranes.

3. Any suggestion of uterine hyperstimulation or hypertonic uterine contractions.

4. Evidence of fetal distress.

5. Evidence of maternal systemic adverse $PGE_2$ effects such as nausea, vomiting hypotension or tachycardia.

6. Prior to starting an intravenous infusion of oxytocin.

**Contra-indications, warnings, etc**

*Contra-indications:* Propess-RS should not be used or left in place:

1. When labour has started.

2. When the membranes have ruptured.

3. When oxytocic drugs are being given.

4. When strong prolonged uterine contraction would be inappropriate such as in patients:

a. who have had previous major uterine surgery.

b. who have had previous surgery to the cervix of the uterus.

c. with a major degree of cephalopelvic disproportion.

d. with fetal malpresentation.

e. with suspicion or evidence of fetal distress.

f. with a history of difficult or traumatic deliveries.

g. who have had more than three full term deliveries.

5. When there is a history of, or current pelvic inflammatory disease, unless adequate prior treatment has been instituted.

6. When there is reason to believe there may be hypersensitivity to $PGE_2$.

7. When there is a multiple pregnancy.

*Precautions and warnings:* The suitability of the patient and the condition of the cervix should be assessed carefully before Propess-RS is used. After insertion, uterine activity and fetal condition must be monitored regularly. If there is any suggestion of maternal or fetal complications or adverse effects, $PGE_2$ delivery should be stopped by removing the pessary from the vagina.

Propess-RS should be used with caution in patients with a previous history of uterine hypertony, glaucoma, or asthma.

Medication with non-steroidal anti-inflammatory drugs, including aspirin, should be stopped before administration of $PGE_2$.

If uterine contractions are prolonged and excessive, there is a possibility of uterine hypertonus or rupture and the pessary should be removed immediately.

It would be prudent to remove the Propess-RS pessary should epidural anaesthesia be given in anticipation of labour before membrane rupture.

High doses of Prostaglandin of the E and F series have been shown to induce bone proliferation in animals at high doses. Similar effects have been observed in neonates exposed to prostaglandins for long periods but no such changes have been seen with the short term administration of Propess-RS for cervical ripening.

*Side-effects:* The occasional effects seen have been those normally associated with intravaginal $PGE_2$ administration.

CTG changes and unspecified fetal distress have been reported during and after administration of intravaginal $PGE_2$. Increased uterine activity with hypertonic contractions with or without fetal distress has been reported and immediate removal of the pessary is recommended. There is a much greater risk of hyperstimulation if the $PGE_2$ source is not removed before administration of oxytocin because prostaglandins are known to potentiate the uterotonic effects of oxytocic drugs.

Gastro-intestinal effects such as nausea, vomiting and diarrhoea have been reported.

$PGE_2$ is known to be responsible for the patency of the ductus arteriosus in pregnancy but there have been no reports of 'blue babies' in the neonatal period after the use of Propess-RS. In a 3 year follow up of 121 babies after labour induction with $PGE_2$, 51 of whom received Propess-RS, there were no adverse effects on physical development or psychomotor evolution in the infants.

*Overdose:* Overdosage or hypersensitivity may lead to hyperstimulation of the uterine muscle or fetal distress. The Propess-RS pessary should be removed immediately and the patient should be managed in accordance with local protocol.

**Pharmaceutical precautions** Propess-RS should be stored unopened, in the foil pack in a refrigerator (2–8°C) until immediately before use.

The opening on one side of the retrieval device is present only to allow the manufacturer to enclose the pessary into the retrieval device during manufacture.

The pessary should NEVER be removed from the retrieval device. On removal of the product, the pessary will have swollen to 2–3 times its original size and be pliable. The whole product should be disposed as clinical waste.

**Legal category** POM.

**Package quantities** Propess-RS is presented in cartons of four individual, sealed aluminium foil/polyethylene laminate sachets.

**Further information** Propess-RS is not approved nor intended for use as an abortifacient.

*Drug delivery system information:* The vaginal pessary is a product designed around the Controlled Therapeutics Delivery System. It is a patented hydrophilic hydrogel polymer which controls the delivery of $PGE_2$ at a near constant rate as it swells in vaginal fluid. In this process the pessary slowly becomes softer and rubbery in consistency, but maintains its physical integrity.

The retrieval system which encloses the pessary is a knitted product made from a polyester which is also used in the manufacture of long-term, vascular implants.

The nature of the device and its retrieval system allow easy and reliable removal of the product when required.

**Product licence number** 8731/0003.

*Product licence holder:* Controlled Therapeutics (Scotland) Limited, East Kilbride G74 5PB.

## VIRORMONE*

**Presentation** Ampoules of 100 mg of Testosterone Propionate BP in ethyl oleate for intramuscular injection.

**Uses** Testosterone is the androgenic hormone of male testis. It is used as replacement therapy in castrated adults and in those who are hypogonadal due to either pituitary or testicular disease.

May also be used for control of carcinoma of the breast in post-menopausal women.

## Dosage and administration
*In the male:* Hypogonadism (adults), delayed puberty, cryptorchidism.

*In the female:* Carcinoma of the breast in post-menopausal women.

| | |
|---|---|
| Hypogonadism | 50 mg 2–3 times weekly |
| Delayed puberty cryptorchidism | 50 mg weekly |
| Carcinoma of the breast | 100 mg 2–3 times weekly |

## Contra-indications, warnings, etc
*Contra-indications:* Breast cancer in men, prostatic carcinoma, pregnancy, breast feeding and nephrosis.

*Interactions:* None stated.

*Effects on ability to drive and use machines:* None stated.

*Other undesirable effects:* None stated.

*Use in pregnancy and lactation:* Contra-indicated.

*Warning:* Tumours of the liver have been reported occasionally in patients subjected to prolonged treatment with androgenic-anabolic steroids. The possibility that these compounds may induce or enhance the development of hepatic tumours cannot at present be excluded and this should be considered when the use of this product is proposed, especially in young people who are not suffering with life threatening disorders.

*Precautions:* Do not use before puberty in males, unless for treatment of delayed puberty. In any case caution is advised since the fusion of the epiphyses is hastened and may lead to short stature.

Use with care in patients with cardiac, renal or hepatic impairment, circulatory failure, hypertension or epilepsy. A reduced dosage may be advisable in elderly male patients since hyperstimulation can occur.

Virilism may occur in female patients on high doses.

*Overdose:* None stated.

*Incompatibilities:* None stated.

**Pharmaceutical precautions**   Protect from light.

**Legal category**   POM.

**Package quantities**   100 mg in 2 ml ampoules. Boxes of 10.

**Further information**   Nil.

**Product licence number**   3194/0064.

## ZOMACTON* INJECTION-12 iu (Somatropin)

**Presentation**   Zomacton Injection-12 iu is presented as a sterile lyophilised powder in a glass vial, with a potency of 3.0 iu per mg. Each vial is supplied with a diluent ampoule of sterile isotonic saline for injection 0.9% w/v (with benzyl alcohol 0.9% w/v preservative).

**Uses**   Zomacton Injection is indicated for the long-term treatment of children who have growth failure due to inadequate secretion of growth hormone.

## Dosage and administration
*Children only:* The dosage and schedule of administration of Zomacton Injection should be individualised for each patient.

The product should be reconstituted using only the diluent supplied. To prevent foaming of the solution, the stream of diluent should be aimed against the side of the vial. The vial must then be swirled with a gentle rotary motion until the contents are completely dissolved and a clear, colourless solution is produced. Since Zomacton Injection is a protein, shaking or vigorous mixing is not recommended. If, after the mixing, the solution is cloudy or contains particulate matter, the contents must be discarded. In the case of cloudiness after refrigeration, the product should be allowed to warm to room temperature. If cloudiness persists, discard the vial and its contents.

Generally a dose of 0.5–0.7 iu/kg bodyweight (corresponding to 0.17 mg/kg–0.23 mg/kg bodyweight or 14.8 iu/m²–20.7 iu/m² body surface area) per week divided into 6–7 subcutaneous injections is recommended (corresponding to a daily injection of 0.07–0.1 iu/kg bodyweight equivalent to 0.023 mg/kg–0.033 mg/kg bodyweight or 2.1–3.0 iu/m² body surface area). The total weekly dose of 0.81 iu/kg bodyweight corresponding to 0.27 mg/kg or 24 iu/m² body surface area should not be exceeded (corresponding to daily injections of up to 0.116 iu/kg equivalent to 0.039 mg/kg). The duration of treatment, usually a period of several years, will depend on maximum achievable therapeutic benefit.

## Contra-indications, warnings, etc
*Contra-indications:* Zomacton Injection should not be used in children with closed epiphyses.

Patients with evidence of progression of an underlying intracranial lesion or other tumour should not receive Zomacton Injection, since the possibility of a tumour growth promoting effect cannot be excluded. Prior to the initiation of therapy with Zomacton Injection, intracranial tumours must be inactive and anti-tumour therapy completed.

Patients with a known sensitivity to benzyl alcohol should not be treated with Zomacton Injection-12 iu.

*Use in pregnancy and lactation:* Zomacton should not be used during pregnancy or lactation. There is no evidence from either human or animal studies of the safety of growth hormone treatment during pregnancy. Also, no information is available as to whether peptide hormones pass into breast milk.

*Special warnings and precautions for use:* Zomacton Injection therapy should be used only under the supervision of a qualified physician, experienced in the management of patients with growth hormone deficiency.

Patients should be observed for evidence of glucose intolerance because growth hormone may induce a state of insulin resistance. Zomacton Injection should be used with caution in patients with diabetes mellitus or a familial predisposition to the disease. Strict monitoring of urine and blood glucose is necessary in these patients. In childen with diabetes mellitus, the dose of insulin may need to be increased to maintain glucose control during Zomacton Injection therapy.

Children with hypopituitarism sometimes experience fasting hypoglycaemia which is improved by therapy with growth hormone. There have been reports that some of these children, when treated with growth hormone injections three times weekly, experience hypoglycaemia on non-treatment days. Thus, in children who have fasting hypoglycaemia associated with hypopituitarism, daily growth hormone administration is recommended.

In patients with growth hormone deficiency secondary to an intracranial lesion, frequent monitoring for progression or recurrence of the underlying disease process is advised. Discontinue Zomacton Injection therapy if progression or recurrence of the lesion occurs.

Fundoscopic examination for papilloedema is recommended at the initiation and periodically during the course of growth hormone treatment, especially if the patients report recurrent headache, visual problems, nausea and/or vomiting which may indicate intracranial hypertension.

Hypothyroidism may develop during treatment with growth hormone. Inadequate treatment of hypothyroidism may prevent optimal response to Zomacton Injection. Therefore, patients should have periodic thyroid function tests and be treated with thyroid hormone when indicated.

Leukaemia has been reported in a small number of growth hormone deficient patients treated with Somatropin as well as in untreated patients. Based on current evidence, experts cannot conclude that Somatropin is responsible for this. If there is any increase in risk to an individual patient it is small.

Slipped capital femoral epiphysis may occur more frequently in patients with endocrine disorders. A patient treated with Zomacton Injection who develops a limp or complains of hip or knee pain should be evaluated by a physician.

*Side-effects:* The subcutaneous administration of growth hormone may lead to the loss or increase of adipose tissue at the injection site. Therefore, injection sites should be changed frequently. Rarely, pain and an itchy rash may develop at the injection site.

Transient headache has been reported. Infrequently, a slight transient oedema may occur during treatment.

Formation of antibodies against Somatropin or *E. coli* has not yet been observed.

In individual cases, especially during the first weeks of growth hormone therapy, a benign intracranial hypertension has been reported. Symptoms usually are headache, nausea and/or vomiting and visual problems requiring fundoscopic examination for papilloedema. In most cases the symptoms resolved without discontinuation of therapy; in severe cases the dose should be reduced or treatment interrupted.

*Interactions:* Glucocorticoid therapy may inhibit the growth promoting effect of Zomacton Injection. Patients with co-existing ACTH deficiency should have their glucocorticoid replacement dose carefully adjusted to avoid impairment of the growth promoting effect of Zomacton Injection.

High doses of androgens, oestrogens or anabolic steroids can accelerate bone maturation and inhibit an increase in growth.

Because human growth hormone can induce a state of insulin resistance, insulin dose may have to be adjusted in the patient receiving concomitant Zomacton Injection.

*Overdose:* The recommended dose of Zomacton Injection should not be exceeded. Acute overdosage may result in an initial hypoglycaemia followed by a subsequent hyperglycaemia.

The effects of long term, repeated use of Zomacton Injection in doses exceeding those recommended, are unknown. However, it is possible that such use might produce signs and symptoms consistent with the known effects of excess human growth hormone (e.g. acromegaly).

**Pharmaceutical precautions**   Zomacton Injection should be stored in the refrigerator at 2°C to 8°C and protected from light. After reconstitution with sterile isotonic saline 0.9% w/v (containing benzyl alcohol preservative 0.9% w/v), Zomacton Injection is stable for 14 days when stored in the refrigerator at 2°C to 8°C and protected from light. Discard any solution left in the vial at the end of this period.

**Legal category**   POM.

**Package quantities**   Each carton contains one vial of Zomacton Injection-12 iu and one diluent ampoule of sterile isotonic saline solution 0.9% w/v 3.5 ml (containing benzyl alcohol preservative 0.9% w/v).

**Further information**   Zomacton Injection contains human growth hormone (Somatropin) produced in a genetically modified Escherichia Coli strain using a recombinant DNA technique. It is chemically identical and biologically equivalent to pituitary-derived Somatropin. It does not contain a terminal methionine residue. The lyophilised powder contains the inactive ingredient mannitol.

**Product licence numbers**
Zomacton Injection   3194/0052
Diluent                      3194/0054.

*Trade Mark

## Forley Ltd

4 Priory Hall
Stillorgan Road
Stillorgan
Co Dublin
Eire

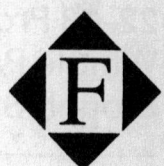

## DIBENYLINE* CAPSULES

**Presentation** Opaque white capsules with clear ruby-red caps, each containing 10 mg phenoxybenzamine hydrochloride as a white powder.

**Uses** Dibenyline is a non-competitive long-acting $\alpha$-adrenergic receptor antagonist.

It is indicated in the short-term management of severe hypertensive episodes associated with phaeochromocytoma. Dibenyline should only be used after careful consideration of the likely benefit of treatment compared with the mutagenic and carcinogenic risk (see *Precautions* below).

### Dosage and administration

*Adults:* The usual starting dose is 10 mg daily. This may be increased by 10 mg daily until control of hypertensive episodes is achieved or postural hypotension occurs. Usually the dosage required is 1 to 2 mg/kg body weight daily in two doses. Concomitant $\beta$-adrenergic blockade may be necessary to control tachycardia and arrhythmias notably when tumours are secreting an appreciable amount of adrenaline as well as noradrenaline.

*Elderly:* Use with caution (see *Contra-indications* and *Precautions* below).

*Children:* There is little experience in children, but doses of 1 to 2 mg/kg daily have been used successfully.

### Contra-indications, warnings, etc

*Contra-indications:* Do not use in patients who have had a cerebrovascular accident; or in the recovery period (usually 3 to 4 weeks) after acute myocardial infarction.

*Precautions:* Use with great caution in patients in whom a fall in blood pressure and/or tachycardia may be undesirable, such as the elderly, or those with severe heart disease, congestive heart failure, cerebrovascular disease or renal damage. The mode of action should be borne in mind if used concurrently with $\alpha$-sympathomimetics or myocardial depressants.

Phenoxybenzamine is carcinogenic in the rat and has shown mutagenic activity in the bacterial Ames test and the mouse lymphoma assay. It should, therefore, be used only after very careful consideration of the risks, in patients in whom alternative treatment is inappropriate.

*Use in pregnancy:* There is little evidence as to the safety of Dibenyline in pregnancy and it should not be used in pregnancy unless essential.

*Adverse reactions:* Side-effects are generally mild and transient, but may include postural hypotension with dizziness and compensatory tachycardia, nasal congestion, inhibition of ejaculation, miosis and lassitude. Gastro-intestinal upset has also been reported.

*Overdosage:* The main effect of overdosage is profound hypotension, which may last several hours, tachycardia and collapse. Treatment consists of the induction of vomiting and/or gastric lavage together with appropriate symptomatic and supportive measures. Treat hypotension with plasma expanders and the 'head down' position. Noradrenaline is of little value when $\alpha$-adrenergic receptors are blocked. Adrenaline should not be used since stimulation of $\beta$-adrenergic receptors will further decrease blood pressure.

**Pharmaceutical precautions** Store in a dry place and protect from light.

**Legal category** POM.

**Package quantities** Opaque blister packs (OP) of 30 (2 × 15) capsules.

**Further information** Treatment should be started as soon as possible after diagnosis and time allowed for stabilisation of the condition before invasive investigations or operations are carried out. Operative cover with intravenous phenoxybenzamine may be given.

In a few inoperable cases, long-term treatment with Dibenyline has been used.

Inactive ingredients include lactose.

**Product licence number** 12300/0007.

## DIBENYLINE* INJECTION

**Presentation** Clear colourless ampoules, each containing 100 mg phenoxybenzamine hydrochloride in 2 ml clear colourless to mid-straw coloured solution.

This solution contains absolute ethyl alcohol, hydrochloric acid and propylene glycol.

**Uses** Phenoxybenzamine is a long-acting, non-competitive, alpha-adrenergic receptor antagonist. By intravenous infusion it is used as part of the investigational, pre-operative and operative management of phaeochromocytoma, and as an adjunct to the treatment of severe shock, not responding to conventional therapy, in the presence of an adequate circulating blood volume.

Dibenyline should only be used after careful consideration of the likely benefit of treatment compared with the mutagenic and carcinogenic risk. See *Precautions* below.

**Dosage and administration** Dibenyline Injection Concentrate *must be diluted* before use. The dose selected should be added aseptically to 200–500 ml 0.9 per cent sodium chloride immediately before use.

*The intravenous route only must be used*, preferably through a large vein. Not more than one dose should be given in 24 hours, infused over at least two hours. It is suggested that one-third of the dose is given over the first hour, and the remaining two-thirds over the second hour if no precipitous fall in blood pressure has occurred. Any solution remaining four hours after dilution should be discarded because of reduced potency.

*Adults:*

*Phaeochromocytoma:* Where alpha-blockade is required as a preparation for investigation or operation in cases of phaeochromocytoma, a daily dose of 1 mg/kg body weight intravenously in 200 ml of physiological saline over two hours has been used, for several days preceding and during the procedure. This dose is a guide and it is often necessary to titrate the dose on a daily basis according to individual response, concomitant beta-receptor blockade may be necessary.

*Shock:* 1 mg/kg body weight in 200 to 500 ml of 0.9 per cent Sodium chloride given over not less than two hours.

*Children:* Dosage in children has not been established.

*Precautions in use:* The patient should be recumbent. Blood pressure must be determined every few minutes during the administration. Facilities for rapid infusion of intravenous fluid should be available. The Dibenyline infusion should be slowed or stopped if there is a precipitous fall in blood pressure. This usually indicates an inadequate circulating blood volume, but occasionally may occur in the presence of an adequate blood volume in hypertensives or in patients with carbon dioxide retention, and in these cases is relatively unresponsive to the administration of intravenous fluids. Nevertheless, if severe hypotension does occur, treatment can be attempted with plasma expanders and the 'head down' position. Noradrenaline may be of little value when alpha-adrenergic receptors are blocked. Adrenaline should not be used since stimulation of beta-adrenergic receptors will further decrease blood pressure. If blood pressure has been stabilised by the administration of appropriate fluids, the Dibenyline infusion may be restarted under close supervision. The blockade produced is often still exerting an effect 24 hours after administration and, even in patients with a favourable response, close attention to their cardiovascular status should be maintained for at least this period. Little can be accomplished by a second administration of

Dibenyline within 24 hours and the drug should not be given more than twice during a 48-hour period.

Care should be taken to avoid extravasation, as the diluted solution is irritant to muscle tissue.

Avoid contamination of the hands with Dibenyline as reactions may occur in sensitive skins.

### Contra-indications, warnings, etc

*Contra-indications:* Do not use in patients who have had a cerebrovascular accident; or in the recovery period (usually 3 to 4 weeks) after acute myocardial infarction. Do not use in the presence of hypovolaemia in patients with severe shock.

*Precautions:* Use with great caution in patients in whom a fall in blood pressure and/or tachycardia may be undesirable, such as the elderly or those with severe ischaemic heart disease, congestive heart failure, extensive arteriosclerosis, cerebrovascular disease or renal damage. The adrenergic blocking effect may aggravate symptoms of respiratory infections. Alpha-sympathomimetics may be ineffective if used concomitantly with phenoxybenzamine. Care should be taken if phenoxybenzamine is used concomitantly with myocardial depressants, e.g. beta-blockers and anti-arrhythmics.

Phenoxybenzamine is carcinogenic in the rat and has shown mutagenic activity in the bacterial Ames test and the mouse lymphoma assay. It should therefore be used only after very careful consideration of the risks, in patients in whom alternative treatment is inappropriate.

*Use in pregnancy:* There is no available evidence as to the safety of Dibenyline in pregnancy and it should not be used in pregnancy or lactation unless essential.

*Adverse reactions:* Dibenyline given intravenously has a sedative effect and patients may become more drowsy or less responsive during the infusion. This may occur in spite of an excellent cardiovascular response and should not be confused with the decreased responsiveness associated with worsening of the shock syndrome.

Other side-effects include orthostatic hypotension with dizziness and compensatory tachycardia, miosis, dry mouth, nasal congestion, decreased sweating and gastrointestinal upset. Convulsions have been reported after rapid infusion.

Some fall in blood pressure is a normal response but an idiosyncratic profound hypotensive effect can occur, usually within five minutes of starting the infusion.

The effect of one dose of Dibenyline on sympathetic motor responses may last 48 hours or more.

*Overdosage:* As described in *Precautions in use*, there may be a precipitous fall in blood pressure even at the recommended dosage. Facilities for rapid infusion of intravenous fluid should therefore be available and in the event of such a severe hypotensive episode, the Dibenyline infusion should be slowed or stopped. Treatment can be attempted with plasma expanders and the 'head down' position. Noradrenaline may be of little value when alpha-adrenergic receptors are blocked and adrenaline is contra-indicated.

**Pharmaceutical precautions** Protect the ampoules from light. Dibenyline solutions should be made up immediately before administration. Any that remains four hours after dilution should be discarded because of reduced potency. A transient clouding of the solution, due to low aqueous solubility of Dibenyline near neutral pH, is unimportant. If markedly discoloured in the ampoule, the preparation should be discarded.

**Legal category** POM.

**Package quantities** Ampoules: 100 mg phenoxybenzamine hydrochloride/2 ml in boxes of 3.

**Further information** Nil.

**Product licence number** 12300/0008.

*Trade Mark

# Fournier Pharmaceuticals Limited
22–23 Progress Business Centre
Whittle Parkway
Slough SL1 6DG

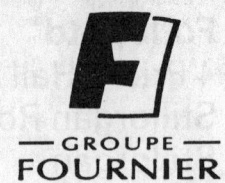

— GROUPE —
**FOURNIER**

## ERECNOS* ▼

### Qualitative and quantitative composition
*Erecnos 10 mg/1 ml:*
Moxisylyte hydrochloride (INN) also known as (thymoxamine hydrochloride (BAN), 10 mg quantity equivalent to moxisylyte 8.85 mg. For one freeze-dried powder.
*Composition of the solution:*
Sodium chloride 9.00 mg
Water for injections qs 1.00 ml
For one prefilled syringe with two compartments.

*Erecnos 20 mg/1 ml:*
Moxisylyte hydrochloride (INN) also known as thymoxamine hydrochloride (BAN), 20 mg quantity equivalent to moxisylyte 17.70 mg. For one freeze-dried powder.
*Composition of the solution:*
Sodium chloride 9.00 mg
Water for injections qs 1.00 ml
For one prefilled syringe with two compartments.

**Pharmaceutical form** Freeze-dried powder and solution for parenteral use (intracavernous injection).

### Clinical particulars
*Therapeutic indications:* Erecnos provides a pharmacological induction of erection.

*Posology and method of administration:*
Intracavernous route only in adult males – *Dosage:* Dosage will be determined by the doctor depending on the patients individual response. The start dose is 10 mg. If the response is insufficient, this dose may be increased to 20 mg at subsequent administrations. The maximum dose per injection is 20 mg.

*Frequency of use:* No more than one dose daily, the maximum number of injections being 3 per week with an interval of at least 48 hours between injections.

*Method of administration:* The first injection must be given under medical supervision. The patient should only administer self-injections into the corpus cavernosum after he has learnt the correct injection technique.
    Once the doctor has taught the patient the injection method, self-injections may be administered by the patient at home. The injection site must be changed at each administration.
    The prescribed dosage MUST NOT be exceeded.

*Injection technique:* Take the penis in the hand, placing the thumb on the mid part on top.
    The injection is given into the corpus cavernosum on the sides of the penis.
    Pierce the skin at right angles, inserting the whole of the needle.
    Gently inject all the product.
    Withdraw the needle and massage the injection site to encourage diffusion of the product.
    The injection is for single use and is to be used immediately after reconstitution.

*Contra-indications:* Should not be injected via the intravenous or intramuscular routes.
    Systolic blood pressure of less than 100 mmHg.
    Patients predisposed to priapism due to underlying medical conditions (e.g. Sickle cell anaemia, Multiple myeloma, leukaemia etc).
    Known allergy to moxisylyte hydrochloride.
    Should not be used in patients with penile implants.
    Women and children because of the therapeutic indication.

*Special warnings and special precautions for use:*
*Warnings:* Treatment by self-injection should be preceded by a learning phase in the doctors surgery. The patient is then strongly recommended to keep with him the telephone number of the medical team responsible for his treatment or that of his nearest casualty unit.
    In some patients moxisylyte hydrochloride may cause transient hypotension therefore patients should remain in a supine position for up to 30 minutes following their injection.
    Moxisylyte hydrochloride is not recommended for patients who have suffered a cardiovascular accident within the previous 3 months (this may include: unstable angina pectoris, acute myocardial infarction or cerebrovascular disease) and whose cardiovascular status has not been stabilised.
    On very rare occasions Erecnos may cause prolonged erections or priapism therefore patients should

be advised to seek immediate medical advice if their erection lasts for more than 3 hours.

*Precautions:* Special counselling should be given to patients with the following disorders before treatment: scarring of the corpus cavernosum (fibrosis/nodule), penile angulation or Peyronie's disease as pain may be experienced at the time of erection.
    Patients using anti-coagulants may have increased levels of bleeding at the injection site. The patient should be advised to exert sufficient pressure on the injection site to encourage coagulation.
    After the first ten injections and at regular intervals thereafter, the doctor should re-assess the treatment to ascertain any local adverse effects and undertake any adjustments of the dosage.
    At the end of the year of treatment physicians should re-consider extension of treatment in the light of information on long term use.

*Interactions with other medicines and other forms of interaction:* Combination of this medicine with other alpha-blockers (alfuzosin, doxazosin, prazosin, terazosin, urapidil) and beta-blockers is not recommended in order to avoid severe orthostatic hypotension.
    Combined administration with any antihypertensives (calcium antagonists, ACE inhibitors) where unavoidable, requires the usual medical precautions to be undertaken in case of potentiation of the antihypertensive effect.
    Should not be used in combination with other drugs for erectile dysfunction.

*Pregnancy and lactation:* Not applicable.

*Effects on ability to drive and use machines:* If the patient suffers from transitory hypotension or dizziness then he should be advised not to drive or operate machinery until this clears.

*Undesirable effects:* The main side effects that were encountered are as follows:
– Pain on injection, haematoma at the injection site.
– Sensation of tiredness with nausea and dizziness associated with transient arterial hypotension.
– Drowsiness, headache, vasomotor flushes.
– Dry mouth, sinus congestion, rhinorrhoea.
– Occasionally priapism and prolonged erection.

*Overdose:* In the event of an overdose, the main complication is priapism. This must be treated by medically trained personnel by aspirating the blood from the corpus cavernosum. The possibility of such an incident occurring means that the patient should always have with him the telephone number of a medical team which can treat him in an emergency.

### Pharmacological properties
*Pharmacodynamic properties:* Alpha-1 blocking peripheral vasodilator.
    Moxisylyte hydrochloride is an adrenergic alpha-blocker acting on the peripheral alpha-1 adrenergic receptors and to a lesser extent on the alpha-2 receptors.
    Its peripheral antagonist action causes myorelaxation of the smooth muscle fibres of the corpus cavernosum, in which the adrenergic receptors are predominant. The result is increased arterial flow and dilatation of the cavernous areolae which are the origin of the erection.

*Pharmacokinetic properties:* After parenteral administration, moxisylyte hydrochloride is deacetylated by plasma and hepatic esterases.
    In Man, 4 metabolites are found in the plasma:
– deacetylmoxisylyte or DAM in its free, glucuroconjugated and sulphoconjugated forms.
– the monodemethyl deacetyl derivative MDAM, in its sulphoconjugated form.
    In species tested (Rats and Dogs) moxisylyte hydrochloride is completely metabolised after intracavernous injection (ICI) or intravenous injection (IVI).
    At equivalent doses, the metabolites found in plasma after ICI and IVI are the same. However, their concentrations after ICI are weaker. The active metabolite (DAM) is no longer measurable in plasma 6 hours after administration.
    After intracavernous injection in Man, elimination of the metabolites is rapid ($t_{\frac{1}{2}}$ of DAM=1 hour) and excretion is primarily via the urinary route. 60–66% of the dose after ICI or IVI is in the form of conjugated DAM and MDAM.
    The peak concentration of DAM is reached 10 to 20

minutes after ICI and is approximately 35 ng/ml following a dose of 10 mg.

*Preclinical safety data:* The intravenous doses of 3 and 3.6 mg/kg/day did not induce toxic effects respectively in the rat and in the dog during 3 months. The local and systemic tolerance after intracavernous injection in the dog was satisfactory. No effect on male rat fertility was observed. Moxisylyte did not show any mutagenic or genotoxic potential (12 tests). Furthermore, no carcinogenic effect in rats was observed after an 18 month treatment by the oral route.

### Pharmaceutical particulars
*List of excipients:* Sodium chloride, water for injections.

*Incompatibilities:* None known.

*Shelf life:* 18 months.

*Special precautions for storage:* To be stored at a temperature of less than 25 degrees centigrade.
    The injection is for single use and is to be used immediately after reconstitution.

*Nature and contents of container:* 10 mg in a dual-compartment, prefilled syringe (glass) mounted with a needle: box of 2.
    20 mg in a dual-compartment, prefilled syringe (glass) mounted with a needle: box of 2.

*Instruction for use/handling:*
    *Preparation of the syringe:* Twist the clear plastic front cap to take it off or it may be easier to place the cap in the fold of the skin between the thumb and forefinger in order to produce better grip before turning and pulling. Do not be surprised if it is difficult to remove: this is a safety feature.
    Release without taking off the rear cap (activator) of the syringe by applying pressure alternately to the sides: the activator should make a snapping sound on release. During release of the activator, the syringe should be held close to the bottom of the barrel and close to the top of the activator. Do not be surprised if it is difficult to release: this a safety feature.
    Hold the syringe vertically with the needle pointing upwards. Push steadily and slowly the lower plunger upwards. This will force the solvent from its compartment into the space containing the moxisylyte powder. After the solvent has been completely forced out of the compartment, continue pushing the plunger until it can go no further.
    Gently shake the syringe until the powder is fully dissolved.
    Remove the protective rear cap by gently grasping and turning.
    Carefully remove the needle cap.
    Expel the air from the syringe.

**Marketing authorisation numbers**
Erecnos 10 mg/1 ml 12509/0009
Erecnos 20 mg/1 ml 12509/0010

**Date of approval/revision of SPC** April 1997.

**Legal category** POM.

## LIPANTIL*

**Presentation** White, hard gelatin capsules each containing 100 mg of fenofibrate.

**Uses** Lipantil reduces elevated serum cholesterol and triglyceride and is of benefit in the treatment of severe hyperlipidaemia in patients in whom dietary measures alone have failed to produce an adequate response. Lipantil is therefore indicated in appropriate cases of hyperlipidaemia (Fredrickson classification types IIa, IIb, III, IV and V ).

| Type | Major Lipid elevated | Lipoproteins elevated |
|------|----------------------|-----------------------|
| IIa | Cholesterol | LDL |
| IIb | Cholesterol, triglyceride | LDL, VLDL |
| III | Cholesterol, triglyceride | LDL, IDL |
| IV | Triglyceride | VLDL |
| V | Triglyceride | Chylomicrons, VLDL |

Lipantil should only be used in patients whose disease is unresponsive to dietary control and in whom a full investigation has been performed to define their abnormality, and where the long-term risks associated with their condition warrant treatment. Other risk factors, such as hypertension and smoking, may also require management.

Epidemiological studies have demonstrated a positive correlation between abnormally increased serum lipid levels and an increased risk of coronary heart disease. The control of such dyslipidaemia forms the rationale for treatment with Lipantil. However, the possible beneficial and adverse long-term consequences of drugs used in the management of hyperlipidaemia are still the subject of scientific discussion. Therefore the presumptive beneficial effect of Lipantil on cardiovascular morbidity and mortality is as yet unproven.

Studies with fenofibrate on lipoprotein fractions show decreases in levels of LDL- and VLDL-cholesterol. HDL-cholesterol levels are frequently increased. LDL- and VLDL-triglycerides are reduced. The overall effect is a decrease in the ratio of low and very low density lipoproteins to high density lipoproteins, which epidemiological studies have correlated with a decrease in atherogenic risk. Apolipoprotein-A and apolipoprotein-B levels are altered in parallel with HDL and LDL and VLDL levels respectively.

Regression of xanthomata has been observed during fenofibrate therapy.

Plasma uric acid levels are increased in approximately 20% of hyperlipidaemic patients, particularly in those with type IV disease. Lipantil has a uricosuric effect and is therefore of additional benefit in such patients.

Patients with raised levels of fibrinogen and Lp(a) have shown significant reducations in these measurements during clinical trials with fenofibrate.

**Dosage and administration** The recommended initial dose is 300 mg daily, taken in divided doses. The normal adult dose is recommended in the elderly. In children the dose level is 5 mg/kg/day. Since it is less well absorbed from an empty stomach, Lipantil should always be taken with food. Dietary restrictions instituted before therapy should be continued.

Response to therapy should be monitored by determination of serum lipid values, and dosage altered within the range 200–400 mg daily as necessary. Rapid reduction of serum lipid levels usually follows Lipantil treatment, but treatment should be discontinued if an adequate response has not been achieved within three months.

**Contra-indications, warnings, etc** Lipantil is contra-indicated in patients with severe liver dysfunction, existing gallbladder disease, severe renal disorders and in patients hypersensitive to fenofibrate. Fenofibrate has not been shown to be teratogenic in animals. However, signs of embryotoxicity have been seen in rats and it is therefore recommended that Lipantil should not be administered to women who are pregnant or are breast-feeding.

In renal dysfunction the dose of Lipantil may need to be reduced, depending on the rate of creatinine clearance (for example to 200 mg daily for a creatinine clearance of 60 ml/minute, and to 100 mg daily for a creatinine clearance of 20 ml/minute). Dose reduction may be considered in elderly patients with impaired renal function.

In common with other hypolipidaemic drugs, chronic administration of fenofibrate to rodents has been associated with hepatic tumour formation. However, liver histology in fenofibrate treated patients shows no evidence of related effects.

In patients receiving oral anti-coagulant therapy, the dose of anti-coagulant should be reduced by about one-third at the commencement of treatment and then gradually adjusted if necessary. No proven clinical interactions of fenofibrate with other drugs have been reported, although in vitro interaction studies suggest displacement of phenylbutazone from plasma protein binding sites. In common with other fibrates, fenofibrate induces microsomal mixed-function oxidases involved in fatty acid metabolism in rodents and may interact with drugs metabolised by these enzymes. Possible interactions with oral hypoglycaemic agents should also be considered.

Adverse reactions observed during Lipantil treatment are infrequent; they are generally minor, transient and do not interfere with treatment. Most commonly reported are mild gastro-intestinal disturbances, skin reactions, headache, fatigue and vertigo.

Sexual asthenia and muscle toxicity (as seen with other systemic lipid modifying drugs) are reported less frequently. Examples of the latter include myositis, myopathy and marked elevations of creatine phosphokinase (CPK). Rhabdomyolysis has also been reported rarely. Patients who develop signs of muscle toxicity should be monitored closely and CPK levels checked. Treatment with fenofibrate should be stopped if myopathy is suspected or if CPK rises to greater than or equal to 10 times the upper limit of normal. The risk of serious muscle toxicity is increased if fenofibrate is used concomitantly with HMG-CoA reductase inhibitors or other fibrates. Combination therapy should be used with caution, and patients monitored closely for signs of muscle toxicity.

There is no evidence of an increased incidence of gallstones. Moderately elevated levels of serum transaminases may be found in some patients, but rarely interfere with treatment. However, it is recommended that serum transaminases should be monitored every three months during the first twelve months of treatment. Treatment should be interrupted in the event of SGPT elevation of more than one hundred international units. Episodes of hepatitis have been reported rarely.

No reports of ill effects from overdosage have been reported. There are no specific antidotes and treatment of acute overdosage should be symptomatic. Gastric lavage and appropriate supportive care may be instituted if necessary.

**Pharmaceutical precautions** Store below 25°C in a dry place. Protect from light.

**Legal category** POM.

**Package quantities** Lipantil is available in blister packs of 84 capsules.

**Further information** Nil.

**Product licence number** 12509/0003.

## LIPANTIL* MICRO 200

**Qualitative and quantitative composition** Each Lipantil Micro 200 capsule contains 200 mg of micronised fenofibrate (INN).

**Pharmaceutical form** Orange, hard gelatin capsule.

**Clinical particulars**

*Therapeutic indications:* Lipantil Micro 200 reduces elevated serum cholesterol and triglyceride and is of benefit in the treatment of severe dyslipidaemia in patients in whom dietary measures alone have failed to produce an adequate response. Lipantil Micro 200 is therefore indicated in appropriate cases of hyperlipidaemia (Fredrickson classification types IIa, IIb, III, IV and V).

| *Type* | *Major lipid elevated* | *Lipoproteins elevated* |
|---|---|---|
| IIa | Cholesterol | LDL |
| IIb | Cholesterol, triglyceride | LDL, VLDL |
| III (rare) | Cholesterol, triglyceride | LDL and Chylomicron Remnants |
| IV | Triglyceride | VLDL |
| V (rare) | Triglyceride | Chylomicrons, VLDL |

Lipantil Micro 200 should only be used in patients whose disease is unresponsive to dietary control and in whom a full investigation has been performed to define their abnormality, and where long-term risks associated with their condition warrant treatment. Other risk factors, such as hypertension and smoking, may also require management.

*Posology and method of administration:*

*Adults:* The recommended initial dose is one capsule taken daily during a main meal. In elderly patients without renal impairment, the normal adult dose is recommended. Since it is less well absorbed from an empty stomach, Lipantil Micro 200 should always be taken with food. Dietary restrictions instituted before therapy should be continued.

Response to therapy should be monitored by determination of serum lipid values. Rapid reduction of serum lipid levels usually follows Lipantil Micro 200 treatment, but treatment should be discontinued if an adequate response has not been achieved within three months.

*Contra-indications:* Lipantil Micro 200 is contra-indicated in children, in patients with severe liver dysfunction, existing gallbladder disease, severe renal disorders and in patients hypersensitive to fenofibrate.

*Special warnings and precautions for use:*

*Renal impairment:* In renal dysfunction the dose of fenofibrate may need to be reduced, depending on the rate of creatinine clearance. In this case, non-micronised fenofibrate (Lipantil capsules) should be used, e.g. 200 mg non-micronised fenofibrate daily for creatinine clearance levels of <60 ml/min and 100 mg non-micronised fenofibrate daily for creatinine clearance levels of <20 ml/min.

Use of Lipantil is also to be preferred in elderly patients with renal impairment where dosage reduction may be required.

*Serum transaminases:* Moderately elevated levels of serum transaminases may be found in some patients but rarely interfere with treatment. However, it is recommended that serum transaminases should be monitored every three months during the first twleve months of treatment. Treatment should be interrupted in the event of SGPT elevation of more than one hundred international units.

*Interactions:*

*Oral anti-coagulants:* In patients receiving oral anti-coagulant therapy, the dose of anti-coagulant should be reduced by about one-third at the commencement of treatment and then gradually adjusted if necessary.

*Other:* No proven clinical interactions of fenofibrate with other drugs have been reported, although *in vitro* interaction studies suggest displacement of phenylbutazone from plasma protein binding sites. In common with other fibrates, fenofibrate induces microsomal mixed-function oxidases involved in fatty acid metabolism in rodents and may interact with drugs metabolised by these enzymes. Possible interactions with oral hypoglycaemic agents should also be considered.

*Pregnancy and lactation:* Fenofibrate has not been shown to be teratogenic in animals. However, signs of embryotoxicity have been seen in rats and it is therefore recommended that Lipantil Micro 200 should not be administered to women who are pregnant or are breast-feeding.

*Effects on ability to drive and use machines:* No effect noted to date.

*Undesirable effects:* Adverse reactions observed during Lipantil Micro 200 treatment are not very frequent; they are generally minor, transient and do not interfere with treatment. Most commonly reported are mild gastro-intestinal disturbances, skin reactions, headache, fatigue and vertigo.

Sexual asthenia and muscle toxicity (as seen with other systemic lipid modifying drugs) are reported less frequently. Examples of the latter include myositis, myopathy and marked elevations of creatine phosphokinase (CPK). Rhabdomyolysis during treatment with fenofibrate has also been reported rarely. Patients who are at risk of developing, or who show signs of muscle toxicity should be monitored closely and CPK levels checked. Treatment with fenofibrate should be stopped if myopathy is suspected or if CPK rises to ≥10 times the upper limit of normal. The risk of serious muscle toxicity is increased if fenofibrate is used concomitantly with HMG-CoA reductase inhibitors or other fibrates. Combination therapy should be used with caution, and patients monitored closely for signs of muscle toxicity.

Gallstones have occasionally been reported during fenofibrate treatment but any causal relationship remains inconclusive.

Moderately elevated levels of serum transaminases may be found in some patients but rarely interfere with treatment (see also *Special warnings and precautions*). Episodes of hepatitis have been reported rarely.

*Overdose:* No reports of ill effects from overdosage have been reported. There are no specific antidotes and treatment of acute overdosage should be symptomatic. Gastric lavage and appropriate supportive care may be instituted if necessary.

**Pharmacological properties**

*Pharmacodynamic properties:* Lipantil Micro 200 is a formulation containing 200 mg of micronised fenofibrate; the administration of this product results in effective plasma concentrations identical to those obtained with 3 capsules of Lipantil containing 100 mg of non-micronised fenofibrate.

Epidemiological studies have demonstrated a positive correlation between abnormally increased serum lipid levels and an increased risk of coronary heart disease. The control of such dyslipidaemia forms the rationale for treatment with Lipantil Micro 200. However the possible beneficial and adverse long term consequences of drugs used in the management of dyslipidaemia are still the subject of scientific discussion. Therefore the presumptive beneficial effect of Lipantil Micro 200 on cardiovascular morbidity and mortality is as yet unproven.

Studies with fenofibrate on lipoprotein fractions show decreases in level of LDL and VLDL cholesterol. HDL cholesterol levels are frequently increased. LDL and VLDL triglycerides are reduced. The overall effect is a decrease in the ratio of low and very low density lipoproteins to high density lipoproteins, which epidemiological studies have correlated with a decrease in atherogenic risk. Apolipoprotein-A and apolipoprotein-B levels are altered in parallel with HDL and LDL and VLDL levels respectively.

Regression of xanthomata has been observed during fenofibrate therapy.

Plasma uric acid levels are increased in approximately 20% of hyperlipidaemic patients, particularly in those with type IV disease. Lipantil Micro 200 has a uricosuric effect and is therefore of additional benefit in such patients.

Patients with raised levels of fibrinogen and Lp(a) have shown significant reductions in these measurements during clinical trials with fenofibrate.

*Pharmacokinetic properties: Absorption:* The unchanged compound is not recovered in the plasma. Fenofibric acid is the major plasma metabolite. Peak plasma concentration occurs after a mean period of 5 hours following dosing. Mean plasma concentration is 15 μg/ml during a total daily dosage of 300 mg of non-micronised fenofibrate (equivalent to 200 mg of micronised fenofibrate). Steady state levels are observed throughout continuous treatments.

Fenofibric acid is highly bound to plasma albumin; it can displace antivitamin K compounds from protein binding sites and may potentiate their anti-coagulant effect.

The plasma half-life of elimination of fenofibric acid is approximately 20 hours.

*Metabolism and excretion:* the product is mainly excreted in the urine; 70% in 24 hours and 88% in 6 days, at which time the total excretion in urine and faeces reaches 93%. Fenofibrate is mainly excreted as fenofibric acid and its derived glucuroconjugate.

## Pharmaceutical particulars

*List of excipients:* Lactose, pregelatinised starch, sodium lauryl sulphate, crospovidone and magnesium stearate.

Composition of the capsule shell: gelatin, titanium dioxide (E171), ferrous oxide (E172) and erythrosine (E127).

*Incompatibilities:* No effect noted to date.

*Shelf life:* 3 years.

*Special precautions for storage:* Store below 25˚C in a dry place. Protect from light.

*Nature and contents of container:* Lipantil Micro 200

is available in a pack containing 3 strips of 10 capsules in blisters.

**Marketing authorisation number**    12509/0001

**Date of approval/revision of SPC**    October 1996.

**Legal category**    POM.

*Trade Mark

**Fujisawa Limited**
CP House, 8th Floor
97–107 Uxbridge Road
London W5 5TL

Fujisawa Limited

## PROGRAF*

**Qualitative and quantitative composition**
*Capsules* containing 1 mg and 5 mg tacrolimus (INN), respectively

*Concentrate for intravenous infusion* containing tacrolimus 5 mg per 1 ml

For excipients see *Pharmaceutical particulars.*

**Pharmaceutical form** Hard gelatin capsules. Concentrate for intravenous infusion.

**Clinical particulars**
*Therapeutic indication:* Primary immunosuppression in liver and kidney allograft recipients and liver and kidney allograft rejection resistant to conventional immunosuppressive regimens.

*Posology and method of administration:*
*General considerations:* The dosage recommendations given below for oral and intravenous administration are intended to act as a guideline. Prograf doses should be adjusted according to individual patient requirements. Only initial dosing is recommended and therefore therapy should be based on clinical judgement aided by measurement of tacrolimus concentrations in blood.

*Route of administration:* Dosing should commence orally, if necessary via an intranasal gastric tube. If the clinical condition of the patient does not allow oral therapy, initial intravenous dosing may be necessary.

*Mode of intake:*
*Prograf Capsules 1 mg/Prograf Capsules 5 mg – Oral Dosing:* It is recommended that the oral daily dose should be taken in two divided doses. The capsules should be swallowed with fluid, preferably water.

Based on pharmacokinetic considerations, the capsules should be taken on an empty stomach or at least 1 hour before or 2–3 hours after a meal to achieve maximal absorption (see *Interactions* and *Pharmacokinetic properties*).

The capsules should be taken out of the blister only immediately before intake. After opening of the aluminium wrapper, the capsules from the blisters must be used within 12 months.

Patients should be cautioned not to swallow desiccant contained within the aluminium wrapper.

*Prograf Concentrate for Infusion 5 mg/ml – Intravenous Dosing: NB:* Prograf Concentrate for Infusion 5 mg/ml must not be injected undiluted. The concentrate for infusion should be diluted in 5% dextrose solution or in physiological saline solution in polyethylene or glass bottles. The concentration of a solution for final infusion produced in this way should be in the range of 0.004 to 0.1 mg/ml. The total volume of infusion during 24 hours should be in the range of 20 to 250 ml. The solution should not be given as a bolus. The content of the concentrate for infusion is not compatible with PVC. The solution for final use should be used up within 24 hours.

*Maximum whole blood concentration levels:* Clinical study analysis suggests that the majority of patients can be successfully managed if the blood concentrations of tacrolimus are maintained below 20 ng/ml.

It is necessary to consider the clinical condition of the patient when interpreting whole blood level concentrations. If the blood levels are below the limit of quantification of the assay and the patient's clinical condition is satisfactory, then the dose should not be adjusted.

In clinical practice, 12 h trough whole blood levels are generally 5–20 ng/ml early post-transplant.

*During of dosing:* For oral dosing the capsules normally have to be taken continually to suppress graft rejection and no limit for therapy duration can be given.

Patients should be converted from intravenous to oral medication as soon as individual circumstances permit. Intravenous therapy should not be continued for more than 7 days.

*Administration with other therapies:* Prograf is normally administered together with other immunosuppressive agents. Prograf should not be given together with cyclosporin.

If allograft rejection or adverse events occur, alteration to the immunosuppressive regimen should be considered.

*Dosage level recommendations:* Initial dose level recommendation.

*Primary immunosuppression dose levels – adults: Liver and kidney transplantation:* Oral tacrolimus therapy should commence at 0.10–0.20 mg/kg/day for liver transplantation and at 0.15–0.30 mg/kg/day for kidney transplantation administered as two divided doses. Administration should start approximately 6 hours after the completion of liver transplant surgery and within 24 hours of kidney transplant surgery.

If the clinical condition of the patient does not allow for oral dosing then intravenous tacrolimus therapy should be initiated as a continuous 24 hour infusion, at 0.01 to 0.05 mg/kg for liver transplants and 0.05 to 0.10 mg/kg for kidney transplants.

*Primary immunosuppression dose levels – paediatric patients:* Paediatric patients generally require doses 1½–2 times higher than the recommended adult doses to achieve the same blood levels. Experience with initial oral administration in paediatric patients is limited.

*Liver and kidney transplantation:* An initial dose of 0.3 mg/kg/day for liver and kidney transplantation should be administered in two divided doses. If the dose cannot be given orally, an initial intravenous dose of 0.05 mg/kg/day for liver transplantation or 0.1 mg/kg/day for kidney transplantation should be administered as a continuous 24-hour infusion.

*Maintenance therapy dose levels:* It is necessary to continue immunosuppression with oral Prograf to maintain graft survival. Dose can frequently be reduced during maintenance therapy. Dosing should be primarily based on clinical assessments of rejection and tolerability in each patient individually. During the course of the post-transplant improvement of the patient, it is likely that the pharmacokinetics of Prograf may be altered, requiring adjustment of the Prograf dose.

If progression of disease occurs (e.g. signs of acute rejection), alteration of the immunosuppressive regimen should be considered. Increase in the amount of corticosteroids, introduction of short courses of mono/polyclonal antibodies and increase in the dose of Prograf have all been used to manage rejection episodes. If signs of toxicity (e.g. pronounced adverse event, see *Undesirable effects*) are noted, the dose of Prograf should be reduced. Patients should be instructed not to decrease the dose without the consent of the treating physician.

When Prograf is administered in combination with a corticosteroid, these may often be reduced and in rare cases the treatment has continued as monotherapy.

*Therapy dose levels for liver and kidney allograft rejection resistant to conventional immunosuppressive regimens:* In patients experiencing rejection episodes which are unresponsive to conventional immunosuppressive therapy, Prograf treatment should begin with the initial dose recommended for primary immunosuppression in that particular allograft.

Co-administration of cyclosporin and Prograf may increase the half-life of cyclosporin and exacerbate any toxic effects. Prograf therapy should be initiated after considering cyclosporin blood concentrations and the clinical condition of the patient. In practice, Prograf therapy has been initiated 12–24 hours after discontinuation of cyclosporin. Monitoring of cyclosporin blood levels should be continued following conversion as the clearance of cyclosporin may be affected.

*Compromised patients*
*Patients with liver impairment:* A dose reduction may be necessary in patients with pre- and/or post-operative impairment, e.g. initial graft dysfunction.

*Patients with renal impairment:* The renal clearance of tacrolimus is low, hence no adjustment in dose is regarded as necessary on pharmacokinetic principles. However, owing to the nephrotoxic potential, careful monitoring of renal function, including serial creatinine estimations, calculations of creatinine clearance and monitoring of urine output, is recommended. The blood concentration of Prograf is not reduced by dialysis.

*Elderly patients:* Limited experience suggests that doses should be the same as for other adults.

*Monitoring of whole blood concentrations:* Various assays have been used to measure blood or plasma levels. Comparison of the levels in published literature with those found in clinical practice should be made with knowledge of the assay methods employed. In current clinical practice, blood levels are monitored using immunoassay methods.

Drug level monitoring is recommended during the early post-transplantation period, following dose adjustment of Prograf therapy after switching from another immunosuppressive regimen or following co-administration of drugs which are likely to lead to a drug to drug interaction. Trough blood levels of Prograf should also be monitored periodically during maintenance therary. The frequency of blood level monitoring should be based on clinical need. As tacrolimus has a long half-life, it can take several days for adjustments in Prograf dosing to be reflected in changes in blood levels.

*Contra-indications:*
Pregnancy
Known hypersensitivity to tacrolimus or other macrolides.
Prograf Capsules 1 mg and Prograf Capsules 5 mg in addition:
Known hypersensitivity to other ingredients of the capsules.
Prograf Concentrate for Infusion 5 mg/ml in addition:
Known hypersensitivity to polyoxyethylated castor oil (HC0–60) or structurally related compounds.

*Special warnings and special precautions for use:* Prograf therapy requires careful monitoring in units equipped and staffed with adequate laboratory and supportive medical resources. The drug should only be prescribed, and changes in immunosuppressive therapy should only be initiated, by physicians experienced in immunosuppressive therapy and the management of transplant patients. The physician responsible for maintenance therapy should have complete information requisite for the follow-up of the patient.

Dose and/or blood level adjustment should only be undertaken by the transplant centre responsible for the transplant patient.

Patients should be thoroughly controlled. In particular during the first months post-transplant, close monitoring of the patient is required.

Regular monitoring of the following parameters should be undertaken on a routine basis: blood pressure, ECG, visual status, blood glucose levels, blood levels of potassium and other electrolytes, creatinine, BUN, haematology parameters, coagulation values and liver function tests. If clinically relevant alterations of these parameters are seen, the dose of tacrolimus should be reviewed.

Renal function tests should be performed at frequent intervals. In particular during the first days post-transplant, monitoring of urinary output should be performed. If necessary the dose should be adjusted.

Several types of neurological and CNS disorders have been reported in association with Prograf therapy. For this reason, patients exhibiting such adverse events should be controlled very carefully. Occurrence of severe CNS symptoms should prompt immediate dose review. It has been reported that in some cases severe tremor and/or motoric (expressive) aphasia may be indicators for severe CNS disorders.

Ventricular hypertrophy or hypertrophy of the septum and rare cases of cardiomyopathy have been reported in association with administration of Prograf. Most of these have been reversible following dose reduction or drug discontinuation, occurring primarily in children having tacrolimus blood trough levels much higher than the recommended maximum levels. Factors which may increase the risk of this condition are pre-existing cardiac disease, corticosteroid usage, hypertension, renal or hepatic dysfunction, infections and fluid overload and oedema. Monitoring of cardiovascular function with echocardiography with or without ECG pre- and post-transplant (e.g. within the first 3 months and then at 9 months to 1 year) is advised for high risk patients. If abnormalities develop, dose reduction of Prograf therapy or discontinuation and change to alternative immunosuppressive therapy should be considered.

As with other potent immunosuppressive compounds, patients treated with Prograf have been reported to develop EBV-associated lymphoproliferative disorders. In patients switched to Prograf, this may be attributable to over-immunosuppression before commencing therapy with this agent. Patients switched to Prograf rescue therapy should not receive concomitantly anti-lymphocyte treatment. Very young (<2 years), EBV-sero-negative children have been reported to have an increased risk of developing a lymphoproliferative disorder. Therefore, in this patient group, EBV serology should be ascertained before starting treatment with Prograf. During treatment, careful monitoring is recommended.

In view of the potential risk of malignancies, patients who spend extended periods in the sun, or are otherwise exposed to UV light, should apply a high protection sun-cream.

If accidentally administered arterially or perivasally, Prograf Concentrate for Infusion 5 mg/ml may cause irritation.

Prograf should not be administered together with cyclosporin.

Prograf Concentrate for Infusion contains polyoxyethylated castor oil which has been reported to cause anaphylactoid reactions. These reactions consist of flushing of the face and upper thorax, acute respiratory distress with dyspnoea and wheezing, blood pressure changes and tachycardia. Caution is therefore necessary in patients who have previously received, by intravenous injection or infusion, preparations containing polyoxyethylated castor oil (such as HCO 60) and patients with an allergenic predisposition. Animal studies have shown that the risk of anaphylaxis may be reduced by slow infusion of polyoxyethylated castor oil containing drugs or by the prior administration of an antihistamine.

*Interactions with other medicaments and other forms of interaction*

*Clinically observed drug interactions:* Imidazole antimycotics (such as clotrimazole [from troches], fluconazole and ketoconazole), macrolide antibiotics (such as clarithromycin and erythromycin, for which up to 10-fold increase in blood trough levels has been observed), danazol and omeprazole have been reported to increase tacrolimus whole blood/plasma levels. Rifampicin has been shown to decrease tacrolimus whole blood and plasma levels.

Concomitant administration of methylprednisolone has been reported to increase and to decrease plasma levels of tacrolimus.

After combination of either amphotericin B or ibuprofen with Prograf enhanced nephrotoxicity has been observed.

*Combination with cyclosporin:* The half-life of cyclosporin has been shown to increase when Prograf is given simultaneously. In addition, synergistic/additive nephrotoxic effects can occur. For these reasons, the combined administration of cyclosporin and Prograf is not recommended and care should be taken when administering tacrolimus to patients who have previously received cyclosporin.

*Drug interactions observed in animals:* In rats, Prograf decreased the clearance and increased the half-life of pentobarbital and antipyrine.

*Potential drug interactions based on the metabolic system for Prograf:* Tacrolimus is cleared by hepatic metabolism. The cytochrome P450 3A4 family of enzymes is responsible for its metabolism. Concomitant use of drugs known to affect the cytochrome P450 3A system requires monitoring of tacrolimus blood levels and possible dose adjustment.

*Drugs inhibiting the cytochrome P450 3A system:* Substances known to inhibit cytochrome P450 3A may decrease the metabolism of Prograf with a resultant increase in tacrolimus blood levels.

Based on *in vitro* studies, the following drugs may be regarded as potential inhibitors of metabolism: bromocriptine, cortisone, dapsone, ergotamine, ethinyloestradiol, gestodene, itraconazole, josamycin, lidocaine, mephenytoin, miconazole, midazolam, nicardipine, nifedipine, nilvadipine, norethindrone, quinidine, tamoxifen, (triacetyl)oleandomycin, verapamil.

Naringenine (flavenoid in grapefruit juice) is known to inhibit the cytochrome P450 3A4 system.

*Drugs inducing the cytochrome P450 3A system:* Drugs known to induce cytochrome P450 3A might theoretically increase the metabolism of Prograf and hence decrease blood levels of tacrolimus. These include barbituates (e.g. phenobarbitone), phenytoin, rifampicin, carbamazepine, metamizole and isoniazide.

*Prograf inhibition of the cytochrome P450 3A system – mediated metabolism of other drugs: In vitro,* Prograf showed a broad and powerful inhibitory effect on cytochrome P450 3A dependent metabolism. Prograf also demonstrated inhibition of cortisone and testosterone metabolism *in vitro.*

As Prograf might interfere with the metabolism of steroidal sexual hormones the efficacy of oral contraception may be decreased.

*Potential drug interactions based on plasma protein binding:* Prograf is extensively bound to plasma proteins. For this reason, possible interactions with other drugs known to have high affinity for plasma proteins (e.g. oral anticoagulants, oral antidiabetics) should be considered.

*Other forms of interaction*

*Vaccines:* During treatment with Prograf, vaccinations may be less effective and the use of live attenuated vaccines should be avoided.

*Compounds with nephrotoxic/neurotoxic effects:* Using Prograf with compounds known to have nephrotoxic or neurotoxic effects, (e.g. aminoglycosides, amphotericin B, gyrase inhibitors, vancomycin, cotrimoxazole and NSAIDs, ganciclovir or aciclovir) may increase toxic effects.

*Potassium:* As Prograf therapy may be associated with hyperkalaemia, or may increase pre-existing hyperkalaemia, high potassium intake or potassium-saving diuretics (e.g. amiloride, triamterene and spironolactone) should be avoided.

*Food:* Administration of Prograf with a meal of moderate fat content has been shown to reduce significantly the oral bioavailability or absorption of the drug. Therefore, it may be preferable to administer Prograf on an empty stomach or at least 1 hour before or 2–3 hours after a meal to achieve maximal absorption.

*Pregnancy and lactation:* Prograf is contra-indicated in pregnancy. In animal studies (rats and rabbits) Prograf has been shown to be teratogenic at doses which also demonstrated maternal toxicity.

Preclinical and human data show that the drug is able to cross the placenta. The possibility of pregnancy should therefore be excluded before initiating Prograf therapy.

As Prograf may alter the metabolism of oral contraceptives, other forms of contraception should be used.

Preclinical data in rats suggest that Prograf is excreted into breast milk. Human data on effects of the drug during the lactation period is limited. As detrimental effects on the newborn cannot be excluded, women should not breast-feed whilst receiving tacrolimus.

*Effects on ability to drive and use machines:* Prograf is associated with visual and neurological disturbances. Patients treated with Prograf who are affected by such disorders should not drive a car or operate dangerous machines. This effect may be enhanced when Prograf is given together with alcohol.

*Undesirable effects:* The adverse drug reactions (ADRs) profile associated with the use of immunosuppressive drugs is often difficult to establish owing to the presence of the mostly severe underlying disease and the concurrent use of many other medications.

There is evidence that many of the ADRs stated below are reversible and respond to dose reduction. Oral administration appears to be associated with a lower incidence of adverse events compared with intravenous use. The ADRs stated below have been arranged according to body system and within these according to frequency.

*Cardiovascular system:*

frequent: hypertension
occasional: angina pectoris, tachycardia, effusion (e.g. pericard, pleural)
rare: hypotension including shock, abnormal ECG, cardiac arrhythmias, including atrial/ventricular fibrillations and cardiac arrest, thrombophlebitis, haemorrhage (e.g. gastrointestinal, cerebral), heart failure, cardiomegaly, bradycardia, ventricular and/or septal hypertrophy (including cardiomyopathy)
isolated: thrombosis, embolus (e.g. pulmonary), ischaemia (e.g. cerebral), infarct (e.g. myocard; kidney; cerebrum), syncope, pericarditis and vascular disease

*Nervous system/sensory system:*

frequent: tremor, headache, insomnia, perception disorder, visual disorders (e.g. cataract, amblyopia)
occasional: depression, neuropathy, nervousness, anxiety, hypertonia, incoordination, emotional lability, amnesia, encephalopathy
rare: migraine, confusion, dizziness, decreased reflexes, somnolence, hallucinations, dream and thinking abnormalities, agitation, psychosis, glaucoma, otological disturbances (e.g. tinnitus, deafness), photophobia
isolated: paralysis (e.g. tetraplegia), coma, convulsion, stupor, speech disorders (e.g. aphasia, dysarthria), refraction disorder, hostility, retinopathy, cortical blindness, taste loss

*Kidney*

frequent: abnormal kidney function (e.g. increase in creatinine, BUN and decrease/increase in urine output)
occasional: lesion of kidney tissue (e.g. tubular necrosis)
rare: dialysis-dependent renal failure, proteinuria, haematuria, hydronephrosis
isolated: HUS, glomerulopathy (glomerulitis, nephritis)

*Digestive system/liver:*

frequent: constipation, diarrhoea, nausea
occasional: cholangitis, vomiting, abnormal liver function test, jaundice, weight and appetite changes, inflammatory disorders (e.g. ulcer), dysfunction of GI-tract (e.g. dyspepsia)
rare: lesion of liver tissue (cirrhosis, necrosis), haematemesis, ileus, ascites, dysphagia
isolated: pancreatitis, hepatomegaly, liver failure, bile duct abnormality

*Metabolism and electrolytes:*

frequent: hypercalaemia, hyperglycaemia, hypophosphataemia
occasional: diabetes mellitus, disorders of acid/base balance, hypervolaemia, hypokalaemia, hyperuricaemia (including gout), increased amylase
rare: decrease in blood concentration of magnesium, calcium, protein, sodium; increase in blood concentration of calcium, phosphate; dehydration, hyperlipidaemia, hypoglycaemia
isolated: hypermagnesaemia, increase of creatine phosphokinase

*Musculoskeletal:*

occasional: cramps
rare: osteoporosis
isolated: myasthenia, avascular bone necrosis, arthritis, myopathy

*Respiratory system:*

occasional: impairment of lung function (e.g. dyspnoea), atelectasis
rare: asthma
isolated: respiratory failure, pulmonary fibrosis

*Skin:*

occasional: alopecia, pruritus, sweating, rash, photosensitivity
rare: gynaecomastia, hirsutism, urticaria
isolated: erythema (e.g. erythema nodosum)

*Haematological and lymphatic system:*

frequent: leucocytosis
occasional: leucopenia, anaemia (e.g. aplastic, haemolytic)
rare: thrombocytopaenia, splenomegaly, eosinophilia, thrombocythaemia
isolated: coagulation disorders, bone marrow depression (incl. pancytopenia), thrombotic thrombocytopenic purpura

*Miscellaneous:*

occasional: oedema in various organ-systems (e.g. CNS, respiratory, cardiovascular), localised pain (e.g. arthralgia, neuralgia, abdominal pain, chest pain), asthenia, fever
isolated: incontinence, prostatic disorder, thyroid and parathyroid disorder

*Malignancies:* Malignancies are known to occur with immunosuppressive therapy. Benign and malignant neoplasms (e.g. of the lymphatic and myeloid system epithelial and mesenchymal tissue) have been reported in isolated cases in association with tacrolimus treatment.

*Autoimmune diseases:* In isolated cases autoimmune processes (e.g. vasculitis, Lyell syndrome, Stevens-Johnson syndrome) were observed in patients receiving tacrolimus.

*Allergic reactions:* Allergic and anaphylactoid reactions were noted in patients being treated with tacrolimus, such as flush, pruritus and anaphylactic shock, in isolated cases.

*Infections:* As with other potent immunosuppressive drugs, the susceptibility to viral, bacterial, fungal and/or protozoal infection is increased in patients receiving tacrolimus. Overall, infections are reported frequently in patients being treated with tacrolimus. The course of pre-existing infectious diseases may also be aggravated. Both generalised (sepsis) and localised infections (abscess, pneumonia) can occur. The risk of over-immunosuppression may be increased if tacrolimus is administered along with other immunosuppressive medication.

*Overdose:* Experience of overdosage is limited.

Early clinical experience (when initial induction doses were 2 or 3 times greater than those currently recommended) suggested that symptoms of overdosage may include, renal, neurological and cardiac disturbances, effects on glucose intolerance, hypertension and electrolyte disorders (e.g. hyperkalaemia). Over-immunosuppression may increase the risk of severe infections.

Isolated reports on overdose of tacrolimus indicate that nausea, vomiting, tremor, increased liver enzyme values, headache, lethargy, urticaria, nephrotoxicity and infections may occur.

Liver function clearly influences all pre- and post-operative pharmacokinetic variables. Patients with failing liver grafts or those switched from other immunosuppressive therapy to Prograf should be monitored carefully to avoid overdosage.

No specific antidote to Prograf therapy is available. If overdosage occurs, general supportive measures and symptomatic treatment should be conducted.

Based on the poor aqueous solubility and extensive erythrocyte and plasma protein binding, it is anticipated that Prograf will not be dialysable. In isolated patients with very high plasma concentrations of tacrolimus, haemofiltration and haemodiafiltration have been reported to considerably decrease the tacrolimus levels. In cases of oral intoxication, gastric lavage and/or the use of absorbents (such as activated charcoal) may be helpful.

**Pharmacological properties**

*Pharmacodynamic properties*

*Pharmacotherapeutic group:* Immunosuppressive macrolide lactone.

*Mechanism of action:* On the molecular level, the effects of tacrolimus appear to be mediated by binding to a cytosolic protein (FKBP12) which is also responsible for the intracellular accumulation of the compound. The FKBP12-tacrolimus complex specifically and competitively binds to and inhibits calcinurin, which leads to a calcium-dependent inhibition of signal transduction pathways in T-cells, thereby preventing transcription of a discrete set of lymphokine genes.

*Pharmacodynamic effects:* Prograf is a highly immunosuppressive agent and has proven activity in both *in vitro* and *in vivo* experiments.

In particular, Prograf inhibits the formation of cytotoxic lymphocytes which are mainly responsible for graft rejection. The drug suppresses T-cell activation and T-helper-cell dependent B-cell proliferation, as well as the formation of lymphokines such as interleukins-2, -3 and γ-interfon and the expression of the interleukin-2 receptor. At the molecular level, the effects of Prograf appear to be mediated by binding to a cytosolic protein (FKBP) which is also responsible for the intracellular accumulation of the compound.

In *in vivo* studies, Prograf has been shown to be efficacious in transplantation of the liver and kidney.

*Pharmacokinetic properties*

*General characteristics*

*Absorption:* Studies in the rat have shown that tacrolimus is absorbed throughout the gastrointestinal tract. The major site of absorption was identified as the upper GI. In man, absorption of tacrolimus from the gastrointestinal tract after oral administration is variable. Peak concentrations ($C_{max}$) of tacrolimus in blood are achieved in approximately 1 to 3 hours. In some patients the drug appears to be continuously absorbed over a prolonged time period yielding more or less a flat absorption profile. Mean (±sd) absorption parameters of tacrolimus are listed in the table below.

After oral administration (0.15 mg/kg/bid) in liver transplant patients, steady state concentrations of tacrolimus were achieved within 3 days in most patients. The oral bioavailability of tacrolimus was reduced when it was administered after food containing a moderate fat content. There was a decrease in AUC (27%), $C_{max}$ (50%) and an increase in $t_{max}$ (173%) in whole blood. Both rate and extent of absorption were reduced when tacrolimus was given with food. Bile does not influence the absorption of tacrolimus and therefore commencement of tacrolimus therapy with an oral dose or early conversion of liver transplant patients from intravenous to oral therapy is possible. There is strong correlation between the area under the curve and the trough whole blood levels at steady state. Thus monitoring of trough whole blood levels provides a good estimate of systemic exposure.

*Distribution and elimination:* In man, the disposition of tacrolimus after intravenous infusion may be described as biphasic. In systemic circulation, tacrolimus binds strongly to erythrocytes resulting in the distribution of whole blood/plasma concentrations of tacrolimus of approximately 20:1. In plasma the drug is highly bound (>98.8%) to plasma proteins, mainly to serum albumin and α-1-acid glycoprotein.

Tacrolimus is extensively distributed in the body. The steady state volume of distribution based on plasma concentrations is approximately 1300 L (healthy subjects). Corresponding data based on whole blood data averaged 47.6 L. The total body clearance (TBC) of tacrolimus from blood is low. In healthy subjects the average TBC was estimated from whole blood concentrations to be 2.43 L/h. In adult liver transplant patients, TBC was 4.1 L/h. In paediatric liver patients, the TBC is approximately double the TBC in adult liver transplant patients. In kidney transplant patients, TBC was 6.7 L/h.

There is evidence that the pharmacokinetics of tacrolimus change with improving clinical condition of the patients. In liver transplant patients, the mean oral dose was decreased by 28% from day 7 to month 6 after transplantation, to maintain similar mean trough levels of tacrolimus. Changes in clearance and/or bioavailability were suggested as probable causes for this effect.

The half-life of tacrolimus is long and variable. In healthy volunteers the main half-life in whole blood is approximately 43 hours. In adult kidney transplant patients, it averaged 12.4 and 11.7 hours respectively. In adult kidney transplant patients, it averaged 15.6 hours.

*Metabolism and biotransformation:* Tacrolimus is cleared by hepatic metabolism. The cytochrome P450 3A4 is primarily responsible for its metabolism. There is also evidence of gastrointestinal metabolism.

Eight metabolites have so far been characterised. Of these, only one metabolite showed significant immunosuppressive activity, in comparison to tacrolimus.

*Excretion:* Following intravenous and oral administration of $^{14}C$-labelled tacrolimus, most of the radioactivity was eliminated in the faeces. Approximately 2% of the radioactivity was eliminated in the urine. Less than 1% of unchanged tacrolimus was detected in the urine and the faeces. This indicates that tacrolimus is almost completely metabolised prior to elimination from the body and that bile is the principal route of elimination.

*Characteristics in patients*

*Relationship between plasma/blood concentrations and therapeutic activity:* As stated in *Posology and method of administration* section, individual dose adjustment controlled by monitoring of Prograf levels in whole blood may be helpful to achieve optimal therapy. Several immunoassays are available for determining Prograf concentrations in whole blood, including a fully automatic microparticle enzyme immunoassay (MEIA). Details are available on request.

*Variations with respect to confounding factors – age, polymorphism, metabolism and concomitant pathological situations (renal failure, hepatic insufficiency):* Based on limited experience, the kinetic properties of Prograf are not altered in elderly patients.

Children require a higher dose of Prograf, approximately 1½ to 2 times higher than that recommended for adults, possibly owing to a higher metabolic turnover.

*Patients with liver dysfunction:* Patients with liver dysfunction tended to have higher Prograf concentrations (and correspondingly longer half-lives and smaller clearance values) compared with patients with a normal liver function.

As the drug is extensively metabolised by the liver, patients with impaired liver function should be carefully monitored, and dose adjustment may be necessary.

*Patients with kidney dysfunction:* Since the drug is nearly completely metabolised, highly lipid-soluble, and has a molecular weight of 822, it is not expected to be dialysable. Also, less than 1% of an administered intravenous dose is excreted in the urine. Therefore, changes to the dosing regimen from the pharmacokinetic point of view are not necessary in patients with renal failure or in patients undergoing dialysis. However, dosage adjustment may be necessary in patients with evidence of drug-induced impairment of kidney function.

| *Population* | *Dose* | *$C^{max}$ (ng/ml)* | *$T^{max}$ (hours)* | *Bioavailability (%)* |
|---|---|---|---|---|
| Healthy subjects (Single dose) | 1×5 mg<br>5×1 mg | 28.6 (8.6)<br>36.2 (13.8) | 1.4 (0.6)<br>1.3 (0.4) | 14.4 (6.0)<br>17.4 (7.0) |
| Adult liver transplant (Steady state) | 0.15 mg/kg/12 h | 74.1 | 3.0 | 21.8 (6.3) |
| Paediatric liver transplant (Steady state) | 0.15 mg/kg/12 h | 37.0 (26.5) | 2.1 (1.3) | 25 (20) |
| Adult kidney transplant (Steady state) | 0.15 mg/kg/12 h | 44.3 (21.9) | 1.5 | 20.1 (11.0) |

*Preclinical safety data*

*Mutagenicity:* Relevant *in vitro* and *in vivo* tests showed no signs of a mutagenic potential of Prograf.

*Carcinogenicity:* In chronic, 1-year toxicity studies (rats and baboons) and in long-term carcinogenicity studies (mouse 18 months and rat 24 months at maximum tolerable dose of 2.5–5 mg/kg/day) no signs of a direct tumorigenic potential of Prograf were seen.

However, as known from other immunosuppressive drugs, malignancies such as lymphomas and skin cancers can be expected but were seen rarely in patients.

*Reproduction toxicity:* In rats, fertility, embryonic and foetal development and the birth as well as the peri- and post-natal development were only impaired when receiving clearly toxic dosages (3.2 mg/kg/day). The only exception was a reversible reduction of the foetal birth weights at a dose of 0.1 mg/kg/day. Furthermore in rabbits, toxic effects on the embryos and on the foetus were observed. Again, these were limited to doses of 1.0 mg/kg/day which showed significant toxicity in maternal animals. Based on these observations, Prograf should not be administered to pregnant women.

**Pharmaceutical particulars**

*List of excipients*

*Prograf Capsules 1 mg/Prograf Capsules 5 mg:* Hydroxypropylmethylcellulose, croscarmellose sodium, lactose, magnesium stearate and titanium dioxide (E 171). Prograf Capsules 5 mg also contain red iron oxide (E 172).

*Prograf Concentrate for Infusion 5 mg/ml:* Polyoxyethylene hydrogenated castor oil, dehydrated alcohol.

*Incompatibilities:* Prograf is not compatible with PVC plastics. Mixed infusions between a solution prepared with Prograf Concentrate for Infusion 5 mg/ml and other drugs should be avoided. In particular mixed infusions with drugs exhibiting a marked alkaline reaction in solution (e.g. aciclovir, ganciclovir) must not be administered as tacrolimus can disintegrate in this condition.

*Shelf life*

*Prograf Capsules 1 mg/Prograf Capsules 5 mg:* Aluminium-wrapped blisters: 24 months when stored at room temperature (15–30°C). After opening of the aluminium wrapper the capsules are stable for 12 months when stored at room temperature.

*Prograf Concentrate for Infusion 5 mg/ml:* 12 months when protected from light and stored at temperatures up to 25°C. To be used within 24 hours when reconstituted with 5% dextrose solution or physiological saline in polyethylene or glass containers.

*Special precautions for storage*

*Prograf Capsules 1 mg/ Prograf Capsules 5 mg:* Once the aluminium wrapper is opened the capsules in the blister strips are stable for 12 months. The individual blister strips should be kept in a dry place. The patients should be instructed accordingly.

*Prograf Concentrate for Infusion 5 mg/ml:* Store below 25°C. Protect from light.

*Nature and contents of container*

*Prograf Capsules 1 mg/Prograf Capsules 5 mg:* Ten capsules per blister sheet. For Prograf Capsules 1 mg three, five or ten blisters and for Prograf Capsules 5 mg three or five blisters are packaged with one dessicant sachet in an aluminium wrapper.

The following pack sizes are currently available on the market:

Prograf Capsules 1 mg: cartons of 50 and 100 capsules

Prograf Capsules 5 mg: cartons of 50 capsules

*Prograf Concentrate for Infusion 5 mg/ml:* Concentrate for Infusion (solution) in transparent glass ampoules.

*Instructions for use/handling:* Tubing, syringes and any other equipment used to administer Prograf should not contain PVC.

*Prograf Capsules 1 mg/Prograf Capsules 5 mg:* To be used as directed. Patients should take the capsules immediately once they are taken out of the blister.

*Prograf Concentrate for Infusion 5 mg/ml:* Prograf Concentrate for Infusion should be prepared for infusion with 5% dextrose solution or physiological saline in polyethylene or glass containers. After constitution, infusion solutions should be used within 24 hours. Opened ampoules should be disposed of immediately, if not used, to avoid contamination.

**Marketing authorisation numbers**

Prograf Capsules 1 mg 13424/0001
Prograf Capsules 5 mg 13424/0002

**Prograf Concentrate for Infusion**
**5 mg/ml**                                    13424/0003

**Date of approval/revision of SPC**   21 July 1997.

**Legal category**   POM.

*Trade Mark

# Galderma (U.K.) Ltd
Leywood House
Woodside Road
Amersham
Bucks HP6 6AA

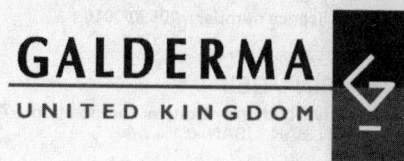

## ACNECIDE* 5% GEL
## ACNECIDE* 10% GEL

**Qualitative and quantitative composition**
Acnecide 5% Gel: Benzoyl Peroxide PhEur 5% w/w.
Acnecide 10% Gel: Benzoyl Peroxide PhEur 10% w/w.

**Pharmaceutical form** Topical gel.

**Clinical particulars**
*Therapeutic indications:* Topical therapy for the treatment of acne vulgaris.

*Posology and method of administration:* For external use only.

*Adults and children:* After washing with a mild cleanser, apply once or twice daily or as directed to the affected areas. Initially Acnecide 5 should be used; treatment may be continued with Acnecide 10 provided Acnecide 5 has been well tolerated. The extent of any drying or peeling may be adjusted by modifying the dosage schedule.

*Contra-indications:* Persons having known sensitivity to benzoyl peroxide.

*Special warnings and special precautions for use:* Avoid contact with the eyes, eyelids, and other mucous surfaces.

*Interaction with other medicaments and other forms of interaction:* None known.

*Pregnancy and lactation:* No known effects. Use at the discretion of the physician.

*Effects on ability to drive and use machines:* Not applicable.

*Undesirable effects:* None known.

*Overdose:* Not applicable.

**Pharmacological properties**
*Pharmacodynamic properties:* Benzoyl peroxide is an established and effective keratolytic agent with antibacterial properties. It has been shown to be effective in reducing the local population of *Propionibacterium acnes* leading to a reduction in the production of irritant fatty acids in the sebaceous glands.

*Pharmacokinetic properties:* Not applicable. Acnecide is a topical preparation.

*Preclinical safety data:* In animal studies by the cutaneous route, benzoyl peroxide is associated with a minimal to moderate skin irritation potential including erythema and oedema. Phototoxic and photoallergic reactions have been reported for benzoyl peroxide therapy.

**Pharmaceutical particulars**
*List of excipients:* Docusate sodium; disodium edetate; poloxamer 182; carbomer 940; propylene glycol; acrylates copolymer or glycerol microsponge; glycerol; silicon dioxide; purified water; and sodium hydroxide to adjust the pH.

*Incompatibilities:* None known.

*Shelf life:* 36 months.

*Special precautions for storage:* Store at room temperature.

*Nature and contents of container:* White low density polyethylene tubes containing 60 g gel.

*Instructions for use/handling:* No special instructions.

**Marketing authorisation numbers**
Acnecide 5% Gel     10590/0006
Acnecide 10% Gel    10590/0007

**Date of approval/revision of SPC** April 1997.

**Legal category** P.

## ALCODERM* CREAM/LOTION

**Presentation**
*Alcoderm cream:* A white, thick smooth cream containing liquid paraffin, purified water, cetyl alcohol, stearyl alcohol, sodium lauryl sulphate, methylparaben, propylparaben, sorbitan monostearate, isopropyl palmitate, Sorbitol solution, cetyl esters wax, perfume, citric acid, sodium hydroxide and silicone fluid.

*Alcoderm lotion:* A creamy white, smooth, viscous lotion containing liquid paraffin, purified water, cetyl alcohol, stearyl alcohol, sodium lauryl sulphate, car-

bomer, triethanolamine, methylparaben, propylparaben, sorbitan monostearate and perfume.

**Uses** Dry, chafed or irritated skin – Alcoderm is indicated in any condition where the moisture content of the horny layer has decreased below the normal level and the skin is no longer soft and pliable.

Also recommended for:
(a) in acute inflammatory conditions where the skin is intact, such as sunburn and windburn.
(b) as a soothing, hydrating agent in certain inflammatory skin conditions where there is dryness and scaling, such as ichthyosis, atopic eczema, winter itch etc.

**Dosage and administration** For external use only.
*Adults, elderly and children:* Apply topically to the skin as required to alleviate the symptoms of dry, chafed or irritated skin conditions, or as directed by a doctor.

**Contra-indications, warnings, etc**
*Contra-indications:* Hypersensitivity to the constituents.

*Warnings:* Avoid contact with the eyes. If symptoms persist consult your physician. In the rare event of a skin reaction, treatment should be discontinued.

*Overdose:* Accidental ingestion is not anticipated to cause any harm to the patient.

**Pharmaceutical precautions** Store below 25°C.

**Legal category** P.

**Package quantities**
Alcoderm Cream:     60 g
Alcoderm Lotion:    200 ml

**Further information** Nil.

**Product licence numbers**
Alcoderm Cream     10590/0004
Alcoderm Lotion    10590/0005

## CALMURID* CREAM

**Presentation** A white cream containing Urea PhEur 10% and Lactic Acid PhEur 5% in a stabilising emulsified base.

**Uses** To be applied topically for the correction of hyperkeratosis and dryness in ichthyosis and allied conditions characterised by dry, rough, scaly skin.

**Dosage and administration** For external use only.
*Adults, elderly and children:* A thick layer of Calmurid is applied twice daily after washing the affected area. The cream is left on the skin for three to five minutes and then lightly rubbed in. Excess cream should be wiped off with a tissue, not washed off. Frequency of application can be reduced as the patient progresses. In hyperkeratosis of the feet, apply Calmurid as above after soaking feet in warm water for 15 minutes and drying with a rough towel.

**Contra-indications, warnings, etc**
*Contra-indications:* Hypersensitivity to any of the constituents of the cream.

*Interactions:* The low pH of the cream might affect the stability of other drugs.

*Other special warnings:* Calmurid is acidic and hypertonic and can cause smarting if applied to raw areas, fissures or mucous membranes. Where this is a barrier to therapy the use of Calmurid diluted 50% with aqueous cream BP for one week should result in freedom from smarting upon use of Calmurid.

*Overdose:* Unlikely. In the case of smarting, wash off cream. Consult doctor or pharmacist.

*Incompatibilities:* The low pH, due to lactic acid, means care in choice of other packages or other drugs admixed.

**Pharmaceutical precautions** Store below 25°C. Do not freeze. Do not put in alloy containers.

**Legal category** P.

**Package quantities** Collapsible plastic tubes of 100 g. Rigid plastic pump dispensers of 500 g.

**Further information** Urea at a concentration of 10%

has keratolytic, anti-microbial, anti-pruritic and hydrating effects on the skin. Lactic acid has keratolytic, hydrating and anti-microbial properties also. Treatment of ichthyotic patients shows a parallel between clinical improvement and increase in the otherwise depressed water binding capacity of the horny layer.

The constituents of the base are: glycerol monostearate, betaine monohydrate, diethanolamine cetyl phosphate ('Amphisol'), adeps solidus (hard fat), cholesterol, sodium chloride, purified water.

**Product licence number** 10590/0009.

## CALMURID HC* CREAM

**Presentation** A smooth, homogenous white oil in water cream containing: Urea PhEur 10% w/w, Lactic Acid PhEur 5% w/w and Hydrocortisone PhEur 1% w/w.

**Uses** To be used topically for the management of atopic eczema, Besniers prurigo, acute and chronic allergic eczema, neurodermatitis and other hyperkeratotic skin conditions with accompanying inflammation.

**Dosage and administration** For external use only.
*Adults, elderly and children:* Apply twice daily to the affected area after bathing or washing. Moist lesions should be treated as to dry them before using Calmurid HC.

**Contra-indications, warnings, etc**
*Contra-indications:* Skin tuberculosis, viral infections accompanied by dermal manifestations e.g. herpes simplex, vaccinia, chicken pox and measles. Syphilitic skin lesions. In concurrent mycotic infections, the cream should be complemented with antimycotic treatment.

*Interactions:* None known.

*Side effects:* If applied to open wounds or mucous membranes the hypertonic and acidic nature of the preparation may produce smarting. Where smarting is a barrier to therapy, dilute with an equal quantity of aqueous cream: after a week of treatment with this material, the normal strength should be tolerated.

*Pregnancy and lactation*
*Pregnancy:* Evidence from animal studies suggests that prolonged intensive therapy with steroids during pregnancy should be avoided.
*Lactation:* Given the slow uptake of hydrocortisone from the skin and the rapid destruction of hydrocortisone by the body, there would seem to be little risk of significant transfer at lactation.

*Precautions and warnings:* In infants, high surface area in relation to mass raises the likelihood of uptake of excessive amounts of steroid from the cream, even without occlusion, thus adrenal suppression is more likely. In infants, long term continuous topical therapy should be avoided.

*Overdose:* The barrier function in the skin to steroid uptake, the low toxicity of hydrocortisone and the natural mechanism for its rapid inactivation make overdose unlikely.

**Pharmaceutical precautions** Store below 25°C. Do not mix with other preparations, as the effect on the stability of each is unknown. Do not pack in alloy containers as they may react with the lactic acid.

**Legal category** POM.

**Package quantities** Collapsible polypropylene tubes of 30 g and 100 g.

**Further information** Urea at a concentration of 10% has keratolytic, anti-microbial, anti-pruritic and hydrating effects on the skin, properties also attributable to lactic acid.

Hydrocortisone 1% is the normal concentration of the drug used as a dermatological anti-inflammatory agent. In some patients with eczema, Calmurid HC cream may be as effective as fluorinated steroid creams.

The constituents of the base are: glycerol monostearate, betaine monohydrate, diethanolamine cetyl phosphate ('Amphisol'), adeps solidus (hard fat), cholesterol, sodium chloride and purified water.

**Product licence number** 10590/0010.

## DIFFERIN* GEL ▼

**Qualitative and quantitative composition** Adapalene (INN, BAN, USAN) 0.1% w/w.

**Pharmaceutical form** Topical gel.

**Clinical particulars**
*Therapeutic indications:* Differin Gel is proposed for the cutaneous treatment of mild to moderate acne where comedones, papules and pustules predominate. Acne of the face, chest or back is appropriate for treatment.

*Posology and method of administration:* Differin Gel should be applied to the acne affected areas once a day before retiring and after washing. A thin film of gel should be applied, with the fingertips, avoiding the eyes and lips (see *Special warnings and special precautions for use*, below). Ensure that the affected areas are dry before application.

Since it is customary to alternate therapies in the treatment of acne, it is recommended that the physician assess the continued improvement of the patient after three months of treatment with Differin Gel.

With patients for whom it is necessary to reduce the frequency of application or to temporarily discontinue treatment, frequency of application may be restored or therapy resumed once it is judged that the patient can again tolerate the treatment. If patients use cosmetics, these should be non-comedogenic and non-astringent. The safety and effectiveness of Differin Gel have not been studied in neonates and young children. Differin Gel should not be used in patients with severe acne.

*Contra-indications:* Hypersensitivity to any ingredient of the product.

*Special warnings and special precautions for use:* If a reaction suggesting sensitivity or severe irritation occurs, use of the medication should be discontinued. If the degree of local irritation warrants, patients should be directed to use the medication less frequently, to discontinue use temporarily, or to discontinue use altogether. Differin Gel should not come into contact with the eyes, mouth, angles of the nose or mucous membranes.

If product enters the eye, wash immediately with warm water. The product should not be applied to either broken (cuts and abrasions) or eczematous skin, nor should it be used in patients with severe acne involving large areas of the body, especially in women of child bearing age who are not on effective contraception.

*Interaction with other medicaments and other forms of interaction:* There are no known interactions with other medications which might be used cutaneously and concurrently with Differin Gel; however, other retinoids or drugs with a similar mode of action should not be used concurrently with adapalene.

Adapalene is essentially stable to oxygen and light and is chemically non-reactive. Whilst extensive studies in animals and man have shown neither phototoxic nor photoallergic potential for adapalene, the safety of using adapalene during repeated exposure to sunlight or UV irradiation has not been established in either animals or man. Exposure to excessive sunlight or UV irradiation should be avoided.

Absorption of adapalene through human skin is low (see *Pharmacokinetic properties*) and therefore interaction with systemic medications is unlikely. There is no evidence that the efficacy of oral drugs such as contraceptives and antibiotics is influenced by the cutaneous use of Differin Gel.

Differin Gel has a potential for mild local irritation, and therefore it is possible that concomitant use of peeling agents, abrasive cleansers, strong drying agents, astringents or irritant products (aromatic and alcoholic agents) may produce additive irritant effects. However, cutaneous antiacne treatment e.g. erythromycin (up to 4%) or clindamycin phosphate (1% as the base) solutions or benzoyl peroxide water based gels up to 10% may be used in the morning when Differin Gel is used at night as there is no mutual degradation or cumulative irritation.

*Pregnancy and lactation:* No information on the effects of Adapalene in pregnant women is available and therefore this product should not be used during pregnancy, unless considered essential by the physician. Because of the risk of teratogenicity shown in animal studies and since there is no information on the use of adapalene in pregnant women, it should not be used in women of child bearing age unless they are using an effective means of contraception.

Adapalene produces teratogenic effects by the oral route in rats and rabbits. At cutaneous doses up to 200-fold the therapeutic dose, producing circulating plasma levels of adapalene at least 35 to 120 times higher than plasma levels demonstrated in therapeutic use, adapalene increased the incidence of additional ribs in rats and rabbits, without increasing the incidence of major malformations.

It is not known whether adapalene is secreted in animal or human milk. In animal studies, infant rats suckled by mother with circulating levels of adapalene at least 300 times those demonstrated in clinical use developed normally.

Its use in women breast feeding infants should be avoided but when it is used in breast feeding women, to avoid contact exposure of the infant, application of adapalene to the chest should be avoided.

*Effects on ability to drive and use machines:* Based upon the pharmacodynamic profile and clinical experience, performance related to driving and using machines should not be affected.

*Undesirable effects:* Side effects include skin irritation, stinging and a feeling of warmth at the site of application.

The major undesirable effect which may occur is irritation of the skin which is reversible when treatment is reduced in frequency or discontinued.

*Overdose:* Differin Gel is not to be taken orally and is for cutaneous use only. If the medication is applied excessively, no more rapid or better results will be obtained and marked redness, peeling or discomfort may occur.

The acute oral dose of Differin Gel required to produce toxic effects in mice and rats is greater than 10 ml/kg. Nevertheless, unless the amount accidentally ingested is small, an appropriate method of gastric emptying should be considered.

**Pharmacological properties**
*Pharmacodynamic properties:* Adapalene is a retinoid-like compound which in, in-vivo and in-vitro models of inflammation, has been demonstrated to possess anti-inflammatory properties. Adapalene is essentially stable to oxygen and light and is chemically non-reactive.

Mechanically, adapalene binds like tretinoin to specific retinoic acid nuclear receptors, but unlike tretinoin, not to cytosolic receptor binding proteins.

Adapalene applied cutaneously is comedolytic in the rhino mouse model and also has effects on the abnormal processes of epidermal keratinisation and differentiation, both of which are present in the pathogenesis of acne vulgaris. The mode of action of adapalene is suggested to be a normalisation of differentiation of follicular epithelial cells resulting in decreased microcomedone formation.

Adapalene is superior to reference retinoids in standard anti-inflammatory assays, both in-vivo and in-vitro. Mechanistically, it inhibits chemotactic and chemokinetic responses of human polymorphonuclear leucocytes and also the metabolism by lipoxidation of arachidonic acid to pro-inflammatory mediators. This profile suggests that the cell mediated inflammatory component of acne may be modified by adapalene.

*Pharmacokinetic properties:* Absorption of adapalene through human skin is low. In clinical trial, measurable plasma adapalene levels were not found following chronic cutaneous application to large areas of acneic skin with an analytical sensitivity of 0.15 ng/ml.

After administration of [$^{14}$C]-adapalene in rats (IV, IP, oral and cutaneous) rabbits (IV, oral and cutaneous) and dogs (IV and oral), radioactivity was distributed in several tissues, the highest levels being found in liver, spleen, adrenals and ovaries. Metabolism in animals has been tentatively identified as being mainly by O-demethylation, hydroxylation and conjugation, and excretion is primarily by the biliary route.

*Preclinical safety data:* In animal studies, adapalene was well tolerated on cutaneous application for periods of up to six months in rabbits and for up to two years in mice. The major symptoms of toxicity found in all animal species by the oral route were related to an hypervitaminosis A syndrome, and included bone dissolution, elevated alkaline phosphatase and a slight anaemia. Large oral doses of adapalene produced no adverse neurological, cardiovascular or respiratory effects in animals. Adapalene is not mutagenic. Lifetime studies with adapalene have been completed in mice at cutaneous doses of 0.6, 2 and 6 mg/kg/day and in rats at oral doses of 0.15, 0.5 and 1.5 mg/kg/day. The only significant finding was a statistically significant increase of benign phaeochromocytomas of the adrenal medulla among male rats receiving adapalene at 1.5 mg/kg/day. These changes are unlikely to be of relevance to the cutaneous use of adapalene.

**Pharmaceutical particulars**
*List of excipients:* Carbomer 940, Methyl Parahydroxybenzoate PhEur, Propylene glycol PhEur, Phenoxyethanol PhEur, Poloxamer 182 PhEur, Sodium Hydroxide PhEur, Disodium Edetate PhEur and Purified Water PhEur.

*Incompatibilities:* None known.

*Shelf life:* The shelf life expiry date shall not exceed two years from the date of its manufacture.

*Special precautions for storage:* Store at room temperature not exceeding 25°C. Warning: do not allow to freeze. Keep out of reach of children.

*Nature and contents of container:* White low density polypropylene tube with a white polypropylene screw cap. Pack size 30 g.

*Instructions for use/handling:* A thin film of the gel should be applied, avoiding eyes, lips and mucous membranes.

**Marketing authorisation number** 10590/0015.

**Date of approval/revision of SPC** August 1996.

**Legal category** POM.

## IONAX* SCRUB

**Presentation** A pale yellow semi-transulcent abradant gel with a fresh odour of lemon. The active ingredients are polyethylene granules 21.87% w/w, benzalkonium chloride solution 0.53% w/w, polyoxyethylene (4) lauryl ether 4.18% w/w, polyoxyethylene (23) lauryl ether 15.42% w/w and denatured alcohol 11.77% w/w in a foaming, aqueous gel base containing propylene glycol, potassium sorbate, silica, lauramine oxide, perfume and colouring.

**Uses** An abradant cleanser for the control and hygiene of acne. For topical application to the skin. To cleanse the skin prior to acne or oily skin treatment.

**Dosage and administration**
*Adults and children:* Use once or twice daily, or as directed by a physician. Apply to wet face. Massage on the skin for one or two minutes, then rinse thoroughly.

**Contra-indications, warnings, etc**
*Warning:* Avoid contact with the eyes. Upon accidental contact, flush with water and avoid rubbing. If the skin becomes too dry or too reddened discontinue use temporarily. For external use only.

**Pharmaceutical precautions** There are no special pharmaceutical precautions.

**Legal category** P.

**Package quantities** 60 g packs in plastic collapsible tubes with plastic screw caps.

**Further information** Nil.

**Product licence number** 10590/0008

## IONIL T* SHAMPOO

**Qualitative and quantitative composition** Coal tar solution 4.25% w/w, salicylic acid 2.0% w/w, benzalkonium chloride 0.2% w/w, polyoxyethylene (4) lauryl ether 7.2% w/w and polyoxyethylene (23) lauryl ether 14.4% w/w.

**Pharmaceutical form** Hydro-alcoholic solution for topical (cutaneous) application as a shampoo.

**Clinical particulars**
*Therapeutic indications:* Psoriasis and seborrhoeic dermatitis of the scalp.

*Posology and method of administration:*
*Adults, elderly and children:* Massage Ionil T Shampoo into wet hair and rinse out (not too much lather will be produced on first application). Apply again, working into a lather, and allow to remain on the hair for five minutes before rinsing.

Repeat the treatment once or twice a week, or as directed by the doctor or pharmacist.

*Contra-indications:* None.

*Special warnings and special precautions for use:* Avoid contact with the eyes. Upon accidental contact, flush with clean, warm water.

*Interaction with other medicaments and other forms of interaction:* None known.

*Pregnancy and lactation:* No special precautions required.

*Effects on ability to drive and use machines:* None.

*Undesirable effects:* None known.

*Overdose:* Not applicable.

**Pharmacological properties**
*Pharmacodynamic properties:* The active constituents of Ionil T Shampoo provide the product with keratolytic, antiseptic and anti-pruritic properties to effect symptomatic relief of psoriasis and seborrhoeic dermatitis of the scalp.

In animal models, coal tar has been demonstrated to suppress epidermal cell DNA synthesis.

*Pharmacokinetic properties:* Not applicable.

*Preclinical safety data:* No specific information is

presented given the widespread use of coal tar preparations on humans over many years.

**Pharmaceutical particulars**

*List of excipients:* Ethyl alcohol, tetrasodium edetate, citric acid and purified water.

*Incompatibilities:* None known.

*Shelf life:* Thirty six (36) months.

*Special precautions for storage:* Ionil T Shampoo should be stored below 25°C and away from direct heat. The product should be stored away from internal preparations and food.

As with all medicines, Ionil T Shampoo should be kept out of the sight and reach of children.

*Nature and contents of container:* White polypropylene flat bottle with a white polypropylene snap or screw cap as the closure; pack sizes 50 ml (physicians sample), 200 ml.

*Instruction for use/handling:* No special instructions.

**Marketing authorisation number** 10590/0003.

**Date of approval/revision of SPC** December 1996.

**Legal category** P.

## NUTRAPLUS* CREAM

**Qualitative and quantitative composition** Urea PhEur 10% w/w.

**Pharmaceutical form** Smooth white, almost odourless cream (water in oil emulsion).

**Clinical particulars**

*Therapeutic indications:* An emollient, moisturising and protective cream for the treatment of dry or damaged skin.

*Posology and method of administration:*

*Adults, elderly and children:* Apply evenly to the dry skin areas two to three times daily, or as directed by the physician or pharmacist.

*Contra-indications:* None.

*Special warnings and special precautions for use:* Avoid contact with the eyes. If irritation occurs, discontinue use temporarily.

*Interaction with other medicaments and other forms of interaction:* None known.

*Pregnancy and lactation:* No known effects. Use at the discretion of the physician or pharmacist.

*Effects on ability to drive and use machines:* Not applicable.

*Undesirable effects:* None known.

*Overdose:* Not applicable.

**Pharmacological properties**

*Pharmacodynamic properties:* Urea is a recognised hydrating agent that has been widely used topically to treat dry or damaged skin.

*Pharmacokinetic properties:* Not applicable. Nutraplus is a topical (cutaneous) preparation.

*Preclinical safety data:* No specific information is presented given the widespread use of topically applied urea on humans over many years.

**Pharmaceutical particulars**

*List of excipients:* Glycerol monostearate, octyl palmitate, myristyl lactate, mineral oil, promulgen D, propylene glycol, propyl parahydroxybenzoate, methyl parahydroxybenzoate, purified water.

*Incompatibilities:* None known.

*Shelf life:* Thirty six months.

*Special precautions for storage:* Nutraplus Cream should be stored below 25°C and away from direct heat. As with all medicines, Nutraplus Cream should be stored out of the sight and reach of children.

*Nature and contents of container:* White, polyethylene tube with a white polypropylene screw cap as the closure. Pack size 100 g.

*Instruction for use/handling:* No special instructions.

**Marketing authorisation number** 10590/0002.

**Date of approval/revision of SPC** 1 March 1996.

**Legal category** P.

## PSORIGEL*

**Qualitative and quantitative composition** Psorigel contains Coal Tar Solution BP 7.5% as the active ingredient.

**Pharmaceutical form** Hydro-alcoholic gel for topical (cutaneous) application.

**Clinical particulars**

*Therapeutic indications:* For the relief and treatment of inflammatory manifestations of tar responsive dermatoses. Among these are eczema, psoriasis, inflammation, erythema, scaling, pruritis and induration that accompany various forms of dermatitis.

Psorigel also helps relieve the itching that accompanies psoriasis and eczema, and helps control flaking and scaling.

For topical use on the affected areas of the skin and scalp.

*Posology and method of administration:* Adults, elderly and children: Rub Psorigel onto the affected areas once or twice daily. The gel may be applied more frequently if necessary. Rub the gel in well, allow it to dry and remove any excess by patting with a paper tissue.

*Contra-indications:* There are no contra-indications to the topical (cutaneous) use of Psorigel.

*Special warnings and special precautions for use:* Avoid contact with the eyes. Upon accidental contact, flush with water.

After using Psorigel, avoid exposure to direct sunlight unless specifically directed by the physician.

The product contains 33% alcohol. Do not use Psorigel on highly inflamed or on broken skin. If undue irritation occurs in use reduce the frequency of use, or discontinue use until the irritation subsides.

The staining potential of the product is minimal but if it does occur, standard laundry procedures will remove most stains.

*Interaction with other medicaments and other forms of interaction:* None known.

*Pregnancy and lactation:* No known effects. Coal tar preparations have been in wide use for many years without apparent deleterious effects. Use at the discretion of the physician or pharmacist.

*Effects on ability to drive and to use machines:* None known.

*Undesirable effects:* None known.

*Overdose:* Not pertinent to this topically applied product.

**Pharmacological properties**

*Pharmacodynamic properties:* The active ingredient of Psorigel is coal tar, which possesses both antipruritic and keratolytic properties. In animal models, coal tar has been demonstrated to suppress epidermal cell DNA synthesis.

*Pharmacokinetic particulars:* Not applicable. Psorigel is a topical (cutaneous) preparation.

*Preclinical safety data:* No specific information is presented given the widespread use of coal tar preparations on humans for many years.

**Pharmaceutical particulars**

*List of excipients:* Carbomer 940, propylene glycol, ethyl alcohol (95.6%), laureth 4, perfume M72-512, di-isopropanolamine, purified water.

*Incompatibilities:* None known.

*Shelf life:* 36 months.

*Special precautions for storage:* Psorigel should be stored below 25°C and away from direct heat. As with all medicines, Psorigel should be kept out of the sight and reach of children.

*Nature and contents of container:* Brown HDPE tube with a polypropylene cap. Pack size 100 g.

*Instructions for use/handling:* No special instructions.

**Marketing authorisation number** 10590/0001

**Date of approval/revision of SPC** 13 April 1996

**Legal category** P.

## ROZEX* GEL

**Qualitative and quantitative composition** Metronidazole PhEur 0.75% w/w.

**Pharmaceutical form** Gel.

**Clinical particulars**

*Therapeutic indications:* Indicated in the treatment of inflammatory papules, pustules and erythema of rosacea.

*Posology and method of administration:* For topical administration only.

*Adults:* Apply and rub in a film of Gel twice daily, morning and evening, to entire affected area after washing.

*Elderly:* The dosage recommended in the elderly is the same as that recommended in adults.

*Children:* Not recommended.

*Contra-indications:* Contra-indicated in individuals with a history of hypersensitivity to metronidazole, parabens or other ingredients of the formulation.

*Special warnings and special precautions for use:* Rozex Gel has been reported to cause lacrimation of the eyes, therefore, contact with the eyes should be avoided. If a reaction suggesting local irritation occurs patients should be directed to use the medication less frequently, discontinue use temporarily or discontinue use until further instructions. Metronidazole is a nitroimidazole and should be used with care in patients with evidence of, or history of, blood dyscrasia. Exposure of treated sites to ultraviolet or strong sunlight should be avoided during use of metronidazole.

*Interaction with other medicaments and other forms of interaction:* Drug interactions are less likely with topical administration but should be kept in mind when Rozex Gel is prescribed for patients receiving anticoagulant treatment. Oral Metronidazole has been reported to potentiate the anti-coagulant effect of dicoumarin and warfarin, resulting in a prolongation of prothrombin time.

*Pregnancy and lactation:* There is no experience to date with the use of Rozex Gel in pregnancy. Metronidazole crosses the placental barrier and rapidly enters the foetal circulation. There is inadequate evidence of the safety of Metronidazole in human pregnancy. In animals, Metronidazole was not teratogenic or embryotoxic unless administered at extremely high doses. Rozex Gel should only be used in pregnancy when there is no safer alternative.

After oral administration, Metronidazole is excreted in breast milk in concentrations similar to those found in the plasma, Metronidazole blood levels from topical administration are significantly lower than those achieved after oral administration. A decision should be made to discontinue nursing or to discontinue the drug, taking into account the importance of the drug to the mother.

*Effects on ability to drive and use machines:* Not applicable.

*Undesirable effects:* Because of the minimal absorption of metronidazole and consequently its insignificant plasma concentration after topical administration, the adverse experiences reported with the oral form of the drug have not been reported with Rozex Gel. Adverse reactions reported with Rozex Gel include watery (tearing) eyes if the gel is applied too closely to this area, transient redness and mild dryness, burning, and skin irritation.

*Overdosage:* There is no human experience with overdosage of Rozex Gel. The acute oral toxicity of Rozex Gel was determined to be greater than 5 g/kg (the highest dose given) in albino rats.

**Pharmacological properties**

*Pharmacodynamic properties:* Metronidazole is an antiprotozoal and antibacterial agent which is active against a wide range of pathogenic micro-organisms. The mechanisms of action of metronidazole in rosacea are unknown but available evidence suggests that the effects may be antibacterial and/or anti-inflammatory.

*Pharmacokinetic properties:* Metronidazole is rapidly and nearly totally absorbed after oral administration. The drug is not significantly bound to serum proteins and distributes well to all body compartments with the lowest concentration found in the fat. Metronidazole is excreted primarily in the urine as parent drug, oxidative metabolites and conjugates.

Bioavailability studies with Rozex Gel in rosacea patients treated with 7.5 mg metronidazole applied topically to the face resulted in maximum serum concentrations of 66 ng/ml which is approximately 100 times less than those attained after a single oral dose of 250 mg. In most patients at most time points after Rozex Gel application, serum concentrations of metronidazole were below the detectable limits of the assay (25 ng/ml).

*Preclinical safety data:* The toxicity studies conducted with the Metronidazole 0.75% Topical Gel formulation demonstrate that the product is non-toxic in rats after acute oral administration of 5 g/kg and produced no ocular irritation in rabbit eyes. The formulation produced no observable effects in rabbits after dermal application of 13 mg/kg for 90 days. No compound-related dermal or systemic effects were observed in a 13-week cutaneous route toxicity study, in which Rozex gel containing Metronidazole 0.75% w/w was applied daily to rabbits at doses ranging between 0.13 and 13 mg/kg. Metronidazole has shown evidence of carcinogenic activity in a number of studies involving chronic, oral administration in mice and rats but not in studies involving hamsters.

One study showed a significant enhancement of UV induced skin tumours in hairless mice treated with Metronidazole intraperitoneally (15 µg per g body weight and per day for 28 weeks). Although the significance of these studies to man is not clear, patients should be advised to avoid or minimise exposure of metronidazole treated sites to sun. Metronidazole has shown mutagenic activity in several in vitro bacterial assay systems. In addition, a dose-response increase in the frequency of micronuclei was observed in mice after intraperitoneal injection and an increase in chromosome aberrations have been reported in patients with Crohn's disease who were treated with 200 to 1200 mg/day of metronidazole for 1 to 24 months. However, no excess chromosomal aberrations in circulating human lymphocytes have been observed in patients treated for 8 months.

## Pharmaceutical particulars

*List of excipients:* Carbomer (Carbopol 940) BP, Disodium Edetate PhEur, Methyl Hydroxybenzoate PhEur, Propyl Hydroxybenzoate PhEur, Propylene Glycol PhEur, Sodium Hydroxide PhEur, Purified Water PhEur.

*Incompatibilities:* None known.

*Shelf life:* Rozex Gel has a shelf life when unopened of 36 months.

*Special precautions for storage:* Store at a temperature not exceeding 25°C, away from direct heat. Do not freeze.

*Nature and contents of container:* Aluminium tubes with epoxy phenolic lining, and white polypropylene or polyethylene screw caps; pack size: 30 g.

*Instructions for use/handling:* Not applicable.

**Marketing authorisation number** 10590/0016

**Date of approval/revision of SPC** July 1996.

**Legal category** POM.

## TETRALYSAL* 300

**Qualitative and quantitative composition** Lymecycline BP 408 mg equivalent to 300 mg tetracycline base.

**Pharmaceutical form** Hard gelatin capsules.

### Clinical particulars

*Therapeutic indications:* Tetralysal 300 contains a broad spectrum antibiotic and is recommended for the treatment of all infections caused by tetracycline-sensitive organisms and may be utilised in all conditions where tetracycline is indicated.

In common with other tetracyclines, it is indicated in penicillin-sensitive patients for the treatment of staphyloccocal infections. Typical indications include: ear, nose and throat infections; acute and chronic bronchitis (including prophylaxis); infections of the gastrointestinal and urinary tracts; non-gonococcal urethritis of chlamydial origin and other chlamydial infections such as trachoma; acne; rickettsial fevers; soft tissue infections.

*Posology and method of administration*

*Adults:* The usual dosage is 1 capsule b.d. If higher doses are required, 3–4 capsules may be given over 24 hours. Lower doses may be given for prophylaxis and for the chronic treatment of acne: in such cases treatment should be continued for at least 8 weeks. In the management of sexually transmitted disease both partners should be treated.

*Elderly:* As with other tetracyclines, no specific dose adjustment is required.

*Children:* Not recommended for children under the age of 12 years. For children over the age of 12 years the adult dosage may be given.

*Contra-indications:* As lymecycline is mainly excreted by the kidneys, Tetralysal 300 should not be administered to patients with overt renal insufficiency. Its use is also contra-indicated in patients hypersensitive to tetracyclines. Children under the age of 8 years.

*Special warnings and precautions for use:* Prolonged use of broad spectrum antibiotics may result in the appearance of resistant organisms and superinfection.

Bulging fontanelles in infants and benign intracranial hypertension in adults has been reported during treatment with tetracyclines. Therefore treatment should cease if evidence of raised intracranial pressure develops during treatment with Tetralysal 300.

*Interactions with other medicaments and other forms of interaction:* The absorption of tetracyclines may be affected by the simultaneous administration of milk, antacids and iron preparations. These products should not be taken within two hours before or after taking Tetralysal 300.

*Pregnancy and lactation:* Tetracyclines are selectively absorbed by developing bones and teeth, and may cause dental staining and enamel hypoplasia. In addition these compounds readily cross the placental barrier and therefore Tetralysal 300 should not be given to pregnant or lactating women.

*Effects on ability to drive and use machine:* None known.

*Undesirable effects:* None known.

*Overdose:* There is no specific treatment, but gastric lavage should be performed as soon as possible. Supportive measures should be instituted as required and a high fluid intake maintained.

## Pharmacological properties

*Pharmacodynamic properties:* Lymecycline has antimicrobial activity and uses similar to those of tetracycline hydrochloride. It acts by interfering with bacterial protein synthesis and is active against a large number of Gram-positive and Gram-negative pathogenic bacteria including some which are resistant to penicillin.

*Pharmacokinetic properties:* Lymecycline is more readily absorbed from the gastro-intestinal tract than tetracycline, with a peak serum concentration of approximately 2 mg/L after 3 hours following a 300 mg dose. In addition, similar blood concentrations are achieved with smaller doses. When the dose is doubled an almost correspondingly higher blood concentration has been reported to occur.

The serum half-life of lymecycline is approximately 10 hours.

*Preclinical safety data:* No specific information is presented given the vast experience gained with the use of tetracyclines in humans over the last forty years.

## Pharmaceutical particulars

*List of excipients:* Silica gel, magnesium stearate, gelatin, glyceryl mon-oleate, purified water.

*Incompatibilities:* None known.

*Shelf life:* Thirty-six (36) months when kept in the original carton (see 'Nature and contents of container').

*Special precautions for storage:* The capsules should be stored in the original container in which they were dispensed at a temperature not exceeding 25°C and protected from light.

As with all medicines, Tetralysal 300 should be kept out of the sight and reach of children.

*Nature and contents of container:* Aluminium-PVC/PVDC calendar blister strips of 14 capsules; two strips per carton, pack size 28 capsules.

*Instruction for use/handling:* No special instructions.

**Marketing authorisation number** 10590/0019

**Date of approval/revision of SPC** 20 June 1996.

**Legal category** POM.

*Trade Mark

# Genus Pharmaceuticals
## (A Wyeth Business)
Huntercombe Lane South
Taplow
Maidenhead, Berks SL6 0PH

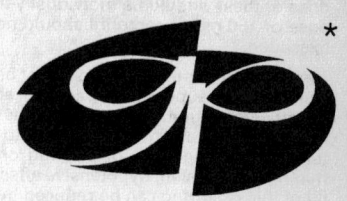

\*

## BENZHEXOL TABLETS 2 mg and 5 mg

### Qualitative and quantitative composition

| Active Constituent | Amount/ tablet | Specification reference |
|---|---|---|
| Benzhexol hydrochloride | 2 mg | BP |
| Benzhexol hydrochloride | 5 mg | BP |

**Pharmaceutical form** Benzhexol Tablets are for oral administration.

*Tablets 2 mg:* Each white scored tablet coded 'Lederle 4434' contains benzhexol hydrochloride 2 mg.

*Tablets 5 mg:* Each white scored tablet coded 'Lederle 4436' contains benzhexol hydrochloride 5 mg.

### Clinical particulars

*Therapeutic indications:* Benzhexol is an antispasmodic drug which exerts a direct inhibitory effect on the parasympathetic nervous system. It also has a relaxing effect on smooth muscle.

It is indicated in all forms of Parkinsonism (postencephalitic, arteriosclerotic and idiopathic). It is often useful as adjuvant therapy when treating these forms of Parkinsonism with levodopa. Benzhexol is effective in reducing the rigidity of muscle spasm, tremor and excessive salivation associated with Parkinsonism. Benzhexol is also indicated to control extrapyramidal disorders (eg akathisia manifested by extreme restlessness and dyskinesia characterised by spastic contractions and involuntary movements) due to central nervous system drugs such as reserpine and the phenothiazines.

*Posology and method of administration:*

*Adults only:* Optimal dosage should always be determined empirically, usually by initiating therapy at a relatively low level and by subsequent graduated increments.

The usual dosage for Parkinsonism is 6–10 mg per day although some patients chiefly in the postencephalitic group may require an average total dose of 12–15 mg daily. It should be given orally either three or four times a day at mealtimes.

Normal dosage for drug-induced Parkinsonism is usually between 5 mg and 15 mg per day, although some cases have been controlled by 1 mg daily.

In all cases, Benzhexol dosage should be increased or decreased only by small increments over a period of several days. In initial therapy the dose should be 1 mg the first day, 2 mg the second day with further increases of 2 mg per day at three to five-day intervals until the optimum dose is reached.

If patients are already being treated with other parasympathetic inhibitors, Benzhexol should be substituted as part of the therapy. When Benzhexol is used concomitantly with levodopa the usual dose of each may need to be reduced. Careful adjustment is necessary, depending on side effects and the degree of symptom control. Benzhexol dosage of 3–6 mg daily in divided doses, is usually adequate.

Benzhexol may be taken before or after meals according to the way the patient reacts. If Benzhexol tends to dry the mouth excessively, it may be better to take it before meals, unless it causes nausea. If taken after meals, induced thirst can be allayed by peppermint, chewing gum or water.

Treatment of drug-induced extrapyramidal disorder: The size and frequency of dose of Benzhexol needed to control extrapyramidal reactions to commonly employed tranquillisers, notably the phenothiazines, thioxanthenes, and butyrophenones must be determined empirically. The total daily dosage usually ranges between 5 and 15 mg, although in some cases, these reactions have been controlled by as little as 1 mg daily.

Satisfactory control may sometimes be more rapidly achieved by temporarily reducing the dosage of both drugs until the desired ataractic effect is retained without concomitant extrapyramidal reactions.

It is sometimes possible to maintain the patient on reduced Benzhexol dosage after the reactions have remained under control for several days. Since these reactions may remain in remission for long periods after discontinuation of Benzhexol therapy, such therapy should be of minimal duration and discontinued after symptoms have subsided for a reasonable period of time.

*Elderly:* Patients over 65 years of age tend to be relatively more sensitive and require smaller amounts of the drug.

*Children:* Not recommended.

*Contra-indications:* None

*Special warnings and special precautions for use:*

*Precautions:* Since the use of Benzhexol may, in some cases, continue indefinitely, the patient should be under careful observation over the long term. It should be administered with care to avoid allergic or other untoward reactions.

Incipient glaucoma may be precipitated by parasympatholytic drugs such as Benzhexol.

Hypertension, cardiac, liver or kidney disorders are not contra-indicated, but such patients should be followed closely. As Benzhexol may provoke or exacerbate tardive dyskinesia, it is not recommended for use in patients with this condition.

Benzhexol should be used with caution in patients with glaucoma, obstructive disease of the gastrointestinal or genito-urinary tracts, and in elderly males with possible prostatic hypertrophy.

Since certain psychiatric manifestations such as confusion, delusions and hallucinations, all of which may occur with any of the atropine-like drugs, have been reported rarely with Benzhexol, it should be used with extreme caution in elderly patients (see Dosage and Administration).

*Warnings:* Benzhexol may be the subject of abuse (on the basis of hallucinogenic or euphoriant properties, common to all anti-cholinergic drugs) if given in sufficient amounts.

*Interaction with other medicaments and other forms of interaction:*

*Drug interactions:* Synergy has been reported between Benzhexol and tricyclic antidepressants, probably because of an additive effect at the receptor site. This can cause dry mouth, constipation and blurred vision. In the elderly, there is a danger of precipitating urinary retention, acute glaucoma or paralytic ileus.

Mono amine oxidase inhibitors can interact with concurrently administered anticholinergic agents including Benzhexol. This can cause dry mouth, blurred vision, urinary hesitancy, urinary retention and constipation.

In general, anticholinergic agents should be used with caution in patients who are receiving tricyclic antidepressants or mono amine oxidase inhibitors. In patients who are already on antidepressant therapy the dose of Benzhexol should be initially reduced and the patient reviewed regularly.

*Pregnancy and lactation:* Not recommended for use in pregnancy or lactation.

*Effects on ability to drive and operate machines:* Can cause blurring of vision, dizziness and mild nausea. Also mental confusion in some cases.

*Undesirable effects:* Minor side-effects such as dryness of mouth, blurring of vision, dizziness, mild nausea or nervousness will be experienced by 30–50% of all patients. These reactions tend to become less pronounced as treatment continues. Euphoria has been reported.

Patients with arteriosclerosis or with a history of other drug idiosyncrasies may exhibit reactions such as mental confusion, agitation, or nausea and vomiting. Such patients should be allowed to develop a tolerance using the smaller initial dose, with gradual increases until the effective level is reached.

*Overdose:* No specific antidote. Gastric lavage, emetic, high enema. Usual general treatment plus cold compresses and forcing of fluid are mandatory. Atropine antagonists may be useful.

### Pharmacological properties

*Pharmacodynamic properties:* Benzhexol hydrochloride is an anticholinergic agent. It is an antispasmodic drug which exerts a direct inhibitory effect on the parasympathetic nervous system. It diminishes salivation, increases the heart rate, dilates the pupils and reduces spasm of smooth muscle.

*Pharmacokinetic properties:* Benzhexol hydrochloride is well absorbed from the gastrointestinal tract. It disappears rapidly from the plasma and tissues and does not accumulate in the body during continued administration of conventional doses.

### Pharmaceutical particulars

*List of excipients:*

*Tablets 2 mg and 5 mg:* Calcium hydrogen phosphate, magnesium stearate, starch pregelatinized, starch

*Incompatibilities:* None

*Shelf life:* 60 months.

*Special precautions for storage:* The products should be stored at controlled room temperature (15°–30°C) in either the original pack or in containers which prevent access of moisture.

*Nature and contents of container:*
Benzhexol Tablets 2 mg     Bottles of 100
Benzhexol Tablets 5 mg     Bottles of 100

*Instructions for use and handling:* None

### Marketing authorisation numbers
Benzhexol Tablets 2 mg     0095/5041R
Benzhexol Tablets 5 mg     0095/5042R

**Date of approval/revision of SPC**   March 1997

**Legal category**   POM

## CAPTOPRIL TABLETS 12.5 mg, 25 mg and 50 mg

**Qualitative and quantitative composition** Captopril tablets 12.5 mg: each tablet contains 12.5 mg captopril. Captopril tablets 25 mg: each tablet contains 25 mg captopril. Captopril tablets 50 mg: each tablet contains 50 mg captopril.

**Pharmaceutical form** Captopril tablets 12.5 mg: white, oval shaped, compressed tablet. Engraved with a vertical line between modified N and 132 on one side and 12.5 on the reverse side.

Captopril tablets 25 mg: white, round bi-convex, compressed tablets. Engraved with quadrisect bar on one side and N over 133 on the reverse side.

Captopril tablets 50 mg: white, capsule shaped, compressed tablet. Engraved with a vertical line between N and 134 on one side and 50 on the other side.

### Clinical particulars

*Therapeutic indications:*
*Hypertension:* Captopril is indicated for the first line treatment of mild to moderate hypertension. In severe hypertension it should be used where standard therapy is ineffective or inappropriate.

*Congestive heart failure:* Captopril is indicated for the treatment of congestive heart failure. The drug should be used together with diuretics and, where appropriate, digitalis.

*Posology and method of administration:*
*Recommended dose and dosage schedule:*

*Hypertension:* Treatment with captopril should be at the lowest effective dose which should be titrated according to the needs of the patient.

*Mild to moderate hypertension:* The starting dose is 12.5 mg twice daily. The usual maintenance dose is 25 mg twice daily which can be increased incrementally, at 2–4 weeks intervals, until a satisfactory response is achieved, to a maximum of 50 mg twice daily.

A thiazide diuretic may be added to captopril if satisfactory response has not been achieved. The dose of diuretic may be increased at 1–2 week intervals to the level of optimum response or until the maximum dose is reached.

*Severe hypertension:* In severe hypertension where standard therapy is ineffective or inappropriate because of adverse effects, the starting dose is 12.5 mg b.d. The dosage may be increased incrementally to a maximum of 50 mg t.i.d. Captopril should be used together with other anti-hypertensive agents but the dose of these should be individually titrated. A daily dose of 150 mg of captopril should not normally be exceeded.

*Heart failure:* Captopril therapy must be started under close medical supervision. Captopril should be introduced when diuretic therapy (such as frusemide 40–80 mg or equivalent) is insufficient to control symptoms. A starting dose of 6.25 mg or 12.5 mg may minimise a transient hypotensive effect. The possibility of this occurring can be reduced by discontinuing or reducing diuretic therapy if possible, prior to initiating captopril. The usual maintenance dose is 25 mg 2 or 3 times a day, which can be increased incrementally, with intervals of at least 2 weeks, until a satisfactory response is achieved. The usual maximum dose is 150 mg daily.

*Elderly:* The dose should be titrated against the blood pressure response and kept as low as possible to achieve adequate control. Since elderly patients may have reduced renal function and other organ dysfunctions, it is suggested that a low dose of captopril be used initially.

*Children:* Captopril is not recommended for the treatment of mild to moderate hypertension in children.

Experience in neonates, particularly premature infants, is limited. Because renal function in infants is not equivalent to that of older children and adults, lower doses of captopril should be used with the patient under close medical supervision.

The starting dose should be 0.3 mg/kg body weight up to a maximum of 6 mg/kg body weight daily, in divided doses. The dose should be individualised according to the response and may be given 2 or 3 times daily.

*Patients with renal impairment:* Captopril in divided doses of 75 to 100 mg/day was well tolerated in patients with diabetic nephropathy and mild to moderate renal impairment (creatinine clearance at least 30 ml/min/1.73 m²).

Patients with severely impaired renal function will take longer to reach steady-state captopril levels and will reach higher steady-state levels for a given daily dose than patients with normal renal function. These patients may therefore respond to smaller or less frequent doses.

Therefore, in patients with severe renal impairment (creatinine clearance less than 30 ml/min/1.73 m²), the initial daily dose should be 12.5 mg b.d. The dose can then be titrated against the response but adequate time should be allowed between dosage adjustments. When concomitant diuretic therapy is required, a loop diuretic rather than a thiazide diuretic should be the diuretic of choice.

Captopril is readily eliminated by haemodialysis.

*Contra-indications:* A history of previous hypersensitivity to the product.

Captopril is contra-indicated in pregnancy and should not be used in women of child bearing potential unless protected by effective contraception.

Because captopril is excreted in breast milk, captopril should not be used in nursing mothers.

See also the section *Use during pregnancy and lactation.*

*Special warnings and precautions for use:* Evaluation of the patient should include assessment of renal function prior to initiation of therapy and at appropriate intervals thereafter. See *Recommended dose and dosage schedule* section.

Captopril should not be used in patients with aortic stenosis or outflow tract obstruction.

As limited experience has been obtained in the treatment of acute hypertensive crises, the use of captopril should be avoided in these patients.

The incidence of adverse reactions to captopril is principally associated with renal function since the drug is excreted primarily by the kidney. The dose should not exceed that necessary for adequate control and should be reduced in patients with impaired renal function.

*Hypotension:* With the first one or two doses some patients may experience symptomatic hypotension. In most instances, symptoms are readily relieved simply by the patient lying down.

In patients with severe and renin dependent hypertension (e.g. renovascular hypertension) or severe congestive heart failure, who are receiving large doses of diuretic, exaggerated hypotensive responses have occurred, usually within one hour of the initial dose of captopril. In these patients, by discontinuing diuretic therapy or significantly reducing the diuretic dose for 4 to 7 days prior to initiating captopril the possibility of this occurrence is reduced. By commencing captopril therapy with small doses (6.25 or 12.5 mg) the duration of any hypotensive effect is lessened. Some patients may benefit from an infusion of saline.

The occurrence of first dose hypotension does not preclude subsequent dose titration with captopril.

Hypotension has been occasionally reported in patients on captopril due to causes of acute volume depletion such as vomiting and diarrhoea.

*Serum potassium:* Since captopril decreases aldosterone production, serum potassium is usually maintained in patients on diuretics. Potassium sparing diuretics or potassium supplements should not therefore be used routinely. In patients with marked renal impairment a significant elevation of serum potassium may occur.

*Renal:* Proteinuria in patients with prior normal renal function is rare.

Where proteinuria has occurred it has usually been in patients with severe hypertension and evidence of prior renal disease. Nephrotic syndrome occurred in some of these patients.

In patients with diabetic nephropathy and proteinuria, who received captopril 75 mg/day for a median of 3 years, there was a consistent reduction in proteinuria. It is unknown whether long-term therapy in patients with other types of renal disease would have similar effects.

Although membranous glomerulopathy was found in biopsies taken from some proteinuric patients, a causal relationship to captopril has not been established.

Some patients with renal disease, particularly those with bilateral renal artery stenosis or unilateral renal stenosis in a single functioning kidney, have developed increased concentrations of blood urea and serum creatinine. Captopril dosage reduction and/or discontinuation of diuretic may be required. For some of these patients it may not be possible to normalise blood pressure and maintain adequate renal perfusion.

Recent clinical observations have shown a high incidence of anaphylactoid-like reactions during haemodialysis with high-flux dialysis membranes (e.g. AN69) in patients receiving ACE inhibitors. Therefore this combination should be avoided.

*Haematological:* Neutropenia/agranulocytosis, thrombocytopenia and anaemia have been reported in patients receiving captopril.

In patients with normal renal function and no other complicating factors, neutropenia occurs rarely. Captopril should be used with extreme caution in patients with collagen vascular disease, immunosuppressant therapy, treatment with allopurinol or procainamide, or a combination of these complicating factors. Some of these patients developed serious infections which in a few instances did not respond to intensive antibiotic therapy.

If captopril is used in such patients, it is advised that white blood cell count and differential counts should be performed prior to therapy, every 2 weeks during the first 3 months of captopril therapy, and periodically thereafter.

During treatment, all patients should be instructed to report any sign of infection (e.g. sore throat, fever), when a differential white blood cell count should be performed. Captopril and other concomitant medication should be withdrawn if neutropenia (neutrophils less than 1000/mm³) is detected or suspected.

In most patients neutrophil counts rapidly returned to normal upon discontinuing captopril.

*Surgery/anaesthesia:* In patients undergoing major surgery, or during anaesthesia with agents which produce hypotension, captopril will block angiotensin-2 formation secondary to compensatory renin release. This may lead to hypotension which can be corrected by volume expansion.

*Clinical chemistry:* Captopril may cause a false-positive urine test for acetone.

*Interactions with other medicaments and other forms of interactions:*
*Diuretics:* Diuretics potentiate the antihypertensive effectiveness of captopril.

Potassium-sparing diuretics (triamterene, amiloride and spironolactone), or potassium supplements may cause significant increase in serum potassium.

*Indomethacin:* A reduction of anti-hypertensive effectiveness may occur. This is probably also the case with other non-steroidal anti-inflammatory drugs.

*Vasodilators:* Captopril has been reported to act synergistically with peripheral vasodilators such as minoxidil. Awareness of this interaction may avert an initial hypotensive response.

*Clonidine:* It has been suggested that the anti-hypertensive effect of captopril can be delayed when patients treated with clonidine are changed to captopril.

*Allopurinol and procainamide:* There have been reports of neutropenia and/or Stevens-Johnson syndrome in patients on captopril plus either allopurinol or procainamide. Although a causal relationship has not been established, these combinations should only be used with caution, especially in patients with impaired renal function.

*Immunosuppressants:* Azathioprine and cyclophosphamide have been associated with blood dyscrasia in patients with renal failure who were also taking captopril.

*Probenecid:* The renal clearance of captopril is reduced in the presence of probenecid.

*Lithium:* Concomitant use of lithium and ACE inhibitors may result in an increase of serum lithium concentration.

*Pregnancy and lactation:* Captopril has been shown to be lethal to rabbit and sheep foetuses. There were no foetotoxic effects to hamster or rat foetuses.

Captopril is contra-indicated in pregnancy and should not be used in women of child bearing potential unless protected by effective contraception.

Exposure of the mother in the second and third trimester of pregnancy has been associated with oligohydramnios and neonatal hypotension and/or anuria.

*Nursing mothers:* Because captopril is excreted in breast milk, captopril should not be used in nursing mothers.

*Effects on ability to drive and use machinery:* An effect on the ability to drive and use machinery cannot be predicted from the pharmacology of this drug. Nevertheless, one should consider the adverse reaction profile of captopril when advising patients on performing these activities.

*Undesirable effects:*
*Idiosyncratic:* Angioedema involving the extremities, face, lips, mucous membranes, tongue, glottis, or larynx has been seen in patients treated with ACE inhibitors, including captopril. In this situation, the ACE inhibitors should be discontinued. Where swelling is confined to the face, lips and mouth the condition will usually resolve without further treatment, although antihistamines may be useful in relieving symptoms. These patients should be followed carefully until the swelling has resolved. However, where there is involvement of the tongue, glottis or larynx, likely to cause airway obstruction, subcutaneous adrenaline (0.5 ml, 1:1000) should be administered promptly where indicated.

*Haematological:* Neutropenia, anaemia and thrombocytopenia (see *Special warnings and precautions for use*). Rarely a positive ANA (antinuclear antibodies) has been reported.

*Renal:* Proteinuria, elevated blood urea and creatinine, elevated serum potassium and acidosis (see *Special warnings and precautions for use*).

*Cardiovascular:* Hypotension (see *Special warnings and precautions for use*), tachycardia.

*Skin:* Rashes, usually pruritic, may occur. They are usually mild, transient and maculopapular, rarely urticarial and disappear within a few days of dosage reduction, short-term treatment with an antihistamine and/or discontinuing therapy. In a few cases the rash has been associated with fever. Pruritus, flushing, vesicular or bullous rash, and photosensitivity have been reported.

*Gastro-intestinal:* Reversible and usually self-limiting taste impairment has been reported. Weight loss may be associated with the loss of taste. Stomatitis, resembling aphthous ulcers, has been reported. Elevation of liver enzymes has been noted in a few patients. Rare cases of hepatocellular injury and cholestatic jaundice have been reported. Gastric irritation and abdominal pain may occur. Pancreatitis has been reported rarely in patients treated with ACE inhibitors; in some cases this has proved fatal.

*Other:* Paraesthesias of the hands, serum sickness, cough, bronchospasm and lymphadenopathy have been reported.

*Overdosage:* In the event of overdosage, blood pressure should be monitored and if hypotension develops volume expansion is the treatment of choice. Captopril is removed by dialysis.

**Pharmacological properties**

*Pharmacodynamic properties:* Captopril is a highly specific competitive inhibitor of angiotensin-1 converting enzyme (ACE), the enzyme responsible for the conversion of angiotensin-1 to angiotensin-2.

ACE is a peptidyldipeptidase which induces the transformation of angiotensin-1 to the vasoconstrictive substance angiotensin-2. Inhibition of ACE leads to a decreased formation of the vasoconstrictive angiotensin-2 in tissue and plasma, which decreases aldosterone secretion and thereby may increase the serum potassium concentration. The plasma renin activity is elevated due to the lack of negative feedback of angiotensin-2 on renin secretion.

ACE degrades bradykinin, a vasodepressor peptide. Therefore inhibition of ACE increases the activity of circulating and local kallikrein-kinin systems (and thereby activates the prostaglandin system). It is possible that this mechanism is part of the hypotensive effect of ACE inhibitors and responsible for some side effects too.

In patients with hypertension captopril leads to a decrease in blood pressure in flat and upright position without compensatory increase of heart rate. Haemodynamic studies revealed a distinct decrease of peripheral arterial resistance during captopril therapy. Usually, no clinically relevant changes of the renal plasma flow and glomerular filtration rate appeared. In most patients the antihypertensive effect started approximately 20–30 minutes after oral administration of captopril. The maximum effect was reached after 60–90 minutes. The maximum hypotensive effect of a defined captopril dose could be demonstrated after 3–4 weeks.

If the advised daily dose is taken, the hypotensive effect remains, even during long-term therapy. No rapid, excessive increase of blood pressure could be observed for short-time therapy discontinuation (rebound effect). Haemodynamic studies in patients with cardiac insufficiency revealed a decrease of the peripheral systemic resistance and an elevation of the venous capacity, resulting in a decrease of preload and afterload of the heart (decrease of the ventricular filling pressure). Cardiac output, stroke work index and exercise capacity increased during captopril therapy as well.

*Pharmacokinetic properties:* After oral administration about 70% of a dose is absorbed from the gastrointestinal tract. Maximum plasma concentrations can be found after approximately 1 hour. Plasma protein binding is approximately 25–30%. Approximately 50% of captopril is metabolised to inactive disulphides. Elimination half life of the unchanged captopril is approximately 1 hour. 95% of captopril is excreted in urine; 40–50% as unchanged drug, the rest as captopril disulphide and captopril cystein disulphide. The excretion rate is decreased in patients with renal impairment. Therefore the captopril dose has to be reduced, or the dosage interval prolonged.

*Bioavailability:* A comparative, open-label, randomised, balanced, 3-way cross-over bioavailability study with the administration of a single oral 50 mg dose of captopril in 27 volunteers was performed. The following data was obtained:

| Parameter/ product | Captopril 50 mg tablet | Reference product B | Reference product C |
|---|---|---|---|
| $C_{max}$ [ng/ml] | 380.59±34.8 | 383.32±35.8 | 391.84±34.8 |
| $t_{max}$ [h] | 0.781±25.5 | 0.792±30.4 | 0.865±25.6 |
| $AUC_{0-infin}$ [ng x h/ml] | 529.8±27.8 | 523.2±24.6 | 537.7±26.9 |

Values as arithmetic mean±standard deviation.

*Pre-clinical safety data:* Acute toxicity (mg/kg body weight):

| Species/ Route | Oral | I.P. | I.V. |
|---|---|---|---|
| Mouse | 6000 | 450 | 1000 |
| Rat | 6000 | 380 | - |

Mice with induced hepatic or renal impairment proved to be twice as sensitive as normal animals.

Single doses over 300 mg/kg body weight orally for dogs and 500 mg/kg body weight orally for monkeys caused vomiting and decreased blood pressure.

*Chronic toxicity:* Studies for chronic toxicity have been carried out in mice, rats, dogs and rhesus monkeys with daily doses up to 1350 mg/kg body weight. Loss of heart weight could be found in mice and rats, as well as hyperplasia of juxtaglomerular cells of the kidney in all investigated species. These changes were a result of the pharmacological effect of captopril.

After 20 months of administration of captopril to rats, a dose-dependent dilatation of retina vessels appeared. Albino rats revealed an increased occurrence of age-related chronic progressive nephrosis. A daily administration 50–200 mg/kg body weight orally over 1 year induced severe bone marrow depression of the myeloid and erythroid cells in Beagle dogs.

*Mutagenicity and carcinogenicity:* Long-term treatment (2 years) with captopril of rats and mice revealed no indication of tumorigenic potential. The mutagenic potential of captopril was investigated insufficiently. Until now, all tests remained negative.

*Reproduction toxicity:* Captopril crosses the placenta and can be found in breast milk. Animal studies revealed no indication of teratogenic characteristics. Toxic effects on the progeny, manifested as an increase of foetal mortality, could mainly be found in the second half of the gestational period. Treatment during peri- and postnatal development of rats brought on growth retardation and increased mortality of the young animals. Fertility of the parental animals was not reduced.

Only little experience concerning the safety of use during pregnancy in humans is available so far. In the past years, cases of a foetal syndrome, marked by severe hypoplasia of cranial bones, intra-uterine growth retardation, oligohydramnios and neonatal anuria, have been described for ACE inhibitors, which may lead to the death of the newly born infant. It is assumed that the hypotensive effect on the foetus during the 2nd and 3rd trimester of pregnancy is the cause. These effects are not expected if therapy is changed well in time to other hypotensives in the first trimester of pregnancy.

**Pharmaceutical particulars**

*List of excipients:* Captopril tablets 12.5 mg: microcrystalline cellulose, pregelatinised starch, sodium starch glycollate, collodial silicium dioxide, sodium lauryl sulphate, magnesium stearate.

Captopril tablets 25 mg: microcrystalline cellulose, pregelatinised starch, sodium starch glycollate, collodial silicium dioxide, sodium lauryl sulphate, magnesium stearate.

Captopril tablets 50 mg: microcrystalline cellulose, pregelatinised starch, sodium starch glycollate, collodial silicium dioxide, sodium lauryl sulphate, magnesium stearate.

*Incompatibilities:* Not applicable.

*Shelf-life:*
Captopril tablets 12.5 mg:     3 years.
Captopril tablets 25 mg:        3 years.
Captopril tablets 50 mg:        3 years.

The expiry date is stated on the pack.

*Special precautions for storage:* Store below 25°C.

*Nature and contents of container:*

*Captopril tablets 12.5 mg:* High density polyethylene container with polypropylene cap, containing 100 tablets and a desiccant bag. Unit dose packages of PVC/paper backed aluminium foil, containing 56 tablets.

*Captopril tablets 25 mg:* High density polyethylene container with polypropylene cap, containing 100 tablets and a desiccant bag. Unit dose packages of PVC/paper backed aluminium foil, containing 56 tablets.

*Captopril tablets 50 mg:* High density polyethylene container with polypropylene cap, containing 100 tablets and a desiccant bag. Unit dose packages of PVC/paper backed aluminium foil, containing 56 tablets.

*Instructions for use/handling:* Do not ingest the desiccant bag.

*Marketing authorisation holder:* Novopharm BV, Netherlands.

**Marketing authorisation numbers**
Captopril tablets 12.5 mg:     14896/0003
Captopril tablets 25 mg:        14896/0004
Captopril tablets 50 mg:        14896/0005

**Date of approval/revision of SPC** 4 February 1997

**Legal category** POM

## ETHAMBUTOL TABLETS

**Presentation** *Tablets 100 mg:* Each yellow coated tablet contains 100 mg ethambutol hydrochloride.

*Tablets 400 mg:* Each grey coated tablet contains 400 mg ethambutol hydrochloride.

**Uses** The primary treatment and re-treatment of tuberculosis and for prophylaxis in cases of inactive tuberculosis or large tuberculin-positive reaction. Ethambutol should only be used in conjunction with other anti-tuberculous drugs to which the patient's organisms are susceptible.

**Dosage and administration** The dosage of Ethambutol must be adjusted according to the body weight of the patient.

*Adults: For primary treatment and prophylaxis:* Ethambutol should be administered in a single daily oral dose of 15 mg/kg, concomitant drugs being maintained at their recommended dosage levels.

*For re-treatment:* For the first 60 days of treatment, Ethambutol should be administered in a single daily oral dose of 25 mg/kg. Thereafter the dosage should be reduced to 15 mg/kg, concomitant drugs being maintained at their recommended dosage levels.

*Children: For primary treatment and re-treatment:* For the first 60 days of treatment, a single daily oral dose of 25 mg/kg. Thereafter the dosage should be reduced to 15 mg/kg, concomitant drugs being maintained at their recommended dosage levels.

*For prophylaxis:* A single daily oral dose of 15 mg/kg, concomitant drugs being used at their recommended dosage levels.

*Elderly:* As for adults. However, patients with decreased renal function may need to have the dosage adjusted as determined by blood levels of Ethambutol. In order to obtain maximum effect due to high serum levels, drug administration should be once daily.

*Administration:* In order to obtain maximum effect due to high serum levels, drug administration should be once daily. Absorption of Ethambutol is not significantly altered by administration with food.

Paediatric doses can be given using an extemporaneously prepared syrup (see Further Information).

A table of dosages is given below.

*Dosage of Ethambutol*
*15 mg/kg (7 mg/lb) schedule:*
*Children*

| Weight range (kg) | Total daily dose (mg) |
|---|---|
| 8 | 120 |
| 17 | 255 |
| 25 | 375 |
| 33 | 495 |

*Adults*

| Weight | | Dose of Ethambutol | Number of tablets | |
|---|---|---|---|---|
| lb | kg | | 100 mg | 400 mg |
| 85–94.5 | 38–42.5 | 600 | 2 plus | 1 |
| 95–109.5 | 43–49.5 | 700 | 3 plus | 1 |
| 110–124.5 | 50–56.5 | 800 | | 2 |
| 125–139.5 | 57–63.5 | 900 | 1 plus | 2 |
| 140–154.5 | 64–70.5 | 1,000 | 2 plus | 2 |
| 155–169.5 | 71–78.5 | 1,100 | 3 plus | 2 |
| 170–184.5 | 79–83.5 | 1,200 | | 3 |
| 185–199.5 | 84–89.5 | 1,300 | 1 plus | 3 |
| 200–214.5 | 90–96.5 | 1,400 | 2 plus | 3 |
| 215 and over | 97 and over | 1,500 | 3 plus | 3 |

*25 mg/kg (11 mg/lb) schedule:*
*Children*

| Weight range kg | Total daily dose (mg) |
|---|---|
| 5 | 125 |
| 10 | 250 |
| 15 | 375 |
| 20 | 500 |
| 25 | 625 |
| 30 | 750 |
| 35 | 875 |

*Adults*

| Weight | | Dose of Ethambutol | Number of tablets | |
|---|---|---|---|---|
| lb | kg | | 100 mg | 400 mg |
| 85–92.5 | 38–41.5 | 1,000 | 2 plus | 2 |
| 93–101.5 | 42–44.5 | 1,100 | 3 plus | 2 |
| 102–109.5 | 45–49.5 | 1,200 | | 3 |
| 110–118.5 | 50–53.5 | 1,300 | 1 plus | 3 |
| 119–128.5 | 54–57.5 | 1,400 | 2 plus | 3 |
| 129–136.5 | 58–61.5 | 1,500 | 3 plus | 3 |
| 137–146.5 | 62–66.5 | 1,600 | | 4 |
| 147–155.5 | 67–70.5 | 1,700 | 1 plus | 4 |
| 156–164.5 | 71–74.5 | 1,800 | 2 plus | 4 |
| 165–173.5 | 75–78.5 | 1,900 | 3 plus | 4 |
| 174–182.5 | 79–82.5 | 2,000 | | 5 |
| 183–191.5 | 83–86.5 | 2,100 | 1 plus | 5 |
| 192–199.5 | 87–90.5 | 2,200 | 2 plus | 5 |
| 200–209.5 | 91–94.5 | 2,300 | 3 plus | 5 |
| 210–218.5 | 95–98.5 | 2,400 | | 6 |
| 219 and over | 99 and over | 2,500 | 1 plus | 6 |

**Contra-indications, warnings, etc**
*Contra-indications:* Ethambutol is contra-indicated in patients who are known to be hypersensitive to the drug. It is also contra-indicated in patients with known optic neuritis unless clinical judgement determines that it may be used.

*Precautions:* Patients with decreased renal function may need to have the dosage adjusted as determined by blood levels of Ethambutol. Animal studies with Ethambutol have shown some teratogenic potential. There have been several reports of the drug having been administered during pregnancy without untoward effect. Nevertheless, it is recommended that the possibility of such effects should be kept in mind when treating women of child-bearing age.

Because this drug has a unique effect on the eye, it is recommended that patients undergo a full ophthalmic examination before starting treatment. This should include visual acuity, colour vision, perimetry and ophthalmoscopy. Many physicians consider that routine ophthalmological examination for adults is not thereafter necessary, but patients should be informed of the importance of reporting any change in vision. However, routine ophthalmological examinations may be considered desirable when treating young children.

*Use in Pregnancy:* Animal studies with Ethambutol have shown some teratogenic potential. There have been several reports of the drug having been administered during pregnancy without untoward effect. Nevertheless, it is recommended that the possibility of such effects should be kept in mind when treating women of child-bearing age.

*Side-effects:* Ethambutol may produce a unique type of visual impairment which is generally reversible and which appears to be due to optic neuritis and to be related to dose and duration of treatment. Less than one per cent of patients undergoing treatment with the higher dose regimen of 25 mg/kg/day for two months, and 15 mg/kg/day thereafter, have exhibited decrease in visual acuity. The change may be unilateral or bilateral and hence both eyes must be tested individually. The effects are generally reversible when administration of the drug is discontinued promptly. In rare cases recovery may be delayed for up to one year or more and the effect may possibly be irreversible in these cases.

Recovery of visual acuity has usually occurred over a period of weeks to months after the drug was discontinued, and patients have then received Ethambutol at lower dosages without toxicity. Hypersensitivity reactions are rare, although rash, pruritus and urticaria have been reported. There are isolated reports of photosensitive lichenoid eruptions, Stevens-Johnson syndrome, epidermal necrolysis, and bullous dermatitis. Interstitial nephritis and anaphylactoid reactions are extremely rare.

Hyperuricaemia has been reported although clinical effects are unlikely. Gastro-intestinal disturbances such as anorexia, nausea, vomiting and diarrhoea have been noted in patients on multiple-drug antituberculous therapy including Ethambutol although not in test patients receiving Ethambutol as sole therapy. Numbness and paraesthesia of the extremities have been reported. Reports of thrombocytopenia are rare.

Hepatic reactions have been reported in patients treated with multiple drug therapy including Ethambutol, and liver function tests should be performed in patients who develop symptoms suggestive of hepatitis or who become generally unwell during treatment.

*Overdosage:* No specific antidote, but gastric lavage should be employed if necessary.

**Pharmaceutical precautions** Ethambutol should be stored at controlled room temperature (15°–30°C) in either the original pack or in containers which prevent access of moisture.

**Legal category** POM

**Package quantities**
Ethambutol 100 mg     Bottles of 100
Ethambutol 400 mg     Bottles of 100

**Further information** Details of a formulation for Ethambutol syrup suitable for paediatric use are available on request from the Medical Information Department. A mixture of Ethambutol syrup and isoniazid elixir BPC should not be prepared as isoniazid is unstable in the presence of sugars.

**Product licence numbers**
Ethambutol 100 mg     0095/0002
Ethambutol 400 mg     0095/0003

# FENBUFEN

## Presentation

*Fenbufen 300 mg Tablets:* Light blue, film coated, capsule shaped tablets, each containing 300 mg of fenbufen and engraved WY050 on one side.

*Fenbufen 300 mg Capsules:* Dark blue capsules, each containing 300 mg of fenbufen and printed WY052 on both the cap and body.

*Fenbufen 450 mg Tablets:* Light blue, film coated, lozenge shaped tablets each containing 450 mg of fenbufen and engraved WY051 on one side.

**Uses** Fenbufen is a non-steroidal, anti-inflammatory drug (NSAID) indicated for the symptomatic treatment of rheumatoid arthritis, osteoarthritis, ankylosing spondylitis and acute musculoskeletal disorders.

**Dosage and administration** *Adults:* 300 mg Tablets or Capsules: One in the morning and two at night.

*450 mg Tablets:* one in the morning and one at night.

*Elderly:* Clinical studies conducted in elderly patients and patients with mild to moderate renal impairment have shown that the pharmacokinetics of Fenbufen are not affected to any clinically relevant extent and the standard adult dose may be used (also see 'Precautions').

*Children:* Not recommended for administration to children under the age of 14.

## Contra-indications, warnings, etc

*Contra-indications:* Active or suspected peptic ulcer or a history of peptic ulceration.

Hypersensitivity to propionic acid anti-inflammatory drugs, or aspirin.

Since the potential exists for cross-sensitivity, Fenbufen should not be used in patients in whom attacks of asthma, urticaria or acute rhinitis are precipitated by aspirin or other NSAIDs.

*Precautions:* As with other NSAID's, Fenbufen should be used with great caution in patients with a history of peptic or intestinal ulceration, and only after other forms of treatment have been carefully considered. Gastrointestinal ulceration, haematemesis or melaena may occur with or without warning symptoms or a previous history.

It is unnecessary to modify the dosage of Fenbufen in mild to moderate renal impairment, however, in common with other NSAID's, there have been a few reports of deterioration in renal function associated with Fenbufen therapy. In view of this, doses in patients with pre-existing renal disease or impaired cardiac or hepatic function should be kept to the minimum necessary to achieve the desired therapeutic effect and renal function should be monitored.

See *Interactions* section for precautions on use with other drugs.

*Use in pregnancy and lactation:* Fenbufen should not be prescribed during pregnancy or lactation, unless there are compelling reasons for doing so and only after careful consideration of the risk/benefit ratio. If absolutely necessary, the lowest effective dose should be used.

*Warnings and adverse effects:* Skin rashes including erythema, maculo-papular, morbilliform and urticaria are the most commonly encountered adverse reactions. Stevens-Johnson syndrome has occasionally been reported. Angioedema, facial oedema, erythema multiforme, epidermal necrolysis, periorbital oedema, pupura, and photosensitivity reactions have all been occasionally reported.

Fenbufen treatment should be discontinued immediately on appearance of a rash. Anti-histamine therapy may help any pruritis associated with the rash. The rash is more common in women and in patients with the rare diagnoses of sero-negative rheumatoid arthritis and psoriatic arthritis. If rash does occur, it will most commonly be seen within the second week of therapy but is very unlikely to occur after two weeks of therapy. The median duration of therapy before a rash occurs is ten days. 80% of eruptions will have resolved after one week of discontinuation of therapy and by two weeks nearly 100% of eruptions will have resolved.

NSAIDs have been reported to cause nephrotoxicity in various forms and their use can lead to interstitial nephritis, nephrotic syndrome and renal failure.

In common with other NSAIDs, allergic interstitial lung disorders (allergic alveolitis, or pulmonary eosinophilia) have been reported rarely; these reactions have resolved within 4–6 weeks of discontinuing therapy.

Vomiting, dyspepsia and nausea are the most commonly encountered gastrointestinal effects. Abdominal pain, diarrhoea, gastritis, haematemesis, gastrointestinal haemorrhage, melaena, constipation, stomatitis, ulcerative stomatitis and anorexia have also occasionally been reported.

Oedema, dizziness, depression, sleep disturbances including vivid dreams, paraesthesia, headache, drowsiness, fatigue, fever and malaise have also occasionally been reported. Increased perspiration and flushing occur rarely. Hypersensitivity reaction such as anaphylaxis and bronchospasm have been reported rarely.

In common with other NSAID's, disturbances of vision and tinnitus have occasionally been reported.

Slight decreases in blood leucocytes, haemoglobin and haematocrit as well as slight increases in prothrombin time and eosinophils have occasionally been recorded. Haematological effects such as agranulocytosis, thrombocytopenia, granulocytopenia, aplastic anaemia, pancytopenia and haemolytic anaemia have been reported rarely. Transient elevations in values of liver function tests have occurred in some patients. Hepatic disorders including hepatitis and jaundice have been reported rarely.

*Drug interactions:* Fenbufen is strongly protein bound – prescribers should be aware of the consequences of increased or decreased blood levels of either drug if Fenbufen is administered with other protein bound drugs such as sulphonylureas, methotrexate, salicylates, hypoglycaemics etc.

Caution should be exercised if NSAIDs and methotrexate are administered within 24 hours of each other, since NSAIDs may increase methotrexate plasma levels resulting in increased toxicity.

In common with other NSAIDs, Fenbufen when administered concurrently with quinolone antibiotics

may cause an increased incidence of quinolone CNS side-effects such as convulsions.

Quinolones should not be administered concurrently with Fenbufen.

Fenbufen produces minor prolongation of prothrombin time in patients taking warfarin. These changes are unlikely to be clinically significant, but patients previously stabilised on oral anticoagulant therapy should be monitored for changes in prothrombin time.

Increases in serum lithium have been reported with some NSAIDs. Serum lithium levels should be monitored if Fenbufen is added to therapy for patients previously stabilised on lithium.

*Overdosage:* Experience of Fenbufen overdosage is limited. There is no specific antidote. Gastric lavage should be performed if appropriate. Otherwise, management should be symptomatic and supportive.

**Pharmaceutical precautions** Store in the original container at room temperature (below 25°C).

**Legal category** POM

**Package quantities**
300 mg Tablets and Capsules: Blister packs of 84 tablets/capsules
450 mg Tablets: Blister packs of 56 tablets.

**Further information** Fenbufen is a pro-drug. It is converted into active metabolites following absorption.

**Product licence numbers**
Fenbufen 300 mg Tablets     0095/0081
Fenbufen 300 mg Capsules    0095/0043
Fenbufen 450 mg Tablets     0095/0092

# LORAZEPAM TABLETS

**Presentation** Lorazepam Tablets are capsule-shaped containing 1 mg or 2.5 mg Lorazepam BP and are approximately 4 x 8 mm. The 1 mg tablets are blue with 'WYETH' on one side and 'WY' breakbar '19' on the other. The 2.5 mg tablets are yellow with 'WYETH' on one side and 'WY' breakbar '20' on the other.

**Uses** Lorazepam is indicated for the short term treatment of moderate and severe anxiety (ie. anxiety that is disabling or subjecting the individual to unacceptable distress). Lorazepam is also indicated for the short term treatment of anxiety in psychosomatic, organic and psychotic illness and the short term treatment of insomnia associated with anxiety. Lorazepam may also be used as premedication before operative dentistry and general surgery.

**Dosage and administration** Dosage and duration of therapy should be individualised. The lowest effective dose should be prescribed for the shortest time possible. Generally, the duration of treatment varies from a few days to 4 weeks including the tapering off process. Extension of the treatment period should not take place without re-evaluation of the need for continued therapy.

Since insomnia is often transient and intermittent, the prolonged administration of Lorazepam is generally unnecessary and is not recommended.

Treatment in all patients should be withdrawn gradually to minimise possible withdrawal symptoms. (See Special Warnings and Precautions for Use).

*Dosage:*
*Adults:*
Moderate to severe anxiety: 1–4 mg daily in divided doses.
Insomnia: 1–2 mg before retiring.
Premedication before operative dentistry or general surgery: 2–3 mg the night before operation. 2–4 mg one to two hours before operation.

*Elderly:* The elderly may respond to lower doses and half the normal adult dose or less may be sufficient.

*Children (aged 5-13 years):* Premedication: 0.5–2.5 mg at 0.05 mg/kg to the nearest 0.5 mg according to weight, not less than one hour before operation.
Lorazepam is not recommended for the treatment of anxiety or insomnia in children.

*Patients with renal or hepatic impairment:* Lower doses may be sufficient in these patients (see Warnings and precautions). Use in patients with severe hepatic insufficiency is contraindicated.

## Contra-indications, warnings, etc
*Contra-indications:*
 – Severe respiratory insufficiency.
 – Sleep apnoea syndrome.
 – Hypersensitivity to benzodiazepines including Lorazepam Tablets or their components.
 – Myasthenia gravis.
 – Severe hepatic insufficiency.

*Pregnancy and lactation:* Benzodiazepines should not be used during pregnancy, especially during the first and last trimesters. Benzodiazepines may cause foetal damage when administered to pregnant women.

If the drug is prescribed to a woman of childbearing potential, she should be warned to contact her physician about stopping the drug if she intends to become, or suspects that she is, pregnant.

Infants of mothers who ingested benzodiazepines for several weeks or more preceding delivery have been reported to have withdrawal symptoms during the postnatal period. Symptoms such as hypoactivity, hypotonia, hypothermia, respiratory depression, apnoea, feeding problems, and impaired metabolic response to cold stress have been reported in neonates born of mothers who have received benzodiazepines during the late phase of pregnancy or at delivery.

There is evidence that Lorazepam is excreted in pharmacologically insignificant amounts in human breast milk. However, Lorazepam should not be administered to nursing women unless the expected benefit to the mother outweighs the potential risk to the infant.

*Warnings and precautions:* Patients should be advised that since their tolerance for alcohol and other CNS depressants will be diminished in the presence of Lorazepam, these substances should either be avoided or taken in reduced dosage.

Lorazepam is not intended for the primary treatment of psychotic illness or depressive disorders, and should not be used alone to treat depressed patients. The use of benzodiazepines may have a disinhibiting effect and may release suicidal tendencies in depressed patients. Therefore, large quantities of Lorazepam should not be prescribed to these patients.

Pre-existing depression may emerge during benzodiazepine use.

The use of benzodiazepines may lead to physical and psychological dependence. The risk of dependence on Lorazepam is low when used at the recommended dose and duration, but increased with higher doses and longer term use. The risk of dependence is further increased in patients with a history of alcoholism or drug abuse, or in patients with significant personality disorders. Therefore, use in individuals with a history of alcoholism or drug abuse should be avoided.

Dependence may lead to withdrawal symptoms, especially if treatment is discontinued abruptly. Therefore, **the drug should always be discontinued gradually.**

Symptoms reported following discontinuation of benzodiazepines include headaches, muscle pain, anxiety, tension, depression, insomnia, restlessness, confusion, irritability, sweating, and the occurrence of 'rebound' phenomena whereby the symptoms that led to treatment with benzodiazepines recur in an enhanced form. These symptoms may be difficult to distinguish from the original symptoms for which the drug was prescribed.

In severe cases the following symptoms may occur: derealisation; depersonalisation; hyperacusis; tinnitus; numbness and tingling of the extremities; hypersensitivity to light, noise, and physical contact; involuntary movements; vomiting; hallucinations; convulsions. Convulsions may be more common in patients with pre-existing seizure disorders or who are taking other drugs that lower the convulsive threshold such as antidepressants.

It may be useful to inform the patient that treatment will be of limited duration and that it will be discontinued gradually. The patient should also be made aware of the possibility of 'rebound' phenomena to minimise anxiety should they occur.

Abuse of benzodiazepines has been reported.

Some loss of efficacy to the hypnotic effects of short-acting benzodiazepines may develop after repeated use for a few weeks.

Anxiety or insomnia may be a symptom of several other disorders. The possibility should be considered that the complaint may be related to an underlying physical or psychiatric disorder for which there is more specific treatment.

Caution should be used in the treatment of patients with acute narrow-angle glaucoma.

Patients with impaired renal or hepatic function should be monitored frequently and have their dosage adjusted carefully according to patient response. Lower doses may be sufficient in these patients. The same precautions apply to elderly or debilitated patients and patients with chronic respiratory insufficiency.

As with all CNS-depressants, the use of benzodiazepines may precipitate encephalopathy in patients with severe hepatic insufficiency. Therefore, use in these patients is contraindicated.

Some patients taking benzodiazepines have developed a blood dyscrasia, and some have had elevations in liver enzymes. Periodic haematologic and liver-function assessments are recommended where repeated courses of treatment are considered clinically necessary.

Transient anterograde amnesia or memory impairment has been reported in association with the use of benzodiazepines. This effect may be advantageous when Lorazepam is used as a premedicant. However, if Lorazepam is used for insomnia due to anxiety, patients should ensure that they will be able to have a period of uninterrupted sleep which is sufficient to allow dissipation of drug effect (e.g., 7-8 hours).

Paradoxical reactions such as restlessness, agitation, irritability, aggressiveness, delusion, rage, nightmares, hallucinations, psychoses, and inappropriate behaviour have been occasionally reported during benzodiazepine use. Such reactions may be more likely to occur in children and the elderly. Should these occur, use of the drug should be discontinued.

Although hypotension has occurred only rarely, benzodiazepines should be administered with caution to patients in whom a drop in blood pressure might lead to cardiovascular or cerebrovascular complications. This is particularly important in elderly patients.

Since Lorazepam Tablets 2.5 mg contain tartrazine (E102), they should not be given to patients who are sensitive to this colouring.

As with all patients on CNS-depressant drugs, patients should be warned not to operate dangerous machinery or motor vehicles until it is known that they do not become drowsy or dizzy from Lorazepam.

*Interactions:* The benzodiazepines, including Lorazepam produce additive CNS depressant effects when co-administered with other medications which themselves produce CNS depression e.g., alcohol, barbiturates, antipsychotics, sedatives/hypnotics, anxiolytics, antidepressants, narcotic analgesics, sedative antihistamines, anticonvulsants, and anaesthetics.

An enhancement of the euphoria induced by narcotic analgesics may occur with benzodiazepine use, leading to an increase in psychic dependence.

Compounds which inhibit certain hepatic enzymes (particularly cytochrome P450) may enhance the activity of benzodiazepines. To a lesser degree this also applies to benzodiazepines which are metabolised only by conjugation.

There have been reports of excessive stupor, significant reduction in respiratory rate and, in one patient, hypotension when Lorazepam and loxapine have been given concomitantly.

There have been reports of marked sedation, excessive salivation, and ataxia when Lorazepam and clozapine have been given concomitantly.

*Side-effects:* Adverse reactions, when they occur, are usually observed at the beginning of therapy and generally decrease in severity or disappear with continued use or upon decreasing the dose.

Most frequently reported adverse reactions associated with benzodiazepines include daytime drowsiness, dizziness, muscle weakness, and ataxia.

Less frequently reported adverse reactions include the following: confusion, depression, fatigue, headache, reduced alertness, numbed emotions, nausea, appetite change, sleep disturbance, dermatological reactions, visual disturbances, change of libido, and gastrointestinal symptoms.

Rarely reported adverse reactions include blood dyscrasia, abnormal liver function tests, transient anterograde amnesia or memory impairment, paradoxical reactions, and hypotension (See Warnings and Precautions).

*Overdose:* In the management of overdosage with any drug, it should be borne in mind that multiple agents may have been taken.

Overdosage of benzodiazepines is usually manifested by degrees of central nervous system depression ranging from drowsiness to coma. In mild cases, symptoms include drowsiness, mental confusion, and lethargy. In more serious cases, and especially when other CNS-depressant drugs or alcohol are ingested, symptoms may include ataxia, hypotension, hypotonia, respiratory depression, coma, and very rarely, death.

If ingestion was recent, induced vomiting and/or gastric lavage should be undertaken followed by general supportive care, monitoring of vital signs and close observation of the patient. If there is no advantage in emptying the stomach, activated charcoal may be effective in reducing absorption. Hypotension, though unlikely, may be controlled with noradrenaline. Lorazepam is poorly dialysable.

The benzodiazepine antagonist, flumazenil may be useful in hospitalised patients for the management of benzodiazepine overdosage. Flumazenil product information should be consulted prior to use.

**Pharmaceutical precautions** Store in a dry place below 25°C.

**Legal category** POM, CD (Sch 4)

**Package quantities** 1 mg and 2.5 mg tablets: boxes of 100 (5 x 20 blister strips).

**Further information** Lorazepam is a benzodiazepine with anxiolytic, sedative and hypnotic properties.

Lorazepam is almost completely absorbed from the gastrointestinal tract and peak serum levels are reached in 2 hours. It is metabolised by a simple one-step process to a pharmacologically inert glucuronide. There are no major active metabolites. The elimination half-life is about 12 hours and there is minimal risk of excessive accumulation.

**Product licence numbers**

| | |
|---|---|
| Lorazepam Tablets 1.0 mg | 0011/0108 |
| Lorazepam Tablets 2.5 mg | 0011/0109 |

## LORMETAZEPAM TABLETS

**Qualitative and quantitative composition** There are two strengths of Lormetazepam Tablets containing 0.5 mg or 1.0 mg lormetazepam.

Lormetazepam (INN, BAN) is chemically defined as 7-chloro-5-(2-chlorophenyl)-1,3-dihydro-3-hydroxy-1-methyl-2H-1,4-benzodiazepin-2-one.

**Pharmaceutical form** Lormetazepam Tablets are round white tablets containing 0.5 mg or 1.0 mg lormetazepam. The 0.5 mg tablets are 6.5 mm in diameter with 'WYETH' embossed on one side and 'WY036' on the other. The 1.0 mg tablets are 6.5 mm in diameter with 'WYETH' on one side and 'WY037' on the other.

**Clinical particulars**

*Therapeutic indications:* Lormetazepam is indicated for the short term treatment of insomnia when it is disabling or subjecting the individual to extreme distress.

*Posology and method of administration:* Dosage and duration of therapy should be individualised. The lowest effective dose should be prescribed for the shortest time possible. Generally, the duration of treatment varies from a few days to 2 weeks, with a maximum of 4 weeks including the tapering off process. Extension of the treatment period should not take place without re-evaluation of the need for continued therapy.

Since insomnia is often transient and intermittent, the prolonged administration of Lormetazepam is generally unnecessary and is not recommended.

Treatment in all patients should be withdrawn gradually to minimise possible withdrawal symptoms (see *Special warnings and precautions for use*).

*Dosage:*

*Adults:* 0.5 mg to 1.5 mg before retiring. Subsequently the initial dosage may be increased in individual cases if this proves necessary

*Elderly:* The lower adult dose is preferable for elderly patients

*Children:* Lormetazepam has not been evaluated for the treatment of children

*Contra-indications:* Severe respiratory insufficiency. Sleep apnoea syndrome. Hypersensitivity to benzodiazepines including Lormetazepam Tablets or their components. Myasthenia gravis. Severe hepatic failure

*Special warnings and precautions for use:* Patients should be advised that since their tolerance for other CNS depressants will be diminished in the presence of Lormetazepam, these substances should either be avoided or taken in reduced dosage. Lormetazepam may enhance the sedative effects of alcohol. Since this effects the ability to drive or use machinery, alcohol should be avoided while taking Lormetazepam.

Lormetazepam is not intended for the primary treatment of psychotic illness or depressive disorders, and should not be used alone to treat depressed patients with associated insomnia. The use of benzodiazepines may have a disinhibiting effect and may release suicidal tendencies in depressed patients. Therefore, large quantities of Lormetazepam should not be prescribed to these patients.

Pre-existing depression may emerge during benzodiazepine use.

The use of benzodiazepines may lead to physical and psychological dependence. The risk of dependence on Lormetazepam is low when used at the recommended dose and duration, but increased with higher doses and longer term use. The risk of dependence is further increased in patients with a history of alcoholism or drug abuse or in patients with significant personality disorders. Therefore, use in individuals with a history of alcoholism or drug abuse should be avoided.

Dependence may lead to withdrawal symptoms, especially if treatment is discontinued abruptly. **Therefore, the drug should always be discontinued gradually.**

Symptoms reported following discontinuation of benzodiazepines include headaches, muscle pain, anxiety, tension, depression, insomnia, restlessness, confusion, irritability, sweating and the occurrence of 'rebound' phenomena whereby the symptoms that led to treatment with benzodiazepines recur in an enhanced form. These symptoms may be difficult to distinguish from the original symptoms for which the drug was prescribed.

In severe cases the following symptoms may occur: derealisation; depersonalisation; hyperacusis; tinnitus; numbness and tingling of the extremities; hypersensitivity to light, noise, and physical contact; involuntary movement; vomiting; hallucinations; convulsions. Convulsions may be more common in patients with pre-existing seizure disorders or who are taking other drugs that lower the convulsive threshold such as antidepressants.

It may be useful to inform the patient that treatment will be of limited duration and that it will be discontinued gradually. The patient should also be made aware of the possibility of 'rebound' phenomena to minimise anxiety should they occur.

Abuse of benzodiazepines has been reported.

Some loss of efficacy to the hypnotic effects of short-acting benzodiazepines may develop after repeated use for a few weeks.

Caution should be used in the treatment of patients with acute narrow-angle glaucoma.

Insomnia may be a symptom of several other disorders. The possibility should be considered that the complaint may be related to an underlying physical or psychiatric disorder for which there is a more specific treatment.

Patients with impaired renal or hepatic function should be monitored frequently and have their dosage adjusted carefully according to patient response. Lower doses may be sufficient in these patients. The same precautions apply to elderly or debilitated patients and patients with chronic respiratory insufficiency.

As with all CNS-depressants, the use of benzodiazepines may precipitate encephalopathy in patients with severe hepatic insufficiency. Therefore, use in these patients is contra-indicated.

Some patients taking benzodiazepines have developed a blood dyscrasia, and some have had elevations in liver enzymes. Periodic haematologic and liver-function assessments are recommended where repeated courses of treatment are considered clinically necessary.

Transient anterograde amnesia or memory impairment has been reported in association with the use of benzodiazepines. This condition, which may be associated with inappropriate behaviour, usually occurs several hours after ingestion. Therefore, patients should ensure that they will be able to have a period of uninterrupted sleep which is sufficient to allow dissipation of drug effect (e.g., 7–8 hours).

Paradoxical reactions such as restlessness, agitation, irritability, aggressiveness, delusion, rage, nightmares, hallucinations, psychoses, and inappropriate behaviour and other adverse behavioural effects have been occassionally reported during benzodiazepine use. Such reactions may be more likely to occur in children and the elderly. Should these occur, use of the drug should be discontinued.

Although hypotension has occurred only rarely, benzodiazepines should be administered with caution to patients in whom a drop in blood pressure might lead to cardiovascular or cerebrovascular complications. This is particulaly important in elderly patients.

*Interactions with other medicaments and other forms of interactions:* The benzodiazepines, including Lormetazepam produce additive CNS depressant effects when co-administered with other medications which themselves produce CNS depression e.g., alcohol, barbiturates, antipsychotics, sedatives/hypnotics, anxiolytics, antidepressants, narcotic analgesics, sedative antihistamines, anticonvulsants, and anaesthetics.

An enhancement of the euphoria induced by narcotic analgesics may occur with benzodiazepine use, leading to an increase in psychic dependence.

Compounds which inhibit certain hepatic enzymes (particularly cytochrome P450) may enhance the activity of benzodiazepines. To a lesser degree this also applies to benzodiazepines which are metabolised only by conjugation.

*Pregnancy and lactation:* Benzodiazepines should not be used during pregnancy, especially during the first and last trimesters. Benzodiazepines may cause foetal damage when administered to pregnant women.

If the drug is prescribed to a woman of childbearing potential, she should be warned to contact her physician about stopping the drug if she intends to become, or suspects that she is, pregnant.

Infants of mothers who ingested benzodiazepines for several weeks or more preceding delivery have been reported to have withdrawal symptoms during the postnatal period. Symptoms such as hypoactivity, hypotonia, hypothermia, respiratory depression, apnoea, feeding problems, and impaired metabolic response to cold stress have been reported in neonates born of mothers who have received benzodiazepines during the late phase of pregnancy or at delivery.

Since limited data indicates that a small proportion of parent drug and its conjugate is excreted in breast milk, Lormetazepam should not be given to breast-feeding women.

*Effects on ability to drive and use machinery:* As with all patients on CNS-depressant drugs, patients should be warned not to operate dangerous machinery or motor vehicles until it is known that they do not become drowsy or dizzy from Lormetazepam.

*Undesirable effects:* Adverse reactions, when they occur, are usually observed at the beginning of therapy and generally decrease in severity or disappear with continued use or upon decreasing the dose.

Most frequently reported adverse reactions associated with benzodiazepines include daytime drowsiness, dizziness, muscle weakness, and ataxia.

Less frequently reported adverse reactions include the following; confusion, depression, fatigue, headache, reduced alertness, numbed emotions, nausea, appetite change, sleep disturbance, dermatological reactions, visual disturbances, change of libido, and gastrointestinal symptoms.

Rarely reported adverse reactions include blood dyscrasia, abnormal liver function tests, transient anterograde amnesia or memory impairment, paradoxical reactions, and hypotension (see also *Special warnings and precautions for use*).

*Overdosage:* In the management of overdosage with any drug, it should be borne in mind that multiple agents may have been taken.

Overdosage of benzodiazepines is usually manifested by degrees of central nervous system depression ranging from drowsiness to coma. In mild cases, symptoms include drowsiness, mental confusion, and lethargy. In more serious cases, and especially when other CNS-depressant drugs or alcohol are ingested, symptoms may include ataxia, hypotension, hypotonia, respiratory depression, coma, and very rarely, death.

If ingestion was recent, induced vomiting and/or gastric lavage should be undertaken followed by general supportive care, monitoring of vital signs and close observation of the patient. If there is no advantage in emptying the stomach, activated charcoal may be effective in reducing absorption. Special attention should be paid to respiratory and cardiovascular functions in intensive care. Hypotension, though unlikely, may be controlled with noradrenaline. Lormetazepam is poorly dialysable.

The benzodiazepine antagonist, flumazenil may be useful in hospitalised patients for the management of benzodiazepine overdosage. Flumazenil product information should be consulted prior to use.

**Pharmacological properties**

*Pharmacodynamic properties:* Lormetazepam is a benzodiazepine with anxiolytic, muscle relaxant, sedative and hypnotic properties. Clinical studies have shown minimal effects on REM sleep and on psychomotor performance on the day after treatment with lormetazepam.

*Pharmacokinetic properties:* Lormetazepam is rapidly absorbed from the gastrointestinal tract and is metabolised by a simple one-step process to a pharmacologically inactive glucuronide. There are no major metabolites and little risk of accumulation. Lormetazepam has a terminal phase half-life of about 11 hours.

*Pre-clinical safety data:* Fertility in male and female rats was not adversely affected by oral lormetazepam.

**Pharmaceutical particulars**

*List of excipients:* Lactose, maize starch, polyvinylpyrrolidone and magnesium stearate.

*Incompatibilities:* None known

*Shelf-life:* 60 months

*Special precautions for storage:* Store in a cool dry place

*Nature and contents of container:* PVC/aluminium foil blister packs. Pack sizes of 30 or 100 tablets.

**Marketing authorisation numbers**

| | |
|---|---|
| Lormetazepam Tablets 0.5 mg | 0011/0068 |
| Lormetazepam Tablets 1.0 mg | 0011/0069 |

**Date of approval/revision** January 1997

**Legal category** CD(Sch 4), POM

## MINOCYCLINE TABLETS 50 mg and 100 mg

**Presentation** *Tablets 50 mg:* Each beige film-coated tablet, embossed M/50 on one face, contains Minocycline hydrochloride equivalent to 50 mg Minocycline base.

*Tablets 100 mg:* Each orange, film-coated tablet, embossed M/100 on one face, contains Minocycline hydrochloride equivalent to 100 mg Minocycline base.

**Uses** Minocycline is a broad spectrum antibiotic used for the treatment of infections caused by tetracycline-sensitive organisms. Some tetracycline-resistant strains of Staphylococci are also sensitive.

*Typical indications include:* Gonorrhoea. Non-gonococcal urethritis. Prostatitis. Acne. Acute and chronic bronchitis. Bronchiectasis. Lung abscess. Pneumonia. Ear, nose and throat infections. Urinary tract infections. Pelvic inflammatory disease (eg salpingitis, oophoritis). Skin and soft tissue infections caused by minocycline sensitive organisms. Ophthalmological infections. Nocardiosis. Prophylactic treatment of asymptomatic meningococcal carriers. Pre- and post-operative prophylaxis of infection.

**Dosage and administration** *Adults:*

1. *Routine antibiotic use:* 200 mg daily in divided doses.
2. *Acne:* 50 mg twice daily, **for a minimum of 6 weeks.**
3. *Gonorrhoea:* In adult males: 200 mg initially, followed by 100 mg every 12 hours for a minimum of 4 days with post-therapy cultures within 2–3 days. Adult females may require more prolonged therapy.
4. *Prophylaxis of asymptomatic meningococcal carriers:* 100 mg bid for five days, usually followed by a course of rifampicin.

*Children:* For children above 12 years of age the recommended dosage for Minocycline is one 50 mg tablet every 12 hours. Minocycline is not recommended for children under 12 years old.

*Elderly:* Minocycline may be used at the normal recommended dosage in elderly patients even with mild to moderate renal impairment, however caution is advised in patients with severe renal impairment.

*Administration:* To reduce the risk of oesophageal irritation and ulceration, the tablets should be swallowed whole with plenty of fluid, while sitting or standing. Unlike earlier tetracyclines, absorption of Minocycline is not significantly impaired by food or moderate amounts of milk.

Treatment of acne should be continued for a minimum of six weeks. If, after six months, there is no satisfactory response Minocycline should be discontinued and other therapies considered. If Minocycline is to be continued for longer than six months, patients should be monitored at least three monthly thereafter for signs and symptoms of hepatitis or SLE (see warnings and precautions).

**Contra-indications, warnings, etc**

*Contra-indications:* Known hypersensitivity to tetracyclines. Use in pregnancy, lactation, children under the age of 12 years, complete renal failure.

*Warnings and precautions:* Minocycline should be used with caution in patients with hepatic dysfunction and in conjunction with alcohol and other hepatotoxic drugs. Rare cases of auto-immune hepatotoxicity and isolated cases of systemic lupus erythematosus (SLE) and also exacerbation of pre-existing SLE have been reported. If patients develop signs or symptoms of SLE or hepatotoxicity, or suffer exacerbation of pre-existing SLE, minocycline should be discontinued. Clinical studies have shown that there is no significant drug accumulation in patients with renal impairment when they are treated with Minocycline in the recommended doses. In cases of severe renal insufficiency, reduction of dosage and monitoring of renal function may be required.

Cross-resistance between tetracyclines may develop in micro-organisms and cross-sensitisation in patients. Minocycline should be discontinued if there are signs/symptoms of overgrowth of resistant organisms, eg enteritis, glossitis, stomatitis, vaginitis, pruritus ani or staphylococcal enteritis.

Patients taking oral contraceptives should be warned that if diarrhoea or breakthrough bleeding occur there is a possibility of contraceptive failure.

*Interactions:* Minocycline should not be used with penicillins. Tetracyclines depress plasma prothrombin activity and reduced doses of concomitant anticoagulants may be necessary.

Absorption of Minocycline is impaired by the concomitant administration of antacids, iron, calcium, magnesium, aluminium and zinc salts. Unlike earlier tetracyclines, absorption of Minocycline is not significantly impaired by food or moderate amounts of milk.

*Use in pregnancy:* Results of animal studies indicate that tetracyclines cross the placenta, are found in foetal tissues and can have toxic effects on the developing foetus (often related to retardation of skeletal development). Evidence of embryotoxicity has also been noted in animals treated early in pregnancy. Minocycline therefore, should not be used in pregnancy unless considered essential.

The use of drugs of the tetracycline class during

tooth development (last half of pregnancy) may cause permanent discolouration of the teeth (yellow-grey-brown). This adverse reaction is more common during long term use of the drugs but has been observed following repeated short term courses. Enamel hypoplasia has also been reported.

*Use in lactation:* Tetracyclines have been found in the milk of lactating women who are taking a drug in this class. Permanent tooth discolouration may occur in the developing infant and enamel hypoplasia has been reported.

*Use in children:* The use of tetracyclines during tooth development in children under the age of 12 years may cause permanent discolouration (see above). Enamel hypoplasia has also been reported.

*Side-effects:* In common with other tetracyclines gastrointestinal disturbances including nausea, anorexia, vomiting and diarrhoea may occur. Dermatological reactions such as erythema multiforme, Stevens Johnson syndrome, exfoliative dermatitis and photosensitivity have been reported, as well as maculopapular and erythematous rashes and, rarely, fixed drug eruptions. Hypersensitivity reactions can include urticaria, fever, arthralgia, pulmonary infiltration, angioneurotic oedema, anaphylaxis and anaphylactoid purpura. Rarely pericarditis and renal failure including interstitial nephritis have been reported. Isolated cases of systemic lupus erythematosus (SLE) and also exacerbation of pre-existing SLE have been reported.

Headache, lightheadedness, dizziness, vertigo and, rarely, impaired hearing have occurred with Minocycline and patients should be warned about the possible hazards of driving or operating machinery during treatment.

As with other tetracyclines bulging fontanelles in infants and benign intracranial hypertension in juveniles and adults have been reported. Treatment should cease if evidence of raised intracranial pressure develops.

Blood: haemolytic anaemia, thrombocytopenia, neutropenia and eosinophilia have been reported with tetracyclines.

In common with other tetracyclines, transient increases in liver function test values and rarely hepatitis and acute liver failure have been reported. Some hepatic reactions have an auto-immune basis, and may occur after several months of Minocycline treatment (see dosage and administration). There have been isolated incidences of pancreatitis.

When given over prolonged periods, tetracyclines have been reported to produce brown-black microscopic discolouration of thyroid tissue. Hyperpigmentation of skin, nails or discolouration of teeth and buccal mucosa have been reported occasionally. These are generally reversible on cessation of therapy. There are isolated cases of discolouration of conjunctiva, lacrimal secretions, breast secretions and perspiration. See also Uses in Pregnancy and Lactation.

*Overdosage:* No specific antidote. Gastric lavage plus appropriate supportive treatment.

**Pharmaceutical precautions** The product should be stored at controlled room temperature (below 30°C) in the original pack or in containers which prevent access of moisture.

Protect from light.

**Legal category** POM

**Package quantities**

| 50 mg Tablets | Blister packs of 84 |
| 100 mg Tablets | Bottles of 50 |

**Further information** Nil

**Product licence numbers**

| 50 mg Tablets | 0095/0062 |
| 100 mg Tablets | 0095/0006 |

## MEPROBAMATE TABLETS

**Presentation** Meprobamate Tablets 400 mg are round white flat tablets with bevelled edges having 'WY035' impressed on one face and 'WYETH' impressed on the opposite face. Each tablet contains 400 mg meprobamate.

**Uses** For use in the short-term treatment of anxiety states, muscle tension and associated conditions where anxiety is present.

**Dosage and administration**

*Route of administration:* Oral

*Adults:* 400 mg three times daily with an additional tablet before retiring.

*Elderly:* The elderly may respond to lower doses and half the normal adult dose or less may be sufficient.

*Children:* Not recommended for children

*Use in pregnancy and lactation:* There is no evidence as to drug safety in human pregnancy, nor is there evidence that it is free from hazard. Do not use during pregnancy, especially during the first three months, unless there are compelling reasons.

Meprobamate should not be used during lactation.

**Contra-indications, warnings, etc**

*Contra-indications:* Use in patients known to be hypersensitive to the active ingredient or to related compounds such as carisoprodol or carbromal.

Use in patients with a known propensity for dependence on drugs including alcohol.

Use in patients susceptible to attacks of acute intermittent porphyria.

Meprobamate should not be used during lactation.

There is no evidence as to drug safety in human pregnancy, nor is there evidence that it is free from hazard. Do not use during pregnancy, especially during the first three months, unless there are compelling reasons.

Acute pulmonary insufficiency

Respiratory Depression

*Warnings and precautions:* This product may cause drowsiness. Patients receiving this medication should not drive or operate machinery unless the drug has been shown not to interfere with physical or mental ability.

Meprobamate may increase the effects of concurrently administered central nervous depressants including alcohol.

Individual response in overdosage is variable but in some cases the symptoms may be severe. It is therefore advisable that caution should be observed in prescribing meprobamate to patients with depression or to others who may be liable to suicidal ideation or intent.

Meprobamate may induce seizures in epileptic patients, and meprobamate withdrawal may precipitate convulsions.

Use with caution in patients with respiratory disease or muscle weakness.

The concurrent use of other CNS depressant drugs should be avoided in hepatic or renal insufficiency.

Like barbiturates, meprobamate causes induction of liver enzymes, so that the availability and blood levels of drugs given concurrently that are metabolised in the liver may be affected. These include the following: coumarin-type anticoagulants, systemic steroids (including oral contraceptives), phenytoin, griseofulvin, rifampicin, phenothiazines (such as chlorpromazine) and tricyclic antidepressants. The clinical importance of the effect of enzyme induction by meprobamate on concurrently administered agents has not been established.

Some degree of dependence may occur in certain cases if dosage recommendations are exceeded. This is more likely in individuals with emotionally unstable personalities if the drug is taken over long periods, or in others liable to alcohol or other drug dependence. Withdrawal reactions have occurred ranging in severity from mild to severe. Severe reactions have been associated with high doses when the drug has been used over a prolonged period and withdrawn abruptly. Symptoms of tremulousness, insomnia, confusion, delirium tremens, convulsions and very occasionally, death have occurred. When the drug has been withdrawn gradually, the withdrawal symptoms, if any, have usually been mild. It is advisable to monitor treatment regularly and to withdraw treatment gradually.

Safety and efficacy of meprobamate have not been established beyond short term use.

*Overdosage:* Acute poisoning with meprobamate produces coma, shock, vasomotor and respiratory collapse. Very few suicide attempts have proved successful and documented fatal doses have ranged from 12 g to 47.6 g. Recovery has occurred after ingestion of similar large amounts (20–40 g). Gastric lavage is only effective within a short period of drug ingestion as meprobamate is rapidly absorbed from the gastrointestinal tract. Blood concentrations may be reduced by a regimen of forced alkaline diuresis or haemodialysis. Respiration may require assistance.

*Side effects:* Drowsiness, dizziness and nausea may be experienced, but these symptoms usually disappear as treatment continues. Ataxia, vomiting, hypotension, paraesthesia and paradoxical excitement may also occur.

Hypersensitivity reactions have been reported in about 2% of patients. These reactions include skin rashes, and may arise after one to four doses of the drug. They may be generalised or local, and include urticaria, itchy maculopapular rashes or erythema. Severe systemic reactions with shaking, chills and fever, nausea and vomiting, hypotension and collapse have occasionally occurred.

Blood disorders including non-thrombocytopenic purpura, and rarely, thrombocytopenia, agranulocytosis, aplastic anaemia and pancytopenia have occurred. Rarely reported reactions, usually occurring as a part of a generalised hypersensitivity reaction include hyperpyrexia, angioneurotic oedema, bronchospasm, oliguria and anuria. Anaphylaxis, ery-

thema multiforme, exfoliative dermatitis, stomatitis, proctitis, Stevens Johnson syndrome and bullous dermatitis have also been reported.

**Pharmaceutical precautions** Store at or below 25°C

**Legal category** CD(Sch 3), POM

**Further information** Safety and efficacy have not been established beyond short-term use.

**Package quantities** Bottles of 84 tablets

**Product licence number** Meprobamate Tablets 400 mg 0011/5010R

## OXAZEPAM TABLETS

**Qualitative and quantitative composition** There are two strengths of oxazepam tablets containing oxazepam 10 mg and 15 mg.

Oxazepam (INN, BAN) is chemically defined as 7-chloro-1,3-dihydro-3-hydroxy-5-phenyl-2H-1,4-benzodiazepine-2-one.

**Pharmaceutical form** Oxazepam Tablets 10 mg are white flat, bevel-edged tablets, 6.5 mm in diameter, marked 'WYETH' on one face and 'WY 012' on the other.

Oxazepam Tablets 15 mg are white, flat, bevel edged tablets, 8.0 mm in diameter, marked 'WYETH' on one face and 'WY 013' on the other.

**Clinical particulars**

*Therapeutic indications:* Oxazepam is indicated for the short term treatment of moderate anxiety ie. anxiety that is disabling or subjecting the individual to unacceptable distress. Oxazepam is also indicated for the short term treatment of anxiety in psychosomatic, organic and psychotic illness and the short term treatment of insomnia associated with anxiety.

*Posology and method of administration:* Dosage and duration of therapy should be individualised. The lowest effective dose should be prescribed for the shortest time possible. Generally, the duration of treatment varies from a few days to 2 weeks, to a maximum of 4 weeks including the tapering off process. Extension of the treatment period should not take place without re-evaluation of the need for continued therapy.

Since insomnia is often transient and intermittent, the prolonged administration of Oxazepam Tablets is generally unnecessary and is not recommended.

Treatment in all patients should be withdrawn gradually to minimise possible withdrawal symptoms. (See Special warnings and precautions for use).

*Dosage:*

*Adults: Moderate anxiety:* one to two 15 mg tablets three (or four) times daily.

*Elderly:* Elderly patients or those who are particularly sensitive to the effects of benzodiazepines; 10–20 mg three or four times daily.

*Insomnia:* Most patients need a dose of 15–25 mg, but some patients may need up to 50 mg. The dose should be taken 1 hour before retiring.

*Children:* Oxazepam is not recommended for the treatment of children.

*Patients with renal or hepatic impairment:* Lower doses may be sufficient in these patients (see *Special warnings and precautions for use*).

*Contra-indications:*

Severe respiratory insufficiency.

Sleep apnoea syndrome.

Hypersensitivity to benzodiazepines including Oxazepam Tablets or their components.

Myasthenia gravis.

Severe hepatic insufficiency.

Oxazepam should not be given to children.

*Special warnings and precautions for use:* Patients should be advised that since their tolerance for alcohol and other CNS depressants will be diminished in the presence of oxazepam, these substances should either be avoided or taken in reduced dosage.

Oxazepam is not intended for the primary treatment of psychotic illness or depressive disorders, and should not be used alone to treat depressed patients. The use of benzodiazepines may have a disinhibiting effect and may release suicidal tendencies in depressed patients. Therefore, large quantities of oxazepam should not be prescribed to these patients.

Pre-existing depression may emerge during benzodiazepine use.

The use of benzodiazepines may lead to physical and psychological dependence. The risk of dependence on Oxazepam is low when used at the recommended dose and duration, but increased with higher doses and longer term use. The risk of dependence is further increased in patients with a history of alcoholism or drug abuse, or in patients with significant personality disorders. Therefore, use in individuals with a history of alcoholism or drug abuse should be avoided.

Dependence may lead to withdrawal symptoms, especially if treatment is discontinued abruptly. Therefore, the drug should always be discontinued gradually.

Symptoms reported following discontinuation of benzodiazepines include headaches, muscle pain, anxiety, tension, depression, insomnia, restlessness, confusion, irritability, sweating, and the occurrence of 'rebound' phenomena whereby the symptoms that led to treatment with benzodiazepines recur in an enhanced form. These symptoms may be difficult to distinguish from the original symptoms for which the drug was prescribed.

In severe cases the following symptoms may occur: derealisation; depersonalisation; hyperacusis; tinnitus; numbness and tingling of the extremities; hypersensitivity to light, noise, and physical contact; involuntary movements; vomiting; hallucinations; convulsions. Convulsions may be more common in patients with pre-existing seizure disorders or who are taking other drugs that lower the convulsive threshold such as antidepressants.

It may be useful to inform the patient that treatment will be of limited duration and that it will be discontinued gradually. The patient should also be made aware of the possibility of 'rebound' phenomena to minimise anxiety should they occur.

Abuse of benzodiazepines has been reported.

Some loss of efficacy to the hypnotic effects of short-acting benzodiazepines may develop after repeated use for a few weeks.

Anxiety may be a symptom of several other disorders. The possibility should be considered that the complaint may be related to an underlying physical or psychiatric disorder for which there is more specific treatment.

Caution should be used in the treatment of patients with acute narrow-angle glaucoma.

Patients with impaired renal or hepatic function should be monitored frequently and have their dosage adjusted carefully according to response. Lower doses may be sufficient in these patients. The same precautions apply to elderly or debilitated patients and patients with chronic respiratory insufficiency.

Patients with severe hepatic impairment may have a decreased ability to clear oxazepam through glucuronidation. Further, as with all CNS-depressants, the use of benzodiazepines may precipitate encephalopathy in patients with severe hepatic insufficiency. Therefore, use in these patients is contraindicated.

Some patients taking benzodiazepines have developed a blood dyscrasia, and some have had elevations in liver enzymes. Periodic haematologic and liver-function assessments are recommended where repeated courses of treatment are considered clinically necessary.

Transient anterograde amnesia or memory impairment has been reported in association with the use of benzodiazepines. This condition usually occurs several hours after ingestion. Therefore, patients receiving Oxazepam for insomnia associated with anxiety should ensure that they will be able to have a period of uninterrupted sleep which is sufficient to allow dissipation of drug effect (e.g., 7–8 hours).

Paradoxical reactions such as restlessness, agitation, irritability, aggressiveness, delusion, rage, nightmares, hallucinations, psychoses, and inappropriate behaviour have been occasionally reported during benzodiazepine use. Such reactions may be more likely to occur in children and the elderly. Should these occur, use of the drug should be discontinued.

Although hypotension has occurred only rarely, benzodiazepines should be administered with caution to patients in whom a drop in blood pressure might lead to cardiovascular or cerebrovascular complications. This is particularly important in elderly patients.

*Interactions with other medicaments and other forms of interactions:* The benzodiazepines, including oxazepam produce additive CNS depressant effects when co-administered with other medications which themselves produce CNS depression e.g., alcohol, barbiturates, antipsychotics, sedatives/hypnotics, anxiolytics, antidepressants, narcotic analgesics, sedative antihistamines, anticonvulsants, and anaesthetics.

An enhancement of the euphoria induced by narcotic analgesics may occur with benzodiazepine use, leading to an increase in psychic dependence.

Compounds which inhibit certain hepatic enzymes (particularly cytochrome P450) may enhance the activity of benzodiazepines. To a lesser degree this also applies to benzodiazepines which are metabolised only by conjugation.

*Pregnancy and lactation:* Benzodiazepines should not be used during pregnancy, especially during the first and last trimesters. Benzodiazepines may cause foetal damage when administered to pregnant women.

If the drug is prescribed to a woman of childbearing potential, she should be warned to contact her physician about stopping the drug if she intends to become, or suspects that she is, pregnant.

Infants of mothers who ingested benzodiazepines for several weeks or more preceding delivery have been reported to have withdrawal symptoms during the postnatal period. Symptoms such as hypoactivity, hypotonia, hypothermia, respiratory depression, apnoea, feeding problems, and impaired metabolic response to cold stress have been reported in neonates born of mothers who have received benzodiazepines during the late phase of pregnancy or at delivery.

The concentration of oxazepam and its conjugate in human breast milk is approximately 10% of the plasma level. Therefore, oxazepam should not be administered to nursing women.

*Effects on ability to drive and use machinery:* As with all patients on CNS-depressant drugs, patients should be warned not to operate dangerous machinery or motor vehicles until it is known that they do not become drowsy or dizzy from oxazepam.

*Undesirable effects:* Adverse reactions, when they occur, are usually observed at the beginning of therapy and generally decrease in severity or disappear with continued use or upon decreasing the dose.

Most frequently reported adverse reactions associated with benzodiazepines include daytime drowsiness, dizziness, muscle weakness, and ataxia.

Less frequently reported adverse reactions include the following: confusion, depression, fatigue, headache, reduced alertness, numbed emotions, nausea, appetite change, sleep disturbance, dermatological reactions, visual disturbances, change of libido, and gastrointestinal symptoms.

Rarely reported adverse reactions include blood dyscrasia, abnormal liver function tests, transient anterograde amnesia or memory impairment, paradoxical reactions, and hypotension (see Special warnings and precautions for use).

*Overdosage:* In the management of overdosage with any drug, it should be borne in mind that multiple agents may have been taken.

Overdosage of benzodiazepines is usually manifested by degrees of central nervous system depression ranging from drowsiness to coma. In mild cases, symptoms include drowsiness, mental confusion, and lethargy. In more serious cases, and especially when other CNS-depressant drugs or alcohol are ingested, symptoms may include ataxia, hypotension, hypotonia, respiratory depression, coma, and very rarely, death.

If ingestion was recent, induced vomiting and/or gastric lavage should be undertaken followed by general supportive care, monitoring of vital signs and close observation of the patient. If there is no advantage in emptying the stomach, activated charcoal may be effective in reducing absorption. Hypotension, though unlikely, may be controlled with noradrenaline. The dialysability of oxazepam is minimal.

The benzodiazepine antagonist, flumazenil may be useful in hospitalised patients for the management of benzodiazepine overdosage. Flumazenil product information should be consulted prior to use.

**Pharmacological properties**

*Pharmacodynamic properties:* Oxazepam is a benzodiazepine with anxiolytic, sedative and hypnotic properties and possibly muscle relaxant and anticonvulsant characteristics.

*Pharmacokinetic properties:* Oxazepam is completely absorbed from the gastrointestinal tract and peak serum levels are reached in 1–5 hours. It is metabolised by a simple one-step process to a pharmacologically inert glucuronide. There are no major active metabolites. The elimination half-life is 6–8 hours and there is minimal risk of excessive accumulation.

*Pre-clinical safety data:* Acute oral $LD_{50}$ in mice is greater than 5000 mg/kg.

Fatty metamorphosis of the liver has been noted in six-week toxicity studies in rats given this product at 0.5% of the diet. Such accumulations of fat are considered reversible, since no liver necrosis or fibrosis is seen.

*In vitro* mutagenicity reports on Oxazepam are inconclusive.

In a carcinogenicity study, oxazepam was administered with diet to rats for two years. Male rats receiving 30 times the maximum human dose showed a statistical increase, when compared to controls, in benign thyroid follicular cell tumours, testicular interstitial cell adenomas, and prostatic adenomas. An earlier published study reported that mice fed dietary dosages of 35 or 100 times the human daily dose of oxazepam for 9 months developed a dose-related increase in liver adenomas. In an independent analysis of some of the microscopic slides from this mouse study, several of these tumours were classified as liver carcinomas. At this time, there is no evidence that clinical use of oxazepam is associated with tumours.

**Pharmaceutical particulars**

*List of excipients:* Calcium hydrogen phosphate, maize starch (dried), methylcellulose, magnesium stearate.

*Incompatibilities:* None known.

*Shelf-life:* 60 months.

*Special precautions for storage:* Store in a dry place below 25°C.

*Nature and contents of container:* 10 mg and 15 mg tablets: Blister packs of PVC backed by hard tempered aluminium foil of 100 tablets.

**Marketing authorisation numbers**
Oxazepam Tablets 10 mg        0011/0110
Oxazepam Tablets 15 mg        0011/0111

**Date of approval/revision of SPC** January 1997

**Legal category**   CD(Sch 4), POM

# PROMAZINE INJECTION BP

**Presentation** Promazine Injection is a clear, colourless aqueous solution containing 50 mg promazine hydrochloride B.P. per millilitre.

**Uses** Promazine is one of the phenothiazine group of antipsychotics which have a wide range of activities arising from the depressant actions on the central nervous system.

*Indications:*

1. As an adjunct to the short term management of moderate to severe psychomotor agitation.
2. Agitation and restlessness in the elderly.
3. Intractable hiccup.
4. Alleviation of nausea and vomiting, including that in labour.

**Dosage and administration**

*Route of administration:* Parenteral. If Promazine is injected intravenously it should be diluted with an equal volume of saline.

*Dosage: Adults:*

*Psychomotor agitation:* 50 mg Promazine intramuscularly. Repeat if necessary after six to eight hours.

*Intractable hiccup:* 50 mg intramuscularly. Repeat if necessary with doses up to 100 mg 4 hourly. The daily dose should not exceed 1 g.

*Labour:* 50 mg Promazine intramuscularly. For convenience, 50 mg Promazine may be mixed with 50 mg pethidine in the same syringe.

*Elderly:* Half the normal dose may be sufficient for a therapeutic response in elderly subjects.

*Children:* Not recommended.

**Contra-indications, warnings etc.**

*Contra-indications:*

1. Use in patients in coma.
2. Bone marrow depression
3. Use in patients hypersensitive to the ingredients or other phenothiazines.
4. Promazine should not be used during lactation
5. Do not use during pregnancy, especially during the first three months, unless there are compelling reasons.

*Precautions and warnings:*

1. Phenothiazines should only be used with great caution in patients with a history of jaundice or with existent liver dysfunction, or blood dyscrasias, coronary insufficiency or cardiac disease.
2. Respiratory depression may occur in patients with severe respiratory disease.
3. Promazine should be used with caution in patients with renal failure.
4. Patients receiving phenothiazines over a prolonged period require regular and careful surveillance with particular attention to: potential for inducing eye changes, effects on haemopoiesis, liver dysfunction, myocardial conduction effects, particularly if other concurrently administered drugs also have potential effects on these systems.
5. Use of phenothiazines at high (relative or absolute) doses may induce extrapyramidal side-effects, dyskinesia, akathisia, dystonia. These are likely to be particularly severe in children. Caution should be exercised in patients with Parkinson's disease. Anti-Parkinsonian agents should not be prescribed routinely because of the risk of aggravating anticholinergic side effects of Promazine, of precipitating toxic-confusional states or of impairing its therapeutic efficacy. They should be given only as required.
6. Prolonged administration of phenothiazines may result in persistent or tardive dyskinesia particularly in the elderly. The risk of developing the syndrome as well as the likelihood of irreversibility, are believed to increase as the duration of treatment and the total

cumulative dose increase. If symptoms of tardive dyskinesia appear, withdrawal of neuroleptic therapy is recommended.

7. Administration by the intravenous route may induce local vascular spasm or thrombophlebitis. The preparation must be diluted before use. Arteriolar spasm and gangrene have been reported following accidental intra-arterial injection of high concentrations.

8. Care should be exercised if Promazine is used for the treatment of patients with cerebral arteriosclerosis, coronary heart disease or other conditions in which a fall in blood pressure might be undesirable.

9. Caution should be observed with patients suffering from epilepsy or conditions predisposing to epilepsy.

10. Personal or family history of narrow angle glaucoma.

11. Phenothiazines may impair body temperature regulation. Caution should be observed in very hot weather.

12. Promazine should be used with caution in the following disease states: hypothyroidism, myasthenia gravis, phaeochromocytoma and prostatic hypertrophy.

13. Antipsychotic drugs may increase prolactin secretion.

14. Phenothiazines may impair alertness and induce drowsiness especially at the start of treatment. Persons taking these drugs should not drive or operate machinery unless the drug has been shown not to interfere with physical or mental ability.

*Use in pregnancy and lactation:* Do not use during pregnancy, especially during the first three months, unless there are compelling reasons. There is insufficient evidence of the safety of promazine in human pregnancy nor is there evidence from animal studies that it is free from hazard.

The use of Promazine during lactation is contra-indicated.

*Interactions:* The concomitant administration of Promazine with other CNS depressants (including alcohol and anaesthetics) or antihypertensives, anticholinergic or dopaminergic drugs may result in accentuation of their effects. Potentiation of action may also occur with monoamine oxidase inhibitors, antidepressants and analgesics. Promazine may impair the effects of anticonvulsants.

Promazine may affect the control of diabetes. Undesirable anti-cholinergic effects may be enhanced by anti-Parkinsonian or other anticholinergic drugs.

*Side-effects:* Promazine is a member of the phenothiazine group of drugs and side effects associated with this group, as well as anticholinergic effects, have been noted.

CNS: Drowsiness, extrapyramidal symptoms, hyperpyrexia, confusional states, and convulsions have been reported. Neuroleptic malignant syndrome (hyperthermia, rigidity autonomic dysfunction and altered consciousness) may occur with any neuroleptic.

Cardiovascular effects such as hypotension and tachycardia may infrequently occur.

The anticholinergic action of Promazine may precipitate symptoms of dry mouth, nasal stuffiness, blurred vision, constipation and also urinary hesitancy or retention in the presence of an enlarged prostate.

Haematological effects have been reported including agranulocytosis and transient leucopenia.

Jaundice and photosensitivity have been reported.

Some individuals may be susceptible to the drug in low dosage and show paradoxical effects of excitement, agitation or insomnia and other minor side effects.

The elderly are particularly susceptible to side effects of Promazine, especially to the sedative, hypotensive and temperature regulation effects. These effects may be dose related.

*Overdose:* Ingestion of large amounts of Promazine is followed by deep sleep, with or without a pronounced fall in blood pressure and without particular change in respiration rate, other than the slowing attendant upon sedation. Occasionally an initial period of excitement may precede coma, followed by grand mal seizures.

In the absence of any specific antidote, treatment should be based on ordinary therapeutic principles with special emphasis on the following measures: 1) treat convulsions if present; 2) correction of acute hypotension if necessary; 3) counteract the effects of an excess of Promazine on the central nervous system; 4) control and natural recovery of hypothermia.

**Pharmaceutical precautions** Promazine Injection BP should not be mixed with other injections with the exception of Pethidine Injection BP.

Store below 25°C and protect from light.

**Legal category** POM

**Package quantities** Boxes of 10 by 1 ml ampoules

**Further information** Nil

**Product licence number** 0011/5043R

# PROMAZINE SUSPENSION

**Qualitative and quantitative composition** Promazine Suspension is an opaque yellow liquid with an odour of pineapple containing 50 mg promazine hydrochloride per 5 ml.

**Pharmaceutical form** Oral suspension

**Clinical particulars**

*Therapeutic indications:*

1. As an adjunct to the short term management of moderate to severe psychomotor agitation.
2. Agitation and restlessness in the elderly.

*Posology and method of administration:*

*Route of administration:* Oral

*Dosage:*
*Psychomotor agitation:*

*Adults:* 100–200 mg four times daily

*Elderly:* Half the normal dose may be sufficient for a therapeutic response in elderly patients.

*Agitation and restlessness:*

*Elderly:* 25 mg initially. Increase if necessary up to 50 mg four times daily.

*Children:* Oral Promazine is not recommended for children.

*Contra-indications:*

1. Use in patients in coma.
2. Use in patients with bone marrow depression.
3. Use in patients hypersensitive to the ingredient or other phenothiazines.
4. Use during lactation.
5. Do not use during pregnancy, especially during the first three months, unless there are compelling reasons.

*Special warnings and precautions for use:*

1. Phenothiazines should only be used with great caution in patients with a history of jaundice or with existent liver dysfunction, or blood dyscrasia, coronary insufficiency or cardiac disease.

2. Respiratory depression may occur in patients with severe respiratory disease.

3. Promazine should be used with caution in patients with renal failure.

4. Patients receiving phenothiazines over a prolonged period require regular and careful surveillance with particular attention to: potential for inducing eye changes, effects on haemopoiesis, liver dysfunction, myocardial conduction effects, particularly if other concurrently administered drugs also have potential effects on these systems.

5. Use of phenothiazines at high (relative or absolute) doses may induce extrapyramidal side-effects, dyskinesia, akathisia, dystonia. These are likely to be particularly severe in children. Caution should be exercised in patients with Parkinson's disease. Anti-Parkinsonian agents should not be prescribed routinely because of the risk of aggravating anticholinergic side effects of Promazine, of precipitating toxic-confusional states, or of impairing its therapeutic efficacy. They should be given only as required.

6. Prolonged administration of phenothiazines may result in persistent or tardive dyskinesia particularly in the elderly. The risk of developing the syndrome, as well as the likelihood of irreversibility, are believed to increase as the duration of treatment, and the total cumulative dose increase. If symptoms of tardive dyskinesia appear, withdrawal of neuroleptic therapy is recommended.

7. Care should be exercised if Promazine is used for the treatment of patients with cerebral arteriosclerosis, coronary heart disease or other conditions in which a fall in blood pressure might be undesirable.

8. Caution should be observed with patients suffering from epilepsy or conditions predisposing to epilepsy.

9. Personal or family history of narrow angle glaucoma.

10. Phenothiazines may impair body temperature regulation. Caution should be observed in very hot weather.

11. Promazine should be used with caution in patients with hypothyroidism, myasthenia gravis, phaeochromocytoma and prostatic hypertrophy.

12. Antipsychotic drugs may increase prolactin secretion.

*Interactions with other medicaments and other forms of interaction:*

1. The concomitant administration of Promazine with other CNS depressants (including alcohol and anaesthetics) or antihypertensives, anticholinergic or dopaminergic drugs may result in accentuation of their effects. Potentiation of action may also occur with monoamine oxidase inhibitors, antidepressants and analgesics.

2. Promazine may impair the effects of anticonvulsants.

3. Promazine suspension is formulated with aluminium hydroxide which may complex tetracyclines if given concomitantly.

4. Promazine may affect the control of diabetes. Undesirable anti-cholinergic effects may be enhanced by anti-Parkinsonian or other anticholinergic drugs.

*Pregnancy and lactation:* Do not use during pregnancy, especially during the first three months, unless there are compelling reasons. There is insufficient evidence of the safety of promazine in human pregnancy nor is there evidence from animal studies that it is free from hazard.

Promazine is contra-indicated in patients who are breastfeeding.

*Effects on the ability to drive and use machines:* Phenothiazines may impair alertness and induce drowsiness especially at the start of treatment. Persons taking these drugs should not drive or operate machinery unless the drug has been shown not to interfere with physical or mental ability.

*Undesirable effects:* Promazine is a member of the phenothiazine class of drugs and side effects associated with this group have been observed.

CNS effects including drowsiness, sedation, extrapyramidal symptoms, hyperpyrexia, confusion, and convulsions have been reported. Neuroleptic malignant syndrome (hyperthermia, rigidity, autonomic dysfunction and altered consciousness) may occur with any neuroleptic.

Cardiovascular effects such as hypotension and tachycardia may occur infrequently.

The anticholinergic action of Promazine may precipitate symptoms of dry mouth, nasal stuffiness, blurred vision, constipation and urinary hesitancy or retention in the presence of an enlarged prostate gland.

Sexual function may be impaired.

Haematological effects have been reported including agranulocytosis and transient leucopenia.

Jaundice, transient abnormalities in liver function without jaundice, allergic skin reactions and photosensitivity have been reported.

Some individuals may be susceptible to the drug in low dosage and show paradoxical effects of excitement, agitation, insomnia and other minor side effects. The elderly are particularly susceptible to side effects of Promazine, especially to the sedative, hypotensive and temperature regulation effects. These effects may be dose related.

*Overdose:* Ingestion of large amounts of promazine is followed by deep sleep, with or without a pronounced fall in blood pressure and without particular change in respiration rate, other than the slowing attendant upon sedation. Occasionally an initial period of excitement may precede coma, followed by grand mal seizures.

In the absence of any specific antidote, treatment should be based on ordinary therapeutic principles with special emphasis on the following measures: 1) gastric lavage; 2) treat convulsions if present; 3) correction of acute hypotension if necessary; 4) counteraction of the effects of an excess of promazine hydrochloride on the central nervous system; 5) control and natural recovery of hypothermia.

**Pharmacological properties**

*Pharmacodynamic properties:* Promazine is one of the phenothiazine group of antipsychotics which have a wide range of activity arising from the depressant actions on the central nervous system. Antipsychotic drugs are considered to act by interfering with dopaminergic transmission in the brain by blocking dopamine receptors. This may give rise to extrapyramidal effects and in addition, hyperprolactinaemia. Antipsychotic drugs also affect to varying degrees cholinergic, alpha adrenergic, histaminergic and tryptaminergic (serotonergic) receptors.

*Pharmacokinetic properties:* Promazine is rapidly absorbed after oral administration. Mean maximum plasma concentration was 13.8 ng/ml at a mean peak time of more than 3 hours. Mean $AUC_{0-48\,hr}$ was 62.3. Terminal half life was 4.5 hours.

*Preclinical safety data:* None stated.

**Pharmaceutical particulars**

*List of excipients:* Embonic acid, A type alumina gel, ammonia solution, antifoam 1520 Dow Corning, ascorbic acid, sodium butyl hydroxybenzoate, sodium methyl hydroxybenzoate, sodium propyl hydroxybenzoate, saccharin sodium, sodium carbonate, sodium metabisulphite, strong sodium hypochlorite solution, sucrose, pineapple flavour, water.

*Incompatibilities:* When required Promazine Suspension may be diluted with syrup BP unpreserved or preserved with p-hydroxybenzoates.

*Shelf life:* 36 months.

*Special precautions for storage:* Store in a cool place. Protect from light.

*Nature and contents of container:* This product will be presented in amber glass bottles with metal screw caps with liners. Bottles size of 150 ml.

*Instructions for use/handling:* None

**Marketing authorisation number** 0011/5045R

**Date of approval/revision** March 1997

**Legal category** POM

## RANITIDINE TABLETS

**Qualitative and quantitative composition** There are two strengths of Ranitidine Tablets containing 150 mg or 300 mg of ranitidine as hydrochloride.

Ranitidine (BAN, INN) is chemically defined as N,N-Dimethyl-5-[2-(1-methylamino-2-nitrovinylamino)ethylthiomethyl]furfurylamine.

**Pharmaceutical form** Ranitidine Tablets are white film-coated tablets containing 150 mg or 300 mg ranitidine.

**Clinical particulars**

*Therapeutic indications:* Ranitidine Tablets are indicated for the following conditions affecting the upper gastro-intestinal tract, where the reduction of secretion of gastric acid is desirable:

- duodenal ulcers including those associated with Helicobacter pylori infection;
- benign gastric ulcers;
- ulcers associated with non-steroidal anti-inflammatory drug therapy;
- oesophageal reflux disease;
- chronic dyspepsia;
- patients with severe gastric acid secretion e.g. Zollinger-Ellison.

Extended or maintenance treatment with ranitidine tablets is indicated for the prevention of recurrent ulcer or management of healed oesophagitis.

Ranitidine Tablets can also be used for prophylaxis of gastrointestinal haemorrhage from stress ulceration, or recurrent haemorrhage from erosions and ulcerations in stomach and duodenum, usually as continuation therapy following intravenous ranitidine. Prophylactic use of Ranitidine Tablets is also indicated for use in patients at risk of acid aspiration e.g. prior to general anesthesia or during labour.

*Posology and method of administration:* Ranitidine Tablets are to be taken whole with some liquid regardless of meals.

*Adults:* The following guidelines apply to adults with a normal renal function:

For the treatment of duodenal ulcers or benign gastric ulcers the usual dosage is 150 mg tablet twice daily to be taken in the morning and evening, or a single dose of 300 mg to be taken in the evening. Treatment should be continued for 4 weeks during which time most ulcers will heal. In patients whose ulcers have not been completely healed after 4 weeks of therapy, treatment should be continued for a further 4 weeks with the same dosage. For those patients responding to short-term therapy or with a history of relapse maintenance treatment of a daily dose of 150 mg to be taken at bedtime is recommended.

In the treatment of duodenal ulcers associated with Helicobacter pylori infection Ranitidine should be administered, as a single dose of 300 mg at bedtime or 150 mg twice daily and given concomitantly with oral amoxicillin or metronidazole (see respective data sheets) for the first two weeks of treatment. Ranitidine treatment should be continued alone for the subsequent two weeks.

For the prophylaxis of duodenal ulcers associated with administration of non-steroidal anti-inflammatory drugs ranitidine 150 mg should be given twice daily. The dose may be increased to 300 mg twice daily if required. The increased dose has not been associated with any increase in the incidence of unwanted effects.

A daily dose of 300 mg is recommended for oesophageal reflux disease, to be taken as 150 mg twice daily or as a single daily dose of 300 mg in the evening. The course of treatment may last up to 8 weeks, and up to 12 weeks if necessary. The dose may be increased to 150 mg four times daily for up to 12 weeks in patients with moderate to severe oesophagitis. Long-term management with ranitidine 150 mg twice daily is recommended for patients with healed oesophagitis only.

A dose of 150 mg twice daily for up to 6 weeks is recommended for symptomatic relief of chronic dyspepsia. Those patients not responding within this time or relapsing shortly after stopping treatment should be re-examined.

For treatment of patients with very severe gastric acid secretion e.g. Zollinger-Ellison syndrome, a higher starting dose of 450 mg daily to be taken as 150 mg three times may be required, and this may be increased to a daily dose of 600-900 mg. If necessary, after analysis of the hydrochloric acid secretion, the patient may be stabilised on higher doses; doses of up to 6 g daily have been tolerated.

Following prophylaxis of stress ulceration or recurrent haemorrhage in the upper gastro-intestinal tract with intravenous ranitidine, Ranitidine Tablets may be substituted at a dose of 150 mg twice daily as soon as the patient is able to take meals again and for as long as the patient is considered to be at risk.

In those patients considered to be at risk of acid aspiration a single dose of 150 mg can be given 2 hours before the induction of general anaesthesia (this may be preceded by a dose of 150 mg the previous evening) or in obstetric patients at the start of labour. While the risk exists this dose may be repeated at 6 hourly intervals if required. If emergency surgery is required once labour has commenced a non-particulate antacid should also be given prior to anaesthesia.

*Children:* The use of ranitidine in children is indicated for peptic ulcer only. The recommended daily dose is 2 mg/kg body weight twice a day, but up to 4 mg/kg twice daily may be given, with a maximum daily dose of 300 mg.

*Patients with renal impairment:* For patients with a creatinine clearance of less than 30 ml/min the recommended daily dose of ranitidine is reduced to 150 mg. A daily dose of 300 mg ranitidine may be given to patients with a creatinine clearance greater than 30 ml/min.

The dose may be increased to 150 mg two times a day if an ulcer has not healed. Maintenance treatment of 150 mg at night may be instituted if deemed necessary.

As ranitidine is dialysable, dialysis patients should be given ranitidine after dialysis has been completed.

*Contra-indications:*

- Hypersensitivity to the active ingredient ranitidine.
- Acute porphyria.

*Special warnings and precautions for use:* As histamine $H_2$-receptor antagonists may alleviate the symptoms or delay the diagnosis of carcinoma of the stomach, care should be taken to exclude the possibility of malignancy in patients presenting with new or recently changed dyspeptic symptoms prior to the institution of treatment with Ranitidine Tablets.

Concomitant use of Ranitidine Tablets with non-steroidal anti-inflammatory drugs prevents ulceration in the duodenum but not in the stomach. It is recommended that these patients, and especially the elderly, should be examined regularly.

As ranitidine is excreted via the kidney, lower doses are recommended for patients with impaired renal function (see *Posology and method of administration*).

*Interactions with other medicaments and other forms of interactions:* As the absorption of ranitidine may be reduced by antacids or sucralfate, it is recommended that with concomitant use of these agents, administration should be separated by two hours.

Although ranitidine would not be expected to raise serum theophylline levels, as seen with cimetidine, there have been several reports of theophylline toxicity developing in patients receiving ranitidine. Therefore serum theophylline levels should be monitored in patients receiving theophylline and ranitidine concomitantly.

As ranitidine may reduce gastric acidity care should be taken when ranitidine is given concomitantly with drugs which have pH-dependent absorption, e.g. ketoconazole.

Ranitidine may increase the effect of alcohol.

Antibiotic associated diarrhoea may occur when amoxycillin or metronidazole are taken with ranitidine.

*Pregnancy and lactation:* As the safety of ranitidine for use during pregnancy has not been established Ranitidine Tablets should only be used during pregnancy if considered absolutely necessary. Studies with ranitidine in animals have not shown any teratogenicity.

Although ranitidine crosses the placental barrier it has been used in therapeutic doses during labour or in patients undergoing caesarean section and appear not to have adverse effects on labour, delivery or the subsequent neonates.

Ranitidine is excreted in human milk and should therefore only be given to breast-feeding women if absolutely necessary due to the possibility of disturbances in the gastric acid secretion of the infant.

*Effects on ability to drive and use machinery:* As ranitidine may induce side effects which can decrease the ability to react (e.g. headache, dizziness or confusion) patients should be warned not to operate dangerous machinery or drive motor vehicles, or work without secure support, until it is known that they know that they are not adversely affected by ranitidine.

*Undesirable effects:* Headaches, tiredness, vertigo, nausea, diarrhoea and constipation occur occasionally during treatment with ranitidine. In most cases these symptoms decrease in severity if treatment is continued.

Severe headaches, mental states of confusion and restlessness, visual disturbances, depression and hallucinations have been reported rarely. These CNS disturbances have occured mainly in elderly or seriously ill patients and have been reversible on discontinuation of ranitidine therapy.

Rare cases of arrythmias, like A-V block, bradycardia and tachycardia, have been reported.

Leucocytopenia and thrombocytopenia have occurred in patients taking ranitidine although these effects are usually reversible on discontinuation of treatment. More rarely, cases of agranulocytosis or pancytopenia, occasionally with bone-marrow hypoplasia or aplasia, have been reported.

Increases in plasma creatinine levels have been observed in some patients taking ranitidine although these were generally insignificant and normalised during treatment.

Changes in liver function have been reported although these effects are transient and recede with continued treatment or on discontinuation of therapy.

Itching and skin rashes, including occasional cases of erythema multiforme, have occurred during treatment with ranitidine. In extremely rare cases an increase in hair loss (alopecia) has been reported.

Rare episodes of hypersensitivity reactions (e.g. urticaria, fever, eosinophilia, angioneurophilia, acute inflammation of the pancreas, angioneurotic oedema, laryngospasm, bronchospasm, chest pains, hypotension, anaphylactic shock have occasionally been reported either during treatment with ranitidine, or occasionally after a single dose.

Although no effects on endocrine or gonadal function have been demonstrated in clinical studies with ranitidine, gynaecomastia and disturbances in sexual behaviour (loss of libido and impotency) have been reported during treatment with ranitidine. A causal connection between ranitidine and these disturbances has not been established.

*Overdosage:* In the management of overdosage with any drug, it should be borne in mind that multiple agents may have been taken.

If ingestion was recent, induced vomiting and/or gastric lavage should be undertaken followed by general supportive care, monitoring of vital signs and close observation of the patient. If there is no advantage in emptying the stomach, activated charcoal may be effective in reducing absorption. If necessary, haemodialysis may be used to remove ranitidine from the plasma.

**Pharmacological properties**

*Pharmacodynamic properties:* Ranitidine is a competitive histamine $H_2$-antagonist which inhibits basal and stimulated gastric acid secretion and acts by reducing both the volume, and the acid and pepsin content, of gastric secretions.

In two studies using a dose of 150 mg twice a day, gastric acid secretion was decreased over 24 hours; by an average of 63% and 69% during the day and by 73% and 90% respectively during the night. In two other studies for prophylaxis of recurrence, a daily dose of 150 mg taken in the evening decreased gastric acid secretion by 42% and 69% over the 24 hours. An evening dose of 300 mg ranitidine administered reduced gastric acid secretion by an average of 50–60% over 24 hours and by 90% during the night.

*Pharmacokinetic properties:* Ranitidine is rapidly absorbed after oral administration with peak blood concentrations achieved within 1 to 3 hours. Oral bioavailability is approximately 50%.

The primary route of elimination of ranitidine and its metabolites is via the kidneys with approximately 30–35% of the oral intake of the active drug excreted unchanged by tubular secretion within the first 24 hours. Small amounts of ranitidine are metabolised in the liver to ranitidine-N-oxide, N-desmethylranitidine and the furane acid derivative. Besides renal elimination, ranitidine is also excreted in faeces.

The elimination half-life of ranitidine is approximately 2–3 hours although in patients with renal impairment this can be increased by 2–3 fold.

*Preclinical safety data:* There is no evidence from extensive studies in animals of any significant toxicological abnormalities, or of any mutagenic potential of ranitidine. No carcinogenicity has been demonstrated in chronic high dose tests in rodents.

Reproductive toxicological studies did not reveal any teratogenic or toxicological effects of ranitidine in rodents.

**Pharmaceutical particulars**

*List of excipients:* Microcrystalline cellulose, croscarmellose sodium, magnesium stearate, ethanol, methanol, hydroxypropylmethyl cellulose, polyethylene glycol, colloidal silicon dioxide, methylene chloride, isopropyl alcohol, titanium dioxide.

*Incompatibilities:* None.

*Shelf-life:* 2 years.

*Special precautions for storage:* Store in a dry place at room temperature below 25°C.
Protect from light.

*Nature and contents of container:* Aluminium foil/PVC blister:
150 mg tablets: Pack sizes 60 tablets
300 mg tablets: Pack sizes 30 tablets

*Marketing authorisation holder:* Novopharm BV, Netherlands.

**Marketing authorisation numbers**
Ranitidine Tablets 150 mg: 14896/0001
Ranitidine Tablets 300 mg: 14896/0002

**Date of approval/revision of SPC** July 1997

**Legal category** POM

## SODIUM CROMOGLYCATE EYE DROPS

**Presentation** A clear colourless aqueous solution of Sodium Cromoglycate BP 2% w/v, with benzalkonium chloride 0.01% w/v.
Inactive ingredients: Benzalkonium Chloride PhEur, Disodium Edetate PhEur.

**Uses** For the relief and treatment of acute allergic conjunctivitis such as hay fever, chronic allergic conjunctivitis and vernal kerato-conjunctivitis. Sodium cromoglycate inhibits the release from sensitised mast cells of mediators of the allergic reaction.

**Dosage and administration** One or two drops to be administered into each eye four times daily, or as prescribed by the doctor.

*Elderly:* There is no evidence to suggest that dosage alteration is required for elderly patients.

**Contra-indications, warnings, etc**
*Contra-indications:* Known hypersensitivity to any ingredient, including sodium cromoglycate, benzalkonium chloride and disodium edetate. Soft contact lenses.

*Use in pregnancy and lactation:* Cumulative experience with sodium cromoglycate suggests that it has no adverse effects on foetal development. However, as with all medicines, caution should be exercised during pregnancy, and should be used in pregnancy only when there is a clear need.

*Side-effects:* Transient stinging and blurring of vision may occur. Patients should be advised not to drive or operate machinery if vision is affected. Other symptoms of local irritation have been reported rarely.

*Overdose:* Overdosage is very unlikely. In the event of accidental ingestion, symptomatic treatment is recommended.

**Pharmaceutical precautions** Store below 25°C. Protect from direct sunlight. Discard any remaining content 4 weeks after opening the bottle.

**Legal category** POM.

**Package quantities** 13.5 ml.

**Further information** Nil.

**Product licence number** 10622/0016.

## TEMAZEPAM ORAL SOLUTION BP

**Presentation** Temazepam Oral Solution BP is a clear, green, lemon-mint flavoured elixir containing 10 mg temazepam per 5 ml.

**Uses** Temazepam Oral Solution B.P. is indicated for the short-term treatment (up to 4 weeks including any tapering off) of insomnia, when it is disabling or subjecting the individual to extreme distress, and for premedication before minor surgery or other procedures, especially when hospital admission is not essential.

**Dosage and administration**

*Route of administration:* Oral

*Insomnia:* Dosage and duration of therapy should be individualised. The lowest effective dose should be prescribed for the shortest time possible. Generally, the duration of treatment varies from a few days to 4 weeks including the tapering off process. Extension of the treatment period should not take place without re-evaluation of the need for continued therapy.

Since insomnia is often transient and intermittent, the prolonged administration of Temazepam Oral Solution BP is generally unnecessary and is not recommended.

Treatment in all patients should be withdrawn gradually to minimise possible withdrawal symptoms (see *Precautions and warnings*).

*Dosage:*

*Adults:* 10–20 mg, but in severe or persistent insomnia, it may be increased up to 40 mg. The solution should be taken up to 30 minutes before going to bed.

*Elderly:* 10 mg. If this dose is not effective, it may be cautiously increased to 20 mg.

*Children:* The safety and efficacy of Temazepam Oral Solution BP in children less than 18 years of age has not been established and such use is not recommended.

*Premedication:*
*Adults:* 20–30 mg taken 30–60 minutes prior to surgery or other procedures.

*Elderly:* Elderly patients are likely to respond to smaller doses, possibly half the normal adult dose.

*Children:* The safety and efficacy of Temazepam Oral Solution B.P. in children less than 18 years of age has not been established and such use is not recommended.

Patients should be accompanied home when Temazepam Oral Solution BP has been used as a premedicant prior to surgery or other procedures on a day attendance basis.

**Contra-indication, warnings, etc**

*Contra-indications:*
Severe respiratory insufficiency
Sleep apnoea syndrome
Hypersensitivity to benzodiazepines including Temazepam Oral Solution B.P. or its components.
Myasthenia gravis
Severe hepatic failure
Temazepam Oral Solution BP should not be given to children

*Use in pregnancy and lactation:* Benzodiazepines should not be used during pregnancy, especially during the first and last trimesters. Benzodiazepines may cause foetal damage when administered to pregnant women.

If the drug is prescribed to a woman of childbearing potential, she should be warned to contact her physician about stopping the drug if she intends to become, or suspects that she is, pregnant.

Infants of mothers who ingested benzodiazepines for several weeks or more preceding delivery have been reported to have withdrawal symptoms during the postnatal period. Symptoms such as hypoactivity, hypotonia, hypothermia, respiratory depression, apnoea, feeding problems, and impaired metabolic response to cold stress have been reported in neonates born of mothers who have received benzodiazepines during the late phase of pregnancy or at delivery.

It is recommended that the use of temazepam be avoided in pregnant women receiving antihistamines (see *Interactions*).

Because it is not known whether Temazepam Oral Solution BP is excreted in human milk, it should not be given to breast-feeding women.

*Precautions and warnings:* As with all patients on CNS-depressant drugs, patients should be warned not to operate dangerous machinery or motor vehicles until it is known that they do not become drowsy or dizzy from Temazepam Oral Solution BP. Patients should be advised that since their tolerance for alcohol and other CNS depressants will be diminished in the presence of Temazepam Oral Solution BP, these substances should either be avoided or taken in reduced dosage.

Temazepam Oral Solution BP is not intended for the primary treatment of psychotic illness or depressive disorders, and should not be used alone to treat depressed patients with associated insomnia. The use of benzodiazepines may have a disinhibiting effect and may release suicidal tendencies in depressed patients. Therefore, large quantities of Temazepam Oral Solution B.P. should not be prescribed to these patients.

Pre-existing depression may emerge during benzodiazepine use.

The use of benzodiazepines may lead to physical and psychological dependence. The risk of dependence on Temazepam Oral Solution B.P. is low when used at the recommended dose and duration, but increases with higher doses and longer term use. The risk of dependence is further increased in patients with a history of alcoholism or drug abuse or in patients with significant personality disorders. Therefore, use in individuals with a history of alcoholism or drug abuse should be avoided.

Dependence may lead to withdrawal symptoms, especially if treatment is discontinued abruptly. Therefore, the drug should always be discontinued gradually.

Symptoms reported following discontinuation of benzodiazepines include headaches, muscle pain, anxiety, tension, depression, insomnia, restlessness, confusion, irritability, sweating, and the occurrence of 'rebound' phenomena whereby the symptoms that led to treatment with benzodiazepines recur in an enhanced form. These symptoms may be difficult to distinguish from the original symptoms for which the drug was prescribed.

In severe cases the following symptoms may occur: derealisation; depersonalisation; hyperacusis; tinnitus; numbness and tingling of the extremities; hypersensitivity to light, noise, and physical contact; involuntary movements; vomiting; hallucinations; convulsions. Convulsions may be more common in patients with pre-existing seizure disorders or who are taking other drugs that lower the convulsive threshold such as antidepressants.

It may be useful to inform the patient that treatment will be of limited duration and that it will be discontinued gradually. The patient should also be made aware of the possibility of 'rebound' phenomena to minimise anxiety should they occur.

Abuse has been reported in poly-drug users.

Some loss of efficacy to the hypnotic effects of short-acting benzodiazepines may develop after repeated use for a few weeks.

Insomnia may be a symptom of several other disorders. The possibility should be considered that the complaint may be related to an underlying physical or psychiatric disorder for which there is more specific treatment.

Caution should be used in the treatment of patients with acute narrow-angle glaucoma.

Patients with impaired renal or hepatic function should be monitored frequently and have their dosage adjusted carefully according to patient response. Lower doses may be sufficient in these patients. The same precautions apply to elderly or debilitated patients and patients with chronic respiratory insufficiency.

As with all CNS-depressants, the use of benzodiazepines may precipitate encephalopathy in patients with severe hepatic insufficiency. Therefore, use in these patients is contraindicated.

Some patients taking benzodiazepines have developed a blood dyscrasia, and some have had elevations in liver enzymes. Periodic haematologic and liver-function assessments are recommended when long-term therapy is clinically necessary.

Transient anterograde amnesia or memory impairment has been reported in association with the use of benzodiazepines. This condition usually occurs several hours after ingestion. Therefore, patients should ensure that they will be able to have a period of uninterrupted sleep which is sufficient to allow dissipation of drug effect (e.g., 7–8 hours).

Paradoxical reactions such as restlessness, agitation, irritability, aggressiveness, delusion, rage, nightmares, hallucinations, psychoses, and inappropriate behaviour have been occasionally reported during benzodiazepines use. Such reactions may be more likely to occur in children and the elderly. Should these occur, use of the drug should be discontinued.

Although hypotension has occurred only rarely, benzodiazepines should be administered with caution to patients in whom a drop in blood pressure might lead to cardiovascular or cerebrovascular complications. This is particularly important in elderly patients.

*Interactions:* The benzodiazepines, including Temazepam Oral Solution B.P., produces additive CNS depressant effects when co-administered with other medications which themselves produce CNS depression e.g., alcohol, barbiturates, antipsychotics, sedative/hypnotics, anxiolytics, antidepressants, narcotic analgesics, sedative antihistamines, anticonvulsants, and anaesthetics.

In animal studies, an increased perinatal mortality has been seen following concomitant administration of temazepam and diphenhydramine to rabbits in the later stages of gestation compared with rabbits that received either drug alone. In humans, one case of stillbirth at term has been reported, occurring 8 hours after a pregnant patient received temazepam and diphenhydramine. Although a causal relationship has not been established it is recommended that the use of temazepam be avoided in pregnant women receiving antihistamines.

*Side effects:* Adverse reactions, when they occur, are usually observed at the beginning of therapy and generally decrease in severity or disappear with continued use or upon decreasing the dose.

Most frequently reported adverse reactions associated with benzodiazepines include daytime drowsiness, dizziness, muscle weakness, and ataxia.

Less frequently reported adverse reactions include the following: confusion, depression, fatigue, headache, reduced alertness, numbed emotions, nausea, appetite change, sleep disturbance, dermatological reactions, visual disturbances, change of libido, and gastrointestinal symptoms.

Rarely reported adverse reactions include blood dyscrasia, abnormal liver function tests, transient anterograde amnesia or memory impairment, paradoxical reactions, and hypotension (see Precautions).

*Overdosage:* In the management of overdosage with

any drug, it should be borne in mind that multiple agents may have been taken.

Overdosage of benzodiazepines is usually manifested by degrees of central nervous system depression ranging from drowsiness to coma. In mild cases, symptoms include drowsiness, mental confusion, and lethargy. In more serious cases, and especially when other CNS-depressant drugs or alcohol are ingested, symptoms may include ataxia, hypotension, hypotonia, respiratory depression, coma, and very rarely, death.

If ingestion was recent, induced vomiting and/or gastric lavage should be undertaken, followed by general supportive care, monitoring of vital signs and close observation of the patient. If there is no advantage in emptying the stomach, activated charcoal may be effective in reducing absorption. Hypotension, though unlikely, may be controlled with noradrenaline. Temazepam is poorly dialysable.

The benzodiazepine antagonist, flumazenil may be useful in hospitalised patients for the management of benzodiazepine overdosage. Flumazenil product information should be consulted prior to use.

**Pharmaceutical precautions** Store below 25°C. Protect from light. Dispense Temazepam Oral Solution B.P. in amber glass bottles.

**Legal category** CD(Sch 3), POM

**Package quantities** Bottles 300 ml.

**Further information** Temazepam is well absorbed and rapidly excreted. Peak plasma levels are usually reached in 20 to 50 minutes. Temazepam has a plasma half life of about ten hours (range 5–15 hours). It is largely metabolised by a simple one-step process to a pharmacologically inert glucuronide. There are no major active metabolites and little risk of accumulation. Clinical studies have shown minimised effects on REM sleep patterns and on psychomotor performance on the day after treatment with Temazepam Oral Solution B.P.

**Product licence number** 0011/0087

## TEMAZEPAM TABLETS

**Presentation** Temazepam tablets are white flat and bevel edged containing 10 mg or 20 mg temazepam. The 10 mg tablets are imprinted WYETH on one side, WY breakbar and 040 on the other. The 20 mg tablets are imprinted WYETH on one side, and WY breakbar and 041 on the other.

**Uses** Temazepam is indicated for the short-term treatment (up to 4 weeks including any tapering off) of insomnia, when it is disabling or subjecting the individual to extreme distress, and for premedication before minor surgery or other procedures, especially when hospital admission is not essential.

**Dosage and administration**

*Route of administration:* Oral

*Insomnia:* Dosage and duration of therapy should be individualised. The lowest effective dose should be prescribed for the shortest time possible. Generally, the duration of treatment varies from a few days to 4 weeks including the tapering off process. Extension of the treatment period should not take place without re-evaluation of the need for continued therapy.

Since insomnia is often transient and intermittent, the prolonged administration of temazepam is generally unnecessary and is not recommended.

Treatment in all patients should be withdrawn gradually to minimise possible withdrawal symptoms. (See *Precautions and warnings*.)

*Dosage*
*Adults:* 10–20 mg, but in severe or persistent insomnia, it may be increased up to 40 mg. The tablets should be taken up to 30 minutes before going to bed.

*Elderly:* 10 mg. If this dose is not effective, it may be cautiously increased to 20 mg.

*Children:* The safety and efficacy of Temazepam in children less than 18 years of age has not been established and such use is not recommended.

*Premedication:*
*Adults:* 20–40 mg taken 30–60 minutes prior to surgery or other procedures.

*Elderly:* Elderly patients are likely to respond to smaller doses, possibly half the normal adult dose.

*Children:* The safety and efficacy of Temazepam in children less than 18 years of age has not been established and such use is not recommended.

Patients should be accompanied home when Temazepam has been used as a premedicant prior to surgery or other procedures on a day attendance basis.

**Contra-indications, warnings, etc**
*Contra-indications:*
  Severe respiratory insufficiency
  Sleep apnoea syndrome
  Hypersensitivity to benzodiazepines including Temazepam tablets or its components.
  Myasthenia gravis
  Severe hepatic failure
  Temazepam should not be given to children

*Use in pregnancy and lactation:* Benzodiazepines should not be used during pregnancy, especially during the first and last trimesters. Benzodiazepines may cause foetal damage when administered to pregnant women.

If the drug is prescribed to a woman of childbearing potential, she should be warned to contact her physician about stopping the drug if she intends to become, or suspects that she is, pregnant.

Infants of mothers who ingested benzodiazepines for several weeks or more preceding delivery have been reported to have withdrawal symptoms during the postnatal period. Symptoms such as hypoactivity, hypotonia, hypothermia, respiratory depression, apnoea, feeding problems, and impaired metabolic response to cold stress have been reported in neonates born of mothers who have received benzodiazepines during the late phase of pregnancy or at delivery.

It is recommended that the use of temazepam be avoided in pregnant women receiving antihistamines (See Interactions).

Because it is not known whether Temazepam is excreted in human milk, it should not be given to breast-feeding women.

*Precautions and warnings:* As with all patients on CNS-depressant drugs, patients should be warned not to operate dangerous machinery or motor vehicles until it is known that they do not become drowsy or dizzy from Temazepam. Patients should be advised that since their tolerance for alcohol and other CNS depressants will be diminished in the presence of Temazepam, these substances should either be avoided or taken in reduced dosage.

Temazepam is not intended for the primary treatment of psychotic illness or depressive disorders, and should not be used alone to treat depressed patients with associated insomnia. The use of benzodiazepines may have a disinhibiting effect and may release suicidal tendencies in depressed patients. Therefore, large quantities of Temazepam tablets should not be prescribed to these patients.

Pre-existing depression may emerge during benzodiazepine use.

The use of benzodiazepines may lead to physical and psychological dependence. The risk of dependence on Temazepam is low when used at the recommended dose and duration, but increases with higher doses and longer term use. The risk of dependence is further increased in patients with a history of alcoholism or drug abuse or in patients with significant personality disorders. Therefore, use in individuals with a history of alcoholism or drug abuse should be avoided.

Dependence may lead to withdrawal symptoms, especially if treatment is discontinued abruptly. Therefore, the drug should always be discontinued gradually.

Symptoms reported following discontinuation of benzodiazepines include headaches, muscle pain, anxiety, tension, depression, insomnia, restlessness, confusion, irritability, sweating, and the occurrence of 'rebound' phenomena whereby the symptoms that led to treatment with benzodiazepines recur in an enhanced form. These symptoms may be difficult to distinguish from the original symptoms for which the drug was prescribed.

In severe cases the following symptoms may occur: derealisation; depersonalisation; hyperacusis; tinnitus; numbness and tingling of the extremities; hypersensitivity to light, noise, and physical contact; involuntary movements; vomiting; hallucinations; convulsions. Convulsions may be more common in patients with pre-existing seizure disorders or who are taking other drugs that lower the convulsive threshold such as antidepressants.

It may be useful to inform the patient that treatment will be of limited duration and that it will be discontinued gradually. The patient should also be made aware of the possibility of 'rebound' phenomena to minimise anxiety should they occur.

Abuse has been reported in poly-drug users.

Some loss of efficacy to the hypnotic effects of short-acting benzodiazepines may develop after repeated use for a few weeks.

Insomnia may be a symptom of several other disorders. The possibility should be considered that the complaint may be related to an underlying physical or psychiatric disorder for which there is more specific treatment.

Caution should be used in the treatment of patients with acute narrow-angle glaucoma.

Patients with impaired renal or hepatic function should be monitored frequently and have their dosage adjusted carefully according to patient response. Lower doses may be sufficient in these patients. The same precautions apply to elderly or debilitated patients and patients with chronic respiratory insufficiency.

As with all CNS-depressants, the use of benzodiazepines may precipitate encephalopathy in patients with severe hepatic insufficiency. Therefore, use in these patients is contraindicated.

Some patients taking benzodiazepines have developed a blood dyscrasia, and some have had elevations in liver enzymes. Periodic haematologic and liver-function assessments are recommended when long-term therapy is clinically necessary.

Transient anterograde amnesia or memory impairment has been reported in association with the use of benzodiazepines. This condition usually occurs several hours after ingestion. Therefore, patients should ensure that they will be able to have a period of uninterrupted sleep which is sufficient to allow dissipation of drug effect (e.g., 7–8 hours).

Paradoxical reactions such as restlessness, agitation, irritability, aggressiveness, delusion, rage, nightmares, hallucinations, psychoses, and inappropriate behaviour have been occasionally reported during benzodiazepines use. Such reactions may be more likely to occur in children and the elderly. Should these occur, use of the drug should be discontinued.

Although hypotension has occurred only rarely, benzodiazepines should be administered with caution to patients in whom a drop in blood pressure might lead to cardiovascular or cerebrovascular complications. This is particularly important in elderly patients.

*Interactions:* The benzodiazepines, including Temazepam, produce additive CNS depressant effects when co-administered with other medications which themselves produce CNS depression e.g., alcohol, barbiturates, antipsychotics, sedative/hypnotics, anxiolytics, antidepressants, narcotic analgesics, sedative antihistamines, anticonvulsants, and anaesthetics.

In animal studies, an increased perinatal mortality has been seen following concomitant administration of temazepam and diphenhydramine to rabbits in the later stages of gestation compared with rabbits that received either drug alone. In humans, one case of stillbirth at term has been reported, occurring 8 hours after a pregnant patient received temazepam and diphenhydramine. Although a causal relationship has not been established it is recommended that the use of temazepam be avoided in pregnant women receiving antihistamines.

*Side effects:* Adverse reactions, when they occur, are usually observed at the beginning of therapy and generally decrease in severity or disappear with continued use or upon decreasing the dose.

Most frequently reported adverse reactions associated with benzodiazepines include daytime drowsiness, dizziness, muscle weakness, and ataxia.

Less frequently reported adverse reactions include the following: confusion, depression, fatigue, headache, reduced alertness, numbed emotions, nausea, appetite change, sleep disturbance, dermatological reactions, visual disturbances, change of libido, and gastrointestinal symptoms.

Rarely reported adverse reactions include blood dyscrasia, abnormal liver function tests, transient anterograde amnesia or memory impairment, paradoxical reactions, and hypotension (see *Precautions and Warnings*).

*Overdose:* In the management of overdosage with any drug, it should be borne in mind that multiple agents may have been taken.

Overdosage of benzodiazepines is usually manifested by degrees of central nervous system depression ranging from drowsiness to coma. In mild cases, symptoms include drowsiness, mental confusion, and lethargy. In more serious cases, and especially when other CNS-depressant drugs or alcohol are ingested, symptoms may include ataxia, hypotension, hypotonia, respiratory depression, coma, and very rarely, death.

If ingestion was recent, induced vomiting and/or gastric lavage should be undertaken, followed by general supportive care, monitoring of vital signs and close observation of the patient. If there is no advantage in emptying the stomach, activated charcoal may be effective in reducing absorption. Hypotension, though unlikely, may be controlled with noradrenaline. Temazepam is poorly dialysable.

The benzodiazepine antagonist, flumazenil may be useful in hospitalised patients for the management of benzodiazepine overdosage. Flumazenil product information should be consulted prior to use.

**Pharmaceutical precautions** Store in a dry place below 25°C.

**Legal category** CD(Sch 3), POM

**Package quantities:** 10 mg Bottles of 50 and securitainers of 500. 20 mg Securitainers of 250.

**Further information** Temazepam is well absorbed and rapidly excreted. Peak plasma levels are usually reached in 20 to 50 minutes. Temazepam has a plasma half life of about ten hours (range 5-15 hours). It is largely metabolised by a simple one-step process to a pharmacologically inert glucuronide. There are no major active metabolites and little risk of accumulation. Clinical studies have shown minimal effects on REM sleep patterns and on psychomotor performance on the day after treatment with Temazepam.

**Product licence numbers**

| | |
|---|---|
| 10 mg Tablets | 0011/0179 |
| 20 mg Tablets | 0011/0180 |

*Trade Mark

# Glaxo Wellcome
Stockley Park West
Middlesex UB11 1BT

*GlaxoWellcome*

## ALKERAN* TABLETS AND INJECTION

**Presentation** *Alkeran Tablets:* White, round, biconvex, compression-coated tablets impressed WELLCOME and A2A, each containing 2 mg Melphalan BP.

White, round, biconvex, compression-coated tablets impressed WELLCOME and B2A, each containing 5 mg Melphalan BP.

*Alkeran Injection:* Alkeran Injection is supplied as a unit pack comprising a vial containing a freeze-dried powder and a vial of solvent-diluent. Each Alkeran vial contains the equivalent of 50 mg of melphalan, in the form of the hydrochloride, as a sterile, white to off-white, freeze-dried powder which includes 20 mg povidone K12. Each vial of solvent-diluent provides 10 ml of buffer solution containing 60% v/v propylene glycol with sodium citrate and ethanol.

**Uses** *Alkeran Tablets* are indicated in the treatment of multiple myeloma and advanced ovarian adenocarcinoma.

*Alkeran Tablets* may be used in the treatment of:
*breast carcinoma:* Alkeran either alone or in combination with other drugs has a significant therapeutic effect in a proportion of patients suffering from advanced breast carcinoma; Alkeran has also been used as an adjuvant to surgery in the management of breast carcinoma.

*polycythaemia rubra vera:* Alkeran is effective in the treatment of a proportion of patients suffering from polycythaemia vera.

*Alkeran Injection,* administered by regional arterial perfusion, is indicated in the treatment of localised malignant melanoma of the extremities and localised soft tissue sarcoma of the extremities.

*Alkeran Injection,* at conventional intravenous dosage, may be used in the treatment of:
*multiple myeloma:* Alkeran Injection, either alone or in combination with other cytotoxic drugs, is as effective as the oral formulation in the treatment of multiple myeloma;
*ovarian cancer:* Alkeran Injection produces an objective response in approximately 50% of the patients with advanced ovarian adenocarcinoma, when given alone, or in combination with other cytotoxic drugs.

Alkeran Injection, at high intravenous dosage, may be used in the treatment of:
*multiple myeloma:* complete remissions have been achieved in up to 50% of patients given high dose Alkeran Injection, with or without autologous bone marrow rescue, either as first line treatment or to consolidate a response to conventional cytoreductive chemotherapy;
*neuroblastoma in childhood:* high dose Alkeran Injection with autologous bone marrow rescue has been used either alone, or combined with radiotherapy and/or other cytotoxic drugs, to consolidate a response to conventional treatment. A significant increase in the duration of disease-free survival was demonstrated in a prospective randomised trial of high dose Alkeran Injection versus no further treatment.

*Mode of action:* Melphalan is a bifunctional alkylating agent. Formation of carbonium intermediates from each of the two bis-2-chloroethyl groups enables alkylation through covalent binding with the 7-nitrogen of guanine on DNA, cross-linking the two DNA strands and thereby preventing cell replication.

*Pharmacokinetics:* The absorption of melphalan was found to be highly variable in 13 patients given 0.6 mg/kg orally, with respect to both the time to first appearance of the drug in plasma (range 0 to 336 minutes) and peak plasma concentration (range 70 to 630 ng/ml). In 5 of the patients who were given an equivalent intravenous dose, the mean bioavailability of melphalan was found to be 56 ± 27%. The terminal plasma half-life was 90 ± 57 minutes with 11% of the drug being recovered in the urine over 24 hours.

The administration of Alkeran Tablets immediately after food delayed the time to achieving peak plasma concentrations and reduced the area under the plasma concentration-time curves by between 39 and 45%.

The pharmacokinetics of intravenous Alkeran given at both conventional and high doses are best described by a bi-exponential, 2-compartment model. In 8 patients given a single bolus dose of 0.5 to 0.6 mg/

kg, the composite initial and terminal half-lives were reported to be 7.7±3.3 minutes and 108±20.8 minutes respectively. Following injection of melphalan, monohydroxymelphalan and dihydroxymelphalan were detected in the patients' plasma, reaching peak levels at approximately 60 minutes and 105 minutes respectively. A similar half-life of 126 ± 6 minutes was seen when melphalan was added to the patients' serum *in vitro* (37°C), suggesting that spontaneous degradation rather than enzymic metabolism may be the major determinant of the drug's half-life in man.

Following administration of a 2 minute infusion of doses ranging from 5 to 23 mg/m² (approximately 0.1 to 0.6 mg/kg) to 10 patients with ovarian cancer or multiple myeloma, the pooled initial and terminal half lives were, respectively, 8.1 ± 6.6 minutes and 76.9 ± 40.7 minutes. In this study, the mean volumes of distribution at steady state and central compartment were 29.1± 13.6 litres and 12.2± 6.5 litres, respectively, and a mean clearance of 342.7 ± 96.8 ml/minute was recorded.

In 15 children and 11 adults given high-dose intravenous Alkeran (140 mg/m²) with forced diuresis, the mean initial and terminal half-lives were found to be 6.5 ± 3.6 minutes and 41.4 ± 16.5 minutes respectively. Mean initial and terminal half-lives of 8.8 ± 6.6 minutes and 73.1 ± 45.9 minutes, respectively, were recorded in 28 patients with various malignancies who were given doses of between 70 and 200 mg/m² as a 2 to 20 minute infusion. The mean volumes of distribution at steady state and central compartment were, respectively, 40.2 ± 18.3 litres and 18.2 ± 11.7 litres, and the mean clearance was 564.6 ± 159.1 ml/minute.

Following hyperthermic (39°C) perfusion of the lower limb with 1.75 mg/kg bodyweight, mean initial and terminal half-lives of 3.6 ± 1.5 minutes and 46.5 ± 17.2 minutes, respectively, were recorded in 11 patients with advanced malignant melanoma. Mean volumes of distribution at steady state and central compartment were, respectively, 2.87 ± 0.8 litres and 1.01 ± 0.28 litres, and a mean clearance of 55.0 ± 9.4 ml/minute was recorded.

**Dosage and administration** Alkeran is a cytotoxic drug which falls into the general class of alkylating agents. It should be prescribed only by physicians experienced in the management of malignant disease with such agents.

Since Alkeran is myelosuppressive, frequent blood counts are essential during therapy and the dosage should be delayed or adjusted if necessary (see *Precautions*).

The absorption of Alkeran after oral administration is variable. Dosage may need to be cautiously increased until myelosuppression is seen, in order to ensure that potentially therapeutic levels have been reached.

*Multiple myeloma: Oral administration:* A typical oral dosage schedule is 0.15 mg/kg bodyweight/day in divided doses for 4 days, repeated at intervals of six weeks. Numerous regimens have, however, been used and the scientific literature should be consulted for details. The administration of oral Alkeran and prednisone maybe more effective than Alkeran alone. The combination is usually given on an intermittent basis. Prolonging treatment beyond one year in responders does not appear to improve results.

*Intravenous administration:* Alkeran Injection has been used on an intermittent basis alone, or in combination with other cytotoxic drugs, at doses varying between 8 mg/m² body surface area and 30 mg/m² body surface area, given at intervals of between 2 to 6 weeks. Additionally, administration of prednisone has been included in a number of regimens. The literature should be consulted for precise details on treatment protocols.

When used as a single agent, a typical intravenous dosage schedule is 0.4 mg/kg bodyweight (16 mg/m² body surface area) repeated at appropriate intervals (e.g. once every 4 weeks), provided there has been recovery of the peripheral blood count during this period.

High-dose regimens generally employ single intravenous doses of between 100 and 200 mg/m² body surface area (approximately 2.5 to 5.0 mg/kg bodyweight), but autologous bone marrow rescue becomes essential following doses in excess of 140 mg/m² body surface area. In cases of renal impairment, the dose should be reduced by 50%

(see *Dosage in renal impairment*). In view of the severe myelosuppression induced by high dose Alkeran Injection, treatment should be confined to specialist centres, with the appropriate facilities, and only be administered by experienced clinicians (see *Precautions*).

*Ovarian adenocarcinoma: Oral administration:* A typical regimen is 0.2 mg/kg bodyweight/day orally for 5 days. This is repeated every 4 to 8 weeks, or as soon as the peripheral blood count has recovered.

*Intravenous administration:* When used intravenously as a single agent, a dose of 1 mg/kg bodyweight (approximately 40 mg/m² body surface area) given at intervals of 4 weeks has often been used.

When combined with other cytotoxic drugs, intravenous doses of between 0.3 and 0.4 mg/kg bodyweight (12 to 16 mg/m² body surface area) have been used at intervals of 4 to 6 weeks.

*Carcinoma of the breast:* Alkeran has been given orally at a dose of 0.15 mg/kg bodyweight or 6 mg/m² body surface area/day for 5 days and repeated every 6 weeks. The dose was decreased if bone marrow toxicity was observed.

*Malignant melanoma:* Hyperthermic regional perfusion with Alkeran has been used as an adjuvant to surgery for early malignant melanoma and as palliative treatment for advanced but localised disease. The scientific literature should be consulted for details of perfusion technique and dosage used. A typical dose range for upper extremity perfusions is 0.6 to 1.0 mg/kg bodyweight and for lower extremity perfusions is 0.8 to 1.5 mg/kg bodyweight.

*Soft tissue sarcoma:* Hyperthermic regional perfusion with Alkeran has been used in the management of all stages of localised soft tissue sarcoma, usually in combination with surgery. Alkeran has also been given with actinomycin D and the scientific literature should be consulted for details of dosage regimens. A typical dose range for upper extremity perfusions is 0.6 to 1.0 mg/kg bodyweight and for lower extremity perfusions is 1 to 1.4 mg/kg bodyweight.

*Polycythaemia rubra vera:* For remission, induction doses of 6 to 10 mg daily for 5 to 7 days have been used, after which 2 to 4 mg daily were given until satisfactory disease control was achieved.

A dose of 2 to 6 mg once per week has been used for maintenance therapy.

In view of the possibility of severe myelosuppression if Alkeran is given on a continuous basis, it is essential that frequent blood counts are taken throughout therapy, with dosage adjustment or breaks in treatment, as appropriate, to maintain careful haematological control.

*Advanced neuroblastoma:* Doses of between 100 and 240 mg/m² body surface area (sometimes divided equally over 3 consecutive days) together with autologous bone marrow rescue, have been used either alone or in combination with radiotherapy and/or other cytotoxic drugs.

*Preparation of Alkeran Injection Solution:* Alkeran Injection should be prepared, AT ROOM TEMPERATURE, by reconstituting the freeze-dried powder with the Solvent-Diluent provided. 10 ml of this vehicle should be added, as a single quantity, and the vial immediately shaken VIGOROUSLY until solution is complete. The resulting solution contains the equivalent of 5 mg per ml anhydrous melphalan and has a pH of approximately 6.5.

Alkeran Injection solution has limited stability and should be prepared immediately before use. Any unused solution should be discarded (see Pharmaceutical precautions).

The reconstituted solution should not be refrigerated as this will cause precipitation.

*Parenteral administration:* Except in cases where regional arterial perfusion is indicated, Alkeran Injection is for intravenous use only.

For intravenous administration it is recommended that Alkeran Injection solution is injected slowly into a fast-running infusion solution via a swabbed injection port.

If direct injection into a fast-running infusion is not appropriate, Alkeran Injection solution may be administered diluted in an infusion bag.

Alkeran is not compatible with infusion solutions containing dextrose, and it is recommended that

ONLY Sodium Chloride Intravenous Infusion 0.9% w/v is used.

When further diluted in an infusion solution, Alkeran Injection has reduced stability and the rate of degradation increases rapidly with rise in temperature. If administration occurs at a room temperature of approximately 25°C, the total time from preparation of the Injection solution to the completion of infusion should not exceed 1.5 hours.

Should any visible turbidity or crystallisation appear in the reconstituted or diluted solutions the preparation must be discarded.

Care should be taken to avoid possible extravasation of Alkeran and in cases of poor peripheral venous access, consideration should be given to use of a central venous line.

If high dose Alkeran Injection is administered with or without autologous bone marrow transplantation, administration *via* a central venous line is recommended.

For regional arterial perfusion, the literature should be consulted for detailed methodology.

*Use in children:* Alkeran, at conventional dosage, is only rarely indicated in children and dosage guidelines cannot be stated.

High dose Alkeran Injection, in association with bone marrow rescue, has been used in childhood neuroblastoma and dosage guidelines based on body surface area, as for adults, may be used.

*Use in the elderly:* Although Alkeran is frequently used at conventional dosage in the elderly, there is no specific information available relating to its administration to this patient sub-group.

Experience in the use of high dose Alkeran in elderly patients is limited. Consideration should therefore be given to ensure adequate performance status and organ function before using high dose Alkeran Injection in elderly patients.

*Dosage in renal impairment:* Alkeran clearance, though variable, is decreased in renal impairment.

Currently available pharmacokinetic data do not justify an absolute recommendation on dosage reduction when administering Alkeran Tablets to patients with renal impairment, but it may be prudent to use a reduced dosage initially until tolerance is established.

When Alkeran Injection is used at conventional intravenous dosage (8 to 40 mg/m² body surface area), it is recommended that the initial dose should be reduced by 50% in patients with moderate to severe renal impairment and subsequent dosage determined according to the degree of haematological suppression.

For high intravenous doses of Alkeran (100 to 240 mg/m² body surface area), the need for dose reduction depends upon the degree of renal impairment, whether autologous bone marrow stem cells are reinfused, and therapeutic need. As a guide, for moderate to severe renal impairment (EDTA clearance 30 to 50 ml/min) a dose reduction of 50% is usual. Adequate hydration and forced diuresis are also necessary. High dose Alkeran is not recommended in patients with more severe renal impairment (EDTA clearance less then 30 ml/min).

### Contra-indications, warnings, etc
*Contra-indications:* Alkeran should not be given to patients who have suffered a previous hypersensitivity reaction to melphalan.

*Precautions:* ALKERAN IS AN ACTIVE CYTOTOXIC AGENT FOR USE UNDER THE DIRECTION OF PHYSICIANS EXPERIENCED IN THE ADMINISTRATION OF SUCH AGENTS.

Alkeran Injection solution may cause local tissue damage should extravasation occur, and consequently it should not be administered by direct injection into a peripheral vein. It is recommended that Alkeran Injection solution is administered by injecting slowly into a fast-running intravenous infusion *via* a swabbed injection port, or *via* a central venous line.

In view of the hazards involved and the level of supportive care required, the administration of high dose Alkeran Injection should be confined to specialist centres, with the appropriate facilities, and only be conducted by experienced clinicians.

In patients receiving high dose Alkeran Injection, consideration should be given to the prophylactic administration of anti-infective agents, the administration of blood products as required, and the maintenance of a high renal output during the period immediately following the administration of Alkeran by the use of hydration and forced diuresis.

Consideration should be given to ensure adequate performance status and organ function before using high dose Alkeran Injection.

*Safe handling of Alkeran:* The handling of Alkeran formulations should follow guidelines for the handling of cytotoxic drugs according to the Royal Pharmaceutical Society of Great Britain Working Party on the Handling of Cytotoxic Drugs.

Provided the outer coating of the tablet is intact, there is no risk in handling Alkeran Tablets.

Alkeran Tablets should not be divided.

*Monitoring:* Since Alkeran is a potent myelosuppressive agent, it is essential that careful attention should be paid to the monitoring of blood counts to avoid the possibility of excessive myelosuppression and the risk of irreversible bone marrow aplasia. Blood counts may continue to fall after treatment is stopped, so at the first sign of an abnormally large fall in leukocyte or platelet counts treatment should be temporarily interrupted. Alkeran should be used with caution in patients who have undergone recent radiotherapy or chemotherapy in view of increased bone marrow toxicity.

*Renal impairment:* Alkeran clearance may be reduced in patients with renal impairment, who may also have uraemic bone marrow suppression. Dose reduction may therefore be necessary (see **Dosage and administration**), and these patients should be closely observed.

Temporary significant elevation of the blood urea has been seen in the early stages of melphalan therapy in myeloma patients with renal damage.

*Mutagenicity:* Melphalan is mutagenic in animals and chromosome aberrations have been observed in patients being treated with the drug.

*Carcinogenicity:* Melphalan, in common with other alkylating agents, may be leukaemogenic in man. There have been reports of acute leukaemia occurring after prolonged melphalan treatment for diseases such as amyloid, malignant melanoma, multiple myeloma, macroglobulinaemia, cold agglutinin syndrome and ovarian cancer.

A comparison of patients with ovarian cancer who received alkylating agents with those who did not showed that the use of alkylating agents, including melphalan, significantly increased the incidence of acute leukaemia.

The leukaemogenic risk must be balanced against the potential therapeutic benefit when considering the use of melphalan.

*Effects on fertility:* Alkeran causes suppression of ovarian function in pre-menopausal women resulting in amenorrhoea in a significant number of patients.

There is evidence from some animal studies that Alkeran can have an adverse effect on spermatogenesis. Therefore, it is possible that Alkeran may cause temporary or permanent sterility in male patients.

*Use in pregnancy and lactation:* The teratogenic potential of Alkeran has not been studied. In view of its mutagenic properties and structural similarity to known teratogenic compounds, it is possible that melphalan could cause congenital defects in the offspring of patients treated with the drug.

As with all cytotoxic chemotherapy, adequate contraceptive precautions should be practised when either partner is receiving Alkeran.

The use of melphalan should be avoided whenever possible during pregnancy, particularly during the first trimester. In any individual case the potential hazard to the fetus must be balanced against the expected benefit to the mother.

Mothers receiving Alkeran should not breast feed.

*Side- and adverse effects:* The most common side-effect is bone marrow depression, leading to leucopenia and thrombocytopenia.

Gastro-intestinal effects such as nausea and vomiting have been reported in up to 30% of patients receiving conventional oral doses of Alkeran.

Stomatitis occurs rarely following conventional doses of Alkeran.

The incidence of diarrhoea, vomiting and stomatitis becomes the dose limiting toxicity in patients given high intravenous doses of Alkeran in association with autologous bone marrow transplantation. Cyclophosphamide pre-treatment appears to reduce the severity of gastro-intestinal damage induced by high dose Alkeran and the literature should be consulted for details.

Allergic reactions to Alkeran such as urticaria, oedema, skin rashes and anaphylactic shock have been reported uncommonly following initial or subsequent dosing, particularly after intravenous administration. Cardiac arrest has also been reported rarely in association with such events.

Maculopapular rashes and pruritus have occasionally been noted.

There have also been case reports of fatal pulmonary fibrosis and haemolytic anaemia occurring after melphalan treatment.

Alopecia has been reported but is uncommon at conventional doses.

A subjective and transient sensation of warmth and/or tingling was described in approximately two thirds of patients with haematological malignancies who were given high dose Alkeran Injection *via* a central line.

*Drug interactions:* Nalidixic acid together with high-dose intravenous melphalan has caused deaths in children due to haemorrhagic enterocolitis.

Impaired renal function has been described in bone marrow transplant patients who were conditioned with high dose intravenous melphalan and who subsequently received cyclosporin to prevent graft-versus-host disease.

*Toxicity and treatment of overdosage:* Gastro-intestinal effects, including nausea, vomiting and diarrhoea are the most likely signs of acute oral overdosage. The immediate effects of acute intravenous overdosage are nausea and vomiting. Damage to the gastro-intestinal mucosa may also ensue, and diarrhoea, sometimes haemorrhagic, has been reported after overdosage. The principal toxic effect is bone marrow suppression, leading to leucopenia, thrombocytopenia and anaemia.

General supportive measures, together with appropriate blood and platelet transfusions, should be instituted if necessary and consideration given to hospitalisation, antibiotic cover, and the use of haematological growth factors.

There is no specific antidote. The blood picture should be closely monitored for at least four weeks following overdosage until there is evidence of recovery.

### Pharmaceutical precautions
*Alkeran Tablets:* Store at 2 to 8°C. Keep dry.
*Injection unit pack:* Store below 30°C. Protect from light.

Alkeran Tablets and Injection surplus to requirements should be destroyed in a manner appropriate to the prevailing local regulatory requirements for the disposal of cytotoxic drugs.

### Legal category POM

### Package quantities
| | |
|---|---|
| Alkeran Tablets 2 mg: | Bottle of 25 |
| Alkeran Tablets 5 mg: | Bottle of 25 |
| Alkeran Injection unit pack: | Vial of Alkeran freeze-dried powder and vial of solvent-diluent. |

### Further information Nil.

### Product licence numbers
| | |
|---|---|
| Alkeran Tablets 2 mg: | 0003/5008R |
| Alkeran Tablets 5 mg: | 0003/5009R |
| Alkeran Injection: | 0003/0323 |
| Alkeran Solvent-Diluent: | 0003/0324 |

## ANECTINE* INJECTION

**Qualitative and quantitative composition** Suxamethonium Chloride Injection BP 100 mg in 2 ml.

### Pharmaceutical form
Injection.

### Clinical particulars
*Therapeutic indications:* Used in anaesthesia as a muscle relaxant to facilitate endotracheal intubation, mechanical ventilation and a wide range of surgical and obstetric procedures.

It is also used to reduce the intensity of muscular contractions associated with pharmacologically or electrically-induced convulsions.

*Posology and method of administration:* Usually by bolus intravenous injection.

*Adults:* The dose is dependent on body weight, the degree of muscular relaxation required, the route of administration, and the response of individual patients.

To achieve endotracheal intubation Anectine is usually administered intravenously in a dose of 1 mg/kg. This dose will usually produce muscular relaxation in about 30 to 60 seconds and has a duration of action of about 2 to 6 minutes. Larger doses will produce more prolonged muscular relaxation, but doubling the dose does not necessarily double the duration of relaxation. Supplementary doses of Anectine of 50% to 100% of the initial dose administered at 5 to 10 minute intervals will maintain muscle relaxation during short surgical procedures performed under general anaesthesia.

For prolonged surgical procedures Anectine may be given by intravenous infusion as a 0.1% to 0.2% solution, diluted in 5% glucose solution or sterile isotonic saline solution, at a rate of 2.5 to 4 mg per minute. The infusion rate should be adjusted according to the response of individual patients.

The total dose of Anectine given by repeated intravenous injection or continuous infusion should *not* exceed 500 mg per hour.

*Children:* Infants and young children are more resistant to Anectine compared with adults.

The recommended intravenous dose of Anectine

for neonates and infants is 2 mg/kg. A dose of 1 mg/kg in older children is recommended.

When Anectine is given as intravenous infusion in children, the dosage is as for adults with a proportionately lower initial infusion rate based on bodyweight.

Anectine may be given intramuscularly to infants at doses up to 4 to 5 mg/kg and in older children up to 4 mg/kg. These doses produce muscular relaxation within about 3 minutes. A total dose of 150 mg should ***not*** be exceeded.

*Use in the elderly:* Dosage requirements of Anectine in the elderly are comparable to those for younger adults.

The elderly may be more susceptible to cardiac arrhythmias, especially if digitalis-like drugs are also being taken. See also *Special warnings and precautions for use.*

*Contra-indications:* Anectine has no effect on the level of consciousness and should not be administered to a patient who is not fully anaesthetised.

Hypersensitivity to suxamethonium may exist in rare instances, and Anectine should not be administered to patients known to be hypersensitive to the drug.

As suxamethonium can act as a trigger of sustained myofibrillar contraction in susceptible individuals, Anectine is contra-indicated in patients with a personal or family history of malignant hyperthermia. If this condition occurs unexpectedly, all anaesthetic agents known to be associated with its development (including Anectine) must be immediately discontinued, and full supportive measures must be immediately instituted. Intravenous dantrolene sodium is the primary specific therapeutic drug and is recommended as soon as possible after the diagnosis is made.

Anectine is contra-indicated in patients known to have an inherited atypical plasma cholinesterase activity.

An acute transient rise in serum potassium often occurs following the administration of Anectine in normal individuals; the magnitude of this rise is of the order of 0.5 mmol/litre. In certain pathological states or conditions this increase in serum potassium following Anectine administration may be excessive and cause serious cardiac arrhythmias and cardiac arrest. For this reason the use of Anectine is contra-indicated in:

- Patients recovering from major trauma, the potential for potassium release is not seen immediately but begins 5 to 15 days after injury. It persists for 2 to 3 months or longer if there is associated sepsis.
- Patients recovering from severe burns; the potential for potassium release is not seen immediately but during the period from about the 10th to 66th day post-burn or longer if there is associated sepsis.
- Patients with neurological deficits involving acute major muscle wasting (upper and/or lower motor neurone lesions); the potential for potassium release occurs within the first 6 months after the acute onset of the neurological deficit and correlates with the degree and extent of muscle paralysis. Patients who have been immobilised for prolonged periods of time may be at similar risk.
- Patients with pre-existing hyperkalaemia. In the absence of hyperkalaemia and neuropathy, renal failure is not a contra-indication to the administration of a normal single dose of Anectine Injection, but multiple or large doses may cause clinically significant rises in serum potassium and should not be used.

Suxamethonium causes a slight transient rise in intra-ocular pressure, and should therefore not be used in the presence of open eye injuries or where an increase in intra-ocular pressure is undesirable unless the potential benefit of its use outweighs the potential risk to the eye.

Anectine should be avoided in patients with congenital myotonic diseases such as myotonia congenita and dystrophia myotonica since its administration may on occasion be associated with severe myotonic spasms and rigidity.

Anectine should be avoided in patients with Duchenne muscular dystrophy since its administration may be associated with rigidity, hyperthermia, hyperkalaemia, myoglobinaemia, cardiac arrest, and post-operative respiratory depression.

*Special warnings and precautions for use:* Anectine should be administered only by or under close supervision of an anaesthetist familiar with its action, characteristics and hazards, who is skilled in the management of artificial respiration and only where there are adequate facilities for immediate endotracheal intubation with administration of oxygen by intermittent positive pressure ventilation.

Anectine should not be mixed in the same syringe with any other agent, espcially thiopentone.

During prolonged administration of Anectine, it is recommended that the patient is fully monitored with a peripheral nerve stimulator in order to avoid overdosage.

Anectine is rapidly hydrolysed by plasma cholinesterase which thereby limits the intensity and duration of the neuromuscular blockade.

Prolonged and intensified neuromuscular blockade following Anectine Injection may occur secondary to reduced plasma cholinesterase activity in the following states or pathological conditions: physiological variation as in pregnancy and the puerperium; genetically determined abnormal plasma cholinesterase; severe generalised tetanus, tuberculosis, other severe or chronic infections; following severe burns; chronic debilitating disease, malignancy, chronic anaemia and malnutrition; end-stage hepatic failure, acute or chronic renal failure; auto-immune diseases: myxoedema, collagen diseases; iatrogenic: following plasma exchange, plasmapheresis, cardiopulmonary bypass, and as a result of concomitant drug therapy (see *Interactions*).

If Anectine is given over a prolonged period, the characteristic depolarising neuromusclar (or Phase I) block may change to one with characteristics of a non-depolarising (or Phase II) block. Although the characteristics of a developing Phase II block resemble those of a true non-depolarising block, the former cannot always be fully or permanently reversed by anticholinesterase agents. When a Phase II block is fully established, its effects will then usually be fully reversible with standard doses of neostigmine accompanied by an anticholinergic agent.

Tachyphylaxis occurs after repeated administration of Anectine.

It is inadvisable to administer Anectine to patients with advanced myasthenia gravis. Although these patients are resistant to suxamethonium they develop a state of Phase II block which can result in delayed recovery. Patients with myasthenic Eaton-Lambert syndrome are more sensitive than normal to Anectine, necessitating dosage reduction.

In healthy adults, Anectine occasionally causes a mild transient slowing of the heart rate on initial administration. Bradycardias are more commonly observed in children and on repeated administration of suxamethonium in both children and adults. Pretreatment with intravenous atropine or glycopyrrolate significantly reduces the incidence and severity of suxamethonium-related bradycardia.

Anectine may induce cardiac arrhythmias. The effects of digitalis may be enhanced with increased ventricular irritability.

*Interaction with other medicaments and other forms of interaction:* Certain drugs or chemicals are known to reduce normal plasma cholinesterase activity and may therefore prolong the neuromuscular blocking effects of Anectine. These include: organophosphorous insecticides and metriphonate; ecothiopate eye drops; trimetaphan; specific anticholinesterase agents: neostigmine, pyridostigmine, physostigmine, edrophonium; cytotoxic compounds; cyclophosphamide, mechlorethamine, triethylene-melamine, and thiotepa; psychiatric drugs: phenelzine, promazine and chlorpromazine; anaesthetic agents and drugs: ketamine, morphine and morphine antagonists, pethidine, pancuronium, propanidid.

Other drugs with potentially deleterious effects on plasma cholinesterase activity include aprotinin, diphenhydramine, promethazine, oestrogens, oxytocin, high-dose steroids, and oral contraceptives.

Certain drugs or substances may enhance or prolong the neuromuscular effects of Anectine by mechanisms unrelated to plasma cholinesterase activity. These include: magnesium salts; lithium carbonate; azathioprine; quinine and chloroquinine; antibiotics such as the aminoglycosides, clindamycin and polymyxins; antiarrhythmic drugs: quinine, procainamide, verapamil, beta-blockers, lignocaine and procaine; volatile inhalational anaesthetic agents: halothane, enflurane, isoflurane, diethylether and methoxyflurane have little effect on the Phase I block of Anectine injection but will accelerate the onset and enhance the intensity of a Phase II suxamethonium-induced block.

*Pregnancy and lactation:* Although Anectine does not readily cross the placental barrier it should not be administered to pregnant women unless the potential benefit outweighs possible hazards.

Plasma cholinesterase levels fall during the first trimester of pregnancy to about 70 to 80% of their pre-pregnancy values; a further fall to about 60 to 70% of the pre-pregnancy levels occurs within 2 to 4 days after delivery. Plasma cholinesterase levels then increase to reach normal over the next 6 weeks. Consequently, a high proportion of pregnant and puerperal patients may exhibit mildly prolonged neuromuscular blockade following Anectine injection.

*Effect on ability to drive and use machines:* Not applicable.

*Undesirable effects:* Muscle pains are frequently experienced after administration of suxamethonium and most commonly occur in ambulatory patients undergoing short surgical procedures under general anaesthesia. There appears to be no direct connection between the degree of visible muscle fasciculation after Anectine administration and the incidence or severity of pain. The use of small doses of non-depolarising muscle relaxants given minutes before suxamethonium administration has been advocated for the reduction of incidence and severity of suxamethonium-associated muscle pains. This technique may require the use of doses of suxamethonium in excess of 1 mg/kg to achieve satisfactory conditions for endotracheal intubation.

The following adverse reactions have been reported after administration of Anectine:

Cardiovascular: bradycardia, tachycardia, hypertension, hypotension, arrhythmias;

Respiratory: bronchospasm, prolonged respiratory depression and apnoea;

Musculoskeletal: muscle fasciculation, post-operative muscle pains, myoglobinaemia, myoglobinuria;

Other: hyperthermia, increased intra-ocular pressure, increased intragastric pressure, rash, excessive salivation.

There are case reports of hyperkalaemia-related cardiac arrests following the administration of suxamethonium to patients with congenital cerebral palsy, tetanus, Duchenne muscular dystrophy, and closed head injury.

*Overdose:* Apnoea and prolonged muscle paralysis are the main serious effects of overdosage. It is essential, therefore, to maintain the airway and adequate ventilation until spontaneous respiration occurs.

The decision to use neostigmine to reverse a Phase II suxamethonium-induced block depends on the judgement of the clinician in the individual case. Valuable information in regard to this decision will be gained by monitoring neuromuscular function. If neostigmine is used its administration should be accompanied by appropriate doses of an anticholinergic agent such as atropine.

**Pharmacological properties**

*Pharmacodynamic properties:* Short-acting depolarising neuromuscular blocking agent.

*Pharmacokinetic properties:* None stated.

*Preclinical safety data:* None relevant to the prescriber additional to that already included in other sections.

**Pharmaceutical particulars**

*List of excipients:* Water for Injections BP.

*Incompatibilities:* None known.

*Shelf life:* 18 months.

*Special precautions for storage:* Store below 4°C. Do not freeze. Protect from light.

*Nature and contents of container:* Neutral glass. 2 ml ampoules.

*Instructions for use/handling:* For intravenous injection under medical direction.

**Marketing authorisation number** 0003/5203R

**Date of approval/revision of SPC** April 1996

**Legal category** POM.

## BETNOVATE* RECTAL OINTMENT

**Presentation** Betnovate Rectal Ointment is a white, translucent preparation containing 0.05% w/w betamethasone valerate, 0.1% w/w phenylephrine hydrochloride, and 2.5% lignocaine hydrochloride.

**Uses** The clinical effectiveness of Betnovate Rectal Ointment is attributable to the marked local anti-inflammatory property of the corticosteroid betamethasone valerate, the analgesic effect of lignocaine, and the vasoconstrictor effect of phenylephrine.

Betnovate Rectal Ointment is indicated for: relief of the symptoms of itching, irritation, discomfort or pain associated with local non-infective anal or peri-anal conditions such as external haemorrhoids.

**Dosage and administration** A course of treatment should be limited to seven days.

Apply a small amount of ointment two or three times a day initially, using the applicator if internal administration is required. When inflammation is subsiding, once-daily application is sufficient in most cases.

**Contra-indications, warnings, etc**

*Contra-indications:* Primary cutaneous viral infections (e.g. herpes simplex, chicken pox). Hypersensitivity to any component of the preparation.

The use of Betnovate Rectal Ointment is not indicated in the treatment of primarily infected skin lesions caused by infection with fungi (e.g. candidiasis, tinea); or bacteria (e.g. impetigo); dermatoses in children under 1 year of age, including dermatitis and napkin eruptions.

*Pregnancy:* There is inadequate evidence of safety in human pregnancy. Topical administration of cortico-steroids to pregnant animals can cause abnormalities of fetal development including cleft palate and intra-uterine growth retardation. There may therefore be a very small risk of such effects in the human fetus.

*Side-effects:* As with all topical corticosteroids, if the Betnovate preparations are used for prolonged periods, the consequences of systemic absorption, e.g. suppression of the HPA axis, should be considered, especially in children.

Prolonged and intensive treatment with active corticosteroid preparations may cause local atrophic changes in the skin.

There are reports of pigmentation changes and hypertrichosis with topical steroids.

*Overdosage:* Acute overdosage is very unlikely to occur, however, in the case of chronic overdosage or misuse the features of hypercorticism may appear and in this situation topical steroids should be discontinued.

**Pharmaceutical precautions** Nil.

**Legal category** POM.

**Package quantities** Tube of 30 g with applicator nozzle.

**Further information** Nil.

**Product licence number** 10949/0024

## BETNOVATE* SCALP APPLICATION

**Presentation** Betnovate Scalp Application is a trans-parent, slightly gelled solution containing 0.1% w/w betamethasone as valerate. The vehicle contains 39.30% w/w isopropyl alcohol, which has antibacterial activity. This preparation complies with the specifica-tion for Betamethasone Valerate Scalp Application BP.

**Uses** Steroid-responsive dermatoses of the scalp, such as psoriasis and seborrhoeic dermatitis.

**Dosage and administration** A small quantity of Betnovate Scalp Application should be applied to the scalp night and morning until improvement is notice-able. It may then be possible to sustain improvement by applying once a day, or less frequently.

**Contra-indications, warnings, etc**
*Contra-indications:* Infections of the scalp. Hypersen-sitivity to the preparation.

Dermatoses in children under one year of age, including dermatitis.

*Precautions:* Care must be taken to keep the prepara-tion away from the eyes. Do not use near a naked flame.

Long-term continuous topical therapy should be avoided where possible, particularly in infants and children, as adrenal suppression can occur even without occlusion.

Topical corticosteroids may be hazardous in psori-asis for a number of reasons including rebound relapses, development of tolerance, risk of generalised pustular psoriasis and development of local or systemic toxicity due to impaired barrier function of the skin. If used in psoriasis careful patient supervision is important.

Development of secondary infection requires withdrawal of topical corticosteroid therapy and commencement of appropriate systemic antimicro-bial therapy.

*Pregnancy:* There is inadequate evidence of safety in human pregnancy. Topical administration of cortico-steroids to pregnant animals can cause abnormalities of fetal development including cleft palate and intra-uterine growth retardation. There may therefore be a very small risk of such effects in the human fetus.

*Side-effects:* Betnovate preparations are usually well tolerated, but if signs of hypersensitivity appear, application should be stopped immediately.

As with other topical corticosteroids, prolonged use of large amounts or treatment of extensive areas can result in sufficient systemic absorption to produce the features of hypercorticism and suppression of the HPA axis. These effects are more likely to occur in infants and children, and if occlusive dressings are used. Local atrophy may occur after prolonged treatment.

There are rare reports of pigmentation changes and hypertrichosis with topical steroids.

In rare instances, treatment of psoriasis with corti-costeroids (or its withdrawal) is thought to have provoked the pustular form of the disease (see *Precautions*).

*Overdosage:* Acute overdosage is very unlikely to occur, however, in the case of chronic overdosage or misuse the features of hypercorticism may appear

and in this situation topical steroids should be discontinued.

**Pharmaceutical precautions** Nil.

**Legal category** POM.

**Package quantities** Plastic squeeze bottles of 100 ml.

**Further information** The least potent corticosteroid which will control the disease should be selected. The viscosity of the scalp application has been adjusted so that the preparation spreads easily without being too fluid. The specially-designed bottle and nozzle allow easy application direct to the scalp through the hair.

**Product licence number** 10949/0045.

## BETNOVATE* SKIN PREPARATIONS

**Presentation** The Betnovate skin preparations contain 0.1% betamethasone as the valerate ester. The Betnovate R.D. (Ready Diluted) skin preparations contain 0.025% betamethasone as the valerate ester.

Betnovate Cream is a smooth, white, water-miscible preparation. It complies with the specification for Betamethasone Valerate Cream BP.

Betnovate Ointment is a white preparation based on soft paraffin. It complies with the specification for Betamethasone Valerate Ointment BP.

Betnovate Lotion is a white, translucent, aqueous fluid. It complies with the specification for Betamethasone Valerate Lotion BP.

Betnovate R.D. Cream and Ointment are ready-diluted 1 in 4 preparations.

**Uses** Betamethasone valerate is an active topical corticosteroid which produces a rapid response in those inflammatory dermatoses that are normally responsive to topical corticosteroid therapy, and is often effective in the less responsive conditions such as psoriasis.

Betnovate preparations are indicated for the treatment of: eczema in children and adults, including atopic and discoid eczemas; prurigo nodularis; psoriasis (excluding widespread plaque psoriasis); neurodermatoses, including lichen simplex, lichen planus; seborrhoeic dermatitis; contact sensitivity reactions; discoid lupus erythematosus and they may be used as an adjunct to systemic steroid therapy in generalised erythroderma.

Betnovate R.D. preparations are indicated for main-tenance treatment when control has been achieved with Betnovate.

**Dosage and administration** A small quantity of Betnovate should be applied to the affected area two or three times daily until improvement occurs. It may then be possible to maintain improvement by applying once a day, or even less often, or by using the appropriate ready-diluted (1 in 4) preparation Betnovate R.D. If no improvement is seen within two or four weeks, reassessment of the diagnosis, or referral, may be necessary.

Betnovate and Betnovate R.D. Creams are especially appropriate for moist or weeping surfaces and Betnovate and Betnovate R.D. Ointments for dry, lichenified or scaly lesions, but this is not invariably so. Betnovate Lotion is particularly suitable when a minimal application to a large area is required.

In the more resistant lesions, such as the thickened plaques of psoriasis on elbows and knees, the effect of Betnovate can be enhanced, if necessary, by occluding the treatment area with polythene film. Overnight occlusion only is usually adequate to bring about a satisfactory response in such lesions; there-after improvement can usually be maintained by regular application without occlusion.

**Contra-indications, warnings, etc**
*Contra-indications:* Rosacea, acne vulgaris and peri-oral dermatitis. Primary cutaneous viral infections (e.g. herpes simplex, chickenpox). Hypersensitivity to the preparation.

The use of Betnovate skin preparations is not indicated in the treatment of primarily infected skin lesions caused by infection with fungi (e.g. candidia-sis, tinea), or bacteria (e.g. impetigo); primary or secondary infections due to yeast; peri-anal and genital pruritus; dermatoses in children under 1 year of age, including dermatitis and napkin eruptions.

*Precautions* Long-term continuous topical therapy should be avoided where possible, particularly in infants and children, as adrenal suppression can occur even without occlusion.

The face, more than other areas of the body, may exhibit atrophic changes after prolonged treatment with potent topical corticosteroids. This must be borne in mind when treating such conditions as psoriasis, discoid lupus erythematosus and severe eczema. If applied to the eyelids, care is needed to ensure that the preparation does not enter the eye, as glaucoma might result.

If used in childhood or on the face, courses should be limited if possible to five days and occlusion should not be used.

Topical corticosteroids may be hazardous in psori-asis for a number of reasons including rebound relapses, development of tolerance, risk or general-ised pustular psoriasis and development of local or systemic toxicity due to impaired barrier function of the skin. If used in psoriasis careful patient supervision is important.

Appropriate antimicrobial therapy should be used whenever treating inflammatory lesions which have become infected. Any spread of infection requires withdrawal of topical corticosteroid therapy and sys-temic administration of antimicrobial agents. Bacterial infection is encouraged by the warm, moist conditions induced by occlusive dressings, and so the skin should be cleansed before a fresh dressing is applied.

*Pregnancy:* There is inadequate evidence of safety in human pregnancy. Topical administration of cortico-steroids to pregnant animals can cause abnormalities of fetal development including cleft palate and intra-uterine growth retardation. There may therefore be a very small risk of such effects in the human fetus.

*Side-effects:* Prolonged and intensive treatment with highly active corticosteroid preparations may cause local atrophic changes in the skin such as striae, thinning, and dilatation of the superficial blood ves-sels, particularly when occlusive dressings are used or when skin folds are involved.

As with other topical corticosteroids, prolonged use of large amounts or treatment of extensive areas can result in sufficient systemic absorption to produce the features of hypercorticism and suppression of the HPA axis. These effects are likely to occur in infants and children, and if occlusive dressings are used. In infants the napkin may act as an occlusive dressing.

There are reports of pigmentation changes and hypertrichosis with topical steroids.

In rare instances, treatment of psoriasis with corticosteroids (or its withdrawal) is thought to have provoked the pustular form of the disease (see *Precautions*).

The Betnovate and Betnovate R.D. preparations are usually well tolerated, but if signs of hypersensitivity appear, application should stop immediately.

Exacerbation of symptoms may occur.

*Overdosage:* Acute overdosage is very unlikely to occur, however, in the case of chronic overdosage or misuse the features of hypercorticism may appear and in this situation topical steroids should be discontinued.

**Pharmaceutical precautions** Nil.

**Legal category** POM.

**Package quantities** Betnovate Cream and Ointment are supplied in 30 and 100 g tubes and in 100 g Pump Dispenser packs.

Betnovate R.D. Cream and Ointment are supplied in 100 g tubes.

Betnovate Lotion is supplied in 100 ml bottles.

**Further information** The least potent corticosteroid which will control the disease should be selected. None of these preparations contain lanolin. Betnovate Cream and Ointment and the correspond-ing R.D. preparations do not contain parabens. Bet-novate Lotion contains parabens.

**Product licence numbers**

| | |
|---|---|
| Betnovate Cream | 10949/0014 |
| Betnovate Cream Pump | 10949/0128 |
| Betnovate R.D. Cream | 10949/0021 |
| Betnovate Ointment | 10949/0020 |
| Betnovate R.D. Ointment | 10949/0022 |
| Betnovate Lotion | 10949/0044 |

## BETNOVATE*-C SKIN PREPARATIONS

**Presentation** The Betnovate-C skin preparations contain 0.1% betamethasone as the valerate ester and 3% clioquinol.

Betnovate-C Cream is a smooth, straw-coloured water-miscible cream.

Betnovate-C Ointment is a pale, straw-coloured to yellow paraffin-based ointment.

**Uses** Betamethasone valerate is an active topical corticosteroid which produces a rapid response in those inflammatory dermatoses that are normally responsive to topical corticosteroid therapy, and is often effective in the less responsive conditions such as psoriasis.

Clioquinol is an anti-infective agent which has both antibacterial and anticandidal activity.

Betnovate-C preparations are indicated for the treatment of the following conditions where secondary bacterial and/or fungal infection is present, suspected, or likely to occur: eczema in children and adults, including atopic and discoid eczemas; prurigo nodularis; psoriasis (excluding widespread plaque psoriasis); neurodermatoses; seborrhoeic dermatitis; contact sensitivity reactions and discoid lupus erythematosus.

Betnovate-C can also be used in the management of secondary infected insect bites and anal and genital intertrigo.

**Dosage and administration** A small quantity should be applied gently to the affected area two or three times daily until improvement occurs. It may then be possible to maintain improvement by applying once a day, or even less often.

Betnovate-C Cream is often appropriate for moist or weeping surfaces and Betnovate-C Ointment for dry, lichenified or scaly lesions, but this is not invariably so.

**Contra-indications, warnings, etc**

*Contra-indications:* Rosacea, acne vulgaris and perioral dermatitis. Primary cutaneous viral infections (e.g. herpes simplex, chickenpox). Hypersensitivity to any component of the preparation or to iodine.

Use of Betnovate-C skin preparations is not indicated in the treatment of primarily infected skin lesions caused by infection with fungi (e.g. candidiasis, tinea); or bacteria (e.g. impetigo); primary or secondary infections due to yeast; perianal or genital pruritus; dermatoses in children under 1 year of age, including dermatitis and napkin eruptions.

*Precautions:* Long-term continuous topical therapy should be avoided where possible, particularly in infants and children, as adrenal suppression can occur even without occlusion.

The face, more than other areas of the body, may exhibit atrophic changes after prolonged treatment with potent topical corticosteroids. This must be borne in mind when treating such conditions as psoriasis, discoid lupus erythematosus and severe eczema with Betnovate. If applied to the eyelids, care is needed to ensure that the preparation does not enter the eye, as glaucoma might result.

If used in childhood, or on the face, courses should be limited to five days and occlusion should not be used.

Topical corticosteroids may be hazardous in psoriasis for a number of reasons including rebound relapses, development of tolerance, risk of generalised pustular psoriasis and development of local or systemic toxicity due to impaired barrier function of the skin. If used in psoriasis careful patient supervision is important.

If infection persists, systemic chemotherapy is required. Any spread of infection requires withdrawal of topical corticosteroid therapy. Bacterial infection is encouraged by the warm, moist conditions induced by occlusive dressings, and the skin should be cleansed before a fresh dressing is applied.

Do not continue for more than 7 days in the absence of clinical improvement, since occult extension of infection may occur due to the masking effect of the steroid.

Betnovate-C may stain hair, skin or fabric, and the application should be covered with a dressing to protect clothing.

Products which contain antimicrobial agents should not be diluted.

*Pregnancy:* There is inadequate evidence of safety in human pregnancy. Topical administration of corticosteroids to pregnant animals can cause abnormalities of fetal development including cleft palate and intrauterine growth retardation. There may therefore be a very small risk of such effects in the human fetus.

*Side-effects:* Prolonged and intensive treatment with highly active corticosteroid preparations may cause local atrophic changes in the skin such as thinning, striae, and dilatation of the superficial blood vessels, particularly when occlusive dressings are used or when skin folds are involved.

As with other topical corticosteroids, prolonged use of large amounts or treatment of extensive areas can result in sufficient systemic absorption to produce the features of hypercorticism and suppression of the HPA axis. These effects are likely to occur in infants and children, and if occlusive dressings are used. In infants the napkin may act as an occlusive dressing.

In rare instances, treatment of psoriasis with corticosteroids (or its withdrawal) is thought to have provoked the pustular form of the disease (see *Precautions*).

There are reports of pigmentation changes and hypertrichosis with topical steroids.

The Betnovate preparations are usually well tolerated, but if signs of hypersensitivity appear, application should be stopped immediately.

Exacerbation of symptoms may occur.

*Overdosage:* Acute overdosage is very unlikely to occur, however, in the case of chronic overdosage or misuse the features of hypercorticism may appear and in this situation topical steroids should be discontinued.

**Pharmaceutical precautions** Nil.

**Legal category** POM.

**Package quantities** Betnovate-C Cream and Ointment are supplied in 30 g tubes.

**Further information** The least potent corticosteroid which will control the disease should be selected. These preparations do not contain lanolin or parabens.

**Product licence numbers**

| | |
|---|---|
| Betnovate-C Cream | 10949/0016 |
| Betnovate-C Ointment | 10949/0017 |

## BETNOVATE*-N SKIN PREPARATIONS

**Presentation** The Betnovate-N skin preparations contain 0.1% betamethasone as the valerate ester and 0.5% neomycin sulphate (3,500 units per gram or per millilitre).

Betnovate-N Cream is a smooth, white, water-miscible cream.

Betnovate-N Ointment is a white, paraffin-based ointment.

**Uses** Betamethasone valerate is an active topical corticosteroid which produces a rapid response in those inflammatory dermatoses that are normally responsive to topical corticosteroid therapy, and is often effective in the less responsive conditions such as psoriasis.

Neomycin sulphate is a broad-spectrum, bactericidal antibiotic effective against the majority of bacteria commonly associated with skin infections.

Betnovate-N preparations are indicated for the treatment of the following conditions where secondary bacterial infection is present, suspected, or likely to occur: eczema in children and adults, including atopic and discoid eczemas; prurigo nodularis; psoriasis (excluding widespread plaque psoriasis); neurodermatoses, seborrhoeic dermatitis; contact sensitivity reactions and they may be used as an adjunct to systemic steroid therapy in generalised erythroderma.

Betnovate-N preparations can also be used in the management of secondarily infected insect bites and anal and genital intertrigo.

**Dosage and administration** A small quantity should be applied gently to the affected area two or three times daily until improvement occurs. It may then be possible to maintain improvement by applying once a day, or even less often.

Betnovate-N Cream is especially appropriate for moist or weeping surfaces, and Betnovate-N Ointment for dry, lichenified or scaly lesions, but this is not invariably so.

**Contra-indications, warnings, etc**

*Contra-indications:* Rosacea, acne vulgaris and perioral dermatitis. Primary cutaneous viral infections (e.g. herpes simplex, chickenpox). Hypersensitivity to any component of the preparation.

Application to large areas especially during pregnancy, in the elderly and in patients with impaired renal function due to a risk of ototoxicity.

Use of Betnovate-N skin preparations is not indicated in the treatment of primarily infected skin lesions caused by infection with fungi (e.g. candidiasis, tinea), or bacteria (e.g. impetigo), primary or secondary infections due to yeast; secondary infections due to Pseudomonas or Proteus species; perianal and genital pruritus; dermatoses in children under 1 year of age, including dermatitis and napkin eruptions.

Preparations containing neomycin should not be used for the treatment of otitis externa when the ear drum is perforated, because of the risk of ototoxicity.

*Precautions:* Long-term continuous topical therapy should be avoided where possible, particularly in infants and children, as adrenal suppression can occur even without occlusion.

The face, more than other areas of the body, may exhibit atrophic changes after prolonged treatment with potent topical corticosteroids. This must be borne in mind when treating such conditions as psoriasis, discoid lupus erythematosus and severe eczema with Betnovate. If applied to the eyelids, care is needed to ensure that the preparation does not enter the eye, as glaucoma might result.

If used in childhood, or on the face, courses should be limited to five days and occlusion should not be used.

Topical corticosteroids may be hazardous in psoriasis for a number of reasons including rebound relapses, development of tolerance, risk of generalised pustular psoriasis and development of local or systemic toxicity due to impaired barrier function of the skin. If used in psoriasis careful patient supervision is important.

Do not continue for more than 7 days in the absence of clinical improvement, since occult extension of infection may occur due to the masking effect of the steroid. If bacterial infection persists, systemic chemotherapy is required. Any spread of infection requires withdrawal of topical corticosteroid therapy. Bacterial infection is encouraged by the warm, moist conditions induced by occlusive dressings, and the skin should be cleansed before a fresh dressing is applied.

Extended or recurrent application may increase the risk of contact sensitisation.

Products which contain antimicrobial agents should not be diluted.

*Pregnancy:* There is inadequate evidence of safety in human pregnancy. Topical administration of corticosteroids to pregnant animals can cause abnormalities of fetal development including cleft palate and intrauterine growth retardation. There may therefore be a very small risk of such effects in the human fetus.

The use of neomycin may be associated with a theoretical risk of fetal ototoxicity (see *Contra-indications*).

*Side-effects:* Prolonged and intensive treatment with highly active corticosteroid preparations may cause local atrophic changes in the skin such as thinning, striae, and dilatation of the superficial blood vessels, particularly when occlusive dressings are used or when skin folds are involved.

As with other topical corticosteroids, prolonged use of large amounts or treatment of extensive areas can result in sufficient systemic absorption to produce the features of hypercorticism and suppression of the HPA axis. These effects are likely to occur in infants and children, and if occlusive dressings are used. In infants the napkin may act as an occlusive dressing.

In rare instances, treatment of psoriasis with corticosteroids (or its withdrawal) is thought to have provoked the pustular form of the disease (see *Precautions*).

There are reports of pigmentation changes and hypertrichosis with topical steroids.

The Betnovate preparations are usually well tolerated, but if signs of hypersensitivity appear application should be stopped immediately.

Exacerbation of symptoms may occur.

*Overdosage:* Acute overdosage is very unlikely to occur, however, in the case of chronic overdosage or misuse the features of hypercorticism may appear and in this situation topical steroids should be discontinued.

**Pharmaceutical precautions** Nil.

**Legal category** POM.

**Package quantities** Betnovate-N Cream and Ointment are supplied in 30 and 100 g tubes.

**Further information** The least potent corticosteroid which will control the disease should be selected. These preparations do not contain lanolin or parabens.

**Product licence numbers**

| | |
|---|---|
| Betnovate-N Cream | 10949/0018 |
| Betnovate-N Ointment | 10949/0019 |

## CEPOREX* ORAL PREPARATIONS

**Presentation** Ceporex Tablets are pink, film-coated tablets, each containing 250 mg, 500 mg or 1 g cephalexin. They are engraved 'Ceporex 250' or 'Ceporex 500' respectively on one side and 'Glaxo' on the reverse. Ceporex Tablets 1 g are engraved with a breakline on one side and 'Glaxo' on the reverse. They comply with the BP specification for Cephalexin Tablets.

Ceporex Capsules are caramel and grey, hard gelatin capsules, each containing 250 mg or 500 mg cephalexin. They are marked 'Ceporex 250' or 'Ceporex 500' respectively and 'Glaxo'. They comply with the BP specification for Cephalexin Capsules.

Ceporex Syrups are prepared by adding water to the granules to give orange-flavoured and coloured suspensions containing 125 mg, 250 mg or 500 mg cephalexin in each 5 ml. All strengths comply with the BP specification for Cephalexin Mixture.

Ceporex Paediatric Drops are prepared by adding water to give 10 ml of orange-flavoured and coloured suspension containing 125 mg cephalexin in each 1.25 ml. The dropper is calibrated at 125 mg and 62.5 mg.

**Uses**

*Indications:* Ceporex is a bactericidal antibiotic of the cephalosporin group which is active against a wide range of Gram-positive and Gram-negative organisms. It is indicated for treatment of the following conditions, when caused by susceptible bacteria.

Respiratory tract infections: Acute and chronic bronchitis and infected bronchiectasis.

Ear, nose and throat infections: Otitis media, mastoiditis, sinusitis, follicular tonsillitis and pharyngitis.

Urinary tract infections: Acute and chronic pyelonephritis, cystitis and prostatitis. Prophylaxis of recurrent urinary tract infection.

Gynaecological and obstetric infections.

Skin, soft-tissue and bone infections.

Gonorrhoea (when penicillin is unsuitable).

Dental procedures: Treatment of dental infections.

As prophylaxis treatment for patients with heart disease undergoing dental treatment as an alternative to penicillin.

**Dosage and administration** Many infections in adults will respond to oral dosage of 1 gram to 2 grams per day in divided doses; however, for most infections, the following simple dosage scheme will be found satisfactory:

*Adults and children over 12 years:* 1 g b.d.

The following additional information should also be considered:

*Adults:* For severe or deep-seated infections, especially when less sensitive organisms are involved, the dosage should be increased to 1 g t.d.s. or 3 g b.d.

For prophylaxis of recurrent urinary tract infections in adults, a dose of 125 mg each night is recommended and may be continued for several months (the 125 mg/5 ml Suspension is suitable for this purpose).

*Children:* Ideally, dosage should be calculated on a bodyweight basis, particularly in infants. The following dosage recommendations for children are derived from a normal dosage of 25 to 60 mg/kg/day. For chronic, severe or deep-seated infections, this should be increased to 100 mg/kg/day (maximum 4 g/day).

Children under 1 year (25 to 60 mg/kg/day) 62.5 to 125 mg b.d.

Children 1-6 years 250 mg–500 mg b.d.

Children 7-12 years 500 mg–1 g b.d.

*Notes:* For most acute infections, treatment should continue for at least two days after signs have returned to normal and symptoms have subsided, but in chronic, recurrent or complicated urinary tract infections, treatment for two weeks (giving 1 g b.d.) is recommended. For gonorrhoea, a single dose of 3 g with 1 g probenecid for males or 2 g with 0.5 g probenecid for females is usually effective. Concurrent administration of probenecid delays excretion of cephalexin and raises the serum levels by 50 to 100%.

Ceporex has not been shown to have a toxic effect on the kidney, but as with other antibiotics which are excreted mainly by the kidneys, unnecessary accumulation may occur in the body when renal function is below about half of normal. Therefore, the maximum recommended dosages (i.e. adults 6 g/day, children 4 g/day) should be reduced proportionately in these patients.

In elderly patients, the possibility of renal impairment should be considered.

Adult patients receiving intermittent dialysis should be given an additional 500 mg Ceporex after each dialysis, i.e., a total dosage of up to 1 g on that day. Children should receive an additional 8 mg per kg.

**Contra-indications, warnings, etc**

*Contra-indications:* Hypersensitivity to any ingredient of the preparation.

*Precautions:* Ceporex is usually well-tolerated by patients allergic to penicillin, but cross-reaction has been encountered rarely.

As with other broad-spectrum antibiotics, prolonged use may result in the overgrowth of non-susceptible organisms (e.g. Candida, Enterococci, *Clostridium difficile*), which may require interruption of treatment. Pseudomembranous colitis has been reported with the use of broad-spectrum antibiotics, therefore, it is important to consider its diagnosis in patients who develop severe diarrhoea during or after antibiotic use.

As with other antibiotics that are excreted mainly by the kidneys, when renal function is poor, dosage of Ceporex should be suitably reduced (see *Dosage and administration*). Laboratory experiments and clinical experience show no evidence of teratogenicity, but it would be wise to proceed with caution during the early months of pregnancy, as with all drugs.

In patients receiving Ceporex, a false-positive reaction for glucose in the urine may be given, with Benedict's or Fehling's solution, or with 'Clinitest' tablets, but not with enzyme-based tests. There are reports of positive Coomb's test.

Ceporex can interfere with the alkaline picrate assay for creatinine, giving a falsely high reading, but the degree of elevation is unlikely to be of clinical importance.

*Side-effects:* A small proportion of patients receiving Ceporex experience gastro-intestinal disturbances such as nausea, vomiting and diarrhoea.

As with other broad-spectrum antibiotics, there have been rare reports of pseudomembranous colitis.

As with other antibiotics, prolonged use may result in the overgrowth of non-susceptible organisms, e.g., Candida. This may present as vulvo-vaginitis.

Reversible neutropenia has occurred in a few patients, but is very rare.

Drug rashes both urticarial and maculopapular.

Ceporex should be used with care in patients with a history of hypersensitivity to drugs.

Severe skin reactions including very rarely toxic epidermal necrolysis (exanthematic necrolysis), and hypersensitivity reactions including angioedema and anaphylaxis.

As with other cephalosporins there have been rare reports of reversible interstitial nephritis.

*Interactions:* Concurrent treatment with high doses of cephalosporins and nephrotoxic drugs such as aminoglycosides or potent diuretics (e.g. Frusemide, ethacrynic acid and piretamide) may adversely affect renal function. Clinical experience has shown that it is not likely to be a problem with Ceporex at the recommended dosage levels.

*Overdosage:* Serum levels of cephalexin can be reduced greatly by peritoneal dialysis or haemodialysis.

**Pharmaceutical precautions** Ceporex Tablets and Capsules should be protected from light.

The reconstituted syrups retain their potency for ten days when kept in a cool place, preferably a refrigerator. The reconstituted syrups may be diluted with water (not Syrup BP), after which they should be used within seven days.

**Legal category** POM.

**Package quantities** Tablets 250 mg and 500 mg: Bottles of 28 (OP), 100 and 500.

Tablets 1 g: Containers of 14 (OP).

Capsules 250 mg and 500 mg: Bottles of 28 (OP), 100, and 500.

Syrup 125 mg/5 ml, 250 mg/5 ml and 500 mg/5 ml: Bottles of 100 ml (OP).

Paediatric Drops 125 mg/1.25 ml: Bottles of 10 ml (OP).

**Further information** Ceporex is resistant to the action of staphylococcal penicillinase, and is therefore active against strains of *Staph. aureus* that are insensitive to penicillin (or ampicillin) through production of that enzyme. Ceporex is also active against the majority of ampicillin-resistant *E. coli*.

Absorption of Ceporex is almost complete, even in the presence of food, and is not adversely affected by coeliac disease, partial gastrectomy, achlorhydria, jaundice or diverticulosis (duodenal or jejunal). Ceporex is excreted in the urine in high concentration.

The serum half-life is normally about one hour, but is longer in the newborn (see *Dosage and administration*). Ceporex has a wide margin of safety.

**Product licence numbers**

| | |
|---|---|
| Ceporex Capsules 250 mg | 10949/0129 |
| Ceporex Capsules 500 mg | 10949/0130 |
| Ceporex Syrup 125 mg | 10949/0131 |
| Ceporex Syrup 250 mg | 10949/0132 |
| Ceporex Syrup 500 mg/ | |
| Ceporex Paediatric Drops | 10949/0133 |
| Ceporex Tablets 250 mg | 10949/0134 |
| Ceporex Tablets 500 mg | 10949/0135 |
| Ceporex Tablets 1 g | 10949/0136 |

# CUTIVATE* CREAM AND OINTMENT

**Presentation** Each gram of Cutivate Cream 0.05% contains fluticasone propionate 500 micrograms in a cream base of propylene glycol, mineral oil, cetostearyl alcohol, polyoxyl 20 cetostearyl ether, isopropyl myristate, dibasic sodium phosphate, citric acid monohydrate, purified water, and imidurea as a preservative.

Each gram of Cutivate Ointment 0.005% contains fluticasone propionate 50 micrograms in a base of propylene glycol, sorbitan sesquioleate, microcrystalline wax, and liquid paraffin.

**Uses** Cutivate skin preparations are indicated for the relief of the inflammatory and pruritic manifestations of corticosteroid-responsive eczema/dermatitis.

**Dosage and administration** Cutivate Cream: Apply a thin film of the Cream to the affected skin areas once daily.

Cutivate Ointment: Apply a thin film to the affected skin areas twice daily.

**Contra-indications, warnings, etc.**

*Contra-indications:*

Rosacea.

Acne vulgaris.

Peri-oral dermatitis.

Primary cutaneous viral infections (e.g., herpes simplex, chickenpox).

Hypersensitivity to any of the ingredients.

Perianal and genital pruritus.

The use of Cutivate skin preparations is not indicated in the treatment of primarily infected skin lesions caused by infection with fungi or bacteria and dermatoses in children under one year of age, including dermatitis and napkin eruptions.

*Precautions:* Fluticasone propionate has a very low propensity for systemic absorption, nevertheless, prolonged application of high doses to large areas of body surface, especially in infants and small children, might lead to adrenal suppression. Children may absorb proportionally larger amounts of topical corticosteroids and thus be more susceptible to systemic toxicity.

The face, more than other areas of the body, may exhibit atrophic changes after prolonged treatment with potent topical corticosteroids. This must be borne in mind when treating severe eczema.

If applied to the eyelids, care is needed to ensure that the preparation does not enter the eye so as to avoid the risk of local irritation or glaucoma.

Appropriate antimicrobial therapy should be used whenever treating inflammatory lesions which have become infected. Any spread of infection requires withdrawal of topical corticosteroid therapy and systemic administration of antimicrobial agents. Bacterial infection is encouraged by the warm, moist conditions induced by occlusive dressing, and so the skin should be cleansed before a fresh dressing is applied.

*Pregnancy:* Topical administration of corticosteroids to pregnant animals can cause abnormalities of fetal development. The relevance of this finding to human beings has not been established; however, administration of fluticasone propionate during pregnancy should only be considered if the expected benefit to the mother is greater than any possible risk to the fetus.

*Lactation:* The excretion of fluticasone propionate into human breast milk has not been investigated. When measurable plasma levels were obtained in lactating laboratory rats following subcutaneous administration there was evidence of fluticasone propionate in the breast milk. However, plasma levels in patients following dermal application of fluticasone propionate at recommended doses are likely to be low.

When fluticasone propionate is used in breast feeding mothers the therapeutic benefits must be weighed against the potential hazards to mother and baby.

*Side-effects:* The fluticasone propionate preparations are usually well tolerated; local burning and pruritus have been reported. If signs of hypersensitivity appear, application should stop immediately.

Prolonged and intensive treatment with potent corticosteroid preparations may cause local atrophic changes in the skin such as thinning, striae, dilatation of the superficial blood vessels, hypertrichosis and hypopigmentation.

Secondary infection, particularly when occlusive dressings are used or when skin folds are involved and allergic contact dermatitis have also been reported with corticosteroid use.

Exacerbation of the signs and symptoms of the dermatoses have been reported with corticosteroid use.

Prolonged use of large amounts of corticosteroids, or treatment of extensive areas, can result in sufficient systemic absorption to produce the features of hypercorticism. This effect is more likely to occur in infants and children, and if occlusive dressings are used. In infants, the napkin may act as an occlusive dressing.

*Overdosage:* Acute overdosage is very unlikely to occur, however, in the case of chronic overdosage or misuse the features of hypercorticism may appear and in this situation, as with any corticosteroid, application should be discontinued. Overdosage by ingestion of fluticasone propionate cream or ointment is extremely unlikely to occur due to the very low oral bioavailability of fluticasone propionate.

**Pharmaceutical precautions** Store below 30°C.

Do not freeze.

**Legal category** POM.

**Package quantities** Cutivate Cream and Ointment are supplied in 15 and 50 g tubes.

**Further information** Fluticasone propionate is a glucocorticoid with high topical anti-inflammatory potency but a low HPA-axis suppressive activity after dermal administration. It therefore has a therapeutic index which is greater than most of the commonly available steroids.

Overt suppression of the HPA-axis (morning plasma cortisol <5 micrograms) is very unlikely to result from therapeutic use of Cutivate skin preparations unless treating more than 50% of an adult's body surface and applying more than 20 g per day; calculation on appropriate dosage for children should allow for their greater surface area to body weight ratio.

Fluticasone propionate has a high degree of selectivity for the glucocorticoid receptor. *In vitro* studies show that fluticasone propionate has a strong affinity for, and agonist activity at, human glucocorticoid receptors. This receptor is believed to be responsible for the anti-inflammatory properties of glucocorticoids.

Pharmacokinetic data for the rat and dog indicate rapid elimination and extensive metabolic clearance.

Distribution studies have shown that only minute traces of orally administered compound reach the systemic circulation, and that any systemically available fluticasone propionate is rapidly eliminated in the bile and excreted in the faeces. Bioavailablility is very low after topical administration, due to limited absorption through the skin and because of extensive hepatic metabolism.

Fluticasone propionate does not persist in any tissue, and does not bind to melanin. The major route of metabolism is hydrolysis to a carboxylic acid, which has very weak glucocorticoid or anti-inflammatory activity. In all test animal species the route of excretion was independent of the route of administration of fluticasone propionate. Excretion is predominantly faecal and is essentially complete within 48 hours.

In man too, metabolic clearance is extensive, and elimination is consequently rapid. Thus drug entering the systemic circulation via the skin will be rapidly inactivated.

**Product licence numbers**

| | |
|---|---|
| Cutivate Cream | 10949/0013 |
| Cutivate Ointment | 10949/0012 |

## CYCLIMORPH* 10 INJECTION CYCLIMORPH* 15 INJECTION

**Qualitative and quantitative composition**
*Ingredients per 1 ml of product:*

| | *10* | *15* |
|---|---|---|
| Morphine Tartrate | 10 mg | 15 mg |
| Cyclizine Tartrate | 39.01 mg | 39.01 mg |

**Pharmaceutical form** Injection.

**Clinical particulars**
*Therapeutic indications:* Cyclimorph Injection is indicated for the relief of moderate to severe pain in all suitable medical and surgical conditions (see *Contra-indications* and *Special warnings and special precautions*) in which reduction of the nausea and vomiting associated with the administration of morphine is required.

*Posology and method of administration:*
*Use by injection in adults:* The usual dose is 10–20 mg morphine tartrate, given subcutaneously, intramuscularly or intravenously.

Additional doses may not be given more frequently than 4-hourly.

Not more than 3 doses (representing 150 mg cyclizine: i.e. 3 ml of Cyclimorph 10 or Cyclimorph 15 Injection) should be given in any 24-hour period.

*Use in the elderly:* Morphine doses should be reduced in elderly patients and titrated to provide optimal pain relief with minimal side effects since:

- Increased duration of pain relief from a standard dose of morphine has been reported in elderly patients.
- A review of pharmacokinetic studies has suggested that morphine clearance decreases and half-life increases in older patients.
- The elderly may be particularly sensitive to the adverse effects of morphine.

*Children:* Cyclimorph Injection should not be used in children under 12 years of age.

*Contra-indications:* Cyclimorph Injection is contra-indicated in individuals with known hypersensitivity to morphine, cyclizine or any of the other constituents.

Cyclimorph Injection, like other opioid-containing preparations, is contra-indicated in patients with respiratory depression. Patients with excessive bronchial secretions should not be given Cyclimorph Injection as morphine diminishes the cough response.

Cyclimorph Injection should not be given during an attack of bronchial asthma or in heart failure secondary to chronic lung disease.

Cyclimorph Injection is contra-indicated in patients with head injury or raised intra-cranial pressure.

*Renal impairment:* Severe and prolonged respiratory depression may occur in patients with renal impairment given morphine; this is attributed to the accumulation of the active metabolite morphine-6-glucuronide. Therefore, Cyclimorph Injection should not be administerd to patients with moderate or severe renal impairment (glomerular filtration rate <20 ml/min).

*Hepatic impairment:* As with other opioid analgesic containing preparations Cyclimorph Injection should not be administered to patients with severe hepatic impairment as it may precipitate coma.

Cyclimorph Injection is contra-indicated in the presence of acute alcohol intoxication. The antiemetic properties of cyclizine may increase the toxicity of alcohol.

Cyclimorph Injection is contra-indicated in individuals receiving monoamine oxidase inhibitors or within 14 days of stopping such treatment.

Cyclimorph Injection, as with other opioid containing preparations, is contra-indicated in patients with ulcerative colitis, since such preparations may precipitate toxic dilation or spasm of the colon.

Cyclimorph Injection is contra-indicated in biliary and renal tract spasm.

*Special warnings and special precautions for use:* In common with the other opioid containing preparations, Cyclimorph Injection has the potential to produce tolerance and physical and psychological dependence in susceptible individuals. Abrupt cessation of therapy after prolonged use may result in withdrawal symptoms.

Cyclimorph Injection should be used with caution in the debilitated since they may be more sensitive to the respiratory depressant effects.

Cyclimorph Injection should be used with caution (including consideration of dose administered) in the presence of the following:

hypothyroidism
adrenocortical insufficiency
hypopituitarism
prostatic hypertrophy
shock
diabetes mellitus

Extreme caution should be exercised when administering Cyclimorph Injection to patients with phaeochromocytoma, since aggravated hypertension has been reported in association with diamorphine.

Cyclizine may cause a fall in cardiac output associated with increases in heart rate, mean arterial pressure and pulmonary wedge pressure. Cyclimorph Injection should therefore be used with caution in patients with severe heart failure.

Because cyclizine has anticholinergic activity it may precipitate incipient glaucoma. It should be used with caution and appropriate monitoring in patients with glaucoma and also in obstructive disease of the gastrointestinal tract.

*Interaction with other medicaments and other forms of interaction:* The central nervous system depressant effects of Cyclimorph Injection may be enhanced by other centrally-acting agents such as phenothiazines, hypnotics, neuroleptics, alcohol and muscle relaxants.

Monoamine oxidase inhibitors (MAOIs) may prolong and enhance the respiratory depressant effects of morphine. Opioids and MAOIs used together may cause fatal hypotension and coma (see *Contra-indications*).

Because of its anticholinergic activity cyclizine may enhance the side effects of other anticholinergic drugs.

The analgesic effect of opioids tends to be enhanced by co-administration of dexamphetamine, hydroxyzine, and some phenothiazines although respiratory depression may also be enhanced by the latter combination.

Morphine may reduce the efficacy of diuretics by inducing the release of antidiuretic hormone.

Propranolol has been reported to enhance the lethality of toxic doses of opioids in animals. Although the significance of this finding is not known for man, caution should be exercised when these drugs are administered concurrently.

*Interference with laboratory tests:* Morphine can react with Folin-Ciocalteau reagent in the Lowry method of protein estimation.

Morphine can also interfere with the determination of urinary 17-ketosteroids due to chemical structure effects in the Zimmerman procedure.

*Use in pregnancy and lactation:*
*Pregnancy:* There is no evidence on the safety of the combination in human pregnancy, nor is there evidence from animal work that the constituents are free from hazard. However, limited data from epidemiological studies of cyclizine and morphine in human pregnancies have found no evidence of teratogenicity. In the absence of definitive human data with the combination the use of Cyclimorph Injection in pregnancy is not advised.

Administration of morphine during labour may cause respiratory depression in the newborn infant.

*Lactation:* Cyclizine is excreted in human milk, however, the amount has not been quantified.

Morphine can significantly suppress lactation. Morphine is excreted in human milk, but the amount is generally considered to be less than 1% of any dose.

*Effects on ability to drive and use machines:* In common with other opioids, morphine may produce orthostatic hypotension and drowsiness in ambulatory patients. Sedation of short duration has been reported in patients receiving intravenous cyclizine. The CNS depressant effects of Cyclimorph Injection may be enhanced by combination with other centrally acting agents (see *Interactions*). Patients should therefore be cautioned against activities requiring vigilance including driving vehicles and operating machinery.

*Undesirable effects:* As Cyclimorph Injection contains morphine and cyclizine, the type and frequency of adverse effects associated with such compounds may be expected.

Adverse reactions attributable to morphine include respiratory depression, raised intra-cranial pressure, orthostatic hypotension, drowsiness, confusion, dysphoria, restlessness, miosis, constipation, nausea, vomiting, skin reactions (e.g. urticaria) biliary tract and renal spasm, vertigo and difficulty with micturition.

Adverse reactions attributable to cyclizine include urticaria, drug rash, drowsiness/sedation, dryness of the mouth, nose and throat, blurred vision, tachycardia, urinary retention, constipation, restlessness, nervousness, insomnia, auditory and visual hallucination and cholestatic jaundice.

A single case of anaphylaxis has been reported following intravenous administration of cyclizine co-administered in the same syringe as propanidid.

Anaphylactic shock is a rare adverse reaction to morphine.

An increase in excitatory phenomena (tremor and muscle movements) has been reported when cyclizine has been given before propanidid and methohexitone anaesthesia. A case of hyperactivity following intravenous administration of morphine during induction of anaesthesia has been reported.

A case of morphine-induced thrombocytopenia has been reported.

Morphine has a depressant effect on gonadal hormone secretion which can result in a reduction of testosterone leading to regression of secondary sexual characteristics in men on long-term therapy.

*Overdose: Signs:* The signs of overdosage with Cyclimorph Injection are those pathognomonic of opioid poisoning i.e. respiratory depression, pin point pupils, hypotension, circulatory failure and deepening coma. Mydriasis may replace miosis as asphyxia intervenes.

Drowsiness, floppiness, miosis and apnoea are signs of opioid overdosage in children as are convulsions.

*Treatment:* It is imperative to maintain and support respiration and circulation.

The specific opioid antagonist naloxone is the treatment of choice for the reversal of coma and restoration of spontaneous respiration, the literature should be consulted for details of appropriate dosage.

The use of a specific opioid antagonist in patients tolerant to morphine may produce withdrawal symptoms.

Patients should be monitored closely for at least 48 hours in case of relapse.

**Pharmacological properties**
*Pharmacodynamic properties:* Cyclizine is a histamine $H_1$ receptor antagonist of the piperazine class. It possesses anticholinergic and antiemetic properties. The exact mechanism by which cyclizine can prevent or suppress both nausea and vomiting from various causes is unknown. Cyclizine increases lower oesophageal sphincter tone and reduces the sensitivity of the labyrinthine apparatus.

Morphine is a competitive agonist at the μ-opioid receptor and is a potent analgesic. It is thought that activity at the μ-receptor subtype may mediate the analgesic and euphoric actions of morphine whilst activity at the μ2-receptor subtype may mediate respiratory depression and inhibition of gut motility. An action at the k-opioid receptor may mediate spinal analgesia.

*Pharmacokinetic properties:* In a healthy adult volunteer the administration of a single oral dose of 50 mg cyclizine resulted in a peak plasma concentration of approximately 70 ng/ml, occurring at about 2 hours after administration. Urine collected over 24 hours contained less than 1% of the total dose administered. In a separate study in one healthy adult volunteer the plasma elimination half-life of cyclizine was approximately 20 hours.

Cyclizine is metabolised to its N-dimethylated derivative norcyclizine, which has little antihistaminic ($H_1$) activity compared to cyclizine.

The mean elimination half-life for morphine in blood and plasma is 2.7 h (range 1.2–4.9 h) and 2.95 (range 0.8–5 h) respectively.

Morphine is extensively metabolised by hepatic biotransformation. In addition, the kidney has been shown to have the capacity to form morphine glucuronides. The major metabolite is morphine-3-glucuronide (approximately 45% of a dose). Morphine-6-glucuronide is a minor metabolite (approx. 5% of the dose) but is highly active. Although renal excretion is a minor route of elimination for unchanged morphine, it constitutes the major mechanism of elimination of conjugated morphine metabolites including the active morphine-6-glucuronide.

Morphine is bound to plasma proteins only to the extent of 25–35% and therefore functions that change the extent of protein binding will have only a minor impact on its pharmacodynamic effects.

*Preclinical safety data:*
*A. Mutagenicity:* Cyclizine was not mutagenic in an Ames test (at a dose level of 100 μg/plate), with or without metabolic activation.

No bacterial mutagenicity studies with morphine have been reported. A review of the literature has indicated that morphine was negative in gene mutation assays in *Drosphilia melanogaster*, but was positive in a mammalian spermatocyte test. The results of another study by the same authors has indicated that morphine causes chromosomal aberrations, in germ cells of male mice when given at dose levels of 10, 20, 40 or 60 mg/kg bodyweight for three consecutive days.

*B. Carcinogenicity:* No long term studies have been conducted in animals to determine whether cyclizine or morphine are potentially carcinogenic.

*C. Teratogenicity:* Some animal studies indicate that cyclizine may be teratogenic at dose levels up to 25 times the clinical dose level. In another study, cyclizine was negative at oral dose levels up to 65 mg/kg in rats and 75 mg/kg in rabbits.

Morphine was not teratogenic in rats when dosed for up to 15 days at 70 mg/kg/day. Morphine given subcutaneously to mice at very high doses (200, 300 or 400 mg/kg/day) on days eight or nine of gestation, resulted in a few cases of exencephaly and axial skeletal fusions. The hypoxic effects of such high doses could account for the defects seen.

Lower doses of morphine (40, 4.0 or 0.4 mg/ml) given to mice as a continuous i.v. infusion (at a dose volume of 0.3 ml/kg) between days seven and ten of gestation, caused soft tissue and skeletal malformations as shown in previous studies.

*D. Fertility:* In a study involving prolonged administration of cyclizine to male and female rats, there was no evidence of impaired fertility after continuous treatment for 90–100 days at dose levels of approximately 15 and 25 mg/kg/day.

Effects of morphine exposure on sexual maturation of male rats, their reproductive capacity and the development of their progeny have been examined. Results indicated that exposure during adolescence led to pronounced inhibition of several indices of sexual maturation (e.g. hormone levels, reduced gonad weights), smaller litters and selective gender specific effects on endocrine function in the offspring.

A disruption in ovulation and amenorrhoea can occur in women given morphine.

**Pharmaceutical particulars**
*List of excipients:* Tartaric acid; sodium metabisulphite; water for injections.

*Incompatibilities:* See drug *Interactions* and *Contra-indications.*

*Shelf life:* 3 years.

*Special precautions for storage:* Store below 30°C. Protect from light. Do not freeze.

*Nature and contents of container:* Ampoules which comply with the requirements of the European Pharmacopoeia for type 1 neutral glass.

*Instructions for use/handling:* No special instructions.

*Pack sizes:* Cyclimorph 10 injection: 1 ml ampoules: Box of 5. Cyclimorph 15 injection: 1 ml ampoules: Box of 5.

**Marketing authorisation numbers**
Cyclimorph 10 Injection 0003/5022
Cyclimorph 15 Injection 0003/5023

**Date of approval/revision of SPC** 28 June 1995

**Legal category** CD (Sch 2), POM.

## DARAPRIM* TABLETS

**Presentation** Each tablet contains 25 mg of Pyrimethamine BP, scored and coded 'WELLCOME A3A' and white in colour.

**Uses** Daraprim is indicated for chemoprophylaxis of malaria due to susceptible strains of plasmodia. However, since resistance to pyrimethamine is increasing worldwide, Daraprim can only be considered suitable for use in individuals who are resident in areas where pyrimethamine is acknowledged to be effective. It is not suitable as a prophylactic for travellers.

**Dosage and administration**
*Adults:* 1 tablet regularly each week.

*Children: Over 10 years:* 1 tablet regularly each week.

*5 to 10 years:* ½ tablet regularly each week.

*Under 5 years:* Formulation not applicable.

Daraprim is rapidly absorbed and therefore prophylactic cover can be expected shortly after the first dose. Prophylaxis should commence before arrival in an endemic area and be continued once weekly. On returning to a non-malarious area, dosage should be maintained for a further four weeks.

*Use in the elderly:* No specific studies have been carried out in the elderly. However, it may be advisable to monitor renal or hepatic function and if there is serious impairment then caution should be exercised.

Daraprim, at the doses recommended for the prevention of Malaria is unlikely to have any adverse effect on older people normally of good health.

**Contra-indications, warnings, etc**
*Contra-indications:* Daraprim should not be given to patients with a history of pyrimethamine sensitivity.

*Precautions:* The recommended dosage should not be exceeded.

Daraprim should be used with caution in patients with hepatic or renal disorders.

During pregnancy and in other conditions predisposing to folate deficiency, a folate supplement should be given.

Daraprim, by its mode of action, may further depress folate metabolism in patients receiving treatment with other folate inhibitors. Occasional reports suggest that individuals taking pyrimethamine as malarial prophylaxis at doses in excess of 25 mg weekly may develop megaloblastic anaemia if co-trimoxazole is prescribed concurrently.

The concurrent administration of lorazepam and Daraprim may induce hepatotoxicity.

Daraprim may exacerbate folate deficiency due to innate disease or malnutrition.

*Side- and adverse effects:* At the recommended dose, side-effects are rare. Occasionally, rashes have been observed which disappeared when the administration of Daraprim was stopped. Excessive doses may produce a macrocytic anaemia resembling that of folic acid deficiency. Insomnia has been reported when pyrimethamine has been given at weekly doses above those recommended.

*Use in pregnancy and lactation:* While there is a theoretical risk of fetal abnormality with all folate inhibitors given during pregnancy, no such adverse effects have been reported with Daraprim in humans. A folate supplement should be given to pregnant women receiving Daraprim. The amount of pyrimethamine excreted in breast milk is insufficient to contra-indicate its use in lactating mothers, but breast-fed infants should not receive other anti-folate agents.

*Toxicity and treatment of overdosage:* Symptoms reported have included vomiting, cyanosis, respiratory distress, convulsions and tachycardia. Routine supportive treatment, including maintenance of a clear airway and control of convulsions, should be given. Adequate fluids should be given to ensure optimal diuresis. Gastric lavage may be of value only if instituted within two hours of ingestion, in view of the rapid absorption of Daraprim. Fresh blood transfusions to counteract blood dyscrasias should be available.

To counteract possible folate deficiency, calcium folinate 9 to 15 mg daily should be given until the signs of toxicity have subsided. There may be a delay of 7 to 10 days before the full leucopenic side-effects become evident, therefore calcium folinate therapy should be continued for the period at risk.

**Pharmaceutical precautions** Store below 35°C. Protect from light.

**Legal category** POM

**Package quantities** 30 tablets as 5 foil strips of 6 tablets.

**Further information** Nil.

**Product licence number** 0003/5026R

## DERMOVATE* CREAM AND OINTMENT

**Presentation** Dermovate Cream and Ointment each contain 0.05% w/w clobetasol propionate. The water-miscible cream and the paraffin-based ointment are both white in appearance.

**Uses** Clobetasol propionate is a very active topical corticosteroid which is of particular value when used in short courses for the treatment of more resistant dermatoses such as psoriasis (excluding widespread plaque psoriasis), recalcitrant eczemas, lichen planus, discoid lupus erythematosus, and other conditions which do not respond satisfactorily to less active steroids.

**Dosage and administration** Apply sparingly to the affected area once or twice daily until improvement occurs. As with other highly active topical steroid preparations, therapy should be discontinued when control is achieved. In the more responsive conditions this may be within a few days.

If no improvement is seen within two to four weeks, reassessment of the diagnosis, or referral, may be necessary.

Repeated short courses of Dermovate may be used to control exacerbations. If continuous steroid treatment is necessary, a less potent preparation should be used.

In very resistant lesions, especially where there is hyperkeratosis, the anti-inflammatory effect of Dermovate can be enhanced, if necessary, by occluding the treatment area with polythene film. Overnight occlusion only is usually adequate to bring about a satisfactory response. Thereafter improvement can usually be maintained by application without occlusion.

**Contra-indications, warnings, etc**
*Contra-indications:* Rosacea, acne vulgaris and perioral dermatitis. Primary cutaneous viral infections (e.g. herpes simplex, chickenpox). Hypersensitivity to the preparation.

The use of Dermovate skin preparations is not indicated in the treatment of primarily infected skin lesions caused by infection with fungi (e.g. candidiasis, tinea), or bacteria (e.g. impetigo); perianal and genital pruritus.

Dermatoses in children under one year of age, including dermatitis and napkin eruptions.

*Precautions:* Long-term continuous topical therapy should be avoided where possible, particularly in infants and children, as adrenal suppression can occur readily even without occlusion.

If used in childhood or on the face, courses should be limited if possible to five days and occlusion should not be used.

The face, more than other areas of the body, may exhibit atrophic changes after prolonged treatment with potent topical corticosteroids. This must be borne in mind when treating such conditions as psoriasis, discoid lupus erythematosus and severe eczema.

If applied to the eyelids, care is needed to ensure that the preparation does not enter the eye, as glaucoma might result.

Topical corticosteroids may be hazardous in psoriasis for a number of reasons including rebound relapses, development of tolerance, risk of generalised pustular psoriasis and development of local or systemic toxicity due to impaired barrier function of the skin. If used in psoriasis careful patient supervision is important.

Appropriate antimicrobial therapy should be used whenever treating inflammatory lesions which have become infected. Any spread of infection requires withdrawal of topical corticosteroid therapy and systemic administration of antimicrobial agents. Bacterial infection is encouraged by the warm, moist conditions induced by occlusive dressings, and so the skin should be cleansed before a fresh dressing is applied.

*Pregnancy:* There is inadequate evidence of safety in human pregnancy. Topical administration of corticosteroids to pregnant animals can cause abnormalities of fetal development including cleft palate and intra-uterine growth retardation. There may therefore be a very small risk of such effects in the human fetus.

*Side-effects:* As with other topical corticosteroids prolonged use of large amounts, or treatment of extensive areas can result in sufficient systemic absorption to produce the features of hypercorticism.

Provided the weekly dosage is less than 50 g in adults, any suppression of the HPA axis is likely to be transient with a rapid return to normal values once the short course of steroid therapy has ceased. The same applies to children given proportionate dosage. Use of occlusive dressing increases the absorption of topical corticosteroids. In infants the napkin may act as an occlusive dressing.

Prolonged and intensive treatment with a highly active corticosteroid preparation may cause local atrophic changes in the skin such as thinning, striae, and dilatation of the superficial blood vessels, particularly when occlusive dressings are used or when skin folds are involved.

In rare instances, treatment of psoriasis with corticosteroids (or its withdrawal) is thought to have provoked the pustular form of the disease (see *Precautions*).

There are reports of pigmentation changes and hypertrichosis with topical steroids.

Dermovate is usually well tolerated, but if signs of hypersensitivity appear, application should be stopped immediately.

Exacerbation of symptoms may occur.

*Overdosage:* Acute overdosage is very unlikely to occur, however, in the case of chronic overdosage or misuse the features of hypercorticism may appear and in this situation topical steroids should be discontinued.

**Pharmaceutical precautions** None.

**Legal category** POM.

**Package quantities** Tubes of 30 and 100 g.

**Further information** The least potent corticosteroid which will control the disease should be selected. Dermovate preparations do not contain lanolin or parabens.

**Product licence numbers**
Dermovate Ointment      10949/0028
Dermovate Cream         10949/0025

## DERMOVATE* SCALP APPLICATION

**Presentation** Dermovate Scalp Application is a transparent, slightly gelled solution containing 0.05% w/w clobetasol propionate. The vehicle contains 50% isopropyl alcohol, which has antibacterial activity.

**Uses** Psoriasis and recalcitrant eczemas of the scalp. Clobetasol propionate is a highly-active topical corticosteroid which is indicated for use in short courses for conditions which do not respond satisfactorily to less active steroids.

**Dosage and administration** Apply sparingly to the scalp night and morning until improvement occurs. As with other highly-active topical steroid preparations, therapy should be discontinued when control is achieved. Repeated short courses of Dermovate Scalp Application may be used to control exacerbations. If continuous steroid treatment is necessary, a less potent preparation should be used.

**Contra-indications, warnings, etc**
*Contra-indications:* Infections of the scalp. Hypersensitivity to the preparation. Dermatoses in children under one year of age, including dermatitis.

*Precautions:* Care must be taken to keep the preparation away from the eyes. Do not use near a naked flame.

Long-term continuous topical therapy should be avoided, particularly in infants and children, as adrenal suppression can occur readily even without occlusion.

Development of secondary infection requires withdrawal of topical corticosteroid therapy and commencement of appropriate systemic antimicrobial therapy.

Topical corticosteroids may be hazardous in psoriasis for a number of reasons including rebound relapses, development of tolerance, risk of generalised pustular psoriasis and development of local or systemic toxicity due to impaired barrier function of the skin. If used in psoriasis careful patient supervision is important.

*Pregnancy:* There is inadequate evidence of safety in human pregnancy. Topical administration of corticosteroids to pregnant animals can cause abnormalities of fetal development including cleft palate and intrauterine growth retardation. There may therefore be a very small risk of such effects in the human fetus.

*Side-effects:* Dermovate preparations are usually well tolerated, but if signs of hypersensitivity appear, application should be stopped immediately.

As with other topical corticosteroids, prolonged use of large amounts or treatment of extensive areas can result in sufficient systemic absorption to produce the features of hypercorticism and suppression of the HPA axis. These effects are more likely to occur in infants and children, and if occlusive dressings are used. Local atrophy may occur after prolonged treatment.

In rare instances, treatment of psoriasis with corticosteroids (or its withdrawal) is thought to have provoked the pustular form of the disease (see *Precautions*).

*Overdosage:* Acute overdosage is very unlikely to occur, however, in the case of chronic overdosage or misuse the features of hypercorticism may appear and in this situation topical steroids should be discontinued.

**Pharmaceutical precautions** None.

**Legal category** POM.

**Package quantities** Plastic squeeze bottle with elongated nozzle containing 30 or 100 ml.

**Further information** The least potent corticosteroid which will control the disease should be selected. The viscosity of the scalp application has been adjusted so that the preparation spreads easily without being too fluid. The specially-designed bottle and nozzle allow easy application direct to the scalp through the hair.

**Product licence number** 10949/0046

## DERMOVATE*-NN SKIN PREPARATIONS

**Presentation** Dermovate-NN skin preparations contain clobetasol propionate 0.05% w/w, neomycin sulphate 0.5% and nystatin 100,000 units per gram.

Dermovate-NN Ointment is a buff paraffin-based ointment.
Dermovate-NN Cream is buff in colour.

**Uses** Clobetasol propionate is a highly active topical corticosteroid which is of particular value when used in short courses for the treatment of recalcitrant eczemas, neurodermatoses, and other conditions which do not respond satisfactorily to less active steroids.

Dermovate-NN is indicated in more resistant dermatoses such as recalcitrant eczemas and psoriasis (excluding widespread plaque psoriasis) where secondary bacterial or candidal infection is present, suspected or likely to occur, as when using occlusive dressings.

**Dosage and administration** Apply sparingly to the affected area once or twice daily until improvement occurs. As with other highly-active topical steroid preparations, therapy should be discontinued when control is achieved. In the more responsive conditions this may be within a few days.

If a longer course is necessary, it is recommended that treatment should not be continued for more than four weeks without the patient's condition being reviewed.

Repeated short courses of Dermovate-NN may be used to control exacerbations. If continuous steroid treatment is necessary, a less potent preparation should be used.

In very resistant lesions, especially where there is hyperkeratosis, the anti-inflammatory effect of Dermovate-NN can be enhanced, if necessary, by occluding the treatment area with polythene. Overnight occlusion only is usually adequate to bring about a satisfactory response, thereafter improvement can usually be maintained by application without occlusion.

**Contra-indications, warnings, etc**
*Contra-indications:* Rosacea, acne vulgaris and perioral dermatitis.

Primary cutaneous viral infections (e.g. herpes simplex, chickenpox).

Hypersensitivity to the preparations.

Use of Dermovate-NN skin preparations is not indicated in the treatment of primarily infected skin lesions caused by infection with fungi (e.g. candidiasis, tinea), bacteria (e.g. impetigo), or yeast; secondary infections due to Pseudomonas or Proteus species; perianal and genital pruritus dermatoses in children under one year of age, including dermatitis and napkin eruptions.

Preparations containing neomycin should not be used for the treatment of otitis externa when the ear drum is perforated, because of the risk of ototoxicity.

Application to large areas especially during pregnancy, in the elderly and in patients with impaired renal function due to a risk of ototoxicity.

*Precautions:* Long-term continuous topical therapy should be avoided where possible, particularly in infants and children, as adrenal suppression can occur readily even without occlusion.

If used in childhood, or on the face, courses should be limited to five days and occlusion should not be used.

The face, more than other areas of the body, may exhibit atrophic changes after prolonged treatment with potent topical corticosteroids. This must be borne in mind when treating such conditions as psoriasis and severe eczema with Dermovate-NN. If applied to the eyelids, care is needed to ensure that the preparation does not enter the eye, as glaucoma might result.

Topical corticosteroids may be hazardous in psoriasis for a number of reasons, including rebound relapses, development of tolerance, risk of generalised pustular psoriasis and development of local or systemic toxicity due to impaired barrier function of the skin. If used in psoriasis careful patient supervision is important.

Do not continue for more than 7 days in the absence of clinical improvement, since occult extension of infection may occur due to the masking effect of the steroid.

If infection persists, systemic chemotherapy is required. Any spread of infection requires withdrawal of topical corticosteroid therapy. Bacterial infection is encouraged by the warm, moist conditions induced by occlusive dressings, and the skin should be cleansed before a fresh dressing is applied.

Extended or recurrent application may increase the risk of contact sensitisation.

Products which contain antimicrobial agents should not be diluted.

*Pregnancy:* There is inadequate evidence of safety in human pregnancy. Topical administration of corticosteroids to pregnant animals can cause abnormalities of fetal development including cleft palate and intrauterine growth retardation. There may therefore be a very small risk of such effects in the human fetus.

The use of neomycin may be associated with a theoretical risk of fetal ototoxicity (see *Contra-indications*).

*Side-effects:* As with other topical corticosteroids prolonged use of large amounts or treatment of extensive areas can result in sufficient systemic absorption to produce the features of hypercorticism.

Provided the weekly dosage is less than 50 g in adults, any suppression of the HPA axis is likely to be transient with a rapid return to normal values once the short course of steroid therapy has ceased. The same applies to children given proportionate dosage. Use of occlusive dressings increases the absorption of topical corticosteroids. In infants the napkin may act as an occlusive dressing.

Prolonged and intensive treatment with highly active corticosteroid preparations may cause local atrophic changes in the skin such as thinning, striae, and dilatation of the superficial blood vessels, particularly when occlusive dressings are used, or when skin folds are involved.

In rare instances, treatment of psoriasis with corticosteroids (or its withdrawal) is thought to have provoked the pustular form of the disease (see *Precautions*).

There are reports of pigmentation changes and hypertrichosis with topical steroids.

Dermovate-NN is usually well tolerated, but if signs of hypersensitivity appear, application should be stopped immediately.

Exacerbation of symptoms may occur.

*Overdosage:* Acute overdosage is very unlikely to occur, however, in the case of chronic overdosage or misuse the features of hypercorticism may appear and in this situation topical steroids should be discontinued.

**Pharmaceutical precautions** None.

**Legal category** POM.

**Package quantities** Tubes of 30 g.

**Further information** The least potent corticosteroid which will control the disease should be selected. Dermovate-NN preparations contain neither lanolin nor parabens.

**Product licence numbers**
Dermovate-NN Ointment      10949/0026
Dermovate-NN Cream         10949/0027

## DICONAL* TABLETS

**Qualitative and quantitative composition** Each tablet contains 10 mg of Dipipanone Hydrochloride BP and 30 mg of Cyclizine Hydrochloride BP, coloured deep pink, scored and coded 'WELLCOME F3A'.

**Pharmaceutical form** Tablet.

**Clinical particulars**
*Therapeutic indications:* Diconal Tablets are indicated for the management of moderate to severe pain in medical and surgical conditions in which morphine may be indicated.

Cyclizine is effective in preventing nausea and vomiting associated with the administration of narcotic analgesics.

*Posology and method of administration:*
*Adults:* The initial dose in all conditions is one tablet every 6 hours. It is unwise to exceed this dose in view of the difficulty in accurately predicting the initial central effects of dipipanone.

Should this dose fail to prove adequate analgesia, as in severe intractable pain or when other potent opioids have been used, it may be increased by half a tablet every six hours.

It is seldom necessary to exceed a dose of 30 mg dipipanone given 6-hourly (i.e. 12 tablets in 24 hours).

*Children:* There is no specific information on the use of Diconal in children. Diconal is very rarely indicated in childen and dosage guidelines cannot be stated.

*Use in the elderly:* There is no specific information on the use of Diconal in elderly patients. In common with opioid drugs, Diconal may be expected to cause confusion in this age group, and careful monitoring is advised (see *Special warnings and precautions*).

*Contra-indications:* Diconal is contra-indicated in individuals who are hypersensitive to dipipanone or cyclizine.

Diconal is generally contra-indicated in patients with respiratory depression, especially in the presence of cyanosis and excessive bronchial secretions.

Diconal should not be given during an attack of bronchial asthma.

Diconal is generally contra-indicated in the presence of acute alcoholism, head injury and raised intracranial pressure.

Diconal is contra-indicated in individuals receiving monoamine oxidase inhibitors, or within 14 days of stopping such treatment.

Diconal is contra-indicated in patients with ulcerative colitis since in common with other narcotic analgesics it may precipitate toxic dilatation or spasm of the colon.

As with all narcotic analgesics Diconal should not be administered to patients with severe hepatic impairment as it may precipitate hepatic encephalopathy.

In severe renal impairment Diconal, in common with all narcotic analgesics, may precipitate coma and should not be administered.

Diconal, in common with morphine and most other narcotics, may cause spasm of the biliary and renal tracts; it is contra-indicated in these conditions.

*Special warnings and precautions for use:* The repeated use of Diconal may lead to tolerance and physical dependence as well as to psychological dependence on the product.

Misuse of Diconal has been reported, particularly by young addicts who have previously been dependent on, or have misused other agents both opiate and non-opiate. Extreme caution is warranted when prescribing Diconal to this group of patients.

Diconal should be used with extreme caution in the presence of the following: hypothyroidism; adreno-cortical insufficiency; prostatic hypertrophy; hypoten-sion secondary to hypovolaemic shock; diabetes mellitus.

Diconal is metabolised in the liver and excreted along with its metabolites in the urine. Where not contra-indicated in patients with impaired hepatic and/or renal function, Diconal should be given at less than the usual recommended dose, and the patient's response used as a guide to further dosage require-ments.

Extreme caution should be exercised when admin-istering Diconal to patients with phaeochromocytoma, since hypertension has been reported in association with other potent opioids.

No data are available as to whether or not dipipa-none has carcinogenic, mutagenic or teratogenic potential. It is not known whether cyclizine has carcinogenic or mutagenic potential. Some animal studies are interpreted as indicating that cyclizine may be teratogenic, but relevance to the human situation is not known.

In a study involving prolonged administration of cyclizine to male and female rats, there was no evidence of impaired fertility after continuous treat-ment for 90–100 days. There are no similar data for dipipanone. There is no information on the effect of Diconal on human fertility.

*Interaction with other medicaments and other forms of interaction:* The central nervous system depressant effects of Diconal may be increased by phenothiazine drugs, alcohol, sedatives and tricyclic antidepres-sants. Concurrent administration of some phenothia-zines increases the respiratory depressant effects of narcotic analgesics and also produces hypotension.

Because of its anticholinergic activity, cyclizine may enhance the side effects of other anticholinergic agents.

Analgesic effects of opioid drugs tend to be en-hanced by co-administration of dexamphetamine, however their use in combination is not recom-mended.

*Pregnancy and lactation:* The use of Diconal during pregnancy is not recommended. No data are available on the therapeutic use of Diconal in human pregnancy. It may be anticipated that if given in the last trimester, Diconal would cause withdrawal symptoms in the neonate.

Diconal is not recommended for use in labour because of its potential to cause respiratory depres-sion in the neonate.

No data are available on the excretion of dipipanone, cyclizine or their metabolites in human milk.

*Effect on ability to drive and use machines:* Ambula-tory patients receiving Diconal should be cautioned against driving cars or operating machinery in view of its tendency to cause drowsiness.

*Undesirable effects:* The adverse effects of dipipanone are common to all opioid agents, and may include: respiratory depression; mental clouding, drowsiness and sedation, confusion, mood changes, euphoria, dysphoria, psychosis, restlessness, miosis and raised intracranial pressure; constipation, nausea and vomiting; sweating, facial flushing and hypotension; urticaria and rashes; difficulty with micturition; biliary and renal tract spasm; vertigo.

In addition, cyclizine may cause drowsiness which is potentiated by other sedative drugs including alcohol. Furthermore dryness of the mouth, nose and throat, blurred vision, tachycardia, urinary retention, restlessness, nervousness, insomnia and auditory and visual hallucinations have been reported, particularly when dosage recommendations have been exceeded. Cholestatic jaundice has occurred in association with cyclizine.

Following cyclizine administration, single case reports have been documented of: fixed drug erup-

tion; generalised chorea; hypersensitivity hepatitis; agranulocytosis.

*Overdose:* The signs of overdosage with Diconal are typically those of opioid poisoning, i.e. respiratory depression, pin-point pupils, hypotension, circulatory failure and deepening coma. Mydriasis may replace miosis as asphyxia intervenes. Drowsiness, floppi-ness, miosis and apnoea have been reported in children, as have convulsions.

General supportive measures should be employed as required. Gastric lavage should be performed if indicated. The specific opioid antagonist naloxone is the treatment of choice for the reversal of coma and the restoration of spontaneous respiration; the litera-ture should be consulted for details of appropriate dosage. Patients should be monitored closely for at least 48 hours after recovery in case of relapse, since the duration of action of the antagonist may be substantially shorter than that of dipipanone.

## Pharmacological properties

*Pharmacodynamic properties:* The onset of analgesic action of dipipanone is approximately one hour and lasts for 4 to 6 hours. Cyclizine produces its anti-emetic effect within 2 hours and lasts for approximately 4 hours.

*Pharmacokinetic properties:* Dipipanone is absorbed from the gastro-intestinal tract. It is metabolised in the liver and excreted in the urine and faeces, although data on the proportions of parent compound and metabolites so excreted are lacking.

In healthy adult volunteers, the administration of a single oral dose of 50 mg cyclizine resulted in a peak plasma concentrations of approximately 70 nano-gram/ml occurring approximately 2 hours after drug administration. The plasma elimination half-life was approximately 20 hours.

The N-demethylated derivative, norcyclizine, has been identified as a metabolite of cyclizine. Norcycli-zine has little antihistaminic ($H_1$) activity compared with cyclizine and has a plasma elimination half life of approximately 20 hours. After a single oral dose of 50 mg cyclizine given to a single adult male volunteer, urine collected over the following 24 hours contained less than 1% of the total dose administered.

*Preclinical safety data:* No additional data of relevance.

## Pharmaceutical particulars

*List of excipients:* Lactose, starches, dye (FD and C Red No 3), gelatin, magnesium stearate. Methylated spirit, ethanol and purified water are all used in the manufacturing process but are not detected in the final formulation.

*Incompatibilities:* None stated.

*Shelf life:* 60 months.

*Special precautions for storage:* Store below 25°C. Protect from light. Keep dry.

*Nature and contents of container:* PVC/aluminium foil blister packs containing 50 tablets.

*Instructions for use/handling:* None stated.

**Marketing authorisation number** 0003/5027R

**Date of approval/revision of SPC** August 1996

**Legal category** POM.

## EFCORTELAN* SKIN PREPARATIONS

**Presentation** Efcortelan Cream contains 0.5%, 1% or 2.5% hydrocortisone in a smooth, white, water-miscible cream base.

Efcortelan Ointment contains 0.5%, 1% or 2.5% hydrocortisone in an off-white, paraffin-based ointment.

Efcortelan Cream 1% complies with the specification for Hydrocortisone Cream BP.

Efcortelan Ointments comply with the specification for Hydrocortisone Ointment BP.

**Uses** Hydrocortisone has topical anti-inflammatory activity of value in the treatment of a wide variety of dermatological conditions, including the following: eczema, including atopic, infantile, discoid and stasis eczemas; prurigo nodularis; neurodermatoses; seborrhoeic dermatitis; intertrigo; contact sensitivity reactions.

Efcortelan preparations can also be used in the management of insect bites and otitis externa.

Efcortelan 0.5% preparations can be used as continuation therapy in mild cases of seborrhoeic or atopic eczema once the acute inflammatory phase has passed.

**Dosage and administration** A small quantity should be applied to the affected area two or three times daily.

Efcortelan Cream is often appropriate for moist or weeping surfaces, and Efcortelan Ointment for dry, lichenified or scaly lesions, but this is not invariably so.

**Contra-indications, warnings, etc**

*Contra-indications:* Skin lesions caused by infection with viruses (e.g. herpes simplex, chickenpox), fungi (e.g. candidiasis, tinea) or bacteria (e.g. impetigo).

Hypersensitivity to the preparations.

*Precautions:* In infants and children, long-term continuous topical therapy should be avoided where possible, as adrenal suppression can occur even without occlusion. In infants, the napkin may act as an occlusive dressing, and increase absorption. Treatment should therefore be limited if possible, to a maximum of seven days.

Appropriate antimicrobial therapy should be used whenever treating inflammatory lesions which have become infected. Any spread of infection requires withdrawal of topical corticosteroid therapy, and systemic administration of antimicrobial agents.

As with all corticosteroids, prolonged application to the face is undesirable.

*Pregnancy:* There is inadequate evidence of safety in human pregnancy. Topical application of cortico-steroids to pregnant animals can cause abnormalities of fetal development including cleft palate and intra-uterine growth retardation. There may, therefore, be a very small risk of such effects in the human fetus.

*Side-effects:* Efcortelan preparations are usually well tolerated, but if signs of hypersensitivity appear, application should stop immediately.

Exacerbation of symptoms may occur.

Local atrophic changes may occur where skin folds are involved, or in areas such as the nappy area in small children, where constant moist conditions favour the absorption of hydrocortisone. Sufficient systemic absorption may also occur in such sites to produce the features of hypercorticism and suppression of the HPA axis after prolonged treat-ment. This effect is more likely to occur in infants and children, and if occlusive dressings are used.

There are reports of pigmentation changes and hypertrichosis with topical steroids.

*Overdosage:* Acute overdosage is very unlikely to occur, however, in the case of chronic overdosage or misuse the features of hypercorticism may appear and in this situation topical steroids should be discontinued.

**Pharmaceutical precautions** None.

**Legal category** POM.

**Package quantities** Efcortelan Cream and Ointment are supplied in 30 g tubes.

**Further information** The least potent corticosteroid which will control the disease should be selected. None of these preparations contain lanolin or parabens.

**Product licence numbers**

| | |
|---|---|
| Efcortelan Cream 0.5% | 10949/0029 |
| Efcortelan Cream 1% | 10949/0030 |
| Efcortelan Cream 2.5% | 10949/0031 |
| Efcortelan Ointment 0.5% | 10949/0032 |
| Efcortelan Ointment 1% | 10949/0033 |
| Efcortelan Ointment 2.5% | 10949/0034 |

## EFCORTESOL* INJECTION

**Presentation** Ampoules of Efcortesol Injection contain an aqueous, ready-prepared buffered solution of hydrocortisone sodium phosphate. Each millilitre contains 100 mg hydrocortisone as the sodium phosphate ester. The solution is clear and colourless or pale yellow. Efcortesol Injection complies with the specification for Hydrocortisone Sodium Phosphate Injection BP.

**Uses** This presentation permits rapid use in emergency situations involving the following conditions.

Status asthmaticus and acute allergic reactions, including anaphylactic reaction to drugs. Efcortesol supplements the action of adrenaline.

Severe shock arising from surgical or accidental trauma or overwhelming infection.

Acute adrenal insufficiency caused by abnormal stress in Addison's disease, hypopituitarism, follow-ing adrenalectomy, and when adrenocortical function has been suppressed by prolonged corticosteroid therapy.

Soft-tissue lesions such as tennis elbow, teno-synovitis and bursitis.

Note: Efcortesol does not replace other forms of therapy for the treatment of shock and status asthmaticus.

**Dosage and administration** Undesirable effects may be minimised by using the lowest effective dose for the minimum period. Frequent patient review is required to appropriately titrate the dose against disease activity (see *Precautions*).

*Systemic therapy in adults:* 100 to 500 mg hydro-cortisone (1 to 5 ml) administered by slow intravenous injection, taking at least half to one minute. This dose can be repeated three or four times in 24 hours, depending upon the condition being treated and the patient's response. Alternatively, Efcortesol Injection may be given as an intravenous infusion. A clinical effect is seen in two to four hours, and it persists for up to eight hours after intravenous injection. The same dose can be given by intramuscular injection, but the response is likely to be less rapid, especially in shock.

*Systemic therapy in children*: As a guide, infants up to 1 year may be given 25 mg hydrocortisone intravenously; children 1 to 5 years, 50 mg; 6 to 12 years, 100 mg (1 ml). This dose can be repeated three or four times in 24 hours depending upon the condition being treated and the patient's response.

*Other uses:* Local treatment of soft-tissue lesions–100 to 200 mg. This daily dose may be repeated on two or three occasions depending upon the patient's response.

Efcortesol Injection is not recommended for intrathecal use.

### Contra-indications, warnings, etc.
*Contra-indications:* Systemic infections, unless specific anti-infective therapy is employed. Live virus immunisation. Hypersensitivity to any component.

Efcortesol Injection should not be injected directly into tendons.

*Precautions:* Suppression of the HPA axis and other undesirable effects may be minimised by using the lowest effective dose for the minimum period (see *Dosage and administration*). The pronounced hormonal effects associated with prolonged corticosteroid therapy will probably not be seen when this injection is used for short term adjunctive therapy in shock. Frequent patient review is required to appropriately titrate the dose against disease activity.

Patients should carry 'Steroid treatment' cards which give clear guidance on the precautions to be taken to minimise risk and which provide details of prescriber, drug, dosage and the duration of treatment. Suppression of the inflammatory response and immune function increases the susceptibility to infections and their severity. The clinical presentation may often be atypical and serious infections such as septicaemia and tuberculosis may be masked and may reach an advanced stage before being recognised.

Chickenpox is of particular concern since this normally minor illness may be fatal in immunosuppressed patients. Patients without a definite history of chickenpox should be advised to avoid close personal contact with chickenpox or herpes zoster and if exposed they should seek urgent medical attention. If the patient is a child, parents must be given the above advice. Passive immunisation with varicella zoster immunoglobulin (VZIG) is needed by exposed non-immune patients who are receiving systemic corticosteroids or who have used them within the previous 3 months; this should be given within 10 days of exposure to chickenpox. If a diagnosis of chickenpox is confirmed, the illness warrants specialist care and urgent treatment. Corticosteroids should not be stopped and the dose may need to be increased.

Live vaccines should not be given to individuals with impaired immune responsiveness. The antibody response to other vaccines may be diminished.

Adrenal cortical atrophy develops during prolonged therapy and may persist for years after stopping treatment. Withdrawal of corticosteroids after prolonged therapy must therefore always be gradual to avoid acute adrenal insufficiency, being tapered off over weeks or months according to the dose and duration of treatment. During prolonged therapy any intercurrent illness, trauma or surgical procedure will require a temporary increase in dosage; if corticosteroids have been stopped following prolonged therapy they may need to be temporarily reintroduced.

Because of the possibility of fluid retention, care must be taken when corticosteroids are administered to patients with renal insufficiency or congestive heart failure.

Corticosteroids may worsen diabetes mellitus, osteoporosis, hypertension, glaucoma and epilepsy and therefore patients with these conditions or a family history should be monitored frequently.

Care is required and frequent patient monitoring necessary where there is a history of severe affective disorders (especially a previous history of steroid psychosis), previous steroid myopathy, peptic ulceration or patients with a history of tuberculosis.

In patients with liver failure, blood levels of corticosteroid may be increased, as with other drugs which are metabolised in the liver and therefore patients should be monitored frequently. Care and monitoring is also required in patients with renal insufficiency.

When treatment is to be discontinued, the dose should be reduced gradually over a period of several weeks or months depending on the dosage and duration of the therapy.

*Pregnancy:* Administration of corticosteroids to pregnant animals can cause abnormalities of fetal development including cleft palate and intra-uterine growth retardation. There may therefore be a very small risk of such effects in the human fetus as such effects have been reported. Hypoadrenalism may occur in the neonate. When corticosteroids are essential however, patients with normal pregnancies may be treated as though they were in the non-gravid state. Patients with pre-eclampsia or fluid retention require close monitoring.

Depression of hormone levels has been described in pregnancy but the significance of this finding is not clear.

*Lactation:* Corticosteroids are excreted in small amounts in breast milk, and infants of mothers taking pharmacological doses of steroids should be monitored carefully for signs of adrenal suppression.

*Use in children:* Corticosteroids cause dose-related growth retardation in infancy, childhood and adolescence, which may be irreversible.

*Use in the elderly:* The common adverse effects of systemic corticosteroids may be associated with more serious consequences in old age, especially osteoporosis, hypertension, hypokalaemia, diabetes, susceptibility to infection and thinning of the skin. Close clinical supervision is required to avoid life-threatening reactions.

*Side-effects:* Paraesthesia may occur following intravenous administration and is probably related to the rate of injection. It is often localised to the genital area but in some cases may radiate over the entire body. The unpleasant and sometimes painful sensation usually passes off within a few minutes and no sequelae have been reported. The effect seems to be related to the sodium phosphate salt of hydrocortisone.

The incidence of predictable undesirable effects, including hypothalamic-pituitary-adrenal suppression correlates with the relative potency of the drug, dosage, timing of administration and the duration of treatment (see *Precautions*).

*Endocrine/metabolic:* Suppression of the hypothalamic-pituitary-adrenal axis, growth suppression in infancy, childhood and adolescence, menstrual irregularity and amenorrhoea. Cushingoid faces, hirsutism, weight gain, impaired carbohydrate tolerance with increased requirement for anti-diabetic therapy. Negative protein and calcium balance. Increased appetite.

*Anti-inflammatory and Immunosuppressive effects:* Increased susceptibility and severity of infections with suppression of clinical symptoms and signs, opportunistic infections, recurrence of dormant tuberculosis (see other special warnings and precautions).

*Musculoskeletal:* Osteoporosis, vertebral and long bone fractures, avascular osteonecrosis, tendon rupture. Proximal myopathy.

*Fluid and electrolyte disturbance:* Sodium and water retention, hypertension, potassium loss, hypokalaemic alkalosis.

*Neuropsychiatric:* Euphoria, psychological dependence, depression, insomnia and aggravation of schizophrenia. Increased intra-cranial pressure with papilloedema in children (pseudotumour cerebri), usually after treatment withdrawal. Aggravation of epilepsy.

*Ophthalmic:* Increased intra-ocular pressure, glaucoma, papilloedema, posterior subcapsular cataracts, corneal or scleral thinning, exacerbation of ophthalmic viral or fungal diseases.

*Gastrointestinal:* Dyspepsia, peptic ulceration with perforation and haemorrhage, acute pancreatitis, candidiasis.

*Dermatological:* Impaired healing, skin atrophy, bruising, telangiectasia, striae, acne.

*General:* Hypersensitivity including anaphylaxis, has been reported. Leucocytosis. Thromboembolism.

*Withdrawal symptoms and signs:* Too rapid a reduction of corticosteroid dosage following prolonged treatment can lead to acute adrenal insufficiency, hypotension and death (see *Precautions*).

A 'withdrawal syndrome' may also occur including, fever, myalgia, arthralgia, rhinitis, conjunctivitis, painful itchy skin nodules and loss of weight.

*Drug interactions:* Rifampicin, rifabutin, carbamazepine, phenobarbitone, phenytoin, primidone, ephedrine and aminoglutethimide enhance the metabolism of corticosteroids and its therapeutic effects may be reduced.

The desired effects of hypoglycaemic agents (including insulin), anti-hypertensives and diuretics are antagonised by corticosteroids, and the hypo-

kalaemic effects of acetazolamide, loop diuretics, thiazide diuretics and carbenoxolone are enhanced.

The efficacy of coumarin anticoagulants may be enhanced by concurrent corticosteroid therapy and close monitoring of the INR or prothrombin time is required to avoid spontaneous bleeding.

The renal clearance of salicylates is increased by corticosteroids and steroid withdrawal may result in salicylate intoxication.

Steroids may reduce the effects of anti-cholinesterases in myasthenia gravis and cholecystographic X-ray media.

**Pharmaceutical precautions** Protect from light.

**Legal category** POM.

**Package quantities** Ampoules 1 ml (100 mg) in box of 5. Ampoules 5 ml (500 mg) in box of 10.

**Further information** It should be noted that 10 ml Efcortesol Injection contains 152 mg (6.6 mmol) sodium and 298 mg (28.2 mmol) phosphate ($PO_4$), it is buffered using dihydrogen phosphate anhydrous and sodium acid phosphate. There is a lack of evidence that use of corticosteroids in septic shock affects mortality in the long term.

**Product licence number** 10949/0098

## EPIVIR* ORAL SOLUTION ▼

**Qualitative and quantitative composition** Epivir contains 10 mg/ml lamivudine in a solution containing 20% (w/v) sucrose, 6% (v/v) ethanol, and preservatives (methyl parahydroxybenzoate and propyl parahydroxybenzoate).

**Pharmaceutical form** Oral solution.

**Clinical particulars**
*Therapeutic indications:* Epivir is indicated in combination with other antiretroviral agents for the treatment of HIV infected adults and children >12 years of age, with progressive immunodeficiency (CD4+ count ≤500 cells/mm³).

Epivir is not recommended for use as monotherapy. Only the combination with zidovudine has been extensively studied in terms of safety and efficacy. Combination studies with other antiretrovirals are in progress.

Lamivudine in combination with zidovudine reduces HIV-1 viral load and increases CD4+ count. A meta-analysis of clinical events in the phase II comparative studies indicates that lamivudine in combination with zidovudine slows the progression of the disease. A study to confirm the effects on AIDS progression and survival is ongoing.

*Posology and method of administration:*
*Adults and children over the age of 12 years:* The recommended dose of Epivir is 150 mg (15 ml) twice daily.

Epivir is also available as a tablet formulation.

Epivir should usually be taken without food. Ingestion with food reduces the $C_{max}$ considerably but does not alter the area under the curve (AUC) (see *Pharmacokinetic properties*). Therefore ingestion with food might be considered when required due to clinical reasons.

The therapy should be initiated by a physician experienced in the management of HIV infection.

*Renal impairment:* Lamivudine levels are increased in patients with moderate–severe renal impairment due to decreased clearance. The dose should therefore be adjusted (see table). Dosing Recommendations:

| Renal function (Clcr, ml/min) | First dose | Maintenance dose |
| --- | --- | --- |
| Clcr≥50 | 150 mg (15 ml) | 150 mg (15 ml) Twice daily |
| 50>Clcr≥30 | 150 mg (15 ml) | 150 mg (15 ml) Once daily |
| 30>Clcr≥15 | 150 mg (15 ml) | 100 mg (10 ml) Once daily |
| 15>Clcr≥5 | 150 mg (15 ml) | 50 mg (5 ml) Once daily |
| 5>Clcr | 50 mg (5 ml) | 25 mg (2.5 ml) Once daily |

*Hepatic impairment:* The influence of hepatic impairment on lamivudine levels is under investigation. Lamivudine clearance is largely renal. Based on preliminary safety data no dosage adjustment is necessary.

*Contra-indications:* The use of Epivir is contra-indicated in patients with known hypersensitivity to lamivudine or to any ingredient of the preparation.

*Special warnings and special precautions for use:*
*Special warnings:* Epivir is not recommended for use as monotherapy.

Cases of pancreatitis have occurred rarely. However it is not clear whether these cases were due to drug treatment or to the underlying HIV disease. Treatment with Epivir should be stopped immediately if clinical signs, symptoms or laboratory abnormalities suggestive of pancreatitis occur.

There are insufficient data on the use of Epivir in children under the age of 12 years.

Administration of Epivir is not recommended during the first 3 months of pregnancy (see *Pregnancy and lactation*).

Patients receiving Epivir or any other antiretroviral therapy may continue to develop opportunistic infections and other complications of HIV infection, and therefore should remain under close clinical observation by physicians experienced in the treatment of patients with associated HIV diseases.

Patients should be advised that current antiretroviral therapy, including Epivir, has not been proven to prevent the risk of transmission of HIV to others through sexual contact or blood contamination. Appropriate precautions should continue to be employed.

*Special precautions for use:* In patients with moderate–severe renal impairment, the terminal plasma half-life of lamivudine is increased due to decreased clearance. The dose should be adjusted (see dosage in renal impairment, *Posology and method of administration*).

Epivir should be used with caution in patients with advanced cirrhotic liver disease due to chronic Hepatitis B infection, as there is a small risk of rebound hepatitis if treatment is discontinued.

Diabetic patients should be advised that each dose (150 mg=15 ml) contains 3 g of sucrose.

Patients should be advised that this medicine contains alcohol.

*Interaction with other medicaments and other forms of interaction:* The likelihood of metabolic interactions is low due to limited metabolism and plasma protein binding and almost complete renal clearance.

A modest increase in $C_{max}$ (28%) was observed for zidovudine when administered with lamivudine, however overall exposure (AUC) is not significantly altered. Zidovudine has no effect on the pharmacokinetics of lamivudine (see *Pharmacokinetic properties*).

The possibility of interactions with other drugs administered concurrently should be considered, particularly when the main route of elimination is active renal secretion via the organic cationic transport system e.g. trimethoprim. Other drugs (e.g. ranitidine, cimetidine) are eliminated only in part by this mechanism and were shown not to interact with lamivudine. The nucleoside analogues (e.g. didanosine and zalcitabine) like zidovudine, are not eliminated by this mechanism and are unlikely to interact with lamivudine.

Administration of prophylactic doses of co-trimoxazole results in a 40% increase in lamivudine exposure, because of the trimethoprim component; the sulphamethoxazole component did not interact. However, unless the patient has renal impairment, no dosage adjustment of lamivudine is necessary (see *Posology and method of administration*). When concomitant administration is warranted, patients should be monitored clinically.

Co-administration of Epivir with high doses of co-trimoxazole for the treatment of Pneumocystis carinii pneumonia (PCP) and toxoplasmosis should be avoided. Lamivudine has no effect on the pharmacokinetics of co-trimoxazole.

Lamivudine metabolism does not involve CYP3A, making interactions with drugs metabolised by this system (e.g. protease inhibitors) unlikely.

Co-administration of Epivir with intravenous ganciclovir or foscarnet is not recommended until further information is available.

*Use during pregnancy and lactation:*
*Pregnancy:* The safety of lamivudine in human pregnancy has not been established. Reproductive studies in animals have not shown evidence of teratogenicity, and showed no effect on male or female fertility. Lamivudine induces early embryolethality when administered to pregnant rabbits at exposure levels comparable to those achieved in man. Lamivudine crosses the placenta in animals but there is no information on placental transfer in humans.

Although animal reproductive studies are not always predictive of the human response, administration during the first three months of pregnancy is not recommended (see *Special warnings and special precautions for use*).

*Lactation:* A study in lactating rats showed that, following oral administration, lamivudine was concentrated four fold and excreted in the milk. It is not known if lamivudine is excreted in human breast milk. Since the drug may pass into breast milk, it is recommended that mothers taking Epivir do not breast feed their infants. Some health experts recommend that HIV infected women do not breast feed

their infants under any circumstances in order to avoid transmission of HIV.

*Effects on ability to drive and use machines:* There have been no studies to investigate the effect of lamivudine on driving performance or the ability to operate machinery. Further, a detrimental effect on such activities cannot be predicted from the pharmacology of the drug. Nevertheless, the clinical status of the patient and the adverse event profile of Epivir should be borne in mind when considering the patient's ability to drive or operate machinery.

*Undesirable effects:* Adverse events have been reported during therapy for HIV disease with Epivir alone and in combination with zidovudine. With many it is unclear whether they are drug related or are as a result of the underlying disease process.

Adverse events which have been commonly reported are headache, malaise, fatigue, nausea, diarrhoea, vomiting, abdominal pain or cramps, insomnia, cough, nasal symptoms and musculoskeletal pain.

Cases of pancreatitis and peripheral neuropathy (or paraesthesia) have been recorded, although no relationship to the dose of Epivir has been noted.

Neutropenia and anaemia (both occasionally severe) have occurred in combination with zidovudine. Thrombocytopenia, transient rises in liver enzymes (AST, ALT) and rises in serum amylase have been reported.

*Overdose:* Administration of lamivudine at very high dose levels in acute animal studies did not result in any organ toxicity. Limited data are available on the consequences of ingestion of acute overdoses in humans. No fatalities occurred, and the patients recovered. No specific signs or symptoms have been identified following such overdose.

If overdosage occurs the patient should be monitored, and standard supportive treatment applied as required. Since lamivudine is dialysable, continuous haemodialysis could be used in the treatment of overdosage, although this has not been studied.

**Pharmacological properties**
*Pharmacodynamic properties:* Pharmacotherapeutic group—nucleoside analogue, ATC Code: J05A B10.

Lamivudine is a nucleoside analogue, Lamivudine is metabolised intracellularly to lamivudine 5'-triphosphate, its main mode of action is as a chain terminator of HIV reverse transcription. The triphosphate has selective inhibitory activity against HIV-1 and HIV-2 replication *in vitro*, it is also active against zidovudine-resistant clinical isolates of HIV.

The relationships between *in vitro* susceptibility of HIV to lamivudine and the clinical response to therapy remain under investigation. *In vitro* sensitivity testing has not been standardised and results may vary according to methodological factors.

Reduced *in vitro* sensitivity to lamivudine has been reported for HIV isolates from patients who have received Epivir therapy.

Lamivudine has been shown to be highly synergistic with zidovudine, inhibiting the replication of HIV in cell culture.

*In vitro* studies indicate that zidovudine-resistant virus isolates can become zidovudine sensitive when they simultaneously acquire resistance to lamivudine. Furthermore, *in vivo*, there is evidence showing that lamivudine plus zidovudine delays the emergence of zidovudine-resistant isolates in individuals with no prior antiretroviral therapy.

*In vitro*, lamivudine demonstrates low cytotoxicity to peripheral blood lymphocytes, to established lymphocyte and monocyte-macrophage cell lines and to a variety of bone marrow progenitor cells *in vitro*. Lamivudine therefore has, *in vitro*, a high therapeutic index.

*Pharmacokinetic properties:*
*Absorption:* Lamivudine is well absorbed from the gut, and the bioavailability of oral lamivudine in adults is normally between 80 and 85%. Following oral administration, the mean time ($t_{max}$) to maximal serum concentrations ($C_{max}$) is about an hour. At therapeutic dose levels i.e. 4 mg/kg/day (as two 12-hourly doses), $C_{max}$ is in the order of 1.5–1.9 mcg/ml.

Co-administration of lamivudine with food results in a delay of $t_{max}$ and a lower $C_{max}$ (decreased by 47%). However, lamivudine bioavailability (based on the AUC) is not influenced.

Co-administration of zidovudine results in a 13% increase in zidovudine exposure and a 28% increase in peak plasma levels. This is not considered to be of significance to patient safety and therefore no dosage adjustments are necessary.

*Distribution:* From intravenous studies, the mean volume of distribution is 1.3 L/kg. The observed half-life of elimination is 5 to 7 hours. The mean systemic clearance of lamivudine is approximately 0.32 L/h/kg, with predominantly renal clearance (>70%) via the organic cationic transport system.

Lamivudine exhibits linear pharmacokinetics over

the therapeutic dose range and displays limited binding to the major plasma protein albumin (<16%–36% to serum albumin in *in vitro* studies).

Limited data shows lamivudine penetrates the central nervous system and reaches the cerebrospinal fluid (CSF). The mean ratio CSF/serum lamivudine concentration 2–4 hours after oral administration was approximately 0.12. The true extent of penetration or relationship with any clinical efficacy is unknown.

*Metabolism:* Lamivudine is predominantly cleared by renal excretion of unchanged drug. The likelihood of metabolic drug interactions with lamivudine is low due to the small extent of hepatic metabolism (5–10%) and low plasma protein binding.

*Elimination:* Studies in patients with renal impairment show lamivudine elimination is affected by renal dysfunction. A recommended dosage regimen for patients with creatinine clearance below 50 ml/min is shown in the dosage section (see *Posology and method of administration*).

An interaction with trimethoprim, a constituent of co-trimoxazole, causes a 40% increase in lamivudine exposure at therapeutic doses. This does not require dose adjustment unless the patient also has renal impairment (see *Interaction with other medicaments and other forms of interaction*, and dosage adjustments in renal impairment in *Posology and method of administration*). Administration of co-trimoxazole with Epivir in patients with renal impairment should be carefully assessed.

*Preclinical safety data:* Administration of lamivudine in animal toxicity studies at high doses was not associated with any major organ toxicity. At the highest dosage levels, minor effects on indicators of liver and kidney function were seen together with occasional reductions in liver weight. The clinically relevant effects noted were a reduction in red blood cell count and neutropenia.

Lamivudine was not mutagenic in bacterial tests but, like many nucleoside analogues, showed activity in an *in vitro* cytogenetic assay and the mouse lymphoma assay. Lamivudine was not genotoxic *in vivo* at doses that gave plasma concentrations around 40–50 times higher than the anticipated clinical plasma levels. As the *in vitro* mutagenic activity of lamivudine could not be confirmed in *in vivo* tests, it is concluded that lamivudine should not represent a genotoxic hazard to patients undergoing treatment.

Long term carcinogenicity studies in animals are ongoing.

**Pharmaceutical particulars**
*List of excipients:* Sucrose PhEur (20% w/v); Ethanol BP (6% v/v); Methyl Parahydroxybenzoate PhEur (E218); Propyl Parahydroxybenzoate PhEur (E216); Citric Acid Anhydrous PhEur; Propylene Glycol PhEur; Disodium Edetate PhEur; Artificial Strawberry Flavour; Artificial Banana Flavour; Water Purified PhEur.

*Incompatibilities:* None reported.

*Shelf life:* 2 years.

*Special precautions for storage:* Store between 2 and 25°C.

*Nature and contents of container:* Cartons containing 240 ml lamivudine 10 mg/ml in a white high density polyethylene (HDPE) bottle, with a child resistant closure. A 10 ml polypropylene oral dosing syringe and a polyethylene adaptor are also included in the pack.

*Instructions for use/handling:* The oral dosing syringe is provided for accurate measurement of the prescribed dose of Oral Solution. Instructions for use are included in the pack.

Discard Oral Solution one month after first opening.

**Marketing authorisation number** EU/1/96/015/002

**Date of approval/revision of SPC** May 1997

**Legal category** POM.

# EPIVIR TABLETS ▼

**Qualitative and quantitative composition** Epivir contains 150 mg lamivudine.

**Pharmaceutical form** Coated tablets. The tablets are white film coated, diamond shaped tablets engraved 'GX CJ7' on one face.

**Clinical particulars**
*Therapeutic indications:* Epivir is indicated in combination with other antiretroviral agents for the treatment of HIV infected adults and children >12 years of age, with progressive immunodeficiency (CD4+ count ≤500 cells/mm³).

Epivir is not recommended for use as monotherapy. Only the combination with zidovudine has been extensively studied in terms of safety and efficacy. Combination studies with other antiretrovirals are in progress.

Lamivudine in combination with zidovudine reduces HIV-1 viral load and increases CD4+ count. A meta-analysis of clinical events in the phase II comparative studies indicates that lamivudine in combination with zidovudine slows the progression of the disease. A study to confirm the effects on AIDS progression and survival is ongoing.

*Posology and method of administration:*
*Adults and children over the age of 12 years:* The recommended dose of Epivir is 150 mg (one tablet) twice daily.

Epivir is also available as an oral solution for those patients for whom the tablets are inappropriate.

Epivir should usually be taken without food. Ingestion with food reduces the $C_{max}$ considerably but does not alter the area under the curve (AUC) (see *Pharmacokinetic properties*). Therefore ingestion with food might be considered when required due to clinical reasons.

The therapy should be initiated by a physician experienced in the management of HIV infection.

*Renal impairment:* Lamivudine levels are increased in patients with moderate–severe renal impairment due to decreased clearance. The dose should therefore be adjusted, using the oral solution presentation of Epivir for patients whose creatinine clearance falls below 30 ml/min (see table).

| Renal function (Clcr, ml/min) | First dose | Maintenance dose |
| --- | --- | --- |
| Clcr≥50 | 150 mg | 150 mg Twice daily |
| 50>Clcr≥30 | 150 mg | 150 mg Once daily |
| Clcr<30 | As doses below 150 mg are needed the use of the oral solution is recommended | |

*Hepatic impairment:* The influence of hepatic impairment on lamivudine levels is under investigation. Lamivudine clearance is largely renal. Based on preliminary safety data no dosage adjustment is necessary.

*Contra-indications:* The use of Epivir is contra-indicated in patients with known hypersensitivity to lamivudine or to any ingredient of the preparation.

*Special warnings and special precautions for use:*
*Special warnings:* Epivir is not recommended for use as monotherapy.

Cases of pancreatitis have occurred rarely. However it is not clear whether these cases were due to drug treatment or to the underlying HIV disease. Treatment with Epivir should be stopped immediately if clinical signs, symptoms or laboratory abnormalities suggestive of pancreatitis occur.

There are insufficient data on the use of Epivir in children under the age of 12 years.

Administration of Epivir is not recommended during the first 3 months of pregnancy (see *Pregnancy and lactation*).

Patients receiving Epivir or any other antiretroviral therapy may continue to develop opportunistic infections and other complications of HIV infection, and therefore should remain under close clinical observation by physicians experienced in the treatment of patients with associated HIV diseases.

Patients should be advised that current antiretroviral therapy, including Epivir, has not been proven to prevent the risk of transmission of HIV to others through sexual conduct or blood contamination. Appropriate precautions should continue to be employed.

*Special precautions for use:* In patients with moderate–severe renal impairment, the terminal plasma half-life of lamivudine is increased due to decreased clearance. The dose should be adjusted. (See dosage in renal impairment, in *Posology and method of administration* section).

Epivir should be used with caution in patients with advanced cirrhotic liver disease due to chronic Hepatitis B infection, as there is a small risk of rebound hepatitis if treatment is discontinued.

*Interaction with other medicaments and other forms of interaction:* The likelihood of metabolic interactions is low due to limited metabolism and plasma protein binding and almost complete renal clearance.

A modest increase in $C_{max}$ (28%) was observed for zidovudine when administered with lamivudine, however overall exposure (AUC) is not significantly altered. Zidovudine has no effect on the pharmacokinetics of lamivudine (see *Pharmacokinetic properties* section).

The possibility of interactions with other drugs administered concurrently should be considered, particularly when the main route of elimination is active renal secretion via the organic cationic transport system e.g. trimethoprim. Other drugs (e.g. ranitidine, cimetidine) are eliminated only in part by this mechanism and were shown not to interact with lamivudine. The nucleoside analogues (e.g.

didanosine and zalcitabine) like zidovudine, are not eliminated by this mechanism and are unlikely to interact with lamivudine.

Administration of prophylactic doses of co-trimoxazole results in a 40% increase in lamivudine exposure, because of the trimethoprim component; the sulphamethoxazole component did not interact. However, unless the patient has renal impairment, no dosage adjustment of lamivudine is necessary (see *Posology and method of administration*). When concomitant administration is warranted, patients should be monitored clinically. Co-administration of Epivir with high doses of co-trimoxazole for the treatment of Pneumocystis carinii pneumonia (PCP) and toxoplasmosis should be avoided. Lamivudine has no effect on the pharmacokinetics of co-trimoxazole.

Lamivudine metabolism does not involve CYP3A, making interactions with drugs metabolised by this system (e.g. protease inhibitors) unlikely.

Co-administration of Epivir with intravenous ganciclovir or foscarnet is not recommended until further information is available.

*Use during pregnancy and lactation:*
*Pregnancy:* The safety of lamivudine in human pregnancy has not been established. Reproductive studies in animals have not shown evidence of teratogenicity, and showed no effect on male or female fertility. Lamivudine induces early embryolethality when administered to pregnant rabbits at exposure levels comparable to those achieved in man. Lamivudine crosses the placenta in animals but there is no information on placental transfer in humans.

Although animal reproductive studies are not always predictive of the human response, administration during the first three months of pregnancy is not recommended (see *Special warnings and special precautions for use*).

*Lactation:* A study in lactating rats showed that, following oral administration, lamivudine was concentrated four fold and excreted in the milk. It is not known if lamivudine is excreted in human breast milk. Since the drug may pass into breast milk, it is recommended that mothers taking Epivir do not breast feed their infants. Some health experts recommended that HIV infected women do not breast feed their infants under any circumstances in order to avoid transmission of HIV.

*Effects on ability to drive and use machines:* There have been no studies to investigate the effect of lamivudine on driving performance or the ability to operate machinery. Further, a detrimental effect on such activities cannot be predicted from the pharmacology of the drug. Nevertheless, the clinical status of the patient and the adverse event profile of Epivir should be borne in mind when considering the patient's ability to drive or operate machinery.

*Undesirable effects:* Adverse events have been reported during therapy for HIV disease with Epivir alone and in combination with zidovudine. With many it is unclear whether they are drug related or are as a result of the underlying disease process.

Adverse events which have been commonly reported are headache, malaise, fatigue, nausea, diarrhoea, vomiting, abdominal pain or cramps, insomnia, cough, nasal symptoms and musculoskeletal pain.

Cases of pancreatitis and peripheral neuropathy (or paraesthesia) have been recorded, although no relationship to the dose of Epivir has been noted.

Neutropenia and anaemia (both occasionally severe) have occurred in combination with zidovudine. Thrombocytopenia, transient rises in liver enzymes (AST, ALT) and rises in serum amylase have been reported.

*Overdose:* Administration of lamivudine at very high dose levels in acute animal studies did not result in any organ toxicity. Limited data are available on the consequences of ingestion of acute overdoses in humans. No fatalities occurred, and the patients recovered. No specific signs or symptoms have been identified following such overdose.

If overdosage occurs the patient should be monitored, and standard supportive treatment applied as required. Since lamivudine is dialysable, continuous haemodialysis could be used in the treatment of overdosage, although this has not been studied.

## Pharmacological properties
*Pharmacodynamic properties:* Pharmacotherapeutic group—nucleoside analogue, ATC Code: J05A B10.

Lamivudine is a nucleoside analogue. Lamivudine is metabolised intracellularly to lamivudine 5′-triphosphate, its main mode of action is as a chain terminator of HIV reverse transcription. The triphosphate has selective inhibitory activity against HIV-1 and HIV-2 replication *in vitro*, it is also active against zidovudine-resistant clinical isolates of HIV.

The relationships between *in vitro* susceptibility of HIV to lamivudine and the clinical response to therapy remain under investigation. *In vitro* sensitivity testing

has not been standardised and results may vary according to methodological factors.

Reduced *in vitro* sensitivity to lamivudine has been reported for HIV isolates from patients who have received Epivir therapy.

Lamivudine has been shown to be highly synergistic with zidovudine, inhibiting the replication of HIV in cell culture.

*In vitro* studies indicate that zidovudine-resistant virus isolates can become zidovudine sensitive when they simultaneously acquire resistance to lamivudine. Furthermore, *in vivo*, there is evidence showing that lamivudine plus zidovudine delays the emergence of zidovudine-resistant isolates in individuals with no prior antiretroviral therapy.

*In vitro*, lamivudine demonstrates low cytotoxicity to peripheral blood lymphocytes, to established lymphocyte and monocyte-macrophage cell lines and to a variety of bone marrow progenitor cells *in vitro*. Lamivudine therefore has, *in vitro*, a high therapeutic index.

*Pharmacokinetic properties:*
*Absorption:* Lamivudine is well absorbed from the gut, and the bioavailability of oral lamivudine in adults is normally between 80 and 85%. Following oral administration, the mean time ($t_{max}$) to maximal serum concentrations ($C_{max}$) is about an hour. At therapeutic dose levels i.e. 4 mg/kg/day (as two 12-hourly doses), $C_{max}$ is in the order of 1.5–1.9 mcg/ml.

Co-administration of lamivudine with food results in a delay of $t_{max}$ and a lower $C_{max}$ (decreased by 47%). However, lamivudine bioavailability (based on the AUC) is not influenced.

Co-administration of zidovudine results in a 13% increase in zidovudine exposure and a 28% increase in peak plasma levels. This is not considered to be of significance to patient safety and therefore no dosage adjustments are necessary.

*Distribution:* From intravenous studies, the mean volume of distribution is 1.3 L/kg. The observed half-life of elimination is 5 to 7 hours. The mean systemic clearance of lamivudine is approximately 0.32 L/h/kg, with predominantly renal clearance (>70%) via the organic cationic transport system.

Lamivudine exhibits linear pharmacokinetics over the therapeutic dose range and displays limited binding to the major plasma protein albumin (<16%–36% to serum albumin in *in vitro* studies).

Limited data shows lamivudine penetrates the central nervous system and reaches the cerebrospinal fluid (CSF). The mean ratio CSF/serum lamivudine concentration 2–4 hours after oral administration was approximately 0.12. The true extent of penetration or relationship with any clinical efficacy is unknown.

*Metabolism:* Lamivudine is predominantly cleared by renal excretion of unchanged drug. The likelihood of metabolic drug interactions with lamivudine is low due to the small extent of hepatic metabolism (5–10%) and low plasma protein binding.

*Elimination:* Studies in patients with renal impairment show lamivudine elimination is affected by renal dysfunction. A recommended dosage regimen for patients with creatinine clearance below 50 ml/min is shown in the dosage section (see *Posology and method of administration*).

An interaction with trimethoprim, a constituent of co-trimoxazole, causes a 40% increase in lamivudine exposure at therapeutic doses. This does not require dose adjustment unless the patient also has renal impairment (see *Interaction with other medicaments and other forms of interaction*, and dosage adjustments in renal impairment in *Posology and method of administration* section). Administration of co-trimoxazole with Epivir in patients with renal impairment should be carefully assessed.

*Preclinical safety data:* Administration of lamivudine in animal toxicity studies at high doses was not associated with any major organ toxicity. At the highest dosage levels, minor effects on indicators of liver and kidney function were seen together with occasional reductions in liver weight. The clinically relevant effects noted were a reduction in red blood cell count and neutropenia.

Lamivudine was not mutagenic in bacterial tests but, like many nucleoside analogues, showed activity in an *in vitro* cytogenetic assay and the mouse lymphoma assay. Lamivudine was not genotoxic *in vivo* at doses that gave plasma concentrations around 40–50 times higher than the anticipated clinical plasma levels. As the *in vitro* mutagenic activity of lamivudine could not be confirmed in *in vivo* tests, it is concluded that lamivudine should not represent a genotoxic hazard to patients undergoing treatment.

Long term carcinogenicity studies in animals are ongoing.

## Pharmaceutical particulars
*List of excipients:* Tablet core: Cellulose, Microcrystal-

line PhEur (E460); Sodium Starch Glycollate BP; Magnesium Stearate PhEur (E572).

Tablet Film Coat: Methylhydroxypropyl Cellulose PhEur (E464); Titanium Dioxide PhEur (E171); Macrogol PhEur; Polysorbate 80 PhEur (E433); Purified Water PhEur.

*Incompatibilities:* None reported.

*Shelf life:* 2 years.

*Special precautions for storage:* Store between 2 and 30°C.

*Nature and contents of container:* Cartons containing 60 coated tablets in a white high density polyethylene (HDPE) bottle, with a child-resistant closure.

*Instructions for use/handling:* None required.

**Marketing authorisation number** EU/1/96/015/001

**Date of approval/revision of SPC** May 1997

**Legal category** POM.

# EUMOVATE* CREAM AND OINTMENT

**Presentation** Eumovate Cream and Ointment contain 0.05% clobetasone butyrate, and are white in appearance. The emollient cream is water-miscible, whilst the ointment has a paraffin base.

**Uses** Clobetasone butyrate is a topically active corticosteroid which provides an exceptional combination of activity and safety. When formulated as Eumovate, it is more effective in the treatment of eczemas than 1% hydrocortisone, or the less-active synthetic steroid preparations that are in common use, yet has little effect on hypothalamic-pituitary-adrenal function. This has been so even when Eumovate was applied to adults in large amounts under whole-body occlusion. All topical corticosteroids can cause cutaneous atrophy if grossly misused. However, studies in animal and human models indicate that Eumovate and hydrocortisone cause less thinning of the epidermis than the other topical steroids tested.

Eumovate is suitable for the treatment of eczema and dermatitis of all types including atopic eczema, photodermatitis, otitis externa, primary irritant and allergic dermatitis (including napkin rash), intertrigo, prurigo nodularis, seborrhoeic dermatitis and insect bite reactions.

Eumovate may be used as maintenance therapy between courses of one of the more active topical steroids.

**Dosage and administration** Eumovate should be applied to the affected area up to four times a day until improvement occurs, when the frequency of application may be reduced.

**Contra-indications, warnings, etc**
*Contra-indications:* Skin lesions caused by infection with viruses (e.g. herpes simplex, chickenpox), fungi (e.g. candidiasis, tinea) or bacteria (e.g. impetigo).

Hypersensitivity to the preparations.

*Precautions:* Although generally regarded as safe, even for long-term administration in adults, there is a potential for overdosage, and in infants and children this may result in adrenal suppression. Extreme caution is required in dermatoses in such patients including napkin eruption (as the napkin may act as an occlusive dressing and increase absorption) and treatment should not normally exceed seven days.

Appropriate antimicrobial therapy should be used whenever treating inflammatory lesions which have become infected. Any spread of infection requires withdrawal of topical corticosteroid therapy, and systemic administration of antimicrobial agents.

As with all corticosteroids, prolonged application to the face is undesirable.

Topical corticosteroids may be hazardous in psoriasis for a number of reasons including rebound relapses, development of tolerance, risk of generalised pustular psoriasis and development of local or systemic toxicity due to impaired barrier function of the skin. If used in psoriasis, careful patient supervision is important.

If applied to the eyelids, care is needed to ensure that the preparation does not enter the eye as glaucoma might result.

*Pregnancy:* There is inadequate evidence of safety in human pregnancy. Topical administration of corticosteroids to pregnant animals can cause abnormalities of fetal development including cleft palate and intrauterine growth retardation. There may therefore be a very small risk of such effects in the human fetus.

*Side-effects:* In the unlikely event of signs of hypersensitivity appearing, application should stop immediately. When large areas of the body are being treated with Eumovate, it is possible that some patients will absorb sufficient steroid to cause transient adrenal suppression despite the low degree of systemic activity associated with clobetasone butyrate.

Local atrophic changes could possibly occur in situations where moisture increases absorption of clobetasone butyrate, but only after prolonged use.

There are reports of pigmentation changes and hypertrichosis with topical steroids.

Exacerbation of symptoms may occur.

*Overdosage:* Acute overdosage is very unlikely to occur, however, in the case of chronic overdosage or misuse the features of hypercorticism may appear and in this situation topical steroids should be discontinued.

**Pharmaceutical precautions** None.

**Legal category** POM.

**Package quantities** Tubes of 30 and 100 g.

**Further information** The least potent corticosteroid which will control the disease should be selected. Neither of these preparations contain lanolin or parabens.

**Product licence numbers**
Eumovate Cream 10949/0035
Eumovate Ointment 10949/0037

# FORTUM* FOR INJECTION

**Qualitative and quantitative composition** Fortum for Injection: Vials contain either 250 mg, 500 mg, 1 g, 2 g or 3 g ceftazidime (as pentahydrate) with sodium carbonate (118 mg per gram of ceftazidime).

Fortum Monovial in a vial containing 2 g ceftazidime pentahydrate.

**Pharmaceutical form** Sterile powder for constitution for injection.

**Clinical particulars**

*Therapeutic indications:*
Single infections
Mixed infections caused by two or more susceptible organisms
Severe infections in general
Respiratory tract infections
Ear, nose and throat infections
Urinary tract infections
Skin and soft tissue infections
Gastrointestinal, biliary and abdominal infections
Bone and joint infections
Dialysis: infections associated with haemo– and peritoneal dialysis and with continuous peritoneal dialysis (CAPD)

In meningitis it is recommended that the results of a sensitivity test are known before treatment with ceftazidime as a single agent. It may be used for infections caused by organisms resistant to other antibiotics including aminoglycosides and many cephalosporins. When appropriate, however, it may be used in combination with an aminoglycoside or other β-lactam antibiotic for example, in the presence of severe neutropenia, or with an antibiotic active against anaerobes when the presence of *Bacteroides fragilis* is suspected. In addition, ceftazidime is indicated in the perioperative prophylaxis of transurethral prostatectomy.

Bacteriology: Ceftazidime is bactericidal in action, exerting its effect on target cell wall proteins and causing inhibition of cell wall synthesis. A wide range of pathogenic strains and isolates associated with hospital-acquired infections are susceptible to ceftazidime *in vitro*, including strains resistant to gentamicin and other aminoglycosides. It is highly stable to most clinically important β-lactamases produced by both gram-positive and gram-negative organisms and consequently is active against many ampicillin- and cephalothin-resistant strains. Ceftazidime has high intrinsic activity *in vitro* and acts within a narrow mic range for most genera with minimal changes in mic at varied inoculum levels. Ceftazidime has been shown to have *in vitro* activity against the following organisms:

Gram-negative: *Pseudomonas aeruginosa,* Pseudomonas spp (other), *Klebsiella pneumoniae,* Klebsiella spp (other), *Proteus mirabilis, Proteus vulgaris, Morganella morganii* (formerly *Proteus morganii), Proteus rettgeri, Providencia* spp, *Escherichia coli,* Enterobacter spp, Citrobacter spp, Serratia spp, Salmonella spp, Shigella spp, *Yersinia enterocolitica, Pasteurella multocida,* Acinetobacter spp, *Neisseria gonorrhoeae, Neisseria meningitidis, Haemophilus influenzae* (including ampicillin-resistant strains), *Haemophilus parainfluenzae* (including ampicillin-resistant strains).

Gram-positive: *Staphylococcus aureus* (methicillin-sensitive strains), *Staphylococcus epidermidis* (methicillin-sensitive strains), Micrococcus spp, *Streptococcus pyogenes,* Streptococcus group b, *Streptococcus pneumoniae, Streptococcus mitis,* Streptococcus spp (excluding *Enterococcus (Streptococcus) faecalis).*

Anaerobic strains: Peptococcus spp, Peptostreptococcus spp, Streptococcus spp, Propionibacterium

spp, *Clostridium perfringens,* Fusobacterium spp, Bacteroides spp (many strains of *Bact. fragilis* are resistant).

Ceftazidime is not active *in vitro* against methicillin-resistant staphylococci, *Enterococcus (Streptococcus) faecalis* and many other enterococci, *Listeria monocytogenes,* Campylobacter spp or *Clostridium difficile.*

*In vitro* the activities of ceftazidime and aminoglycoside antibiotics in combination have been shown to be at least additive; there is evidence of synergy in some strains tested. This property may be important in the treatment of febrile neutropenic patients.

*Posology and method of administration:* Ceftazidime is to be used by the parenteral route, the dosage depending upon the severity, sensitivity and type of infection and the age, weight and renal function of the patient.

*Adults:* The adult dosage range for ceftazidime is 1 to 6 g per day 8 or 12 hourly (i.m. or i.v.). In the majority of infections, 1 g 8-hourly or 2 g 12-hourly should be given. In urinary tract infections and in many less serious infections, 500 mg or 1 g 12-hourly is usually adequate. In very severe infections, especially immunocompromised patients, including those with neutropenia, 2 g 8 or 12-hourly or 3 g 12-hourly should be administered.

When used as a prophylactic agent in prostatic surgery 1 g (from the 1 g vial) should be given at the induction of anaesthesia. A second dose should be considered at the time of catheter removal.

*Elderly:* In view of the reduced clearance of ceftazidime in acutely ill elderly patients, the daily dosage should not normally exceed 3 g, especially in those over 80 years of age.

*Cystic fibrosis:* In fibrocystic adults with normal renal function who have pseudomonal lung infections, high doses of 100 to 150 mg/kg/day as three divided doses should be used. In adults with normal renal function 9 g/day has been used.

*Infants and children:* The usual dosage range for children aged over two months is 30 to 100 mg/kg/day, given as two or three divided doses.

Doses up to 150 mg/kg/day (maximum 6 g daily) in three divided doses may be given to infected immunocompromised or fibrocystic children or children with meningitis.

*Neonates and children up to 2 months of age:* Whilst clinical experience is limited, a dose of 25 to 60 mg/kg/day given as two divided doses has proved to be effective. In the neonate the serum half-life of ceftazidime can be three to four times that in adults.

*Dosage in impaired renal function:* Ceftazidime is excreted by the kidneys almost exclusively by glomerular filtration. Therefore, in patients with impaired renal function it is recommended that the dosage of ceftazidime should be reduced to compensate for its slower excretion, except in mild impairment, i.e. glomerular filtration rate (GFR) greater than 50 ml/min. In patients with suspected renal insufficiency, an initial loading dose of 1 g of ceftazidime may be given. An estimate of GFR should be made to determine the appropriate maintenance dose.

*Renal impairment:* For patients in renal failure on continuous arteriovenous haemodialysis or high-flux haemofiltration in intensive therapy units, it is recommended that the dosage should be 1 g daily in divided doses. For low-flux haemofiltration it is recommended that the dosage should be that suggested under impaired renal function.

Recommended maintenance doses are shown below:

*Recommended maintenance doses of ceftazidime in renal insufficiency:*

| Creatinine clearance ml/min | Approx. serum creatinine* µmol/l (mg/dl) | Recommended unit dose of ceftazidime (g) | Frequency of dosing (hourly) |
|---|---|---|---|
| 50-31 | 150-200 (1.7-2.3) | 1 | 12 |
| 30-16 | 200-350 (2.3-4.0) | 1 | 24 |
| 15-6 | 350-500 (4.0-5.6) | 0.5 | 24 |
| <5 | >500 (>5.6) | 0.5 | 48 |

* These values are guidelines and may not accurately predict renal function in all patients especially in the elderly in whom the serum creatinine concentration may overestimate renal function.

In patients with severe infections, especially in neutropenics, who would normally receive 6 g of ceftazidime daily were it not for renal insufficiency, the unit dose given in the table above may be increased by 50% or the dosing frequency increased appropriately. In such patients it is recommended that ceftazidime serum levels should be monitored and trough levels should not exceed 40 mg/litre.

When only serum creatinine is available, the following

formula (Cockcroft's equation) may be used to estimate creatinine clearance. The serum creatinine should represent a steady state of renal function:

Males:
Creatinine clearance (ml/min) =

$$\frac{\text{Weight (kg)} \times (140-\text{age in years})}{72 \times \text{serum creatinine (mg/dl)}}$$

Females:
0.85 x above value.
To convert serum creatinine in µmol/litre into mg/dl divide by 88.4.
In children the creatinine clearance should be adjusted for body surface area or lean body mass and the dosing frequency reduced in cases of renal insufficiency as for adults.
The serum half-life of ceftazidime during haemodialysis ranges from 3 to 5 hours. The appropriate maintenance dose of ceftazidime should be repeated following each haemodialysis period.
Dosage in peritoneal dialysis: Ceftazidime may also be used in peritoneal dialysis and continuous ambulatory peritoneal dialysis (CAPD). As well as using ceftazidime intravenously, it can be incorporated into the dialysis fluid (usually 125 to 250 mg for 2L of dialysis fluid).
Administration: Ceftazidime may be given intravenously or by deep intramuscular injection into a large muscle mass such as the upper outer quadrant of the gluteus maximus or lateral part of the thigh.

Contra-indications: Ceftazidime is contra-indicated in patients with known hypersensitivity to cephalosporin antibiotics.

Special warnings and special precautions for use:
Hypersensitivity reactions: As with other β-lactam antibiotics, before therapy with ceftazidime is instituted, careful inquiry should be made for a history of hypersensitivity reactions to ceftazidime, cephalosporins, penicillins or other drugs. Ceftazidime should be given only with special caution to patients with type I or immediate hypersensitivity reactions to penicillin. If an allergic reaction to ceftazidime occurs, discontinue the drug. Serious hypersensitivity reactions may require epinephrine (adrenaline), hydrocortisone, antihistamine or other emergency measures.
Renal function: Cephalosporin antibiotics at high dosage should be given with caution to patients receiving concurrent treatment with nephrotoxic drugs, e.g. aminoglycoside antibiotics, or potent diuretics such as frusemide, as these combinations are suspected of affecting renal function adversely. Clinical experience with ceftazidime has shown that this is not likely to be a problem at the recommended dose levels. There is no evidence that ceftazidime adversely affects renal function at normal therapeutic doses: however, as for all antibiotics eliminated via the kidneys, it is necessary to reduce the dosage according to the degree of reduction in renal function to avoid the clinical consequences of elevated antibiotic levels, e.g. neurological sequelae, which have occasionally been reported when the dose has not been reduced appropriately (see Dosage in Impaired Renal Function).
Overgrowth of non-susceptible organisms: As with other broad spectrum antibiotics, prolonged use of ceftazidime may result in the overgrowth of non-susceptible organisms (e.g. Candida, Enterococci) which may require interruption of treatment or adoption of appropriate measures. Repeated evaluation of the patient's condition is essential.

Interaction with other medicaments and other forms of interaction: Ceftazidime does not interfere with enzyme-based tests for glycosuria. Slight interference with copper reduction methods (Benedict's, Fehling's, Clinitest) may be observed. Ceftazidime does not interfere in the alkaline picrate assay for creatinine. The development of a positive Coombs' test associated with the use of ceftazidime in about 5% of patients may interfere with the cross-matching of blood.
Chloramphenicol is antagonistic in vitro with ceftazidime and other cephalosporins. The clinical relevance of this finding is unknown, but if concurrent administration of ceftazidime with chloramphenicol is proposed, the possibility of antagonism should be considered.

Pregnancy and lactation: There is no experimental evidence of embryopathic or teratogenic effects attributable to ceftazidime but, as with all drugs, it should be administered with caution during the early months of pregnancy and in early infancy. Use in pregnancy requires that the anticipated benefit be weighed against the possible risks.
Ceftazidime is excreted in human milk in low concentrations and consequently caution should be exercised when ceftazidime is administered to a nursing mother.

Effects on ability to drive and use machines: None reported.

Undesirable effects: Clinical trial experience has shown that ceftazidime is generally well tolerated.
Adverse reactions are infrequent and include:
Local: phlebitis or thrombophlebitis with i.v. administration, pain and/or inflammation after i.m. injection.
Hypersensitivity: maculopapular or urticarial rash, fever, pruritus, and very rarely angioedema and anaphylaxis (including bronchospasm and/or hypotension).
As with other cephalosporins, there have been rare reports of toxic epidermal necrolysis.
Gastrointestinal: diarrhoea, nausea, vomiting, abdominal pain, and very rarely oral thrush or colitis. As with other cephalosporins, colitis may be associated with Clostridium difficile and may present as pseudomembranous colitis.
Other adverse events which may be related to ceftazidime therapy or of uncertain aetiology include:
Genito-urinary: Candidiasis, vaginitis.
Central nervous system: Headache, dizziness, paraesthesiae and bad taste. There have been reports of neurological sequelae including tremor, myoclonia, convulsions, and encephalopathy in patients with renal impairment in whom the dose of ceftazidime has not been appropriately reduced.
Laboratory test changes noted transiently during ceftazidime therapy include: eosinophilia, positive Coombs' test, very rarely haemolytic anaemia, thrombocytosis and elevations in one or more of the hepatic enzymes, ALT (SGPT), AST (SGOT), LDH, GGT and alkaline phosphatase.
As with some other cephalosporins, transient elevation of blood urea, blood urea nitrogen and/or serum creatinine have been observed occasionally. Very rarely, leucopenia, neutropenia, agranulocytosis, thrombocytopenia and lymphocytosis have been seen.

Overdose: Overdosage can lead to neurological sequelae including encephalopathy, convulsions and coma.
Serum levels of ceftazidime can be reduced by dialysis.

**Pharmacological properties**

Pharmacodynamic properties: Ceftazidime is a bactericidal cephalosporin antibiotic which is resistant to most β-lactamases and is active against a wide range of gram-positive and gram-negative bacteria.

Pharmacokinetic properties: Ceftazidime administered by the parenteral route reaches high and prolonged serum levels in man. After intramuscular administration of 500 mg and 1 g, serum mean peak levels of 18 and 37 mg/litre respectively are rapidly achieved. Five minutes after an intravenous bolus injection of 500 mg, 1 g or 2 g, serum mean levels are respectively 46, 87 and 170 mg/litre.
Therapeutically effective concentrations are still found in the serum 8 to 12 hours after both intravenous and intramuscular administration. The serum half-life is about 1.8 hours in normal volunteers and about 2.2 hours in patients with apparently normal renal function. The serum protein binding of ceftazidime is low at about 10%.
Ceftazidime is not metabolised in the body and is excreted unchanged in the active form into the urine by glomerular filtration. Approximately 80 to 90% of the dose is recovered in the urine within 24 hours. Less than 1% is excreted via the bile, significantly limiting the amount entering the bowel.
Concentrations of ceftazidime in excess of the minimum inhibitory levels for common pathogens can be achieved in tissues such as bone, heart, bile, sputum, aqueous humour, synovial and pleural and peritoneal fluids. Transplacental transfer of the antibiotic readily occurs. Ceftazidime penetrates the intact blood brain barrier poorly and low levels are achieved in the csf in the absence of inflammation. Therapeutic levels of 4 to 20 mg/litre or more are achieved in the csf when the meninges are inflamed.

Preclinical safety data: No additional data of relevance.

**Pharmaceutical particulars**

List of excipients: Sodium carbonate (anhydrous sterile).

Incompatibilities: Ceftazidime is less stable in Sodium Bicarbonate Injection than other intravenous fluids. It is not recommended as a diluent.
Ceftazidime and aminoglycosides should not be mixed in the same giving set or syringe.
Precipitation has been reported when vancomycin has been added to ceftazidime in solution. It is recommended that giving sets and intravenous lines are flushed between administration of these two agents.

Shelf life: Three years when stored below 25˚C and protected from light. Two years for Fortum Monovials when stored below 30˚C and protected from light.

Special precautions for storage: Fortum for Injection should be stored below 25˚C and Fortum Monovial should be stored below 30˚C. Protect from light.

Nature and contents of container: Individually cartoned vials containing 250 mg, 500 mg or 1 g ceftazidime (as pentahydrate) for intramuscular or intravenous use in packs of 5.
Individually cartoned vials containing 2 g ceftazidime (as pentahydrate) for intravenous use in packs of 5.
Individually cartoned vials containing 2 g ceftazidime (as pentahydrate) for intravenous infusion in packs of 5.
Individually cartoned Monovials containing 2 g ceftazidime (as pentahydrate) for intravenous infusion.
Individually cartoned vials containing 3 g ceftazidime (as pentahydrate) for intravenous and intravenous infusion use.
Individually packaged Fortum Saline Infusion Kit containing 2 g ceftazidime (as pentahydrate) with sodium carbonate (118 mg per gram ceftazidime), a 50 ml infusion bag of Sodium Chloride Intravenous Infusion, a transfer needle, a pre-injection swab, a sealing cap and a label for the infusion bag.

Instructions for use/handling: Instructions for constitution: See table for addition volumes and solution concentrations, which may be useful when fractional doses are required.

### Preparation of solution

| Vial size | | Amount of Diluent to be added (ml) | Approximate Concentration (mg/ml) |
|---|---|---|---|
| 250 mg | Intramuscular | 1.0 | 210 |
| 250 mg | Intravenous | 2.5 | 90 |
| 500 mg | Intramuscular | 1.5 | 260 |
| 500 mg | Intravenous | 5.0 | 90 |
| 1 g | Intramuscular | 3.0 | 260 |
| 1 g | Intravenous | 10.0 | 90 |
| 2 g | Intravenous bolus | 10.0 | 170 |
| 2 g | Intravenous Infusion | 50.0* | 40† |
| 3 g | Intravenous bolus | 15.0 | 170 |
| 3 g | Intravenous Infusion | 75.0* | 40† |

*Note: Addition should be in two stages unless using the infusion kit (see text).

†Note: Use Sodium Chloride Injection 0.9%, Dextrose Injection 5% or other approved diluent (see Pharmaceutical particulars) as Water for Injections produces hypotonic solutions at this concentration.

All sizes of vials as supplied are under reduced pressure. As the product dissolves, carbon dioxide is released and a positive pressure develops. For ease of use, it is recommended that the following techniques of reconstitution are adopted.

250 mg i.m./i.v., 500 mg i.m./i.v., 1 g i.m./i.v., and 2 g and 3 g i.v. bolus vials:
1. Insert the syringe needle through the vial closure and inject the recommended volume of diluent. The vacuum may assist entry of the diluent. Remove the syringe needle.
2. Shake to dissolve: carbon dioxide is released and a clear solution will be obtained in about 1 to 2 minutes.
3. Invert the vial. With the syringe plunger fully depressed, insert the needle through the vial closure and withdraw the total volume of solution into the syringe (the pressure in the vial may aid withdrawal). Ensure that the needle remains within the solution and does not enter the head space. The withdrawn solution may contain small bubbles of carbon dioxide; they may be disregarded.

2 g and 3 g i.v. infusion vials:
This vial may be constituted for short intravenous infusion (e.g. up to 30 minutes) as follows:
1. Insert the syringe needle through the vial closure and inject 10 ml of diluent for 2 g vial and 15 ml for 3 g vial. The vacuum may assist entry of the diluent. Remove the syringe needle.
2. Shake to dissolve: carbon dioxide is released and a clear solution obtained in about 1 to 2 minutes.
3. Insert a gas relief needle through the vial closure to relieve the internal pressure and, with the gas relief in position, add a further 40 ml of diluent for 2 g vial and 60 ml for 3 g vial. Remove the gas relief needle and syringe needle; shake the vial and set up for infusion use in the normal way.

NOTE: To preserve product sterility, it is important that a gas relief needle is not inserted through the vial closure before the product has dissolved.

2 g i.v. infusion kit:

Throughout the reconstitution procedure, aseptic technique should be used.

1) Remove the overwrap from the infusion bag. Remove the plastic dust cover from the vial and disinfect the rubber closure by using the Glaxo pre-injection swab.

Break tip off red plastic protector of infusion bag additive port.

2) Grasp transfer needle by central collar and remove either cap from the transfer needle.

3) Keeping the bag uppermost, hold the bag by the additive port and insert the exposed end of the transfer needle into the drug additive port. Please ensure that the bag is not squeezed as this may allow non-sterile air to enter the bag or solution to be expelled.

4) Keeping the bag uppermost, hold the collar of the transfer needle and remove the cover from the other needle of the transfer device. Insert the exposed end of the transfer needle into the vial closure.

5) Hold the bag uppermost and approximately one-third fill the vial by repeatedly squeezing and releasing the bag.

The vial is supplied under reduced pressure.

6) Hold vial/bag assembly centrally and shake, or repeatedly invert to dissolve the powder in the vial. As the antibiotic dissolves, carbon dioxide is released causing frothing which clears quickly. The carbon dioxide will pressurise the bag and vial.

7) Invert the assembly so that the vial is held above the bag and return the solution to the bag by repeatedly squeezing and releasing the bag. Repeat steps 5, 6 and 7 to rinse the inside of the vial.

8) Remove the transfer needle and vial from the bag as a single unit, replace the needle guards and dispose of safely. Squeeze the bag to inspect for minute leaks and examine the solution for visible particles. If in doubt, consult hospital pharmacy.

9) Place clear plastic guard over additive port and push firmly to close. The additive port is now sealed.

10) Complete the patient and drug information label and apply to the unprinted side of the reconstituted infusion bag.

11) Twist off the plastic strip which covers the solution administration set port of the bag and insert a solution administration set connector into the port. Prepare solution administration set according to manufacturers' instructions. The bag will contain a larger gas space than is usually present in an infusion bag. This gas can be carefully vented in a laminar flow cabinet before the solution administration set is attached. If the infusion is given without venting the bag, care should be taken to ensure the infusion is stopped before the gas enters the i.v. line.

Fortum Monovial:

The contents of the Monovial are added to small volume infusion bags containing 0.9% Sodium Chloride Injection or 5% Dextrose Injection, or another compatible fluid.

The 2 g presentation must be constituted in not less than 100 ml infusion bag.

1) Peel off the removable top part of the label and remove the cap.

2) Insert the needle of the Monovial into the additive port of the infusion bag.

3) To activate, push the plastic needle holder of the Monovial down onto the vial shoulder until a 'click' is heard.

4) Holding it upright, fill the vial to approximately two-thirds capacity by squeezing the bag several times.

5) Shake the vial to reconstitute the Fortum.

6) On constitution, the Fortum will effervesce slightly.

7) With the vial uppermost, transfer the reconstituted Fortum into the infusion bag by squeezing and releasing the bag.

8) Repeat the steps 4 to 7 to rinse the inside of the vial. Dispose of the empty Monovial safely. Check that the powder is completely dissolved and that the bag has no leaks.

Fortum Monovial is for i.v. infusion only.

These solutions may be given directly into the vein or introduced into the tubing of a giving set if the patient is receiving parenteral fluids. Ceftazidime is compatible with the most commonly used intravenous fluids.

Vials of Fortum for Injection and Fortum Monovials as supplied are under reduced pressure; a positive pressure is produced on constitution due to the release of carbon dioxide.

Vials of Fortum for Injection should be stored at a temperature below 25°C.

Vials of Fortum for Injection do not contain any preservatives and should be used as single-dose preparations.

The combination pack is intended solely for the preparation of a saline infusion of ceftazidime.

In keeping with good pharmaceutical practice, it is preferable to use freshly constituted solutions of Fortum for Injection. If this is not practicable, satisfactory potency is retained for 24 hours in the refrigerator (2–8°C) when prepared in Water for Injections BP or any of the injections listed below.

At ceftazidime concentrations between 1 mg/ml and 40 mg/ml in:

0.9% Sodium Chloride Injection BP

M/6 Sodium Lactate Injection BP

Compound Sodium Lactate Injection BP (Hartmann's Solution)

5% Dextrose Injection BP

0.225% Sodium Chloride and 5% Dextrose Injection BP

0.45% Sodium Chloride and 5% Dextrose Injection BP

0.9% Sodium Chloride and 5% Dextrose Injection BP

0.18% Sodium Chloride and 4% Dextrose Injection BP

10% Dextrose Injection BP

Dextran 40 Injection BP 10% in 0.9% Sodium Chloride Injection BP

Dextran 40 Injection BP 10% in 5% Dextrose Injection BP

Dextran 70 Injection BP 6% in 0.9% Sodium Chloride Injection BP

Dextran 70 Injection BP 6% in 5% Dextrose Injection BP

(Ceftazidime is less stable in Sodium Bicarbonate Injection than in other intravenous fluids. It is not recommended as a diluent.)

At concentrations of between 0.05 mg/ml and 0.25 mg/ml in Intraperitoneal Dialysis Fluid (Lactate) BPC 1973.

When reconstituted for intramuscular use with: 0.5% or 1% Lignocaine Hydrochloride Injection BP.

When admixed at 4 mg/ml with (both components retain satisfactory potency):

Hydrocortisone (hydrocortisone sodium phosphate) 1 mg/ml in 0.9% Sodium Chloride Injection BP or 5% Dextrose Injection BP

Cefuroxime (cefuroxime sodium) 3 mg/ml in 0.9% Sodium Chloride Injection BP

Cloxacillin (cloxacillin sodium) 4 mg/ml in 0.9% Sodium Chloride Injection BP

Heparin 10u/ml or 50u/ml in 0.9% Sodium Chloride Injection BP

Potassium Chloride 10 mEq/L or 40 Eq/L in 0.g% Sodium Chloride Injection BP

The contents of a 500 mg vial of Fortum for Injection, constituted with 1.5 ml water for injections, may be added to metronidazole injection (500 mg in 100 ml) and both retain their activity.

Solutions range from light yellow to amber depending on concentration, diluent and storage conditions used. Within the stated recommendations, product potency is not adversely affected by such colour variations.

*Marketing authorisation holders:* Fortum: Glaxo Operations UK Ltd, Greenford, Middlesex UB6 OHE

Sodium chloride intravenous infusion: Galen Research Ltd, Craigavon, Northern Ireland BT63 5UA

**Marketing authorisation numbers**

| | |
|---|---|
| 250 mg vials | 0004/0304 |
| 500 mg vials | 0004/0292 |
| 1 gram vials | 0004/0293 |
| 2 and 3 gram vials | 0004/0294 |
| Sodium Chloride Intravenous Infusion | 3460/0015 |

**Date of approval/revision of SPC** 4 October, 1995

**Legal category** POM.

## GRISOVIN* TABLETS

**Presentation** Grisovin Tablets contain 125 mg or 500 mg of the antibiotic griseofulvin in fine particle form. Both are white, film-coated biconvex tablets engraved 'GRISOVIN 125' or 'GRISOVIN 500' on one side as appropriate and 'Glaxo' on the other. They comply with the specification for Griseofulvin Tablets BP, BNF.

**Uses** The treatment of fungal infections of the skin, scalp, hair or nails where topical therapy is considered inappropriate or has failed.

*Mode of action:* Griseofulvin is an antifungal antibiotic which is active *in vitro* against common dermatophytes. It exerts its antifungal effect by disrupting the cell division spindle apparatus of fungal cells, thereby arresting cell division.

When griseofulvin is given orally for systemic treatment of fungal infections, it enables newly-formed keratin of the skin, hair and nails to resist attack by the fungi. As the new keratin extends, the old infected keratin is shed. Grisovin is effective against the dermatophytes causing ringworm (tinea), including: *Microsporum canis* and *T. verrucosum*.

Grisovin is not effective in infections caused by Candida albicans (monilia), Aspergilli, *Malassezia furfur (Pityriasis versicolor)* and Nocardia species.

**Dosage and administration** Doses should be taken after meals, otherwise absorption is likely to be inadequate.

*Adults:* Normally 500 to 1,000 mg daily, but not less than 10 mg/kg bodyweight daily. A single dose daily is often satisfactory, but divided doses may be more effective in patients who respond poorly.

*Children:* Usually 10 mg per kg (5 mg/lb) bodyweight daily in divided doses.

*Duration of treatment:* This depends upon the thickness of keratin at the site of infection. For hair or skin at least four weeks' treatment is required, whereas toe or finger nails may need six to twelve months' treatment. Therapy should be continued for at least two weeks after all signs of infection have disappeared.

**Contra-indications, warnings, etc**

*Contra-indications:* Porphyria or severe liver disease. Griseofulvin may cause liver disease to deteriorate, and liver function should be monitored in such conditions.

*Systemic lupus erythematosus:* Griseofulvin has been reported to exacerbate the condition.

Hypersensitivity to any ingredient of the preparation.

There is no evidence of the safety of Grisovin in human pregnancy. Griseofulvin is teratogenic in animals and some case reports of human fetal abnormalities have been observed. Therefore, Grisovin should not be used in pregnancy, or in women intending to become pregnant within one month following cessation of treatment.

Males should not father children within six months of treatment with Grisovin.

Long term administration of high doses of griseofulvin with food has been reported to induce hepatomas in mice and thyroid tumours in rats but not hamsters. The clinical significance of these findings in man is not known. In view of these data, Grisovin Tablets should not be used prophylactically.

*Contraception/Pregnancy:* Concurrent treatment with griseofulvin may reduce the effectiveness of oral contraceptives, so additional contraceptive precautions should be taken during griseofulvin treatment and for a month after stopping griseofulvin. There is no evidence of its safety in human pregnancy (see *Contra-indications*). Griseofulvin is teratogenic in animals and some case reports suggest that it produces human fetal abnormalities.

As Grisovin is capable of inducing aneuploidy (abnormal segregation of chromosomes following cell division) in mammalian cells exposed to the compound *in vitro* and *in vivo*, women should be warned that they should not take the drug during pregnancy or become pregnant within one month following cessation of treatment.

Additionally, males should not father children within six months of treatment.

*Lactation:* It is not known if griseofulvin is excreted in human milk. Safety in children of mothers who are breast-feeding has not been established.

*Precautions:* Griseofulvin may decrease the effect of the coumarin anti-coagulants.

Absorption of griseofulvin is inhibited when phenobarbitone is taken concurrently. The blood level, and hence efficacy, of griseofulvin may also be impaired as the result of concurrent administration of substances such as phenylbutazone and sedative and hypnotic drugs which induce metabolising enzymes.

Patients should be warned that an enhancement of the effects of alcohol by griseofulvin has been reported.

*Side-effects:* Headache and gastric discomfort sometimes occur, but usually disappear as treatment continues. On rare occasions urticarial reactions, skin rashes and precipitation of systemic lupus erythematosus have been reported.

Toxic epidermal necrolysis and erythema multiforme have been reported.

There have been reports of central nervous system effects e.g. confusion, dizziness, impaired co-ordination and peripheral neuropathy.

Leucopenia with neutropenia has been reported.

Photosensitivity reactions can occur on exposure to intense natural or artificial sunlight.

In those rare cases where individuals are affected by drowsiness while taking griseofulvin, they should not drive vehicles or operate machinery.

*Overdosage:* Treatment is unlikely to be required in cases of acute overdosage.

**Pharmaceutical precautions** None.

*Pharmacokinetics* The absorption of griseofulvin from the gastrointestinal tract is variable and incomplete. On average, less than 50% of the oral dose is absorbed, but fatty foods and a reduction in particle size will increase the rate and extent of the absorption.

After oral dosing there is a phase of rapid absorption followed by slower prolonged absorption. Peak plasma levels (0.5–1.5 micrograms after a 500 mg oral dose) are achieved by 4 hours and are maintained for 10–20 hours. The terminal plasma half-life ranges from 9.5–21 hours, there being considerable intersubject variability. In plasma, griseofulvin is approximately 84% bound to plasma proteins, predominantly albumin.

The absorbed griseofulvin is excreted in the urine mainly as 6-desmethylgriseofulvin or its glucuronide conjugate.

There is selective deposition of griseofulvin in newly-formed keratin of hair, nails and skin, which gradually moves to the surface of these appendages.

**Legal category** POM.

**Package quantities** *125 mg Tablets:* Bottles of 100 tablets (OP). *500 mg Tablets*: Bottles of 100 tablets (OP).

**Further information** Customary hygienic measures should be adopted to minimise the risk of re-infection, and concurrent use of a topical fungicide may be helpful to minimise any spread of infective material.

**Product licence numbers**
Grisovin Tablets 125 mg 10949/0100
Grisovin Tablets 500 mg 10949/0101

## IMIGRAN* INJECTION

**Presentation** Imigran Subcutaneous Injection: Pre-filled syringes containing 6 mg of sumatriptan base, as the succinate salt, in an isotonic solution of 0.5 ml. The syringes should be used in conjunction with an auto-injector.

**Uses**
*Indications:* Imigran Subcutaneous Injection is indicated for the acute relief of migraine attacks, with or without aura, and for the acute treatment of cluster headache. Imigran should only be used where there is a clear diagnosis of migraine or cluster headache.

*Mode of action/pharmacology:* Sumatriptan has been demonstrated to be a specific and selective 5-hydroxytryptamine$_1$ (5-HT$_1$) receptor agonist with no effect on other 5-HT receptor subtypes. This receptor is found predominantly in cranial blood vessels, and, in animals, sumatriptan selectively constricts the carotid arterial circulation but does not alter cerebral blood flow. The carotid arterial circulation supplies blood to the extracranial and intracranial tissues, such as the meninges. Dilatation of these vessels is thought to be the underlying mechanism of migraine in man. Clinical response begins 10 to 15 minutes following subcutaneous injection.

**Dosage and administration** Imigran should not be used prophylactically.

It is recommended to start the treatment at the first sign of a migraine headache or associated symptoms such as nausea, vomiting or photophobia. The efficacy of sumatriptan is independent of the duration of the attack when starting treatment.

Imigran Injection should be injected subcutaneously using an auto-injector.

Patients should be advised to observe strictly the instruction leaflet for the Imigran auto-injector especially regarding the safe disposal of syringes and needles.

*Migraine:* The recommended adult dose of Imigran is a single 6 mg subcutaneous injection. Patients who do not respond to this dose should not take a second dose of Imigran for the same attack. Imigran may be taken for subsequent attacks. Patients who respond initially but whose migraine returns may take a further dose at any time in the next 24 hours provided that one hour has elapsed since the first dose. The maximum dose in 24 hours is two 6 mg injections (12 mg).

Imigran is recommended as monotherapy for the acute treatment of migraine and should not be given concomitantly with other acute migraine therapies. If a patient fails to respond to a single dose of Imigran there are no reasons, either on theoretical grounds or from limited clinical experience, to withhold products containing aspirin or non-steroidal anti-inflammatory drugs or paracetamol for further treatment of the attack.

*Cluster headache:* The recommended adult dose is a single 6 mg subcutaneous injection for each cluster attack. The maximum dose in 24 hours is two 6 mg injections (12 mg) with a minimum interval of one hour between the two doses.

*Children:* The safety and effectiveness of Imigran in children has not yet been established.

*Use in patients aged more than 65 years:* Experience of the use of Imigran in patients aged over 65 years is limited. The pharmacokinetics do not differ significantly from a younger population but, until further clinical data are available, the use of Imigran in patients aged over 65 years is not recommended.

**Contra-indications, warnings, etc**
*Contra-indications:* Hypersensitivity to any component of the preparation.
Ischaemic heart disease.
Previous myocardial infarction.
Prinzmetal's angina/coronary vasospasm.
Uncontrolled hypertension.

Concomitant use of ergotamine or derivatives of ergotamine and sumatriptan.

Concurrent administration of selective 5-HT re-uptake inhibitors, lithium and monoamine oxidase inhibitors, or use within two weeks of discontinuation of MAOI therapy is contraindicated.

*Warnings:* Imigran should only be used where there is a clear diagnosis of migraine or cluster headache.

The recommended doses of Imigran should not be exceeded.

Imigran Injection should not be given intravenously because of its potential to cause vasospasm.

Before treating headaches in patients not previously diagnosed as migraineurs, and in migraineurs who present with atypical symptoms, care should be taken to exclude other potentially serious neurological conditions. There have been rare reports where patients received sumatriptan for severe headaches which subsequently were shown to have been secondary to an evolving neurological lesion (cerebrovascular accident, subarachnoid haemorrhage). In this regard, it should be noted that migraineurs may be at risk of certain cerebrovascular events (e.g. cerebrovascular accident, transient ischaemic attack).

If a patient does not respond to the first dose a second dose should not be given for the same attack but the opportunity should be taken to review the diagnosis.

Following administration, sumatriptan can be associated with transient symptoms including chest pain and tightness which may be intense and involve the throat. These symptoms may mimic angina pectoris but, in patients in whom cardiac investigations have been performed, they have only rarely been found to be the result of coronary vasospasm. The vasospasm may result in arrhythmias, ischaemic ECG changes or myocardial infarction. If the patient experiences symptoms which are severe or persistent or are consistent with angina, further doses should not be taken until appropriate investigations have been carried out to check for the possibility of ischaemic changes.

Imigran should therefore not be given to patients in whom unrecognised cardiac disease is likely without a prior evaluation for underlying cardiovascular disease. Such patients include post-menopausal women, males over 40 and patients with risk factors for coronary artery disease.

Rare cases of anaphylaxis have been reported and this should be considered as an alternative basis for such symptoms which mimic angina pectoris.

Drowsiness may occur as a result of migraine or its treatment with Imigran. Caution is recommended in patients performing skilled tasks, e.g., driving or operating machinery.

*Precautions:* Sumatriptan may cause short-lived elevation of blood pressure and peripheral vascular resistance. Prolonged vasospastic reactions have been reported with ergotamine. As these effects may be additive, 24 hours should elapse before sumatriptan can be taken following any ergotamine-containing preparation. Conversely, ergotamine-containing preparations should not be taken until 6 hours have elapsed following sumatriptan administration.

Imigran should be administered with caution to patients with conditions which may affect significantly the absorption, metabolism or excretion of the drug e.g. impaired hepatic or renal function.

Imigran should be used with caution in patients with a history of epilepsy or structural brain lesions.

Patients with known hypersensitivity to sulphonamides may exhibit an allergic reaction following administration of Imigran. Reactions may range from cutaneous hypersensitivity to anaphylaxis.

*Pregnancy:* No teratogenic effects have been seen in rats or rabbits and sumatriptan had no effect on the post-natal development of rats.

When administered to pregnant rabbits throughout the period of organogenesis sumatriptan has occasionally caused embryolethality at doses which were sufficiently high to produce maternal toxicity.

In a rat fertility study oral doses of sumatriptan resulting in plasma levels approximately 150 times those seen in man after a 6 mg subcutaneous dose were associated with a reduction in the success of insemination. This effect did not occur during a subcutaneous study where maximum plasma levels achieved approximately 100 times those in man by the subcutaneous route.

As yet, experience of the use of sumatriptan during human pregnancy is limited. Although animal reproduction studies are not always predictive of human response, administration of this drug is not recommended during pregnancy unless the expected benefit to the mother is greater than any possible risk to the fetus.

*Lactation:* Sumatriptan is excreted in breast milk in animals. No data exist in humans. Caution should therefore be exercised when considering the administration of Imigran to a nursing woman.

*Side-effects:* The most common side effect associated with treatment with Imigran administered subcutaneously is transient pain at the site of injection.

Other side effects which have been reported include the following: pain, sensations of tingling, heat, heaviness, pressure or tightness. These symptoms are usually transient and may be intense and can affect any part of the body including the chest and throat. Flushing, dizziness, paraesthesia, and feelings of weakness. These are mostly mild to moderate in intensity and transient. Fatigue and drowsiness have been reported. Nausea and vomiting occurred in some patients but the relationship to Imigran is not clear. Transient increases in blood pressure arising soon after treatment have been recorded. Minor disturbances in liver function tests have occasionally been observed. There have been rare reports of seizures, the majority of these patients have a previous history of epilepsy or structural lesions predisposing to epilepsy. Hypotension and bradycardia have been rarely reported. Hypersensitivity reactions ranging from cutaneous hypersensitivity to, in rare cases, anaphylaxis. Tachycardia and palpitations. In extremely rare cases serious coronary events have been reported which have included cardiac arrhythmias, ischaemic ECG changes or myocardial infarction.

*Interactions:* Studies in healthy subjects show that Imigran does not interact with propranolol, pizotifen or alcohol. Sumatriptan has the potential to interact with lithium, MAOIs, 5-HT re-uptake inhibitors, ergotamine and derivatives of ergotamine (see also *Contra-indications*).

Prolonged vasospastic reactions have been reported with ergotamine. As these effects may be additive, 24 hours should elapse before sumatriptan can be taken following any ergotamine-containing preparation. Conversely, ergotamine-containing preparations should not be taken until 6 hours have elapsed following sumatriptan administration.

*Overdosage:* There have been some reports of overdosage with Imigran Injection. Patients have received single injections of up to 12 mg subcutaneously without significant adverse effects. Doses up to 16 mg subcutaneously were not associated with side effects other than those mentioned. There is no experience of doses greater than these.

If overdosage with Imigran occurs, the patient should be monitored for at least ten hours and standard supportive treatment applied as required.

It is unknown what effect haemodialysis or peritoneal dialysis has on the plasma concentrations of Imigran.

**Pharmaceutical precautions** Imigran Injection should be stored below 30°C and protected from light.

**Legal category** POM.

**Package quantities** *Treatment pack:* 2 pre-filled syringes (in cases) plus an auto-injector, in a plastic tray within a carton.
*Refill pack:* 2 pre-filled syringes (in cases) in a carton.

**Further information**
*Pharmacokinetics:* Following subcutaneous injection, Imigran has a high mean bioavailability (96%) with peak serum concentrations occurring in 25 minutes. Average peak serum concentration after a 6 mg subcutaneous dose is 72ng/ml. The elimination phase half-life is approximately two hours. Plasma protein binding is low (14 to 21%), mean volume of distribution is 170 litres. Mean total plasma clearance is approximately 1, 160 ml/min and the mean renal plasma clearance is approximately 260 ml/min. Non-renal clearance accounts for about 80% of the total clearance suggesting that sumatriptan is eliminated primarily by metabolism. The major metabolite, the indole acetic acid analogue of sumatriptan, is mainly excreted in the urine where it is present as a free acid and the glucuronide conjugate. It has no known 5-HT$_1$ or 5-HT$_2$ activity. Minor metabolites have not been identified.

In a pilot study no significant differences were found in the pharmacokinetic parameters between the elderly and young healthy volunteers.

**Product licence number** Imigran Injection 10949/0113

## IMIGRAN* 20 NASAL SPRAY ▼

**Qualitative and quantitative composition** Imigran 20 Nasal Spray: Unit dose spray device for intranasal administration. The device delivers 20 mg of sumatriptan in 0.1 ml of an aqueous buffered solution.

**Pharmaceutical form** Nasal spray.

**Clinical particulars**

*Therapeutic indications:* Imigran Nasal Spray is indicated for the acute treatment of migraine attacks with or without aura.

*Posology and method of administration:* Imigran Nasal Spray should not be used prophylactically.

Imigran is recommended as monotherapy for the acute treatment of a migraine attack and should not be given concomitantly with ergotamine or derivatives of ergotamine (including methysergide) (see *Contra-indications*).

It is advisable that Imigran be given as early as possible after the onset of a migraine headache. It is equally effective at whatever stage of the attack it is administered.

*Adults:* The optimal dose of Imigran Nasal Spray is 20 mg for administration into one nostril. Although, due to inter/intra patient variability of both the migraine attacks and the absorption of sumatriptan, 10 mg may be effective in some patients.

If a patient does not respond to the first dose of Imigran, a second dose should not be taken for the same attack. However, the attack can be treated with paracetamol, aspirin or non-steroidal anti-inflammatory drugs. Imigran may be taken for subsequent attacks.

If the patient has responded to the first dose, but the symptoms recur, a second dose may be given in the next 24 hours, provided that there is a minimum interval of two hours between the two doses.

No more than two Imigran 20 mg Nasal Sprays to be used in any 24 hour period.

*Children (under 18 years of age):* The safety and effectiveness of Imigran Nasal Spray in children has not yet been established.

*Elderly (over 65):* There is no experience of the use of Imigran Nasal Spray in patients over 65. The kinetics in elderly patients have not been sufficiently studied. Therefore, the use of sumatriptan is not recommended until further data is available.

*Contra-indications:* Hypersensitivity to any component of the preparation.

Sumatriptan should not be given to patients who have had myocardial infarction or have ischaemic heart disease, coronary vasospasm (Prinzmetal's angina), peripheral vascular disease or patients who have symptoms or signs consistent with ischaemic heart disease.

Sumatriptan should not be administered to patients with a history of cerebrovascular accident (CVA) or transient ischaemic attack (TIA).

Sumatriptan should not be administered to patients with severe hepatic impairment.

The use of sumatriptan in patients with uncontrolled hypertension is contra-indicated.

The concomitant administration of ergotamine, or derivatives of ergotamine (including methysergide) is contra-indicated (see *Interactions*).

Concurrent administration of monoamine oxidase inhibitors and sumatriptan is contra-indicated.

Imigran must not be used within two weeks of discontinuation of therapy with monoamine oxidase inhibitors.

*Special warnings and special precautions for use:* Imigran Nasal Spray should only be used where there is a clear diagnosis of migraine. Sumatriptan is not indicated for use in the management of hemiplegic, basilar or ophthalmoplegic migraine.

As with other acute migraine therapies, before treating headaches in patients not previously diagnosed as migraineurs, and in migraineurs who present with atypical symptoms, care should be taken to exclude other potentially serious neurological conditions.

It should be noted that migraineurs may be at increased risk of certain cerebrovascular events (e.g. CVA, TIA).

Following administration, sumatriptan can be associated with transient symptoms including chest pain and tightness which may be intense and involve the throat (see *Side effects*). Where such symptoms are thought to indicate ischaemic heart disease, appropriate evaluation should be carried out.

Sumatriptan should not be given to patients in whom unrecognised cardiac disease is likely without a prior evaluation for underlying cardiovascular disease. Such patients include post-menopausal women, males over 40 and patients with risk factors for coronary artery disease.

Sumatriptan should be administered with caution to patients with controlled hypertension as transient increases in blood pressure and peripheral vascular resistance have been observed in a small proportion of patients.

There have been rare postmarketing reports describing patients with weakness, hyper-reflexia, and inco-ordination following the use of a selective serotonin reuptake inhibitor (SSRI) and sumatriptan. If concomitant treatment with sumatriptan and an SSRI is clinically warranted, appropriate observation of the patient is advised.

Sumatriptan should be administered with caution to patients with conditions which may affect significantly the absorption, metabolism or excretion of the drug, e.g. impaired hepatic or renal function.

Patients with known hypersensitivity to sulphonamides may exhibit an allergic reaction following administration of sumatriptan. Reactions may range from cutaneous hypersensitivity to anaphylaxis.

The recommended dose of Imigran should not be exceeded.

*Interaction with other medicaments and other forms of interaction:* There is no evidence of interactions with propranolol, flunarizine, pizotifen or alcohol.

There are limited data on an interaction with ergotamine containing preparations. The increased risk of coronary vasospasm is a theoretical possibility and concomitant administration is contra-indicated.

The period of time that should elapse between the use of sumatriptan and ergotamine containing preparations is not known. This will also depend on the doses and type of ergotamine containing products used. The effects may be additive. It is advised to wait at least 24 hours following the use of ergotamine containing preparations before administering sumatriptan. Conversely, it is advised to wait at least six hours following use of sumatriptan before administering an ergotamine containing product (see *Contra-indications*).

An interaction may occur between sumatriptan and MAOIs and concomitant administration is contra-indicated (see *Contra-indications*). Rarely an interaction may occur between sumatriptan and SSRIs.

*Pregnancy and lactation:* The safety of this medicinal product for use in human pregnancy has not been established. Evaluation of experimental animal studies does not indicate direct teratogenic effects or harmful effects on peri- and postnatal development.

However, embryofetal viability might be affected in the rabbit. Because animal reproduction studies are not always predictive of human response, administration of this drug should only be considered if the expected benefit to the mother is greater than any possible risk to the fetus.

It has been demonstrated that following subcutaneous administration sumatriptan is secreted into breast milk. Infant exposure can be minimised by avoiding breast feeding for 24 hours after treatment.

*Effects on ability to drive and use machines:* No data are available. Drowsiness may occur as a result of migraine or its treatment with sumatriptan. This may influence the ability to drive and to operate machinery.

*Undesirable effects:*

*General:* The most frequently reported side effect following the use of Imigran Nasal Spray is its taste.

Following administration of Imigran Nasal Spray mild, transient irritation or a burning sensation in the nose or throat or epistaxis have been reported.

The following symptoms are usually transient and may be intense and can affect any part of the body including the chest and throat: pain, sensations of tingling, heat, heaviness, pressure or tightness.

The following symptoms are mostly mild to moderate in intensity and transient: flushing, dizziness, and feelings of weakness.

Fatigue and drowsiness have been reported.

*Cardiovascular:* Hypotension, bradycardia, tachycardia, palpitations.

Transient increases in blood pressure arising soon after treatment have been recorded.

In extremely rare cases serious coronary events have been reported which have included cardiac arrhythmias, transient ischaemic ECG changes or myocardial infarction.

*Gastrointestinal:* Nausea and vomiting occurred in some patients but the relationship to sumatriptan is not clear.

*CNS:* There have been rare reports of seizures, following use of sumatriptan. Although some have occurred in patients with either a history of seizures or concurrent conditions predisposing to seizures, there are also reports in patients where no such predisposing factors are apparent.

*Eye disorders:* Patients treated with Imigran rarely exhibit visual disorders like flickering and diplopia. Additionally cases of nystagmus, scotoma and reduced vision have been observed. Very rarely a transient loss of vision has been reported. However, visual disorders may also occur during a migraine attack itself.

*Hypersensitivity/Skin:* Hypersensitivity reactions ranging from cutaneous hypersensitivity to rare cases of anaphylaxis.

*Laboratory values:* Minor disturbances in liver function tests have occasionally been observed.

*Overdose:* Single doses, of sumatriptan, up to 40 mg intranasally and in excess of 16 mg subcutaneously and 400 mg orally have not been associated with side effects other than those mentioned.

In clinical studies volunteers have received 20 mg of sumatriptan by the intranasal route three times a day for a period of 4 days without significant adverse effects.

If overdosage occurs, the patient should be monitored for at least ten hours and standard supportive treatment applied as required. It is unknown what effect haemodialysis or peritoneal dialysis has on the plasma concentrations of sumatriptan.

**Pharmacological properties**

*Pharmacodynamic properties:* Pharmacotherapeutic group: Analgesics: Other antimigraine preparations. ATC code: N02CX04.

Sumatriptan has been demonstrated to be a selective vascular 5-hydroxytryptamine-1-($5HT_{1d}$) receptor agonist with no effect at other 5HT receptor ($5HT_2$-$5HT_7$) subtypes. The vascular $5HT_{1d}$ receptor is found predominantly in cranial blood vessels and mediates vasoconstriction. In animals sumatriptan selectively constricts the carotid arterial circulation, the carotid arterial circulation supplies blood to the extracranial and intracranial tissues such as the meninges and dilatation and/or oedema formation in these vessels is thought to be the underlying mechanism of migraine in man. In addition, evidence from animal studies suggests that sumatriptan inhibits trigeminal nerve activity. Both these actions (cranial vasoconstriction and inhibition of trigeminal nerve activity) may contribute to the anti-migraine action of sumatriptan in humans.

Clinical response begins 15 minutes following a 20 mg dose given by intra-nasal administration.

Because of its route of administration Imigran Nasal Spray may be particularly suitable for patients who suffer with nausea and vomiting during an attack.

*Pharmacokinetic properties:* After intranasal administration, sumatriptan is rapidly absorbed, maximum plasma concentration occurring in 1–1.5 hours. After a 20 mg dose, the mean maximum concentration is 13 ng/ml. Mean intranasal bioavailability, relative to subcutaneous administration is about 16%, partly due to pre-systemic metabolism.

Following oral administration, pre-systemic clearance is reduced in patients with hepatic impairment resulting in increased plasma levels of sumatriptan, a similar increase would be expected following intra-nasal administration.

Plasma protein binding is low (14–21%), the mean total volume of distribution is 170 litres. The elimination half-life is approximately 2 hours. The mean plasma clearance is approximately 1160 ml/min and the mean renal plasma clearance is approximately 260 ml/min. Non-renal clearance accounts for about 80% of the total clearance. Sumatriptan is eliminated primarily by oxidative metabolism mediated by monoamine oxidase A. The major metabolite, the indole acetic acid analogue of sumatriptan is mainly excreted in urine, where it is present as a free acid and the glucuronide conjugate. It has no known $5HT_1$ or $5HT_2$ activity. Minor metabolites have not been identified. The pharmacokinetics of intra-nasal sumatriptan do not appear to be significantly affected by migraine attacks.

The kinetics in the elderly have been insufficiently studied to justify a statement on possible differences in kinetics between elderly and young volunteers.

*Preclinical safety data:* In studies carried out to test for local and ocular irritancy, following administration of sumatriptan nasal spray, there was no nasal irritancy seen in laboratory animals and no ocular irritancy observed when the spray was applied directly to the eyes of rabbits.

In a rat fertility study a reduction in success of insemination was seen at exposures sufficiently in excess of the maximum human exposure. In rabbits embryolethality, without marked teratogenic defects, was seen. The relevance for humans of these findings is unknown.

Sumatriptan was devoid of genotoxic and carcinogenic activity *in vitro* systems and animal studies.

**Pharmaceutical particulars**

*List of excipients:* Potassium Dihydrogen Phosphate PhEur, Dibasic Sodium Phosphate Anhydrous USP, Sulphuric Acid BP, Sodium Hydroxide PhEur, Purified Water PhEur.

*Incompatibilities:* None reported.

*Shelf life:* 2 years.

*Special precautions for storage:* Imigran Nasal Spray should be stored between 2–30˚C. It should be kept in the sealed blister, preferably in the box, to protect from light.

*Nature and contents of container:* The container

consists of a vial with rubber stopper and applicator. Imigran Nasal 20 mg: unit dose spray device containing 0.1 ml solution. Pack with 2 sprays.

*Instructions for use/handling: See patient information leaflet.*

**Marketing authorisation number**   10949/0261

**Date of approval/revision of SPC**   November 1996

**Legal category**   POM.

## IMIGRAN* TABLETS

**Presentation**   Imigran Tablets 100 mg: white, capsule-shaped, biconvex film-coated tablets engraved 'Imigran' on one face and 'Glaxo' on the other. Each tablet contains 100 mg sumatriptan base (as the succinate salt).

Imigran Tablets 50 mg: pink, capsule-shaped, biconvex film-coated tablets engraved 'Imigran' on one face and '50' on the other. Each tablet contains 50 mg sumatriptan base (as the succinate salt). The 50 mg tablets may also be marked with '50' on one side and blank on the other.

### Uses
*Indications:* Imigran Tablets are indicated for the acute relief of migraine attacks, with or without aura. Imigran should only be used where there is a clear diagnosis of migraine.

*Mode of action/pharmacology:* Sumatriptan has been demonstrated to be a selective 5-hydroxytryptamine$_1$ (5-HT$_1$) receptor agonist with no effect on other 5-HT receptor subtypes. This receptor is found predominantly in cranial blood vessels, and in animals sumatriptan selectively constricts the carotid arterial circulation but does not alter cerebral blood flow. The carotid arterial circulation supplies blood to the extracranial and intracranial tissues such as the meninges. Dilatation of these vessels is thought to be the underlying mechanism of migraine in man. Clinical response begins around 30 minutes following oral administration.

Although the recommended dose of oral Imigran is 50 mg, migraine attacks vary in severity both within and between patients. Doses of 25–100 mg have shown greater efficacy than placebo in clinical trials, but 25 mg is statistically significantly less effective than 50 and 100 mg.

**Dosage and administration**   Imigran should not be used prophylactically.

Imigran should be given as early as possible after the onset of an attack of migraine but it is equally effective at whatever stage of the attack it is administered.

The recommended dose of oral Imigran is a single 50 mg tablet. Some patients may require 100 mg. If symptoms recur, further doses may be given at any time in the next 24 hours provided that not more than 300 mg is taken in any 24-hour period.

Patients who do not respond to the prescribed dose of Imigran should not take a second dose for the same attack.

Imigran is recommended as monotherapy for the acute treatment of migraine and should not be given concomitantly with other acute migraine therapies. If a patient fails to respond to a single dose of Imigran there are no reasons, either on theoretical grounds or from limited clinical experience, to withhold products containing aspirin or non-steroidal anti-inflammatory drugs or paracetamol for further treatment of the attack.

The tablets should be swallowed whole with water.

*Children:* The safety and effectiveness of Imigran in children has not yet been established.

*Use in patients aged more than 65 years:* Experience of the use of Imigran in patients aged over 65 years is limited. The pharmacokinetics do not differ significantly from a younger population but until further clinical data are available, the use of Imigran in patients aged over 65 years is not recommended.

### Contra-indications, warnings, etc
*Contra-indications:*   Hypersensitivity   to   any component of the preparation.
  Ischaemic heart disease.
  Previous myocardial infarction.
  Prinzmetal's angina/coronary vasospasm.
  Uncontrolled hypertension.
  Concomitant use of ergotamine or derivatives of ergotamine and sumatriptan.
  Concurrent administration of selective 5-HT re-uptake inhibitors, lithium and monoamine oxidase inhibitors, or use within two weeks of discontinuation of MAOI therapy is contra-indicated.

*Warnings:* Imigran should only be used where there is a clear diagnosis of migraine.

The recommended doses of Imigran should not be exceeded.

Before treating headaches in patients not previously diagnosed as migraineurs, and in migraineurs who present with atypical symptoms, care should be taken to exclude other potentially serious neurological conditions. There have been rare reports where patients received sumatriptan for severe headaches which subsequently were shown to have been secondary to an evolving neurological lesion (cerebrovascular accident, subarachnoid haemorrhage). In this regard, it should be noted that migraineurs may be at risk of certain cerebrovascular events (e.g. cerebrovascular accident, transient ischaemic attack).

If a patient does not respond to the first dose a second dose should not be given for the same attack but the opportunity should be taken to review the diagnosis.

Following administration, sumatriptan can be associated with transient symptoms including chest pain and tightness which may be intense and involve the throat. These symptoms may mimic angina pectoris but, in patients in whom cardiac investigations have been performed, they have only rarely been found to be the result of coronary vasospasm. The vasospasm may result in arrhythmias, ischaemic ECG changes or myocardial infarction. If the patient experiences symptoms which are severe or persistent or are consistent with angina, further doses should not be taken until appropriate investigations have been carried out to check for the possibility of ischaemic changes.

Imigran should therefore not be given to patients in whom unrecognised cardiac disease is likely without a prior evaluation for underlying cardiovascular disease. Such patients include post-menopausal women, males over 40 and patients with risk factors for coronary artery disease.

Rare cases of anaphylaxis have been reported and this should be considered as an alternative basis for symptoms which mimic angina pectoris.

Drowsiness may occur as a result of migraine or its treatment with Imigran. Caution is recommended in patients performing skilled tasks, e.g. driving or operating machinery.

*Precautions:* Sumatriptan may cause short-lived elevation of blood pressure and peripheral vascular resistance. Prolonged vasospastic reactions have been reported with ergotamine. As these effects may be additive, 24 hours should elapse before sumatriptan can be taken following any ergotamine containing preparation. Conversely, ergotamine containing preparations should not be taken until 6 hours have elapsed following sumatriptan administration.

Imigran should be administered with caution to patients with conditions which may affect significantly the absorption, metabolism or excretion of the drug e.g. impaired hepatic or renal function. A 50 mg dose should be considered in patients with hepatic impairment.

Imigran should be used with caution in patients with a history of epilepsy or structural brain lesions. Patients with known hypersensitivity to sulphonamides may exhibit an allergic reaction following administration of Imigran. Reactions may range from cutaneous hypersensitivity to anaphylaxis.

*Pregnancy:* No teratogenic effects have been seen in rats or rabbits and sumatriptan had no effect on the post-natal development of rats.

When administered to pregnant rabbits throughout the period of organogenesis sumatriptan has occasionally caused embryolethality at doses which were sufficiently high to produce maternal toxicity.

In a rat fertility study oral doses of sumatriptan resulting in plasma levels approximately 200 times those seen in man after a 100 mg oral dose were associated with a reduction in the success of insemination. This effect did not occur during a subcutaneous study where maximum plasma levels achieved approximately 150 times those in man by the oral route.

As yet, experience of the use of sumatriptan during human pregnancy is limited. Although animal reproduction studies are not always predictive of human response, administration of this drug is not recommended during pregnancy unless the expected benefit to the mother is greater than any possible risk to the fetus.

*Lactation:* Sumatriptan is excreted in breast milk in animals. No data exist in humans. Caution should therefore be exercised when considering the administration of Imigran to a nursing woman.

*Side-effects:* Side-effects which have been reported include the following: pain, sensations of tingling, heat, heaviness, pressure or tightness. These symptoms are usually transient and may be intense and can affect any part of the body including the chest and throat. Flushing, dizziness, paraesthesia, and feelings of weakness. These are mostly mild to moderate in intensity and transient. Fatigue and drowsiness have been reported. Nausea and vomiting occurred in some patients but the relationship to Imigran is not clear. Transient increases in blood pressure arising soon after treatment have been recorded. Minor disturbances in liver function tests have occasionally been observed. There have been rare reports of seizures, the majority of these patients have a previous history of epilepsy or structural lesions predisposing to epilepsy. Hypotension and bradycardia have been rarely reported. Hypersensitivity reactions ranging from cutaneous hypersensitivity to, in rare cases, anaphylaxis. Tachycardia and palpitations. In extremely rare cases serious coronary events have been reported which have included cardiac arrhythmias, ischaemic ECG changes or myocardial infarction.

*Interactions:* Studies in healthy subjects show that Imigran does not interact with propranolol, pizotifen or alcohol. Sumatriptan has the potential to interact with lithium, MAOIs, 5-HT re-uptake inhibitors, ergotamine and derivatives of ergotamine (see also *Contra-indications*).

Prolonged vasospastic reactions have been reported with ergotamine. As these effects may be additive, 24 hours should elapse before sumatriptan can be taken following any ergotamine-containing preparation. Conversely, ergotamine-containing preparations should not be taken until 6 hours have elapsed following sumatriptan administration.

*Overdosage:* There have been no reports of overdosage with Imigran Tablets. Doses up to 400 mg orally were not associated with side effects other than those mentioned. There is no experience of doses greater than these.

If overdosage with Imigran occurs, the patient should be monitored for at least ten hours and standard supportive treatment applied as required.

It is unknown what effect haemodialysis or peritoneal dialysis has on the plasma concentrations of Imigran.

**Pharmaceutical precautions**   Imigran Tablets should be stored below 30°C.

**Legal category** POM.

**Package quantities**   Imigran Tablets: A double foil blister pack of 2, 3, 6, or 12 tablets in a wallet with an outer carton.

### Further information
*Pharmacokinetics:* Following oral administration, Imigran is rapidly absorbed, 70% of maximum concentration occurring at 45 minutes. After 100 mg dose the mean maximum plasma concentration is 54 ng/ml. Mean absolute oral bioavailability is 14% partly due to pre-systemic metabolism and partly due to incomplete absorption. The elimination phase half-life is approximately 2 hours, although there is an indication of a longer terminal phase. Plasma protein binding is low (14-21%), mean volume of distribution is 170 litres. Mean total plasma clearance is approximately 1160 ml/min and the mean renal plasma clearance is approximately 260 ml/min. Non-renal clearance accounts for about 80% of the total clearance suggesting that sumatriptan is eliminated primarily by metabolism. The major metabolite, the indole acetic acid analogue of sumatriptan is mainly excreted in the urine, where it is present as a free acid and the glucuronide conjugate. It has no known 5HT$_1$ or 5HT$_2$ activity. Minor metabolites have not been identified. The pharmacokinetics of oral sumatriptan do not appear to be significantly affected by migraine attacks.

In a pilot study no significant differences were found in the pharmacokinetic parameters between the elderly and young healthy volunteers.

**Product licence numbers**
Imigran Tablets 100 mg 10949/0231
Imigran Tablets 50 mg  10949/0222

*Product licence holder:* Glaxo Wellcome UK Limited, Stockley Park West, Uxbridge, Middlesex UB11 1BT.

## IMURAN* TABLETS AND INJECTION

**Presentation**   Yellow, round, biconvex, film-coated tablets, scored and impressed 'WELLCOME K7A' and containing 50 mg Azathioprine BP in each tablet.

Orange, round, biconvex, film-coated tablets, scored and impressed 'L3C' and containing 25 mg Azathioprine BP in each tablet.

*Injection:* A yellow to amber, sterile, freeze-dried powder supplied in clear glass vials containing 50 mg Azathioprine BP as the sodium salt.

The sodium ion content is approximately 4.5 mg (4.5 mEq).

**Uses**   Imuran is used as an immunosuppressant antimetabolite either alone or, more commonly, in combination with other agents (usually corticosteroids) and procedures which influence the immune response. Therapeutic effect may be evident only after weeks or months and can include a steroid-sparing effect, thereby reducing the toxicity associated with high dosage and prolonged usage of corticosteroids.

Imuran, in combination with corticosteroids and/or other immunosuppressive agents and procedures, is indicated to enhance the survival of organ transplants, such as renal transplants, cardiac transplants, and hepatic transplants; and to reduce the corticosteroid requirements of renal transplant recipients.

Imuran, either alone or more usually in combination with corticosteroids and/or other drugs and procedures, has been used with clinical benefit (which may include reduction of dosage or discontinuation of corticosteroids) in a proportion of patients suffering from the following:

severe rheumatoid arthritis;

systemic lupus erythematosus;

dermatomyositis and polymyositis;

auto-immune chronic active hepatitis;

pemphigus vulgaris;

polyarteritis nodosa;

auto-immune haemolytic anaemia;

chronic refractory idiopathic thrombocytopenic purpura.

**Dosage and administration** Imuran Injection should be used ONLY when the oral route is impractical, and should be discontinued as soon as oral therapy is tolerated. It must be administered only by the intravenous route.

Specialist medical literature should be consulted for guidance as to clinical experience in particular conditions.

*Dosage in transplantation–adults and children:* Depending on the immunosuppressive regimen employed, a dosage of up to 5 mg/kg bodyweight/day may be given on the first day of therapy, either orally or intravenously.

Maintenance dosage should range from 1 to 4 mg/kg bodyweight/day and must be adjusted according to clinical requirements and haematological tolerance.

Evidence indicates that Imuran therapy should be maintained indefinitely, even if only low doses are necessary, because of the risk of graft rejection.

*Dosage in other conditions–adults and children:* In general, starting dosage is from 1 to 3 mg/kg bodyweight/day, and should be adjusted, within these limits, depending on the clinical response (which may not be evident for weeks or months) and haematological tolerance.

When therapeutic response is evident, consideration should be given to reducing the maintenance dosage to the lowest level compatible with the maintenance of that response. If no improvement occurs in the patient's condition within 3 months, consideration should be given to withdrawing Imuran.

The maintenance dosage required may range from less than 1 mg/kg bodyweight/day to 3 mg/kg bodyweight/day, depending on the clinical condition being treated and the individual patient response, including haematological tolerance.

In patients with renal and/or hepatic insufficiency, dosages should be given at the lower end of the normal range (see *Precautions* for further details).

*Use in the elderly:* (see *Renal and/or hepatic insufficiency*): There is limited experience of the administration of Imuran to elderly patients. Although the available data do not provide evidence that the incidence of side effects among elderly patients is higher than that among other patients treated with Imuran, it is recommended that the dosages used should be at the lower end of the range.

Particular care should be taken to monitor haematological response and to reduce the maintenance dosage to the minimum required for clinical response.

*Reconstitution and dilution of Imuran Injection:* Precautions should always be taken when handling Imuran Injection (see *Safe handling of Imuran*).

No antimicrobial preservative is included. Therefore, reconstitution and dilution must be carried out under full aseptic conditions, preferably immediately before use. Any unused solution should be discarded.

The contents of each vial should be reconstituted by the addition of 5 ml to 15 ml of Water for Injections BP. The reconstituted solution is stable for up to 5 days when stored between 5°C and 25°C.

When diluted on the basis of 5 ml of reconstituted solution to a volume of between 20 ml and 200 ml of one of the following infusion solutions, Imuran is stable for up to 24 hours at room temperature (15°C to 25°C):

Sodium Chloride Intravenous Infusion BP (0.45% w/v and 0.9% w/v).

Sodium Chloride (0.18% w/v) and Glucose (4.0% w/v) Intravenous Infusion BP.

Should any visible turbidity or crystallisation appear in the reconstituted or diluted solution the preparation must be discarded.

Imuran Injection should ONLY be reconstituted with the recommended volume of Water for Injections BP and should be diluted as specified above. Imuran Injection should not be mixed with other drugs or fluids, except those specified above, before administration.

*Administration of Imuran Injection:* Imuran Injection, when reconstituted as directed, is a very irritant solution with a pH of 10–12.

When the reconstituted solution is diluted as directed above, the pH of the resulting solution may be expected to be within the range pH 8.0 to 9.5 (the greater the dilution, the lower the pH).

Where dilution is not practicable, the reconstituted solution should be injected slowly over a period of not less than one minute and followed immediately by not less than 50 ml of one of the recommended infusion solutions.

Care must be taken to avoid perivenous injection which may produce tissue damage.

*Safe handling of Imuran Injection:* Health professionals who handle Imuran Injection should follow guidelines for the handling of cytotoxic drugs (for example, the Royal Pharmaceutical Society of Great Britain Working Party Report on the Handling of Cytotoxic Drugs, 1983).

Imuran Injection should be prepared for administration either by or under the direct supervision of a pharmacist, or by another specially trained person, who is familiar with its properties and has expertise in the safe handling of similar preparations.

Imuran Injection should be prepared for use in the aseptic unit of a pharmacy, which is equipped with a suitable vertical laminar flow cabinet designed to ensure adequate protection of both operator and product and, preferably, reserved solely for cytotoxic preparations. Where such a facility does not exist, a specially designated side room of a ward or clinic may be used.

Personnel involved with the preparation of Imuran Injection should wear the following protective clothing:

Polyvinylchloride disposable gloves of a suitable quality (rubber gloves are not adequate);

Surgical facemask of suitable quality;

Protective goggles or glasses which should be washed thoroughly with water after use;

Disposable apron.

In an aseptic facility, other suitable clothing will be required.

Any spillage should be dealt with immediately, by mopping with damp, disposable paper towels which are placed in a high-risk waste disposal bag after use. Contaminated surfaces should be washed with copious quantities of water.

Should Imuran Injection solution come into contact with the skin, the skin should be washed thoroughly with soap and plenty of cold water.

If the eyes are contaminated, **immediate** irrigation with sodium chloride eye wash should be carried out and medical attention sought without delay. If sodium chloride solution is not available, large volumes of clean tap water may be used.

*Administration:* The patient's eyes, skin and mucous membranes should be protected from contact with the reconstituted or diluted solution; care should be taken, however, to ensure that the patient is not made unduly anxious by the procedures used.

The patient's clothing, body and bedding should be protected by use of an absorbent disposable layer on top of a waterproof layer.

*Disposal:* Imuran Injection solution should be disposed of in an appropriate manner (for example, deep burial or high-temperature incineration) according to local regulatory requirements.

Disposal of sharp objects, such as needles, syringes, administration sets and ampoules should be in rigid containers labelled with a suitable hazard warning seal. Personnel involved in disposal should be aware of the precautions to be observed, and the material should be destroyed in accordance with local regulatory requirements which may include incineration.

*Safe handling of Imuran Tablets:* Provided that the film-coating is intact, there is no risk in handling film-coated Imuran Tablets. Imuran Tablets should not be divided and, provided the coating is intact, no additional precautions are required when handling them.

**Contra-indications, warnings, etc**

*Contra-indications:* Imuran is contra-indicated in patients known to be hypersensitive to azathioprine. Hypersensitivity to 6-mercaptopurine (6-MP) should alert the prescriber to probable hypersensitivity to Imuran.

Imuran therapy should not be initiated in patients who may be pregnant, or who are likely to become pregnant in the near future (see *Precautions* ).

*Precautions: Monitoring:* There are potential hazards in the use of Imuran. It should be prescribed only if the patient can be adequately monitored for toxic effects throughout the duration of therapy.

It is suggested that during the first 8 weeks of therapy, complete blood counts, including platelets, should be performed weekly or more frequently if high dosage is used or if severe renal and/or hepatic disorder is present. The blood count frequency may be reduced later in therapy, but it is suggested that complete blood counts are repeated monthly, or at least at intervals of not longer than 3 months.

Patients receiving Imuran should be instructed to report immediately any evidence of infection, unexpected bruising or bleeding or other manifestations of bone marrow depression.

There are rare individuals with an inherited deficiency of the enzyme thiopurine methyltransferase (TPMT) who may be unusually sensitive to the myelosuppressive effect of azathioprine and prone to developing rapid bone marrow depression following the initiation of treatment with Imuran.

*Renal and/or hepatic insufficiency:* It has been suggested that the toxicity of Imuran may be enhanced in the presence of renal insufficiency, but controlled studies have not supported this suggestion. Nevertheless, it is recommended that the dosages used should be at the lower end of the normal range and that haematological response should be carefully monitored. Dosage should be further reduced if haematological toxicity occurs.

Caution is necessary during the administration of Imuran to patients with hepatic dysfunction, and regular complete blood counts and liver function tests should be undertaken. In such patients the metabolism of Imuran may be impaired, and the dosage of Imuran should therefore be reduced to the lower end of the recommended range. Dosage should be further reduced if hepatic or haematological toxicity occurs.

Limited evidence suggests that Imuran is not beneficial to patients with hypoxanthine-guanine-phosphoribosyltransferase deficiency (Lesch-Nyhan syndrome). Therefore, given the abnormal metabolism in these patients, it is not prudent to recommend that these patients should receive Imuran.

*Mutagenicity:* Chromosomal abnormalities have been demonstrated in both male and female patients treated with Imuran. It is difficult to assess the role of Imuran in the development of these abnormalities.

Chromosomal abnormalities, which disappear with time, have been demonstrated in lymphocytes from the offspring of patients treated with Imuran. Except in extremely rare cases, no overt physical evidence of abnormality has been observed in the offspring of patients treated with Imuran. Azathioprine and long-wave ultraviolet light have been shown to have a synergistic clastogenic effect in patients treated with azathioprine for a range of disorders.

*Teratogenicity:* Studies in pregnant rats, mice and rabbits using azathioprine in dosages from 5 to 15 mg/kg bodyweight/day over the period of organogenesis have shown varying degrees of fetal abnormalities. Teratogenicity was evident in rabbits at 10 mg/kg bodyweight/day.

Evidence of the teratogenicity of Imuran in man is equivocal. As with all cytotoxic chemotherapy, adequate contraceptive precautions should be advised when either partner is receiving Imuran.

*Carcinogenicity:* There is no clear evidence that, in therapeutic doses, Imuran *per se* is oncogenic in man, but the issue remains unresolved.

The risk of developing post-transplant lymphomas is increased in patients who receive aggressive treatment with immunosuppressive drugs, and such therapy should be maintained at the lowest effective levels. The increased risk of developing lymphomas in immunosuppressed rheumatoid arthritis patients compared with the general population appears to be related at least in part to the disease itself. There have been reports of increased incidences of skin cancers in renal transplant recipients compared with the general population, which may be in part associated with immunosuppressive therapy.

*Effects on fertility:* Relief of chronic renal insufficiency by renal transplantation involving the administration of Imuran has been accompanied by increased fertility in both male and female transplant recipients.

*Drug interactions: Allopurinol/oxipurinol/thiopurinol:* Xanthine oxidase activity is inhibited by allopurinol, oxipurinol and thiopurinol which results in reduced conversion of biologically active 6-thioinosinic acid to biologically inactive 6-thiouric acid. When allopurinol, oxipurinol and/or thiopurinol are given concomitantly with 6-mercaptopurine or azathioprine, the dose of 6-mercaptopurine and azathioprine should be reduced to one-quarter of the original dose.

*Neuromuscular blocking agents:* Imuran can potentiate the neuromuscular blockade produced by depolarising agents such as succinylcholine and can reduce the blockade produced by non-depolarising agents such as tubocurarine. There is considerable variation in the potency of this interaction.

*Warfarin:* Inhibition of the anticoagulant effect of warfarin, when administered with azathioprine, has been reported.

*Cytostatic/myelosuppressive agents:* Where possible, concomitant administration of cytostatic drugs, or drugs which may have a myelosuppressive effect, such as penicillamine, should be avoided. There are conflicting clinical reports of interactions, resulting in serious haematological abnormalities, between Imuran and co-trimoxazole.

There has been a case report suggesting that haematological abnormalities may develop due to the concomitant administration of Imuran and captopril.

It has been suggested that cimetidine and indomethacin may have myelosuppressive effects which may be enhanced by concomitant administration of Imuran.

*Other interactions:* Frusemide has been shown to impair the metabolism of azathioprine by human hepatic tissue *in vitro.* The clinical significance is unknown.

*Vaccines:* The immunosuppressive activity of Imuran could result in an atypical and potentially deleterious response to live vaccines and so the administration of live vaccines to patients receiving Imuran therapy is contra-indicated on theoretical grounds.

A diminished response to killed vaccines is likely and such a response to hepatitis B vaccine has been observed among patients treated with a combination of azathioprine and corticosteroids.

A small clinical study has indicated that standard therapeutic doses of Imuran do not deleteriously affect the response to polyvalent pneumococcal vaccine, as assessed on the basis of mean anti-capsular specific antibody concentration.

*Side- and adverse effects: Hypersensitivity reactions:* Several different clinical syndromes, which appear to be idiosyncratic manifestations of hypersensitivity, have been described occasionally following administration of Imuran. Clinical features include general malaise, dizziness, nausea, vomiting, diarrhoea, fever, rigors, exanthema, rash, myalgia, arthralgia, renal dysfunction and hypotension. In many cases, rechallenge has confirmed an association with Imuran.

Immediate withdrawal of azathioprine and institution of circulatory support where appropriate have led to recovery in the majority of cases. Other marked underlying pathology has contributed to the very rare deaths reported.

Following a hypersensitivity reaction to Imuran, the necessity for continued administration of Imuran should be carefully considered on an individual basis.

*Haematopoiesis:* Therapeutic use of Imuran may be associated with a dose-related, generally reversible, depression of bone marrow function, most frequently expressed as leucopenia, but also sometimes as anaemia and thrombocytopenia.

Reversible, dose-related increases in mean corpuscular volume and red cell haemoglobin content have occurred in association with Imuran therapy. Megaloblastic bone marrow changes have also been observed but severe megaloblastic anaemia and erythroid hypoplasia are rare.

Failure to reduce the dosage of Imuran in the presence of allopurinol can result in severe bone marrow suppression and pancytopenia.

*Susceptibility to infection:* Transplant recipients receiving Imuran and corticosteroids have shown increased susceptibility to viral, fungal and bacterial infections evident both in skin and other body systems. The use of Imuran in other conditions does not appear to give rise to a marked increase in susceptibility to such infections.

*Gastro-intestinal reactions:* A minority of patients experience nausea when first given Imuran. This appears to be relieved by administering the tablets after meals.

Serious complications, including colitis, diverticulitis and bowel perforation, have been described in transplant recipients receiving immunosuppressive therapy. However, the aetiology is not clearly established and high-dose corticosteroids may be implicated. Severe diarrhoea, recurring on rechallenge, has been reported in patients treated with Imuran for inflammatory bowel disease. The possibility that exacerbation of symptoms might be drug-related should be borne in mind when treating such patients.

Pancreatitis has been reported in a small percentage of patients on Imuran therapy, particularly in renal transplant patients and those diagnosed as having inflammatory bowel disease. There are difficulties in relating the pancreatitis to the administration of one particular drug, although rechallenge has confirmed an association with Imuran on occasions.

Cholestasis and deterioration of liver function have occasionally been reported in association with Imuran therapy and are usually reversible on withdrawal of therapy.

A rare, but life-threatening hepatic veno-occlusive disease associated with chronic administration of azathioprine has been described, primarily in transplant patients. In some cases withdrawal of azathioprine has resulted in either a temporary or permanent improvement in liver histology and symptoms.

*Pulmonary reactions:* Reversible pneumonitis has been described very rarely.

*Alopecia:* Hair loss has been described on a number of occasions in patients receiving azathioprine and other immunosuppressive agents. In many instances the condition resolved spontaneously despite continuing therapy. The relationship between alopecia and azathioprine treatment is uncertain.

*Use in pregnancy and lactation:* Imuran should not be given during pregnancy without careful assessment of risk versus benefit.

Azathioprine and/or its metabolites have been found in low concentrations in foetal blood and amniotic fluid after maternal administration of azathioprine.

Leucopenia and/or thrombocytopenia have been reported in a proportion of neonates whose mothers took azathioprine throughout their pregnancies. Extra care in haematological monitoring is advised during pregnancy.

6-mercaptopurine has been identified in the colostrum and breast-milk of women receiving azathioprine treatment.

*Toxicity and treatment of overdosage: Symptoms and signs:* Unexplained infection, ulceration of the throat, bruising and bleeding are the main signs of overdosage with Imuran and result from bone marrow depression which may be maximal after 9 to 14 days. These signs are more likely to be manifest following chronic overdosage, rather than after a single acute overdose. There has been a report of a patient who ingested a single overdose of 7.5 g of azathioprine. The immediate toxic effects of this overdose were nausea, vomiting and diarrhoea, followed by mild leucopenia and mild abnormalities in liver function. Recovery was uneventful.

*Treatment:* There is no specific antidote. Gastric lavage has been used. Subsequent monitoring, including haematological monitoring, is necessary to allow prompt treatment of any adverse effects which may develop. The value of dialysis in patients who have taken an overdose of Imuran is not known, though azathioprine is partially dialysable.

**Pharmaceutical precautions**
*Tablets:* Store below 25°C. Protect from light.
*Injection:* Store below 25°C. Protect from light. Keep dry.

**Legal category** POM.

**Package quantities** Imuran Tablets 25 mg: Blister packs of 100 as 10 blister strips of 10 tablets.

Imuran Tablets 50 mg: Blister packs of 100 as 10 blister strips of 10 tablets and 1000 tablets.

Imuran Injection: Single vials.

**Further information**
*Mode of action:* While the precise modes of action remain to be elucidated, some suggested mechanisms include:
1. the release of 6-MP which acts as a purine antimetabolite.
2. the possible blockade of -SH groups by alkylation.
3. the inhibition of many pathways in nucleic acid biosynthesis, hence preventing proliferation of cells involved in determination and amplification of the immune response.
4. damage to deoxyribonucleic acid (DNA) through incorporation of purine thio-analogues.
Because of these mechanisms, the therapeutic effect of Imuran may be evident only after several weeks or months of treatment.

Imuran appears to be well absorbed from the upper gastro-intestinal tract.

Studies in mice with $^{35}$S-azathioprine showed no unusually large concentration in any particular tissue, but there was very little $^{35}$S found in brain.

Plasma levels of azathioprine and 6-mercaptopurine do not correlate well with the therapeutic efficacy or toxicity of Imuran.

*Pharmacology:* Azathioprine is an imidazole derivative of 6-mercaptopurine (6-MP). It is rapidly broken down *in vivo* into 6-MP and a methylnitroimidazole moiety. The 6-MP readily crosses cell membranes and is converted intracellularly into a number of purine thioanalogues, which include the main active nucleotide, thioinosinic acid. The rate of conversion varies from one person to another. Nucleotides do not traverse cell membranes and therefore do not circulate in body fluids. Irrespective of whether it is given directly or is derived *in vivo* from azathioprine, 6-MP is eliminated mainly as the inactive oxidised metabolite thiouric acid. This oxidation is brought about by xanthine oxidase, an enzyme which is inhibited by allopurinol. The activity of the methylnitroimidazole moiety has not been defined clearly. However, in several systems it appears to modify the activity of azathioprine as compared with that of 6-MP. Determinations of plasma concentrations of azathioprine or 6-MP have no prognostic value as regards effectiveness or toxicity of these compounds.

**Product licence numbers**
Imuran Tablets 25 mg: 0003/0225
Imuran Tablets 50 mg: 0003/0226
Imuran Injection: 0003/5043R

## LANVIS* TABLETS

**Presentation** Each pale greenish yellow biconvex tablet, scored and coded 'WELLCOME U3B', contains 40 mg Thioguanine BP.

**Uses** Lanvis is indicated primarily for the treatment of acute leukaemias, especially acute myelogenous leukaemia and acute lymphoblastic leukaemia.

Lanvis is also used in the treatment of chronic granulocytic leukaemia.

*Mode of action:* Thioguanine is a sulphydryl analogue of guanine and behaves as a purine antimetabolite. It is activated to its nucleotide, thioguanylic acid. Thioguanine metabolites inhibit *de novo* purine synthesis and purine nucleotide interconversions. Thioguanine is also incorporated into nucleic acids and DNA (deoxyribonucleic acid) incorporation is claimed to contribute to the agent's cytotoxicity. Cross resistance usually exists between thioguanine and mercaptopurine, and it is not to be expected that patients resistant to one will respond to the other.

**Dosage and administration** The exact dose and duration of administration will depend on the nature and dosage of other cytotoxic drugs given in conjunction with Lanvis.

Lanvis is variably absorbed following oral administration and plasma levels may be reduced following emesis or intake of food.

*Induction therapy:* For *adults,* the usual dosage of Lanvis is between 100 and 200 mg/m² body surface area, per day on a single or twice-daily dosing regimen over a period of 5 to 20 days.

For *children,* similar dosages to those used in adults, with appropriate correction for body surface area, have been used, although lower dosages of 60 to 75 mg/m² body surface area have been employed in some regimens.

*Maintenance:* For both adults and children, intermittent or continuous daily maintenance doses of between 60 and 200 mg/m² body surface area have been used.

*Use in the elderly:* There are no specific dosage recommendations in elderly patients (see *Dosage in renal or hepatic impairment*).

Lanvis has been used in various combination chemotherapy schedules in elderly patients with acute leukaemia at equivalent doses to those used in younger patients.

*Dosage in renal or hepatic impairment:* Consideration should be given to reducing the dosage in patients with impaired hepatic or renal function.

**Contra-indications, warnings, etc**
*Contra-indications:* In view of the seriousness of the indications there are no absolute contra-indications.

*Precautions:* Lanvis is an active cytotoxic agent for use only under the direction of physicians experienced in the administration of such agents.

During remission induction, full blood counts must be carried out frequently.

The main side-effect of treatment with Lanvis is bone marrow suppression leading to leucopenia and thrombocytopenia. Patients must be carefully monitored during therapy. The leucocyte and platelet counts continue to fall after treatment is stopped, so at the first sign of an abnormally large fall in these counts, treatment should be temporarily discontinued. Bone marrow suppression is readily reversible if Lanvis is withdrawn early enough. During remission induction in acute myelogenous leukaemia the patient may frequently have to survive a period of relative bone marrow aplasia and it is important that adequate supportive facilities are available.

Patients on myelosuppressive chemotherapy are particularly susceptible to a variety of infections.

During remission induction particularly, when rapid cell lysis is occurring, adequate precautions should be taken to avoid hyperuricaemia and/or hyperuricosuria and the risk of uric acid nephropathy.

In view of its action on cellular DNA, thioguanine is potentially mutagenic and carcinogenic.

It is recommended that the handling of Lanvis Tablets follows the 'Guidelines for the Handling of Cytotoxic Drugs' issued by the Royal Pharmaceutical Society of Great Britain Working Party on the Handling of Cytotoxic Drugs.

If halving of a tablet is required, care should be taken not to contaminate the hands or inhale the drug.

Since the enzyme hypoxanthine guanine phosphoribosyl transferase is responsible for the conversion of

Lanvis to its active metabolite, it is possible that patients deficient in this enzyme, such as those suffering from Lesch-Nyhan syndrome, may be resistant to the drug. Resistance to azathioprine (Imuran*), which has one of the same active metabolites as Lanvis, has been demonstrated in two children with Lesch-Nyhan syndrome.

*Side-and adverse effects:* Lanvis is usually one component of combination chemotherapy and, consequently, it is not possible to ascribe the side effects unequivocally to this drug alone.

The following side effects have been reported during treatment with thioguanine-containing regimens: gastro-intestinal intolerance; stomatitis; intestinal necrosis and perforation; liver function abnormalities and jaundice, which may be reversible if therapy is withdrawn; veno-occlusive disease (VOD) of the liver which, in most cases, was reversible on withdrawal of chemotherapy; one case of centrilobular hepatic necrosis in a patient who had been treated for acute myelogenous leukaemia with high cumulative doses of Lanvis and cytosine arabinoside. This patient was also taking oral contraceptives.

*Drug interactions:* The combination of busulphan and Lanvis has resulted in the development of nodular regenerative hyperplasia, portal hypertension and oesophageal varices.

*Use in pregnancy and lactation:* Lanvis, like other cytotoxic agents, is potentially teratogenic. There have been isolated cases where men, who have received combinations of cytotoxic agents including Lanvis, have fathered children with congenital abnormalities. Its use should be avoided whenever possible during pregnancy, particularly during the first trimester. In any individual case the potential hazard to the fetus must be balanced against the expected benefit to the mother.

As with all cytotoxic chemotherapy, adequate contraceptive precautions should be advised when either partner is receiving Lanvis.

There are no reports documenting the presence of Lanvis or its metabolites in maternal milk. It is suggested that mothers receiving Lanvis should not breast feed.

*Toxicity and treatment of overdosage:* The principal toxic effect is on the bone marrow, and haematological toxicity is likely to be more profound with chronic overdosage than with a single ingestion of Lanvis. As there is no known antidote the blood picture should be closely monitored and general supportive measures, together with appropriate blood transfusion instituted if necessary.

**Pharmaceutical precautions** Store below 25°C. Protect from light. Keep dry.

**Legal category** POM

**Package quantities** Bottle of 25 tablets.

**Further information** The concomitant use of Zyloric* (allopurinol) to inhibit uric acid formation does not necessitate reduction of dosage of Lanvis as is necessary with Puri-Nethol* (6–mercaptopurine) and Imuran* (azathioprine).

**Product licence number** 0003/0083.

## LEUKERAN* TABLETS

**Presentation** 2 mg Chlorambucil BP, coded 'WELLCOME C2A'. Coloured yellow with white core.
5 mg Chlorambucil BP, coded 'WELLCOME H2A'. Coloured yellow with white core.

**Uses** Cytotoxic agent.
Leukeran is indicated in the treatment of Hodgkin's disease, certain forms of non-Hodgkin's lymphoma, chronic lymphocytic leukaemia, Waldenstrom's macroglobulinaemia and advanced ovarian adeno-carcinoma. Leukeran has a significant therapeutic effect in a proportion of patients with breast cancer.

**Dosage and administration**
*Adults: Hodgkin's disease:* Used as a single agent a typical dosage is 0.2 mg/kg/day for 4 to 8 weeks. Leukeran is usually included in combination therapy and a number of regimes have been used. Leukeran has been used as an alternative to nitrogen mustard with a reduction in toxicity but similar therapeutic results.

*Non-Hodgkin's lymphoma:* Used as a single agent the usual dosage is 0.1 to 0.2 mg/kg/day for 4 to 8 weeks initially. Maintenance therapy is then given either by a reduced daily dosage or intermittent courses of treatment. Leukeran is useful in the management of patients with advanced diffuse lymphocytic lymphoma and those who have relapsed after radio-therapy. There is no significant difference in the overall response rate obtained with chlorambucil as a single agent and combination chemotherapy in patients with advanced non-Hodgkin's lymphocytic lymphoma.

*Chronic lymphocytic leukaemia:* Treatment with Leukeran is usually started after the patient has developed symptoms or when there is evidence of impaired bone marrow function (but not marrow failure) as indicated by the peripheral blood count. Initially, Leukeran is given at a dosage of 0.15 mg/kg/day until the total leucocyte count has fallen to 10,000 per microlitre. Treatment may be resumed 4 weeks after the end of the first course and continued at a dosage of 0.1 mg/kg/day.

In a proportion of patients, usually after about 2 years of treatment, the blood leucocyte count is reduced to the normal range, enlarged spleen and lymph nodes become impalpable and the proportion of lymphocytes in the bone marrow is reduced to less than 20%. Patients with evidence of bone marrow failure should first be treated with prednisolone and evidence of marrow regeneration should be obtained before commencing treatment with Leukeran. Intermittent high dose therapy has been compared with daily Leukeran but no significant difference in therapeutic response or frequency of side effects was observed between the two treatment groups.

*Waldenstrom's macroglobulinaemia:* Leukeran is the treatment of choice in this indication. Starting doses of 6 to 12 mg daily until leucopenia occurs are recommended followed by 2 to 8 mg daily indefinitely.

*Ovarian carcinoma:* Used as a single agent a typical dosage is 0.2 mg/kg/day for 4 to 6 weeks. A dosage of 0.3 mg/kg/day has been given until leucopenia had been induced. Maintenance dosage of 0.2 mg/kg/day has been given aiming to keep the total leucocyte count below 4,000/mm³. In practice, maintenance courses tend to last 2 to 4 weeks with intervals of 2 to 6 weeks between each course.

*Advanced breast cancer:* Used as a single agent a typical dosage is 0.2 mg/kg bodyweight per day for 6 weeks. Leukeran may be given in combination with prednisolone at a dose range of 14 to 20 mg daily, regardless of bodyweight, over 4 to 6 weeks provided there is no serious haemopoietic depression. Leukeran may be given in combination with methotrexate, 5–fluorouracil, and prednisolone at a dosage of 5 to 7.5 mg/m²/day.

*Children:* Leukeran may be used in the management of Hodgkin's disease and non-Hodgkin's lymphomas in children. The dosage regimens are similar to those used in adults.

*Use in the elderly:* No specific studies have been carried out in the elderly. However, it may be advisable to monitor renal or hepatic function and if there is serious impairment then caution should be exercised.

**Contra-indications, warnings, etc**
*Contra-indications:* In view of the seriousness of the indications there are no absolute contra-indications.

*Precautions:* Leukeran is an active cytotoxic agent for use only under the direction of physicians experienced in the administration of such agents.

*Safe handling of Leukeran Tablets:* The handling of Leukeran Tablets should follow guidelines for the handling of cytotoxic drugs according to prevailing local recommendations and/or regulations (for example, Royal Pharmaceutical Society of Great Britain Working Party on the Handling of Cytotoxic Drugs).

Provided that the outer coating of the tablet is intact, there is no risk in handling Leukeran Tablets. Leukeran Tablets should not be divided.

Since Leukeran is capable of producing irreversible bone marrow suppression, blood counts should be closely monitored in patients under treatment.

At therapeutic dosage Leukeran depresses lymphocytes and has less effect on neutrophil and platelet counts and on haemoglobin levels. Discontinuation of Leukeran is not necessary at the first sign of a fall in neutrophils but it must be remembered that the fall may continue for 10 days or more after the last dose.

Leukeran should not be given to patients who have recently undergone radiotherapy or received other cytotoxic agents.

When lymphocytic infiltration of the bone marrow is present or the bone marrow is hypoplastic, the daily dose should not exceed 0.1 mg/kg bodyweight.

Patients with evidence of impaired renal function should be carefully monitored as they are prone to additional myelosuppression associated with azotaemia.

The metabolism of Leukeran is still under investigation and consideration should be given to dose reduction in patients with gross hepatic dysfunction.

Leukeran has been shown to cause chromatid or chromosome damage in man. Development of acute leukaemia after Leukeran therapy for chronic lymphocytic leukaemia has been reported. However, it was not clear whether the acute leukaemia was part of the natural history of the disease or if the chemotherapy was the cause.

A comparison of patients with ovarian cancer who received alkylating agents with those who did not, showed that the use of alkylating agents, including Leukeran, significantly increased the incidence of acute leukaemia.

Acute myelogenous leukaemia has been reported in a small proportion of patients receiving Leukeran as long-term adjuvant therapy for breast cancer.

The leukaemogenic risk must be balanced against the potential therapeutic benefit when considering the use of Leukeran.

Chlorambucil may cause suppression of ovarian function and amenorrhoea has been reported following chlorambucil therapy.

Azoospermia has been observed as a result of therapy with Leukeran although it is estimated that a total dose of at least 400 mg is necessary.

Varying degrees of recovery of spermatogenesis have been reported in patients with lymphoma following treatment with Leukeran in total doses of 410 to 2,600 mg. Patients receiving phenylbutazone may require a reduced dose of Leukeran.

*Drug interactions:* Animal studies indicate that patients who receive phenylbutazone may require a reduction of the standard chlorambucil doses because of the possibility of enhanced chlorambucil toxicity.

*Side- and adverse effects:* The most common side-effect is bone marrow suppression. Although this frequently occurs, it is usually reversible if Leukeran is withdrawn early enough. However, irreversible bone marrow failure has been reported.

Gastro-intestinal disturbances such as nausea and vomiting, diarrhoea and oral ulceration occur infrequently. Other side-effects may be encountered but usually only when the therapeutic dosage has been exceeded.

Severe interstitial pulmonary fibrosis has occasionally been reported in patients with chronic lymphocytic leukaemia on long-term Leukeran therapy. However, this may be reversible on withdrawal of Leukeran.

Hepatotoxicity and jaundice have been reported after Leukeran treatment.

Skin rashes are uncommon but have on very rare occasions been reported to progress to serious conditions including Stevens-Johnson syndrome and toxic epidermal necrolysis.

Other reported adverse reactions include fever, peripheral neuropathy, interstitial pneumonia and sterile cystitis.

Seizures have occurred in children with nephrotic syndrome treated with Leukeran and dose-related focal fits in adults have been reported.

*Use in pregnancy and lactation:* As with other cytotoxic agents Leukeran is potentially teratogenic. The use of Leukeran should be avoided whenever possible during pregnancy, particularly during the first trimester. In any individual case, the potential hazard to the fetus must be balanced against the expected benefit to the mother.

As with all cytotoxic chemotherapy, adequate contraceptive precautions should be advised when either partner is receiving Leukeran.

Mothers receiving Leukeran should not breast feed.

*Toxicity and treatment of overdosage:* Reversible pancytopenia was the main finding of inadvertent overdoses of Leukeran. Neurological toxicity ranging from agitated behaviour and ataxia to multiple grand mal seizures has also occurred. As there is no known antidote the blood picture should be closely monitored and general supportive measures should be instituted, together with appropriate blood transfusion if necessary.

**Pharmaceutical precautions** Store at 2 to 8°C in a dry place.

**Legal category** POM

**Package quantities**
2 mg: Bottle of 25 tablets
5 mg: Bottle of 25 tablets

**Further information** Leukeran has the pharmacological properties of the nitrogen mustard compounds. The drug is only partly radiomimetic, affecting chiefly the lymphoid tissues. Experimental studies have shown that chlorambucil is well absorbed and well tolerated by the oral route.

**Product licence numbers**
Leukeran Tablets 2 mg: 0003/5264R
Leukeran Tablets 5 mg: 0003/5265R

## MALARONE* ▼

**Qualitative and quantitative composition** Each tablet contains: Atovaquone 250 mg and proguanil hydrochloride 100 mg.

**Pharmaceutical form** Round, biconvex, pink film

coated tablets containing 250 mg atovaquone and 100 mg proguanil hydrochloride.

**Clinical particulars**
*Therapeutic indications:* Malarone is a fixed dose combination of atovaquone and proguanil hydrochloride which acts as a blood schizonticide. It is indicated for: Treatment of acute, uncomplicated *Plasmodium falciparum* malaria.

Because Malarone is effective against drug sensitive and drug resistant *P. falciparum* it is especially recommended for acute, uncomplicated *P. falciparum* malaria acquired in areas where the pathogen may be resistant to other antimalarials, such as chloroquine, halofantrine, mefloquine, amodiaquine and chloroquine plus pyrimethimene/sulphadoxine.

*Posology and method of administration:* The daily dose should be taken with food or a milky drink at the same time each day.

In the event of vomiting within 1 hour of dosing a repeat dose should be taken.

*Dosage in adults:* Four tablets as a single dose for three consecutive days.

*Dosage in children:*
11–20 kg bodyweight: One tablet daily for three consecutive days.
21–30 kg bodyweight: Two tablets as a single dose for three consecutive days.
31–40 kg bodyweight: Three tablets as a single dose for three consecutive days.
>40 kg bodyweight: Dose as for adults.

*Dosage in the elderly:* Although no studies have been carried out in the elderly, no special precautions or dosage adjustment are anticipated in this age group.

*Dosage in hepatic impairment:* Although no studies have been carried out, no special precautions or dosage adjustment are anticipated.

*Dosage in renal impairment:* Proguanil, and hence Malarone, should be administered with caution to patients with acute renal failure (see *Special warnings and precautions for use*).

*Contra-indications:* Malarone is contra-indicated in individuals with known hypersensitivity to atovaquone or proguanil hydrochloride or any component of the formulation.

*Special warnings and precautions for use:* Malarone has not been evaluated for the treatment of cerebral malaria or other severe manifestations of complicated malaria including hyperparasitaemia, pulmonary oedema or renal failure.

Parasite relapse occurred commonly when *P. vivax* malaria was treated with Malarone alone.

In the event of recrudescent infections due to *P. falciparum*, patients should be treated with a different blood schizonticide.

Because absorption of atovaquone may be reduced in patients with diarrhoea and vomiting, alternative therapy should be considered in such patients. If Malarone is used in these patients parasitaemia should be closely monitored.

Parasitaemia should be closely monitored in patients receiving concurrent metoclopramide or tetracycline (see *Interactions*).

The concomitant administration of Malarone and rifampicin is not recommended (see *Interactions*).

Proguanil, and hence Malarone, should be administered with caution to patients with acute renal failure (see *Posology and method of administration*).

*Interaction with other medicaments and other forms of interaction:* Concomitant treatment with metoclopramide and tetracycline have been associated with significant decreases in plasma concentrations of atovaquone (see *Special warnings and precautions for use*).

Concomitant administration of rifampicin is known to reduce atovaquone levels by approximately 50% (see *Special warnings and precautions for use*).

Atovaquone is highly protein bound (>99%) but does not displace other highly protein bound drugs *in vitro*, indicating significant drug interactions arising from displacement are unlikely.

*Pregnancy and lactation:* The safety of atovaquone and proguanil hydrochloride when administered concurrently for use in human pregnancy has not been established.

There is no evidence of teratogenicity in reproductive studies in rats with atovaquone alone. Segment II studies in rats with proguanil and atovaquone in combination up to a dose of atovaquone: proguanil (50:20) mg/kg/day show no indication of teratogenic effects.

However, as animal studies are not always predictive of human response the use of Malarone in pregnancy should only be considered if the expected benefit to the mother outweighs the risk to the fetus.

*Lactation:* The atovaquone concentrations in milk, in a rat study, were 30% of the concurrent atovaquone concentrations in maternal plasma. It is not known whether atovaquone is excreted in human milk.

Proguanil is excreted in human milk in small quantities.

It is not recommended that mothers receiving Malarone breast feed their babies.

*Effects on ability to drive and use machines:* There have been no studies to investigate the effect of Malarone on driving performance or the ability to operate machinery but a detrimental effect on such activities is not predicted from the pharmacology of the component drugs.

*Undesirable effects:* As Malarone contains atovaquone and proguanil hydrochloride, the type and severity of adverse reactions associated with each of the compounds may be expected. However, at the doses employed for the treatment of malaria, they are generally mild and of limited duration.

In a database comprising approximately 500 patients abdominal pain, headache, anorexia, nausea, vomiting, diarrhoea and coughing were the most commonly reported adverse experiences.

The only abnormalities noted in laboratory tests were occasional reversible abnormalities in liver function tests which were not associated with untoward clinical events.

*Overdose:* There have been no reports of overdosage with Malarone. In cases of suspected overdosage symptomatic and supportive therapy should be given as appropriate.

**Pharmacological properties**
*Pharmacodynamic properties:* Pharmacotherapeutic group – Antimalarials: biguanides–proguanil combinations. ATC Code: P01B B51.

*Mode of action:* The constituents of Malarone, atovaquone and proguanil hydrochloride, interfere with two different pathways involved in the biosynthesis of pyrimidines required for nucleic acid replication. Atovaquone is a selective and potent inhibitor of parasite mitochondrial electron transport. Proguanil hydrochloride primarily exerts its effect by means of the metabolite cycloguanil, a dihydrofolate reductase inhibitor. Inhibition of dihydrofolate reductase in the malaria parasite disrupts deoxythymidylate synthesis. These two mechanisms are believed to be the prime explanation of the synergy seen when used in combination.

*Microbiology:* Atovaquone has potent activity against *Plasmodium spp in vitro* $IC_{50}$ against *P. falciparum* 0.23–1.43 ng/ml.

The animalarial activity of proguanil is exerted via the primary metabolite cycloguanil (*in vitro* $IC_{50}$ against various *P. falciparum* strains of 4–20 ng/ml; some activity of proguanil and another metabolite, 4-chlorophenylbiguanide, is seen *in vitro* at 600–3000 ng/ml).

In *in vitro* studies of *P. falciparum* the combination of atovaquone and proguanil was shown to be synergistic. This enhanced efficacy was also demonstrated in clinical studies in both immune and non-immune patients.

*Pharmacokinetic properties:* There are no pharmacokinetic interactions between atovaquone and proguanil at the recommended dose.

*Absorption:* Atovaquone is a highly lipophilic compound with low aqueous solubility. The bioavailability of atovaquone shows considerable inter-individual variability. Dietary fat taken with atovaquone increases the rate and extent of absorption, increasing AUC 2–3 times and $C_{max}$ 5 times over fasting. Patients are recommended to take Malarone tablets with food (see *Posology and method of administration*).

Proguanil hydrochloride is rapidly and extensively absorbed regardless of food intake.

*Distribution:* Atovaquone is highly protein bound (>99%) but does not displace other highly protein bound drugs *in vitro*, indicating significant drug interactions arising from displacement are unlikely.

The volume of distribution of atovaquone is 0.62±0.19 l/kg.

Proguanil is 75% protein bound.

In human plasma the binding of atovaquone and proguanil were unaffected by the presence of the other.

*Metabolism:* There is no evidence that atovaquone is metabolised and there is negligible excretion of atovaquone in urine with the parent drug being predominantly (>90%) eliminated unchanged in faeces.

Proguanil hydrochloride is partially metabolised with less than 40% being excreted unchanged in the urine. Its metabolites cycloguanil and 4-chlorophenylbiguanide are also excreted in the urine.

During treatment of malaria with Malarone at recommended doses proguanil metabolism status appears to have no implications for treatment.

*Elimination:* The elimination half-life of atovaquone is about 2–3 days in adults and 1–2 days in children.

The clearance of atovaquone is 0.15±0.09 ml/min/kg.

The elimination half lives of proguanil and cycloguanil are about 12–15 hours in both adults and children.

*Preclinical safety data:*
*Repeat dose toxicity:* Results of repeat dose studies in rats and dogs at dosages of atovaquone: proguanil hydrochloride up to 100:40 mg/kg/day for 30 days either singly or in combination revealed reversible toxicity attributable to proguanil alone. There was no additional animal toxicity attributable to atovaquone alone or to the combination. Dosages of atovaquone: proguanil hydrochloride of 50:20 mg/kg/day was the no-effect dose.

*Reproductive toxicity studies:* Reproduction toxicity studies in animals did not indicate any teratogenic potential at dosages of atovaquone: proguanil hydrochloride of up to 50:20 mg/kg/day (see *Pregnancy and lactation*). In rabbits given atovaquone alone at dosages up to 1200 mg/kg/day, an increased incidence of resorptions and decreased length and weight of fetuses was noted. These effects were likely to be secondary to toxicity of atovaquone in maternal animals.

*Mutagenicity:* A wide range of mutagenicity tests have shown no evidence that atovaquone or proguanil have mutagenic activity as single agents.

Mutagenicity studies have not been performed with atovaquone in combination with proguanil.

*Carcinogenicity:* Oncogenicity studies of atovaquone alone in mice showed an increased incidence of hepatocellular adenomas and carcinomas. No such findings were observed in rats and mutagenicity tests were negative. These findings appear to be due to the inherent susceptibility of mice to atovaquone and are considered of no relevance in the clinical situation.

Oncogenicity studies on proguanil alone or in combination with atovaquone have not been undertaken.

**Pharmaceutical particulars**
*List of excipients: Core:* Poloxamer 188 BP; Microcrystalline Cellulose PhEur; Low-substituted Hydroxypropyl Cellulose USNF; Povidone K30 PhEur; Sodium Starch Glycollate PhEur; Magnesium Stearate PhEur.

*Coating:* Methylhydroxypropyl Cellulose PhEur; Titanium Dioxide PhEur; Iron Oxide Red E172; Macrogol 400 PhEur; Polyethylene Glycol 8000 USNF.

*Incompatibilities:* None known.

*Shelf life:* 3 years.

*Special precautions for storage:* None.

*Nature and contents of container:* PVC aluminium foil blister packs containing 12 tablets.

*Instructions for use/handling:* None.

**Marketing authorisation number** 10949/0258

**Date of approval/revision of SPC** 18 April 1997

**Legal category** POM

## MIVACRON* INJECTION

**Presentation** Mivacron Injection is a clear, pale yellow, sterile aqueous solution, in glass ampoules, containing 2 mg/ml mivacurium as mivacurium chloride. Each 5 ml ampoule contains 10 mg mivacurium and each 10 ml ampoule contains 20 mg mivacurium.

**Uses** Mivacron is a highly selective, short-acting, non-depolarising, neuromuscular blocking agent with a fast recovery profile. Mivacron is used as an adjunct to general anaesthesia to relax skeletal muscles and to facilitate tracheal intubation and mechanical ventilation.

This formulation contains no antimicrobial preservative and is intended for single patient use.

*Pharmacokinetics:* Mivacurium chloride is a mixture of three stereoisomers. The trans-trans and cis-trans stereoisomers comprise 92% to 96% of mivacurium chloride and when studied in cats their neuromuscular blocking potencies are not significantly different from each other or from mivacurium chloride. The cis-cis isomer has been estimated from studies in cats to have one-tenth of the neuromuscular blocking potency of the other two stereoisomers. Enzymatic hydrolysis by plasma cholinesterase is the primary mechanism for inactivation of mivacurium and yields a quaternary alcohol and a quaternary monoester metabolite. Pharmacological studies in cats and dogs have shown that the metabolites possess insignificant neuromuscular, autonomic or cardiovascular activity at concentrations higher than seen in man.

**Dosage and administration**
*Use by injection in adults:* Mivacron is administered

by intravenous injection. The mean dose required to produce 95% suppression of the adductor pollicis single twitch response to ulnar nerve stimulation ($ED_{95}$) is 0.07 mg/kg (range 0.06 to 0.09) in adults receiving narcotic anaesthesia.

The recommended bolus dose range for healthy adults is 0.07 to 0.25 mg/kg. The duration of neuromuscular blockade is related to the dose. Doses of 0.07, 0.15, 0.20 and 0.25 mg/kg produce clinically effective block for approximately 13, 16, 20 and 23 minutes respectively.

Doses of up to 0.15 mg/kg may be administered over 5 to 15 seconds. Higher doses should be administered over 30 seconds in order to minimise the possibility of occurrence of cardiovascular effects.

The following dosage regimens are recommended for tracheal intubation:

i) A dose of 0.2 mg/kg, administered over 30 seconds, produces good to excellent conditions for tracheal intubation within 2 to 2.5 minutes.

ii) A dose of 0.25 mg/kg administered as a divided dose (0.15 mg/kg followed 30 seconds later by 0.1 mg/kg), produces good to excellent conditions for tracheal intubation within 1.5 to 2.0 minutes of completion of administration of the first dose portion.

With Mivacron, significant train-of-four fade is not seen during onset. It is often possible to intubate the trachea before complete abolition of the train-of-four response of the adductor pollicis muscle has occurred.

Full block can be prolonged with maintenance doses of Mivacron. Doses of 0.1 mg/kg administered during narcotic anaesthesia each provide approximately 15 minutes of additional clinically effective block. Successive supplementary doses do not give rise to accumulation of neuromuscular blocking effect.

The neuromuscular blocking action of Mivacron is potentiated by isoflurane or enflurane anaesthesia. If steady-state anaesthesia with isoflurane or enflurane has been established, the recommended initial Mivacron dose should be reduced by up to 25%. Halothane appears to have only a minimal potentiating effect on Mivacron and dose reduction is probably not necessary.

Once spontaneous recovery is underway it is complete in approximately 15 minutes and is independent of the size of the Mivacron dose administered.

The neuromuscular block produced by Mivacron can be reversed with standard doses of anticholinesterase agents. However, because spontaneous recovery after mivacurium is rapid, reversal may not be routinely required since it shortens recovery time by only 5 to 6 minutes.

*Use as an infusion in adults:* Continuous infusion of Mivacron may be used to maintain neuromuscular block. Upon early evidence of spontaneous recovery from an initial Mivacron dose, an infusion rate of 8 to 10 microgram/kg/min (0.5 to 0.6 mg/kg/hr) is recommended. The initial infusion rate should be adjusted according to the patient's response to peripheral nerve stimulation and clinical criteria. Adjustments of the infusion rate should be made in increments of approximately 1 microgram/kg/min (0.06 mg/kg/hr). In general, a given rate should be maintained for at least 3 minutes before a rate change is made. On average, an infusion rate of 6 to 7 microgram/kg/min will maintain neuromuscular block within the range of 89% to 99% for extended periods in adults receiving narcotic anaesthesia. During steady-state isoflurane or enflurane anaesthesia, reduction in the infusion rate by up to 40% should be considered. With halothane, smaller reductions in infusion rate may be required.

Spontaneous recovery after Mivacron infusion is independent of the duration of infusion and comparable to recovery reported for single doses.

Continuous infusion of Mivacron has not been associated with the development of tachyphylaxis or cumulative neuromuscular blockade.

Mivacron (2 mg/ml) may be used undiluted for infusion.

Mivacron is compatible with the following infusion fluids:

Sodium Chloride Intravenous Infusion (0.9% w/v)
Glucose Intravenous Infusion (5% w/v)
Sodium Chloride (0.18% w/v) and Glucose (4% w/v) Intravenous Infusion
Lactated Ringer's Injection, USP

When diluted with the listed infusion solutions in the proportion of 1 plus 3 (i.e. to give 0.5 mg/ml) Mivacron Injection has been shown to be chemically and physically stable for at least 48 hours at 30°C. However, since the product contains no antimicrobial preservative, dilution should be carried out immediately prior to use, administration should commence as soon as possible thereafter, and any remaining solution should be discarded.

*Dose in children aged 2 months to 12 years:* Mivacron has a faster onset, shorter clinically effective duration of action and more rapid spontaneous recovery in infants and children than in adults.

The $ED_{95}$ in infants aged 2 to 6 months is approximately 0.07 mg/kg; and in infants and children aged 7 months to 12 years is approximately 0.1 mg/kg.

Pharmacodynamic data for recommended initial doses in infants and children are summarised in the following table:

| *Age* | *Dose for Tracheal Intubation* | *Time to Maximum Neuromuscular Block (Min)* | *Duration of Clinically Effective Block (Min)* |
|---|---|---|---|
| 2 to 6 Months[A] | 0.15 mg/kg | 1.4 | 9 |
| 7 Months to12 Years[B] | 0.2 mg/kg | 1.7 | 9 |

[A] Data obtained during halothane anaesthesia.
[B] Data obtained during halothane or narcotic anaesthesia.

Since maximum block is usually achieved within 2 minutes following administration of these doses, tracheal intubation should be possible within this time.

Infants and children generally require more frequent maintenance doses and higher infusion rates than adults. Pharmacodynamic data for maintenance doses are summarised in the table below together with recommended infusion rates:

| *Age* | *Maintenance Dose* | *Duration of Clinically Effective Block (Min)* | *Average Infusion Rate Required to Maintain 89–99% Neuromuscular Block* |
|---|---|---|---|
| 2 Months–12 Years[A] | 0.1 mg/kg | 6–9 | 11–14 micrograms/kg/min (0.7–0.9 mg/kg/hr) |

[A] Data obtained during halothane or narcotic anaesthesia.

Once spontaneous recovery is underway, it is complete in approximately 10 minutes.

*Dose in neonates and infants under 2 months of age:* No dose recommendations for neonates and infants under 2 months of age can be made until further information becomes available.

*Dose in the elderly:* In elderly patients receiving single bolus doses of Mivacron, the onset time, duration of action and recovery rate may be extended relative to younger patients by 20 to 30%. Elderly patients may also require decreased infusion rates or smaller or less frequent maintenance bolus doses.

*Dose in patients with cardiovascular disease:* In patients with clinically significant cardiovascular disease, the initial dose of Mivacron should be administered over 60 seconds. Mivacron has been administered in this way with minimal haemodynamic effects to patients undergoing cardiac surgery.

*Dose in patients with reduced renal function:* In patients with end-stage renal failure, the clinically effective duration of block produced by 0.15 mg/kg is approximately 1.5 times longer than in patients with normal renal function. Subsequently, dosage should be adjusted according to individual clinical response.

*Dose in patients with reduced hepatic function:* In patients with end-stage liver failure the clinically effective duration of block produced by 0.15 mg/kg is approximately 3 times longer than in patients with normal hepatic function. This prolongation is related to the markedly reduced plasma cholinesterase activity seen in these patients. Subsequently, dosage should be adjusted according to individual clinical response.

*Dose in patients with reduced plasma cholinesterase activity:* Mivacurium is metabolised by plasma cholinesterase. Plasma cholinesterase activity may be diminished in the presence of genetic abnormalities of plasma cholinesterase (e.g. patients heterozygous or homozygous for the atypical plasma cholinesterase gene), in various pathological conditions and by the administration of certain drugs (see *Drug interactions*).

The possibility of prolonged neuromuscular block following administration of Mivacron must be considered in patients with reduced plasma cholinesterase activity. Mild reductions (i.e. within 20% of the lower limit of the normal range) are not associated with clinically significant effects on duration. In patients heterozygous for the atypical plasma cholinesterase gene, the clinically effective duration of block of 0.15 mg/kg Mivacron is approximately 10 minutes longer than in control patients.

*Dose in obese patients:* In obese patients (those weighing 30% or more above their ideal bodyweight for height), the initial dose of Mivacron should be based upon ideal bodyweight and not actual bodyweight.

*Monitoring:* In common with all neuromuscular blocking agents, monitoring of neuromuscular function is recommended during the use of Mivacron in order to individualise dosage requirements.

**Contra-indications, warnings, etc**

*Contra-indications:* Mivacron should not be administered to patients known to have an allergic hypersensitivity to the drug.

Mivacron is contra-indicated in pregnancy since there is no information on the use of Mivacron in pregnant women.

Mivacron is contra-indicated in patients known or suspected of being homozygous for the atypical plasma cholinesterase gene (see *Precautions*).

*Precautions:* In common with all the other neuromuscular blocking agents, Mivacron paralyses the respiratory muscles as well as other skeletal muscles but has no effect on consciousness. Mivacron should be administered only by or under close supervision of an experienced anaesthetist with adequate facilities for endotracheal intubation and artificial ventilation.

In common with suxamethonium/succinylcholine, adult and paediatric patients homozygous for the atypical plasma cholinesterase gene (1 in 2,500 patients) are extremely sensitive to the neuromuscular blocking effect of Mivacron. In three such adult patients, a small dose of 0.03 mg/kg (approximately the $ED_{10-20}$ in genotypically normal patients) produced complete neuromuscular block for 26 to 128 minutes. Once spontaneous recovery had begun, neuromuscular block in these patients was antagonised with conventional doses of neostigmine (see *Dosage and administration* and *Use in patients with reduced plasma cholinesterase activity*).

In adults, doses of Mivacron of ≥0.2 mg/kg (≥3 x $ED_{95}$) have been associated with histamine release when administered by rapid bolus injection. However, the slower administration of the 0.2 mg/kg Mivacron dose and the divided administration of the 0.25 mg/kg Mivacron dose (see *Dosage and administration*) minimise the cardiovascular effects of these doses. Cardiovascular safety did not appear to be compromised in children given a rapid bolus dose of 0.2 mg/kg in clinical studies.

Caution should be exercised in administering Mivacron to patients with a history suggestive of an increased sensitivity to the effects of histamine, e.g. asthma. If Mivacron is used in this group of patients it should be administered over 60 seconds.

Mivacron should be administered over a period of 60 seconds to patients who may be unusually sensitive to falls in arterial blood pressure, for example those who are hypovolaemic.

Mivacron does not have significant vagal or ganglion blocking properties in the recommended dosage range. Recommended doses of Mivacron consequently have no clinically significant effects on heart rate and will not counteract the bradycardia produced by many anaesthetic agents or by vagal stimulation during surgery.

In common with other non-depolarising neuromuscular blocking agents, increased sensitivity to Mivacron can be expected in patients with myasthenia gravis, other forms of neuromuscular disease and cachectic patients. Severe acid-base or electrolyte abnormalities may increase or reduce sensitivity to Mivacron.

Mivacron solution is acidic (approximately pH 4.5) and should not be mixed in the same syringe or administered simultaneously through the same needle with highly alkaline solutions (e.g. barbiturate solutions). It has been shown to be compatible with some commonly used peri-operative drugs supplied as acidic solutions, e.g. fentanyl, alfentanil, sufentanil, droperidol and midazolam. Where other anaesthetic agents are administered through the same indwelling needle or cannula as used for Mivacron, and compatibility has not been demonstrated, it is recommended that each drug is flushed through with physiological saline.

Studies in malignant hyperthermia-susceptible pigs, indicated that Mivacron does not trigger this syndrome. Mivacron has not been studied in malignant hyperthermia-susceptible patients.

Patients with burns may develop resistance to non-depolarising neuromuscular blocking agents and require increased doses. However, such patients may also have reduced plasma cholinesterase activity, requiring dose reduction. Consequently, burn patients should be given a test dose of 0.015 to 0.020 mg/kg Mivacron followed by appropriate dosing guided by monitoring of block with a nerve stimulator.

No data are available on the long-term use of Mivacron in patients undergoing mechanical ventilation in the intensive care unit.

Mivacron has been evaluated in four short-term mutagenicity tests. Mivacron was non-mutagenic in the Ames Salmonella assay, the mouse lymphoma assay, the human lymphocyte assay and the *in vivo* rat bone marrow cytogenetic assay.

There is no information available on whether mivacurium has carcinogenic potential.

Fertility studies have not been performed.

*Side- and adverse effects:* Associated with the use of Mivacron there have been reports of skin flushing, erythema, urticaria, mild transient hypotension, transient tachycardia or bronchospasm which have been attributed to histamine release. These effects are dose–related and more common following initial doses of ≥ 0.2 mg/kg or more when given rapidly and are reduced if Mivacron is injected over 30 to 60 seconds or in divided doses over 30 seconds.

*Use in pregnancy and lactation:* Animal studies have indicated that mivacurium has no adverse effect on fetal development.

There is no information on the use of Mivacron in pregnant women (see *Contra-indications*).

There has been no experience with the use of Mivacron during Caesarean section.

It is not known whether Mivacron is excreted in human milk.

*Drug interactions:* The neuromuscular block produced by mivacurium may be increased by the concomitant use of inhalational anaesthetics such as enflurane, isoflurane and halothane.

Mivacron has been safely administered following suxamethonium-facilitated tracheal intubation. Evidence of spontaneous recovery from suxamethonium should be observed prior to administration of Mivacron.

In common with all non-depolarising neuromuscular blocking agents, the magnitude and/or duration of non-depolarising neuromuscular block may be increased and infusion requirements may be reduced as a result of interaction with: antibiotics, including the aminoglycosides, polymyxins, spectinomycin, tetracyclines, lincomycin and clindamycin; anti arrhythmic drugs: propranolol, calcium channel blockers, lignocaine, procainamide and quinidine; diuretics: frusemide and possibly thiazides, mannitol and acetazolamide; magnesium salts; ketamine; lithium salts; ganglion blocking drugs: trimetaphan, hexamethonium.

Drugs that may reduce plasma cholinesterase activity may also prolong the neuromuscular blocking action of Mivacron. These include anti-mitotic drugs, monoamine oxidase inhibitors, ecothiopate iodide, pancuronium, organophosphates, anticholinesterases, certain hormones, bambuterol.

Rarely, certain drugs may aggravate or unmask latent myasthenia gravis or actually induce a myasthenic syndrome; increased sensitivity to Mivacron would be consequent on such a development. Such drugs include various antibiotics, β-blockers, (propranolol, oxprenolol), anti-arrhythmic drugs (procainamide, quinidine), anti-rheumatic drugs (chloroquine, D-penicillamine), trimetaphan, chlorpromazine, steroids, phenytoin and lithium.

In common with other non-depolarising neuromuscular blocking agents, the onset of block is likely to be lengthened and the duration of block shortened in patients receiving chronic phenytoin or carbamazepine therapy.

A depolarising muscle relaxant such as suxamethonium chloride should not be administered to prolong the neuromuscular blocking effects of non-depolarising agents, as this may result in a prolonged and complex block which can be difficult to reverse with anticholinesterase drugs.

*Toxicity and treatment of overdosage:* Prolonged muscle paralysis and its consequences are the main signs of overdosage with neuromuscular blocking agents. However, the risk of haemodynamic side-effects especially decreases in blood pressure, may be increased.

It is essential to maintain a patent airway together with assisted positive pressure ventilation until spontaneous respiration is adequate. Full sedation will be required since consciousness is not impaired. Recovery may be hastened by the administration of anticholinesterase agents accompanied by atropine or glycopyrrolate, once evidence of spontaneous recovery is present. Cardiovascular support may be provided by proper positioning of the patient and administration of fluids or vasopressor agents as required.

**Pharmaceutical precautions** Store below 25°C. Do not freeze. Protect from light.

Since no antimicrobial preservative is included, Mivacron must be used under full aseptic conditions and any dilution carried out immediately before use. Any unused solution in open ampoules should be discarded.

Mivacron Injection is acidic (approximately pH 4.5) and should not be mixed with highly alkaline solutions (e.g. barbiturates). Mivacron Injection has been shown to be compatible with some commonly used peri-operative drugs supplied as acidic solutions. Where such agents are administered through the same indwelling needle or cannula as used for Mivacron Injection, and compatibility has not been demonstrated, it is recommended that each drug is flushed through with physiological saline.

**Legal category** POM

**Package quantities** Ampoules of 5 ml and 10 ml in packs of 5.

**Further information** The termination of the neuromuscular blocking action of Mivacron is mainly dependent on hydrolysis by plasma pseudocholinesterase, which is present at high levels in human plasma.

Multiple degradation/elimination pathways appear to exist for Mivacron (e.g. hydrolysis by liver esterases, elimination in bile and renal excretion).

**Product licence number** 0003/0325.

## MYLERAN* TABLETS 0.5 mg

**Qualitative and quantitative composition** Busulphan 0.5 mg per tablet.

**Pharmaceutical form** Tablet.

**Clinical particulars**

*Therapeutic indications:* Myleran is indicated for the palliative treatment of the chronic phase of chronic granulocytic leukaemia. Although not curative, Myleran is very effective in reducing the total granulocyte mass, relieving the symptoms of disease and improving the clinical state of the patient.

Myleran has been shown to be superior to splenic irradiation when judged by survival times and maintenance of haemoglobin levels and is as effective in controlling spleen size.

Myleran is ineffective once blast transformation has occurred.

Myleran is effective in producing prolonged remission in polycythaemia vera, particularly in cases with marked thrombocytosis.

Myleran may be useful in selected cases of essential thrombocythaemia and myelofibrosis.

Oral administration.

*Posology and method of administration:*

*Induction in adults:* Treatment is usually initiated as soon as the condition is diagnosed. The dose is 0.06 mg/kg/day, with an initial daily maximum of 4 mg, which may be given as a single dose.

There is individual variation in the response to Myleran and in a small proportion of patients the bone marrow may be extremely sensitive (see *Special warnings and precautions for use*).

The blood count must be monitored at least weekly during the induction phase and it may be helpful to plot counts on semilog graph paper.

The dose should be increased only if the response is inadquate after three weeks.

Treatment should be continued until the total leucocyte count has fallen to between 15 and $25 \times 10^9$ per litre (typically 12 to 20 weeks). Treatment may then be interrupted, following which a further fall in the leucocyte count may occur over the next two weeks. Continued treatment at the induction dose after this point, or following depression of the platelet count to below $100 \times 10^9$ per litre is associated with a significant risk of prolonged and possibly irreversible bone marrow aplasia.

*Maintenance in adults:* Control of the leukaemia may be achieved for long periods without further Myleran treatment; further courses are usually given when the leucocyte count rises to $50 \times 10^9$ per litre, or symptoms return.

Some clinicians prefer to give continuous maintenance therapy. Continuous treatment is more practical when the duration of unmaintained remissions is short. The usual maintenance dosage is 0.5 to 2 mg/day, but individual requirements may be much less. The aim is to maintain a leucocyte count of 10 to $15 \times 10^9$ per litre and blood counts must be performed at least every 4 weeks. The maintenance dose may also be adjusted by reducing the number of treatment days per week.

Lower doses of Myleran should be used if it is administered in conjunction with other cytotoxic agents (see also *Undesirable effects* and *Drug interactions*).

*Children:* Chronic granulocytic leukaemia is rare in the paediatric age group. Myleran may be used to treat Philadelphia chromosome positive (Ph' positive) disease, but the Ph' negative juvenile variant responds poorly.

*Polycythaemia vera:* The usual dose is 4 to 6 mg daily, continued for 4 to 6 weeks, with careful monitoring of the blood count, particularly the platelet count.

Further courses are given when relapse occurs; alternatively, maintenance therapy may be given using approximately half the induction dose.

If the polycythaemia is controlled primarily by venesection, short courses of Myleran may be given solely to control the platelet count.

*Myelofibrosis:* The usual initial dose is 2 to 4 mg daily.

Very careful haematological control is required because of the extreme sensitivity of the bone marrow in this condition.

*Essential thrombocythaemia:* The usual dose is 2 to 4 mg per day.

Treatment should be interrupted if the total leucocyte count falls below $5 \times 10^9$ per litre or the platelet count below $500 \times 10^9$ per litre.

*Use in the elderly:* No special comment.

*Contra-indications:* Myleran should not be used in patients whose disease has demonstrated resistance to busulphan.

Myleran should not be given to patients who have previously suffered a hypersensitivity reaction to the drug.

*Special warnings and precautions for use:* Myleran is an active cytotoxic agent for use **only** under the direction of physicians experienced in the administration of such agents.

Myleran should be discontinued if lung toxicity develops (see *Side-effects*).

Myleran should not generally be given in conjunction with or soon after radiotherapy.

If anaesthesia is required in patients with possible pulmonary toxicity, the concentration of inspired oxygen should be kept as low as safely as possible and careful attention given to post-operative respiratory care.

Hyperuricaemia and/or hyperuricosuria are not uncommon in patients with chronic granulocytic leukaemia and should be corrected before starting treatment with Myleran. During treatment, hyperuricaemia and the risk of uric nephropathy should be prevented by adequate prophylaxis, including adequate hydration and the use of allopurinol.

Very careful consideration should be given to the use of Myleran for the treatment of polycythaemia vera and essential thrombocythaemia in view of the drug's carcinogenic potential. The use of Myleran for these indications should be avoided in younger or asymptomatic patients. If the drug is considered necessary, treatment courses should be kept as short as possible.

**Careful attention must be paid to monitoring the blood counts throughout treatment to avoid the possibility of excessive myelosuppression and the risk of irreversible bone marrow aplasia.**

It is recommended that the handling of Myleran Tablets follows the 'Guidelines for the Handling of Cytotoxic Drugs' issued by the Royal Pharmaceutical Society of Great Britain Working Party on the Handling of Cytotoxic Drugs.

If halving of a tablet is required, care should be taken not to contaminate the hands or inhale the drug.

Busulphan has been shown to be mutagenic in various experimental systems, including bacteria, fungi, *Drosophila* and cultured mouse lymphoma cells.

*In vivo* cytogenetic studies in rodents have shown an increased incidence of chromosome aberrations in both germ cells and somatic cells after busulphan treatment.

Various chromosome aberrations have been noted in cells from patients receiving Myleran.

On the basis of short-term tests, Myleran has been classified as potentially carcinogenic by the IARC. The World Health Association has concluded that there is a causal relationship between busulphan exposure and cancer.

Widespread epithelial dysplasia has been observed in patients treated with long-term Myleran, with some of the changes resembling precancerous lesions.

A number of malignant tumours have been reported in patients who have received Myleran treatment.

The evidence is growing that Myleran, in common with other alkylating agents, is leukaemogenic. In a controlled prospective study in which 2 years' Myleran treatment was given as an adjuvant to surgery for lung cancer, long-term follow-up showed an increased incidence of acute leukaemia compared with the placebo-treated group. The incidence of solid tumours was not increased.

Although acute leukaemia is probably part of the natural history of polycythaemia vera, prolonged alkylating agent therapy may increase the incidence.

Ovarian suppression and amenorrhoea with menopausal symptoms commonly occur in pre-menopausal patients. In one case, recovery of ovarian function has been reported with continuing treatment.

Myleran treatment in a pre-adolescent girl prevented the onset of puberty due to ovarian failure.

Bulsulphan interferes with spermatogenesis in

experimental animals, and there have been clinical reports of sterility, azoospermia and testicular atrophy in male patients.

*Interaction with other medicaments and other forms of interaction:* The combination of Myleran and thioguanine has resulted in the development of nodular regenerative hyperplasia, portal hypertension and oesophageal varices.

The effects of other cytotoxics producing pulmonary toxicity may be additive.

*Pregnancy and lactation:* As with all cytotoxic chemotherapy, adequate contraceptive precautions should be advised when either partner is receiving Myleran.

Busulphan is teratogenic in animal studies and potentially teratogenic in humans. A few cases of congenital abnormalities, not necessarily attributable to busulphan, have been reported and third trimester exposure may be associated with impaired intrauterine growth. However, there have also been many reported cases of apparently normal children born after exposure to Myleran *in utero*, even during the first trimester.

The use of Myleran should be avoided whenever possible during pregnancy, particularly during the first trimester. In every individual case the expected benefit of treatment to the mother must be weighed against the possible risks to the fetus.

It is not known whether Myleran or its metabolites are excreted in human breast milk, Mothers receiving Myleran should not breast feed their infants.

*Effect on ability to drive and use machines:* None known.

*Undesirable effects:* The main adverse reaction of Myleran treatment is bone marrow depression, particularly thrombocytopenia.

Gastro-intestinal effects such as nausea, vomiting and diarrhoea have been reported rarely at normal therapeutic doses and may possibly be ameliorated by using divided doses.

Diffuse interstitial pulmonary fibrosis, with progressive dyspnoea and a persistent, non-productive cough has occurred rarely, usually after prolonged treatment over a number of years.

Histological features include atypical changes of the alveolar and bronchiolar epithelium and the presence of giant cells with large hyperchromatic nuclei. Once pulmonary toxicity is established the prognosis is poor despite Myleran withdrawal and three is little evidence that corticosteroids are helpful. The onset is usually insidious but may also be acute. The lung pathology may be complicated by superimposed infections. Pulmonary ossification and dystrophic calcification have also been reported. It is possible that subsequent radiotherapy can augment subclinical lung injury caused by Myleran. Other cytotoxic agents may cause additive lung toxicity.

Hyperpigmentation is the most common skin reaction and occurs in 5 to 10% of patients, particularly those with a dark complexion. It is often most marked on the neck, upper trunk, nipples, abdomen and palmar creases. In a few cases following prolonged Myleran therapy, hyperpigmentation occurs as a part of a clinical syndrome resembling adrenal insufficiency (Addison's disease). It is characterised by weakness, severe fatigue, anorexia, weight loss, nausea and vomiting and hyperpigmentation of the skin, but without biochemical evidence of adrenal impairment or mucous membrane hyperpigmentation or hair loss. The syndrome has sometimes resolved when Myleran has been withdrawn.

Other rare skin reactions include urticaria, erythema multiforme, erythema nodosum, alopecia, porphyria cutanea tarda, an 'allopurinol-type' rash and excessive dryness and fragility of the skin with complete anhydrosis, dryness of the oral mucous membranes and cheilosis. Sjogren's syndrome has also been reported.

An increased cutaneous radiation effect has been observed in patients receiving radiotherapy soon after high-dose Myleran.

There have been occasional reports of cholestatic jaundice and liver function abnormalities, but Myleran is not generally considered to be significantly hepatotoxic at normal therapeutic doses. However, retrospective review of post-mortem reports of patients who had been treated with low-dose Myleran for at least two years for chronic granulocytic leukaemia showed evidence of centrilobular sinusoidal fibrosis. The combination of Myleran and thioguanine is associated with significant hepatotoxicity.

Hyperbilirubinaemia, jaundice, hepatic veno-occlusive disease and centrilobular sinusoidal fibrosis with hepatoceullular atrophy and necrosis have been observed after high-dose Myleran treatment.

Lens changes and cataracts, which may be bilateral, have been reported during Myleran therapy. Corneal thinning has been reported after bone marrow transplantation preceded by high-dose Myleran treatment.

Convulsions have been observed in adults who have received high-dose Myleran.

Gynaecomastia has been reported as a side effect of Myleran, as have myasthenia gravis and haemorrhagic cystitis.

Many histological and cytological changes have been observed in patients treated with Myleran, including widespread dysplasia affecting uterine cervical, bronchial and other epithelia. Most reports relate to long-term treatment but transient epithelial abnormalities have been observed following short-term high-dose treatment.

*Overdose:* The acute dose-limiting toxicity of Myleran in man is myelosuppression. If high-dose Myleran is used in association with bone marrow transplantation. The dose-limiting toxicity is then gastro-intestinal with mucositis, nausea, vomiting, diarrhoea and anorexia. The main effect of chronic overdosage is bone marrow depression and pancytopenia.

There is no known antidote to Myleran. There are no data about the possible value of dialysis. Appropriate supportive treatment should be given during the period of haematological toxicity.

**Pharmacological properties**

*Pharmacodynamic properties:* Busulphan (1,4-Butanediol Dimethanesulfonate) is a bifunctional alkylating agent. Binding to DNA is believed to play a role in its mode of action and di-guanyl derivatives have been isolated but interstrand crosslinking has not been conclusively demonstrated.

The basis for the uniquely selective effect of busulphan on granulocytopoiesis is not fully understood.

*Pharmacokinetic properties:* Early studies were carried out with radioactive labelled bulsuphan. More recently, gas liquid chromatography with selected ion monitoring has been used to quantitate busulphan in biological fluids. Busulphan doses of 2 to 6 mg were well absorbed and the kinetic data could be fitted to a zero-order absorption, one-compartment open model. The mean half-life for drug elimination was 2.57 hours.

The pharmacokinetics of busulphan have also been studied in patients following high-dose administration (1 mg/kg every 6 hours for 4 days). Drug was assayed either using gas liquid chromatography with electron capture detection or by high-performance liquid chromatography (HPLC). Using the former technique, the mean elimination half-life was found to be 2.3 hours after the final busulphan dose, but 3.4 hours after the first dose.

This suggests that busulphan may increase its own metabolic rate on repeated treatment.

The mean steady-state plasma concentration was 1.1 microgram/ml after dosing. Due to the variable absorption kinetics observed, it was not possible to evaluate the order of kinetics.

Using HPLC, steady-state plasma levels of busulphan were found to range from 2 to 8 microM (approximately 0.5 to 2 microgram/ml respectively). Peak plasma levels ranged from 3.1 to 5.9 microgram/ml in a patient treated with total dose of 16 mg/kg, or from 3.8 to 9.7 microgram/ml in two patients treated with a total of 20 mg/kg.

The urinary metabolites of busulphan have been identified as 3-hydroxsulpholane, tetrahydrothiophene 1-oxide and sulpholane, in patients treated with high-dose busulphan. Very little busulphan is excreted unchanged in the urine. After low- and high-dose administration, values of 1 and 2% respectively of unchanged drug has been observed.

Busulphan given in high doses has recently been shown to enter the cerebrospinal fluid (CSF) in concentrations comparable to those found in plasma, with a mean CSF: plasma ratio of 1.3:1. The saliva: plasma distribution of busulphan was found to be 1.1:1.

The level of busulphan bound reversibly to plasma proteins has been variably reported to be insignificant or approximately 55%. Irreversible binding of drug to blood cells and plasma proteins has been reported to be 47% and 32% respectively.

*Preclinical safety data:* There are no preclinical data of relevance to the prescriber which are additional to that in other sections of this SPC.

**Pharamceutical particulars**

*List of excipients:* Lactose PhEur; Maize Starch PhEur; Povidone BP; Magnesium Stearate PhEur; Erythrosine, E127 – Aluminium Lake HSE; Industrial Methylated Spirit BP or Ethanol BP; Gelatine PhEur; Purified Water PhEur.

*Incompatibilities:* None known.

*Shelf life:* 3 years.

*Special precautions for storage:* Store between 2–8°C. Keep dry.

*Nature and contents of container:* Amber glass bottles with low-density polyethylene snap-fit closures. Pack size of 25 tablets per bottle.

*Instructions for use/handling:* No special instructions.

**Marketing authorisation numbers**

| | |
|---|---|
| Myleran Tablets 0.5 mg | 0003/5113R |
| Myleran Tablets 2 mg | 0003/5112R |

**Date of approval/revision of SPC** 27 March 1996

**Legal category** POM.

## NARAMIG* TABLETS 2.5 mg ▼

**Qualitative and quantitative composition** Tablets containing 2.5 mg of naratriptan as naratriptan hydrochloride.

**Pharmaceutical form** Tablets

**Clinical particulars**

*Therapeutic indications:* Naramig Tablets are indicated for the acute treatment of migraine attacks with or without aura.

*Posology and method of administration:* Naramig Tablets are recommended as monotherapy for the acute treatment of a migraine attack.

Naramig Tablets should not be used prophylactically.

Naramig Tablets should be swallowed whole with water.

*Adults (18–65 years of age):* The recommended dose of Naramig Tablets is a single 2.5 mg tablet.

The total dose should not exceed two 2.5 mg tablets in any 24-hour period.

If symptoms of migraine should recur, following an initial response, a second dose may be taken provided that there is a minimum interval of four hours between the two doses.

If a patient does not respond to a first dose of Naramig Tablets a second dose should not be taken for the same attack, as it is unlikely to be of benefit. However, Naramig Tablets may be used for subsequent migraine attacks.

*Adolescents (12–17 years of age):* Efficacy of Naramig Tablets at single doses of 0.25, 1.0 and 2.5 mg was not demonstrated to be greater than placebo-controlled study in adolescents (12 to 17 years). Therefore, the use of Naramig Tablets in patients under 18 years of age is not recommended.

*Children (under 12 years of age):* There are no data available on the use of naratriptan in children under 12 years of age, therefore its use in this age group is not recommended.

*Elderly (over 65 years of age):* The safety and effectiveness of naratriptan in individuals over age 65 have not been evaluated and, therefore, its use in this age group cannot be recommended. There is a moderate decrease in clearance with age (see *Pharmacokinetics*).

*Renal impairment:* Naramig should be used with caution in patients with renal impairment. The maximum dose in any 24-hour treatment period is a single 2.5 mg tablet. The use of Naramig is contra-indicated in patients with severe renal impairment (creatinine clearance <15 ml/min) (see *Contra-indications* and *Pharmacokinetics*).

*Hepatic impairment:* Naramig should be used with caution in patients with hepatic impairment. The maximum dose in any 24-hour treatment period is a single 2.5 mg tablet. The use of Naramig is contra-indicated in patients with severe hepatic impairment (Child-Pugh grade C) (see *Contra-indications* and *Pharmacokinetics*).

*Contra-indications:* Hypersensitivity to any component of the preparation.

As with other 5-hydroxytryptamine$_1$ (5-HT$_1$) receptor agonists naratriptan should not be used in patients who have had a myocardial infarction or have ischaemic heart disease, or Prinzmetal's angina/coronary vasospasm, peripheral vascular disease or patients who have symptoms or signs consistent with ischaemic heart disease.

Naratriptan should not be administered to patients with a history of cerebrovascular accident (CVA) or transient ischaemic attack (TIA).

The use of naratriptan in patients with uncontrolled hypertension is contra-indicated.

As with other 5-HT$_1$ receptor agonists the concomitant use of naratriptan and other 5HT$_1$ agonists is contra-indicated.

Naratriptan is contra-indicated in patients with severely impaired renal or hepatic function.

*Special warnings and precautions for use:* Naratriptan should only be used where there is a clear diagnosis of migraine.

Naratriptan is not indicated for use in the management of hemiplegic, basilar or ophthalmoplegic migraine.

As with other acute migraine therapies, before treating headaches in patients not previously diagnosed as migraineurs, and in migraineurs who present with atypical symptoms, care should be taken to exclude other potentially serious neurological conditions. It should be noted that migraineurs may be at risk of certain cerebrovascular events (e.g. CVA or TIA).

As with other 5-$HT_1$ receptor agonists, naratriptan should not be given to patients in whom unrecognised cardiac disease is likely without a prior evaluation for underlying cardiovascular disease. Such patients include postmenopausal women, males over 40 and patients with risk factors for coronary artery disease.

If symptoms consistent with ischaemic heart disease occur appropriate evaluation should be carried out.

The concomitant administration of ergotamine and derivatives of ergotamine (including methysergide) with naratriptan is not recommended.

Naratriptan contains a sulphonamide component. Therefore, there is a theoretical risk of a hypersensitivity reaction in patients with known hypersensitivity to sulphonamides.

The recommended dose of naratriptan should not be exceeded.

*Interactions with other medicaments and other forms of interaction:* There is no evidence of interactions with β-blockers, tricyclic antidepressants, selective serotonin reuptake inhibitors, alcohol or food.

Co-administration of naratriptan with ergotamine, dihydroergotamine, or sumatriptan did not result in clinically significant effects on blood pressure, heart rate or ECG or affect naratriptan exposure.

Naratriptan does not exhibit monoamine oxidase enzymes; therefore interactions with monoamine oxidase inhibitors are not anticipated. In addition, the limited metabolism of naratriptan and the wide range of cytochrome P450 isoenzymes involved suggest that significant drug interactions with naratriptan are unlikely (see *Pharmacokinetics*).

*Pregnancy and lactation:* The safe use of naratriptan in pregnant women has not been established. Evaluation of experimental animal studies does not indicate any direct teratogenic effects or harmful effects on peri- and postnatal development.

Because animal reproduction studies are not always predictive of human response administration of naratriptan should only be considered if the expected benefit to the mother is greater than any possible risk to the fetus.

Naratriptan and/or drug related metabolites are secreted into the milk of lactating rats. Caution should be exercised when considering administration of naratriptan to nursing women.

*Effects on ability to drive and use machines:* Caution is recommended in patients performing skilled tasks (e.g. driving or operating machinery) as drowsiness may occur as a result of migraine. Drowsiness was no more apparent with naratriptan than with placebo in clinical trials.

*Undesirable effects:* Naramig is well tolerated.

At therapeutic doses of naratriptan the incidence of side effects reported in clinical trials was similar to placebo.

Some of the symptoms may be part of the migraine attack.

Frequent (>1/100)

*General:* The following symptoms are usually transient, may be intense and can affect any part of the body including the chest and throat: sensations of tingling or heat. Malaise/fatigue, dizziness, drowsiness.

*Gastrointestinal:* Nausea, vomiting.

Less frequent (<1/100)

*General:* The following symptoms are usually transient, may be intense and can affect any part of the body including the chest and throat: pain, sensations of heaviness, pressure or tightness.

*Cardiovascular:* Bradycardia, tachycardia, palpitations.

*Eye:* Visual disturbance.

*Overdosage:* There is no experience of accidental overdosage. However, administration of a high dose of 25 mg naratriptan in one healthy male subject increased blood pressure by up to 71 mmHg and resulted in adverse events including light-headedness, tension in the neck, tiredness and a loss of co-ordination. Blood pressure returned to baseline by 8 hours after dosing without other pharmacological intervention.

It is unknown what effect haemodialysis or peritoneal dialysis has on the plasma concentrations of naratriptan.

*Treatment:* If overdosage with naratriptan occurs, the patient should be monitored for at least 24 hours and standard supportive treatment applied as required.

**Pharmacological properties**

*Pharmacodynamic properties:* Naratriptan has been shown to be a selective agonist for 5 hydroxytryptamine$_1$ (5-$HT_1$) receptors mediating vascular contraction. This receptor is found predominantly in intracranial (cerebral and dural) blood vessels. Naratriptan has high affinity for human cloned 5-$HT_{1B}$ and 5-$HT_{1D}$ receptors, the human 5-$HT_{1B}$ receptor is thought to correspond to the vascular 5-$HT_1$ receptor mediating contraction of intracranial blood vessels. Naratriptan has little or no effect at other 5-HT receptor (5-$HT_2$, 5-$HT_3$, 5-$HT_4$ and 5-$HT_7$) subtypes.

In animals, naratriptan selectively constricts the carotid arterial circulation. This circulation supplies blood to the extracranial and intracranial tissues such as the meninges, and dilatation and/or oedema formation in these vessels is thought to be the underlying mechanism of migraine in man. In addition, experimental evidence suggests that naratriptan inhibits trigeminal nerve activity. Both these actions may contribute to the anti-migraine action of naratriptan in humans.

In man, a meta-analysis of BP recordings in 15 studies showed that the population average maximum increases in systolic and diastolic blood pressure after a 2.5 mg dose of naratriptan tablets would be less than 5 mmHg and 3 mmHg respectively. The blood pressure response was unaffected by age, weight, hepatic or renal impairment.

*Pharmacokinetic properties:*

*Absorption, distribution, metabolism and elimination:* Following oral administration, naratriptan is rapidly absorbed with maximum plasma concentrations observed at 2–3 hours. After administration of a 2.5 mg naratriptan tablet $C_{max}$ is approximately 8.3 ng/ml (95% CI:6.5 to 10.5 ng/ml) in women and 5.4 ng/ml (95% CI: 4.7 to 6.1 ng/ml) in men.

The oral bioavailability is 74% in women and 63% in men with no differences in efficacy and tolerability in clinical use. Therefore, a gender-related dose adjustment is not required.

Naratriptan is distributed in a volume of 170 l. Plasma protein binding is low (29%).

The mean elimination half-life ($t_{1/2}$) is 6 hours.

Mean clearance after intravenous administration was 470 ml/min in men and 380 ml/min in women. Renal clearance is similar in men and women at 220 ml/min and is higher than the glomerular filtration rate suggesting that naratriptan is actively secreted in the renal tubules. Naratriptan is predominantly excreted in the urine with 50% of the dose recovered as unchanged naratriptan and 30% recovered as inactive metabolites. *In vitro*, naratriptan was metabolised by a wide range of cytochrome P450 isoenzymes. Consequently, significant metabolic drug interactions with naratriptan are not anticipated (see *Interactions*).

*Special patient populations:*

*Elderly:* In healthy elderly subjects (n=12), clearance was decreased by 26% when compared to healthy young subjects (n=12) in the same study (see *Posology and method of administration*).

*Gender:* The naratriptan AUC and $C_{max}$ were approximately 35% lower in males compared to females however, with no differences in efficacy and tolerability in clinical use. Therefore, a gender-related dose adjustment is not required (see *Posology and method of administration*).

*Renal impairment:* Renal excretion is the major route for the elimination of naratriptan. Accordingly exposure to naratriptan may be increased in patients with renal disease.

In a study in male and female renally-impaired patients (creatinine clearance 18 to 115 ml/min; n=15) matched for sex, age and weight with healthy subjects (n=8); renally-impaired patients had an approximately 80% increase in $t_{1/2}$ and an approximately 50% reduction in clearance (see *Posology and method of administration*).

*Hepatic impairment:* The liver plays a lesser role in the clearance of orally administered naratriptan. In a study in male and female hepatically-impaired patients (Child-Pugh grade A or B n=8) matched for sex, age and weight with healthy subjects who received oral naratriptan; hepatically-impaired patients had an approximately 40% increase in $t_{1/2}$ and an approximately 30% reduction in clearance (see *Posology and method of administration*).

*Preclinical safety data:* No clinically relevant findings were observed in preclinical studies.

**Pharmaceutical particulars**

*List of excipients:*

*Tablet core:* Microcrystalline cellulose; Anhydrous lactose; Croscarmellose sodium; Magnesium stearate.

*Film coat:* Methylhydroxypropylcellulose; Titanium dioxide (E171); Triacetin; Iron oxide yellow (E172); Indigo carmine aluminium lake (E132).

*Incompatibilities:* None reported.

*Shelf life:* 24 months.

*Special precautions for storage:* Store below 30°C.

*Nature and contents of container:* 2, 4 or 6 tablets in a double-foil blister pack.

*Instructions for use/handling:* None.

**Marketing authorisation number** 10949/0273

**Date of approval/revision of SPC** April 1997

**Legal category** POM

## NIMBEX INJECTION 2 mg/ml NIMBEX [FORTE] INJECTION 5 mg/ml

**Qualitative and quantitative composition** A sterile solution containing 2 mg cisatracurium (bis-cation) per ml as cisatracurium besilate (BAN, pINN). The product contains no antimicrobial preservative and is supplied in an ampoule.

A sterile solution containing 5 mg cisatracurium (bis-cation) per ml as cisatracurium besilate (BAN, pINN). The product contains no antimicrobial preservative and is supplied in a vial.

*Chemical description:* Nimbex (cisatracurium besilate), (1R, 1'R, 2R, 2'R,)-2,2'-(3, 11-Dioxo-4,10-dioxatridecamethylene) bis (1,2,3,4-tetrahydro-6,7-dimethoxy-2-methyl-1-veratryisoquinolinium) dibenzenesulfonate.

Cisatracurium besilate is one of the ten isomeric components of atracurium besilate comprising about 15% of the mixture.

**Pharmaceutical form** Solution for injection.

**Clinical particulars** Nimbex is an intermediate-duration, non-depolarising neuromuscular blocking agent for intravenous administration.

*Therapeutic indications:* Nimbex is indicated for use during surgical and other procedures and in intensive care. Nimbex can be used as an adjunct to general anaesthesia, or sedation in the Intensive Care Unit (ICU) to relax skeletal muscles, and to facilitate tracheal intubation and mechanical ventilation.

*Posology and method of administration:* Please note that Nimbex should not be mixed in the same syringe or administered simultaneously through the same needle as propofol injectable emulsion or with alkaline solutions such as sodium thiopentone (please refer to *Incompatibilities* section).

Nimbex contains no antimicrobial preservative and is intended for single patient use.

*Monitoring advice:* As with other neuromuscular blocking agents, monitoring of neuromuscular function is recommended during the use of Nimbex in order to individualise dosage requirements.

Use by intravenous bolus injection.

*Dosage in adults:* Tracheal Intubation. The recommended intubation dose of Nimbex for adults is 0.15 mg/kg (body weight). This dose produced good to excellent conditions for tracheal intubation 120 seconds after administration of Nimbex, following induction of anaesthesia with propofol.

Higher doses will shorten the time to onset of neuromuscular block.

Table 1 summarises mean pharmacodynamic data when Nimbex was administered at doses of 0.1 to 0.4 mg/kg/(body weight) to healthy adult patients during opioid (thiopentone/fentanyl/midazolam) or propofol anaesthesia.

Enflurane or isoflurane anaesthesia may extend the clinically effective duration of an initial dose of Nimbex by as much as 15%.

*Maintenance:* Neuromuscular block can be extended with maintenance doses of Nimbex. A dose of 0.03 mg/kg (body weight) provides approximately 20 minutes of additional clinically effective neuromuscular block during opioid or propofol anaesthesia.

Consecutive maintenance doses do not result in progressive prolongation of effect.

*Spontaneous recovery:* Once spontaneous recovery from neuromuscular block is underway, the rate is independent of the Nimbex dose administered. During opioid or propofol anaesthesia, the median times from 25 to 75% and from 5 to 95% recovery are approximately 13 and 30 minutes, respectively.

*Reversal:* Neuromuscular block following Nimbex administration is readily reversible with standard doses of anticholinesterase agents. The mean times from 25 to 75% recovery and to full clinical recovery ($T_4$:$T_1$ ratio ³0.7) are approximately 4 and 9 minutes respectively, following administration of the reversal agent at an average of 10% $T_1$ recovery.

*Dosage in children aged 2 to 12 years:* The recommended initial dose of Nimbex in children aged 2 to 12 years, during opioid anaesthesia, is 0.1 mg/kg (bodyweight) administered over 5 to 10 seconds. Table 2 summarises mean pharmacodynamic data obtained during opioid or halothane anaesthesia. A dose of 0.1 mg/kg (bodyweight) has a faster onset time, a shorter clinically effective duration and a faster spontaneous recovery profile than those observed in adults under similar anaesthetic conditions.

Based on the tabulated data, halothane may be expected to potentiate the neuromuscular blocking

Table 1

| Initial Nimbex dose mg/kg (bodyweight) | Anaesthetic background | Time to 90% $T_1$† suppression min | Time to maximum $T_1$† suppression min | Time to 25% spontaneous $T_1$† recovery min |
|---|---|---|---|---|
| 0.1 | Opioid | 3.4 | 4.8 | 45 |
| 0.15 | Propofol | 2.6 | 3.5 | 55 |
| 0.2 | Opioid | 2.4 | 2.9 | 65 |
| 0.4 | Opioid | 1.5 | 1.9 | 91 |

†T, Single twitch response as well as the first component of the Train-of-four response of the adductor pollicis muscle following supramaximal electrical stimulation of the ulnar nerve.

Table 2

| Initial Nimbex dose mg/kg (bodyweight) | Anaesthetic background | Time to 90% $T_1$† suppression min | Time to maximum $T_1$† suppression min | Time to 25% spontaneous $T_1$† recovery min |
|---|---|---|---|---|
| 0.1 | Opioid | 1.7 | 2.8 | 28 |
| 0.08 | Halothane | 1.7 | 2.5 | 31 |

Table 3

*Infusion delivery rate of Nimbex injection 2 mg/ml*

| Patient (bodyweight) (kg) | Dose (µ/kg/min) | | | | Infusion rate |
|---|---|---|---|---|---|
| | 1.0 | 1.5 | 2.0 | 3.0 | |
| 20 | 0.6 | 0.9 | 1.2 | 1.8 | ml/hr |
| 70 | 2.1 | 3.2 | 4.2 | 6.3 | ml/hr |
| 100 | 3.0 | 4.5 | 6.0 | 9.0 | ml/hr |

Table 4

*Infusion delivery rate of Nimbex FORTE injection 5 mg/ml*

| Patient (bodyweight) (kg) | Dose (µ/kg/min) | | | | Infusion rate |
|---|---|---|---|---|---|
| | 1.0 | 1.5 | 2.0 | 3.0 | |
| 70 | 0.8 | 1.2 | 1.7 | 2.5 | ml/hr |
| 100 | 1.2 | 1.8 | 2.4 | 3.6 | ml/hr |

effect of Nimbex by approximately 20%. No information is available on the use of Nimbex in children during isoflurane or enflurane anaesthesia but these agents may also be expected to extend the clinically effective duration of a dose of Nimbex by approximately 15–20%.

*Tracheal intubation:* Although intubation has not been specifically studied in this age group, onset is faster than in adults and therefore intubation should also be possible within 2 minutes of administration. No dosage recommendation for intubation in children can be made until further information becomes available.

*Maintenance:* Neuromuscular block can be extended with maintenance doses of Nimbex. A dose of 0.02 mg/kg (body weight) provides approximately 9 minutes of additional clinically effective neuromuscular block during halothane anaesthesia. Consecutive maintenance doses do not result in progressive prolongation of effect.

*Spontaneous Recovery:* During opioid anaesthesia, the median times from 25 to 75% and from 5 to 95% recovery are approximately 10 and 25 minutes, respectively.

*Reversal:* Neuromuscular block following Nimbex administration is readily reversible with standard doses of anti-cholinesterase agents. The mean times from 25 to 75% recovery and to full clinical recovery ($T_4$:$T_1$ ratio $^3$0.7) are approximately 2 and 5 minutes respectively, following administration of the reversal agent at an average of 13% $T_1$ recovery.

*Use by intravenous infusion:*
*Dosage in adults and children aged 2 to 12 years:* Maintenance of neuromuscular block may be achieved by infusion of Nimbex. An initial infusion rate of 3 mg/kg (bodyweight)/min (0.18 mg/kg/hr) is recommended to restore 89 to 99% $T_1$ suppression following evidence of spontaneous recovery. After an initial period of stabilisation of neuromuscular block, a rate of 1 to 2 mg/kg (body weight)/min (0.06 to 0.12 mg/kg/hr) should be adequate to maintain block in this range in most patients.

Reduction of the infusion rate by up to 40% may be required when Nimbex is administered during isoflurane or enflurane anaesthesia (see *Interactions* section).

The infusion rate will depend upon the concentration of cisatracurium in the infusion solution, the desired degree of neuromuscular block, and the patient's weight. Tables 3 and 4 provide guidelines for delivery of undiluted Nimbex.

Steady rate continuous infusion of Nimbex is not associated with a progressive increase or decrease in neuromuscular blocking effect.

Following discontinuation of infusion of Nimbex, spontaneous recovery from neuromuscular block proceeds at a rate comparable to that following administration of a single bolus.

*Dosage in children aged less than 2 years:* No dosage recommendation for paediatric patients under 2 years of age can be made until further information becomes available.

*Dosage in elderly patients:* No dosing alterations are required in elderly patients. In these patients Nimbex has a similar pharmacodynamic profile to that observed in young adult patients but, as with other neuromuscular blocking agents, it may have a slightly slower onset.

*Dosage in patients with renal impairment:* No dosing alterations are required in patients with renal failure. In these patients Nimbex has a similar pharmacodynamic profile to that observed in patients with normal renal function but it may have a slightly slower onset.

*Dosage in patients with hepatic impairment:* No dosing alterations are required in patients with end-stage liver disease. In these patients Nimbex has a similar pharmacodynamic profile to that observed in patients with normal hepatic function but it may have a slightly faster onset.

*Dosage in patients with cardiovascular disease:* Nimbex has been administered by rapid bolus injection in doses of up to 0.1 mg/kg to patients undergoing coronary artery bypass graft (CABG) surgery, and was not associated with clinically significant cardiovascular effects.

*Dosage in intensive care unit (ICU) patients:* Nimbex may be administered by bolus dose and/or infusion to adult patients in the ICU. An initial infusion rate of Nimbex of 3 mg/kg (body weight)/min (0.18 mg/kg/hr) is recommended for adult ICU patients. There may be wide interpatient variation in dosage requirements and these may increase or decrease with time. In clinical studies the average infusion rate was 3 mg/kg/min [range 0.5 to 10.2 mg/kg (body weight)/min (0.03 to 0.6 mg/kg/hr)].

The median time to full spontaneous recovery following long-term (up to 6 days) infusion of Nimbex in ICU patients was approximately 50 minutes.

The recovery profile after infusions of Nimbex to ICU patients is independent of duration of infusion.

*Contra-indications:* Nimbex is contra-indicated in patients known to be hypersensitive to cisatracurium, atracurium, or benzenesulfonic acid.

Nimbex is contra-indicated in pregnancy since there is no information on the use of Nimbex in pregnant women.

Nimbex is contra-indicated in children under 2 years

of age since it has not been studied in this patient population.

*Special warnings and special precautions for use:* Cisatracurium paralyses the respiratory muscles as well as other skeletal muscles but has no known effect on consciousness or pain threshold. Nimbex should be only administered by or under the supervision of anaesthetists or other clinicians who are familiar with the use and action of neuromuscular blocking agents. Facilities for tracheal intubation, and maintenance of pulmonary ventilation and adequate arterial oxygenation have to be available.

Great caution should be exercised when administering Nimbex to patients who have shown allergic hypersensitivity to other neuromuscular blocking agents since cross-reactivity between neuromuscular blocking agents has been reported.

Cisatracurium does not have significant vagolytic or ganglion-blocking properties.

Consequently, Nimbex has no clinically significant effect on heart rate and will not counteract the bradycardia produced by many anaesthetic agents or by vagal stimulation during surgery.

Patients with myasthenia gravis and other forms of neuromuscular disease have shown greatly increased sensitivity to non-depolarising blocking agents. An initial dose of not more than 0.02 mg/kg Nimbex is recommended in these patients.

Severe acid-base and/or serum electrolyte abnormalities may increase or decrease the sensitivity of patients to neuromuscular blocking agents.

Cisatracurium has not been studied in patients with a history of malignant hyperthermia. Studies in malignant hyperthermia-susceptible pigs indicated that cisatracurium does not trigger this syndrome.

There have been no studies of cisatracurium in patients undergoing surgery with induced hypothermia (25 to 28°C). As with other neuromuscular blocking agents the rate of infusion required to maintain adequate surgical relaxation under these conditions may be expected to be significantly reduced.

Cisatracurium has not been studied in patients with burns; however, as with other non-depolarising neuromuscular blocking agents, the possibility of increased dosing requirements and shortened duration of action must be considered if Nimbex injection is administered to these patients.

Nimbex is hypotonic and must not be applied into the infusion line of a blood transfusion.

*Interaction with other medicaments and other forms of interaction:* Many drugs have been shown to influence the magnitude and/or duration of action of non-depolarising neuromuscular blocking agents, including the following:

*Increased effect:* By anaesthetic agents such as enflurane, isoflurane, halothane (see *Posology and method of administration*) and ketamine, by other non-depolarising neuromuscular blocking agents or by other drugs such as antibiotics (including the aminoglycosides, polymyxins, spectinomycin, tetracyclines, lincomycin and clindamycin); anti-arrhythmic drugs (including propranolol, calcium channel blockers, lignocaine, procainamide and quinidine); diuretics, (including frusemide and possibly thiazides, mannitol and acetazolamide); magnesium and lithium salts and ganglion blocking drugs (trimetaphan, hexamethonium).

A decreased effect is seen after prior chronic administration of phenytoin or carbamazepine.

Prior administration of suxamethonium has no effect on the duration of neuromuscular block following bolus doses of Nimbex or on infusion rate requirements.

Administration of suxamethonium to prolong the effects of non-depolarising neuromuscular blocking agents may result in a prolonged and complex block which can be difficult to reverse with anticholinesterases.

Rarely, certain drugs may aggravate or unmask latent myasthenia gravis or actually induce a myasthenic syndrome; increased sensitivity to non-depolarising neuromuscular blocking agents might result. Such drugs include various antibiotics, β-blockers (propranolol, oxprenolol), anti-arrhythmic drugs (procainamide, quinidine), anti-rheumatic drugs (chloroquine, D-penicillamine), trimetaphan, chlorpromazine, steroids, phenytoin and lithium.

*Pregnancy and lactation:* Nimbex is contra-indicated in pregnancy since there is no information on the use of Nimbex in pregnant women. Fertility studies have not been performed. Reproduction studies in rats have not revealed any adverse effects on fetal development of cisatracurium. The relevance of these studies is limited due to species differences in metabolism and low systemic exposure levels.

It is not known whether cisatracurium or its metabolites are excreted in human milk.

*Effect on ability to drive and use machines:* This

precaution is not relevant to the use of Nimbex. However the usual precautions relating to performance of tasks following general anaesthesia still apply.

*Undesirable effects:* Adverse effects recorded following administration of Nimbex were cutaneous flushing or rash, bradycardia, hypotension and bronchospasm (see *Dosage in intensive care unit (ICU) patients* and *Pharmacodynamic properties*).

*Overdosage:* Symptoms and signs: Prolonged muscle paralysis and its consequences are expected to be the main signs of overdosage with Nimbex.

Management: It is essential to maintain pulmonary ventilation and arterial oxygenation until adequate spontaneous respiration returns. Full sedation will be required since consciousness is not impaired by Nimbex. Recovery may be accelerated by the administration of anti-cholinesterase agents once evidence of spontaneous recovery is present.

**Pharmacological properties**

*Pharmacodynamic properties:* Cisatracurium is an intermediate-duration, non-depolarising benzylisoquinolinium skeletal muscle relaxant.

Clinical studies in man indicated that Nimbex is not associated with dose-dependent histamine release even at doses up to and including 8×$ED_{95}$.

*Mode of action:* Cisatracurium binds to cholinergic receptors on the motor end-plate to antagonise the action of acetylcholine, resulting in a competitive block of neuromuscular transmission. This action is readily reversed by anti-cholinesterase agents such as neostigmine or edrophonium.

The $ED_{95}$ (dose required to produce 95% depression of the twitch response of the adductor pollicis muscle to stimulation of the ulnar nerve) of cisatracurium is estimated to be 0.05 mg/kg bodyweight during opioid anaesthesia (thiopentone/fentanyl/midazolam).

The $ED_{95}$ of cisatracurium in children during halothane anaesthesia is 0.04 mg/kg.

*Pharmacokinetic properties:* Cisatracurium undergoes degradation in the body at physiological pH and temperature by Hofmann elimination (a chemical process) to form laudanosine and the monoquaternary acrylate metabolite. The monoquaternary acrylate undergoes hydrolysis by non-specific plasma esterases to form the monoquaternary alcohol metabolite. Elimination of cisatracurium is largely organ independent but the liver and kidneys are primary pathways for the clearance of its metabolites.

These metabolites do not possess neuromuscular blocking activity.

Pharmacokinetics in adult patients: Non-compartmental pharmacokinetics of cisatracurium are independent of dose in the range studied (0.1 to 0.2 mg/kg, i.e. 2 to 4×$ED_{95}$).

Population pharmacokinetic modelling confirms and extends these findings up to 0.4 mg/kg (8×$ED_{95}$). Pharmacokinetic parameters after doses of 0.1 and 0.2 mg/kg Nimbex administered to healthy adult surgical patients are summarised in the table below:

| *Parameter* | *Range of mean values* |
|---|---|
| Clearance | 4.7 to 5.7 ml/min/kg |
| Volume of distribution at steady state | 121 to 161 ml/kg |
| Elimination half-life | 22 to 29 min |

*Pharmacokinetics in elderly patients:* There are no clinically important differences in the pharmacokinetics of cisatracurium in elderly and young adult patients. The recovery profile is also unchanged.

*Pharmacokinetics in patients with renal/hepatic impairment:* There are no clinically important differences in the pharmacokinetics of cisatracurium in patients with end-stage renal failure or end stage liver disease and in healthy adult patients. Their recovery profiles are also unchanged.

*Pharmacokinetics during infusions:* The pharmacokinetics of cisatracurium after infusions of Nimbex are similar to those after single bolus injection. The recovery profile after infusion of Nimbex is independent of duration of infusion and is similar to that after single bolus injection.

*Pharmacokinetics in intensive care unit (ICU) patients:* The pharmacokinetics of cisatracurium in ICU patients receiving prolonged infusions are similar to those in healthy surgical adults receiving infusions or single bolus injections. The recovery profile after infusions of Nimbex in ICU patients is independent of duration of infusion.

*Preclinical safety data: Acute toxicity:* Meaningful acute studies with cisatracurium could not be performed. For symptoms of toxicity see *Overdosage.*

*Subacute toxicity:* Studies with repeated administration for three weeks in dogs and monkeys showed no compound specific toxic signs.

*Mutagenicity:* Cisatracurium was not mutagenic in an in vitro microbial mutagenicity test at concentrations up to 5000 mg/plate.

In an *in vivo* cytogenetic study in rats, no significant chromosomal abnormalities were seen at s.c doses up to 4 mg/kg.

Cisatracurium was mutagenic in an in vitro mouse lymphoma cell mutagenicity assay, at concentrations of 40 mg/ml and higher.

A single positive mutagenic response for a drug used infrequently and/or briefly is of questionable clinical relevance.

*Carcinogenicity:* Carcinogenicity studies have not been performed.

*Local tolerance:* The result of an intra-arterial study in rabbits showed that Nimbex injection is well tolerated and no drug related changes were seen.

**Pharmaceutical particulars**

*List of excipients:* Benzenesulfonic Acid solution 32% w/v (Wellcome specification); Water for Injections (PhEur).

*Incompatibilities:* Degradation of cisatracurium besilate has been demonstrated to occur more rapidly in lactated Ringer's Injection and 5% Dextrose and lactated Ringer's Injection than in the infusion fluids listed in *Instructions for use/handling* section.

Therefore it is recommended that lactated Ringer's Injection and 5% Dextrose and lactated Ringer's Injection are not used as the diluent in preparing solutions of Nimbex for infusion.

Since Nimbex is stable only in acidic solutions it should not be mixed in the same syringe or administered simultaneously through the same needle with alkaline solutions, e.g., sodium thiopentone. It is compatible with ketorolac trometamol or propofol injectable emulsion.

*Shelf life:* Shelf-life of the medicinal product as packaged for sale: 24 months at 2–8°C.

Shelf-life after dilution according to directions: The product contains no antimicrobial preservative and therefore should be used immediately on dilution, or failing this the aseptically prepared dilution should be stored at 2–8°C for no more than 24 hrs, after which time unused solution should be discarded.

Shelf-life after the first time the pack is opened: The pack is designed for use on a single occasion, injected or diluted immediately after opening, any remaining solution should be discarded.

*Special precautions for storage:* Do not freeze. Protect from light.

*Nature and contents of container:* Nimbex injection 2 mg/ml comes in boxes of 5×2.5 ml, 5 ml or 10 ml ampoules, 2×25 ml ampoules and Nimbex [Forte] injeciton 5 mg/ml as 1×30 ml vial.

Type I, clear, neutral glass ampoules.

Type I, clear, neutral glass vial with a polymeric coated synthetic bromobutyl rubber stopper and aluminium collar with plastic flip-top cover.

*Instructions for use/handling:* Use only clear and almost colourless up to slightly yellow/greenish yellow coloured solutions.

Diluted Nimbex is physically and chemically stable for at least 24 hours at 5°C and 25°C at concentrations between 0.1 and 2 mg/ml in the following infusion fluids, in either polyvinyl chloride or polypropylene containers:

Sodium Chloride (0.9% w/v) Intravenous Infusion.
Glucose (5% w/v) Intravenous Infusion.
Sodium Chloride (0.18% w/v) and Glucose (4% w/v) Intravenous Infusion.
Sodium Chloride (0.45% w/v) and Glucose (2.5% w/v) Intravenous Infusion.

However, since the product contains no antimicrobial preservative, dilution should be carried out immediately prior to use, or failing this be stored as directed under *Special precautions for storage.*

Nimbex has been shown to be compatible with the following commonly used peri-operative drugs, when mixed in conditions simulating administration into a running intravenous infusion via a Y-site injection port: alfentanil hydrochloride, droperidol, fentanyl citrate, midazolam hydrochloride and sufentanil citrate. Where other drugs are administered through the same indwelling needle or cannula as Nimbex, it is recommended that each drug be flushed through with an adequate volume of a suitable intravenous fluid, e.g. Sodium Chloride Intravenous Infusion (0.9% w/v).

As with other drugs administered intravenously, when a small vein is selected as the injection site, Nimbex should be flushed through the vein with a suitable intravenous fluid, e.g. sodium chloride intravenous infusion (0.9% w/v).

**Marketing authorisation numbers**

| | |
|---|---|
| Nimbex Injection 2 mg/ml | 0003/0364 |
| Nimbex (Forte) Injection 5 mg/ml | 0003/0365 |

**Date of approval/revision of SPC** 7 August 1995

**Legal category** POM.

# PHYSEPTONE* INJECTION PHYSEPTONE* TABLETS

**Presentation** Physeptone Injection contains 10 mg Methadone Hydrochloride BP in each ml.

Physeptone Tablets each contain 5 mg Methadone Hydrochloride BP, scored, coded 'WELLCOME L4A' and white in colour.

**Uses** For use as an analgesic for moderate to severe pain.

**Dosage and administration**

*Adults:* Usual single dose 5 to 10 mg by mouth, subcutaneous or intramuscular injection.

Owing to its long plasma half-life caution with repeated dosage should be observed in the very ill or elderly. The usual initial dose should be 5 to 10 mg, 6 to 8 hourly, later adjusted to the degree of pain relief obtained.

*Children:* Not suitable.

*Use in the elderly:* Use caution with repeated dosage in elderly and ill patients.

**Contra-indications, warnings, etc**

*Contra-indications:* Respiratory depression and obstructive airways disease. Concurrent administration with monoamine oxidase inhibitors, or within 2 weeks of discontinuation of treatment with them. Obstetric use is not recommended.

*Precautions:* Tolerance and dependence of the morphine type may occur.

Methadone can produce drowsiness and clouding of consciousness; patients should therefore be warned not to drive or use machines while taking the drug.

*Side- and adverse effects:* Nausea, vomiting and dizziness may occur, particularly in ambulant patients. Nausea and vomiting appear to be more frequent after oral administration than after injection.

*Use in pregnancy and lactation:* There is inadequate evidence of safety in human pregnancy but the drug has been widely used for many years without apparent ill-consequence and animal studies have not shown any hazard. From theoretical considerations methadone is likely to be excreted in breast milk.

*Drug interactions:* Monoamine oxidase inhibitors (MAOIs) may prolong and enhance the respiratory depressant effects of methadone.

The general depressant effects of methadone may be enhanced by other agents with central nervous system depressant activity such as alcohol, phenothiazines, tricyclic antidepressants and barbiturates.

Rifampicin has been reported to reduce circulating levels of methadone and to increase its urinary excretion.

Phenytoin has been reported to enhance the metabolism of methadone.

*Toxicity and treatment of overdosage:* The cardinal signs of methadone overdose are coma, depressed respiration, pinpoint pupils, hypotension and pulmonary oedema. The presence of signs of drug abuse supports the diagnosis. In children, methadone overdose produces drowsiness, floppiness, pinpoint pupils and apnoea.

Treatment consists of the establishment of a patent airway together with other supportive measures, and the administration of a specific opioid antagonist, preferably naloxone, given in a dose of 0.4 mg by intravenous injection repeated 2 or 3 times after 2 to 3 minutes. Reversal of coma and respiratory depression is seen within two minutes of naloxone administration. Naloxone should be administered to children in doses of 5 to 10 micrograms per kilogram body weight and to neonates in doses of 10 micrograms per kilogram body weight. Repeated treatment with naloxone may be required to prevent recurrence of coma because the duration of action of naloxone is shorter than that of methadone. Patients should be monitored for signs of relapse for at least 48 hours.

**Pharmaceutical precautions**

*Injection:* Store below 25°C, protect from light.
*Tablets:* Store below 25°C.

**Legal category** CD (Sch 2), POM

**Package quantities**

*Physeptone Injection:* 10 mg in 1 ml ampoules. Boxes of 5 and 100 ampoules.

*Physeptone Tablets:* Blister pack of 50 tablets as 5 blister strips of 10 tablets.

**Further information** Nil.

**Product licence numbers**

| | |
|---|---|
| Physeptone Injection: | 0003/5100R |
| Physeptone Tablets: | 0003/5099R |

# PREDNESOL* TABLETS

**Presentation** Small, pink, soluble tablets engraved 'Prednesol Glaxo' on one side and scored on the reverse. Each tablet contains 5 mg prednisolone as the sodium phosphate ester.

**Uses** Prednisolone is a glucocorticosteroid which is four times as active as hydrocortisone on a weight-for-weight basis.

Prednisolone sodium phosphate is very soluble in water, and is therefore less likely to cause local gastric irritation than prednisolone alcohol, which is only slightly soluble. This is important when high dosages are required, as in immuno-suppressive therapy.

A wide variety of diseases may sometimes require corticosteroid therapy. Some of the principal indications are:

bronchial asthma, severe hypersensitivity reactions, anaphylaxis;

rheumatoid arthritis, systemic lupus erythematosus, dermatomyositis, mixed connective tissue disease (excluding systemic sclerosis), polyarteritis nodosa;

inflammatory skin disorders, including pemphigus vulgaris, bullous pemphigoid and pyoderma gangrenosum;

minimal change nephrotic syndrome, acute interstitial nephritis;

ulcerative colitis, Crohn's disease; sarcoidosis; rheumatic carditis;

haemolytic anaemia (autoimmune), acute and lymphatic leukaemia, malignant lymphoma, multiple myeloma, idiopathic thrombocytopenic purpura; immunosuppression in transplantation.

**Dosage and administration** Prednesol Tablets are best taken dissolved in water, but they can be swallowed whole without difficulty.

The lowest dosage that will produce an acceptable result should be used (see *Precautions*); when it is possible to reduce the dosage, this must be accomplished by stages. During prolonged therapy any intercurrent illness, trauma or surgical procedure will require a temporary increase in dosage; if corticosteroids have been stopped following prolonged therapy they may need to be temporarily re-introduced.

*Adults:* The dose used will depend upon the disease, its severity, and the clinical response obtained. The following regimens are for guidance only. Divided dosage is usually employed.

*Short-term treatment:* 20 to 30 mg daily for the first few days, subsequently reducing the daily dosage by 2.5 or 5 mg every two to five days, depending upon the response.

*Rheumatoid arthritis:* 7.5 to 10 mg daily. For maintenance therapy the lowest effective dosage is used.

*Most other conditions:* 10 to 100 mg daily for one to three weeks, then reducing to the minimum effective dosage.

*Children:* Fractions of the adult dosage may be used (e.g. 75% at 12 years, 50% at 7 years and 25% at 1 year) but clinical factors must be given due weight.

**Contra-indications, warnings, etc.**
*Contra-indications:* Systemic infections, unless specific anti-infective therapy is employed. Live virus immunisation. Hypersensitivity to any component of the tablets.

*Precautions:* Patients should carry 'Steroid treatment' cards which give clear guidance on the precautions to be taken to minimise risk and which provide details of prescriber, drug, dosage and the duration of treatment.

Adrenal cortical atrophy develops during prolonged therapy and may persist for years after stopping treatment. Withdrawal of corticosteroids after prolonged therapy must therefore always be gradual to avoid acute adrenal insufficiency, being tapered off over weeks or months according to the dose and duration of treatment. During prolonged therapy any intercurrent illness, trauma or surgical procedure will require a temporary increase in dosage; if corticosteroids have been stopped following prolonged therapy they may need to be temporarily re-introduced.

Suppression of the HPA axis and other undesirable effects may be minimised by using the lowest effective dose for the minimum period, and by administering the daily requirement as a single morning dose or, whenever possible, as a single morning dose on alternate days. Frequent patient review is required to appropriately titrate the dose against disease activity (see *Dosage*).

Suppression of the inflammatory response and immune function increases the susceptibility to infections and their severity. The clinical presentation may often be atypical and serious infections such as septicaemia and tuberculosis may be masked and may reach an advanced stage before being recognised.

Chickenpox is of particular concern since this normally minor illness may be fatal in immunosuppressed patients. Patients without a definite history of chickenpox should be advised to avoid close personal contact with chickenpox or herpes zoster and if exposed they should seek urgent medical attention. If the patient is a child parents must be given the above advice. Passive immunisation with varicella zoster immunoglobulin (VZIG) is needed by exposed non-immune patients who are receiving systemic corticosteroids or who have used them within the previous 3 months; this should be given within 10 days of exposure to chickenpox. If a diagnosis of chickenpox is confirmed, the illness warrants specialist care and urgent treatment. Corticosteroids should not be stopped and the dose may need to be increased.

Live vaccines should not be given to individuals with impaired immune responsiveness. The antibody response to other vaccines may be diminished.

Because of the possibility of fluid retention, care must be taken when corticosteroids are administered to patients with renal insufficiency or hypertension or congestive heart failure.

Corticosteroids may worsen diabetes mellitus, osteoporosis, hypertension, glaucoma and epilepsy and therefore patients with these conditions or a family history of them should be monitored frequently.

Care is required and frequent patient monitoring necessary where there is a history of severe affective disorders (especially a previous history of steroid psychosis), previous steroid myopathy, peptic ulceration or patients with a history of tuberculosis.

In patients with liver failure, blood levels of corticosteroid may be increased, as with other drugs which are metabolised in the liver. Frequent patient monitoring is therefore necessary.

*Use in children:* Corticosteroids cause dose-related growth retardation in infancy, childhood and adolescence, which may be irreversible.

*Use in the elderly:* The common adverse effects of systemic corticosteroids may be associated with more serious consequences in old age, especially osteoporosis, hypertension, hypokalaemia, diabetes, susceptibility to infection and thinning of the skin. Close clinical supervision is required to avoid life-threatening reactions.

*Pregnancy:* Administration of corticosteroids to pregnant animals can cause abnormalities of fetal development including cleft palate and intra-uterine growth retardation. There may therefore be a very small risk of such effects in the human fetus. Hypoadrenalism may occur in the neonate. When corticosteroids are essential however, patients with normal pregnancies may be treated as though they were in the non-gravid state. Patients with pre-eclampsia or fluid retention require close monitoring.

Depression of hormone levels has been described in pregnancy but the significance of this finding is not clear.

*Lactation:* Corticosteroids are excreted in small amounts in breast milk and infants of mothers taking pharmacological doses of steroids should be monitored carefully for signs of adrenal suppression.

*Side-effects:* The incidence of predictable undesirable effects, including hypothalamic-pituitary-adrenal suppression correlates with the relative potency of the drug, dosage, timing of administration and the duration of treatment (see *Precautions*).

*Endocrine/metabolic:* Suppression of the hypothalamic-pituitary-adrenal axis, growth suppression in infancy, childhood and adolescence, menstrual irregularity and amenorrhoea. Cushingoid faces, hirsutism, weight gain, impaired carbohydrate tolerance with increased requirement for anti-diabetic therapy. Negative protein and calcium balance. Increased appetite.

*Anti-inflammatory and immunosuppressive effects:* Increased susceptibility and severity of infections with suppression of clinical symptoms and signs, opportunistic infections, recurrence of dormant tuberculosis (see *Precautions*).

*Musculoskeletal:* Osteoporosis, vertebral and long bone fractures, avascular osteonecrosis particularly of the femoral head may occur after prolonged corticosteroid therapy or after repeat short courses involving high doses, tendon rupture. Proximal myopathy.

*Fluid and electrolyte disturbance:* Sodium and water retention, hypertension, potassium loss, hypokalaemic alkalosis.

*Neuropsychiatric:* Euphoria, psychological dependence, depression, insomnia and aggravation of schizophrenia. Increased intra-cranial pressure with papilloedema in children (pseudotumour cerebri), usually after treatment withdrawal. Aggravation of epilepsy.

*Ophthalmic:* Increased intra-ocular pressure, glaucoma, papilloedema, posterior subcapsular cataracts, corneal or scleral thinning, exacerbation of ophthalmic viral or fungal diseases.

*Gastrointestinal:* Dyspepsia, peptic ulceration with perforation and haemorrhage, acute pancreatitis, candidiasis.

*Dermatological:* Impaired healing, skin atrophy, bruising, telangiectasia, striae, acne.

*General:* Hypersensitivity including anaphylaxis, has been reported. Leucocytosis. Thromboembolism.

*Withdrawal symptoms and signs:* Too rapid a reduction of corticosteroid dosage following prolonged treatment can lead to acute adrenal insufficiency, hypotension and death (see *Precautions*).

A 'withdrawal syndrome' may also occur including, fever, myalgia, arthralgia, rhinitis, conjunctivitis, painful itchy skin nodules and loss of weight.

*Drug interactions:* Rifampicin, rifabutin, carbamazepine, phenobarbitone, phenytoin, primidone, ephedrine and aminoglutethimide enhance the metabolism of corticosteroids and its therapeutic effects may be reduced.

The desired effects of hypoglycaemic agents (including insulin), anti-hypertensives and diuretics are antagonised by corticosteroids, and the hypokalaemic effects of acetazolamide, loop diuretics, thiazide diuretics and carbenoxolone are enhanced.

The efficacy of coumarin anticoagulants may be enhanced by concurrent corticosteroid therapy and close monitoring of the INR or prothrombin time is required to avoid spontaneous bleeding.

The renal clearance of salicylates is increased by corticosteroids and steroid withdrawal may result in salicylate intoxication.

Steroids may reduce the effects of anticholinesterases in myasthenia gravis and cholecystographic X-ray media.

*Overdosage:* Treatment is unlikely to be needed in cases of acute overdosage.

**Pharmaceutical precautions** Protect from light.

**Legal category** POM.

**Package quantities** The tablets are strip-packed in cartons of 100 (OP).

**Further information** Prednesol Tablets do not contain carbohydrates.

**Product licence number** 10949/0107

# PROPADERM* SKIN PREPARATIONS

**Presentation** Propaderm Cream and Ointment are topical preparations of Beclomethasone Dipropionate BP. Beclomethasone Dipropionate BP is a potent anti-inflammatory steroid when applied topically to the skin.

Propaderm Cream: Beclomethasone Dipropionate BP 0.025% in a cream base.

Propaderm Ointment: Beclomethasone Dipropionate BP 0.025% in an ointment base.

Propaderm Cream is white in colour; Propaderm Ointment is yellowish.

**Uses** Propaderm Cream and Ointment are indicated for the treatment of the various forms of eczema in children and adults including atopic and discoid eczemas; primary irritant and allergic dermatitis; psoriasis (excluding widespread plaque psoriasis); neurodermatoses including lichen simplex; intertrigo; discoid lupus erythematosus.

Propaderm Cream is often appropriate for moist or weeping surfaces and Propaderm Ointment for dry, lichenified or scaly lesions but this is not invariably so.

**Dosage and administration** Propaderm preparations should be applied thinly over the whole of the affected area and gently rubbed in. Initially, application should be made twice daily, but when improvement is seen, the intervals between applications may be extended and treatment eventually stopped. If no improvement is seen within two to four weeks, reassessment of the diagnosis, or referral may be necessary. After cessation of treatment, should the condition recur, twice daily treatment should be re-instituted. However, when improvement is seen again, the intervals between application may be gradually extended until maintenance dosing of application every third or fourth day is achieved. This is likely to avoid subsequent reappearance of the condition. The beneficial effects may be enhanced by preliminary use of hot soaks, or by intermittent applications or occlusive dressings.

**Contra-indications, warnings, etc.**
*Contra-indications:* Propaderm should not be applied to the eyes. Rosacea, acne vulgaris; peri-oral

dermatitis. Primary cutaneous viral infections (e.g. herpes simplex, chickenpox). Hypersensitivity to the preparation. Varicose ulcers or any other stasis ulcers.

Use of Propaderm preparations is not indicated in the treatment of primarily infected skin lesions caused by infection with fungi (e.g. candidiasis, tinea) or bacteria (e.g. impetigo); primary or secondary infections due to yeasts; perianal and genital pruritus; dermatoses in children under 1 year of age, including dermatitis and napkin eruptions.

*Precautions:* Long-term continuous therapy should be avoided where possible, particularly in infants and children, as adrenal suppression can occur even without occlusion.

The face, more than the other areas of the body, may exhibit atrophic changes after prolonged treatment with potent topical corticosteroids. This must be borne in mind when treating such conditions as psoriasis, discoid lupus erythematosus and severe eczema. If applied to the eyelids, care is needed to ensure that the preparation does not enter the eye, as glaucoma might result.

If used in childhood, or on the face, courses should be limited if possible to five days and occlusion should not be used.

Topical corticosteroids may be hazardous in psoriasis for a number of reasons including rebound relapses, development of tolerance, risk of generalised pustular psoriasis and development of local or systemic toxicity due to impaired barrier function of the skin. If used in psoriasis careful patient supervision is important.

Appropriate antimicrobial therapy should be used whenever treating inflammatory lesions which have become infected. Any spread of infection requires withdrawal of topical corticosteroid therapy and systemic administration of antimicrobial agents.

Bacterial infection is encouraged by the warm, moist conditions induced by occlusive dressings, and so the skin should be cleansed before a fresh dressing is applied.

*Pregnancy:* There is inadequate evidence of safety in human pregnancy. Topical administration of corticosteroids to pregnant animals can cause abnormalities of fetal development including cleft palate and intrauterine growth retardation. There may therefore be a very small risk of such effects in the human fetus.

*Side-effects:* Prolonged and intensive treatment with highly active corticosteroid preparations may cause local atrophic changes in the skin such as thinning, striae, and dilatation of the superficial blood vessels, particularly when occlusive dressings are used or when skin folds are involved.

As with other topical corticosteroids, prolonged use of large amounts, or treatment of extensive areas, can result in sufficient systemic absorption to produce the features of hypercorticism. The effect is more likely to occur in infants and children, and if occlusive dressings are used. In infants, the napkin may act as an occlusive dressing.

Should systemic corticosteroid effects arise from application of Propaderm preparations topical treatment should be discontinued. If adrenal function is impaired the patient will need to be protected from any harmful effects of stress with oral corticosteroid preparations until normal adrenal function is established.

There are reports of pigmentation changes and hypertrichosis with topical steroids.

In rare instances, treatment of psoriasis with corticosteroids (or its withdrawal) is thought to have provoked the pustular form of the disease (see *Precautions*).

Propaderm Cream and Ointment are usually well tolerated, but if signs of hypersensitivity appear, application should stop immediately.

Exacerbation of symptoms may occur.

*Overdosage:* Acute overdosage is very unlikely to occur. However, in the case of chronic overdosage or misuse the features of hypercorticism may appear and in this situation topical steroids should be discontinued.

**Pharmaceutical precautions**
*Storage:* All Propaderm preparations should be stored at a temperature below 25˚C and protected from light.
*Dilution:* Propaderm Cream may be diluted, if necessary, with Cetomacrogol Cream Formula A BPC. For Propaderm Ointment, dilution can be effected with White Soft Paraffin BP.

**Legal category** POM.

**Package quantities** Propaderm Cream is available in tubes of 30 g; Propaderm Ointment in tubes of 30 g.

**Further information** No Propaderm preparation contains lanolin or parabens.

**Product licence numbers**
Propaderm Cream       10949/0038
Propaderm Ointment    10949/0039

## PURI-NETHOL* TABLETS

**Presentation** Each pale-yellow tablet contains 50 mg Mercaptopurine BP, and is scored and coded 'WELLCOME 04A'.

**Uses** Cytotoxic agent.

Puri-Nethol is indicated for the treatment of acute leukaemia. It is of value in remission induction and is particularly indicated for maintenance therapy in acute lymphoblastic leukaemia and acute myelogenous leukaemia. Puri-Nethol is also used in the treatment of chronic granulocytic leukaemia.

*Mode of action:* 6–mercaptopurine is an analogue of adenine, one of the bases required for nucleic acid biosynthesis, and of the purine base hypoxanthine. Hence Puri-Nethol acts as an antimetabolite and interferes with the synthesis of nucleic acids in proliferating cells. Its metabolites are also pharmacologically active.

*Pharmacokinetics:* Absorption of an oral dose of Puri-Nethol is incomplete and variable averaging about 50% of the administered dose. The half-life of 6–mercaptopurine in the circulation is of the order of 90 minutes. It is extensively metabolised and excreted *via* the kidneys and the active metabolites have a longer half-life than the parent drug. 6–mercaptopurine has pKa's of 7.7 and 11.0.

**Dosage and administration** *For adults and children* the usual dose is 2.5 mg/kg bodyweight per day, but the dose and duration of administration depend on the nature and dosage of other cytotoxic agents given in conjunction with Puri-Nethol. The dosage should be carefully adjusted to suit the individual patient. Puri-Nethol has been used in various combination therapy schedules for acute leukaemia and the literature should be consulted for details. Consideration should be given to reducing the dosage in patients with impaired hepatic or renal function. When Zyloric* (allopurinol) and mercaptopurine are administered concomitantly it is essential that only a quarter of the usual dose of mercaptopurine is given since Zyloric (allopurinol) decreases the rate of catabolism of mercaptopurine.

*Use in the elderly:* No specific studies have been carried out in the elderly. However, it is advisable to monitor renal and hepatic function in these patients, and if there is any impairment consideration should be given to reducing Puri-Nethol dosage.

**Contra-indications, warnings, etc**
*Contra-indications:* In view of the seriousness of the indications there are no absolute contra-indications.

*Precautions:* Puri-Nethol is an active cytotoxic agent for use only under the direction of physicians experienced in the administration of such agents.

Since Puri-Nethol is strongly myelosuppressive, full blood counts must be taken daily during remission induction. Patients must be carefully monitored during therapy.

Treatment with Puri-Nethol causes bone marrow suppression leading to leucopenia and thrombocytopenia.

The leucocyte and platelet counts continue to fall after treatment is stopped, so at the first sign of an abnormally large fall in the counts, treatment should be interrupted immediately.

Bone marrow suppression is reversible if Puri-Nethol is withdrawn early enough.

During remission induction in acute myelogenous leukaemia the patient may frequently have to survive a period of relative bone marrow aplasia and it is important that adequate supportive facilities are available.

Puri-Nethol is hepatotoxic and liver function tests should be monitored weekly during treatment. More frequent monitoring may be advisable in those with pre-existing liver disease or receiving other potentially hepatotoxic therapy. The patient should be instructed to discontinue Puri-Nethol immediately if jaundice becomes apparent.

During remission induction when rapid cell lysis is occurring, uric acid levels in blood and urine should be monitored as hyperuricaemia and/or hyperuricosuria may develop, with the risk of uric acid nephropathy.

Puri-Nethol in common with other antimetabolites is potentially mutagenic and chromosome damage has been reported in rats and man. Increases in chromosomal aberrations were observed in the peripheral lymphocytes of leukaemic patients and in a hypernephroma patient who received an unstated dose of 6–mercaptopurine.

In view of its action on cellular deoxyribonucleic acid (DNA) 6–mercaptopurine is potentially carcinogenic and consideration should be given to the theoretical risk of carcinogenesis with this treatment. Three cases have been documented of the occurrence of acute nonlymphatic leukaemia in patients who received 6–mercaptopurine for non-neoplastic disorders.

A patient with Hodgkin's disease treated with 6–mercaptopurine and multiple additional cytotoxic agents developed acute myelogenous leukaemia. Twelve and a half years after 6–mercaptopurine treatment for myasthenia gravis a female patient developed chronic myeloid leukaemia.

It is advised that care be taken when handling or halving these tablets so as not to contaminate hands or to inspire drug.

*Side- and adverse effects:* The main side-effect of treatment with Puri-Nethol is bone marrow suppression leading to leucopenia and thrombocytopenia. Puri-Nethol is hepatotoxic in animals and man. The histological findings in man have shown hepatic necrosis and biliary stasis. The incidence of hepatotoxicity varies considerably and can occur with any dose but more frequently when the recommended dose of 2.5 mg/kg bodyweight daily is exceeded. Monitoring of liver function tests may allow early detection of liver toxicity. This is usually reversible if Puri-Nethol therapy is stopped soon enough, but fatal liver damage has occurred.

Anorexia, nausea and vomiting have occasionally been noted.

Oral ulceration has been reported during Puri-Nethol therapy and rarely intestinal ulceration has occurred.

Rare complications are drug fever and skin rash.

Pancreatitis has been reported in association with the unlicensed use of 6–mercaptopurine in the treatment of inflammatory bowel disease.

*Drug interactions:* When Zyloric (allopurinol) and Puri-Nethol are administered concomitantly it is essential that only a quarter of the usual dose of Puri-Nethol is given since Zyloric decreases the rate of catabolism of Puri-Nethol.

Inhibition of the anticoagulant effect of warfarin, when given with Puri-Nethol, has been reported.

*Use in pregnancy and lactation:* Puri-Nethol is embryotoxic in rats. This effect is dose dependent.

Normal offspring have been born after Puri-Nethol therapy during human pregnancy, but abortion, prematurity and malformation have been reported. A leukaemia patient treated with 6–mercaptopurine 100 mg/day (plus splenic irradiation) throughout pregnancy gave birth to a normal, premature baby. A second baby, born to the same mother, who was treated as before together with busulphan 4 mg/day, had multiple severe abnormalities, including corneal opacities, microphthalmia, cleft palate and hypoplasia of the thyroid and ovaries.

The small numbers involved do not allow an evaluation of the degree of risk of Puri-Nethol therapy during pregnancy and the possible hazard to the fetus must be balanced against the expected benefit in any individual case.

Transient profound oligospermia was observed in a young man who received 6–mercaptopurine 150 mg/day plus prednisone 80 mg/day for acute leukaemia. Two years after cessation of the chemotherapy he had a normal sperm count and fathered a normal child.

Mothers receiving Puri-Nethol should not breast feed.

*Toxicity and treatment of overdosage:* The principal toxic effects on the bone marrow and haematological toxicity is likely to be more profound with chronic overdosage than with a single ingestion of Puri-Nethol. The risk of overdosage is also increased when Zyloric is being given concomitantly with Puri-Nethol. As there is no known antidote the blood picture should be closely monitored and general supportive measures, together with appropriate blood transfusion, instituted if necessary.

**Pharmaceutical precautions** Store below 25˚C. Keep dry, protect from light.

**Legal category** POM

**Package quantities** Bottle of 25 tablets.

**Further information** Puri-Nethol is an analogue of adenine and hypoxanthine, and microbiological studies have shown it to be an antagonist of these; its mode of action differs thus from that of the folic antagonists.

**Product licence number** 0003/5227R

## PYLORID* TABLETS ▼

**Qualitative and quantitative composition** Each tablet contains 400 mg of ranitidine bismuth citrate (INN).

**Pharmaceutical form** Light blue, film-coated, octagonal capsule-shaped tablets.

**Clinical particulars**
*Therapeutic indications:* Treatment of duodenal ulcer and benign gastric ulcer.

Eradication of *Helicobacter pylori* and prevention of

relapse of duodenal ulcer when administered in conjunction with clarithromycin or amoxycillin.

*Posology and method of administration:* The recommended dose should be taken twice daily, in the morning and evening, preferably with food.

*Treatment of peptic ulcer disease:*
Duodenal ulcer: Pylorid 400 mg b.d. for 4 weeks. Treatment may be extended for a further 4 weeks. Benign gastric ulcer: Pylorid 400 mg b.d. for 8 weeks.

*Eradication of Helicobacter pylori and prevention of relapse of duodenal ulcer:* Since eradication rates for *Helicobacter pylori* after monotherapy with Pylorid were very low, Pylorid should be used in combination with clarithromycin in one of the following regimens:

Pylorid 400 mg b.d. with clarithromycin 500 mg b.d. for the first 2 weeks of treatment, followed by Pylorid tablets 400 mg b.d. for a further 2 weeks. Alternatively, clarithromycin 500 mg may be given t.d.s. with Pylorid 400 mg b.d. for the initial 2-week period.

Treatment with Pylorid in combination with amoxycillin resulted in lower eradication rates than with clarithromycin. However, in cases where clarithromycin cannot be given, amoxycillin may be given as a second alternative in the following regimen:

Pylorid 400 mg b.d. with amoxycillin 500 mg q.d.s. for the first 2 weeks of treatment, followed by Pylorid Tablets 400 mg b.d. for a further 2 weeks.

Pylorid is not indicated for long-term (maintenance) therapy; more than two 8-week courses in any one year should be avoided because of the possibility of accumulation of bismuth. If 4-week courses of therapy are given, up to a maximum of 16 weeks of treatment may be given in any one year.

*Elderly patients:* Ranitidine and bismuth exposure is increased in elderly patients as a result of decreased renal clearance (see *Renal impairment* and *Contra-indications*).

*Children:* There are no data available on the use of Pylorid Tablets in children. Therefore, they are not recommended for use in children.

*Renal impairment:* Ranitidine and bismuth exposure is increased in patients with renal impairment as a result of decreased clearance. As with other bismuth-containing drugs, Pylorid should not be used in patients with moderate to severe renal impairment i.e., creatinine clearance typically <25 ml/min (see *Contra-indications*).

*Hepatic impairment:* There is no information regarding the use of Pylorid Tablets in patients with hepatic impairment. However, as ranitidine and bismuth in the systemic circulation are eliminated mainly by renal clearance, no dosage adjustment is necessary in hepatically-impaired patients.

*Contra-indications:* Pylorid Tablets are contra-indicated in patients known to have hypersensitivity to any of the ingredients.

Pylorid is contra-indicated for long-term (maintenance) therapy.

As with other bismuth-containing drugs, Pylorid should not be used in patients with moderate to severe renal impairment i.e., creatinine clearance typically <25 ml/min.

*Special warnings and precautions for use:* The possibility of malignancy should be excluded before commencement of therapy in patients with gastric ulcer, as treatment with Pylorid Tablets may mask symptoms of gastric carcinoma.

Pylorid Tablets should be avoided in patients with a history of acute porphyria.

When co-prescription of clarithromycin or amoxycillin is clinically indicated, the relevant prescribing information should be consulted prior to initiation of therapy.

*Interaction with other medicaments and other forms of interaction:* An increase in median trough plasma bismuth concentrations has been observed when Pylorid is co-administered with clarithromycin. However, this has not been associated with any adverse clinical sequelae in clinical trials. Clarithromycin levels are unaffected by the administration of ranitidine bismuth citrate, although systemic exposure to the active metabolite of clarithromycin is increased. The ranitidine absorption from Pylorid Tablets is increased when co-administered with clarithromycin. This enhanced ranitidine exposure is of no clinical concern due to the wide therapeutic index of ranitidine.

Food causes a decrease in bismuth absorption which is not of any clinical relevance. Limited data suggest increased ulcer healing when Pylorid Tablets are administered with food (see *Posology and method of administration*).

The co-administration of antacids with Pylorid Tablets does not result in any clinically relevant effect.

*Pregnancy and lactation:* The safety of ranitidine bismuth citrate in human pregnancy has not been established. As animal reproductive studies are not always predictive of human response, Pylorid Tablets should not be used in pregnancy.

It has been demonstrated in animal reproductive studies that during repeat dosing, low levels of ranitidine and bismuth cross the placenta. There was no evidence that ranitidine bismuth citrate induced any major malformations in either fetal rats or rabbits after maternal administration at high dose levels. Embryo/fetal lethality in rabbits, as a consequence of the maternal susceptibility to antimicrobial agents, together with minor effects of skeletal development in both rats and rabbits, were a result of dose levels considerably in excess of clinical exposure and were related to maternal toxicity.

It has been demonstrated that during repeat dosing of ranitidine bismuth citrate in the lactating rat, low levels of ranitidine and bismuth are secreted in the milk with consequent exposure of the pups. The passage of ranitidine bismuth citrate into human breast milk has not been evaluated.

Consequently, Pylorid Tablets should not be used by women who are breast feeding.

*Effects on ability to drive and use machines:* None reported.

*Undesirable effects:* Blackening of the stools is frequently reported with bismuth-containing drugs.

As with other medicines containing bismuth, ranitidine bismuth citrate may cause blackening of the tongue.

There have been rare reports of hypersensitivity reactions including pruritus, skin rash and anaphylaxis.

Gastro-intestinal disturbances, including diarrhoea, abdominal discomfort, and gastric pain may occur.

Headache.

Treatment with Pylorid Tablets may cause transient changes in the liver enzymes SGPT (ALT) and SGOT (AST).

Mild anaemia has been reported.

The following have been reported as adverse events in patients treated with ranitidine. Because ranitidine is used for longer treatment periods, their relevance to the clinical use of Pylorid Tablets is unknown.

There have been occasional reports of hepatitis (hepatocellular, hepatocanalicular or mixed) with or without jaundice. These were usually reversible. Acute pancreatitis has been rarely reported. Blood count changes (leucopenia, thrombocytopenia) have occurred in a few patients.

These are usually reversible. Rare cases of agranulocytosis or pancytopenia, sometimes with marrow hypoplasia or aplasia have been reported. As with other H₂-receptor antagonists, there have been rare reports of bradycardia and A-V Block. Dizziness has been reported in a very small proportion of patients. Rare cases of reversible mental confusion, depression and hallucinations have been reported, predominantly in severely ill and elderly patients. Rare cases of erythema multiforme have been reported. Musculoskeletal symptoms such as arthralgia and myalgia have been reported rarely. There have been a few reports of breast symptoms in men taking ranitidine.

*Overdose:* Administration of ranitidine bismuth citrate in acute animal studies at very high dosages has been associated with nephrotoxicity. In cases of overdose, gastric lavage and appropriate supportive therapy would be indicated. The ranitidine and bismuth components may be removed from the plasma by haemodialysis.

**Pharmacological properties**
*Pharmacodynamic properties: Pharmaco-therapeutic group:* Pylorid Tablets are histamine H₂-receptor antagonists, with anti-*H. pylori*, and mucosal protective activity.

*Mechanism of action:* Ranitidine bismuth citrate inhibits basal and stimulated secretion of gastric acid, reducing both the volume and the acid and pepsin content of the secretion, is bactericidal to *Helicobacter pylori* in vitro, and has gastric mucosal-protective actions.

These pharmacodynamic properties depend on the dissociation of ranitidine bismuth citrate into ranitidine and bismuth components. The biological and anti-*H. pylori* activity of the latter is related to the solubility of dissociated bismuth from ranitidine bismuth citrate. As the absorption of bismuth from ranitidine bismuth citrate is minimal (see *Pharmacokinetic properties*) the *H. pylori* activity is a local effect. Even in acidic conditions, which lead to precipitation of bismuth, sufficient bismuth from ranitidine bismuth citrate remains soluble to inhibit the growth of *H. pylori*.

*Pharmacokinetic properties:* Bismuth absorption from Pylorid Tablets is less than 1% of the bismuth dose administered, and is similar in healthy volunteers, male and female subjects, patients with peptic ulcer disease and gastritis patients. The rate of absorption of ranitidine and bismuth is rapid, the time to peak plasma levels typically being 1–3 h and 15–60 min, respectively. The absorption of bismuth from Pylorid Tablets is dependent on intragastric pH and increases if the intragastric pH is raised to ≥6 prior to dosing.

However, the co-administration of antacids has no clinically relevant effect (see *Interactions*).

Ranitidine is cleared primarily by renal clearance (approximately 500 ml/min). This accounts for approximately 70% of the total clearance, which is approximately 700 ml/min. Ranitidine is rapidly eliminated from the body, with a half-life of about 3 hours after oral dosing; and does not accumulate in the plasma with twice daily dosing.

Bismuth in the systemic circulation is cleared from the body mainly by renal clearance (approximately 50 ml/min). Multiple half-lives describe the distribution and elimination of bismuth. The mean terminal plasma half-life of bismuth is 20.7 days and the mean terminal half-life of bismuth urinary excretion is 45.1 days. Bismuth accumulates in plasma upon twice daily dosing with Pylorid Tablets. Within 3 months of completing a 4- or 8-week course of treatment with Pylorid, plasma concentrations and urinary excretion of bismuth have returned to pre-treatment levels in most patients.

Ranitidine and bismuth exposure is increased in patients with renal impairment and the elderly as a result of decreased renal clearance.

Patients with moderate to severe renal impairment (creatinine clearance typically <25 ml/min) should not be given Pylorid Tablets (see *Posology and method of administration* and *Contra-indications*).

*Preclinical safety data:* In acute animal studies at high dosages, nephrotoxicity was observed in all species studied.

In local tolerance studies ranitidine bismuth citrate was slightly irritating to abraded guinea pig skin. It was also a weak skin contact sensitiser in the guinea pig "split adjuvant" test.

No mutagenic activity was seen in standard genotoxicity tests with ranitidine bismuth citrate. A weak clastogenic effect was seen *in vitro*. This can be accounted for as an effect of a bismuth containing compound as it also occurred with bismuth citrate, at bismuth equivalent concentrations of 33 mcg/ml for ranitidine bismuth citrate compared to 26 mcg/ml for bismuth citrate. As no genotoxic activity was demonstrated *in vivo* these findings are not considered to be of any clinical significance.

Evidence of bismuth accumulation in tissues to steady state was observed following long-term repeat dosing in animal studies. To avoid the possibility of bismuth accumulation, ranitidine bismuth citrate is not indicated for maintenance therapy in man.

**Pharmaceutical particulars**
*List of excipients: Tablet core:* Sodium carbonate (anhydrous) USNF; Microcrystalline cellulose PhEur; Polyvidone K30 PhEur; Magnesium stearate PhEur.

*Tablet film coat:* Hydroxypropylmethyl cellulose PhEur (E464); Titanium dioxide PhEur (E171); Triacetin USP; Indigo carmine aluminium lake (E132).

*Incompatibilities:* None reported.

*Shelf life:* 3 years.

*Special precautions for storage:* Store Pylorid Tablets below 30°C.

*Nature and contents of container:* Cartons containing 14, 28 or 56 tablets in a double-foil blister pack.

The tablets are light blue, film-coated, octagonal capsule-shaped tablets identified by a logo on one face, containing 400 mg of ranitidine bismuth citrate.

*Instructions for use/handling:* None.

**Marketing authorisation number** 14213/0001

**Date of approval/revision of SPC** 14 April 1997

**Legal category** POM

# RETROVIR* IV FOR INFUSION

**Qualitative and quantitative composition** Zidovudine 200 mg.

**Pharmaceutical form** Retrovir IV for Infusion is a clear, nearly colourless, sterile aqueous solution in an amber glass vial containing 10 mg zidovudine per ml, with a pH of approximately 5.5. Each 20 ml vial contains 200 mg zidovudine.

**Clinical particulars**
*Therapeutic indications:* Retrovir IV for Infusion is indicated for the short-term management of serious manifestations of Human Immunodeficiency Virus (HIV) infection in patients with the Acquired Immune Deficiency syndrome (AIDS) or AIDS-related complex (ARC) who are unable to take Retrovir Oral Formulations. Evidence of efficacy has been demonstrated in AIDS patients who have recovered from their first episode of *Pneumocystis carinii* pneumonia within 4 months and ARC patients with multiple signs of HIV infection, including mucocutaneous candidiasis, weight loss (more than 10% or 14 pounds), lymphadenopathy and unexplained fever.

Retrovir should be considered for use in HIV-positive pregnant women (over 14 weeks of gestation) and their newborn infants as it has been shown to reduce the rate of maternal-foetal transmission of HIV.

*Posology and method of administration:* The required dose of Retrovir IV for Infusion must be administered by slow intravenous infusion of the diluted product *over a one-hour period.*

Retrovir IV for Infusion must *NOT* be given intramuscularly.

*Dilution:* Retrovir IV for Infusion must be diluted prior to administration.

The required dose (see *Dosage*) should be added to and mixed with Glucose Intravenous Infusion (5% w/v) to give a final zidovudine concentration of either 2 mg/ml or 4 mg/ml. These dilutions are chemically and physically stable for up to 48 hours at both 5°C and 25°C.

Since no antimicrobial preservative is included, dilution must be carried out under full aseptic conditions, preferably immediately prior to administration, and any unused portion of the vial should be discarded. Should any visible turbidity appear in the product either before or after dilution or during infusion, the preparation should be discarded.

*Dosage in adults:* A dose for Retrovir IV for Infusion of 1 or 2 mg zidovudine/kg bodyweight every 4 hours approximately corresponds to an oral dose of 1.5 or 3.0 mg zidovudine/kg every 4 hours (600 or 1200 mg/day for a 70 kg patient).

The effectiveness of lower dosage in the treatment or prevention of HIV-associated neurological dysfunction and malignancies is unknown. Patients should receive Retrovir IV for Infusion only until oral therapy can be administered (see *Undesirable effects*).

*Dosage adjustments in patients with haematological adverse reactions:* Dosage adjustments may be necessary in patients with haematological adverse reactions. This is more likely in patients with poor bone marrow reserve prior to treatment. If the haemoglobin level falls to between 7.5 g/decilitre (4.65 mmol/litre) and 9 g/decilitre (5.59 mmol/litre) or the neutrophil count falls to between $0.75\times10^9$/litre and $1.0\times10^9$/litre, the daily dosage may be reduced until there is evidence of marrow recovery; alternatively, recovery may be enhanced by brief (2 to 4 weeks) interruption of Retrovir therapy. If dosage reduction is considered, the daily dosage may, for example, be halved and subsequently increased, depending on patient tolerance, up to the original dosage.

Therapy with Retrovir IV for Infusion should be discontinued if the haemoglobin level falls below 7.5 g/decilitre (4.65 mmol/litre) or if the neutrophil count falls to less than $0.75\times10^9$/litre. Marrow recovery is usually observed within 2 weeks after which time Retrovir therapy at a reduced dosage may be reinstituted. After a further 2 to 4 weeks the dosage of zidovudine may be gradually increased, depending on patient tolerance until the original dosage is reached, although data on the use of intravenous Retrovir for periods in excess of 2 weeks are limited.

*Dosage in children:* Limited data are available on the use of Retrovir IV for Infusion in children. A range of dosages between 80–160 mg/m² every 6 hours (320–640 mg/m²/day) has been used. Exposure following the 120 mg/m² dose every 6 hours approximately corresponds to the recommended oral dose of 180 mg/m² every 6 hours.

*Dosage in the prevention of maternal-foetal transmission:* Although the optimal dosage schedule has not been identified the following dosage regimen has been shown to be effective. Pregnant women (over 14 weeks of gestation) should be given 500 mg/day orally (100 mg five times a day) until the beginning of labour. During labour and delivery Retrovir should be administered intravenously at 2 mg/kg bodyweight given over 1 hour followed by a continuous intravenous infusion at 1 mg/kg/h until the umbilical cord is clamped. The newborn infants should be given 2 mg/kg bodyweight orally every 6 hours starting within 12 hours after birth and continuing until 6 weeks-old. Infants unable to receive oral dosing should be given Retrovir intravenously at 1.5 mg/kg bodyweight infused over 30 minutes every 6 hours.

IN CASE OF PLANNED CAESAREAN, THE INFUSION SHOULD BE STARTED 4 HOURS BEFORE THE OPERATION.

In the event of a false labour, the Retrovir infusion should be stopped and oral dosing restarted.

*Dosage in the elderly:* No data are available, however special care is advised in this age group due to age-associated changes such as the decrease in renal functions and alterations in haematological parameters.

*Dosage in renal impairment:* Compared to healthy subjects, patients with advanced renal failure have a 50% higher maximum plasma concentration after oral

administration. Systemic exposure (measured as area under the zidovudine concentration time curve) is increased 100%; the half-life is not significantly altered. In renal failure there is substantial accumulation of the major glucuronide metabolite but this does not appear to cause toxicity. Patients with advanced renal failure should receive Retrovir at the lower end of the dosage range. Haematological parameters and clinical response, may influence the need for subsequent dosage adjustment. Haemodialysis and peritoneal dialysis have no significant effect on zidovudine elimination whereas elimination of the glucuronide metabolite is increased.

*Dosage in hepatic impairment:* Limited data in patients with cirrhosis given oral Retrovir suggest that accumulation of zidovudine may occur in patients with hepatic impairment because of decreased glucuronidation. Dosage adjustments may be necessary but precise recommendations cannot be made at present. If monitoring of plasma zidovudine levels is not feasible, physicians will need to pay particular attention to signs of intolerance and increase the interval between doses as appropriate.

*Contra-indications:* Retrovir IV for Infusion is contra-indicated in patients known to be hypersensitive to zidovudine, or to any of the components of the formulation.

Retrovir IV for infusion should not be given to patients with abnormally low neutrophil counts (less than $0.75\times10^9$/litre) or abnormally low haemoglobin levels (less than 7.5 g/decilitre or 4.65 mmol/litre).

Retrovir is contra-indicated in newborn infants with hyperbilirubinaemia requiring treatment other than phototherapy, or with increased transaminase levels of over five times the upper limit of normal.

*Special warnings and precautions for use:* Retrovir is not a cure for HIV infection and patients remain at risk of developing illnesses which are associated with immune suppression, including opportunistic infections and neoplasm. Whilst it has been shown to reduce the risk of opportunistic infections, data on the development of neoplasms, including lymphomas, are limited. The available data on patients treated for advanced HIV disease indicate that the risk of lymphoma development is consistent with that observed in untreated patients. In patients with early HIV disease on long term treatment the risk of lymphoma development is unknown. Retrovir should be administered under the supervision of a doctor with experience of treating patients with HIV infection or AIDS/ARC. An appropriate treatment procedure requires access to suitable facilities e.g. for performing haematological monitoring investigations, including determination of CD4+ lymphocytes and for provision of blood transfusions if necessary.

*Haematological adverse reactions:* Anaemia (usually occurring after 6 weeks of Retrovir therapy but occasionally earlier), neutropenia (usually occurring at any time after 4 weeks' therapy but sometimes earlier) and leucopenia (usually secondary to neutropenia) can be expected to occur frequently in patients receiving Retrovir IV for Infusion; therefore, haematological parameters should be carefully monitored. It is recommended that blood tests are performed at least weekly in patients receiving Retrovir IV for Infusion. Particular care should be taken in patients with pre-existing bone marrow compromise (e.g. haemoglobin less than 9 g/decilitre (5.59 mmol/litre) or neutrophil count less than $1.0\times10^9$/litre). Lower daily dosages from the start of treatment may be appropriate for some such patients.

If severe anaemia or myelosuppression occurs dosage adjustments are suggested (see *Posology and method of administration*). Such abnormalities are usually rapidly reversible on stopping therapy. In patients with significant anaemia, dosage adjustments do not necessarily eliminate the need for transfusions.

*Lactic acidosis and severe hepatomegaly with steatosis:* Rare occurrences of lactic acidosis, in the absence of hypoxaemia, and severe hepatomegaly with steatosis have been reported and are potentially fatal; it is not known whether these events are causally related to Retrovir, but they have been reported in HIV-positive patients without AIDS. Treatment with Retrovir should be suspended in the setting of rapidly elevating aminotransferase levels, progressive hepatomegaly, or metabolic/lactic acidosis of unknown aetiology (see *Undesirable effects*).

Caution should be exercised when administering Retrovir to any patient, particularly obese women, with hepatomegaly, hepatitis or other known risk factor for liver disease. These patients should be followed closely while on therapy with Retrovir.

Patients should be cautioned about the concomitant use of self-administered medications (see *Interaction with other medicaments*).

Patients should be advised that zidovudine therapy has not been shown to reduce the risk of transmission

of HIV to others through sexual contact or blood contamination.

*Interaction with other medicaments and other forms of interaction:* As experience of drug with interactions with Retrovir is still limited, care should be taken when combining with other drug regimens. The interactions listed below should not be considered exhaustive but are representative of the classes of drug where caution should be exercised.

Phenytoin blood levels have been reported to be low in some patients receiving Retrovir, while in one patient a high level was noted. These observations suggest that phenytoin levels should be carefully monitored in patients receiving both drugs.

Paracetamol use during treatment with Retrovir in a placebo-controlled trial was associated with an increased incidence of neutropenia especially following chronic therapy. However, the available pharmacokinetic data indicate that paracetamol does not increase plasma levels of zidovudine nor of its glucuronide metabolite.

Other drugs including but not limited to aspirin, codeine, morphine, indomethacin, ketoprofen, naproxen, oxazepam, lorazepam, cimetidine, clofibrate, dapsone and isoprinosine may alter the metabolism of zidovudine by competitively inhibiting glucuronidation or directly inhibiting hepatic microsomal metabolism. Careful thought should be given to the possibilities of drug interactions before using such drugs, particularly for chronic therapy, in combination with Retrovir IV for Infusion.

Concomitant therapy especially acute therapy with potentially nephrotoxic or myelosuppressive drugs (e.g. systemic pentamidine, dapsone, pyrimethamine, co-trimoxazole, amphotericin, flucytosine, ganciclovir, interferon, vincristine, vinblastine and doxorubicin) may also increase the risk of adverse reactions with Retrovir IV for Infusion. If concomitant therapy with any of these drugs is necessary then extra care should be taken in monitoring renal function and haematological parameters and if required, the dosage of one or more agents should be reduced.

The nucleoside analogue ribavirin antagonises the *in vitro* antiviral activity of zidovudine and so concomitant use of such drugs should be avoided.

Since some patients receiving Retrovir may continue to experience opportunistic infections, concomitant use of prophylactic antimicrobial therapy may have to be considered. Such therapy has included co-trimoxazole, aerosolised pentamidine, pyrimethamine and acyclovir. Limited data from controlled clinical trials do not indicate a significantly increased risk of adverse reactions to Retrovir with these drugs.

Limited data suggest that probenecid increases the mean half life and area under the plasma concentration curve of zidovudine by decreasing glucuronidation. Renal excretion of the glucuronide (and possibly zidovudine itself) is reduced in the presence of probenecid.

*Use during pregnancy and lactation:*
*Pregnancy:* The use of Retrovir in pregnant women over 14 weeks of gestation, with subsequent treatment of their newborn infants, has been shown to significantly reduce the rate of maternal-fetal transmission of HIV based on viral cultures in infants.

Interim analysis of the pivotal US placebo-controlled study indicated that Retrovir reduced maternal-fetal transmission by approximately 70%. In this study, pregnant women had CD4+ cell counts of 200 to 1818/mm³ (median in treated group 560/mm³) and began treatment therapy between weeks 14 and 34 of gestation and had no clinical indications for Retrovir therapy; their newborn infants received Retrovir until 6-weeks old. A decision to reduce the risk of maternal transmission of HIV should be based on the balance of potential benefits and potential risk. Pregnant women considering the use of Retrovir during pregnancy for prevention of HIV transmission to their infants should be advised that transmission may still occur in some cases despite therapy.

The efficacy of zidovudine to reduce the maternal-fetal transmission in women with previously prolonged treatment with zidovudine or other anti-Retroviral agents or women infected with HIV strains with reduced sensitivity to zidovudine is unknown.

It is unknown whether there are any long-term consequences of *in utero* and infant exposure to Retrovir. Based on the animal carcinogenicity/mutagenicity findings a carcinogenic risk to humans cannot be excluded (see *Preclinical safety data*). Zidovudine has been shown to be mutagenic in some, but not all, standard *in vitro* and *in vivo* assays. Although the predictive value of rodent carcinogenicity studies for humans is uncertain, late-occurring vaginal tumours (appearing after 19 months of continuous daily oral dosing) have been seen in rodents following lifetime dosing with zidovudine. The relevance of these findings to both infected and uninfected infants exposed to Retrovir is unknown. However, pregnant women considering using Retrovir during pregnancy should be made aware of these findings.

Given the limited data on the general use of Retrovir in pregnancy, Retrovir should only be used prior to the 14th week of gestation when the potential benefit to the mother outweighs the risk to the fetus. Studies in pregnant rats and rabbits given zidovudine orally at dosage levels up to 450 and 500 mg/kg/day respectively during the major period of organogenesis have revealed no evidence of teratogenicity. There was, however, a statistically significant increase in fetal-resorptions in rats given 150 to 450 mg/kg/day and in rabbits given 500 mg/kg/day. A separate study, reported subsequently, found that rats given a dosage of 3000 mg/kg/day, which is very near the oral median lethal dose (3683 mg/kg), caused marked maternal toxicity and an increase in the incidence of fetal malformations. No evidence of teratogenicity was observed in this study at the lower dosages tested (600 mg/kg/day or less).

*Lactation:* Limited data indicate that zidovudine is excreted in animal milk. It is not known if zidovudine is excreted in human milk.

Since the drug may pass into breast milk it is recommended that mothers taking Retrovir do not breast feed their infants.

*Fertility:* It is not known whether zidovudine can effect human fertility. There are no data on the effect of Retrovir on human female fertility. In men, Retrovir has not been shown to affect sperm count, morphology or motility.

*Effects on ability to drive and use machines:* Retrovir IV for Infusion is generally used in an in-patient hospital population and information on ability to drive and use machinery is not usually relevant. There have been no studies to investigate the effect of Retrovir on driving performance or the ability to operate machinery. Further, a detrimental effect on such activities cannot be predicted from the pharmacology of the drug. Nevertheless, the clinical status of the patient and the adverse events profile of Retrovir should be borne in mind when considering the patient's ability to drive or operate machinery.

*Undesirable effects:* The most serious adverse reactions include anaemia (which may require transfusions), neutropenia and leucopenia. These occur more frequently at higher doses (1200–1500 mg/day) and in AIDS than in ARC patients (especially when there is poor bone marrow reserve prior to treatment), and particularly in patients with CD4+ cell counts less than 100/mm³. Dosage reduction or cessation of therapy may become necessary (see *Posology and method of administration*). The incidence of neutropenia was also increased in those patients whose neutrophil counts, haemoglobin levels and vitamin B12 levels were low at the start of Retrovir therapy, and in those patients taking paracetamol concurrently (see *Interaction with other medicaments*).

Other frequent adverse events reported in a large placebo-controlled clinical trial of Retrovir included nausea, vomiting, anorexia, abdominal pain, headache, rash, fever, myalgia, paraesthesiae, insomnia, malaise, asthenia and dyspepsia. Apart from nausea, severe headaches, myalgia and insomnia, which were significantly more common in patients receiving Retrovir, the incidence of the other adverse events was only slightly higher than in the placebo recipients.

Other reported adverse events included, somnolence, diarrhoea, dizziness, sweating, dyspnoea, flatulence, taste perversion, chest pain, loss of mental acuity, anxiety, urinary frequency, depression, generalised pain, chills, cough, urticaria, pruritus and influenza-like syndrome. The incidence of these and other less frequent adverse events was generally similar in Retrovir and placebo-treated patients. The available data from studies of Retrovir Oral Formulations indicate that the incidence of nausea and other frequently reported clinical adverse revents consistently decreases over time during the first few weeks of therapy with Retrovir.

The following events have been reported in patients treated with Retrovir. They may also occur as part of the underlying disease process or as a result of the wide range of drugs used in the management of HIV disease. The relationship between these events and use of Retrovir may therefore be difficult to evaluate, particularly in the medically complicated situations which characterise advanced HIV disease. If the severity of the symptoms warrants it, a reduction or suspension of Retrovir therapy may assist in the assessment and management of these conditions:

- myopathy;
- pancytopenia with marrow hypoplasia and isolated thrombocytopenia;
- lactic acidosis in the absence of hypoxaemia, liver disorders such as severe hepatomegaly with steatosis, raised blood levels of liver enzymes and bilirubin;
- pancreatitis;
- nail, skin and oral mucosa pigmentation.

Convulsions and other cerebral events have also been reported in patients receiving open-label therapy with Retrovir. However, the relationship between these events and the use of Retrovir is difficult to evaluate. Furthermore, the weight of evidence indicates an overall beneficial effect of Retrovir on HIV-associated neurological disorders.

Experience with Retrovir IV for Infusion treatment for periods in excess of 2 weeks is limited, although some patients have received treatment for up to 12 weeks. The most frequent adverse events were anaemia, neutropenia and leucopenia. Local reactions were infrequent.

*Children:* Limited data from open labelled studies in children, involving intravenous administration of a limited duration, do not contradict the adverse event profile of zidovudine in adults.

In a placebo-controlled trial, overall clinical adverse events and laboratory test abnormalities were similar for women in the Retrovir and placebo groups. However, there was a trend for mild and moderate anaemia to be seen more commonly prior to delivery in the zidovudine treated women.

In the same trial, haemoglobin concentrations in infants exposed to Retrovir for this indication were marginally lower than in infants in the placebo group, but transfusion was not required. Anaemia resolved within 6 weeks after completion of Retrovir therapy. Other clinical adverse events and laboratory test abnormalities were similar in the Retrovir and placebo groups. The long term consequences of *in utero* and infant exposure to Retrovir are unknown.

*Overdosage: symptoms and signs:* Dosages as high as 7.5 mg/kg by infusion every 4 hours for 2 weeks have been administered to 5 patients. One patient experienced an anxiety reaction while the other 4 had no untoward effects.

Limited data are available on the consequences of ingestion of acute oral overdoses in both adults and children. No fatalities occurred and all patients recovered. The highest recorded blood level of zidovudine was 185 µM (49.4 mcg/ml). No specific symptoms or signs have been identified following such overdosage.

*Treatment:* Patients should be observed closely for evidence of toxicity (see *Undesirable effects*) and given the necessary supportive therapy.

Haemodialysis and peritoneal dialysis appear to have a limited effect on elimination of zidovudine but enhances the elimination of the glucuronide metabolite.

**Pharmacological properties**
*Pharmacodynamic properties:*
(a) *Mode of action:* Zidovudine is an antiviral agent which is highly active *in vitro* against Retroviruses including the Human Immunodeficiency Virus (HIV).

Zidovudine is phosphorylated in both infected and uninfected cells to the monophosphate (MP) derivative by cellular thymidine kinase. subsequent phosphorylation of zidovudine-MP to the diphosphate (DP), and then the triphosphate (TP) derivative is catalysed by cellular thymidylate kinase and non-specific kinases respectively. Zidovudine-TP acts as an inhibitor of and substrate for the viral reverse transcriptase. The formation of further proviral DNA is blocked by incorporation of zidovudine-TP into the chain and subsequent chain termination.

Competition by zidovudine-TP for HIV reverse transcriptase is approximately 100-fold greater than for cellular DNA polymerase alpha.

(b) *Microbiology:* The relationships between *in vitro* susceptibility of HIV to zidovudine and clinical response to therapy remain under investigation. *In vitro* sensitivity testing has not been standardised and results may therefore vary according to methodological factors.

Reduced *in vitro* sensitivity to zidovudine has been reported for HIV isolates from patients who have received prolonged courses of Retrovir therapy. The available information indicates that the early HIV disease, the frequency and the degree of reduction of *in vitro* sensitivity is notably less than for advanced disease.

*Pharmacokinetic properties:*
(a) *Pharmacokinetics in adults:* Dose-independent kinetics were observed in patients receiving one-hour infusions of 1 to 5 mg/kg 3 to 6 times daily. Mean steady state peak ($C^{ss}max$) and trough ($C^{ss}min$) plasma concentrations in adults following a one-hour infusion of 2.5 mg/kg every 4 hours were 4.0 and 0.4 µM, respectively (or 1.1 and 0.1 mcg/ml).

The mean terminal plasma half life was 1.1 hours, the mean total body clearance was 27.1 ml/min/kg and the apparent volume of distribution was 1.6 litres/kg. Renal clearance of zidovudine greatly exceeds creatinine clearance, indicating significant tubular secretion takes place.

The 5'-glucuronide of zidovudine is the major metabolite in both plasma and urine accounting for approximately 50–80% of the administered dose eliminated by renal excretion. 3'-amino-3'-deoxy-thymidine (AMT) has been identified as a metabolite of zidovudine following intravenous dosing.

There are limited data concerning the pharmacokinetics of zidovudine in patients with renal or hepatic impairment (see *Posology and method of administration*). There are also limited data on the pharmacokinetics of zidovudine in pregnant women. No specific data are available on the pharmacokinetics of zidovudine in the elderly.

(b) *Pharmacokinetics in children:* In children over the age of 5–6 months, the pharmacokinetic profile of zidovudine is similar to that in adults. $C^{ss}max$ levels were 1.46 mcg/ml following an intravenous dose of 80 mg zidovudine/m² body surface area, 2.26 mcg/ml following 120 mg/m² and 2.96 mcg/ml following 160 mg/m².

With intravenous dosing, the mean terminal plasma half-life and total body clearance were 1.5 hours and 30.9 ml/min/kg respectively. The major metabolite is the 5'-glucuronide. After intravenous dosing, 29% of the dose was recovered unchanged in the urine and 45% excreted as the glucuronide. Renal clearance of zidovudine greatly exceeds creatinine clearance indicating that significant tubular secretion takes place.

The limited data available on the pharmacokinetics in neonates and young infants indicate that glucuronidation of zidovudine is reduced with a consequent increase in bioavailability, reduction in clearance and longer half-life in infants less than 14 days-old but thereafter the pharmacokinetics appear similar to those reported in adults.

(c) *Distribution:* In adults the average cerebrospinal fluid/plasma zidovudine concentration ratio 2 to 4 hours after chronic intermittent oral dosing was found to be approximately 0.5. Limited data indicate that zidovudine crosses the placenta and is found in amniotic fluid and fetal blood. Zidovudine has also been detected in semen.

In children the mean cerebrospinal fluid/plasma zidovudine concentration ratio ranged from 0.52–0.85 as determined during oral therapy 0.5 to 4 hours after dosing and was 0.87 as determined during intravenous therapy 1–5 hours after a 1 hour infusion. During continuous intravenous infusion the mean steady-state cerebrospinal fluid/plasma concentration ratio was 0.24.

Plasma protein binding is relatively low (34 to 38%) and drug interactions involving binding site displacement are not anticipated.

*Preclinical safety data:*
(a) *Mutagenicity:* No evidence of mutagenicity was observed in the Ames test. However, zidovudine was weakly mutagenic in a mouse lymphoma cell assay and was positive in an *in vitro* cell transformation assay. Clastogenic effects (chromosome damage) were observed in an *in vitro* study in human lymphocytes and in *in vivo* oral repeat dose micronucleus studies in rats and mice. An *in vivo* cytogenetic study in rats did not show chromosomal damage. A study of peripheral blood lymphocytes of eleven AIDS patients showed a higher chromosome breakage frequency in those who had received Retrovir than in those who had not. The clinical significance of these findings is unclear.

(b) *Carcinogenicity:* Zidovudine was administered orally at three dosage levels to separate groups of mice and rats (60 females and 60 males in each group). Initial single daily doses were 30, 60 and 120 mg/kg/day and 80, 220 and 600 mg/kg/day in mice and rats, respectively. The doses in mice were reduced to 20, 30 and 40 mg/kg/day after Day 90 because of treatment-related anaemia, whereas in rats only the high dose was reduced (to 450 and then 300 mg/kg/day on Days 91 and 279, respectively).

In mice, seven late-appearing (after 19 months) vaginal neoplasms (5 squamous cell carcinomas, one squamous cell papilloma and one squamous polyp) occurred at the highest dose. One late-appearing squamous cell papilloma occurred in the vagina of a middle-dose animal. No vaginal tumours were found at the lowest dose.

In rats, two late-appearing (after 20 months) vaginal squamous cell carcinomas occurred in animals given the highest dose. No vaginal tumours occurred at the middle or low doses in rats.

There were no other drug-related tumours observed in either sex of either species.

The predictive value of rodent carcinogenicity studies for humans is uncertain and thus the clinical significance of these findings is unclear.

(c) *Teratogenicity:* Use during pregnancy and lactation.

(d) *Fertility:* Zidovudine did not impair male or female fertility in rats given oral dosages up to 450 mg/kg/day.

## Pharmaceutical particulars

*List of excipients:* Hydrochloric acid; sodium hydroxide; water for injections.

*Incompatibilities:* None.

*Shelf life:* 3 years.

*Special precautions for storage:* Store below 30°C. Protect from light.

*Nature and contents of container:* Glass vial containing 20 ml.

*Instructions for use/handling:* No special instructions are required.

**Marketing authorisation number** 0003/0332

**Date of approval/revision of SPC** October 1994

**Legal category** POM.

# RETROVIR* CAPSULES AND SYRUP

## Qualitative and quantitative composition

*Retrovir Capsules:* Ingredients per capsule:

|  | 100 mg capsules | 250 mg capsule |
|---|---|---|
| Zidovudine | 100.0 mg | 250.0 mg |

*Retrovir Oral Solution:* Ingredients per 5 ml:
Zidovudine 50.0 mg.

*Retrovir Tablets:* In one 300 mg tablet:
Zidovudine 300.0 mg.

## Pharmaceutical form

*Retrovir 100 mg Capsules:* Hard gelatin capsules with opaque white cap and body and a central dark-blue band, printed 'Wellcome', '100' and coded 'Y9C' and each containing 100 mg zidovudine.

*Retrovir 250 mg Capsules:* Hard gelatin capsules with opaque blue cap, opaque white body and a central dark-blue band, printed 'Wellcome', '250' and coded H2F and each containing 250 mg zidovudine.

*Retrovir Syrup:* A clear, pale yellow, strawberry-flavoured, sugar-free oral solution containing 50 mg zidovudine in each 5 ml.

The pack contains a 10 ml oral-dosing syringe which should be fitted to the bottle before use and closed with the cap provided.

*Retrovir 300 mg Tablets:* White, round, biconvex, film-coated tablets, with a white to beige core scored and branded 'WELLCOME X4F' and each containing 300 mg zidovudine.

## Clinical particulars

*Therapeutic indications:* Retrovir Oral Formulations are indicated for the management of patients with advanced HIV disease, such as those with the Acquired Immune Deficiency Syndrome (AIDS) or AIDS-related complex (ARC).

In adult patients with HIV infection, Retrovir Oral Formulations are also indicated:
– in early symptomatic patients with CD4 counts of less than 500/mm³,
– or in asymptomatic patients with markers indicating risk of progressive disease including repeated CD4 counts of less than 200/mm³, or with CD4 counts between 500/mm³ and 200/mm³ which are rapidly falling.

Retrovir is also indicated for HIV-infected children who have HIV-related symptoms or who are asymptomatic with markers indicating significant HIV-related immune suppression.

Retrovir should be considered for use in HIV-positive pregnant women (over 14 weeks of gestation) and their newborn infants as it has been shown to reduce the rate of maternal-foetal transmission of HIV.

*Posology and method of administration:*
*Dosage in adults:* Although a broad range of dosage regimens has been employed, 500 or 600 mg/day in two to five divided doses has been commonly used worldwide. Alternatively, a daily dosage of 1,000 mg in two divided doses has been used in clinical trials. The effectiveness of lower dosages in the treatment or prevention of HIV-associated neurological dysfunction and malignancies is unknown.

*Dosage in children:* In children over the age of 3 months the recommended starting dose is 180 mg/m² body surface area every six hours (720 mg/m²/day). The maximum dosage should not exceed 200 mg every 6 hours.

The optimum dosage regimen remains to be determined and may vary from patient to patient. A range of dosages, generally between 120 and 180 mg/m² body surface area every 6 hours (between 480 and 720 mg/m²/day), has been used. The effectiveness of lower dosages in the treatment or prevention of HIV-associated neurological dysfunction and malignancies in children is unknown. The effectiveness of less frequent dosing in children remains to be established.

In children under the age of 3 months the limited data available are insufficient to propose specific

dosage recommendations (see *Pharmacokinetic properties).*

*Dosage in the prevention of maternal-foetal transmission:* Although the optimal dosage schedule has not been identified the following dosage regimen has been shown to be effective. Pregnant women (over 14 weeks of gestation) should be given 500 mg/day orally (100 mg five times per day) until the beginning of labour. During labour and delivery Retrovir should be administered intravenously at 2 mg/kg bodyweight given over 1 hour followed by a continuous intravenous infusion at 1 mg/kg/h until the umbilical cord is clamped. The newborn infant should be given 2 mg/kg bodyweight orally every 6 hours starting within 12 hours after birth and continuing until 6-weeks-old. Infants unable to receive oral dosing should be given Retrovir intravenously at 1.5 mg/kg bodyweight infused over 30 minutes every 6 hours.

IN CASE OF PLANNED CAESAREAN, THE INFUSION SHOULD BE STARTED 4 HOURS BEFORE THE OPERATION.

In the event of a false labour, the Retrovir infusion should be stopped and oral dosing restarted.

*Dosage adjustments in patients with haematological adverse reactions:* Dosage adjustments may be necessary in patients with haematological adverse reactions. This is more likely in patients with poor bone marrow reserve prior to treatment, particularly in patients with advanced HIV disease. If the haemoglobin level falls to between 7.5 g/decilitre (4.65 mmol/litre) and 9 g/decilitre (5.59 mmol/litre) or the neutrophil count falls to between 0.75× 10⁹/litre and 1.0×10⁹/litre, the daily dosage may be reduced until there is evidence of marrow recovery; alternatively, recovery may be enhanced by a brief (2 to 4 weeks) interruption of Retrovir therapy. If dosage reduction is considered, the daily dosage may, for example, be halved and subsequently increased, depending on patient tolerance, up to the original dosage. Therapy with Retrovir should be interrupted if the haemoglobin level falls below 7.5 g/decilitre (4.65 mmol/litre) or the neutrophil count falls to less than 0.75×10⁹/litre. Marrow recovery is usually observed within two weeks after which time Retrovir therapy at a reduced dosage may be reinstituted. After a further 2 to 4 weeks the dosage may be gradually increased, depending on patient tolerance, up to the original dosage.

*Dosage in the elderly:* No specific data are available; however special care is advised in this age group due to age-associated changes such as the decrease in renal function and alterations in haematological parameters.

*Dosage in renal impairment:* Compared to healthy subjects, patients with advanced renal failure have a 50% higher maximum plasma concentration of zidovudine. Systemic exposure (measured as area under the zidovudine concentration-time curve) is increased 100%; the half life is not significantly altered. In renal failure there is substantial accumulation of the major, glucuronide metabolite but this does not appear to cause toxicity. Patients with advanced renal failure should receive Retrovir at the lower end of the dosage range. Haematological parameters and clinical response response may influence the need for subsequent dosage adjustment. Haemodialysis and peritoneal dialysis have no signficant effect on zidovudine elimination whereas elimination of the glucuronide metabolite is increased.

*Dosage in hepatic impairment:* Limited data in patients with cirrhosis suggest that accumulation of zidovudine may occur in patients with hepatic impairment because of decreased glucuronidation. Dosage adjustments may be necessary but precise recommendations cannot be made at present. If monitoring of plasma zidovudine levels is not feasible, physicians will need to pay particular attention to signs of intolerance and increase the interval between doses as appropriate.

*Contra-indications:* Retrovir Oral Formulations are contra-indicated in patients known to be hypersensitive to zidovudine, or to any of the components of the formulations. Retrovir Oral Formulations should not be given to patients with abnormally low neutrophil counts (less than 0.75×10⁹/litre) or abnormally low haemoglobin levels (less than 7.5 g/decilitre or 4.65 mmol/litre).

Retrovir is contra-indicated in new born infants with hyperbilirubinaemia requiring treatment other than phototherapy, or with increased transaminase levels of over five times the upper limit of normal.

*Special warnings and special precautions for use:* Retrovir is not a cure for HIV infection and patients remain at risk of developing illnesses which are associated with immune suppression, including opportunistic infections and neoplasms. Whilst it has been shown to reduce the risks of opportunistic infections, data on the development of neoplasms, including lymphomas, are limited. The available data

on patients treated for advanced HIV disease indicate that the risk of lymphoma development is consistent with that observed in untreated patients. In patients with early HIV disease on long-term treatment the risk of lymphoma development is unknown.

Retrovir should be administered under the supervision of a doctor with experience of treating patients with HIV infection or AIDS/ARC. An appropriate treatment procedure requires access to suitable facilities e.g. for performing haematological monitoring investigations, including determination of CD4+ lymphocytes and for provision of blood transfusions if necessary.

*Haematological adverse reactions:* Anaemia (usually not observed before six weeks of Retrovir therapy but occasionally occurring earlier), neutropenia (usually not observed before four weeks' therapy but sometimes occurring earlier) and leucopenia (usually secondary to neutropenia) can be expected to occur in patients with advanced symptomatic HIV disease receiving Retrovir; therefore haematological parameters should be carefully monitored. For patients with advanced symptomatic HIV disease it is generally recommended that blood tests are performed at least every two weeks for the first three months of therapy and at least monthly thereafter.

Particular care should be taken in patients with pre-existing bone marrow compromise (e.g. haemoglobin less than 9 g/decilitre (5.59 mmol/litre) or neutrophil count less than 1.0×10⁹/litre). Lower daily dosages from the start of treatment may be appropriate for some such patients.

In patients with early HIV disease (where bone marrow reserve is generally good), haematological adverse reactions are infrequent. Depending on the overall condition of the patient, blood tests may be performed less often, for example every one to three months. Decreases in the haemoglobin level of more than 25% from baseline and falls in the neutrophil count of more than 50% from baseline may require more frequent monitoring.

If severe anaemia or myelosuppression occurs, dosage adjustments are suggested (see *Posology and method of administration).* Such abnormalities are usually rapidly reversible on stopping therapy. In patients with significant anaemia, dosage adjustments do not necessarily eliminate the need for transfusions.

*Lactic acidosis and severe hepatomegaly with steatosis:* Rare occurrences of lactic acidosis, in the absence of hypoxaemia, and severe hepatomegaly with steatosis have been reported and are potentially fatal; it is not known whether these events are causally related to Retrovir, but they have been reported in HIV-positive patients without AIDS. Treatment with Retrovir should be suspended in the setting of rapidly elevating aminotransferase levels, progressive hepatomegaly, or metabolic/lactic acidosis of unknown aetiology (see *Undesirable effects).*

Caution should be exercised when administering Retrovir to any patient, particularly obese women, with hepatomegaly, hepatitis, or other known risk factor for liver disease. These patients should be followed closely while on therapy with Retrovir.

Patients should be cautioned about the concomitant use of self-administered medications (see *Interactions with other medicaments and other forms of interaction).*

Patients should be advised that Retrovir therapy has not been proven to prevent the transmission of HIV to others through sexual contact or blood contamination.

*Use in elderly and in patients with renal or hepatic impairment:* See *Posology and method of administration.*

*Interaction with other medicaments and other forms of interaction:* As experience of drug interactions with Retrovir is limited, care should be taken when combining other drug regimens. The interactions listed below should not be considered exhaustive but are representative of the classes of drug where caution should be exercised.

Phenytoin blood levels have been reported to be low in some patients receiving Retrovir, while in one patient a high level was noted. These observations suggest that phenytoin levels should be carefully monitored in patients receiving both drugs.

Paracetamol use during treatment with Retrovir in a placebo-controlled trial was associated with an increased incidence of neutropenia especially following chronic therapy. However, the available pharmacokinetic data indicate that paracetamol does not increase plasma levels of zidovudine nor of its glucuronide metabolite.

Other drugs, including but not limited to, aspirin, codeine, morphine, indomethacin, ketoprofen, naproxen, oxazepam, lorazepam, cimetidine, clofibrate, dapsone and isoprinosine, may alter the metabolism of zidovudine by competitively inhibiting glucuronidation or directly inhibiting hepatic microsomal metabolism. Careful thought should be given to the possibilities of drug interaction before using such drugs, particularly for chronic therapy, in combination with Retrovir.

Concomitant treatment, especially acute therapy, with potentially nephrotoxic or myelosuppressive drugs (e.g. systemic pentamidine, dapsone, pyrimethamine, co-trimoxazole, amphotericin, flucytosine, ganciclovir, interferon, vincristine, vinblastine and doxorubicin) may also increase the risk of adverse reactions to Retrovir. If concomitant therapy with any of these drugs is necessary then extra care should be taken in monitoring renal function and haematological parameters and, if required, the dosage of one or more agents should be reduced.

The nucleoside analogue ribavirin antagonises the in vitro antiviral activity of zidovudine and so concomitant use of this drug should be avoided.

Since some patients receiving Retrovir may continue to experience opportunistic infections, concomitant use of prophylactic antimicrobial therapy may have to be considered. Such prophylaxis has included co-trimoxazole, aerosolised pentamidine, pyrimethamine and acyclovir. Limited data from clinical trials do not indicate a significantly increased risk of adverse reactions to Retrovir with these drugs.

Limited data suggest that probenecid increases the mean half-life and area under the plasma concentration curve of zidovudine by decreasing glucuronidation. Renal excretion of the glucuronide (and possibly zidovudine itself) is reduced in the presence of probenecid.

*Use during pregnancy and lactation:*
*Pregnancy:* The use of Retrovir in pregnant women over 14 weeks of gestation, with subsequent treatment of their newborn infants, has been shown to significantly reduce the rate of maternal-fetal transmission of HIV based on viral cultures in infants.

Interim analysis of the pivotal U.S. placebo-controlled study indicated that Retrovir reduced maternal-fetal transmission by approximately 70%. In this study, pregnant women had CD4+cell counts of 200 to 1818/mm³ (median in treated group 560/mm³) and began treatment therapy between weeks 14 and 34 of gestation and had no clinical indications for Retrovir therapy; their newborn infants received Retrovir until 6-weeks old.

A decision to reduce the risk of maternal transmission of HIV should be based on the balance of potential benefits and potential risk. Pregnant women considering the use of Retrovir during pregnancy for prevention of HIV transmission to their infants should be advised that transmission may still occur in some cases despite therapy.

The efficacy of zidovudine to reduce the maternal-fetal transmission in women with previously prolonged treatment with zidovudine or other anti-Retroviral agents or women infected with HIV strains with reduced sensitivity to zidovudine is unknown.

It is unknown whether there are any long-term consequences of in utero and infant exposure to Retrovir. Based on the animal carcinogenicity/mutagenicity findings a carcinogenic risk to humans cannot be excluded (see *Preclinical safety data*). Zidovudine has been shown to be mutagenic in some, but not all, standard in vitro and in vivo assays. Although the predictive value of rodent carcinogenicity studies for humans is uncertain, late-occurring vaginal tumours (appearing after 19 months of continuous daily oral dosing) have been seen in rodents following lifetime dosing with zidovudine. The relevance of these findings to both infected and uninfected infants exposed to Retrovir is unknown. However, pregnant women considering using Retrovir during pregnancy should be made aware of these findings. Given the limited data on the general use of Retrovir in pregnancy, Retrovir should only be used prior to the 14th week of gestation when the potential benefit to the mother outweighs the risk to the fetus. Studies in pregnant rats and rabbits given zidovudine orally at dosage levels up to 450 and 500 mg/kg/day respectively during the major period of organogenesis have revealed no evidence of teratogenicity. There was, however, a statistically significant increase in fetal resorptions in rats given 150 to 450 mg/kg/day and in rabbits given 500 mg/kg/day. A separate study, reported subsequently, found that rats given a dosage of 3000 mg/kg/day, which is very near the oral median lethal dose (3683 mg/kg), caused marked maternal toxicity and an increase in the incidence of fetal malformations. No evidence of teratogenicity was observed in this study at the lower dosages tested (600 mg/kg/day or less).

*Fertility:* Zidovudine did not impair male or female fertility in rats given oral doses of up to 450 mg/kg/day.

There are no data on the effect of Retrovir on human female fertility. In men, Retrovir has not been shown to affect sperm count, morphology or motility.

*Lactation:* Limited data indicate that zidovudine is excreted in animal milk. It is not known if zidovudine is excreted in human milk.

Since the drug may pass into breast milk, it is recommended that mothers taking Retrovir do not breast feed their infants.

*Effects on ability to drive and use machines:* There have been no studies to investigate the effect of Retrovir on driving performance or the ability to operate machinery. Further, a detrimental effect on such activities cannot be predicted from the pharmacology of the drug. Nevertheless, the clinical status of the patient and the adverse event profile of Retrovir should be borne in mind when considering the patient's ability to drive or operate machinery.

*Undesirable effects:*
*Adults:* The most serious adverse reactions include anaemia (which may require transfusions), neutropenia and leucopenia. These occur more frequently at higher dosages (1200–1500 mg/day) and in patients with advanced HIV disease (especially when there is poor bone marrow reserve prior to treatment), and particularly in patients with CD4+cell counts less than 100/mm³. Dosage reduction or cessation of therapy may become necessary (see *Posology and method of administration*). The incidence of neutropenia was also increased in those patients whose neutrophil counts, haemoglobin levels and serum vitamin B₁₂ levels were low at the start of Retrovir therapy and in those patients taking paracetamol concurrently (see *Interaction with other medicaments and other forms of interaction*).

Other frequent adverse events reported in large placebo-controlled clinical trials included nausea, vomiting, anorexia, abdominal pain, headache, rash, fever, myalgia, paraesthesiae, insomnia, malaise, asthenia and dyspepsia. Apart from the adverse reaction of nausea, which was significantly more common in all studies in patients receiving Retrovir, the other adverse events were not consistently reported to be more common than in the placebo recipients. Severe headache, myalgia and insomnia were more common in Retrovir-treated patients with advanced HIV disease, whilst vomiting, anorexia, malaise and asthenia were more common in Retrovir-treated patients with early HIV disease. Other adverse events recorded included somnolence, diarrhoea, dizziness, sweating, dyspnoea, flatulence, taste perversion, chest pain, loss of mental acuity, anxiety, urinary frequency, depression, generalised pain, chills, cough, urticaria, pruritius and an influenza-like syndrome. The incidence of these and other less frequent adverse events was similar in both Retrovir and placebo-treated patients.

The available data from both placebo-controlled and open-labelled studies indicate that the incidence of nausea and other frequently reported clinical adverse events consistently decreases over time during the first few weeks of therapy with Retrovir.

The following events have been reported in patients treated with Retrovir. They may also occur as part of the underlying disease process or as a result of the wide range of drugs used in the management of HIV disease. The relationship between these events and use of Retrovir is therefore difficult to evaluate, particularly in the medically complicated situations which characterise advanced HIV disease. If the severity of the symptoms warrants it, a reduction or suspension of Retrovir therapy may assist in the assessment and management of these conditions:

– myopathy;
– pancytopenia with marrow hypoplasia and isolated thrombocytopenia;
– lactic acidosis in the absence of hypoxaemia, liver disorders such as severe hepatomegaly with steatosis;
– raised blood levels of liver enzymes and bilirubin;
– pancreatitis;
– nail, skin and oral mucosa pigmentation.

Convulsions and other cerebral events have also been reported in patients receiving open-label therapy with Retrovir. However, the relationship between these events and the use of Retrovir is difficult to evaluate. Furthermore, the weight of evidence indicates an overall beneficial effect of Retrovir on HIV-associated neurological disorders.

*Children:* Because of the absence of placebo-controlled studies, there are only limited data from open-label studies in children with symptomatic HIV infection.

As in adults, the most serious adverse reactions include anaemia (which may require transfusions), neutropenia and leucopenia. Dosage adjustments may become necessary (see *Posology and method of administration*). The adverse event profile in children and adults receiving Retrovir appears similar.

*Adverse reactions with Retrovir for the prevention of maternal-fetal transmission:* In a placebo-controlled trial, overall clinical adverse events and laboratory test abnormalities were similar for women in the Retrovir and placebo groups. However, there was a trend for mild and moderate anaemia to be seen more commonly prior to delivery in the zidovudine treated women.

In the same trial, haemoglobin concentrations in infants exposed to Retrovir for this indication were marginally lower than in infants in the placebo group, but transfusion was not required. Anaemia resolved within 6 weeks after completion of Retrovir therapy. Other clinical adverse events and laboratory test abnormalities were similar in the Retrovir and placebo groups. The long term consequences of in utero and infant exposure to Retrovir are unknown.

*Overdosage: Symptoms and signs:* Limited data are available on the consequences of ingestion of acute overdoses in both adults and children. No fatalities occurred and all patients recovered. The highest recorded blood level of zidovudine was 185 µM (49.4 mcg/ml). No specific symptoms or signs have been identified following such overdosage.

Dosages as high as 1250 mg Retrovir orally every four hours for four weeks have been administered to two patients with advanced HIV disease. One experienced anaemia and neutropenia while the other had no untoward effects.

*Treatment:* Patients should be observed closely for evidence of toxicity (see *Undesirable effects*) and given the necessary supportive therapy.

Haemodialysis and peritoneal dialysis appear to have a limited effect on elimination of zidovudine but enhance the elimination of the glucuronide metabolite.

## Pharmacological properties
*Pharmacodynamic properties:*
*A. Mode of action:* Zidovudine is an antiviral agent which is highly active in vitro against Retroviruses including the Human Immunodeficiency Virus (HIV).

Zidovudine is phosphorylated in both infected and uninfected cells to the monophosphate (MP) derivative by cellular thymidine kinase. Subsequent phosphorylation of zidovudine-MP to the diphosphate (DP), and then the triphosphate (TP) derivative is catalysed by cellular thymidylate kinase and non-specific kinases respectively. Zidovudine-TP acts as an inhibitor of and substrate for the viral reverse transcriptase. The formation of further proviral DNA is blocked by incorporation of zidovudine-TP into the chain and subsequent chain termination.

Competition by zidovudine-TP for HIV reverse transcriptase is approximately 100-fold greater than for cellular DNA polymerase alpha.

*B. Microbiology:* The relationships between in vitro susceptibility of HIV to zidovudine and clinical response to therapy remain under investigation. In vitro sensitivity testing has not been standardised and results may therefore vary according to methodological factors.

Reduced in-vitro sensitivity to zidovudine has been reported for HIV isolates from patients who have received prolonged courses of Retrovir therapy. The available information indicates that for early HIV disease, the frequency and degree of reduction of in-vitro sensitivity is notably less than for advanced disease.

*Pharmacokinetic properties:*
*A. Pharmacokinetics in adults:* Zidovudine is well absorbed from the gut and, at all dose levels studied, the bioavailability was 60–70%. From a Phase I study, mean steady state peak (C$^{ss}$max) and trough (C$^{ss}$min) plasma concentrations following oral administration of Retrovir (in solution) at doses of 5 mg/kg every four hours were 71. and 0.4 microMolar (µM) (or 1.9 and 0.1 microgram (mcg/ml) respectively. From a bioequivalence study, mean C$^{ss}$max and C$^{ss}$min levels following oral administration of Retrovir Capsules every 4 hours and dose normalised to 200 mg were 4.5 µM (or 1.2 mcg/ml) and 0.4 µM (or 0.1 mcg/ml) respectively.

From studies with intravenous Retrovir, the mean terminal plasma half-life was 1.1 hours, the mean total body clearance was 27.1 ml/min/kg and the apparent volume of distribution was 1.6 Litres/kg. Renal clearance of zidovudine greatly exceeds creatinine clearance, indicating that significant tubular secretion takes place.

The 5'-glucuronide of zidovudine is the major metabolite in both plasma and urine, accounting for approximately 50–80% of the administered dose eliminated by renal excretion. 3'-amino-3'-deoxythymidine (AMT) has been identified as a metabolite of zidovudine following intravenous dosing. There are limited data on the pharmacokinetics of zidovudine in patients with renal or hepatic impairment (see *Posology and method of administration*). There are also limited data on the pharmacokinetics of zidovudine in pregnant women.

No specific data are available on the pharmacokinetics of zidovudine in the elderly.

*B. Pharmacokinetics in children:* In children over the age of 5–6 months, the pharmacokinetic profile of zidovudine is similar to that in adults.

Zidovudine is well absorbed from the gut and, at all

dose levels studied, its bioavailability was 60–74% with a mean of 65%. C$^{ss}$max levels were 4.45 µM (1.19 mcg/ml) following a dose of 120 mg Retrovir (in solution)/m² body surface area and 7.7 µM (2.06 mcg/ml) at 180 mg/m² body surface area. Dosages of 180 mg/m² four times daily in children produced similar systemic exposure (24 hour AUC 40.0 hr µM or 10.7 hr mcg/ml) as doses of 200 mg six times daily in adults (40.7 hr µM or 10.9 hr mcg/ml).

With intravenous dosing, the mean terminal plasma half-life and total body clearance were 1.5 hours and 30.9 ml/min/kg respectively. The major metabolite was 5'-glucuronide. After intravenous dosing, 29% of the dose was recovered unchanged in the urine and 45% excreted as the glucuronide. Renal clearance of zidovudine greatly exceeds creatinine clearance indicating that signficiant tubular secretion take place.

The limited data available on the pharmacokinetics in neonates and young infants indicate that glucuronidation of zidovudine is reduced with a consequent increase in bioavailability, reduction in clearance and longer half life in infants less than 14 days old but thereafter the pharmacokinetics appear similar to those reported in adults.

*C. Distribution:* In adults, the average cerebrospinal fluid/plasma zidovudine concentration ratio 2 to 4 hours after dosing was found to be approximately 0.5. Limited data indicate that zidovudine crosses the placenta and is found in amniotic fluid and fetal blood. Zidovudine has also been detected in semen. In children the mean cerebrospinal fluid/plasma zidovudine concentration ratio ranged from 0.52–0.85, as determined during oral therapy 0.5 to 4 hours after dosing and was 0.87 as determined during intravenous therapy 1–5 hours after a 1 hour infusion. During continuous intravenous infusion, the mean steady-state cerebrospinal fluid/plasma concentration ratio was 0.24.

Plasma protein binding is relatively low (34 to 38%) and drug interactions involving binding site displacement are not anticipated.

*Preclinical safety data:*
*Mutagenicity:* No evidence of mutagenicity was observed in the Ames test. However, zidovudine was weakly mutagenic in a mouse lymphoma cell assay and was positive in an *in vitro* cell transformation assay. Clastogenic effects were observed in an *in vitro* study in human lymphocytes and in *in vivo* oral repeat dose micronucleus studies in rats and mice. An *in vivo* cytogenetic study in rats did not show chromosomal damage. A study of the peripheral blood lymphocytes of eleven AIDS patients showed a higher chromosome breakage frequency in those who had received Retrovir than in those who had not. The clinical significance of these findings is unclear.

*Carcinogenicity:* Zidovudine was administered orally at three dosage levels to separate groups of mice and rats (60 females and 60 males in each group). Initial single daily doses were 30, 60 120 mg/kg/day and 80, 220 and 600 mg/kg/day in mice and rats, respectively. The doses in mice were reduced to 20, 30 and 40 mg/kg/day after Day 90 because of treatment-related anaemia, whereas in rats only the high dose was reduced (to 450 and then 300 mg/kg/day on Days 91 and 279, respectively). In mice, seven late-appearing (after 19 months) vaginal neoplasms (five squamous cell carcinomas, one squamous cell papilloma and one squamous polyp) occurred at the highest dose. One late-appearing squamous cell papilloma occurred in the vagina of a middle-dose animal. No vaginal tumours were fund at the lowest dose.

In rats, two late-appearing (after 20 months) vaginal squamous cell carcinomas occurred in animals given the highest dose. No vaginal tumours occurred at the middle or low doses in rats.

There were no other drug-related tumours observed in either sex of either species.

The predictive value of rodent carcinogenicity studies for humans is uncertain and thus the clinical significance of these findings is unclear.

*Teratogenicity:* See *Use during pregnancy and lactation.*

**Phamaceutical particulars**
List of excipients:
*Retrovir Capsules:* Starches; microcrystalline cellulose; sodium starch glycollate; magnesium stearate.

*Retrovir Tablets:* Microcrystalline cellulose; sodium starch glycollate; povidone K30; magnesium stearate; colour concentrate OY-7300; white (hypromellose, titanium dioxide, polyethylene glycol 400); polyethylene glycol 8000.

*Retrovir Syrup:* Hydrogenated glucose syrup; glycerol; citric acid; sodium benzoate; saccharin sodium; flavour strawberry, flavour white sugar; purified water.

*Incompatibilities:* None.

*Shelf life:*
Retrovir Capsules 100 mg and 250 mg: 5 years
Retrovir Tablets 300 mg: 3 years
Retrovir Syrup: 2 years

*Special precautions for storage:*
*Retrovir Capsules* 100 mg and 250 mg: Store below 30°C. Keep dry. Protect from light.

*Retrovir Tablets* 300 mg:
Store below 30°C. Protect from light.

*Retrovir Syrup:* Store below 30°C.

*Nature and contents of container:*
*Retrovir Capsules 100 mg:* glass bottle containing 100 capsules.

*Retrovir Capsules 250 mg:* PVC/aluminium foil blister pack containing 40 capsules.

*Retrovir Tablets 300 mg:* PVC/aluminium foil blister packs of 28 and 60 tablets. Amber glass bottle containing 28 tablets.

*Retrovir Syrup:* 200 ml amber glass bottle with metal roll-on closure and polyethylene wad and with a 10 ml oral-dosing syringe in the pack which should be fitted to the bottle before use and closed with the cap provided.

*Instructions for use/handling:* No special instructions are required.

**Marketing authorisation numbers**
Retrovir Capsules 100 mg    0003/0239
Retrovir Capsules 250 mg    0003/0240
Retrovir Tablets 300 mg     0003/0357
Retrovir Syrup              0003/0288

**Date of approval/revision of SPC**  13 January 1997.

**Legal category**  POM.

# SEPTRIN* FOR INFUSION
## Strong Sterile Co-trimoxazole Solution
## To make Co-trimoxazole Intravenous Infusion BP

**Presentation** Septrin for Infusion contains 80 mg Trimethoprim BP and 400 mg Sulphamethoxazole BP in each 5 ml ampoule. The infusion is a faintly yellow aqueous solution and contains 45% w/v propylene glycol together with ethyl alcohol. It has a pH of approximately 10.

**Uses** Septrin is an antibacterial agent. Septrin is effective *in vitro* against a wide range of Gram-positive and Gram-negative organisms. It is not active against *Mycobacterium tuberculosis, Mycoplasma,* or *Treponema pallidum. Pseudomonas aeruginosa* is usually insensitive.

In general, the indications for the use of Septrin for Infusion are the same as those for oral presentations.

It is intended that Septrin for Infusion should be used only during such a period as the patient is unable to accept oral therapy, where initiation of treatment is particularly urgent or for convenience if the patient is already receiving intravenous fluids. Although intravenous co-trimoxazole is useful in critically ill patients, there may be no therapeutic advantage over the oral preparation.

Septrin for Infusion has been investigated clinically in the following indications amongst others:
*Respiratory tract infections:* Pneumonia and *Pneumocystis carinii* pneumonitis.
*Genito-urinary infections*
*Gastro-intestinal tract infections:* Shigellosis and typhoid fever.
*Other bacterial infections caused by sensitive organisms:* Brucellosis, septicaemia, intra-abdominal sepsis, meningitis, osteoarticular infections, paediatric soft tissue and skeletal infections.

*In vitro activity:* Sulphamethoxazole competitively inhibits the utilisation of para-aminobenzoic acid in the synthesis of dihydrofolate by the bacterial cell resulting in bacteriostasis. Trimethoprim reversibly inhibits bacterial dihydrofolate reductase (DHFR), an enzyme in the folate metabolic pathway converting dihydrofolate to tetrahydrofolate. Depending on the conditions the effect may be bactericidal. Thus, trimethoprim and sulphamethoxazole block two consecutive steps in the biosynthesis of purines and therefore nucleic acids essential to many bacteria. This action produces marked potentiation of activity *in vitro* between the two agents.

Trimethoprim binds to plasmodial DHFR but less tightly than to the bacterial enzyme. Its affinity for mammalian DHFR is some 50,000 times less than for the corresponding bacterial enzyme.

The majority of common pathogenic bacteria are sensitive *in vitro* to trimethoprim and sulphamethoxazole at concentrations well below those reached in blood, tissue fluids and urine after the administration of recommended doses. These organisms include:

Gram Negative
*Bordetella pertussis*
Brucella spp.
Citrobacter spp.
*Escherichia coli* (including enterotoxigenic strains)
*Haemophilus ducreyi*
*Haemophilus influenzae* (including ampicillin-resistant strains)
Klebsiella/Enterobacter spp.
*Legionella pneumophila*
*Morganella morganii* (previously *Proteus morganii*)
Neisseria spp.
Proteus spp.
Providencia spp. (including previously *Proteus rettgeri*)
Certain Pseudomonas spp. except *aeruginosa*
Salmonella spp. including *S. typhi* and *paratyphi*
*Serratia marcescens*
Shigella spp.
*Vibrio cholerae*
Yersinia spp.

Gram Positive
*Listeria monocytogenes*
Nocardia spp.
*Staphylococcus aureus*
*Staphylococcus epidermidis* and *saprophyticus*
*Streptococcus faecalis*
*Streptococcus pneumoniae*
*Streptococcus pyogenes*
*Streptococcus viridans*
Many strains of *Bacteroides fragilis* are sensitive. Some strains of *Campylobacter fetus* subsp. *jejuni* and *Chlamydia* are sensitive without evidence of synergy. Some varieties of non-tuberculous mycobacteria are sensitive to sulphamethoxazole but not trimethoprim. Mycoplasmas, *Ureaplasma urealyticum, Mycobacterium tuberculosis* and *Treponema pallidum* are insensitive.

Satisfactory sensitivity testing is achieved only with recommended media, free from inhibitory substances especially thymidine and thymine.

*Pharmacokinetics:* Peak plasma levels of trimethoprim and sulphamethoxazole are higher and achieved more rapidly after one hour of intravenous infusion of Septrin for Infusion than after oral administration of an equivalent dose of a Septrin oral presentation. Plasma concentrations, elimination half-life and urinary excretion rates show no significant differences following either the oral or intravenous route of administration.

Trimethoprim is a weak base with a pKa of 7.3. It is lipophilic. Tissue levels of trimethoprim are generally higher than corresponding plasma levels, the lungs and kidneys showing especially high concentrations. Trimethoprim concentrations exceed those in plasma in the case of bile, prostatic fluid and tissue, sputum, and vaginal secretions. Levels in the aqueous humor, breast milk, cerebrospinal fluid, middle ear fluid, synovial fluid and tissue (interstitial) fluid are adequate for antibacterial activity. Trimethoprim passes into amniotic fluid and fetal tissues reaching concentrations approximating those in maternal serum.

Approximately 50% of trimethoprim in the plasma is protein bound. The half-life in man is in the range 8.6 to 17 hours in the presence of normal renal function. It is increased by a factor of 1.5 to 3.0 when the creatinine clearance is less than 10 ml/minute. There appears to be no significant difference in the elderly compared with young patients.

The principal route of excretion of trimethoprim is renal and approximately 50% of the dose is excreted in the urine within 24 hours as unchanged drug. Several metabolites have been identified in the urine. Urinary concentrations of trimethoprim vary widely.

Sulphamethoxazole is a weak acid with a pKa of 6.0. The concentration of active sulphamethoxazole in amniotic fluid, aqueous humor, bile, cerebrospinal fluid, middle ear fluid, sputum, synovial fluid and tissue (interstitial) fluid is of the order of 20 to 50% of the plasma concentration. Approximately 66% of sulphamethoxazole in the plasma is protein bound. The half-life in man is approximately 9 to 11 hours in the presence of normal renal function. There is no change in the half-life of active sulphamethoxazole with a reduction in renal function but there is prolongation of the half-life of the major, acetylated metabolite when the creatinine clearance is below 25 ml/minute.

The principal route of excretion of sulphamethoxazole is renal; between 15% and 30% of the dose recovered in the urine is in the active form. In elderly patients there is a reduced renal clearance of sulphamethoxazole.

**Dosage and administration**
*Administration:* Septrin for Infusion is for administration ONLY by the intravenous route and MUST BE DILUTED before administration.
DILUTION SHOULD BE CARRIED OUT IMMEDIATELY BEFORE USE.
After adding Septrin for Infusion to the infusion solution, shake thoroughly to ensure complete mix-

ing. If visible turbidity or crystallisation appears at any time before or during an infusion, the mixture should be discarded.

It is recommended that Septrin for Infusion is diluted according to the following schedules:

One ampoule Septrin for Infusion (5 ml) to 125 ml infusion solution.

Two ampoules Septrin for Infusion (10 ml) to 250 ml infusion solution.

Three ampoules Septrin for Infusion (15 ml) to 500 ml infusion solution.

Septrin for Infusion is known to be compatible, when diluted as schedules above, with the following fluids:

Glucose Intravenous Infusion BP (5% w/v and 10% w/v).

Sodium Chloride Intravenous Infusion BP (0.9% w/v).

Sodium Chloride (0.18% w/v) and Glucose (4% w/v) Intravenous Infusion BP.

Dextran 70 Injection BP (6% w/v) in glucose (5% w/v) or normal saline.

Dextran 40 Injection BP (10% w/v) in glucose (5% w/v) or normal saline.

Ringer's Solution for Injection BPC 1959.

NO OTHER SUBSTANCE SHOULD BE MIXED WITH THE INFUSION.

The duration of the infusion should be approximately 1 to 1½ hours, but this should be balanced against the fluid requirements of the patient.

When fluid restriction is necessary, Septrin for Infusion may be administered at a higher concentration, 5 ml diluted with 75 ml of glucose 5% w/v in water. The resultant solution, whilst being clear to the naked eye, may on occasion exceed the BP limits set for particulate matter in large volume parenterals. The solution should be infused over a period not exceeding one hour. Discard any unused diluted solution.

*Acute Infections: Adults and children over 12 years:* Standard dosage: 2 ampoules (10 ml) every 12 hours.

*Children aged 12 years and under:* The recommended dosage is approximately 6 mg trimethoprim and 30 mg sulphamethoxazole per kg bodyweight per 24 hours, given in two equally divided doses. As a guide the following schedules may be used, diluted as described above.

*6 weeks to 5 months:* 1.25 ml every 12 hours.

*6 months to 5 years:* 2.5 ml every 12 hours.

*6 to 12 years:* 5.0 ml every 12 hours.

For severe infections in all age groups dosage may be increased by 50%.

Treatment should be continued until the patient has been symptom free for two days; the majority will require treatment for at least 5 days.

*Special Dosage Recommendations:*

*Dosage recommendations in impaired renal function:*

Adults and children over 12 years (no information is available for children under 12 years of age):

| Creatinine clearance (ml/min) | Serum creatinine (µmol/l) | Recommended Dosage |
|---|---|---|
| Above 25 | men < 265 women < 175 | STANDARD DOSAGE. |
| 15 to 25 | men 265 to 620 women 175 to 400 | STANDARD DOSAGE for maximum of 3 days followed by half the standard daily dosage. |
| Below 15 | men > 620 women > 400 | Not recommended unless haemodialysis facilities are available when half the standard daily dosage may be given. |

Measurements of plasma concentrations of sulphamethoxazole at intervals of 2 to 3 days are recommended in samples obtained 12 hours after administration of Septrin for Infusion. If the concentration of total sulphamethoxazole exceeds 150 microgram/ml then treatment should be interrupted until the value falls below 120 microgram/ml (see Further information).

*Dosage in Pneumocystis carinii pneumonitis:* *Treatment:* 20 mg trimethoprim and 100 mg sulphamethoxazole per kg bodyweight per day in two or more divided doses. Therapy should be changed to the oral route as soon as possible and continued for a total treatment period of two weeks. The aim is to obtain peak plasma or serum levels of trimethoprim of ≥ 5 micrograms/ml *(see Side- and adverse effects)*.

*Prevention:* STANDARD DOSAGE (i.v. or oral as appropriate) for the duration of the period at risk.

*Acute brucellosis:* It may be advisable to use a *higher* than STANDARD DOSAGE initially when the intravenous route may be preferred. Treatment should continue for a period of at least four weeks and repeated courses may be beneficial.

*Use in the elderly:* No specific studies have been carried out in the elderly, although Septrin has been widely used in older people. See *Precautions* for further information.

**Contra-indications, warnings, etc**

*Contra-indications:* Septrin should not be given to patients with a history of hypersensitivity to sulphonamides, trimethoprim or co-trimoxazole.

Septrin for Infusion is contra-indicated in patients showing marked liver parenchyma damage.

Except under careful supervision Septrin for Infusion should not be given to patients with serious haematological disorders. Co-trimoxazole has been given to patients receiving cytotoxic therapy with little or no additional effect on the bone marrow or peripheral blood.

Septrin for Infusion is contra-indicated in severe renal insufficiency where repeated measurements of the plasma concentration cannot be performed.

Septrin for Infusion should not be given to premature babies nor to full-term infants during the first six weeks of life.

*Precautions:* Septrin for Infusion should be discontinued if a skin rash appears.

Septrin for Infusion contains sulphite. This may cause allergic-type reactions including anaphylactic symptoms and life-threatening or less severe asthmatic episodes in susceptible individuals.

Fluid overload is possible, especially when very high doses are being administered to patients with underlying cardiopulmonary disease.

An adequate urinary output should be maintained at all times. Evidence of crystalluria *in vivo* is rare, although sulphonamide crystals have been noted in cooled urine from treated patients. In patients suffering from malnutrition the risk may be increased.

For patients with known renal impairment special measures should be adopted (see *Dosage recommendations in impaired renal function*).

Regular monthly blood counts are advisable when Septrin is given for long periods since there exists a possibility of asymptomatic changes in haematological laboratory indices due to lack of available folate. These changes may be reversed by administration of folinic acid (5 to 10 mg/day) without interfering with the antibacterial activity.

Particular care is always advisable when treating elderly patients because, as a group, they are more susceptible to adverse reactions and more likely to suffer serious side effects as a result.

Special care should be exercised in treating elderly or suspected folate-deficient patients; folate supplementation should be considered.

A folate supplement should also be considered with prolonged high dosage of Septrin.

In treatment of tonsillo-pharyngitis due to Group A β-haemolytic streptococci, eradication of these organisms from the oropharynx is less effective than with penicillin.

Trimethoprim has been noted to impair phenylalanine metabolism but this is of no significance in phenylketonuric patients on appropriate dietary restriction.

The administration of Septrin to patients known or suspected to be at risk of acute porphyria should be avoided. Both trimethoprim and sulphonamides (although not specifically sulphamethoxazole) have been associated with clinical exacerbation of porphyria.

*Drug interactions:* Co-trimoxazole has been shown to potentiate the anticoagulant activity of warfarin *via* stereo-selective inhibition of its metabolism. Sulphamethoxazole may displace warfarin from plasmaalbumin protein-binding sites *in vitro*. Careful control of the anticoagulant therapy during treatment with Septrin is advisable.

Co-trimoxazole prolongs the half-life of phenytoin and if co-administered the prescriber should be alert for excessive phenytoin effect. Close monitoring of the patient's condition and serum phenytoin levels is advisable.

Interaction with sulphonylurea hypoglycaemic agents is uncommon but potentiation has been reported.

Concurrent use of rifampicin and Septrin results in a shortening of the plasma half-life of trimethoprim after a period of about one week. This is not thought to be of clinical significance.

Reversible deterioration in renal function has been observed in patients treated with co-trimoxazole and cyclosporin following renal transplantation.

Occasional reports suggest that patients receiving pyrimethamine as malarial prophylaxis at doses in excess of 25 mg weekly may develop megaloblastic anaemia should co-trimoxazole be prescribed concurrently.

In elderly patients concurrently receiving diuretics, mainly thiazides, there appears to be an increased risk of thrombocytopenia with or without purpura.

When trimethoprim is administered simultaneously

with drugs that form cations at physiological pH, and are also partly excreted by active renal secretion (e.g. procainamide, amantadine), there is the possibility of competitive inhibition of this process which may lead to an increase in plasma concentration of one or both of the drugs.

Concomitant use of trimethoprim with digoxin has been shown to increase plasma digoxin levels in a proportion of elderly patients.

If Septrin is considered appropriate therapy in patients receiving other anti-folate drugs such as methotrexate, a folate supplement should be considered (see *Precautions*).

*Side- and adverse effects:* As Septrin contains trimethoprim and a sulphonamide, the type and frequency of adverse reactions associated with such compounds may be expected. At the recommended dosages Septrin is usually well tolerated.

Of the reported adverse reactions most are mild and comprise nausea, with or without vomiting, and skin rashes.

More severe skin sensitivity reactions such as erythema multiforme bullosa (Stevens-Johnson syndrome), and toxic epidermal necrolysis (Lyell syndrome) have occurred rarely; the latter condition carries a high mortality.

Haematological changes have been reported, the majority being mild and reversible when treatment was stopped. The changes are mainly leucopenia, neutropenia, thrombocytopenia and, less commonly, agranulocytosis, megaloblastic anaemia and purpura. Although most of the changes cause no clinical symptoms they may become severe in isolated cases, especially in the elderly, in those with hepatic or renal dysfunction or in those with poor folate status; such patients should be observed carefully. Septrin may induce haemolysis in certain susceptible glucose-6-phosphate dehydrogenase deficient patients but this does not appear to be dose-related.

Aseptic meningitis has been reported in association with the administration of co-trimoxazole. The condition was rapidly reversible on withdrawal of the drug, but recurred in a number of cases on re-exposure to either co-trimoxazole or to trimethoprim alone.

Hepatic changes including cholestatic jaundice and hepatic necrosis have been reported rarely and may be fatal.

Local thrombophlebitis may occasionally be a problem at the site of injection.

Diarrhoea, glossitis and stomatitis are uncommon. Pseudomembranous colitis has been reported rarely.

Monilial overgrowth is also very rare.

Impaired renal function has been reported rarely following the administration of co-trimoxazole, but its relationship to therapy remains unproven.

Allergic reactions including serum sickness and mild anaphylaxis have been reported rarely.

There have been a few reports of subjective experiences such as headache, depression, dizziness and hallucinations but their relationship to therapy remains unproven.

At the high dosages used for the therapy of *Pneumocystis carinii* pneumonitis in patients with Acquired Immune Deficiency Syndrome, rash, fever, neutropenia, thrombocytopenia and raised liver enzymes have been reported, necessitating cessation of therapy. Concomitant administration of intravenous diphenhydramine may permit continued infusion.

*Use in pregnancy and lactation:* The safety of Septrin in human pregnancy has not been established. The drug should not be given during pregnancy. Animal studies have shown teratogenic effects typical of a folate antagonist in rats but not rabbits at high doses; these were prevented by administration of dietary folates. Sulphonamide-containing products should not be administered in late pregnancy because of the risk of kernicterus.

The usual caution in prescribing any drug for women of child-bearing age should be exercised with Septrin.

Despite the excretion of sulphamethoxazole into breast milk, the administration of Septrin to lactating women represents a negligible risk to the suckling infant.

*Toxicity and treatment of overdosage:* The maximum tolerated dose in humans is unknown.

Nausea, vomiting, dizziness and confusion are likely symptoms of overdosage.

In cases of known, suspected or accidental overdosage, stop therapy.

Acidification of the urine will increase the elimination of trimethoprim. Inducing diuresis plus alkalinisation of urine will enhance the elimination of sulphamethoxazole. Alkalinisation will reduce the rate of elimination of trimethoprim. Calcium folinate (5 to 10 mg/day) will reverse any folate deficiency effect of trimethoprim on the bone marrow should this occur. General supportive measures are recommended.

Both trimethoprim and active sulphamethoxazole are dialysable by renal dialysis.

**Pharmaceutical precautions** Store below 30°C. Protect from light.

**Legal category** POM

**Package quantities** Box of 10 ampoules.

**Further information** Septrin does not affect incubating syphilis.

Trimethoprim may interfere with the estimation of serum/plasma creatinine when the alkaline picrate reaction is used. This may result in overestimation of the order of 10%. Functional inhibition of the renal tubular secretion of creatinine may produce a spurious fall in the estimated rate of creatinine clearance.

Trimethoprim does not induce its own metabolism and therefore no dose modification is required on this account during long-term treatment.

Trimethoprim interferes with assays for serum methotrexate when dihydrofolate reductase from *Lactobacillus casei* is used in the assay.

Co-trimoxazole may affect the results of thyroid function tests but this is probably of little or no clinical significance.

Plasma or serum levels of sulphamethoxazole and trimethoprim may be determined by high-performance liquid chromatography.

**Product licence number**    0003/0095

## SEPTRIN* TABLETS
## SEPTRIN* DISPERSIBLE TABLETS
## SEPTRIN* FORTE TABLETS
## SEPTRIN* ADULT SUSPENSION
## SEPTRIN* PAEDIATRIC SUSPENSION

**Presentation**
*Septrin Tablets* (Co-trimoxazole Tablets BP) each containing 80 mg Trimethoprim BP and 400 mg Sulphamethoxazole BP. White, biconvex scored tablets, coded 'Y2B WELLCOME'.

*Septrin Dispersible Tablets* (Dispersible Co-trimoxazole Tablets BP) each containing 80 mg Trimethoprim BP and 400 mg Sulphamethoxazole BP. Coded Septrin 'Y2B WELLCOME'. Orange in colour.

*Septrin Forte Tablets* (Co-trimoxazole Tablets BP) each containing 160 mg Trimethoprim BP and 800 mg Sulphamethoxazole BP. White, biconvex, elongated tablets, scored and coded 'O2C WELLCOME'.

*Septrin Adult Suspension* (Co-trimoxazole Mixture BP) contains 80 mg Trimethoprim BP and 400 mg Sulphamethoxazole BP in each 5 ml. Off-white in colour.

*Septrin Paediatric Suspension (Paediatric Co-trimoxazole Mixture BP) contains 40 mg Trimethoprim BP and 200 mg Sulphamethoxazole BP in each 5 ml. Off-white in colour. Sugar free.*

**Uses**    Septrin should only be used where, in the judgement of the physician, the benefits of treatment outweigh any possible risks; consideration should be given to the use of a single effective antibacterial agent.

The *in vitro* susceptibility of bacteria to antibiotics varies geographically and with time; the local situation should always be considered when selecting antibiotic therapy.

Treatment and prevention of *Pneumocystis carinii* pneumonitis (see *Dosage and administration* and *Side- and adverse effects*).

Treatment and prophylaxis of toxoplasmosis, treatment of nocardiosis.

*Urinary tract infections: Acute uncomplicated urinary tract infections:* Treatment of urinary tract infections where there is bacterial evidence of sensitivity to co-trimoxazole and good reason to prefer this combination to a single antibiotic.

*Respiratory tract infections: Otitis media:* Acute treatment of otitis media, where there is good reason to prefer co-trimoxazole to a single antibiotic.

Treatment of acute exacerbations of chronic bronchitis, where there is bacterial evidence of sensitivity to co-trimoxazole and good reason to prefer this combination to a single antibiotic.

**Dosage and administration**    It may be preferable to take Septrin with some food or drink to minimise the possibility of gastrointestinal disturbances.

*Acute infections: Adults and children over 12 years:*
Standard dosage

| Tablets/Dispersible Tablets | Forte Tablets | Adult Suspension |
|---|---|---|
| 2 every 12 hours | 1 every 12 hours | 10 ml every 12 hours. |

*Children aged 12 years and under:*
Standard dosage

| Age | Paediatric Suspension |
|---|---|
| 6 to 12 years | 10 ml every 12 hours |
| 6 months to 5 years | 5 ml every 12 hours |
| 6 weeks to 5 months | 2.5 ml every 12 hours. |

This dosage approximates to 6 mg trimethoprim and 30 mg sulphamethoxazole per kilogram body weight per 24 hours.

Treatment should be continued until the patient has been symptom free for two days; the majority will require treatment for at least 5 days. If clinical improvement is not evident after 7 days' therapy, the patient should be reassessed.

As an alternative to *standard dosage* for acute uncomplicated lower urinary tract infections, short-term therapy of 1 to 3 days' duration has been shown to be effective.

*Use in the elderly:* Particular care is *always* advisable when treating elderly patients because, as a group, they are more susceptible to adverse reactions and more likely to suffer serious effects as a result particularly when complicating conditions exist, e.g. impaired kidney and/or liver function and/or concomitant use of other drugs.

*Special dosage recommendations:* Unless otherwise specified *standard dosage* applies.

Where dosage is expressed as 'tablets' this refers to the adult tablet, i.e. 80 mg Trimethoprim BP and 400 mg Sulphamethoxazole BP. If other formulations are to be used appropriate adjustment should be made.

*Impaired renal function: Adults and children over 12 years:* (no information is available for children under 12 years of age).

| Creatinine clearance (ml/min) | Recommended Dosage |
|---|---|
| >30 | standard dosage |
| 15 to 30 | Half the standard dosage |
| <15 | Not recommended |

Measurements of plasma concentration of sulphamethoxazole at intervals of 2 to 3 days are recommended in samples obtained 12 hours after administration of Septrin. If the concentration of total sulphamethoxazole exceeds 150 microgram/ml then treatment should be interrupted until the value falls below 120 microgram/ml.

*Pneumocystis carinii pneumonitis: Treatment:* 20 mg trimethoprim and 100 mg sulphamethoxazole per kg bodyweight per day in two or more divided doses for two weeks. The aim is to obtain peak plasma or serum levels of trimethoprim of ≥5 microgram/ml (verified in patients receiving 1-hour infusions of intravenous Septrin) (see *Side- and adverse effects*).

*Prevention: Adults:* The following dose schedules may be used:
160 mg trimethoprim/800 mg sulphamethoxazole daily 7 days per week.
160 mg trimethoprim/800 mg sulphamethoxazole three times per week on alternate days.
320 mg trimethoprim/1,600 mg sulphamethoxazole per day in two divided doses three times per week on alternate days.

*Children:* Standard dosage for the duration of the period at risk – either given 7 days per week or three days per week (on consecutive days).

This dosage approximates to 150 mg trimethoprim/m²/day and 750 mg sulphamethoxazole/m²/day to be given in equally divided doses twice a day. The total daily dose should not exceed 320 mg trimethoprim and 1,600 mg sulphamethoxazole.

*Nocardiosis:* There is no consensus on the most appropriate dosage. Adult doses of 6 to 8 tablets daily for up to 3 months have been used.

*Toxoplasmosis:* There is no consensus on the most appropriate dosage for the treatment or prophylaxis of this condition. The decision should be based on clinical experience. For prophylaxis, however, the dosages suggested for prevention of PCP may be appropriate.

**Contra-indications, warnings, etc**
*Contra-indications:* Septrin should not be given to patients with a history of hypersensitivity to sulphonamides, trimethoprim or co-trimoxazole.

Contra-indicated in patients showing marked liver parenchymal damage.

Contra-indicated in severe renal insufficiency where repeated measurements of the plasma concentration cannot be performed.

Except under careful supervision Septrin should not be given to patients with serious haematological disorders (see *Side- and adverse effects*). Co-trimoxazole has been given to patients receiving cytotoxic therapy with little or no additional effect on the bone marrow or peripheral blood.

Septrin should not be given to premature babies nor to full-term infants during the first 6 weeks of life except for the treatment/prophylaxis of PCP in infants 4 weeks of age or greater.

*Precautions:* Fatalities, although rare, have occurred due to severe reactions including Stevens-Johnson syndrome, Lyell syndrome (toxic epidermal necrolysis), fulminant hepatic necrosis, agranulocytosis, aplastic anaemia, other blood dyscrasias and hypersensitivity of the respiratory tract.

Septrin should be discontinued at the first appearance of skin rash (see *Side- and adverse effects*).

Particular care is *always* advisable when treating elderly patients because, as a group, they are more susceptible to adverse reactions and more likely to suffer serious effects as a result particularly when complicating conditions exist, e.g. impaired kidney and/or liver function and/or concomitant use of other drugs.

Special care should be exercised in treating elderly or suspected folate-deficient patients; folate supplementation should be considered.

An adequate urinary output should be maintained at all times. Evidence of crystalluria *in vivo* is rare, although sulphonamide crystals have been noted in cooled urine from treated patients. In patients suffering from malnutrition the risk may be increased.

Regular monthly blood counts are advisable when Septrin is given for long periods since there exists a possibility of asymptomatic changes in haematological laboratory indices due to lack of available folate. These changes may be reversed by administration of folinic acid (5 to 10 mg/day) without interfering with the antibacterial activity.

A folate supplement should also be considered with prolonged high dosage of Septrin (see *Drug interactions*).

In glucose-6-phosphate dehydrogenase (G-6-PD) deficient patients haemolysis may occur.

Septrin should be given with caution to patients with servere allergy or bronchial asthma.

Septrin should not be used in the treatment of streptococcal pharyngitis due to Group A haemolytic streptococci; eradication of these organisms from the oropharynx is less effective than with penicillin.

Trimethoprim has been noted to impair phenylalanine metabolism but this is of no significance in phenylketonuric patients on appropriate dietary restriction.

The administration of Septrin to patients known or suspected to be at risk of acute porphyria should be avoided. Both trimethoprim and sulphonamides (although not specifically sulphamethoxazole) have been associated with clinical exacerbation of porphyria.

*Use in pregnancy and lactation:* The safety of Septrin in human pregnancy has not been established and as trimethoprim and sulphamethoxazole may interfere with folic acid metabolism, co-trimoxazole should not be used during pregnancy unless in the judgement of the clinician the potential benefit to the mother justifies the potential risk to the foetus.

At doses greatly in excess of the recommended human therapeutic dose, trimethoprim has been reported to be teratogenic in rats with effects typical of a folate antagonist and preventable by administration of dietary folate. No significant drug-related malformations have been demonstrated in rabbits but at doses approximately ten times in excess of the human therapeutic dose in increase in foetal deaths was noted.

Trimethoprim and sulphamethoxazole are excreted into breast milk, however, the administration of Septrin to lactating women represents a negligible risk to the suckling infant.

*Side- and adverse effects:* As Septrin contains trimethoprim and a sulphonamide the type and frequency of adverse reactions associated with such compounds may be expected. At the recommended dosages Septrin is usually well tolerated.

Of the reported adverse reactions most are mild and comprise nausea, with or without vomiting, and skin rashes.

*Skin effects:* Skin rashes with photosensitivity also reported. More severe skin sensitivity reactions such as exfoliative dermatitis, erythema multiforme, Stevens-Johnson syndrome and Lyell syndrome (toxic epidermal necrolysis) have occurred rarely; the last condition carries a high mortality.

*Allergic effects:* Other allergic reactions including serum sickness, anaphylaxis, allergic myocarditis, angioedema and drug fever have been reported rarely. Periarteritis nodosa and systemic lupus erythematosus have also been documented.

*Effects associated with PCP management:* At the high dosages used for the therapy of *Pneumocystis carinii* pneumonitis in patients with acquired immune deficiency syndrome (AIDS), rash, fever, neutropenia, thrombocytopenia, raised liver enzymes, hyperkalaemia and hyponatremia have been reported, necessitating cessation of therapy. If signs of bone marrow depression occur, the patient should be given calcium folinate supplementation (5 to 10 mg/day). Severe hypersensitivity reactions have also been reported in HIV-infected patients on re-exposure to co-trimoxazole, sometimes after a dosage interval of a few days.

*Haematological effects:* Haematological changes have been reported, the majority being mild and reversible when treatment was stopped. The changes are mainly leucopenia, neutropenia, thrombocytopenia and, less commonly, agranulocytosis, megaloblastic anaemia, aplastic anaemia, haemolytic anaemia and methaemoglobinaemia. Although most of the changes cause no clinical symptoms they may become severe in isolated cases especially in the elderly, in those with hepatic or renal dysfunction or in those with poor folate status. Fatalities have been recorded in at-risk patients and such patients should be observed carefully (see *Contra-indications*). Septrin may induce haemolysis in certain susceptible G-6-PD deficient patients.

*Gastro-intestinal effects:* Hepatic changes including elevation of serum transaminases and bilirubin levels. Cholestatic jaundice and hepatic necrosis have been reported rarely and may be fatal.

Diarrhoea, glossitis and stomatitis are uncommon. Anorexia has been reported. Pseudomembranous colitis and pancreatitis have been reported rarely.

*Neurological effects:* Aseptic meningitis has been reported in association with the administration of co-trimoxazole. The condition was rapidly reversible on withdrawal of the drug, but recurred in a number of cases on re-exposure to either co-trimoxazole or to trimethoprim alone.

Convulsions, peripheral neuritis, ataxia, vertigo, and tinnitus have also been reported. There have also been a few reports of subjective experiences such as headache, depression, dizziness and hallucinations.

*Genito-urinary effects:* Impaired renal function, including cases of interstitial nephritis, has been reported rarely following the administration of co-trimoxazole.

*Respiratory effects:* Cough, shortness of breath and pulmonary infiltrates have been reported. These may be early indicators of respiratory hypersensitivity which, while rare, has been fatal.

*Metabolic effects:* Hyperkalaemia and hyponatraemia have been reported occasionally in association with elderly patients or in patients taking high doses.

*Musculoskeletal effects:* Arthralgia and myalgia have been reported.

*Miscellaneous:* Monilial overgrowth is very rare.

*Drug interactions:* In elderly patients concurrently receiving diuretics, mainly thiazides, there appears to be an increased risk of thrombocytopenia.

Occasional reports suggest that patients receiving pyrimethamine at doses in excess of 25 mg weekly may develop megaloblastic anaemia should co-trimoxazole be prescribed concurrently.

Reversible deterioration in renal function has been observed in patients treated with co-trimoxazole and cyclosporin following renal transplantation.

Co-trimoxazole has been shown to potentiate the anticoagulant activity of warfarin via stereo-selective inhibition of its metabolism. Sulphamethoxazole may displace warfarin from plasma-albumin protein-binding sites *in vitro*. Careful control of the anticoagulant therapy during treatment with Septrin is advisable.

Co-trimoxazole prolongs the half-life of phenytoin and if co-administered could result in excessive phenytoin effect. Close monitoring of the patient's condition and serum phenytoin levels are advisable.

Interaction with sulphonylurea hypoglycaemic agents is uncommon but potentiation has been reported.

Concurrent use of rifampicin and Septrin results in a shortening of the plasma half-life of trimethoprim after a period of about one week. This is not thought to be of clinical significance.

When trimethoprim is administered simultaneously with drugs that form cations at physiological pH, and are also partly excreted by active renal secretion (e.g. procainamide, amantadine), there is the possibility of competitive inhibition of this process which may lead to an increase in plasma concentration of one or both of the drugs.

Concomitant use of trimethoprim with digoxin has been shown to increase plasma digoxin levels in a proportion of elderly patients.

If Septrin is considered appropriate therapy in patients receiving other anti-folate drugs such as methotrexate, a folate supplement should be considered (see *Precautions*).

*Toxicity and treatment of overdosage:* Nausea, vomiting, dizziness and confusion are likely signs/symptoms of overdosage. Bone marrow depression has been reported in acute trimethoprim overdosage.

If vomiting has not occurred, induction of vomiting may be desirable. Gastric lavage may be useful, though absorption from the gastrointestinal tract is normally very rapid and complete within approximately two hours. This may not be the case in gross overdosage. Dependant on the status of renal function administration of fluids is recommended if urine output is low.

Both trimethoprim and active sulphamethoxazole are moderately dialysable by haemodialysis. Peritoneal dialysis is not effective.

**Further information** *In vitro activity:* Sulphamethoxazole competitively inhibits the utilisation of para-aminobenzoic acid in the synthesis of dihydrofolate by the bacterial cell resulting in bacteriostasis. Trimethoprim reversibly inhibits bacterial dihydrofolate reductase (DHFR), an enzyme active in the folate metabolic pathway converting dihydrofolate to tetrahydrofolate. Depending on the conditions the effect may be bactericidal. Thus, trimethoprim and sulphamethoxazole block two consecutive steps in the biosynthesis of purines and therefore nucleic acids essential to many bacteria. This action produces marked potentiation of activity *in vitro* between the two agents.

Trimethoprim binds to plasmodial DHFR but less tightly than to the bacterial enzyme. Its affinity for mammalian DHFR is some 50,000 times less than for the corresponding bacterial enzyme.

Many of common pathogenic bacteria are sensitive *in vitro* to trimethoprim and sulphamethoxazole at concentrations well below those reached in blood, tissue fluids and urine after the administration of recommended doses. In common with other antibiotics, however, *in vitro* activity does not necessarily imply that clinical efficacy has been demonstrated and it must be noted that satisfactory sensitivity testing is achieved only with recommended media, free from inhibitory substances especially thymidine and thymine.

*Pharmacokinetics:* After oral administration, trimethoprim and sulphamethoxazole are rapidly and nearly completely absorbed. The presence of food does not appear to delay absorption. Peak levels in the blood occur between one and four hours after ingestion and the level attained is dose related. Effective levels persist in the blood for up to 24 hours after a therapeutic dose.

Trimethoprim is a weak base with a pKa of 7.4. It is lipophilic. Tissue levels of trimethoprim are generally higher than corresponding plasma levels, the lungs and kidneys showing especially high concentrations.

Approximately 50% of trimethoprim in the plasma is protein bound and the principal route of excretion of trimethoprim is renal. The half life in man is in the range 8.6 to 17 hours in the presence of normal renal function. It is increased by a factor of 1.5 to 3.0 when the creatinine clearance is less than 10 ml/minute. There appears to be no significant difference in the elderly compared with young patients.

Sulphamethoxazole is a weak acid with a pKa of 6.0. The concentration of active sulphamethoxazole in a variety of body fluids is of the order of 20 to 50% of the plasma concentration.

Approximately 66% of sulphamethoxazole in the plasma is protein bound and the principal route of excretion of sulphamethoxazole is renal. The half-life in man is approximately 9 to 11 hours in the presence of normal renal function. There is no change in the half-life of active sulphamethoxazole with a reduction in renal function but there is prolongation of the half life of the major, acetylated metabolite when the creatinine clearance is below 25 ml/minute.

In elderly patients there is a reduced renal clearance of sulphamethoxazole.

**Pharmaceutical precautions**

*Tablets:* Store below 25˚C. Protect from light.

*Dispersible Tablets:* Store below 25˚C. Keep dry. Protect from light.

*Adult and Paediatric Suspension:* Store below 25˚C. Protect from light.

**Legal category** POM.

**Package quantities**

| | |
|---|---|
| Septrin Tablets: | Packs of 100 tablets. |
| Septrin Dispensible Tablets: | Packs of 100 tablets. |
| Septrin Forte Tablets: | Packs of 100 tablets. |
| Septrin Adult Suspension: | Bottle of 100 ml. |
| Septrin Paediatric Suspension: | Bottle of 100 ml. |

**Further information** Trimethoprim interferes with assays for serum methotrexate when dihydrofolate reductase from *Lactobacillus casei* is used in the assay. No interference occurs if methotrexate is measured by radioimmune assay.

Trimethoprim may interfere with the estimation of serum/plasma creatinine when the alkaline picrate reaction is used. This may result in overestimation of serum/plasma creatinine of the order of 10%. Functional inhibition of the renal tubular secretion of creatinine may produce a spurious fall in the estimated rate of creatinine clearance.

**Product licence numbers**

| | |
|---|---|
| Tablets: | 0003/0109R |
| Dispersible Tablets: | 0003/0099R. |
| Forte Tablets: | 0003/0121 |
| Adult Suspension: | 0003/5223R |
| Paediatric Suspension: | 0003/5222R |

## TRACRIUM* INJECTION

**Presentation** Tracrium Injection is a clear, faintly yellow, sterile aqueous solution in a glass ampoule containing 10 mg atracurium besylate per ml. Each 2.5 ml ampoule contains 25 mg atracurium besylate, each 5 ml ampoule contains 50 mg atracurium besylate and each 25 ml ampoule contains 250 mg atracurium besylate.

**Uses** Tracrium is a highly selective, competitive or non-depolarising neuromuscular blocking agent. It is used as an adjunct to general anaesthesia or sedation in the intensive care unit (ICU), to relax skeletal muscles, and to facilitate tracheal intubation and mechanical ventilation.

**Dosage and administration**

*Use by injection in adults:* Tracrium is administered by intravenous injection.

The dosage range recommended for adults is 0.3 to 0.6 mg/kg (depending on the duration of full block required) and will provide adequate relaxation for about 15 to 35 minutes.

Endotracheal intubation can usually be accomplished within 90 seconds from the intravenous injection of 0.5 to 0.6 mg/kg.

Full block can be prolonged with supplementary doses of 0.1 to 0.2 mg/kg as required. Successive supplementary dosing does not give rise to accumulation of neuromuscular blocking effect.

Spontaneous recovery from the end of full block occurs in about 35 minutes as measured by the restoration of the tetanic response to 95% of normal neuromuscular function.

The neuromuscular block produced by Tracrium can be rapidly reversed by standard doses of anticholinesterase agents, such as neostigmine and edrophonium, accompanied or preceded by atropine, with no evidence of recurarisation.

*Use as an infusion in adults:* After an initial bolus dose of 0.2 to 0.6 mg/kg, Tracrium can be used to maintain neuromuscular block during long surgical procedures by administration as a continuous infusion at rates of 0.3 to 0.6 mg/kg/hour.

Tracrium can be administered by infusion during cardiopulmonary bypass surgery at the recommended infusion rates. Induced hypothermia to a body temperature of 25˚ to 26˚C reduces the rate of inactivation of atracurium, therefore full neuromuscular block may be maintained by approximately half the original infusion rate at these low temperatures.

Tracrium is compatible with the following infusion solutions for the times stated below:

| Infusion solution | Period of stability |
|---|---|
| Sodium Chloride Intravenous Infusion BP (0.9% w/v) | 24 hours |
| Glucose Intravenous Infusion BP (5% w/v) | 8 hours |
| Ringer's Injection USP | 8 hours |
| Sodium Chloride (0.18% w/v) and Glucose (4% w/v) Intravenous Infusion BP | 8 hours |
| Compound Sodium Lactate Intravenous Infusion BP (Hartmann's Solution for Injection) | 4 hours. |

When diluted in these solutions to give atracurium besylate concentrations of 0.5 mg/ml and above, the resultant solutions will be stable in daylight for the stated periods at temperatures of up to 30˚C.

*Use in children:* The dosage in children over the age of one month is similar to that in adults on a bodyweight basis.

*Use in neonates:* There are insufficient data to recommend a dose for use in neonates. However, this patient group is known to have increased sensitivity to non-depolarising muscle relaxants.

*Use in the elderly:* Tracrium may be used at standard dosage in elderly patients. It is recommended, however, that the initial dose be at the lower end of the range and that it be administered slowly.

*Use in patients with reduced renal and/or hepatic function:* Tracrium may be used at standard dosage at all levels of renal or hepatic function, including end stage failure.

*Use in patients with cardiovascular disease:* In patients with clinically significant cardiovascular disease, the initial dose of Tracrium should be administered over a period of 60 seconds.

*Use in intensive care unit (ICU) patients:* After an optional initial bolus dose of Tracrium of 0.3 to 0.6 mg/kg, Tracrium can be used to maintain neuromuscular block by administering a continous infusion at rates of between 11 and 13 microgram/kg/min (0.65 to 0.78 mg/kg/hr). There may be wide inter-patient variability in dosage requirements and these may increase or decrease with time. Infusion rates as low as 4.5 microgram/kg/min (0.27 mg/kg/hr) or as high as 29.5 microgram/kg/min (1.77 mg/kg/hr) are required in some patients.

The rate of spontaneous recovery from neuromuscular block after infusion of Tracrium in ICU patients is independent of the duration of administration.

Spontaneous recovery to a train-of-four ratio >0.75 (the ratio of the height of the fourth to the first twitch in a train-of-four) can be expected to occur in approximately 60 minutes. A range of 32 to 108 minutes has been observed in clinical trials.

*Monitoring:* In common with all neuromuscular blocking agents, monitoring of neuromuscular function is recommended during the use of Tracrium in order to individualise dosage requirements.

**Contra-indications, warnings, etc**
*Contra-indications:* Tracrium should not be administered to patients known to have an allergic hypersensitivity to the drug.

*Precautions:* In common with all the other neuromuscular blocking agents, Tracrium paralyses the respiratory muscles as well as other skeletal muscles but has no effect on consciousness. Tracrium should be administered only with adequate general anaesthesia and only by or under the close supervision of an experienced anaesthetist with adequate facilities for endotracheal intubation and artificial ventilation.

In common with other neuromuscular blocking agents, the potential for histamine release exists in susceptible patients during Tracrium administration. Caution should be exercised in administering Tracrium to patients with a history suggestive of an increased sensitivity to the effects of histamine.

Monitoring of serial creatinine phosphate (cpk) values should be considered in asthmatic patients receiving high dose corticosteroids and neuromuscular blocking agents in ICU.

Tracrium does not have significant vagal or ganglionic blocking properties in the recommended dosage range. Consequently, Tracrium has no clinically significant effects on heart rate in the recommended dosage range and it will not counteract the bradycardia produced by many anaesthetic agents or by vagal stimulation during surgery.

In common with other non-depolarising neuromuscular blocking agents, increased sensitivity to atracurium may be expected in patients with myasthenia gravis and other forms of neuromuscular disease.

As with other neuromuscular blocking agents severe acid-base and/or serum electrolyte abnormalities may increase or decrease the sensitivity of patients to atracrium.

As with other non-depolarising neuromuscular blockers hypophosphataemia may prolong recovery. Recovery may be hastened by correcting this condition.

Tracrium should be administered over a period of 60 seconds to patients who may be unusually sensitive to falls in arterial blood pressure, for example those who are hypovolaemic.

Tracrium is inactivated by high pH and so must not be mixed in the same syringe with thiopentone or any alkaline agent.

When a small vein is selected as the injection site, Tracrium should be flushed through the vein with physiological saline after injection. When other anaesthetic drugs are administered through the same indwelling needle or cannula as Tracrium it is important that each drug is flushed through with an adequate volume of physiological saline.

Studies in malignant hyperthermia in susceptible animals (swine), and clinical studies in patients susceptible to malignant hyperthermia indicate that Tracrium does not trigger this syndrome.

In common with other non-depolarising neuromuscular blocking agents, resistance may develop in patients suffering from burns. Such patients may require increased doses, dependent on the time elapsed since the burn injury and the extent of the burn.

One metabolite of atracurium, laudanosine, when administered alone to laboratory animals, has been associated with cerebral excitatory effects. Although seizures have been seen in ICU patients receiving atracurium, none have been considered attributable to laudanosine or atracurium even after weeks of prolonged infusion.

*Carcinogenicity:* Carcinogenicity studies have not been performed.

*Teratogenicity:* Animal studies have indicated that Tracrium has no significant effects on fetal development.

*Fertility:* Fertility studies have not been performed.

*Drug interactions:* The neuromuscular block produced by Tracrium may be increased by the concomitant use of inhalational anaesthetics such as halothane, isoflurane and enflurane.

In common with all non-depolarising neuromuscular blocking agents the magnitude and/or duration of a non-depolarising neuromuscular block may be increased as a result of interaction with: antibiotics, including the aminoglycosides, polymyxins, spectinomycin, tetracyclines, lincomycin and clindamycin; antiarrhythmic drugs, propranolol, calcium channel blockers, lignocaine, procainamide and quinidine; diuretics: frusemide and possibly mannitol, thiazide diuretics and acetazolamide; magnesium sulphate, ketamine, lithium salts, ganglion blocking agents, trimetaphan, hexamethonium.

Rarely, certain drugs may aggravate or unmask latent myasthenia gravis or actually induce a myasthenic syndrome; increased sensitivity to Tracrium would be consequent on such a development. Such drugs include various antibiotics, β-blockers (propranolol, oxprenolol), antiarrhythmic drugs (procainamide, quinidine), antirheumatic drugs (chloroquine, D-penicillamine), trimetaphan, chlorpromazine, steroids, phenytoin and lithium.

The onset of non-depolarising neuromuscular block is likely to be lengthened and the duration of block shortened in patients receiving chronic anticonvulsant therapy.

The administration of combinations of non-depolarising neuromuscular blocking agents in conjunction with Tracrium may produce a degree of neuromuscular blockage in excess of that which might be expected were an equipotent total dose of Tracrium administered. Any synergistic effect may vary between different drug combinations.

A depolarising muscle relaxant such as suxamethonium chloride should not be administered to prolong the neuromuscular blocking effects of non-depolarising blocking agents such as atracurium, as this may result in a prolonged and complex block which can be difficult to reverse with anticholinesterase drugs.

*Side- and adverse effects:* Associated with the use of Tracrium there have been reports of skin flushing, and mild transient hypotension or bronchospasm, which have been attributed to histamine release. Very rarely, severe anaphylactoid reactions have been reported in patients receiving Tracrium in conjunction with one or more anaesthetic agents.

There have been rare reports of seizures in ICU patients who have been receiving atracurium concurrently with several other agents. These patients usually had one or more medical conditions predisposing to seizures (e.g. cranial trauma, cerebral oedema, viral encephalitis, hypoxic encephalopathy, uraemia). In clinical trials, there appears to be no correlation between plasma laudanosine concentration and the occurrence of seizures.

*Use in pregnancy and lactation:* In common with all neuromuscular blocking agents, Tracrium should be used during pregnancy only if the potential benefit to the mother outweighs any potential risk to the foetus.

Tracrium is suitable for maintenance of muscle relaxation during Caesarean section as it does not cross the placenta in clinically significant amounts following recommended doses.

It is not known whether Tracrium is excreted in human milk.

*Toxicity and treatment of overdosage: Signs:* Prolonged muscle paralysis and its consequences are the main signs of overdosage.

*Treatment:* It is essential to maintain a patent airway together with assisted positive pressure ventilation until spontaneous respiration is adequate. Full sedation will be required since consciousness is not impaired. Recovery may be hastened by the administration of anticholinesterase agents accompanied by atropine or glycopyrrolate, once evidence of spontaneous recovery is present.

**Pharmaceutical precautions** Store at 2°to 8°C. Protect from light. Do not freeze. Any unused Tracrium from opened ampoules should be discarded.

Short periods at temperatures up to 30°C are permissible but ONLY to allow transportation or temporary storage outside of a cold store. It is estimated that an 8% loss of potency would occur if Tracrium Injection was stored at 30°C for one month.

**Legal category** POM.

**Package quantities** Box of 5×2.5 ampoules (each ampoule containing 25 mg atracurium besylate).

Box of 5×5 ml ampoules (each ampoule containing 50 mg atracurium besylate).

Box of 2×25 ml ampoules (each containing 250 mg atracurium besylate).

**Further information** Tracrium is inactivated by Hofmann elimination, a non-enzymatic process which occurs at physiological pH and temperature, and by ester hydrolysis catalysed by non-specific esterases.

The termination of the neuromuscular blocking action of Tracrium is not dependent on its hepatic or renal metabolism or excretion. Its duration of action, therefore, is unlikely to be affected by impaired renal, hepatic or circulatory function.

Tests with plasma from patients with low levels of pseudochlolinesterase show that the inactivation of Tracrium proceeds unaffected.

Tracrium has no direct effect on intra-ocular pressure, and is therefore suitable for use in ophthalmic surgery.

Variations in the blood pH and body temperature of the patient within the physiological range will not significantly alter the duration of action of Tracrium.

Haemofiltration and haemodiafiltration have a minimal effect on plasma levels of atracurium and its metabolites, including laudanosine. The effects of haemodialysis and haemoperfusion on plasma levels of atracurium and its metabolites are unknown.

**Product licence number** 0003/0166.

## TRIMOVATE* CREAM

**Qualitative and quantitative composition** Trimovate Cream is a yellow water-miscible cream containing clobetasone butyrate 0.05% w/w, oxytetracycline 3.0% w/w as calcium oxytetracycline and nystatin 100,000 units per gram.

**Pharmaceutical form** Cream for topical administration.

**Clinical particulars**
*Therapeutic indications:* Clobetasone butyrate is a topically active corticosteroid which provides an exceptional combination of activity and safety. Topical formulations have been shown to be more effective in the treatment of eczemas than 1% hydrocortisone, yet to have little effect on hypothalamic-pituitary-adrenal function.

The combination of the topically active antibiotics, nystatin and oxytetracycline, provides a broad spectrum of antibacterial and anticandidal activity against many of the organisms associated with infected dermatoses. Trimovate is indicated for the treatment and management of steroid responsive dermatoses where candidal or bacterial infection is present, suspected or likely to occur and the use of a more potent topical corticosteroid is not required. These include infected eczemas, intertrigo, napkin rash, anogenital pruritus and seborrhoeic dermatitis.

*Posology and method of administration:* Apply to the affected area up to four times a day.

Suitable for treating infants, children and adults.

*Contra-indications:* Primary cutaneous infections caused by viruses (e.g. herpes simplex, chickenpox) fungi and bacteria. Secondary infections due to dermatophytes, Pseudomonas or Proteus species.

Hypersensitivity to the preparation.

*Special warnings and special precautions for use:* Although generally regarded as safe, even for long term administration in adults, there is a potential for overdosage, and in children this may result in adrenal suppression. Extreme caution is required in dermatoses in such patients and treatment should not normally exceed seven days. In infants, the napkin may act as an occlusive dressing, and increase absorption.

If infection persists, systemic chemotherapy is likely to be required. Any spread of infection requires withdrawal of topical corticosteroid therapy. Bacterial infection is encouraged by the warm, moist conditions induced by occlusive dressings, and the skin should be cleansed before a fresh dressing is applied. Do not continue for more than seven days in the absence of clinical improvement, since occult extension of infection may occur due to the masking effect of the steroid.

As with all corticosteroids, prolonged application to the face is undesirable. If applied to the eyelids, care is needed to ensure that the preparation does not enter the eye, as glaucoma might result.

Trimovate may cause slight staining of hair, skin or fabric, but this can be removed by washing. The application may be covered with a non-occlusive dressing to protect clothing.

Extended or recurrent application may increase the risk of contact sensitisation.

Products which contain antimicrobial agents should not be diluted.

*Interaction with other medicaments and other forms of interaction:* None reported.

*Pregnancy and lactation:* There is inadequate evidence of safety in human pregnancy. Topical administration of corticosteroids to pregnant animals can cause abnormalities of fetal development including cleft palate and intra-uterine growth retardation. There may therefore be a very small risk of such effects in the human fetus.

*Effects on ability to drive and use machines:* None stated.

*Undesirable effects:* In the unlikely event of signs of hypersensitivity appearing, application should be stopped immediately.

If large areas of the body were to be treated with Trimovate, it is possible that some patients would absorb sufficient steroid to cause transient adrenal suppression despite the low degree of systemic activity associated with clobetasone butyrate.

Local atrophic changes could possibly occur in situations where moisture increases absorption of clobetasone butyrate, but only after prolonged use.

There are reports of pigmentation changes and hypertrichosis with topical steroids. Exacerbation of symptoms may occur with extensive use.

*Overdose:* Acute overdosage is very unlikely to occur, however, in the case of chronic overdosage or misuse the features of hypercorticism may appear and in this situation topical steroids should be discontinued.

### Pharmacological properties

*Pharmacodynamic properties:* Clobetasone butyrate is a topically active corticosteroid.

Clobetasone butyrate is less potent than other available corticosteroid preparations and has been shown not to suppress the hypothalamic-pituitary-adrenal axis in patients treated for psoriasis or eczema. Pharmacological studies in man and animals have shown that clobetasone butyrate has a relatively high level of topical activity accompanied by a low level of systemic activity.

The use of nystatin in the local treatment of candidal infections of the skin and of the tetracyclines in localised bacterial infections is well known. Nystatin is included in Trimovate at the standard concentration recommended by the British Pharmaceutical codex for the topical preparation nystatin ointment (100,000 units/g), and oxytetracycline calcium is included at a concentration to give approximately the same level of activity as recommended for Oxytetracycline Ointment BPC (3.0% w/w).

The principle action of the preparation is based on the anti-inflammatory activity of the corticosteroid. The broad spectrum antibacterial and anti-candidal activity provided by the combination of oxytetracycline and nystatin allow this effect to be utilised in the treatment of conditions which are or are likely to become infected.

*Pharmacokinetic properties:* Trimovate has been shown to have a satisfactory pharmacokinetic profile by many years of successful clinical experience.

*Preclinical safety data:* No additional data of relevance.

### Pharmaceutical particulars

*List of excipients:* Titanium dioxide, glyceryl monostearate, cetostearyl alcohol, white soft paraffin, polyoxyl 40 stearate, dimethicone 20, glycerol, chlorocresol, sodium metabisulphite, sodium acid phosphate, disodium hydrogen phosphate anhydrous, purified water.

*Incompatibilities:* None reported.

*Shelf-life:* 18 months.

*Special precautions for storage:* Store below 25°C.

*Nature and contents of container:* Collapsible latex-banded aluminium tube, internally coated with epoxy resin-based lacquer with polypropylene cap.

*Instructions for use/handling:* None stated.

**Marketing authorisation number** 10949/0040

**Date of approval/revision of SPC** March 1996

**Legal category** POM.

## ULTIVA* FOR INJECTION ▼

**Qualitative and quantitative composition** Ultiva is a sterile, endotoxin-free, preservative-free, white to off white, lyophilised powder, to be reconstituted before use.

When reconstituted as directed, solutions of Ultiva are clear and colourless and contain 1 mg/ml of remifentanil base as remifentanil hydrochloride.

Ultiva for injection is available as glass vials containing 1 mg, 2 mg or 5 mg of remifentanil base.

**Pharmaceutical form** Lyophilised powder for reconstitution for intravenous administration.

### Clinical particulars

*Therapeutic indications:* Ultiva is indicated as an analgesic agent for use during induction and/or maintenance of general anaesthesia under close supervision.

*Posology and method of administration:* Ultiva should be administered only in a setting fully equipped for the monitoring and support of respiratory and cardio-vascular function, and by persons specifically trained in the use of anaesthetic drugs and the recognition and management of the expected adverse effects of potent opioids, including respiratory and cardiac resuscitation. Such training must include the establishment and maintenance of a patent airway and assisted ventilation.

Ultiva is for intravenous use only and must not be administered by epidural or intrathecal injection (see *Contra-indications*).

Ultiva is stable for 24 hours at room temperature after reconstitution and further dilution to concentrations of 20 to 250 mcg/ml with one of the following i.v. fluids listed below: 50 mcg/ml is the recommended dilution for general anaesthesia.

Sterilised Water for Injections
5% Dextrose Injection
5% Dextrose and 0.9% Sodium Chloride Injection
0.9% Sodium Chloride Injection
0.45% Sodium Chloride Injection

(See *Instructions for use/handling* for additional information, including tables to help titrate Ultiva to the patient's anaesthetic needs.)

The administration of Ultiva must be individualised based on the patient's response.

The table below summarises the starting infusion rates and dose range.

At the doses recommended below, remifentanil significantly reduces the amount of hypnotic agent required to maintain anaesthesia. Therefore, isoflurane and propofol should be administered as recommended above to avoid excessive depth of anaesthesia (see *Concomitant medication*).

*Induction of anaesthesia:* Ultiva should be administered with a hypnotic agent, such as propofol, thiopental, or isoflurane, for the induction of anaesthesia. Administering Ultiva after a hypnotic agent will reduce the incidence of muscle rigidity. Ultiva can be administered at an infusion rate of 0.5 to 1 mcg/kg/min, with or without an initial bolus infusion of 1 mcg/kg given over not less than 30 seconds. If endotracheal intubation is to occur more than 8 to 10 minutes after the start of the infusion of Ultiva, then a bolus infusion is not necessary.

*Maintenance of anaesthesia:* After endotracheal intubation, the infusion rate of Ultiva should be decreased, according to anaesthetic technique, as indicated in the table below. Due to the fast onset and short duration of action of Ultiva, the rate of administration during anaesthesia can be titrated upward in 25% to 100% increments or downward in 25% to 50% decrements, every 2 to 5 minutes to attain the desired level of μ-opioid response. In response to light anaesthesia, supplemental bolus infusions may be administered every 2 to 5 minutes.

*Guidelines for discontinuation:* Due to the very rapid offset of action of Ultiva no residual opioid activity will be present within 5 to 10 minutes after discontinuation. For those patients undergoing surgical procedures where post-operative pain is anticipated, analgesics should be administered prior to discontinuation of Ultiva. Sufficient time must be allowed to reach the maximum effect of the longer acting analgesic. The choice of analgesic should be appropriate for the patient's surgical procedure and the level of post-operative care.

Care should be taken to avoid inadvertent administration of Ultiva remaining in i.v. lines and cannulae (see *Special warnings and precautions for use*).

*Concomitant medication:* Ultiva decreases the amounts or doses of inhaled anaesthetics, hypnotics and benzodiazepines required for anaesthesia (see *Special warnings and precautions for use* and *Interaction with other medicaments and other forms of interaction*).

Doses of the following agents used in anaesthesia: isoflurane, thiopentone, propofol and temazepam have been reduced by up to 75% when used concurrently with remifentanil.

*Spontaneous ventilation anaesthesia:* In spontaneous ventilation anaesthesia respiratory depression is likely to occur. Special care is needed to adjust the dose to the patient and ventilatory support may be required. The recommended starting dose is 0.04 mcg/kg/min with titration to effect. A range of infusion rates from 0.025 to 0.1 mcg/kg/min has been studied. Bolus doses are not recommended.

*Children (2–12 years of age):* There are no data available on use in children under 2 years of age.

The pharmacokinetics of remifentanil in children 2 to 12 years of age are similar to those seen in adults after correction for body weight differences.

Clinical experience in a limited number of children 2 to 12 years of age has shown that doses required are similar to those recommended for adults on a weight-related basis. In the studies performed, remifentanil was only given after the children had been induced with an inhalation agent, intubated and had received an anti-cholinergic drug.

*Elderly (over 65 years of age):* Caution should be exercised in the administration of Ultiva in this population. The initial starting dose of Ultiva administered to patients over 65 should be half the recommended adult dose and then titrated to individual patient need as an increased sensitivity to the pharmacodynamic effects of remifentanil has been seen in this patient population.

*ASA III/IV patients:* As the haemodynamic effects of potent opioids can be expected to be more pronounced in ASA III/IV patients, caution should be exercised in the administration of Ultiva in this population. Initial dosage reduction and subsequent titration to effect is therefore recommended.

*Obese patients:* It is recommended that for obese patients the dosage of Ultiva should be reduced and based upon ideal bodyweight as the clearance and volume of distribution of remifentanil are better correlated with ideal bodyweight than actual bodyweight.

*Renal impairment:* No dosage adjustment, relative to that used in healthy adults, is necessary as the pharmacokinetic profile of remifentanil is unchanged in this patient population.

*Hepatic impairment:* No adjustment of the initial dose, relative to that used in healthy adults, is necessary as the pharmacokinetic profile of remifentanil is unchanged in this patient population. However, patients with severe hepatic impairment may be slightly more sensitive to the respiratory depressant effects of remifentanil. These patients should be closely monitored and the dose of Ultiva titrated to individual patient need.

*Long-term use in the Intensive Care Unit (ICU):* No data are available on the long-term (longer than 24 hours) use of Ultiva in ICU patients.

*Contra-indications:* As glycine is present in the formulation Ultiva is contra-indicated for epidural and intrathecal use.

Ultiva is contra-indicated in patients with known hypersensitivity to any component of the preparation and other fentanyl analogues.

Ultiva is contra-indicated for use as the sole agent for induction of anaesthesia.

*Special warnings and precautions for use:* Ultiva should be administered only in a setting fully equipped for the monitoring and support of respiratory and cardiovascular function, and by persons specifically trained in the use of anaesthetic drugs and the recognition and management of the expected adverse effects of potent opioids, including respiratory and cardiac resuscitation. Such training must include the establishment and maintenance of a patent airway and assisted ventilation.

*Inadvertent administration:* A sufficient amount of Ultiva may be present in the dead space of the i.v. line and/or cannula to cause respiratory depression, apnoea and/or muscle rigidity if the line is flushed with i.v. fluids or other drugs. This may be avoided by administering Ultiva into a fast flowing i.v. line or via a dedicated i.v. line which is removed when Ultiva is discontinued.

*Muscle rigidity – prevention and management:* At the doses recommended muscle rigidity may occur. As with other opioids, the incidence of muscle rigidity is related to the dose and rate of administration. Therefore, bolus infusions should be administered over not less than 30 seconds.

Muscle rigidity induced by remifentanil must be treated in the context of the patient's clinical condition with appropriate supporting measures including ventilatory support. Excessive muscle rigidity occurring

### Dosing guidelines for Ultiva-based anaesthesia

| Indication | Bolus infusion (mcg/kg) | Continuous infusion (mcg/kg/min) | |
| --- | --- | --- | --- |
| | | Starting rate | Range |
| Induction of anaesthesia | 1 (give over not less than 30 seconds)† | 0.5 to 1 | — |
| Maintenance of anaesthesia in ventilated patients | | | |
| • Nitrous oxide (66%) | 0.5 to 1 | 0.4 | 0.1 to 2 |
| • Isoflurane (starting dose 0.5 MAC) | 0.5 to 1 | 0.25 | 0.05 to 2 |
| • Propofol (starting dose 100 mcg/kg/min) | 0.5 to 1 | 0.25 | 0.05 to 2 |

† When given by bolus infusion at induction Ultiva should be administered over not less than 30 seconds.

during the induction of anaesthesia should be treated by the administration of a neuromuscular blocking agent and/or additional hypnotic agents. Muscle rigidity seen during the use of remifentanil as an analgesic may be treated by stopping or decreasing the rate of administration of remifentanil. Resolution of muscle rigidity after discontinuing the infusion of remifentanil occurs within minutes.

*Respiratory depression – management:* As with all potent opioids, profound analgesia is accompanied by marked respiratory depression. Therefore, remifentanil should only be used in areas where facilities for monitoring and dealing with respiratory depression are available. The appearance of respiratory depression should be managed appropriately, including decreasing the rate of infusion by 50%, or a temporary discontinuation of the infusion. Unlike other fentanyl analogues, remifentanil has not been shown to cause recurrent respiratory depression even after prolonged administration. However, as many factors may affect post-operative recovery it is important to ensure that full consciousness and adequate spontaneous ventilation are achieved before the patient is discharged from the recovery area.

*Cardiovascular effects:* Hypotension and bradycardia may be managed by reducing the rate of infusion of Ultiva or the dose of concurrent anaesthetics or by using i.v. fluids, vasopressor or anticholinergic agents as appropriate.

Debilitated, hypovolaemic, and elderly patients may be more sensitive to the cardiovascular effects of remifentanil.

*Rapid offset of action:* Due to the very rapid offset of action of Ultiva, no residual opioid activity will be present within 5–10 minutes after the discontinuation of Ultiva. For those patients undergoing surgical procedures where post-operative pain is anticipated, analgesics should be administered prior to discontinuation of Ultiva. Sufficient time must be allowed to reach the maximum effect of the longer acting analgesic. The choice of analgesic should be appropriate for the patient's surgical procedure and the level of post-operative care.

*Drug abuse:* As with other opioids remifentanil may produce dependency.

*Interaction with other medicaments and other forms of interaction:* Remifentanil is not metabolised by plasmacholinesterase, therefore, interactions with drugs metabolised by this enzyme are not anticipated.

As with other opioids remifentanil decreases the amounts or doses of inhaled and i.v. anaesthetics, and benzodiazepines required for anaesthesia (see *Posology and method of administration*).

*Pregnancy and lactation:* There are no adequate and well-controlled studies in pregnant women. Ultiva should be used during pregnancy only if the potential benefit justifies the potential risk to the fetus.

It is not known whether remifentanil is excreted in human milk. However, because fentanyl analogues are excreted in human milk and remifentanil-related material was found in rat milk after dosing with remifentanil, caution should be exercised when remifentanil is administered to a nursing mother.

*For a summary of the reproductive toxicity study findings please refer to Preclinical safety data.*

*Labour and delivery:* The safety profile of remifentanil during labour or delivery has not been demonstrated.

*Effects on the ability to drive and use machines:* If an early discharge is envisaged, following treatment using anaesthetic agents, patients should be advised not to drive or operate machinery.

*Undesirable effects:* The most common adverse events associated with remifentanil are direct extensions of μ-opioid agonist pharmacology. These are acute respiratory depression, bradycardia, hypotension and/or skeletal muscle rigidity. These adverse events resolve within minutes of discontinuing or decreasing the rate of remifentanil administration.

Post-operative shivering, nausea and vomiting have also been reported.

*Overdose:* As with all potent opioid analgesics, overdose would be manifested by an extension of the pharmacologically predictable actions of remifentanil. Due to the very short duration of action of Ultiva, potential for deleterious effects due to overdose are limited to the immediate time period following drug administration. Response to discontinuation of the drug is rapid, with return to baseline within ten minutes.

In the event of overdose, or suspected overdose, take the following actions: discontinue administration of Ultiva; maintain a patent airway; initiate assisted or controlled ventilation with oxygen; maintain adequate cardiovascular function. If depressed respiration is associated with muscle rigidity, a neuromuscular blocking agent may be required to facilitate assisted or controlled respiration. Intravenous fluids and vasopressor for the treatment of hypotension and other supportive measures may be employed.

Intravenous administration of an opioid antagonist such as naloxone may be given as a specific antidote in addition to ventilatory support to manage severe respiratory depression. The duration of respiratory depression following overdose with Ultiva is unlikely to exceed the duration of action of the opioid antagonist.

**Pharmacological properties**

*Pharmacodynamic properties:* Remifentanil is a selective μ-opioid agonist with a rapid onset and very short duration of action. The μ-opioid activity, of remifentanil, is antagonised by narcotic antagonists, such as naloxone.

Assays of histamine in patients and normal volunteers have shown no elevation in histamine levels after administration of remifentanil in bolus doses up to 30 mcg/kg.

*Pharmacokinetic properties:* Following administration of the recommended doses of remifentanil, the effective biological half-life is 3–10 minutes. The average clearance of remifentanil in young healthy adults is 40 ml/min/kg, the central volume of distribution is 100 ml/kg and the steady-state volume of distribution is 350 ml/kg. Blood concentrations of remifentanil are proportional to the dose administered throughout the recommended dose range. For every 0.1 mcg/kg/min increase in infusion rate, the blood concentration of remifentanil will rise 2.5 ng/ml. Remifentanil is approximately 70% bound to plasma proteins.

*Metabolism:* Remifentanil is an esterase metabolised opioid that is susceptible to metabolism by non-specific blood and tissue esterases. The metabolism of remifentanil results in the formation of an essentially inactive carboxylic acid metabolite (1/4600th as potent as remifentanil). The half-life of the metabolite in healthy adults is 2 hours. Approximately 95% of remifentanil is recovered in the urine as the carboxylic acid metabolite. Remifentanil is not a substrate for plasma cholinesterase.

*Renal impairment:* The pharmacokinetics of remifentanil are not changed in patients with severe renal impairment (creatinine clearance<10 ml/minute). In

### Table 1: Ultiva for Injection Infusion Rates (ml/kg/h)

| Drug Delivery Rate (mcg/kg/min) | Infusion Delivery Rate (ml/kg/h) for Solution Concentrations of | | |
|---|---|---|---|
| | 25 mcg/ml 1 mg/40 ml | 50 mcg/ml 1 mg/20 ml | 250 mcg/ml 10 mg/40 ml |
| 0.0125 | 0.03 | 0.015 | not recommended |
| 0.025 | 0.06 | 0.03 | not recommended |
| 0.05 | 0.12 | 0.06 | 0.012 |
| 0.075 | 0.18 | 0.09 | 0.018 |
| 0.1 | 0.24 | 0.12 | 0.024 |
| 0.15 | 0.36 | 0.18 | 0.036 |
| 0.2 | 0.48 | 0.24 | 0.048 |
| 0.25 | 0.6 | 0.3 | 0.06 |
| 0.5 | 1.2 | 0.6 | 0.12 |
| 0.75 | 1.8 | 0.9 | 0.18 |
| 1.0 | 2.4 | 1.2 | 0.24 |
| 1.25 | 3.0 | 1.5 | 0.3 |
| 1.5 | 3.6 | 1.8 | 0.36 |
| 1.75 | 4.2 | 2.1 | 0.42 |
| 2.0 | 4.8 | 2.4 | 0.48 |

### Table 2: Ultiva for Injection Infusion Rates (ml/h) for a 25 mcg/ml Solution

| Infusion Rate (mcg/kg/min) | Patient Weight (kg) | | | | | | | |
|---|---|---|---|---|---|---|---|---|
| | 30 | 40 | 50 | 60 | 70 | 80 | 90 | 100 |
| 0.0125 | 0.9 | 1.2 | 1.5 | 1.8 | 2.1 | 2.4 | 2.7 | 3.0 |
| 0.025 | 1.8 | 2.4 | 3.0 | 3.6 | 4.2 | 4.8 | 5.4 | 6.0 |
| 0.05 | 3.6 | 4.8 | 6.0 | 7.2 | 8.4 | 9.6 | 10.8 | 12.0 |
| 0.075 | 5.4 | 7.2 | 9.0 | 10.8 | 12.6 | 14.4 | 16.2 | 18.0 |
| 0.1 | 7.2 | 9.6 | 12.0 | 14.4 | 16.8 | 19.2 | 21.6 | 24.0 |
| 0.15 | 10.8 | 14.4 | 18.0 | 21.6 | 25.2 | 28.8 | 32.4 | 36.0 |
| 0.2 | 14.4 | 19.2 | 24.0 | 28.8 | 33.6 | 38.4 | 43.2 | 48.0 |

### Table 3: Ultiva for Injection Infusion Rates (ml/h) for a 50 mcg/ml Solution

| Infusion Rate (mcg/kg/min) | Patient Weight (kg) | | | | | | | |
|---|---|---|---|---|---|---|---|---|
| | 30 | 40 | 50 | 60 | 70 | 80 | 90 | 100 |
| 0.025 | 0.9 | 1.2 | 1.5 | 1.8 | 2.1 | 2.4 | 2.7 | 3.0 |
| 0.05 | 1.8 | 2.4 | 3.0 | 3.6 | 4.2 | 4.8 | 5.4 | 6.0 |
| 0.075 | 2.7 | 3.6 | 4.5 | 5.4 | 6.3 | 7.2 | 8.1 | 9.0 |
| 0.1 | 3.6 | 4.8 | 6.0 | 7.2 | 8.4 | 9.6 | 10.8 | 12.0 |
| 0.15 | 5.4 | 7.2 | 9.0 | 10.8 | 12.6 | 14.4 | 16.2 | 18.0 |
| 0.2 | 7.2 | 9.6 | 12.0 | 14.4 | 16.8 | 19.2 | 21.6 | 24.0 |
| 0.25 | 9.0 | 12.0 | 15.0 | 18.0 | 21.0 | 24.0 | 27.0 | 30.0 |
| 0.5 | 18.0 | 24.0 | 30.0 | 36.0 | 42.0 | 48.0 | 54.0 | 60.0 |
| 0.75 | 27.0 | 36.0 | 45.0 | 54.0 | 63.0 | 72.0 | 81.0 | 90.0 |
| 1.0 | 36.0 | 48.0 | 60.0 | 72.0 | 84.0 | 96.0 | 108.0 | 120.0 |
| 1.25 | 45.0 | 60.0 | 75.0 | 90.0 | 105.0 | 120.0 | 135.0 | 150.0 |
| 1.5 | 54.0 | 72.0 | 90.0 | 108.0 | 126.0 | 144.0 | 162.0 | 180.0 |
| 1.75 | 63.0 | 84.0 | 105.0 | 126.0 | 147.0 | 168.0 | 189.0 | 210.0 |
| 2.0 | 72.0 | 96.0 | 120.0 | 144.0 | 168.0 | 192.0 | 216.0 | 240.0 |

### Table 4: Ultiva for Injection Infusion Rates (ml/h) for a 250 mcg/ml Solution

| Infusion Rate (mcg/kg/min) | Patient Weight (kg) | | | | | | | |
|---|---|---|---|---|---|---|---|---|
| | 30 | 40 | 50 | 60 | 70 | 80 | 90 | 100 |
| 0.1 | 0.72 | 0.96 | 1.20 | 1.44 | 1.68 | 1.92 | 2.16 | 2.40 |
| 0.15 | 1.08 | 1.44 | 1.80 | 2.16 | 2.52 | 2.88 | 3.24 | 3.60 |
| 0.2 | 1.44 | 1.92 | 2.40 | 2.88 | 3.36 | 3.84 | 4.32 | 4.80 |
| 0.25 | 1.80 | 2.40 | 3.00 | 3.60 | 4.20 | 4.80 | 5.40 | 6.00 |
| 0.5 | 3.60 | 4.80 | 6.00 | 7.20 | 8.40 | 9.60 | 10.80 | 12.00 |
| 0.75 | 5.40 | 7.20 | 9.00 | 10.80 | 12.60 | 14.40 | 16.20 | 18.00 |
| 1.0 | 7.20 | 9.60 | 12.00 | 14.40 | 16.80 | 19.20 | 21.60 | 24.00 |
| 1.25 | 9.00 | 12.00 | 15.00 | 18.00 | 21.00 | 24.00 | 27.00 | 30.00 |
| 1.5 | 10.80 | 14.40 | 18.00 | 21.60 | 25.20 | 28.80 | 32.40 | 36.00 |
| 1.75 | 12.60 | 16.80 | 21.00 | 25.20 | 29.40 | 33.60 | 37.80 | 42.00 |
| 2.0 | 14.40 | 19.20 | 24.00 | 28.80 | 33.60 | 38.40 | 43.20 | 48.00 |

anephric patients, the half-life of the carboxylic acid metabolite increases to approximately 30 hours. However, in light of the estimated potency ratio of the metabolite compared with the parent molecule (1:4,600), pharmacokinetic simulations indicate that the carboxylic acid metabolite will not accumulate to clinically active concentrations after remifentanil infusions of up to 2 mcg/kg/min for up to 12 hours.

*Hepatic impairment:* The pharmacokinetics of remifentanil are not changed in patients with severe hepatic impairment awaiting liver transplant, or during the anhepatic phase of liver transplant surgery. Patients with severe hepatic impairment may be slightly more sensitive to the respiratory depressant effects of remifentanil. These patients should be closely monitored and the dose of remifentanil should be titrated to the individual patient need.

*Children:* The pharmacokinetics of remifentanil in children 2–12 years of age are similar to those seen in adults after correcting for differences in body weight.

*Elderly:* The clearance of remifentanil is slightly reduced (approximately 25%) in elderly patients (>65 years) compared to young patients. The pharmacodynamic activity of remifentanil increases with increasing age. Elderly patients have a remifentanil EC50 for formation of delta waves on the electroencephalogram (EEG) that is 50% lower than young patients; therefore, the initial dose of remifentanil should be reduced by 50% in elderly patients and then carefully titrated to meet the individual patient need.

*Preclinical safety data:* Intrathecal administration of the glycine formulation without remifentanil to dogs caused agitation, pain and hind limb dysfunction and inco-ordination. These effects are believed to be secondary to the glycine excipient. Glycine is a commonly used excipient in intravenous products and this finding has no relevance for intravenous administration of Ultiva.

*Reproductive toxicity studies:* Remifentanil has been shown to reduce fertility in male rats when administered daily by intravenous injection for at least 70 days at a dose of 0.5 mg/kg, or approximately 250 times the maximum recommended human bolus dose of 2 mcg/kg. The fertility of female rats was not affected at doses up to 1 mg/kg when administered for at least 15 days prior to mating. No teratogenic effects have been observed with remifentanil at doses up to 5 mg/kg in rats and 0.8 mg/kg in rabbits. Administration of remifentanil to rats throughout late gestation and lactation at doses up to 5 mg/kg i.v. had no significant effect on the survival, development, or reproductive performance of the $F_1$ generation.

*Genotoxicity:* Remifentanil was devoid of genotoxic activity in bacteria and in rat liver or mouse bone marrow cells *in vivo.* However, a positive response was seen *in vitro* in different mammalian cell systems in the presence of a metabolic activation system. This activity was seen only at concentrations more than three orders of magnitude higher than therapeutic blood levels.

**Pharmaceutical particulars**

*List of excipients:* Glycine PhEur; Hydrochloric acid PhEur.

*Incompatibilities:* Ultiva should only be admixed with those infusion solutions recommended (see *Instructions for use/handling*).

It should not be admixed with Lactated Ringer's Injection or Lactated Ringer's and 5% Dextrose Injection.

Ultiva should not be mixed with propofol in the same intravenous admixture solution.

Administration of Ultiva into the same intravenous line with blood/serum/plasma is not recommended. Non-specific esterase in blood products may lead to the hydrolysis of remifentanil to its inactive metabolite.

Ultiva should not be mixed with other therapeutic agents prior to administration.

*Shelf life:* Two years.

*Special precautions for storage:* Store at or below 25°C.

The reconstituted solution of Ultiva is chemically and physically stable for 24 hours at room temperature. However, Ultiva does not contain an antimicrobial preservative and thus care must be taken to assure the sterility of prepared solutions. Reconstituted product should be used promptly, and any unused material discarded.

*Nature and contents of container:* Ultiva Injection for intravenous use is available as:

1 mg Remifentanil lyophilised powder in 3 ml vials in cartons of 5.

2 mg Remifentanil lyophilised powder in 5 ml vials in cartons of 5.

5 mg Remifentanil lyophilised powder in 10 ml vials in cartons of 5.

*Instructions for use/handling:* Ultiva is stable for 24 hours at room temperature after reconstitution and further dilution to concentrations of 20 to 250 mcg/ml

with one of the following i.v. fluids listed below: 50 mcg/ml is the recommended dilution for general anaesthesia.

Sterilised Water for Injections
5% Dextrose Injection
5% Dextrose and 0.9% Sodium Chloride Injection
0.9% Sodium Chloride Injection
0.45% Sodium Chloride Injection

Ultiva has been shown to be compatible with the following intravenous fluids when administered into a running i.v. catheter:

Lactated Ringer's Injection
Lactated Ringer's and 5% Dextrose Injection

Ultiva has been shown to be compatible with propofol when administered into a running i.v. catheter.

The tables on the previous page give guidelines for infusion rates of Ultiva.

**Marketing authorisation numbers**
Ultiva for Injection 1 mg    14213/0002
Ultiva for Injection 2 mg    14213/0003
Ultiva for Injection 5 mg    14213/0004

**Date of approval/revision of SPC**   October 1996

**Legal category**  POM

## VASOXINE* INJECTION

**Qualitative and quantitative composition**   Methoxamine Hydrochloride BP 2% w/v.

**Pharmaceutical form**   Injection.

**Clinical particulars**

*Therapeutic indications:* Methoxamine hydrochloride is a direct stimulant of α-adrenergic receptors and is indicated for counteraction of systemic hypotension. The most common clinical application for methoxamine is the prevention or correction of hypotension associated with the use of spinal anaesthetics or antihypertensive drugs.

Methoxamine hydrochloride can be used to increase blood pressure during cyclopropane anaesthesia for it does not increase the irritability of the cyclopropane-sensitised heart.

*Posology and method of administration:*

*Adults:* The usual intravenous dose for emergencies is 3–5 mg (0.15–0.25 ml) Vasoxine intravenously injected slowly (e.g. at a rate of 1 mg methoxamine hydrochloride/min). Intravenous doses may be supplemented by intramuscular injection of 10–15 mg (0.5–0.75 ml Vasoxine Injection), to provide a more prolonged effect.

For use shortly before or during administration of spinal anaesthesia, a dose of methoxamine hydrochloride of 10–20 mg (0.5–1.0 ml Vasoxine Injection) intramuscularly may be given to prevent or correct systemic hypotension. For a low spinal block, a 10 mg dose of methoxamine hydrochloride may be adequate. For a high spinal block with extensive sympathetic blockade, the tendency for blood pressure to fall is greater and so a dose of 15–20 mg methoxamine hydrochloride may be required. Repeated doses may be necessary, but about 15 minutes should be allowed for the previous intramuscular dose to act.

For cases of only moderate hypotension, 5–10 mg methoxamine hydrochloride (0.25–0.5 ml Vasoxine Injection) intramuscularly may be adequate.

*Children up to 12 years of age:* The efficacy of methoxamine in children has not been established.

However, if required, a dose of 40–70 mcg Vasoxine Injection/kg bodyweight administered intravenously or 70–280 mcg Vasoxine Injection/kg bodyweight by intramuscular injection would be considered appropriate.

*Use in the elderly:* No specific information is available on the use of methoxamine in the elderly. However, see precautions and warning and adverse reactions.

*Route of administration:* Intravenous or intramuscular.

*Contra-indications:*   Known hypersensitivity to methoxamine. Vasoxine is contra-indicated in cases of pre-existent severe hypertension.

*Special warnings and precautions for use:* Methoxamine should not be administered unless facilities are available to make frequent measurements of systemic blood pressure.

The effect of increased arterial pressure on a patient with pre-existing vascular disease or impairment of myocardial function should be considered before administering Vasoxine.

Vasoxine Injection should be used with care in hyperthyroidism for there may be a marked pressor response.

When administered intravenously, large veins are preferred to prevent extravasation of Vasoxine Injection. Extravasation may cause necrosis and sloughing

of surrounding tissue. The infusion site should be monitored closely for free flow.

Vasoxine should not be used in combination with local anaesthetics to prolong their action at local sites.

Use Vasoxine Injection with care in patients with poor left ventricular function as the increase in peripheral resistance which is brought about by methoxamine may cause or exacerbate cardiac failure.

The use of Vasoxine Injection is not a substitute for replacement of lost intravascular fluid and care should be taken to ensure adequate provision of intravenous fluid, plasma or blood before or during recourse to Vasoxine Injection.

There are no data available on whether or not methoxamine has a carcinogenic or mutagenic potential, or whether it may affect fertility.

*Interaction with other medicaments and other forms of interaction:* Concomitant use of Vasoxine with sympathomimetic agents, such as decongestants, some appetite suppressants and amphetamine-like psychostimulants may cause an exaggerated response to methoxamine.

The systemic pressor effect of methoxamine can be markedly potentiated in patients who are taking or who have taken monoamine oxidase inhibitors in the preceding two weeks. This effect may also occur in patients who are taking tricyclic antidepressants, ergot alkaloids, some oxytoxic drugs, β-adrenergic blocking agents, guanethidine or reserpine.

*Pregnancy and lactation:* It is reported that vasopressors with strong α-adrenergic activity diminish uterine blood flow and may adversely affect the fetus. Use of Vasoxine Injection to prevent and treat hypotension during spinal anaesthesia in obstetric patients cannot be recommended.

In the absence of adequate experience of administration to pregnant women, Vasoxine Injection should not be used during pregnancy unless the potential benefit to the mother outweighs any possible risk to the fetus.

It is not known if methoxamine is excreted in human milk.

*Effects on ability to drive and use machines:* None known.

*Undesirable effects:* Subjective effects reported by patients receiving methoxamine include dull headaches, feelings of cold and other skin sensations resulting from piloerection, sensation of fullness in neck and chest and desire to micturate.

Reflex bradycardia may occur with methoxamine which can be countered with standard doses of atropine given intravenously.

Vomiting and headache have been reported without severe hypertension.

*Overdose:* The hypertension caused by an overdose of Vasoxine Injection should be managed with an α-adrenergic blocking agent such as phentolamine, administered intravenously and repeated as necessary. Clinically significant bradycardia should be treated with intravenous atropine.

**Pharmacological properties**

*Pharmacodynamic properties:* Methoxamine is a vasopressor agent which produces a prompt and prolonged rise in blood pressure after parenteral administration. It acts by exclusively stimulating α-adrenergic receptors and hence causing vasoconstriction.

*Pharmacokinetic properties:* The usual time of onset of activity is one minute after intravenous injections and twenty minutes after the intramuscular injections. The usual duration of activity is about one hour after intravenous and somewhat longer after intramuscular administration. Actual plasma concentrations attained have never been measured, so the disposition and elimination rate have to be inferred from observation of biological activity. Methoxamine is not active after oral administration.

*Preclinical safety data:* There are no preclinical data of relevance to the prescriber which are additional to that in other sections of the SPC.

**Pharmaceutical particulars**

*List of excipients:* Sodium Chloride HSE*; Sodium Chloride PhEur*; Water for Injections PhEur.

* These ingredients are alternatives.

*Incompatibilities:* None known.

*Shelf life:* 60 months.

*Special precautions for storage:* Store at 25°C. Do not freeze.

*Nature and contents of container:* Neutral glass ampoules. 1 ml nominal fill volume. Pack size: 1.

*Instructions for use/handling:* Not applicable.

**Marketing authorisation number** 0003/5066R

**Date of approval/revision of SPC** September 1996.

**Legal category** POM.

## WELLFERON* INJECTION

**Qualitative and quantitative composition**
*Active ingredient:* Human lymphoblastoid interferon, 3 Mega Units, 5 Mega Units or 10 Mega Units in 1 ml in each vial, (1 Mega Unit (MU) = $1 \times 10^6$ International Units of lymphoblastoid interferon by reference to the WHO International Reference Preparation of lymphoblastoid interferon Ga 23–901–532).

**Pharmaceutical form** A clear colourless solution which is administered by intramuscular or subcutaneous injection.

**Clinical particulars**
*Therapeutic indication:* Wellferon is indicated for the treatment of patients with hairy cell leukaemia.

Wellferon is indicated for the treatment of patients with chronic myeloid leukaemia in the chronic phase. Treatment has been shown to result in an improvement in overall survival when compared with conventinal cytotoxic chemotherapy. (Median survival 59 versus 38 months; overall survival $p=0.001$.)

Wellferon is indicated for the treatment of adult patients with chronic active hepatitis B, who have markers for viral replication, e.g. those who are positive for HBV-DNA, DNA polymerase or HBeAg.

Wellferon is indicated for the treatment of patients with chronic hepatitis C (non A non B) infection. Efficacy has been established on the basis of normalisation of serum aminotransferases, clearance of serum HCV-RNA and improvements in liver histology.

*Posology and method of administration for adults and children:* The site of injection should be changed in succeeding injections.

Some patients appear to be less troubled by interferon-related side effects if the dose is administered in the evening.

The subcutaneous route is more acceptable and convenient for patient self-administration than the intramuscular route.

*Dosage in adults*
*Hairy cell leukaemia:* For remission induction, the dose recommended is 3 MU given daily by subcutaneous or intramuscular injection.

After initial improvement in peripheral haematological indices (commonly 12 to 16 weeks), the dose may be administered thrice weekly during which time further improvement in the bone marrow is to be anticipated.

Haematological recovery is to be expected in patients who have failed splenectomy as well as in those with palpable splenomegaly in whom a reduction in spleen size is to be anticipated.

Alternative dosage regimens have also been used with effect. A randomised study comparing dosing at 2.0 MU/m² body surface area daily for one month and then thrice weekly, and 0.2 MU/m² body surface area according to the same schedule, has shown a greater anti-leukaemic effect at one year using the higher dosage regimen, although side effects were less using the lower dose. See also Special Warnings.

Prolonged treatment for 6 months or more may be required to clear hairy cells from the bone marrow. Studies have suggested a broad correlation between the degree of reponse achieved and cumulative dose administered.

*Chronic myeloid leukaemia:* Wellferon treatment should be started once initial control of the white cell count has been achieved to a level of 4 to $20 \times 10^9$/l for a period of a least 4 weeks using cytotoxic chemotherapy e.g. conventional doses of busulphan or hydroxyurea. If busulphan is used for this purpose, there should be an interval of at least 4 weeks between stopping busulphan and starting Wellferon therapy. If either the leucocyte or platelet count is still falling after this interval the start of Wellferon treatment should be further delayed until the count is stable.

For the first 3 weeks of therapy, the dose recommended is 3 MU given daily by subcutaneous injection.

After 3 weeks, the dose is adjusted to achieve a leucocyte count between 2 and $5 \times 10^9$/l. Dose adjustment may be made by altering the daily dose and also by varying the number of days each week on which the dose is administered.

The median average weekly dose in long term clinical studies was approximately 21 MU per week.

In the event of intolerance or severe cytopenia the total weekly dose should be reduced.

If the leucocyte count falls below $2 \times 10^9$/l, the total dose per week should be reduced. Wellferon should be stopped if the leucocyte count falls below $1 \times 10^9$/l and restarted when the count exceeds $2 \times 10^9$/l.

If the platelet count falls below $50 \times 10^9$/l, the total dose per week should be reduced. Wellferon should be stopped if the platelet count falls below $25 \times 10^9$/l and restarted when the count exceeds $50 \times 10^9$/l.

If the leucocyte count rises above $30 \times 10^9$/l, chemotherapy with either hydroxyurea or busulphan at conventional dosage should be given in addition to Wellferon until the leucocyte count has re-established between 4 and $20 \times 10^9$/l for a period of 4 weeks. Chemotherapy is then discontinued, but administration is repeated in the same manner whenever the leucocyte count exceeds $30 \times 10^9$/l. Weekly blood counts are recommended when initiating combination treatment with Wellferon and cytotoxic drugs and if significant chemotherapy-related myelosuppression occurs, chemotherapy should be discontinued and withheld until haematological recovery in accordance with normal clinical practice. (See prescribing information for busulphan and hydroxyurea.)

Wellferon is continued indefinitely until the leucocyte count is no longer controlled (even despite additional chemotherapy), or evidence of acceleration or blast transformation is apparent.

Although there is limited clinical experience, doses of 3 MU or 6 MU (occasionally 9 MU) daily have been successfully used to achieve initial control of the white cell count. In the event of intolerance, dose reduction along the lines of those discussed above should be considered.

Prolonged treatment of at least 6 months and frequently longer, may be required to achieve a cytogenetic response in terms of suppression of the philadephia chromosome (PH) positive cells in the bone marrow.

*Chronic hepatitis B infection:* A twelve week course of thrice weekly subcutaneous or intramuscular injections of 10 to 15 MU (up to 7.5 MU/m² body surface area) is generally recommended.

Longer periods of treatment for up to six months at lower doses (5 to 10 MU or up to 5 MU/m² of body surface area thrice weekly) have been employed and may be preferred for patients who do not tolerate higher doses.

An initial period, employing escalating daily doses, usually over five days (but up to 28 days with the longer treatment), may be a convenient way of introducing treatment.

*Chronic hepatitis C infection (non A non B):* The optimal treatment schedule with Interferons for chronic hepatitis C (non A non B) has not yet been established.

A 48 week course of thrice weekly subcutaneous (or intramuscular) injection of 5 MU is recommended. A good response may still be achieved in some patients with an alternative dose such as 3 MU thrice weekly for 48 weeks. The 3 MU thrice weekly regimen may also be more appropriate in patients where tolerance of the higher dose is in doubt.

Clinical experience indicates that Wellferon therapy can result in an ALT response at the end of treatment in up to 50% of patients. Approximately half of these patients will maintain a sustained ALT response, post-treatment.

Almost 50% of HCV infected patients treated with Wellferon show sustained improvement in liver inflammation on histological examination.

*Dosage in children:*
*Hairy cell leukaemia:* Not known to occur in children.

*Chronic Myeloid leukaemia:* Wellferon has been used in the management of PH positive chronic myeloid leukaemia in children, using the adult dosing regimen, although data are limited.

*Chronic hepatitis B infection:* Up to 10 MU/m² body surface area has been administered to children with chronic hepatitis B. However, efficacy of therapy has not yet been demonstrated.

*Chronic hepatitis C infection (non A non B):* Chronic hepatitis C (non A non B) is rare in children. No information on treatment is available.

*Dosage in the elderly:* Elderly patients may be less tolerant of the side effects of interferon, particularly those effects which are cumulative. These patients should be seen frequently whilst receiving treatment; Wellferon dosage should be reduced or even stopped if patients are unduly sensitive to side effects.

Whilst vigilance is necessary in treating elderly Chronic Myeloid Leukaemia (CML) patients (≥65 years) clinical experience indicates that they gain simiilar survival benefit with comparable treatment tolerance to that of younger patients.

*Contra-indications:* Hairy cell leukaemia and phase chronic myeloid leukaemia: Wellferon should not be given to patients known to be hypersensitive to the preparation or any of its components. Other than known hypersensitivity there are no contra-indications to the use of Wellferon in hairy cell leukaemia or chronic myeloid leukaemia.

Chronic hepatitis B infection and chronic hepatitis C: A history of hypersensitivity to interferon alpha-nl (lns), or any component of the preparation.

Severe pre-existing cardiac disease.

Severe renal or hepatic dysfunction.

Epilepsy and/or compromised central nervous system function.

Chronic hepatitis with advanced decompensated cirrhosis of the liver.

Chronic hepatitis in patients who are being or have recently been treated with immunosuppressive agents excluding short term 'steroid withdrawal'.

*Special warnings and special precautions for use:* Extreme caution is advised when using alpha interferons in the treatment of patients with concurrent renal, cardiovascular or severe hepatic disease, central nervous system disease, or patients with a history of pre-existing mental disturbance. In view of rare cases of cardiac arrhythmia or infarction occurring in patients receiving Wellferon it is prudent to perform an ECG before starting and during treatment in patients with pre-existing heart disease. Consideration should be given to dose reduction or temporary cessation of dosing if problems are encountered when treating patients suffering from concurrent diseases such as these.

It is important to monitor the blood count closely in patients during the first 6 weeks of treatment for hairy cell leukaemia, following which the suppressive effects of alpha interferons on the bone marrow will be overtaken by the improving leukaemic state, leading towards a normalisation of haematological parameters. In patients with profound or potentially life-threatening neutropenia or thrombocytopenia at the outset it may be preferable to initiate treatment with a lower dose of Wellferon, particularly for out-patients who are remote from immediate medical care.

During Wellferon treatment of chronic myeloid leukaemia the blood count should be monitored weekly in the first 3 weeks and thereafter at least once a month or more frequently if cytopenias occur. In the event of dose escalation above 3 MU daily the patient should be seen weekly until tolerance has been assessed.

Severe cytopenias, with or without bone marrow aplasia, have been observed very occasionally in patients with chronic myeloid leukaemia treated with Wellferon directly after busulphan therapy. Careful monitoring of the blood count in patients in whom busulphan induction is used is important to ensure that the leucocyte and platelet counts have stabilised before starting treatment with Wellferon.

Caution is advised if either busulphan or hydroxyurea is reintroduced in combination with Wellferon and weekly blood counts are recommended.

During Wellferon treatment of chronic hepatitis B infection and chronic hepatitis C infection it is similarly important to monitor blood count and liver function throughout treatment.

Care should be exercised in treating patients with certain pre-existing autoimmune diseases e.g. thyroid disorders, as rare occurrences of exacerbation of disease have been reported.

Efficacy against hepatitis B virus and hepatitis C (non A non B) virus infections has not yet been demonstrated in patients whose immune systems are compromised (e.g. by current or recent therapy with immunosuppressive drugs (excluding short term steroid pre treatment) or due to human immunodeficiency virus (HIV) infection).

As with other alpha interferon preparations, care should be exercised when using Wellferon in combination with vinblastine. With relatively high doses of vinblastine and Wellferon, life-threatening (rarely fatal) myelosuppression has been reported.

Care should be exercised in treating patients with asthma, as exacerbation of the disease has been reported on isolated occasions following alpha interferon administration.

It is prudent to ensure maintenance of adequate hydration.

*Interaction with other medicaments and other forms of interaction:* Alpha-interferons may alter the activity of certain enzymes. In particular, they reduce the activity of P-450 cytochromes. The metabolism of drugs such as cimetidine, phenytoin, warfarin, theophylline, diazepam and propranolol by these enzyme systems may therefore be impaired in patients receiving alpha interferon. Several cytotoxic drugs e.g. cyclophosphamide, are also metabolised by these enzymes.

Concurrent administration of a combination of relatively high doses of vinblastine with Wellferon has been shown to produce severe myelosuppression.

In the treatment of chronic myeloid leukaemia, the use of Wellferon immediately following busulphan has occasionally resulted in bone marrow aplasia and the combination should therefore be regarded as potentially severely myelotoxic. If chemotherapy is administered concurrently with Wellferon to maintain control of the leucocyte count the blood count should be checked frequently to ensure that severe myelosuppression does not occur.

In the treatment of chronic hepatitis B infection, the occurrence of an acute, hepatitis-like illness presents the theoretical risk of additive interaction with hepatotoxic drugs and of further impairment of hepatic drug metabolish.

Progressive renal failure has been reported in patients receiving concurrent high dose acyclovir. Concurrent administration of interferon with drugs which act on the central nervous system has occasionally resulted in unexpectedly severe changes in mental state.

Concurrent administration of immunosuppressive drugs (including corticosteroids), which may enhance viral replication, should be avoided during treatment of chronic hepatitis B infection with Wellferon.

*Pregnancy and lactation:* Offspring from pregnant rhesus monkeys given daily Wellferon dosages of up to 2.5 MU/kg bodyweight (from Day 21 through to Day 50 in one group and from Day 51 through to Day 130 in the second group) did not reveal teratogenic or other adverse effects, although there was an increased incidence of abortion and stillbirth in those animals who received the highest dose (2.5 MU/kg bodyweight daily).

No studies have been performed in animals to determine whether Wellferon may affect fertility.

No information is available on the use of Wellferon in human pregnancy. In view of the profound effects of the drug on human metabolism and physiology however, Wellferon should be considered as a drug which might result in damage to the fetus and patients should therefore be advised accordingly. The expected clinical benefit of treatment to the patient must be balanced against any possible hazard to the developing fetus. Adequate contraceptive precautions should be advised if either partner is receiving Wellferon. In view of the long clinical course of chronic hepatitis B infection and the availability of hepatitis B immunisation for the neonate, use of Wellferon to treat chronic hepatitis B infection during human pregnancy is not recommended.

There is no information on the excretion of interferon in human breast milk, following Wellferon therapy. In consequence lactating women should be advised accordingly and the possible risks balanced against the advantages of treatment.

*Effects on ability to drive and use machines:* As alpha interferons may effect central nervous system functions, patients should be warned not to drive a vehicle or operate machinery until their tolerance of treatment has been assessed.

*Undesirable effects:* Wellferon in common with other alpha-interferons is a highly active mediator of biological events and its use may be associated with severe side effects, particularly when large doses are administered.

The most frequently reported side effects of Wellferon and other alpha interferon preparations consist of fever, chills, occasionally rigors, headache, malaise and myalgia, all reminiscent of an attack of influenza. These acute side effects can usually be reduced or eliminated by concurrent administration of paracetamol and tend to diminish with continuing therapy. In contrast however, continuing therapy can lead to lethargy, weakness, arthralgia, and fatigue accompanied by anorexia and weight loss.

Alpha-interferons have a suppressive effect on the bone marrow leading to a fall in the white blood count, particularly the granulocytes, the platelet count and, less commonly, the haemoglobin concentration. Additionally, abnormalities in the blood-clotting mechanism have occurred. These effects can lead to an increased risk of infection and haemorrhage.

Marked effects on the central nervous system may occur; these include abnormal electroencephalograms with excess slow wave activity, severe depression, confusion, apathy and coma. Occasionally seizures occur which may be precipitated by fever in children. A few reports of movement disorders (including extrapyramidal and cerebellar dysfunction) have been reported in cancer patients receiving Wellferon.

The administration of alpha-interferons may give rise to hypotension, hypertension or arrhythmias in certain individuals. Severe cardiovascular events reported in patients receiving alpha interferons include myocardial infarction, cerebrovascular accident and peripheral ischaemia.

Nausea, vomiting and diarrhoea have occurred during therapy with alpha-interferons.

Alpha interferons can lead to an elevation in liver-related enzymes; this is usually transient but occasionally is marked and persistent. Hepatic necrosis has been reported on very rare occasions.

On rare occasions elevations of serum creatinine levels have been seen in Wellferon treated patients.

In patients with myelomatosis, there have been rare reports of renal failure/and or nephrotic syndrome in patients treated with Wellferon, all had varying degrees of prior renal dysfunction.

After repeated very high doses (100–200 MU) intravenously by infusion, hypocalcaemia and hyperkalaemia have occurred.

Reactions at injection sites have been reported in some patients.

Alopecia occurs occasionally as a late side effect.

Other uncommon events which have been reported in patients receiving alpha-interferons include Raynaud's phenomenon, dyspnoea, urticaria, erythema nodosum, skin rashes, pruritus, psoriasis, mucositis, isolated peripheral nerve defects, and disturbances of antidiuretic hormone levels.

Isolated cases of various autoimmune phenomena e.g. immune thrombocytopenia, haemolytic anaemia, hypothyroidism have occurred following alpha-interferon administration. In some patients with pre-existing autoimmune phenomena, isolated cases of exacerbation have been seen.

*Overdose:* There have been no reports of overdosage but repeated large doses of alpha interferons are associated with profound lethargy, fatigue, prostration and coma. Such patients should be hospitalised for observation, and appropriate supportive treatment given.

**Pharmacological properties**

*Pharmacodynamic properties:* The mode of action of alpha-interferon in hairy cell leukaemia is not understood. The rapid rate of clearance of hairy cells from the blood on commencing treatment suggests a direct effect of interferon following cellular binding, particularly since malignant hairy cells are known to bear prolific inteferon receptors on their surface membranes. The resulting anti-leukaemic effect may be brought about by a reduction in the sensitivity of hairy cells to stimulation by growth factors produced by the same cells (autocrine loop) or different cells (paracrine loop) a change towards a more differentiated state and a decrease in cell proliferation.

The mechanism of action of alpha-interferon in chronic myeloid leukaemia is not fully understood. Possibilities include inhibition of the late progenitor cell stage of chronic myeloid leukaemia, either directly or by interruption of an autocrine feedback loop, enhancement of T-cells to inhibit the proliferation of chronic myeloid leukaemia cells and modulation of interactions between chronic myeloid leukaemia progenitor cells and bone marrow stromal cells, leading to growth arrest and repopulation of the marrow with normal progenitors.

The mode of action of alpha-interferon in the treatment of chronic hepatitis B is poorly understood but seems to consist of both a direct antiviral effect and immuno-modulatory actions.

The mode of action of alpha-interferon in the treatment of chronic hepatitis C (non A non B) has not yet been determined; however, it is currently thought to consist mainly of an antiviral effect supported by immunomodulatory effects.

*Antibodies to Wellferon:* Neutralising antibodies occur infrequently in patients receiving Wellferon which therefore appears to have low immunogenicity. An overall anti-interferon antibody incidence of 2.0% was found in follow-up sera from more than 1500 patients who had received Wellferon for benign and malignant diseases.

*Pharmacokinetic properties:* There is considerable inter-patient variability in the handling of alpha-interferons; furthermore, absolute serum levels may be less meaningful as a measure of alpha-interferon biological activity than the induction of certain cellular enzymes such as 2′,-5′-oligoadenylate synthetase (2-5A synthetase) or human Mx protein. Following intramuscular or subcutaneous administration, maximum serum levels are usually reached within 4 to 8 hours, but may merge into a plateau phase as a result of rate-limited absorption from the site of administration.

The measured serum half-life also varies considerably as a result of this, being in the approximate range of 4 to 12 hours although the true elimination half life can be estimated to be about 3 to 4 hours. Similar serum alpha-interferon levels and pharmacokinetics are found after intramuscular and subcutaneous administration of Wellferon. When Wellferon is administered at the recommended daily dose for the treatment of hairy cell leukaemia, steady state accumulation results in maximum serum values lying in the approximate range of 30 to 90 IU per ml. The range of doses suggested for the treatment of chronic hepatitis B infection can be expected to result in maximum serum concentrations of 200 to 300 IU per ml. Alpha-interferon is not detectable in the urine except rarely in cases of severe renal disease. In a study of 20 patients aged 29–81 years, with estimated creatinine clearances of 15 to >100 ml/min, there were no apparent effects of renal function or age on Wellferon pharmacokinetic parameters in the range 3 MU to 100 MU. Total body clearance estimates, uncorrected for bioavailability (CL/b), have been calculated for Wellferon; from two different studies mean values were found to be 57 ml/min/m², and approximately 2 ml/min/kg respectively.

*Preclinical safety data:* The alpha interferons are unusually restricted in their species specificity. Additionally administration of a heterologous protein to primates and rodents results in the production of circulating antibodies. These factors greatly limit the predictive value of pre-clinical information. The studies conducted in animals have not demonstrated any particular toxic or pharmacologic effects.

*Carcinogenicity:* No studies have been conducted in animals to determine whether Wellferon has carcinogenic potential.

*Mutagenicity:* Wellferon was not mutagenic in the Ames test.

**Pharmaceutical particulars**

*List of excipients:* Sodium Chloride PhEur; Tris (Tromethamine) USP; Glycine BP; Human Albumin Solution (equivalent to total protein) PhEur; Water for Injection PhEur.

*Incompatibilities:* Not applicable.

*Shelf life:* 3 years at 2–8°C. Wellferon contains no preservative, therefore any partly used vials should be discarded immediately after withdrawal of the required dose.

*Special precautions for storage:* Store between 2 and 8°C. Protect from light.

*Nature and contents of container:* Wellferon is filled in nominal 1 ml volumes into Ph.Eur. Type 1 glass (white neutral) vials, plugged with red butyl/natural rubber closures with an aluminium collar and polypropylene flip-off cap.

*Instructions for use/handling:* Not applicable.

**Marketing authorisation number** 0003/0221

**Date of approval/revision of SPC** November 1996.

**Legal category** POM.

## WELLVONE* SUSPENSION ▼

**Qualitative and quantitative composition** Atovaquone 150 mg/ml. A unit dose of 5 ml contains 750 mg atovaquone.

**Pharmaceutical form** A bright yellow oral suspension containing 150 mg atovaquone/ml.

**Clinical particulars**

*Therapeutic indications:* Wellvone suspension is indicated for: Acute treatment of mild to moderate *Pneumocystis carinii* pneumonia (PCP) (alveolar-arterial oxygen tension difference $[A\text{-}a)DO_2] \leq 45$ mmHg (6 kPa) and oxygen tension in arterial blood $(PaO_2) \geq 60$ mmHg (8 kPa) breathing room air) in patients who are intolerant of co-trimoxazole therapy (see *Special warnings and precautions for use*).

*Posology and method of administration:* The importance of taking the full prescribed dose of Wellvone **with food** should be stressed to patients. The presence of food, particularly high fat food, increases bioavailability by two to three fold.

*Dosage in adults: Pneumocystis carinii* pneumonia: The recommended oral dose is 750 mg twice a day (1×5 ml morning and evening) administered with food each day for 21 days.

Higher doses may be more effective and will be investigated (see *Pharmacokinetic properties*).

*Dosage in children:* Clinical efficacy has not been studied.

*Dosage in the elderly:* There have been no studies of Wellvone in the elderly (see *Special warnings and precautions for use).*

*Renal or hepatic impairment:* Wellvone has not been specifically studied in patients with significant hepatic or renal impairment (see *Pharmacokinetics in adults*). If it is necessary to treat such patients with Wellvone, caution is advised and administration should be closely monitored.

*Contra-indications:* Wellvone suspension is contra-indicated in individuals with known hypersensitivity to atovaquone or to any components of the formulation.

*Special warnings and precautions for use:* Diarrhoea at the start of treatment has been shown to be associated with significantly lower atovaquone plasma levels. These in turn correlated with a higher incidence of therapy failures and a lower survival rate. Therefore, alternative therapies should be considered for such patients and for patients who have difficulty taking Wellvone with food.

The concomitant administration of atovaquone and

rifampicin is not recommended (see *Interaction with other medicaments*).

The efficacy of Wellvone has not been systematically evaluated (i) in patients failing other PCP therapy, including co-trimoxazole, (ii) for treatment of severe episodes of PCP [(A-a) $DO_2$>45 mmHg 6kPa] or (iii) as a prophylactic agent for PCP or (iv) versus intravenous pentamidine for treatment of PCP.

No data are available in non-HIV immunocompromised patients suffering with PCP.

As HIV infection is rarely observed in elderly patients, no clinical experience of atovaquone treatment has been gained. Therefore use in the elderly should be closely monitored.

Patients with pulmonary disease should be carefully evaluated for causes of disease other than PCP and treated with additional agents as appropriate. Wellvone is not expected to be effective therapy for other fungal, bacterial, mycobacterial or viral diseases.

*Interaction with other medicaments and other forms of interaction:* As experience is limited, care should be taken when combining other drugs with Wellvone.

Concomitant administration of rifampicin is known to reduce atovaquone levels by approximately 50% and could result in subtherapeutic plasma concentrations in some patients (see *Special warnings and precautions for use*).

Concomitant treatment with metoclopramide has been associated with significant decreases in plasma concentrations of atovaquone. Caution should be exercised in prescribing this drug with Wellvone until the potential interaction has been further studied.

In clinical trials of Wellvone small decreases in plasma concentrations of atovaquone (mean <3 mcg/ml) were associated with concomitant administration of paracetamol, benzodiazepines, acyclovir, opiates, cephalosporins, anti-diarrhoeals and laxatives. The causal relationship between the change in plasma concentrations of atovaquone and the administration of the drugs mentioned above is unknown.

Clinical trials have evaluated the interaction of Wellvone Tablets with:

*Zidovudine* – Zidovudine does not appear to affect the pharmacokinetics of atovaquone. However, pharmacokinetic data have shown that atovaquone appears to decrease the rate of metabolism of zidovudine to its glucuronide metabolite (steady state AUC of zidovudine was increased by 33% and peak plasma concentration of the glucuronide was decreased by 19%). At zidovudine dosages of 500 or 600 mg/day it would seem unlikely that a three week, concomitant course of Wellvone for the treatment of acute PCP would result in an increased incidence of adverse reactions attributable to higher plasma concentrations of zidovudine.

*Didanosine (ddl)* – ddl does not affect the pharmacokinetics of atovaquone as determined in a prospective multidose interaction study of atovaquone and ddl. However, there was a 24% decrease in the AUC for ddl when co-administered with atovaquone which is unlikely to be of clinical significance.

Nevertheless, the modes of interaction being unknown, the effects of atovaquone administration on zidovudine and ddl may be greater with atovaquone suspension. The higher concentrations of atovaquone possible with the suspension might induce greater changes in the AUC values for zidovudine or ddl than those observed. Patients receiving atovaquone and zidovudine should be regularly monitored for zidovudine associated adverse effects.

There are no data available for interaction of atovaquone with other anti-retroviral drugs.

In clinical trials of Wellvone the following medications were not associated with a change in steady state plasma concentrations of atovaquone: fluconazole, clotrimazole, ketoconazole, antacids, systemic corticosteroids, non-steroidal anti-inflammatory drugs, anti-emetics (excluding metoclopramide) and $H_2$-antagonists.

Atovaquone is highly bound to plasma proteins and caution should be used when administering Wellvone concurrently with other highly plasma protein bound drugs with narrow therapeutic indices. Atovaquone does not affect the pharmacokinetics, metabolism or extent of protein binding of phenytoin *in vivo. In vitro* there is no plasma protein binding interaction between atovaquone and quinine, phenytoin, warfarin, sulphamethoxazole, indomethacin or diazepam.

*Pregnancy and lactation:* There is no information on the effects of atovaquone administration during human pregnancy. Atovaquone should not be used during pregnancy unless the benefit of treatment to the mother outweighs any possible risk to the developing fetus.

Insufficient data are available from animal experiments to assess the possible risk to reproductive potential or performance.

It is not known whether atovaquone is excreted in human milk, and therefore breast feeding is not recommended.

*Effects on ability to drive and use machines:* There have been no studies to investigate the effect of Wellvone on driving performance or the ability to operate machinery but a detrimental effect on such activities is not predicted form the pharmacology of the drug.

*Undesirable effects:* Patients participating in clinical trials with Wellvone have often had complications of advanced Human Immunodeficiency Virus (HIV) disease and therefore the causal relationship between the adverse experiences and atovaquone is difficult to evaluate.

The most common adverse experiences reported while receiving treatment with Wellvone, regardless of attributability, are: rash, nausea, diarrhoea, headache, vomiting, fever and insomnia.

The most common abnormalities in laboratory parameters reported in patients receiving Wellvone, regardless of attributability, are: elevated liver enzyme levels, elevated amylase levels, hyponatraemia, neutropenia and anaemia.

*Overdose:* There have been no reports of overdosage from the administration of Wellvone in humans.

In the case of overdosage, treatment should be symptomatic.

**Pharmacological properties**

*Pharmacodynamic properties:*

*(a) Mode of action:* Atovaquone belongs to a new therapeutic class with a novel mechanism of action. It is a selective and potent inhibitor of the eukaryotic mitochondrial electron transport chain in a number of parasitic protozoa. The site of action appears to be the cytochrome bcl complex (complex III). The ultimate metabolic effect of such blockade is likely to be inhibition of nucleic acid and ATP synthesis.

*(b) Microbiology:* Atovaquone has potent antiprotozoal activity, both *in vitro* and in animal models, particularly against the parasitic protozoan-life fungus *Pneumocystis carinii* ($IC_{50}$ 0.1–1.0 mcg/ml).

*Pharmacokinetic properties:* Atovaquone is a highly lipophilic compound with a low aqueous solubility. It is 99.9% bound to plasma proteins. The bioavailability of the drug demonstrates a relative decrease with single doses above 750 mg, and it shows considerable inter-individual variability. Average absolute bioavailability of a 750 mg single dose of atovaquone suspension administered with food to adult HIV positive males is 47% (compared to 23% for Wellvone tablets). Following the intravenous administration, the volume of distribution and clearance were calculated to be 0.62±0.19 l/kg and 0.15±0.09 ml/min/kg, respectively.

The bioavailability of atovaquone is greater when administered with food than in the fasting state. In healthy volunteers, a standardised breakfast (23 g fat; 610 kCal) increased bioavailability two to three-fold following a single 750 mg dose. The mean area under the atovaquone plasma concentration-time curve (AUC) was increased 2.5 fold and the mean $C_{max}$ was increased 3.4 fold. The mean (±SD) AUC values for suspension were 324.3 (±115.0) mcg/ml.h fasted and 800.6 (±319.8) mcg/ml.h with food.

In a safety and pharmacokinetic study in patients with PCP, the following results were obtained.

| Dose regimen | 750 mg twice daily | 1000 mg twice daily |
|---|---|---|
| Number of patients | 18 | 9 |
| C avg. ss (range) | 22 mcg/ml (6–41) | 25.7 mcg/ml (15–36) |
| % of patients with C Avg. ss>15 mcg/ml | 67% | 100% |

Average steady state concentrations above 15 mcg/ml are predictive of a high (>90%) success rate.

In healthy volunteers and patients with AIDS atovaquone has a half-life of 2 to 3 days.

In healthy volunteers there is no evidence that the drug is metabolised and there is negligible excretion of atovaquone in the urine, with parent drug being predominantly (>90%) excreted unchanged in faeces.

*Preclinical safety data:*

*(a) Carcinogenicity:* Oncogenicity studies in mice showed an increased incidence of hepatocellular adenomas and carcinomas without determination of the no observed adverse effect level. No such findings were observed in rats and mutagenicity tests were negative. These findings appear to be due to the inherent susceptibility of mice to atovaquone and are not predictive of a risk in the clinical situation.

*(b) Reproductive toxicity:* In the dosage range of 600 to 1200 mg/kg studies in rabbits gave indications of maternal and embryotoxic effects.

**Pharmaceutical particulars**

*List of excipients:* Benzyl alcohol; xanthan gum; poloxamer 188; saccharin sodium; tutti frutti flavour (Firmenich 51.880/A); purified water.

*Incompatibilities:* None.

*Shelf life:* 2 years (after first opening, the suspension may be stored for up to 21 days).

*Special precautions for storage:* Store below 25°C. Do not freeze.

*Nature and contents of container:* A 240 ml high density polyethylene bottle with child resistant closure, containing 226 ml of atovaquone suspension.

A 5 ml measuring spoon (polypropylene) is included.

*Instructions for use/handling:* Do not dilute.

**Marketing authorisation number** 10949/0271

**Date of approval/revision of SPC** March 1997.

**Legal category** POM.

## WELLVONE* TABLETS

**Qualitative and quantitative composition** Atovaquone 250 mg per tablet.

**Pharmaceutical form** Round, biconvex pale yellow film-coated tablets coded P7F and branded 'Wellcome' and each containing 250 mg atovaquone.

**Clinical particulars**

*Therapeutic indications:* Wellvone Tablets are indicated for: Acute treatment of mild to moderate *Pneumocystis carinii* pneumonia (PCP) (alveolar-arterial oxygen tension difference [(A-a)$DO_2$]≤45 mmHg (6kPa) and oxygen tension in arterial blood ($PaO_2$)≥60 mmHg (8kPa) breathing room air) in patients who are intolerant of co-trimoxazole therapy. (See *Special warnings and precautions for use.*)

*Posology and method of administration:* The importance of taking the full prescribed dose of Wellvone *with food* should be stressed to patients. The presence of food particularly high fat food, increases bioavailability by two to three fold.

*Dosage in adults: Pneumocystis carinii* pneumonia: The recommended oral dose is 750 mg (three 250 g tablets) administered with food three times daily for 21 days.

*Dosage in children:* Clinical efficacy has not been studied.

*Dosage in the elderly:* There have been no studies of Wellvone in the elderly (see *Special warnings and precautions for use.*)

*Renal or hepatic impairment:* Wellvone has not been specifically studied in patients with significant hepatic or renal impairment (see *Pharmocokinetics in adults*). If it is necessary to treat such patients with Wellvone, caution is advised and administration should be closely monitored.

*Contra-indications:* Wellvone tablets are contra-indicated in individuals with known hypersensitivity to atovaquone or to any components of the formulation.

*Special warnings and precautions for use:* Absorption of atovaquone is limited but can be significantly increased when the drug is taken with food (see *Pharmacokinetics in adults*). Diarrhoea at the start of treatment has been shown to be associated with significantly lower atovaquone plasma levels. These in turn correlated with a higher incidence of therapy failures and a lower survival rate. Therefore, alternative therapies should be considered for such patients and for patients who have difficulty taking Wellvone with food.

The concomitant administration of atovaquone and rifampicin is not recommended (see *Interaction with other medicaments*).

The efficacy of Wellvone has not been systematically evaluated (i) in patients failing other PCP therapy, including co-trimoxazole; (ii) for treatment of severe episodes of PCP [(A-a)$DO_2$]>45 mmHg (6kPa)]; (iii) as a prophylactic agent for PCP or (iv) versus intravenous pentamidine for treatment of PCP.

No data are available in non-HIV immunocompromised patients suffering with PCP.

As HIV infection is rarely observed in elderly patients, no clinical experience of atovaquone treatment has been gained. Therefore use in the elderly should be closely monitored.

Patients with pulmonary disease should be carefully evaluated for causes of disease other than PCP and treated with additional agents as appropriate. Wellvone is not expected to be effective therapy for concurrent fungal, bacterial, mycobacterial or viral diseases.

*Interaction with other medicaments and other forms of interaction:* As experience is limited, care should be taken when combining other drugs with Wellvone.

Concomitant administration of rifampicin is known to reduce atovaquone levels by approximately 50% and could result in subtherapeutic plasma concentrations in some patients (see *Special warnings and precautions for use*).

Concomitant treatment with metoclopramide has been associated with significant decreases in plasma concentrations of atovaquone. Caution should be exercised in prescribing this drug with Wellvone until the potential interaction has been further studied.

In clinical trials of Wellvone small decreases in plasma concentrations of atovaquone (mean <3 mcg/ml) were associated with concomitant administration of paracetamol, benzodiazepines, aciclovir, opiates, cephalosporins, anti-diarrhoeals and laxatives. The causal relationship between the change in plasma concentrations of atovaquone and the administration of the drugs mentioned above is unknown.

Zidovudine does not appear to affect the pharmacokinetics of atovaquone. However, pharmacokinetic data have shown that atovaquone appears to decrease the rate of metabolism of zidovudine to its glucuronide metabolite (steady state AUC of zidovudine was increased by 33% and peak plasma concentration of the glucuronide was decreased by 19%). At zidovudine dosages of 500 or 600 mg/day it would seem unlikely that a three week, concomitant course of Wellvone for the treatment of acute PCP would result in an increased incidence of adverse reactions attributable to higher plasma concentrations of zidovudine. There are no data available for ddI (didanosine) or ddC (zalcitabine).

In clinical trials of Wellvone the following medications were not associated with a change in steady state plasma concentrations of atovaquone: fluconazole, clotrimazole, ketoconazole, antacids, systemic corticosteroids, non-steroidal anti-inflammatory drugs, anti-emetics (excluding metoclopramide) and $H_2$-antagonists.

Atovaquone is highly bound to plasma proteins and caution should be used when administering Wellvone concurrently with other highly plasma protein bound drugs with narrow therapeutic indices. Atovaquone does not affect the pharmacokinetics, metabolism or extent of protein binding of phenytoin *in vivo. In vitro* there is no plasma protein binding interaction between atovaquone and quinine, phenytoin, warfarin, sulphamethoxazole, indomethacin or diazepam.

*Use during pregnancy and lactation:* There is no information on the effects of atovaquone administration during human pregnancy. Atovaquone should not be used during pregnancy unless the benefit of treatment to the mother outweighs any possible risk to the developing fetus.

Insufficient data are available from animal experiments to assess the possible risk to reproductive potential or performance.

It is not known whether atovaquone is excreted in human milk, and therefore breast feeding is not recommended.

*Effects on ability to drive and use machines:* There have been no studies to investigate the effect of Wellvone on driving performance or the ability to operate machinery but a detrimental effect on such activities is not predicted from the pharmacology of the drug.

*Undesirable effects:* Patients participating in clinical trials with Wellvone have often had complications of advanced Human Immunodeficiency Virus (HIV) disease and therefore the causal relationship between the adverse experiences and atovaquone is difficult to evaluate.

The most common adverse experiences reported while receiving treatment with Wellvone, regardless of attributability, are: rash, nausea, diarrhoea, headache, vomiting, fever and insomnia.

The most common abnormalities in laboratory parameters reported in patients receiving Wellvone, regardless of attributability, are: elevated liver enzyme levels, elevated amylase levels, hyponatraemia, neutropenia and anaemia.

*Overdose:* There have been no reports of overdosage from the administration of Wellvone in humans. In the case of overdosage, treatment should be symptomatic.

**Pharmacological properties**

*Pharmacodynamic properties:*

*(a) Mode of action:* Atovaquone belongs to a new therapeutic class with a novel mechanism of action. It is a selective and potent inhibitor of the eukaryotic mitochondrial electron transport chain in a number of parasitic protozoa. The site of action appears to be the cytochrome bcl complex (complex III). The ultimate metabolic effect of such blockade is likely to be inhibition of nucleic acid and ATP synthesis.

*(b) Microbiology:* Atovaquone has potent antiprotozoal activity, both *in vitro* and in animal models, particularly against the parasitic protozoan-like fungus *Pneumocystis carinii* ($IC_{50}$ 0.1–1.0 mcg/ml).

*Pharmacokinetic properties:*

*Pharmocokinetics in adults:* Atovaquone is a highly lipophilic compound with a low aqueous solubility. It is 99.9% bound to plasma proteins. The bioavailability of the drug is low and demonstrates a relative decrease with single doses above 750 mg. It shows considerable inter-individual variability. The absolute bioavailability of a 750 mg single dose of atovaquone (3×250 mg tablets) administered with food, to adult HIV positive males is 21%. (90% CI 17% to 27%.)

The bioavailability of atovaquone is greater when administered with food than in fasting state. In healthy volunteers, a standardised breakfast (23 g fat; 610 kCal) increased bioavailability two to three-fold following a single 750 mg dose. The mean (±SD) area under the atovaquone plasma concentration-time curve (AUC) values were 150 (±59.5) and 391.5 (±186.4) mcg/ml.h in fasted and fed volunteers respectively. Following administration of a single 500 mg dose to volunteers who had received either no food, a low-fat meal (23 g fat) or high-fat meal (46 g fat), mean AUC values increased 2.7 and 4-fold with the low and high-fat content meal respectively, compared with the fasting control.

Significant differences in the bioavailability of atovaquone have been observed between healthy volunteers, HIV-infected asymptomatic volunteers and people with Acquired Immune Deficiency Syndrome (AIDS). Steady-state atovaquone plasma concentrations in people with AIDS ranged from one third to one half of the levels achieved in asymptomatic HIV-infected volunteers. For example, in subjects with AIDS a dose of 3,000 mg once daily produced a mean (±SD) steady-state plasma concentration of 16.2±6.6 mcg/ml, compared with asymptomatic HIV-infected subjects who achieved mean steady state concentrations of 48.8±21.6 mcg/ml after 3,000 mg once daily.

In the controlled efficacy trial for the treatment of PCP, where patients with AIDS received 750 mg Wellvone three times daily with food, the mean (±SD) steady-state plasma concentration was 13.9±6.9 mcg/ml (n=191).

In healthy volunteers and patients with AIDS atovaquone has a half-life of 2 to 3 days.

In healthy volunteers there is no evidence that the drug is metabolised and there is negligible excretion of atovaquone in the urine, with parent drug being predominantly (>90%) excreted unchanged in faeces.

*Preclinical safety data:*

*(a) Carcinogenicity:* Oncogenicity studies in mice showed an increased incidence of hepatocellular adenomas and carcinomas without determination of the no observed adverse effect level. No such findings were observed in rats and mutagenicity tests were negative. These findings appear to be due to the inherent susceptibility of mice to atovaquone and are not predictive of a risk in the clinical situation.

*(b) Reproductive toxicity:* In the dosage range of 600 to 1,200 mg/kg studies in rabbits gave indications of maternal and embryotoxic effects.

**Pharmaceutical particulars**

**List of excipients:** Cores: low-substituted hydroxypropyl cellulose; microcrystalline cellulose; povidone K30; sodium starch glycollate; magnesium stearate.

Film coat: colour concentrate OY-S-7914 yellow.

Polish: polyethylene glycol 8000.

*Incompatibilities:* None.

*Shelf life:* 2 years.

*Special precautions for storage:* Store below 30°C.

*Nature and contents of container:* Amber glass bottle with low density polyethylene snap fit closure containing 189 tablets.

**Marketing authorisation number** 0003/0337.

**Date of approval/revision of SPC** November 1996.

**Legal category** POM.

## ZANTAC* INJECTION

**Presentation** Zantac Injection: 2 ml ampoules each containing 50 mg ranitidine (as hydrochloride) in 2 ml aqueous solution for intravenous or intramuscular administration.

2 ml Zantac Injection contains 2.82 mg (0.122 mmol) sodium.

**Uses**

*Indications:* Zantac Injection is indicated for the treatment of duodenal ulcer, benign gastric ulcer, post-operative ulcer, oesophageal reflux disease, Zollinger-Ellison syndrome, and the following conditions where reduction of gastric secretion and acid output is desirable: the prophylaxis of gastro-intestinal haemorrhage from stress ulceration in seriously ill patients; the prophylaxis of recurrent haemorrhage in patients with bleeding peptic ulcers and before general anaesthesia in patients considered to be at risk of acid aspiration (Mendelson's syndrome), particularly obstetric patients during labour.

For appropriate cases Zantac Tablets are also available (see separate Data Sheet).

*Mode of action:* Zantac is a specific, rapidly acting histamine $H_2$-antagonist. It inhibits basal and stimulated secretion of gastric acid, reducing both the volume and the acid and pepsin content of the secretion.

**Dosage and administration**

*Adults and elderly:* Zantac Injection may be given either as a slow (over a period of at least two minutes) intravenous injection of 50 mg, after dilution to a volume of 20 ml per 50 mg dose, which may be repeated every six to eight hours; or as an intermittent intravenous infusion at a rate of 25 mg per hour for two hours; the infusion may be repeated at six to eight hour intervals; or as an intramuscular injection of 50 mg (2 ml) every six to eight hours.

In the prophylaxis of haemorrhage from stress ulceration in seriously ill patients or the prophylaxis of recurrent haemorrhage in patients bleeding from peptic ulceration, parenteral administration may be continued until oral feeding commences. Patients considered to be still at risk may then be treated with Zantac Tablets 150 mg twice daily (see separate Data Sheet).

In the prophylaxis of upper gastro-intestinal haemorrhage from stress ulceration in seriously ill patients a priming dose of 50 mg as a slow intravenous injection followed by a continuous intravenous infusion of 0.125-0.250 mg/kg/hr may be preferred.

In patients considered to be at risk of developing acid aspiration syndrome Zantac Injection 50 mg may be given intramuscularly or by slow intravenous injection 45 to 60 minutes before induction of general anaesthesia.

*Children:* The use of Zantac Injection in children has not been evaluated.

**Contra-indications, warnings, etc.**

*Contra-indications:* Ranitidine is contra-indicated for patients known to have hypersensitivity to any component of the preparation.

*Precautions:* Treatment with a histamine $H_2$-antagonist may mask the symptoms associated with carcinoma of the stomach and may therefore delay diagnosis of the condition. Accordingly, where gastric ulcer is suspected the possibility of malignancy should be excluded before therapy with Zantac is instituted.

Ranitidine is excreted via the kidney and so plasma levels of the drug are increased in patients with severe renal impairment. Accordingly, it is recommended in such patients that Zantac be administered in doses of 25 mg.

Bradycardia in association with rapid administration of Zantac Injection has been reported rarely, usually in patients with factors predisposing to cardiac rhythm disturbances. Recommended rates of administration should not be exceeded.

It has been reported that the use of higher than recommended doses of intravenous $H_2$-antagonists has been associated with rises in liver enzymes when treatment has been extended beyond five days.

Zantac crosses the placenta but therapeutic doses administered to obstetric patients in labour or undergoing caesarean section have been without any adverse effect on labour, delivery or subsequent neonatal progress. Zantac is also excreted in human breast milk. Like other drugs, Zantac should only be used during pregnancy and nursing if considered essential.

Although clinical reports of acute intermittent porphyria associated with ranitidine administration have been rare and inconclusive, ranitidine should be avoided in patients with a history of this condition.

*Side-effects:* The following have been reported as events in clinical trials or in the routine management of patients treated with ranitidine. The relationship to ranitidine therapy has not been established in many cases.

Transient and reversible changes in liver function tests can occur. There have been occasional reports of hepatitis (hepatocellular, hepatocanalicular or mixed) with or without jaundice. These were usually reversible. Acute pancreatitis has been reported rarely.

Leucopenia and thrombocytopenia have occurred rarely in patients. These are usually reversible. Rare cases of agranulocytosis or of pancytopenia, sometimes with marrow hypoplasia, or aplasia have been reported.

Hypersensitivity reactions (urticaria, angioneurotic oedema, fever, bronchospasm, hypotension, anaphylactic shock) have been seen rarely following the parenteral and oral administration of ranitidine. These reactions have occasionally occurred after a single dose.

As with other $H_2$-receptor antagonists there have been rare reports of bradycardia, A-V Block and asystole.

Headache, sometimes severe, and dizziness have been reported in a very small proportion of patients. Rare cases of reversible mental confusion, depression and hallucinations have been reported, predominantly in severely ill and elderly patients.

Skin rash has been reported, including rare cases of erythema multiforme. Musculoskeletal symptoms such as arthralgia and myalgia have been reported rarely.

No clinically significant interference with endocrine or gonadal function has been reported. There have been a few reports of breast symptoms (swelling and/ or discomfort) in men taking ranitidine; some cases have resolved on continued ranitidine treatment. Discontinuation of therapy may be necessary in order to establish the underlying cause.

*Overdosage:* Zantac is very specific in action and accordingly no particular problems are expected following overdosage with the drug. Symptomatic and supportive therapy should be given as appropriate. If need be, the drug may be removed from the plasma by haemodialysis.

**Pharmaceutical precautions** Zantac Injection has been shown to be compatible with the following intravenous infusion fluids:

0.9% Sodium Chloride BP; 5% Dextrose BP; 0.18% Sodium Chloride and 4% Dextrose BP; 4.2% Sodium Bicarbonate BP and Hartmann's Solution. Although compatibility studies have only been undertaken in polyvinyl chloride infusion bags (in glass for Sodium Bicarbonate BP) and a polyvinyl chloride administration set it is considered that adequate stability would be conferred by the use of a polyethylene infusion bag. All unused admixtures of Zantac Injection with infusion fluids should be discarded 24 hours after preparation.

Store below 25°C. Protect from light. Zantac Injection should not be autoclaved.

**Legal category** POM.

**Package quantities** Zantac Injection: 2 ml ampoules, boxes of five.

**Further information**

*Drug interactions:* Ranitidine does not inhibit the hepatic cytochrome P450-linked mixed function oxygenase system. Accordingly, ranitidine does not potentiate the actions of drugs which are inactivated by this enzyme; these include diazepam, lignocaine, phenytoin, propranolol, theophylline and warfarin.

*Pharmacokinetics:* Absorption of ranitidine after intramuscular injection is rapid and peak plasma concentrations are usually achieved within 15 minutes of administration. Ranitidine is not extensively metabolised. Elimination of the drug is primarily by tubular secretion. The elimination half-life of ranitidine is 2-3 hours. In balance studies with 150 mg 3H-ranitidine 93% of an intravenous dose was excreted in urine and 5% in faeces. Analysis of urine excreted in the first 24 hours after dosing showed that 70% of the intravenous dose was eliminated unchanged. About 6% of the dose is excreted in the urine as the N-oxide, 2% as the S-oxide, 2% as desmethyl ranitidine and 1-2% as the furoic acid analogue.

*Use in renal transplants:* Zantac has been used in patients with renal transplants.

**Product licence number** 10949/0109

## ZANTAC* TABLETS AND SYRUP

**Presentation** Zantac Tablets 150 mg: 5-sided, white, film-coated, biconvex circular tablet, engraved on one face with ZANTAC 150 and on the other with GLAXO plus two linear lines. Each tablet contains ranitidine 150 mg (as hydrochloride).

Zantac Tablets 300 mg: White, capsule-shaped, film-coated tablet, engraved ZANTAC 300 on one face and GLAXO on the other. Each tablet contains ranitidine 300 mg (as hydrochloride).

Zantac Syrup: A peppermint flavoured, sugar-free syrup, free from artificial colouring. Each 10 ml contains ranitidine 150 mg (as hydrochloride).

Zantac Effervescent Tablets 150 mg: White to pale yellow, round, flat, bevel-edged tablets which effervesce on dissolution in water to give a clear, grapefruit/orange flavoured solution. Each tablet contains ranitidine 150 mg (as hydrochloride) and 14.3 mEq (328 mg) of sodium.

Zantac Effervescent Tablets 300 mg: White to pale yellow, round, flat, bevel-edged tablets which effervesce on dissolution in water to give a clear, grapefruit/orange flavoured solution. Each tablet contains ranitidine 300 mg (as hydrochloride) and 20.8 mEq (479 mg) of sodium.

**Uses**

*Indications:* Zantac Tablets and Syrup are indicated for the treatment of duodenal ulcer and benign gastric ulcer, including that associated with non-steroidal anti-inflammatory agents. In addition, Zantac Tablets and Syrup are indicated for the prevention of NSAID associated duodenal ulcers. Zantac Tablets are indicated for the treatment of duodenal ulcers associated with *Helicobacter pylori* infection.

Zantac Tablets and Syrup are also indicated for the treatment of post-operative ulcer, Zollinger-Ellison syndrome, and oesophageal reflux disease including the long term management of healed oesophagitis as well as the symptomatic relief of gastro-oesophageal reflux disease. Other patients with chronic episodic dyspepsia, characterised by pain (epigastric or retrosternal) which is related to meals or disturbs sleep but is not associated with the preceding conditions may benefit from ranitidine treatment. Zantac Tablets and Syrup are indicated for the following conditions where reduction of gastric secretion and acid output is desirable: the prophylaxis of gastrointestinal haemorrhage from stress ulceration in seriously ill patients; the prophylaxis of recurrent haemorrhage in patients with bleeding peptic ulcers and before general anaesthesia in patients considered to be at risk of acid aspiration (Mendelson's syndrome), particularly obstetric patients during labour. For appropriate cases Zantac Injection is also available (see separate Data Sheet).

*Mode of action:* Zantac is a specific, rapidly acting histamine $H_2$-antagonist. It inhibits basal and stimulated secretion of gastric acid, reducing both the volume and the acid and pepsin content of the secretion. Zantac has a relatively long duration of action and so a single 150 mg dose effectively suppresses gastric acid secretion for twelve hours.

**Dosage and administration** Zantac Effervescent Tablets should be placed in half a glass of water (minimum 75 ml) and allowed to dissolve completely before swallowing. The effervescent tablets contain aspartame.

*Adults:* The usual dosage is 150 mg twice daily, taken in the morning and evening. Alternatively, patients with duodenal ulceration, gastric ulceration or oesophageal reflux disease may be treated with a single bedtime dose of 300 mg. It is not necessary to time the dose in relation to meals. In most cases of duodenal ulcer, benign gastric ulcer and post operative ulcer, healing occurs in four weeks. Healing usually occurs after a further four weeks of treatment in those patients whose ulcers have not fully healed after the initial course of therapy.

In ulcers following non-steroidal anti-inflammatory drug therapy or associated with continued non-steroidal anti-inflammatory drugs, eight week's treatment may be necessary.

For the prevention of non-steroidal anti-inflammatory drug-associated duodenal ulcers ranitidine 150 mg twice daily may be given concomitantly with non-steroidal anti-inflammatory drug therapy. In duodenal ulcer 300 mg twice daily for 4 weeks results in healing rates which are higher than those at 4 weeks with ranitidine 150 mg twice daily or 300 mg nocte. The increased dose has not been associated with an increased incidence of unwanted effects.

For duodenal ulcers associated with *Helicobacter pylori* infection Zantac 300 mg at bedtime or 150 mg twice daily may be given with oral amoxycillin 750 mg three times daily and metronidazole 500 mg three times daily for two weeks. Therapy with Zantac should continue for a further 2 weeks. This dose regimen significantly reduces the frequency of duodenal ulcer recurrence.

Maintenance treatment at a reduced dosage of 150 mg at bedtime is recommended for patients who have responded to short-term therapy, particularly those with a history of recurrent ulcer.

In patients with gastro-oesophageal reflux disease, a dose regimen of 150 mg twice daily for 2 weeks is recommended and this can be repeated in patients in whom the initial symptomatic response is inadequate.

In the management of oesophageal reflux disease, the recommended course of treatment is either 150 mg twice daily or 300 mg at bedtime for up to 8 weeks or if necessary 12 weeks.

In patients with moderate to severe oesophagitis, the dosage of ranitidine may be increased to 150 mg four times daily for up to twelve weeks.

The increased dose has not been associated with an increased incidence of unwanted effects. For the long-term treatment of healed oesophagitis, the recommended adult oral dose is 150 mg twice daily. Long-term treatment is not indicated in the management of patients with unhealed oesophagitis, with or without Barrett's epithelium.

In patients with Zollinger-Ellison syndrome, the starting dose is 150 mg three times daily and this may be increased as necessary. Patients with this syndrome have been given increasing doses up to 6 g per day and these doses have been well tolerated.

For patients with chronic episodic dyspepsia the recommended course of treatment is 150 mg twice daily for up to six weeks. Anyone not responding or relapsing shortly afterwards should be investigated.

In the prophylaxis of haemorrhage from stress ulceration in seriously ill patients or the prophylaxis of recurrent haemorrhage in patients bleeding from peptic ulceration, treatment with Zantac Tablets or Syrup 150 mg twice daily may be substituted for Zantac Injection (see separate Data Sheet) once oral feeding commences in patients considered to be still at risk from these conditions.

In patients thought to be at risk of acid aspiration syndrome an oral dose of 150 mg can be given 2 hours before induction of general anaesthesia, and preferably also 150 mg the previous evening. Alternatively, Zantac Injection for intravenous and intramuscular use is also available (see separate Data Sheet).

In obstetric patients at commencement of labour, an oral dose of 150 mg may be given followed by 150 mg at six-hourly intervals. It is recommended that since gastric emptying and drug absorption are delayed during labour, any patient requiring emergency general anaesthesia should be given, in addition, a non-particulate antacid (e.g. sodium citrate) prior to induction of anaesthesia. The usual precautions to avoid acid aspiration should also be taken.

*Children:* The recommended oral dose for treatment of peptic ulcer in children is 2 mg/kg to 4 mg/kg twice daily to a maximum of 300 mg ranitidine per day.

**Contra-indications, warnings, etc**

*Contra-indications:* Ranitidine is contra-indicated for patients known to have hypersensitivity to any component of the preparation.

*Precautions:* Treatment with a histamine $H_2$-antagonist may mask symptoms associated with carcinoma of the stomach and may therefore delay diagnosis of the condition. Accordingly, where gastric ulcer has been diagnosed or in patients of middle age and over with new or recently changed dyspeptic symptoms the possibility of malignancy should be excluded before therapy with Zantac Tablets or Syrup is instituted.

Ranitidine is excreted via the kidney and so plasma levels of the drug are increased in patients with severe renal impairment. Accordingly, it is recommended that the therapeutic regimen for Zantac in such patients be 150 mg at night for 4 to 8 weeks. The same dose should be used for maintenance treatment should this be deemed necessary. If an ulcer has not healed after treatment the standard dosage regimen of 150 mg twice daily should be instituted, followed, if need be, by maintenance treatment of 150 mg at night.

Regular supervision of patients who are taking non-steroidal anti-inflammatory drugs concomitantly with ranitidine is recommended, especially in the elderly. Current evidence shows that ranitidine protects against NSAID associated ulceration in the duodenum and not in the stomach.

Zantac crosses the placenta but therapeutic doses administered to obstetric patients in labour or undergoing caesarean section have been without any adverse effect on labour, delivery or subsequent neonatal progress. Zantac is also excreted in human breast milk.

Like other drugs, Zantac should only be used during pregnancy and nursing if considered essential.

Although clinical reports of acute intermittent porphyria associated with ranitidine administration have been rare and inconclusive, ranitidine should be avoided in patients with a history of this condition.

Zantac Effervescent Tablets contain sodium (see Presentation section). Care should therefore be taken in treating patients in whom sodium restriction is indicated. As Zantac Effervescent Tablets contain aspartame they should be used with caution in patients with phenylketonuria.

*Side-effects:* The following have been reported as events in clinical trials or in the routine management of patients treated with ranitidine. The relationship to ranitidine therapy has not been established in many cases.

Transient and reversible changes in liver function tests can occur. There have been occasional reports of hepatitis (hepatocellular, hepatocanalicular or mixed) with or without jaundice. These were usually reversible. Acute pancreatitis has been reported rarely.

Leucopenia and thrombocytopenia have occurred rarely in patients. These are usually reversible. Rare cases of agranulocytosis or of pancytopenia, sometimes with marrow hypoplasia, or aplasia have been reported.

Hypersensitivity reactions (urticaria, angioneurotic oedema, fever, bronchospasm, hypotension, anaphylactic shock) have been seen rarely following the parenteral and oral administration of ranitidine. These reactions have occasionally occurred after a single dose.

As with other $H_2$-receptor antagonists, there have been rare reports of bradycardia and A-V block.

Headache, sometimes severe, and dizziness have been reported in a very small proportion of patients. Rare cases of reversible mental confusion, depression and hallucinations have been reported, predominantly in severely ill and elderly patients.

Skin rash has been reported, including rare cases

of erythema multiforme. Musculoskeletal symptoms such as arthralgia and myalgia have been reported rarely.

No clinically significant interference with endocrine or gonadal function has been reported. There have been a few reports of breast symptoms (swelling and/or discomfort) in men taking ranitidine; some cases have resolved on continued ranitidine treatment. Discontinuation of therapy may be necessary in order to establish the underlying cause.

Antibiotic associated diarrhoea may occur when amoxycillin and metronidazole are taken with ranitidine.

*Use in elderly patients:* Rates of healing of ulcers in clinical trial patients aged 65 and over have not been found to differ from those in younger patients. Additionally, there was no difference in the incidence of adverse effects.

*Overdosage:* Zantac is very specific in action and accordingly no particular problems are expected following overdosage. In the case of the effervescent formulations, clinicians should be aware of the sodium content (see Presentation section). Symptomatic and supportive therapy should be given as appropriate. If need be, the drug may be removed from the plasma by haemodialysis.

**Pharmaceutical precautions** Zantac Syrup should be stored at a temperature not exceeding 25°C. Zantac Syrup should not be diluted or admixed with other liquid preparations.

Effervescent products should be stored below 30°C in a dry place.

**Legal category** POM.

**Package quantities**
Zantac Tablets 150 mg: Carton of 60 tablets, foil-wrapped (OP).
Zantac Tablets 300 mg: Carton of 30 tablets, foil-wrapped (OP).
Zantac Syrup: Bottles of 300 ml (OP).
Zantac Effervescent Tablets 150 mg: Carton of 4 polypropylene tubes, each containing 15 tablets (OP).
Zantac Effervescent Tablets 300 mg: Carton of 2 polypropylene tubes, each containing 15 tablets (OP).

**Further information**
*Drug interactions:* Ranitidine does not inhibit the hepatic cytochrome P450-linked mixed function oxygenase system. Accordingly, ranitidine does not potentiate the actions of drugs which are inactivated by this enzyme; these include amoxycillin, diazepam, lignocaine, phenytoin, metronidazole, propranolol, theophylline and warfarin. There is no evidence of an interaction between ranitidine and amoxycillin or metronidazole.

*Pharmacokinetics:* The bioavailability of ranitidine is consistently about 50%. Absorption of ranitidine after oral administration is rapid and peak plasma concentrations are usually achieved 2-3 hours after administration. Absorption is not significantly impaired by food or antacids. Ranitidine is not extensively metabolised. Elimination of the drug is primarily by tubular secretion. The elimination half-life of ranitidine is 2-3 hours. In balance studies with 150 mg 3H-ranitidine 60-70% of an oral dose was excreted in urine and 26% in faeces. Analysis of urine excreted in the first 24 hours after dosing showed that 35% of the oral dose was eliminated unchanged. About 6% of the dose is excreted as the N-oxide, 2% as the S-oxide, 2% as desmethyl ranitidine and 1-2% as the furoic acid analogue.

*Use in renal transplants:* Zantac has been used in patients with renal transplants.

*Duodenal ulcers associated with Helicobacter pylori:* Helicobacter pylori infects about 95% of patients with duodenal ulcer and 80% of patients with gastric ulcer.

Clinical evidence has shown that ranitidine combined with amoxycillin and metronidazole eradicates *Helicobacter pylori* in approximately 90% of patients. This combination therapy has been shown to significantly reduce duodenal ulcer recurrence.

Zantac Syrup contains 7.5% w/v ethanol.

**Product licence numbers**
Zantac Tablets 150 mg          10949/0042
Zantac Tablets 300 mg          10949/0043
Zantac Syrup                   10949/0108
Zantac Effervescent 150 mg Tablets   10949/0139
Zantac Effervescent 300 mg Tablets   10949/0140

## ZINACEF*

**Qualitative and quantitative composition** Vials contain either 250 mg, 750 mg or 1.5 g cefuroxime (as sodium).

**Pharmaceutical form** Cefuroxime is a white to cream powder to which appropriate amounts of water are added to prepare an off-white suspension for intra-muscular use or a yellowish solution for intravenous administration.

**Clinical particulars**
*Therapeutic indications:* Zinacef is a bactericidal cephalosporin antibiotic which is resistant to most β-lactamases and is active against a wide range of Gram-positive and Gram-negative organisms. It is indicated for the treatment of infections before the infecting organism has been identified or when caused by sensitive bacteria. In addition, it is an effective prophylactic against post-operative infection in a variety of operations. Usually Zinacef will be effective alone, but when appropriate it may be used in combination with an aminoglycoside antibiotic, or in conjunction with metronidazole, orally or by suppository or injection.

In situations where mixed aerobic and anaerobic infections are encountered or suspected (e.g. peritonitis, aspiration pneumonia, abscesses in the lung, pelvis and brain), or are likely to occur (e.g. in association with colorectal or gynaecological surgery) it is appropriate to administer Zinacef in combination with metronidazole.

Most of these infections will respond to an i.v. regimen of Zinacef (750 mg) plus metronidazole injection (500 mg/100 ml) administered eight-hourly for which the Zinacef/Metronidazole Infusion Kit may be appropriate. In more severe or well established mixed infections, an i.v. regimen of Zinacef (1.5 g) plus metronidazole injection (500 mg/100 ml) eight-hourly may be indicated. For the prophylaxis of infection in surgery (e.g. colorectal and gynaecological) a single dose of 1.5 g Zinacef plus metronidazole injection (500 mg/100 ml) is appropriate. Alternatively, this may be followed by two 750 mg doses of Zinacef plus metronidazole.

Indications include:
*Respiratory tract infections* for example, acute and chronic bronchitis, infected bronchiectasis, bacterial pneumonia, lung abscess and post operative chest infections.
*Ear, nose and throat infections* for example, sinusitis, tonsillitis and pharyngitis.
*Urinary tract infections* for example, acute and chronic pyelonephritis, cystitis and asymptomatic bacteriuria.
*Soft-tissue infections* for example, cellulitis, erysipelas, peritonitis and wound infections.
*Bone and joint infections* for example, osteomyelitis and septic arthritis.
*Obstetric and gynaecological infections* pelvic inflammatory diseases.
*Gonorrhoea* particularly when penicillin is unsuitable.
*Other infections* including septicaemia and meningitis.
*Prophylaxis* against infection in abdominal, pelvic, orthopaedic, cardiac, pulmonary, oesophageal and vascular surgery where there is increased risk from infection.

*Posology and method of administration:*
*Intramuscular:* Add 1 ml water for injections to 250 mg Zinacef or 3 ml water for injections to 750 mg Zinacef. Shake gently to produce an opaque suspension.

*Intravenous:* Dissolve Zinacef in water for injections using at least 2 ml for 250 mg, at least 6 ml for 750 mg or 15 ml for 1.5 g. For short intravenous infusion (e.g. up to 30 minutes), 1.5 g may be dissolved in 50 ml water for injections. These solutions may be given directly into the vein or introduced into the tubing of the giving set if the patient is receiving parenteral fluids.

*Adults:* Many infections will respond to 750 mg t.i.d. by i.m. or i.v. injection. For more severe infections, this dose should be increased to 1.5 g t.i.d. i.v. The frequency of i.m. or i.v. injection can be increased to six-hourly if necessary, giving total doses of 3 g to 6 g daily.

*Infants and children:* Doses of 30 to 100 mg/kg/day given as three or four divided doses. A dose of 60 mg/kg/day will be appropriate for most infections.

*Neonates:* Doses of 30 to 100 mg/kg/day given as two or three divided doses. In the first weeks of life the serum half-life of cefuroxime can be three to five times that in adults.

*Elderly:* See dosage in adults.

*Other recommendations:*
*Gonorrhoea:* 1.5 g should be given as a single dose. This may be given as 2×750 mg injections into different sites, e.g. each buttock.

*Meningitis:* Zinacef is suitable for sole therapy of bacterial meningitis due to sensitive strains. The following dosages are recommended:

*Infants and children:* 200 to 240 mg/kg/day i.v. in three or four divided doses. This dosage may be reduced to 100 mg/kg/day i.v. after three days or when clinical improvement occurs.

*Neonates:* 3 g i.v. every eight hours. Data are not yet sufficient to recommend a dose for intrathecal administration.

*Adults:* 3 g i.v. every eight hours. Data are not yet sufficient to recommend a dose for intrathecal administration.

*Prophylaxis:* The usual dose is 1.5 g i.v. with induction of anaesthesia for abdominal, pelvic and orthopaedic operations, but may be supplemented with two 750 mg i.m. doses eight and sixteen hours later. In cardiac, pulmonary, oesophageal and vascular operations, the usual dose is 1.5 g i.v. with induction of anaesthesia continuing with 750 mg i.m. t.d.s. for a further 24 to 48 hours.

In total joint replacement, 1.5 g cefuroxime powder may be mixed dry with each pack of methyl methacrylate cement polymer before adding the liquid monomer.

*Dosage in impaired renal function:* Cefuroxime is excreted by the kidneys. Therefore, as with all such antibiotics, in patients with markedly impaired renal function it is recommended that the dosage of Zinacef should be reduced to compensate for its slower excretion. However, it is not necessary to reduce the dose until the creatinine clearance falls below 20 ml/min. In adults with marked impairment (creatinine clearance 10-20 ml/min) 750 mg b.d. is recommended and with severe impairment (creatinine clearance <10 ml/min) 750 mg once daily is adequate. For patients on haemodialysis a further 750 mg dose should be given at the end of each dialysis. When continuous peritoneal dialysis is being used, a suitable dosage is usually 750 mg twice daily.

For patients in renal failure on continuous arterio-venous haemodialysis or high-flux haemofiltration in intensive therapy units a suitable dosage is 750 mg twice daily. For low-flux haemofiltration follow the dosage recommended under impaired renal function.

*Contra-indications:* Hypersensitivity to cephalosporin antibiotics.

*Special warnings and precautions for use:* Cephalosporin antibiotics may in general be given safely to patients who are hypersensitive to penicillins, although cross-reactions have been reported. Especial care is indicated in patients who have experienced an anaphylactic reaction to penicillin.

There may be some variation on the results of biochemical tests of renal function, but these do not appear to be of clinical importance. As a precaution, renal function should be monitored if this is already impaired.

*Interaction with other medicaments and other forms of interaction:* Cephalosporin antibiotics at high dosage should be given with caution to patients receiving concurrent treatment with potent diuretics such as frusemide and aminoglycosides, as these combinations are suspected of adversely affecting renal function. Clinical experience with Zinacef has shown that this is not likely to be a problem at the recommended dose levels.

Zinacef does not interfere in enzyme-based tests for glycosuria. Slight interference with copper reduction methods (Benedict's, Fehling's, Clinitest) may be observed. However, this should not lead to false-positive results, as may be experienced with some other cephalosporins.

It is recommended that either the glucose oxidase or hexokinase methods are used to determine blood/plasma glucose levels in patients receiving Zinacef. This antibiotic does not interfere in the alkaline picrate assay for creatinine.

*Pregnancy and lactation:* There is no experimental evidence of embryopathic or tetratogenic effects attributable to Zinacef but, as with all drugs, it should be administered with caution during the early months of pregnancy.

Cefuroxime is excreted in human milk, and consequently caution should be exercised when Zinacef is administered to a nursing mother.

*Effect on ability to drive and use machines:* None reported.

*Undesirable effects:* Adverse reactions to Zinacef have occurred relatively infrequently and have been generally mild and transient in nature.

Hypersensitivity reactions have been reported; these include skin rashes (maculopapular and urticarial), drug fever and very rarely anaphylaxis.

As with other antibiotics, prolonged use may result in the overgrowth of non-susceptible organisms, e.g. candida. Gastrointestinal disturbance, including, very rarely, symptoms of pseudomembranous colitis may occur during or after treatment. The principal changes in haematological parameters seen in some patients have been of decreased haemoglobin concentration and of eosinophilia, leukopenia and neutropenia. A positive Coombs' test has been found in some patients treated with cefuroxime — this phenomenon can interfere with the cross-matching of blood.

Although there are sometimes transient rises in serum liver enzymes or serum bilirubin, particularly in patients with pre-existing liver disease, there is no evidence of hepatic involvement.

Transient pain may be experienced at the site of intramuscular injection. This is more likely to occur with higher doses. However, it is unlikely to be a cause for discontinuation of treatment. Occasionally, thrombophlebitis may follow intravenous injection.

As with other cephalosporins, there have been very rare reports of thrombocytopenia.

*Overdose:* Overdosage of cephalosporins can cause cerebral irritation leading to convulsions. Serum levels of cefuroxime can be reduced by haemodialysis or peritoneal dialysis.

**Pharmacological properties**

*Pharmacodynamic properties:* Cefuroxime is a bactericidal cephalosporin antibiotic which is resistant to most β-lactamases and is active against a wide range of Gram-positive and Gram-negative organisms.

It is highly active against *Staphylococcus aureus*, including strains which are resistant to penicillin (but not the rare methicillin-resistant strains), *Staph. epidermidis, Haemophilus influenzae,* Klebsiella spp, Enterobacter spp, *Streptococcus pyogenes, Escherichia coli, Str. mitis (viridans group),* Clostridium spp, *Proteus mirabilis, Pr. rettgeri, Salmonella typhi, S. typhimurium* and other Salmonella spp, Shigella spp, Neisseria spp (including β-lactamase producing strains of *N. gonorrhoea*) and *Bordetella pertussis.* It is also moderately active against strains of *Pr. vulgaris, Morganella morganii* (formerly *Proteus morganii*) and *Bacteroides fragilis.*

The following organisms are not susceptible to cefuroxime: *Clostridium difficile,* Pseudomonas spp, Campylobacter spp, *Acinetobacter calcoaceticus,* Legionella spp and methicillin-resistant strains of *Staph. aureus* and *Staph. epidermidis.* Some strains of the following genera have also been found not to be susceptible to Zinacef: *Strep. faecalis, Morganella morganii, Proteus vulgaris,* Enterobacter spp, Citrobacter spp, Serratia spp and *Bacteroides fragilis.*

*In vitro* the activities of Zinacef and aminoglycoside antibiotics in combination have been shown to be at least additive with occasional evidence of synergy.

Metronidazole is active against a wide range of pathogenic micro-organisms notably species of Bacteroides, Fusobacteria, Clostridia, Eubacteria and anaerobic cocci. It is also active against *Gardnerella vaginalis, Trichomonas, Entamoeba histolytica, Giardia lamblia* and *Balantidium coli.*

*Pharmacokinetic properties:* Peak levels of cefuroxime are achieved within 30 to 45 minutes after intramuscular administration. The serum half-life after either intrasmuscular or intravenous injection is approximately 70 minutes. Concurrent administration of probenecid prolongs the excretion of the antibiotic and produces an elevated peak serum level. There is almost complete recovery of unchanged cefuroxime in the urine within 24 hours of administration, the major part being eliminated in the first six hours. Approximately 50% is excreted through the renal tubules and approximately 50% by glomerular filtration. Concentrations of cefuroxime in excess of the minimum inhibitory levels for common pathogens can be achieved in bone, synovial fluid and aqueous humor. Cefuroxime passes the blood-brain barrier when the meninges are inflamed.

**Pharmaceutical particulars**

*List of excipients:* None.

*Incompatibilities:* Cefuroxime is compatible with most commonly used intravenous fluids and electrolyte solutions.

The pH of 2.74% w/v Sodium Bicarbonate Injection BP considerably affects the colour of solutions and therefore this solution is not recommended for the dilution of Zinacef. However, if required, for patients receiving sodium bicarbonate injection by infusion, the Zinacef may be introduced into the tube of the giving set.

Zinacef should not be mixed in the syringe with aminoglycoside antibiotics.

*Shelf life:* Two years when stored below 25°C and protected from light.

*Special precautions for storage:* Store below 25°C and protect from light.

After constitution, Zinacef should be stored at 2 to 8°C for no longer than 24 hours.

*Nature and contents of container:*

*(1) Moulded glass (type I or III) vials with fluoro-resin laminated closures containing either 250 mg, 750 mg or 1.5 g Zinacef.*

*(2) A kit containing 1 vial of Zinacef 750 mg and 1×50 ml infusion of normal saline (PL3460/0015), a transfer needle for the preparation of an intravenous infusion and a swab (Zinacef/saline infusion kit).*

*(3) A kit containing 1 vial of Zinacef 750 mg and 1×500 mg/100 ml infusion of metronidazole (PL4515/0035) a transfer needle, a port stopper and a swab; for the preparation of an intravenous infusion (Zinacef/metronidazole infusion kit).*

*(4) A bulk pack of 100 vials.*

*(5) Monovial containing either 750 mg or 1.5 g Zinacef with transfer needle.*

**Marketing authorisation number** 0004/0263

**Date of approval/revision of SPC** 8 May 1997.

**Legal category** POM

## ZINNAT* TABLETS AND SUSPENSION

**Presentation** Zinnat Tablets 125 mg: white, film-coated, capsule-shaped tablets engraved with 'Glaxo' on one side and '125' on the other. Each tablet contains cefuroxime 125 mg (as cefuroxime axetil).

Zinnat Tablets 250 mg: white, film-coated, capsule-shaped tablets engraved with 'Glaxo' on one side and '250' on the other. Each tablet contains cefuroxime 250 mg (as cefuroxime axetil).

Zinnat Suspension 125 mg: granules for oral suspension in multidose bottles and sachets. Constitution of the multidose bottles as directed yields a suspension containing 125 mg of cefuroxime (as cefuroxime axetil) in each 5 ml. Constitution of the contents of the sachets gives a suspension containing 125 mg of cefuroxime (as cefuroxime axetil).

**Uses** Cefuroxime axetil is an oral prodrug of the bactericidal cephalosporin antibiotic cefuroxime, which is resistant to most β-lactamases and is active against a wide range of Gram-positive and Gram-negative organisms. It is indicated for the treatment of infections caused by sensitive bacteria.

*Indications include:*

*Lower respiratory tract infections:* for example, acute bronchitis, acute exacerbations of chronic bronchitis and pneumonia.

*Upper respiratory tract infections:* for example, ear, nose, throat infections, such as otitis media, sinusitis, tonsillitis and pharyngitis.

*Genito-urinary tract infections:* for example, pyelonephritis, cystitis and urethritis.

*Skin and soft-tissue infections:* for example, furunculosis, pyoderma and impetigo.

*Gonorrhoea:* acute uncomplicated gonococcal urethritis, and cervicitis.

*Treatment of early Lyme disease and subsequent prevention of late Lyme disease:* in adults and children over 12 years old.

*Microbiology:* Cefuroxime axetil owes its *in vivo* bactericidal activity to the parent compound, cefuroxime. Cefuroxime is a well-characterised and effective antibacterial agent which has broad-spectrum bactericidal activity against a wide range of common pathogens, including β-lactamase-producing strains. Cefuroxime has good stability to bacterial β-lactamase and consequently, is active against many ampicillin-resistant and amoxycillin-resistant strains. The bactericidal action of cefuroxime results from inhibition of cell-wall synthesis by binding to essential target proteins.

Cefuroxime is usually active against the following organisms *in vitro*:

Aerobes, Gram-negative: *Haemophilus influenzae* (including ampicillin-resistant strains); *Haemophilus parainfluenzae; Moraxella catarrhalis; Escherichia coli;* Klebsiella spp; *Proteus mirabilis; Proteus inconstans;* Providencia spp; *Proteus rettgeri* and *Neisseria gonorrhoeae* (including penicillinase and non-penicillinase-producing strains).

Some strains of *Morganella morganii,* Enterobacter spp and Citrobacter spp have been shown by *in vitro* tests to be resistant to cefuroxime and other β-lactam antibiotics.

Aerobes, Gram-positive: *Staphylococcus aureus* (including penicillinase-producing strains but excluding methicillin-resistant strains); *Staphylococcus epidermidis* (including penicillinase producing strains but excluding methicillin-resistant strains); *Streptococcus pyogenes* (and β-haemolytic streptococci), *Streptococcus pneumoniae;* Streptococcus Group B (*Streptococcus agalactiae*) and Propionibacterium spp. Certain strains of enterococci, e.g. *Streptococcus faecalis,* are resistant.

Anaerobes, Gram-positive and Gram-negative cocci (including Peptococcus and Peptostreptococcus spp); Gram-positive bacilli (including Clostridium spp) and Gram-negative bacilli (including Bacteroides and Fusobacterium spp). Most strains of *Bacteroides fragilis* are resistant.

Other organisms, *Borrelia burgdorferi.*

Pseudomonas spp, Campylobacter spp, *Acinetobacter calcoaceticus, Listeria monocytogenes,* Legionella spp and most strains of Serratia and *Proteus vulgaris* and *Clostridium difficile* are resistant to many cephalosporins including cefuroxime.

**Dosage and administration**

*Adults:* Most infections will respond to 250 mg b.d. In mild to moderate lower respiratory tract infections e.g. bronchitis 250 mg b.d. should be given. For more severe lower respiratory tract infections, or if pneumonia is suspected then 500 mg b.d. should be given. For urinary tract infections a dose of 125 mg b.d. is usually adequate; in pyelonephritis the recommended dose is 250 mg b.d. A single dose of one gram is recommended for the treatment of uncomplicated gonorrhoea. Lyme disease in adults and children over the age of 12 years: the recommended dose is 500 mg b.d. for 20 days.

*Children:* The usual dose is 125 mg b.d. (1 x 125 mg tablet or 5 ml of suspension or 1 x 125 mg sachet), or 10 mg/kg b.d. to a maximum of 250 mg daily. For otitis media, in children less than 2 years of age the usual dosage is 125 mg b.d. (1 x 125 mg tablet or 5 ml of suspension or 1 x 125 mg sachet), or 10 mg/kg b.d. to a maximum of 250 mg daily and in children over 2 years of age, 250 mg b.d. (1 x 250 mg tablet or 10 ml of suspension or 2 x 125 mg sachets), or 15 mg/kg b.d. to a maximum of 500 mg daily. There is no experience in children under 3 months of age.

Zinnat Tablets should not be crushed. Therefore, in younger children the suspension is more appropriate.

No special precautions are necessary in patients with renal impairment or on renal dialysis or in the elderly at dosages up to the normal maximum of 1 g per day.

The usual course of therapy is seven days.

Zinnat should be taken after food for optimum absorption.

**Contra-indications, warnings, etc**

*Contra-indications:* Hypersensitivity to cephalosporin antibiotics.

*Precautions:* Cephalosporin antibiotics may in general be given safely to patients who are hypersensitive to penicillins, although cross-reactions have been reported. Special care is indicated in patients who have experienced an anaphylactic reaction to penicillins.

As with other antibiotics, prolonged use of cefuroxime axetil may result in the overgrowth of non-susceptible organisms (e.g. Candida, Enterococci, *Clostridium difficile*), which may require interruption of treatment. Pseudomembranous colitis has been reported with the use of broad-spectrum antibiotics, therefore, it is important to consider its diagnosis in patients who develop serious diarrhoea during or after antibiotic use.

There is no experimental evidence of embryopathic or teratogenic effects attributable to cefuroxime axetil but, as with all drugs, it should be administered with caution during early months of pregnancy. Cefuroxime is excreted in human milk, and consequently caution should be exercised when cefuroxime axetil is administered to a nursing mother.

It is recommended that either the glucose oxidase or hexokinase methods are used to determine blood/plasma glucose levels in patients receiving cefuroxime axetil. This antibiotic does not interfere in the alkaline picrate assay for creatinine.

The Jarisch-Herxheimer reaction has been seen following Zinnat treatment of Lyme disease. It results from the bactericidal activity of Zinnat on the causative organism of Lyme disease, the spirochaete *Borrelia burgdorferi.* Patients should be reassured that this is a common and usually self-limited consequence of antibiotic treatment of Lyme disease.

*Side-effects:* Adverse reactions to cefuroxime axetil have been generally mild and transient in nature.

As with other cephalosporins, there have been rare reports of erythema multiforme, Stevens-Johnson syndrome, toxic epidermal necrolysis (exanthematic necrolysis) and hypersensitivity reactions including skin rashes, urticaria, pruritus, drug fever, serum sickness, and very rarely anaphylaxis.

Gastrointestinal disturbances including diarrhoea and nausea and vomiting have been reported. Diarrhoea, although uncommon, is more likely to be associated with higher doses.

As with other broad-spectrum antibiotics, there have been occasional reports of pseudomembranous colitis.

Headache has also been reported.

Eosinophilia and transient increases of hepatic enzyme levels [ALT (SGPT), AST (SGOT) and LDH] have been noted during Zinnat therapy. As with other cephalosporins, jaundice has been reported very rarely. A positive Coombs' test has been reported during treatment with cephalosporins–this phenomenon can interfere with cross-matching of blood.

*Overdosage:* Overdosage of cephalosporins can cause cerebral irritancy leading to convulsions.

Serum levels of cefuroxime can be reduced by haemodialysis or peritoneal dialysis.

**Pharmaceutical precautions** Zinnat Tablets should be stored below 30C.

Zinnat Suspension granules should be stored below 30C.

*Directions for constituting suspension in bottles:* Shake the bottle to loosen dry granules, add water as directed on the label and replace cap. INVERT bottle and shake granules down into water using a rocking action. Continue to shake the bottle until the suspension is well dispersed. If using a dosing syringe, allow the constituted suspension to stand for at least one hour before taking the first dose.

If desired the dose of the constituted suspension may be added to children's cold drinks such as fruit drinks or cold milk immediately prior to administration.

*Directions for constituting suspension from sachets:* Empty granules from sachet into a glass, add 10 ml water, or 10 ml children's cold drinks such as fruit drinks or milk, stir well and drink straight away.

The constituted suspension (in multidose bottles) should be stored below 25°C and preferably in a refrigerator. The constituted suspension (from sachets) and the further diluted suspension from multidose bottles in children's cold drinks should be taken immediately.

The constituted suspension (in multidose bottles) retains potency for up to 10 days when stored below 25°C.

Zinnat granules should not be constituted in hot drinks. The constituted suspension should not be mixed with hot drinks.

**Legal category** POM.

**Package quantities** Zinnat Tablets, both 125 mg and 250 mg strengths, are supplied in foil strips of 14 and 50.

Zinnat Suspension, 125 mg/5 ml, granules for oral suspension are supplied in multidose bottles of 70 ml and in 125 mg sachets packed in cartons of 14.

**Further information** After oral administration, cefuroxime axetil is absorbed from the gastrointestinal tract and rapidly hydrolysed in the intestinal mucosa and blood to release cefuroxime into the circulation. Optimum absorption occurs when it is administered after a meal. Peak serum cefuroxime levels occur approximately two to three hours after oral dosing. The serum half life is about 1.2 hours. Approximately 50% of serum cefuroxime is protein bound. Cefuroxime is not metabolised and is excreted by glomerular filtration and tubular secretion. Concurrent administration of probenecid increases the area under the mean serum concentration time curve by 50%. Serum levels of cefuroxime are reduced by dialysis.

Cefuroxime is also available as the sodium salt (Zinacef) for parenteral administration. This permits parenteral therapy with cefuroxime to be followed by oral therapy in situations where a change from parenteral to oral treatment is clinically indicated.

**Product licence numbers**
Zinnat Tablets 125 mg 10949/0095
Zinnat Tablets 250 mg 10949/0096
Zinnat Suspension 125 mg 10949/0094

## ZOFRAN* INJECTION
## ZOFRAN* FLEXI-AMP INJECTION

**Qualitative and quantitative composition** Zofran Injection 2 mg/ml: 2 ml glass ampoules each containing 4 mg ondansetron (as hydrochloride dihydrate) in aqueous solution for intramuscular or intravenous administration. 4 ml glass ampoules each containing 8 mg ondansetron (as hydrochloride dihydrate) in aqueous solution for intravenous or intramuscular administration.

Zofran Flexi-amp injection 2 mg/ml: 2 ml plastic ampoules each containing 4 mg ondansetron (as hydrochloride dihydrate) in aqueous solution for intramuscular or intravenous administration. 4 ml plastic ampoules each containing 8 mg ondansetron (as hydrochloride dihydrate) in aqueous solution for intravenous or intramuscular administration.

**Pharmaceutical form** Injection (aqueous solution).

**Clinical particulars**
*Therapeutic indications:* Zofran is indicated for the management of nausea and vomiting induced by cytotoxic chemotherapy and radiotherapy, and for the prevention and treatment of post-operative nausea and vomiting (PONV).

*Posology and method of administration:*
*Chemotherapy and radiotherapy*
*Adults:* The emetogenic potential of cancer treatment varies according to the doses and combinations of chemotherapy and radiotherapy regimens used. The route of administration and dose of Zofran should be flexible in the range of 8 to 32 mg a day and selected as shown below.

*Emetogenic chemotherapy and radiotherapy.* For most patients receiving emetogenic chemotherapy or radiotherapy, Zofran 8 mg should be administered as a slow intravenous injection immediately before treatment, or orally 1 to 2 hours before treatment, followed by 8 mg orally twelve hourly.

To protect against delayed or prolonged emesis after the first 24 hours, Zofran should be continued orally, 8 mg twice daily for up to 5 days after a course of treatment.

*Highly emetogenic chemotherapy:* For patients receiving highly emetogenic chemotherapy, e.g. high-dose cisplatin. Zofran has been shown to be equally effective in the following dose schedules over the first 24 hours of chemotherapy.

A single dose of 8 mg by slow intravenous injection immediately before chemotherapy.

A dose of 8 mg by slow intravenous injection immediately before chemotherapy, followed by two further intravenous doses of 8 mg two to four hours apart, or by a constant infusion of 1 mg/hour for up to 24 hours.

A single dose of 32 mg diluted in 50 to 100 ml of saline or other compatible infusion fluid (see *Instructions for use/handling*) and infused over not less than 15 minutes immediately before chemotherapy.

The selection of dose regimen should be determied by the severity of the emetogenic challenge.

The efficacy of Zofran in highly emetogenic chemotherapy may be enhanced by the addition of a single intravenous dose of dexamethasone sodium phosphate, 20 mg administered prior to chemotherapy.

To protect against delayed or prolonged emesis after the first 24 hours, Zofran should be continued orally, 8 mg twice daily for up to 5 days after a course of treatment.

*Children:* Zofran may be administered as a single intravenous dose of 5 mg/m$^2$ immediately before chemotherapy, followed by 4 mg orally twelve hours later. 4 mg orally twice daily should be continued for up to 5 days after a course of treatment.

*Elderly:* Zofran is well tolerated by patients over 65 years and no alteration of dosage, dosing frequency or route of administration are required.

*Patients with renal impairment:* No alteration of daily dosage or frequency of dosing, or route of administration are required.

*Patients with hepatic impairment:* Clearance of Zofran is significantly reduced and serum half-life significantly prolonged in subjects with moderate or severe impairment of hepatic function. In such patients a total daily dose of 8 mg should not be exceeded.

*Post-operative nausea and vomiting (PONV): Adults:* For the prevention of PONV Zofran may be administered as a single dose of 4 mg given by intramuscular or slow intravenous injection at induction of anaesthesia or as a single dose of 16 mg given orally one hour prior to anaesthesia.

For treatment of established PONV a single dose of 4 mg given by intramuscular or slow intravenous injection is recommended.

*Children (aged 2 years and over):* For prevention of PONV in paediatric patients having surgery performed under general anaesthesia, ondansetron may be administered by slow intravenous injection at a dose of 0.1 mg/kg up to a maximum of 4 mg either prior to, at or after induction of anaesthesia.

For treatment of established PONV in paediatric patients, ondansetron may be administered by slow intravenous injection at a dose of 0.1 mg/kg up to a maximum of 4 mg.

There is limited data on the use of Zofran in the prevention and treatment of PONV in children under 2 years of age.

*Elderly:* There is limited experience in the use of Zofran in the prevention and treatment of PONV in the elderly, however, Zofran is well tolerated in patients over 65 years receiving chemotherapy.

*Patients with renal impairment:* No alteration of daily dosage or frequency of dosing, or route of administration are required.

*Patients with hepatic impairment:* Clearance of Zofran is significantly reduced and serum half life significantly prolonged in subjects with moderate or severe impairment of hepatic function. In such patients a total daily dose of 8 mg should not be exceeded.

*Patients with poor sparteine/debrisoquine metabolism:* The elimination half-life of ondansetron is not altered in subjects classified as poor metabolisers of sparteine and debrisoquine. Consequently in such patients repeat dosing will give drug exposure levels no different from those of the general population. No alteration of daily dosage or frequency of dosing are required.

*Contra-indications:* Hypersensitivity to any component of the preparation.

*Special warnings and precautions for use:* None.

*Interaction with other medicaments and other forms of interaction:* There is no evidence that ondansetron either induces or inhibits the metabolism of other drugs commonly co-administered with it. Specific studies have shown that ondansetron does not interact with alcohol, temazepam, frusemide, tramadol and propofol.

*Pregnancy and lactation:* Zofran is not teratogenic in animals. There is no experience in humans. As with other medications Zofran should not be used during pregnancy, especially during the first trimester, unless the expected benefit to the patient is thought to outweigh any possible risk to the fetus.

Tests have shown that ondansetron passes into the milk of lactating animals. It is therefore recommended that mothers receiving Zofran should not breast-feed their babies.

*Effects on ability to drive and use machines:* In psychomotor testing ondansetron does not impair performance nor cause sedation.

*Undesirable effects:* Ondansetron is known to increase large bowel transit time and may cause constipation in some patients. The following side effects can occur: headache, a sensation of flushing or warmth, hiccups and occasional transient, asymptomatic increases in aminotransferases. There have been rare reports of immediate hypersensitivity reactions, sometimes severe, including anaphylaxis. Rare cases of transient visual disturbances (e.g. blurred vision) and dizziness have been reported during rapid intravenous administration of ondansetron. There have been rare reports suggestive of involuntary movement disorders without definitive evidence of persistent clinical sequelae and seizures have been rarely observed although no known pharmacological mechanism can account for ondansetron causing these effects. Chest pain, cardiac arrhythmias, hypotension and bradycardia have been rarely reported.

*Overdose:* Little is at present known about overdosage with ondansetron. However, two patients who received doses of 84 and 145 mg intravenously reported only mild side-effects and required no active therapy. In cases of suspected overdose, symptomatic and supportive therapy should be given as appropriate.

**Pharmacological properties**
*Pharmacodynamic properties:* Ondansetron is a potent, highly selective 5HT$_3$ receptor-antagonist. Its precise mode of action in the control of nausea and vomiting is not known. Chemotherapeutic agents and radiotherapy may cause release of 5HT in the small intestine initiating a vomiting reflex by activating vagal afferents via 5HT$_3$ receptors. Ondansetron blocks the initiation of this reflex. Activation of vagal afferents may also cause a release of 5HT in the area postrema, located on the floor of the fourth ventricle, and this may also promote emesis through a central mechanism. Thus, the effect of ondansetron in the management of the nausea and vomiting induced by cytotoxic chemotherapy and radiotherapy is probably due to antagonism of 5HT$_3$ receptors on neurons located both in the peripheral and central nervous system. The mechanisms of action in post-operative nausea and vomiting are not known but there may be common pathways with cytotoxic-induced nausea and vomiting.

Ondansetron does not alter plasma prolactin concentrations.

The role of ondansetron in opiate-induced emesis is not yet established,

*Pharmacokinetic properties:* The disposition of ondansetron following oral, intramuscular or intravenous dosing is similar with a terminal elimination half-life of about 3 hours and steady state volume of distribution of about 140 L. A 4 mg intravenous infusion of ondansetron given over five minutes results in peak plasma concentrations of about 65 ng/ml. Following 4 mg intramuscular administration of ondansetron, peak plasma concentrations of about 25 ng/ml are attained within 10 minutes of injection. Equivalent systemic exposure is achieved after 4 mg intramuscular and intravenous administration of ondansetron. Ondansetron is not highly protein bound (70–76%). Ondansetron is cleared from the systemic circulation predominantly by hepatic metabolism through multiple enzymatic pathways. Less than 5% of the absorbed dose is excreted unchanged in the urine. the absence of the enzyme CYP2D6 (the debrisoquine polymorphism) has no effect on ondansetron's pharmacokinetics. The pharmacokinetic properties of ondansetron are unchanged on repeat dosing.

Studies in healthy elderly volunteers have shown slight, but clinically insignificant, age-related increases in both oral bioavailability (65%) and half-life (5 h) of ondansetron. Gender differences were shown in the disposition of ondansetron, with females having a greater rate and extent of absorption following an oral dose and reduced systemic clearance and volume of distribution (adjusted for weight).

In a study of 21 paediatric patients aged between 3 and 12 years undergoing elective surgery with general anaesthesia, the absolute values for both the clearance and volume of distribution of ondansetron following a single intravenous dose of 2 mg (3–7 years old) or 4 mg (8–12 years old) were reduced. The magnitude of the change was age-related, with clearance falling from about 300 ml/min at 12 years of age to 100 ml/min at 3 years. Volume of distribution fell from about 75 L at 12 years to 17 L at 3 years. Use of weight-based dosing (0.1 mg/kg up to 4 mg maximum) compensates for these changes and is effective in normalising systemic exposure in paediatric patients.

In patients with renal impairment (creatinine clearance > 15 ml/min), both systemic clearance and volume of distribution are reduced, resulting in a slight, but clinically insignificant, increase in elimination half-life (5.4 h). A study in patients with severe renal impairment who required regular haemodialysis (studied between dialyses) showed ondansetron's pharmacokinetics to be essentially unchanged.

In patients with severe hepatic impairment, ondansetron's systemic clearance is markedly reduced with prolonged elimination half-lives (15–32 h).

*Preclinical safety data:* No additional data of relevance.

**Pharmaceutical particulars**
*List of excipients:* Citric acid monohydrate, sodium citrate, sodium chloride, Water for Injections.

*Incompatibilities:* Zofran injection should not be administered in the same syringe or infusion as any other medication.

*Shelf life:* 36 months (unopened). 24 hours (dilutions stored 2–8°C).

*Special precautions for storage:* Protect from light. Store below 30°C.

Dilutions of Zofran Injection in compatible intravenous infusion fluids are stable under normal room lighting conditions or daylight for at least 24 hours, thus no protection from light is necessary while infusion takes place.

*Nature and contents of container:* Zofran Injection: Type I clear glass snap-ring ampoules.

Zofran Flexi-amp Injection: Polypropylene blow-fill-sealed ampoules with a twist-off top and overwrapped in a double foil blister.

Five ampoules are packed in a carton.

*Instructions for use/handling:* Zofran Injection and Zofran Flexi-amp Injection should not be autoclaved.

*Compatibility with intravenous fluids:* Zofran Injection should only be admixed with those infusion solutions which are recommended:
Sodium Chloride Intravenous Infusion BP 0.9% w/v
Glucose Intravenous Infusion BP 5% w/v
Mannitol Intravenous Infusion BP 10% w/v
Ringers Intravenous Infusion
Potassium Chloride 0.3% w/v and Sodium Chloride 0.9% w/v Intravenous Infusion BP
Potassium Chloride 0.3% w/v and Glucose 5% w/v Intravenous Infusion BP

In keeping with good pharmaceutical practice dilutions of Zofran injection in intravenous fluids should be prepared at the time of infusion or stored at 2–8°C for no more than 24 hours before the start of administration.

Compatibility studies have been undertaken in polyvinyl chloride infusion bags and polyvinyl chloride administration sets. It is considered that adequate stability would also be conferred by the use of polyethylene infusion bags or Type 1 glass bottles. Dilutions of Zofran in sodium chloride 0.9% w/v or in glucose 5% w/v have been demonstrated to be stable in polypropylene syringes. It is considered that Zofran Injection diluted with other compatible infusion fluids would be stable in polypropylene syringes.

*Compatibility with other drugs:* Zofran may be administered by intravenous infusion at 1 mg/hour, e.g. from an infusion bag or syringe pump. The following drugs may be administered via the Y-site of the Zofran giving set for ondansetron concentrations of 16 to 160 micrograms/ml (e.g. 8 mg/500 ml and 8 mg/50 ml respectively):

*Cisplatin:* Concentrations up to 0.48 mg/ml (e.g. 240 mg in 500 ml) administered over one to eight hours.

*5-Fluorouracil:* Concentrations up to 0.8 mg/ml (e.g. 2.4 g in 3 litres or 400 mg in 500 ml) administered at a rate of at least 20 ml per hour (500 ml per 24 hours). Higher concentrations of 5-fluorouracil may cause precipitation of ondansetron. The 5-fluorouracil infusion may contain up to 0.045% w/v magnesium chloride in addition to other excipients shown to be compatible.

*Carboplatin:* Concentrations in the range 0.18 mg/ml to 9.9 mg/ml (e.g. 90 mg in 500 ml to 990 mg in 100 ml), administered over ten minutes to one hour.

*Etoposide:* Concentrations in the range 0.14 mg/ml to 0.25 mg/ml (e.g. 72 mg in 500 ml to 250 mg in 1 litre), administered over thirty minutes to one hour.

*Ceftazidime:* Doses in the range 250 mg to 2,000 mg reconstituted with Water for Injections BP as recommended by the manufacturer (e.g. 2.5 ml for 250 mg and 10 ml for 2 g ceftazidime) and given as an intravenous bolus injection over approximately five minutes.

*Cyclophosphamide:* Doses in the range 100 mg to 1 g, reconstituted with Water for Injections BP, 5 ml per 100 mg cyclophosphamide, as recommended by the manufacturer and given as an intravenous bolus injection over approximately five minutes.

*Doxorubicin:* doses in the range 10–100 mg reconstituted with Water for Injections BP, 5 ml per 10 mg doxorubicin, as recommended by the manufacturer and given as an intravenous bolus injection over approximately 5 minutes.

*Dexamethasone:* Dexamethasone sodium phosphate 20 mg may be administered as a slow intravenous injection over 2–5 minutes via the Y-site of an infusion set delivering 8 or 32 mg of ondansetron diluted in 50–100 ml of a compatible infusion fluid over approximately 15 minutes. Compatibility between dexamethasone sodium phosphate and ondansetron has been demonstrated supporting administration of these drugs through the same giving set resulting in concentrations in line of 32 microgram – 2.5 mg/ml for dexamethasone sodium phosphate and 8 microgram – 1 mg/ml for ondansetron.

**Marketing authorisation number** 0004/0375.

**Date of approval/revision of SPC** January 1997.

**Legal category** POM.

## ZOFRAN* SUPPOSITORIES 16 mg ▼

**Qualitative and quantitative composition** White, torpedo-shaped suppositories containing 16 mg of ondansetron.

**Pharmaceutical form** Suppositories.

**Clinical particulars**
*Therapeutic indications* The management of nausea and vomiting induced by cytotoxic chemotherapy and radiotherapy.

*Posology and method of administration:*
*Adults (including the elderly):* The emetogenic potential of cancer treatment varies according to the doses and combinations of chemotherapy and radiotherapy regimens used. The route of administration and dose of Zofran should be flexible and selected as shown below.

*Emetogenic chemotherapy and radiotherapy:* Zofran can be given either by rectal, oral (tablets or syrup) or intravenous administration.

For rectal administration: One suppository (16 mg ondansetron) 1–2 hours before treatment.

To protect against delayed or prolonged emesis after the first 24 hours, oral or rectal treatment with Zofran should be continued for up to 5 days after a course of treatment.

The recommended dose for rectal administration is one suppository daily.

*Highly emetogenic chemotherapy (e.g. high-dose cisplatin):* Zofran can be given either by rectal or intravenous administration.

For rectal administration: One suppository (16 mg ondansetron) 1–2 hours before treatment.

The efficacy of Zofran in highly emetogenic chemotherapy may be enhanced by the addition of a single intravenous dose of dexamethasone sodium phosphate 20 mg, administered prior to chemotherapy.

To protect against delayed or prolonged emesis after the first 24 hours, oral or rectal treatment with Zofran should be continued for up to 5 days after a course of treatment.

The recommended dose for rectal administration is one suppository daily.

*Children:* The use of Zofran Suppositories in children is not recommended.

Zofran may be administered as a single intravenous dose of 5 mg/m² immediately before chemotherapy, followed by 4 mg orally twelve hours later. 4 mg orally twice daily should be continued for up to 5 days after a course of treatment.

*Patients with renal impairment:* No special requirements.

*Patients with hepatic impairment:* Clearance of Zofran is significantly reduced and serum half-life significantly prolonged in subjects with moderate or severe impairment of hepatic function. In such patients a total daily dose of 8 mg should not be exceeded and therefore intravenous or oral administration is recommended.

*Patients with poor sparteine/debrisoquine metabolism:* The elimination half-life of ondansetron is not altered in subjects classified as poor metabolisers of sparteine and debrisoquine. Consequently, in such patients repeat dosing will give drug exposure levels no different from those of the general population. No alteration of daily dosage or frequency of dosing are required.

*Contra-indications:* Hypersensitivity to any ingredient.

*Special warnings and precautions for use:* None.

*Interaction with other medicaments and other forms of interaction:* There is no evidence that ondansetron either induces or inhibits the metabolism of other drugs commonly co-administered with it. Specific studies have shown that ondansetron does not interact with alcohol, temazepam, frusemide, tramadol and propofol.

*Pregnancy and lactation:* Zofran is not teratogenic in animals. There is no experience in humans. As with other medications Zofran should not be used during pregnancy, especially during the first trimester, unless the expected benefit to the patient is thought to outweigh any possible risk to the fetus.

Tests have shown that ondansetron passes into the milk of lactating animals. It is therefore recommended that mothers receiving Zofran should not breast-feed their babies.

*Effect on ability to drive and use machines:* None reported.

*Undesirable effects:* There have been rare reports of immediate hypersensitivity reactions, sometimes severe, including anaphylaxis.

Chest pain, cardiac arrhythmias, hypotension and bradycardiac have been rarely reported.

There have been rare reports suggestive of involuntary movement disorders without definitive evidence of persistent clinical sequelae, and seizures have been rarely observed, although no known pharmacological mechanism can account for ondansetron causing these effects.

Ondansetron is known to increase large bowel transit time and may cause constipation in some patients.

The following side effects can occur: headache, a sensation of flushing or warmth, hiccups and occasional transient, asymptomatic increases in aminotransferases.

There have been rare reports of a local anal/rectal burning sensation following insertion of a suppository.

*Overdose:* Little is at present known about overdosage with ondansetron. However, two patients who received doses of 84 and 145 mg intraveneously reported only mild side-effects and required no active therapy. In cases of suspected overdose, symptomatic and supportive therapy should be given as appropriate.

The use of Ipecacuanha to treat overdose with ondansetron is not recommended as patients are unlikely to respond due to the anti-emetic action of Zofran itself.

**Pharmacological properties**
*Pharmacodynamic properties:* Ondansetron is a potent, highly selective $5HT_3$ receptor-antagonist. The precise mode of action in the control of nausea and vomiting is not known. Chemotherapeutic agents and radiotherapy may cause release of 5HT in the small intestine initiating a vomiting reflex by activating vagal afferents via $5HT_3$ receptors. Ondansetron blocks the initiation of this reflex. Activation of vagal afferents may also cause a release of 5HT in the area postrema, located on the floor of the fourth ventricle, and this may also promote emesis through a central mechanism. Thus, the effect of ondansetron in the management of the nausea and vomiting induced by cytotoxic chemotherapy and radiotherapy is probably due to antagonism of $5HT_3$ receptors on neurons located both in the peripheral and central nervous system. The mechanisms of action in post-operative nausea and vomiting are not known but there may be common pathways with cytotoxic-induced nausea and vomiting.

Ondansetron does not alter plasma prolactin concentrations.

The role of ondansetron in opiate-induced emesis is not yet established.

*Pharmacokinetic properties:* Following rectal administration, plasma ondansetron concentrations become detectable between 15 and 60 minutes after dosing. Concentrations rise in an essentially linear fashion, until peak concentrations of 20–30 ng/ml are attained, typically 6 hours after dosing. Plasma concentrations then fall, but at a slower rate than observed following oral dosing due to continued absorption of ondansetron. The half-life of the elimination phase is determined by the rate of ondansetron absorption, not systemic clearance, and is approximately 6 hours. Females show a small, clinically insignificant, increase in half-life in comparison with males. The absolute bioavailability of ondansetron from the suppository is approximately 60% and is not affected by gender.

Ondansetron is not highly protein bound (70–76%), and is cleared from the systemic circulation predominantly by hepatic metabolism through multiple enzymatic pathways. Less than 5% of the absorbed dose is excreted unchanged in the urine. The absence of the enzyme CYP2D6 (the debrisoquine polymorphism) has no effect on the pharmacokinetics. The pharmacokinetic properties of ondansetron are unchanged on repeat dosing.

Studies in healthy elderly volunteers show slight age-related increases in both oral bioavailability (65%) and half-life (5 h) of ondansetron. In patients with renal impairment (creatinine clearance >15 ml/min), systemic clearance and volume of distribution are reduced following i.v. administration of ondansetron, resulting in a slight, but clinically insigificant increase in elimination half-life (5.4 h). A study in patients with severe renal impairment who required regular haemodialysis (studied between dialyses) showed the pharmacokinetics to be essentially unchanged following intraveneous administration.

Specific studies in the elderly or patients with renal impairment have been limited to i.v. and oral administration. However, it is anticipated that the half-life of ondansetron after rectal administration, in these populations will be similar to that seen in healthy volunteers since the rate of elimination of ondansetron following rectal administration is not determined by systemic clearance.

The pharmacokinetics of ondansetron following administration as a suppository have not been evaluated in patients with hepatic impairment.

*Preclinical safety data:* No additional data of relevance.

**Pharmaceutical particulars**
*List of excipients:* Witepsol S58.

*Incompatibilities:* None reported.

*Shelf life:* 2 years.

*Special precautions for storage:* Store below 30°C.

*Nature and contents of container:* Each suppository is in an individually sealed cavity enclosed in a perforated cardboard mount and packed into a carton.

*Instructions for use/handling:* Insert into the rectum.

For detailed instructions see the patient information leaflet included in every pack.

**Marketing authorisation number** 10949/0247.

**Date of approval/revision of SPC** January 1997.

**Legal category** POM.

## ZOFRAN* SYRUP ▼

**Qualitative and quantitative composition** Sugar-free strawberry flavoured liquid.

Each 5 ml contains 4 mg of ondansetron as the hydrochloride dihydrate.

**Pharmaceutical form** Oral solution.

**Clinical particulars**
*Therapeutic indications:* The management of nausea and vomiting induced by cytotoxic chemotherapy and radiotherapy, and for the prevention of post-operative nausea and vomiting in adults.

*Posology and method of administration:*
*Chemotherapy and radiotherapy-induced nausea and vomiting – Adults (including the elderly):* The emetogenic potential of cancer treatment varies according to the doses and combinations of chemotherapy and radiotherapy regimens used. The route of administration and dose of Zofran should be flexible and selected as shown below.

*Emetogenic chemotherapy and radiotherapy:* Zofran can be given either by rectal, oral (tablets or syrup) or intravenous administration.

For oral administration: 8 mg 1–2 hours before treatment, followed by 8 mg 12 hours later.

To protect against delayed or prolonged emesis after the first 24 hours, oral or rectal treatment with Zofran should be continued for up to 5 days after a course of treatment.

The recommended dose for oral administration is 8 mg twice daily.

*Highly emetogenic chemotherapy (e.g. high dose cisplatin):* Zofran can be given either by rectal or intravenous administration.

To protect against delayed or prolonged emesis after the first 24 hours, oral or rectal treatment with Zofran should be continued for up to 5 days after a course of treatment.

The recommended dose for oral administration is 8 mg twice daily.

*Children:* Zofran may be administered as a single intravenous dose of 5 mg/m$^2$ immediately before chemotherapy, followed by 4 mg orally twelve hours later. 4 mg orally twice daily should be continued for up to 5 days after a course of treatment.

*Post operative nausea and vomiting* (PONV):
*Adults: For the prevention of PONV:* Zofran can be administered orally or by intravenous or intramuscular injection.

For oral administration: 16 mg one hour prior to anaesthesia. Alternatively, 8 mg one hour prior to anaesthesia followed by two further doses of 8 mg at eight-hourly intervals.

*For the treatment of established PONV:* Intravenous or intramuscular administration is recommended.

*Children (aged 2 years and over):* For the prevention and treatment of PONV: Slow intravenous injection is recommended.

*Elderly:* There is limited experience in the use of Zofran in the prevention and treatment of PONV in the elderly. However Zofran is well tolerated in patients over 65 years receiving chemotherapy.

**For both indications**
*Patients with renal impairment:* No special requirements.

*Patients with hepatic impairment:* Clearance of Zofran is significantly reduced and serum half-life significantly prolonged in subjects with moderate or severe impairment of hepatic function. In such patients a total daily dose of 8 mg should not be exceeded.

*Patients with poor sparteine/debrisoquine metabolism:* The elimination half-life of ondansetron is not altered in subjects classified as poor metabolisers of sparteine and debrisoquine. Consequently, in such patients repeat dosing will give drug exposure levels no different from those of the general population. No alteration of daily dosage or frequency of dosing are required.

*Contra-indications:* Hypersensitivity to any ingredient.

*Special warnings and precautions for use:* None.

*Interaction with other medicaments and other forms of interaction:* There is no evidence that ondansetron either induces or inhibits the metabolism of other drugs commonly co-administered with it. Specific studies have shown that ondansetron does not interact with alcohol, temazepam, frusemide, tramadol and propofol.

*Pregnancy and lactation:* Zofran is not teratogenic in animals. There is no experience in humans. As with other medications Zofran should not be used during pregnancy, especially during the first trimester, unless the expected benefit to the patient is thought to outweigh any possible risk to the fetus.

Tests have shown that ondansetron passes into the milk of lactating animals. It is therefore recommended that mothers receiving Zofran should not breast-feed their babies.

*Effect on ability to drive and use machines:* None reported.

*Undesirable effects:* There have been rare reports of immediate hypersensitivity reactions, sometimes severe, including anaphylaxis.

Chest pain, cardiac arrhythmias, hypotension and bradycardiac have been rarely reported.

There have been rare reports suggestive of involuntary movement disorders without definitive evidence of persistent clinical sequelae, and seizures have been rarely observed, although no known pharmacological mechanism can account for ondansetron causing these effects.

Ondansetron is known to increase large bowel transit time and may cause constipation in some patients.

The following side effects can occur: headache, a sensation of flushing or warmth, hiccups and occasional transient, asymptomatic increases in aminotransferases.

*Overdose:* Little is at present known about overdosage with ondansetron. However, two patients who received doses of 84 and 145 mg intraveneously reported only mild side-effects and required no active therapy. In cases of suspected overdose, symptomatic and supportive therapy should be given as appropriate.

The use of Ipecacuanha to treat overdose with ondansetron is not recommended as patients are unlikely to respond due to the anti-emetic action of Zofran itself.

**Pharmacological properties**
*Pharmacodynamic properties:* Ondansetron is a potent, highly selective $5HT_3$ receptor-antagonist. Its precise mode of action in the control of nausea and vomiting is not known. Chemotherapeutic agents and radiotherapy may cause release of 5HT in the small intestine initiating a vomiting reflex by activating vagal afferents via $5HT_3$ receptors. Ondansetron blocks the initiation of this reflex. Activation of vagal afferents may also cause a release of 5HT in the area postrema, located on the floor of the fourth ventricle, and this may also promote emesis through a central mechanism. Thus, the effect of ondansetron in the management of the nausea and vomiting induced by cytotoxic chemotherapy and radiotherapy is probably due to antagonism of $5HT_3$ receptors on neurons located both in the peripheral and central nervous system. The mechanisms of action in post-operative nausea and vomiting are not known but there may be common pathways with cytotoxic-induced nausea and vomiting.

Ondansetron does not alter plasma prolactin concentrations.

The role of ondansetron in opiate-induced emesis is not yet established.

*Pharmacokinetic properties:* Following oral administration of ondansetron, absorption is rapid with maximum peak plasma concentrations of about 30 ng/ml being attained and achieved in approximately 1.5 hours after an 8 mg dose. The syrup and tablet formulations are bioequivalent and have an absolute oral bioavailability of 60%. The disposition of ondansetron following oral, intravenous and intramuscular dosing is similar with a terminal elimination half-life of approximately 3 hours and a steady-state volume of distribution of about 140 L. Ondansetron is not highly protein bound (70–76%) and is cleared from the systemic circulation predominantly by hepatic metabolism through multiple enzymatic pathways. Less than 5% of the absorbed dose is excreted unchanged in the urine. The absence of the enzyme CYP2D6 (the debrisoquine polymorphism) has no effect on the pharmacokinetics of ondansetron. The pharmacokinetic properties of ondansetron are unchanged on repeat dosing.

Studies in healthy elderly volunteers have shown slight, but clinically insignificant, age-related increases in both oral bioavailability (65%) and half-life (5 h) of ondansetron. General differences were shown in the disposition of ondansetron, with females having a greater rate and extent of absorption following an oral dose and reduced systemic clearance and volume of distribution (adjusted for weight).

In a study of 21 paediatric patients aged between 3 and 12 years undergoing elective surgery with general anaesthesia, the absolute values for both the clearance and volume of distribution of ondansetron following a single intravenous dose of 2 mg (3–7 years old) or 4 mg (8–12 years old) were reduced. The magnitude of the change was age-related, with clearance falling from about 300 ml/min at 12 years of age to 100 ml/min at 3 years. Volume of distribution fell from about 75 L at 12 years to 17 L at 3 years. Use of weight-based dosing (0.1 mg/kg up to 4 mg maximum) compensates for these changes and is effective in normalising systemic exposure in paediatric patients.

In patients with renal impairment (creatinine clearance >15 ml/min), systemic clearance and volume of distribution are reduced, resulting in a slight, but clinically insignificant increase in elimination half-life (5.4 h). A study in patients with severe renal impairment who required regular haemodialysis (studied between dialyses) showed ondansetron's pharmacokinetics to be essentially unchanged.

In patients with severe hepatic impairment, systemic clearance is markedly reduced with prolonged elimination half-lives (15–32 h) and an oral bioavailability approaching 100% because of reduced presystemic metabolism.

*Preclinical safety data:* No additional data of relevance.

**Pharmaceutical particulars**
*List of excipients:* Citric acid; sodium citrate dihydrate; sodium benzoate; sorbitol solution; strawberry flavour; purified water.

*Incompatibilities:* None reported.

*Shelf life:* 2 years.

*Special precautions for storage:* Store upright below 30°C. Do not refrigerate.

*Nature and contents of container:* 60 ml amber glass bottle with a child-resistant cap containing 50 ml of Zofran Syrup.

*Instructions for use/handling:* For oral administration. For detailed information see the patient information leaflet included in every pack.

**Marketing authorisation number** 10949/0246.

**Date of approval/revision of SPC** September 1996.

**Legal category** POM.

## ZOFRAN* TABLETS 4 mg

**Qualitative and quantitative composition** Each Zofran Tablet 4 mg is a yellow, oval, film-coated tablet engraved 'GLAXO' on one face and '4' on the other. Each tablet contains ondansetron 4 mg (as hydrochloride dihydrate).

**Pharmaceutical form** Film-coated tablet.

**Clinical particulars**
*Therapeutic indications:* Zofran is indicated for the management of nausea and vomiting induced by cytotoxic chemotherapy and radiotherapy, and for the prevention and treatment of post-operative nausea and vomiting.

*Posology and method of administration:*
*Chemotherapy and radiotherapy-induced nausea and vomiting: Adults:* The emetogenic potential of cancer treatment varies according to the doses and combinations of chemotherapy and radiotherapy regimens used. The route of administration and dose of Zofran should be flexible in the range of 8–32 mg a day and selected as shown below.

*Emetogenic chemotherapy and radiotherapy:* For most patients receiving emetogenic chemotherapy or radiotherapy, Zofran 8 mg should be administered as a slow intravenous injection immediately before treatment, or orally 1–2 hours before treatment, followed by 8 mg orally twelve hourly.

To protect against delayed or prolonged emesis after the first 24 hours, Zofran should be continued orally, 8 mg twice daily for up to 5 days after a course of treatment.

*Highly emetogenic chemotherapy:* For patients receiving highly emetogenic chemotherapy, e.g. high-dose cisplatin, Zofran has been shown to be equally effective in the following dose schedules over the first 24 hours of chemotherapy:

A single dose of 8 mg by slow intravenous injection immediately before chemotherapy.

A dose of 8 mg by slow intravenous injection immediately before chemotherapy, followed by two further intravenous doses of 8 mg two to four hours apart, or by a constant infusion of 1 mg/hour for up to 24 hours.

A single dose of 32 mg diluted in 50–100 ml of saline or other compatible infusion fluid and infused over not less than 15 minutes immediately before chemotherapy.

The selection of dose regimen should be determined by the severity of the emetogenic challenge.

The efficacy of Zofran in highly emetogenic chemotherapy may be enhanced by the addition of a single intravenous dose of dexamethasone sodium phosphate, 20 mg administered prior to chemotherapy.

To protect against delayed or prolonged emesis after the first 24 hours, Zofran should be continued orally, 8 mg twice daily for up to 5 days after a course of treatment.

*Children:* Zofran may be administered as a single intravenous dose of 5 mg/m² immediately before chemotherapy, followed by 4 mg orally twelve hours later. 4 mg orally twice daily should be continued for up to 5 days after a course of treatment.

*Elderly:* Zofran is well tolerated by patients over 65 years and no alteration of dosage, dosing frequency or route of administration are required.

*Patients with renal impairment:* No alteration of daily dosage or frequency of dosing, or route of administration are required.

*Patients with hepatic impairment:* Clearance of Zofran is significantly reduced and serum half-life significantly prolonged in subjects with moderate or severe impairment of hepatic function. In such patients a total daily dose of 8 mg should not be exceeded.

*Post operative nausea and vomiting (PONV): Adults:* For the prevention of PONV Zofran may be administered orally at a dose of 8 mg given one hour prior to anaesthesia followed by two further doses of 8 mg at eight-hourly intervals. Alternatively, a single dose of 16 mg may be given orally one hour prior to anaesthesia or 4 mg by intramuscular or slow intravenous injection at induction of anaesthesia.

For the treatment of established PONV a single dose of 4 mg given by intramuscular or slow intravenous injection is recommended.

*Children:* For the prevention and treatment of PONV, slow intravenous injection is recommended.

*Elderly:* There is limited experience in the use of Zofran in the prevention and treatment of PONV in the elderly. However Zofran is well tolerated in patients over 65 years receiving chemotherapy.

*Patients with renal impairment:* No alteration of daily dosage or frequency of dosing, or route of administration are required.

*Patients with hepatic impairment:* Clearance of Zofran is significantly reduced and serum half-life significantly prolonged in subjects with moderate or severe impairment of hepatic function. In such patients a total daily dose of 8 mg should not be exceeded.

*Patients with poor sparteine/debrisoquine metabolism:* The elimination half-life of ondansetron is not altered in subjects classified as poor metabolisers of sparteine and debrisoquine. Consequently, in such patients repeat dosing will give drug exposure levels no different from those of the general population. No alteration of daily dosage or frequency of dosing are required.

*Contra-indications:* Hypersensitivity to any component of the preparation.

*Special warnings and precautions for use:* None.

*Interaction with other medicaments and other forms of interaction:* None known.

*Pregnancy and lactation:* Zofran is not teratogenic in animals. There is no experience in humans. As with other medications Zofran should not be used during pregnancy, especially during the first trimester, unless the expected benefit to the patient is thought to outweigh any possible risk to the fetus.

Tests have shown that ondansetron passes into the milk of lactating animals. It is therefore recommended that mothers receiving Zofran should not breast-feed their babies.

*Effect on ability to drive and use machines:* In psychomotor testing ondansetron does not impair performance nor cause sedation.

*Undesirable effects:* Ondansetron is known to increase large bowel transit time and may cause constipation in some patients. The following side effects can occur: headache, a sensation of flushing or warmth, hiccups and occasional transient, asymptomatic increases in aminotransferases. There have been rare reports of immediate hypersensitivity reactions sometimes severe including anaphylaxis. Rare cases of transient visual disturbances (e.g. blurred vision) and dizziness have been reported during rapid intravenous administration of ondansetron. There have been rare reports suggestive of involuntary movement disorders without definitive evidence of persistent clinical sequelae and seizures have been rarely observed although no known pharmacological mechanism can account for ondansetron causing these effects. Chest pain, cardiac arrhythmias, hypotension and bradycardiac have been rarely reported.

*Overdose:* Little is at present known about overdosage with ondansetron. However, two patients who received doses of 84 and 145 mg intravenously reported only mild side-effects and required no active therapy. In cases of suspected overdose, symptomatic and supportive therapy should be given as appropriate.

**Pharmacological properties**
*Pharmacodynamic properties:* Ondansetron is a potent, highly selective $5HT_3$ receptor-antagonist. Its precise mode of action in the control of nausea and vomiting is not known. Chemotherapeutic agents and radiotherapy may cause release of 5HT in the small intestine initiating a vomiting reflex by activating vagal afferents via $5HT_3$ receptors. Ondansetron blocks the initiation of this reflex. Activation of vagal afferents may also cause a release of 5HT in the area postrema, located on the floor of the fourth ventricle, and this may also promote emesis through a central mechanism. Thus, the effect of ondansetron in the management of the nausea and vomiting induced by cytotoxic chemotherapy and radiotherapy is probably due to antagonism of $5HT_3$ receptors on neurons located both in the peripheral and central nervous system. The mechanisms of action in post-operative nausea and vomiting are not known but there may be common pathways with cytotoxic-induced nausea and vomiting.

Ondansetron does not alter plasma prolactin concentrations.

*Pharmacokinetic properties:* Following oral administration of ondansetron, absorption is rapid with maximum peak plasma concentrations of about 30 ng/ml being attained and achieved in approximately 1.5 hours after an 8 mg dose. Similar concentrations are achieved within approximately 10 minutes of a 4 mg intramuscular dose. The absolute bioavailability of the drug is approximately 60%. Equivalent systemic exposure is achieved following intramuscular and intravenous administration. The disposition of ondansetron following oral, intravenous and intramuscular dosing is similar with a terminal elimination half-life of approximately 3 hours and a steady-state volume of distribution of about 140 L, though this may be prolonged to about 5 hours in the elderly. Ondansetron is cleared from the systemic circulation predominantly by metabolism with less than 5% of a dose excreted unchanged in the urine. Studies in healthy elderly volunteers have shown a slightly increased oral bioavailability (65%) for ondansetron. In patients with severe hepatic impairment, systemic clearance is markedly reduced with prolonged elimination half-lives (15–32 h) and an oral bioavailability approaching 100% because of reduced pre-systemic metabolism. There is no evidence that ondansetron either induces or inhibits the metabolism of other drugs commonly co-administered with it, although specific studies have shown that ondansetron does not interact with alcohol, temazepam, frusemide, tramadol and propofol. The plasma protein binding is 70–76%.

*Preclinical safety data:* No additional data of relevance.

**Pharmaceutical particulars**
*List of excipients:* Lactose, microcrystalline cellulose, pre-gelatinised maize starch, magnesium stearate, methylhydroxypropylcellulose, titanium dioxide (E171), iron oxide (E172).

*Incompatibilities:* None reported.

*Shelf life:* 36 months.

*Special precautions for storage:* Store below 30°C.

*Nature and contents of container:* Blister packs of 30 tablets comprising PVC film and aluminium foil lidding.

*Instructions for use/handling:* None stated.

**Marketing authorisation number** 10949/0110.

**Date of approval/revision of SPC** March 1996.

**Legal category** POM.

## ZOFRAN* TABLETS 8 mg

**Qualitative and quantitative composition** Each Zofran Tablet 8 mg is a yellow, oval, film-coated tablet engraved 'GLAXO' on one face and '8' on the other. Each tablet contains ondansetron 8 mg (as hydrochloride dihydrate).

**Pharmaceutical form** Film-coated tablet.

**Clinical particulars**
*Therapeutic indications:* Zofran is indicated for the management of nausea and vomiting induced by cytotoxic chemotherapy and radiotherapy, and for the prevention and treatment of post-operative nausea and vomiting.

*Posology and method of administration:*
*Chemotherapy and radiotherapy-induced nausea and vomiting: Adults:* The emetogenic potential of cancer treatment varies according to the doses and combinations of chemotherapy and radiotherapy regimens used. The route of administration and dose of Zofran should be flexible in the range of 8–32 mg a day and selected as shown below.

*Emetogenic chemotherapy and radiotherapy:* For most patients receiving emetogenic chemotherapy or radiotherapy, Zofran 8 mg should be administered as a slow intravenous injection immediately before treatment, or orally 1–2 hours before treatment, followed by 8 mg orally twelve hourly.

To protect against delayed or prolonged emesis after the first 24 hours, Zofran should be continued orally, 8 mg twice daily for up to 5 days after a course of treatment.

*Highly emetogenic chemotherapy:* For patients receiving highly emetogenic chemotherapy, e.g. high-dose cisplatin, Zofran has been shown to be equally effective in the following dose schedules over the first 24 hours of chemotherapy:

A single dose of 8 mg by slow intravenous injection immediately before chemotherapy.

A dose of 8 mg by slow intravenous injection immediately before chemotherapy, followed by two further intravenous doses of 8 mg two to four hours apart, or by a constant infusion of 1 mg/hour for up to 24 hours.

A single dose of 32 mg diluted in 50–100 ml of saline or other compatible infusion fluid and infused over not less than 15 minutes immediately before chemotherapy.

The selection of dose regimen should be determined by the severity of the emetogenic challenge.

The efficacy of Zofran in highly emetogenic chemotherapy may be enhanced by the addition of a single intravenous dose of dexamethasone sodium phosphate, 20 mg administered prior to chemotherapy.

To protect against delayed or prolonged emesis after the first 24 hours, Zofran should be continued orally, 8 mg twice daily for up to 5 days after a course of treatment.

*Children:* Zofran may be administered as a single intravenous dose of 5 mg/m² immediately before chemotherapy, followed by 4 mg orally twelve hours later. 4 mg orally twice daily should be continued for up to 5 days after a course of treatment.

*Elderly:* Zofran is well tolerated by patients over 65 years and no alteration of dosage, dosing frequency or route of administration are required.

*Patients with renal impairment:* No alteration of daily dosage or frequency of dosing, or route of administration are required.

*Patients with hepatic impairment:* Clearance of Zofran is significantly reduced and serum half-life significantly prolonged in subjects with moderate or severe impairment of hepatic function. In such patients a total daily dose of 8 mg should not be exceeded.

*Post operative nausea and vomiting (PONV): Adults:* For the prevention of PONV Zofran may be administered orally at a dose of 8 mg given one hour prior to anaesthesia followed by two further doses of 8 mg at eight-hourly intervals. Alternatively, a single dose of 16 mg may be given orally one hour prior to anaesthesia or 4 mg by intramuscular or slow intravenous injection at induction of anaesthesia.

For the treatment of established PONV a single dose of 4 mg given by intramuscular or slow intravenous injection is recommended.

*Children:* For the prevention and treatment of PONV, slow intravenous injection is recommended.

*Elderly:* There is limited experience in the use of Zofran in the prevention and treatment of PONV in the elderly. However Zofran is well tolerated in patients over 65 years receiving chemotherapy.

*Patients with renal impairment:* No alteration of daily dosage or frequency of dosing, or route of administration are required.

*Patients with hepatic impairment:* Clearance of Zofran is significantly reduced and serum half-life significantly prolonged in subjects with moderate or severe impairment of hepatic function. In such patients a total daily dose of 8 mg should not be exceeded.

*Patients with poor sparteine/debrisoquine metabolism:* The elimination half-life of ondansetron is not altered in subjects classified as poor metabolisers of sparteine and debrisoquine. Consequently, in such patients repeat dosing will give drug exposure levels no different from those of the general population. No alteration of daily dosage or frequency of dosing are required.

*Contra-indications:* Hypersensitivity to any component of the preparation.

*Special warnings and precautions for use:* None.

*Interaction with other medicaments and other forms of interaction:* None known.

*Pregnancy and lactation:* Zofran is not teratogenic in animals. There is no experience in humans. As with other medications Zofran should not be used during pregnancy, especially during the first trimester, unless the expected benefit to the patient is thought to outweigh any possible risk to the fetus.

Tests have shown that ondansetron passes into the milk of lactating animals. It is therefore recommended that mothers receiving Zofran should not breast-feed their babies.

*Effect on ability to drive and use machines:* In psychomotor testing ondansetron does not impair performance nor cause sedation.

*Undesirable effects:* Ondansetron is known to increase large bowel transit time and may cause constipation in some patients. The following side effects can occur: headache, a sensation of flushing or warmth, hiccups and occasional transient, asymptomatic increases in aminotransferases. There have been rare reports of immediate hypersensitivity reactions sometimes severe including anaphylaxis. Rare cases of transient visual disturbances (e.g. blurred vision) and dizziness have been reported during rapid intravenous administration of ondansetron. There have been rare reports suggestive of involuntary movement disorders without definitive evidence of persistent clinical sequelae and seizures have been rarely observed although no known pharmacological mechanism can account for ondansetron causing these effects. Chest pain, cardiac arrhythmias, hypotension and bradycardia have been rarely reported.

*Overdose:* Little is at present known about overdosage with ondansetron. However, two patients who received doses of 84 and 145 mg intraveneously reported only mild side-effects and required no active therapy. In cases of suspected overdose, symptomatic and supportive therapy should be given as appropriate.

**Pharmacological properties**
*Pharmacodynamic properties:* Ondansetron is a potent, highly selective $5HT_3$ receptor-antagonist. Its precise mode of action in the control of nausea and vomiting is not known. Chemotherapeutic agents and radiotherapy may cause release of 5HT in the small intestine initiating a vomiting reflex by activating vagal afferents via $5HT_3$ receptors. Ondansetron blocks the initiation of this reflex. Activation of vagal afferents may also cause a release of 5HT in the area postrema, located on the floor of the fourth ventricle, and this may also promote emesis through a central mechanism. Thus, the effect of ondansetron in the management of the nausea and vomiting induced by cytotoxic chemotherapy and radiotherapy is probably due to antagonism of $5HT_3$ receptors on neurons located both in the peripheral and central nervous system. The mechanisms of action in post-operative nausea and vomiting are not known but there may be common pathways with cytotoxic-induced nausea and vomiting.

Ondansetron does not alter plasma prolactin concentrations.

*Pharmacokinetic properties:* Following oral administration of ondansetron, absorption is rapid with maximum peak plasma concentrations of about 30 ng/ml being attained and achieved in approximately 1.5 hours after an 8 mg dose. Similar concentrations are achieved within approximately 10 minutes of a 4 mg intramuscular dose. The absolute bioavailability of the drug is approximately 60%. Equivalent systemic exposure is achieved following intramuscular and intravenous administration. The disposition of ondansetron following oral, intravenous and intramuscular dosing is similar with a terminal elimination half-life of approximately 3 hours and a steady-state volume of distribution of about 140 L, though this may be prolonged to about 5 hours in the elderly. Ondansetron is cleared from the systemic circulation predominantly by metabolism with less than 5% of a dose excreted unchanged in the urine. Studies in healthy elderly volunteers have shown a slightly increased oral bioavailability (65%) for ondansetron. In patients with severe hepatic impairment, systemic clearance is markedly reduced with prolonged elimination half-lives (15–32 h) and an oral bioavailability approaching 100% because of reduced pre-systemic metabolism. There is no evidence that ondansetron either induces or inhibits the metabolism of other drugs commonly co-administered with it, although specific studies have shown that ondansetron does not interact with alcohol, temazepam, frusemide, tramadol and propofol. The plasma protein binding is 70–76%.

*Preclinical safety data:* No additional data of relevance.

**Pharmaceutical particulars**
*List of excipients:* Lactose, microcrystalline cellulose, pre-gelatinised maize starch, magnesium stearate, methylhydroxypropylcellulose, titanium dioxide (E171), iron oxide (E172).

*Incompatibilities:* None reported.

*Shelf life:* 36 months.

*Special precautions for storage:* Store below 30°C.

*Nature and contents of container:* Blister packs of 10 tablets comprising PVC film and aluminium foil lidding.

*Instructions for use/handling:* None stated.

**Marketing authorisation number** 10949/0111.

**Date of approval/revision of SPC** March 1996.

**Legal category** POM.

*\*Trade Mark*

# Glenwood Laboratories Ltd
Jenkins Dale
Chatham
Kent ME4 5RD

## MYOTONINE*

**Qualitative and quantitative composition** 10 mg tablet weighs 400 mg; active ingredient 10 mg Bethanechol Chloride USPXXII.

25 mg tablet weighs 450 mg; active ingredient 25 mg Bethanechol Chloride USPXXII.

Other ingredients: see *List of excipients.*

### Pharmaceutical form
Tablet: 10 mg white, flat bevelled edge and single scored.

Tablet: 25 mg white, flat bevelled edge and cross scored.

### Clinical particulars
*Therapeutic indications:* Urinary retention: acute postoperative, postpartum and neurogenic. Reflux oesophagitis.

*Posology and method of administration:* Administration orally by tablets.

*Adults:* 10 mg–25 mg 3–4 times daily. Taken $\frac{1}{2}$ hr before food. Occasionally it may be felt necessary to initiate therapy with a 50 mg dose.

*Children:* The experience with children is limited; therefore no recommended dose is given.

*Elderly:* Adult dosage administered with caution.

*Contra-indications:* Intestinal or urinary obstruction, recent myocardial infarction, recent intestinal anastomosis.

*Special warnings and special precautions for use:* A severe cholinergic reaction is likely to occur if Bethanechol Chloride is administered IV or IM. This reaction has also rarely occurred in cases of hypersensitivity or overdose.

*Interaction with other medicaments and other forms of interaction:* Pharmacological interactions may occur with the following when bethanechol is administered.

Quinidine and procainamide which may antagonise cholinergic effects, cholinergic drugs which may have an additive effect, particularly cholinesterase inhibitors.

When administered to patients receiving ganglionic compounds, a critical fall in blood pressure may occur preceded by severe abdominal symptoms.

*Pregnancy and lactation:* Should not be used during pregnancy or lactation.

*Effects on ability to drive and use machines:* In some cases the ability to drive and operate machinery may be impaired.

*Undesirable effects:* Nausea, vomiting, sweating and intestinal colic.

*Overdose:*

*Symptoms:* Include nausea, salivation, lachrymation, eructation, involuntary defecation and urination, transient dyspnoea, palpitation, bradycardia and peripheral vasodilation leading to hypertension, transient heart block and a feeling of constriction under the sternum.

*Procedure:* The stomach should be emptied by aspiration and lavage. Give atropine sulphate 1–2 mg intravenously, intramuscularly or subcutaneously to control muscarinic effects. This dose may be repeated every 2–4 hours as necessary. Supportive treatment includes intravenous administration of diazepam 5–10 mg; muscle twitching may be controlled by small doses of tubocurarine (together with assisted respiration); oxygen may be required.

### Pharmacological properties
*Pharmacodynamic properties:* Bethanechol is a synthetic choline ester of carbamic acid which possesses a significant acetylcholine-like activity. It is active after oral administration. As a consequence of the very slow hydrolysation by acetylcholinesterase, bethanechol has a prolonged action as has been demonstrated on the urinary tract.[1] The onset of action after oral administration of bethanechol chloride occurs within an hour.[2,3]

The major pharmacological effects of bethanechol result from interaction of the drug with muscarinic receptor sites of smooth muscles, especially those of the urinary bladder and gastrointestinal tract.[1,4,5] In addition, minor but important nicotine effects have been noted.

In usual therapeutic doses, bethanechol does not cross the blood brain barrier.[6] Studies addressing pharmacokinetic-pharmacodynamic association are not available.

*References*
1. Draper J.W., Zorgniotta A.W. The effects of banthine and similar agents on the urinary tract. N.Y. State *J. Med.* 1954; 54; 77.
2. Boas E., Comarr A.E. *Neurological Urology.* Baltimore, University Park Press 1971; 215.
3. Lapides J., Friend C.R., Ajemian E.P., Sonda L.P. Comparison of action of oral and parenteral bethanechol chloride upon the urinary bladder. *Invest. Urol.* 1963; 1:94.
4. Paul D.A., Icardi J.A., Parkman H.P., Ryan J.P. Development changes in gastric fundus smooth muscle contractility and involvement of extracellular calcium in foetal and adult guinea pigs. *Paediatr. Res.* 1994; 36:642–646.
5. Ursillo R.C. Rationale for drug therapy in bladder dysfunction. In. Boyarsk s. *The Neurogenic Bladder.* Baltimore, The Williams and Wilkins CO. 1967; 187.
6. Goodman Gilman. *The Pharmacological Basis of Therapeutics.* Editors: Goodman, Gilman A; Rale T.W., Nies A.S., Taylor P., New York. Pergamon Press. 8th Edition 1991.

**Preclinical safety data** Not applicable.

### Pharmaceutical particulars
*List of excipients:* Calcium Sulphate Hemihydrate BP; Maize Starch BP; Talc BP (iron free); Magnesium Stearate BP.

*Incompatibilities:* Major – none known.

*Shelf life:* The shelf life of Myotonine tablets is currrently two years from date of manufacture.

*Storage:* Store below 20°C. Keep out of reach of children and away from direct heat or light sources. Store in areas free from the risk of dampness.

*Nature and contents of container:* The container is of polypropylene with a tamper-evident polyethylene cap and closure. A filla may be inserted to reduce the risk of tablet breakage due to ullage.

Each container is filled with 100 tablets.

**Marketing authorisation number**
Myotonine 10 mg    00245/5009R
Myotonine 25 mg    00245/5010R.

**Date of approval/revision of SPC** April 1996.

**Legal category** POM.

## POTABA*

**Presentation** Potaba is pure potassium para-aminobenzoate. It is available in the following presentations:
Potaba envules. Single dose sachets, each containing 3 g Potaba.
Potaba tablets – White concave tablets each containing 500 mg Potaba.
Potaba capsules – All white capsules each containing 500 mg Potaba.

### Uses
*Mode of Action:* Potaba is an antifibrosis agent. It has been suggested that the antifibrosis activity of Potaba is brought about by the drug increasing oxygen uptake at the tissue level. Fibrosis is believed to occur from either too much serotonin or too little monoamine oxidase activity over a period of time. The activity of monoamine oxidase is dependent upon an adequate oxygen supply. By increasing oxygen supply at the tissue level Potaba enhances monoamine oxidase activity thereby preventing or bringing about regression of fibrosis.

*Indications:* Scleroderma. Peyronie's disease (Induratio penis plastica).

**Dosage and administration** The usual adult daily dose of Potaba is 12 g, given in four to six divided doses, usually with food. Potaba Envules each contain 3 g which can be dissolved in any desired drink – citrus juices are excellent – and taken four times daily with food. Alternatively, the 0.5 g tablets or capsules should be taken at the rate of 4 tablets/capsules 6 times daily with food or taken at the rate of 6 tablets/capsules 4 times daily with food. Tablets must be dissolved in an appropriate amount of liquid to avoid gastro-intestinal upset.

**Contra-indications, warnings, etc** Potaba should not be administered to patients taking sulphonamides, as it will inactivate this medication.

*Precautions:* Treatment with Potaba should be interrupted during periods of low food intake (eg, during fasting, anorexia, nausea). This is to avoid the possible development of hypoglycaemia.

Potaba should be given cautiously to patients with renal impairment.

Potaba treatment should be discontinued if a hypersensitivity reaction occurs.

*Side effects:* No serious adverse effects have been reported in patients treated with Potaba. Anorexia, nausea, fever and rash occur infrequently and subside with omission of the drug. Desensitisation can often be accomplished and treatment with Potaba resumed.

*Overdose:* No particular problems are expected following overdosage with Potaba. Symptomatic and supportive therapy should be given as appropriate.

**Pharmaceutical precautions** Potaba preparations should be stored in a cool place.

**Legal category** P.

**Package quantities** Potaba Envules – Box of 40 envules. Potaba tablets – Containers of 120 and 1000 tablets. Potaba capsules – Containers of 240 capsules.

**Further information** It is necessary to continue treatment with Potaba at the full recommended dose (12 g daily) for up to twelve months or longer to effect regression of the fibrous plaque in the penis. Patients should be instructed not to interrupt treatment, except during periods of low food intake (see precautions above).

Para–aminobenzoate is considered to be a member of the vitamin B complex. Small amounts are found in yeast, cereal, eggs, milk and meats. Detectable amounts are normally present in human blood and other biological fluids.

**Product licence numbers**
Envules    0245/5000R
Capsules   0245/5001R
Tablets    0245/5002R

*Trade Mark

# Goldshield Pharmaceuticals Ltd
## NLA Tower
## 12–16 Addiscombe Road
## Croydon
## CR0 0XT

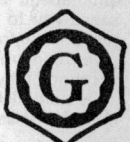

## DINDEVAN* TABLETS

**Presentation**
*Dindevan Tablets 10 mg:* White tablets engraved D10, each tablet containing Phenindione BP 10 mg.

*Dindevan Tablets 25 mg:* Green tablets engraved D25, each tablet containing Phenindione BP 25 mg.

*Dindevan Tablets 50 mg:* White tablets engraved D50, each tablet containing Phenindione BP 50 mg.

**Uses** Dindevan (Phenindione BP) is a synthetic anticoagulant which acts by interfering with the formation of clotting factors II, VII, IX and X. It produces its effect in 36 to 48 hours after the initial dose: the effect wanes over a period of 48 to 72 hours after Dindevan is stopped.

Anticoagulant therapy can be initiated with heparin and Dindevan together.

*Indications:* Prophylaxis of systemic embolisation in patients with rheumatic heart disease and atrial fibrillation.

Prophylaxis after insertion of prosthetic heart valves. Prophylaxis and treatment of venous thrombosis and pulmonary embolism.

**Dosage and administration** *Initial loading dose:* Usually 200 mg, followed on the second day with a dose of 100 mg.

*Maintenance therapy:* Dosage must be adjusted, from the third day, in accordance with the results of appropriate coagulation tests. Concomitant heparin therapy affects the results of control tests and should be discontinued at least six hours before the first test is carried out.

Control tests must be made at regular intervals and the dosage further adjusted according to the results obtained. As a general guide, a maintenance dosage of between 50 and 150 mg per day will prove satisfactory in most cases. Occasionally, a resistant patient may need 200 mg or more per day; on the other hand a sensitive patient may need less than 50 mg per day.

**Contra-indications, warnings, etc**
*Contra-indications:* Pregnancy. Infants should not be fed with breast milk from mothers being treated with Dindevan. Known hypersensitivity to phenindione. Dindevan should not be given in the presence of severe hepatic or renal disease, bacterial endocarditis, actual or potential haemorrhagic conditions, or to patients with uncontrolled hypertension. Its use within 24 hours following surgery or labour should be undertaken with caution, if at all.

*Precautions:* (See Drug interactions) The following factors may exaggerate the effects of Dindevan and necessitate a reduction in dosage: loss in weight; elderly subject; acute illness, impaired renal function; decreased dietary intake of vitamin K and administration of certain drugs (see 'Drug interactions').

Factors which may call for an increase in maintenance dosage include weight gain, diarrhoea and vomiting, increased intake of vitamin K, fats and oils and administration of certain drugs (see 'Drug interactions').

Administration of vitamin K can lead to resistance to the action of Dindevan for some days. For this reason, fresh-frozen plasma should be administered to patients with prosthetic heart valves where haemorrhage has occurred.

*Pregnancy:* Oral anticoagulants should not be used in pregnancy particularly because of possible teratogenicity and the risk of foetal haemorrhage near term. It is therefore suggested that heparin (which does not cross the placenta) be used during the first trimester and after 37 weeks gestation. However, the use of heparin in pregnancy is not absolutely safe and specialist guidance is advisable for those who are pregnant and who need anti-coagulant therapy. Women of child-bearing age who are receiving treatment with Dindevan should be cautioned about the possible complications of pregnancy. Infants should not be fed with breast milk from mothers being treated with Dindevan.

*Side-effects:* The following effects have been reported: hypersensitivity including skin rashes, alopecia, exanthema, skin necrosis, exfoliative dermatitis, fever, leucopenia and agranulocytosis, diarrhoea, vomiting, hepatitis and renal damage with tubular necrosis. Micro-adenopathy, jaundice, albuminuria, eosinophilia, a leukaemoid blood picture or cytopenia or haemothorax may also be observed. If any of these are observed administration of Dindevan should stop immediately and full investigations of blood and of liver and kidney function should be carried out. Possible sensitivity to other drugs should be considered. Other anticoagulants, such as warfarin, are usually tolerated by patients sensitive to Dindevan. If therapy is controlled as recommended then bleeding due to overdosage of anticoagulant is rare. An episode of bleeding occurring during anticoagulant therapy must therefore be investigated fully and not regarded automatically as a manifestation of overdosage.

*NB.* The metabolites of Dindevan often colour the urine pink or orange. This may be distinguished from discolouration caused by haemoglobin by the addition of a few drops of dilute acetic acid to the urine. If the colour is due to Dindevan it will disappear immediately.

*Drug interactions:* Care is required in the concomitant use of all drugs in patients receiving oral anticoagulant therapy. Known interactions include the following, but prescribers of other or newly available medicines should refer to the manufacturers prescribing information or the appropriate monograph. The following may exaggerate the effects of Dindevan: ACTH, allopurinol, amiodarone, amitriptyline/nortriptyline, anabolic steroids, azapropazone, aztreonam, broad spectrum antibiotics, ciprofloxacin, cimetidine, clofibrate, corticosteroids, co-trimoxazole, dextropropoxyphene, diflunisal, dipyridamole, disulfiram, feprazone, flurbiprofen, gemfibrozil, glucagon, hepato-toxic drugs, indomethacin, metronidazole, NSAIDS, oxyphenbutazone, phenformin, phenylbutazone, quinidine, salicylates, sulindac, sulphinpyrazone, thyroid compounds, tolbutamide. Monitoring and reduction of the dose of Dindevan may be necessary.

The following may reduce the effects of Dindevan: alcohol in large amounts, carbamazepine, cholestyramine, dichloralphenazone, glutethimide, griseofulvin, phenobarbitone, phenytoin, rifampicin. Monitoring and increase of the dose of Dindevan may be necessary.

*Overdosage:* If haemorrhage occurs or a potential bleeding state arises, excessive depression of the coagulation activity can be corrected by temporary withdrawal of Dindevan accompanied, if necessary, by infusion of fresh-frozen plasma or whole blood. Vitamin K, 5 to 10 mg intravenously, may be required to supplement specific treatment with factor concentrates.

**Pharmaceutical precautions** No special requirements or precautions.

**Legal category** POM.

**Package quantities** Dindevan Tablets 10 mg, 25 mg and 50 mg are each available in containers of 100 tablets (OP).

**Further information** Also contains Lactose BP.

**Product licence numbers**
| | |
|---|---|
| Dindevan Tablets 10 mg | 10972/0037 |
| Dindevan Tablets 25 mg | 10972/0038 |
| Dindevan Tablets 50 mg | 10972/0039 |

## ELTROXIN* TABLETS

**Presentation** Small white tablets engraved 'Eltroxin 50' or 'Eltroxin 100' containing 50 micrograms (0.05 mg) or 100 micrograms (0.1 mg) anhydrous thyroxine sodium respectively. The lower-strength tablets are scored. Eltroxin Tablets comply with the specification for Thyroxine Tablets BP.

**Uses** Hypothyroidism.

**Dosage and administration** *Adults:* Initially 50 to 100 micrograms daily, preferably taken before breakfast, and adjusted at three to four weeks intervals by 50 micrograms until normal metabolism is steadily maintained; this may require doses of 100 to 200 micrograms daily. With patients aged over 50 years, it is not advisable to exceed 50 micrograms a day initially, and where there is cardiac disease, 25 micrograms daily, or 50 micrograms on alternate days, is more suitable. In this condition the daily dosage may be increased by 25 micrograms at intervals of perhaps four weeks.

In younger patients, and in the absence of heart disease, a serum thyroxine (T4) level of about 70 to 160 nanomols per litre, or a serum thyrotrophin level of less than 5 milli-units per litre, should be aimed at. In those aged over 50, and/or in the presence of heart disease, clinical response is probably a more acceptable criterion of dosage than serum levels.

A pre-therapy ECG is valuable, as changes induced by hypothyroidism may be confused with ECG evidence of ischaemia. If too rapid an increase of metabolism is produced (causing diarrhoea, nervousness, rapid pulse, insomnia, tremors and sometimes anginal pain where there is latent myocardial ischaemia), dosage must be reduced or withheld for a day or two, then begun again at a lower level.

*Congenital hypothyroidism and juvenile myxoedema:* The largest dose consistent with freedom from toxic effects should be given. The dosage is guided by clinical response, growth assessment and appropriate thyroid function tests – clinically normal pulse rate and absence of diarrhoea or constipation are the most useful indicators.

Thyrotrophin levels may remain elevated during the first year of life in children with neonatal hypothyroidism due to re-setting of the hypothalamic-pituitary axis. For infants with congenital hypothyroidism, a suitable starting dose is 25 micrograms Eltroxin daily, with increments of 25 micrograms every two to four weeks until mild toxic symptoms appear. Dosage is then slightly reduced. The same applies to juvenile myxoedema, except that the starting dose for children older than one year may be 2.5 to 5 micrograms/kg/day.

**Contra-indications, warnings, etc**
*Contra-indications:* Thyrotoxicosis. Hypersensitivity to any component of the preparation.

*Precautions:* Patients with panhypopituitarism or other causes predisposing to adrenal insufficiency may react unfavourably to thyroxine treatment, and it is advisable to initiate corticosteroid therapy before giving thyroxine in these cases.

Special care is needed in the elderly and in patients with symptoms of myocardial insufficiency or ECG evidence of myocardial infarction.

Thyroid replacement therapy may result in an increase in dosage requirement of insulin or other antidiabetic therapy. Care is needed in patients with diabetes mellitus or diabetes insipidus.

*Use in pregnancy and lactation:* The safety of thyroxine during pregnancy is unknown but any possible risk of congenital abnormalities should be weighed up against the risk to the foetus of untreated hypothyroidism.

Thyroxine is excreted into breast milk in low concentrations and it is contentious whether this may interfere with neonatal screening programs.

*Side-effects:* The following effects are indicative of excessive dosage and usually disappear on reduction of dosage or withdrawal of treatment for a few days. Anginal pain, cardiac arrhythmias, palpitation, and cramps in skeletal muscle; also tachycardia, diarrhoea, vomiting, tremors, restlessness, excitability, insomnia, headache, flushing, sweating, excessive loss of weight and muscular weakness.

*Drug interactions:* Thyroxine increases the effect of anticoagulants and it may be necessary to reduce the dose of anticoagulant if excessive hypoprothrombinaemia and bleeding are to be avoided. Phenytoin levels may be increased by thyroxine. Anticonvulsants such as carbamazepine and phenytoin enhance the metabolism of thyroid hormones and may displace them from plasma proteins.

Initiation or discontinuation of anticonvulsant therapy may alter thyroxine dose requirements.

If co-administered with cardiac glycosides, adjustment of dosage of cardiac glycoside may be necessary. The effect of sympathomimetic agents is also enhanced. Thyroxine raises blood sugar levels and this may upset the stability of patients receiving antidiabetic agents. Thyroxine increases receptor sensitivity to catecholamines thus accelerating the response to tricyclic antidepressants. Cholestyramine given concurrently reduces the gastrointestinal absorption of thyroxine.

Co-administration of oral contraceptives may result in an increased dosage requirement of thyroid therapy.

A number of drugs may affect thyroid function tests and this should be borne in mind when monitoring a patient on thyroxine therapy.

*Overdosage:* Gastric lavage or emesis is required if the patient is seen within several hours of taking the dose. In addition to exaggeration of side effects the following symptoms may be seen: agitation, confusion, irritability, hyperactivity, sweating, mydriasis, tachycardia, arrhythmias, tachypnoea, pyrexia, increased bowel movements and convulsions. The appearance of clinical hyperthyroidism may be delayed for up to five days.

Treatment is symptomatic, and tachycardia has been controlled in an adult by 40 mg doses of propranolol given every six hours and other symptoms by diazepam and/or chlorpromazine as appropriate.

**Pharmaceutical precautions**  Protect from light.

**Legal category**  POM.

**Package quantities**  Bottles of 100 and 1,000 tablets.

**Further information** · 100 micrograms thyroxine is equivalent in activity to 20 to 30 micrograms liothyronine or 60 mg Thyroid BP. Also contains Lactose BP.

**Product licence numbers**
Tablets 50 micrograms      10972/0031
Tablets 100 micrograms     10972/0032

## MAREVAN* TABLETS

**Presentation**  Marevan Tablets are Warfarin Tablets BP.

*Marevan Tablets 1 mg:* Brown tablets engraved M1, each tablet containing Warfarin Sodium BP 1 mg.

*Marevan Tablets 3 mg:* Blue tablets engraved M3, each tablet containing Warfarin Sodium BP 3 mg.

*Marevan Tablets 5 mg:* Pink tablets engraved M5, each tablet containing Warfarin Sodium BP 5 mg.

**Uses**  Marevan is a synthetic anti-coagulant of the coumarin series and acts by inhibiting the formation of active clotting factors II, VII, IX and X. An effect on prothrombin time is produced in 24 to 36 hours after the initial dose. This reaches a maximum in 36 to 48 hours and is maintained for 48 hours or more after administration is stopped.

*Indications:* Prophylaxis of systemic embolisation in patients with rheumatic heart disease and atrial fibrillation.

Prophylaxis after insertion of prosthetic heart valves. Prophylaxis and treatment of venous thrombosis and pulmonary embolism.

Transient cerebral ischaemic attacks.

**Dosage and administration**  *Adults and the elderly:* The typical induction dose of Marevan is 10 mg daily for 2 days, but this should be tailored to individual requirement.

The daily maintenance dose of Marevan is usually 3 to 9 mg taken at the same time each day. The exact maintenance dose for an individual is dependent on the prothrombin time or other appropriate coagulation tests.

The maintenance dose is omitted if the prothrombin time is excessively prolonged. Once the maintenance dose is stabilised in the therapeutic range, it is rarely necessary to alter it.

In emergencies, anticoagulant therapy should be initiated with heparin and Marevan together. Where there is less urgency, as in patients disposed to or at special risk of thromboembolism, anticoagulant therapy may be initiated with Marevan alone.

Concomitant heparin therapy affects the results of control tests and should be discontinued at least six hours before the first test is carried out.

Control tests must be made at regular intervals and Marevan maintenance dosage further adjusted according to the results obtained.

*Children:* The dosage of Marevan which may be used in children has not yet been established.

**Contra-indications, warnings, etc**

*Contra-indications:* Pregnancy (see below). Known hypersensitivity to warfarin. Marevan should not be given in the presence of severe hepatic or renal disease, bacterial endocarditis, actual or potential haemorrhagic conditions, eg. peptic ulcer, or to patients with uncontrolled hypertension. Its use within 24 hours following surgery or labour should be undertaken with caution, if at all.

*Precautions:* The following factors may exaggerate the effects of Marevan and necessitate a reduction in dosage; loss of weight, elderly subject, acute illness, deficient renal function, decreased dietary intake of vitamin K, administration of certain drugs (see 'Drug interactions').

Factors which may call for an increase in maintenance dosage include weight gain, diarrhoea and vomiting, increased intake of vitamin K, fats and oils, and the administration of certain drugs (see 'Drug interactions').

Careful additional laboratory control is necessary if the patient is to be changed from one formulation to another.

Reversal of warfarin anticoagulation by vitamin K takes several days. In emergency situations fresh-frozen plasma should be given.

*Pregnancy:* Oral anticoagulants should not be used in pregnancy particularly because of possible teratogenicity and the risk of foetal haemorrhage near term. It is therefore suggested that heparin (which does not cross the placenta) be used during the first trimester and after 37 weeks gestation. However, the use of heparin in pregnancy is not absolutely safe and specialist guidance is advisable for those who are pregnant and who need anticoagulant therapy. Women of child bearing age who are receiving treatment with Marevan should be cautioned about the possible complications of pregnancy.

*Side-effects:* The following effects have been reported: hypersensitivity, skin rashes, alopecia, diarrhoea, an unexplained drop in haematocrit, a 'purple toes' syndrome, jaundice and hepatic dysfunction.

Skin necrosis within a few days of starting treatment has been infrequently reported. Most subjects are obese, elderly women. The first sign is an erythematous swollen patch. Administration of vitamin K at this stage may prevent the development of ecchymosis and infarction.

Purpura, fever, nausea, vomiting, pancreatitis, haemothorax and epistaxis may also be observed. If any of these are observed administration of Marevan should stop immediately. Possible sensitivity to other drugs should be considered. Other anticoagulants are often tolerated by patients sensitive to Marevan. If therapy is controlled as recommended then bleeding due to overdosage of anticoagulant is rare. An episode of bleeding occurring during anticoagulant therapy

must therefore be investigated fully and not regarded automatically as a manifestation of overdosage.

*Drug interactions:* Care is required in the concomitant use of all drugs in patients receiving oral anticoagulant therapy. Known interactions include the following, but prescribers of other or newly available medicines should refer to the manufacturer's information or appropriate monograph.

The activity of warfarin may be potentiated by amiodarone, amitriptyline/nortriptyline, anabolic steroids, azapropazone, bezafibrate, cephamandole, chloral hydrate, chloramphenicol, cimetidine, clofibrate, co-trimoxazole, danazol, dextropropoxyphene, dextrothyroxine, dipyridamole, erythromycin, feprazone, glucagon, latamoxef, metronidazole, miconazole, neomycin, oxyphenbutazone, phenformin, phenylubutazone, phenyramidol, quinidine, salicylates, sulphonamides (eg. sulphaphenazole, sulphinpyrazone), tamoxifen, tolbutamide and tricolofos.

Potentiation may also occur with the following drugs, aztreonam, ciprofloxacin, diflunisel, fluconazole, flurbiprofen, fluroxamine, gemfibrocil, indomethacin, mefenamic acid, piroxicam, sulindac and possibly other anti-inflammatory analgesics, ketoconazole, nalidixic acid, norfloxacin, omeprazole, propafenone, tetracyclines and other broad spectrum antibiotics.

Anticoagulant activity may be possibly increased by allopurinol, disulfiram, methylphenidate, paracetamol, thyroid drugs, and any potentially hepatoxic drug.

Both potentiation and inhibition of anticoagulant effect have been reported with phenytoin, ACTH and corticosteroids.

Anticoagulant activity may also be increased with large amounts of chronic ingestion of alcohol, particularly in patients with impaired liver function.

Warfarin absorption is impaired and activity decreased by cholestyramine and sulcralfate. Cholestyramine, however, may also decrease absorption of vitamin K and thus increase coumarin anticoagulant activity. Anticoagulant effect may be decreased by administration of vitamin K (eg. as a constituent of some enteral feeds).

The anticoagulant activity of warfarin may be inhibited by drugs which induce liver enzymes such as aminoglutethimide, barbiturates, carbamazepine, ethchlorvynol, glutethimide, primidone, griseofulvin, dichloralphenazone, rifampicin and oral contraceptives.

*Overdosage:* If haemorrhage occurs or a potential bleeding state arises, excessive depression of the coagulation activity can be corrected by temporary withdrawal of Marevan accompanied, if necessary, by infusion of fresh-frozen plasma or whole blood. Vitamin K, 5 to 10 mg orally or intravenously, may be required to supplement specific treatment with factor concentrates.

**Pharmaceutical precautions**  Replace cap securely and protect from light.

**Legal category**  POM.

**Package quantities**  Marevan Tablets 1 mg are available in containers of 100 (OP) and 500.

Marevan Tablets 3 mg are available in containers of 100 (OP) and 500.

Marevan Tablets 5 mg are available in containers of 100 (OP) and 500.

**Further information**  Also contains Lactose BP.

**Product licence numbers**
Marevan Tablets 1 mg    10972/0034
Marevan Tablets 3 mg    10972/0035
Marevan Tablets 5 mg    10972/0036

*Trade Mark

# Hoechst Marion Roussel Ltd
Broadwater Park
Denham
Uxbridge
Middlesex UB9 5HP

# Hoechst Marion Roussel

## Hoechst ■

Hoechst Marion Roussel
The Pharmaceutical Company of Hoechst

## ACTINAC*

**Presentation** Actinac is presented as a pale yellow dry powder, together with a solvent for the preparation of a lotion for topical application. Each gram of powder contains:

| | |
|---|---|
| Chloramphenicol BP | 40 mg |
| Hydrocortisone Acetate PhEur | 40 mg |
| Butoxyethyl nicotinate | 24 mg |
| Allantoin | 24 mg |
| Precipitated Sulphur BP | 320 mg |

The solvent is Purified Water, containing a bacteriostat.

**Uses** Actinac is for use in the topical treatment of acne vulgaris and other acneiform conditions. It is formulated to control local infection and suppress inflammation with its consequent scarring effects.

**Dosage and administration** The lotion is applied to the affected area each night and morning for the first four days, after this it is applied only at night and continued for three nights after the lesions have disappeared.

**Contra-indications, warnings, etc** Actinac is contra-indicated in patients who have a known hypersensitivity to any of the ingredients.

Avoid Actinac coming into contact with the eyes and mouth.

Early in the course of treatment, erythema may occur at the site of application and the patient may experience a sensation of warmth due to the vasodilator action of the nicotinate. In the unlikely event of a severe reaction, the patient is instructed to consult the doctor before further use of Actinac.

In pregnant animals, systemic and topical administration of corticosteroids can cause abnormalities of foetal development. The relevance of this finding to human beings has not been established. However, topical steroids should not be used extensively in pregnancy, i.e. in large amounts or for long periods.

**Pharmaceutical precautions** Store below 15˚C. The lotion when constituted will remain active for 21 days. Any lotion remaining after this time must be discarded and a fresh supply of lotion prepared.

**Legal category** POM.

**Package quantities** Each pack of Actinac contains two bottles of powder (each 6.25 g), two bottles of solvent (each 20 ml) and an instruction leaflet for the patient.

**Further information** Actinac powder contains Tragacanth, Myrj 53, Syloid 244, Purified Talc, Titanium Dioxide. The solvent contains benzoic acid.

It is advisable to remove jewellery before applying the lotion.

**Product licence number** 0109/0037.

*Product licence holder:* Roussel Laboratories Limited, Broadwater Park, Denham, Uxbridge.

## ALTACITE PLUS* (Approved name: Co-Simalcite)

**Presentation** *Suspension:* Viscous, slightly off-white aqueous suspension, flavoured with spearmint. Each 5 ml of suspension contains co-simalcite 500/125 (500 mg of hydrotalcite and 125 mg of activated dimethicone).

*Tablets:* White, circular, flat, bevel-edged tablets of 19 mm diameter having a peppermint flavour. Each tablet contains 500 mg of hydrotalcite and 250 mg of activated dimethicone.

**Uses** Altacite Plus has antacid, mucosal protective and anti-flatulent properties. As an antacid, Altacite Plus buffers in the optimal range of pH 3-5 for over two hours.

It is indicated for symptomatic relief in the following conditions: dyspepsia; flatulence and abdominal distension; hyperacidity; gastritis; peptic ulceration; heartburn, especially when associated with reflux oesophagitis or hiatus hernia; and heartburn in pregnancy.

**Dosage and administration**

*Suspension:*
*Adults:* 10 ml suspension between meals and at bedtime or as directed by the physician.
*Elderly:* No specific recommendations in the elderly.
*Children (8-12 years):* Half the adult dose.

*Tablets:*
*Adults:* 2 tablets between meals and at bedtime, or as directed by the physician. *Children (8-12 years):* Half the adult dose.

The tablets should be chewed or crushed before swallowing.

**Contra-indications, warnings , etc** There are no known contra-indications to Altacite Plus, but it is wise to avoid any drug, including antacids, during the first trimester of pregnancy. They may be used whilst breast feeding. As with other compounds containing aluminium or magnesium, Altacite Plus may reduce intestinal absorption of tetracycline. Side-effects are uncommon. Diarrhoea and vomiting have been reported but have ceased on withdrawal of therapy.

**Pharmaceutical precautions** Store below 25˚C

**Legal category** P.

**Package quantities** *Altacite Plus Suspension:* Polyethylene laminate bottle containing 500 ml and glass bottles containing 100 ml. *Altacite Plus Tablets:* Tube of 20 tablets.

**Further information** There is no evidence of absorption of hydrotalcite in man. Investigations in healthy human volunteers have shown no elevation of serum aluminium or magnesium levels on administration of hydrotalcite at therapeutic dosage for a continuous period of 28 days.

The sodium content of Altacite Plus suspension is low (0.078 mmol/5 ml).

Altacite Plus Tablets contain Lactose (anhydrous).

**Product licence numbers**
| | |
|---|---|
| Altacite Plus Suspension | 0109/0062 |
| Altacite Plus Tablets | 0109/0056 |

*Product licence holder:* Roussel Laboratories Limited, Broadwater Park, Denham, Uxbridge.

## ASPAV*

**Presentation** White, circular, flat bevelled-edge tablets, with the identifying letters 'AP' on one face; or as an alternative, plain tablets devoid of surface markings. Each tablet containing the equivalent of Aspirin PhEur 500 mg and 7.71 mg Papaveretum BP (equivalent to 5 mg anhydrous morphine).

**Uses** For the relief of moderate to severe pain in post-operative states and the relief of chronic pain associated with inoperable carcinoma.

**Dosage and administration**
*Adults* (not recommended for children under 12 years); One or two tablets dispersed in water every 4-6 hours. (Not more than eight tablets in any 24 hour period).

**Contra-indications, warnings, etc**
*Contra-indications:* Not recommended for children under 12 years. Should not be administered to patients with known sensitivity to aspirin or papaveretum. Aspav should not be given to patients with respiratory depression, or obstructive airways disease and should not be given to patients receiving concurrent therapy with monoamine oxidase inhibitors, or within two weeks of their withdrawal.

*Warnings:* Aspirin may give rise to hypersensitivity reactions, asthma and may induce gastro-intestinal haemorrhage (occasionally major). Aspirin may precipitate bronchospasm and may induce attacks of asthma in susceptible subjects. Reduced dosage is advised in elderly and debilitated patients, hypothyroid patients and those with head injuries or chronic hepatic disease. As with all narcotics, patients taking Aspav should avoid alcohol.

*Precautions:* Aspav should be given with care to patients known to have a lesion of the gastric mucosa. Aspav may also modify patients' reactions and they should be advised against driving or performing other complex manual tasks.

*Use in pregnancy and lactation:* There is clinical and epidemiological evidence for the safety of aspirin in human pregnancy; nevertheless, the safety of the combination has not been established. Although Aspav has been used clinically for many years without noticeable ill consequences, the principle of using only essential drugs in the early months of pregnancy should be observed. Aspirin may prolong labour and contribute to maternal and neonatal bleeding; its use is best avoided at term.

*Tolerance:* Repeated administration of Aspav may give rise to tolerance and dependence of the morphine type.

*Side-effects:* These include asthma or difficulty in breathing, allergic reactions (such as rash or swelling), bleeding in the stomach which can be severe. Aspav may modify patients reactions and they should be advised against driving or performing other complex manual tasks.

*Interactions:* Papaveretum is an analgesic with CNS depressant properties; these properties may be enhanced when Aspav is taken in combination with other CNS depressants and/or alcohol. Aspirin may enhance the activity of coumarin anticoagulants and oral hypoglycaemic agents. The activity of methotrexate may be markedly enhanced and its toxicity increased; the toxicity of sulphonamides may also be increased. Aspirin diminishes the effect of uricosuric agents such as probenecid and sulphinpyrazone.

*Effects of overdosage:* Side-effects of overdosage are similar to those with morphine, but occur to a lesser extent; they may include pin-point pupils, depressed respiration and coma. In severe poisoning there may be dilatation of the pupils, shock, severe respiratory depression and pulmonary oedema.

Gastric lavage should be performed soon after ingestion, and oxygen, intravenous fluids and other intensive supportive therapy carried out, as necessary. Levallorphan tartrate 1–2 mg IV, naloxone or nalorphine are suitable antidotes for opioid analgesics.

**Pharmaceutical precautions** Aspav Tablets should be stored in a cool dry place, in a tightly closed container, and protected from light.

**Legal category** POM.

**Package quantities** Securitainers of 100 tablets.

**Further information** Aspav has advantages over morphine combinations, as papaveretum has intrinsic spasmolytic activity in addition to its analgesic properties. Aspav is not subject to the prescribing regulations of the Misuse of Drugs Act. Each tablet contains 1607 mg Lactose BP.

**Product licence number** 0142/5597

*Product licence holder:* AH Cox & Co Ltd, Whiddon Valley, Devon.

## CEFROM* ▼

**Presentation** Cefrom is supplied as a dry white to pale yellow crystalline powder in vials containing 250 mg, 500 mg, 1 g and 2 g cefpirome (as sulphate) for intravenous injection and bottles containing 1 g and 2 g cefpirome (as sulphate) for intravenous infusion. Anhydrous sodium carbonate is also included (approximately 242 mg per gram of cefpirome) to improve solubility and adjust the pH to within the physiological pH range.

When Cefrom is dissolved in Water for Injections effervescence occurs and a faint yellow to yellow solution is formed. Each gram of Cefrom contains approximately 107 mg (4.7 meq) of sodium.

**Uses**
*Properties:* Cefrom is a bactericidal β-lactamase-stable cephalosporin antibiotic. As a β-lactam, Cefrom acts by disturbing the synthesis of the main bacterial cell-wall polymer, peptidoglycan. It is bactericidal at low concentrations against an extremely broad spectrum of Gram-negative and Gram-positive pathogens. Cefrom penetrates the cell wall of bacteria extremely

rapidly and binds to the target enzymes (penicillin-binding proteins) with high affinity. This has been demonstrated in numerous *in vitro* studies with hospital- and community-acquired pathogens throughout the world, and recent studies show no change in the pattern of sensitivity. Many strains resistant to other injectable cephalosporins, penicillins and aminoglycosides are sensitive to Cefrom.

*Indications:* Cefrom is indicated for the treatment of infections, either before the infecting organism has been identified or when caused by bacteria of established sensitivity, as follows:

Lower respiratory tract infections (bronchopneumonia and lobar pneumonia).

Complicated upper (pyelonephritis) and lower urinary tract infections.

Skin and soft tissue infections (cellulitis, skin abscess and wound infections).

Infections in neutropenic patients.

Bacteraemia/septicaemia.

Severe infections, as listed above.

*Bacteriology:* Most strains of the following species show sensitivity to Cefrom *in vitro*.

Gram-Positive: *Staphylococcus aureus* (including penicillin-resistant strains), coagulase-negative *Staphylococcus* spp. (including penicillin-resistant but not methicillin-resistant strains), *Streptococcus* Group A (*Streptococcus pyogenes*), B (*Streptococcus agalactiae*), C, F and G, *Streptococcus mitis*, *Streptococcus sanguis*, *Streptococcus viridans*, *Streptococcus pneumoniae*, *Propionibacterium acnes*, *Peptostreptococcus anaerobius*, *Corynebacterium diphtheriae*, *Corynebacterium pyogenes*, *Clostridium* spp.

Gram-Negative: *Citrobacter* spp., *Escherichia coli*, *Salmonella* spp., *Shigella* spp., *Klebsiella* spp. (indole-positive and indole-negative), *Enterobacter* spp., *Hafnia alvei*, *Serratia* spp., *Proteus mirabilis*, *Proteus vulgaris*, *Proteus rettgeri*, *Morganella morganii*, *Providencia* spp., *Yersinia enterocolitica*, *Pasteurella multocida*, *Haemophilus influenzae*, *Haemophilus ducreyi*, *Moraxella catarrhalis*, *Neisseria meningitidis*, *Neisseria gonorrhoeae*, *Aeromonas hydrophila*, *Pseudomonas aeruginosa*, *Pseudomonas* spp. (non-aeruginosa), *Bacteroides fragilis* (non-β-lactamase-producing strains).

Most strains of the following species are resistant to Cefrom *in vitro*:

Gram-Positive: *Enterococcus faecium*, *Listeria monocytogenes*, *Clostridium difficile*.

Gram-Negative: *Xanthomonas maltophilia*, *Fusobacterium varium*, *Bacteroides fragilis* (β-lactamase-producing strains).

Cefpirome shows synergistic activity with aminoglycosides against many bacteria.

Infections caused by the following pathogens have been successfully treated in clinical trials:

Gram-Positive: *Staphylococcus aureus* and coagulase-negative *Staphylococcus* spp. (*Staphylococcus epidermidis*, *Staphylococcus saprophyticus*, *Staphylococcus hominis*, *Staphylococcus warneri*), haemolytic and non-haemolytic streptococci, *Streptococcus pyogenes* (Group A), streptococci of serogroups B, F, *Streptococcus pneumoniae*, *Streptococcus agalactiae*, streptococci of the viridans group, *Corynebacterium* spp.

Gram-negative: *Escherichia coli*, *Enterobacter* spp., indole-positive and indole-negative *Klebsiella* spp. and *Proteus* spp., *Morganella morganii*, *Providencia* spp., *Citrobacter* spp., *Salmonella* spp., *Hafnia alvei*, *Serratia marcescens*, *Pasturella multocida*, *Haemophilus influenzae* and other *Haemophilus* species, *Moraxella catarrhalis*, *Neisseria* spp., *Alcaligenes* spp., *Pseudomonas aeruginosa* and other *Pseudomonas* species, *Bacteroides* spp.

**Dosage and administration** Cefrom is to be administered by i.v. injection or infusion, the dosage, mode of administration and duration of treatment depending upon the severity of the infection, sensitivity of the pathogens, condition of the patient and renal function. The following dosages are recommended for moderate to severe infections in patients with normal renal function:

*Adults:*

**Cefrom dosage**

| Indication | Unit dose (g) | Dosage interval (hours) | Total daily dose (g) |
|---|---|---|---|
| Complicated upper and lower urinary tract infections | 1 | 12 | 2 |
| Skin and soft tissue infections | 1 | 12 | 2 |
| Lower respiratory tract infections | 1 or 2 | 2 | 2 or 4 |
| Bacteraemia/Septicaemia and severe infections | 2 | 12 | 4 |
| Infections in neutropenic patients | 2 | 12 | 4 |

For urinary tract and skin soft tissue infections, the unit dose may be increased to 2 g in very severe cases.

*Elderly:* No dosage adjustment is required, unless renal impairment is present.

*Children:* There is insufficient evidence on which to base an appropriate dosage regimen in children under 12 years of age. Therefore, Cefrom is not recommended for this age group.

*Dosage in patients with impaired renal function:* Cefrom is excreted principally by the kidney. The dose must therefore be reduced in patients with impaired renal function to compensate for the slower excretion. The following doses are recommended:

| Creatinine clearance | Recommended dose in normal renal function | |
|---|---|---|
| >50 ml/min | 1.0 g b.i.d. | 2.0 g b.i.d. |
| | Dose Adjustment | |
| | 1.0 g loading dose then | 2.0 g loading dose then |
| 50–20 ml/min | 0.5 g b.i.d. | 1.0 g b.i.d. |
| 20–5 ml/min | 0.5 g once daily | 1.0 g once daily |
| <5 ml/min (haemodialysis patients) | 0.5 g daily+0.25 g immediately after dialysis | 1.0 g daily+0.5 g immediately after dialysis |

Cefrom may interfere with some creatinine assays (see Interactions).

*Administration:*

*Intravenous injection:* The contents of one vial of 1 or 2 g Cefrom are dissolved in 10 or 20 ml sterile Water for Injections respectively, and then injected over 3–5 minutes either directly into a vein or into the distal section of a clamped-off infusion tube. For patients with renal impairment, 0.25 or 0.5 g Cefrom are dissolved in 2 or 5 ml Water for Injections respectively. To obtain these fractional doses from the 1 g vial, see the table below.

| Vial size (g) | Volume of Water for Injection to be added (ml) | Approx. available volume (ml) | Fractional dose: Volume required (ml) | Approx. concentration (mg/ml) |
|---|---|---|---|---|
| 1 g | 10 ml | 10.7 ml | 0.5 g:5.4 ml 0.25 g:2.8 ml | 93.5 mg/ml |

*Short intravenous infusion:* The contents of one 1 or 2 g bottle of Cefrom are dissolved in 100 ml sterile Water for Injections (or one of the infusion solutions described in *Pharmaceutical precautions*) and then infused over 20–30 minutes.

*Instructions for use/handling:* The vials are manufactured under slight negative pressure. The negative pressure facilitates the addition of the solvent. Carbon dioxide is released when the solvent and the powder for reconstitution are mixed, and an increase in pressure occurs. The solution may still contain bubbles of carbon dioxide, but these have no adverse effects on efficacy. The vials containing the solvent and powder for reconstitution should be held horizontal when preparing the infusion solution, and the needle should be inserted rapidly.

Effervescence occurs on dissolution of Cefrom and the vial or bottle has to be tipped gently from side to side for approximately 1 minute before Cefrom is completely dissolved.

Cefrom should not be administered in sodium bicarbonate solution.

**Contra-indications, warnings, etc**

*Contra-indications:* Hypersensitivity to cephalosporins.

Preliminary enquiry as to previous hypersensitivity to β-lactam antibiotics is required.

The use of Cefrom is strictly contra-indicated in subjects with a previous history of immediate hypersensitivity to cephalosporins. In any doubt, it is essential that a physician is present at the first administration in order to treat any possible anaphylactic reaction.

*Cross-sensitivity:* As there is cross allergy between penicillin and cephalosporins in 5 to 10% of cases, use of cefpirome should be undertaken with extreme care in penicillin sensitive patients. Careful surveillance is necessary from the first administration. Hypersensitivity reactions (anaphylaxis) occurring with these two classes of antibiotic may be serious or even fatal.

Occurrence of a hypersensitivity reaction requires treatment to be stopped.

*Blood constituents:* For courses of treatment lasting longer than 10 days, blood count should be monitored and in the event of neutropenia developing treatment should be discontinued.

*Precautions:*

*Renal function:* Caution should be exercised if cefpirome is administered together with aminoglycosides or loop diuretics; renal function must be monitored in all such cases.

*Pseudomembranous colitis:* Severe and persistent diarrhoea has been observed during treatment with antibiotics of several different classes. This may be symptomatic of pseudomembranous colitis (in most cases due to *Clostridium difficile*) which may be fatal. This is a rare complication with cephalosporins. Once pseudomembranous colitis is suspected as the diagnosis, confirmed by sigmoidoscopy, cefpirome treatment must be stopped immediately and specific antibiotic therapy must be started (e.g. vancomycin or metronidazole). The administration of products which may cause faecal stasis is contra-indicated.

*Drug interactions:* Drug interactions have not been observed with Cefrom. Although there is no evidence that Cefrom adversely affects renal function at normal therapeutic doses, cephalosporin antibiotics may potentiate the nephrotoxic effects of certain drugs (e.g. aminoglycosides) if administered concomitantly.

Probenicid interferes with renal tubular transfer of cefpirome, delaying its excretion and increasing the plasma concentration.

*Other interactions:* A false-positive Coombs test result may be obtained in rare cases during treatment with Cefrom. Glycosuria should be determined by enzymatic methods during treatment as non-enzymatic methods may give a false-positive result.

Cefrom gives a strong, creatinine-like reaction in creatinine assays based on the picrate method. The use of an enzyme method is recommended to avoid falsely high levels of creatinine. If an enzyme method is not available, blood sampling should be done immediately before the next administration of cefpirome because if the recommended dosage and dosage intervals are followed, the serum level of cefpirome at that time is expected to be below the interference limit.

*Pregnancy:* The safety of this medicinal product for use in human pregnancy has not been established. Cefrom should therefore not be used during pregnancy. An evaluation of experimental animal studies has not indicated direct or indirect harmful effects with respect to reproduction, development of the embryo or foetus, the course of gestation and perinatal and postnatal development.

*Lactation:* As cefpirome is excreted in human breast milk, either Cefrom treatment should be discontinued or breast feeding ceased.

*Side-effects:* The following may be observed during treatment with cephalosporins:

*Hypersensitivity reactions:* Allergic skin reactions: rash, urticaria, pruritis; drug fever; severe acute allergic reactions (anaphylaxis) may occur and require emergency treatment.

Interstitial nephritis has been observed in rare instances during treatment with other cephalosporins.

*Effects on the gastro-intestinal tract:* Nausea and vomiting; diarrhoea; in very rare cases, pseudomembranous colitis (see Precautions).

*Effects on liver function:* Increase in liver enzymes in the serum (ASAT{GOT}, ALAT{GPT}, alkaline phosphatase), Gamma GT, LDH and/or bilirubin.

*Effects on renal function:* Slight increases in serum creatinine and urea may be observed, but are only rarely a reason for discontinuing treatment.

*Changes in blood constituents:* Thrombocytopenia; eosinophilia; very rarely, haemolytic anaemia. As with other β-lactam antibiotics, granulocytopenia and, more rarely, agranulocytosis may develop during treatment with Cefrom, particularly if given over long periods.

*Local reactions:* Inflammatory irritation of the venous wall and pain at the site of injection.

*Other:* Superinfections; taste disturbances shortly after injection; headache.

*Effects on ability to drive and use machines:* There is no evidence that Cefrom impairs the ability to drive or operate machines.

*Overdosage:* So far, there has been no clinical experience with overdoses of Cefrom. Serum levels of Cefrom can be reduced by peritoneal dialysis and haemodialysis.

**Pharmaceutical precautions**

*Vials (sterile powder):* Protect from light; do not store drug product at above 25°C. Some intensification of colour may occur on storage. However, provided the recommended storage conditions are observed, this does not indicate a change in potency or safety.

*Reconstituted solutions:* In keeping with good pharmaceutical practice, it is preferable to use freshly constituted solutions of Cefrom. Cefrom can be stored for up to 24 hrs refrigerated (2–8°C) when prepared in Water for Injections BP.

Cefrom is compatible with several other commonly

used intravenous infusion fluids and will retain satisfactory potency for up to 24 hrs when refrigerated (2–8°C) in the following fluids:

Water for Injections BP, 0.9% Sodium Chloride Injection BP, 5% glucose solution, 10% glucose solution, 5% fructose solution, Ringers Solutions BPC.

Some intensification of colour may occur on storage. However, provided the recommended storage conditions are observed, this does not indicate a change in potency or safety.

No data is yet available to support the mixing of reconstituted cefpirome with any other drugs or infusion solutions other than those specified above.

**Legal category** POM.

**Package quantities** Individually packed vials containing 250 mg, 500 mg, 1 g or 2 g cefpirome (as sulphate) for intravenous injection in packs of 5.

Individually packed bottles containing 1 g or 2 g cefpirome (as sulphate) for intravenous infusion in packs of 5.

**Further information** *Bioavailability and absorption:* Bioavailability after i.m. administration is greater than 90%.

*Distribution:* The average peak ($C_{5\,min}$) serum level after single i.v. doses of 1 g is 80–90 mg/l. Pharmacokinetics are dose linear. The volume of distribution is 14–19 L. No accumulation is seen after multiple dosing. The elimination half-life in serum is 1.8–2.2 hours. Serum protein binding is lower than 10% and is dose independent. Rapid penetration into the following body tissues and fluids has been observed.

**Cefrom tissue distribution**

| Tissue/fluid | Dose (g) | Mean concentration | | |
|---|---|---|---|---|
| | | 2 h | <8 h | 12 h |
| Tissue (mg/kg) | | | | |
| Prostate | 1 | 12.9 | 6.1 | 1.7 |
| Bronchial mucosa | 1 | 33.0 | 15.7 | — |
| Fluid (mg/l) | | | | |
| Interstitial | 1 | 32.9 | 13.3 | 2.9 |
| Peritoneal | 1 | 46.3 | 10.6 | — |
| Meninges | | | | |
| Inflamed | 2 | 2.7 | 3.6 | 2.3 |
| Non-inflamed | 2 | 0.5 | 0.8 | — |

**Cefrom tissue to serum or fluid to serum ratio**

| Tissue/fluid | Dose (g) | Tissue:serum or fluid:serum ratio | | |
|---|---|---|---|---|
| | | 2 h | <8 h | 12 h |
| Tissue (mg/kg) | | | | |
| Prostate | 1 | 0.3 | 0.4 | 0.6 |
| Bronchial mucosa | 1 | 0.6 | 0.6 | — |
| Fluid (mg/l) | | | | |
| Interstitial | 1 | 1.9 | 2.3 | 3.0 |
| Peritoneal | 1 | 1.1 | 1.0 | — |
| Meninges | | | | |
| Inflamed | 2 | 0.05 | 0.9 | 0.7 |
| Non-inflamed | 2 | 0.01 | 0.13 | — |

Peak plasma levels are above the MICs for all commonly encountered pathogens.

*Biotransformation and excretion:* Cefrom is principally eliminated by the kidney; 80–90% of the administered drug is recovered in the urine. Radioactive counts recovered in the urine consist of 98–99% unchanged Cefrom. Approximately 30% of a 1 g dose is eliminated by haemodialysis.

*Special groups:* Elderly (>65 years): The mean $C_{5\,min}$ serum level after a single i.v. dose of 2 g to healthy subjects is 174 mg/l. The elimination half-life in serum is 3.4 hours and urinary excretion of the unchanged product is 71% after 24 hours. In patients older than 65 years $C_{5\,min}$ after i.v. doses of 1 and 2 g amounts to 127.1 and 231.1 mg/l respectively. The elimination half-lives after the same doses amounts to 4.4±1.4 and 4.5±1.6 hours respectively.

*Renally impaired patients:* The average elimination half-lives after single doses of 2 g i.v. to patients with different degrees of renal impairment are as follows:

**Cefrom elimination in renally impaired patients**

| | Creatinine clearance (ml/min) | | | |
|---|---|---|---|---|
| | >50 | 20–50 | 10–20 | <10 |
| Elimination half-life (h) | 2.6 | 9.2 | 9.8 | 14.5 |

Dose adjustments are required in renally impaired patients only at creatinine clearance levels below 50 ml/min (see *Dosage and administration*).

**Product licence numbers**

| | |
|---|---|
| 250 mg i.v. injection | 0109/0242 |
| 500 mg i.v. injection | 0109/0243 |
| 1 g i.v. injection | 0109/0244 |
| 2 g i.v. injection | 0109/0245 |
| 1 g i.v. infusion | 0109/0246 |
| 2 g i.v. infusion | 0109/0247 |

*Product licence holder:* Roussel Laboratories Limited, Broadwater Park, Denham, Uxbridge.

# CIDOMYCIN* CREAM

**Qualitative and quantitative composition** Cream containing Gentamicin Sulphate 0.3% w/w.

**Pharmaceutical form** Cream

**Clinical particulars**

*Therapeutic indications:* Cidomycin is a wide-spectrum antibiotic and is recommended for the treatment of primary and secondary skin infections due to susceptible bacteria.

*Primary infections:* Superficial folliculitis.

*Secondary infections:* Infected, contact, seborrhoeic and eczematoid dermatitis, pustular acne and paronychia.

*Posology and method of administration:*
*Route of administration:* Cutaneous.

*Adults and children:* A small amount of cream should be applied to the lesions three or four times daily or as prescribed. If necessary this may be covered with a dressing. Elderly: As adults.

*Contra-indications:* Cidomycin is contra-indicated when there is a known hypersensitivity to any ingredient of the preparation, including aminoglycosides.

*Special warnings and precautions for use:* Ototoxicity has been recorded following the use of gentamicin. Groups at special risk include patients with impaired renal function and possibly the elderly and children.

*Interactions with other medicaments and other forms of interaction:* None known.

*Use in pregnancy and lactation:* There are no proven cases of intrauterine damage caused by gentamicin. However, in common with most drugs known to cross the placenta, usage in pregnancy should only be considered in life threatening situations where expected benefits outweigh possible risks. In the absence of gastro-intestinal inflammation, the amount of gentamicin ingested from the milk is unlikely to result in significant blood levels in breast-fed infants.

*Effects on ability to drive and to use machines:* None known.

*Undesirable effects (frequency and seriousness):* If irritation, sensitisation or super-infection develop, treatment with Cidomycin should be discontinued and appropriate therapy instituted. With application to large wounds, ototoxicity may be a hazard in children and the elderly.

*Overdose:* Haemodialysis or peritoneal dialysis will aid the removal of gentamicin from the blood.

**Pharmacological properties**

*Pharmacodynamic properties:* Gentamicin is a mixture of antibiotic substances produced by the growth of *Micromonospora purpurea*. It is bactericidal with greater antibacterial activity than streptomycin, neomycin or kanamycin.

Gentamicin exerts a number of effects on cells of susceptible bacteria. It affects the integrity of the plasma membrane and the metabolism of RNA, but its most important effects is inhibition of protein synthesis at the level of the 30s ribosomal subunit.

*Pharmacokinetic properties:* The literature states that the absorption rate has been low however if applied on a large area or on the day of burning, the absorption of the drug into the blood stream was significant. This absorption has rarely been of clinical significance. (See undesirable effects section).

*Preclinical safety data:* Not applicable.

**Pharmaceutical particulars**

*List of excipients:* The cream contains acid, propylene glycol monostearate, isopropyl myristate, tween 40, butyl hydroxybenzoate, methyl hydroxybenzoate, sorbitol, propylene glycol and purified water.

*Incompatibilities:* In order to preserve its antibacterial activity, Cidomycin Cream should not be diluted by the addition of excipient.

*Shelf-life:* 2 years.

*Special precautions for storage:* Store below 25°C.

*Nature and contents of container:* A 30 g collapsible aluminium tube containing the cream.

*Instructions for use/handling:* None.

*Marketing authorisation holder:* Roussel Laboratories Ltd., Broadwater Park, Denham, Uxbridge, Middlesex UB9 5HP

**Marketing authorisation number**
Cidomycin Cream          0109/5063R

**Date of approval/revision of SPC** May 1997

**Legal category** POM

# CIDOMYCIN* EYE/EAR DROPS
# CIDOMYCIN* EYE OINTMENT

**Presentation**

*Drops:* Each millilitre of drops contains Gentamicin Sulphate BP equivalent to 0.3% w/v gentamicin base in sterile buffered isotonic aqueous solution.

*Ointment:* Each gram of ointment contains Gentamicin Sulphate BP equivalent to 0.3% w/v gentamicin base in Plastibase*.

**Uses** Cidomycin (gentamicin) is an aminoglycoside antibiotic with broad spectrum bactericidal activity against most Gram–positive and Gram-negative bacteria.

*In the eye:* Cidomycin drops and ointment are indicated in the topical treatment of external bacterial infections of the eye, including conjunctivitis, blepharitis, styes, corneal ulcers and for prophylaxis in trauma.

*In the ear:* Cidomycin drops may also be used effectively in the treatment of external ear infections due to sensitive organisms.

**Dosage and administration** For adults and children.

*In the eye:* 1 to 3 drops should be instilled into the affected eye three or four times daily, or as required; alternatively, the ointment may be used applying it to the affected area three or four times daily, or as required.

*In the ear:* Following cleansing of the affected ear, 2 to 4 drops should be instilled three or four times daily and at night.

No specific recommendations for the elderly.

**Contra-indications, warnings, etc** The product is contra-indicated where there is known hypersensitivity to any of the ingredients. If irritation, sensitisation or superinfection develop, treatment with Cidomycin should be discontinued and appropriate therapy instituted. Use in the ear is contra-indicated if the drum is perforated.

*Interactions:* Gentamicin is pharmaceutically incompatible with amphotericin, cephalosporins, erythromycin, heparin, penicillins, sodium bicarbonate, and sulphadiazine sodium.

Potent diuretics such as ethacrynic acid and frusemide are believed to enhance any risk of ototoxicity. Amphotericin B, cisplatin and cyclosporin are potential enhancers of nephrotoxicity. Neuromuscular blockade and respiratory paralysis have been reported from the administration of aminoglycosides to patients who have received curare-type muscle relaxants during anaesthesia.

*Effects on ability to drive and to use machines:* Topical eye preparations may cause transient blurring of vision on instillation. Patients should be warned not to drive or operate hazardous machinery unless vision is clear.

*Other undesirable effects:* Gentamicin drops or ointment may cause transient eye irritation. Severe dose-related ototoxicity can occur with gentamicin in susceptible patients, particularly those with renal impairment. Vestibular damage is more common than hearing loss.

Reversible nephrotoxicity may occur and acute nerve failure has been reported, often in association with concurrent administration of cephalosporins.

*Use in pregnancy and lactation:* There are no proven cases of intrauterine damage caused by gentamicin. However, as with most drugs known to cross the placenta, usage in pregnancy should be considered where benefits outweigh possible risks. In the absence of gastro-intestinal inflammation, the amount of gentamicin ingested from breast milk is unlikely to result in significant blood levels in infants.

*Other special warnings and precautions:* If irritation, sensitisation, or super-infection develop, treatment with Cidomycin should be discontinued and appropriate therapy instituted.

*Overdose:* In the unlikely event of over dosage haemodialysis or peritoneal dialysis will aid the removal of gentamicin from the blood.

**Pharmaceutical precautions** Eye/Ear Drops: Store below 25°C.

Eye Ointment: Store below 30°C.

**Legal category** POM.

**Package quantities** Cidomycin Eye/Ear Drops–8 ml in ophthalmic dispenser.

Cidomycin Eye Ointment–5 g tube (fitted with ophthalmic nozzle).

**Further information** Cidomycin eye/ear drops contain disodium edetate, benzalkonium chloride solution, sodium metabisulphite, sodium phosphate, sodium acid phosphate and Purified Water.

**Product licence numbers**
Cidomycin Eye/Ear Drops 0109/0114
Cidomycin Eye Ointment 0109/0115

*Product licence holder:* Roussel Laboratories Limited, Broadwater Park, Denham, Uxbridge.

## CIDOMYCIN* INJECTIONS

**Presentation** Cidomycin for parenteral use is available as:

Cidomycin Adult Injectable in 2 ml vials or ampoules each containing the equivalent of 80 mg gentamicin base as Gentamicin Sulphate BP.

Cidomycin Paediatric Injectable in 2 ml vials each containing the equivalent of 20 mg gentamicin base as Gentamicin Sulphate BP.

Cidomycin Intrathecal Injection in 1 ml ampoules each containing 5 mg gentamicin base as Gentamicin Sulphate BP.

**Uses** Gentamicin is an aminoglycoside antibiotic with broad-spectrum bactericidal activity. It is usually active against most strains of the following organisms: *Escherichia coli, Klebsiella* spp., *Proteus* spp. (indole positive and indole negative), *Pseudomonas aeruginosa,* staphylococci, *Enterobacter* spp., *Citrobacter* spp and *Providencia* spp.

Gentamicin injection and gentamicin paediatric injection are indicated in urinary-tract infections, chest infections, bacteraemia, septicaemia, severe neonatal infections, and other systemic infections due to sensitive organisms.

Gentamicin intrathecal injection is indicated as a supplement to systemic therapy in bacterial meningitis, ventriculitis and other bacterial infections of the central nervous system.

**Dosage and administration**

*Gentamicin intramuscular/intravenous injection:*

*Adults: Serious infections:* If renal function is not impaired, 5 mg/kg daily in divided doses at six or eight hourly intervals. The total daily dose may be subsequently increased or decreased as clinically indicated.

*Systemic infections.* If renal function is not impaired, 3-5 mg/kg/day in divided doses according to severity of infection, adjusting according to clinical response and body weight.

*Urinary-tract infections:* As 'Systemic infections'. Or, if renal function is not impaired, 160 mg once daily may be used.

*Children:* Premature infants or full term neonates up to 2 weeks of age: 3 mg/kg 12-hourly. 2 weeks to 12 years: 2 mg/kg 8-hourly.

*The elderly:* There is some evidence that elderly patients may be more susceptible to aminoglycoside toxicity whether secondary to previous eighth nerve impairment or borderline renal dysfunction. Accordingly, therapy should be closely monitored by frequent determination of gentamicin serum levels, assessment of renal function and signs of ototoxicity.

*Gentamicin intrathecal injection:* Bacterial meningitis and ventriculitis: the starting dose of gentamicin intrathecal injection for both children and adults is 1 mg daily, intrathecally or intraventricularly, together with 1 mg/kg every eight hours intramuscularly. The MIC of the infecting organism in the CSF should be assessed and, if necessary, the intrathecal/intraventricular dose increased to 5 mg daily, whilst keeping the intramuscular dose at 1 mg/kg eight-hourly. Treatment should be continued for at least seven days but longer if necessary. Periodic serum and CSF gentamicin assays should be carried out to ensure that adequate antibiotic levels are maintained and that serum and CSF levels do not exceed 10 mg/l.

*Renal impairment:* Gentamicin is excreted by simple glomerular filtration and therefore reduced dosage is necessary where renal function is impaired. Nomograms are available for the calculation of dose, which depends on the patient's age, weight and renal function. The following table may be useful when treating adults.

| Blood urea (mg/100 ml) | Blood urea (mmol/l) | Creatinine clearance (GFR) (ml/min) | Dose and frequency of administration |
|---|---|---|---|
| <40 | 6–7 | >70 | 80 mg* 8-hourly |
| 40–100 | 6–17 | 30–70 | 80 mg* 12-hourly |
| 100–200 | 17–34 | 10–30 | 80 mg* daily |
| >200 | >34 | 5–10 | 80 mg* every 48 hours |
| Twice-weekly intermittent haemodialysis | | <5 | 80 mg* after dialysis |

*60 mg if body weight <60 kg. Frequency of dosage in hours may also be approximated as serum creatinine (mg%)× weight or in SI units, as serum creatinine (micromol/l) divided by 11. If these dosage guides are used peak serum levels must be measured. Peak levels of gentamicin occur approximately one hour after intramuscular injection and intravenous injection. Trough levels are measured just prior to the next injection. Assay of peak serum levels gives confirmation of adequacy of dosage and also serves to detect levels above 10 mg/l, at which the possibility of ototoxicity should be considered. One-hour concentrations of gentamicin should not exceed 10 mg/l (but should reach 4 mg/l), while the pre-dose trough concentration should be less than 2 mg/l.

The recommended dose and precautions for intramuscular and intravenous administration are identical. Gentamicin when given intravenously should be injected directly into a vein or into the drip set tubing over no less than three minutes. If administered by infusion, this should be over no longer than 20 minutes and in no greater volume of fluid than 100 ml.

**Contra-indications, warnings, etc**

*Contra-indications:* Hypersensitivity; myasthenia gravis.

*Warnings:* Ototoxicity has been recorded following the use of gentamicin. Groups at special risk include patients with impaired renal function and possibly the elderly. Consequently, renal, auditory and vestibular functions should be monitored in these patients and serum levels determined so as to avoid peak concentrations above 10 mg/l and troughs above 2 mg/l. As there is some evidence that risk of both ototoxicity and nephrotoxicity is related to the level of total exposure, duration of therapy should be the shortest possible compatible with clinical recovery. In some patients with impaired renal function there has been a transient rise in blood-urea-nitrogen which has usually reverted to normal during or following cessation of therapy. It is important to adjust the frequency of dosage according to the degree of renal function (see table).

*Pregnancy and lactation:* There are no proven cases of intrauterine damage caused by gentamicin. However, in common with most drugs known to cross the placenta, usage in pregnancy should only be considered in life-threatening situations where the expected benefits outweigh possible risks. In the absence of gastro-intestinal inflammation, the amount of gentamicin ingested from the milk is unlikely to result in significant blood levels in breast-fed infants.

*Interaction with other substances:* Concurrent administration of gentamicin and other potentially ototoxic or nephrotoxic drugs should be avoided. Potent diuretics such as ethacrynic acid and frusemide are believed to enhance the risk of ototoxicity whilst amphotericin B, cisplatin and cyclosporin are potential enhancers of nephrotoxicity. Any potential nephrotoxicity of cephalosporins, and in particular cephaloridine, may also be increased in the presence of gentamicin. Consequently, if this combination is used monitoring of kidney function is advised.

Neuromuscular blockade and respiratory paralysis have been reported from administration of aminoglycosides to patients who have received curare-type muscle relaxants during anaesthesia.

*Overdosage:* Haemodialysis and peritoneal dialysis will aid removal from blood but the former is probably more efficient. Calcium salts given intravenously have been used to counter the neuromuscular blockade caused by gentamicin.

**Pharmaceutical precautions** Cidomycin Adult Injectable and Paediatric Injectable: Store at room temperature (15 to 25°C). Do not refrigerate. Cidomycin Intrathecal injection: Store below 25°C. Gentamicin is a remarkably stable antibiotic and does not require refrigeration.

In general gentamicin injection should not be mixed. In particular the following are incompatible in mixed solution with gentamicin injection: penicillins, cephalosporins, erythromycin, heparins, sodium bicarbonate (Carbon dioxide may be liberated on addition of the two solutions. Normally this will dissolve in the solution but under some circumstances small bubbles may form). Dilution in the body will obviate the danger of physical and chemical incompatibility and enable gentamicin to be given concurrently with the drugs listed above either as a bolus injection into the drip tubing, with adequate flushing, or at separate sites. In the case of carbenicillin, administration should only be at a separate site.

**Legal category** POM.

**Package quantities** Cidomycin Adult Injectable: Packs of 25×2 ml vials or ampoules.

Cidomycin Paediatric Injectable: Packs of 5×2 ml vials.

Cidomycin Intrathecal Injection: Packs of 5×1 ml ampoules.

**Further information** Cidomycin Adult Injectable and Paediatric Injectable contains methylhydroxybenzoate, Propylhydroxybenzoate and disodium edetate. Cidomycin Intrathecal Injection contains sodium chloride.

**Product licence numbers**
Cidomycin Adult Injectable 0109/5065R
Cidomycin Paediatric Injectable 0109/5066R
Cidomycin Intrathecal Injection 0109/0057R

*Product licence holder:* Roussel Laboratories Limited, Broadwater Park, Denham, Uxbridge.

## CLAFORAN*

**Qualitative and quantitative composition** Claforan is supplied as a white to slightly creamy powder, which when dissolved in Water for Injections PhEur forms a straw-coloured solution suitable for IV or IM injection. Variations in the intensity of colour of the freshly prepared solution do not indicate a change in potency or safety.

500 mg vial: Contains cefotaxime sodium equivalent to 500 mg cefotaxime base.
1 g vial: Contains cefotaxime sodium equivalent to 1 g cefotaxime base.
2 g vial: Contains cefotaxime sodium equivalent to 2 g cefotaxime base.

Each gram of Claforan contains approximately 48 mg (2.09 mmol) of sodium.

**Pharmaceutical form** Vials containing powder to be dissolved in Water for Injections PhEur

**Clinical particulars**

*Therapeutic indications:* Claforan is a broad-spectrum bactericidal cephalosporin antibiotic. Claforan is exceptionally active in vitro against Gram-negative organisms sensitive or resistant to first or second generation cephalosporins. It is similar to other cephalosporins in activity against Gram-positive organisms.

Claforan is indicated in the treatment of the following infections either before the infecting organism has been identified or when caused by bacteria of established sensitivity.

*Septicaemias.*

*Respiratory tract infections:* such as acute and chronic bronchitis, bacterial pneumonia, infected bronchiectasis, lung abscess and post-operative chest infections.

*Urinary tract infections:* such as acute and chronic pyelonephritis, cystitis and asymptomatic bacteriuria.

*Soft-tissue infections:* such as cellulitis, peritonitis and wound infections.

*Bone and joint infections:* such as osteomyelitis, septic arthritis.

*Obstetric and gynaecological infections:* such as pelvic inflammatory disease.

*Gonorrhoea:* particularly when penicillin has failed or is unsuitable.

*Other bacterial infections:* meningitis and other sensitive infections suitable for parenteral antibiotic therapy.

*Prophylaxis:* The administration of Claforan prophylactically may reduce the incidence of certain post-operative infections in patients undergoing surgical procedures that are classified as contaminated or potentially contaminated or in clean operations where infection would have serious effects.

Protection is best ensured by achieving adequate local tissue concentrations at the time contamination is likely to occur. Claforan should therefore be administered immediately prior to surgery and if necessary continued in the immediate post-operative period.

Administration should usually be stopped within 24 hours since continuing use of any antibiotic in the majority of surgical procedures does not reduce the incidence of subsequent infection.

*Bacteriology:* The following organisms have shown in vitro sensitivity to Claforan.

Gram positive: Staphylococci, including coagulase-positive, coagulase-negative and penicillinase-producing strains. β-haemolytic and other streptococci such as *Streptococcus mitis* (*viridans*) (many strains of enterococci, e.g. *Streptococcus faecalis,* are relatively resistant). *Streptococcus* (Diplococcus) *pneumoniae. Clostridium* spp.

Gram negative: *Escherichia coli, Haemophilus influenzae* including ampicillin resistant strains, *Klebsiella* spp, *Proteus* spp (both indole positive and indole negative), *Enterobacter* spp, *Neisseria* spp. (including β-lactamase producing strains of *N. gonorrhoeae*), *Salmonella* spp. (including *S typhi*), *Shigella* spp, *Providencia* spp, *Serratia* spp, *Citrobacter* spp. Claforan has frequently exhibited useful in vitro activity against *Pseudomonas* and *Bacteroides* species although some strains of *Bacteroides fragilis* are resistant.

There is in vitro evidence of synergy between Claforan and aminoglycoside antibiotics such as gentamicin against some species of Gram-negative bacteria including some strains of *Pseudomonas.* No in vitro antagonism has been noted. In severe infections caused by *Pseudomonas* spp. the addition of an aminoglycoside antibiotic may be indicated.

*Posology and method of administration:* Claforan may

be administered intravenously or by bolus injection or infusion or intramuscularly. The dosage, route and frequency of administration should be determined by the severity of infection, the sensitivity of causative organisms and condition of the patient. Therapy may be initiated before the results of sensitivity tests are known.

*Adults:* The recommended dosage for mild to moderate infections is 1 g 12 hourly. However, dosage may be varied according to the severity of the infection, sensitivity of causative organisms and condition of the patient. Therapy may be initiated before the results of sensitivity tests are known.

In severe infections dosage may be increased up to 12 g daily given in 3 or 4 divided doses. For infections caused by sensitive *Pseudomonas* spp. daily doses of greater than 6 g will usually be required.

*Children:* The usual dosage range is 100-150 mg/kg/day in 2 to 4 divided doses. However, in very severe infections doses of up to 200 mg/kg/day may be required.

*Neonates:* The recommended dosage is 50 mg/kg/day in 2 to 4 divided doses. In severe infections 150-200 mg/kg/day, in divided doses, have been given.

*Dosage in Gonorrhoea:* A single injection of 1 g may be administered intramuscularly or intravenously.

*Dosage in renal impairment:* Because of extra-renal elimination, it is only necessary to reduce the dosage of Claforan in severe renal failure (GFR < 5 ml/min = serum creatinine approximately 751 micromol/litre). After an initial loading dose of 1 g, daily dose should be halved without change in the frequency of dosing, i.e. 1 g 12 hourly becomes 0.5 g 12 hourly, 1 g 8 hourly becomes 0.5 g 8 hourly, 2 g 8 hourly becomes 1 g 8 hourly etc. As in all other patients, dosage may require further adjustment according to the course of the infection and the general condition of the patient.

*Intravenous and Intramuscular Administration:* Reconstitute Claforan with Water for Injection PhEur as given in the Dilution Table. Shake well until dissolved and then withdraw the entire contents of the vial into the syringe and use immediately.

Dilution table:

| Vial size | Diluent to be added | Approx available volume |
|---|---|---|
| 500 mg | 2 ml | 2.2 ml |
| 1 g | 4 ml | 4.5 ml |
| 2 g | 10 ml | 11.2 ml |

*Intravenous Infusion:* Claforan may be administered by intravenous infusion. 1-2 g are dissolved in 40-100 ml of Water for Injection PhEur or in the infusion fluids listed under *Pharmaceutical particulars.* The prepared infusion may be administered over 20-60 minutes.

*Contra-indications:* Known or suspected allergy to cephalosporins.

*Special warnings and precautions for use:* Cephalosporin antibiotics may usually be given safely to patients who are hypersensitive to penicillins, although cross reactions have been reported. Special care is indicated in patients who have had an anaphylactic response to penicillin.

Patients with severe renal dysfunction should be placed on the dosage schedule recommended under *Posology and method of administration.*

*Interactions with other medicaments and other forms of interaction:* Cephalosporin antibiotics at high dosage should be given with caution to patients receiving aminoglycoside antibiotics or potent diuretics such as frusemide as these combinations are suspected to adversely affect renal function. However, at the recommended doses, enhancement of nephrotoxicity is unlikely to be a problem with Claforan.

Interference with Laboratory Tests: A positive Coombs test may be seen during treatment with cephalosporins. This phenomenon may occur during treatment with cefotaxime.

A false positive reaction to glucose may occur with reducing substances but not with the use of specific glucose oxidase methods.

*Pregnancy and lactation:* Although studies in animals have not shown an adverse effect on the developing foetus, the safety of Claforan in human pregnancy has not been established. Consequently, Claforan should not be administered during pregnancy especially during the first trimester, without carefully weighing the expected benefit against possible risks.

Claforan is excreted in the milk.

*Effects on ability to drive and use machines:* Not applicable.

*Undesirable effects:* Adverse reactions to Claforan have occurred relatively infrequently and have generally been mild and transient. Effects reported include candidiasis, rashes, fever, transient rises in liver transaminase and/or alkaline phosphatase and diarrhoea.

As with all cephalosporins, pseudomembranous colitis may rarely occur during treatment. If this occurs the drug should be stopped and specific treatment instituted.

As with other cephalosporins, changes in renal function have been rarely observed with high doses of cefotaxime. Administration of high doses of cephalosporins, particularly in patients with renal insufficiency may result in encephalopathy.

Hypersensitivity reactions have been reported, these include skin rashes, drug fever and very rarely anaphylaxis.

As with other β-lactam antibiotics, granulocytopenia and more rarely agranulocytosis may develop during treatment with cefotaxime, particularly if given over long periods. A few cases of eosinophilia and neutropenia have been observed, reversible when treatment is ceased. Some cases of rapidly reversible eosinophilia and thrombocytopenia on stopping treatment have been reported. Rare cases of haemolytic anaemia have been reported. For cases of treatment lasting longer than 10 days, blood count should, therefore, be monitored.

Transient pain may be experienced at the site of injection. This is more likely to occur with higher doses. Occasionally, phlebitis has been reported in patients receiving intravenous Claforan. However, this has rarely been a cause for discontinuation of treatment.

*Overdose:* Serum levels of Claforan may be reduced by peritoneal dialysis or haemodialysis. In the case of overdosage, particularly in renal insufficiency there is a risk of reversible encephalopathy.

**Pharmacological properties**

*Pharmacodynamic properties:* Claforan is a broad spectrum bactericidal cephalosporin antibiotic. Claforan is exceptionally active in vitro against Gram-negative organisms sensitive or resistant to first or second generation cephalosporins. It is similar to other cephalosporins in activity against Gram-positive bacteria.

*Pharmacokinetic properties:* After a 1000 mg intravenous bolus, mean peak plasma concentrations of cefotaxime usually range between 81 and 102 microgram/ml. Doses of 500 mg and 2000 mg produce plasma concentrations of 38 and 200 microgram/ml, respectively. There is no accumulation following administration of 1000 mg intravenously or 500 mg intramuscularly for 10 or 14 days.

The apparent volume of distribution at steady-state of cefotaxime is 21.6 litres/1.73 m² after 1 g intravenous 30 minute infusion.

Concentrations of cefotaxime (usually determined by non-selective assay) have been studied in a wide range of human body tissues and fluids. Cerebrospinal fluid concentrations are low when the meninges are not inflamed, but are between 3 and 30 microgram/ml in children with meningitis. Cefotaxime usually passes the blood-brain barrier in levels above the MIC of common sensitive pathogens when the meninges are inflamed. Concentrations (0.2-5.4 microgram/ml), inhibitory for most Gram-negative bacteria, are attained in purulent sputum, bronchial secretions and pleural fluid after doses of 1 or 2 g. Concentrations likely to be effective against most sensitive organisms are similarly attained in female reproductive organs, otitis media effusions, prostatic tissue, interstitial fluid, renal tissue, peritoneal fluid and gall bladder wall, after usual therapeutic doses. High concentrations of cefotaxime and desacetyl-cefotaxime are attained in bile.

Cefotaxime is partially metabolised prior to excretion. The principal metabolite is the microbiologically active product, desacetyl-cefotaxime. Most of a dose of cefotaxime is excreted in the urine about 60% as unchanged drug and a further 24% as desacetyl-cefotaxime. Plasma clearance is reported to be between 260 and 390 ml/minute and renal clearance 145 to 217 ml/minute.

After intravenous administration of cefotaxime to healthy adults, the elimination half-life of the parent compound is 0.9 to 1.14 hours and that of the desacetyl metabolite, about 1.3 hours.

In neonates the pharmacokinetics are influenced by gestational and chronological age, the half-life being prolonged in premature and low birth weight neonates of the same age.

In severe renal dysfunction the elimination half-life of cefotaxime itself is increased minimally to about 2.5 hours, whereas that of desacetyl-cefotaxime is increased to about 10 hours. Total urinary recovery of cefotaxime and its principal metabolite decreases with reduction in renal function.

*Preclinical safety data:* Not applicable.

**Pharmaceutical particulars**

*List of excipients:* None.

*Incompatibilities:* None stated.

*Shelf life:* Finished Product: 24 months. Reconstituted Solution: 24 hours.

*Special precautions for storage:* Finished Product: Store below 25˚C. Protect from light.

Reconstituted Solution: Whilst it is preferable to use only freshly prepared solutions for both intravenous and intramuscular injection, Claforan is compatible with several commonly used intravenous infusion fluids and will retain satisfactory potency for up to 24 hours refrigerated in the following:

Water for Injections PhEur
Sodium Chloride Injection BP
5% Dextrose Injection BP
Dextrose and Sodium Chloride Injection BP
Compound Sodium Lactate Injection BP (Ringer-lactate Injection).

After 24 hours any unused solution should be discarded.

Claforan is also compatible with 1% lignocaine, however freshly prepared solutions should be used.

Claforan is also compatible with metronidazole infusion (500 mg/100 ml) and both will maintain potency when refrigerated for up to 24 hours. Some increase in colour of prepared solutions may occur on storage. However, provided the recommended storage conditions are observed, this does not indicate change in potency or safety.

*Nature and contents of container:* Claforan is supplied in tubular or moulded glass vials PhEur, closed with a grey elastomer stopper and sealed with an aluminium cap fitted with a detachable flip top.

The bottles are boxed individually and in packs of 1, 10, 25 or 50.

*Instruction for use/handling:* Not applicable.

*Marketing authorisation holder:* Roussel Laboratories Ltd, Broadwater Park, Denham, Uxbridge, Middlesex UB9 5HP UK

**Marketing authorisation number** 0109/0074

**Date of approval/revision of SPC** December 1995

**Legal category** POM

## CLOMID*

**Presentation** Beige, round, flat, bevelled tablet. A scored bisect line on one side and the other engraved 'M' within two circles. Each tablet contains 50 mg Clomiphene Citrate BP.

**Uses**

*Action:* The ovulatory response to cyclic Clomid therapy appears to be mediated through increased output of pituitary gonadotrophins, which in turn stimulates the maturation and endocrine activity of the ovarian follicle and the subsequent development and function of the corpus luteum. The role of the pituitary is indicated by increased urinary excretion of gonadotrophins and the response of the ovary is manifested by increased urinary oestrogen excretion.

*Indications:* Clomid is indicated for the treatment of ovulatory failure in women desiring pregnancy.

Clomid is indicated only for patients in whom ovulatory dysfunction is demonstrated, who meet the conditions described in this data sheet. Other causes of infertility must be excluded or adequately treated before giving Clomid.

Good levels of endogenous oestrogen (as estimated from vaginal smears, endometrial biopsy, assay of urinary oestrogen, or endometrial bleeding in response to progesterone) provide a favourable prognosis for ovulatory response induced by Clomid. A low level of oestrogen, although clinically less favourable, does not preclude successful outcome of therapy.

Clomid therapy is ineffective in patients with primary pituitary or primary ovarian failure. Clomid therapy cannot substitute for specific treatment of other causes of ovulatory failure, such as thyroid or adrenal disorders. For hyperprolactinaemia there is other preferred treatment.

Clomid is not first line treatment for low-weight related amenorrhoea, with infertility, and has no value if a high FSH blood level is observed following an early menopause.

**Dosage and administration**

*General considerations:* The work-up and treatment should be supervised by physicians experienced in management of gynaecological or endocrine disorders. Patients should be chosen for therapy with Clomid only after careful diagnostic evaluation. The plan of therapy should be outlined in advance. Other causes of infertility should be excluded or adequately treated before giving Clomid.

Many patients will respond to 50 mg daily for 5 days. In the determination of a starting dose efficacy must be balanced against potential adverse effects. For example, the data available suggest that ovulation and pregnancy are slightly more attainable on 100 mg/day for 5 days than on 50 mg/day for 5 days. As the dosage is increased, however, ovarian hyperstimulation and other adverse effects may increase. Furthermore, although the data do not yet establish a relationship between dosage and multiple births, it would seem reasonable on pharmacological grounds that such a relationship does exist.

For these reasons it would seem prudent to begin treatment with the lower dose, 50 mg daily for 5 days, and to increase the dose only in patients who do not respond to the first course. Special care with lower dosage or duration of treatment for the first course is particularly recommended if unusual sensitivity to pituitary gonadotrophin is suspected, such as in patients with polycystic ovary syndrome.

*Recommended dosage:* The recommended dose for the first course of Clomid is 50 mg (1 tablet) daily for 5 days. Therapy may be started at any time in the patient who has had no recent uterine bleeding. If progestin-induced bleeding is planned, or if spontaneous uterine bleeding occurs before therapy, the regimen of 50 mg daily for 5 days should be started on or about the fifth day of the cycle. When ovulation occurs at this dosage, there is no advantage to increasing the dose in subsequent cycles of treatment.

If ovulation appears not to have occurred after the first course of therapy, a second course of 100 mg daily (two 50 mg tablets given as a single daily dose) for five days should be given. This course may be started as early as 30 days after the previous one. *Increase of the dosage or duration of therapy beyond 100 mg/day for 5 days should not be undertaken.*

The majority of patients who are going to respond will respond to the first course of therapy, and 3 courses should constitute an adequate therapeutic trial. If ovulatory menses have not yet occurred, the diagnosis should be re-evaluated. Treatment beyond this is not recommended in the patient who does not exhibit evidence of ovulation.

*Pregnancy:* The importance of properly timed coitus cannot be over-emphasised (i.e. at about the time of ovulation). For regularity of cyclic ovulatory response it is also important that each course of Clomid be started on or about the fifth cycle day, once ovulation has been established. Clomid therapy follows the rule of diminishing returns, such that likelihood of conception diminishes with each succeeding course of therapy. Before starting treatment, patients and their male partners should be advised of the possibility of multiple pregnancy and its potential hazards if conception occurs in relationship to Clomid therapy.

*Long-term cyclic therapy:* Not recommended.

The relative safety of long-term cyclic therapy has not been conclusively demonstrated, and since the majority of patients will ovulate following 3 courses, long-term cyclic therapy is not recommended, i.e. beyond a total of about 6 cycles (including 3 ovulatory cycles).

**Contra-indications, warnings, etc**

*Contra-indications:*

*Use in pregnancy:* Clomid is not indicated during pregnancy. Although there is no evidence that Clomid has a harmful effect on the human foetus, there is evidence that Clomid has a deleterious effect on rat and rabbit foetuses when given in high doses to the pregnant animal. To avoid inadvertent Clomid administration during early pregnancy, appropriate tests should be utilised during each treatment cycle to determine whether ovulation occurs. The patient should have a pregnancy test before the next course of Clomid therapy.

*Liver disease:* Clomid therapy is contra-indicated in patients with liver disease or a history of liver dysfunction.

*Abnormal uterine bleeding:* Clomid is contra-indicated in patients with hormone-dependant tumours or in patients with abnormal uterine bleeding of undetermined origin.

*Ovarian cyst:* Clomid should not be given in the presence of an ovarian cyst, except polycystic ovary, since further enlargement of the cyst may occur. Patients should be evaluated for the presence of ovarian cyst prior to each course of treatment.

*Warnings:*

*Ovarian hyperstimulation syndrome:* Ovarian hyperstimulation syndrome (OHSS) has been reported in patients receiving Clomid therapy for ovulation induction. In some cases, OHSS occurred following the cyclic use of Clomid therapy or when Clomid was used in combination with gonadotrophins. The following symptoms have been reported in association with this syndrome during Clomid therapy: pericardial effusion, anasarca, hydrothorax, acute abdomen, renal failure, pulmonary oedema, ovarian haemorrhage, deep venous thrombosis, torsion of the ovary and acute respiratory distress. If conception results, rapid progression to the severe form of the syndrome may occur.

To minimise the hazard of the abnormal ovarian enlargement associated with Clomid therapy, the lowest dose consistent with expectation of good results should be used.

The patient should be instructed to inform the physician of any abdominal or pelvic pain, weight gain, discomfort or distension after taking Clomid. Maximal enlargement of the ovary may not occur until several days after discontinuation of the course of Clomid. Some patients with polycystic ovary syndrome who are unusually sensitive to gonadotrophin may have an exaggerated response to usual doses of Clomid.

The patient who complains of abdominal or pelvic pain, discomfort, or distension after taking Clomid should be examined because of the possible presence of an ovarian cyst or other cause. Due to fragility of enlarged ovaries in severe cases, abdominal and pelvic examination should be performed very cautiously. If abnormal enlargement occurs, Clomid should not be given until the ovaries have returned to pre-treatment size. Ovarian enlargement and cyst formation associated with Clomid therapy usually regress spontaneously within a few days or weeks after discontinuing treatment. Most of these patients should be managed conservatively. The dosage and/or duration of the next course of treatment should be reduced.

*Visual symptoms:* Patients should be advised that blurring or other visual symptoms may occasionally occur during or shortly after therapy with Clomid. Patients should be warned that visual symptoms may render such activities as driving a car or operating machinery more hazardous than usual, particularly under conditions of variable lighting. The significance of these visual symptoms is not understood. If the patient has any visual symptoms, treatment should be discontinued and ophthalmological evaluation performed.

*Precautions:*

*Multiple pregnancy:* There is an increased chance of multiple pregnancy when conception occurs in relationship to Clomid therapy. During the clinical investigation studies, the incidence of multiple pregnancy was 7.9% (186 of 2369 Clomid associated pregnancies on which outcome was reported). Among these 2369 pregnancies, 2183 (92.1%) were single, 165 (6.9%) twin, 11 (0.5%) triplet, 7 (0.3%) quadruplet and 3 (0.13%) quintuplet. Of the 165 twin pregnancies for which sufficient information was available, the ratio of monozygotic to dizygotic twins was 1:5.

*Ectopic pregnancy:* There is an increased chance of ectopic pregnancy (including tubal and ovarian sites) in women who conceive following Clomid therapy. Ectopic pregnancy associated with Clomid involves a multiple pregnancy with coexisting extrauterine and intrauterine gestations.

*Uterine fibroids:* Caution should be exercised when using Clomid in patients with uterine fibroids due to the potential for further enlargement of the fibroids.

*Pregnancy wastage and birth anomalies:* The overall incidence of reported birth anomalies from pregnancies associated with maternal Clomid ingestion (before or after conception) during the investigational studies was within the range of that reported in published references for the general population. Among the birth anomalies spontaneously reported in the published literature as individual cases, the proportion of neural tube defects has been high among pregnancies associated with ovulation induced by Clomid, but this has not been supported by data from population-based studies.

The physician should explain so that the patient understands the assumed risk of any pregnancy whether the ovulation was induced with the aid of Clomid or occurred naturally.

The patient should be informed of the greater pregnancy risks associated with certain characteristics or conditions of any pregnant woman e.g. age of female and male partner, history of spontaneous abortions, Rh genotype, abnormal menstrual history, infertility history (regardless of cause), organic heart disease, diabetes, exposure to infectious agents such as rubella, familial history of birth anomaly, and other risk factors that may be pertinent to the patient for whom Clomid is being considered. Based upon the evaluation of the patient, genetic counselling may be indicated. Population-based reports have been published on possible elevation of risk of Down's Syndrome in ovulation induction cases and of increase in trisomy defects among spontaneously aborted foetuses from subfertile women receiving ovulation inducing drugs (no woman with Clomid alone without additional inducing drugs). However, as yet, the reported observations are too few to confirm or not to confirm the presence of an increased risk that would justify amniocentesis, other than for the usual indications because of age and family history.

The experience from patients of all diagnoses during clinical investigation of Clomid shows a pregnancy (single and multiple) wastage or foetal loss rate of 21.4% (abortion rate of 19%), ectopic pregnancies 1.18%, hydatidiform mole 0.17%, foetus papyraceous 0.04% and of pregnancies with one or more stillbirths 1.01%.

Clomid therapy after conception was reported for 158 of the 2369 delivered and reported pregnancies in the clinical investigations. Of these 158 pregnancies, 8 infants (born of 7 pregnancies) were reported to have birth defects.

There was no difference in reported incidence of birth defects whether Clomid was given before the 19th day after conception or between the 20th and 35th day after conception. This incidence is within the anticipated range of the general population.

*Lactation:* It is not known whether Clomid is excreted in human milk.

*Ovarian cancer:* There have been rare reports of ovarian cancer with fertility drugs; infertility itself is a primary risk factor. Epidemiological data suggest that prolonged use of Clomid may increase this risk. Therefore the recommended duration of treatment should not be exceeded (see *Dosage and administration*).

*Side-effects*

*Symptoms/signs/conditions:* Adverse effects appeared to be dose related, occurring more frequently at higher dose and with the longer courses of treatment used in investigational studies. At recommended dosage, adverse effects are not prominent and infrequently interfere with treatment.

During investigational studies, the more common reported adverse effects included ovarian enlargement (13.6%), vasomotor flushes (10.4%), abdominal-pelvic discomfort (distension, bloating) (5.5%), nausea and vomiting (2.2%), breast discomfort (2.1%), visual symptoms (1.5%), headache (1.3%) and intermenstrual spotting or menorrhagia (1.3%).

*Ovarian enlargement:* At recommended dosage, abnormal ovarian enlargement is infrequent, although the usual cyclic variation in ovarian size may be exaggerated. Similarly, cyclic ovarian pain (Mittelschmerz) may be accentuated. With higher or prolonged dosage, more frequent ovarian enlargement and cyst formation may occur, and the luteal phase of the cycle may be prolonged.

Rare instances of massive ovarian enlargement are recorded. Such an instance has been described in a patient with polycystic ovary syndrome whose Clomid therapy consisted of 100 mg daily for 14 days. Abnormal ovarian enlargement usually regresses spontaneously, most of the patients with this condition should be treated conservatively.

*Eye/visual symptoms:* Symptoms described usually as 'blurring' or spots or flashes (scintillating scotomata), increase in incidence with increasing total dose and usually disappear within periods ranging from a few days to a few weeks after Clomid is discontinued.

These symptoms appear to be due to intensification and prolongation of after-images. After-images as such have also been reported. Symptoms often first appear or are accentuated with exposure to bright-light environment.

Ophthalmologically definable scotomata, phosphenes and reduced visual actuity have been reported.

There are rare reports of cataracts and optic neuritis.

*Genito-urinary:* There are reports of new cases of endometriosis and exacerbation of pre-existing endometriosis during Clomid therapy.

Multiple pregnancies, including simultaneous intrauterine and extrauterine pregnancies, have been reported.

*Tumours/neoplasms:* Isolated reports have been received of the occurrence of endocrine-related or dependent neoplasms or their aggravation. Ovarian cancer: See Precautions.

*Central nervous system:* Convulsions have been reported. Patients with a history of seizures may be predisposed. In investigational patients, CNS symptoms/signs/conditions of dizziness, light-headedness/vertigo (0.9%), nervous tension/insomnia (0.8%), and fatigue/depression (0.7%) were reported. After prescription availability, there were isolated additional reports of these conditions and also reports of other conditions such as syncope/fainting, cerebrovascular accident, cerebral thrombosis, psychotic reactions including paranoid psychosis, neurologic impairment, disorientation and speech disturbance.

*Dermatosis:* Dermatitis and rash were reported by investigational patients. Conditions such as rash and urticaria were the most common ones reported after prescription availability but also reported were conditions such as allergic reaction, erythema multiforme, ecchymosis and angioneurotic oedema. Hair thinning has been reported very rarely.

*Liver function:* Bromsulphalein (BSP) retention of greater than 5% was reported in 32 of 141 patients in whom it was measured, including 5 of 43 patients who took approximately the dose of Clomid now recommended. Retention was usually minimal unless associated with prolonged continuous Clomid administration or with apparently unrelated liver disease. Other liver function tests were usually normal. In a later study in which patients were given 6 consecutive monthly courses of Clomid (50 or 100 mg daily for 3 days) or matching placebo, BSP tests were done on 94 patients. Values in excess of 5% retention were recorded in 11 patients, 6 of whom had taken drug and 5 placebo.

In a separate report, one patient taking 50 mg of Clomid daily developed jaundice on the 19th day of treatment; liver biopsy revealed bile stasis without evidence of hepatitis.

*Overdosage:* Toxic effects of acute overdosage of Clomid have not been reported but the number of overdose cases recorded is small. In the event of overdose, appropriate supportive measures should be employed.

**Pharmaceutical precautions** Clomid tablets should be protected from light, moisture and excessive heat.

**Legal category** POM.

**Package quantities** Clomid is obtainable in packs of 30 and 100 tablets in blister packs.

**Further information** Clomid is prescribable under the supervision of an appropriate specialist.

Orally administered $^{14}$C labelled clomiphene citrate was readily absorbed when administered to humans. Cumulative excretion of the $^{14}$C label by way of the urine and faeces averaged about 50% of the oral dose after 5 days in 6 subjects, with mean urinary excretion of 7.8% and mean faecal excretion of 42.4%. A mean rate of excretion of 0.73% per day of the $^{14}$C dose after 31 days to 35 days and 0.45% per day of the $^{14}$C dose after 42 days to 45 days was seen in faecal and urine samples collected from 6 subjects for 14 to 53 days after clomiphene citrate $^{14}$C administration. The remaining drug/metabolites may be slowly excreted from a sequestered enterohepatic recirculation pool.

**Product licence number** 4425/5900

*Product licence holder:* Marion Merrell Ltd, Broadwater Park, Denham Uxbridge, Middlesex UB9 5HP.

## CLORHEXITULLE*

**Presentation** Clorhexitulle is a sterile, open-mesh gauze dressing impregnated with White Soft Paraffin BP containing 0.5% micronised chlorhexidine acetate.

Each dressing is enclosed between two pieces of vegetable parchment and presented in individual heat sealed sachets to maintain sterility until opened.

**Uses** Properties: Chlorhexidine acetate is a potent antiseptic which is bactericidal to a wide range of Gram-positive and Gram-negative organisms. It also has some activity against yeasts such as *Candida* and other fungi.

Clorhexitulle is indicated as a bactericidal dressing for the prevention and control of existing infections in a wide range of surgical, traumatic and ulcerative conditions such as: varicose, diabetic and tropical ulcer; lacerations, abrasions, bites, puncture wounds, crush injuries; burns and scalds; pressure sores including bedsores; skin grafts (donor and recipient sites), avulsion of finger and/or toe nails, circumcision, suture lines; secondarily infected skin conditions (e.g. eczema, dermatitis, herpes zoster), colostomies, ileostomies, tracheostomies, incised abscesses, incised perionychia.

**Dosage and administration** A single layer of Clorhexitulle should be applied to the cleansed lesion, and changed as necessary according to the amount of exudation.

Clorhexitulle is suitable for use on adults, children and infants.

**Contra-indications, warnings, etc**
*Contra-indications:* Known allergy to chlorhexidine.

*Precautions:* Avoid Clorhexitulle coming into contact with the eyes. Clorhexitulle should not be applied to more than 40% of the body surface in adults. In infants, because of the difference in the ratio of surface area to body weight, the maximal area covered should not exceed 20%.

*Side-effects:* Although no adverse reactions to Clorhexitulle have been recorded, skin sensitivity to chlorhexidine has occasionally been reported.

*Use in pregnancy and lactation:* The safety of using Clorhexitulle during pregnancy and lactation has not been established. Consequently, Clorhexitulle should not be used during the first trimester of pregnancy without weighing the expected benefits against the possible risks.

*Incompatibilities:* Chlorhexidine is incompatible with soaps and other anionic detergents. Chlorhexidine acetate is incompatible with potassium iodide.

**Pharmaceutical precautions** Clorhexitulle should be stored flat at or below 25°C.

**Legal category** P.

**Package quantities** Cellophane wrapped packs of 10 sachets, each sachet contains one sterile, antiseptic gauze dressing (10 cm×10 cm) placed between layers of parchment.

**Further information** Nil.

**Product licence number** 0109/0085

*Product licence holder:* Roussel Laboratories Ltd, Broadwater Park, Denham, Uxbridge, Middlesex UB9 5HP.

## DAONIL* TABLETS
## SEMI-DAONIL* TABLETS

**Presentation** Daonil Tablets each contain 5 mg Glibenclamide BP. Daonil is presented as white oblong tablets, scored in the middle, one half bearing the Hoechst insignia, the other bearing the letters LDI. The tablet is 10 mm in length and 5 mm wide.

Semi-Daonil Tablets each contain 2.5 mg Glibenclamide BP. Semi-Daonil is presented as white circular biplanar tablets, 6 mm in diameter, one side bearing the Hoechst insignia, the other scored and bearing the letters LBG on either side of the score mark.

Excipients include lactose.

**Uses** Daonil is a hypoglycaemic agent, indicated for the oral treatment of patients with non-insulin dependent diabetes who respond inadequately to dietary measures alone.

**Dosage and administration**
1. *Treatment of previously untreated diabetics:* Stabilisation can be started with one 5 mg tablet of Daonil daily. The dose should be taken by mouth, with or immediately after breakfast or the first main meal. Where control is satisfactory, 1 tablet is continued as the maintenance dose. If control is unsatisfactory, the dose can be adjusted by increments of 2.5 or 5 mg at weekly intervals. The total daily dosage rarely exceeds 15 mg and increasing the daily dosage above this does not generally produce any additional effect. The total daily requirement should normally be administered as a single dose at breakfast, or with the first main meal; due consideration should be given to the patient's dietary habits and daily activity in apportioning the dosage.

*Elderly:* In debilitated or aged patients, who may be more liable to hypoglycaemia, treatment should be initiated with one Semi-Daonil tablet daily.

2. *Change-over from other oral anti-diabetics:* The change over to Daonil from other drugs with a similar mode of action can be carried out without any break in therapy. Daonil treatment should be started with one 5 mg tablet daily and adjusted by increments of 2.5-5 mg to achieve control. For patients not adequately controlled on other oral agents, treatment is commenced with the equivalent dose of Daonil, without exceeding an initial dose of 10 mg. If response is inadequate, the dose can be raised in a stepwise fashion to 15 mg daily. One 5 mg tablet of Daonil is approximately equivalent to 1 g tolbutamide or glymidine, 250 mg chlorpropamide or tolazamide, 500 mg acetohexamide, 25 mg glibornuride or 5 mg glipizide.

3. *Change-over from biguanides:* Daonil treatment should be started with 1 tablet of Semi-Daonil (2.5 mg) and the biguanide withdrawn. The dosage should then be adjusted by increments of 2.5 mg to achieve control.

*Combination with biguanides:* If adequate control is not possible with diet and 15 mg of Daonil, control can often be re-established by combined administration of Daonil and a biguanide derivative.

4. *Change-over from insulin:* While it is appreciated that most patients who are on insulin therapy will continue to need it, there may be a few patients, particularly those on low daily doses, who will remain stabilised if transferred from insulin to Daonil.

The tablets should always be taken with, or immediately after, the first main meal.

*Children:* As non-insulin dependent diabetes is not usually a disease of childhood, Daonil is not recommended for use in children.

**Contra-indications, warnings, etc**
*Contra-indications:* Daonil should not be used in patients who have or have ever had diabetic ketoacidosis or diabetic/coma pre-coma or in patients who have insulin-dependant diabetes mellitus, serious impairment of renal, hepatic or adrenocortical function, in patients who are hypersensitive to glibenclamide, or in circumstances of unusual stress, e.g. surgical operations or during pregnancy, when dietary measures and insulin are essential.

*Warnings:* The hypoglycaemic effect of glibenclamide may be enhanced by ACE inhibitors, anabolic steroids, beta-adrenergic blocking agents, benzafibrate, chloramphenicol, clofibrate, coumarin derivatives, cyclophosphamide, disopyramide, fenfluramine, fluoxetine, guanethidine, MAO inhibitors, miconazole, phenylbutazone, probenecid, quinolone antibacterials, salicylates, sulphinpyrazone, sulphonamides and tetracycline compounds or diminished by clonidine, corticosteroids, diazoxide, diuretics, glucagon, laxative abuse, nicotinic acid (high dose), oral contraceptives, phenothiazine derivatives, phenytoin, sympathomimetic agents and thyroid hormones.

Both a potentiation and a reduction in the blood sugar-lowering effect have been reported in patients treated concomitantly with clonidine or H2 receptor antagonists.

The warning symptoms of a hypoglycaemic attack may be masked during concomitant treatment with beta-adrenergic blocking agents, clonidine or guanethidine.

There is no information on the use of Daonil in human pregnancy but it has been in wide, general use for many years without apparent ill consequence. Animal studies have shown no hazard.

*Nursing mothers:* It has not yet been established whether glibenclamide is transferred to human milk. However, other sulphonylureas have been found in milk and there is no evidence to suggest that glibenclamide differs from the group in this respect.

*Overdosage:* Hypoglycaemia may be treated in the conscious patient by the administration of glucose, or three to four lumps of table sugar with water. This may be repeated as necessary.

If the patient is comatose, glucose should be administered as an intravenous infusion and the patient monitored. Bolus glucose injections are not recommended because of the possibility of rebound hypoglycaemia which may be delayed. Alternatively, glucagon may be administered in a dose of 1 mg subcutaneously or intramuscularly to restore consciousness.

*Side-effects:* Adverse reactions serious enough to warrant discontinuation of treatment are uncommon, but mild gastro-intestinal or allergic skin reactions have occurred. Cross sensitivity to sulphonamides or their derivatives may occur. Transient visual disturbances may occur at the start of treatment. Reversible leucopenia and thrombocytopenia have been reported but are rare. Agranulocytosis, pancytopenia and haemolytic anaemia have been reported very rarely. Treatment with sulphonylureas has been associated with occasional disturbances of liver function and cholestatic jaundice. If hepatitis or cholestatic jaundice occurs, glibenclamide should be discontinued. Hypoglycaemic symptoms have occasionally been reported when the dose has been administered without due regard to the patient's dietary habits.

**Pharmaceutical precautions** Daonil Tablets should be stored in a cool, dry place protected from light and in containers similar to those of the manufacturer.

**Legal category** POM.

**Package quantities** Daonil and Semi-Daonil Tablets are available in blister (calendar) packs of 28 (OP).

**Further information** Orally administered Daonil is rapidly absorbed. It is substantially metabolised prior to its excretion in urine and bile. Some of the metabolites have hypoglycaemic activity, markedly reduced in comparison with the parent compound and usually without clinical significance.

**Product licence numbers**
Daonil Tablets 5 mg     0086/5002.
Semi-Daonil Tablets 2.5 mg   0086/0068.

*Product licence holder:* Hoechst UK Ltd., Hoechst House, Salisbury Road, Middlesex TW4 7JH

## DIMETRIOSE*

**Qualitative and quantitative composition** Gestrinone capsules 2.5 mg.

**Pharmaceutical form** Hard white, size no. 4 gelatin capsules containing a white to slightly yellow powder. The capsule will be printed "Roussel" and logo.

**Clinical particulars**

*Therapeutic Indications:* Therapeutic treatment of endometriosis.

*Posology and method of administration:*
Adults: Gestrinone is for oral administration to adult females only. The dose is one capsule twice a week. To ensure that pregnant patients are not treated, it is essential that **the first dose is taken on the first day of the menstrual cycle.**

The second dose should be taken three days later. Thereafter, Gestrinone capsules should be taken on the same two days of the week (preferably at the same time) every week for the duration of the treatment, which will normally be six months.

Should one dose be missed, then a capsule should be taken as soon as possible and the original sequence maintained.

Should two or more doses be missed, treatment should be discontinued and therapy re-started on the first day of the new cycle, following a negative pregnancy test and according to the usual dosage schedule.

Children & Elderly Adults: Treatment with Gestrinone is not appropriate.

*Contra-indications:* Pregnancy. Lactation. Severe cardiac, renal or hepatic insufficiency. Metabolic and/or vascular disorders during previous oestrogen and/or progestogen therapy.

*Special warnings and precautions for use:* The possibility of pregnancy must be ruled out before starting treatment, especially in the case of pre-existing amenorrhoea.

Gestrinone, at the recommended dose, may inhibit ovulation in some women but, pregnancies can occur with this treatment and gestrinone must **not** be relied on for contraception.

As concurrent administration of oral contraceptives may modify the action of gestrinone, it is, therefore, essential that barrier methods are used throughout treatment as the use of gestrinone is totally contraindicated in pregnancy.

Because gestrinone may occasionally cause some degree of fluid retention, patients with cardiac or renal dysfunction require close monitoring.

Monitor ALAT, ASAT, cholesterol fractions in hyperlipidaemic subjects and blood sugar levels in diabetics.

Gestrinone will cause a decrease in the concentration of thyroid-binding globulin. Hence there will be a decrease in serum total thyroxine levels. This is without clinical significance as free thyroxine levels remain within the reference range as do thyroid-stimulating hormone levels.

*Interactions with other medicaments and other forms of interaction:* Concomitant administration of anti-epileptic drugs or rifampicin may result in accelerated metabolism of gestrinone.

*Use in pregnancy and lactation:* Gestrinone is specifically contraindicated in pregnancy and lactation.

Administration should be discontinued if a patient is found to be pregnant as animal studies have shown embryotoxicity in some species, albeit at doses well in excess of those used clinically.

*Effects on ability to drive and to use machines:* None stated.

*Undesirable effects (frequency and seriousness):* Spotting has been reported in some patients both during the first few weeks and throughout treatment.

Acne, oily skin, fluid retention, weight gain, hirsutism, voice change and other androgen-type effects have been reported by some patients.

Other unwanted reactions recorded during gestrinone therapy include transient increases in liver transaminases, headache, gastro-intestinal disturbance, change in libido, hot flushes, decrease in breast size, nervousness and depression, cramp and change in appetite.

*Overdose:* Acute toxicity studies in animals indicate that serious reactions are unlikely as an immediate result of a single excessive dose.

In the case of acute overdosage, the drug should be removed by emesis or gastric lavage if ingestion is recent and the patient kept under observation in case of delayed reaction.

**Pharmacological properties**

*Pharmacodynamic properties:* Gestrinone, a synthetic steroid hormone, is an antiprogestin: it is not an oestrogen-progestogen combination. Gestrinone has an inhibitory effect on endometrial tissue. It is believed to act by direct inhibition of the synthesis-release mechanisms of pituitary gonadotrophins and a direct antagonist action on endometrial tissues.

*Pharmacokinetic properties:* Gestrinone shows linear pharmacokinetics after oral administration of 1.25 mg, 2.5 or 5 mg. The peak concentration appears between 2.8 and 3.1 hours after administration.

The plasma half life is about 24 hours.

Three days after administration blood levels are only 5% of the maximum plasma concentration. The steady state is reached since the second administration, which is three days after the initial dose, therefore there is virtually no risk of accumulation under normal conditions of use.

Investigation of the absolute bioavailability in a subject after gestrinone administration demonstrates that after oral administration, absorption is virtually complete and the first pass metabolism is negligible.

Gestrinone undergoes important hepatic metabolism, essentially through hydroxylation processes, resulting in the formation of conjugated metabolites.

**Pharmaceutical particulars**

*List of excipients:* The product contains Colloidal Silicon Dioxide, Maize Starch, Microcrystalline Cellulose, Lactose, Magnesium Stearate, and Talc.

The white opaque capsule shell contains Titanium Dioxide and Gelatin.

*Incompatibilities:* None stated.

*Shelf life:* 48 Months.

*Special precautions for storage:* Store below 25°C protected from light.

*Nature and contents of container:* Dimetriose capsules are supplied in blister packs of 8 capsules.

*Instructions for use/handling:* None.

*Marketing authorisation holder:* Roussel Laboratories Ltd., Broadwater Park, Denham, Uxbridge, Middlesex UB9 5HP. UK

**Marketing authorisation number** 0109/0207

**Date of revision/approval of SPC** May 1997

**Legal category** POM

## EUGLUCON*

**Qualitative and quantitative composition** Each Euglucon tablet contains: either 2.5 mg or 5 mg of Glibenclamide.

**Pharmaceutical form** Tablets for oral use.

**Clinical particulars**

*Therapeutic indications:* Euglucon is indicated for the treatment of maturity-onset diabetes which is not adequately controlled by dietary measures alone.

*Posology and method of administration:*
*Adults and the elderly:* Euglucon should be taken with or immediately after food. The total daily dosage is preferably given as a single dose at breakfast or with the first main meal, but due consideration should be given to the patient's meal habits and daily activity when apportioning dosage.

*New Diabetics:* In maturity-onset diabetes of mild to moderate severity, treatment should be started with 5 mg daily or 2.5 mg in debilitated or elderly patients. If this dosage is not sufficient for proper control it should be increased by 2.5 mg at intervals of one week or as directed by the clinician. The total daily dose of Euglucon rarely exceeds 15 mg. Increasing dosage beyond this point is unlikely to produce further response.

*Transfer from other sulphonylureas:* Transfer to Euglucon can usually be carried out without any break in therapy. Euglucon treatment should be started with 5 mg daily and, if necessary, adjusted in steps of 2.5 mg or 5 mg. A dose of 5 mg Euglucon is approximately equivalent to 1000 mg tolbutamide, 250 mg chlorpropamide, 25 mg glibornuride or 5 mg glipizide.

*Change-over from biguanides:* Euglucon treatment should be started with 2.5 mg of Euglucon and the biguanide withdrawn. The dosage should then be adjusted by increments of 2.5 mg to achieve control.

*Combination with Biguanides:* If adequate control is not possible with diet and 15 mg of Euglucon, control can often be re-established by combination of Euglucon and a biguanide derivative.

*Euglucon and Insulin:* While it is appreciated that most patients who are on insulin therapy will continue to need it, there may be a few patients, particularly those on low daily dosages, who will remain stabilised if transferred to Euglucon.

No dosage recommendations are made for the administration of Euglucon to children.

*Contra-indications:* Euglucon is contra-indicated in:

1. The treatment of juvenile or unstable diabetes.
2. Patients who have had serious metabolic decompensation with ketosis and, in particular, in diabetic pre-coma and coma.
3. Serious impairment of renal, hepatic, thyroid or adrenocortical function.
4. Pregnancy, after delivery, Euglucon therapy can be started or resumed.
5. Hypersensitivity to Glibenclamide.

*Special warnings and precautions for use:* None

*Interactions with other medicaments and other forms of interaction:* The hypoglycaemic action of oral antidiabetic agents including Euglucon may be enhanced by sulphonamides, salicylates, phenylbutazone, coumarin derivatives, beta-blocking agents, mono-amine oxidase inhibitors, cyclophosphamide, benza-fibrate, clofibrate, fenfluramine, tetracyclines, sulphinpyrazone and chloramphenicol. Conversely, thiazide diuretics, frusemide, ethacrynic acid, oral contraceptives containing oestrogens/gestagens phenothiazine derivatives, nicotinic acid (high dosage), sympathomimetics, thyroid hormones and corticosteroids may diminish hypoglycaemic activity. Hypoglycaemic activity may also be affected by tuberculostatics.

In patients suffering from intercurrent infections or trauma, the dosage of Euglucon may need to be increased. If such complications are severe, diabetic control may be lost necessitating withdrawal of Euglucon and maintenance of diabetic control with insulin. Euglucon should be re-introduced when the patient has recovered from the infection or trauma.

*Pregnancy and lactation:* Pregnancy: There is no information on the use of Euglucon in human pregnancy but is has been in wide, general use for many years without apparent ill consequence. Animal studies have shown no hazard.

Nursing mothers: It has not been established whether glibenclamide is excreted in human milk. Other sulphonylureas have been found in milk. There is no evidence that glibenclamide differs from the group in this respect.

*Effects on ability to drive and to use machines:* No adverse effect on the ability to drive or use machines is expected in well controlled patients but patients should be warned about the possible adverse effects of hypoglycaemia.

*Undesirable effects (frequency and seriousness):* Euglucon is well tolerated and side effects serious enough to necessitate withdrawal are uncommon. Gastro-intestinal symptoms (nausea, anorexia and diarrhoea) are uncommon and allergic skin reactions are seldom encountered.

Reversible leucopenia and thrombocytopenia have been reported but are rare. Treatment with sulphonylureas has been associated with occasional disturbances of liver function and cholestatic jaundice. If hepatitis or cholestatic jaundice occurs, glibenclamide should be discontinued. As with other agents, hypoglycaemia can occur with Euglucon, but is not usually prolonged and responds to appropriate therapeutic measures.

*Overdose:* If a hypoglycaemic reaction should occur, the conscious patient may be treated with dextrose or 3–4 lumps of table sugar with water. This may be repeated, if necessary, in 15 minutes.

If the patient is comatose, sucrose or dextrose may be given by stomach tube or dextrose given intravenously. Glucagon may be administered in a dose of 1 mg subcutaneously or intramuscularly to produce consciousness.

**Pharmacological properties**

*Pharmacodynamic properties:* Euglucon is an oral hypoglycaemic agent of the sulphonylurea type.

*Pharmacokinetic properties:* Absorption studies in healthy human volunteers using labelled glibenclamide formulated as Euglucon tablets showed a mean absorption of 84 ± 9%.

The half-life is about 10 hours

Excretion was approximately 50% in the urine and 50% in the faeces. Absorbed glibenclamide was completely metabolised and the three isolated metabolites in the concentrations found had no significant hypoglycaemic activity.

**Pharmaceutical particulars**

*List of excipients:* The product contains: Lactose, Maize Starch, Aerosil, (Colloidal Silicon Dioxide) , Talc, Magnesium Stearate, Purified Water

*Incompatibilities:* None

*Shelf life:* 60 Months

*Special precautions for storage:* Store below 25°C.

*Nature and contents of container:* Euglucon 2.5 mg and 5 mg tablets are supplied in blister packs of 28.

*Instructions for use/handling:* None.

*Marketing authorisation holder:* Roussel Laboratories Ltd., Broadwater Park, North Orbital Road, Denham, Uxbridge, Middlesex UB9 5HP

**Marketing authorisation numbers**

| | |
|---|---|
| Euglucon 2.5 mg | 0109/0073 |
| Euglucon 5 mg | 0109/5023R |

**Date of approval/revision of SPC** May 1997

**Legal category** POM

## FERTIRAL*

**Presentation** Fertiral contains Gonadorelin BP (luteinising hormone releasing hormone) 500 micrograms in 1 ml aqueous solution presented as a 2 ml ampoule containing 1000 micrograms. The solution also contains sodium chloride, sodium dihydrogen phosphate and benzyl alcohol as excipients.

**Uses** Amenorrhoea and infertility associated with:

1. Hypogonadotrophic hypogonadism.
2. Multifollicular ovaries: where this finding implies that pulse frequency and amplitude of endogenous LHRH are abnormal, e.g. in patients in whom weight related amenorrhoea has been corrected.

**Dosage and administration** Gonadorelin is given by means of an intermittent pulsatile pump, a pulse being delivered every 90 minutes over the entire 24 hour period. Treatment should be initiated by subcutaneous infusion but in some patients intravenous therapy may be required. Dosage should be determined individually but a starting dose of 10–20 micrograms given over 1 minute every 90 minutes is recommended. Treatment should be continued until conception occurs, or for a maximum of 6 months. Ultrasound of ovary or oestradiol or urinary oestrogen levels or basal body temperature measurements may be used to monitor treatment (see also *Pharmaceutical Precautions*).

**Contra-indications, warnings, etc** Gonadorelin should not be used in patients with endometriotic cysts or polycystic disease of the ovaries. Treatment with gonadorelin should not be started in women with weight related amenorrhoea until the weight has been corrected and the ponderal index is above 19.5. Gonadorelin may be discontinued once evidence of conception has been obtained. Pituitary adenoma is a relative contra-indication.

*Side-effects:* Side-effects are very rare. Skin rashes have been reported at the infusion site. The following reactions have been reported after treatment with the high dose diagnostic preparation of gonadorelin: Abdominal pain, nausea, headache and increased menstrual bleeding.

*Overdosage:* Treatment of overdose should be symptomatic.

**Pharmaceutical precautions** Gonadorelin should be infused using a pulsatile pump e.g. Graseby MS 27 with an infusion set of minimum volume e.g. Butterfly 25 or Butterfly 19 cannulae (Abbott). For intravenous administration heparin is added to the gonadorelin solution at a concentration of 150 IU/ml.

Store below 25°C. Use normal saline to dilute if necessary; use immediately after dilution. The solution is stable in the pump, at about body temperature, for 4 days.

Fertiral contains benzyl alcohol 1% as a preservative.

**Legal category** POM.

**Package quantities** Fertiral is available in packs of 5×2 ml ampoules.

**Further information** Results from clinical studies show a rate of multiple pregnancy very similar to that of the normal population.

**Product licence number** 0086/0093

*Product licence holder:* Hoechst UK Ltd., Hoechst House, Salisbury Road, Middlesex TW4 7JH

## FRISIUM*

**Qualitative and quantitative composition** Clobazam 10 mg

**Pharmaceutical form** Tablet

### Clinical particulars

*Therapeutic indications:* Frisium is a 1,5–benzodiazepine indicated for the short-term relief (2–4 weeks) only of anxiety that is severe, disabling or subjecting the individual to unacceptable distress, occurring alone or in association with insomnia or short-term psychosomatic, organic or psychotic illness. The use of Frisium to treat short-term "mild" anxiety is inappropriate and unsuitable. Frisium may be used as adjunctive therapy in epilepsy.

*Posology and method of administration:* The usual anxiolytic dose for adults is 20–30 mg daily in divided doses or as a single dose given at night. Doses of up to 60 mg daily have been used in the treatment of adult in-patients with severe anxiety.

The lowest dose that can control symptoms should be used. It should not be used for longer than 4 weeks. Long term chronic use as an anxiolytic is not recommended. Treatment should always be withdrawn gradually. Patients who have taken Frisium for a long time may require a longer period during which doses are reduced.

*Epilepsy:* In epilepsy a starting dose of 20–30 mg/day is recommended, increasing as necessary up to a maximum of 60 mg daily. A break in therapy may be beneficial if drug exhaustion develops, recommencing therapy at a low dose.

*Elderly:* Doses of 10–20 mg daily in anxiety may be used in the elderly, who are more sensitive to the effects of psychoactive agents.

*Children:* When prescribed for children over three years of age, dosage should not exceed half the recommended adult dose. There is insufficient experience of the use of Frisium in children under three years of age to enable any dosage recommendation to be made.

Benzodiazepines should be used in reduced doses in patients with impaired renal or hepatic function.

*Contra-indications:* Frisium should not be used in patients known to be hypersensitive to benzodiazepines, or any of the excipients or in patients with a history of drug dependence.

Frisium should not be used in phobic and obsessional states or for the treatment of chronic psychosis.

It should not be used alone to treat depression or anxiety associated with depression as suicide may be precipitated in such patients.

*Special warnings and special precautions for use:* Amnesia may occur with benzodiazepines. In cases of loss or bereavement psychological adjustment may be inhibited by benzodiazepines.

Special caution is necessary if Frisium is used in patients with myasthenia gravis, spinal or cerebellar ataxia or sleep apnoea.

Disinhibiting effects may be manifested in various ways. Suicide may be precipitated in patients who are depressed and aggressive behaviour towards self and others may be precipitated. Extreme caution should therefore be used in prescribing benzodiazepines in patients with personality disorders.

Withdrawal from benzodiazepines may be associated with physiological and psychological symptoms. Withdrawal symptoms occur with benzodiazepines following normal therapeutic doses given for short periods of time.

Respiratory function should be monitored in patients with acute severe respiratory insufficiency.

*Interactions with other medicaments and other forms of interaction:* Frisium is a benzodiazepine derivative and, in common with other members of this group, may potentiate the effects of central nervous system depressant drugs, such as alcohol, analgesics, hypnotics and neuroleptics.

Addition of Frisium to established anticonvulsant medication may cause a change in plasma levels of these drugs. If used as an adjuvant in epilepsy the dosage of Frisium should be determined by monitoring the EEG and the plasma levels of the drugs checked

The effects of muscle relaxants, analgesics and nitrous oxide may be enhanced.

Concurrent treatment with drugs that inhibit the mono-oxygenase system (e.g. cimetidine) may enhance the effect of clobazam.

*Pregnancy and lactation:* There is little information on the use of Frisium in early pregnancy but no untoward effects have been found in animal studies. However, there are reports of a possible association between malformations in infants and the administration of other benzodiazepines in early pregnancy. Frisium should not be used in the first trimester of pregnancy and in the later stages only if there are strong indications for its use.

Clobazam has been detected in the breast milk of nursing mothers, but the effect on the neonate is not known. However, breast feeding should be stopped during clobazam treatment.

*Effects on ability to drive and use machines:* The ability to drive or operate machinery may be impaired in individuals who are particularly sensitive to the effects of Frisium or in patients taking high doses.

*Undesirable effects:* Side-effects such as drowsiness, dizziness or dryness of the mouth, constipation, loss of appetite, nausea, or a fine tremor of the fingers have been reported. These are more likely to occur at the beginning of treatment and often disappear with continued treatment or a reduction in dose. Paradoxical reactions, such as restlessness, irritability or difficulty in sleeping, may occur. Isolated cases of skin reactions, such as rashes or urticaria, have been observed.

Slowing of reaction time, ataxia, confusion and headaches may occasionally occur.

After prolonged use of benzodiazepines, impairment of consciousness, sometimes combined with respiratory disorders, has been reported in very rare cases, particularly in elderly patients: it sometimes persists for some length of time. These disorders have not been seen so far under clobazam treatment.

When used as an adjuvant in the treatment of epilepsy, this preparation may in rare cases cause restlessness and muscle weakness.

As with other benzodiazepines, the therapeutic benefit must be balanced against the risk of habituation and dependence during prolonged use.

*Overdose:* Muscle weakness, ataxia, drowsiness and sedation may occur and, after very high doses, the patient may lose consciousness. The treatment of overdosage is symptomatic. The stomach should be emptied as soon as possible by gastric lavage and general supportive measures should be undertaken as necessary. Forced diuresis or haemodialysis are ineffective.

### Pharmacological properties

*Pharmacodynamic properties:* Clobazam is a 1,5-benzodiazepine. In single doses up to 20 mg or in divided doses up to 30 mg, clobazam does not affect psychomotor function, skilled performance, memory or higher mental functions.

*Pharmacokinetic properties:* Absorption of clobazam is virtually complete after oral administration. Approximately 85% is protein bound in man. It is metabolised

by demethylation and hydroxylation. It is excreted unchanged and as metabolites in the urine (87%) and feces.

*Preclinical safety data:* None applicable

**Pharmaceutical particulars**

*List of excipients:* Lactose monohydrate, maize starch, colloidal silicon dioxide, talc, magnesium stearate.

*Incompatibilities:* None

*Shelf life:* Five years

*Special precautions for storage:* Store below 25°C

*Nature and contents of container:* Blister pack containing 30 tablets

*Instruction for use/handling:* None

*Marketing authorisation holder:* Hoechst UK Ltd., Hoechst House, Salisbury Road, Hounslow, Middlesex TW4 7JH

**Marketing authorisation number** 0086/0202

**Date of approval/revision of SPC** 8 May 1997

**Legal category** POM

## HAEMACCEL* INFUSION SOLUTION

**Presentation** 3.5% colloidal infusion solution for plasma substitution.
Composition:

| Haemaccel contains | Per 500 ml bottle | Per 1,000 ml |
|---|---|---|
| Polygeline (degraded and modified gelatin of average molecular weight 30,000) | 17.50 g | 35.00 g |
| Cations | | |
| Na$^+$ | 72.50 mmol | 145.00 mmol |
| K$^+$ | 2.55 mmol | 5.10 mmol |
| Ca$^{++}$ | 3.13 mmol | 6.25 mmol |
| Anions | | |
| Cl$^-$ | 72.50 mmol | 145.00 mmol |
| PO$_4^{---}$ and SO$_4^{--}$ | traces | traces |

Isoionic equilibrium is made up by the polypeptides.

There are no preservatives.

*Physico-chemical properties:*

| | |
|---|---|
| Viscosity ratio | 1.7–1.8 |
| Dynamic viscosity (at 37°C) | 1.15–1.20 kPa.s (cP) |
| Iso-electric point | pH 4.7±0.3 |
| pH of the infusion solution | 7.3±0.3 |
| Colloid osmotic pressure (at 37°C) | 3.432–3.824 kPa (350-390 mmH$_2$O) |
| Gel point | below + 3°C |
| Appearance | straw-coloured |
| Nitrogen equivalent of polygeline | 3.15 g in 500 ml |

**Uses**

1. As a plasma volume substitute in the initial treatment of hypovolaemic shock due to:
   a. Haemorrhage (visible or concealed)
   b. Burns, peritonitis, pancreatitis, crush injuries
2. Fluid replacement in plasma exchange.
3. Extra-corporeal circulation.
4. Isolated organ perfusion.
5. As a carrier solution for insulin.

**Dosage and administration** Haemaccel should be administered intravenously in a volume approximately equal to the estimated blood loss.

In common with all intravenous infusion solutions, Haemaccel should, if possible, be warmed to body temperature before use. However, in emergencies, it may be infused at ambient temperatures. For technical reasons there is a residual air volume in the container. Thus, pressure infusions with the plastic infusion bottle must be carried out under controlled conditions only, as the risk of air embolism cannot be excluded.

*Infusion rate:* The rate of infusion is determined by the condition of the patient. Normally 500 ml will be infused in not less than 60 minutes, but in emergencies Haemaccel can be rapidly infused. Losses of up to 25% of the blood volume can be replaced by Haemaccel alone.

*Plastic infusion bottle:* It is advisable to disinfect the bottle top then pull out the plastic ring. A hole will be exposed through which the piercing needle of an infusion set can be pushed. There is no need to disinfect the cap further.

*Hypovolaemic shock:* 500–1,000 ml Haemaccel should be infused intravenously initially. Up to 1,500 ml blood loss can be replaced entirely by Haemaccel. For between 1,500 ml and 4,000 ml blood loss, fluid replacement should be with equal volumes of Haemaccel and blood, given separately (see Pharmaceutical precautions). For losses over 4,000 ml the separate infusions should be in the ratio of two parts blood to one part Haemaccel. The haematocrit should not be allowed to fall below 25%.

*Burns:* It is suggested that at least 1 ml Haemaccel be infused per kg body weight, multiplied by the % of body surface burned for each 24 hours for two days, e.g. if a 70 kg person has burns covering 10% of body surface, then the dosage of Haemaccel should be at least 1 (ml) x 70 (kg) x 10(%) = 700 ml/24 hours. Additional crystalloid solutions should be given to cover the normal fluid loss, i.e. about 2,000 ml per 24 hours. In severe burns, additional protein and vitamin therapy may be required. The volume of colloid and crystalloid given should be varied according to the clinical response of the patient, the urine volume, its specific gravity and osmolality, etc.

*Plasma exchange:* Haemaccel should be given either alone or in combination with other replacement fluids in a volume adequate to replace the plasma removed. Up to 2 litres have been given as sole replacement fluid.

**Contra-indications, warnings, etc**
*Contra-indications:* Known hypersensitivity to constituents of the preparation. Existing anaphylactoid reactions.

*Warnings:* In the following cases, Haemaccel should be administered with caution:

All conditions in which an increase in intravascular volume and its consequences (e.g. increased stroke volume, elevated blood pressure), or an increase in interstitial fluid volume, or haemodilution could represent a special risk for the patient. Examples of such conditions are: congestive heart failure, hypertension, oesophageal varices, pulmonary oedema, haemorrhagic diathesis, renal and post-renal anuria.

In all patients at an increased risk of histamine release (e.g. allergic persons and patients with a history of histamine response; also patients who in the previous 7 days have received a drug which releases histamine). In the latter cases, Haemaccel may be given only after taking appropriate prophylactic steps. Reactions caused by histamine release can be avoided by the prophylactic use of H1 or H2 receptor antagonists.

Inappropriately rapid administration of Haemaccel, especially to normovolaemic patients, may cause the release of vasoactive substances. The exact mechanism of such histamine release has not been clearly defined.

*Side-effects:* During or after the infusion of volume-expanding solutions, transient urticarial skin reactions (wheals), hypotension, tachycardia, bradycardia, nausea/vomiting, dyspnoea, increases in temperature and/or shivering may occasionally occur.

Rare cases of severe hypersensitivity reactions including shock have been observed. Treatment will depend on the nature and severity of the reaction.

*Mild reactions:* Administer corticosteroids and antihistamines.

In the event of anaphylactic shock, the infusion should be discontinued and adrenaline (5–10 ml of 1:10,000 by slow intravenous injection or 0.5–1.0 ml of 1:1,000 by i.m./s.c. injection) should immediately be given. Administration of adrenaline should be repeated every 15 minutes until improvement occurs. Circulatory collapse requires volume replacement, preferably monitored by a central venous pressure line. Large volumes of electrolyte solution may be necessary because, in severe anaphylactic shock, plasma loss may constitute up to 40% of the plasma volume. A slow intravenous injection of an H₁ antagonist such as 10–20 mg chlorpheniramine may be given.

Histamine release has been shown to be a cause of anaphylactic side-effects associated with infusions of Haemaccel.

These reactions may occur as a result of the cumulative effect of several histamine-releasing drugs (e.g. anaesthetics, muscle relaxants, analgesics, ganglion blockers and anticholineric drugs).

*Interactions with other agents:* Haemaccel contains calcium ions and caution should be observed in patients being treated with cardiac glycosides.

Due to the calcium content of Haemaccel, the serum calcium concentrations may be found to be slightly elevated for a temporary period–especially when large amounts of Haemaccel are administered by rapid infusion. So far, no reports have been received of cases involving clinical signs of hypercalcaemia resulting from an infusion of Haemaccel.

The infusion of Haemaccel may result in a temporary increase in the erythrocyte sedimentation rate.

*Pregnancy:* Haemorrhage around the time of childbirth or blood loss during other obstetric or gynaecological procedures may necessitate plasma volume replacement. Haemaccel has been used for many years for the initial treatment in such cases without apparent ill consequence. If plasma volume replace-

ment is needed during pregnancy, Haemaccel may be used if blood is not available.

**Pharmaceutical precautions** There are no special storage requirements. Haemaccel will gel below 3°C; however, warming will reverse this. Freezing does not alter its physico-chemical characteristics in any way. Haemaccel contains no preservatives; any unused fluid should be discarded once a bottle has been opened.

Haemaccel may be mixed with other infusion solutions (e.g. saline, dextrose, Ringer's solution, etc.) or with heparinised blood. Sterility must be maintained. Compatible water-soluble drugs may be infused in Haemaccel, e.g. insulin, streptokinase, etc. Any additive should be injected into the bottle through the small hole located next to the pull-ring.

Citrated blood should *not* be mixed with Haemaccel since clotting of the blood may occur due to the presence of calcium ions in Haemaccel. However, citrated blood may be infused before or after Haemaccel provided that there is adequate flushing of the infusion set.

Do not use Haemaccel if the seal has been broken or if the contents are cloudy.

Haemaccel has a shelf life of five years at storage temperatures of up to 25°C.

**Legal category** POM.

**Package quantities** Available in 500 ml plastic bottles.

**Further information** Haemaccel is of particular value as a volume replacement as it promotes a demonstrable osmotic diuresis, thereby protecting the kidneys. Provided that the recipient's red cells are suspended in saline rather than serum it does not interfere with subsequent blood grouping and cross matching, nor does it interfere with the coagulation system. It is non-immunogenic and does not induce antibody formation.

**Product licence number** 0086/0040

*Product licence holder:* Hoechst UK Ltd., Hoechst House, Salisbury Road, Middlesex TW4 7JH

## HYDROTALCITE

**Qualitative and quantitative composition** Each 5 ml of suspension contains 500 mg of Hydrotalcite light. Each tablet contains 500 mg Hydrotalcite BP.

**Pharmaceutical form**   Suspension / Tablet

**Clinical particulars**

*Therapeutic indications:* Use as an antacid. Hydrotalcite is indicated for symptomatic relief in the following conditions: peptic ulceration; dyspepsia; hyperacidity; gastritis; heartburn, especially when associated with oesophagitis or hiatus hernia and heartburn in pregnancy.

*Posology and method of administration:*
Adults: 10 ml or 2 tablets between meals and at bedtime or as directed by the physician.
Elderly: No specific recommendations.
Children (6-12 years): Half the adult dose.
Children under 6 years: Not recommended.
Route of Administration: Oral. The tablets should be chewed or crushed before swallowing.

*Contra-indications:* None known.

*Special warnings and precautions for use:* None stated.

*Interactions with other medicaments and other forms of interaction:* Hydrotalcite may interfere with the intestinal absorption of tetracyclines.

*Use in pregnancy and lactation:* It is wise to avoid any drugs, including antacids during the first trimester of pregnancy.

*Effects on ability to drive and to use machines:* None known.

*Undesirable effects (frequency and seriousness):* Side effects are uncommon, diarrhoea and vomiting have been reported.

*Overdose:* There is no evidence of absorption of hydrotalcite in man. Investigations in healthy human volunteers have shown no elevation of serum aluminium or magnesium levels on administering of hydrotalcite at therapeutic dosage for a continuous period of 28 days.

**Pharmacological properties**

*Pharmacodynamic properties:* Raising the pH of gastric contents to above 3.5 significantly reduces the pain and discomfort of acid associated symptoms, especially heartburn, dyspepsia, peptic ulceration, gastritis, reflux oesophagitis, hydrotalcite, buffering in the range of pH 3.5 over two hours, combines those properties of magnesium and aluminium based antacids in producing effective rises in pH over a considerable period.

*Pharmacokinetic properties:* Not applicable.

*Preclinical Safety Data:* Not applicable.

**Pharmaceutical particulars**

*List of excipients:* Hydrotalcite Suspension also contains Sorbitol, Carmellose Sodium, Veegum Regular, Sodium Propyl Hydroxybenzoate, Sodium Butyl Hydroxybenzoate, Hydrogen Peroxide 30% solution PhEur*, Creme de menthe 1951 and purified water.
*Quantity includes an overage of 70 PPM.

Hydrotalcite Tablets also contain mannitol, magnesium stearate, talc, sodium saccharin, lactose and buttermint flavouring.

*Incompatibilities:* None known.

*Shelf-life:* Hydrotalcite Suspension: 24 months; Hydrotalcite Tablets: 60 months.

*Special precautions for storage:* Hydrotalcite Suspension: Store between 4°C and 25°C. Hydrotalcite Tablets: Store in a cool, dry place below 25°C.

*Nature and contents of container:* The suspension is in a white pigmented plastic bottle with HDPE as the internal layer and sealed by a white pigmented polypropylene tamper evident closure. Bottle of 500 ml.

The tablets are in a PVC/blister pack inside a secondary cardboard carton containing 56 tablets.

*Instructions for use/handling:* Not applicable.

*Marketing authorisation holder:* Roussel Laboratories Ltd., Broadwater Park, Denham, Uxbridge, Middlesex UB9 5HP

**Marketing authorisation number**
Hydrotalcite Tablets     0109/0040
Hydrotalcite Suspension  0109/0041R

**Date of approval/revision of SPC** May 1997

**Legal category** POM

## KOLANTICON* GEL

**Presentation**   Kolanticon Gel is a white, viscous, peppermint-flavoured suspension, each 5 ml containing:
Dicyclomine Hydrochloride BP     2.5 mg
Dried Aluminium Hydroxide Gel BP   200 mg
Light Magnesium Oxide BP      100 mg
Simethicone USP          20 mg

**Uses**  Kolanticon is an antacid-antiflatulent-anti-spasmodic-demulcent indicated for the treatment and prophylaxis of symptoms of peptic ulcer and functional dyspepsia especially in patients in whom gastric distress results from hyperacidity, smooth muscle spasm and flatulence. Also indicated for symptomatic relief in oesophagitis, hiatus hernia, gastritis and iatrogenic gastritis.

**Dosage and administration**  Two to four 5 ml spoonfuls every four hours as required.

**Contra-indications, warnings, etc**
*Contra-indications:* Known idiosyncrasy to any of the ingredients. Should not be used in patients with obstructive uropathy, obstructive disease of the gastro-intestinal tract, paralytic ileus and intestinal atony, severe ulcerative colitis, and myasthenia gravis.

*Precautions:* In the presence of renal insufficiency magnesium salts may cause central nervous system depression. Aluminium hydroxide in the presence of low phosphorous diets may cause phosphorous deficiency. Aluminium hydroxide may reduce absorption of tetracyclines when given concomitantly. Products containing dicyclomine hydrochloride should be used with caution in any patient with or suspected of having glaucoma or prostatic hypertrophy. Use with care in patients with hiatus hernia associated with reflux oesophagitis because anticholinergic drugs may aggravate this condition.

*Use in pregnancy and lactation:* Epidemiological studies in pregnant women with products containing dicyclomine hydrochloride (at doses up to 40 mg/day) have not shown that dicyclomine increases the risk of foetal abnormalities if administered during the first trimester of pregnancy. Reproduction studies have been performed in rats and rabbits at doses of up to 100 times the maximum recommended dose (based on 60 mg per day for an adult person) and have revealed no evidence of impaired fertility or harm to the foetus due to dicyclomine.

Since risk of teratogenicity cannot be excluded with absolute certainty for any product, the drug should be used during pregnancy only if clearly needed.

It is not known whether dicyclomine is secreted into human milk. Because many drugs are excreted in human milk, caution should be exercised when dicyclomine is administered to a nursing woman.

*Side-effects:* In particularly sensitive patients dicyclomine hydrochloride may cause atropine-like side-effects such as dry mouth, blurred vision, urinary retention or constipation.

*Overdosage:* Signs and symptoms of dicyclomine hydrochloride overdose include: headache, nausea and vomiting, blurred vision, dilated pupils, hot dry skin, dizziness, vertigo, dryness of mouth, difficulty in swallowing and CNS stimulation.

Treatment may include emetics, gastric lavage and symptomatic therapy if indicated.

**Pharmaceutical precautions** Store in a cool place. Shake well before use.

**Legal category** P

**Package quantities** Amber glass bottles of 200 ml and 500 ml (original pack).

**Further information** Nil.

**Product licence number** 4425/0032

*Product licence holder:* Marion Merrell Ltd., Broadwater Park, Denham, Uxbridge, Middlesex UB9 5HP

## LASIKAL* TABLETS

**Presentation** Lasikal Tablets each contain 20 mg Frusemide BP and 750 mg (10 mmol $K^+$) slow-release potassium chloride. They are presented as film-coated, biconvex, twin-layered tablets, 12.5 mm in diameter, marked 'LK' on one side. The frusemide layer is white and the slow-release potassium chloride layer is yellow.

Excipients include lactose and Sunset Yellow.

**Uses** Lasikal contains a short-acting diuretic and a slow-release potassium supplement. It is intended for the treatment of oedema in patients who require potassium supplementation.

**Dosage and administration** The recommended initial adult dose is 2 tablets (40 mg frusemide and 20 mmol K+) to be taken each morning. This may be increased to four tablets daily, to be taken as 2 tablets each morning and evening, or may be decreased to 1 tablet each morning, according to clinical response.

Lasikal tablets must be swallowed whole.

*Children:* Lasikal tablets cannot be sub-divided and are unsuitable for paediatric use.

*Elderly:* Frusemide and potassium may both be excreted more slowly in the elderly.

**Contra-indications, warnings, etc**
*Contra-indications:* Lasikal is contra-indicated in anuria, hyperkalaemia, precomatose states associated with liver cirrhosis, Addison's disease and in patients taking potassium-sparing diuretics. Hypersensitivity to frusemide or sulphonamides is also a contra-indication.

*Warnings:* Patients with prostatic hypertrophy or impairment of micturition have an increased risk of developing acute retention.

Where indicated, steps should be taken to correct hypotension or hypovolaemia before commencing therapy.

The dosage of concurrently administered cardiac glycosides or antihypertensive agents may require adjustment.

ACE inhibitors should not be used in combination with Lasikal as serum potassium levels may be increased.

The toxic effects of nephrotoxic antibiotics may be increased by concomitant administration of potent diuretics such as frusemide.

Latent diabetes may become manifest or the insulin requirements of diabetic patients may increase.

Care should be exercised when treating patients with renal insufficiency because of the risk of hyperkalaemia.

In common with other diuretics, serum lithium levels may be increased when lithium is given concomitantly with frusemide, necessitating adjustment of the lithium dosage.

Certain non-steroidal anti-inflammatory agents have been shown to antagonise the action of diuretics such as frusemide and may cause renal failure in cases of pre-existing hypovolaemia.

Frusemide may sometimes attenuate the effects of other drugs (e.g. the effects of antidiabetics and of pressor amines) and sometimes potentiate them (e.g. the effects of salicylates, theophylline, lithium and curare-type muscle relaxants).

Interactions have also been reported with ototoxic antibiotics. In cases of concomitant glucocorticoid therapy or abuse of laxatives, the risk of an increased potassium loss should be borne in mind.

*Precautions:* Results of animal work, in general, show no hazardous effect of frusemide in pregnancy. There is clinical evidence of safety of the drug in the third trimester of human pregnancy; however, frusemide should be used in pregnancy only if strictly indicated and for short term treatment.

*Nursing mothers:* As frusemide may inhibit lactation or pass into breast milk, it should be used with caution in nursing mothers.

*Overdosage:* In cases of overdose there is a danger of dehydration and electrolyte depletion due to excessive diuresis. Treatment should therefore be aimed at fluid replacement and correction of the electrolyte imbalance.

*Side-effects:* Lasikal is generally well tolerated. Side-effects of a minor nature such as nausea, malaise or gastric upset may occur but are not usually severe enough to necessitate withdrawal of treatment.

As with other diuretics, electrolytes and water balance may be disturbed as a result of diuresis after prolonged therapy. This may cause symptoms such as headache, hypotension or muscle cramps.

Serum calcium levels may be reduced; in very rare cases tetany has been observed. Nephrocalcinosis has been reported in premature infants.

Isolated cases of acute pancreatitis have been reported after long-term diuretic (including frusemide) treatment. Disorders of hearing after frusemide are rare and, in most cases reversible. They may occur if frusemide is injected too rapidly, particularly in patients with renal insufficiency.

As with other diuretics a transient rise in creatinine and urea levels has also been reported with frusemide.

The incidence of allergic reactions, such as skin rash, photosensitivity, vasculitis, fever or interstitial nephritis, is very low, but when these occur treatment should be withdrawn.

In common with other sulphonamide-based diuretics, hyperuricaemia may occur and, in rare cases, clinical gout may be precipitated.

Serum cholesterol and triglyceride levels may rise during frusemide treatment. During long term therapy they will usually return to normal within six months.

Bone marrow depression has been reported as a rare complication and necessitates withdrawal of treatment.

Pre-existing metabolic alkalosis (e.g. in decompensated cirrhosis of the liver) may be aggravated by frusemide treatment.

Reduced mental alertness may impair ability to drive or operate dangerous machinery.

**Pharmaceutical precautions** Lasikal should be stored below 25°C in a dry place, protected from light, in the original container or in containers similar to those of the manufacturer. Lasikal tablets should be dispensed in moisture-tight containers which offer protection from light.

**Legal category** POM.

**Package quantities** Lasikal is available in containers of 100 tablets.

**Further information** Frusemide produces a prompt and effective diuresis which lasts for approximately four hours following oral administration. The potassium chloride in Lasikal tablets is contained in an inert matrix which allows slow release of potassium ions, thereby helping to avoid high local $K^+_{ion}$ concentrations in the intestine.

Ghost tablets may appear in the patient's faeces.

**Product licence number** 0086/0060

*Product licence holder:* Hoechst UK Ltd., Hoechst House, Salisbury Road, Middlesex TW4 7JH

## LASILACTONE* CAPSULES

**Presentation** Lasilactone Capsules each contain 20 mg of Frusemide BP and 50 mg Spironolactone BP. They are presented as hard gelatin capsules with a light blue opaque cap and white opaque body. Excipients include lactose.

**Uses** Lasilactone contains a short-acting diuretic and a long-acting aldosterone antagonist. It is indicated in the treatment of resistant oedema where this is associated with secondary hyperaldosteronism; conditions include chronic congestive cardiac failure and hepatic cirrhosis.

Treatment with Lasilactone should be reserved for cases refractory to a diuretic alone at conventional dosage.

This fixed ratio combination should only be used if titration with the component drugs separately indicates that this product is appropriate.

The use of Lasilactone in the management of essential hypertension should be restricted to patients with demonstrated hyperaldosteronism. It is recommended that in these patients also, this combination should only be used if titration with the component drugs separately indicates that this product is appropriate.

**Dosage and administration** In accordance with the recommendations on usage given above the dosage of Lasilactone will normally be in the range of 1 to 4 capsules daily (20–80 mg Lasix and 50–200 mg spironolactone).

*Children:* The product is not suitable for use in children.

*Elderly:* Frusemide and spironolactone may both be excreted more slowly in the elderly.

**Contra-indications, warnings, etc**
*Contra-indications:* Lasilactone should not be given in acute renal failure, renal insufficiency (creatinine clearance <30 ml/minute ≡serum creatinine of about 1.8–2.0 mg/100 ml), anuric states, hyperkalaemia, Addison's disease or in patients hypersensitive to frusemide, spironolactone or sulphonamides.

*Warnings:* Patients with prostatic hypertrophy or impairment of micturition have an increased risk of developing acute retention. Caution should also be exercised in the presence of liver disease as hepatic coma may be precipitated in susceptible cases. Administration of Lasilactone should be avoided in the presence of hyperkalaemia and hyponatraemia. Concomitant administration of triamterene, amiloride or potassium supplements or non-steroidal anti-inflammatory drugs is not recommended as hyperkalaemia may result. Where indicated, steps should be taken to correct hypotension, hypovolaemia and severe hypokalaemia before starting therapy.

The dosage of concurrently administered cardiac glycosides or hypotensive agents may require adjustment.

ACE inhibitors should not be used in combination with Lasilactone as serum potassium levels may be increased.

The toxic effects of nephrotoxic antibiotics may be potentiated by concurrent administration of potent diuretics such as frusemide.

Latent diabetes may become manifest or the insulin requirements of diabetic patients may increase.

In common with other diuretics, serum lithium levels may be increased when lithium is given concomitantly with frusemide, necessitating adjustment of the lithium dosage.

Certain non-steroidal anti-inflammatory agents have been shown to antagonise the action of diuretics such as frusemide and may cause renal failure in cases of pre-existing hypovolaemia. Frusemide may sometimes attenuate the effects of other drugs (e.g. the effects of antidiabetics and of pressor amines) and sometimes potentiate them (e.g. the effects of salicylates, theophylline, lithium and curare-type muscle relaxants). Salicylates may attenuate the effect of spironolactone. Concomitant glucocorticoid medication or abuse of laxatives may lead to potassium deficiency. In the presence of potassium deficiency the effect of cardiac glycosides may be enhanced.

Interactions have also been reported with carbenoxolone and with ototoxic antibiotics.

Concurrent administration of Lasilactone and sucralfate should be avoided as sucralfate decreases the absorption of frusemide.

*Carcinogenicity:* Spironolactone has been shown to produce tumours in rats when administered at high doses over a long period of time. The significance of these findings with respect to clinical use is not certain. However, the long-term use of spironolactone in young patients requires careful consideration of the benefits and the potential hazard involved.

*Precautions:* Caution should be observed in patients liable to electrolyte deficiency.

Results of animal work, in general, show no hazardous effect of frusemide in pregnancy. There is clinical evidence of the safety of the drug in the third trimester of human pregnancy; however, frusemide should be used in pregnancy only if strictly indicated and for short term treatment.

Spironolactone or its metabolites may cross the placental barrier.

*Nursing mothers:* Lasilactone is contra-indicated in nursing mothers because canrenone, a metabolite of the spironolactone component of this preparation, appears in breast milk. (Frusemide may inhibit lactation or pass into breast milk).

*Overdosage:* In cases of overdosage with Lasilactone there is a danger of severe electrolyte disturbance and dehydration due to excessive diuresis. Signs of overdosage may include drowsiness, mental confusion, nausea, vomiting, dizziness or diarrhoea. Electrolyte disturbances such as hyperkalaemia and hyponatraemia may be induced. Hyperkalaemia may be manifested clinically by paraesthesia, weakness, flaccid paralysis or muscle spasm and may be difficult to distinguish from hypokalaemia. Electrocardiographic changes may be the earliest signs of potassium disturbances.

Treatment should be aimed at the replacement of fluid and the correction of any electrolyte imbalance.

*Side-effects:* Frusemide is generally well tolerated. Side-effects of a minor nature such as nausea, malaise or gastric upset may occur but are not usually severe enough to necessitate withdrawal of treatment.

As with other diuretics, electrolytes and water balance may be disturbed as a result of diuresis after prolonged therapy. This may cause symptoms such as headache, hypotension or muscle cramps.

Calcium depletion may occur. Nephrocalcinosis has been reported in premature infants treated with frusemide.

The incidence of allergic reactions, such as skin rashes (including photosensitivity reactions), vasculitis, fever or interstitial nephritis, is very low, but when these occur treatment should be withdrawn.

Auditory disorders and acute pancreatitis have been reported with high dose parenteral frusemide.

A transient rise in creatinine and urea levels has also been reported. In common with other sulphonamide-based diuretics, the administration of frusemide may induce a rise in serum uric acid; in rare cases, clinical gout may be precipitated.

Serum cholesterol and triglyceride levels may rise during frusemide treatment. During long term therapy they will usually return to normal within six months.

Bone marrow depression has been reported as a rare complication of Lasix therapy and necessitates withdrawal of treatment.

Spironolactone has been reported to induce gastro-intestinal intolerance. Stomach ulcers (sometimes with bleeding) have been reported rarely. Eosinophilia may occur occasionally. Spironolactone may also cause drowsiness, headache, ataxia, lethargy and mental confusion. Dose-dependent mastodynia and reversible gynaecomastia may occur in both sexes. Urticaria may occur occasionally. Maculopapular or erythematous cutaneous eruptions have been reported rarely. In women, dose dependent menstrual irregularities and hirsuitism may be seen and in men impairment of potency. Spironolactone may cause vocal changes in the form of hoarseness and deepening of the voice in women and increase in the pitch in men. These vocal changes in both sexes may be irreversible. Therefore, this risk should be carefully considered for patients whose voice is of professional importance e.g. singers, teachers, actors.

Reduced mental alertness may impair the ability to drive or operate dangerous machinery.

**Pharmaceutical precautions** Lasilactone should be stored at ambient temperature, protected from light, in the original container or in containers similar to those of the manufacturer.

**Legal category** POM.

**Package quantities** Lasilactone is available in blister (calendar) packs of 28 capsules (original packs).

**Further information** Frusemide is an effective short-acting diuretic; diuresis usually commences within one hour and lasts for four to six hours.

Spironolactone is a competitive inhibitor of aldosterone and thus increases sodium excretion whilst reducing potassium loss at the distal renal tubule. It has a slow and prolonged action, maximum response being usually attained after 2–3 days' treatment.

**Product licence number** 0086/0039

*Product licence holder:* Hoechst UK Ltd., Hoechst House, Salisbury Road, Middlesex TW4 7JH

## LASIX* TABLETS 20 mg

**Qualitative and quantitative composition** Lasix Tablets 20 mg each contain 20 mg Frusemide BP

**Pharmaceutical form** Uncoated tablets

**Clinical particulars**

*Therapeutic indications:* Lasix is a diuretic recommended for use in all indications when a prompt and effective diuresis is required.

Lasix Tablets 20 mg are indicated for the maintenance therapy of mild oedema of any origin.

*Posology and method of administration:* Lasix has an exceptionally wide therapeutic range, the effect being proportional to the dosage. Lasix is best given as a single dose either daily or on alternate days.

The usual initial daily dose is 40 mg. This may require adjustment until the effective dose is achieved. In mild cases, 20 mg daily or 40 mg on alternate days may be sufficient, whereas in cases of resistant oedema, daily doses of 80 mg and above may be used.

*Children:* Oral doses for children range from 1 to 3 mg/kg body weight daily up to a maximum total dose of 40 mg/day.

*Elderly:* In the elderly, frusemide is generally eliminated more slowly. Dosage should be titrated until the required response is achieved.

*Contra-indications:* Lasix is contra-indicated in anuria, electrolyte deficiency and pre-comatose states associated with liver cirrhosis. Hypersensitivity to frusemide or sulphonamides.

*Special warnings and special precautions for use:* Patients with prostatic hypertrophy or impairment of micturition have an increased risk of developing acute retention.

Where indicated, steps should be taken to correct hypotension or hypovolaemia before commencing therapy.

Latent diabetes may become manifest or the insulin requirements of diabetic patients may increase.

Caution should be observed in patients liable to electrolyte deficiency.

*Interaction with other medicaments and other forms of interaction:* The dosage of concurrently administered cardiac glycosides or anti-hypertensive agents may require adjustment. A marked fall in blood pressure may be seen when ACE inhibitors are added to frusemide therapy. The dose of frusemide should be reduced, or the drug stopped, before initiating the ACE inhibitor.

The toxic effects of nephrotoxic antibiotics may be increased by concomitant administration of potent diuretics such as frusemide.

In common with other diuretics, serum lithium levels may be increased when lithium is given concomitantly with frusemide, necessitating adjustment of the lithium dosage.

Certain non-steroidal anti-inflammatory agents (e.g. indomethacin, acetylsalicylic acid) may attenuate the action of frusemide and may cause renal failure in cases of pre-existing hypovolaemia. Frusemide may sometimes attenuate the effects of other drugs (e.g. the effects of antidiabetics and of pressor amines) and sometimes potentiate them (e.g. the effects of salicylates, theophylline, lithium and curare-type muscle relaxants).

Interactions have also been reported with ototoxic antibiotics. In cases of concomitant gluco-corticoid therapy or abuse of laxatives, the risk of an increased potassium loss should be borne in mind.

*Pregnancy and lactation:* Results of animal work, in general, show no hazardous effect of Lasix in pregnancy. There is clinical evidence of safety of the drug in the third trimester of human pregnancy; however, Lasix should be used in pregnancy only if strictly indicated and for short term treatment.

As Lasix may inhibit lactation or may pass into the breast milk it should be used with caution in nursing mothers.

*Effects on ability to drive and use machines:* Reduced mental alertness may impair ability to drive or operate dangerous machinery.

*Undesirable effects:* Lasix is generally well tolerated. Side-effects of a minor nature such as nausea, malaise or gastric upset may occur but are not usually severe enough to necessitate withdrawal of treatment.

As with other diuretics, electrolytes and water balance may be disturbed as a result of diuresis after prolonged therapy. This may cause symptoms such as headache, hypotension or muscle cramps.

Serum calcium levels may be reduced; in very rare cases tetany has been observed. Nephrocalcinosis has been reported in premature infants.

Isolated cases of acute pancreatitis have been reported after long-term diuretic (including frusemide) treatment. Disorders of hearing after frusemide are rare and, in most cases reversible. They may occur if frusemide is injected too rapidly, particularly in patients with renal insufficiency.

As with other diuretics a transient rise in creatinine and urea levels has also been reported with frusemide.

The incidence of allergic reactions, such as skin rashes, photosensitivity, vasculitis, fever or interstitial nephritis, is very low, but when these occur treatment should be withdrawn.

In common with other sulphonamide-based diuretics, hyperuricaemia may occur and, in rare cases, clinical gout may be precipitated.

Serum cholesterol and triglyceride levels may rise during frusemide treatment. During long term therapy they will usually return to normal within six months.

Bone marrow depression has been reported as a rare complication and necessitates withdrawal of treatment.

Pre-existing metabolic alkalosis (e.g. in decompensated cirrhosis of the liver) may be aggravated by frusemide treatment.

*Overdose:* In cases of overdose there is a danger of dehydration and electrolyte depletion due to excessive diuresis. Treatment should therefore be aimed at fluid replacement and correction of the electrolyte imbalance.

**Pharmacological properties**

*Pharmacodynamic properties:* The evidence from many experimental studies suggests that frusemide acts along the entire nephron with the exception of the distal exchange site. The main effect is on the ascending limb of the loop of henle with a complex effect on renal circulation. Blood-flow is diverted from the juxta-medullary region to the outer cortex the principal renal action of frusemide is to inhibit active chloride transport in the thick ascending limb. Re-absorption of sodium chloride from the nephron is reduced and a hypotonic or isotonic urine produced.

It has been established that prostaglandin (PG) biosynthesis and the renin-angiotensin system are affected by frusemide administration and that frusemide alters the renal permeability of the glomerulus to serum proteins.

*Pharmacokinetic properties:* Frusemide is a weak carboxylic acid which exists mainly in the dissociated form in the gastro-intestinal tract. Frusemide is rapidly but incompletely absorbed (60–70%) on oral administration and its effect is largely over within four hours. The optimal absorption site is the upper duodenum at pH 5.0. Regardless of route of administration, 69–97% of activity from a radio-labelled dose is excreted in the first 4 hours after the drug is given. Frusemide is bound to plasma albumin and little biotransformation takes place. Frusemide is mainly eliminated via the kidneys (80–90%); a small fraction of the dose undergoes biliary elimination and 10–15% of the activity can be recovered from the faeces.

*a) In renal/hepatic impairment:* Where liver disease is present, biliary elimination is reduced. Up to 50% renal impairment has little effect on the elimination rate of Lasix, but less than 20% residual renal function increases the elimination time.

*b) The Elderly:* The elimination of frusemide is delayed in the elderly where a certain degree of renal impairment is present.

*c) New-born:* A sustained diuretic effect is seen, possibly due to immature tubular function.

*Preclinical safety data:* No further information provided.

**Pharmaceutical particulars**

*List of excipients:* Lactose, maize starch, talc, magnesium stearate and colloidal silicon dioxide.

*Incompatibilities:* None

*Shelf-life:* Five years

*Special precautions for storage:* Store protected from light in the manufacturers containers or similar.

*Nature and contents of container:* Lasix Tablets 20 mg are available in blister packs of 28.

*Instructions for use/handling:* None

*Marketing authorisation holder:* Hoechst UK Ltd, Hoechst House, Salisbury Road, Hounslow, Middlesex, TW4 7JH

**Marketing authorisation number** 0086/0017

**Date of approval/revision of SPC** 16 March 1996

**Legal category** POM

## LASIX* TABLETS 40 mg

**Presentation** Lasix Tablets 40 mg each contain 40 mg Frusemide BP. They are presented as flat white tablets with bevelled edges, 8 mm in diameter, one face bearing the Hoechst logo, the other face with a break line, each half marked DLI.

Excipients include lactose.

**Uses** Lasix is a diuretic recommended for use in all indications when a prompt and effective diuresis is required. Indications for Lasix Tablets 40 mg include cardiac, pulmonary, hepatic and renal oedema, peripheral oedema due to mechanical obstruction or venous insufficiency and hypertension.

**Dosage and administration** Lasix has an exceptionally wide therapeutic range, the effect being proportional to the dosage. Lasix is best given as a single dose either daily or on alternate days.

The usual initial daily dose is 40 mg. This may require adjustment until the effective dose is achieved. In mild cases, 20 mg daily or 40 mg on alternate days may be sufficient, whereas in cases of resistant oedema, daily doses of 80 mg and above may be used.

*Children:* Oral doses for children range from 1 to 3 mg/kg body weight daily up to a maximum total dose of 40 mg/day.

*Elderly:* In the elderly, frusemide is generally eliminated more slowly. Dosage should be titrated until the required response is achieved.

**Contra-indications, warnings, etc**

*Contra-indications:* Lasix is contra-indicated in anuria, electrolyte deficiency and pre-comatose states associated with liver cirrhosis. Hypersensitivity to frusemide or sulphonamides.

*Warnings:* Patients with prostatic hypertrophy or impairment of micturition have an increased risk of developing acute retention.

Where indicated, steps should be taken to correct hypotension or hypovolaemia before commencing therapy.

The dosage of concurrently administered cardiac glycosides or anti-hypertensive agents may require adjustment. A marked fall in blood pressure may be seen when ACE inhibitors are added to frusemide therapy. The dose of frusemide should be reduced, or the drug stopped, before initiating the ACE inhibitor.

The toxic effects of nephrotoxic antibiotics may be increased by concomitant administration of potent diuretics such as frusemide.

Latent diabetes may become manifest or the insulin requirements of diabetic patients may increase.

In common with other diuretics, serum lithium levels may be increased when lithium is given concomitantly with frusemide, necessitating adjustment of the lithium dosage.

Certain non-steroidal anti-inflammatory agents (e.g. indomethacin, acetylsalicylic acid) may attenuate the action of frusemide and may cause renal failure in cases of pre-existing hypovolaemia. Frusemide may sometimes attenuate the effects of other drugs (e.g. the effects of antidiabetics and of pressor amines) and sometimes potentiate them (e.g. the effects of salicylates, theophylline, lithium and curare-type muscle relaxants).

Interactions have also been reported with ototoxic antibiotics. In cases of concomitant glucocorticoid therapy or abuse of laxatives, the risk of an increased potassium loss should be borne in mind.

*Precautions:* Caution should be observed in patients liable to electrolyte deficiency.

Results of animal work, in general, show no hazardous effect of Lasix in pregnancy. There is clinical evidence of safety of the drug in the third trimester of human pregnancy; however, Lasix should be used in pregnancy only if strictly indicated and for short term treatment.

*Nursing mothers:* As Lasix may inhibit lactation or may pass into the breast milk it should be used with caution in nursing mothers.

*Overdosage:* In cases of overdose there is a danger of dehydration and electrolyte depletion due to excessive diuresis. Treatment should therefore be aimed at fluid replacement and correction of the electrolyte imbalance.

*Side-effects:* Lasix is generally well tolerated. Side-effects of a minor nature such as nausea, malaise or gastric upset may occur but are not usually severe enough to necessitate withdrawal of treatment.

As with other diuretics, electrolytes and water balance may be disturbed as a result of diuresis after prolonged therapy. This may cause symptoms such as headache, hypotension or muscle cramps.

Serum calcium levels may be reduced; in very rare cases tetany has been observed. Nephrocalcinosis has been reported in premature infants.

Isolated cases of acute pancreatitis have been reported after long-term diuretic (including frusemide) treatment. Disorders of hearing after frusemide are rare and, in most cases reversible. They may occur if frusemide is injected too rapidly, particularly in patients with renal insufficiency.

As with other diuretics a transient rise in creatinine and urea levels has also been reported with frusemide.

The incidence of allergic reactions, such as skin rashes, photosensitivity, vasculitis, fever or interstitial nephritis, is very low, but when these occur treatment should be withdrawn.

In common with other sulphonamide-based diuretics, hyperuricaemia may occur and, in rare cases, clinical gout may be precipitated.

Serum cholesterol and triglyceride levels may rise during frusemide treatment. During long term therapy they will usually return to normal within six months.

Bone marrow depression has been reported as a rare complication and necessitates withdrawal of treatment.

Pre-existing metabolic alkalosis (e.g. in decompensated cirrhosis of the liver) may be aggravated by frusemide treatment.

Reduced mental alertness may impair ability to drive or operate dangerous machinery.

**Pharmaceutical precautions** Lasix tablets should be stored protected from light, in the manufacturer's containers or similar.

**Legal category** POM.

**Package quantities** Lasix Tablets 40 mg are available in packs of 28 and 250 (The pack size of 28 is an original pack).

**Further information** Lasix produces a prompt and effective diuresis which lasts for approximately four hours following oral administration. Therefore the time of administration can be adjusted to suit the patient's requirements.

**Product licence number** 0086/5011R

*Product licence holder:* Hoechst UK Ltd., Hoechst House, Salisbury Road, Middlesex TW4 7JH

## LASIX* INJECTION 20 mg/2 ml

**Presentation** Lasix Injection 20 mg contains 20 mg Frusemide BP in 2 ml aqueous solution. The solution also contains sodium chloride and sodium hydroxide as excipients.

**Uses** Lasix is a diuretic recommended for use when a prompt and effective diuresis is required. The intravenous formulation is appropriate for use in emergencies or when oral therapy is precluded. Indications include cardiac, pulmonary, hepatic and renal oedema.

**Dosage and administration** Lasix injection *must* always be given slowly. The diuretic effect of Lasix is proportional to the dosage. Doses of 20–50 mg intramuscularly or intravenously may be given initially. If larger doses are required, they should be given by slow infusion and titrated according to the response.

*Children:* Parenteral doses for children range from 0.5–1.5 mg/kg body weight daily up to a maximum total daily dose of 20 mg.

*Elderly:* In the elderly, frusemide is generally eliminated more slowly. Dosage should be titrated until the required response is achieved.

**Contra-indications, warnings, etc** Intravenous injections of Lasix *must* always be given slowly, i.e. at a rate not exceeding 4 mg/minute.

*Contra-indications:* Lasix is contra-indicated in anuria, electrolyte deficiency and pre-comatose states associated with liver cirrhosis. Hypersensitivity to frusemide or sulphonamides.

*Warnings:* Patients with prostatic hypertrophy or impairment of micturition have an increased risk of developing acute retention.

Where indicated, steps should be taken to correct hypotension or hypovolaemia before commencing therapy.

The dosage of concurrently administered cardiac glycosides or antihypertensive agents may require adjustment. A marked fall in blood pressure may be seen when ACE inhibitors are added to frusemide therapy. The dose of frusemide should be reduced, or the drug stopped, before initiating the ACE inhibitor.

The toxic effects of nephrotoxic antibiotics may be increased by concomitant administration of potent diuretics such as frusemide.

Latent diabetes may become manifest or the insulin requirements of diabetic patients may increase.

In common with other diuretics, serum lithium levels may be increased when lithium is given concomitantly with frusemide, necessitating adjustment of the lithium dosage.

Certain non-steroidal anti-inflammatory agents (e.g. indomethacin, acetylsalicylic acid) may attenuate the action of frusemide and may cause renal failure in cases of pre-existing hypovolaemia. Frusemide may sometimes attenuate the effects of other drugs (e.g. the effects of antidiabetics and of pressor amines) and sometimes potentiate them (e.g. the effects of salicylates, theophylline, lithium and curare-type muscle relaxants).

Interactions have also been reported with ototoxic antibiotics and parenteral cisplatin. In cases of concomitant glucocorticoid therapy or abuse of laxatives, the risk of an increased potassium loss should be borne in mind.

*Precautions:* Caution should be observed in patients liable to electrolyte deficiency.

Results of animal work, in general, show no hazardous effect of Lasix in pregnancy. There is clinical evidence of safety of the drug in the third trimester of human pregnancy; however, Lasix should be used in pregnancy only if strictly indicated and for short term treatment.

*Nursing mothers:* As Lasix may inhibit lactation or may pass into breast milk, it should be used with caution in nursing mothers.

*Overdosage:* In cases of overdose there is a danger of dehydration and electrolyte depletion due to excessive diuresis. Treatment should therefore be aimed at fluid replacement and correction of the electrolyte imbalance.

*Side-effects:* Lasix is generally well tolerated. Side-effects of a minor nature such as nausea, malaise or gastric upset may occur but are not usually severe enough to necessitate withdrawal of treatment. Serum calcium levels may be reduced; in very rare cases tetany has been observed. Nephrocalcinosis has been reported in premature infants.

The incidence of allergic reactions, such as skin rashes, photosensitivity, vasculitis, fever, interstitial nephritis or shock, is very low but when these occur, treatment should be withdrawn. Standard measures for the treatment of shock should be taken if necessary.

Isolated cases of acute pancreatitis have been reported after long-term diuretic (including frusemide) treatment. Disorders of hearing after frusemide are rare and, in most cases reversible. They may occur if frusemide is injected too rapidly, particularly in patients with renal insufficiency.

As with other diuretics a transient rise in creatinine and urea levels has been reported with frusemide.

In common with other sulphonamide-based diuretics hyperuricaemia may occur and, in rare cases, clinical gout may be precipitated.

Serum cholesterol and triglyceride levels may rise during frusemide treatment. During long term therapy they will usually return to normal within six months.

Bone marrow depression has been reported as a rare complication and necessitates withdrawal of treatment.

Pre-existing metabolic alkalosis (e.g. in decompensated cirrhosis of the liver) may be aggravated by frusemide treatment.

Reduced mental alertness may impair ability to drive or operate dangerous machinery.

**Pharmaceutical precautions** Lasix injections should be stored in a cool dry place, protected from light. Frusemide may precipitate out of solution in fluids of low pH (e.g. dextrose solutions) Injections of Lasix should not be mixed with any other preparations. Opened ampoules should be used immediately and any remainder discarded.

**Legal category** POM.

**Package quantities** Lasix ampoules 20 mg are available in packs of 5×2 ml.

**Further information** Lasix 20 mg injection contains approximately 0.14 mmol Na$^+$/ml.

**Product licence number** 0086/5012R
*Product licence holder:* Hoechst UK Ltd., Hoechst House, Salisbury Road, Middlesex TW4 7JH

## LASIX* PAEDIATRIC LIQUID

**Qualitative and quantitative composition** Lasix contains Frusemide BP as active ingredient. When reconstituted, Lasix Paediatric Liquid contains 1 mg Frusemide BP in 1 ml of liquid.

**Pharmaceutical form** Granules for reconstitution to oral solution.

**Clinical particulars**
*Therapeutic indications:* Lasix Paediatric Liquid is a diuretic for treatment of oedema in children or in patients unable to take solid oral dosage forms of Lasix.

*Posology and method of administration:* Children: Dosage 1-3 mg/kg body weight daily. (1-3 ml/kg as reconstituted liquid).
*Adults:* Substitution for oral tablet therapy, dosage 20-80 mg (20-80 ml) daily. Lasix Paediatric Liquid contains sorbitol and may cause flatulence, abdominal distension or diarrhoea if given in large quantities to adults who are unable to take solid oral dose forms of Lasix. (see *Special warnings and precautions*).

*Elderly:* The dose range for adults applies but in the elderly, frusemide is generally eliminated more slowly. Dosage should be titrated until the required response is achieved.

*Contra-indications:* Electrolyte deficiency and pre-comatose states associated with liver cirrhosis. Hypersensitivity to frusemide or sulphonamides.

*Special warnings and precautions for use:* Lasix Paediatric Liquid contains sorbitol and may cause flatulence, abdominal distension or diarrhoea if given in large quantities to adults who are unable to take solid oral dosage forms of Lasix.

Patients with prostatic hypertrophy or impairment of micturition have an increased risk of developing acute retention.

Where indicated steps should be taken to correct hypotension or hypovolaemia before commencing therapy.

Latent diabetes may become manifest or the insulin requirements of diabetic patients may increase.

Caution should be observed in patients liable to electrolyte deficiency.

*Interactions with other medicaments and other forms of interaction:* The dosage of concurrently administered cardiac glycosides or antihypertensive agents may require adjustment. A marked fall in blood pressure may be seen when ACE inhibitors are added to frusemide therapy. The dose of frusemide should be reduced or the drug stopped, before initiating the ACE inhibitor.

The toxic effects of nephrotoxic antibiotics may be increased by concomitant administration of potent diuretics such as frusemide.

In common with other diuretics, serum lithium levels may be increased when lithium is given concomitantly with frusemide, necessitating adjustment of the lithium dosage.

Certain non-steroidal anti-inflammatory agents have been shown to antagonise the action of diuretics such as frusemide and may cause renal failure in cases of pre-existing hypovolaemia.

Interactions have also been reported with ototoxic

antibiotics and parenteral cisplatin. In cases of concomitant glucocorticoid therapy or abuse of laxatives, the risk of an increased potassium loss should be borne in mind.

Frusemide may sometimes attenuate the effects of other drugs (e.g the effects of antidiabetics and pressor amines) and some times potentiate them (e.g the effects of salicylates, theophylline and curare-type muscle relaxants.

*Pregnancy and lactation:* Results of animal work in general show no hazardous effect of Lasix in pregnancy. There is clinical evidence of the safety of the drug in the third trimester of pregnancy in humans. However, Lasix should be used in pregnancy only if strictly indicated and for short-term treatment.

As Lasix may inhibit lactation, it should be used with caution in nursing mothers.

*Effects on ability to drive and use machines:* Reduced mental alertness may impair ability to drive or operate dangerous machinery.

*Undesirable effects:* Lasix is generally well-tolerated. Nausea, malaise or gastric upset may occur but are not usually severe enough to necessitate withdrawal of treatment.

As with other diuretics, electrolytes and water balance may be disturbed as a result of diuresis after prolonged therapy. This may cause symptoms such as headache, hypotension or muscle cramps.

Flatulence, abdominal distension or diarrhoea may occur following the ingestion of large quantities of Lasix Paediatric Liquid, due to its sorbitol content.

Serum calcium levels may be reduced; in very rare cases tetany has been observed. Nephrocalcinosis has been reported in premature infants.

The incidence of allergic reactions, such as skin rashes, photosensitivity, vasculitis, fever or interstitial nephritis, is very low but treatment should be withdrawn when these occur.

Isolated cases of acute pancreatitis have been reported after long term diuretic (including frusemide) treatment. Disorders of hearing after frusemide are rare, and in most cases reversible. They may occur if frusemide is injected too rapidly, particularly in patients with renal insufficiency.

A transient rise in creatinine and urea levels has been reported with frusemide, as with other diuretics.

In common with other sulphonamide-based diuretics, hyperuricaemia may occur and in rare cases, clinical gout be precipitated.

Bone marrow depression has been reported as a rare complication and necessitates withdrawal of treatment.

Pre-existing metabolic alkalosis (e.g in decompensated cirrhosis of the liver) may be aggravated by frusemide treatment.

Serum cholesterol and triglyceride levels may rise during frusemide treatment. During long term therapy they will usually return to normal levels within six months.

*Overdose:* In cases of overdose there is a danger of dehydration and electrolyte depletion due to excessive diuresis. Treatment should be aimed at fluid replacement and correction of the electrolyte imbalance.

**Pharmacological properties**

*Pharmacodynamic properties:* The evidence from many experimental studies suggests that frusemide acts along the entire nephron with the exception of the distal exchange site. The main effect is on the ascending limb of the loop of henle with a complex effect on renal circulation. Blood-flow is diverted from the juxta-medullary region to the outer cortex. The principle renal action of frusemide is to inhibit active chloride transport in the thick ascending limb. Reabsorption of sodium chloride from the nephron is reduced and a hypotonic or isotonic urine produced. It has been established that prostaglandin (PG) biosynthesis and the renin-angiotensin system are affected by frusemide administration and that frusemide alters the renal permeability of the glomerulus to serum proteins.

*Pharmacokinetic properties:* Frusemide is a weak carboxylic acid which exists mainly in the dissociated form in the gastrointestinal tract. Frusemide is rapidly but incompletely absorbed (60-70%) on oral administration and its effect is largely over within 4 hours. The optimal absorption site is the upper duodenum at pH 5.0. Regardless of route of administration 69-97% of activity from a radio-labelled dose is excreted in the first 4 hours after the drug is given. Frusemide is bound to plasma albumin and little biotransformation takes place. Frusemide is mainly eliminated via the kidneys (80-90%); a small fraction of the dose undergoes biliary elimination and 10-15% of the activity can be recovered from the faeces.

(A) In Renal/Hepatic Impairment: Where liver disease is present, biliary elimination is reduced up to 50%, renal impairment has little effect on the elimination rate of Lasix. But less than 20% residual renal function increases the elimination time.

(B) The Elderly: The elimination of frusemide is delayed in the elderly where a certain degree of renal impairment is present.

(C) Newborn: A sustained diuretic effect is seen in the newborn, possibly due to immature tubular function.

*Preclinical safety data:* None stated.

**Pharmaceutical particulars**

*List of excipients:* Sorbitol, disodium hydrogen orthophosphate, sodium sulphite, disodium edetate, sodium hydroxide, nipasept sodium, vanilla flavour and saccharin sodium distilled water (not detected in finished product).

*Incompatibilities:* Frusemide should not be mixed with fluids of low pH.

*Shelf life:* Three years unopened, 30 days after reconsitutution.

*Special precautions for storage:* Store in a dry place at ambient temperature, protected from light in the original container.

Reconstituted liquid should be stored in a cool place e.g. in a refrigerator at 5°C, protected from light.

*Nature and contents of container:* Lasix Paediatric Liquid is available in amber glass bottles, which on reconsitutution of the product contain 150 ml.

*Instruction for use/handling:* The granulate should only be reconstituted with 142 ml of distilled water. The use of sterile distilled water is recommended when the product is intended for administration to neonates.

*Marketing authorisation holder:* Hoechst UK Ltd, Hoechst House, Salisbury Road, Hounslow, Middlesex, TW4 7JH.

**Marketing authorisation number** 0086/0063R

**Date of approval/revision of SPC** July 1995

**Legal category** POM

## LASORIDE* (co-amilofruse 5/40)

**Qualitative and quantitative composition** Each tablet contains, as active ingredients, 40 mg frusemide and 5 mg amiloride hydrochloride.

**Pharmaceutical form** Oblong, biconvex yellow tablets

**Clinical particulars**

*Therapeutic indications:* Where a prompt diuresis is required and where potassium conservation is important

*Posology and method of administration:* The adult dose is one to two tablets, to be taken in the morning. *Elderly:*The elderly are more likely to experience hyperkalaemia since renal reserve may be reduced. The dosage should be adjusted according to renal function, blood electrolytes and diuretic response.

*Children:* Not recommended for use in children (see contraindications).

*Contra-indications:* Hyperkalaemia (serum potassium > 5.3 mmol/litre), Addison's disease, acute renal failure, anuria, severe progressive renal disease, electrolyte imbalance, precomatose states associated with cirrhosis, concomitant potassium supplements, spironolactone or triamterene, known sensitivity to frusemide or amiloride.

Lasoride is contra-indicated in children as safety in this age group has not been established.

*Special warnings and precautions for use:*

*Warnings:* Hyperkalaemia has been observed in patients receiving amiloride hydrochloride.

Frusemide may cause latent diabetes to become manifest. It may be necessary to increase the dose of hypoglycaemic agents in diabetic patients.

Lasoride should be discontinued before a glucose tolerance test.

Patients with prostatic hypertrophy or impairment of micturition have an increased risk of developing acute urinary retention during diuretic therapy.

Serum uric acid levels may rise during treatment with Lasoride and acute attacks of gout may be precipitated.

*Precautions:* Patients who are being treated with the preparation require regular supervision, with monitoring of fluid and electrolyte states to avoid excessive loss of fluid.

Lasoride should be used with particular caution in elderly patients or those with potential obstruction in the urinary tract or disorders rendering electrolyte balance precarious.

Hyponatraemia, hypochloraemia and raised blood urea nitrogen may occur during vigorous diuresis, especially in seriously ill patients or the elderly. Careful monitoring of serum electrolytes and urea should therefore be undertaken in these patients.

*Interactions with other medicaments and other forms of interaction:* The dosage of concurrently administered cardiac glycosides or antihypertensive agents may require adjustment.

The toxic effects of nephrotoxic antibiotics may be increased by concomitant administration of potent diuretics such as Lasoride.

In common with other diuretics, serum lithium levels may be increased when lithium is given concomitantly with frusemide, necessitating adjustment of the lithium dosage.

ACE inhibitors should not be used in combination with Lasoride as serum potassium levels may be increased.

Certain non-steroidal anti-inflammatory agents (e.g. indomethacin, acetylsalicylic acid) may attenuate the action of diuretics such as frusemide and may cause renal failure in cases of pre-existing hypovolaemia. Frusemide may sometimes attenuate the effects of other drugs (e.g. the effect of antidiabetics and of pressor amines) and sometimes potentiate them (e.g. the effects of salicylates, theophylline, lithium and curare-type muscle relaxants).

Interactions have also been reported with ototoxic antibiotics. In cases of concomitant corticosteroid therapy or abuse of laxatives, the risk of an increased potassium loss should be borne in mind.

*Pregnancy and lactation:* The safety of Lasoride use during pregnancy and lactation has not been established.

*Effects on ability to drive and to operate machinery:* Reduced mental alertness may impair ability to drive or operate dangerous machinery.

*Undesirable effects:* Malaise, gastric upset, nausea, vomiting, diarrhoea, and constipation may occur.

If skin rashes or pruritus occur, treatment should be withdrawn.

Serum calcium levels may be reduced; in very rare cases tetany has been observed.

Serum cholesterol and triglyceride levels may rise during frusemide treatment but will usually return to normal within six months.

Rare complications may include minor psychiatric disturbances and disturbances in liver function tests. Isolated cases of acute pancreatitis have been reported after long-term diuretic (including frusemide) treatment.

Disorders of hearing after frusemide are rare and, in most cases reversible. They may occur if frusemide is injected too rapidly, particularly in patients with renal insufficiency.

Bone marrow depression occasionally complicates treatment, necessitating withdrawal of the product. The haematopoietic state should be regularly monitored during treatment.

*Overdosage:* Treatment of overdosage should be aimed at reversing dehydration and correcting electrolyte imbalance, particularly hyperkalaemia. Emesis should be induced or gastric lavage performed. Treatment is symptomatic and supportive. If hyperkalaemia is seen, appropriate measures to reduce serum potassium must be instituted.

**Pharmacological properties**

*Pharmacodynamic properties:* Frusemide: Frusemide is a potent diuretic acting on the loop of Henle to inhibit electrolyte re-absorption, excretion of sodium, potassium and chloride ions is increased and water excretion enhanced.

Amiloride: Amiloride is a mild diuretic acting mainly on distal renal tubules. It increase excretion of sodium and chloride and reduces excretionof potassium. It is mainly used as an adjunct to the thiazides, frusemide and similar diuretics

*Pharmacokinetic properties:* Frusemide: Frusemide is rapidly absorbed from the gastrointestinal tract after oral administration. It has a biphasic half-life in the plasma with a terminal elimination of about 1.5 hours.

It is up to 99% bound to plasma proteins..

Amiloride: Amiloride is relatively well absorbed from the gastro-intestinal tract after oral administration.

Peak serum concentration are attained 3 to 4 hours after administration. It is estimated to have a serum half-life of about 9–10 hours.

**Pharmaceutical particulars**

*List of excipients:* Lactose, maize starch, talc, colloidal silicon dioxide, magnesium stearate and colouring agent E104 (dispersed quinoline yellow lake).

*Incompatibilities:* Not applicable.

*Shelf life:* 3 years

*Special precautions for storage:* Protect from light.

*Nature and contents of the container:* Amber glass bottles of 50 and 100 tablets and securitainers of 50, 100 and 1000 tablets.

Also blister pack of 28 tablets in a calendar pack.

*Instructions for use/handling:* Not applicable

*Marketing authorisation holder:* Hoechst UK Ltd.,

Hoechst House, Salisbury Road, Hounslow, Middx., TW4 6JH

**Marketing authorisation number** 0086/0120

**Date of approval/revision of SPC** 12 May 1992

**Legal category** POM

## LOPRAZOLAM TABLETS 1 mg

**Presentation** Loprazolam tablets 1 mg. Pale yellow, biconvex tablets, 7 mm in diameter, marked Dormonoct* 1 on one face with breakline on reverse. Each tablet contains loprazolam mesylate equivalent to 1 mg loprazolam.

**Uses** Loprazolam is indicated for the short-term treatment of insomnia including difficulty in falling asleep and/or frequent nocturnal awakenings. Benzodiazepines should be used to treat insomnia only when it is severe, disabling or subjecting the individual to extreme distress. An underlying cause for insomnia should be sought before deciding upon the use of benzodiazepines for symptomatic relief.

**Dosage and administration**

*Adults:* The recommended dose is 1 mg at bedtime. This may be increased to 1.5 mg or 2 mg if necessary.

*Elderly:* Dosage in the elderly should be limited to 1 mg at bedtime.

*Frail, debilitated or aged patients:* A starting dose of a half tablet may be appropriate. Dosage should not exceed 1 mg.

Treatment should if possible be intermittent.

The lowest dose to control symptoms should be used. Treatment should not normally be continued beyond 4 weeks.

Long-term chronic use is not recommended.

Treatment should always be tapered off gradually.

Patients who have taken benzodiazepines for a long time may require a longer period during which doses are reduced.

*Children:* There is insufficient evidence to recommend the use of Loprazolam in children.

**Contra-indications, warnings, etc**

*Contra-indications:* Sensitivity to benzodiazepines, acute pulmonary insufficiency, myasthenia gravis, alcohol intake, phobic or obsessional states, monotherapy in depression or anxiety associated with depression and chronic psychosis.

*Pregnancy and lactation:* The use of loprazolam during pregnancy should be avoided. The possibility of loprazolam being excreted in the milk should also be considered in nursing mothers.

*Precautions:* As with all CNS-active drugs, patients should be warned of the possible hazard of driving or operating machinery. Loprazolam may be potentiated by or with cisapride, alcohol, or other drugs acting on the CNS. Additive synergy has been observed with neuromuscular depressants (curare-like drugs and muscle relaxants). Disinhibiting effects may be manifested in various ways. Suicide may be precipitated in patients who are depressed and aggressive behaviour towards self and others may be precipitated. Extreme caution should therefore be used in prescribing benzodiazepines in patients with personality disorders.

In general, the dependence potential of benzodiazepines is low but this increases when high doses are attained, especially when given over long periods, and particularly in patients with a history of alcoholism or drug abuse. However, withdrawal symptoms occur even with normal therapeutic doses given for short periods of time. Withdrawal from benzodiazepines may be associated with physiological and psychological symptoms of withdrawal including depression. Patients receiving benzodiazepines should be regularly monitored.

Loprazolam should be used with caution in chronic pulmonary insufficiency, cerebrovascular disease and chronic renal or hepatic impairment.

*Side-effects:* In general, loprazolam is very well tolerated. However, the common side effects of benzodiazepines, including headaches, nausea, drowsiness, hypotonia, blurring of vision, dizziness and ataxia may occur on the following day, particularly in unusually sensitive patients or when dosage has been excessive.

Rare behavioural adverse effects of benzodiazepines include paradoxical aggressive outbursts, excitement, confusion, and the uncovering of depression with suicidal tendencies. Even more rare side effects reported with some benzodiazepines have been hypotension, gastrointestinal and visual disturbances, skin rashes, urinary retention, changes in libido, blood dyscrasias and jaundice. Amnesia may occur. In cases of loss or bereavement psychological adjustment may be inhibited by benzodiazepines.

*Overdosage:* As with other benzodiazepines, overdosage does not usually present a threat to life. Treatment is symptomatic and gastric lavage may be of use if performed shortly after ingestion. Use of a specific antidote such as flumazenil in association with symptomatic treatment in hospital should be considered.

**Pharmaceutical precautions** Store below 25°C in a dry place. Protect from light.

**Legal category** CD(Sch 4) POM.

**Package quantities** Loprazolam Tablets 1 mg are blister packed and presented in OP cartons of 28.

**Further information** Loprazolam is an intermediate acting benzodiazepine. There are no long-lived sedative metabolites. Therefore there is a reduced likelihood of the occurrence of daytime drowsiness or impairment in the performance of skilled tasks, associated with the long acting products. Equally, there is less likelihood of rebound insomnia, which may occur with the ultra-short acting benzodiazepines.

Loprazolam was previously known as Dormonoct*. Loprazolam tablets contain lactose.

**Product licence number** 0109/0080.

*Product licence holder:* Roussel Laboratories Ltd., Broadwater Park, Denham, Uxbridge, Middlesex UB9 5HP

## MERBENTYL* SYRUP

**Presentation** Merbentyl Syrup is colourless, and raspberry flavoured. Each 5 ml contains 10 mg Dicyclomine Hydrochloride BP.

**Uses** Merbentyl is a smooth muscle antispasmodic primarily indicated for the treatment of functional conditions involving smooth muscle spasm of the gastro-intestinal tract. The commonest of these is irritable colon (mucous colitis, spastic colon).

**Dosage and administration** *Adults:* One to two 5 ml spoonfuls (10–20 mg) three times daily before or after meals.

*Children (2–12 years):* One 5 ml spoonful (10 mg) three times daily.

*Children (6 months–2 years):* 5–10 mg three or four times daily, 15 minutes before feeds. Do not exceed a daily dose of 40 mg. If it is necessary to dilute Merbentyl syrup this may be done using Syrup BP or, if diluted immediately prior to use, with water.

**Contra-indications, warnings, etc**

*Contra-indications:* Known idiosyncrasy to dicyclomine hydrochloride. Infants under 6 months of age.

*Precautions:* Products containing dicyclomine hydrochloride should be used with caution in any patient with, or suspected of having, glaucoma or prostatic hypertrophy. Use with care in patients with hiatus hernia associated with reflux oesophagitis because anticholinergic drugs may aggravate the condition.

There are rare reports of infants, 3 months of age and under, administered dicyclomine hydrochloride syrup, who have evidenced respiratory symptoms (breathing difficulty, shortness of breath, breathlessness, respiratory collapse, apnoea), as well as seizures, syncope, asphyxia, pulse rate fluctuations, muscular hypotonia and coma. The above symptoms have occurred within minutes of ingestion and lasted 20–30 minutes. The symptoms were reported in association with dicyclomine hydrochloride syrup therapy but the cause and effect relationship has neither been disproved nor proved. The timing and nature of the reactions suggest that they were a consequence of local irritation and/or aspiration, rather than to a direct pharmacological effect. Although no causal relationship between these effects, observed in infants, and dicyclomine administration has been established, dicyclomine hydrochloride is contra-indicated in infants under 6 months of age. See 'Contra-indications' above.

*Use in pregnancy and lactation:* Epidemiological studies in pregnant women with products containing dicyclomine hydrochloride (at doses up to 40 mg/day) have not shown that dicyclomine hydrochloride increases the risk of foetal abnormalities if administered during the first trimester of pregnancy. Reproduction studies have been performed in rats and rabbits at doses of up to 100 times the maximum recommended dose (based on 60 mg per day for an adult person) and have revealed no evidence of impaired fertility or harm to the foetus due to dicyclomine.

Since the risk of teratogenicity cannot be excluded with absolute certainty for any product, the drug should be used during pregnancy only if clearly needed.

It is not known whether dicyclomine is secreted in human milk. Because many drugs are excreted in human milk, caution should be exercised when dicyclomine is administered to a nursing woman.

*Side-effects:* Side-effects seldom occur with Merbentyl. However, in susceptible individuals, dry mouth, thirst and dizziness may occur. On rare occasions, fatigue, sedation, blurred vision, rash, constipation, anorexia, nausea and vomiting, headache, and dysuria have also been reported.

*Overdosage:* Symptoms of Merbentyl overdosage are headache, dizziness, nausea, dry mouth, difficulty in swallowing, dilated pupils and hot dry skin. Treatment may include emetics, gastric lavage and symptomatic therapy if indicated.

**Pharmaceutical precautions** Should be stored and dispensed in amber glass bottles.

**Legal category** POM

P – Preparations of Dicyclomine Hydrochloride for internal use with a maximum dose of 10 mg and a maximum daily dose of 60 mg.

**Package quantities** Amber glass bottle of 500 ml.

**Further information** Nil.

**Product licence number** 4425/0047

*Product licence holder:* Marion Merrell Ltd., Broadwater Park, Denham, Uxbridge, Middlesex UB9 5HP

## MERBENTYL* AND MERBENTYL 20* TABLETS

**Presentation**

*Merbentyl Tablets:* White, round, plain biconvex tablets, stamped 'M' in two concentric circles, containing Dicyclomine Hydrochloride BP 10 mg.

*Merbentyl 20 Tablets:* White, biconvex, oval tablets stamped MERBENTYL 20 containing Dicyclomine Hydrochloride BP 20 mg.

**Uses** Merbentyl is a smooth muscle antispasmodic primarily indicated for the treatment of functional conditions involving smooth muscle spasm of the gastro-intestinal tract.

**Dosage and administration** *Adults:* 10–20 mg three times daily before or after meals.

*Children: (2–12 years):* 10 mg three times daily.

**Contra-indications, warnings, etc**

*Contra-indications:* Known idiosyncrasy to dicyclomine hydrochloride.

*Precautions:* Products containing dicyclomine hydrochloride should be used with caution in any patient with, or suspected of having glaucoma or prostatic hypertrophy. Use with care in patients with hiatus hernia associated with reflux oesophagitis because anticholinergic drugs may aggravate the condition.

*Use in pregnancy and lactation:* Epidemiological studies in pregnant women with products containing dicyclomine hydrochloride (at doses up to 40 mg/day) have not shown that dicyclomine hydrochloride increases the risk of foetal abnormalities if administered during the first trimester of pregnancy. Reproduction studies have been performed in rats and rabbits at doses of up to 100 times the maximum recommended dose (based on 60 mg per day for an adult person) and have revealed no evidence of impaired fertility or harm to the foetus due to dicyclomine.

Since the risk of teratogenicity cannot be excluded with absolute certainty for any product, the drug should be used during pregnancy only if clearly needed.

It is not known whether dicyclomine is secreted in human milk. Because many drugs are excreted in human milk, caution should be exercised when dicyclomine is administered to a nursing woman.

*Side-effects:* Side-effects seldom occur with Merbentyl. However, in susceptible individuals, dry mouth, thirst and dizziness may occur. On rare occasions, fatigue, sedation, blurred vision, rash, constipation, anorexia, nausea and vomiting, headache and dysuria have also been reported.

*Overdosage:* Symptoms of Merbentyl overdosage are headache, dizziness, nausea, dry mouth, difficulty in swallowing, dilated pupils and hot dry skin. Treatment may include emetics, gastric lavage and symptomatic therapy if indicated.

**Pharmaceutical precautions** None.

**Legal category** POM.

P – Preparations of Dicyclomine Hydrochloride for internal use with a maximum dose of 10 mg and a maximum daily dose of 60 mg.

**Package quantities** Merbentyl Tablets: Blister pack of 100 tablets. Merbentyl 20 Tablets: Original pack of 84 tablets.

**Further information** Nil.

**Product licence numbers**

Merbentyl Tablets 4425/0035
Merbentyl 20 Tablets 4425/0081

*Product licence holder:* Marion Merrell Ltd., Broadwater Park, Denham, Uxbridge, Middlesex UB9 5HP

# MERBENTYL 20* TABLETS

**Qualitative and quantitative composition** Dicyclomine hydrochloride BP 20 mg

**Pharmaceutical form** White oval biconvex tablets, stamped MERBENTYL 20.

## Clinical particulars

*Therapeutic indications:* Smooth muscle antispasmodic primarily indicated for treatment of functional conditions involving smooth muscle spasm of the gastrointestinal tract.

*Posology and method of administration:* Route of administration: Oral.
*Adults and children over 12 years:* 1 tablet three times a day before or after meals.

*Contra-indications:* Known idiosyncrasy to dicyclomine hydrochloride.

*Special warnings and special precautions for use:* Products containing dicyclomine hydrochloride should be used with caution in any patient with or suspected of having glaucoma or prostatic hypertrophy. Use with care in patients with hiatus hernia associated with reflux oesophagitis because anticholinergic drugs may aggravate the condition.

*Interaction with other medicaments and other forms of interaction:* None stated.

*Pregnancy and lactation:* Epidemiological studies in pregnant women with products containing dicyclomine hydrochloride (at doses up to 40 mg/day) have not shown that dicyclomine hydrochloride increases the risk of foetal abnormalities if administered during the first trimester of pregnancy. Reproduction studies have been performed in rats and rabbits at doses of up to 100 times the maximum recommended dose (based on 60 mg per day for an adult person) and have revealed no evidence of impaired fertility or harm to the foetus due to dicyclomine. Since the risk of teratogenicity cannot be excluded with absolute certainty for any product, the drug should be used during pregnancy only if clearly needed.

It is not known whether dicyclomine is secreted in human milk. Because many drugs are excreted in human milk, caution should be exercised when dicyclomine is administered to a nursing woman.

*Effects on ability to drive and use machines:* None stated.

*Undesirable effects:* Side-effects seldom occur with Merbentyl tablets. However, in susceptible individuals, dry mouth, thirst and dizziness may occur. On rare occasions, fatigue, sedation, blurred vision, rash, constipation, anorexia, nausea and vomiting, headache and dysuria have also been reported.

*Overdose:* Symptoms of Merbentyl overdosage are headache, dizziness, nausea, dry mouth, difficulty in swallowing, dilated pupils and hot dry skin. Treatment may include emetics, gastric lavage and symptomatic therapy if indicated.

## Pharmacological properties

*Pharmacodynamic properties:* Dicyclomine hydrochloride relieves smooth muscle spasm of the gastrointestinal tract.

Animal studies indicate that this action is achieved via a dual mechanism: (1) a specific anticholinergic effect (antimuscarinic at the ACh-receptor sites) and (2) a direct effect upon smooth muscle (musculotropic).

*Pharmacokinetic properties:* After a single oral 20 mg dose of dicyclomine hydrochloride in volunteers, peak plasma concentration reached a mean value of 58 ng/ml in 1 to 1.5 hours. $^{14}$C labelled studies demonstrated comparable bioavailability from oral and intravenous administration. The principal route of elimination is via the urine.

*Preclinical safety data:* None stated.

## Pharmaceutical particulars

*List of excipients:*

| | Per Tablet |
|---|---|
| Lactose BP | 126.50 mg |
| Calcium Hydrogen Phosphate BP | 51.00 mg |
| Icing Sugar* | 49.50 mg |
| Maize Starch BP | 32.20 mg |
| Glucose Liquid** | 6.10 mg |
| Magnesium Stearate BP | 3.0 mg |
| Purified Water BP | ND |

* mixture of Sucrose 97% BP, Starch 3% BP

** equivalent to 4.8 mg Glucose Solids

*Incompatibilities:* None stated.

*Shelf-life:* 5 years.

*Special precautions for storage:* None stated.

*Nature and contents of container:* Container: Opaque blue 250 micron PVC blisters with aluminium foil 20 micron. Pack Size: 84 tablets.

*Instructions for use/handling:* None stated.

*Marketing authorisation holder:* Marion Merrell Ltd, Broadwater Park, Denham, Uxbridge, Middlesex, UB9 5HP

**Marketing authorisation number** 4425/0081

**Date of approval/revision of SPC** January 1996

**Legal category** POM

# METENIX* 5 TABLETS

**Qualitative and quantitative composition** Metolazone 5 mg.

**Pharmaceutical form** Tablet.

## Clinical particulars

*Therapeutic indications:* Metenix 5 is a diuretic for use in the treatment of mild and moderate hypertension. Metenix 5 may be used in conjunction with non-diuretic antihypertensive agents and, in these circumstances, it is usually possible to achieve satisfactory control of blood pressure with a reduced dose of the non-diuretic agent. Patients who have become resistant to therapy with these agents may respond to the addition of Metenix 5 to their antihypertensive regimen.

Metenix 5 may also be used for the treatment of cardiac, renal and hepatic oedema, ascites or toxaemia of pregnancy.

*Posology and method of administration:* For oral administration:
*Hypertension:* The recommended initial dose in mild and moderate hypertension is 5 mg daily. After three to four weeks, the dose may be reduced if necessary to 5 mg on alternate days as maintenance therapy.
*Oedema:* In oedematous conditions, the normal recommended dose is 5–10 mg daily, given as a single dose. In resistant conditions, this may be increased to 20 mg daily or above. However, no more than 80 mg should be given in any 24–hour period.
*Children:* There is insufficient knowledge of the effects of Metenix 5 in children for any dosage recommendations to be made.
*Elderly:* Metolazone may be excreted more slowly in the elderly.

*Contra-indications:* Metenix 5 is contra-indicated in electrolyte deficiency states, anuria, coma or pre-comatose states associated with liver cirrhosis; also in patients with known allergy or hypersensitivity to metolazone.

*Special warnings and special precautions for use:* Because of the antihypertensive effects of metolazone the dosage of concurrently administered non-diuretic antihypertensive agents may need to be reduced.

Caution should be exercised during Metenix 5 therapy in patients liable to electrolyte deficiency.

Chloride deficit, hyponatraemia and a low salt syndrome may also occur, particularly when the patient is also on a diet with restricted salt intake. Hypomagnesaemia has been reported as a consequence of prolonged diuretic therapy.

Prolonged therapy with Metenix 5 may result in hypokalaemia. Serum potassium levels should be determined at regular intervals and, if necessary, potassium supplementation should be instituted.

Fluid and electrolyte balance should be carefully monitored during therapy especially if Metenix 5 is used concurrently with other diuretics. In particular, Metenix 5 may potentiate the diuresis produced by frusemide and, if the two agents are used concurrently, patients should be carefully monitored.

*Interactions with other medicaments and other forms of interaction:* The dosage of concurrently administered cardiac glycosides may require adjustment. Metenix 5 may aggravate the increased potassium excretion associated with steroid therapy or diseases such as cirrhosis or severe ischaemic heart disease. Latent diabetes may become manifest or the insulin requirements of diabetic patients may increase.

Non steroidal anti-inflammatory drugs (e.g. Indomethacin, Sulindac) may attenuate the action of Metolazone.

Prolongation of bleeding time has been reported during concomitant administration of Metenix and warfarin.

*Pregnancy and lactation:* There is little evidence of safety of the drug in human pregnancy, but it has been in wide, general use for many years without apparent ill consequence, animal studies having shown no hazard.

If Metenix 5 is given to nursing mothers, metolazone may be present in the breast milk.

*Effects on ability to drive and use machines:* None known.

*Undesirable effects:* Metenix 5 is generally well tolerated. There have been occasional reports of headache, anorexia, vomiting, abdominal discomfort, muscle cramps and dizziness. There have been isolated reports of urticaria, leucopenia, tachycardia, chills and chest pain.

Hyperuricaemia or azotaemia may occur during treatment with Metenix 5, particularly in patients with impaired renal function. On rare occasions, clinical gout has been reported.

*Overdose:* In cases of overdose there is a danger of dehydration and electrolyte depletion. Treatment should therefore be aimed at fluid replacement and correction of the electrolyte imbalance.

## Pharmacological properties

*Pharmacodynamic properties:* Metolazone is a substituted quinazolinone diuretic.

*Pharmacokinetic properties:* Diuresis and saluresis begin within one hour of administration of Metenix 5 tablets, reaching a maximum in two hours and continuing for 12–24 hours according to dosage.

*Preclinical safety data:* None applicable

## Pharmaceutical particulars

*List of excipients:* Microcrystalline cellulose, magnesium stearate, F and D C blue no 2 lake (E132)

*Incompatibilities:* None

*Shelf life:* 5 years

*Special precautions for storage:* Metenix 5 tablets should be stored protected from light, in the original container or in containers similar to those of the manufacturer.

*Nature and contents of container:* Blister pack of 30 or 100 tablets.

*Instruction for use/handling:* None

*Marketing authorisation holder:* Hoechst UK Ltd, Hoechst House, Salisbury Road, Hounslow, Middlesex TW4 7JH

**Marketing authorisation number** 0086/0056

**Date of approval/revision of SPC** December 1996

**Legal category** POM

# MOLIPAXIN*

**Presentation** Molipaxin (trazodone hydrochloride) is available as:

*Molipaxin CR 150 mg tablets:* blue, controlled release, film coated octagonal tablet embossed 'Molipaxin' on one face and 'CR 150' on the other, approximately 10 mm in diameter. Each tablet contains 150 mg trazodone hydrochloride in a special formulation providing a controlled release.

*Molipaxin Capsules 50 mg:* Size No. 3, opaque violet/green capsules printed R365B and ▲. Each capsule contains 50 mg trazodone hydrochloride.

*Molipaxin Capsules 100 mg:* Size No. 2, opaque violet/fawn capsules printed R365C and ▲. Each capsule contains 100 mg trazodone hydrochloride.

*Molipaxin Tablets 150 mg:* Salmon-pink film coated, round biconvex tablets, approximately 11 mm in diameter with a white core. The tablet is embossed with 'Molipaxin' and '150' on one face and a breakline on the other face.

*Molipaxin Liquid:* For oral use, a clear, colourless solution with an orange odour and taste. Each 5 ml contains 50 mg trazodone hydrochloride.

## Uses

*Properties:* Molipaxin is a potent antidepressant. It also has anxiety reducing activity. Molipaxin is a triazolopyridine derivative chemically unrelated to known tricyclic, tetracyclic and other antidepressant agents. The available data show that at low, sub-therapeutic doses trazodone acts as a 5-HT antagonist and at higher, therapeutic doses inhibits 5-HT reuptake. These effects and the effects of trazodone on noradrenergic transmission probably underlie the antidepressant actions of Molipaxin. The importance of the effects on each transmitter is unknown.

*Indications:* Relief of symptoms in all types of depressive illness including depressive illness accompanied by anxiety. Symptoms of depressive illness likely to respond to the first week of treatment include depressed mood, insomnia, anxiety, somatic symptoms and hypochondriasis.

## Dosage and administration

*Adults:* The starting dose of Molipaxin is 150 mg/day. This may be taken as:

– Molipaxin CR, 150 mg tablet, single dose,

  or

– Molipaxin capsules or liquid, divided doses,

  or

– Molipaxin capsules, tablets or liquid, single dose on retiring.

Dosage may be increased to 300 mg/day, the major

portion of which is preferably taken on retiring. In hospitalised patients, dosage may be further increased to 600 mg/day in divided doses.

*Elderly:* Dosage in the elderly or frail should be started at 100 mg/day in divided doses or as a single dose on retiring. This may be taken as Molipaxin Capsules, Tablets or Liquid.

Dosage may be increased, under supervision, according to efficacy and tolerability. Doses above 300 mg/day are unlikely to be required.

Molipaxin CR tablets should be swallowed whole and not chewed.

Tolerability may be improved by taking Molipaxin after food.

In conformity with current psychiatric opinion, it is suggested that Molipaxin be continued for several months after remission. Cessation of Molipaxin treatment should be gradual.

*Children:* There are insufficient data to recommend the use of Molipaxin in children.

### Contra-indications, warnings, etc

*Contra-indications:* Known hypersensitivity to trazodone.

*Precautions:* As with all other drugs acting on the central nervous system, patients should be warned against the risk of handling machinery and driving.

Although no untoward effects have been reported, Molipaxin may enhance the effects of muscle relaxants and volatile anaesthetics. Similar considerations apply to combined administration with sedative and antidepressant drugs, including alcohol. Molipaxin has been well tolerated in depressed schizophrenic patients receiving standard phenothiazine therapy and also in depressed parkinsonian patients receiving therapy with levodopa.

Possible interactions with monoamine oxidase inhibitors have occasionally been reported, therefore, concurrent administration with MAOIs is not recommended. Giving Molipaxin within two weeks of stopping MAOIs or giving MAOIs within one week of stopping Molipaxin is not recommended.

Since Molipaxin is only a very weak inhibitor of noradrenaline re-uptake and does not modify the blood pressure response to tyramine, interference with the hypotensive action of guanethidine-like compounds is unlikely. However, studies in laboratory animals suggest that Molipaxin may inhibit most of the acute actions of clonidine. In the case of other types of antihypertensive drug, although no clinical interactions have been reported, the possibility of potentiation should be considered.

Concurrent use with trazodone may result in elevated serum levels of digoxin or phenytoin. Monitoring of these serum levels should be considered in these patients.

Current clinical experience suggests that Molipaxin does not cause seizures. Nevertheless, care should be exercised when administering Molipaxin to patients suffering epilepsy, avoiding in particular, abrupt increases or decreases in dosage.

Molipaxin should be administered with care in patients with severe hepatic, renal or cardiac disease.

*Pregnancy and lactation:* Although studies in animals have not shown any direct teratogenic effect, the safety of Molipaxin in human pregnancy has not been established. On basic principles, therefore, its use during the first trimester should be avoided. The possibility of Molipaxin being excreted in the milk should also be considered in nursing mothers.

*Side-effects:* Molipaxin is a sedative antidepressant, but the drowsiness sometimes experienced during the first days of treatment usually disappears on continued therapy.

Anticholinergic-like symptoms do occur but the incidence is similar to placebo. The following symptoms, most of which are commonly reported in cases of untreated depression, have also been recorded in small numbers of patients receiving Molipaxin therapy: dizziness, headache, nausea and vomiting, weakness, decreased alertness, weight loss, tremor, dry mouth, bradycardia, tachycardia, postural hypotension, oedema, constipation, diarrhoea, blurred vision, restlessness, confusional states, insomnia and skin rash.

Blood dyscrasias, including agranulocytosis, thrombocytopenia and anaemia, have been reported on rare occasions. Adverse effects on hepatic function, including jaundice and hepatocellular damage, sometimes severe, have been rarely reported. Should such effects occur, Molipaxin should be discontinued immediately.

As with other drugs with alpha-adrenolytic activity, Molipaxin has been associated with priapism. This may be treated with an intracavernosum injection of an alpha adrenergic agent such as adrenaline or metaraminol. However, there are reports of trazodone induced priapism which have required surgical intervention or led to permanent sexual dysfunction.

Patients developing this suspected adverse reaction should cease Molipaxin therapy immediately.

*Overdosage:* The most frequently reported reactions to overdose have included drowsiness, dizziness and vomiting. There is no specific antidote to Molipaxin. The stomach should be emptied as quickly as possible followed by the oral administration of activated charcoal. Treatment should be symptomatic and supportive in the case of hypotension and excessive sedation.

**Pharmaceutical precautions** Molipaxin CR: Store below 25°C in a dry place. Protect from light.
Molipaxin Capsules: Store in a dry place.
Molipaxin Tablets: Store in a dry place.
Molipaxin Liquid: Protect from light and store below 25°C.
*NB.* Molipaxin Liquid is primarily intended for in-patient use. If dispensed for out-patient use a standard childproof cap should be fitted.

**Legal category** POM.

**Package quantities**
*Molipaxin CR:* 150 mg tablets presented in blister strips of 14 in a pack size of 28.
*Molipaxin Capsules:* Molipaxin 50 mg and 100 mg capsules are presented in blister strips of 14 in pack sizes of 84 and 56, respectively.
*Molipaxin Tablets:* Molipaxin 150 mg in blister strips of 14 in a pack size of 28 tablets.
*Molipaxin Liquid:* Bottle of 150 ml oral liquid.

**Further information** In contrast to the tricyclic antidepressants, Molipaxin is devoid of anticholinergic activity. Consequently troublesome side effects such as dry mouth, blurred vision and urinary hesitancy have occurred no more frequently than in patients receiving placebo therapy. This may be of importance when treating depressed patients who are at risk from conditions such as glaucoma, urinary retention and prostatic hypertrophy.

Studies in animals have shown that Molipaxin is less cardiotoxic than the tricyclic antidepressants and clinical studies suggest that the drug may be less likely to cause cardiac arrhythmias in man. Clinical studies in patients with pre-existing cardiac disease indicate that trazodone may be arrhythmogenic in some patients in that population. Arrhythmias identified include isolated premature ventricular contractions, ventricular couplets, and short episodes (3–4 beats) of ventricular tachycardia.

Molipaxin has no effect on arterial blood $pCO_2$ or $pO_2$ levels in patients with severe respiratory insufficiency due to chronic bronchial or pulmonary disease.
Molipaxin CR tablets contain caster sugar, E132, E171
Molipaxin capsules contain E171, E127, E132, E172
Molipaxin tablets contain lactose, E172, E171
Molipaxin liquid contains Benzoic Acid

**Product licence numbers**
| | |
|---|---|
| Molipaxin CR 150 mg | 0109/0214 |
| Molipaxin 50 mg | 0109/0045 |
| Molipaxin 100 mg | 0109/0046 |
| Molipaxin 150 mg | 0109/0133 |
| Molipaxin Liquid 50 mg/5 ml | 0109/0117 |

*Product licence holder:* Roussel Laboratories Limited, Broadwater Park, Denham, Uxbridge.

## NORPLANT* ▼

**Presentation** Norplant consists of six flexible closed capsules for subdermal implantation designed to release the progestin, levonorgestrel, over a period of five years. The capsules are made of a medical grade elastomer (polydimethylsiloxane), measure about 34 mm in length and 2.44 mm in diameter and each contains 38 mg Levonorgestrel BP.

**Uses** Contraception. Norplant is a long term (up to five years) reversible contraceptive system. The efficacy of Norplant in preventing pregnancy is comparable to or greater than that of other hormonally based and non-hormonally based reversible methods of contraception. The efficacy of Norplant does not depend on patient compliance but may be reduced in heavier women.

**Dosage and administration** Norplant is recommended for insertion into women aged from 18 to 40 years.
*Norplant should be inserted or removed only by a Health Care Professional who has completed, (or is participating under supervision in), a training programme such as that leading to a Letter of Competence in subdermal contraceptive implants offered by the Faculty of Family Planning and Reproductive Healthcare of the Royal College of Obstetricians and Gynaecologists.*
One Norplant set consists of six capsules in a sterile pouch. Insertion is performed using a trocar to place the capsules under the skin. Strict asepsis must be observed. The capsules should be inserted in the

inner aspect of the upper non-dominant arm approximately 6-8 cm above the fold in the elbow. Prior to insertion the skin should be cleansed: the insertion area should be anaesthetised with local anaesthetic: a 2 mm transverse incision should be made in the skin using a scalpel. At the first insertion, using the trocar provided, the capsules should be placed subdermally in the direction of the axilla and in a fan shape. The skin incision should be cleansed and dressed. Care should be taken that capsules are not nicked, cut or broken during insertion or removal. Further information on insertion is contained in a leaflet in the package and is also available from the product licence holder.

*Starting Norplant:* Norplant should be inserted ideally on day 1 of a menstrual cycle, but may be inserted from days 2 to 5 of the menstrual cycle and, additional non-hormonal contraceptive precautions must be used for 7 days afterwards.

If Norplant is inserted at any other time, pregnancy must be excluded prior to insertion and additional non-hormonal contraceptive cover used for 7 days afterwards.

*After abortion:* Norplant should be inserted immediately post-abortion and not more than 5 days later. If inserted after this time additional non-hormonal contraceptive precautions must be used for 7 days afterwards.

*After childbirth:* In line with the recommendations for other progestogen-only contraceptive methods, Norplant may be inserted from day 21 after birth. If inserted after this time, additional non-hormonal contraceptive precautions must be used for 7 days afterwards.

*Removing Norplant:* Norplant should be removed within 5 years of insertion. Removal may be done at any time in the menstrual cycle. Loss of contraceptive effect should be viewed in practice as immediate and a new method commenced as appropriate. After the skin has been cleaned local anaesthetic should be infiltrated. A 4 mm skin incision should be made with a scalpel over the apex of the fan according to the requirements of the specific technique that you have been trained to use. The capsules should be removed using small forceps (e.g. mosquito's). Removal usually takes 20-30 minutes. On rare occasions one or more of the capsules may prove difficult to remove. If it is not possible to remove all 6 capsules at once, further visits may be required when the area has healed (4–6 weeks later). In overseas experience removal difficulties have been observed in approximately 5% of cases. If the patient wishes to continue using the method, a new set of Norplant capsules can be inserted through the same incision, but in the opposite direction.

### Contra-indications, warnings etc

*Contra-indications:* Known or suspected pregnancy, sensitivity to levonorgestrel; undiagnosed vaginal bleeding; known or suspected sex hormone dependent neoplasia; acute liver disease; benign or malignant liver tumours; existence or past history of thromboembolic disease; past history or evidence of severe arterial disease; risk of ischaemic heart disease (family history and plasma cholesterol above 6.5 mmol/l); recent trophoblastic disease before levels of human chorionic gonadotrophin have returned to normal.

*Warnings:* In patients with a history of thromboembolic disease Norplant should only be used if other methods are unsuitable and after careful assessment of risk benefit ratio. Patients who develop arterial thrombolic or embolic disease should have Norplant capsules removed.

The effects of Norplant on clotting factors and plasma lipids have been inconsistent. Caution should be observed when using Norplant in patients with recognised risk factors for or any predisposition to arterial disease or any form of migraine. If focal or crescendo migraine develop or become worse during use, removal of Norplant capsules should be considered.

Women who become significantly depressed or have a history of depression, should be carefully observed and removal of Norplant considered.

Benign intracranial hypertension has been reported on rare occasions in Norplant users. Although a causal relationship to the use of Norplant has not been established, this diagnosis should be considered if significant episodes of headache or visual disturbance occur. If the diagnosis is confirmed, Norplant should be removed.

Variation in menstrual bleeding patterns may occur. Irregular menstrual bleeding, intermenstrual bleeding, prolonged episodes of bleeding and spotting and amenorrhoea occur in some women. Overall these irregularities diminish with continuing use. Significant blood loss is rare and haemoglobin concentrations normally rise slightly in Norplant users.

Since some users of Norplant experience periods of amenorrhoea, missed menstrual periods should not be relied on as the sole means of diagnosing pregnancy. Pregnancy tests should be performed whenever a pregnancy is suspected. Six or more weeks of amenorrhoea after a period of regular menses may indicate pregnancy. The capsules must be removed if pregnancy occurs.

Ectopic pregnancies have been reported among Norplant users. The incidence of ectopic pregnancies in Norplant users was however, below that estimated to occur in the United Kingdom in non-contraceptive users. The risk of ectopic pregnancy may be increased in years 4 and 5 after Norplant insertion and possibly in heavier women. Any patient who presents with lower abdominal pain or pregnancy should be evaluated to exclude ectopic pregnancy.

When follicular development occurs with Norplant, atresia of the follicle is sometimes delayed and the follicle may continue to grow beyond the normal size. In the majority of women enlarged follicles will disappear spontaneously. Rarely they may cause abdominal pain by, for example twisting or rupturing. Even in the presence of symptoms conservative management is indicated but ectopic pregnancy must be excluded. Only in unusual circumstances is surgical intervention warranted.

*Precautions:* Any hormonally-based method of contraception should only be used under regular medical supervision. Examination of the pelvic organs and breasts and blood pressure measurements should be made at suitable intervals.

*Major or minor surgery:* As with other methods of contraception which have no oestrogen component, Norplant may be continued during surgical procedures but in cases of high risk of thrombosis consideration should be given to standard prophylactic measures.

*Drug interactions:* As is the case with combined and progestogen-only contraceptive pills the efficacy of Norplant may be reduced by carbamazepine, barbiturates, phenytoin, primidone, phenylbutazone, rifampicin and griseofulvin. Though not established for non-oral systemically administered contraceptive steroids, these and other hepatic enzyme inducers must be presumed to increase the risk of method failure. This will normally mean that the method is inappropriate in long term users of such drugs. A supplementary contraceptive method should be used during short term treatment with such drugs and for seven days thereafter, rising to 28 days if the drug was used more than four weeks or at all in the case of rifampicin.

Antibiotics, except rifampicin and griseofulvin, are thought not to reduce the effectiveness of Norplant.

*Use during pregnancy and lactation:* There have been reports of fetal congenital malformations when progestogens have been used in pregnant women. If pregnancy occurs Norplant capsules must be removed. Levonorgestrel is excreted in breast milk in small quantities. The long-term effects on the nursing infant are unknown.

*Side-effects:* Frequent irregular or prolonged menstrual bleeding; spotting; amenorrhoea. Pain or itching near implant site; infection at implant site; difficulty in removal. Controlled clinical trials suggest the following adverse effects are associated with the use of Norplant: headache, nervousness, nausea, dizziness, adnexal enlargement, dermatitis, acne, change of appetite, mastalgia, weight changes, hirsutism, hypertrichosis and scalp hair loss. Other events possibly associated with the use of Norplant include breast discharge, cervicitis, mood changes, depression, musculoskeletal pain, abdominal discomfort, vaginitis and vaginal discharge.

Hypertension has occurred in a small percentage of women taking oral hormonal contraceptives. This is usually reversible on discontinuing treatment.

Although there is evidence that combined oral contraceptives may increase the risk of arterial thrombosis, such as myocardial or cerebral infarction, the association of progestogen-only methods, like Norplant, to this risk is not known.

*Overdosage:* There is no experience of overdose with Norplant.

**Pharmaceutical precautions** Store below 25˚C, protected from light and moisture.

**Legal category** POM

**Package quantities** Each carton includes a sterile pack containing six capsules each filled with 38 mg of levonorgestrel for use by a single patient.

**Product licence number** 0109/0249

*Product licence holder:* Roussel Laboratories Ltd., Broadwater Park, Denham, Uxbridge, Middlesex UB9 5HP

## ODRIK*

**Qualitative and quantitative composition**
0.5 mg capsule contains 0.5 mg of Trandolapril.

1.0 mg capsule contains 1.0 mg of Trandolapril.
2.0 mg capsule contains 2.0 mg of Trandolapril.

**Pharmaceutical form**
0.5 mg opaque red/yellow capsules.
1.0 mg opaque red/orange capsules.
2.0 mg opaque red/red capsules.

**Clinical particulars**

*Therapeutic Indications:* Mild or moderate hypertension. Left ventricular dysfunction after myocardial infarction.

It has been demonstrated that Odrik improves survival following myocardial infarction in patients with left ventricular dysfunction (ejection fraction ≤ 35 percent), with or without symptoms of heart failure, and/or, with or without residual ischaemia. Long-term treatment with Odrik significantly reduces overall cardiovascular mortality. It significantly decreases the risk of sudden death and the occurrence of severe or resistant heart failure.

*Posology and method of administration:*
*Adults: Mild or moderate hypertension:* For adults not taking diuretics, without congestive heart failure and without renal or hepatic insufficiency; the recommended initial dosage is 0.5 mg as a single daily dose. A 0.5 mg dose will only achieve a therapeutic response in a minority of patients. Dosage should be doubled incrementally at intervals of 2 to 4 weeks, based on patient response, up to a maximum of 4 mg as a single daily dose. The usual maintenance dose range is 1 to 2 mg as a single daily dose. If the patient response is still unsatisfactory at a dose of 4 mg Odrik, combination therapy should be considered.

*Left ventricular dysfunction after myocardial infarction:* Following a myocardial infarction, therapy may be initiated as early as on the third day. Treatment should be initiated at a daily dose of 0.5 mg. The dose should be progressively increased to a maximum of 4 mg as a single daily dose. Depending upon the tolerability such as symptomatic hypotension, this forced titration can be temporarily suspended.

In the event of hypotension, all concomitant hypotensive therapies such as vasodilators including nitrates, diuretics, must be carefully checked and if possible their dose reduced.

The dose of Odrik should be lowered only if the previous measures are not effective or not feasible.

*Elderly:* The dose in elderly patients is the same as in adults. There is no need to reduce the dose in elderly patients with normal renal and hepatic function. Caution in elderly patients with concomitant use of diuretics, congestive heart failure or renal or hepatic insufficiency. The dose should be titrated according to the need for the control of blood pressure.

*Prior diuretic treatment:* In patients who are at risk from a stimulated renin-angiotensin system (e.g. patients with water and sodium depletion) the diuretic should be discontinued 2-3 days before beginning therapy with 0.5 mg trandolapril to reduce the likelihood of symptomatic hypotension. The diuretic may be resumed later if required.

*Cardiac failure:* In hypertensive patients who also have congestive heart failure, with or without associated renal insufficiency, symptomatic hypotension has been observed after treatment with ACE inhibitors. In these patients therapy should be started at a dose of 0.5 mg Odrik once daily under close medical supervision in hospital.

*Dosage adjustment in renal impairment:* For patients with mild or moderate renal impairment (creatinine clearance of 10-70 ml/min) the usual adult and elderly doses are recommended.

For patients with severe renal impairment (creatinine clearance of <10 ml/min) the usual adult and elderly starting doses are also recommended but the maximum daily dose should not exceed 2 mg. In these patients therapy should be under close medical supervision.

*Dialysis:* It is not known for certain if trandolapril or trandolaprilat are removed by dialysis. However, it would be expected that dialysis could remove the active moiety, trandolaprilat, from the circulation, resulting in a possible loss of control of blood pressure. Therefore careful monitoring of the patient's blood pressure during dialysis is required, and the dosage of trandolapril adjusted if needed.

*Dosage adjustment in hepatic impairment:* In patients with severely impaired liver function a decrease in the metabolic clearance of the parent compound trandolapril and the active metabolite trandolaprilat results in a large increase in plasma trandolapril levels and to a lesser extent an increase in trandolaprilat levels. Treatment with Odrik should therefore be initiated at a dose of 0.5 mg once daily under close medical supervision.

*Children:* Odrik has not been studied in children and therefore use in this age group is not recommended.

*Contra-indications:* Known hypersensitivity to trandolapril. History of angioneurotic oedema associated with administration of an ACE inhibitor. Hereditary/idiopathic angioneurotic oedema. Pregnancy or lactation. Use in children.

*Special warnings and precautions for use:* Odrik should not be used in patients with aortic stenosis or outflow obstruction.
*Assessment of renal function:* Evaluation of the patient should include assessment of renal function prior to initiation of therapy and during treatment. Proteinuria may occur if renal impairment is present prior to therapy or relatively high doses are used.
*Impaired renal function:* Patients with severe renal insufficiency may require reduced doses of Odrik; their renal function should be closely monitored. In the majority, renal function will not alter. In patients with renal insufficiency, congestive heart failure or unilateral or bilateral renal artery stenosis, in the single kidney as well as after renal transplantation, there is a risk of impairment of renal function. If recognised early, such impairment of renal function is reversible upon discontinuation of therapy.

Some hypertensive patients with no apparent preexisting renal disease may develop minor and usually transient increases in blood urea nitrogen and serum creatinine when Odrik is given concomitantly with a diuretic. Dosage reduction of Odrik and/or discontinuation of the diuretic may be required. Additionally, in patients with renal insufficiency the risk of hyperkalaemia should be considered and the patient's electrolyte status checked regularly.
*Impaired liver function:* As trandolapril is a prodrug metabolised to its active moiety in the liver, particular caution and close monitoring should be applied to patients with impaired liver function.
*Symptomatic hypotension:* In patients with uncomplicated hypertension, symptomatic hypotension has been observed rarely after the initial dose of Odrik as well as after increasing the dose of Odrik. It is more likely to occur in patients who have been volume- and salt-depleted by prolonged diuretic therapy, dietary salt restriction, dialysis, diarrhoea or vomiting. Therefore, in these patients, diuretic therapy should be discontinued and volume and/or salt depletion should be corrected before initiating therapy with Odrik.

If symptomatic hypotension occurs, the patient should be placed in a supine position and, if necessary, receive an intravenous infusion of physiological saline. Intravenous atropine may be necessary if there is associated bradycardia. Treatment with Odrik may usually be continued following restoration of effective blood volume and blood pressure.
*Surgery/anaesthesia:* In patients undergoing surgery or during anaesthesia with agents producing hypotension, Odrik may block angiotensin II formation secondary to compensatory renin release. If hypotension occurs and is considered to be due to this mechanism, it can be corrected by appropriate treatment.

*Agranulocytosis and bone marrow depression:* In patients on angiotensin converting enzyme inhibitors, agranulocytosis and bone marrow depression have been seen rarely. They are more frequent in patients with renal impairment, especially if they have a collagen vascular disease. However, regular monitoring of white blood cell counts and protein levels in urine should be considered in patients with collagen vascular disease (e.g. lupus erythematosus and scleroderma), especially associated with impaired renal function and concomitant therapy particularly with corticosteroids and antimetabolites.
*Hyperkalaemia:* Elevated serum potassium has been observed very rarely in hypertensive patients. Risk factors for the development of hyperkalaemia include renal insufficiency, potassium sparing diuretics, the concomitant use of agents to treat hypokalaemia, diabetes mellitus and/or left ventricular dysfunction after myocardial infarction.
*Angioneurotic oedema:* Rarely, ACE inhibitors (such as trandolapril) may cause angioneurotic oedema that includes swelling of the face, extremities, tongue, glottis and/or larynx. Patients experiencing angioneurotic oedema must immediately discontinue Odrik therapy and be monitored until oedema resolution.

Angioneurotic oedema to the face will usually resolve spontaneously. Oedema involving not only the face but also the glottis may be life-threatening because of the risk of airway obstruction.

Angioneurotic oedema involving the tongue, glottis or larynx requires immediate sub-cutaneous administration of 0.3-0.5 ml of adrenaline solution (1:1000) along with other therapeutic measures as appropriate.

Caution must be exercised in patients with a history of idiopathic angioneurotic oedema and Odrik is contraindicated if angioneurotic oedema was an adverse reaction to an ACE inhibitor (see *Contraindications* section).
*Cough:* During treatment with an ACE inhibitor, a dry and non-productive cough may occur which disappears after discontinuation.

*Interactions with other medicaments and other forms of interaction:* Combination with diuretics or other antihypertensive agents may potentiate the antihypertensive response to Odrik. Adrenergic-blocking drugs should only be combined with trandolapril under careful supervision.

Potassium sparing diuretics (spironolactone, amiloride, triamterene) or potassium supplements may increase the risk of hyperkalaemia particularly in renal failure. Odrik may attenuate the potassium loss caused by thiazide-type diuretics. If concomitant use of these agents is indicated, they should be given with caution and serum potassium should be monitored regularly.

*Antidiabetic agents:* As with all ACE-inhibitors, concomitant use of antidiabetic medicines (insulin or oral hypoglycaemic agents) may cause an increased blood glucose lowering effect with greater risk of hypoglycaemia. Therefore, blood glucose should be closely monitored in diabetics treated with a hypoglycaemic agent and trandolapril, particularly when starting or increasing the dose of ACE-inhibitor, or in patients with impaired renal function.

*Combinations necessitating a warning:* In some patients already receiving diuretic treatment, particularly if this treatment has been recently instituted, the fall in blood pressure on initiation of treatment with Odrik may be excessive. The risk of symptomatic hypotension may be reduced by stopping the diuretic a few days before starting treatment with Odrik. If it is necessary to continue the diuretic treatment, the patient should be monitored, at least after the initial administration of Odrik. As with all antihypertensives, combination with a neuroleptic or tricyclic antidepressant increases the risk of orthostatic hypotension. Odrik may reduce the elimination of lithium and serum levels of lithium should be monitored.

Anaphylactoid reactions to high-flux polyacrylonitrile membranes used in haemodialysis have been reported in patients treated with ACE inhibitors. As with other antihypertensives of this chemical class this combination should be avoided when prescribing ACE inhibitors to renal dialysis patients.

The effects of certain anaesthetics may be enhanced by ACE inhibitors.

Allopurinol, cytostatic or immunosuppresive agents, systemic corticosteroids or procainamide may increase the risk of leucopenia, if used concomitantly with ACE inhibitors.

The antihypertensive effect of ACE inhibitors may be reduced by the administration of NSAIDs. an additive effect on serum potassium increase has been described when NSAIDs and ACE inhibitors have been used concomitantly, while renal function may be reduced.

Antacids cause reduced bioavailability of ACE inhibitors.

The antihypertensive effects of ACE inhibitors may be reduced by sympathomimetics, patients should be carefully monitored.

No clinical interaction has been observed in patients with left ventricular dysfunction after myocardial infarction when Odrik has been concomitantly administered with thrombolytics, aspirin, beta blockers, calcium channel blockers, nitrates, anticoagulants, diuretics or digoxin.

*Use in pregnancy and lactation:* The use of Odrik is contra-indicated in pregnancy and lactation. Pregnancy should be excluded before start of treatment and avoided during treatment. Exposure of the mother to ACE inhibitors in mid or late pregnancy has been associated with oligohydramnios and neonatal hypotension with anuria or renal failure.

In the rat and particularly in the rabbit, trandolapril caused maternal toxicity together with fetotoxicity at high doses. Neither embryotoxicity nor teratogenicity was observed in the rat, rabbit or monkey.

*Effects on ability to drive and to use machines:* Given the pharmacological properties of Odrik, no particular effect is expected. However, in some individuals, ACE inhibitors may affect the ability to drive or operate machinery particularly at the start of treatment, when changing over from other medication or during concomitant use of alcohol. Therefore, after the first dose, or subsequent increases in dose it is not advisable to drive or operate machinery for several hours.

*Undesirable effects (frequency and seriousness):* The following adverse events have been reported with ACE inhibitors as a class. Not all will have been reported in association with Odrik.

In long term studies the most frequently reported adverse events were cough, headaches, asthenia and dizziness.

*Respiratory:* Dyspnoea, sinusitis, rhinitis, glossitis, bronchitis and bronchospasm have been reported, but rarely in association with treatment with ACE inhibitors.

*Cardiovascular:* Tachycardia, palpitations, arrhythmias, angina pectoris, myocardial infarction, transient ischaemic attacks and cerebral haemorrhage have been reported in association with hypotension during treatment with ACE inhibitors.

*Gastrointestinal:* Nausea, vomiting, abdominal pain, indigestion, diarrhoea, constipation and dry mouth have occurred occasionally during treatment with ACE inhibitors.

There have been reports of individual incidents of cholestatic jaundice, hepatitis, pancreatitis and ileus connected with the use of ACE inhibitors.

*Hypersensitivity:* Allergic hypersensitivity reactions such as pruritis and rash have been reported. Urticaria, erythema multiform, Stevens-Johnson Syndrome, toxic epidermal necrolysis, psoriasis-like efflorescences and alopecia, which may be accompanied by fever, myalgia, arthralgia, eosinophilia and/or increased ANA (anti-nuclear antibody)-titres have been occasionally reported with ACE inhibitor treatment.

*Angioneurotic oedema:* In very rare cases angioneurotic oedema has occurred. If laryngeal stridor or angioedema of the face, tongue or glottis occurs treatment with Odrik must be discontinued and appropriate therapy instituted immediately.

*Renal:* Deterioration of renal function and acute renal failure have been reported with the use of ACE inhibitors.

*Drug/laboratory parameters:* Reversible (on stopping treatment) increases in blood urea and plasma creatinine may result, particularly if renal insufficiency, severe heart failure or renovascular hypertension are present.

Decreased haemoglobin, haematocrit, platelets and white cell count, and individual cases of agranulocytosis or pancytopenia, have been reported with ACE inhibitor treatment : also evaluate liver enzymes and serum bilirubin. Haemolytic anaemia has been reported in some patients with a congenital deficiency concerning g-6 PDH (glucose-6-phosphate dehydrogenase) during treatment with ACE inhibitors.

*Overdose:* Symptoms expected with ACE inhibitors are severe hypotension, shock, stupor, bradycardia, electrolyte disturbance and renal failure. In the event of overdosage following recent ingestion, consideration should be given to emptying the stomach contents. Blood pressure should be monitored and if hypotension develops, volume expansion should be considered.

**Pharmacological properties**

*Pharmacodynamic properties:* Odrik capsules contain the prodrug trandolapril, a non-peptide angiotensin converting enzyme (ACE) inhibitor with a carboxyl group but without a sulphydryl group. Trandolapril is rapidly absorbed and then non-specifically hydrolysed to its potent, long-acting active metabolite, trandolaprilat.

Trandolaprilat binds tightly and in a saturable manner to ACE.

The administration of trandolapril causes decreases in the concentrations of angiotensin II, aldosterone and atrial natriuretic factor and increases in plasma renin activity and concentrations of angiotensin I. Odrik thus modulates the renin-angiotensin-aldosterone system which plays a major part in regulating blood volume and blood pressure and consequently has a beneficial antihypertensive effect.

The administration of usual therapeutic doses of Odrik to hypertensive patients produces a marked reduction of both supine and erect blood pressure. The antihypertensive effect is evident after 1 hour, with a peak effect between 8 and 12 hours, persisting for at least 24 hours.

The properties of trandolapril might explain the results obtained in the regression of cardiac hypertrophy with improvement of diastolic function, and improvement of arterial compliance in humans. In addition a decrease in vascular hypertrophy has been shown in animals.

*Pharmacokinetic properties:* Trandolapril is very rapidly absorbed after oral administration. The amount absorbed is equivalent to 40 to 60% of the administered dose and is not affected by food consumption.

The peak plasma concentration of trandolapril is observed 30 minutes after administration. Trandolapril disappears rapidly from the plasma with a half-life of less than one hour.

Trandolapril is hydrolysed to trandolaprilat, a specific angiotensin converting enzyme inhibitor. The amount of trandolaprilat formed is not modified by food consumption. The peak plasma concentration of trandolaprilat is reached after 4 to 6 hours.

In the plasma trandolaprilat is more than 80% protein-bound. It binds saturably, with a high affinity, to angiotensin converting enzyme. The major proportion of circulating trandolaprilat is also non-saturably bound to albumin.

After repeated administration of Odrik in a single daily dose, steady state is reached on average in four days, both in healthy volunteers and in young or elderly hypertensives. The effective half-life of trandolaprilat is between 16 and 24 hours. The terminal half life of elimination is between 47 and 98 hours, depending on dose. This terminal phase probably represents binding/dissociation kinetics of the trandolaprilat/ACE complex.

Trandolaprilat eliminated in the urine in the unchanged form accounts for 10 to 15% of the dose of trandolapril administered. After oral administration of the labelled product in man, 33% of the radioactivity is found in the urine and 66% in the faeces.

The renal clearance of trandolaprilat is proportional to the creatinine clearance. The plasma concentrations of trandolaprilat are significantly higher in patients with a creatinine clearance less than or equal to 30 ml/min. However, after repeated dosing in patients with chronic renal failure steady state is also reached on average in four days, whatever the degree of renal failure.

*Preclinical safety data:* Acute oral toxicity studies of trandolapril and its active metabolite, trandolaprilat, in rats and mice showed both compounds to be non-toxic with respective $LD_{50}$ values of > 4000 mg/kg and > 5000 mg/kg.

Repeat dose oral toxicity was evaluated in the rat and dog with studies of up to 18 and 12 months duration respectively. The principal observations in these studies were of anaemia (doses of 20 mg/kg/day and above in the rat 30 day study and 25 mg/kg/day and above in the dog 6 month study), gastric irritation and ulceration (doses of 20 mg/kg/day and above in the rat 30 day study and 125 mg/kg/day in the dog 6 month study) and renal lesions (20 mg/kg/day and above in the rat 30 day study and 10 mg/kg/day in the dog 30 day study): renal lesions were also seen in the 6 month studies in the rat and dog (from doses of 0.25 and 25 mg/kg/day respectively)–these were reversible on cessation of treatment.

Reproduction toxicity studies showed effects on renal development in offspring with increased incidence of renal pelvic dilation; this was seen at doses of 10 mg/kg/day and above in the rat but these changes did not affect the normal development of the offspring.

Trandolapril was not mutagenic or carcinogenic.

**Pharmaceutical particulars**

*List of excipients:* Corn starch, lactose, povidone, sodium stearyl fumarate and printing ink (shellac, industrial methylated spirit, purified water, soya lecithin, 2-ethoxyethanol, dimethyl polysiloxane and black iron oxide).

*Incompatibilities:* None.

*Shelf life:*

| | |
|---|---|
| Odrik 0.5 mg: | |
| PVC/Al blister pack | 24 months |
| Aluminium blister pack | 24 months |
| Colourless glass bottle | 24 months |
| Odrik 1 mg & 2 mg: | |
| PVCA/Al blister pack | 36 months |
| Aluminium blister pack | 36 months |
| Colourless glass bottle | 36 months |

*Special precautions for storage:* For PVCA/Aluminium blisters: Store in a dry place

*Nature and contents of container:* Blister packs containing 28 or 56 capsules

*Instructions for use/handling:* None.

*Marketing authorisation holder:* Roussel Laboratories Ltd., Broadwater Park, Denham, Uxbridge, Middlesex UB9 5HP

**Marketing authorisation numbers**

| | |
|---|---|
| Odrik 0.5 mg capsule | 0109/0237 |
| Odrik 1 mg capsule | 0109/0238 |
| Odrik 2 mg capsule | 0109/0239 |

**Date of approval/revision of SPC** May 1997

**Legal category** POM

# OESTROGEL* PUMP-PACK

**Qualitative and quantitative composition** Oestrogel contains oestradiol as active ingredient, 0.06% w/w.

**Pharmaceutical form** Hydro-alcoholic gel.

**Clinical particulars**

*Therapeutic indications:* As oestrogen replacement therapy for the relief of symptoms due to natural or surgically induced menopause, such as vasomotor symptoms (hot flushes and sweating), atrophic vaginitis and atrophic urethritis.

*Posology and method of administration:*

*Adults and the elderly:* Each measure from the dispenser is 1.25 g of Oestrogel. Two measures (2.5 g) of Oestrogel once daily (1.5 mg 17β-oestradiol) is the usual starting dose, which in the majority of women will provide effective relief of symptoms. If after one month's treatment effective relief is not obtained, the dosage may be increased accordingly to a maximum of four measures (5 g) of Oestrogel daily (3.0 mg 17β-oestradiol).

The lowest effective dose should be used for maintenance therapy. In women with an intact uterus the recommended dose of a progestogen should be administered for 12 days of each month, in accordance with the manufacturers recommendations. Oestrogel should be administered daily on a continuous basis.

The correct dose of gel should be dispensed and applied to clean, dry, intact areas of skin e.g. on the arms and shoulders, or inner thighs. The area of application should be at least 750 cm², twice the area of the template provided. One measure from the dispenser, or half the prescribed dose, should be applied to each arm/shoulder (or thigh). Oestrogel should NOT be applied on or near the breasts or on the vulval region.

Oestrogel should be allowed to dry for 5 minutes before covering the skin with clothing.

*Children:* Not recommended for children.

*Contra-indications:* Pregnancy and lactation. Known or suspected cancer of the breast, genital tract or other oestrogen dependent neoplasia. Severe hepatic, renal or cardiac disease. Porphyria. Active deep vein thrombosis, thromboembolic disorders, or a confirmed history of these conditions. Endometrial hyperplasia, undiagnosed vaginal bleeding.

*Special warnings and precautions for use:* Before commencing any oestrogen therapy, the patient should have a complete physical and gynaecological examination, including blood pressure, breasts, abdomen and pelvic organs, and endometrial assessment where necessary. This should be repeated at regular intervals.

Prolonged use of unopposed oestrogens may increase the risk of endometrial carcinoma. In women with an intact uterus the addition of a progestogen is therefore considered essential. Caution should be exercised in prescribing oestrogens for patients with mastopathy or a strong family history of breast cancer.

In patients with hypertension, or a history of it, blood pressure should be monitored at regular intervals. If hypertension develops in patients receiving oestrogens, treatment should be discontinued.

Epidemiological studies have suggested that hormone replacement therapy (HRT) is associated with an increased relative risk of developing venous thromboembolism (VTE) i.e. deep vein thrombosis or pulmonary embolism. The studies find a 2-3 fold increase for users compared with non-users which for healthy women amounts to a low risk of one extra case of VTE each year for every 5000 patients taking HRT.

Generally recognised risk factors for VTE include a personal or family history and severe obesity (Body Mass Index >30 kg/m²). In women with these factors the benefits of treatment with HRT need to be carefully weighed against risks.

The risk of VTE may be temporarily increased with prolonged immobilisation, major trauma or major surgery. In women on HRT scrupulous attention should be given to prophylactic measures to prevent VTE following surgery. Where prolonged immobilisation is liable to follow elective surgery, particularly abdominal or orthopaedic surgery to the lower limbs, consideration should be given to temporarily stopping HRT 4 weeks earlier.

If venous thromboembolism develops after initiating therapy the drug should be discontinued.

Care should be taken with patients with cholelithiasis, a history of endometriosis, diabetes mellitus, migraine, otosclerosis or any other condition which is known to deteriorate during pregnancy.

The gel should be applied by the patient herself, not by anyone else, and skin contact, particularly with a male partner, should be avoided for one hour after application. Washing the skin or contact with other skin products should be avoided until at least one hour after application of Oestrogel.

*Interactions with other medicaments and other forms of interaction:* Treatment with surface active agents (e.g. sodium lauryl sulphate), or other drugs which alter barrier structure or function, could remove drug bound to the skin, altering transdermal flux. Therefore patients should avoid the use of strong skin cleansers and detergents (e.g. benzalkonium or benzothonium chloride products), skin care products of high alcoholic content (astringents, sunscreens) and keratolytics (e.g. salicylic acid, lactic acid).

The use of any concomitant skin medication which alters skin production (e.g. cytotoxic drugs) should be avoided.

*Pregnancy and lactation:* Use is contra-indicated in pregnancy and during lactation.

*Effects on ability to drive and use machines:* None known.

*Undesirable effects:* Irritation, reddening of the skin or mild and transient erythema at the site of application have been occasionally reported. In this instance a different site of application should be used, but if the topical side-effects continue, consideration should be given to discontinuation of treatment.

Systemic side-effects with Oestrogel are rare but

---

the following have been reported with oral oestrogen therapy:

*Genito-urinary tract:* increase in the size of uterine fibromyomata, excessive production of cervical mucus.

*Breast:* pain, enlargement and secretion.

*Gastrointestinal tract:* nausea

*CNS:* headache, migraine and mood changes.

*Overdose:* Pain in the breasts or excessive production of cervical mucus may be indicative of too high a dosage, but acute overdosage has not been reported and is unlikely to be a problem. Overdosages of oestrogen may cause nausea, and withdrawal bleeding may occur. There are no specific antidotes and treatment should be symptomatic.

**Pharmacological properties**

*Pharmacodynamic properties:* As the major oestrogen secreted by the human ovary, oestradiol is crucial to the development and maintenance of the female reproductive system and secondary sex characteristics, it promotes growth and development of the vagina, uterus and fallopian tubes, and enlargement of the breasts. Indirectly it contributes to the shaping of the skeleton, maintenance of tone and elasticity of urogenital structures, changes in the epiphyses of the long bones that allow for pubertal growth spurt and its termination, growth of axillary and pubic hair and pigmentation of the nipples and genitals.

The onset of menopause results from a decline in the secretion of oestradiol and other oestrogens by the ovary resulting initially in the cessation of menstruation, followed by menopausal symptoms such as vasomotor symptoms (hot flushes and sweating), muscle cramps, myalgias, arthralgias, anxiety, atrophic vaginitis and kraurosis vulvae. Oestrogens are also an important factor in preventing bone loss and after the menopause women lose bone mineral content at an average rate of 15-20% in a ten year period.

*Pharmacokinetic properties:* Pharmacokinetic studies indicate that, when applied topically to a large area of skin in a volatile solvent, approximately 10% of the oestradiol is percutaneously absorbed into the vascular system, regardless of the age of the patient. Daily application of 2.5 g or 5 g Oestrogel over a surface area of 400-750cm² results in a gradual increase in oestrogen blood levels to steady state after approximately 3-5 days and provides circulating levels of both oestradiol and oestrone equivalent in absolute concentrations and in their respective ratio to those obtained during the early-mid follicular phase of the menstrual cycle.

Avoidance of first pass metabolism by the percutaneous route not only results in a physiologic ratio of oestradiol and oestrone, but also reduces the impact on hepatic biosynthesis of protein that has been demonstrated with orally administered oestrogens.

*Preclinical safety data:* Not applicable.

**Pharmaceutical particulars**

*List of excipients:* Ethanol, carbomer, triethanolamine and purified water.

*Incompatibilities:* None known.

*Shelf life:* 18 months

*Special precautions for storage:* Store below 25°C.

*Nature and contents of container:* Rigid plastic container enclosing a LDPE bag fitted with a metering valve and closed with a polypropylene cap, containing 80 g.

*Instruction for use/handling:* Not applicable.

*Marketing authorisation holder:* Hoechst UK Ltd., Hoechst House, Salisbury Road, Hounslow, Middlesex. TW4 6JH.

**Marketing authorisation number**   0086/0211

**Date of approval/revision of SPC**   1 September 1997

**Legal category**   POM

## ORELOX*   ▼

**Presentation**   Biconvex, cylindrical white tablets which on breaking show a pale yellow core surrounded by a white film coating. Each Orelox tablet contains 130 mg of cefpodoxime proxetil (equivalent to 100 mg cefpodoxime).

**Uses**

*Indications:* Orelox is a bactericidal cephalosporin antibiotic active against a wide range of Gram-negative and Gram-positive organisms. It is indicated for the treatment of the following infections either before the infecting organism has been identified or when caused by bacteria of established sensitivity.

Indications include:

*Upper respiratory tract infections,* including sinusitis, caused by organisms sensitive to cefpodoxime. In tonsillitis and pharyngitis, Orelox should be reserved for recurrent or chronic infections, or for infections

---

where the causative organism is known or suspected to be resistant to commonly used antibiotics.

*Lower respiratory tract infections* caused by organisms sensitive to cefpodoxime, including acute bronchitis and relapses or exacerbations of chronic bronchitis, and bacterial pneumonia, including patients at risk or compromised by other underlying illnesses.

*Properties:* Orelox (cefpodoxime proxetil) is a beta-lactam antibiotic, a 3rd generation oral cephalosporin. It is the prodrug of cefpodoxime.

Following oral administration, Orelox is taken up by the gastro-intestinal wall where it is rapidly hydrolysed to cefpodoxime, a bactericidal antibiotic, which is then absorbed systemically.

The mechanism of action of cefpodoxime is based on inhibition of bacterial cell wall synthesis. It is stable to numerous beta-lactamases.

*Bacteriology:* Cefpodoxime has been shown to possess in vitro bactericidal activity against numerous Gram-positive and Gram-negative bacteria.

It is highly active against the Gram-positive organisms: *Streptococcus pneumoniae,* streptococci of groups A *(S. pyogenes),* B *(S. agalactiae),* C, F and G, other streptococci *(S. mitis, S. sanguis and S. salivarius),* *Corynebacterium diphtheriae.*

*Gram-negative organisms:* *Haemophilus influenzae* (beta-lactamase and non beta-lactamase producing strains), *Haemophilus para-influenzae* (beta-lactamase and non beta-lactamase producing strains), *Moraxella (Branhamella) catarrhalis* (beta-lactamase and non beta-lactamase producing strains), *Neisseria meningitidis, Escherichia coli, Klebsiella pneumoniae, Klebsiella oxytoca.*

It is moderately active against: Methicillin-sensitive staphylococci, penicillinase and non-penicillinase producing strains *(S. aureus* and *S. epidermidis).*

In addition, as with many cephalosporins, the following are resistant to cefpodoxime: Methicillin-resistant staphylococci *(S. aureus* and *S. epidermidis), Staphylococcus saprophyticus, Pseudomonas aeruginosa* and *Pseudomonas* spp., *Clostridium difficile, Bacteroides fragilis* and related species.

As with all antibiotics, sensitivity should be confirmed by in-vitro testing whenever possible.

**Dosage and administration**

*Adults:*

*Upper respiratory tract infections:* For upper respiratory tract infections, including sinusitis, caused by organisms sensitive to cefpodoxime. In tonsillitis and pharyngitis, Orelox should be reserved for recurrent or chronic infections, or for infections where the causative organism is known or suspected to be resistant to commonly used antibiotics. Sinusitis: 200 mg twice daily. Other upper respiratory tract infections: 100 mg twice daily.

*Lower respiratory tract infections:* For lower respiratory tract infections caused by organisms sensitive to cefpodoxime, including acute bronchitis, relapses or exacerbations of chronic bronchitis and bacterial pneumonia; 100-200 mg twice daily, dependent on the severity of the infection.

Tablets should be taken during meals for optimum absorption (morning and evening).

*Elderly:* In the elderly, provided renal function is normal, it is not necessary to modify the dosage.

*Children:* Orelox Paediatric is available to treat infants (over 15 days old) and children. Please refer to separate data sheet for details.

*Renal impairment:* The dosage of Orelox does not require modification if creatinine clearance exceeds 40 ml/min. Below this value, pharmacokinetic studies indicate an increase in plasma elimination half life and maximum plasma concentrations, and hence the dosage should be adjusted appropriately.

| Creatinine clearance (ml/min) | |
|---|---|
| 39–10 | Unit dose administered as a single dose every 24 hours. |
| <10 | Unit dose administered as a single dose every 48 hours. |
| Haemodialysis patients | Unit dose administered after each dialysis session. |

*Hepatic impairment:* The dosage does not require modification in cases of hepatic impairment.

**Contra-indications, warnings, etc**

*Contra-indications:* Hypersensitivity to cephalosporin antibiotics.

*Precautions:* Preliminary enquiry about allergy is necessary before prescribing cephalosporins since cross-allergy to penicillins occurs in 5%-10% of cases. Particular care will be needed in patients sensitive to penicillin. Strict medical surveillance is necessary from the very first administration. Where there is doubt, medical assistance should be available at the initial administration in order to treat any anaphylactic episode. In patients who are allergic to other cephalosporins, the possibility of cross allergy to Orelox should be borne in mind. Orelox should not be given to those patients with a previous history of immediate type hypersensitivity to cephalosporins. Hypersensitivity reactions (anaphylaxis) observed with beta lactam antibiotics can be serious and occasionally fatal.

The onset of any manifestation of hypersensitivity indicates that treatment should be stopped.

Orelox is not the preferred antibiotic for the treatment of staphylococcal pneumonia and should not be used in the treatment of atypical pneumonia caused by organisms such as *Legionella, Mycoplasma* and *Chlamydia.*

In cases of severe renal insufficiency it may be necessary to reduce the dosage regimen dependent on the creatinine clearance.

Possible side-effects include gastrointestinal disorders such as nausea, vomiting and abdominal pain. Antibiotics should always be prescribed with caution in patients with a history of gastrointestinal disease, particularly colitis. Orelox may induce diarrhoea, antibiotic associated colitis and pseudomembranous colitis. These side effects, which may occur more frequently in patients receiving higher doses for prolonged periods, should be considered as potentially serious. The presence of *C. difficile* should be investigated. In all potential cases of colitis, the treatment should be stopped immediately. The diagnosis should be confirmed by sigmoidoscopy, and specific antibiotic therapy (vancomycin) substituted if considered clinically necessary. The administration of products which cause faecal stasis must be avoided. Although any antibiotic may cause pseudomembranous colitis, the risk may be higher with broad-spectrum drugs, such as the cephalosporins. As with all beta-lactam antibiotics, neutropenia, and more rarely agranulocytosis may develop, particularly during extended treatment, for cases of treatment lasting longer than 10 days, blood count should therefore be monitored, and treatment discontinued if neutropenia is found. Changes in renal function have been observed with antibiotics of the same class particularly when given concurrently with potentially nephrotoxic drugs such as aminoglycosides and/or potent diuretics. In such cases, renal function should be monitored.

*Effects on the ability to drive and use machinery:* Attention should be drawn to the risk of dizzy sensations.

*Pregnancy:* Studies carried out in several animal species have not shown any teratogenic or fetotoxic effects. However, the safety of Orelox in pregnancy has not been established, as with all drugs, it should be administered with caution during the early months of pregnancy.

*Lactation:* Cefpodoxime is excreted in human milk. Either breastfeeding or treatment of the mother should be stopped.

*Side-effects.* Possible side-effects include gastrointestinal disorders such as diarrhoea, nausea, vomiting and abdominal pain. Occasional cases have been reported of headaches and rare cases of allergic reactions including hypersensitivity, mucocutaneous reactions, skin rashes and pruritus. Occasional cases of bullous reactions such as Stevens Johnson Syndrome, toxic epidermal necrolysis and erythema multiforme have also been received. Transient moderate elevations of ASAT, ALAT and alkaline phosphatases have been reported, as have slight increases in blood urea and creatinine. Exceptionally rare are the occurrence of haematological disorders such as thrombocytosis, thrombocytopenia, leucopenia and eosinophilia.

*Interactions:* No clinically significant drug interactions have been reported during the course of clinical studies.

As with other cephalosporins, isolated cases showing development of a positive Coombs test have been reported.

An increase in gastric pH, caused by the administration of Histamine H blocking drugs or antacids, will result in decreased bioavailability. In contrast a decrease in gastric pH will increase bioavailability.

A false positive reaction for glucose in the urine may occur with Benedicts or Fehlings solutions or with copper sulphate test tablets, but not with tests based on enzymatic glucose oxidase reactions.

The bioavailability increases if the product is administered during meals.

*Treatment of overdosage:* In the event of overdosage with Orelox, supportive and symptomatic therapy is indicated.

In cases of overdosage, particularly in patients with renal insufficiency, encephalopathy may occur. The encephalopathy is usually reversible once cefpodoxime plasma levels have fallen.

*Incompatibilities.* None known.

**Pharmaceutical precautions:** Store below 25°C.

**Legal category** POM

**Package quantities** Orelox tablets in blister packs of 10.

**Further information** Orelox is absorbed in the intestine and is hydrolysed to the active metabolite cefpodoxime. Concentrations of cefpodoxime in excess of the minimum inhibitory levels for common pathogens can be achieved in lung parenchyma, bronchial mucosa, pleural fluid, tonsils and interstitial fluid. The volume of distribution is 32.3 litres and peak plasma levels of cefpodoxime occur 2.3 hours after dosing. The main route of excretion is renal. Orelox tablets contain lactose and ethyl alcohol, E171.

**Product licence number** 0109/0231

*Product licence holder:* Roussel Laboratories Ltd., Broadwater Park, Denham, Uxbridge, Middlesex UB9 5HP

# ORELOX* PAEDIATRIC SUSPENSION ▼

**Presentation** Bottles of granules for the preparation of an oral suspension. When reconstituted each 5 ml volume contains 52 mg of cefpodoxime proxetil (equivalent to 40 mg cefpodoxime).

## Uses

*Indications:* Orelox is a bactericidal cephalosporin antibiotic active against a wide range of Gram-negative and Gram-positive organisms. It is indicated for the treatment of the following infections either before the infecting organism has been identified or when caused by bacteria of established sensitivity. Indications include:

Upper respiratory tract infections caused by organisms sensitive to cefpodoxime, including acute otitis media, sinusitis, tonsillitis and pharyngitis.

Orelox should be reserved for recurrent or chronic infections, or for infections where the causative organism is known or suspected to be resistant to commonly used antibiotics.

Lower respiratory tract infections caused by organisms sensitive to cefpodoxime, including pneumonia, acute bronchitis and when bacterial super-infection complicates bronchiolitis.

*Properties:* Orelox (cefpodoxime proxetil) is a beta-lactam antibiotic, a 3rd generation oral cephalosporin. It is the prodrug of cefpodoxime.

Following oral administration, Orelox is taken up by the gastro-intestinal wall where it is rapidly hydrolysed to cefpodoxime, a bactericidal antibiotic, which is then absorbed systemically.

The mechanism of action of cefpodoxime is based on inhibition of bacterial cell wall synthesis. It is stable to numerous beta-lactamases.

*Bacteriology:* Cefpodoxime has been shown to possess in vitro bactericidal activity against numerous Gram-positive and Gram-negative bacteria.

It is highly active against the Gram-positive organisms: *Streptococcus pneumoniae,* streptococci of groups A *(S. pyogenes),* B *(S. agalactiae),* C, F and G, other streptococci *(S. mitis, S. sanguis* and *S. salivarius),* Proprionibacterium acnes, *Corynebacterium diphtheriae.* Gram-negative organisms: *Haemophilus influenzae* (beta-lactamase and non beta-lactamase producing strains), *Haemophilus parainfluenzae* (beta-lactamase and non beta-lactamase producing strains), *Moraxella catarrhalis* (beta-lactamase and non beta-lactamase producing strains), *Escherichia coli* and *Klebsiella pneumoniae*

It is moderately active against: Methicillin-sensitive staphylococci, penicillinase and non-penicillinase producing strains *(S. aureus* and *S. epidermidis).*

In addition, as with many cephalosporins, the following are resistant to cefpodoxime: Methicillin-resistant staphylococci *(S. aureus* and coagulase-negative staphylococci), *Staphylococcus saprophyticus, Pseudomonas aeruginosa, Pseudomonas* spp., *Clostridium difficile, Bacteroides fragilis* and related species.

As with all antibiotics, sensitivity should be confirmed by *in-vitro* testing whenever possible.

## Dosage and administration

*Adults and elderly:* Not applicable for this product.

*Children:* The recommended mean dosage for children is 8 mg/kg/day administered in two divided doses at 12 hour intervals. The following dosage regimen is proposed as a guide to prescribing:

### Orelox dosage in children

| Age | Dosage |
| --- | --- |
| Below 6 months | 8 mg/kg/day in 2 divided doses |
| 6 months–2 years | 5 ml twice daily |
| 3–8 years | 10 ml twice daily |
| Above 9 years | 12.5 ml twice daily or 100 mg tablet twice daily |

Orelox should not be used in infants less than 15 days old, as no experience yet exists in this age group.

A measuring spoon (5 ml) with 2.5 ml graduation is provided with the bottle to aid correct dosing. One measuring spoon (5 ml) contains the equivalent of 40 mg cefpodoxime.

The product should be taken during meals for optimal absorption.

*Renal impairment:* The dosage of Orelox does not require modification if creatinine clearance exceeds 40 ml/min/1.73 m².

Below this value, pharmacokinetic studies indicate an increase in plasma elimination half-life and the maximum plasma concentration, and hence the dosage should be adjusted appropriately.

### Orelox in renal impairment

| Creatinine clearance | Dosage |
| --- | --- |
| For values of 10–39 ml/min/1.73 m² | Every 24 hrs the unit dose should be administered as a single dose. |
| For values of <10 ml/min/1.73 m² | Every 48 hrs the unit dose should be administered as a single dose. |
| Haemodialysis patients | After each dialysis session, the unit dose should be administered. |

*Hepatic impairment:* The dosage does not require modification in cases of hepatic impairment.

*Instructions for reconstitution:* Before preparing the suspension the silica gel dessicant contained in the capsule inside the cap must be removed and disposed of. The suspension is prepared by adding water to the bottle up to the calibrated mark and shaking thoroughly to obtain an evenly dispersed suspension.

### Contra-indications, warnings, etc

*Contra-indications:* Patients with hypersensitivity to cephalosporin antibiotics.

Patients with phenylketonuria since the product contains aspartame.

*Precautions:* Preliminary enquiry about allergy to penicillin is necessary before prescribing cephalosporins since cross-allergy to penicillins occurs in 5–10% of cases.

Particular care will be needed in patients sensitive to penicillin: strict medical surveillance is necessary from the very first administration. Where there is doubt, medical assistance should be available at the initial administration in order to treat any anaphylactic episode.

In patients who are allergic to other cephalosporins, the possibility of cross allergy to Orelox should be borne in mind. Orelox should not be given to those patients with a previous history of immediate type hypersensitivity to cephalosporins.

Hypersensitivity reactions (anaphylaxis) observed with beta lactam antibiotics can be serious and occasionally fatal. The onset of any manifestation of hypersensitivity indicates that treatment should be stopped.

Orelox is not the preferred antibiotic for the treatment of staphylococcal pneumonia and should not be used in the treatment of atypical pneumonia caused by organisms such as *Legionella, Mycoplasma* and *Chlamydia.*

In cases of severe renal insufficiency it may be necessary to reduce the dosage regimen dependent on the creatinine clearance.

Antibiotics should always be prescribed with caution in patients with a history of gastrointestinal disease, particularly colitis. Orelox may induce diarrhoea, antibiotic associated colitis and pseudomembraneous colitis. These side-effects, which may occur more frequently in patients receiving higher doses for prolonged periods, should be considered as potentially serious. The presence of *C. difficile* should be investigated. In all potential cases of colitis, the treatment should be stopped immediately. The diagnosis should be confirmed by sigmoidoscopy and specific antibiotic therapy (vancomycin) substituted if considered clinically necessary. The administration of products which cause faecal stasis must be avoided. Although any antibiotic may cause pseudomembraneous colitis, the risk may be higher with broad-spectrum drugs, such as the cephalosporins.

As with all beta-lactam antibiotics, neutropenia, and more rarely agranulocytosis may develop, particularly during extended treatment. For cases of treatment lasting longer than 10 days, blood count should therefore be monitored, and treatment discontinued if neutropenia is found.

The product should not be used in infants less than 15 days old as no clinical trial data in this age group yet exists.

Changes in renal function have been observed with antibiotics of the same class, particularly when given concurrently with potentially nephrotoxic drugs such as aminoglycosides and/or potent diuretics. In such cases, renal function should be monitored.

*Pregnancy:* Not applicable.

*Lactation:* Not applicable.

*Side-effects.* These consist principally of gastrointestinal disorders such as diarrhoea, nausea, vomiting and abdominal pain and rash, urticaria and itching.

Occasional cases have been reported of headaches, dizziness, tinnitus, paresthesia, asthenia and malaise. Rare cases of allergic reactions including hypersensitivity, mucocutaneous reactions, skin rashes and pruritus. Occasional cases of bullous reactions such as Stevens Johnson Syndrome, toxic epidermal necrolysis and erythema multiforme have also been received. Transient moderate elevations of ASAT, ALAT and alkaline phosphatases have been reported, as have slight increases in blood urea and creatinine. Exceptionally rare are the occurrence of liver damage and of haematological disorders such as reduction in haemoglobin, thrombocytosis, thrombocytopenia and eosinophilia. As with other cephalosporins there have been rare reports of anaphylactic reactions, bronchospasm, purpura and angiodema.

*Interactions:* No clinically significant drug interactions have been reported during the course of clinical studies. However, studies have shown that bioavailability is decreased by approximately 30% when Orelox is administered with drugs which neutralise gastric pH or inhibit acid secretions. Therefore, such drugs as antacids of the mineral type and $H_2$ blockers such as ranitidine, which cause an increase in gastric pH, should be taken 2 to 3 hours after Orelox administration. In contrast, drugs which decrease gastric pH, such as pentagastrin will increase bioavailability. The clinical consequences remain to be established.

The bioavailability increases if the product is administered during meals.

As with other cephalosporins, isolated cases showing development of a positive Coombs test have been reported.

A false positive reaction for glucose in the urine may occur with Benedicts or Fehlings solutions or with copper sulphate test tablets, but not with tests based on enzymatic glucose oxidase reactions.

*Treatment of overdosage:* In the event of overdosage with Orelox, supportive and symptomatic therapy is indicated.

In cases of overdosage, particularly in patients with renal insufficiency, encephalopathy may occur. The encephalopathy is usually reversible once cefpodoxime plasma levels have fallen.

*Incompatibilities:* None reported during clinical studies.

**Pharmaceutical precautions** *Bottles:* Unreconstituted product should be stored below 25°C.

Reconstituted suspension can be stored for up to 10 days refrigerated (2–8°C).

**Legal category** POM.

**Package quantities** Calibrated amber glass bottles containing granules for the preparation of 50 ml or 100 ml of suspension. A plastic spoon is supplied with the bottles.

**Further information** Orelox is taken up in the intestine and is hydrolysed to the active metabolite cefpodoxime. Concentrations of cefpodoxime in excess of the minimum inhibitory levels for common pathogens can be achieved in lung parenchyma, bronchial mucosa, pleural fluid, tonsils and interstitial fluid. When cefpodoxime proxetil is administered orally to fasting subjects as a tablet corresponding to 100 mg of cefpodoxime, 40 to 50% is absorbed. The volume of distribution is 30–35 l in young healthy adults, and peak levels of cefpodoxime occur 2 to 3 hrs after dosing. Cefpodoxime is very slightly metabolised, the main route of excretion is renal (80% is liberated unchanged in the urine), the elimination half life is approximately 2.4 hours.

Repeat dose pharmacokinetic studies indicate no accumulation of the active principle.

The percentage of cefpodoxime plasma protein binding is about 40% and is mainly to albumin. This binding is non saturable.

In renal insufficiency corresponding to a creatinine clearance of less than 40 ml/min, an increase in the plasma elimination half-life and the maximum plasma concentrations means that the dose should be reduced in accordance with the degree of renal insufficiency.

In hepatic insufficiency, the slight pharmacokinetic changes observed do not justify any specific modification of the dose regimen.

In children, studies have shown the maximum plasma concentration occurs approximately 2–4 hours after dosing. A single 5 mg/kg dose in 4–12 year olds produced a maximum concentration similar to that in adults given a 200 mg dose.

In patients below 2 years of age, receiving repeated doses of 5 mg/kg every 12 hours, the average plasma concentrations, 2 hours post dose, are between 2.7 mg/l (1 month–6 months) and 2.0 mg/l (7 months–2 years).

In patients between 1 month and 12 years of age, after repeated doses of 5 mg/kg every 12 hours, the residual plasma concentrations of cefpodoxime at steady state, are between 0.2 to 0.3 mg/l (1 month–2 years) and 0.1 mg/l (2 years–12 years).

**Product licence number** 0109/0254.
*Product licence holder:* Roussel Laboratories Ltd., Broadwater Park, Denham, Uxbridge, Middlesex UB9 5HP

## PERFAN* INJECTION

**Presentation** Perfan Injection is a 5 mg/ml solution of enoximone presented in ampoules containing 20 ml.

Other ingredients are alcohol (95%), sodium hydroxide, propylene glycol and Water for Injections.

Perfan Injection is a sterile, clear yellow solution (pH approximately 12.0) for intravenous administration, which must be diluted before use. Containers of diluted product are intended for single use only.

**Uses**
*Actions:* Perfan has positive inotropic and vasodilator properties.

*Indications:* Perfan Injection is indicated for the treatment of congestive heart failure, typically where cardiac output is reduced and filling pressures increased, in patients who require intravenous therapy and who can be closely monitored. The duration of therapy should depend on the patient's continued positive and beneficial response. Sustained haemodynamic and clinical effects have been observed in patients treated for up to 48 hours.

**Dosage and administration** Perfan Injection must be diluted before use. Dilutions should be used immediately and any unused portion discarded.

*Dilution:* The pH of Perfan Injection is approximately 12.0. Perfan Injection must be diluted with an equal volume of 0.9% Sodium Chloride Injection or Water for Injections before administration.

Do not use more dilute solutions or other diluents, particularly dextrose injection, as crystal formation may occur.

Since crystal formation has been observed within approximately 1 hour after mixing Perfan Injection in glass containers or syringes, only plastic containers or syringes should be used for dilutions.

*Administration:* The following procedure is recommended for the administration of the diluted Perfan Injection.

*Initial therapy:* Therapy should be initiated with a dose of 0.5–1.0 mg/kg given as a slow injection (not faster than 12.5 mg/min); further doses of 0.5 mg/kg may be given similarly every 30 minutes until a satisfactory response is achieved or a total initial dose of 3.0 mg/kg is reached. Alternatively, treatment may be initiated as an infusion at a rate of 90 micrograms/kg/minute administered over 10 to 30 minutes until the required haemodynamic response is achieved.

*Maintenance therapy:* To maintain the effects of Perfan Injection the initial dose (not more than 3.0 mg/kg) may be repeated as required every 3–6 hours and adjusted according to the response of the patient. Alternatively, a continuous or intermittent infusion at a rate of 5 to 20 micrograms/kg/minute may be instituted. Total dose over 24 hours should not normally exceed 24.0 mg/kg. In patients with renal impairment the dosage or dosage frequency may need to be reduced.

Precautions should be taken to avoid venous extravasation during administration.

This dosing regimen will produce, in the majority of patients, a 30% or greater increase in cardiac output and/or decreases in pulmonary capillary wedge pressure of about 30% and right atrial pressure of about 40%. It should be noted that the initial haemodynamic response determines the subsequent rate of administration as well as the duration of treatment.

*Use in children:* Safety and effectiveness in children have not been established.

**Contra-indications, warnings, etc**
*Contra-indications:* Perfan Injection is contra-indicated in patients with a known hypersensitivity to Perfan or its components.

*Use in pregnancy and lactation:* There is no evidence of animal teratogenicity with oral therapy. Reproduction studies performed in rats at doses up to 300 mg/kg/day and 100 mg/kg/day have revealed reductions in maternal food consumption, maternal body weight gain and in pup weight at weaning and sexual maturity when enoximone was administered throughout pregnancy and lactation. Sexual behaviour and reproductive capability were unaltered by enoximone treatment. There are no adequate and well-controlled studies in pregnant women. Perfan Injection should be used during pregnancy only if the potential benefit justifies the potential risk. It is not known whether this drug is excreted in human milk. Because many drugs are excreted in human milk, caution should be exercised when Perfan Injection is administered to a nursing mother.

*Precautions:* Perfan Injection should be used cautiously when heart failure is associated with hypertrophic cardiomyopathy, stenotic or obstructive valvular disease or other outlet obstruction.

During treatment with Perfan Injection the following parameters should be monitored: blood pressure, heart rate, ECG, central venous pressure and fluid and electrolyte status; monitoring of platelet counts and hepatic enzyme levels is recommended.

*Drug/laboratory interactions:* No clinical manifestations of untoward drug interaction were observed in patients receiving Perfan Injection most of whom concomitantly received one or more of the following: diuretics (amiloride, triamterene, frusemide and spironolactone), digitalis glycosides (digoxin), potassium supplements, antiarrhythmics (diltiazem, propranolol, lignocaine, nifedipine, procainamide and quinidine), vasodilators (captopril, hydralazine, nitroprusside and nitrates), anticoagulants (warfarin and heparin), analgesics (acetylsalicylic acid, paracetamol and codeine), sedatives (chloral hydrate, diazepam and lorazepam) and positive inotropic agents (dobutamine and dopamine).

In general, administration of Perfan Injection has not been associated with clinically significant alterations in laboratory tests. However, some changes have been noted in platelet counts (reduction in a small percentage of patients) and hepatic enzyme levels (a few patients with minor abnormalities). Monitoring of these parameters is recommended.

*Side-effects:* Whilst Perfan Injection has not been shown to be arrhythmogenic in electrophysiological studies, ectopic beats have been observed in some patients during or after Perfan Injection administration. Ventricular tachycardias or supraventricular arrhythmias have been reported less frequently and are more likely to occur in patients with pre-existing arrhythmias. Perfan Injection may induce hypotension as a consequence of its vasodilator activity. Temporary discontinuation of treatment or a reduction in dosage will usually reverse these conditions.

Other side-effects reported include headache, insomnia, nausea and/or vomiting, and diarrhoea.

Isolated cases of chills, oliguria, fever, urinary retention and upper and lower extremity pain have also been reported.

*Overdosage:* Intravenous administration of Perfan Injection has been shown to produce reductions in blood pressure with occasional instances of hypotensive symptoms. If symptomatic hypotension is observed, administration of Perfan Injection should be reduced or discontinued. No specific antidote is known, but general measures for circulatory support should be taken.

**Pharmaceutical precautions** Store at or below 20°C. Use only 0.9% Sodium Chloride Injection or Water for Injections as diluents.

After dilution, use immediately and discard unused portion. If immediate administration is not possible, do not refrigerate dilutions as crystal formation may occur.

Do not administer unless diluted product is a clear yellow solution.

Other drugs should not be mixed in the same container as Perfan Injection.

**Legal category** POM.

**Package quantities** Ampoules of 20 ml in cartons of 10 ampoules.

**Further information** Nil.

**Product licence number** 4425/0086.
*Product licence holder:* Marion Merrell Ltd., Broadwater Park, Denham, Uxbridge, Middlesex UB9 5HP

## PROCTOSEDYL*

**Presentation** Proctosedyl is available as smooth, off-white suppositories and as an odourless, yellowish-white, translucent, greasy ointment. Each suppository or gram of ointment contains the following active ingredients:
Cinchocaine Hydrochloride BP      5 mg
Hydrocortisone BP      5 mg

**Uses** The local anaesthetic cinchocaine relieves pain and relaxes sphincteric spasm. Pruritus and inflammation are relieved by hydrocortisone, which also decreases serous discharge.

Proctosedyl is therefore useful for the short term relief (not more than 7 days) of pain, irritation and pruritus associated with haemorrhoids and pruritus ani.

**Dosage and administration** A suppository is inserted morning and evening, and after each stool.

Apply the ointment in small quantities with the finger, on the painful or pruritic area, morning and evening and after each stool. For deep application attach cannula to tube, insert to full extent and squeeze tube gently from lower end whilst withdrawing.

The ointment may be used separately or concurrently with the suppositories.

**Contra-indications, warnings, etc.**
*Contra-indications.* Known hypersensitivity to any of the ingredients. Not for use in the presence of infection.

*Pregnancy.* In pregnant animals, administration of corticosteroids can cause abnormalities of fetal development. The relevance of this finding to human beings has not been established. However, topical steroids should not be used extensively in pregnancy, i.e. in large amounts or for long periods.

*Precautions.* Apply only to the region of the rectum and anus and surrounding skin. Hydrocortisone can cause thinning and damage of the skin especially of the face. As with all preparations containing topical corticosteroids, the possibility of systemic absorption should be considered. In particular, long-term continuous therapy should be avoided in infants. Adrenal suppression can occur even without occlusion.

*Side-effects.* In persons sensitive to any of the ingredients, skin rash may occur. Although less likely to cause adrenal suppression when applied topically, Hydrocortisone, applied to a large enough area, especially of damaged skin for long enough, or if under occlusive dressing, may have this adverse effect.

**Pharmaceutical precautions** Ointment: Store below 25°C. Suppositories: Store below 25°C.

**Legal category** POM.

**Package quantities** Proctosedyl Suppositories: Packs of 12. Proctosedyl Ointment: Tubes of 30 g (with cannula).

**Further information** Proctosedyl ointment contains white soft paraffin, liquid paraffin and wool fat. Proctosedyl suppositories contain Suppocire AM.

**Product licence numbers**
Proctosedyl Ointment          0109/5038R
Proctosedyl Suppositories     0109/5039R

*Product licence holder:* Roussel Laboratories Ltd., Broadwater Park, Denham, Uxbridge, Middlesex UB9 5HP

# RASTINON* TABLETS 500 mg

**Presentation** Rastinon Tablets each contain 500 mg Tolbutamide BP. They are presented as uncoated white, circular, scored tablets, 13 mm in diameter, one side bearing the Hoechst insignia, the other bearing the marks 'Rastinon' above and '0.5' below the score mark.

**Uses** Rastinon is a hypoglycaemic agent, indicated for the oral treatment of patients with non-insulin dependent diabetes (maturity-onset or type II diabetes) who respond inadequately to dietary treatment alone. Rastinon is particularly suitable for elderly patients.

**Dosage and administration**
1. *Treatment of previously untreated diabetics:* Stabilisation can be achieved by commencing with 2 tablets daily. The subsequent dosage must depend on the patient's individual response. The average daily dose is 1-3 tablets which can be taken as a single or divided dose as required. Generally, patients who do not respond to 4 tablets (2 g) daily will not respond to higher doses.

2. *Change-over from other oral antidiabetics:* The change-over to Rastinon, from other drugs with a similar mode of action, can be carried out without any break in therapy, even with chlorpropamide despite the long persistence of this agent in the body.

Stabilisation can be achieved by commencing with 2 tablets daily, subsequent dosage depending on the patient's individual response.

3. *Combination with biguanides:* If adequate control is not possible with diet and 4 tablets of Rastinon daily, control can often be re-established by combined administration of Rastinon and a biguanide derivative.

4. *Change-over from insulin:* Some cases of non-insulin dependent diabetes, previously treated with insulin, can be changed to Rastinon. Low insulin doses (less than 20 units) can be replaced immediately. With higher doses a gradual change is advisable by giving insulin and Rastinon concurrently and reducing the dose of insulin.

The tablets may be taken by mouth as a single dose with or immediately after the first main meal of the day, or as a divided dose.

*Children:* As non-insulin dependent diabetes is not usually a disease of childhood, Rastinon is not recommended for use in children.

*Elderly:* Rastinon is particularly suitable for elderly patients. However, since this patient group may be more liable to sulphonylurea-induced hypoglycaemia, treatment should be initiated at lower dosage.

**Contra-indications, warnings, etc**
*Contra-indications:* Rastinon should not be used in patients with insulin-dependent type I diabetes mellitus, diabetic coma, breakdown of control of diabetes (e.g. diabetic ketoacidosis, precoma), who have severe impairment of renal, hepatic, adrenocortical or thyroid function, known hypersensitivity to tolbutamide, acute porphyria, or in circumstances of unusual stress, e.g. surgical operations or during pregnancy and lactation, when dietary treatment and insulin are essential.

Rastinon should not be used during the first trimester of pregnancy. There is some evidence of harmful effects in pregnancy in animals and isolated reports which suggest a hazard in human pregnancy.

*Nursing mothers:* Tolbutamide has been detected in breast milk in small quantities; the effect of this low dose on the neonate is unknown.

*Precautions:* Caution is required in patients with impaired liver function.

*Warnings:* Debilitated or aged patients may be more liable to hypoglycaemia. Rastinon may be used in mild to moderate renal impairment at a reduced dose.

*Interactions:* The hypoglycaemic effect of tolbutamide may be enhanced by ACE inhibitors, anabolic agents, beta-adrenergic blocking agents, bezafibrate, biguanide preparations, chloramphenicol, clofibrate, coumarin derivatives, fenfluramine, fenyramidol, fluoxetine, guanethidine, monoamine oxidase inhibitors, miconazole, para-aminosalicylic acid, high-dose parenteral oxpentifylline, phenylbutazone, phosphamides, probenecid, salicylates, sulphinpyrazone, sulphonamides, tetracyclines and cyclophosphamide. In patients receiving treatment with beta-blockers, clonidine, guanethidine or reserpine the warning signs of a hypoglycaemic attack may be masked.

Attenuation of the blood-sugar-lowering action of Rastinon may result from the concomitant use of adrenaline, lithium, rifampicin, acetazolamide, corticosteroids, diazoxide, thiazide diuretics, glucagon, indomethacin, nicotinates (in high doses), phenothiazine derivatives, phenytoin, oral contraceptives/sex hormones (progestogens, oestrogens), sympathomimetic agents, thyroid hormones.

Both potentiation and attenuation of effect have been reported in patients treated concomitantly with clonidine and reserpine.

Alcohol may potentiate the blood-sugar-lowering action of Rastinon. Chronic alcoholism and chronic abuse of laxatives may lead to deterioration of control of diabetes.

*Overdosage:* Hypoglycaemia may be treated in the conscious patient by the administration of glucose or 3–4 lumps of table sugar with water. This may be repeated as necessary.

If the patient is comatose, up to 50 ml of a 50% glucose solution should be given as a rapid intravenous injection. This may be followed by a continuous infusion of a more dilute (10%) glucose solution at a rate that will maintain the blood glucose at a level about 5.6 mmol/l (100 mg/dl). The patient should be monitored closely for 24–48 hours for any recurrence of hypoglycaemia. Alternatively, glucagon may be administered in a dose of 1 mg subcutaneously or intramuscularly to restore consciousness.

*Side-effects:* Transient visual disturbances may occur at the commencement of treatment.

Adverse reactions serious enough to warrant discontinuation of treatment are uncommon but mild reactions affecting the gastro-intestinal tract such as nausea, sensation of pressure or repletion in the epigastrium and diarrhoea have been observed in exceptional instances. Hypersensitivity reactions involving the skin, including photosensitivity reactions have occurred in isolated cases. Cross-sensitivity to sulphonamides or their derivatives is a possibility.

The adverse reactions described below are very rare, but can be life-threatening in occasional instances:

There have been reports of anaemia, agranulocytosis, pancytopenia and transient changes in liver enzyme concentrations and liver function tests during treatment with tolbutamide, but these effects are not known to be directly attributable to the drug. Haemolytic anaemia, cholestatic jaundice and vasculitis, though not common, have been reported.

Alcohol intolerance has been observed only in exceptional cases.

**Pharmaceutical precautions** Rastinon tablets should be stored below 25°C.

**Legal category** POM.

**Package quantities** Rastinon is available in packs of 100 tablets.

**Further information** Orally administered Rastinon is rapidly absorbed. It is extensively metabolised in the liver prior to excretion in the urine. Both of its metabolites possess some hypoglycaemic activity; this, however, is less pronounced than that of the parent compound.

**Product licence number** 0086/5016R
*Product licence holder:* Hoechst UK Ltd., Hoechst House, Salisbury Road, Middlesex TW4 7JH

# RELEFACT* LH-RH INFECTION

**Qualitative and quantitative composition** Gonadorelin 100 microgram

**Pharmaceutical form** Solution for Injection

**Clinical particulars**

*Therapeutic indications:* Intravenous injection of Relefact LH-RH causes release of LH (luteinizing hormone) and FSH (follicle-stimulating hormone) from the pituitary gland. It provides a means of assessing the reserve of LH and FSH in the pituitary glands of patients with suspected pituitary impairment. In addition, Relefact LH-RH may be of value in the differential diagnosis of delayed puberty and hypogonadism.

*Posology and method of administration:* Relefact LH-RH should be administered intravenously to adults or children as a single dose of 100 microgram. The test is based upon the pituitary response to this dose measured as serum LH and FSH levels. Qualitative data may be obtained from a single test but each laboratory must establish its own normal range for values of serum LH and FSH to obtain quantitative assessment of pituitary reserve.

*Contra-indications:* Relefact LH-RH should not be administered in pregnancy. There is a theoretical possibility of induction of ovulation following the administration of LH-RH. Pituitary adenoma is a relative contra-indication.

*Special warnings and special precautions for use:* None known

*Interactions with other medicaments and other forms of interaction:* None known

*Pregnancy and lactation:* Relefact LH-RH should not be administered in pregnancy

*Effects on ability to drive and use machines:* None known

*Undesirable effects:* Side-effects of any description are rare, but the following reactions have been reported in isolated cases in healthy women: abdominal pain, nausea, headache and increased menstrual bleeding.

*Overdose:* Overdosage with Relefact LH-RH has never been reported and is unlikely to be a problem.

**Pharmacological properties**

*Pharmacodynamic properties:* LH-RH, a decapeptide, is a hypothalamic releasing hormone which stimulates the synthesis of follicle-stimulating hormone and luteinising hormone in the anterior lobe of the pituitary as well as their release. LH-RH secretion is controlled by several factors including circulating sex hormones.

Hence, it is used in the assessment of the reserve of LH and FSH in the pituitary glands of patients with suspected pituitary impairment. In addition, it may be of value in the differential diagnosis of delayed puberty and hypogonadism.

*Pharmacokinetic properties:* LH-RH is rapidly hydrolysed in plasma ($t_\frac{1}{2}$ = 4 minutes) and about half of the dose has been detected in the urine as metabolites within the hour.

*Preclinical safety data:* Not applicable

**Pharmaceutical particulars**

*List of excipients:* Mannitol, sodium dihydrogen phosphate, sodium chloride and water for injections

*Incompatibilities:* Do not dilute or mix with any additive

*Shelf life:* Three years

*Special precautions for storage:* Store in a cool place

*Nature and contents of container:* 1 ml glass ampoule containing 100 microgram gonadorelin in 1 ml aqueous solution

Available in packs of 10 ampoules

*Instruction for use/handling:* Test procedure:
1. Obtain venous blood sample for control value of LH and, if facilities are available for its measurement, FSH.

2. Rapid intravenous injection of 100 microgram Relefact LH-RH.

3. Obtain venous blood sample 20 minutes after injection for measurement of LH/FSH response.

Interpretation of results:

1. *Normal response:* Following the administration of Relefact LH-RH there is a rise in serum LH within two minutes of injection; the response is dose-dependent. Peak levels are achieved 20–30 minutes after injection and baseline levels are approached six hours after a dose of 100 microgram. The FSH response is similar but of lesser magnitude (except (a) prior to puberty when, in both sexes, the FSH response is higher than the LH response and (b) in some patients with hypothalamic-pituitary dysfunction, e.g. anorexia nervosa). The normal female response to Relefact LH-RH shows cyclical variation, the response in the luteal phase being about twice that seen in the early follicular phase.

It is important for each laboratory to establish its own normal ranges of LH and FSH according to the time of the menstrual cycle before attempting to obtain quantitative results.

2. *Assessment of pituitary function:* Relefact LH-RH is a very sensitive index of pituitary function. Consequently, many patients with pituitary tumours, who do not respond to other dynamic tests of pituitary function (such as the growth hormone response to hypoglycaemia), will show a normal response to Relefact LH-RH; others will show an impaired or absent response. A normal response to the Relefact LH-RH test in clinically hypogonadal patients with pituitary abnormalities indicates that their pituitary glands are capable of producing LH and FSH in response to therapy. Similar responses may be seen in patients with hypothalamic tumours such as craniopharyngiomas.

3. *Assessment of primary and secondary hypogonadism:* Patients with primary hypogonadism resulting from gonadal failure or gonadal dysgenesis will have an exaggerated response to Relefact LH-RH. The majority of these patients will also have elevated basal values. The test is of particular value in those cases where basal levels are normal.

The majority of patients with congenital hypogonadotrophic hypogonadism with or without hyposmia (Kallman's syndrome) show a normal or impaired response to single doses of Relefact LH-RH.

These results indicate that, in most cases of isolated pituitary gonadotrophin deficiency, there is a reduced output of hypothalamic hormone releasing factor. An absent response to a single injection, however, is not necessarily indicative of pituitary failure, as more than one injection may be required in order to produce a response.

4. *Assessment of delayed puberty:* In simple delayed puberty the LH and FSH responses are within the normal range, whereas patients with hypogonadotrophic hypogonadism or hypopituitarism have an absent or impaired response. Patients with primary gonadal failure will have an exaggerated response

*Marketing authorisation holder:* Hoechst UK Ltd., Salisbury Road, Hounslow, Middx., TW4 6JH

**Marketing authorisation number** 0086/0019

**Date of approval/revision of SPC 17 December 1991**

**Legal category** POM

# RIFADIN*

**Presentation**

*Rifadin capsules 150 mg:* Blue and red containing 150 mg Rifampicin PhEur and marked 'R-150'.

*Rifadin capsules 300 mg:* Red containing 300 mg Rifampicin PhEur and marked 'R-300'.

*Rifadin syrup:* Raspberry colour and flavour, containing 100 mg Rifampicin PhEur in each 5 ml.

**Uses**

*Mode of action:* Rifadin is a semi-synthetic antibiotic with bactericidal activity against most Mycobacteria and Gram-positive organisms. Rifadin is also active against Gram-negative organisms at higher concentrations.

*Indications:*

*Tuberculosis:* Rifadin, used in combination with other active anti-tuberculosis drugs, is indicated in the treatment of all forms of tuberculosis, including fresh, advanced, chronic and drug-resistant cases. Rifadin is also effective against most atypical strains of Mycobacteria.

*Leprosy:* Rifadin, used in combination with at least one other active anti-leprosy drug, is indicated in the management of multibacillary and paucibacillary leprosy to effect conversion of the infectious state to a non-infectious state.

*Other Infections:* Rifadin is indicated in the treatment of Brucellosis, Legionnaires Disease, and serious staphylococcal infections. To prevent emergence of resistant strains of the infecting organisms, Rifadin

should be used in combination with another antibiotic appropriate for the infection.

*Prophylaxis of meningococcal meningitis:* Rifadin is indicated for the treatment of asymptomatic carriers of *N. meningitidis* to eliminate meningococci from the nasopharynx.

*Haemophilus influenzae:* Rifadin is indicated for the treatment of asymptomatic carriers of *H. influenzae* and as chemoprophylaxis of exposed children, 4 years of age or younger.

**Dosage and administration** The daily dose of Rifadin, calculated from the patient's body weight, should preferably be taken at least 30 minutes before a meal or 2 hours after a meal to ensure rapid and complete absorption.

*Tuberculosis:* Rifadin should be given with other effective anti-tuberculosis drugs to prevent the possible emergence of rifampicin-resistant strains of Mycobacteria.

*Adults:* The recommended single daily dose in tuberculosis is 8–12 mg/kg.

*Usual daily dose:* Patients weighing less than 50 kg – 450 mg. Patients weighing 50 kg or more – 600 mg.

*Children:* In children, oral doses of 10–20 mg/kg body weight daily are recommended, although a total daily dose should not usually exceed 600 mg.

*Leprosy:* 600 mg doses of rifampicin should be given once per month. Alternatively, a daily regimen may be used. The recommended single daily dose is 10 mg/kg.

*Usual daily dose:* Patients weighing less than 50 kg – 450 mg. Patients weighing 50 kg or more – 600 mg.

In the treatment of leprosy, rifampicin should always be used in conjunction with at least one other antileprosy drug.

*Brucellosis, Legionnaires Disease or serious staphylococcal infections:*

*Adults:* The recommended daily dose is 600 – 1200 mg given in 2 to 4 divided doses, together with another appropriate antibiotic to prevent the emergence of resistant strains of the infecting organisms.

*Prophylaxis of meningococcal meningitis:*

*Adults:* 600 mg twice daily for 2 days.

*Children (1–12 years):* 10 mg/kg twice daily for 2 days.

*Children (3 months–1 year):* 5 mg/kg twice daily for 2 days.

*Prophylaxis of Haemophilus influenzae*

*Adults and children:* For members of households exposed to *H. influenzae* B disease when the household contains a child 4 years of age or younger, it is recommended that all members (including the child) receive rifampicin 20 mg/kg once daily (maximum daily dose 600 mg) for 4 days.

Index cases should be treated prior to discharge from hospital.

*Neonates (1 month):* 10 mg/kg daily for 4 days.

*Impaired liver function:* A daily dose of 8 mg/kg should not be exceeded in patients with impaired liver function.

*Use in the elderly:* In elderly patients, the renal excretion of rifampicin is decreased proportionally with physiological decrease of renal function; due to compensatory increase of liver excretion, the terminal half-life in serum is similar to that of younger patients. However, as increased blood levels have been noted in one study of rifampicin in elderly patients, caution should be exercised in using rifampicin in such patients, especially if there is evidence of impaired liver function.

**Contra-indications, warnings, etc**

*Contra-indications:* Rifadin is contra-indicated in the presence of jaundice, and in patients who are hypersensitive to the rifamycins.

*Use in pregnancy and lactation:* At very high doses in animals rifampicin has been shown to have teratogenic effects. There are no well controlled studies with rifampicin in pregnant women. Therefore, Rifadin should be used in pregnant women or in women of child bearing potential only if the potential benefit justifies the potential risk to the foetus. When Rifadin is administered during the last few weeks of pregnancy it may cause post-natal haemorrhages in the mother and infant for which treatment with Vitamin K1 may be indicated.

Rifampicin is excreted in breast milk, patients receiving rifampicin should not breast feed unless in the physician's judgement the potential benefit to the patient outweighs the potential risk to the infant.

*Precautions:* Patients with impaired liver function should only be given rifampicin in cases of necessity, and then with caution and under close medical supervision. In these patients, lower doses of rifampicin are recommended and careful monitoring of liver function, especially serum glutamic pyruvic transaminase (SGPT) and serum glutamic oxaloacetic transaminase (SGOT) should be carried out prior to

therapy and then every two to four weeks during therapy. If signs of hepatocellular damage occur, rifampicin should be withdrawn. In patients with impaired liver function, elderly patients, malnourished patients, and possibly, children under two years of age, caution is particularly recommended when instituting therapeutic regimens in which isoniazid is to be used concurrently with Rifadin. It is rarely necessary, in the absence of clinical findings, to increase the frequency of performing routine liver function tests in patients with normal pretreatment liver function.

In some patients hyperbilirubinaemia can occur in the early days of treatment. This results from competition between rifampicin and bilirubin for hepatic excretion.

An isolated report showing a moderate rise in bilirubin and/or transaminase level is not in itself an indication for interrupting treatment; rather the decision should be made after repeating the tests, noting trends in the levels and considering them in conjunction with the patient's clinical condition.

Because of the possibility of immunological reaction (see *Side-effects*) occurring with intermittent therapy (less than 2 to 3 times per week) patients should be closely monitored. Patients should be cautioned against interrupting treatment.

Rifampicin has enzyme-inducing properties including induction of delta amino levulinic acid synthetase. Isolated reports have associated porphyria exacerbation with rifampicin administration.

*Drug/laboratory interactions:* Rifampicin has been shown in animals and man to have liver enzyme inducing properties and may reduce the activity of anticoagulants, corticosteroids, cyclosporin, digitalis preparations, oral contraceptives, oral hypoglycaemic agents, dapsone, phenytoin, quinidine, narcotics and analgesics. It may be necessary to adjust the dosage of these drugs if they are given concurrently with Rifadin, particularly when it is initiated or withdrawn.

Patients on oral contraceptives should be advised to use alternative, non-hormonal methods of birth control during Rifadin therapy. Also diabetes may become more difficult to control.

If *p*-aminosalicylic acid and rifampicin are both included in the treatment regimen, they should be given not less than eight hours apart to ensure satisfactory blood levels.

Therapeutic levels of rifampicin have been shown to inhibit standard microbiological assays for serum folate and Vitamin B12. Thus alternative assay methods should be considered. Transient elevation of BSP and serum bilirubin have been reported. Therefore, these tests should be performed before the morning dose of rifampicin.

*Side-effects:* Reactions occurring with either daily or intermittent dosage regimens include:

*Cutaneous reactions* which are mild and self-limiting and do not appear to be hypersensitivity reactions. Typically they consist of flushing and itching with or without a rash.

*Gastro-intestinal reactions* consist of anorexia, nausea, vomiting, abdominal discomfort, and diarrhoea. Pseudomembranous colitis has been reported with rifampicin therapy.

*Hepatitis* can be caused by rifampicin and liver function tests should be monitored (see Precautions).

*Thrombocytopenia* with or without purpura may occur, usually associated with intermittent therapy, but is reversible if drug is discontinued as soon as purpura occurs. Cerebral haemorrhage and fatalities have been reported when rifampicin administration has been continued or resumed after the appearance of purpura.

Eosinophilia, leucopenia, oedema, muscle weakness and myopathy have been reported to occur in a small percentage of patients treated with rifampicin.

Reactions usually occurring with intermittent dosage regimens and probably of immunological origin include:

– 'Flu Syndrome' consisting of episodes of fever, chills, headache, dizziness, and bone pain appearing most commonly during the 3rd to the 6th month of therapy. The frequency of the syndrome varies but may occur in up to 50% of patients given once-weekly regimens with a dose of rifampicin of 25 mg/kg or more.

– Shortness of breath and wheezing.

– Decrease in blood pressure and shock.

– Acute haemolytic anaemia.

– Acute renal failure usually due to acute tubular necrosis or acute interstitial nephritis.

If serious complications arise, e.g. renal failure, thrombocytopenia or haemolytic anaemia, rifampicin should be stopped and never restarted.

Occasional disturbances of the menstrual cycle have been reported in women receiving long term anti-tuberculosis therapy with regimens containing rifampicin.

Rifampicin may produce a reddish discolouration

of the urine, sputum and tears. The patient should be forewarned of this. Soft contact lenses may be permanently stained.

*Overdosage:* In cases of overdosage with Rifadin, gastric lavage should be performed as soon as possible. Intensive supportive measures should be instituted and individual symptoms treated as they arise.

**Pharmaceutical precautions** Rifadin syrup should not be diluted. It should be dispensed in clear or amber glass bottles. Store below 30°C.

Rifadin capsules should be protected from light and moisture and stored below 25°C.

**Legal category** POM

**Package quantities** Rifadin capsules 150 mg: Blister packs of 100 capsules.

Rifadin capsules 300 mg: Blister packs of 100 capsules.

Rifadin syrup 100 mg/5 ml: Bottles of 120 ml.

**Further information** An oral dose of 450–600 mg Rifadin produces therapeutically effective levels in the blood, with the peak concentrations being observed approximately 2 hours after administration. There is a good distribution of rifampicin into body tissues and fluids including lung, bone, lymph nodes and inflammatory exudates. Rifampicin is excreted mainly in the bile and urine, and high concentrations are reached in both these fluids. No cross resistance has been shown between Rifadin and other anti-Mycobacteria agents.

**Product licence numbers**

| | |
|---|---|
| Rifadin capsules 150 mg | 4425/5915R |
| Rifadin capsules 300 mg | 4425/5916R |
| Rifadin syrup | 4425/5917R |

*Product licence holder:* Marion Merrell Ltd., Broadwater Park, Denham, Uxbridge, Middlesex UB9 5HP

## RIFADIN* FOR INFUSION

**Presentation** 20 ml vial containing 600 mg Rifampicin BP (red lyophilised powder) and 10 ml ampoule of clear colourless solvent solution (pyrogen free water plus polysorbate 81).

**Uses**

*Mode of action:* Rifadin is a semi-synthetic antibiotic with bactericidal activity against most Mycobacteria and Gram-positive organisms. Rifadin is also active against Gram-negative organisms at higher concentrations.

*Indications:* Rifadin for Infusion is indicated for acutely ill patients who are unable to tolerate oral therapy e.g. post operative or comatose patients or patients in whom gastrointestinal absorption is impaired.

Oral therapy should be used where possible. As soon as patients are able to accept oral medication, they should be transferred to Rifadin Capsules or Syrup.

*Tuberculosis:* Rifadin, used in combination with other active anti-tuberculosis drugs, is indicated in the treatment of all forms of tuberculosis, including fresh, advanced, chronic and drug-resistant cases. Rifadin is also effective against most atypical strains of Mycobacteria.

*Leprosy:* Rifadin, used in combination with at least one other active anti-leprosy drug, is indicated in the management of multibacillary and paucibacillary leprosy to effect conversion of the infectious state to a non-infectious state.

*Other infections:* Rifadin is indicated in the treatment of Brucellosis, Legionnaires Disease, and serious staphylococcal infections. To prevent emergence of resistant strains of the infecting organisms, Rifadin should be used in combination with another antibiotic appropriate for the infection.

*Preparation of infusion:* Rifadin for Infusion is prepared by aseptically adding the solvent to the vial of rifampicin powder and shaking vigorously and continuously for about 30 seconds. When the powder has completely dissolved, the solution should be immediately diluted in 500 ml 5% glucose solution, or other suitable infusion fluid (see 'Pharmaceutical precautions'). It is suggested that the infusion is administered over a period of 2–3 hours. Rifadin solution should be used within 6 hours of preparation.

**Dosage and administration** Treatment with Rifadin for Infusion should include concomitant use of other appropriate antibacterials to prevent the emergence of resistant strains of the causative organism.

*Tuberculosis:*

*Adults:* A single daily administration of 600 mg given by intravenous infusion over 2 to 3 hours has been found to be effective and well tolerated for adult patients. Serum concentrations following this dosage regimen are similar to those obtained after 600 mg by mouth.

*Children:* The usual paediatric regimen is a single daily dose of up to 20 mg/kg bodyweight; the total daily dose should not normally exceed 600 mg.

*Leprosy:* The recommended daily dose is 10 mg/kg.

*Usual daily dose:* Patients weighing less than 50 kg – 450 mg. Patients weighing 50 kg or more – 600 mg. Alternatively, 600 mg doses of rifampicin may be given once per month.

In the treatment of leprosy, rifampicin should always be used in conjunction with at least one other antileprosy drug.

*Brucellosis, Legionnaires Disease or serious staphylococcal infections:*

*Adults:* The recommended daily dose is 600 – 1200 mg given in 2 to 4 divided doses, together with another antibacterial agent with similar properties to prevent the emergence of resistant strains.

*Impaired liver function:* A daily dose of 8 mg/kg should not be exceeded in patients with impaired liver function.

*Use in the elderly:* In elderly patients, the renal excretion of rifampicin is decreased proportionally with physiological decrease of renal function; due to compensatory increase of liver excretion, the serum terminal half-life is similar to that of younger patients. However, as increased blood levels have been noted in one study of rifampicin in elderly patients, caution should be exercised in using rifampicin in such patients, especially if there is evidence of liver function impairment.

**Contra-indications, warnings, etc**

*Contra-indications:* Rifadin for Infusion is contraindicated in patients who are hypersensitive to rifamycins.

Although not recommended for use in patients with jaundice, the therapeutic benefit of Rifadin for Infusion should be weighed against the possible risks.

*Use in pregnancy and lactation:* At very high doses in animals rifampicin has been shown to have teratogenic effects. There are no well controlled studies with rifampicin in pregnant women. Therefore, Rifadin for Infusion should be used in pregnant women or in women of child bearing potential only if the potential benefit justifies the potential risk to the foetus. When rifampicin is administered during the last few weeks of pregnancy it may cause post-natal haemorrhages in the mother and infant for which treatment with Vitamin K1 may be indicated.

Rifampicin is excreted in breast milk and patients receiving rifampicin should not breast feed unless in the physician's judgement the potential benefit to the patient outweighs the potential risk to the infant.

*Precautions:* Patients with impaired liver function should only be given rifampicin in cases of necessity, and then with caution and under close medical supervision. In these patients, lower doses of rifampicin are recommended and careful monitoring of liver function, especially serum glutamic pyruvic transaminase (SGPT) and serum glutamic oxaloacetic transaminase (SGOT) should be carried out. If signs of hepatocellular damage occur, rifampicin should be withdrawn. In patients with impaired liver function, elderly patients, malnourished patients, and possibly, children under two years of age, caution is particularly recommended when instituting therapeutic regimens in which isoniazid is to be used concurrently with rifampicin.

It is rarely necessary, in the absence of clinical findings, to increase the frequency of performing routine liver function tests in patients with normal pretreatment liver function. In the presence of complete renal failure, rifampicin is excreted entirely in the bile: provided hepatic function is not impaired the dosage of rifampicin need not be adjusted.

In some patients hyperbilirubinaemia resulting from competition between rifampicin and bilirubin for excretory pathways of the liver at the cell level can occur in the early days of treatment. An isolated report showing a moderate rise in bilirubin and/or transaminase level is not in itself an indication for interrupting treatment; rather the decision should be made after repeating the tests, noting trends in the levels and considering them in conjunction with the patient's clinical condition.

Rifampicin has enzyme-inducing properties including induction of delta amino levulinic acid synthetase. Isolated reports have associated porphyria exacerbation with rifampicin administration.

*Drug/laboratory interactions:* Rifampicin has been shown in animals and man to have liver enzyme inducing properties and may reduce the activity of anticoagulants, corticosteroids, cyclosporin, digitalis preparations, oral contraceptives, oral hypoglycaemic agents, dapsone, phenytoin, quinidine, narcotics and analgesics. It may be necessary to adjust the dosage of these drugs if they are given concurrently with Rifadin, particularly when it is initiated or withdrawn.

Therapeutic levels of rifampicin have been shown to inhibit standard microbiological assays for serum folate and Vitamin B12. Thus alternative assay methods should be considered. Transient elevation of BSP and serum bilirubin have been reported. Therefore, these tests should be performed before the daily administration of Rifadin for Infusion.

*Side-effects:* Rifadin for Infusion is generally well tolerated and accepted by patients, although hypersensitivity reactions have been described and occasionally patients have experienced fever, skin rashes and nausea/vomiting.

Occasional instances of phlebitis and pain at the infusion site have been reported.

Reactions occurring with either daily or intermittent dosage regimens include:

*Cutaneous reactions* which are mild and self-limiting may occur and do not appear to be hypersensitivity reactions. Typically they consist of flushing and itching with or without a rash.

*Gastro-intestinal reactions* consist of anorexia, nausea, vomiting, abdominal discomfort, and diarrhoea. Pseudomembranous colitis has been reported with rifampicin therapy.

*Hepatitis* can be caused by rifampicin and liver function tests should be monitored (see Precautions).

*Thrombocytopenia* with or without purpura may occur, usually associated with intermittent therapy, but is reversible if the drug is discontinued as soon as purpura occurs. Cerebral haemorrhage and fatalities have been reported when rifampicin administration has been continued or resumed after the appearance of purpura.

Eosinophilia, leucopenia, oedema, muscle weakness and myopathy have been reported to occur in a small percentage of patients treated with rifampicin.

Reactions usually occurring with intermittent dosage regimens and probably of immunological origin include:

– 'Flu Syndrome' consisting of episodes of fever, chills, headache, dizziness, and bone pain appearing most commonly during the 3rd to the 6th month of therapy. The frequency of the syndrome varies but may occur in up to 50% of patients given once-weekly regimens with a dose of rifampicin of 25 mg/kg or more.
– Shortness of breath and wheezing.
– Decrease in blood pressure and shock.
– Acute haemolytic anaemia.
– Acute renal failure usually due to acute tubular necrosis or acute interstitial nephritis.

If serious complications arise, (renal failure, thrombocytopenia or haemolytic anaemia), rifampicin should be stopped and never restarted.

Occasional disturbances of the menstrual cycle have been reported in women receiving long term anti-tuberculosis therapy with regimens containing rifampicin.

Rifampicin may produce a reddish discolouration of the urine, sputum and tears. The patient should be forewarned of this. Soft contact lenses may be permanently stained.

*Overdose:* In cases of overdosage with rifampicin, intensive supportive measures should be instituted and individual symptoms treated as they arise.

**Pharmaceutical precautions** Rifadin for Infusion should be freshly prepared.

*Compatibilities:* Rifadin for Infusion is compatible with the following infusion solutions for up to 6 hours: Mannitol 10% and 20%, Macrodex with Saline Solution, Macrodex with Glucose Solution, Rheomacrodex, Sodium Bicarbonate 1.4%, Laevulose 5% and 10%, Ringer Lactate, Ringer Acetate, Dextrose 5% and 10%, Saline Solution.

*Incompatibilities:* Rifadin for Infusion is incompatible with the following: Perfudex, Sodium Bicarbonate 5%, Sodium Lactate 0.167M, Ringer Acetate with Dextrose.

**Legal category** POM

**Package quantities** Combined pack of one vial containing 600 mg Rifampicin BP, and one ampoule containing 10 ml solvent.

**Further information** Nil.

**Product licence number** 4425/0051

*Product licence holder:* Marion Merrell Ltd., Broadwater Park, Denham, Uxbridge, Middlesex UB9 5HP

## RIFATER*

**Presentation** Smooth, round, shiny, light pink, sugar coated tablets containing Isoniazid PhEur 50 mg, Pyrazinamide PhEur 300 mg and Rifampicin PhEur 120 mg.

**Uses** Rifater is indicated in the treatment of pulmonary tuberculosis.

**Dosage and administration** Rifater is recommended in the initial intensive phase of the short-course treatment of pulmonary tuberculosis. During this phase, which lasts for 2 months, Rifater should be administered on a daily continuous basis. The concomitant administration of ethambutol or intramuscular streptomycin over the same period of time is advised.

Each Rifater tablet contains isoniazid (INH), pyrazinamide (Z) and rifampicin (RAMP) in such a ratio that the administration of 9–12 mg/kg RAMP, 4–5 mg/kg INH and 23–30 mg/kg Z can be achieved by giving 3 tablets daily to patients weighing less than 40 kg, 4 tablets to patients weighing 40–49 kg, 5 tablets to patients weighing 50–64 kg and 6 tablets to patients weighing 65 kg or more.

Rifater should be given as a single dose and preferably on an empty stomach at least 30 minutes before a meal or 2 hours after a meal to ensure rapid and complete absorption.

Once the initial intensive phase of treatment has been completed treatment can be continued with the combination rifampicin-isoniazid (Rifinah*) always on a daily basis.

This regimen, if correctly applied, is 100% effective with very few, if any, relapses. The clinical evidence indicates that these occur generally in the first 6 months after stopping treatment with bacilli fully sensitive to the drugs employed, so that changes in the drugs to be utilised for further treatment are not required. The regimen has been found to be fully effective also in the presence of a bacillary population resistant to isoniazid, to streptomycin or to both drugs.

*Children:* The ratio of the three drugs in Rifater may not be appropriate in children (e.g. higher mg/kg doses of INH are usually given in children than in adults). Rifater can be used only in special cases, after careful consideration of the mg/kg dose of each component.

*Use in the elderly:* Caution should be exercised in such patients, in view of the possible decrease of the excretory function of the kidney and of the liver.

**Contra-indications, warnings, etc**
*Contra-indications:* Rifater is contra-indicated in patients who are hypersensitive to any one of the components of the combination. Rifater is contra-indicated in the presence of jaundice.

*Use in pregnancy and lactation:* At very high doses in animals rifampicin has been shown to have teratogenic effects. There are no well controlled studies with Rifater in pregnant women. Therefore, Rifater should be used in pregnant women or in women of child-bearing potential only if the potential benefit justifies the potential risk to the foetus. When administered during the last few weeks of pregnancy, Rifater may cause post-natal haemorrhages in the mother and infant, for which treatment with Vitamin K1 may be indicated.

Rifampicin and isoniazid are excreted in breast milk and patients receiving Rifater should not breast feed unless in the physician's judgement the potential benefit to the patient outweighs the potential risk to the infant.

*Precautions:* The precautions for the use of Rifater are the same as those considered when a triple individual administration of rifampicin, isoniazid and pyrazinamide is required. Each of these drugs has been associated with liver dysfunction. Patients with impaired liver function should only be given Rifater in cases of necessity and then with caution and under strict medical supervision. In these patients, careful monitoring of liver function, especially serum glutamic pyruvic transaminase (SGPT) and serum glutamic oxaloacetic transaminase (SGOT) should be carried out prior to therapy and then every two to four weeks during therapy. If signs of hepatocellular damage occur, Rifater should be withdrawn. Care should be exercised in the treatment of elderly or malnourished patients who may also require Vitamin B6 supplementation with the isoniazid therapy.

In some cases hyperbilirubinaemia resulting from competition between rifampicin and bilirubin for excretory pathways of the liver at the cell level can occur in the early days of treatment. An isolated report showing a moderate rise in bilirubin and/or transaminase level is not in itself an indication for interrupting treatment; rather, the decision should be made after repeating the tests, noting trends in the levels and considering them in conjunction with the patient's clinical condition.

Rifater should be used with caution in patients with a history of gout. If hyperuricaemia accompanied by an acute gouty arthritis occurs, the patient should be transferred to a regimen not containing pyrazinamide (e.g. Rifinah 150 or 300).

The possibility of pyrazinamide having an adverse effect on blood clotting time or vascular integrity should be borne in mind in patients with haemoptysis.

Because of the possibility of immunological reaction (see 'Side-effects') occurring with intermittent rifampicin therapy (less than 2 to 3 per week) patients

should be closely monitored. Patients should be cautioned against interruption of dosage regimens since these reactions may occur.

*Drug/laboratory interactions:* Rifampicin has liver enzyme-inducing properties and may reduce the activity of a number of drugs including anticoagulants, corticosteroids, cyclosporin, digitalis preparations, quinidine, oral contraceptives, oral hypoglycaemic agents, dapsone, narcotics and analgesics. It may be necessary to adjust the dosage of these drugs if they are given concurrently with Rifater.

Patients using oral contraceptives should be advised to change to non-hormonal methods of birth control during Rifater therapy. Also diabetes may become more difficult to control.

If p-aminosalicylic acid and rifampicin are both included in the treatment regimen, they should be given not less than eight hours apart to ensure satisfactory blood levels.

Therapeutic levels of rifampicin have been shown to inhibit standard microbiological assays for serum folate and Vitamin B12. Thus alternative assay methods should be considered. Transient elevation of BSP and serum bilirubin have been reported. Therefore, these tests should be performed before the morning dose of rifampicin. Isoniazid may decrease the excretion of phenytoin or may enhance its effects. Appropriate adjustment of the anti-convulsant dose should be made.

*Side-effects: Rifampicin:* Reactions occurring with either daily or intermittent dosage regimens include: *Cutaneous reactions* which are mild and self-limiting and do not appear to be hypersensitivity reactions. Typically they consist of flushing and itching with or without a rash.

*Gastro-intestinal reactions* consist of anorexia, nausea, vomiting, abdominal discomfort, and diarrhoea. Pseudomembranous colitis has been reported with rifampicin therapy.

*Hepatitis* can be caused by rifampicin and liver function tests should be monitored. (See 'Precautions').

*Thrombocytopenia* with or without purpura may occur, usually associated with intermittent therapy, but is reversible if drug is discontinued as soon as purpura occurs. Cerebral haemorrhage and fatalities have been reported when rifampicin administration has been continued or resumed after the appearance of purpura.

Eosinophilia, leucopenia, oedema, muscle weakness and myopathy have been reported to occur in a small percentage of patients treated with rifampicin.

Reactions usually occurring with intermittent dosage regimens and probably of immunological origin include:

- 'Flu Syndrome' consisting of episodes of fever, chills, headache, dizziness, and bone pain appearing most commonly during the 3rd to the 6th month of therapy. The frequency of the syndrome varies but may occur in up to 50% of patients given once-weekly regimens with a dose of rifampicin of 25 mg/kg or more.
- Shortness of breath and wheezing.
- Decrease in blood pressure and shock.
- Acute haemolytic anaemia.
- Acute renal failure usually due to acute tubular necrosis or to acute interstitial nephritis.

If serious complications arise, (renal failure, thrombocytopenia or haemolytic anaemia), Rifater should be stopped and never restarted.

Occasional disturbances of the menstrual cycle have been reported in women receiving long term anti-tuberculosis therapy with regimens containing rifampicin.

Rifampicin may produce a reddish discolouration of the urine, sputum and tears. The patient should be forewarned of this. Soft contact lenses may be permanently stained.

*Isoniazid:* Severe and sometimes fatal hepatitis may occur with isoniazid therapy. Polyneuritis associated with isoniazid, presenting as paraesthesia, muscle weakness, loss of tendon reflexes, is unlikely to occur with the recommended daily dose of Rifater. Various haematological disturbances have been identified during treatment with isoniazid, including eosinophilia, agranulocytosis, and anaemia. High doses of isoniazid can cause convulsions. The possibility that the frequency of seizures may be increased in patients with epilepsy should be borne in mind.

*Pyrazinamide:* Adverse reactions, other than hepatic reactions, which have been attributed to pyrazinamide are active gout (pyrazinamide has been reported to reduce urate excretion), sideroblastic anaemia, arthralgia, anorexia, nausea and vomiting, dysuria, malaise, fever, urticaria and aggravation of peptic ulcer. The hepatic reaction is the most common adverse reaction and varies from a symptomless abnormality of hepatic cell function detected only through laboratory liver function tests, through a mild

syndrome of fever, malaise and liver tenderness, to more serious reactions such as clinical jaundice and rare cases of acute yellow atrophy and death.

*Overdosage:* In cases of overdosage with Rifater, gastric lavage should be performed as soon as possible. Intensive supportive measures should be instituted and individual symptoms treated as they arise. Parenteral pyridoxine (Vitamin B6) should be given. Symptoms are more likely to be related to isoniazid, including coma, respiratory distress, hyperglycaemia and metabolic ketoacidosis.

**Pharmaceutical precautions**   None.

**Legal category**   POM.

**Package quantities**   Blister strips of 20's in packs of 100's.

**Further information**   Nil.

**Product licence number** 4425/0060.
*Product licence holder:* Marion Merrell Ltd., Broadwater Park, Denham, Uxbridge, Middlesex UB9 5HP

# RIFINAH*

## Presentation
*Rifinah 300:* orange, capsule-shaped sugar coated tablets containing 300 mg Rifampicin PhEur and 150 mg Isoniazid PhEur.

*Rifinah 150:* cyclamen, round biconvex sugar coated tablets containing 150 mg Rifampicin PhEur and 100 mg Isoniazid PhEur.

**Uses**   Rifinah 300 and Rifinah 150 are indicated in the treatment of all forms of tuberculosis, including fresh, advanced and chronic cases.

**Dosage and administration**   Another anti-tuberculosis drug may be given concurrently with Rifinah until the susceptibility of the infecting organism to rifampicin and isoniazid has been confirmed.

*Adults:* Patients should be given the following single daily dose preferably on an empty stomach at least 30 minutes before a meal or 2 hours after a meal:
*Rifinah 150:* Patients weighing less than 50 kg – 3 tablets.
*Rifinah 300:* Patients weighing 50 kg or more – 2 tablets.

*Use in the elderly:* Caution should be exercised in such patients especially if there is evidence of liver impairment.

**Contra-indications, warnings, etc**
*Contra-indications:* Rifinah 300 and Rifinah 150 are contra-indicated in the presence of jaundice. Rifinah 300 and Rifinah 150 are contra-indicated in patients who are hypersensitive to rifamycins or isoniazid.

*Use in pregnancy and lactation:* Rifampicin has been shown to be teratogenic in rodents when given in large doses. There are no well controlled studies with Rifinah in pregnant women. Therefore, Rifinah should be used in pregnant women or in women of child bearing potential only if the potential benefit justifies the potential risk to the foetus.

When administered during the last few weeks of pregnancy, rifampicin can cause post-natal haemorrhages in the mother and infant, for which treatment with Vitamin K1 may be indicated.

Rifampicin and isoniazid are excreted in breast milk and patients receiving Rifinah should not breast feed unless in the physician's judgement the potential benefit to the patient outweighs the potential risk to the infant.

*Precautions:* Rifinah is a combination of 2 drugs, each of which has been associated with liver dysfunction. Patients with impaired liver function should only be given Rifinah in cases of necessity, and then with caution and under close medical supervision. In these patients, careful monitoring of liver function, especially serum glutamic pyruvic transaminase (SGPT) and serum glutamic oxaloacetic transaminase (SGOT) should be carried out prior to therapy and then every two to four weeks during therapy. Similar care should be exercised in elderly patients, malnourished patients and children under two years of age. If signs of hepatocellular damage occur, Rifinah should be withdrawn. Care should be exercised in the treatment of elderly or malnourished patients who may also require Vitamin B6 supplementation with the isoniazid therapy.

In some cases hyperbilirubinaemia resulting from competition between rifampicin and bilirubin for excretory pathways of the liver at the cell level can occur in the early days of treatment. An isolated report showing a moderate rise in bilirubin and/or transaminase level is not in itself an indication for interrupting treatment; rather the decision should be made after repeating the tests, noting trends in the levels and considering them in conjunction with the patient's clinical condition.

Because of the possibility of immunological reaction

(see 'Side-effects') occurring with intermittent rifampicin therapy (less than 2 to 3 times per week) patients should be closely monitored. Patients should be cautioned against interruption of dosage regimens since these reactions may occur.

*Drug/laboratory interactions:* Rifampicin has liver enzyme inducing properties and may reduce the activity of a number of drugs including anticoagulants, corticosteroids, cyclosporin, digitalis preparations, quinidine, oral contraceptives, oral hypoglycaemic agents, dapsone, narcotics and analgesics. It may be necessary to adjust the dosage of these drugs if they are given concurrently with Rifinah. Patients using oral contraceptives should be advised to change to non-hormonal methods of birth control during Rifinah therapy. Also, diabetes may become more difficult to control. When rifampicin is taken with para-aminosalicylic acid (P.A.S.), rifampicin levels in the serum may decrease. Therefore the drugs should be taken at least eight hours apart. Therapeutic levels of rifampicin have been shown to inhibit standard microbiological assays for serum folate and Vitamin B12. Thus, alternative assay methods should be considered. Transient elevation of BSP and serum bilirubin have been reported. Therefore, these tests should be performed before the morning dose of rifampicin. Isoniazid may decrease the excretion of phenytoin or may enhance its effects. Appropriate adjustments of the anticonvulsant dose should be made.

*Side-effects:*

*Rifampicin:* Reactions to rifampicin occurring with either daily or intermittent dosage regimens include:

*Cutaneous reactions* which are mild and self-limiting and do not appear to be hypersensitivity reactions. Typically they consist of flushing and itching with or without a rash. More serious hypersensitivity cutaneous reactions occur but are uncommon.

*Gastro-intestinal reactions* consist of anorexia, nausea, vomiting, abdominal discomfort, and diarrhoea. Pseudomembranous colitis has been reported with rifampicin therapy.

*Hepatitis* can be caused by rifampicin and liver function tests should be monitored (see *Precautions*).

*Thrombocytopenia* with or without purpura may occur, usually associated with intermittent therapy, but is reversible if drug is discontinued as soon as purpura occurs. Cerebral haemorrhage and fatalities have been reported when rifampicin administration has been continued or resumed after the appearance of purpura.

Eosinophilia, leucopenia, oedema, muscle weakness and myopathy have been reported to occur in a small percentage of patients treated with rifampicin.

Reactions usually occurring with intermittent dosage regimens and probably of immunological origin include:

- 'Flu Syndrome' consisting of episodes of fever, chills, headache, dizziness, and bone pain appearing most commonly during the 3rd to the 6th month of therapy. The frequency of the syndrome varies but may occur in up to 50% of patients given once-weekly regimens with a dose of rifampicin of 25 mg/kg or more.
- Shortness of breath and wheezing.
- Decrease in blood pressure and shock.
- Acute haemolytic anaemia.
- Acute renal failure usually due to acute tubular necrosis or to acute interstitial nephritis.

If serious complications arise (renal failure, thrombocytopenia or haemolytic anaemia) rifampicin should be stopped and never restarted.

Occasional disturbances of the menstrual cycle have been reported in women receiving long term antituberculosis therapy with regimens containing rifampicin.

Rifampicin may produce a reddish discolouration of the urine, sputum and tears. The patient should be forewarned of this. Soft contact lenses may be permanently stained.

*Isoniazid:* Severe and sometimes fatal hepatitis may occur with isoniazid therapy. Polyneuritis associated with isoniazid, presenting as paraesthesia, muscle weakness, loss of tendon reflexes, is unlikely to occur with the recommended daily dose of Rifinah. Various haematological disturbances have been identified during treatment with isoniazid, including eosinophilia, agranulocytosis, and anaemia. High doses of isoniazid can cause convulsions. The possibility that the frequency of seizures may be increased in patients with epilepsy should be borne in mind.

*Overdosage:* In cases of overdosage with Rifinah 300 or Rifinah 150, gastric lavage should be performed as soon as possible. Intensive supportive measures should be instituted and individual symptoms treated as they arise. Parenteral pyridoxine (Vitamin B6) should be given. Symptoms are more likely to be related to isoniazid, including coma, respiratory distress, hyperglycaemia and metabolic ketoacidosis.

**Pharmaceutical precautions** Store below 25°C.

If it proves necessary to open a blister pack, Rifinah 300 and Rifinah 150 should be dispensed in amber glass or plastic containers. Protect from moisture.

**Legal category** POM.

**Package quantities** Rifinah 300: Original packs of 56 tablets (4 weeks calendar packs); Blister packs of 100 tablets.

Rifinah 150: Original packs of 84 tablets (4 weeks calendar packs); Blister packs of 100 tablets.

**Further information** The recommended daily dose of Rifinah 300 or Rifinah 150 produces therapeutically effective blood levels of rifampicin and isoniazid, two of the most powerful antituberculosis drugs. Serum concentrations and the biological half-life of the two component drugs do not differ significantly from values obtained when the drugs are given alone.

**Product licence numbers**
Rifinah 150 4425/0041
Rifinah 300 4425/0042

*Product licence holder:* Marion Merrell Ltd., Broadwater Park, Denham, Uxbridge, Middlesex UB9 5HP

## RYTHMODAN* CAPSULES RYTHMODAN* RETARD TABLETS RYTHMODAN* INJECTION

**Presentation**

*Oral:*

*Rythmodan Capsules:* Capsules with opaque green cap and opaque beige body with 'RY' and 'RL' printed in black, containing 100 mg of disopyramide base.

Capsules with opaque white cap and body with 'RY' and '150' printed in black, containing 150 mg disopyramide base.

*Rythmodan Retard Tablets:* White, circular biconvex tablets, 12 mm in diameter, film-coated with a break line. Tablets are marked 'RY' and 'R' on one side and [logo] on the reverse. Each tablet contains disopyramide phosphate equivalent to 250 mg disopyramide base in a sustained release formulation.

*Intravenous Injection:*

*Rythmodan Injection:* Ampoules for intravenous use only. 5 ml ampoules containing disopyramide phosphate equivalent to 50 mg disopyramide base in solution.

**Uses** *Properties:* Rythmodan is able to prevent and control a wide variety of cardiac arrhythmias, probably by slowing conduction in the His-Purkinje system and by increasing the effective refractory period of the atria and ventricles.

*Indications:* Oral Rythmodan is indicated in:

1. Maintenance of normal rhythm following conversion by Rythmodan Injection, other parenteral drugs or electroconversion.
2. Prevention of arrhythmias after myocardial infarction.
3. Treatment of persistent ventricular and atrial extrasystoles, paroxysmal supraventricular tachycardia, Wolff-Parkinson-White syndrome.
4. Suppression of arrhythmias during surgical procedures.
5. Control of arrhythmias following the use of digitalis or similar glycosides.

Rythmodan Injection is intended for intravenous use only and is indicated in the following conditions:

1. Conversion of ventricular and supraventricular arrhythmias after myocardial infarction, including those not responding to lignocaine or other I.V. treatment.
2. Control of ventricular and atrial extrasystoles, supraventricular tachycardia, and Wolff-Parkinson-White syndrome.
3. Control of arrhythmias following digitalis or similar glycosides when Rythmodan cannot be administered orally.

**Dosage and administration**

*Oral Rythmodan Capsules:* The recommended daily dosage in adults is 300–800 mg in divided doses adjusted according to the response of the patient.

*Heart failure:* In determining the intervals between administration of Rythmodan capsules it should be borne in mind that whilst the elimination half-life in normal volunteers is approximately seven hours, in patients with heart failure, half-life values of 12 hours or more have been recorded.

*Impaired renal function* (Disease state or the elderly): Standard capsules should be used in patients in renal failure. A reduced dosage, preferably accompanied by assay of disopyramide plasma levels in cases of severe renal failure (creatinine clearance <8 ml/min) is recommended. The following table may be helpful as a guide.

| *Creatinine clearance (ml/min)* | *Dosage 100 or 150 mg capsules* |
|---|---|
| Normal | Normal dosage |
| 20–60 | 100 mg 8-hourly or 150 mg 12-hourly |
| 8–20 | 100 mg 12-hourly |
| <8 | 150 mg daily |

*Rythmodan Retard Tablets:* The recommended dose for stabilised patients or those receiving Rythmodan for the first time is 1 to 1½ tablets (250-375 mg) twice daily. Patients being transferred from intravenous therapy with Rythmodan should be stabilised on standard Rythmodan capsules for the first 24 hours (see below). Tablets should be swallowed and not crushed or chewed.

Intravenous Injection: *Rythmodan Injection:* The recommended dosage can be given by two different regimes.

1. An initial direct intravenous injection of 2 mg/kg (but not exceeding 150 mg (15 ml) irrespective of body weight) should be given SLOWLY OVER NOT LESS THAN FIVE MINUTES, i.e. the rate of injection must not exceed 30 mg (3 ml) per minute in order to reduce or avoid unwanted haemodynamic effects. If conversion occurs during this time the injection should be stopped. If the arrhythmia is to respond to Rythmodan it will usually do so within 10-15 minutes after completion of the injection.

Transfer to oral maintenance therapy is accomplished by giving 200 mg orally, immediately on cessation of intravenous administration, followed by 200 mg every 8 hours for 24 hours. Most patients may be maintained subsequently on a daily dosage of 500-750 mg of Rythmodan, preferably administered as 1 to 1½ Rythmodan Retard tablets (250-375 mg) twice daily. Where the need for lower dosage outweighs the convenience of twice daily administration, appropriate doses of conventional capsules (100 or 150 mg) may be administered.

If conversion is achieved by intravenous Rythmodan but the arrhythmia subsequently recurs, a further slow direct intravenous injection over not less than five minutes may be administered cautiously and preferably under ECG control. The total administration by the intravenous route should not exceed 4 mg/kg (maximum 300 mg) in the first hour, nor should the combined administration by the intravenous and oral routes exceed 800 mg in 24 hours.

2. An initial direct intravenous injection as above, i.e. over not less than five minutes, maintained by intravenous infusion by drip of 20-30 mg/hour (or 0.4 mg/kg/hour) up to a maximum of 800 mg daily. This regime should be employed if the patient is unable to take oral medication or in particularly serious arrhythmias being treated in *coronary care units*.

*Children:* There are insufficient data to recommend the use of Rythmodan in children.

**Contra-indications, warnings, etc**

*Contra-indications:* Disopyramide is contra-indicated in second or third degree heart block and sinus node disease if no pacemaker is present, cardiogenic shock and severe uncompensated heart failure and hypersensitivity to disopyramide. Patients with renal impairment should not be treated with sustained release dysopyramide.

*Warnings and precautions:* There have been reports of ventricular tachycardia or ventricular fibrillation or Torsade de Pointes in patients receiving disopyramide. These have been usually, but not always, associated with significant widening of the QRS complex or prolonged QT interval. If these ECG changes or arrhythmias develop the drug should be discontinued.

Disopyramide should be used only with caution in patients with atrial flutter or atrial tachycardia with block as conversion of a partial AV block to a 1:1 response may occur. Accordingly, the need for prior digitalisation should be considered.

Owing to its negative inotropic effect, disopyramide should be used with caution in patients suffering from significant cardiac failure. Such patients should be fully digitalised or controlled with other therapy before initiating treatment with disopyramide.

The occurrence of hypotension following disopyramide administration, which has been observed especially in patients with cardiomyopathy or inadequately compensated congestive heart failure, requires prompt discontinuation of the drug. Any resumption of therapy should be at a lower dose with close patient monitoring.

*Interactions:* Combination with other negative inotropic drugs such as beta-adrenoceptor blockers or verapamil may result in summation of negative inotropic effects, especially in patients with AV nodal or bundle branch conduction defects. Disopyramide may also summate with other class 1 anti-arrhythmic agents such as lignocaine, phenytoin and procainamide.

The concomitant use of erythromycin may result in cardiac arrhythmias.

In view of the serious nature of many of the conditions being treated it is suggested that *Rythmodan Injection should only be used when facilities exist for cardiac monitoring or defibrillation, should the need arise.*

Disopyramide should be used with caution in patients receiving concurrent therapy with diuretics likely to give rise to hypokalaemia since this may reduce patient response to disopyramide.

Disopyramide should be used with caution in the treatment of digitalis intoxication.

Due to its anticholinergic properties, patients with glaucoma, a tendency to urinary retention, or any patient receiving a drug with anticholinergic activity may be unsuitable for Rythmodan therapy.

Care should be taken when prescribing disopyramide for patients with bundle branch block as the effect of disopyramide in this condition is unpredictable. If first degree heart block develops in a patient receiving disopyramide, dosage should be reduced and may require discontinuation if the block persists.

Since disopyramide is eliminated predominantly by glomerular filtration the dose administered to patients with significant renal impairment may require adjustment. Patients with renal impairment should not be treated with sustained release disopyramide.

Hypoglycaemia has been reported in association with Rythmodan administration. Impaired renal function and cardiac function may be predisposing factors in such patients. Strict adherence to the dosing recommendations is advised and consideration should be given to monitoring blood glucose levels, and if hypoglycaemia occurs treatment with Rythmodan should be stopped.

Hepatic impairment causes an increase in the plasma half-life of Rythmodan and a reduced dosage may be required.

*Pregnancy:* Although Rythmodan has undergone animal tests for teratogenicity without evidence of any effect on the developing foetus, its safety in human pregnancy has not been established. Disopyramide has been reported to stimulate contractions of the pregnant uterus. The drugs should only be used during pregnancy if benefits clearly outweigh the possible risks to the mother and foetus.

*Lactation:* No data for Rythmodan Injection, but studies have shown that oral disopyramide is secreted in breast milk although no adverse effects to the infant have been noted. However, clinical experience is limited and disopyramide should only be used in lactation if, in the clinicians judgement, it is essential for the welfare of the patient. The infant should be closely supervised, particularly for anti-cholinergic effects and drug levels determined if necessary. Ideally, if the drug is considered essential an alternative method of feeding should be used.

*Side-effects:* The principal side-effects of Rythmodan largely relate to the drugs significant inotropic effects which have been on occasion associated with hypotension and cardio-vascular collapse. Most common side effects (dry mouth, blurred vision, urinary hesitancy) are attributable to the drug's mild anticholinergic action. Exceptionally this may be marked. Gastrointestinal irritation may also occur. Very rarely, disopyramide therapy has been associated with acute psychosis, cholestatic jaundice and hypoglycaemia. Side effects usually disappear rapidly with reduction of dosage or cessation of therapy. Profuse sweating may indicate too rapid intravenous injection.

*Overdosage:* Animal studies indicate that overdosage may lead to cardiac arrest or atrio-ventricular block or to disorders of ventricular excitability leading to terminal ventricular fibrillation. Intracardiac conduction defects and ventricular hyperexcitability may be controlled by general intensive supportive therapy.

Infusion studies in dogs and man have shown the effectiveness of isoprenaline and dopamine in restoring any marked fall in blood pressure.

**Pharmaceutical precautions** Rythmodan injection: Store below 25°C. Rythmodan Retard: Store below 30°C.

Rythmodan Injection is physically compatible with the following: Sodium Chloride Injection BP, Dextrose Injection BP, Compound Sodium Chloride Injection BPC, Compound Sodium Lactate Injection BP.

**Legal category** POM.

**Package quantities**

| | |
|---|---|
| Rythmodan Capsules 100 mg | OP packs of 84 |
| Rythmodan Capsules 150 mg | OP packs of 84 |
| Rythmodan Retard 250 mg | OP packs of 56 |
| Rythmodan Injection 50 mg/5 ml | Packs of 5 ampoules |

**Further information** Rythmodan Retard Tablets contain caster sugar and titanium dioxide E171. Rythmodan Injection contains benzyl alcohol, sorbitol and purified water.

**Product licence numbers**

| | |
|---|---|
| Rythmodan Capsules 100 mg | 0109/0022 |
| Rythmodan Capsules 150 mg | 0109/0075 |
| Rythmodan Retard Tablets 250 mg | 0109/0094 |
| Rythmodan Injection | 0109/0060 |

*Product licence holder:* Roussel Laboratories Ltd., Broadwater Park, Denham, Uxbridge, Middlesex UB9 5HP

## SABRIL* SACHETS

**Qualitative and quantitative composition** Each sachet contains vigabatrin 0.5 mg

**Pharmaceutical form** Powder

**Clinical particulars**

*Therapeutic indications:* Recommended for the treatment of epilepsy which is not satisfactorily controlled by another antiepileptic drug.

Recommended as monotherapy for management of Infantile Spasms (West's syndrome).

*Posology and method of administration:* Sabril is for oral administration once or twice daily and may be taken before or after meals.

Sabril should be added to the patient's current therapeutic regimen.

*Adults:* Maximal efficacy is usually seen in the 2–4 g/day range. A starting dose of 1 g daily should be added to the patient's current anti-epileptic drug regimen. The daily dose should then be titrated in 0.5 g increments at weekly intervals depending on clinical response and tolerability. Although a slight increase in efficacy has been observed in some patients treated with up to a maximum of 6 g/day, this dose has been associated with an increased incidence of adverse effects. Doses above 4 g/day should only be used in exceptional circumstances with close monitoring for adverse effects.

There is no direct correlation between plasma concentration and efficacy. The duration of the effects of the drug are dependent on the rate of enzyme resynthesis rather than the concentration of the drug in the plasma.

*Children:* The recommended starting dose in children is 40 mg/kg/day increasing to 80–100 mg/kg/day depending on response. Convenient recommendations in relation to body weight are:

Bodyweight:
10–15 kg ½–1 g/day
15–30 kg 1–1½ g/day
30–50 kg 1½–3 g/day
>50 kg 2–4 g/day

*Infants:* Monotherapy for Infantile Spasms (West's Syndrome): The recommended dose is between 60–100 mg/kg/day depending on the severity of the spasms. This may be titrated over a period of one week if necessary. Doses of up to 150 mg/kg/day have been used with good tolerability.

*Elderly and patients with renal impairment:* Since vigabatrin is eliminated in the kidney, caution should be exercised when administering the drug to the elderly and more particularly in patients with creatinine clearance less than 60 ml/min. Adjustment of dose or frequency of administration should be considered. Such patients may respond to a lower maintenance dose.

*Contra-indications:* Pregnant women (see 'Pregnancy and lactation') and patients who have a history of hypersensitivity to vigabatrin or its product components.

*Special warnings and special precautions for use:* Animal safety studies indicate that vigabatrin causes intramyelinic oedema in the brain white matter tracts. Currently there is no evidence to suggest that this effect occurs in man. However it is recommended that patients treated with Sabril are closely observed for adverse effects on neurological function: details of animal findings are given in 'Preclinical safety data'.

As with other antiepileptic drugs abrupt withdrawal may lead to rebound seizures. If a patient is to be withdrawn from Sabril treatment, it is recommended that this is done gradually by reducing the dose over 2–4 weeks.

Sabril should be used with caution in patients with a history of psychosis or behavioural problems.

*Interaction with other medicaments and other forms of interaction:* As Sabril is neither metabolised, nor protein bound and is not an inducer of hepatic cytochrome P450 drug-metabolising enzymes, interactions with other drugs are unlikely. However, during controlled clinical studies a gradual reduction of about 20% in the plasma concentrations of phenytoin has been observed. The exact nature of this interaction is presently not understood, however, in the majority of cases it is unlikely to be of therapeutic significance.

The plasma concentrations of carbamazepine, phenobarbitone and sodium valproate have also been monitored during controlled clinical trials and no clinically significant interactions have been detected.

*Pregnancy and lactation:* As little data are available on the use of Sabril during pregnancy, it is currently contra-indicated in pregnant women.

Studies in animals have shown that vigabatrin does not adversely affect fertility, foetal development or pup development, nor is it teratogenic in the rat at doses up to 150 mg/kg or the rabbit at doses up to 100 mg/kg. However, in the rabbit at doses of 150 and 200 mg/kg, a slight increase in the incidence of cleft palate was observed.

There are no adequate and well-controlled studies in pregnant women. Congenital anomalies have been reported in the off-spring of mothers using vigabatrin during pregnancy. No trends in the type of abnormal pregnancy outcome are evident from the available data.

In the absence of data on the excretion of vigabatrin in human milk, breast feeding during Sabril treatment is not recommended.

*Effects on ability to drive and use machines:* As a general rule, uncontrolled epileptic patients are not allowed to drive or handle potentially dangerous machinery. In view of the fact that drowsiness has been observed in clinical trials with Sabril, patients should be warned of this possibility at the start of treatment.

*Undesirable effects:* Adverse reactions are mainly CNS related and probably a secondary consequences of the increase in GABA caused by Sabril. The most commonly reported adverse reactions are drowsiness and fatigue except in children where excitation/agitation are more frequent. Other CNS-related reactions that have been reported include dizziness, nervousness, irritability, headache, nystagmus, ataxia, tremor, paraesthesia, impaired or decreased concentration or alertness and less commonly confusion, memory disturbance and vision complaints such as diplopia. Rare instances of visual field defect, photophobia and retinal disorders (such as peripheral retinal atrophy) have been observed.

Psychiatric reactions (agitation, aggression, depression, abnormal thinking, paranoid reactions) have been reported during vigabatrin therapy. These reactions occurred in patients with and without psychiatric history and were usually reversible when vigabatrin doses were reduced or gradually discontinued (see *Special warnings and special precautions for use*). Depression was a common psychiatric reaction but seldom required discontinuation of vigabatrin. Less common reactions included psychotic symptoms. Hypomania and mania have been reported rarely.

The sedative effect of vigabatrin usually decreases with continuing treatment. However, rare instances of patients developing marked sedation/stupor/confusion in association with non-specific slow wave activity on electroencephalogram have been described soon after the introduction of vigabatrin. Such reactions have been fully reversible following dose reduction or discontinuation of vigabatrin.

Other adverse reactions reported include weight gain, oedema, minor gastro-intestinal side-effects and alopecia. Allergic reactions such as rash and urticaria have been reported rarely.

As with other antiepileptic drugs, some patients may experience an increase in seizure frequency with vigabatrin. Patients with myoclonic seizures may be particularly liable to this effect.

Laboratory data indicate that Sabril treatment does not lead to renal or hepatic toxicity. Decreases in SGOT or SGPT, which are considered to be a result of inhibition of these transaminases by Sabril, have been observed. Chronic treatment with Sabril may be associated with a slight decrease in haemoglobin which rarely attains clinical significance.

*Overdose:* There is no specific antidote and the usual supportive measures should be employed. Vigabatrin overdose has been reported. When provided, doses were most commonly between 7.5 g to 30 g; however ingestions up to 65 g have been reported. Nearly half of the cases involved multiple drug ingestions. None of the overdoses resulted in death.

Activated charcoal has been shown not to significantly absorb vigabatrin in an *in-vitro* study. The effectiveness of haemodialysis in the treatment of vigabatrin overdose is unknown.

**Pharmacological properties**

*Pharmacodynamic properties:* Sabril is an antiepileptic drug with a clearly defined mechanism of action. Treatment with Sabril leads to an increase in the concentration of GABA (gamma amino butyric acid), the major inhibitory neurotransmitter in the brain. This is because vigabatrin, the active ingredient in Sabril, was designed rationally as a selective reversible inhibitor of GABA-transaminase, the enzyme responsible for the breakdown of GABA.

Controlled and long-term clinical trials have shown that Sabril is an effective anticonvulsant agent when given as add-on therapy in patients with epilepsy not controlled satisfactorily by conventional therapy. This efficacy is particularly marked in patients with seizures of partial origin.

*Pharmacokinetic properties:* Vigabatrin is a water soluble compound. The absorption of Sabril is rapid and complete, with the presence of food having no effect. The drug is widely distributed with an apparent volume of distribution slightly greater than total body water. Plasma and CSF concentrations are linearly related to dose over the recommended dosage range.

There is no direct correlation between plasma concentration and efficacy. This is a consequence of the mechanism of action of vigabatrin, the duration of the effects of the drug being dependent on the rate of enzyme resynthesis rather than on the concentration of drug in the plasma.

Sabril is eliminated from the plasma with a terminal half-life of 5–8 hours with approximately 70% of a single oral dose being recovered as unchanged drug in the urine in the first 24 hours post-dose. No metabolites have been identified.

Sabril does not induce the hepatic cytochrome P450 enzymes nor is it metabolised or protein bound. Therefore drug interactions are unlikely.

*Preclinical safety data:* Animal safety studies carried out in the rat, mouse, dog and monkey indicated that vigabatrin has no significant adverse effects on the liver, kidney, lung, heart or gastrointestinal tract. In the brain, microvacuolation has been observed in white matter tracts of rat, mouse and dog at doses of 30–50 mg/kg/day.

In the monkey these lesions are minimal or equivocal. This effect is caused by a separation of the outer lamellar sheath of myelinated fibres, a change characteristic of intramyelinic oedema. In both rat and dog the intramyelinic oedema was reversible on stopping vigabatrin treatment and even with continued treatment histologic regression was observed. However, in rodents, minor residual changes consisting of swollen axons (eosinophilic spheroids) and mineralised microbodies have been observed. In the dog, the results of an electrophysiological study indicate that intramyelinic oedema is associated with an increase in the latency of the somatosensory evoked potential which is reversible when the drug is withdrawn.

In humans, there is no evidence of intramyelinic oedema. Tests done to confirm lack of significant adverse effect on neurological function include evoked potentials, CAT scans, magnetic resonance imaging, CSF analyses and in a small number of cases, neuropathological examinations of brain specimens.

## Pharmaceutical particulars

*List of excipients:* Polyvinylpyrrolidone PhEur

*Incompatibilities:* Not applicable

*Shelf life:* 3 years

*Special precautions for storage:* None stated

*Nature and contents of the container:* Containers: Sachets (paper, polythene/aluminium foil/laminated) packed in cardboard cartons. Pack size: 50 sachets.

*Instructions for use/handling:* Not applicable

*Marketing authorisation holder:* Marion Merrell Ltd., Broadwater Park, Denham, Uxbridge, Middlesex UB9 5HP

**Marketing authorisation number** 4425/0119

**Date of approval/revision of SPC** April 1997

**Legal category** POM

## SABRIL* TABLETS AND SACHETS

**Presentation**
*Sabril Tablets:* White, oval, biconvex tablets with a breakline on one side and SABRIL on the other. Each tablet contains 500 mg vigabatrin.

*Sabril Sachets:* Sachets containing 500 mg vigabatrin as a white to off-white granular powder. The contents should be dissolved in water or a soft drink immediately prior to oral administration. Inactive ingredients: polyvinyl pyrrolidone.

**Uses**
*Mode of action:* Vigabatrin is a selective, irreversible inhibitor of GABA-transaminase. Treatment with Sabril leads to an increase in brain levels of GABA (gamma aminobutyric acid), the major inhibitory neurotransmitter in the brain.

*Indications:* Sabril is indicated for the treatment of epilepsy which is not satisfactorily controlled by another antiepileptic drug.

Sabril is recommended as monotherapy for the management of infantile spasms (West's Syndrome).

**Dosage and administration** Sabril is for oral administration once or twice daily and may be taken before or after meals. It should be added to the patient's current therapeutic regimen.

*Adults:* Maximal efficacy is usually seen in the 2–4 g/day range. A starting dose of 1 g (2 tablets or sachets) daily should be added to the patient's current antiepileptic drug regimen. The daily dose should then be titrated in 0.5 g increments at weekly intervals depending on clinical response and tolerability. Although a slight increase in efficacy has been observed in some patients treated with up to a maximum of 6 g/day, this dose has been associated with an increased incidence of adverse effects. Doses above 4 g/day should only be used in exceptional circumstances with close monitoring for adverse effects.

There is no direct correlation between plasma concentration and efficacy. The duration of the effects of the drug are dependent on the rate of enzyme resynthesis rather than the concentration of drug in the plasma.

*Children:* The recommended starting dose in children is 40 mg/kg/day increasing to 80–100 mg/kg/day depending on response. Convenient whole tablet/sachet recommendations are:

Bodyweight:
10–15 kg 1–2 tablets or sachets/day
15–30 kg 2–3 tablets or sachets/day
30–50 kg 3–6 tablets or sachets/day
> 50 kg 4–8 tablets or sachets/day (adult dose)

*Infants:* Monotherapy for infantile spasms (West's Syndrome): The recommended dose is between 60–100 mg/kg/day depending on the severity of the spasms. This may be titrated over a period of one week if necessary. Doses of up to 150 mg/kg/day have been used with good tolerability.

*Elderly and patients with renal impairment:* Since vigabatrin is eliminated via the kidney, caution should be exercised when administering the drug to the elderly and more particularly in patients with creatinine clearance less than 60 ml/min. Adjustment of dose or frequency of administration should be considered. Such patients may respond to a lower maintenance dose.

**Contra-indications, warnings, etc**
*Contra-indications:* Pregnant women (see *Use in pregnancy and lactation*); patients who have a history of hypersensitivity to vigabatrin or its product components.

*Use in pregnancy and lactation:* As little data are available on the use of Sabril during pregnancy, it is currently contra-indicated in pregnant women.

Studies in animals have shown that vigabatrin does not adversely affect fertility, foetal development or pup development, nor is it teratogenic in rat at doses up to 150 mg/kg or the rabbit at doses up to 100 mg/kg. However, in the rabbit at doses of 150 and 200 mg/kg, a slight increase in the incidence of cleft palate was observed.

There are no adequate and well controlled studies in pregnant women. Congenital anomalies have been reported in the off-spring of some mothers using vigabatrin during pregnancy. No trends in the type of abnormal pregnancy outcome are evident from available data.

In the absence of data on the excretion of vigabatrin in human milk, breast-feeding during Sabril treatment is not recommended.

*Precautions:* As with other antiepileptic drugs abrupt withdrawal may lead to rebound seizures. If treatment is to be discontinued it is recommended that this is done by gradually reducing the dose over 2–4 weeks.

Sabril should be used with caution in patients with a history of psychosis or behavioural problems (see *Side-effects*).

Sabril is eliminated via the kidney and should be used with care in the elderly and patients with impaired renal function (see *Dosage*).

*Warning:* Animal safety studies indicate that vigabatrin causes intramyelinic oedema in the brain white matter tracts. Currently there is no evidence to suggest that this effect occurs in man. However, it is recommended that patients treated with Sabril are closely observed for adverse effects on neurological function. Details of animal findings are given under 'Further Information'.

*Effects on driving ability:* Drowsiness has been observed in clinical trials and patients should be warned of this possibility before treatment. Special care should be taken by patients driving, operating machinery or performing any hazardous task.

*Side-effects:* Adverse reactions are mainly CNS related and probably a secondary consequence of the increase in GABA caused by Sabril. The most commonly reported adverse reactions are drowsiness and fatigue except in children where excitation/agitation are more frequent. Other CNS-related reactions that have been reported include dizziness, nervousness, irritability, headache, nystagmus, ataxia, tremor, paraesthesia, impaired or decreased concentration or alertness and less commonly confusion, memory disturbance and vision complaints such as diplopia. Rare instances of visual field defect, photophobia and retinal disorders (such as peripheral retinal atrophy) have been observed.

Psychiatric reactions (agitation, aggression, depression, abnormal thinking, paranoid reactions) have been reported during vigabatrin therapy. These reactions occurred in patients with and without a psychiatric history and were usually reversible when vigabatrin doses were reduced or gradually discontinued (See *Precautions*). Depression was a common psychiatric reaction but seldom required discontinuation of vigabatrin. Less common reactions included psychotic symptoms. Hypomania and mania have been reported rarely.

The sedative effect of vigabatrin usually decreases with continuing treatment. However, rare instances of marked sedation/stupor/confusion, in association with non-specific slow wave activity on electroencephalogram have been described soon after the introduction of vigabatrin. Such reactions have been fully reversible following dose reduction or discontinuation of vigabatrin.

Other adverse reactions reported include weight gain, oedema, minor gastrointestinal side-effects and alopecia. Allergic reactions such as rash and urticaria have been reported rarely.

As with other antiepileptic drugs, some patients may experience an increase in seizure frequency with vigabatrin. Patients with myoclonic seizures may be particularly liable to this effect.

Laboratory data indicate that Sabril treatment does not lead to renal or hepatic toxicity. Decreases in SGOT and SGPT have been observed and may be a result of inhibition of these transaminases by Sabril. Chronic treatment with Sabril may be associated with a slight decrease in haemoglobin which rarely attains clinical significance.

*Drug interactions:* Sabril is not metabolised, or protein bound and does not induce hepatic cytochrome P450 or drug metabolising enzymes so interactions with other drugs are unlikely. In clinical studies a gradual reduction of about 20% in plasma phenytoin concentration has been observed. The mechanism is not understood but this is unlikely to be of therapeutic significance. No clinically significant interactions have been seen with carbamazepine, phenobarbitone or sodium valproate in clinical trials.

*Overdose:* There is no specific antidote and the usual supportive measures should be employed. Vigabatrin overdose has been reported. When provided, doses were most commonly between 7.5 g to 30 g; however, ingestions up to 65 g have been reported. Nearly half of the cases involved multiple drug ingestions. None of the overdoses resulted in death.

Activated charcoal has been shown not to significantly absorb vigabatrin in an *in-vitro* study. The effectiveness of haemodialysis in the treatment of vigabatrin overdose is unknown.

**Pharmaceutical precautions** None.

**Legal category** POM.

**Package quantities** Sabril Tablets: Blister strips of 10 in cartons of 100.
Sabril Sachets: Packs of 50.

**Further information** Animal safety studies carried out in rat, mouse, dog and monkey have indicated that vigabatrin has no significant adverse effects on the liver, kidney, lung, heart or gastrointestinal tract. In the brain, microvacuolation has been observed in white matter tracts of rat, mouse and dog at doses of 30–50 mg/kg/day. In the monkey these lesions are minimal or equivocal. This effect is caused by a separation of the outer lamellar sheath of myelinated fibres, a change characteristic of intramyelinic oedema. In both rat and dog the intramyelinic oedema was reversible on stopping vigabatrin treatment and even with continued treatment histologic regression was observed. However, in rodents, minor residual changes consisting of swollen axons (eosinophilic spheroids) and mineralised microbodies have been observed. In the dog, the results of an electrophysiological study indicate that intramyelinic oedema is associated with an increase in the latency of the somatosensory evoked potential which is reversible when the drug is withdrawn.

In humans, there is no evidence of intramyelinic oedema. Tests done to confirm lack of significant adverse effect on neurological function include evoked potentials, CAT scans, magnetic resonance imaging, CSF analysis and in a small number of cases, neuropathological examinations of brain specimens.

**Product licence numbers**
Sabril Tablets    4425/0098
Sabril Sachets    4425/0119

*Product licence holder:* Marion Merrell Ltd., Broadwater Park, Denham, Uxbridge, Middlesex UB9 5HP

# SOFRADEX* EAR/EYE DROPS AND OINTMENT

## Qualitative and quantitative composition

Ear/eye ointment containing 0.5% w/w Framycetin Sulphate, 0.05% w/w Dexamethasone and 0.005% w/w Gramicidin.

Ear/eye drop bottles containing 0.5% w/v of Framycetin Sulphate, Dexamethasone Sodium Metasulphobenzoate (equivalent to 0.05% w/v of Dexamethasone) and 0.005% w/v of Gramicidin.

**Pharmaceutical form** Ear/eye ointment. Sterile clear colourless ear/eye drops.

## Clinical particulars

*Therapeutic indications:*

1. In the eye: For the short-term treatment of steroid responsive conditions of the eye when prophylactic antibiotic treatment is also required, after excluding the presence of fungal and viral disease.
2. In the ear: Otitis externa.
3. Application to the eyelid: Blepharitis.(Eye ointment only)

*Posology and method of administration:* Route of administration: Auricular and ocular use.

*Adults (and the elderly) and children:*

*Ear/Eye Ointment:* In the eye: Apply sparingly two or three times daily, or at night if drop treatment is given during the day. In the ear: Apply once or twice daily.

*Ear/Eye Drops:* In the Eye: One or two drops applied to each affected eye up to six times daily or more frequently if required. In the Ear: Two or three drops instilled into the ear three or four times daily

*Contra-indications:* Viral, fungal, tuberculous or purulent conditions of the eye. Use is contraindicated if glaucoma is present or herpetic keratitis (e.g. dendritic ulcer) is considered a possibility. Use of topical steroids in the latter condition can lead to extension of the ulcer and marked visual deterioration.

Otitis externa should not be treated when the eardrum is perforated because of the risk of ototoxicity.

Hypersensitivity to the preparation.

*Special warnings and precautions for use:* Topical corticosteroids should never be given for an undiagnosed red eye as inappropriate use is potentially blinding.

Treatment with corticosteroid/antibiotic combinations should not be continued for more than 7 days in the absence of any clinical improvement, since prolonged use may lead to occult extension of infection due to the masking effect of the steroid. Prolonged use may also lead to skin sensitisation and the emergence of resistant organisms.

Prolonged use may lead to the risk of adrenal suppression in infants.

Treatment with corticosteroid preparations should not be repeated or prolonged without regular review to exclude raised intraocular, pressure, cataract formation or unsuspected infections.

Aminoglycoside antibiotics may cause irreversible, partial or total deafness when given systemically or when applied topically to open wounds or damaged skin. This effect is dose related and is enhanced by renal or hepatic impairment. Although this effect has not been reported following topical ocular use, the possibility should be considered when high dose topical treatment is given to small children or infants.

*Interactions with other medicaments and other forms of interaction:* Non relevant to topical use.

*Use in pregnancy and lactation:* Safety for use in pregnancy and lactation has not been established. There is inadequate evidence of safety in human pregnancy. Topical administration of corticosteroids to pregnant animals can cause abnormalities of foetal development including cleft palate and intrauterine growth retardation. There may therefore be a very small risk of such effects in the human foetus. There is a risk of foetal ototoxicity if aminoglycoside antibiotic preparations are administered during pregnancy.

*Effects on ability to drive and to use machines:* Will cause blurring of vision on application. Warn patients not to drive or operate hazardous machinery unless vision is clear.

*Undesirable effects (frequency and seriousness):* Hypersensitivity reactions, usually of the delayed type, may occur leading to irritation, burning, stinging, itching and dermatitis.

Topical steroid use may result in increased intraocular pressure leading to optic nerve damage, reduced visual acuity and visual field defects.

Intensive or prolonged use of topical corticosteroids may lead to formation of posterior subcapsular cataracts.

In those diseases causing thinning of the cornea or sclera, corticosteroid therapy may result in thinning of the globe leading to perforation.

*Overdosage:* Long-term intensive topical use may lead to systemic effects.

Oral ingestion of the contents of one bottle (up to 10 ml) of the eye drops, is unlikely to lead to any serious adverse effects.

## Pharmacological properties

*Pharmacodynamic properties:* Framycetin sulphate is an aminoglycoside antibiotic with a spectrum of activity similar to that of neomycin, this includes *Staphylococcus aureus* and most clinically significant gram negative organisms.

Gramicidin is an antimicrobial cyclic polypeptide active in vitro against many gram positive bacteria. It is used for the local treatment of susceptible infections, sometimes in combination with other antimicrobial agents and frequently with a corticosteroid.

Dexamethasone is a synthetic glucocorticoid and has the same general properties as other corticosteroids.

*Pharmacokinetic properties:* Framycetin sulphate absorption occurs from inflamed skin and wounds. Once absorbed it is rapidly excreted by the kidneys in active form. It has been reported to have a half life of 2-3 hours.

Gramicidin has properties similar to those of tyrothricin and is too toxic to be administered systemically.

Dexamethasone is readily absorbed from the gastrointestinal tract. It has a biological half-life in plasma of about 190 minutes.

*Preclinical safety data:* Not applicable.

## Pharmaceutical particulars

*List of excipients:* The ointment contains Plastibase 30w. The drops contain citric acid, sodium citrate, lithium chloride, phenylethyl alcohol, industrial methylated spirit, polysorbate 80, purified water.

*Incompatibilities:* None known.

*Shelf life:* Sofradex Ear/Eye Ointment: 5 years. Sofradex Ear/Eye Drops: 24 Months

*Special precautions for storage:* Store below 25°C, do not refrigerate.

*Nature and contents of container:* Ear/ Eye Ointment: 5 g white pigment plasticised PVC tube with tamper evident seal or white pigment multilaminated tube (Aluminium Foil Barrier/Inner Coating HDPE) with tamper evident seal.

Ear/ Eye Drops: Glass bottle fitted with a special dropper attachment, in pack sizes of 8 or 10 ml. Plastic dropper bottle, in a pack of 10 ml.

*Instructions for use/handling:* None.

*Marketing authorisation holder:* Roussel Laboratories Ltd., Broadwater Park, Denham, Uxbridge, Middlesex UB9 5HP

**Marketing authorisation numbers**
Sofradex Ear/Eye Drops          0109/0030R
Sofradex Ear/Eye Ointment       0109/0031R

**Date of approval/revision of SPC**   May 1997

**Legal category** POM

# SOFRAMYCIN* STERILE EYE DROPS/ OINTMENT

**Presentation** Soframycin is available as a sterile eye ointment and as colourless, sterile eye drops.

Each gram of ointment contains Framycetin Sulphate BP (Soframycin) 5 mg in Plastibase*.

Each millilitre of drops contains Framycetin Sulphate BP (Soframycin) 5 mg in a sterile, buffered, isotonic, aqueous solution.

**Uses** Soframycin is used for the topical treatment of bacterial eye infections due to sensitive organisms, including conjunctivitis, blepharitis, styes and infected corneal abrasions, burns and ulcers. It may also be used prophylactically in patients undergoing removal of ocular foreign bodies.

**Dosage and administration** *Soframycin Drops:* For rapid effect, preferably during the daytime, one or two drops should be applied to each affected eye every one or two hours or more frequently if required. Severe infections may require one or two drops every 15-20 minutes initially, reducing the frequency of instillation gradually as the infection is controlled.

*Soframycin Ointment:* For continued effect, Soframycin ointment should be applied, to each affected eye two or three times daily, or before retiring if drops have been used during the day.

**Contra-indications, warnings, etc.**

*Contra-indications:* Known hypersensitivity to Framycetin or to any component of the preparation.

*Interactions:* None relevant to topical use.

*Effects on ability to drive and to use machines:* Topical eye preparations may cause transient blurring of vision on instillation. Patients should be warned not to drive or operate hazardous machinery unless vision is clear.

*Other undesirable effects:* Hypersensitivity reactions, usually of the delayed type, may occur with local treatment with Framycetin (cross-sensitivity with other aminoglycoside antibiotics may occur). Irritation, stinging or burning, itching and dermatitis may sometimes occur.

*Use in pregnancy and lactation:* There is inadequate evidence for the safety of Framycetin in pregnancy and lactation. However, it has been used for many years with no direct evidence of ill consequences. Use should be only when considered essential by the physician.

*Other special warnings and precautions:*

1. Prolonged use should be avoided as it may lead to skin sensitisation and the emergence of resistant organisms.
2. Contact lenses should be removed during the period of treatment.
3. Aminoglycosides have been reported to cause irreversible partial or total deafness when given systemically, topically to open wounds or broken skin, or intraperitoneally. These effects have not been reported with topical ocular administration of Framycetin. However, the possibility should be considered when using high dose topical treatment in small children, or those patients with renal or hepatic impairment.
4. In cases of severe infections the topical use of Framycetin should be supplemented with appropriate systemic treatment.

*Overdosage:* Not applicable.

**Pharmaceutical precautions** Soframycin Eye Drops: Store below 25°C. Protect from light. Soframycin ointment: Store cool.

**Legal category** POM.

**Package quantities** *Soframycin Eye Drops:* 10 ml bottle. *Soframycin Eye Ointment:* Tubes of 5 g (fitted with ophthalmic nozzle).

**Further information** Soframycin Eye Drops contain Citric Acid, Sodium Chloride, Sodium Citrate, Benzalkonium Chloride Solution and Purified Water.

**Product licence numbers**
Soframycin Eye Drops        0109/0140
Soframycin Eye Ointment     0109/5041R

*Product licence holder:* Roussel Laboratories Ltd., Broadwater Park, North Orbital Road, Denham, Uxbridge, Middlesex UB9 5HP

# SOFRA-TULLE*

**Qualitative and quantitative composition** Each unit is impregnated with Framycetin Sulphate BP 1% (Soframycin).

**Pharmaceutical form** A sterile, lightweight, lanoparaffin gauze dressing 10 x 10 cm impregnated with Framycetin Sulphate BP 1% (Soframycin).

**Clinical particulars**

*Therapeutic Indications:* Sofra-tulle has a wide range of antibacterial activity and is an ideal dressing for immediate use in a variety of infected lesions.

*Thermal:* Burns, scalds.

*Traumatic:* Lacerations, abrasions, bites, puncture, wounds, crush injuries.

*Ulcerative:* Varicose, diabetic, decubitus and tropical ulcers.

*Elective:* Skin grafts (donor and receptors sites) avulsion of finger and/or toe nails, circumcision, suture lines.

*Miscellaneous:* Secondary infected skin conditions (e.g. eczema, dermatitis, herpes zoster), colostomies, ileostomies, tracheostomies, incised abscesses, incised perionychia.

*Posology and method of administration:*

Adults, Children and the Elderly: If necessary, the lesion should first be cleansed, then a single layer of Sofra-tulle applied and covered with a suitable dressing.

When dressing ulcers, the tulle should be shaped to fit the ulcer crater.

If the lesion exudes profusely it is advisable to change the dressings at least once a day.

*Contra-indications:* Sofra-tulle is contra-indicated where there is known allergy to lanolin or to Soframycin, or where organisms are known to be resistant to the latter.

*Special warnings and special precautions for use:* In most cases, absorption of the antibiotic is negligible. However, where large body areas are involved e.g. 30% or more body burns, the possibility of ototoxicity being produced by prolonged applications should be borne in mind.

*Interactions with other medicaments and other forms of interaction:* None

*Use in pregnancy and lactation:* There is inadequate evidence of safety in human pregnancy.

*Effects on ability to drive and to use machines:* None

*Undesirable effects (frequency and seriousness):* Cross-sensitisation to Soframycin may occur in patients known to be allergic to streptomyces-derived antibiotics (neomycin, paramomycin, kanamycin).

*Overdose:* Unlikely to occur (refer to Special warnings and special precautions for use).

## Pharmacological properties

*Pharmacodynamic properties:* Framycetin Sulphate has broad spectrum bactericidal activity against most Gram-positive and Gram-negative rods and many Gram-positive and Gram-negative cocci including some but not all streptococci.

Like other aminoglycoside antibiotics framycetin sulphate interferes with protein synthesis by specifically and irreversibly binding to the 30S subunit of sensitive 70S ribosomes resulting in misreading of m RNA. The precise mechanisms are unknown.

*Pharmacokinetic properties:* Absorption is negligible through the skin except for large burn areas. If there is absorption of framycetin sulphate, it is excreted unchanged in the urine by glomerular filtration.

*Preclinical safety data:* Not applicable.

## Pharmaceutical particulars

*List of Excipients:* The product contains lanolin and white soft paraffin.

*Incompatibilities:* Not applicable

*Shelf-life:* 36 Months

*Special precautions for storage:* Store flat below 25°C.

*Nature and contents of container:* Each unit pack contains one sterile antibiotic gauze dressing 10 cm x 10 cm packed in cartons of 10 and 50 units.

*Instructions for use/handling:* None.

*Marketing authorisation holder:* Roussel Laboratories Ltd., Broadwater Park, North Orbital Road, Denham, Uxbridge, Middlesex UB9 5HP

**Marketing authorisation number** 0109/5047R

**Date of approval/revision of SPC** May 1997

**Legal category** POM

# STREPTASE* INJECTION 250000 IU

**Qualitative and quantitative composition** Streptase Injection contains purified streptokinase as active ingredient. Each vial contains 250,000 International Units.

**Pharmaceutical form** Freeze dried powder for reconstitution into solution for infusion.

## Clinical particulars

*Therapeutic indications:* Intravascular dissolution of thrombi and emboli in: extensive deep vein thrombosis; pulmonary embolism; acute or sub-acute occlusion of peripheral arteries; central retinal venous or arterial thrombosis.

*Posology and method of administration:* Streptase should be given by intravenous infusion in physiological saline, Haemaccel, 5% glucose, 5% fructose or ringer-lactate solution.

*Loading dose:* Since human exposure to streptococci is common, antibodies to streptokinase(streptokinase resistance) are found normally. Thus, a loading dose of Streptase sufficient to neutralise the resistance is required. A dose of 250,000 units of Streptase infused into a peripheral vein over 30 minutes has been found appropriate in over 90% of patients.

*Maintenance dose:* A maintenance dose infusion of 100,000 units/hour is given following the loading dose. Administer the maintenance dose of 100,000 units per hour for 72 hours for the treatment of deep vein thrombosis, for 24 hours for the treatment of pulmonary embolism (up to 72 hours if concurrent deep vein thrombosis is suspected), for 24–72 hours for the treatment of arterial thrombosis and for up to 12 hours for central retinal thrombosis.

*Control of therapy:* If the thrombin time of any other parameter of lysis after 4 hours of therapy is less than approximately 1.5 times the normal control value, discontinue Streptase as excessive resistance to streptokinase is present.

*Children:* In children, in whom it is always advisable to estimate the initial dose by means of the streptokinase resistance test, the recommended maintenance dose per hour is 20 units/ml blood volume.

*Patient monitoring:* Before commencing thrombolytic therapy, it is desirable to obtain a thrombin time (TT), activated partial thromboplastin time (aPTT),

haematocrit and platelet count to obtain the haemostatic status of the patient. If heparin has been given, it should be discontinued and the TT or aPTT should be less than twice the normal control value before thrombolytic therapy is started.

In patients previously treated with coumarin derivatives, the INR (International Normalised Ratio) should be below 1.7 before starting therapy with streptokinase.

During the infusion, decreases in the plasminogen and fibrinogen level and an increase in the level of fibrin degradation products (FDP) (the latter two serving to prolong the clotting times of coagulation tests) will generally confirm the existence of a lytic state. Therefore therapy can be monitored by performing the TT or aPTT approximately 4 hours after initiation of therapy.

*Anticoagulation after terminating intravenous streptokinase therapy:* At the end of Streptase therapy, treatment with heparin by continuous intravenous infusion is recommended to prevent recurrent thrombosis. Heparin treatment (without a loading dose) should not begin until the thrombin time has decreased to less than twice the normal control value (approximately 3 to 4 hours). (See manufacturer's prescribing information for proper use of heparin). This should be followed by oral anticoagulation in the conventional manner.

*Contra-indications:* Contra-indications to Streptase treatment include all conditions that are likely to be associated with existing or very recent haemorrhage, for example:
– active internal bleeding
– recent cerebrovascular accident
– intracranial or intraspinal surgery
– known intracranial neoplasm
– recent trauma to the head
– severe uncontrollable hypertension
– uncontrollable clotting disorders
– previous severe allergic reactions, including vasculitic purpura, to streptokinase or streptokinase-containing products.

Other contra-indications include: Existing or very recent haemorrhage associated with:
– all forms of reduced blood coagulability, in particular spontaneous fibrinolysis
– local lesions with risk of bleeding (e.g. gastrointestinal conditions with existing haemorrhage, previous translumbar aortography, puncture of large arteries, intramuscular injection, indwelling catheters or endotracheal tubes)
– recent operations (up to the 6th post-operative day, depending on the extent of the procedure) and recent severe trauma
– recent abortion or delivery
– diseases of the urogenital tract with existing or potential sources of bleeding.
– recent streptococcal infections which have produced high anti-streptokinase titres (e.g. acute rheumatic fever, acute glomerulonephritis), or recent streptokinase therapy more than 5 days and less than 12 months previously.
– subacute bacterial endocarditis.
– pericarditis. In isolated cases pericarditis has been misdiagnosed as an acute myocardial infarction and treated with Streptase leading to pericardial effusions and cardiac tamponade.
– severe hypertension with systolic values over 200 mmHg or diastolic values over 100 mmHg or hypertensive retinal changes Grades III/IV.
– severe liver or kidney damage.
– disorders of cerebral blood flow or recent cerebral haemorrhage.
– pulmonary disease with cavitation (e.g. open tuberculosis) or severe bronchitis.
– acute pancreatitis.
– advanced age with suspicion of arteriosclerotic degeneration.
– septic thrombotic disease.
– pregnancy (see *Pregnancy and lactation*).

*Special warnings and special precautions for use:* Caution is necessary in patients with mitral valve defects or atrial fibrillation because of the danger of cerebral embolisation from the left side of the heart.

The risks of therapy must be weighed against the dangers of the disease.

Caution is necessary in patients with diabetic retinopathy as there may be an increased risk of local bleeding.

Streptokinase is unlikely to be effective in the following conditions:
– deep vein thrombosis more than 14 days old
– occlusion of central retinal artery more than 6-8 hours old and thrombosis of retinal vein

*Interaction with other medicaments and other forms of interaction:* There is an increased risk of haemorrhage in patients who are receiving or have recently been treated with anticoagulants or any drugs which affect platelet formation or function. Simultaneous treatment with dextrans also increases the danger of

haemorrhage. The effects of drugs which act upon platelet formation or function should be allowed to subside before starting long-term lysis with Streptase (see 'Patient monitoring').

If the patient has been given heparin, its effects can be neutralised by giving protamine sulphate.

In patients previously treated with coumarin derivatives, the INR should be below 1.7 before starting treatment with streptokinase.

*Pregnancy and lactation:* Streptase is contra-indicated in pregnancy.

There is no evidence of the drug's safety in pregnancy nor is there any evidence from animal work that it is free from hazard. Bleeding and anaphylactic reactions might cause abortion and fetal death, especially when Streptase is given within the first 18 weeks of pregnancy. Use only when there is no safer alternative and when the disease (as, for example, in individual cases of massive pulmonary embolism) carries a high risk for the mother.

*Effects on ability to drive and use machines:* Not applicable.

*Undesirable effects:*
*Early reactions:* Fever and chills, asthenia, malaise, headache, gastrointestinal symptoms or musculoskeletal pain may occur but usually respond well to symptomatic therapy.

If hypotension occurs, it can usually be controlled temporarily slowing the infusion rate. Tachycardia or bradycardia have been observed occasionally.

Patients may develop allergic reactions (e.g. rash, flushing, dyspnoea, bronchospasm). Allergic reactions can be largely avoided by giving the initial intravenous dose slowly. Corticosteroids can also be given prophylactically (e.g. 100–250 mg methylprednisolone ten minutes before starting streptokinase therapy). If an allergic reaction occurs the infusion should be discontinued and the patient given intravenous corticosteroids together with adrenaline and an antihistamine. Once the symptoms have subsided treatment can be continued.

Streptokinase administration has been associated with low back pain. This may indicate an allergic response, and it may be appropriate to discontinue the infusion. In some cases, without other features of allergy, infusion has been continued with analgesic cover, without adverse consequence.

Anaphylactic reactions have been observed rarely. If an anaphylactic reaction occurs discontinue the infusion immediately and give adrenaline immediately by slow intravenous injection. In addition high doses of corticosteroids by slow intravenous injection may be given.

*Haemorrhage:* Minor bleeding may occur at infusion sites. Discontinuation of treatment is not necessary.

In serious haemorrhagic complications, streptokinase therapy should be discontinued and a proteinase inhibitor, e.g. aprotinin should be given in the following dosages:

Initially inject 500,000 KIU to one million KIU by slow intravenous injection or infusion (maximum rate 5 ml/min). If necessary, this should be followed by 200,000 KIU four-hourly until the bleeding stops.

In addition, combination with synthetic antifibrinolytics is recommended. If necessary, clotting factors can be substituted.

Severe haemorrhages including gastrointestinal and liver haemorrhages, splenic rupture, urogenital haemorrhages, rare cases of intracranial haemorrhages with their complications (also with fatal outcome) or retroperitoneal haemorrhages have been observed.

During thrombolytic treatment of acute myocardial infarction, haemorrhages into the pericardium including myocardial rupture can occur in individual cases.

Haemorrhage can occur in any tissue and organ in the body, and can present with symptoms affecting any body system, including the abdomen and cardiovascular, joints and CNS. Haemorrhage should be considered as a potential cause of unusual symptoms occurring after administration.

*Other reactions:* In a few sporadic cases, neuroallergic symptoms (Guillane-Barre syndrome, polyneuropathy) have been reported in temporal coincidence with Streptase administration.

Uveitis has been reported in temporal association with streptokinase administration.

Serum sickness has been reported but is rare. Arthritis, vasculitis and nephritis have been reported in temporal association with streptokinase administration.

Persistent angina pectoris and cardiac failure, possibly leading to cardiac and respiratory arrest, may occur during thrombolytic therapy of acute myocardial infarction.

The risk of pulmonary embolis in patients with deep vein thrombosis is not greater during treatment with streptokinase than during treatment with heparin alone. If acute or recurrent pulmonary embolism occurs during the treatment, the course of streptokinase should be continued as originally planned so as to lyse the emboli.

Non-cardiogenic pulmonary oedema has been observed in a few cases, mainly after intracoronary thrombolytic therapy in patients with extensive myocardial infarction.

Transient increases in liver function tests or bilirubin have been reported. Jaundice may occur as a consequence of bilirubin increase. A few cases of cholesterol embolism have been described in temporal coincidence with thrombolytic therapy, particularly in patients undergoing angiography.

Individual cases of cerebral convulsions have been reported under thrombolytic therapy, and in temporal coincidence with cardiovascular hypoxia and cerebral haemorrhage.

*Overdose:* Long term overdose of streptokinase may induce the risk of rethrombosis by prolonged decrease of plasminogen. (See also *Side-effects, haemorrhages*).

## Pharmacological properties

*Pharmacodynamic properties:* Streptokinase is an enzyme obtained from β haemolytic streptococci of the lancefield group C. It is a potent activator of the fibrinolytic enzyme system in man and it acts directly by complexing with plasminogen to form an activator complex which then reacts with plasminogen to form plasmin.

*Pharmacokinetic properties:* Streptokinase has a very short half-life, the first rapid clearance from the plasma is due to the formation of the complex between streptokinase and streptokinase antibody. The complex is biochemically inert and is cleared rapidly from the circulation. Once the antibody has been neutralised, the streptokinase activates plasminogen and the resulting complex acts on non complexed plasminogen to form plasmin. During these events the streptokinase is proteolytically modified into several lower molecular weight fragments.

Peak fibrinolytic activity is found in the blood about 20 minutes after dosing activity is detected in the urine 2 hours after dosing.

*Preclinical safety data:* Extensive studies in different species of laboratory animals have shown that multiple human doses do not have an acute toxic dose.

## Pharmaceutical particulars

*List of excipients:* Human albumin, sodium-L-hydrogen glutamate monohydrate and polygeline.

*Incompatibilities:* Other drugs should not be added to the infusion solution.

*Shelf-life:* Three years.

*Special precautions for storage:* Streptase should be stored below 25°C. Once dissolved in physiological saline Streptase can be stored for 24 hours at +2 to +8°C without loss of activity.

*Nature and contents of container:* 5 ml multidose glass vials, containing 250,000 International Units of streptokinase.

*Instructions for use/handling:* To ensure that the contents of the vial are rapidly and completely dissolved, 5 ml physiological saline should be injected into the vial and the residual vacuum.

*Marketing authorisation holder:* Hoechst UK Ltd, Hoechst House, Salisbury Road, Hounslow, Middlesex, TW4 7JH

**Marketing authorisation number**  0086/5020R

**Date of approval/revision of SPC**  February 1997

**Legal category**  POM

## STREPTASE* INJECTION 750000 IU

**Qualitative and quantitative composition** Streptase Injection contains purified streptokinase as active ingredient. Each vial contains 750,000 International Units.

**Pharmaceutical form** Freeze dried powder for reconstitution into solution for infusion.

## Clinical particulars

*Therapeutic indications:* Intravascular dissolution of thrombi and emboli in: extensive deep vein thrombosis; pulmonary embolism; acute or sub-acute occlusion of peripheral arteries; central retinal venous or arterial thrombosis.

*Posology and method of administration:* Streptase should be given by intravenous infusion in physiological saline, Haemaccel, 5% glucose, 5% fructose or ringer-lactate solution.

*Loading dose:* Since human exposure to streptococci is common, antibodies to streptokinase (streptokinase resistance) are found normally. Thus, a loading dose of Streptase sufficient to neutralise the resistance is required. A dose of 250,000 units of Streptase infused

into a peripheral vein over 30 minutes has been found appropriate in over 90% of patients.

*Maintenance dose:* A maintenance dose infusion of 100,000 units/hour is given following the loading dose. Administer the maintenance dose of 100,000 units per hour for 72 hours for the treatment of deep vein thrombosis, for 24 hours for the treatment of pulmonary embolism (up to 72 hours if concurrent deep vein thrombosis is suspected), for 24-72 hours for the treatment of arterial thrombosis and for up to 12 hours for central retinal thrombosis.

*Control of therapy:* If the thrombin time of any other parameter of lysis after 4 hours of therapy is less than approximately 1.5 times the normal control value, discontinue Streptase as excessive resistance to streptokinase is present.

*Children:* In children, in whom it is always advisable to estimate the initial dose by means of the streptokinase resistance test, the recommended maintenance dose per hour is 20 units/ml blood volume.

*Patient Monitoring:* Before commencing thrombolytic therapy, it is desirable to obtain a thrombin time (TT), activated partial thromboplastin time (aPTT), haematocrit and platelet count to obtain the haemostatic status of the patient. If heparin has been given, it should be discontinued and the TT or aPTT should be less than twice the normal control value before thrombolytic therapy is started.

In patients previously treated with coumarin derivatives, the INR (International Normalised Ratio) should be below 1.7 before starting therapy with streptokinase.

During the infusion, decreases in the plasminogen and fibrinogen level and an increase in the level of fibrin degradation products (FDP) (the latter two serving to prolong the clotting times of coagulation tests) will generally confirm the existence of a lytic state. Therefore therapy can be monitored by performing the TT or aPTT approximately 4 hours after initiation of therapy.

*Anticoagulation after terminating intravenous streptokinase therapy:*

At the end of Streptase therapy, treatment with heparin by continuous intravenous infusion is recommended to prevent recurrent thrombosis. Heparin treatment (without a loading dose) should not begin until the thrombin time has decreased to less than twice the normal control value (approximately 3 to 4 hours). (See manufacturer's prescribing information for proper use of heparin). This should be followed by oral anticoagulation in the conventional manner.

*Contra-indications:* Contra-indications to Streptase treatment include all conditions that are likely to be associated with existing or very recent haemorrhage, for example:

– active internal bleeding
– recent cerebrovascular accident
– intracranial or intraspinal surgery
– known intracranial neoplasm
– recent trauma to the head
– severe uncontrollable hypertension
– uncontrollable clotting disorders
– previous severe allergic reactions, including vasculitic purpura, to streptokinase or streptokinase-containing products.

Other contraindications include: Existing or very recent haemorrhage associated with:

– all forms of reduced blood coagulability, in particular spontaneous fibrinolysis
– local lesions with risk of bleeding (e.g. gastrointestinal conditions with existing haemorrhage, previous translumbar aortography, puncture of large arteries, intramuscular injection, indwelling catheters or endotracheal tubes)
– recent operations (up to the 6th post-operative day, depending on the extent of the procedure) and recent severe trauma
– recent abortion or delivery
– diseases of the urogenital tract with existing or potential sources of bleeding.
– Recent streptococcal infections which have produced high anti-streptokinase titres (e.g. acute rheumatic fever or acute glomerulonephritis), or recent streptokinase therapy more than 5 days and less than 12 months previously.
– Subacute bacterial endocarditis.
– Pericarditis. In isolated cases pericarditis has been misdiagnosed as an acute myocardial infarction and treated with Streptase, leading to pericardial effusions and cardiac tamponade.
– Severe hypertension with systolic values over 200 mmHg or diastolic values over 100 mmHg or hypertensive retinal changes Grades III/IV.
– Severe liver or kidney damage.
– Disorders of cerebral blood flow or recent cerebral haemorrhage.
– Pulmonary disease with cavitation (e.g. open tuberculosis) or severe bronchitis.
– Acute pancreatitis.
– Advanced age with suspicion of arteriosclerotic degeneration.

– Septic thrombotic disease.
– pregnancy (see *Pregnancy and lactation*).

*Special warnings and special precautions for use:* Caution is necessary in patients with mitral valve defects or atrial fibrillation because of the danger of cerebral embolisation from the left side of the heart.

The risks of therapy must be weighed against the dangers of the disease.

Caution is necessary in patients with diabetic retinopathy as there may be an increased risk of local bleeding.

Streptokinase is unlikely to be effective in the following conditions:

– deep vein thrombosis more than 14 days old
– occlusion of central retinal artery more than 6–8 hours old and thrombosis of retinal vein more than 10 days old

*Interaction with other medicaments and other forms of interaction:* There is an increased risk of haemorrhage in patients who are receiving or have recently been treated with anticoagulants or any drugs which affect platelet formation or function. Simultaneous treatment with dextrans also increases the danger of haemorrhage. The effects of drugs which act upon platelet formation or function should be allowed to subside before starting long-term lysis with Streptase (see *Patient monitoring*).

If the patient has been given heparin, its effects can be neutralised by giving protamine sulphate.

In patients previously treated with coumarin derivatives, the INR should be below 1.7 before starting treatment with streptokinase.

*Pregnancy and lactation:* Streptase is contra-indicated in pregnancy.

There is no evidence of the drug's safety in pregnancy nor is there any evidence from animal work that it is free from hazard. Bleeding and anaphylactic reactions might cause abortion and fetal death, especially when Streptase is given within the first 18 weeks of pregnancy. Use only when there is no safer alternative and when the disease (as, for example, in individual cases of massive pulmonary embolism) carries a high risk for the mother.

*Effects on ability to drive and use machines:* Not applicable.

*Undesirable effects:*
*Haemorrhage:* Minor bleeding may occur at infusion sites. Discontinuation of treatment is not necessary.

In serious haemorrhagic complications, streptokinase therapy should be discontinued and a proteinase inhibitor, e.g. aprotinin should be given in the following dosages:

Initially inject 500,000 KIU to one million KIU by slow intravenous injection or infusion (maximum rate 5 ml/min). If necessary, this should be followed by 200,000 KIU four-hourly until the bleeding stops.

In addition, combination with synthetic antifibrinolytics is recommended. If necessary, clotting factors can be substituted.

Severe haemorrhages including gastrointestinal and liver haemorrhages, splenic rupture, urogenital haemorrhages, rare cases of intracranial haemorrhages with their complications (also with fatal outcome) or retroperitoneal haemorrhages have been observed.

During thrombolytic treatment of acute myocardial infarction, haemorrhages into the pericardium including myocardial rupture can occur in individual cases.

Haemorrhage can occur in any tissue and organ in the body, and can present with symptoms affecting any body system, including the abdomen and cardiovascular, joints and CNS. Haemorrhage should be considered as a potential cause of unusual symptoms occurring after administration.

*Other Reactions:* In a few sporadic cases, neuroallergic symptoms (Guillane-Barre syndrome, polyneuropathy) have been reported in temporal coincidence with Streptase administration.

Uveitis has been reported in temporal association with streptokinase administration.

Serum sickness has been reported but is rare. Arthritis, vasculitis and nephritis have been reported in temporal association with streptokinase administration.

Persistent angina pectoris and cardiac failure, possibly leading to cardiac and respiratory arrest, may occur during thrombolytic therapy of acute myocardial infarction.

The risk of pulmonary embolis in patients with deep vein thrombosis is not greater during treatment with streptokinase than during treatment with heparin alone. If acute or recurrent pulmonary embolism occurs during the treatment, the course of streptokinase should be continued as originally planned so as to lyse the emboli.

Non-cardiogenic pulmonary oedema has been observed in a few cases, mainly after intracoronary thrombolytic therapy in patients with extensive myocardial infarction.

Transient increases in liver function tests or bilirubin have been reported. Jaundice may occur as a consequence of bilirubin increase. A few cases of cholesterol embolism have been described in temporal coincidence with thrombolytic therapy, particularly in patients undergoing angiography.

Individual cases of cerebral convulsions have been reported under thrombolytic therapy, and in temporal coincidence with cardiovascular hypoxia and cerebral haemorrhage.

*Overdose:* Long term overdose of streptokinase may induce the risk of rethrombosis by prolonged decrease of plasminogen. (See also side-effects, haemorrhages).

### Pharmacological properties

*Pharmacodynamic properties:* Streptokinase is an enzyme obtained from β-haemolytic streptococci of the lancefield group C. It is a potent activator of the fibrinolytic enzyme system in man and it acts directly by complexing with plasminogen to form an activator complex which then reacts with plasminogen to form plasmin.

*Pharmacokinetic properties:* Streptokinase has a very short half-life, the first rapid clearance from the plasma is due to the formation of the complex between streptokinase and streptokinase antibody. The complex is biochemically inert and is cleared rapidly from the circulation. Once the antibody has been neutralised , the streptokinase activates plasminogen and the resulting complex acts on non complexed plasminogen to form plasmin. During these events the streptokinase is proteolytically modified into several lower molecular weight fragments.

Peak fibrinolytic activity is found in the blood about 20 minutes after dosing, activity is detected in the urine 2 hours after dosing.

*Preclinical safety data:* Extensive studies in different species of laboratory animals have shown that multiple human doses have no acute toxic dose.

### Pharmaceutical particulars

*List of excipients:* Human albumin, sodium-L-hydrogen glutamate monohydrate and polygeline.

*Incompatibilities:* Other drugs should not be added to the infusion solution.

*Shelf-life:* Three years.

*Special precautions for storage:* Streptase should be stored below 25°C. Once dissolved in physiological saline Streptase can be stored for 24 hours at +2 to +8°C without loss of activity.

*Nature and contents of container:* 5 ml multidose glass vials, containing 750,000 International Units of streptokinase .

*Instructions for use/handling:* To ensure that the contents of the vial are rapidly and completely dissolved, 5 ml physiological saline should be injected into the vial and the residual vacuum.

*Marketing authorisation holder:* Hoechst UK Ltd, Hoechst House, Salisbury Road, Hounslow, Middlesex, TW4 7JH

**Marketing authorisation number**  0086/5021R

**Date of approval/revision of SPC**  February 1997.

**Legal category** POM

## STREPTASE* INJECTION 1.5 Million IU

**Qualitative and quantitative composition** Streptase contains purified streptokinase as active ingredient. Each vial contains 1.5 million International Units.

**Pharmaceutical form**  Freeze dried powder for reconstitution into solution for infusion.

### Clinical particulars

*Therapeutic indication:*  Treatment of acute myocardial infarction

*Posology and method of administration:*
*Adults:* Streptase should be given by intravenous infusion in 50-200 ml physiological saline
or 5% glucose, 5% fructose, Ringer-lactate solution or Haemaccel as soon as
possible after the onset of symptoms. The efficacy of Streptase therapy is diminished if treatment is delayed. The benefit/risk profile of treatment initiated more than 12 hours after the onset of a myocardial infarction is uncertain. A single dose of 1.5 million IU streptokinase
should be infused over one hour.  No laboratory controls are necessary.
*Children:* There are no recommendations for the use of Streptase in acute myocardial
infarction in children.
*Adjuvant therapy:* Treatment with aspirin (150 mg daily) for at least 4 weeks is recommended for prophylaxis after streptokinase therapy for acute myocardial infarction.

The first dose should be given as soon as possible after the myocardial infarction.

*Contra-indications:* Contra-indications to Streptase treatment include all conditions that are likely to be associated with existing or very recent haemorrhage. Absolute contra-indications include:

- Active internal bleeding
- Recent cerebrovascular accident
- Intracranial or intra-spinal surgery
- Recent trauma to the head
- Known intracranial neoplasm
- Severe uncontrollable hypertension
- Uncontrollable clotting disorders (with the exception of consumption coagulopathy)
- Previous severe allergic reactions, including vasculitic purpura, to streptokinase or streptokinase-containing products

The following conditions would normally be considered to be contraindications to Streptase
therapy. However, in certain situations the benefits of treatment may be considered to outweigh the potential risks. 'Relative' contraindications of this nature include:
Existing or very recent haemorrhage:
- All forms of reduced blood coagulability, in particular spontaneous fibrinolysis.
- Local lesions with risk of bleeding (e.g. gastrointestinal conditions with existing haemorrhage, previous translumbar aortography, puncture of large arteries, intramuscular injections, indwelling catheters or endotracheal tubes).
- Recent operations (up to the 6th post-operative day, depending on the extent of the procedure) and recent severe trauma
- Recent abortion or delivery.
- Diseases of the urogenital tract with existing or potential sources of bleeding.
- Recent streptococcal infections which have produced high anti-streptokinase titres (e.g. acute rheumatic fever, acute glomerulonephritis), or recent streptokinase therapy more than 5 days and less than 12 months previously.

Subacute bacterial endocarditis.
Pericarditis. In isolated cases pericarditis has been misdiagnosed as an acute myocardial infarction and treated with Streptase, leading to pericardial effusions and cardiac tamponade.
Severe hypertension with systolic values over 200 mm/Hg or diastolic values over 100 mg/Hg
or hypertensive retinal changes grades III/IV.
Severe liver or kidney damage.
Disorders of cerebral blood flow or recent cerebral haemorrhage.
Pulmonary diseases with cavitation (e.g. open tuberculosis) or severe bronchitis.
Acute pancreatitis.
Advanced age with suspicion or arteriosclerotic degeneration.
Septic thrombotic disease.
Pregnancy (see 'Pregnancy and lactation).

*Special warnings and special precautions for use:* Caution is necessary in patients with mitral valve defects or atrial fibrillation, because of the danger of cerebral embolisation from the left side of the heart.
The risk of therapy must be weighed against the dangers of the disease.
Caution is necessary in patients with diabetic retinopathy as there may be an increased risk of local bleeding.

*Interaction with other medicaments and other forms of interaction:* There is an increased risk of haemorrhage in patients who are receiving or who have recently been treated with anticoagulants or any drugs which affect platelet formation or function.
Simultaneous treatment with dextrans also increased the danger of haemorrhage.
If the patient has previously been receiving heparin, its effects can be neutralised by giving
protamine sulphate.
In patients previously treated with coumarin derivatives, the INR should be below 1.7 before starting treatment with streptokinase.

*Pregnancy and lactation:* Streptase is contra-indicated in pregnancy. There is no evidence of the drug's safety in pregnancy, nor is there evidence from animal work that it is free from hazard. Bleeding and anaphylactic reactions might cause abortion and fetal death, especially when Streptase is given within the first 18 weeks of pregnancy.   Use only when there is no safer alternative.

*Effects on ability to drive and use machines:* Not applicable.

*Undesirable effects:*
*Haemorrhages:* Minor bleeding may occur at infusion sites. Discontinuation of treatment is not necessary.
In serious haermorrhagic complications, streptokinase therapy should be discontinued and a proteinase

inhibitor, e.g. aprotinin should be given in the following dosages:
Initially inject 500,000 KIU to one million KIU by slow intravenous injection of infusion
(maximum rates 5 ml/min). If necessary, this should be followed by 200,000 KIU four-hourly
until the bleeding stops.
In addition, combination with synthetic antifibrinolytics is recommended. If necessary, clotting factors can be substituted.
Severe haemorrhages including gastrointestinal and liver haemorrhages, splenic rupture, urogenital haemorrhages, rare cases of intracranial haemorrhages with their complications (also with fatal outcome) or retroperitoneal haemorrhages have been observed.
During thrombolytic treatment of acute myocardial infarction, haemorrhages into the pericardium including myocardial rupture can occur in individual cases.
Haemorrhage can occur in any tissue and organ in the body and can present with symptoms affecting any body system, including the abdomen and cardiovascular system, joints and CNS.
Haemorrhage should be considered as a potential cause of unusual symptoms occurring after administration.
*Early reactions:* Early reactions such as fever and chills, asthenia, malaise, headache, gastrointestinal symptoms or musculoskeletal pain are less likely to occur after a single infusion of Streptase than during prolonged therapy. Such reactions usually respond well to symptomatic therapy.
Patients may develop allergic reactions (e.g. rash, flushing, dyspnoea, bronchospasm). Allergic reactions can be largely avoided by giving the initial intravenous dose slowly. Corticosteroids can also be given prophylactically (e.g. 100–250 mg methylprednisolone 10 minutes before starting streptokinase treatment). If an allergic reaction occurs the infusion should be discontinued and the patient given intravenous corticosteroids together with adrenaline and an antihistamine. Once the symptoms have subsided, treatment can be continued.
Streptokinase administration has been associated with low back pain. This may indicate an allergic response, and it may be appropriate to discontinue the infusion. In some cases, without other features of allergy, infusion has been continued with analgesic cover, without adverse consequence.
Anaphylactic reactions have been observed rarely. If an anaphylactic reaction occurs discontinue the infusion immediately and give adrenaline immediately by slow intravenous injection. In addition, high doses of corticosteroids by slow intravenous injection may be given.
*Other reactions:* In a few sporadic cases, neuroallergic symptoms (Guillane-Barre Syndrome, polyneuropathy) have been reported in temporal coincidence with Streptase administration.
Uveitis has been reported in temporal association with streptokinase administration.
Serum sickness has been reported but is rare. Arthritis, vasculitis and nephritis have been reported in temporal association with streptokinase administration.
Arrhythmias and transient hypotension have been noted, particularly after high dose, short-term therapy. Tachycardia and bradycardia have been observed occasionally.
Persistent angina pectoris and cardiac failure, possibly leading to cardiac and respiratory arrest, may occur during thrombolytic therapy of acute myocardial infarction.
Non-cardiogenic pulmonary oedema has been observed in a few cases, mainly after intracoronary thrombolytic therapy in patients with extensive myocardial infarction.
Transient increases in liver function tests or bilirubin have been reported. Jaundice may occur as a consequence of bilirubin increase. A few cases of cholesterol embolism have been described in temporal coincidence with thrombo-lytic therapy, particularly in patients undergoing angiography.
Individual cases of cerebral convulsion were reported under thrombolytic therapy, and in temporal coincidence with cardiovascular hypoxia and cerebral haemorrhage.

*Overdose:* Long-term overdosage of streptokinase may induce the risk of rethrombosis by prolonged decrease of plasminogen. See also side-effects, haermorrhages.

### Pharmacological properties

*Pharmacodynamic properties:* Strepokinase is an enzyme obtained from β haemolytic streptococci of Lancefield group C. It is a potent activator of the fibrinolytic enzyme system in man and it acts indirectly by complexing with plasminogen to form an activator complex which then reacts with more plasminogen to form plasmin.

*Pharmacokinetic properties:* Streptokinase has a very

short half-life, the first rapid clearance from the plasma is due to the formation of the complex between stretokinase and stretokinase antibody. This complex is biochemically inert and is cleared rapidly from the circulation. Once the antibody has been neutralised, the streptokinase activates plasminogen and the resulting complex acts on non complexed plasminogen to form plasmin. During these events the streptokinase is proteolytically modified into several lower molecular weight fragments.

Peak fibrinolytic activity is found in the blood about 20 minutes after dosing activity is detected in the urine 2 hours after dosing.

*Preclinical safety data:* Extensive studies in different species of laboratory animals have shown that the multiple human doses have no acute toxic effect.

### Pharmaceutical particulars

*List of excipients:* Human albumin, sodium-L-hydrogen glutamate monohydrate, polygeline

*Incompatibilities:* Other drugs should not be added to the infusion solution.

*Shelf-life:* Three years

*Special precautions for storage:* Streptase is to be stored below 25°C. Once dissolved in sterile physiological saline Streptase can be stored for 24 hours at +2 to +8°C without loss of activity.

*Nature and contents of container:* Multidose glass vial sealed with rubber infusion stopper, plastic disc and aluminium cap, containing 1.5 million International Units of streptokinase.

*Instructions for use/handling:* For rapid, complete reconstitution, inject 5 ml of physiological saline into the vacuum vial and remove the residual vacuum by briefly loosening the needle from the syringe.

*Marketing authorisation holder:* Hoechst UK Ltd, Hoechst House, Salisbury Road, Hounslow, Middlesex, TW4 7JH

**Marketing authorisation number**　0086/0127

**Date of approval/revision of SPC**　February 1997

**Legal category** POM

## SURGAM* SA CAPSULES 300 mg

**Qualitative and quantitative composition**　Each capsule contains 300 mg tiaprofenic acid.

**Pharmaceutical form**　Capsules containing a pellet formulation providing sustained release.

### Clinical particulars

*Therapeutic indications:* Rheumatoid arthritis, osteoarthritis, ankylosing spondylitis, low back pain, musculo-skeletal disorders such as fibrositis, capsulitis, epicondylitis and other soft-tissue inflammatory conditions, sprains and strains, post-operative inflammation and pain and other soft tissue injuries.

*Posology and method of administration:* For oral administration. Tablets to be swallowed whole.
*Adults:* Two capsules (600 mg tiaprofenic acid) once daily.
*Elderly:* As for adults (see *Special warnings and precautions*). NSAIDs should be used with particular caution in older patients who generally are more prone to adverse reactions.
In cases of renal, cardiac or hepatic impairment, the dosage should be kept as low as possible. It is suggested that in such cases, the dosage be reduced to 200 mg twice daily.
*Children:* There are insufficient data to recommend use of Surgam in children.

*Contra-indications:*

- Active gastroduodenal ulceration or history of gastroduodenal ulceration.
- Active bladder or prostatic disease or symptoms.
- History of recurrent urinary tract disorders.
- Hypersensitivity to tiaprofenic acid and to any of the ingredients in the drug.
- History of asthma, rhinitis or urticaria whether or not induced by aspirin and other NSAIDs.
- Pregnancy (see *Pregnancy and lactation*)
- Severe renal or hepatic insufficiency.

*Special warnings and precautions for use:* As with other NSAIDs, Surgam should be used with care in the elderly and in patients with renal, cardiac or hepatic insufficiency as the use of these drugs may result in the deterioration of renal function. The dose should be kept as low as possible and renal function should be monitored in these patients. Renal function should also be monitored in patients on diuretics. Tiaprofenic acid should be used with caution in patients with arterial hypertension.

Tiaprofenic acid can cause cystitis which may become severe if the treatment is continued after the onset of urinary symptoms. If urinary symptoms such as frequency, urgency, dysuria, nocturia or haematu-

ria occur, tiaprofenic acid should be stopped immediately and urinalysis and urine culture performed. Patients should be warned about the onset of urinary symptoms which may suggest cystitis and are advised to stop taking the drug and seek medical advice if these occur.

Because of the risk of serious gastrointestinal side effects, especially in patients on anticoagulant treatment, special attention should be paid to the appearance of any gastrointestinal symptoms; treatment should be stopped immediately in the event of gastrointestinal haemorrhage.

*Interactions with other medicaments and other forms of interaction:* Since Surgam is highly protein-bound, it is not recommended for co-administration with other highly protein-bound drugs such as heparin. Modification of the dosage may be necessary with hypoglycaemic agents, phenytoin and diuretics.

Concomitant use of Surgam with corticosteroids and other NSAIDs including high-dose salicylates and high dose methotrexate should be avoided. Caution should be exercised when administered with cardiac glycosides, low dose methotrexate and sulphonamides. As with other NSAIDs, careful patient monitoring is suggested if Surgam and an oral anticoagulant are administered together.

NSAIDs have been reported to increase steady state plasma levels of lithium and it is therefore recommended that these are carefully monitored in patients receiving Surgam therapy.

The use of aspirin and other NSAIDs should be avoided for at least 8 -12 days after taking mifepristone.

NSAIDs may cause sodium and fluid retention and may interfere with the natriuretic action of diuretic agents thus reducing the effects of these and other antihypertensive drugs (e.g. β-blockers, ACE inhibitors and anti-angiotensin II receptor inhibitors). This should be borne in mind in patients with incipient or actual congestive heart failure and/or hypotension. The risk of nephrotoxicity may be increased if NSAIDs are given with cyclosporins. Convulsions may occur due to an interaction with quinolone antibiotics.

*Pregnancy and lactation: Pregnancy:* Tiaprofenic acid crosses the placental barrier.

Although animal studies have not revealed evidence of teratogenicity, safety in human pregnancy and lactation cannot be assumed and, in common with other NSAIDs, administration during the first trimester should be avoided.
*Lactation:* The level of Surgam in mother's milk has been studied and the total daily exposure is very small; approximately 0.2% of the administered dose and is unlikely to be of pharmacological significance. Breast feeding or treatment of the mother should be stopped as necessary.

*Effects on ability to drive and use machines:* None known.

*Undesirable effects:*
*Gastrointestinal tract:* Reported reactions include dyspepsia, nausea, vomiting, abdominal pain, anorexia, indigestion, heartburn, constipation, gastritis, flatulence and diarrhoea. In common with NSAIDs, gastroduodenal ulcers, perforation and overt or occult gastrointestinal haemorrhage resulting in anaemia have occasionally been reported and in exceptional case may have been associated with fatalities.
*Muco-cutaneous:* Rash, urticaria, pruritus, purpura, alopecia and very rarely erythema multiforme and bullous eruptions ( Stevens Johnson Syndrome or exceptionally toxic epidermal necrolysis) have been reported. Very rarely photosensitivity reactions and aphthous stomatitis.
*Hypersensitivity reactions:* Asthmatic attacks, especially in subjects allergic to aspirin and other NSAIDs, angio-oedema. Anaphylactic shock has also been reported.
*Haematological:* Thrombocytopenia , prolongation of bleeding time may occur.
*Nervous system:* Headaches, dizziness, tinnitus and drowsiness.
*Urinary system:* Bladder pain, dysuria, frequency and cystitis have been reported with tiaprofenic acid and other NSAIDs. On the basis of spontaneous reports, tiaprofenic acid appears to have a greater propensity than other NSAIDs to cause urinary disorders. Although generally reversible, in some cases where tiaprofenic acid treatment has continued after the onset of urinary symptoms and an association with tiaprofenic acid not recognised, serious consequences requiring surgical intervention have resulted. Therefore, treatment with tiaprofenic acid should be discontinued immediately if urinary disorders develop
*Renal:* Sodium and water retention (see *Special warnings and precautions*). NSAIDs have been reported to cause nephrotoxicity in various forms. As with other NSAIDs, isolated cases of acute interstitial nephritis, nephrotic syndrome and renal failure have also been reported with tiaprofenic acid.
*Hepatic:* Liver test abnormalities

*Overdose:* In the event of overdosage with Surgam, supportive and symptomatic therapy is indicated.

### Pharmacological properties
*Pharmacodynamic properties:* Tiaprofenic acid is a propionic acid derivative having anti-inflammatory and analgesic properties.

The effects of tiaprofenic acid on articular cartilage have been investigated in in-vitro experiments and in ex-vivo studies using different animal models of arthritis. Ex-vivo experiments on human chondrocyte cultures have also been conducted. In these experiments, tiaprofenic acid, in concentrations equivalent to the therapeutic dose, did not depress the biosynthesis of proteoglycans and did not alter the differentiation of proteoglycans secreted. The degradation of proteoglycan aggregates was inhibited. These results suggest a neutral or possibly beneficial effect of tiaprofenic acid on joint cartilage under experimental conditions. The clinical significance of these findings has been studied in a long-term double-blind controlled study in which tiaprofenic acid did not significantly increase the rate of radiological deterioration of joint space in patients with osteoarthritis of the knee.

*Pharmacokinetic properties:* Surgam SA (600 mg) gives a Cmax of 28.1 mg/1 which is not significantly different from 300 mg conventional Surgam (37.3 mg/1).

The plasma concentration remains above 10 mg/1 for 6-8 hours, against 2 to 3 hours with the conventional tablet.

Despite these differences in profile, there was no significant difference in the amount of Tiaprofenic acid absorbed as measured by areas under the plasma concentration curve and quantities eliminated in the urine.

*Preclinical safety data:* Not applicable

### Pharmaceutical particulars
*List of excipients: Pellets:* Glyceryl monostearate; Microcrystalline Cellulose; Purified Talc
　*Capsule shell–CAP:* Erythrosine E127; Titanium Dioxide E171; Indigo carmine 132
　*Capsule shell–BODY:* Erythrosine E127; Indigo carmine E132; Gelatin

*Incompatibilities:* None known

*Shelf life:* 60 months from date of manufacture.

*Special precautions for storage:* Store below 25°C in a dry place and protect from light.

*Nature and contents of container:* Blister packs of 56 tablets manufactured from 250 micrometer PVC/20 micrometer aluminium foil.

*Instruction for use/handling:* Not applicable

*Marketing authorisation holder:* Roussel Laboratories Ltd., Broadwater Park, Denham, Uxbridge, Middlesex UB9 5HP UK

**Marketing authorisation number**　0109/0167

**Date of approval/revision of SPC**　July 1997

**Legal category**　POM

## SURGAM* TABLETS 200 mg

**Qualitative and quantitative composition**　Each tablet contains 200 mg tiaprofenic acid.

**Pharmaceutical form**　Tablets.

### Clinical particulars
*Therapeutic indications:* Rheumatoid arthritis, osteoarthritis, ankylosing spondylitis, low back pain, musculo-skeletal disorders such as fibrositis, capsulitis, epicondylitis and other soft-tissue inflammatory conditions, sprains and strains, post-operative inflammation and pain and other soft tissue injuries.

*Posology and method of administration:* For oral administration.
*Adults:* 600 mg daily in divided doses. 300 mg twice a day. Alternatively 200 mg three times a day.
*Elderly:* As for adults (see *Special warnings and precautions*). NSAIDs should be used with particular caution in older patients who generally are more prone to adverse reactions.
In cases of renal, cardiac or hepatic impairment, the dosage should be kept as low as possible. It is suggested that in such cases, the dosage be reduced to 200 mg twice daily.
*Children:* There are insufficient data to recommend use of Surgam in children.

*Contra-indications:*

- Active gastroduodenal ulceration or history of gastroduodenal ulceration.
- Active bladder or prostatic disease or symptoms.
- History of recurrent urinary tract disorders.
- Hypersensitivity to tiaprofenic acid and to any of the ingredients in the drug.

- History of asthma, rhinitis or urticaria whether or not induced by aspirin and other NSAIDs.
- Pregnancy (see *Pregnancy and lactation*).
- Severe renal or hepatic insufficiency.

*Special warnings and precautions for use:* As with other NSAIDs, Surgam should be used with care in the elderly and in patients with renal, cardiac or hepatic insufficiency as the use of these drugs may result in the deterioration of renal function. The dose should be kept as low as possible and renal function should be monitored in these patients. Renal function should also be monitored in patients on diuretics. Tiaprofenic acid should be used with caution in patients with arterial hypertension.

Tiaprofenic acid can cause cystitis which may become severe if the treatment is continued after the onset of urinary symptoms. If urinary symptoms such as frequency, urgency, dysuria, nocturia or haematuria occur, tiaprofenic acid should be stopped immediately and urinalysis and urine culture performed. Patients should be warned about the onset of urinary symptoms which may suggest cystitis and are advised to stop taking the drug and seek medical advice if these occur.

Because of the risk of serious gastrointestinal side effects, especially in patients on anticoagulant treatment, special attention should be paid to the appearance of any gastrointestinal symptoms; treatment should be stopped immediately in the event of gastrointestinal haemorrhage.

*Interactions with other medicaments and other forms of interaction:* Since Surgam is highly protein-bound, it is not recommended for co-administration with other highly protein-bound drugs such as heparin. Modification of the dosage may be necessary with hypoglycaemic agents, phenytoin and diuretics.

Concomitant use of Surgam with corticosteroids and other NSAIDs including high-dose salicylates and high dose methotrexate should be avoided. Caution should be exercised when administered with cardiac glycosides, low dose methotrexate and sulphonamides. As with other NSAIDs, careful patient monitoring is suggested if Surgam and an oral anticoagulant are administered together.

NSAIDs have been reported to increase steady state plasma levels of lithium and it is therefore recommended that these are carefully monitored in patients receiving Surgam therapy.

The use of aspirin and other NSAIDs should be avoided for at least 8-12 days after taking mifepristone.

NSAIDs may cause sodium and fluid retention and may interfere with the natriuretic action of diuretic agents thus reducing the effects of these and other antihypertensive drugs (e.g. β-blockers, ACE inhibitors and anti-angiotensin II receptor inhibitors). This should be borne in mind in patients with incipient or actual congestive heart failure and/or hypotension. The risk of nephrotoxicity may be increased if NSAIDs are given with cyclosporins. Convulsions may occur due to an interaction with quinolone antibiotics.

*Pregnancy and lactation: Pregnancy:* Tiaprofenic acid crosses the placental barrier.

Although animal studies have not revealed evidence of teratogenicity, safety in human pregnancy and lactation cannot be assumed and, in common with other NSAIDs, administration during the first trimester should be avoided.

*Lactation:* The level of Surgam in mother's milk has been studied and the total daily exposure is very small; approximately 0.2% of the administered dose and is unlikely to be of pharmacological significance. Breast feeding or treatment of the mother should be stopped as necessary.

*Effects on ability to drive and use machines:* None known.

*Undesirable effects:*
*Gastrointestinal tract:* Reported reactions include dyspepsia, nausea, vomiting, abdominal pain, anorexia, indigestion, heartburn, constipation, gastritis, flatulence and diarrhoea. In common with NSAIDs, gastroduodenal ulcers, perforation and overt or occult gastrointestinal haemorrhage resulting in anaemia have occasionally been reported and in exceptional case may have been associated with fatalities.

*Muco-cutaneous:* Rash, urticaria, pruritus, purpura, alopecia and very rarely erythema multiforme and bullous eruptions (Stevens Johnson Syndrome or exceptionally toxic epidermal necrolysis) have been reported. Very rarely photosensitivity reactions and aphthous stomatitis.

*Hypersensitivity reactions:* Asthmatic attacks, especially in subjects allergic to aspirin and other NSAIDs, angio-oedema. Anaphylactic shock has also been reported.

*Haematological:* Thrombocytopenia , prolongation of bleeding time may occur.

*Nervous system:* Headaches, dizziness, tinnitus and drowsiness.

*Urinary system:* Bladder pain, dysuria, frequency and cystitis have been reported with tiaprofenic acid

and other NSAIDs. On the basis of spontaneous reports, tiaprofenic acid appears to have a greater propensity than other NSAIDs to cause urinary disorders. Although generally reversible, in some cases where tiaprofenic acid treatment has continued after the onset of urinary symptoms and an association with tiaprofenic acid not recognised, serious consequences requiring surgical intervention have resulted. Therefore, treatment with tiaprofenic acid should be discontinued immediately if urinary disorders develop
*Renal:* Sodium and water retention (see *Special warnings and precautions*).

NSAIDs have been reported to cause nephrotoxicity in various forms. As with other NSAIDs, isolated cases of acute interstitial nephritis, nephrotic syndrome and renal failure have also been reported with tiaprofenic acid.

*Hepatic:* Liver test abnormalities
*Overdose:* In the event of overdosage with Surgam, supportive and symptomatic therapy is indicated.

**Pharmacological properties**
*Pharmacodynamic properties:* Non-steroidal anti-inflammatory drug.

The effects of tiaprofenic acid on articular cartilage have been investigated in in-vitro experiments and in ex-vivo studies using different animal models of arthritis. Ex-vivo experiments on human chondrocyte cultures have also been conducted. In these experiments, tiaprofenic acid, in concentrations equivalent to the therapeutic dose, did not depress the biosynthesis of proteoglycans and did not alter the differentiation of proteoglycans secreted. The degradation of proteoglycan aggregates was inhibited. These results suggest a neutral or possibly beneficial effect of tiaprofenic acid on joint cartilage under experimental conditions. The clinical significance of these findings has been studied in a long-term double-blind controlled study in which tiaprofenic acid did not significantly increase the rate of radiological deterioration of joint space in patients with osteoarthritis of the knee.

*Pharmacokinetic properties: Single dose studies:* Following oral administration (max. at 90 mins). Plasma level zero at 24 hours.
$t\frac{1}{2}$ = 1.5 to 2 hours.
*Repeated dose studies:* Surgam is rapidly eliminated and there is no accumulation after repeated doses of 600 mg/day in divided doses. Steady state after first day. No impairment of absorption in patients with RA undergoing long term therapy. There is no evidence of different pharmacokinetics in the elderly.
*Protein binding* = 97-98%
*Plasma clearance* = 6 litres/hour
*Elimination* = 60% of urine remainder in bile
*Metabolites* = there are two main metabolites which account for about 10% of urinary excretion and have low pharmacological activity. The parent compound is excreted mostly in the form of acrylglucuronide.

*Preclinical safety data:* Not applicable

**Pharmaceutical particulars**
*List of excipients:* Maize starch, pluronic F68, magnesium stearate and talc.

*Incompatibilities:* None known

*Shelf life:* 60 months

*Special precautions for storage:* Store below 25°C. Protect from light.

*Nature and contents of container:* Blister packs sealed with aluminium foil in a cardboard carton in packs of 84.

*Instruction for use/handling:* Not applicable.

*Marketing authorisation holder:* Roussel Laboratories Ltd., Broadwater Park, Denham, Uxbridge, Middlesex UB9 5HP UK

**Marketing authorisation number**   0109/0108

**Date of approval/revision of SPC**   July 1997

**Legal category**   POM

## SURGAM* TABLETS 300 mg

**Qualitative and quantitative composition**   Each tablet contains 300 mg tiaprofenic acid.

**Pharmaceutical form**   Tablets.

**Clinical particulars**
*Therapeutic indications:* Rheumatoid arthritis, osteoarthritis, ankylosing spondylitis, low back pain, musculo-skeletal disorders such as fibrositis, capsulitis, epicondylitis and other soft-tissue inflammatory conditions, sprains and strains, post-operative inflammation and pain and other soft tissue injuries.

*Posology and method of administration:* For oral administration.
*Adults:* 600 mg daily in divided doses. 300 mg twice a day, alternatively 200 mg three times a day. *Elderly:* As for adults (see *Special warnings and precautions*).

NSAIDs should be used with particular caution in older patients who generally are more prone to adverse reactions.

In cases of renal, cardiac or hepatic impairment, the dosage should be kept as low as possible. It is suggested that in such cases, the dosage be reduced to 200 mg twice daily.
*Children:* There are insufficient data to recommend use of Surgam in children.

*Contra-indications:*
- Active gastroduodenal ulceration or history of gastroduodenal ulceration.
- Active bladder or prostatic disease or symptoms.
- History of recurrent urinary tract disorders.
- Hypersensitivity to tiaprofenic acid and to any of the ingredients in the drug.
- History of asthma, rhinitis or urticaria whether or not induced by aspirin and other NSAIDs.
- Pregnancy ( see *Pregnancy and lactation*)
- Severe renal or hepatic insufficiency.

*Special warnings and precautions for use:* As with other NSAIDs, Surgam should be used with care in the elderly and in patients with renal, cardiac or hepatic insufficiency as the use of these drugs may result in the deterioration of renal function. The dose should be kept as low as possible and renal function should be monitored in these patients. Renal function should also be monitored in patients on diuretics. Tiaprofenic acid should be used with caution in patients with arterial hypertension.

Tiaprofenic acid can cause cystitis which may become severe if the treatment is continued after the onset of urinary symptoms. If urinary symptoms such as frequency, urgency, dysuria, nocturia or haematuria occur, tiaprofenic acid should be stopped immediately and urinalysis and urine culture performed. Patients should be warned about the onset of urinary symptoms which may suggest cystitis and are advised to stop taking the drug and seek medical advice if these occur.

Because of the risk of serious gastrointestinal side effects, especially in patients on anticoagulant treatment, special attention should be paid to the appearance of any gastrointestinal symptoms; treatment should be stopped immediately in the event of gastrointestinal haemorrhage.

*Interactions with other medicaments and other forms of interaction:* Since Surgam is highly protein-bound, it is not recommended for co-administration with other highly protein-bound drugs such as heparin. Modification of the dosage may be necessary with hypoglycaemic agents, phenytoin and diuretics.

Concomitant use of Surgam with corticosteroids and other NSAIDs including high-dose salicylates and high dose methotrexate should be avoided. Caution should be exercised when administered with cardiac glycosides, low dose methotrexate and sulphonamides. As with other NSAIDs, careful patient monitoring is suggested if Surgam and an oral anticoagulant are administered together.

NSAIDs have been reported to increase steady state plasma levels of lithium and it is therefore recommended that these are carefully monitored in patients receiving Surgam therapy.

The use of aspirin and other NSAIDs should be avoided for at least 8-12 days after taking mifepristone.

NSAIDs may cause sodium and fluid retention and may interfere with the natriuretic action of diuretic agents thus reducing the effects of these and other antihypertensive drugs (e.g. β-blockers, ACE inhibitors and anti-angiotensin II receptor inhibitors). This should be borne in mind in patients with incipient or actual congestive heart failure and/or hypotension. The risk of nephrotoxicity may be increased if NSAIDs are given with cyclosporins. Convulsions may occur due to an interaction with quinolone antibiotics.

*Pregnancy and lactation: Pregnancy:* Tiaprofenic acid crosses the placental barrier.

Although animal studies have not revealed evidence of teratogenicity, safety in human pregnancy and lactation cannot be assumed and, in common with other NSAIDs, administration during the first trimester should be avoided.

*Lactation:* The level of Surgam in mother's milk has been studied and the total daily exposure is very small; approximately 0.2% of the administered dose and is unlikely to be of pharmacological significance. Breast feeding or treatment of the mother should be stopped as necessary.

*Effects on ability to drive and use machines:* None known.

*Undesirable effects:*
*Gastrointestinal tract:* Reported reactions include dyspepsia, nausea, vomiting, abdominal pain, anorexia, indigestion, heartburn, constipation, gastritis, flatulence and diarrhoea. In common with NSAIDs, gastroduodenal ulcers, perforation and overt or occult gastrointestinal haemorrhage resulting in anaemia have occasionally been reported and in exceptional case may have been associated with fatalities.

*Muco-cutaneous:* Rash, urticaria, pruritus, purpura, alopecia and very rarely erythema multiforme and bullous eruptions (Stevens Johnson Syndrome or exceptionally toxic epidermal necrolysis) have been reported. Very rarely photosensitivity reactions and aphthous stomatitis.

*Hypersensitivity reactions:* Asthmatic attacks, especially in subjects allergic to aspirin and other NSAIDs, angio-oedema. Anaphylactic shock has also been reported.

*Haematological:* Thrombocytopenia , prolongation of bleeding time may occur.

*Nervous system:* Headaches, dizziness, tinnitus and drowsiness.

*Urinary system:* Bladder pain, dysuria, frequency and cystitis have been reported with tiaprofenic acid and other NSAIDs. On the basis of spontaneous reports, tiaprofenic acid appears to have a greater propensity than other NSAIDs to cause urinary disorders. Although generally reversible, in some cases where tiaprofenic acid treatment has continued after the onset of urinary symptoms and an association with tiaprofenic acid not recognised, serious consequences requiring surgical intervention have resulted. Therefore, treatment with tiaprofenic acid should be discontinued immediately if urinary disorders develop.

*Renal:* Sodium and water retention ( see *Special warnings and precautions*).

NSAIDs have been reported to cause nephrotoxicity in various forms. As with other NSAIDs, isolated cases of acute interstitial nephritis, nephrotic syndrome and renal failure have also been reported with tiaprofenic acid.

*Hepatic:* Liver test abnormalities

*Overdose:* In the event of overdosage with Surgam, supportive and symptomatic therapy is indicated.

### Pharmacological properties

*Pharmacodynamic properties:* Non-steroidal anti-inflammatory drug.

The effects of tiaprofenic acid on articular cartilage have been investigated in in-vitro experiments and in ex-vivo studies using different animal models of arthritis. Ex-vivo experiments on human chondrocyte cultures have also been conducted. In these experiments, tiaprofenic acid, in concentrations equivalent to the therapeutic dose, did not depress the biosynthesis of proteoglycans and did not alter the differentiation of proteoglycans secreted. The degradation of proteoglycan aggregates was inhibited. These results suggest a neutral or possibly beneficial effect of tiaprofenic acid on joint cartilage under experimental conditions. The clinical significance of these findings has been studied in a long-term double-blind controlled study in which tiaprofenic acid did not significantly increase the rate of radiological deterioration of joint space in patients with osteoarthritis of the knee.

*Pharmacokinetic properties: Single dose studies:* Following oral administration (max. at 90 mins). Plasma level zero at 24 hours.

$t\frac{1}{2}$ = 1.5 to 2 hours.

*Repeated dose studies:* Surgam is rapidly eliminated and there is no accumulation after repeated doses of 600 mg/day in divided doses. Steady state after first day. No impairment of absorption in patients with RA undergoing long term therapy. There is no evidence of different pharmacokinetics in the elderly.

Protein binding = 97–98%

Plasma clearance = 6 litres/hour

Elimination = 60% of urine remainder in bile

Metabolites = there are two main metabolites which account for about 10% of urinary excretion and have low pharmacological activity. The parent compound is excreted mostly in the form of acrylglucuronide.

*Preclinical safety data:* Not applicable

### Pharmaceutical particulars

*List of excipients:* Maize starch, pluronic F68, magnesium stearate and talc.

*Incompatibilities:* None known

*Shelf life:* 60 months

*Special precautions for storage:* Store below 25°C. Protect from light.

*Nature and contents of container:* Blister packs sealed with aluminium foil in a cardboard carton in packs of 56.

*Instruction for use/handling:* Not applicable.

*Marketing authorisation holder:* Roussel Laboratories Ltd., Broadwater Park, Denham, Uxbridge, Middlesex UB9 5HP UK

**Marketing authorisation number** 0109/0109

**Date of approval/revision of SPC** July 1997

**Legal category** POM

# TARGOCID*

**Presentation** For intravenous or intramuscular injection or intravenous infusion.

*Targocid 200 mg:* Each vial provides 200 mg teicoplanin presented as a lyophilisate for reconstitution. Each pack contains an ampoule of diluent (Water for Injections PhEur).

*Targocid 400 mg:* Each vial provides 400 mg teicoplanin presented as a lyophilisate for reconstitution. Each pack contains an ampoule of diluent (Water for Injections PhEur).

The vials do not contain any preservative.

## Uses

*Properties:* Teicoplanin is a bactericidal, glycopeptide antibiotic, produced by fermentation of *Actinoplanes teichomyceticus.* It is active against both aerobic and anaerobic Gram-positive bacteria.

Species usually sensitive (MIC less than or equal to 16 mg/l): *Staphylococcus aureus* and coagulase negative staphylococci (sensitive or resistant to methicillin), streptococci, enterococci, *Listeria monocytogenes*, micrococci, *Eikenella corrodens*, group JK corynebacteria and Gram-positive anaerobes including *Clostridium difficile*, and peptococci.

Species usually resistant (MIC superior to 16 mg/l): *Nocardia asteroides, Lactobacillus* spp, *Leuconostoc* and all Gram-negative bacteria. Bactericidal synergy has been demonstrated *in vitro* with aminoglycosides against group D streptococci and staphylococci. *In vitro* combinations of teicoplanin with rifampicin or fluorinated quinolones show primarily additive effects and sometimes synergy.

One-step resistance to teicoplanin could not be obtained *in vitro* and multi-step resistance was only reached *in vitro* after 11–14 passages.

Teicoplanin does not show cross-resistance with other classes of antibiotics.

*Susceptibility testing:* Sensidiscs are charged with 30 micrograms of teicoplanin. Strains showing an inhibition zone diameter of 14 mm or more are susceptible, and those of 10 mm or less are resistant.

*Indications:* Targocid is indicated in potentially serious Gram-positive infections including those which cannot be treated with other antimicrobial drugs, e.g. penicillins and cephalosporins.

Targocid is useful in the therapy of serious staphylococcal infections in patients who cannot receive or who have failed to respond to the penicillins and cephalosporins, or who have infections with staphylococci resistant to other antibiotics.

The effectiveness of teicoplanin has been documented in the following infections: Skin and soft tissue infections, urinary tract infections, lower respiratory tract infections, joint and bone infections, septicaemia, endocarditis and peritonitis related to continuous ambulatory peritoneal dialysis.

Targocid may be used for antimicrobial prophylaxis in orthopaedic surgery at risk of Gram-positive infection.

## Dosage and administration

*Preparation of injection:* The entire contents of the water ampoule should be slowly added to the vial of Targocid and the vial rolled gently until the powder is completely dissolved, taking care to avoid formation of foam. If the solution does become foamy then allow to stand for about 15 minutes for the foam to subside.

A calculated excess is included in each vial of Targocid so that, when prepared as described above, a full dose of 200 mg or 400 mg (depending on the strength of the vial) will be obtained if all the reconstituted solution is withdrawn from the vial by a syringe. The concentration of teicoplanin in these injections will be 100 mg in 1.5 ml (from the 200 mg vial) and 400 mg in 3 ml (from the 400 mg vial).

*Administration:* The reconstituted Targocid injection may be administered directly either intravenously or intramuscularly. The intravenous injection may be administered either as a bolus or as a 30 minute infusion. Dosage is usually once daily but, in cases of severe infection, a second injection should be administered on the first day in order to reach more rapidly the required serum concentrations. The majority of patients with infections caused by organisms sensitive to the antibiotic show a therapeutic response within 48–72 hours. The total duration of therapy is determined by the type and severity of the infection and the clinical response of the patient. In endocarditis and osteomyelitis, treatment for three weeks or longer is recommended.

Determination of teicoplanin serum concentrations may optimise therapy. In severe infections, trough serum concentrations should not be less than 10 mg/l (see *Further information*). Peak concentrations measured one hour after a 400 mg intravenous dose are usually in the range of 20–50 mg/l; peak serum concentrations of up to 250 mg/l have been reported after intravenous doses of 25 mg/kg. A relationship

between serum concentration and toxicity has not been established.

*Therapeutic dosage:*

*Adult or elderly patients with normal renal function:*

*Prophylaxis:* 400 mg intravenously as a single dose at induction of anaesthesia.

*Moderate infections:* skin and soft tissue infection, urinary tract infection, lower respiratory tract infection.

*Loading dose:* one single i.v. or i.m. injection of 400 mg on the first day.

*Maintenance dose:* a single i.v. or i.m. injection of 200 mg daily.

*Severe infections:* joint and bone infection, septicaemia, endocarditis.

*Loading dose:* three 400 mg i.v. injections administered 12 hours apart.

*Maintenance dose:* a single i.v. or i.m. injection of 400 mg daily.

In some clinical situations, such as infected, severely burned patients or *Staphylococcus aureus* endocarditis, unit maintenance doses of up to 12 mg/kg have been administered (intravenously).

*NB:* Standard doses of 200 and 400 mg equate respectively to mean doses of 3 and 6 mg/kg. In patients weighing more than 85 kg it is recommended to adapt the dosage to the weight following the same therapeutic schedule: moderate infection 3 mg/kg, severe infection 6 mg/kg.

*Children:* Teicoplanin can be used to treat Gram positive infections in children from the age of 2 months. For severe infections and neutropenic patients the recommended dose is 10 mg/kg every 12 hours for the first three doses; thereafter a dose of 10 mg/kg should be administered by either intravenous or intramuscular injection as a single dose each day. For moderate infections the recommended dose is 10 mg/kg by intravenous injection every twelve hours for the first three doses; thereafter a dose of 6 mg/kg should be administered by either intravenous or intramuscular injection as a single dose each day.

*Neonates:* The recommended dosage for neonates is a loading dose of 16 mg/kg followed by a daily maintenance dose of 8 mg/kg. The doses should be given as intravenous infusion over thirty minutes.

*Adults and elderly patients with renal insufficiency:* For patients with impaired renal function, reduction of dosage is not required until the fourth day of Targocid treatment. Measurement of the serum concentration of teicoplanin may optimise therapy (see section 'Administration').

*From the fourth day of treatment:*

*In mild renal insufficiency:* Creatinine clearance between 40 and 60 ml/min, Targocid dose should be halved, either by administering the initial unit dose every two days, or by administering half of this dose once a day.

*In severe renal insufficiency:* Creatinine clearance less than 40 ml/min, and in haemodialysed patients, Targocid dose should be one third of the normal either by administering the initial unit dose every third day, or by administering one third of this dose once a day. Teicoplanin is not removed by dialysis. *In continuous ambulatory peritoneal dialysis:* After a single loading iv dose of 400 mg if the patient is febrile, the recommended dosage is 20 mg/l per bag in the first week, 20 mg/l in alternate bags in the second week, and 20 mg/l in the overnight dwell bag only during the third week.

## Contra-indications, warnings, etc

*Contra-indications:* Teicoplanin is contra-indicated in patients who have exhibited previous hypersensitivity to the drug.

*Warnings:* Targocid should be administered with caution in patients known to be hypersensitive to vancomycin since cross hypersensitivity may occur. However, a history of the 'Red Man Syndrome' that can occur with vancomycin is not a contra-indication to Targocid.

Thrombocytopenia has been reported with teicoplanin, especially at higher doses than those usually recommended. It is advisable for periodic haematological studies to be performed during treatment. Liver and renal function tests are advised during treatment.

Serial renal and auditory function tests should be undertaken in the following circumstances:

- prolonged treatment in patients with renal insufficiency.
- concurrent and sequential use of other drugs which may have neurotoxic and/or nephrotoxic properties. These include aminoglycosides, colistin, amphotericin B, cyclosporin, cisplatin, frusemide and ethacrynic acid.

However, there is no evidence of synergistic toxicity with combinations with Targocid.

Dosage must be adapted in patients with renal impairment (see *Dosage*).

The use of Targocid may result in overgrowth of non-susceptible organisms. If new infections due to bacteria or fungi appear during treatment appropriate measures should be taken.

*Use in pregnancy:* Animal reproduction studies have not shown evidence of impairment of fertility or teratogenic effects. At high doses in rats there was an increased incidence of stillbirths and neonatal mortality. It is recommended that Targocid should not be used during confirmed or presumed pregnancy or during lactation unless a physician considers that the potential benefits outweigh any possible risk. There is no information about the excretion of teicoplanin in milk or placental transfer of the drug.

*Interactions:* In clinical trials teicoplanin has been administered to many patients already receiving various medications including other antibiotics, antihypertensives, anaesthetic agents, cardiac drugs, and antidiabetic agents without evidence of adverse interaction. In particular, in patients treated with concomitant aminoglycosides there was no evidence of synergistic oto- or nephrotoxicity. Animal studies have shown lack of interaction with diazepam, thiopentone, morphine, neuromuscular blocking agents or halothane.

*Side-effects:* Targocid is generally well tolerated. Side-effects rarely require cessation of therapy and are generally mild and transient; serious side-effects are rare. The following adverse events have been reported:
*Local reactions:* erythema, local pain, thrombophlebitis.
  *Allergic:* rash, pruritus, fever, bronchospasm, anaphylactic reactions.
  *Gastro-intestinal:* nausea, vomiting, diarrhoea.
  *Blood:* eosinophilia, leucopenia, thrombocytopenia, thrombocytosis.
  *Liver function:* increases in serum transaminases and/or serum alkaline phosphatase.
  *Renal function:* transient elevations of serum creatinine.
  *Central nervous system:* dizziness and headache.
  *Other reported events with an unknown causal relationship:* Mild hearing loss, tinnitus and vestibular disorder.

*Overdosage:* Targocid is not removed by haemodialysis. Treatment of overdosage should be symptomatic. Several overdoses of 100 mg/kg day have been administered in error to two neutropenic paediatric patients, aged 4 and 8 years. Despite high plasma concentrations of teicoplanin up to 300 mg/l, there were no symptoms or laboratory abnormalities.

**Pharmaceutical precautions** In keeping with good clinical and pharmaceutical practice reconstituted vials of Targocid should be used immediately and any unused portion discarded. On the few occasions when changing circumstances make this impracticable reconstituted solutions should be kept at 4°C and discarded within 24 hours.

The reconstituted solution may be injected directly, or alternatively diluted with: 0.9% Sodium Chloride Injection; Compound Sodium Lactate Injection (Ringer-Lactate Solution, Hartmanns Solution); 5% Dextrose Injection; 0.18% Sodium Chloride and 4% Dextrose Injection; Peritoneal dialysis solution containing 1.36% or 3.86% Dextrose.
Solutions of teicoplanin and aminoglycosides are incompatible when mixed directly and should not be mixed before injection.
Vials of dry Targocid should be stored below 25°C.

**Legal category** POM.

**Package quantities**
*Targocid 200 mg:* Combined pack of one vial providing 200 mg teicoplanin and one ampoule containing Water for Injections, PhEur.
  *Targocid 400 mg:* Combined pack of one vial providing 400 mg teicoplanin and one ampoule containing Water for Injections, PhEur.

**Further information**
*Pharmacokinetics:* Following injection teicoplanin rapidly penetrates into tissues, including skin, fat and bone, and reaches the highest concentrations in the kidney, trachea, lungs and adrenals. Teicoplanin does not readily penetrate into the cerebrospinal fluid (CSF).
In man the plasma level profile after intravenous administration indicates a biphasic distribution (with a rapid distribution phase having a half life of about 0.3 hour, followed by a more prolonged distribution phase having a half life of about 3 hours), followed by slow elimination (with a terminal elimination half life of about 150 hours). At 6 mg/kg administered intravenously at 0, 12, 24 hours and every 24 hours thereafter as a 30 minute infusion, a predicted trough serum concentration of 10 mg/l would be reached by Day 4. The steady state volume of distribution after 3 to 6 mg/kg intravenously ranges from 0.94 l/kg to 1.4

l/kg. The volume of distribution in children is not substantially different from that in adults.
Approximately 90–95% teicoplanin is bound with weak affinity to plasma proteins. Teicoplanin penetrates readily into blister exudates and into joint fluid; it penetrates neutrophils and enhances their bactericidal activity; it does not penetrate red blood cells.
No metabolites of teicoplanin have been identified; more than 97% of the administered teicoplanin is excreted unchanged.
The elimination of teicoplanin from the plasma is prolonged with a terminal half life of elimination in man of about 150 hours. Teicoplanin is excreted mainly in the urine.

**Product licence numbers**
Targocid 200 mg vial    4425/0088
    400 mg vial    4425/0089
Water for Injections PhEur 4425/0090

*Product licence holder:* Marion Merrell Ltd., Broadwater Park, Denham, Uxbridge, Middlesex UB9 5HP

## TARIVID* I.V. INFUSION 2 mg/ml

**Presentation** Tarivid I.V. infusion contains 100 mg ofloxacin (as 110 mg ofloxacin hydrochloride) in 50 ml clear, greenish-yellow solution, or 200 mg ofloxacin (as 220 mg ofloxacin hydrochloride) in 100 ml greenish-yellow solution.

**Uses** Ofloxacin is a synthetic 4-fluoroquinolone antibacterial agent with bactericidal activity against a wide range of Gram-negative and Gram-positive organisms. It is indicated for the treatment of the following infections when caused by sensitive organisms:
Lower respiratory tract: Acute and chronic infections.
Upper and lower urinary tract: Acute and chronic lower urinary tract infections; acute and chronic upper urinary tract infections (pyelonephritis).
Septicaemia.
Skin and soft tissue infections.
Microbiological results indicate that the following pathogens may be regarded as sensitive: *Staphylococcus aureus* (including methicillin resistant staphylococci), *Staphylococcus epidermidis*, *Neisseria* species, *Escherichia coli, Citrobacter, Klebsiella, Enterobacter, Hafnia, Proteus* (indole-negative and indole-positive strains), *Salmonella, Shigella, Acinetobacter, Yersinia enterocolitica, Campylobacter jejuni, Aeromonas, Plesiomonas, Vibrio cholerae, Vibrio parahaemolyticus, Haemophilus influenzae, Chlamydiae, Legionella*.
Variable sensitivity is shown by Streptococci, *Serratia marcescens, Pseudomonas aeruginosa* and Mycoplasmas.
Anaerobic bacteria (e.g. *Fusobacterium* species, *Bacteroides* species, *Eubacterium* species, Peptococci, Peptostreptococci) are normally resistant.
Tarivid is not active against *Treponema pallidum*.

**Dosage and administration** General dosage recommendations: The dose of ofloxacin is determined by the type and severity of the infection.
*Adults:* The usual intravenous dosages in adults are:
Complicated urinary tract infection: 200 mg daily.
Lower respiratory tract infection: 200 mg twice daily
Septicaemia: 200 mg twice daily.
Skin and soft tissue infections: 400 mg twice daily.
The infusion time for Tarivid I.V. should not be less than 30 minutes for 200 mg. Generally, individual doses are to be given at approximately equal intervals.
The dose may be increased to 400 mg twice daily in severe or complicated infections.

*Impaired renal function:* Following a normal initial dose, dosage should be reduced in patients with impairment of renal function. When creatinine clearance is 20–50 ml/minute (serum creatinine 1.5–5.0 mg/dl) the dosage should be reduced by half (100–200 mg daily). If creatinine clearance is less than 20 ml/minute (serum creatinine greater than 5 mg/dl) 100 mg should be given every 24 hours. In patients undergoing haemodialysis or peritoneal dialysis, 100 mg should be given every 24 hours.

*Impaired liver function:* The excretion of ofloxacin may be reduced in patients with severe hepatic dysfunction.

*Children:* Ofloxacin is not indicated for use in children or growing adolescents.

*Elderly:* No adjustment of dosage is required in the elderly, other than that imposed by consideration of renal or hepatic function.

*Duration of treatment:* The duration of treatment is determined according to the response of the causative organisms and the clinical picture. As with all antibacterial agents, treatment with Tarivid should be continued for at least 3 days after the body temperature has returned to normal and the symptoms have subsided.

In most cases of acute infection, a course of treatment lasting 7 to 10 days is sufficient.
Once the patient's condition has improved, the mode of administration should be changed from parenteral to oral, normally at the same total daily dose.
Treatment should not exceed 2 months duration.

**Contra-indications, warnings, etc**
*Contra-indications:* Ofloxacin should not be used in patients with known hypersensitivity to 4-quinolone antibacterials, or any of the excipients.
Ofloxacin should not be used in patients with a past history of tendinitis.
Ofloxacin, like other 4-quinolones, is contra-indicated in patients with a history of epilepsy or with a lowered seizure threshold. Ofloxacin is contra-indicated in children or growing adolescents, and in pregnant or breast-feeding women, since animal experiments do not entirely exclude the risk of damage to the cartilage of joints in the growing subject.
Patients with latent or actual defects in glucose-6-phosphate dehydrogenase activity may be prone to haemolytic reactions when treated with quinolone antibacterial agents.

*Precautions:* Patients being treated with ofloxacin should not expose themselves unnecessarily to strong sunlight and should avoid UV rays (sunlamps, solaria). Caution is recommended if the drug is to be used in psychotic patients or in patients with a history of psychiatric disease.

*Warnings:* Sudden reductions in blood pressure may occur when Tarivid I.V. is administered with hypotensive agents. In such cases, or if the drug is given concomitantly with barbiturate anaesthetics, cardiovascular function should be monitored.
Administration of antibiotics, especially if prolonged, may lead to proliferation of resistant microorganisms. The patient's condition must therefore be checked at regular intervals. If a secondary infection occurs, appropriate measures must be taken.

*Use in pregnancy and lactation:* The safety of this medicinal product for use in human pregnancy has not been established. Reproduction studies performed in rats and rabbits did not reveal any evidence of teratogenicity, impairment of fertility or impairment of peri- and post-natal development. However, as with other quinolones, ofloxacin has been shown to cause arthropathy in immature animals and therefore its use during pregnancy is not recommended. Studies in rats have indicated that ofloxacin is secreted in milk. It should therefore not be used during lactation.

*Interactions:* Prolongation of bleeding time has been reported during concomitant administration of Tarivid and anticoagulants.
There may be a further lowering of the cerebral seizure threshold when quinolones are given concurrently with other drugs which lower the seizure threshold e.g. theophylline. However, ofloxacin is not thought to cause a pharmacokinetic interaction with theophylline, unlike some other fluoroquinolones.
Further lowering of the cerebral seizure threshold may also occur with certain nonsteroidal antiinflammatory drugs.
Ofloxacin may cause a slight increase in serum concentrations of glibenclamide administered concurrently; patients treated with this combination should be closely monitored.
With high doses of quinolones, impairment of excretion and an increase in serum levels may occur when co-administered with other drugs that undergo renal tubular secretion (e.g. probenecid, cimetidine, frusemide and methotrexate).

*Interactions with laboratory tests:* Determination of opiates or porphyrins in urine may give false-positive results during treatment with ofloxacin.

*Side-effects:* In rare cases after i.v. infusion, a reduction in blood pressure may occur. If this effect is marked, the infusion should be stopped. Pain, reddening of the infusion site and thrombophlebitis have been reported in rare cases.
The overall frequency of adverse reactions from the clinical trial data base is about 7%. The commonest events involved the gastrointestinal system (about 5.0%) and the nervous system (about 2.0%).
The following provides a tabulation based on post marketing experience where occasional represents a frequency of 0.1-1.0%, rare <0.1%, very rare <0.01% and isolated cases <<0.01%.
*Digestive and liver side effects:* Occasional: Nausea and vomiting, diarrhoea, abdominal pain, gastric symptoms. (Diarrhoea may sometimes be a symptom of enterocolitis which may, in some cases, be haemorrhagic).
Rare: Loss of appetite, increase in liver enzymes and/or bilirubin.
Very rare: cholestatic jaundice, hepatitis or severe liver damage may develop. A particular form of enterocolitis that can occur with antibiotics is pseudomembranous colitis (in most cases due to *Clostrid-*

ium difficile). Even if *Clostridium difficile* is only suspected, administration of ofloxacin should be discontinued immediately and appropriate treatment given. Drugs that inhibit peristalsis should not be administered in such cases.

*Central nervous system:* Occasional: Headache, dizziness, sleep disorders, restlessness.

Rare: Confusion, nightmares, anxiety, depression, hallucinations and psychotic reactions, drowsiness, unsteady gait and tremor (due to disorders of muscular co-ordination), neuropathy, numbness and paraesthesia, or hypaesthesiae, visual disturbances, disturbances of taste and smell (including, in exceptional cases, loss of function), extrapyramidal symptoms.

Very rare: Convulsions, hearing disorders (including, in exceptional cases, loss of hearing).

These reactions have occurred in some patients after the first dose of ofloxacin. In such cases, discontinue treatment immediately.

*Cardiovascular system:* Tachycardia and a temporary decrease in blood pressure have been reported.

Rare: circulatory collapse (due to pronounced drop in blood pressure).

*Haematological side effects:* Very rare: anaemia, leucopenia (including agranulocytosis), thrombocytopenia, pancytopenia. Only in some cases are these due to bone marrow depression. In very rare cases, haemolytic anaemia may develop.

*Renal side effects:* Rare: Disturbances of kidney function.

Isolated cases: Acute interstitial nephritis or an increase in serum creatinine, which may progress to acute renal failure.

*Allergic and skin side effects:* Occasional: Skin rash, itching.

Very rare: Rash on exposure to strong sunlight, other severe skin reactions. Hypersensitivity reactions, immediate or delayed, usually involving the skin (e.g. erythema multiforme, Stevens-Johnson syndrome, Lyell's syndrome and vasculitis) may occur. In exceptional circumstances, vasculitis can lead to skin lesions including necrosis and may involve internal organs. There are rarely other signs of anaphylaxis such as tachycardia, fever, dyspnoea, shock, angioneurotic oedema, vasculitic reactions, eosinophilia. In these cases treatment should be discontinued immediately and where appropriate, supportive treatment given.

Isolated cases: Pneumonitis.

*Other side effects:* Rare: Malaise.

Very rare: Excessive rise or fall in blood-sugar levels. Weakness, joint and muscle pains (in isolated cases these may be symptoms of rhabdomyolysis).

Isolated cases: Tendon discomfort, including inflammation and rupture of tendons (e.g. the Achilles tendon) particularly in patients treated concurrently with corticosteroids. In the event of signs of inflammation of a tendon, treatment with Tarivid must be halted immediately and appropriate treatment must be initiated for the affected tendon.

The possibility cannot be ruled out that ofloxacin may trigger an attack of porphyria in predisposed patients.

Except in very rare instances (e.g. isolated cases of smell, taste and hearing disorders) the adverse effects observed subsided after discontinuation of ofloxacin.

*Ability to drive:* Since there have been occasional reports of somnolence, impairment of skills, dizziness and visual disturbances, patients should know how they react to Tarivid before they drive or operate machinery. These effects may be enhanced by alcohol.

*Overdosage:* The most important signs to be expected following acute overdosage are CNS symptoms such as confusion, dizziness, impairment of consciousness and convulsive seizures, as well as gastrointestinal reactions such as nausea and mucosal erosions.

Elimination of ofloxacin may be increased by forced diuresis.

**Pharmaceutical precautions** Tarivid I.V. should be stored at ambient temperature in a dry place. It should be protected from light and kept in its cardboard box until immediately before use. Once the infusion bottle has been opened, the solution should be used immediately.

Tarivid I.V. should be administered alone unless compatibility with other infusion fluids has been demonstrated. Compatible infusion solutions include isotonic sodium chloride solution, Ringer's solution and 5% glucose solution. Heparin and ofloxacin are incompatible.

**Legal category** POM.

**Package quantities** Tarivid I.V. is available in packs of 50 or 100 ml solution.

**Further information.** Crystalluria has not been reported with ofloxacin.

**Product licence number** 0086/0145
*Product licence holder:* Hoechst UK Ltd., Hoechst House, Salisbury Road, Middlesex TW4 7JH

## TARIVID* TABLETS 200 mg and 400 mg

**Presentation** Tarivid tablets contain ofloxacin. The 200 mg tablet is film coated, yellowish-white, oblong (14 x 7 mm), biconvex with a score line marked with MXI and the Hoechst logo on either side of the score line. The 400 mg tablet is film coated, yellow, oblong (18 x 8 mm), biconvex with a score mark. Excipients include lactose.

**Uses** Ofloxacin is a synthetic 4-fluoroquinolone antibacterial agent with bactericidal activity against a wide range of Gram-negative and Gram-positive organisms. It is indicated for the treatment of the following infections when caused by sensitive organisms: Upper and lower urinary tract infections; lower respiratory tract infections; uncomplicated urethral and cervical gonorrhoea; non-gonococcal urethritis and cervicitis; skin and soft-tissue infections.

Microbiological results indicate that the following pathogens may be regarded as sensitive: *Staphylococcus aureus* (including methicillin resistant staphylococci), *Staphylococcus epidermidis, Neisseria* species, *Escherichia coli, Citrobacter, Klebsiella, Enterobacter, Hafnia, Proteus* (indole-negative and indole-positive strains), *Haemophilus influenzae,* Chlamydiae, *Legionella, Gardnerella.*

Variable sensitivity is shown by Streptococci, *Serratia marcescens, Pseudomonas aeruginosa* and Mycoplasmas.

Anaerobic bacteria (e.g. *Fusobacterium* species, *Bacteroides* species, *Eubacterium* species, Peptococci, Peptostreptococci) are normally resistant.

Tarivid is not active against *Treponema pallidum.*

**Dosage and administration:** General dosage recommendations: The dose of ofloxacin is determined by the type and severity of the infection. The dosage range for adults is 200 mg to 800 mg daily. Up to 400 mg may be given as a single dose, preferably in the morning, larger doses should be given as two divided doses. Generally, individual doses are to be given at approximately equal intervals. Tarivid tablets should be swallowed with liquid; they should not be taken within two hours of magnesium/aluminium containing antacids, sucralfate or iron preparations since reduction of absorption of ofloxacin can occur.

Lower urinary tract infection: 200–400 mg daily.

Upper urinary tract infection: 200–400 mg daily increasing, if necessary, to 400 mg twice a day.

Lower respiratory tract infection: 400 mg daily increasing, if necessary, to 400 mg twice daily.

Uncomplicated urethral and cervical gonorrhoea: A single dose of 400 mg.

Non-gonococcal urethritis and cervicitis: 400 mg daily in single or divided doses.

Skin and soft tissue infections: 400 mg twice a day.

*Impaired renal function:* Following a normal initial dose, dosage should be reduced in patients with impairment of renal function. When creatinine clearance is 20–50 ml/minute (serum creatinine 1.5–5.0 mg/dl) the dosage should be reduced by half (100–200 mg daily). If creatinine clearance is less than 20 ml/minute (serum creatinine greater than 5 mg/dl) 100 mg should be given every 24 hours. In patients undergoing haemodialysis or peritoneal dialysis, 100 mg should be given every 24 hours.

*Impaired liver function:* The excretion of ofloxacin may be reduced in patients with severe hepatic dysfunction.

*Children:* Ofloxacin is not indicated for use in children or growing adolescents.

*Elderly:* No adjustment of dosage is required in the elderly, other than that imposed by consideration of renal or hepatic function.

*Duration of treatment:* Duration of treatment is dependent on the severity of the infection and the response to treatment. The usual treatment period is 5–10 days except in uncomplicated gonorrhoea, where a single dose is recommended.

Treatment should not exceed 2 months duration.

**Contra-indications, warnings, etc**

*Contra-indications:* Ofloxacin should not be used in patients with known hypersensitivity to 4-quinolone antibacterials, or any of the tablet excipients.

Ofloxacin should not be used in patients with a past history of tendinitis.

Ofloxacin, like other 4-quinolones, is contra-indicated in patients with a history of epilepsy or with a lowered seizure threshold. Ofloxacin is contra-indicated in children or growing adolescents, and in pregnant or breast-feeding women, since animal experiments do not entirely exclude the risk of damage to the cartilage of joints in the growing subject.

Patients with latent or actual defects in glucose-6-phosphate dehydrogenase activity may be prone to haemolytic reactions when treated with quinolone antibacterial agents.

*Warnings and precautions:* Patients being treated with ofloxacin should not expose themselves unnecessarily to strong sunlight and should avoid UV rays (sunlamps, solaria). Caution is recommended if the drug is to be used in psychotic patients or in patients with a history of psychiatric disease.

Administration of antibiotics, especially if prolonged, may lead to proliferation of resistant microorganisms. The patient's condition must therefore be checked at regular intervals. If a secondary infection occurs, appropriate measures must be taken.

*Use in pregnancy and lactation:* The safety of this medicinal product for use in human pregnancy has not been established. Reproduction studies performed in rats and rabbits did not reveal any evidence of teratogenicity, impairment of fertility or impairment of peri- and post-natal development. However, as with other quinolones, ofloxacin has been shown to cause arthropathy in immature animals and therefore its use during pregnancy is not recommended. Studies in rats have indicated that ofloxacin is secreted in milk. It should therefore not be used during lactation.

*Interactions:* Co-administered magnesium/aluminium antacids, sucralfate or iron preparations can reduce absorption. Therefore, ofloxacin should be taken 2 hours before such preparations. Prolongation of bleeding time has been reported during concomitant administration of Tarivid and anticoagulants.

There may be a further lowering of the cerebral seizure threshold when quinolones are given concurrently with other drugs which lower the seizure threshold, (e.g. theophylline). However, ofloxacin is not thought to cause a pharmacokinetic interaction with theophylline, unlike some other fluoroquinolones.

Further lowering of the cerebral seizure threshold may also occur with certain nonsteroidal anti-inflammatory drugs.

Ofloxacin may cause a slight increase in serum concentrations of glibenclamide administered concurrently; patients treated with this combination should be closely monitored.

With high doses of quinolones, impairment of excretion and an increase in serum levels may occur when co-administered with other drugs that undergo renal tubular secretion (e.g. probenecid, cimetidine, frusemide and methotrexate).

*Interactions with laboratory tests:* Determination of opiates or porphyrins in urine may give false-positive results during treatment with ofloxacin.

*Side-effects:* The overall frequency of adverse reactions from the clinical trial data base is about 7%. The commonest events involved the gastrointestinal system (about 5%) and the nervous system (about 2%).

The following provides a tabulation based on post marketing experience where occasional represents a frequency of 0.1-1%, rare <0.1%, very rare <0.01% and isolated cases <<0.01%.

*Digestive and liver side effects:* Occasional: Nausea and vomiting, diarrhoea, abdominal pain, gastric symptoms. (Diarrhoea may sometimes be a symptom of enterocolitis which may, in some cases, be haemorrhagic). Rare: Loss of appetite, increase in liver enzymes and/or bilirubin. Very rare: cholestatic jaundice; hepatitis or severe liver damage may develop. A particular form of enterocolitis that can occur with antibiotics is pseudomembranous colitis (in most cases due to *Clostridium difficile*). Even if *Clostridium difficile* is only suspected, administration of ofloxacin should be discontinued immediately, and appropriate treatment given. Drugs that inhibit peristalsis should not be administered in such cases.

*Central nervous system:* Occasional: Headache, dizziness, sleep disorders, restlessness. Rare: Confusion, nightmares, anxiety, depression, hallucinations and psychotic reactions, drowsiness, unsteady gait and tremor (due to disorders of muscular co-ordination), neuropathy, numbness and paraesthesia or hypaesthesia, visual disturbances, disturbance of taste and smell (including, in exceptional cases, loss of function), extrapyramidal symptoms. Very rare: Convulsions, hearing disorders (including, in exceptional cases, loss of hearing). These reactions have occurred in some patients after the first dose of ofloxacin. In such cases, discontinue treatment immediately.

*Cardiovascular system:* Tachycardia and a temporary decrease in blood pressure have been reported. Rare: Circulatory collapse (due to pronounced drop in blood pressure).

*Haematological side effects:* Very rare: anaemia, leucopenia (including agranulocytosis), thrombocytopenia, pancytopenia. Only in some cases are these due to bone marrow depression. In very rare cases, haemolytic anaemia may develop.

*Renal side effects:* Rare: Disturbances of kidney function. Isolated cases: Acute interstitial nephritis, or an increase in serum creatinine, which may progress to acute renal failure.

*Allergic and skin side effects:* Occasional: Skin rash, itching. Very rare: Rash on exposure to strong sunlight, other sever skin reactions. Hypersensitivity reactions, immediate or delayed, usually involving the skin (e.g. erythema multiforme, Stevens-Johnson syndrome, Lyell's syndrome and vasculitis) may occur. In exceptional circumstances, vasculitis can lead to skin lesions including necrosis and may also involve internal organs. There are rarely other signs of anaphylaxis such as tachycardia, fever, dyspnoea, shock, angioneurotic oedema, vasculitic reactions, eosinophilia. In these cases treatment should be discontinued immediately and where appropriate, supportive treatment given.

Isolated cases: Pneumonitis.

*Other side effects:* Rare: Malaise. Very rare: Excessive rise or fall in blood-sugar levels. Weakness, joint and muscle pains (in isolated cases these may be symptoms of rhabdomyolysis). Isolated cases: Tendon discomfort including inflammation and rupture of tendons (e.g. the Achilles tendon) particularly in patients treated concurrently with corticosteroids. In the event of signs of inflammation of the tendon, treatment with Tarivid must be halted immediately and appropriate treatment must be initiated for the affected tendon.

The possibility cannot be ruled out that ofloxacin may trigger an attack of porphyria in predisposed patients.

Except in very rare instances (e.g. isolated cases of smell, taste and hearing disorders) the adverse effects observed subsided after discontinuation of ofloxacin.

*Ability to drive:* Since there have been occasional reports of somnolence, impairment of skills, dizziness and visual disturbances, patients should know how they react to Tarivid before they drive or operate machinery. These effects may be enhanced by alcohol.

*Overdosage:*The most important signs to be expected following acute overdosage are CNS symptoms such as confusion, dizziness, impairment of consciousness and convulsive seizures, as well as gastrointestinal reactions such as nausea and mucosal erosions.

In the case of overdose steps to remove any unabsorbed ofloxacin e.g. gastric lavage, administration of adsorbants and sodium sulphate, if possible during the first 30 minutes are recommended; antacids are recommended for the protection of the gastric mucosa.

Elimination of ofloxacin may be increased by forced diuresis.

**Pharmaceutical precautions** Keep medicines out of the reach of children. Store in a dry place.

**Legal category** POM.

**Package quantities** Blister packs of 10, 20 and 100 tablets (200 mg) and 5, 10 and 50 tablets (400 mg).

**Further information** Crystalluria has not been reported with ofloxacin.

**Product licence numbers**
Tarivid 200 mg    0086/0139
Tarivid 400 mg    0086/0150

*Product licence holder:* Hoechst UK Ltd., Hoechst House, Salisbury Road, Middlesex TW4 7JH

# TELFAST* 120 & 180 ▼

## Qualitative and quantitative composition
Telfast 120: Active ingredient: fexofenadine base 112 mg (as fexofenadine hydrochloride 120 mg).
Telfast 180: Active ingredient: fexofenadine base 168 mg (as fexofenadine hydrochloride 180 mg).

## Pharmaceutical form
Telfast 120: Peach, modified capsule-shaped, film-coated tablets.
Telfast 180: Peach, capsule-shaped, film-coated tablets.

## Clinical particulars

*Therapeutic indications:*
Telfast 120: Relief of symptoms associated with seasonal allergic rhinitis.
Telfast 180: Relief of symptoms associated with chronic idiopathic urticaria.

*Posology and method of administration:*
*Adults and children aged 12 years and over:*
Telfast 120: The recommended dose of fexofenadine hydrochloride for adults and children aged 12 years and over is 120 mg once daily.
Telfast 180:The recommended dose of fexofenadine hydrochloride for adults and children aged 12 years and over is 180 mg once daily.
Fexofenadine is a pharmacologically active metabolite of terfenadine.
*Children under 12 years of age:* The efficacy and safety of fexofenadine hydrochloride has not been studied in children under 12.
*Special risk groups:* Studies in special risk groups (elderly, renally or hepatically impaired patients) indicate that it is not necessary to adjust the dose of fexofenadine hydrochloride in these patients.

*Contra-indications:* The product is contraindicated in patients with known hypersensitivity to any of its ingredients.

*Special warnings and precautions for use:* As with most new drugs there is only limited data in the elderly and renally or hepatically impaired patients. Fexofenadine hydrochloride should be administered with care in these special groups.

*Interaction with other medicaments and other forms of interaction:*Fexofenadine does not undergo hepatic biotransformation. Coadministration of fexofenadine hydrochloride with erythromycin or ketoconazole has been found to result in a 2-3 times increase in the level of fexofenadine in plasma. The changes were not accompanied by any effects on the QT interval and were not associated with any increase in adverse events compared to the drugs given singly.

Animal studies have shown that the increase in plasma levels of fexofenadine observed after coadministration of erythromycin or ketoconazole, appears to be due to an increase in gastrointestinal absorption and either a decrease in biliary excretion or gastrointestinal secretion, respectively.

No interaction between fexofenadine and omeprazole was observed. However, the administration of an antacid containing aluminium and magnesium hydroxide gels 15 minutes prior to fexofenadine hydrochloride caused a reduction in bioavailability, most likely due to binding in the gastrointestinal tract. It is advisable to leave 2 hours between administration of fexofenadine hydrochloride and aluminium and magnesium hydroxide containing antacids.

*Pregnancy and lactation:* No animal reproduction studies have been performed with fexofenadine hydrochloride. Supportive pharmacokinetic studies with terfenadine have been performed and show adequate extent of exposure to fexofenadine at the high dose level in animal reproduction studies performed with terfenadine. In these studies no evidence of teratogenicity or effects on male fertility were observed. Effects on female fertility and on peri and post natal development were seen only at maternally toxic doses.

There is no experience with fexofenadine hydrochloride in pregnant women. As with other medications fexofenadine hydrochloride should not be used during pregnancy unless the expected benefit to the patient outweighs any possible risk to the foetus.

There are no data on the content of human milk after administering fexofenadine hydrochloride. However, when terfenadine was administered to nursing mothers fexofenadine was found to cross into human breast milk. Therefore fexofenadine hydrochloride is not recommended for mothers breast feeding their babies.

*Effects on ability to drive and use machines:* On the basis of the pharmacodynamic profile and reported adverse events it is unlikely that fexofenadine hydrochloride tablets will produce an effect on the ability to drive or use machines. In objective tests, Telfast has been shown to have no significant effects on central nervous system function. This means that patients may drive or perform tasks that require concentration. However, in order to identify sensitive people who have an unusual reaction to drugs, it is advisable to check the individual response before driving or performing complicated tasks.

*Undesirable effects:* In controlled clinical trials the most commonly reported adverse events were headache (7.3%), drowsiness (2.3%), nausea (1.5%), dizziness (1.5%) and fatigue (0.9%). The incidence of these events observed with fexofenadine was similar to that observed with placebo.

*Overdose:* There has been no reported case of an acute overdose of fexofenadine hydrochloride. Standard measures should be considered to remove any unabsorbed drug. Haemodialysis does not effectively remove fexofenadine hydrochloride from blood.

**Pharmacological properties**

*Pharmacodynamic properties:* Fexofenadine hydrochloride is a non-sedating $H_1$ antihistamine. Fexofenadine is a pharmacologically active metabolite of terfenadine.

Human histamine wheal and flare studies following single and twice daily doses of fexofenadine hydrochloride demonstrate that the drug exhibits an antihistaminic effect beginning within one hour, achieving maximum at 6 hours and lasting 24 hours. There was no evidence of tolerance to these effects after 28 days of dosing. A positive dose-response relationship between doses of 10 mg to 130 mg taken orally was found to exist. In this model of antihistaminic activity, it was found that doses of at least 130 mg were required to achieve a consistent effect that was maintained over a 24 hour period. Maximum inhibition in skin wheal and flare areas were greater than 80%.

No significant differences in $QT_c$ intervals were observed in seasonal allergic rhinitis patients given

fexofenadine hydrochloride up to 240 mg twice daily for 2 weeks when compared to placebo. Also, no significant change in $QT_c$ intervals was observed in healthy subjects given fexofenadine hydrochloride up to 60 mg twice daily for 6 months, 400 mg twice daily for 6.5 days and 240 mg once daily for 1 year, when compared to placebo. Fexofenadine at concentrations 32 times greater than the therapeutic concentration in man had no effect on the delayed rectifier K+ channel cloned from human heart.

Fexofenadine hydrochloride (5-10 mg/kg p.o.) inhibited antigen induced bronchospasm in sensitised guinea pigs and inhibited histamine release at supratherapeutic concentrations (10-100 micromolar) from peritoneal mast cells.

*Pharmacokinetic properties:*Fexofenadine hydrochloride is rapidly absorbed into the body following oral administration, with $T_{max}$ occurring at approximately 1-3 hours post dose. The mean $C_{max}$ value was approximately 427 ng/ml following the administration of a 120 mg dose once daily and approximately 494 ng/ml following the administration of a 180 mg dose once daily.

Fexofenadine is 60-70% plasma protein bound. Fexofenadine undergoes negligible metabolism, as it was the only major compound identified in urine and faeces of animals and man. The plasma concentration profiles of fexofenadine follow a bi-exponential decline with a terminal elimination half-life ranging from 11 to 15 hours after multiple dosing. The single and multiple dose pharmacokinetics of fexofenadine are linear between 40 mg and 240 mg taken daily. The major route of elimination is believed to be via biliary excretion while up to 10% of ingested dose is excreted unchanged through the urine.

*Preclinical safety data:* Dogs tolerated 450 mg/kg administered twice daily for 6 months and showed no toxicity other than occasional emesis. Also, in single dose dog and rodent studies, no treatment-related gross findings were observed following necropsy.

Radiolabelled fexofenadine hydrochloride in tissue distribution studies of the rat indicated that fexofenadine did not cross the blood brain barrier.

Fexofenadine hydrochloride was found to be non-mutagenic in various *in vitro* and *in vivo* mutagenicity tests.

The carcinogenic potential of fexofenadine hydrochloride was assessed using terfenadine studies with supporting pharmacokinetic studies showing fexofenadine hydrochloride exposure (via plasma AUC values). No evidence of carcinogenicity was observed in rats and mice given terfenadine (up to 150 mg/kg/day).

**Pharmaceutical particulars**

*List of excipients:* Tablet core: Microcrystalline Cellulose, Pregelatinised Maize Starch, Croscarmellose Sodium, Magnesium Stearate

Film coat: Hydroxypropyl Methylcellulose, Povidone, Titanium Dioxide (E171), Colloidal Anhydrous Silica, Macrogol 400, Iron oxide (E172).

*Incompatibilities:* None

*Shelf life:* 18 months

*Special precautions for storage:* None

*Nature and contents of container:* Blue or white opaque polyvinylchloride blisters (pharmaceutical grade) 200 micrometers thick with a polyvinylidine chloride coating of 90 g/m² on the internal surface of the blister. The PVC/PE/PVDC is sealed to hard tempered aluminium foil 20 micrometer thick with a vinyl heat seal coating. The blisters are packaged into cardboard boxes.

*Instructions for use/handling:* No special instructions.

*Marketing authorisation holder:* Marion Merrell Ltd., Broadwater Park, Denham, Uxbridge, Middlesex, UB9 5HP

**Marketing authorisation numbers**
Telfast 120:          4425/0157
Telfast 180:          4425/0158

**Date of approval/revision of SPC** May 1997.

**Legal category** POM.

# TRENTAL 400

**Qualitative and quantitative composition** Oxpentifylline 400 mg

**Pharmaceutical form** Slow release sugar coated tablet

**Clinical particulars**

*Therapeutic indications:* Trental 400 is indicated in the treatment of peripheral vascular disease, including intermittent claudication and rest pain.

*Posology and method of administration:* The recommended initial dose is 1 tablet (400 mg) three times daily; two tablets daily may prove sufficient in some patients, particularly for maintenance therapy. Tablets should be taken with or immediately after meals, and swallowed whole with plenty of water.

*Elderly:* No special dosage requirements.

*Children:* Trental 400 is not suitable for use in children.

*Special cases:* In patients with impairment of renal function (creatinine clearance below 30 ml/min) a dose reduction by approximately 30% to 50% may be necessary guided by individual tolerance.

*Contra-indications:* Trental 400 is contra-indicated in cases where there is known hypersensitivity to the active constituent, oxpentifylline other methyl xanthines or any of the excipients. Also in patients with cerebral haemorrhage, extensive retinal haemorrhage, acute myocardial infarction and severe cardiac arrhythmias.

*Special warnings and special precautions for use:* In patients with hypotension or severe coronary artery disease, Trental 400 should be used with caution, as a transient hypotensive effect is possible and, in isolated cases, might result in a reduction in coronary artery perfusion.

Particularly careful monitoring is required in patients with impaired renal function. In patients with a creatinine clearance of less than 30 ml/min it may be necessary to reduce the daily dose of Trental 400 to one or two tablets to avoid accumulation. In patients with severely impaired liver function the dosage may need to be reduced.

*Interactions with other medicaments and other forms of interaction:* High doses of Trental injection have been shown, in rare cases, to intensify the hypoglycaemic action of insulin and oral hypoglycaemic agents. However, no effect on insulin release has been observed with Trental following oral administration.

Trental 400 may potentiate the effect of anti-hypertensive agents and the dosage of the latter may need to be reduced.

Trental 400 should not be given concomitantly with ketorolac as there is increased risk of bleeding and/or prolongation of prothrombin time.

Concomitant administration of oxpentifylline and theophylline may increase theophylline levels in some patients. Therefore there may be an increase in and intensification of adverse effects of theophylline.

*Pregnancy and lactation:* There is no information on the use of Trental in pregnancy but no untoward effects have been found in animal studies. Trental 400 should not be administered during pregnancy.

Oxpentifylline passes into breast milk in minute quantities. Because insufficient experience has been gained, the possible risks and benefits must be weighed before administration of Trental 400 to breast feeding mothers.

*Effects on ability to drive and use machines:* No effect known.

*Undesirable effects:* Gastrointestinal side-effects (e.g. nausea, vomiting, diarrhoea), may occur which, in individual cases, could necessitate discontinuation of treatment. Headache, dizziness, agitation and sleep disorders may occasionally occur as well as, in isolated cases intrahepatic cholestasis and transaminase elevation.

There have been reports of flushing, occasionally tachycardia and rarely angina pectoris and hypotension, particularly if using high doses of oxpentifylline. In such cases a discontinuation of the medication or a reduction of the daily dosage is required.

Hypersensitivity reactions such as pruritus, rash, urticaria, anaphylactic or anaphylactoid reactions with angioneurotic edema or bronchospasm may occur in isolated cases and usually disappear rapidly after discontinuation of the drug treatment

A few very rare events of bleeding (e.g. skin, mucosa) have been reported in patients treated with Trental with and without anticoagulants or platelet aggregation inhibitors. The serious cases are predominantly concentrated in the gastrointestinal, genitourinary, multiple site and surgical wound areas and are associated with bleeding risk factors. A causal relationship between Trental therapy and bleeding has not been established. Thrombocytopenia has occurred in isolated cases.

*Overdose:* The treatment of overdosage should be symptomatic with particular attention to supporting the cardiovascular system.

**Pharmacological properties**

*Pharmacodynamic properties:* Leukocyte properties of haemorrheologic importance have been modified in animal and in vitro human studies. Oxpentifylline has been shown to increase leukocyte deformability and to inhibit neutrophil adhesion and activation.

*Pharmacokinetic properties:* The half life of absorption of Trental 400 is 4-6 hours. Oxpentifylline is extensively metabolised, mainly in the liver. Sixty percent of a single dose of Trental 400 is eliminated via the kidney over 24 hours.

*Preclinical safety data:* Nothing of clinical relevance.

**Pharmaceutical particulars**

*List of excipients:* Hydroxyethyl cellulose, polyvinylpyrrolidone, talc, magnesium stearate, sucrose, gum arabic, polyethylene glycol 6000, erythrosine (E127), titanium dioxide (E171).

*Incompatibilities:* None known.

*Shelf life:* 5 years.

*Special precautions for storage:* Store below 25°C in a dry place.

*Nature and contents of container:* Blister Pack (Alu/PVC) of 10 and 90 tablets, amber glass bottles of 100 and 250 tablets, plastic pots of 100 and 250 tablets.

*Instruction for use/handling:* None

*Marketing authorisation holder:* Hoechst UK Ltd, Hoechst House, Salisbury Road, Hounslow, Middlesex, TW4 7JH.

**Marketing authorisation number**   0086/0058

**Date of approval/revision of SPC**   31 January 97.

**Legal category** POM

# TRILUDAN* TABLETS
# TRILUDAN* FORTE TABLETS
# TRILUDAN* SUSPENSION

**Presentation**

*Triludan Tablets:* White to off white, round, flat faced, bevel edged tablets with 'M' in two concentric circles on one side and a scored bisect line on the other. Each tablet contains 60 mg terfenadine.

*Triludan Forte Tablets:* White to off white, convex, capsule shaped tablets with inscribed 'T', 'F' and scoreline on one face. Each tablet contains 120 mg terfenadine.

*Triludan Suspension:* A white, oral, sugar-free suspension with a banana flavour containing 30 mg terfenadine in 5 ml.

**Uses**   Triludan is an antihistamine, indicated for the symptomatic relief of hay fever, allergic rhinitis and allergic skin conditions.

**Dosage and administration**

*Adults and children over 12 years:* The following may be given as a single dose or in two divided doses. *Allergic skin conditions:* 120 mg per day. Hayfever, allergic rhinitis: Starting dose is 60 mg daily, increasing to 120 mg daily if required.

*Children: Allergic skin conditions, hayfever, allergic rhinitis:*

6–12 years: 30 mg twice daily.

3–6 years: 15 mg twice daily.

Do not exceed the maximum recommended dose.

**Contra-indications, warnings, etc**

*Contra-indications:* Concomitant administration of terfenadine with azole antifungals or macrolide antibiotics.

Patients with significant hepatic dysfunction.

Patients with known hypersensitivity to terfenadine or any of the ingredients of the formulation.

*Warnings:* QT prolongation and/or ventricular arrhythmias, including torsades de pointes have been reported at doses higher than those recommended and at normal doses in patients in whom terfenadine metabolism is impaired by drugs or by liver disease (see Contra-indications).

If syncope occurs, terfenadine should be discontinued and the patient evaluated for potential arrhythmias.

*Precautions:* Terfenadine is not recommended in patients in whom electrolyte imbalance or prolonged QT interval are known or suspected.

Concomitant use of terfenadine is not recommended in patients receiving potentially arrhythmogenic drugs (such as antiarrhythmic agents, neuroleptics, tricyclic antidepressants), and those producing electrolyte imbalance (e.g. diuretics); astemizole. Although evidence is lacking, the risk of arrhythmia might be increased (see *Warnings*).

*Use in pregnancy and lactation:* Although animal studies have not indicated adverse effects, terfenadine, like most medicines, should not be used during pregnancy unless, in the opinion of the physician, the potential benefits outweigh any potential risks.

The carboxylic acid metabolite is detectable in human breast milk after terfenadine administration. Therefore, infants should not be fed breast milk by a patient receiving terfenadine unless in the opinion of the physician, the potential benefits outweigh the potential risks to the infant.

*Drug interactions:* Terfenadine undergoes extensive metabolism in the liver: there are recognised interactions with drugs which are potent inhibitors of hepatic metabolism: (see *Warnings*).

Concomitant administration of azole antifungals with terfenadine is contra-indicated. Pharmacokinetic data indicate that ketoconazole and itraconazole inhibit the metabolism of terfenadine.

Concomitant administration of macrolide antibiotics with terfenadine is contra-indicated. Pharmacokinetic data indicate that most macrolides inhibit the metabolism of terfenadine. Two studies reported no interaction with concomitant terfenadine and azithromycin at the doses studied. However, because of the chemical similarity of azithromycin to the other macrolides, use with terfenadine is not recommended.

Concurrent use of terfenadine with drugs with arrhythmogenic potential and with those causing electrolyte imbalance is not recommended (see *Precautions*).

Terfenadine should not be taken with grapefruit juice because its metabolism may be inhibited.

*Side-effects:* In controlled clinical studies the incidence of adverse reactions in patients receiving terfenadine was similar to that reported in patients receiving placebo.

These adverse reactions included drowsiness, headache, gastrointestinal distress, fatigue, dizziness, dry mouth and skin eruption or itching (including rash and urticaria).

Other side-effects that have been reported spontaneously during marketing of terfenadine include: anaphylaxis, angioedema, arrhythmias, bronchospasm, confusion, depression, erythema multiforme, galactorrhoea, hair loss or thinning, insomnia, jaundice, liver dysfunction (including transaminase elevations) and rare cases of hepatitis, menstrual disorders, (including dysmenorrhoea), musculoskeletal symptoms, nightmares, palpitations, paraesthesia, photosensitivity, prolonged QT interval, seizures, sweating, syncope (see *Warnings*), thrombocytopenia, tremor, urinary frequency, ventricular tachyarrhythmias, (ventricular tachycardia, ventricular fibrillation and torsade de pointes) and visual disturbances.

*Effects on ability to drive and to use machines:* In objective tests Triludan has been shown to be free from central nervous system side-effects. Reports of drowsiness are extremely rare. This means that patients usually may drive or perform tasks requiring concentration. However, in order to identify sensitive people who have unusual reaction to drugs, it is advisable to check the individual response before driving or performing complicated tasks.

In actual driving tests, Triludan does not impair performance nor is there a change in mood.

*Overdosage:* Several cases of overdosage have been reported. Generally signs and symptoms were absent or mild. However, arrhythmias including ventricular tachycardia or fibrillation or torsades de pointes have been reported at overdoses greater than the recommended dose and have occurred up to 15 hours after the dose. Therefore, in cases of overdosage, cardiac monitoring for at least 24 hours is recommended along with standard measures to remove any unabsorbed drug. Temporary cardiac pacing is the suggested mode of therapy in persistent torsades de pointes. Haemodialysis or haemoperfusion does not effectively remove the major metabolite of terfenadine from blood.

**Pharmaceutical precautions**   None.

**Legal category**   POM

**Package quantities**   *Triludan Tablets:* Packs of 60 and 10 tablets.

*Triludan Forte Tablets:* Packs of 30 and 7 tablets.

*Triludan Suspension:* Amber glass bottles of 200 ml.

**Product licence numbers**

| | |
|---|---|
| Triludan Tablets | 4425/0024 |
| Triludan Forte Tablets | 4425/0091 |
| Triludan Suspension | 4425/0057 |

*Product licence holder:* Marion Merrell Ltd., Broadwater Park, Denham, Uxbridge, Middlesex UB9 5HP

# TRITACE*

**Qualitative and quantitative composition**

1.25 mg ramipril
2.5 mg ramipril
5.0 mg ramipril

**Pharmaceutical form**

1.25 mg: Yellow opaque/white opaque hard gelatin capsules.

2.5 mg: Orange opaque / white opaque hard gelatin capsules.

5.0 mg: Scarlet opaque / white opaque hard gelatin capsules.

Capsules are marked with the strength and the Hoechst logo.

**Clinical particulars**

*Therapeutic indications:* Tritace is indicated in the treatment of mild to moderate hypertension.

Congestive heart failure as adjunctive therapy to diuretics with or without cardiac glycosides.

Tritace has been shown to reduce mortality when administered to patients surviving acute myocardial infarction with clinical evidence of heart failure.

*Posology and method of administration:*
*Hypertension:* The recommended initial dosage in patients not on diuretics and without congestive heart failure is 1.25 mg Tritace once a day. Dosage should be increased incrementally at intervals of 1–2 weeks, based on patient response, up to a maximum of 10 mg once a day.

A 1.25 mg dose will only achieve a therapeutic response in a minority of patients. The usual effective dose range is 2.5–5 mg as a single daily dose. If the patient response is still unsatisfactory at a dose of 10 mg Tritace, combination treatment is recommended.

*Diuretic-treated patients:* The diuretic should be discontinued 2–3 days before beginning therapy with Tritace to reduce the likelihood of symptomatic hypotension. It may be resumed later if required.

*Cardiac failure:* In hypertensive patients who also have congestive heart failure, with or without associated renal insufficiency, symptomatic hypotension has been observed after treatment with ACE inhibitors. In these patients therapy should be started at a dose of 1.25 mg under close medical supervision in hospital.

*Congestive heart failure:* Recommended initial dose: In patients stabilised on diuretic therapy the initial dose is 1.25 mg once daily. Depending on the patient's response, the dose may be increased. It is recommended that the dose, if increased, be doubled at intervals of 1 to 2 weeks. If a daily dose of 2.5 mg or more is required, this may be taken as a single dose or as two divided doses. Maximum permitted daily dose: 10 mg.

In order to minimise the possibility of symptomatic hypotension, patients on previous high dose diuretics should have the diuretic dose reduced before starting Tritace.

*Post myocardial infarction:* Initiation of therapy: treatment must be started in hospital between day 3 and day 10 following AMI the starting dose is 2.5 mg twice a day which is increased to 5 mg twice a day after 2 days. If the initial 2.5 mg dose is not tolerated a dose of 1.25 mg twice a day should be given for two days before increasing to 2.5 mg and 5.0 mg twice a day. If the dose cannot be increased to 2.5 mg twice a day treatment should be withdrawn.

*Maintenance dose:* 2.5 to 5.0 mg twice a day.

*Dosage adjustment in renal impairment:* The usual dose of Tritace is recommended for patients with a creatinine clearance >30 ml/min (serum creatinine <165 micromol/litre). For patients with a creatinine clearance <30 ml/min (serum creatinine >165 micromol/litre) the initial dose is 1.25 mg Tritace once daily and the maximum dose 5 mg Tritace once daily.

In patients with severe renal impairment (creatinine clearance <10 ml/min and serum creatinine of 400-650 micromol/litre), the recommended initial dose is also 1.25 mg Tritace once a day, but the maintenance dose should not exceed 2.5 mg Tritace once a day.

*Dosage in hepatic impairment:* In patients with impaired liver function the metabolism of the parent compound ramipril, and therefore the formation of the bioactive metabolite ramiprilat, is delayed due to diminished activity of esterases in the liver, resulting in elevated plasma ramipril levels. Treatment with Tritace should therefore be initiated at a dose of 1.25 mg under close medical supervision in patients with impaired liver function.

*Elderly:* Caution in elderly patients with concomitant use of diuretics, congestive heart failure or renal or hepatic insufficiency. The dose should be titrated according to need for the control of blood pressure.

*Children:* Tritace has not been studied in children, and therefore use in this age group is not recommended.

Tritace should be taken with a glass of water. Food intake has no marked effect on the extent of absorption.

*Contra-indications:* Hypersensitivity to ramipril or any of the excipients. History of angioneurotic oedema, haemodynamically relevant renal artery stenosis, hypotensive or haemodynamically unstable patients. Pregnancy. Lactation.

*Special warnings and special precautions for use:* Tritace should not be used in patients with aortic or mitral valve stenosis or outflow obstruction.

*Precautions:* Assessment of renal function: Evaluation of the patient should include assessment of renal function prior to initiation of therapy and during treatment.

*Impaired renal function:* Patients with renal insufficiency may require reduced or less frequent doses of Tritace; their renal function should be closely monitored. In the majority, renal function will not alter. There is a risk of impairment of renal function, particularly in patients with renal insufficiency, congestive heart failure, bilateral renal artery stenosis and unilateral renal artery stenosis in the single kidney as well as after renal transplantation. If recognised early, such impairment of renal function is reversible upon discontinuation of therapy.

Patients haemodialysed using high flux polyacrylonitrile ('AN69') membranes are highly likely to experience anaphylactoid reactions if they are treated with ACE inhibitors. This combination should therefore be avoided, either by use of alternative antihypertensive drugs or alternative membranes for dialysis.

Similar reactions have been observed during low-density lipoprotein apheresis with dextran sulphate. This method should, therefore, not be used in patients treated with ACE inhibitors.

Some hypertensive patients with no apparent pre-existing renal disease, may develop minor and usually transient increases in blood urea nitrogen and serum creatinine when Tritace is given, in particular concomitantly with a diuretic. Dosage reduction of Tritace and/or discontinuation of the diuretic may be required. Additionally, in patients with renal insufficiency, there is a risk of hyperkalaemia.

*Impaired liver function:* As ramipril is a prodrug metabolised to its active moiety in the liver, particular caution and close monitoring should be applied to patients with impaired liver function. The metabolism of the parent compound, and therefore the formation of the bioactive metabolite ramiprilat, may be diminished resulting in markedly elevated plasma levels of the parent compound (due to the reduced activity of esterases in the liver).

*Symptomatic hypotension:* In patients with uncomplicated hypertension, symptomatic hypotension has been observed rarely after the initial dose of Tritace as well as after increasing the dose of Tritace. It is more likely to occur in patients who have been volume-and salt-depleted by prolonged diuretic therapy, dietary salt restriction, dialysis, diarrhoea, vomiting or in patients with severe heart failure. Therefore, in these patients, diuretic therapy should be discontinued and volume and/or salt depletion should be corrected before initiating therapy with Tritace.

If symptomatic hypotension occurs, the patient should be placed in a supine position and, if necessary, receive an intravenous infusion of physiological saline. Intravenous atropine may be necessary if there is associated bradycardia. Treatment with Tritace may usually be continued following restoration of effective blood volume and blood pressure.

*Surgery/anaesthesia:* In patients undergoing surgery or during anaesthesia with agents producing hypotension, Tritace may block angiotensin II formation secondary to compensatory renin release. If hypotension occurs and is considered to be due to this mechanism, it can be corrected by appropriate treatment.

*Agranulocytosis and bone marrow depression:* In patients on angiotensin converting enzyme inhibitors agranulocytosis and bone marrow depression have been seen rarely, as well as a reduction in red cell count, haemoglobin content and platelet count. They are more frequent in patients with renal impairment, especially if they have a collagen vascular disease. Regular monitoring of white blood cell counts and protein levels in urine should be considered in patients with collagen vascular disease (e.g. lupus erythematosus and scleroderma), especially associated with impaired renal function and concomitant therapy particularly with corticosteroids and antimetabolites. Patients on allopurinol, immunosuppressants and other substances that may change the blood picture also have increased likelihood of other blood picture changes.

*Hyperkalaemia:* Elevated serum potassium has been observed very rarely in hypertensive patients. Risk factors for the development of hyperkalaemia include renal insufficiency, potassium sparing diuretics and the concomitant use of agents to treat hypokalaemia.

*Interactions with other medicaments and other forms of interaction:* Combination with diuretics or other antihypertensive agents may potentiate the antihypertensive response to Tritace. Adrenergic-blocking drugs should only be combined with ramipril under careful supervision.

Potassium sparing diuretics (spironolactone, amiloride, triamterene) or potassium supplements may increase the risk of hyperkalaemia. Tritace may attenuate the potassium loss caused by thiazide-type diuretics. If concomitant use of these agents is indicated, they should be given with caution and serum potassium should be monitored regularly.

When antidiabetic agents (insulin and sulphonylurea derivatives) are used concurrently, the possibility of increased blood-sugar reduction must be considered.

If Tritace is given with lithium, an increase in serum lithium concentration may occur.

When ACE inhibitors are administered simultaneously with non-steroidal anti-inflammatory drugs (e.g. acetylsalicylic acid and indomethacin), attenuation of the antihypertensive effect may occur.

The protein binding of ramipril is about 73% and of ramiprilat about 56%.

*Pregnancy and lactation:* Pregnancy should be excluded before start of treatment with Tritace and avoided during treatment; exposure of the mother to ACE inhibitors in mid or late pregnancy has been associated with oligohydramnios and neonatal hypotension with anuria or renal failure.

From animal experiments it is known that use of ramipril may cause a decreased utero-placental perfusion. There is also a potential risk of fetal or post-natal effect as ACE inhibitors also influence the local renin-angiotensin system. In peri-post natal studies increased renal pelvic dilatation was observed in the first generation offspring. However, ramipril was not fetotoxic in our studies although ACE inhibitors have shown fetotoxicity in some species.

Tritace should not be used during lactation.

*Effects on ability to drive and use machines:* In individual cases, treatment with Tritace may affect the ability to drive and operate machinery. This occurs especially at the start of treatment, when changing over from other preparations and during concomitant use of alcohol. After the first dose or subsequent increases in dose it is not advisable to drive or operate machinery for several hours.

*Undesirable effects:* Generally, adverse reactions have been mild and transient, and have not required discontinuation of therapy. The most frequently reported adverse reactions are nausea, dizziness and headache.

*Cardiovascular:* Symptomatic hypotension accompanied by dizziness, weakness and nausea may occur after the initial dose of Tritace and after an increase in the dose of Tritace. It has been rarely observed, but may occur in severely salt/volume-depleted patients such as those treated with diuretics, patients on dialysis and in patients with severe congestive heart failure. Syncope has also been observed rarely.

Myocardial infarction or cerebrovascular accident possibly secondary to severe hypotension in high risk patients, chest pain, palpitations, rhythm disturbances, angina pectoris may occur.

*Renal:* Treatment with Tritace may impair renal function.

*Gastrointestinal:* Treatment with Tritace may be associated with symptoms in the digestive tract, e.g. dryness of the mouth, irritation or inflammation of the oral mucosa, digestive disturbances, constipation, diarrhoea, nausea, and vomiting, (gastritis-like) stomach pain, upper abdominal discomfort (sometimes with increased levels of pancreatic enzymes), increases in hepatic enzymes and/or serum bilirubin, jaundice due to impaired excretion of bile pigment (cholestatic jaundice), other forms of impaired liver function, and hepatitis.

Pancreatitis has been reported rarely in patients treated with ACE inhibitors; in some cases this has proved fatal.

*Allergic:* Hypersensitivity reactions accompanied by pruritus, rash, shortness of breath and sometimes fever may occur, but usually resolve spontaneously after withdrawal of Tritace.

In addition, the following cutaneous and mucosal reaction may occur: reddening of skin areas with accompanying heat sensation, conjunctivitis, itching, urticaria, other skin or mucosal eruptions (maculopapular and lichenoid exanthema and enanthema, erythema multiforme), sometimes pronounced hair loss, and precipitation or intensification of Raynaud's phenomenon. With other ACE inhibitors psoriasiform and pemphigoid exanthema and enanthema), hypersensitivity of the skin to light, and onycholysis have been observed.

Vasculitis, muscle and joint pains, fever, or eosinophilia may occur. Raised titres of antinuclear antibodies have been seen with other ACE inhibitors.

*Angioneurotic oedema:* In very rare cases angioneurotic oedema has occurred during therapy with ACE inhibitors including Tritace. If laryngeal stridor or angioedema of the face, tongue or glottis occurs, treatment with Tritace must be discontinued and appropriate therapy instituted immediately.

*Respiratory tract:* A dry tickling cough may occur. This is possibly due to the desired ACE inhibition as are the following adverse effects: rhinitis, sinusitis, bronchitis and, especially in patients with tickling cough, bronchospasm.

*Other adverse reactions:* Disturbances of balance, headache, nervousness, restlessness, tremor, sleep disorders, confusion, loss of appetite, depressed mood, feeling of anxiety, paraesthesiae, taste change, taste reduction and sometimes loss of taste, muscle cramps, erectile impotence and reduced sexual desire may occur.

*Laboratory test findings:* Increases in blood urea nitrogen and serum creatinine may occur, in particular with renal insufficiency or in patients pretreated with a diuretic. Pre-existing proteinuria may deteriorate.

Serum sodium levels may decrease. Elevation of serum potassium may occur, since Tritace leads to a decrease in aldosterone secretion; potassium-sparing diuretics (spironolactone, amiloride, triamterene) or potassium supplements should therefore be avoided.

*Overdose:* In case of overdosage prolonged hypotension is to be expected. Treatment with an intravenous infusion of physiological saline and/or angiotensin II may be required.

## Pharmacological properties

*Pharmacodynamic properties:* Ramipril is a prodrug which, after absorption from the gastrointestinal tract, is hydrolysed in the liver to form the active angiotensin converting enzyme (ACE) inhibitor, ramiprilat which is a potent and long acting ACE inhibitor. Administration of ramipril causes an increase in plasma renin activity and a decrease in plasma concentrations of angiotensin II and aldosterone. The beneficial haemodynamic effects resulting from ACE inhibition are a consequence of the reduction in angiotensin II causing dilatation of peripheral vessels and reduction in vascular resistance. There is evidence suggesting that tissue ACE particularly in the vasculature, rather than circulating ACE, is the primary factor determining the haemodynamic effects.

Angiotensin converting enzyme is identical with kininase II, one of the enzymes responsible for the degradation of bradykinin. There is evidence that ACE inhibition by ramiprilat appears to have some effects on the kallikrein-kinin-prostaglandin systems. It is assumed that effects on these systems contribute to the hypotensive and metabolic activity of ramipril.

Administration of Tritace to hypertensive patients results in reduction of both supine and standing blood pressure. The antihypertensive effect is evident within one to two hours after the drug intake; peak effect occurs 3-6 hours after drug intake and has been shown to be maintained for at least 24 hours after usual therapeutic doses.

*Pharmacokinetic properties:* Following oral administration ramipril is rapidly absorbed from the gastrointestinal tract, peak plasma concentrations of ramipril are reached within one hour. Peak plasma concentrations of the active metabolite, ramiprilat, are reached within 2–4 hours.

Plasma concentrations of ramiprilat decline in a polyphasic manner. The effective half-life of ramiprilat after multiple once daily administration of ramipril is 13–17 hours for 5–10 mg ramipril and markedly longer for lower doses, 1.25–2.5 mg ramipril. This difference is related to the long terminal phase of the ramiprilat concentration time curve observed at very low plasma concentrations. This terminal phase is independent of the dose, indicating a saturable capacity of the enzyme to bind ramiprilat. Steady-state plasma concentrations of ramiprilat after once daily dosing with the usual doses of ramipril are reached by about the fourth day of treatment.

Ramipril is almost completely metabolised and the metabolites are excreted mainly via the kidneys. In addition to the bioactive metabolite, ramiprilat, other, inactive metabolites have been identified, including diketopiperazine ester, diketopiperazine acid and conjugates.

*Preclinical safety data:* Reproduction toxicology studies in the rat, rabbit and monkey did not disclose any teratogenic properties. Fertility was not impaired either in male or in female rats. The administration of ramipril to female rats during the fetal period and lactation produced irreversible renal damage (dilatation of the renal pelvis) in the offspring at daily doses of 50 mg/kg body weight and higher.

## Pharmaceutical particulars

*List of excipients:* Pregelatinised starch, Gelatin, Colours include: E171, E 172 (1.25 mg); E127, E171, E172 (2.5 mg); E127, E131, E171 (5 mg) in the capsule shell.

*Incompatibilities:* None known

*Shelf Life:* 2 years (1.25 mg capsule); 3 years (2.5 and 5 mg capsules)

*Special precautions for storage:* Tritace capsules should be stored below 25˚C. They should be kept away from children.

*Nature and contents of container:* Blister (calendar) pack of 28 capsules

*Instruction for use/handling:* None.

*Marketing authorisation holder:* Hoechst UK Limited, Hoechst House, Salisbury Road, Hounslow, Middlesex, TW4 6JH

**Marketing authorisation numbers**
1.25 mg capsules   0086/0130
2.5 mg capsules   0086/0131
5.0 mg capsules   0086/0132

**Date of approval/revision of SPC** 16 October 1996

**Legal category**   POM

*\*Trade Mark*

# ICN Pharmaceuticals Ltd
Mallard House
Peregrine Business Park
Gomm Road
High Wycombe
Bucks HP13 7DL

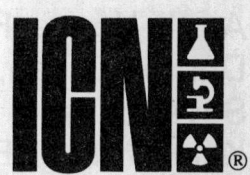

## VIRAZID* (RIBAVIRIN) AEROSOL

**Qualitative and quantitative composition** Ribavirin 6 g

International non-proprietary name (INN): Ribavirin
Chemical name: 1-Beta-D-Ribofuranosyl-1H,2,4-triazole-3-carboxamide

**Pharmaceutical form** Powder for inhalation solution.

*Therapeutic indications:* Virazid is indicated in the treatment of infants and children with severe respiratory syncytial virus (RSV) bronchiolitis.

*Important:* Ribavirin aerosol is more effective when instituted within the first 3 days of the treatment of bronchiolitis. Treatment early in the course of the disease may be necessary to achieve efficacy.

Treatment with Virazid must be accompanied by, and does not replace, standard supportive respiratory and fluid management for infants and children with severe respiratory tract infection.

Nebulised bronchodilators, when clinically indicated, should be administered with the SPAG generator turned off.

*Posology and method of administration:* Ribavirin aerosol is only recommended for use in infants and children.

Aerosol administration or nebulisation should be carried out in a small particle aerosol generator (SPAG). Before use read the SPAG Operator's Manual for instructions.

Treatment is carried out for 12-18 hours per day for at least 3 and no more than 7 days and is part of a total treatment programme.

The daily dose is prepared by dissolving 6 g of Ribavirin in a minimum of 75 ml Water for Injection BP. Shake well. Transfer dissolved drug and dilute to a total volume of 300 ml of distilled water in the reservoir of the aerosol generator.

The concentration of ribavirin in the reservoir is 20 mg/ml in the SPAG unit and the average concentration for a 7 hour period is 190 micrograms/l of air

*Method of administration:* Please see *Instructions for use/handling* for instructions on preparation of the aerosol solution.

The aerosol is delivered to an infant oxygen hood from the SPAG aerosol generator. Administration by face mask or oxygen tent may be necessary if a hood cannot be employed (see SPAG Operator's Manual). However, the volume of distribution and condensation area are larger in a tent and the efficacy of this method of administration has been evaluated only in a small number of patients.

*Contra-indications:* Ribavirin is contra-indicated in females who are or may become pregnant and it should be noted that ribavirin can be detected in human blood even four weeks after oral administration has ceased.

*Special warnings and special precautions for use:* Precipitation of the drug in respiratory equipment and consequent accumulation of fluid in the tubing has caused difficulties for patients requiring assisted ventilation.

In infants requiring assisted ventilation, Virazid should only be used when there is constant monitoring of both patients and equipment.

Directions for use during assisted ventilation are given in the SPAG manual which should be read carefully before such administration.

The teratogenic risk of Virazid to humans is unknown. As a precaution, women who are pregnant or trying to become pregnant should avoid exposure to the Virazid aerosol. Health care workers directly providing care to patients receiving aerosolized Virazid, should be aware that ribavirin has been shown to be teratogenic in rabbits and rodents but not in baboons. However no reports of teratogenicity in the offspring of mothers who were exposed to Virazid aerosol during pregnancy have been confirmed.

Nebulised Virazid may potentially escape into the hospital environment during therapy. However, ribavirin was not detected in the erythrocytes, plasma or urine of subjects exposed for a mean of 25 hours during 5 consecutive days.

It is good practice to avoid unnecessary occupational exposure to chemicals whenever possible. Several methods have been employed to lower environmental exposure during Virazid use. The most practical of these is to turn the SPAG device off for 5 to 10 minutes prior to prolonged contact.

*Interactions with other medicaments and other forms of interaction* None known.

*Pregnancy and lactation:* Ribavirin is contra-indicated in females who are or may become pregnant, and in nursing mothers. Ribavirin can be detected in human blood four weeks after administration has ceased. Although there are no pertinent human data, oral ribavirin has been found to be teratogenic in tested rodent species. Pregnant baboons given up to 120 mg/kg/day orally over a 4 week period and within 20 days of gestation failed to exhibit any teratogenic effects.

*Effects on ability to drive and use machines:* None known.

*Undesirable effects (frequency and seriousness)*
*Side-effects:* Several serious adverse events occurred in severely ill infants with life-threatening underlying disease, many of whom required assisted ventilation. These events included worsening of respiratory status, bacterial pneumonia and pneumothorax. The role of ribavirin aerosol in these events has not been determined.

Anaemia (often of a haemolytic variety) and reticulocytosis have been reported with oral and intravenous administration. Rarely, cases of non-specific anaemia and haemolysis have been reported spontaneously in association with the aerosol administration of Virazid.

*Overdose:* No overdoses have been reported.

### Pharmacological properties

*Pharmacodynamic properties:* Ribavirin has anti-viral inhibitory activity in vitro against respiratory syncytial virus, influenza virus and herpes simplex virus. Ribavirin is also active against respiratory syncytial virus in experimentally infected cotton rats.

The inhibitory activity of ribavirin on RSV in cell cultures is selective. The mechanism of action is unknown, but there is evidence that ribavirin interferes with protein translation by mRNA of several other RNA viruses, possibly the result of interference with formation of the 5¹ cap structure of mRNA.

*Pharmacokinetic properties:* Assay for ribavirin in human materials is by a radioimmunoassay which detects ribavirin and at least one metabolite.

Ribavirin administered by aerosol is absorbed systemically. Four paediatric patients inhaling ribavirin aerosol administered by face mask for 2.5 hours each day had plasma concentrations ranging from 0.44 to 1.44µM, with a mean concentration of 0.76µM. The plasma half-life was reported to be 9.5 hours. Three paediatric patients inhaling ribavirin aerosol administered by face mask or mist tent for 20 hours each day for 5 days had plasma concentrations ranging from 1.5 to 14.3µM, with a mean concentration of 6.8µM.

It is likely that the concentration of ribavirin in respiratory tract secretions is much higher than plasma concentrations in view of the route of administration.

The bioavailability of ribavirin is unknown and may depend on the mode of aerosol delivery. After aerosol treatment, peak plasma concentrations are less than the concentration that reduced RSV plaque formation in tissue cultures by 85 to 98%. After aerosol treatment, respiratory tract secretions are likely to contain ribavirin in concentrations many fold higher than those required to reduce plaque formation. However, RSV is an intracellular virus and serum concentrations may better reflect intracellular concentrations in the respiratory tract than respiratory secretion concentrations.

*Preclinical safety data:* Pertinent information is included in the *Pregnancy and Lactation* section.

### Pharmaceutical particulars

*List of excipients:* Not applicable.

*Incompatibilities:* None known.

*Shelf life:* 5 years. After reconstitution in Water for Injections, Virazid should be used within 24 hours.

*Special precautions for storage:* Store in a dry place at 15-25°C.

*Nature and contents of containers::* 100 ml Type 1 glass serum bottle with butyl rubber closure and aluminium seal with tear-off septum. Each bottle contains 6 g ribavirin as a lyophilised white cake. Virazid is packaged in cartons of three bottles.

*Instructions for use/handling:* By aseptic technique dissolve the powder in a minimum of 75 ml Water for Injections BP in the 100 ml vial. The solution should be adequately mixed to ensure complete dissolution. Shake well. It is not recommended that this solution is heated during dissolution. Transfer to the clean, sterilised 500 ml flask and dilute to a final volume of 300 ml with Water for Injections BP. The final concentration should be 20 mg/ml.

The Water for Injections BP used to make up the Virazid solution should not have any antimicrobial agent or any other substance added and all solutions should be inspected for particulate matter and discoloration prior to administration.

See guidelines for avoiding unwanted exposure to Virazid aerosol under *Special warnings and special precautions for use.*

**Marketing authorisation number** 15142/0001

**Date of revision/approval of SPC** May 1996.

**Legal category** POM

*Trade Mark

# Immuno Ltd
Arctic House, Rye Lane,
Dunton Green,
Sevenoaks,
Kent TN14 5HB

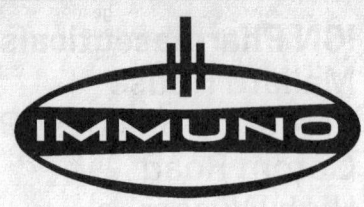

## FEIBA* IMMUNO
(Factor VIII Inhibitor Bypassing
Fraction Human) Vapour Heated

**Presentation** FEIBA in its lyophilised form is an amorphous powder. After reconstitution with Water for Injections BP it is a clear yellowish solution.

It is produced from pooled human venous plasma. Only plasma units which are non reactive in tests for HBsAg and antibody to HIV1, HIV2 and HCV are used in the manufacture of FEIBA. All plasma units are further tested for ALT.

The product is subjected to in-process virus inactivation where vapour is first applied for 10 hours at 60°C ± 0.5°C and an excess pressure of 190 ± 20 mbar followed by one hour at 80°C ± 0.5°C and an excess pressure of 370 ± 30 mbar.

FEIBA contains an anti-inhibitor coagulant complex with standardised FEIB-activity (Factor Eight Inhibitor Bypassing Activity):

1 mg of protein contains 0.7 to 2.5 units FEIBA.

FEIBA also contains factors II, IX and X mainly in non-activated form as well as activated factor VII: factor VIII coagulant antigen (FVIII C:Ag) is present in a concentration of up to 0.1 U/1 U FEIBA. The factors of the kallikrein-kinin system are present in trace amounts or absent.

1 unit of FEIBA is defined as that amount of factor VIII inhibitor bypassing activity which shortens the activated partial thromboplastin time (APTT) of a high titre factor VIII inhibitor plasma to 50% of the buffer value (blank).

The state of the art suggests that it cannot be precluded with certainty that both known or unknown viruses, which may occur in plasma, are transmitted through factor concentrates.

**Uses** FEIBA is indicated for the control of bleeding episodes in haemophilia A patients with Factor VIII Inhibitors and also in patients with acquired Factor VIII Inhibitors.

**Dosage and administration** FEIBA should only be administered intravenously. Do not exceed an injection/infusion rate of 2 units of FEIBA per kg bodyweight per minute.

As a general guide a dose of 50 to 100 units of FEIBA per kg bodyweight is recommended, however, not exceeding a daily dose of 200 U/kg bodyweight.

Dosage is independent of the patient's inhibitor titre. Since the response to treatment may differ from patient to patient the dosage recommendations are only guidelines.

Coagulation tests such as the whole blood clotting time (WBCT), the thromboelastogram (TEG, r-value), and the APTT usually show only a minor shortening and need not correlate with clinical improvement. For this reason these tests have only very limited value for monitoring FEIBA therapy.

### 1. SPONTANEOUS BLEEDING
*Joint muscle and soft tissue haemorrhage:* For minor to moderate bleeds a dose of 50–75 U/kg bodyweight is recommended at 12-hour intervals. Treatment should be continued until clear signs of clinical improvement appear, such as relief of pain, reduction of swelling or mobilisation of the joint.

For major muscle and soft tissue haemorrhage, such as retroperitoneal bleeding, doses of 100 U/kg bodyweight at 12 hour intervals are recommended.

*Mucous membrane bleeding:* A dose of 50 U/kg bodyweight is recommended to be given every 6 hours with careful monitoring of the patient (visible bleeding site, repeated measurements of haematocrit). Again if haemorrhage does not stop, the dose may be increased to 100 U/kg bodyweight taking care not to exceed the maximum daily dose of 200 U/kg bodyweight.

*Other severe haemorrhage:* Severe haemorrhage, such as CNS bleeding has been effectively treated with doses of 100 U/kg bodyweight at 12 hour intervals. In individual cases FEIBA may be given at intervals of 6 hours until clear clinical improvement is achieved. (Do not exceed the maximum daily dose).

### 2. SURGERY
Taking care not to exceed the maximum daily dose,
50–100 U/kg bodyweight should be given at intervals of up to 6 hours.

The above dosage schedule applies equally to children and the elderly.

*Use in the elderly:*
No specific precautions have to be taken into account when using FEIBA in the elderly. Attention is, however, drawn to the fact that in patients with a tentative or definitive diagnosis of coronary heart disease the use of FEIBA is only indicated in life-threatening bleeding events.

*Use in pregnancy:*
Animal reproduction studies have not been conducted with FEIBA. It is also not known whether the product can cause fetal harm when administered to a pregnant woman or can affect reproduction capacity.

### Contra-indications, warnings, etc

*Contra-indications:*
*Disseminated intravascular coagulation (DIC):* Laboratory and/or clinical symptoms which are clearly indicative of DIC.

Laboratory, histological and/or clinical signs of liver damage: due to the delayed clearance of activated coagulation factors such patients are at an increased risk of developing DIC.

*Myocardial infarction, acute thrombosis and/or embolism:* Except in cases of life threatening bleeding where no other form of therapy is likely to bring about satisfactory results.

*Precautions and warnings:* In rare cases allergic reactions such as fever, urticarial rashes, nausea and retching as well as other anaphylactoid reactions of varying severity have been observed after administration of FEIBA. Severe allergic and anaphylactoid reactions may necessitate the interruption of substitution treatment. Mild reactions can be managed with antihistamines: severe reactions require immediate intervention. In patients with a history of hypersensitivity reactions to plasma derivatives the prophylactic administration of antihistamines may be indicated.

In individual instances myocardial infarction was found to occur after high doses and/or prolonged administration and/or in the presence of risk factors predisposing to cardiovascular disease.

Single doses of 100 units FEIBA per kg bodyweight and daily doses of 200 units FEIBA per kg bodyweight should not be exceeded. Patients given single doses of 100 units FEIBA per kg bodyweight should be monitored for the development of DIC or symptoms of acute coronary ischaemia.

High doses of FEIBA should be given only as long as absolutely necessary to stop bleeding.

*Disseminated intravascular coagulation (DIC):* After administration of high doses (single doses of more than 100 units FEIBA per kg bodyweight, and daily doses of more than 200 units per kg bodyweight) laboratory signs such as the presence of fibrinopeptide A, Fibrin/Fibrinogen degradation products, or prolonged activated partial thromboplastin time (APTT), thrombin time and prothrombin time indicative of DIC were observed in a few cases.

If clinical signs of intravascular coagulation occur, which include changes in blood pressure, pulse rate, respiratory distress, chest pain and cough, the infusion should be stopped immediately and the patient monitored for DIC by appropriate laboratory tests.

*Laboratory tests and clinical efficacy:* In vitro tests to control efficacy such as APTT, whole blood clotting time and thromboelastogram (TEG) need not correlate with clinical improvement. For this reason, attempts at normalising these values by increasing the dose of FEIBA may not be successful and are strongly discouraged because of the potential hazard of producing DIC by overdosage.

*Significance of platelet count:* In case of inadequate or reduced response to FEIBA treatment it is recommended that a platelet count be performed, since a sufficient number of functionally intact platelets is considered to be necessary for the efficacy of FEIBA.

*Antifibrinolytics:* If treatment with both antifibrinolytics such as epsilon-aminocaproic acid and FEIBA is to be carried out, the interval between the administration of either product should be a least 6 hours.

*Treatment of overdosage:* Occasionally biological and/or clinical signs of DIC have been observed following the administration of high doses of FEIBA.

In such cases administration of the product should be stopped promptly.

If the coagulation parameters indicative of DIC do not quickly return to normal once administration of FEIBA is halted, it should be attempted to control the consumption reaction with Heparin or with antifibrinolytics in the case of secondary hyperfibrinolysis.

**Pharmaceutical precautions** FEIBA must be stored between +2°C and +8°C when it will have a shelf life of 2 years. The product may be stored at room temperature (maximum 25°C) for six months within the two year shelf life period.

**Legal category** POM

**Package quantities** FEIBA is supplied in packs containing 500 and 1000 FEIBA units together with a separate vial containing 20 ml Water for Injections BP as solvent. All packs contain sufficient equipment for reconstitution and administration.

**Further information**
*1. Effect on laboratory tests:* Inherent in its mechanism of action FEIBA causes a shortening of the following clotting times: activated partial thromboplastin time (APTT), whole blood clotting time (WBCT), activated clotting time (ACT), thromboelastogram (TEG).

Coagulation tests measuring the extrinsic coagulation system such as the prothrombin time, which is usually normal in haemophiliacs remained unchanged after treatment with FEIBA. Overdosage of the product may result in laboratory signs of DIC such as the presence of fibrinopeptide A, fibrin/fibrinogen degradation products, a fall in fibrinogen, a prolonged APTT, thrombin time and prothrombin time.

*2. Interactions:* It is not recommended to use antifibrinolytics such as epsilon-aminocaproic acid in combination with FEIBA treatment (see *Precautions and warnings*).

*3.* FEIBA is only available to Haemophilia Treatment Centres.

**Product licence numbers** 0215/0021-22

## GAMMABULIN*
### Normal Immunoglobulin Injection BP

**Presentation** Gammabulin is a concentrate of antibodies present in the IgG fraction of human plasma. It is produced from pooled human plasma of venous origin. Only plasma units which are non-reactive in tests for HBsAg and antibodies to HIV1, HIV2 and HCV are used in the manufacture of Gammabulin. All plasma units are further tested for ALT.

Gammabulin is a clear pale yellow to light brown solution.

Gammabulin has a protein content of 16% of which 90% is gamma globulin. Glycine is added as a stabiliser at a concentration of 2.25%. There is no preservative added to the product.

**Uses** Gammabulin is used in the treatment of:
Antibody deficiency syndrome and recurring bacterial infections in dys-, hypo- and agammaglobulinaemia.

Hepatitis A prophylaxis.

Prevention or modification of measles infection.

Treatment of susceptible pregnant women exposed to Rubella infection in whom continuing pregnancy places the fetus at risk.

**Dosage and administration** Gammabulin must be administered by the intramuscular route.

All recommendations and doses given below refer to the 16% solution and are expressed in ml.

*Antibody deficiency syndrome in dys-, hypo- and agammaglobulinaemia:* By intramuscular administration of Gammabulin antibody concentrate the frequency and severity of recurring bacterial infections can be reduced. For treatment of immunoglobulin deficiency, it is necessary to achieve and maintain an immunoglobulin level of approximately 200 mg per 100 ml serum.

*Initial dosage:* 1.8 ml per kg bodyweight, e.g. in three

single administrations of 0.6 ml/ kg bodyweight each at intervals of 24 hours.

*Maintenance dose:* 0.6 ml per kg bodyweight monthly.

*Hepatitis A:* Gammabulin is an efficient agent for the prevention or modification of Hepatitis A. It must be pointed out that after immunoglobulin administration an anicteric course of Hepatitis has been observed. Because of this, regular monitoring of transaminase levels may be warranted.

*Dosage for children:* 0.02-0.04 ml per kg bodyweight. If exposure continues, repeat the dose after 4-6 months.

*Dosage for adults:* (a) for a short period of exposure of less than 2 months: 0.02 to 0.04 ml per kg bodyweight. (b) for longer periods of exposure: 0.08 to 0.12 ml per kg bodyweight. If exposure continues, repeat the dose after 4 to 6 months.

*Note:* No benefit may be expected if administered after the onset of clinical symptoms.

*Measles:* Gammabulin should be given as soon as possible at a dose of 0.25 ml/ kg bodyweight to prevent or modify measles in a susceptible person exposed less than six days previously. Gammabulin may be especially indicated for susceptible household contacts of measles patients, particularly with children under one year of age or children who are immunosuppressed or have an immune deficiency disease and should not receive measles vaccine or any other live viral vaccine.

*Prophylaxis:* 0.2 ml per kg bodyweight. With continued or repeated exposure repeat after 3 weeks.

*Mitigation without influence on the immunising effect:* 0.04 ml per kg bodyweight.

*Rubella (German Measles):* The routine use of Gammabulin prophylaxis of Rubella in early pregnancy is of dubious value and cannot be justified. Some studies suggest that the use of Gammabulin in exposed, susceptible women can lessen the likelihood of infection and fetal damage, therefore 20 ml of Gammabulin may benefit those women in whom continuing pregnancy places the fetus at risk.

*Use in the elderly:* No special precautions need to be observed in the elderly.

*Use in pregnancy:* See *Interactions* with live vacines e.g. Rubella. According to present knowledge, no influence of immunoglobulin administrations in temporal connection with Rho prophylaxis with anti-D immunoglobulin can be proved. The diaplacental passage of administered immunoglobulin G into the fetus may be assumed.

**Contra-Indications, warnings, etc** Gammabulin is generally well tolerated without reactions. On very rare occasions (e.g. in special forms of a- or hypogammaglobulinaemia) anaphylactoid reactions may occur in patients who have antibodies against Immunoglobulin A (IgA) or who have shown atypical reaction after blood transfusion or following administration of blood derivatives.

Gammabulin must be not administered intravenously.

*Treatment of overdosage:* Gammabulin is a homologous protein, the antibody spectrum and protein structure of which corresponds qualitatively to that of an average donor population. Overdosage need not be expected to lead to more frequent or more severe adverse reactions than the recommended dose.

**Pharmaceutical precautions** Gammabulin should be stored between +2°C and +8°C when it will have a shelf life of 3 years. Gammabulin should be protected from the light.

**Legal category** POM

**Package quantitites** Rubber capped vials containing 2 ml, 5 ml or 10 ml.

**Further information** Gammabulin should be used immediately after drawing up the vial contents. Gammabulin vials are intended for single dose use only.

*Effect on laboratory tests:* Laboratory tests, as far as antibody determinations are concerned, are influenced inasmuch as the application of Gammabulin may lead to an increased or new appearance of types of antibodies (e.g. antibacterial, antiviral or antitoxic antibodies). In cases of very high doses, determinations of serum complement may give reduced values (consumption). Phagocytosis (phagocytosis index) may be increased.

*Interactions:* Active immunization with live virus vaccines (e.g. measles, mumps or rubella) should be postponed until 3 months after the last administration of Gammabulin, as the efficacy of the live virus vaccines may be impaired.

Administration of Gammabulin should be postponed until 2-4 weeks after the first complete cycle of immunization with live virus vaccines and 2 weeks after booster injection.

**Product licence number** 0215/0018

## HUMAN ALBUMIN SOLUTION 4.5% BP IMMUNO*

**Presentation** Human Albumin Solution 4.5% BP Immuno is a sterile solution of protein for intravenous administration prepared from human plasma of venous origin. Only plasma units which are non reactive in tests for HBsAg and antibodies to HIV1, HIV2 and HCV are used in the manufacture of Human Albumin Solution 4.5% BP Immuno. All plasma units are further tested for ALT. It is heat treated for 10 hours at 60°C in the final container in accordance with international guidelines. The product contains a minimum of 96% albumin and is stabilised with 3.6 mmol/l sodium caprylate and sodium acetyltryptophanate.

**Uses** Human Albumin Solution 4.5% BP Immuno is indicated for volume replacement in hypovolaemic shock, as a replacement fluid during therapeutic plasmapheresis and in hypoalbuminaemia associated with an oncotic deficit.

**Dosage and administration**

*Hypovolaemic shock:* The dosage is largely determined by the duration and severity of hypovolaemia.

*Adults:* 500 ml/hr (125 drops/ min) in severe shock up to 1000 ml/hour (rapid infusion).

*Children:* For shock due to hypovolaemia and/or dehydration 20-30 ml/ kg bodyweight infused at a rate of 5-10 ml/ min.

If the haematocrit drops below 25%, packed red cells or whole blood should be given in conjunction with Human Albumin Solution 4.5% B.P. Immuno to maintain the oxygen transport capacity of the blood.

*Hypoalbuminaemia with oncotic deficit:*

*Adults:* 3.5–7.0 ml/ kg bodyweight daily infused at a rate of 250-500 ml/hr.

*Children:* 5–10 ml/ kg bodyweight per day given slowly.

*Use in the elderly:* In elderly patients careful haemodynamic and respiratory monitoring is essential throughout the administration of Human Albumin Solution 4.5% B.P. Immuno as a circulatory overload may lead to decompensation of the haemodynamic system.

In dehydrated patients only low concentrated protein solutions (up to 5% protein content) should be administered.

*Use in pregnancy:* As some patients show renal insufficiency during pregnancy, concentrated human albumin should be administered only when absolutely indicated and with utmost caution. Based on a persisting hypertension careful haemodynamic monitoring is essential to avoid an overloading syndrome which may lead to cardiac decompensation.

**Contra-indications, warnings, etc** Do not use if the solution is cloudy or contains a deposit.

Once the container has been penetrated the contents should be used within three hours and any unused preparation discarded.

Adequate precautions should be taken against circulatory overload. If symptoms of hypervolaemia develop the rate of infusion should be slowed or even halted.

Though side effects are extremely rare, such reactions as flushing, chills, fever, tachycardia, hypotension, urticarial skin rash and nausea may occur.

In these cases, the infusion of Human Albumin Solution 4.5% BP Immuno should be interrupted (or replaced by Ringer's solution) and antihistamines and/or corticosteroids should be administered intravenously (e.g. 50-200 mg prednisolone).

Human Albumin has been reported to contain trace amounts of Aluminium. In accordance with the limits laid down by the British Pharmacopoeia Human Albumin Solution 4.5% BP Immuno contains less than 200 micrograms per litre. It is therefore suitable for use in patients undergoing dialysis and premature infants.

Nevertheless, accumulation of Aluminium in patients with chronic renal insufficiency has led to toxic effects such as hypercalcaemia, Vitamin D refractory osteodystrophy, anaemia and severe progressive encephalopathy.

When large volumes of Human Albumin solutions are contemplated for administration to such patients the potential risks as compared to the expected benefits should be carefully evaluated.

*Treatment of overdosage:* Interrupt infusion immediately and carefully watch the patient's haemodynamic parameters.

The half life of human albumin in the tissue is approximately 16-18 days. The disappearance rate of intravascular albumin depends on the permeability of the vascular system and on the catabolic rate.

**Pharmaceutical precautions** Human Albumin Solution 4.5% BP Immuno should be stored between +2°C and +25°C. It must be protected from light. The shelf life is 3 years.

**Legal category** POM

**Package quantities** Human Albumin Solution 4.5% BP Immuno is supplied in 50 ml, 100 ml, and 400 ml infusion bottles.

**Further information** Human Albumin Solution 4.5% BP Immuno is compatible with whole blood or packed red cells as well as the usual electrolyte and carbohydrate solutions intended for intravenous use. However, it should not be mixed with protein hydrolysates, amino acid mixtures or solutions containing alcohol. Human Albumin Solution 4.5% BP Immuno must not be given through infusion sets which have been used, or are intended, for simultaneous infusion of protein hydrolysates, amino acid mixtures, or solutions containing alcohol. Only clear solutions of slightly yellowish colour should be administered.

*Effect on Laboratory Tests:* As a consequence of haemodilution patients' blood samples taken during or shortly after infusion show lower laboratory test results (e.g. haematocrit) corresponding to the amount of Human Albumin Solution 4.5% BP Immuno administered to the patient (calculation based on isotonic solutions). Human Albumin Solution 4.5% BP Immuno does not interfere with the determination of patients' Rh-factors nor is there any adverse effect on thrombocyte function or blood coagulation.

**Product licence number** 0215/0002

## HUMAN ALBUMIN SOLUTION 20% BP IMMUNO*

**Presentation** Human Albumin Solution 20% BP Immuno is a solution in water of human albumin containing a low proportion of salt and is described as Salt Poor Albumin. It is a clear liquid varying in colour from amber to orange-brown and is presented as a solution for intravenous injection or infusion. It is prepared from pooled human plasma of venous origin. Only plasma units which are non reactive in tests for HBsAg and antibodies to HIV1, HIV2 and HCV are used in the manufacture of Human Albumin Solution 20% BP Immuno. All plasma units are further tested for ALT. The product contains 20% protein of which at least 96% is albumin, the rest being thermostable alpha and beta globulins.

It is stabilised with 16 mmol/l sodium caprylate and 16 mmol/l sodium acetyltryptophanate and heat treated for 10 hours at 60°C in the final container in accordance with international guidelines. There is no preservative added to the solution.

**Uses** Human Albumin Solution 20% BP Immuno is administered as an injection or an infusion in the treatment of acute oedema: hypoalbuminaemia. For the treatment of the acute phase of burns or haemorrhagic shock, Human Albumin Solution 20% BP Immuno is diluted 1:4 with dextrose 5% or isotonic electrolyte solutions and the resulting 5% solution administered by infusion.

**Dosage and administration**

*Acute oedema:* There is an increased tendency for oedema to occur in patients with hypoalbuminaemia. Attempts should be made to bring about diuresis using the appropriate dose of Human Albumin Solution 20% BP Immuno. A reduction in oedema may then result.

*Recommended dosage: Adults* 100 ml Human Albumin Solution 20% BP Immuno (20 g). *Children* 2 ml Human Albumin Solution 20% BP Immuno (0.4 g) per kg bodyweight.

*Pre- and post-operative hypoproteinaemia:* In debilitated patients stabilisation of the protein balance with Human Albumin Solution 20% B.P. Immuno may considerably improve the pre-operative condition of the patient. The catabolism of albumin can be severely disturbed after operations on the gastro-intestinal tract and hypoproteinaemia may result. The normal average albumin breakdown of 70 g per week may be enhanced under pathological conditions. Additional loss of protein and diminished albumin synthesis might lead to severe albumin deficiency.

Repeated post-operative infusions of Human Albumin Solution 20% B.P. Immuno can be most valuable in such cases.

*Recommended dosage for pre- and post-operative hypoproteinaemia: Adults* 100 to 200 ml Human Albumin Solution 20% BP Immuno (20 to 40 g) daily in concentrated or diluted form depending on the plasma volume and serum albumin level of the patient. The dosage and duration of this substitution therapy depends on the amount of protein lost and should be continued until the serum concentration returns to normal. *Children* 1.5 to 3 ml Human Albumin Solution 20% BP Immuno (0.3 to 0.6 g) per kg bodyweight daily in concentrated form or diluted to a 5% solution. In hypoproteinaemia multiple administration of albumin might be necessary until the plasma protein level has returned to normal.

Attention must be paid to the oncotic activity of albumin which may lead to an increased blood volume.

See *Precautions*.

*Other hypoalbuminaemia*

(a) Hepatic cirrhosis with diffuse loss of parenchyma leads to diminished production of albumin and a resulting hypoalbuminaemia which, as a consequence, enhances the formation of ascites and oedema. Treatment with albumin results in the disappearance of oedema and a reduction of ascites.

*Recommended dosage: Adults* 100 to 200 ml Human Albumin Solution 20% BP Immuno (20 to 40 g) daily. *Children and Infants* 1.5 to 3 ml Human Albumin Solution 20% BP Immuno (0.3 to 0.6 g) per kg bodyweight.

(b) Nephrotic Syndrome. In cases of nephrotic syndrome particularly with patients who do not respond at all, or only slightly, to diuretics, the administration of Human Albumin Solution 20% BP Immuno will induce diuresis and therefore bring about a reduction of the oedema.

*Recommend dosage: Adults* 200 to 400 ml Human Albumin Solution 20% BP Immuno (40 to 80 g) daily. *Children and Infants* 3 to 6 ml Human Albumin Solution 20% BP Immuno (0.6 to 1.2 g) per kg bodyweight in concentrated form.

The dose should be infused over a period of 60 to 90 minutes.

*Shock:* Shock due to blood loss should be treated with whole blood, red cell concentrates, fresh frozen plasma, or with albumin diluted with isotonic electrolyte and/or dextrose solution 5%. *Adults* 50 to 200 ml Human Albumin Solution 20% BP Immuno (10 to 40 g) diluted 1:4 with isotonic electrolyte and/or dextrose solution 5%. *Children* 1 to 2 ml Human Albumin Solution 20% BP Immuno (0.2 g to 0.4 g) per kg bodyweight diluted 1:4 with isotonic electrolyte and/or dextrose solution 5%.

*Burns:* Return of fluid from the extravascular compartment to the circulation must be ensured in cases of burns with associated hypoalbuminaemia.

In these cases hyperoncotic Human Albumin Solution 20% BP Immuno can be used with careful control of the oncotic pressure and the haemodynamic parameters.

*Recommended dosage: Adults* 50 to 200 ml Human Albumin Solution 20% BP Immuno (10 to 40 g). *Children* 1 to 2 ml Human Albumin Solution 20% BP Immuno (0.2 to 0.4 g) per kg bodyweight.

The initial dose should be infused over a period of 5 to 15 minutes.

In cases of extensive and severe burns with an increased haematocrit value, normalisation of the circulatory conditions can be achieved very effectively with Human Albumin Solution 20% BP Immuno diluted with dextrose 5% and/or isotonic electrolyte solutions.

*Recommended initial dosage: Adults* 200 to 400 ml Human Albumin Solution 20% BP Immuno (40 to 80 g) diluted 1:4 corresponding to 800 to 1600 ml of a 5% albumin solution. *Children* 4 ml Human Albumin Solution 20% BP Immuno per kg bodyweight diluted 1:4 corresponding to 16 ml of a 5% albumin solution.

The total dosage over the first 24 hours can be determined in accordance with the formula: 2 ml × bodyweight (kg) × % of surface burned + 1500 ml.

After the acute stage has been brought under control, considerable protein deficiency, largely of albumin, may occur. This hypoalbuminaemia can be corrected by administration of the following doses: *Adults* 50 ml Human Albumin Solution 20% BP Immuno (10 g) twice a day. *Children* 1 ml Human Albumin Solution 20% BP Immuno (0.2 g) per kg bodyweight twice a day.

*Use in the elderly:* In elderly patients careful haemodynamic and respiratory monitoring is essential throughout the administration of Human Albumin Solution 20% BP Immuno as a circulatory overload may lead to decompensation of the haemodynamic system.

In dehydrated patients only low concentrated protein solutions (up to 5% protein content) should be administered.

*Use in pregnancy:* As some patients show renal insufficiency during pregnancy, concentrated human albumin should be administered only when absolutely indicated and with utmost caution. Based on a persisting hypertension, monitoring is essential to avoid an overloading syndrome which may lead to cardiac decompensation.

**Contra-indications, warnings, etc**

1. Human Albumin Solution 20% BP Immuno must not be used if the solution is cloudy or contains a deposit.

Once the container has been penetrated, the contents must be used within 3 hours and any unused preparation discarded.

2. With patients suffering from hypertension or in cases of latent or manifest cardiac insufficiency, caution is indicated in the administration of Human Albumin Solution 20% BP Immuno. The single doses should be reduced to relatively small amounts and the infusion given slowly. A careful watch must be kept for the possible development of pulmonary oedema. If pulmonary oedema occurs, the infusion must be stopped immediately.

3. In all cases of considerable blood loss, whole blood or packed red cells must be given in addition to Human Albumin Solution 20% BP Immuno.

4. Intolerance reactions are extremely rare with Human Albumin Solution 20% BP Immuno.

5. Human Albumin has been reported to contain trace amounts of Aluminium. In accordance with the limits laid down by the British Pharmacopoeia Human Albumin Solution 20% BP Immuno contains less than 200 micrograms per litre. It is therefore suitable for use in patients undergoing dialysis and premature infants.

Nevertheless, accumulation of Aluminium in patients with chronic renal insufficiency has led to toxic effects such as hypercalcaemia, Vitamin D refractory osteodystrophy, anaemia and severe progressive encephalopathy.

When large volumes of Human Albumin solutions are contemplated for administration to such patients the potential risks as compared to the expected benefits should be carefully evaluated.

*Treatment of overdosage:* Interrupt infusion immediately and carefully watch the patient's haemodynamic parameters.

The half life of human albumin in the tissue is approximately 16–18 days. The disappearance rate of intravascular albumin depends on the permeability of the vascular system and on the catabolic rate.

**Pharmaceutical precautions** Human Albumin Solution 20% BP Immuno should be stored between + 2°C and + 8°C. It must be protected from light. The shelf life is 3 years.

**Legal category:** POM

**Package quantities** Human Albumin Solution 20% BP Immuno is supplied in rubber capped vials of 10 ml, 50 ml and 100 ml.

**Further information** Human Albumin Solution 20% BP Immuno is compatible with whole blood or packed red cells as well as the usual electrolyte and carbohydrate solutions intended for intravenous use. However, it should not be mixed with protein hydrolysates, amino acid mixtures or solutions containing alcohol. Human Albumin Solution 20% BP Immuno must not be given through infusion sets which have been used, or are intended, for simultaneous infusion of protein hydrolysates, amino acid mixtures, or solutions containing alcohol. Only clear solutions of slightly yellowish colour should be administered.

*Effect on laboratory tests:* As a consequence of haemodilution patients' blood samples taken during or shortly after infusion show lower laboratory test results (e.g. haematocrit) corresponding to the amount of Human Albumin Solution 20% BP Immuno administered to the patient (calculation based on isotonic solutions). Human Albumin Solution 20% BP Immuno does not interfere with the determination of patients' Rh-factors nor is there any adverse effect on thrombocyte function or blood coagulation.

**Product licence number** 0215/0009

## PARTOBULIN* Anti-D(Rho) Immunoglobulin Injection BP

**Presentation** Partobulin is a clear liquid varying in colour from pale yellow to light brown. Each preloaded syringe contains 1,250 iu (250 micrograms) Anti-D in 1 ml of solution. It is prepared from pooled human venous plasma with a high content of Anti-D antibodies. Only plasma units which are non reactive in tests for HBsAg and antibodies to HIV1, HIV2 and HCV are used in the manufacture of Partobulin. All plasma units are further tested for ALT. Glycine and Sodium Chloride are added as stabilisers. There is no preservative added to the product.

**Uses** Partobulin is used for the prevention of $D(Rh_o)$ sensitisation.

**Dosage and administration** Partobulin must be administered by the intramuscular route. Partobulin is indicated to prevent $D(Rh_o)$ sensitisation in the situations described below when the blood groups of mother/recipient and fetus/child/transfused blood are as follows or when the rhesus factor of the fetus/child is unknown or cannot be determined:

| Mother/recipient | *Fetus/child/transfused blood* |
|---|---|
| *$D(Rh_o)$-negative* | *$D(Rh_o)$-positive* |
| *$D(Rh_o)$-negative* | *$D^u$-positive* |
| *$D^u$-positive* | *$D(Rh_o)$-positive* |

*(a) Abortion and miscarriage:* Following every abortion or miscarriage where $D(Rh_o)$ sensitisation may be expected, 1,250 iu should be administered immediately or at the latest within 72 hours.

*(b) Antenatal prophylaxis:* As sensitisation can also occur during preganacy, 1,250 iu may be administered during weeks 28 and 34 of pregnancy in $D(Rh_o)$ negative or $D^u$ positive mothers.

In addition, after any potentially sensitising episode such as amniocentesis, external cephalic version, abdominal trauma, antepartum haemorrhage, ectopic pregnancy or chorionic villus sampling, 1,250 iu should be administered immediately or at the latest within 72 hours.

Note: Where antenatal prophylaxis has been given, a further dose should routinely be administered to the mother within 72 hours of birth.

*(c) Parturition:* In first deliveries and all subsequent deliveries where $D(Rh_o)$ sensitisation may be expected 1,250 iu should be administered immediately or at the latest within 72 hours.

*(d) Macrotransfusion:* In all deliveries where a transplacental haemorrhage of more than 25 ml fetal blood (1% of fetal erythrocytes according to the elution method of Kleihauer and Betke) into the maternal blood occurs and a $D(Rh_o)$ incompatibility exists, a dose of 5,000 iu (i.e. 4 preloaded syringes of Partobulin) or 50 iu per ml of fetal blood is recommended.

Such macroinfiltrations occur in less than 1% of cases.

*(e) $D(Rh_o)$ incompatible blood transfusion:* Following the transfusion of $D(Rh_o)$ incompatible blood an i.m. injection of 50 to 100 iu Anti-$D(Rh_o)$ Immunoglobulin per ml of transfused blood is recommended. Recent findings underline the necessity of starting the treatment as soon as possible. Some authors are using considerably higher doses and monitoring the disappearance of $D(Rh_o)$ positive cells and also determining the antibody excess.

*Use in the elderly:* Use in the elderly is normally limited to the prevention of sensitisation following incompatible transfusion. Under these circumstances no special precautions or dosage amendments need to be observed in the elderly.

*Use in pregnancy:* The use of Partobulin during pregnancy as described under Indications and Dosage does not usually produce antibody titres in the maternal circulation that might threaten the fetus. Exceptions are possible, for example, if anti-D immunoglobulin is given repeatedly at short intervals. In general, the antibody titre in the maternal blood should not exceed 1:2 (Coombs Test).

**Contra-indications, warnings, etc** Partobulin must not be administered intravenously. Partobulin must not be administered to $D(Rh_o)$ positive individuals or $D(Rh_o)$ positive newborns.

Partobulin is generally well tolerated without reactions. On very rare occasions (e.g. in special forms of a- or Hypo-gammaglobulinaemia), anaphylactoid reactions may occur in people who have antibodies against immune globulin A (IgA) or have shown atypical reaction after blood transfusion or following administration of blood derivatives.

*Interactions:* Active Immunisation with live virus vaccines (e.g. Measles, Mumps or Rubella) should be postponed until 3 months after the last administration of Partobulin, as the efficacy of the live virus vaccine may be impaired.

If Partobulin needs to be administered within 2-4 weeks of a live virus vaccination, then the efficacy of such a vaccination may be impaired.

*Treatment of overdosage:* In rhesus negative individuals overdosage need not be expected to lead to more frequent or more severe adverse reactions than the normal dose. It has been observed that even an accidental injection of the preparation into the newborn does not necessarily lead to adverse reaction.

**Pharmaceutical precautions** Partobulin should be stored between +2°C and +8°C when it will have a shelf life of three years.

**Legal category** POM

**Package quantities** Pre-loaded syringes containing 1,250 iu (250 micrograms) Anti-D in 1 ml.

**Further information** Partobulin should be administered immediately following removal of the protective needle cover. Partobulin syringes are intended for single dose use only.

*Effect on laboratory tests:* Passively introduced $D(Rh_o)$ antibodies may be detected in the blood of the mother several weeks and even months after an injection of Partobulin. Therefore, any previous administration of

Partobulin must be taken into account when examining maternal blood for its content of D(Rh₀) antibody and when evaluating these tests.

The presence of additional antibodies (e.g. Rubella) in Partobulin may lead to false positive reactions in tests for such antibodies.

**Product licence number** 0215/0026

# TETABULIN*
## Tetanus Immunoglobulin BP Immuno

### Qualitative and quantitative composition
*Active ingredient:* Tetanus antitoxin

*Quantitative composition:* 1 ml of solution contains Tetanus antitoxin 250iu

**Pharmaceutical form** Solution for intramuscular administration.

### Clinical particulars

*Therapeutic indications:* Prophylaxis in persons with recent injuries who have no immunity, incomplete or unknown immunity against tetanus.

Therapy of clinically manifest tetanus.

*Posology and method of administration:*
*Posology:* Passive immunisation against tetanus is recommended in all cases of injury where a risk of tetanus infection is involved and where active protection against tetanus is insufficient, i.e. when immunisation is incomplete, when the immune response is reduced or following severe loss of blood or plasma. Tetanus Immunoglobulin BP Immuno is also indicated when the status of immunisation is unknown or when active immunisation is contraindicated.

Besides thorough debridement and cleansing of the wound along with the injection of Tetanus Immunoglobulin BP Immuno, active immunisation with tetanus vaccine should be started simultaneously at a separate injection site unless active immunisation is contraindicated.

It is recommended that the physician determines if a minor wound is 'tetanus-prone', based on the likelihood that *Clostridium tetani* was present on the object which caused the wound.

The same dose applies to both children and adults.

a. *Prophylaxis of tetanus:* 250 iu by intramuscular injection

This dose should be doubled in cases where the wound is heavily contaminated or older than 12 hours and in patients weighing more than 90 kg. Patients with antibody deficiency syndrome such as dys-, hypo- or agammaglobulinaemia or with a reduced capacity of antibody formation (after radiotherapy or steroid treatment, burns, etc.) should receive another dose of Tetanus Immunoglobulin BP Immuno 3 to 4 weeks after the first dose as a prophylaxis against the delayed onset of tetanus.

A further dose should also be given after 3 to 4 weeks where simultaneous vaccination is contraindicated.

b. *Therapy of tetanus:* Several studies suggest the value of HTIG in the treatment of active tetanus using doses of between 30 and 300iu per kg bodyweight i.m. in combination with other appropriate clinical procedures.

The absence of thiomersal as a preservative theoretically allows intrathecal administration although efficacy and safety in children and adults have not yet been definitely assessed.

*Method of administration:* Slow injection by the i.m. route only.

If large doses (>5 ml) are required, it is advisable to administer them in divided doses at different sites.

*Contra-indications:* The lethal risk associated with tetanus rules out any potential contraindication (see *Warnings* below).

*Special warnings and special precautions for use:* The warnings and precautions described for human normal immunoglobulin (i.m.) may be applied for Tetanus Immunoglobulin BP Immuno and are described below.

Do not give this product intravascularly (possibility of shock). Therefore, it is necessary to verify that the needle has not penetrated a blood vessel.

Give with caution in highly allergic individuals due to the potential risk of hypersensitivity reactions such as anaphylactoid shock.

Measures against allergic and anaphylactoid reactions require immediate discontinuation of the injection. If allergic reactions persist after discontinuation of the injection, then appropriate treatment with, for example, antihistamines and/or corticosteroids is recommended.

In anaphylactoid shock, treatment should follow the guidelines of shock therapy.

*Interaction with other medicaments and other forms of interaction:*
*Live attenuated virus vaccines:* If the patient has received live attenuated virus vaccines (measles, rubella, mumps, varicella) within the two previous weeks, an assay of protective post-vaccinal antibodies may be of value before giving a possible booster.

After injection of immunoglobulin, wait at least 6 weeks (and preferably 3 months) prior to administering any live attenuated virus vaccines (measles, rubella, mumps, varicella).

The efficacy of the virus vaccines may be impaired by the antibodies contained in the immunoglobulin preparation.

*Interpretation of blood typing and antibody testing:* After injection of immunoglobulin, take into account the possible and transitory cross-reactions of the antibodies administered which may lead to false-positive results in serological testing.

*Pregnancy and lactation:* The safety of this medicinal product for use in pregnancy has not been established in controlled clinical trials. Long lasting clinical experience with immunoglobulin, in particular the routine administration of anti-D immunoglobulin, does indicate that no harmful effects on the course of pregnancy, on the fetus and the neonate are to be expected (category A).

Experimental animal studies are inappropriate with respect to the product which is heterologous for animals (immunological incompatibility).

Immunoglobulins are excreted into the milk and may contribute to the transfer of protective antibodies to the neonate.

*Effects on ability to drive and use machines:* There are no known restrictions.

*Undesirable effects:* The undesirable effects described for human normal immunoglobulin (i.m.) may be applied for Tetanus Immunoglobulin BP Immuno and are described below.

Pain and discomfort may be observed at the site of administration; this local pain can be prevented by giving smaller volumes more frequently.

Occasionally, fever, cutaneous reactions, chills may occur. In rare instances nausea, vomiting, hypotension, tachycardia, allergic reactions have been reported.

Serious effects such as anaphylactoid shock have been observed in isolated cases.

*Overdose:* Overdosage with Tetanus Immunoglobulin BP Immuno is not known.

### Pharmacological properties

*Pharmacodynamic properties:* Tetanus Immunoglobulin BP Immuno is a sterile preparation that contains antibodies to tetanus toxin.

Tetanus Immunoglobulin BP Immuno is prepared from pooled plasma containing specific antibodies against the toxin of *Clostridium tetani*.

*Pharmacokinetic properties:* Measurable levels of antibodies are obtained approximately 20 minutes after i.m. injection. Peak serum levels are usually achieved 2 to 3 days later.

The half-life is 3 to 4 weeks.

*Preclinical safety data:*
*Viral safety:* The respective national guidelines on the collection of human plasma in their effective versions are observed. In addition, several steps of the manufacturing process contribute to the viral safety of human immunoglobulins. They result in extensive partitioning and/or inactivation of potentially contaminating viruses.

*Toxicological properties:* Immunoglobulins are normal constituents of the human body. Repeated dose toxicity testing in animals is impracticable due to interference with developing antibodies.

Tetanus Immunoglobulin BP Immuno has not been reported to be associated with embryo-fetal toxicity, oncogenic or mutagenic potential.

### Pharmaceutical particulars

*List of excipients:* 1 ml of solution contains:

| | |
|---|---|
| Protein (>90% gamma globulin) | 100–170 mg |
| Glycine | 22.5 mg |
| Sodium Chloride | 3.0 mg |

*Incompatibilities:* Tetanus Immunoglobulin BP Immuno must not be mixed with other pharmaceutical products.

*Shelf life:* 3 years when stored between +2°C and +8°C.

Once a container has been opened, its contents should be used immediately.

*Special precautions for storage:* Store at a temperature of between +2°C and +8°C. Protect from light. Do not freeze. Do not use after the expiry date indicated on the label.

*Nature and contents of container:* Preloaded syringe of neutral glass, hydrolytic type 1, each containing 1 ml of solution.

*Instructions for use/handling:* Tetanus Immunoglobulin BP Immuno should be administered immediately following removal of the protective needle cover from the preloaded syringe. Tetanus Immunoglobulin BP Immuno syringes are intended for single dose use only. Do not use solutions which are cloudy or have deposits.

**Marketing authorisation number** 0215/0030

**Date of approval/revision** August 1993

**Legal category** POM

*Trade Mark

# International Medication Systems (UK) Ltd

Evans House
Regent Park
Kingston Road
Leatherhead
Surrey KT22 7PQ

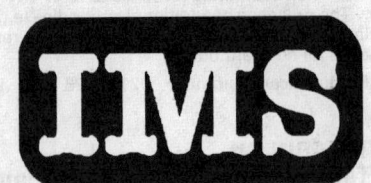

## EPINEPHRINE (ADRENALINE) INJECTION 1:1000 MINIJET*

**Qualitative and quantitative composition** Epinephrine USP 1 mg per ml.

**Pharmaceutical form** Sterile aqueous solution for intramuscular or subcutaneous administration.

### Clinical particulars

*Therapeutic indications:* Emergency treatment of anaphylaxis or acute angioneurotic oedema with airways obstruction, or acute allergic reactions.

*Posology and method of administration:* For the relief of life-threatening angioneurotic oedema and anaphylactic shock, epinephrine should be administered by intramuscular injection.

For acute allergic reactions due to insect stings etc: Intramuscular or subcutaneous injection.

*Adults:* 0.5 to 1.0 ml (0.5-1.0 mg), administered slowly. The dose may be repeated every 5 to 15 minutes as needed.

*Elderly:* As for adults, use with caution.

*Children (up to age of 12):* 0.01 ml/kg bodyweight (0.01 mg/kg), up to a maximum of 0.5 ml. This can be repeated twice at 15 minute intervals, then every 4 hours as needed. The actual amount varies according to whether the child is small, medium or large for his/her age:

Volume of epinephrine 1:1,000 for intramuscular injection in anaphylactic shock:

| Age | Volume of epinephrine (ml) |
| --- | --- |
| Under 1 year | 0.05 |
| 1 year | 0.1 |
| 2 years | 0.2 |
| 3-4 years | 0.3 |
| 5 years | 0.4 |
| 6-12 years | 0.5 |

These doses are for robust children. If underweight use half these doses.

*Contra-indications:* Contra-indications are relative as this product is intended for use in life-threatening emergencies.

Other than in the emergency situation, the following contra-indications should be considered: hyperthyroidism, hypertension, ischaemic heart disease, diabetes mellitus and closed angle glaucoma.

*Special warnings and precautions for use:* These special warnings and precautions are relative as this product is intended for use in life-threatening situations.

Administer slowly with caution to elderly patients and to patients with ischaemic heart disease, hypertension, diabetes mellitus, hyperthyroidism or psychoneurosis. Anginal pain may be induced when coronary insufficiency is present. Use with caution in patients with closed angle glaucoma.

*Interaction with other medicaments and other forms of interaction:* The effects of epinephrine may be potentiated by tricyclic antidepressants. Halothane and other anaesthetics such as cyclopropane and trichloroethylene, increase the risk of epinephrine-induced ventricular arrhythmias and acute pulmonary oedema, if hypoxia is present. Severe hypertension and bradycardia may occur with non-selective beta-blocking drugs, such as propranolol. Propranolol also inhibits the bronchodilator effect of epinephrine. The risk of cardiac arrhythmias is higher when epinephrine is given to patients receiving digoxin or quinidine. Epinephrine-induced hypoglycaemia may lead to loss of blood-sugar control in diabetic patients treated with hypoglycaemic agents.

*Pregnancy and lactation :* Epinephrine crosses the placenta. There is some evidence of a slightly increased incidence of congenital abnormalities. Injection of epinephrine may cause foetal tachycardia, cardiac irregularities, extrasystoles and louder heart sounds. In labour, epinephrine may delay the second stage. Epinephrine should only be used in pregnancy if the potential benefits outweigh the risks to the foetus.

Epinephrine is excreted in breast milk but, as pharmacologically active plasma concentrations are not achieved by the oral route, the use of epinephrine in breast-feeding mothers is presumed to be safe.

*Effect on ability to drive and use machinery:* Not applicable; this preparation is intended for use only in emergencies.

*Undesirable effects:* The potentially severe adverse effects of epinephrine arise from its effect upon blood pressure and cardiac rhythm. Ventricular fibrillation may occur and severe hypertension may lead to cerebral haemorrhage and pulmonary oedema. Symptomatic adverse effects are anxiety, dyspnoea, restlessness, palpitations, tachycardia, tremor, weakness, dizziness, headache and cold extremities. Biochemical effects include inhibition of insulin secretion and hypoglycaemia (even with low doses), gluconeogenesis, glycolysis, lipolysis and ketogenesis.

*Overdose:*

*Symptoms:* cardiac arrhythmias leading to ventricular fibrillation and death, severe hypertension leading to pulmonary oedema and cerebral haemorrhage.

*Treatment:* combined alpha- and beta-adrenergic blocking agents such as labetalol may counteract the effects of epinephrine, or a beta-blocking agent may be used to treat any supraventricular arrhythmias and phentolamine to control the alpha-mediated effects on the peripheral circulation. Rapidly acting vasodilators such as nitrates and sodium nitroprusside may also be helpful.

Immediate resuscitation support must be available.

### Pharmacological properties

*Pharmacodynamic properties:* Epinephrine is a direct-acting sympathomimetic agent exerting its effect on alpha- and beta-adrenoceptors. Major effects are increased systolic blood pressure, reduced diastolic pressure, tachycardia, hyperglycaemia and hypokalaemia. It is a powerful cardiac stimulant. It has vasopressor properties and is a bronchodilator.

*Pharmacokinetic properties:* Epinephrine is rapid in onset and of short duration and is rapidly distributed to the heart, spleen, several glandular tissues and adrenergic nerves. It crosses the placenta and is excreted in breast milk. It is approximately 50% bound to plasma proteins. The onset of action is rapid and after intravenous infusion, the half-life is approximately 5-10 minutes.

Epinephrine is rapidly metabolised in the liver and tissues by oxidative deamination and O-methylation followed by reduction or by conjugation with glucuronic acid or sulphate. Up to 90% of the intravenous dose is excreted in the urine as metabolites.

*Preclinical safety data:* Not applicable since Epinephrine (Adrenaline) Injection has been used in clinical practice for many years and its effects in man are well known.

### Pharmaceutical particulars

*List of excipients:* Citrate Acid Monohydrate USP, Sodium Citrate Dihydrate USP, Sodium Chloride USP, Sodium Bisulphite USP, Hydrochloric Acid 10% w/v USP, Water for Injection USP.

*Incompatibilities:* Epinephrine should not be mixed with sodium bicarbonate; the solution is oxidised to adrenochrome and then forms polymers.

*Shelf life:* 9 months.

*Special precautions for storage:* Store below 25°C. Protect from light.

*Nature and contents of container:* The solution is contained in a USP type I glass vial with an elastomeric closure which meets all the relevant USP specifications. The product is available either as 0.5 ml or 1 ml.

*Instructions for use/handling:* The container is specially designed for use with the IMS Minijet injector.

**Marketing authorisation number** 3265/0030

**Date of approval/revision of SPC** May 1997

**Legal category** POM

*Trade Mark

# Invicta Pharmaceuticals
## A division of Pfizer Limited
## Sandwich
## Kent CT13 9NJ

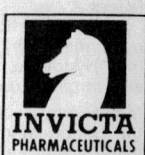

## CARDURA*

**Qualitative and quantitative composition** Doxazosin mesylate:
1.213 mg equivalent to 1 mg doxazosin,
2.43 mg equivalent to 2 mg doxazosin,
4.86 mg equivalent to 4 mg doxazosin.

**Pharmaceutical form** Tablets for oral administration.
1 mg pentagonal tablets: marked DXP1 on one side and 'PFIZER' on the other.
2 mg ovoid tablets: marked DXP2 on one side and 'PFIZER' on the other.
4 mg square tablets: marked DXP4 on one side and 'PFIZER' on the other.

### Clinical particulars
*Therapeutic indications:*
*Hypertension:* Cardura is indicated for the treatment of hypertension and can be used as the sole agent to control blood pressure in the majority of patients. In patients inadequately controlled on single antihypertensive therapy, Cardura may be used in combination with a thiazide diuretic, beta-adrenoceptor blocking agent, calcium antagonist or an angiotensin-converting enzyme inhibitor.

*Benign prostatic hyperplasia:* Cardura is indicated for the treatment of urinary outflow obstruction and symptoms associated with benign prostatic hyperplasia (BPH).

*Posology and method of administration:*
*Hypertension:* Cardura is used in a once daily regimen: the initial dose is 1 mg. Dosage may then be increased after one or two weeks of therapy to 2 mg and thereafter, if necessary to 4 mg. The majority of patients who respond to Cardura will do so at a dose of 4 mg or less. Dosage can be further increased if necessary to 8 mg or the maximum recommended dose of 16 mg.

*Benign prostatic hyperplasia:* The initial dosage of Cardura is 1 mg given once daily. Depending on the individual patient's response dosage may then be increased to 2 mg and thereafter to 4 mg and up to the maximum recommended dose of 8 mg. The recommended titration interval is 1–2 weeks. The usual recommended dose is 2–4 mg daily.

*Children:* There is insufficient exprience to recommend the use of Cardura in children.

*Elderly:* Normal adult dosage.

*Patients with renal impairment:* Since there is no change in pharmacokinetics in patients with impaired renal function the usual adult dose of Cardura is recommended. Cardura is not dialysable.

*Patients with hepatic impairment:* There have been no pharmacokinetic studies in patients with liver impairment, nor in patients taking drugs known to influence hepatic metabolism (e.g. cimetidine). Cardura should be used with care in such patients.

*Contra-indications:* Cardura is contra-indicated in patients with a known hypersensitivity to quinazolines.

*Use during lactation:* Animal studies have shown that doxazosin accumulates in breast milk. The clinical safety of Cardura during lactation has not been established, consequently Cardura is contra-indicated in nursing mothers.

*Special warnings and precautions for use:*
*Impaired liver function:* As with any drug wholly metabolised by the liver, Cardura should be administered with caution to patients with evidence of impaired hepatic function (see *Pharmacokinetic properties*).

*Interactions with other medicaments and other forms of interaction:* Doxazosin is highly bound to plasma proteins (98%). *In vitro* data in human plasma indicates that doxazosin has no effect on protein binding of the drugs tested (digoxin, phenytoin, warfarin or indomethacin). No adverse drug interactions have been observed with thiazide diuretics, frusemide, beta-blocking agents, non-steroidal anti-inflammatory drugs, antibiotics, oral hypoglycaemic drugs, uricosuric agents, or anticoagulants.

*Pregnancy and lactation*
*Use during pregnancy:* Although no teratogenic effects were seen in animal testing, reduced fetal survival was observed in animals at extremely high doses. These doses were approximately 300 times the maximum recommended human dose. As there are no adequate and well controlled studies in pregnant women, the safety of Cardura's use during pregnancy has not yet been established. Accordingly, Cardura should be used only when, in the opinion of the physician, potential benefit outweighs potential risk.

*Use during lactation:* Contra-indicated (see *Contra-indications*).

*Effects on ability to drive and use machines:* The ability to drive or use machinery may be impaired, especially when initiating therapy.

*Undesirable effects:*
*Hypertension:* In clinical trials involving patients with hypertension, the most common reactions associated with Cardura therapy were of a postural type (rarely associated with fainting) or non-specific and included: dizziness, headache, fatigue/malaise, postural dizziness, vertigo, oedema, asthenia, somnolence, nausea and rhinitis.

Extremely rare cases of urinary incontinence were reported; this may be related to Cardura's pharmacological action.

Isolated reports of priapism have been reported to be associated with alpha-1-antagonists, including Cardura.

The following additional adverse events have been reported in marketing experience among patients treated for hypertension. In general, these are not distinguishable from symptoms that might have occurred in the absence of exposure to Cardura: tachycardia, palpitations, chest pain, angina pectoris, myocardial infarction, cerebrovascular accidents and cardiac arrhythmias.

*Benign prostatic hyperplasia:* Experience in controlled clinical trials in BPH indicates a similar adverse event profile to that seen in hypertension.

*Overdose:* Should overdosage lead to hypotension, the patient should be immediately placed in a supine, head down position. Other supportive measures may be appropriate in individual cases. Since Cardura is highly protein bound, dialysis is not indicated.

### Pharmacological properties
*Pharmacodynamic properties:* Doxazosin is a potent and selective post-junctional alpha-1-adrenoceptor antagonist. This action results in a decrease in systemic blood pressure. Cardura is appropriate for oral administration in a once daily regimen in patients with essential hypertension.

Cardura has been shown to be free of adverse metabolic effects and is suitable for use in patients with co-existent diabetes mellitus, gout and insulin resistance.

Cardura is suitable for use in patients with co-existent asthma, left ventricular hypertrophy and in elderly patients. Treatment with Cardura has been shown to result in regression of left ventricular hypertrophy, inhibition of platelet aggregation and enhanced activity of tissue plasminogen activator. Additionally, Cardura improves insulin sensitivity in patients with impairment.

Cardura in addition to its antihypertensive effect, has in long term studies produced a modest reduction in plasma total cholesterol, LDL-cholesterol and triglyceride concentrations and therefore may be of particular benefit to hypertensive patients with concomitant hyperlipidaemia.

Administration of Cardura to patients with symptomatic BPH results in a significant improvement in urodynamics and symptoms. The effect in BPH is thought to result from selective blockade of the alpha-adrenoceptors located in the prostatic muscular stroma, capsule and bladder neck.

*Pharmacokinetic properties:* Following oral administration in humans (young male adults or the elderly of either sex), doxazosin is well absorbed and approximately two thirds of the dose is bioavailable. The mean plasma elimination half life is 22 hours thus making the drug suitable for once daily administration.

Doxazosin is extensively metabolised in man and in the animal species tested, with the faeces being the predominant route of excretion.

After oral administration of Cardura the plasma concentrations of the metabolites are low. The most active (6' hydroxy) metabolite is present in man at one fortieth of the plasma concentration of the parent compound which suggests that the antihypertensive activity is in the main due to doxazosin.

*Preclinical safety data:* None stated.

### Pharmaceutical particulars
*List of excipients:* Lactose, magnesium stearate, microcrystalline cellulose, sodium lauryl sulphate and sodium starch glycolate.

*Incompatibilities:* None stated.

*Shelf life:* 5 years.

*Special precautions for storage:* Store below 30°C.

*Nature and contents of container:* Cardura 1 mg, 2 mg and 4 mg Tablets are available as calendar packs of 28 tablets. Aluminium/PVC/PVdC blister strips, 14 tablets/strip, 2 strips in a carton box.

*Instruction for use/handling:* No special requirements.

**Marketing authorisation numbers**
Cardura 1 mg    0057/0276
Cardura 2 mg    0057/0277
Cardura 4 mg    0057/0278

**Date of approval/revision of SPC** April 1997.

**Legal category** POM.

## HYPOVASE*

**Presentation** Hypovase is available in tablets containing prazosin hydrochloride BP equivalent to the following quantities of prazosin:

500 microgram white tablets, unscored: marked 'Pfizer' on one side.
1 mg scored orange tablets: marked HYP/1 on one side.
2 mg scored white tablets: marked HYP/2 on one side and 'Pfizer' on the other.

*Inactive excipients:* Tablets (all strengths): avicel pH 101, calcium phosphate dibasic anhydrous, magnesium stearate, maize starch, sodium lauryl sulphate. In addition, the 1 mg tablet contains the azo-dye, sunset yellow E110.

### Uses
*Actions:* Hypovase causes a decrease in total peripheral vascular resistance thought to be mediated by selective inhibition of post-synaptic alpha-1-adrenoceptors in vascular smooth muscle. The results of forearm plethysmographic studies in humans demonstrate that the resultant peripheral vasodilatation is a balanced effect on both resistance vessels (arterioles) and capacitance vessels (veins).

In hypertensive patients, blood pressure is lowered in both the supine and standing positions; this effect is more pronounced on the diastolic blood pressure. Tolerance to the antihypertensive effect has not been observed in long-term clinical use; relatively little tachycardia or change in renin levels has been noted. Rebound elevation of blood pressure does not occur following abrupt cessation of Hypovase therapy.

The therapeutic efficacy of Hypovase in patients with congestive heart failure is ascribed to a reduction in left ventricular filling pressure, reduction in cardiac impedance and an augmentation of cardiac output. The use of Hypovase in congestive heart failure does not provoke a reflex tachycardia and blood pressure reduction is minimal in normotensive patients.

Hypovase has been found to successfully reduce the severity of the signs, symptoms, frequency and duration of attacks, in patients with Raynaud's disease.

In low dosage, antagonism of alpha-1-receptors on prostatic and urethral smooth muscle has been shown to improve the urinary pressure profile in men and to improve symptoms of benign prostatic hypertrophy.

Clinical studies have shown that Hypovase therapy is not associated with adverse changes in the serum lipid profile.

Following oral administration in normal volunteers and hypertensive patients, plasma concentrations reach a peak in one to two hours, with a plasma half-life of two to three hours. Pharmacokinetic data in a limited number of patients with congestive heart failure, most of whom showed evidence of hepatic congestion, indicates that peak plasma concentrations are reached in 2.5 hours and plasma half-life is approximately 7 hours. Hypovase is highly bound to plasma protein. Studies indicate that Hypovase is extensively metabolised, primarily by demethylation and conjugation, and excreted mainly via bile and faeces.

Renal blood flow and glomerular filtration rate are not impaired by long term oral administration and thus Hypovase can be used with safety in patients with impaired renal function.

*Indications:* Hypertension: Hypovase is indicated in the treatment of all grades of essential (primary) hypertension and of all grades of secondary hypertension of varied aetiology. It can be used as the initial and sole agent or it may be employed in a treatment regimen in conjunction with a diuretic and/or other antihypertensive drug as needed for proper patient response.

Congestive heart failure: Hypovase may be used alone or added to the therapeutic regimen in those patients with congestive heart failure who are resistent or refractory to conventional therapy with diuretics, and/or cardiac glycosides.

Raynaud's phenomenon and Raynaud's disease: Hypovase is indicated for the symptomatic treatment of patients with Raynaud's phenomenon and Raynaud's disease.

Benign prostatic hyperplasia: Hypovase is indicated as an adjunct in the symptomatic treatment of urinary obstruction caused by benign prostatic hyperplasia, and may therefore be of value in patients awaiting prostatic surgery.

## Dosage and administration

*Hypertension:* The dosage range is from 500 micrograms – 20 mg daily. It is recommended that therapy be initiated at the lowest dose, 500 micrograms, twice or three dimes daily for three to seven days, with the starting dose administered in the evening. This dose should be increased to 1 mg twice or three times daily for a further three to seven days. Thereafter, the daily dose should be increased gradually as determined by the patients response to the blood pressure lowering effect. Most patients are likely to be maintained on a dosage regimen of Hypovase alone of up to 15 mg daily in divided doses. Maximum recommended daily dosage: 20 mg in divided doses.

The b.d. starter pack is available for the convenience of prescribers to initiate treatment up to 2 mg twice daily.

Patients receiving other antihypertensive therapy but with inadequate control: The dosage of the other drug should be reduced to a maintenance level and Hypovase initiated at 500 micrograms in the evening, then continuing with 500 micrograms twice or three times daily. Subsequent dosage increase, should be made gradually depending upon the patient's response.

There is evidence that adding Hypovase to angiotensin converting enzyme inhibitor, beta-adrenergic antagonist or calcium antagonist therapy may bring about a substantial reduction in blood pressure. Therefore, the low initial dosage regimen is recommended.

*Congestive cardiac failure:* The recommended starting dose is 500 micrograms two, three or four times daily, increasing to 4 mg in divided doses. Dosage should be adjusted according to the patient's clinical response, based on careful monitoring of cardiopulmonary signs and symptoms, and when indicated, haemodynamic studies. Dosage may be adjusted as often as every two or three days in patients under close medical supervision. In severely ill, decompensated patients, rapid dosage adjustment over one to two days may be indicated and is best done when haemodynamic monitoring is available. In clinical studies, the therapeutic dosages ranged from 4 mg to 20 mg daily in divided doses. Adjustment of dosage may be required in the course of Hypovase therapy in some patients to maintain optimal clinical improvement.

Usual daily maintenance dosage: 4 mg to 20 mg in divided doses.

*Raynaud's phenomenon and Raynaud's disease:* The recommended starting dosage is 500 micrograms twice daily given for a period of three to seven days and should be adjusted according to the patient's clinical repsonse. Usual maintenance dosage 1 mg or 2 mg twice daily.

*Benign prostatic hyperplasia:* The recommended dosage is 500 micrograms twice daily for a period of 3 to 7 days, with the initial dose administered in the evening. The dosage should then be adjusted according to clinical response. The usual maintenance dosage is 2 mg twice daily. This dose should not be exceeded, unless the patient requires Hypovase as antihypertensive therapy.

Patients with BPH receiving antihypertensive therapy: It is recommended that patients receiving antihypertensive therapy are administered Hypovase for BPH only under supervision of the practitioner responsible for treating the patient's hypertension.

Patients with moderate to severe grades of renal impairment: Evidence to date shows that Hypovase does not further compromise renal function when

used in patients with renal impairment. As some patients in this category have responded to small doses of Hypovase, it is recommended that therapy be initiated at 500 micrograms daily and that dosage increases be instituted cautiously.

Patients with hepatic dysfunction: No information is available on the use of Hypovase in this patient group, however, since Hypovase normally undergoes substantial first pass metabolism and subsequent metabolism and excretion by the liver, it is recommended that therapy be initiated at 500 micrograms daily and that dosage increases be instituted cautiously.

*Use in the elderly:* Since the elderly may be more susceptible to hypotension, therapy should be initiated with the lowest possible dose.

*Use in children:* Hypovase is not recommended for the treatment of children under the age of 12 years since safe conditions for its use have not been established.

## Contra-indications, warnings, etc

*Contra-indications:* Sensitivity to Hypovase or related quinazolines.

*Warnings:*

*Use in pregnancy or lactation:* Although no teratogenic effects were seen in animal testing, the safety of Hypovase during pregnancy has not yet been established. The use of prazosin and a beta-blocker for the control of severe hypertension in 44 pregnant women revealed no drug-related foetal abnormalities or adverse effects. Therapy with prazosin was continued for as long as 14 weeks.

Prazosin has also been used alone or in combination with other hypotensive agents in severe hypertension of pregnancy. No foetal or neonatal abnormalities have been reported with the use of prazosin.

Studies to date are inadequate to establish the safety of Hypovase in pregnancy, accordingly, it should be used only when, in the opinion of the physician, potential benefit outweighs potential risk. Hypovase has been shown to be excreted in small amounts in human milk. Caution should be exercised when Hypovase is administered to nursing mothers.

*In patients with congestive cardiac failure:* Hypovase is not recommended in the treatment of congestive cardiac failure due to mechanical obstruction such as aortic valve stenosis, mitral valve stenosis, pulmonary embolism and restrictive pericardial disease. Adequate data are not yet available to establish efficacy in patients with heart failure due to recent myocardial infarction.

*Benign prostatic hyperplasia:* Hypovase is not recommended for patients with a history of micturition syncope.

*Precautions:*

*In patients with hypertension:* A very small percentage of patients may respond in an abrupt and exaggerated manner to the initial dose of Hypovase. Postural hypotension evidenced by dizziness and weakness, or rarely loss of consciousness, has been reported, particularly with the commencement of therapy, but this effect is readily avoided by initiating treatment with a low dose of Hypovase and with small increases in dosage during the first one to two weeks of therapy. The effect when observed, is not related to the severity of hypertension, is self-limiting and in most patients does not recur after the initial period of therapy or during subsequent dosage increments.

When instituting therapy with any effective antihypertensive agent, the patient should be advised how to avoid symptoms resulting from postural hypotension and what measures to take should they develop.

*In patients with congestive cardiac failure:* When Hypovase is initially administered to patients with congestive cardiac failure who have undergone vigorous diuretic or other vasodilator treatment, particularly in higher than the recommended starting dose, the resultant decrease in left ventricular filling pressure may be associated with a significant fall in cardiac output and systemic blood pressure. In such patients, observance of the recommended starting dose of Hypovase followed by gradual dosage increase is particularly important (see 'Dosage and administration').

The clinical efficacy of Hypovase in congestive cardiac failure has been reported to diminish after several months of treatment, in a proportion of patients. In these patients there is usually evidence of weight gain or peripheral oedema indicating fluid retention. Since spontaneous deterioration may occur in such severely ill patients a causal relationship to prazosin therapy has not been established. Thus, as with all patients with congestive cardiac failure, careful adjustment of diuretic dosage according to the patient's clinical condition is required to prevent excessive fluid retention and consequent relief of symptoms.

In those patients without evidence of fluid retention,

when clinical improvement has diminished, an increase in the dosage of Hypovase will usually restore clinical efficacy.

*Raynaud's phenomenon and Raynaud's disease:* Because Hypovase decreases peripheral vascular resistance, careful monitoring of blood pressure during initial administration and during subsequent dosage increments of Hypovase is suggested. Close observation is especially recommended for patients already taking medications that are known to lower blood pressure.

*Benign prostatic hyperplasia:* Hypovase decreases peripheral vascular resistance and since many patients with this disorder are elderly, careful monitoring of blood pressure during initial administration and during adjustment of dosage is recommended. The possibility of postural hypotension, or rarely, loss of consciousness, as reported in other patient groups should be borne in mind. Hypovase may augment the efficacy of antihypertensive therapy, consequently, close observation is especially recommended for patients taking medications that are known to lower blood pressure. Hypovase should not normally be administered to patients already receiving another alpha-1-antagonist.

*Driving/use of machinery:* The patient should be advised that the ability to drive or use machinery may be impaired should dizziness or weakness occur during the initiation of Hypovase therapy.

*Drug interactions:* Hypovase has been administered without any adverse drug interaction in clinical experience to date with the following:

(1) cardiac glycosides – digitalis and digoxin;
(2) hypoglycaemic agents – insulin, chlorpropamide, phenformin, tolazamide and tolbutamide;
(3) tranquillizers and sedatives – chlordiazepoxide, diazepam and phenobarbitone;
(4) agents for treatment of gout – allopurinol, colchicine and probenecid;
(5) anti-arrhythmic agents – procainamide and quinidine;
(6) analgesic, antipyretic, and anti-inflammatory agents – dextropropoxyphene, aspirin, indomethacin and phenylbutazone;

There is evidence that adding Hypovase to beta-adrenergic antagonist or calcium antagonist therapy may produce a substantial reduction in blood pressure. Therefore, the low initial dosage regimen is recommended.

*Drug/laboratory test interactions:* False positive results may occur in screening tests for phaeochromocytoma (urinary vanillylmandelic acid (VMA) and methoxyhydroxyphenyl glycol (MHPG) metabolites of noradrenaline) in patients who are being treated with Hypovase.

*Side-effects:* In patients with hypertension: The most common side-effects associated with Hypovase therapy are: dizziness, headache, drowsiness, lack of energy, weakness, nausea, and palpitations. In most instances side-effects will disappear with continued therapy or may be tolerated with no decrease in dosage of the drug.

In addition, the following reactions have been associated with Hypovase therapy: vomiting, diarrhoea, constipation, abdominal discomfort and/or pain, liver function abnormalities, pancreatitis, oedema, dyspnoea, faintness, transient temporary loss of consciousness, tachycardia, nervousness, vertigo, hallucinations, depression, paraesthesia, rash, pruritus, alopecia, lichen planus, urinary frequency, impotence, incontinence, priapism, blurred vision, reddended sclera, epistaxis, tinnitus, dry mouth, nasal congestion, diaphoresis, fever, positive ANA titre and arthralgia.

Some of these reactions have occurred rarely, and in many instances the exact causal relationships have not been established.

Literature reports exist associating Hypovase therapy with a worsening of pre-existing narcolepsy. A causal relationship is uncertain in these cases.

*In patients with congestive cardiac failure:* The following side-effects have been observed when Hypovase is used in conjunction with cardiac glycosides and diuretics: drowsiness, dizziness, postural hypotension, blurred vision, oedema, dry mouth, palpitations, nausea, diarrhoea, impotence, headache, and nasal congestion. In most instances these occurrences have been mild to moderate in severity and have resolved with continued therapy or have been tolerated with no decrease in drug dosage.

*Raynaud's phenomenon and Raynaud's disease:* The most common, although infrequently reported side-effect, is mild dizziness.

*Benign prostatic hyperplasia:* The most common, although infrequently reported side-effect, is dizziness.

*Overdosage:* Should overdosage lead to hypotension, support of the cardiovascular system is of first importance. Restoration of blood pressure and normalisation of heart rate may be accomplished by keeping the patient in the supine position. If this measure is inadequate, shock should first be treated with volume expanders. If necessary, vasopressors including angiotensin should then be used. Renal function should be monitored and supported as needed. Laboratory data indicate Hypovase is not dialysable because it is protein bound.

**Pharmaceutical precautions**   Store below 30°C.

**Legal category**   POM.

**Package quantities**   b.d. starter pack, for the convenience of patients initiating Hypovase therapy, containing 8×500 microgram Hypovase tablets and 32×1 mg Hypovase tablets (see 'Further information').

Hypovase 500 microgram: Original packs of 56 tablets (in blister strips of 4×14 tablets).

Hypovase 1 mg: Original packs of 56 tablets (in blister strips of 4×14 tablets).

Hypovase 2 mg: Original packs of 56 tablets (in blister strips of 4×14 tablets).

**Further information**   The two week b.d. starter pack has the following instructions to the patient:

'Step 1 (500 micrograms tablets) – evening day 1 to morning day 5
Step 2 (1 mg tablets) – evening day 5 to morning day 9
Step 3 (2×1 mg tablets) – evening day 9 to morning day 15
Your doctor will wish you to follow further dosage instructions beyond Step 3 and you should follow those instructions or see your doctor before the end of Step 3.'

The tablets (500 microgram and 1 mg) are carefully packed in sequence, in blister strips to ensure correct usage.

**Product licence numbers**

| | |
|---|---|
| 500 microgram tablet | 0057/0149R |
| 1 mg tablet | 0057/0106R |
| 2 mg tablet | 0057/0107R |

# LUSTRAL*

**Qualitative and quantitative composition**   Sertraline hydrochloride equivalent to 50 mg or 100 mg sertraline.

**Pharmaceutical form**   50 mg white, capsular shaped, film-coated tablets coded 'LTL-50' on one side and 'PFIZER' on the other.
100 mg white, capsular shaped, film-coated tablets coded 'LTL-100' on one side and 'PFIZER' on the other.

**Clinical particulars**
*Therapeutic indications:* Lustral is indicated for the treatment of symptoms of depressive illness, including accompanying symptoms of anxiety. Following satisfactory response, continuation with Lustral therapy is effective in preventing relapse of the initial episode of depression or recurrence of further depressive episodes, including accompanying symptoms of anxiety.

*Posology and method of administration:*
*Adults:* Lustral should be given as a single daily dose. Lustral tablets can be administered with or without food. The starting dose is 50 mg daily and the usual therapeutic dose is 50 mg daily.

In some patients doses higher than 50 mg daily may be required. In patients with incomplete response but good toleration at lower doses, dosage adjustments should be made in 50 mg increments over a period of weeks to a maximum of 200 mg daily.

Once optimal therapeutic response is achieved the dose should be reduced, depending on therapeutic response, to the lowest effective level. Doses of 150 mg or more should not be used for periods exceeding 8 weeks. Dosage during prolonged maintenance therapy should be kept at the lowest effective level, with subsequent adjustments depending on therapeutic response. The onset of therapeutic effect may be seen within 7 days, although 2–4 weeks are usually necessary for full antidepressant activity.

Lustral tablets are for oral administration only.

*Use in patients with renal or hepatic impairment:* As with many other medications, sertraline should be used with caution in patients with renal and hepatic impairment (see *Contra-indications, precautions*).

*Use in children:* The use of Lustral in children is not recommended as safety and efficacy have not been established.

*Use in the elderly:* No special precautions are required. The usual adult dose is recommended. Several hundred elderly patients have participated in clinical studies with Lustral. The pattern and incidence of adverse reactions in the elderly is similar to that in younger patients.

*Contra-indications:* Lustral is contra-indicated in patients with a known hypersensitivity to sertraline.

Concomitant use in patients taking monoamine oxidase inhibitors (MAOIs) is contra-indicated (see *Special warnings and precautions for use*).

*Use in hepatic impairment:* Sertraline is extensively metabolised by the liver. A single dose pharmacokinetic study in subjects with mild, stable cirrhosis demonstrated a prolonged elimination half-life and increased AUC in comparison to normal subjects.

There is insufficient clinical experience in patients with significant hepatic dysfunction and accordingly Lustral should not be used in such patients.

*Special warnings and special precautions for use:*
*Monoamine oxidase inhibitors:* Cases of serious reactions have been reported in patients receiving Lustral in combination with a monoamine oxidase inhibitor (MAOI), including the selective MAOI selegiline and the reversible MAOI (reversible inhibitor of monoamine oxidase RIMA), moclobemide. Some cases presented with features resembling the serotonin syndrome. Similar cases, sometimes fatal, have been reported with other antidepressants during combined treatment with a MAOI and in patients who have recently discontinued an antidepressant drug and have been started on a MAOI. Symptoms of a drug interaction between an SSRI and a MAOI include: hyperthermia, rigidity, myoclonus, autonomic instability with possible rapid fluctuations of vital signs, mental status changes that include confusion, irritability and extreme agitation progressing to delirium and coma. Therefore, Lustral should not be used in combination with a MAOI or within 14 days of discontinuing treatment with a MAOI. Similarly, at least 14 days should elapse after discontinuing Lustral treatment before starting a MAOI.
*Electroconvulsive therapy (ECT):* There are no clinical studies establishing the risks or benefits of the combined use of ECT and Lustral.
*Activation of mania/hypomania:* As with other antidepressants, activation of mania/hypomania has been reported in a small proportion of patients.
*Seizures:* Seizures are a potential risk with antidepressant drugs. Lustral should be avoided in patients with unstable epilepsy and patients with controlled epilepsy should be carefully monitored. The drug should be discontinued in any patient who develops seizures.
*Suicide:* Since the possibility of a suicide attempt is inherent in depression and may persist until significant remission occurs, patients should be closely supervised during the early course of therapy.

*Use in renal insufficiency:* Since sertraline is extensively metabolised, excretion of unchanged drug in urine is a minor route of elimination. In patients with mild to moderate renal impairment (creatinine clearance 20–50 ml/min) or severe renal impairment (creatinine clearance <20 ml/min), single dose pharmacokinetic parameters were not significantly different compared with controls. However, steady state pharmacokinetics of sertraline have not been adequately studied in this patient population and caution is advised when treating patients with renal impairment.

*Use in the elderly:* Several hundred elderly patients have participated in clinical studies with Lustral. The pattern and incidence of adverse reactions in the elderly is similar to that in younger patients.

*Interactions with other medicaments and other forms of interaction:*
*Monoamine oxidase inhibitors:* (see *Special warnings and special precautions for use*).
*Centrally active medication:* Caution is advised if Lustral is administered with other centrally active medication.
*Alcohol:* In 11 healthy subjects administered Lustral (200 mg daily) for 9 days, there was no adverse effect on cognitive or psychomotor performance relative to placebo, following a single dose of 500 mg/kg alcohol. However, the concomitant use of Lustral and alcohol in depressed patients is not recommended.
*Lithium:* In placebo-controlled trials in normal volunteers, the co-administration of Lustral and lithium did not significantly alter lithium pharmacokinetics, however it is recommended that plasma lithium levels be monitored following initiation of lithium therapy.
Co-administration of Lustral with lithium did result in an increase in tremor relative to placebo, indicating a possible pharmacodynamic interaction. As with other SSRIs, caution is recommended when co-administering sertraline with medications, such as lithium, which may act via serotonergic mechanisms.
*Serotonergic drugs:* There is limited controlled experience regarding the optimal timing of switching from other antidepressant drugs to Lustral. Care and prudent medical judgment should be exercised when switching, particularly from long-acting agents. The duration of washout period which should intervene before switching from one selective serotonin reuptake inhibitor (SSRI) to another has not been established.
Until further data are available, serotonergic drugs,

such as tryptophan, sumatriptan or fenfluramine, should not be used concomitantly with Lustral.
*Other drug interactions:* Since Lustral is bound to plasma proteins, the potential of Lustral to interact with other plasma protein bound drugs should be borne in mind.
Formal drug interaction studies have been performed with Lustral. Co-administration of Lustral (200 mg daily) with diazepam or tolbutamide resulted in small, statistically significant changes in some pharmacokinetic parameters. Co-administration with cimetidine caused a substantial decrease in sertraline clearance. The clinical significance of these changes is unknown. Lustral had no effect on the beta-adrenergic blocking ability of atenolol. No interaction with Lustral (200 mg daily) was observed with glibenclamide or digoxin.
Co-administration of Lustral (200 mg daily) with warfarin resulted in a small but statistically significant increase in prothrombin time, the clinical significance of which is unknown. Accordingly, prothrombin time should be carefully monitored when Lustral therapy is initiated or stopped.
Lustral (200 mg daily), did not potentiate the effects of carbamazepine, haloperidol or phenytoin on cognitive and psychomotor performance in healthy subjects.

*Pregnancy and lactation:*
*Use in pregnancy:* Reproduction studies have been performed in rats and rabbits at doses up to approximately 20 times and 10 times the maximum daily human dose, respectively. There was no evidence of teratogenicity or embryotoxicity at any dose level. At the dose level corresponding to approximately 2.5 to 10 times the maximum daily human dose, however, sertraline was associated with delayed ossification in foetuses, probably secondary to effects on the dams.
There was decreased neonatal survival following maternal administration of sertraline at doses approximately 5 times the maximum human dose. Similar effects on neonatal survival have been described for other antidepressant drugs. The clinical significance of these effects is unknown.
There are no adequate and well-controlled studies in pregnant women. Since animal reproduction studies are not always predictive of human response, Lustral should be used during pregnancy only if the perceived benefits outweigh the risks. Women of childbearing potential should employ an adequate method of contraception if taking Lustral.

*Use during lactation:* Limited data concerning sertraline levels in breast milk are available, hence use in nursing mothers is not recommended.

*Effects of ability to drive and use machines:* Since antidepressant drugs may impair the abilities required to perform potentially hazardous tasks such as driving a car or operating machinery, the patient should be cautioned accordingly. Lustral should not be administered with benzodiazepines or other tranquillizers in patients who drive or operate machinery.

*Undesirable effects:* In multiple dose studies involving dose escalation based on the patients' response, side-effects which occurred significantly more frequently with Lustral than placebo were: nausea, diarrhoea/loose stools, dyspepsia, tremor, dizziness, insomnia, somnolence, increased sweating, dry mouth and male sexual dysfunction (principally ejaculatory delay).
Spontaneous reports of malaise and rash (including rare reports of erythema multiforme) have been reported with Lustral.
Asymptomatic elevations in serum transaminases (AST and ALT) have been reported infrequently (approximately 0.8%) in association with Lustral administration. The abnormalities usually occurred within the first 1 to 9 weeks of drug treatment and promptly diminished upon drug discontinuation.
Seizures: See *Special warnings and special precautions for use.* Lustral should be discontinued in a patient who develops seizures.
There have been isolated reports of movement disorders, such as extrapyramidal symptoms and gait abnormalities, with Lustral and their association with the drug is not proven. Most of these have occurred in patients on concomitant neuroleptic medication or with pre-existing movement disorder.
There have been isolated reports of hyperprolactinaemia, galactorrhoea and menstrual irregularities with Lustral. Association with the drug is not proven.
Rare cases of hyponatraemia have been reported and appeared to be reversible when Lustral was discontinued. Some cases were possibly due to the syndrome of inappropriate antidiuretic hormone secretion. The majority of reports were associated with older patients and patients taking diuretics or other medications. Rare cases of withdrawal reaction have been reported.

*Overdose:* On the evidence available, Lustral has a wide margin of safety in overdose. Overdoses of Lustral alone of up to 8 g have been reported. Deaths involving overdoses of Lustral in combination with other drugs and/or alcohol have been reported. Therefore, any overdosage should be treated aggressively.

No specific therapy is recommended and there are no specific antidotes to Lustral. Establish and maintain an airway, ensure adequate oxygenation and ventilation. Activated charcoal, which may be used with sorbitol, may be as or more effective than emesis or lavage, and should be considered in treating overdose. Cardiac and vital signs monitoring is recommended along with general symptomatic and supportive measures. Due to the large volume of distribution of sertraline, forced diuresis, dialysis, haemoperfusion and exchange transfusion are unlikely to be of benefit.

**Pharmacological properties**
*Pharmacodynamic properties:* Sertraline is a potent and specific inhibitor of neuronal serotonin (5-HT) uptake *in vitro* and *in vivo*, but is without affinity for muscarinic, serotonergic, dopaminergic, adrenergic, histaminergic, GABA or benzodiazepine receptors.

Sertraline is devoid of stimulant, sedative or anticholinergic activity or cardiotoxicity in animals.

Unlike tricyclic antidepressants, no weight gain is observed with treatment for depression.

Lustral has not been observed to produce physical or psychological dependence.

*Pharmacokinetic properties:* Sertraline exhibits dose proportional pharmacokinetics over a range of 50–200 mg. After oral administration of sertraline in man, peak blood levels occur at about 4.5–8.4 hours. Daily doses of sertraline achieve steady-state after one week. Sertraline has a plasma half-life of approximately 26 hours with a mean half-life for young and elderly adults ranging from 22–36 hours. Sertraline is approximately 98% bound to plasma proteins. The principal metabolite, N-desmethylsertraline, is inactive in *in vivo* models of depression and has a half-life of approximately 62–104 hours. Sertraline and N-desmethylsertraline are both extensively metabolised in man and the resultant metabolites excreted in faeces and urine in equal amounts. Only a small amount (<0.2%) of unchanged sertraline is excreted in the urine.

The pharmacokinetics of sertraline in elderly patients are similar to younger adults.

Food does not significantly change the bioavailability of Lustral tablets.

*Preclinical safety data:* Extensive chronic safety evaluation studies in animals show that sertraline is generally well tolerated at doses that are appreciable multiples of those that are clinically effective.

**Pharmaceutical particulars**
*List of excipients:* Sertraline tablets include the following inert ingredients: calcium hydrogen phosphate, microcrystalline cellulose, hydroxypropylcellulose, sodium starch glycollate, magnesium stearate, hydroxypropylmethylcellulose, polyethylene glycol, polysorbate-80, titanium dioxide (E171).

*Incompatibilities:* None.

*Shelf life:* Current stability data for tablets supports a shelf life of 5 years.

*Special precautions for storage:* None.

*Nature and contents of container:* Lustral is available as: Calendar packs of 28 tablets. Aluminium/PVC blister strips, 14 tablets/strip, 2 strips in a carton box.

*Instructions for use/handling:* No special requirements.

**Marketing authorisation numbers**
Lustral Tablets 50 mg     0057/0308
Lustral Tablets 100 mg    0057/0309

**Date of approval/revision of SPC**   February 1996.

**Legal category**   POM.

# VIBRAMYCIN*
# VIBRAMYCIN* 50
# VIBRAMYCIN*-D

## Qualitative and quantitative composition
*Active ingredient:* doxycycline.
Vibramycin 50 Capsules contain 50 mg doxycycline as doxycycline hyclate PhEur.
Vibramycin Capsules contain 100 mg doxycycline as doxycycline hyclate PhEur.
Vibramycin-D Dispersible Tablets contain 100 mg doxycycline PhEur.

## Pharmaceutical form
Vibramycin 50 capsules are green and ivory, coded 'Pfizer' and 'VBM 50'.
Vibramycin capsules 100 mg are green, coded 'Pfizer' and 'VBM 100'.
Vibramycin-D Dispersible Tablets are off-white buff tablets coded 'D 9' on one side and 'Pfizer' on the other.

## Clinical particulars
*Therapeutic indications:* Vibramycin has been found clinically effective in the treatment of a variety of infections caused by susceptible strains of Gram-positive and Gram-negative bacteria and certain other micro-organisms.

*Respiratory tract infections:* Pneumonia and other lower respiratory tract infections due to susceptible strains of *Streptococcus pneumoniae, Haemophilus influenzae, Klebsiella pneumoniae* and other organisms. *Mycoplasma pneumoniae* pneumonia. Treatment of chronic bronchitis, sinusitis.

*Urinary tract infections* caused by susceptible strains of Klebsiella species, Enterobacter species, *Escherichia coli, Streptococcus faecalis* and other organisms.

*Sexually transmitted diseases:* Infections due to *Chlamydia trachomatis* including uncomplicated urethral, endocervical or rectal infections. Non-gonococcal urethritis caused by *Ureaplasma urealyticum* (T-mycoplasma). Vibramycin is also indicated in chancroid, granuloma inguinale and lymphogranuloma venereum. Vibramycin is an alternative drug in the treatment of gonorrhoea and syphilis.

*Skin infections:* Acne vulgaris, when antibiotic therapy is considered necessary.

Since Vibramycin is a member of the tetracycline series of antibiotics, it may be expected to be useful in the treatment of infections which respond to other tetracyclines, such as:

*Ophthalmic infections:* Due to susceptible strains of gonococci, staphylococci and Haemophilus influenzae. Trachoma, although the infectious agent, as judged by immunofluorescence, is not always eliminated. Inclusion conjunctivitis may be treated with oral Vibramycin alone or in combination with topical agents.

*Rickettsial infections:* Rocky Mountain spotted fever, typhus group, Q fever, Coxiella endocarditis and tick fevers.

*Other infections:* Psittacosis, brucellosis (in combination with streptomycin), cholera, bubonic plague, louse and tick-borne relapsing fever, tularaemia, glanders, meliodosis, chloroquine-resistant falciparum malaria and acute intestinal amoebiasis (as an adjunct to amoebicides).

Vibramycin is an alternative drug in the treatment of leptospirosis, gas gangrene and tetanus.

Vibramycin is indicated for prophylaxis in the following conditions: Scrub typhus, travellers' diarrhoea (enterotoxigenic *Escherichia coli*), leptospirosis.

*Posology and method of administration*
*Dosage:*
*Adults:* The usual dose of Vibramycin for the treatment of acute infections in adults is 200 mg on the first day (as a single dose or in divided doses) followed by a maintenance dose of 100 mg/day. In the management of more severe infections, 200 mg daily should be given throughout treatment.

Capsules and Dispersible Tablets are for oral administration only.

Vibramycin-D tablets are administered by drinking a suspension of the tablets in a small amount of water.

Vibramycin capsules should be administered with adequate amounts of fluid. This should be done in the sitting or standing position and well before retiring at night to reduce the risk of oesophageal irritation and ulceration. If gastric irritation occurs, it is recommended that Vibramycin be given with food or milk. Studies indicate that the absorption of Vibramycin is not notably influenced by simultaneous ingestion of food or milk.

Exceeding the recommended dosage may result in an increased incidence of side effects. Therapy should be continued for at least 24 to 48 hours after symptoms and fever have subsided.

When used in streptococcal infections, therapy should be continued for 10 days to prevent the development of rheumatic fever or glomerulonephritis.

*Dosage recommendations in specific infections:*
*Acne vulgaris:* 50 mg daily with food or fluid for 6 to 12 weeks.

*Sexually transmitted diseases:* 100 mg twice daily for 7 days is recommended in the following infections: uncomplicated gonococcal infections (except anorectal infections in men); uncomplicated urethral, endocervical or rectal infection caused by *Chlamydia trachomatis*; non-gonococcal urethritis caused by *Ureaplasma urealyticum*. Acute epididymo-orchitis caused by *Chlamydia trachomatis* or *Neisseria gonorrhoea* 100 mg twice daily for 10 days. Primary and secondary syphilis: 300 mg a day in divided doses for at least 10 days.

*Louse- and tick-borne relapsing fevers:* A single dose of 100 or 200 mg according to severity.

*Chloroquine-resistant falciparum malaria:* 200 mg daily for at least 7 days. Due to the potential severity of the infection, a rapid-acting schizonticide such as quinine should always be given in conjunction with Vibramycin; quinine dosage recommendations vary in different areas.

*For the prevention of scrub typhus:* 200 mg as a single dose.

*For the prevention of travellers' diarrhoea in adults:* 200 mg on the first day of travel (administered as a single dose or as 100 mg every 12 hours) followed by 100 mg daily throughout the stay in the area. Data on the use of the drug prophylactically are not available beyond 21 days.

*For the prevention of leptospirosis:* 200 mg once each week throughout the stay in the area and 200 mg at the completion of the trip. Data on the use of the drug prophylactically are not available beyond 21 days.

*Use in children:* See under *Contra-indications.*

*Use in the elderly:* Vibramycin may be prescribed in the elderly in the usual dosages with no special precautions. No dosage adjustment is necessary in the presence of renal impairment. The Vibramycin-D dispersible tablet may be preferred for the elderly since it is less likely to be associated with oesophageal irritation and ulceration.

*Use in patients with impaired hepatic function:* See under *Special warnings/precautions.*

*Use in patients with renal impairment:* Studies to date have indicated that administration of Vibramycin at the usual recommended doses does not lead to accumulation of the antibiotic in patients with renal impairment, see under *Special warnings/precautions.*

*Contra-indications:* Persons who have shown hypersensitivity to any of the tetracyclines. The use of drugs of the tetracycline class during tooth development (pregnancy, infancy and childhood to the age of 12 years) may cause permanent discolouration of the teeth (yellow-grey-brown). This adverse reaction is more common during long-term use of the drugs but has been observed following repeated short-term courses. Enamel hypoplasia has also been reported. Vibramycin is therefore contra-indicated in these groups of patients.

*Pregnancy:* Vibramycin is contra-indicated in pregnancy. It appears that the risks associated with the use of tetracyclines during pregnancy are predominantly due to effects on teeth and skeletal development. (See above about use during tooth development).

*Nursing mothers:* Tetracyclines are excreted into milk and are therefore contra-indicated in nursing mothers. (See above about use during tooth development.)

*Children:* Vibramycin is contra-indicated in children under the age of 12 years. As with other tetracyclines, Vibramycin forms a stable calcium complex in any bone-forming tissue. A decrease in the fibula growth rate has been observed in prematures given oral tetracyclines in doses of 25 mg/kg every 6 hours. This reaction was shown to be reversible when the drug was discontinued. (See above about use during tooth development.)

*Special warnings and special precautions for use*
*Use in patients with impaired hepatic function:* Vibramycin should be administered with caution to patients with hepatic impairment or those receiving potentially hepatotoxic drugs.

*Use in patients with renal impairment:* Excretion of doxycycline by the kidney is about 40%/72 hours in individuals with normal renal function. This percentage excretion may fall to a range as low as 1–5%/72 hours in individuals with severe renal insufficiency (creatinine clearance below 10 ml/min). Studies have shown no significant difference in the serum half-life of doxycycline in individuals with normal and severely impaired renal function. Haemodialysis does not alter the serum half-life of doxycycline. The anti-anabolic action of the tetracyclines may cause an increase in blood urea. Studies to date indicate that this does not occur with the use of Vibramycin in patients with impaired renal function.

*Photosensitivity:* Photosensitivity manifested by an exaggerated sunburn reaction has been observed in some individuals taking tetracyclines. Patients likely to be exposed to direct sunlight or ultraviolet light should be advised that this reaction can occur with tetracycline drugs and treatment should be discontinued at the first evidence of skin erythema.

*Microbiological overgrowth:* The use of antibiotics may occasionally result in the overgrowth of nonsusceptible organisms including Candida. If a resistant organism appears, the antibiotic should be discontinued and appropriate therapy instituted.

*Venereal disease:* When treating venereal disease, where co-existent syphilis is suspected, proper diagnostic procedures including dark-field examinations should be utilised. In all such cases monthly serological tests should be made for at least four months.

*Beta-haemolytic streptococci infections:* Infections due to group A beta-haemolytic streptococci should be treated for at least 10 days.

*Interaction with other medicaments and other forms of treatment:* The absorption of doxycycline may be impaired by concurrently administered antacids containing aluminium, calcium or magnesium; oral zinc, iron salts or bismuth preparations.

Since bacteriostatic drugs may interfere with the bactericidal action of penicillin, it is advisable to avoid giving Vibramycin in conjunction with penicillin.

Tetracyclines depress plasma prothrombin activity and reduced doses of concomitant anticoagulants may be necessary.

The serum half-life of doxycycline may be shortened when patients are concurrently receiving barbiturates, carbamazepine or phenytoin. An increase in the daily dosage of Vibramycin should be considered.

Alcohol may decrease the half-life of doxycycline.

A few cases of pregnancy or breakthrough bleeding have been attributed to the concurrent use of tetracycline antibiotics with oral contraceptives.

*Pregnancy and lactation:* See under *Contra-indications.*

*Effects on ability to drive and use machines:* Vibramycin has to date not been associated with effects on the ability to drive and to use machinery.

*Undesirable effects:* Due to virtually complete absorption of Vibramycin gastro-intestinal side-effects are infrequent. The following adverse reactions have been observed in patients receiving tetracyclines.

*Gastro-intestinal:* Gastro-intestinal symptoms are usually mild and seldom necessitate discontinuation of treatment. Anorexia, nausea, vomiting, diarrhoea, glossitis, dysphagia, enterocolitis and inflammatory lesions (with candidial overgrowth) in the anogenital region. Rare instances of oesophagitis and oesophageal ulceration have been reported in patients receiving Vibramycin. A significant proportion of these occurred with the hyclate salt in the capsule form. Most of the patients took medication immediately before going to bed.

*Hepatic toxicity:* Abnormal hepatic function has been reported.

*Skin:* Maculopapular and erythematous rashes occur, but were uncommon in clinical trials. Exfoliative dermatitis has been reported but is uncommon. Photosensitivity is discussed under *Special warnings and special precautions for use.*

*Hypersensitivity reactions:* Urticaria, angioneurotic oedema, anaphylaxis, anaphylactoid purpura, pericarditis, and exacerbation of systemic lupus erythematosus.

Bulging fontanelles in infants and benign intracranial hypertension in adults have been reported in individuals receiving full therapeutic dosages of tetracyclines. These conditions disappeared rapidly when the drug was discontinued.

*Blood:* Haemolytic anaemia, thrombocytopenia, neutropenia and eosinophilia have been reported with tetracyclines.

When given over prolonged periods, tetracyclines have been reported to produce brown-black microscopic discolouration of thyroid tissue. No abnormalities of thyroid function are known to occur.

*Overdose:* Acute overdosage with antibiotics is rare. In the event of overdosage discontinue medication. Gastric lavage plus appropriate supportive treatment is indicated.

Dialysis does not alter serum half-life and thus would not be of benefit in treating cases of overdosage.

## Pharmacological properties

*Pharmacodynamic properties:* Vibramycin is primarily bacteriostatic and is believed to exert its antimicrobial effect by the inhibition of protein synthesis. Vibramycin is active against a wide range of Gram-positive and Gram-negative bacteria and certain other microorganisms.

*Pharmacokinetic properties:* Tetracyclines are readily absorbed and are bound to plasma proteins in varying degrees. They are concentrated by the liver in the bile and excreted in the urine and faeces at high concentrations and in a biologically active form. Doxycycline is virtually completely absorbed after oral administration. Studies reported to date indicate that the absorption of doxycycline, unlike certain other tetracyclines, is not notably influenced by the ingestion of food or milk. Following a 200 mg dose, normal adult volunteers averaged peak serum levels of 2.6 micrograms/ml of doxycycline at 2 hours decreasing to 1.45 micrograms/ml at 24 hours. Doxycycline has a high degree of lipid solubility and a low affinity for calcium. It is highly stable in normal human serum. Doxycycline will not degrade into an epianhydro form.

## Pharmaceutical particulars

*List of excipients:* Vibramycin 100 mg capsules: Maize Starch PhEur, Lactose PhEur, alginic acid, magnesium stearate NF, Sodium Lauryl Sulphate PhEur. The capsule shell contains: gelatin BP, titanium dioxide (E171), patent blue V (E131) and quinoline yellow (E104).

Vibramycin 50 mg capsules: Maize Starch PhEur, Lactose PhEur, alginic acid, magnesium stearate NF, Sodium Lauryl Sulphate PhEur. In addition the capsule shell cap contains: gelatin BP, titanium dioxide (E171), patent blue V (E131) and quinoline yellow (E104) and the body contains yellow iron oxide (E172), indigotine (E132) and titanium dioxide (E171).

Vibramycin D Dispersible tablets: Colloidal silicon dioxide PhEur, microcrystalline cellulose PhEur and Magnesium Stearate PhEur.

*Incompatibilities:* None stated.

*Shelf life:* Vibramycin 50 and 100 mg capsules 48 months.

Vibramycin-D Dispersible tablets 48 months.

*Special precautions for storage:* Store below 25°C.

*Nature and contents of container:* Vibramycin Capsules 100 mg are available as: Packs of 8 capsules. Aluminium/PVC blister strips, a single strip of 8 capsules in a carton box.

Vibramycin 50 Capsules 50 mg are available as: Calendar packs of 28 capsules. Aluminium/PVC blister strips, 14 capsules per strip, 2 strips in a carton box.

Vibramycin-D Dispersible Tablets 100 mg are available as: Packs of 8 tablets. Aluminium/PVC blister strips, a single strip of 8 tablets in a carton box.

*Instructions for use/handling:* No special requirements.

*Marketing authorisation holder:* Pfizer Limited (trading as Invicta Pharmaceuticals), Ramsgate Road, Sandwich.

## Marketing authorisation numbers

| | |
|---|---|
| Vibramycin Capsules 100 mg | 0057/5059R |
| Vibramycin Capsules 50 mg | 0057/0238 |
| Vibramycin-D Dispersible Tablets 100 mg | 0057/0188 |

**Date of approval/revision of SPC**  August 1996.

**Legal category**  POM.

*\*Trade Mark*

# Janssen-Cilag Ltd
Saunderton
High Wycombe
Bucks HP14 4HJ

## ANQUIL*

**Presentation** White, uncoated tablets marked 'JANS-SEN' on one side and 'A/0.25' on the reverse. Each tablet contains 0.25 mg benperidol. The tablets also contain lactose.

**Uses** Anquil is a neuroleptic of the butyrophenone series for the control of deviant anti-social sexual behaviour.

**Dosage and administration** Anquil is intended for oral administration to adults only. The recommended daily dose is 0.25-1.5 mg in divided doses. Dosage is best initiated and adjusted under close clinical supervision, as individual response to neuroleptic drugs is variable.

In determining dosage, consideration should be given to the patient's age, severity of symptoms and previous response to other neuroleptic drugs.

In adolescents a lower dose may be advisable.

*Use in children:* Not recommended.

*Use in the elderly:* Patients who are elderly or debilitated, or those with previously reported adverse reactions to neuroleptic drugs, may require less Anquil, and half the normal starting dose may be sufficient for therapeutic response.

**Contra-indications, warnings, etc**
*Contra-indications:* Comatose states, patients with extrapyramidal symptoms, CNS depression, hypersensitivity to any of the ingredients of Anquil or other butyrophenones, depressive disorders or Parkinson's disease.

*Precautions:* Rare cases of sudden and unexplained death have been reported in psychiatric patients receiving antipsychotic drugs. However, Anquil has not been clearly implicated in any case.

Acute withdrawal symptoms, including nausea, vomiting and insomnia, have very rarely been described after abrupt cessation of high doses of antipsychotic drugs. Relapse may also occur and gradual withdrawal is advisable.

Where prolonged treatment with Anquil is envisaged, it would be a reasonable precaution to carry out regular blood counts and tests of liver function.

Caution is advised in patients with liver disease, renal failure, cardiovascular disease, epilepsy, and conditions predisposing to epilepsy or convulsions.

*Use during pregnancy and lactation:* The safety of Anquil in pregnancy has not been established, although studies in animals have not demonstrated teratogenic effects. As with other drugs, it is not advisable to administer Anquil in pregnancy.

Butyrophenones are excreted in breast milk and are not recommended during lactation. If the use of Anquil is considered essential, breast feeding should be discontinued.

*Effects on driving ability and operation of machinery:* Anquil may interfere with activities requiring mental alertness. Therefore, patients should be advised not to drive or operate machinery until their individual susceptibility is known.

*Interactions:* In common with all neuroleptics, Anquil can increase the central nervous system depression produced by other CNS-depressant drugs, including alcohol, hypnotics, sedatives, strong analgesics or sedating antihistamines and may antagonise the action of adrenaline and other sympathomimetic agents.

Certain agents (eg phenobarbitone, carbamazepine, phenytoin), as well as smoking and alcohol consumption, which stimulate metabolising enzymes in the liver, may theoretically enhance the metabolic breakdown of neuroleptics, necessitating an increased dose.

Anquil may impair the anti-Parkinson effects of levodopa and other dopamine agonists. The dosage of anti-convulsants may need to be increased to take account of the lowered seizure threshold.

The risk of hypotension with antihypertensive drugs may be increased when Anquil is given concomitantly.

Enhanced CNS effects when combined with methyldopa have been reported for some butyrophenones.

*Adverse effects:*
*Central nervous system:* In common with all neuroleptics, extrapyramidal symptoms may occur. Acute dystonias may occur early in treatment. Parkinsonian rigidity, tremor and akathisia tend to appear less rapidly. Oculogyric crises and laryngeal dystonias have been reported.

Anti-Parkinson agents should only be given as required; they should not be prescribed routinely because of the possible risk of impairing the therapeutic efficacy of Anquil.

Tardive dyskinesia may occur during administration or after withdrawal of neuroleptic drugs, including Anquil. The syndrome is common among patients treated with moderate to high doses of anti-psychotic drugs for prolonged periods of time and may prove irreversible, particularly in patients over the age of 50.

It is unlikely to occur in the short-term when low or moderate doses of Anquil are used as recommended, but the risk increases with age and increasing dosage. Anquil should be given in the minimal effective dose for the minimum possible time.

The potential seriousness and unpredictability of tardive dyskinesia and the fact that it has occasionally been reported to occur when neuroleptic anti-psychotic drugs have been prescribed for relatively short periods in low dosage means that the prescribing of such agents requires especially careful assessment of risks versus benefit. Tardive dyskinesia can be precipitated or aggravated by anti-Parkinson drugs. Tardive dyskinesias may occur after abrupt drug withdrawal.

It has been reported that fine vermicular movements of the tongue may be an early sign of tardive dyskinesia and that the full syndrome may not develop if the medication is stopped at that time. If signs and symptoms of tardive dyskinesia appear, the discontinuation of all neuroleptic drugs should be considered.

As with other neuroleptics, rare cases of Neuroleptic Malignant Syndrome, an idiosyncratic response characterised by hyperthermia, muscle rigidity, autonomic instability, altered consciousness, coma and elevated CPK levels, have been reported. Signs of autonomic dysfunction such as tachycardia, labile arterial pressure and sweating may precede the onset of hyperthermia, acting as early warning signs. Antipsychotic treatment should be withdrawn immediately and appropriate supportive therapy and careful monitoring instituted.

Anquil, even in low dosage in susceptible (especially non-psychotic) individuals, may cause unpleasant subjective feelings of being mentally dulled or slowed down, dizziness, headache, or paradoxical effects of excitement, agitation or insomnia.

Depression and seizures have been reported rarely. A causal relationship with Anquil has not been unequivocally established.

Confusional or agitated states have been reported rarely.

*Gastrointestinal system:* Nausea, vomiting, loss of appetite, constipation and dyspepsia have been reported.

*Endocrinological system:* Hormonal effects of antipsychotic neuroleptic drugs include hyper-prolactinaemia, which may cause galactorrhoea, gynaecomastia and oligo- or amenorrhoea.

*Cardiovascular system:* Dose-related hypotension is uncommon but can occur, particularly in the elderly who are more susceptible to the sedative and hypotensive effects. Benign tachycardia has occasionally been reported.

*Other adverse reactions:* Jaundice or transient abnormalities of liver function in the absence of jaundice have been reported. The following effects have been reported rarely: oedema, skin rashes or hypersensitivity reactions such as exanthema and pruritus. Blood dyscrasias, including granulocytopenia, have been reported occasionally. Weight changes may occur. Isolated cases of excessive salivation have been reported.

*Overdosage:*
*Symptoms:* In general, the manifestations of Anquil overdosage are an extension of its pharmacological action. In patients who have received daily doses of 160 mg, the most prominent side-effects were extrapyramidal symptoms such as oculogyric crisis, excessive salivation, muscle rigidity, akinesia and akathisia. Drowsiness or paradoxical excitement may occur.

*Treatment:* There is no specific antidote to Anquil. Treatment consists of supportive and symptomatic measures combined with standard measures to remove any unabsorbed drug. Extrapyramidal symptoms should be treated with anti-Parkinson drugs as required.

**Pharmaceutical precautions** Protect from light.

**Legal category** POM.

**Package quantities** Anquil tablets, each containing 0.25 mg benperidol, are supplied in packs of 100.

**Further information** Nil.

**Product licence number** 0242/0014R.

## BINOVUM*

**Qualitative and quantitative composition** BiNovum are tablets for oral administration.

Each white tablet contains norethisterone PhEur 0.5 mg and ethinyloestradiol PhEur 0.035 mg.

Each peach coloured tablet contains norethisterone PhEur 1.0 mg and ethinyloestradiol PhEur 0.035 mg.

**Pharmaceutical form** Tablets.

The white tablets are small, round and engraved C 535 on both faces.

The peach-coloured tablets are small, round and engraved C 135 on both faces.

**Clinical particulars**
*Therapeutic indications:* Contraception and the recognised indications for such oestrogen/progestogen combinations.

*Posology and method of administration:*
*Adults:* It is preferable that tablet intake from the first pack is started on the first day of menstruation in which case no extra contraceptive precautions are necessary.

If menstruation has already begun (that is 2, 3 or 4 days previously), tablet taking should commence on day 5 of the menstrual period. In this case additional contraceptive precautions must be taken for the first 7 days of tablet taking.

If menstruation began more than 5 days previously then the patient should be advised to wait until her next menstrual period before starting to take BiNovum.

*How to take BiNovum:* One tablet is taken daily at the same time (preferably in the evening) without interruption for 21 days, followed by a break of 7 tablet-free days. (A white tablet is taken every day for 7 days, then a peach coloured tablet is taken every day for 14 days, then 7 tablet-free days). Each subsequent pack is started after the 7 tablet-free days have elapsed. Additional contraceptive precautions are not then required.

*Elderly:* Not applicable.

*Children:* Not recommended.

*Contra-indications:*
*Absolute contra-indications:*
– pregnancy or suspected pregnancy (that cannot yet be excluded).
– circulatory disorders (cardiovascular or cerebrovascular) such as thrombophlebitis and thromboembolic processes (or a history of these conditions), moderate to severe hypertension, hyperlipoproteinaemia. In addition the presence of more than one of the risk factors for arterial disease.
– severe liver disease, cholestatic jaundice or hepatitis (viral or non-viral) or a history of these conditions if the results of liver function tests have failed to return to normal, and for 3 months after liver function tests have been found to be normal; a history of jaundice of pregnancy or jaundice due to the use of steroids, Rotor syndrome and Dubin-Johnson syndrome, hepatic cell tumours and porphyria.
– cholelithiasis.
– known or suspected oestrogen-dependent tumours; endometrial hyperplasia; undiagnosed vaginal bleeding.
– systemic lupus erythematosus or a history of this condition.
– a history during pregnancy or previous use of steroids of:
– severe pruritus
– herpes gestationis
– a manifestation or deterioration of otosclerosis

*Relative contra-indications:* If any relative contra-indications listed below are present, the benefits of oestrogen/progestogen containing preparations must be weighed against the possible risk for each individual case and the patient kept under close supervision. In case of aggravation or appearance of any of these conditions whilst the patient is taking the pill, its use should be discontinued.

– conditions implicating an increasing risk of developing venous thrombo-embolic complications, e.g. severe varicose veins or prolonged immobilisation or major surgery. Disorders of coagulation.

– presence of any risk factor for arterial disease e.g. smoking, hyperlipidaemia or hypertension.

– other conditions associated with an increased risk of circulatory disease such as latent or overt cardiac failure, renal dysfunction, or a history of these conditions.

– epilepsy or a history of this condition.

– migraine or a history of this condition.

– a history of cholelithiasis.

– presence of any risk factor for oestrogen-dependent tumours; oestrogen-sensitive gynaecological disorders such as uterine fibromyomata and endometriosis.

– diabetes mellitus.

– severe depression or a history of this condition. If this is accompanied by a disturbance in tryptophan metabolism, administration of vitamin B6 might be of therapeutic value.

– sickle cell haemoglobinopathy, since under certain circumstances, e.g. during infections or anoxia, oestrogen containing preparations may induce thromboembolic process in patients with this condition.

– if the results of liver function tests become abnormal, use should be discontinued.

*Special warnings and special precautions for use:*
*Post partum administration:* Following a vaginal delivery, oral contraceptive administration to non-breast-feeding mothers can be started 21 days post-partum provided the patient is fully ambulant and there are no puerperal complications. No additional contraceptive precautions are required. If post partum administration begins more than 21 days after delivery, additional contraceptive precautions are required for the first 7 days of pill-taking.

If intercourse has taken place post-partum, oral contraceptive use should be delayed until the first day of the first menstrual period.

After miscarriage or abortion administration should start immediately in which case no additional contraceptive precautions are required.

*Changing from a 21 day pill or another 22 day pill to BiNovum:* All tablets in the old pack should be finished. The first BiNovum tablet is taken the next day i.e. no gap is left between taking tablets nor does the patient need to wait for her period to begin. Tablets should be taken as instructed in 'How to take BiNovum'. Additional contraceptive precautions are not required. The patient will not have a period until the end of the first BiNovum pack, but this is not harmful, nor does it matter if she experiences some bleeding on tablet-taking days.

*Changing from a combined every day pill (28 day tablet) to BiNovum:* BiNovum should be started after taking the last active tablet from the 'Every day Pill' pack (i.e. after taking 21 or 22 tablets). The first BiNovum tablet is taken the next day i.e. no gap is left between taking tablets nor does the patient need to wait for her period to begin. Tablets should be taken as instructed in 'How to take BiNovum'. Additional contraceptive precautions are not required. Remaining tablets from the every day (ED) pack should be discarded.

The patient will not have a period until the end of the first BiNovum pack, but this is not harmful, nor does it matter if she experiences some bleeding on tablet-taking days.

*Changing from a progestogen-only pill (POP or mini pill) to BiNovum:* The first BiNovum tablet should be taken on the first day of the period, even if the patient has already taken a mini pill on that day. Tablets should be taken as instructed in 'How to take BiNovum'. Additional contraceptive precautions are not required. All the remaining progestogen-only pills in the mini pill pack should be discarded.

If the patient is taking a mini pill, then she may not always have a period, especially when she is breast-feeding. The first BiNovum tablet should be taken on the day after stopping the mini pill. All remaining pills in the mini pill packet must be discarded. Additional contraceptive precautions must be taken for the first 7 days.

*To skip a period:* To skip a period, a new pack of BiNovum should be started on the day after finishing the current pack (the patient skips the tablet-free days). Tablet-taking should be continued in the usual way.

During the use of the second pack she may experience slight spotting or break-through bleeding but contraceptive protection will not be diminished provided there are no tablet omissions.

The next pack of BiNovum is started after the usual 7 tablet-free days, regardless of whether the period has completely finished or not.

*Reduced reliability:* When BiNovum is taken according to the directions for use the occurrence of pregnancy is highly unlikely. However the reliability of oral contraceptives may be reduced under the following circumstances:
*Forgotten tablets:* If the patient forgets to take a tablet, she should take it as soon as she remembers and take the next one at the normal time. This may mean that two tablets are taken in one day. Provided she is less than 12 hours late in taking her tablet, BiNovum will still give contraceptive protection during this cycle and the rest of the pack should be taken as usual.

If she is more than 12 hours late in taking one or more tablets then she should take the last missed pill as soon as she remembers but leave the other missed pills in the pack. She should continue to take the rest of the pack as usual but must use extra precautions (e.g. sheath, diaphragm, plus spermicide) and follow the '7-day rule' (see *Further information* for the 7 day rule).

If there are 7 or more pills left in the pack after the missed and delayed pills then the usual 7-day break can be left before starting the next pack. If there are less than 7 pills left in the pack after the missed and delayed pills then when the pack is finished the next pack should be started the next day. If withdrawal bleeding does not occur at the end of the second pack then a pregnancy test should be performed.

*Vomiting or diarrhoea:* If after tablet intake vomiting or diarrhoea occurs, a tablet may not be absorbed properly by the body. If the symptoms disappear within 12 hours of tablet-taking, the patient should take an extra tablet from a spare pack and continue with the rest of the pack as usual.

However, if the symptoms continue beyond those 12 hours, additional contraceptive precautions are necessary for any sexual intercourse during the stomach or bowel upset and for the following 7 days (the patient must be advised to follow the '7-day rule').

*Change in bleeding pattern:* If after taking BiNovum for several months there is a sudden occurrence of spotting or breakthrough bleeding (not observed in previous cycles) or the absence of withdrawal bleeding, contraceptive effectiveness may be reduced. If withdrawal bleeding fails to occur and none of the above mentioned events have taken place, pregnancy is highly unlikely and oral contraceptive use can be continued until the end of the next pack.

(If withdrawal bleeding fails to occur at the end of the second cycle, tablet intake should be discontinued and pregnancy excluded before oral contraceptive use can be resumed). However, if withdrawal bleeding is absent and any of the above mentioned events has occurred, tablet intake should be discontinued and pregnancy excluded before oral contraceptive use can be resumed.

*Medical examination/consultation:* A complete medical history and physical examination should be taken prior to the initiation or reinstitution of oral contraceptives and should be repeated periodically.

These physical examinations should include special reference to blood pressure, breasts, abdomen and pelvic organs, including cervical cytology and, where indicated by the medical or family history, relevant laboratory tests. Caution should be observed when prescribing oral contraceptives to young women whose cycles are not yet stabilised.

*Surgery, varicose veins or immobilisation:* In patients using oestrogen-containing preparations the risk of deep vein thrombosis may be temporarily increased when undergoing a major operation (e.g. abdominal, orthopaedic), and surgery to the legs, medical treatment for varicose veins or prolonged immobilisation. Therefore, it is advisable to discontinue oral contraceptive use at least 4 to 6 weeks prior to these procedures if performed electively and to (re)start not less than 2 weeks after full ambulation. The latter is also valid with regard to immobilisation after an accident or emergency surgery. In case of emergency surgery, thrombotic prophylaxis is usually indicated e.g. with subcutaneous heparin.

*Chloasma:* Chloasma may occasionally occur, especially in women with a history of chloasma gravidarum. Women with a tendency to chloasma should avoid exposure to the sun or ultraviolet radiation whilst taking this preparation. Chloasma is often not fully reversible.

*Laboratory tests:* The use of steroids may influence the results of certain laboratory tests. In the literature, at least a hundred different parameters have been reported to possibly be influenced by oral contraceptive use, predominantly by the oestrogenic component. Among these are: biochemical parameters of the liver, thyroid, adrenal and renal function, plasma levels of (carrier) proteins and lipid/lipoprotein fractions and parameters of coagulation and fibrinolysis.

*Further information:*
*Additional contraceptive precautions:* When additional contraceptive precautions are required the patient should be advised either not to have sex, or to use a cap plus spermicide or for her partner to use a condom. Rhythm methods should not be advised as the pill disrupts the usual cyclical changes associated with the natural menstrual cycle e.g. changes in temperature and cervical mucus.

*The 7-day rule:* If any one tablet is forgotten for more than 12 hours.

If the patient has vomiting or diarrhoea for more than 12 hours.

If the patient is taking any of the drugs listed under 'Interactions':

The patient should continue to take her tablets as usual and:

– Additional contraceptive precautions must be taken for the next 7 days.

*But–if these 7 days run beyond the end of the current pack,* the next pack must be started as soon as the current one is finished, i.e. no gap should be left between packs. (This prevents an extended break in tablet taking which may increase the risk of the ovaries releasing an egg and thus reducing contraceptive protection). The patient will not have a period until the end of 2 packs but this is not harmful nor does it matter if she experiences some bleeding on tablet taking days.

*Interactions:* Irregular cycles and reduced reliability of oral contraceptives may occur when these preparations are used concomitantly with drugs such as anticonvulsants, barbiturates, antibiotics, (e.g. tetracyclines, ampicillin, rifampicin, etc), griseofulvin, activated charcoal and certain laxatives. Special consideration should be given to patients being treated with antibiotics for acne. They should be advised to use a non-hormonal method of contraception, or to use an oral contraceptive containing a progestogen showing minimal androgenicity, which have been reported as helping to improve acne without using an antibiotic. Oral contraceptives may diminish glucose tolerance and increase the need for insulin or other antidiabetic drugs in diabetics.

*Pregnancy and lactation:* BiNovum is contra-indicated for use during pregnancy or suspected pregnancy, since it has been suggested that combined oral contraceptives, in common with many other substances, might be capable of affecting the normal development of the child in the early stages of pregnancy. It can be concluded, however, that, if a risk of abnormality exists at all, it must be very small.

Mothers who are breast-feeding should be advised not to use the combined pill since this may reduce the amount of breast-milk, but may be advised instead to use a progestogen-only pill (POP).

*Effects on ability to drive and to use machines:* Not applicable.

*Undesirable effects:* Various adverse reactions have been associated with oral contraceptive use. The first appearance of symptoms indicative of any one of these reactions necessitates immediate cessation of oral contraceptive use while appropriate diagnostic and therapeutic measures are undertaken.

*Serious adverse reactions:*
– There is a general opinion, based on statistical evidence that users of combined oral contraceptives experience more often than non-users various disorders of the coagulation. How often these disorders occur in users of modern low-oestrogen oral contraceptives is unknown, but there are reasons for suggesting that they may occur less often than with the older types of pill which contain more oestrogen.

– Various reports have associated oral contraceptive use with the occurrence of deep venous thrombosis, pulmonary embolism and other embolisms. Other investigations of these oral contraceptives have suggested an increased risk of oestrogen and/or progestogen dose-dependent coronary and cerebrovascular accidents, predominantly in heavy smokers. Thrombosis has very rarely been reported to occur in other veins or arteries, e.g. hepatic, mesenteric, renal or retinal.

– It should be noted that there is no consensus about often contradictory findings obtained in early studies. The physician should bear in mind the possibility of vascular accidents occurring and that there may not be full recovery from such disorders and they may be fatal. The physician should take into account the presence of risk factors for arterial disease and deep venous thrombosis when prescribing oral contraceptives. Risk factors for arterial disease include smoking, the presence of hyperlipidaemia, hypertension or diabetes.

– Signs and symptoms of a thrombotic event may include: sudden severe pain in the chest, whether or not reaching to the left arm; sudden breathlessness; and unusual severe, prolonged headache, especially if it occurs for the first time or gets progressively worse, or is associated with any of the following symptoms: sudden partial or complete loss of vision or diplopia, aphasia, vertigo, a bad fainting attack or collapse with or without focal epilepsy, weakness or very marked numbness suddenly affecting one side or one part of the body, motor disturbances; severe pain in the calf of one leg; acute abdomen.

– Cigarette smoking increases the risk of serious cardiovascular adverse reactions to oral contraceptive use. The risk increases with age and with heavy smoking and is more marked in women over 35 years of age. Women who use oral contraceptives should be strongly advised not to smoke.

– The use of oestrogen-containing oral contraceptives may promote growth of existing sex steroid dependent tumours. For this reason, the use of these oral contraceptives in patients with such tumours is contra-indicated. Numerous epidemiological studies have been reported on the risk of ovarian, endometrial, cervical and breast cancer in women using combined oral contraceptives.

– The evidence is clear that combined oral contraceptives offer substantial protection against both ovarian and endometrial cancer. An increased risk of cervical cancer in long term users of combined oral contraceptives has been reported in some studies, but there continues to be controversy about the extent to which this is attributable to the confounding effects of sexual behaviour and other factors.

– The evidence linking combined oral contraceptive use and breast cancer remains inconclusive. The results of some studies suggest an increased risk of breast cancer presenting below the age of about 35, the risk rising with duration of use. Any possible increased risk of breast cancer with combined oral contraceptives is however likely to be small, and may be expected to be less with low dose pills.

– This possible risk should be weighed against the many benefits of combined oral contraceptives, including their protective effects against ovarian and endometrial cancers.

– Malignant hepatic tumours have been reported on rare occasions in long-term users of oral contraceptives. Benign hepatic tumours have also been associated with oral contraceptive usage. A hepatic tumour should be considered in the differential diagnosis when upper abdominal pain, enlarged liver or signs of intra-abdominal haemorrhage occur.

– The use of oral contraceptives may sometimes lead to the development of cholestatic jaundice or cholelithiasis.

– On rare occasions the use of oral contraceptives may trigger or reactivate systemic lupus erythematosus.

– A further rare complication of oral contraceptive use is the occurrence of chorea which can be reversed by discontinuing the pill. The majority of cases of oral contraceptive-induced chorea show a pre-existing predisposition which often relates to acute rheumatism.

*Other adverse reactions:*

*Cardiovascular system:* Rise of blood pressure. If hypertension develops, treatment should be discontinued.

*Genital tract:* Intermenstrual bleeding, post-medication amenorrhoea, changes in cervical secretion, increase in size of uterine fibromyomata, aggravation of endometriosis, certain vaginal infections, e.g. candidiasis.

*Breast:* Tenderness, pain, enlargement, secretion.

*Gastro-intestinal tract:* Nausea, vomiting, cholelithiasis, cholestatic jaundice.

*Skin:* Erythema nodosum, rash, chloasma, erythema multiforme, hirsutism, loss of scalp hair.

*Eyes:* Discomfort of the cornea if contact lenses are used.

*CNS:* Headache, migraine, mood changes, depression.

*Metabolic:* Fluid retention, change in body weight, reduced glucose tolerance.

*Other:* Changes in libido, leg cramp, premenstrual-like syndrome.

*Overdose:* There have been no reports of serious ill-health from overdosage even when a considerable number of tablets have been taken by a small child. In general, it is therefore unnecessary to treat overdosage. However, if overdosage is discovered within two or three hours and is large, then gastric lavage can be safely used. There are no antidotes and further treatment should be symptomatic.

### Pharmacological properties

*Pharmacodynamic properties:* BiNovum Oral Contraceptive Tablets act through the mechanism of gonadotrophin suppression by the oestrogenic and progestational actions of the ethinyloestradiol and norethisterone. The primary mechanism of action is inhibition of ovulation, but alterations to the cervical mucus and to the endometrium may also contribute to the efficacy of the product.

*Pharmacokinetic properties:* Norethisterone and ethi-

nyloestradiol are absorbed from the gastro-intestinal tract and metabolised in the liver. To obtain maximal contraceptive effectiveness the tablet should be taken as directed and at approximately the same time each day.

Because the active ingredients are metabolised in the liver, reduced contraceptive efficacy has been associated with concomitant use of oral contraceptives and rifampicin. A similar association has been suggested with oral contraceptives and barbiturates, phenytoin sodium, phenylbutazone, griseofulvin and ampicillin.

*Preclinical safety data:* The toxicology of norethisterone and ethinyloestradiol has been extensively investigated in animal studies and through long term clinical experience with widespread use in contraceptives.

### Pharmaceutical particulars

*List of excipients:* Lactose; magnesium stearate; pregelatinised starch; methanol (does not appear in final product); purified water (peach coloured tablets only; does not appear in final product); FD & C yellow No 6 (peach coloured tablets only).

*Incompatibilities (major):* Not applicable.

*Shelf life:* Three years.

*Special precautions for storage:* Store at room temperature (below 25°C). Protect from light.

*Nature and contents of container:* Carton containing 3 PVC/foil blister strips of 21 tablets each.

**Marketing authorisation number**   0242/0208

**Date of approval/revision of SPC**   18 March 1996

**Legal category** POM

## CILEST* 250/35 ORAL CONTRACEPTIVE TABLETS

**Qualitative and quantitative composition** Cilest are tablets for oral administration.

Each tablet contains norgestimate 0.25 mg and ethinyloestradiol 0.035 mg.

**Pharmaceutical form** Tablets (small, round, dark blue, engraved 'C 250' on both faces).

### Clinical particulars

*Therapeutic indications:* Contraception and the recognised indications for such oestrogen/progestogen combinations.

*Posology and method of administration:* For oral administration.

*Adults:* It is preferable that tablet intake from the first pack is started on the first day of menstruation in which case no extra contraceptive precautions are necessary.

If menstruation has already begun (that is 2, 3 or 4 days previously), tablet taking should commence on day 5 of the menstrual period. In this case additional contraceptive precautions must be taken for the first 7 days of tablet taking.

If menstruation began more than 5 days previously then the patient should be advised to wait until her next menstrual period before starting to take Cilest.

*How to take Cilest:* One tablet is taken daily at the same time (preferably in the evening) without interruption for 21 days, followed by a break of 7 tablet-free days. Each subsequent pack is started after the 7 tablet-free days have elapsed. Additional contraceptive precautions are not then required.

*Elderly:* Not applicable.

*Children:* Not recommended.

*Absolute contra-indications:*

– pregnancy or suspected pregnancy (that cannot yet be excluded).

– circulatory disorders (cardiovascular or cerebrovascular) such as thrombophlebitis and thromboembolic processes (or a history of these conditions), moderate to severe hypertension, hyperlipoproteinaemia. In addition the presence of more than one of the risk factors for arterial disease.

– severe liver disease, cholestatic jaundice or hepatitis (viral or non-viral) or a history of these conditions if the results of liver function tests have failed to return to normal, and for 3 months after liver function tests have been found to be normal; a history of jaundice of pregnancy or jaundice due to the use of steroids, Rotor syndrome and Dubin-Johnson syndrome, hepatic cell tumours and porphyria.

– cholelithiasis.

– known or suspected oestrogen-dependent tumours; endometrial hyperplasia; undiagnosed vaginal bleeding.

– systemic lupus erythematosus or a history of this condition.

– a history during pregnancy or previous use of steroids of:

– severe pruritus.

– herpes gestationis.

– a manifestation or deterioration of otosclerosis.

*Relative contra-indications:* If any relative contra-indications listed below is present, the benefits of oestrogen/progestogen-containing preparations must be weighed against the possible risk for each individual case and the patient kept under close supervision. In case of aggravation or appearance of any of these conditions whilst the patient is taking the pill, its use should be discontinued.

– conditions implicating an increasing risk of developing venous thrombo-embolic complications, e.g. severe varicose veins or prolonged immobilisation or major surgery.

– disorders of coagulation.

– presence of any risk factor for arterial disease e.g. smoking, hyperlipidaemia or hypertension.

– other conditions associated with an increased risk of circulatory disease such as latent or overt cardiac failure, renal dysfunction, or a history of these conditions.

– epilepsy or a history of this condition.

– migraine or a history of this condition.

– a history of cholelithiasis.

– presence of any risk factor for oestrogen-dependent tumours; oestrogen-sensitive gynaecological disorders such as uterine fibromyomata and endometriosis.

– diabetes mellitus.

– severe depression or a history of this condition. If this is accompanied by a disturbance in tryptophan metabolism, administration of vitamin B6 might be of therapeutic value.

– sickle cell haemoglobinopathy, since under certain circumstances, e.g. during infections or anoxia, oestrogen-containing preparations may induce thromboembolic process in patients with this condition.

– if the results of liver function tests become abnormal, use should be discontinued.

*Special warnings and special precautions for use:*

*Post partum administration:* Following a vaginal delivery, oral contraceptive administration to non-breast-feeding mothers can be started 21 days postpartum provided the patient is fully ambulant and there are no puerperal complications. No additional contraceptive precautions are required. If post-partum administration begins more than 21 days after delivery, additional contraceptive precautions are required for the first 7 days of pill-taking.

If intercourse has taken place post-partum, oral contraceptive use should be delayed until the first day of the first menstrual period.

After miscarriage or abortion administration should start immediately in which case no additional contraceptive precautions are required.

*Changing from a 21 day pill or another 22 day pill to Cilest:* All tablets in the old pack should be finished. The first Cilest tablet is taken the next day i.e. no gap is left between taking tablets nor does the patient need to wait for her period to begin. Tablets should be taken as instructed in 'How to take Cilest'. Additional contraceptive precautions are not required. The patient will not have a period until the end of the first Cilest pack, but this is not harmful, nor does it matter if she experiences some bleeding on tablet-taking days.

*Changing from a combined every day pill (28 day tablets) to Cilest:* Cilest should be started after taking the last active tablet from the 'Every day Pill' pack (i.e. after taking 21 or 22 tablets). The first Cilest tablet is taken the next day i.e. no gap is left between taking tablets nor does the patient need to wait for her period to begin. Tablets should be taken as instructed in 'How to take Cilest'. Additional contraceptive precautions are not required. Remaining tablets from the every day (ED) pack should be discarded.

The patient will not have a period until the end of the first Cilest pack, but this is not harmful, nor does it matter if she experiences some bleeding on tablet-taking days.

*Changing from a progestogen-only pill (POP or mini pill) to Cilest:* The first Cilest tablet should be taken on the first day of the period, even if the patient has already taken a mini pill on that day. Tablets should be taken as instructed in 'How to take Cilest'. Additional contraceptive precautions are not required. All the remaining progestogen-only pills in the mini pill pack should be discarded.

If the patient is taking a mini pill, then she may not always have a period, especially when she is breast-feeding. The first Cilest tablet should be taken on the day after stopping the mini pill. All remaining pills in the mini pill packet must be discarded. Additional contraceptive precautions must be taken for the first 7 days.

*To skip a period:* To skip a period, a new pack of Cilest should be started on the day after finishing the current pack (the patient skips the tablet-free days). Tablet-taking should be continued in the usual way.

During the use of the second pack she may experience slight spotting or break-through bleeding but contraceptive protection will not be diminished provided there are no tablet omissions.

The next pack of Cilest is started after the usual 7 tablet-free days, regardless of whether the period has completely finished or not.

*Reduced reliability:* When Cilest is taken according to the directions for use the occurrence of pregnancy is highly unlikely. However, the reliability of oral contraceptives may be reduced under the following circumstances:

*Forgotten tablets:* If the patient forgets to take a tablet, she should take it as soon as she remembers and take the next one at the normal time. This may mean that two tablets are taken in one day. Provided she is less than 12 hours late in taking her tablet, Cilest will still give contraceptive protection during this cycle and the rest of the pack should be taken as usual.

If she is more than 12 hours late in taking one or more tablets then she should take the last missed pill as soon as she remembers but leave the other missed pills in the pack. She should continue to take the rest of the pack as usual but must use extra precautions (e.g. sheath, diaphragm, plus spermicide) and follow the '7-day rule' (see Further Information for the 7 day rule).

If there are 7 or more pills left in the pack after the missed and delayed pills then the usual 7-day break can be left before starting the next pack. If there are less than 7 pills left in the pack after the missed and delayed pills then when the pack is finished the next pack should be started the next day. If withdrawal bleeding does not occur at the end of the second pack then a pregnancy test should be performed.

*Vomiting or diarrhoea:* If after tablet intake vomiting or diarrhoea occurs, a tablet may not be absorbed properly by the body. If the symptoms disappear within 12 hours of tablet-taking, the patient should take an extra tablet from a spare pack and continue with the rest of the pack as usual.

However, if the symptoms continue beyond those 12 hours, additional contraceptive precautions are necessary for any sexual intercourse during the stomach or bowel upset and for the following 7 days (the patient must be advised to follow the '7-day rule').

*Change in bleeding pattern:* If after taking Cilest for several months there is a sudden occurrence of spotting or breakthrough bleeding (not observed in previous cycles) or the absence of withdrawal bleeding, contraceptive effectiveness may be reduced. If withdrawal bleeding fails to occur and none of the above mentioned events has taken place, pregnancy is highly unlikely and oral contraceptive use can be continued until the end of the next pack.

(If withdrawal bleeding fails to occur at the end of the second cycle, tablet intake should be discontinued and pregnancy excluded before oral contraceptive use can be resumed). However, if withdrawal bleeding is absent and any of the above mentioned events has occurred, tablet intake should be discontinued and pregnancy excluded before oral contraceptive use can be resumed.

*Medical examination/consultation:* A complete medical history and physical examination should be taken prior to the initiation or reinstitution of oral contraceptives and should be repeated periodically.

These physical examinations should include special reference to blood pressure, breasts, abdomen and pelvic organs, including cervical cytology and, where indicated by the medical or family history, relevant laboratory tests. Caution should be observed when prescribing oral contraceptives to young women whose cycles are not yet stabilised.

*Surgery, varicose veins or immobilisation:* In patients using oestrogen-containing preparations the risk of deep vein thrombosis may be temporarily increased when undergoing a major operation (e.g. abdominal, orthopaedic), and surgery to the legs, medical treatment for varicose veins or prolonged immobilisation. Therefore, it is advisable to discontinue oral contraceptive use at least 4 to 6 weeks prior to these procedures if performed electively and to (re)start not less than 2 weeks after full ambulation. The latter is also valid with regard to immobilisation after an accident or emergency surgery. In case of emergency surgery, thrombotic prophylaxis is usually indicated e.g. with subcutaneous heparin.

*Chloasma:* Chloasma may occasionally occur, especially in women with a history of chloasma gravidarum. Women with a tendency to chloasma should avoid exposure to the sun or ultraviolet radiation whilst taking this preparation. Chloasma is often not fully reversible.

*Laboratory tests:* The use of steroids may influence the results of certain laboratory tests. In the literature, at least a hundred different parameters have been reported to possibly be influenced by oral contraceptive use, predominantly by the oestrogenic component. Among these are: biochemical parameters of the liver, thyroid, adrenal and renal function, plasma levels of (carrier) proteins and lipid/lipoprotein fractions and parameters of coagulation and fibrinolysis.

*Further information:*

*Additional contraceptive precautions:* When additional contraceptive precautions are required the patient should be advised either not to have sex, or to use a cap plus spermicide or for her partner to use a condom. Rhythm methods should not be advised as the pill disrupts the usual cyclical changes associated with the natural menstrual cycle e.g. changes in temperature and cervical mucus.

*The 7-day rule:* If any one tablet is forgotten for more than 12 hours.

If the patient has vomiting or diarrhoea for more than 12 hours.

If the patient is taking any of the drugs listed under *Interactions:*

The patient should continue to take her tablets as usual and:

– Additional contraceptive precautions must be taken for the next 7 days.

*But–if these 7 days run beyond the end of the current pack,* the next pack must be started as soon as the current one is finished, i.e. no gap should be left between packs. (This prevents an extended break in tablet taking which may increase the risk of the ovaries releasing an egg and thus reducing contraceptive protection). The patient will not have a period until the end of 2 packs but this is not harmful nor does it matter if she experiences some bleeding on tablet taking days.

*Interactions with other medicaments and other forms of interaction:* Irregular cycles and reduced reliability of oral contraceptives may occur when these preparations are used concomitantly with drugs such as anticonvulsants, barbiturates, antibiotics, (e.g. tetracyclines, ampicillin, rifampicin, etc), griseofulvin, activated charcoal and certain laxatives. Special consideration should be given to patients being treated with antibiotics for acne. They should be advised to use a non-hormonal method of contraception, or to use an oral contraceptive containing a progestogen showing minimal androgenicity, which have been reported as helping to improve acne without using an antibiotic. Oral contraceptives may diminish glucose tolerance and increase the need for insulin or other antidiabetic drugs in diabetics.

*Pregnancy and lactation*: Cilest is contra-indicated for use during pregnancy or suspected pregnancy, since it has been suggested that combined oral contraceptives, in common with many other substances, might be capable of affecting the normal development of the child in the early stages of pregnancy. It can be definitely concluded, however, that, if a risk of abnormality exists at all, it must be very small.

Mothers who are breast-feeding should be advised not to use the combined pill since this may reduce the amount of breast-milk, but may be advised instead to use a progestogen-only pill (POP).

*Effects on ability to drive and to use machines:* Not applicable.

*Undesirable effects:* Various adverse reactions have been associated with oral contraceptive use. The first appearance of symptoms indicative of any one of these reactions necessitates immediate cessation of oral contraceptive use while appropriate diagnostic and therapeutic measures are undertaken.

*Serious adverse reactions:* There is a general opinion, based on statistical evidence, that users of combined oral contraceptives experience more often than non-users various disorders of the coagulation. How often these disorders occur in users of modern low-oestrogen oral contraceptives is unknown, but there are reasons for suggesting that they may occur less often than with the older types of pill which contain more oestrogen.

Various reports have associated oral contraceptive use with the occurrence of deep venous thrombosis, pulmonary embolism and other embolisms. Other investigations of these oral contraceptives have suggested an increased risk of oestrogen and/or progestogen dose-dependent coronary and cerebrovascular accidents, predominantly in heavy smokers. Thrombosis has very rarely been reported to occur in other veins or arteries, e.g. hepatic, mesenteric, renal or retinal.

It should be noted that there is no consensus about often contradictory findings obtained in early studies. The physician should bear in mind the possibility of vascular accidents occurring and that there may not be full recovery from such disorders and they may be fatal. The physician should take into account the presence of risk factors for arterial disease and deep venous thrombosis when prescribing oral contraceptives. Risk factors for arterial disease include smoking, the presence of hyperlipidaemia, hypertension or diabetes.

Signs and symptoms of a thrombotic event may include: sudden severe pain in the chest, whether or not reaching to the left arm; sudden breathlessness; and unusual severe, prolonged headache, especially if it occurs for the first time or gets progressively worse, or is associated with any of the following symptoms: sudden partial or complete loss of vision or diplopia, aphasia, vertigo, a bad fainting attack or collapse with or without focal epilepsy, weakness or very marked numbness suddenly affecting one side or one part of the body, motor disturbances; severe pain in the calf of one leg; acute abdomen.

Cigarette smoking increases the risk of serious cardiovascular adverse reactions to oral contraceptive use. The risk increases with age and with heavy smoking and is more marked in women over 35 years of age. Women who use oral contraceptives should be strongly advised not to smoke.

The use of oestrogen-containing oral contraceptives may promote growth of existing sex steroid dependent tumours. For this reason, the use of these oral contraceptives in patients with such tumours is contra-indicated. Numerous epidemiological studies have been reported on the risk of ovarian, endometrial, cervical and breast cancer in women using combined oral contraceptives. The evidence is clear that combined oral contraceptives offer substantial protection against both ovarian and endometrial cancer. An increased risk of cervical cancer in long term users of combined oral contraceptives has been reported in some studies, but there continues to be controversy about the extent to which this is attributable to the confounding effects of sexual behaviour and other factors.

The evidence linking combined oral contraceptive use and breast cancer remains inconclusive. The results of some studies suggest an increased risk of breast cancer presenting below the age of about 35, the risk rising with duration of use. Any possible increased risk of breast cancer with combined oral contraceptives is however likely to be small, and may be expected to be less with low dose pills. This possible risk should be weighed against the many benefits of combined oral contraceptives, including their protective effects against ovarian and endometrial cancers.

Malignant hepatic tumours have been reported on rare occasions in long-term users of oral contraceptives. Benign hepatic tumours have also been associated with oral contraceptive usage. A hepatic tumour should be considered in the differential diagnosis when upper abdominal pain, enlarged liver or signs of intra-abdominal haemorrhage occur.

The use of oral contraceptives may sometimes lead to the development of cholestatic jaundice or cholelithiasis.

On rare occasions the use of oral contraceptives may trigger or reactivate systemic lupus erythematosus.

A further rare complication of oral contraceptive use is the occurrence of chorea which can be reversed by discontinuing the pill. The majority of cases of oral contraceptive-induced chorea show a pre-existing predisposition which often relates to acute rheumatism.

*Other adverse reactions:*

*Cardiovascular system:* Rise of blood pressure. If hypertension develops, treatment should be discontinued.

*Genital tract:* Intermenstrual bleeding, post-medication amenorrhoea, changes in cervical secretion, increase in size of uterine fibromyomata, aggravation of endometriosis, certain vaginal infections, e.g. candidiasis.

*Breast:* Tenderness, pain, enlargement, secretion.

*Gastro-intestinal tract:* Nausea, vomiting, cholelithiasis, cholestatic jaundice.

*Skin:* Erythema nodosum, rash, chloasma, erythema multiforme.

*Eyes:* Discomfort of the cornea if contact lenses are used.

*CNS:* Headache, migraine, mood changes, depression.

*Metabolic:* Fluid retention, change in body weight, reduced glucose tolerance.

*Other:* Changes in libido.

*Overdose:* There have been no reports of serious ill-health from overdosage even when a considerable number of tablets have been taken by a small child. In general, it is therefore unnecessary to treat overdosage. However, if overdosage is discovered within two or three hours and is large, then gastric lavage can be safely used. There are no antidotes and further treatment should be symptomatic.

**Pharmacological properties**

*Pharmacodynamic properties:* Cilest acts through the mechanism of gonadotrophin suppression by the oestrogenic and progestational actions of ethinyloestradiol and norgestimate. The primary mechanism of action is inhibition of ovulation, but alterations to the cervical mucus and to the endometrium may also contribute to the efficacy of the product.

*Pharmacokinetic properties:* Norgestimate and ethinyloestradiol are absorbed from the gastro-intestinal tract and metabolised in the liver. To obtain maximal contraceptive effectiveness the tablets should be taken as directed and at approximately the same time each day.

Because the active ingredients are metabolised in the liver, reduced contraceptive efficacy has been associated with concomitant use of oral contraceptives and rifampicin. A similar association has been suggested with oral contraceptives and barbiturates, phenytoin sodium, phenylbutazone, griseofulvin and ampicillin.

*Preclinical safety data:* The toxicology of norgestimate and ethinyloestradiol has been extensively investigated in animal studies and through long term clinical experience with widespread use in contraceptives.

**Pharmaceutical particulars**

*List of excipients:* Lactose (anhydrous); magnesium stearate; pregelatinised starch; F.D. & C. Blue No. 2 Lake; methanol (does not appear in final product).

*Incompatibilities (major):* Not applicable.

*Shelf life:* Three years.

*Special precautions for storage:* Store at room temperature (below 25°C). Protect from light.

*Nature and contents of container:* Carton containing 3 PVC/foil blister strips of 21 tablets each.

**Marketing authorisation number**    0242/0209

**Date of approval/revision of SPC**    18 November 1995.

**Legal category** POM.

## DAKTACORT* CREAM AND OINTMENT

**Qualitative and quantitative composition**    *Cream and ointment:* Miconazole nitrate 2% w/w and hydrocortisone 1% w/w.

**Pharmaceutical form**    *Cream:* White, homogeneous cream. *Ointment:* White, odourless, fatty ointment.

**Clinical particulars**
*Therapeutic indications:* For the topical treatment of inflamed dermatoses where infection by susceptible organisms and inflammation co-exist, eg intertrigo and infected eczema.

Moist or dry eczema or dermatitis including atopic eczema, primary irritant or contact allergic eczema or seborrhoeic eczema including that associated with acne.

Intertriginous eczema including inflammatory intertrigo, perianal and genital dermatitis.

Organisms which are susceptible to miconazole are dermatophytes and pathogenic yeasts (eg *Candida* spp.). Also many Gram-positive bacteria including most strains of *Streptococcus* and *Staphylococcus.*

The properties of Daktacort indicate it particularly for the initial stages of treatment. Once the inflammatory symptoms have disappeared (after about 7 days), treatment can be continued where necessary with Daktarin Cream or Daktarin Powder.

*Posology and method of administration:* For topical administration.

*Cream:* Apply the cream two or three times a day to the affected area, rubbing in gently until the cream has been absorbed by the skin.

*Ointment:* Daktacort ointment should be applied topically two or three times daily.

The same dosage applies to both adults and children.

*Use in elderly:* Natural thinning of the skin occurs in the elderly, hence corticosteroids should be used sparingly and for short periods of time.

In infants, long term continuous topical corticosteroid therapy should be avoided.

If after about 7 days' application, no improvement has occurred, cultural isolation of the offending organism should be followed by appropriate local or systemic antimicrobial therapy.

*Contra-indications:* True hypersensitivity to any of the ingredients. Tubercular or viral infections of the skin or those caused by Gram-negative bacteria.

*Special warnings and special precautions for use:* As with any topical corticosteroid, care is advised with infants and children when Daktacort is to be applied to extensive surface areas or under occlusive dressings including baby napkins; similarly, application to the face should be avoided.

In infants, long term continuous topical corticosteroid therapy should be avoided. Adrenal suppression can occur even without occlusion.

*Interactions with other medicaments and other forms of interaction:* None known.

*Pregnancy and lactation:* In animals, miconazole nitrate has shown no teratogenic effects but is foetotoxic at high oral doses and administration of corticosteroids to pregnant animals can cause abnormalities of foetal development. The relevance of these findings to humans has not been established. However, combinations of topical steroids with imidazoles should be used in pregnant women only if the practitioner considers it to be necessary.

*Effects on ability to drive and use machines:* None known.

*Undesirable effects:* Rarely, local sensitivity may occur requiring discontinuation of treatment.

*Overdose:* Topically applied corticosteroids can be absorbed in sufficient amounts to produce systemic effects. If accidental ingestion of large quantities of the product occurs, an appropriate method of gastric emptying may be used if considered necessary.

**Pharmacological properties**
*Pharmacodynamic properties:* Miconazole nitrate is active against dermatophytes and pathogenic yeasts, and many Gram-positive bacteria. Hydrocortisone has anti-inflammatory activity.

*Pharmacokinetic properties:* Not applicable.

*Preclinical safety data:* Not applicable.

**Pharmaceutical particulars**
*List of excipients:*
Cream: PEG-6, PEG-32 and glycol stearate; polyoxyethylene glycol glycerides; mineral oil; benzoic acid; disodium edetate; butylated hydroxyanisole; purified water.
Ointment: Plastibase 50W.

*Incompatibilities:* None.

*Shelf life:* 36 months.

*Special precautions for storage: Cream:* Store in a refrigerator (2–8°C).
*Ointment:* Store at room temperature.

*Nature and contents of container:* Aluminium tube with polypropylene cap.
*Cream:* Each tube contains 30 g cream.
*Ointment:* Each tube contains 30 g ointment.

*Instructions for use/handling:* None.

**Marketing authorisation numbers**
Daktacort Cream    0242/0042
Daktacort Ointment    0242/0130

**Date of approval/revision of SPC**
*Cream:*      April 1997.
*Ointment:*    February 1997.

**Legal category**    POM.

## DAKTARIN* CREAM

**Presentation**    White, non-staining, water miscible cream containing miconazole nitrate Ph Eur 2% w/w. The cream also contains macrogol stearate, glycol stearate, peglicol 5 oleate, liquid paraffin, benzoic acid (E210), butylated hydroxyanisole (E320) and purified water.

**Uses**    Miconazole nitrate is a synthetic imidazole antifungal agent with a broad spectrum of activity against pathogenic fungi (including yeasts and dermatophytes) and Gram-positive bacteria (*Staphylococcus* and *Streptococcus* spp.). Daktarin cream and powder are used for the topical treatment of fungal infections of the skin and super infections due to Gram-positive bacteria.

These include athlete's foot, ringworm (tinea infections), intertrigo, candida nappy rash, paronychia, erythrasma, fungal infection of the outer ear and pityriasis versicolor. Daktarin cream may also be used for nail infections.

**Dosage and administration**    The dosage is the same for all ages.

*Cream:* In skin infections, apply to the affected area twice daily. In nail infections, apply to the infected nail(s) once or twice daily.

To prevent relapse, treatment should be continued for ten days after all the lesions have disappeared.

*Use in elderly:* As above.

**Contra-indications, warnings, etc**
*Contra-indications:* None stated.

*Use in pregnancy:* In animals, miconazole nitrate has shown no teratogenic effects but is foetotoxic at high oral doses. Only small amounts of miconazole nitrate are absorbed following topical administration. However, as with other imidazoles, miconazole nitrate should be used with caution during pregnancy.

*Side-effects:* Occasionally irritation has been reported. Rarely local sensitisation or hypersensitivity may occur in which case administration of the product should be discontinued.

*Overdosage:* Daktarin cream is intended for topical use. If accidental ingestion of large quantities of the product occurs, an appropriate method of gastric emptying may be used if considered desirable.

**Pharmaceutical precautions**    Store away from direct heat.

**Legal category**   P.

**Package quantities**    15 g and 30 g tubes.

Daktarin cream is also available as a Twin Pack, containing Daktarin cream 30 g tube plus Daktarin powder 30 g pack (PL 0242/0017).

**Further information**    Daktarin twin pack is particularly indicated for those infections involving moist areas of the body, especially athlete's foot.

A leaflet outlining to the patient the hygiene routines to be observed and the correct method of application of Daktarin is included in each pack of cream and in the twin pack.

**Product licence number** 0242/0016

## DAKTARIN* ORAL GEL

**Presentation**    Sugar-free, orange-flavoured oral gel containing miconazole 2% w/w.

**Uses**    The active ingredient, miconazole, is a synthetic imidazole antifungal agent with a broad spectrum of activity against pathogenic fungi (including yeasts and dermatophytes) and Gram-positive bacteria (*Staphylococcus* and *Streptococcus* spp.). It may act by interfering with the permeability of fungal cell membranes.

When administered orally, miconazole is incompletely absorbed from the gastro-intestinal tract.

Daktarin oral gel is indicated for the treatment and prevention of fungal infections of the oropharynx and gastrointestinal tract and of superinfections due to Gram-positive bacteria. This includes oral candidosis and denture stomatitis. Daktarin oral gel may be used prophylactically in the management of patients at high risk from opportunistic fungal infection. Patients likely to benefit from this treatment include those who are immunosuppressed such as transplant patients, cancer patients (particularly those undergoing cytotoxic therapy) and patients suffering from congenital immunological abnormalities.

Daktarin oral gel may also be used for the eradication of fungi from gut reservoirs when necessary (such as prior to relevant surgery or as an adjunct to local treatment of vulvo-vaginitis).

**Dosage and administration**    Daktarin oral gel should be taken after meals. Dosage is based on 15 mg/kg/day (one 5 ml spoonful contains 125 mg miconazole).

*Adults:* One to two spoonfuls (5–10 ml) of gel four times daily.

*Children aged 6 years and over:* One spoonful (5 ml) of gel four times daily.

*Children aged 2–6 years:* One spoonful of gel (5 ml) twice daily.

*Infants under 2 years:* Half spoonful (2.5 ml) of gel twice daily.

Alternatively, for localised lesions of the mouth, a small amount of gel may be applied directly to the affected area with a clean finger, two to four times a day.

For best results in the treatment of oral lesions, miconazole should be kept in contact with the affected area for as long as possible. This can be achieved by retaining the gel in the mouth for the maximum time possible.

Treatment should be continued for up to two days after symptoms have cleared.

For oral candidosis, dental prosthesis should be removed at night and brushed with the gel.

*Use in elderly:* As for adults.

**Contra-indications, warnings, etc.**
*Contra-indications:* Known hypersensitivity to miconazole or to any of the ingredients. Liver dysfunction.

The drugs terfenadine, astemizole and cisapride should not be given concurrently with Daktarin oral gel (see also *Interactions*).

*Precautions and warnings:* If the concomitant use of Daktarin and anticoagulants is envisaged, the anticoagulant effect should be carefully monitored and titrated. It is advisable to monitor miconazole and phenytoin levels, if they are used concomitantly.

Miconazole can inhibit the metabolism of drugs metabolised by the cytochrome P450-3A and -2C9 families. This can result in an increase and/or prolongation of their effects, including side effects. Examples are:

- terfenadine, astemizole and cisapride. The metabolism of these drugs was inhibited by miconazole in in vitro studies. Therefore, they should not be used in patients treated with Daktarin oral gel.

- oral anticoagulants, cyclosporin, phenytoin, oral hypoglycaemics and possibly tacrolimus. It is advisable to reduce the dosage of such drugs, if necessary.

*Use in pregnancy:* In animals, miconazole has shown no teratogenic effects but is foetotoxic at high oral doses. The significance of this to man is unknown. However, as with other imidazoles, Daktarin oral gel should be avoided in pregnant women if possible. The potential hazards should be balanced against the possible risks.

It is not known whether miconazole is excreted in human milk. Caution should be exercised when prescribing Daktarin oral gel to nursing mothers.

*Effects on ability to drive and use machinery:* Daktarin should not affect alertness or driving ability.

*Side-effects:* Occasionally, nausea and vomiting have been reported, and with long term treatment, diarrhoea. In rare instances allergic reactions have been reported. There are isolated reports of hepatitis, for which the causal relationship with Daktarin has not been established.

*Overdosage: Symptoms:* In general miconazole is not highly toxic. In the event of accidental overdosage, vomiting and diarrhoea may occur.
*Treatment:* Treatment is symptomatic and supportive. A specific antidote is not available.

**Pharmaceutical precautions** Nil.

**Legal category** POM.

**Package quantities** Daktarin oral gel is supplied in 80 g tubes with a 5 ml plastic spoon, marked with a 2.5 ml graduation.

**Further information** Oral miconazole is also available as Daktarin oral tablets, supplied in blister packs of 20 tablets each containing miconazole base 250 mg. For details of dosage and administration refer to separate data sheet. Daktarin oral gel contains alcohol and glycerine.

**Product licence number** 0242/0048.

## DAKTARIN* ORAL TABLETS

**Presentation** White, cross-scored tablets marked with 'Janssen' and M250 containing miconazole 250 mg. The tablets also contain lactose and sucrose.

**Uses** The active ingredient, miconazole, is a synthetic imidazole anti-fungal agent with a broad spectrum of activity against pathogenic fungi (including yeasts and dermatophytes) and Gram-positive bacteria (*Staphylococcus* and *Streptococcus* spp.). It may act by interfering with the permeability of fungal cell membranes.

Miconazole is incompletely absorbed from the gastro-intestinal tract.

Daktarin oral tablets are for the treatment (including prophylaxis) of fungal infections of the oropharynx and gastrointestinal tract and of superinfections due to Gram-positive bacteria.

Daktarin oral tablets may be used prophylactically in the management of patients at high risk from opportunistic fungal infection. Patients likely to benefit from this treatment include those who are immunosuppressed such as transplant patients, cancer patients (particularly those undergoing cytotoxic therapy) and patients suffering from congenital immunological abnormalities. Daktarin oral tablets may also be used for the eradication of fungi from gut reservoirs when necessary (such as prior to relevant surgery).

**Dosage and administration** Daktarin oral tablets should be taken after meals.
Dosage is based on 15 mg/kg/day.

*Adults:* One 250 mg tablet four times/day for 10 days or for up to 2 days after the symptoms have cleared.

*Children:* Use Daktarin oral gel.

*Use in elderly:* As for adults.
Topical treatment of the oropharynx may be achieved by sucking the tablet, allowing it to dissolve slowly in the mouth.
Treatment should be continued for up to 2 days after symptoms have cleared.

### Contra-indications, warnings, etc
*Contra-indications:* Known hypersensitivity to miconazole or to any of the ingredients. Liver dysfunction.
The drugs terfenadine, astemizole and cisapride should not be given concurrently with Daktarin oral tablets (see also *Interactions*).

*Precautions and warnings:* If the concomitant use of Daktarin and anticoagulants is envisaged, the anticoagulant effect should be carefully monitored and titrated. It is advisable to monitor miconazole and phenytoin levels, if they are used concomitantly.

Miconazole can inhibit the metabolism of drugs metabolised by the cytochrome P450-3A and -2C9 families. This can result in an increase and/or prolongation of their effects, including side effects. Examples are:

- terfenadine, astemizole and cisapride. The metabolism of these drugs was inhibited by miconazole in in vitro studies. Therefore, they should not be used in patients treated with Daktarin oral tablets.

- oral anticoagulants, cyclosporin, phenytoin, oral hypoglycaemics and possibly tacrolimus. It is advisable to reduce the dosage of such drugs, if necessary.

*Use in pregnancy:* In animals, miconazole has shown no teratogenic effects but is foetotoxic at high oral doses. The significance of this to man is unknown. However, as with other imidazoles, Daktarin oral tablets should be avoided in pregnant women if possible. The potential hazards should be balanced against the possible risks.

It is not known whether miconazole is excreted in human milk. Caution should be exercised when prescribing Daktarin oral gel to nursing mothers.

*Effects on ability to drive and use machinery:* Daktarin should not affect alertness or driving ability.

*Side-effects:* Occasionally, nausea and vomiting have been reported, and with long term treatment, diarrhoea. In rare instances allergic reactions have been reported. There are isolated reports of hepatitis, for which the causal relationship with Daktarin has not been established.

*Overdosage: Symptoms:* In general miconazole is not highly toxic. In the event of accidental overdosage, vomiting and diarrhoea may occur.
*Treatment:* Treatment is symptomatic and supportive. A specific antidote is not available.

**Pharmaceutical precautions** Nil.

**Legal category** POM.

**Package quantities** Daktarin oral tablets are supplied in blister packs of 20.

**Further information** Oral miconazole is also available as a sugar-free orange flavoured gel containing miconazole base 2% w/w (25 mg/ml). Daktarin Oral Gel is supplied in a 80 g tube. For details of dosage and administration refer to separate data sheet.

**Product licence number**
Daktarin Oral Tablets 0242/0047

## DAKTARIN* POWDER

**Qualitative and quantitative composition** Daktarin powder contains miconazole nitrate PhEur 2.0% w/w.

**Pharmaceutical form** Topical powder.

### Clinical particulars

*Therapeutic indications:* For the treatment of mycotic infections of the skin and superinfections due to Gram positive bacteria.

*Posology and method of administration:* Daktarin powder is for topical administration.
*Adults:* Twice daily application of powder to the lesions, treatment being prolonged for some 10 days after all lesions have disappeared to prevent relapse.
*Elderly and children:* As for adults.

*Contra-indications:* The powder should not be recommended for the treatment of infections of the hair and nails.

*Special warnings and special precautions for use:* None.

*Interactions with other medicaments and other forms of interaction:* None known.

*Pregnancy and lactation:* In animals, miconazole nitrate has shown no teratogenic effects but is foetotoxic at high oral doses. Only small amounts of miconazole nitrate are absorbed following topical administration. However, as with other imidazoles, miconazole nitrate should be used with caution during pregnancy.

*Effects on ability to drive and use machines:* None known.

*Undesirable effects:* Hypersensitivity has rarely been recorded, if it should occur the treatment should be discontinued

*Overdose:* Daktarin powder is intended for topical use. If accidental ingestion of large quantities of product occurs, an appropriate method of gastric emptying may be used if considered desirable.

### Pharmacological properties

*Pharmacodynamic properties:* Miconazole is an imidazole antifungal agent and may act by interfering with the permeability of the fungal cell membrane. It possesses a wide antifungal spectrum and has some antibacterial activity.

*Pharmacokinetic properties:* There is little absorption through skin or mucous membranes when miconazole nitrate is applied topically.

When administered orally miconazole is incompletely absorbed from the gastro-intestinal tract. Peak plasma concentrations occur at about 4 hours after administration. Miconazole disappears from the plasma in a triphasic manner with a biological half life of about 24 hours. Over 90% is reported to be bound to plasma proteins.

*Preclinical safety data:* Not applicable.

### Pharmaceutical particulars

*List of excipients:* Talc; zinc oxide; colloidal silicon dioxide.

*Incompatibilities:* Not applicable.

*Shelf life:* Five years.

*Special precautions for storage:* Store at room temperature.

*Nature and contents of container:* High density polyethylene bottle with a polypropylene dredger-cap and screw-cap containing 20 gram of powder.

*Instructions for use/handling:* Not applicable.

**Marketing authorisation number** 0242/0017.

**Date of approval/revision of SPC** 21 May 1996.

**Legal category** P.

## DELFEN* CONTRACEPTIVE FOAM

**Qualitative and quantitative composition** Contains 12.5% w/w of nonoxynol-9.

**Pharmaceutical form** Foam.

### Clinical particulars
*Therapeutic indications:* For use as a spermicidal contraceptive in conjunction with barrier methods of contraception.

*Posology and method of administration:* For topical intravaginal administration.
For use by adult females only.
Insert one applicatorful intravaginally prior to coitus. A fresh application of foam must be made if intercourse is repeated or delayed for more than one hour. The diaphragm must be allowed to remain *in situ* for at least six to eight hours after coitus.
Douching is not recommended, but if desired it should be deferred for at least six hours after intercourse.

*Contra-indications:* Hypersensitivity to nonoxynol-9 or to any component of the preparation.
Patients with absent vaginal sensation, eg paraplegics and quadriplegics.

*Special warnings and special precautions for use:* Spermicidal intravaginal preparations are intended for use in conjunction with barrier methods of contraception such as condoms, diaphragms and caps.
Where avoidance of pregnancy is important the choice of contraceptive method should be made in consultation with a doctor or a family planning clinic.
If vaginal or penile irritation occurs discontinue use. If symptoms worsen or continue for more than 48 hours medical advice should be sought.

*Interactions with other medicaments and other forms of interaction:* None known.

*Pregnancy and lactation:* There is no evidence from animal and human studies that nonoxynol-9 is teratogenic. Human epidemiological studies have not shown any firm evidence of adverse effects on the foetus, however some studies have shown that nonoxynol-9 may be embryotoxic in animals. This product should not be used if pregnancy is suspected or confirmed. Animal studies have detected nonoxynol-9 in milk after intravaginal administration. Use by lactating women has not been studied.

*Effects on ability to drive and use machines:* None known.

*Undesirable effects:* May cause irritation of the vagina or penis.

*Overdose:* If taken orally the surfactant properties of this preparation may cause gastric irritation. General supportive therapy should be carried out. Hepatic and renal function should be monitored if medically indicated.

### Pharmacological properties
*Pharmacodynamic properties:* The standard in vitro test (Sander-Cramer) evaluating the effect of nonoxynol-9 on sperm motility has shown the compound to be a potent spermicide.
The site of action of nonoxynol-9 has been determined as the sperm cell membrane. The lipoprotein

membrane is disrupted, increasing permeability, with subsequent loss of cell components and decreased motility. A similar effect on vaginal epithelial and bacterial cells is also found.

*Pharmacokinetic properties:* The intravaginal absorption and excretion of radiolabelled ($^{14}$C) nonoxynol-9 has been studied in non-pregnant rats and rabbits and in pregnant rats. No appreciable difference was found in the extent or rate of absorption in pregnant and non-pregnant animals. Plasma levels peaked at about one hour and recovery from urine as unchanged nonoxynol-9 accounted for approximately 15-25% and faeces approximately 70% of the administered dose as unchanged nonoxynol-9. Less than 0.3% was found in the milk of lactating rats. No metabolites were detected in any of the samples analysed.

*Preclinical safety data:* Not applicable.

### Pharmaceutical particulars

*List of excipients:* Acetic acid glacial; benzoic acid (E 210); cetyl alcohol; methyl parahydroxybenzoate (E 218); phosphoric acid; polyvinyl alcohol; propylene glycol; sodium carboxymethylcellulose; stearic acid; diethylaminoethyl stearamide; Van Dyke Perfume No. 6301; purified water; isobutane (propellant).

*Incompatibilities:* Not applicable.

*Shelf life:* 3 years.

*Special precautions for storage:* Store at room temperature (at or below 25°C). Caution: contents under pressure, with flammable propellant. Do not burn or puncture.

*Nature and contents of container:* Aluminium aerosol can containing a minimum of 20 doses of Delfen foam. An applicator is also provided in the pack.

*Instructions for use/handling:* Not applicable.

**Marketing authorisation number**  0242/0211

**Date of approval/revision of SPC**  October 1996.

**Legal category**  GSL.

# DROLEPTAN*

**Presentation**  *Injection:* Clear, colourless, aqueous injection in 2 ml ampoules. Each millilitre contains 5 mg droperidol. Injection also contains mannitol, lactic acid and water for injection.

*Tablets:* Yellow, uncoated, scored tablets marked 'JANSSEN' on one side and D above 10 on the reverse. Each tablet contains 10 mg droperidol. Tablets also contain lactose and E104.

*Liquid:* Clear, colourless, odourless liquid containing 1 mg droperidol/ml for oral administration. Liquid also contains methyl and propyl parabens.

## Uses

*Properties:* Droleptan is a butyrophenone neuroleptic. Its pharmacological profile is characterised mainly by dopamine-blocking and $\alpha_1$-adrenolytic effects. Droleptan is devoid of anticholinergic and antihistaminic activity.

*Indications:* Droleptan is a major tranquilliser with the following indications:

1. In anaesthesia:

a. in conjunction with a narcotic analgesic in the technique of neuroleptanalgesia (iv or im);
b. either alone or in combination with a narcotic analgesic for premedication;
c. for post-operative nausea and vomiting (iv or im).

2. For treatment of chemotherapy-induced nausea and vomiting (iv or im).

3. In psychiatry for rapidly calming the manic, agitated patient.

## Dosage and administration

*Neuroleptanalgesia:*
*Adults:* 5–15 mg iv at induction of anaesthesia with a narcotic analgesic.
   *Children:* 0.2–0.3 mg/kg iv.

*Premedication in anaesthesia:*
*Adults:* Up to 10 mg im or oral.
   *Children:* 0.2–0.5 mg/kg im or 0.3–0.6 mg/kg oral.

*Anti-emetic:*
   Post-operative
   *Adults:* 5 mg iv or im;
   *Children:* Doses used have ranged between 0.02–0.075 mg/kg im or iv dependent on emetic stimulus.

*In cancer chemotherapy:*
*Adults:* Out-patients or those on mildly emetic therapy should receive the lowest recommended dose. Patients on more aggressive chemotherapy may require doses in the upper range of those recommended. Dosage must always be determined individually.

A loading dose of 1–10 mg im or iv should be given 30 minutes before commencement of therapy, followed either by a continuous infusion of 1–3 mg/hr or 1–5 mg im or iv every 1–6 hours as required.

*Children:* Doses used have ranged between 0.02–0.075 mg/kg im or iv depending on emetic stimulus. Dosage must be determined individually using minimum effective dose.

*In psychiatry:*
*Adults:* 5–15 mg iv; up to 10 mg im; 5–20 mg oral. The dosage may be repeated at intervals of 4–6 hours (im or iv) or 4–8 hours (oral).
*Children:* 0.5–1 mg/day im or oral adjusted according to response.

In psychiatry, dosage should be individually determined and is best initiated and titrated under close clinical supervision. To determine the initial dose, consideration should be given to the patient's age, severity of symptoms, and previous response to other neuroleptic drugs.

Patients who are elderly or debilitated or those with previously reported adverse reactions to neuroleptic drugs, may require less Droleptan and half the normal starting dose in psychiatry may be sufficient for therapeutic response. The optimal response in such patients is usually obtained with more gradual titration and at lower dose levels. In adolescents a lower starting dose may be advisable.

## Contra-indications, warnings, etc

*Contra-indications:* Droleptan is contra-indicated in patients with known hypersensitivity to the product, in patients with severe depression, in comatose individuals or in patients with Parkinson's disease.

*Use in pregnancy and lactation:* The safety of Droleptan in pregnancy has not been established, although studies in animals have not demonstrated teratogenic effects. As with other drugs, it is not advisable to administer Droleptan in pregnancy.

Butyrophenones are excreted in breast milk and are not recommended during lactation. If the use of Droleptan is essential, breast feeding should be discontinued.

*Effects on driving ability and operation of machinery:* Some degree of sedation or impairment of alertness may occur, particularly with higher doses and at the start of treatment and may be potentiated by alcohol. Patients should be advised not to drive or operate machinery during treatment until their susceptibility is known, or on the day following administration if early discharge is envisaged.

*Precautions and warnings:* Caution is advised in patients with liver disease, renal failure, epilepsy, and conditions predisposing to epilepsy or convulsions.

In anaesthesia, intravenous induction agents will generally be required in lower dosage where Droleptan is used as part of the anaesthetic technique, and the effects of heavy sedative premedication may be potentiated. When using Droleptan at induction of anaesthesia, provision should be made for rapid infusion of intravenous fluid to correct any large fall in blood pressure, which, if it occurs, is due to relative hypovolaemia and is more common in the elderly or untreated hypertensives.

Mild to moderate hypotension and occasionally (reflex) tachycardia have been observed following administration of Droleptan. This reaction usually subsides spontaneously. However, should hypotension persist, the possibility of hypovolaemia should be considered and appropriate fluid replacement administered.

Since there is a risk of QT prolongation, Droleptan should only be used with caution in patients with hypokalaemia or in patients with pre-existing prolonged QT-interval.

Acute withdrawal symptoms, including nausea, vomiting and insomnia, have very rarely been described after abrupt cessation of high doses of antipsychotic drugs. Relapse may also occur and gradual withdrawal is advisable.

*Interactions:* In common with all neuroleptics, Droleptan can increase the central nervous system depression produced by other CNS-depressant drugs, including alcohol, hypnotics, sedatives or strong analgesics; and may antagonise the action of adrenaline and other sympathomimetic agents. Droleptan may potentiate the action of antihypertensive agents, so that orthostatic hypotension may ensue.

Since droperidol blocks dopamine receptors, it may inhibit the action of dopamine agonists, such as bromocriptine, lisuride and levodopa.

The dosage of anti-convulsants may need to be increased to take account of the lowered seizure threshold.

Enhanced CNS effects, when combined with methyldopa, have been reported for some butyrophenones.

Theoretically, certain agents (e.g. phenobarbitone, carbamazepine, phenytoin), as well as smoking and alcohol consumption, which stimulate metabolizing enzymes in the liver, may enhance the metabolic breakdown of neuroleptics, possibly necessitating adjustment of the dose.

*Adverse effects:* In common with all neuroleptics, extrapyramidal symptoms may occur. Acute dystonias may occur early in treatment. Parkinsonian rigidity, tremor and akathisia tend to appear less rapidly. Oculogyric crises and laryngeal dystonias have been reported. Extrapyramidal symptoms are less common at the low single doses used in anaesthesia or as an anti-emetic.

Anti-Parkinson agents should only be given as required; they should not be prescribed routinely because of the possible risk of impairing the therapeutic efficacy of Droleptan.

Tardive dyskinesia may occur during administration or after withdrawal of neuroleptic drugs, including Droleptan, and can be precipitated or aggravated by anti-Parkinson drugs. Tardive dyskinesia has not been reported following anti-emetic or anaesthetic uses of Droleptan.

The syndrome is unlikely to occur in the short-term when low or moderate doses of Droleptan are used as recommended, but since its occurrence may be related to duration of treatment, as well as daily dose, Droleptan should be given in the minimum effective dose for the minimum possible time.

The potential seriousness and unpredictability of tardive dyskinesia, and the fact that it has occasionally been reported to occur when neuroleptic anti-psychotic drugs have been prescribed for relatively short periods in low doses, means that the prescribing of such agents requires especially careful assessment of risks versus benefits.

It has been reported that fine vermicular movements of the tongue may be an early sign of tardive dyskinesia and that the full syndrome might not develop if medication is stopped at that time.

Gastrointestinal symptoms, nausea, loss of appetite and dyspepsia, have been reported.

Hormonal effects of anti-psychotic neuroleptic drugs include hyper-prolactinaemia, which may cause galactorrhoea, gynaecomastia and oligo- or amenorrhoea.

Dose-related mild to moderate hypotension and occasionally (reflex) tachycardia have been observed following administration of droperidol (see precautions and warnings), particularly in the elderly, who are more susceptible to the sedative and hypotensive effects. As with other neuroleptics, isolated cases of arrhythmia and sudden death have been reported during the acute parenteral use of high doses of Droleptan in psychiatric patients.

Droleptan, even in low dosage in susceptible (especially non-psychotic) individuals, may cause unpleasant subjective feelings of being mentally dulled or slowed down, dizziness, headache, or paradoxical effects of excitement, agitation or insomnia.

In common with other antipsychotics, Droleptan may be associated with rare cases of neuroleptic malignant syndrome, an idiosyncratic response characterised by hyperthermia, muscle rigidity, autonomic instability, altered consciousness, coma and elevated creatine phosphokinase levels. Signs of autonomic dysfunction such as tachycardia, labile arterial pressure and sweating may precede the onset of hyperthermia, acting as early warning signs. In such cases, Droleptan treatment should be discontinued immediately and appropriate supportive therapy initiated. Recovery usually occurs within five to seven days of antipsychotic withdrawal. Affected patients should be carefully monitored. Dantrolene sodium, bromocriptine mesylate and ECT have all been reported as offering benefit in some patients with neuroleptic malignant syndrome.

The following effects have been reported rarely: oedema, various skin rashes and reactions, hypersensitivity, jaundice or transient abnormalities of liver function in the absence of jaundice; anxiety or confusional states or epileptic fits, vision disturbances, sweating.

Blood dyscrasias have been reported very rarely.

*Overdosage:*
*Symptoms:* In general, the manifestations of Droleptan overdosage are an extension of its pharmacological actions, the most prominent of which would be severe extrapyramidal symptoms, hypotension and psychic indifference with a transition to sleep. The risk of cardiac arrhythmias should be considered. The patient may appear comatose with respiratory depression and hypotension which could be severe enough to produce a shock-like state. Convulsions may also occur.

*Treatment:* There is no specific antidote to droperidol. A patent airway should be established and maintained with mechanically assisted ventilation if necessary. In view of isolated observations of arrhythmia following high doses of droperidol, ECG monitoring is mandatory. Hypotension and circulatory collapse should be treated by plasma volume expansion and other appropriate measures. Adrenaline should not be used. The patient should be monitored carefully for 24 hours or longer, body warmth and adequate fluid intake should be maintained.

**Pharmaceutical precautions** Droleptan preparations should be protected from light.

Droleptan is chemically incompatible with the induction agents thiopentone and methohexitone, because of the wide difference in pH.

**Legal category** POM.

**Package quantities** Droleptan injection is supplied in 2 ml ampoules (5 mg/ml) in packs of 10.

Droleptan tablets each containing 10 mg droperidol are supplied in packs of 50.

Droleptan liquid is supplied in amber glass bottles of 100 ml and 500 ml (1 mg/ml).

**Further information** The relative bioavailability of the oral form is 75% compared with iv administration, the peak concentration being reached after 1–2 hours.

The action of a single intramuscular and intravenous dose commences 3–10 minutes after administration, although the peak effect may not be apparent for up to 30 minutes. The tranquillising and sedative effects tend to persist for 2 to 4 hours, although alertness may be affected for up to 12 hours.

**Product licence numbers**

Droleptan injection    0242/5003R
Droleptan tablets    0242/5004R
Droleptan liquid    0242/0080

# DUROGESIC*

**Presentation** Durogesic is a transdermal drug delivery system comprising a transparent, self-adhesive patch containing a drug reservoir of fentanyl. Each system is designed to release fentanyl into the systemic circulation over a period of 72 hours. There are four different strengths:

Durogesic 25, with a delivery rate of approximately 25 micrograms/hour fentanyl (active surface area 10 cm², fentanyl content 2.5 mg, and printed 'Durogesic 25µg fentanyl/h' in pink)

Durogesic 50, with a delivery rate of approximately 50 micrograms/hour fentanyl (active surface area 20 cm², fentanyl content 5 mg, and printed 'Durogesic 50µg fentanyl/h' in green)

Durogesic 75, with a delivery rate of approximately 75 micrograms/hour fentanyl (active surface area 30 cm², fentanyl content 7.5 mg, and printed 'Durogesic 75µg fentanyl/h' in blue)

Durogesic 100, with a delivery rate of approximately 100 micrograms/hour fentanyl (active surface area 40 cm², fentanyl content 10 mg, and printed 'Durogesic 100µg fentanyl/h' in grey)

The drug reservoir also contains ethanol BP, hydroxyethylcellulose Ph Eur and purified water Ph Eur. The contact adhesive is silicone medical adhesive.

## Uses

*Indications:* Durogesic is indicated in the management of chronic intractable pain due to cancer.

*Properties:* Fentanyl is an opioid analgesic with a high affinity for the µ-opioid receptor.

Durogesic provides continuous systemic delivery of fentanyl over the 72 hour administration period. After the first Durogesic application, serum fentanyl concentrations increase gradually, generally levelling off between 12 and 24 hours and remaining relatively constant for the remainder of the 72-hour application period. Peak serum levels of fentanyl generally occur between 24 and 72 hours after the first application. The serum fentanyl concentrations attained are proportional to the Durogesic patch size. For all practical purposes by the second 72-hour application, a steady state serum concentration is reached and is maintained during subsequent applications of a patch of the same size.

After Durogesic is removed, serum fentanyl concentrations decline gradually, falling approximately 50% in 17 (range 13–22) hours. Continued absorption of fentanyl from the skin accounts for a slower disappearance of the drug from the serum than is seen after an iv infusion. Fentanyl is metabolised primarily in the liver. Around 75% of fentanyl is excreted into the urine, mostly as metabolites, with less than 10% as unchanged drug. About 9% of the dose is recovered in the faeces, primarily as metabolites. The major metabolite, norfentanyl, is inactive. Mean values for unbound fractions of fentanyl in plasma are estimated to be between 13 and 21%.

**Dosage and administration** Durogesic should be applied to non-irritated and non-irradiated skin on a flat surface of the torso or upper arm. A non-hairy area should be selected. If the site of Durogesic application requires to be cleansed prior to application of the system, this should be done with water. Soaps, oils, lotions or any other agent that might irritate the skin or alter its characteristics should not be used. The skin should be completely dry before the system is applied.

Durogesic should be applied immediately after removal from the sealed pouch. Following removal of the protective layer, the transdermal system should

be pressed firmly in place with the palm of the hand for approximately 30 seconds, making sure the contact is complete, especially around the edges.

Durogesic should be worn continuously for 72 hours. A new system should then be applied to a different skin site after removal of the previous transdermal system. Several days should elapse before a new patch is applied to the same area of skin.

*Adults:*

*Initial dose selection* The initial Durogesic dose should be based on the patient's opioid history, including the degree of opioid tolerance, if any, as well as on the current general condition and medical status of the patient.

*In strong opioid-naive patients* The lowest Durogesic dose, 25 micrograms/h, should be used as the initial dose.

*In opioid-tolerant patients* The initial dose of Durogesic should be based on the previous 24 hour opioid analgesic requirement. A recommended conversion scheme from oral morphine to Durogesic is given below:

| Oral 24-hour morphine (mg/day) | Durogesic (micrograms/h) |
| --- | --- |
| <135 | 25 |
| 135-224 | 50 |
| 225-314 | 75 |
| 315-404 | 100 |
| 405-494 | 125 |
| 495-584 | 150 |
| 585-674 | 175 |
| 675-764 | 200 |
| 765-854 | 225 |
| 855-944 | 250 |
| 945-1034 | 275 |
| 1035-1124 | 300 |

For both strong opioid-naive and opioid-tolerant patients, the initial evaluation of the analgesic effect of Durogesic should not be made before the system has been worn for 24 hours due to the gradual increase in serum fentanyl concentrations up to this time. Previous analgesic therapy should therefore be phased out gradually from the time of the first patch application until analgesic efficacy with Durogesic is attained.

*Dose titration and maintenance therapy:* The Durogesic patch should be replaced every 72 hours. The dose should be titrated individually until analgesic efficacy is attained. If analgesia is insufficient at the end of the initial application period the dose may be increased. Dose adjustment, when necessary, should normally be performed in 25 micrograms/h increments, although the supplementary analgesic requirements (oral morphine 90 mg/day ≈ Durogesic 25 micrograms/h) and pain status of the patient should be taken into account. More than one Durogesic system may be used for doses greater than 100 micrograms/h. Patients may require periodic supplemental doses of a short-acting analgesic for 'breakthrough' pain. Additional or alternative methods of analgesia should be considered when the Durogesic dose exceeds 300 micrograms/h.

*Discontinuation of Durogesic:* If discontinuation of Durogesic is necessary, any replacement with other opioids should be gradual, starting at a low dose and increasing slowly. This is because fentanyl levels fall gradually after Durogesic is removed; it may take 17 hours or more for the fentanyl serum concentration to decrease by 50%. As a general rule, the discontinuation of opioid analgesia should be gradual.

*Use in elderly patients:* Data from intravenous studies with fentanyl suggest that elderly patients may have reduced clearance, a prolonged half-life and they may be more sensitive to the drug than younger patients. Studies of Durogesic in elderly patients demonstrated fentanyl pharmacokinetics which did not differ significantly from young patients although serum concentrations tended to be higher. Elderly, cachectic, or debilitated patients should be observed carefully for signs of fentanyl toxicity and the dose reduced if necessary.

*Use in children:* The safety and efficacy of Durogesic in children has not been established and is therefore not recommended.

## Contra-indications, warnings, etc

*Contra-indications:* Durogesic is contra-indicated in patients with known hypersensitivity to fentanyl or to the adhesive in the system.

Durogesic is a sustained-release preparation indicated for the treatment of chronic intractable cancer pain and is contra-indicated in acute pain because of the lack of opportunity for dosage titration in the short term and the resultant possibility of significant respiratory depression.

*Warnings and precautions:* Patients who have experienced serious adverse events should be monitored

for up to 24 hours after Durogesic removal since serum fentanyl concentrations decline gradually and are reduced by about 50% in approximately 17 (range 13-22) hours.

Durogesic should be kept out of the reach of children at all times before and after use.

*Respiratory depression:* As with all potent opioids, some patients may experience significant respiratory depression with Durogesic; patients must be observed for these effects. Respiratory depression may persist beyond the removal of the Durogesic system. The incidence of respiratory depression increases as the Durogesic dose is increased. See also 'Overdosage' concerning respiratory depression. CNS active drugs may increase the respiratory depression (see 'Interactions').

*Chronic pulmonary disease:* Fentanyl, like other opioids, may have more severe adverse effects in patients with chronic obstructive or other pulmonary disease. In such patients, they may decrease respiratory drive and increase airway resistance.

*Drug dependence:* Tolerance and physical and psychological dependence may develop upon repeated administration of opioids such as fentanyl. Iatrogenic addiction following opioid administration is rare.

*Increased intracranial pressure:* Durogesic should be used with caution in patients who may be particularly susceptible to the intracranial effects of $CO_2$ retention such as those with evidence of increased intracranial pressure, impaired consciousness or coma. Durogesic should be used with caution in patients with brain tumours.

*Cardiac disease:* Fentanyl may produce bradycardia and Durogesic should therefore be administered with caution to patients with bradyarrhythmias.

*Hepatic disease:* Because fentanyl is metabolised to inactive metabolites in the liver, hepatic disease might delay its elimination. In patients with hepatic cirrhosis, the pharmacokinetics of a single application of Durogesic were not altered although serum concentrations tended to be higher in these patients. Patients with hepatic impairment should be observed carefully for signs of fentanyl toxicity and the dose of Durogesic reduced if necessary.

*Renal disease:* Less than 10% of fentanyl is excreted unchanged by the kidney and, unlike morphine, there are no known active metabolites eliminated by the kidney. Data obtained with intravenous fentanyl in patients with renal failure suggest that the volume of distribution of fentanyl may be changed by dialysis. This may affect serum concentrations. If patients with renal impairment receive Durogesic, they should be observed carefully for signs of fentanyl toxicity and the dose reduced if necessary.

*Patients with fever/external heat:* Patients who develop fever should be monitored for opioid side effects since significant increases in body temperature can potentially increase fentanyl delivery rate.

Patients should also be advised to avoid exposing the Durogesic application site to direct external heat sources such as heating pads, hot water bottles, electric blankets, heat lamps, saunas or hot whirlpool spa baths while wearing the system, since there is potential for temperature dependent increases in release of fentanyl from the system.

*Pregnancy and lactation:* The safety of fentanyl in pregnancy has not been established. Durogesic should not be used in women of child-bearing potential without adequate contraception unless in the judgement of the doctor the potential benefits outweigh the possible hazards.

Fentanyl is excreted into breast milk hence Durogesic should not be used by women who are breast-feeding.

*Effects on driving and operating machinery:* Durogesic may impair the mental or physical ability required to perform potentially hazardous tasks such as driving or operating machinery.

*Drug interactions:* The concomitant use of other CNS depressants, including opioids, anxiolytics, hypnotics, general anaesthetics, antipsychotics, skeletal muscle relaxants, sedating antihistamines and alcoholic beverages may produce additive depressant effects; hypoventilation, hypotension and profound sedation or coma may occur. Therefore, the use of concomitant CNS active drugs requires special care and observation.

*Patch disposal:* Used patches may contain significant residues of active substance. After removal, therefore, used patches should be folded firmly in half, adhesive side inwards, so that the release membrane is not exposed, and then discarded safely and out of the reach of children according to the instructions in the pack.

*Side effects:* The most serious adverse reaction, as with all potent opioids, is hypoventilation. Other opioid-related adverse reactions include: nausea; vomiting; constipation; hypotension; somnolence; confusion; hallucinations; euphoria; pruritus and urinary retention.

Local skin reactions such as rash, erythema and itching have occasionally been reported. These reactions usually resolve within 24 hours of removal of the patch.

*Overdosage: Symptoms*: The symptoms of fentanyl overdosage are an extension of its pharmacological actions, the most serious effect being respiratory depression.

*Treatment*: For management of respiratory depression, immediate countermeasures include removing Durogesic and physically or verbally stimulating the patient. These actions can be followed by administration of a specific opioid antagonist such as naloxone. The interval between iv opioid antagonist doses should be carefully chosen and repeated administration or a continuous infusion of naloxone may be necessary because of continued absorption of fentanyl from the skin after patch removal, which may result in prolonged respiratory depression. Reversal of the narcotic effect may result in acute onset of pain and release of catecholamines.

A patent airway should be established and maintained. An oropharyngeal airway or endotracheal tube and oxygen should be administered and respiration assisted or controlled, as appropriate. Adequate body temperature and fluid intake should be maintained.

If severe or persistent hypotension occurs, hypovolaemia should be considered, and the condition should be managed with appropriate parenteral fluid therapy.

**Pharmaceutical precautions**   Store below 25˚C.

**Legal category** CD (Sch 2), POM

**Package quantities**   Durogesic 25, 50, 75, 100: Cartons of 5 patches individually packaged in pouches.

**Further information**   None.

**Product licence numbers**

| Durogesic 25 | 0242/0192 |
| Durogesic 50 | 0242/0193 |
| Durogesic 75 | 0242/0194 |
| Durogesic 100 | 0242/0195 |

## EVOREL* CONTI AND SEQUI

**Qualitative and quantitative composition** Evorel Conti and Sequi are both Transdermal Delivery Systems (TDS). Evorel Conti contains: 3.2 mg of estradiol hemihydrate and 11.2 mg of norethisterone acetate.

Evorel Sequi consists of:

(a) 4 Evorel 50 TDSs, each containing: 3.2 mg of estradiol hemihydrate.

(b) 4 Evorel Conti TDSs, each containing: 3.2 mg of estradiol hemihydrate and 11.2 mg of noresthisterone acetate.

**Pharmaceutical form**   Evorel 50, Evorel Conti and Evorel Sequi are Transdermal Delivery Systems (TDS), or transdermal patches, composed of a flat two-layer laminate which is 0.1 mm in thickness. The first layer is a flexible, translucent, and nearly colourless backing film. The second layer is a monolayer adhesive film (matrix) composed of acrylic adhesive and guar gum and contains the hormones. This system is protected by a polyester foil release liner, which is affixed to the adhesive matrix and is removed prior to application of the patch to the skin. The polyester foil used is coated with silicone on both sides. The release liner has a S-shaped opening to facilitate its removal prior to use. Each TDS is enclosed in a protective, hermetically-sealed sachet.

Evorel Conti has a surface area of 16 sq cm and contains 3.2 mg of estradiol corresponding to a nominal release of 50 micrograms of estradiol per 24 hours and 11.2 mg of norethisterone acetate corresponding to a nominal release of 170 micrograms of norethisterone acetate per 24 hours. Each TDS is marked in the centre of the lower margin on the outside of the backing film: CEN1.

Evorel 50 has a surface area of 16 sq cm and contains 3.2 mg of estradiol corresponding to a nominal release of 50 micrograms of estradiol per 24 hours. The release liner of Evorel 50 is aluminised on one side. Each TDS is marked in the centre of the lower margin of the outside of the backing film: CE50.

**Clinical particulars**

*Therapeutic indications:* Hormone replacement therapy for the relief of menopausal symptoms.

*Posology and method of administration:*
*Adults*
*Evorel Conti:* Evorel Conti TDS should be applied individually without interruption.

Each Evorel Conti TDS should be applied twice weekly, every three to four days, to the trunk below the waist.

Insufficient data are available to guide dose adjustments for patients with severe liver or kidney function impairment.

*Evorel Sequi:* Evorel Sequi comprises four Evorel 50 TDSs and four Evorel Conti TDSs.

Evorel 50 and Evorel Conti should be applied individually in the following sequence: four Evorel 50 TDSs followed by four Evorel Conti TDSs. This cycle should be repeated without interruption. TDSs should be applied twice weekly, every three to four days, to the trunk below the waist.

Insufficient data are available to guide dose adjustments for patients with severe liver or kidney function impairment.

It is important that the TDS be used in the correct sequence to ensure regular cyclic bleeding. Most patients will experience vaginal bleeding after the start of the progestogen therapy.

*Children:* Evorel Conti and Evorel Sequi (Evorel 50 and Evorel Conti) are not indicated in children.

*Elderly:* Data are insufficient in regard to the use of Evorel Conti and Evorel Sequi in the elderly (>65 years old).

*Administration:* The sachet containing one TDS should be opened and one part of the protective foil removed at the S-shaped incision. The TDS should be applied to clean, dry, healthy, intact skin as soon as it is removed from the sachet. The patient should avoid contact between fingers and the adhesive part of the TDS during application. Each application should be made to a different area of the skin, on the trunk below the waist. **Evorel Conti and Sequi should not be applied on or near the breasts.**

Should a TDS fall off, it should be replaced immediately with a new equivalent Evorel 50 or Evorel Conti TDS. However the usual day of changing TDSs should be maintained.

*Contra-indications:*

– Hypersensitivity to any component of this product.
– Malignant tumours of the breast.
– Genital tract or other oestrogen-dependent neoplasia.
– Undiagnosed vaginal bleeding.
– Pregnancy or lactation.
– Severe hepatic or renal disease.
– Active thrombophlebitis or thromboembolic disorders.
– Endometriosis

*Special warnings and special precautions for use:* Prior to commencing, and periodically during oestrogen replacement therapy, it is recommended that the patient be given a thorough physical and gynaecological examination. A complete medical and family history should be taken. Repeated breakthrough bleeding, unexplained vaginal bleeding, and changes noticed during breast examination require further evaluation.

At the present time, the results of epidemiological studies suggest an increase in the relative risk of breast cancer in postmenopausal women receiving long-term hormone replacement therapy. Concurrent progestogen does not appear to protect for this risk. Therefore, a careful appraisal of the risk/benefit ratio should be undertaken before the initiation of long-term treatment.

Published studies suggest that there is no increased risk of thromboembolic disease, including myocardial infarction, stroke and thrombophlebitis with oestrogen replacement therapy at the current recommended low dosage in apparently normal women. However, treatment should be discontinued immediately following the occurrence of an acute thromboembolic event. There is no evidence that a history of deep vein thrombosis, pulmonary embolism, stroke or myocardial infarction associated with recognised risk factors such as immobilisation or the post-operative period should be a contra-indication to oestrogen replacement therapy. However, in the absence of specific data, Evorel Conti and Evorel Sequi should be used with caution in these patients.

Appropriate monitoring is recommended in patients with cardiac impairment, epilepsy, diabetes mellitus, hypertension, disturbances or impairment of liver or kidney function, mastopathy, a family history of breast cancer, or a history of cholestatic jaundice.

Administration of unopposed oestrogen in patients with an intact uterus has been reported to increase the risk of endometrial hyperplasia and of endometrial carcinoma. Therefore, oestrogen in combination with continuous administration of progestogen as in Evorel Conti, or with sequential administration of a progestogen as in Evorel Sequi, is recommended in women with an intact uterus in order to reduce the risk of hyperplasia or endometrial carcinoma.

Evorel Conti and Evorel Sequi are not to be used as contraception.

The TDSs should be kept away from children and pets.

*Interactions with other medicaments and other forms of interaction:* Drugs which induce microsomal liver enzyme activity may alter oestrogen and progestogen metabolism. Examples of such drugs are barbiturates, hydantoins, carbamazepine, meprobamate, phenylbutazone, and rifampicin. On a theoretical basis, the effects of liver enzyme induction on the metabolism of transdermally administered estradiol and norethisterone acetate should be minimised by the avoidance of the first pass liver metabolism.

*Pregnancy and lactation:* The use of Evorel Conti and Evorel Sequi is contra-indicated in pregnancy and lactation.

*Effects on ability to drive and use machines:* There are no known data on the effects of Evorel Conti and Evorel Sequi on the ability to drive or use machinery.

*Undesirable effects:* The most commonly reported adverse events reported in clinical trials with Evorel Conti and Evorel Sequi include vaginal bleeding, spotting, breast tenderness, headache, and abdominal cramps/bloating. These adverse events reflect the known profile of oestrogen or oestrogen/progestogen therapy.

Skin reactions reported include transient erythema and irritation with or without pruritus at the site of TDS application. Very rarely, contact dermatitis, reversible post-inflammatory pigmentation, generalised pruritus, and exanthema occurred in studies with Evorel 50.

Rare adverse events reported in association with **oral** progestogen or oestrogen replacement therapy include: thromboembolic events, cholestasis, benign or malignant breast disease, uterine carcinoma, aggravation of epilepsy, liver adenoma and galactorrhoea. If such events occur, Evorel Conti and Evorel Sequi should be discontinued immediately.

*Overdose:* Symptoms of overdose of oestrogen and progestogen therapy may include nausea, break-through bleeding, breast tenderness, abdominal cramps and/or bloating. These symptoms can be reversed by removing the TDS.

**Pharmacological properties**

*Pharmacodynamic properties:* Evorel Conti and Evorel Sequi belong to pharmacotherapeutic class G 03 F A 01, according to the ATC classification.

The active hormone of Evorel Conti and Evorel Sequi is 17β-estradiol, the biologically most potent oestrogen produced by the ovary. Its synthesis in the ovarian follicles is regulated by pituitary hormones. Like all steroid hormones, estradiol diffuses freely into target cells, where it binds to specific macromolecules (receptors). The estradiol-receptor complex then interacts with genomic DNA to alter transcriptional activity. This results in increases or decreases in protein synthesis and in changes of cellular functions.

Estradiol is secreted at different rates during the menstrual cycle. The endometrium is highly sensitive to estradiol, which regulates endometrial proliferation during the follicular phase of the cycle and together with progesterone, induces secretory changes during the luteal phase. Around the menopause estradiol secretion becomes irregular and eventually ceases altogether. The absence of estradiol is associated with menopausal symptoms such as vasomotor instability, sleep disturbances, depressive mood, signs of vulvovaginal and urogenital atrophy and with increased bone loss. In addition, there is growing evidence for an increased incidence in cardiovascular disease in the absence of oestrogen.

Oestrogen replacement therapy has been found effective in most postmenopausal women to compensate for the endogenous oestrogen depletion. It has been demonstrated that transdermal estradiol administration of 50 micrograms per day is effective in the treatment of menopausal symptoms and of postmenopausal bone loss.

In postmenopausal women, Evorel Conti and Evorel Sequi increases estradiol to early follicular levels, with a consequent significant decrease in hot flushes, improvement in Kupperman Index and beneficial changes in vaginal cytology.

However, there is substantial evidence that oestrogen replacement therapy is associated with an increase in endometrial cancer. There is also compelling evidence that adjunctive progestogen treatment protects against oestrogen-induced endometrial cancer. Therefore, women with a uterus should receive combination oestrogen-progestogen hormone replacement therapy.

Norethisterone acetate, used in Evorel Conti and Evorel Sequi, is rapidly hydrolysed to norethisterone, a synthetic 19-nortestosterone derivative of the 13-methyl gonane group, with potent progestational activity. Transdermal norethisterone acetate administration prevents oestrogen-related endometrial proliferation. Combined 17β-estradiol-norethisterone acetate therapy is effective in treating the deficits associated with menopause.

*Pharmacokinetic properties:* Estradiol is readily absorbed from the gastrointestinal tract and is extensively metabolised by the intestinal mucosa and the liver during the first hepatic passage. Transdermal delivery of estradiol is sufficient to cause a systemic effect.

Estradiol distributes widely in body tissues and is bound to albumin (~60-65%) and sex-hormone-binding globulin (~35-45%) in serum. Serum protein-binding fractions remain unaltered following transdermal delivery of estradiol. Estradiol is promptly eliminated from the systemic circulation. The elimination half-life is ~1 hour following intravenous administration. Estradiol is metabolised principally into the less pharmacologically active estrone and its conjugates. Estradiol, estrone and estrone sulphate are interconverted to each other and are excreted in urine as glucuronides and sulphates. The skin metabolises estradiol only to a small extent.

In a single and multiple application study in postmenopausal women, serum estradiol concentrations increased rapidly from pretreatment levels (~ 5 pg/ml) after application of a Evorel Conti TDS. At four hours after application, the mean serum estradiol concentration was ~19 pg/ml. A mean peak serum estradiol concentration of ~41 pg/ml above the pretreatment level was observed at about 23 hours following application. Serum estradiol concentrations remained elevated for the 3.5-day application period. Concentrations returned rapidly to pretreatment levels within 24 hours following removal of the TDS. A serum half-life of ~6.6 hours was determined following removal of the TDS, indicative of the skin depot effect. Multiple application of the Evorel Conti TDS resulted in little or no accumulation of estradiol in the systemic circulation.

Higher circulating levels of estradiol were attained from Evorel 50. Both formulations were shown to be effective in achieving serum estradiol concentration typically seen in premenopausal women. Prior to treatment, the mean serum estradiol to estrone concentration ratio ($E_2/E_1$) was less than 0.3 in the postmenopausal women studied. During use of Evorel Conti TDS the $E_2/E_1$ ratios increased rapidly and were maintained at physiological levels that approximated 1. The $E_2/E_1$ ratios returned to pretreatment levels within 24 hours after removal of the TDS. An average $E_2/E_1$ ratio that approximated 1 was also maintained over an entire 3.5-day application period following Evorel 50 application.

Norethisterone acetate is rapidly hydrolysed to the active progestogen, norethisterone. After oral administration, norethisterone is subject to pronounced first-pass metabolism which reduces the bioavailability. Transdermal delivery of norethisterone acetate produces a sustained and effective level of norethisterone in the systemic circulation.

Norethisterone distributes widely in body tissues and is bound to albumin (~61%) and sex-hormone-binding globulin (~36%) in serum. The elimination half-life is ~6 to 12 hours following oral administration which is not altered following long-term therapy. Norethisterone is primarily metabolised in the liver by reduction of the α,β-unsaturated ketone structure in ring A of the molecule. Among the four possible stereoisomeric tetrahydrosteroids, the 5β-, 3α-hydroxy-derivative appears to be the predominant metabolite. These compounds are primarily excreted in urine and faeces as sulphate and glucuronide conjugates.

In a single and multiple application study in postmenopausal women, serum norethisterone concentrations rose within 1 day after application of a Evorel Conti TDS to a mean steady-state level of ~199 pg/ml. Mean steady-state serum norethisterone concentrations ranging between ~141 to 224 pg/ml were maintained for the entire 3.5-day application period following multiple application. Mean concentrations declined rapidly to the lower limit of assay quantitation at 24 hours after removal of the TDS. A serum half-life of ~15 hours was determined following removal of the TDS, indicative of the skin depot effect. As expected from transdermal delivery of most drugs, only a transient and limited increase in serum norethisterone concentrations was observed following multiple application of the TDS.

*Preclinical safety data:* Estradiol is a naturally occurring hormone and norethisterone acetate is a synthetic derivative of 19-nortestosterone. The pharmacology and toxicology of estradiol and norethisterone acetate are well documented.

Additional toxicity studies which include local tolerance studies in rabbits and dermal sensitisation studies in guinea pigs have been conducted to support registration of Evorel Conti and Evorel Sequi. These studies indicate that Evorel Conti TDS caused mild local skin irritation. It is recognised that test studies on rabbits over-predict skin irritation which occurs in humans. Evorel Conti appeared to be a weak sensitiser

to the guinea pig model. Clinical trial experience with a duration of TDS use over more than one year revealed no evidence of a clinically relevant sensitisation potential in humans.

**Pharmaceutical particulars**

*List of excipients:* Adhesive: acrylate-vinylacetate copolymer (Duro-Tak 387-2287); guar gum. Backing film: polyethylene terephthalate foil (Hostaphan MN19). Release liner: siliconised polyethylene terephthalate foil, is removed before application.

*Incompatibilities:* No creams, lotions, or powders should be applied to the skin area where the TDS is to be applied to prevent interference with the adhesive properties of Evorel 50 and Evorel Conti TDS.

*Shelf life:* Evorel Conti and Evorel Sequi have a shelf-life of 24 months, when stored at or below 25°C. The product can be used until the expiration date mentioned on the container.

*Special precautions for storage:* Store at room temperature, at or below 25°C, within the original sachet and box.

Keep out of reach of children. This also applies to used and disposed TDSs.

*Nature and contents of container: Evorel Conti:* Each carton box has 8 TDSs in individual foil-lined sachets. The sachet comprises a 4 layer laminate including:

– surlyn-ionomer film on the inside,
– then aluminium foil,
– then polyethylene film,
– with a layer of bleached reinforced paper on the outside.

*Evorel Sequi:* Each carton box has 8 TDSs in individual foil-lined sachets. The sachet comprises a 4 layer laminate including:

– surlyn-ionomer film on the inside,
– then aluminium foil,
– then polyethylene film,
– with a layer of bleached reinforced paper on the outside.

One Evorel Sequi box contains 4 Evorel 50 TDSs and 4 Evorel Conti TDSs.

*Instructions for use/handling:* The TDSs should be placed on a clean, dry area of skin on the trunk of the body below the waist. Creams, lotions, or powders may interfere with the adhesive properties of the Evorel Conti and Evorel Sequi TDS. The TDS should not be applied on or near to the breasts. The area of application should be changed, with an interval of at least one week allowed between applications to a particular site. The skin area selected should not be damaged or irritated. The waistline should not be used because excessive rubbing of the TDS may occur.

The TDS should be used immediately after opening the sachet. Remove one part of the protecting foil. Apply the exposed part of adhesive to the application site from the edge to the middle; avoid wrinkling of the TDS. The second part of the protective foil should now be removed and the freshly exposed adhesive applied. Wrinkling should again be avoided and the palm of the hand used to press the TDS onto the skin and to bring the TDS to skin temperature, at which the adhesive effect is optimised. Do not touch the adhesive part of the TDS.

When using Evorel Sequi for the first two weeks, one of the Evorel 50 TDSs should be applied and changed twice weekly. During the following two weeks of Evorel Sequi, one of the Evorel Conti TDSs should be applied, also to be changed twice weekly. The patient then starts again with a new box of Evorel Sequi.

To remove the Evorel TDS, peel away an edge of the patch and pull smoothly away from the skin.

Any gum that remains on the skin after removal of Evorel TDS may be removed by rubbing it off with the fingers or washing with soap and water.

The TDSs should be disposed of in household waste (do not flush down the toilet).

**Marketing authorisation numbers**
Evorel Conti     0242/0319
Evorel Sequi     0242/0320

**Date of approval/revision of SPC**   May 1997.

**Legal category** POM.

# EVOREL* PAK

**Presentation**   Evorel Pak is a calendar pack comprising:

8 'Evorel 50' patches–each patch is a square shaped, transparent, self-adhesive transdermal delivery system of surface area 16 sq cm and 0.2 mm thickness, for application to the skin surface. Each consists of a monolayered adhesive matrix throughout which 17β-estradiol is uniformly distributed and each contains 3.2 mg of estradiol corresponding to a release rate of

50 micrograms of estradiol in 24 hours. Patches are marked 'CE 50'.

12 white tablets each containing 1 mg norethisterone. The tablets are round with C over 1 engraved on both faces.

**Uses** Hormone replacement therapy for the symptomatic relief of menopausal symptoms.

*Mode of action:* Oestrogen substitution effectively prevents the characteristic symptomatic, metabolic and atrophic changes associated with loss of ovarian function due to natural or surgical menopause.

Evorel releases estradiol transdermally into the circulation. In post-menopausal women Evorel increases estradiol levels to early and mid-follicular phase levels.

Norethisterone tablets, an oral progestogen, is used to oppose the oestrogenic effects on the endometrium by converting the oestrogen primed proliferative endometrium into secretory endometrium which, on withdrawal of norethisterone at the end of each cycle, causes a withdrawal bleed in most patients thus eliminating the possibility of endometrial hyperplasia.

*Pharmacokinetics:* With Evorel therapeutic serum estradiol levels are achieved approximately four hours after application to the skin. From 10 hours onwards, the serum levels remain stable and at early to mid-follicular levels throughout the duration of the application (3 to 4 days).

Twenty four hours following removal of Evorel estradiol levels return to baseline.

Norethisterone is rapidly and completely absorbed from the gastrointestinal tract; mean peak plasma levels are observed at 1 to 2 hours post-dose and the elimination half-life is 7 to 9 hours.

**Dosage and administration**

*Adults:* Evorel should be applied twice weekly on a continuous basis, each patch being removed after 3 to 4 days and a fresh patch applied. One norethisterone tablet should be taken by mouth daily for the last 12 days ie days 15–26 of each 28 day cycle of oestrogen replacement therapy. Therapy should be started with one 'Evorel 50' patch (delivering 50 micrograms of estradiol/24 hours) and the dose adjusted after the first month if necessary depending on efficacy and signs of over oestrogenisation (eg breast tenderness). For maintenance therapy the lowest effective dose should be used; a maximum dose of 100 micrograms of estradiol/24 hours should not be exceeded.

Evorel should be applied to the skin as soon as it is removed from the wrapper. Recommended application sites are on clean, dry, healthy, intact skin and each application should be made to a slightly different area of skin on the trunk below waistline. **Evorel should not be applied on or near the breasts.** Evorel should remain in place during bathing and showering. Should it fall off during bathing or showering the patient should wait until cutaneous vasodilation ceases before applying a replacement patch to avoid potential excessive absorption. Should a patch fall off at other times it should be replaced immediately.

Patients can be advised to use baby oil to help remove any gum/glue which may remain on their skin after patch removal.

*Children:* Evorel Pak is not indicated in children.

*Use in pregnancy and lactation:* Evorel Pak is contra-indicated in pregnancy or lactation.

**Contra-indications, warnings, etc.**
*Contra-indications:* Known or suspected malignant tumours of the breast, genital tract or other oestrogen dependent neoplasia. Undiagnosed vaginal bleeding, known or suspected pregnancy and lactation, severe hepatic, renal or cardiac disease, Rotor syndrome or Dubin-Johnson syndrome, active thrombophlebitis or thromboembolic disorders, endometriosis, hypersensitivity to any of the excipients. History during pregnancy of idiopathic jaundice, severe pruritus or pemphigoid gestationis.

*Precautions and warnings:* At the present time there is suggestive evidence of an overall change in the relative risk of breast cancer in post menopausal women receiving hormone replacement therapy. Some studies have reported an increased risk of breast cancer in long-term users, others, however, have shown no such increase. It is not known whether concurrent progestogen use influences the risk of breast cancer. A careful appraisal of the risk/benefit ratio should be undertaken before treating for longer than 5 years.

Administration of unopposed oestrogen therapy in patients with an intact uterus has been reported to increase the risk of endometrial hyperplasia. Consequently, prior to commencing and periodically during oestrogen replacement therapy, it is recommended that the patient should be given a thorough physical and gynaecological examination and a complete medical and family history taken. Repeated breakthrough bleeding should be investigated, including endometrial biopsy.

There is no indication from published studies that the risk of thromboembolic disease, including myocardial infarction, stroke and thrombophlebitis is increased with oestrogen replacement therapy at the current recommended low dosage in apparently normal women. However, treatment should be discontinued immediately following the occurrence of an acute vascular thromboembolic event during therapy. There is no evidence that a history of deep vein thrombosis, pulmonary embolism, stroke or myocardial infarction should be a contra-indication to oestrogen replacement therapy when associated with recognised risk factors such as prolonged immobilisation, post-partum, post-trauma or post-operatively (eg in particular after pelvic surgery) but in the absence of specific data, hormone replacement therapy should be used with caution.

Close monitoring is recommended in patients with epilepsy, diabetes or hypertension (as oestrogens may cause fluid retention), disturbances or impairment of liver function, mastopathy or a strong family history of breast cancer, fibrocystic disease, uterine fibromyomata, cholelithiasis, otosclerosis, multiple sclerosis, systemic lupus erythematosus, porphyria, melanoma, migraine, asthma, as these conditions may be worsened by oestrogen therapy.

Consideration should be given to discontinuing treatment at least four weeks prior to surgery or during periods of prolonged immobilisation. Also, if hypertension develops after initiating therapy, consider discontinuing Evorel Pak while the cause is investigated.

*Drug interactions:* Barbiturates, hydantoins, carbamazepine, meprobamate, phenylbutazone, antibiotics (including rifampicin) and activated charcoal, may impair the activity of oestrogen and progestogens (irregular bleeding and recurrence of symptoms may occur). In transdermal administration of estradiol, a first pass effect via the liver is avoided.

Evorel Pak is not to be used for contraception.

*Side-effects:* Minor effects of oestrogen and combined oestrogen/progestogen hormone replacement therapy which do not usually preclude continuation of therapy include headaches, nausea and breast-tenderness. The following side effects have been reported with oestrogen/progestogen therapy:

*Genito-urinary system:* Pre-menstrual-like syndrome, increase in size of uterine fibromyomata, vaginal candidiasis, change in cervical erosion and degree of cervical secretion, cystitis-like syndrome.

*Breasts:* Tenderness, enlargement, secretion.

*Gastrointestinal:* Nausea, vomiting, abdominal cramps, bloating, cholestatic jaundice.

*Skin:* Chloasma which may persist when drug is discontinued, erythema multiforme, erythema nodosum, haemorrhagic eruption, loss of scalp hair, hirsutism.

*Eyes:* Steepening of corneal curvature, intolerance to contact lenses.

*CNS:* Headaches, migraine, dizziness, mental depression, chorea.

*Miscellaneous:* Increase or decrease in weight, reduced carbohydrate tolerance, aggravation of porphyria, oedema, changes in libido, leg cramps.

In clinical studies with 'Evorel 50' patches, the following side effects were seen: breast tenderness (less than 2%), bleeding (less than 2%) and intermittent bleeding/spotting (less than 5%). None were serious and they reflect the known profile of oestrogen or oestrogen/progestogen therapy. Skin reactions were reported by less than 6% of patients over six treatment cycles.

*Overdosage:* There have been no reports of serious ill-effects from overdosage with Evorel or norethisterone and treatment is usually unnecessary. Nausea and vomiting may occur in the event of a norethisterone overdosage. There is no special antidote and treatment should be symptomatic. The most commonly observed symptoms of overdose with oestrogen therapy are breast tenderness, nausea and breakthrough bleeding. Effects of Evorel overdosage can be reversed by removal of the patch.

**Pharmaceutical precautions** Protect from light. Store below 25°C.

**Legal category** POM.

**Package quantities** Evorel Pak contains: 8 'Evorel 50' patches, each presented in a sealed protective pouch; 12 norethisterone 1 mg tablets; Patient Information Booklet.

**Further information** Nil.

**Product licence numbers** 0242/0223 and 0242/0241

## EVOREL* 25, EVOREL 50, EVOREL 75 AND EVOREL 100 PATCH

**Name of medicinal product** Evorel 25, Evorel 50, Evorel 75 and Evorel 100 Patch.

**Qualitative and quantitative composition** Each 25 patch contains estradiol 1.60 mg, each 50 patch contains 3.2 mg oestradiol, each 75 patch contains estradiol 4.80 mg and each 100 patch contains estradiol 6.40 mg.

**Pharmaceutical form** Evorel is a square shaped, transparent, self-adhesive transdermal delivery system (patch) of 0.2 mm thickness for application to the skin surface. It consists of a monolayered adhesive matrix throughout which 17β oestradiol is uniformly distributed. The adhesive matrix is protected on the outside surface (from clothes etc) by a polyethylene teraphthalate backing foil, while the adhesive surface of the patch is covered by a polyester sheet (the release liner) which is removed before placing the patch on the body surface. This release liner has an S-shaped incision which facilitates easy removal from the patch.

Evorel is available in four sizes corresponding to four different concentrations:

Evorel 25 is marked 'CE25', has a surface area of 8 sq cm and contains 1.6 mg oestradiol corresponding to a release rate of 25 micrograms of oestradiol in 24 hours.

Evorel 50 is marked 'CE50', has a surface area of 16 sq cm and contains 3.2 mg oestradiol corresponding to a release rate of 50 micrograms of oestradiol in 24 hours.

Evorel 75 is marked 'CE75', has a surface area of 24 sq cm and contains 4.8 mg oestradiol corresponding to a release rate of 75 micrograms of oestradiol in 24 hours.

Evorel 100 is marked 'CE100', has a surface area of 32 sq cm and contains 6.4 mg oestradiol corresponding to a release rate of 100 micrograms of oestradiol in 24 hours.

### Clinical particulars

*Therapeutic indications:* Oestrogen replacement for the symptomatic relief of menopausal symptoms.

*Posology and method of administration:*
*Adults:* Evorel should be applied twice weekly on a continuous basis, each patch being renewed after 3 to 4 days and a fresh patch applied. Therapy should be started with one Evorel patch (delivering 50 micrograms of estradiol/24 hours) and the dose adjusted after the first month if necessary depending on efficacy and signs of over-oestrogenisation (eg breast tenderness). For maintenance therapy the lowest effective dose should be used; a maximum dose of 100 micrograms of estradiol/24 hours should not be exceeded. Evorel should be applied to the skin as soon as it is removed from the wrapper.

Recommended application sites are on clean, dry, healthy, intact skin and each application should be made to a slightly different area of skin on the trunk below waistline. **Evorel should not be applied on or near the breasts.** Evorel should remain in place during bathing and showering. Should it fall off during bathing or showering the patient should wait until cutaneous vasodilation ceases before applying a replacement patch to avoid potential excessive absorption. Should a patch fall off at other times it should be replaced immediately.

Patients can be advised to use baby oil to help remove any gum/glue which may remain on their skin after patch removal.

Unopposed oestrogen therapy is not recommended unless the patient has had hysterectomy. Where a progestogen is considered necessary, the appropriate dose should be administered for not less than 12 days each month.

*Children:* Evorel is not indicated in children.

*Contra-indications:* Known or suspected malignant tumours of the breast, genital tract or other oestrogen dependent neoplasia. Undiagnosed vaginal bleeding, known or suspected pregnancy and lactation, severe hepatic, renal or cardiac disease, Rotor syndrome or Dubin-Johnson syndrome, active thrombophlebitis or thromboembolic disorders, endometriosis, hypersensitivity to any of the excipients.

*Special warnings and special precautions for use:* At the present time there is suggestive evidence of an overall change in the relative risk of breast cancer in the post menopausal women receiving hormone replacement therapy. A careful appraisal of the risk/benefit ratio should be undertaken before treating for longer than 5 years.

Administration of unopposed oestrogen therapy in patients with an intact uterus has been reported to increase the risk of endometrial hyperplasia. Consequently, prior to commencing and periodically during oestrogen replacement therapy, it is recommended that the patient should be given a thorough physical and gynaecological examination and a complete medical and family history taken. Repeated breakthrough bleeding should be investigated, including endometrial biopsy.

Close monitoring is recommended in patients with: epilepsy, diabetes or hypertension (as oestrogens may cause fluid retention), disturbances or impairment of liver function, mastopathy or a strong family history of breast cancer, fibrocystic disease, uterine fibromyomata, cholelithiasis, otosclerosis, multiple sclerosis, systemic lupus erythematosus, porphyria, melanoma, migraine, and asthma, as these conditions may be worsened by oestrogen therapy.

Consideration should be given to discontinuing treatment at least four weeks prior to surgery or during periods of prolonged immobilisation. Also, if hypertension develops after initiating therapy, consider discontinuing Evorel while the cause is investigated.

There is no indication from published studies that the risk of thromboembolic disease, including myocardial infarction, stroke and thrombophlebitis is increased with oestrogen replacement therapy at the current recommended low dosage in apparently normal women. However, treatment should be discontinued immediately following the occurrence of an acute vascular thromboembolic event during therapy. There is no evidence that a history of deep vein thrombosis, pulmonary stroke or myocardial infarction should be a contra-indication to oestrogen replacement therapy when associated with recognised risk factors such as prolonged immobilisation, post-partum, post-trauma or post-operatively (eg in particular after pelvic surgery) but in the absence of specific data, Evorel should be used with caution.

Evorel is not to be used for contraception.

*Interactions with other medicaments and other forms of interaction:* Drugs which cause liver enzyme induction may alter oestrogen action. Examples of such drugs include barbiturates, hydantoins, carbamazepine, meprobamate, phenylbutazole and rifampicin. In transdermal administration of estradiol, a first pass effect via the liver is avoided.

There have been no reports of interaction with Evorel although the clinical exposure has been very limited.

*Pregnancy and lactation:* Evorel is contra-indicated in pregnancy and lactation.

*Effects on ability to drive and use machines:* In normal use, Evorel would not be expected to have any effect on the ability to drive or use machinery.

*Undesirable effects:* Although side effects are rare, minor effects which do not usually preclude continuation of therapy include headaches, nausea, breast tenderness, and intermittent bleeding.

In clinical studies with Evorel (50 μg/24 hours) the following side effects were seen: breast tenderness (less than 2%), bleeding (less than 21%), and intermittent bleeding/spotting (less than 5%). None were serious, reflecting the known profile of oestrogen or oestrogen/progestogen therapy. Skin reactions were reported by less than 6% of patients over six treatment cycles. Rarely, dizziness, bloating, oedema, weight gain and leg cramps may occur.

*Overdose:* By virtue of the mode of administration of Evorel, overdosage is unlikely, but effects can if necessary be reversed by removal of the patch. The most commonly observed symptoms of overdose with oestrogen therapy are breast tenderness, nausea and breakthrough bleeding.

### Pharmacological properties
*Pharmacodynamic properties:* Estradiol is a naturally occurring oestrogenic hormone. It is formed in the ovarian follicles under the influence of the pituitary gland. In the female it stimulates the accessory reproductive organs and causes development of the secondary sexual changes in the endometrium during the first half of the menstrual cycle.

Estradiol is readily and completely absorbed from the gastro-intestinal tract through the skin and mucous membranes. Metabolism is primarily in the liver. Excretion of the less active metabolites, primarily oestrone and oestriol is via the urine.

Evorel releases estradiol transdermally into the circulation in pre-menopausal physiological amounts.

In post-menopausal women Evorel increased estradiol levels to early and mid-follicular phase levels. The transcutaneous route avoids the first pass hepatic effect seen with orally administered oestrogens.

In contrast with oral oestrogens, stimulation of hepatic protein synthesis is largely avoided with consequent lack of effect on circulating levels of renin substrate, thyroid binding globulin, sex hormone binding globulin and cortisol binding globulin. Similarly coagulation factors also appear to be unaffected (eg fibrinopeptide A etc). Transdermal estradiol does not affect circulating levels of renin.

Studies with Evorel have shown a significant decrease in hot flushes, improvement in Kupperman Index and vaginal cytology.

Local tolerance with Evorel has been very good. The adhesive matrix used has a low irritation index.

*Pharmacokinetic properties:*
*General characteristics:* Oestrogens are in general readily absorbed from the gastro-intestinal tract,

through the skin and mucous membranes. Absorption from the gastro-intestinal tract is prompt and complete. Transdermal absorption of oestrogens is sufficient to cause a systemic effect. Inactivation of oestrogens is related to first pass hepatic metabolism and not to poor absorption. A certain proportion of oestrogen is excreted into the bile and then reabsorbed from the intestine. During the enterohepatic circulation, estradiol is readily oxidised to the less pharmacologically active oestrone which may in turn then be hydrated to form oestriol (also pharmacologically less than estradiol). Estradiol circulates in the blood in association with sex hormone-binding globulin and albumin.

*Characteristics in patients:* With Evorel therapeutic serum estradiol levels are achieved approximately four hours after application to the skin. From 10 hours onwards, the serum levels remain stable and at early to mid-follicular levels throughout the duration of the application (3 to 4 days).

Twenty four hours following removal of the transdermal therapeutic system estradiol levels return to baseline.

*Preclinical safety data:* Not applicable.

### Pharmaceutical particulars

*List of excipients:* Adhesive acrylic polymer (Duro-Tak 387-2287); guar gum (meyprogat 90); Hostaphan MN19 (polyester film–removed before application).

*Incompatibilities:* None known.

*Shelf life:* Evorel 25, 75 patch and 100 patch 18 months for the product as packed for sale.

Evorel 50 patch: 24 months for the product as packed for sale.

*Special precautions for storage:* Store below 25°C.

*Nature and contents of container:* Each Evorel patch size is presented in a sealed protective pouch. The pouches are packed in a cardboard carton.

*Instructions for use/handling:* None.

### Marketing authorisation numbers

| | |
|---|---|
| Evorel 25 | 0242/0293 |
| Evorel 50 | 0242/0223 |
| Evorel 75 | 0242/0294 |
| Evorel 100 | 0242/0295 |

**Date of approval/revision of SPC** December 1994

**Legal category** POM.

## GYNO-DAKTARIN* 1

**Qualitative and quantitative composition** Miconazole nitrate 1200 mg.

**Pharmaceutical form** White, egg-shaped soft gelatin Scherer capsule.

### Clinical particulars

*Therapeutic indications:* For the local treatment of vulvovaginal candidosis and superinfections due to gram-positive bacteria.

*Posology and method of administration:* Gyno-Daktarin 1 is for intravaginal administration.
*Adults and elderly:* One ovule to be inserted high in the vagina at night, as a single dose.
*Children:* Not recommended.

*Contra-indications:* None known.

*Special warnings and special precautions for use:* None known.

*Interactions with other medicaments and other forms of interaction:* Contact should be avoided between contraceptive diaphragms or sheaths and Gyno-Daktarin 1 since the rubber may be damaged by the emollient base.

*Pregnancy and lactation:* In animals, miconazole nitrate has shown no teratogenic effects but is foetotoxic at high oral doses. The significance of this to man is unknown as there is no evidence of increased risk when taken in human pregnancy. However, as with other imidazoles, Gyno-Daktarin 1 should be used in pregnant women only if the practitioner considers it to be necessary.

*Effects on ability to drive and use machines:* None.

*Undesirable effects:* Occasionally, irritation has been reported. Rarely, local sensitisation may occur requiring discontinuation of treatment.

*Overdose:* Gyno-Daktarin 1 is for intravaginal use only. If accidental ingestion of large quantities occurs, an appropriate method of gastric emptying may be used if considered desirable.

### Pharmacological properties

*Pharmacodynamic properties:* Miconazole is a synthetic imidazole antifungal agent with a broad spectrum of activity against pathogenic fungi (including yeasts and dermatophytes) and gram-positive bacteria (*Staphylococcus* and *Streptococcus* spp).

*Pharmacokinetic properties:* There is little absorption through mucous membranes when miconazole nitrate is applied topically.

*Preclinical safety data:* Not applicable.

### Pharmaceutical particulars

*List of excipients:* Liquid paraffin; white petrolatum; lecithin. The capsule itself contains: Gelatin; glycerol; titanium dioxide; sodium ethylparahydroxybenzoate; sodium propyl parahydroxybenzoate.

*Incompatibilities:* None known.

*Shelf life:* 60 months.

*Special precautions for storage:* Store at room temperature.

*Nature and contents of container:* Blister packs.

*Instructions for use/handling:* None.

**Marketing authorisation number** 0242/0121

**Date of approval/revision of SPC** January 1997

**Legal category** POM.

## GYNO-DAKTARIN*

**Presentation** *Cream:* White, non-staining, water miscible cream containing miconazole nitrate 2% w/w. Cream also contains benzoic acid (E210), butylated hydroxyanisole (E320), liquid paraffin, macrogol 6-32 stearate, glycol stearate, peglicol 5 oleate and purified water.

*Combi-pack:* White, non-staining pessaries each containing 100 mg miconazole nitrate plus white, non-staining, water miscible cream containing miconazole nitrate 2% w/w.

**Uses** Miconazole is a synthetic imidazole antifungal agent with a broad spectrum of activity against pathogenic fungi (including yeasts and dermatophytes) and gram-positive bacteria (*Staphylococcus* and *Streptococcus* spp).

Gyno-Daktarin is for the local treatment of vulvovaginal candidosis and superinfection due to susceptible gram-positive bacteria.

Gyno-Daktarin cream may also be used for treatment of mycotic balanitis.

**Dosage and administration** Gyno-Daktarin cream may be used in both adults and children. Gyno-Daktarin pessaries are for use in adults only.

*Pessary:* One pessary to be inserted high into the vagina as a single dose at night.

*Cream:* 5 g once daily into vagina for 10–14 days or twice daily for 7 days. For vulvitis and balanitis the cream should be applied topically twice daily.

Continue treatment for a few days after symptomatic relief has been achieved.

**Contra-indications, warnings, etc**
*Contra-indications:* None known.

*Use in pregnancy:* In animals miconazole nitrate has shown no teratogenic effects but is foetotoxic at high oral doses. The significance of this to man is unknown as there is no evidence of an increased risk when taken in human pregnancy. However as with other imidazoles, Gyno-Daktarin should be used in pregnant women only if the practitioner considers it to be necessary.

*Side-effects:* Occasionally, irritation has been reported. Rarely, local sensitisation may occur requiring discontinuation of treatment.

*Precautions:* Contact should be avoided between contraceptive diaphragms or sheaths and Gyno-Daktarin pessaries since the rubber may be damaged by the emollient base.

*Overdosage:* Gyno-Daktarin preparations are for intravaginal or topical use only. If accidental ingestion of large quantities occurs, an appropriate method of gastric emptying may be used if considered desirable.

**Pharmaceutical precautions** *Cream:* Store away from direct heat. *Pessaries:* Store in a cool place.

**Legal category** POM.

**Package quantities** *Cream:* supplied in 78 g tubes with disposable applicators – seven days' treatment. *Combi-pack:* Gyno-Daktarin combi-pack consists of 14 pessaries plus 15 g topical cream.

**Further information** Gyno-Daktarin may be used in 'problem vaginitis' as seen in diabetic patients and in women using oral contraceptives.

A leaflet instructing the patient on the correct use is included in each package of Gyno-Daktarin.

**Product licence numbers**

| | |
|---|---|
| Gyno-Daktarin Cream | 0242/0015 |
| Gyno-Daktarin Combi-Pack | 0242/0015 |
| | 0242/0037 |

## GYNO-DAKTARIN* PESSARIES

**Qualitative and quantitative composition** Miconazole nitrate 100 mg.

**Pharmaceutical form** Vaginal pessary.

### Clinical particulars

*Therapeutic indications:* For the local treatment of vulvovaginal candidosis and superinfections due to gram-positive bacteria.

*Posology and method of administration:*
*Adults and elderly:* One pessary to be inserted in the vagina once daily for 14 days or 1 pessary twice daily for 7 days.
*Children:* Not recommended.

*Method of administration:* Vaginal administration.

*Contra-indications:* None known.

*Special warnings and special precautions for use:* None.

*Interactions with other medicaments and other forms of interaction:* Contact should be avoided between contraceptive diaphragms or sheaths and Gyno-Daktarin pessaries since the rubber may be damaged by the emollient base.

*Pregnancy and lactation:* In animals, miconazole nitrate has shown no teratogenic effects but is foetotoxic at high oral doses. The significance of this to man is unknown as there is no evidence of increased risk when taken in human pregnancy. However, as with other imidazoles, Gyno-Daktarin should be used in pregnant women only if the practitioner considers it to be necessary.

*Effects on ability to drive and use machines:* None.

*Undesirable effects:* Occasionally, irritation has been reported. Rarely, local sensitisation may occur requiring discontinuation of treatment.

*Overdose:* Gyno-Daktarin pessaries are for intravaginal use only. In the unlikely event of oral ingestion, an appropriate method of gastric emptying may be used if considered desirable.

### Pharmacological properties

*Pharmacodynamic properties:* Miconazole is a synthetic imidazole antifungal agent with a broad spectrum of activity against pathogenic fungi (including yeasts and dermatophytes) and gram-positive bacteria (*Staphylococcus* and *Streptococcus* spp).

*Pharmacokinetic properties:* There is little absorption through mucous membranes when miconazole nitrate is applied topically.

*Preclinical safety data:* Not applicable.

### Pharmaceutical particulars

*List of excipients:* Hard fat.

*Incompatibilities:* Not applicable.

*Shelf life:* 60 months.

*Special precautions for storage:* Store in a cool place.

*Nature and contents of container:* Cardboard cartons containing 14 pessaries packed in PVC-polyethylene strips.

*Instructions for use/handling:* None.

**Marketing authorisation number** 0242/0037

**Date of approval/revision of SPC** September 1995.

**Legal category** POM.

## GYNO-PEVARYL* CREAM

**Presentation** A white non-perfumed cream containing 1% w/w econazole nitrate.

**Uses** For the treatment of mycotic vulvovaginitis and mycotic balanitis.

### Dosage and administration

*Females:* One applicatorful (approximately 5 g) intravaginally once daily at night for not less than 14 days. The cream should also be applied to the vulva. The full 14 days treatment should be carried out even if the symptoms of vaginal itching or discharge have disappeared. The sexual partner should also be treated.

**Contra-indications, warnings, etc.** Hypersensitivity to any imidazole preparation (or other vaginal antifungal products).

*Side-effects:* Rarely, transient local mild irritation may occur immediately after application.

*Precautions:* Hypersensitivity has rarely been recorded, if it should occur, administration should be discontinued.

Gyno-Pevaryl Cream should be used only by those women who have symptoms of candidosis, and think that they might have candidosis.

If they believe or suspect that they might have some

other sexually transmitted disease, either as well as, or instead of, candidosis, they should consult a Genitourinary Medicine Clinic or their own doctor.

The preparation should not be used if they are pregnant, or think that they might be pregnant, without first consulting a doctor.

It should not be used by those under 16 years of age or over 60 years without first consulting a doctor.

The woman should see her doctor if, after treatment:

– There is not complete relief of symptoms within 7 days.
– There is recurrence of symptoms within 4 weeks of treatment.
– She has more than two episodes of infection within a 6 month period, even if it completely resolves with treatment.
– Adverse effects such as redness, irritation or swelling, associated with the treatment occur.
– Self medication should not be undertaken if the woman has:
– Any abnormal or irregular vaginal bleeding.
– Any blood staining of a vaginal discharge.
– Any vulval or vaginal sores, ulcers or blisters.
– Any associated lower abdominal pain or dysuria.

In all of these cases she should consult her doctor.
Contact between contraceptive diaphragms and this product must be avoided since the rubber may be damaged by this preparation.

In animals, econazole nitrate has shown no teratogenic effects, but is foetotoxic at high doses. The significance of this to man is unknown as there is no evidence of increased risk when taken in human pregnancy. However, as with other imidazoles, econazole should only be used in pregnancy if the practitioner considers it to be necessary.

*Overdosage:* Gyno-Pevaryl Cream is intended for intravaginal/penile use. If accidental ingestion of large quantities of the product occurs, an appropriate method of gastric emptying may be used if considered desirable.

**Pharmaceutical precautions**   Store at room temperature, not exceeding 25°C.

**Legal category**   P.

**Package quantities**   Tubes of 15 g and 30 g. An applicator is not included in the pack. It can be purchased separately.

**Further information** Anogenital hygiene is important to help prevent reinfection.

**Product licence number**   0242/0229.


## GYNO-PEVARYL* 1 VAGINAL PESSARY
## GYNO-PEVARYL* 1 VAGINAL PESSARY AND CREAM C.P. PACK

**Presentation** *Pessary:* Light beige bullet shaped pessary containing 150 mg econazole nitrate.

*C.P. Pack:* A combination pack comprising a Gyno-Pevaryl 1 Vaginal Pessary (containing 150 mg econazole nitrate) and a 15 g tube of Gyno-Pevaryl Cream (containing 1% w/w econazole nitrate).

**Uses** *Pessary:* Vaginitis due to *Candida albicans* and other yeasts.
*C.P. Pack:* Pessary as above; cream to treat mycotic vulvovaginitis and mycotic balanitis.

**Dosage and administration**
*Pessary:* The pessary should be inserted as high as possible into the vagina in the evening prior to retiring.
*C.P. Pack:* Pessary as above. The cream should also be applied to the area around the vaginal opening and the vulva. The full 14 days treatment should be carried out even if the symptoms of vaginal itching or discharge have disappeared. The sexual partner should also be treated with the cream.

**Contra-indications, warnings, etc**
*Contra-indications:* Hypersensitivity to any imidazole preparation (or other vaginal antifungal products).

*Side-effects:* Rarely, transient local mild irritation may occur immediately after application.

*Precautions:* Hypersensitivity has rarely been recorded, if it should occur, administration of the product should be discontinued.

Gyno-Pevaryl should be used only by those women who have symptoms of candidosis, and think that they might have candidosis.

If they believe or suspect that they might have some other sexually transmitted disease, either as well as, or instead of, candidosis, they should consult a Genitourinary Medicine Clinic or their own doctor.

The preparation should not be used if they are pregnant, or think that they might be pregnant, without first consulting a doctor.

It should not be used by those under 16 years of age or over 60 years without first consulting a doctor.

The woman should see her doctor if, after treatment:

– There is not complete relief of symptoms within 7 days.
– There is recurrence of symptoms within 4 weeks of treatment.
– She has more than two episodes of infection within a 6 month period, even if it completely resolves with treatment.
– Adverse effects such as redness, irritation or swelling, associated with the treatment occur.
– Self medication should not be undertaken if the woman has:
– Any abnormal or irregular vaginal bleeding.
– Any blood staining of a vaginal discharge.
– Any vulval or vaginal sores, ulcers or blisters.
– Any associated lower abdominal pain or dysuria.

In all of these cases she should consult her doctor.
Contact between contraceptive diaphragms and Gyno-Pevaryl must be avoided since the rubber may be damaged by this preparation.

In animals econazole nitrate has shown no teratogenic effects, but is foetotoxic at high doses. The significance of this in man is unknown as there is no evidence of an increased risk when taken in human pregnancy. However, as with other imidazoles, econazole should be used in pregnancy only if the practitioner considers it to be necessary.

*Overdosage:* Gyno-Pevaryl 1 Vaginal Pessary and Cream are intended for intravaginal use. Cream is also for penile use. If accidental ingestion of large quantities of the product occurs, an appropriate method of gastric emptying may be used if considered desirable.

**Pharmaceutical precautions**   Store at room temperature, not exceeding 25°C.

**Legal category**   P.

**Package quantities**   *Pessaries:* Each pack contains one pessary with a plastic vaginal applicator and a patient instruction leaflet. The pessary is individually sealed in a white plastic strip marked Gyno-Pevaryl 1.

*C.P. Pack:* Each pack contains one pessary, a 15 g tube of cream and a patient instruction leaflet.

**Further information**   Anogenital hygiene is important to help prevent re-infection.

Due to the differing nature of the pessary base of Gyno-Pevaryl 1, substitution of a single Gyno-Pevaryl 150 pessary from the three pessary treatment must not be made.

**Product licence numbers**
Gyno-Pevaryl         0242/0226
Combipack            0242/0226 and 0242/0229


## GYNO-PEVARYL*150 VAGINAL PESSARIES
## GYNO-PEVARYL*150 VAGINAL PESSARIES AND CREAM COMBIPACK

**Presentation**   *Pessaries:* White egg-shaped pessaries each containing 150 mg econazole nitrate and melting at 37°C.

*Combipack:* A combination pack comprising 3 Gyno-Pevaryl vaginal pessaries (each containing 150 mg econazole nitrate) plus a 15 g tube of Gyno-Pevaryl cream (containing 1% w/w econazole nitrate).

**Uses** *Pessaries:* Vaginitis due to *Candida albicans* and other yeasts.
*Combipack:* Pessaries as above; cream to treat mycotic vulvovaginitis and mycotic balanitis.

**Dosage and administration**   *Pessaries:* One pessary should be inserted high into the vagina each evening for three consecutive days.

*Combipack:* Pessaries as above. The cream should also be applied to the area around the vaginal opening and the vulva. The full 14 days treatment should be carried out even if the symptoms of vaginal itching or discharge have disappeared. The sexual partner should also be treated with the cream.

**Contra-indications, warnings, etc.**
*Contra-indications:* Hypersensitivity to any imidazole preparation (or other vaginal antifungal products).

*Side-effects:* Rarely, transient local mild irritation may occur immediately after application.

*Precautions:* Hypersensitivity has rarely been recorded, if it should occur, administration should be discontinued.

Gyno-Pevaryl cream should be used only by those women who have symptoms of candidosis, and think that they might have candidosis.

If they believe or suspect that they might have some other sexually transmitted disease, either as well as, or instead of, candidosis, they should consult a Genitourinary Medicine Clinic or their own doctor.

The preparation should not be used if they are pregnant, or think that they might be pregnant, without first consulting a doctor.

It should not be used by those under 16 years of age or over 60 years without first consulting a doctor.

The woman should see her doctor if, after treatment:

– There is not complete relief of symptoms within 7 days.
– There is recurrence of symptoms within 4 weeks of treatment.
– She has more than two episodes of infection within a 6 month period, even if it completely resolves with treatment.

Adverse effects such as redness, irritation or swelling, associated with the treatment occur.

Self medication should not be undertaken if the woman has:

Any abnormal or irregular vaginal bleeding.
Any blood staining of a vaginal discharge.
Any vulval or vaginal sores, ulcers or blisters.
Any associated lower abdominal pain or dysuria.

In all of these cases she should consult her doctor.
Contact between contraceptive diaphragms and Gyno-Pevaryl must be avoided since the rubber may be damaged by this preparation.

In animals econazole nitrate has shown no teratogenic effects, but is foetotoxic at high doses. The significance of this in man is unknown as there is no evidence of an increased risk when taken in human pregnancy. However, as with other imidazoles, econazole should be used in pregnancy only if the practitioner considers it to be necessary.

*Overdosage:* Gyno-Pevaryl Vaginal Pessaries and Cream are intended for intravaginal use. If accidental ingestion of large quantities of the product occurs, an appropriate method of gastric emptying may be used if considered desirable.

**Pharmaceutical precautions**   Store at room temperature, not exceeding 25°C.

**Legal category**   P.

**Package quantities**   *Pessaries:* Each pack contains 3 pessaries and a patient instruction leaflet. The pessaries are individually sealed in a white plastic strip marked Gyno-Pevaryl 150 at regular intervals. *Combipack:* Each pack contains 3 pessaries, a 15 g tube of cream and a patient instruction leaflet.

**Further information**   Anogenital hygiene is important to help prevent re-infection.

**Product licence numbers**
Gyno-Pevaryl Pessaries   0242/0227
Combipack                0242/0227 and 0242/0229


## GYNOL* II CONTRACEPTIVE JELLY

**Qualitative and quantitative composition**   The gel contains 2.0% w/w of nonoxynol-9.

**Pharmaceutical form**   Vaginal jelly.

**Clinical particulars**

*Therapeutic indications:* For use as a spermicidal contraceptive in conjunction with barrier methods of contraception.

*Posology and method of administration:* For topical intravaginal administration.

For use by adult females only.

The gel should be spread over the surface of the diaphragm which will be in contact with the cervix, and on the rim. The diaphragm and spermicide must be allowed to remain undisturbed for at least six to eight hours after coitus. A fresh application of gel or other spermicides eg Orthoforms Contraceptive pessaries must be made prior to any subsequent acts of coitus within this period of time, without removing the diaphragm. (A vaginal applicator should be used for inserting more jelly).

Douching is not recommended, but if desired it should be deferred for at least six hours after intercourse.

*Contra-indications:* Hypersensitivity to nonoxynol-9 or to any component of the preparation. Patients with absent vaginal sensation eg paraplegics and quadriplegics.

*Special warnings and special precautions for use:* Spermicidal intravaginal preparations are intended for use in conjunction with barrier methods of contraception such as condoms, diaphragms and caps.

Where avoidance of pregnancy is important the choice of contraceptive method should be made in consultation with a doctor or a family planning clinic.

If vaginal or penile irritation occurs discontinue use. If symptoms worsen or continue for more than 48 hours medical advice should be sought.

*Interactions with other medicaments and other forms of interaction:* None known.

*Pregnancy and lactation:* There is no evidence from

animal and human studies that nonoxynol-9 is teratogenic. Human epidemiological studies have not shown any firm evidence of adverse effects on the foetus, however some studies have shown that nonoxynol-9 may be embryotoxic in animals. This product should not be used if pregnancy is suspected or confirmed. Animal studies have detected nonoxynol-9 in milk after intravaginal administration. Use by lactating women has not been studied.

*Effects on ability to drive and use machines:* None known.

*Undesirable effects:* May cause irritation of the vagina or penis.

*Overdose:* If taken orally the surfactant properties of this preparation may cause gastric irritation. General supportive therapy should be carried out. Hepatic and renal function should be monitored if medically indicated.

**Pharmacological properties**

*Pharmacodynamic properties:* The standard in vitro test (Sander-Cramer) evaluating the effect of nonoxynol-9 on animal sperm motility has shown the compound to be a potent spermicide.

The site of action of nonoxynol-9 has been determined as the sperm cell membrane. The lipoprotein membrane is disrupted, increasing permeability, with subsequent loss of cell components and decreased motility. A similar effect on vaginal epithelial and bacterial cells is also found.

*Pharmacokinetic properties:* The intravaginal absorption and excretion of radiolabelled ($^{14}C$) nonoxynol-9 has been studied in non-pregnant rats and rabbits and in pregnant rats. No appreciable difference was found in the extent or rate of absorption in pregnant and non-pregnant animals. Plasma levels peaked at about one hour and recovery from urine as unchanged nonoxynol-9 accounted for approximately 15-25% and faeces approximately 70% of the administered dose as unchanged nonoxynol-9. Less than 0.3% was found in the milk of lactating rats. No metabolites were detected in any of the samples analysed.

*Preclinical safety data:* Not applicable.

**Pharmaceutical particulars**

*List of excipients:* Methyl parahydroxybenzoate (E 218); sorbitol solution (E 420); lactic acid; povidone K30; propylene glycol; sodium carboxymethylcellulose; sorbic acid (E 200); purified water.

*Incompatibilities:* Not applicable.

*Shelf life:* 2 years.

*Special precautions for storage:* Store at room temperature (at or below 25°C).

*Nature and contents of container:* Epoxy resin lined aluminium tubes with polyethylene caps. Available in 81 gram packs; an applicator is available separately if required.

*Instructions for use/handling:* Not applicable.

**Marketing authorisation number** 0242/0225

**Date of approval/revision of SPC** July 1996

**Legal category** GSL.

## HALDOL*

**Presentation** Pale blue, cross scored, uncoated tablets, marked Janssen on one side, containing 5 mg haloperidol BP. The tablets also contain lactose and E132 as inactive ingredients.

Clear, colourless, odourless liquid containing 2 mg haloperidol BP per ml for oral administration. The liquid also contains methyl paraben as an inactive ingredient.

Amber glass ampoules containing 5 mg haloperidol BP in 1 ml aqueous solution for injection also containing lactic acid and water for injection as inactive ingredients.

Amber glass ampoules containing 10 mg haloperidol BP in 2 ml aqueous solution for injection also containing lactic acid and water for injection as inactive ingredients.

**Uses** Haldol is a neuroleptic butyrophenone drug with a wide range of actions, indicated in the following conditions:

*Adults:*

- Schizophrenia: treatment of symptoms and prevention of relapse (oral and im).
- Other psychoses, especially paranoid (oral and im).
- Mania and hypomania (oral and im).
- Mental or behavioural problems such as aggression, hyperactivity and self-mutilation in the mentally retarded and in patients with organic brain damage (oral and im).
- As an adjunct to short-term management of moderate to severe psychomotor agitation, excitement, violent or dangerously impulsive behaviour (oral and im).
- Intractable hiccup (oral).
- Restlessness and agitation in the elderly (oral).
- Gilles de la Tourette syndrome and severe tics (oral).
- Nausea and vomiting (im).

*Children* (oral administration only):

- Childhood behavioural disorders especially when associated with hyperactivity and aggression.
- Gilles de la Tourette syndrome.
- Childhood schizophrenia.

**Dosage and administration** Dosage for all indications should be individually determined and is best initiated and titrated under close clinical supervision. To determine the initial dose, consideration should be given to the patient's age, severity of symptoms and previous response to other neuroleptics.

Patients who are elderly or debilitated or those with previously reported adverse reactions to neuroleptic drugs may require less haloperidol. The normal starting dose should be halved, followed by a gradual titration to achieve optimal response.

*Oral administration:*
*Adults:*

*Schizophrenia, Psychoses, Mania and Hypomania, Mental or Behavioural Problems, Psychomotor Agitation, Excitement, Violent or Dangerously Impulsive Behaviour, Organic Brain Damage.*

Initial dosage: Moderate symptomatology 1.5-3.0 mg bd. or tds.

Severe symptomatology/resistant patients 3.0-5.0 mg bd or tds.

The same starting doses may be employed in adolescents, who, in certain cases, may require up to 30 mg or, exceptionally, up to 60 mg/day.

In resistant schizophrenics, daily dosages up to 100 mg (or rarely up to 120 mg) may be necessary to achieve an optimal response.

Maintenance dosage: Once satisfactory control of symptoms has been achieved dosage, should be gradually reduced to the lowest effective maintenance dose, often as low as 5 or 10 mg/day. Too rapid a dosage reduction should be avoided.

*Restlessness or Agitation in the Elderly:* Initial dose 1.5-3.0 mg bd or tds titrated as required, to attain an effective maintenance dose (1.5-50 mg daily).

*Gilles de la Tourette Syndrome, Severe Tics, Intractable Hiccup:* Starting dose 1.5 mg tds. adjusted according to response. A daily maintenance dose of 10 mg may be required in Gilles de la Tourette syndrome.

*Children*

*Childhood Behavioural Disorders/Schizophrenia:* Total daily maintenance dose of 0.025-0.05 mg/kg/day. Half the total dose should be given in the morning and the other half in the evening, up to a maximum of 10 mg daily.

*Gilles de la Tourette Syndrome:* Oral maintenance doses of up to 10 mg/day in most patients.

*Parenteral administration*
*Adults*

*Schizophrenia, Psychoses, Mania and Hypomania, Mental or Behavioural Problems, Psychomotor Agitation, Excitement, Violent or Dangerously Impulsive Behaviour, Organic Brain Damage:* For control of acutely agitated patients with moderate symptoms: 2-10 mg im.

Depending on the response of the patient, subsequent doses may be given every 4-8 hours, although it may be given every hour, if necessary, until sufficient symptom control is achieved or up to a maximum of 60 mg/day.

Infrequently, severely disturbed patients may require an initial dose of up to 30 mg.

Oral treatment should succeed intramuscular administration as soon as practicable. Bioavailability from the oral route is about 60% of that from the im route, and readjustment of dose may be required.

Haldol can also be administered by the iv route.

*Nausea and vomiting:* 1-2 mg im.

*Children:* Not recommended for parenteral use in children.

**Contra-indications, warnings etc.**
*Contra-indications:* Comatose states; CNS depression; Parkinson's disease; known hypersensitivity to haloperidol; lesions of the basal ganglia.

*Use in pregnancy and lactation:* The safety of haloperidol in pregnancy has not been established. There is some evidence of harmful effects in some but not all animal studies. There have been a number of reports of birth defects following foetal exposure to haloperidol for which a causal role for haloperidol cannot be excluded. Haldol should be used during pregnancy only if the anticipated benefit outweighs the risk and the administered dose and duration of treatment should be as low and as short as possible.

Haloperidol is excreted in breast milk. There have been isolated cases of extrapyramidal symptoms in breast-fed children. If the use of Haldol is essential, the benefits of breast feeding should be balanced against its potential risks.

*Effects on ability to drive and use machines:* Some degree of sedation or impairment of alertness may occur, particularly with higher doses and at the start of treatment, and may be potentiated by alcohol or other CNS depressants. Patients should be advised not to undertake activities requiring alertness such as driving or operating machinery during treatment, until their susceptibility is known.

*Precautions and warnings:* Please also refer to *Drug nteractions* section.

Caution is advised in patients with liver disease, renal failure, phaeochromocytoma, epilepsy, and conditions predisposing to epilepsy (eg alcohol withdrawal and brain damage) or convulsions. Haloperidol should only be used with great caution in patients with disturbed thyroid function. Antipsychotic therapy in those patients must always be accompanied by adequate management of the underlying thyroid dysfunction.

Cases of sudden death have been reported in psychiatric patients receiving antipsychotic drugs, including haloperidol. The risk-benefit of haloperidol treatment should be fully assessed before treatment is commenced and patients with risk factors for ventricular arrhythmias such as cardiac disease, subarachnoid haemorrhage, metabolic abnormalities such as hypokalaemia, hypocalcaemia or hypomagnesemia, starvation, alcohol abuse or those receiving concomitant therapy with other drugs known to prolong the QT interval, should be monitored carefully (ECGs and potassium levels), particularly during the initial phase of treatment, to obtain steady plasma levels.

Acute withdrawal symptoms including nausea, vomiting and insomnia have very rarely been described after abrupt cessation of high doses of antipsychotic drugs. Relapse may also occur and gradual withdrawal is advisable.

In schizophrenia, the response to antipsychotic drug treatment may be delayed. If drugs are withdrawn, recurrence of symptoms may not become apparent for several weeks or months.

As with all antipsychotic agents, haloperidol should not be used alone where Depression is predominant. It may be combined with antidepressants to treat those conditions in which Depression and psychosis coexist. Haloperidol may impair the metabolism of tricyclic antidepressants (clinical significance unknown).

If concomitant antiparkinson medication is required, it may have to be continued after haloperidol is discontinued to take account of any differences in excretion rates. The physician should keep in mind the possible anticholinergic effects associated with antiparkinson agents.

*Drug interactions:* In common with all neuroleptics, haloperidol can increase the central nervous system depression produced by other CNS-depressant drugs, including alcohol, hypnotics, sedatives or strong analgesics. An enhanced CNS effect, when combined with methyldopa, has been reported.

Haloperidol may antagonise the action of adrenaline and other sympathomimetic agents and reverses the blood pressure lowering effects of adrenergic-blocking agents such as guanethidine.

The dosage of anticonvulsants may need to be increased to take account of the lowered seizure threshold. Coadministration of enzyme-inducing drugs such as carbamazepine, phenobarbitone and rifampicin with haloperidol may result in a significant reduction of haloperidol plasma levels. The haloperidol dose may therefore need to be increased, according to the patient's response. After stopping such drugs, it may be necessary to readjust the dosage of haloperidol.

Haloperidol may impair the metabolism of tricyclic antidepressants (clinical significance unknown) and the antiparkinson effects of levodopa.

In pharmacokinetic studies, increased haloperidol levels have been reported when haloperidol was given concomitantly with the following drugs: quinidine, buspirone and fluoxetine. Haloperidol plasma levels should therefore be monitored and reduced if necessary.

Antagonism of the effect of phenindione has been reported.

In rare cases, an encephalopathy-like syndrome has been reported in combination with lithium and haloperidol. It remains controversial whether these cases represent a distinct clinical entity or whether they are in fact cases of NMS and/or lithium toxicity. Signs of encephalopathy-like syndrome include confusion, disorientation, headache, disturbances of balance and drowsiness. One report showing symptomless EEG abnormalities on the combination has suggested that EEG monitoring might be advisable. When lithium and haloperidol therapy are used concomitantly, haloperidol should be given in the lowest effective dosage and lithium levels should be monitored and kept below 1 mmol/l. If symptoms of encephalopathy-like syndrome occur, therapy should be stopped immediately.

*Adverse effects: Central nervous system:* In common with all neuroleptics, extrapyramidal symptoms may occur, eg tremor, rigidity, hypersalivation, bradykinesia, akathisia, acute dystonia, oculogyric crisis and laryngeal dystonia. Anti-Parkinson agents should not be prescribed routinely.

As with all antipsychotic agents, tardive dyskinesia may appear in some patients on long-term therapy or after drug discontinuation.

The syndrome is mainly characterised by rhythmical involuntary movements of the tongue, face, mouth or jaw. The manifestations may be permanent in some patients. The syndrome may be masked when treatment is reinstituted, when the dosage is increased or when a switch is made to a different antipsychotic drug. Treatment should be discontinued as soon as possible.

However since its occurrence may be related to duration of treatment, as well as daily dose, Haldol should be given in the minimum effective dose for the minimum possible time, unless it is established that long term administration for the treatment of schizophrenia is required.

It has been reported that fine vermicular movements of the tongue may be an early sign of tardive dyskinesia and that the full syndrome may not develop if the medication is stopped at that time.

The following effects have been reported rarely: confusional states or epileptic fits, depression, sedation, agitation, drowsiness, insomnia, headache, vertigo and apparent exacerbation of psychotic symptoms.

In common with other antipsychotic drugs, haloperidol has been associated with rare cases of neuroleptic malignant syndrome (CMS), an idiosyncratic response characterised by hyperthermia, generalised muscle rigidity, autonomic instability, altered consciousness, coma and elevated CPK. Signs of autonomic dysfunction such as tachycardia, labile arterial pressure and sweating may precede the onset of hyperthermia, acting as early warning signs. Antipsychotic treatment should be withdrawn immediately and appropriate supportive therapy and careful monitoring instituted.

Haloperidol, even in low dosage in susceptible (especially non-psychotic) individuals, may cause unpleasant subjective feelings of being mentally dulled or slowed down, dizziness, headache or paradoxical effects of excitement, agitation or insomnia.

*Gastrointestinal system:* Gastrointestinal symptoms, nausea, loss of appetite, constipation and dyspepsia have been reported.

*Endocrinological system:* Hormonal effects of antipsychotic neuroleptic drugs include hyperprolactinaemia, which may cause galactorrhoea, gynaecomastia and oligo- or amenorrhoea. Hypoglycaemia and the syndrome of inappropriate antidiuretic hormone secretion have been reported rarely. Impairment of sexual function including erection and ejaculation has also been occasionally reported.

*Cardiovascular system:* Tachycardia and dose related hypotension are uncommon, but can occur, particularly in the elderly, who are more susceptible to the sedative and hypotensive effects. Less commonly hypertension has also been reported. Cardiac effects such as QT-interval prolongation, Torsade de Pointes and/or ventricular arrhythmias have been reported rarely. They may occur more frequently with high doses, intravenous administration and in predisposed patients (see *Precautions and Warnings*).

*Autonomic nervous system:* Dry mouth as well as excessive salivation, blurred vision, urinary retention and hyperhidrosis have been reported.

*Dermatological system:* The following effects have been reported rarely: oedema, various skin rashes and reactions including urticaria, exfoliative dermatitis and erythema multiforme. Photosensitive skin reactions have been reported very rarely.

*Other adverse reactions:* The following effects have been reported rarely: jaundice, cholestatic hepatitis or transient abnormalities of liver function in the absence of jaundice; priapism and weight changes may occur. Temperature disorders may also occur, characteristically hyperthermia associated with NMS, although hypothermia has also been reported.

The following have been reported very rarely: blood dyscrasias, including agranulocytosis, thrombocytopenia and transient leucopenia; hypersensitivity reactions including anaphylaxis.

*Overdose*
*Symptoms:* In general, the manifestations of haloperidol overdosage are an extension of its pharmacological actions, the most prominent of which would be severe extrapyramidal symptoms, hypotension and psychic indifference with a transition to sleep. The risk of ventricular arrhythmias possibly associated

with QT-prolongation should be considered. The patient may appear comatose with respiratory depression and hypotension which could be severe enough to produce a shock-like state. Paradoxically hypertension rather than hypotension may occur. Convulsions may also occur.

*Treatment:* There is no specific antidote to haloperidol. A patent airway should be established and maintained with mechanically assisted ventilation if necessary. In view of isolated reports of arrhythmia ECG monitoring is strongly advised. Hypotension and circulatory collapse should be treated by plasma volume expansion and other appropriate measures. Adrenaline should not be used. The patient should be monitored carefully for 24 hours or longer, body temperature and adequate fluid intake should be maintained.

In cases of severe extrapyramidal symptoms, appropriate antiparkinson medication should be administered.

**Pharmaceutical precautions** Store tablets in a cool dry place. Haldol oral liquid should be stored at room temperature. Ampoules should be protected from light.

**Legal category** POM.

**Further information** Haldol is rapidly absorbed after oral administration with a mean bioavailability of 44-74% (approximately 60%). Variable bioavailability is likely due to inter-individual differences in GI absorption and extent of first-pass hepatic metabolism.

Distribution is rapid to extravascular tissues, especially liver and adipose tissue. It is approximately 92% bound to plasma proteins. Haloperidol crosses the blood-brain barrier and is excreted in human breast milk.

Haloperidol is extensively metabolised by oxidative dealkylation, and ultimately conjugated with glycine. Half life is approximately 20 hours.

A 10 mg iv dose of haloperidol given over 2 minutes produced a peak serum concentration of 34 µg/ml at the end of infusion, declining to 1 µg/ml by 40 hours. Following im administration of 2 mg, peak plasma concentrations were similar to after oral, ie 10 µg/ml, but are reached within 20 minutes.

**Package quantities**

| | |
|---|---|
| 5.0 mg tablet | packs of 100 tablets |
| 5 mg/ml injectable solution | 5 × 1 ml ampoules |
| 10 mg/2 ml injectable solution | 5 × 2 ml ampoules |
| 2 mg/ml oral solution | 100 ml amber glass bottles with calibrated pipette |

**Product licence numbers**

| | |
|---|---|
| 5.0 mg tablet | 0242/0031R |
| 5 mg/ml injectable solution | 0242/0036R |
| 10 mg/2 ml injectable solution | 0242/0036R |
| 2 mg/ml oral liquid | 0242/0035R |

# HALDOL* TABLETS 10 mg

**Qualitative and quantitative composition** Haloperidol 10 mg.

**Pharmaceutical form** Tablets.

**Clinical particulars**
*Therapeutic indications:*
 Adults:
  Schizophrenia: treatment of symptoms and prevention of relapse.
  Other psychoses: especially paranoid.
  Mania and hypomania.
  Mental or behavioural problems such as aggression, hyperactivity and self mutilation in the mentally retarded and in patients with organic brain damage.
  As an adjunct to short term management of moderate to severe psychomotor agitation, excitement, violent or dangerously impulsive behaviour.
  Intractable hiccup.
  Restlessness and agitation in the elderly.
  Gilles de la Tourette Syndrome and severe tics.

*Children (oral administration only):*
  Childhood behavioural disorders, especially when associated with hyperactivity and aggression.
  Gilles de la Tourette Syndrome.
  Childhood schizophrenia.

*Posology and method of administration:* Dosage for all indications should be individually determined and is best initiated and titrated under close clinical supervision. To determine initial dose, consideration should be given to the patient's age, severity of symptoms and previous response to neuroleptic drugs.

Patients who are elderly or debilitated or those with previously reported adverse reactions to neuroleptic drugs may require less Haldol. The normal starting dose should be halved, followed by a gradual titration to achieve optimal response.

Oral administration.

*Adults*
*Schizophrenia, Psychoses, Mania and Hypomania, Mental or Behavioural Problems, Psychomotor Agitation, Excitement, Violent or Dangerously Impulsive Behaviour, Organic Brain Damage.*
 *Initial dose:*
 Moderate symptomatology–1.5–3.0 mg bd or tds.
 Severe symptomatology/resistant patients–3.0–5.0 mg bd or tds.
 The same starting dose may be employed in adolescents, who in certain cases, may require up to 30 mg or exceptionally, up to 60 mg/day. In resistant schizophrenics daily dosages up to 100 mg (or rarely up to 120 mg) may be necessary to achieve an optimal response.

 *Maintenance dosage:* Once satisfactory control of symptoms has been achieved dosage should be gradually reduced to the lowest effective maintenance dose, often as low as 5 or 10 mg/day. Too rapid a dosage reduction should be avoided.

*Restlessness or agitation in the elderly:* Initial dose: 1.5–3.0 mg bd or tds titrated as required, to attain an effective maintenance dose (1.5-50 mg daily).

*Gilles de la Tourette Syndrome, Severe Tics, Intractable Hiccup:* Starting dose 1.5 mg tds adjusted according to response. A daily maintenance dose of 10 mg may be required in Gilles de la Tourette Syndrome.

*Children*
*Childhood Behavioural Disorders and Schizophrenia:* Total daily maintenance dose of 0.025-0.05 mg/kg/day. Half the total dose should be given in the morning and the other half in the evening, up to a maximum of 10 mg daily.

*Gilles de la Tourette Syndrome:* Oral maintenance doses up to 10 mg/day in most patients.

*Contra-indications:*Comatose states, CNS depression, Parkinson's disease, known hypersensitivity to haloperidol, lesions of basal ganglia.

*Special warnings and special precautions for use:* Caution is advised in patients with liver disease, renal failure, phaeochromocytoma, epilepsy, and conditions predisposing to epilepsy (eg alcohol withdrawal and brain damage) or convulsions. Haloperidol should only be used with great caution in patients with disturbed thyroid function. Antipsychotic therapy in those patients must always be accompanied by adequate management of the underlying thyroid dysfunction.

Cases of sudden death have been reported in psychiatric patients receiving antipsychotic drugs, including haloperidol. The risk-benefit of haloperidol treatment should be fully assessed before treatment is commenced and patients with risk factors for ventricular arrhythmias such as cardiac disease, subarachnoid haemorrhage, metabolic abnormalities such as hypokalaemia, hypocalcaemia or hypomagnesemia, starvation, alcohol abuse or those receiving concomitant therapy with other drugs known to prolong the QT interval, should be monitored carefully (ECGs and potassium levels), particularly during the initial phase of treatment, to obtain steady plasma levels.

Acute withdrawal symptoms including nausea, vomiting and insomnia have very rarely been described after abrupt cessation of high doses of antipsychotic drugs. Relapse may also occur and gradual withdrawal is advisable.

In schizophrenia, the response to antipsychotic drug treatment may be delayed. If drugs are withdrawn, recurrence of symptoms may not become apparent for several weeks or months.

As with all antipsychotic agents, haloperidol should not be used alone where depression is predominant. It may be combined with antidepressants to treat those conditions in which depression and psychosis coexist. Haloperidol may impair the metabolism of tricyclic antidepressants (clinical significance unknown).

If concomitant antiparkinson medication is required, it may have to be continued after haloperidol is discontinued to take account of any differences in excretion rates. The physician should keep in mind the possible anticholinergic effects associated with antiparkinson agents.

*Interactions with other medicaments and other forms of interaction:* In common with all neuroleptics, haloperidol can increase the central nervous system depression produced by other CNS-depressant drugs, including alcohol, hypnotics, sedatives or strong analgesics.

Haloperidol may antagonise the action of adrenaline and other sympathomimetic agents and reverses the blood pressure lowering effects of adrenergic-blocking agents such as guanethidine.

Haloperidol may impair the antiparkinson effects of levodopa. In pharmacokinetic studies, increased haloperidol levels have been reported when haloperidol was given concomitantly with the following drugs: quinidine, buspirone and fluoxetine. Haloperidol plasma levels should therefore be monitored and reduced if necessary. The dosage of anticonvulsants may need to be increased to take account of the lowered seizure threshold.

Coadministration of enzyme-inducing drugs such as carbamazepine, phenobarbitone and rifampicin with haloperidol may result in a significant reduction of haloperidol plasma levels. The haloperidol dose may therefore need to be increased, according to the patient's response. After stopping such drugs, it may be necessary to readjust the dosage of haloperidol.

An enhanced CNS effect, when combined with methyldopa, has been reported.

In rare cases, an encephalopathy-like syndrome has been reported in combination with lithium and haloperidol. It remains controversial whether these cases represent a distinct clinical entity or whether they are in fact cases of NMS and/or lithium toxicity. Signs of encephalopathy-like syndrome include confusion, disorientation, headache, disturbances of balance and drowsiness. One report showing symptomless EEG abnormalities on the combination has suggested that EEG monitoring might be advisable. When lithium and haloperidol therapy are used concomitantly, haloperidol should be given in the lowest effective dosage and lithium levels should be monitored and kept below 1 mmol/l. If symptoms of encephalopathy-like syndrome occur, therapy should be stopped immediately.

Haloperidol may impair the metabolism of tricyclic antidepressants (clinical significance unknown). Antagonism of the effect of phenindione has been reported.

*Pregnancy and lactation:* The safety of haloperidol in pregnancy has not been established. There is some evidence of harmful effects in some, but not all animal studies. There have been a number of reports of birth defects following foetal exposure to haloperidol for which a causal role for haloperidol cannot be excluded. Haldol should be used during pregnancy only if the anticipated benefit outweighs the risk and the administered dose and duration of treatment should be as low and as short as possible.

Haloperidol is excreted in breast milk. There have been isolated cases of extrapyramidal symptoms in breast-fed children. If the use of Haldol is essential, the benefits of breast feeding should be balanced against its potential risks.

*Effects on ability to drive and use machines:* Some degree of sedation or impairment of alertness may occur, particularly with higher doses and at the start of treatment, and may be potentiated by alcohol or other CNS depressants. Patients should be advised not to undertake activities requiring alertness such as driving or operating machinery during treatment, until their susceptibility is known.

*Undesirable effects:*
*Central nervous system:* In common with all neuroleptics, extrapyramidal symptoms may occur, eg tremor, rigidity, hypersalivation, bradykinesia, akathisia, acute dystonia, oculogyric crisis and laryngeal dystonia.

Anti-Parkinson agents should not be prescribed routinely.

As with all antipsychotic agents, tardive dyskinesia may appear in some patients on long-term therapy or after drug discontinuation.

The syndrome is mainly characterised by rhythmical involuntary movements of the tongue, face, mouth or jaw. The manifestations may be permanent in some patients. The syndrome may be masked when treatment is reinstituted, when the dosage is increased or when a switch is made to a different antipsychotic drug. Treatment should be discontinued as soon as possible.

However, since its occurrence may be related to duration of treatment, as well as daily dose, haloperidol should be given in the minimum effective dose for the minimum possible time, unless it is established that long term administration for the treatment of schizophrenia is required.

It has been reported that fine vermicular movements of the tongue may be an early sign of tardive dyskinesia and that the full syndrome may not develop if the medication is stopped at that time.

The following effects have been reported rarely: confusional states or epileptic fits, depression, sedation, agitation, drowsiness, insomnia, headache, vertigo and apparent exacerbation of psychotic symptoms.

In common with other antipsychotic drugs, haloperidol has been associated with rare cases of neuroleptic malignant syndrome (NMS), an idiosyncratic response characterised by hyperthermia, generalised muscle rigidity, autonomic instability, altered consciousness, coma and elevated CPK. Signs of autonomic dysfunction such as tachycardia, labile arterial pressure and sweating may precede the onset of hyperthermia, acting as early warning signs. Antipsychotic treatment should be withdrawn immediately and appropriate supportive therapy and careful monitoring instituted.

Haloperidol, even in low dosage in susceptible (especially non-psychotic) individuals, may cause unpleasant subjective feelings of being mentally dulled or slowed down, dizziness, headache or paradoxical effects of excitement, agitation or insomnia.

*Gastrointestinal system:* Gastrointestinal symptoms, nausea, loss of appetite, constipation and dyspepsia have been reported.

*Endocrinological system:* Hormonal effects of antipsychotic neuroleptic drugs include hyper-prolactinaemia, which may cause galactorrhoea, gynaecomastia and oligo- or amenorrhoea. Hypoglycaemia and the syndrome of inappropriate antidiuretic hormone secretion have been reported rarely. Impairment of sexual function including erection and ejaculation has also been occasionally reported.

*Cardiovascular system:* Tachycardia and dose related hypotension is uncommon, but can occur, particularly in the elderly, who are more susceptible to the sedative and hypotensive effects. Less commonly hypertension has also been reported. Cardiac effects such as QT-interval prolongation, Torsade de Pointes and/or ventricular arrhythmias have been reported rarely. They may occur more frequently with high doses, intravenous administration and in predisposed patients (see Precautions and Warnings).

*Autonomic nervous system:* Dry mouth as well as excessive salivation, blurred vision, urinary retention and hyperhidrosis have been reported.

*Dermatological system:* The following effects have been reported rarely: oedema, various skin rashes and reactions including urticaria, exfoliative dermatitis and erythema multiforme. Photosensitive skin reactions have been reported very rarely.

*Other adverse reactions:* The following effects have been reported rarely: jaundice, cholestatic hepatitis or transient abnormalities of liver function in the absence of jaundice; priapism and weight changes. Temperature disorders may also occur, characterisically hyperthermia associated with NMS, although hypothermia has also been reported.

The following have been reported very rarely: blood dyscrasias, including agranulocytosis, thrombocytopenia and transient leucopenia; hypersensitivity reactions including anaphylaxis.

*Overdose:*
*Symptoms:* In general, the manifestations of haloperidol overdosage are an extension of its pharmacological actions, the most prominent of which would be severe extrapyramidal symptoms, hypotension and psychic indifference with a transition to sleep. The risk of ventricular arrhythmias possibly associated with QT-prolongation should be considered. The patient may appear comatose with respiratory depression and hypotension which could be severe enough to produce a shock-like state. Paradoxically hypertension rather than hypotension may occur. Convulsions may also occur.

*Treatment:* There is no specific antidote to haloperidol. A patent airway should be established and maintained with mechanically assisted ventilation if necessary. In view of isolated reports of arrhythmia ECG monitoring is strongly advised. Hypotension and circulatory collapse should be treated by plasma volume expansion and other appropriate measures. Adrenaline should not be used. The patient should be monitored carefully for 24 hours or longer, body temperature and adequate fluid intake should be maintained.

In cases of severe extrapyramidal symptoms, appropriate antiparkinsonian medication should be administered.

**Pharmacological properties**
*Pharmacodynamic properties:* Haloperidol acts as a central and peripheral dopamine receptor antagonist it also has some anticholinergic activity and binds to opiate receptors.

*Pharmacokinetic properties:* Haloperidol is rapidly absorbed after oral administration with a bioavailability of 44-74% (mean 60%) after tablets. Variable bioavailability is likely due to inter-individual differences in GI absorption and extent of first-pass hepatic metabolism.

Distribution is rapid to extravascular tissue, haloperidol crosses the blood-brain barrier and is excreted in human breast milk.

Metabolism is by oxidative dealkylation. The elimination half-life is approximately 20 hours, with considerable diurnal variation.

*Preclinical safety data:* Not applicable.

**Pharmaceutical particulars**
*List of excipients:* Calcium phosphate dihydrate; corn starch; calcium stearate; quinoline yellow (E104); purified water *

\* not present in final product.

*Incompatibilities:* Not applicable.

*Shelf life:* 60 months.

*Special precautions for storage:* Store in a cool, dry place.

*Nature and contents of container:* Blister packs of aluminium foil and polyvinylchloride genotherm glass clear.

The strips are packed in cardboard cartons containing 100 tablets per pack.

*Instructions for use/handling:* None specific.

**Marketing authorisation number** 0242/0039R

**Date of approval/revision of SPC** May 1997

**Legal category** POM.

## HALDOL\* DECANOATE

**Presentation** Straw coloured, viscous solution presented in 1 ml brown glass ampoules equivalent to 100 mg/ml haloperidol (as decanoate ester) and in 1 ml brown glass ampoules containing haloperidol 50 mg/ml (as decanoate ester). Both solutions also contain benzyl alcohol and sesame oil as inactive ingredients.

**Uses** Haldol Decanoate is an ester of the potent butyrophenone neuroleptic, haloperidol. The active agent is slowly released from an intramuscular depot injection of Haldol Decanoate. Haldol Decanoate is indicated where long term maintenance treatment with a neuroleptic is required; for example in schizophrenia, other psychoses (especially paranoid), and other mental or behavioural problems where maintenance treatment is clearly indicated.

**Dosage and administration** Haldol Decanoate is for use in adults only and has been formulated to provide one month's therapy for most patients following a single deep intramuscular injection in the gluteal region. Haldol Decanoate should not be administered intravenously.

Since individual response to neuroleptic drugs is variable, dosage should be individually determined and is best initiated and titrated under close clinical supervision.

The size of the initial dose will depend on both the severity of the symptomatology and the amount of oral medication required to maintain the patient before starting depot treatment.

An initial dose of 50 mg every four weeks is recommended, increasing if necessary by 50 mg increments to 300 mg every four weeks. If, for clinical reasons, 2-weekly administration is preferred, these doses should be halved.

In patients with severe symptomatology, or in those who required large oral doses as maintenance therapy, higher doses of Haldol Decanoate will be required. However, clinical experience with Haldol Decanoate at doses greater than 300 mg per month is limited.

Routine administration of volumes greater than 3 mls at any one injection site is not recommended as larger volumes of injection are uncomfortable for the patient.

Haldol Decanoate should be administered by deep intramuscular injection using an appropriate needle, preferably 2-2.5 inch long of at least 21 gauge. Local reactions and medication oozing from the injection site may be reduced by the use of a good injection technique, eg the 'z-track' method. As with all oily injections, it is important to ensure, by aspiration before injection, that intravenous entry has not occurred.

For patients previously maintained on oral neuroleptics, an approximate guide to the starting dose of Haldol Decanoate is as follows: 500 mg of chlorpromazine a day is equivalent to 100 mg of Haldol Decanoate monthly.

The approximate equivalence for transferring patients previously maintained on fluphenazine decanoate or flupenthixol decanoate is as follows: 25 mg of fluphenazine decanoate 2-weekly or 40 mg of flupenthixol decanoate 2-weekly is equivalent to 100 mg of Haldol Decanoate monthly. This dose should be adjusted to suit the individual patient's response.

*Use in elderly:* It is recommended to start with low doses, for example 12.5 mg–25 mg every 4 weeks, only increasing the dose according to the individual patient's response.

**Contra-indications, warnings, etc**
*Contra-indications:* Comatose states; CNS depression; Parkinson's disease; known hypersensitivity to haloperidol; lesions of the basal ganglia.

*Use in pregnancy and lactation:* The safety of haloperidol in pregnancy has not been established. There is some evidence of harmful effects in some but not all animal studies. There have been a number of reports of birth defects following foetal exposure to haloperidol for which a causal role for haloperidol cannot be excluded. Haldol Decanoate should be used during pregnancy only if the anticipated benefit outweighs the risk and the administered dose and duration of treatment should be as low and as short as possible.

Haloperidol is excreted in breast milk. There have been isolated cases of extrapyramidal symptoms in breast-fed children. If the use of Haldol Decanoate is essential, the benefits of breast feeding should be balanced against its potential risks.

*Effects on ability to drive and use machines:* Some degree of sedation or impairment of alertness may occur, particularly with higher doses and at the start of treatment, and may be potentiated by alcohol or other CNS depressants. Patients should be advised not to undertake activities requiring alertness such as driving or operating machinery during treatment, until their susceptibility is known.

*Precautions and warnings:* Please also refer to *Drug interactions* section.

Caution is advised in patients with liver disease, renal failure, phaeochromocytoma, epilepsy, and conditions predisposing to epilepsy (eg alcohol withdrawal and brain damage) or convulsions. Haloperidol should only be used with great caution in patients with disturbed thyroid function. Antipsychotic therapy in those patients must always be accompanied by adequate management of the underlying thyroid dysfunction.

Cases of sudden death have been reported in psychiatric patients receiving antipsychotic drugs, including haloperidol. The risk-benefit of Haldol Decanoate treatment should be fully assessed before treatment is commenced and patients with risk factors for ventricular arrhythmias such as cardiac disease, subarachnoid haemorrhage, metabolic abnormalities such as hypokalaemia, hypocalcaemia or hypomagnesemia, starvation, alcohol abuse or those receiving concomitant therapy with other drugs known to prolong the QT interval, should be monitored carefully (ECGs and potassium levels), particularly during the initial phase of treatment, to obtain steady plasma levels.

In schizophrenia, the response to antipsychotic drug treatment may be delayed. If drugs are withdrawn, recurrence of symptoms may not become apparent for several weeks or months.

As with all antipsychotic agents, haloperidol should not be used alone where depression is predominant. It may be combined with antidepressants to treat those conditions in which depression and psychosis coexist. Haloperidol may impair the metabolism of tricyclic antidepressants (clinical significance unknown).

If concomitant antiparkinson medication is required, it may have to be continued after haloperidol is discontinued to take account of any differences in excretion rates. The physician should keep in mind the possible anticholinergic effects associated with antiparkinson agents.

*Drug interactions:* In common with all neuroleptics, haloperidol can increase the central nervous system depression produced by other CNS-depressant drugs, including alcohol, hypnotics, sedatives or strong analgesics. An enhanced CNS effect, when combined with methyldopa, has been reported.

Haloperidol may antagonise the action of adrenaline and other sympathomimetic agents and reverses the blood pressure lowering effects of adrenergic-blocking agents such as guanethidine.

The dosage of anticonvulsants may need to be increased to take account of the lowered seizure threshold. Coadministration of enzyme-inducing drugs such as carbamazepine, phenobarbitone and rifampicin with haloperidol may result in a significant reduction of haloperidol plasma levels. The haloperidol dose may therefore need to be increased or the dosage interval reduced, according to the patient's response. After stopping such drugs, it may be necessary to readjust the dosage of haloperidol decanoate.

Haloperidol may impair the metabolism of tricyclic antidepressants (clinical significance unknown) and the antiparkinson effects of levodopa.

In pharmacokinetic studies, increased haloperidol levels have been reported when Haldol Decanoate was given concomitantly with the following drugs: quinidine, buspirone and fluoxetine. Haloperidol plasma levels should therefore be monitored and reduced if necessary.

Antagonism of the effect of phenindione has been reported.

In rare cases, an encephalopathy-like syndrome has been reported in combination with lithium and Haldol Decanoate. It remains controversial whether these cases represent a distinct clinical entity or whether they are in fact cases of NMS and/or lithium toxicity. Signs of encephalopathy-like syndrome include confusion, disorientation, headache, disturbances of balance and drowsiness. One report showing symptomless EEG abnormalities on the combination has suggested that EEG monitoring might be advisable. When lithium and haloperidol therapy are used

concomitantly, haloperidol should be given in the lowest effective dosage and lithium levels should be monitored and kept below 1 mmol/l. If symptoms of encephalopathy-like syndrome occur, therapy should be stopped immediately.

*Adverse effects: Central nervous system:* In common with all neuroleptics, extrapyramidal symptoms may occur eg tremor, rigidity, hypersalivation, bradykinesia, akathisia, acute dystonia, oculogyric crisis and laryngeal dystonia. Anti-Parkinson agents should not be prescribed routinely. Preliminary results suggest that withdrawal of anti-Parkinson medication may be attempted following transfer from oral medication to monthly depot injections of Haldol Decanoate.

As with all antipsychotic agents, tardive dyskinesia may appear in some patients on long-term therapy or after drug discontinuation.

The syndrome is mainly characterised by rhythmical involuntary movements of the tongue, face, mouth or jaw. The manifestations may be permanent in some patients. The syndrome may be masked when treatment is reinstituted, when the dosage is increased or when a switch is made to a different antipsychotic drug. Treatment should be discontinued as soon as possible.

However since its occurrence may be related to duration of treatment, as well as dose, haloperidol should be given in the minimum effective dose for the minimum possible time, unless it is established that long term administration for the treatment of schizophrenia is required.

It has been reported that fine vermicular movements of the tongue may be an early sign of tardive dyskinesia and that the full syndrome may not develop if the medication is stopped at that time.

The following effects have been reported rarely with haloperidol: confusional states or epileptic fits, depression, sedation, agitation, drowsiness, insomnia, headache, vertigo and apparent exacerbation of psychotic symptoms.

In common with other antipsychotic drugs, haloperidol has been associated with rare cases of neuroleptic malignant syndrome (NMS), an idiosyncratic response characterised by hyperthermia, generalised muscle rigidity, autonomic instability, altered consciousness, coma and elevated CPK. Signs of autonomic dysfunction such as tachycardia, labile arterial pressure and sweating may precede the onset of hyperthermia, acting as early warning signs. Antipsychotic treatment should be withdrawn immediately and appropriate supportive therapy and careful monitoring instituted.

Haloperidol, even in low dosage in susceptible (especially non-psychotic) individuals, may cause unpleasant subjective feelings of being mentally dulled or slowed down, dizziness, headache or paradoxical effects of excitement, agitation or insomnia.

*Gastrointestinal system:* Gastrointestinal symptoms, nausea, loss of appetite, constipation and dyspepsia have been reported with haloperidol.

*Endocrinological system:* Hormonal effects of antipsychotic neuroleptic drugs include hyperprolactinaemia, which may cause galactorrhoea, gynaecomastia and oligo- or amenorrhoea. Hypoglycaemia and the syndrome of inappropriate antidiuretic hormone secretion have been reported rarely. Impairment of sexual function including erection and ejaculation has also been occasionally reported.

*Cardiovascular system:* Tachycardia and dose related hypotension are uncommon, but can occur with haloperidol, particularly in the elderly, who are more susceptible to the sedative and hypotensive effects. Less commonly hypertension has also been reported. Cardiac effects such as QT-interval prolongation, Torsade de Pointes and/or ventricular arrhythmias have been reported rarely. They may occur more frequently with high doses, intravenous administration and in predisposed patients(see Precautions and Warnings).

*Autonomic nervous system:* Dry mouth as well as excessive salivation, blurred vision, urinary retention and hyperhidrosis have been reported with haloperidol.

*Dermatological system:* The following effects have been reported rarely with haloperidol: oedema, various skin rashes and reactions including urticaria, exfoliative dermatitis and erythema multiforme. Photosensitive skin reactions have been reported very rarely.

*Other adverse reactions:* The following effects have been reported rarely with haloperidol: jaundice, cholestatic hepatitis or transient abnormalities of liver function in the absence of jaundice; priapism and weight changes may occur. Temperature disorders may also occur, characteristically hyperthermia associated with NMS, although hypothermia has also been reported.

The following have been reported very rarely with haloperidol: blood dyscrasias, including agranulocytosis, thrombocytopenia and transient leucopenia; hypersensitivity reactions including anaphylaxis. Oc-

casional local reactions such as erythema, swelling or tender lumps have been reported.

*Overdose:*
*Symptoms:* In general, the manifestations of haloperidol overdosage are an extension of its pharmacological actions, the most prominent of which would be severe extrapyramidal symptoms, hypotension and psychic indifference with a transition to sleep. The risk of ventricular arrhythmias possibly associated with QT-prolongation should be considered. The patient may appear comatose with respiratory depression and hypotension which could be severe enough to produce a shock-like state. Paradoxically hypertension rather than hypotension may occur. Convulsions may also occur.

*Treatment:* There is no specific antidote to haloperidol. A patent airway should be established and maintained with mechanically assisted ventilation if necessary. In view of isolated reports of arrhythmia ECG monitoring is strongly advised. Hypotension and circulatory collapse should be treated by plasma volume expansion and other appropriate measures. Adrenaline should not be used. The patient should be monitored, body temperature and adequate fluid intake should be maintained.

In cases of severe extrapyramidal symptoms, appropriate antiparkinson medication should be administered.

**Pharmaceutical precautions** Haldol Decanoate should be protected from light and stored at room temperature. In common with other depot neuroleptics, if stored for long periods in the cold, precipitation may occur which may clear on storage at room temperature. If precipitate does not clear, the contents of the ampoule should be discarded. Do not store below room temperature.

**Legal category**　POM.

**Package quantities**　100 mg/ml ampoules: 1 ml ampoules in packs of 5. 50 mg/ml ampoules: 1 ml ampoules in packs of 5.

**Further information**　Haloperidol decanoate in solution is slowly released from the injection site and enters the systemic circulation, where it is hydrolysed by esterases to haloperidol. After an initial dose of 30–300 mg of haloperidol decanoate plasma concentrations ranged from 0.8–3.2 ng/ml. After the second dose they were raised to 2.8 ng/ml which was steady state. A monthly dose of approximately 20 times the previous oral maintenance dose has been shown to be approximately clinically equivalent. Blood levels will vary considerably between patients.

**Product licence numbers**
50 mg/ml　　0242/0094
100 mg/ml　　0242/0095

## HISMANAL*

**Presentation**　White, biconvex, half-scored, uncoated tablets. Each tablet is marked 'Janssen' on one side and 'Ast/10' on the reverse, and contains astemizole 10 mg. Hismanal tablets also contain lactose.

White suspension with a fruity flavour containing astemizole 1 mg/ml in 200 ml amber glass bottles. Hismanal suspension also contains sorbitol and alcohol.

**Uses**　Hismanal is a long acting antihistamine ($H_1$-antagonist) characterised by a lack of sedative potential.

Hismanal is indicated for allergic rhinitis and conjunctivitis and other conditions normally responsive to antihistamines, including allergic skin reactions (urticaria).

**Dosage and administration**

*Adults and children over 12 years:* The daily dose is 10 mg (one tablet or 10 ml) as a single intake, which should not be exceeded.

*Children 6–12 years:* The daily dose is 5 mg ($\frac{1}{2}$ a tablet or 5 ml), which should not be exceeded.

*Children under 6 years:* There have been no specific studies in children under 6 years, therefore the drug is not indicated in this age group.

*Use in elderly:* There have been no specific studies in the elderly.

**Contra-indications, warnings, etc**

*Contra-indications:* Pregnancy; known hypersensitivity to astemizole or any of the inactive ingredients; concomitant administration of erythromycin or oral forms of ketoconazole, itraconazole or miconazole, or therapeutic doses of quinine; significant liver dysfunction; pre-existing prolongation of the QT interval; hypokalaemia; concurrent use of other medications which may predispose to arrhythmias (such as anti-arrhythmic agents, neuroleptics, tricyclic antidepressants, terfenadine).

*Precautions:* Because of the risk of developing serious

ventricular arrhythmias at high doses, the recommended dose of Hismanal should not be exceeded.

Because of the potential of some diuretics to produce hypokalaemia, care should be taken if it is proposed to administer diuretics concurrently with Hismanal.

Adequate contraceptive precautions should be taken by women of childbearing potential during therapy, and, in view of the prolonged half-life, for several weeks after stopping treatment.

*Interactions:* Concomitant administration of oral forms of ketoconazole, itraconazole or miconazole and of therapeutic doses of quinine may decrease the metabolism of astemizole and result in elevated plasma levels. The concomitant use of these substances orally with astemizole is therefore contra-indicated.

Astemizole may also interact with other drugs with arrhythmogenic potential (see contra-indications).

Arrhythmias have been reported rarely in association with the combination of erythromycin and astemizole. The mechanism of interaction is unclear but this combination of drugs should be avoided (see contra-indications). Limited information is available on the possible interaction between astemizole and other macrolide antibiotics, however, *in vitro* studies suggest that an interaction between astemizole and clarithromycin or azithromycin is less likely.

*Use in pregnancy:* Like many other antihistamines, Hismanal has been associated with adverse effects on the maintenance of pregnancy in rats. No teratogenic effects were observed in animal studies with Hismanal.

The safety of Hismanal in human pregnancy has not been established. Therefore it is contra-indicated during pregnancy.

Since astemizole is excreted in breast milk, it should not be used by nursing mothers.

*Adverse reactions:* Ventricular arrhythmias have occurred at high doses including QT-prolongation and Torsades de Pointes. In some cases, severe arrhythmias have been preceded by or associated with one or more episodes of syncope. Therefore, syncope in patients receiving astemizole should lead to immediate discontinuation of treatment and appropriate clinical evaluation, including electrocardiography.

As might be expected with Hismanal's lack of sedative potential, sedation has been reported extremely rarely. It should be recognised that, in controlled clinical trials, the incidence of sedation with Hismanal has been no greater than that with placebo. Weight gain has occasionally been reported.

Rare cases, spontaneously reported from post-marketing experience with Hismanal include hypersensitivity reactions such as angio-oedema, bronchospasm, photosensitivity, pruritus, rash and anaphylactoid reactions. There have also been isolated cases of convulsions, benign paraesthesias, myalgia/arthralgia, oedema, mood disturbances, insomnia, nightmares, transaminase elevation and hepatitis. In most cases, a causal relationship with Hismanal is unclear.

*Overdosage: Symptoms:* In patients exceeding the recommended dose, cases of serious, life-threatening cardiovascular adverse events including QT-prolongation, Torsades de Pointes, and other ventricular arrhythmias have been observed. While the majority of such events have occurred following substantial overdoses of astemizole, arrhythmias, including Torsades de Pointes, have very rarely occurred at reported doses as low as 20-30 mg daily (2-3 times the recommended daily dose).
*Treatment:* Supportive measures including gastric lavage and emesis should be employed, followed by the administration of activated charcoal. In these patients the ECG should be carefully monitored. If the QT-interval is prolonged the monitoring should continue as long as it remains prolonged. The terminal half-life is 1-2 days for astemizole and 9-13 days for desmethylastemizole (the active metabolite). Studies in patients with renal insufficiency suggest that haemodialysis does not increase the clearance of the drug.

**Pharmaceutical precautions** Nil.

**Legal category** POM.

**Package quantities** Supplied in packs of 30 tablets. Amber glass bottles containing 200 ml suspension (1 mg/ml).

**Further information** Although clinical trials have shown no interaction between Hismanal and diazepam or alcohol, care should be taken to caution the patient against excessive alcohol intake while on medication. Controlled clinical trials with placebo and reference antihistamines have demonstrated that Hismanal is non-sedative, and should not therefore interfere with activities requiring mental alertness, for example, driving or operating machinery. Nevertheless as with other medications, patients should exert

caution when undertaking such activities following the first dose of Hismanal.

Pharmacokinetic studies in man demonstrate that astemizole is rapidly absorbed, peak plasma concentrations are attained within 1-2 hours. There is extensive first-pass metabolism and significant tissue distribution. At steady state, the average peak plasma concentration of astemizole plus its metabolite desmethylastemizole (considered together to represent the pharmacologically active fraction in plasma) is 3-5 ng/ml. The terminal half-life is 1-2 days for astemizole and 9-13 days for desmethylastemizole.

Astemizole is excreted as metabolites mainly within the bile.

Receptor binding studies have shown that astemizole, at pharmacological doses, provides complete occupancy of peripheral, $H_1$-receptors and does not reach the $H_1$-receptors in the brain, because the drug does not readily cross the blood-brain barrier.

In spite of the long half-life of astemizole and its metabolites, the pharmacokinetics are linear after single and chronic dosing.

Astemizole does not induce human liver enzymes.

**Product licence numbers**
Hismanal tablets          0242/0086
Hismanal suspension       0242/0111

## HYPNOMIDATE*

**Presentation** Clear colourless solution containing 2 mg/ml etomidate. The aqueous vehicle contains 35% propylene glycol and water for injection.

**Uses**
*Indications:* Intravenous induction of anaesthesia.

*Properties:* Hypnomidate is a short-acting hypnotic agent. It is an imidazole-derivative, chemically unrelated to other intravenous hypnotics.

**Dosage and administration** Adults: A dose of 0.3 mg/kg given intravenously at induction of anaesthesia gives sleep lasting from 6 to 10 minutes.

*Elderly:* A dose of 0.15-0.2 mg/kg bodyweight should be given and the dose should be further adjusted according to effects.

*Children up to 15 years old:* The dosage may be increased by up to 30% of the adult dose because it is sometimes necessary in order to obtain the same depth and duration of sleep.

Since Hypnomidate has no analgesic action, appropriate analgesics should be used in procedures involving painful stimuli.

Do not exceed a total dose of 30 ml (3 ampoules).

Hypnomidate should only be given by slow intravenous injection.

Hypnomidate may be diluted with sodium chloride infusion BP or dextrose infusion BP but it is not compatible with compound sodium lactate infusion BP (Hartmann's solution). Combinations with pancuronium bromide may show a very slight opalescence; for this reason the two should not be mixed together.

**Contra-indications, warnings, etc**
*Contra-indications:* Hypnomidate is contra-indicated in patients with known hypersensitivity to etomidate.

*Warnings:* Hypnomidate should not be administered to patients with evidence, or suggestion of, reduced adrenal cortical function.

Reduced serum cortisol levels, unresponsive to ACTH injections, have been reported in some patients during induction of anaesthesia but particularly during maintenance of anaesthesia with etomidate; for this reason etomidate should not be used for maintenance. However when etomidate is used for induction, the post-operative rise in serum cortisol which has been observed after thiopentone induction is delayed for approximately 3-6 hours.

In cases of adrenocortical gland dysfunction and during very long surgical procedures, a prophylactic cortisol supplement may be required (for example 50 to 100 mg hydrocortisone).

Convulsions may occur in unpremedicated patients.

In patients with liver cirrhosis, or in those who have already received neuroleptic, opiate or sedative agents, the dose of etomidate should be reduced.

When Hypnomidate is used, resuscitation equipment should be readily available to manage apnoea.

*Precautions:* Hypnomidate should only be given by slow intravenous injection.

*Side effects:* The use of narcotic analgesics or diazepam as premedication and during surgery will reduce the uncontrolled spontaneous muscle movements shown by some patients after Hypnomidate administration.

Pain can occur after injection into the small veins of the dorsum of the hand. Use of larger veins or an intravenous application of a small dose of fentanyl 1 to 2 minutes before induction reduces pain on injection.

Nausea and/or vomiting may occur although these

are mainly as a result of concurrent use of opiates. Coughing, hiccough and/or shivering may also be experienced. Allergic reactions, including rare cases of bronchospasm and anaphylactoid reactions, have been reported. Rare cases of laryngospasm, cardiac arrhythmias and convulsions have also been reported.

A slight and transient drop in blood pressure may occur due to a reduction of the peripheral vascular resistance. In vulnerable patients, special care should be exercised to minimise this effect.

Respiratory depression and apnoea may occur.

*Interactions:* Sedative drugs potentiate the hypnotic effect of Hypnomidate.

Hypnomidate is pharmacologically compatible with the muscle relaxants, premedicant drugs and inhalation anaesthetics in current clinical use.

*Use in pregnancy:* Hypnomidate has no primary effect on fertility, nor primary embryotoxic or teratogenic effects. At maternally toxic doses in rats, decreased survival was noted. Safety in human pregnancy has not been established. As with other drugs, the possible risks should be weighed against the potential benefits before the drug is administered during pregnancy. Hypnomidate may cross the placental barrier during obstetric anaesthesia.

*Lactation:* It is not known whether hypnomidate is excreted in human milk. However, caution should be exercised when Hypnomidate is administered to a nursing mother.

*Effects on ability to drive and use machinery:* Not applicable but no effects likely. After very short surgical procedures (up to 15 minutes) the patient regains normal alertness 30 to 60 minutes after waking. After long operations, normal alertness is regained after 4 to 24 hours, depending on the duration of the operation.

*Overdosage:* Overdosing is likely to result in prolonged anaesthesia with the possibility of respiratory depression and even arrest. Hypotension has also been observed. General supportive measures and close observation are recommended. In addition, administration of 50-100 mg hydrocortisone (not ACTH) may be required for depression of cortisol secretion.

**Pharmaceutical precautions** Store at room temperature.

**Legal category** POM.

**Package quantities** Hypnomidate is supplied as 10 ml ampoules in packs of 10.

**Further information** Hypnomidate is rapidly metabolised and eliminated and recovery of consciousness from a single dose is rapid and complete.

**Product licence number** 0242/0019.

## IMODIUM* CAPSULES AND SYRUP

**Qualitative and quantitative composition** *Capsules:* Loperamide hydrochloride 2 mg.
*Syrup:* Loperamide hydrochloride 0.2 mg/ml.

**Pharmaceutical form** Capsules and syrup for oral administration.

**Clinical particulars**
*Therapeutic indications:*
*Capsules and syrup: P Classification:* For the symptomatic treatment of acute diarrhoea in adults and children aged 12 years and over.
*Capsules: POM Classification:* For the symptomatic treatment of acute diarrhoea of any aetiology including acute exacerbations of chronic diarrhoea for periods of up to 5 days in adults and children over 8 years. For the symptomatic treatment of chronic diarrhoea in adults.
*Syrup: POM Classification:* For the symptomatic treatment of acute diarrhoea of any aetiology including acute exacerbations of chronic diarrhoea for periods of up to 5 days in adults and children over 4 years. For the symptomatic treatment of chronic diarrhoea in adults.

*Posology and method of administration:*
*Acute diarrhoea*
*Adults:* Two capsules or four 5 ml spoonfuls initially, followed by one capsule or two 5 ml spoonfuls after each loose stool. The usual dose is 3-4 capsules a day. The total daily dose should not exceed eight capsules or sixteen spoonfuls.
*Children:* The following doses should not be exceeded.
*Children over 8 years:* One capsule or two 5 ml spoonfuls four times daily until diarrhoea is controlled (up to 5 days).
*Children 4-8 years:* Use syrup: One 5 ml spoonful three or four times daily with the duration limited to 3 days.
Not recommended for children under 4 years of age.

Further investigation into the cause of the diarrhoea should be considered if there is no improvement within two days of starting treatment with Imodium.

*Chronic diarrhoea*
*Adults:* Patients may need widely differing amounts of Imodium. The starting dose should be between two and four capsules, or four and eight 5 ml spoonfuls per day in divided doses, depending on severity. If required this dose can be adjusted up to a maximum of eight capsules or sixteen 5 ml spoonfuls daily.

Having established the patient's daily maintenance dose, Imodium may be administered on a twice daily regimen. Tolerance has not been observed and therefore subsequent dosage adjustment should be unnecessary.

*Use in elderly:* As for adults.

*Method of administration:* Oral use.

*Contra-indications:* Imodium should not be used in children less than 4 years of age. Imodium must not be used when inhibition of peristalsis is to be avoided, in particular when ileus or constipation are present or when abdominal distension develops particularly in severely dehydrated children or in patients with acute ulcerative colitis or pseudomembranous colitis associated with broad spectrum antibiotics. Imodium should not be used **alone** in acute dysentery, which is characterised by blood in stools and elevated body temperatures.

*Special warnings and special precautions for use:* In patients with diarrhoea, especially young children, fluid and electrolyte depletion may occur. Use of Imodium does not preclude the administration of appropriate fluid and electrolyte replacement therapy.

Since persistent diarrhoea can be an indicator of potentially more serious conditions, Imodium should not be used for prolonged periods until the underlying cause of the diarrhoea has been investigated.

Imodium must be used with caution when the hepatic function necessary for the drug's metabolism is defective (eg in cases of severe hepatic disturbance), as this might result in a relative overdose.

*Also for P use only:* If symptoms persist for more than 24 hours, consult your doctor.

*Interactions with other medicaments and other forms of interaction:* None stated.

*Pregnancy and lactation:* Safety in human pregnancy has not been established although studies in animals have not demonstrated any teratogenic effects. As with other drugs, it is not advisable to administer Imodium in pregnancy. Although the fraction of Imodium secreted in human breast milk is extremely low, caution is advised if Imodium is to be administered to a nursing mother.

*Effects on ability to drive and use machines:* None stated.

*Undesirable effects:* Abdominal cramps, nausea, vomiting, tiredness, drowsiness, dizziness, dry mouth and skin reactions, including urticaria have been reported. *Also for POM use only:* On occasions paralytic ileus, bloating and constipation have been reported.

*Overdose:* In case of overdosage the following effects may be observed: constipation, ileus and neurological symptoms (myosis, muscular hypertonia, somnolence and bradypnoea). If intoxication is suspected, naloxone may be given as an antidote. Since the duration of action of Imodium is longer than that of naloxone, the patient should be kept under constant observation for at least 48 hours in order to detect any possible depression of the central nervous system. Children, and patients with hepatic dysfunction, may be more sensitive to CNS effects. Gastric lavage, or induced emesis and /or enema or laxatives may be recommended.

**Pharmacological properties**
*Pharmacodynamic properties:* Loperamide binds to the opiate receptor in the gut wall, reducing propulsive peristalsis and increasing intestinal transit time. Loperamide increases the tone of the anal sphincter.

*Pharmacokinetic properties:* The half-life of loperamide in man is 10.8 hours with a range of 9–14 hours. Studies on distribution in rats show high affinity for the gut wall with preference for binding to the receptors in the longitudinal muscle layer. Loperamide is well absorbed from the gut, but is almost completely extracted and metabolised by the liver where it is conjugated and excreted via the bile. Due to its high affinity for the gut wall and its high first pass metabolism, very little loperamide reaches the systemic circulation.

*Preclinical safety data:* Not applicable.

**Pharmaceutical particulars**
*List of excipients:*
    Capsules: Lactose; maize starch; talc; magnesium stearate
    Capsule cap: Titanium dioxide; yellow ferric oxide; indigotindisulphonate sodium; gelatin

Capsule body: Titanium dioxide; black ferrous oxide; indigotindisulphonate sodium; erythrosin; gelatin

Syrup: Glycerol; sodium saccharin; methyl parahydroxybenzoate; propyl parahydroxybenzoate; cochineal red A ; raspberry flavour; red currant flavour; alcohol; citric acid monohydrate; purified water.

*Incompatibilities:* Not applicable.

*Shelf life:* 60 months.

*Special precautions for storage:* None.

*Nature and contents of container: Capsules:* Blister packs consisting of aluminium foil, hermetalu and polyvinyl chloride genotherm glass clear.
The blister strips are packed in cardboard cartons to contain 30 capsules.
OR
Tubs of capsules containing 250 capsules.
*Syrup:* Amber glass bottle with either a pilfer-proof aluminium screw cap coated on the inside with PVC or a child resistant polypropylene screw cap lined inside with an LDPE insert and a 5 ml or 10 ml polypropylene measuring cup. Imodium Syrup is supplied in bottles of 100 ml.

*Instructions for use/handling:* Not applicable.

**Marketing authorisation numbers**
Imodium Capsules        0242/0028
Imodium Syrup           0242/0040

**Date of approval/revision of SPC** *Capsules:* July 1995. *Syrup:* December 1995.

**Legal category** POM/P.

# LEUSTAT* INJECTION

**Qualitative and quantitative composition** Leustat (cladribine) Injection is a synthetic antineoplastic agent for continuous intravenous infusion. It is a clear, colourless, sterile, preservative-free, isotonic solution. Leustat Injection is available in single-use vials containing 10 mg (1 mg/ml) of 2-chloro-2'-deoxy-β-D-adenosine, or cladribine, a chlorinated purine nucleoside analogue. Each millilitre of Leustat Injection contains 1 mg of the active ingredient, cladribine, and 9 mg (0.15 mEq) of sodium chloride as an inactive ingredient. The solution has pH range of 5.5 to 8.0. Phosphoric acid and/or dibasic sodium phosphate may have been added to adjust the pH.
The chemical name of cladribine is 2-chloro-6-amino-9 (2-deoxy-β-D-erythropento-furanosyl) purine.

**Pharmaceutical form** A sterile, buffered solution in vials containing 10 mg (1 mg/ml) of 2-chloro-2'-deoxy-β-D-adenosine (cladribine) for dilution and subsequent continuous intravenous infusion.

**Clinical particulars**

*Therapeutic indications:* Leustat Injection is indicated for the primary or secondary treatment of patients with Hairy Cell Leukaemia (HCL).

*Posology and method of administration:*
*Usual dose*
*Adults and elderly:* The recommended treatment for Hairy Cell Leukaemia is a single course of Leustat given by continuous intravenous infusion for 7 consecutive days at a dose of 0.09 mg/kg/day (3.6 mg/m²/ day). Deviations from this dosage regimen are not advised. Physicians should consider delaying or discontinuing the drug if neurotoxicity or renal toxicity occurs.
*Children:* Safety and efficacy in children have not been established.
Specific risk factors predisposing to increased toxicity from Leustat have not been defined. In view of the known toxicities of agents of this class, it would be prudent to proceed carefully in patients with known or suspected renal insufficiency or severe bone marrow impairment of any aetiology. Patients should be monitored closely for haematological and renal and hepatic toxicity.
*Preparation and administration of intravenous solutions:* Leustat Injection must be diluted with the designated diluent prior to administration. Since the drug product does not contain any anti-microbial preservative or bacteriostatic agent, aseptic technique and proper environmental precautions must be observed in preparation of a solution of Leustat. For full details concerning preparation of an infusion solution, see Instructions for Use/Handling.

*Contra-indications:* Leustat Injection is contra-indicated in those patients who are hypersensitive to this drug or any of its components. Leustat is contra-indicated in pregnant women and nursing mothers.

*Special warnings and special precautions for use:* Leustat Injection is a potent antineoplastic agent with potentially significant toxic side effects. It should be administered under the supervision of a qualified

physician experienced in the use of antineoplastic therapy.
*Bone marrow suppression:* Suppression of bone marrow function should be anticipated. This is usually reversible and appears to be dose dependent. Severe bone marrow suppression, including neutropenia, anaemia and thrombocytopenia, has been commonly observed in patients treated with Leustat, especially at high doses. At initiation of treatment, most patients in the clinical studies had haematological impairment as a manifestation of active Hairy Cell Leukaemia. Following treatment with Leustat, further haematological impairment occurred before recovery of peripheral blood counts began. During the first two weeks after treatment initiation, mean platelet count, absolute neutrophil count (ANC), and haemoglobin concentration declined and then subsequently increased with normalisation of mean counts by day 15, week 5 and week 8, respectively. The myelosuppressive effects of Leustat were most notable during the first month following treatment. Forty three percent (43%) of patients received transfusions with RBCs and 13% received transfusions with platelets during month 1. Careful haematological monitoring, especially during the first 4 to 8 weeks after treatment with Leustat is recommended (see *Undesirable effects*).
*Neurotoxicity:* Serious neurological toxicity (including irreversible paraparesis and quadraparesis) has been reported in patients who received Leustat Injection by continuous infusion at high doses (4 to 9 times the recommended dose for hairy cell leukaemia). Neurological toxicity appears to demonstrate a dose relationship; however, neurological toxicities have been reported with the recommended dose. Physicians should consider delaying or discontinuing therapy if neurotoxicity occurs.
*Fever/infection:* Fever (temperature greater than or equal to 37.8°C) was associated with the use of Leustat in approximately 72% (89/124) of patients. Most febrile episodes occurred during the first month. Although seventy percent (70%) of patients were treated empirically with parenteral antibiotics, less than a third of febrile events were associated with documented infection. Since the majority of fevers occurred in neutropenic patients, patients should be closely monitored during the first month of treatment and empirical antibiotics should be initiated as clinically indicated. Given the known myelosuppressive effects of Leustat, practitioners should carefully evaluate the risks and benefits of administering this drug to patients with active infections. Since fever may be accompanied by increased fluid loss, patients should be kept well hydrated (see *Undesirable effects*).
Rare cases of tumour lysis syndrome have been reported in patients with haematological malignancies having a high tumour burden.
*Effect on renal and hepatic function:* Acute renal insufficiency has developed in some patients receiving high doses of Leustat. In addition, there are inadequate data on dosing of patients with renal or hepatic insufficiency. Until more information is available, caution is advised when administering the drug to patients with known or suspected renal or hepatic insufficiency. All patients should have their renal and hepatic function monitored regularly (see *Effects of high doses*).
Leustat Injection must be diluted in a designated intravenous solution prior to administration (See Instructions for use/handling for full details concerning preparation of an infusion solution).
*Laboratory tests:* During and following treatment, the patient's haematological profile should be monitored regularly to determine the degree of haematopoietic suppression. After peripheral counts have normalised, bone marrow aspiration and biopsy should be performed to confirm response to treatment with Leustat. Febrile events should be investigated with appropriate laboratory and radiological studies. As with other potent chemotherapeutic agents, monitoring of renal and hepatic function should be performed as clinically indicated, especially in patients with underlying kidney or liver dysfunction.
*Carcinogenesis/mutagenesis:* No animal carcinogenicity studies have been conducted with Leustat. Cladribine is mutagenic in mammalian cells in culture. Cladribine was not mutagenic to bacteria and did not induce unscheduled DNA synthesis in primary rat hepatocyte cultures.
*Impairment of fertility:* When administered intravenously to Cynomolgus monkeys, Leustat (cladribine) has been shown to cause suppression of rapidly generating cells, including testicular cells. The effect on human fertility is unknown.
*Extravasation:* Should the drug accidentally be given extravenously, local tissue damage is unlikely. If extravasation occurs, the administration should be stopped immediately and restarted in another vein. Other recommended local measures include elevating the arm and applying an ice pack to reduce swelling.

*Interactions with other medicaments and other forms of interaction:* Caution should be exercised if Leustat

Injection is administered following or in conjunction with other drugs known to cause myelosuppression. Following administration of Leustat Injection, caution should be exercised before administering other immunosuppressive or myelosuppresive therapy. (See Bone marrow suppression)

*Pregnancy and lactation:* Leustat Injection is teratogenic in mice and rabbits and consequently has the potential to cause foetal harm when administered to a pregnant woman. There are no human data, but Leustat Injection is contra-indicated in pregnancy.

A significant increase in foetal variations was observed in mice receiving 1.5 mg/kg/day (4.5 mg/m²) and increased resorptions, reduced litter size and increased foetal malformations were observed when mice received 3.0 mg/kg/day (9 mg/m²). Foetal death and malformations were observed in rabbits that received 3.0 mg/kg/day (33.0 mg/m²). No foetal effects were seen in mice at 0.5 mg/kg/day (1.5 mg/m²) or in rabbits at 1.0 mg/kg/day (11.0 mg/m²).

Although there is no evidence of teratogenicity in humans due to Leustat, other drugs which inhibit DNA synthesis (eg methotrexate and aminopterin) have been reported to be teratogenic in humans. Leustat has been shown to be embryotoxic in mice when given at doses equivalent to the recommended dose.

It is not known whether this drug is excreted in human milk. Because it may be excreted in human milk and because there is potential for serious adverse reactions in nursing infants, Leustat should not be given to a nursing mother.

*Effects on ability to drive and use machines:* Given the patients underlying medical condition and the safety profile of Leustat Injection, caution should be exercised when a patient is performing activities requiring substantial physical well-being (See Undesirable effects).

*Undesirable effects:*

*Overview:* The following safety data are based on 124 patients with HCL enrolled in the pivotal studies. Severe neutropenia was noted in 70% of patients in month 1; fever in 72% at anytime; and infection was documented in 31% of patients in month 1. Other adverse experiences reported frequently during the first 14 days after initiating treatment included: fatigue (49%), nausea (29%), rash (31%), headache (23%) and decreased appetite (23%). Most non-haematological adverse experiences were mild to moderate in severity.

During the first 14 days, events reported by greater than 5% but less than 20% of patients included:

Body as a whole: Chills (13%), asthenia (11%), diaphoresis (11%), malaise (8%), trunk pain (7%).

Gastro-intestinal: Vomiting (14%), constipation (14%), diarrhoea (12%), abdominal pain (8%), flatulence (7%).

Haemic/lymphatic: Purpura (12%), petechia (9%).

Nervous system: Dizziness (13%), insomnia (8%), anxiety (7%).

Cardiovascular system: Oedema (8%), tachycardia (8%), heart murmur (7%).

Respiratory system: Abnormal breath sounds (14%), cough (12%), abnormal chest sounds (12%), shortness of breath (7%).

Skin/subcutaneous tissue: Injection site reaction (15%), pruritus (9%), pain (9%), erythema (8%).

Musculoskeletal system: Myalgia (8%).

Injection site reactions (ie redness, swelling, pain), thrombosis and phlebitis appear usually to be related to the infusion procedure and/or indwelling catheter, rather than to the medication or the vehicle.

From day 15 to the last day of follow-up, the following effects were reported in greater than 5% of patients: fatigue (14%), rash (10%), headache (7%), oedema (7%), arthralgia (7%), malaise (6%), diaphoresis (6%).

*Bone marrow suppression:* Myelosuppression was frequently observed during the first month after starting treatment with Leustat Injection. Neutropenia (ANC less than 500 x 10⁶/L) was noted in 69% of patients, compared with 25% in whom it was present initially. Severe anaemia (haemoglobin less than 8.5 g/dL) occurred in 41.1% of patients, compared with 12% initially and thrombocytopenia (platelets less than 20x10⁹/L) occurred in 15% of patients, compared to 5% in whom it was noted initially.

Analysis of lymphocyte subsets indicates that treatment with cladribine is associated with prolonged depression of the CD4 counts. Prior to treatment, the mean CD4 count was 766/µl. The mean CD4 count nadir, which occurred 4 to 6 months following treatment, was 272/µl. Fifteen (15) months after treatment, mean CD4 counts remained below 500/µl. CD8 counts behaved similarly, though increasing counts were observed after 9 months. There were no serious opportunistic infections reported during this time. The clinical significance of the prolonged CD4 lymphopenia is unclear.

Prolonged bone marrow hypocellularity (< 35%) was observed. It is not known whether the hypocellularity is the result of disease related marrow fibrosis or Leustat Injection toxicity.

*Fever/infection:* As with other agents having known immunosuppressive effects, opportunistic infections have occurred in the acute phase of treatment due to the immunosuppression mediated by cladribine. Fever was a frequently observed side effect during the first month of study.

During the first month, 12% of patients experienced severe fever (i.e. greater than or equal to 40°C). Documented infections were noted in fewer than one-third of all febrile episodes. Of the 124 patients treated, 11 were noted to have a documented infection in the month prior to treatment. In the month following treatment, 31% of patients had a documented infection: 13.7% of patients had bacterial infection, 6.5% had viral and 6.5% had fungal infections. Seventy percent (70%) of these patients were treated empirically with antibiotics.

During the first month, serious infections (eg septicaemia, pneumonia), were reported in 7% of all patients; the remainder were mild or moderate. During the second month, the overall rate of documented infection was 8%; these infections were mild to moderate and no severe systemic infections were seen. After the third month, the monthly incidence of infection was either less than or equal to that of the months immediately preceding Leustat therapy.

*Effects of high doses:* In a Phase 1 study with 31 patients in which Leustat Injection was administered at high doses (4 to 9 times that recommended for hairy cell leukaemia) for 7 to 14 days in conjunction with cyclophosphamide and total body irradiation as preparation for bone marrow transplantation, acute nephrotoxicity, delayed onset neurotoxicity, severe bone marrow suppression with neutropenia, anaemia, and thrombocytopenia and gastrointestinal symptoms were reported.

*Nephrotoxicity:* Six patients (19%) developed manifestations of acute renal dysfunction/insufficiency (eg acidosis, anuria, elevated serum creatinine, etc) within 7 to 13 days after starting treatment with Leustat, 5 of the affected patients required dialysis. Renal insufficiency was reversible in 2 of these patients. Evidence of tubular damage was noted at autopsy in 2 (of 4) patients whose renal function had not recovered at the time of death. Several of these patients had also been treated with other medications having known nephrotoxic potential.

*Neurotoxicity:* Eleven patients (35%) experienced delayed onset neurological toxicity. In the majority, this was characterised by progressive irreversible motor weakness, of the upper and/or lower extremities (paraparesis/quadraparesis), noted 35 to 84 days after starting high dose therapy.

Non-invasive neurological testing was consistent with demyelinating disease.

*Post-marketing experience:* The following additional adverse events have been reported since the drug became commercially available. These adverse events have been reported primarily in patients who received multiple courses of Leustat Injection:

Haematological: bone marrow suppression with prolonged pancytopenia, including some reports of aplastic anaemia; haemolytic anaemia, which was reported in patients with lymphoid malignancies, occurring within the first few weeks following treatment.

Hepatic: reversible, generally mild, increases in bilirubin and transaminases.

Nervous system: neurological toxicity.

Respiratory system: pulmonary interstitial infiltrates, in most cases an infectious aetiology was identified.

Opportunistic infections have occurred in the acute phase of treatment due to the immunosuppression mediated by Leustat Injection.

*Overdose:* High doses of Leustat have been associated with serious neurological toxicity (including irreversible paraparesis/quadraparesis), acute nephrotoxicity, and severe bone marrow suppression resulting in neutropenia, anaemia and thrombocytopenia. (See Special warnings and special precautions for use). There is no known specific antidote to overdosage. It is not known whether the drug can be removed from the circulation by dialysis or haemofiltration. Treatment of overdosage consists of discontinuation of Leustat Injection, careful observation and appropriate supportive measures.

**Pharmacological properties**

*Pharmacodynamic properties:* Leustat Injection (also known as 2-chloro-2′-deoxy-β-D-adenosine or 2-CdA or cladribine) is a synthetic antineoplastic agent.

*Cellular resistance and sensitivity:* The selective toxicity of 2-chloro-2′-deoxy-β-D-adenosine towards certain normal and malignant lymphocyte and monocyte populations is based on the relative activities of deoxycytidine kinase, deoxynucleotidase and adenosine deaminase. It is postulated that cells with high deoxycytidine kinase and low deoxynucleotidase activities will be selectively killed by 2-chloro-2′-deoxy-β-D-adenosine as toxic deoxynucleotides accumulate intracellularly.

Cells containing high concentrations of deoxynucleotides are unable to properly repair single-strand DNA breaks. Leustat Injection can be distinguished from other chemotherapeutic agents affecting purine metabolism in that it is cytotoxic to both actively dividing and quiescent lymphocytes and monocytes, inhibiting both DNA synthesis and repair.

*Pharmacokinetic properties:* When Leustat Injection was given by continuous intravenous infusion over 7 days the mean steady-state serum concentration was estimated to be 6 ng/ml with an estimated systemic clearance of 640 ml/h/kg. Accumulation of Leustat over the seven day treatment period was not noted.

Plasma concentrations are reported to decline multi-exponentially after intravenous infusions with terminal half-lives ranging from approximately 3-22 hours. In general, the apparent volume of distribution of cladribine is very large (mean approximately 9l/kg), indicating an extensive distribution of cladribine in body tissues. The mean half-life of cladribine in leukaemic cells has been reported to be 23 hours.

There is little information available on the metabolism or route of excretion of cladribine in man. Based on animal data, it is expected that cladribine is cleared by the kidneys. However, information on the contribution of renal clearance to total body clearance is not available. The effect of renal and hepatic impairment on the elimination of cladribine has not been investigated in humans.

Cladribine penetrates into cerebrospinal fluid. One report indicates that concentrations are approximately 25% of those in plasma.

Cladribine is bound approximately 20% to plasma proteins.

*Preclinical safety data:* Preclinical safety data has been included in specific sections of SPC.

**Pharmaceutical particulars**

*List of excipients:* 9.0 mg (0.15 mEq) of sodium chloride as an inactive ingredient. Phosphoric acid and/or dibasic sodium phosphate to adjust the pH to a range of 5.5 to 8.0.

*Incompatibilities:* Since limited compatibility data are available, adherence to the recommended diluents and infusion systems is advised.

Solutions containing Leustat Injection should not be mixed with other intravenous drugs or additives or infused simultaneously via a common intravenous line, since compatibility testing has not been performed.

If the same intravenous line is used for sequential infusion of several different drugs, the line should be flushed with a compatible diluent before and after infusion of Leustat.

The use of 5% dextrose as a diluent is not recommended because of increased degradation of cladribine.

*Shelf life:* When stored in refrigerated conditions between 2° to 8°C (36° to 46°F) protected from light, unopened vials of Leustat Injection are stable until the expiration date indicated on the package. Freezing does not adversely affect the solution.

If freezing occurs, thaw naturally to room temperature. DO NOT heat or microwave. Once thawed, the vial of Leustat Injection is stable until expiry if refrigerated. *DO NOT REFREEZE.*

Once diluted, solutions containing Leustat Injection should be administered promptly or stored in the refrigerator (2° to 8°C) for no more than 8 hours prior to start of administration.

*Special precautions for storage:* Store refrigerated at 2° to 8°C (36° to 46°F). Protect from light during storage.

*Nature and contents of container:* Leustat Injection is supplied as a sterile, preservative-free, isotonic solution containing 10 mg (1 mg/ml) of cladribine (as 10 ml) in a single-use, flint glass 20 ml vial.

*Instructions for use/handling:* Preparation and administration of intravenous solutions: Leustat Injection must be diluted with the designated diluent prior to administration. Since the drug product does not contain any anti-microbial preservative or bacteriostatic agent, aseptic technique and proper environmental precautions must be observed in preparation of a solution of Leustat.

Parental drug products should be inspected visually for particulate matter and discoloration prior to administration, whenever solution and container permit. A precipitate may occur during the exposure of Leustat to low temperatures; it may be resolubilised by allowing the solution to warm naturally to room temperature and by shaking vigorously. *DO NOT HEAT OR MICROWAVE.*

Care must be taken to assure the sterility of prepared solutions. Once diluted, solutions of Leustat Injection should be administered promptly or stored in the refrigerator (2° to 8°C) for no more than 8 hours prior to start of administration. Vials of Leustat Injection are for single-use only. Any unused portion should be discarded in an appropriate manner.

The potential hazards associated with cytotoxic agents are well established and proper precautions should be taken when handling, preparing, and administering Leustat Injection. The use of disposable gloves and protective garments is recommended. If Leustat Injection contacts the skin or mucous membranes, wash the involved surface immediately with copious amounts of water.

*Preparation of a single daily dose:* Add the calculated dose for a 24 hours period (0.09 mg/kg or 0.09 ml/kg or 3.6 mg/m²) of Leustat Injection to an infusion bag containing 100 ml to 500 ml of 0.9% sodium chloride injection (PhEur). Infuse intravenously continuously over 24 hours. Repeat daily for a total of 7 consecutive days. The use of 5% dextrose as a diluent is not recommended because of increased degradation of cladribine. Admixtures of Leustat Injection are chemically and physically stable for at least 24 hours at room temperature under normal room fluorescent light in most commonly available PVC infusion containers.

| | Dose of Leustat | Recommended diluent | Quantity of diluent |
|---|---|---|---|
| 24-hour infusion method | 1 (day) x 0.09 mg/kg | 0.9% sodium chloride injection PhEur | 100 ml to 500 ml |

*Name and address of marketing authorisation holder:* Janssen-Cilag Limited, Saunderton, High Wycombe, Buckinghamshire HP14 4HJ.

**Marketing authorisation number** 0242/0232

**Date of approval/revision of SPC** May 1996

**Legal category** POM.

## MICRONOR* HRT

**Presentation** Micronor HRT tablets are round white tablets engraved C over 1 on both faces. Each tablet contains 1 mg of norethisterone.

**Uses** The progestogenic opposition of menopausal oestrogen replacement therapy.

*Mode of Action:* Micronor HRT tablets convert the oestrogen primed proliferative endometrium into secretory endometrium which, on withdrawal of norethisterone at the end of each cycle, causes a withdrawal bleed in most patients thus eliminating endometrial hyperplasia.

**Dosage and administration**
*Adult females:* One tablet should be taken by mouth each day on days 15-26 of each 28 day cycle of oestrogen replacement therapy.

*Children:* Micronor HRT tablets are not indicated for use in children.

*Use in pregnancy and lactation:* Micronor HRT is contra-indicated.

**Contra-indications, warnings etc**

*Contra-indications:* Micronor HRT tablets should not be used for contraception. Use is not recommended during pregnancy or lactation, severe disturbance of liver function, Dubin-Johnson and Rotor Syndromes, history during pregnancy of idiopathic jaundice, severe pruritus or pemphigoid gestationis.

*Warnings and precautions:* Prior to commencing and regularly during oestrogen replacement therapy, it is recommended that the patient should be given a thorough physical and gynaecological examination and a complete medical and family history should be taken. Close monitoring is recommended in patients with epilepsy, diabetes or hypertension, disturbances or impairment of liver function, mastopathy, or a strong family history of mammary cancer, uterine fibroids, cholelithiasis, multiple sclerosis, systemic lupus erythematosus, porphyria, melanoma and asthma. Repeated breakthrough bleeding should be investigated including endometrial biopsy.

At present there is suggestive evidence of an overall change in the relative risk of breast cancer in the post menopausal women receiving hormone replacement therapy. Some studies have reported an increased risk of breast cancer in long-term users, others, however, have shown no such increase. It is not known whether concurrent progestogen use influences the risk of breast cancer. A careful appraisal of the risk-benefit ratio should be undertaken before treatment for longer than 5 years. Administration of unopposed oestrogen therapy in patients with an intact uterus has been reported to increase the risk of endometrial hyperplasia.

There is no indication from published studies that the risk of thromboembolic disease, including myocardial infarction, stroke and thrombophlebitis is increased with hormone replacement therapy at the current recommended low dosage in apparently normal women. However, treatment should be discontinued immediately following the occurrence of an acute vascular thromboembolic event during therapy. There is no evidence that a past history of deep vein thrombosis, pulmonary embolism, stroke, or myocardial infarction should be a contra-indication to hormone replacement therapy when associated with recognised risk factors such as immobilisation (e.g. post-partum or post-trauma) or post-operative (e.g. in particular after pelvic surgery) but in the absence of specific data, hormone replacement therapy should be used with caution.

*Drug interactions:* Barbiturates, hydantoins, carbamazepine, meprobamate, phenylbutazone, antibiotics, (including rifampicin) and activated charcoal, may impair the activity of oestrogen and progestogens (irregular bleeding and recurrence of symptoms may occur).

*Side-effects:* Minor effects of oestrogen and combined oestrogen/progestogen hormone replacement therapy which do not usually preclude continuation of therapy include headaches, nausea and breast-tenderness. The following side effects have been reported with oestrogen/progestogen therapy:
*Genito-urinary system:* Pre-menstrual-like syndrome, increase in size of uterine fibromyomata, vaginal candidiasis, change in cervical erosion and degree of cervical secretion, cystitis-like syndrome.
*Breasts:* Tenderness, enlargement, secretion.
*Gastrointestinal:* Nausea, vomiting, abdominal cramps, bloating, cholestatic jaundice.
*Skin:* Chloasma which may persist when drug is discontinued, erythema multiforme, erythema nodosum, haemorrhagic eruption, loss of scalp hair, hirsutism.
*Eyes:* Steepening of corneal curvature, intolerance to contact lenses.
*CNS:* Headaches, migraine, dizziness, mental depression, chorea.
*Miscellaneous:* Increase or decrease in weight, reduced carbohydrate tolerance, aggravation of porphyria, oedema, changes in libido, leg cramps.

*Overdosage:* There have been no reports of serious ill-effects from overdosage with norethisterone and treatment is usually unnecessary. Nausea and vomiting may occur.

There is no special antidote and treatment should be symptomatic.

**Pharmaceutical precautions** Protect from light. Store at room temperature (at or below 25°C).

**Legal category** POM.

**Package quantities** Carton containing 3 aluminium/PVC blister strips of 12 tablets each.

**Further information** Nil.

**Product licence number** 0242/0241.

## MICRONOR* ORAL CONTRACEPTIVE TABLETS

**Presentation** White, ¼ inch diameter, circular tablets with flat faces and bevelled edges, bearing on each face the engraving C over 035. Micronor Oral Contraceptive Tablets each contain 350 micrograms Norethisterone.

**Uses** Contraception.

**Action** Micronor has a progestational effect on the endometrium and on the cervical mucus. The exact mechanism of how it prevents conception has not been confirmed.

**Dosage and administration** Tablet intake from the first pack is started on the first day of menstruation; no extra contraceptive precautions are necessary. One tablet is taken at the same time each day, every day of the year, whether menstruation occurs or not.

*Changing from another progestogen-only pill or from a combined oral contraceptive:* Start Micronor on the day following completion of the previous oral contraceptive pack without a break (or, in the case of the ED pill, omitting the inactive pills). No extra contraceptive precautions are required.

*Post-partum administration:* Micronor can be started on the 21st day after childbirth. This will ensure the patient is protected immediately. If there is any delay in taking the first dose, contraception may not be established until 7 days after the first tablet has been taken. In these circumstances patients should be advised that extra contraceptive precautions (non-hormonal methods) are necessary.

*After miscarriage or abortion:* Patients can take Micronor on the day after miscarriage or abortion, in which case no additional contraceptive precautions are required.

**Contra-indications, warnings, etc**

*Contra-indications:* Existing thrombophlebitis, existing thromboembolic disorders, cerebrovascular disease or a past history of this condition, myocardial infarction or a past history of this condition. Markedly impaired liver function. Known or suspected hormone dependent neoplasia. Known or suspected carcinoma of the breast. Undiagnosed abnormal genital tract bleeding. Known or suspected pregnancy. Cholestatic jaundice of pregnancy or jaundice with prior pill use. Hepatic adenomas or carcinomas.

*Warnings and precautions:* There is a general opinion, based on statistical evidence, that users of **combined** oral contraceptives (ie oestrogen plus progestogen) experience more often than non-users various disorders of the circulation of blood, including strokes (blood clots in, and haemorrhages from, the blood vessels of the brain), heart attacks (coronary thromboses) and blood clots obstructing the arteries of the lungs (pulmonary emboli).

There may not be a full recovery from such disorders and it should be realised that in a few cases they may be fatal.

To date no association between these disorders and progestogen only oral contraceptives (such as Micronor Oral Contraceptive Tablets) has been shown. However there is a risk that the users of such progestogen only oral contraceptives will (like users of the combined oral contraceptive) be exposed to an increased risk of suffering from these disorders.

Because of a possible increased risk of post surgery thromboembolic complications in oral contraceptive users, therapy should be discontinued six weeks prior to elective surgery.

When Micronor is administered during the post-partum period, the increased risk of thromboembolic disease associated with the post-partum period must be considered.

Masculinisation of the female foetus has occurred when progestogens have been used in pregnant women, although this has been observed at doses much higher than that contained in Micronor. Pregnancy should be ruled out before continuing administration of Micronor to patients who have gone 45 days without a menstrual period.

A small fraction of the active ingredients in oral contraceptives has been identified in the milk of mothers receiving these drugs. The effects, if any, on the breast-fed child have not been determined. If possible the use of oral contraceptives should be deferred until the infant is weaned.

Malignant hepatic tumours have been reported on rare occasions in long-term users of oral contraceptives. Benign hepatic tumours have also been associated with oral contraceptive usage. A hepatic tumour should be considered in the differential diagnosis when upper abdominal pain, enlarged liver or signs of intra-abdominal haemorrhage occur.

Pregnancies in progestogen-only pill (POP) users are more likely to be ectopic than are pregnancies occurring in the general population since POPs offer less protection against ectopic pregnancy than against intra-uterine pregnancy.

Reduced efficacy and increased incidence of breakthrough bleeding have been associated with concomitant use of oral contraceptives and rifampicin. A similar association has been suggested with oral contraceptives and barbiturates, phenytoin sodium, ampicillin, tetracycline and griseofulvin.

*Missed tablets:* If a tablet is missed within 3 hours of the correct dosage time, then the missed tablet should be taken as soon as possible; this will ensure that contraceptive protection is maintained. If one (for longer than 3 hours) or more tablets are missed, it is recommended that the patient takes the last missed tablet as soon as possible and continues to take the rest of the tablets as usual. Additional means of contraception (non-hormonal) should be used for the next seven days.

If the patient does not have a period within 45 days of her last period, Micronor should be discontinued and pregnancy should be excluded.

*Vomiting and diarrhoea:* Additional contraceptive measures (non-hormonal) should be employed during the period of gastrointestinal upset and for the next seven days.

*Reasons for stopping oral contraceptives immediately:* Early manifestations of thrombotic or thromboembolic disorders, thrombophlebitis, cerebrovascular disorders (including haemorrhage), myocardial infarction, pulmonary embolism. Gradual or sudden, partial or complete loss of vision. Proptosis or diplopia. Onset or aggravation of migraine or development of headaches of a new pattern which are recurrent, persistent or severe. Papilloedema or any evidence of retinal vascular lesions. During periods of immobility (eg after accidents). Pregnancy. Manifestations of liver tumours.

Examination of the pelvic organs, breasts and blood pressure should precede the prescribing of any oral contraceptive and should be repeated regularly. The following are some of the medical conditions reported to be influenced by the combined pill, and may be affected by Micronor. The physician will have to exercise medical judgement to commence, continue or discontinue therapy as appropriate. The worsening or first appearance of any of these conditions may indicate that Micronor should be discontinued.

(a) Pre-existing uterine fibromyomata may increase in size.

(b) A decrease in glucose tolerance in a significant number of women.

(c) An increase in blood pressure in a small but significant number of women.

(d) Cholestatic jaundice. Patients with a history of cholestatic jaundice of pregnancy are more likely to develop cholestatic jaundice during oral contraceptive therapy.

(e) Amenorrhoea during and after oral contraceptive therapy. Temporary infertility after discontinuation of treatment.

(f) Depression.

(g) Fluid retention. Conditions which might be influenced by this factor include epilepsy, migraine, asthma, cardiac or renal dysfunction.

(h) Varicose veins.

(I) Multiple sclerosis.

(j) Porphyria.

(k) Tetany.

(l) Intolerance to contact lenses or any condition that is prone to worsen during pregnancy.

The following laboratory determinations may be altered in patients using oral contraceptives.

*Hepatic:* Increased BSP retention and other tests.

*Coagulation:* Increased prothrombin, Factors VII, VIII, IX and X, decreased antithrombin III, increased platelet aggregability.

*Endocrine:* Increased PBI and butanol extractable protein bound iodine and decreased T3 uptake, increased glucose blood levels.

*Others:* Increased phospholipids and tri-glycerides, decreased serum folate values and disturbance in tryptophan metabolism, decreased pregnanediol excretion, reduced response to metyrapone test.

These tests usually return to pre-therapy values after discontinuing oral contraceptive use. However, the physician should be aware that these altered determinations may mask an underlying disease.

*Side-effects:* Micronor has been found to be a well tolerated drug. Side-effects are usually self-limiting and of relatively short duration. Amongst the symptoms reported are headaches/migraine, nausea, vomiting, breast changes, change in weight, changes in libido, chloasma, breakthrough bleeding and spotting, rash, depression, irregular cycle length (particularly in the early cycles of therapy). It is important that patients should be advised that whilst on Micronor therapy they may experience variation in cycle length and that they should continue taking a tablet every day whether they have a period or not. However, patients should be advised to discontinue Micronor and to consult their doctor if they have gone 45 days without having a period.

*Overdosage:* Serious ill effects have not been reported following acute ingestion of large doses of oral contraceptives by young children. Overdosage may cause nausea, and withdrawal bleeding may occur in females. An appropriate method of gastric emptying may be used if considered desirable.

**Pharmaceutical precautions** Store at room temperature (below 25°C); protect from light.

**Legal category** POM.

**Package quantities** Carton containing 3 pushpaks each of 28 tablets–sufficient for 3 cycles.

**Further information** Nil.

**Product licence number** 0242/0234.

## NIZORAL* TABLETS

**Qualitative and quantitative composition** Ketoconazole 200 mg.

**Pharmaceutical form** Tablet.

**Clinical particulars**

*Therapeutic indications:* Systemic mycoses, eg systemic candidosis, paracoccidioidomycosis, coccidioidomycosis, histoplasmosis.

Serious chronic mucocutaneous candidosis (including exceptionally disabling paronychia) not responsive to other therapy or when the organism is resistant to other therapy.

Serious mycoses of the gastrointestinal tract not responsive to other therapy or when organisms are resistant to other therapy.

Chronic vaginal candidosis not responsive to other therapy.

Prophylactic treatment to prevent mycotic infection in patients with reduced immune responses, eg in

cancer, during treatment with immunosuppressive medication, or with burns.

Culturally determined dermatophyte infections of skin or finger nails which have failed to respond to adequate dose regimes of conventional anti-dermatophyte agents (excluding fungal infection of toe nails). Nizoral is not indicated for pityriasis versicolour, usually an asymptomatic skin rash.

*Posology and method of administration:* Nizoral tablets should be taken orally with meals to ensure maximum absorption.

*Adults:*
*Mycoses and dermatophyte infections (except vaginal infections):* One tablet once daily, usually for 14 days.

If an adequate response has not been achieved after 14 days, treatment can be continued until at least one week after symptoms have cleared and cultures have become negative. The dose may also be increased to 400 mg once daily if necessary.

As nail infections always require long term therapy, they should only be treated when a clinical rather than a purely cosmetic problem exists and only after alternative treatment has failed.

*Prophylaxis and maintenance treatment:* One tablet daily.

*Chronic vaginal candidosis:* Two tablets once daily for 5 days.

*Children:* Dosage should be reduced to 50 or 100 mg depending on body weight (ie approximately 3 mg/kg), for example:
Age 1–4 years: 50 mg
Age 5–12 years: 100 mg

*Elderly:* In the absence of specific data, chronic vaginal candidosis–as for adults; All other indications–200 mg daily.

*Method of administration:* oral.

*Contra-indications:* Nizoral should not be used in patients with a known hypersensitivity to ketoconazole or to any other imidazole antifungal.

Since it cannot be excluded that patients with pre-existing liver disease may be at greater risk of developing hepatic damage, oral ketoconazole treatment is contra-indicated in these patients. In patients suspected of having pre-existing liver disease, liver function tests should be performed prior to treatment and ketoconazole should not be used if significant abnormalities are observed. When administered in high doses (>80 mg/kg) to pregnant rats, ketoconazole has been shown to cause abnormalities of foetal development. The relevance of this finding to humans has not been established and consequently Nizoral is contra-indicated in pregnancy.

Astemizole, cisapride or terfenadine should not be given concurrently with oral ketoconazole.

*Special warnings and special precautions for use:* Hepatitis has been reported. The risk of hepatitis is greater in patients on long term treatment (>14 days). In patients receiving long term treatment, the benefits must be weighed against the possible risks.

In patients in whom long term treatment (ie >14 days) with ketoconazole is indicated, LFTs should be performed prior to starting treatment.

Asymptomatic elevations in serum transaminase can occur early during treatment with ketoconazole. These may either be insignificant and transient, or can represent early evidence of hepatotoxicity. Patients should therefore be monitored clinically and biochemically with serum transaminase determinations after the first 2 weeks of treatment, at 4 weeks and at monthly intervals thereafter. If significantly elevated levels are observed, liver function tests (LFTs) should be performed at weekly intervals until transaminase levels return to normal. If significant progressive elevation occurs or the patient develops symptoms of hepatitis (malaise, fever, dark urine, pale stools or jaundice), treatment with ketoconazole should be stopped immediately. The patient should then be monitored both clinically and biochemically for at least 2 months or until enzyme levels return to normal. Patients should also be told to consult their doctor if any of the above symptoms develop.

Hepatic damage has usually been reversible on discontinuation of treatment. Rarely, however, fatalities have been reported following ketoconazole treatment, usually where therapy has been continued despite development of symptoms of hepatitis.

The risk factors for the development of hepatitis includes age over 50 (especially women), known drug intolerance or prior administration of potentially hepatotoxic agents and history of liver disease.

*Interactions with other medicaments and other forms of interaction:* The concomitant administration of terfenadine, cisapride or astemizole, with oral ketoconazole is contra-indicated. Ketoconazole is extensively bound to plasma proteins. Since ketoconazole inhibits certain hepatic oxidase enzymes, it may decrease the elimination of co-administered drugs whose metabolism depends on such enzymes. Increased levels of such drugs, when used together with ketoconazole, have been associated with an increase in side-effects. Known examples of serious interactions include those with cyclosporin, tacrolimus, astemizole, terfenadine, cisapride, anticoagulants, corticosteroids, alfentanil, taxanes and, possibly, busulphan. The plasma levels or effects of cyclosporin, anticoagulants, corticosteroids and busulphan should be carefully monitored, if co-administered with oral ketoconazole, and the dosage reduced if necessary. The concomitant use of ketoconazole and alfentanil may significantly inhibit the latter's clearance and increase the risk of prolonged or delayed respiratory depression. Taxanes should be used carefully with ketoconazole because the potential interaction may enhance toxicity. Terfenadine, cisapride or astemizole should not be taken concomitantly with oral ketoconazole (see contra-indications). Exceptional cases of a disulfiram-like reaction to alcohol, characterised by flushing, rash, peripheral oedema, nausea and headache, have been reported. All symptoms resolved completely within a few hours.

Concomitant use of rifampicin with ketoconazole may reduce the blood levels of both drugs. Similarly concomitant isoniazid treatment reduces the plasma levels of ketoconazole. If these combinations are to be used plasma levels should be carefully monitored.

Concomitant use of ketoconazole and phenytoin may alter the metabolism of one or both drugs.

Absorption of ketoconazole is maximal when taken during a meal, as it depends on stomach acidity. Concomitant treatment with agents that reduce gastric secretion (anti-cholinergic drugs, antacids, H$_2$ antagonists, proton pump inhibitors) should be avoided and, if indicated, such drugs should be taken not less than two hours after Nizoral.

*Pregnancy and lactation:* Nizoral is contra-indicated in pregnancy. Nizoral may be excreted in breast milk and therefore it is not advisable to breast feed whilst being treated with Nizoral.

*Effects on ability to drive and use machines:* None known.

*Undesirable effects:* Alterations in liver function tests have occurred in patients on ketoconazole; these changes may be transient, cases of hepatitis have been reported (see Warnings section). In rare cases, anaphylactoid reactions have been reported after the first dose. Hypersensitivity reactions including urticaria and angio-oedema have also been reported. The most commonly observed side effects are gastric upsets (nausea, vomiting, abdominal pain), rash, urticaria, pruritus and headache. Thrombocytopenia, paraesthesia, photophobia, exanthema, dizziness and alopecia have been reported rarely. Ketoconazole, 200 mg once daily, produces a transient decrease in plasma testosterone levels during the first 4–6 hours after intake of the drug. During long-term therapy at this dose, testosterone levels are usually not significantly different from controls. In rare instances, gynaecomastia and oligospermia have been reported. A few cases of menstrual irregularities have been reported when ketoconazole has been co-administered with the oral contraceptive. Although impaired response of plasma cortisol to ACTH has been described, clinically significant symptoms of adrenal insufficiency are unlikely to occur at recommended doses. However, patients with impaired adrenal function, or who may be under periods of stress (eg major surgery, intensive care, etc), should have their adrenal function monitored.

*Overdose:* Cases should be treated symptomatically with supportive measures or gastric lavage as necessary.

**Pharmacological properties**

*Pharmacodynamic properties:* Ketoconazole is an imidazole-dioxolane anti-mycotic which is effective after oral administration and has a broad spectrum of activity against dermatophytes, yeasts and other pathogenic fungi.

*Pharmacokinetic properties:* Ketoconazole is incompletely absorbed by the gastro-intestinal tract; absorption is reduced when gastric acidity is reduced. Peak plasma levels are obtained 2 hours after oral administration.

Ketoconazole is extensively bound to plasma proteins. Penetration into cerebrospinal fluid is poor. Ketoconazole is extensively metabolised in the body and is excreted in the urine as inactive metabolites and unchanged drug. It is also excreted in the faeces.

*Preclinical safety data:* Not applicable.

**Pharmaceutical particulars**
*List of excipients:* Maize starch; lactose; polyvidone; microcrystalline cellulose; colloidal anhydrous silica; magnesium stearate; purified water*.

* Not present in final product

*Incompatibilities:* None.

*Shelf life:* Five years.

Special precautions for storage: Store in a dry place. Store between 15°C and 30°C.

*Nature and contents of container:* Blister packs containing 30 tablets.

*Instructions for use/handling:* Not applicable.

**Marketing authorisation number** 0242/0083

**Date of approval/revision of SPC** June 1996.

**Legal category** POM.

## NIZORAL* SUSPENSION

**Presentation** Pink, cherry flavoured suspension in 100 ml amber glass bottles containing 20 mg ketoconazole per ml. The suspension also contains microcrystalline cellulose, carboxymethylcellulose sodium, sodium saccharin dihydrate and erythrosine sodium (E127).

**Uses** Nizoral is an imidazole-dioxolane antimycotic which is effective after oral administration and has a broad spectrum of activity against dermatophytes, yeasts and other pathogenic fungi. The indications for Nizoral are:

*In adults and children:*

1. Systemic mycoses, e.g. systemic candidosis, paracoccidioidomycosis, coccidioidomycosis, histoplasmosis.
2. Serious chronic mucocutaneous candidosis (including exceptionally disabling paronychia) not responsive to other therapy or when the organism is resistant to other therapy.
3. Serious mycoses of the gastrointestinal tract not responsive to other therapy or when organisms are resistant to other therapy.
4. Chronic vaginal candidosis not responsive to other therapy.
5. Prophylactic treatment to prevent mycotic infection in patients with reduced immune responses, e.g. in cancer, during treatment with immunosuppressive medication, or with burns.
6. Dermatophyte infections confirmed by culture of skin or finger nails which have failed to respond to adequate dose regimes of conventional anti-dermatophyte agents (excluding fungal infection of toe nails). Nizoral suspension, unlike the shampoo and cream formulations, is not indicated for pityriasis versicolor.

**Dosage and administration** Nizoral is for oral administration and should always be taken with meals.

The risk of hepatitis (see *Warnings*) may increase in relation to the duration of treatment, if therapy is continued for more than 14 days the benefits must be weighed against the possible risks.

*In adults:*
*Mycoses and dermatophyte infections (except vaginal candidosis):* Two 5 ml doses of suspension (200 mg) once daily, with food, usually for 14 days.

If an adequate response has not been achieved after 14 days, treatment may be continued until at least one week after symptoms have cleared and cultures have become negative. The dose may be increased to 400 mg once daily if necessary.

As nail infections always require long term therapy they should only be treated when a clinical rather than a purely cosmetic problem exists and only after alternative treatment has failed.

*Prophylaxis and maintenance treatment:* Two 5 ml doses of suspension (200 mg) once daily with food.

*Chronic vaginal candidosis:* Four 5 ml doses of suspension (400 mg) once daily with food for 5 days.

*Use in children:* Dosage should be reduced to 50 or 100 mg depending on bodyweight (ie approximately 3 mg/kg), for example:
Age 1–4 years—2.5 ml (50 mg) daily with food
Age 5–12 years—5 ml (100 mg) daily with food

*Use in elderly:* In the absence of specific data, chronic vaginal candidosis – as for adults; all other indications – 2 × 5 ml doses of suspension (200 mg) daily with food.

**Contra-indications, warnings, etc**
*Contra-indications:* Nizoral should not be used in patients with a known hypersensitivity to ketoconazole or to any other imidazole antifungal.

Since it cannot be excluded that patients with pre-existing liver disease may be at greater risk of developing hepatic damage, oral ketoconazole treatment is contra-indicated in these patients.

In patients suspected of having pre-existing liver disease, liver function tests should be performed prior to treatment and ketoconazole should not be used if significant abnormalities are observed.

Nizoral is contra-indicated in pregnancy (see *Use in pregnancy* section).

Astemizole, cisapride or terfenadine should not be given concurrently with oral ketoconazole.

*Warnings and precautions:* Hepatitis has been reported. The risk of developing hepatitis is greater in patients on long term treatment (>14 days). In patients receiving long term treatment, the benefits must be weighed against possible risks.

In patients in whom long term treatment (ie >14 days) with ketoconazole is indicated, LFTs should be performed prior to starting treatment.

Asymptomatic elevations in serum transaminase can occur early during treatment with ketoconazole. These may either be insignificant and transient, or can represent early evidence of hepatotoxicity. Patients should therefore be monitored clinically and biochemically with serum transaminase determinations after the first 2 weeks of treatment, at 4 weeks and at monthly intervals thereafter. If significantly elevated levels are observed, liver function tests (LFTs) should be performed at weekly intervals until transaminase levels return to normal. If significant progressive elevation occurs or the patient develops symptoms of hepatitis (malaise, fever, dark urine, pale stools or jaundice), treatment with ketoconazole should be stopped immediately. The patient should then be monitored both clinically and biochemically for at least 2 months or until enzyme levels return to normal. Patients should also be told to consult their doctor if any of the above symptoms develop.

The risk factors for the development of hepatitis include age over 50 (especially women), known drug intolerance or prior administration of potentially hepatotoxic agents and history of liver disease.

Hepatic damage has usually been reversible on discontinuation of treatment. Rarely, however, fatalities have been reported following ketoconazole treatment, usually where therapy has been continued despite development of symptoms of hepatitis.

*Drug interactions:* The concomitant administration of terfenadine, cisapride or astemizole with oral ketoconazole is contra-indicated.

Absorption of Nizoral is maximal when taken during a meal, as it depends on stomach acidity. Concomitant treatment with agents that reduce gastric secretion (anti-cholinergic drugs, antacids, $H_2$ antagonists, proton pump inhibitors) should be avoided and, if indicated, such drugs should be taken not less than two hours after Nizoral.

Ketoconazole is extensively bound to plasma proteins.

Since ketoconazole inhibits certain hepatic oxidase enzymes, it may decrease the elimination of co-administered drugs whose metabolism depends on such enzymes. Increased levels of such drugs, when used together with ketoconazole, have been associated with an increase in side-effects. Known examples of serious interactions include those with cyclosporin, tacrolimus, astemizole, terfenadine, cisapride, anticoagulants, corticosteroids, alfentanil, taxanes and, possibly, busulphan. The plasma levels or effects of cyclosporin, anticoagulants, corticosteroids and busulphan should be carefully monitored, if co-administered with oral ketoconazole, and the dosage reduced if necessary. The concomitant use of ketoconazole and alfentanil may significantly inhibit the latter's clearance and increase the risk of prolonged or delayed respiratory depression. Taxanes should be used carefully with ketoconazole because the potential interaction may enhance toxicity. Terfenadine, cisapride or astemizole should not be taken concomitantly with oral ketoconazole (see contra-indications). Exceptional cases of a disulfiram-like reaction to alcohol, characterised by flushing, rash, peripheral oedema, nausea and headache have been reported. All symptoms resolved completely within a few hours.

Concomitant use of rifampicin with ketoconazole may reduce the blood levels of both drugs. Similarly, concomitant isoniazid treatment reduces the plasma levels of ketoconazole. If these combinations are to be used, plasma levels should be carefully monitored.

Concomitant use of ketoconazole and phenytoin may alter the metabolism of one or both drugs.

*Use in pregnancy and lactation:* When administered in high doses (>80 mg/kg) to pregnant rats, Nizoral has been shown to cause abnormalities of foetal development. The relevance of this finding to humans has not been established, although Nizoral is contra-indicated in pregnancy.

Nizoral may be excreted in breast milk and therefore it is not advisable to breast feed whilst being treated with Nizoral.

*Side-effects:* Alterations in liver function tests have occurred in patients on ketoconazole; these changes may be transient. Cases of hepatitis have been reported (see 'Warnings' section).

In rare cases, anaphylactoid reactions have been reported after the first dose. Hypersensitivity reactions including urticaria and angio-oedema have also been reported. The most commonly observed side-effects are gastric upsets (nausea, vomiting, abdominal pain), rash, urticaria, pruritus and headache. Thrombocytopenia, paraesthesia, photophobia, exanthema, dizziness and alopecia have been reported rarely.

Ketoconazole, 200 mg once daily, produces a transient decrease in plasma levels of testosterone during the first 4–6 hours after intake of the drug. During long term therapy at this dose, testosterone levels are usually not significantly different from controls. In rare instances, gynaecomastia and oligospermia have been reported. A few cases of menstrual irregularities have been reported when ketoconazole has been co-administered with the oral contraceptive. Although impaired response of plasma cortisol to ACTH has been described, clinically significant symptoms of adrenal insufficiency are unlikely to occur at recommended doses. However, patients with impaired adrenal function, or who may be under periods of stress (eg major surgery, intensive care, etc) should have their adrenal function monitored.

*Overdosage:* In the event of overdosage, cases should be treated symptomatically with supportive measures or gastric lavage as necessary.

**Pharmaceutical precautions** None.

**Legal category** POM.

**Package quantities** Nizoral suspension is supplied 100 ml bottles.

**Further information** Nil.

**Product licence number** 0242/0101

## NIZORAL* CREAM

**Presentation** White, non-staining, water miscible cream containing ketoconazole 2% w/w. The cream also contains propylene glycol, cetyl alcohol and stearyl alcohol, sorbitan monostearate, polysorbate 60 and 80, sodium sulphite, isopropyl myristate and water.

**Uses** Nizoral has a potent antimycotic activity against dermatophytes and yeasts. Nizoral cream acts rapidly on pruritus which is commonly seen in dermatophyte and yeast infections. This symptomatic improvement often occurs before the first signs of healing are observed.

After topical application, Nizoral is not systemically absorbed and does not produce detectable plasma concentrations.

Nizoral cream is indicated for topical application in the treatment of dermatophyte infections of the skin such as tinea corporis, tinea cruris, tinea manus and tinea pedis infections due to *Trichophyton* spp, *Microsporum* spp. and *Epidermophyton* spp.

Nizoral cream is also indicated for the treatment of cutaneous candidosis (including external application in vulvitis), pityriasis versicolor, and seborrhoeic dermatitis caused by *Pityrosporum* spp.

**Dosage and administration** Nizoral cream should be applied to the infected areas once or twice daily, depending on the severity of the infection.

The treatment should be continued until a few days after the disappearance of all signs and symptoms. The usual duration of treatment is: pityriasis versicolor 2–3 weeks, tinea corporis 3–4 weeks, tinea pedis 4–6 weeks.

The diagnosis should be reconsidered if no clinical improvement is noted after 4 weeks. General measures in regard to hygiene should be observed to control sources of infection or reinfection.

Seborrhoeic dermatitis is a chronic condition and relapse is highly likely.

**Contra-indications, warnings, etc**
*Contra-indications:* Nizoral cream is contra-indicated in patients who have shown hypersensitivity to any of the ingredients or to ketoconazole itself.

*Warnings:* Not for ophthalmic use.

If a potent topical corticosteroid has been used previously in the treatment of seborrhoeic dermatitis, a recovery period of 2 weeks should be allowed before using Nizoral cream, as an increased incidence of steroid induced skin sensitization has been reported when no recovery period is allowed.

*Side-effects:* A few instances of irritation, dermatitis, and burning sensation have been observed during treatment with Nizoral cream.

*Use in pregnancy:* After topical application, Nizoral cream is not systemically absorbed and does not produce detectable plasma concentrations. However as with any medication, Nizoral cream should only be used in pregnant women if its use is considered essential.

*Overdosage:* If accidental ingestion of Nizoral cream occurs, an appropriate method of gastric emptying may be used if considered appropriate.

**Pharmaceutical precautions** Store at 25°C or below.

**Legal category** POM.

**Package quantities** 30 g tubes.

**Further information** Dermatophytes and yeast infections of the skin such as tinea corporis, tinea cruris, tinea manus, tinea pedis, pityriasis versicolor, seborrhoeic dermatitis and cutaneous candidosis, are common infections in patients with HIV infection and AIDS. These patients may also be treated with Nizoral cream.

**Product licence number** 0242/0107.

## NIZORAL* SHAMPOO

**Presentation** 120 ml viscous pink liquid in plastic bottles containing ketoconazole 20 mg/ml. Nizoral shampoo also contains sodium lauryl ether sulphate, disodium monolauryl ether sulphosuccinate, coconut fatty acid diethanolamide, laurdimonium hydrolysed animal collagen, macrogol 120 methyl glucose dioleate, sodium chloride, sodium hydroxide, imidurea, hydrochloric acid, erythrosine (E127) and purified water.

**Uses:** Ketoconazole has a potent antimycotic activity against pathogenic dermatophytes and yeasts including *Pityrosporum* spp. Nizoral shampoo rapidly relieves the scaling and pruritus usually associated with seborrhoeic dermatitis, pityriasis capitis (dandruff) and pityriasis versicolor.

Nizoral shampoo is not systemically absorbed after topical administration, as blood levels are not detectable after chronic use. Nizoral shampoo is indicated for the prevention and treatment of seborrhoeic dermatitis, dandruff and pityriasis versicolor.

**Dosage and administration**
*Adults and children:* Shake the bottle well. Wash the hair or affected areas of the skin with Nizoral shampoo. Leave in contact for 3-5 minutes before rinsing thoroughly.

*Seborrhoeic dermatitis and dandruff: Treatment:* Use Nizoral shampoo twice weekly for 2-4 weeks.
*Prophylaxis:* Use Nizoral shampoo once every 1-2 weeks.

*Pityriasis versicolor: Treatment:* Use Nizoral shampoo once daily for a maximum of 5 days.
*Prophylaxis:* As patches of pityriasis versicolor become more apparent on exposure to the sun, Nizoral shampoo may be used once daily for a maximum of 3 days in a single treatment course before exposure to sunshine.

**Contra-indications, warnings, etc**
*Contra-indications:* Hypersensitivity to any of the ingredients.

*Interactions:* To prevent a rebound effect after stopping prolonged treatment with topical corticosteroids, it is recommended to continue applying the topical corticosteroid together with Nizoral shampoo and to subsequently and gradually withdraw the steroid therapy over a period of 2-3 weeks.

*Precautions:* Seborrhoeic dermatitis and dandruff are often associated with increased hair shedding, and this has also been reported, although rarely, with the use of Nizoral shampoo.

Keep out of the eyes. If the shampoo should get into the eyes, they should be bathed with cold water.

*Use in pregnancy:* Since no ketoconazole is detected in plasma following topical administration, pregnancy and lactation are not a contra-indication for the use of Nizoral shampoo.

*Side-effects:* As with other shampoos, a local burning sensation, itching, irritation and oily/dry hair may occur, but are rare, when using Nizoral shampoo. In rare instances, mainly in patients with chemically damaged hair or grey hair, a discolouration of the hair has been observed.

*Accidental ingestion:* In the event of accidental ingestion, only supportive measures should be carried out. In order to avoid aspiration, neither emesis nor gastric lavage should be instigated.

**Pharmaceutical precautions** Store at 25°C or below.

**Legal category** POM.

**Package quantities** 120 ml bottles.

**Further information** Seborrhoeic dermatitis, pityriasis capitis (dandruff) and pityriasis versicolor are common infections in patients with HIV infection and AIDS. These patients may also be treated with Nizoral shampoo.

**Product licence number** 0242/0139

## ORAP*

**Presentation** White, scored, uncoated tablets marked 'JANSSEN' on one side and 0/2 on the other, each contains 2 mg pimozide. The tablets also contain lactose and sucrose as inactive ingredients.

Pale green, cross-scored, uncoated tablets marked 'JANSSEN' on one side, each contains 4 mg pimozide. The tablets also contain E132, E172 as inactive ingredients.

White, scored, uncoated tablets marked 'JANSSEN' on one side and 0/10 on the other, each contains 10 mg pimozide. The tablets also contain lactose, as an inactive ingredient.

**Uses** Orap is an anti-psychotic of the diphenylbutylpiperidine series and is indicated in:

Chronic schizophrenia, for the treatment of symptoms and prevention of relapse.

Other psychoses, especially paranoid and monosymptomatic hypochondriacal psychoses (eg delusional parasitosis).

**Dosage and administration** Orap is intended for once daily oral administration in adults and children over 12 years of age.

Since individual response to anti-psychotic drugs is variable, dosage should be individually determined and is best initiated and titrated under close clinical supervision. In determining the initial dose, consideration should be given to the patient's age, severity of symptoms and previous response to other neuroleptic drugs. Dose increases should be made at weekly intervals or longer, and by increments of 2–4 mg in the daily dose.

The patients should be reviewed regularly to ensure the minimum effective dose is being used.

*Chronic schizophrenia:* The dose ranges between 2 and 20 mg daily, with 2 mg as a starting dose. This may be increased according to response and tolerance to achieve an optimum dose.

*Paranoid states and monosymptomatic hypochondriacal psychosis (MHP):* An initial dose of 4 mg daily which may then be gradually increased, if necessary, according to response to a maximum of 16 mg daily.

*Use in elderly:* Elderly patients require half the normal starting dose of pimozide.

**Contra-indications, warnings, etc**
*Contra-indications:* In common with several other neuroleptics, pimozide has been reported to prolong the QT interval. It is, therefore, contra-indicated in patients with a pre-existing congenital prolongation of QT and in patients with a history of cardiac arrhythmias.

Orap is also contra-indicated in patients with severe central nervous system depression and in patients with a known hypersensitivity to pimozide or other diphenylbutyl-piperidine derivatives. Orap should not be used in patients with depression or Parkinson's syndrome.

*Use in pregnancy and lactation:* The safety of Orap in human pregnancy has not been established. Studies in animals have not demonstrated teratogenic effects. As with other drugs, it is not advisable to administer Orap in pregnancy.

Orap may be excreted in breast milk. If the use of Orap is considered essential, breast feeding should be discontinued.

*Precautions and warnings:* Please also refer to the drug interactions section.

Caution is advised in patients with hepatic or renal dysfunction, phaeochromocytoma, thyrotoxicosis, epilepsy and conditions predisposing to epilepsy (e.g. alcohol withdrawal and brain damage).

It is recommended that a baseline ECG is undertaken in all patients prior to commencing treatment with pimozide in view of the cardiac contra-indications and in order to identify possible subsequent electrocardiographic changes. It is further recommended that an ECG is repeated annually or earlier if clinically indicated. Periodic assessment of cardiac function should be undertaken in those patients receiving pimozide in excess of 16 mg daily. If repolarisation changes (prolongation of QT interval, T-wave or U-wave changes) appear or arrhythmias develop, treatment should be reviewed and either gradually withdrawn or the dose reduced under close supervision.

There is potentially an increased risk of inducing cardiac rhythm disorders when pimozide is combined with macrolides and therefore concomitant use is not recommended.

Drugs which may prolong the QT interval (such as certain anti-malarials, anti-arrhythmics and certain anti-histamines) or cause electrolyte disturbances are not recommended in patients receiving long-term pimozide (please also refer to the drug interactions section).

Electrolyte disturbances, notably hypokalaemia, should also be considered a risk factor.

As with other neuroleptics, cases of sudden unexpected death have been rarely reported with pimozide (generally in doses in excess of the current recommended maximum of 20 mg per day). Whilst the cause of death in these cases is not known with certainty, it is postulated that the QT prolongation seen with pimozide in some patients may have made the patients susceptible to some form of fatal arrhythmia (e.g. Torsades de Pointes). Whilst some of these patients were taking pimozide as a sole therapy, the remainder were also taking other drugs, including neuroleptics, implicated in the aetiology of arrhythmias.

In schizophrenia, the response to antipsychotic drug treatment may be delayed. If drugs are withdrawn, recurrence of symptoms may not become apparent for several weeks or months.

Acute withdrawal symptoms, including nausea, vomiting and insomnia, have very rarely been described after abrupt cessation of high doses of antipsychotic drugs. Gradual withdrawal is advisable.

*Effects on driving ability and use of machinery:* Orap may impair alertness, especially at the start of treatment. These effects may be potentiated by alcohol. Patients should be warned of the risks of sedation and advised not to drive or operate machinery during treatment until their susceptibility is known.

*Drug interactions:* Please also refer to the precautions and warnings section. As with all neuroleptics, Orap may increase the central nervous system depression produced by other CNS depressant drugs, including alcohol, hypnotics, sedatives or strong analgesics.

Orap may impair the antiparkinson effect of levodopa. The dosage of anticonvulsants may need to be increased to take account of the lowered seizure threshold.

Concurrent treatment with neuroleptics should be kept to a minimum as they may predispose to the cardiotoxic effects of pimozide. Particular care should be exercised in patients who are using depot neuroleptics. Low potency neuroleptics such as chlorpromazine and thioridazine should not be used concomitantly with pimozide.

Concurrent use of pimozide with drugs which also have arrhythmogenic potential (such as antiarrhythmic agents and tricyclic antidepressants) is not recommended.

Concurrent use of pimozide with macrolides such as erythromycin, clarithromycin and azithromycin is not recommended.

Drugs which may prolong the QT interval, such as quinine and mefloquine; amiodarone, bretylium, disopyramide, procainamide, quinidine and sotalol; terfenadine and astemizole, are not recommended in patients receiving long-term pimozide treatment.

Concurrent use of drugs causing electrolyte imbalance is not recommended and hypokalaemia should be avoided. Diuretics should be avoided but if necessary, potassium-sparing diuretics are preferred.

*Side-effects:* In common with all neuroleptics, extrapyramidal symptoms may occur. Antiparkinson agents should not be prescribed routinely because of the possible risk of impairing the efficacy of Orap. They should only be given as required.

Tardive dyskinesia is common among patients treated with moderate to high doses of antipsychotic drugs for prolonged periods of time and may prove irreversible, particularly in patients over 50 years of age.

The potential seriousness and unpredictability of tardive dyskinesia and the fact that it has occasionally been reported to occur when neuroleptic antipsychotic drugs have been prescribed for a relatively short period in low dosage means that the prescribing of such agents requires especially careful assessment of risk versus benefit. Tardive dyskinesia can be precipitated or aggravated by antiparkinson drugs. Short-term dyskinesias may occur after abrupt drug withdrawal.

Epileptic fits have been reported even in low dosage. The elderly may be more liable to experience adverse effects.

Dose-related side effects, including drowsiness, insomnia, anxiety, and gastrointestinal symptoms, such as nausea, constipation or dyspepsia may occur. Dizziness, vertigo, weakness, excessive sweating, headache, dry mouth, loss of libido, impotence and hypotension have been reported, but autonomic symptoms are infrequent. QT-interval prolongation and/or ventricular arrhythmias have rarely been reported, and predominantly with high doses and in predisposed patients. Hypersensitivity reactions such as skin rash, itching, shortness of breath or swollen face have also rarely been reported.

Hormonal effects of antipsychotic neuroleptic drugs include hyperprolactinaemia, which may cause galactorrhoea, gynaecomastia and oligo- or amenorrhoea. Very rarely, cases have been reported of hyponatraemia, either due to polydipsia or to the Syndrome of Inappropriate Secretion of Anti-Diuretic Hormone. Neuroleptics may very rarely be associated with body temperature dysregulation.

Glycosuria has been reported.

In common with other antipsychotics, pimozide has been associated with rare cases of neuroleptic malignant syndrome, an idiosyncratic response characterised by hyperthermia, muscle rigidity, autonomic instability, altered consciousness and coma. Signs of autonomic dysfunction such as tachycardia, labile arterial pressure and sweating may precede the onset of hyperthermia, acting as early warning signs. Recovery usually occurs within five to seven days of antipsychotic withdrawal. Affected patients should be carefully monitored. Dantrolene sodium, bromocriptine mesylate and ECT have all been reported as offering benefit in some patients with neuroleptic malignant syndrome.

*Overdosage:* In general, the signs and symptoms of overdosage with Orap would be an exaggeration of known pharmacological effects, the most prominent of which would be severe extrapyramidal symptoms, hypotension or sedation. The risk of cardiac arrhythmias, possibly associated with QT-prolongation, should be considered. The patient may appear comatose with respiratory depression and hypotension which could be severe enough to produce a shock-like state.

*Treatment:* There is no specific antidote to pimozide. Gastric lavage, establishment of a patent airway and, if necessary, mechanically assisted respiration are advised. Electrocardiographic monitoring should commence immediately and continue until the ECG returns to normal. Hypotension and circulatory collapse may be counteracted by the use of intravenous fluids, plasma or concentrated albumin, and vasopressor agents such as noradrenaline. Adrenaline should not be used.

In cases of severe extrapyramidal symptoms, antiparkinson medication should be administered.

Because of the long half life of pimozide, patients who have taken an overdose should be observed for at least 4 days.

**Pharmaceutical precautions** Nil.

**Legal category** POM.

**Package quantities** Orap tablets each containing 2 mg pimozide are supplied in packs of 100.

Orap tablets each containing 4 mg pimozide are supplied in packs of 100.

Orap tablets each containing 10 mg pimozide are supplied in packs of 100.

**Further information** The mean serum elimination half-life of pimozide in schizophrenic patients is approximately 55 hours. This is highly variable and may be as long as 150 hours in some individuals. There is a 13-fold interindividual difference in the area under the serum pimozide concentration-time curve and an equivalent degree of variation in peak serum levels among patients studied. The significance of this is unclear since there are few correlations between plasma levels and clinical findings.

**Product licence numbers**

| | |
|---|---|
| Orap 2 mg | 0242/5010R |
| Orap 4 mg | 0242/0038R |
| Orap 10 mg | 0242/0069R |

## ORTHO* DIENOESTROL CREAM

**Presentation** A white non-staining cream containing 0.01% w/w dienoestrol.

**Uses** For intravaginal use only. Indicated in the treatment of atrophic vaginitis and kraurosis vulvae in post menopausal women, and for the treatment of pruritus vulvae and dyspareunia when associated with the atrophic vaginal epithelium.

**Dosage and administration** Given for short term use only. The lowest dose that will control symptoms should be chosen and medication should be discontinued as promptly as possible.

Attempts to discontinue or taper medication should be made at three to six month intervals, following physical examination. The usual dosage range is one or two applicatorfuls per day for one or two weeks, then gradually reduced to one half initial dosage for a similar period. A maintenance dose of one applicatorful, one to three times a week, may be used after restoration of the vaginal mucosa has been achieved. If the treatment is continued, treated patients with an intact uterus should be monitored closely for signs of endometrial cancer and appropriate diagnostic measures should be taken to rule out malignancy in the event of persistent or recurring abnormal vaginal bleeding.

Studies of the addition of a progestin for seven or more days of a cycle of oestrogen administration have reported a lowered incidence of endometrial hyperplasia. Morphological and biochemical studies of endometrium suggest that 10 to 13 days of progestin are needed to provide maximal maturation of the endometrium and to eliminate any hyperplastic changes.

In women with an intact uterus the addition of a progestogen is essential. There are possible additional risks which may be associated with the inclusion of progestin in oestrogen replacement regimens. The potential risks include adverse effects on carbohydrate and lipid metabolism.

As a general rule it is advisable that patients receiving any form of oestrogen replacement therapy should have a complete physical examination at least once a year.

**Contra-indications, warnings, etc** Pregnancy is an absolute contra-indication to the use of Dienoestrol cream since it may be harmful to the developing foetus.

Oestrogens should not be used in women with any of the other following conditions: known or suspected oestrogen-dependent neoplasia; endometrial hyperplasia; uterine fibromyomata; undiagnosed abnormal genital bleeding; cardiovascular disorders, eg thrombophlebitis, thrombosis or thromboembolic disorders; severe liver disease; porphyria, hypersensitivity to peanuts or arachis oil.

*Thromboembolic disorders:* While an increased rate of thromboembolic and thrombotic disease in post-menopausal users of oestrogen has not been found this does not rule out the possibility that such an increase may be present or that subgroups of women who have underlying risk factors or who are receiving relatively large doses of oestrogen may have increased risk. Therefore oestrogens should not be used in persons with active thrombophlebitis or thromboembolic disorders, and they should not be used (except in treatment of malignancy) in persons with a history of such disorders. If any signs of thrombosis develop, whether cardiovascular or cerebrovascular, in patients receiving oestrogen, discontinue treatment. Oestrogen treatment should be stopped before surgery in order to decrease the risk of deep vein thrombosis.

Prolonged exposure to unopposed oestrogen may increase the risk of development of endometrial carcinoma, induction of other malignant neoplasms, and the risk of cancer of the breast: long term continuous administration of natural and synthetic oestrogens in certain animal species increases the frequency of carcinomas of the breast, cervix, vagina and liver. There is now evidence that oestrogens increase the risk of carcinoma of the endometrium in humans. At the present time there is no satisfactory evidence that oestrogens given to post-menopausal women increase the risk of cancer of the breast, although a recent long-term follow up of a single physician has raised this possibility. However, because of animal data there is a need for caution in prescribing oestrogens for women with a strong family history of breast cancer or who have breast nodules, fibrocystic disease, or abnormal mammograms.

*Gall bladder disease:* A recent study has reported a two to three-fold increase in the risk of surgically confirmed gall bladder disease in women receiving post-menopausal oestrogens, similar to the two-fold increase previously noted in users of oral contraceptives.

*Hepatic adenoma:* Benign hepatic adenomas appear to be associated with the use of oral contraceptives. Although benign, and rare, these may rupture and may cause death through intra-abdominal haemorrhage. Such lesions have not yet been reported in association with other oestrogen or progestogen preparations but should be considered in oestrogen users having abdominal pain and tenderness, abdominal mass, or hypovolemic shock.

*Elevated blood pressure:* It has been reported that this may occur with the use of oestrogens in the menopause and blood pressure should be monitored with oestrogen use, especially if high doses are used. Treatment should be discontinued with emergent or increasing hypertension.

*Precautions:* A complete medical and family history should be taken prior to the initiation of any oestrogen therapy. The pretreatment and periodic physical examinations should include special reference to blood pressure, breasts, abdomen, and pelvic organs, and should include a Papanicolaou smear.

A pathologist should be advised of oestrogen therapy when relevant specimens are submitted. Certain endocrine and liver function tests may be affected by oestrogen containing products. These are:

Increased BSP retention.

Increased prothrombin and factors VII, VIII, IX, and X; decreased antithrombin 3, increased norepinephrine-induced platelet aggregability.

Impaired glucose tolerance.

Increased thyroid binding globulin (TBG) leading to increased circulating total thyroid hormone, as measured by PBI, T4 by column or T4 by RIA. Free T3 resin uptake is decreased, reflecting the elevated TRG; free T4 is unaltered.

Decreased pregnanediol excretion.

Reduced response to metyrapone.

Reduced serum folate concentration.

Increased serum triglyceride and phospholipid concentration.

Certain patients may develop undesirable manifestations of excessive oestrogenic stimulations, such as abnormal or excessive uterine bleeding, mastodynia, etc. Pre-existing uterine fibroids may increase in size during oestrogen use.

Patients with a past history of jaundice during pregnancy have an increased risk of recurrence of jaundice while receiving oestrogen. The medication should be discontinued while the cause is investigated.

Oestrogens may cause fluid retention. Conditions possibly affected by this factor such as epilepsy, migraine and cardiac or renal dysfunction require careful monitoring.

Oestrogens should be used with caution in patients with:

Metabolic bone diseases that are associated with hypercalcaemia.

Impaired liver function.

A history of mental depression.

Diabetes.

Contact lenses.

Oestrogens should be used judiciously in patients in whom bone growth is not complete.

Ortho Dienoestrol is generally well tolerated. There have been occasional reports of burning, itching and irritation. The doctor should also be aware of those adverse reactions reported to occur with systemic administration of oestrogens.

*Genito-urinary tract:* intermenstrual bleeding, increase in the size of uterine fibromyomata, change in amount of cervical secretion.

*Breast:* tenderness, enlargement, secretion.

*Gastrointestinal tract:* nausea, vomiting, cholestatic jaundice.

*Skin:* erythema nodosum, rash, chloasma.

*Eyes:* corneal discomfort if contact lenses are used.

*CNS:* headache, migraine, mood changes.

*Metabolic:* reduced glucose tolerance and changes in body weight.

Other events normally associated with the use of oral contraceptives may result from prolonged use of unopposed oestrogens.

*Overdosage:* Ortho Dienoestrol Cream is intended for intravaginal use. If accidental ingestion of large quantities of the product occurs, an appropriate method of gastric emptying may be used if considered desirable. Overdosage may cause nausea, and in females withdrawal bleeding may occur.

**Pharmaceutical precautions** Store at room temperature, not exceeding 25°C.

**Legal category** POM.

**Package quantities** Tube containing 78 g with the Ortho Plastic Vaginal Applicator.

**Further information** Nil.

**Product licence number** 0242/0244.

## ORTHO-GYNEST* CREAM AND PESSARIES

**Presentation** Cream: White to faint yellowish cream with fat like odour containing 0.01% w/w oestriol. Pessaries: White pessaries each containing 0.5 mg oestriol and melting at 37°C.

**Uses** Oestriol is a naturally occurring oestrogen which exerts specific actions on the vulva, vagina and cervix.

Ortho-Gynest Cream and Pessaries are indicated for the treatment of atrophic vaginitis and kraurosis vulvae in post menopausal women, and for the treatment of pruritus vulvae and dyspareunia when associated with atrophic vaginal epithelium.

For intravaginal use only.

**Dosage and administration** The lowest dose that will control symptoms should be chosen and medication should be discontinued as promptly as possible. Attempts to taper and discontinue medication should be made at three to six month intervals following initiation of therapy and in conjunction with physical examination.

The recommended initial daily dose is one applicatorful or one pessary inserted high into the vagina, preferably in the evening.

A maintenance dose of one applicatorful or one pessary twice a week may be used after restoration of the vaginal mucosa has been achieved.

**Contra-indications, warnings, etc.** Prolonged exposure to unopposed oestrogens may increase the risk of development of endometrial carcinoma. Although publications indicate that oestriol may occupy a somewhat different position with respect to mammary and endometrial carcinomas than other oestrogens, contra-indications for treatment with Ortho-Gynest Cream and Pessaries should be the same as for other oestrogen products.

*Oestrogens should not be used in women with any of the following conditions:* known or suspected cancer of the breast, known or suspected oestrogen-dependent neoplasia, undiagnosed abnormal genital bleeding, active thrombophlebitis or thromboembolic disorders, a past history of thrombophlebitis, thrombosis or thromboembolic disorders. Markedly impaired liver function. Congenital or existing disorders of lipid metabolism. History during pregnancy of idiopathic jaundice, severe pruritus, herpes gestationis or otosclerosis. Dubin-Johnson syndrome. Rotor syndrome. Ortho-Gynest Cream is contraindicated in women with hypersensitivity to arachis oil or peanuts.

Ortho-Gynest Cream and Pessaries are contraindicated in pregnancy; therapy should be discontinued immediately pregnancy is suspected.

An increased risk of gall-bladder disease has been reported in women receiving post-menopausal oestrogens, similar to the increase noted in users of oral contraceptives.

Benign hepatic adenomas appear to be associated with the use of oral contraceptives and although rare, these may rupture and cause death, through intra-abdominal haemorrhage. Such lesions have not yet been reported in association with other oestrogen or progestogen preparations but should be considered in oestrogen users having abdominal pain and tenderness, abdominal mass or hypovolemic shock.

It has been reported that elevated blood pressure may occur with the use of oestrogens in menopausal women and blood pressure should be monitored with oestrogen use.

*Precautions:* A complete medical and family history should be taken prior to the initiation of any oestrogen therapy. The pre-treatment and periodic physical examinations should include special reference to blood pressure, breasts, abdomen, and pelvic organs and should include a Papanicolaou smear.

A pathologist should be advised of oestrogen therapy when relevant specimens are submitted.

Certain patients may develop undesirable manifestations of excessive oestrogenic stimulation such as abnormal or excessive uterine bleeding, mastodynia etc. Bleeding occurring during therapy should be investigated to exclude serious concomitant pathology. Pre-existing uterine fibroids may increase in size during oestrogen use.

Oestrogen may aggravate cases of porphyria.

Patients with a past history of jaundice during pregnancy have an increased risk of recurrence of jaundice while receiving oestrogen therapy. If jaundice develops in any patient receiving oestrogen, the medication should be discontinued while the cause is investigated.

Oestrogens should be used with caution in patients with endometriosis.

*Overdosage:* Ortho-Gynest Cream and Pessaries are intended for intravaginal use. If accidental ingestion of large quantities of the product occurs, an appropriate method of gastric emptying may be used if considered desirable.

**Pharmaceutical precautions** Store at room temperature (not exceeding 25°C).

**Legal category** POM.

**Package quantities** *Cream:* Tube containing 80 g with the Ortho* Plastic Vaginal Applicator.

*Pessaries:* Pack of 15 individually sealed pessaries.

**Further information** Nil.

**Product licence numbers**

| | |
|---|---|
| Cream | 0242/0249 |
| Pessaries | 0242/0250 |

## ORTHO*GYNE-T* 380 SLIMLINE INTRAUTERINE COPPER CONTRACEPTIVE DEVICE

**Presentation** Each device consists of a polyethylene 'T' shaped support with 180 mg pure copper wire (providing a surface area of 320 mm²) wound around the vertical section of the 'T' and one collar with 70 mg pure copper providing an exposed surface area of 30 mm² on the distal portion of each transverse arm. The support is impregnated with a radiopaque substance and has a polyethylene suture attached to the base of the 'T'.

**Uses** Contraception.

**Dosage and administration** One device is inserted by its introducer into the uterus preferably at the end of the menstrual period. The device should be removed after eight years of use. If continued contraception is required a new device may be inserted.

**Contra-indications, warnings, etc.**

*Contra-indications: Absolute Contra-indications:*

(i)   Pregnancy or suspected pregnancy.
(ii)  Known or suspected malignancy of the genital tract including undiagnosed vaginal bleeding or an unresolved abnormal cervical smear.
(iii) Active pelvic inflammatory disease.
(iv)  Copper allergy or Wilson's disease.

*Relative contra-indications:*

(i)    Nulliparity.
(ii)   Previous ectopic pregnancy.
(iii)  History of pelvic inflammatory disease or pregnancy related infection.
(iv)   Congenital or acquired uterine abnormalities resulting in uterine cavity distortion, including fibroids, previous uterine incision or perforation, or tubal surgery.
(v)    Unresolved lower genital tract infection.
(vi)   Menorrhagia.
(vii)  Significant anaemia.
(viii) Severe dysmenorrhoea.
(ix)   Immunosuppression of any cause, including chronic corticosteroid therapy.
(x)    History of multiple sexual partners or sexually transmitted diseases.
(xi)   Valvular heart disease.
(xii)  Anticoagulant therapy.

*NB:* Nulliparity in combination with any of:
1. Previous pelvic inflammatory disease;
2. Previous ectopic pregnancy; or
3. History of multiple sexual partners or sexually transmitted diseases.
May be considered as an absolute contra-indication to the use of an IUCD.

*Warnings and precautions:*

*Prior to insertion:* A thorough history and physical examination, including a pelvic examination and cervical cytology (if a smear has not recently been taken) should be performed, to exclude pregnancy, infection, other abnormalities of the uterus and to determine the size and position of the uterus.

Vaginal or cervical infection should be appropriately treated before insertion is considered.

IUCDs should also be used with caution in patients with hypermenorrhoea, or receiving coagulopathy.

It has been reported that IUCDs may be less effective in insulin-dependent diabetics.

*Insertion:* Insertion should be as early as possible in the menstrual cycle unless alternative methods of effective contraception have been used throughout the cycle.

If the device is being inserted into a patient with known or suspected cardiac abnormalities then antibiotic cover is required both at insertion and removal.

The possibility of a seizure being precipitated in an epileptic, at or shortly after insertion should be borne in mind.

Insertion of an IUCD into a uterine cavity measuring less than 6.5 cm by sounding may increase the incidence of expulsion, bleeding pain and perforation. Expulsion rate can also be increased when insertions are made before normal uterine involution occurs following delivery.

*Precautions in use:* The patient should be re-examined 3 months after insertion, and thereafter at yearly intervals to ensure the device is still in place.

The patient should be advised to contact her doctor immediately if she misses a menstrual period, has any other reason to think she may be pregnant, or if any other unwanted symptoms develop.

Abnormal bleeding in an established IUCD user is not necessarily due to the device and should always be fully investigated to exclude other pathology.

Medical diathermy or ultrasonic therapy must not be applied to the user's abdomen or sacral region, since heating of the copper may cause injury.

*Removal of Ortho Gyne-T 380 Slimline:* Ideally, to avoid the risk of pregnancy, the device should not be removed between the end of a menstrual cycle and the 20th day of a 28 day cycle unless immediate replacement by a new device is required, or unless an additional contraceptive has been used for the previous 7 days. If removal is essential (e.g. to treat severe pelvic infection) post-coital contraception should be considered.

The device should be removed for the following reasons:

(i)   Excessive and persistent bleeding or cramping.
(ii)  Perforation of the uterus and location of the device outside the uterine cavity. In this case, hospital investigation and surgical removal will be required.
(iii) Partial downward displacement of the device within the cervical canal.
(iv)  Development of either a Papanicolaou smear class III or higher, or treatment resistant cervical erosions, or suspected dysplasia or neoplasia of the genital tract.
(v)   Pelvic infection resistant to treatment.

(vi)  Menorrhagia producing significant anaemia or intractable pain.
(vii) For women who have reached the menopause the IUCD should be removed one year after the last period.

*Lost threads:* The patient should check periodically, particularly after menstruation to ensure that the threads still protrude from the cervix. She should return to her doctor if she becomes aware that the device has been expelled.

In the absence of a detectable thread, a uterine sound should be introduced into the endometrial cavity following the same technique as for insertion. In most cases the IUCD can be detected by the sound. If the threads have retracted into the uterine cavity, they may be brought back down through the cervix and into the vagina. In such cases there is usually no need to replace the device providing there is no evidence of infection.

If the device cannot be detected by the sound, ultrasound or X-ray techniques may be required.

*Pregnancy and lactation:* Use is contra-indicated in pregnancy, suspicion of pregnancy or patients with a history of ectopic pregnancy.

Should intra-uterine pregnancy occur with a device in situ there is an increased risk of spontaneous abortion which may become infected. If pregnancy occurs, the IUCD should be removed provided there is no difficulty in doing so, as this will reduce the risk of abortion and subsequent complications.

If the thread is not visible then it is recommended that the device is left in-situ until the pregnancy goes to term or a decision is made to terminate the pregnancy.

The risk of ectopic pregnancy and the increased incidence of septic abortion (associated in some instances with septicaemia, septic shock and death) are reportedly higher in women who become pregnant with an IUCD in situ.

Such patients should be closely observed under specialist care and told to report immediately all abnormal occurrences such as 'flu-like' symptoms, fever, cramp-like pain, bleeding or excessive discharge, as onset of septicaemia associated with septic abortion may be insidious with general symptoms rather than initial signs of spontaneous abortion.

The long term effects of copper on the foetus are not known.

May be used during lactation.

*Side-effects:* Side-effects include uterine or cervical perforation, displacement, pelvic infection, heavy menses, dysmenorrhoea, and allergy. On insertion some pain and bleeding may occur, with epileptic seizure, or vasovagal attack occurring occasionally.

*On insertion:* Perforation may rarely occur at the time of insertion. Partial penetration of the uterine wall may occur, allowing complete penetration days or weeks later. This may lead to pelvic haematoma or abscess, or peritonitis. Suspicion of such events requires urgent gynaecological referral.

Pain and bleeding may occur on insertion and removal of the device. Syncope or bradycardia may occur in some women during insertion or removal of an IUCD. In the event of early signs of vasovagal attack, insertion may need to be abandoned or the device removed. The women should be kept supine, the head lowered and the legs elevated to the vertical position if necessary in order to restore cerebral blood flow. A clear airway must be maintained. Persistent bradycardia may be controlled with intravenous atropine.

If oxygen is available it may be administered.

Uterine pain during the days following insertion usually responds to simple analgesics.

*After insertion:* Partial or complete expulsion of the device may occur.

An increased incidence of pelvic inflammatory disease associated with the use of IUCDs has been reported. Patients experiencing abdominal pain should be investigated further to find the cause, as this may be a sign of pelvic infection.

Bleeding and spotting often occur during the first cycle post insertion with prolongation of menstruation and increased menstrual flow experienced by some women.

In addition, the following adverse reactions have rarely been reported: Dysmenorrhoea may occur or be aggravated. Amenorrhoea, or delayed menses. Pelvic infection (with a consequent risk of future infertility), backache, pains in the legs, dyspareunia, infections of the genito-urinary tract and reproductive organs. Increased risk of septic abortion or septicaemia, ectopic pregnancy and urticarial allergic skin reactions. Difficult removal, uterine embedment, neurovascular episodes. Fragmentation of the IUCD and breakage of the string may also occur.

Very rarely weight fluctuation, nervousness, anaemia, cervical erosion and cystic masses in the pelvis have been reported.

*Overdosage:* Not applicable.

**Pharmaceutical precautions** If the seal of the sterile pack is broken the device inside should not be used.

**Legal category** POM. Also available through Family Planning Clinics.

**Package quantities** Each sterile Ortho Gyne-T 380 Slimline Intrauterine Copper Contraceptive Device unit is supplied in a sealed transparent envelope. Full fitting instructions and advice for the patient are supplied with each device.

**Further information** Nil.

**Product licence number** 0076/0093.

## ORTHO-CREME* CONTRACEPTIVE CREAM

**Qualitative and quantitative composition** Contains 2.0% w/w of nonoxynol-9.

**Pharmaceutical form** Cream.

**Clinical particulars**
*Therapeutic indications:* For use as a spermicidal contraceptive in conjunction with barrier methods of contraception.

*Posology and method of administration:* For topical intravaginal administration.

For use by adult females only.

The cream should be spread over the surface of the diaphragm which will be in contact with the cervix and on the rim. The diaphragm must be allowed to remain *in situ* for at least six to eight hours after coitus. A fresh application of cream or other spermicides, e.g. Orthoforms Contraceptive Pessaries, must be made prior to any subsequent act of coitus within this period of time, without removing the diaphragm. (A vaginal applicator should be used for inserting more cream.)

Douching is not recommended, but if it is desired it should be deferred for at least six hours after intercourse.

*Contra-indications:* Hypersensitivity to nonoxynol-9 or to any component of the preparation.

Patients with absent vaginal sensation, eg paraplegics and quadriplegics.

*Special warnings and special precautions for use:* Spermicidal intravaginal preparations are intended for use in conjunction with barrier methods of contraception such as condoms, diaphragms and caps.

Where avoidance of pregnancy is important the choice of contraceptive method should be made in consultation with a doctor or a family planning clinic.

If vaginal or penile irritation occurs discontinue use. If symptoms worsen or continue for more than 48 hours medical advice should be sought.

*Interactions with other medicaments and other forms of interaction:* None known.

*Pregnancy and lactation:* There is no evidence from animal and human studies that nonoxynol-9 is teratogenic. Human epidemiological studies have not shown any firm evidence of adverse effects on the foetus. However some studies have shown that nonoxynol-9 may be embryotoxic in animals. This product should not be used if pregnancy is suspected or confirmed. Animal studies have detected nonoxynol-9 in milk after intravaginal administration. Use by lactating women has not been studied.

*Effects on ability to drive and use machines:* None known.

*Undesirable effects:* May cause irritation of the vagina or penis.

*Overdose:* If taken orally the surfactant properties of this preparation may cause gastric irritation. General supportive therapy should be carried out. Hepatic and renal function should be monitored if medically indicated.

**Pharmacological properties**
*Pharmacodynamic properties:* The standard *in vitro* test (Sander-Cramer) evaluating the effect of nonoxynol-9 on animal sperm motility has shown the compound to be a potent spermicide.

The site of action of nonoxynol-9 has been determined as the sperm cell membrane. The lipoprotein membrane is disrupted, increasing permeability, with subsequent loss of cell components and decreased motility. A similar effect on vaginal epithelial and bacterial cells is also found.

*Pharmacokinetic properties:* The intravaginal absorption and excretion of radiolabelled ($^{14}$C) nonoxynol-9 has been studied in non-pregnant rats and rabbits and in pregnant rats. No appreciable difference was found in the extent or rate of absorption in pregnant and non-pregnant animals. Plasma levels peaked at about one hour and recovery from urine as unchanged nonoxynol-9 accounted for approximately 15-25% and faeces approximately 70% of the administered dose as unchanged nonoxynol-9. Less than 0.3% was found in the milk of lactating rats. No metabolites were detected in any of the samples analysed.

*Preclinical safety data:* Not applicable.

**Pharmaceutical particulars**
*List of excipients:* Benzoic acid (E 210); cetyl alcohol; lavender compound 13091; methyl hydroxybenzoate (E218); propyl hydroxybenzoate (E216); propylene glycol; sodium carboxymethylcellulose; sodium lauryl sulphate; stearic acid; triethanolmine; acetic acid glacial; castor oil; potassium hydroxide; sorbic acid (E200); purified water.

*Incompatibilities:* Not applicable.

*Shelf life:* 3 years.

*Special precautions for storage:* Store at room temperature (at or below 25°C).

*Nature and contents of container:* Epoxy-resin lined aluminium tubes of 70 g with polyethylene cap.

*Instructions for use/handling:* Not applicable.

**Marketing authorisation number** 0242/0248

**Date of approval/revision of SPC** October 1996

**Legal category** GSL.

## ORTHO-NOVIN* 1/50 ORAL CONTRACEPTIVE TABLETS

**Presentation** Ortho-Novin oral contraceptive tablets are white, 1/4 inch diameter, circular tablets with flat faces and bevelled edges, engraved C over 150 on each face. Each tablet contains 1.0 mg norethisterone and 50 μg mestranol.

**Uses** Contraception and the recognised indications for such oestrogen/progestogen combinations.

*Action:* Through the mechanism of gonadotrophin suppression by the oestrogenic and progestational actions of the ingredients.

Although the primary mechanism of action is inhibition of ovulation, alterations to the cervical mucus and to the endometrium may also contribute to the efficacy of the product.

**Dosage and administration** It is preferable that tablet intake from the first pack is started on the first day of menstruation in which case no extra contraceptive precautions are necessary.

If menstruation has already begun (that is 2, 3 or 4 days previously), tablet taking should commence on day 5 of the menstrual period. In this case additional contraceptive precautions must be taken for the first 7 days of tablet taking. (See further information for additional contraceptive precautions).

If menstruation began more than 5 days previously then the patient should be advised to wait until her next menstrual period before starting to take Ortho-Novin.

*How to take Ortho-Novin:* One tablet is taken daily at the same time (preferably in the evening) without interruption for 21 days, followed by a break of 7 tablet-free days. Each subsequent pack is started after the 7 tablet-free days have elapsed. Additional contraceptive precautions are not then required.

*Use during pregnancy:* Ortho-Novin is contra-indicated for use during pregnancy or suspected pregnancy, since it has been suggested that combined oral contraceptives, in common with many other substances, might be capable of affecting the normal development of the child in the early stages of pregnancy. It can be definitely concluded, however, that, if a risk of abnormality exists at all, it must be very small.

*Post-partum administration:* Following a vaginal delivery, oral contraceptive administration to non-breast feeding mothers can be started 21 days post-partum, provided the patient is fully ambulant and there are no puerperal complications. No additional contraceptive precautions are required. If post-partum administration begins more than 21 days after delivery, additional contraceptive precautions are required for the first 7 days of pill-taking. If intercourse has taken place post-partum, oral contraceptive use should be delayed until the first day of the first menstrual period.

*N.B.* Mothers who are breast feeding should be advised not to use the combined pill since this may reduce the amount of breast-milk, but may be advised instead to use a progestogen-only pill (POP).

After miscarriage or abortion administration should start immediately in which case no additional contraceptive precautions are required.

*Changing from a 21 day pill or another 22 day pill to Ortho-Novin:* All tablets in the old pack should be finished. The first Ortho-Novin tablet is taken the next day i.e. no gap is left between taking tablets nor does the patient need to wait for her period to begin. Tablets should be taken as instructed in 'How to take Ortho-Novin'. Additional contraceptive precautions are not required. The patient will not have a period until the end of the first Ortho-Novin pack, but this is not harmful, nor does it matter if she experiences some bleeding on tablet-taking days.

*Changing from a combined Every Day Pill (28 day tablets) to Ortho-Novin:* Ortho-Novin should be started after taking the last active tablet from the 'Every Day Pill' pack (i.e. after taking 21 or 22 tablets). The first Ortho-Novin tablet is taken the next day i.e. no gap is left between taking tablets nor does the patient need to wait for her period to begin. Tablets should be taken as instructed in 'How to take Ortho-Novin'. Additional contraceptive precautions are not required. Remaining tablets from the Every Day (ED) pack should be discarded. The patient will not have a period until the end of the first Ortho-Novin pack, but this is not harmful, nor does it matter if she experiences some bleeding on tablet-taking days.

*Changing from a Progestogen-only Pill (POP or Mini Pill) to Ortho-Novin:* The first Ortho-Novin tablet should be taken on the first day of the period, even if the patient has already taken a mini pill on that day. Tablets should be taken as instructed in 'How to take Ortho-Novin'. Additional contraceptive precautions are not required. All the remaining progestogen-only pills in the mini pill pack should be discarded.

If the patient is taking a (mini) pill, then she may not always have a period, especially when she is breast feeding. The first Ortho-Novin tablet should be taken on the day after stopping the mini pill. All remaining pills in the mini pill packet must be discarded. Additional contraceptive precautions must be taken for the first 7 days.

*To skip a period:* To skip a period, a new pack of Ortho-Novin should be started on the day after finishing the current pack (the patient skips the tablet-free days). Tablet-taking should be continued in the usual way. During the use of the second pack she may experience slight spotting or break-through bleeding but contraceptive protection will not be diminished provided there are no tablet omissions.

The next pack of Ortho-Novin is started after the usual 7 tablet-free days, regardless of whether the period has completely finished or not.

*Reduced reliability:* The reliability of Ortho-Novin may be reduced under the following circumstances.

*Forgotten tablets:* For further advice on the above please see precautions and warnings.

*Vomiting or diarrhoea:* For further advice on the above, please see precautions and warnings.

*Interactions:* For further advice on the above, please see precautions and warnings.

**Contra-indications, warnings, etc**
*Absolute contra-indications:* Pregnancy or suspected pregnancy (that cannot yet be excluded).

Circulatory disorders (cardiovascular or cerebrovascular) such as thrombophlebitis and thromboembolic processes (or a history of these conditions), moderate to severe hypertension, hyperlipoproteinaemia. In addition the presence of more than one of the risk factors for arterial disease which are discussed under 'Serious adverse reactions'.

Severe liver disease, cholestatic jaundice or hepatitis (viral or non-viral) or a history of these conditions if the results of liver function tests have failed to return to normal, and for 3 months after liver function tests have been found to be normal; a history of jaundice of pregnancy or jaundice due to the use of steroids, Rotor syndrome and Dubin-Johnson syndrome, hepatic cell tumours and porphyria.

Cholelithiasis.

Known or suspected oestrogen-dependent tumours, (see 'Serious Adverse Reactions'); endometrial hyperplasia; undiagnosed vaginal bleeding.

Systemic lupus erythematosus or a history of this condition.

A history during pregnancy or previous use of steroids of: severe pruritus; herpes gestationis; a manifestation or deterioration of otosclerosis.

*Relative contra-indications:* If any of the relative contra-indications listed below is present, the benefits of oestrogen/progestogen-containing preparations must be weighed against the possible risk for each individual case and the patient kept under close supervision. In case of aggravation or appearance of any of these conditions whilst the patient is taking the pill, its use should be discontinued.

– Conditions implicating an increasing risk of developing venous thromboembolic complications, e.g. severe varicose veins or prolonged immobilisation or major surgery (see *Precautions and warnings*).
– Disorders of coagulation.
– Presence of any risk factor for arterial disease e.g.

smoking, hyperlipidaemia or hypertension (see *Serious adverse reactions*).
– Other conditions associated with an increased risk of circulatory disease such as latent or overt cardiac failure, renal dysfunction, or a history of these conditions.
– Epilepsy or a history of this condition.
– Migraine or a history of this condition.
– A history of cholelithiasis.
– Presence of any risk factor for oestrogen-dependent tumours; oestrogen-sensitive gynaecological disorders such as uterine fibromyomata and endometriosis (see also under *Serious adverse reactions*).
– Diabetes mellitus.
– Severe depression or a history of this condition. If this is accompanied by a disturbance in tryptophan metabolism, administration of vitamin B6 might be of therapeutic value.
– Sickle cell haemoglobinopathy, since under certain circumstances, e.g. during infections or anoxia, oestrogen-containing preparations may induce thromboembolic process in patients with this condition.
– If the results of liver function tests become abnormal, use should be discontinued.

*Precautions and warnings:*
*Reduced reliability:* When Ortho-Novin is taken according to the directions for use the occurrence of pregnancy is highly unlikely. However, the reliability of oral contraceptives may be reduced under the following circumstances:

*Forgotten tablets:* If the patient forgets to take a tablet, she should take it as soon as she remembers and take the next one at the normal time. This may mean that two tablets are taken in one day. Provided she is less than 12 hours late in taking her tablet, Ortho-Novin will still give contraceptive protection during this cycle and the rest of the pack should be taken as usual.
If she is more than 12 hours late in taking one or more tablets then she should take the last missed pill as soon as she remembers but leave the other missed pills in the pack. She should continue to take the rest of the pack as usual but must use extra precautions (e.g. sheath, diaphragm plus spermicide) and follow the '7-day rule' (see further information for 7-day rule). If there are 7 or more pills left in the pack after the missed and delayed pills then the usual 7-day break can be left before starting the next pack. If there are less than 7 pills left in the pack after the missed and delayed pills then when the pack is finished the next pack should be started the next day. If withdrawal bleeding does not occur at the end of the second pack then a pregnancy test should be performed.

*Vomiting or diarrhoea:* If after tablet intake vomiting or diarrhoea occurs, a tablet may not be absorbed properly by the body. If the symptoms disappear within 12 hours of tablet-taking, the patient should take an extra tablet from a spare pack and continue with the rest of the pack as usual.
However, if the symptoms continue beyond those 12 hours, additional contraceptive precautions are necessary for any sexual intercourse during the stomach or bowel upset and for the following 7 days (the patient must be advised to follow the '7-day rule').

*Change in bleeding pattern:* If after taking Ortho-Novin for several months there is a sudden occurrence of spotting or break-through bleeding (not observed in previous cycles) or the absence of withdrawal bleeding, contraceptive effectiveness may be reduced. If withdrawal bleeding fails to occur and none of the above mentioned events has taken place, pregnancy is highly unlikely and oral contraceptive use can be continued until the end of the next pack.
(If withdrawal bleeding fails to occur at the end of the second cycle, tablet intake should be discontinued and pregnancy excluded before oral contraceptive use can be resumed). However, if withdrawal bleeding is absent and any of the above mentioned events has occurred, tablet intake should be discontinued and pregnancy excluded before oral contraceptive use can be resumed.

*Interactions:* Irregular cycles and reduced reliability of oral contraceptives may occur when these preparations are used concomitantly with drugs such as anticonvulsants, barbiturates, antibiotics, (e.g. tetracyclines, ampicillin, rifampicin, etc.), griseofulvin, activated charcoal and certain laxatives. Special consideration should be given to patients being treated with antibiotics for acne. They should be advised to use a non-hormonal method of contraception, or to use an oral contraceptive containing a progestogen showing minimal androgenicity, which have been reported as helping to improve acne without using an antibiotic. Oral contraceptives may diminish glucose tolerance and increase the need for insulin or other antidiabetic drugs in diabetics.

*Medical examination/consultation:* A complete medical history and physical examination should be taken prior to the initiation or reinstitution of oral contraceptives and should be repeated periodically.
These physical examinations should include special reference to blood pressure, breasts, abdomen and pelvic organs, including cervical cytology and, where indicated by the medical or family history, relevant laboratory tests. Caution should be observed when prescribing oral contraceptives to young women whose cycles are not yet stabilised.

*Surgery, varicose veins or immobilisation:* In patients using oestrogen-containing preparations the risk of deep vein thrombosis may be temporarily increased when undergoing a major operation (eg abdominal, orthopaedic), any surgery to the legs, medical treatment for varicose veins or prolonged immobilisation. Therefore, it is advisable to discontinue oral contraceptive use at least 4 to 6 weeks prior to these procedures if performed electively and to (re)start not less than 2 weeks after full ambulation. The latter is also valid with regard to immobilisation after an accident or emergency surgery. In case of emergency surgery, thrombotic prophylaxis is usually indicated e.g. with subcutaneous heparin.

*Chloasma:* Chloasma may occasionally occur, especially in women with a history of chloasma gravidarum. Women with a tendency to chloasma should avoid exposure to the sun or ultraviolet radiation whilst taking this preparation. Chloasma is often not fully reversible.

*Laboratory tests:* The use of steroids may influence the results of certain laboratory tests. In the literature, at least a hundred different parameters have been reported to possibly be influenced by oral contraceptive use, predominantly by the oestrogenic component. Among these are: biochemical parameters of the liver, thyroid, adrenal and renal function, plasma levels of (carrier) proteins and lipid/lipoprotein fractions and parameters of coagulation and fibrinolysis.

*Adverse reactions:* Various adverse reactions have been associated with oral contraceptive use. The serious reactions are dealt with in more detail. The first appearance of symptoms indicative of any one of these reactions necessitates immediate cessation of oral contraceptive use while appropriate diagnostic and therapeutic measures are undertaken.

*Serious adverse reactions:* There is a general opinion, based on statistical evidence that users of combined oral contraceptives experience more often than non-users various disorders of the circulation. How often these disorders occur in users of modern low-oestrogen oral contraceptives is unknown, but there are reasons for suggesting that they may occur less often than with the older types of pill which contain more oestrogen.
Various reports have associated oral contraceptive use with the occurrence of deep venous thrombosis, pulmonary embolism and other embolisms. Other investigations of these oral contraceptives have suggested an increased risk or oestrogen and/or progestogen dose-dependent coronary and cerebrovascular accidents, predominantly in heavy smokers. Thrombosis has very rarely been reported to occur in other veins or arteries, e.g. hepatic, mesenteric, renal or retinal.
It should be noted that there is no consensus about the often contradictory findings obtained in early studies. The physician should bear in mind the possibility of vascular accidents occurring and that there may not be full recovery from such disorders and they may be fatal. The physician should take into account the presence of risk factors for arterial disease and deep venous thrombosis when prescribing oral contraceptives. Risk factors for arterial disease include smoking, the presence of hyperlipidaemia, hypertension or diabetes.
Signs and symptoms of a thrombotic event may include: sudden severe pain in the chest, whether or not reaching to the left arm; sudden breathlessness; any unusual severe, prolonged headache, especially if it occurs for the first time or gets progressively worse, or is associated with any of the following symptoms: sudden partial or complete loss of vision or diplopia, aphasia, vertigo, a bad fainting attack or collapse with or without focal epilepsy, weakness or very marked numbness suddenly affecting one side or one part of the body, motor disturbances; severe pain in the calf of one leg; acute abdomen.
Cigarette smoking increases the risk of serious cardiovascular adverse reactions to oral contraceptive use. The risk increases with age and with heavy smoking and is more marked in women over 35 years of age. Women who use oral contraceptives should be strongly advised not to smoke.
The use of oestrogen-containing oral contraceptives may promote growth of existing sex steroid dependent tumours. For this reason, the use of these oral contraceptives in patients with such tumours is contra-indicated. Numerous epidemiological studies have been reported of the risk or ovarian, endometrial, cervical and breast cancer in women using combined oral contraceptives.
The evidence is clear that combined oral contraceptives offer substantial protection against both ovarian and endometrial cancer. An increased risk of cervical cancer in long term users of combined oral contraceptives has been reported in some studies, but there continues to be controversy about the extent to which this is attributable to the confounding effects of sexual behaviour and other factors.
The evidence linking combined oral contraceptive use and breast cancer remains inconclusive. The results of some studies suggest an increased risk of breast cancer presenting below the age of about 35, the risk rising with duration of use. Any possible increased risk of breast cancer with combined oral contraceptives is however likely to be small, and may be expected to be less with low dose pills. This possible risk should be weighed against the many benefits of combined oral contraceptives, including their protective effects against ovarian and endometrial cancers.
Malignant hepatic tumours have been reported on rare occasions in long-term users of oral contraceptives. Benign hepatic tumours have also been associated with oral contraceptive usage. A hepatic tumour should be considered in the differential diagnosis when upper abdominal pain, enlarged liver or signs of intra-abdominal haemorrhage occur.
The use of oral contraceptives may sometimes lead to the development of cholestatic jaundice or cholelithiasis.
On rare occasions the use of oral contraceptives may trigger or reactivate systemic lupus erythematosus.
A further rare complication of oral contraceptive use is the occurrence of chorea which can be reversed by discontinuing the pill. The majority of cases of oral-contraceptive-induced chorea show a pre-existing predisposition which often relates to acute rheumatism.

*Other adverse reactions:*
*Cardiovascular System:* Rise of blood pressure. If hypertension develops, treatment should be discontinued
*Genital Tract:* Intermenstrual bleeding, post-medication amenorrhoea, changes in cervical secretion, increase in size of uterine fibromyomata, aggravation of endometriosis, certain vaginal infections, e.g. candidiasis.
*Breast:* Tenderness, pain, enlargement, secretion.
*Gastro Intestinal Tract:* Nausea, vomiting, cholelithiasis, cholestatic jaundice.
*Skin:* Erythema nodosum, rash, chloasma, erythema multiforme, hirsutism, loss of scalp hair.
*Eyes:* Discomfort of the cornea if contact lenses are used.
*CNS:* Headache, migraines, mood changes, depression
*Metabolic:* Fluid retention, change in body weight, reduced glucose tolerance.
*Other:* Changes in libido, leg cramps.

*Overdosage:* There have been no reports of serious ill-health from overdosage even when a considerable number of tablets have been taken by a small child. In general, it is therefore unnecessary to treat overdosage. However, if overdosage is discovered within 2 or 3 hours and is large, then gastric lavage can be safely used. There are no antidotes and further treatment should be symptomatic.

**Further information**
*Additional contraceptive precautions:* When additional contraceptive precautions are required the patient should be advised either not to have sex, or to use a cap plus spermicide or for her partner to use a condom. Rhythm methods should not be advised as the pill disrupts the usual cyclical changes associated with the natural menstrual cycle e.g. changes in temperature and cervical mucus.

*The 7-day rule:* If any one tablet is forgotten for more than 12 hours:
If the patient has vomiting or diarrhoea for more than 12 hours:
If the patient is taking any of the drugs listed under 'Interactions':
The patient should continue to take her tablets as usual and additional contraceptive precautions must be taken for the next 7 days.

BUT–if these 7 days run beyond the end of the current pack, the next pack must be started as soon as the current one is finished, i.e. no gap should be left between packs. (This prevents an extended break in tablet taking which may increase the risk of the ovaries releasing an egg and thus reducing contraceptive protection.) The patient will not have a period until the end of 2 packs but this is not harmful nor does it matter if she experiences some bleeding on tablet taking days.

**Pharmaceutical precautions** Store at room temperature (below 25°C). Protect from light.

**Legal category** POM.

**Package quantities** Carton containing 3 push packs of 21 tablets–sufficient for 3 cycles.

**Product licence number** 0242/0252.

## ORTHOFORMS* CONTRACEPTIVE PESSARIES

**Qualitative and quantitative composition** Nonoxynol-9, 5.0% w/w.

**Pharmaceutical form** Pessary.

**Clinical particulars**

*Therapeutic indications:* For use as a spermicide contraceptive in conjunction with barrier methods of contraception.

*Posology and method of administration:* For topical intravaginal administration.

For use by adult females only.

The Orthoforms Contraceptive Pessary should be inserted as high as possible into the vagina approximately 10 minutes before intercourse to permit the pessary to melt.

Any subsequent acts of intercourse should not be undertaken before the insertion of an additional pessary.

*Contra-indications:* Hypersensitivity to nonoxynol-9 or to any component of the preparation.

Patients with absent vaginal sensation e.g. paraplegics and quadriplegics.

*Special warnings and special precautions for use:* Spermicidal intravaginal preparations are intended for use in conjunction with barrier methods of contraception such as condoms, diaphragms and caps.

Where avoidance of pregnancy is important the choice of contraceptive method should be made in consultation with a doctor or family planning clinic.

If vaginal or penile irritation occurs, discontinue use. If symptoms worsen or continue for more than 48 hours, medical advice should be sought.

*Interactions with other medicaments and other forms of interaction:* None known.

*Pregnancy and lactation:* There is no evidence from animal or human studies that nonoxynol-9 is teratogenic. Human epidemiological studies have not shown any firm evidence of adverse effects on the foetus. However, some studies have shown that nonoxynol-9 may be embryotoxic in animals. This product should not be used if pregnancy is suspected or confirmed.

Animal studies have detected nonoxynol-9 in milk after intravaginal administration. Use by lactating women has not been studied.

*Effects on ability to drive and use machines:* None known.

*Undesirable effects:* Orthoforms Contraceptive Pessaries may cause irritation of the vagina or penis.

*Overdose:* If taken orally, the surfactant properties of this preparation may cause gastric irritation. General supportive therapy should be carried out. Hepatic and renal function should be monitored if medically indicated.

**Pharmacological properties**

*Pharmacodynamic properties:* The standard *in vitro* test (Sander-Cramer) evaluating the effect of nonoxynol-9 on animal sperm motility has shown the compound to be a potent spermicide.

The site of action of nonoxynol-9 has been determined as the sperm cell membrane. The lipoprotein membrane is disrupted, increasing permeability, with subsequent loss of cell components and decreased motility. A similar effect on vaginal epithelial and bacterial cells is also found.

*Pharmacokinetic properties:* The intravaginal absorption and excretion of radiolabelled ($^{14}$C) nonoxynol-9 has been studied in non-pregnant rats and rabbits and in pregnant rats. No appreciable difference was found in the extent or rate of absorption in pregnant and non-pregnant animals. Plasma levels peaked at about one hour and recovery from urine as unchanged nonoxynol-9 accounted for approximately 15-25% and faeces approximately 70% of the administered dose as unchanged nonoxynol-9. Less than 0.3% was found in the milk of lactating rats. No metabolites were detected in any of the samples analysed.

*Preclinical safety data:* See 'Pregnancy and lactation'.

**Pharmaceutical particulars**

*List of excipients:* Cetomacrogol 1000 BP; citric acid monohydrate PhEur; polyethylene glycol 1500; polyethylene glycol 1000 BP; purified water PhEur.

*Incompatibilities:* None known.

*Shelf life:* 36 months.

*Special precautions for storage:* Store in a cool place (8-15°C).

*Nature and contents of container:* Immediate container: polyvinylchloride/polyethylene laminate moulds.

Three strips of 5 pessaries are packed in an outer cardboard carton.

*Instructions for use/handling:* None stated.

**Marketing authorisation number** 0242/0247

**Date of approval/revision of SPC** October 1996.

**Legal category** GSL.

## OVYSMEN* ORAL CONTRACEPTIVE TABLETS

**Qualitative and quantitative composition** Ovysmen are tablets for oral administration.

Each tablet contains norethisterone 0.5 mg and ethinyloestradiol 0.035 mg.

**Pharmaceutical form** Tablets.

**Clinical particulars**

*Therapeutic indications:* Contraception and the recognised indications for such oestrogen/progestogen combinations.

*Posology and method of administration:* For oral administration.

*Adults:* It is preferable that tablet intake from the first pack is started on the first day of menstruation in which case no extra contraceptive precautions are necessary.

If menstruation has already begun (that is 2, 3 or 4 days previously), tablet taking should commence on day 5 of the menstrual period. In this case additional contraceptive precautions must be taken for the first 7 days of tablet taking.

If menstruation began more than 5 days previously then the patient should be advised to wait until her next menstrual period before starting to take Ovysmen.

*How to take Ovysmen:* One tablet is taken daily at the same time (preferably in the evening) without interruption for 21 days, followed by a break of 7 tablet-free days. Each subsequent pack is started after the 7 tablet-free days have elapsed. Additional contraceptive precautions are not then required.

*Elderly:* Not applicable.

*Children:* Not recommended.

*Contra-indications:*

*Absolute contra-indications:*

- pregnancy or suspected pregnancy (that cannot yet be excluded).
- circulatory disorders (cardiovascular or cerebrovascular) such as thrombophlebitis and thromboembolic processes (or a history of these conditions), moderate to severe hypertension, hyperlipoproteinaemia.

In addition the presence of more than one of the risk factors for arterial disease.

- severe liver disease, cholestatic jaundice or hepatitis (viral or non-viral) or a history of these conditions if the results of liver function tests have failed to return to normal, and for 3 months after liver function tests have been found to be normal; a history of jaundice of pregnancy or jaundice due to the use of steroids, Rotor syndrome and Dubin--Johnson syndrome, hepatic cell tumours and porphyria.

- cholelithiasis.
- known or suspected oestrogen-dependent tumours; endometrial hyperplasia; undiagnosed vaginal bleeding.
- systemic lupus erythematosus or a history of this condition.
- a history during pregnancy or previous use of steroids of: severe pruritus; herpes gestationis; a manifestation or deterioration of otosclerosis.

*Relative contra-indications:* If any relative contra-indications listed below is present, the benefits of oestrogen/progestogen-containing preparations must be weighed against the possible risk for each individual case and the patient kept under close supervision. In case of aggravation or appearance of any of these conditions whilst the patient is taking the pill, its use should be discontinued.

- conditions implicating an increasing risk of developing venous thrombo-embolic complications, e.g. severe varicose veins or prolonged immobilisation or major surgery. Disorders of coagulation.

- presence of any risk factor for arterial disease e.g. smoking, hyperlipidaemia or hypertension.

- other conditions associated with an increased risk of circulatory disease such as latent or overt cardiac failure, renal dysfunction, or a history of these conditions.

- epilepsy or a history of this condition.
- migraine or a history of this condition.
- a history of cholelithiasis.
- presence of any risk factor for oestrogen-dependent tumours; oestrogen-sensitive gynaecological disorders such as uterine fibromyomata and endometriosis.
- diabetes mellitus.
- severe depression or a history of this condition. If this is accompanied by a disturbance in tryptophan metabolism, administration of vitamin B6 might be of therapeutic value.
- sickle cell haemoglobinopathy, since under certain circumstances, eg during infections or anoxia, oestrogen-containing preparations may induce thromboembolic process in patients with this condition.
- if the results of liver function tests become abnormal, use should be discontinued.

*Special warnings and special precautions for use:*

*Post partum administration:* Following a vaginal delivery, oral contraceptive administration to non-breast-feeding mothers can be started 21 days post-partum provided the patient is fully ambulant and there are no puerperal complications. No additional contraceptive precautions are required. If post-partum administration begins more than 21 days after delivery, additional contraceptive precautions are required for the first 7 days of pill-taking.

If intercourse has taken place post-partum, oral contraceptive use should be delayed until the first day of the first menstrual period.

After miscarriage or abortion administration should start immediately in which case no additional contraceptive precautions are required.

*Changing from a 21 day pill or another 22 day pill to Ovysmen:* All tablets in the old pack should be finished. The first Ovysmen tablet is taken the next day, ie no gap is left between taking tablets nor does the patient need to wait for her period to begin. Tablets should be taken as instructed in 'How to take Ovysmen'. Additional contraceptive precautions are not required. The patient will not have a period until the end of the first Ovysmen pack, but this is not harmful, nor does it matter if she experiences some bleeding on tablet-taking days.

*Changing from a combined every day pill (28 day tablets) to Ovysmen:* Ovysmen should be started after taking the last active tablet from the 'Every day Pill' pack (i.e. after taking 21 or 22 tablets). The first Ovysmen tablet is taken the next day, ie no gap is left between taking tablets nor does the patient need to wait for her period to begin. Tablets should be taken as instructed in 'How to take Ovysmen' (see *Posology and method of administration*). Additional contraceptive precautions are not required. Remaining tablets from the every day (ED) pack should be discarded.

The patient will not have a period until the end of the first Ovysmen pack, but this is not harmful, nor does it matter if she experiences some bleeding on tablet-taking days.

*Changing from a progestogen-only pill (POP or mini pill) to Ovysmen:* The first Ovysmen tablet should be taken on the first day of the period, even if the patient has already taken a mini pill on that day. Tablets should be taken as instructed in 'How to take Ovysmen'. Additional contraceptive precautions are not required. All the remaining progestogen-only pills in the mini pill pack should be discarded.

If the patient is taking a mini pill, then she may not always have a period, especially when she is breast-feeding. The first Ovysmen tablet should be taken on the day after stopping the mini pill. All remaining pills in the mini pill packet must be discarded. Additional contraceptive precautions must be taken for the first 7 days.

*To skip a period:* To skip a period, a new pack of Ovysmen should be started on the day after finishing the current pack (the patient skips the tablet-free days). Tablet-taking should be continued in the usual way.

During the use of the second pack she may experience slight spotting or break-through bleeding but contraceptive protection will not be diminished provided there are no tablet omissions.

The next pack of Ovysmen is started after the usual 7 tablet-free days, regardless of whether the period has completely finished or not.

*Reduced reliability:* When Ovysmen is taken according to the directions for use the occurrence of pregnancy is highly unlikely. However, the reliability of oral contraceptives may be reduced under the following circumstances:

*(i) Forgotten tablets:* If the patient forgets to take a tablet, she should take it as soon as she remembers and take the next one at the normal time. This may mean that two tablets are taken in one day. Provided she is less than 12 hours late in taking her tablet, Ovysmen will still give contraceptive protection during

this cycle and the rest of the pack should be taken as usual.

If she is more than 12 hours late in taking one or more tablets then she should take the last missed pill as soon as she remembers but leave the other missed pills in the pack. She should continue to take the rest of the pack as usual but must use extra precautions (eg sheath, diaphragm, plus spermicide) and follow the '7-day rule' (see *Further Information* for the 7 day rule).

If there are 7 or more pills left in the pack after the missed and delayed pills then the usual 7-day break can be left before starting the next pack. If there are less than 7 pills left in the pack after the missed and delayed pills then when the pack is finished the next pack should be started the next day. If withdrawal bleeding does not occur at the end of the second pack then a pregnancy test should be performed.

*(ii) Vomiting or diarrhoea:* If after tablet intake vomiting or diarrhoea occurs, a tablet may not be absorbed properly by the body. If the symptoms disappear within 12 hours of tablet-taking, the patient should take an extra tablet from a spare pack and continue with the rest of the pack as usual.

However, if the symptoms continue beyond those 12 hours, additional contraceptive precautions are necessary for any sexual intercourse during the stomach or bowel upset and for the following 7 days (the patient must be advised to follow the '7-day rule').

*(iii) Change in bleeding pattern:* If after taking Ovysmen for several months there is a sudden occurrence of spotting or breakthrough bleeding (not observed in previous cycles) or the absence of withdrawal bleeding, contraceptive effectiveness may be reduced. If withdrawal bleeding fails to occur and none of the above mentioned events has taken place, pregnancy is highly unlikely and oral contraceptive use can be continued until the end of the next pack. (If withdrawal bleeding fails to occur at the end of the second cycle, tablet intake should be discontinued and pregnancy excluded before oral contraceptive use can be resumed). However, if withdrawal bleeding is absent and any of the above mentioned events has occurred, tablet intake should be discontinued and pregnancy excluded before oral contraceptive use can be resumed.

*Medical examination/consultation:* A complete medical history and physical examination should be taken prior to the initiation or reinstitution of oral contraceptives and should be repeated periodically.

These physical examinations should include special reference to blood pressure, breasts, abdomen and pelvic organs, including cervical cytology and, where indicated by the medical or family history, relevant laboratory tests. Caution should be observed when prescribing oral contraceptives to young women whose cycles are not yet stabilised.

*Surgery, varicose veins or immobilisation:* In patients using oestrogen-containing preparations the risk of deep vein thrombosis may be temporarily increased when undergoing a major operation (e.g. abdominal, orthopaedic), and surgery to the legs, medical treatment for varicose veins or prolonged immobilisation. Therefore, it is advisable to discontinue oral contraceptive use at least 4 to 6 weeks prior to these procedures if performed electively and to (re)start not less than 2 weeks after full ambulation. The latter is also valid with regard to immobilisation after an accident or emergency surgery. In case of emergency surgery, thrombotic prophylaxis is usually indicated eg with subcutaneous heparin.

*Chloasma:* Chloasma may occasionally occur, especially in women with a history of chloasma gravidarum. Women with a tendency to chloasma should avoid exposure to the sun or ultraviolet radiation whilst taking this preparation. Chloasma is often not fully reversible.

*Laboratory tests:* The use of steroids may influence the results of certain laboratory tests. In the literature, at least a hundred different parameters have been reported to possibly be influenced by oral contraceptive use, predominantly by the oestrogenic component. Among these are: biochemical parameters of the liver, thyroid, adrenal and renal function, plasma levels of (carrier) proteins and lipid/lipoprotein fractions and parameters of coagulation and fibrinolysis.

*Further information:*
*Additional contraceptive precautions:* When additional contraceptive precautions are required the patient should be advised either not to have sex, or to use a cap plus spermicide or for her partner to use a condom. Rhythm methods should not be advised as the pill disrupts the usual cyclical changes associated with the natural menstrual cycle, eg changes in temperature and cervical mucus.

*The 7-day rule*
If any one tablet is forgotten for more than 12 hours.

If the patient has vomiting or diarrhoea for more than 12 hours.

If the patient is taking any of the drugs listed under *Interactions*:

The patient should continue to take her tablets as usual and:
- Additional contraceptive precautions must be taken for the next 7 days.

*But - if these 7 days run beyond the end of the current pack*, the next pack must be started as soon as the current one is finished, ie no gap should be left between packs. (This prevents an extended break in tablet taking which may increase the risk of the ovaries releasing an egg and thus reducing contraceptive protection.) The patient will not have a period until the end of 2 packs but this is not harmful nor does it matter if she experiences some bleeding on tablet taking days.

*Interactions with other medicaments and other forms of interaction:* Irregular cycles and reduced reliability of oral contraceptives may occur when these preparations are used concomitantly with drugs such as anticonvulsants, barbiturates, antibiotics (eg tetracyclines, ampicillin, rifampicin, etc), griseofulvin, activated charcoal and certain laxatives. Special consideration should be given to patients being treated with antibiotics for acne. They should be advised to use a non-hormonal method of contraception, or to use an oral contraceptive containing a progestogen showing minimal androgenicity, which have been reported as helping to improve acne without using an antibiotic. Oral contraceptives may diminish glucose tolerance and increase the need for insulin or other antidiabetic drugs in diabetics.

*Pregnancy and lactation:* Ovysmen is contra-indicated for use during pregnancy or suspected pregnancy, since it has been suggested that combined oral contraceptives, in common with many other substances, might be capable of affecting the normal development of the child in the early stages of pregnancy. It can be definitely concluded, however, that, if a risk of abnormality exists at all, it must be very small.

Mothers who are breast-feeding should be advised not to use the combined pill since this may reduce the amount of breast-milk, but may be advised instead to use a progestogen-only pill (POP).

*Effects on ability to drive and use machines:* Not applicable.

*Undesirable effects:* Various adverse reactions have been associated with oral contraceptive use. The first appearance of symptoms indicative of any one of these reactions necessitates immediate cessation of oral contraceptive use while appropriate diagnostic and therapeutic measures are undertaken.

*Serious adverse reactions:* There is a general opinion, based on statistical evidence, that users of combined oral contraceptives experience more often than non-users various disorders of the coagulation. How often these disorders occur in users of modern low-oestrogen oral contraceptives is unknown, but there are reasons for suggesting that they may occur less often than with the older types of pill which contain more oestrogen.

Various reports have associated oral contraceptive use with the occurrence of deep venous thrombosis, pulmonary embolism and other embolisms. Other investigations of these oral contraceptives have suggested an increased risk of oestrogen and/or progestogen dose-dependent coronary and cerebrovascular accidents, predominantly in heavy smokers. Thrombosis has very rarely been reported to occur in other veins or arteries, eg hepatic, mesenteric, renal or retinal.

It should be noted that there is no consensus about often contradictory findings obtained in early studies. The physician should bear in mind the possibility of vascular accidents occurring and that there may not be full recovery from such disorders and they may be fatal. The physician should take into account the presence of risk factors for arterial disease and deep venous thrombosis when prescribing oral contraceptives. Risk factors for arterial disease include smoking, the presence of hyperlipidaemia, hypertension or diabetes.

Signs and symptoms of a thrombotic event may include: sudden severe pain in the chest, whether or not reaching to the left arm; sudden breathlessness; and unusual severe, prolonged headache, especially if it occurs for the first time or gets progressively worse, or is associated with any of the following symptoms: sudden partial or complete loss of vision or diplopia, aphasia, vertigo, a bad fainting attack or collapse with or without focal epilepsy, weakness or very marked numbness suddenly affecting one side or one part of the body, motor disturbances; severe pain in the calf of one leg; acute abdomen.

Cigarette smoking increases the risk of serious cardiovascular adverse reactions to oral contraceptive

use. The risk increases with age and with heavy smoking and is more marked in women over 35 years of age. Women who use oral contraceptives should be strongly advised not to smoke.

The use of oestrogen-containing oral contraceptives may promote growth of existing sex steroid dependent tumours. For this reason, the use of these oral contraceptives in patients with such tumours is contra-indicated. Numerous epidemiological studies have been reported on the risk of ovarian, endometrial, cervical and breast cancer in women using combined oral contraceptives. The evidence is clear that combined oral contraceptives offer substantial protection against both ovarian and endometrial cancer. An increased risk of cervical cancer in long term users of combined oral contraceptives has been reported in some studies, but there continues to be controversy about the extent to which this is attributable to the confounding effects of sexual behaviour and other factors.

The evidence linking combined oral contraceptive use and breast cancer remains inconclusive. The results of some studies suggest an increased risk of breast cancer presenting below the age of about 35, the risk rising with duration of use. Any possible increased risk of breast cancer with combined oral contraceptives is however likely to be small, and may be expected to be less with low dose pills. This possible risk should be weighed against the many benefits of combined oral contraceptives, including their protective effects against ovarian and endometrial cancers.

Malignant hepatic tumours have been reported on rare occasions in long-term users of oral contraceptives. Benign hepatic tumours have also been associated with oral contraceptive usage. A hepatic tumour should be considered in the differential diagnosis when upper abdominal pain, enlarged liver or signs of intra-abdominal haemorrhage occur.

The use of oral contraceptives may sometimes lead to the development of cholestatic jaundice or cholelithiasis.

On rare occasions the use of oral contraceptives may trigger or reactivate systemic lupus erythematosus.

A further rare complication of oral contraceptive use is the occurrence of chorea which can be reversed by discontinuing the pill. The majority of cases of oral contraceptive-induced chorea show a pre-existing predisposition which often relates to acute rheumatism.

*Other adverse reactions:*
*Cardiovascular system:* Rise of blood pressure. If hypertension develops, treatment should be discontinued.

*Genital tract:* Intermenstrual bleeding, post-medication amenorrhoea, changes in cervical secretion, increase in size of uterine fibromyomata, aggravation of endometriosis, certain vaginal infections, eg candidiasis.

*Breast:* Tenderness, pain, enlargement, secretion.
*Gastro-intestinal tract:* Nausea, vomiting, cholelithiasis, cholestatic jaundice.

*Skin:* Erythema nodosum, rash, chloasma, erythema multiforme, hirsutism, loss of scalp hair.

*Eyes:* Discomfort of the cornea if contact lenses are used.

*CNS:* Headache, migraine, mood changes, depression.

*Metabolic:* Fluid retention, change in body weight, reduced glucose tolerance.

*Other:* Changes in libido, leg cramps.

*Overdose:* There have been no reports of serious ill-health from overdosage even when a considerable number of tablets have been taken by a small child. In general, it is therefore unnecessary to treat overdosage. However, if overdosage is discovered within two or three hours and is large, then gastric lavage can be safely used. There are no antidotes and further treatment should be symptomatic.

**Pharmacological properties**

*Pharmacodynamic properties:* Ovysmen acts through the mechanism of gonadotrophin suppression by the oestrogenic and progestational actions of ethinyloestradiol and norethisterone. The primary mechanism of action is inhibition of ovulation, but alterations to the cervical mucus and to the endometrium may also contribute to the efficacy of the product.

If a patient misses more than one tablet she should begin taking tablets again as soon as remembered and an additional reliable method of contraception used until the next withdrawal bleed. The patient should be advised that during the first 14 days of the first course of tablets, she should use an additional reliable non-hormonal form of contraception.

*Pharmacokinetic properties:* Norethisterone and ethinyloestradiol are absorbed from the gastro-intestinal tract and metabolised in the liver. To obtain maximal contraceptive effectiveness the tablets should be taken as directed and at approximately the same time each day. If the patient has vomiting or diarrhoea absorption of the hormones will be impaired, making it advisable to use an additional reliable method of contraception until her next menstrual period.

Because the active ingredients are metabolised in the liver, reduced contraceptive efficacy has been associated with concomitant use of oral contraceptives and rifampicin. A similar association has been suggested with oral contraceptives and barbiturates, phenytoin sodium, phenylbutazone, griseofulvin and ampicillin.

*Preclinical safety data:* The toxicology of norethisterone and ethinyloestradiol has been extensively investigated in animal studies and through long term clinical experience with widespread use in contraceptives.

### Pharmaceutical particulars

*List of excipients:* Lactose (anhydrous); magnesium stearate; pregelatinised starch; methanol (does not appear in final product).

*Incompatibilities:* Not applicable.

*Shelf life:* Three years.

*Special precautions for storage:* Store at room temperature (below 25°C). Protect from light.

*Nature and contents of container:* Carton containing 3 PVC/foil blister strips of 21 tablets each.

*Instructions for use/handling:* Not applicable.

**Marketing authorisation number** 0242/0253

**Date of approval/revision of SPC** May 1997

**Legal category** POM.

## PANCREASE* CAPSULES

**Presentation** Hard, white, gelatin capsules printed 0095 on the body, containing enteric coated microspheres of porcine Pancrelipase USP. Each capsule has a protease activity of not less than 330 BP Units, an amylase activity of not less than 2,900 BP Units and lipase activity of not less than 5,000 BP Units.

**Uses** Exocrine pancreatic enzyme deficiency as in cystic fibrosis, chronic pancreatitis, post-pancreatectomy, post-gastrointestinal bypass surgery (e.g. Billroth II gastroenterostomy), ductal obstruction from neoplasm (e.g. of the pancreas or common bile duct).

The enzymes catalyse the hydrolysis of fats into glycerol and fatty acids, protein into proteoses and derived substances and starch into dextrins and sugars.

**Dosage and administration** For adults and children 1 or 2 capsules during each meal and one capsule with snacks. Occasionally a third capsule with meals may be required depending upon individual requirements. Where swallowing of capsules is difficult, they may be opened and the microspheres taken with liquids or soft foods which do not require chewing. To protect the enteric coating the microspheres should not be crushed or chewed.

**Contra-indications, warnings, etc** Hypersensitivity to pork protein. The safety of Pancrease during pregnancy has not yet been established. Such use is not recommended.

The most frequently reported adverse reactions to Pancrease Capsules are gastrointestinal in nature. Less frequently allergic-type reactions have also been observed.

Extremely high doses of exogenous pancreatic enzymes have been associated with hyperuricosuria and hyperuricaemia.

Contact of the microspheres with food having a pH higher than 5.5 can dissolve the protective enteric shell.

**Pharmaceutical precautions** Keep bottle tightly closed. Store at room temperature in a dry place. Do not refrigerate.

**Legal category** P.

**Package quantities** Containers of 100 capsules.

**Further information** The enteric coated Pancrease microspheres resist gastric inactivation and deliver predictable, high levels of biologically active enzymes into the duodenum.

**Product licence number** 0242/0254.

## PANCREASE* HL CAPSULES

**Presentation** Hard, size 0 elongated white opaque gelatin capsules with a red band and the letters HL in red on the body and cap. Each capsule contains light brown, homogeneous enterically coated minitablets of Pancreatin BP with an enzyme activity (which is higher than standard preparations) of not less than 25000 BP units lipase, 22500 BP units amylase and 1250 BP units Protease per capsule.

**Uses** Exocrine pancreatic enzyme deficiency as in cystic fibrosis, chronic pancreatitis, post pancreatectomy, post gastrointestinal bypass surgery (eg Billroth II gastroenterostomy), and ductal obstruction from neoplasm (eg of the pancreas or common bile duct). The enzymes catalyse the hydrolysis of fats into glycerol and fatty acids, protein into proteoses and derived substances and starch into dextrins and sugars.

**Dosage and administration** For adults and children 1 or 2 capsules during each meal and 1 capsule with snacks. The interindividual response to Pancreatin supplements is variable and the number of capsules may need to be titrated to the individual based upon parameters of steatorrhoea and symptomatology. Further dose increases, if required, should be added slowly, with careful monitoring of response and symptomology.

Where patients are already in receipt of lower unit dose enteric coated Pancreatin supplements then Pancrease HL may be substituted at one third of the number of capsules normally consumed with the previous preparation.

Where swallowing of capsules is difficult then they may be opened and the minitablets taken with liquids or soft foods which do not require chewing. To protect the enteric coating the minitablets should not be crushed or chewed.

It is important to ensure adequate hydration of patients at all times while dosing with Pancrease HL Capsules.

Patients who are taking or have been given in excess of 10,000 units of lipase/kg/day are at risk of developing colon damage. The dose of Pancrease HL should usually not exceed this dose.

**Contra-indications, warnings, etc** Hypersensitivity to pork protein or any excipients. Children aged 15 years or under with cystic fibrosis. The safety of Pancrease HL during pregnancy has not been established. Consequently use of Pancrease HL in pregnancy and lactation is not recommended.

Contact of the minitablets with food having a pH higher than 5.5 can dissolve the protective coating and will reduce the efficacy of the product.

*Adverse reactions:* The most frequently reported adverse reactions to Pancreatin supplements are gastrointestinal in nature such as abdominal discomfort, nausea, vomiting, perianal irritation or inflammation. Less frequently allergic-type reactions generally of the skin have also been observed. Very high doses of pancreatic enzymes have been associated with hyperuricosuria and hyperuricaemia. This has been virtually eliminated with enteric coated preparations.

Stricture of the ileo-caecum and large bowel and colitis have been reported in children with cystic fibrosis taking Pancrease HL.

Abdominal symptoms (not usually experienced by the patient) or changes in abdominal symptoms should be reviewed to exclude the possibility of colonic damage, especially if the patient is taking in excess of 10,000 units of lipase/kg/day.

*Overdosage:* Overdosage is unlikely and has not been experienced to date with Pancrease HL. Inappropriately large doses could result in symptoms such as abdominal discomfort, nausea, vomiting, perianal irritation or inflammation.

**Pharmaceutical precautions** Keep container tightly closed. Store at room temperature (10–25°C) in a dry place. Do not refrigerate.

**Legal category** POM.

**Package quantities** Containers of 100 or 500 capsules.

**Further information** The enteric coated minitablets in Pancrease HL capsules resist gastric inactivation and deliver therapeutic levels of biologically active enzymes into the duodenum. The higher Lipase content per capsule may enable a reduction in previous capsule consumption of approximately one third but it is important that the individual's response is monitored during the first weeks of therapy with Pancrease HL and dosage adjusted if necessary.

**Product licence number** 0242/0255.

## PEVARYL* TOPICAL CREAM
## PEVARYL* TOPICAL LOTION

**Presentation** *Cream:* A soft, white, water-miscible cream containing 1% w/w econazole nitrate.

*Lotion:* A milky white homogeneous lotion containing 1% econazole nitrate.

**Uses** For the treatment of fungal infections of the skin.

**Dosage and administration** *Cream:* Apply to the affected area 2 times daily and rub in gently. Continue the application until all skin lesions are healed.

In nail infections, apply once daily and cover with an occlusive dressing.

*Lotion:* As for Pevaryl Cream.

In order to prevent relapse, treatment should be continued for 2 weeks after clinical cure.

**Contra-indications, warnings, etc**
*Contra-indications: Lotion and cream:* Care should be taken in the presence of eczematous dermatitis.

*Side-effects:* Rarely, transient local mild irritation may occur immediately after application.

*Precautions: Cream and Lotion:* Hypersensitivity has rarely been recorded, if it should occur, administration of the product should be discontinued.

*Incompatibilities:* None known.

*Overdosage:* Pevaryl Topical Cream and Lotion are intended for topical application only. If accidental ingestion of large quantities of the product occurs, an appropriate method of gastric emptying may be used if considered desirable.

*Use in pregnancy:* Only small amounts of the drug are absorbed through the skin and no teratogenic effects have been observed in animals. Hence, the product may be used with caution during pregnancy.

**Pharmaceutical precautions** *Cream and lotion:* None.

**Legal category** P

**Package quantities** *Cream:* Each tube contains 30 g. *Lotion:* Each bottle contains 30 ml.

**Further information** Nil.

**Product licence numbers**
Cream              0242/0259
Lotion             0242/0260

## PEVARYL* TC CREAM

**Presentation** Pevaryl TC cream is a soft white water-miscible cream containing 1% w/w econazole nitrate and 0.1% w/w triamcinolone acetonide.

**Uses** For the topical treatment of inflammatory dermatomycoses and inflammatory skin conditions complicated by or threatened by bacterial or fungal skin infection.

Econazole nitrate is a broad spectrum antifungal agent with activity against many gram positive bacteria.

Triamcinolone acetonide is a potent corticosteroid with anti-inflammatory, antipruritic and antiallergic activity.

**Dosage and administration** The cream should be applied by gently rubbing into the skin with the finger twice daily for 14 days OR apply twice daily to the affected area OR as directed by your doctor.

**Contra-indications, warnings, etc**
*Contra-indications:* Like all preparations containing corticosteroids, Pevaryl TC cream should not be used on tubercular or luetic skin infections or in viral diseases (e.g. herpes, vaccinia, varicella). Pevaryl TC cream should not be administered to patients who have previously exhibited hypersensitivity to imidazoles or corticosteroids.

Long-term continuous steroid therapy should be avoided since adrenal suppression can occur, particularly when infants or children are treated or when occlusive dressings are applied. In addition, long term therapy with corticosteroids can cause skin lesions such as atrophy, telangiectasia and striae.

*Pregnancy:* Topical administration of corticosteroids to pregnant animals can cause foetal abnormalities. The relevance of this finding to human beings has not been established. However, topical steroids should not be used extensively in pregnancy, ie in large amounts or for prolonged periods.

*Side-effects:* Transient local mild irritation at the application site has been reported. Hypersensitivity has rarely been reported. Discontinuation of therapy usually results in cessation of the symptoms.

**Pharmaceutical precautions** Store at room temperature (at or below 25°C).

**Legal category** POM.

**Package quantities** 15 g tube.

**Further information** Nil.

**Product licence number** 0242/0263.

## PREPULSID*

**Presentation** *Tablets:* White, biconvex, scored tablets, engraved CIS/10 on one side and JANSSEN on the reverse. Each tablet contains cisapride monohydrate equivalent to 10 mg of cisapride. The tablets contain lactose.

*Suspension:* White, cherry-flavoured suspension containing cisapride monohydrate equivalent to cisapride 5 mg per 5 ml. The suspension also contains sucrose, methyl and propyl parabens.

## Uses
*Properties:* Prepulsid is a gastrointestinal prokinetic agent which stimulates lower oesophageal, gastric, small intestinal and colonic motility.

Prepulsid probably acts by enhancing the release of acetylcholine at the level of the myenteric plexus in the gut wall, and therefore its effects on motility can largely be abolished by atropine. The mechanism by which acetylcholine release is enhanced is unclear. There is no direct evidence of antidopaminergic or direct cholinergic effects.

Prepulsid has no effect on prolactin release or gastric secretion.

In patients with gastro-oesophageal reflux, Prepulsid increases the resting tone of the lower oesophageal sphincter, and increases the amplitude of lower oesophageal contractions. Prepulsid has also been shown, by using pH monitoring, to reduce the duration of reflux episodes.

In patients with dyspepsia, impaired gastric emptying and GORD, Prepulsid improves gastric emptying of liquid and solid meals, and shortens mouth to caecum transit time.

Prepulsid also stimulates colonic propulsive peristalsis and accelerates colonic transit.

*Indications:* Treatment of symptoms (e.g. heartburn, regurgitation) and mucosal lesions associated with gastro-oesophageal reflux. Prepulsid may also be used for the maintenance treatment of reflux oesophagitis.

The management of symptoms of dyspepsia (e.g. epigastric pain or burning, early satiety, bloating), where peptic ulcer or other lesions have been excluded from the diagnosis.

Relief of symptoms (e.g. nausea, early satiety, anorexia, bloating, epigastric pain) of impaired gastric motility secondary to disturbed and delayed gastric emptying associated with diabetes, systemic sclerosis and autonomic neuropathy.

**Dosage and administration** Prepulsid should preferably be taken 15-30 minutes before a meal in order to ensure maximum plasma levels immediately after food intake.

*Adults and children aged 12 years and over*

*Dyspepsia:* 10 mg Prepulsid three times daily. The usual course of treatment is 4 weeks.

*Gastro-oesophageal reflux:* 10 mg Prepulsid three times daily. Night time symptoms can be treated with an extra 10 mg dose at bedtime. Alternatively, 20 mg Prepulsid twice daily (before breakfast and at bedtime). Healing of oesophageal lesions has been reported following treatment with 10 mg qds or 20 mg bd. A 12 week course of treatment is recommended to give maximum benefit.

For maintenance treatment, 20 mg Prepulsid once daily (at bedtime) or 10 mg Prepulsid twice daily (before breakfast and at bedtime) is recommended. It may be necessary to increase this dose to 20 mg Prepulsid twice daily in patients whose lesions were initially very severe.

Impaired gastric motility: 10 mg Prepulsid three or four times daily. An initial course of 6 weeks is recommended, but longer periods of treatment may be required.

*Use in children:* Clinical experience with Prepulsid in children younger than 12 years is limited. Hence the drug can only be recommended for use in children aged 12 years and older.

*Use in elderly:* Repeated dosing in elderly patients with Prepulsid produced steady state plasma levels which were generally higher than those reported in younger patients, due to a moderate prolongation of the elimination half life. Therapeutic doses, however, are similar to those used in younger patients. Therefore it is recommended that when Prepulsid is used in elderly patients, a starting dose similar to that used in other adults is prescribed initially. This can then be adapted depending on the therapeutic effects or possible side effects of the treatment.

*Abnormal renal or liver function:* Because of the importance of the hepatic metabolism and renal excretion of Prepulsid, the dosage should initially be halved in patients with hepatic or renal insufficiency. Subsequently the dose can be adapted depending on individual clinical response.

## Contra-indications, warnings etc
*Contra-indications:* Prepulsid is contra-indicated in pregnancy (see Use in pregnancy section) and in patients in whom gastrointestinal stimulation might be dangerous, eg gastrointestinal haemorrhage, mechanical obstruction or perforation. Concomitant administration of Prepulsid and oral or parenteral (but not topical) formulations of ketoconazole, itraconazole, miconazole, fluconazole, erythromycin, clarith-

romycin and nefazodone or protease inhibitors such as ritonavir is also contra-indicated (see drug interactions section). Prepulsid is also contra-indicated in patients known to be hypersensitive to the product.

*Warnings:* Abnormal renal or liver function (see dosage section).

Isolated cases of QT-interval prolongation and/or Torsades de Pointes have been reported in patients receiving multiple other medications and/or who have pre-existing cardiac disease or risk factors for arrhythmia. A causal relationship with Prepulsid has not been established. The recommended dose of Prepulsid should not be exceeded and it should be used with caution in patients with conditions leading to QT-interval prolongation, such as uncorrected electrolyte disturbances (particularly hypokalaemia and hypomagnesaemia), congenital QT-interval prolongation or in patients who are taking medication known to prolong QT interval.

*Drug interactions:* Since Prepulsid accelerates gastric emptying, the absorption from the stomach of concomitantly administered drugs may be diminished, whereas absorption of drugs from the small intestine may be accelerated. For drugs that require careful individual titration, such as anticonvulsants, it may be useful to measure their plasma concentration.

Prepulsid does not affect psychomotor performance nor does it induce sedation or drowsiness. However, the sedative effects of benzodiazepines and alcohol may be accelerated when administered concomitantly with Prepulsid.

The beneficial effects of Prepulsid on gastrointestinal motility are largely antagonised by anticholinergic drugs.

In patients receiving anticoagulants, the prothrombin time may be increased. It is advisable to check the prothrombin time within the first few days of initiating or discontinuing Prepulsid treatment, and to adapt the dose of anticoagulant if necessary.

The drug exhibits extensive binding to plasma proteins, mainly to albumin.

Prepulsid is metabolised mainly via the cytochrome P450 3A4 enzyme. Available human pharmacokinetic data indicate that oral ketoconazole significantly inhibits the metabolism of Prepulsid, resulting in markedly elevated plasma levels of Prepulsid. Data suggest that co-administration of Prepulsid and oral ketoconazole can result in QT-interval prolongation, which can lead to ventricular arrhythmias (see warnings section). *In vitro* data suggest that itraconazole, miconazole and nefazodone or protease inhibitors such as ritonavir may also markedly inhibit the metabolism of Prepulsid. Post-marketing experience suggests that this may also apply to fluconazole, erythromycin and clarithromycin. Therefore, Prepulsid should not be co-administered in patients requiring oral or parenteral ketoconazole, itraconazole, miconazole, fluconazole, erythromycin, clarithromycin and nefazodone or protease inhibitors such as ritonavir.

Cimetidine co-administration leads to an increased peak plasma concentration and AUC of Prepulsid. There is no effect on Prepulsid absorption when it is co-administered with ranitidine. The gastrointestinal absorption of cimetidine and ranitidine is accelerated when they are co-administered with Prepulsid. The level of change is unlikely to be clinically significant.

*Use in pregnancy:* In animals Prepulsid has shown no teratogenic or primary foetotoxic effects. Nevertheless, the safety of Prepulsid in human pregnancy has not been established and therefore, as with other drugs, it is contra-indicated in pregnancy.

*Use in lactation:* Although the excretion of Prepulsid in human breast milk is minimal (milk to serum ratio of 0.045), it is not advisable to breast feed while taking Prepulsid.

*Side-effects:* The most frequent side effects reported with Prepulsid are gastrointestinal: abdominal cramps, borborygmi and diarrhoea. They are mainly transient and rarely require discontinuation of treatment. Should severe abdominal cramps occur with single administrations of 20 mg Prepulsid, it is recommended that the dose per administration is halved and the frequency of dosing doubled so that the total daily dose is unaltered.

Less frequent side-effects include headaches and lightheadedness. Cases of hypersensitivity have occasionally been reported. Reports of convulsions, extrapyramidal effects and dose related increase in urinary frequency have been received. Exceptional cases of reversible liver function abnormalities, with or without cholestasis, have been reported. Cases of gynaecomastia and galactorrhoea have also been reported, however, in large scale surveillance studies the incidence (<0.1%) has not exceeded that commonly reported in the general population. A causal relationship with Prepulsid has not been unequivocally established.

*Overdosage:* The symptoms that occur most frequently after overdosing are abdominal cramping and

increased stool frequency. Rare cases of QT-interval prolongation have been reported. In infants*, mild sedation, apathy and atony were also observed.

* (< 1 year of age)

In case of overdosage, the administration of activated charcoal and close observation of the patient are recommended. It is also recommended that patients are evaluated for possible QT-interval prolongation and for factors such as electrolyte disturbances (especially hypokalaemia) and bradycardia that can predispose to the occurrence of Torsades de Pointes.

**Pharmaceutical precautions** *Tablets:* Store at room temperature in a dry place and protect from light.
*Suspension:* Store at room temperature (below 25°C).

**Legal category** POM.

**Package quantities** 10 mg tablets: packs of 120 tablets.
Suspension: bottles of 500 ml.

**Further information** Prepulsid is rapidly absorbed, with peak plasma levels 1 to 2 hours after dosing, and an elimination half-life of approximately 10 hours.

It undergoes extensive first-pass metabolism in the liver and gut wall, with the main metabolic pathways being oxidative N-dealkylation and aromatic hydroxylation. Excretion is mainly as metabolites (90%) with approximately equal amounts in both urine and faeces.

**Product licence numbers**
Prepulsid 10 mg tablets 0242/0136
Prepulsid suspension 0242/0157

## RAPIFEN*

**Presentation** Clear, colourless, preservative-free, aqueous injection presented in 2 ml and 10 ml ampoules. Each millilitre contains 500 micrograms of alfentanil as the hydrochloride. Rapifen also contains sodium chloride and water for injection.

**Uses** Rapifen is a potent, opioid analgesic with a very rapid and short-lived action. This makes it especially suitable for use as an adjunct to anaesthesia in short operative procedures and out-patient surgery, requiring spontaneous respiration.

Rapifen may also be administered to ventilated patients undergoing longer operative procedures, either as a bolus followed by iv increments or infusion, or as an iv infusion throughout.

**Dosage** Rapifen by the intravenous route can be administered to both adults and children. The dosage of Rapifen should be individualised according to age, bodyweight, physical status, underlying pathological condition, use of other drugs and type of surgery and anaesthesia. The usual recommended dosage regimen is as follows:

| | Initial | Supplemental |
| --- | --- | --- |
| **Adults** | | |
| Spontaneous respiration | up to 500 mcg | 250 mcg |
| Assisted ventilation | 30-50 mcg/kg | 15 mcg/kg |
| **Children** | | |
| Assisted ventilation | 30-50 mcg/kg | 15 mcg/kg |

In spontaneously breathing patients, the initial bolus dose should be given slowly over about 30 seconds (dilution may be helpful).

*Use in children:* Children may require higher or more frequent dosing owing to a shorter half life of Rapifen in this age group.

*Use in elderly and debilitated patients:* Lower or less frequent dosing may be required owing to a longer half life (dilution may be helpful).

After intravenous administration in unpremedicated adult patients, 1 ml Rapifen may be expected to have a peak effect in 90 seconds and to provide analgesia for 5-10 minutes. Periods of more painful stimuli may be overcome by the use of small increments of Rapifen. For procedures of longer duration additional increments will be required.

In ventilated patients undergoing longer procedures, Rapifen may be infused at a rate of 0.5-1 microgram/kg/minute. Adequate plasma concentrations of alfentanil will only be achieved rapidly if this infusion is preceded by a loading dose of 50-100 micrograms/kg given as a bolus or fast infusion over 10 minutes. Even lower doses may be adequate, for example, in geriatric patients or where anaesthesia is being supplemented by other agents. The infusion should be discontinued up to 30 minutes before the anticipated end of surgery. Increasing the infusion rate may prolong recovery. Therefore supplementation of the anaesthetic if required is best managed by extra bolus doses of Rapifen (1-2 ml) or low concentrations of a volatile agent for brief periods. In ventilated patients, the last bolus dose should not be given later than about 10 minutes before the end of surgery to avoid the continuation of respiratory depression after surgery is complete.

Also see precautions and drug interactions.

### Contra-indications, warnings, etc.

*Contra-indications:* Obstructive airways disease or respiratory depression if not ventilating.

Concurrent administration with monoamine oxidase inhibitors or within 2 weeks of their discontinuation.

Administration in labour or before clamping of the cord during Caesarean section due to the possibility of respiratory depression in the new-born infant.

Patients with a known intolerance to alfentanil or other morphinomimetics.

*Warnings:* Following administration of Rapifen, a transient fall in blood pressure may occur. The magnitude of this effect may be exaggerated in the hypovolaemic patient or in the presence of concomitant sedative medication. Appropriate measures to maintain a stable arterial pressure should be taken.

Significant respiratory depression will occur following administration of Rapifen in doses in excess of 1 mg. This and the other pharmacological effects of Rapifen are usually of short duration and can be reversed by specific opioid antagonists (eg naloxone). Additional doses of the antagonists may be necessary because the respiratory depression may last longer than the duration of action of the opioid antagonist.

Like other opioids, alfentanil may cause bradycardia, an effect that may be marked and rapid in onset but which can be antagonised by atropine. Particular care must be taken following treatment with drugs which may depress the heart or increase vagal tone, such as anaesthetic agents or beta-blockers since they may predispose to bradycardia or hypotension. Heart rate and blood pressure should therefore be monitored carefully. If hypotension or bradycardia occur, appropriate measures should be instituted.

Asystole following bradycardia has been reported on very rare occasions in non-atropinised patients. Therefore it is advisable to be prepared to administer an anticholinergic drug.

*Precautions:* It is wise to reduce the dosage in the elderly and debilitated patients. In hypothyroidism, pulmonary disease, decreased respiratory reserve, alcoholism and liver or renal impairment the dosage should be titrated with care and prolonged monitoring may be required.

Patients on chronic opioid therapy or with a history of opioid abuse may require higher doses.

Rapifen may induce muscle rigidity during induction. Rigidity, which may also involve the thoracic muscles, can be avoided by the following measures:

- slow iv injection (usually sufficient for lower doses);
- premedication with a benzodiazepine;
- administration of a muscle relaxant just prior to administration of Rapifen;

As with all potent opioids, profound analgesia is accompanied by marked respiratory depression, which may persist into or recur in the early postoperative period. Care should be taken after infusions or large doses of alfentanil to ensure that adequate spontaneous breathing has been established and maintained in the absence of stimulation before discharging the patient from the recovery area. Resuscitation equipment and narcotic antagonists should be readily available. Hyperventilation during anaesthesia may alter the patient's response to $CO_2$, thus affecting respiration postoperatively.

The use of rapid bolus injections of opioids should be avoided in patients with compromised intracerebral compliance; in such patients a transient decrease in the mean arterial pressure has occasionally been accompanied by a transient reduction of the cerebral perfusion pressure.

*Drug interactions:* The concomitant use of cimetidine or erythromycin with Rapifen can significantly inhibit alfentanil clearance and may increase the risk of prolonged or delayed respiratory depression. Therefore smaller doses may be required and the duration of action may be extended. Theoretically similar considerations may apply to other enzyme inhibitors.

Treatment with drugs which may depress the heart or increase vagal tone, such as beta-blockers and anaesthetic agents, may predispose to bradycardia or hypotension. Bradycardia and possibly asystole can occur when Rapifen is combined with non-vagolytic muscle relaxants.

The use of opioid premedication, barbiturates, benzodiazepines, neuroleptics, halogenic gases and other non-selective CNS depressants may enhance or prolong the respiratory depressant effects of alfentanil.

If other narcotic or CNS depressant drugs are used concurrently with alfentanil, the effects of the drugs can be expected to be additive. When patients have received such drugs the dose of alfentanil required

will be less than usual. Likewise, following the administration of alfentanil, the dose of other CNS-depressant drugs should be reduced.

*Effects on driving ability and operation of machinery:* Where early discharge is envisaged patients, should be advised not to drive or operate machinery for 24 hours following administration.

*Side-effects:* The most common adverse reactions reported with alfentanil are respiratory depression, apnoea and bradycardia.

Nausea and vomiting and dizziness have been reported.

In patients receiving doses of Rapifen large enough to require assisted ventilation, myoclonic movements and muscle rigidity (possibly involving the thoracic muscles) have rarely been reported shortly after the administration of Rapifen.

Other reported adverse reactions are laryngospasm, slight transient hypotension, allergic reactions (such as anaphylaxis, bronchospasm and urticaria), asystole and arrhythmias.

*Use in pregnancy and lactation:* Safety in human pregnancy has not been established although studies in animals have not demonstrated teratogenic or acute embryotoxic effects. As with other drugs, risk should be weighed against potential benefit to the patient.

Limited data suggest that alfentanil may appear in breast milk. It is therefore recommended that breast feeding is not initiated within 24 hours of treatment.

*Overdosage:* The manifestations of alfentanil overdose are generally an extension of its pharmacological action, which include the following:

*Action:*

Bradycardia: Anticholinergics such as atropine or glycopyrrolate;

Hypoventilation or apnoea: $O_2$ administration, assisted or controlled respiration and an opioid antagonist may be required;

Muscle rigidity: Intravenous neuromuscular blocking agent may be given.

A specific opioid antagonist (e.g. naloxone) should be available to treat respiratory depression. If hypotension is severe or persists, the possibility of hypovolaemia should be considered and controlled with appropriate parenteral fluid administration.

The suggested treatments given above do not preclude the use of other clinically indicated countermeasures.

Body temperature and adequate fluid intake should be maintained and the patient observed for 24 hours.

### Pharmaceutical precautions

If desired, Rapifen can be mixed with Sodium Chloride Injection BP, Dextrose Injection BP or Compound Sodium Lactate Injection BP (Hartmann's Solution). Such dilutions are compatible with plastic bags and giving sets. These dilutions should be used within 24 hours of preparation.

Rapifen should be stored at room temperature.

### Legal category

CD (Sch 2), POM.

### Package quantities

Rapifen is supplied in 2 ml ampoules (0.5 mg/ml) in packs of 10 and in 10 ml ampoules (0.5 mg/ml) in packs of 10.

### Further information

The analgesic potency of Rapifen is one quarter that of fentanyl. The duration of action of Rapifen is one third that of an equianalgesic dose of fentanyl and is clearly dose-related. Its depressant effects on respiratory rate and alveolar ventilation are also of shorter duration than those of fentanyl.

The onset of action of Rapifen is four times more rapid than that of an equianalgesic dose of fentanyl. The peak analgesic and respiratory depressant effects occur within 90 seconds.

### Product licence number

0242/0091.

## RAPIFEN* INTENSIVE CARE

### Presentation

Clear, colourless, preservative-free, aqueous injection presented in 1 ml ampoules. Each millilitre contains 5 mg of alfentanil as the hydrochloride. Rapifen Intensive Care also contains sodium chloride and water for injection.

### Uses

Rapifen Intensive Care is a potent, opioid analgesic with a very rapid onset of action. It is indicated for analgesia and suppression of respiratory activity and to provide analgesic cover for painful manoeuvres in mechanically ventilated patients on intensive care. It will aid compliance with mechanical ventilation, and tolerance of the endotracheal tube. Intravenous bolus doses of Rapifen (0.5 mg/ml) may be used to provide additional pain relief during brief painful procedures in intensive care such as physiotherapy, endotracheal suction etc.

Patients may appear to be awake in the presence of adequate analgesia. At the proposed doses, Rapifen Intensive Care has no sedative activity. Therefore supplementation with an appropriate hypnotic or

sedative agent is recommended. As alfentanil and the sedative drug need to be titrated separately admixture of the two drugs is not recommended.

Alfentanil given by infusion should only be used in areas where facilities are available to deal with respiratory depression and where continuous monitoring is performed. Alfentanil should only be prescribed by physicians familiar with the use of potent opioids when given by continuous iv infusion.

### Dosage and administration

Once the patient has been intubated, mechanical ventilation can be initiated using the following dosage regimes:

The recommended initial infusion rate for mechanically ventilated adult patients is 2 mg per hour (equivalent to 0.4 mls per hour of undiluted Rapifen Intensive Care). The product should be diluted using the standard infusion solutions. For a 70 kg patient, this corresponds to approximately 30 micrograms/kg/ hour. More rapid control may initially be gained by using a loading dose. For example, a dose of 5 mg may be given in divided doses over a period of 10 minutes, during which time careful monitoring of blood pressure and heart rate should be performed. If hypotension or bradycardia occur, the rate of administration should be reduced accordingly and other appropriate measures instituted.

The dose to produce the desired effects should then be individually determined and reassessed regularly to ensure that the optimum dose is being used. In clinical trials, patient requirements have generally been met with doses of 0.5 to 10 mg alfentanil per hour.

Additional bolus doses of 0.5–1.0 mg alfentanil may be given to provide analgesia during short painful procedures.

Elderly and debilitated patients may require lower doses. In hypothyroidism, pulmonary disease, decreased respiratory reserve, alcoholism and liver impairment the dosage should be titrated with care and prolonged monitoring may be required.

Present data suggest that clearance of alfentanil is unaltered in renal failure. However there is an increased free fraction and hence dosage requirements may be less than in the patient with normal renal function.

Patients on chronic opioid therapy or with a history of opioid abuse may require higher doses. Obese patients may require a dose based on their lean body mass.

Adolescents and young adults will require higher than average doses. There is little experience of use of alfentanil to treat children in intensive care.

The maximum recommended duration of treatment with alfentanil infusions is 4 days.

See also precautions and drug interactions.

### Contra-indications, warnings, etc

*Contra-indications:* Known intolerance to alfentanil or other morphinomimetics.

*Warnings:* Following administration of Rapifen Intensive Care, a transient fall in blood pressure may occur. The magnitude of this effect may be exaggerated in the hypovolaemic patient or in the presence of concomitant sedative medication. Appropriate measures to maintain a stable arterial pressure should be taken.

Like other opioids, alfentanil may cause bradycardia, an effect which may be marked and rapid in onset but which can be antagonised by atropine. Particular care must be exerted following treatment with drugs which may depress the heart or increase vagal tone, such as anaesthetic agents or beta blockers which may predispose to bradycardia or hypotension. Heart rate and blood pressure should therefore be monitored carefully. If hypotension or bradycardia occur, the rate of administration of alfentanil should be reduced and other appropriate measures instituted.

Asystole following bradycardia has been reported on very rare occasions in non-atropinised patients. Therefore it is advisable to be prepared to administer an anticholinergic drug.

Care must be taken if the patient has received monoamine oxidase inhibitors within the previous 2 weeks.

Significant respiratory depression will occur following administration of alfentanil in doses in excess of 1 mg. If necessary for assessment purposes, naloxone or other specific antagonists may be administered to reverse the opioid respiratory depression and other pharmacological effects of alfentanil. More than one dose of naloxone may be required in view of its short half life.

Muscle rigidity (morphine-like effect) may occur, in which case neuromuscular blocking drugs may be helpful.

*Precautions:* It is wise to reduce the dosage in the elderly and debilitated patient. In hypothyroidism, pulmonary disease, decreased respiratory reserve, alcoholism and liver or renal impairment the dosage should be titrated with care and prolonged monitoring may be required.

Patients on chronic opioid therapy or with a history of opioid abuse may require higher doses.

As with all potent opioids, profound analgesia is accompanied by marked respiratory depression, which may persist into or recur in the early post infusion period. Care should therefore be taken throughout the weaning period and adequate spontaneous respiration should be established and maintained in the absence of stimulation or ventilatory support. Following cessation of the infusion the patient should be closely observed for at least six hours. Prior use of opioid premedication may enhance or prolong the respiratory depressant effects of alfentanil.

The use of rapid bolus injections of opioids should be avoided in patients with compromised intracerebral compliance; in such patients a transient decrease in the mean arterial pressure has occasionally been accompanied by a transient reduction of the cerebral perfusion pressure.

*Effects on driving ability and operation of machinery:* Where early discharge is envisaged, patients should be advised not to drive or operate machinery for the 24 hours following administration.

*Drug interactions:* The concomitant use of cimetidine or erythromycin with Rapifen Intensive Care can significantly inhibit alfentanil clearance and may increase the risk of prolonged or delayed respiratory depression. Therefore smaller doses may be required and the duration of action may be extended. Theoretically similar considerations may apply to other enzyme inhibitors.

Treatment with drugs which may depress the heart or increase vagal tone, such as beta-blockers and anaesthetic agents, may predispose to bradycardia or hypotension. Bradycardia and possibly asystole can occur when Rapifen Intensive Care is combined with non-vagolytic muscle relaxants.

Prior use of opioid premedication, barbiturates, benzodiazepines, neuroleptics, halogenic gases and other non-selective CNS depressants may enhance or prolong the respiratory depressant effects of alfentanil.

If other narcotic or CNS depressant drugs are used concurrently with alfentanil, the effects of the drugs can be expected to be additive. When patients have received such drugs, the dose of alfentanil required will be less than usual. Likewise, following the administration of alfentanil, the dose of other CNS-depressant drugs should be reduced.

*Side-effects:* The most common adverse reactions reported with alfentanil are respiratory depression, apnoea and bradycardia.

Nausea and vomiting and dizziness have been reported.

In patients receiving doses of alfentanil large enough to require assisted ventilation, myoclonic movements and muscle rigidity (possibly involving the thoracic muscles) have rarely been reported shortly after the administration of alfentanil.

Other reported adverse reactions are laryngospasm, slight transient hypotension, allergic reactions (such as anaphylaxis, bronchospasm and urticaria), asystole and arrhythmias.

*Use in pregnancy and lactation:* Safety in human pregnancy has not been established although studies in animals have not demonstrated teratogenic or acute embryotoxic effects. As with other drugs possible risk should be weighed against potential benefit to the patient.

Limited data suggest that alfentanil may appear in breast milk. It is therefore recommended that breast feeding is not initiated within 24 hours of treatment.

*Overdosage:* The manifestations of alfentanil overdose are generally an extension of its pharmacological action, which include the following:
*Action:*
Bradycardia: Anticholinergics such as atropine or glycopyrrolate;
Hypoventilation or apnoea: O₂ administration, assisted or controlled respiration and an opioid antagonist may be required;
Muscle rigidity: Intravenous neuromuscular blocking agent may be given.

A specific opioid antagonist (e.g. naloxone) should be available to treat respiratory depression. If hypotension is severe or persists, the possibility of hypovolaemia should be considered and controlled with appropriate parenteral fluid administration.

The suggested treatments given above do not preclude the use of other clinically indicated counter measures.

Body temperature and adequate fluid intake should be maintained and the patient observed for 24 hours.

**Pharmaceutical precautions** Rapifen Intensive Care should be diluted with Sodium Chloride Intravenous Infusion BP, Glucose Intravenous Infusion BP or Compound Sodium Lactate Intravenous Infusion BP (Hartmann's solution). Such dilutions are compatible

with plastic bags and giving sets. These dilutions should be used within 24 hours of preparation.

Store at room temperature.

**Legal category** CD (Sch 2), POM.

**Package quantities** Rapifen Intensive Care 5 mg/ml is supplied in 1 ml ampoules in packs of 10 ampoules.

**Further information** Nil.

**Product licence number** 0242/0137.

## RETIN-A* LOTION, GEL, CREAM

**Presentation** Retin-A is available as either a clear yellow solution of 0.025% w/w tretinoin BP supplied in amber bottles or in tubes of tretinoin BP gel 0.01% w/w or tretinoin BP cream 0.025% w/w or gel 0.025% w/w.

**Uses** For topical application in the treatment of acne vulgaris in which comedones, papules and pustules predominate.

Retin-A Lotion is best suited for large areas such as the back.

Retin-A Gel is best suited for severe acne, for initial therapy and for oily and dark skin.

Retin-A Cream is best suited for use on dry and fair skin.

**Dosage and administration** Retin-A should be applied once or twice daily to the area of skin where acne lesions occur. Only apply sufficient to cover the affected areas lightly, using a gauze swab, cotton wool or the tips of clean fingers. Avoid over-saturation to the extent that excess medication could run into the eyes, angles of the nose or other areas where treatment is not intended.

Initial application may cause transitory stinging and a feeling of warmth. The correct frequency of administration should produce a slight erythema similar to that of mild sunburn.

It is also possible to apply Retin-A and benzoyl peroxide alternately. The suggested regimens are either benzoyl peroxide in the morning and Retin-A in the evening or the preparations should be used on alternate days.

If Retin-A is applied excessively, no more rapid or better results will be obtained and marked redness, peeling or discomfort may occur. Should this occur accidentally or through over-enthusiastic use, application should be discontinued for a few days.

Patience is needed in this treatment, since the therapeutic effects will not usually be observed until after 6-8 weeks of treatment. During the early weeks of treatment, an apparent exacerbation of inflammatory lesions may occur. This is due to the action of the medication on deep, previously unseen comedones and papules. Once the acne lesions have responded satisfactorily, it should be possible to maintain the improvement with less frequent applications.

Moisturisers and cosmetics may be used during treatment with Retin-A but should not be applied to the skin at the same time. The skin should be thoroughly washed before application of Retin-A. Astringent toiletries should be avoided.

*Children:* Safety and effectiveness of Retin-A in children has not been established.

**Contra-indications, warnings, etc**
*Contra-indications:* History of sensitivity/hypersensitivity reactions to any of the components, pregnancy, personal or familial history of cutaneous epithelioma.

*Special warnings and special precautions for use:*

*Local irritation:* The presence of cutaneous irritative signs (e.g. erythema, peeling, pruritus, sunburn, etc) should prohibit initiation or recommencement of treatment with Retin-A until the symptoms resolve.

In certain sensitive individuals, topical use may induce severe local erythema, swelling, pruritus, warmth, burning or stinging, blistering, crusting and/or peeling at the site of application. If the degree of local irritation warrants, the patient should be directed to apply the medication less frequently or discontinue its use temporarily. If a patient experiences severe or persistent irritation, the patient should be advised to discontinue application of Retin-A completely and, if necessary, consult a physician.

Weather extremes, such as wind or cold, also may be irritating to patients being treated with Retin-A.

Tretinoin has been reported to cause severe irritation on eczematous skin and should be used with utmost caution in patients with this condition.

*Exposure to sunlight:* Exposure to sunlight, including ultraviolet sunlamps, should be avoided or minimised during the use of tretinoin. Patients with sunburn should be advised not to use the product until fully recovered because of potential severe irritation to skin. A patient who experiences considerable sun exposure due to occupational duties and/or anyone inherently sensitive to the sun should exercise particular caution., When exposure to sunlight cannot be

avoided, use of sunscreen products and protective clothing over treated areas is recommended.

*General precautions for use:* Before application of Retin-A areas to be treated should be cleansed thoroughly.

Abstain from washing the treated area frequently: twice daily is sufficient. Use of mild soap is recommended. Dry skin without rubbing.

Avoid contact with eyes, eyelids, nostrils, mouth and mucous membranes. If contact in these areas occurs, careful washing with water is recommended.

*Warning:* The weight of evidence indicates that topical tretinoin is not carcinogenic. In a lifetime study of CD-1 mice, a low incidence of skin tumours was seen at 100 and 200 times the estimated clinical dose but, although no such tumours were seen in the study controls, the incidence in these treated animals was within the historic control range for CD-1 mice. Studies in hairless albino mice suggest that tretinoin may accelerate the tumorigenic potential of UVB light from a solar simulator. In other studies, when lightly pigmented hairless mice treated with tretinoin were exposed to carcinogenic doses of UVB light, the photocarcinogenic effects of tretinoin were not observed. Due to significantly different experimental conditions, no strict comparison of this disparate data is possible. Although the significance of these studies in man is not clear, patients should avoid or minimise exposure to sunlight.

The weight of evidence indicates that topical tretinoin is not mutagenic. The mutagenic potential of tretinoin was evaluated in the Ames assay and the *in-vivo* mouse micronucleus assay, both of which showed negative findings.

*Interactions with other medicaments and other forms of interaction:* Retin-A should be used with caution in the presence of:
- Concomitant topical medications
- Toiletry preparations having a strong drying, abrasive or desquamative effect.

Following prolonged use of a peeling agent it is advisable to 'rest' a patients skin until the effects of the peeling agent subside before the use of Retin-A is begun. When Retin-A and peeling agents are alternated contact dermatitis may result and the frequency of application may have to be reduced.

*Pregnancy and lactation:* The topical human dose used in a 50 kg adult applying a maximum volume of 500 mg of 0.05% Retin-A cream is 0.005 mg/kg. In animal reproductive studies, oral tretinoin is known to be teratogenic and has been shown to be foetotoxic in rats when given in doses 500 times the topical human dose. In reproduction studies in rats and rabbits, topical tretinoin, when used at doses 500 and 320 times the topical human dose, respectively, induced minor skeletal abnormalities, e.g. irregularly contoured or partially ossified skull bones. These changes may be considered variants of normal development and are usually corrected after weaning. Retin-A should not be used during pregnancy.

It is not known whether tretinoin is excreted in human milk, therefore caution should be exercised when Retin-A is administered to a nursing mother.

*Effects on ability to drive and use machinery:* Retin-A is administered topically and is unlikely to have an effect on one's ability to drive or operate machinery.

*Undesirable effects:* Local reactions frequently reported during therapy included: dry or peeling skin, burning, stinging, warmth, erythema, pruritus, rash and temporary hypo- and hyper-pigmentation. These skin reactions were usually mild to moderate and were generally well-tolerated. They usually occurred early in therapy and, except for dry or peeling skin which persisted during therapy, generally decreased over the course of therapy. Rarely reported undesirable effects are blistering and crusting of the skin, eye irritation and oedema.

True contact allergy to topical tretinoin is rarely encountered. Heightened susceptibility to either sunlight or other sources of UVB light has been reported.

*Overdose:* Excessive application of Retin-A does not improve the results of treatment and may induce marked irritation, e.g. erythema, peeling, pruritus, etc. Oral ingestion of Retin-A may lead to the same effects associated with excessive oral intake of vitamin A (e.g. pruritus, dry skin, arthralgias, anorexia, vomiting). In the event of accidental ingestion, if the ingestion is recent an appropriate method of gastric emptying should be used as soon as possible.

**Pharmaceutical precautions** Store in a cool place. The 100 ml bottle of lotion should be protected from light and any remaining medicine discarded on completion of treatment.

**Legal category** POM.

**Package quantities** *Lotion:* Amber glass bottle containing 100 ml.
*Gel and Cream:* Tubes containing 60 g.

**Further information** Nil.

**Product licence numbers**

| | |
|---|---|
| Lotion | 0242/0269 |
| Gel 0.01% | 0242/0268 |
| Cream | 0242/0266 |
| Gel 0.025% | 0242/0265 |

## RETINOVA*

**Qualitative and quantitative composition** Retinova contains the active ingredient tretinoin 0.05% w/w in a water-in-oil emulsion for topical use only.

**Pharmaceutical form** Emollient Cream.

### Clinical particulars

*Therapeutic indication:* For the topical treatment of mottled hyperpigmentation, roughness and fine wrinkling of photodamaged skin due to chronic sun exposure.

*Posology and method of administration:* Retinova should be applied to affected areas once at night daily. Only sufficient quantity to cover the areas lightly should be used. Application of Retinova may cause transitory stinging and a feeling of warmth. The correct frequency of administration normally produces a slight transient erythema similar to that of mild sunburn. No more rapid or better results will be obtained with excessive use of Retinova and local side effects such as redness, peeling or discomfort may occur. Should this occur treatment should be discontinued for a few days. (See Local Irritation).

Care should be taken to avoid contact with the eyes, nostrils, mouth or other areas where treatment is not intended.

*Duration of treatment:* Improvements in the signs of photodamage with Retinova are not immediate but occur gradually over the course of therapy, hence patience is needed during this treatment. Onset of visible improvements varied across clinical studies, however, in general, effects emerged within 3-4 months of commencing treatment. Six months of treatment may be required before definite beneficial effects are seen.

Once the maximum beneficial effects have been achieved, they can be maintained with application of Retinova once to thrice weekly. If maintenance therapy is not used, the beneficial effect achieved will diminish over time.

Moisturisers and cosmetics may be used during treatment with Retinova but should not be applied to the skin at the same time. The skin should be thoroughly washed before application of Retinova. (See Special Warnings and Special Precautions for use). Patients should be advised on the importance of sun avoidance, use of sunscreens, moisturising products and protective clothing.

*Contra-indications:* History of sensitivity/hypersensitivity reactions to any of the components, pregnancy, personal or familial history of cutaneous epithelioma.

*Special warnings and special precautions for use:*

*Local irritation:* The presence of cutaneous irritative signs (e.g. erythema, peeling, pruritus, sunburn, etc) should prohibit initiation or recommencement of treatment with Retinova until the symptoms resolve.

In certain sensitive individuals, topical use may induce severe local erythema, swelling, pruritus, warmth, burning or stinging, blistering, crusting and/ or peeling at the site of application. If the degree of local irritation warrants, the patient should be directed to apply the medication less frequently or discontinue its use temporarily. If a patient experiences severe or persistent irritation, the patient should be advised to discontinue application of Retinova completely and, if necessary, consult a physician. (See Posology and Method of Administration).

Caution should be exercised during concomitant therapy with other local irritants, especially those having an abrasive, drying or desquamative effect (See Interaction with Other Medicaments and other forms of interaction).

Weather extremes, such as wind or cold, also may be irritating to patients being treated with Retinova (Also see: Exposure to sunlight).

Tretinoin has been reported to cause severe irritation on eczematous skin and should be used with utmost caution in patients with this condition.

*Exposure to sunlight:* Exposure to sunlight, including ultraviolet sunlamps, should be avoided or minimised during the use of tretinoin. Patients with sunburn should be advised not to use the product until fully recovered because of potential severe irritation to skin. A patient who experiences considerable sun exposure due to occupational duties and/or anyone inherently sensitive to the sun should exercise particular caution. When exposure to sunlight cannot be avoided, use of sunscreen products and protective clothing over treated areas is recommended.

*General precautions for use:* Before application of Retinova, areas to be treated should be cleansed thoroughly.

Abstain from washing the treated area frequently: twice daily is sufficient. Use of a mild soap is recommended. Dry skin without rubbing.

Avoid contact with eyes, eyelids, nostrils, mouth and mucous membranes. If contact in these areas occurs, careful washing with water is recommended.

*Warning:* The weight of evidence indicates that topical tretinoin is not carcinogenic. In a lifetime study of CD-1 mice, a low incidence of skin tumours was seen at 100 and 200 times the estimated clinical dose but, although no such tumours were seen in the study controls, the incidence in these treated animals was within the historic control range for CD-1 mice. Studies in hairless albino mice suggest that tretinoin may accelerate the tumorigenic potential of UVB light from a solar simulator. In other studies, when lightly pigmented hairless mice treated with tretinoin were exposed to carcinogenic doses of UVB light, the photocarcinogenic effects of tretinoin were not observed. Due to significantly different experimental conditions, no strict comparison of this disparate data is possible. Although the significance of these studies in man is not clear, patients should avoid or minimise exposure to sunlight (see *Exposure to sunlight*).

The weight of evidence indicates that topical tretinoin is not mutagenic. The mutagenic potential of tretinoin was evaluated in the Ames assay and the *in vivo* mouse micronucleus assay, both of which showed negative findings.

*Paediatric use:* Safety and effectiveness of Retinova in children have not been established.

*Interaction with other medicaments and other forms of interaction:* Use Retinova with caution in the presence of:
- concomitant topical medications
- toiletry preparations having a strong drying, abrasive or desquamative effect.

*Pregnancy and lactation:* In clinical trials with Retinova, the topical human dose used in a 50 kg adult applying a maximum volume of 500 mg of 0.05% cream was 0.005 mg/kg. In animal reproductive studies, oral tretinoin is known to be teratogenic and has been shown to be foetotoxic in rats when given in doses 500 times the topical human dose. In reproduction studies in rats and rabbits, topical tretinoin, when used at doses 500 and 320 times the topical human dose, respectively, induced minor skeletal abnormalities, e.g. irregularly contoured or partially ossified skull bones. These changes may be considered variants of normal development and are usually corrected after weaning.

Retinova should not be used during pregnancy.

It is not known whether tretinoin is excreted in human milk, therefore caution should be exercised when Retinova is administered to a nursing mother.

*Effects on ability to drive and use machinery:* Retinova is administered topically and is unlikely to have an effect on one's ability to drive or operate machinery.

*Undesirable effects:* Local reactions frequently reported during therapy included: dry or peeling skin, burning, stinging, warmth, erythema and pruritus and temporary hypo-pigmentation and hyper-pigmentation. These skin reactions were usually mild to moderate and were generally well-tolerated. They usually occurred early in therapy and, except for dry or peeling skin which persisted during therapy, generally decreased over the course of therapy (see *Local irritation*).

Clinical studies with Retinova showed no incidence of true allergic contact sensitivity. Heightened susceptibility to either sunlight or other sources of UVB light has been reported.

*Overdose:* Excessive application of Retinova does not improve the results of treatment and may induce marked irritation, e.g. erythema, peeling, pruritus, etc. Oral ingestion of Retinova may lead to the same side effects associated with excessive oral intake of vitamin A (e.g. pruritus, dry skin, arthralgias, anorexia, vomiting).

### Pharmacological properties

*Pharmacodynamic properties:* The mechanism of action of topical tretinoin as a treatment for photodamage is not completely understood. However, it is known that tretinoin activates gene transcription for many important proteins by binding to specific retinoid receptors in the cell nucleus. Studies employing light microscopy show an increase in Type 1 collagen, while ultrastructural studies show an increased number of anchoring fibrils in the papillary dermis of tretinoin-treated photodamaged skin. These molecular events, coupled with the characteristic histologic effects of tretinoin, i.e. increased epidermal and granular layer thickness with changes in stratum corneum morphology, indicate a specific effect rather than one induced by irritation, as has been previously suggested.

*Pharmacokinetic properties:* Upon topical application of Retinova, tretinoin penetrates both the epidermis and dermis. Percutaneous absorption of tretinoin in an emollient cream formulation was assessed in healthy male subjects after a single application and after repeated daily applications. The mean percutaneous absorption was less than 2% and endogenous concentrations of tretinoin and its major metabolites were unaltered.

*Preclinical safety data:* See sections *Warning* and *Pregnancy and lactation.*

### Pharmaceutical particulars

*List of excipients:* Light mineral oil; sorbitol solution (E420); hydroxyoctacosanyl hydroxystearate; methoxy PEG-22/dodecyl glycol copolymer; PEG-45/dodecyl glycol copolymer; stearoxytrimethylsilane and stearyl alcohol; dimethicone 50 cs; fragrance; methylparahydroxybenzoate (E218); edetate disodium; Quaternium-15; butylated hydroxytoluene (E321); citric acid (monohydrate); purified water.

*Incompatibilities:* None pertinent.

*Shelf-life:* 18 months.

*Special precautions for storage:* Store at or below 25°C (77°F). DO NOT FREEZE.

*Nature and content of container:* Blind ended, lined aluminium tube with opaque white polyethylene cap, containing 20 g of cream.

*Instructions for use/handling:* Discard any remaining medicine upon completion of treatment.

**Marketing authorisation number** 0242/0264

**Date of approval/revision of SPC** January 1995.

**Legal category** POM.

## RISPERDAL*

**Qualitative and quantitative composition** *Tablets:* risperidone 1, 2, 3, 4 and 6 mg.
*Liquid:* risperidone 1 mg/ml.

**Pharmaceutical form** Coated tablets.

| | |
|---|---|
| 1 mg: | White, oblong tablets, marked Ris\|1. |
| 2 mg: | Pale orange, oblong tablets, marked Ris\|2. |
| 3 mg: | Yellow, oblong tablets, marked Ris\|3. |
| 4 mg: | Green, oblong tablets, marked Ris\|4. |
| 6 mg: | Yellow, circular tablets, marked Ris\|6. |

Oral liquid

### Clinical particulars

*Therapeutic indications:* Risperdal is indicated for the treatment of acute and chronic schizophrenic psychoses, and other psychotic conditions, in which positive symptoms (such as hallucinations, delusions, thought disturbances, hostility, suspiciousness), and/or negative symptoms (such as blunted affect, emotional and social withdrawal, poverty of speech) are prominent. Risperdal also alleviates affective symptoms (such as depression, guilt feelings, anxiety) associated with schizophrenia.

*Posology and method of administration:* 1 ml of Risperdal liquid contains 1 mg risperidone. If necessary Risperdal liquid may be diluted with mineral water, orange juice or black coffee. When diluted in this way, the product should be used immediately. The liquid should not be mixed with tea (see *Pharmaceutical particulars*).

Switching from other antipsychotics: where medically appropriate, gradual discontinuation of the previous treatment while Risperdal therapy is initiated is recommended. Where medically appropriate when switching patients from depot antipsychotics, consider initiating Risperdal therapy in place of the next scheduled injection. The need for continuing existing antiparkinson medication should be re-evaluated periodically.

*Adults:* Risperdal may be given once or twice daily. Patients should be titrated to 6 mg/day gradually over three days. All patients, whether acute or chronic, should start with 2 mg/day Risperdal. The dosage should be increased to 4 mg/day on the second day and 6 mg/day on the third day. However, some patients such as first episode patients may benefit from a slower rate of titration. From then on the dosage can be maintained unchanged, or further individualised, if needed. The usual effective dosage is 4 to 8 mg/day although in some patients an optimal response may be obtained at lower doses.

Doses above 10 mg/day generally have not been shown to provide additional efficacy to lower doses and may increase the risk of extrapyramidal symptoms. Doses above 10 mg/day should only be used in individual patients if the benefit is considered to outweigh the risk. Doses above 16 mg/day have not been extensively evaluated for safety and therefore should not be used.

*Elderly:* A starting dose of 0.5 mg bd is recommended. This dosage can be individually adjusted with 0.5 mg bd increments to 1 to 2 mg bd.

Risperdal is well tolerated by the elderly.

*Children:* Not recommended in children aged less than 15 years.

*Renal and liver disease:* A starting dose of 0.5 mg bd is recommended. This dosage can be individually adjusted with 0.5 mg bd increments to 1 to 2 mg bd.

Risperdal should be used with caution in this group of patients until further experience is gained.

*Method of administration:* Oral use.

*Contra-indications:* Risperdal is contra-indicated in patients with a known hypersensitivity to the product.

*Special warnings and precautions for use:* Due to the alpha-blocking activity of Risperdal, orthostatic hypotension can occur, especially during the initial dose-titration period. Risperdal should be used with caution in patients with known cardiovascular disease. A dose reduction should be considered if hypotension occurs.

If further sedation is required, an additional drug (such as a benzodiazepine) should be administered rather than increasing the dose of Risperdal.

Drugs with dopamine receptor antagonistic properties have been associated with the induction of tardive dyskinesia, characterised by rhythmical involuntary movements, predominantly of the tongue and/or face. It has been reported that the occurrence of extrapyramidal symptoms is a risk factor for the development of tardive dyskinesia. If signs and symptoms of tardive dyskinesia appear, the discontinuation of all antipsychotic drugs should be considered.

It is recommended to halve both the starting dose and the subsequent dose increments in geriatric patients and in patients with renal or liver insufficiency.

Caution should also be exercised when prescribing Risperdal to patients with Parkinson's disease since, theoretically, it may cause a deterioration of the disease.

Classical neuroleptics are known to lower the seizure threshold. Caution is recommended when treating patients with epilepsy.

As with other antipsychotics, patients should be advised of the potential for weight gain.

*Interactions with other medicaments and other forms of interaction:* Possible interactions of Risperdal with other drugs have not been systematically evaluated. Given the primary CNS effects of Risperdal it should be used with caution in combination with other centrally acting drugs.

Risperdal may antagonise the effect of levodopa and other dopamine-agonists.

Carbamazepine has been shown to decrease the plasma levels of the antipsychotic fraction of Risperdal. A similar effect might be anticipated with other drugs which stimulate metabolising enzymes in the liver. On initiation of carbamazepine or other hepatic enzyme-inducing drugs, the dosage of Risperdal should be re-evaluated and increased if necessary. Conversely, on discontinuation of such drugs, the dosage of Risperdal should be re-evaluated and decreased if necessary.

Phenothiazines, tricyclic antidepressants and some beta-blockers may increase the plasma concentrations of risperidone but not those of the antipsychotic fraction. Based on *in vitro* studies, the same interaction may occur with haloperidol and fluoxetine.

When Risperdal is taken together with other highly protein-bound drugs, there is no clinically relevant displacement of either drug from the plasma proteins.

Food does not affect the absorption of Risperdal.

*Pregnancy and lactation:* Although, in experimental animals, risperidone did not show direct reproductive toxicity, some indirect, prolactin- and CNS-mediated effects were observed, typically delayed oestrus and changes in mating and nursing behaviour in rats. No teratogenic effect of risperidone was noted in any study. The safety of Risperdal for use during human pregnancy has not been established. Therefore, Risperdal should only be used during pregnancy if the benefits outweigh the risks.

In animal studies, risperidone and 9-hydroxyrisperidone are excreted in the milk. It is not known whether Risperdal is excreted in human milk. Therefore, women receiving Risperdal should not breast feed.

*Effects on ability to drive and use machines:* Risperdal may interfere with activities requiring mental alertness. Therefore, patients should be advised not to drive or operate machinery until their individual susceptibility is known.

*Undesirable effects:* Risperdal is generally well tolerated and in many instances it has been difficult to differentiate adverse events from symptoms of the underlying disease. Adverse events observed in association with the use of Risperdal include:

Common: insomnia, agitation, anxiety, headache.

Less common: somnolence, fatigue, dizziness, impaired concentration, constipation, dyspepsia, nausea/vomiting, abdominal pain, blurred vision, priapism, erectile dysfunction, ejaculatory dysfunction, orgasmic dysfunction, urinary incontinence, rhinitis, rash and other allergic reactions.

The incidence and severity of extrapyramidal symptoms are significantly less than with haloperidol. However, in some cases the following extrapyramidal symptoms may occur: tremor, rigidity, hypersalivation, bradykinesia, akathisia, acute dystonia. If acute in nature, these symptoms are usually mild and are reversible upon dose reduction and/or administration of antiparkinson medication, if necessary.

As with other neuroleptics, rare cases of neuroleptic malignant syndrome, characterised by hyperthermia, muscle rigidity, autonomic instability, altered consciousness and elevated CPK levels, have been reported. In such an event, all antipsychotic drugs, including Risperdal, should be discontinued.

Occasionally, orthostatic dizziness, hypotension including orthostatic, tachycardia including reflex tachycardia and hypertension have been observed following administration of Risperdal.

Risperdal can induce a dose-dependent increase in plasma prolactin concentration. Possible associated manifestations are: galactorrhoea, gynaecomastia, disturbances of the menstrual cycle and amenorrhoea.

Weight gain, oedema and increased hepatic enzyme levels have been observed during treatment with Risperdal.

A mild fall in neutrophil and/or thrombocyte count has been reported.

As with classical neuroleptics, rare cases of the following have been reported in schizophrenic patients: water intoxication with hyponatraemia, either due to polydipsia or to the syndrome of inappropriate secretion of antidiuretic hormone; tardive dyskinesia, body temperature dysregulation and seizures.

*Overdose:* Overdosages of up to 360 mg have been reported. In general, reported signs and symptoms have been those resulting from an exaggeration of the drug's known pharmacological effects. These include drowsiness and sedation, tachycardia and hypotension, and extrapyramidal symptoms. A prolonged QT interval was reported in a patient with concomitant hypokalaemia who had ingested 360 mg. The patient made an uneventful recovery. In case of acute overdosage, the possibility of multiple drug involvement should be considered.

Establish and maintain a clear airway, and ensure adequate oxygenation and ventilation. Gastric lavage (after intubation, if the patient is unconscious) and administration of activated charcoal together with a laxative should be considered. Cardiovascular monitoring should commence immediately and should include continuous electrocardiographic monitoring to detect possible arrhythmias.

There is no specific antidote to Risperdal. Therefore appropriate supportive measures should be instituted. Hypotension and circulatory collapse should be treated with appropriate measures such as intravenous fluids and/or sympathomimetic agents. In case of severe extrapyramidal symptoms, anticholinergic medication should be administered. Close medical supervision and monitoring should continue until the patient recovers.

**Pharmacological properties**

*Pharmacodynamic properties:* Risperdal is a novel antipsychotic belonging to a new class of antipsychotic agents, the benzisoxazole-derivatives.

Risperdal is a selective monoaminergic antagonist with a high affinity for both serotonergic 5-$HT_2$ and dopaminergic $D_2$ receptors. Risperdal binds also to alpha$_1$-adrenergic receptors and, with lower affinity, to $H_1$-histaminergic and alpha$_2$-adrenergic receptors. Risperdal has no affinity for cholinergic receptors. Although Risperdal is a potent $D_2$ antagonist, an activity which is considered to improve the positive symptoms of schizophrenia, it causes less depression of motor activity and induction of catalepsy than classical neuroleptics. Balanced central serotonin and dopamine antagonism may reduce the tendency to cause extrapyramidal side effects, and extend the therapeutic activity to the negative and affective symptoms of schizophrenia.

*Pharmacokinetic properties:* Risperdal is completely absorbed after oral administration, reaching peak plasma concentrations within 1 to 2 hours. The absorption is not affected by food.

The most important route of metabolism of Risperdal is hydroxylation to 9-hydroxy-risperidone which has a similar pharmacological activity to risperidone. This hydroxylation is subject to debrisoquine-type genetic polymorphism but this does not affect the active antipsychotic fraction since this consists of risperidone and its active metabolite 9-hydroxyrisperidone. After oral administration, the elimination half-life of the active antipsychotic fraction is 24 hours.

A single-dose study showed higher active plasma concentrations and a slower elimination of Risperdal in the elderly and in patients with renal insufficiency. Risperdal plasma concentrations were normal in patients with liver insufficiency.

*Preclinical safety data:* Not applicable.

**Pharmaceutical particulars**

*List of excipients: Tablets:* All four tablet strengths contain the following excipients: Lactose; maize starch; microcrystalline cellulose; hypromellose 2910 15 mPa.s; magnesium stearate; colloidal anhydrous silica; sodium lauryl sulphate; purified water*.

* not present in the final product.

In addition, the tablets also contain the following excipients:

1 mg: Hypromellose 2910 5 mPa.s, propylene glycol.

2 mg: Hypromellose 2910 5 mPa.s, titanium dioxide, talc, propylene glycol, orange yellow S (E110) aluminium lake.

3 mg: Hypromellose 2910 5 mPa.s, titanium dioxide (E171), talc, propylene glycol, quinoline yellow (E104).

4 mg: Hypromellose 2910 5 mPa.s, titanium dioxide (E171), talc, propylene glycol, quinoline yellow (E104), indigotine disulphonate (E132), aluminium lake.

6 mg: Titanium dioxide (E171), talc, propylene glycol, quinoline yellow (E104), orange yellow S(E110).

Liquid: Tartaric acid, benzoic acid, sodium hydroxide, purified water.

*Incompatibilities: Tablets:* Not applicable.
*Liquid:* Risperdal Liquid should only be diluted with those beverages listed in Posology and method of administration.

*Shelf life: Tablets:* 1, 2, 3 & 4 mg tablets: 36 months. 6 mg tablets: 24 months.

*Liquid:* The unopened bottles have a shelf life of 36 months. Once opened, the contents of the bottle should be used within 3 months.

*Special precautions for storage: Tablets:* Store below 30°C.
*Liquid:* Store below 30°C; protect from freezing.

*Nature and contents of container: Tablets:* Blister strips consisting of polyvinylchloride (PVC)/low density polyethylene (LDPE)/polyvinylidene chloride (PVDC) and aluminium foil. The strips are packed in cardboard cartons to contain either 6 (1 mg tablets only), 20 (1 mg tablets only), 60 tablets (2, 3 and 4 mg tablets) or 28 tablets (6 mg tablets) per pack.
*Liquid:* Amber glass bottle with a plastic child-resistant and tamper-evident cap. Each bottle contains 100 ml.

*Instructions for use/handling: Tablets:* Not applicable.
*Liquid:* A special dosing pipette is supplied with each pack of Risperdal Liquid.

*Instructions for using the pipette with Risperdal liquid:*

1. Remove the child-proof cap from the bottle by pushing down on the cap while turning it anticlockwise (Fig. 1)

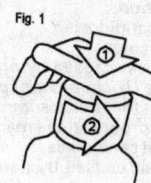

Fig. 1

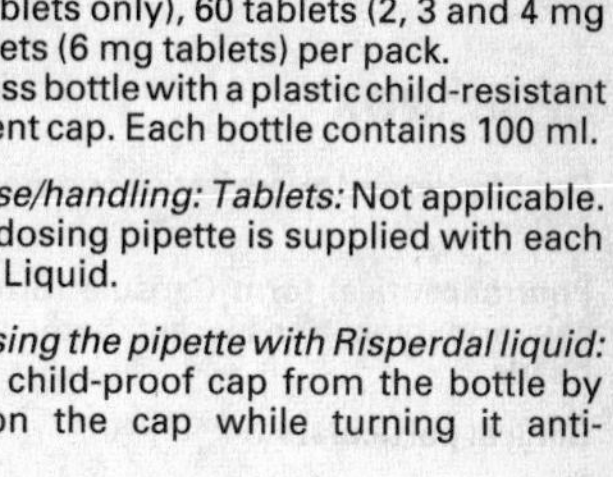


2. Place the bottle on a flat surface.
3. Pull the pipette out of its case (Fig. 2).

Fig. 2

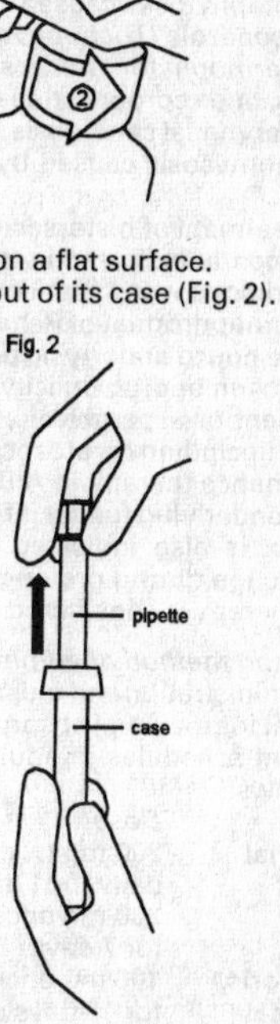


4. Insert the pipette into the liquid in the bottle.
5. While holding the lower ring, pull the top ring upwards until the mark that matches the number of mg or ml to be taken is just visible (Fig. 3).

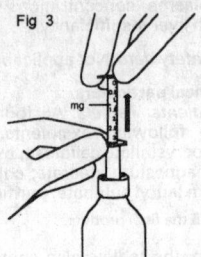

Fig 3

6. Holding the lower ring, remove the whole pipette from the bottle (Fig. 4).

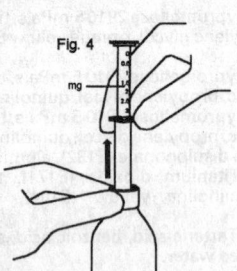

Fig. 4

7. To empty the pipette, push down on the top ring while still holding the lower ring.

8. The contents of the pipette may be emptied directly into the mouth or into a drink of mineral water, orange juice or black coffee.

9. Put the empty pipette back in its case.

10. Replace the child-proof cap on the bottle by screwing it down clockwise.

**Marketing authorisation numbers**

| | |
|---|---|
| 1 mg tablets | 0242/0186 |
| 2 mg tablets | 0242/0187 |
| 3 mg tablets | 0242/0188 |
| 4 mg tablets | 0242/0189 |
| 6 mg tablets | 0242/0317 |
| 1 mg/ml liquid | 0242/0199 |

**Date of approval/revision of SPC** May 1997

**Legal category** POM.

## SPORANOX*

**Qualitative and quantitative composition** Itraconazole 100 mg.

**Pharmaceutical form** Capsule (Size 0): opaque blue cap and pink transparent body containing coated beads.

**Clinical particulars**

*Therapeutic indications:*
1. Vulvovaginal candidosis.
2. Pityriasis versicolor.
3. Dermatophytoses caused by organisms susceptible to itraconazole *(Trichophyton* spp., *Microsporum* spp., *Epidermophyton floccosum)* eg tinea pedis, tinea cruris, tinea corporis, tinea manuum.
4. Oropharyngeal candidosis.
5. Onychomycosis caused by dermatophytes and/or yeasts.
6. The treatment of histoplasmosis.
7. Sporanox is indicated in the following systemic fungal conditions when first-line systemic anti-fungal therapy is inappropriate or has proved ineffective. This may be due to underlying pathology, insensitivity of the pathogen or drug toxicity.
- Treatment of aspergillosis, candidosis and cryptococcosis (including cryptococcal meningitis);
- Maintenance therapy in AIDS patients to prevent relapse of underlying fungal infection.
Sporanox is also indicated in the prevention of fungal infection during prolonged neutropenia when standard therapy is considered inappropriate.

*Posology and method of administration:* Sporanox is for oral administration and must be taken immediately after a meal for maximal absorption.
Treatment schedules in adults for each indication are as follows:

| Indication | Dose | Remarks |
|---|---|---|
| Vulvovaginal candidosis | 200 mg twice daily for 1 day | |
| Pityriasis versicolor | 200 mg once daily for 7 days | |
| Tinea corporis, tinea cruris | 100 mg once daily for 15 days or 200 mg once daily for 7 days | |
| Tinea pedis, tinea manuum | 100 mg once daily for 30 days | |
| Oropharyngeal candidosis | 100 mg once daily for 15 days | Increase dose to 200 mg once daily for 15 days in AIDS or neutropenic patients because of impaired absorption in these groups. |
| Onychomycosis | 200 mg once daily for 3 months | |

For skin, vulvovaginal and oropharyngeal infections, optimal clinical and mycological effects are reached 1-4 weeks after cessation of treatment and for nail infections, 6–9 months after the cessation of treatment. This is because elimination of itraconazole from skin, nails and mucous membranes is slower than from plasma.
The length of treatment for systemic fungal infections should be dictated by the mycological and clinical response to therapy:

| Indication | Dose | Remarks |
|---|---|---|
| Aspergillosis | 200 mg once daily | Increase dose to 200 mg twice daily in case of invasive or disseminated disease |
| Candidosis | 100-200 mg once daily | Increase dose to 200 mg twice daily in case of invasive or disseminated disease |
| Non-meningeal cryptococcosis | 200 mg twice daily | |
| Cryptococcal meningitis | 200 mg twice daily | |
| Histoplasmosis | 200 mg once daily - 200 mg twice daily | |
| Maintenance in AIDS | 200 mg once daily | See note on impaired absorption below |
| Prophylaxis in neutropenia | 200 mg once daily | See note on impaired absorption below |

Impaired absorption in AIDS and neutropenic patients may lead to low itraconazole blood levels and lack of efficacy. In such cases blood level monitoring and if necessary an increase in itraconazole dose to 200 mg twice daily is indicated.

*In children (below 12 years):* There are inadequate data on Sporanox in children for its use to be recommended, unless the potential benefits outweigh the risks.

*In elderly:* As for use in children.

*Contra-indications:* When administered at high doses to pregnant rats (40 mg/kg/day) and mice (80 mg/kg/day), itraconazole was shown to cause abnormalities of foetal development. No data are available in human pregnancy, and itraconazole is therefore contra-indicated in pregnancy. Adequate contraceptive precautions should be taken by women of childbearing potential during therapy and for one menstrual cycle after stopping therapy.
Itraconazole is also contra-indicated in patients who have shown hypersensitivity to itraconazole, other azole antifungal agents or any of the excipients.
The drugs terfenadine, astemizole, cisapride, HMG-CoA reductase inhibitors such as simvastatin, oral midazolam or triazolam should not be given concurrently with itraconazole (see also interactions).

*Special warnings and special precautions for use:* Absorption is impaired when gastric acidity is decreased. In patients also receiving acid neutralising medicines (eg aluminium hydroxide) these should be administered at least 2 hours after the intake of Sporanox. In patients with achlorhydria such as certain AIDS patients and patients on secretion supressors (eg H2-antagonists, proton-pump inhibitors), it is advisable to administer Sporanox with a cola beverage.
Rarely cases of hepatitis and cholestatic jaundice have been reported, mainly in patients treated for longer than one month. It is therefore advisable to monitor liver function in patients receiving continuous treatment of more than one month's duration. Additionally, if during treatment (other than single-day therapy for vulvovaginal candidosis) patients develop symptoms suggestive of hepatitis such as anorexia, nausea, vomiting, fatigue, abdominal pain or dark urine, liver enzymes should be monitored promptly. If these are abnormal, treatment should be stopped. In patients with raised liver enzymes, or with a known history of liver disease, or who have experienced liver toxicity with other drugs, treatment should not be started unless the expected benefit exceeds the risk of hepatic injury. In such instances liver enzyme monitoring is necessary.
Itraconazole is predominantly metabolised in the liver. A slight decrease in oral bioavailability in cirrhotic patients has been observed, although this was not of statistical significance. The terminal half-life was however significantly increased. It is advised to monitor the itraconazole plasma concentrations in such patients and to adapt the dose when necessary.
The oral bioavailability of itraconazole may be lower in some patients with renal insufficiency (e.g. those receiving continuous ambulatory peritoneal dialysis). Monitoring of the itraconazole plasma levels and dose adaptation are advisable.
Isolated cases of peripheral neuropathy have been reported, predominantly during long-term treatment and in severely compromised patients. The causal relationship to Sporanox was uncertain. If neuropathy occurs which may be attributable to Sporanox, treatment should be discontinued.
In systemic candidosis, if fluconazole-resistant strains of *Candida* species are suspected, it cannot be assumed that these are sensitive to itraconazole, hence their sensitivity should be tested before the start of Sporanox therapy.

*Interaction with other medicaments and other forms of interaction:*
*Drug-interactions:* Enzyme-inducing drugs such as rifampicin and phenytoin significantly reduce the oral bioavailability of itraconazole. Consequently, monitoring of the itraconazole plasma concentration is advised when enzyme-inducing agents are co-administered.
Itraconazole can inhibit the metabolism of drugs metabolised by the cytochrome 3A family. This can result in an increase and/or a prolongation of their effects, including side effects. Known examples are:
- Terfenadine, astemizole and cisapride, resulting in increased plasma levels of these drugs and predisposing to serious arrhythmias. Combination of itraconazole with terfenadine, astemizole or cisapride is contra-indicated.
- Midazolam and triazolam, resulting in increased plasma levels of these drugs. Combination of itraconazole with oral midazolam or triazolam is contra-indicated. If midazolam is administered intravenously (eg as premedication in surgical or investigative procedures) special care should be observed since the sedative effect may be prolonged.
- HMG-CoA reductase inhibitors such as simvastatin. These drugs should not be used during treatment with Sporanox.
- Oral anticoagulants, digoxin, cyclosporin A, systemic methylprednisolone, vinca-alkaloids and possibly tacrolimus. Co-administration of itraconazole and digoxin has led to increased levels of the latter drug. A rise in cyclosporin levels has also been reported in patients treated with high doses of itraconazole for several weeks. Plasma levels of digoxin and cyclosporin should therefore be monitored during concomitant administration of itraconazole and the doses adjusted accordingly. *In vitro* studies indicate that a similar interaction may occur with tacrolimus. With respect to oral anticoagulants, similar interactions have been reported and it is advisable to monitor prothrombin time and reduce the dosage of oral anticoagulants if necessary. Co-administration of itraconazole and vinca-alkaloids may potentiate the toxic effects of the latter drugs and should this occur, co-administration of these drugs should be reconsidered.
- Dihydropyridine calcium channel blockers and quinidine. Patients should be monitored for side effects, eg oedema and tinnitus/decreased hearing, respectively. If necessary, the dose of these drugs should be reduced.
Despite the fact that itraconazole is 99.8% bound to plasma proteins, there are no *in vitro* interactions on the plasma protein binding between itraconazole and imipramine, propanolol, diazepam, cimetidine, indomethacin, tolbutamide or sulphadimidine.
Itraconazole does not appear to affect the metabolism of ethinyloestradiol and norethisterone. Reports suggest that there is no interaction of itraconazole with the oral pharmacokinetics of AZT (zidovudine).

*Pregnancy and lactation:*
*Pregnancy:* Sporanox is contra-indicated in pregnancy (see Contra-indications section for further details).
*Lactation:* Only small amounts of itraconazole are excreted in human milk. The expected benefits of therapy should be weighed against the risks to the infant.

*Effects on ability to drive and use machines:* None known.

*Undesirable effects:* The most frequently reported adverse experiences in association with the use of Sporanox are of gastro-intestinal origin, such as dyspepsia, nausea, abdominal pain and constipation. Less frequently reported adverse experiences include headache, reversible increases in hepatic enzymes, menstrual disorder, dizziness and allergic reactions (such as pruritus, rash, urticaria and angio-oedema). Isolated cases of peripheral neuropathy and of Stevens-Johnson syndrome have also been reported; a causality for the latter was not established.

Mainly in patients receiving prolonged treatment (ie approximately one month), most of whom had major underlying pathology and multiple concomitant medications, cases of hypokalaemia, oedema and hair loss have been observed. Hepatitis and cholestatic jaundice have been reported rarely, mainly in patients treated for longer than one month.

*Overdose:* In the event of overdosage, patients should be treated symptomatically with supportive measures and gastric lavage as necessary. No specific antidote is available. Itraconazole cannot be removed by haemodialysis.

### Pharmacological properties

*Pharmacodynamic properties:* Itraconazole is a substituted triazole antimycotic with a broad spectrum of activity against *Candida* spp and other yeasts, dermatophytes and pathogenic fungi. It acts by impairing the synthesis of ergosterol in fungal cell membranes.

*Pharmacokinetic properties:* Peak plasma concentrations of itraconazole in the region of 1 mcg equiv/ml are reached 1.5-3 hrs after administration. In man the elimination half life is about 20 hrs. Oral intake immediately after a meal doubled the peak level 3–4 hrs after intake.

Peak concentrations of itraconazole in keratinous tissues, especially skin, are up to 3 times higher than in plasma. Therapeutic levels in the skin persist for up to 2–4 weeks after stopping treatment as elimination is related to epidermal regeneration, rather than redistribution into the systemic circulation. Itraconazole is extensively metabolised by the liver to a large number of metabolites, which constitute 40% of the excreted dose. Faecal excretion of parent drug varies from 3-18% of the dose, and urinary excretion of unchanged drug is less than 0.03%.

*Preclinical safety data:* Not applicable.

### Pharmaceutical particulars

*List of excipients:* Sugar spheres; hypromellose 2910 5 mPa.s; macrogol 20000. Capsule shell: Titanium dioxide; indigo carmine; gelatin; erythrosine.

*Incompatibilities:* None known.

*Shelf life:* 36 months.

*Special precautions for storage:* Protect from light. Store in a dry place. Store between 15°C and 30°C.

*Nature and contents of container:* Perlalux tristar blister–plastic foil consisting of 3 layers:
Polyvinylchloride on the out side;
Low density polyethylene in the middle;
Polyvinylidenechloride on the inside.
Aluminium foil (thickness 20 µm) coated on the inner side with colourless heat-seal Lacquer: pvc mixed polymers with acrylates, 6 g/m².
or
PVC blister consisting of -
Polyvinylchloride 'genotherm' glass clear, thickness 250 µm;
Aluminium foil (thickness 20 µm) coated on the inner side with a colourless heat-seal Lacquer: pvc mixed polymers with acrylates, 6 g/m².
Pack sizes: 4, 15, 60 capsules.

*Instructions for use/handling:* Not applicable.

**Marketing authorisation number** 0242/0142.

**Date of approval/revision of SPC**  February 1997.

**Legal category** POM.

## SPORANOX* LIQUID

**Qualitative and quantitative composition**  Itraconazole 10 mg/ml.

**Pharmaceutical form**  Oral solution containing 10 mg itraconazole/ml.

### Clinical particulars
*Therapeutic indications:* Sporanox liquid is indicated for the treatment of oral and/or oesophageal candidosis in HIV-positive or other immunocompromised patients.

*Posology and method of administration:* For optimal absorption, Sporanox liquid should be taken without food. The liquid should be swished around the oral cavity and swallowed. There should be no rinsing after swallowing.

Treatment of oral and/or oesophageal candidosis: 200 mg (2 measuring cups) per day in one or two

intakes for 1 week. If there is no response after 1 week, treatment should be continued for another week.

Treatment of fluconazole resistant oral and/or oesophageal candidosis: 200 to 400 mg (2–4 measuring cups) daily in one or two intakes for 2 weeks. If there is no response after 2 weeks, treatment should be continued for another 2 weeks.

*Contra-indications:* Sporanox liquid is contra-indicated in patients who have shown hypersensitivity to the drug or its excipients.

Sporanox liquid should only be given to pregnant women in life-threatening cases and when in these cases the potential benefit outweighs the potential harm to the foetus. Adequate contraceptive precautions should be taken by women of childbearing potential using Sporanox liquid until the next menstrual period following the end of Sporanox therapy.

*Special warnings and special precautions for use:*

*Paediatric use:* Since clinical data on the use of Sporanox liquid in paediatric patients is limited, it is advised to use Sporanox liquid in these patients only if the potential benefit outweighs the potential risks.

*Use in elderly:* Since clinical data of the use of Sporanox liquid in elderly patients is limited, it is advised to use Sporanox liquid in these patients only if the potential benefit outweighs the potential risks.

It is advisable to monitor liver function in patients receiving continuous treatment of more than one month and promptly in patients developing symptoms suggestive of hepatitis such as anorexia, nausea, vomiting, fatigue, abdominal pain or dark urine. If abnormal, treatment should be stopped. In patients with raised liver enzymes or an active liver disease, or who have experienced liver toxicity with other drugs, treatment should not be started unless the expected benefit exceeds the risk of hepatic injury. In such cases, liver enzyme monitoring is necessary.

*Hepatic impairment:* Itraconazole is predominantly metabolised in the liver. The terminal half-life of itraconazole in cirrhotic patients is somewhat prolonged. A decrease in the oral bioavailability of itraconazole from Sporanox capsules was observed in cirrhotic patients. This can also be expected with Sporanox liquid. It is advised to monitor the itraconazole plasma concentrations and to adapt the dose when necessary.

*Renal impairment:* A decrease in the oral bioavailability of itraconazole from Sporanox capsules was observed in some patients with renal insufficiency. This can also be expected with Sporanox liquid. It is advised to monitor the itraconazole plasma concentrations and to adapt the dose when necessary.

If neuropathy occurs that may be attributable to Sporanox liquid, the treatment should be discontinued.

There is no information regarding cross hypersensitivity between itraconazole and other azole antifungal agents. Caution should be used in prescribing Sporanox liquid to patients with hypersensitivity to other azoles.

*Interactions with other medicaments and other forms of interaction:* Enzyme-inducing drugs such as rifampicin and phenytoin significantly reduce the oral bioavailability of itraconazole. Consequently, monitoring of the itraconazole plasma concentrations is advised when enzyme-inducing agents are co-administered.

Itraconazole can inhibit the metabolism of drugs metabolised by the cytochrome 3A family. This can result in an increase and/or a prolongation of their effects, including side effects. Known examples are:
Terfenadine, astemizole, cisapride, HMG-CoA reductase inhibitors such as simvastatin, oral midazolam and triazolam. These agents should not be used by patients during treatment with Sporanox liquid. If midazolam is administered IV, special care is required since the sedative effects may be prolonged.
Oral-anticoagulants digoxin, Cyclosporin A, systemic methylprednisolone, vinca-alkaloids and possibly tacrolimus. The plasma levels or the effects of these drugs should be monitored. Their dosage, if co-administered with itraconazole, should be reduced if necessary.
Dihydropyridine calcium channel blockers and quinidine. Patients should be monitored for side effects, e.g. oedema and tinnitus/decreased hearing, respectively. If necessary, the dose of these drugs should be reduced.
*In vitro* studies have shown that there are no interactions on the plasma protein binding between itraconazole and imipramine, propranolol, diazepam, cimetidine, indomethacin, tolbutamide and sulfamethazine.
No interaction of itraconazole with AZT (zidovudine) has been observed.
No inducing effects of itraconazole on the metabolism of ethinyloestradiol and norethisterone were observed.

*Pregnancy and lactation:* When administered at high doses to pregnant rats (40 mg/kg/day or higher) and mice (80 mg/kg/day or higher), itraconazole was shown to increase the incidence of foetal abnormalities and did produce adverse effects on the embryo.

No studies are available on the use of Sporanox liquid in pregnant women. Therefore, Sporanox liquid should only be given in life-threatening cases and when in these cases the potential benefit outweighs the potential harm to the foetus.

Only a very small amount of itraconazole is excreted in human milk. The expected benefits of treatment with Sporanox liquid should therefore be weighed against the potential risk of breast-feeding. In case of doubt the patient should not breast-feed.

*Effects on ability to drive and use machines:* No effects have been observed.

*Undesirable effects:* Adverse experiences reported in association with the use of Sporanox liquid:
The most frequently reported were of gastro-intestinal origin, such as diarrhoea, nausea, abdominal pain and vomiting. Less frequently reported adverse experiences include headache, reversible increases in hepatic enzymes, dizziness and allergic reactions (such as pruritus, rash, urticaria and angio-oedema).

Adverse experiences reported in association with the use of Sporanox 100 mg capsules. The most frequently reported were of a gastro-intestinal origin, such as dyspepsia, nausea, abdominal pain and constipation. Less frequently reported adverse experiences include headache, reversible increases in hepatic enzymes, menstrual disorder, dizziness and allergic reactions (such as pruritus, rash, urticaria and angio-oedema).

Isolated cases of peripheral neuropathy and of Stevens-Johnson syndrome have also been reported; a causality for the latter was not established.

Especially in patients receiving prolonged (= approximately 1 month) treatment, most of whom had major underlying pathology and multiple concomitant medications, cases of hypokalaemia, oedema, hepatitis and hair loss have been observed

*Overdose:* No data are available. In the event of accidental overdosage, supportive measures should be employed. Within the first hour after ingestion, gastric lavage may be performed. Activated charcoal may be given if considered appropriate. Itraconazole cannot be removed by haemodialysis. No specific antidote is available.

### Pharmacological properties
*Pharmacodynamic properties:* Itraconazole, a triazole derivative, has a broad spectrum of activity. With respect to *Candida* spp, its activity includes *C. albicans, C. glabrata* and *C. krusei.*
*In vitro* studies have demonstrated that itraconazole impairs the synthesis of ergosterol in fungal cells. Ergosterol is a vital cell membrane component in fungi. Impairment of its synthesis ultimately results in an anti-fungal effect.

*Pharmacokinetic properties:* The oral bioavailability of Sporanox liquid is maximal when it is taken without food. During chronic administration, steady-state is reached after 1–2 weeks. Peak plasma levels are observed 2 hours (fasting) to 5 hours (with food) following the oral administration. After repeated once a day administration of itraconazole 200 mg in fasting condition, steady-state plasma concentrations of itraconazole fluctuate between 1 and 2 µg/ml (trough to peak). When the oral solution is taken with food, steady-state plasma concentrations of itraconazole are about 25% lower.

The plasma protein binding of itraconazole is 99.8%. Itraconazole is extensively distributed into tissues which are prone to fungal invasion. Concentrations in lung, kidney, liver, bone, stomach, spleen and muscle were found to be two to three times higher than the corresponding plasma concentration.

Itraconazole is extensively metabolised by the liver into a large number of metabolites. One of the metabolites is hydroxy-itraconazole, which has *in vitro* a comparable antifungal activity to itraconazole. Plasma levels of hydroxy-itraconazole are about twice as high as those of itraconazole.

After repeated oral administration, elimination of itraconazole from plasma is biphasic with a terminal half-life of 1.5 days. Faecal excretion of the parent drug varies between 3-18% of the dose. Renal excretion of the parent drug is less than 0.03% of the dose. About 35% of the dose is excreted as metabolites in the urine within 1 week.

*Preclinical safety data:* All preclinical safety data relevant to the prescriber have been included in the appropriate sections.

### Pharmaceutical particulars
*List of excipients:* Hydroxypropyl-β-cyclodextrin; sorbitol; propylene glycol; hydrochloric acid; cherry flavour 1; cherry flavour 2; caramel; sodium saccharin; sodium hydroxide; purified water.

*Incompatibilities:* None known.

*Shelf life:* 12 months as packaged for sale.
3 months after first opening the container.

*Special precautions for storage:* Store at 25°C or below.

*Nature and contents of container:* 150 ml amber glass bottle.

*Instructions for use/handling:* Sporanox liquid is supplied in bottles with a child-proof cap, and should be opened as follows: push the plastic screw cap down while turning it counter clockwise.

**Marketing authorisation number** 0242/0307

**Date of approval/revision of SPC** January 1997

**Legal category** POM.

## SPORANOX*-PULSE

**Qualitative and quantitative composition** Itraconazole 100 mg.

**Pharmaceutical form** Capsule (Size 0): opaque blue cap and pink transparent body containing cream coloured coated beads.

**Clinical particulars**
*Therapeutic indications:* Onychomycosis caused by dermatophytes and/or yeasts.
Tinea pedis and/or tinea manuum.

*Posology and method of administration:* Sporanox-Pulse is for oral administration and must be taken immediately after a meal for maximal absorption.
Treatment schedules in adults are as follows:

| *Indication* | *Dose* | *Remarks* |
|---|---|---|
| Tinea pedis and/ or tinea manuum | 1 pulse treatment | A pulse treatment consists of 200 mg bd for 7 days. |
| Onychomycosis–fingernails<br>Onychomycosis–toenails | 2 pulse treatments | Pulse treatments are separated by a 3-week drug-free interval |

Impaired absorption in AIDS and neutropenic patients may lead to low itraconazole blood levels and lack of efficacy. In such cases blood level monitoring is indicated.

*In children (below 12 years):* There are inadequate data on Sporanox-Pulse in children for its use to be recommended, unless the potential benefits outweigh the risks.

*In elderly:* As for use in children.

*Contra-indications:* When administered at high doses to pregnant rats (40 mg/kg/day) and mice (80 mg/kg/day), itraconazole was shown to cause abnormalities of foetal development. No data are available in human pregnancy, and itraconazole is therefore contra-indicated in pregnancy. Adequate contraceptive precautions should be taken by women of childbearing potential during therapy and for one menstrual cycle after stopping therapy.

Itraconazole is also contra-indicated in patients who have shown hypersensitivity to itraconazole, other azole antifungal agents or any of the excipients.

The drugs terfenadine, astemizole, cisapride, HMG-CoA reductase inhibitors such as simvastatin, oral midazolam or triazolam should not be given concurrently with itraconazole (see also *Interactions*).

*Special warnings and special precautions for use:* Absorption is impaired when the gastric acidity is decreased. In patients also receiving acid neutralising medicines (eg aluminium hydroxide) these should be administered at least 2 hours after the intake of Sporanox-Pulse. In patients with achlorhydria such as certain AIDS patients and patients on secretion suppressors (eg $H_2$-antagonists, proton-pump inhibitors) it is advisable to administer Sporanox-Pulse with a cola beverage.

Rarely cases of hepatitis and cholestatic jaundice have been reported, mainly in patients treated for longer than one month. It is therefore advisable to monitor liver function in patients receiving continuous treatment of more than one month's duration. If during treatment patients develop symptoms suggestive of hepatitis such as anorexia, nausea, vomiting, fatigue, abdominal pain or dark urine, liver enzymes should be monitored promptly. If these are abnormal, treatment should be stopped. In patients with raised liver enzymes, or with a known history of liver disease, or who have experienced liver toxicity with other drugs, treatment should not be started unless the expected benefit exceeds the risk of hepatic injury. In such instances liver enzyme monitoring is necessary.

Itraconazole is predominantly metabolised in the liver. A slight decrease in oral bioavailability in cirrhotic patients has been observed, although this was not of statistical significance. The terminal half-life was however significantly increased. It is advised to monitor the itraconazole plasma concentrations in such patients and to adapt the dose when necessary.

The oral bioavailability of itraconazole may be lower in some patients with renal insufficiency (eg those receiving continuous ambulatory peritoneal dialysis). Monitoring of the itraconazole plasma levels and dose adaptation are advisable.

Isolated cases of peripheral neuropathy have been reported, predominantly during long-term treatment and in severely compromised patients. The causal relationship to itraconazole was uncertain. If neuropathy occurs which may be attributable to Sporanox-Pulse, treatment should be discontinued.

*Interactions with other medicaments and other forms of interaction: Drug-interactions:* Enzyme-inducing drugs such as rifampicin and phenytoin significantly reduce the oral bioavailability of itraconazole. Consequently, monitoring of the itraconazole plasma concentration is advised when enzyme-inducing agents are co-administered.

Itraconazole can inhibit the metabolism of drugs metabolised by the cytochrome 3A family. This can result in an increase and/or a prolongation of their effects, including side effects. Known examples are:
– Terfenadine, astemizole and cisapride, resulting in increased plasma levels of these drugs and predisposing to serious arrhythmias. Combination of itraconazole with terfenadine, astemizole or cisapride is contra-indicated.
– Midazolam and triazolam, resulting in increased plasma levels of these drugs. Combination of itraconazole with oral midazolam or triazolam is contra-indicated. If midazolam is administered intravenously (eg as premedication in surgical or investigative procedures) special care should be observed since the sedative effect may be prolonged.
– HMG-CoA reductase inhibitors such as simvastatin. These drugs should not be used during treatment with Sporanox-Pulse.
– Oral anticoagulants, digoxin, Cyclosporin A, systemic methylprednisolone, vinca-alkaloids and possibly tacrolimus. Co-administration of itraconazole and digoxin has led to increased levels of the latter drug. A rise in cyclosporin levels has also been reported in patients treated with high doses of itraconazole for several weeks. Plasma levels of digoxin and cyclosporin should therefore be monitored during concomitant administration of itraconazole and the doses adjusted accordingly. *In vitro* studies indicate that a similar interaction may occur with tacrolimus. With respect to oral anticoagulants, similar interactions have been reported and it is advisable to monitor prothrombin time and reduce the dosage of oral anticoagulants if necessary. Co-administration of itraconazole and vinca-alkaloids may potentiate the toxic effects of the latter drugs and should this occur, co-administration of these drugs should be reconsidered.
– Dihydropyridine calcium channel blockers and quinidine. Patients should be monitored for side effects, eg oedema and tinnitus/decreased hearing, respectively. If necessary, the dose of these drugs should be reduced.

Despite the fact that itraconazole is 99.8% bound to plasma proteins, there are no *in vitro* interactions on the plasma protein binding between itraconazole and imipramine, propanolol, diazepam, cimetidine, indomethacin, tolbutamide or sulphadimidine.

Itraconazole does not appear to affect the metabolism of ethinyloestradiol and norethisterone. Reports suggest that there is no interaction of itraconazole with the oral pharmacokinetics of AZT (zidovudine).

*Pregnancy and lactation:*
*Pregnancy:* Sporanox-Pulse is contra-indicated in pregnancy (see Contra-indications section for further details).

*Lactation:* Only small amounts of itraconazole are excreted in human milk. The expected benefits of therapy should be weighed against the risks to the infant.

*Effects on ability to drive and use machines:* None known.

*Undesirable effects:* The most frequently reported adverse experiences in association with the use of Sporanox-Pulse are of gastro-intestinal origin, such as dyspepsia, nausea, abdominal pain and constipation. Less frequently reported adverse experiences include headache, reversible increases in hepatic enzymes, menstrual disorder, dizziness and allergic reactions (such as pruritus, rash, urticaria and angio-oedema). Isolated cases of peripheral neuropathy and of Stevens-Johnson syndrome have also been reported; a causality for the latter was not established.

Mainly in patients receiving prolonged treatment (ie approximately one month), most of whom had major underlying pathology and multiple concomitant medications, cases of hypokalaemia, oedema and hair loss have been observed. Hepatitis and cholestatic jaundice have been reported rarely, mainly in patients treated for longer than one month.

*Overdose:* In the event of overdosage, patients should be treated symptomatically with supportive measures and gastric lavage as necessary. No specific antidote is available. Itraconazole cannot be removed by haemodialysis.

**Pharmacological properties**
*Pharmacodynamic properties:* Itraconazole is a substituted triazole antimycotic with a broad spectrum of activity against *Candida* spp and other yeasts, dermatophytes and pathogenic fungi. It acts by impairing the synthesis of ergosterol in fungal cell membranes.

*Pharmacokinetic properties:* Peak plasma concentrations of itraconazole in the region of 1 mcg equiv/ml are reached 1.5–3 hrs after administration. In man the elimination half life is about 20 hrs. Oral intake immediately after a meal doubled the peak level 3–4 hrs after intake.

Peak concentrations of itraconazole in keratinous tissues, especially skin, are up to 3 times higher than in plasma. Therapeutic levels in the skin persist for up to 2–4 weeks after stopping treatment as elimination is related to dermal regeneration, rather than redistribution into the systemic circulation.

Itraconazole is extensively metabolised by the liver to a large number of metabolites, which constitute 40% of the excreted dose. Faecal excretion of parent drug varies from 3–18% of the dose, and urinary excretion of unchanged drug is less than 0.03%.

*Preclinical safety data:* No relevant information additional to that contained elsewhere in the Summary of Product Characteristics.

**Pharmaceutical particulars**
*List of excipients:* Sugar spheres NF; Hypromellose 2910 5 mPa.s PhEur; Macrogol 20000 PhEur. Capsule shell: Titanium dioxide E171; indigo carmine E132; Gelatin PhEur; erythrosine E127.

*Incompatibilities:* None known.

*Shelf life:* 36 months.

*Special precautions for storage:* Protect from light. Store in a dry place. Store between 15°C and 30°C.

*Nature and contents of container:* Perlalux tristar blister–plastic foil consisting of 3 layers:
– Polyvinylchloride 200 μm on the inner side;
– Low density polyethylene 25 μm in the middle;
– Polyvinylidenechloride 90 g/m² at the outside.

Aluminium foil (thickness 20 μm) coated on the inner side with colourless heat-seal Lacquer: PVC mixed polymers with acrylates, 6 g/m².

or:

PVC blister consisting of:

Polyvinylchloride 'genotherm' glass clear, thickness 250 μm;

Aluminium foil (thickness 20 μm) coated on the inner side with a colourless heat-seal Lacquer: PVC mixed polymers with acrylates, 6 g/m².

Pack size: 28 capsules.

*Instructions for use/handling:* Not applicable.

**Marketing authorisation number** 0242/0334

**Date of approval/revision of SPC** March 1997

**Legal category** POM.

## STUGERON*

**Presentation** White, uncoated, scored tablets marked 'JANSSEN' on one side and S above 15 on the reverse. Each tablet contains 15 mg cinnarizine. Stugeron tablets also contain lactose and sucrose but do not contain any colours.

**Uses** Stugeron is used for the control of vestibular disorders such as vertigo, tinnitus, nausea and vomiting as seen in Meniere's disease.

**Dosage and administration** Stugeron is for oral administration and may be sucked, chewed or swallowed whole by both adults and children according to the following dosage regimen:

*Vestibular symptoms: Adults and children over 12:* 2 tablets three times a day.

*Children 5-12 years:* one half the adult dose.

*Use in elderly:* As for adults.

Stugeron should preferably be taken after meals. These doses should not be exceeded.

**Contra-indications, warnings, etc**
*Contra-indications:* Stugeron should not be given to patients with known hypersensitivity to cinnarizine.

*Warnings:* As with other antihistamines, Stugeron may cause epigastric discomfort; taking it after meals may diminish gastric irritation. In patients with Parkinson's disease, Stugeron should only be given if the advantages outweigh the possible risk of aggravating this disease.

Stugeron may cause drowsiness especially at the start of treatment; patients affected in this way should not drive or operate machinery.

*Drug interactions:* Concurrent use of alcohol, CNS depressants or tricyclic antidepressants may potentiate the sedative effects of either these drugs or of Stugeron.

Because of its antihistamine effect, Stugeron may prevent an otherwise positive reaction to dermal reactivity indicators if used within 4 days prior to skin testing.

*Use in pregnancy:* The safety of Stugeron in human pregnancy has not been established although studies in animals have not demonstrated teratogenic effects. As with other drugs, it is not advisable to administer Stugeron in pregnancy.

*Use in lactation:* There are no data on the excretion of Stugeron in human breast milk: use of Stugeron is not recommended in nursing mothers.

*Side-effects:* Drowsiness and gastro-intestinal disturbances may occur. These are usually transient.

In rare cases, headache, dry mouth, weight gain, perspiration or allergic reactions may occur. Very rare cases of lichen planus, lupus-like skin reactions and cholestatic jaundice have been reported.

Rare cases of aggravation or appearance of extrapyramidal symptoms (sometimes associated with depressive feelings) have been described, predominantly in elderly people during prolonged therapy. The treatment should be discontinued in such cases.

*Overdosage:* Vomiting, drowsiness, coma, tremor and hypotonia may occur.

There is no specific antidote to Stugeron but in the event of overdosage, gastric lavage and the administration of activated charcoal may help.

**Pharmaceutical precautions** Store at room temperature.

**Legal category** P.

**Package quantities** Stugeron tablets each containing 15 mg cinnarizine are supplied in packs of 100.

**Further information** Nil.

**Product licence number** 0242/5009R.

**Legal category** P.

## STUGERON* FORTE 75 mg

**Presentation** Hard gelatin capsule (No 4) with an orange cap and yellow body: each capsule contains cinnarizine 75 mg. The capsules also contain lactose, erythrosine (E127), titanium dioxide (E171), sunset yellow (E110) and yellow ferric oxide (E172).

**Uses** Stugeron Forte is indicated for the long term management of the symptoms of peripheral arterial disease, including intermittent claudication, rest pain, muscular cramps and vasospastic disorders, eg Raynaud's disease.

*Actions:* Cinnarizine's action in the treatment of peripheral vascular disease is due to its anti-vasoconstrictor properties, its action on blood hyperviscosity and its anti-ischaemic effect. Anti-vasoconstriction is thought to be through a calcium blocker mechanism, and is evident selectively in vascular smooth muscle. Increased peripheral muscle blood flow may be mediated by prevention of calcium entry into ischaemic erythrocytes, thereby preserving flexibility.

**Dosage and administration** Stugeron Forte is for oral administration to adults.

The recommended starting dose is 1 capsule three times daily. The maintenance dose is 1 capsule two or three times daily according to the response.

Stugeron Forte should preferably be taken after meals. These doses should not be exceeded.

Peripheral arterial disease is slow to improve with any form of drug treatment. Maximum benefit with Stugeron Forte will not be seen until after several weeks of continuous treatment although significant improvement in blood flow has frequently been demonstrated after 1 week.

*Use in elderly:* as above.

*Use in children:* not recommended.

**Contra-indications, warnings, etc**

*Contra-indications:* Stugeron Forte should not be given to patients with known hypersensitivity to cinnarizine.

*Warnings:* Stugeron Forte has not been found to reduce blood pressure significantly. However, the drug should be used with reasonable caution in hypotensive patients.

As with other antihistamines, Stugeron Forte may cause epigastric discomfort; taking it after meals may diminish gastric irritation. In patients with Parkinson's disease, Stugeron Forte should only be given if the

advantages outweigh the possible risk of aggravating this disease.

Stugeron Forte may cause drowsiness especially at the start of treatment; patients affected in this way should not drive or operate machinery.

*Drug interactions:* Concurrent use of alcohol, CNS depressants or tricyclic antidepressants may potentiate the sedative effects of either these drugs or of Stugeron Forte.

Because of its antihistamine effect, Stugeron Forte may prevent an otherwise positive reaction to dermal reactivity indicators if used within 4 days prior to skin testing.

*Use in pregnancy:* The safety of Stugeron Forte in human pregnancy has not been established although studies in animals have not demonstrated teratogenic effects. As with other drugs, it is not advisable to administer Stugeron Forte in pregnancy.

*Use in lactation:* There are no data on the excretion of Stugeron Forte in human breast milk: use of Stugeron Forte is not recommended in nursing mothers.

*Side effects:* Drowsiness and gastro-intestinal disturbances may occur. These are usually transient.

In rare cases, headache, dry mouth, weight gain, perspiration or allergic reactions may occur. Very rare cases of lichen planus, lupus-like skin reactions and cholestatic jaundice have been reported.

Rare cases of aggravation or appearance of extrapyramidal symptoms (sometimes associated with depressive feelings) have been described, predominantly in elderly people during prolonged therapy. The treatment should be discontinued in such cases.

*Overdosage:* Vomiting, drowsiness, coma, tremor and hypotonia may occur.

There is no specific antidote to Stugeron Forte but in the event of overdosage, gastric lavage and the administration of activated charcoal may help.

**Pharmaceutical precautions** Store between 15°C and 30°C.

**Legal category** P.

**Package quantities** Stugeron Forte is supplied in packs of 100 capsules.

**Further information** Animal studies have shown that cinnarizine protects the arterial wall from arteriosclerotic degeneration due to hypertension.

**Product licence number** 0242/0008.

## SUBLIMAZE*

**Qualitative and quantitative composition** Fentanyl citrate 78.5 micrograms equivalent to 50 micrograms per ml fentanyl base.

**Pharmaceutical form** Injection.

**Clinical particulars**

*Therapeutic indications:* Sublimaze is a narcotic analgesic used:

a. In low doses to provide analgesia during short surgical procedures.

b. In high doses as an analgesic/respiratory depressant in patients requiring assisted ventilation.

c. In combination with a neuroleptic in the technique of neuroleptanalgesia.

d. In the treatment of severe pain, such as the pain of myocardial infarction.

*Posology and method of administration:*

*Route of administration*

Intravenous administration either as a bolus or by infusion.

Intramuscular administration.

Sublimaze, by the intravenous route, can be administered as a bolus or as an infusion to both adults and children. The dose of Sublimaze should be individualised according to age, body weight, physical status, underlying pathological condition, use of other drugs and type of surgery and anaesthesia. The usual dose is as follows:

| | ADULTS | | CHILDREN | |
|---|---|---|---|---|
| | Initial | Supplemental | Initial | Supplemental |
| Spontaneous respiration | 50-200 mcg | 50 mcg | 3-5 mcg/kg | 1 mcg/kg |
| Assisted ventilation | 300-3500 mcg | 100-200 mcg | 15 mcg/kg | 1-3 mcg/kg |

Doses in excess of 200 mcg are for use in anaesthesia only. As a premedicant, 1-2 ml Sublimaze may be given intramuscularly 45 minutes before induction of anaesthesia.

After intravenous administration in unpremedicated adult patients 2 ml Sublimaze may be expected to provide sufficient analgesia for 10–20 minutes in surgical procedures involving low pain intensity. 10 ml

Sublimaze injected as a bolus gives analgesia lasting about one hour. The analgesia produced is sufficient for surgery involving moderately painful procedures. Giving a dose of 50 mcg/kg Sublimaze will provide intense analgesia for some four to six hours, for intensely stimulating surgery.

Sublimaze may also be given as an infusion. In ventilated patients, a loading dose of Sublimaze may be given as a fast infusion of approximately 1 mcg/kg/min for the first 10 minutes followed by an infusion of approximately 0.1 mcg/kg/min. Alternatively the loading dose of Sublimaze may be given as a bolus. Infusion rates should be titrated to individual patient response, lower infusion rates may be adequate. Unless it is planned to ventilate post-operatively, the infusion should be terminated at about 40 minutes before the end of surgery.

Lower infusion rates eg 0.05–0.08 mcg/kg/minute are necessary if spontaneous ventilation is to be maintained. Higher infusion rates (up to 3 mcg/kg/minute) have been used in cardiac surgery.

When judging the dose it is important to assess the likely degree of surgical stimulation, the effect of premedicant drugs, and the duration of the procedure.

Use in elderly and debilitated patients: It is wise to reduce the dosage in the elderly and debilitated patients. The effect of the initial dose should be taken into account in determining supplemental doses.

*Contra-indications:* Respiratory depression, obstructive airways disease. Concurrent administration with monoamine inhibitors, or within 2 weeks of their discontinuation. Known intolerance to fentanyl or other morphinomimetics.

*Special warnings and special precautions for use:* Tolerance and dependence may occur. Following intravenous administration of fentanyl, a transient fall in blood pressure may occur, especially in hypovolaemic patients. Appropriate measures to maintain a stable arterial pressure should be taken.

Significant respiratory depression will occur following the administration of fentanyl in doses in excess of 200 mcg. This, and the other pharmacological effects of fentanyl, can be reversed by specific narcotic analgesics (eg naloxone). Additional doses of the latter may be necessary because the respiratory depression may last longer than the duration of action of the opioid antagonist.

Bradycardia and possibly asystole can occur in nonatropinised patients, and can be antagonised by atropine.

Muscular rigidity (morphine-like effect) may occur. Rigidity, which may also involve the thoracic muscles, can be avoided by the following measures:

- Slow iv injection (usually sufficient for lower doses).

- Premedication with benzodiazepines.

- Use of muscle relaxants.

As with all opioid analgesics, care should be observed when administering fentanyl to patients with Myasthenia Gravis.

It is wise to reduce dosage in the elderly and debilitated patients.

In hypothyroidism, pulmonary disease, decreased respiratory reserve, alcoholism and liver or renal impairment the dosage should be titrated with care and prolonged monitoring may be required.

Patients on chronic opioid therapy or with a history of opioid abuse may require higher doses.

Administration in labour may cause respiratory depression in the new born infant.

As with all potent opioids, profound analgesia is accompanied by marked respiratory depression, which may persist into or recur in the early postoperative period. Care should be taken after large doses or infusions of fentanyl to ensure that adequate spontaneous breathing has been established and maintained before discharging the patient from the recovery area.

Resuscitation equipment and opioid antagonists should be readily available. Hyperventilation during anaesthesia may alter the patients response to CO2, thus affecting respiration postoperatively.

The use of rapid bolus injections of opioids should be avoided in patients with compromised intracerebral compliance; in such patients the transient decrease in the mean arterial pressure has occasionally been accompanied by a transient reduction of the cerebral perfusion pressure.

*Interactions with other medicaments and other forms of interaction:* The use of opioid premedication, barbiturates, benzodiazepines, neuroleptics, halogenic gases and other non-selective CNS depressants (e.g. alcohol) may enhance or prolong the respiratory depression of fentanyl.

When patients have received CNS-depressants, the dose of fentanyl required will be less than usual. Likewise, following the administration of fentanyl the dose of other CNS-depressant drugs should be reduced.

Bradycardia and possibly asystole can occur when

fentanyl is combined with non-vagolytic muscle relaxants.

The concomitant use of droperidol can result in a higher incidence of hypotension.

*Pregnancy and lactation:* Although no teratogenic or acute embryotoxic effects have been observed in animal experiments, insufficient data are available to evaluate any harmful effects in humans. As with other drugs, possible risks should be weighed against potential benefits to the patient.

Administration during childbirth (including caesarean section) is not recommended because fentanyl crosses the placenta and the foetal respiratory centre is particularly sensitive to opioids. If fentanyl is nevertheless administered, an antidote for the child should always be at hand.

Fentanyl may enter the maternal milk. It is therefore recommended that breast feeding is not initiated within 24 hours of treatment.

*Effects on ability to drive and use machines:* Where early discharge is envisaged, patients should be advised not to drive or operate machinery for 24 hours following administration.

*Undesirable effects:* The side effects are those associated with intravenous opioids e.g. respiratory depression, apnoea, muscular rigidity (which may also involve thoracic muscles), myoclonic movements, bradycardia, transient hypotension, nausea, vomiting and dizziness.

Other less frequently reported adverse reactions are:

- laryngospasm;
- allergic reactions (eg anaphylaxis, bronchospasm, pruritus, urticaria) and asystole although it is uncertain whether there is a causal relationship as several drugs were co-administered;
- secondary rebound respiratory depression has rarely been reported.

When a neuroleptic such as droperidol is used with fentanyl, the following adverse reactions may be observed: chills and/or shivering, restlessness, postoperative hallucinatory episodes and extrapyramidal symptoms.

*Overdose:*
*Symptoms:* The manifestations of fentanyl overdosage are generally an extension of its pharmacological action. Depending on the individual sensitivity, the clinical picture is determined primarily by the degree of respiratory depression, which varies from bradypnoea to apnoea.

*Treatment:*
- hypoventilation or apnoea: O$_2$ administration, assisted or controlled respiration.
- respiratory depression: Specific narcotic antagonist (eg naloxone). This does not preclude the use of immediate countermeasures.
- muscular rigidity: Intravenous neuromuscular blocking agent.

The patient should be carefully observed; body warmth and adequate fluid intake should be maintained. If hypotension is severe or if it persists, the possibility of hypovolaemia should be considered, and if present, it should be controlled with appropriate parenteral fluid administration.

**Pharmacological properties**
*Pharmacodynamic properties:* Fentanyl is a synthetic opiate with a clinical potency of 50 to 100 times that of morphine. Its onset of action is rapid and its duration of action is short. In man, a single iv dose of 0.5-1 mg/70 kg body weight immediately produces a pronounced state of surgical analgesia, respiratory depression, bradycardia and other typical morphine-like effects. The duration of action of the peak effects is about 30 minutes. All potent morphine-like drugs produce relief from pain, ventilatory depression, emesis, constipation, physical dependence, certain vagal effects and varying degrees of sedation. Fentanyl, however, differs from morphine not only by its short duration of action but also by its lack of emetic effect and minimal hypotensive activity in animals.

*Pharmacokinetic properties:* Some pharmacokinetic parameters for fentanyl are as follows:
Urinary excretion = 8%
Bound in plasma = 80%
Clearance (ml . min$^{-1}$ . kg$^{-1}$) = 13±2
Volume of distribution (litres/kg) = 4.0±0.4
Half life (hours) = 3.7±0.4

*Preclinical safety data:* Not applicable.

**Pharmaceutical particulars**
*List of excipients:* Sodium chloride; water for injections; sodium hydroxide; hydrochloric acid.

*Incompatibilities:* The product is chemically incompatible with the induction agents thiopentone and methohexitone because of the wide differences in pH.

*Shelf life:* 36 months.

*Special precautions for storage:* Protect from light.

*Nature and contents of container:* Colourless glass ampoules (PhEur, USP Type 1).
Pack size: packs of 10 of 2 ml and 10 ml ampoules.

*Instructions for use/handling:* Not applicable (store as a CD).

**Marketing authorisation number** 0242/5001R

**Date of approval/revision of SPC** March 1997

**Legal category** POM.

## SULTRIN* TRIPLE SULFA CREAM

**Presentation** A white, non-staining cream containing sulphathiazole 3.42% w/w, sulphacetamide 2.86% w/w and sulphabenzamide 3.70% w/w.

**Uses** For the treatment of infections caused by *Haemophilus vaginalis.*

**Dosage and administration** One applicatorful intravaginally twice daily for 10 days. The dosage may then be reduced to once a day if necessary.

**Contra-indications, warnings, etc**
*Contra-indications:*
- Known hypersensitivity to sulphonamides or any of the excipients.
- Known hypersensitivity to peanuts.
- Renal disease.

*Warnings:* The safety and effectiveness for use in children have not been established. Since the primary route of excretion of sulphonamides is renal, caution should be used in prescribing the product to elderly patients who potentially may have impaired renal function.

Treatment should be stopped if local sensitisation or an allergic reaction develops.

General hygiene measures should be observed to control sources of infection and reinfection. Appropriate treatment should be used if the sexual partner is also infected.

*Pregnancy:* There is no evidence as to the safety of Sultrin Triple Sulfa cream in human pregnancy nor is there evidence from animal work that sulphonamides administered vaginally are free from hazard. Therefore, although no reports of adverse effects of Sultrin in pregnancy have been documented, as with any drug in this category, use in pregnancy should be avoided.

*Side-effects:* Local irritation and/or allergy have occasionally been reported. As sulphonamides may be absorbed from the vaginal mucosa, the following adverse effects associated with such compounds should be borne in mind:
- Hypersensitivity reactions: skin rashes; severe and potentially fatal skin reactions such as toxic epidermal necrolysis (Lyell's Syndrome) and erythema multiforme bullosa (Stevens-Johnson Syndrome).
- Blood dyscrasias: including agranulocytosis and aplastic anaemia.
- Renal failure.

*Overdosage:* Sultrin Triple Sulfa Cream is intended for intravaginal use. If accidental ingestion of large quantities of the product occurs, an appropriate method of gastric emptying may be used if considered desirable. Elimination of sulphonamides in the urine may be assisted by giving alkalis such as sodium bicarbonate and increasing fluid intake.

**Pharmaceutical precautions** Store at room temperature (below 25°C).

**Legal category** POM.

**Package quantities** Tube containing 8O g with the Ortho Plastic Vaginal Applicator.

**Product licence number** 0242/0273.

## TOPAMAX* ▼

**Qualitative and quantitative composition** Topamax (topiramate) is available in tablets for oral administration containing 25, 50, 100 and 200 mg of topiramate.

**Pharmaceutical form** Topamax is available as embossed, round, coated tablets in the following strengths and colours: 25 mg white, 50 mg light yellow, 100 mg yellow and 200 mg salmon. The tablets will be imprinted as follows:

25 mg "TOP" on one side; "25" on the other
50 m "TOP" on one side; "50" on the other
100 mg "TOP" on one side; "100" on the other
200 mg "TOP" on one side; "200" on the other

**Clinical particulars**

*Therapeutic indications:* Adjunctive therapy of partial seizures, with or without secondarily generalised seizures, in patients who are inadequately controlled on conventional first line antiepileptic drugs.

*Posology and method of administration:* The minimal effective dose is 200 mg per day. The usual total daily dose is 200 mg to 400 mg in two divided doses. Some patients may require doses up to 800 mg per day which is the maximum recommended dose. It is recommended that therapy be initiated at a low dose, followed by titration to an effective dose.

Titration should begin at 100 mg daily for one week. A lower dose may be used. The daily dose should then be increased by 100 mg and taken in two divided doses for a further week. Subsequent dose increments should be made at weekly intervals and should be 200 mg taken in two divided doses. If the patient is unable to tolerate the titration regimen then lower increments or longer intervals between increments may be used. Dose titration should be guided by clinical outcome.

Tablets should not be broken. Topamax can be taken without regard to meals.

It is not necessary to monitor topiramate plasma concentrations to optimise Topamax therapy.

These dosing recommendations apply to all adults, including the elderly, in the absence of underlying renal disease (see *Special warnings and special precautions for use*).

Since Topamax is removed from plasma by haemodialysis, a supplemental dose of Topamax equal to approximately one-half the daily dose should be administered on haemodialysis days. The supplemental dose should be administered in divided doses at the beginning and completion of the haemodialysis procedure. The supplemental dose may differ based on the characteristics of the dialysis equipment being used.

Use in children is not recommended because there are only limited data in this age group and the safe and effective dose has not been defined.

*Contra-indications:* Hypersensitivity to any component of this product.

*Special warnings and special precautions for use:* Antiepileptic drugs, including Topamax, should be withdrawn gradually to minimise the potential of increased seizure frequency. In clinical trials, dosages were decreased by 100 mg/day at weekly intervals. In some patients, withdrawal was accelerated without complications.

The major route of elimination of unchanged topiramate and its metabolites is via the kidney. Renal elimination is dependent on renal function and is independent of age. Patients with moderate or severe renal impairment may take 10 to 15 days to reach steady-state plasma concentrations as compared to 4 to 8 days in patients with normal renal function. As with all patients, the titration schedule should be guided by clinical outcome (ie seizure control, avoidance of side effects) with the knowledge that subjects with known renal impairment may require a longer time to reach steady state at each dose.

Some patients, especially those with a predisposition to nephrolithiasis, may be at increased risk for renal stone formation. Adequate hydration is recommended to reduce this risk.

Risk factors for nephrolithiasis include prior stone formation, a family history of nephrolithiasis and hypercalciuria. None of these risk factors can reliably predict stone formation during topiramate treatment. In addition, patients taking other medication associated with nephrolithiasis may be at increased risk.

*Interactions with other medicaments and other forms of interaction:*
*Effects of Topamax on other antiepileptic drugs:* The addition of Topamax to other antiepileptic drugs (phenytoin, carbamazepine, valproic acid, phenobarbital, primidone) has no clinically significant effect on their steady-state plasma concentrations, except in some patients where the addition of Topamax to phenytoin may result in an increase of plasma concentrations of phenytoin. Consequently, it is advised that any patient on phenytoin should have phenytoin levels monitored.

*Effects of other antiepileptic drugs on Topamax:* Phenytoin and carbamazepine decrease the plasma concentration of topiramate. The addition or withdrawal of phenytoin or carbamazepine to Topamax therapy may require an adjustment in dosage of the latter. This should be done by titrating to clinical effect.

The addition or withdrawal of valproic acid does not produce clinically significant changes in plasma concentrations of topiramate and, therefore, does not warrant dosage adjustment of Topamax.

The results of these interactions are summarised in the following table:

| AED Coadministered | AED Concentration | Topiramate Concentration |
|---|---|---|
| Phenytoin | <->** | ↓ |
| Carbamazepine (CBZ) | <-> | ↓ |
| Valproic Acid | <-> | <-> |
| Phenobarbital | <-> | NS |
| Primidone | <-> | NS |

<-> = No effect on plasma concentration

** = Plasma concentrations increase in some patients
↓ = Plasma concentrations decrease
NS = Not studied
AED= antiepileptic drug

*Other drug interactions:*
*Digoxin:* In a single-dose study, serum digoxin area under plasma concentration curve (AUC) decreased 12% due to concomitant administration of Topamax. The clinical relevance of this observation has not been established. When Topamax is added or withdrawn in patients on digoxin therapy, careful attention should be given to the routine monitoring of serum digoxin.

*Oral contraceptives:* In an interaction study with a combined oral contraceptive, Topamax increased plasma clearance of the oestrogenic component significantly. Consequently, and bearing in mind the potential risk of teratogenicity, patients should receive a preparation containing not less than 50 µg of oestrogen or use some alternative non-hormonal method of contraception. Patients taking oral contraceptives should be asked to report any change in their bleeding patterns.

*Others:* Topamax, when used concomitantly with other agents predisposing to nephrolithiasis, may increase the risk of nephrolithiasis. While using Topamax, agents like these should be avoided since they may create a physiological environment that increases the risk of renal stone formation. The interaction with benzodiazepines has not been studied.

*Pregnancy and lactation:* As with other antiepileptic drugs, topiramate was teratogenic in mice, rats and rabbits. In rats, topiramate crosses the placental barrier.
There are no studies using Topamax in pregnant women. However, Topamax should not be used during pregnancy unless, in the opinion of the physician, the potential benefit outweighs the potential risk to the foetus. It is recommended that women of child bearing potential use adequate contraception. Topamax should not be used during breast feeding.

*Effects on ability to drive and use machines:* As with all antiepileptic drugs, Topamax may produce central nervous system related adverse events. Drowsiness is likely and Topamax may be more sedating than other antiepileptic drugs. These adverse events could potentially be dangerous in patients driving a vehicle or operating machinery, particularly until such time as the individual patient's experience with the drug is established.

*Undesirable effects:* Since Topamax has most frequently been co-administered with other antiepileptic agents, it is not possible to determine which agents, if any, are associated with adverse effects. In placebo-controlled double-blind trials in which there was a rapid titration period, the following adverse events were reported to be probably or definitely related to topiramate in 5% or more of patients: ataxia, concentration impaired, confusion, dizziness, fatigue, paraesthesia, somnolence and thinking abnormal. Topamax may cause agitation and emotional lability (which may manifest as abnormal behaviour) and depression. Other less common adverse effects include amnesia, anorexia, aphasia, diplopia, nausea, nystagmus, speech disorder, taste perversion, vision abnormal and weight decrease. Isolated cases of venous thromboembolic events have been reported. A causal association with the drug has not been established.
Topamax increases the risk of nephrolithiasis especially in those with a predisposition (see *Special warnings and special precautions for use*). In the initial clinical trials none of the calculi required open surgery and three-quarters were passed spontaneously. Most of the patients opted to continue treatment despite nephrolithiasis.

*Overdose:* In acute overdose with Topamax, if the ingestion is recent, the stomach should be emptied immediately by lavage or by induction of emesis. *In vitro*, activated charcoal has not been shown to absorb topiramate, therefore, its use in overdosage is not recommended. Supportive treatment should be used as appropriate. Haemodialysis is an effective means of removing topiramate from the body. However, in cases of acute overdosage, including doses of over 20 g in one individual, haemodialysis has not been necessary.

## Pharmacological properties
*Pharmacodynamic properties:* Topiramate is a novel antiepileptic agent classified as a sulphamate-substituted monosaccharide. Three pharmacological properties of topiramate have been identified that may contribute to its anticonvulsant activity:
Topiramate reduces the frequency at which action potentials are generated when neurones are subjected to a sustained depolarisation indicative of a state-dependent blockade of voltage-sensitive sodium channels.
Topiramate markedly enhances the activity of GABA at some types of GABA receptors but has no apparent effect on the activity of N-methyl-D-aspartate (NMDA) at the NMDA receptor subtype.
Topiramate weakly antagonises the excitatory activity of kainate/AMPA subtype of glutamate receptor.
In addition, topiramate inhibits some isoenzymes of carbonic anhydrase. This pharmacologic effect is much weaker than that of acetazolamide, a known carbonic anhydrase inhibitor, and is not thought to be a major component of topiramate's antiepileptic activity.

*Pharmacokinetic properties:* Topiramate is rapidly and well absorbed. Based on recovery of radioactivity from the urine, the mean extent of absorption of a 100 mg dose of $^{14}$C topiramate was at least 81%. There is no clinically significant effect of food on topiramate. Generally 13-17% of topiramate is bound to plasma proteins. The mean apparent volume of distribution has been measured as 0.55-0.8 L/kg for single doses up to 1200 mg. There is an effect of gender on the volume of distribution. Values for females are circa 50% of those for males.
Topiramate is not extensively metabolised (≈20%) in healthy volunteers. Topiramate is metabolised up to 50% in patients receiving concomitant antiepileptic therapy with known inducers of drug metabolising enzymes. Six metabolites have been isolated, characterised and identified from plasma, urine and faeces of humans. Two metabolites, which retained most of the structure of topiramate, were tested and found to have little or no anticonvulsant activity.
In humans, the major route of elimination of unchanged topiramate and its metabolites is via the kidney. Overall, plasma clearance is approximately 20 to 30 ml/min in humans following oral administration.
Topiramate exhibits low intersubject variability in plasma concentrations and, therefore, has predictable pharmacokinetics. The pharmacokinetics of topiramate are linear with plasma clearance remaining constant and area under the plasma concentration curve increasing in a dose-proportional manner over a 100 to 400 mg single oral dose range in healthy subjects. Patients with normal renal function may take 4 to 8 days to reach steady-state plasma concentrations. The mean Cmax following multiple, twice a day oral doses of 100 mg to healthy subjects was 6.76 µg/ml. Following administration of multiple doses of 50 mg and 100 mg of topiramate twice a day, the mean plasma elimination half-life was approximately 21 hours.
The plasma and renal clearance of topiramate are decreased in patients with impaired renal function ($CL_{CR}$ ≤ 60 ml/min), and the plasma clearance is decreased in patients with end-stage renal disease.
Plasma clearance of topiramate is unchanged in elderly subjects in the absence of underlying renal disease.
Plasma clearance of topiramate is decreased in patients with moderate to severe hepatic impairment.

*Preclinical safety data:* Acute and long-term exposure of mice, rats, dogs and rabbits to topiramate was well-tolerated.
As with other antiepileptic drugs, topiramate was teratogenic in mice, rats and rabbits. Overall numbers of fetal malformations in mice were increased for all drug-treated groups, but no significant differences or dosage-response relationships were observed for overall or specific malformations, suggesting that other factors such as maternal toxicity may be involved.
In a battery of *in vitro* and *in vivo* mutagenicity assays, topiramate did not show genotoxic potential.

**Pharmaceutical particulars**
*List of excipients:* Topamax contains the following inactive ingredients: Lactose Hydrous PhEur; Pregelatinized starch (modified) PhEur; Pregelatinized starch PhEur; purified water; Carnauba wax PhEur; Microcrystalline cellulose PhEur; Sodium starch glycolate PhEur; Magnesium stearate PhEur; OPADRY White, Yellow, Pink, Red (depending on the colour, contains hydroxypropyl methylcellulose, titanium dioxide, polyethylene glycol, synthetic iron oxide and polysorbate 80).

*Incompatibilities:* None known.

*Shelf life:* 36 months.

*Special precautions for storage:* Store in a dry place at or below 25°C.

*Nature and contents of container:* Available in opaque containers with tamper-evident closures containing 60 tablets.

*Instructions for use/handling:* Not applicable

**Marketing authorisation number**
Topamax 25 mg    0242/0301
Topamax 50 mg    0242/0302
Topamax 100 mg    0242/0303
Topamax 200 mg    0242/0304

**Date of approval/revision** February 1997.

**Legal category** POM.

## TRINOVUM* ORAL CONTRACEPTIVE TABLETS

**Presentation** Trinovum oral contraceptive tablets are 1/4 inch diameter, circular tablets with flat faces and bevelled edges. The 7 white tablets contain 500 µg norethisterone and 35 µg ethinyloestradiol and are engraved C over 535 on each face. The 7 light peach coloured tablets contain 750 µg norethisterone and 35 µg ethinyloestradiol and are engraved C over 735 on each face. The 7 peach coloured tablets contain 1.0 mg norethisterone PhEur and 35 µg ethinyloestradiol and are engraved C over 135 on each face.

**Uses** Contraception and the recognised indications for such oestrogen/progestogen combinations.

**Action** Through the mechanism of gonadotrophin suppression by the oestrogenic and progestational actions of the ingredients.
Although the primary mechanism of action is inhibition of ovulation, alterations to the cervical mucus and to the endometrium may also contribute to the efficacy of the product.

**Dosage and administration** It is preferable that tablet intake from the first pack is started on the first day of menstruation in which case no extra contraceptive precautions are necessary.
If menstruation has already begun (that is 2, 3 or 4 days previously), tablet taking should commence on day 5 of the menstrual period. In this case additional contraceptive precautions must be taken for the first 7 days of tablet taking. (See further information for additional contraceptive precautions).
If menstruation began more than 5 days previously then the patient should be advised to wait until her next menstrual period before starting to take Trinovum.

*How to take Trinovum:* One tablet is taken daily at the same time (preferably in the evening) without interruption for 21 days, followed by a break of 7 tablet-free days (a white tablet is taken every day for 7 days, then a pale peach coloured tablet every day for 7 days, then a peach coloured tablet every day for 7 days, then 7 tablet-free days). Each subsequent pack is started after the 7 tablet-free days have elapsed. Additional contraceptive precautions are not then required.

*Use during pregnancy:* Trinovum is contra-indicated for use during pregnancy or suspected pregnancy, since it has been suggested that combined oral contraceptives, in common with many other substances, might be capable of affecting the normal development of the child in the early stages of pregnancy. It can be definitely concluded, however, that, if a risk of abnormality exists at all, it must be very small.

*Post-partum administration:* Following a vaginal delivery, oral contraceptive administration to non-breast feeding mothers can be started 21 days post-partum, provided the patient is fully ambulant and there are no puerperal complications. No additional contraceptive precautions are required. If post-partum administration begins more than 21 days after delivery, additional contraceptive precautions are required for the first 7 days of pill-taking. If intercourse has taken place post-partum, oral contraceptive use should be delayed until the first day of the first menstrual period.

*N.B.* Mothers who are breast feeding should be advised not to use the combined pill since this may reduce the amount of breast-milk, but may be advised instead to use a progestogen-only pill (POP).
After miscarriage or abortion administration should start immediately in which case no additional contraceptive precautions are required.

*Changing from a 21 day pill or another 22 day pill to Trinovum:* All tablets in the old pack should be finished. The first Trinovum tablet is taken the next day i.e. no gap is left between taking tablets nor does the patient need to wait for her period to begin. Tablets should be taken as instructed in 'How to take Trinovum'. Additional contraceptive precautions are not required. The patient will not have a period until the end of the first Trinovum pack, but this is not harmful, nor does it matter if she experiences some bleeding on tablet-taking days.

*Changing from a combined Every Day Pill (28 day tablets) to Trinovum:* Trinovum should be started after taking the last active tablet from the 'Every Day Pill' pack (ie after taking 21 or 22 tablets). The first Trinovum tablet is taken the next day ie no gap is left between taking tablets nor does the patient need to wait for her period to begin. Tablets should be taken as instructed in 'How to take Trinovum'. Additional contraceptive precautions are not required. Remaining tablets from the Every Day (ED) pack should be discarded. The patient will not have a period until the end of the first Trinovum pack, but this is not harmful, nor does it matter if she experiences some bleeding on tablet-taking days.

*Changing from a Progestogen-only Pill (POP or Mini Pill) to Trinovum:* The first Trinovum tablet should be taken on the first day of the period, even if the patient has already taken a mini pill on that day. Tablets should be taken as instructed in 'How to take Trinovum'. Additional contraceptive precautions are not required. All the remaining progestogen-only pills in the mini pill pack should be discarded.

If the patient is taking a (mini) pill, then she may not always have a period, especially when she is breast feeding. The first Trinovum tablet should be taken on the day after stopping the mini pill. All remaining pills in the mini pill packet must be discarded. Additional contraceptive precautions must be taken for the first 7 days.

*To skip a period:* To skip a period, a new pack of Trinovum should be started on the day after finishing the current pack (the patient skips the tablet-free days). Tablet-taking should be continued in the usual way. During the use of the second pack she may experience slight spotting or break-through bleeding but contraceptive protection will not be diminished provided there are no tablet omissions.

The next pack of Trinovum is started after the usual 7 tablet-free days, regardless of whether the period has completely finished or not.

*Reduced reliability:* The reliability of Trinovum may be reduced under the following circumstances.
*Forgotten tablets:* For further advice on the above please see precautions and warnings.
  *Vomiting or diarrhoea:* For further advice on the above, please see precautions and warnings.
  *Interactions:* For further advice on the above, please see precautions and warnings.

### Contra-indications, warnings, etc
*Absolute contra-indications:* Pregnancy or suspected pregnancy (that cannot yet be excluded).

Circulatory disorders (cardiovascular or cerebrovascular) such as thrombophlebitis and thromboembolic processes (or a history of these conditions), moderate to severe hypertension, hyperlipoproteinaemia. In addition the presence of more than one of the risk factors for arterial disease which are discussed under 'Serious adverse reactions'.

Severe liver disease, cholestatic jaundice or hepatitis (viral or non-viral) or a history of these conditions if the results of liver function tests have failed to return to normal, and for 3 months after liver function tests have been found to be normal; a history of jaundice of pregnancy or jaundice due to the use of steroids, Rotor syndrome and Dubin-Johnson syndrome, hepatic cell tumours and porphyria.

Cholelithiasis.

Known or suspected oestrogen-dependent tumours (see *Serious adverse reactions*); endometrial hyperplasia; undiagnosed vaginal bleeding.

Systemic lupus erythematosus or a history of this condition.

A history during pregnancy or previous use of steroids of: severe pruritus; herpes gestationis; a manifestation or deterioration of otosclerosis.

*Relative contra-indications:* If any of the relative contra-indications listed below is present, the benefits of oestrogen/progestogen-containing preparations must be weighed against the possible risk for each individual case and the patient kept under close supervision. In case of aggravation or appearance of any of these conditions whilst the patient is taking the pill, its use should be discontinued.

- Conditions implicating an increasing risk of developing venous thromboembolic complications, eg severe varicose veins or prolonged immobilisation or major surgery (see *Precautions and warnings*).
- Disorders of coagulation.
- Presence of any risk factor for arterial disease eg smoking, hyperlipidaemia or hypertension (see *Serious adverse reactions*).
- Other conditions associated with an increased risk of circulatory disease such as latent or overt cardiac failure, renal dysfunction, or a history of these conditions.
- Epilepsy or a history of this condition.
- Migraine or a history of this condition.
- A history of cholelithiasis.
- Presence of any risk factor for oestrogen-dependent tumours; oestrogen-sensitive gynaecological disorders such as uterine fibromyomata and endometriosis (see also under *Serious adverse reactions*).
- Diabetes mellitus.
- Severe depression or a history of this condition. If this is accompanied by a disturbance in tryptophan metabolism, administration of vitamin B6 might be of therapeutic value.
- Sickle cell haemoglobinopathy, since under certain circumstances, e.g. during infections or anoxia, oestrogen-containing preparations may induce

thromboembolic process in patients with this condition.

If the results of liver function tests become abnormal, use should be discontinued.

*Precautions and warnings:*
*Reduced reliability:* When Trinovum is taken according to the directions for use the occurrence of pregnancy is highly unlikely. However, the reliability of oral contraceptives may be reduced under the following circumstances:

*Forgotten tablets:* If the patient forgets to take a tablet, she should take it as soon as she remembers and take the next one at the normal time. This may mean that two tablets are taken in one day. Provided she is less than 12 hours late in taking her tablet, Trinovum will still give contraceptive protection during this cycle and the rest of the pack should be taken as usual.

If she is more than 12 hours late in taking one or more tablets then she should take the last missed pill as soon as she remembers but leave the other missed pills in the pack. She should continue to take the rest of the pack as usual but must use extra precautions (e.g. sheath, diaphragm plus spermicide) and follow the '7-day rule' (see further information for 7-day rule). If there are 7 or more pills left in the pack after the missed and delayed pills then the usual 7-day break can be left before starting the next pack. If there are less than 7 pills left in the pack after the missed and delayed pills then when the pack is finished the next pack should be started the next day. If withdrawal bleeding does not occur at the end of the second pack then a pregnancy test should be performed.

*Vomiting or diarrhoea:* If after tablet intake vomiting or diarrhoea occurs, a tablet may not be absorbed properly by the body. If the symptoms disappear within 12 hours of tablet-taking, the patient should take an extra tablet from a spare pack and continue with the rest of the pack as usual.

However, if the symptoms continue beyond those 12 hours, additional contraceptive precautions are necessary for any sexual intercourse during the stomach or bowel upset and for the following 7 days (the patient must be advised to follow the '7-day rule').

*Change in bleeding pattern:* If after taking Trinovum for several months there is a sudden occurrence of spotting or break-through bleeding (not observed in previous cycles) or the absence of withdrawal bleeding, contraceptive effectiveness may be reduced. If withdrawal bleeding fails to occur and none of the above mentioned events has taken place, pregnancy is highly unlikely and oral contraceptive use can be continued until the end of the next pack.

(If withdrawal bleeding fails to occur at the end of the second cycle, tablet intake should be discontinued and pregnancy excluded before oral contraceptive use can be resumed). However, if withdrawal bleeding is absent and any of the above mentioned events has occurred, tablet intake should be discontinued and pregnancy excluded before oral contraceptive use can be resumed.

*Interactions:* Irregular cycles and reduced reliability of oral contraceptives may occur when these preparations are used concomitantly with drugs such as anticonvulsants, barbiturates, antibiotics, (eg tetracyclines, ampicillin, rifampicin, etc), griseofulvin, activated charcoal and certain laxatives. Special consideration should be given to patients being treated with antibiotics for acne. They should be advised to use a non-hormonal method of contraception, or to use an oral contraceptive containing a progestogen showing minimal androgenicity, which have been reported as helping to improve acne without using an antibiotic. Oral contraceptives may diminish glucose tolerance and increase the need for insulin or other antidiabetic drugs in diabetics.

*Medical examination/consultation:* A complete medical history and physical examination should be taken prior to the initiation or reinstitution of oral contraceptives and should be repeated periodically.

These physical examinations should include special reference to blood pressure, breasts, abdomen and pelvic organs, including cervical cytology and, where indicated by the medical or family history, relevant laboratory tests. Caution should be observed when prescribing oral contraceptives to young women whose cycles are not yet stabilised.

*Surgery, varicose veins or immobilisation:* In patients using oestrogen-containing preparations the risk of deep vein thrombosis may be temporarily increased when undergoing a major operation (e.g. abdominal, orthopaedic), any surgery to the legs, medical treatment for varicose veins or prolonged immobilisation. Therefore, it is advisable to discontinue oral contraceptive use at least 4 to 6 weeks prior to these procedures if performed electively and to (re)start not less than 2 weeks after full ambulation. The latter is also valid with regard to immobilisation after an accident or emergency surgery. In case of emergency

surgery, thrombotic prophylaxis is usually indicated e.g. with subcutaneous heparin.

*Chloasma:* Chloasma may occasionally occur, especially in women with a history of chloasma gravidarum. Women with a tendency to chloasma should avoid exposure to the sun or ultraviolet radiation whilst taking this preparation. Chloasma is often not fully reversible.

*Laboratory tests:* The use of steroids may influence the results of certain laboratory tests. In the literature, at least a hundred different parameters have been reported to possibly be influenced by oral contraceptive use, predominantly by the oestrogenic component. Among these are: biochemical parameters of the liver, thyroid, adrenal and renal function, plasma levels of (carrier) proteins and lipid/lipoprotein fractions and parameters of coagulation and fibrinolysis.

*Adverse reactions:* Various adverse reactions have been associated with oral contraceptive use. The serious reactions are dealt with in more detail. The first appearance of symptoms indicative of any one of these reactions necessitates immediate cessation of oral contraceptive use while appropriate diagnostic and therapeutic measures are undertaken.

*Serious adverse reactions:* There is a general opinion, based on statistical evidence that users of combined oral contraceptives experience more often than non-users various disorders of the circulation. How often these disorders occur in users of modern low-oestrogen oral contraceptives is unknown, but there are reasons for suggesting that they may occur less often than with the older types of pill which contain more oestrogen.

Various reports have associated oral contraceptive use with the occurrence of deep venous thrombosis, pulmonary embolism and other embolisms. Other investigations of these oral contraceptives have suggested an increased risk or oestrogen and /or progestogen dose-dependent coronary and cerebrovascular accidents, predominantly in heavy smokers. Thrombosis has very rarely been reported to occur in other veins or arteries, e.g. hepatic, mesenteric, renal or retinal.

It should be noted that there is no consensus about the often contradictory findings obtained in early studies. The physician should bear in mind the possibility of vascular accidents occurring and that there may not be full recovery from such disorders and they may be fatal. The physician should take into account the presence of risk factors for arterial disease and deep venous thrombosis when prescribing oral contraceptives. Risk factors for arterial disease include smoking, the presence of hyperlipidaemia, hypertension or diabetes.

Signs and symptoms of a thrombotic event may include: sudden severe pain in the chest, whether or not reaching to the left arm; sudden breathlessness; any unusual severe, prolonged headache, especially if it occurs for the first time or gets progressively worse, or is associated with any of the following symptoms: sudden partial or complete loss of vision or diplopia, aphasia, vertigo, a bad fainting attack or collapse with or without focal epilepsy, weakness or very marked numbness suddenly affecting one side or one part of the body, motor disturbances; severe pain in the calf of one leg; acute abdomen.

Cigarette smoking increases the risk of serious cardiovascular adverse reactions to oral contraceptive use. The risk increases with age and with heavy smoking and is more marked in women over 35 years of age. Women who use oral contraceptives should be strongly advised not to smoke.

The use of oestrogen-containing oral contraceptives may promote growth of existing sex steroid dependent tumours. For this reason, the use of these oral contraceptives in patients with such tumours is contra-indicated. Numerous epidemiological studies have been reported of the risk or ovarian, endometrial, cervical and breast cancer in women using combined oral contraceptives.

The evidence is clear that combined oral contraceptives offer substantial protection against both ovarian and endometrial cancer. An increased risk of cervical cancer in long term users of combined oral contraceptives has been reported in some studies, but there continues to be controversy about the extent to which this is attributable to the confounding effects of sexual behaviour and other factors.

The evidence linking combined oral contraceptive use and breast cancer remains inconclusive. The results of some studies suggest an increased risk of breast cancer presenting below the age of about 35, the risk rising with duration of use. Any possible increased risk of breast cancer with combined oral contraceptives is however likely to be small, and may be expected to be less with low dose pills. This possible risk should be weighed against the many benefits of combined oral contraceptives, including their protective effects against ovarian and endometrial cancers.

Malignant hepatic tumours have been reported on rare occasions in long-term users of oral contraceptives. Benign hepatic tumours have also been associated with oral contraceptive usage. A hepatic tumour should be considered in the differential diagnosis when upper abdominal pain, enlarged liver or signs of intra-abdominal haemorrhage occur.

The use of oral contraceptives may sometimes lead to the development of cholestatic jaundice or cholelithiasis.

On rare occasions the use of oral contraceptives may trigger or reactivate systemic lupus erythematosus.

A further rare complication of oral contraceptive use is the occurrence of chorea which can be reversed by discontinuing the pill. The majority of cases of oral-contraceptive-induced chorea show a pre-existing predisposition which often relates to acute rheumatism.

*Other adverse reactions:*
*Cardiovascular system:* Rise of blood pressure. If hypertension develops, treatment should be discontinued
*Genital tract:* Intermenstrual bleeding, post-medication amenorrhoea, changes in cervical secretion, increase in size of uterine fibromyomata, aggravation of endometriosis, certain vaginal infections, e.g. candidiasis.
*Breast:* Tenderness, pain, enlargement, secretion.
*Gastro intestinal tract:* Nausea, vomiting, cholelithiasis, cholestatic jaundice.
*Skin:* Erythema nodosum, rash, chloasma, erythema multiforme, hirsutism, loss of scalp hair.
*Eyes:* Discomfort of the cornea if contact lenses are used.
*CNS:* Headache, migraines, mood changes, depression
*Metabolic:* Fluid retention, change in body weight, reduced glucose tolerance.
*Other:* Changes in libido, leg cramps, premenstrual-like syndrome.

*Overdosage:* There have been no reports of serious ill-health from overdosage even when a considerable number of tablets have been taken by a small child. In general, it is therefore unnecessary to treat overdosage. However, if overdosage is discovered within 2 or 3 hours and is large, then gastric lavage can be safely used. There are no antidotes and further treatment should be symptomatic.

**Further information**
*Additional contraceptive precautions:* When additional contraceptive precautions are required the patient should be advised either not to have sex, or to use a cap plus spermicide or for her partner to use a condom. Rhythm methods should not be advised as the pill disrupts the usual cyclical changes associated with the natural menstrual cycle e.g. changes in temperature and cervical mucus.

*The 7-day rule:* If any one tablet is forgotten for more than 12 hours:
If the patient has vomiting or diarrhoea for more than 12 hours:
If the patient is taking any of the drugs listed under 'Interactions':
The patient should continue to take her tablets as usual and additional contraceptive precautions must be taken for the next 7 days.

BUT–if these 7 days run beyond the end of the current pack, the next pack must be started as soon as the current one is finished, i.e. no gap should be left between packs. (This prevents an extended break in tablet taking which may increase the risk of the ovaries releasing an egg and thus reducing contraceptive protection.) The patient will not have a period until the end of 2 packs but this is not harmful nor does it matter if she experiences some bleeding on tablet taking days.

**Pharmaceutical precautions** Store at room temperature (below 25°C). Protect from light.

**Legal Category** POM.

**Package quantities** Carton containing 3 push packs of 21 tablets–sufficient for 3 cycles.

**Product licence number** 0242/0279.

# VERMOX* TABLETS

**Qualitative and quantitative composition** Mebendazole 100 mg.

**Pharmaceutical form** Tablet.

**Clinical particulars**
*Therapeutic indications:* For the treatment of *trichuris trichiura* (whipworm), *enterobius vermicularis* (pinworm), *ascaris lumbricoides* (roundworm), *ancylostoma duodenale* (common hookworm), *necator americanus* (American hookworm) in single or mixed infections.

*Posology and method of administration:*
*Adults and children over 2 years:* For the control of trichuriasis, ascaris and hookworm infections, one tablet bd for three consecutive days.
For the control of enterobiasis a single tablet is administered. It is highly recommended that a second tablet is taken after two weeks, if reinfection is suspected.

*Method of administration:* Oral.

*Contra-indications:* Vermox is contra-indicated in pregnancy and in patients who have shown hypersensitivity to the product or any components.

*Special warnings and special precautions for use:* Not recommended in the treatment of children under 2 years.

*Interactions with other medicaments and other forms of interaction:* Concomitant treatment with cimetidine may inhibit the metabolism of mebendazole in the liver, resulting in increased plasma concentrations of the drug especially during prolonged treatment.

*Pregnancy and lactation:*
*Pregnancy:* Since Vermox is contra-indicated in pregnancy patients who think they are or may be pregnant should not take this preparation.
*Lactation:* As it is not known whether Vermox is excreted in human milk it is not advisable to breast feed following administration of Vermox.

*Effects on ability to drive and use machines:* None stated.

*Undesirable effects:* Side effects reported for Vermox have been minor. Transient abdominal pain and diarrhoea have been reported, only rarely, in cases of massive infestation and expulsion of worms. Hypersensitivity reactions including exanthema, rash, urticaria and angio-oedema have rarely been observed.

*Overdose:* In the event of accidental overdosage, abdominal cramps, nausea, vomiting and diarrhoea may occur. Cases should be treated symptomatically with supportive measures and gastric lavage with activated charcoal as necessary. Although the maximum treatment duration of Vermox is limited to three days there have been rare reports of reversible liver function disturbances, hepatitis and neutropenia described in patients who were treated for hydatid disease with large doses for prolonged periods of time.

**Pharmacological properties**
*Pharmacodynamic properties: In vitro* and *in vivo* work suggests that mebendazole blocks the uptake of glucose by adult and larval forms of helminths, in a selective and irreversible manner. Inhibition of glucose uptake appears to lead to endogenous depletion of glycogen stores within the helminth. Lack of glycogen leads to decreased formation of ATP and ultrastructural changes in the cells.

*Pharmacokinetic properties:* Using a tracer dose of $^3$H-mebendazole the pharmacokinetics and bioavailability of a solution and iv drug have been examined. After oral administration the half life was 0.93 hours. Absorption of this tracer dose was almost complete but low availability indicated a high first pass effect. At normal therapeutic doses it is very hard to measure levels in the plasma.

*Preclinical safety data:* Not applicable.

**Pharmaceutical particulars**
*List of excipients:* Microcrystalline cellulose; sodium starch glycolate; talc; maize starch; sodium saccharin; magnesium stearate; hydrogenated vegetable oil; orange flavour; colloidal anhydrous silica; sodium lauryl sulphate; orange yellow S; purified water*; 2-propanol*.

* Not present in the final product.

*Incompatibilities:* Not applicable.

*Shelf life:* 60 months.

*Special precautions for storage:* None.

*Nature and contents of container:* Blister strips of PVC genotherm glass clear aluminium foil coated on the inside with a heat seal lacquer.
Pack sizes: 1 and 6 tablet packs.

*Instructions for use/handling:* Not applicable.

**Marketing authorisation number** 0242/0011

**Date of approval/revision of SPC** June 1996

**Legal category** POM.

# VERMOX* SUSPENSION

**Presentation** White, banana flavoured suspension of mebendazole 2% w/v. Each 5 ml contains mebendazole 100 mg. Vermox suspension also contains sucrose and methyl and propyl parabens.

**Uses** Vermox is a broad spectrum anthelmintic indicated for the treatment of:

Enterobius vermicularis  } (Threadworm/Pinworm)
Oxyuris vermicularis
Trichuris trichiura          (Whipworm)
Ascaris lumbricoides     (Large Roundworm)
Ancylostoma duodenale  (Common Hookworm)
Necator americanus       (American Hookworm)

in single or mixed infestations.

**Dosage and administration** Vermox suspension is for oral administration.

The same dosage applies to adults and children aged two years and above. No special procedures such as purging, use of laxatives and/or dietary changes are required.
(a) Threadworm (*Enterobius vermicularis*)
A single dose of 5 ml suspension. Care should be taken to avoid re-infection and it is strongly recommended that all members of the family are treated simultaneously. The efficacy of Vermox in threadworm infestations is such that treatment failures will be rare. If re-infection is suspected, it is highly recommended that a second dose is administered after two weeks.
(b) Whipworm (*Trichuris trichiura*)
Large Roundworm (*Ascaris lumbricoides*)
Common Hookworm (*Ancylostoma duodenale*)
5 ml suspension twice daily (morning and evening) for three consecutive days.

*Use in elderly:* As above.

**Contra-indications, warnings, etc**
*Contra-indications:* Vermox is contra-indicated in pregnancy (see 'use in pregnancy' section), and in patients who have shown hypersensitivity to the product or any of its components.

*Use in pregnancy:* Vermox has shown embryotoxic and teratogenic activity in rats at single oral doses. No such findings have been reported in the rabbit, dog, sheep, or horse. Since there is a risk that Vermox could produce foetal damage if administered during pregnancy, *it is contra-indicated in women who are thought to be or may be pregnant.*

*Use in lactation:* As it is not known whether Vermox is excreted in human milk it is not advisable to breast feed following the administration of Vermox.

*Use in infants:* Vermox has not been studied extensively in children under two years of age – for this reason it is not currently recommended in the treatment of children under two years.

*Drug interactions:* Concomitant treatment with cimetidine may inhibit the metabolism of mebendazole in the liver, resulting in increased plasma concentrations of the drug especially during prolonged treatment.

*Side-effects:* Side-effects reported for Vermox have been minor. Transient abdominal pain and diarrhoea have been reported, only rarely, in cases of massive infestation and expulsion of worms. Hypersensitivity reactions including exanthema, rash, urticaria and angio-oedema have rarely been observed.

*Overdosage:* In the event of accidental overdosage, abdominal cramps, nausea, vomiting and diarrhoea may occur. Cases should be treated symptomatically with supportive measures and gastric lavage with activated charcoal as necessary. Although the maximum treatment duration of Vermox is limited to three days there have been rare reports of reversible liver function disturbances, hepatitis and neutropenia described in patients who were treated for hydatid disease with large doses for prolonged periods of time.

**Pharmaceutical precautions** Vermox suspension should be shaken before use.

**Legal category** POM.

**Package quantities** 30 ml bottle.

**Further information** Nil.

**Product licence number** 0242/0050

*Trade Mark

# JHC Healthcare Ltd
## 5 Lower Merrion Street
## Dublin 2
## Eire

**JHC**

## MYOCRISIN*

**Qualitative and quantitative composition** Sodium aurothiomalate BP 50 mg in 0.5 ml (10%), Sodium aurothiomalate BP 10 mg in 0.5 ml (2%) and Sodium aurothiomalate BP 20 mg in 0.5 ml (4%).

**Pharmaceutical form** Injection.

**Clinical particulars**

*Therapeutic indications:* Myocrisin is used in the management of active progressive rheumatoid arthritis and progressive juvenile chronic arthritis especially if polyarticular or seropositive.

*Posology and method of administration:* Do not use a darkened solution (more than pale yellow).

Myocrisin should be administered only by deep intramuscular injection followed by gentle massage of the area. The patient should remain under medical observation for a period of 30 minutes after drug administration.

*Adults:* An initial test dose of 10 mg should be given in the first week followed by weekly doses of 50 mg until signs of remission occur. At this point 50 mg doses should be given at two week intervals until full remission occurs. With full remission the interval between injections should be increased progressively to three, four and then, after 18 months to 2 years, to six weeks.

If after reaching a total dose of 1 g (excluding the test dose), no major improvement has occurred and the patient has not shown any signs of gold toxicity, six 100 mg injections may be administered at weekly intervals. If no sign of remission occurs after this time other forms of treatment are to be considered.

*Elderly:* There are no specific dosage recommendations. Elderly patients should be monitored with extra caution.

*Children:* Progressive juvenile chronic arthritis:
Weekly doses of 1 mg/kg should be given but not exceeding a maximum weekly dose of 50 mg. Depending on urgency, this dose may be preceded by a smaller test dose such as 1/10 or 1/5 of the full dose for 2-3 weeks. Continue weekly doses until signs of remission appear then increase the intervals between injections to two weeks. With full remission increase the interval to three then four weeks. In the absence of signs of remission after twenty weeks consider raising the dose slightly or changing to another therapy.

Treatment should be continued for six months. Response can be expected at the 300-500 mg level. If patients respond, maintenance therapy should be continued with the dosage administered over the previous 2-4 weeks, for 1-5 years.

*Contra-indications:* Pregnancy (see *Pregnancy and lactation*)

Myocrisin is contraindicated in patients with gross renal or hepatic disease, a history of blood dyscrasias, exfoliative dermatitis or systemic lupus erythematosus.

The absolute contraindications should be positively excluded before considering gold therapy.

*Special warnings and special precautions for use:* As with other gold preparations, reactions which resemble anaphylactoid effects have been reported. These effects may occur after any course of therapy within the first ten minutes following drug administration (see administration). If anaphylactoid effects are observed, treatment with Myocrisin should be discontinued.

Myocrisin should be administered with extra caution in the elderly and in patients with a history of urticaria, eczema or colitis. Extra caution should also be exercised if phenylbutazone or oxyphenbutazone are administered concurrently.

Before starting treatment and again before each injection, the urine should be tested for protein, the skin inspected for rash and a full blood count performed, including a numerical platelet count (not an estimate) and the readings plotted. Blood dyscrasias are most likely to occur when between 400 mg and 1 g of gold have been given, or between the 10th and 20th week of treatment, but can also occur with much lower doses or after only 2-4 weeks of therapy.

The presence of albuminura, pruritus or rash, or an eosinophilia, are indications of developing toxicity. The Myocrisin should be withheld for one or two weeks until all signs have disappeared when the course may be restarted on a test dose followed by a decreased frequency of gold injections.

A complaint of sore throat, glossitis, buccal ulceration and/or easy bruising or bleeding, demands an immediate blood count, followed if indicated, by appropriate treatment for agranunulocytosis, aplastic anaemia and/or thrombocytopenia. Every patient treated with Myocrisin should be warned to report immediately the appearance of pruritis, metallic taste, sore throat or tongue, buccal ulceration or easy bruising, purpura, epistaxis, bleeding gums, menorrhagia or diarrhoea.

*Interaction with other medicaments and other forms of interaction:* Concurrent gold administration may exacerbate aspirin-induced hepatic dysfunction. Caution should be exercised if phenylbutazone or oxyphenbutazone are administered concurrently.

*Pregnancy and lactation:* The safety of Myocrisin in the foetus and the new-born has not been established. Female patients receiving Myocrisin should be instructed to avoid pregnancy. Pregnant patients should not be treated with Myocrisin. Lactating mothers under treatment with Myocrisin excrete significant amounts of gold in their breast milk and should not breast feed their infants.

*Effects on ability to drive and use machines:* None

*Undesirable effects:* Hepatotoxicity with cholestatic jaundice is a rare complication which may occur early in the course of treatment. It subsides on withdrawing Myocrisin. A rare but severe form of enterocolitis has been described.

Diffuse unilateral or bilateral pulmonary fibrosis very rarely occurs. This progressive condition usually responds to drug withdrawal and steroid therapy. An annual x-ray is recommended and attention should be paid to unexplained breathlessness and dry cough.

Side effects may be largely avoided by the indicated careful titration of dosage. Minor reactions, usually manifest as skin rashes are the most frequent and commonly benign, but as such reactions may be the forerunners of severe gold toxicity they must never be treated lightly. Significant skin complications are almost exclusively pruritic. Irreversible skin pigmentation can occur in sun-exposed areas after prolonged treatment with Myocrisin. Rare reports of alopecia exist. Nephrotic syndrome has been rarely reported.

*Overdose:* Minor side effects resolve spontaneously on withdrawal of Myocrisin. Symptomatic treatment of pruritus with antihistamines may be helpful. Major skin lesions and serious blood dyscrasias demand hospital admission when dimercaprol or penacillamine may be used to enhance gold excretion. Fresh blood and/or platelet transfusions, corticosteroids and androgenic steroids may be required in the management of severe blood dyscrasias

**Pharmacological properties**

*Pharmacological properties:* The precise mode of action of sodium aurothiomalate is not yet known. Treatment with gold has been shown to be accompanied by a fall in ESR and C-reactive protein, an increase in serum histidine and sulphydryl levels and a reduction in serum immunoglobulins, rheumatoid factor titres and Clq-binding activity.

Numerous experimental observations have been recorded including physico-chemical changes in collagen and interference with complement activation, gammaglobulin aggregation, prostaglandin biosythesis, inhibition of cathepsin and production of superoxide radicals by activated polymophonuclear leukocytes.

*Pharmacokinetics properties:* Sodium aurothiomalate is absorbed readily after intramuscular injection and becomes bound to plasma proteins. With doses of 50 mg weekly the steady-state serum concentration of gold is about 3 to 5 microgram per ml. It is widely distributed and accumulates in the body. Concentrations in synovial fluid have been shown to be similar or slightly less than those in plasma. Sodium aurothiomalate is mainly excreted in the urine with smaller amounts in the faeces. The serum half-life of gold clearance is about 5 or 6 days but after a course of treatment, gold may be found in the urine for up to a year or more owing to its presence in deep body compartments.

Gold has been detected in the foetus following administration of sodium aurothiomalate to the mother. Gold has been detected in the breast fed child where the mother has received sodium aurothiomalate.

*Preclinical safety data:* No additional pre-clinical data of relevance to the prescriber.

**Pharmaceutical particulars**
*List of excipients:* Phenylmercuric nitrate BP, Water for Injections BP.

*Incompatibilities:* None Known

*Shelf life:* 36 months

*Special precautions for storage:* Store below 25°C. Protect from light

*Nature and contents of container:* Boxes of 10 x 10 mg, 20 mg and 50 mg ampoules

*Instructions for use/handling:* None stated

**Marketing authorisation numbers**
Injection 10 mg   16186/0007
Injection 20 mg   16186/0008
Injection 50 mg   16186/0009

**Date of approval/revision of SPC** March 1997

**Legal category** POM

## NEULACTIL* TABLETS

**Qualitative and quantitative composition**
Pericyazine 10 mg
Pericyazine 2.5 mg

**Pharmaceutical form**
2.5 mg–Circular, very pale lime-yellow tablet, with one face impressed 'Neulactil' just inside the perimeter, breakline on reverse
10 mg–Circular, very pale lime-yellow tablet, with one face impressed 'Neulactil' just inside the perimeter around a central '10'. Breakline on reverse

**Clinical particulars**
*Therapeutic indications:* In adults with schizophrenia or other psychoses, for the treatment of symptoms or prevention of relapse.

In anxiety, psychomotor agitation, violent or dangerously impulsive behaviour. Neulactil is used as an adjunct to the short-term management of these conditions.

*Posology and method of administration:*

*Route of administration:* Oral.

Dosage requirement varies with the individual and the severity of the condition being treated. Initial dosage should be low with progressive increases until the desired response is obtained, after which dosage should be adjusted to maintain control of the symptoms.

*Severe conditions: Schizophrenia and other psychoses. Adults:* Initially 75 mg per day in divided doses. Dosage should be increased by 25 mg per day at weekly intervals until the optimum effect is achieved. Maintenance therapy would not normally be expected to exceed 300 mg per day. *Elderly:* Initially 15-30 mg per day in divided doses. If this is well tolerated the dosage may be increased if necessary for optimum control of behaviour.

*Mild or moderate conditions: In anxiety: Adults:* Initially 15-30 mg daily, divided into two portions with a larger dose being given in the evening. *Elderly:* 5-10 mg per day is suggested as a starting dose. It may be divided so that a larger portion is given in the evening. Half or quarter the normal adult dose may be sufficient for maintenance therapy.

Neulactil tablets are not recommended for children.

*Contra-indications:* See use in pregnancy below.

*Special warnings and precautions for use:* Neuroleptics should be avoided in patients with liver or renal dysfunction, epilepsy, Parkinson's disease, hypothyroidism, cardiac failure, phaeochromocytoma, myasthenia gravis, prostrate hypertrophy. It should be avoided in patients known to be hypersensitive to phenothiazines or with a history of narrow angle glaucoma. It should be used with caution in the elderly, particularly during very hot or very cold weather (risk of hyper-hypothermia).

*Interactions with other medicaments and other forms of interaction:* The following interactions are common to all phenothiazine neuroleptics. These interactions are a theoretical nature and are not serious.

The CNS depressant actions of neuroleptic agents may be intensified (additively) by alcohol, barbiturates and other sedatives. Respiratory depression may occur.

The hypotensive effect of most antihypertensive drugs, especially alpha adrenoceptor blocking agents may be exaggerated by neuroleptics.

The mild anticholinergic effect of neuroleptics may be exchanged by other anticholinergic drugs, possibly leading to constipation, heat stroke, etc.

The action of some drugs may be opposed by neuroleptics; these include amphetamine, levodopa, clonidine, guanethidine, adrenaline.

Anticholinergic agents may reduce the antipsychotic effect of neuroleptics.

Some drugs interfere with absorption of neuroleptic agents: antacids, anti-Parkinson drugs, lithium. Increases or decreases in the plasma concentrations of a number of drugs, eg: propranolol, phenobarbitone have been observed but were not of clinical significance.

High doses of neuroleptics may reduce the response to hypoglycaemic agents the dosage of which might have been raised.

Adrenaline must not be used in patients overdosed with neuroleptics. Most of the above interactions are of a theoretical nature and not serious.

Simultaneous administration of desferrioxamine and prochlorperazine has been observed to induce a transient metabolic encephalopathy characterised by loss of consciousness for 48-72 hours. It is possible this may occur with 'Neulactil' since it shares many of the pharmacological properties of prochlorperazine.

*Pregnancy and lactation:* There is inadequate evidence of the safety of Neulactil in human pregnancy but it has been widely used for many years without apparent ill consequence. There is evidence with some neuroleptics of harmful effects in animals. Like other drugs 'Neulactil' should be avoided in pregnancy unless the physician considers it essential. It may occasionally prolong labour and at such a time should be withheld until the cervix is dilated 3-4cm. Possible adverse effects on the foetus include lethargy or paradoxical hyperexcitability, tremor and low Apgar score.

Phenothiazines may be excreted in milk, therefore breastfeeding should be suspended during treatment.

*Effects on ability to drive and use machines:* Patients should be warned about drowsiness during early days of treatment, and advised not to drive or operate machinery. The elderly are particularly susceptible to postural hypotension

*Undesirable effects:* Liver function: jaundice, occurs in a very small percentage of patients taking neuroleptics. A premonitory sign may be a sudden onset of fever after one to three weeks of treatment followed by the development of jaundice. Neuroleptic jaundice has the biochemical and other characteristics of obstructive jaundice and is associated with obstruction of the canaliculi by bile thrombi; the frequent presence of an accompanying eosinophilia indicates the allergic nature of this phenomenon. Treatment should be withheld on the development of jaundice. Cardiorespiratory: hypotension, usually postural, commonly occurs. Elderly or volume depleted subjects are particularly susceptible. Cardiac arrhythmias, including atrial arrhythmia, A-V block, ventricular tachycardia and fibrillation have been reported during neuroleptic therapy, possibly related to dosage. Pre-existing cardiac disease, old age, hypokalaemia and concurrent tricyclic anti-depressants may predispose. ECG changes, usually benign, include widened QT interval, ST depression, U-waves and T-wave changes. Respiratory depression is possible in susceptible patients. Blood picture: A mild leukopenia occurs in up to 30% of patients on prolonged high dosage of neuroleptics: Agranulocytosis may occur rarely; it is not dose related. The occurrence of unexplained infections or fever requires immediate haematological investigation. Extraphyramidal: acute dystonias or dyskinesias, usually transitory are commoner in children and young adults, and usually occur within the first four days of treatment or after dosage increases. Akathisia characteristically occurs after large initial doses. Parkinsonism is commoner in adults and the elderly. It usually develops after weeks or months of treatment. One or more of the following may be seen: tremor, rigidity, akinesia, or other features of Parkinsonism. Commonly just tremor. Tardive dyskinesia: if this occurs it is usually, but not necessarily after prolonged or high dosage. It can even occur after treatment has been stopped. Dosage should therefore be kept low whenever possible. Skin and eyes: contact skin sensitation is a serious but rare complication in those frequently handling preparations of phenothiazines; The greatest care must be taken to avoid contact of the drug with the skin. Skin rashes of various kinds

may also be seen in patients treated with the drug. Patients on high dosage should be warned that they may develop photosensitivity in sunny weather and should avoid exposure to direct sunlight. *Endocrine:* hyperprolactinaemia which may result in galactorrhoea, gynaecomastia, amenorrhoea; impotence. Neuroleptic malignant syndrome (hyperthermia, rigidity autonomic dysfunction and altered consciousness) may occur with any neuroleptic. Minor side effects are nasal stuffiness, dry mouth, insomnia, agitation

*Overdose: Toxicity and treatment of overdosage:* Symptoms of neuroleptic overdosage include drowsiness or loss of consciousness, hypotension, tachycardia, ECG changes, ventricular arrhythmias and hypothermia. Severe extra-pyramidal dyskinesias may occur. If the patient is seen sufficiently soon (up to 6 hours) after ingestion of a toxic dose, gastric lavage may be attempted. Pharmacological induction of emesis is unlikely to be of any use. Activated charcoal should be given. There is no specific antidote. Treatment is supportive. Generalised vasodilatation may result in circulatory collapse; raising the patient's legs may suffice, in severe cases, volume expansion by intravenous fluids may be needed; infusion fluids should be warmed before administration in order not to aggravate hypothermia. Positive inotropic agents such as dopamine may be tried if fluid replacement is insufficient to correct the circulatory collapse. Peripheral vasoconstrictor agents are not generally recommended; avoid the use of adrenaline. Ventricular or supraventricular tachy-arrhythmias usually respond to restoration of normal body temperature and correction of circulatory or metabolic disturbances. If persistent or life threatening, appropriate anti-arrhythmic therapy may be considered. Avoid lignocaine, and as far as possible long acting, anti-arrhythmic drugs. Pronounced central nervous system depression requires airway maintenance or, in extreme circumstances, assisted respiration. Severe dystonic reactions usually respond to procyclidine (5-10 mg) or orphenedrine (20-40 mg) administered intramuscularly or intravenously. Convulsions should be treated with intravenous diazepam. Neuroleptic malignant syndrome should be treated with cooling. Dantrolene sodium may be tried.

## Pharmacological properties

*Pharmacodynamic properties:* Pericyazine is a neuroleptic with cardiovascular and antihistamine effects similar to those of chlorpromazine, but it has a stronger antiserotonin effect and a powerful central sedative effect.

*Pharmacokinetic properties:* Kinetics: there is little information about plasma concentrations, distribution and excretion in humans. The rate of metabolism and excretion of phenothiazines decreases in old age.

*Preclinical safety data:* There are no pre-clinical data of relevance to the prescriber which are additional to that already included in other sections of the SPC.

*List of excipients:* Lactose Anhydrous USP, Microcrystalline cellulose (E460), Sodium starch glycollate, Magnesium sterateBP, Colloidal silicon dioxide (E551), Methylhydroxybenzoate BP (E218)

*Incompatibilities:* None known.

*Shelf-life:* 60 months

*Special precautions for storage:* Protect from light.

*Nature and contents of container:* Containers of 84×2.5 mg (OP) and 10 mg tablets.

*Instructions for use in handling:* None stated

### Marketing authorisation numbers
Tablets 2.5 mg  16186/0003
Tablets 10 mg   16186/0004

**Date of approval/revision of SPC:** February 1997

**Legal category** POM

## NEULACTIL FORTE SYRUP

**Qualitative and quantitative composition** Pericyazine 10 mg/5 ml.

**Pharmaceutical form** Forte Syrup, clear orange brown syrupy liquid.

**Clinical particulars**
*Therapeutic indications:* In adults with schizophrenia or other psychoses, for the treatment of symptoms or prevention of relapse.

In anxiety, psychomotor agitation, violent or dangerously impulsive behaviour. Neulactil is used as an adjunct to the short-term management of these conditions.

In children with behaviour disorders or schizophrenia.

*Posology and method of administration:*
*Route of administration:* Oral. Dosage requirement varies with the individual and the severity of the

condition being treated. Initial dosage should be low with progressive increases until the desired response is obtained, after which dosage should be adjusted to maintain control of the symptoms.

*Schizophrenia and other psychoses: Adults:* Initially 75 mg per day in divided doses. Dosage should be increased by 25 mg per day at weekly intervals until the optimum effect is achieved. Maintenance therapy would not normally be expected to exceed 300 mg per day. *Elderly:* Initially 15-30 mg per day in divided doses. If this is well tolerated the dosage may be increased if necessary for optimum control of behaviour. *Children* The initial daily dose should be calculated on bodyweight. A child weighing 10 kg should receive 0.5 milligram and this initial dose should be increased by 1 mg for each additional 5 kg of bodyweight up to a total daily dose of 10 mg daily. This dosage may be gradually increased until the desired effect is achieved, but the daily maintenance dose should not exceed twice the initial amount.

Neulactil is not recommended for use in children below 1 year of age.

*Anxiety, psychomotor agitation, violent or dangerously impulsive behaviour.: Adults:* Initially 15-30 mg daily, divided into two portions with a larger dose being given in the evening. *Elderly:* 5–10 mg per day is suggested as a starting dose. It may be divided so that a larger portion is given in the evening. Half or quarter the normal adult dose may be sufficient for maintenance therapy. *Children: Not recommended for children.*

*Contra-indications:* None stated

*Special warnings and precautions for use:* Neuroleptics should be avoided in patients with liver or renal dysfunction, epilepsy, Parkinson's disease, hypothyroidism, cardiac failure, phaeochromocytoma, myasthenia gravis, prostrate hypertrophy. It should be avoided in patients known to be hypersensitive to phenothiazines or with a history of narrow angle glaucoma. It should be used with caution in the elderly, particularly during very hot or very cold weather (risk of hyper-hypothermia).

*Interactions with other medicaments and other forms of interaction:* The following interactions are common to all phenothiazine neuroleptics. These interactions are mainly of a theoretical nature and not serious.

The CNS depressant actions of neuroleptic agents may be intensified (additively) by alcohol, barbiturates and other sedatives. Respiratory depression may occur.

The hypotensive effect of most antihypertensive drugs, especially alpha adrenoceptor blocking agents may be exaggerated by neuroleptics.

The mild anticholinergic effect of neuroleptics may be enhanced by other anticholinergic drugs, possibly leading to constipation, heat stroke, etc.

The action of some drugs may be opposed by neuroleptics; these include amphetamine, levodopa, clonidine, guanethidine, adrenaline.

Anticholinergic agents may reduce the antipsychotic effect of neuroleptics.

Some drugs interfere with absorption of neuroleptic agents: antacids, anti-Parkinson drugs, lithium. Increases or decreases in the plasma concentrations of a number of drugs, eg: propranolol, phenobarbitone have been observed but were not of clinical significance.

High doses of neuroleptics may reduce the response to hypoglycaemic agents the dosage of which might have been raised.

Adrenaline must not be used in patients overdosed with neuroleptics.

Simultaneous administration of desferrioxamine and prochlorperazine has been observed to induce a transient metabolic encephalopathy characterised by loss of consciousness for 48-72 hours. It is possible this may occur with Neulactil since it shares many of the pharmacological properties of prochlorperazine

*Pregnancy and lactation:* There is inadequate evidence of the safety of Neulactil in human pregnancy but it has been widely used for many years without apparent ill consequence. There is evidence with some neuroleptics of harmful effects in animals. Like other drugs Neulactil should be avoided in pregnancy unless the physician considers it essential. It may occasionally prolong labour and at such a time should be withheld until the cervix is dilated 3-4cm. Possible adverse effects on the foetus include lethargy or paradoxical hyperexcitability, tremor and low Apgar score.

Phenothiazines may be excreted in milk, therefore breastfeeding should be suspended during treatment.

*Effects on ability to drive and use machines:* Patients should be warned about drowsiness during early days of treatment, and advised not to drive or operate machinery. The elderly are particularly susceptible to postural hypotension

*Undesirable effects: Liver function:* jaundice occurs in a very small percentage of patients taking neuroleptics. A premonitory sign may be a sudden onset of fever after one to three weeks of treatment followed by the development of jaundice. Neuroleptic jaundice has the biochemical and other characteristics of obstructive jaundice and is associated with obstruction of the canaliculi by bile thrombi; the frequent presence of an accompanying eosinophilia indicates the allergic nature of this phenomenon. Treatment should be withheld on the development of jaundice. *Cardiorespiratory:* hypotension, usually postural, commonly occurs. Elderly or space depleted subjects are particularly susceptible. Cardiac arrhythmias, including atrial arrhythmia, A-V block, ventricular tachycardia and fibrillation have been reported during neuroleptic therapy, possibly related to dosage. Pre-existing cardiac disease, old age, hypokalaemia and concurrent tricyclic anti-depressants may predispose. ECG changes, usually benign, include widened QT interval, ST depression, U-waves and T-wave changes. Respiratory depression is possible in susceptible patients. *Blood picture:* A mild leukopenia occurs in up to 30% of patients on prolonged high dosage of neuroleptics: Agranulocytosis may occur rarely; it is not dose-related. The occurrence of unexplained infections or fever requires immediate haematological investigation. *Extrapyramidal:* acute dystonias or dyskinesias, usually transitory are commoner in children and young adults, and usually occur within the first four days of treatment or after dosage increases. Akathisia characteristically occurs after large initial doses. Parkinsonism is commoner in adults and the elderly. It usually develops after weeks or months of treatment. One or more of the following may be seen: tremor, rigidity, akinesia, or other features of Parkinsonism. Commonly just tremor. *Tardive dyskinesia:* if this occurs it is usually, but not necessarily after prolonged or high dosage. It can even occur after treatment has been stopped. Dosage should therefore be kept low whenever possible. *Skin and eyes:* Skin rashes of various kinds may also be seen in patients treated with the drug. Patients on high dosage should be warned that they may develop photosensitivity in sunny weather and should avoid exposure to direct sunlight. *Endocrine:* hyperprolactinaemia which may result in galactorrhoea, gynaecomastia, amenorrhoea; impotence. Neuroleptic malignant syndrome (hyperthermia, rigidity autonomic dysfunction and altered consciousness) may occur with any neuroleptic. Minor side effects are nasal stuffiness, dry mouth, insomnia, agitation.

*Overdose:* Symptoms of neuroleptic overdosage include drowsiness or loss of consciousness, hypotension, tachycardia, ECG changes, ventricular arrhythmias and hypothermia. Severe extra-pyramidal dyskinesias may occur.

If the patient is seen sufficiently soon (up to 6 hours) after ingestion of a toxic dose, gastric lavage may be attempted. Pharmacological induction of emesis is unlikely to be of any use. Activated charcoal should be given. There is no specific antidote. Treatment is supportive.

Generalised vasodilatation may result in circulatory collapse; raising the patient's legs may suffice, in severe cases, volume expansion by intravenous fluids may be needed; infusion fluids should be warmed before administration in order not to aggravate hypothermia.

Positive inotropic agents such as dopamine may be tried if fluid replacement is insufficient to correct the circulatory collapse. Peripheral vasoconstrictor agents are not generally recommended; avoid the use of adrenaline.

Ventricular or supraventricular tachy-arrhythmias usually respond to restoration of normal body temperature and correction of circulatory or metabolic disturbances. If persistent or life threatening, appropriate anti-arrhythmic therapy may be considered. Avoid lignocaine, and as far as possible long acting, anti-arrhythmic drugs.

Pronounced central nervous system depression requires airway maintenance or, in extreme circumstances, assisted respiration. Severe dystonic reactions usually respond to procyclidine (5-10 mg) or orphenedrine (20-40 mg) administered intramuscularly or intravenously. Convulsions should be treated with intravenous diazepam.

Neuroleptic malignant syndrome should be treated with cooling. Dantrolene sodium may be tried.

**Pharmacological properties**

*Pharmacodynamic properties:* Pericyazine is a neuroleptic with cardiovascular and antihistamine effects similar to those of chlorpromazine, but it has a stronger antiserotonin effect and a powerful central sedative effect.

*Pharmacokinetic properties:* Kinetics: there is little information about plasma concentrations, distribution and excretion in humans. The rate of metabolism and excretion of phenothiazines decreases in old age.

*Preclinical safety data:* There are no pre-clinical data of relevance to the prescriber which are additional to that already included in other sections of the SPC.

**Pharmaceutical particulars**

*List of excipients:* Sugar, Caramel Flavour, Spearmint Oil, Peppermint Oil, Fruit cup 868, 'Tween' 20 (Polysorbate 20), Citric acid anhydrous, Sodium citrate gran., Sodium sulphite anhydrous, Sodium metabisulphite powder, Ascorbic acid, Sodium benzoate, Demineralised water BP(E218)

*Incompatibilities:* None known

*Shelf-life:* 24 months unopened, 1 month after opening.

*Special precautions for storage:* Protect from light

*Nature and contents of container:* Amber glass bottle containing 100 ml. HDPE/polypropylene child resistant cap with tamper evident band or rolled on pilfer proof aluminium cap and a PVDC emulsion coated wad.

*Instructions for use in handling:* Care must be taken to avoid contact of the drug with skin. Contact sensitisation is a serious but rare complication in those frequently handling preparations of phenothiazines.

**Marketing authorisation number** 16186/0005

**Date of approval/revision of SPC** May 1997

**Legal category** POM

## PENTACARINAT*

**Qualitative and quantitative composition** Pentacarinat 300 mg contain Pentamidine Isethionate BP 300 mg (Equivalent to 172.4 mg pentamidine base)

**Pharmaceutical form** Sterile powder for use after reconstitution

**Clinical particulars**

*Therapeutic indications:* Pentamidine is indicated in the treatment of: Pneumonia due to Pneumocystis carinii (PCP), Leishmaniasis including visceral and cutaneous, Early phase African sleeping sickness caused by Trypanosoma gambiense, All indications can be treated by deep intramuscular injection or intravenous injection.

Pneumocystis carinii pneumonia can also be treated by the inhalation route.

Pentacarinat is also indicated in the prevention of Pneumocystis carinii pneumonia in patients infected by the human immunodeficiency virus (HIV) who have experienced a previous episode of PCP. Administration is by the inhalation route.

*Posology and method of administration:* Pentamidine powder is reconstituted before use with Water for Injections BP. For intravenous use the required dose of pentamidine isethionate is diluted further in 50-250 ml of glucose intravenous infusion BP or 0.9% (normal) Sodium Chloride Injection BP.

The following dosage regimens are recommended for adults, children and infants.

*Treatment: Pneumocystis carinii pneumonia:* By slow iv infusion, 4 mg/kg bodyweight of pentamidine isethionate once daily for at least 14 days. If administered by inhalation, two 300 mg vials are dissolved in 6 ml of water for injection and the resultant solution administered by a suitable nebuliser once daily for three weeks.

*Leishmaniasis:* Visceral: 3-4 mg/kg bodyweight of pentamidine isethionate on alternate days to a maximum of 10 injections, preferably by im injection. A repeat course may be necessary. Cutaneous: 3-4 mg/kg bodyweight, once or twice weekly by im injection until the condition resolves.

*Trypanosomiasis:* 4 mg/kg bodyweight of pentamidine isethionate once daily or on alternate days to a total of 7-10 injections. The im or iv infusion route may be used.

There are no specific dosage recommendations for the elderly.

In renal failure the following recommendations are made for a creatinine clearance of less than 10 ml/min.:

*P. carinii pneumonia:* in life threatening cases, 4 ml/kg bodyweight once daily for 7 to 10 days, then 4 mg/kg bodyweight on alternate days, to complete the course of at least 14 doses. In less severe cases, 4 mg/kg bodyweight on alternate days, to complete the course of at least 14 doses.

No dosage reductions are necessary in renally impaired patients with leishmaniasis or trypanosomiasis.

Hepatic failure: no specific dosage recommendations.

*Prevention:* Dissolve the contents of one pentacarinat vial (300 mg pentamidine isethionate) in 4-6 ml water for injections BP. In the prophylaxis of P. carinii pneumonia, the adult dosage is 300 mg every 4 weeks or 150 mg every 2 weeks.

*Contra-indications:* The drug should not be administered to patients with a known hypersensitivity to pentamidine.

*Special warnings and precautions for use:* Pentamidine isethionate should be used with particular caution in patients with hepatic and/or renal dysfunction, hypertension or hypotension, hyperglycaemia or hypoglycaemia, leucopenia, thrombocytopenia or anaemia. Fatalities due to severe hypotension, hypoglycaemia, acute pancreatitis and cardiac arrhythmias have been reported in patients treated with pentamidine isethionate, by both the intramuscular and intravenous routes. Baseline blood pressure should be established and patients should receive the drug lying down. Blood pressure should be closely monitored during administration and at regular intervals until treatment is concluded. Therefore patients receiving pentamidine by inhalation should be closely monitored for the development of severe adverse reactions.

Laboratory monitoring: The following tests should be carried out before, during and after therapy by the parenteral route:

Blood urea, nitrogen and serum creatinine daily during therapy.

Complete blood and platelet counts daily during therapy.

Fasting blood glucose measurements daily during therapy, and at regular intervals after completion of therapy. Hyperglycaemia and diabetes mellitus, with or without preceding hypoglycaemia have occurred up to several months after cessation of therapy.

Liver function tests (LFTS) including bilirubin, alkaline phosphatase, aspartate aminotransferase (AST/GOT), and alkaline aminotransferase (ALT/GPT). If baseline measurements are normal and remain so during therapy, test weekly. When there is baseline elevation in LFTS and/or LFTS increase during therapy, continue monitoring weekly unless the patient is on other hepatotoxic agents, when monitoring every 3-5 days is appropriate.

Serum calcium, test weekly.

Electrocardiograms at regular intervals.

The benefit of aerosolised pentamidine therapy in patients at high risk of a pneumothorax should be weighed against the clinical consequences of such a manifestation.

*Interactions with other medicaments and other forms of interaction:* There are no documented interactions with other medicaments.

*Pregnancy and lactation:* There is no evidence of the safety of pentamidine isethionate in human pregnancy. A miscarriage within the first trimester of pregnancy has been reported following aerosolised prophylactic administration. Pentamidine isethionate should not be administered to pregnant patients unless considered essential. *Lactation:* The use of pentamidine isethionate is contra-indicated in breast feeding mothers unless considered essential by the physician.

*Effects on ability to drive and use machines:* Pentamidine has no known effect on the ability to drive and use machines.

*Undesirable effects: Parenteral Route:* Severe reactions which may be life threatening include hypotension, hypoglycaemia, pancreatitis, cardiac arrythmias, leucopenia, thrombocytopenia, acute renal failure, hypocalcaemia. A possible case of Stevens-Johnson syndrome has been reported.

Less severe reactions include azotemia, abnormal liver function tests, leucopenia, anaemia, thrombocytopenia, hyperkalaemia, nausea and vomiting, hypotension, dizziness, syncope, flushing, hypoglycaemia, hyperglycaemia, rash, taste disturbances.

Local reactions can occur ranging in severity from discomfort and pain to induration, abscess formation and muscle necrosis.

Reversible renal side effects occur with the highest frequency (over 20% of patients) with a slightly lower frequency of local reactions.

Side effects including metabolic disturbances, hepatic, haematological, or hypotensive episodes occur much less frequently (5-10% patients).

*Inhalation route:* Bronchospasm has been reported to occur following use of the nebuliser. This has been particularly noted in patients who have a history of smoking or asthma. This can usually be controlled by prior use of bronchodilators.

The occurrence of cases of pneumothorax has been reported in patients presenting a history of PCP. Although the aetiology of the pneumothorax was not linked primarily to the aerosolised administration of pentamidine in the majority of cases, a causal relationship to pentamidine cannot be ruled out.

Local reactions involving the upper respiratory tract can occur ranging in severity from cough, shortness of breath and wheezing to bronchospasms.

Other side effects reported were hypotention, hypoglycaemia, acute pancreatitis, renal insufficiency rash, fever, decrease in appetite, taste disturbances, fatigue, light-headedness and nausea.

*Overdosage:* Treatment is symptomatic. No cases of overdosage have been recorded with pentamidine isethionate.

**Pharmacological properties**
*Pharmacodynamic properties:* Pentamidine isethionate is an aromatic diamine. It is an antiprotozoal agent which acts by interfering with DNA and folate transformation, and by the inhibition of RNA and protein synthesis.

*Pharmacokinetic properties:* After intravenous infusion, plasma levels of pentamidine fall rapidly during the first two hours to one twentieth of peak levels, followed by a much slower decline thereafter. After intramuscular administration, the apparent volume of distribution of pentamidine is significantly greater (>3 times) than that observed following intravenous administration.

Elimination of half-lives after parenteral administration were estimated to be about 6 hours after intravenous infusion in patients with a normal renal function. The elimination of half-life following intramuscular injection was found to be about 9 hours.

Following parenteral administration, pentamidine appears to be widely distributed in the body and probably accumulates in tissue, particularly the liver and kidney. Only a small amount is excreted unchanged in the urine.

When administered by the use of a nebuliser, human kinetic studies revealed significant differences when compared to parenteral administration. Aerosol administration resulted in a 10-fold increase in bronchial alveolar lavage (BAL) supernatant fluid and an 80-fold increase in BAL sediment concentrations in comparison with those seen with equivalent intravenous doses.

Limited data suggests that the half-life of pentamidine in BAL fluid is greater than 10 to 14 days. Peak plasma concentrations after inhalation therapy were found to be approximately 10% of those observed with equivalent intramuscular doses and less than 5% of those observed following intravenous administration. This suggests that systemic effects by the inhalation route are less likely.

Long term pulmonary parenchymal effects of aerosolised pentamidine are not known. Lung volume and alveolar capillary diffusion, however, have not been shown to be affected by high doses of pentamidine administered by inhalation to AIDS patients.

*Preclinical safety data:* No additional data of relevance to the prescriber

**Pharmaceutical particulars**
*List of excipients:* Not applicable.

*Incompatibilities:* Pentamidine isethionate solution should not be mixed with any injection solutions other than Water for Injections BP, Glucose Intravenous Infusion BP and 0.9% (normal) Sodium Chloride Injection BP.

*Shelf life:* 60 months when unopened. After reconstitution 24 hours.

*Special precautions for storage:* Store the dry product below 30°C.

Store the reconstituted product (for intravenous infusion) at 2-8°C. Use within 24 hours.

*Nature and contents of container:* Cardboard carton containing 5 x 10 ml glass vials each with rubber bung and aluminium ring. Each vial contains 300 mg Pentamidine Isethionate BP.

*Instructions for use/handling:* This product should be reconstituted in a fume cupboard. Store the dry product below 30°C. Store dilute reconstituted drug solutions between 2-8°C, and discard all unused portions within 24 hours of preparation. Concentrated solutions for administration by the inhalation or intramuscular routes should be used immediately.

After reconstitution with Water for Injections BP, pentacarinat should not be mixed with any injection solutions other than Glucose Intravenous Infusion 5% BP and 0.9% (normal) Sodium Chloride Injection BP.

The optimal particle size for alveolar deposition is between 1 and 2 microns.

The freshly prepared solution should be administered by inhalation using a suitable nebuliser such as a Respirgard II (trade mark of Marquest Medical Products Inc.), Modified Acorn system 22 (trade mark of Medic-Aid) or an equivalent device with either a compressor or piped oxygen at a flow rate of 6 to 10 Litres/Minute.

The nebuliser should be used in a vacated , well ventilated room. Only staff wearing adequate protective clothing (mask, goggles, gloves) should be in the room when nebulisers are being used.

A suitable well fitted one-way system should be employed such that the nebuliser stores the aerosolised drug during exhalations and disperses exhaled pentamidine into a reservoir. A filter should be fitted to the exhaust line to reduce atmospheric pollution. It is advisable to use a suitable exhaust tube which vents directly through a window to the external atmosphere. Care should be taken to ensure that passers-by will not be exposed to the exhaust.

All bystanders including medical personnel, women of child bearing potential, pregnant women, children, and people with a history of asthma, should avoid exposure to atmospheric pentamidine resulting from nebuliser usage.

Dosage equivalence: 4 mG of pentamidine isethionate contains 2.3 mG pentamidine base; 1 mg of pentamidine base is equivalent to 1.74 mG pentamidine isethionate.

Displacement value: 300 mG of pentamidine isethionate displace approximately 0.15 ml of water.

**Marketing authorisation number** 16186/0001

**Date of approval/revision of SPC** February 1997

**Legal category** POM

## PENTACARINAT* READY-TO-USE SOLUTION

**Presentation** A clear colourless, solution, supplied in a 10 ml unit-dose container, containing 300 mg pentamidine isethionate. The solution also contains glucose and sodium acetate buffer.

**Uses** Pentacarinat Ready-to-Use Solution is indicated in the treatment of *Pneumocystis carinii* pneumonia (PCP)in the patients infected by the human immunodeficiency virus (HIV).

Pentacarinat Ready-to-Use Solution is also indicated for the prevention of Pneumocystis carinii pneumonia in patients infected by the human immunodeficiency virus who have experienced a previous episode of PCP.

*Kinetics:* When administered by the use of a nebuliser, human kinetic studies revealed significant differences compared to parenteral administration. Aerosol administration resulted in a 10-fold increase in bronchial alveolar lavage (BAL) supernatant fluid, and an 80-fold increase in BAL sediment concentrations in comparison with those seen with equivalent parenteral doses.

Limited data suggest that the half-life of pentamidine in BAL fluid is greater than 10 to 14 days.

Long-term pulmonary parenchymal effects of aerosolised pentamidine are not known. Lung volume and alveolar capillary diffusion, however, have not been shown to be affected by high doses of pentamidine administered by inhalation to AIDS patients.

**Dosage and administration**
*Treatment:* For the treatment of P. carinii pneumonia, the dosage is 600 mg (two bottles of solution), given once daily for 3 weeks.

*Prophylaxis:* For prevention of P. carinii pneumonia, the dosage is 300 mg once a month or 150 mg every two weeks.

The solution containing the required dosage should be administered by inhalation using a suitable nebuliser such as a Respirgard II*, modified Acorn System 22* or an equivalent device with either a compressor or piped oxygen at a flow rate of 6 to 10 litres/minute.

The nebuliser should be used in a vacated, well ventilated room. Only staff wearing adequate protective clothing (mask, goggles, gloves) should be in the room when nebulisers are being used.

The optimal particle size for alveolar deposition is between 1 and 2 microns.

A suitable, well fitted one-way system should be employed such that the nebuliser stores the aerosolised drug during exhalations and disperses exhaled pentamidine into a reservoir. A filter should be fitted to the exhaust line to reduce atmospheric pollution. It is advisable to use a suitable exhaust tube which vents directly through a window to the external atmosphere. Care should be taken to ensure that passers-by will not be exposed to the exhaust.

*Elderly:* No specific dosage recommendations.

*Hepatic failure:* No information available.

**Contra-indications, warnings, etc** The drug should not be administered to patients with a known hypersensitivity to pentamidine.

*Pregnancy:* There is no evidence of the safety of aerosolised pentamidine in human pregnancy. A miscarriage within the first trimester of pregnancy has been reported following aerosolised prophylactic administration. Pentamidine isethionate should not be administered to pregnant patients unless considered essential.

*Lactation:* The use of pentamidine isethionate is contra-indicated in breast-feeding mothers unless considered essential by the physician.

*Precautions:* Fatalities due to severe hypotension, hypoglycaemia, acute pancreatitis and cardiac arrhythmias have been reported in patients treated with pentamidine isethionate, by both the intramuscular and intravenous routes. Therefore patients receiving pentamidine by inhalation should be closely monitored for the development of severe adverse reactions.

Pentamidine Isethionate should be used with particular caution in patients with hepatic and/or renal dysfunction, hypertension, hyperglycaemia, hypoglycaemia, leucopenia, thrombocytopenia or anaemia. Bronchospasm has been reported to occur following the use of the nebuliser. This has been particularly noted in patients who have a history of smoking or asthma. This can be controlled by prior use of bronchodilators.

The benefit of aerosolised pentamidine therapy in patients at high risk of a pneumothorax should be weighed against the clinical consequences of such an occurrence.

*Interactions:* None known.

*Adverse effects:* Cases of pneumothorax have been reported in patients with a history of PCP. Although the aetiology of the pneumothorax was not linked primarily to the aerosolised administration of pentamidine in the majority of cases, a causal relationship cannot be ruled out. Local reactions involving the respiratory tract can occur ranging in severity from cough, shortness of breath and wheezing to bronchospasms. Other adverse effects reported with the use of aerosolised pentamidine are rash, hypotension, hypoglycaemia, acute pancreatitis, renal insufficiency, fever, decrease in appetite, taste disturbances, fatigue, light-headedness and nausea.

A miscarriage within the first trimester of pregnancy has been reported following prophylactic administration of aerosolised pentamidine.

*Treatment of overdosage:* No cases of overdosage have been recorded with pentamidine. Should overdosage occur treatment should be symptomatic.

**Pharmaceutical precautions** Store between 15°C–25°C. Any solid material should be redissolved by gentle warming before use.

**Legal category** POM.

**Package quantities** 10×300 mg bottles.

**Further information** Pentamidine isethionate is an aromatic diamidine. It is an antiprotozoal agent which acts by interfering with DNA and folate transformation, and by inhibition of RNA and protein synthesis. Dosage equivalence: 4 mg of pentamidine isethionate contains 2.3 mg pentamidine base; 1 mg of pentamidine base is equivalent to 1.74 mg pentamidine isethionate.

All bystanders including medical personnel, women of child bearing potential, pregnant women, children and people with a history of asthma, should avoid exposure to atmospheric pentamidine resulting from nebuliser usage.

**Product licence number** 16186/0002.

## PIPORTIL* DEPOT INJECTION

**Qualitative and quantitative composition:** pipothiazine palmitate HSE 5.0% w/v

**Pharmaceutical form:** Depot injection.

**Clinical particulars**
*Therapeutic indications:* For the maintenance treatment of schizophrenia and paranoid psychoses and prevention of relapse, especially where compliance with oral medication is a problem

*Posology and method of administration:* Patients should be stabilised on Piportil Depot under psychiatric supervision. Administration should be by deep intramuscular injection into the gluteal region. Wide variation of response can be expected. The following dosage recommendations are suitable for either indication.

*Adults:* Initially 25 mg should be given to assess the response of the patient to the drug. Further doses should be administered at appropriate intervals, increasing by increments of 25 or 50 mg until a satisfactory response is obtained. In clinical practice, Piportil Depot has been shown to have a long duration of action, allowing intervals of 4 weeks between injections for maintenance therapy. Dosage should be adjusted under close supervision to suit each individual patient in order to obtain the best therapeutic response compatible with tolerance. The duration of action depends on the dose administered, allowing dosage intervals to be varied to suit individual circumstances. Most patients respond favourably to a dose of 50-100 mg every 4 weeks, the maximum recommended dose is 200 mg every four weeks.

*Elderly:* Neuroleptics should be used cautiously in the elderly: A reduced starting dose is recommended, ie 5-10 mg might be considered.

*Children:* Not recommended for use in children.

*Contra-indications:* Piportil Depot should not be administered to patients in a comatose state or with marked cerebral atherosclerosis, phaeochromocytoma, renal or liver failure, severe cardiac insufficiency or hypersensitivity to other phenothiazine derivatives.

*Special warnings and special precautions for use:* Piportil Depot should be used with caution in patients suffering from or who have a history of, the following conditions: severe respiratory disease, epilepsy, alcohol withdrawal symptoms, brain damage, Parkinson's disease or marked extrapyramidal symptoms with previously used neuroleptics, personal or family history of narrow angle glaucoma, hypothyroidism, myasthenia gravis, prostatic hypertrophy, thyrotoxicosis. Care is required in very hot or very cold weather particularly in elderly frail patients.

*Interactions with other medicaments and other forms of interaction:* The CNS depressant actions of neuroleptic agents may be intensified (additively) by alcohol, barbiturates and other sedatives. Respiratory depression may occur.

The hypotensive effect of most antihypertensive drugs especially alpha adrenoceptor blocking agents may be exaggerated by neuroleptics.

The mild anticholinergic effect of neuroleptics may be enhanced by other anticholinergic drugs possibly leading to constipation, heat stroke, etc.

The action of some drugs may be opposed by phenothiazine neuroleptics; these include amphetamine, levodopa, clonidine, guanethidine, adrenaline.

Anticholinergic agents may reduce the antipsychotic effect of neuroleptics.

Some drugs interfere with absorption of neuroleptic agents: antacids, anti-Parkinson drugs, lithium. Increases or decreases in the plasma concentrations of a number of drugs, e.g. propranolol, phenobarbitone have been observed but were not of clinical significance.

High doses of neuroleptics reduce the response to hypoglycaemic agents, the dosage of which might have to be raised.

Adrenaline must not be used in patients overdosed with phenothiazine neuroleptics. Most of the above interactions are of a theoretical nature and not dangerous.

Simultaneous administration of desferrioxamine and prochlorperazine has been observed to induce a transient metabolic encephalopathy characterised by loss of consciousness for 48–72 hours.

It is possible that this may occur with Piportil since it shares many of the pharmacological properties of prochlorperazine.

*Pregnancy:* There is inadequate evidence of safety of Piportil Depot in human pregnancy, although animal studies have shown no hazard. The drug should not be used during pregnancy or lactation unless the physician considers it essential.

*Effect on ability to drive and use machines:* None stated

*Undesirable effects:* Minor side effects of neuroleptics are nasal stuffiness, dry mouth, insomnia, agitation and weight gain. Other possible adverse effects are listed below.

Liver function: jaundice, usually transient, occurs in a very small percentage of patients taking neuroleptics. A premonitory sign may be a sudden onset of fever after one to three weeks of treatment followed by the development of jaundice. Neuroleptic jaundice has the biochemical and other characteristics of obstructive jaundice and is associated with obstructions of the canaliculi by bile thrombi; the frequent presence of an accompanying eosinophilia indicates the allergic nature of this phenomenon. Treatment should be withheld on the development of jaundice.

Cardiorespiratory: Hypotension, usually postural, commonly occurs. Elderly or volume depleted subjects are particularly susceptible; it is more likely to occur after intramuscular administration.

Cardiac arrhythmias, including atrial arrhythmia, A-V block, ventricular tachycardia and fibrillation have been reported during neuroleptic therapy, possibly related to dosage. Pre-existing cardiac disease, old age, hypokalaemia and concurrent tricyclic antidepressants may predispose. ECG changes, usually benign, include widened QT interval, ST depression, U-waves and T-wave changes.

Respiratory depression is possible in susceptible patients.

Blood picture: A mild leukopenia occurs in up to 30% of patients on prolonged high dosage of neuroleptics. Agranulocytosis may occur rarely; it is not dose-related. The occurrence of unexplained infections or fever requires immediate haematological investigation.

Extrapyramidal: Acute dystonias or dyskinesias, usually transitory, are commoner in children and young adults, and usually occur within the first 4 days of treatment or after dosage increases. Akathisia characteristically occurs after large initial doses. Parkinsonism is commoner in adults and the elderly. It usually develops after weeks or months of treatment. One or more of the following may be seen: tremor, rigidity, akinesia or other features of Parkinsonism. Commonly just tremor. Tardive dyskinesia: If this occurs it is usually, but not necessarily, after prolonged or high dosage. It can even occur after treatment has been stopped. Dosage should therefore be kept low whenever possible.

Skin and eyes: contact skin sensitisation is a serious but rare complication in those frequently handling preparations of phenothiazines; the greatest care must be taken to avoid contact of the drug with the skin. Skin rashes of various kinds may also be seen in patients treated with these drugs. Patients on high dosage should be warned that they may develop photosensitivity in sunny weather and should avoid exposure to direct sunlight.

Ocular changes and the development of a metallic greyish-mauve coloration of exposed skin have been noted in some individuals mainly females, who have received chlorpromazine continuously for long periods (four to eight years). Other neuroleptics have been implicated but less frequently.

Endocrine: hyperprolactinaemia which may result in galactorrhoea, gynaecomastia, amenorrhoea; impotence.

Neuroleptic malignant syndrome (hyperthermia, rigidity, autonomic dysfunction and altered consciousness) may occur with any neuroleptic.

*Overdose:* Symptoms of phenothiazine overdosage include drowsiness or loss of consciousness, hypotension, tachycardia, ECG changes, ventricular arrhythmias and hypothermia. Severe extrapyramidal dyskinesias may occur.

Generalised vasodilatation may result in circulatory collapse; raising the patient's legs may suffice, in severe cases, volume expansion by intravenous fluids may be needed; infusion fluids should be warmed before administration in order not to aggravate hypothermia.

Positive inotropic agents such as dopamine may be tried if fluid replacement is insufficient to correct the circulatory collapse. Peripheral vasoconstrictor agents are not generally recommended; avoid the use of adrenaline.

Ventricular or supraventricular tachy-arrhythmias usually respond to restoration of normal body temperature and correction of circulatory or metabolic disturbances. If they are persistent or life threatening, appropriate anti-arrhythmic therapy may be considered. Avoid lignocaine and, as far as possible, long acting anti-arrhythmic drugs.

Pronounced central nervous system depression requires airway maintenance or, in extreme circumstances, assisted respiration. Severe dystonic reactions usually respond to procyclidine (5–10 mg) or orphenadrine (20–40 mg) administered intramuscularly or intravenously. Convulsions should be treated with intravenous diazepam.

Neuroleptic malignant syndrome should be treated with cooling. Dantrolene sodium may be tried.

**Pharmacological particulars**

*Pharmacodynamic properties:* Slow release phenothiazine neuroleptic.

*Pharmacokinetics properties:* There is little information about blood levels, distribution and excretion in humans. The rate of metabolism and excretion of phenothiazines decreases in old age

*Preclinical safety data:* There are no pre-clinical data of relevance to the prescriber which are additional to that already included in other sections of the SPC.

**Pharmaceutical particulars**

List of excipients: Sesame oil (peroxide-free).

*Incompatibilities:* Piportil Depot injection should not be admixed with any other substance.

*Shelf-life:* 60 months.

*Special precautions for storage:* Protect from light.

*Nature and contents of container:* 1 and 2 ml clear glass ampoules- pack containing 10 ampoules.

*Instructions for Use/handling:* None stated.

**Marketing authorisation number** 16186/0006

**Date of approval/revision of SPC** February 1997

**Legal category** POM

*Trade Mark

# Knoll Limited
## 9 Castle Quay
## Castle Boulevard
## Nottingham NG7 1FW

## AKINETON*

**Presentation** White tablets each containing 2 mg biperiden hydrochloride, quartered by score lines on one side with the Knoll logo on the reverse side.

Akineton is also available in 1 ml ampoules containing 5 mg of Biperiden Lactate BP.

**Uses** Akineton is an anticholinergic drug used for the treatment of drug–induced extrapyramidal symptoms and all other types of parkinsonism.

### Dosage and administration
*Adults*
*Tablets:* Initially half a tablet (1 mg) twice daily, increasing gradually to 1 tablet three times daily. After maintenance at this level for a few days, increase the dose gradually until no further symptomatic improvement is obtained. Decrease cautiously to lowest dose which adequately controls symptoms. The optimum maintenance dose varies from 3–12 mg daily. If a reduction in salivation occurs, the tablets are best taken after meals. Otherwise, tablets should be taken during meals.
*Ampoules:* 0.5–1 ampoule as a single dose to a maximum of 4 ampoules in one day, by intramuscular or slow intravenous injection.

*Children:* Not recommended.

### Contra-indications, warnings, etc
*Contra-indications:* Akineton is absolutely contra-indicated in the presence of untreated narrow angle glaucoma, mechanical stenoses in the gastrointestinal tract and in megacolon. Prostatic adenoma and diseases that can lead to perilous tachycardia are relative contra-indications. The use of Akineton is also contra-indicated in patients hypersensitive to Akineton or any of the inactive ingredients.

*Interactions with other medicaments and other forms of interaction:* The administration of Akineton in combination with other anticholinergic psychotropic drugs, antihistamines, antiparkinsonian drugs and antispasmodics can potentiate the CNS and peripheral side effects. The concomitant intake of quinidine may potentiate the anticholinergic effect (especially AV conduction). The concurrent administration of levodopa and Akineton may potentiate dyskinesia. Tardive dyskinesia induced by neuroleptics may be intensified by Akineton. Parkinsonian symptoms in the presence of existing tardive dyskinesia are occasionally so serious as to mandate continued anticholinergic therapy.

As a centrally-acting drug, Akineton may potentiate the effect of alcohol.

The effect of metoclopramide and compounds with similar activity on the gastrointestinal tract is attenuated by anticholinergics such as Akineton.

*Effects on ability to drive and to use machines:* Occasionally, drowsiness may occur. These effects may possibly be enhanced by the additional administration of other antiparkinsonism drugs, antihistamines, tricyclic antidepressants, neuroleptics or quinidine. Patients who drive a car or operate potentially dangerous machinery which requires concentration should be warned that side-effects of this type are a possibility.

*Other undesirable effects (frequency and seriousness):* Central nervous system side-effects may take the form of fatigue, dizziness and drowsiness; at higher doses, restlessness and confusion, occasionally impairment of memory and in rare cases, hallucinations. Peripheral side-effects include dry mouth, disturbances of accommodation, hypohidrosis, constipation, gastric symptoms and an increase in heart rate; very rarely, a decrease in heart rate. Parenteral administration may be followed by a fall in blood pressure. Allergic skin rash and dyskinesia have also been observed occasionally following the administration of Akineton. In some cases, especially in patients with prostatic adenoma, Akineton may cause micturition difficulties (a dose reduction is recommended) and, more rarely, retention of urine (antidote: carbachol).

*Use in pregnancy and lactation:* There is no evidence to suggest that Akineton presents a particular teratogenic risk. In view of the lack of experience with the use of Akineton in pregnancy, the drug should only be used with great caution in such cases, especially during the first trimester.

Anticholinergics can inhibit lactation. No data on this subject are available for Akineton. Akineton transfers to human milk, and concentrations equal to those found in the maternal plasma may be reached. Since the type and extent of metabolism in neonates are not known and since pharmacological/toxicological effects cannot be excluded, breast-feeding is not generally recommended.

*Other special warnings and precautions:* Side-effects occur especially in the early stages of treatment and if the dose is increased too rapidly. Except in the case of vital complications, abrupt discontinuation of the drug is to be avoided due to the risk of excessive counter-regulation. Elderly patients, particularly those with cerebral lesions of a vascular or degenerative nature, may frequently exhibit increased sensitivity even to therapeutic doses of the substance. As the results of animal studies have demonstrated, centrally-acting anticholinergic drugs like Akineton may lead to an increased tendency to cerebral seizure. Physicians should therefore take account of this fact in the management of predisposed persons.

Akineton abuse has been observed.

Especially when Akineton is taken in combination with other centrally-acting drugs, anticholinergics or alcohol, central nervous and peripheral side-effects may impair the ability to drive and to operate machinery.

*Combined treatment:* In some cases, the response of tremor to Akineton alone may be inadequate. In such cases, combined therapy with an additional preparation effective against tremor should be considered.

*Overdosage (symptoms, emergency procedures, antidotes):* The symptoms of overdose are anticholinergic effects such as mydriasis, dryness of mucous membranes, flushing, rise in heart rate, reduction of bowel motility, reduction in ureter and bladder tone, increased temperature, excitation, confusion, clouding of consciousness and/or hallucinations. In severe overdose, cardiac and respiratory depression may occur.

*Treatment:* Gastric lavage or emesis should be considered. As an antidote, anticholinesterase inhibitors are recommended. Vital signs should be closely monitored and appropriate supportive measures taken. Artificial ventilation, reduction of fever, and the application of a bladder-emptying catheter may be necessary. In the event of cardiac depression, a cardiac stimulant drug such as dobutamine may be considered.

*Incompatibilities:* None.

**Pharmaceutical precautions** Store in a cool place, protected from light.

**Legal category** POM

**Package quantities** Akineton 2 mg tablets in blister packs of 100 tablets. Akineton 5 mg/ml ampoules in boxes of 5 x 1 ml ampoules.

**Further information** Metabolisable carbohydrate content: Approx. 0.16 g per tablet. Sodium content: 0.13 mmol per ampoule (0.13 mmol per ml).

**Product licence numbers**
Tablets          0169/0009
Ampoules     0169/0010

## APRINOX*

### Qualitative and quantitative composition
Aprinox Tablets 2.5 mg:   Bendrofluazide BP 2.5 mg:
Aprinox Tablets 5.0 mg.   Bendrofluazide BP 5.0 mg.

**Pharmaceutical form** White tablets.

### Clinical particulars

*Therapeutic indications:* For the treatment of oedema and hypertension. Aprinox may also be used to suppress lactation.

*Posology and method of administration:* For oral administration.
Diuretic: Initially 5 to 10 mg once daily or on alternate days. Maintenance: 5 to 10 mg once or twice weekly. The dose should be taken early in the morning so as to complete diuresis by bedtime.

Antihypertensive: 2.5 to 5 mg once daily. When Aprinox is used concurrently with other antihypertensive agents, the dose of the latter should be halved.
Suppression of lactation: 5 mg in the morning and 5 mg at midday for about five days.
Children: Dosage in children may be up to 400 microgram/kg bodyweight initially, reducing to 50–100 microgram/kg bodyweight daily for maintenance.
Elderly: The dosage of thiazide diuretics may need to be reduced in the elderly, particularly when renal function is impaired, because of the possibility of electrolyte imbalance.

*Contra-indications:* Aprinox is contra-indicated in severe renal failure and in patients with known hypersensitivity to thiazides.

*Special warnings and special precautions for use:* Bendrofluazide should be used with caution in patients with Addison's disease, hypercalcaemia and hepatic or renal impairment. Renal function should be continuously monitored during thiazide therapy. Thiazide diuretics may exacerbate or activate systemic lupus erythematosus in susceptible patients.

All thiazide diuretics can produce a degree of electrolyte imbalance, especially in patients with renal or hepatic impairment or when dosage is high or prolonged. Serum electrolytes should be checked for abnormalities, particularly hypokalaemia, and the latter corrected by the addition of a potassium supplement to the regimen.

*Interaction with other medicaments and other forms of interaction:* Sensitivity to digitalis glycosides may be increased by the hypokalaemic effect of concurrent bendrofluazide. Patients should be observed for signs of digitalis intoxication, in particular arrhythmias, and if these appear, the dosage of the digitalis glycoside should be temporarily reduced and a potassium supplement given to restore stability.

Serum lithium concentrations may be increased by concurrent use of thiazide diuretics.

Non-steroidal anti-inflammatory agents may blunt the diuretic and antihypertensive effects of thiazide diuretics.

ACTH, corticosteroids, acetazolamide and carbenoxolone may exacerbate the hypokalaemia associated with thiazide use. Thiazide diuretics may enhance the neuromuscular blocking effects of the non-depolarising muscle relaxants, e.g. tubocurarine.

Thiazides may enhance the effects of antihypertensive agents, while postural hypotension associated with therapy may be enhanced by concomitant ingestion of alcohol, barbiturates or opioids.

Bendrofluazide may interfere with a number of laboratory tests, including estimation of serum protein-bound iodine and tests of parathyroid function.

*Pregnancy and lactation:* Diuretics are best avoided for the management of oedema of pregnancy or hypertension in pregnancy as their use may be associated with hypokalaemia, increased blood viscosity and reduced placental perfusion.

There is inadequate evidence of safety in human pregnancy and foetal bone marrow depression and thrombocytopenia have been described. Foetal and neonatal jaundice have also been described.

As diuretics pass into breast milk and bendrofluazide can suppress lactation, its use should be avoided in mothers who wish to breast feed.

*Effects on ability to drive and use machines:* No adverse effects known.

*Undesirable effects:* All thiazide diuretics can produce a degree of electrolyte imbalance, e.g. hypokalaemia.

Thiazide diuretics may raise the serum uric acid levels with subsequent exacerbation of gout in susceptible subjects.

Thiazide diuretics sometimes lower carbohydrate tolerance and the insulin dosage of the diabetic patient may require adjustment. Care is necessary when bendrofluazide is administered to those with a known predisposition to diabetes.

Rarely, blood dyscrasias, including agranulocytosis, aplastic anaemia, thrombocytopenia and leucopenia, and pancreatitis have been reported with long term therapy. Skin rashes and impotence have occasionally been reported.

*Overdose:* Symptoms of overdosage include anorexia, nausea, vomiting, diarrhoea, diuresis, dehydration, hypotension, dizziness, weakness, muscle cramps, paraesthesia, tetany, gastrointestinal bleeding, hyponatraemia, hypo- or hyperglycaemia, hypokalaemia and metabolic alkalosis. Initial treatment consists of either emesis or gastric lavage, if appropriate. Otherwise treatment should be symptomatic and supportive including the correction of fluid and electrolyte imbalance. Blood pressure should also be monitored. There is no specific antidote.

**Pharmacological properties**

*Pharmacodynamic properties:* Bendrofluazide is a thiazide diuretic which reduces the absorption of electrolytes from the renal tubules, thereby increasing the excretion of sodium and chloride ions, and consequently of water. The excretion of other electrolytes, notably potassium and magnesium, is also increased. The excretion of calcium is reduced. Thiazides also reduce carbonic anhydrase activity so that bicarbonate excretion is increased, but this effect is generally small and does not appreciably alter the acid-base balance or the pH of the urine. Thiazides also have a hypotensive effect, due to a reduction in peripheral resistance and enhance the effects of other antihypertensive agents.

*Pharmacokinetic properties:* Bendrofluazide is completely absorbed from the gastrointestinal tract and it is fairly extensively metabolised. About 30% is excreted unchanged in the urine. The onset of diuretic action of the thiazides following oral administration occurs within two hours and the peak effect between three and six hours after administration. The duration of the diuretic action of bendrofluazide is between 18 and 24 hours. The onset of the hypotensive action is generally three or four days.

*Preclinical safety data:* Not applicable.

**Pharmaceutical particulars**

*List of excipients:* Lactose, maize starch, stearic acid, French chalk for tablets.

*Incompatibilities:* Not applicable.

*Shelf life:* 36 months.

*Special precautions for storage:* None.

*Nature and contents of container:* Amber glass bottle having a tin-plate cap with a waxed aluminium-faced pulpboard liner. Pack sizes: 500 tablets.

*Instructions for use/handling:* None.

**Marketing authorisation numbers**
Aprinox Tablets 2.5 mg 00169/0045
Aprinox Tablets 5.0 mg 00169/0046.

**Date of approval/revision of SPC** February 1996.

**Legal category** POM.

## ARYTHMOL*

**Qualitative and quantitative composition** Each film-coated tablet contains 150 mg propafenone hydrochloride or 300 mg propafenone hydrochloride.

**Pharmaceutical form** Film-coated tablets for oral use.

**Clinical particulars**
*Therapeutic indications:*

1. The prophylaxis and treatment of paroxysmal supraventricular tachyarrhythmias which include paroxysmal atrial flutter/fibrillation and paroxysmal re-entrant tachycardias involving the AV node or accessory bypass tracts when standard therapy has failed or is contra-indicated.
2. The prophylaxis and treatment of ventricular arrhythmias.

*Posology and method of administration:* It is recommended that Arythmol therapy should be initiated under hospital conditions, by a physician experienced in the treatment of arrhythmias. The individual maintenance dose should be determined under cardiological surveillance, including ECG monitoring and blood pressure control. If the QRS interval is prolonged by more than 20%, the dose should be reduced or discontinued until the ECG returns to normal limits.

*Adults:* Initially 150 mg three times daily, increasing at a minimum of three-day intervals to 300 mg twice daily and, if necessary, to a maximum of 300 mg three times daily.

The tablets should be swallowed whole and taken with a drink after food. A reduction in the total daily dose is recommended for patients below 70 kg bodyweight.

*Elderly patients:* Higher plasma concentrations of propafenone have been noted during treatment. Elderly patients may therefore respond to a lower dose.

*Children:* A suitable dosage form of Arythmol for children is not available.

*Dosage in impaired liver function:* Propafenone is extensively metabolised via a saturable hepatic oxidative pathway. In view of the increased bioavailability and elimination half-life of propafenone, a reduction in the recommended dose may be necessary.

*Dosage in impaired renal function:* Although the elimination of propafenone and its major metabolite is not affected by renal impairment, Arythmol should be administered cautiously.

*Contra-indications:* Uncontrolled congestive heart failure, cardiogenic shock (except arrhythmia-induced), severe bradycardia, uncontrolled electrolyte disturbances, severe obstructive pulmonary disease, marked hypotension.

Arythmol may worsen myasthenia gravis.

Unless patients are adequately paced (see Precautions), Arythmol should not be used in the presence of sinus node dysfunction, atrial conduction defects, second degree or greater AV block, bundle branch block or distal block. Minor prolongation of PR interval and intraventricular conduction defects (QRS duration of less than 20%) are to be expected during treatment with Arythmol and do not warrant dose reduction or drug withdrawal.

*Special warnings and precautions for use:* The weak negative inotropic effect of Arythmol may assume importance in patients predisposed to cardiac failure. In common with other anti-arrhythmic drugs, Arythmol has been shown to alter sensitivity and pacing threshold. In patients with pacemakers, appropriate adjustments may be required. Because of the beta-blocking effect, care should be exercised in the treatment of patients with obstructive airways disease or asthma. Patients with structural heart disease may be predisposed to serious adverse effects.

*Interaction with other medicaments and other forms of interaction:* The effects of propafenone may be potentiated if it is given in combination with other local anaesthetic agents or agents which depress myocardial activity.

Propafenone has been shown to increase the plasma levels of digoxin and caution should be exercised with regard to digitalis toxicity.

Propafenone has been shown to increase the plasma levels of warfarin with an accompanying increase in prothrombin time, which may require reduction of the dose of warfarin.

Plasma levels of propafenone may be increased by concomitant administration of cimetidine.

Increased propranolol and metoprolol plasma levels have been observed when these beta-blockers were used concurrently with propafenone. Thus, dose reduction of these beta-blockers may be required. Details of interactions with other beta-blockers are not known.

Concomitant administration of propafenone and quinidine may result in decreased oral clearance with an increase in the steady-state plasma concentration of propafenone. There has been a report of the lowering of propafenone levels by rifampicin, via the hepatic mixed oxidase system. This reduction may lead to breakthrough arrhythmias.

Cases of possible interactions with cyclosporin (levels increased with deterioration in renal function), theophylline (levels increased), desipramine (levels increased) have also been reported.

Due to the arrhythmogenic effects of tricyclic and related antidepressants, and/or neuroleptics, these drugs may interact adversely when used concomitantly with antiarrhythmic drugs including propafenone.

*Pregnancy and lactation:* Animal studies have not shown any teratogenic effects but, as there is no experience of the use of the drug in human pregnancy, Arythmol should not be used during pregnancy and lactation.

Propafenone may be excreted in breast milk. The use of Arythmol tablets in nursing women should therefore also be given critical consideration.

*Effects on ability to drive and use machines:* Blurred vision, dizziness, fatigue and postural hypotension may affect the patient's speed of reaction and impair the individual's ability to operate machinery or motor vehicles.

*Undesirable effects:* Arythmol may produce minor nervous system and cardiovascular side-effects but is generally well tolerated. Occasionally and particularly with higher doses, gastrointestinal disorders (i.e. anorexia, bloating, nausea and vomiting, constipation, diarrhoea, retching), dizziness, fatigue, bitter taste, headache, blurred vision, dry mouth and vertigo have been reported. Very rarely, fatigue, restlessness, nightmares, sleep disorders, psychological disorders such as states of anxiety and confusion, and extrapyramidal symptoms may occur. Allergic skin reactions such as reddening, pruritus, exanthema or urticaria may occur infrequently. Postural hypotension is occasionally seen, particularly in the elderly. These effects disappear after reduction of the dose or discontinuation of the drug. Bradycardia, sinoatrial, atrioventricular or intraventricular block may occur (see Overdosage). In common with other anti-arrhythmic drugs, there is a small risk of proarrhythmic effects. Convulsions have been observed extremely rarely in cases of overdosage. Rare cases of individual hypersensitivity reactions (manifested by cholestasis, blood dyscrasias, lupus syndrome) and seizures have been reported. All were reversible on discontinuation of treatment. In some cases, a diminution of potency and a drop in sperm count have been observed after high doses of Arythmol. This phenomenon is reversible when treatment is discontinued. However, since treatment with Arythmol may be vital, the drug must not be discontinued due to this adverse reaction without consulting the attending physician. Very rarely, a fully reversible decrease of the white cell, granulocyte and platelet counts has been observed. Isolated cases of agranulocytosis have been reported.

*Overdose:* Experience with overdosage is limited. No specific antidote is known. Procedures to enhance drug elimination from the body by haemodialysis or haemoperfusion are unlikely to succeed because of the large volume of drug distribution. The usual emergency measures for acute cardiovascular collapse should be applied. In severe conduction disturbance associated with a compromised cardiac function, atropine, isoprenaline or pacemaker therapy may be required. If electrical stimulation is not possible, an attempt should be made to shorten the QRS duration and increase the heart rate with high doses of isoprenaline. Bundle branch block by itself is not an indication for isoprenaline. Hypotension may require inotropic support. Convulsions should be treated with I.V. diazepam.

**Pharmacological properties**
*Pharmacodynamic properties:* Propafenone is a class 1c anti-arrhythmic agent.

It has a stabilising action on myocardial membranes, reduces the fast inward current carried by sodium ions with a reduction of depolarisation rate, and prolongs the impulse conduction time in the atrium, AV node and, primarily, in the His-Purkinje system.

Impulse conduction through accessory pathways, as in WPW syndrome, is inhibited either by a prolongation of the refractory period or by a blockade of the conduction pathway, both in anterograde but mostly retrograde direction.

At the same time, spontaneous excitability is reduced by an increase of the myocardial stimulus threshold while electrical excitability of the myocardium is decreased by an increase of the ventricular fibrillation threshold.

*Anti-arrhythmic effects:* Slowing of upstroke velocity of the action potential, decrease of excitability, homogenisation of conduction rates, suppression of ectopic automaticity, lowered myocardial disposition to fibrillation.

Propafenone has moderate $\beta_1$ sympatholytic activity without clinical relevance. However, the possibility exists that high daily doses (900–1200 mg) may trigger a sympatholytic (anti-adrenergic) effect.

In the ECG, propafenone causes a slight prolongation of P, PR and QRS intervals while the $QT_c$ interval remains unaffected as a rule.

In digitalised patients with an ejection fraction of 35–50%, contractility of the left ventricle is slightly decreased. In patients with acute transmural infarction and heart failure, the intravenous administration of propafenone may markedly reduce the left ventricular ejection fraction but to an essentially lesser extent in patients in the acute stages of infarction without heart failure. In both cases, pulmonary arterial pressure is minimally raised. Peripheral arterial pressure does not show any significant changes. This demonstrates that propafenone does not exert an unfavourable effect on left ventricular function which would be of clinical relevance. Clinically-relevant reduction of left ventricular function is to be expected only in patients with pre-existing poor ventricular function.

Untreated heart failure might then deteriorate, possibly resulting in decompensation.

*Pharmacokinetic properties:* Following oral administration, propafenone is nearly completely absorbed in the gastrointestinal tract in a dose-dependent manner and distributed rapidly in the body. After a single dose of one tablet, bioavailability is about 50%. With repeated doses, plasma concentration and bioavailability rise disproportionately due to saturation of the first-pass metabolism in the liver. Steady state is reached after 3 or 4 days when bioavailability is increased to about 100%.

Therapeutic plasma levels are in the range of 150 ng/ml to 1500 ng/ml. In the therapeutic concentration range, more than 95% of propafenone is bound to plasma proteins. Comparing cumulative urinary excretion over 24 hours demonstrated that 1.3% of intravenous (70 mg) and 0.65% of oral (600 mg) propafenone is excreted unchanged in the urine, i.e. propafenone is almost exclusively metabolised in the liver. Even in the presence of impaired renal function, reduced elimination of propafenone is not likely, which is confirmed by case reports and single kinetic studies in patients undergoing chronic haemodialysis: clinical chemistry values did not differ from those of patients with uncompromised kidneys.

The terminal elimination half-life in patients is 5–7 hours, 12 hours in single cases, following repeated doses. A close positive correlation between plasma level and AV conduction time was seen in the majority of both healthy volunteers and patients.

At a concentration of 500 ng/ml, the PR interval is statistically significantly prolonged as compared to baseline values which allows for dose titration and monitoring of the patients with the help of ECG readings. The frequency of ventricular extrasystoles decreases as plasma concentrations increase. Adequate anti-arrhythmic activity has in single cases been observed at plasma levels as low as <500 ng/ml.

*Preclinical safety data:* Intravenous administration of propafenone at doses within the toxic range has caused reversible disorders of spermatogenesis at irregular intervals in monkeys, dogs and rabbits.

### Pharmaceutical particulars

*List of excipients:* Maize starch, vinyl pyrolidone – vinyl acetate copolymer, talc, magnesium stearate, hydroxypropyl methylcellulose, polyethylene glycol 6000, titanium dioxide E171, sodium lauryl sulphate.

*Incompatibilities:* None.

*Shelf-life:* The recommended shelf-life is 5 years.

*Special precautions for storage:* Store at room temperature (i.e. below 25°C).

*Nature and contents of container:* PVC/aluminium blister. Arythmol 150 mg tablets: pack of 90. Arythmol 300 mg tablets: pack of 60.

*Instructions for use/handling:* Due to the bitter taste and local anaesthetic action of propafenone, the tablets should be taken whole together with some liquid after meals.

### Marketing authorisation numbers

150 mg    0169/0015
300 mg    0169/0016

**Date of approval/revision of SPC**   March 1996.

**Legal category**   POM.

## BRUFEN*

**Presentation**   *Tablets:* Brufen is available as sugar-coated tablets containing either 200 mg or 400 mg (Brufen 400) Ibuprofen BP. It is also available as Brufen 600, film-coated tablets each containing 600 mg of Ibuprofen BP.

The tablets are light magenta in colour. The 200 mg tablets bear the overprint 'Brufen' in black; the 400 mg tablets are overprinted 'Brufen 400' and the 600 mg tablets 'Brufen 600', also in black.

*Granules:* Brufen Granules are packed in sachets, each one containing 600 mg of Ibuprofen BP. One sachet dispersed in water makes an effervescent, orange-flavoured drink.

*Syrup:* For children, and for adults who have difficulty in swallowing tablets, Brufen is presented as Brufen Syrup, an orange-flavoured liquid containing 100 mg of Ibuprofen BP in each 5 ml.

*Inactive ingredients:* Brufen (200 mg) – sodium benzoate; sucrose; erythrosine. Brufen 400 – sodium benzoate; sucrose; erythrosine. Brufen 600 – erythrosine. Brufen Granules – sucrose; microcrystalline cellulose; saccharin. Brufen Syrup – sucrose; sorbitol; methyl hydroxybenzoate; propyl hydroxybenzoate; sodium benzoate; sunset yellow.

**Uses**   Brufen is indicated for its analgesic and anti-inflammatory effects in the treatment of rheumatoid arthritis (including juvenile rheumatoid arthritis or Still's disease), ankylosing spondylitis, osteoarthritis and other non-rheumatoid (seronegative) arthropathies.

In the treatment of non-articular rheumatic conditions, Brufen is indicated in periarticular conditions such as frozen shoulder (capsulitis), bursitis, tendinitis, tenosynovitis and low back pain; Brufen can also be used in soft-tissue injuries such as sprains and strains.

Brufen is indicated for its analgesic effect in the relief of mild to moderate pain such as dysmenorrhoea, dental and post-operative pain and for the symptomatic relief of headache including migraine headache.

### Dosage and administration

*Adults:* The recommended dosage of Brufen is 1200–1800 mg daily in divided doses. Some patients can be maintained on 600–1200 mg daily. In severe or acute conditions, it can be advantageous to increase the dosage until the acute phase is brought under control, provided that the total daily dosage does not exceed 2400 mg in divided doses.

*Children:* The daily dosage of Brufen is 20 mg/kg of bodyweight in divided doses. This can be achieved as follows using the syrup:

1–2 years: One 2.5 ml spoonful (50 mg) three to four times a day.

3–7 years: One 5 ml spoonful (100 mg) three to four times a day.

8–12 years: Two 5 ml spoonfuls (200 mg) three to four times a day.

In juvenile rheumatoid arthritis, up to 40 mg/kg of bodyweight daily in divided doses may be taken in severe cases. Not recommended for children weighing less than 7 kg.

Brufen Granules are not recommended for children under 12 years of age.

*Elderly:* No special dosage modifications are required for elderly patients, unless renal or hepatic function is impaired, in which case dosage should be assessed individually.

### Contra-indications, warnings, etc

*Contra-indications:* Brufen should not be administered to patients with a history of, or active, peptic ulceration (see *Adverse events*).

Brufen is contra-indicated in patients who have previously shown hypersensitivity reactions (e.g. asthma, rhinitis or urticaria) in response to ibuprofen, aspirin or other non-steroidal anti-inflammatory drugs (NSAIDs; see *Adverse events*).

*Precautions:* Caution is required if Brufen is administered to patients suffering from, or with a previous history of, bronchial asthma since ibuprofen has been reported to cause bronchospasm in such patients (see *Adverse events*).

Brufen should only be given with care to patients with a history of gastrointestinal disease (see *Adverse events*).

Caution is required in patients with renal, hepatic or cardiac impairment since the use of NSAIDs may result in deterioration of renal function (see *Adverse events*). The dose should be kept as low as possible and renal function should be monitored in these patients.

Brufen should be given with care to patients with a history of heart failure or hypertension since oedema has been reported in association with ibuprofen administration (see *Adverse events*).

Each Brufen Granules sachet contains 197 mg (approximately 9 mEq) sodium. This should be considered in patients whose overall intake of sodium must be markedly restricted.

*Adverse events:*

*Gastrointestinal:* The most commonly-observed adverse events are gastrointestinal in nature. Nausea, vomiting, diarrhoea, dyspepsia, abdominal pain, melaena, haematemesis, ulcerative stomatitis and gastrointestinal haemorrhage have been reported following ibuprofen administration. Less frequently, gastritis, duodenal ulcer, gastric ulcer and gastrointestinal perforation have been observed. Epidemiological data indicate that of the seven most widely used oral, non-aspirin NSAIDs, ibuprofen presents the lowest risk of upper gastrointestinal toxicity.

*Hypersensitivity:* Hypersensitivity reactions have been reported following treatment with ibuprofen. These may consist of (a) non-specific allergic reaction and anaphylaxis, (b) respiratory tract reactivity comprising asthma, aggravated asthma, bronchospasm or dyspnoea, or (c) assorted skin disorders, including rashes of various types, pruritus, urticaria, purpura, angioedema and, less commonly, bullous dermatoses (including epidermal necrolysis and erythema multiforme).

*Cardiovascular:* Oedema has been reported in association with ibuprofen treatment.

*Other adverse events reported less commonly and for which causality has not necessarily been established include:*

*Renal:* Nephrotoxicity in various forms, including interstitial nephritis, nephrotic syndrome and renal failure.

*Hepatic:* Abnormal liver function, hepatitis and jaundice.

*Neurological and special senses:* Visual disturbances, optic neuritis, headaches, paraesthesia, depression, confusion, hallucinations, tinnitus, vertigo, dizziness, malaise, fatigue and drowsiness.

*Haematological:* Thrombocytopenia, neutropenia, agranulocytosis, aplastic anaemia and haemolytic anaemia.

*Dermatological:* Photosensitivity (see *Hypersensitivity* for other skin reactions).

*Use in pregnancy and lactation:* Whilst no teratogenic effects have been demonstrated in animal toxicology studies, the use of ibuprofen during pregnancy should, if possible, be avoided. Congenital abnormalities have been reported in association with ibuprofen administration in man; however, these are low in frequency and do not appear to follow any discernible pattern. In view of the known effects of NSAIDs on the foetal cardiovascular system (closure of ductus arteriosus), use in late pregnancy should be avoided.

In the limited studies so far available, ibuprofen appears in the breast milk in very low concentrations and is unlikely to adversely affect the breast-fed infant.

*Drug interactions:* Care should be taken in patients treated with any of the following drugs as interactions have been reported in some patients.

Antihypertensives: Reduced antihypertensive effect.

Diuretics: Reduced diuretic effect. Diuretics can increase the risk of nephrotoxicity of NSAIDs.

Cardiac glycosides: NSAIDs may exacerbate cardiac failure, reduce GFR and increase plasma cardiac glycoside levels.

Lithium: Decreased elimination of lithium.

Methotrexate: Decreased elimination of methotrexate.

Cyclosporin: Increased risk of nephrotoxicity with NSAIDs.

Mifepristone: NSAIDs should not be used for 8–12 days after mifepristone administration as NSAIDs can reduce the effects of mifepristone.

Other analgesics: Avoid concomitant use of two or more NSAIDs.

Corticosteroids: Increased risk of gastrointestinal bleeding.

Anticoagulants: Enhanced anticoagulant effect.

Quinolone antibiotics: Animal data indicate that NSAIDs can increase the risk of convulsions associated with quinolone antibiotics. Patients taking NSAIDs and quinolones may have an increased risk of developing convulsions.

*Treatment of overdosage:* Gastric lavage and, if necessary, correction of serum electrolytes and appropriate supportive measures. There is no specific antidote to ibuprofen.

**Pharmaceutical precautions**   Brufen 600 (600 mg tablets), Brufen Granules and Brufen Syrup should be stored below 25°C. Brufen Syrup should be protected from light.

**Legal category**   POM.

### Package quantities

Brufen Tablets (200 mg): Pack of 100.
Brufen 400 (400 mg tablets): Pack of 100; pack of 250.
Brufen 600 (600 mg tablets): Pack of 100.
Brufen Granules (600 mg sachets): Box of 20 sachets.
Brufen Syrup: Bottle of 500 ml.

**Further information**   Taken on an empty stomach, peak serum levels of ibuprofen occur 45 minutes after ingestion whereas, taken after a meal, the peak may occur up to 90 minutes post-ingestion. Since most people can take Brufen on an empty stomach without gastric discomfort, the initial dose of the day will be more rapidly effective if taken before food. This is particularly valuable in providing relief of the morning stiffness associated with arthritis.

### Product licence numbers

Brufen Tablets 200 mg    0169/0049
Brufen Tablets 400 mg    0169/0050
Brufen Tablets 600 mg    0169/0051
Brufen Granules    0169/0047
Brufen Syrup    0169/0048

## BRUFEN* RETARD

**Presentation**   Brufen Retard is a white, pillow-shaped, film-coated tablet containing 800 mg of Ibuprofen BP in a sustained-release form. Each tablet is overprinted 'Brufen Retard' in red.

*Other ingredients:* Xanthan gum; povidone; hydroxypropylmethylcellulose; stearic acid; titanium dioxide; colloidal silicon dioxide; talc; shellac; red iron oxide; soya lecithin; dimethylpolysiloxane.

**Uses**   Brufen Retard is indicated for its analgesic and anti-inflammatory effects in the treatment of rheumatoid arthritis (including juvenile rheumatoid arthritis or Still's disease in children over 12 years), ankylosing spondylitis, osteoarthritis and other non-rheumatoid (seronegative) arthropathies.

In the treatment of non-articular rheumatic conditions, Brufen Retard is indicated in periarticular conditions such as frozen shoulder (capsulitis); bursitis, tendinitis, tenosynovitis and low back pain; Brufen Retard can also be used in soft-tissue injuries such as sprains and strains.

Brufen Retard is indicated for its analgesic effect in the relief of mild to moderate pain such as dysmenorrhoea, dental and post-operative pain and for the symptomatic relief of headache and migraine headache.

### Dosage and administration

*Adults:* The recommended daily dosage is two tablets as a single dose, preferably in the early evening, well before retiring to bed. The tablets should be swallowed whole with plenty of fluid. In severe or acute conditions, the total daily dosage may be increased to three tablets taken in two divided doses.

*Children:* Brufen Retard is not recommended for children under 12 years.

*Elderly:* No special dosage modifications are required for elderly patients, unless renal or hepatic function is impaired, in which case dosage should be assessed individually.

**Contra-indications, warnings, etc**

*Contra-indications:* Brufen Retard should not be administered to patients with a history of, or active, peptic ulceration (see *Adverse events*).

Brufen Retard is contra-indicated in patients who have previously shown hypersensitivity reactions (e.g. asthma, rhinitis or urticaria) in response to ibuprofen, aspirin or other non-steroidal anti-inflammatory drugs (NSAIDs; see *Adverse events*).

*Precautions:* Caution is required if Brufen Retard is administered to patients suffering from, or with a previous history of, bronchial asthma since ibuprofen has been reported to cause bronchospasm in such patients (see *Adverse events*).

Brufen Retard should only be given with care to patients with a history of gastrointestinal disease (see *Adverse events*).

Caution is required in patients with renal, hepatic or cardiac impairment since the use of NSAIDs may result in deterioration of renal function (see *Adverse events*). The dose should be kept as low as possible and renal function should be monitored in these patients.

Brufen Retard should be given with care to patients with a history of heart failure or hypertension since oedema has been reported in association with ibuprofen administration (see *Adverse events*).

*Adverse events:*

*Gastrointestinal:* The most commonly-observed adverse events are gastrointestinal in nature. Nausea, vomiting, diarrhoea, dyspepsia, abdominal pain, melaena, haematemesis, ulcerative stomatitis and gastrointestinal haemorrhage have been reported following ibuprofen administration. Less frequently, gastritis, duodenal ulcer, gastric ulcer and gastrointestinal perforation have been observed. Epidemiological data indicate that of the seven most widely used oral, non-aspirin NSAIDs, ibuprofen presents the lowest risk of upper gastrointestinal toxicity.

*Hypersensitivity:* Hypersensitivity reactions have been reported following treatment with ibuprofen. These may consist of (a) non-specific allergic reaction and anaphylaxis, (b) respiratory tract reactivity comprising asthma, aggravated asthma, bronchospasm or dyspnoea, or (c) assorted skin disorders, including rashes of various types, pruritus, urticaria, purpura, angioedema and, less commonly, bullous dermatoses (including epidermal necrolysis and erythema multiforme).

*Cardiovascular:* Oedema has been reported in association with ibuprofen treatment.

*Other adverse events reported less commonly and for which causality has not necessarily been established include:*

*Renal:* Nephrotoxicity in various forms, including interstitial nephritis, nephrotic syndrome and renal failure.

*Hepatic:* Abnormal liver function, hepatitis and jaundice.

*Neurological and special senses:* Visual disturbances, optic neuritis, headaches, paraesthesia, depression, confusion, hallucinations, tinnitus, vertigo, dizziness, malaise, fatigue and drowsiness.

*Haematological:* Thrombocytopenia, neutropenia, agranulocytosis, aplastic anaemia and haemolytic anaemia.

*Dermatological:* Photosensitivity (see *Hypersensitivity* for other skin reactions).

*Use in pregnancy and lactation:* Whilst no teratogenic effects have been demonstrated in animal toxicology studies, the use of ibuprofen during pregnancy should, if possible, be avoided. Congenital abnormalities have been reported in association with ibuprofen administration in man; however, these are low in frequency and do not appear to follow any discernible pattern. In view of the known effects of NSAIDs on the foetal cardiovascular system (closure of ductus arteriosus), use in late pregnancy should be avoided.

In the limited studies so far available, ibuprofen appears in the breast milk in very low concentrations and is unlikely to adversely affect the breast-fed infant.

*Drug interactions:* Care should be taken in patients treated with any of the following drugs as interactions have been reported in some patients.

Antihypertensives: Reduced antihypertensive effect.

Diuretics: Reduced diuretic effect. Diuretics can increase the risk of nephrotoxicity of NSAIDs.

Cardiac glycosides: NSAIDs may exacerbate cardiac failure, reduce GFR and increase plasma cardiac glycoside levels.

Lithium: Decreased elimination of lithium.

Methotrexate: Decreased elimination of methotrexate.

Cyclosporin: Increased risk of nephrotoxicity with NSAIDs.

Mifepristone: NSAIDs should not be used for 8–12 days after mifepristone administration as NSAIDs can reduce the effects of mifepristone.

Other analgesics: Avoid concomitant use of two or more NSAIDs.

Corticosteroids: Increased risk of gastrointestinal bleeding.

Anticoagulants: Enhanced anticoagulant effect.

Quinolone antibiotics: Animal data indicate that NSAIDs can increase the risk of convulsions associated with quinolone antibiotics. Patients taking NSAIDs and quinolones may have an increased risk of developing convulsions.

*Treatment of overdosage:* Gastric lavage may be of value for a considerable time after ingestion. The tablets may not be totally retrieved. If necessary, correct serum electrolytes. There is no specific antidote to ibuprofen.

**Pharmaceutical precautions** Store below 25°C in a cool dry place.

**Legal category** POM.

**Package quantities** Pack of 56.

**Further information** Nil.

**Product licence number** 0169/0053

# CHYMODIACTIN 4000 UNITS

**Warning** Chymodiactin should only be used in a hospital setting by clinicians experienced in the diagnosis and management of all spinal disorders and who have received specialised training in chemonucleolysis.

The proper selection of patients for the appropriate use of Chymodiactin in chemonucleolysis requires precise diagnosis in order to eliminate conditions other than herniated lumbar discs which may produce similar signs and symptoms of nerve root compression.

Chymodiactin should be used only in facilities where supporting personnel as well as clinicians are qualified and equipped to diagnose and manage all potential complications in the use of Chymodiactin, including anaphylaxis.

**Presentation** Chymodiactin is a sterile lyophilised powder of the proteolytic enzyme chymopapain. The product is available in 2 ml vials exhibiting 4000 picoKatals activity (=4,000 Smith BAPNA assay units) of chymopapain with 1·4 mg L-cysteine hydrochloride monohydrate as activator.

The proteolytic enzyme chymopapain is derived from the crude latex of Carica papaya and is purified by column chromatography.

*Other ingredients:* Sodium hydroxide and/or hydrochloric acid as pH adjusters.

**Uses** Chymodiactin Injection is indicated for the treatment of patients with clinically-confirmed herniated lumbar intervertebral discs whose symptoms and signs have not responded to an adequate period or periods of conservative therapy.

**Dosage and administration**

*Adults:* The lumbar intervertebral disc should be treated with a single injection of Chymodiactin on one occasion directly into the nucleus pulposus (see under 'Procedure').

Vials of Chymodiactin Injection 4000 picoKatals are reconstituted with 2 ml Water for Injections BP, the resulting solution containing 2000 picoKatals chymopapain per ml.

Recommended dosage is 2000–4000 picoKatals (1–2 ml) per disc, preferably 3000 picoKatals (1·5 ml) per disc. The maximum dose in a single patient with multiple disc herniation is 8000 picoKatals (4 ml).

*Children:* The safety and efficacy of Chymodiactin has not been studied in paediatric patients. Its use is therefore not recommended in this patient group.

*Elderly:* There is insufficient evidence to recommend use in patients over the age of 60 years.

**Contra-indications, warnings, etc**

*Contra-indications:* Chymodiactin is contra-indicated in patients with a known sensitivity to chymopapain, papaya or other papaya derivatives. It is also contra-indicated in severe spondylolisthesis, progressive paralysis or other increasing neurological dysfunction, and in patients with evidence of spinal cord tumour or a cauda equina lesion.

Chymopapain is a foreign protein and, as such, its injection has the potential to generate an immunological response. Therefore, patients who have previously received an injection of chymopapain must not be re-injected with Chymodiactin.

Patients with congestive cardiac failure, coronary artery disease or respiratory failure should be excluded from chymopapain therapy because of the cardiovascular risk in shock should an anaphylactic reaction occur. Additionally, patients on beta-blockers should be excluded due to the blocking effects on rescue adrenaline, should this be required, and because such agents significantly potentiate the liberation of chemical mediators of anaphylaxis.

Chymodiactin is contra-indicated in patients in whom a pre-operative sensitivity screening test is performed and found to be positive.

*Warnings and precautions:* 1. Anaphylactic reactions have been observed in a small proportion of patients after injection with Chymodiactin. In post-marketing surveillance conducted in the USA, such reactions occurred in 0.5% of cases overall, but a major European survey has revealed an incidence of 0.14% in contemporary clinical practice.

The reaction can be immediate or delayed for up to one hour after injection and may be life-threatening if not treated promptly. At least one open intravenous line must always be in place for such an occurrence. The reaction may commence with almost immediate hypotension and/or bronchospasm, the former being more common.

Subsequently, laryngeal oedema, cardiac arrhythmia/arrest, coma and death may ensue. Speed in diagnosis and treatment is critical since the clinical signs, severity of progression and duration of an anaphylactic reaction are highly unpredictable. Other signs of allergic response must be watched for, e.g. erythema, pilomotor erection, rash, pruritus, urticaria, conjunctivitis, vasomotor rhinitis, angioedema and various gastrointestinal disturbances, which may herald the imminent onset of a major reaction.

Post-marketing surveillance data from the United States indicates that females are more likely to develop anaphylactic reactions than males, the rates being 0.9% and 0.3%, respectively. There was a statistically significant difference in the frequency of anaphylaxis dependent on whether local or general anaesthesia was used for the procedure, rates of 0.4% and 0.6% being noted, respectively. However, such a difference was not confirmed in the European survey, as both forms of anaesthesia were associated with a recorded incidence of 0.14%.

2. Acute transverse myelitis/acute transverse myelopathy has been reported in association with the injection of chymopapain at a rate of about 1 in 18,000 patients. Although a cause/effect relationship to the injection of chymopapain itself has not been established, the reported rate is significantly higher than the background incidence reported in the medical literature. These patients are characterised clinically by the delayed (2–3 weeks) onset of paraplegia or paraparesis without prior signs or symptoms. Patients receiving injections at more than one disc space appear to be at increased risk.

Paraplegia, cerebral haemorrhage and other serious neurological complications have been reported soon after chymopapain injection in a small number of patients. Causal relationships to the drug when properly injected have not been established. Needle trauma and/or introduction of chymopapain and contrast media into the spinal fluid may be causal in some of these cases. Less severe neurological reactions have included sacral burning, leg pain, hypalgesia, leg weakness, bilateral cramp, pain in the opposite leg and paraesthesia.

3. The drug is extremely toxic when injected intrathecally in animals. Therefore, great caution must be exercised in ensuring that Chymodiactin is not introduced into the dural canal either directly or by leakage.

4. Several deaths have been reported in association with Chymodiactin injection. These have been related to complications secondary to anaphylaxis, to staphylococcal meningitis with disc abscess or of unknown aetiology. The mortality rate associated with Chymodiactin is estimated at 1 in 4,500 patients (0·02%).

5. Discitis, both bacterial and aseptic, has been reported in several patients.

6. Less severe, but more frequent, adverse reactions include back pain/stiffness/soreness in approximately 50% of treated patients and/or back spasm in approximately 30%. Less frequent adverse reactions include rash, itching, urticaria, nausea, paralytic ileus, urinary retention, headache and dizziness.

7. Certain radio-opaque contrast media are neurotoxic. It has been suggested that the toxicity of these materials may be enhanced by the co-administration of Chymodiactin. Intrathecal administration of Chymodiactin results in capillary disruption and bleeding which may again potentiate the neurotoxicity of contrast agents.

Consequently, it is recommended that discography is not performed as part of the chemonucleolysis procedure unless the operating surgeon determines that the risks of discography are outweighed by the benefits in a particular clinical situation.

8. *Pregnancy and lactation:* As adequate studies have not been performed in either pregnant or lactating

women, Chymodiactin is not recommended for use in these patient groups.

*Procedure*

*1. Pre-Treatment:* Because of the possibility of anaphylaxis during chemonucleolysis with Chymodiactin, a careful history should be conducted to determine if the patient has multiple allergies, especially a known allergy to papaya or papaya derivatives.

Pre-dose sensitivity testing to detect patients likely to be hypersensitive to Chymodiactin is recommended prior to Chymodiactin chemonucleolysis. Skin and serum testing methods are available.

The following pre-treatment may reduce the incidence, or decrease the severity, of any anaphylactic reaction.

(a) H$_1$ antagonist – e.g. chlorpheniramine – 4 mg orally, 6 hourly for 24 hours prior to chemonucleolysis to block H$_1$ effects.

(b) H$_2$ antagonist – e.g. cimetidine – 4–5 mg/kg bodyweight orally 2 hours prior to chemonucleolysis to block H$_2$ effects.

(c) Adequate hydration should be maintained throughout the procedure. A secure, wide-bore venous access must be established pre-operatively and maintained for at least one hour after injection of the enzyme, to facilitate emergency intervention if required.

(d) Corticosteroid – e.g. hydrocortisone – orally or intravenously immediately prior to injection may stabilise membranes, decrease permeability and mediator release. Doses from 500–1,000 mg have been recommended.

(a), (b) and (c) are recommended and (d) is optional.

*2. Anaesthesia:* The choice of anaesthesia for a specific patient should be made by the attending surgeon and anaesthetist. However, **it is recommended that supplemented local anaesthesia be used for chemonucleolysis whenever possible.**

*Local anaesthesia:* The use of supplemented local anaesthesia in preference to general anaesthesia provides an awake patient, more likely to be alert to pain, particularly if the needle impinges on nerve tissue. In addition, it is likely that a patient under local anaesthetic will not tolerate an excessive number of attempts to place the needle.

*General anaesthesia:* The advantages of general anaesthesia are thought to be: ease of airway management if anaphylaxis should develop; more precise patient positioning for injection; less patient discomfort.

If halothane anaesthesia is used, it should be noted that if adrenaline is required for treatment of an anaphylactic reaction, there is a potential for arrhythmogenic interaction of the two drugs.

*3. Needle placement:* Needle placement for the intradiscal administration of Chymodiactin should be made by clinicians experienced in needle placement. Needle placement should be via the lateral approach to avoid puncture of the dura mater. Serious neurological toxicity has been reported using a posterior transdural approach. Therefore, this latter method should not be used.

Great care must be taken to ensure that the dura is not penetrated and that chymopapain or contrast agents (if used) do not enter the subarachnoid space. If there is any question regarding needle tip location within the nucleus of the disc, or if the contrast agent extravasates into the subarachnoid space, the procedure should be abandoned and chymopapain should not be injected.

Prior to injection of Chymodiactin, visualisation of the needle tip position in the disc must be confirmed using an X-ray image intensifier for both the anteroposterior and lateral views.

As an additional aid to needle tip visualisation, surgeons performing chemonucleolysis may wish to consider the injection of saline or water into the nucleus pulposus (saline or water acceptance test). The use of this procedure does not supplant careful evaluation of high quality anteroposterior and lateral X-ray views of the disc.

**Discography is not recommended at the time of the Chymodiactin injection unless the attending surgeon considers the risks to be outweighed by the benefits in the particular clinical situation.** If, however, discography is considered to be essential, it should be performed using non-ionic water soluble contrast media. At least 15 minutes should elapse after the administration of the radio-opaque contrast medium to allow for diffusion and absorption of the medium before injection of Chymodiactin through the same needle after removal of the obturator.

A volume of less than 0·5 ml of the contrast medium is ordinarily sufficient in determining the location of the needle tip.

If high quality X-ray equipment including an image intensifier is not available to perform chemonucleolysis, the procedure should not be carried out. If there is any question about satisfactory needle placement or if needle placement is difficult, requiring repeated attempts, the procedure should be abandoned.

*4. Injection:* (a) For 3 minutes prior to Chymodiactin injection, 100% oxygen (O$_2$) may be administered to the patient by the anaesthetist to maximise oxygenation in case of anaphylaxis.

(b) Based on the increased frequency of neurological adverse reactions in patients with two or more disc level injections, **chemonucleolysis should be limited to the one disc producing the patient's symptoms unless definitive signs, symptoms and diagnostic procedure indicate that more than one disc is at fault.**

*Treatment of anaphylaxis:* Clinical judgement, speed of therapy and choice of agents all enter into the treatment of anaphylaxis. It must be emphasised that adrenaline is the definitive therapeutic agent in the immediate treatment of the condition. Beta-blocker therapy may antagonise the action of adrenaline, and if halothane is used for general anaesthesia, there is a potential for an arrhythmogenic interaction with adrenaline.

The recommended treatment for severe anaphylactic reaction includes the immediate administration of a vasopressor such as 0·5–1·0 ml of 1:1,000 adrenaline, generally by the intramuscular route. Aminophylline and corticosteroids may be administered intravenously to relieve bronchospasm.

The severe manifestations of anaphylaxis include a sudden fall in blood pressure due to generalised vasodilation and increased capillary permeability, angioedema (including laryngeal oedema), and bronchospasm. Milder signs and symptoms include rhinitis, pruritus, urticaria, vomiting, diarrhoea and abdominal pain. The fall in cardiac output which accompanies a reduced venous return may cause secondary myocardial and tissue hypoxia, with cardiac arrhythmias and a metabolic acidosis completing a vicious circle in severe cases.

*Immediate therapy of acute reaction:* (a) The keystone of effective treatment is adrenaline. As soon as the reaction is recognised 500–1000 micrograms (0·5 to 1·0 ml of 1:1,000 solution) should be injected intramuscularly (not subcutaneously).

(b) Intramuscular injections of adrenaline should be repeated every 15 minutes until improvement occurs.

(c) A slow intravenous injection of 20 mg of the H$_1$ antagonist, chlorpheniramine should be given immediately after intramuscular adrenaline and repeated over the subsequent 24 to 48 hours to prevent relapse.

Intravenous corticosteroids (e.g. hydrocortisone) have little place in the immediate management. Their beneficial effects are delayed for several hours. In severely ill patients, however, early administration may help prevent deterioration after the primary treatment has been given. Most patients respond to the combination of intramuscular adrenaline and an intravenous H$_1$-antagonist.

*Continuation therapy:* Continuing deterioration with circulatory collapse, bronchospasm or laryngeal oedema requires further treatment. Circulatory collapse requires volume replacement by intravenous fluids monitored, if possible, by a central venous pressure line. If electrolyte solutions are used, large volumes may be necessary because in severe anaphylactic shock the plasma loss may constitute 20–40% of the plasma volume. Colloid solutions such as plasma protein fraction or dextran are theoretically preferable but may themselves release histamine, though in severe anaphylaxis intracellular stores of histamine are likely to have been depleted. Bronchospasm refractory to intramuscular adrenaline requires treatment with intravenous aminophylline, a nebulised beta$_2$-agonist (such as salbutamol or terbutaline), oxygen, and (if necessary) assisted ventilation. Respiratory obstruction due to laryngeal oedema may require emergency tracheostomy.

Effective treatment of anaphylactic shock clearly depends on the severity of the clinical condition and the circumstances under which it occurs.

**Pharmaceutical precautions** Chymodiactin lyophilised powder should be stored under refrigeration (2–8°C), although it is stable at room temperature (25°C) for periods of time up to 18 months without loss of potency.

The drug should be used within 2 hours of its reconstitution. A vial should be used for only one patient and unused drug discarded and not stored for future use.

Since inactivation of the enzyme will occur with some bacteriostatic agents in common use, diluents containing such agents should not be used.

**Legal category** POM.

**Package quantities** Cartons containing 1 vial of Chymodiactin Injection 4000 picoKatals together with a leaflet for the information of the medical profession and a patient information leaflet.

**Further information** Chymodiactin has been shown to dissolve the nucleus pulposus of dogs and rabbits at doses as low as 50 units/disc and 100 units/disc, respectively. Doses of 3,000 units/disc cause thinning

of the inner portion of the annulus in rabbits but do not penetrate the entire structure, while doses as high as 24,000 units/disc in dogs resulted in no apparent significant change in the peripheral portion of the annulus. In vitro studies demonstrated that chymopapain solubilised the glycosaminoglycan protein complex of human nucleus pulposus, but did not attack the collagen of this structure.

When chymopapain was injected into dogs and rabbits, doses up to 100 times greater than that required to remove the nucleus pulposus were well tolerated when injected intravenously, intradiscally and epidurally. The drug is extremely toxic when injected intrathecally; the approximate LD$_{50}$ is 15 units/kg in rabbits, 150 units/kg in dogs and 200 units/kg in baboons. Therefore, great caution must be exercised to ensure that Chymodiactin is not injected intrathecally into the dural canal in the human.

In experiments in baboons, the serial injection of contrast agents (Renografin, Conray or Amipaque) into the spinal fluid, followed by Chymodiactin 15 minutes later produced serious neurotoxicity, including weakness, paralysis and death in doses that were harmless or only slightly toxic when administered as single agents. This information supports the clinical observation that the documented entry of contrast agent and presumed entry of chymopapain into the spinal fluid can produce serious neurotoxicity including paraplegia and cerebral haemorrhage.

**Product licence number** 0169/0055

## DELTASTAB* INJECTION

**Presentation** Deltastab Injection is a sterile suspension of 25 mg/ml Prednisolone Acetate BP 1963.

*Other ingredients:* Water for injections; benzyl alcohol; sodium carboxymethylcellulose; polysorbate 80; sodium chloride; with sodium hydroxide and/or hydrochloric acid as pH adjusters.

**Uses** Prednisolone is a glucocorticoid which has anti-inflammatory activity. Deltastab Injection is intended for the local treatment by intra-articular or periarticular injection of the following conditions: rheumatoid arthritis, osteoarthritis, synovitis not associated with infection, tennis elbow, golfer's elbow, bursitis.

Deltastab Injection is suitable for administration by the intramuscular route in conditions requiring systemic corticosteroids, e.g. suppression of inflammatory and allergic disorders such as bronchial asthma, anaphylaxis, ulcerative colitis and Crohn's disease.

**Dosage and administration**

*Adults:* For articular injection: 5–25 mg depending upon the size of the joint. The injections may be repeated when relapse occurs. Not more than three joints should be treated in any one day.

For intramuscular injection: dosage will depend upon the clinical circumstances and the judgement of the physician. Suggested dose 25–100 mg once or twice weekly.

*Children:* Corticosteroids cause growth retardation in infancy, childhood and adolescence, which may be irreversible. Treatment should be limited to the minimum dosage for the shortest possible time.

*Elderly:* Steroids should be used cautiously in the elderly since adverse effects are enhanced by old age (see Warnings).

Note: When long-term treatment is to be discontinued, the dose administered should be gradually reduced over a period of weeks or months depending on dosage and duration of therapy (see Warnings).

Undesirable effects may be minimised by using the lowest effective dose for the minimum period, and by administering the daily requirement as a single morning dose or whenever possible as a single morning dose on alternate days. Frequent patient review is required to appropriately titrate the dose against disease activity.

**Contra-indications, warnings, etc**

*Contra-indications:* Deltastab Injection is contra-indicated in patients with known hypersensitivity to any of the ingredients, and in patients with systemic infections, unless specific anti-infective therapy is employed. It is also contra-indicated in patients vaccinated with live vaccines (see Warnings).

Intra-articular and periarticular injections of Deltastab Injection are contra-indicated when the joint or surrounding tissues are infected. The presence of infection also precludes injection into tendon sheaths and bursae. Deltastab Injection must not be injected directly into tendons, nor should it be injected into the spinal or other non-diarthrodial joints.

*Precautions:* A patient information leaflet should be supplied with this product.

Intra-articular corticosteroids are associated with a substantially increased risk of inflammatory response in the joint, particularly bacterial infection introduced with the injection. Great care is required that all intra-articular steroid injections should be undertaken under aseptic conditions.

*Warnings:*

*Adrenal suppression:* Adrenal cortical atrophy develops during prolonged therapy and may persist for years after stopping treatment. Withdrawal of corticosteroids after prolonged therapy must therefore always be gradual to avoid acute adrenal insufficiency, being tapered off over weeks or months according to the dose and duration of treatment. During prolonged therapy, any intercurrent illness, trauma or surgical procedure will require a temporary increase in dosage. If corticosteroids have been stopped following prolonged therapy they may need to be temporarily reintroduced.

Patients should carry 'Steroid Treatment' cards which give clear guidance on the precautions to be taken to minimise risk and which provide details of prescriber, drug, dosage and the duration of treatment.

*Anti-inflammatory/immunosuppressive effects and infection:* Suppression of inflammatory response and immune function increases the susceptibility to infections and their severity. The clinical presentation may often be atypical and serious infections such as septicaemia and tuberculosis may be masked and may reach an advanced stage before being recognised. New infections may appear during the use of corticosteroids.

Chickenpox is of particular concern since this normally minor illness may be fatal in immunosuppressed patients. Patients (or parents of children) without a definite history of chickenpox should be advised to avoid close personal contact with chickenpox or herpes zoster and if exposed they should seek urgent medical attention. Passive immunisation with varicella zoster immunoglobulin (VZIG) is needed by exposed non-immune patients who are receiving systemic corticosteroids or who have used them within the previous 3 months. This should be given within 10 days of exposure to chickenpox. If a diagnosis of chickenpox is confirmed, the illness warrants specialist care and urgent treatment. Corticosteroids should not be stopped and the dose may need to be increased.

Live vaccines should not be given to individuals with impaired immune responsiveness. Killed vaccines or toxoids may be given though their effects may be attenuated.

Particular care is required when prescribing systemic corticosteroids in patients with the following conditions and frequent patient monitoring is necessary:

(a) Osteoporosis (post-menopausal females are particularly at risk).

(b) Hypertension or congestive heart failure.

(c) Existing or previous history of severe affective disorders (especially previous history of steroid psychosis).

(d) Diabetes mellitus (or a family history of diabetes).

(e) Previous history of tuberculosis or characteristic appearance on chest X-ray. The emergence of active tuberculosis can, however, be prevented by the prophylactic use of antituberculous therapy.

(f) Glaucoma (or a family history of glaucoma).

(g) Previous corticosteroid-induced myopathy.

(h) Liver failure.

(i) Renal insufficiency.

(j) Epilepsy.

(k) Peptic ulceration.

During treatment, the patient should be observed for psychotic reactions, muscular weakness, electrocardiographic changes, hypertension and untoward hormonal effects.

Corticosteroids should be used with caution in patients with hypothyroidism.

*Drug interactions:* The effectiveness of anticoagulants may be increased or decreased with concurrent corticosteroid therapy, and close monitoring of the INR or prothrombin time is required to avoid spontaneous bleeding.

Serum levels of salicylates may increase considerably if corticosteroid therapy is withdrawn, possibly causing intoxication. Since both salicylates and corticosteroids are ulcerogenic, it is possible that there will be an increased rate of gastrointestinal ulceration.

The desired actions of hypoglycaemic drugs (including insulin), antihypertensives and diuretics will be antagonised by corticosteroids.

The potassium-depleting effects of amphotericin, carbenoxolone and diuretics (acetazolamide, loop diuretics and thiazides) are enhanced by corticosteroids and signs of hypokalaemia should be looked for during their concurrent use.

There is a small amount of evidence that use of corticosteroids and methotrexate simultaneously may cause increased methotrexate toxicity and possibly death, although this combination of drugs has been used very successfully.

The metabolism of corticosteroids may be enhanced and the therapeutic effects reduced by certain barbiturates (e.g. phenobarbitone) and by phenytoin, rifampicin, rifabutin, primidone, carbamazepine and aminoglutethimide.

*Use in pregnancy and lactation:* There is evidence of harmful effects in pregnancy in animals.

There may be a small risk of cleft palate and intra-uterine growth retardation in the foetus. Hypoadrenalism may occur in the neonate.

When corticosteroids are essential, however, patients with normal pregnancies may be treated as though they were in the non-gravid state. Patients with pre-eclampsia or fluid retention require close monitoring.

Corticosteroids are excreted in small amounts in breast milk and infants of mothers taking pharmacological doses of steroids should be monitored carefully for signs of adrenal suppression.

The decision to use Deltastab Injection during pregnancy and lactation must be made by weighing up the relative risks associated with the use of the drug against the potential benefits in maternal disease.

*Use in children:* Corticosteroids cause growth retardation in infancy, childhood and adolescence, which may be irreversible. Treatment should be limited to the minimum dosage for the shortest possible time, in order to minimise suppression of the hypothalamo-pituitary-adrenal axis and growth retardation.

*Use in the elderly:* The common adverse effects of systemic corticosteroids may be associated with more serious consequences in old age, especially osteoporosis, hypertension, hypokalaemia, diabetes, susceptibility to infection and thinning of the skin. Close clinical supervision is required to avoid life-threatening reactions.

*Undesirable effects:* With intra-articular or other local injections, the principal side-effect encountered is a temporary local exacerbation with increased pain and swelling. Normally this subsides after a few hours.

The incidence of predictable undesirable effects, including hypothalamic-pituitary-adrenal suppression, correlates with the relative potency of the drug, dosage, timing of administration and the duration of treatment (see Warnings).

The following side-effects may be associated with the long-term systemic use of corticosteroids.

*Anti-inflammatory and immunosuppressive effects:* Increased susceptibility and severity of infections with suppression of clinical symptoms and signs, opportunistic infections, recurrence of dormant tuberculosis (see Warnings).

*Gastrointestinal:* Dyspepsia, peptic ulceration with perforation and haemorrhage, abdominal distension, oesophageal ulceration, candidiasis, acute pancreatitis.

*Musculoskeletal:* Proximal myopathy, osteoporosis, vertebral and long bone fractures, avascular osteonecrosis, tendon rupture.

*Fluid and electrolyte disturbance:* Sodium and water retention, hypertension, potassium loss, hypokalaemic alkalosis.

*Dermatological:* Impaired healing, skin atrophy, bruising, striae, acne, telangiectasia.

*Endocrine/metabolic:* Suppression of the hypothalamo-pituitary-adrenal axis, growth suppression in infancy, childhood and adolescence, menstrual irregularity and amenorrhoea. Cushingoid facies, hirsutism, weight gain, impaired carbohydrate tolerance with increased requirement for antidiabetic therapy. Negative protein and calcium balance. Increased appetite.

*Neuropsychiatric:* Euphoria, psychological dependence, depression, insomnia and aggravation of schizophrenia. Increased intracranial pressure with papilloedema in children (pseudotumour cerebri), usually after treatment withdrawal. Aggravation of epilepsy.

*Ophthalmic:* Increased intra-ocular pressure, glaucoma, papilloedema, posterior subcapsular cataracts, corneal or scleral thinning, exacerbation of ophthalmic viral or fungal diseases.

*General:* Hypersensitivity, including anaphylaxis has been reported. Nausea, malaise, leucocytosis, thromboembolism.

*Withdrawal symptoms and signs:* Too rapid a reduction of corticosteroid dosage following prolonged treatment can lead to acute adrenal insufficiency, hypotension and death (see Warnings).

A 'withdrawal syndrome' may also occur including fever, myalgia, arthralgia, rhinitis, conjunctivitis, painful itchy skin nodules and loss of weight.

*Treatment of overdosage:* Overdosage is unlikely with Deltastab Injection but there is no specific antidote available. Treatment should be symptomatic.

**Pharmaceutical precautions** Store between 15°C and 25°C. Protect from light. Shake well before use.

**Legal category** POM.

**Package quantities** 10 ampoules of 1 ml. Each pack contains a leaflet for the information of the medical profession and a patient information leaflet.

**Further information** Nil.

**Product licence number** 0169/0058.

## DIMERCAPROL INJECTION BP

**Qualitative and quantitative composition** Dimercaprol PhEur 5.0% w/v (50 mg/ml)

**Pharmaceutical form** Solution for injection.

**Clinical particulars**

*Therapeutic indications:* Dimercaprol Injection is indicated in the treatment of acute poisoning by certain heavy metals: arsenic, mercury, gold, bismuth, antimony and possibly thallium. Although dimercaprol has not been successful in the treatment of lead poisoning when used alone, there is evidence that used in conjunction with sodium calcium edetate, it can be used successfully in the treatment of lead poisoning, particularly in children.

*Posology and method of administration:* For intramuscular injection.

Adults: 400–800 mg, in divided doses, on the first day. 200–400 mg, in divided doses, on the second and third days. 100–200 mg, in divided doses, on subsequent days.

Within the above dose range, individual dosage should be calculated on a bodyweight basis and will depend upon the severity of symptoms and the causative agent. As a general guide, single doses should not exceed 3 mg/kg bodyweight. However, in severe acute poisoning, single doses up to 5 mg/kg bodyweight may be required initially.

Children: Dimercaprol Injection is well tolerated by children and the dosage should be calculated on the basis of bodyweight, using the same unit dose/kg of bodyweight as for an adult under similar clinical circumstances.

Elderly: There are no specific data on the use of dimercaprol in the elderly but since it is eliminated via the kidney, it should be used with caution in this age group.

*Contra-indications:* Dimercaprol Injection is contra-indicated in poisoning by iron, cadmium or selenium, in the presence of impaired hepatic function unless due to arsenic poisoning and in patients hypersensitive to dimercaprol.

*Special warnings and special precautions for use:* Dimercaprol Injection should be used with care in patients with hypertension or impaired renal function. It should be discontinued or continued with extreme caution if acute renal insufficiency develops during therapy. Dimercaprol Injection may not be effective in cases of concomitant renal failure, e.g. in arsine poisoning and some cases of arsenic poisoning. Any abnormal reaction (e.g. pyrexia) occurring after the initial injection of dimercaprol should be assessed before continuing treatment. The use of Dimercaprol Injection does not eliminate the need for the general treatment of poisoning due to the particular heavy metal.

*Interaction with other medicaments and other forms of interaction:* Iron supplements must not be taken during dimercaprol therapy as iron forms toxic complexes with it.

*Pregnancy and lactation:* Dimercaprol Injection has been used in Wilson's disease with successful full-term pregnancies, but since there is no other experience of its use in pregnancy or lactation, it should be prescribed with caution during these periods.

*Effects on ability to drive and use machines:* No adverse effects known.

*Undesirable effects:* Side effects are relatively frequent, but at the therapeutic dosage employed, are seldom severe enough to warrant cessation of treatment and are almost invariably reversible. There is some evidence to indicate that 30–60 mg of ephedrine sulphate by mouth, given half an hour before each injection of dimercaprol, will reduce these reactions. Also, a minimum interval of four hours between doses appears to reduce side effects. Dimercaprol may cause the following side effects, particularly at the higher dosage levels: elevation of blood pressure accompanied by tachycardia, nausea and possibly vomiting, burning sensation of the lips, mouth, throat and eyes, salivation and lacrimation, conjunctivitis, rhinorrhoea, muscle pain and spasm, abdominal pain, headache, tingling of the hands and other extremities, a feeling of constriction in the chest and throat, sweating of the forehead and hands. Local pain may occur at the site of injection and gluteal abscess has occasionally been encountered.

A side effect apparently peculiar to children is a fever which develops after the second or third injection, and persists until treatment with dimercaprol is terminated.

*Overdose:* Symptoms of overdosage include malaise, nausea, vomiting, lacrimation and salivation, burning sensation of lips, mouth, throat and eyes with headache. A sense of constriction of the throat and chest. Increased blood pressure maximal after 15–20 minutes. Transient effects lasting about four hours.

Treatment consists of the subcutaneous administration of diphenhydramine 50 mg or ephedrine 30 mg or ephedrine in a dosage of 30–60 mg orally if time permits.

### Pharmacological properties

*Pharmacodynamic properties:* Dimercaprol is a chelating agent used in the treatment of acute poisoning by heavy metals. The sulphydryl groups of dimercaprol compete with endogenous sulphydryl groups on proteins such as enzymes to combine with these metals; chelation by dimercaprol therefore prevents or reverses any inhibition of the sulphydryl enzymes by the metal and the dimercaprol-metal complex formed is readily excreted by the kidney.

*Pharmacokinetic properties:* After intramuscular injection, maximum plasma concentrations of dimercaprol may be attained within one hour. Dimercaprol is rapidly metabolised and the metabolites and dimercaprol-metal chelates are excreted in the urine and bile. Elimination is essentially complete within four hours of a single dose.

*Preclinical safety data:* Not applicable.

### Pharmaceutical particulars

*List of excipients:* Benzyl benzoate, arachis oil, 5N alcoholic ammonia, nitrogen.

*Incompatibilities:* None known.

*Shelf life:* 36 months.

*Special precautions for storage:* Store at 2°–25°C. Protect from light.

*Nature and contents of container:* A 2 ml clear neutral glass ampoule with ceramic breakring. Pack size: 10 ampoules packed in a polystyrene pack within a cardboard sleeve.

*Instructions for use/handling:* Special precautions for disposal: react with weak aqueous solution (up to 15% of calcium hypochlorite). Leave for 24 hours. Neutralise and discharge to drain with copious quantities of water.

**Marketing authorisation number** 00169/0061

**Date of approval/revision of SPC** October 1995

**Legal category** POM

## FROBEN*

**Presentation** Yellow, sugar-coated tablets containing either 50 mg or 100 mg of Flurbiprofen BP. The 50 mg tablets are overprinted 'F50' in black; the 100 mg tablets are overprinted 'F100' in black.

White wax suppositories containing 100 mg of flurbiprofen.

*Inactive ingredients: Tablets –* lactose; sucrose; sunset yellow; quinoline yellow; sodium benzoate; glucose; titanium dioxide. *Suppository –* Witepsol.

**Uses** Froben is a non-steroidal anti-inflammatory drug (NSAID) which has significant anti-inflammatory, analgesic and antipyretic properties and is indicated in the treatment of rheumatoid disease, osteoarthritis, ankylosing spondylitis, musculoskeletal disorders and trauma such as periarthritis, frozen shoulder, bursitis, tendinitis, tenosynovitis, low back pain, sprains and strains. Froben is also indicated for its analgesic effect in the relief of mild to moderate pain, in conditions such as dental pain, post-operative pain, dysmenorrhoea and migraine.

### Dosage and administration

*Adults:* The recommended daily dose is 150–200 mg in divided doses.

In patients with severe symptoms or disease of recent origin, or during acute exacerbations, the total daily dosage may be increased to 300 mg in divided doses.

*Dysmenorrhoea:* A dosage of 100 mg (in the form of tablets or suppositories) to be administered at the start of symptoms, followed by 50 or 100 mg (in the form of tablets) given at 4–6 hourly intervals. The maximum total daily dosage should not exceed 300 mg.

*Children:* Not recommended for use in children under 12 years.

*Elderly:* Although Froben is generally well tolerated in the elderly, some patients, especially those with

impaired renal function, may eliminate NSAIDs more slowly than normal. In these cases, Froben should be used with caution and dosage should be assessed individually.

**Contra-indications, warnings, etc** Froben is contra-indicated in patients with peptic ulceration, gastrointestinal haemorrhage and ulcerative colitis.

Froben should not be given to patients with a history of asthma or to patients who have experienced bronchospasm, anaphylactic reactions, angioedema or other hypersensitivity-type reactions from use of aspirin or other NSAIDs.

Froben Suppositories are contra-indicated in patients with inflammatory diseases of the rectum and peri-anal area.

Caution is necessary if given to patients with a history of heart failure, hypertension or non-allergic asthma.

As it has been shown that Froben may prolong bleeding time, it should be used with caution in patients with a potential for abnormal bleeding.

NSAIDs have been reported to cause nephrotoxicity in various forms, including interstitial nephritis, nephrotic syndrome and renal failure. In patients with renal, cardiac or hepatic impairment, caution is required since the use of NSAIDs may result in deterioration of renal function. The dose should be kept as low as possible and renal function should be monitored in these patients.

*Side-effects:* Dyspepsia, nausea, vomiting, gastrointestinal haemorrhage, diarrhoea, mouth ulcers, fluid retention and oedema have been reported. Exacerbation of peptic ulceration and perforation have also been reported.

Urticaria, angioedema and rashes of varying description have been reported.

Very rarely, cholestatic jaundice and thrombocytopenia have been reported. These are usually reversible on withdrawal of the drug.

Very rarely, aplastic anaemia and agranulocytosis have been reported in association with the use of flurbiprofen but causality has not been established.

Occasional symptoms due to local irritation with the suppositories may occur, e.g. diarrhoea and pruritus.

*Use in pregnancy and lactation:* Preclinical studies have not revealed any teratogenic effects, although Froben should not be prescribed during pregnancy unless the benefits outweigh the possible risks. If Froben is used during early pregnancy, the lowest effective dosage should be employed. During the third trimester of pregnancy, regular use of NSAIDs has been associated with delayed and prolonged parturition and premature closure of the foetal ductus arteriosus in utero and possibly persistent pulmonary hypertension of the newborn.

The amounts of flurbiprofen secreted into the breast milk during lactation are considered to be too small to be harmful and therefore, breast feeding would not be contra-indicated.

*Drug interactions:* The diuretic response to frusemide can occasionally be reduced by flurbiprofen. Similarly, interference with the action of anticoagulants has occasionally been reported.

Other studies have failed to show any interaction between flurbiprofen and digoxin, tolbutamide or antacids.

*Interference with laboratory tests:* There is no evidence that flurbiprofen interferes with standard laboratory tests.

*Treatment of overdosage:* Gastric lavage and, if necessary, correction of serum electrolytes. There is no specific antidote to flurbiprofen.

**Pharmaceutical precautions** Suppositories: Store in a cool place.

**Legal category** POM.

### Package quantities

*50 mg Tablets:* Packs of 100 (strips of 10).
*100 mg Tablets:* Packs of 100 (strips of 10).
*100 mg Suppositories:* Packs of 12 (strips of 6).

**Further information** Flurbiprofen is a potent inhibitor of prostaglandin synthetase which most probably explains its pharmacological effects.

### Product licence numbers

| | |
|---|---|
| Froben 50 mg Tablets | 0169/0066 |
| Froben 100 mg Tablets | 0169/0067 |
| Froben 100 mg Suppositories | 0169/0064 |

## FROBEN SR*

**Presentation** A hard gelatin capsule with a yellow opaque cap and a transparent yellow body containing white to off-white beads, printed 'FSR' in black. Each capsule contains 200 mg flurbiprofen in sustained-release form.

*Inactive ingredients:* Microcrystalline cellulose; quinoline yellow; titanium dioxide.

**Uses** Froben SR is a non-steroidal anti-inflammatory drug (NSAID) which has significant analgesic and anti-inflammatory properties and is indicated in the treatment of osteoarthritis, rheumatoid disease, ankylosing spondylitis, musculoskeletal disorders and trauma such as periarthritis, frozen shoulder, bursitis, tendinitis, tenosynovitis, low back pain, sprains and strains.

### Dosage and administration

*Adults:* The recommended daily dose is one 200 mg capsule, taken preferably in the evening, after food.

*Children:* Froben SR is not recommended for children under 12 years.

*Elderly:* Although flurbiprofen is well tolerated in the elderly, some patients, especially those with impaired renal function, may eliminate NSAIDs more slowly than normal. In these cases, Froben SR should be used with caution and dosage should be assessed individually, using the standard formulation if necessary.

**Contra-indications, warnings, etc** Froben SR is contra-indicated in patients with peptic ulceration, gastrointestinal haemorrhage and ulcerative colitis.

Froben SR should not be given to patients with a history of asthma or to patients who have experienced bronchospasm, anaphylactic reactions, angioedema or other hypersensitivity-type reactions from use of aspirin or other NSAIDs.

Caution is necessary if given to patients with a history of heart failure, hypertension or non-allergic asthma.

As it has been shown that flurbiprofen may prolong bleeding time, it should be used with caution in patients with a potential for abnormal bleeding.

NSAIDs have been reported to cause nephrotoxicity in various forms, including interstitial nephritis, nephrotic syndrome and renal failure. In patients with renal, cardiac or hepatic impairment, caution is required since the use of NSAIDs may result in deterioration of renal function. The dose should be kept as low as possible and renal function should be monitored in these patients.

*Side-effects:* Dyspepsia, nausea, vomiting, gastrointestinal haemorrhage, diarrhoea, mouth ulcers, fluid retention and oedema have been recorded with flurbiprofen. Exacerbation of peptic ulceration and perforation have also been reported.

Urticaria, angioedema and rashes of varying description have been reported.

Very rarely, cholestatic jaundice and thrombocytopenia have been reported. These are usually reversible on withdrawal of the drug.

Very rarely, aplastic anaemia and agranulocytosis have been reported in association with the use of flurbiprofen but causality has not been established.

*Use in pregnancy and lactation:* Preclinical studies have not revealed any teratogenic effects, although Froben SR should not be prescribed during pregnancy unless the benefits outweigh the possible risks. During the third trimester of pregnancy, regular use of NSAIDs has been associated with delayed and prolonged parturition and premature closure of the foetal ductus arteriosus in utero and possibly persistent pulmonary hypertension of the newborn.

The amounts of flurbiprofen secreted into the breast milk during lactation are considered to be too small to be harmful and therefore, breast feeding would not be contra-indicated.

*Drug interactions:* The diuretic response to frusemide can occasionally be reduced by flurbiprofen. Similarly, interference with the action of anticoagulants has occasionally been reported.

Other studies have failed to show any interaction between flurbiprofen and digoxin, tolbutamide or antacids.

*Interference with laboratory tests:* There is no evidence that flurbiprofen interferes with standard laboratory tests.

*Treatment of overdosage:* Gastric lavage and, if necessary, correction of serum electrolytes. There is no specific antidote to flurbiprofen.

**Pharmaceutical precautions** No special storage conditions are necessary.

**Legal category** POM.

**Package quantities** HDPE bottle of 30 capsules.

**Further information** Flurbiprofen is a potent inhibitor of prostaglandin synthetase which most probably explains its pharmacological effects.

Taken once a day, preferably in the evening, Froben SR is particularly suitable for those patients where compliance may be a problem and for better control of morning stiffness.

**Product licence number** 0169/0068.

# FURAMIDE*

**Qualitative and quantitative composition** Diloxanide Furoate BP 500 mg

**Pharmaceutical form** A flat, white tablet, scored and with a characteristic engraving E/F on one face.

## Clinical particulars

*Therapeutic indications:* For the treatment of acute and chronic intestinal amoebiasis.

*Posology and method of administration:* For oral administration.

Adults: One tablet three times daily for ten days.

Children: 20 mg/kg bodyweight daily in divided doses for ten days. Furamide is not suitable for use in children weighing less than 25 kg.

Elderly: There is no need for a dosage reduction in the elderly.

If required, a second course of treatment may be prescribed.

*Contra-indications:* Hypersensitivity to diloxanide furoate.

*Special warnings and special precautions for use:* None.

*Interaction with other medicaments and other forms of interaction:* No clinically-significant drug interactions known.

*Pregnancy and lactation:* The safety of Furamide during pregnancy and lactation has not been established and use during these periods should therefore be avoided.

*Effects on ability to drive and use machines:* No adverse effects known.

*Undesirable effects:* No serious side effects have been reported and the bacterial flora of the gut is not upset. Flatulence sometimes occurs but may usually be disregarded. Occasionally, vomiting, pruritus and urticaria may occur.

*Overdose:* Furamide tablets are unlikely to constitute a hazard in overdosage. In severe overdosage, early gastric lavage is recommended. There is no specific antidote. Treatment should be symptomatic and supportive.

## Pharmacological properties

*Pharmacodynamic properties:* Diloxanide furoate is a luminal amoebicide acting principally in the bowel lumen, although its mode of action is not known.

*Pharmacokinetic properties:* In the gut, diloxanide furoate is largely, if not wholly, hydrolysed into diloxanide and furoic acid under the combined action of bacterial and gut esterases. After absorption, diloxanide is very rapidly conjugated to form a glucuronide. In circulating blood, it is present to about 99% as a glucuronide and 1% as free diloxanide. Diloxanide is predominantly excreted in the urine. It is believed that the unabsorbed diloxanide is the active anti-amoebic substance, up to 10% remaining in the gut which is subsequently excreted as diloxanide in the faeces.

*Preclinical safety data:* Not applicable.

## Pharmaceutical particulars

*List of excipients:* Maize starch, pregelatinized maize starch, dried maize starch, magnesium stearate, purified water.

*Incompatibilities:* None known.

*Shelf life:* 36 months.

*Special precautions for storage:* None.

*Nature and contents of container:* A white aluminium tube with a polythene foam disc and a white aluminium screw cap with flowed-in PVC. Pack size: 15 tablets.

*Instructions for use/handling:* Not applicable.

**Marketing authorisation number** 00169/0070

**Date of approval/revision of SPC** October 1995

**Legal category** POM

# GOPTEN*

## Qualitative and quantitative composition
Gopten Capsules 0.5 mg    Trandolapril 0.5 mg
Gopten Capsules 1.0 mg    Trandolapril 1.0 mg
Gopten Capsules 2.0 mg    Trandolapril 2.0 mg

## Pharmaceutical form
Gopten Capsules 0.5 mg    Opaque red/yellow capsules

Gopten Capsules 1.0 mg    Opaque red/orange capsules

Gopten Capsules 2.0 mg    Opaque red/red capsules

## Clinical particulars

*Therapeutic indications:* Mild or moderate hypertension.

Left ventricular dysfunction after myocardial infarction.

It has been demonstrated that Gopten improves survival following myocardial infarction in patients with left ventricular dysfunction (ejection fraction ≤35 percent), with or without symptoms of heart failure, and/or with or without residual ischaemia.

Long-term treatment with Gopten significantly reduces the overall cardiovascular mortality. It significantly decreases the risk of sudden death and the occurrence of severe or resistant heart failure.

*Posology and method of administration:* For oral administration.

Hypertension: For adults not taking diuretics, without congestive heart failure and without renal or hepatic insufficiency, the recommended initial dosage is 0.5 mg as a single daily dose. A 0.5 mg dose will only achieve a therapeutic response in a minority of patients. Dosage should be doubled incrementally at intervals of 2 to 4 weeks, based on patient response, up to a maximum of 4 mg as a single daily dose.

The usual maintenance dose range is 1 to 2 mg as a single daily dose. If the patient response is still unsatisfactory at a dose of 4 mg Gopten, combination therapy should be considered.

Left ventricular dysfunction after myocardial infarction: Following a myocardial infarction, therapy may be initiated as early as the third day. Treatment should be initiated at a daily dose of 0.5 mg. The dose should be progressively increased to a maximum of 4 mg as a single daily dose. Depending upon the tolerability such as symptomatic hypotension, this forced titration can be temporarily suspended.

In the event of hypotension, all concomitant hypotensive therapies such as vasodilators, including nitrates and diuretics must be carefully checked and if possible, their dose reduced.

The dose of Gopten should be lowered only if the previous measures are not effective or not feasible.

Elderly: The dose in elderly patients is the same as in adults. There is no need to reduce the dose in elderly patients with normal renal and hepatic function. Caution is required in elderly patients with concomitant use of diuretics, congestive heart failure or renal or hepatic insufficiency. The dose should be titrated according to the need to control blood pressure.

Prior diuretic treatment: In patients who are at risk from a stimulated renin-angiotensin system (e.g. patients with water and sodium depletion), the diuretic should be discontinued 2–3 days before beginning therapy with 0.5 mg trandolapril to reduce the likelihood of symptomatic hypotension. The diuretic may be resumed later if required.

Cardiac failure: In hypertensive patients who also have congestive heart failure, with or without associated renal insufficiency, symptomatic hypotension has been observed after treatment with ACE inhibitors. In these patients, therapy should be started at a dose of 0.5 mg Gopten once daily under close medical supervision in hospital.

Dosage adjustment in renal impairment: For patients with mild or moderate renal impairment (creatinine clearance of 10–70 ml/min), the usual adult and elderly doses are recommended. For patients with severe renal impairment (creatinine clearance of <10 ml/min), the usual adult and elderly starting doses are also recommended but the maximum daily dose should not exceed 2 mg. In these patients, therapy should be under close medical supervision.

Dialysis: It is not known for certain if trandolapril or trandolaprilat are removed by dialysis. However it would be expected that dialysis could remove the active moiety, trandolaprilat, from the circulation, resulting in a possible loss of control of blood pressure. Therefore careful monitoring of the patient's blood pressure during dialysis is required, and the dosage of trandolapril adjusted if needed.

Dosage adjustment in hepatic impairment: In patients with severely impaired liver function, a decrease in the metabolic clearance of the parent compound, trandolapril and the active metabolite, trandolaprilat results in a large increase in plasma trandolapril levels and to a lesser extent, an increase in trandolaprilat levels. Treatment with Gopten should therefore be initiated at a dose of 0.5 mg once daily under close medical supervision.

Children: Gopten has not been studied in children and therefore use in this age group is not recommended.

*Contra-indications:* Known hypersensitivity to trandolapril. History of angioneurotic oedema associated with administration of an ACE inhibitor. Hereditary/idiopathic angioneurotic oedema. Pregnancy or lactation. Use in children.

*Special warnings and special precautions for use:*

Gopten should not be used in patients with aortic stenosis or outflow obstruction.

Assessment of renal function: Evaluation of the patient should include assessment of renal function prior to initiation of therapy and during treatment. Proteinuria may occur if renal impairment is present prior to therapy or relatively high doses are used.

Impaired renal function: Patients with severe renal insufficiency may require reduced doses of Gopten; their renal function should be closely monitored. In the majority, renal function will not alter. In patients with renal insufficiency, congestive heart failure or unilateral or bilateral renal artery stenosis, in the single kidney as well as after renal transplantation, there is a risk of impairment of renal function. If recognised early, such impairment of renal function is reversible upon discontinuation of therapy.

Some hypertensive patients with no apparent pre-existing renal disease may develop minor and usually transient increases in blood urea nitrogen and serum creatinine when Gopten is given concomitantly with a diuretic. Dosage reduction of Gopten and/or discontinuation of the diuretic may be required. Additionally, in patients with renal insufficiency, the risk of hyperkalaemia should be considered and the patient's electrolyte status checked regularly.

Impaired liver function: As trandolapril is a prodrug metabolised to its active moiety in the liver, particular caution and close monitoring should be applied to patients with impaired liver function.

Symptomatic hypotension: In patients with uncomplicated hypertension, symptomatic hypotension has been observed rarely after the initial dose of Gopten, as well as after increasing the dose of Gopten. It is more likely to occur in patients who have been volume- and salt-depleted by prolonged diuretic therapy, dietary salt restriction, dialysis, diarrhoea or vomiting. Therefore, in these patients, diuretic therapy should be discontinued and volume and/or salt depletion should be corrected before initiating therapy with Gopten.

If symptomatic hypotension occurs, the patient should be placed in a supine position and, if necessary, receive an intravenous infusion of physiological saline. Intravenous atropine may be necessary if there is associated bradycardia. Treatment with Gopten may usually be continued following restoration of effective blood volume and blood pressure.

Surgery/anaesthesia: In patients undergoing surgery or during anaesthesia with agents producing hypotension, Gopten may block angiotensin II formation secondary to compensatory renin release. If hypotension occurs and is considered to be due to this mechanism, it can be corrected by appropriate treatment.

Agranulocytosis and bone marrow depression: In patients on ACE inhibitors, agranulocytosis and bone marrow depression have been seen rarely. They are more frequent in patients with renal impairment, especially if they have a collagen vascular disease. However, regular monitoring of white blood cell counts and protein levels in urine should be considered in patients with collagen vascular disease (e.g. lupus erythematosus and scleroderma), especially associated with impaired renal function and concomitant therapy, particularly with corticosteroids and antimetabolites.

Hyperkalaemia: Elevated serum potassium has been observed very rarely in hypertensive patients. Risk factors for the development of hyperkalaemia include renal insufficiency, potassium-sparing diuretics, the concomitant use of agents to treat hypokalaemia, diabetes mellitus and/or left ventricular dysfunction after myocardial infarction.

Angioneurotic oedema: Rarely, ACE inhibitors (such as trandolapril) may cause angioneurotic oedema that includes swelling of the face, extremities, tongue, glottis, and/or larynx. Patients experiencing angioneurotic oedema must immediately discontinue Gopten therapy and be monitored until oedema resolution.

Angioneurotic oedema to the face will usually resolve spontaneously. Oedema involving not only the face but also the glottis may be life-threatening because of the risk of airway obstruction.

Angioneurotic oedema involving the tongue, glottis or larynx requires immediate subcutaneous administration of 0.3–0.5 ml of adrenaline solution (1:1000) along with other therapeutic measures as appropriate.

Caution must be exercised in patients with a history of idiopathic angioneurotic oedema, and Gopten is contra-indicated if angioneurotic oedema was an adverse reaction to an ACE inhibitor (see Contra-indications).

Cough: During treatment with an ACE inhibitor, a dry and non-productive cough may occur which disappears after discontinuation.

*Interaction with other medicaments and other forms of interaction:* Drug interactions: Combination with diuretics or other antihypertensive agents may potentiate the antihypertensive response to Gopten. Adrenergic-blocking drugs should only be combined with trandolapril under careful supervision.

Potassium-sparing diuretics (spironolactone, amiloride, triamterene) or potassium supplements may increase the risk of hyperkalaemia, particularly in renal failure. Gopten may attenuate the potassium loss caused by thiazide-type diuretics. If concomitant use of these agents is indicated, they should be given with caution and serum potassium should be monitored regularly.

Antidiabetic agents: As with all ACE inhibitors, concomitant use of antidiabetic medicines (insulin or oral hypoglycaemic agents) may cause an increased blood glucose lowering effect with greater risk of hypoglycaemia. Therefore, blood glucose should be closely monitored in diabetics treated with a hypoglycaemic agent and Gopten, particularly when starting or increasing the dose of ACE inhibitor, or in patients with impaired renal function.

Combinations necessitating a warning: In some patients already receiving diuretic treatment, particularly if this treatment has been recently instituted, the fall in blood pressure on initiation of treatment with Gopten may be excessive. The risk of symptomatic hypotension may be reduced by stopping the diuretic a few days before starting treatment with Gopten. If it is necessary to continue the diuretic treatment, the patient should be monitored, at least after the initial administration of Gopten. As with all antihypertensives, combination with a neuroleptic or tricyclic antidepressant increases the risk of orthostatic hypotension. Gopten may reduce the elimination of lithium and serum levels of lithium should be monitored.

Anaphylactoid reactions to high-flux polyacrylonitrile membranes used in haemodialysis have been reported in patients treated with ACE inhibitors. As with other antihypertensives of this chemical class, this combination should be avoided when prescribing ACE inhibitors to renal dialysis patients.

The effects of certain anaesthetics may be enhanced by ACE inhibitors .

Allopurinol, cytostatic or immunosuppressive agents, systemic corticosteroids or procainamide may increase the risk of leucopenia , if used concomitantly with ACE inhibitors.

The antihypertensive effect of ACE inhibitors may be reduced by the administration of NSAIDs. An additive effect on serum potassium increase has been described when NSAIDs and ACE inhibitors have been used concomitantly, while renal function may be reduced.

Antacids cause reduced bioavailability of ACE inhibitors.

The antihypertensive effects of ACE inhibitors may be reduced by sympathomimetics. Patients should be carefully monitored.

No clinical interaction has been observed in patients with left ventricular dysfunction after myocardial infarction when Gopten has been concomitantly administered with thrombolytics, aspirin, beta-blockers, calcium channel blockers, nitrates, anticoagulants, diuretics or digoxin.

*Pregnancy and lactation:* The use of Gopten is contraindicated in pregnancy and lactation. Pregnancy should be excluded before start of treatment and avoided during treatment. Exposure of the mother to ACE inhibitors in mid or late pregnancy has been associated with oligohydramnios and neonatal hypotension with anuria or renal failure.

In the rat and particularly in the rabbit, trandolapril caused maternal toxicity together with foetotoxicity at high doses. Neither embryotoxicity nor teratogenicity was observed in the rat, rabbit or monkey.

*Effects on ability to drive and use machines:* Given the pharmacological properties of Gopten, no particular effect is expected. However, in some individuals, ACE inhibitors may affect the ability to drive or operate machinery, particularly at the start of treatment, when changing over from other medication or during concomitant use of alcohol. Therefore, after the first dose or subsequent increases in dose, it is not advisable to drive or operate machinery for several hours.

*Undesirable effects:* The following adverse events have been reported with ACE inhibitors as a class. Not all will have been reported in association with Gopten.

In long-term studies with Gopten, the most frequently reported adverse events were cough, headaches, asthenia and dizziness.

Respiratory: Dyspnoea, sinusitis, rhinitis, glossitis, bronchitis and bronchospasm have been reported, but rarely in association with treatment with ACE inhibitors.

Cardiovascular: Tachycardia, palpitations, arrhythmias, angina pectoris, myocardial infarction, transient ischaemic attacks and cerebral haemorrhage have been reported in association with hypotension during treatment with ACE inhibitors.

Gastrointestinal: Nausea, vomiting, abdominal pain, indigestion, diarrhoea, constipation and dry mouth have occurred occasionally during treatment with ACE inhibitors.

There have been reports of individual incidents of cholestatic jaundice, hepatitis, pancreatitis, and ileus connected with the use of ACE inhibitors.

Hypersensitivity: Allergic hypersensitivity reactions such as pruritus and rash have been reported. Urticaria, erythema multiforme, Stevens-Johnson syndrome, toxic epidermal necrolysis, psoriasis-like efflorescences and alopecia, which may be accompanied by fever, myalgia, arthralgia, eosinophilia and/or increased ANA (anti-nuclear antibody)-titres have been occasionally reported with ACE inhibitor treatment.

Angioneurotic oedema: In very rare cases, angioneurotic oedema has occurred. If laryngeal stridor or angioedema of the face, tongue or glottis occurs, treatment with Gopten must be discontinued and appropriate therapy instituted immediately.

Renal: Deterioration of renal function and acute renal failure have been reported with the use of ACE inhibitors.

Drug/Laboratory parameters: Reversible (on stopping treatment) increases in blood urea and plasma creatinine may result, particularly if renal insufficiency, severe heart failure, or renovascular hypertension are present.

Decreased haemoglobin, haematocrit, platelets and white cell count, and individual cases of agranulocytosis or pancytopenia, have been reported with ACE inhibitor treatment; also evaluate liver enzymes and serum bilirubin. Haemolytic anaemia has been reported in some patients with a congenital deficiency concerning G-6-PDH (glucose-6-phosphate dehydrogenase) during treatment with ACE inhibitors.

*Overdose:* Symptoms expected with ACE inhibitors are severe hypotension, shock, stupor, bradycardia, electrolyte disturbance and renal failure. In the event of overdosage following recent ingestion, consideration should be given to emptying the stomach contents. Blood pressure should be monitored and if hypotension develops, volume expansion should be considered.

**Pharmacological properties**

*Pharmacodynamic properties:* Gopten capsules contain the prodrug, trandolapril, a non-peptide ACE inhibitor with a carboxyl group but without a sulphydryl group. Trandolapril is rapidly absorbed and then non-specifically hydrolysed to its potent, long-acting active metabolite, trandolaprilat.

Trandolaprilat binds tightly and in a saturable manner to ACE. The administration of trandolapril causes decreases in the concentrations of angiotensin II, aldosterone and atrial natriuretic factor and increases in plasma renin activity and concentrations of angiotensin I. Gopten thus modulates the renin-angiotensin-aldosterone system which plays a major part in regulating blood volume and blood pressure and consequently has a beneficial antihypertensive effect.

The administration of usual therapeutic doses of Gopten to hypertensive patients produces a marked reduction in both supine and erect blood pressure. The antihypertensive effect is evident after 1 hour, with a peak effect between 8 and 12 hours, persisting for at least 24 hours.

The properties of trandolapril might explain the results obtained in the regression of cardiac hypertrophy with improvement of diastolic function, and improvement of arterial compliance in humans. In addition, a decrease in vascular hypertrophy has been shown in animals.

*Pharmacokinetic properties:* Trandolapril is very rapidly absorbed after oral administration. The amount absorbed is equivalent to 40 to 60% of the administered dose and is not affected by food consumption.

The peak plasma concentration of trandolapril is observed 30 minutes after administration. Trandolapril disappears rapidly from the plasma with a half-life of less than one hour.

Trandolapril is hydrolysed to trandolaprilat, a specific ACE inhibitor. The amount of trandolaprilat formed is not modified by food consumption. The peak plasma concentration of trandolaprilat is reached after 4 to 6 hours.

In the plasma, trandolaprilat is more than 80% protein-bound. It binds saturably, with a high affinity, to ACE. The major proportion of circulating trandolaprilat is also non-saturably bound to albumin.

After repeated administration of Gopten in a single daily dose, steady state is reached on average in four days, both in healthy volunteers and in young or elderly hypertensives. The effective half-life of trandolaprilat is between 16 and 24 hours. The terminal half-life of elimination is between 47 hours and 98 hours depending on dose. This terminal phase probably represents binding/dissociation kinetics of the trandolaprilat/ACE complex.

Trandolaprilat eliminated in the urine in the unchanged form accounts for 10 to 15% of the dose of trandolapril administered. After oral administration of the labelled product in man, 33% of the radioactivity is found in the urine and 66% in the faeces.

The renal clearance of trandolaprilat is proportional to the creatinine clearance. The plasma concentrations of trandolaprilat are significantly higher in patients with a creatinine clearance less than or equal to 30 ml/min. However, after repeated dosing in patients with chronic renal failure, steady state is also reached on average in four days, whatever the degree of renal failure.

*Preclinical safety data:* Acute oral toxicity studies of trandolapril and its active metabolite, trandolaprilat, in rats and mice showed both compounds to be non-toxic with respective LD50 values of > 4000 mg/kg and > 5000 mg/kg.

Repeat dose oral toxicity was evaluated in the rat and dog with studies of up to 18 and 12 months' duration, respectively. The principal observations in these studies were of anaemia (doses of 20 mg/kg/day and above in the rat 30-day study and 25 mg/kg/day and above in the dog 6-month study), gastric irritation and ulceration (doses of 20 mg/kg/day and above in the rat 30-day study and 125 mg/kg/day in the dog 6-month study) and renal lesions (20 mg/kg/day and above in the rat 30-day study and 10 mg/kg/day in the dog 30-day study). Renal lesions were also seen in the 6-month studies in the rat and dog (from doses of 0.25 and 25 mg/kg/day, respectively); these were reversible on cessation of treatment.

Reproduction toxicity studies showed effects on renal development in offspring with increased incidence of renal pelvic dilation; this was seen at doses of 10 mg/kg/day and above in the rat but these changes did not affect the normal development of the offspring.

Trandolapril was not mutagenic or carcinogenic.

**Pharmaceutical particulars**

*List of excipients:* Corn starch PhEur, lactose PhEur, povidone PhEur, sodium stearyl fumarate USNF, printing ink (shellac, industrial methylated spirit, purified water, soya lecithin, 2-ethoxyethanol, dimethylpolysiloxane, black iron oxide), E171 (titanium dioxide), E127 (erythrosine), E172 (yellow iron oxide), gelatin.

*Incompatibilities:* None.

*Shelf life:* Gopten 0.5 mg: 24 months. Gopten 1.0 mg, 2.0 mg: 36 months.

*Special precautions for storage:* PVC/Al pack: Store in a dry place. Aluminium pack: None.

*Nature and contents of container:* Gopten 0.5 mg: PVC/Al or Aluminium calendar pack containing 14 capsules. Gopten 1.0 mg, 2.0 mg: PVC/Al or Aluminium calendar pack containing 28 capsules.

*Instructions for use/handling:* None.

**Marketing authorisation number**
Gopten Capsules 0.5 mg   00169/0031
Gopten Capsules 1.0 mg   00169/0030
Gopten Capsules 2.0 mg   00169/0029

**Date of approval/revision of SPC**   January 1997

**Legal category**   POM

# HYDRENOX*

**Qualitative and quantitative composition** Hydroflumethiazide BP 50 mg

**Pharmaceutical form** White tablets, scored on one side and marked with the letter 'H' on the reverse.

**Clinical particulars**

*Therapeutic indications:* For the treatment of oedema and hypertension.

*Posology and method of administration:* For oral administration.

*Diuretic:* 50 to 200 mg daily, depending upon the severity of the oedema, as a single dose in the morning. The daily dose should be given early enough to complete diuresis by bedtime. Doses of 25 to 50 mg on alternate days are usually adequate for maintenance therapy.

*Antihypertensive:* 25 to 50 mg daily. When Hydrenox is used concurrently with other antihypertensive agents, the dose of the latter should be halved.

*Children:* Dosage in children is at the discretion of the physician. 1 mg/kg of bodyweight has been suggested as suitable for most cases.

*Elderly:* The dosage of thiazide diuretics may need to be reduced in the elderly, particularly when renal function is impaired, because of the possibility of electrolyte imbalance.

*Contra-indications:* Hydrenox is contra-indicated in severe renal failure and in patients with known hypersensitivity to thiazides.

*Special warnings and special precautions for use:* Hydroflumethiazide should be used with caution in patients with Addison's disease, hypercalcaemia and hepatic or renal impairment. Renal function should be continuously monitored during thiazide therapy. Thiazide diuretics may exacerbate or activate systemic lupus erythematosus in susceptible patients.

All thiazide diuretics can produce a degree of electrolyte imbalance, especially in patients with renal or hepatic impairment or when dosage is high or prolonged. Serum electrolytes should be checked for abnormalities, particularly hypokalaemia, and the latter corrected by the addition of a potassium supplement to the regimen.

*Interaction with other medicaments and other forms of interaction:* Sensitivity to digitalis glycosides may be increased by the hypokalaemic effect of concurrent hydroflumethiazide. Patients should be observed for signs of digitalis intoxication, in particular arrhythmias, and if these appear, the dosage of the digitalis glycoside should be temporarily reduced and a potassium supplement given to restore stability.

Serum lithium concentrations may be increased by concurrent use of thiazide diuretics.

Non-steroidal anti-inflammatory agents may blunt the diuretic and antihypertensive effects of thiazide diuretics.

ACTH, corticosteroids, acetazolamide and carbenoxolone may exacerbate the hypokalaemia associated with thiazide use. Thiazide diuretics may enhance the neuromuscular blocking effects of the non-depolarising muscle relaxants, e.g. tubocurarine.

Thiazides may enhance the effects of antihypertensive agents, while postural hypotension associated with therapy may be enhanced by concomitant ingestion of alcohol, barbiturates or opioids.

Hydroflumethiazide may interfere with a number of laboratory tests, including estimation of serum protein-bound iodine and tests of parathyroid function.

*Pregnancy and lactation:* Diuretics are best avoided for the management of oedema of pregnancy or hypertension in pregnancy as their use may be associated with hypokalaemia, increased blood viscosity and reduced placental perfusion.

There is inadequate evidence of safety in human pregnancy and foetal bone marrow depression and thrombocytopenia have been described. Foetal and neonatal jaundice have also been described.

As diuretics pass into breast milk and hydroflumethiazide can suppress lactation, its use should be avoided in mothers who wish to breast feed.

*Effects on ability to drive and use machines:* No adverse effects known.

*Undesirable effects:* All thiazide diuretics can produce a degree of electrolyte imbalance, e.g. hypokalaemia.

Thiazide diuretics may raise the serum uric acid levels with subsequent exacerbation of gout in susceptible subjects.

Thiazide diuretics sometimes lower carbohydrate tolerance and the insulin dosage of the diabetic patient may require adjustment. Care is necessary when hydroflumethiazide is administered to those with a known predisposition to diabetes.

Rarely, blood dyscrasias, including agranulocytosis, aplastic anaemia, thrombocytopenia and leucopenia, and pancreatitis have been reported with long-term therapy. Skin rashes and impotence have occasionally been reported.

*Overdose:* Symptoms of overdosage include anorexia, nausea, vomiting, diarrhoea, diuresis, dehydration, hypotension, dizziness, weakness, muscle cramps, paraesthesia, tetany, gastrointestinal bleeding, hyponatraemia, hypo- or hyperglycaemia, hypokalaemia and metabolic alkalosis. Initial treatment consists of either emesis or gastric lavage, if appropriate. Otherwise treatment should be symptomatic and supportive including the correction of fluid and electrolyte imbalance. Blood pressure should also be monitored. There is no specific antidote.

**Pharmacological properties**

*Pharmacodynamic properties:* Hydroflumethiazide is a thiazide diuretic which reduces the absorption of electrolytes from the renal tubules, thereby increasing the excretion of sodium and chloride ions, and consequently of water. The excretion of other electrolytes, notably potassium and magnesium, is also increased. The excretion of calcium is reduced. Thiazides also reduce carbonic anhydrase activity so that bicarbonate excretion is increased, but this effect is generally small and does not appreciably alter the acid-base balance or the pH of the urine. Thiazides also have a hypotensive effect, due to a reduction in peripheral resistance and enhance the effects of other antihypertensive agents.

*Pharmacokinetic properties:* Hydroflumethiazide is incompletely but fairly rapidly absorbed from the gastrointestinal tract. It has a metabolite which is reported to be extensively bound to red blood cells. Hydroflumethiazide is excreted in the urine. Its metabolite has also been detected in the urine.

*Preclinical safety data:* Not applicable.

**Pharmaceutical particulars**

*List of excipients:* Lactose, maize starch, stearic acid, talc.

*Incompatibilities:* Not applicable.

*Shelf life:* 36 months.

*Special precautions for storage:* None.

*Nature and contents of container:* Amber glass bottle with a tin-plate screw cap with a waxed aluminium-faced pulpboard liner. Pack sizes: 100.

*Instructions for use/handling:* None.

**Marketing authorisation number**   0169/0072

**Date of approval/revision of SPC**   July 1995

**Legal category**   POM

## HYDROCORTISTAB* INJECTION

**Qualitative and quantitative composition**   Hydrocortisone Acetate PhEur 2.5% w/v (25 mg/ml)

**Pharmaceutical form**   Suspension for injection.

**Clinical particulars**

*Therapeutic indications:* Hydrocortistab Injection is indicated for the local treatment, by intra-articular or periarticular injection, of arthritic conditions such as rheumatoid arthritis and osteoarthritis when few joints are involved. It is also suitable for the symptomatic treatment, by local injection, of certain non-articular inflammatory conditions such as inflamed tendon sheaths and bursae.

Hydrocortistab Injection is not suitable for the production of systemic effects.

*Posology and method of administration:* For intra-articular or periarticular injection. Hydrocortistab Injection may also be injected into non-articular tissues (e.g. tendon sheaths/bursae).

Adults: 5–50 mg, depending on the size of the joint.
Children: 5–30 mg, daily in divided doses.
Elderly: Steroids should be used cautiously in the elderly, since adverse effects are enhanced in old age.

No more than three joints should be treated in one day. The injection may be repeated at intervals of about three weeks.

*Contra-indications:* Hydrocortistab Injection is contra-indicated in patients with known hypersensitivity to any of the ingredients, and in patients with systemic infections, unless specific anti-infective therapy is employed.

Intra-articular and periarticular injections of Hydrocortistab Injection are contra-indicated when the joint or surrounding tissues are infected. The presence of infection also precludes injection into tendon sheaths and bursae. Hydrocortistab Injection must not be injected directly into tendons, nor should it be injected into spinal or other non-diarthrodial joints.

*Special warnings and special precautions for use:* Since joints and tissues injected with corticosteroids have an increased susceptibility to infection, local injections of Hydrocortistab should be carried out with full aseptic precautions.

Caution is necessary when prescribing corticosteroids in patients with the following conditions:

(a) Previous history of tuberculosis or characteristic appearance on chest X-ray. The emergence of active tuberculosis can, however, be prevented by the prophylactic use of antituberculous therapy.

(b) Diabetes mellitus (or a family history of diabetes).

(c) Osteoporosis (postmenopausal females are particularly at risk).

(d) Hypertension.

(e) History of severe affective disorders (especially previous history of steroid psychosis).

(f) Glaucoma (or a family history of glaucoma).

(g) Previous steroid myopathy.

(h) Peptic ulceration.

(i) Epilepsy.

(j) Vaccination with live vaccines.

Use in children: Corticosteroids cause growth retardation in infancy, childhood and adolescence. Treatment should be limited to the minimum dosage for the shortest possible time, in order to minimise suppression of the hypothalamo-pituitary-adrenal axis and growth retardation.

Use in the elderly: Treatment of elderly patients, particularly if long-term, should be planned bearing in mind the more serious consequences of the common side effects of corticosteroids in old age, especially osteoporosis, diabetes, hypertension, susceptibility to infection and thinning of the skin.

*Interaction with other medicaments and other forms of interaction:* The effectiveness of anticoagulants may be increased or decreased with concurrent corticosteroid therapy.

Serum levels of salicylates may increase considerably if corticosteroid therapy is withdrawn, possibly causing intoxication. Since both salicylates and corticosteroids are ulcerogenic, it is possible that there will be an increased rate of gastrointestinal ulceration.

The actions of hypoglycaemic drugs will be antagonised by the hyperglycaemic actions of corticosteroids.

Since amphotericin, diuretics (acetazolamide, loop diuretics and thiazides) and corticosteroids have potassium-depleting effects, signs of hypokalaemia should be looked for during their concurrent use.

There is a small amount of evidence that the simultaneous use of corticosteroids and methotrexate may cause increased methotrexate toxicity and possibly death, although this combination of drugs has been used very successfully.

The therapeutic effects of corticosteroids may be reduced by certain barbiturates (particularly when given at high doses), phenytoin and rifampicin.

The concurrent use of corticosteroids with antacids, cimetidine or theophylline appears to have no effect on the therapeutic use of either drug.

*Pregnancy and lactation:* There is evidence of harmful effects in pregnancy in animals.

There is inadequate evidence of safety in human pregnancy and there may be a very small risk of cleft palate and intra-uterine growth retardation in the foetus.

Trace amounts of hydrocortisone have been measured in breast milk but it is doubtful if these amounts are clinically significant. However, in lactation, continuous therapy with high doses could possibly affect the child's adrenal function. Monitor carefully.

The decision to use Hydrocortistab Injection during pregnancy and lactation must be made by weighing up the relative risks associated with the use of the drug against the potential benefits in maternal disease.

*Effects on ability to drive and use machines:* No adverse effects known.

*Undesirable effects:* With intra-articular or other local injections, the principal side effect encountered is a temporary local exacerbation with increased pain and swelling. This normally subsides after a few hours.

In certain circumstances, particularly after high or prolonged local dosage, corticosteroids can be absorbed in amounts sufficient to produce systemic effects.

The following side effects may be associated with the long-term systemic use of corticosteroids.

Gastrointestinal: Dyspepsia, peptic ulceration with perforation and haemorrhage, abdominal distension, oesophageal ulceration, oesophageal candidiasis, acute pancreatitis.

Musculoskeletal: Proximal myopathy, osteoporosis, vertebral and long bone fractures, avascular osteonecrosis, tendon rupture.

Fluid and electrolyte disturbance: Sodium and water retention, hypertension, hypokalaemic alkalosis.

Dermatological: Impaired healing, skin atrophy, bruising, striae, acne, telangiectasia.

Endocrine/metabolic: Suppression of the hypothalamo-pituitary-adrenal axis, growth suppression in childhood and adolescence, menstrual irregularity and amenorrhoea. Cushingoid facies, hirsutism, weight gain, impaired carbohydrate tolerance with increased requirement for antidiabetic therapy, negative nitrogen balance.

Neuropsychiatric: Euphoria, psychological dependence, depression, insomnia. Intracranial hypertension in children. Aggravation of schizophrenia.

Ophthalmic: Increased intra-ocular pressure, glaucoma, papilloedema, cataracts, corneal or scleral thinning, exacerbation of ophthalmic viral disease.

General: Opportunistic infection, recurrence of dormant tuberculosis, leucocytosis, hypersensitivity, thromboembolism, increased appetite, nausea, malaise.

Withdrawal symptoms and signs: Fever, myalgia, arthralgia, adrenal insufficiency.

*Overdose:* Overdosage is unlikely with Hydrocortistab Injection but there is no specific antidote available. Treatment should be symptomatic.

**Pharmacological properties**

*Pharmacodynamic properties:* Hydrocortisone has both glucocorticoid and mineralocorticoid activity.

*Pharmacokinetic properties:* Absorption following intra-articular or soft tissue injection is slow. Systemic absorption occurs slowly after local, intra-articular injection. Hydrocortisone is more than 90% bound to plasma proteins. Hydrocortisone is metabolised in the liver and most body tissues to hydrogenated and degraded forms, such as tetrahydrocortisone and tetrahydrocortisol. These are excreted in the urine, mainly conjugated as glucuronides, together with a very small proportion of unchanged hydrocortisone.

*Preclinical safety data:* Not applicable.

**Pharmaceutical particulars**

*List of excipients:* Water for injections, benzyl alcohol, sodium chloride for injections, sodium carboxymethylcellulose, polysorbate 80, with sodium hydroxide and/or hydrochloric acid as pH adjusters.

*Incompatibilities:* Not applicable.

*Shelf life:* 36 months.

*Special precautions for storage:* Store at 15–25°C and protect from light. Do not freeze.

*Nature and contents of container:* Glass ampoules. Pack size: 10×1 ml ampoules.

*Instructions for use/handling:* Shake the ampoule well before use. Do not freeze.

**Marketing authorisation number** 00169/0074

**Date of approval/revision of SPC** April 1996

**Legal category** POM

## KAODENE*

**Presentation** Kaodene is an aqueous suspension containing Codeine Phosphate PhEur 10 mg and Light Kaolin BP 3 g in each 10 ml. It is an off-white liquid with the odour and flavour of aniseed.

*Other ingredients:* Purified water; chloroform; xanthan gum; blanose sodium carboxymethylcellulose; vanilla essence; methyl hydroxybenzoate; anise oil; propyl hydroxybenzoate; sodium saccharin; peppermint oil.

**Uses** Kaodene is indicated for the symptomatic relief of simple diarrhoea.

**Dosage and administration** *Adults, elderly and children over 12 years:* 20 ml three or four times daily.

*Children from 5 to 12 years:* 10 ml three or four times daily.
*Children under 5 years:* Not recommended.

**Contra-indications, warnings, etc** Kaodene is contraindicated in patients with pseudomembranous colitis, diverticular disease or respiratory depression.

It should be used with caution in patients with ulcerative colitis and hepatic or renal dysfunction.

The long-term administration of Kaodene, particularly in the elderly, is not recommended.

It cannot be used as a substitute for rehydration therapy.

Codeine phosphate is a narcotic analgesic and, given in large doses, may induce tolerance and psychological and physical dependence.

It may occasionally cause drowsiness, nausea, vomiting and constipation.

Large doses of codeine may cause drowsiness and CNS depression, but this should not be a problem with the recommended doses of Kaodene.

*Effects on ability to drive and use machines:* Kaodene may cause drowsiness and may therefore influence the ability to drive and use machines.

*Use in pregnancy and lactation:* The safety of Kaodene during pregnancy has not been established and therefore use of the product during this period should be avoided, unless under medical supervision. In limited studies, codeine appears in the breast milk in very low concentrations and is unlikely to affect the breast-fed infant adversely.

*Drug interactions:* Kaodene may interfere with the absorption of some drugs from the gastrointestinal tract, including certain antibiotics and digoxin. The depressant effects of codeine are enhanced by alcohol. May interact with monoamine oxidase inhibitors.

*Interference with laboratory tests:* Administration of Kaodene may interfere with laboratory estimations of serum amylase and certain liver function tests.

*Overdosage:* Symptoms of overdosage include the adverse effects given above. In addition, large overdoses may produce respiratory depression, hypotension, circulatory failure and deepening coma. Initial treatment includes emptying the stomach by aspiration and lavage. Intensive supportive therapy may be required to correct respiratory failure and shock. In addition the narcotic antagonist, naloxone hydrochloride, may be used to counteract very rapidly the severe respiratory depression and coma. A dose in adults of 0.4–2 mg is given intravenously or intramuscularly, repeated at intervals of 2–3 minutes if necessary up to 10 mg. In children, doses of naloxone of 5–10 micrograms/kg bodyweight may be given intravenously or intramuscularly.

**Pharmaceutical precautions** No special storage conditions are necessary.

**Legal category** CD (Sch 5), P.

**Package quantities** Bottle of 250 ml.

**Further information** Nil.

**Product licence number** 0169/0078.

## MUSTINE HYDROCHLORIDE FOR INJECTION BP

**Presentation** Synonyms: Chlormethine Hydrochloride (INN); Nitrogen Mustard; Mustargen Hydrochloride.

Mustine hydrochloride is di (2-chloroethyl) methylamine hydrochloride. It is a white or almost white hygroscopic, vesicant, crystalline powder or mass and is very soluble in water.

Mustine hydrochloride is supplied in sterile vials each containing 10 mg of the powder. The injection is prepared by dissolving this in Sodium Chloride Injection BP 0.9% w/v or Water for Injections BP.

**Uses** Mustine Hydrochloride BP is a powerful cytotoxic agent used in the treatment of several neoplastic conditions. It is an alkylating agent and also possesses immunosuppressant properties.

The principal use of mustine hydrochloride is as part of combination treatment for Hodgkin's disease. It is sometimes used in non-Hodgkin's lymphomas and carcinoma of bronchus, ovary and breast. It may be applied locally for the treatment of mycosis fungoides.

**Dosage and administration** *Routes of administration:* Intravenous injection or topical application.

*Intravenous injection*

*Recommended dose and dosage schedule:* Single doses of 0.4 mg/kg bodyweight or a course of 4 daily doses of 0.1 mg/kg given by intravenous injection. The term 'bodyweight' is defined, in this case, as the actual bodyweight at the time of treatment except in cases where the weight has been artificially increased by oedema, ascites, or other fluid collections. The weight of the body before the increase is used in such cases.

UNDER NO CIRCUMSTANCES SHOULD MUSTINE BE GIVEN INTRAMUSCULARLY.

A repeat course of mustine therapy should not be undertaken for at least 6 weeks or until the bone marrow has recovered its haemopoietic activity.

*Preparation of intravenous injection:* A fresh solution is prepared by dissolving 10 mg of mustine hydrochloride in 10 ml of Sodium Chloride Injection BP 0.9% w/v, or Water for Injections BP. The best method of administration is to set up an intravenous drip of Sodium Chloride Injection BP 0.9% w/v or Dextrose Injection BP 5% w/v; the required dose of mustine, prepared as above, is then injected into the tubing. This avoids the hazards of extravasation during injection. The drip rate should be fast at approximately 60 drops per minute and the injection of mustine should be carried out over 2 minutes. The drip rate should then be reduced to 20 drops per minute.

Alternatively, the concentrated solution of mustine hydrochloride is freshly prepared as above and transferred aseptically to 500 ml of sterile Sodium Chloride Injection BP 0.9% w/v.

*Topical use:* Mycosis fungoides may be treated by topical application of a dilute solution of mustine hydrochloride. Various strengths of mustine hydrochloride have been used but 20 mg in 100 ml of 0.9% w/v Sodium Chloride Injection BP or Water for Injections BP is frequently recommended.

This solution is applied to the affected cutaneous area using a gauze pad. The person applying the solution should wear polyvinylchloride gloves to give protection.

*Elderly:* Elderly patients with generalised vascular disease may be more prone to local vascular and extravascular toxicity.

**Contra-indications, warnings, etc** Mustine should not be given during pregnancy or during lactation to mothers who are breast-feeding. The drug possesses foetotoxic and teratogenic potential.

Mustine should not be used in patients with severe leucopenia, thrombocytopenia or anaemia and in co-existent or suspected granuloma.

*Precautions and warnings*
1. *Extravasation:* Extravasation during injection should be avoided as this may cause severe tissue necrosis. Infusion should be stopped immediately if local pain is experienced. Where doubt occurs as to whether significant leakage has occurred, the infusion should be discontinued and the cannula resited in another vein. If extravasation does occur during injection, the involved area should be infiltrated with isotonic sodium thiosulphate injection followed by the application of an ice compress intermittently for six to twelve hours. Management of extravasation must be carried out quickly because of mustine's rapid local toxic effects.

2. *Handling:*
(a) Trained personnel should reconstitute the drug.
(b) This should be performed in a designated area, which has good general and local ventilation.
(c) The work surface should be covered with disposable plastic-backed absorbent paper.
(d) Protective gloves should be worn – polyvinylchloride gloves give adequate protection whereas rubber and polyethylene gloves have been shown to be ineffective.
(e) Mustine hydrochloride is a potent vesicant and local irritant to skin and mucous membranes. It can cause severe damage to eyes and the vapour irritates the respiratory tract. Precautions should be taken to prevent accidental contact with skin, eyes and clothing. Avoid ingestion and inhalation.

*First aid measures:*
(i) Eyes – Immediately irrigate with large amounts of water or 2% solution of sodium bicarbonate for at least 10 minutes and obtain urgent medical attention. The person concerned should then be seen by an ophthalmologist.
(ii) Skin – Wash away immediately with large amounts of water or, if at hand, sodium carbonate solution or an isotonic solution of sodium thiosulphate.
(iii) If accidentally ingested, wash out the mouth thoroughly with water and give water to drink.
(iv) If inhaled – remove to fresh air.
Urgent medical attention should be sought after any of these occurrences.
(f) Mustine hydrochloride should not be handled by pregnant staff.
(g) Adequate care and precautions should be taken in the disposal of items (syringes, needles, etc.) used to reconstitute cytotoxic drugs.
(h) After treatment with mustine all apparatus, including PVC gloves should be washed thoroughly. A 2.5% solution of sodium carbonate is particularly suitable for the lavage or the use of the following solution:

*Decontamination solution:* Distilled water 3 litres; Caustic soda solution SG 1.50–1 litre; Industrial Methylated Spirit (IMS) 66 OP–4.5 litres. This solution should be prepared at least 24 hours before use and placed under work bench near ventilation exhaust. Decontamination procedure – bottles (including caps), equipment, etc., must be dismantled as far as possible and immersed in the decontamination solution for at least 48 hours. The solution should then be decanted to the sluice and bottles, equipment, etc. washed three times with clean water prior to disposal. Note: Bottles, equipment, etc. may be temporarily stored awaiting decontamination on a suitable tray which is then placed inside a plastic bag and securely tied.
(i) Use Luèr-lock fittings on all syringes and sets. Large bore needles are recommended to minimise pressure and the possible formation of aerosols. The latter may also be reduced by the use of a venting needle.

3. *Side-effects:* Intravenous use: Nausea, emesis, fever and/or leucopenia are the most common side-effects. Nausea and vomiting often occur during the eight hours following injection and appropriate sedation and anti-emetics should be prescribed 10–30 minutes before mustine is injected. Transient anorexia and occasional diarrhoea may occur and peptic ulcers have been reported.

Neurological disturbances including lightheadedness, headache, drowsiness, tinnitus and deafness may occur. Skin rashes, alopecia and herpes zoster in patients with latent herpes infection have been reported.

Severe bone marrow depression may follow mustine therapy, with lymphocytopenia, granulocytopenia and occasionally, agranulocytosis. These conditions are more likely to occur in patients when the total dose in a single course of therapy exceeds 0.4 mg/kg bodyweight and in those who have had previous treatment with other antineoplastic agents or recent radiotherapy. Severe anaemia and thrombocytopenia may occur. Peripheral blood counts should be checked prior to each treatment. Leucocytes and platelet counts in peripheral blood start to fall about one week after treatment with a nadir between 14 and 18 days. During the same period there is a fall in haemoglobin levels. Both leucocyte and platelet counts return to normal before the end of the fourth week. Vein irritation leading to discolouration may occur, even in the absence of extravasation. Thrombophlebitis and venous thrombosis are potential complications of mustine therapy.

Subsequent to mustine administration, extensive and rapid development of amyloidosis may occur in the presence of acute and chronic suppurative inflammation.

In non-pregnant women, delayed menstruation or temporary amenorrhoea may follow the treatment. In males, a reduction of active spermatogenesis has been reported. Hyperuricaemia may develop in patients with large tumour masses.

Prolonged use of alkylating agents, particularly when combined with extensive radiation, is associated with a marked increase in the incidence of acute non-lymphocytic leukaemia.

Topical use: When mustine is applied topically, patients may develop a contact dermatitis, but systemic side-effects have not been reported.

4. *Treatment of overdose:* Sodium thiosulphate will neutralise an injection of mustine hydrochloride BUT ONLY IF GIVEN IMMEDIATELY AFTERWARDS. Each 10 mg mustine requires 640 mg sodium thiosulphate given as an isotonic solution. This is equivalent to approximately 1.5 ml of a 50% injection of sodium thiosulphate diluted with 20 ml 0.9% sodium chloride injection or approximately 21 ml of 3% sodium thiosulphate injection.

*Drug interactions:* No clinically-significant drug interactions are known.

*Effects on ability to drive and use machines:* No adverse effects known.

**Pharmaceutical precautions** Store at 2° to 15°C.

*Stability of reconstituted solution:* Whenever possible, mustine injection should be reconstituted immediately before use. A study has been conducted to investigate the stability of mustine hydrochloride (1 mg/ml) in Sodium Chloride 0.9% Injection or Water for Injections, using an HPLC assay specific for mustine. The results suggest that to minimise accumulation of degradation products of mustine, reconstituted solutions should be used within 4 hours when stored at room temperature or 6 hours at 4°C. Solutions stored at –20°C in syringes degraded by about 5% in 4 weeks.

*Incompatibilities:* A 0.2% solution of mustine hydrochloride in water has a pH of 3 to 5 and it is recommended that mustine injection is administered in 0.9% sodium chloride or 5% dextrose since it is rapidly unstable in alkaline solutions.

**Legal category** POM.

**Package quantities** Pack of 10 vials.

**Further information** Following intravenous injection or infusion, mustine hydrochloride is rapidly converted to an ethyleneimmonium ion which alkylates and cross links guanine bases in the deoxyribonucleic acid of the chromosomes thus arresting cell division. Although its cytotoxic and growth-inhibitory action affects all cells, it has a special affinity for rapidly multiplying cells, including certain neoplastic growths, bone marrow and lymphatic tissues. The aim of treatment is, therefore, to build up maximal concentrations in the neoplastic tissues and permit minimal amounts to reach the normal tissues.

Mustine usually disappears from the blood within approximately 10 minutes. Less than 0.1% of the drug is excreted unchanged in the urine.

**Product licence number** 0169/0081.

## NIVEMYCIN*

**Qualitative and quantitative composition** Each tablet contains an amount of Neomycin Sulphate PhEur equivalent to 550 mg of material having a potency of 700 units/mg.

**Pharmaceutical form** Tablets.

**Clinical particulars**

*Therapeutic indications:* Nivemycin (Neomycin Sulphate PhEur) is indicated for pre-operative sterilisation of the bowel and may be useful in the treatment of impending hepatic coma, including portal systemic encephalopathy.

*Posology and method of administration:* For oral administration.

Pre-operative sterilisation of the bowel:
Adults: Two tablets every hour for 4 hours, then 2 tablets every 4 hours for two or three days before the operation.
Children over 12 years: Two tablets every 4 hours for two or three days before the operation.
Children from 6 to 12 years: A half to one tablet every 4 hours for two or three days before the operation.
For practical reasons, use of the tablets in children under 6 years is not recommended.
In hepatic coma, the adult dose is 4–12 g/day in divided doses for a period of 5–7 days. For children, 50–100 mg/kg/day in divided doses appears appropriate. Chronic hepatic insufficiency may require up to 4 g/day over an indefinite period.
The elderly dose is the same as for adults.

*Contra-indications:* Nivemycin should not be given when intestinal obstruction is present. Hypersensitivity to aminoglycosides. Infants under 1 year.

*Special warnings and special precautions for use:* The absorption of neomycin is poor from the alimentary

tract, with about 97% of an orally-administered dose being excreted unchanged in the faeces. However, impaired GI motility may increase absorption of the drug and it is therefore possible, as with other broad-spectrum antibiotics, that prolonged therapy could result in ototoxicity and nephrotoxicity, particularly in patients with a degree of renal failure.

When used as an adjunct in the management of hepatic coma, care should be taken that administration is of the minimal period necessary, since prolonged exposure to the drug may result in malabsorption. Neomycin should be used with caution in patients with neuromuscular disorders and parkinsonism. There is almost complete cross-resistance between neomycin, kanamycin, paromomycin and framycetin. Cross-resistance with gentamicin has also been reported.

Since prolonged therapy may result in the overgrowth of non-sensitive organisms, treatment should not be continued longer than necessary to prevent superinfection due to the overgrowth of non-sensitive organisms.

*Interaction with other medicaments and other forms of interaction:* Neomycin may impair absorption of other drugs including phenoxymethylpenicillin and digoxin. The efficacy of oral contraceptives may be reduced. Care should be taken when considering the use of neomycin concurrently with drugs with a potential to cause nephrotoxicity or ototoxicity and with drugs with neuromuscular-blocking activity.

*Pregnancy and lactation:* The use of neomycin in pregnancy is not recommended unless the benefits outweigh the potential risks.

There are no reports linking the use of neomycin to congenital defects. However, small amounts of the drug are absorbed when given orally and neomycin and other aminoglycosides may have harmful effects on the foetus following oral absorption during pregnancy.

In some circumstances, neomycin may enter the breast milk of lactating mothers. There is little risk of ototoxicity in the infant, but abnormal development of the gut flora may occur. The use of neomycin in lactating mothers is not recommended unless the benefits outweigh the potential risks.

*Effects on ability to drive and use machines:* Not applicable.

*Undesirable effects:* Nausea, vomiting, diarrhoea, increased salivation, stomatitis, nephrotoxicity, ototoxicity, rise in serum levels of hepatic enzymes and bilirubin, blood dyscrasias, haemolytic anaemia, confusion, paraesthesia, disorientation, nystagmus, hypersensitivity reactions including dermatitis, pruritus, drug fever and anaphylaxis.

*Overdose:* In overdose, exacerbation of the adverse events reported for neomycin (nausea, diarrhoea, nephrotoxicity, ototoxicity etc) is expected.

Monitor renal and auditory function. If these are impaired, haemodialysis is indicated. Prolonged assisted ventilation may also be required.

**Pharmacological properties**

*Pharmacodynamic properties:* Neomycin is an aminoglycoside antibiotic. Neomycin acts by binding to polysomes, inhibiting protein synthesis and generating errors in the transcription of the genetic code.

*Pharmacokinetic properties:* The absorption of neomycin from the alimentary tract is poor: only ~3% of an oral dose is absorbed. Neomycin is rapidly excreted by the kidneys in the unchanged form. The plasma half-life in healthy adults is approximately 2–3 hours. Oral doses of 3 g produce peak plasma concentrations of up to 4 microgram/ml.

*Preclinical safety data:* Not applicable.

**Pharmaceutical particulars**

*List of excipients:* Plasdone K29-32, isopropyl alcohol, calcium stearate.

*Incompatibilities:* Not applicable.

*Shelf life:* 3 years.

*Special precautions for storage:* Store below 30°C in a dry place. Protect from light.

*Nature and contents of container:* An amber glass bottle having a tin-plate screw cap with a waxed aluminium-faced pulpboard liner. The ullage is filled with cotton wool. Pack size: 100 tablets.

*Instructions for use/handling:* Not applicable.

**Marketing authorisation number** 00169/0083

**Date of approval/revision of SPC** January 1996

**Legal category** POM

## PHENYLEPHRINE INJECTION BP
## 10 mg/ml

**Qualitative and quantitative composition** Phenylephrine Hydrochloride PhEur 1.0% w/v.

**Pharmaceutical form** Sterile solution.

**Clinical particulars**

*Therapeutic indications:* For the treatment of hypotensive states, e.g. circulatory failure, during spinal anaesthesia or drug-induced hypotension.

*Posology and method of administration:* For subcutaneous, intramuscular, slow intravenous injection or intravenous infusion.
Adults: Phenylephrine Injection may be administered subcutaneously or intramuscularly in a dosage of 2 to 5 mg with further doses of 1 to 10 mg if necessary according to response, or in a dose of 100 to 500 micrograms by slow intravenous injection as a 0.1% solution, repeated as necessary after at least 15 minutes.

Alternatively, 10 mg in 500 ml of glucose 5% injection or sodium chloride 0.9% injection may be infused intravenously, initially at a rate of up to 180 micrograms per minute, reduced according to response to 30–60 micrograms per minute.
*Children:* 100 microgram/kg bodyweight subcutaneously or intramuscularly.
*Elderly:* There is no need for dosage reduction in the elderly.

*Contra-indications:* Patients taking monoamine oxidase inhibitors, or within 14 days of ceasing such treatment. Severe hypertension and hyperthyroidism.

*Special warnings and special precautions for use:* Great care should be exercised in administering Phenylephrine Injection to patients with pre-existing cardiovascular disease such as ischaemic heart disease, arrhythmias, occlusive vascular disease including arteriosclerosis, hypertension or aneurysms. Anginal pain may be precipitated in patients with angina pectoris.

Care is also required when given to patients with diabetes mellitus or closed-angle glaucoma.

*Interaction with other medicaments and other forms of interaction:* Phenylephrine may interact with cyclopropane and halothane and other halogenated inhalational anaesthetics, to induce ventricular fibrillation. An increased risk of arrhythmias may also occur if Phenylephrine Injection is given to patients receiving cardiac glycosides, quinidine or tricyclic antidepressants.

Phenylephrine may increase blood pressure and consequently reverse the action of many antihypertensive agents. Interactions of phenylephrine with alpha- and beta-receptor blocking drugs may be complex.

*Pregnancy and lactation:* The safety of phenylephrine during pregnancy and lactation has not been established. Administration of phenylephrine in late pregnancy or labour may cause foetal hypoxia and bradycardia. Excretion of phenylephrine in breast milk appears to be minimal.

*Effects on ability to drive and use machines:* No adverse effects known.

*Undesirable effects:* Extravasation of Phenylephrine Injection may cause tissue necrosis. Phenylephrine will cause a rise in blood pressure with headache and vomiting and this may produce cerebral haemorrhage and pulmonary oedema. There may also be a reflex bradycardia or tachycardia, other cardiac arrhythmias, anginal pain, palpitations and cardiac arrest, hypotension with dizziness, and fainting and flushing. Phenylephrine may induce difficulty in micturition and urinary retention, dyspnoea, altered metabolism including disturbances of glucose metabolism, sweating, hypersalivation, transient tingling and coolness of the skin and temporary fullness of the head. Phenylephrine is without significant stimulating effects on the central nervous system at usual doses.

*Overdose:* Symptoms of overdosage include headache, vomiting, hypertension and reflex bradycardia and other cardiac arrhythmias.

Treatment should consist of symptomatic and supportive measures. The hypertensive effects may be treated with an alpha-adrenoceptor blocking drug, such as phentolamine, 5 to 60 mg i.v. over 10–30 minutes, repeated as necessary.

**Pharmacological properties**
*Pharmacodynamic properties:* Phenylephrine Injection is a sympathomimetic agent with mainly direct effects on adrenergic receptors. It has predominantly alpha-adrenergic activity and is without significant stimulating effects on the central nervous system at usual doses. After injection it produces peripheral vasoconstriction and increased arterial pressure. It also causes reflex bradycardia.

*Pharmacokinetic properties:* When injected subcutaneously or intramuscularly, phenylephrine takes 10 to 15 minutes to act. Subcutaneous and intramuscular injections are effective for up to about one hour and two hours, respectively. Intravenous injections are effective for up to about 20 minutes. Phenylephrine is metabolised in the liver by monoamine oxidase. The metabolites, their route and rate of excretion have not been identified.

*Preclinical safety data:* Not applicable.

**Pharmaceutical particulars**
*List of excipients:* N/1 sodium hydroxide for SP, N/1 hydrochloric acid for SP, Water for Injections PhEur, sterile N/1 sodium hydroxide for SP, sterile N/1 hydrochloric acid for SP.

*Incompatibilities:* Phenylephrine Injection has been stated to be incompatible with alkalis, ferric salts, phenytoin sodium and oxidising agents.

*Shelf life:* 24 months.

*Special precautions for storage:* Store at 2–25˚C. Protect from light.

*Nature and contents of container:* 1 ml neutral glass ampoule with ceramic breakring. Pack size: 10 ampoules.

*Instructions for use/handling:* Not applicable.

**Marketing authorisation number** 00169/0084

**Date of approval/revision of SPC** August 1995

**Legal category** POM

## PROTAMINE SULPHATE INJECTION BP 1%

**Qualitative and quantitative composition** Protamine Sulphate Injection BP 1% contains protamine sulphate 10 mg/ml in sodium chloride 0.9% w/v.

**Pharmaceutical form** Sterile solution for injection.

**Clinical particulars**
*Therapeutic indications:* Protamine sulphate neutralises the anticoagulant action of heparin. It is given by intravenous injection to restore the original coagulation time of the blood in patients receiving heparin, and in the treatment of haemorrhage due to heparin overdosage.

*Posology and method of administration:* For intravenous injection.

The dose is calculated from the results of determinations of the amount required to produce an acceptable blood clotting time in the patient.

Protamine sulphate is given by slow intravenous injection, being administered at the rate of 5 ml of the 1% solution over a period of ten minutes. 1 ml of Protamine Sulphate Injection BP 1% is required to neutralise the anticoagulant activity of approximately 850 Units of heparin (lung) or 1100 Units of heparin (mucous) that has been injected within the previous fifteen minutes.

As more time elapses after the heparin injection, so proportionately less protamine sulphate is required. Ideally, the dosage of protamine sulphate should be controlled by serial measurements of the patient's coagulation time. This helps to avoid an excess of protamine sulphate which, having some anticoagulant effect itself, can prolong coagulation time.

The anticoagulant effect of Heparin Retard injection can be counteracted by the intravenous injection of up to 5 ml of Protamine Sulphate Injection BP 1% over ten minutes. Because of the prolonged action of Heparin Retard, the dosage of protamine sulphate is best controlled by measurements of coagulation time.

*Contra-indications:* Protamine Sulphate Injection is contra-indicated in patients who are known to be hypersensitive to protamine.

*Special warnings and special precautions for use:* Protamine sulphate should be used with caution in patients with a known hypersensitivity to fish, in vasectomised or infertile males, and in patients who have received protamine-containing insulin or previous protamine sulphate therapy.

Not more than 50 mg of protamine sulphate, ie 5 ml of Protamine Sulphate Injection BP 1%, should usually be given at any one time. Protamine sulphate is a specific antidote to heparin and is not suitable for reversing the action of indirect anticoagulants such as coumarin and indanedione derivatives.

Care is also required when given to patients with diabetes mellitus or closed-angle glaucoma.

*Interaction with other medicaments and other forms of interaction:* Protamine sulphate may increase the magnitude and/or duration of action of non-depolarising neuromuscular blocking agents.

*Pregnancy and lactation:* The safety of protamine sulphate during pregnancy and lactation has not been established.

Neither animal nor human reproduction studies

have been conducted, and therefore the drug should only be used during pregnancy when clearly needed. It is not known whether protamine sulphate is distributed into breast milk and the drug should be used with caution during lactation.

*Effects on ability to drive and use machines:* No adverse effects known.

*Undesirable effects:* Intravenous injections of protamine sulphate, particularly if given rapidly, may cause hypotension, bradycardia and dyspnoea. A sensation of warmth, transitory flushing, nausea, vomiting and lassitude may also occur. Occasionally, hypersensitivity reactions including urticaria, angioedema, pulmonary oedema, anaphylaxis and anaphylactoid reactions have been reported.

*Overdose:* Protamine sulphate is a weak anticoagulant and overdosage may theoretically result in bleeding. Usually, no specific therapy is required.

**Pharmacological properties**
*Pharmacodynamic properties:* Protamine sulphate is strongly basic and acts as a heparin antagonist by complexing with the strongly acidic heparin sodium or heparin calcium to form a stable complex.

*Pharmacokinetic properties:* Protamine sulphate has a rapid onset of action. Following intravenous administration, neutralisation of heparin occurs within 5 minutes. Although the metabolic fate of the protamine-heparin complex is not known, it appears that the complex is partially degraded, thus freeing heparin.

*Preclinical safety data:* Not applicable.

**Pharmaceutical particulars**
*List of excipients:* Water for injections, sodium chloride for injections, sodium hydroxide and/or hydrochloric acid as pH adjusters.

*Incompatibilities:* Protamine sulphate is incompatible with certain antibiotics, including several penicillins and cephalosporins.

*Shelf life:* 36 months.

*Special precautions for storage:* Store at 15 to 25˚C. Do not refrigerate.

*Nature and contents of container:* One point cut ampoule. Pack size: 6×10 ml ampoules.

*Instructions for use/handling:* None.

**Marketing authorisation number** 00169/0085

**Date of approval/revision of SPC** April 1996

**Legal category** POM

## PROTHIADEN*

**Qualitative and quantitative composition** Each Prothiaden tablet contains 75 mg Dothiepin Hydrochloride BP. Each Prothiaden capsule contains 25 mg Dothiepin Hydrochloride BP.

**Pharmaceutical form** Red, sugar-coated tablets, bearing the overprint 'P75' in white; red/brown, hard gelatin capsules bearing the overprint 'P25' in white.

**Clinical particulars**
*Therapeutic indications:* Prothiaden is indicated in the treatment of symptoms of depressive illness, especially where an anti-anxiety effect is required.

*Posology and method of administration:* For oral administration.

Adults: Initially 75 mg/day in divided doses or as a single dose at night, increasing to 150 mg/day. In certain circumstances, *e.g.* in hospital use, dosages up to 225 mg daily have been used.

Suggested regimens: 25 or 50 mg three times daily or, alternatively, 75 or 150 mg as a single dose at night. Should the regimen of 150 mg as a single nighttime dose be adopted, it is better to give a smaller dose for the first few days.

Elderly: 50 to 75 mg daily initially. As with any antidepressant, the initial dose should be increased with caution under close supervision. Half the normal adult dose may be sufficient to produce a satisfactory clinical response.

Children: Not recommended.

*Contra-indications:* Prothiaden is contra-indicated following recent myocardial infarction, and in patients with any degree of heart block or other cardiac arrhythmias. It is also contra-indicated in mania and severe liver disease.

*Special warnings and special precautions for use:* It may be two to four weeks from the start of treatment before there is an improvement in the patient's depression; the subject should be monitored closely during this period. The anxiolytic effect may be observed within a few days of commencing treatment.

The elderly are particularly liable to experience adverse effects with antidepressants, especially agi-

tation, confusion and postural hypotension. Patients posing a high risk of suicide require close supervision.

Prothiaden should be avoided in patients with a history of epilepsy and in patients with narrow-angle glaucoma or symptoms suggestive of prostatic hypertrophy. Use with caution in patients with cardiovascular disorders.

Tricyclic antidepressants potentiate the central nervous depressant action of alcohol. Anaesthetics given during tri/tetracyclic antidepressant therapy may increase the risk of arrhythmias and hypotension. If surgery is necessary, the anaesthetist should be informed that a patient is being so treated.

On stopping treatment, it is recommended that antidepressants should be withdrawn gradually, wherever possible.

*Interaction with other medicaments and other forms of interaction:* Prothiaden should not be given concurrently with a monoamine oxidase inhibitor, nor within fourteen days of ceasing such treatment. The concomitant administration of Prothiaden and SSRIs should be avoided since increases in plasma tricyclic antidepressant levels have been reported following the co-administration of some SSRIs.

Prothiaden may alter the pharmacological effect of some concurrently administered drugs including CNS depressants such as alcohol and narcotic analgesics; the effect of these will be potentiated as will be the effects of adrenaline and noradrenaline (some local anaesthetics contain these sympathomimetics). Anaesthetics given during tri/tetracyclic antidepressant therapy may increase the risk of arrhythmias and hypotension.

Prothiaden has quinidine-like actions on the heart. For this reason, its concomitant use with other drugs which may affect cardiac conduction (*e.g.* sotalol, terfenadine, astemizole, halofantrine) should be avoided.

The hypotensive activity of certain antihypertensive agents (*e.g.* bethanidine, debrisoquine, guanethidine) may be reduced by Prothiaden. It is advisable to review all antihypertensive therapy during treatment with tricyclic antidepressants.

Barbiturates may decrease and methylphenidate may increase the serum concentration of dothiepin and thus affect its antidepressant action.

There is no evidence that dothiepin interferes with standard laboratory tests.

*Pregnancy and lactation:* Treatment with Prothiaden should be avoided during pregnancy, unless there are compelling reasons. There is inadequate evidence of safety of the drug during human pregnancy.

There is evidence that dothiepin is secreted in breast milk but this is at levels which are unlikely to cause problems.

*Effects on ability to drive and use machines:* Initially, Prothiaden may impair alertness; patients likely to drive vehicles or operate machinery should be warned of this possibility.

*Undesirable effects:* The following adverse effects, although not necessarily all reported with dothiepin, have occurred with other tricyclic antidepressants:

Atropine-like side effects including dry mouth, disturbances of accommodation, tachycardia, constipation and hesitancy of micturition are common early in treatment, but usually lessen.

Other adverse effects include drowsiness, sweating, postural hypotension, tremor and skin rashes. Interference with sexual function may occur.

Potentially serious adverse effects are rare. These include depression of the bone marrow, agranulocytosis, hepatitis (including altered liver function), cholestatic jaundice, convulsions and inappropriate ADH secretion.

Psychotic manifestations, including mania and paranoid delusions, may be exacerbated during treatment with tricyclic antidepressants.

Withdrawal symptoms may occur on abrupt cessation of tricyclic therapy and include insomnia, irritability and excessive perspiration. Similar symptoms in neonates whose mothers received tricyclic antidepressants during the third trimester have also been reported.

Cardiac arrhythmias and severe hypotension are likely to occur with high dosage or in deliberate overdosage. They may also occur in patients with pre-existing heart disease taking normal dosage.

*Overdose:* Symptoms of overdosage may include dryness of the mouth, excitement, ataxia, drowsiness, loss of consciousness, muscle twitching, convulsions, widely dilated pupils, hyperreflexia, sinus tachycardia, cardiac arrhythmias, hypotension, hypothermia, depression of respiration, visual hallucinations, delirium, urinary retention, paralytic ileus, and respiratory or metabolic alkalosis.

Treatment should consist of gastric lavage. When the patient is unconscious or the cough reflex depressed, the lungs should be protected by a cuffed endotracheal tube. Repeated gastric/intestinal aspiration or repeated administration of activated charcoal may remove drug and metabolites excreted into the gut via the bile. Continuous ECG monitoring is advisable. Abnormalities of cardiac rhythm and epileptic convulsions may occur and should be treated accordingly. Forced diuresis is not recommended. Bed rest is advisable, even after recovery.

**Pharmacological properties**

*Pharmacodynamic properties:* Dothiepin is a tricyclic antidepressant which acts by increasing transmitter levels at central synapses, so producing a clinical antidepressant effect.

Dothiepin, in common with other tricyclics, inhibits the reuptake of noradrenaline and 5-hydroxytryptamine, with a significantly greater action on the reuptake of noradrenaline. In addition, dothiepin inhibits the neuronal uptake of dopamine.

As a consequence of its effects on monoamine levels, dothiepin appears to produce adaptive changes in the brain by reducing or down-regulating both noradrenaline receptor numbers and noradrenaline-induced cyclic-AMP formation.

*Pharmacokinetic properties:* Dothiepin is readily absorbed from the gastrointestinal tract and extensively metabolised in the liver. Metabolites include northiaden, dothiepin-S-oxide and northiaden-S-oxide. Dothiepin is excreted in the urine, mainly in the form of metabolites; appreciable amounts are also excreted in the faeces. A half-life of about 50 hours has been reported for dothiepin and its metabolites.

*Preclinical safety data:* Not applicable.

**Pharmaceutical particulars**

*List of excipients:* Tablets: Refined sugar, tricalcium phosphate, maize starch, talc, povidone, liquid glucose, magnesium stearate, sandarac or sandarac tablet varnish, ponceau 4R, sunset yellow, titanium dioxide, shellac, white beeswax, sodium benzoate, polydimethylsiloxane, soya lecithin.

Capsules: Maize starch, magnesium stearate, gelatin, glycerin, ponceau 4R, yellow iron oxide, black iron oxide, red iron oxide, titanium dioxide, shellac, polydimethylsiloxane, soya lecithin.

*Incompatibilities:* Not applicable.

*Shelf life:* Tablets: 36 months. Capsules: 36 months.

*Special precautions for storage:* Tablets: None. Capsules: None.

*Nature and contents of container:* Tablets: Blister pack containing 28 tablets. Plastic bottle containing 500 tablets. Capsules: Amber glass bottle containing 100 or 600 tablets.

*Instructions for use/handling:* None.

**Marketing authorisation numbers**
Prothiaden Tablets 75 mg     00169/0087
Prothiaden Capsules 25 mg    00169/0086

**Date of approval/revision of SPC**   February 1996

**Legal category** POM

# PROTIUM*  ▼

**Qualitative and quantitative composition** Pantoprazole sodium sesquihydrate 45.1 mg (equivalent to pantoprazole 40 mg).

**Pharmaceutical form** Enteric-coated tablet for oral use.

**Clinical particulars**
*Therapeutic indications:* For symptomatic improvement and healing of gastrointestinal diseases which require a reduction in acid secretion:
– duodenal ulcer
– gastric ulcer
– moderate and severe reflux oesophagitis.

Note: Prior to treatment of gastric ulcer, the possibility of malignancy should be excluded as treatment with Protium may alleviate the symptoms of malignant ulcers and can thus delay diagnosis.

*Posology and method of administration:* The recommended oral dosage is one enteric-coated tablet per day. Protium should not be chewed or crushed, and should be swallowed whole with water either before or during breakfast.

In most patients, freedom from symptoms is achieved rapidly.

As sufficient experience with long-term administration in man is lacking, the length of a course of treatment with Protium should not exceed 8 weeks.

*Duodenal ulcer:* Duodenal ulcers generally heal within 2 weeks. If a 2-week period of treatment is not sufficient, healing will be achieved in almost all cases within a further 2 weeks.

*Gastric ulcer:* A 4-week period is usually required for the treatment of gastric ulcers. If this is not sufficient, healing will usually be achieved within a further 4 weeks.

*Gastro-oesophageal reflux:* A 4-week period is usually required for the treatment of gastro-oesopha-

geal reflux. If this is not sufficient, healing will usually be achieved within a further 4 weeks.

*Elderly:* No dose adjustment is necessary in the elderly.

*Patients with impaired renal function:* No dose adjustment is necessary in patients with renal impairment.

*Patients with hepatic cirrhosis:* Due to an increased AUC and a modified metabolism of pantoprazole in patients with hepatic cirrhosis, the dose regimen should be reduced to one tablet every other day.

*Children:* There is no information on the use of pantoprazole in children. Therefore Protium should not be used in children.

*Contra-indications:* Protium may not be used in cases of known hypersensitivity to any of its constituents.

*Special warnings and precautions for use:* None.

*Interactions with other medicaments and other forms of interaction:* No drug interactions have been reported so far (see also *Pharmacokinetic properties*).

*Pregnancy and lactation:*
*Use during pregnancy:* There is no information about the safety of pantoprazole during pregnancy in humans. Animal experiments have revealed no signs of foetal damage, but reproduction studies have revealed reduced litter weight and delayed development of the skeleton at doses above 15 mg/kg.

During pregnancy, Protium should not be used unless the benefit exceeds the potential risk.

*Use during lactation:* There is no information about the safety of pantoprazole during breast-feeding in humans. In the rat, not more than 0.02% of the administered dose is excreted via the breast milk.

During breast-feeding, Protium should not be used unless the benefit exceeds the potential risk.

*Effects on ability to drive and use machines:* Pantoprazole does not affect the ability to drive and use machines.

*Undesirable effects:* Treatment with Protium can occasionally lead to headache (1.3%) or diarrhoea (1.5%).

Skin rashes (0.4%), pruritus (0.5%) and dizziness (0.7%) were observed rarely.

*Overdose:* There are no known symptoms of overdosage in man. However, pantoprazole is very specific in action and no particular problems are anticipated.

Doses of up to 240 mg i.v. were administered without obvious adverse effects.

As pantoprazole is extensively protein bound, it is not readily dialysable. Apart from symptomatic and supportive treatment, no specific therapeutic recommendations can be made.

**Pharmacological properties**
*Pharmacodynamic properties:* Pantoprazole is a proton pump inhibitor, i.e. it inhibits specifically and dose-proportionally the gastric $H^+/K^+$-ATPase enzyme which is responsible for acid secretion in the parietal cells of the stomach.

The substance is a substituted benzimidazole which accumulates in the acidic environment of the parietal cells after absorption. There it is converted into the active form, a cyclic sulphenamide, which binds to the $H^+/K^+$-ATPase, thus inhibiting the proton pump and causing potent and long-lasting suppression of basal and stimulated gastric acid secretion. As pantoprazole acts distally to the receptor level, it can inhibit gastric acid secretion irrespective of the nature of the stimulus (acetylcholine, histamine, gastrin).

Pantoprazole's selectivity is due to the fact that it can only exert its full effect in a strongly acidic environment (pH<3), remaining mostly inactive at higher pH values. As a result, its complete pharmacological and thus therapeutic effect can only be achieved in the acid-secretory parietal cells. By means of a feedback mechanism, this effect is diminished at the same rate as acid secretion is inhibited.

Pantoprazole has the same effect whether administered orally or intravenously.

Following intravenous or oral administration, pantoprazole inhibits the pentagastrin-stimulated gastric acid secretion. In volunteers, acid secretion was inhibited by 56% following the first i.v. administration of 30 mg and by 99% after 5 days. With an oral dose of 40 mg, inhibition was 51% on day 1 and 85% on day 7. Basal 24 hour acidity was reduced by 37% and 98%, respectively.

The fasting gastrin values increased under pantoprazole but in most cases they did not exceed the normal upper limit. Following completion of a course of oral treatment, the median gastrin levels clearly declined again.

*Pharmacokinetic properties:*
*General pharmacokinetics:* Pantoprazole is rapidly absorbed and the maximal plasma concentration is achieved even after one single 40 mg oral dose. On average, the maximum plasma concentrations are approximately 2–3 microgram/ml about 2.5 hours

post-administration and these values remain constant after multiple administration. Terminal half-life is about 1 hour. Volume of distribution is about 0.15 L/kg and clearance is about 0.1 L/h/kg. There were a few cases of subjects with delayed elimination. Because of the specific activation within the parietal cell, the elimination half-life does not correlate with the much longer duration of action (inhibition of acid secretion).

Pharmacokinetics do not vary after single or repeated administration.

The plasma kinetics of pantoprazole are linear after both oral and intravenous administration.

Studies with pantoprazole in humans reveal no interaction with the cytochrome P450-system of the liver. There was no induction of the P450-system seen as tested after chronic administration with antipyrine as a marker. Also, no inhibition of metabolism was observed after concomitant administration of pantoprazole with either antipyrine, diazepam, phenytoin, nifedipine, theophylline, digoxin or oral contraceptives. Concomitant administration of pantoprazole with warfarin has no influence on warfarin's effect on the coagulation factors.

The absolute bioavailability of the tablet is about 77%. Concomitant intake of food or antacids had no influence on AUC, maximum plasma concentrations and thus bioavailability.

Pantoprazole's plasma protein binding is about 98%. The substance is almost exclusively metabolised in the liver. Renal elimination represents the major route of excretion (about 80%) for the metabolites of pantoprazole; the rest are excreted in the faeces. The main metabolite in both the plasma and urine is desmethylpantoprazole which is conjugated with sulphate. The half-life of the main metabolites (about 1.5 hours) is not much longer than that of pantoprazole.

*Characteristics in patients/special groups of subjects:* Although for patients with hepatic cirrhosis (classes A and B according to Child) the half-life values increased to between 7 and 9 hours and the AUC values increased by a factor of 5 to 7, the maximum plasma concentration only increased slightly by a factor of 1.5 compared with healthy subjects. Therefore the dose regimen in patients with hepatic cirrhosis should be reduced to one tablet every other day.

No dose reduction is required when pantoprazole is administered to patients with impaired kidney function (including dialysis patients). As with healthy subjects, pantoprazole's half-life is short. Only very small amounts of pantoprazole are dialysed. Although the main metabolite has a moderately delayed half-life (2–3 hours), excretion is still rapid and thus accumulation does not occur.

A slight increase in AUC and $C_{max}$ in elderly volunteers compared with younger counterparts is also not clinically relevant.

*Preclinical safety data:*
*Acute toxicity:* In acute toxicity studies in mice, the $LD_{50}$ values were found to be 370 mg/kg bodyweight for i.v. administration and around 700 mg/kg bodyweight for oral administration.

In the rat, the corresponding values were around 240 mg/kg for i.v. administration and 900 mg/kg for oral administration.

*Chronic toxicity:* Hypergastrinaemia and morphologic changes of the mucosa were observed in studies investigating repeated administration for up to 12 months in the rat and dog. Most of the effects were reversible and attributable solely to the drug action, i.e. suppression of acid secretion.

In long-term studies in the rat and dog, there was an increase in stomach and liver weights, the increase being reversible after the substance was discontinued. The increase in liver weight following highly toxic doses was seen as a result of the induction of drug-metabolising enzymes.

Thyroid activation in two rat experiments is due to the rapid metabolism of thyroid hormones in the liver and has also been described in a similar form for other drugs. Changes in the thyroid and associated reduced degradation of cholesterol have been observed in one-year studies in the rat and dog. Hypertrophy of the thyroid and increases in cholesterol levels are reversible.

In studies in the dog, a species-specific pulmonary oedema was observed. The animal-specific metabolite which was responsible for the oedema could not be identified in man.

*Carcinogenicity:* In a 2-year carcinogenicity study in rats – which corresponds to lifetime treatment for rats – ECL cell carcinoids were found. The mechanism leading to the formation of gastric carcinoids by substituted benzimidazoles has been carefully investigated and allows the conclusion that it is a secondary reaction to the massively elevated serum gastrin levels occurring in the rat during treatment. In addition, rats have more ECL cells in the mucosa of the glandular stomach than man, so that a larger number of responder cells for the increased gastrin values can become active.

ECL cell neoplasms were not observed in either a study in mice (24 months) or in long-term studies in the dog. In clinical studies (40–80 mg for 1 year), ECL cell density slightly increased.

In the two-year studies, an increased number of neoplastic changes of the liver was observed in rats and female mice and was interpreted as being due to pantoprazole's high metabolic rate in the liver.

A slight increase in neoplastic changes of the thyroid was observed in the group of rats receiving the highest dose. The occurrence of these neoplasms is associated with the pantoprazole-induced changes in the breakdown of thyroxine in the rat liver. In man, no changes in the thyroid hormones T3, T4 and TSH were observed. This high dose phenomenon in the rat is therefore not relevant for man.

*Mutagenicity:* In mutagenicity studies, there were no indications of a mutagenic action *in vivo* or *in vitro*.

*Reproduction toxicology:* Investigations revealed no evidence of impaired fertility or teratogenic effects. Penetration of the placenta was investigated in the rat and was found to increase with advanced gestation. As a result, the concentration of pantoprazole in the foetus is increased shortly before birth regardless of the route of administration.

In humans, there is no experience of the use of the drug during pregnancy.

### Pharmaceutical particulars

*List of excipients:* Crospovidone, mannitol, hydroxy-propyl methylcellulose, poly (ethylacrylate, methacrylic acid) 1:1, anhydrous sodium carbonate, propylene glycol, polyvidone K90, calcium stearate, triethyl citrate, polyvidone K25, titanium dioxide (E 171), polysorbate 80, sodium lauryl sulphate, yellow iron oxide (E 172).

*Incompatibilities:* None.

*Shelf life:* Protium tablets are stable over a period of 3 years.

*Special precautions for storage:* Store below 30°C.

*Nature and contents of container:* Protium is presented as a patient pack of 28 tablets, available in PE bottles packed in carton boxes.

*Instructions for use/handling:* None.

*Marketing authorisation holder:* Byk Gulden, Lomberg Chemische Fabrik GmbH, Byk Gulden Straße 2, D-78467 Konstanz, Germany.

**Marketing authorisation number** 04889/0010.

**Date of approval/revision of the SPC** July 1996.

**Legal category** POM.

# SECURON*

**Presentation** Securon tablets containing 40 mg Verapamil Hydrochloride PhEur are white, film-coated tablets impressed with 40 on one side and the Knoll logo on the other.

Securon tablets containing 80 mg Verapamil Hydrochloride PhEur are white, film-coated tablets impressed with SECURON 80 on one side and KNOLL above the score-line on the other.

Securon tablets containing 120 mg Verapamil Hydrochloride PhEur are white, film-coated tablets impressed with Securon 120 on one side and KNOLL above the score-line on the other.

Inactive ingredients: Lactose.

**Uses** Securon is a calcium antagonist which blocks the inward movement of calcium ions in cardiac muscle cells, in smooth muscle cells of the coronary and systemic arteries and in the cells of the intracardiac conduction system. Securon lowers peripheral vascular resistance with no reflex tachycardia. Its efficacy in reducing both raised systolic and diastolic blood pressure is thought to be due to this mode of action. The decrease in systemic and coronary vascular resistance and the sparing effect on intracellular oxygen consumption appear to explain the anti-anginal properties of the drug. Because of its effect on the movement of calcium in the intracardiac conduction system, Securon reduces automaticity, decreases conduction velocity and increases the refractory period.

Securon is indicated for

(1) the treatment of mild to moderate hypertension;

(2) the treatment and prophylaxis of chronic stable angina, vasospastic angina and unstable angina;

(3) the treatment and prophylaxis of paroxysmal supraventricular tachycardia and the reduction of ventricular rate in atrial flutter/fibrillation. Verapamil should not be used when atrial flutter/fibrillation complicates Wolff-Parkinson-White syndrome (see Precautions).

### Dosage and administration
*Adults*

*Hypertension:* Initially 120 mg b.d. increasing to 160 mg b.d. when necessary. In some cases, dosages of up to 480 mg daily, in divided doses, have been used. A further reduction in blood pressure may be obtained by combining Securon with other antihypertensive agents, in particular diuretics. For concomitant administration with beta-blockers see Precautions.

*Angina:* 120 mg t.d.s. is recommended. 80 mg t.d.s. can be completely satisfactory in some patients with angina of effort. Less than 120 mg t.d.s. is not likely to be effective in variant angina.

*Supraventricular tachycardias:* 40–120 mg t.d.s. according to the severity of the condition.

*Children:* Up to 2 years: 20 mg, 2–3 times a day.
2 years and above: 40–120 mg, 2-3 times a day, according to age and effectiveness.

*Elderly patients:* The adult dose is recommended unless liver or renal function is impaired (see Precautions).

### Contra-indications, warnings etc
*Contra-indications:* Cardiogenic shock; acute myocardial infarction complicated by bradycardia, hypotension or left ventricular failure; second or third degree atrioventricular block; sino-atrial block; sick sinus syndrome; uncompensated heart failure; bradycardia of less than 50 beats/minute; hypotension of less than 90 mmHg systolic.

*Interactions with other medicaments and other forms of interaction:* Interactions between verapamil and the following medications have been reported:

*Digoxin:* Verapamil has been shown to increase the serum concentration of digoxin and caution should be exercised with regard to digitalis toxicity. The digitalis level should be determined and the glycoside dose reduced, if required.

*Beta-blockers, anti-arrhythmic agents or inhaled anaesthetics:* The combination with Securon may lead to additive cardiovascular effects (e.g. AV block, bradycardia, hypotension, heart failure). Intravenous beta-blockers should not be given to patients under treatment with Securon.

*Carbamazepine, cyclosporin and theophylline:* Use of verapamil has resulted in increased serum levels of these medications, which could lead to increased side-effects.

*Rifampicin, phenytoin and phenobarbitone:* Serum levels of verapamil reduced.

*Lithium:* Serum levels of lithium may be reduced (pharmacokinetic effect); there may be increased sensitivity to lithium causing enhanced neurotoxicity (pharmacodynamic effect).

*Cimetidine:* Increase in verapamil serum level is possible.

*Neuromuscular blocking agents employed in anaesthesia:* The effects may be potentiated.

The effects of Securon may be additive to other hypotensive agents.

*Effects on the ability to drive and use machines:* Depending on individual susceptibility, the patient's ability to drive a vehicle or operate machinery may be impaired. This is particularly true in the initial stages of treatment, or when changing over from another medication. Like many other common medicines, verapamil has been shown to increase the blood levels of alcohol and slow its elimination. Therefore, the effects of alcohol may be exaggerated.

*Other undesirable effects (frequency and seriousness):* Particularly when given in high doses or in the presence of previous myocardial damage, some cardiovascular effects of verapamil may occasionally be greater than therapeutically desired: bradycardic arrhythmias, such as sinus bradycardia, sinus arrest with asystole, second and third degree AV block, bradyarrhythmia in atrial fibrillation, hypotension, development or aggravation of heart failure.

Securon is generally well tolerated. Side-effects are usually mild and transient and discontinuation of therapy is rarely necessary. Constipation may occur. Flushing is observed occasionally and headaches, nausea, vomiting, dizziness, fatigue and ankle oedema have been reported rarely. Allergic reactions (e.g. erythema, pruritus, urticaria, Quincke's oedema, Stevens-Johnson syndrome) are very rarely seen. A reversible impairment of liver function, characterised by an increase in transaminase and/or alkaline phosphatase may occur on very rare occasions during verapamil treatment and is most probably a hypersensitivity reaction.

On very rare occasions, gynaecomastia has been observed in elderly male patients under long-term verapamil treatment, which was fully reversible in all cases when the drug was discontinued.

Gingival hyperplasia may very rarely occur when the drug is administered over prolonged periods, and is fully reversible when the drug is discontinued. Erythromelalgia and paraesthesia may occur. In very rare cases, there may be myalgia and arthralgia. Rises in prolactin levels have been reported.

*Use in pregnancy and lactation:* Although animal studies have not shown any teratogenic effects, verapamil should not be given during the first trimester of pregnancy unless, in the clinician's judgement, it is essential for the welfare of the patient.

Verapamil is excreted into the breast milk in small amounts and is unlikely to be harmful. However, rare hypersensitivity reactions have been reported with verapamil and, therefore, it should only be used during lactation if, in the clinician's judgement, it is essential for the welfare of the patient.

*Other special warnings and precautions:* Since verapamil is extensively metabolised in the liver, careful dose titration of verapamil is required in patients with liver disease. The disposition of verapamil in patients with renal impairment has not been fully established and therefore careful patient monitoring is recommended. Verapamil is not removed during dialysis.

Verapamil may affect impulse conduction and therefore Securon should be used with caution in patients with first degree AV block. Patients with atrial flutter/fibrillation in association with an accessory pathway (e.g. WPW syndrome) may develop increased conduction across the anomalous pathway and ventricular tachycardia may be precipitated. Securon may affect left ventricular contractility; this effect is small and normally not important but cardiac failure may be precipitated or aggravated. In patients with incipient cardiac failure, therefore, Securon should be given only after such cardiac failure has been controlled with appropriate therapy, e.g. digitalis. When treating hypertension with verapamil, monitoring of the patient's blood pressure at regular intervals is required.

*Overdosage (symptoms, emergency procedures, antidotes):* The course of symptoms in verapamil intoxication depends on the amount taken, the point in time at which detoxification measures are taken and myocardial contractility (age-related). The main symptoms are as follows: blood pressure fall (at times to values not detectable), shock symptoms, loss of consciousness, 1st and 2nd degree AV block (frequently as Wenckebach's phenomenon with or without escape rhythms), total AV block with total AV dissociation, escape rhythm, asystole, sinus bradycardia, sinus arrest. The therapeutic measures to be taken depend on the point in time at which verapamil was taken and the type and severity of intoxication symptoms. Gastric lavage, taking the usual precautionary measures may be appropriate. The usual intensive resuscitation measures, such as extrathoracic heart massage, respiration, defibrillation and/or pacemaker therapy. Specific measures to be taken: Elimination of cardiodepressive effects, hypotension or bradycardia. The specific antidote is calcium, e.g. 10–20 ml of a 10% calcium gluconate solution administered intravenously (2.25–4.5 mmol), repeated if necessary or given as a continuous drip infusion (e.g. 5 mmol/hour). The following measures may also be necessary: In case of 2nd or 3rd degree AV block, sinus bradycardia, asystole: atropine, isoprenaline, orciprenaline or pacemaker therapy. In case of hypotension after appropriate positioning of the patient: dopamine, dobutamine, noradrenaline. If there are signs of continuing myocardial failure: dopamine, dobutamine, cardiac glycosides or if necessary, repeated calcium gluconate injections.

*Incompatibilities:* None.

**Pharmaceutical precautions** Store in a dry place at room temperature (below 25°C).

**Legal category** POM

**Package quantities** Securon 120 mg tablets: blister pack of 60 tablets.

Securon 80 mg, 40 mg tablets: blister packs of 100 tablets.

**Further information** Nil.

**Product licence numbers**
Securon tablets 40 mg    0169/0003
Securon tablets 80 mg    0169/0004
Securon tablets 120 mg   0169/0005

# SECURON* IV

**Presentation** Securon IV is an aqueous solution of Verapamil Hydrochloride BP in a concentration of 2.5 mg/ml. Each ampoule contains 5 mg of Verapamil Hydrochloride BP in 2 ml of intravenous injection solution.

**Uses** Securon is a calcium antagonist which blocks the inward movement of calcium ions in cardiac muscle cells, in smooth muscle cells of the coronary and systemic arteries and in the cells of the intracardiac conduction system. Because of its effect on the movement of calcium in the intracardiac conduction system, Securon reduces automaticity, decreases conduction velocity, and increases the refractory period.

Securon IV is indicated in the treatment of paroxysmal supraventricular tachycardia and the reduction of ventricular rate in atrial flutter/fibrillation. Verapamil should not be used when atrial flutter/fibrillation complicates Wolff-Parkinson-White syndrome (see 'Contra-indications').

**Dosage and administration**
*Adults:* 5–10 mg by slow intravenous injection over a period of 2 minutes. The patient should be observed continuously preferably under ECG and blood pressure control. If necessary, e.g. in paroxysmal tachycardia, a further 5 mg may be given after 5–10 minutes.

*Children:* Securon IV must always be administered under ECG monitoring in young patients.

0–1 year: 0.1–0.2 mg/kg bodyweight (usual single dose range 0.75–2 mg).

1–15 years: 0.1–0.3 mg/kg bodyweight (usual single dose range 2–5 mg).

The dose may be repeated after 30 minutes if necessary. Many cases are controlled by doses at the lower end of the range. The injection should be stopped at the onset of the desired effect.

*Elderly:* The dosage should be administered over 3 minutes to minimise the risk of adverse effects.

*Dosage in impaired liver and renal function:* Significant hepatic and renal impairment should not increase the effects of a single intravenous dose but may prolong its duration of action.

For use with beta-blocker therapy see 'Contra-indications' and 'Precautions'.

**Contra-indications, warnings, etc**
*Contra-indications:* Cardiogenic shock; acute myocardial infarction complicated by bradycardia, marked hypotension or left ventricular failure; second or third degree AV block; sino-atrial block; sick sinus syndrome; uncompensated heart failure; marked bradycardia of less than 50 beats/minute; marked hypotension of less than 90 mmHg systolic; patients with atrial flutter/fibrillation in the presence of an accessory pathway (e.g. WPW syndrome) may develop increased conduction across the anomalous pathway and ventricular tachycardia may be precipitated; simultaneous administration of intravenous beta-blockers.

*Interactions with other medicaments and other forms of interaction:* Interactions between verapamil and the following medications have been reported:

*Digoxin:* Verapamil has been shown to increase the serum concentration of digoxin and caution should be exercised with regard to digitalis toxicity. The digitalis level should be determined and the glycoside dose reduced, if required.

*Beta-blockers, anti-arrhythmic agents, inhaled anaesthetics:* The effect of Securon IV, beta-blockers, anti-arrhythmic agents and inhaled anaesthetics may be additive both with respect to conduction and contraction. Securon IV should not be given in combination with intravenous beta-blocker therapy and care must be exercised if Securon IV is combined with oral beta-blocker therapy or anti-arrhythmic agents by any route.

*Carbamazepine, cyclosporin and theophylline:* Use of verapamil has resulted in increased serum levels of these medications, which could lead to increased side-effects.

*Rifampicin, phenytoin and phenobarbitone:* Serum levels of verapamil reduced.

*Lithium:* Serum levels of lithium may be reduced (pharmacokinetic effect); there may be increased sensitivity to lithium causing enhanced neurotoxicity (pharmacodynamic effect).

*Cimetidine:* Increase in verapamil serum level is possible.

*Neuromuscular blocking agents employed in anaesthesia:* The effects may be potentiated.

The effects of Securon IV may be additive to other hypotensive agents.

After intravenous administration of Securon IV, hypotensive reactions have been observed in individual patients receiving quinidine therapy.

*Effects on the ability to drive and use machines:* It is not expected that patients receiving Securon IV will be driving or using machines. However, it should be noted that depending on individual susceptibility, the patient's ability to drive a vehicle or operate machinery may be impaired. This is particularly true in the initial stages of treatment or when changing over from another medication. Like many other common medicines, verapamil has been shown to increase the levels of alcohol and slow its elimination. Therefore, the effects of alcohol may be exaggerated.

*Other undesirable effects (frequency and seriousness):* Securon IV is generally well tolerated but due to the drug's mode of action, undesired cardiovascular effects may occur, particularly at high doses and in patients with AV block and/or impaired myocardial function. Decreased heart rate, hypotension and decreased myocardial contractility have been reported. On rare occasions, second or third degree AV block may occur and, in extreme cases, this may lead to asystole. The asystole is usually of short duration and cardiac action returns spontaneously after a few seconds, usually in the form of sinus rhythm. If necessary, the procedures for the treatment of overdosage should be followed as described below. A slight transient fall in blood pressure, due to a reduction in peripheral resistance, may be seen. In rare cases this may lead to severe hypotension. On rare occasions, headache, vertigo and flushing have been reported. Allergic reactions (erythema, pruritus, urticaria, bronchospasm, Quincke's oedema, Stevens-Johnson syndrome) are extremely rare.

*Use in pregnancy and lactation:* Although animal studies have not shown any teratogenic effects, verapamil should not be given during the first trimester of pregnancy unless, in the clinician's judgement, it is essential for the welfare of the patient.

Verapamil is excreted into the breast milk in small amounts and is unlikely to be harmful. However, rare hypersensitivity reactions have been reported with verapamil and, therefore, it should only be used during lactation if, in the clinician's judgement, it is essential for the welfare of the patient.

*Other special warnings and precautions:* Verapamil may affect impulse conduction and therefore Securon IV should be used with caution in patients with first degree AV block. Securon IV may affect left ventricular contractility; this effect is small and normally not important but cardiac failure may be precipitated or aggravated. In patients with incipient cardiac failure, therefore, Securon IV should only be given after cardiac failure has been controlled with appropriate therapy, e.g. digitalis and/or diuretics.

*Overdose (symptoms, emergency procedures, antidotes):* The symptoms of overdosage include hypotension, shock, loss of consciousness, first and second degree AV block (frequently as Wenckebach's phenomenon with or without escape rhythms), total AV block with total AV dissociation, escape rhythm, asystole, sinus bradycardia, sinus arrest.

Treatment of overdosage depends on the type and severity of symptoms. The specific antidote is calcium, e.g. 10–20 ml of 10% calcium gluconate solution i.v. (2.25–4.5 mmol) if necessary by repeated injection or continuous infusion (e.g. 5 mmol/hr). The usual emergency measures for acute cardiovascular collapse should be applied and followed by intensive care. Similarly in the case of second and third degree AV block, atropine, orciprenaline, isoprenaline and, if required, pacemaker therapy should be considered. If there are signs of myocardial insufficiency, dopamine, dobutamine, cardiac glycosides or calcium gluconate (10–20 ml of a 10% solution) can be administered.

In the case of hypotension, after appropriately positioning the patient, dopamine, dobutamine or noradrenaline may be given.

*Incompatibilities:* Securon IV is incompatible with alkaline solutions.

**Pharmaceutical precautions** Store at room temperature. Protect from light.

**Legal category** POM

**Package quantities** 5x2 ml ampoule.

**Further information** Each ampoule contains 17 mg sodium chloride (8.5 mg/ml).

Following intravenous infusion in man, verapamil is eliminated bi-exponentially with a rapid distribution phase (half-life about 4 mins) and a slower terminal elimination phase (half-life 2–5 hours).

**Product licence number** 0169/0017.

## SECURON SR*
## HALF SECURON SR*

**Qualitative and quantitative composition** Securon SR: Verapamil Hydrochloride PhEur 240 mg.

Half Securon SR: Verapamil Hydrochloride PhEur 120 mg.

**Pharmaceutical form** Film-coated, sustained-release tablets.

Securon SR tablets are oblong, pale green, scored and embossed with two Knoll logos (triangles) on one side. Half Securon SR tablets are round, white, unscored and embossed with 'KNOLL' on one side and '120 SR' on the reverse.

**Clinical particulars**
*Therapeutic indications:* Securon SR and Half Securon SR are indicated for the treatment of mild to moderate hypertension and the treatment and prophylaxis of angina pectoris.

Secondary prevention of re-infarction after an acute myocardial infarction in patients without heart failure, and not receiving diuretics (apart from low-dose diuretics when used for indications other than heart failure), and where beta-blockers are not appropriate. Treatment is to be started at least one week after an acute myocardial infarction.

*Posology and method of administration:* For oral administration.

Securon SR and Half Securon SR tablets should not be chewed. Securon SR tablets are scored and may be halved without damaging the sustained-release formulation.

Adults: Hypertension: One tablet of Securon SR (240 mg) daily. For patients new to verapamil therapy, the physician should consider halving the initial dose to 120 mg (Half Securon SR). Most patients respond to 240 mg daily (one tablet Securon SR) given as a single dose. If control is not achieved after a period of at least one week, the dosage may be increased to a maximum of two Securon SR tablets daily (one in the morning and one in the evening at an interval of about twelve hours). A further reduction in blood pressure may be achieved by combining Securon SR tablets with other antihypertensive agents, in particular diuretics. Half Securon SR tablets may be used for dose titration purposes.

Angina pectoris: One tablet of Securon SR twice daily. A small number of patients respond to a lower dose and where indicated, adjustment down to one tablet of Securon SR daily could be made. Half Securon SR tablets may be used for dose titration purposes.

Secondary prevention of re-infarction after an acute myocardial infarction in patients without heart failure, and not receiving diuretics (apart from low-dose diuretics when used for indications other than heart failure), and where beta-blockers are not appropriate: Treatment is to be started at least one week after an acute myocardial infarction. 360 mg/day in divided doses, to be taken either as one Half Securon SR (120 mg) three times daily, or as one Securon SR (240 mg) to be taken in the morning and one Half Securon SR (120 mg) tablet in the evening, on a daily basis.

Elderly patients: The adult dose is recommended unless liver or renal function is impaired (see Precautions).

Children: Securon SR and Half Securon SR tablets are not recommended for children.

*Contra-indications:* Cardiogenic shock; acute myocardial infarction complicated by bradycardia, marked hypotension, left ventricular failure; second or third degree atrioventricular block; sino-atrial block; sick sinus syndrome; uncompensated heart failure; bradycardia of less than 50 beats/minute; hypotension of less than 90 mmHg systolic.

Concomitant ingestion of grapefruit juice.

*Special warnings and special precautions for use:* Since verapamil is extensively metabolised in the liver, careful dose titration of verapamil is required in patients with liver disease. The disposition of verapamil in patients with renal impairment has not been fully established and therefore careful patient monitoring is recommended. Verapamil is not removed during dialysis.

Verapamil may affect impulse conduction and should therefore be used with caution in patients with first degree atrioventricular block. Patients with atrial flutter/fibrillation in association with an accessory pathway (e.g. WPW-syndrome) may develop increased conduction across the anomalous pathway and ventricular tachycardia may be precipitated. Verapamil may affect left ventricular contractility. This effect is small and normally not important but cardiac failure may be precipitated or aggravated. In patients with incipient cardiac failure, therefore, verapamil should be given only after such cardiac failure has been controlled with appropriate therapy, e.g. digitalis.

When treating hypertension with verapamil, monitoring of the patient's blood pressure at regular intervals is required.

*Interaction with other medicaments and other forms of interaction:* Verapamil has been shown to increase the serum concentration of digoxin and caution should be exercised with regard to digitalis toxicity. The digitalis level should be determined and the glycoside dose reduced, if required. The combination of verapamil and beta-blockers, anti-arrhythmic agents or inhaled anaesthetics may lead to additive cardiovascular effects (e.g. AV block, bradycardia, hypotension, heart failure). Intravenous beta-blockers should not be given to patients under treatment with verapamil. The effects of verapamil may be additive to other hypotensive agents.

Interactions between verapamil and the following have been reported:

Carbamazepine, cyclosporin and theophylline: Use of verapamil has resulted in increased serum levels of these medications, which could lead to increased side effects.

Rifampicin, phenytoin and phenobarbitone: Serum levels of verapamil reduced.

Lithium: Serum levels of lithium may be reduced (pharmacokinetic effect); there may be increased sensitivity to lithium causing enhanced neurotoxicity (pharmacodynamic effect).

Cimetidine: Increase in verapamil serum level is possible.

Neuromuscular blocking agents employed in anaesthesia: The effects may be potentiated.

Grapefruit juice: Increase in verapamil serum level has been reported.

Alcohol: Increase in blood alcohol has been reported.

*Pregnancy and lactation:* Although animal studies have not shown any teratogenic effects, verapamil should not be given during the first trimester of pregnancy unless, in the clinician's judgement, it is essential for the welfare of the patient.

Verapamil is excreted into the breast milk in small amounts and is unlikely to be harmful. However, rare hypersensitivity reactions have been reported with verapamil and, therefore, it should only be used during lactation if, in the clinician's judgement, it is essential for the welfare of the patient.

*Effects on ability to drive and use machines:* Depending on individual susceptibility, the patient's ability to drive a vehicle or operate machinery may be impaired. This is particularly true in the initial stages of treatment, or when changing over from another drug. Like many other common medicines, verapamil has been shown to increase the blood levels of alcohol and slow its elimination. Therefore, the effects of alcohol may be exaggerated.

*Undesirable effects:* Particularly when given in high doses or in the presence of previous myocardial damage, some cardiovascular effects of verapamil may occasionally be greater than therapeutically desired: bradycardic arrhythmias, such as sinus bradycardia, sinus arrest with asystole, second and third degree AV block, bradyarrhythmia in atrial fibrillation, hypotension, development or aggravation of heart failure.

Securon SR and Half Securon SR tablets are generally well tolerated. Side-effects are usually mild and transient and discontinuation of therapy is rarely necessary. Constipation may occur. There have been rare reports of flushing, headache, nausea, vomiting, dizziness, fatigue and ankle oedema. Allergic reactions (e.g. erythema, pruritus, urticaria, Quincke's oedema, Stevens-Johnson syndrome) are very rarely seen. A reversible impairment of liver function, characterised by an increase of transaminases and/or alkaline phosphatase may occur on very rare occasions during verapamil treatment and is most probably a hypersensitivity reaction.

On very rare occasions, gynaecomastia has been observed in elderly male patients under long-term verapamil treatment, which was fully reversible in all cases when the drug was discontinued.

Gingival hyperplasia may very rarely occur when the drug is administered over prolonged periods, and is fully reversible when the drug is discontinued.

Erythromelalgia and paraesthesia may occur. In very rare cases, there may be myalgia and arthralgia. Rises in prolactin levels have been reported.

*Overdose:* The course of symptoms in verapamil intoxication depends on the amount taken, the point in time at which detoxication measures are taken and myocardial contractility (age-related). The main symptoms are as follows: blood pressure fall (at times to values not detectable), shock symptoms, loss of consciousness, 1st and 2nd degree AV block (frequently as Wenckebach's phenomenon with or without escape rhythms), total AV block with total AV dissociation, escape rhythm, asystole, sinus bradycardia, sinus arrest. The therapeutic measures to be taken depend on the point in time at which verapamil was taken and the type and severity of intoxication symptoms. In intoxications with large amounts of slow-release preparations (Securon SR and Half Securon SR), it should be noted that the release of the active drug and the absorption in the intestine may take more than 48 hours. Depending on the time of ingestion, it should be taken into account that there may be some lumps of incompletely-dissolved tablets along the entire length of the gastrointestinal tract, which function as active drug depots.

General measures to be taken: gastric lavage with the usual precautions, even later than 12 hours after ingestion, if no gastrointestinal motility (peristaltic sounds) is detectable. Where intoxication by Securon SR or Half Securon SR tablets is suspected, extensive elimination measures are indicated, such as induced vomiting, removal of the contents of the stomach and the small intestine under endoscopy, intestinal lavage, laxative, high enemas. The usual intensive resuscitation measures, such as extrathoracic heart massage, respiration, defibrillation and/or pacemaker therapy.

Specific measures to be taken: elimination of cardiodepressive effects, hypotension or bradycardia. The specific antidote is calcium, e.g. 10–20 ml of a 10% calcium gluconate solution administered intravenously (2.25–4.5 mmol), repeated if necessary or given as a continuous drip infusion (e.g. 5 mmol/hour).

The following measures may also be necessary: in case of 2nd or 3rd degree AV block, sinus bradycardia, asystole: atropine, isoprenaline, orciprenaline or pacemaker therapy. In case of hypotension: dopamine, dobutamine, noradrenaline. If there are signs of continuing myocardial failure: dopamine, dobutamine, if necessary repeated calcium injections.

## Pharmacological properties

*Pharmacodynamic properties:* Verapamil, a phenylalkylamine calcium antagonist, has a balanced profile of cardiac and peripheral effects. It lowers heart rate, increases myocardial perfusion and reduces coronary spasm. In a clinical study in patients after myocardial infarction, verapamil reduced total mortality, sudden cardiac death and reinfarction rate.

Verapamil reduces total peripheral resistance and lowers high blood pressure by vasodilation without reflex tachycardia. Because of its use-dependent action on the voltage-operated calcium channel, the effects of verapamil are more pronounced on high than on normal blood pressure.

As early as day one of treatment, blood pressure falls; the effect is found to persist also in long-term therapy. Verapamil is suitable for the treatment of all types of hypertension: for monotherapy in mild to moderate hypertension; combined with other antihypertensives (in particular with diuretics and, according to more recent findings, with ACE inhibitors) in more severe types of hypertension. In hypertensive diabetic patients with nephropathy, verapamil in combination with ACE inhibitors led to a marked reduction of albuminuria and to an improvement of creatinine clearance.

*Pharmacokinetic properties:* Absorption: More than 90% of an orally-administered dose of verapamil is absorbed. Due to an intensive hepatic first-pass metabolism, the absolute bioavailability is about 22%, with a variability of about 10–35%. Under multiple dosing, bioavailability increases by about 30%. Bioavailability is not affected by food consumption.

Distribution/Biotransformation/Elimination: Plasma concentrations reach their peak 4–8 hours after drug intake. Plasma protein binding of verapamil is more than 90%. The elimination half-life is about 5–8 hours. The mean residence time of sustained-release verapamil is 13 hours. After repeated single daily doses, steady-state conditions are reached between 3–4 days.

Within 5 days, approximately 70% of an orally-administered dose is excreted in the urine and about 16% with the faeces. Only 3–4% is eliminated renally as unchanged drug. Norverapamil, one of the 12 metabolites identified in urine, which represents about 6% of the dose eliminated, has 10–20% of the activity of verapamil. Norverapamil can reach steady-state plasma concentrations approximately equal to those of verapamil itself.

At-risk Patients: In patients with liver cirrhosis, bioavailability is increased and elimination half-life is prolonged. In patients with compensated hepatic insufficiency, no influence on the kinetics of verapamil was observed. The disposition of verapamil in patients with renal impairment has not been fully established.

*Preclinical safety data:* Not applicable.

## Pharmaceutical particulars

*List of excipients:* Securon SR: Sodium alginate, microcrystalline cellulose, povidone, purified water, talc, titanium dioxide (E171), hydroxypropyl methylcellulose, magnesium stearate, polyethylene glycol 400, polyethylene glycol 6000, montan glycol wax, L-green lake (E104, E132).

*Half Securon SR:* Sodium alginate, microcrystalline cellulose, povidone, purified water, talc, titanium dioxide (E171), hydroxypropyl methylcellulose, magnesium stearate, polyethylene glycol 400, polyethylene glycol 6000, montan glycol wax.

*Incompatibilities:* There are no major incompatibilities listed.

*Shelf life:* 60 months from date of manufacture.

*Special precautions for storage:* Store in a dry place, away from direct sunlight, below 25°C.

*Nature and contents of container:* PVC/PVDC blister packs, in a cardboard outer container, containing 28 tablets.

*Instructions for use/handling:* There are no special instructions for use/handling.

**Marketing authorisation numbers**
Securon SR                00169/0007
Half Securon SR           00169/0026

**Date of approval/revision of SPC** April 1997

**Legal category** POM

*\*Trade Mark*

# Kyowa Hakko UK Ltd
## CP House
## 97–107 Uxbridge Road
## London W5 5TL

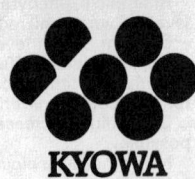

## MITOMYCIN-C KYOWA*

**Presentation** Purple crystalline powder for intravenous injection containing Mitomycin-C Kyowa 2 mg potency with 48 mg sodium chloride, 10 mg potency with 240 mg sodium chloride, 20 mg potency with 480 mg sodium chloride for reconstitution with water for injections using the volume recommended for each strength.

**Uses** Mitomycin-C Kyowa is an antitumour antibiotic that is activated in the tissues to an alkylating agent which disrupts deoxyribonucleic acid (DNA) in cancer cells by forming a complex with DNA and also acts by inhibiting division of cancer cells by interfering with the biosynthesis of DNA. *In vivo*, Mitomycin-C Kyowa is rapidly cleared from the serum after intravenous administration. The time required to reduce the serum concentration by 50 per cent after a 30 mg bolus injection is 17 minutes. After injection of 30 mg, 20 mg, or 10 mg intravenously, the maximal serum concentrations were 2.4 micrograms/ml, 1.7 micrograms/ml and 0.52 micrograms/ml respectively. Clearance is effected primarily by metabolism in the liver but metabolism occurs in other tissues as well. The rate of clearance is inversely proportional to the maximal serum concentration because, it is thought, of saturation of the degradative pathways. Approximately 10 per cent of a dose of Mitomycin-C Kyowa is excreted unchanged in the urine. Since metabolic pathways are saturated at relatively low doses, the percentage dose excreted in the urine increases with increasing dose. In children, excretion of intravenously administered Mitomycin-C Kyowa is similar to that in adults.

*Clinical indications:* Antimitotic and Cytotoxic.

Mitomycin-C Kyowa is recommended for certain types of cancer in combination with other drugs or after primary therapy has failed. It has been successfully used to improve subjective and objective symptoms in a wide range of neoplastic conditions.

As a single agent in the treatment of superficial bladder cancer. In addition it has been shown that post-operative instillations of Mitomycin-C Kyowa can reduce recurrence rates in newly diagnosed patients with superficial bladder cancer.

As a single agent and in combination with other drugs in metastatic breast cancer.

In combination with other agents in advanced squamous cell carcinoma of the uterine cervix.

It shows a degree of activity as part of combination therapy in carcinoma of the stomach, pancreas and lung (particularly non-small cell).

It shows a degree of activity as a single agent and in combination in liver cancer when given by the intra-arterial route.

It has a possible role in combination with other cytotoxic drugs in colorectal cancer.

It shows a degree of activity as a single agent or part of combination therapy in cancer of the head and neck.

It shows a degree of activity as a single agent in cancer of the prostate.

It has a possible role in skin cancer.

It has a degree of activity in leukaemia and non-solid tumours.

It has a possible role in sarcomas.

It has been successfully used in combination with surgery, pre-operatively (oesophageal, squamous cell carcinoma) and post-operatively (gastric cancer).

It has been shown to be effective when used in combination with radiotherapy.

**Dosage and administration** Intravenously, the dose should be given with great care in order to avoid extravasation.

The usual dose is in the range of 4 to 10 mg potency (0.06 to 0.15 mg/kg) given at 1 to 6 weekly intervals depending on whether other drugs are given in combination and on bone marrow recovery.

In a number of combination schedules, the dose is 10 mg potency/m² of body surface area, the course being repeated at intervals for as long as required. A course ranging from 40 to 80 mg potency (0.58 to 1.2 mg/kg) is often required for a satisfactory response when used alone or in combination.

A higher dosage course may be given when used alone or as part of a particular combination schedule and total cumulative doses exceeding 2 mg/kg have been given.

For administration into specific tissues, Mitomycin-C Kyowa can be given by the intra-arterial route directly into the tumours.

Because of cumulative myelosuppression, patients should be fully re-evaluated after each course and the dose reduced if the patient has experienced any toxic effects. Individual doses greater than 0.06 mg/kg have not been shown to be more effective and are more toxic than lower doses.

*Treatment of superficial urinary bladder tumours:* In the treatment of superficial bladder tumours, the usual dose is 20 to 40 mg potency dissolved in 20 to 40 ml of Water for Injections, instilled into the bladder through a urethral catheter, weekly or three times a week for a total of 20 doses.

In the prevention of recurrent superficial bladder tumours, various doses have been used. These include 20 mg in 20 ml of Water for Injections every two weeks and 40 mg in 40 ml of Water for Injections monthly or three monthly. The dose is instilled into the bladder through a urethral catheter.

In both cases the dose should be adjusted in accordance with the age and condition of the patient.

### Contra-indications, warnings, etc

*Contra-indications:* Mitomycin-C Kyowa is contra-indicated in patients who have demonstrated a hypersensitive or idiosyncratic reaction to it in the past.

*Precautions:* Mitomycin-C Kyowa should be administered under the supervision of a physician experienced in cytotoxic cancer chemotherapy. Patients should be monitored closely during each course of treatment, paying particular attention to peripheral blood count including platelet count.

No repeat dosage should be given until leucocyte count has returned to 3.0×10⁹ per litre and platelet count to 90.0×10⁹ per litre. If disease progression continues after two courses of treatment, the drug should be stopped since the chances of response are then minimal.

The person administering the injection of Mitomycin-C Kyowa should not allow the solution to come into contact with his or her skin.

*Side and adverse effects:* The principal toxicity of Mitomycin-C Kyowa is bone marrow suppression, particularly thrombocytopenia and leucopenia. The nadir is usually around four weeks after treatment and toxicity is cumulative, with increasing risk after each course of treatment.

Severe renal toxicity has occasionally been reported after treatment and renal function should be monitored before starting treatment and again after each course. Nausea and vomiting are sometimes experienced immediately after treatment but these are usually mild and of short duration. Local ulceration and cellulitis may be caused by tissue extravasation during intravenous injection and utmost care should be taken in administration. In the event of extravasation following an intravenous injection of Mitomycin-C Kyowa it is recommended that 5 ml of sodium bicarbonate 8.4% solution is immediately infiltrated into the area where extravasation has occurred, followed by an injection of 4 mg dexamethasone. In addition a systemic injection of 200 mg vitamin B6 may be of some value in promoting the regrowth of tissues that have been damaged.

*Use in pregnancy and lactation:* Mitomycin-C Kyowa should not normally be administered to patients who are pregnant or to mothers who are breast feeding. Teratological changes have been noted in animal studies. The effect of Mitomycin-C Kyowa on fertility is unknown.

*Treatment of skin or eye contact:* Any Mitomycin-C Kyowa substance or solution in contact with the skin should be washed several times with 8.4% sodium bicarbonate solution, followed by washing with soap and water. Use of handcreams or other emollient preparations is inappropriate as this may assist the penetration of any traces of Mitomycin-C Kyowa into the epidermal tissue.

Contact with the eye. The eye should be rinsed several times with sodium bicarbonate eye lotion and the eye examined for several days after contact for evidence of corneal damage. If this occurs, appropriate treatment should be instituted.

**Pharmaceutical precautions** The contents of the vial should be reconstituted with water for injections or 20% dextrose solution, 5 ml for the 2 mg vial, at least 10 ml for the 10 ml vial and at least 20 ml for the 20 mg vial.

Unreconstituted Mitomycin-C Kyowa remains stable for four years after manufacture when stored at room temperature. Reconstitution, as directed, should be accomplished using aseptic technique and the resulting solutions are best used immediately. If reconstituted Mitomycin-C Kyowa must be stored prior to use, it should be protected from light and kept in a cool place – it should not be refrigerated. Solutions stored in this way should be discarded if unused after 24 hours.

When reconstituted solution is added to infusion fluids, especially where these contain dextrose, the resulting solution should be used immediately.

**Legal category** POM.

**Package quantities** 2 mg, 10 mg and 20 mg vials for intravenous injection, in packs of ten, one and one respectively.

**Further information** Mitomycin-C Kyowa vials are available through hospital pharmacies and can be supplied to retail pharmacists for dispensing against prescriptions for patients whose treatment has been initiated in hospital practice.

**Product licence numbers**

| | |
|---|---|
| 2 mg | 12196/0001 |
| 10 mg | 12196/0002 |
| 20 mg | 12196/0003. |

*Trade Mark

# Laboratories for Applied Biology Limited
91 Amhurst Park
London N16 5DR

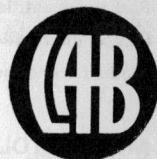

## CERUMOL* EAR DROPS

**Presentation** A clear oily preparation containing:

| | |
|---|---|
| Arachis (Peanut) oil BP | 57.3% w/v |
| Chlorbutol BP | 5.0% w/v |
| p-Dichlorobenzene | 2.0% w/v |

**Uses** Occlusion or partial occlusion of external auditory meatus by either a collection of soft wax or a harder wax plug.

**Dosage and administration** *At home:* With the head inclined, 5 drops are put into the ear. This may cause a harmless tingling sensation. A plug of cotton wool moistened with Cerumol should then be applied to retain the liquid. One hour later, or the next morning, the plug is removed. The procedure is repeated twice a day for three days; the loosened wax may then come out on its own making syringing unnecessary. If any wax remains the doctor should be consulted so that syringing of the softened residue may be carried out.
*At the surgery:* If there has been no prior treatment with Cerumol, 5 drops are instilled as described above and left for at least 20 minutes. Then syringing or a probe tipped with cotton wool may be employed.

**Contra-indications, warnings, etc** Otitis externa, seborrhoeic dermatitis, eczema affecting the external ear and perforated ear drum. Arachis Oil BP is a refined oil free of protein and is extremely unlikely to cause a reaction in subjects with peanut allergy. Such individuals did not react to Arachis Oil BP given by mouth in a randomised double-blind trial. There have not been any reports of reactions to Cerumol by subjects with peanut allergy; individuals with this allergy might nevertheless not wish to use Cerumol.
*Use in pregnancy:* No side-effects have been reported.
*Other special warnings:* Not to be taken internally. Do not use for more than three days. If the condition persists consult your doctor.
*Overdosage:* As the product is applied topically, overdosage as such is not possible. In the case of accidental ingestion, the amounts of the majority of ingredients in the 11 ml bottle are too small to give rise to toxic effects. The 550 mg of chlorbutol in the whole bottle might cause excessive sedation in a child.

**Pharmaceutical precautions** No special storage precautions.

**Legal category** P

**Package quantities** 11 ml vial with separate dropper.

**Further information** Nil.

**Product licence number** 0118/0013.

## EMESIDE* CAPSULES AND SYRUP

**Presentation** Soft orange gelatin capsules each containing 250 mg of Ethosuximide BP.
Blackcurrant or orange-flavoured syrup containing 250 mg of Ethosuximide BP per 5 ml.

**Uses** Emeside gives selective control of absence seizures (petit-mal) even when complicated by grandmal. It is also indicated for myoclonic seizures. The reduction of seizure frequency is thought to be achieved by depression of the motor cortex and elevation of the threshold to convulsive stimuli as seen by the suppression of the characteristic spike and wave EEG pattern. Emeside may be prescribed together with other anticonvulsants such as phenobarbitone, phenytoin, primidone or sodium valproate where grandmal or other forms of epilepsy may require additional treatment.

**Dosage and administration** *Adults and children over 6 years:* Start with a small dose – 500 mg daily with increments of 250 mg every five to seven days until control is achieved usually with 1,000–1,500 mg (4–6 capsules) daily. Occasionally 2,000 mg daily in divided dose may be necessary.
The half life of ethosuximide in the plasma is about 60 hours in adults but the daily dose if large is more comfortably divided between morning and evening.
If Emeside is being substituted for another antiepileptic drug the latter must not be withdrawn abruptly but the replacement made gradually with overlap of the preparations otherwise petit mal may break through; the slow withdrawal applies to Emeside when another drug is to replace it.

*Children and infants under six years:* Begin with a daily dose of 250 mg (5 ml syrup) and increase the dose gradually by small increments every few days until control is achieved, the maximum dose should be 1,000 mg.
Peak concentrations occur in plasma 1–7 hours after ingestion and the plasma half life is about 30 hours in children and 60 hours in adults. Plasma levels of ethosuximide to be effective lie between 40 and 85 microgram per ml but the clinical response should be the criterion for regulation of dosage. Because young children metabolise ethosuximide more rapidly than adults higher and more frequent doses may be necessary.

**Contra-indications, warnings, etc** Plasma concentrations are not accurately predictable and since compliance is variable, monitoring of plasma concentrations can be of value in unresponsive cases. Known hypersensitivity to succinimides. Exercise caution with regular appropriate tests in patients with hepatic or renal disease and monitor drug plasma concentrations. Porphyrias. Ethosuximide may be excreted into breast milk. Mothers receiving the drug should not breastfeed. There is a recognised small increase in the incidence of congenital malformations in children born to mothers receiving anti-convulsants. For women planning pregnancy or who are already pregnant the risk should be weighed carefully against the benefit of treatment.
As with all syrups it is advisable to brush the teeth or rinse the mouth after taking Emeside syrup.
*Side Effects:* Nausea, vomiting, anorexia and epigastric pain are common at first and generally subside. High dosage may cause sedation or confusion. Unusual symptoms are headache, fatigue, drowsiness, dizziness, ataxia, dyskinesia, hiccough, photophobia, depression and skin rash. Isolated reports have been made of erythema nodosum, erythema multiforme, agranulocytosis, aplastic anaemia. In some instances, patients who become leucopenic on other anticonvulsant therapy have been treated satisfactorily with ethosuximide. Lupus-like reactions have been reported in children given ethosuximide. They vary in severity from systemic immunological disorders, which include the nephrotic syndrome, to the asymptomatic presence of antinuclear antibodies.
*Drug Interaction:* The plasma concentrations of ethosuximide are reduced by carbamazepine and increased by isoniazid, phenytoin and sodium valproate.
*Overdosage:* Where more than 2 g has been thought to be ingested gastric lavage may be employed, if the time lapse is less than four hours.
Routine observation of respiration and circulation will indicate the need for supportive measures.

**Pharmaceutical precautions** Store in a cool dry place. Recommended diluent – unpreserved Syrup BP; use within 14 days.

**Legal category** POM.

**Package quantities** *Capsules:* 112.
*Syrup (blackcurrant or orange flavour):* Bottles of 200 ml.

**Further information** As with all syrups it is advisable to brush the teeth or rinse the mouth after taking Emeside syrup.

**Product licence numbers**

| | |
|---|---|
| Emeside Capsules | 0118/5002 |
| Emeside Syrup orange | 0118/5003 |
| Emeside Syrup blackcurrant | 0118/5004. |

## HALYCITROL* VITAMIN EMULSION

**Presentation** Orange flavoured emulsion containing 27,600 microgram (92,000 iu)/100 ml Vitamin A and 190 microgram (7,600 iu) Vitamin D per 100 ml. This is equivalent to 1,380 microgram (4,600 iu) of Vitamin A and 9.5 microgram (380 iu) of Vitamin D in a 5 ml daily dose.

**Uses** For prevention of vitamin A and D deficiency.

**Dosage and administration** *Adults and children above 6 months:* 5 ml daily.
*Infants up to six months:* 2.5 ml daily.
*Pregnancy:* Vitamin A supplements should only be taken during pregnancy when deficiency is demon-

strated or anticipated, e.g. due to malabsorption or restricted diets.

**Contra-indications, warnings, etc** Prolonged excessive ingestion of vitamins A and D can lead to hypervitaminosis states.
*Hypervitaminosis A:* Symptoms include dry rough skin, painful joint swellings, anorexia and vomiting.
*Hypervitaminosis D:* Infants already receiving vitamin D from such sources as vitaminised margarine and cereals can develop infantile hypercalcaemia from excessive vitamin D intake.
In children and adults the symptoms of hypercalcaemia are weakness, anorexia, abdominal pain, constipation, thirst and polyuria with the development of nephrocalcinosis, renal stones and renal failure. Individuals with renal disease and Sarcoidosis are particularly susceptible.

**Pharmaceutical precautions** Store in a cool place.

**Legal category** GSL.

**Package quantities** Bottles of 114 ml.

**Further information** This is a preparation of fish oil devoid of any fish odour or taste.

**Product licence number** 0118/0015.

## LABITON* TONIC

**Presentation** A brown liquid containing vitamin B₁ 0.75 mg, dried extract of kola nuts 6.05 mg, alcohol 2.8 ml, caffeine (total) 7 mg per 10 ml.

**Uses** The kola nut contains complex catechine-caffeinates which give central stimulation, increase muscular performance and reduce fatiguability. Vitamin B₁ is included to make up deficiency resulting from recent illness or anorexia. Labiton is indicated for use as a tonic for fatigue, anorexia and debility in convalescence after infections such as influenza and after operations.

**Dosage and administration** 10–20 ml twice daily, before or after meals, with or without water.
Not intended for administration to children.

**Contra-indications, warnings, etc** Undesirable in cases of hepatitis and patients taking sedatives. Car drivers should be made aware of the presence of alcohol and should be advised not to exceed the recommended dosage, especially if taking tranquillisers or remedies for allergies that have sedative side effects.
*Drug interactions:* Alcohol can cause flushing or a disulfiram-like reaction with metronidazole and chlorpropamide; this is dose-related in susceptible individuals. Interaction with Labiton has not been reported with any drug and is unlikely with correct dosage. With excessive dosage there could be potentiation of CNS depressants and potentiation of the hypoglycaemic effect of insulin.
*Overdosage:* Treatment is that for alcohol with correction of dehydration, attendance to the airway and other supportive measures for coma.

**Pharmaceutical precautions** Store in a cool place. Use within nine months of opening.

**Legal category** GSL.

**Package quantities** Supplied in bottles of 200 ml and 1 litre.

**Further information** Nil.

**Product licence number** 0118/5005.

## LABOSEPT* PASTILLES

**Presentation** Hexagonal red pastilles each containing Dequalinium Chloride BP 0.25 mg in a slow dissolving gelatine base.

**Uses** For bacterial and fungal infections of the mouth and throat.

**Dosage and administration** *Adults and children:* To be sucked slowly every three or four hours. For maximum benefit pastilles should be lodged comfortably between gum and cheek rather than be chewed. The daily dose should not exceed eight pastilles.

**Contra-indications, warnings, etc** Side effects and ill-effects from overdosage have not been reported.

**Pharmaceutical precautions** No special precautions.

**Legal category** P.

**Package quantities**    Carton containing 20 pastilles.

**Further information**    Contains no sugar.

**Product licence number**    0118/0012.

## MONPHYTOL*

**Presentation**    A colourless, rapidly drying, non-greasy paint containing chlorbutol 3%, methyl undecylenate 5%, propyl undecylenate 0.7%, salicylic acid 3%, methyl salicylate 25%, and propyl salicylate 5%.

**Uses**    Monphytol is indicated for tinea pedis, tinea unguium, tinea circinata, erosio interdigitalis, intertrigo.

**Dosage and administration**    *Adults over 12:* Twice daily moisten brush with Monphytol and apply to the affected parts, reaching gently into the folds of the skin. Treatment should be repeated from time to time after the condition has subsided to prevent reinfection.

*Children under 12, pregnant and lactating women:* The safety of this product has not been demonstrated for these groups. Its use must be at the physician's discretion.

**Contra-indications, warnings, etc**    Monphytol may sting sensitive weeping areas of acutely inflamed skin. Other treatment (to reduce inflammation and exudation) may first be necessary. Monphytol should not be used on bleeding areas.

**Pharmaceutical precautions**    During use avoid contact of liquid with plastics. Store away from heat.

**Legal category**    P.

**Package quantities**    Bottles containing 18 ml.

**Further information**    Nil.

**Product licence number**    0118/5010R.

*Trade Mark

# Lagap Pharmaceuticals Ltd
Woolmer Way
Bordon
Hants GU35 9QE

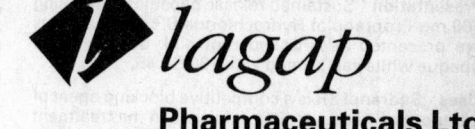

## BACLOFEN TABLETS BP 10 mg
**Qualitative and quantitative composition** Each tablet contains Baclofen BP 10 mg.

**Pharmaceutical form** Tablets.

**Clinical particulars**
*Therapeutic indications:* Baclofen is indicated for the relief of spasticity of voluntary muscle resulting from such disorders as: multiple sclerosis, other spinal lesions e.g.: tumours of the spinal cord, syringomyelia, motor neurone disease, transverse myelitis, traumatic partial section of the cord.

Baclofen is also indicated in adults and children for the relief of spasticity of voluntary muscle arising from e.g.: cerebrovascular accidents, cerebral palsy, meningitis, traumatic head injury.

Patient selection is most important when initiating baclofen therapy; it is likely to be of most benefit in patients whose spasticity constitutes a handicap to activities and/or physiotherapy. Treatment should not be commenced until the spastic state has been stabilised.

*Posology and method of administration:* Oral administration.

The possible extent of clinical improvement to the patient should be assessed prior to the initiation of baclofen therapy. Titrated doses should be carefully administered in gradually increasing quantities until the patient's condition is stable (this is particularly important in elderly patients). If the dosage is too high or has been increased too quickly, side effects may ensue, especially in patients who are mobile to minimise muscle weakness in unaffected limbs or where some degree of spasticity is required.

*Adults:* The following slowly increasing dosage regimen is suggested, but may be adjusted to suit the patient.

5 mg 3 times a day for 3 days.
10 mg 3 times a day for 3 days.
15 mg 3 times a day for 3 days.
20 mg 3 times a day for 3 days.

Doses up to 60 mg a day usually provide satisfactory control of symptoms, though careful adjustment according to the requirements of each patient is frequently necessary. Small, more frequent doses of baclofen may prove better in some cases than larger, less frequent doses. If required, the dose may be increased slowly. A maximum daily dose of more than 100 mg is not recommended, unless the patient is hospitalised and under close supervision. Once this maximum recommended dose is reached, if the therapeutic effects are not evident in 6 weeks, it may not be of benefit for the patient to continue on baclofen therapy.

Some patients may benefit from the use of baclofen just at night to oppose painful flexor spasm. Also, a single dose about an hour before carrying out tasks like dressing, washing, shaving and physiotherapy will often augment a patient's motility.

*Elderly:* The elderly may be more susceptible to side effects, especially when first introducing baclofen. Initially, small doses are advised, with gradual adjustment under careful supervision. The eventual average maximum dose is as for adults, but caution should be exercised especially in patients with impaired renal function (see below).

*Children:* Dosages in the range of 0.75 to 2 mg/kg body weight should be used. In children over 10 years of age, a maximum daily dosage of 2.5 mg/kg body weight may be given. Treatment usually commences with 2.5 mg 4 times a day. Dosage should be cautiously raised at approximately 3 day intervals until the child's individual requirements are met.

*Maintenance therapy:*
Children aged 12 months to 2 years: 10 to 20 mg
Children aged 2 to 6 years: 20 to 30 mg
Children aged 6 to 10 years: 30 to 60 mg.

*Patients with impaired renal function:* A low dosage of baclofen should be given, i.e. approximately 5 mg a day, in patients with impaired renal function or who are undergoing chronic haemodialysis.

*Patients with spastic states of cerebral origin:* A very cautious dosage schedule should be adopted and patients should be carefully monitored as unwanted effects are more likely to occur in these patients.

*Contra-indications:* Peptic ulceration and hypersensitivity to baclofen.

*Special warnings and special precautions for use:* Psychotic disorders, confusional states or schizophrenia may be worsened by treatment with baclofen. Therefore, patients with these conditions should be kept under close observation and treatment should be administered cautiously.

Epileptic manifestations may be exacerbated with baclofen treatment, but may be used if appropriate supervision and anticonvulsive therapy are maintained.

Caution should be exercised with baclofen therapy in patients suffering from renal, hepatic or respiratory impairment or who have had a cerebrovascular accident.

Patients with neurogenic disturbances affecting emptying of the bladder may show improvement in their condition whilst taking baclofen. However, patients with pre-existing sphincter hypertonia may suffer with acute urine retention during treatment with baclofen; as a result it should be used cautiously in these patients.

Appropriate laboratory tests should be carried out on patients with hepatic dysfunction or diabetes mellitus to make sure that no drug-induced changes to the underlying diseases have resulted with concomitant baclofen therapy as, rarely, elevated SGOT, alkaline phosphatase and glucose levels in serum have been recorded.

Baclofen therapy should always be gradually discontinued, unless serious adverse effects have occurred, by reducing the dose over a period of 1–2 weeks. Anxiety, confusion, hallucinations, psychosis, mania, paranoia, convulsions, tachycardia, and, as a rebound phenomenon, temporary aggravation of spasticity, have all been reported on abrupt withdrawal.

*Interactions with other medicaments and other forms of interaction:* There have been reports of hallucinations, agitation and mental confusion with the use of baclofen with levodopa and carbidopa in Parkinson's disease.

Use of tricyclic antidepressants and baclofen may result in the potentiation of the effect of baclofen, resulting in pronounced muscular hypotonia.

Baclofen excretion may be reduced by drugs which produce renal insufficiency, e.g. ibuprofen, resulting in toxic effects.

Concomitant use of drugs acting on the CNS or alcohol with baclofen may lead to increased sedation.

Fentanyl induced analgesia may be extended by pretreatment with baclofen.

Hyperkinetic symptoms in patients receiving lithium may be exacerbated by baclofen.

Antihypertensive therapy may require adjustment as an increased fall in blood pressure may result with concomitant treatment with baclofen.

*Pregnancy and lactation:* Not recommended in pregnancy as fetal malformations have been reported as having occurred in rats but not mice or rabbits. Where treatment is necessary, the benefits for the mother should be carefully considered against the possible risks to the child, particularly in the first trimester when baclofen should only be used if essential. Baclofen is not recommended whilst breast-feeding as it is known to be present in the milk.

*Effects on ability to drive and use machines:* Patients taking baclofen should not take charge of vehicles, other means of transport, or machinery where loss of attention may lead to accidents.

*Undesirable effects:* Undesirable effects occur predominantly with initial treatment, with large doses, if the dose is increased too quickly or in the treatment of the elderly. These effects rarely necessitate withdrawal of the medication and are frequently of short duration. Modifying the dosage may lessen or eliminate the effects.

It may be difficult to distinguish between drug-induced undesirable effects and those caused by the diseases being treated.

*Gastro-intestinal tract:* Mild gastro-intestinal disturbances such as constipation or diarrhoea may occasionally occur. Dry mouth, nausea and vomiting have also been reported. Should nausea continue despite reduced dosage, baclofen should be taken with food or a milk drink.

*Genito-urinary tract:* Increased frequency of micturition, dysuria and enuresis have rarely been reported.

*Cardio-respiratory system:* Hypotension and cardiovascular or respiratory depression have been reported occasionally.

*Central nervous system:* Especially at the beginning of treatment, effects including drowsiness and daytime sedation may occur with occasional reports of lassitude, exhaustion, light-headedness, confusion, dizziness, headache and insomnia.

A lower convulsion threshold and seizures may occur, particularly in patients with epilepsy.

Other neurological effects which have been reported include paraesthesiase, muscle weakness, myalgia, ataxia, tremor, nystagmus and accommodation disorders. Reported psychiatric effects include euphoria, hallucinations, nightmares and depressive states.

*Other unwanted effects:* There have been very rare reports of skin rash, hyperhidrosis, visual disturbance, changes in taste sensation and a deterioration in liver function tests.

Increased spasticity as a contradictory response to the medication has been reported in some patients.

Some patients may experience greater difficulty in walking or coping for themselves as a result of excessive hypotonia. This may be alleviated by altering the dosage schedule.

*Overdosage: Symptoms:* Primarily, these are signs of central nervous depression: including drowsiness, consciousness impairment, respiratory depression, coma. Also likely are confusion, agitation, hallucinations, eye accommodation disorders, absent pupillary reflex, generalised muscular hypotonia, myoclonia, hyporeflexia or areflexia, convulsions, peripheral vasodilatation, hypotension, bradycardia, hypothermia, nausea, vomiting, diarrhoea, hypersalivation and elevated LDH, SGOT and AP values.

Deterioration in the condition may occur if various substances/drugs acting on the CNS, e.g. alcohol, tricyclic antidepressants or diazepam, have been taken at the same time.

*Treatment:* No specific antidote is known. Removal of the drug from the gastro-intestinal tract should be attempted by inducing vomiting or gastric lavage. Comatose patients need to be intubated prior to gastric lavage. Activated charcoal or, if necessary, a saline aperient may be given. In respiratory depression, artificial respiration and measures to support cardiovascular functions should be applied. Large quantities of fluid should be given, possibly with a diuretic, since baclofen is excreted mainly through the kidneys. If convulsions occur, intravenous diazepam should be administered.

**Pharmacological properties**
*Pharmacodynamic properties:* Baclofen is an analogue of aminobutyric acid. Its mode of action is not fully understood. It inhibits monosynaptic and polysynaptic transmission at the spinal level and also depresses the CNS.

*Pharmacokinetic properties:* The following mean values were obtained for Baclofen Tablets 10 mg in healthy volunteers.

| | |
|---|---|
| $T_{\frac{1}{2}}$ (hours) | 3.301 |
| $T_{max}$ (hours) | 1.549 |
| $C_{max}$ (ng/ml) | 102 |
| AUC (ng/ml hours) | 674 |

**Pharmaceutical particulars**
*List of excipients:* Lactose, potato starch, microcrystalline cellulose, sodium starch glycollate and magnesium stearate.

*Incompatibilities:* Not known.

*Shelf life:* 3 years.

*Special precautions for storage:* Store in a cool dry place and protect from light.

*Nature and contents of container:* Securitainer with polyethylene closure. Pack size: 100.

*Instructions for use/handling:* Not applicable.

**Marketing authorisation number** 4416/0160.

**Date of revision of SPC** 21 May 1997.

**Legal category** POM.

# BEDRANOL* SR 160 MG CAPSULES

**Presentation** Sustained release capsules containing 160 mg Propranolol Hydrochloride BP. The capsules are presented as a transparent pink body with an opaque white cap printed with 160 SR 45.

**Uses** Bedranol SR is a competitive blocking agent of adrenergic β-receptor sites. It is used in the treatment of hypertension and angina.

## Dosage and administration

*Adults:* Hypertension. The initial dose is one capsule daily taken orally in the morning or evening. An adequate response is seen by most patients at this dosage. If necessary, the dose can be increased to 2 capsules. A further reduction in blood pressure may be achieved by combining Bedranol SR with other antihypertensive agents.

Angina. Most patients will respond to one capsule daily taken orally in the morning or evening.

*Children:* Bedranol SR is not intended for use in children.

*Elderly:* The evidence concerning the relationship between blood level and age is conflicting. For patients already established on 160 mg propranolol daily, one capsule of Bedranol SR may be given. It is suggested that elderly patients being started off on propranolol treatment may need smaller initial doses and in these circumstances an alternative preparation should be used.

## Contra-indications, warnings, etc

*Contra-indications:* Bedranol SR should not be used in the presence of second or third degree heart block; in patients with cardiogenic shock; if there is a history of bronchospasm; after prolonged fasting and in metabolic acidosis.

*Precautions:* Patients with a history of wheezing or asthma should not take propranolol, unless it is considered essential. The label will carry the following warning: 'Do not take this medicine if you have a history of wheezing or asthma'. The patient information leaflet will state: 'Do not take this medicine if you have a history of wheezing or asthma. Consult your doctor or pharmacist first.'

Withdrawal of the drug for any reason should be gradual.

Bedranol SR should be used with caution in patients whose cardiac reserve is poor. It should be avoided in overt heart failure but may be used where the signs of heart failure are controlled.

One of the pharmacological actions of propranolol is to reduce the heart rate. In the rare instance when symptoms may be attributable to the slow heart rate, the dose may be reduced.

Care should be exercised when treating patients with renal impairment as it has been suggested that a reduced initial dosage is given.

Hepatic metabolism is a major route of elimination and therefore patients with liver disease may need to be given a reduced dosage. In these circumstances this preparation is not recommended.

In patients with ischaemic heart disease treatment should not be discontinued abruptly. Either the equivalent dose of another beta-blocker may be substituted or the withdrawal of Bedranol SR should be gradual. This can be done by substituting the equivalent dose in propranolol 40 mg tablets and then reducing the dose.

In patients with portal hypertension, liver function will deteriorate and there is a risk of developing hepatic encephalopathy.

Caution should be exercised when transferring patients from clonidine to beta-adrenoceptor blocking drugs.

Bedranol SR should not impair ability to drive and use machines.

*Interactions:* If Bedranol SR and clonidine are given concurrently, clonidine should not be discontinued until several days after withdrawal of the beta-blocker.

Propranolol modifies the tachycardia of hypoglycaemia. Caution should be exercised in the concurrent use of Bedranol SR and hypoglycaemic therapy in diabetic patients. Propranolol may prolong the hypoglycaemic response to insulin.

Care should be taken in the parenteral administration of preparations containing adrenaline to patients taking beta-adrenoceptor blocking drugs as, in rare cases, vasoconstriction, hypertension and bradycardia may result.

Care should be taken in prescribing a beta-adrenoceptor blocking drug with Class 1 antidysrhythmic agents such as disopyramide.

Beta-adrenoceptor blocking drugs should be used with caution in combination with verapamil in patients with impaired ventricular function. The combination should not be given to patients with conduction abnormalities. Neither drug should be administered intravenously within 48 hours of discontinuing the other.

As with all beta-blocking drugs it may be necessary to withdraw Bedranol SR before surgery. Twenty-four hours should be allowed to elapse between the last dose and anaesthesia. If Bedranol SR treatment is continued throughout surgery the anaesthetist should be informed and care should be taken when using anaesthetic agents such as ether, cyclopropane and trichloroethylene. Vagal dominance if it occurs may be corrected by 1–2 mg I.V. atropine.

*Interference with laboratory tests:* Propranolol has been reported to interfere with the estimation of serum bilirubin by the diazo method and with the determination of catecholamines by methods using fluorescence.

*Pregnancy and lactation:* Although there is no evidence that propranolol is teratogenic, Bedranol SR should not be used in pregnancy unless absolutely necessary. It is excreted in breast milk but the quantity is small and should not affect the infant.

*Side-effects:* Minor side-effects such as cold extremities, nausea, insomnia, lassitude, diarrhoea and muscle fatigue are usually transient. Isolated cases of paraesthesia of the hands have been reported. There have been reports of skin rashes and/or dry eyes associated with the use of beta-adrenergic blocking drugs. The reported incidence is small and in most cases, the symptoms have cleared when treatment is withdrawn. Cases of bradycardia, thrombocytopenia and purpura have rarely been recorded. A low incidence of CNS symptoms, including hallucinations have been reported. If these symptoms are not attributed to some other cause, Bedranol SR should be withdrawn.

Rare cases of blood dyscrasias have been reported.

Bradycardia and hypotension are usually a sign of overdosage but may rarely be due to intolerance of the drug in which case it should be withdrawn.

*Overdosage:* Excessive bradycardia can be countered with 1–2 mg I.V. atropine, followed if necessary by a bolus dose of glucagon 10 mg I.V. This may be repeated if necessary or followed by an intravenous infusion of glucagon 1–10 mg/hour depending on response. If glucagon is unavailable a beta-receptor stimulant such as isoprenaline 25 micrograms I.V. or orciprenaline 500 micrograms I.V. may be given by slow intravenous injection.

**Pharmaceutical precautions** Store in a cool dry place and protect from light.

**Legal category** POM.

**Package quantities** Pack of 100 capsules.

**Further information** Nil.

**Product licence number** 4416/0068.

# CAPTOPRIL TABLETS BP

**Qualitative and quantitative composition** Each Captopril Tablet contains Captopril BP 12.5 mg, 25 mg or 50 mg.

**Pharmaceutical form** Uncoated tablets.

## Clinical particulars

*Therapeutic indications:*

*Hypertension:* For the treatment of mild to moderate hypertension. Captopril may be used in severe hypertension when standard therapy is inadequate or ineffective.

*Congestive heart failure:* In the treatment of congestive heart failure, Captopril should be used in association with diuretics and, if appropriate, digitalis.

*Myocardial infarction:* Following myocardial infarction in patients with left ventricular dysfunction, Captopril may be used to improve prognosis. Cardiac function should be assessed by echocardiography or radionuclide studies before starting treatment with Captopril.

*Posology and method of administration:* For oral administration only.

*Hypertension:* Captopril may be used alone or in combination with other therapies for the treatment of hypertension. Treatment should be started at a low dose and increased gradually at 2 to 4 week intervals until an adequate effect is achieved. The starting dose should be 12.5 mg twice daily and, in order to avoid a precipitous drop in blood pressure in some patients, the first dose should be given at bedtime. If possible, diuretics should be discontinued for a few days before commencing Captopril. In those patients who are still on diuretics, or who are elderly or have renal impairment, the starting dose should be 6.25 mg twice daily.

The maintenance dose is usually 25 mg to 50 mg twice daily but in more severe cases, up to 50 mg three times daily may be needed.

*Congestive heart failure:* In the treatment of heart failure, Captopril should be started under close medical supervision. A low initial dose of 6.25 mg or 12.5 mg twice daily will minimise hypotensive effects. The dose should be gradually increased at intervals of not less than 14 days until a satisfactory therapeutic response is attained. The maximum daily dose is usually 50 mg three times a day.

*Myocardial infarction:* A starting dose of 6.25 mg should be increased to a maximum of 150 mg daily over several weeks. The patient's tolerance will determine the dose used but symptomatic hypotension indicates the need to reduce the dose. Captopril may be used in conjunction with other post-infarction treatments including thrombolytics, aspirin and beta-blockers.

*In renal impairment:* As Captopril is largely excreted via the kidneys, the dosage and dose frequency should be reduced in patients with renal impairment (creatinine clearance of less than 30 ml/min or plasma creatinine above 150 μmol/l). As ACE inhibitors may reduce or abolish glomerular filtration in patients with renovascular disease they should not be used in such patients unless careful monitoring of renal function is available.

Captopril is removed by haemodialysis.

*Elderly patients:* The lowest dose of Captopril which achieves a satisfactory therapeutic effect should be used in elderly patients, particularly those with evidence of renal or other organ dysfunction.

*Children:* The use of Captopril is not recommended for the treatment of mild to moderate hypertension in children.

Experience in neonates, particularly premature infants, is limited. Because renal function in infants is not equivalent to that of older children and adults lower doses of Captopril should be used with the patients under close medical supervision. The starting dose may be 0.3 mg/kg bodyweight daily increasing to a maximum of 6 mg/kg in two or three divided doses.

*Contra-indications:* Hypersensitivity to Captopril, other ACE inhibitors or any of the tablet ingredients. Captopril is contra-indicated in pregnancy and lactation.

*Special warnings and precautions for use:* Captopril should not be used in patients with aortic stenosis or outflow tract obstruction. Renal function should be assessed before starting treatment with Captopril and at intervals during the course of therapy. Patients with bilateral renovascular disease should not be treated with ACE inhibitors except under very careful supervision. It is considered that patients with peripheral vascular disease or generalised atherosclerosis may be at higher risk of renovascular disease and care should be taken in those with systemic lupus erythematosus or scleroderma.

Hypotensive episodes may occur after the first one or two doses and this is usually relieved by lying the patient down or starting therapy at bedtime. Patients with severe hypertension or those with renin dependent hypertension may be more likely to develop hypotensive episodes and a lower starting dose may be appropriate. In patients on diuretics, reduction of the dose or withdrawal of the diuretic for a few days prior to starting treatment with Captopril may reduce the chance of hypotension occurring.

Potassium supplements or potassium sparing diuretics should not normally be used with ACE inhibitors because they decrease aldosterone production. A rise in serum potassium levels may occur in patients with renal impairment.

Anaphylactoid reactions have been reported in patients on ACE inhibitors undergoing renal dialysis using polyacrylonitrile membranes. The combined use of such membranes and ACE inhibitors should be avoided.

*Interactions with other medicaments and other forms of interaction:* Diuretics potentiate the anti-hypertensive action of Captopril. Potassium sparing diuretics or potassium supplements may cause an increase in serum potassium.

The response to other vasodilator drugs may be enhanced by Captopril and this should be borne in mind when adding Captopril to existing therapy.

Patients previously treated with clonidine may have a delayed response when they are changed to Captopril.

Indomethacin may reduce the anti-hypertensive effect of Captopril and this may occur with other non-steroidal anti-inflammatory drugs.

Probenecid reduces the renal clearance of Captopril.

Lithium serum levels may be increased when lithium is given with Captopril.

Allopurinol and procainamide have been reported to cause neutropenia and/or Stevens-Johnson syndrome when given concomitantly with Captopril. Care should be taken when using such combinations of drugs, particularly in patients with impaired renal function.

Azathioprine and cyclophosphamide given with Captopril have been associated with blood dyscrasias, especially in patients with renal failure.

A false-positive test for acetone in the urine may be caused by Captopril.

Polyacrylonitrile dialysis membranes have been associated with anaphylactoid reactions in patients taking ACE inhibitors.

Hypotension occurring during surgery or general anaesthesia as a result of angiotensin II blockade in patients treated with Captopril should be corrected by volume expansion.

*Pregnancy and lactation:* Captopril is contra-indicated in pregnancy. Captopril is known to be fetotoxic in some animal species and has been associated with oligohydramnios and hypotension and/or anuria in the neonate when given to pregnant women in the second or third trimesters. Women of child-bearing potential should take adequate contraceptive precautions if being treated with Captopril.

Captopril is excreted in breast milk and therefore should not be given to nursing mothers.

*Effects on ability to drive and use machines:* Patients should be warned to avoid driving or operating machinery if they experience any dizziness or fatigue when taking Captopril.

*Undesirable effects:* Adverse effects are usually dose related and more frequent in patients with impaired renal function. The more common side effects include skin rashes which occur with pruritus, hypotension; cough; taste disturbance and renal side effects. Reports in the literature indicate that the incidence of occurrence of these side effects varies up to 5%. The main exception to this is the incidence of rash occurring and up to 7% has been recorded for patients with impaired renal function.

*Renal:* proteinuria, hyperkalaemia. Some deterioration in renal function has been seen with raised blood urea and creatinine levels and reversible renal failure may occur in patients with existing renovascular disease.

*Cardiovascular:* tachycardia and hypotention may occur, particularly early in treatment, in patients with heart failure or volume or salt depleted such as those already on diuretics.

*Gastro-intestinal:* stomatitis, gastric irritation or abdominal pain, weight loss associated with taste disturbance. Transient increases in liver enzymes have been noted and, rarely, cholestatic jaundice or hepatocellular injury has occurred. Pancreatitis has been rarely reported in patients on ACE inhibitors.

*Haematological:* neutropenia, agranulocytosis, thrombocytopenia, anaemia and aplastic anaemia have been reported, more often in patients with renal impairment. Patients should be warned to report any unexpected bleeding, bruising or sore throats and appropriate haematological tests should be performed.

*Dermatological:* itchy skin rashes, urticaria, and vesicular or bullous rashes have been reported. Photosensitivity has occurred.

*Other effects:* headache, angioedema, paraesthesiae of extremities, serum sickness, lymphadenopathy, bronchospasm have been reported with Captopril.

*Overdose:* Blood pressure should be monitored and, if necessary, hypotension can be corrected by volume expansion. Captopril is readily eliminated by haemodialysis.

**Pharmacological properties**

*Pharmacodynamic properties:* Captopril is a highly specific competitive inhibitor of angiotensin I converting enzyme thus reducing angiotensin II levels. It reduces peripheral vascular resistance, lowering blood pressure, and by reducing both pre-load and after-load it is useful in the treatment of heart failure.

*Pharmacokinetic properties:* Captopril is fairly well absorbed and although blood levels are reduced when taken with food, its antihypertensive effect does not seem to be altered. There is some reversible binding to plasma proteins. About 50% is metabolised and the drug is mostly excreted via the kidneys either as metabolites or unchanged drug within about 6 hours. There is some accumulation with chronic dosing and renal impairment reduces clearance.

*Preclinical safety data:* It is reported that studies carried out in rabbits revealed that captopril had an embryocidal effect. However, no teratogenic or carcinogenic effects were observed. Captopril is reported to have a lethal effect in sheep foetuses. No toxic effects have been observed in hamster or rat foetuses.

It is reported that studies carried out in dogs revealed that bone marrow suppression occurred which was dose related. Anaemia is reported to have occurred at lower doses while leucopenia and thrombocytopenia were observed at higher doses only. Studies carried out in monkeys, rats and mice have shown anaemia to occur at very high doses which exceed the maximum dose in humans.

**Pharmaceutical particulars**

*List of excipients:* Lactose PhEur; Maize Starch PhEur; Microcrystalline Cellulose PhEur; Stearic Acid BP.

*Incompatibilities:* Not applicable.

*Shelf life:* 3 years.

*Special precautions for storage:* Store at a temperature not exceeding 25°C.

*Nature and contents of container:* Captopril tablets are available in blister strips composed of PVC/Aluminium.
Pack size: 56 tablets.

*Instructions for use/handling:* Not applicable.

**Marketing authorisation numbers**
Captopril Tablets BP 12.5 mg    4416/0271
Captopril Tablets BP 25 mg      4416/0272
Captopril Tablets BP 50 mg      4416/0273

**Date of approval/revision of SPC**   14 October 1996.

**Legal category**   POM.

# CARBO-DOME* CREAM

**Qualitative and quantitative composition**   Each 100 g of cream contain Coal Tar Solution BP 10 g.

**Pharmaceutical form**   Cream.

**Clinical particulars**
*Therapeutic indications:* The coal tar solution in Carbo-Dome Cream has a keratoplastic and antipruritic effect in psoriasis.
*Indications:* Psoriasis.

*Posology and method of administration:* For topical application only. Apply to the affected areas two or three times daily. This dosage is recommended for both children and adults.

*Contra-indications:* Coal tar should not be used when a patient has known sensitivity to coal tar or any of the other ingredients. It should not be used on broken or highly inflamed skin.

*Special warnings and precautions for use:* For topical administration only.
Coal tar should be used with caution on the face (avoiding the eyes), skin flexures or genitalia. If it gets in the eyes, rinse them thoroughly with water.
Avoid exposure to direct sunlight and UV lamps after applying, unless its action is specifically required – see *Interactions* below.

*Interactions with other medicaments and other forms of interaction:* Ultraviolet-B (UVB) light increases the effect of coal tar in the treatment of psoriasis.

*Pregnancy and lactation:* Although there is no direct evidence of the safety of coal tar used topically in pregnancy and lactation, has been used over many years without known ill effects.

*Effects on ability to drive and use machines:* None known.

*Undesirable effects:* Coal tar may cause photosensitivity and patients should be warned to avoid exposure to sunlight or UV lamps after treatment (unless this is specifically intended).
Coal tar may cause irritation, acneiform eruptions or folliculitis, and may cause staining.

*Overdosage:* Not applicable.

**Pharmacological properties**
*Pharmacodynamic properties:* Coal tar as presented in this product is an antipruritic keratoplastic and weak antiseptic.

*Pharmacokinetic properties:* The product is designed for external use only. Absorption of the coal tar is not reported in 'Martindale' and therefore the pharmacokinetics is not addressed.

*Preclinical safety data:* There are no pre-clinical data of relevance to the prescriber which are additional to that already included in other sections of the SPC.

**Pharmaceutical particulars**
*List of excipients:* Dehydag wax SX, beeswax, white soft paraffin, light liquid paraffin, glycerol, sodium lauryl sulphate, methyl-p-hydroxybenzoate and purified water.

*Incompatibilities:* None recorded.

*Shelf life:* 36 months.

*Special precautions for storage:* Store in cool place.

*Nature and contents of container:* Tubes (aluminium). Pack sizes: 30 g and 100 g.

*Instructions for use/handling:* Not applicable.

**Marketing authorisation number**   4416/0106.

**Date of revision of SPC**   March 1996.

**Legal category**   GSL.

# CO-AMILOFRUSE TABLETS BP

**Qualitative and quantitative composition**   Each tablet contains Frusemide BP 40 mg and Amiloride Hydrochloride BP equivalent to anhydrous amiloride hydrochloride 5 mg.

**Pharmaceutical form**   Tablet.

**Clinical particulars**
*Therapeutic indications:* For the treatment of oedematous conditions where rapid diuresis with potassium conservation is required.
This includes congestive cardiac failure, oedema due to renal disease, corticosteroid therapy, and ascites associated with cirrhosis.

*Posology and method of administration:*
*Adults:* The normal dose is one tablet a day, to be taken in the morning. This can be increased to two tablets daily, if necessary.

*Elderly:* The dose may require adjustment according to the patient's diuretic response. If necessary, a lower dose (e.g. half a tablet) may be taken. Creatinine and serum electrolytes should be monitored carefully.

*Children:* Not recommended for use in children.

Oral administration.

*Contra-indications:* Known sensitivity to frusemide, amiloride hydrochloride or any of the other ingredients, acute renal failure or severe progressive renal disease. Addison's disease, hyperkalaemia (serum potassium >5.3 mmol/litre), anuria, electrolyte imbalance, precomatose states associated with cirrhosis, concomitant potassium supplements or potassium sparing diuretics. Co-amilofruse is also contra-indicated in children as safety has not been established.

*Special warnings and precautions for use:* Tests should be performed to monitor kidney function and serum electrolyte levels. This is particularly important in the treatment of the elderly, patients with impaired kidney function, potential obstruction of the urinary tract or fragile electrolyte balance, where a reduced dosage may be required.
Frusemide may cause latent diabetes to become manifest. It may be necessary to increase the dose of hypoglycaemic agents in diabetic patients. Patients suffering from diabetes mellitus are at an increased risk of developing hyperkalaemia. Treatment with co-amilofruse should be discontinued three days prior to glucose tolerance tests.
Co-amilofruse should be used with caution in patients with prostatic hypertrophy or impaired micturition as acute urinary retention may occur.

*Interactions with other medicaments and other forms of interaction:* Concurrent use of ACE inhibitors, non-steroidal anti-inflammatory drugs, cyclosporin, trilostane, potassium salts and hypoglycaemic agents may lead to an increased risk of hyperkalaemia.
The potential risk of nephrotoxicity may be increased when cephaloridine, NSAIDs, or aminoglycoside antibiotics are used concurrently. Ototoxicity may also occur with concurrent use of aminoglycoside antibiotics.
The dosage of cardiac glycosides, lithium, non-depolarising muscle relaxants, antihypertensive agents and hypoglycaemic agents may require adjustment.

*Pregnancy and lactation:* Use in pregnancy and lactation should be avoided as safety has not been established.

*Effects on ability to drive and use machines:* Reduced mental alertness and confusion may affect ability to drive. Other activities requiring full alertness should be avoided.

*Undesirable effects:* Side effects which may occur include nausea, vomiting, abdominal pain, diarrhoea or constipation, parasthesia, thirst, dizziness, skin rash (although rare may be severe), pruritus, weakness, muscle cramps, headache and minor psychiatric or visual changes.
Tinnitus and deafness and hypersensitivity reactions including interstitial nephritis occur rarely.
Hyperuricaemia may occur, precipitating attacks of gout in some patients. Pancreatitis has been reported with high doses and cholestatic jaundice has also been reported.
Bone marrow depression has occurred rarely: agranulocytosis, thrombocytopenia and leucopenia have been reported. The patients haematopoetic state should be regularly monitored throughout treatment.

*Overdose:* Symptoms of overdosage include dehydration, electrolyte imbalance (particularly hyperkalaemia). If possible, emesis should be induced or gastric lavage performed. In order to correct electrolyte changes and dehydration, sodium chloride and water should be administered. If there is evidence of hyperkalaemia, measures should be taken to reduce serum potassium levels.

**Pharmacological properties**
*Pharmacodynamic properties:* Frusemide is a high ceiling diuretic which acts on the ascending limb of the loop of Henle, inhibiting sodium and chloride reabsorption. It causes an increase in urinary excretion of sodium, chloride, water, potassium, calcium and magnesium. It also increases the excretion of bicarbonate, resulting in a rise in urinary pH.
Frusemide increases ammonia excretion via the

kidney and decreases the secretion of uric acid, resulting in increased blood urate levels, which may precipitate gout.

Amiloride is a diuretic acting primarily in the distal tubule and promotes the excretion of sodium in the urine without decreasing the potassium levels in plasma. When excretion of potassium is increased by other diuretics, amiloride causes a noticeable decrease in potassium excretion. Amiloride also decreases urinary excretion of calcium and magnesium.

*Pharmacokinetic properties:* Frusemide is readily absorbed from the gastro-intestinal tract and is about 60% bioavailable. It is extensively bound to plasma proteins. The elimination half-life is approximately 1–2 hours and produces a duration of action of 3–6 hours. Approximately 50% of an oral dose of amiloride is absorbed which is not significantly bound to plasma protein. Absorption is reduced by food and the elimination half-life is 6–9 hours with peak serum levels at 3–4 hours.

*Preclinical safety data:* Not relevant.

**Pharmaceutical particulars**

*List of excipients:* Lactose, polyvinylpyrrolidone, orange E110 soluble, orange E110 insoluble, microcrystalline cellulose, sodium starch glycollate, magnesium stearate and purified water.

*Incompatibilities:* Not known.

*Shelf life:* 36 months.

*Special precautions for storage:* Store in dry place. Protect from light.

*Nature and contents of container:* Pack sizes: 28 and 56 tablets.

Blister strips composed of: 250 µm PVC/PVdC coated foil, 20 µm aluminium foil. Blister strips will be packed in cartons.

*Instructions for use/handling:* Not applicable.

**Marketing authorisation number** 04416/0267.

**Date of approval/revision of SPC** April 1996.

**Legal category** POM.

## DIAZEPAM SYRUP 2 mg/5 ml
## DIAZEPAM FORTE SYRUP 5 mg/5 ml

**Presentation** Bottles contain either diazepam BP 2 mg in 5 ml or diazepam BP 5 mg in 5 ml. The non-active ingredients include ethanol, sucrose, microcrystalline cellulose, ponceau 4R (E124), potassium sorbate, flavour, and methylhydroxybenzoate and propylhydroxybenzoate as preservatives.

**Uses** Diazepam has anticonvulsant, anxiolytic, sedative, muscle relaxant and amnesic properties. It is indicated:

*Adults:*

(i) for the short-term relief (2–4 weeks only) of anxiety that is severe, disabling or subjecting the individual to unacceptable distress, occurring alone or in association with insomnia or short-term psychosomatic, organic or psychotic illness;

(ii) as a sedative and premedicant;

(iii) as an anticonvulsant in the management of status epilepticus, febrile convulsions and poisoning;

(iv) in the control of muscle spasms as in tetanus;

(v) in the management of alcohol withdrawal symptoms;

(vi) in selected cases it may be useful in the management of cerebral spasticity.

*Children:*

(i) night terrors and somnambulism;

(ii) premedication;

(iii) in the control of muscle spasms as in tetanus;

(iv) in selected cases, it may be useful in controlling tension and irritabilty in cerebral spasticity.

The use of diazepam to treat short-term anxiety is inappropriate and unsuitable. Diazepam should be used to treat insomnia only when it is severe, disabling or subjecting the individual to extreme stress.

**Dosage and administration** For oral administration.

The lowest dose that can control the symptoms should be used and treatment should not be continued beyond 4 weeks.

*Adults:* Anxiety states: 2 mg three times daily up to 30 mg daily in divided doses.

Insomnia associated with anxiety: 5 mg to 15 mg before retiring.

Muscle spasms: 2 mg to 15 mg daily in divided doses up to 60 mg in severe spastic disorders such as cerebral spasticity, epilepsy and muscle spasms associated with upper-motor neurone disease.

In the control of muscle spasms as in tetanus: 3 mg to 10 mg/kg bodyweight daily.

Alcohol withdrawal symptoms: 5 mg to 20 mg repeated within 2 to 4 hours if necessary.

Premedication in dental patients: 5 mg the night before, 5 mg on waking and another 5 mg two hours before the appointment.

*Children:* Night terrors and somnabulism: 1 mg to 5 mg daily before retiring.

Premedication: 2 mg to 10 mg.

Management of cerebral spasticity: 2 mg to 40 mg daily in divided doses.

In the control of muscle spasms in tetanus: 3 mg to 10 mg/kg bodyweight daily.

*Elderly or debilitated patients:* The dosage should be half that recommended in adults.

Doses should be repeated only on medical advice. Long-term chronic use is not recommended and treatment should always be tapered off gradually. When a benzodiazepine is used as a hypnotic, treatment should, if possible, be intermittent.

**Contra-indications, warnings, etc**

*Contra-indications:* Patients with a known sensitivity to benzodiazepines; acute pulmonary insufficiency; respiratory depression.

*Use in pregnancy and lactation:* The use of diazepam is not recommended during pregnancy, especially during the first and last trimesters. During labour, diazepam given in single high or repeated low doses has been reported to produce hypotonia, hypothermia and poor suckling in the neonate and irregularities of foetal heart rate. Diazepam has been detected in breast milk and is, therefore, not recommended during lactation.

*Warnings:* The lowest dose that can control the symptoms should be used and treatment should not be continued beyond 4 weeks. The risk of dependence increases when high dosages are attained, especially when given over long periods. This is particularly so in patients with a history of alcoholism, drug abuse or in patients with marked personality disorders.

Treatment should always be tapered off gradually. Sudden cessation of treatment can result in symptoms such as depression, nervousness, rebound insomnia, irritability, sweating and diarrhoea even in patients receiving normal therapeutic doses for short periods of time. Abrupt withdrawal following high dosage may produce confusion, toxic psychosis, convulsions or a condition resembling delirium tremens.

Diazepam should not be used to treat chronic psychoses or phobic or obsessional states. Because diazepam-induced disinhibition may precipitate suicidal or aggressive behaviour, it should not be used alone to treat depression or anxiety related depression. Caution must be exercised when treating patients with personality disorders.

Elderly or debilitated patients may be more prone to adverse effects and care must be taken in patients with impaired liver or kidney function. Care is also required in patients with organic brain disease (particularly arteriosclerosis).

Diazepam should be avoided in cases of loss or bereavement as psychological adjustment may be inhibited by benzodiazepines.

Patients should be advised to avoid driving or operating machinery as diazepam, particularly when combined with alcohol, can reduce alertness and performance of skilled tasks.

*Interactions:* Sedation, or respiratory or cardiovascular depression may be enhanced if diazepam is combined with centrally acting drugs such as alcohol, anaesthetics, analgesics, antidepressants, hypnotics, neuroleptics and tranquillisers. Diazepam is primarily metabolised by hepatic microsomal oxidation and drugs which affect liver enzymes, such as cimetidine and phenobarbitone, may alter its pharmacokinetics. Diazepam has been reported to be displaced from protein-binding sites by sodium valproate.

*Side-effects:* Diazepam may cause drowsiness, sedation, blurring of vision, unsteadiness and ataxia. These may occur after a single as well as repeated doses and persist to the following day. Less common effects include vertigo, headache, confusion, slurred speech, visual disturbance, tremor, changes in libido, skin rashes and gastro-intestinal upset. Jaundice or blood dyscrasias have been reported rarely. High doses may be associated with respiratory depression or hypotension.

Abnormal psychological reactions to benzodiazepines have been reported. Rare behavioural adverse effects include paradoxical aggressive outbursts, excitement, confusion and the uncovering of depression with suicidal tendencies.

*Overdosage:* The symptoms of overdosage may include drowsiness, ataxia and dysarthria with coma or cardio-respiratory depression in very severe cases. Treatment should be symptomatic. Flumazenil is a specific antidote for use in emergency situations under close hospital supervision.

**Pharmaceutical precautions** Store in a cool place and protect from light.

**Legal category** CD (Sch 4), POM.

**Package quantities** Syrup 2 mg/5 ml: Bottles of 100 ml and 500 ml

Forte Syrup 5 mg/5 ml: Bottles of 100 ml

**Further information** Nil.

**Product licence numbers**

| | |
|---|---|
| Syrup 2 mg/5 ml | 4416/0026 |
| Forte Syrup 5 mg/5 ml | 4416/0067 |

## DIAZEPAM RECTAL TUBES

**Presentation** Polyethylene tube containing 5 mg or 10 mg diazepam, in approximately 2.5 ml volume. The non-active ingredients include benzoic acid, sodium benzoate, ethanol, propylene glycol, benzyl alcohol and water.

*Actions:* Diazepam has a anticonvulsant, anxiolytic, sedative, muscle relaxant and amnesic properties.

It is indicated:

(i) for the short-term relief (2–4 weeks only) of anxiety that is severe, disabling or subjecting the individual to unacceptable distress, occurring alone or in association with insomnia or short-term psychosomatic, organic or psychotic illness;

(ii) as a sedative and premedicant;

(iii) as an anticonvulsant in the management of status epilepticus, febrile convulsions and poisoning;

(iv) in the control of muscle spasms as in tetanus;

(v) in the management of alcohol withdrawal symptoms.

The use of diazepam to treat short-term anxiety is inappropriate and unsuitable. Diazepam should be used to treat insomnia only when it is severe, disabling or subjecting the individual to extreme stress.

**Dosage and administration** For rectal administration only. Tubes are for single use only.

The lowest dose that can control the symptoms should be used and treatment should not be continued beyond 4 weeks.

*Adults and children over 3 years:* One 10 mg tube. If a child is particularly small, then consideration should be given to reducing the dose to one 5 mg tube and reducing the depth of insertion.

*Children 1 to 3 years:* One 5 mg tube. Insert the tube to about half-nozzle length (approx 2.5 cm).

*Children under 1:* Not recommended.

*Elderly and debilitated patients:* The dosage should be half that recommended for adults.

For acute muscle spasm, acute anxiety or agitation use 10 mg and repeat if necessary after 4 hours.

For sedative cover during dental or other surgical and medical procedures, give a dose dependent on patient's response using 0.2 mg/kg body weight as a guide.

Doses should be repeated only on medical advice. Long-term chronic use is not recommended and treatment should always be tapered off gradually. When a benzodiazepine is used as a hypnotic, treatment should, if possible, be intermittent.

**Contra-indications, warnings, etc**

*Contra-indications:* Patients with a known sensitivity to benzodiazepines; acute pulmonary insufficiency; respiratory depression.

*Use in pregnancy and lactation:* The use of diazepam is not recommended during pregnancy, especially during the first and last trimesters. During labour, diazepam given in single high or repeated low doses has been reported to produce hypotonia, hypothermia and poor suckling in the neonate and irregularities of fetal heart rate. Diazepam has been detected in breast milk and is, therefore, not recommended during lactation.

*Warnings:* The lowest dose that can control the symptoms should be used and treatment should not be continued beyond 4 weeks. The risk of dependence increases when high dosages are attained, especially when given over long periods. This is particularly so in patients with a history of alcoholism, drug abuse or in patients with marked personality disorders.

Treatment should always be tapered off gradually. Sudden cessation of treatment can result in symptoms such as depression, nervousness, rebound insomnia, irritability, sweating and diarrhoea even in patients receiving normal therapeutic doses for short periods of time. Abrupt withdrawal following high dosage may produce confusion, toxic psychosis, convulsions or a condition resembling delirium tremens.

Diazepam should not be used to treat chronic psychoses or phobic or obsessional states. Because diazepam-induced disinhibition may precipitate suicidal or aggressive behaviour, it should not be used alone to treat depression or anxiety related depression. Cautioin must be exercised when treating patients with personality disorders.

Elderly or debilitated patients may be more prone to adverse effects an care must be taken in patients with impaired liver or kidney function. Care is also required in patients with organic brain disease (particularly arteriosclerosis).

Diazepam should be avoided in cases of loss or bereavement as psychological adjustment may be inhibited by benzodiazepines.

Patients should be advised to avoid driving or operating machinery as diazepam, particularly when combined with alcohol, can reduce alertness and performance of skilled tasks.

*Interactions:* Sedation, or respiratory or cardio-vascular depression may be enhanced if diazepam is combined with centrally acting drugs such as alcohol, anaesthetics, analgesics, antidepressants, hypnotics, neuroleptics and tranquillisers. Diazepam is primarily metabolised by hepatic microsomal oxidation and drugs which affect liver enzymes, such as cimetidine and phenobarbitone, may alter its pharmacokinetics. Diazepam has been reported to be displaced from protein-binding sites by sodium valproate.

*Side-effects:* Diazepam may cause drowsiness, sedation, blurring of vision, unsteadiness and ataxia. These may occur after a single as well as repeated doses and persist to the following day. Less common effects include vertigo, headache, confusion, slurred speech, visual disturbance, tremor, changes in libido, skin rashes and gastro-intestinal upset. Jaundice or blood dyscrasias have been reported rarely. High doses may be associated with respiratory depression or hypotension.

Abnormal psychological reactions to benzodiazepines have been reported. Rare behavioural adverse effects include paradoxical aggressive outbursts, excitement, confusion and the uncovering of depression with suicidal tendencies.

*Overdosage:* The symptoms of overdosage may include drowsiness, ataxia and dysarthia with coma or cardio-respiratory depression in very severe cases. Treatment should be symptomatic. Flumazenil is a specific antidote for use in emergency situations under close hospital supervision.

**Pharmaceutical precautions** Store in cool dry place below 22°C.

**Legal category** CD (Sch 4), POM.

**Package quantities** Pack of 5 tubes.

**Further information** Nil.

**Product licence numbers**

| | |
|---|---|
| 5 mg rectal tube | 4416/0027 |
| 10 mg rectal tube | 4416/0028 |

## DOXYLAR* CAPSULES BP 50 mg

**Presentation** Dark green and white capsules printed LAGAP DOX 50, containing Doxycycline Hydrochloride BP equivalent to 50 mg Doxycycline.

**Uses**

*Indications:* Doxycycline is clinically useful in the treatment of a variety of infections caused by susceptible strains of gram-positive and gram-negative bacteria and certain other micro-organisms. These include: Respiratory tract infections: lower respiratory tract infections including pneumonia, due to susceptible strains of *Haemophilis influenzae, Klebsiella pneumoniae, Streptococcus pneumoniae* and other organisms. *Mycoplasma pneumoniae* pneumonia. The treatment of chronic bronchitis and sinusitis.

Dermatological infections: Doxycycline can be used in the treatment of acne vulgaris in cases where antibiotic therapy is considered necessary.

Urinary infections: Infections caused by susceptible strains of klebsiella, enterobacter, *Escherichia coli, Streptococcus faecalis* and other organisms.

Sexually transmitted diseases: Infections including uncomplicated urethral, endocervical or rectal infections due to *Chlamydia trachomatis,* non-gonoccal urethritis, caused by *Ureaplasma urealyticulum* (T-mycoplasma). Doxycycline can also be used to treat chancroid and infections due to *Calymmatobacterium granulomatis* or as an alternative drug for the treatment of gonorrhoea and syphilis.

As a member of the tetracycline group of antibiotics, doxycycline may be useful in the treatment of infections due to other tetracycline-sensitive micro-organisms such as: Ophthalmic infections: Due to *Haemophilus influenzae* and susceptible strains of gonococci and staphylococci. Doxycycline is indicated in the treatment of trachoma. Inclusion conjunctivitis may be treated with oral doxycycline alone, or in combination with topical medication.

Rickettsial infections: Tick Fevers, Q Fever, Rocky Mountain Spotted Fever, Coxiella endocarditis and typhus group.

Prophylaxis: Doxycycline is also indicated in the prophylactic treatment of leptospirosis, scrub typhus and travellers' diarrhoea (entero-toxigenic *Escherichia coli*).

Miscellaneous: Psittacosis, leptospirosis, cholera, meliodosis, other infections due to susceptible strains of yersinia species, brucella species (in combination with streptomycin), clostridium species, *Francisella tularensis* and chloroquine-resistant falciparam malaria.

**Dosage and administration**

*Recommended doses:*

*Adults:* 200 mg on the first day (administered as a single dose or divided into 2 equal doses with a 12 hour interval) followed by a maintenance dose of 100 mg/day. For more severe infections (particularly chronic infections of the urinary tract) 200 mg should be given throughout the treatment.

*Children (over 12 years of age):* Normal adult dose should be given. Not recommended for use for children under 12 years of age (see *Contra-indications*).

*Elderly:* Doxycyline may be prescribed in the usual dose with no special precautions. No dosage adjustment is necessary in the presence of renal impairment.

It is recommended that patients over 70 years of age are specifically instructed regarding the administration of doxycycline.

An adequate volume of fluid should be taken when administering doxycycline capsules; this should preferably be taken in an upright position and *not* immediately before going to bed.

If gastric irritation occurs doxycyline should be given with food or milk.

Treatment should be continued at least 24 to 48 hours after fever and symptoms have subsided. When used in streptococcal infections, therapy should be continued for 10 days to prevent the development of rheumatic fever or glomerulo-nephritis.

*Specific infections:* Acne vulgaris: 50 mg daily with food or fluid for 6 to 12 weeks.

Sexually transmitted diseases: For the treatment of uncomplicated gonococcal infections (except anorectal infections in males), uncomplicated urethral, endocervical or rectal infections caused by *Chlamydia trachomatis,* or non-gonococcal urethritis caused by *Ureaplasma urealyticum,* 100 mg should be taken twice daily for 7 days.

For the treatment of acute epididymo-orchitis caused by *Chlamydia trachomatis* or *Neisseria gonorrhoeae;* 100 mg twice daily for 10 days.

For the treatment of primary and secondary syphilis: 300 mg a day in divided doses for at least 10 days.

Louse and tick-borne relapsing fevers: A single dose of 100 mg or 200 mg according to severity.

Chloroquine-resistant falciparam malaria: 200 mg to be taken daily for at least 7 days. A quick-acting schizonticide such as quinine should be used in conjunction with doxycycline because of the potential severity of the infection. Recommended dosages for quinine vary in different areas.

Prophylaxis: For the prevention of travellers' diarrhoea in adults: 200 mg on the first day of travel (administered as a single dose or as 100 mg every 12 hours), followed by 100 mg daily throughout the stay in the area.

For the prevention of scrub typhus: 200 mg to be taken as a single dose.

For the prevention of leptospirosis: 200 mg to be taken once a week throughout the stay in the area and 200 mg at the end of the trip.

**Contra-indications, warnings, etc**

*Contra-indications:* Doxycycline should not be administered to patients who have shown hypersensitivity to tetracyclines.

Doxycycline is also contra-indicated in pregnancy, infancy and childhood up to 12 years of age. The use of tetracyclines during tooth development may cause permanent discolouration of the teeth (yellow-grey-brown). This reaction is more common during long term use of the drug but has been observed following repeated short term courses. Enamel hypoplasia has also been reported.

As for other tetracyclines, doxycyline forms a stable calcium complex in any bone-forming tissue. A decrease in the fibula growth has been observed in prematures given oral tetracycline in doses of 25 mg/kg every 6 hours. This reaction was shown to be reversible when the drug was discontinued.

*Interactions with other medicaments and other forms of interaction:* Patients on anticoagulant therapy may require a reduction in anticoagulant dosage as tetracyclines have been shown to depress plasma prothrombin activity.

Since bacteriostatic drugs may interfere with the bacteriocidal action of penicillin, doxycycline should not be administered in conjunction with penicillins.

Antacids containing aluminium, calcium, magnesium or zinc, bismuth chelates, sucralfate or iron-containing compounds impair absorption and should therefore not be given to patients taking doxycycline.

The concurrent use of tetracyclines and methoxyflurane has been reported to result in fatal renal toxicity.

Barbiturates, carbamazepine, primidone and phenytoin have been reported to decrease the half-life of doxycycline.

A few cases of pregnancy or breakthrough bleeding have been attributed to the concurrent use of tetracycline or oxytetracycline with oral contraceptives.

Doxycycline used concurrently with cyclosporins has been reported to decrease the half-life of doxycycline.

*Effects on ability to drive and to use machines:* Nausea has been reported.

*Other undesirable effects:* Doxycycline is almost completely absorbed and therefore gastro-intestinal side-effects are infrequent. The following undesirable effects have been observed in patients receiving tetracyclines.

Gastro-intestinal: Nausea, vomiting, anorexia, dysphagia, glossitis, diarrhoea, enterocolitis and inflammatory lesions with monilial overgrowth in the ano-genital region. Oesophagitis and oesophageal ulceration have also been reported. A high proportion of these occurrences involved the hydrochloride salt in capsule form and taking medication immediately before going to bed.

Skin: Maculo papular and erythematous rashes. Skin photosensitivity is addressed under *Other special warnings and precautions.* Exfoliative dermatitis has been reported but is uncommon.

Renal: An apparently dose related rise in blood urea has been reported with tetracyclines.

Blood: Thrombocytopenia, neutropenia, haemolytic anaemia and eosinophilis have been reported with tetracyclines.

Hypersensitivity Reactions: Exacerbation of systemic lupus erythematosus, anaphylaxis, anaphylactoid purpura, pericarditis, urticaria and angioneurotic oedema.

Other: Bulging fontanelles in infants and benign intracranial hypertension in adults has been reported with the use of tetracyclines. Treatment should cease if evidence of raised intracranial pressure develops. These conditions disappeared rapidly when the drug was discontinued.

Brown-black microscopic discolouration of thyroid tissue has been reported with long-term use of tetracyclines. Thyroid function is normal.

*Use in pregnancy and lactation:* Use of doxycycline is contra-indicated during pregnancy as it can have toxic effects on the developing foetus.

Tetracyclines are also found in the milk of lactating women receiving doxycycline therapy and should therefore not be used in nursing mothers (see *Contra-indications* about tooth development).

*Other special warnings and precautions:* Doxycycline should be administered with caution to patients with hepatic impairment or those receiving potentially hepatotoxic drugs.

Care should be taken in the treatment of patients with myasthenia gravis who may be at risk of neuromuscular blockade.

Patients taking doxycycline should be warned that exposure to strong sunlight or ultraviolet light may experience photosensitivity appearing as a severe sunburn reaction. Treatment should cease at the first sign of skin erythema.

In the treatment of venereal disease where co-existent syphilis is suspected, formal diagnostic procedures including dark-field examinations should be employed and monthly serological tests should be conducted for at least 4 months.

Infections due to a group A beta haemolytic streptococci should be treated for at least 10 days.

Overgrowth of non-susceptible organisms may occur when using antibiotics. Continued observation of the patient is necessary and if a resistant organism appears, antibiotic therapy should be discontinued and appropriate measures instituted.

*Overdose:* Acute overdosage with antibiotics is rare. In the event of overdosage, gastric lavage and other supportive measures are indicated.

*Incompatibilities:* Not known.

**Pharmaceutical precautions** Store in a dry place.

**Legal category** POM.

**Package quantities** Packs of 28, 30, 56, 60, 84, 100, 150, 168 and 200 capsules.

**Further information** Nil.

**Product licence number** 4416/0264.

## DOXYLAR* CAPSULES BP 100 mg

**Presentation** Dark green capsules printed LAGAP DOX 100, containing Doxycycline Hydrochloride BP equivalent to 100 mg Doxycycline.

**Uses**

*Indications:* Doxycycline is clinically useful in the treatment of a variety of infections caused by susceptible strains of gram-positive and gram-negative bacteria and certain other micro-organisms. These include:

Respiratory tract infections: lower respiratory tract infections including pneumonia, due to susceptible strains of *Haemophilus influenzae, Klebsiella pneumoniae, Streptococcus pneumoniae* and other organisms. *Mycoplasma pneumoniae* pneumonia. The treatment of chronic bronchitis and sinusitis.

Urinary infections: Infections caused by susceptible strains of klebsiella, enterobactor, *Escherichia coli, Streptococcus faecalis* and other organisms.

Sexually transmitted diseases: Infections including uncomplicated urethral, endocervical or rectal infections due to *Chlamydia trachomatis*, non-gonoccal urethritis, caused by *Ureaplasma urelyticulum* (T-mycoplasma). Doxycycline can also be used to treat chancroid and infections due to *Calymmatobacterium granulomatis* or as an alternative drug for the treatment of gonorrhoea and syphilis.

As a member of the tetracycline group of antibiotics, doxycycline may be useful in the treatment of infections due to other tetracycline-sensitive microorganisms such as:

Ophthalmic infections: Due to *Haemophilus influenzae* and susceptible strains of gonococci and staphylococci. Doxycycline is indicated in the treatment of trachoma. Inclusion conjunctivitis may be treated with oral doxycycline alone, or in combination with topical medication.

Rickettsial infections: Tick Fevers, Q Fever, Rocky Mountain Spotted Fever, Coxiella endocarditis and typhus group.

Prophylaxis: Doxycycline is also indicated in the prophylactic treatment of leptospirosis, scrub typhus and travellers' diarrhoea (entero-toxigenic *Escherichia coli*).

Miscellaneous: Psittacosis, leptospirosis, cholera, meliodosis, other infections due to susceptible strains of yersinia species, brucella species (in combination with streptomycin), clostridum species, *Francisella tularensis* and chloroquine-resistant falciparam malaria.

**Dosage and administration**
*Recommended doses:*
*Adults:* 200 mg on the first day (administered as a single dose or divided into 2 equal doses with a 12 hour interval) followed by a maintenance dose of 100 mg/day. For more severe infections (particularly chronic infections of the urinary tract) 200 mg should be given throughout the treatment.

*Children (over 12 years of age):* Normal adult dose should be given. Not recommended for use for children under 12 years of age (see *Contra-indications*).

*Elderly:* Doxycyline may be prescribed in the usual dose with no special precautions. No dosage adjustment is necessary in the presence of renal impairment.

It is recommended that patients over 70 years of age are specifically instructed regarding the administration of doxycycline.

An adequate volume of fluid should be taken when administering doxycycline capsules; this should preferably be taken in an upright position and *not* immediately before going to bed.

If gastric irritation occurs doxycyline should be given with food or milk.

Treatment should be continued at least 24 to 48 hours after fever and symptoms have subsided. When used in streptococcal infections, therapy should be continued for 10 days to prevent the development of rheumatic fever or glomerulo-nephritis.

*Specific infections:* Sexually transmitted diseases: For the treatment of uncomplicated gonococcal infections (except anorectal infections in males), uncomplicated urethral, endocervical or rectal infections caused by *Chlamydia trachomatis*, or non-gonococcal urethritis caused by *Ureaplasma urealyticum*, 100 mg should be taken twice daily for 7 days.

For the treatment of acute epididymo-orchitis caused by *Chlamydia trachomatis* or *Neisseria gonorrhoeae*; 100 mg twice daily for 10 days.

For the treatment of primary and secondary syphillis: 300 mg a day in divided doses for at least 10 days.

Louse and tick-borne relapsing fevers: A single dose of 100 mg or 200 mg according to severity.

Chloroquine-resistant falciparam malaria: 200 mg to be taken daily for at least 7 days. A quick-acting schizonticide such as quinine should be used in conjunction with doxycycline because of the potential severity of the infection. Recommended dosages for quinine vary in different areas.

Prophylaxis: For the prevention of travellers' diarrhoea in adults: 200 mg on the first day of travel (administered as a single dose or as 100 mg every 12 hours), followed by 100 mg daily throughout the stay in the area.

For the prevention of scrub typhus: 200 mg to be taken as a single dose.

For the prevention of leptospirosis: 200 mg to be taken once a week throughout the stay in the area and 200 mg at the end of the trip.

**Contra-indications, warnings, etc**
*Contra-indications:* Doxycycline should not be administered to patients who have shown hypersensitivity to tetracyclines.

Doxycycline is also contra-indicated in pregnancy, lactation, infancy and childhood up to 12 years of age. The use of tetracyclines during tooth development may cause permanent discolouration of the teeth (yellow-grey-brown). This reaction is more common during long term use of the drug but has been observed following repeated short term courses. Enamel hypoplasia has also been reported.

As for other tetracyclines, doxycyline forms a stable calcium complex in any bone-forming tissue. A decrease in the fibula growth has been observed in prematures given oral tetracyclines in doses of 25 mg/kg every 6 hours. This reaction was shown to be reversible when the drug was discontinued.

*Interactions with other medicaments and other forms of interaction:* Patients on anticoagulant therapy may require a reduction in anticoagulant dosage as tetracyclines have been shown to depress plasma prothrombin activity.

Since bacteriostatic drugs may interfere with the bacteriocidal action of penicillin, doxycycline should not be administered in conjunction with penicillins.

Antacids containing aluminium, calcium, magnesium or zinc, bismuth chelates, sucralfate or iron-containing compounds impair absorption and should therefore not be given to patients taking doxycycline.

The concurrent use of tetracyclines and methoxyflurane has been reportd to result in fatal renal toxicity.

Barbiturates, carbamazepine, primidone and phenytoin have been reported to decrease the half-life of doxycycline.

A few cases of pregnancy or breakthrough bleeding have been attributed to the concurrent use of tetracycline or oxytetracycline with oral contraceptives.

Doxycycline used concurrently with cyclosporins has been reported to increase the plasma concentration of cyclosporin.

*Effects on ability to drive and to use machines:* Nausea has been reported.

*Other undesirable effects:* Doxycycline is almost completely absorbed and therefore gastro-intestinal side-effects are infrequent. The following undesirable effects have been observed in patients receiving tetracyclines.

Gastro-intestinal: Nausea, vomiting, anorexia, dysphagia, glossitis, diarrhoea, enterocolitis and inflammatory lesions with monilial overgrowth in the ano-genital region. Oesophagitis and oesophageal ulceration have also been reported. A high proportion of these occurrences involved the hydrochloride salt in capsule form and taking medication immediately before going to bed.

Skin: Maculo papular and erythematous rashes. Skin photosensitivity is addressed under *Other special warnings and precautions.* Exfoliative dermatitis has been reported but is uncommon.

Renal: An apparently dose related rise in blood urea has been reported with tetracyclines.

Blood: Thrombocytopenia, neutropenia, haemolytic anaemia and eosinophilia have been reported with tetracyclines.

Hypersensitivity reactions: Exacerbation of systemic lupus erythematosus, anaphylaxis, anaphylactoid purpura, pericarditis, urticaria and angioneurotic oedema.

Other: Bulging fontanelles in infants and benign intracranial hypertension in adults has been reported with the use of tetracyclines. Treatment should cease if evidence of raised intracranial pressure develops. These conditions disappeared rapidly when the drug was discontinued.

Brown-black microscopic discolouration of thyroid tissue has been reported with long-term use of tetracyclines. Thyroid function is normal.

*Use in pregnancy and lactation:* Use of doxycycline is contra-indicated during pregnancy as it can have toxic effects on the developing foetus.

Tetracyclines are also found in the milk of lactating women receiving doxycycline therapy and should therefore not be used in nursing mothers (see *Contra-indications* about tooth development).

*Other special warnings and precautions:* Doxycycline should be administered with caution to patients with hepatic impairment, acute porphyria or those receiving potentially hepatotoxic drugs.

Care should be taken in the treatment of patients with myasthenia gravis who may be at risk of neuromuscular blockade.

Patients taking doxycycline should be warned that exposure to strong sunlight or ultraviolet light may experience photosensitivity appearing as a severe sunburn reaction. Treatment should cease at the first sign of skin erythema.

In the treatment of venereal disease where co-existent syphilis is suspected, formal diagnostic procedures including dark-field examinations should be employed and monthly serological tests should be conducted for at least 4 months.

Infections due to a group A beta haemolytic streptococci should be treated for at least 10 days.

Overgrowth of non-susceptible organisms may occur when using antibiotics. Continued observation of the patient is necessary and if a resistant organism appears, antibiotic therapy should be discontinued and appropriate measures instituted.

*Overdose:* Acute overdosage with antibiotics is rare. In the event of overdosage, gastric lavage and other supportive measures are indicated.

*Incompatibilities:* Not known.

**Pharmaceutical precautions** Store in a cool dry place. Protect from light.

**Legal category** POM.

**Package quantities** Packs of 50 capsules.

**Further information** Nil.

**Product licence number** 4416/0007.

## HYPOLAR* RETARD 20

**Qualitative and quantitative composition** Each tablet contains 20 mg nifedipine PhEur in a modified release formulation.

**Pharmaceutical form** Modified release tablets.

**Clinical particulars**
*Therapeutic indications:* Hypolar Retard 20 tablets are indicated for the treatment of hypertension and the prophylaxis of chronic stable angina pectoris.

Hypolar Retard 20 has no therapeutic antiarrhythmic effect.

*Posology and route of administration:* These tablets should be swallowed with a glass of water. They must be swallowed whole and not broken or chewed.

*Adults:* The recommended starting dose of nifedipine is 10 mg every 12 hours swallowed with water with subsequent titration of dosage according to response. The dose may be adjusted to 40 mg every 12 hours.

*Elderly:* The pharmacokinetics of nifedipine are altered in the elderly so that lower maintenance doses of nifedipine may be required compared to younger patients.

Nifedipine is metabolised primarily by the liver and therefore patients with liver dysfunction should be carefully monitored. Patients with renal impairment should not require adjustment of dosage.

Treatment with Hypolar Retard 20 may be continued long term.

*Children:* Nifedipine is not recommended for use in children.

*Route of administration:* Oral.

*Contra-indications:* Nifedipine has been shown to be teratogenic in animals and therefore Hypolar Retard 20 tablets should not be administered to women who are pregnant or may become pregnant and to nursing mothers.

Other contra-indications:

- Patients with cardiogenic shock.
- Hypersensitivity to nifedipine or other dihydropyridines because of the theoretical risk of cross reactivity.
- Nifedipine should not be used in clinically significant aortic stenosis, unstable angina, or during or within one month of a myocardial infarction.
- Nifedipine should not be used for the treatment of acute attacks of angina.
- The safety of nifedipine in malignant hypertension has not been established.
- Nifedipine should not be used for secondary prevention of myocardial infarction.
- Nifedipine should not be administered concomitantly with rifampicin since effective plasma levels of nifedipine may not be achieved owing to enzyme induction.

*Special warnings and special precautions for use:* Hypolar Retard 20 should be used with caution in patients with severe hypotension and in patients whose cardiac reserve is poor.

Cardiac ischaemic pain has been reported to have occurred in some patients within 1 to 4 hours of receiving nifedipine. In such cases treatment should be discontinued.

Caution should be exercised when Hypolar Retard 20 is given to diabetic patients as they may require adjustment of their diabetic therapy.

In patients with malignant hypertension and hypovolaemia who are on dialysis, a significant decrease in blood pressure can occur.

*Interactions with other medicaments and other forms of interaction:* Hypolar Retard 20 may be used in combined therapy with other antihypertensive agents including beta-blockers where an additive or synergistic hypotensive effect is to be expected. Withdrawal of any previous antihypertensive agents should be gradual as nifedipine will not compensate for any possible rebound effects.

As with other dihydropyridines, nifedipine should not be taken with grapefruit juice because bioavailability is increased.

Cimetidine may potentiate the antihypertensive effect of Hypolar Retard 20 if it is administered simultaneously.

Nifedipine should not be administered concomitantly with rifampicin since effective plasma levels of nifedipine, may not be achieved owing to enzyme induction (see Contra-indications).

It is reported that serum quinidine levels have been shown to be reduced when it is used in combination with nifedipine.

The simultaneous administration of nifedipine and digoxin may lead to reduced digoxin clearance and hence an increase in the plasma digoxin. Digoxin levels should be monitored and, if necessary, the digoxin dose reduced.

Other reactions reported include increased plasma levels of theophylline and phenytoin when used in combination with nifedipine and the enhanced effect of non-polarising muscle relaxants such as tubocurarine.

Pregnancy and lactation: As nifedipine has been shown to be teratogenic in animals, Hypolar Retard 20 should not be administered to women who are pregnant or may become pregnant and to nursing mothers.

Effects on ability to drive and use machines: Nausea, headaches, lethargy and dizziness have been reported to occur and therefore the patient should be warned of these possible effects.

Undesirable effects: Exacerbation of angina pectoris may occur rarely at the start of treatment with modified relase formulations of nifedipine. The occurrence of myocardial infarction has been described although it is not possible to distinguish such an event from the natural course of ischaemic heart disease.

The most common side effects reported are dizziness, flushing, headaches, hypotension, tachycardia and palpitations and ankle swelling. Other less common side effects include gastrointestinal disturbances, increased micturition, rash, pruritus and urticaria, nausea, lethargy, paraesthesiae, myalgia, tremor and visual disturbances. Gingival hyperplasia has been reported to occur, and in older men gynaecomastia following long term therapy, however both these conditions are reversible on withdrawal of the drug.

There have been reports of rare cases of hypersensitivity-type jaundice. Liver function disturbances such as intra-hepatic cholestasis may also occur. Discontinuation of therapy will result in regression of these side effects.

Overdosage: This may be associated with severe hypotension, tachycardia or bradycardia and unconsciousness although there are few reports and the symptoms are not necessarily dose-related.

The metabolic disturbances which can occur include hyperglycaemia, metabolic acidosis and hypo- or hyperkalaemia. The cardiac effects which may occur include heart block, AV dissociation and asystole and cardiogenic shock with pulmonary oedema.

Other effects include drowsiness, dizziness, confusion, nausea, vomiting, lethargy, flushing and hypoxia.

In the treatment of overdosage it is important to restore stable cardiovascular conditions as soon as possible and achieve total elimination of nifedipine.

Gastric lavage and charcoal instillation may be of assistance if the patient is found early after the overdose. Gastric lavage may be necessary in combination with irrigation of the small intestine. Ipecacuanha should be given to children.

Activated charcoal should be given in 4 hourly doses of 25 g for adults and 10 g for children. The patient should be carefully monitored.

Hypotension should be treated by placing the patient in the supine position with the feet raised and the use of plasma expanders, as appropriate. If necessary, intravenous administration of 10% calcium gluconate 10–20 ml over a period of 5–10 minutes may be appropriate. Beta-sympathomimetics may be given e.g.: isoprenaline. If the blood pressure response is inadequate with calcium and isoprenaline, vasoconstricting sympathomimetics such as dopamine or noradrenaline should be administered. The patient's response should determine the dosage of these drugs.

If bradycardia persists the patient may be treated with atropine, beta-sympathomimetics or a temporary cardiac pacemaker.

It has also been reported that the use of metaraminol combined with calcium salts has been beneficial.

Care should be exercised with any additional fluids given to avoid cardiac overload.

## Pharmacological properties

Pharmacodynamic properties: Nifedipine is a dihydro-

pyridine and is a potent antagonist of calcium influx through the slow channel of the cell membrane of cardiac and smooth muscle cells. Nifedipine also binds to intracellular calcium binding proteins. Calcium is normally released from the sarcoplasmic reticulum intracellularly and this combined with the influx of extracellular calcium results in enhanced binding calcium to calmodulin. Calcium channel blockers such as nifedipine act as arteriolar dilators by inhibiting this calcium entry in to the channel. The effects are more pronounced on vascular smooth muscle because depolarisation of cardiac muscle cells is dependent on both sodium ion influx and calcium ion influx and also nifedipine has little effect on the rate of recovery of the slow calcium channel.

Nifedipine is known to be an effective and relatively well tolerated treatment for angina and mild to severe hypertension.

The antihypertensive effects of nifedipine are achieved by causing periperal vasodilatation resulting in a reduction in peripheral resistance. Nifedipine reduces blood pressure in hypertension but has little or no effect in normotensive individuals.

Nifedipine produces its effects in the treatment of angina by reducing peripheral and coronary vascular resistance, leading to an increase in coronary blood flow, cardiac output and stroke volume and causing a decrease in after-load.

Pharmacokinetic properties: Nifedipine is rapidly and almost completely absorbed from the gastro-instestinal tract after oral administration, however due to extensive hepatic first pass metabolism the resultant bioavailability lies between 45% and 75%.

Hypolar Retard 20 is a modified release preparation designed to release Nifedipine over a period of time. Following a pharmacokinetic study in volunteers it was found that the average time to reach maximum plasma concentration was 2.2 hours and the mean peak plasma concentration was found to be 58.5 ng/ml. The average elimination half-life was found to be 17.3 hours. Nifedipine is highly bound to plasma protein.

Preclinical safety data: Not required.

### Pharmaceutical particulars

List of excipients: Microcrystalline cellulose, lactose, corn starch, talc, hydroxypropyl methyl cellulose, magnesium stearate, polysorbate 80, polyethylene glycol 4000, iron oxide (E172), and titanium dioxide (E171).

Incompatibilities: None reported.

Shelf life: 2 years.

Special precautions for storage: Store in dry place below 25°C. Protect from light.

Nature and contents of container: Blister strips composed of PVC foil 250 μm±5%, PVdC 25 μm±5%, aluminium foil 25 μm±8%, PVdC 20 μm±10%.
Pack size: 56.

Instructions for use/handling: Not applicable.

Marketing authorisation number  4416/0245.

Date of revision of SPC  May 1997.

Legal category  POM.

## INDOLAR* SR

**Presentation**  Blue/colourless capsules containing white sustained release beads. Each capsule containing 75 mg Indomethacin BP.

Inactive ingredients: Sucrose; Lactose.

**Uses**  Non-steroidal analgesic and anti-inflammatory agent indicated in active rheumatoid arthritis, osteoarthritis, ankylosing spondylitis, degenerative joint disease of the hip, acute musculo-skeletal disorders and low back pain. Also indicated in periarticular disorders such as bursitis, tendinitis, synovitis, tenosynovitis and capsulitis. Also indicated in inflammation, pain and oedema following orthopaedic procedures and the treatment of pain and associated symptoms of primary dysmenorrhoea.

**Dosage and administration**  Indolar SR Capsules should always be given with food or milk to reduce the chance of gastro-intestinal disturbance.

To minimise the evolution of unwanted reactions it is helpful in chronic conditions to start the therapy with a low dosage, increasing as required.

Adults: One capsule once or twice daily, depending on patient needs and response.

Dosage in dysmenorrhoea: One capsule a day, starting with the onset of cramps or bleeding, and continuing for as long as symptoms usually last.

Children: Safety in children has not been established.

Elderly: Particular care should be taken with older patients who are more susceptible to side-effects from indomethacin.

### Contra-indications, warnings, etc

Contra-indications: Patients with angioneurotic oedema or who have, with aspirin or other non-steroidal anti-inflammatory drugs experienced acute asthmatic attacks, urticaria or rhinitis.

Active peptic ulcer, a history of recurrent gastrointestinal lesions, sensitivity to indomethacin or to aspirin.

Not to be used during pregnancy or during lactation as indomethacin is secreted in breast milk.

Safety in children has not been established.

Side-effects: The most common side-effects are headache, dizziness and dyspepsia; patients should be warned that they may experience dizziness and should therefore avoid driving or undertaking other activities which require full alertness. If headache persists even after dosage reduction indomethacin should be withdrawn.

Gastro-intestinal disorders which occur can be reduced by giving indomethacin with food, milk or antacids. Ulceration of the oesophagus, stomach or duodenum may also occur, accompanied by haemorrhage and perforation (a few fatalities have been reported).

Intestinal ulceration has rarely been associated with stenosis and obstruction. Also, bleeding without obvious ulceration and perforation of pre-existing sigmoid lesions (such as a diverticulum or carcinoma) have occurred; and increased abdominal pain in patients with ulcerative colitis (or the development of this condition) and regional ileitis have been rarely reported. If gastro-intestinal bleeding does occur treatment with indomethacin should be discontinued.

Blood dyscrasias, particularly thrombocytopenia have been reported.

Oedema and increased blood pressure also sometimes occur, as does haematuria.

Hypersensitivity reactions include pruritus, urticaria, angiitis, erythema nodosum. Skin rash and hair loss may also occur.

Acute respiratory distress, including sudden dyspnoea and asthma, have been reported on rare occasions. Bronchospasm may be precipitated in patients suffering from, or with a previous history of, bronchial asthma or allergic disease.

Indomethacin should be used with caution in patients with hepatic or renal dysfunction. Hepatitis and jaundice have been reported rarely.

Non-steroidal anti-inflammatory drugs may precipitate renal decompensation in those with renal or hepatic dysfunction, diabetes mellitus, advanced age, extracellular volume depletion, congestive cardiac failure, sepsis or concomitant use of other nephrotoxic drugs. Also, there have been reports of acute interstitial nephritis with haematuria, proteinuria and occasionally the nephrotic syndrome in long-term therapy with indomethacin.

In common with other anti-inflammatory analgesic antipyretic agents, indomethacin may mask the signs and symptoms of infectious disease and this should be borne in mind in order to avoid delay in starting treatment for infection.

Indomethacin should be used with caution in patients with an existing, albeit controlled infection.

Particular care should be taken with older patients who are more susceptible to side-effects from indomethacin.

Interactions: Co-administration of diflunisal with Indomethacin increases the plasma level of Indomethacin by about a third with a concomitant decrease in renal clearance. Fatal gastro-intestinal haemorrhage has occurred. The combination should not be used.

Use of indomethacin with aspirin or other salicylates is not recommended because there is no enhancement of therapeutic effect while the incidence of gastro-intestinal side-effects is increased. Moreover, co-administration of aspirin may decrease the blood concentration of indomethacin.

Indomethacin may decrease the tubular secretion of methotrexate thus potentiating toxicity; simultaneous use should be undertaken with caution.

Patients receiving anticoagulants should be observed carefully for alteration of prothrombin time even though clinical studies suggest no influence from indomethacin on hypoprothrombinaemia induced by anticoagulants.

Indomethacin can inhibit platelet aggregation – an effect which disappears within 24 hours of discontinuation; the bleeding time may be prolonged and this effect may be exaggerated in patients with an underlying haemostatic defect.

Indomethacin and triamterene should not be administered together since reversible renal failure may be induced.

Co-administration of probenecid may increase plasma levels of Indomethacin.

Because Indomethacin may reduce the antihypertensive effect of beta-blockers, patients receiving dual therapy should have the antihypertensive effect of their therapy reassessed.

If the patient is receiving corticosteroids concomitantly, a reduction in dosage of these may be possible, but should only be effected slowly under supervision.

Indomethacin is an inhibitor of prostaglandin synthesis and therefore the following drug interactions may occur; Indomethacin may raise plasma lithium levels and reduce renal lithium clearance in subjects with steady state plasma lithium concentrations. At the onset of such combined therapy, plasma lithium concentration should be monitored more frequently.

Indomethacin may reduce the diuretic and antihypertensive effect of thiazides and frusemide in some patients. Indomethacin may cause blocking of the frusemide-induced increase in plasma renin activity.

It is reported that a few patients receiving non-steroidal anti-inflammatory drugs manifest borderline elevations in liver function test results; if these persist or worsen or symptoms of liver disease, a rash or eosinophilia develop, treatment with indomethacin should be stopped. Periodic assessments to detect, at an early stage, unwanted effects on peripheral blood (anaemia) and liver function are advisable. The dexamethasone suppression test may give false negative results. An increase in plasma potassium concentration (including hyperkalaemia) has been reported even in the absence of renal impairment. Since indomethacin is eliminated primarily by the kidney, patients with impaired renal function should be monitored closely and a lower daily dosage may be needed to avoid accumulation.

*Warnings and adverse reactions:*

CNS: Headache, dizziness or lightheadedness, depression, vertigo and fatigue are not uncommon; infrequently there may be confusion, anxiety or other psychiatric disturbance, drowsiness, convulsions, neuropathy or paraesthesia, involuntary movements, insomnia, aggravation of epilepsy or Parkinsonism. All are often transient and likely to abate or disappear with reduced or ceased dosage.

Gastro-intestinal: Nausea, anorexia, vomiting, epigastric discomfort or abdominal pain, constipation or diarrhoea all have been reported; more rarely, stomatitis, flatulence, ulceration at any point in the gastro-intestinal tract (even with resultant stenosis and obstruction), bleeding (even without obvious ulceration or from a diverticulum) and perforation of pre-existing sigmoid lesions have all been reported.

Hepatic: Rarely hepatitis and jaundice (some fatalities have been reported).

Cardiovascular/renal: Oedema, increased blood pressure, hypotension, tachycardia, chest pain, arrhythmia, palpitations, congestive cardiac failure, elevation of blood urea and haematuria all have been reported infrequently.

In patients with renal, cardiac or hepatic impairment caution is required since the use of non-steroidal anti-inflammatory drugs may result in deterioration of renal function. The dose should be kept as low as possible and renal function should be monitored.

Non-steroidal anti-inflammatory drugs have been reported to cause nephrotoxicity in various forms and their use can lead to interstitial nephritis, nephrotic syndrome and renal failure.

Dermatological/hypersensitivity: Itching, urticaria, angioneurotic oedema, angiitis, erythema nodosum, rash and exfoliative dermatitis all have been reported infrequently – as have Stevens Johnson syndrome, erythema multiforme, toxic epidermal necrolysis, hair loss, acute anaphylaxis (including acute loss of blood pressure) and acute respiratory distress (including sudden dyspnoea, asthma and pulmonary oedema). There may be bronchospasm in patients with a history of bronchial asthma or other allergic disease.

Haematological: Blood dyscrasias (thrombocytopenia, leucopenia, petechiae, ecchymosis, purpura, aplastic or haemolytic anaemia, agranulocytosis and bone marrow depression, disseminated intravascular coagulation) may occur infrequently.

Ocular: Blurred vision and orbital and peri-orbital pain are seen infrequently. Corneal deposits and retinal disturbances have been reported in some patients with rheumatoid arthritis on prolonged therapy with indomethacin, and ophthalmic examinations are desirable in patients given prolonged treatment.

Aural: Tinnitus, or hearing disturbance (rarely deafness) have been reported.

Genito-urinary: Proteinuria, nephrotic syndrome, interstitial nephritis, renal insufficiency or failure all have been reported.

Other: Hyperglycaemia, glycosuria, hyperkalaemia, vaginal bleeding, epistaxis, breast changes (enlargement, tenderness, gynaecomastia), flushing, sweating and ulcerative stomatitis all have been reported rarely.

*Overdosage:* Many of the unwanted symptoms associated with indomethacin therapy may be seen. Treatment is symptomatic and supportive – emptying the stomach by induction of vomiting and/or lavage and use of activated charcoal. Antacid therapy may be useful. Close monitoring thereafter is required because intestinal ulceration may develop. It can be noted that indomethacin has a biphasic plasma elimination with the terminal phase showing a half-life ranging between 2 and 12 hours.

**Pharmaceutical precautions** Store in a cool, dry place and protect from light.

**Legal category** POM.

**Package quantities** 100 capsules.

**Further information** Nil.

**Product licence number** 4416/0066.

## KETOPROFEN CAPSULES BP

**Qualitative and quantitative composition** Each capsule contains Ketoprofen BP 50 mg or 100 mg.

**Pharmaceutical form** Capsule.

**Clinical particulars**

*Therapeutic indications:* Ketoprofen capsules are recommended for the management of rheumatoid arthritis, osteoarthritis, ankylosing spondylitis, acute articular and periarticular disorders, fibrositis, cervical spondylitis, low back pain, painful musculoskeletal conditions and dysmenorrhoea. Ketoprofen reduces joint pain and inflammation, and facilitates increase in mobility and functional independence. As with other non-steroidal anti-inflammatory agents, it does not cure the underlying disease.

*Posology and method of administration:* Ketoprofen capsules should always be taken with food to reduce the occurrence of gastrointestinal disturbance.

*Adults:* 50–100 mg twice daily. The dosage can be altered depending on the patient weight and on the severity of symptoms.

*Dysmenorhoea:* 50 mg up to 3 times a day. Three to 4 days treatment is normally required from the outset of menstruation or symptoms of dysmenorrhoea.

*Children:* Dosage has not been established.

*Contra-indications:* Ketoprofen should not be given to patients sensitive to aspirin or other non-steroidal anti-inflammatory agents. In such patients and in those suffering from, or with a history of, bronchial asthma or allergic disease, severe bronchospasm might be precipitated.

Ketoprofen is contra-indicated in patients with active peptic ulceration, a history of recurrent peptic ulceration or chronic dyspepsia, severe renal dysfunction.

*Special warnings and special precautions for use:* Ketoprofen capsules should always be given with food to limit gastrointestinal disturbance.

Ketoprofen should be used with caution in patients with renal impairment. Inhibition of renal prostaglandin synthesis by non-steroidal anti-inflammatory agents may interfere with renal function especially in the presence of existing renal disease.

*Interactions with other medicaments and other forms of interaction:* Ketoprofen is highly protein-bound. If used concomitantly with other protein-binding drugs such as anticoagulants, sulphonamides or hydantoins an alteration in dosage level may be required to avoid increased levels of such drugs resulting from competition for plasma protein-binding sites. Similar acting drugs such as aspirin or other non-steroidal anti-inflammatory agents should not be administered concomitantly with ketoprofen as the potential for adverse reactions is increased.

Serious interactions have been recorded after the use of non-steroidal anti-inflammatory agents including ketoprofen with high dose methotrexate.

*Pregnancy and lactation:* Studies in animals have not demonstrated any embryopathic effects. It is recommended to avoid ketoprofen unless considered absolutely essential, in which case it is advised to discontinue treatment within one week of expected confinement when non-steroidal anti-inflammatory drugs might cause premature closure of the ductus arteriosus or persistent pulmonary hypertension in the neonate. Labour could also be delayed. Trace amounts of ketoprofen are also excreted in breast milk.

The use of ketoprofen during pregnancy and lactation should be avoided unless considered essential.

*Effects on ability to drive and use machines:* Dizziness, mild confusion, vertigo and drowsiness have been reported, therefore patients who drive or operate machinery should be advised of this.

*Undesirable effects:* Adverse effects reported are frequently transient and are mainly gastrointestinal effects such as indigestion, dyspepsia, nausea, constipation, diarrhoea, heartburn and various types of abdominal discomfort. Other minor effects such as headache, dizziness, mild confusion, vertigo, drowsiness, oedema, mood change and insomnia have been reported to occur less commonly.

Major gastrointestinal adverse effects such as peptic ulceration, haemorrhage or perforation may rarely occur.

Major adverse effects involving other organ systems such as haematological reactions including thrombocytopenia, renal and hepatic damage, dermatological reactions, bronchospasm and anaphylaxis are rare.

It is advisable in all cases of major adverse effects for ketoprofen to be withdrawn at once.

*Overdosage:* Ketoprofen is of low toxicity in overdosage, symptoms after acute ketoprofen intoxication are largely limited to drowsiness, abdominal pain and vomiting, but adverse effects seen after overdosage with propionic acid derivatives such as hypotension, bronchospasm and gastrointestinal haemorrhage should be anticipated.

Treatment is otherwise supportive and symptomatic.

**Pharmacological properties**

*Pharmacodynamic properties:* Ketoprofen is a potent non-steroidal anti-inflammatory analgesic agent and is a strong inhibitor of prostaglandin synthetase.

*Pharmacokinetic properties:* In a bioequivalence study in healthy volunteers the following values were obtained for Ketoprofen Capsules 50 mg:

$C_{max}$ 12.27±4.96 mg/l

$T_{max}$ 1.17±0.48 hours.

*Preclinical safety data:* Not relevant.

**Pharmaceutical particulars**

*List of excipients:* Magnesium stearate and lactose. The 50 mg capsule shells contain gelatin, erythrosine (E127), indigotine (E132), titanium dioxide (E171) and quinoline yellow (E104). The 100 mg capsule shells contain gelatin, red iron oxide (E172) and titanium dioxide (E171).

*Incompatibilities:* Not recorded.

*Shelf life:* 60 months.

*Special precautions for storage:* Store in a dry place not above 25°C.

*Nature and contents of container:* Amber glass bottles. Ketoprofen 50 mg capsules – pack size: 100. Ketoprofen 100 mg capsules – pack size 100.

*Instructions for use/handling:* Not applicable.

**Marketing authorisation numbers**

Ketoprofen Capsules BP 50 mg 4416/0139

Ketoprofen Capsules BP 100 mg 4416/0140

**Date of approval/revision of SPC** 21 May 1997.

**Legal category** POM.

## LARAFEN* CR CAPSULES

**Presentation** Gelatin capsule with opaque pink cap and transparent body printed LAGAP on one half with KET200CR on the other half in black ink. Each capsule contains 200 mg Ketoprofen BP in whitish pH-sensitive controlled-release pellets.

**Uses** Larafen CR is an analgesic, anti-inflammatory and antipyretic; and is recommended for the treatment of rheumatoid arthritis, osteoarthritis, ankylosing spondylitis and other musculoskeletal conditions including bursitis, capsulitis, synovitis and tendinitis, fibrositis and low back pain. It is also useful to relieve the pain of sciatica, acute gout and dysmenorrhoea.

*Pharmacokinetics:* Larafen CR Capsule is a controlled release formulation which is designed to release Ketoprofen over a period of time. Following a pharmacokinetic study in volunteers it was found that the average time to achieve maximum plasma concentration was 6.9 hours. The average half-life was found to be 7.4 hours, with a range of 5.5 to 8.0 hours. The average mean residence time was about 14 hours with an average clearance of 2.4 litres per hour. The study carried out over a five day period at the proposed dosage of once daily indicates that there is no accumulation on continued daily dosing. Ketoprofen is very highly bound to plasma protein.

**Dosage and administration**

*Adults:* One 200 mg Larafen CR capsule to be taken orally once daily with a little food.

*Elderly:* As for adult dosage as there is no evidence that that the pharmacokinetics of ketoprofen are altered in the elderly.

*Children:* There are no recommendations for the use of Larafen CR in children.

**Contra-indications, warnings, etc**

*Contra-indications:* Larafen CR should not be given to patients with active peptic ulceration or a history of recurrent peptic ulceration or chronic dyspepsia; known hypersensitivity to Ketoprofen, aspirin or other non-steroidal anti-inflammatory agents; severe renal dysfunction.

*Warnings:* Some patients with a history of bronchial asthma or allergic disease may suffer bronchospasm, particularly those with a history of allergy to Ketoprofen and related compounds. As non-steroidal anti-inflammatory agents can inhibit renal prostaglandin synthesis and interfere with renal function, care should be taken when using Larafen CR in patients with renal impairment. NSAIDs have been reported to cause nephrotoxicity in various forms; interstitial nephritis, nephrotic syndrome and renal failure. In patients with renal cardiac or hepatic impairment caution is required since the use of NSAIDs may result in deterioration of renal function: the dose should be kept as low as possible and renal function should be monitored. As with other drugs in the same therapeutic category, patients should be advised to take Larafen CR with food.

*Interactions:* The active ingredient of Larafen CR, ketoprofen, is highly protein bound, therefore alteration of the dosage of other protein bound drugs such as anticoagulants, sulphonamides and hydantoins such as phenytoin may be necessary when taken together. Serious interactions have been reported with methotrexate, digoxin, lithium and diuretics. To avoid the risk of increased side-effects, Larafen CR should not be given with other non-steroidal anti-inflammatory agents.

*Pregnancy and lactation:* There is no evidence of teratogenic effects of ketoprofen but as with all drugs, administration during pregnancy should be avoided unless essential. Because Ketoprofen interferes with prostaglandin synthesis, there may be premature closure of the ductus arteriosus or persistent pulmonary hypertension in the neonate, or delay in labour if Larafen CR is administered within a few days before the delivery. Small amounts of ketoprofen are excreted in breast milk so use in nursing mothers should be avoided.

*Side-effects:* The most common adverse effects relate to the gastrointestinal tract, mainly indigestion, dyspepsia, heartburn, various types of abdominal discomfort, nausea, constipation and diarrhoea. Other effects such as headache, dizziness, confusion, drowsiness, oedema, change of mood and insomnia occur less commonly. Peptic ulceration, perforation and gastrointestinal haemorrhage may rarely occur. Other rare adverse events reported include haematological reactions such as thrombocytopenia, hepatic or renal damage, dermatological reactions, bronchospasm and anaphylaxis. Should any severe adverse event occur, treatment with Larafen CR should be stopped immediately. Patients should be warned of the potential side effects.

*Overdosage:* As with other propionic acid derivatives, ketoprofen demonstrates less toxicity than aspirin or paracetamol. The most likely symptoms of overdosage are drowsiness, abdominal pain and vomiting but hypotension, bronchospasm and gastro-intestinal haemorrhage may occur. Because Larafen CR is a controlled release preparation, continued absorption from capsules in the gastro-intestinal tract, may be expected. Treatment should be symptomatic and may include gastric washout and the use of activated charcoal.

**Pharmaceutical precautions** Store in a dry place below 25°C. Protect from light.

**Legal category** POM.

**Package quantities** Blister packs of 28.

**Further information** Nil.

**Product licence number** 4416/0221

## METROLYL*

**Presentation** *Metrolyl Tablets* containing 200 mg and 400 mg Metronidazole BP. 200 mg – white, breakline on one side, LAGAP on reverse. 400 mg – white, marked 11 breakline 400 on one side, LAGAP on reverse.

*Metrolyl Suppositories* containing 500 mg Metronidazole BP and 1 g Metronidazole BP.

*Metrolyl Injection* (for intravenous infusion) 0.5 per cent w/v in 100 ml PVC minibags (500 mg metronidazole per 100 ml).

*Inactive ingredients:* Metrolyl Tablets – Lactose; Metrolyl Injection – Sodium Chloride; Metrolyl Suppositories – Witepsol.

**Uses** 1. Treatment of infections in which anaerobic bacteria have been identified or are suspected as pathogens, particularly *Bacteroides fragilis* and other species of bacteroides and including other species for which metronidazole is bactericidal e.g. fusobacteria, eubacteria, clostridia and anaerobic cocci.

Metrolyl can be used in septicaemia, bacteraemia, brain abscess, necrotising pneumonia, osteomyelitis, puerperal sepsis, pelvic abscess, peritonitis and post operative wound infection from which one or more of these anaerobes have been isolated.

2. Prevention of post operative infections due to anaerobic bacteria.

3. Use in treatment of acute ulcerative gingiritis and acute dental, pericoronitis and apical infections.

4. Trichomonas infections.

5. Amoebiasis.

6. Giardiasis.

**Dosage and administration** Seven days treatment should be satisfactory for most patients. Prolonged treatment can be used if the physician considers it to be necessary. Metrolyl tablets should be swallowed with water, during or after a meal.

*1. Treatment of anaerobic infections*

A. *Oral medication:* Metrolyl tablets may be given alone or in association with other appropriate bactericidal agents. Adults and children over 10 years: 400 mg three times daily. Children under 10 years: 7.5 mg per kg body weight three times daily.

B. *Rectal medication:* Rectal administration using Metrolyl Suppositories can be used in patients for whom oral medication is not possible or is contraindicated. The suppositories may be administered alone or concurrently with other bacteriologically appropriate antibacterial agents.

Treatment of anaerobic infections: Adults and children over 10 years: 1 gram suppository inserted into the rectum eight-hourly for three days. If rectal medication must be continued for more than three days the suppositories should be inserted at 12-hourly intervals. Children (5 to 10 years): As for adults *but* with 500 mg suppositories three times daily. Infants and children under five years: As for children of 5 to 10 years *but* with appropriate reduction in dosage of suppositories (one-half of a 500 mg suppository for one to five years and one-quarter of a 500 mg suppository for under one year).

C. *Intravenous medication:* Intravenous medication can be used in patients with severe anaerobic infections for whom oral medication is not possible: it is particularly useful in emergencies and is indicated in patients needing surgery who:

Have anaerobic sepsis such as septicaemia, peritonitis, subphrenic or pelvic abscesses.

At operation show signs of established or impending anaerobic sepsis.

Undergo operations in which contamination occurs with anaerobes from the gastro intestinal or female genital tract or the oropharynx.

In infants and other patients maintained on intravenous fluids, Metrolyl Injection may be diluted with appropriate volumes of normal saline, dextrose-saline, dextrose 5% w/v or potassium chloride injections (20 mmol and 40 mmol.)

*Treatment:* Adults and children over 10 years: 100 ml (500 mg metronidazole) by intravenous injection eight hourly. Injection should be infused intravenously at the rate of 5 ml per minute but may be administered alone or concurrently (but separately) with other appropriate antibacterial agents in parenteral dosage forms. Oral medication (400 mg 3 times daily) should be substituted as soon as possible.

Children under 10 years: As for adults *but* single dose is based on 1.5 ml (7.5 mg metronidazole) per kg body weight every eight hours and the oral dose at 7.5 mg/kg body weight.

*2. Prevention of anaerobic infections*

A. *Oral medication:*

(a) Gynaecological surgery: Adults: 1 gram orally as a single dose followed by 200 mg orally 3 times daily until pre-operative withholding of solids and liquids by mouth becomes necessary. Oral medication with 200 mg 3 times daily should be resumed after the operation and for up to 7 days.

(b) Pre-operative medication for elective colonic surgery: Adults: 200 mg orally six hourly co-administered with an aminoglycoside antibiotic for 3 days before surgery; or 400 mg orally 8 hourly with phthalylsulphathiazole (2.5 g six hourly) for 4 days before surgery.

B. *Rectal medication:* In appendicectomy: Adults and children over 10 years: 1 gram suppository inserted into the rectum two hours before surgery and repeated

### Oral dosage regime for Metrolyl

| | Adults/Children over 10yrs | Children 7–10 yrs | Children 3–7 yrs | Children 1–3 yrs |
|---|---|---|---|---|
| Urogenital trichomoniasis (treat sexual partners concurrently) | 200 mg tds×7 d or 800 mg morning +1200 mg evening ×2 d or 2 g once | 100 mg tds×7 d | 100 mg bd×7 d | 50 mg tds×7 d |
| Bacterial vaginosis | 400 mg bds×7 d or 2 g once | | | |
| Amoebiasis: (a) invasive intestinal disease in susceptible subjects | 800 mg tds×5 d | 400 mg tds×5 d | 200 mg qds×5 d | 200 mg tds×5 d |
| (b) intestinal disease in less susceptible subjects and chronic amoebic hepatitis | 400 mg tds×5–10 d | 200 mg tds×5–10 d | 100 mg qds×5–10 d | 100 mg tds×5–10 d |
| (c) amoebic liver abscess+other forms of extra-intestinal amoebiasis | 400 mg tds×5 d | 200 mg tds×5 d | 100 mg qds×5 d | 100 mg tds×5 d |
| (d) symptomless cyst passers | 400 mg–800 mg tds×5–10 d | 200 mg–400 mg tds×5–10 d | 100 mg–200 mg qds×5–10 d | 100 mg–200 mg tds×5–10 d |
| Giardiasis: | 2000 mg od×3 d | 1000 mg od×3 d | 600 mg–800 mg od×3 d | 500 mg od×3 d |
| Acute ulcerative gingivitis: | 200 mg tds×3 d | 100 mg tds×3 d | 100 mg bd×3 d | 50 mg tds×3 d |
| Acute dental infections: | 200 mg tds×3–7 d | | | |
| Leg ulcers and pressure sores | 400 mg tds×7 d | | | |

Proportionately smaller dosages should be given to children and babies weighing less than 10 kg.

at eight-hourly intervals. If rectal medication is necessary after the third post-operative day, the frequency of administration should be reduced to 12-hourly.

Children (5 to 10 years): 500 mg suppositories administered as for adults.

*C. Intravenous medication:* Adults and children over 10 years: 100 ml (500 mg) by intravenous infusion immediately before, during or after operation, followed by the same dose eight hourly until oral medication (200 to 400 mg 3 times daily) can be given to complete a seven day course.

Children under 10 years: As for adults *but* the single intravenous dose is based on 1.5 ml (7.5 mg metronidazole) per kg body weight and the oral dose on 3.7 to 7.5 mg per kg body weight.

**Contra-indications, warnings, etc** There are no known absolute contra-indications for the use of Metrolyl. However, known sensitivity to metronidazole is an absolute contra-indication.

*Precautions:* Recommended doses are given as a guideline based on experience. If therapy is to continue for longer than 10 days clinical and laboratory monitoring is advised.

Clinicians considering continuous therapy for relief of chronic conditions are advised to consider the therapeutic benefit against risk of peripheral neuropathy.

Underlying gonococcal infection may persist after elimination of Trichomonas vaginalis.

*Pregnancy:* The safety of use of metronidazole in pregnancy has not been established and its use should be avoided; if essential, short high-dose regimes should *not* be used. Metronidazole is excreted in milk and no adverse effects in the newborn have been reported; the intake by the suckling infant of a mother receiving normal dosage is less than a therapeutic dose for the infants.

No dose modification is needed in renal failure since the elimination half-life of metronidazole is unchanged in this condition. The clinical significance of retained metabolites is not known; their efficient removal occurs during dialysis so that metronidazole should be re-administered after haemodialysis. No dosage adjustment is needed for patients undergoing intermittent or continuous ambulatory peritoneal dialysis.

Impairment of metronidazole clearance may occur in patients with advanced hepatic insufficiency since the drug is mainly metabolized by hepatic oxidation. High concentrations of metronidazole may contribute to the symptoms of hepatic encephalopathy – a condition in which significant cumulation may occur. Dose reduction to one-third once daily may be needed.

The consumption of alcohol during metronidazole therapy should be avoided since there could be a disulfiram-like reaction.

Potentiation of warfarin-type (but not heparin) anticoagulant therapy has been reported so that dose adjustment of the anticoagulant may be needed.

Lithium retention with evidence of possible renal damage has been reported where this compound and metronidazole have been used concurrently; preferably, apart from monitoring lithium, creatinine and electrolyte concentrations, lithium therapy should be tapered and/or withdrawn before use of metronidazole.

The half-life of metronidazole is reduced from 7–8 hours to about 3 hours in patients receiving phenobarbitone.

In patients taking metronidazole, the assay of aspartate amino transferase may give spuriously low values; this depends on the method used.

Metronidazole has no activity against aerobic or facultative anaerobic bacteria.

*Adverse effects:* Serious reactions are rare.

An unpleasant taste in the mouth, furred tongue, nausea, vomiting or other gastro-intestinal disturbance have been reported. There is evidence that metronidazole has been associated with abnormal liver function tests, cholestatic hepatitis and jaundice which may be reversed upon drug withdrawal.

Urticaria, skin rash, pruritus, angioedema and rarely anaphylaxis have occurred.

Erythema multiforme has been reported but this resolves on drug withdrawal.

Drowsiness, dizziness, headache, ataxia and darkening of the urine (due to metabolites) have been reported rarely.

Peripheral neuropathy and/or transient epileptiform seizures have occurred during prolonged or intensive treatment but in most cases neuropathy disappears on cessation of therapy.

There have been reports of bone marrow depression disorder such as agranulocytosis, leucopenia, neutropenia, thrombocytopenia and pancytopenia which may be reversed on drug withdrawal, although fatalities have been reported.

*Overdosage:* There is no specific treatment and uneventful recovery has followed ingestion of up to 12 g.

**Pharmaceutical precautions** Store in a cool dry place, protect from light. The injection is not intended for multi-dose use.

**Legal category** POM.

**Package quantities** 200 mg tablets – packs of 250. 400 mg tablets – packs of 100. 500 mg suppository – packs of 10. 1 g suppository – packs of 10. 100 ml PVC minibag containing 500 mg metronidazole BP – packs of 10.

**Product licence numbers**

| | |
|---|---|
| Metrolyl 200 mg Tablets | 4416/0060 |
| Metrolyl 400 mg Tablets | 4416/0061 |
| Metrolyl 500 mg Suppositories | 4416/0053 |
| Metrolyl 1 g Suppositories | 4416/0054 |
| Metrolyl Injection 500 mg/100 ml | 4416/0010 |

## MODISAL 60 XL*

**Qualitative and quantitative composition** Isosorbide-5-mononitrate 60 mg.

**Pharmaceutical form** Tablets (modified release).

**Clinical particulars**

*Therapeutic indications:* Prophylactic treatment of angina pectoris.

*Posology and method of administration:*

*Adults:* One tablet (60 mg) once daily given in the morning. The dose may be increased to two tablets (120 mg), the whole dose to be given together. The dose can be titrated to minimise the possibility of headache by initiating treatment with half a tablet (30 mg) for the first two to four days. The tablets should not be chewed or crushed and should be swallowed with half a glass of fluid.

*Children:* The safety and efficacy of Modisal 60 XL modified release tablets has not been established.

*Elderly:* No need for routine dosage adjustment in the elderly has been found, but special care may be needed in those with increased susceptibility to hypotension or marked hepatic or renal insufficiency.

*Contra-indications:* Severe cerebrovascular insufficiency. Hypotension.

*Special warnings and precautions for use:* Modisal 60 XL modified release tablets are not indicated for relief of acute anginal attacks; in the event of an acute attack, sublingual or buccal glyceryl trinitrate tablets should be used.

*Interactions with other medicaments and other forms of interaction:* There is a possibility that ISMN may enhance the hypotensive effect of hydrazaline.

*Pregnancy and lactation:* The safety and efficacy of Modisal 60 XL modified release tablets during pregnancy or lactation has not been established.

*Effects on ability to drive and use machines:* The patient should be warned not to drive or operate machinery if hypotension or dizziness occurs.

*Undesirable effects:* Headache may occur when treatment is initiated, but usually disappears after 1–2 weeks of treatment. Hypotension with symptoms such as dizziness or nausea has occasionally been reported. These symptoms generally disappear during long-term treatment.

*Overdose:* Treatment should be symptomatic. The main symptom is likely to be hypotension.

**Pharmacological properties**

*Pharmacodynamic properties:* Organic nitrates (including GTN, ISDN and ISMN) are potent relaxers of smooth muscle. They have a powerful effect on vascular smooth muscle with less effect on bronchiolar, gastrointestinal, ureteral and uterine smooth muscle. Low concentrations dilate both arteries and veins.

Venous dilatation pools blood in the periphery leading to a decrease in venous return, central blood volume, and ventricular filling volumes and pressures. Cardiac output may remain unchanged or it may decline as a result of the decrease in venous return. Arterial blood pressure usually declines secondary to a decrease in cardiac output or arteriolar vasodilatation, or both. A modest reflex increase in heart rate results from the decrease in arterial blood pressure. Nitrates can dilate epicardial coronary arteries including atherosclerotic stenoses.

The cellular mechanism of nitrate-induced smooth muscle relaxation has become apparent in recent years. Nitrates enter the smooth muscle cell and are cleaved to inorganic nitrate and eventually to nitric oxide. This cleavage requires the presence of sulphydryl groups, which apparently come from the amino acid cysteine. Nitric oxide undergoes further reduction to nitrosothiol by further interaction with sulphydryl groups. Nitrosothiol activates guanylate cyclase in the vascular smooth muscle cells, thereby generating cyclic guanosine monophosphate (CGMP). It is this latter compound, CGMP, that produces smooth muscle relaxation by accelerating the release of calcium from these cells.

*Pharmacokinetic properties:*

*Absorption:* Isosorbide-5-mononitrate is readily absorbed from the gastro-intestinal tract.

*Distribution:* Following administration of conventional tablets, peak plasma levels are reached in about 1 hour. Unlike isosorbide dinitrate, ISMN does not undergo first-pass hepatic metabolism and bioavailability is 100%. ISMN has a volume of distribution of about 40 litres and is not significantly protein bound.

*Elimination:* ISMN is metabolised to inactive metabolites including isosorbide and isosorbide glucuronide. The pharmacokinetics are unaffected by the presence of heart failure, renal or hepatic insufficiency. Only 20% of ISMN is excreted unchanged in the urine. An elimination half life of about 4–5 hours has been reported.

*Preclinical safety data:* Not applicable.

**Pharmaceutical particulars**

*List of excipients:* Stearic acid, carnauba wax, hydroxypropylmethylcellulose, lactose, magnesium stearate, talc, purified siliceous earth, polyethylene glycol 4000, E171, E172.

*Incompatibilities:* None known.

*Shelf life:* 3 years.

*Special precautions for storage:* Store in a dry place at or below 25°C. Protect from light.

*Nature and contents of container:* The tablets are packed in aluminium foil/PVC blisters packed in boxes of 28 oval, cream-coloured tablets, half-scored on both sides and marked 60 on one side.

*Instructions for use/handling:* The tablets should be swallowed whole with half a glass of water. They must not be chewed or crushed.

*Marketing authorisation holder:* Valpharma s.a., Via Ranco 112, 47031 Serravalle, Republic of San Marino.

**Marketing authorisation number** 11102/0007.

**Date of approval/revision of SPC** October 1996.

**Legal category** P.

## MONOVENT* SYRUP

**Qualitative and quantitative composition** Each 5 ml spoonful of syrup contains Terbutaline Sulphate BP 1.5 mg.

**Pharmaceutical form** Syrup.

**Clinical particulars**

*Therapeutic indications:* Terbutaline sulphate is a selective $\beta_2$-adrenergic agonist recommended for use in the following indications: prophylactic treatment and relief of an acute attack of allergic, intrinsic and exercise-induced asthma; chronic bronchitis; emphysema; other bronchopulmonary disorders in which bronchospasm is a complicating factor; for the management of uncomplicated premature labour.

*Posology and method of administration:*

*Use in bronchospasm:* Monovent Syrup has a duration of action of 7 to 8 hours. Therefore, the minimum recommended dosage interval is 7 hours.

*Adults and elderly patients:* The starting dose should be 2×5 ml spoonfuls, 3 times in 24 hours. This may be increased to 3×5 ml spoonfuls, 3 times in 24 hours, if necessary.

*Children:* A dosage of 0.075 mg (0.25 ml) per kilogram of the child's weight, 3 times in a 24 hour period, is recommended, e.g.

| *Body weight (kg)* | *Dosage* |
|---|---|
| 14 | 3.5 ml×3 |
| 16 | 4 ml×3 |
| 18 | 4.5 ml×3 |
| 20 | 5 ml×3 |
| 24 | 6 ml×3 |
| 28 | 7 ml×3 |
| 32 | 8 ml×3 |
| 36 | 9 ml×3 |
| 40 | 10 ml×3 |

*Use in the management of labour:*

*Adults:* Oral treatment should not be used initially in an attempt to arrest premature labour.

After contractions have been controlled by intravenous infusion or subcutaneous injections of terbutaline sulphate, maintenance therapy may be continued with Monovent Syrup at a dose of 5 mg, 3 times in a 24 hour period. Oral treatment may be continued for as long as the doctor considers it necessary to delay labour or delivery.

*Route of administration:* Oral.

*Contra-indications:* Monovent is contra-indicated in patients with a history of hypersensitivity to any of its constituents.

Although Monovent can be used in the management of uncomplicated premature labour, its use in the following conditions is contra-indicated: any condition of the mother or foetus in which prolongation of the pregnancy is hazardous, e.g. severe toxaemia, ante-partum haemorrhage, intra-uterine infection, ablatio placentae, threatened abortion during the first and second trimesters, or cord compression.

*Special warnings and precautions for use:* Care should be taken with patients suffering from myocardial insufficiency or thyrotoxicosis.

Due to the hyperglycaemic effects of $\beta_2$-stimulants, additional blood glucose controls are initially recommended when Monovent therapy is commenced in diabetic patients.

If treatment becomes less effective or shorter acting the patient's general condition should be reviewed.

Potentially serious hypokalaemia may result from $\beta_2$ agonist therapy. Particular caution is advised in severe asthma as this effect may be potentiated by concomitant treatment with xanthine derivatives, steroids, diuretics and by hypoxia. It is recommended that serum potassium levels are monitored in such situations.

Due to the positive inotropic effect of $\beta_2$-agonists, terbutaline sulphate should not be used in patients with hypertrophic cardiomyopathy.

During infusion treatment in pregnant women with $\beta_2$-stimulants, in combination with corticosteroids, a rare complication with a pathological picture resembling pulmonary oedema, has been reported.

An increased tendency to uterine bleeding in connection with Caesarean section has been reported. This can be stopped effectively by administering 1–2 mg of propranolol intravenous injection.

*Interactions with other medicaments and other forms of interaction:* Non-selective β-blocking agents such as propranolol may partially or totally inhibit the effect of β-stimulants. Therefore Monovent Syrup and non-selective β-blockers should not normally be administered concurrently. Monovent should be used with caution in patients receiving other sympathomimetics.

*Pregnancy and lactation:* Although no teratogenic effects have been reported in animals or in patients Monovent should only be administered with caution during the first trimester of pregnancy.

Terbutaline sulphate is secreted via breast milk but influence on the infant is unlikely at therapeutic doses.

*Effects on ability to drive and use machines:* In view of tht fact that tremor and palpitations have been reported it is felt that patients who drive or operate machinery should be advised of this.

*Undesirable effects:* The frequency of side-effects is low at the recommended doses. Side-effects which have been recorded such as tremor, headache, tonic cramp and palpitations are all characteristic of sympathomimetic amines. A few patients feel tense; this is also due to the effects on skeletal muscle and not to direct CNS stimulation. Whenever these side-effects have occurred the majority have usually been spontaneously reversible within the first week of treatment. Urticaria and exanthema may occur.

In children, sleep and behavioural disturbances have been seen.

Potentially serious hypokalaemia may result from $\beta_2$-agonist therapy.

*Overdose:* Possible symptoms and signs: headache, anxiety, tremor, tonic cramp, palpitations, arrhythmia. A fall in blood pressure sometimes occurs. Laboratory findings: hypokalaemia, hyperglycaemia and lacto-acidosis sometimes occur.

*Treatment:* (a) Mild and moderate cases: Reduce the dose. Then increase the dose more slowly if the bronchodilator effect is insufficient.

(b) Severe cases: Gastric lavage, activated charcoal. Determination of acid-base balance, blood sugar and electrolytes. Monitoring of heart rate and rhythm and blood pressure. Metabolic changes should be corrected. A cardioselective β-blocker (e.g. metoprolol) is recommended for the treatment of arrhythmias causing a haemodynamic deterioration. The β-blocker should be used with care because of the possibility of inducing bronchoconstriction. If the $\beta_2$-medicated reduction in peripheral vascular resistance significantly contributes to the fall in blood pressure, a volume expander should be given.

**Pharmacological properties**

*Pharmacodynamic properties:* Terbutaline sulphate is a selective $\beta_2$-adrenergic agonist.

*Pharmacokinetic properties:* Terbutaline sulphate is incompletely absorbed from the gastro-intestinal tract and is also subject to fairly extensive first-pass metabolism by sulphate (and some glucuronide) conjugation in the liver and possibly gut wall. It is excreted in the urine partly as the inactive conjugates and partly as unchanged terbutaline the ratio of this depends on the method of administration.

*Preclinical safety data:* Not relevant.

**Pharmaceutical particulars**

*List of excipients:* Citric acid, disodium edetate, ethanol, glycerol, sodium hydroxide, sorbitol, sodium benzoate, lemon limette flavouring, raspberry flavouring, purified water.

*Incompatibilties:* No other major incompatibilities are reported.

*Shelf life:* 36 months.

*Special precautions for storage:* Store below 25°C.

*Nature and contents of container:* Amber glass bottle with plastic cap or plastic bottle and cap. Pack size: 300 ml.

*Instructions for use/handling:* Not applicable.

**Marketing authorisation number** 4416/0100

**Date of approval/revision of SPC** October 1996.

**Legal category** POM.

## NYSTATIN ORAL SUSPENSION BP

**Qualitative and quantitative composition** Each ml contains 100,000 I.U. Nystatin BP.

**Pharmaceutical form** Oral suspension.

**Clinical particulars**

*Therapeutic indications:* Suspension for the prevention and treatment of candidal infections of the oral cavity, oesophagus and intestinal tract. It provides effective prophylaxis against oral candidosis in those born of mothers with vaginal candidosis.

*Posology and method of administration:*

*Adults:* For the treatment of denture sores, and oral infections in adults caused by *Candida albicans*. 1 ml of the suspension should be dropped into the mouth four times daily; it shoud be kept in contact with the affected areas as long as possible.

For the treatment of intestinal candidosis 5 ml of the suspension should be dropped into the mouth four times daily.

For prophylaxis a total daily dosage of 1 million units has been found to suppress the overgrowth of *Candida albicans* in patients receiving broad-spectrum antibiotic therapy.

Administration should be continued for 48 hours after clinical cure to prevent relapse.

*Children:* In intestinal and oral candidosis (thrush) in infants and children 1 ml should be dropped into the mouth four times a day. The longer the suspension is kept in contact with the affected area in the mouth before swallowing, the greater will be its effect.

Administration should be continued for 48 hours after clinical cure to prevent relapse.

For prophylaxis in the newborn the suggested dose is 1 ml once daily.

*Elderly:* No specific dosage recommendation or precautions.

*Route of administration:* Oral.

*Contra-indications:* Known sensitivity to any of the ingredients.

*Special warnings and special precautions for use:* Side effects: Nausea, vomiting and diarrhoea have occasionally been reported with doses of nystatin exceeding 4 to 5 million units daily. No systemic effects or allergic reactions have been assoiciated with its oral use.

The label states the following warnings:

Caution – do not use if seal is broken.
Shake well before use.
Store in a cool place. Avoid freezing.
Caution – contains sugar – should not be given to children with disaccharide intolerance.

The product should be protected from light.
The product should not be diluted.

*Interactions with other medicaments and other forms of interaction:* Not known.

*Pregnancy and lactation:* Absorption of Nystatin from the gastro-intestinal tract is negligible, therefore no special precautions apply in pregnancy.

*Effects on ability to drive and use machines:* No known effects.

*Undesirable effects:* Nystatin Oral Suspension BP contains sugar and should not be given to children with disaccharide intolerance.

*Overdosage:* Since the absorption of Nystatin from the gastro-intestinal tract is negligible, overdosage causes no systemic toxicity.

**Pharmacological properties**

*Pharmacodynamic properties:* Nystatin is a mixture of antifungal polyenes produced by the growth of certain strains of *Streptomyces noursei*, or by any other means. It consists largely of Nystatin $A_1$.

*Pharmacokinetic properties:* Nystatin is a tetraene macrolide. There is no data available on the pharmacokinetics as it is not absorbed from the gastro-intestinal tract, skin or vagina and most of the use is topical. Microbial growth-inhibiting concentrations have been shown to be in the range 3–6 mg/l.

*Preclinical safety data:* Not required.

**Pharmaceutical particulars**

*List of excipients:* Sodium carboxymethylcellulose, methyl p-hydroxybenzoate, propyl p-hydroxybenzoate, sodium metabisulphite, sucrose, saccharin sodium, sodium citrate, permaseal aniseed flavour, purified water.

*Incompatibilities:* Not known.

*Shelf life:* 36 months.

*Special precautions for storage:* Store in a cool place – avoid freezing.

*Nature and contents of container:* 30 g amber glass bottle fitted with a

(i) phenolic resin plastic cap and tin-foil covered melinex liner *or*
(ii) child-resistant cap.

Pack size: 30 ml.

*Instructions for use/handling:* Shake well before use.

**Marketing authorisation number** 4416/0161

**Date of approval/revision of SPC** September 1996.

**Legal category** POM.

## RHUMALGAN* CR 75 AND RHUMALGAN* CR 100

**Presentation**

*Rhumalgan CR 100:* Pale, red, round tablets, containing 100 mg diclofenac sodium BP in a controlled release formulation.

*Rhumalgan CR 75:* White, triangular tablets, containing 75 mg diclofenac sodium BP in a controlled release formulation.

**Uses**

*Action:* Diclofenac sodium is a non-steroidal anti-inflammatory drug (NSAID) with analgesic and antipyretic properties. It is an inhibitor of prostaglandin synthetase.

*Indications:* Rheumatoid arthritis; osteoarthritis; ankylosing spondylitis; acute gout; low back pain; relief of pain in fractures; acute musculo-skeletal disorders and trauma including periarthritis (particularly frozen shoulder), bursitis, tendinitis, tenosynovitis, dislocations, sprains and strains; and the control of pain and inflammation in orthopaedic, dental and other minor surgery.

*Pharmacokinetics:* Rhumalgan CR tablets are extended release preparations designed to release diclofenac over a period of time. Following a pharmacokinetic study with the 100 mg tablets in volunteers it was found that the average time to reach maximum plasma concentration was 6.05 hours. The average elimination half life was found to be 6.75 hours. The average maximum plasma concentration was found to be 262 ng/ml. Diclofenac sodium is highly protein bound.

**Dosage and administration** For oral administration.

*Adults:* One 100 mg tablet a day or one 75 mg tablet once or twice a day. Tablets should be swallowed whole preferably with food.

*Children:* Not suitable for use in children.

*Elderly:* Care should be used when treating patients who are frail or have a low body weight as they will in general be more susceptibel to adverse reactions. The lowest effective dose should be used in these patients. The standard adult dose may be used for other elderly patients.

**Contra-indications, warnings, etc**

*Contra-indications:* Hypersensitivity to diclofenac sodium. Active or suspected peptic ulcer; gastro-intestinal bleeding. Patients who when taking aspirin or other non-steroidal anti-inflammatory drugs suffer attacks of asthma, urticaria or acute rhinitis.

*Pregnancy:* Diclofenac sodium should only be used during pregnancy and lactation if considered essential.

Diclofenac sodium is reported to cross the placenta in mice and rats but there have not been any studies reported of humans.

*Precautions:* Patients with a history of gastro-intestinal ulceration, haematemesis, or melaena, should be carefully observed, and care should be taken when treating patients with ulcerative colitis, Crohn's disease, haematological abnormalities, or bleeding diathesis. Elderly patients and those with renal, hepatic or cardiac impairment should also be monitored as renal function may be reduced by NSAID therapy. Renal function should be monitored and the lowest effective dose used.

In patients with impairment of cardiac or renal

function, those recovering from major surgery or those being treated with diuretics, prostaglandins are important for the maintenance of renal blood flow. The possibility of inhibition of prostaglandins synthetase should be considerd when giving diclofenac to these patients. On stopping diclofenac, effects on renal function are usually reversible.

Diclofenac should be stopped if liver function tests show abnormalities which persist or worsen, or if liver disease develops or if other symptoms such as eosinophilia or rash occur.

Diclofenac sodium may trigger an attack in patients with hepatic porphyria.

Monitoring of renal function, hepatic function (elevation of liver enzymes may occur) and blood counts should be performed on long-term NSAID patients, as a precautionary measure.

Patients should not drive or operative machinery if they experience dizziness or other central nervous system disturbances.

*Interactions:* Diclofenac may increase plasma concentrations of lithium (by the impairment of its excretion from the kidneys) and digoxin.

Methotrexate and NSAIDs should only be administered within 24 hours of each other if given with extreme caution. NSAIDs are reported to increase the plasma levels of methotrexate resulting in increased toxicity.

If other NSAIDs are given concomitantly with diclofenac sodium the frequency of side effects may be increased.

NSAIDs may increase cyclosporin nephrotoxcity as a result of their effect on renal prostaglandins.

There is an increased risk of convulsions if quinolone antibiotics are given while NSAIDs are being taken, and caution is advised when considering their use.

The activity of diuretics may be inhibited by some NSAIDs. Increased serum potassium levels may result when diclofenac is given concomitantly with potassium-sparing diuretics. Serum potassium levels should therefore be monitored.

Care is required when giving anticoagulants with NSAIDs as diclofenac may reversibly inhibit platelet aggregation. Monitoring is recommended to ensure the desired response to the anticoagulant is maintained as there are rare reports of increased risk of haemorrhage with combined diclofenac and anticoagulant therapy.

It has been reported that hypo- and hyperglycaemic effects have occurred rarely when diclofenac and oral antidiabetic agents have been given together and adjustment of the hypoglycaemic may be required.

*Side-effects:* Common side effects include nausea, headaches, diarrhoea, epigastric pain, anorexia, dyspepsia, flatulence, abdominal cramps, vertigo and dizziness. Serious effects such as peptic ulcer, gastrointestinal bleeding and bloody diarrhoea have occasionally been reported, and there are reports of isolated cases of lower gut disorders (exacerbations of ulcerative colitis or Crohn's proctocolitis and nonspecific haemorrhagic colitis), glossitis, constipation, pancreatitis, oesophageal lesions and aphthous stomatitis.

Skin rashes and eruptions have occasionally been reported and rarely urticaria. There are also rare reports of erythema multiforme, Stevens-Johnson syndrome, Lyell's syndrome, bullous reactions, eczema, erythroderma, hair loss, photosensitivity reactions and purpura.

Isolated effects on the central nervous system include drowsiness, tiredness, impaired hearing, insomnia, convulsions, irritability, anxiety, depression, psychotic reactions, tremors, memory disturbance, vertigo, disturbance of sensation, disorientation, disturbance of vision, tinnitus, nightmares and taste alterations.

Occasional effects on the kidney include acute renal insufficiency, urinary abnormalities (e.g. haematuria, proteinuria), nephrotic syndrome, papillary necrosis and interstitial nephritis.

Effects on the liver include occasional reports of elevation of serum aminotransferase enzymes (ALT, AST) and rarely, liver function disorders including hepatitis with or without jaundice.

Leucopenia, haemolytic anaemia, thrombocytopenia, aplastic anaemia and agranulocytosis have rarely been reported. Other rarely reported reactions include hypersensitivity reactions (anaphylactic/analphylactoid systemic reactions, hypotension, bronchospasm), oedema, palpitation, impotence, chest pain and hypertension.

*Overdosage:* Gastric lavage and treatment with activated charcoal should be used as soon as possible after overdosage in order to prevent absorption of the drug.

Further treatment is supportive and symptomatic. Complications that might be encountered include renal failure, hypotension, convulsions, respiratory depression, and gastro-intestinal irritation.

**Pharmaceutical precautions** Store in a dry place below 25˚C. Protect from light.

**Legal category** POM.

**Package quantities**
Rhumalgan CR 75: Blister packs of 28 and 56.
Rhumalgan CR 100: Calendar packs of 28.

**Further information** Other ingredients include the colours: titanium dioxide, (E171) used for both strengths and iron oxide, (E172) used for the 100 mg CR tablets only.

**Product licence numbers**
Rhumalgan CR 75     4416/0242
Rhumalgan CR 100    4416/0243.

# TEMAZEPAM TABLETS

**Qualitative and quantitative composition** Each tablet contains: 10 mg or 20 mg Temazepam BP.

**Pharmaceutical form** Tablet.

**Clinical particulars**
*Therapeutic indications:* For the short-term treatrment of insomnia in cases where it is severe, disabling or subjecting the individual to extreme distress. Temazepam is also indicated for pre-operative medication prior to minor surgery or other similar procedures.

*Posology and method of administration:* The recommended doses are as follows:

*Insomnia:*
*Adults* – 10–20 mg. In extreme cases this may be increased to 30–40 mg.
*Elderly* – 10 mg. In extreme cases this may be increased to 20 mg.
Tablets should be taken approximately 30 minutes before retiring to bed.

*Premedication:*
*Adults* – The normal dose is 20–40 mg, half an hour to an hour before the procedure.
*Elderly* – 10–20 mg.

*Children:* Temazepam tablets are not recommended for use in children.

The lowest possible dose should be used. Treatment should not be continued beyond four weeks and treatment should be tapered off gradually (see *Special warnings and precautions*).

Oral administration.

*Contra-indications:* Temazepam is contra-indicated in the treatment of patients suffering from severe respiratory or hepatic insufficiency, myasthenia gravis or sleep apnoea syndrome. It is also contra-indicated for use in those who have previously experienced hypersensitivity to this or other benzodiazepines.

*Special warnings and precautions for use:* The cause for insomnia should be determined prior to the use of temazepam, and it should not be used for first line treatment of psychotic illness. Temazepam should also not be used on its own to treat depression or anxiety accompanying depression.

The duration of treatment should be as short as possible (less than 4 weeks) including the tapering off process. More long-term treatment is not advised without re-assessment of the condition. Treatment should be discontinued gradually to minimise the risk of withdrawal or rebound phenomena where the symptoms requiring the treatment recur in an enhanced form.

Temazepam should also be used cautiously in patients with a history of alcohol or drug abuse, or severe hepatic or renal insufficiency.

When used to treat insomnia patients should ensure that they will be able to have 7–8 hours of uninterrupted sleep in order to reduce the risk of anterograde amnesia occurring. If insufficient sleep does occur, this could lead to impaired alertness. Sedation, amnesia, impaired concentration and impaired muscular function may adversely affect the ability to drive or to use machines.

When temazepam is used for pre-medication, patients should be accompanied home afterwards.

There is a risk of drug dependency developing with the use of temazepam. This risk increases in severity with increasing dose and duration of treatment. There is also a greater risk in patients with a history of alcohol or drug abuse, or personality disorder.

If dependence does develop, abrupt discontinuation of treatment will be accompanied by withdrawal symptoms. These may consist of headaches, muscle pain, extreme anxiety, tension, restlessness, confusion and irritability.

The use of benzodiazepines in patients also suffering from depression may unveil suicidal tendencies. Amnesia may occur and in cases of loss and bereavement, psychological adjustment may be inhibited by benzodiazepines.

*Interactions with other medicaments and other forms of interaction:* The concomitant use of temazepam and alcohol may enhance the sedative effect and is therefore not recommended.

Concurrent use of antipsychotics, antidepressants, narcotic analgesics, hypnotics, anxiolytics/sedatives, sedative antihistamines, anaesthetics and antiepileptic drugs may further enhance the central depressive effect.

Ehanced euphoria may also occur with combined use of temazepam and narcotic analgesics, therefore possibly increasing the risk of dependence.

*Pregnancy and lactation:* The use of temazepam during pregnancy and lactation is not recommended as safety in these patient groups has not been established.

Should a patient become pregnant while taking temazepam, she should contact her doctor regarding the discontinuation of treatment with temazepam.

If temazepam is used during the latter stages of pregnancy or during labour because the perceived benefit to the patient outweighs the risk to the neonate, the possibility of hypothermia, hypotonia and moderate respiratory depression should be borne in mind.

If a patient has however had longer-term treatment with temazepam, the possibility of physical dependence and therefore risk of withdrawal symptoms of the child should be considered.

*Effects on ability to drive and use machines:* Temazepam may result in impaired alertness, if this occurs, patients should avoid driving or operating machinery.

*Undesirable effects:* At the start of treatment patients may suffer from drowsiness, reduced alertness, dizziness, confusion, fatigue, muscle weakness, numbed emotions, headache, ataxia or double vision. These will normally disappear with continued treatment.

More rarely, vivid dreams/nightmares, restless sleep, palpitations, change in libido, skin reactions, sedation, impaired muscular function, dry mouth and gastrointestinal disturbances may occur.

Pre-existing depression may be unmasked during treatment with temazepam.

Blood dyscrasias, urinary retention, increased liver enzymes, jaundice and visual disturbances have also been reported to occur occasionally. If any of these effects do occur, treatment should be discontinued.

Other effects, including delusions, psychoses, hallucinations, irritability and restlessness, aggressiveness and rages or other inappropriate behaviour have also been reported to occur, predominantly in elderly patients. If any of these effects occur, treatment should be discontinued.

*Overdose:* Overdose of temazepam usually results in some form of central nervous system depression ranging from drowsiness to coma.

Flumazenil may be used as antidote therapy.

Overdose with temazepam on its own should not present a threat to life. Temazepam overdose combined with the use of other CNS depressants or alcohol should be treated immediately.

Vomiting or gastric lavage should be induced within one hour. If emptying of the stomach is not advantageous then activated charcoal should be administered to reduce absorption of the drug.

In intensive care treatment, special attention should be given to respiratory and cardiovascular functions.

**Pharmacological properties**
*Pharmacodynamic properties:* Temazepam is known to have hypnotic/sedative and anxiolytic properties. It therefore results in anxiolysis, muscle relaxation and central nervous system sedation. It has been suggested that a close molecular association between the sites and action for gamma-aminobutyric acid (GABA) and benzodiazepines and potentiation of GABA may be responsible for these effects.

Other neurotransmitters may also be affected.

*Pharmacokinetic properties:* Temazepam is readily and almost completely absorbed from the gastrointestinal tract and has been reported to be relatively extensively bound to plasma proteins (75–95%). Peak plasma concentrations are reached approximately one hour after dosing. The majority of a dose of temazepam is metabolised to inactive glucuronides, which are then excreted in the urine.

*Preclinical safety data:* Not relevant.

**Pharmaceutical particulars**
*List of excipients:* Lactose monohydrate, maize starch, pregelled starch, sodium starch glycollate, microcrystalline cellulose and magnesium stearate.

*Incompatibilities:* Not known.

*Shelf life:* 24 months.

*Special precautions for storage:* Store at or below 25˚C in a dry place. Protect from light.

*Nature and contents of container:* 10 mg strength: packs of 500 tablets. 20 mg strength: packs of 250. Polypropylene plastic tablet container, with tamper evident lid.

*Instructions for use/handling:* Not applicable.

**Marketing authorisation numbers**

Temazepam Tablets 10 mg     4416/0269

Temazepam Tablets 20 mg     4416/0270

**Date of approval/revision of SPC**    January 1997.

**Legal category**    CD (Sch 3), POM.

# VERAPAMIL HYDROCHLORIDE TABLETS BP

## Presentation

*Tablets 40 mg:* Yellow, biconvex, film-coated tablets each containing 40 mg Verapamil Hydrochloride BP.

*Tablets 80 mg:* Yellow, biconvex, film-coated tablets each containing 80 mg Verapamil Hydrochloride BP.

*Tablets 120 mg:* Yellow, biconvex, film-coated tablets each containing 120 mg Verapamil Hydrochloride BP and embossed with $\frac{75}{120}$ on one side.

## Uses

*Actions:* Verapamil is a calcium antagonist which blocks the inward movement of calcium in cardiac muscle cells, in smooth muscle cells of the coronary and systemic arteries and in the cells of the intracardiac conduction system.

*Indications:* Verapamil Hydrochloride is useful in: the treatment and prophlyaxis of angina pectoris, and variant angina: the treatment and prophylaxis of paroxysmal supraventricular tachycardia and atrial flutter/filbrillation (Verapamil should not be used when atrial flutter/fibrillation complicates Wolf-Parkinson-White syndrome): and the treatment of mild to moderate hypertension.

## Dosage and administration

*Angina:*

*Adults:* 120 mg three times daily is recommended.

Some patients with angina of effort may respond to 80 mg three times daily, but this dose is not likely to be effective in angina at rest and variant angina.

*Supraventricular tachycardias:*

*Adults:* 40–120 mg three times daily according to the severity of the condition.

*Children 2 years and above:* 40–120 mg 2–3 times daily, according to age and effectiveness.

*Hypertension:*

*Adults:* 160 mg twice daily. A small number of patients may be controlled successfully on 120 mg twice daily, whereas others may require up to 480 mg daily, given in divided doses.

A further reduction in blood pressure may be obtained by combining Verapamil tablets with other antihypertensive agents, eg thiazide diuretics. For concomitant use with beta-blockers see 'Interactions' below.

*Children:* Up to 10 mg/kg/day in divided doses according to the severity of the condition.

*Elderly:* No special dosage recommendations, except in patients with impaired liver function or cardiac conduction problems, where a reduced dosage may be necessary.

## Contra-indications, warnings, etc

*Contra-indications:* Hypotension, cardiogenic shock, marked bradycardia (less than 50 beats/minute), second or third degree atrioventricular block, sinoatrial block, sick sinus syndrome, uncompensated heart failure. Combination with β-blockers is contra-indicated in patients with poor ventricular function. Concomitant ingestion of grapefruit juice.

*Interactions:* Verapamil Hydrochloride and beta-blockers may be additive, both with respect to conduction and contraction. Verapamil Hydrochloride should, therefore, be given with care to those who are receiving beta-blockers.

Intravenous beta-blockers should not be given to patients on Verapamil.

Verapamil hydrochloride has been shown to increase the serum concentration of digoxin, therefore care should be exercised with regard to digitalis toxicity.

Verapamil may have an additive effect when given with other antihypertensive drugs, and a reduction in the dosage of the other antihypertensive drug could be possible.

Long-term verapamil treatment may give rise to potentiation of neuromuscular blocking agents during anaesthesia.

The concomitant use of verapamil and anti-arrhythmic agents or inhaled anaesthetics may lead to additive cardiovascular effects.

It is reported that the effects of carbamazepine are potentiated by verapamil, and rifampicin attentuates the effects of verapamil.

It has been reported that the concomitant administration of verapamil and grapefruit juice can lead to an increase in verapamil serum level.

Other reported interactions include those with cyclosporin and theophylline (increased plasma levels), and with lithium (neurotoxic interactions have been reported).

*Side-effects:* Verapamil is generally well tolerated. Constipation may occur. Other less common side effects reported include flushing, nausea, fatigue, dizziness and headaches. On rare occasions vomiting and allergic reactions have been reported. On very rare occasions, a reversible impairment of liver function, characterised by an increase in transaminases and/or alkaline phosphatase may occur during verapamil hydrochloride treatment.

There have been rare reports of gynaecomastia in elderly male patients and gingival hyperplasia. These were observed in patients on long term therapy and were reversible when the drug was discontinued.

*Use in pregnancy and lactation:* Verapamil is excreted in breast milk in small amounts. Although animal studies have not shown any teratogenic effects, verapamil hydrochloride should not be administered during pregnancy or lactation, unless in the clinician's judgement it is considered essential for the patient's welfare.

*Warnings:* Verapamil hydrochloride may affect impulse conduction and should be used carefully in patients with first degree atrioventricular block.

Patients with atrial fibrillation/flutter and an accessory pathway (e.g. Wolf-Parkinson-White syndrome) may rarely develop increased conduction across the anomalous pathway and ventricular tachycardia may be precipitated.

Verapamil hydrochloride may affect left ventricular contractility. This effect is small, but cardiac failure may be precipitated or aggravated if it exists. In cases with poor ventricular function, verapamil hydrochloride should only be given after appropriate therapy for cardiac failure such as digitalis, etc.

Caution should be observed in the acute phase of myocardial infarction.

In patients with impaired liver function, a reduction in dosage may be required due to the decrease in drug metabolism.

The effect of verapamil in patients with renal impairment is unknown and therefore careful patient monitoring is recommended. Verapamil is not removed during dialysis.

*Overdosage:* Usual emergency measures for acute cardiovascular side-effects should be applied, eg in the case of cardiac arrest, heart massage, mechanical respiration, followed by appropriate intensive care; in the case of second and third degree A.V. block, atropine, isoprenaline and, if required, pace-maker therapy. In the case of myocardial insufficiency, dopamine, dobutamine, cardiac glycosides or calcium gluconate (10–20 ml of a 10% solution); and in the case of hypotension, appropriate positioning of the patient with dopamine, dobutamine or noradrenaline, as required.

**Pharmaceutical precautions**    Store in a cool, dry place.

**Legal category**    POM.

**Package quantities**    40 mg tablets 28, 30, 56, 84, 90, 100, 112 and 120 in securitainers.

   80 mg tablets: 100 in securitainers.

   120 mg tablets: 100 in securitainers.

**Further information**    Nil.

**Product licence numbers**

   40 mg tablets    4416/0121

   80 mg tablets    4416/0122

   120 mg tablets    4416/0123

*\*Trade Mark*

**Lederle Laboratories**
Cyanamid of Great Britain Limited
Fareham Road
Gosport, Hants PO13 OAS

**Please refer to Wyeth Laboratories.**

# Leo Laboratories Limited
Longwick Road
Princes Risborough
Bucks. HP27 9RR

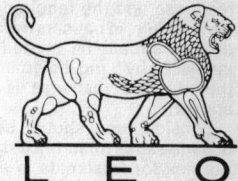

## BETIM* TABLETS

**Presentation** White, flat circular tablets engraved with '102' on the scored face and with an Assyrian lion on the reverse. Each tablet contains Timolol Maleate PhEur 10 mg.

### Uses

*Mode of action:* Betim is a beta-adrenergic receptor blocking agent. The competitive antagonism of adrenergic transmitters at beta receptors blocks beta-sympathomimetic activity particularly in the heart, the bronchi and blood vessels.

Betim has been shown to be a highly specific beta-adrenergic blocking drug and it does not block the chronotropic or inotropic effects of calcium, glucagon, theophylline or digitalis. It does not have significant local anaesthetic or direct myocardial depressant activity nor any significant intrinsic beta-adrenergic stimulant effect.

Betim reduces heart rate and force of myocardial contraction and therefore myocardial oxygen consumption. Modification of the cardiovascular responses to stress or exercise is therapeutically useful in the treatment of angina pectoris.

The beta blocking action of Betim is also of therapeutic value in hypertension although the exact mechanism of action is unclear.

Timolol maleate is rapidly and nearly completely absorbed following oral administration. Beta blocking activity is apparent within 30 minutes of administration and the duration of action, though dependent on dose, has been shown to last for up to 24 hours. Dose proportionality has been established. Plasma half life is approximately 2.7–5.0 hours with a peak plasma concentration occurring approximately 2 hours post dose. Timolol undergoes significant hepatic metabolism, but 'first pass metabolism' is low.

5% of timolol is excreted unchanged by the kidneys. These pharmacokinetic parameters are unchanged in hypertensive patients and following multiple dosages.

The rate of timolol metabolism varies between individuals; poor metabolisers (approximately 10%) show higher plasma levels and slower elimination of timolol than extensive metabolisers. Within individuals, however, plasma concentrations and half-life are reproducible. As the therapeutic response and some adverse effects are related to plasma concentrations of timolol, poor metabolisers may require lower than normal doses.

*Indications:* Betim is indicated in angina pectoris due to ischaemic heart disease, for the treatment of hypertension and to reduce mortality and reinfarction in patients surviving acute myocardial infarction. Betim is also indicated in the prophylactic treatment of migraine in order to reduce the number of attacks.

### Dosage and administration

*For angina:* The recommended dose range is 5–30 mg twice daily. The initial dose should be 5 mg twice daily, increasing the daily dose by 10 mg every 3–4 days to achieve optimum results.

*Hypertension:* The recommended dose range is 10–60 mg daily.

Most hypertensive patients will be controlled by 10–30 mg timolol which can be administered once daily or in two divided doses if preferred. Doses in excess of 30 mg daily should be given in two equally divided doses. The dose of Betim may need adjustment when used in conjunction with other antihypertensive drugs.

*After myocardial infarction:* Start with 5 mg (½ tablet) twice daily for two days. If there are no adverse effects, increase dosage to 10 mg twice daily and maintain at this dose.

*For the prophylactic treatment of migraine:* 10 to 20 mg once daily or in two divided doses.

*Dosage in the elderly:* Initiate treatment with lowest adult dose and thereafter adjust according to response.

*Children:* Safety and efficacy in children has not been established.

### Contra-indications, warnings, etc

*Contra-indications:* Heart failure, unless adequately controlled. Sinus bradycardia or heart block. Cardiogenic shock. Bronchial asthma, chronic obstructive pulmonary disease. Patients receiving monoamine oxidase inhibitors. Pregnancy. Sick sinus syndrome, severe peripheral vascular disease or Raynaud's disease, hypersensitivity to timolol or any other ingredients.

*Precautions:* Although Betim has no direct myocardial depressant activity, the continued depression of sympathetic drive through beta blockade may lead to cardiac failure. All patients should be observed for evidence of cardiac failure; if it occurs, then treatment with beta blockers should be gradually withdrawn. If it is not possible to withdraw beta blocker treatment, then digitalisation and diuretic therapy should be considered.

Betim may be used safely in diabetes. It may however interfere with the cardiovascular and possibly the metabolic responses to hypoglycaemia and therefore should be used with caution in diabetic patients treated with insulin or oral hypoglycaemic agents as well as in patients subject to spontaneous hypoglycaemia.

Betim should be administered with caution to patients with impaired renal function or impaired hepatic function.

*Drug interactions:* Caution is recommended when Betim is administered to patients on catecholamine depleting drugs such as reserpine or guanethidine.

The bioavailability of Betim will be increased by co-administration with cimetidine and reduced with rifampicin.

Some non-steroidal anti-inflammatory agents have been shown to impair the anti-hypertensive effect of beta blocking drugs.

Betim may be prescribed with vasodilators, but increased gastro-intestinal blood flow may affect absorption and metabolism of timolol.

Betim should be used with caution in patients already receiving other hypotensive drugs, including clonidine.

The effect of sympathomimetic agents, eg isoprenaline, salbutamol, will be reduced by concomitant use of beta blockers.

The depressant effect of beta blocking drugs on myocardial contractility and on intracardiac conduction may be increased by concomitant use with other drugs having similar effects. Serious effects have been reported with verapamil, disopyramide, lignocaine and tocainide and may be anticipated with any of the Class 1 antiarrhythmic agents. Special care is necessary when any of these agents are given intravenously in patients who are beta blocked.

The adverse vasoconstrictor effects of ergot preparations may be potentiated during the treatment of migraine with beta blocking drugs.

*Anaesthesia:* The withdrawal of beta blocking drugs prior to surgery is not necessary in the majority of patients. However, anaesthetic agents such as ether, cyclopropane and trichloroethylene should not be used whereas halothane, isoflurane, nitrous oxide, intravenous induction agents, muscle relaxants, narcotic analgesics and local anaesthetic agents are all compatible with beta adrenergic blockade. Local anaesthetics with added vasoconstrictors, eg adrenaline, should be avoided.

*Use in pregnancy:* Betim is contraindicated in pregnancy. Timolol maleate appears in breast milk (milk: plasma ratio 0.8) and its use by nursing mothers requires caution. The neonate should be observed for any side-effects.

*Side-effects:* Betim is usually well tolerated in normal use. General symptoms resulting from beta blockade include fatigue and weakness.

Cardiovascular: bradycardia, heart failure, coldness of the limb extremities, hypotension, heart block.

Digestive: epigastric distress, nausea and vomiting.

CNS: dizziness, disorientation, vertigo, paraesthesiae, headache, hallucinations, nightmares, insomnia, somnolence, depression.

Respiratory: Dyspnoea, broncho-spasm.

Retroperitoneal fibrosis, allergic skin reactions, including erythematous or psoriaform rashes and arthralgia, have been rarely reported.

*Warning:* There have been reports of skin rashes and/or dry eyes associated with the use of beta-adrenergic blocking drugs. The reported incidence is rare and in most cases the symptoms have cleared when treatment was withdrawn.

Discontinuance of the drug should be considered if any such reaction is not otherwise explicable. Cessation of therapy with the beta-blocker should be gradual although withdrawal symptoms with timolol are infrequent.

*Overdosage:* Poisoning due to an overdose of Betim may lead to severe hypotension, sinus bradycardia, atrioventricular block, cardiogenic shock, cardiac arrest, bronchospasm, impairment of consciousness, coma, occasionally, hyperkalaemia. The first manifestations usually appear 20 minutes to 2 hours after drug ingestion.

Treatment should include close monitoring of cardiovascular, respiratory and renal function, and blood glucose and electrolytes. Further absorption may be prevented by induction of vomiting, gastric lavage or administration of activated-charcoal if ingestion is recent. Cardiovascular complications should be treated symptomatically, which may require the use of sympathomimetic agents (eg noradrenaline, metariminol), atropine or inotropic agents, (eg dopamine, dobatamine). Temporary pacing may be required for AV block. Glucagon can reverse the effects of excessive beta-blockage, given in a dose of 1–10 mg intravenously. Intravenous $B_2$-stimulants, eg terbutaline may be required to relieve bronchospasm.

Timolol cannot be effectively removed by haemo-dialysis.

**Pharmaceutical precautions** Nil.

**Legal category** POM.

**Package quantities** Packs of 100 tablets.

**Further information** Nil.

**Product licence number** 0043/0035R.

## BURINEX* TABLETS

**Presentation** *Tablets 1 mg:* Each tablet contains 1 mg bumetanide – a white, flat, circular, uncoated tablet marked with the number 133 on the scored face and with an Assyrian Lion on the reverse.

*Tablets 5 mg:* Each tablet contains 5 mg bumetanide – a white, flat, circular, uncoated, bevelled-edge tablet marked with a score line and '5 mg' on one face.

### Uses

*Mode of action:* Burinex (bumetanide) is a potent, high ceiling loop diuretic with a rapid onset and a short duration of action. The primary site of action is the ascending limb of the Loop of Henlé where it exerts inhibiting effects on electrolyte reabsorption causing the diuretic and natriuretic action observed.

After oral administration of 1 mg Burinex, diuresis begins within 30 minutes with a peak effect between one and two hours. The diuretic effect is virtually complete in three hours after a 1 mg dose.

*Pharmacokinetics:* Burinex is well absorbed after oral administration with the bioavailability reaching between 80 and 95%. The elimination half life ranges from between 0.75 to 2.6 hours. No active metabolites are known. Renal excretion accounts for approximately half the clearance with hepatic excretion responsible for the other half. There is an increase in half-life and a reduced plasma clearance in the presence of renal or hepatic disease. In patients with chronic renal failure the liver takes more importance as an excretory pathway although the duration of action is not markedly prolonged.

*Indications:* Burinex is indicated whenever diuretic therapy is required in the treatment of oedema, e.g. that associated with congestive heart failure, cirrhosis of the liver and renal disease including the nephrotic syndrome.

In oedema of cardiac or renal origin where high doses of a potent short acting diuretic are required, Burinex 5 mg tablets may be used.

### Dosage and administration

*Burinex 1 mg tablets:* Most patients require a daily dose of 1 mg which can be given as a single morning or early evening dose. Depending on the patient's response, a second dose can be given six to eight hours later. In refractory cases, the dose can be increased until a satisfactory diuretic response is obtained, or infusions of Burinex can be given.

*Burinex 5 mg tablets:* The dose should be carefully

titrated in each patient according to the patient's response and the required therapeutic activity. As a general rule, in patients not controlled on lower doses, dosage should be started at 5 mg daily and then increased by 5 mg increments every 12–24 hours until the required response is obtained or side-effects appear.

Consideration should be given to a twice daily dosage rather than once daily. Direct substitution of Burinex for frusemide in a 1:40 ratio at high doses should be avoided. Treatment should be initiated at a lower equivalent dose and gradually increased in 5 mg increments.

*Children:* Not recommended for children under 12 years of age.

*Dosage in the elderly:* Adjust dosage according to response; a dose of 0.5 mg bumetanide per day may be sufficient in some elderly patients.

### Contra-indications, warnings, etc

*Contra-indications:* Although Burinex can be used to induce diuresis in renal insufficiency, any marked increase in blood urea or the development of oliguria or anuria during treatment of severe progressing renal disease are indications for stopping treatment with Burinex.

Hypersensitivity to Burinex. Burinex is contra-indicated in hepatic coma and care should be taken in states of severe electrolyte depletion.

As with other diuretics, Burinex should not be administered concurrently with lithium salts. Diuretics can reduce lithium clearance resulting in high serum levels of lithium.

*Precautions:* Excessively rapid mobilisation of oedema particularly in elderly patients, may give rise to sudden changes in cardiovascular pressure-flow relationships with circulatory collapse. This should be borne in mind when Burinex is given in high doses intravenously or orally. Electrolyte disturbances may occur particularly in those patients taking a low-salt diet. Regular checks of serum electrolytes, in particular sodium, potassium, chloride and bicarbonate should be performed and replacement therapy instituted where indicated.

Like other diuretics, Burinex shows a tendency to increase the excretion of potassium which can lead to an increase in the sensitivity of the myocardium to the toxic effects of digitalis. Thus the dose may need adjustment when given in conjunction with cardiac glycosides.

Burinex may potentiate the effects of antihypertensive drugs. Therefore, the dose of the latter may need adjustment when Burinex is used to treat oedema in hypertensive patients.

As with other diuretics, Burinex may cause an increase in blood uric acid. Periodic checks on urine and blood glucose should be made in diabetics and patients suspected of latent diabetes.

Patients with chronic renal failure on high doses of Burinex should remain under constant hospital supervision.

Certain non-steroidal anti-inflammatory drugs have been shown to antagonise the action of diuretics.

*Warnings:* Encephalopathy may be precipitated in patients with pre-existing hepatic impairment.

Burinex should be used with caution in patients already receiving nephrotoxic or ototoxic drugs.

*Use in pregnancy and lactation:* Although tests in four animal species have shown no teratogenic effects, the ordinary precaution of avoiding use of Burinex in the first trimester of pregnancy should at present be observed.

Since it is not known whether bumetanide is distributed into breast milk, a nursing mother should either stop breast feeding or observe the infant for any adverse effects if the drug is absolutely necessary for the mother.

*Adverse effects:* Reported reactions include abdominal pain, vomiting, dyspepsia, diarrhoea, stomach and muscle cramps, arthralgia, dizziness, fatigue, hypotension, headache, nausea, encephalopathy (in patients with pre-existing hepatic disease), fluid and electrolyte depletion, dehydration, hyperuricaemia, raised blood urea and serum creatinine, hyperglycaemia, abnormalities of serum levels of hepatic enzymes, skin rashes, pruritis, urticaria, thrombocytopenia, gynaecomastia and painful breasts. Bone marrow depression associated with the use of Burinex has been reported rarely but it has not been proven definitely to be attributed to the drug. Hearing disturbance after administration of Burinex is rare and reversible.

*High dose therapy:* In patients with severe chronic renal failure given high doses of Burinex, there have been reports of severe, generalised, musculoskeletal pain sometimes associated with muscle spasm, occurring one to two hours after administration and lasting up to 12 hours. The lowest reported dose causing this type of adverse reaction was 5 mg by intravenous injection and the highest was 75 mg

orally in a single dose. All patients recovered fully and there was no deterioration in their renal function. The cause of this pain is uncertain but it may be a result of varying electrolyte gradients at the cell membrane level.

Experience suggests that the incidence of such reactions is reduced by initiating treatment at 5–10 mg daily and titrating upwards using a twice daily dosage regimen at doses of 20 mg per day or more.

*Overdosage:* Symptoms would be those caused by excessive diuresis. Empty stomach by gastric lavage or emesis. General measures should be taken to restore blood volume, maintain blood pressure and correct electrolyte disturbance.

**Pharmaceutical precautions** Burinex is presented in amber glass containers to protect against deterioration due to exposure to light.

**Legal category** POM.

**Package quantities**
1 mg tablets – calendar pack of 28 (OP).
5 mg tablets – calendar pack of 28 (OP).

**Further information** Burinex is also available as Burinex K tablets, each containing 0.5 mg bumetanide and 573 mg potassium chloride in a slow release core.

**Product licence numbers**
Burinex 1 mg    0043/0021R
Burinex 5 mg    0043/0043R

## BURINEX* INJECTION

**Presentation** A solution containing 0.5 mg bumetanide per ml in amber glass ampoules of 2 ml, 4 ml and 10 ml, each ampoule containing 1 mg, 2 mg and 5 mg bumetanide respectively. Other ingredients: xylitol, disodium hydrogen phosphate dihydrate, sodium dihydrogen phosphate dihydrate and water for injections.

**Uses**    *Mode of action:* Burinex (bumetanide) is a potent high ceiling diuretic with a rapid onset and a short duration of action.

After intravenous injection, diuresis usually starts within a few minutes and ceases in about two hours.

In most patients 1 mg of Burinex produces a similar diuretic effect to 40 mg of frusemide.

Burinex excretion in the urine shows a good correlation with the diuretic response. In patients with chronic renal failure, the liver takes more importance as an excretory pathway, although the duration of action in such patients is not markedly prolonged.

*Indications:* Burinex is indicated whenever diuretic therapy is required in the treatment of oedema, e.g. that associated with congestive heart failure, cirrhosis of the liver and renal disease including the nephrotic syndrome.

For those oedematous conditions where a prompt diuresis is required, Burinex Injection may be used, e.g. acute pulmonary oedema, acute and chronic renal failure, salicylate or barbiturate poisoning. Burinex Injection can be given intravenously or intramuscularly to those patients who are unable to take Burinex tablets or who fail to respond satisfactorily to oral therapy.

**Dosage and administration**
*Pulmonary oedema:* Initially 1–2 mg by intravenous injection. This can be repeated, if necessary, 20 minutes later.

In those conditions in which an infusion is appropriate, 2–5 mg may be given in 500 ml infusion fluid over 30–60 minutes. (See pharmaceutical precautions.)

When intramuscular administration is considered appropriate, a dose of 1 mg should be given initially and the dose then adjusted according to diuretic response.

*Children:* Not recommended for children under 12 years of age.

*Dosage in the elderly:* Adjust dosage according to response; a dose of 0.5 mg bumetanide per day may be sufficient in some elderly patients.

**Contra-indications, warnings, etc**
*Contra-indications:* Although Burinex can be used to induce diuresis in renal insufficiency, any marked increase in blood urea or the development of oliguria or anuria during treatment of severe progressing renal disease are indications for stopping treatment with Burinex.

Hypersensitivity to Burinex. Burinex is contra-indicated in hepatic coma and care should be taken in states of severe electrolyte depletion.

As with other diuretics, Burinex should not be administered concurrently with lithium salts. Diuretics can reduce lithium clearance resulting in high serum levels of lithium.

*Precautions:* Excessively rapid mobilisation of oedema particularly in elderly patients, may give rise to

sudden changes in cardiovascular pressure-flow relationships with circulatory collapse. This should be borne in mind when Burinex is given in high doses intravenously or orally. Electrolyte disturbances may occur, particularly in those patients taking a low-salt diet. Regular checks of serum electrolytes, in particular sodium, potassium, chloride and bicarbonate should be performed and replacement therapy instituted where indicated.

Like other diuretics, Burinex shows a tendency to increase the excretion of potassium which can lead to an increase in the sensitivity of the myocardium to the toxic effects of digitalis. Thus the dose may need adjustment when given in conjunction with cardiac glycosides.

Burinex may potentiate the effects of antihypertensive drugs. Therefore, the dose of the latter may need adjustment when Burinex is used to treat oedema in hypertensive patients.

As with other diuretics, Burinex may cause an increase in blood uric acid. Periodic checks on urine and blood glucose should be made in diabetics and patients suspected of latent diabetes.

Patients with chronic renal failure on high doses of Burinex should remain under constant hospital supervision.

*Pregnancy:* Although tests in four animal species have shown no teratogenic effects, the ordinary precaution of avoiding use of Burinex in the first trimester of pregnancy should at present be observed. Since it is not known whether bumetanide is distributed into breast milk, a nursing mother should either stop breast feeding or observe the infant for any adverse reactions if the drug is absolutely necessary for the mother.

*Adverse Reactions:* Reported reactions include skin rashes and muscular cramps in the legs, abdominal discomfort, thrombocytopenia and gynaecomastia. Bone marrow depression associated with the use of Burinex has been reported rarely, but it has not been proven definitely to be attributed to the drug. Hearing disturbance after administration of Burinex is rare and reversible. The possibility of hearing disturbance must be considered, particularly when Burinex is injected too quickly and in high doses.

*High Dose Therapy:* In patients with severe chronic renal failure given high doses of Burinex, there have been reports of severe, generalised, musculoskeletal pain sometimes associated with muscle spasm, occurring one to two hours after administration and lasting up to 12 hours. The lowest reported dose causing this type of adverse reaction was 5 mg by intravenous injection and the highest was 75 mg orally in a single dose. All patients recovered fully and there was no deterioration in their renal function.

The cause of this pain is uncertain but it may be a result of varying electrolyte gradients at the cell membrane level.

Experience suggests that the incidence of such reactions is reduced by initiating treatment at 5–10 mg daily and titrating upwards using a twice daily dosage regimen at doses of 20 mg per day or more.

*Overdosage:* Symptoms would be those caused by excessive diuresis. General measures should be taken to restore blood volume, maintain blood pressure and correct electrolyte disturbance.

**Pharmaceutical precautions** Burinex is presented in amber glass containers to protect against deterioration due to exposure to light.

When an intravenous infusion is required, Burinex Injection may be added to Dextrose Injection BP, Sodium Chloride Injection BP or Sodium Chloride and Dextrose Injection BP.

When 25 mg bumetanide (as Burinex Injection) was added to 1 litre of these infusion fluids, no evidence of precipitation was observed over a period of 72 hours. Higher concentrations of Burinex in these infusion fluids may cause precipitation. It is good practice to inspect all infusion fluids containing Burinex from time to time. Should cloudiness appear, the infusion should be discarded.

**Legal category** POM.

**Package quantities** Packs of 5×2 ml, 5×4 ml and 5×10 ml.

**Further information** Nil.

**Product licence number** 0043/0060

## BURINEX* LIQUID

**Presentation** An opalescent, pale green, viscous, aqueous solution for oral administration containing 1 mg bumetanide in 5 ml (0.2 mg per ml).

**Uses**
*Mode of action:* Burinex (bumetanide) is a potent high ceiling diuretic with a rapid onset and a short duration of action. After oral administration of 1 mg Burinex, diuresis begins within 30 minutes with a peak effect

between one and two hours. The diuretic effect is virtually complete in three hours after a 1 mg dose.

In most patients 1 mg of Burinex produces a similar diuretic effect to 40 mg frusemide.

Burinex is well absorbed after oral administration. Burinex excretion in the urine shows good correlation with the diuretic response. In patients with chronic renal failure the liver takes more importance as an excretory pathway although the duration of action in such patients is not markedly prolonged.

*Indications:* Burinex is indicated whenever diuretic therapy is required in the treatment of oedema, e.g. that associated with congestive heart failure, cirrhosis of the liver and renal disease including the nephrotic syndrome.

Burinex liquid may be more appropriate in patients who have difficulty swallowing tablets.

**Dosage and administration** Usually 1 mg (5 ml) as a single oral dose given morning or early evening. The dosage should be adjusted according to the patient's response.

*Children:* Not recommended for children under 12 years of age.

*Dosage in the elderly:* Adjust dosage according to response; a dose of 0.5 mg bumetanide per day may be sufficient in some elderly patients.

**Contra-indications, warnings, etc**
*Contra-indications:* Although Burinex can be used to induce diuresis in renal insufficiency, any marked increase in blood urea or the development of oliguria or anuria during treatment of severe progressing renal disease are indications for stopping treatment with Burinex.

Burinex is contra-indicated in hepatic coma and care should be taken in states of severe electrolyte depletion.

As with other diuretics, Burinex should not be administered concurrently with lithium salts. Diuretics can reduce lithium clearance resulting in high serum levels of lithium.

*Precautions:* Excessively rapid mobilisation of oedema particularly in elderly patients may give rise to sudden changes in cardiovascular pressure flow relationships with circulatory collapse. This should be borne in mind when Burinex is given in high doses intravenously or orally. Electrolyte disturbances may occur, particularly in those patients taking a low salt diet. Regular checks of serum electrolytes, in particular sodium, potassium, chloride and bicarbonate should be performed and replacement therapy instituted where indicated.

Like other diuretics, Burinex shows a tendency to increase the excretion of potassium which can lead to an increase in the sensitivity of the myocardium to the toxic effects of digitalis. Thus the dose may need adjustment when given in conjunction with cardiac glycosides.

Burinex may potentiate the effects of antihypertensive drugs. Therefore, the dose of the latter may need adjustment when Burinex is used to treat oedema in hypertensive patients.

As with other diuretics, Burinex may cause an increase in blood uric acid. Periodic checks on urine and blood glucose should be made in diabetics and patients suspected of latent diabetes.

Patients with chronic renal failure on high doses of Burinex should remain under constant hospital supervision.

*Pregnancy:* Although tests in four animal species have shown no teratogenic effects, the ordinary precaution of avoiding use of Burinex in the first trimester of pregnancy should at present be observed.

*Adverse reactions:* Reported reactions include skin rashes and muscular cramps in the legs, abdominal discomfort, thrombocytopenia, and gynaecomastia.

*High dose therapy:* In patients with severe chronic renal failure given high doses of Burinex, there have been reports of severe, generalised, musculoskeletal pain sometimes associated with muscle spasm, occurring one or two hours after administration and lasting up to 12 hours. The lowest reported dose causing this type of adverse reaction was 5 mg by intravenous injection and the highest was 75 mg orally in a single dose. All patients recovered fully and there was no deterioration in their renal function.

The cause of this pain is uncertain but it may be a result of varying electrolyte gradients at the cell membrane level.

Experience suggests that the incidence of such reactions is reduced by initiating treatment at 5–10 mg daily and titrating upwards using a twice daily dosage regimen at doses of 20 mg per day or more.

*Overdosage:* Symptoms would be those caused by excessive diuresis. Empty stomach by gastric lavage or emesis. General measures should be taken to restore blood volume, maintain blood pressure and correct electrolyte disturbance.

**Pharmaceutical precautions** Burinex is presented in amber glass containers to protect against deterioration due to exposure to light. Do not refrigerate.

**Legal category** POM.

**Package quantities** Bottles of 150 ml (OP). A measure-spoon graduated at 2.5 ml and 5 ml is supplied.

**Further information** Nil.

**Product licence number** 0043/0075

## BURINEX* A TABLETS

**Presentation** Cream, oval tablets, flat with bevelled edge, engraved with a number (149) on the scored face and with an Assyrian lion on the reverse. Each tablet contains 1 mg bumetanide and 5 mg amiloride hydrochloride.

**Uses**
*Mode of action:* Burinex A combines the potent loop diuretic bumetanide with the mild potassium sparing diuretic amiloride.

The action of bumetanide starts within 30 minutes and is virtually complete within 3 hours. The addition of amiloride will reduce any tendency towards hypokalaemia and its mild natriuretic effect will be additive to that of bumetanide.

*Indications:* Burinex A is indicated where a prompt diuresis is required. It is particularly of value in conditions where potassium conservation is important.

**Dosage and administration** The normal adult dose is 1 to 2 tablets daily. The dose may be adjusted according to response.

*The elderly:* The dose should be adjusted according to needs and serum electrolytes and urea should be monitored carefully.

*Children:* Not recommended for use in children.

**Contra-indications, warnings, etc**
*Contra-indications:* Hyperkalaemia (serum potassium >5.3 mmol/litre), severe electrolyte imbalance, acute renal insufficiency, severe progressive renal disease, anuria, severe liver disease, adrenocortical insufficiency (Addison's Disease), precomatose states associated with cirrhosis, known sensitivity to bumetanide or amiloride. Burinex A should not be given concurrently with potassium supplements or potassium-sparing agents. Burinex A is contraindicated in children as safety in this age group has not been established.

Hypersensitivity to Burinex. Burinex is contra-indicated in hepatic coma and care should be taken in states of severe electrolyte depletion.

*Warnings:* Serum uric acid levels may be increased and acute attacks of gout may be precipitated. Patients with prostatic hypertrophy or impaired micturition may be at risk of developing acute retention. Burinex A should be discontinued before a glucose tolerance test. Burinex A may cause latent diabetes to become manifest. It may be necessary to increase the dose of hypoglycaemic agents in diabetic patients.

*Precautions:* Patients who are being treated with this preparation require regular supervision with monitoring of fluid and electrolyte status to avoid excessive fluid loss.

In common with other potent diuretics, Burinex A should be used with caution in elderly patients or those with disorders rendering electrolyte balance precarious. Hyponatraemia, hypochloraemia and raised blood urea may occur during vigorous diuresis especially in seriously ill patients. Careful monitoring of serum electrolytes and urea should be undertaken in these patients.

*Side-effects:* Bumetanide and amiloride are generally well tolerated. Side effects which may occur include: Abdominal pain, nausea and vomiting, dyspepsia, diarrhoea, stomach and muscle cramps, arthralgia, dizziness, fatigue, hypotension, headache, encephalopathy (in patients with pre-existing hepatic disease), fluid and electrolyte depletion, dehydration, hyperuricaemia, increased blood urea and serum creatinine, hyperglycaemia, abnormalities of serum levels of hepatic enzymes, skin rashes, pruritis, urticaria, thrombocytopenia, gynaecomastia and painful breasts. Bone marrow depression associated with the use of Burinex has been reported rarely but it has not been proven definitely to be attributed to the drug.

*Use during pregnancy and lactation:* The safety of the use of Burinex A during pregnancy has not been established. Since it is not known whether bumetanide or amiloride are distributed into breast milk, a nursing mother should either stop breast feeding or stop taking Burinex A. The decision depends on the importance of the drug to the mother.

*Drug interactions:* Hyperkalaemia has been observed in patients receiving amiloride and therefore concurrent use of Burinex A with potassium conserving diuretics is not recommended.

In common with other diuretics serum lithium levels may be increased when lithium is given concurrently with Burinex A necessitating adjustment of the lithium dosage. As ACE inhibitors may elevate serum potassium levels, especially in the presence of renal impairment, combination with Burinex A is best avoided in elderly patients or in those in whom renal function may be compromised. If use of the combination is considered essential the clinical condition and serum electrolytes must be carefully and continuously monitored.

Burinex A may enhance the nephrotoxicity of cephalosporin and aminoglycoside antibiotics. The dose of cardiac glycosides or hypotensive agents may require adjustment.

*Overdosage:* Symptoms would be those caused by excessive diuresis such as dehydration, electrolyte imbalance, particularly hyperkalaemia, and hypotension and treatment should be aimed at reversing these. No specific antidote is available. Treatment is symptomatic and supportive. If hyperkalaemia is present appropriate measures must be instituted to reduce serum potassium.

**Pharmaceutical precautions** Nil.

**Legal category** POM.

**Package quantities** Calendar pack of 2×14 tablets (OP).

**Further information** Nil.

**Product licence number** 0043/0161.

## BURINEX* K TABLETS

**Qualitative and quantitative composition** Each tablet contains Bumetanide BP 0.5 mg and Potassium Chloride PhEur 573 mg.

**Pharmaceutical form** Tablet.

**Clinical particulars**
*Therapeutic indications:* For the treatment of oedema where potassium supplementation is necessary.

*Posology and method of administration:* For oral administration.

*Adults:* The recommended initial dose is 2 tablets to be taken once daily (morning or evening). This may be increased up to 4 tablets daily (given as a single dose or in divided doses if preferred), or reduced to 1 tablet daily according to clinical response. If more than 4 tablets are to be taken daily, it is preferred to administer the diuretic and potassium supplement as two separate preparations.

*Elderly:* Adjust dosage according to response. A dose of 1 tablet per day may be sufficient in some elderly patients.

Burinex K tablets must be swallowed whole and never chewed. The tablets should be swallowed whole with at least 100 ml of water.

*Children:* Not recommended in children under 12 years.

*Contra-indications:* The product should not be used with potassium-sparing diuretics (e.g. spironolactone, triamterene or amiloride) or in patients with renal insufficiency.

As with other diuretics, Burinex K should not be administered concurrently with lithium salts. Diuretics can reduce lithium clearance resulting in high serum levels of lithium.

All solid forms of potassium medication are contra-indicated in the presence of obstruction in the digestive tract (e.g. resulting from compression of the oesophagus due to dilation of the left atrium or from stenosis of the gut).

Anuria, Crohns Disease, hyperkalaemia, precomatose states associated with liver cirrhosis, Addison's Disease, known hypersensitivity to bumetanide or Burinex.

*Special warnings and special precautions for use:* The 15.4 mmol of potassium included in the usual dose of Burinex K (2 tablets daily) should help to prevent hypokalaemia in many patients. Certain patients, however, as for example those with hepatic ascites or those on a very low potassium diet, may require considerably more potassium than this. Periodic checks should, therefore, be made on the serum potassium level in patients on long-term therapy.

The diuretic in Burinex K may potentiate the effect of antihypertensive drugs, increase blood uric acid and (though rarely) affect carbohydrate metabolism. Certain non-steroidal anti-inflammatory drugs have been shown to antagonise the action of diuretics.

Non-specific small bowel lesions characterised by stenosis and possibly accompanied by ulceration have been associated with the oral administration of tablets and capsules containing potassium salts. Symptoms and signs which indicate ulceration or obstruction of the small bowel in patients taking tablets or capsules containing potassium salts are indications for stopping treatment with such preparations immediately.

Patients with prostatic hypertrophy or impairment of micturition have an increased risk of developing acute retention. Where indicated, steps should be taken to correct hypotension or hyperkalaemia before commencing therapy. ACE inhibitors should not be used with combination diuretic potassium products, such as Burinex K, as serum potassium levels may be increased. The toxic effects of nephrotoxic antibiotics may be increased by concomitant administration of potent diuretics such as bumetanide.

*Interactions with other medicaments and other forms of interaction:* See Special warnings and special precautions for use above.

*Pregnancy and lactation:* Although tests in four animal species have shown no teratogenic effects, the ordinary precaution of avoiding use of Burinex in the first trimester of pregnancy should at present be observed.

Since it is not known whether bumetanide is distributed into breast milk, a nursing mother should either stop breast feeding or observe the infant for any adverse effects if the drug is absolutely necessary for the mother.

*Effects on ability to drive and use machines:* None known.

*Undesirable effects:* Reported reactions include skin rashes and muscular cramps in the legs, abdominal discomfort, thrombocytopenia and gynaecomastia. As with other diuretics, fluid and electrolyte balance may be disturbed as a result of diuresis after prolonged therapy. This may cause symptoms such as headache, hypotension and myalgia.

Bone marrow depression associated with the use of Burinex has been reported rarely but it has not been proven definitely to be attributed to the drug. Hearing disturbance after administration of Burinex is rare and reversible.

*Overdosage:* General measures should be taken to restore blood volume and maintain blood pressure. Any electrolyte imbalance should be corrected.

### Pharmacological properties

*Pharmacodynamic properties:* Burinex K combines the very potent high-ceiling diuretic bumetanide with a slow-release potassium chloride supplement. Bumetanide has a rapid onset and a short duration of action. As with most diuretics, long-term therapy may be associated with potassium depletion.

*Pharmacokinetic properties:* The potassium supplement in Burinex K will help to maintain normal levels of potassium, especially in those patients whose dietary intake of potassium is inadequate.

The formulation of Burinex K presents the following advantages. The diuretic is coated around the tablet from which it is rapidly released. The diuretic and saluretic effects begin within 30 minutes after oral administration, peak at one to two hours, and are largely complete within three hours. In contrast, the potassium chloride, which is included in an inert wax core, is released only slowly over a period of six hours after oral ingestion. This slow-release minimises the risk of gastro-intestinal intolerance as well as that of ulceration and stenosis resulting from localised high concentrations of potassium salts in the small bowel.

*Preclinical safety data:* There are no pre-clinical data of relevance to the prescriber which are additional to that already included in other sections of the SPC.

### Pharmaceutical particulars

*List of excipients:* Ethyl cellulose, ferric oxide brown, glycerol, magnesium stearate, stearyl alcohol, hydroxypropylmethylcellulose, polyvidone K25, sucrose, talc, titanium dioxide.

*Incompatibilities:* None known.

*Shelf life:* 3 years.

*Special precautions for storage:* None.

*Nature and contents of container:* Blister packs of 28.

*Instructions for use/handling:* None.

**Marketing authorisation number** 0043/0027R.

**Date of approval/revision of SPC** December 1996.

**Legal category** POM.

## DOVONEX* CREAM

**Presentation** Dovonex Cream contains 50 micrograms calcipotriol per g (as the hydrate) in a smooth, soft, white cream base.

Other ingredients: cetomacrogol 1000, cetostearyl alcohol, chloroallylhexaminium chloride, disodium edetate, disodium phosphate dihydrate, glycerol 85%, liquid paraffin, purified water, white soft paraffin.

### Uses

*Mode of action:* Calcipotriol is a vitamin D derivative. *In vitro* data suggest that calcipotriol induces differentiation and suppresses proliferation of keratino-

cytes. This is the proposed basis for its effect in psoriasis.

*Indications:* Dovonex Cream is indicated for the topical treatment of mild to moderate plaque psoriasis (psoriasis vulgaris) affecting up to 40% of skin area.

### Dosage and administration

*Adults:* Dovonex Cream should be applied to the affected area twice daily. Maximum weekly dose should not exceed 100 g.

*Children over 12 years:* Dovonex Cream should be applied to the affected area twice daily. Maximum weekly dose should not exceed 75 g.

*Children aged 6 to 12 years:* Dovonex Cream should be applied to the affected area twice daily. Maximum weekly dose should not exceed 50 g.

*Children under 6 years:* There is limited experience of the use of Dovonex in this age group. A maximum safe dose has not been established.

These dose recommendations are based on extensive experience in adults. In respect of children, clinical experience in children has shown Dovonex to be safe and effective over eight weeks at a mean dose of 15 g per week but with wide variability in dose among patients. Individual dose requirement depends on the extent of psoriasis but should not exceed the above recommendations.

### Contra-indications, warnings, etc

*Contra-indications:* Dovonex Cream is contraindicated in patients with known disorders of calcium metabolism. As with other topical preparations, Dovonex Cream is contraindicated in patients with hypersensitivity to any of the ingredients.

*Precautions:* Dovonex Cream should not be used on the face. Patients should be advised to wash their hands after applying the cream and to avoid inadvertent transfer to other body areas, especially the face. Care should be exercised in patients with other types of psoriasis, since hypercalcaemia, which rapidly reversed on cessation of treatment, has been reported in patients with generalised pustular or erythrodermic exfoliative psoriasis.

*Side-effects:* The most common side-effect is transient local irritation which seldom requires discontinuation of treatment. Other local reactions may occur including dermatitis, pruritus, erythema, aggravation of psoriasis, photosensitivity. Facial or perioral dermatitis may occur rarely.

*Use during pregnancy and lactation:* Safety for use during human pregnancy has not yet been established, although studies in experimental animals have not shown teratogenic effects. Avoid use in pregnancy unless there is no safer alternative. It is not known whether calcipotriol is excreted in breast milk.

*Drug interactions:* There is no interaction between calcipotriol and sunlight or UV light. There is no experience of concomitant therapy with other antipsoriatic products applied to the same skin area.

*Overdose:* Hypercalcaemia should not occur at the recommended dose of Dovonex Cream. Excessive use may cause elevated serum calcium which rapidly subsides when the treatment is discontinued.

**Pharmaceutical precautions** Store below 25°C.

**Legal category** POM.

**Package quantities** Tubes of 30 g (OP), 60 g (OP) and 120 g (OP).

**Further information** Nil.

**Product licence number** 0043/0188.

## DOVONEX* OINTMENT

### Qualitative and quantitative composition
Calcipotriol 50 micrograms/g.

**Pharmaceutical form** Ointment.

### Clinical particulars
*Therapeutic indications:* Dovonex Ointment is indicated for the topical treatment of mild to moderate plaque psoriasis (psoriasis vulgaris) affecting up to 40% of skin area.

*Posology and method of administration:*
*Adults:* Dovonex Ointment should be applied to the affected area once or twice daily. For maximum benefit use the ointment twice daily. Maximum weekly dose should not exceed 100 g.

*Children over 12 years:* Dovonex Ointment should be applied to the affected area twice daily. Maximum weekly dose should not exceed 75 g.

*Children aged 6 to 12 years:* Dovonex Ointment should be applied to the affected area twice daily. Maximum weekly dose should not exceed 50 g.

*Children under 6 years:* There is limited experience of the use of Dovonex Ointment in this age group. A maximum safe dose has not been established.

These dose recommendations are based on exten-

sive experience in adults. In respect of children, clinical experience in children has shown Dovonex to be safe and effective over eight weeks at a mean dose of 15 g per week but with wide variability in dose among patients. Individual dose requirement depends on the extent of psoriasis but should not exceed the above recommendations.

*Contra-indications:* Dovonex Ointment is contraindicated in patients with known disorders of calcium metabolism. As with other topical preparations, Dovonex Ointment is contra-indicated in patients with hypersensitivity to any of its constituents.

*Special warnings and special precautions for use:* Dovonex Ointment should not be used on the face. Patients should be advised to wash their hands after applying the ointment and to avoid inadvertent transfer to other body areas, especially the face. Patients should be advised to use no more than the recommended dose (see section on *Posology and method of administration*) since hypercalcaemia, which rapidly reverses on cessation of treatment, may occur.

*Interaction with other medicaments and other forms of interaction:* There is no interaction between calcipotriol and sunlight or UV light. There is no experience of concomitant therapy with other antipsoriatic products applied to the same skin area.

*Pregnancy and lactation:* Safety for use during human pregnancy has not yet been established, although studies in experimental animals have not shown teratogenic effects. Avoid use in pregnancy unless there is no safer alternative. It is not known whether calcipotriol is excreted in breast milk.

*Effects on ability to drive and use machines:* Not applicable.

*Undesirable effects:* The most common side-effect is transient local irritation which seldom requires discontinuation of treatment. Other local reactions may occur including dermatitis, pruritus, erythema, aggravation of psoriasis, photosensitivity. Facial or perioral dermatitis may occur rarely.

*Overdose:* Hypercalcaemia may occur in patients with plaque psoriasis who use more than the recommended dose of Dovonex Ointment weekly and has been reported at lower doses in patients with generalised pustular or erythrodermic exfoliative psoriasis.

### Pharmacological properties
*Pharmacodynamic properties:* Calcipotriol is a vitamin D derivative. *In vitro* data suggest that calcipotriol induces differentiation and suppresses proliferation of keratinocytes. This is the proposed basis for its effect in psoriasis.

*Pharmacokinetic properties:* Data from a single study containing 5 evaluable patients with psoriasis treated with 0.3–1.7 g of a 50 micrograms/g tritium labelled calcipotriol ointment suggested that less than 1% of the dose was absorbed.

However, total recovery of the tritium label over a 96 hour period ranged from 6.7 to only 32.6%, figures maximised by uncorrected chemiluminescence. There were no data on $^3$H tissue distribution or excretion from the lungs.

*Preclinical safety data:* The effect on calcium metabolism is approximately 100 times less than that of the hormonally active form of vitamin $D_3$.

### Pharmaceutical particulars
*List of excipients:* Disodium edetate, disodium phosphate dihydrate, DL-α-tocopherol, liquid paraffin, polyoxyethylene-(2)-stearyl ether, propylene glycol, purified water and white soft paraffin.

*Incompatibilities:* Not applicable.

*Shelf life:* 2 years.

*Special precautions for storage:* Store below 25°C.

*Nature and contents of container:* Lacquered aluminium tube with polypropylene screw cap. Pack sizes: 30, 60, 120 g.

*Instructions for use/handling:* None.

**Marketing authorisation number** 0043/0177.

**Date of approval/revision of SPC** June 1997.

**Legal category** POM.

## DOVONEX* SCALP SOLUTION

### Qualitative and quantitative composition
Calcipotriol 50 micrograms per ml (as the hydrate).

**Pharmaceutical form** Solution.

### Clinical particulars
*Therapeutic indications:* Dovonex Scalp Solution is indicated for the topical treatment of scalp psoriasis.
*Posology and method of administration:*
*Adults:* Dovonex Scalp Solution should be applied twice daily (morning and evening) to the affected areas. Maximum weekly dose should not exceed 60 ml.

When used together with Dovonex Cream or Ointment, the total dose of calcipotriol should not exceed 5 mg in any week, e.g. 60 ml of Scalp Solution plus one 30 g tube of Cream or Ointment, or 30 ml of Scalp

Solution plus 60 g (two 30 g tubes) of Cream or Ointment.

*Children:* Not recommended as there is no experience of the use of Dovonex Scalp Solution in children.

*Contra-indications:* Dovonex Scalp Solution is contra-indicated in patients with known disorders of calcium metabolism. As with other topical preparations, Dovonex Scalp Solution is contra-indicated in patients with hypersensitivity to any of its constituents.

*Special warnings and special precautions for use:* Application of Dovonex to the face may cause local irritation. Dovonex Scalp Solution should not therefore be applied directly to the face. Patients should be advised to wash their hands after applying the scalp solution and to avoid inadvertent transfer to the face. Patients should be advised to use no more than the maximum weekly dose since hypercalcaemia, which rapidly reverses on cessation of treatment, may occur.

*Interaction with other medicaments and other forms of interaction:* There is no interaction between calcipotriol and UV light. There is no experience of concomitant therapy with other antipsoriatic products applied to the same area.

*Pregnancy and lactation:* Safety for use during human pregnancy has not yet been established, although studies in experimental animals have not shown teratogenic effects. Avoid use in pregnancy unless there is no safer alternative. It is not known whether calcipotriol is excreted in breast milk.

*Effects on ability to drive and use machines:* Not applicable.

*Undesirable effects:* The most common side-effect is local irritation on the scalp or face. Facial or perioral dermatitis may occur. Other local reactions may occur. Reactions which have been reported with Dovonex Ointment include dermatitis, pruritus, erythema, aggravation of psoriasis, photosensitivity, and rarely hypercalcaemia or hypercalciuria.

*Overdose:* Hypercalcaemia may occur in patients with plaque psoriasis who use more than 100 g of Dovonex Ointment weekly and has been reported at lower doses in patients with generalised pustular or erythrodermic exfoliative psoriasis.

**Pharmacological properties**
*Pharmacodynamic properties:* Calcipotriol is a vitamin D derivative. *In vitro* data suggest that calcipotriol induces differentiation and suppresses proliferation of keratinocytes. This effect is the proposed basis for its effect in psoriasis.

*Pharmacokinetic properties:* Not applicable.

*Preclinical safety data:* The effect on the calcium metabolism is approximately 100 times less than that of the hormonally active form of vitamin $D_3$.

**Pharmaceutical particulars**
*List of excipients:* Hydroxypropyl cellulose, isopropanol, levomenthol, sodium citrate, propylene glycol, purified water.

*Incompatibilities:* None known.

*Shelf life:* 2 years.

*Special precautions for storage:* Store below 25°C. The alcohol base is flammable.

*Nature and contents of container:* 60 ml polyethylene bottle with nozzle.

*Instructions for use/handling:* None.

**Marketing authorisation number** 0043/0190.

**Date of approval/revision of SPC** February 1996.

**Legal category** POM.

## FUCIDIN* TABLETS FUCIDIN* SUSPENSION

**Presentation**
*Fucidin Tablets:* White, oval film coated tablet with an Assyrian lion on one side and the number 121 on the other. Each tablet contains 250 mg Sodium Fusidate BP (equivalent to 240 mg fusidic acid). Sodium fusidate is the sodium salt of fusidic acid.

*Fucidin Suspension:* Each 5 ml of white to off-white, banana-flavoured aqueous suspension contains 250 mg Fusidic Acid BP.

**Uses**
*Mode of action:* Fusidic acid and its salts are potent anti-staphylococcal agents with unusual ability to penetrate tissue. Bactericidal levels have been assayed in bone and necrotic tissue. Blood levels are cumulative, reaching concentrations of 20–35 micrograms/ml after oral administration of 250 mg twice daily for seven days and 50–100 microgram/ml after oral administration of 1.5 g daily for three to four days. Concentrations of 0.03–0.12 micrograms/ml inhibit nearly all strains of *Staphylococcus aureus.* Fusidic acid is active against *Staphylococcus epidermidis* and methicillin resistant staphylococci.

Fucidin is excreted mainly in the bile, little or none being excreted in the urine.

In severe or deep-seated infections and when prolonged therapy may be required, systemic Fucidin should generally be given concurrently with other anti-staphylococcal antibiotic therapy.

*Indications:* Fucidin is indicated in the treatment of all staphylococcal infections due to susceptible organisms, such as: cutaneous infections; osteomyelitis; pneumonia; septicaemia; wound infections; endocarditis; superinfected cystic fibrosis.

Fucidin should be administered intravenously whenever oral therapy is inappropriate, which includes cases where absorption from the gastro-intestinal tract is unpredictable.

**Dosage and administration**
*Fucidin Tablets:* For staphylococcal cutaneous infections:
*Adult:* standard dose: 250 mg (one tablet) sodium fusidate (equivalent to 240 mg fusidic acid) twice daily for 5–10 days.

For staphylococcal infections such as osteomyelitis; pneumonia; septicaemia; wound infections; endocarditis; superinfected cystic fibrosis:
*Adult:* standard dose: 500 mg (two tablets) sodium fusidate (equivalent to 480 mg fusidic acid/three times daily.

In severe cases of fulminating infections, the dosage may be doubled or appropriate combined therapy may be used.

*Fucidin Suspension:* For all staphylococcal infections. Each 5 ml of Fucidin Suspension is therapeutically equivalent to 175 mg of sodium fusidate owing to its lower oral bioavailability. Therefore the following dosages are recommended:

*Adult dose:* 15 ml three times daily.

*Children:* 0–1 year: 1 ml/kg bodyweight daily, divided into 3 equal doses.
1–5 years: 5 ml three times daily.
5–12 years: 10 ml three times daily.

Since Fucidin is excreted in the bile, no dosage modifications are needed in renal impairment.

The dosage in patients undergoing haemodialysis needs no adjustment as Fucidin is not significantly dialysed.

*Dosage in the elderly:* No dosage alterations are necessary in the elderly.

**Contra-indications, warnings, etc**
*Contra-indications:* Contra-indicated in patients with known hypersensitivity to fusidic acid and its salts.

*Precautions:* Caution should be exercised with other antibiotics which have similar biliary excretion pathways, e.g. lincomycin and rifampicin. Periodic liver function tests should be carried out when high oral doses are used, when the drug is given for prolonged periods and in patients with liver dysfunction.

Fucidin displaces bilirubin from its albumin binding site *in vitro.* The clinical significance of this finding is uncertain and kernicterus has not been observed in neonates receiving Fucidin. However, this observation should be borne in mind when the drug is given to pre-term, jaundiced, acidotic or seriously ill neonates.

*Pregnancy and lactation:* There is inadequate evidence of safety in human pregnancy. Animal studies and many years of clinical experience suggest that fusidic acid is devoid of teratogenic effects. There is evidence to suggest that when given systemically fusidic acid can cross the placental barrier. If the administration of Fucidin to pregnant patients is considered essential, its use requires that the potential benefits be weighed against the possible hazards to the foetus.

Safety in nursing mothers has not been established. When fusidic acid (as the sodium salt) has been given systemically, levels have been detected in the breast milk. Caution is, therefore, required when Fucidin is used in mothers who wish to breast feed.

*Adverse reactions:* In some patients given Fucidin, particularly the young and elderly, a reversible jaundice has been reported. Jaundice has been seen most frequently in patients receiving intravenous Fucidin in high dosage, or where the drug has been infused too rapidly or at too high a concentration in the infusion fluid. In some instances instituting oral therapy may be beneficial.

If the jaundice persists Fucidin should be withdrawn, following which the serum bilirubin will invariably return to normal.

Reported reactions are gastro-intestinal upsets and, rarely, skin rashes.

*Overdosage:* There has been no experience of overdosage with Fucidin. Treatment should be restricted to symptomatic and supportive measures. Dialysis is of no benefit, since the drug is not significantly dialysed.

**Pharmaceutical precautions**
*Fucidin Tablets:* Nil.

*Fucidin Suspension:* Protect from direct sunlight and heat. The Suspension should be shaken before use and dilution is not recommended.

**Legal category** POM.

**Package quantities** *Tablets:* Bottles of 100.
*Suspension:* Bottles of 50 ml (OP).

**Further information** Both oral and intravenous Fucidin have been given concurrently with other antibiotics, e.g. cloxacillin, flucloxacillin, ampicillin, methicillin and erythromycin.

Fusidic acid and its salts exhibit no cross hypersensitivity or cross resistance with other antibiotics in clinical use.

Despite many years of clinical use, resistance to fusidic acid amongst *Staphylococcus aureus* remains low.

**Product licence numbers**
Tablets 0043/5000R
Suspension 0043/5014R

## FUCIDIN* FOR INTRAVENOUS INFUSION

**Presentation** A pack of 2 vials. One vial contains Sodium Fusidate BP, 500 mg (equivalent to 480 mg fusidic acid) as a dry powder. The second vial of 10 ml sterile phosphate-citrate buffer solution (pH 7.4–7.6), contains disodium hydrogen phosphate, citric acid, disodium edetate and water for injections. When reconstituted contains 3.1 mMol sodium and 1.1 mMol phosphate.

**Uses**
*Mode of action:* Fusidic acid and its salts are potent anti-staphylococcal agents with unusual ability to penetrate tissue. Bactericidal levels have been assayed in bone and necrotic tissue. Concentrations of 0.03–1.12 micrograms/ml inhibit nearly all strains of *Staphylococcus aureus.* Fusidic acid is active against *Staphylococcus epidermidis* and methicillin-resistant staphylococci.

In severe or deep-seated infections and when prolonged therapy may be required, systemic Fucidin should generally be given concurrently with other anti-staphylococcal antibiotic therapy.

*Pharmacokinetics:* 500 mg of sodium fusidate given as a single infusion over 2 hours results in a Cmax of 52 micrograms/ml. Blood levels are cumulative, reaching concentrations of 60–120 micrograms/ml after repeated infusion of 500 mg sodium fusidate every 8 hours for 2–3 days.

The plasma half-life is approximately 10–15 hours.

Fucidin is excreted mainly in the bile, little or none being excreted in the urine.

*Indications:* Fucidin is indicated in the treatment of all staphylococcal infections due to susceptible organisms such as: osteomyelitis, pneumonia, septicaemia, wound infections, endocarditis, superinfected cystic fibrosis, cutaneous infections.

Fucidin should be administered intravenously whenever oral therapy is inappropriate, which includes cases where absorption from the gastro-intestinal tract is unpredictable.

**Dosage and administration**
*Adults weighing more than 50 kg:* 500 mg sodium fusidate three times daily.

*Children and adults weighing less than 50 kg:* 6–7 mg sodium fusidate per kg bodyweight three times daily.

*Recommended procedure:* To reconstitute, dissolve the contents of one vial containing 500 mg sodium fusidate powder (equivalent to 480 mg of fusidic acid) in the 10 ml buffer provided.

*For adults weighing more than 50 kg:* Add the 10 ml fusidate/buffer solution to 500 ml of infusion fluid.

*For children and adults weighing less than 50 kg:* Add the 10 ml fusidate/buffer solution to 500 ml of infusion fluid. Each dose corresponds to 6–7 ml of the resulting solution per kg bodyweight.

The diluted fluid should be infused via a central venous line over 2 hours. If a superficial vein is employed a more prolonged period of at least 6 hours is advisable.

Since Fucidin is excreted in the bile, no dosage modifications are needed in renal impairment.

The dosage in patients undergoing haemodialysis needs no adjustment as Fucidin is not significantly dialysed.

*Dosage in the elderly:* No dosage alterations are necessary in the elderly.

If additional antibacterial therapy is to be employed, it is recommended that for parenteral administration, separate infusion fluids be used.

**Contra-indications, warnings, etc**
*Contra-indications:* Contraindicated in patients with known hypersensitivity to fusidic acid and its salts. Intravenous Fucidin should not be infused with amino acid solutions or in whole blood. Due to local tissue

injury, Fucidin should not be administered intramuscularly or subcutaneously.

*Precautions:* Caution should be exercised with other antibiotics which have similar biliary excretion pathways, e.g. lincomycin and rifampicin. Periodic liver function tests should be carried out when high oral doses are used, when the drug is given for prolonged periods and in patients with liver dysfunction.

Fucidin displaces bilirubin from its albumin binding site in vitro. The clinical significance of this finding is uncertain and kernicterus has not been observed in neonates receiving Fucidin. However, this observation should be borne in mind when the drug is given to pre-term, jaundiced, acidotic or seriously ill neonates.

*Pregnancy and lactation:* There is inadequate evidence of safety in human pregnancy. Animal studies and many years of clinical experience suggest that fusidic acid is devoid of teratogenic effects. There is evidence to suggest that when given systemically, fusidic acid can cross the placental barrier. If the administration of Fucidin to pregnant patients is considered essential, it requires that the potential benefits be weighed against the possible hazards to the foetus.

Safety in nursing mothers has not been established. When fusidic acid (as the sodium salt) has been given systemically, levels have been detected in the breast milk. Caution is, therefore, required when Fucidin is used in mothers who wish to breast feed.

*Adverse reactions:* In some patients given Fucidin, particularly the young and elderly, a reversible jaundice has been reported. Jaundice has been seen most frequently in patients receiving intravenous Fucidin in high dosage, or where the drug has been infused too rapidly or at too high a concentration in the infusion fluid. In some instances, instituting oral therapy may be beneficial. If the jaundice persists, Fucidin should be withdrawn, following which the serum bilirubin will invariably return to normal. Reported reactions are thrombophlebitis and, rarely, skin rashes.

*Overdosage:* There has been no experience of overdosage with Fucidin. Treatment should be restricted to symptomatic and supportive measures. Dialysis is of no benefit since the drug is not significantly dialysed.

**Pharmaceutical precautions** Fucidin dry powder is stable for 3 years when stored at room temperature (below 25˚C) and protected from light. When the buffer solution is transferred to the powder vial, this vial should be regarded as a unit dose. The required amount of Fucidin/buffer solution should be used once only and any unused portion discarded.

In vitro compatibility studies of Fucidin for Intravenous Infusion with commonly used infusion solutions have been carried out.

The results showed that sodium fusidate reconstituted at 50 mg/ml in buffer solution is physically and chemically compatible for at least 24 hours at room temperature with the following infusion solutions (the figure in parenthesis shows the concentration of sodium fusidate in the final admixture):

Sodium Chloride Intravenous Infusion BP 0.9% (1–2 mg/ml)

Dextrose Intravenous Infusion BP 5% (1–2 mg/ml)

Compound Sodium Lactate Intravenous Infusion ("Ringer-Lactate Solution") (1 mg/ml)

Sodium Lactate Intravenous Infusion BP (1 mg/ml)

Sodium Chloride (0.18%) and Dextrose (4%) Intravenous Infusion BP (1 mg/ml)

Potassium Chloride (0.3%) and Dextrose (5%) Intravenous Infusion BP (1 mg/ml)

Sodium Fusidate reconstituted at 50 mg/ml in buffer solution is physically incompatible with infusion fluids containing 20% or more of dextrose, lipid infusions and peritoneal dialysis fluids. Precipitation may occur in dilutions which result in a pH of less than 7.4.

**Legal category** POM.

**Package quantities** Pack containing a single pair of vials.

**Further information** Fucidin should be administered intravenously into a wide bore vein with a good blood flow. Excessive doses may cause venospasm and haemolysis of erthrocytes. Both oral and intravenous Fucidin have been given concurrently with other antibiotics, e.g. cloxacillin, flucloxacillin, ampicillin, methicillin and erythromycin.

Fusidic acid and its salts exhibit no cross hypersensitivity or cross resistance with other antibiotics in clinical use.

Despite many years of clinical use, resistance to fusidic acid amongst *Staphylococcus aureus* remains low.

**Product licence number** 0043/0184.

## FUCIDIN* CREAM
## FUCIDIN* OINTMENT
## FUCIDIN* GEL
## FUCIDIN* INTERTULLE

**Presentation** *Fucidin Cream* contains Fusidic Acid BP 2% in a cream base. Other ingredients: potassium sorbate 0.27% as preservative, butylated hydroxyanisole, cetyl alcohol, glycerol, liquid paraffin, polysorbate 60, purified water and white soft paraffin.

*Fucidin Ointment* contains Fusidic Acid, as the sodium salt, BP 2% in an ointment base (no preservative). Other ingredients: cetyl alcohol, lanolin, liquid paraffin and white soft paraffin.

*Fucidin Gel* contains Fusidic Acid BP 2% in a water-miscible base. Other ingredients: methyl paraben 0.27% and propyl paraben 0.03% as preservatives, carbomer, dimeticone, polysorbate 80, trolamine and water for injections.

*Fucidin Intertulle:* Sterile gauze squares each impregnated with Fusidic Acid, as the sodium salt, BP 2% (Fucidin Ointment) in an ointment base and enclosed between two leaves of sterile parchment in a sealed foil pack.

**Uses** *Mode of Action:* Fusidic acid is a potent topical antibacterial agent. Fusidic acid and its salts show fat and water solubility and strong surface activity and exhibit unusual ability to penetrate intact skin. Concentrations of 0.03–0.12 microgram/ml inhibit nearly all strains of *Staphylococcus aureus*. Topical application of fusidic acid is also effective against Streptococci, Corynebacteria, Neisseria and certain Clostridia.

*Indications:* Indicated either alone or in combination with systemic therapy, in the treatment of primary and secondary skin infections caused by sensitive strains of *Staphylococcus aureus*, Streptococcus spp and *Corynebacterium minutissimum*. Primary skin infections that may be expected to respond to treatment with fusidic acid applied topically include: impetigo contagiosa, superficial folliculitis, furunculosis, sycosis barbae, hidradenitis axillaris, abscesses, carbuncles, paronychia and erythrasma; also such secondary skin infections as infected eczematoid dermatitis, infected contact dematitis, infected wounds, infected burns, infected ulcers and other bacterial superinfections.

**Dosage and administration** *Fucidin Cream, Fucidin Gel and Fucidin Ointment: Adults and children:* Uncovered lesions – apply gently, three or four times daily. Covered lesions – less frequent applications may be adequate.

*Fucidin Intertulle:* Usually, once a day application but frequency of application will vary with clinical circumstances. The intertulle should be covered with a suitable dressing which should be renewed frequently.

**Contra-indications, warnings, etc**

*Contra-indications:* Infection caused by non-susceptible organisms, in particular, *Pseudomonas aeruginosa*.

Fucidin Cream, Ointment, Gel and Intertulle are contra-indicated in patients with hypersensitivity to fusidic acid and its salts.

*Precautions:* Bacterial resistance has been reported to occur with the use of fusidic acid applied topically. As with all topical antibiotics extended or recurrent application may increase the risk of contact sensitisation and the development of antibiotic resistance.

Fusidic acid does not appear to cause conjunctival irritation in experimental animals. Caution should, however, still be exercised when using Fucidin Cream or Gel near the eye. The sodium salt of fusidic acid has been shown to cause conjunctival irritation. The Ointment and Intertulle should not be used in or near the eye.

*Pregnancy and lactation:* There is inadequate evidence of safety in human pregnancy. Animal studies and many years of clinical experience have suggested that fusidic acid is devoid of teratogenic effects. There is evidence to suggest that when given systemically, fusidic acid can penetrate the placental barrier. The use of topical Fucidin in pregnancy requires that the potential benefits be weighed against the possible hazards to the foetus.

Safety in nursing mothers has not been established. When fusidic acid (as the sodium salt) has been given systemically, levels have been detected in breast milk but with topical use the possible amount of drug present is unlikely to affect the infant.

*Adverse reactions:* Hypersensitivity reactions to the active ingredient in the form of skin rashes and mild stinging and irritation on application, have been reported rarely.

*Overdosage:* Not applicable.

**Pharmaceutical precautions** *Fucidin Cream and Ointment:* Nil.

*Fucidin Gel:* Store below 25˚C but do not freeze.
*Fucidin Intertulle:* Store below 25˚C.

**Legal category** POM.

**Package quantities** *Fucidin Cream, Fucidin Ointment and Fucidin Gel:* Tubes of 15 g (OP) and 30 g (OP).
*Fucidin Intertulle:* Box of 10 foil packs, each containing one tulle piece (10 cm × 10 cm) (OP).

**Further information** Fusidic acid and its salts exhibit no cross hypersensitivity with other antibiotics in clinical use.

Despite many years of clinical use, resistance to fusidic acid amongst *Staphylococcus aureus*, remains low.

The ointment base contains lanolin.

The gel base is non-staining and contains no lanolin or other fatty constituents.

The cream base is a vanishing base and contains no lanolin.

**Product licence numbers**

| | |
|---|---|
| Fucidin Cream | 0043/0065 |
| Fucidin Ointment | 0043/5005R |
| Fucidin Gel | 0043/5018R |
| Fucidin Intertulle | 0043/5007R |

## FUCIDIN* H CREAM
## FUCIDIN* H OINTMENT
## FUCIDIN* H GEL

**Presentation** Fucidin H cream contains Fusidic Acid BP 2% and Hydrocortisone Acetate PhEur 1% in a cream base. Other ingredients: potassium sorbate 0.27% as preservative, butylated hydroxyanisole, cetyl alcohol, glycerol, liquid paraffin, polysorbate 60, purified water and white soft paraffin.

Fucidin H Ointment contains Fusidic Acid, as the sodium salt BP 2% and Hydrocortisone Acetate PhEur 1% in an ointment base. Other ingredients: cetyl alcohol, lanolin, liquid paraffin and white soft paraffin.

Fucidin H Gel contains Fusidic Acid BP 2% and Hydrocortisone Acetate PhEur 1% in a water-miscible gel base. Other ingredients: methyl paraben 0.27% and propyl paraben 0.03% as preservatives, carbomer, dimeticone, polysorbate 80, trolamine and water for injections.

**Uses** *Mode of Action:* Fucidin H Cream, H Ointment and H Gel combine the potent topical antibacterial action of fusidic acid with the anti-inflammatory and antipruritic effects of hydrocortisone. Concentrations of 0.03–0.12 microgram fusidic acid per ml inhibit nearly all strains of *Staphylococcus aureus*. Topical application of fusidic acid is also effective against Streptococci, Corynebacteria, Neisseria and certain Clostridia.

*Indications:* Fucidin H Cream, H Ointment and H Gel are indicated in eczema and dermatitis with secondary bacterial infections, including atopic eczema, primary irritant dermatitis and allergic and seborrhoeic dermatitis where the organisms responsible are known to be or believed to be sensitive to fusidic acid.

**Dosage and administration** *Adults and children:* Uncovered lesions – apply gently, three or four times daily. Covered lesions – less frequent applications may be adequate.

**Contra-indications, warnings, etc**

*Contra-indications:* As with other topical corticosteroid preparations, Fucidin H Cream, H Ointment and H Gel are contra-indicated in primary bacterial, viral and fungal skin infections.

Fucidin H Cream, H Ointment and H Gel are contra-indicated in patients with hypersensitivity to fusidic acid and its salts.

*Precautions:* Fucidin H Ointment should not be used in or near the eye, as sodium fusidate causes conjunctival irritation.

Fusidic acid does not appear to cause conjunctival irritation in experimental animals. Caution should still be exercised, however, when Fucidin H Cream or Fucidin H Gel is used near the eye.

Steroid-antibiotic combinations should not be continued for more than 7 days in the absence of any clinical improvement since in this situation occult extension of the infection may occur due to the masking of the steroid. Similarly, steroids may also mask hypersensitivity reactions.

Bacterial resistance has been reported to occur with the use of fusidic acid applied topically. As with all topical antibiotics, extended or recurrent application may increase the risk of contact sensitisation and the development of antibiotic resistance.

*Pregnancy and lactation:* There is inadequate evidence of safety in human pregnancy.

Topical administration of corticosteroids to pregnant animals can cause abnormalities of foetal development including cleft palate and intra-uterine growth retardation. There may, therefore, be a very small risk of such effects in the human foetus.

Animal studies and many years of clinical experience have suggested that fusidic acid is devoid of teratogenic effects. There is evidence to suggest that when given systemically, fusidic acid can penetrate the placental barrier. The use of topical Fucidin in pregnancy requires that the potential benefits be weighed against the possible hazards to the foetus.

Safety in nursing mothers has not been established. When fusidic acid (as the sodium salt) has been given systemically, levels have been detected in breast milk, but with topical use the possible amount of drug present is unlikely to affect the infant.

In infants, long-term continuous topical therapy with corticosteroids should be avoided. Adrenal suppression can occur even without occlusion.

*Adverse reactions:* Hypersensitivity reactions to the active ingredient in the form of skin rashes and mild stinging and irritation on application, have been reported rarely.

*Overdosage:* Not applicable.

**Pharmaceutical precautions** *Fucidin H Cream and H Ointment:* Nil. *Fucidin H Gel:* Store below 25°C but do not freeze.

**Legal category** POM.

**Package quantities** Tubes of 15 g (OP) and 30 g (OP).

**Further information** Fusidic acid and its salts exhibit no cross hypersensitivity with other antibiotics in clinical use.

Despite many years of clinical use, resistance to fusidic acid amongst *Staphylococcus aureus*, remains low.

The ointment base contains lanolin.

The gel base is non-staining and contains no lanolin or other fatty constituents.

The cream base is a vanishing base and contains no lanolin.

**Product licence numbers**
Fucidin H Cream        0043/0093
Fucidin H Gel          0043/0024R
Fucidin H Ointment     0043/5012R

## FuciBET* CREAM

**Presentation** FuciBET cream contains betamethasone 0.1% (as the valerate ester) and Fusidic Acid PhEur 2% in a smooth white to off-white water miscible base. Other ingredients: chlorocresol 0.1% as preservative, cetomacrogol 1000, cetostearyl alcohol, liquid paraffin, purified water, sodium dihydrogen phosphate and white soft paraffin.

**Uses** FuciBET combines the well-known anti-inflammatory and antipruritic effects of betamethasone with the potent topical antibacterial action of fusidic acid.

Betamethasone valerate is a topical steroid rapidly effective in those inflammatory dermatoses which normally respond to this form of therapy. More refractory conditions can often be treated successfully.

When applied topically, fusidic acid is effective against *Staphylococcus aureus*, Streptococci, Corynebacteria, Neisseria and certain Clostridia and Bacteroides. Concentrations of 0.03 to 0.12 microgram per ml inhibit nearly all strains of *S. aureus*. The antibacterial activity of fusidic acid is not diminished in the presence of betamethasone.

*Indications:* FuciBET is indicated for the treatment of eczematous dermatoses including atopic eczema, infantile eczema, discoid eczema, stasis eczema, contact eczema and seborrhoeic eczema when secondary bacterial infection is confirmed or suspected.

**Dosage and administration** A small quantity should be applied to the affected area two or three times daily until a satisfactory response is obtained. It may then be possible to maintain improvement by less frequent application or by the use of a less potent topical steroid/antibacterial preparation such as Fucidin H Ointment or Fucidin H Gel.

In the more resistant lesions the effect of FuciBET can be enhanced by occlusion with polythene film. Overnight occlusion is usually adequate.

**Contra-indications, warnings, etc**
*Contra-indications:* Acne rosacea and peri-oral dermatitis. Skin lesions of viral, fungal or bacterial origin. Hypersensitivity to the preparation.

*Precautions:* Long-term continuous topical therapy should be avoided, particularly in infants and children. Adrenal suppression can occur even without occlusion. Atrophic changes may occur on the face and to a lesser degree in other parts of the body, after prolonged treatment with potent topical steroids.

Caution should be exercised if FuciBET is used near the eye. Glaucoma might result if the preparation enters the eye. Systemic chemotherapy is required if bacterial infection persists.

*Pregnancy:* Topical administration of any corticosteroid to pregnant animals can cause abnormalities of foetal development. The relevance of this finding to human beings has not been established; however, topical steroids should not be used extensively in pregnancy, i.e. in large amounts or for prolonged periods.

*Adverse reactions:* Prolonged and intensive treatment with potent corticosteroids may cause local atrophic changes in the skin, including striae, thinning and dilation of superficial blood vessels, particularly when applied to the flexures or when occlusion is employed.

As with other topical corticosteroids sufficient systemic absorption to produce hypercorticism can occur with prolonged or extensive use. Infants and children are at particular risk, more so if occlusive dressings are used. A napkin may act as an occlusive dressing in infants.

Hypersensitivity reactions to fusidic acid are rare and FuciBET does not contain lanolin. However, if signs of hypersensitivity occur, treatment should be withdrawn.

*Overdosage:* Not applicable.

**Pharmaceutical precautions** Nil.

**Legal category** POM.

**Package quantities** Tubes of 15 g (OP), 30 g (OP) and 60 g (OP).

**Further information** The least potent corticosteroid, which controls the disease, should be used.

**Product licence number** 0043/0091.

## FUCITHALMIC*

**Presentation** Sterile viscous drops of a 1% aqueous sustained release formulation of Fusidic Acid PhEur preserved with benzalkonium chloride. Other ingredients: disodium edetate, mannitol, carbomer, sodium hydroxide and water for injections.

**Uses**
*Mode of action:* Fucithalmic is active against a wide range of Gram-positive organisms, particularly *Staphylococcus aureus*. Other species against which Fucithalmic has been shown to have *in-vitro* activity include *Streptococcus, Neisseria, Haemophilus, Moraxella* and *Corynebacteria*.

The sustained release formulation of Fucithalmic ensures a prolonged contact with the conjunctival sac. Twice daily application provides sufficient fusidic acid concentrations in all relevant tissues of the eye. Fusidic acid penetrates well into the aqueous humour.

*Indications:* Fucithalmic is indicated for the topical treatment of bacterial conjunctivitis where the organism is known to be sensitive to the antibiotic.

**Dosage and administration** For all ages: One Fucithalmic drop to be instilled into the eye twice daily. Treatment should be continued for at least 48 hours after the eye returns to normal.

**Contra-indications, warnings, etc**
*Contra-indications:* Hypersensitivity to any of its components.

*Precautions:* Should not be used when contact lenses are being worn.

*Side-effects:* Transient stinging after application has been encountered. Hypersensitivity may occur.

*Overdosage:* Not applicable.

**Pharmaceutical precautions** Store below 25°C. Keep the tube tightly closed. The tube should be discarded one month after opening.

**Legal category** POM.

**Package quantities** Available in 5 g tubes (OP).

**Further information** Nil.

**Product licence number** 0043/0137.

## HEPARIN (MUCOUS) INJECTION BP

**Presentation** Heparin (Mucous) Injection BP 1,000 units per ml: each ml contains 1,000 units sodium heparin. (Presented in 5 ml vials with 1% benzyl alcohol, 0.1% methylparahydroxybenzoate and 0.02% propylparahydroxybenzoate as preservatives. Also contains sodium citrate, sodium chloride and water for injections.)

Heparin (Mucous) Injection BP 5,000 units per ml: each ml contains 5,000 units sodium heparin. (Presented in 5 ml vials with 1% benzyl alcohol, 0.1% methylparahydroxybenzoate and 0.02% propylparahydroxybenzoate as preservatives. Also contains sodium citrate, sodium chloride and water for injections.)

Heparin (Mucous) Injection BP 25,000 units per ml: each ml contains 25,000 units sodium heparin. (Presented in 5 ml vials with 1% benzyl alcohol, 0.1% methylparahydroxybenzoate and 0.02% propyl-

parahydroxybenzoate as preservatives. Also contains sodium citrate and water for injections.)

**Uses** *Mode of action:* Heparin is a naturally occurring anticoagulant which prevents the coagulation of blood *in vivo* and *in vitro*. It potentiates the inhibition of several activated coagulation factors, including thrombin and factor X.

*Indications:* Treatment of thrombo-embolic disorders such as deep vein thrombosis, acute arterial embolism or thrombosis, thrombophlebitis, pulmonary embolism and fat embolism.

Prophylaxis against deep vein thrombosis and thromboembolic events in susceptible patients.

**Dosage and administration**
*Treatment dosage*

*Intravenous administration:* 5,000–10,000 units every 4 hours or 500 units/kg bodyweight daily as a continuous infusion in sodium chloride injection or dextrose injection. The dose should be individually adjusted according to coagulation tests.

*Subcutaneous administration:* The initial dose is 250 units/kg bodyweight. Further doses should be given every 12 hours and individually adjusted according to coagulation tests.

*Dosage adjustment:* It is recommended that dosages be adjusted to maintain a thrombin clotting time, whole blood clotting time or activated partial thromboplastin time 1.5–2 times that of control on blood withdrawn 4–6 hours after the first injection or commencement of infusion and at similar intervals until the patient is stabilised.

*Prophylactic dosage*
Administration is by subcutaneous injection.

*Patients undergoing major elective surgery:* 5,000 units should be given 2 hours pre-operatively and then every 8–12 hours post-operatively for 10–14 days or until the patient is ambulant whichever is the longer.

*Following myocardial infarction:* 5,000 units should be given twice daily for 10 days or until the patient is mobile.

*Other patients:* 5,000 units should be given every 8–12 hours.

These standard prophylactic regimens do not require routine control.

*Dosage in children*

*Treatment dosage:* Standard treatment dosages should be given initially. Subsequent dosages and/or dosage intervals should be individually adjusted according to changes in thrombin clotting time, whole blood clotting time and/or activated partial thromboplastin time.

*Dosage in the elderly*

*Treatment dosage:* Lower treatment dosages may be required, however, standard treatment dosages should be given initially and then subsequent dosages and/or dosage intervals should be individually adjusted according to changes in thrombin clotting time, whole blood clotting time and/or activated partial thromboplastin time.

*Prophylactic dosage:* Dosage alterations are unnecessary for prophylaxis in the elderly.

*Pregnancy*

*Treatment dosage:* Standard treatment dosages should be given initially by continuous intravenous infusion or every 12 hours by subcutaneous injection. Intermittent intravenous injections are not advised. Subsequent dosages and/or dosage intervals should be individually adjusted according to changes in thrombin clotting time, whole blood clotting time and/or activated partial thromboplastin time.

*Prophylactic dosage:* It is recommended that plasma heparin levels be maintained below 0.4 units/ml, as determined by specific anti-Xa assay. A suggested dosage is 5,000 units every 12 hours in early pregnancy, increasing to 10,000 units every 12 hours in the last trimester. The dosage should be reduced during labour and the standard prophylactic dosage is suitable in the puerperium.

**Contra-indications, warnings, etc**
*Contra-indications:* Haemorrhagic disorders and patients with an actual or potential bleeding site e.g. peptic ulcer.

*Precautions:* Heparin therapy should be given with caution to patients with impaired renal or hepatic function.

Oral anticoagulants or drugs which interfere with platelet function, eg aspirin and dextran solutions should be administered with caution.

*Pregnancy and lactation:* Although animal studies have not been performed, epidemiological studies indicate that if drug therapy is needed in pregnancy, the use of heparin in the recommended dosage is acceptable. Heparin does not cross the placenta or appear in breast milk.

*Adverse reactions:* Hypersensitivity and acute reversible thrombocytopenia may occur rarely. Osteoporosis and alopecia have been reported after prolonged therapy.

*Overdosage:* The effect of heparin can be reversed immediately by intravenous administration of a 1% protamine sulphate solution. The dose of protamine sulphate required for neutralisation should be determined accurately by titrating the patient's plasma. It is important to avoid overdosage of protamine sulphate because protamine itself has anticoagulant properties. A single dose of protamine sulphate should never exceed 50 mg. Intravenous injection of protamine may cause a sudden fall in blood pressure, bradycardia, dyspnoea and transitory flushing, but these may be avoided or diminished by slow and careful administration.

**Pharmaceutical precautions** Store below 25°C. Heparin has been reported to be incompatible in aqueous solutions with certain substances, eg, some antibiotics, hydrocortisone, phenothiazines, narcotic analgesics and some antihistamines.

**Legal category** POM.

**Package quantities** *Heparin 1,000 units per ml:* 5 ml vials. Packs of 10.
*Heparin 5,000 units per ml:* 5 ml vials. Packs of 10.
*Heparin 25,000 units per ml:* 5 ml vials. Packs of 5.

**Further information** Nil.

**Product licence numbers**
1,000 units (with preservative)    0043/0041R
5,000 units (with preservative)    0043/0038R
25,000 units (with preservative)   0043/0039R

## HEP-FLUSH*

**Presentation** Heparin flush solution, each ml containing 100 units sodium heparin in saline. Also contains 1% benzyl alcohol, 0.1% methylparahydroxybenzoate and 0.02% propylparahydroxybenzoate as preservatives, sodium citrate and water for injections. Available as ampoules of 200 units in 2 ml.

**Uses**
*Mode of action:* Heparin is a naturally occurring anticoagulant which prevents the coagulation of blood *in vivo* and *in vitro.* It potentiates the inhibition of several activated coagulation factors, including thrombin and factor X.

*Indications:* To maintain the patency of in-dwelling intravenous lines. It is not recommended for therapeutic use.

**Dosage and administration** For routine use, 2 ml containing 200 units of heparin should be administered into the catheter/cannula every 4 to 8 hours or as required.

**Contra-indications, warnings, etc** When used as recommended the low dose of heparin reaching the blood should have no systemic effects.

**Pharmaceutical precautions** Store below 25°C. Hep-Flush is compatible with normal saline. Heparin has been reported to be incompatible in aqueous solution with certain substances, e.g. some antibiotics, hydrocortisone, phenothiazines, narcotic analgesics and antihistamines.

**Legal category** POM.

**Package quantities** Packs of 10×2 ml ampoules.

**Further information** Nil.

**Product licence number** 0043/0057

## HEPLOK*

**Presentation** Heparin flush solution; 5 ml ampoule, each ml containing 10 units sodium heparin in saline (no preservative), (i.e. 50 units per ampoule).

**Uses**
*Mode of action:* Heparin is a naturally occurring anticoagulant which prevents the coagulation of blood *in vivo* and *in vitro.* It potentiates the inhibition of several activated coagulation factors, including thrombin and factor X.

*Indications:* To maintain the patency of in-dwelling intravenous lines. It is not recommended for therapeutic use.

**Dosage and administration** For routine use 1–5 ml (10–50 units heparin) should be administered into the catheter/cannula every 4 to 8 hours or as required.

**Contra-indications, warnings, etc** When used as recommended the low dose of heparin reaching the blood should have no systemic effects.

**Pharmaceutical precautions** Store below 25°C.

Heplok is compatible with normal saline. Heparin has been reported to be incompatible in aqueous solution with certain substances, e.g. some antibiotics, hydrocortisone, phenothiazines, narcotic analgesics and antihistamines.

**Legal category** POM.

**Package quantities** Packs of 10×5 ml ampoules.

**Further information** Nil.

**Product licence number** 0043/0092.

## INNOHEP* SYRINGE 20,000 IU/ML ▼

**Qualitative and quantitative composition** Tinzaparin sodium 20,000 anti-Factor Xa IU/ml.

**Pharmaceutical form** Solution for injection.

**Clinical particulars**
*Therapeutic indications:* Treatment of deep-vein thrombosis.

*Posology and method of administration:* Administration is by subcutaneous injection only.

*Adults:* 175 anti-Factor Xa IU/kg bodyweight once daily, for at least 6 days and until adequate oral anticoagulation is established. There is no need to monitor the Innohep treatment.

*Use in the elderly:* No dose modifications are necessary.

*Use in children:* There is no experience of use in children.

*Contra-indications:* Known hypersensitivity to constituents. Generalised haemorrhagic tendency, uncontrolled severe hypertension, active peptic ulcer, septic endocarditis. Thrombocytopenia in patients with a positive *in vitro* aggregation test in the presence of tinzaparin.

*Special warnings and precautions for use:* Care should be taken when Innohep is administered to patients with severe liver or kidney insufficiency. In such cases a dose reduction should be considered.

Innohep should not be administered by intramuscular injection due to the risk of haematoma.

Innohep should be used with caution in patients with a history of asthma due to the presence of sodium bisulphite.

Care should be taken when Innohep is administered to patients who have recently suffered from cerebral haemorrhage, trauma and/or had recent surgery to the central nervous system.

Innohep should be used with caution in patients with hypersensitivity to heparin or to other low molecular weight heparins.

*Interaction with other medicaments and other forms of interaction:* Any drug which affects platelet function, aggregation or blood coagulation, e.g. salicylates, non-steroidal anti-inflammatory drugs, vitamin K antagonists (such as warfarin) and dextran, should be used with caution in patients receiving Innohep.

*Pregnancy and lactation:* No transplacental passage of Innohep was found (assessed by anti-Factor Xa and anti-Factor IIa activity) in patients given a dose of 35–40 anti-Factor Xa IU/kg in the second trimester of pregnancy. In rabbits, no transplacental passage of anti-Factor Xa or anti-Factor IIa activity was observed after doses of 1750 anti-Factor Xa IU/kg. Toxicological studies in rats have shown no embryotoxic or teratogenic effects, although a lower birthweight was found.

Although these animal studies show no hazard, as a precaution Innohep should not be used in pregnancy unless no safer alternative is available.

It is not known whether Innohep is excreted in breast milk. However, patients are advised to stop breast-feeding while receiving Innohep.

*Effects on ability to drive and use machines:* No adverse effects to be expected.

*Undesirable effects:* Skin rashes and minor bruising at the site of injection have occurred occasionally. Systemic allergic reactions have been reported extremely rarely.

Innohep, like heparin, has been shown to increase the risk of haemorrhage. However, at the recommended dose this risk is low. As with heparin, thrombocytopenia may occur rarely.

As for heparin, a transient increase in aminotransferase levels is frequently seen. Cessation of treatment is not usually required.

*Overdose:* Overdose of Innohep may result in bleeding. The effect of Innohep can be reversed by giving protamine sulphate. There is no clinical experience of overdose with Innohep, but animal studies indicate a higher neutralising dose of protamine sulphate for Innohep than for unfractionated heparin. APTT (activated partial thromboplastin time) should be monitored. Excess bleeding is not seen in animal experiments when the APTT is brought within the normal range. Transfusion of fresh plasma may be used if necessary. Plasma anti-Factor Xa and anti-

Factor IIa activity should be measured during the management of overdose situations.

**Phamacological properties**
*Pharmacodynamic properties:* Innohep is an antithrombotic agent. It potentiates the inhibition of several activated coagulation factors, especially Factor Xa, its activity being mediated via antithrombin III.

*Pharmacokinetic properties:* The pharmacokinetics/pharmacodynamic activity of Innohep is monitored by anti-Factor Xa activity. Following subcutaneous injection of Innohep, anti-Factor Xa activity reaches a maximum at 4–6 hours (peak anti-Factor Xa activity, after administration of 175 anti-Factor Xa IU/kg bodyweight once daily, is approximately 0.5–1.0 IU/ml). Detectable anti-Factor Xa activity persists for 24 hours.

*Preclinical safety data:* There are no preclinical data of relevance to the prescriber which are additional to that already included in other sections of the SPC.

**Pharmaceutical particulars**
*List of excipients:* Sodium metabisulphite, sodium hydroxide, water for injections.

*Incompatibilities:* Innohep should be given by subcutaneous injection only. It should not be mixed with any other injection.

*Shelf life:* 2 years.

*Special precautions for storage:* To be stored at room temperature.

*Nature and contents of container:* A prefilled variable dose graduated syringe containing:
  0.5 ml (10,000 anti-Factor Xa IU)
  0.7 ml (14,000 anti-Factor Xa IU)
  0.9 ml (18,000 anti-Factor Xa IU)
in packs of 2 and 6 syringes.

*Instructions for use/handling:* Contains no bactericide, any portion of the contents not used at once should be discarded together with the syringe.

**Marketing authorisation number** 0043/0197.

**Date of approval/revision of SPC** September 1996.

**Legal category** POM.

## INNOHEP* 20,000 IU/ML ▼

**Presentation** Innohep contains tinzaparin sodium (low molecular weight heparin) in a sterile solution for subcutaneous injection, presented in vials. Each vial contains tinzaparin sodium 40,000 anti-Factor Xa IU in 2 ml.

Other ingredients: benzyl alcohol, sodium bisulphite, sodium hydroxide and water for injections.

**Uses**
*Mode of action:* Innohep is an antithrombotic agent. It potentiates the inhibition of several activated coagulation factors, especially Factor Xa, its activity being mediated via Antithrombin III.

*Pharmacokinetics:* The pharmacokinetics/pharmacodynamic activity of Innohep is monitored by anti-Factor Xa activity. Following subcutaneous injection of Innohep, anti-Factor Xa activity reaches a maximum at 4–6 hours (peak anti-Factor Xa activity, after administration of 175 anti-Factor Xa IU/kg bodyweight once daily, is approximately 0.5–1.0 IU/ml). Detectable anti-Factor Xa activity persists for 24 hours.

*Indications:* For the treatment of deep vein thrombosis.

**Dosage and administration** Administration is by subcutaneous injection.

*Adults:* 175 anti-Factor Xa IU/kg bodyweight once daily, for at least 6 days and until adequate oral anticoagulation is established.

There is no need to monitor the Innohep treatment.

*Use in the elderly:* No dose modifications are necessary.

*Use in children:* There is no experience of use in children.

**Contra-indications, warnings, etc**
*Contra-indications:* Known hypersensitivity to constituents. Generalised haemorrhagic tendency, uncontrolled severe hypertension, active peptic ulcer, septic endocarditis.

*Precautions:* Care should be taken when Innohep is administered to patients with severe liver or kidney insufficiency. In such cases a dose reduction should be considered.

Innohep should not be administered by intramuscular injection due to the risk of haematoma.

Innohep should be used with caution in patients with a history of asthma due to the presence of sodium bisulphite.

*Interactions:* Any drug which affects platelet function or coagulation e.g. salicylates, vitamin K antagonists and dextran should be used with caution in patients receiving Innohep.

*Use in pregnancy and lactation:* No transplacental

passage of Innohep was found (assessed by anti-Factor Xa and anti-Factor IIa activity) in patients given a dose of 35–40 anti-Factor Xa IU/kg in the second trimester of pregnancy. In rabbits, no transplacental passage of anti-Factor Xa or anti-Factor IIa activity was observed after doses of 1750 anti-Factor Xa IU/kg. Toxicological studies in rats have shown no embryotoxic or teratogenic effects, although a lower birthweight was found.

Although these animal studies show no hazard, as a precaution Innohep should not be used in pregnancy unless no safer alternative is available.

It is not known whether Innohep is excreted in breast milk. However, patients are advised to stop breast-feeding while receiving Innohep.

*Side-effects:* Skin rashes and minor bruising at the site of injection have occurred occasionally. Systemic allergic reactions have not been reported although this is a potential rare side-effect.

Innohep, like heparin, has been shown to increase the risk of haemorrhage. However, at the recommended dose this risk is low. As with heparin, thrombocytopenia may occur rarely.

As for heparin, a transient increase in aminotransferase levels is frequently seen. Cessation of treatment is not usually required.

*Overdosage:* Overdose of Innohep may result in bleeding. The effect of Innohep can be reversed by giving protamine sulphate. There is no clinical experience of overdose with Innohep, but animal studies indicate a higher neutralising dose of protamine sulphate for Innohep than for unfractionated heparin. APTT (Activated Partial Thromboplastin Time) should be monitored. Excess bleeding is not seen in animal experiments when the APTT is brought within the normal range. Transfusion of fresh plasma may be used if necessary.

**Pharmaceutical precautions** Store at room temperature. The vial should be discarded 14 days after first use.

**Legal category** POM.

**Package quantities** Innohep 20,000 IU/ml in 2 ml vials – pack of 1.

**Further information** Nil.

**Product licence number** 0043/0192.

## INNOHEP* SYRINGE 3,500 ANTI-FACTOR Xa IU IN 0.3 ML
## INNOHEP* 5,000 IU IN 0.5 ML

**Presentation** Innohep contains tinzaparin sodium (low molecular weight heparin) in a sterile solution for subcutaneous injection, presented in unit dose syringes and ampoules.

Innohep unit dose syringes contain tinzaparin 3,500 anti-Factor Xa IU in 0.3 ml without preservative. Other ingredients: sodium bisulphite, sodium hydroxide and water for injections.

Innohep unit dose ampoules contain tinzaparin sodium 5,000 anti-Factor Xa IU in 0.5 ml (10,000 anti-Factor Xa IU/ml) without preservative. Other ingredients: sodium bisulphite, sodium hydroxide and water for injections.

**Uses**
*Mode of action:* Innohep is an antithrombotic agent. It potentiates the inhibition of several activated coagulation factors, especially Factor Xa, its activity being mediated via Antithrombin III.

*Pharmacokinetics:* The pharmacokinetics/pharmaco-dynamics of Innohep are monitored by anti-Factor Xa activity. Innohep has a bioavailability of around 90% following subcutaneous injection. The absorption half-life is 200 minutes, peak plasma activity being observed after 4–6 hours. The elimination half-life is about 90 minutes. There is a linear dose response relationship between plasma activity and the dose administered.

*Indications:* For the prevention of thromboembolic events including deep vein thrombosis in patients undergoing general and orthopaedic surgery.

**Dosage and administration** Administration is by subcutaneous injection.

*Adults*
*Patients undergoing general surgery:* 3,500 anti-Factor Xa IU 2 hours before surgery and then once daily for 7–10 days, post-operatively.

*Patients undergoing orthopaedic surgery:* In this high risk group the dose should be based on body weight. The recommended dose is 50 anti-Factor Xa IU/kg body weight (3,500 anti-Factor Xa IU for a 70 kg adult) 2 hours before surgery and then once daily for 7–10 days, post-operatively.

*Use in the elderly:* No dose modifications are necessary.

*Use in children:* There is no experience of use in children.

**Contra-indications, warnings, etc**
*Contra-indications:* Known hypersensitivity to constituents. Generalised haemorrhagic tendency, uncontrolled severe hypertension, active peptic ulcer, septic endocarditis.

*Precautions:* Care should be taken when Innohep is administered to patients with severe liver or kidney insufficiency. In such cases a dose reduction should be considered.

Innohep should not be administered by intramuscular injection due to the risk of haematoma.

Innohep should be used with caution in patients with a history of asthma due to the presence of sodium bisulphite.

*Interactions:* Any drug which affects platelet function or coagulation e.g. salicylates, vitamin K antagonists and dextran should be used with caution in patients receiving Innohep.

*Use in pregnancy and lactation:* No transplacental passage of Innohep was found (assessed by anti-factor Xa and anti-Factor IIa activity) in patients given a dose of 35–40 anti-Factor Xa IU/kg in the second trimester of pregnancy. In rabbits, no transplacental passage of anti-Factor Xa or anti-Factor IIa activity was observed after doses of 1750 anti-Factor Xa IU/kg. Toxicological studies in rats have shown no embryotoxic or teratogenic effects, although a lower birthweight was found.

Although these animal studies show no hazard, as a precaution Innohep should not be used in pregnancy unless no safer alternative is available.

It is not known whether Innohep is excreted in breast milk, however patients are advised to stop breast-feeding while receiving Innohep.

*Side effects:* Skin rashes and minor bruising at the site of injection have occurred occasionally. Systemic allergic reactions have not been reported although this is a potential rare side-effect.

Innohep, like heparin, has been shown to increase the risk of haemorrhage. However, at the recommended dose this risk is low and haemorrhagic complications were rare in the clinical trial programme. Compared to placebo, Innohep has not caused a fall in thrombocyte count, however, as with heparin, thrombocytopenia may occur rarely.

As for heparin, a transient increase in aminotransferase levels is frequently seen. Cessation of treatment is not usually required.

*Overdosage:* Overdose of Innohep may result in bleeding. The effect of Innohep can be reversed by giving protamine sulphate. There is no clinical experience of overdose with Innohep, but animal studies indicate a higher neutralising dose of protamine sulphate for Innohep than for unfractionated heparin. APTT (Activated Partial Thromboplastin Time) should be monitored. Excess bleeding is not seen in animal experiments when the APTT is brought within the normal range. Transfusion of fresh plasma may be used if necessary.

**Pharmaceutical precautions** Store at room temperature. Any portion of the contents not used at once should be discarded.

**Legal category** POM.

**Package quantities** Innohep 3,500 anti-Factor Xa IU in 0.3 ml unit dose syringe—packs of 10. Innohep 5,000 IU in 0.5 ml ampoule—packs of 10.

**Further information** Nil.

**Product licence numbers**
Innohep syringe 3,500 anti-Factor Xa IU/0.3 ml 0043/0167.
Innohep 5,000 IU/0.5 ml 0043/0166.

## INNOHEP* 5,000 ANTI-FACTOR Xa IU IN 5 ML ▼

**Presentation** Innohep contains tinzaparin sodium (low molecular weight heparin) in a sterile solution for injection, presented in ampoules. Each ampoule contains tinzaparin sodium 5,000 anti-Factor Xa IU in 5 ml without preservative.

Other ingredients: sodium citrate, sodium chloride, sodium bisulphite and water for injections.

**Uses**
*Mode of action:* Innohep is an antithrombotic agent. It potentiates the inhibition of several activated coagulation factors, especially Factor Xa, its activity being mediated via Antithrombin III.

*Pharmacokinetics:* The pharmacokinetics/pharmaco-dynamics of Innohep are monitored by anti-Factor Xa activity. The half life of Innohep in patients with renal insufficiency given a bolus intravenous dose of 2,500 anti-Factor Xa IU is about 2.5 hours. There is a linear

dose response relationship between plasma activity and the dose administered.

*Indications:* For the prevention of clotting in the extracorporeal circuit during haemodialysis in patients with chronic renal insufficiency.

**Dosage and administration** For haemodialysis the dose of Innohep should be given into the arterial side of the dialyser or intravenously. The dialyser can be primed by flushing with 500–1000 ml isotonic sodium chloride (9 mg/ml) containing 5000 anti-Factor Xa IU Innohep per litre.

*Adults:* In chronic renal insufficiency.
   (a) Short-term haemodialysis – duration of haemodialysis up to 4 hours.
   A bolus dose of 2,000–2,500 anti-Factor Xa IU into the arterial side of the dialyser (or intravenously).
   (b) Long-term haemodialysis – duration of haemodialysis more than 4 hours.
   A bolus dose of 2,500 anti-Factor Xa IU into the arterial side of the dialyser (or intravenously), followed by 750 anti-Factor Xa IU/hour infused into the extracorporeal circuit.

*Dose adjustment:* The bolus Innohep dose may be adjusted (increased or decreased) by 250–500 anti-Factor Xa IU until a satisfactory response is obtained.

   Additional Innohep (500–1000 anti-Factor Xa IU) may be given if concentrated red cells or blood transfusions (which may increase the likelihood of clotting in the dialyser) are given during dialysis or additional treatment beyond the normal dialysis duration is employed.

*Dose monitoring:* Determination of plasma anti-Factor Xa may be used to monitor the Innohep dose. Plasma anti-Factor Xa, 1 hour after dosing, should be within the range 0.4–0.5 IU/ml.

*Use in the elderly:* No dose modifications are necessary.

*Use in children:* There is no experience of use in children.

**Contra-indications, warnings, etc**
*Contra-indications:* Known hypersensitivity to constituents. Generalised haemorrhagic tendency, uncontrolled severe hypertension, active peptic ulcer, septic endocarditis.

*Precautions:* Care should be taken when Innohep is administered to patients with severe liver insufficiency. In such cases a dose reduction should be considered.

Innohep should not be administered by intramuscular injection due to the risk of haematoma.

Innohep should be used with caution in patients with a history of asthma due to the presence of sodium bisulphite.

*Interactions:* Any drug which affects platelet function or coagulation e.g. salicylates, vitamin K antagonists and dextran should be used with caution in patients receiving Innohep.

Innohep does not appear to interact with other drugs used widely in chronic renal failure, including vitamin B supplements, aluminium hydroxide, calcium supplements, alfacalcidol, ranitidine, vitamin C supplements, ferrous sulphate, folic acid, nifedipine, erythropoietin and azatadine.

*Use in pregnancy and lactation:* No transplacental passage of Innohep was found (assessed by anti-Factor Xa and anti-Factor IIa activity) in patients given a dose of 35–40 anti-Factor Xa IU/kg in the second trimester of pregnancy. In rabbits, no transplacental passage of anti-Factor Xa or anti-Factor IIa activity was observed after doses of 1750 anti-Factor Xa IU/kg. Toxicological studies in rats have shown no embryotoxic or teratogenic effects, although a lower birthweight was found.

Although these animal studies show no hazard, as a precaution Innohep should not be used in pregnancy unless no safer alternative is available.

It is not known whether Innohep is excreted in breast milk. However, patients are advised to stop breast-feeding while receiving Innohep.

*Side-effects:* Bleeding may occur at high dosages. Systemic allergic reactions have not been reported although this is a potential rare side-effect. Innohep, like heparin, has been shown to increase the risk of haemorrhage. However, at the recommended dose this risk is low. As with heparin, thrombocytopenia may occur rarely.

As for heparin, a transient increase in aminotransferase levels is frequently seen. Cessation of treatment is not usually required.

*Overdosage:* Overdose of Innohep may result in bleeding. The effect of Innohep can be reversed by giving protamine sulphate. There is no clinical experience of overdose with Innohep, but animal studies indicate a higher neutralising dose of protamine sulphate for Innohep than for unfractionated heparin. APTT (Activated Partial Thromboplastin Time) should be monitored. Excess bleeding is not seen in animal experiments when the APTT is brought within the normal range. Transfusion of fresh plasma may be used if necessary.

**Pharmaceutical precautions** Store at room temperature. Any portion of the contents not used at once should be discarded.

**Legal category** POM.

**Package quantities** Innohep 5,000 anti-Factor Xa IU in 5 ml ampoule – packs of 10.

**Further information** Nil.

**Product licence number** 0043/0191.

## MINIHEP*
## MINIHEP* SYRINGES

**Presentation**
*Minihep:* Heparin (Mucous) Injection BP. Single dose ampoules containing sodium heparin 5,000 iu in 0.2 ml (no preservative). Other ingredients: water for injections.
*Minihep Syringes:* Heparin (Mucous) Injection BP. Single dose syringes containing sodium heparin 5,000 iu in 0.2 ml (no preservative). Other ingredients: water for injections.

**Uses**
*Mode of action:* Heparin is a naturally occurring anticoagulant which prevents the coagulation of blood *in vivo* and *in vitro*. It potentiates the inhibition of several activated coagulation factors, including thrombin and factor X.
*Indications:* Prophylaxis against deep vein thrombosis and thromboembolic events in susceptible patients.

**Dosage and administration** Administration is by subcutaneous injection.
*Patients undergoing major elective surgery:* 5,000 iu in 0.2 ml should be given two hours pre-operatively and then every 8–12 hours post-operatively for 10–14 days, or until the patient is ambulant, whichever is the longer.
*Following myocardial infarction:* 5,000 iu in 0.2 ml should be given twice daily for 10 days, or until the patient is mobile.
*Other patients:* 5,000 iu in 0.2 ml should be given every 8–12 hours.
These standard dosage regimens do not require routine control.
*Dosage in the elderly:* Dosage alterations are unnecessary for prophylaxis in the elderly.
*Pregnancy:* It is recommended that plasma heparin levels be maintained below 0.4 iu/ml as determined by specific anti-Xa assay. A suggested dosage is 5,000 units every 12 hours in early pregnancy increasing to 10,000 iu every 12 hours in the last trimester. The dosage should be reduced during labour and the standard prophylactic dosage is suitable in the puerperium.

**Contra-indications, warnings, etc**
*Contra-indications:* Haemorrhagic disorders and patients with an actual or potential bleeding site, e.g. peptic ulcer.
*Precautions:* Heparin therapy should be given with caution to patients with impaired renal or hepatic function.
Oral anticoagulants or drugs which interfere with platelet function, e.g. aspirin and dextran solutions, should be administered with caution.
*Pregnancy and lactation:* Although animal studies have not been performed, epidemiological studies indicate that if drug therapy is needed in pregnancy, the use of heparin in the recommended dosage is acceptable. Heparin does not cross the placenta or appear in breast milk.
*Adverse reactions:* Hypersensitivity and acute reversible thrombocytopenia may occur rarely. Osteoporosis and alopecia have been reported after prolonged therapy.
*Overdosage:* The effect of heparin can be reversed immediately by intravenous administration of a 1% protamine sulphate solution. The dose of protamine sulphate required for neutralisation should be determined accurately by titrating with the patient's plasma.
It is important to avoid overdosage of protamine sulphate because protamine itself has anticoagulant properties. A single dose of protamine sulphate should never exceed 50 mg. Intravenous injection of protamine may cause a sudden fall in blood pressure, bradycardia, dyspnoea and transitory flushing, but these may be avoided or diminished by slow and careful administration.

**Pharmaceutical precautions** Store below 25°C.

**Legal category** POM.

**Package quantities**
Packs of 10×0.2 ml ampoules.
Packs of 10×0.2 ml syringes.

**Further information** Nil.

**Product licence numbers**
Minihep             0043/0088.
Minihep Syringes     0043/0164.

## MINIHEP* CALCIUM
## MINIHEP* CALCIUM SYRINGE

**Presentation**
*Minihep Calcium:* Heparin (Mucous) Injection BP Single dose ampoules containing calcium heparin 5,000 iu in 0.2 ml, without preservative. Other ingredients: water for injections.
*Minihep Calcium Syringe:* Heparin (Mucous) Injection BP Single dose syringes containing calcium heparin 5,000 iu in 0.2 ml, without preservative. Other ingredients: sodium acetate and water for injections.

**Uses**
*Mode of action:* Heparin is a naturally occurring anticoagulant which prevents the coagulation of blood *in vivo* and *in vitro*. It potentiates the inhibition of several activated coagulation factors, including thrombin and factor X.
*Indications:* Prophylaxis against deep vein thrombosis and thromboembolic events in susceptible patients.

**Dosage and administration** Administration is by subcutaneous injection.
*Patients undergoing major elective surgery:* 5,000 iu in 0.2 ml should be given 2 hours pre-operatively and then every 8–12 hours post-operatively for 10–14 days or until the patient is ambulant, whichever is the longer.
*Following myocardial infarction:* 5,000 iu in 0.2 ml should be given twice daily for 10 days or until the patient is mobile.
*Other patients:* 5,000 iu in 0.2 ml should be given every 8–12 hours.
These standard dosage regimens do not require routine control.
*Dosage in the elderly:* Dosage alterations are unnecessary for prophylaxis in the elderly.
*Pregnancy:* It is recommended that plasma heparin levels be maintained below 0.4 iu/ml as determined by specific anti-Xa assay. A suggested dosage is 5,000 iu every 12 hours in early pregnancy, increasing to 10,000 iu every 12 hours in the last trimester.
The dosage should be reduced during labour and the standard prophylactic dosage is suitable in the puerperium.

**Contra-indications, warnings, etc**
*Contra-indications:* Haemorrhagic disorders and patients with an actual or potential bleeding site, e.g. peptic ulcer.
*Precautions:* Heparin therapy should be given with caution to patients with impaired renal or hepatic function.
Oral anticoagulants or drugs which interfere with platelet function, e.g. aspirin and dextran solutions, should be administered with caution.
*Pregnancy and lactation:* Although animal studies have not been performed, epidemiological studies indicate that if drug therapy is needed in pregnancy the use of heparin in the recommended dosage is acceptable. Heparin does not cross the placenta or appear in breast milk.
*Adverse reactions:* Hypersensitivity and acute reversible thrombocytopenia may occur rarely. Osteoporosis and alopecia have been reported after prolonged therapy.
*Overdosage:* The effect of heparin can be reversed immediately by intravenous administration of a 1% protamine sulphate solution. The dose of protamine sulphate required for neutralisation should be determined accurately by titrating with the patient's plasma.
It is important to avoid overdosage of protamine sulphate because protamine itself has anticoagulant properties. A single dose of protamine sulphate should never exceed 50 mg. Intravenous injection of protamine may cause a sudden fall in blood pressure, bradycardia, dyspnoea and transitory flushing, but these may be avoided or diminished by slow and careful administration.

**Pharmaceutical precautions** Store below 25°C.

**Legal category** POM.

**Package quantities**
Packs of 10×0.2 ml ampoules.
Packs of 10×0.2 ml syringes.

**Further information** Nil.

**Product licence numbers**
Minihep Calcium          0043/0051.
Minihep Calcium Syringe    0043/0165.

## ONE-ALPHA* INJECTION

**Presentation** One-Alpha Injection is a clear, colourless solution containing 2 micrograms/ml of alfacalcidol. Available in amber glass ampoules containing 0.5 ml or 1.0 ml to provide dose units of 1 microgram and 2 micrograms, respectively. Other ingredients: citric acid, ethanol, sodium citrate, propylene glycol and water for injections.

**Uses**
*Mode of action:* Alfacalcidol (One-Alpha) is converted rapidly in the liver to 1,25 dihydroxyvitamin D. This is the metabolite of vitamin D which acts as a regulator of calcium and phosphate metabolism. Since this conversion is rapid, the clinical effects of One-Alpha and 1,25 dihydroxyvitamin D are very similar.
Impaired 1α hydroxylation by the kidneys reduces endogenous 1,25 dihydroxyvitamin D production. This contributes to the disturbances in mineral metabolism found in several disorders, including renal bone disease, hypoparathyroidism, neonatal hypocalcaemia and vitamin D dependent rickets. These disorders, which require high doses of parent vitamin D for their correction, will respond to small doses of One-Alpha.
The delay in response and high dosage required in treating these disorders with parent vitamin D makes dosage adjustment difficult. This can result in unpredictable hypercalcaemia which may take weeks or months to reverse. The major advantage of One-Alpha is the more rapid onset of response, which allows a more accurate titration of dosage. Should inadvertent hypercalcaemia occur it can be reversed within days of stopping treatment.
*Indications:* One-Alpha is indicated in all conditions where there is a disturbance of calcium metabolism due to impaired 1α hydroxylation such as when there is reduced renal function. The main indications are:
(a) Renal osteodystrophy
(b) Hyperparathyroidism (with bone disease)
(c) Hypoparathyroidism
(d) Neonatal hypocalcaemia
(e) Nutritional and malabsorptive rickets and osteomalacia
(f) Pseudo-deficiency (D dependent) rickets and osteomalacia
(g) Hypophosphataemic vitamin D resistant rickets and osteomalacia

**Dosage and administration** One-Alpha Injection should be administered intravenously as a bolus over approximately 30 seconds.
The dosage of One-Alpha Injection is the same as for One-Alpha in its oral presentations.
*Initial dose*
Adults: 1 microgram/day
Dosage in the elderly: 0.5 microgram/day
Neonates and premature infants: 0.05–0.1 microgram/kg/day
Children under 20 kg bodyweight: 0.05 microgram/kg/day
Children over 20 kg bodyweight: 1 microgram/day
The dose of One-Alpha should be adjusted thereafter to avoid hypercalcaemia according to the biochemical response.
Indices of response include plasma levels of calcium (ideally corrected for protein binding), alkaline phosphatase, parathyroid hormone, as well as radiographic and histological investigations.
Maintenance doses are generally in the range of 0.25–1 microgram/day.
When administered as intravenous injection to patients undergoing haemodialysis the initial dosage for adults is 1 microgram per dialysis. The maximum dose recommended is 6 micrograms per dialysis and not more than 12 micrograms per week. The injection should be administered into the return line from the haemodialysis machine at the end of each dialysis.
*(a) Renal bone disease:* Patients with relatively high initial plasma calcium levels may have autonomous hyperparathyroidism, often unresponsive to One-Alpha. Other therapeutic measures may be indicated.
Before and during treatment with One-Alpha, phosphate binding agents should be considered to prevent hyperphosphataemia. It is particularly important to make frequent plasma calcium measurements in patients with chronic renal failure because prolonged hypercalcaemia may aggravate the decline of renal function.
*(b) Hyperparathyroidism:* In patients with primary or tertiary hyperparathyroidism about to undergo parathyroidectomy, pre-operative treatment with One-Alpha for 2–3 weeks alleviates bone pain and myopathy without aggravating pre-operative hypercalcaemia. In order to decrease post-operative hypocalcaemia, One-Alpha should be continued until plasma alkaline phosphatase levels fall to normal or hypercalcaemia occurs.
*(c) Hypoparathyroidism:* In contrast to the response to parent vitamin D, low plasma calcium levels are restored to normal relatively quickly with One-Alpha.

Severe hypocalcaemia is corrected more rapidly with higher doses of One-Alpha (eg 3–5 micrograms) together with calcium supplements.

*(d) Neonatal hypocalcaemia:* Although the normal starting dose of One-Alpha is 0.05–0.1 microgram/kg/day (followed by careful titration) in severe cases doses of up to 2 microgram/kg/day may be required. Whilst ionised serum calcium levels may provide a guide to response, measurement of plasma alkaline phosphatase activity may be more useful. Levels of alkaline phosphatase approximately 7.5 times above the adult range indicates active disease.

*(e) Nutritional and malabsorptive rickets and osteomalacia:* Nutritional rickets and osteomalacia can be cured rapidly with One-Alpha. Malabsorptive osteomalacia (responding to large doses of IM or IV parent vitamin D) will respond to small doses of One-Alpha.

*(f) Pseudo-deficiency (D-dependent) rickets and osteomalacia:* Although large doses of parent vitamin D would be required, effective doses of One-Alpha are similar to those required to heal nutritional Vitamin D deficiency rickets and osteomalacia.

*(g) Hypophosphataemic vitamin D-resistant rickets and osteomalacia:* Neither large doses of parent vitamin D nor phosphate supplements are entirely satisfactory. Treatment with One-Alpha at normal dosage rapidly relieves myopathy when present and increases calcium and phosphate retention. Phosphate supplements may also be required in some patients.

### Contra-indications, warnings, etc
*Precautions:* During treatment with One-Alpha Injection serum calcium should be monitored regularly.

One-Alpha Injection should be avoided in patients with known sensitivity to injections containing propylene glycol and it should be used with caution in small premature infants.

*Drug interactions:* Patients taking barbiturates or anticonvulsants may require larger doses of One-Alpha to produce the desired effect.

*Pregnancy and lactation:* There is inadequate evidence of safety of One-Alpha in human pregnancy but it has been in wide use for many years without apparent ill consequences. Animal studies have shown no hazard. If drug therapy is needed in pregnancy, One-Alpha can be used if there is no alternative.

Although it has not been established, it is likely that increased amounts of 1,25 dihydroxyvitamin D will be found in the milk of lactating mothers treated with One-Alpha. This may influence calcium metabolism in the infant.

*Side-effects:* Rarely hypercalcaemia occurs during treatment with One-Alpha Injection. This can be rapidly corrected by stopping treatment until plasma calcium levels return to normal (about 1 week). Treatment may then be restarted at a reduced dose.

*Overdosage:* Hypercalcaemia is treated by stopping One-Alpha. Severe hypercalcaemia may be additionally treated with a "loop" diuretic and intravenous fluids, or with corticosteroids.

**Pharmaceutical precautions**  Store in a cool place (below 15°C).

**Legal category**  POM.

**Package quantities**  Amber glass ampoules containing 0.5 ml or 1 ml solution. Packs of 10 ampoules of 0.5 ml or 10 ampoules of 1 ml.

**Further information**  Nil.

**Product licence number**  0043/0183.

## ONE-ALPHA* CAPSULES
## ONE-ALPHA* SOLUTION

**Presentation**  *One-Alpha Capsules:* Capsules contain alfacalcidol (1α hydroxy-vitamin D) in two strengths: Brown capsule – contains 1 microgram alfacalcidol; white capsule – contains 0.25 microgram alfacalcidol. *One-Alpha Solution:* A clear or slightly opalescent solution, one ml contains 0.2 microgram alfacalcidol.

### Uses
*Action:* Alfacalcidol (One-Alpha) is converted rapidly in the liver to 1,25 dihydroxyvitamin D. This is the metabolite of vitamin D which acts as a regulator of calcium and phosphate metabolism. Since this conversion is rapid, the clinical effects of One-Alpha and 1,25 dihydroxyvitamin D are very similar.

Impaired 1α hydroxylation by the kidneys reduces endogenous 1,25 dihydroxyvitamin D production. This contributes to the disturbances in mineral metabolism found in several disorders, including renal bone disease, hypoparathyroidism, neonatal hypocalcaemia and vitamin D dependent rickets. These disorders, which require high doses of parent vitamin D for their correction, will respond to small doses of One-Alpha.

The delay in response and high dosage required in treating these disorders with parent vitamin D makes dosage adjustment difficult. This can result in unpredictable hypercalcaemia which may take weeks or months to reverse. The major advantage of One-Alpha is the more rapid onset of response, which allows a more accurate titration of dosage. Should inadvertent hypercalcaemia occur it can be reversed within days of stopping treatment.

*Indications:* One-Alpha is indicated in all conditions, where there is disturbance of calcium metabolism due to impaired 1α hydroxylation such as when there is reduced renal function.

The main indications are:

(a) Renal osteodystrophy
(b) Hyperparathyroidism (with bone disease)
(c) Hypoparathyroidism
(d) Neonatal hypocalcaemia
(e) Nutritional and malabsorptive rickets and osteomalacia
(f) Pseudo-deficiency (D dependent) rickets and osteomalacia
(g) Hypophosphataemic vitamin D resistant rickets and osteomalacia

**Dosage and administration**  One-Alpha may be administered as capsules or solution. One-Alpha Solution should be administered using the enclosed oral dispenser. Initial dose for all indications:

| | |
|---|---|
| Adults | 1 microgram/day |
| Dosage in the elderly | 0.5 microgram/day |
| Neonates and premature infants | 0.05–0.1 microgram/kg/day |
| Children under 20 kg bodyweight | 0.05 microgram/kg/day |
| Children over 20 kg bodyweight | 1 microgram/day |

The dose of One-Alpha should be adjusted thereafter to avoid hypercalcaemia according to the biochemical response.

Indices of response include plasma levels of calcium (ideally corrected for protein binding), alkaline phosphatase, parathyroid hormone, as well as radiographic and histological investigations.

Plasma levels should initially be measured at weekly intervals. The daily dose of One-Alpha may be increased by increments of 0.25–0.5 microgram. When the dose is stabilised, measurements may be taken every 2–4 weeks.

Most adult patients respond to doses between 1 and 3 micrograms per day. When there is biochemical or radiographic evidence of bone healing (and in hypoparathyroid patients when normal plasma calcium levels have been attained), the dose generally decreases. Maintenance doses are generally in the range of 0.25 to 1 microgram per day. If hypercalcaemia occurs, One-Alpha should be stopped until plasma calcium returns to normal (approximately 1 week) then restarted at half the previous dose.

*(a) Renal bone disease:* Patients with relatively high initial plasma calcium levels may have autonomous hyperparathyroidism, often unresponsive to One-Alpha. Other therapeutic measures may be indicated.

Before and during treatment with One-Alpha, phosphate binding agents should be considered to prevent hyperphosphataemia. It is particularly important to make frequent plasma calcium measurements in patients with chronic renal failure because prolonged hypercalcaemia may aggravate the decline of renal function.

*(b) Hyperparathyroidism:* In patients with primary or tertiary hyperparathyroidism about to undergo parathyroidectomy, pre-operative treatment with One-Alpha for 2–3 weeks alleviates bone pain and myopathy without aggravating pre-operative hypercalcaemia. In order to decrease post-operative hypocalcaemia, One-Alpha should be continued until plasma alkaline phosphatase levels fall to normal or hypercalcaemia occurs.

*(c) Hypoparathyroidism:* In contrast to the response to parent vitamin D, low plasma calcium levels are restored to normal relatively quickly with One-Alpha. Severe hypocalcaemia is corrected more rapidly with higher doses of One-Alpha (e.g. 3–5 micrograms) together with calcium supplements.

*(d) Neonatal hypocalcaemia:* Although the normal starting dose of One-Alpha is 0.05–0.1 microgram/kg/day (followed by careful titration) in severe cases doses of up to 2 microgram/kg/day may be required. Whilst ionised serum calcium levels may provide a guide to response, measurement of plasma alkaline phosphatase activity may be more useful. Levels of alkaline phosphatase approximately 7.5 times above the adult range indicates active disease.

A dose of 0.1 microgram/kg/day of One-Alpha has proven effective as prophylaxis against early neonatal hypocalcaemia in premature infants.

*(e) Nutritional and malabsorptive rickets and osteomalacia:* Nutritional rickets and osteomalacia can be cured rapidly with One-Alpha. Malabsorptive osteomalacia (responding to large doses of IM or IV parent vitamin D) will respond to small doses of One-Alpha.

*(f) Pseudo-deficiency (D-dependent) rickets and osteomalacia:* Although large doses of parent vitamin D would be required, effective doses of One-Alpha are similar to those required to heal nutritional Vitamin D deficiency rickets and osteomalacia.

*(g) Hypophosphataemic vitamin D-resistant rickets and osteomalacia:* Neither large doses of parent vitamin D nor phosphate supplements are entirely satisfactory. Treatment with One-Alpha at normal dosage rapidly relieves myopathy when present and increases calcium and phosphate retention. Phosphate supplements may also be required in some patients.

### Contra-indications, warnings, etc
*Precautions and side-effects:* If hypercalcaemia occurs during treatment with One-Alpha this can be rapidly corrected by stopping treatment until plasma calcium levels return to normal (about 1 week). One-Alpha may then be restarted at half the previous dose.

Patients taking barbiturates or anticonvulsants may require larger doses of One-Alpha to produce the desired effect.

*Pregnancy and lactation:* There is inadequate evidence of safety of One-Alpha in human pregnancy but it has been in wide use for many years without apparent ill consequences. Animal studies have shown no hazard. If drug therapy is needed in pregnancy, One-Alpha can be used if there is no alternative.

Although it has not been established, it is likely that increased amounts of 1,25 dihydroxyvitamin D will be found in the milk of lactating mothers treated with One-Alpha. This may influence calcium metabolism in the infant.

*Overdosage:* Hypercalcaemia is treated by stopping One-Alpha. Severe hypercalcaemia may be additionally treated with a 'loop' diuretic and intravenous fluids, or with corticosteroids.

**Pharmaceutical precautions**  One-Alpha capsules: Protect from direct sunlight.

One-Alpha solution: Protect from direct sunlight and store in a cool place (below 15°C).

**Legal category**  POM.

**Package quantities**  Capsules: Bottles of 100 capsules. Solution: Amber glass bottle of 60 ml (OP); an oral dispenser is enclosed.

**Further information**  One-Alpha Solution is sugar free and contains no colouring agents.

**Product licence numbers**
| | |
|---|---|
| Capsules 1 microgram | 0043/0050 |
| Capsules 0.25 microgram | 0043/0052 |
| Solution | 0043/0133 |

## PONDOCILLIN* TABLETS
## PONDOCILLIN* SUSPENSION

**Presentation**  *Tablets:* Each tablet contains 500mg pivampicillin – a white film-coated ovoid tablet with the number 128 printed on one side and an Assyrian lion on the other.

*Suspension:* Bottles containing an off-white to pale yellow granulate for the preparation of 50 ml and 100 ml suspension. When reconstituted each 5 ml contains 175 mg pivampicillin. Also contains sorbitol, aspartame, polyparahydroxybenzoate, sodium chloride, banana and vanilla dry flavour.

**Uses**  Pondocillin (pivampicillin) is the pivaloyloxymethyl ester of ampicillin, and is rapidly hydrolysed in the body to ampicillin by non-specific enzymes present in serum, gastro-intestinal mucosa and other tissues.

After oral administration of Pondocillin, the plasma levels of ampicillin are 2–3 times higher than those obtained with equimolar doses of oral ampicillin. A peak level generally occurs after 1 hour compared to approximately 2 hours with oral ampicillin. These levels are comparable to those obtained with an equimolar dose of intramuscular ampicillin.

Concentrations achieved in the urine are similarly raised. Generally, twice the amount of antibiotic can be recovered after treatment with Pondocillin when compared with equimolar doses of oral ampicillin. Whereas between 30–40% of the administered dose appears in the urine in the first 6 hours after oral administration of ampicillin, 70% can be recovered after an equimolar dose of Pondocillin.

Pondocillin is stable in the presence of gastric acid, and, unlike oral ampicillin, absorption is not affected by the presence of food. Plasma concentrations achieved in the post-prandial state do not differ significantly when compared with the fasting state. Like ampicillin, Pondocillin is destroyed by penicillinase-producing bacteria.

*Indications:* Like ampicillin, Pondocillin has a broad

spectrum of activity against both gram-negative and gram-positive organisms. It is particularly indicated for the treatment of infections caused by susceptible strains of *Shigella, Salmonella, N. gonorrhoea, Esch. coli, H. influenzae, Pr. mirabilis* and is also indicated for pneumococcal, streptococcal and non-penicillinase-producing staphylococcal infections.

Specific infections include:

(a) Acute and chronic bronchitis
(b) Pneumonia
(c) Ear, nose and throat infections
(d) Gynaecological infections
(e) Urinary tract infections
(f) Skin and soft tissue infections
(g) Gonorrhoea

**Dosage and administration** *Tablets:* Usual dosage for adults: 500 mg pivampicillin to be administered twice daily. Dosage may be doubled in cases of severe infection. Gonorrhoea: 1.5–2 g pivampicillin as a single dose. 1 g probenecid can be given concurrently as desired. The medication may be taken with food or fluids.

*Suspension: Infants under 1 yr:* 40–60 mg/Kg bodyweight per day.

*Children aged 1–5 yrs:* 10–15 ml per day

*Children aged 6–10 yrs:* 15–20 ml per day

*Adults and children over 10 yrs:* 30ml per day.

The daily dosage may be given either as 2 or 3 equal divided doses.

Dosage may be doubled where appropriate.

*Dosage in the elderly:* Renal excretion of ampicillin is delayed in the elderly but significant accumulation of the drug is not likely at the recommended adult dosage of Pondocillin.

**Contra-indications, warnings, etc**
*Contra-indications:* Pondocillin is contra-indicated in any patient with a history of hypersensitivity to any of the penicillins or cephalosporins. Because of the high frequency of exanthemata associated with ampicillin therapy in infectious mononucleosis, treatment with Pondocillin is contra-indicated in this disease. Pondocillin is contra-indicated in patients with known carnitine deficiency, in patients with Reye's or Reye-like syndromes, and infants under 3 months.

Pondocillin is also contra-indicated in infections caused by penicillinase-producing bacteria.

*Precautions:* Care should be exercised when treating patients with a history of sensitivity to a variety of allergens, since serious hypersensitivity (anaphylactic) reactions are more likely to occur. If lymphatic leukaemia is treated with Pondocillin then caution is urged because of the frequency of exanthemata associated with ampicillin therapy.

The use of concurrent antacid therapy with Pondocillin is not recommended, since it reduces absorption of the antibiotic, and may cause underdosing.

During long-term therapy and in patients with severe renal or hepatic impairment it is advisable to carry out routine liver and kidney function tests.

Pondocillin should be used with caution for long-term or frequently repeated treatment, due to the possibility of carnitine depletion. Concurrent treatment with valproic acid, valproate or other medication liberating pivalic acid should be avoided.

*Pregnancy:* In keeping with current practice use during pregnancy should be avoided. Ampicillin crosses the placenta and small amounts have been detected in breast milk.

*Adverse Reactions:* Pondocillin is a compound of low toxicity. Like ampicillin, skin rashes of two types have been noted: a non-specific erythema which usually disappears during treatment, and urticaria which may cause withdrawal of the drug. As with other penicillins, fever, joint pains, angioedema and anaphylactic shock in hypersensitive patients may occur.

Upper gastro-intestinal disturbances, such as nausea, vomiting, retrosternal pain and flatulence have occurred more frequently when a dose has been given on an empty stomach. Diarrhoea has been reported, but less frequently than with ampicillin. This observation underlines the importance of giving Pondocillin with or just after a meal. None of these effects appear to be dose-related. Other side effects reported are dizziness and pruritis. Reduction in serum and total body carnitine has been reported.

*Warning:* Pondocillin suspension is not recommended for the treatment of *severe* infections in infancy.

*Overdosage:* There is no experience of overdosage with Pondocillin. However, excessive doses of Pondocillin are likely to induce nausea, vomiting and gastritis. Treatment should be restricted to symptomatic and supportive measures.

**Pharmaceutical precautions** *Tablets:* Nil.
*Suspension:* Pondocillin suspension when reconstituted, is stable for 14 days at room temperature or for 4 weeks when kept in a refrigerator.

**Legal category** POM.

**Package quantities** *Tablets:* Bottles of 100 tablets.

*Suspension:* Available in amber bottles making 100 ml (OP) suspension when dispensed.

**Further information** Nil.

**Product licence numbers**
Tablets 0043/0067
Suspension 0043/0031R

## PRESTIM* TABLETS
## PRESTIM* FORTE TABLETS

**Presentation** *Prestim:* White, flat, petal-shaped tablets engraved with 132 on the scored face and with an Assyrian lion on the reverse. Each tablet contains Timolol Maleate PhEur 10 mg and Bendrofluazide PhEur 2.5 mg.

*Prestim Forte:* White, flat, petal-shaped tablets engraved with 146 on the scored face and with an Assyrian lion on the reverse. Each tablet contains Timolol Maleate PhEur 20 mg and Bendrofluazide PhEur 5 mg.

**Uses** *Mode of Action:* Bendrofluazide, a thiazide diuretic, has an established action in the treatment of hypertension.

Timolol maleate is a beta-adrenergic receptor blocking agent with marked hypotensive activity lasting up to 24 hours.

It has been shown that the combination of a beta-blocking agent with a thiazide diuretic gives an enhanced antihypertensive effect. This means that a relatively lower dose of the beta-blocker is required.

*Indications:* For the treatment of mild to moderate hypertension.

**Dosage and administration** The recommended dosage range is:

*For Prestim Tablets:* 1–4 tablets daily. Most patients are controlled on 1 or 2 tablets.

*For Prestim Forte Tablets:* ½–2 tablets daily.

The dosage can be taken in the morning or in two divided doses, morning and evening.

If blood pressure control is not achieved on 4 tablets Prestim daily or 2 tablets Prestim Forte daily, consideration should be given to titrating timolol and bendrofluazide separately or adding another agent with hypotensive activity.

*Dosage in the elderly:* Initiate treatment with 1 tablet Prestim or ½ tablet Prestim Forte daily and thereafter adjust according to response.

**Contra-indications, warnings, etc**
*Contra-indications:* Anuria. Prestim should not be used in patients with renal failure or with a history of hypersensitivity to the thiazides.

Uncontrolled heart failure, bradycardia, cardiogenic shock, bronchial asthma, chronic obstructive pulmonary disease, patients receiving adrenergic augmenting drugs (monoamine oxidase inhibitors and tricyclic antidepressants).

Anaesthesia with agents that produce myocardial depression, such as chloroform and ether.

Pregnancy.

As with other diuretics, Prestim should not be administered concurrently with lithium salts. Diuretics can reduce lithium clearance resulting in high serum levels of lithium.

*Precautions:* The continued depression of sympathetic drive through beta blockade may lead to cardiac failure, and, if it occurs, digitalisation should be considered.

Caution should be exercised in patients with diabetes mellitus, spontaneous hypoglycaemia, impaired renal or hepatic function and in patients receiving catecholamine depleting drugs, such as reserpine or guanethidine.

*Adverse Reactions:* Side-effects associated with beta blockade, e.g. gastro-intestinal symptoms, dizziness, insomnia, sedation, depression, weakness, dyspnoea, bradycardia, heart block, bronchospasm and heart failure.

Thiazide diuretics may cause excessive depletion of fluid and electrolytes during prolonged or intense use. Symptoms are muscle pain or fatigue, thirst and oliguria. With thiazide diuretics hypokalaemia is more severe in patients already depleted of potassium, as in renal or hepatic insufficiency. Coma may be precipitated in hepatic cirrhosis.

The thiazides may induce hyperglycaemia and glycosuria in diabetic and other susceptible patients. The thiazides increase blood urea, which is most pronounced in patients with renal disease and pre-existing retention of nitrogen. Hyperuricaemia sometimes can occur.

Reports of other adverse reactions to the thiazides include skin rashes with associated photosensitivity,

necrotising vasculitis, acute pancreatitis, blood dyscrasias and aggravation of pre-existing myopia.

*Warning:* There have been reports of skin rashes and/or dry eyes associated with the use of beta-adrenergic blocking drugs. The reported incidence is small and in most cases the symptoms have cleared when treatment was withdrawn. Discontinuance of the drug should be considered if any such reaction is not otherwise explicable. Cessation of therapy with the beta-blocker should be gradual.

*Overdosage:* The most common signs of overdosage are bradycardia, hypotension, bronchospasm and acute cardiac failure. Suggested treatments are as follows:

*Severe bradycardia:* I.V. atropine sulphate 0.25–2 mg. If bradycardia persists, I.V. isoprenaline 25 micrograms may be given.

*Severe hypotension:* I.V. noradrenaline or adrenaline.

*Bronchospasm:* Isoprenaline hydrochloride, orciprenaline or salbutamol.

*Acute cardiac failure:* Digitalis, diuretics and oxygen. In refractory cases I.V. aminophylline and I.V. glucagon 0.5–1 mg have been reported useful.

General measures should be taken to restore blood volume, maintain blood pressure and correct electrolyte imbalance.

**Pharmaceutical precautions** Nil.

**Legal category** POM.

**Package quantities** Prestim: Glass bottles of 100 and 500 tablets.
Prestim Forte: Glass bottles of 100 tablets.

**Further information** Both constituents cross the placenta and appear in breast milk.

**Product licence numbers**
Prestim 0043/0047
Prestim Forte 0043/0084

## PUMP-HEP*
## Heparin for Continuous Infusion

**Presentation** Heparin (Mucous) Injection BP 1000 units/ml. Single dose ampoules of 20 ml, 10 ml or 5 ml containing 1,000 units sodium heparin per ml without preservative (i.e. 20,000, 10,000 or 5,000 units per ampoule respectively). Other ingredients: sodium chloride, sodium citrate and water for injections.

**Uses**
*Mode of action:* Heparin is a naturally occurring anticoagulant which prevents the coagulation of blood *in vivo* and *in vitro*. It potentiates the inhibition of several activated coagulation factors, including thrombin and factor X.

*Indications:* Treatment of thrombo-embolic disorders such as: deep vein thrombosis, acute arterial embolism or thrombosis, thrombophlebitis, pulmonary embolism, fat embolism.

**Dosage and administration** Pump-Hep may be used when heparin is being administered intravenously as an alternative to diluting heparin taken from multidose vials.

500 units/kg bodyweight daily or 5,000–10,000 units every 4 hours as a continuous infusion in sodium chloride injection or dextrose injection. The dose should be individually adjusted according to coagulation tests.

*Dosage adjustment:* It is recommended that the dosages be adjusted to maintain a thrombin clotting time, whole blood clotting time or activated partial thromboplastin time 1.5 to 2 times that of control on blood withdrawn 4–6 hours after commencement of infusion and at similar intervals until the patient is stabilised.

*Dosage in the elderly:* Lower dosages may be required, however, standard dosages should be given initially and then subsequent dosages and/or dosage intervals should be individually adjusted according to changes in thrombin clotting time, whole blood clotting time and/or activated partial thromboplastin time.

*Pregnancy:* Standard dosages should be given initially. Intermittent intravenous injections are not advised. Subsequent dosages and/or dosage intervals should be individually adjusted according to changes in thrombin clotting time, whole blood clotting time and/or activated partial thromboplastin time.

**Contra-indications, warnings, etc**
*Contra-indications:* Haemorrhagic disorders and patients with an actual or potential bleeding site, eg, peptic ulcer.

*Precautions:* Heparin therapy should be given with caution to patients with impaired renal or hepatic functions.

Oral anticoagulants or drugs which interfere with

platelet function, eg aspirin and dextran solutions should be administered with caution.

*Pregnancy and lactation:* Although animal studies have not been performed, epidemiological studies indicate that if drug therapy is needed in pregnancy, the use of heparin in the recommended dosage is acceptable. Heparin does not cross the placenta or appear in breast milk.

*Adverse reactions:* Hypersensitivity and acute thrombocytopenia may occur rarely. Osteoporosis and alopecia have been reported after prolonged therapy.

*Overdosage:* The effect of heparin can be reversed immediately by intravenous administration of a 1% protamine sulphate solution. The dose of protamine sulphate required for neutralisation should be determined accurately by titrating the patient's plasma.

It is important to avoid overdosage of protamine sulphate because protamine itself has anticoagulant properties. A single dose of protamine should never exceed 50 mg. Intravenous injection of protamine may cause a sudden fall in blood pressure, bradycardia, dyspnoea and transitory flushing, but these may be avoided or diminished by slow and careful administration.

**Pharmaceutical precautions** Store below 25˚C.

Heparin has been reported to be incompatible in aqueous solutions with certain substances, eg some antibiotics, hydrocortisone, phenothiazines, narcotic analgesics and some antihistamines.

**Legal category** POM.

**Package quantities** Packs of 10×20 ml ampoules; 10×10 ml ampoules; 10×5 ml ampoules.

**Further information** Nil.

**Product licence number** 0043/0149.

# UNIHEP* LEO 1,000
# UNIHEP* LEO 5,000
# UNIHEP* LEO 10,000
# UNIHEP* LEO 25,000

**Presentation**
*Unihep Leo 1,000:* Heparin (Mucous) Injection BP 1,000 units per ml. Single dose ampoules containing sodium heparin 1,000 units in 1 ml (no preservative). Other ingredients: sodium chloride, sodium citrate and water for injections.

*Unihep Leo 5,000:* Heparin (Mucous) Injection BP 5,000 units per ml. Single dose ampoules containing sodium heparin 5,000 units in 1 ml (no preservative). Other ingredients: water for injections.

*Unihep Leo 10,000:* Heparin (Mucous) Injection BP 10,000 units per ml. Single dose ampoules containing sodium heparin 10,000 units in 1 ml (no preservative). Other ingredients: water for injections.

*Unihep Leo 25,000:* Heparin (Mucous) Injection BP 25,000 units per ml. Single dose ampoules containing sodium heparin 25,000 units in 1 ml (no preservative). Other ingredients: water for injections.

**Uses**
*Mode of action:* Heparin is a naturally occurring anticoagulant which prevents the coagulation of blood *in vivo* and *in vitro*. It potentiates the inhibition of several activated coagulation factors, including thrombin and factor X.

*Indications:* Treatment of thromboembolic disorders such as: deep vein thrombosis, acute arterial embolism or thrombosis, thrombophlebitis, pulmonary embolism, fat embolism.

Prophylaxis against deep vein thrombosis and thromboembolic events in susceptible patients.

**Dosage and administration**
*Treatment dosage*
*Intravenous administration:* 5,000–10,000 units every 4 hours or 500 units/kg bodyweight daily as a continuous infusion in sodium chloride injection or dextrose injection. Doses should be individually adjusted according to coagulation tests.

*Subcutaneous administration:* The initial dose is 250 units/kg bodyweight. Further doses should be given every 12 hours and individually adjusted according to coagulation tests.

*Dosage adjustment:* It is recommended that dosages be adjusted to maintain a thrombin clotting time, whole blood clotting time or activated partial thromboplastin time 1.5 to 2 times that of control on blood withdrawn 4–6 hours after the first injection or commencement of infusion, and at similar intervals until the patient is stabilised.

*Prophylactic dosage*
Administration is by subcutaneous injection.

*Patients undergoing major elective surgery:* 5,000 units should be given 2 hours pre-operatively and then every 8–12 hours post-operatively for 10–14

days or until the patient is ambulant whichever is the longer.

*Following myocardial infarction:* 5,000 units should be given twice daily for 10 days or until the patient is mobile.

*Other patients:* 5,000 units should be given every 8–12 hours.

These standard prophylactic regimens do not require routine control.

*Dosage in children*
*Treatment dosage:* Standard treatment dosages should be given initially. Subsequent dosages and/or dosage intervals should be individually adjusted according to changes in thrombin clotting time, whole blood clotting time and/or activated partial thromboplastin time.

*Dosage in the elderly*
*Treatment dosage:* Lower treatment dosages may be required, however, standard treatment dosages should be given initially and then subsequent dosages and/or dosage intervals should be individually adjusted according to changes in thrombin clotting time, whole blood clotting time and/or activated partial thromboplastin time.

*Prophylactic dosage:* Dosage alterations are unnecessary for prophylaxis in the elderly.

*Pregnancy*
*Treatment dosage:* Standard treatment dosages should be given initially by continuous intravenous infusion or every 12 hours by subcutaneous injection. Intermittent intravenous injections are not advised. Subsequent dosages and/or dosage intervals should be individually adjusted according to changes in thrombin clotting time, whole blood clotting time and/or activated partial thromboplastin time.

*Prophylactic dosage:* It is recommended that plasma heparin levels be maintained below 0.4 units/ml, as determined by specific anti-Xa assay. A suggested dosage is 5,000 units every 12 hours in early pregnancy increasing to 10,000 units every 12 hours in the last trimester. The dosage should be reduced during labour and the standard prophylactic dosage is suitable in the puerperium.

**Contra-indications, warnings, etc**
*Contra-indications:* Haemorrhagic disorders and patients with an actual or potential bleeding site, e.g. peptic ulcer.

*Precautions:* Heparin therapy should be given with caution to patients with impaired renal or hepatic function.

Oral anticoagulants or drugs which interfere with platelet function, e.g. aspirin and dextran solutions should be administered with caution.

*Pregnancy and lactation:* Although studies have not been performed, epidemiological studies indicate that if drug therapy is needed in pregnancy, the use of heparin in the recommended dosage is acceptable. Heparin does not cross the placenta or appear in breast milk.

*Adverse reactions:* Hypersensitivity and acute reversible thrombocytopenia may occur rarely. Osteoporosis and alopecia have been reported after prolonged therapy.

*Overdosage:* The effect of heparin can be reversed immediately by intravenous administration of a 1% protamine sulphate solution. The dose of protamine sulphate required for neutralisation should be determined accurately by titrating with the patient's plasma.

It is important to avoid overdosage of protamine sulphate because protamine itself has anticoagulant properties. A single dose of protamine sulphate should never exceed 50 mg. Intravenous injection of protamine may cause a sudden fall in blood pressure, bradycardia, dyspnoea and transitory flushing but these may be avoided or diminished by slow and careful administration.

**Pharmaceutical precautions** Store below 25˚C. Heparin has been reported to be incompatible in aqueous solutions with certain substances, e.g. some antibiotics, hydrocortisone, phenothiazines, narcotic analgesics and some antihistamines.

**Legal category** POM.

**Package quantities**

| | |
|---|---|
| Unihep Leo 1,000: | Packs of 5×10 ampoules |
| Unihep Leo 5,000: | Packs of 5×10 ampoules |
| Unihep Leo 10,000: | Packs of 10 ampoules |
| Unihep Leo 25,000: | Packs of 10 ampoules |

**Further information** Nil.

**Product licence numbers**

| | |
|---|---|
| Unihep Leo 1,000 | 0043/0085 |
| Unihep Leo 5,000 | 0043/0086 |
| Unihep Leo 10,000 | 0043/0064 |
| Unihep Leo 25,000 | 0043/0087 |

# UROKINASE

**Presentation** Urokinase 5,000 and urokinase 25,000 are available in single vials containing 5,000 and 25,000 International Units (IU) of urokinase in a sterile, white, freeze-dried powder form. Excipients: Mannitol, disodium edetate, disodium hydrogen phosphate.

**Uses** Urokinase is an enzyme extracted from human adult male urine. As urokinase is of human origin, it is not antigenic in man.

*Mode of action:* Urokinase brings about the dissolution of blood clots by promoting the activation of plasminogen; the latter is the inactive precursor of plasmin, the proteolytic enzyme responsible for the breakdown of fibrin into small soluble peptides which are dispersible through the blood stream.

Urokinase is indicated for the lysis of clots in the following conditions:

(i) Thromboembolic occlusive vascular disease such as deep vein thrombosis (DVT), pulmonary embolism (PE) and peripheral vascular occlusion.

(ii) Hyphaema (haemorrhage into the anterior chamber of the eye).

(iii) Arterio-venous haemodialysis shunts and intravenous cannulae which are blocked by fibrin clots.

**Dosage and administration** Urokinase should be reconstituted with a small amount of sterile Water for Injections or saline and then further diluted with normal saline to the desired volume for administration.

*Adults:*
*(i) Thromboembolic occlusive vascular disease*
*Deep vein thrombosis:* A recommended dosage regimen consists of an initial loading dose of 4,400 IU/kg body weight in 15 ml solution, given over 10 minutes followed by an intravenous infusion of 4,400 IU/kg/hour for 12–24 hours.

*Pulmonary embolism:* A recommended dosage regimen consists of an initial loading dose of 4,400 IU/kg body weight in 15 ml solution, given over 10 minutes followed by an intravenous infusion of 4,400 IU/kg/hour for 12 hours.

Alternatively, a 50 ml bolus injection of urokinase into the pulmonary artery, repeated for up to 3 doses, at 24 hour intervals, has been employed. The initial dosage of 15,000 IU/kg/body weight may be adjusted if necessary for subsequent injections, dependent upon the plasma fibrinogen concentration produced by the previous injection.

*Peripheral vascular occlusion:* A recommended dosage regimen involves the infusion of a 2,500 IU/ml solution of urokinase (500,000 IU in 200 ml) into the clot, using angiography to monitor the progress of treatment. Urokinase should be infused into the clot at a dose rate of 4,000 IU/minute (96 ml/hr) for 2 hours followed by repeat angiography. The catheter is then advanced into the remaining occluded segment and urokinase infused at 4,000 IU/min for a further 2 hours; this may be repeated up to 4 times if antegrade flow has not occurred. After lysing a channel through the occlusion the catheter is withdrawn until it is proximal to the remaining clot lining the vessel wall. Urokinase is given at a dose rate of 1,000 IU/min (0.4 ml) until the clot has completely lysed. A dose of 500,000 IU given over approximately 8 hours should be sufficient to achieve this.

If the clot is not reduced in length by more than 25% after the initial infusion of 500,000 IU and by an incremental 10% by subsequent infusions of 500,000 IU, consideration should be given to discontinuation of treatment.

After fibrinolytic therapy has been completed, treatment may be continued with suitable anticoagulant therapy.

*(ii) Hyphaema:* When saline irrigation is unsuccessful in removing the blood clot, urokinase may be considered for the management of hyphaema, particularly when the clot completely fills the anterior chamber and there is an accompanying rise in intra-ocular pressure. The following general technique is used: an incision of about 3 mm is made inside the temporal limbus of the cornea. 5,000 IU urokinase is dissolved in Sodium Chloride Injection (2 ml) and drawn up into a syringe fitted with a suitable irrigator. The tip of the irrigator is introduced through the incision so as to be over the iris rather than the pupillary space (thus avoiding risk of damage to the lens), with the aperture directed towards the corneal endothelium or parallel to the plane of the iris. The solution is injected and withdrawn repeatedly with minimal pressure. Clot disintegration commonly begins within five minutes, facilitating injection of the solution and aspiration of the clot. The chamber is then washed out with saline. If residual clot remains, a small quantity of the solution (e.g. 0.3 ml) may be left in the anterior chamber to facilitate further dissolution of the clot over the next 24–48 hours.

*(iii) Clotted arterio-venous shunts:* Generally, 5,000–25,000 IU urokinase in 2–3 ml Sodium Chloride Injec-

tion is instilled into the affected limb of the shunt which is then clamped off for 2–4 hours. The lysate is then aspirated. This may be repeated if necessary. For the venous side an infusion of 5,000 IU in 200 ml, run in over 30 minutes, has been used but this may be less satisfactory than the use of more concentrated solutions.

*Dosage in the elderly:* Initially no dosage alterations are recommended, however, thereafter, the dosage should be adjusted as necessary, according to response.

*Dosage in children:* Initially no dosage alterations are recommended, however, thereafter, the dosage should be adjusted as necessary, according to response.

*Use in pregnancy:* The use of urokinase is contra-indicated in pregnancy and the immediate post-partum period.

*Monitoring of treatment:* The need for haematological monitoring arises only when urokinase is used systemically to induce a state of whole-body fibrinolysis (e.g. in the treatment of thromboembolic occlusion). Several tests may be needed to give an overall picture of the coagulation status, because there is no simple way of measuring an induced thrombolytic state.

Suitable tests include: measurement of euglobin lysis time, assay of thrombolytic state using [131]I-fibrinogen; assay for plasminogen and fibrinogen; measurements of thrombin clotting time; prothrombin time; platelet counts and detection of fibrin degradation products.

Local use of urokinase in 'closed situations' does not require haematological monitoring.

**Contra-indications, warnings, etc**

*Contra-indications:* Urokinase is contra-indicated in any situation where bleeding has occurred, or is likely to occur.

Recent surgery (including biopsy): administration of urokinase for thromboembolic occlusive vascular disease is not recommended for 72 hours following surgery because of the risk of bleeding from the operation site.

Severe hypertension (with systolic bp > 200 mmHg and/or diastolic bp > 120 mmHg): in patients with severe hypertension, administration of urokinase carries the risk of cerebral haemorrhage.

Pregnancy: Urokinase is contra-indicated in pregnancy and the immediate post-partum period.

Severe hepatic or renal insufficiency.

When used in 'local' situations, the above contra-indications may not be relevant.

*Warnings:* If bleeding occurs following systemic use, the infusion should be stopped immediately. However, this contra-indication is relative. The benefits of the continued use of urokinase must be weighed against the risks of stopping therapy, for example, in the situation where vascular occlusion can be life-threatening. For treatment of bleeding see 'Overdosage'.

When used in the eye, a normal gonioscopy result should be evident.

*Precautions:* Systemic urokinase should be used with caution in patients with gastrointestinal lesions such as peptic ulceration, which may be prone to haemorrhage, and in patients who have had multiple intracardiac and intravascular punctures as a consequence of cardio-pulmonary resuscitation.

*Interactions:* In glucose solution there is a measurable (< 10%) reduction in the activity of urokinase after 8 hours. Concomitant administration of dextran sulphate may prolong the activity of urokinase.

*Side-effects:* The following side-effects have been associated with urokinase use in the listed indications.
Hyphaema—none reported.

Arteriovenous shunts—warmth, initial severe pain and dull ache in shunt limb have been reported occasionally.

Thromboembolic occlusive vascular disease—overt bleeding, haemorrhagic complications may occur. Temporary increase in temperature (when a high yield of lysis degradation products are produced) and haematuria have been reported occasionally.

*Overdosage:* If severe haemorrhage occurs, treatment with urokinase must be stopped. Aprotinin and synthetic inhibitors such as epsilon-aminocaproic acid, tranexamic acid or p-aminomethylbenzoic acid can be used to inhibit the fibrinolytic action of urokinase. In serious cases, human fibrinogen, Factor XIII, Cohn-Fraction I, packed red cells or whole blood can be given, as appropriate.

**Pharmaceutical precautions** Urokinase in the lyophilised form should be stored below 25°C. When reconstituted, urokinase is stable for 24 hours when stored below 25°C.

**Legal category** POM.

**Package quantities** Single vials of 5,000 and 25,000 IU.

**Further information** Nil.

**Product licence numbers**
Urokinase 5,000 IU 3400/0001R
Urokinase 25,000 IU 3400/0026R
*Product licence holder:* Serono Laboratories (UK) Ltd.

*\*Trade Mark*

# Eli Lilly and Company Limited
## Kingsclere Road
## Basingstoke
## Hants. RG21 6XA

 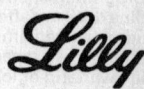

1996
THE QUEEN'S AWARD
FOR EXPORT ACHIEVEMENT

## AXID*

**Presentation** Capsules (pale yellow and dark yellow, coded 3144) containing 150 mg nizatidine INN.

Capsules (pale yellow and brown, coded 3145) containing 300 mg nizatidine INN.

**Uses** For the treatment of the following diseases where reduction of gastric acid is indicated: Duodenal ulcer; benign gastric ulcer; prevention of duodenal or benign gastric ulcer recurrence; gastric oesophageal reflux disease (including erosions, ulcerations and associated heartburn); gastric and/or duodenal ulcer associated with concomitant use of non-steroidal anti-inflammatory drugs.

**Dosage and administration** Axid is administered orally.

*Adults:* For treatment of duodenal ulcer, the recommended daily dose is 300 mg in the evening. Treatment should continue for four weeks, although this period may be reduced if healing is confirmed earlier by endoscopy. Most ulcers will heal within four weeks, but if complete ulcer healing has not occurred after four weeks therapy, patients should continue therapy for a further four weeks.

For the treatment of benign gastric ulcer, the recommended daily dose is 300 mg in the evening for four or, if necessary, eight weeks. Prior to treatment with nizatidine, care should be taken to exclude the possibility of gastric cancer.

If preferred, the 300 mg daily dose for the treatment of duodenal or benign gastric ulcer may be given as two divided doses of 150 mg in the morning and evening.

For the prevention of duodenal or benign gastric ulcer recurrence (prophylactic maintenance therapy) the recommended daily dose is 150 mg in the evening. Treatment may continue for up to one year.

For the treatment of gastric oesophageal reflux disease, the recommended dosage is from 150 mg twice daily, up to 300 mg twice daily. Therapy for up to 12 weeks is indicated for erosions and ulcerations, and associated heartburn.

For the treatment of gastric and/or duodenal ulcer associated with concomitant use of non-steroidal anti-inflammatory drugs, the recommended daily dose is 300 mg daily (either 300 mg at bedtime or 150 mg twice daily, in the morning and in the evening) for up to 8 weeks. In most patients, the ulcers will heal within 4 weeks. During treatment, the use of non-steroidal anti-inflammatory drugs may continue.

*The elderly:* Age does not significantly influence efficacy or safety. Normally dosage modification is not required except in patients who have moderate to severe renal impairment (creatinine clearance less than 50 ml/min).

*Children:* Not recommended, as safety and efficacy have not been established.

*Patients with impaired renal function:* Nizatidine is principally excreted via the kidneys.

For patients who have moderate renal impairment (creatinine clearance less than 50 ml/min) or patients who have severe renal impairment (creatinine clearance less than 20 ml/min), the dosage should be reduced as follows:

### DOSAGE RECOMMENDED

| No Renal Impairment | Moderate Renal Impairment (Reduce Dose By 50%) | Severe Renal Impairment (Reduce Dose By 75%) |
|---|---|---|
| 600 mg | 150 mg twice daily | 150 mg daily |
| 300 mg | 150 mg in the evening | 150 mg on alternate days |
| 150 mg | 150 mg on alternate days | 150 mg every third day |

**Contra-indications, warnings, etc**
*Contra-indication:* Known hypersensitivity to H₂-receptor antagonists.

*Warnings*

*Usage in pregnancy:* The safety of nizatidine for use during pregnancy has not been established. Animal studies have shown no evidence of impaired fertility or teratogenicity attributable to nizatidine. Nizatidine should only be used in pregnant women, or in those planning pregnancy, if considered absolutely necessary, and then with caution.

*Usage in lactation:* Studies conducted in lactating women have shown that 0.1% of the administered oral dose of nizatidine is secreted in human milk in proportion to plasma concentrations. Because of the growth depression in pups reared by lactating rats treated with nizatidine, Axid should be administered to nursing mothers only if considered absolutely necessary.

*Drug interactions:* There is evidence that nizatidine does not affect the serum levels of concomitantly administered aminophylline, theophylline, chlordiazepoxide, diazepam, lignocaine, phenytoin, ibuprofen, metoprolol, warfarin or lorazepam. Nizatidine does not inhibit the hepatic cytochrome P450-linked drug metabolising enzyme system, but may increase absorption of salicylates when they are used in very high dosage. Approximately 35 per cent of nizatidine is bound to plasma protein. Warfarin, diazepam, paracetamol, propantheline, phenobarbitone and propranolol did not affect plasma protein binding of nizatidine *in vitro*.

Absorption of nizatidine is not clinically significantly affected by food intake, anticholinergic agents or antacids.

*Precautions:* As nizatidine is partially metabolised by the liver and principally excreted by the kidneys, patients with impaired liver or kidney function should be treated with caution. (See *Dosage and administration* section.)

Symptomatic response to nizatidine therapy does not preclude the presence of gastric malignancy.

*Side-effects:* In large scale clinical trials, anaemia, sweating and urticaria were significantly more common in nizatidine treated patients when compared with placebo. In these trials, 1.9 per cent of treated patients experienced somnolence, compared to 1.6 per cent of placebo patients (non-significant).

In the same trials, patients treated with both nizatidine and placebo had mild, transient, asymptomatic elevations of transaminases or alkaline phosphatase; rare instances of marked elevations (>500 iu/l) occurred in nizatidine treated patients. The overall rate of occurrences of elevated liver enzymes and elevations to 3 times the upper limit of normal, however, did not differ significantly from placebo. All abnormalities were reversible after discontinuation of nizatidine. Since introduction hepatitis and jaundice have been reported. Rare cases of cholestatic or mixed hepatocellular and cholestatic injury with jaundice have been reported, with reversal of the abnormalities after discontinuation.

The following effects have also been rarely reported, although a causal relationship has not always been established: thrombocytopenic purpura, fatal thrombocytopenia, exfoliative dermatitis, vasculitis, gynaecomastia, impotence, hyperuricaemia, fever, nausea and reversible mental confusion.

Rare episodes of hypersensitivity reactions (e.g. bronchospasm, laryngeal oedema, rash, pruritus and eosinophilia), serum sickness and anaphylaxis have been reported.

*Overdosage:* There is little experience of overdose in humans. Tested at very high doses in animals, nizatidine has been shown to be relatively non-toxic. Animal studies suggest that cholinergic-type effects, including lacrimation, salivation, emesis, miosis and diarrhoea, may occur following very large oral doses. *Treatment:* Symptomatic and supportive therapy is recommended. Activated charcoal, emesis or lavage may reduce nizatidine absorption. The ability of haemodialysis to remove nizatidine from the body has not been conclusively demonstrated. However, this method is not expected to be efficient, since nizatidine has a large volume of distribution.

**Pharmaceutical precautions** Store below 25°C.

**Legal category** POM.

**Package quantities**
Capsules 150 mg: Blister packs of 30
Capsules 150 mg: Blister packs of 28 (hospitals only)
Capsules 300 mg: Blister packs of 30
Capsules 300 mg: Blister packs of 28 (hospitals only)

**Further information** Nizatidine is a potent, selective, competitive and fully reversible histamine H₂-receptor antagonist with a rapid onset of action. It significantly decreases acid concentration together with the volume of basal and stimulated gastric secretion. In clinical trials, nizatidine usually abolished ulcer pain within the first week of therapy. Nizatidine 300 mg at bedtime significantly reduced overnight gastric secretion, but did not increase subsequent basal or meal stimulated gastrin production. Intrinsic factor is not decreased in subjects administered nizatidine.

Nizatidine has no significant effect on the serum concentrations of gonadotrophins, prolactin, growth hormone, antidiuretic hormone, cortisol, tri-iodothyronine, thyroxine, testosterone, 5a-dihydrotestosterone, androstenedione or oestradiol.

Experience in clinical trials indicates that nizatidine has no greater potential than placebo for antiandrogenic effects.

**Product licence numbers**
Capsules 150 mg: 0006/0230
Capsules 300 mg: 0006/0231

## AXID* INJECTION

**Presentation** Ampoules containing 100 mg nizatidine in 4 ml.

Nizatidine solution is a clear and colourless to yellow liquid that tends to darken slightly. It has a pH of 6.5 to 7.5. Each 1 ml contains 25 mg nizatidine.

**Uses** Nizatidine injection is indicated in hospitalised patients as an alternative to the oral dosage form, for short-term use in peptic ulcer patients until oral medication is indicated.

For appropriate cases the oral dosage form, Axid capsules, is also available (see separate data sheet).

**Dosage and administration**
*Continuous intravenous infusion:* Dilute 300 mg (12 ml) in 150 ml of compatible i.v. solution and infuse the solution at a rate to achieve a dose of 10 mg/hr.

*Intermittent intravenous infusion:* Dilute 100 mg (4 ml) in 50 ml of compatible i.v. solution and infuse over a 15 minute period three times daily.

The total daily dose of nizatidine should not exceed 480 mg. To maintain gastric pH ≥4, a continuous infusion of 10 mg/hr is recommended. Nizatidine should not be given by rapid i.v. infusion.

Compatible solutions include 0.9% Sodium Chloride Intravenous Infusion BP, 5% Dextrose Intravenous Infusion BP, Compound Sodium Lactate Intravenous Infusion BP or 5% Sodium Bicarbonate Intravenous Infusion BP.

*The elderly:* Age does not significantly influence efficacy or safety. Normally dosage modification is not required except in patients who have moderate to severe renal impairment (creatinine clearance less than 50 ml/min).

*Children:* Not recommended, as safety and efficacy have not been established.

*Patients with impaired renal function:* Nizatidine is principally excreted via the kidneys. For patients with moderate renal impairment (creatinine clearance 20-50 ml/min), the dose should be reduced to 120-150 mg daily. For patients with severe renal impairment (creatinine clearance less than 20 ml/min), the dose should be reduced to 75 mg daily. The clinical effects of this dosage reduction, in patients with renal failure, have not been evaluated.

**Contra-indications, warnings, etc**
*Contra-indication:* Known hypersensitivity to H₂-receptor antagonists.

*Warnings*

*Usage in pregnancy:* The safety of nizatidine for use during pregnancy has not been established. Animal studies have shown no evidence of impaired fertility or teratogenicity attributable to nizatidine. Nizatidine should only be used in pregnant women, or in those planning pregnancy, if considered absolutely necessary, and then with caution.

*Usage in lactation:* Studies conducted in lactating women have shown that 0.1% of the administered oral dose of nizatidine is secreted in human milk in proportion to plasma concentrations. Because of the growth depression in pups reared by lactating rats treated with nizatidine, Axid should be administered to nursing mothers only if considered absolutely necessary.

*Drug interactions:* There is evidence that oral nizatidine does not affect the serum levels of concomitantly administered aminophylline, theophylline, chlordiazepoxide, diazepam, lignocaine, phenytoin, metoprolol, warfarin or lorazepam. Nizatidine does not inhibit the hepatic cytochrome P450-linked drug metabolising enzyme system, but may increase absorption of salicylates when they are used in very high dosage. Approximately 35 per cent of nizatidine is bound to plasma protein. Warfarin, diazepam, paracetamol, propantheline, phenobarbitone and propranolol did not affect plasma protein binding of nizatidine *in vitro.*

*Precautions:* As nizatidine is partially metabolised by the liver and principally excreted by the kidneys, patients with impaired liver or kidney function should be treated with caution. (See *Dosage and administration* section.)

Symptomatic response to nizatidine therapy does not preclude the presence of gastric malignancy.

*Side-effects:* Pain and minor bruising at the injection site were reported in clinical trials.

In large scale clinical trials, anaemia, sweating and urticaria were significantly more common in patients treated with oral nizatidine when compared with placebo. In these trials, 1.9 per cent of treated patients experienced somnolence, compared to 1.6 per cent of placebo patients (non-significant).

In the same trials, patients treated with both nizatidine and placebo had mild, transient, asymptomatic elevations of transaminases or alkaline phosphatase; rare instances of marked elevations (>500iu/l) occurred in nizatidine treated patients. The overall rate of occurrences of elevated liver enzymes and elevations to 3 times the upper limit of normal, however, did not differ significantly from placebo. All abnormalities were reversible after discontinuation of nizatidine. Since introduction hepatitis and jaundice have been reported. Rare cases of cholestatic or mixed hepatocellular and cholestatic injury with jaundice have been reported, with reversal of the abnormalities after discontinuation.

Intravenous nizatidine was not associated with abnormalities in liver test results.

Rare occurrences of tachycardia, bradycardia, postural hypotension and syncope were reported with rapid i.v. injection.

The following effects have also been rarely reported, although a causal relationship has not always been established: thrombocytopenic purpura, fatal thrombocytopenia, exfoliative dermatitis, vasculitis, gynaecomastia, impotence, hyperuricaemia, fever, nausea and reversible mental confusion.

Rare episodes of hypersensitivity reactions (e.g. bronchospasm, laryngeal oedema, rash, pruritus and eosinophilia), serum sickness and anaphylaxis have been reported.

*Overdosage:* There is little experience of overdose in humans. Tested at very high doses in animals, nizatidine has been shown to be relatively non-toxic. Animal studies suggest that cholinergic-type effects, including lacrimation, salivation, emesis, miosis and diarrhoea, may occur following very large oral doses.
*Treatment:* Symptomatic and supportive therapy is recommended. The ability of haemodialysis to remove nizatidine from the body has not been conclusively demonstrated. However, this method is not expected to be efficient, since nizatidine has a large volume of distribution.

**Pharmaceutical precautions**
*Unreconstituted ampoules:* Store below 25°C. Protect from light.

*Reconstituted ampoules:* Nizatidine injection is stable for 24 hours at 2–8°C when added to, or diluted with, an appropriate solution (see *Dosage and administration*). In accordance with recognised practices, infusion fluids containing nizatidine should not be used after this period.

Parenteral drug products should be inspected visually for particulate matter and discolouration before administration, whenever solution and container permit. Nizatidine injection tends to darken but this does not adversely affect potency.

**Legal category** POM.

**Package quantity** 100 mg ampoules in packs of 5.

**Further information** Nizatidine is a potent, selective, competitive and fully reversible histamine $H_2$-receptor antagonist with a rapid onset of action. It significantly decreases acid concentration together with the volume of basal and stimulated gastric secretion. Intrinsic factor is not decreased in subjects administered nizatidine.

Nizatidine has no significant effect on the serum concentrations of gonadotrophins, prolactin, growth hormone, antidiuretic hormone, cortisol, tri-iodothyronine, thyroxine, testosterone, 5a–dihydrotestosterone, androstenedione or oestradiol.

Experience in clinical trials indicates that nizatidine has no greater potential than placebo for antiandrogenic effects.

**Product licence number** 0006/0256.

## BRIETAL* Sodium

**Presentation** Brietal Sodium (methohexitone sodium for injection), in crystalline form, is supplied as follows: 500 mg (with anhydrous Sodium Carbonate BP 30 mg) in 50 ml rubber-stoppered vials.

**Uses**
*Action:* Methohexitone sodium is a rapid, ultrashort-acting barbiturate anaesthetic agent.

*Indications:* Brietal Sodium is an intravenous anaesthetic agent for the induction of anaesthesia. It is used alone for short surgical procedures, or in combination with other agents for more prolonged anaesthesia.

**Dosage and administration** Pre-anaesthetic medication is generally advisable. Brietal Sodium may be used with any recognised pre-anaesthetic medications, but the phenothiazines are less satisfactory than the combination of an opiate and a belladonna derivative.

This drug should be administered by persons qualified in the use of intravenous anaesthetics. Facilities for assisting respiration and administering oxygen are necessary adjuncts for intravenous anaesthesia. Since cardiorespiratory arrest may occur, patients should be observed carefully during and after use of Brietal Sodium. Resuscitative equipment (i.e. intubation and cardioversion equipment, oxygen, suction and a secure intravenous line) and personnel qualified in its use must be immediately available.

Brietal Sodium is administered by intravenous injection (not infusion), usually in a 1% solution (10 mg per ml). Higher concentrations markedly increase the incidence of muscular movements and irregularities in respiration and blood pressure. Higher concentrations should normally be avoided.

*Adults:* As an initial guide, an injection rate of 1 ml of a 1% solution (10 mg) in five seconds may be used – although a faster rate than this is preferred by some anaesthetists. The dose usually ranges between 5 and 12 ml (50–120 mg, with an average of about 70 mg), but it must be adjusted to the needs of the individual patient. The induction dose maintains unconsciousness for about five to seven minutes.

*The elderly:* Onset of anaesthesia may be slow due to sluggish circulation, therefore methohexitone should be injected slowly.

*Children:* The dose should be adjusted for age and/or weight. Doses of approximately 1 mg/kg are usually satisfactory.

*Maintenance:* Brietal Sodium is best used simply as an induction agent. If further injection for maintenance is needed the dose must be individualised; but, as a guide, 2–4 ml of a 1% solution (20 to 40 mg) every four to seven minutes may be used. Other parenteral agents, usually narcotic analgesics, are usually employed with methohexitone during longer procedures.

*Preparation of solutions:* The recommended diluent for Brietal Sodium is Water for Injections PhEur. Solutions may also be prepared in Sodium Chloride Intravenous Infusion BP or 5% Dextrose Intravenous Infusion BP. Brietal Sodium is not compatible with Compound Sodium Lactate Intravenous Infusion BP or diluents containing bacteriostats.

For a 1% solution (10 mg per ml) vial contents should be diluted as follows:
100 mg: Add 10 ml diluent.
500 mg: Add 50 ml diluent.

**Contra-indications, warnings, etc**
*Contra-indications:* Hypersensitivity to barbiturates. When general anaesthesia is contra–indicated, Brietal Sodium should not be used. Patients with latent or manifest porphyria should not receive barbiturates in any form.

*Warnings:* Because the liver is involved in demethylation and oxidation of methohexitone and because barbiturates may enhance pre-existing circulatory depression, severe hepatic dysfunction, severe cardiovascular instability, or a shock-like condition, may be reason for selecting another induction agent.

Methohexitone is not recommended for use in patients in status asthmaticus or in individuals with a history of epilepsy. Psychomotor seizures may be elicited in susceptible individuals.

*Danger of intra-arterial injection:* Unintended intra-arterial injection of barbiturate solutions may be followed by the production of platelet aggregates and thrombosis, starting in arterioles distal to the site of injection. The resulting necrosis may lead to gangrene, which may require amputation. The first sign in conscious patients may be a complaint of fiery burning that roughly follows the injected artery. If noted, the injection should be stopped immediately. *Transient* bleaching *may* or may not be noted very early. Blotchy cyanosis and dark discolouration may then be the first sign in anaesthetised patients. There is no established treatment, other than prevention. Animal experiments and published individual cases concerned with a variety of arteriolar irritants, including barbiturates, suggest that one or more of the following *may* be of benefit in reducing the area of necrosis: (a) arterial injection of heparin at the site of injury, followed by systemic anticoagulation; (b) sympathetic blockade (or brachial plexus blockade in the arm); (c) intra-arterial glucocorticoid injection at the site of injury, followed by systemic steroids; (d) a case report of non-barbiturate injury suggested that intra-arterial urokinase may promote fibrinolysis, even if administered late in treatment.

If extravasation occurs, the injection should be discontinued. Local irritation may result; subcutaneous swelling may also serve as a sign of arterial or periarterial placement of the catheter.

*Drug interactions:* Barbiturates may influence the absorption and elimination of other concomitantly used drugs, such as diphenylhydantoin, halothane, anticoagulants, corticosteroids, ethanol and propylene glycol-containing solutions.

The central nervous system depressant effect of methohexitone may be additive with that of other CNS depressants, including alcohol and antihistamines.

Prolonged administration may result in cumulative effects, including extended somnolence, protracted unconsciousness and respiratory and cardiovascular depression. Respiratory depression in the presence of an impaired airway may lead to hypoxia, cardiac arrest and death.

*Usage in pregnancy:* The safety of methohexitone sodium for use during pregnancy has not been established. Brietal Sodium should not be used in the pregnant patient unless, in the opinion of the clinician, the expected benefit outweighs the possible risk. Animal studies have shown no evidence of teratogenicity or of impaired fertility.

*Labour and delivery:* Methohexitone sodium has been used in caesarean section delivery but, because of its solubility, it readily and rapidly traverses the placenta and may therefore cause respiratory depression in the newly delivered baby. The obstetrician and paediatrician should be aware of this fact.

*Nursing mothers:* Caution should be exercised when methohexitone is administered to a nursing woman.

*Precautions:* Brietal Sodium should be administered only by persons who are experienced in general anaesthesia and who have appropriate equipment on hand for the prevention and treatment of anaesthetic emergencies. Respiratory depression, laryngospasm, apnoea, hypotension or cardiorespiratory arrest may occur owing to individual variations in tolerance or to the physical status of the patient. Caution should be exercised in debilitated patients, in those with severe anaemia or extreme obesity, or in those with impaired function of respiratory, circulatory, renal, hepatic or endocrine systems. It is essential that a free airway be maintained at all times. As with any potent anaesthetic agent, pulmonary ventilation should be maintained if prolonged apnoea occurs. Too rapid induction, inadequate dosage, or insufficient or unsuitable pre-anaesthetic medication may result in skeletal muscle hyperactivity, laryngospasm, cough, sneezing or hiccups. Hiccups, coughing and/or muscle twitching may also impair pulmonary ventilation.

Following induction, temporary hypotension and tachycardia may occur.

The patient's stomach should be empty. The usual pre-anaesthetic medications may be administered for the production of sedation and inhibition of secretions. If increased muscular relaxation is required for the performance of certain surgical procedures, it may be accomplished by the concomitant use of Brietal Sodium and skeletal muscle relaxants.

Postanaesthetic shivering may occur.

When appropriate, patients should be instructed as to the hazards of drowsiness that may follow use of methohexitone sodium. Outpatients should be released in the company of another individual, and no skilled activities, such as operating machinery or driving a motor vehicle, should be engaged in for at least 24 hours.

Liver function studies may be influenced by administration of a single dose of barbiturates.

Excretion occurs via the kidneys through glomerular filtration.

*Side-effects:* Side-effects associated with methohexitone sodium are extensions of pharmacological effects and include:
*Cardiovascular:* Circulatory depression, thrombophle-

bitis, hypotension, peripheral vascular collapse and convulsions in association with cardiorespiratory arrest.

*Respiratory:* Respiratory depression (including apnoea), cardiorespiratory arrest, laryngospasm, bronchospasm, hiccups and dyspnoea.

*Neurological:* Skeletal-muscle hyperactivity (twitching), injury to nerves adjacent to injection site, and seizures.

*Psychiatric:* Emergence delirium, restlessness and anxiety may occur, especially in the presence of postoperative pain.

*Gastro-intestinal:* Nausea, emesis and abdominal pain.

*Allergic:* Erythema, pruritus, urticaria and cases of anaphylaxis have been reported rarely.

*Other:* Other adverse reactions include pain at injection site, salivation, headache and rhinitis.

*Drug abuse and dependence:* Methohexitone sodium may be habit forming.

*Overdosage:* The onset of toxicity following an overdose of intravenously administered methohexitone will be within seconds. If methohexitone is administered rectally or is ingested, the onset of toxicity may be delayed. The manifestations include central nervous system depression, respiratory depression, hypotension, loss of peripheral vascular resistance, and muscular hyperactivity ranging from twitching to convulsive-like movements or actual convulsions. Other findings may include allergic reactions. Following massive exposure to any barbiturate, pulmonary oedema, circulatory collapse with loss of peripheral vascular tone, and cardiac arrest may occur.

*Management:* No specific antidote is known. Treatment consists of the usual life supporting measures.

**Pharmaceutical precautions** The pH of a 1% solution of Brietal Sodium is between 10 and 11. Owing to differences in pH, solutions of Brietal Sodium should not be mixed with acid solutions such as atropine sulphate, tubocurarine and succinylcholine chloride.

Do not use solvents containing bacteriostats, as these may cause precipitation.

Vials of Brietal Sodium should be stored below 25°C.

*After reconstitution:* Solutions of methohexitone sodium should be freshly prepared and used promptly. Reconstituted solutions are chemically stable at room temperature (15°–25°C) for 24 hours.

Parenteral drug products should be inspected visually for particulate matter and discolouration prior to administration, whenever solution and container permit.

**Legal category** POM.

**Package quantity**
500 mg in 50 ml vial:       Single vials.

**Further information** Nil.

**Product licence number**
500 mg:      0006/5051

# CEFUROXIME

**Qualitative and quantitative composition** Each vial contains, as the active ingredient, Cefuroxime Sodium for Injection equivalent to 250 mg, 750 mg or 1.5 g of cefuroxime.

**Pharmaceutical form** Vials containing an off-white to slightly yellow sterile powder for reconstitution for injection or infusion.

**Clinical particulars**

*Therapeutic indications:* Cefuroxime is indicated for the treatment of infections caused by susceptible strains of the designated micro-organisms, or before the infecting organism has been identified, in the diseases listed below.

*Respiratory tract infections,* for example, acute and chronic bronchitis, infected bronchiectasis, bacterial pneumonia, lung abscess and post operative chest infections.

*Ear, nose and throat infections,* for example, sinusitis, tonsillitis and pharyngitis.

*Urinary tract infections,* for example, acute and chronic pyelonephritis, cystitis and asymptomatic bacteriuria.

*Soft tissue infections,* for example, cellulitis, erysipelas, peritonitis and wound infections.

*Bone and joint infections,* for example, osteomyelitis and septic arthritis.

*Obstetric and gynaecological infections,* pelvic inflammatory disease.

*Gonorrhoea,* particularly if penicillin is unsuitable.

*Other infections,* including septicaemia and meningitis.

*Prophylaxis* against infection in abdominal, pelvic, orthopaedic, cardiac, pulmonary, oesophageal and vascular surgery where there is increased risk from infection.

*Posology and method of administration:* Usually cefuroxime is effective when administered alone, but when appropriate it may be used in combination with metronidazole or an aminoglycoside.

*General dosage:*
*Adults:* Many infections will respond to 750 mg three times daily by intramuscular or intravenous injection. For more severe infections this dose should be increased to 1.5 g three times daily intravenously. The frequency of dosage may be increased to six-hourly injections, intramuscular or intravenous, giving total daily doses of 3 g to 6 g.

*Infants and children:* Doses of 30 to 100 mg/kg/day given in three or four divided doses. A dose of 60 mg/kg/day will be appropriate for most infections.

*Neonates:* Doses of 30 to 100 mg/kg/day given in two or three divided doses. In the first weeks of life the serum half-life of cefuroxime can be three to five times that in adults.

*Gonorrhoea:* 1.5 g should be given as a single dose or as two 750 mg injections into different sites, eg, each buttock.

*Meningitis:* Cefuroxime therapy is suitable for sole therapy of bacterial meningitis due to sensitive strains. *Infants and children:* 200 to 240 mg/kg/day intravenously in three or four divided doses. This dosage may be reduced to 100 mg/kg/day after three days or when clinical improvement occurs.

*Neonates:* The initial dosage should be 100 mg/kg/day intravenously. This dosage may be reduced to 50 mg/kg/day after three days or when clinical improvement occurs.

*Adults:* 3 g intravenously every eight hours. No data is currently available to recommend a dose for intrathecal administration.

*Prophylaxis:* The usual dose is 1.5 g intravenously with induction of anaesthesia. For orthopaedic, pelvic and abdominal operations this may be followed with two 750 mg doses 8 and 16 hours later. For vascular, cardiac, oesophageal and pulmonary operations this may be supplemented with 750 mg intramuscularly three times a day for a further 24 to 48 hours.

In total joint replacement, 1.5 g cefuroxime powder may be mixed dry with each pack of methyl methacrylate cement polymer before adding the liquid monomer.

*Dosage in impaired renal function:* As cefuroxime is excreted by the kidneys, the dosage should be reduced to allow for slower excretion in patients with impaired renal function, once creatinine clearance falls below 20 ml/min, as follows.

| | |
|---|---|
| Marked impairment (creatinine clearance 10 to 20 ml/min) | 750 mg twice daily |
| Severe impairment (creatinine clearance of less than 10 ml/min)* | 750 mg once daily |
| Continuous peritoneal dialysis | 750 mg twice daily |
| Renal failure on continuous arteriovenous haemodialysis or high-flux haemofiltration in intensive therapy units | 750 mg twice daily |
| Low-flux haemofiltration | As for impaired renal function |

*For patients on haemodialysis, a further 750 mg should be given at the end of each dialysis session.

*Contra-indications:* Contra-indicated in patients hypersensitive to the cephalosporin group of antibiotics.

*Special warnings and precautions for use:* Cephalosporin antibiotics may, in general, be given safely to patients who are hypersensitive to penicillins, although cross-reactions have been reported. Special care is indicated in patients who have experienced an anaphylactic reaction to penicillin.

Cephalosporin antibiotics at high dosage should be given with caution to patients receiving potent diuretics or aminoglycosides, as these combinations are suspected of adversely affecting renal function. Clinical experience has shown that this is not likely to be a problem at the recommended dose levels.

*Interactions with other medicaments and other forms of interaction:* Concurrent administration of probenecid prolongs the excretion of cefuroxime and produces an elevated peak serum level.

*Interference with laboratory tests:* Slight interference may occur with the copper reduction methods (Fehling's, Benedict's) but this should not lead to false-positive results. Cefuroxime does not interfere with the enzyme based tests for glycosuria, or with the alkaline picrate method for creatinine. It is recommended that either the hexokinase or glucose oxidase methods are used for determination of blood/plasma glucose levels.

*Pregnancy and lactation:* Studies in animals revealed no evidence of embryopathic or teratogenic effects due to cefuroxime, but, as with all drugs, it should be used with caution during pregnancy.

Since cefuroxime is excreted in human milk, caution should be exercised when administering this antibiotic to a nursing mother.

*Effects on ability to drive and use machines:* Cefuroxime is not known to affect the ability to drive or use machines.

*Undesirable effects:* Cefuroxime is generally well tolerated. Adverse reactions have been infrequent, generally mild and transient.

*Hypersensitivity reactions:* Including skin rashes (maculopapular and urticarial), fever and, very rarely, anaphylaxis. As with any antibiotic, prolonged use may lead to overgrowth of non-susceptible organisms, eg, Candida.

*Gastro-intestinal disturbance:* Including, very rarely, pseudomembranous colitis, which has been reported with most broad spectrum antibiotics.

*Haematological:* A decrease in haemoglobin concentration, eosinophilia, leucopenia and neutropenia have been observed. Positive Coombs' test have been reported. As with other cephalosporins, thrombocytopenia has been reported rarely.

*Hepatic:* Transient rises in liver enzymes or serum bilirubin have been observed, particularly in patients with pre-existing liver disease, but there is no evidence of hepatic involvement.

*Renal:* There may be some variation in the results of biochemical tests or renal function, but these results do not appear to be of clinical significance.

*Other:* Transient pain may be experienced at the site of intramuscular injection. Occasionally thrombophlebitis may occur at the site of intravenous injection.

*Overdose:* Overdosage of cephalosporins can lead to cerebral irritation and seizures. With seizures the drug should be discontinued and appropriate anticonvulsive and supportive therapy administered. Serum levels of cefuroxime can be reduced by haemodialysis or peritoneal dialysis.

**Pharmacological properties**

*Pharmacodynamic properties:* Cefuroxime (cefuroxime sodium) is a semi-synthetic, broad spectrum cephalosporin antibiotic exerting its bactericidal action by inhibition of cell wall synthesis. This antibiotic is resistant to most beta-lactamases and is active against the following pathogens.

*Gram-negative: Haemophilus influenzae, Neisseria* spp (including *Neisseria gonorrhoeae*), *Escherichia coli, Klebsiella* spp (including *Klebsiella pneumoniae*), *Enterobacter* spp, *Bordetella pertussis, Salmonella* spp (including *Salmonella typhi* and *Salmonella typhimurium*), *Shigella* spp, *Proteus mirabilis, Proteus rettgeri, Proteus vulgaris, Morganella morganii* (formerly *Proteus morganii*).

*Gram-positive: Staphylococcus aureus* (including strains resistant to penicillin), *Staphylococcus epidermidis* and certain strains of streptococci, e.g. *Streptococcus pyogenes* and *Streptococcus mitis* (viridans group).

*Anaerobic organisms: Clostridium* spp, *Bacteroides fragilis.*

*Resistant strains: Pseudomonas* and *Campylobacter* spp, *Acinetobacter calcoaceticus, Clostridium difficile, Legionella* spp and methicillin-resistant strains of *Staphylococcus aureus* and *Staphylococcus epidermidis.* Some strains of *Streptococcus faecalis, Morganella morganii, Proteus vulgaris, Bacteroides fragilis, Serratia* spp, *Enterobacter* spp and *Citrobacter* spp.

*In vitro* the activities of cefuroxime and aminoglycoside antibiotics in combination have been shown to be at least additive with occasional evidence of synergy.

*Pharmacokinetic properties:* The serum half-life after either intramuscular or intravenous administration is approximately 70 minutes. After intramuscular injection the peak serum level occurs after about 45 minutes.

The antibiotic can be found in bone, synovial fluid and aqueous humour above the minimum inhibitory levels for common pathogens. The blood-brain barrier can be passed by cefuroxime when the meninges are inflamed.

Cefuroxime is excreted approximately 50% by glomerular filtration and 50% through the renal tubules. Cefuroxime is almost completely recovered unchanged in the urine within 24 hours, most being excreted within six hours.

*Preclinical safety data:* There is no experimental evidence of embryopathic or teratogenic effects attributable to cefuroxime.

**Pharmaceutical particulars**

*List of excipients:* Each vial contains only the active ingredient, cefuroxime sodium.

*Incompatibilities:* Cefuroxime should not be mixed in the syringe with aminoglycoside antibiotics.

*Shelf life:*
*Before reconstitution:* 18 months when stored below 25°C.

In keeping with good pharmaceutical practice, freshly constituted suspensions or solutions should be used immediately. If this is not practicable then solution may be stored for up to 24 hours under refrigerated conditions (2-8°C).

*Special precautions for storage:* Protect from light. Before reconstitution store below 25°C. After reconstitution the product may be stored in a refrigerator for up to 24 hours.

*Nature and contents of container:* Type III flint glass vial, stoppered with halobutyl closures and sealed with aluminium seals that may be combined with a polypropylene cap.

*Package quantities:*
Vials 250 mg: Single vials
Vials 750 mg: Single vials
Vials 1.5 g: Single vials

*Instructions for use/handling:*
*Intramuscular injection:* Add 1 ml of Water for Injections to 250 mg or 3 ml of Water for Injections to 750 mg. Shake gently to produce a suspension.

*Intravenous administration:* Dissolve cefuroxime in Water for Injections using at least 2 ml for 250 mg, at least 6 ml for 750 mg and at least 15 ml for 1.5 g. For short intravenous infusion, 1.5 g may be dissolved in 50 ml of Water for Injections. Reconstituted solutions may be diluted with:
   5% or 10% Dextrose
   5% Dextrose containing 0.2%, 0.225%, 0.45% or 0.9% Sodium Chloride Injection
   5% Dextrose containing 20 mEq Potassium Chloride
   0.9% Sodium Chloride Injection
   M/6 Sodium Lactate Injection
   Ringer's Injection
   Lactated Ringer's Injection
   Heparin (10 and 50 units/ml) in 0.9% Sodium Chloride Injection
   10 mEq Potassium Chloride in 0.9% Sodium Chloride Injection
These solutions may be given directly into a vein or introduced into the tubing of the giving set if the patient is receiving parenteral fluids.

**Marketing authorisation numbers**
Cefuroxime Sodium for Injection      0006/0318
250 mg
Cefuroxime Sodium for Injection      0006/0332
750 mg
Cefuroxime Sodium for Injection      0006/0333
1.5 g

**Date of approval/revision of SPC**   28 January 1997

**Legal category**  POM

## CELANCE*

**Presentation**  Tablets (ivory, modified rectangle shaped, scored, marked Lilly 4131) containing 50 micrograms pergolide base.

Tablets (green, modified rectangle shaped, scored, marked Lilly 4133) containing 250 micrograms pergolide base.

Tablets (pink, modified rectangle shaped, scored, marked Lilly 4135) containing 1000 micrograms pergolide base.

**Uses**  Pergolide mesylate is indicated as adjunctive treatment to levodopa in the management of the signs and symptoms of Parkinson's disease. Pergolide mesylate is a dopamine receptor agonist at both $D_1$ and $D_2$ receptor sites.

**Dosage and administration**  For oral administration to adults only.

Administration of pergolide mesylate should be initiated with a daily dosage of 50 micrograms for the first 2 days. The dosage should then be gradually increased by 100 or 150 micrograms/day every third day over the next 12 days of therapy. The dosage may then be increased by 250 micrograms/day every third day until an optimal therapeutic dosage is achieved.

Pergolide mesylate is usually administered in divided doses 3 times per day. During dosage titration, the dosage of concurrent *l*-dopa may be cautiously decreased.

In clinical studies, the mean therapeutic daily dosage of pergolide mesylate was 3 mg/day (3000 micrograms/day). The average concurrent daily dosage of *l*-dopa/carbidopa (expressed as *l*-dopa) was approximately 650 mg/day. The efficacy of pergolide mesylate at doses above 5 mg/day (5000 micrograms/day) has not been systematically evaluated.

*Children:* Safety and effectiveness have not been established.

The major route of excretion is via the kidney.

**Contra-indications, warnings, etc**
*Contra-indication:* Hypersensitivity to this drug or other ergot derivatives.

*Warnings:* Patients should be warned to begin therapy with low doses and to increase dosage in carefully adjusted increments over a period of 3 to 4 weeks (see *Dosage and administration*) to minimise the risk of symptomatic postural and/or sustained hypotension. With gradual dosage titration, tolerance to the hypotension usually develops (but see *Drug interactions*).

In controlled trials, pergolide mesylate with *l*-dopa caused hallucinosis in about 14 per cent of patients, as opposed to 3 per cent taking placebo with *l*-dopa. This was of sufficient severity to cause discontinuation of treatment in about 3 per cent of those enrolled. Tolerance to this untoward effect was not observed.

In the placebo-controlled trial, 2 of 187 patients treated with placebo died, as compared with 1 of 189 patients treated with pergolide mesylate. Of the 2299 patients treated with pergolide mesylate in pre-marketing studies evaluated in October 1988, 6.2 per cent died while on the drug or shortly after discontinuation. The patient population under evaluation was elderly, ill and at high risk for death. A case-by-case review of the patients who died failed to disclose any unique set of signs, symptoms, or laboratory results that would suggest that treatment with pergolide caused these deaths.

Caution should be exercised when administering to patients prone to cardiac dysrhythmias or with significant underlying cardiac disease.

In a placebo-controlled study, patients taking pergolide mesylate had significantly more episodes of atrial premature contractions (APCs) and sinus tachycardia.

Pergolide should be used with caution in patients with a history of pleuritis, pleural effusion, pleural fibrosis, pericarditis, pericardial effusion, retroperitoneal fibrosis or similar conditions which may have occurred in association with the use of ergot derivatives. There have been rare reports of these conditions in patients receiving pergolide, and in some cases there had been similar events during prior exposure to bromocriptine. Patients with a history of such events should be carefully monitored clinically and with appropriate radiographic and laboratory studies whilst taking pergolide.

*Precautions:* Use in patients on *l*-dopa may cause and/or exacerbate pre-existing states of confusion and hallucinations (see *Warnings*). Abrupt discontinuation of pergolide mesylate, in patients receiving it chronically as an adjunct to *l*-dopa, may precipitate the onset of hallucinations and confusion; these may occur within a span of several days. Discontinuation of pergolide should be undertaken gradually, even if the patient is to remain on *l*-dopa.

Administration to patients receiving *l*-dopa may cause and/or exacerbate pre-existing dyskinesia.

Patients and their families should be informed of the common adverse consequences of the use of pergolide mesylate and the risk of hypotension.

Patients should be advised to tell their doctor if they become pregnant or intend to become pregnant during therapy. They should also tell their doctor if they are breast feeding.

No specific laboratory tests are essential for the management of patients. Periodic routine evaluation is appropriate.

*Drug interactions:* Dopamine antagonists, such as the neuroleptics (phenothiazines, butyrophenones, thioxanthines) or metoclopramide, ordinarily should not be administered concurrently with pergolide mesylate (a dopamine agonist); these agents may diminish the effectiveness of pergolide mesylate.

Because pergolide mesylate is approximately 90 per cent associated with plasma proteins, caution should be exercised if it is co-administered with other drugs known to affect protein binding.

There are no studies involving the concomitant administration of pergolide and warfarin. When these two drugs are co-prescribed, careful monitoring of anticoagulation should be performed, with adjustments of dosage as necessary.

Because of the risk of postural and/or sustained hypotension in patients taking pergolide, caution should be exercised if it is co-administered with antihypertensive agents.

*Carcinogenesis, mutagenesis and impairment of fertility:* Two year carcinogenicity studies in mice and rats used doses up to 340 and 12 times the maximum human oral dose (6 mg or 6000 micrograms/day equivalent to 120 micrograms/kg/day). A low incidence of uterine neoplasms occurred in both rats and mice. Endometrial adenomas and carcinomas were observed in rats. Endometrial sarcomas were observed in mice. These occurrences are probably attributable to the high oestrogen/progesterone ratio, which would occur in rodents as a result of the prolactin-inhibiting action of pergolide mesylate.

These endocrine mechanisms are not present in humans. However, there are no human data with pergolide to substantiate this conclusion concerning the lack of potential for human risk.

Mutagenic potential was evaluated in a battery of tests. A weak response was noted in one test but the other three tests were negative. The relevance to humans is unknown.

Impaired fertility was observed in mice at the highest dose (5.6 mg or 5600 micrograms/kg/day). This may be related to depressed prolactin levels.

*Pregnancy:* In animal studies there was no evidence of harm to the foetus due to pergolide mesylate. There are, however, no adequate and well-controlled studies in pregnant women. In pre-marketing studies there were 33 pregnancies that resulted in healthy babies and 6 pregnancies that resulted in congenital abnormalities, although a causal relationship has not been established. This drug should be used during pregnancy only if clearly needed.

*Nursing mothers:* It is not known whether pergolide is excreted in human milk. The pharmacological action of pergolide mesylate suggests it may interfere with lactation. A decision should be made whether to discontinue nursing or the drug, taking into account the importance of the drug to the mother.

*Side-effects:* The following adverse events, which are listed in decreasing order of frequency under body system, were observed during placebo-controlled clinical trials at a frequency of one per cent or greater and at a significantly higher incidence than placebo (*P* value ≤0.05):
   *Body as a whole:* Pain, abdominal pain.
   *Digestive system:* Nausea, dyspepsia.
   *Nervous system:* Dyskinesia, hallucinations, somnolence.
   *Respiratory system:* Rhinitis, dyspnoea. Following market introduction, there have been reports of cases of serosal inflammatory conditions, such as pleuritis, pleural effusion, pleural fibrosis, pericarditis, pericardial effusion and retroperitoneal fibrosis, in patients taking pergolide (see 'Warnings').
   *Special senses:* Diplopia.

Other events that have been reported include insomnia, confusion, dizziness, constipation, diarrhoea, abnormal liver function tests, orthostatic hypotension, syncope, atrial premature contractions, sinus tachycardia, rash and fever.

The more common events that caused discontinuation were related to the nervous system, primarily hallucinations and confusion.

Rare post-marketing spontaneous reports of neuroleptic malignant syndrome have been received but no clear causal relationship with the drug has been established.

*Overdosage:* There is no clinical experience with massive overdosage. Overdoses of 60 mg on one day, 19 mg/day for 3 days, or 14 mg/day for 23 days have occurred. Symptoms and signs included vomiting, hypotension, agitation, severe hallucinations, severe involuntary movements and tingling sensations. Another patient who inadvertently received 7 mg, instead of the prescribed 0.7 mg (700 micrograms), experienced palpitations, hypotension and ventricular extrasystoles. The highest daily dose (prescribed for several patients with refractory Parkinson's disease) has exceeded 30 mg.

In animals, manifestations of overdosage include nausea, vomiting, convulsions, decreased blood pressure and CNS stimulation.

*Treatment:* Symptomatic supportive therapy and cardiac monitoring is recommended.

Arterial blood pressure should be maintained. An antiarrhythmic agent may be necessary. If signs of CNS stimulation are present, a phenothiazine, or other butyrophenone neuroleptic agent, may be indicated.

Activated charcoal may be considered instead of, or in addition to, gastric emptying.

Dialysis or haemoperfusion are unlikely to be of benefit.

**Pharmaceutical precautions**  Store at room temperature.

**Legal category**  POM.

**Package quantities**
Tablets 50 micrograms:      Blister packs of 100.
Tablets 250 micrograms:     Blister packs of 100.
Tablets 1000 micrograms:    Blister packs of 100.
Starter packs of 75 × 50 microgram tablets and 6 × 250 microgram tablets.

**Further information**  Nil.

**Product licence numbers**
Tablets 50 micrograms:      0006/0250
Tablets 250 micrograms:     0006/0251
Tablets 1000 micrograms:    0006/0252

## CINOBAC*

**Presentation**  Capsules (green and orange, coded 3056) containing 500 mg (1.9 mmol) cinoxacin.

**Uses** Cinoxacin, a quinolone, has *in vitro* activity against many gram-negative aerobic bacteria, particularly strains of *Enterobacteriaceae.* Cinoxacin inhibits bacterial DNA synthesis, is bactericidal, and is active across the entire urinary pH range.

Cinoxacin is indicated for acute, recurrent and chronic upper and lower urinary tract infections (including cystitis, pyelonephritis or pyelitis and asymptomatic bacteriuria) caused by susceptible micro-organisms.

A single dose of 500 mg, taken at bedtime, for up to 5 months, has been shown to be effective as preventive therapy in women with a history of recurrent urinary tract infections.

Cinoxacin is active against most strains of the following organisms: *Enterobacter* spp. (including *Ent. aerogenes, Ent. cloacae* and *Ent. hafniae), Escherichia coli, Klebsiella* spp., *Proteus mirabilis,* and *Pr. vulgaris.*

Cinoxacin is also active against approximately 50 per cent of strains of *Pr. rettgeri, Providencia* and *Serratia* species.

*In vitro* susceptibility testing should be performed prior to administration of the drug and, when clinically indicated, during treatment.

Using NCCLS recommended methods for sensitivity testing, the criteria for dilution methods are:

MIC ≤ 16 micrograms/ml: susceptible
MIC = 32 micrograms/ml: intermediate
MIC ≥ 64 micrograms/ml: resistant.

Standard cinoxacin powder should give an MIC range of 2.0–8.0 micrograms/ml with *E. coli* ATCC 25922.

For the standard disc test using a 100 microgram cinoxacin disc, zone diameters are:

Zone ≥ 19 mm: susceptible
Zone 15–18 mm: intermediate
Zone ≤ 14 mm: resistant.

Certain strains of *Enterobacteriaceae* exhibit heterogeneity of resistance to cinoxacin by producing isolated colonies within the inhibition zone. The clear inhibition zone should be measured within such isolated colonies.

The 100 microgram disc should give a 26–32 mm zone diameter with *E. coli* ATCC 25922. Other quinolone discs should not be substituted.

*Enterococcus* species, *Pseudomonas* species and *Staphylococcus* species are resistant.

Cross-resistance with nalidixic acid has been demonstrated. Conventional chromosomal resistance to cinoxacin taken at recommended doses has been reported to emerge in approximately 4 per cent of patients during treatment. However, bacterial resistance to cinoxacin has not been shown to be transferable via R factor.

**Dosage and administration** The usual adult dose is 1 g daily, administered orally as 500 mg b.d. for seven to fourteen days.

For prophylactic use, a single dose of 500 mg daily, taken at bedtime.

Not recommended for use in children, and growing adolescents, under the age of 18 years.

*The elderly:* As for adults, unless renal function is impaired (see *Precautions*).

*Renal impairment:* A reduced dosage must be employed. After an initial dose of 500 mg, use the following maintenance dose schedule:

| Renal Function | Dosage |
|---|---|
| Moderate impairment | 500 mg once daily |
| Marked impairment (creatinine clearance < 20 ml/min/1.73m²) | Not recommended |

Cinoxacin may be taken with or without meals.

**Contra-indications, warnings, etc**
*Contra-indication:* Hypersensitivity to cinoxacin or other quinolones.

*Warnings:* Since cinoxacin, like other quinolones, causes arthropathy in immature animals, its use during pregnancy or for children, and growing adolescents, under 18 years of age is not recommended.

*Usage in pregnancy or lactation:* Cinoxacin should not be administered during pregnancy or to the nursing mother unless the potential benefit justifies the potential risk to the foetus or infant. Reproduction studies in rats and rabbits, at doses up to 10 times the daily human dose, have revealed no evidence of impaired fertility or harm to the foetus. However, there are no well controlled studies in pregnant women. It is not known whether cinoxacin is excreted in human milk.

Convulsions and abnormal electroencephalograms have been reported with quinolones, although no causal relationship has been established. Convulsions, increased intracranial pressure, toxic psychoses and CNS stimulation (tremors, restlessness, lightheadedness, confusion and hallucinations) have been reported with other quinolones. Cinoxacin should be used with caution in patients with CNS disorders,

such as severe cerebral arteriosclerosis, epilepsy, or other factors that predispose to seizures. If such reactions occur discontinue treatment and give appropriate therapy.

Serious and, occasionally, fatal hypersensitivity (anaphylactoid) reactions, some following the first dose, have been reported in patients during quinolone therapy. Some reactions were accompanied by cardiovascular collapse, loss of consciousness, tingling, pharyngeal and facial oedema, dyspnoea, urticaria and itching. Only a few patients had a history of hypersensitivity reactions. If an allergic reaction or skin rash occurs, discontinue the drug. Appropriate supportive therapy is recommended.

*Precautions:* Since cinoxacin is eliminated primarily by the kidney, dosage should be reduced in patients with reduced renal function (see 'Dosage and Administration'). Administration of cinoxacin is not recommended for patients with severely impaired renal function (creatinine clearance < 20 ml/min/1.73 m²). Although crystalluria is not expected to occur with the usually recommended dosages of cinoxacin, patients should be well hydrated and alkalinisation of the urine should be avoided. Patients should be advised to drink fluids liberally.

Moderate to severe phototoxicity reactions have been observed in patients who were exposed to direct sunlight while receiving some quinolones. Patients should be advised to avoid excessive sunlight. Discontinue the drug if phototoxicity occurs.

Since cinoxacin can cause dizziness and lightheadedness, patients should be sure they are not adversely affected before driving, operating machinery, or engaging in other activities requiring mental alertness or co-ordination.

Periodic assessment of renal, hepatic and haematopoietic function is advisable during prolonged therapy.

*Drug interactions:* Cinoxacin may enhance the effects of oral anticoagulants, such as warfarin. When concomitant administration cannot be avoided, daily coagulation tests are essential.

Elevated plasma levels of theophylline and theophylline-related side-effects have been reported with concomitant quinolone use. Therefore, the monitoring of theophylline plasma levels should be considered, and theophylline dosage adjusted as required.

Quinolones have been shown to reduce the clearance of caffeine and prolong caffeine's half-life.

Antacids or sucralfate interfere with the absorption of some quinolones, resulting in low urine levels. Concomitant administration of quinolones, with products containing iron or multi vitamins containing zinc, may also result in low urine levels.

Elevated cyclosporin serum levels have been reported with the concomitant use of quinolones and cyclosporin.

Seizures have been reported in patients taking another quinolone antimicrobial and fenbufen concurrently.

*Side-effects:* The most frequently reported adverse events in postmarketing surveillance have been nausea, hypersensitivity reactions, headache and dizziness.

*Gastro-intestinal:* Nausea, anorexia, vomiting, abdominal cramps, perverse taste and diarrhoea have been reported.

*Hypersensitivity:* Rash, pruritus, urticaria, oedema, angio-oedema and eosinophilia. Anaphylaxis, anaphylactoid reactions and toxic epidermal necrolysis have been reported rarely. Erythema multiforme, and Stevens-Johnson syndrome.

*Haematological:* Thrombocytopenia has been reported rarely.

*Nervous system:* Dizziness, headache, insomnia, drowsiness, tingling sensation, perineal burning, photophobia and tinnitus.

*Laboratory values:* Transient changes in blood urea, AST, ALT, serum creatinine and alkaline phosphatase have been observed occasionally. Reduction in haematocrit/haemoglobin.

Although not observed in clinical studies of cinoxacin involving 1,118 patients, the following side-effects have been reported for drugs in the same class: restlessness, nervousness, change in colour perception, difficulty in focusing, decrease in visual acuity, double vision, weakness, constipation, erythema and bullae, disorientation, agitation, acute anxiety, palpitation, gum soreness, joint stiffness, swelling of extremities, toxic psychoses or, rarely, convulsions.

*Overdosage*
*Signs and symptoms:* May include anorexia, nausea, vomiting, epigastric distress and diarrhoea. The severity of epigastric distress and diarrhoea are dose related. Headache, dizziness, insomnia, photophobia, tinnitus and tingling sensation have also been reported.

*Treatment:* Patients should be kept well hydrated to prevent crystalluria. Symptomatic and supportive therapy is recommended. Activated charcoal should

be considered instead of, or in addition to, gastric emptying. Forced diuresis, peritoneal dialysis, haemodialysis, or charcoal haemoperfusion have not been established as beneficial.

**Pharmaceutical precautions** Store at room temperature (15°–25°C).

**Legal category** POM.

**Package quantity** Blister pack of 14.

**Further information** Nil.

**Product licence number** 0006/0124.

# CYCLOSERINE

**Qualitative and quantitative composition** Each capsule contains as active ingredient 250 mg of cycloserine.

**Pharmaceutical form** Capsules, red and grey, coded F04.

**Clinical particulars**
*Therapeutic indications:*
*Actions:* Cycloserine inhibits cell wall synthesis in susceptible strains of Gram-positive and Gram-negative bacteria and in *Mycobacterium tuberculosis.*

*Indications:* Cycloserine is indicated in the treatment of active pulmonary and extra-pulmonary tuberculosis (including renal disease) when the organisms are susceptible to this drug and after failure of adequate treatment with the primary medications (streptomycin, isoniazid, rifampicin and ethambutol). Like all anti-tuberculous drugs, cycloserine should be administered in conjunction with other effective chemotherapy and not as the sole therapeutic agent.

Cycloserine may be effective in the treatment of acute urinary tract infections caused by susceptible strains of Gram-positive and Gram-negative bacteria, especially *Klebsiella/Enterobacter* species and *Escherichia coli.* It is generally no more and may be less effective than other antimicrobial agents in the treatment of urinary tract infections caused by bacteria other than mycobacteria. Use of cycloserine in these infections should be considered only when the more conventional therapy has failed and when the organism has been demonstrated to be sensitive to the drug.

*Posology and method of administration:*
*Adults:* The usual dosage is 500 mg to 1 g daily in divided doses, monitored by blood level determinations. The initial adult dosage most frequently given is 250 mg twice daily at 12-hour intervals for the first two weeks. A daily dosage of 1 g should not be exceeded.

*Children:* The usual starting dose is 10 mg/kg/day, then adjusted according to blood levels obtained and therapeutic response.

*The elderly:* As for adults but reduce dosage if renal function is impaired.

*Contra-indications:* Cycloserine is contra-indicated in the presence of any of the following: hypersensitivity to cycloserine; epilepsy; depression, severe anxiety or psychosis; severe renal insufficiency; alcohol abuse.

*Special warnings and special precautions for use:* Administration of cycloserine should be discontinued or the dosage reduced if the patient develops allergic dermatitis or symptoms of central nervous system toxicity such as convulsions, psychosis, somnolence, depression, confusion, hyper-reflexia, headache, tremor, vertigo, paresis or dysarthria.

Toxicity is usually associated with blood levels of greater than 30 mg/l, which may be the result of high dosage or inadequate renal clearance. The therapeutic index for this drug is low. The risk of convulsions is increased in chronic alcoholics (see below).

Patients should be monitored by haematological, renal excretion, blood level and liver function studies.

Before treatment with cycloserine is begun, cultures should be taken and the susceptibility of the organism to the drug should be established. In tuberculous infections, sensitivity to the other anti-tuberculous agents in the regimen should also be demonstrated.

Blood levels should be determined at least weekly for patients having reduced renal function, for individuals receiving a daily dosage of more than 500 mg, and for those showing signs and symptoms suggestive of toxicity. The dosage should be adjusted to keep the blood level below 30 mg/l.

Anticonvulsant drugs or sedatives may be effective in controlling symptoms of central nervous system toxicity, such as convulsions, anxiety or tremor. Patients receiving more than 500 mg of cycloserine daily should be closely observed for such symptoms. The value of pyridoxine in preventing CNS toxicity from cycloserine has not been proved.

Administration of cycloserine and other anti-tuberculous drugs has been associated in a few instances with vitamin B$_{12}$ and/or folic acid deficiency, megaloblastic anaemia and sideroblastic anaemia. If evidence of anaemia develops during treatment, appropriate investigations and treatment should be carried out.

*Interaction with other medicaments and other forms of interaction:*
*Drug interactions:* Concurrent administration of ethionamide has been reported to potentiate neurotoxic side-effects. Alcohol and cycloserine are incompatible, especially during a regimen calling for large doses of the latter. Alcohol increases the possibility and risk of epileptic episodes. Patients receiving cycloserine and isoniazid should be monitored for signs of CNS toxicity, such as dizziness and drowsiness, as these drugs have a combined toxic action on the CNS. Dosage adjustments may be necessary.

*Pregnancy and lactation:*
*Usage in pregnancy:* Concentrations in fetal blood approach those found in the serum. A study in 2 generations of rats given doses up to 100 mg/kg/day demonstrated no teratogenic effect in offspring. It is not known whether cycloserine can cause fetal harm when administered to a pregnant woman or can affect reproduction capacity. Cycloserine should be given to a pregnant woman only if clearly needed.
*Usage in nursing mothers:* Concentrations in the mother's milk approach those found in the serum. A decision should be made whether to discontinue nursing or to discontinue the drug, taking into account the importance of the drug to the mother.

*Effects on ability to drive and use machines:* None known.

*Undesirable effects:* Most side-effects occurring during treatment with cycloserine involve the nervous system or are manifestations of drug hypersensitivity. The following side-effects have been observed: nervous system manifestations, which appear to be related to higher dosages of drug, ie, more than 500 mg daily, can be convulsions, drowsiness, somnolence, headache, tremor, dysarthria, vertigo, confusion and disorientation with loss of memory, psychosis, possibly with suicidal tendencies, character changes, hyperirritability, aggression, paresis, hyper-reflexia, paraesthesiae, major and minor localised clonic seizures and coma.

Other reported side-effects include allergy, rash, megaloblastic anaemia and elevated serum aminotransferases, especially in patients with pre-existing liver disease.

Sudden development of congestive heart failure, in patients receiving 1 to 1.5 g of cycloserine daily, has been reported.

*Overdose:*
*Signs and symptoms:* Acute toxicity can occur if more than 1 g is ingested by an adult. Chronic toxicity is dose related and can occur if more than 500 mg is administered daily. For patients with renal impairment see *Contra-indications* and *Special warnings and special precautions for use.* Toxicity commonly affects the central nervous system. Effects may include headache, vertigo, confusion, drowsiness, hyperirritability, paraesthesias, dysarthria and psychosis. Following larger ingestions, paresis, convulsions and coma often occur. Ethanol may increase the risk of seizures.
*Treatment:* Symptomatic and supportive therapy is recommended. Activated charcoal may be more effective in reducing absorption than emesis or lavage. In adults, many neurotoxic effects can be both treated and prevented with 200-300 mg of pyridoxine daily. Haemodialysis removes cycloserine from the bloodstream but should be reserved for life-threatening toxicity.

**Pharmacological properties**
*Pharmacodynamic properties:*
*Actions:* Cycloserine inhibits cell wall synthesis in susceptible strains of Gram-positive and Gram-negative bacteria and in *Mycobacterium tuberculosis.*
*Indications:* Cycloserine is indicated in the treatment of active pulmonary and extra-pulmonary tuberculosis (including renal disease) when the organisms are susceptible to this drug and after failure of adequate treatment with the primary medications (streptomycin, isoniazid, rifampicin and ethambutol). Like all anti-tuberculous drugs, cycloserine should be administered in conjunction with other effective chemotherapy and not as the sole therapeutic agent.

Cycloserine may be effective in the treatment of acute urinary tract infections caused by susceptible strains of Gram-positive and Gram-negative bacteria, especially *Klebsiella/Enterobacter* species and *Escherichia coli.* It is generally no more and may be less effective than other antimicrobial agents in the treatment of urinary tract infections caused by bacteria other than mycobacteria. Use of cycloserine in these infections should be considered only when the more conventional therapy has failed and when the organism has been demonstrated to be sensitive to the drug.
*Pharmacokinetic properties:* Cycloserine is rapidly absorbed from the GI tract after oral administration,

giving detectable levels in plasma within an hour. It is widely distributed throughout body fluids and tissues.

There is no appreciable blood-brain barrier, and CSF levels are approximately the same as plasma levels. It is found in the sputum of tuberculous patients and has been detected in pleural and ascitic fluids, bile, amniotic fluid and fetal blood, breast milk, lung and lymph tissues.

Cycloserine is excreted into the urine, levels appearing within half an hour of oral ingestion. Approximately 66 per cent of a dose appears unchanged in the urine in 24 hours. A further 10 per cent is excreted over the next 48 hours. It is not significantly excreted in the faeces. Approximately 35 per cent is metabolised, but the metabolites have not yet been identified.

The half-life of cycloserine is in the range 8-12 hours.

*Preclinical safety data:* A study in two generations of rats given doses up to 100 mg/kg/day demonstrated no teratogenic effect in offspring.

**Pharmaceutical particulars**
*List of excipients:* Talc; liquid paraffin; amaranth; erythrosine; sunset yellow; titanium dioxide; black iron oxide; gelatin.

*Incompatibilities:* None known.

*Shelf life:* Twelve months when stored appropriately.

*Special precautions for storage:* Keep tightly closed. Protect from moisture. Store below 25°C.

*Nature and contents of container:* HDPE bottles of 100 capsules.

*Instructions for use/handling:* For oral administration.

**Marketing authorisation number**   0006/5045R

**Date of approval/revision of SPC**   20 July 1995

**Legal category**   POM

# DOBUTREX*

**Presentation**   Dobutrex (dobutamine hydrochloride for injection) is available as: Dobutrex Solution: Vials containing 20 ml of sterile solution, for intravenous use only. Each ml contains 12.5 mg dobutamine, 0.24 mg sodium metabisulphite and water for injection.

**Uses**
*Actions:* The primary action of dobutamine is to augment cardiac contractility by stimulating the beta-1 receptors of the heart. It is a direct-acting agent.

*Indications:* Dobutrex is indicated for adults who require inotropic support in the treatment of low output cardiac failure associated with myocardial infarction, open heart surgery, cardiomyopathies, septic shock and cardiogenic shock. Dobutrex can also increase or maintain cardiac output during positive end expiratory pressure (PEEP) ventilation.

Dobutrex may also be used for cardiac stress testing as an alternative to exercise in patients for whom routine exercise testing cannot be satisfactorily performed. This use of dobutamine should only be undertaken in units which already perform exercise stress testing and all normal care and precautions required for such testing are also required when using dobutamine for this purpose.

**Dosage and administration**   For intravenous administration only.

Dobutrex Solution must be further diluted to at least 50 ml prior to administration in an i.v. container with one of the intravenous solutions listed below:

Sodium Chloride Intravenous Infusion BP
5% Glucose Intravenous Infusion BP
5% Glucose + 0.9% Sodium Chloride Intravenous Infusion BP
5% Glucose + 0.45% Sodium Chloride Intravenous Infusion BP
Sodium Lactate Intravenous Infusion BP

If diluting to 250 ml or 500 ml, dilution will give a concentration for administration as follows:

250 ml contains 1,000 micrograms/ml of dobutamine
500 ml contains 500 micrograms/ml of dobutamine

The prepared solution should be used within 24 hours.

*Administration:* Due to its short half-life, Dobutrex must be administered as a continuous intravenous infusion. After dilution, Dobutrex should be administered intravenously through an intravenous needle or catheter. An i.v. drip chamber or other suitable metering device is essential for controlling the rate of flow in drops per minute.

*Recommended dosage for adults and the elderly:* Most patients will respond satisfactorily to doses ranging from 2.5 to 10 micrograms/kg/minute. Occasionally, however, a dose as low as 0.5 micrograms/kg/minute will elicit a response. Rarely, a dose as high as 40 micrograms/kg/minute is required.

The rate of administration and the duration of therapy should be adjusted according to the patient's response as determined by heart rate, blood pressure, urine flow, and, if possible, measurement of cardiac output.

Rather than abruptly discontinuing therapy with Dobutrex, it is often advisable to decrease the dosage gradually.

Side-effects, which are dose-related, are infrequent when Dobutrex is administered at rates below 10 micrograms/kg/minute. Rates as high as 40 micrograms/kg/minute have been used occasionally without significant adverse effects.

The final volume administered should be determined by the fluid requirements of the patient. Concentrations as high as 5,000 micrograms/ml have been used in patients on a restricted fluid intake. High concentrations of dobutamine should only be given with an infusion pump, to ensure accurate dosage.

*Cardiac stress testing:* When used as an alternative to exercise for cardiac stress testing the recommended dose is an incremental increase of 5 micrograms/kg/min from 5 up to 20 micrograms/kg/min, each dose being infused for 8 minutes. Continuous ECG monitoring is essential and the infusion terminated in the event of >3 mm ST segment depression or any ventricular arrhythmia. The infusion should also be terminated if heart rate reaches the age/sex maximum, systolic blood pressure rises above 220 mm Hg or any side-effects occur – see *Side-effects.*

*Paediatric use:* The safety and efficacy of dobutamine for use in children have not been established.

**Contra-indications, warnings, etc**
*Contra-indication:* Previous hypersensitivity to dobutamine.

*Warnings:* If tachycardia or an undue increase in systolic blood pressure occurs or if an arrhythmia is precipitated, the dose of dobutamine should be reduced or the drug should be discontinued temporarily.

Dobutamine may precipitate or exacerbate ventricular ectopic activity; rarely has it caused ventricular tachycardia or fibrillation. Because dobutamine facilitates atrioventricular conduction, patients with atrial flutter or fibrillation may develop rapid ventricular responses.

Particular care should be exercised when dobutamine is used in patients with acute myocardial infarction because any significant increase in heart rate or excessive increases in arterial pressure that occur may intensify ischaemia and cause anginal pain and ST segment elevation.

Inotropic agents, including dobutamine, do not improve haemodynamics in most patients with mechanical obstruction that hinders either ventricular filling or outflow, or both. Inotropic response may be inadequate in patients with markedly reduced ventricular compliance. Such conditions are present in cardiac tamponade, valvular aortic stenosis, and idiopathic hypertrophic subaortic stenosis.

The use of dobutamine as an alternative to exercise for cardiac stress testing is not recommended for patients with unstable angina, bundle branch block, valvular heart disease, aortic outflow obstruction or any cardiac condition that could make them unsuitable for exercise stress testing.

*Usage in pregnancy and lactation:* Reproduction studies performed in rats and rabbits have revealed no evidence of harm to the foetus or teratogenic effects due to dobutamine. Animal studies to evaluate effects on fertility have not been conducted. As there are no adequate and well-controlled studies in pregnant women, and as animal reproduction studies are not always predictive of human response, dobutamine should not be used during pregnancy unless the potential benefits outweigh the potential risks to the foetus.

It is not known whether this drug is excreted in human milk, so caution should be exercised. If a mother requires dobutamine treatment, breast feeding should be discontinued for the duration of treatment.

*Precautions:* During the administration of dobutamine, as with any parenteral catecholamine, heart rate and rhythm, arterial blood pressure, and infusion rate should be monitored closely. When initiating therapy, electrocardiographic monitoring is advisable until a stable response is achieved.

Precipitous decreases in blood pressure (hypotension) have occasionally been described in association with dobutamine therapy. Decreasing the dose or discontinuing the infusion typically results in rapid return of blood pressure to baseline values, but rarely intervention may be required and reversibility may not be immediate.

Dobutamine should be used with caution in the presence of severe hypotension complicating cardiogenic shock (mean arterial pressure less than 70 mm Hg).

Hypovolaemia should be corrected when necessary with whole blood or plasma before dobutamine is administered.

If arterial blood pressure remains low or decreases progressively during administration of dobutamine despite adequate ventricular filling pressure and cardiac output, consideration may be given to the concomitant use of a peripheral vasoconstrictor agent, such as dopamine or noradrenaline.

Dobutrex contains sodium metabisulphite. Sulphites may cause allergic-type reactions, including anaphylactic symptoms and life-threatening or less severe asthmatic episodes in certain susceptible people. Sulphite sensitivity is seen more frequently in asthmatic than in non–asthmatic people.

*Drug interactions:* The potency of dobutamine may be decreased if the patient is given beta-adrenergic receptor antagonists. In such a case, the unopposed alpha-agonist effects of dobutamine may become apparent, including peripheral vasoconstriction and hypertension. Conversely, alpha-adrenergic blockade may make the beta-1 and beta-2 effects apparent, resulting in tachycardia and vasodilatation.

*Side-effects:* For cardiovascular effects, see *Warnings* and *Precautions* sections.

*Reactions at site of intravenous infusion:* Phlebitis has occasionally been reported. Local inflammatory changes have been described following inadvertent infiltration. Isolated cases of cutaneous necrosis have been reported.

The following side-effects have been reported rarely: nausea, headache, anginal pain, non-specific chest pain, palpitations, shortness of breath, and reactions suggestive of hypersensitivity, including rash, fever, eosinophilia and bronchospasm. Isolated cases of thrombocytopenia have been reported.

As with other catecholamines, decreases in serum potassium concentrations have occurred, rarely to hypokalaemic values. Consideration should be given to monitoring serum potassium.

*Long-term safety:* Infusions for up to 72 hours have revealed no adverse effects other than those seen with shorter infusions. There is evidence that partial tolerance develops with continuous infusions of dobutamine for 72 hours or more; therefore, higher doses may be required to maintain the same effects.

*Overdosage:* Overdoses of dobutamine have been reported rarely. The symptoms of toxicity may include anorexia, nausea, vomiting, tremor, anxiety, palpitations, headache, shortness of breath and anginal and non–specific chest pain. The positive inotropic and chronotropic effects of dobutamine may cause hypertension, tachyarrhythmias, myocardial ischaemia and ventricular fibrillation. Hypotension may result from vasodilatation.

The duration of action of dobutamine hydrochloride is generally short (half-life, approximately 2 minutes). Temporarily discontinue dobutamine until the patient's condition stabilises. The patient should be monitored and any appropriate resuscitative measures initiated promptly.

Forced diuresis, peritoneal dialysis, haemodialysis, or charcoal haemoperfusion have not been established as beneficial.

If the product is ingested, unpredictable absorption may occur from the mouth and gastrointestinal tract.

**Pharmaceutical precautions**
*Undiluted vials of Dobutrex Solution:* Store below 25°C.

Prepared intravenous solutions are stable for 24 hours at room temperature.

Do not add Dobutrex to 5% Sodium Bicarbonate Intravenous Infusion BP or to any other strongly alkaline solutions. Because of potential physical incompatibilities, it is recommended that dobutamine hydrochloride not be mixed with other drugs in the same solution.

Dobutamine hydrochloride should not be used with other agents or diluents containing both sodium metabisulphite and ethanol.

Solutions containing Dobutrex may turn pink; the colour may intensify with time. This colour change is due to slight oxidation of the drug, but there is no significant loss of potency during the recommended storage period.

**Legal category** POM.

**Package quantity** Single 20 ml vials containing 250 mg dobutamine as the hydrochloride salt.

**Further information** Nil.

**Product licence number** 0006/0180.

# DOLOXENE*

**Qualitative and quantitative composition** Each capsule contains, as active ingredient, 100 mg Dextropropoxyphene Napsylate BP (approximately equivalent to 65 mg dextropropoxyphene hydrochloride or 60 mg dextropropoxyphene base).

**Pharmaceutical form** Capsules, opaque pink, coded Lilly H64.

**Clinical particulars**

*Therapeutic indications:*
*Actions:* Dextropropoxyphene is a mild narcotic analgesic structurally related to methadone.
*Indications:* For the relief of mild to moderate pain.

*Posology and method of administration:* For oral administration to adults only. The usual dose is one capsule three or four times daily, and should not normally be exceeded. Consideration should be given to a reduced total daily dosage in patients with hepatic or renal impairment.
*The elderly:* There is evidence of prolonged half-life in the elderly, so reduction in dosage should be considered.
*Children:* Dextropropoxyphene is not recommended for use in children.

*Contra-indications:* Hypersensitivity to dextropropoxyphene.
Use in patients who are suicidal or addiction-prone.

*Special warnings and special precautions for use:*
*Warnings:* PATIENTS SHOULD BE ADVISED NOT TO EXCEED THE RECOMMENDED DOSE AND TO AVOID ALCOHOL.

Dextropropoxyphene products in excessive doses, either alone or in combination with other CNS depressants, including alcohol, are a major cause of drug-related deaths. Fatalities within the first hour of overdosage are not uncommon and can occur within 15 minutes. Some deaths have occurred as a consequence of the accidental ingestion of excessive quantities of dextropropoxyphene alone, or in combination with other drugs.

Dextropropoxyphene should be prescribed with caution for those patients whose medical condition requires the concomitant administration of sedatives, tranquillisers, muscle relaxants, antidepressants or other CNS-depressant drugs. Patients should be advised of the additive depressant effects of these combinations. Doloxene should also be prescribed with caution in patients who use alcohol in excess.

*Drug dependence:* Dextropropoxyphene, when taken in higher than recommended doses over long periods of time, can produce drug dependence.

*Precautions:* Dextropropoxyphene should be administered with caution to patients with hepatic or renal impairment since higher serum concentrations or delayed elimination may occur.

*Interaction with other medicaments and other forms of interaction:*
*Drug interactions:* The CNS-depressant effect of dextropropoxyphene is additive with that of other CNS depressants, including alcohol.

Dextropropoxyphene may interfere with the metabolism of antidepressants, anticonvulsants and warfarin-like drugs. Severe neurological signs, including coma, have occurred with concomitant use of carbamazepine.

*Pregnancy and lactation:*
*Pregnancy:* Safety in pregnancy has not been established relative to possible adverse effects on foetal development. Withdrawal symptoms in neonates have been reported following use during pregnancy. Therefore, dextropropoxyphene should not be used in pregnant women unless, in the judgment of the physician, the potential benefits outweigh the possible hazards.
*Nursing mothers:* Low levels of dextropropoxyphene have been detected in human milk. In postpartum studies involving nursing mothers who were given dextropropoxyphene, no adverse effects were noted in the infants.

*Effects on the ability to drive and use machines:*
*Ambulatory patients:* Dextropropoxyphene may impair abilities required for tasks such as driving a car or operating machinery. The patient should be cautioned accordingly.

*Undesirable effects:* The most frequently reported have been dizziness, sedation, nausea and vomiting. Some of these side-effects may be alleviated if the patient lies down.

Other side-effects include constipation, abdominal pain, rashes, light-headedness, headache, weakness, euphoria, dysphoria, hallucinations and minor visual disturbances.

Dextropropoxyphene therapy has been associated with abnormal liver function tests and, more rarely, with instances of reversible jaundice (including cholestatic jaundice).

Subacute painful myopathy has occurred following chronic dextropropoxyphene overdosage.

Chronic ingestion of dextropropoxyphene in doses exceeding 720 mg per day has caused toxic psychoses and convulsions.

*Overdose:* Initial consideration should be given to the management of the CNS effects of dextropropoxyphene overdosage. Resuscitative measures should be initiated promptly.

In the acute phase dextropropoxyphene produces symptoms typical of narcosis, with somnolence or coma and respiratory depression, sometimes with convulsions. Blood pressure falls and cardiac performance deteriorates. Cardiac arrhythmias and conduction delay may be present. A combined respiratory-metabolic acidosis occurs, which may be severe if large amounts of salicylates have also been ingested. Death may occur.

Naloxone will reduce the respiratory depression and 0.4-2 mg IV should be administered promptly. (This may be repeated at 2-3 minute intervals, but if there is no response after 10 mg of naloxone the diagnosis should be questioned.) The duration of antagonism may be brief and need repeating for up to 24 hours. Mechanical ventilation, with oxygen, may be required, and PEEP ventilation is desirable if pulmonary oedema is present.

Blood gases, pH and electrolytes should be monitored and electrocardiographic monitoring is essential. Ventricular fibrillation or cardiac arrest may occur. Respiratory acidosis rapidly subsides as ventilation is restored and hypercapnoea eliminated, but lactic acidosis may require IV bicarbonate for prompt correction. In addition to the use of a narcotic antagonist, the patient may require titration with an anti-convulsant to control convulsions. Gastric lavage may be useful and activated charcoal can absorb a significant amount of ingested dextropropoxyphene.

*Treatment of dextropropoxyphene overdose in children:* See general comments above. Naloxone at 0.01 mg/kg body weight IV should be administered promptly. If there is no response a dose of 0.1 mg/kg IV may be used.

**Pharmacological properties**

*Pharmacodynamic properties:* Propoxyphene is a mild centrally acting analgesic agent structurally related to methadone. The potency of propoxyphene hydrochloride is from two-thirds to equal that of codeine. The combination of propoxyphene with a mixture of aspirin and caffeine produces greater analgesia than that produced by either propoxyphene or aspirin and caffeine administered alone.

*Pharmacokinetic properties:* Equimolar doses of propoxyphene hydrochloride or napsylate provide similar plasma concentrations. Following administration of 65, 130 or 195 mg of propoxyphene hydrochloride, the bioavailability of propoxyphene is equivalent to that of 100, 200 or 300 mg, respectively, of propoxyphene napsylate. Peak plasma concentrations of propoxyphene are reached in two to two and one-half hours. After a 65 mg oral dose of propoxyphene hydrochloride, peak plasma levels of 0.05 to 0.1 mcg/ml are achieved.

Repeated doses of propoxyphene at six-hour intervals lead to increasing plasma concentrations, with a plateau after the ninth dose at 48 hours.

Propoxyphene is metabolised in the liver to yield norpropoxyphene. Propoxyphene has a half-life of six to twelve hours, whereas that of norpropoxyphene is 30 to 36 hours. Norpropoxyphene has substantially less central-nervous-system-depressant effect than propoxyphene but a greater local anaesthetic effect, which is similar to that of amitriptyline and antiarrhythmic agents, such as lignocaine and quinidine.

*Preclinical safety data:* Animal toxicology studies indicate that, on a molar basis, the napsylate salt of dextropropoxyphene is less toxic than the hydrochloride. This may be due to its relative insolubility and retarded absorption.

**Pharmaceutical particulars**

*List of excipients:* Starch; Dimethicone; Gelatin; Titanium dioxide; Red Iron Oxide; Black Edible Printing Ink.

*Incompatibilities:* Not applicable.

*Shelf life:* Two years.

*Special precautions for storage:* Store below 25°C.

*Nature and contents of container:* Blister packs of 100 (10 strips of 10 capsules).

*Instructions for use/handling:* No special instructions.

**Marketing authorisation number** 0006/5068R

**Date of approval/revision of SPC** 7 November 1996

**Legal category** CD (Sch 5), POM

# DOLOXENE* COMPOUND

**Qualitative and quantitative composition**

| | Quantity/Dose Unit |
|---|---|
| Dextropropoxyphene napsylate | 100.0 mg |
| Acetylsalicylic acid | 375.0 mg |
| Caffeine | 30.0 mg |

**Pharmaceutical form**    Capsules (light grey opaque cap, red opaque body), coded H91.

**Clinical particulars**

*Therapeutic indications:*
*Actions:* Dextropropoxyphene is a mild narcotic analgesic structurally related to methadone.

*Indication:* For the relief of mild to moderate pain.

*Posology and method of administration:* For oral administration to adults only. The usual dose is one capsule three or four times daily, and should not normally be exceeded.

The maximum dose of dextropropoxyphene napsylate is 600 mg/day.

Consideration should be given to a reduced total daily dosage in patients with hepatic or renal impairment.

*The elderly:* There is evidence of prolonged half-life in the elderly, so reduction in dosage should be considered. The elderly are more likely to experience gastric side-effects and tinnitus with aspirin.

*Children:* Doloxene compound is not recommended for use in children.

*Contra-indications:* Hypersensitivity to any of the constituents, hypoprothrombinaemia, haemophilia and active peptic ulceration.

Use in patients who are suicidal or addiction-prone.

*Special warnings and special precautions for use:* Patients should be advised not to exceed the recommended dose and to avoid alcohol.

Dextropropoxyphene products in excessive doses, either alone or in combination with other CNS depressants, including alcohol, are a major cause of drug-related deaths. Fatalities within the first hour of overdosage are not uncommon and can occur within 15 minutes. Some deaths have occurred as a consequence of the accidental ingestion of excessive quantities alone, or in combination with other drugs.

Doloxene Compound should be prescribed with caution for those patients whose medical condition requires the concomitant administration of sedatives, tranquillisers, muscle relaxants, antidepressants or other CNS-depressant drugs; patients should be advised of the additive depressant effects of these combinations. Doloxene Compound should also be prescribed with caution in patients who use alcohol in excess.

Salicylates should be used with caution in patients with a history of peptic ulceration or coagulation abnormalities. They may also induce gastro-intestinal haemorrhage, occasionally major.

In large doses, salicylates may also decrease insulin requirements.

High doses of caffeine may cause tremors and palpitations.

*Drug dependence:* Dextropropoxyphene, when taken in higher than recommended doses over long periods of time, can produce drug dependence.

Dextropropoxyphene should be administered with caution to patients with hepatic or renal impairment since higher serum concentrations or delayed elimination may occur.

*Interaction with other medicaments and other forms of interaction:*
*Drug interactions:* The CNS depressant effect of dextropropoxyphene is additive with that of other CNS depressants, including alcohol.

Dextropropoxyphene may interfere with the metabolism of antidepressants, anticonvulsants and warfarin-like drugs. Severe neurological signs, including coma, have occurred with concurrent use of carbamazepine.

Aspirin may enhance the effect of anticoagulants, inhibit uricosuric agents, precipitate bronchospasm or induce asthma in susceptible individuals.

*Pregnancy and lactation:*
*Pregnancy:* Safety in pregnancy has not been established relative to possible adverse effects on foetal development. Instances of withdrawal symptoms in the neonate have been reported following usage of dextropropoxyphene. Aspirin does not appear to have teratogenic effects. However, prolonged pregnancy and labour, with increased bleeding before and after delivery, decreased birth weight and increased rate of stillbirth were reported with high blood salicylate levels. Therefore, Doloxene Compound should not be used in pregnant women unless, in the judgment of the physician, the potential benefits outweigh the possible hazards and it should be avoided during the last 3 months of pregnancy.

*Nursing mothers:* Low levels of dextropropoxyphene have been detected in human milk. In postpartum studies involving nursing mothers who were given dextropropoxyphene, no adverse effects were noted in the infants. Aspirin is also excreted in breast milk.

*Effects on ability to drive and use machines:*
*Ambulatory patients:* Dextropropoxyphene may impair abilities required for tasks such as driving a car

or operating machinery. The patient should be cautioned accordingly.

*Undesirable effects:* The most frequently reported have been dizziness, sedation, nausea and vomiting. Some of these side-effects may be alleviated if the patient lies down.

Other side-effects include constipation, abdominal pain, rashes, light-headedness, headache, weakness, euphoria, dysphoria, hallucinations and minor visual disturbances.

Dextropropoxyphene therapy has been associated with abnormal liver function tests and, more rarely, with instances of reversible jaundice (including cholestatic jaundice).

Renal papillary necrosis may result from chronic aspirin use, particularly when the dosage is greater than recommended and when combined with paracetamol.

Subacute painful myopathy has occurred following chronic dextropropoxyphene overdosage.

Chronic ingestion of dextropropoxyphene in doses exceeding 720 mg per day has caused toxic psychoses and convulsions.

Salicylates may induce hypersensitivity, asthma, urate kidney stones, chronic gastro-intestinal blood loss, tinnitus, nausea and vomiting.

*Overdose:* Initial consideration should be given to the management of the CNS effects of dextropropoxyphene overdosage. Resuscitative measures should be initiated promptly.

*Dextropropoxyphene:* In the acute phase dextropropoxyphene produces symptoms typical of narcosis, with somnolence or coma and respiratory depression, sometimes with convulsions. Blood pressure falls and cardiac performance deteriorates. Cardiac arrhythmias and conduction delay may be present. A combined respiratory-metabolic acidosis occurs, which may be severe if large amounts of salicylates have also been ingested. Death may occur.

Naloxone will reduce the respiratory depression and 0.4–2 mg IV should be administered promptly. (This may be repeated at 2-3 minute intervals, but if there is no response after 10 mg of naloxone the diagnosis should be questioned.) The duration of antagonism may be brief and need repeating for up to 24 hours. Mechanical ventilation, with oxygen, may be required, and PEEP ventilation is desirable if pulmonary oedema is present.

Blood gases, pH and electrolytes should be monitored and electrocardiographic monitoring is essential. Ventricular fibrillation or cardiac arrest may occur. Respiratory acidosis rapidly subsides as ventilation is restored and hypercapnoea eliminated, but lactic acidosis may require IV bicarbonate for prompt correction. In addition to the use of a narcotic antagonist, the patient may require titration with an anti-convulsant to control convulsions. Gastric lavage may be useful and activated charcoal can absorb a significant amount of ingested dextropropoxyphene.

*Treatment of dextropropoxyphene overdose in children:* See general comments above. Naloxone at 0.01 mg/kg body weight IV should be administered promptly. If there is no response a dose of 0.1 mg/kg IV may be used.

*Aspirin:* Symptoms include central nausea and vomiting, tinnitus and deafness, vertigo and headaches, mental dullness and confusion, diaphoresis, rapid pulse, and increased respiration and respiratory alkalosis.

Treatment includes minimising drug absorption, promoting kidney elimination, and correcting metabolic derangements affecting body temperature, hydration, acid-base balance, and electrolyte balance.

If the patient is seen within 4 hours of ingestion, the stomach should be emptied by inducing vomiting or by gastric lavage.

The nomogram of Done is a useful prognostic guide in which the expected severity of salicylate intoxication is based on serum salicylate levels and the time interval between ingestion and taking the blood sample.

Exchange transfusion is most feasible for a small infant. Intermittent peritoneal dialysis is useful for cases of moderate severity in adults. Intravenous fluids alkalinised by the addition of sodium bicarbonate or potassium citrate are helpful. Haemodialysis with the artificial kidney is the most effective means of removing salicylate and is indicated for the very severe cases of salicylate intoxication.

**Pharmacological properties**

*Pharmacodynamic properties:* Propoxyphene is a mild centrally acting analgesic agent structurally related to methadone. The potency of propoxyphene hydrochloride is from two-thirds to equal that of codeine. The combination of propoxyphene with a mixture of aspirin and caffeine produces greater analgesia than that produced by either propoxyphene or aspirin and caffeine administered alone.

*Pharmacokinetic properties:* Equimolar doses of propoxyphene hydrochloride or napsylate provide similar

plasma concentrations. Following administration of 65, 130 or 195 mg of propoxyphene hydrochloride, the bioavailability of propoxyphene is equivalent to that of 100, 200 or 300 mg, respectively, of propoxyphene napsylate. Peak plasma concentrations of propoxyphene are reached in two to two and one-half hours. After a 65 mg oral dose of propoxyphene hydrochloride, peak plasma levels of 0.05 to 0.1 mcg/ml are achieved.

Repeated doses of propoxyphene at six-hour intervals lead to increasing plasma concentrations, with a plateau after the ninth dose at 48 hours.

Propoxyphene is metabolised in the liver to yield norpropoxyphene. Propoxyphene has a half-life of six to twelve hours, whereas that of norpropoxyphene is 30 to 36 hours. Norpropoxyphene has substantially less central-nervous-system-depressant effect than propoxyphene but a greater local anaesthetic effect, which is similar to that of amitriptyline and antiarrhythmic agents, such as lignocaine and quinidine.

*Preclinical safety data:* Not applicable.

**Pharmaceutical particulars**

*List of excipients:* Dimethicone; Starch Flowable; Black Iron Oxide; Titanium Dioxide; Erythrosine; Quinoline Yellow; Gelatin; Edible Printing Ink, E172.

*Incompatibilities:* Not applicable.

*Shelf life:* 3 years.

*Special precautions for storage:* Store below 25°C.

*Nature and contents of container:* Blister pack containing 100 capsules (10 strips of 10 capsules).

*Instructions for use/handling:* Not applicable.

**Marketing authorisation number**    0006/0091R

**Date of approval/revision of SPC**    18 September 1995

**Legal category**    CD (Sch 5), POM

## ELDISINE*

> **WARNING**
> THIS PRODUCT IS **NOT**
> FOR INTRATHECAL USE

**Presentation**    Vials containing 5 mg Eldisine (vindesine sulphate for injection) and 25 mg Mannitol BP. (Supplied in a combination package with an accompanying vial of diluting solution, 5 ml containing 45 mg Sodium Chloride PhEur with 2% Benzyl Alcohol BP as a preservative.)

**Uses**    Eldisine is an anti–neoplastic drug for intravenous use which can be used alone or in combination with other oncolytic drugs. Information available at present suggests that Eldisine as a single agent may be useful for the treatment of: acute lymphoblastic leukaemia of childhood resistant to other drugs; blastic crises of chronic myeloid leukaemia; malignant melanoma unresponsive to other forms of therapy; advanced carcinoma of the breast, unresponsive to appropriate endocrine surgery and/or hormonal therapy.

**Dosage and administration**    This preparation is for intravenous use only. It should be administered only by individuals experienced in vindesine administration.

> Fatal if given intrathecally
> (see *Warnings* for treatment).

Extreme care must be used in calculating and administering the dose of vindesine, since overdosage may have a very serious or fatal outcome.

It is recommended that the drug be administered intravenously in a single rapid bolus injection at weekly intervals. The size of the dose is determined by body surface area. In adults and the elderly, the recommended starting dose is 3 mg/m², and children may be started at 4 mg/m². Thereafter, granulocyte counts should be made prior to each subsequent dose to determine the patient's sensitivity to the drug. Provided there is no granulocytopenia or other toxicity (see *Adverse reactions*) the dosage may be increased in 0.5 mg/m² steps at weekly intervals.

In adults, the maximum total weekly dosage for which data exists is 4 mg/m². The optimum dose of vindesine is that which produces mild to modest granulocytopenia. Sustained granulocyte counts lower than 2,500 cells/mm³ are to be avoided.

Those with decreased marrow function from leukaemia infiltration or replacement will require full doses to attempt to restore marrow function. This must be done under close supervision.

The dose should not be increased after that dose which: (i) reduces the granulocyte count to below 1,500 cells/mm³ or, on rare occasions, (ii) reduces the platelet count to below 100,000/mm³; (iii) causes acute abdominal pain (see under *Precautions*).

On each of the above occasions there should be full recovery before administering the next dose, which should be reduced from the one causing the adverse reaction. For most patients, however, the weekly dosage will prove to be in the range of 3.0 to 4.0 mg/$m^2$ in adults and 4.0 to 5.0 mg/$m^2$ in children.

The use of small amounts of vindesine daily for long periods is not advised, even though the resulting total weekly dosage may be similar to that recommended. Little or no added therapeutic advantage has been demonstrated when such regimens have been used, and side-effects are increased. Strict adherence to the recommended dosage schedule is very important.

As vindesine is excreted principally by the liver, it may be necessary to reduce initial doses in the presence of significantly impaired hepatic or biliary function.

The metabolism of vinca alkaloids has been shown to be mediated by hepatic cytochrome P450 isoenzymes in the CYP 3A subfamily. This metabolic pathway may be impaired in patients with hepatic dysfunction or who are taking concomitant potent inhibitors of these isoenzymes. (See *Precautions*.)

To prepare a solution containing 1 mg/ml add the 5 ml of accompanying diluting solution to the 5 mg of Eldisine in the sterile vial. The drug dissolves rapidly to give a clear solution.

The dose of Eldisine solution (calculated to provide the desired number of milligrams per square metre of the patient's surface area) may be injected either into the tubing of a running intravenous infusion (*compatible infusions are 5% Dextrose Intravenous Infusion BP, Sodium Chloride Intravenous Infusion BP and dextrose/saline infusions*) or directly into a vein.

The latter procedure is readily adaptable to outpatient therapy. In either case, the injection should be completed in 1 to 3 minutes. If care is taken to ensure that the needle is securely within the vein and that no solution containing vindesine is spilled extravascularly, cellulitis and/or phlebitis is unlikely to occur.

Because of the enhanced possibility of thrombosis, it is considered inadvisable to inject a solution into an extremity in which the circulation is impaired, or potentially impaired, by such conditions as compressing or invading neoplasm, phlebitis or varicosity.

*Caution:* It is extremely important to choose the largest accessible vein and to be certain that the needle is properly positioned in the vein before any vindesine is injected. If leakage into surrounding tissues should occur during intravenous administration, it may cause considerable irritation. The injection should be discontinued as soon as leakage occurs, and any remaining portion of the dose should then be introduced into another vein. Local injection of hyaluronidase and the application of moderate heat to the area of leakage help disperse the drug and are thought to minimise discomfort and the possibility of cellulitis.

**Contra-indications, warnings, etc**

*Contra-indications*

| |
|---|
| Intrathecal administration has resulted in death (see *Warnings* for treatment). |

Use in patients who have drug-induced severe granulocytopenia (less than 1,500 granulocytes per $mm^3$) or severe thrombocytopenia. Vindesine should not be used in the presence of bacterial infection. Such infections must be brought under control with antiseptics or antibiotics before using vindesine.

Patients with the demyelinating form of Charcot-Marie-Tooth syndrome should not be given vindesine.

*Warning:* Syringes containing this product should be labelled 'FATAL IF GIVEN INTRATHECALLY. FOR INTRAVENOUS USE ONLY.' An auxiliary sticker is provided in the pack with this warning.

Extemporaneously prepared syringes containing this product must be packaged in an overwrap which is labelled 'DO NOT REMOVE COVERING UNTIL MOMENT OF INJECTION. FATAL IF GIVEN INTRATHECALLY. FOR INTRAVENOUS USE ONLY.'

The following treatment successfully arrested progressive paralysis in a single patient mistakenly given the related vinca alkaloid, vincristine sulphate, intrathecally. This treatment should be initiated immediately after the intrathecal injection:

1. Removal of as much CSF as is safely possible.
2. Flushing with Lactated Ringer's solution by continuous infusion at 150 ml/h, through a catheter in a cerebral lateral ventricle and removed through lumbar access, until fresh frozen plasma became available.
3. Fresh frozen plasma, 25 ml, diluted with 1 l of Lactated Ringer's was then infused similarly at 75 ml/h. The rate of infusion should be adjusted to maintain a spinal fluid protein level of 150 mg/dl. Repeat this procedure using a second litre of diluted fresh frozen plasma.
4. Glutamic acid, 10 gm, was given i.v. over 24 hours, followed by 500 mg t.d.s. by mouth for 1 month. Glutamic acid may not be essential.

*Usage in pregnancy or lactation:* The safety of this product for use during pregnancy has not been established. Animal studies with vindesine suggest that teratogenic effects may occur. The benefit-to-risk ratio must be carefully considered before use in pregnant patients. Eldisine should not normally be given to mothers who are breast feeding.

*Precautions:* Clinically, the dose–limiting toxicity of vindesine is granulocytopenia, although in general oncolytic activity is obtained at doses causing little or no effect on the granulocytes. Individual patient variation has been observed with respect to the severity of side-effects, including neurotoxicity, granulocytopenia, alopecia, and decrease in bowel motility.

When granulocytopenia occurs, the nadir in the granulocyte count may be expected to occur 3–5 days after the last day of drug administration. Recovery of the granulocyte count is rapid thereafter and is usually complete within 7–10 days after the last dose.

The thrombocyte count is usually either unaffected or increased by weekly therapy with vindesine. However, significant thrombocytopenia has occurred occasionally, particularly when doses are given more frequently than once a week. It is probably more likely to occur when patients are thrombocytopenic (less than 100,000 cells/$mm^3$) prior to therapy with vindesine.

The effect of vindesine upon the red blood cell count and haemoglobin concentration is usually insignificant when other treatment does not complicate the picture. It should be remembered, however, that patients with malignant disease may exhibit anaemia even in the absence of any treatment.

If granulocytopenia with less than 1,000 granulocytes/$mm^3$ occurs following a dose of vindesine, the patient should be watched carefully for evidence of infection until the granulocyte count has returned to a safe level.

While neurotoxicity is not usually dose–limiting, there have been instances in which neurotoxicity has made it necessary to reduce the dosage or temporarily discontinue use of vindesine. Neurotoxicity induced by vindesine is believed to be generally less severe and less progressive in nature than the effects observed with vincristine.

Particular attention should be given to dosage and neurological side–effects if vindesine is administered to patients with pre–existing neuromuscular disease, and also when other drugs with neurotoxic potential are being used. The neurotoxicity associated with vindesine therapy may be additive.

Care should be exercised when vindesine has been the cause of acute abdominal pain, as paralytic ileus may be a significant risk if further doses of vindesine are given, particularly if the dose is increased. Prophylactic measures should be taken to prevent obstipation that may result from a decrease in bowel motility.

When chemotherapy is being given in conjunction with radiation therapy through portals which include the liver, the use of vindesine should be delayed until radiation therapy has been completed.

Acute shortness of breath and severe bronchospasm have been reported following the administration of vindesine. These reactions have been encountered most frequently when vindesine was used in combination with mitomycin–C and may be serious when there is pre–existing pulmonary dysfunction. The onset may be within minutes, or several hours after the drug is injected and may occur up to 2 weeks after a dose of mitomycin–C. Progressive dyspnoea, requiring chronic therapy, may occur. Vindesine should not be re–administered.

The simultaneous oral or intravenous administration of phenytoin and anti-neoplastic chemotherapy combinations have been reported to have reduced blood levels of the anticonvulsant and to have increased seizure activity. Although the contribution of the vinca alkaloids has not been established, dosage adjustment of phenytoin may need to be made when used in combination with vindesine.

Caution should be exercised in patients concurrently taking drugs known to inhibit drug metabolism by hepatic cytochrome P450 isoenzymes in the CYP 3A subfamily, or in patients with hepatic dysfunction. Concurrent administration of vindesine sulphate with an inhibitor of this metabolic pathway may cause an earlier onset and/or an increased severity of side-effects.

Extreme care should be exercised to prevent injection outside the vein. Extravasation during intravenous injection will cause cellulitis and phlebitis. If the amount of extravasation is great, sloughing will occur. Healing of such wounds may require several weeks and be attended by severe pain. The discomfort may persist after healing of the ulcer.

Care must be taken to avoid contamination of the eye with concentrations of vindesine used clinically. If accidental contamination occurs, severe irritation and/or corneal ulceration may result. The eye should be washed immediately and thoroughly with water or saline.

*Adverse reactions:* Prior to the use of the drug, patients and/or their parents/guardians should be advised of the possibility of untoward symptoms. Acute toxicity appears to be dose related and is more likely to occur if doses above 4 mg/$m^2$ are employed. Granulocytopenia is usually the dose–limiting factor. Neurotoxicity is common and appears to be related to the cumulative total dose given.

The following side–effects have been reported:

*Gastro–intestinal:* Nausea, vomiting, constipation, stomatitis, ileus, diarrhoea, anorexia, abdominal pain, dysphagia, dyspepsia, perforated duodenal ulcer (nausea and vomiting usually may be controlled by anti-emetic agents).

*Neurological:* Numbness and tingling of hands/feet (paraesthesia), peripheral neuritis, jaw pain, mental depression, loss of deep–tendon reflexes, foot drop, headache, convulsions. Cortical blindness has been reported in patients treated with multiple–agent chemotherapy that has included vindesine. The contribution of vindesine to this reaction is unknown. Treatment with vinca alkaloids has resulted rarely in both vestibular and auditory damage to the eighth cranial nerve. Manifestations include partial or total deafness, which may be temporary or permanent, and difficulties with balance, including dizziness, nystagmus and vertigo. Particular caution is warranted when vindesine sulphate is used in combination with other agents known to be ototoxic, such as the platinum-containing oncolytics.

*Haematological:* Granulocytopenia, thrombocytopenia, thrombocytosis, mild anaemia.

*Pulmonary:* See under 'Precautions'.

*Cutaneous:* Alopecia from mild to total is the commonest side–effect. Regrowth of hair may occur while still on therapy. Maculopapular rashes, cellulitis with extravasation. Injection site reaction (see *Dosage and administration – Caution*).

*Miscellaneous:* Generalised musculoskeletal pain, malaise, chills and fevers, asthenia.

*Overdosage:* Side–effects following the use of vindesine are dose related. Therefore, following administration of more than the recommended dose, patients can be expected to experience these effects in an exaggerated fashion.

Supportive care should include: (a) daily blood counts for guidance in transfusion requirement; (b) prevention of the side–effects that result from the syndrome of inappropriate secretion of antidiuretic hormone. This includes restriction of fluid intake and, perhaps, the use of a diuretic drug acting on the loop of Henle and distal tubule function; (c) use of cathartics to prevent ileus; (d) administration of an anticonvulsant; (e) monitoring the patient's cardiovascular system.

The use of folinic acid in addition to the other supportive measures recommended may be considered although, unlike vincristine, studies have not been conducted to confirm its protective action. Clinical experience of vindesine overdosage is extremely limited, with only one published case.

**Pharmaceutical precautions**

*Special dispensing information:* When dispensing vindesine sulphate in other than the original container, it is imperative that it be packaged in an overwrap bearing the statement 'DO NOT REMOVE COVERING UNTIL MOMENT OF INJECTION. FATAL IF GIVEN INTRATHECALLY. FOR INTRAVENOUS USE ONLY.' A syringe containing a specific dose must be labelled, using the auxiliary sticker provided in the pack, with this warning.

*Guidelines for the safe handling of anti-neoplastic agents:* Cytotoxic preparations should not be handled by pregnant staff.

Trained personnel should reconstitute the drug. This should be performed in a designated area. The work surface should be covered with disposable plastic-backed absorbent paper.

Adequate protective gloves, masks and clothing should be worn. Precautions should be taken to avoid the drug accidentally coming into contact with the eyes. If accidental contamination occurs, the eye should be washed with water or saline thoroughly and immediately.

Use Luer-lock fittings on all syringes and sets. Large bore needles are recommended to minimise pressure and the possible formation of aerosols. The latter may also be reduced by the use of a venting needle.

Adequate care and precaution should be taken in the disposal of items (syringes, needles, etc) used to reconstitute cytotoxic drugs.

Vials of Eldisine should be stored in a refrigerator between 2°and 8°C.

*After reconstitution:* After a portion of the solution has been removed from a vial, the remainder of the contents of the vial may be stored in a refrigerator for future use for 30 days without significant loss of potency. When the reconstituted vial of Eldisine is to be stored for more than 48 hours, it is essential to use the accompanying diluting solution or a diluent which contains a preservative.

Eldisine should never be mixed with any other drug.

**Legal category** POM.

**Package quantities** Vials 5 mg: Single vials.

**Further information** Nil.

**Product licence numbers**
Vials 5 mg: 0006/0137
Diluent: 0006/5174

# GEMZAR* ▼

**Qualitative and quantitative composition** Gemcitabine hydrochloride equivalent to 200 mg gemcitabine.

Gemcitabine hydrochloride equivalent to 1 g gemcitabine.

Gemcitabine (INN) is 2'-deoxy-2',2'-difluorocytidine monohydrochloride (β-isomer).

**Pharmaceutical form** Vials containing sterile lyophilised powder for reconstitution for intravenous use.

## Clinical particulars

*Therapeutic indications:* Gemcitabine is indicated for the palliative treatment of adult patients with locally advanced or metastatic non-small cell lung cancer.

Gemcitabine is indicated for the treatment of adult patients with locally advanced or metastatic adenocarcinoma of the pancreas. Gemcitabine is indicated for patients with 5-FU refractory pancreatic cancer.

*Posology and method of administration:*

*Non-small cell lung cancer*
*Adults:* The recommended dose of gemcitabine is 1,000 mg/m², given by 30 minute intravenous infusion. This should be repeated once weekly for three weeks, followed by a one week rest period. This four week cycle is then repeated. Dosage reduction is applied based upon the amount of toxicity experienced by the patient.

*Pancreatic cancer*
*Adults:* The recommended dose of gemcitabine is 1,000 mg/m², given by 30 minute intravenous infusion. This should be repeated once weekly for up to 7 weeks, followed by a week of rest. Subsequent cycles should consist of injections once weekly for 3 consecutive weeks out of every 4 weeks. Dosage reduction is applied based upon the amount of toxicity experienced by the patient.

Patients receiving gemcitabine should be monitored prior to each dose for platelet, leucocyte and granulocyte counts and, if necessary, the dose of gemcitabine may be either reduced or withheld in the presence of haematological toxicity, according to the following scale:

| Absolute granulocyte count (× 10⁶/l) | | Platelet count (× 10⁶/l) | % of full dose |
|---|---|---|---|
| >1,000 | and | >100,000 | 100 |
| 500-1,000 | or | 50,000-100,000 | 75 |
| <500 | or | <50,000 | hold |

Periodic checks of liver and kidney functions, including transaminases and serum creatinine, should also be performed in patients receiving gemcitabine.

Gemcitabine is well tolerated during the infusion, with only a few cases of injection site reaction reported. There have been no reports of injection site necrosis. Gemcitabine can be easily administered on an outpatient basis.

*Elderly patients:* Gemcitabine has been well tolerated in patients over the age of 65. There is no evidence to suggest that dose adjustments are necessary in the elderly, although gemcitabine clearance and half-life are affected by age.

*Children:* Gemcitabine has not been studied in children.

*Hepatic and renal impairment:* Gemcitabine should be used with caution in patients with hepatic insufficiency or with impaired renal function. No studies have been done in patients with significant hepatic or renal impairment.

*Radical radiotherapy:* Gemcitabine should not be used concurrently with radical radiotherapy (see 'Special Warnings and Special Precautions for Use').

*Contra-indications:* Gemcitabine is contra-indicated in those patients with a known hypersensitivity to the drug.

*Special warnings and special precautions for use:*
*Warnings:* Prolongation of the infusion time and increased dosing frequency have been shown to increase toxicity.

Gemcitabine can suppress bone marrow function as manifested by leucopenia, thrombocytopenia and anaemia. However, myelosuppression is short lived and usually does not result in dose reductions and rarely in discontinuation (see *Posology and method of administration* and *Undesirable effects*).

Gemcitabine should be discontinued at the first signs of any evidence of microangiopathic haemolytic anaemia such as rapidly falling haemoglobin with concomitant thrombocytopenia, elevation of serum bilirubin, serum creatinine, blood urea nitrogen, or LDH, which may indicate development of haemolytic uraemic syndrome (see *Undesirable effects*).

Gemcitabine should not be given with concurrent radical, as opposed to palliative, radiotherapy. In a clinical trial, where gemcitabine, at a dose of 1,000 mg/m² was administered concurrently for up to 6 consecutive weeks with radical thoracic radiation (ie, radiation doses and field sizes for possible cure) to patients with non-small cell lung cancer, significant toxicity in the form of severe, and potentially life-threatening, oesophagitis and pneumonitis was observed, particularly in patients receiving radical radiotherapy over a large field.

*Precautions:*
*General:* Patients receiving therapy with gemcitabine must be monitored closely. Laboratory facilities should be available to monitor patient status. Treatment for a patient compromised by drug toxicity may be required.

*Laboratory tests:* Therapy should be started cautiously in patients with compromised bone marrow function. As with other oncolytics, the possibility of cumulative bone marrow suppression when using combination or sequential chemotherapy should be considered.

Patients receiving gemcitabine should be monitored prior to each dose for platelet, leucocyte and granulocyte counts. Suspension or modification of therapy should be considered when drug-induced marrow depression is detected. Guidelines regarding dose modifications are provided in 'Posology and method of administration' above. Peripheral blood counts may continue to fall after the drug is stopped.

*Interaction with other medicaments and other forms of interaction:* No interactions have been reported.

*Pregnancy and lactation:* The safety of this medicinal product for use in human pregnancy has not been established. Evaluation of experimental animal studies has shown reproductive toxicity, eg, birth defects or other effects on the development of the embryo or fetus, the course of gestation or peri and postnatal development. The use of gemcitabine should be avoided in pregnant or nursing women because of the potential hazard to the fetus or infant.

*Effects on ability to drive and use machines:* Gemcitabine has been reported to cause mild to moderate somnolence. Patients should be cautioned against driving or operating machinery until it is established that they do not become somnolent.

*Undesirable effects:*
*Haematological:* Because gemcitabine is a bone marrow suppressant, anaemia, leucopenia and thrombocytopenia can occur as a result of administration of gemcitabine. Myelosuppression is usually mild to moderate, and is more pronounced for the granulocyte count.

Thrombocythaemia is also commonly reported.

*Gastro-intestinal:* Abnormalities of liver transaminase enzymes occur in about two-thirds of patients, but they are usually mild, non-progressive and rarely necessitate stopping treatment. However, gemcitabine should be used with caution in patients with impaired liver function (see *Posology and method of administration*).

Nausea and nausea accompanied by vomiting are each reported in one-third of patients, respectively. This adverse event requires therapy in about 20% of patients, is rarely dose-limiting, and is easily manageable with standard anti-emetics.

*Renal:* Mild proteinuria and haematuria are reported in approximately half the patients, but are rarely clinically significant, and are not usually associated with any change in serum creatinine or blood urea nitrogen. However, a few cases of renal failure of uncertain aetiology have been reported, including, in very rare instances, cases of haemolytic uraemic syndrome (signs of microangiopathic haemolytic anaemia such as rapidly falling haemoglobin with concomitant thrombocytopenia, elevation of serum bilirubin, serum creatinine, blood urea nitrogen, or LDH, see 'Special warnings and special precautions for use'). Hence, gemcitabine should be used with caution in patients with impaired renal function.

*Allergic:* A rash is seen in approximately 25% of patients and is associated with pruritus in about 10% of patients. The rash is usually mild, not dose-limiting, and responds to local therapy. Desquamation, vesiculation and ulceration have been reported rarely. Anaphylaxis has been reported rarely.

Bronchospasm after gemcitabine infusion has been reported in less than 1% of patients. Bronchospasm is usually mild and transient, but parenteral therapy may be required. Gemcitabine should not be administered to patients with a known hypersensitivity to this drug (see 'Contra-indications').

Dyspnoea occurring within hours following gemcitabine injection is reported by approximately 8% of patients. This dyspnoea is usually mild, short-lived, rarely dose-limiting, and usually abates without any specific therapy. The mechanism of this event is unknown and the relationship to gemcitabine is not clear.

Interstitial pneumonitis (with associated pulmonary infiltrates) has been seen in less than 1% of patients. If this occurs gemcitabine should be discontinued. Steroids may ameliorate the condition.

*Other effects:* An entity resembling influenza is reported by approximately 20% of patients. This is usually mild, short-lived, and rarely dose-limiting. Fever, headache, back pain, chills, myalgia, asthenia and anorexia are the most commonly reported symptoms. Cough, rhinitis, malaise, sweating and insomnia are also commonly reported. Fever and asthenia are also reported frequently as isolated symptoms. The mechanism of this toxicity is unknown. Reports received indicate that paracetamol may produce symptomatic relief.

Oedema/peripheral oedema is reported by approximately 30% of patients. Some cases of facial oedema have also been reported. Pulmonary oedema was reported infrequently (1%). Oedema/peripheral oedema is usually mild to moderate, rarely dose-limiting, is sometimes reported as painful and is usually reversible after stopping gemcitabine treatment. The mechanism of this toxicity is unknown. It is not associated with any evidence of cardiac, hepatic or renal failure.

The following adverse effects are also commonly reported: alopecia (usually minimal hair loss), 13% of patients; somnolence, 10%; diarrhoea, 8%; oral toxicity (mainly soreness and erythema), 7%; and constipation, 6%.

Radiation toxicity (see *Special warnings and special precautions for use*).

A few cases of hypotension were reported. Some cases of myocardial infarction, congestive heart failure and arrhythmia have been reported in studies, but there is no clear evidence that gemcitabine causes cardiac toxicity.

*Overdose:* There is no antidote for overdosage of gemcitabine. Single doses as high as 5.7 g/m² have been administered by IV infusion over 30 minutes every two weeks with clinically acceptable toxicity. In the event of suspected overdose, the patient should be monitored with appropriate blood counts and should receive supportive therapy, as necessary.

## Pharmacological properties

*Pharmacodynamic properties:*
*Cytotoxic activity in cell culture models:* Gemcitabine exhibits significant cytotoxicity activity against a variety of cultured murine and human tumour cells. It exhibits cell phase specificity, primarily killing cells undergoing DNA synthesis (S-phase) and under certain conditions blocking the progression of cells through the G1/S-phase boundary. *In vitro* the cytotoxic action of gemcitabine is both concentration and time dependent.

*Antitumour activity in preclinical models:* In animal tumour models, the antitumour activity of gemcitabine is schedule dependent. When administered daily gemcitabine causes death in animals with minimal antitumour activity. However, when an every third or fourth day dosing schedule is used, gemcitabine can be given at non-lethal doses that have excellent antitumour activity against a broad range of mouse tumours.

*Cellular metabolism and mechanisms of action:* Gemcitabine (dFdC) is metabolised intracellularly by nucleoside kinases to the active diphosphate (dFdCDP) and triphosphate (dFdCTP) nucleosides. The cytotoxic action of gemcitabine appears to be due to inhibition of DNA synthesis by two actions of dFdCDP and dFdCTP. First, dFdCDP inhibits ribonucleotide reductase which is uniquely responsible for catalysing the reactions that generate the deoxynucleoside triphosphates for DNA synthesis. Inhibition of this enzyme by dFdCDP causes a reduction in the concentrations of deoxynucleosides in general, and especially in that of dCTP. Second, dFdCTP competes with dCTP for incorporation into DNA (self-potentiation). Likewise, a small amount of gemcitabine may also be incorporated into RNA. Thus, the reduction in the intracellular concentration of dCTP potentiates the incorporation of dFdCTP into DNA. DNA polymerase epsilon is essentially unable to remove gemcitabine and repair the growing DNA strands. After gemcitabine is incorporated into DNA, one additional nucleotide is added to the growing DNA strands. After this addition there is essentially a complete inhibition in further DNA synthesis (masked chain termination). After incorporation into DNA, gemcitabine then appears to induce the programmed cellular death process known as apoptosis.

*Pharmacokinetic properties:*
*Gemcitabine pharmacokinetics:* The pharmacokinet-

ics of gemcitabine have been examined in 353 patients in seven studies. The 121 women and 232 men ranged in age from 29 to 79 years. Of these patients, approximately 45% had non-small cell lung cancer and 35% were diagnosed with pancreatic cancer. The following pharmacokinetic parameters were obtained for doses ranging from 500 to 2592 mg/m² that were infused from 0.4 to 1.2 hours. Peak plasma concentrations (obtained within 5 minutes of the end of the infusion): 3.2 to 45.5µg/ml.

Volume of distribution of the central compartment: 12.4 l/m² for women and 17.5 l/m² for men (interindividual variability was 91.9%). Volume of distribution of the peripheral compartment: 47.4 l/m². The volume of the peripheral compartment was not sensitive to gender.

*Plasma protein binding:* Negligible.

*Systemic clearance:* Ranged from 29.2 l/hr/m² to 92.2 l/hr/m² depending on gender and age (interindividual variability was 52.2%). Clearance for women is approximately 25% lower than the values for men. Although rapid, clearance for both men and women appears to decrease with age. For the recommended gemcitabine dose of 1,000 mg/m² given as a 30 minute infusion, lower clearance values for women and men should not necessitate a decrease in the gemcitabine dose.

*Urinary excretion:* Less than 10% is excreted as unchanged drug.

*Renal clearance:* 2 to 7 l/hr/m².

*Half-life:* Ranged from 42 to 94 minutes depending on age and gender. For the recommended dosing schedule, gemcitabine elimination should be virtually complete within 5 to 11 hours of the start of the infusion. Gemcitabine does not accumulate when administered once weekly.

*Metabolism:* Gemcitabine is rapidly metabolised by cytidine deaminase in the liver, kidney, blood and other tissues.

Intracellular metabolism of gemcitabine produces the gemcitabine mono, di and triphosphates (dFdCMP, dFdCDP and dFdCTP) of which dFdCDP and dFdCTP are considered active. These intracellular metabolites have not been detected in plasma or urine.

The primary metabolite, 2'-deoxy-2',2'-difluorouridine (dFdU), is not active and is found in plasma and urine.

*dFdCTP kinetics:* This metabolite can be found in peripheral blood mononuclear cells and the information below refers to these cells.

*Half-life of terminal elimination:* 0.7-12 hours.

Intracellular concentrations increase in proportion to gemcitabine doses of 35-350 mg/m²/30 min, which give steady state concentrations of 0.4-5µg/ml. At gemcitabine plasma concentrations above 5µg/ml, dFdCTP levels do not increase, suggesting that the formation is saturable in these cells. Parent plasma concentrations following a dose of 1,000 mg/m²/30 min are greater than 5µg/ml for approximately 30 minutes after the end of the infusion, and greater than 0.4 µg/ml for an additional hour.

*dFdU kinetics*

*Peak plasma concentrations (3-15 minutes after end of 30 minute infusion, 1,000 mg/m²):* 28-52µg/ml.

*Trough concentration following once weekly dosing:* 0.07-1.12µg/ml, with no apparent accumulation.

Triphasic plasma concentration versus time curve, mean half-life of terminal phase - 65 hours (range 33-84 hr).

*Formation of dFdU from parent compound:* 91%-98%.

*Mean volume of distribution of central compartment:* 18 l/m² (range 11-22 l/m²).

*Mean steady state volume of distribution (Vss):* 150 l/m² (range 96-228 l/m²).

*Tissue distribution:* Extensive.

*Mean apparent clearance:* 2.5 l/hr/m² (range 1-4 l/hr/m²).

*Urinary excretion:* All.

*Overall elimination:* Amount recovered in one week: 92%-98%, of which 99% is dFdU, 1% of the dose is excreted in faeces.

*Preclinical safety data:* In repeat dose studies of up to 6 months in duration in mice and dogs, the principal finding was haematopoietic suppression. These effects were related to the cytotoxic properties of the drug and were reversible when treatment was withdrawn. The degree of the effect was schedule and dose-dependent.

*Carcinogenesis, mutagenesis, fertility:* Chromosomal damage, including chromatid breaks, has been produced by gemcitabine in *in vitro* studies. Gemcitabine caused a reversible, dose and schedule dependent hypospermatogenesis in male mice. Although animal studies have shown an effect of gemcitabine on male fertility, no effect has been seen on female fertility. Long-term animal studies have not been conducted to evaluate the carcinogenic potential of gemcitabine.

**Pharmaceutical particulars**

*List of excipients:* Mannitol; Sodium Acetate.

*Incompatibilities:* Compatibility with other drugs has not been studied.

*Shelf life:* 2 years for the lyophilised powder.

*Special precautions for storage:* Store at room temperature (15 to 25°C).

Solutions of reconstituted gemcitabine, in sterile Sodium Chloride Injection BP, should be kept at controlled room temperature (15 to 25°C). Reconstituted solutions should be used as soon as possible, and no later than six hours after reconstitution. Solutions should not be refrigerated, as crystallisation may occur.

*Nature and content of container:* Glass vial.

**Package quantities**

Vials 200 mg:  Single vials
Vials 1 g:  Single vials

**Instructions for use/handling**

*Reconstitution:* Gemzar has only been shown to be compatible with Sodium Chloride Injection BP. Accordingly, only this diluent should be used for reconstitution. Compatibility with other drugs has not been studied, therefore, it is not recommended to mix Gemzar with other drugs when reconstituted. Due to solubility considerations, the maximum concentration for gemcitabine upon reconstitution is 40 mg/ml. Reconstitution at concentrations greater than 40 mg/ml may result in incomplete dissolution, and should be avoided.

To reconstitute, add at least 5 ml of Sodium Chloride Injection BP to the 200 mg vial or at least 25 ml of Sodium Chloride Injection BP to the 1 g vial. Shake to dissolve. The appropriate amount of drug may be administered as prepared or further diluted with Sodium Chloride Injection BP.

Parenteral drugs should be inspected visually for particulate matter and discoloration, prior to administration, whenever solution and container permit.

*Guidelines for the safe handling of antineoplastic agents:* Cytotoxic preparations should not be handled by pregnant staff. Trained personnel should reconstitute the drug. This should be performed in a designated area. The work surface should be covered with disposable plastic-backed absorbent paper.

Adequate protective gloves, masks and clothing should be worn. Precautions should be taken to avoid the drug accidentally coming into contact with the eyes. If accidental contamination occurs, the eye should be washed with water thoroughly and immediately.

Use Luer-lock fittings on all syringes and sets. Large bore needles are recommended to minimise pressure and the possible formation of aerosols. The latter may also be reduced by the use of a venting needle.

Adequate care and precaution should be taken in the disposal of items used to reconstitute Gemzar. Any unused dry product or contaminated materials should be placed in a high risk waste bag. Sharp objects (needles, syringes, vials, etc) should be placed in a suitable rigid container. Personnel concerned with the collection and disposal of this waste should be aware of the hazard involved. Waste material should be destroyed by incineration. Any excess drug solution should be flushed directly into a drain with copious amounts of water.

**Marketing authorisation numbers**

200 mg vial: 0006/0301
1 g vial:  0006/0302

**Date of approval/revision of SPC** 10 January 1997

**Legal category** POM

# GLUCAGON

**Qualitative and quantitative composition** Vials containing 1 unit (1.09 mg) of glucagon as the hydrochloride.

**Pharmaceutical form** Parenteral injection. The product is in lyophilised form and is supplied with an accompanying diluting solution.

**Clinical particulars**

*Therapeutic indications:*

*Indications:* Glucagon is useful in counteracting severe hypoglycaemic reactions.

Glucagon is indicated as a diagnostic aid in the radiological examination of the stomach, duodenum, small bowel and colon, when a hypotonic state would be advantageous.

Glucagon is as effective for this examination as the anticholinergic drugs, but it has fewer side-effects. When glucagon is administered concomitantly with an anticholinergic agent, the response is not significantly greater than when either drug is used alone. However, the addition of the anticholinergic agent results in increased side-effects.

*Posology and method of administration:* The diluent is provided for use only in the preparation of glucagon

for *intermittent* parenteral injection and for no other use.

Glucagon should not be used at concentrations greater than 1 unit/ml (1 mg/ml).

Glucagon may be given by subcutaneous, intramuscular or intravenous injection. Administration as a continuous intravenous infusion for long periods is not recommended.

*Dosage in the elderly:* As for adults.

*Directions for the use of glucagon in hypoglycaemia:*

1. Dissolve the lyophilised glucagon in the accompanying diluent.
2. For *adults* and children weighing more than 20 kilograms, give 1 unit (1 mg) by subcutaneous, intramuscular or intravenous injection.
3. For *children* weighing less than 20 kilograms, give 0.5 unit (0.5 mg) or a dose equivalent to 20-30 microgram/kilogram.
4. The patient will normally awaken in 15 minutes. If the response is delayed, there is no contraindication to the administration of 1 or 2 additional doses of glucagon: however, in view of the deleterious effects of cerebral hypoglycaemia and depending on the duration and depth of coma, the use of parenteral glucose *must* be considered.
5. Intravenous glucose *must* be given if the patient fails to respond to glucagon.
6. When the patient responds, give supplementary carbohydrate to restore the liver glycogen and prevent secondary hypoglycaemia.

It is important that the patient be aroused as quickly as possible, because prolonged hypoglycaemic reactions may result in cortical damage. Glucagon or intravenous glucose will awaken the patient sufficiently so that oral carbohydrates may be taken.

Although the patient or family members may use glucagon for the treatment of hypoglycaemia during an emergency, a doctor must still be notified when hypoglycaemic reactions occur so that the treatment regimen may be adjusted if necessary.

Instructions describing the method of using this preparation are included in the vial carton. It is advisable for the patient and family members to become familiar with the technique of preparing Glucagon for Injection before an emergency arises. Patients are instructed to use 1 unit (1 mg) for adults and, if recommended by a doctor, 0.5 unit (0.5 mg) for children weighing less than 20 kilograms.

*For use as a diagnostic aid:* Dissolve the lyophilised glucagon in the accompanying diluting solution. Glucagon should not be used at concentrations greater than 1 unit/ml (1 mg/ml).

The following doses may be administered for relaxation of the stomach, duodenum, and small bowel, depending on the time of onset of action and the duration of effect required for the examination. Since the stomach is less sensitive to the effect of glucagon, 0.5 unit (0.5 mg) IV or 2 units (2 mg) im are recommended.

| Dose† | Route of Administration | Time of Onset of Action | Approximate Duration of Effect |
|---|---|---|---|
| 0.25–0.5 units | IV | 1 minute | 9–17 minutes |
| 1 unit | im | 8–10 minutes | 12–27 minutes |
| 2 units* | IV | 1 minute | 22–25 minutes |
| 2 units* | im | 4–7 minutes | 21–32 minutes |

*2-unit (2 mg) doses are associated with a higher incidence of nausea and vomiting than lower doses.
 †1 unit equals 1 mg.

For examination of the colon, it is recommended that a 2 unit dose be administered intramuscularly approximately 10 minutes prior to initiation of the procedure. Relaxation of the colon and reduction of discomfort to the patient will allow the radiologist to perform a more satisfactory examination.

*Contra-indications:* Hypersensitivity to glucagon. Patients with phaeochromocytoma, where glucagon can cause the tumour to release catecholamines, which result in sudden and marked hypertension.

*Special warnings and special precautions for use:*
*Warnings:* Glucagon should be administered cautiously to patients with known or suspected insulinoma. In these patients intravenous administration of glucagon will produce an initial increase in blood glucose but, because of its insulin-releasing effect, may subsequently cause severe hypoglycaemia. A patient developing symptoms of hypoglycaemia after a dose of glucagon should be given glucose orally, intravenously, or by gavage, whichever is more appropriate.

Exogenous glucagon also stimulates the release of catecholamines. In the presence of phaeochromocytoma, glucagon can cause the tumour to release catecholamines, which results in a sudden and marked increase in blood pressure. Five to 10 mg of phentolamine mesylate may be administered IV in an attempt to control the blood pressure.

*Precautions:* Glucagon is helpful in hypoglycaemia only if liver glycogen is available. Because glucagon is of little or no help in states of starvation, adrenal insufficiency, or chronic hypoglycaemia, glucose should be considered for the treatment of hypoglycaemia.

Blood glucose determinations should be obtained to follow the patient in hypoglycaemic shock until he is asymptomatic.

Glucagon should be used with caution as a diagnostic aid in diabetic patients.

*Interaction with other medicaments and other forms of interaction:* Glucagon may enhance the anticoagulant effect of warfarin.

*Pregnancy and lactation:*
*Usage in pregnancy:* Animal reproduction studies have revealed no evidence of impaired fertility or foetal harm due to glucagon. However, in the absence of adequate human studies, glucagon should be used during pregnancy only if clearly needed.

*Usage in nursing mothers:* It is not known whether this drug is excreted in human milk. Although the plasma half-life is only 3 to 6 minutes and it is not active when taken orally, caution should be exercised when glucagon is administered to a nursing woman.

*Effects on ability to drive and use machines:* Not applicable.

*Undesirable effects:* Glucagon is relatively free of adverse reactions, except for occasional nausea and vomiting, which may also occur with hypoglycaemia. Diarrhoea and hypokalaemia have rarely been reported, as well as generalised allergic reactions, including urticaria, respiratory distress and hypotension.

*Overdose:*
*Signs and symptoms:* Although there is a lack of human experience and glucagon is generally well tolerated, nausea, vomiting, gastric hypotonicity and diarrhoea would be expected. Intravenous glucagon has positive inotropic and chronotropic effects. Increases in blood pressure and pulse might be more severe in patients taking beta-blockers and might require therapy in patients with phaeochromocytoma, insulinomas or coronary artery disease. When large doses (0.5-16 mg/hour by continuous infusion for periods of 5-166 hours) were given to cardiac patients, positive inotropy occurred and side-effects included nausea, vomiting and decreasing serum potassium.

As a polypeptide, glucagon would be rapidly destroyed if ingested.

*Treatment:* The plasma half-life of glucagon is approximately 3-6 minutes. Symptomatic and supportive therapy might include supplemental potassium for hypokalaemia, or phentolamine if a dramatic increase in blood pressure occurs. Forced diuresis, peritoneal dialysis, haemodialysis, or charcoal haemoperfusion have not been established as beneficial.

**Pharmacological properties**

*Pharmacodynamic properties:*
*Actions:* Glucagon causes an increase in blood glucose concentrations and is used in the treatment of hypoglycaemic states. It is effective in small doses. Glucagon acts only on liver glycogen, converting it to glucose, and is therefore helpful only if liver glycogen is available. It is of little or no help in states of starvation, adrenal insufficiency or chronic hypoglycaemia. The patient with Type I diabetes does not have as great a response in blood glucose levels as does the Type II stable diabetic, therefore, supplementary carbohydrate should be given as soon as possible, especially to juvenile patients.

Parenteral administration of glucagon produces relaxation of the smooth muscle of the stomach, duodenum, small bowel and colon.

*Pharmacokinetic properties:* The half-life of glucagon in plasma is approximately 3-6 minutes, which is similar to that of insulin.

*Preclinical safety data:* There are no preclinical data of relevance to the prescriber in addition to that summarised in other sections of the summary of product characteristics.

**Pharmaceutical particulars**

*List of excipients:*
Lyophilised product: Lactose
Diluting solution: Glycerin; Phenol; Sodium hydroxide*; Hydrochloric acid*; Water for injection.
*May have been added during manufacture to adjust the pH.

*Incompatibilities:* Not applicable.

*Shelf life:*
*Prior to reconstitution:* 3 years.
Reconstituted solutions should be used immediately.

*Special precautions for storage:*
*Prior to reconstitution:* Store below 25°C.

*Nature and contents of container:* Glass vial (No. 666), containing 1 unit (1.09 mg) of glucagon as the hydrochloride, accompanied by glass vial (No. 667), containing 1 ml of diluent.

*Instructions for use/handling:* Crystalline glucagon is a white powder containing less than 0.05% zinc. It is relatively insoluble in water but is soluble at a pH of less than 3 or more than 9.5. Glucagon is stable in lyophilised form at room temperatures.

Use accompanying diluent solution for reconstitution.

After reconstitution, solutions should be used immediately. Glucagon solutions should not be used unless they are clear and of a water-like consistency.

If glucagon is to be given at doses higher than 2 units (2 mg), it should be reconstituted with Sterile Water for Injection, instead of the diluting solution supplied, and used immediately.

**Marketing authorisation numbers**
Vials 1 unit: 0006/5110
Vials diluting solution: 0006/5112

**Date of approval/revision of SPC** October 1995

**Legal category** POM

## HUMAJECT* PENS
## HUMULIN* PREFILLED INSULIN PENS
## HUMAJECT* S (Soluble)
## HUMAJECT* I (Isophane)
## HUMAJECT* M1 (Mixture 1)
## HUMAJECT* M2 (Mixture 2)
## HUMAJECT* M3 (Mixture 3)
## HUMAJECT* M4 (Mixture 4)

**Qualitative and quantitative composition**

| *Active Ingredient* | *Quantity per ml* |
|---|---|
| Human Insulin (recombinant DNA origin) | 100IU |

Humulin Soluble is a sterile, clear, colourless, aqueous solution of human insulin adjusted to a pH range of 7.0 to 7.8.

Humulin Soluble is a rapidly acting insulin preparation.

Humulin Isophane is a sterile suspension of a white, crystalline precipitate of isophane human insulin in an isotonic phosphate buffer adjusted to a pH range of 6.9 to 7.5.

Humulin Isophane is an intermediate acting insulin preparation.

Humulin Mixture 1, Mixture 2, Mixture 3 and Mixture 4 are sterile suspensions of human insulin in the proportion of 10%, 20%, 30%, 40% and 50% soluble insulin to 90%, 80%, 70%, 60% and 50% isophane insulin, respectively, adjusted to a pH range of 6.9 to 7.5.

Humulin Mixtures are intermediate acting insulin preparations.

**Pharmaceutical form** A solution or suspension for injection filled into *cartridges* administered via a non-reusable device.

Humaject is a disposable injector containing a 3.0 ml cartridge prefilled with human insulin for parenteral administration.

**Clinical particulars**

*Therapeutic indications:* For the treatment of patients with diabetes mellitus who require insulin for the maintenance of glucose homeostasis. Humulin is also indicated for the initial control of diabetes mellitus and diabetes mellitus in pregnancy.

*Posology and method of administration:* The dosage should be determined by the physician, according to the requirement of the patient.

Humulin Soluble, Humulin Isophane and Mixtures in cartridge presentations should be given by subcutaneous injection but may, although not recommended, also be given by intramuscular injection. These formulations should not be administered intravenously.

Subcutaneous administration should be in the upper arms, thighs, buttocks or abdomen. Use of injection sites should be rotated so that the same site is not used more than approximately once a month.

Care should be taken when injecting any Humulin insulin preparations to ensure that a blood vessel has not been entered. After any insulin injection, the injection site should not be massaged.

Humulin Isophane may be administered in combination with Humulin Soluble (see *Special warnings and special precautions for use - Mixing of insulins*).

Humulin Mixture formulations are ready-made defined mixtures of Humulin Soluble and Humulin Isophane insulin, designed to avoid the need for the patient to mix insulin preparations. A patient's treatment regimen should be based on their individual metabolic requirements.

*Contra-indications:* Hypoglycaemia.

Hypersensitivity to Humulin or to the formulation excipients.

Under no circumstances should any Humulin formulation, other than Humulin Soluble in vials, be given intravenously.

*Special warnings and special precautions for use:*
*Transferring from other insulins:* A small number of patients transferring from insulins of animal origin may require a reduced dosage and/or a change in the ratio of soluble to intermediate preparations, especially if they are very tightly controlled and bordering on hypoglycaemia. The dosage reduction may occur immediately after transfer or be a gradual process lasting for several weeks. There is a risk of hypoglycaemia if insulin requirement is decreased, and both the physician and the patient should be aware of this possibility. The risk can be considered minimal if the daily dosage is less than 40IU. Insulin-resistant patients receiving more than 100IU daily should be referred to hospital for transfer.

A few patients who experienced hypoglycaemic reactions after transfer to human insulin have reported that the early warning symptoms were less pronounced or different from those experienced with their previous animal insulin. Patients whose blood glucose control is greatly improved, eg, by intensified insulin therapy, may lose some or all of the warning symptoms of hypoglycaemia and should be advised accordingly. Other conditions which may make the early warning symptoms of hypoglycaemia different or less pronounced include long duration of diabetes, diabetic nerve disease, or medications such as beta blockers. Uncorrected hypoglycaemic and hyperglycaemic reactions can cause loss of consciousness, coma or death.

Insulin requirements may change significantly in diseases of the adrenal, pituitary or thyroid glands and in the presence of renal or hepatic impairment.

Insulin requirements may be increased during illness or emotional disturbances.

Adjustment of insulin dosage may also be necessary if patients undertake increased physical activity or change their usual diet.

*Mixing of insulins:* Separate cartridges of Humulin Soluble and Isophane can be used for administration of the correct amount of each formulation.

*Interaction with other medicaments and other forms of interaction:* The patient should check with their physician when using other medicines in addition to Humulin.

Insulin requirements may be reduced by the concurrent administration of drugs with hypoglycaemic activity, eg, alcohol, monoamine oxidase inhibitors and beta-adrenergic blockers or aspirin.

Insulin requirements may be increased by concurrent administration of drugs, eg, oral contraceptives, corticosteroids or thyroid hormone replacement therapy.

The effects of mixing human insulin with insulins of animal origin have not been studied and this practice is not recommended.

*Pregnancy and lactation:* It is essential to maintain good control of the insulin treated (insulin-dependent or gestational diabetes) patient throughout pregnancy. Insulin requirements usually fall during the first trimester and increase during the second and third trimesters. Patients with diabetes should be advised to inform their doctors if they are pregnant or are contemplating pregnancy.

Diabetic patients who are lactating may require adjustments in insulin dose and/or diet.

*Effects on ability to drive and use machines:* Use of the correct therapeutic dose has no known effect on driving or the use of machinery.

*Undesirable effects:* Lipodystrophy, insulin resistance and hypersensitivity reactions are among the side-effects associated with insulins of animal origin. However, the incidence of such side-effects with Humulin is minimal. In the rare event of a severe allergy to Humulin, treatment is required immediately. A change of insulin or desensitisation may be required.

Hypoglycaemia is the most frequent undesirable effect that a diabetic may suffer. Severe hypoglycaemia may lead to loss of consciousness, and in extreme cases, death.

*Overdose:* Insulin has no specific overdose definitions, because serum glucose concentrations are a result of complex interactions between insulin levels, glucose availability and other metabolic processes. Hypoglycaemia may occur as a result of an excess of insulin relative to food intake and energy expenditure.

Hypoglycaemia may be associated with listlessness, confusion, palpitations, headache, sweating and vomiting.

Mild hypoglycaemic episodes will respond to oral administration of glucose or sugar products.

Correction of moderately severe hypoglycaemia can be accomplished by intramuscular or subcutaneous administration of glucagon, followed by oral carbohydrate when the patient recovers sufficiently. Patients who fail to respond to glucagon must be given glucose solution intravenously.

If the patient is comatose, glucagon should be administered intramuscularly or subcutaneously. However, glucose solution must be given intravenously if glucagon is not available or if the patient fails to respond to glucagon. The patient should be given a meal as soon as consciousness is recovered.

### Pharmacological properties

*Pharmacodynamic properties:* The prime activity of insulin is the regulation of glucose metabolism.

In addition, insulin has several anabolic and anti-catabolic actions on a variety of different tissues. Within muscle tissue this includes increasing glycogen, fatty acid, glycerol and protein synthesis, and amino acid uptake, while decreasing glycogenolysis, gluconeogenesis, ketogenesis, lipolysis, protein catabolism and amino acid output.

The typical activity profile (glucose utilisation curve) following subcutaneous injection is illustrated below by the heavy line. Variations that a patient may experience in timing and/or intensity of insulin activity are illustrated by the shaded area. Individual variability will depend on factors such as size of dose, site of injection, temperature and physical activity of the patient.

*Pharmacokinetic properties:* The pharmacokinetics of insulin do not reflect the metabolic action of that hormone. Therefore, it is more appropriate to examine glucose utilisation curves (as discussed above) when considering the activity of insulin.

*Preclinical safety data:* Humulin is human insulin produced by recombinant technology. No serious events have been reported in subchronic toxicology studies.

### Pharmaceutical particulars
*List of excipients:*

*For Humulin Soluble preparations:*Each will contain Human Insulin (recombinant DNA origin) and the following excipients:

(a) *m*-Cresol distilled, 2.5 mg/ml; (b) glycerol; (c) water for injections; (d) hydrochloric acid; and (e) sodium hydroxide.

These are included as:

(a) preservative; (b) tonicity modifier; (c) solvent; (d) pH adjustment; and (e) pH adjustment, respectively.

Hydrochloric acid and/or sodium hydroxide may have been used during manufacture to adjust the pH.

*For Humulin Isophane and Mixture preparations:*Each will contain Human Insulin (recombinant DNA origin) and the following excipients:

(a) *m*-Cresol distilled, 1.6 mg/ml; (b) glycerol; (c) phenol, 0.65 mg/ml; (d) protamine sulphate; (e) dibasic sodium phosphate; (f) zinc oxide; (g) water for injections; (h) hydrochloric acid; and (i) sodium hydroxide.

These are included as:

(a) preservative; (b) tonicity modifier; (c) preservative; (d) complexes with insulin to prolong its action; (e) buffer; (f) adjust zinc content; (g) solvent; (h) pH adjustment; and (i) pH adjustment, respectively.

Hydrochloric acid and/or sodium hydroxide may have been used during manufacture to adjust the pH.

*Incompatibilities:* Humulin products should not be mixed with either animal insulins or human insulin preparations produced by other manufacturers.

*Shelf life:* The shelf life for Humulin Soluble, Isophane and Mixture presentations is two years when stored under appropriate conditions.

The in-use shelf life for all Humaject pens is 28 days.

*Special precautions for storage:* Humulin preparations should be stored in a refrigerator between 2° and 8°C. They should not be frozen or exposed to excessive heat or sunlight.

When in-use the Humaject pens may be kept at room temperature for up to 28 days:

*Nature and contents of container:*
*Humaject pens:* The product is filled in cartridges that comply with the requirements of the Ph Eur for Type I flint glass, and sealed with rubber closures consisting of a plunger head at the bottom and a disk seal at the top of the cartridge.

*Package quantities:*Humaject pens, each containing 3.0 ml Humulin, in packs of 5.

*Instructions for use/handling:*
*(a) Preparing a dose:* Humaject containing Humulin Soluble formulation does not require resuspension and should only be used if it is clear, colourless, with no solid particles visible and if it is of water-like appearance.

Humaject containing Humulin Isophane and Mixture formulations should be rolled in the palms of the hands ten times and inverted 180° ten times immediately before use to resuspend the insulin until it appears uniform cloudy or milky. Do not shake vigorously as this may cause frothing which may interfere with the correct measurement of the dose.

The cartridges should be examined frequently and should not be used if clumps of material are present or if solid white particles stick to the bottom or wall of the cartridge or vial, giving a frosted appearance.

Humulin cartridges are not designed to allow any other insulin to be mixed in the cartridge. Cartridges are not designed to be refilled.

*Cartridges:* Non-reusable device - Humaject.

### Preparing a dose
**1. Mixing Insulin Suspensions.** Remove pen cap. Roll the pen back and forth in your hands 10 times. Then, turn the pen up and down 10 times until insulin is evenly mixed.

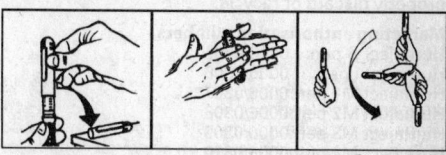

**2. Resetting the pen.** Before each injection the **star** (★) must appear in the dose window. If the **star** (★) is not in the dose window, while holding the white cylinder firmly, turn the **CLEAR PLASTIC BARREL IN THE DIRECTION OF THE ARROWS**. Turn until the **star** (★) appears in the dose window. (Do **NOT** turn the white dose set/plunger knob to reset to **star** (★).)

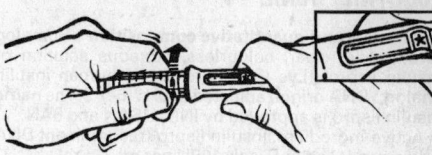

**3. Putting on the B-D pen needle.** Wipe rubber seal with alcohol. Remove paper tab from needle. Screw capped needle onto the end of the pen until tight.

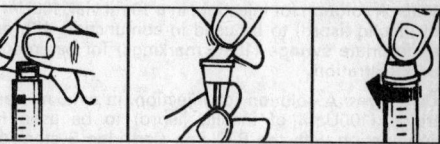

**4. Clearing air bubbles.**
a) Turn the dose set/plunger knob in direction of the arrow until a '2' shows in the dose display window. You will hear one click.
b) Hold pen upright. Remove outer needle cap and cover.
c) Depress plunger knob to remove any large air bubbles.
A small drop of insulin should appear at the tip of the needle. If insulin does not appear, repeat step a, b and c above.
d) Replace outer needle cap.

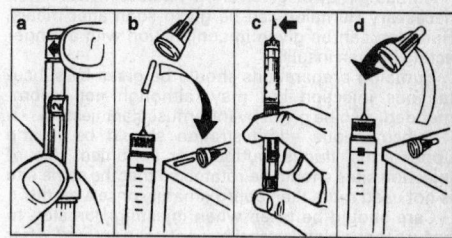

**5. Reset Pen so the star (★) appears in the dose window. SEE STEP 2.**

**6. Setting Your Dose.** To set your dose, turn the dose set/plunger knob in the direction of the arrow. Turn until your dose appears in the dose window. Pen will click once for each 2 units dialled. This knob can be moved back and forth to adjust your dose.

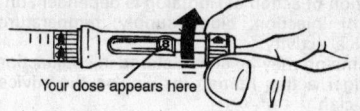

Your dose appears here

*(b) Injecting a dose*
Cartridges:
1. Wash your hands.
2. Choose a site for the injection.
3. Clean the skin with an alcohol swab.
4. Remove outer needle cap.
5. Stabilise the skin by spreading it or pinching up a large area. Insert the needle as instructed by your doctor.
6. To inject insulin via a Humaject pen, push the dose knob down with the thumb until a click is heard. Wait 5 seconds.
7. Pull the needle straight out of the skin and apply

## Time Action Profiles

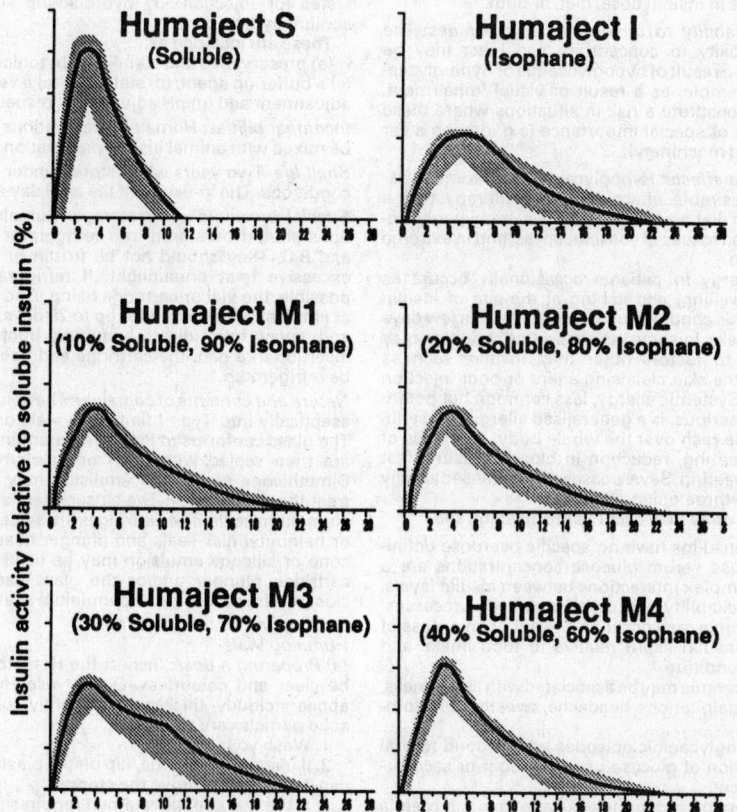

### Humaject S
(Soluble)

### Humaject I
(Isophane)

### Humaject M1
(10% Soluble, 90% Isophane)

### Humaject M2
(20% Soluble, 80% Isophane)

### Humaject M3
(30% Soluble, 70% Isophane)

### Humaject M4
(40% Soluble, 60% Isophane)

Insulin activity relative to soluble insulin (%)

Time (hours)

gentle pressure over the injection site for several seconds. Do not rub the area.
8. Using the outer needle cap, unscrew the needle immediately after injection and dispose of it safely. Removing the needle immediately after injection ensures sterility, prevents leakage and re-entry of air and potential needle clogs.
9. Replace the cap on the pen.

*(c) Disposal of used containers and needles:*
Do not reuse needles. Dispose of the needle in a responsible manner. Needles and pens must not be shared. Humaject pens can be used until empty, then properly discard or recycle.

**Marketing authorisation numbers**
Humaject S pen: 0006/0305
Humaject I pen: 0006/0306
Humaject M1 pen: 0006/0307
Humaject M2 pen: 0006/0308
Humaject M3 pen: 0006/0309
Humaject M4 pen: 0006/0310

**Date of approval/revision of SPC** 13 December 1994

**Legal category** P

## HUMALOG* VIALS AND CARTRIDGES 100U/ML, 10ML ▼

**Qualitative and quantitative composition** Humalog is a sterile, clear, colourless, aqueous solution of insulin lispro ([Lys (B28), Pro (B29)] human insulin analog, rDNA origin) adjusted to pH 7.0–7.8. The name insulin lispro is approved by INN, USAN and BAN.

Active ingredient: Insulin lispro (recombinant DNA origin produced in *E. coli*) 100U per ml.

The concentration of insulin lispro is 3.5 mg insulin lispro per ml for the 100U/ml product.

**Pharmaceutical forms**
*Vials:* A solution for injection, in a 10 ml vial (100U/ml of insulin lispro) to be used in conjunction with an appropriate syringe (100U markings) for parenteral administration.

*Cartridges:* A solution for injection, in a 1.5 ml cartridge (100U/ml of insulin lispro) to be used in conjunction with the B–D Pen Cartridge System or Lilly–Diapen pen injection delivery systems for parenteral subcutaneous administration.

**Clinical particulars**
*Therapeutic indication:* For the treatment of patients with diabetes mellitus who require insulin for the maintenance of normal glucose homeostasis. Humalog is also indicated for the initial stabilisation of diabetes mellitus.

*Posology and method of administration:* The dosage should be determined by the physician, according to the requirement of the patient.

Humalog may be given shortly before meals. When necessary Humalog can be given soon after meals. Humalog can be given in conjunction with a longer acting human insulin.

Humalog preparations should be given by subcutaneous injection but may, although not recommended, also be given by intramuscular injection.

Subcutaneous administration should be in the upper arms, thighs, buttocks or abdomen. Use of injection sites should be rotated so that the same site is not used more than approximately once a month.

Care should be taken when injecting Humalog to ensure that a blood vessel has not been entered. After injection, the site of injection should not be massaged.

Humalog takes effect rapidly and has a shorter duration of activity (2 to 5 hours) as compared with soluble insulin. This rapid onset of activity allows Humalog to be given very close to mealtime. The time course of action of any insulin may vary considerably in different individuals or at different times in the same individual. As with all insulin preparations, the duration of action of Humalog is dependent on dose, site of injection, blood supply, temperature and physical activity.

Humalog may be administered in conjunction with a longer acting human insulin, on the advice of a physician.

*Contra-indications:* Hypoglycaemia. Hypersensitivity to insulin lispro or one of its excipients.

*Special warnings and special precautions for use:* Transferring a patient to another type or brand of insulin should be done under strict medical supervision. Changes in strength, brand (manufacturer), type (soluble, isophane, lente, etc), species (animal, human, human insulin analog) and/or method of manufacture (recombinant DNA versus animal-source insulin) may result in the need for a change in dosage.

Vials: The shorter acting Humalog should be drawn into the syringe first, to prevent contamination of the vial by the longer acting insulin. Mixing of the insulins ahead of time or just before the injection should be on the advice of the physician. However, a consistent routine must be followed.

Patients taking Humalog may require a change in dosage from that used with their usual insulins. If an adjustment is needed, it may occur with the first dose or during the first several weeks or months.

Patients whose blood glucose is greatly improved, eg, by intensified insulin therapy, may lose some or all of the warning symptoms of hypoglycaemia and should be advised accordingly.

A few patients who have experienced hypoglycaemic reactions after transfer from animal–source insulin to human insulin have reported that the early warning symptoms of hypoglycaemia were less pronounced or different from those experienced with their previous insulin. Uncorrected hypoglycaemic or hyperglycaemic reactions can cause loss of consciousness, coma or death.

Insulin requirements may be reduced in the presence of renal or hepatic impairment.

Insulin requirements may be increased during illness or emotional disturbances.

Adjustment of dosage may also be necessary if patients undertake increased physical activity or change their usual diet. Exercise taken immediately after a meal may increase the risk of hypoglycaemia.

Administration of insulin lispro to children should be considered only in case of an expected benefit when compared to soluble insulin.

*Interaction with other medicaments and other forms of interaction:* Insulin requirements may be increased by drugs with hyperglycaemic activity, such as oral contraceptives, corticosteroids, or thyroid replacement therapy, danazol, beta 2 stimulants (ritodrine, salbutamol, terbutaline).

Insulin requirements may be reduced in the presence of drugs with hypoglycaemic activity, such as oral hypoglycaemics, salicylates (for example, aspirin), sulpha antibiotics, and certain antidepressants, certain angiotensin converting enzyme inhibitors (captopril, enalapril), beta blockers, octreotide, alcohol.

Humalog should not be mixed with animal insulins.

The physician should be consulted when using other medications in addition to Humalog.

*Use in pregnancy and lactation:* There is no significant experience with Humalog in pregnancy.

It is essential to maintain good control of the insulin–treated (insulin–dependent or gestational diabetes) patient throughout pregnancy. Insulin requirements usually fall during the first trimester and increase during the second and third trimesters. Patients with diabetes should be advised to inform their doctor if they are pregnant or are contemplating pregnancy. Careful monitoring of glucose control, as well as general health, is essential in pregnant patients with diabetes.

Patients with diabetes who are lactating may require adjustments in insulin dose, diet, or both.

*Effects on ability to drive and use machines:* The patient's ability to concentrate and react may be impaired as a result of hypoglycaemia or hyperglycaemia, for example, as a result of visual impairment. This may constitute a risk in situations where these abilities are of special importance (e.g. driving a car or operating machinery).

*Undesirable effects:* Hypoglycaemia is the most frequent undesirable effect of insulin therapy that a patient with diabetes may suffer. Severe hypoglycaemia may lead to loss of consciousness, and in extreme cases, death.

Local allergy in patients occasionally occurs as redness, swelling, and itching at the site of insulin injection. This condition usually resolves in a few days to a few weeks. In some instances, this condition may be related to factors other than insulin, such as irritants in the skin cleansing agent or poor injection technique. Systemic allergy, less common but potentially more serious, is a generalised allergy to insulin. It may cause rash over the whole body, shortness of breath, wheezing, reduction in blood pressure, fast pulse, or sweating. Severe cases of generalised allergy may be life–threatening.

Lipodystrophy may occur at the injection site.

*Overdose:* Insulins have no specific overdose definitions because serum glucose concentrations are a result of complex interactions between insulin levels, glucose availability and other metabolic processes. Hypoglycaemia may occur as a result of an excess of insulin or insulin lispro relative to food intake and energy expenditure.

Hypoglycaemia may be associated with listlessness, confusion, palpitations, headache, sweating and vomiting.

Mild hypoglycaemic episodes will respond to oral administration of glucose or other sugar or saccharated products.

Correction of moderately severe hypoglycaemia can be accomplished by intramuscular or subcutaneous administration of glucagon, followed by oral carbohydrate when the patient recovers sufficiently. Patients who fail to respond to glucagon must be given glucose solution intravenously.

If the patient is comatose, glucagon should be administered intramuscularly or subcutaneously. However, glucose solution must be given intravenously if glucagon is not available or if the patient fails to respond to glucagon. The patient should be given a meal as soon as consciousness is recovered.

**Pharmacological properties**
*Pharmacodynamic properties:* Pharmaco–therapeutic group: fast acting human insulin analogue.

The primary activity of insulin lispro is the regulation of glucose metabolism.

In addition, insulins have several anabolic and anti–catabolic actions on a variety of different tissues. Within muscle tissue this includes increasing glycogen, fatty acid, glycerol and protein synthesis and amino acid uptake, while decreasing glycogenolysis, glyconeogenesis, ketogenesis, lipolysis, protein catabolism and amino acid output.

Humalog has a rapid onset of action (approximately 15 minutes), thus allowing it to be given closer to a meal (within zero to 15 minutes of the meal) when compared to soluble insulin (30 to 45 minutes before). Humalog takes effect rapidly and has a shorter duration of activity (2 to 5 hours) when compared to soluble insulin. As with all insulin preparations, the time course of Humalog action may vary in different individuals or at different times in the same individual and is dependent on site of injection, blood supply, temperature and physical activity. The typical activity profile following subcutaneous injection is illustrated below. The representation below reflects the relative amount of glucose over time required to maintain subject's whole blood glucose concentrations near fasting levels and is an indicator of the effect of these insulins on glucose metabolism over time.

*Pharmacokinetic properties:* The pharmacokinetics of Humalog reflect a compound that is rapidly absorbed, and achieves peak blood levels 30 to 70 minutes following subcutaneous injection. When considering the clinical relevance of these kinetics, it is more appropriate to examine the glucose utilisation curves (as discussed in *Pharmacodynamic properties*).

*Preclinical safety:* In *in vitro* tests, including binding to insulin receptor sites and effects on growing cells, Humalog behaved in a manner that closely resembled human insulin. Studies also demonstrate that the dissociation of binding to the insulin receptor of Humalog is equivalent to human insulin. Acute, one month and twelve month toxicology studies produced no significant toxicity findings.

**Pharmaceutical particulars**
*List of excipients:* Each vial or cartridge will contain insulin lispro and the following excipients:

(a) *m*-cresol distilled [3.15 mg/ml]; (b) glycerol; (c) dibasic sodium phosphate.$7H_2O$; (d) zinc oxide; (e) water for injection; (f) hydrochloric acid and (g) sodium hydroxide.

These are included as:

(a) preservative and stabiliser; (b) tonicity modifier; (c) a buffering agent; (d) stabiliser; (e) a vehicle; (f) pH adjustment and (g) pH adjustment, respectively.

*Incompatibilities:* Humalog preparations should not be mixed with animal insulin preparations.

*Shelf life:* Two years when stored under appropriate conditions. The in-use shelf life is 28 days.

*Special precautions for storage:* Humalog preparations should be stored in a refrigerator between 2° and 8°C. They should not be frozen or exposed to excessive heat or sunlight. If refrigeration is not possible, the vial or cartridge being used can be kept at ambient temperature for up to 28 days, below 30°C and away from direct heat and light. Following insertion in a pen, the cartridge and pen should not be refrigerated.

*Nature and contents of container:* The solution is filled aseptically into Type I flint glass vials or cartridges. The glass conforms to PhEur requirements. The vials are then sealed with butyl or halobutyl stoppers. Dimethicone or silicone emulsion may be used to treat the vial stopper. The closures are secured with aluminium seals. The cartridges are sealed with butyl or halobutyl disk seals and plunger heads. Dimethicone or silicone emulsion may be used to treat the cartridge plunger and/or the glass cartridge. The closures are secured with aluminium seals.

*Instructions for use/handling:*
*Humalog Vials*
*(a) Preparing a dose:* Inspect the Humalog. It should be clear and colourless. Do not use Humalog if it appears cloudy, thickened or slightly coloured, or if solid particles are visible.

1. Wash your hands.

2. If using a new bottle, flip off the plastic protective cap, but **do not remove the stopper**.

3. If the therapeutic regimen requires the injection of basal insulin and Humalog at the same time, the two can be mixed in the syringe. If mixing insulins,

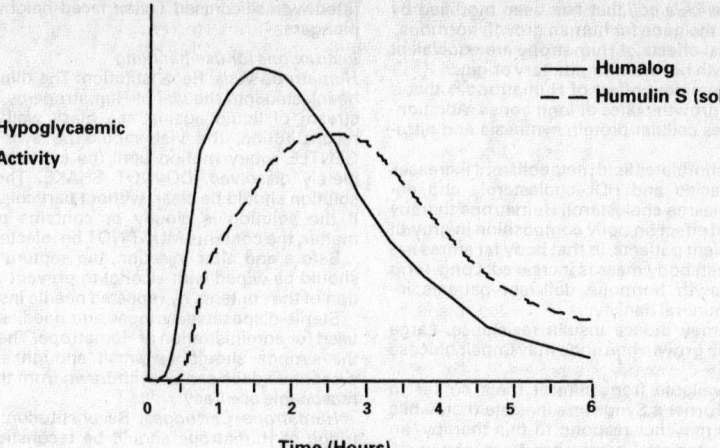

Hypoglycaemic Activity

— Humalog
-- Humulin S (soluble)

Time (Hours)

refer to the instructions for mixing that follow in Section (b).

4. Draw air into the syringe equal to the prescribed Humalog dose. Wipe the top of the bottle with an alcohol swab. Put the needle through rubber top of the Humalog bottle and inject the air into the bottle.

5. Turn the bottle and syringe upside down. Hold the bottle and syringe firmly in one hand.

6. Making sure the tip of the needle is in the Humalog, withdraw the correct dose into the syringe.

7. Before removing the needle from the bottle, check the syringe for air bubbles that reduce the amount of Humalog in it. If bubbles are present, hold the syringe straight up and tap its side until the bubbles float to the top. Push them out with the plunger and withdraw the correct dose.

8. Remove the needle from the bottle and lay the syringe down so that the needle does not touch anything.

*(b) Mixing Humalog with longer-acting human insulins*

1. Humalog should be mixed with longer–acting human insulins only on the advice of a doctor.

2. Draw air into the syringe equal to the amount of longer–acting insulin being taken. Insert the needle into the longer–acting insulin bottle and inject the air. Withdraw the needle.

3. Now inject air into the Humalog bottle in the same manner, but **do not** withdraw the needle.

4. Turn the bottle and syringe upside down.

5. Making sure the tip of the needle is in the Humalog, withdraw the correct dose of Humalog into the syringe.

6. Before removing the needle from the bottle, check the syringe for air bubbles that reduce the amount of Humalog in it. If bubbles are present, hold the syringe straight up and tap its side until the bubbles float to the top. Push them out with the plunger and withdraw the correct dose.

7. Remove the needle from the bottle of Humalog and insert it into the bottle of the longer–acting insulin. Turn the bottle and syringe upside down. Hold the bottle and syringe firmly in one hand and shake gently. Making sure the tip of the needle is in the insulin, withdraw the dose of longer–acting insulin.

8. Remove the needle and lay the syringe down so that the needle does not touch anything.

*(c) Mixing insulins:* Do not mix insulins in vials with insulins in cartridges.

*Humalog Cartridges*

(a) *Preparing a dose:* Inspect the Humalog. It should be clear and colourless. Do not use Humalog if it appears cloudy, thickened or slightly coloured, or if solid particles are visible.

The manufacturer's instructions for the B–D Pen Cartridge System or Lilly–Diapen pen injection delivery systems should be followed for loading the cartridge, attaching the needle and administering the insulin injection. The following description is a general one and the manufacturer's instructions with each individual pen must be followed.

(b) *Injecting a dose:*

1. Wash your hands.

2. Choose a site for injection.

3. Clean the skin with an alcohol swab.

4. Remove outer needle cap.

5. Stabilise the skin by spreading it or pinching up a large area. Insert the needle as instructed.

6. Press the knob.

7. Pull the needle out and apply gentle pressure over the injection site for several seconds. Do not rub the area.

8. Using the outer needle cap, unscrew the needle and dispose of it safely.

9. Use of injection sites should be rotated so that the same site is not used more than approximately once a month.

(c) *Mixing insulins:* Do not mix insulins in vials with insulins in cartridges.

*Marketing authorisation holder:* Eli Lilly Nederland BV, Krijtwal 17–23, 3432 ZT Nieuwegein, Netherlands.

**Marketing authorisation numbers**
Vials: EU/1/96/007/002
Cartridges: EU/1/96/007/003

**Date of approval/revision of SPC** November 1997

**Legal category** P

**Package quantities** 10 ml glass vials – single vials. 1.5 ml glass cartridges – packs of 5.

# HUMATROPE* VIALS AND CARTRIDGES

## Qualitative and quantitative composition
*Humatrope Vials*
*4iu product* (a) Humatrope: Each vial of powder for injection contains 1.48 mg somatropin equivalent to 4iu. The vial also contains mannitol, glycine and dibasic sodium phosphate.

(b) Diluent: Each vial contains 2 ml. The diluent contains Water for Injection and glycerol with 3.15 mg/ml *m*–cresol as a preservative.

*16iu product* (a) Humatrope: Each vial of powder for injection contains 5.92 mg somatropin equivalent to 16iu. The vial also contains mannitol, glycine and dibasic sodium phosphate.

(b) Diluent: Each vial contains 8 ml. The diluent contains Water for Injection and glycerol with 3.15 mg/ml *m*–cresol as a preservative.

*Humatrope Cartridges*
(a) Humatrope: Three presentations of Humatrope cartridges are available, containing 6.66 mg, 13.32 mg or 26.64 mg of somatropin, equivalent to 18, 36 or 72iu somatropin, respectively. Each cartridge also contains mannitol, glycine and dibasic sodium phosphate.

(b) Diluent: Each cartridge is supplied in a combination package with an accompanying syringe containing 3.15 ml of diluting solution. The diluent contains Water for Injection; 0.3% *m*–cresol as a preservative; and 1.7%, 0.29% and 0.29% glycerine in the 18iu, 36iu and 72iu cartridges, respectively.

(c) Humatro-Pen II: The pen allows the dose to be dialled in increments of 0.04 ml. The maximum volume that can be administered as a single injection is 0.6 ml. The incremental concentration and maximum injectable dose for each cartridge are shown in the following table.

| Cartridge | Humatrope/ 0.04 ml | Maximum injectable dose |
| --- | --- | --- |
| 18iu | 0.25iu | 3.75iu |
| 36iu | 0.50iu | 7.50iu |
| 72iu | 1.00iu | 15.00iu |

**Pharmaceutical form** Vials and Cartridges of Humatrope for subcutaneous or intramuscular injection following reconstitution.

## Clinical particulars
*Therapeutic indications*
*Paediatric patients:* Humatrope is indicated for the long–term treatment of children who have growth failure due to an inadequate secretion of normal endogenous growth hormone.

Humatrope is also indicated for the treatment of short stature in children with Turner's Syndrome, confirmed by chromosome analysis.

*Adult patients:* Humatrope is indicated for replacement therapy in adults with pronounced growth hormone deficiency as diagnosed in 2 different dynamic tests for growth hormone deficiency.

Patients must also fulfil the following criteria:

*Childhood onset:* Patients who were diagnosed as growth hormone deficient during childhood, must be retested and their growth hormone deficiency confirmed before replacement therapy with Humatrope is started.

*Adult onset:* Patients must have growth hormone deficiency as a result of hypothalamic or pituitary disease and at least one other hormone deficiency diagnosed (except for prolactin) and adequate replacement therapy instituted, before replacement therapy using growth hormone may begin.

*Posology and method of administration:* The dosage and administration schedule should be personalised for each individual, however, for

*Growth hormone deficient paediatric patients:* The recommended dosage is 0.5iu/kg of body weight per week by subcutaneous or intramuscular injection. This is equivalent to approximately 12iu/m² per week. This weekly dosage should be divided into 6 to 7 injections, administered daily.

*Growth hormone deficient adult patients:* The recommended dosage at the start of therapy is 0.125iu/kg per week, given as a daily subcutaneous injection. This dose should be gradually increased, according to individual patient requirements, to a maximum of 0.25iu/kg per week. Side–effects of the patients, as well as determination of insulin–like growth factor (IGF–1) in serum, should be used as guidance for dose titration. The minimum effective dose should be used and dose requirements may decline with increasing age.

*Patients with Turner's Syndrome:* The recommended dosage is 0.8 to 0.9iu/kg per week. This is equivalent to approximately 24 to 28iu/m² per week. This weekly dosage should be divided into 6 to 7 subcutaneous injections to be administered preferably in the evening.

The subcutaneous injection sites should be varied in order to avoid lipo–atrophy.

*Contra-indications*
(a) Humatrope should not be used when there is any evidence of activity of a tumour. Intracranial lesions must be inactive and antitumour therapy complete prior to the institution of growth hormone therapy. Humatrope should be discontinued if there is evidence of tumour growth.

(b) Humatrope should not be reconstituted with the supplied diluent for patients with a known sensitivity to either *m*–cresol or glycerol.

(c) Humatrope should not be used for growth promotion in children with closed epiphyses.

*Special warnings and special precautions for use:* (a) Previous paediatric subjects who had been treated with growth hormone during childhood until final height was attained, should be re-evaluated for growth hormone deficiency after epiphyseal closure, before replacement therapy is commenced at the doses recommended for adults.

(b) If sensitivity to the accompanying diluent occurs, the vials may be reconstituted with Sterile Water for Injection. When Humatrope is reconstituted in this manner, use only one reconstituted dose per vial, discard any unused portion. Refrigerate the solution at 2-8°C if it is not to be used immediately after reconstitution. Use the reconstituted dose within 24 hours.

(c) Diagnosis and therapy with Humatrope should be initiated and monitored by physicians who are appropriately qualified and experienced in the diagnosis and management of patients with growth hormone deficiency.

(d) Patients with growth hormone deficiency secondary to an intracranial lesion should be examined frequently for progression or recurrence of the underlying disease process.

(e) In cases of severe or recurrent headache, visual problems, nausea and/or vomiting, a fundoscopy for papilloedema is recommended. If papilloedema is confirmed, a diagnosis of benign intracranial hypertension should be considered and, if appropriate, the growth hormone treatment should be discontinued.

At present there is insufficient evidence to guide clinical decision making in patients with resolved intracranial hypertension. If growth hormone treatment is restarted, careful monitoring for symptoms of intracranial hypertension is necessary.

(f) Patients with endocrine disorders, including growth hormone deficiency, may develop slipped capital epiphyses more frequently. Any child with the onset of a limp during growth hormone therapy should be evaluated.

(g) If injected subcutaneously, the injection sites should be rotated to minimise the risk of lipo-atrophy occurring.

(h) A state of hypothyroidism may develop during somatropin treatment. In patients with (pan)hypopituitarism, standard replacement therapy must be closely monitored.

(i) For paediatric patients, the treatment should be continued until the end of growth has been reached. It is advisable not to exceed the recommended dosage in view of the potential risks of acromegaly, hyperglycaemia and glucosuria.

(j) After intramuscular injection, hypoglycaemia may appear. Therefore, the recommended dosage should be accurately checked in cases of intramuscular injection.

(k) Experience with patients above 60 years is lacking.

(l) Experience with prolonged treatment in adults is lacking.

*Interaction with other medicaments and other forms of interaction*

(a) Because human growth hormone may induce a state of insulin resistance, patients should be monitored for evidence of glucose intolerance.

(b) Subjects with diabetes mellitus should be carefully monitored during treatment with Humatrope. An adjustment of the insulin dose may be required.

(c) Excessive glucocorticoid therapy will inhibit the growth promoting effect of human growth hormone. Patients with coexisting ACTH deficiency should have their glucocorticoid replacement dose carefully adjusted to avoid an inhibitory effect on growth.

*Pregnancy and lactation:* Animal reproduction studies have not been conducted with Humatrope. It is not known whether Humatrope can cause foetal harm when administered to a pregnant woman or can affect reproduction capacity. Humatrope should be given to a pregnant woman only if clearly needed.

There have been no studies conducted with Humatrope in nursing mothers. It is not known whether this drug is excreted in human milk. Because many drugs are excreted in human milk, caution should be exercised when Humatrope is administered to a nursing woman.

*Effects on the ability to drive and use machines:* Humatrope has no known effect on ability to drive or use machines.

*Undesirable effects*

*Paediatric patients:* In clinical trials with growth hormone deficient patients, approximately 2% of the patients developed antibodies to growth hormone. In trials in Turner's Syndrome where higher doses were used, up to 8% of patients developed antibodies to growth hormone. The binding capacity of these antibodies was low and growth rate was not affected adversely. Testing for antibodies to growth hormone should be carried out in any patient who fails to respond to therapy.

In clinical studies in which high doses of Humatrope were administered to healthy adult volunteers, the following events occurred infrequently: headache, localised muscle pain, weakness, mild hyperglycaemia, and glucosuria.

In studies with growth hormone deficient children, injection site pain was reported infrequently. A mild and transient oedema, which appeared in 2.5% of patients, was observed early during the course of treatment.

Leukaemia has been reported in a small number of children who have been treated with growth hormone of pituitary origin and somatrem and Humatrope. The relationship, if any, between leukaemia and growth hormone therapy is uncertain.

Some rare cases of benign intracranial hypertension have been reported.

*Adult patients:* Side-effects, possibly related to the biological action or dosage of growth hormone, include: oedema (local and generalised), joint pain and disorder, muscle pain, paraesthesia and hypertension.

In patients with adult onset growth hormone deficiency, oedema, muscle pain and joint pain and disorder, were reported early in therapy and tended to be transient.

Adult patients treated with growth hormone, following diagnosis of growth hormone deficiency in childhood, reported side-effects less frequently than those with adult onset growth hormone deficiency.

*Overdose:* Acute overdose could lead initially to hypoglycaemia and subsequently to hyperglycaemia. Long-term overdosage could result in signs and symptoms of acromegaly consistent with the known effects of excess human growth hormone.

**Pharmacological properties**

*Pharmacodynamic properties:* Humatrope is a polypeptide hormone of recombinant DNA origin. It has 191 amino acid residues and a molecular weight of 22,125 daltons. The amino acid sequence of the product is identical to that of human growth hormone of pituitary origin. Humatrope is synthesised in a strain of *Escherichia coli* that has been modified by the addition of the gene for human growth hormone.

The biological effects of Humatrope are equivalent to human growth hormone of pituitary origin.

The most prominent effect of Humatrope is that it stimulates the growth plates of long bones. Additionally, it promotes cellular protein synthesis and nitrogen retention.

Humatrope stimulates lipid metabolism: it increases plasma fatty acids and HDL-cholesterols and decreases total plasma cholesterol. Humatrope therapy has a beneficial effect on body composition in growth hormone deficient patients, in that body fat stores are reduced and lean body mass is increased. Long-term therapy in growth hormone deficient patients increases bone mineral density.

Humatrope may induce insulin resistance. Large doses of human growth hormone may impair glucose tolerance.

The data available from clinical trials so far in patients with Turner's Syndrome indicate that, while some patients may not respond to this therapy, an increase over predicted height has been observed, the average being 3.3 ± 3.9cm. The results indicate that patients who are very small at the start of therapy may be the better responders.

*Pharmacokinetic properties:* The bioavailability of Humatrope is the same whether presented in vials or cartridges. A dose of 100 micrograms/kg to adult male volunteers will give a peak serum level ($C_{max}$) of about 55ng/ml, a half-life ($t^1/_2$) of nearly four hours and maximal absorption (AUC [0 to ∞]) of about 475ng/hr/ml.

*Preclinical safety data:* Humatrope is human growth hormone produced by recombinant technology. No serious events have been reported in subchronic toxicology studies. Long-term animal studies for carcinogenicity and impairment of fertility with this human growth hormone (Humatrope) have not been performed. There has been no evidence to date of Humatrope induced mutagenicity.

**Pharmaceutical particulars**

*List of excipients*

*Humatrope Vials: Humatrope:* In addition to somatropin, each vial will contain (a) mannitol, (b) glycine, (c) dibasic sodium phosphate, (d) phosphoric acid and (e) sodium hydroxide.

These are included respectively as (a) carrier and stabiliser, (b) stabiliser, (c) buffering agent, (d) and (e) adjustment of pH during manufacture if necessary.

*Diluent:* Each diluent vial will contain (a) glycerol, (b) *m*-cresol, (c) Water for Injection, (d) hydrochloric acid and (e) sodium hydroxide.

These are included respectively as (a) tonicity modifier, (b) preservative, (c) solvent, (d) and (e) adjustment of pH during manufacture if necessary.

*Humatrope Cartridges: Humatrope:* Each cartridge will contain a lyophilised plug composed of somatropin and the following excipients: (a) glycine, (b) mannitol, (c) dibasic sodium phosphate, (d) acidic adjustment of pH.

These are included respectively as (a) stabiliser, (b) carrier and stabiliser, (c) buffering agent.

*Diluent:* Each diluent syringe will contain (a) glycerol, (b) *m*-cresol, (c) Water for Injection, (d) acidic or alkaline adjustment of pH.

These are included respectively as (a) tonicity modifier, (b) preservative, (c) solvent.

*Incompatibilities:* There are no known incompatibilities with Humatrope.

*Shelf life*

*Humatrope Vials: Before reconstitution:* The combination pack of Humatrope and diluent has a shelf life of 24 months when stored at 2 to 8°C.

*After reconstitution:* Vials of Humatrope are stable for up to 14 days when reconstituted with diluent for Humatrope and stored at 2 to 8°C.

*Humatrope Cartridges: Before reconstitution:* Cartridge: 24 months at 2-8°C. Diluent: 24 months at temperatures up to 30°C.

*After reconstitution:* Cartridges of Humatrope are stable for up to 21 days when reconstituted with diluent for Humatrope and stored at 2 to 8°C.

*Special precautions for storage:* Avoid freezing the diluent and reconstituted drug.

*Nature and contents of container*

*Humatrope Vials:* Vials: Humatrope is presented in Type I flint glass vials with rubber stoppers.

Diluent: The diluent is presented in Type I flint glass with rubber stoppers.

*Humatrope Cartridges:* Cartridges: Humatrope is presented in Type I flint glass syringes that have been siliconised. The cartridges are fitted with a siliconised rubber plunger and a halobutyl rubber closure, which are secured in place with a plastic lyocap.

Diluent: The diluent is presented in Type I flint glass syringes that have been siliconised. The syringes are fitted with siliconised Teflon faced halobutyl rubber plungers.

*Instructions for use/handling*

*Humatrope Vials:* Reconstitution: The diluent should be injected into the vial of Humatrope by aiming the stream of liquid against the glass wall. Following reconstitution, the vial should be swirled with a GENTLE rotary motion until the contents are completely dissolved. DO NOT SHAKE. The resulting solution should be clear, without particulated matter. If the solution is cloudy or contains particulated matter, the contents MUST NOT be injected.

Before and after injection, the septum of the vial should be wiped with alcohol to prevent contamination of the contents by repeated needle insertions.

Sterile disposable syringes and needles should be used for administration of Humatrope. The volume of the syringe should be small enough so that the prescribed dose can be withdrawn from the vial with reasonable accuracy.

*Humatrope Cartridges:* Reconstitution: Each cartridge of Humatrope should be reconstituted using the accompanying diluent syringe and the diluent connector. To reconstitute, attach the diluent connector to the cartridge and then inject the entire contents of the pre-filled diluent syringe into the cartridge. The diluent connector automatically aims the stream of liquid against the glass wall of the cartridge. Following reconstitution, the cartridge should be gently rocked back and forth until the contents are completely dissolved. DO NOT SHAKE. The resulting solution should be clear, without particulate matter. If the solution is cloudy or contains particulate matter, the contents MUST NOT be injected.

The cartridges have been designed for use only with the Humatro-Pen II. The diluent connector is for single use only. Discard it after use. A sterile needle should be used for each administration of Humatrope.

**Marketing authorisation numbers**

| | |
|---|---|
| Vials 4iu: | 0006/0237 |
| Vials 16iu: | 0006/0263 |
| Cartridges 18iu: | 0006/0297 |
| Cartridges 36iu: | 0006/0298 |
| Cartridges 72iu: | 0006/0299 |
| Diluent: | 0006/0254 |
| Diluent (36 and 72iu): | 0006/0300 |

**Date of approval/revision of SPC** 21 July 1995

**Legal category** POM

**Package quantities** Single vials and cartridges.

## HUMULIN* VIALS AND CARTRIDGES
## HUMULIN* S (Soluble)
## HUMULIN* I (Isophane)
## HUMULIN* LENTE
## HUMULIN* ZN (Zinc)
## HUMULIN* M1 (Mixture 1)
## HUMULIN* M2 (Mixture 2)
## HUMULIN* M3 (Mixture 3)
## HUMULIN* M4 (Mixture 4)
## HUMULIN* M5 (Mixture 5)

**Qualitative and quantitative composition**

| *Active Ingredient* | *Quantity per ml* |
|---|---|
| Human Insulin (recombinant DNA origin) | 100IU |

Humulin Soluble is a sterile, clear, colourless, aqueous solution of human insulin adjusted to a pH range of 7.0 to 7.8.

Humulin Soluble is a rapidly acting insulin preparation.

Humulin Isophane is a sterile suspension of a white, crystalline precipitate of isophane human insulin in an isotonic phosphate buffer adjusted to a pH range of 6.9 to 7.5.

Humulin Isophane is an intermediate acting insulin preparation.

Humulin Mixture 1, Mixture 2, Mixture 3, Mixture 4 and Mixture 5 are sterile suspensions of human insulin in the proportion of 10%, 20%, 30%, 40% and 50% soluble insulin to 90%, 80%, 70%, 60% and 50% isophane insulin respectively, adjusted to a pH range of 6.9 to 7.5.

Humulin Mixtures are intermediate acting insulin preparations.

Humulin Lente is a sterile suspension of human insulin zinc suspension in the proportion of 30% amorphous and 70% crystalline, adjusted to a pH range of 7.0 to 7.8.

Humulin Lente is an intermediate acting insulin preparation.

Humulin Zinc is a sterile, white suspension of crystalline human insulin zinc suspension, adjusted to a pH range of 7.0 to 7.8.

Humulin Zinc is a longer acting insulin preparation.

**Pharmaceutical form** A solution or suspension for injection filled into:

A. *Cartridges* administered via a reusable device.

The 1.5 ml prefilled cartridge to be used in conjunction with the BD pen or Lilly-Diapen pen injection delivery systems, the 3.0 ml cartridge to be used in conjunction with the BD pen+, all designed to deliver human insulin by parenteral administration.

B. *Vials*

A 10 ml vial of human insulin for parenteral administration.

**Clinical particulars**

*Therapeutic indications:* For the treatment of patients with diabetes mellitus who require insulin for the maintenance of glucose homeostasis. Humulin is also indicated for the initial control of diabetes mellitus and diabetes mellitus in pregnancy.

*Posology and method of administration:* The dosage should be determined by the physician, according to the requirement of the patient.

Humulin Soluble should be given by subcutaneous injection but may, although not recommended, also be given by intramuscular injection. It may also be administered intravenously.

Humulin Isophane, Mixtures, Lente and Zinc in vials and Humulin Isophane and Mixtures in cartridge presentations should be given by subcutaneous injection but may, although not recommended, also be given by intramuscular injection. These formulations should not be administered intravenously.

Subcutaneous administration should be in the upper arms, thighs, buttocks or abdomen. Use of injection sites should be rotated so that the same site is not used more than approximately once a month.

Care should be taken when injecting any Humulin insulin preparations to ensure that a blood vessel has not been entered. After any insulin injection, the injection site should not be massaged.

Humulin Isophane, Humulin Lente and Humulin Zinc may be administered in combination with Humulin Soluble. (See *Special warnings and special precautions for use - Mixing of insulins.*)

Humulin Mixture formulations are ready-made defined mixtures of Humulin Soluble and Humulin Isophane insulin designed to avoid the need for the patient to mix insulin preparations. A patient's treatment regimen should be based on their individual metabolic requirements.

*Contra-indications:* Hypoglycaemia.

Hypersensitivity to Humulin or to the formulation excipients.

Under no circumstances should any Humulin formulation, other than Humulin Soluble, be given intravenously.

*Special warnings and special precautions for use:*
*Transferring from other insulins:* A small number of patients transferring from insulins of animal origin may require a reduced dosage and/or a change in the ratio of soluble to intermediate preparations, especially if they are very tightly controlled and bordering on hypoglycaemia. The dosage reduction may occur immediately after transfer or be a gradual process lasting for several weeks. There is a risk of hypoglycaemia if insulin requirement is decreased, and both the physician and the patient should be aware of this possibility. The risk can be considered minimal if the daily dosage is less than 40IU. Insulin-resistant patients receiving more than 100IU daily should be referred to hospital for transfer.

A few patients who experienced hypoglycaemic reactions after transfer to human insulin have reported that the early warning symptoms were less pronounced or different from those experienced with their previous animal insulin. Patients whose blood glucose control is greatly improved, eg, by intensified insulin therapy, may lose some or all of the warning symptoms of hypoglycaemia and should be advised accordingly. Other conditions which may make the early warning symptoms of hypoglycaemia different or less pronounced include long duration of diabetes, diabetic nerve disease, or medications such as beta blockers. Uncorrected hypoglycaemic and hyperglycaemic reactions can cause loss of consciousness, coma or death.

Insulin requirements may change significantly in diseases of the adrenal, pituitary or thyroid glands, and in the presence of renal or hepatic impairment.

Insulin requirements may be increased during illness or emotional disturbances.

Adjustment of insulin dosage may also be necessary if patients undertake increased physical activity or change their usual diet.

*Mixing of insulins:* The shorter acting insulin should be drawn into the syringe first, to prevent contamination of the vial by the longer acting preparation. It is advisable to inject directly after mixing. However, if a delay is necessary, a consistent routine must be followed.

Alternatively a separate syringe, or separate cartridges of Humulin Soluble and Isophane, can be used for administration of the correct amount of each formulation.

*Interactions with other medicaments and other forms of interaction:* The patient should check with their physician when using other medicines in addition to Humulin.

Insulin requirements may be reduced by the concurrent administration of drugs with hypoglycaemic activity e.g. alcohol, monoamine oxidase inhibitors and beta-adrenergic blockers or aspirin.

Insulin requirements may be increased by concurrent administration of drugs, e.g. oral contraceptives, corticosteroids or thyroid hormone replacement therapy.

The effects of mixing human insulin with insulins of animal origin have not been studied and this practice is not recommended.

*Pregnancy and lactation:* It is essential to maintain good control of the insulin treated (insulin-dependent or gestational diabetes) patient throughout pregnancy. Insulin requirements usually fall during the first trimester and increase during the second and third trimesters. Patients with diabetes should be advised to inform their doctors if they are pregnant or are contemplating pregnancy.

Diabetic patients who are lactating may require adjustments in insulin dose and/or diet.

*Effects on ability to drive and use machines:* Use of the correct therapeutic dose has no known effect on driving or the use of machinery.

*Undesirable effects:* Lipodystrophy, insulin resistance and hypersensitivity reactions are among the side-effects associated with insulins of animal origin. However, the incidence of such side-effects with Humulin is minimal. In the rare event of a severe allergy to Humulin, treatment is required immediately. A change of insulin or desensitisation may be required.

Hypoglycaemia is the most frequent undesirable

## TIME-ACTION PROFILES

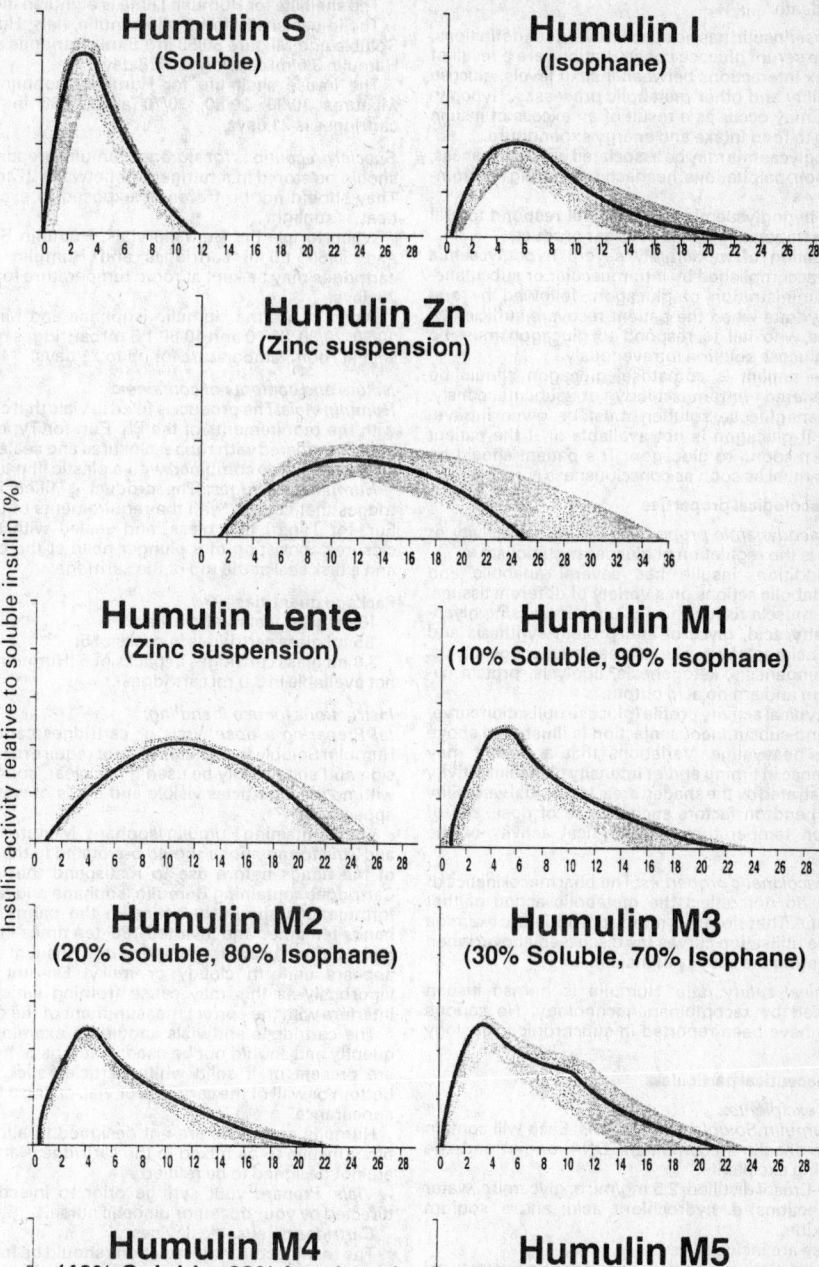

Time (hours)

effect that a diabetic may suffer. Severe hypoglycaemia may lead to loss of consciousness, and in extreme cases, death.

*Overdose:* Insulin has no specific overdose definitions, because serum glucose concentrations are a result of complex interactions between insulin levels, glucose availability and other metabolic processes. Hypoglycaemia may occur as a result of an excess of insulin relative to food intake and energy expenditure.

Hypoglycaemia may be associated with listlessness, confusion, palpitations, headache, sweating and vomiting.

Mild hypoglycaemic episodes will respond to oral administration of glucose or sugar products.

Correction of moderately severe hypoglycaemia can be accomplished by intramuscular or subcutaneous administration of glucagon, followed by oral carbohydrate when the patient recovers sufficiently. Patients who fail to respond to glucagon must be given glucose solution intravenously.

If the patient is comatose, glucagon should be administered intramuscularly or subcutaneously. However, glucose solution must be given intravenously if glucagon is not available or if the patient fails to respond to glucagon. The patient should be given a meal as soon as consciousness is recovered.

### Pharmacological properties

*Pharmacodynamic properties:* The prime activity of insulin is the regulation of glucose metabolism.

In addition, insulin has several anabolic and anti-catabolic actions on a variety of different tissues. Within muscle tissue this includes increasing glycogen, fatty acid, glycerol and protein synthesis and amino acid uptake, while decreasing glycogenolysis, glyconeogenesis, ketogenesis, lipolysis, protein catabolism and amino acid output.

The typical activity profile (glucose utilisation curve) following subcutaneous injection is illustrated above by the heavy line. Variations that a patient may experience in timing and/or intensity of insulin activity are illustrated by the shaded area. Individual variability will depend on factors such as size of dose, site of injection temperature and physical activity of the patient.

*Pharmacokinetic properties:* The pharmacokinetics of insulin do not reflect the metabolic action of that hormone. Therefore, it is more appropriate to examine glucose utilisation curves (as discussed above) when considering the activity of insulin.

*Preclinical safety data:* Humulin is human insulin produced by recombinant technology. No serious events have been reported in subchronic toxicology studies.

### Pharmaceutical particulars

*List of excipients:*
*For Humulin Soluble preparations:* Each will contain Human Insulin (recombinant DNA origin) and the following excipients:
a. *m*-Cresol distilled, 2.5 mg/ml; b. glycerol; c. water for injections; d. hydrochloric acid; and e. sodium hydroxide.

These are included as:
a. preservative; b. tonicity modifier; c. solvent; d. pH adjustment; and e. pH adjustment, respectively.

Hydrochloric acid and/or sodium hydroxide may have been used during manufacture to adjust the pH.

*For Humulin Isophane and Mixture preparations:* Each will contain Human Insulin (recombinant DNA origin) and the following excipients:
a. *m*-Cresol distilled, 1.6 mg/ml; b. glycerol; c. phenol, 0.65 mg/ml; d. protamine sulphate; e. dibasic sodium phosphate; f. zinc oxide; g. water for injections; h. hydrochloric acid; and i. sodium hydroxide.

These are included as:
a. preservative; b. tonicity modifier; c. preservative; d. complexes with insulin to prolong its action; e. buffer; f. adjust zinc content; g. solvent; h. pH adjustment; and i. pH adjustment, respectively.

Hydrochloric acid and/or sodium hydroxide may have been used during manufacture to adjust the pH.

*For Humulin Lente and Zinc preparations:* Each will contain Human Insulin (recombinant DNA origin) and the following excipients:
a. Sodium acetate; b. sodium chloride; c. methyl parahydroxybenzoate, 1 mg/ml; d. water for injections; e. zinc oxide; f. hydrochloric acid; and g. sodium hydroxide.

These are included as:
a. buffering agent; b. tonicity modifier; c. preservative; d. solvent; e. adjust zinc content; f. pH adjustment; and g. pH adjustment, respectively.

Hydrochloric acid and/or sodium hydroxide may have been used during manufacture to adjust the pH.

*Incompatibilities:* Humulin products should not be mixed with either animal insulins or human insulin preparations produced by other manufacturers.

*Shelf life:* The shelf life for Humulin Soluble, Isophane,

Zinc and Mixture presentations is two years when stored under appropriate conditions.

The shelf life for Humulin Lente is eighteen months.

The in-use shelf life for all Humulin vials, Humulin Soluble and Mixture 50/50 in 1.5 ml cartridges and all Humulin 3.0 ml cartridges is 28 days.

The in-use shelf life for Humulin Isophane and Mixtures 10/90, 20/80, 30/70 and 40/60 in 1.5 ml cartridges is 21 days.

*Special precautions for storage:* Humulin preparations should be stored in a refrigerator between 2° and 8°C. They should not be frozen or exposed to excessive heat or sunlight.

When in use the Humulin vials, Humulin Soluble and 50/50 1.5 ml cartridges and Humulin 3.0 ml cartridges may be kept at room temperature for up to 28 days.

When in use the Humulin Isophane and Mixtures 10/90, 20/80, 30/70 and 40/60 1.5 ml cartridges may be kept at room temperature for up to 21 days.

*Nature and contents of container:*
*Humulin vials:* The product is filled in vials that comply with the requirements of the Ph. Eur. for Type I flint glass, stoppered with rubber closures and sealed with aluminium seals combined with a plastic 'flip top'.

*Humulin cartridges:* The product is filled in cartridges that comply with the requirements of the Ph. Eur. for Type I flint glass, and sealed with rubber closures consisting of a plunger head at the bottom and a disk seal at the top of the cartridge.

### Package quantities
10 ml glass vials - single vials.
1.5 ml glass cartridges in packs of 5.
3.0 ml glass cartridges in packs of 5 (Humulin M5 is not available in 3.0 ml cartridges).

*Instructions for use /handling:*
(a) Preparing a dose: Vials or cartridges containing Humulin Soluble formulation do not require resuspension and should only be used if it is clear, colourless, with no solid particles visible and if it is of water-like appearance.

Vials containing Humulin Isophane, Mixtures, Lente and Zinc formulations should be rotated in the palms of the hands before use to resuspend the insulin. Cartridges containing Humulin Isophane and Mixture formulations should be rolled in the palms of the hands ten times and inverted 180° ten times immediately before use to resuspend the insulin until it appears uniform cloudy or milky. Do not shake vigorously as this may cause frothing which may interfere with the correct measurement of the dose.

The cartridges and vials should be examined frequently and should not be used if clumps of material are present or if solid white particles stick to the bottom or wall of the cartridge or vial, giving a frosted appearance.

Humulin cartridges are not designed to allow any other insulin to be mixed in the cartridge. Cartridges are not designed to be refilled.

*Vials:* Prepare your syringe prior to injection, as directed by your doctor or diabetic nurse.
*Cartridges:* Reusable devices.
The manufacturer's instructions should be followed for loading the cartridge and attaching the needle.

(b) Injecting a dose:
*Vials:* Inject the correct dose of insulin, as directed by your doctor or diabetic nurse.
*Cartridges:*

1. Wash your hands.
2. Choose a site for the injection.
3. Clean the skin with an alcohol swab.
4. Remove outer needle cap.
5. Stabilise the skin by spreading it or pinching up a

large area. Insert the needle as instructed by your doctor.
6. Inject the insulin according to the instructions of the pen manufacturer.
7. Pull the needle straight out of the skin and apply gentle pressure over the injection site for several seconds. Do not rub the area.
8. Using the outer needle cap, unscrew the needle immediately after injection and dispose of it safely. Removing the needle immediately after injection ensures sterility, prevents leakage and re-entry of air and potential needle clogs.
9. Replace the cap on the pen.

(c) Disposal of used containers and needles
Do not reuse needles. Dispose of the needle in a responsible manner. Needles and pens must not be shared. Vials and cartridges can be used until empty, then properly discard or recycle.

### Marketing authorisation numbers

| | |
|---|---|
| Humulin S vial: | 0006/0216 |
| Humulin I vial: | 0006/0228 |
| Humulin Lente vial: | 0006/0224 |
| Humulin Zn vial: | 0006/0226 |
| Humulin M1 vial: | 0006/0220 |
| Humulin M2 vial: | 0006/0222 |
| Humulin M3 vial: | 0006/0233 |
| Humulin M4 vial: | 0006/0235 |
| Humulin M5 vial: | 0006/0270 |
| Humulin S cartridge: | 0006/0242 |
| Humulin I cartridge: | 0006/0257 |
| Humulin M1 cartridge: | 0006/0258 |
| Humulin M2 cartridge: | 0006/0259 |
| Humulin M3 cartridge: | 0006/0260 |
| Humulin M4 cartridge: | 0006/0261 |
| Humulin M5 cartridge: | 0006/0312 |

**Date of approval/revision of SPC** 13 December 1994

**Legal category** P

## KEFADIM*

### Qualitative and quantitative composition

| | Vial size | | |
|---|---|---|---|
| | 500 mg | 1 g | 2 g |
| *Active constituent:* | | | |
| Ceftazidime pentahydrate | 580 mg | 1.16 g | 2.33 g |
| equivalent to ceftazidime | 500 mg | 1.0 g | 2.0 g |
| *Other constituents:* | | | |
| Sodium carbonate | 59 mg | 118 mg | 236 mg |

**Pharmaceutical form** Powder for injection.

### Clinical particulars

*Therapeutic indications:* Kefadim is indicated in the treatment of the following infections when due to susceptible micro-organisms:

Lower respiratory tract infections
Skin and soft tissue infections
Bone and joint infections
Urinary tract infections
Gynaecological infections
Intra-abdominal infections, including peritonitis
Septicaemia
Central nervous system infections, including meningitis. In meningitis, it is recommended that the results of a sensitivity test are known before treatment with ceftazidime as a single agent.

Kefadim may be used alone in cases of confirmed or suspected sepsis. It may also be used concomitantly with other antibiotics, such as aminoglycosides, in severe and life-threatening infections and in the immunocompromised patient.

*Posology and method of administration:* Ceftazidime may be given intravenously or by deep intramuscular

*Table 1:* Recommended Dosage Schedule for Kefadim

| | DOSE | FREQUENCY |
|---|---|---|
| **Adults** | | |
| Usual recommended dose | 1 g IV or im | q 8 or 12 h |
| Uncomplicated urinary tract infections | 250 mg IV or im | q 12 h |
| Bone and joint infections | 2 g IV | q 12 h |
| Complicated urinary tract infections | 500 mg IV or im | q 8 or 12 h |
| Uncomplicated pneumonia; mild skin and skin-structure infections | 500 mg-1 g IV or im | q 8 h |
| Serious gynaecological and intra-abdominal infections | 2 g IV | q 8 h |
| Meningitis | 2 g IV | q 8 h |
| Very severe life-threatening infections, especially in immunocompromised patients | 2 g IV | q 8 h |
| Pseudomonal lung infections in patients with cystic fibrosis with normal renal function* | 30-50 mg/kg IV to a maximum of 6 g/day | q 8 h |
| Neonates and children up to 2 months | 12.5-30 mg/kg IV | q 12 h |
| Infants and children (2 months to 12 years of age) | 17-50 mg/kg IV to a maximum of 6 g/day† | q 8 h |

*Although clinical improvement has been shown, complete eradication of infecting organisms cannot be expected in patients with chronic respiratory disease and cystic fibrosis.

†The higher dose should be reserved for immunocompromised children or children with cystic fibrosis or meningitis.

injection into a large muscle mass (such as the upper outer quadrant of the gluteus maximus, or lateral part of the thigh).

The guidelines for dosage of Kefadim are listed in *Table 1*.

*Adults and the elderly:* The usual dosage range for ceftazidime is 500 mg to 2 g every eight to twelve hours. The dosage and route of administration should be determined by the susceptibility of the causative organisms, the severity of infection, and the condition and renal function of the patient.

In view of the reduced clearance of ceftazidime in acutely ill elderly patients, the daily dosage should not normally exceed 2 g, especially in those over 80 years of age (*Table 2*).

*Infants and children over 2 months of age:* The dosage range is 50-150 mg/kg/day IV, in three divided doses, with a maximum of 6 g/day. The higher dose should be reserved for immunocompromised children, or children with cystic fibrosis or meningitis.

*Neonates and children up to 2 months of age:* The dosage range is 25 to 60 mg/kg/day, given as two divided doses. In the neonate, the serum half-life of ceftazidime can be three to four times that in adults.

*Dosage in impaired renal function:* Ceftazidime is excreted by the kidneys almost exclusively by glomerular filtration. Therefore, in patients with impaired renal function (GFR <50 ml/min), it is recommended that the dose of ceftazidime should be reduced to compensate for its slower excretion. In patients with suspected renal insufficiency, an initial loading dose of 1 g may be given. An estimate of GFR should be made to determine the appropriate maintenance dose. The recommended dosage is shown in *Table 2*.

*Table 2:* Recommended Maintenance Dosage of Kefadim in Patients with Renal Insufficiency

| CREATININE CLEARANCE (ML/MIN) | RECOMMENDED DOSE OF KEFADIM | FREQUENCY |
| --- | --- | --- |
| 50-31 | 1 g | q 12 h |
| 30-16 | 1 g | q 24 h |
| 15-6 | 500 mg | q 24 h |
| <5 | 500 mg | q 48 h |

When only serum creatinine is available, the following formula (Cockcroft's equation) may be used to estimate creatinine clearance. The serum creatinine should represent a steady state of renal function:

*Males:*

$$\text{Creatinine clearance (ml/min)} = \frac{\text{Weight (kg)} \times (140 - \text{age in years})}{72 \times \text{serum creatinine (mg/dl)}}$$

*Females:*

0.85 x above value

In patients with severe infections who would normally receive 6 g of Kefadim daily, were it not for renal insufficiency, the dose in *Table 2* may be increased by 50% or the dosing frequency increased appropriately. Continued dosage should be determined by further monitoring of creatinine clearance, severity of the infection, and susceptibility of the causative organism. In such patients, it is recommended that ceftazidime serum levels should be monitored and trough levels should not exceed 40 mg/ litre.

In children, as for adults, the creatinine clearance should be adjusted for body surface area or lean body mass and the dosing frequency reduced in cases of renal insufficiency.

The serum half-life of ceftazidime during haemodialysis ranges from 3 to 5 hours.

In patients undergoing haemodialysis, a loading dose of 1 g of Kefadim is recommended, followed by 1 g after each haemodialysis period. Kefadim can also be used in patients undergoing intraperitoneal and continuous ambulatory peritoneal dialysis (CAPD). In such patients, a loading dose of 1 g of Kefadim may be given, followed by 500 mg every 24 hours. In addition to intravenous use, Kefadim can be incorporated in the dialysis fluid at a concentration of 250 mg for 2 litres of dialysis fluid.

NOTE: Kefadim should generally be continued for 2 days after the signs and symptoms of infection have disappeared, however, in complicated infections, longer therapy may be required.

*Intramuscular administration:* Kefadim should be reconstituted with Water for Injections PhEur or 0.5% or 1% Lignocaine Hydrochloride Injection BP. Refer to *Table 3*.

*Intravenous administration:* For direct intermittent intravenous administration, reconstitute Kefadim with Water for Injections PhEur (see *Table 3*). Slowly inject the solution directly into the vein over a period of 3 to 5 minutes or give through the tubing of a giving set. Ceftazidime is compatible with the most commonly used intravenous fluids (see *Pharmaceutical particulars*).

*Table 3:* Preparation of Solutions of Kefadim

| | AMOUNT OF DILUENT TO BE ADDED (ML) | APPROXIMATE AVAILABLE VOLUME (ML) | APPROXIMATE CEFTAZIDIME CONCENTRATION (MG/ML) |
| --- | --- | --- | --- |
| Intramuscular | | | |
| 500 mg | 1.5 | 1.8 | 280 |
| 1 g | 3.0 | 3.6 | 280 |
| Intravenous | | | |
| 500 mg | 5 | 5.3 | 100 |
| 1 g | 10 | 10.6 | 100 |
| 2 g | 10 | 11.2 | 180 |
| Infusion (100 ml) | | | |
| 2 g | 100* | 100 | 20 |

*Note: Addition should be in 2 stages (see *Instructions for reconstitution* below).

When Kefadim is dissolved, carbon dioxide is released and a positive pressure develops. For ease of use, please follow the recommended techniques of reconstitution described below.

For intravenous infusion, reconstitute the 2 g infusion (100 ml) vial with 100 ml Water for Injections PhEur or one of the compatible intravenous fluids. Alternatively, reconstitute the 500 mg, 1 g or 2 g vial, and add an appropriate quantity of the resulting solution to an IV container with one of the compatible intravenous fluids.

Intermittent intravenous infusion with a Y-type giving set can be accomplished with compatible solutions. However, during infusion of a solution containing ceftazidime, it is desirable to discontinue the other solution.

*Instructions for reconstitution:*

For 500 mg im/IV, 1 g im/IV, and 2 g IV vials:

1. Inject the diluent and shake well to dissolve. The vials may contain a vacuum to assist injection of the diluent.
2. Carbon dioxide is released as the antibiotic dissolves, generating pressure within the vial. The solution will become clear within 1 to 2 minutes.
3. Invert the vial, and completely depress the syringe plunger prior to insertion.
4. Insert the needle through the vial stopper. Be sure the needle remains within the solution, and withdraw contents of the vial in the usual manner. Pressure in the vial may aid withdrawal.
5. The withdrawn solution may contain carbon dioxide bubbles which should be expelled from the syringe before injection.

For 2 g infusion vials:

1. Inject 10 ml of the diluent and shake to dissolve. The vials may contain a vacuum to assist injection of the diluent.
2. Carbon dioxide is released as the antibiotic dissolves, generating pressure within the vial. The solution will become clear within 1 to 2 minutes.
3. Insert a vent needle to release pressure before adding additional diluent to the vial. Add diluent and then remove the vent needle.
4. Additional pressure that may develop in the vial, especially after storage, should be relieved prior to administration to the patient.

NOTE: To preserve product sterility, it is important that a gas relief needle is *not* inserted through the vial closure before the product has dissolved.

*Contra-indications:* Ceftazidime is contra-indicated in patients with known hypersensitivity to ceftazidime or cephalosporin antibiotics.

*Special warnings and precautions for use:*
*Warnings:* Before therapy with ceftazidime is instituted, careful inquiry should be made to determine whether the patient has had previous hypersensitivity reactions to ceftazidime, cephalosporins, penicillins, or other drugs. Ceftazidime should be given only with special caution to patients with type 1 or immediate hypersensitivity reactions to penicillin. If an allergic reaction to ceftazidime occurs, discontinue the drug. Serious acute hypersensitivity reactions may require adrenaline, hydrocortisone, antihistamine or other emergency measures.

Pseudomembranous colitis has been reported with the use of ceftazidime, other cephalosporins, and virtually all broad-spectrum antibiotics, therefore, it is important to consider its diagnosis in patients who develop diarrhoea in association with antibiotic use. Such colitis may range in severity from mild to life-threatening. Symptoms can appear during or after treatment.

Mild cases of pseudomembranous colitis usually respond to drug discontinuance alone. In moderate to severe cases, appropriate measures should be taken.

*Precautions:* Kefadim has not been shown to be nephrotoxic, however, because high and prolonged serum antibiotic concentrations can occur from usual doses in patients with transient or persistent reduction of urinary output because of renal insufficiency, the total daily dosage should be reduced when ceftazidime is administered to such patients to avoid the clinical consequences, eg, seizures due to elevated levels of antibiotics (see *Posology and method of administration*). Continued dosage should be determined by degree of renal impairment, severity of infection and susceptibility of causative organisms.

As with other antibiotics, prolonged use of Kefadim may result in the overgrowth of non-susceptible organisms. Repeated evaluation of the patient's condition is essential. If superinfection occurs during therapy, appropriate measures should be taken.

Kefadim should be used with caution in individuals with a history of gastro-intestinal disease, particularly colitis.

Ceftazidime does not interfere with enzyme-based tests for glycosuria. Slight interference with copper reduction methods (Benedict's, Fehling's, Clinitest) may be observed.

*Interaction with other medicaments and other forms of interaction:* Nephrotoxicity has been reported following concomitant administration of cephalosporins and aminoglycoside antibiotics or potent diuretics, such as frusemide. Renal function should be carefully monitored, especially if higher dosages of the aminoglycosides are to be administered or if therapy is prolonged, because of the potential nephrotoxicity and ototoxicity of aminoglycoside antibiotics. Nephrotoxicity and ototoxicity were not noted when Kefadim was given alone in clinical trials.

*Pregnancy and lactation:* Reproduction studies have been performed in mice and rats at doses up to 40 times the human dose and have revealed no evidence of impaired fertility or harm to the foetus due to Kefadim. There are, however, no controlled studies in pregnant women. As animal reproduction studies are not always predictive of human response, this drug should be used during pregnancy only if clearly needed.

Ceftazidime is excreted in human milk in low concentrations and consequently caution should be exercised when ceftazidime is administered to a nursing woman.

*Effects on ability to drive and use machines:* Not applicable.

*Undesirable effects:* Clinical trial experience has shown that Kefadim is generally well tolerated. The most common side-effects were local reactions following intravenous injection and allergic and gastro-intestinal reactions.

*Local effects:* Phlebitis or thrombophlebitis, and inflammation at the site of injection.

*Hypersensitivity:* Pruritus, rash and fever. Angioedema and anaphylaxis (bronchospasm and/or hypotension) have been reported very rarely.

*Gastro-intestinal:* Diarrhoea, nausea, vomiting and abdominal pain, pseudomembranous colitis (see *Warnings*). Very rarely, oral thrush.

*Central nervous system:* Headache, dizziness, paraesthesias and bad taste. There have been reports of neurological sequelae, including tremor, myoclonica, convulsions and encephalopathy, in patients with renal impairment in whom the dose of ceftazidime has not been appropriately reduced.

*Miscellaneous:* Candidiasis and vaginitis.

*Laboratory test changes (usually transient):* Eosinophilia, positive Coombs' test without haemolysis, thrombocytosis, and slight elevations in one or more hepatic enzymes: AST (SGOT), ALT (SGPT), LDH, GGT and alkaline phosphatase. Transient elevations of blood urea, blood urea nitrogen, and/or serum creatinine have been observed occasionally. Transient leucopenia, neutropenia, agranulocytosis, thrombocytopenia and lymphocytosis have been seen very rarely.

*Overdose:*
*Signs and symptoms:* Toxic signs and symptoms

following an overdose of ceftazidime may include pain, inflammation, and phlebitis at the injection site. Overdosage can lead to neurological sequelae, including encephalopathy, convulsions and coma.

The administration of inappropriately large doses of parenteral cephalosporins may cause dizziness, paraesthesias, and headaches. Seizures may occur following overdosage with some cephalosporins, particularly in patients with renal impairment in whom accumulation is likely to occur.

Laboratory abnormalities that may occur after an overdose include elevations in creatinine, BUN, liver enzymes and bilirubin, a positive Coombs' test, thrombocytosis, thrombocytopenia, eosinophilia, leucopenia, and prolongation of the prothrombin time.

The subcutaneous median lethal dose in rats and mice ranged from 5.8 to 20 g/kg and the intravenous median lethal dose in rabbits was >2 g/kg.

*Treatment:* If seizures occur, the drug should be discontinued promptly; anti-convulsant therapy may be administered if clinically indicated. An airway should be established. Cardiac and vital signs monitoring is recommended, along with general symptomatic and supportive measures.

In cases of severe overdosage, especially in a patient with renal failure, combined haemodialysis and haemoperfusion may be considered if response to more conservative therapy fails.

**Pharmacological properties**

*Pharmacodynamic properties:* Ceftazidime is a semi-synthetic, beta-lactam antibiotic, for parenteral administration.

*In vitro* tests demonstrate that ceftazidime is bactericidal. It acts against a wide range of gram-negative organisms, including strains resistant to gentamicin and other aminoglycosides. It is also active against Gram-positive organisms, and is highly stable to most clinically important beta-lactamases, whether plasmid or chromosomally mediated.

Ceftazidime has been shown to have *in vitro* activity against the following organisms:

*Pseudomonas* spp. (including *Pseudomonas aeruginosa*); *Klebsiella* spp. (including *Klebsiella pneumoniae*); *Proteus mirabilis* and *Proteus vulgaris*; *Morganella morganii* (formerly *Proteus morganii*); *Providencia* spp. (including *Providencia rettgeri*, formerly *Proteus rettgeri*); *Escherichia coli*; *Enterobacter* spp.; *Citrobacter* spp.; *Serratia* spp.; *Salmonella* spp.; *Shigella* spp.; *Yersinia enterocolitica*; *Pasteurella multocida*; *Acinetobacter* spp.; *Neisseria gonorrhoeae*; *Neisseria meningitidis*; *Haemophilus influenzae* (including amipicillin-resistant strains); *Haemophilus parainfluenzae* (including ampicillin-resistant strains); *Staphylococcus aureus* (methicillin-sensitive strains); *Staphylococcus epidermidis* (methicillin-sensitive strains); *Streptococcus pyogenes*; *Streptococcus* Group B; *Streptococcus pneumoniae*; *Streptococcus* spp.; *Peptococcus* spp.; *Peptostreptococcus* spp.; *Clostridium* spp; (but not *C. difficile*); *Bacteroides* spp. (but most strains of *B. fragilis* are resistant).

Using the ICS agar dilution method (or its equivalent) for susceptibility testing, the criteria for dilution methods are:

| | |
|---|---|
| MIC <16 mg/litre: | Susceptible |
| MIC >16 but <64 mg/litre: | Moderately susceptible (ie, susceptible to high dosage or if infection confined to tissues or fluids [eg, urine] in which high antibiotic levels are attained) |
| MIC ≥64 mg/litre: | Resistant |

and for the standard disc test using a 30 microgram ceftazidime disc, are (zone diameters):

| | |
|---|---|
| Zone ≥18 mm: | Susceptible |
| Zone 15-17 mm: | Moderately susceptible |
| Zone ≤14 mm: | Resistant |

Ceftazidime is not active *in vitro* against methicillin-resistant staphylococci; *Streptococcus faecalis* and many other enterococci; *Listeria monocytogenes*; *Campylobacter* spp. or *C. difficile*.

Ceftazidime and the aminoglycosides have been shown to be synergistic *in vitro* against some strains of *P. aeruginosa* and the *Enterobacteriaceae*. Ceftazidime and carbenicillin have also been shown to be synergistic *in vitro* against *P. aeruginosa*.

*Pharmacokinetic properties:* After intravenous administration of 500 mg or 1 g of ceftazidime, over 5 minutes, to normal adults, mean peak serum concentrations were 45 mg/litre and 90 mg/litre, respectively. Following intravenous infusion of 500 mg, 1 g and 2 g of ceftazidime, over 20 to 30 minutes, to normal adults, mean peak serum concentrations of 42, 69 and 170 mg/litre, respectively, were achieved. The average serum concentrations in these adults, over an 8 hour period, are given in *Table 4*.

*Table 4:* Ceftazidime Concentrations in Serum

| CEFTAZIDIME DOSAGE (IV) | SERUM CONCENTRATIONS (MG/LITRE) | | | | |
|---|---|---|---|---|---|
| | 0.5h | 1h | 2h | 4h | 8h |
| 500 mg | 42 | 25 | 12 | 6 | 2 |
| 1 g | 60 | 39 | 23 | 11 | 3 |
| 2 g | 129 | 75 | 42 | 13 | 5 |

Following intramuscular administration of 500 mg and 1 g ceftazidime to normal adults, mean peak serum concentrations at approximately 1 hour were 17 mg/litre and 39 mg/litre, respectively. Serum concentrations remained above 4 mg/litre for 6 and 8 hours after the intramuscular administration of 500 mg and 1 g doses, respectively.

The half-life of ceftazidime was approximately 1.9 hours after intravenous administration and 2 hours after intramuscular administration.

Less than 10% of ceftazidime was protein bound and the degree of protein binding was independent of concentration.

Following multiple intravenous doses of 1 g and 2 g every 8 hours for 10 days, there was no evidence of accumulation of ceftazidime in the serum of individuals with normal renal function.

The presence of hepatic dysfunction had no effect on the pharmacokinetics of ceftazidime in individuals who received 2 g intravenously every 8 hours for 5 days. Therefore, dosage adjustment is not required for patients with hepatic dysfunction, unless renal function is also impaired.

Approximately 80% to 90% of a dose of ceftazidime is excreted unchanged by the kidneys over a 24 hour period. The elimination of ceftazidime by the kidneys resulted in high urinary concentrations.

Concentrations of ceftazidime in excess of the minimum inhibitory levels of common pathogens can be achieved in tissues such as bone, heart, bile, sputum, aqueous humour, synovial, pleural and peritoneal fluids.

Transplacental transfer of the antibiotic readily occurs.

Ceftazidime penetrates the intact blood-brain barrier poorly and low levels are achieved in the CSF in the absence of inflammation. Therapeutic levels of 4 to 20 mg/litre or more are achieved in the CSF when the meninges are inflamed.

*Preclinical safety data:* Long-term studies in animals have not been performed to evaluate carcinogenic potential. However, a mouse micronucleus test and an Ames test were both negative for mutagenic effects.

**Pharmaceutical particulars**

*List of excipients:* Sodium carbonate.

*Incompatibilities:* Solutions of Kefadim, like those of most beta-lactam antibiotics, should not be added to solutions of aminoglycoside antibiotics because of potential interaction. However, if concurrent therapy with Kefadim and an aminoglycoside is indicated, each of these antibiotics should be administered in different sites.

Precipitation has been reported when vancomycin has been added to ceftazidime in solution. Therefore, it would be prudent to flush giving sets and intravenous lines between administration of these two agents.

Kefadim is less stable in Sodium Bicarbonate Injection than in other intravenous fluids. Sodium Bicarbonate Injection is not recommended as a diluent. Solutions of Kefadim in 5% Dextrose or 0.9% Sodium Chloride Injection are stable for at least 6 hours at room temperature in plastic tubing, drip chambers, and volume control devices of common intravenous infusion sets.

*Shelf life:*
*Unreconstituted vials:* 2 years.

*Reconstituted vials:* It is good practice to reconstitute immediately prior to use. If this is not feasible, Kefadim should be stored in a refrigerator and used within 24 hours. After reconstitution, protection from light is not necessary. The pH of freshly reconstituted solutions ranges from 5.0 to 7.5.

*Special precautions for storage:*
*Unreconstituted vials:* Protect from light. Store at room temperature (15°-25°C).

*Nature and contents of container:* Kefadim is supplied as a sterile dry powder in single-dose flint Type I or III glass vial with a rubber closure and aluminium seal containing 500 mg, 1 g and 2 g ceftazidime (as pentahydrate) with sodium carbonate (118 mg per gram of ceftazidime).

Kefadim is also supplied as a sterile dry powder, in 100 ml vials, for infusion, containing 2 g ceftazidime.

The total sodium content of the mixture is approximately 54 mg (2.3 mEq) per gram of ceftazidime.

**Package quantities**

500 mg/10 ml: Single vials in packs of 10
1 g/20 ml: Single vials in packs of 10
2 g/50 ml: Single vials in packs of 10
2 g/100 ml: Single vials in packs of 1

*Instructions for use/handling:* Solutions of Kefadim range from light yellow to amber, depending on the diluent and concentration.

Kefadim is compatible with the more commonly used intravenous infusion fluids. Solutions at concentrations between 1 mg/ml and 40 mg/ml in the following infusion fluids may be stored for up to 24 hours at room temperature: 0.9% Sodium Chloride Injection BP; M/6 Sodium Lactate Injection BP; Ringer's Injection USP; Lactated Ringer's Injection USP; 5% Dextrose Injection BP; 0.225% Sodium Chloride and 5% Dextrose Injection BP; 0.45% Sodium Chloride and 5% Dextrose Injection BP; 0.9% Sodium Chloride and 5% Dextrose Injection BP; 10% Dextrose Injection BP; and 10% Invert Sugar in Water for Injection.

At a concentration of 4 mg/ml, Kefadim has been found compatible for 24 hours at room temperature in 0.9% Sodium Chloride Injection or 5% Dextrose Injection when admixed with cefuroxime sodium, 3 mg/ml; heparin, 10u/ml or 50u/ml; or potassium chloride, 10 mEq/l or 40 mEq/l.

Parenteral drug products should be inspected visually and cloudy solutions should be discarded.

Kefadim powder and solutions will darken, depending on storage conditions. However, product potency is not adversely affected if storage conditions and storage periods are observed.

**Marketing authorisation numbers**

| | |
|---|---|
| Vials 500 mg: | 0006/0239 |
| Vials 1 g: | 0006/0240 |
| Vials 2 g: | 0006/0241 |

**Date of approval/revision of SPC** 26 November 1993

**Legal category** POM

## KEFLEX*

**Qualitative and quantitative composition** Each tablet contains, as the active ingredient, cephalexin monohydrate equivalent to 250 mg or 500 mg of cephalexin base.

Each capsule contains, as the active ingredient, cephalexin monohydrate equivalent to 250 mg or 500 mg of cephalexin base.

Each bottle, when prepared as directed, contains, as the active ingredient, cephalexin monohydrate equivalent to 125 mg/5 ml or 250 mg/5 ml of cephalexin base.

**Pharmaceutical form**

Tablets 250 mg: 9.5 mm diameter, peach, marked Lilly U57.

Tablets 500 mg: Pillow-shaped, 16 mm long, scored, peach, marked Lilly U49.

Capsules 250 mg: Green and white, coded H69.

Capsules 500 mg: Pale green and dark green, coded H71.

Granules for suspension 125 mg: Pink granules.

Granules for suspension 250 mg: Orange granules.

**Clinical particulars**

*Therapeutic indications:* Cephalexin is indicated in the treatment of the following infections due to susceptible micro-organisms:

Respiratory tract infections
Otitis media
Skin and soft tissue infections
Bone and joint infections
Genito-urinary tract infections, including acute prostatitis
Dental infections

*Posology and method of administration:* Cephalexin is administered orally.

*Adults:* The adult dosage ranges from 1-4 g daily in divided doses; most infections will respond to a dosage of 500 mg every 8 hours. For skin and soft tissue infections, streptococcal pharyngitis and mild, uncomplicated urinary tract infections, the usual dosage is 250 mg every 6 hours, or 500 mg every 12 hours.

For more severe infections or those caused by less susceptible organisms, larger doses may be needed. If daily doses of cephalexin greater than 4 g are required, parenteral cephalosporins, in appropriate doses, should be considered.

*The elderly and patients with impaired renal function:* As for adults. Reduce dosage if renal function is markedly impaired (see *Precautions*).

*Children:* The usual recommended daily dosage for children is 25-50 mg/kg (10-20 mg/lb) in divided doses. For skin and soft tissue infections, streptococcal pharyngitis and mild, uncomplicated urinary tract infections, the total daily dose may be divided and administered every 12 hours. For most infections the following schedule is suggested:

*Children under 5 years:* 125 mg every 8 hours.
*Children 5 years and over:* 250 mg every 8 hours.

In severe infections, the dosage may be doubled. In the therapy of otitis media, clinical studies have shown that a dosage of 75 to 100 mg/kg/day in 4 divided doses is required.

In the treatment of beta-haemolytic streptococcal infections, a therapeutic dose should be administered for at least 10 days.

*Contra-indications:* Cephalexin is contra-indicated in patients with known allergy to the cephalosporin group of antibiotics.

*Special warnings and special precautions for use:* Before instituting therapy with cephalexin, every effort should be made to determine whether the patient has had previous hypersensitivity reactions to the cephalosporins, penicillins or other drugs. Cephalexin should be given cautiously to penicillin-sensitive patients. There is some clinical and laboratory evidence of partial cross-allergenicity of the penicillins and cephalosporins. Patients have had severe reactions (including anaphylaxis) to both drugs.

Pseudomembranous colitis has been reported with virtually all broad-spectrum antibiotics, including macrolides, semisynthetic penicillins and cephalosporins. It is important, therefore, to consider its diagnosis in patients who develop diarrhoea in association with the use of antibiotics. Such colitis may range in severity from mild to life-threatening. Mild cases of pseudomembranous colitis usually respond to drug discontinuance alone. In moderate to severe cases, appropriate measures should be taken.

If an allergic reaction to cephalexin occurs, the drug should be discontinued and the patient treated with the appropriate agents.

Prolonged use of cephalexin may result in the overgrowth of non-susceptible organisms. Careful observation of the patient is essential. If superinfection occurs during therapy, appropriate measures should be taken.

Cephalexin should be administered with caution in the presence of markedly impaired renal function. Careful clinical and laboratory studies should be made because safe dosage may be lower than that usually recommended.

Positive direct Coombs' tests have been reported during treatment with the cephalosporin antibiotics. In haematological studies, or in transfusion cross-matching procedures when antiglobulin tests are performed on the minor side, or in Coombs' testing of newborns whose mothers have received cephalosporin antibiotics before parturition, it should be recognised that a positive Coombs' test may be due to the drug.

A false positive reaction for glucose in the urine may occur with Benedict's or Fehling's solutions or with copper sulphate test tablets.

*Interactions with other medicaments and other forms of interaction:* None known.

*Pregnancy and lactation:*
*Usage in pregnancy:* Although laboratory and clinical studies have shown no evidence of teratogenicity, caution should be exercised when prescribing for the pregnant patient.

*Usage in nursing mothers:* The excretion of cephalexin in human breast milk increased up to 4 hours following a 500 mg dose. The drug reached a maximum level of 4 micrograms/ml, then decreased gradually and had disappeared 8 hours after administration. Caution should be exercised when cephalexin is administered to a nursing woman.

*Effects on ability to drive and use machines:* None known.

*Undesirable effects:*
*Gastro-intestinal:* Symptoms of pseudomembranous colitis may appear either during or after antibiotic treatment. Nausea and vomiting have been reported rarely. The most frequent side-effect has been diarrhoea. It was very rarely severe enough to warrant cessation of therapy. Dyspepsia and abdominal pain have also occurred. As with some penicillins and some other cephalosporins, transient hepatitis and cholestatic jaundice have been reported rarely.

*Hypersensitivity:* Allergic reactions have been observed in the form of rash, urticaria, angioedema and, rarely, erythema multiforme, Stevens-Johnson syndrome and toxic epidermal necrolysis. These reactions usually subsided upon discontinuation of the drug, although in some cases supportive therapy may be necessary. Anaphylaxis has also been reported.

*Other:* These have included genital and anal pruritus, genital candidiasis, vaginitis and vaginal discharge, dizziness, fatigue, headache, agitation, confusion, hallucinations, arthralgia, arthritis and joint disorder. Reversible interstitial nephritis has been reported rarely. Eosinophilia, neutropenia, thrombocytopenia and slight elevations in AST and ALT have been reported.

*Overdose:* Symptoms of oral overdose may include nausea, vomiting, epigastric distress, diarrhoea and haematuria.

In the event of severe overdosage, general supportive care is recommended, including close clinical and laboratory monitoring of haematological, renal and hepatic functions, and coagulation status until the patient is stable. Forced diuresis, peritoneal dialysis, haemodialysis, or charcoal haemoperfusion have not been established as beneficial for an overdose of cephalexin. It would be extremely unlikely that one of these procedures would be indicated.

Unless 5 to 10 times the normal total daily dose has been ingested, gastro-intestinal decontamination should not be necessary.

There have been reports of haematuria, without impairment of renal function, in children accidentally ingesting more than 3.5 g of cephalexin in a day. Treatment has been supportive (fluids) and no sequelae have been reported.

## Pharmacological properties

*Pharmacodynamic properties:*
*Microbiology: In vitro* tests demonstrate that the Cephalosporins are bactericidal because of their inhibition of cell-wall synthesis.

Cephalexin is active against the following organisms *in vitro:*
  Beta-haemolytic streptococci
  Staphylococci, including coagulase-positive, coagulase-negative and penicillinase-producing strains.
  *Streptococcus pneumoniae*
  *Escherichia coli*
  *Proteus mirabilis*
  *Klebsiella* species
  *Haemophilus influenzae*
  *Branhamella catarrhalis*
  Most strains of enterococci (*Streptococcus faecalis*) and a few strains of staphylococci are resistant to cephalexin. It is not active against most strains of *Enterobacter* species, *Morganella morganii* and *Pr. vulgaris.* It has no activity against *Pseudomonas* or *Herellea* species. When tested by *in vitro* methods, staphylococci exhibit cross-resistance between cephalexin and methicillin-type antibiotics.

*Pharmacokinetic properties:*
*Human pharmacology:* Cephalexin is acid stable and may be given without regard to meals. It is rapidly absorbed after oral administration. Following doses of 250 mg, 500 mg and 1 g, average peak serum levels of approximately 9, 18 and 32 mg/l, respectively, were obtained at 1 hour. Measurable levels were present 6 hours after administration. Cephalexin is excreted in the urine by glomerular filtration and tubular secretion. Studies showed that over 90% of the drug was excreted unchanged in the urine within 8 hours. During this period, peak urine concentrations following the 250 mg, 500 mg and 1 g doses were approximately 1000, 2200 and 5000 mg/l, respectively.

Cephalexin is almost completely absorbed from the gastro-intestinal tract, and 75-100% is rapidly excreted in active form in the urine. Absorption is slightly reduced if the drug is administered with food. The half-life is approximately 60 minutes in patients with normal renal function. Haemodialysis and peritoneal dialysis will remove cephalexin from the blood.

Peak blood levels are achieved one hour after administration, and therapeutic levels are maintained for 6-8 hours. Approximately 80% of the active drug is excreted in the urine within 6 hours. No accumulation is seen with dosages above the therapeutic maximum of 4 g/day.

The half-life may be increased in neonates due to their renal immaturity, but there is no accumulation when given at up to 50 mg/kg/day.

*Preclinical safety data:* The daily oral administration of cephalexin to rats in doses of 250 or 500 mg/kg prior to and during pregnancy, or to rats and mice during the period of organogenesis only, had no adverse effect on fertility, foetal viability, foetal weight, or litter size.

Cephalexin showed no enhanced toxicity in weanling and newborn rats as compared with adult animals.

The oral $LD_{50}$ of cephalexin in rats is 5,000 mg/kg.

## Pharmaceutical particulars

*List of excipients:*
The tablets contain the following excipients: Sodium Starch Glycollate Type A; Magnesium Stearate; Povidone; Methylhydroxypropylcellulose; Glycerol; Talc; Titanium Dioxide; Methyl Cellulose; Iron Oxide Yellow; Iron Oxide Red.

The capsules contain the following excipients: Cellulose with Sodium Carboxymethyl Cellulose; Dimethicone; Magnesium Stearate; Patent Blue V; Quinoline Yellow; Titanium Dioxide; Gelatin.

The granules contain the following excipients: Sucrose; Imitation Guarana Flavour; Erythrosine Aluminium Lake (125 mg suspension only); Sunset Yellow (250 mg suspension only).

*Incompatibilities:* None known.

*Shelf life:*
*Tablets or capsules:* When stored appropriately, 3 years.
  *Suspension:* When stored appropriately,
Unreconstituted product:        3 years.
Bottles of reconstituted
  product:                      10 days.
Sachets:                        For immediate use.

*Special precautions for storage:* Store below 30°C. Keep containers tightly closed.

After mixing, Keflex Suspensions should be stored in a cool place (6°C-15°C) or in a refrigerator (2°C-8°C) and be used within 10 days. Where dilution is unavoidable, Syrup BP should be used after the suspension has been prepared according to the manufacturer's instructions.

*Nature and contents of container:*
*Tablets:* The products are filled into HDPE bottles of 100 or 500 tablets, or blister strips of 28 tablets consisting of UPVC with aluminium foil backing. Additionally, the 500 mg product may be packed into blisters of 21 tablets.

*Capsules:* The products are filled into HDPE bottles of 100 or 500 capsules, or blister strips of 28 capsules consisting of UPVC with aluminium foil backing. Additionally, the 500 mg product may be packed into blisters of 21 capsules.

*Suspension:* The product is filled into 100 ml HDPE bottles with screw caps, or sachet packs (unit dose) consisting of paper/polythene/aluminium foil/polythene.

## Package quantities
Tablets 250 mg: Bottles of 100 and 500, blister packs of 28.
Tablets 500 mg: Bottles of 100 and 500, blister packs of 21 and 28.
Capsules 250 mg: Bottles of 100 and 500, blister packs of 28.
Capsules 500 mg: Bottles of 100 and 500, blister packs of 21 and 28.
Suspension 125 mg/5 ml: Bottles of 100 ml.
Suspension 250 mg/5 ml: Bottles of 100 ml.

*Instructions for use/handling:* For oral use.
*Suspension:* To the bottle containing granules, is added a total of 60 ml water in two portions, shaking after each addition until suspended. If dilution is unavoidable, Syrup BP should be used after the suspension has been prepared as described.
Shake well before use.

## Marketing authorisation numbers
Tablets:                  0006/0073, 5096
Capsules:                 0006/0076, 5103
Suspension 125 mg/5 ml:   0006/5097
Suspension 250 mg/5 ml:   0006/5098

**Date of approval/revision of SPC**   17 June 1996

**Legal category**   POM

# KEFZOL*

**Qualitative and quantitative composition**   Kefzol is supplied in rubber-stoppered vials containing the equivalent of 500 mg and 1 g cephazolin as the sodium salt.

**Pharmaceutical form**   Powder for injections.

**Clinical particulars**
*Therapeutic indications:* Kefzol is indicated in the treatment of the following infections due to susceptible micro-organisms:
  Respiratory tract infections
  Genito-urinary tract infections
  Skin and soft tissue infections
  Bone and joint infections
  Septicaemia
  Endocarditis
  Biliary tract infections
*Prophylactic use:* Perioperative administration of cephazolin may reduce the incidence of postoperative infections in patients undergoing contaminated or potentially contaminated surgical procedures associated with a high risk of infection, or where the occurrence of a postoperative infection could be especially serious.

Cephazolin is active against the following organisms *in vitro:*
  *Staphylococcus aureus* (penicillin-sensitive and penicillin-resistant)
  *Staphylococcus epidermidis*
  Group A beta-haemolytic streptococci and other strains of streptococci (many strains of enterococci are resistant)
  *Streptococcus pneumoniae*
  *Escherichia coli*
  *Klebsiella* species
  *Proteus mirabilis*
  *Haemophilus influenzae*
  *Enterobacter aerogenes*

*Posology and method of administration:* After reconstitution, Kefzol may be administered intramuscularly or intravenously.

*Intramuscular administration:* Reconstitute with Water for Injections PhEur, 0.9% Sodium Chloride Intravenous Infusion BP, or 5% Dextrose Intravenous Infusion BP, according to Table 1. Shake well until dissolved. Kefzol should be injected into a large muscle mass.

Table 1: Dilution table

| Vial Size | Diluent to be Added | Approximate Available Volume | Approximate Average Concentration |
|---|---|---|---|
| 500 mg | 4.0 ml | 4.1 ml | 125 mg/ml |
| 500 mg | 2.0 ml | 2.2 ml | 225 mg/ml |
| 1 g* | 2.5 ml | 3.0 ml | 330 mg/ml |

*The 1 g vial should be reconstituted only with Water for Injections PhEur.

*Intravenous administration:* Kefzol may be administered by intravenous injection or by continuous or intermittent infusion. Total daily dosages are the same as for intramuscular injection.

*Intermittent intravenous infusion:* Kefzol may be administered along with primary intravenous fluid management programmes in a volume control set or in a separate secondary IV bottle. Reconstituted 500 mg or 1 g of Kefzol may be diluted in 50 to 100 ml of Water for Injections PhEur or one of the following intravenous solutions:

  0.9% Sodium Chloride Intravenous Infusion BP
  5% or 10% Dextrose Intravenous Infusion BP
  5% Dextrose in Compound Sodium Lactate Intravenous Infusion BP
  0.9% Sodium Chloride and 5% Dextrose Intravenous Infusion BP
  0.45% Sodium Chloride and 5% Dextrose Intravenous Infusion BP
  Compound Sodium Lactate Intravenous Infusion BP
  5% or 10% Invert Sugar in Water for Injections PhEur

*Direct intravenous injection:* Dilute 500 mg or 1 g of reconstituted Kefzol in a minimum of 10 ml of Water for Injections PhEur and inject solution slowly over a period of three to five minutes. Do not inject in less than 3 minutes. The injection may be made directly into a vein or, for patients receiving the above parenteral fluids, through the tubing.

*Dosage:* The usual adult dosages are given in Table 2.

Table 2: Usual adult dosage

| Type of Infection | Dose | Frequency |
|---|---|---|
| Pneumococcal pneumonia | 500 mg | q 12 h |
| Mild infections caused by susceptible Gram-positive cocci | 250 mg to 500 mg | q 8 h |
| Acute uncomplicated urinary tract infections | 1 g | q 12 h |
| Moderate to severe infections | 500 mg to 1 g | q 6 to 8 h |
| Severe, life-threatening infections (e.g. endocarditis and septicaemia)* | 1 g to 1.5 g | q 6 h |

*In rare instances, doses up to 12 g cephazolin per day have been used.

In adults with renal impairment, cephazolin is not readily excreted. After a loading dose appropriate to the severity of the infection, the following recommendations (Table 3) may be used as a guide.

In patients undergoing peritoneal dialysis (2 l/h), mean serum levels of cephazolin were approximately 10 and 30 micrograms/ml after 24 hours' instillation of a dialysing solution containing 50 mg/l and 150 mg/l, respectively.

*The elderly:* As for adults.

Table 3: Dosage of Kefzol in Adults With Reduced Renal Function

| Creatinine Clearance (ml/min) | Serum Creatinine (mg %) | Dosage Reduction |
|---|---|---|
| ≥55 | ≤1.5 | None |
| 35–54 | 1.6 to 3.0 | None q 8 + hrs |
| 11–34 | 3.1–4.5 | 50% q 12 hrs |
| ≤10 | ≥4.6 | 50% q 18–24 hrs |

*Paediatric dosage:* In children, a total daily dosage of 25 to 50 mg/kg of body weight, divided into three or four equal doses, is effective for most mild to moderately severe infections (Table 4). Total daily dosage may be increased to 100 mg/kg of body weight for severe infections.

Table 4: Paediatric Dosage Guide

| Weight kg | 25 mg/kg/day Divided into 3 doses | | 25 mg/kg/day Divided into 4 doses | |
|---|---|---|---|---|
| | Approximate single dose (q 8 h) | Volume needed with dilution of 125 mg/ml | Approximate single dose (q 6 h) | Volume needed with dilution of 125 mg/ml |
| 4.5 | 40 mg | 0.35 ml | 30 mg | 0.25 ml |
| 9.0 | 75 mg | 0.6 ml | 55 mg | 0.45 ml |
| 13.5 | 115 mg | 0.9 ml | 85 mg | 0.7 ml |
| 18.0 | 150 mg | 1.2 ml | 115 mg | 0.9 ml |
| 22.5 | 190 mg | 1.5 ml | 140 mg | 1.1 ml |

| Weight kg | 50 mg/kg/day Divided into 3 doses | | 50 mg/kg/day Divided into 4 doses | |
|---|---|---|---|---|
| | Approximate single dose (q 8 h) | Volume needed with dilution of 225 mg/ml | Approximate single dose (q 6 h) | Volume needed with dilution of 225 mg/ml |
| 4.5 | 75 mg | 0.35 ml | 55 mg | 0.25 ml |
| 9.0 | 150 mg | 0.7 ml | 110 mg | 0.5 ml |
| 13.5 | 225 mg | 1.0 ml | 170 mg | 0.75 ml |
| 18.0 | 300 mg | 1.35 ml | 225 mg | 1.0 ml |
| 22.5 | 375 mg | 1.7 ml | 285 mg | 1.25 ml |

In children with mild to moderate renal impairment (creatinine clearance of 70-40 ml/min), 60% of the normal daily dose given in divided doses q 12 h should be sufficient. In children with moderate impairment (creatinine clearance of 40-20 ml/min), 25% of the normal daily dose in divided doses q 12 h should be adequate. In children with marked impairment (creatinine clearance of 20-5 ml/min), 10% of the normal daily dose given q 24 h should be sufficient. All dosage recommendations apply after an initial loading dose.

Since safety for use in premature infants and in infants under 1 month of age has not been established, the use of cephazolin in these patients is not recommended.

*Prophylactic use:* The following doses are recommended for perioperative use:

*Adults:* 1 g intravenously or intramuscularly one-half to one hour prior to surgical incision, followed by 0.5 to 1 g intravenously or intra-muscularly every six to eight hours for 24 hours postoperatively. Additionally, for lengthy operative procedures (e.g. two hours or more), 0.5 to 1 g intravenously or intramuscularly during surgery.

The prophylactic administration of cephazolin should usually be discontinued within a 24 hour period after the surgical procedure. For patients undergoing open-heart surgery or implantation of prosthetic devices, administration may be continued for three to five days.

*Contra-indications:* Cephazolin is contra-indicated in patients with known allergy to the cephalosporin group of antibiotics.

*Special warnings and special precautions for use:*
*Warnings:* Before instituting therapy with cephazolin, every attempt should be made to determine if the patient has had previous hypersensitivity reactions to the cephalosporins, penicillins, or other drugs, in which case this product should be given cautiously. Serious acute hypersensitivity reactions may require adrenaline and other emergency measures.

There is some evidence of partial cross-allergenicity between the penicillins and the cephalosporins. Patients have been reported to have had severe reactions (including anaphylaxis) to both drugs.

Antibiotics should be administered cautiously to any patient who has demonstrated some form of allergy, particularly to drugs.

Cephalosporins may be absorbed onto the surface of red cell membranes and react with antibodies directed against the drug. This can produce a positive Coombs' test and very rarely a haemolytic anaemia. Cross-reactivity may occur with penicillins for this reaction.

Pseudomembranous colitis has been reported with virtually all broad-spectrum antibiotics, so it is important to consider this diagnosis in patients who develop diarrhoea in association with the use of antibiotics. Severity ranges from mild to life-threatening; mild cases usually respond to drug discontinuance alone. In moderate to severe cases, appropriate measures should be taken.

*Precautions:* If an allergic reaction to cephazolin occurs, the drug should be discontinued and the patient treated with the usual agents (e.g. adrenaline or other pressor amines, antihistamines, or corticosteroids).

Broad-spectrum antibiotics should be prescribed with caution in individuals with a history of gastrointestinal disease, particularly colitis.

Prolonged use of cephazolin may result in the overgrowth of non-susceptible organisms. Careful observation of the patient is essential. If superinfection occurs during therapy, appropriate measures should be taken.

When cephazolin is administered to patients with impaired renal function, the daily dosage should be reduced to avoid toxicity (see *Posology and method of administration*).

*Interaction with other medicaments and other forms of interaction:* Probenecid may decrease renal tubular secretion of cephalosporins when used concurrently, which results in increased and more prolonged cephalosporin blood levels.

The results of experimental studies in animals given cephalosporins suggest that the concurrent use of potent diuretics, such as frusemide or ethacrynic acid, may increase the risk of renal toxicity.

A false positive reaction for glucose in the urine may occur with Benedict's or Fehling's solutions or with copper sulphate test tablets.

Positive direct and indirect antiglobulin (Coombs') tests have occurred; these may also occur in neonates whose mothers received cephalosporins before delivery.

*Pregnancy and lactation:*
*Usage in pregnancy:* Although animal studies have shown no evidence of impaired fertility or teratogenicity, there are no adequate and well-controlled studies in pregnant women. Therefore, caution should be exercised when prescribing for the pregnant patient. When cephazolin has been administered prior to caesarean section, drug levels in cord blood have been approximately one-fourth to one-third of maternal drug levels. The drug appeared to have no adverse effect on the fetus.

*Usage in nursing mothers:* Caution is required when cephazolin is administered to a nursing woman, as very low concentrations of cephazolin have been found in breast milk.

*Usage in neonates:* The safety of this product for use in prematures and infants under one month of age has not been established.

*Effects on ability to drive and use machines:* Not applicable.

*Undesirable effects:* The following side-effects have been reported:
*Gastro-intestinal:* Symptoms of pseudomembranous colitis may appear either during or after treatment. Nausea, anorexia, vomiting, diarrhoea and oral candidiasis have been reported.

*Hypersensitivity:* Drug fever, rash, vulvar pruritus, eosinophilia and anaphylaxis.

*Haematological:* Neutropenia, leucopenia, thrombocythaemia, and positive direct and indirect Coombs' tests.

*Neurological:* Convulsions have occasionally been reported, especially after administration of high doses to patients with marked renal impairment.

*Renal:* Transient rise in blood urea nitrogen levels has been observed without clinical evidence of renal impairment. Interstitial nephritis and other renal disorders have been reported rarely. Most patients experiencing these reactions have been seriously ill and were receiving multiple drug therapies. The role of cephazolin has not been determined.

*Hepatic:* Transient rises in AST, ALT and ALP levels have been observed rarely. As with some penicillins and some other cephalosporins, transient hepatitis and cholestatic jaundice have been reported rarely.

*Other:* Pain on intramuscular injection, sometimes with induration, has occurred infrequently. Phlebitis at the site of intravenous injection has been noted. Other side-effects have included genital and anal pruritus, genital candidiasis and vaginitis.

*Overdose:*
*Signs and symptoms:* May include pain, inflammation and phlebitis at the injection site.

The administration of inappropriately large doses of parenteral cephalosporins may cause dizziness, paraesthesiae and headaches. Seizures may occur with some cephalosporins, particularly in patients with renal impairment in whom accumulation is likely to occur.

Laboratory abnormalities may include elevations in creatinine, BUN, liver enzymes and bilirubin, a positive Coombs' test, thrombocytosis, thrombocytopenia, eosinophilia, leucopenia and prolongation of prothrombin time.

*Treatment:* In the event of serious overdosage, general supportive care is recommended, with monitoring of haematological, renal and hepatic functions and coagulation status until the patient is stable. If seizures occur, the drug should be discontinued promptly. Anticonvulsant therapy may be clinically indicated. General supportive therapy is recommended.

In cases of severe overdosage, especially in a patient with renal failure, combined haemodialysis and haemoperfusion may be considered, although supporting data are not available.

### Pharmacological properties

*Pharmacodynamic properties:* Cephazolin is a bactericidal antibiotic which interferes with the final stage of bacterial cell wall synthesis of Gram-negative and Gram-positive bacteria.

*Pharmacokinetic properties:* Cephazolin is poorly absorbed from the gastrointestinal tract and is therefore given parenterally. Following 500 mg intramuscularly, peak plasma levels of 30 micrograms/ml are obtained in 1 hour. Cephazolin is 90% bound to plasma proteins. The half life with normal renal function is 1.8 hours. It is excreted unchanged in the urine, approximately 80% being recoverable in the 24 hours following injection.

*Preclinical safety data:* There are no preclinical data of relevance to the prescriber in addition to that summarised in other sections of the summary of product characteristics.

### Pharmaceutical particulars

*List of excipients:* Not applicable.

*Incompatibilities:* Extemporaneous mixtures with other antibiotics (including aminoglycosides) are not recommended.

*Shelf life:*
Unreconstituted vials: 2 years.
*After reconstitution:* If stored below 25°C, use within 24 hours. If kept in a refrigerator (2°–8°C), use within 96 hours.

*Special precautions for storage:*
Unreconstituted vials: Protect from light.

*Nature and contents of container:*
500 mg vials: Glass vials in packs of 10
1 g vials: Glass vials in packs of 10

*Instructions for use/handling:* Prior to administration, parenteral drug products should be inspected visually for particulate matter and discolouration, whenever solution and container permit.

**Marketing authorisation number**  0006/0078R

**Date of approval/revision of SPC**  6 December 1991

**Legal category**  POM

# NEBCIN*

**Presentation**  Nebcin is presented in vials in the following strengths:

1 ml vials containing tobramycin sulphate equivalent to 40 mg tobramycin base.
2 ml vials containing tobramycin sulphate equivalent to 80 mg tobramycin base.
2 ml vials containing tobramycin sulphate equivalent to 20 mg tobramycin base.

Also containing 0.5% w/v Phenol BP with sodium bisulphite and Disodium Edetate BP.

**Uses**  Nebcin is indicated for the treatment of the following infections caused by susceptible microorganisms:

Central nervous system infections, including meningitis, septicaemia and neonatal sepsis.
Gastro-intestinal infections, including peritonitis, and other significant infections such as complicated and recurrent urinary tract infections, including pyelonephritis and cystitis.
Lower respiratory tract infections, including pneumonia, bronchopneumonia and acute bronchitis.
Skin, bone and soft tissue infections, including burns.

Nebcin may be considered in serious staphylococcal infections for which penicillin or other less potentially toxic drugs are contra-indicated and when bacterial susceptibility testing and clinical judgement indicate its use.

Tobramycin is usually active against most strains of the following organisms:

*Pseudomonas aeruginosa*
*Proteus* species (indole-positive and indole-negative), including *Pr. mirabilis, Pr. rettgeri* and *Pr. vulgaris*
*Morganella morganii*
*Escherichia coli*
*Klebsiella-Enterobacter-Serratia* species
*Citrobacter* species
*Providencia* species
Staphylococci including *Staphylococcus aureus* (coagulase-positive and coagulase-negative).

Most strains of enterococci demonstrate *in vitro* resistance. The combination of penicillin G and tobramycin results in a synergistic bactericidal effect *in vitro* against certain strains of *Enterococcus faecalis* (formerly *Streptococcus faecalis*). However, this combination is not synergistic against other closely related

organisms, e.g. *E. faecium* (formerly *S. faecium*). Speciation of enterococci alone cannot be used to predict susceptibility. Susceptibility testing and tests for antibiotic synergism are emphasised.

Cross-resistance between aminoglycosides occurs and depends largely on inactivation by bacterial enzymes.

The combination of tobramycin and carbenicillin is synergistic *in vitro* against most strains of *Ps. aeruginosa.* Other Gram-negative organisms may be affected synergistically by the combination of tobramycin and a cephalosporin.

**Dosage and administration**  Nebcin may be given intramuscularly or intravenously. The patient's pretreatment body weight should be obtained for calculation of correct dosage.

The intramuscular dose is the same as the intravenous dose.

It is recommended that both peak and trough serum levels should be determined whenever possible to ensure the correct dosage is given. Blood levels should always be determined in patients with chronic infections such as cystic fibrosis, or where longer duration of treatment may be necessary, or in patients with decreased renal function.

*Patients with normal renal function: Adults:* The usual recommended dosage for adults with serious infections is 3 mg/kg/day, administered in three equal doses every eight hours (see Table 1). For life-threatening infections, dosages up to 5 mg/kg/day may be administered in three or four equal doses. The dosage should be reduced to 3 mg/kg/day as soon as clinically indicated. To prevent increased toxicity due to excessive blood levels, dosage should not exceed 5 mg/kg/day unless serum levels are monitored (see 'Warnings' and 'Precautions').

To achieve therapeutic serum levels in patients with cystic fibrosis, it may be necessary to administer up to 8 to 10 mg/kg/day in equally divided doses. Because serum concentrations of tobramycin vary from one patient to another, serum levels should be monitored.

Table 1: Dosage Schedule Guide for Adults with Normal Renal Function (Dosage at 8–hour intervals)

| Patient weight (kg) | Usual dose for serious infections 1 mg/kg q 8 h (total 3 mg/kg/day) | | Maximum dose for life–threatening infections (reduce as soon as possible) 1.66 mg/kg q 8 h (total 5 mg/kg/day unless monitored) | |
|---|---|---|---|---|
| | mg/dose | ml/dose* | mg/dose | ml/dose* |
| 120 | 120 | 3.0 | 200 | 5.0 |
| 100 | 100 | 2.5 | 166 | 4.0 |
| 80 | 80 | 2.0 | 133 | 3.0 |
| 60 | 60 | 1.5 | 100 | 2.5 |
| 40 | 40 | 1.0 | 66 | 1.6 |

*Applicable to 40 mg/ml product forms.

In adults with normal renal function, mild to moderate infections of the urinary tract have responded to a dosage of 2–3 mg/kg/day administered as a single intramuscular injection.

*The elderly:* As for adults, but see recommendations for patients with impaired renal function.

*Children:* The recommended dosage is 6–7.5 mg/kg/day, administered in three or four equally divided doses. In some patients it may be necessary to administer higher doses.

*Premature or full-term neonates:* Dosages of up to 4 mg/kg/day may be administered in two equal doses every 12 hours, for those between 1.5 and 2.5 kg body weight.

The usual duration of treatment is 7 to 10 days. A longer course of therapy may be necessary in difficult and complicated infections. In such cases, monitoring of renal, auditory and vestibular functions is advised, because neurotoxicity is more likely to occur when treatment is extended for longer than 10 days.

*Obese patients:* The appropriate dose may be calculated using the patient's estimated lean body weight, plus 40% of the excess, as the weight on which to determine mg/kg.

*Patients with impaired renal function:* Following a loading dose of 1 mg/kg, subsequent dosage in these patients must be adjusted, either with lower doses administered at eight–hour intervals or with normal doses at prolonged intervals (see Table 2). Both of these regimens are suggested as guides to be used when serum levels of tobramycin cannot be measured directly. They are based on either the creatinine clearance or the serum creatinine of the patient, because these values correlate with the half–life of tobramycin. Neither regimen should be used when dialysis is being performed.

*Reduced dosage at eight-hour intervals (Regimen I):* An appropriately reduced dosage range can be found in the accompanying table (Table 2) for any patient for whom the blood urea, creatinine clearance or serum creatinine values are known. The choice of dose within the indicated range should be based on the severity of the infection, the sensitivity of the pathogen, and individual patient considerations, especially renal function. An alternative rough guide for determining reduced dosage at eight-hour intervals (for patients whose steady-state serum creatinine values are known) is to divide the normally recommended dose by the patient's serum creatinine value (mg/100 ml).

*Normal dosage at prolonged intervals (Regimen II):* Recommended intervals between doses are given in the accompanying table (Table 2). As a general rule, the dosage frequency in hours can be determined by multiplying the patient's serum creatinine level (mg/100 ml) by six.

The dosage schedules derived from either method should be used in conjunction with careful clinical and laboratory observations of the patient and should be modified as necessary (see *Warnings*).

*Intramuscular administration:* Nebcin may be administered by withdrawing the appropriate dose directly from the vial.

*Intravenous administration:* For intravenous administration, the usual volume of diluent (0.9% Sodium Chloride Intravenous Infusion BP or 5% Dextrose Intravenous Infusion BP) for adult doses is 50–100 ml. For children, the volume of diluent should be proportionately less than for adults. The diluted solution should be infused over a period of 20–60 minutes avoiding admixture with any other drug. Nebcin may be administered slowly by direct intravenous injection or into the tubing of a drip set. When given in this way, serum levels may exceed 12 mg/l for a short time (see *Contra-indications, warnings, etc.*).

### Contra-indications, warnings, etc

*Contra-indications:* Intrathecal administration. Hypersensitivity to any aminoglycoside is a contra–indication to the use of tobramycin because of the known cross–allergenicity of drugs in this class.

*Warnings:* Nebcin contains sodium bisulphite which may cause allergic–type reactions, including anaphylactic symptoms and life–threatening or less severe asthmatic episodes, in certain susceptible people. The overall prevalence of sulphite sensitivity in the general population is unknown and probably low, but it occurs more frequently in asthmatic patients.

Patients treated with tobramycin should be under close observation because tobramycin and other aminoglycoside antibiotics have an inherent potential for causing nephrotoxicity and ototoxicity.

Both vestibular and auditory ototoxicity can occur. The auditory changes are irreversible, are usually bilateral, and may be partial or total. Eighth cranial nerve impairment may develop in patients with pre-existing renal damage and if tobramycin is administered for longer periods or in higher doses than those recommended. Other manifestations of neurotoxicity may include numbness, skin tingling, muscle twitching and convulsions. The risk of aminoglycoside-induced hearing loss increases with the degree of exposure to either high peak or high trough serum concentrations. Patients who develop cochlear damage may not have symptoms during therapy to warn them of eighth-nerve toxicity, and partial or total irreversible bilateral deafness may continue to develop after the drug has been discontinued. Rarely, nephrotoxicity may not become manifest until the first few days after cessation of therapy. Aminoglycoside-induced nephrotoxicity is usually reversible.

Therefore, renal and eighth cranial nerve function should be closely monitored in patients with known or suspected renal impairment and also in those whose renal function is initially normal but who develop signs of renal dysfunction during therapy. Evidence of impairment in renal, vestibular and/or auditory function requires discontinuation of the drug or dosage adjustment.

Monitoring of renal function is particularly important in elderly patients who may have reduced renal function that may not be evident in the results of routine screening tests, such as blood urea or serum creatinine. A creatinine clearance determination may be more useful.

Serum concentrations should be monitored when feasible, and prolonged concentrations above 12 mg/l should be avoided. Rising trough levels (above 2 mg/l) may indicate tissue accumulation. A useful guideline would be to perform serum level assays after two or three doses, so that the dosage could be adjusted if necessary, and also at three to four day intervals during therapy. In the event of changing renal function, more frequent serum levels should be obtained and the dosage or dosage intervals adjusted according to the guidelines provided in the *Dosage and administration* section. In order to measure the peak level, a serum sample should be drawn about 30 minutes

Table 2. Two maintenance regimens based on renal function and body weight following an initial dose of 1 mg/kg†

| *Renal function‡* | | | | | *Regimen I* — *Adjusted doses at 8-hour intervals* | *or* | *Regimen II* — *Normal dosage at prolonged intervals* |
|---|---|---|---|---|---|---|---|
| *Blood urea* | | *Serum creatinine* | | *Creatinine clearance* | *Weight* | | *Weight/Dose* 50–60 kg: 60 mg; 60–80 kg: 80 mg |
| *mg/100 ml* | *mmol/l* | *mg/100 ml* | *mcmol/l* | *ml/min* | *50–60 kg* | *60–80 kg* | |
| Normal: | | | | | | | |
| < 42 | < 7.0 | < 1.3 | < 114.9 | > 70 | 60 mg | 80 mg | q 8 h |
| 42–74 | 7.0–12.3 | 1.4–1.9 | 123.8–168 | 69–40 | 30–60 mg | 50–80 mg | q 12 h |
| 75–105 | 12.5–17.5 | 2.0–3.3 | 176.8–291.7 | 39–20 | 20–25 mg | 30–45 mg | q 18 h |
| 106–140 | 17.7–23.3 | 3.4–5.3 | 300.6–468.5 | 19–10 | 10–18 mg | 15–24 mg | q 24 h |
| 141–160 | 23.5–26.7 | 5.4–7.5 | 477.4–663 | 9–5 | 5–9 mg | 7–12 mg | q 36 h |
| > 160 | > 26.7 | > 7.6 | > 671.8 | < 4 | 2.5–4.5 mg | 3.5–6 mg | q 48 h§ |

†For life-threatening infections, dosages 50% above those normally recommended may be used. The dosages should be reduced as soon as possible when improvement is noted.
‡If used to estimate degree of renal impairment, blood urea and serum creatinine concentrations should reflect a steady state of renal uraemia.
§When dialysis is not being performed.

following intravenous infusion or at one hour after intramuscular injection. Trough levels are measured by obtaining serum samples at eight hours or just prior to the next dose of tobramycin.

Urine should be examined for increased excretion of protein, cells and casts. Serum creatinine or creatinine clearance (preferred over blood urea) should be measured periodically. When feasible, it is recommended that serial audiograms be obtained in patients old enough to be tested, particularly high-risk patients.

The risk of toxic reactions is low in patients with normal renal function who do not receive tobramycin in higher doses or for longer periods of time than those recommended.

Patients with reduced renal function, however, are particularly prone to the potential ototoxic and nephrotoxic effects of this drug, so dosage should be adjusted carefully on the basis of regular monitoring of serum drug concentrations and of renal function.

Concurrent and/or sequential use of other potentially neurotoxic and/or nephrotoxic drugs, particularly other aminoglycosides (e.g. amikacin, streptomycin, neomycin, kanamycin, gentamicin and paromomycin), amphotericin B, cephaloridine, viomycin, polymyxin B, colistin, cisplatin and vancomycin, requires careful monitoring. Other factors that may increase patient risk are advanced age and dehydration.

Tobramycin should not be given concurrently with potent diuretics. Some diuretics themselves cause ototoxicity, and intravenously administered diuretics enhance aminoglycoside toxicity by altering antibiotic concentrations in serum and tissue.

*Usage in pregnancy:* Aminoglycosides can cause foetal harm when administered to a pregnant woman. Aminoglycoside antibiotics cross the placenta, and there have been several reports of total irreversible bilateral congenital deafness in children whose mothers received streptomycin during pregnancy. Serious side-effects to mother, foetus, or newborn have not been reported in the treatment of pregnant women with other aminoglycosides, but tobramycin should not be administered to the pregnant patient unless the potential benefits clearly outweigh any potential risk. If tobramycin is used during pregnancy or if the patient becomes pregnant whilst taking tobramycin, she should be informed of the potential hazard to the foetus.

*Usage in nursing mothers:* Tobramycin is excreted in the breast milk and should be avoided in nursing women.

*Precautions*

*Use in neonates:* Tobramycin should be used with caution in premature and neonatal infants because of their renal immaturity and the resulting prolongation of serum half-life of the drug.

*General:* Serum calcium, magnesium, and sodium should be monitored. It is particularly important to monitor serum levels closely in patients with known renal impairment.

In patients with extensive burns, altered pharmacokinetics may result in reduced serum concentrations of aminoglycosides. In such patients treated with tobramycin, measurement of serum concentration is especially recommended as a basis for determination of appropriate dosage.

Aminoglycosides may be absorbed in significant quantities from body surfaces after local irrigation or application and may cause neurotoxicity and nephrotoxicity.

Although not indicated for intraocular and/or subconjunctival use, there have been reports of macular necrosis following this type of injection.

Aminoglycosides should be used with caution in patients with muscular disorders, such as myasthenia gravis or parkinsonism, since these drugs may aggravate muscle weakness because of their potential curare-like effect on neuromuscular function.

Neuromuscular blockade or respiratory paralysis may occur following rapid intravenous administration of many aminoglycosides and have been reported in cats receiving very high doses of tobramycin (40 mg/kg). The possibility of prolonged secondary apnoea should be considered if tobramycin is administered to anaesthetised patients who are also receiving neuromuscular blocking agents such as succinylcholine, tubocurarine or decamethonium, or to patients receiving massive transfusions of citrated blood. If neuromuscular blockade occurs, it may be reversed by the administration of calcium salts.

The inactivation of tobramycin by beta-lactam antibiotics (penicillins or cephalosporins) has been demonstrated *in vitro* and in patients with severe renal impairment. Such inactivation has not been found in patients with normal renal function if the drugs are administered by separate routes.

If overgrowth of non-susceptible organisms occurs, appropriate therapy should be initiated.

*Side-effects:* Renal function changes, as shown by rising blood urea and serum creatinine and by oliguria, cylindruria and increased proteinuria, have been reported, especially in patients with a history of renal impairment who are treated for longer periods or with higher doses than those recommended. These changes can occur in patients with initially normal renal function.

Side-effects on both vestibular and auditory branches of the eighth cranial nerve have been reported, especially in patients receiving high doses or prolonged therapy, in those given previous courses of therapy with an ototoxin, and in cases of dehydration. Symptoms include dizziness, vertigo, tinnitus, roaring in the ears and hearing loss. Hearing loss is usually irreversible and is manifested initially by diminution of high-tone acuity.

Other reported side-effects, possibly related to tobramycin, include increased AST, ALT, and serum bilirubin; decreased serum calcium, magnesium, sodium and potassium; anaemia, granulocytopenia, thrombocytopenia, leucopenia, leucocytosis and eosinophilia; and fever, rash, exfoliative dermatitis, itching, urticaria, nausea, vomiting, diarrhoea, headache, lethargy, pain at the injection site, mental confusion and disorientation.

*Overdosage:* Severity of the manifestations of a tobramycin overdose depend on the dose, the patient's renal function, state of hydration, age and whether concurrent medication with similar toxicities is being given. Toxicity may occur in patients treated for more than 10 days, given more than 5 mg/kg/day, children given more than 7.5 mg/kg/day, or patients with reduced renal function whose dose has not been appropriately adjusted.

Nephrotoxicity following the parenteral administration of an aminoglycoside is most closely related to the AUC of serum concentration versus time. Nephrotoxicity is more likely if trough levels fail to fall below 2 mg/l and is also proportional to the average blood concentration. Patients who are elderly, have renal impairment, are receiving other nephrotoxic or ototoxic drugs, or are volume depleted, are at greater risk for developing acute tubular necrosis. Auditory and vestibular toxicities have been associated with aminoglycoside overdose. These toxicities occur in patients treated longer than 10 days, in patients with abnormal renal function, in dehydrated patients, or in patients on other ototoxic drugs. These patients may not have signs or symptoms, or may experience dizziness, tinnitus, vertigo and a loss of high-tone acuity. Signs and symptoms may not occur until long after the drug has been discontinued.

Neuromuscular blockade or respiratory failure may occur following rapid intravenous administration of many aminoglycosides. These reactions and prolonged respiratory paralysis may occur more commonly in patients with myasthenia gravis or Parkinson's disease, or those receiving decamethonium, tubocurarine or succinylcholine. Neuromuscular blockade may be reversed by the administration of calcium salts, but mechanical assistance may be necessary.

Toxicity from ingested tobramycin is unlikely because aminoglycosides are poorly absorbed from an intact gastro-intestinal tract.

*Treatment:* Resuscitative measures should be initiated promptly if respiratory paralysis occurs. Neuromuscular blockade may be reversed by giving calcium salts. Fluid balance, creatinine clearance and tobramycin plasma levels should be carefully monitored until the tobramycin level falls below 2 mg/l. Haemodialysis or peritoneal dialysis will help remove tobramycin from the blood. Between 25% and 70% of the administered dose may be removed, depending on the duration and type of dialysis employed; haemodialysis is the more effective method.

**Pharmaceutical precautions** *Undiluted vials:* Store below 25°C. Nebcin should not be physically premixed with other drugs but should be administered separately according to the recommended dose and route.

Prior to administration, parenteral drug products should be inspected visually for particulate matter and discolouration whenever solution and container permit.

**Legal category** POM.

**Package quantity** Boxes of 10 rubber-stoppered injection vials.

**Further information** Nil.

**Product licence numbers**
40 mg per 1 ml: 0006/0084
10 mg per 1 ml: 0006/0085

## NU-SEALS 75*
## NU-SEALS 300*

**Presentation** Enteric sealed tablets of aspirin. Nu-Seals Aspirin is available as 75 mg tablets (coded 75, in red) or as 300 mg tablets (coded 300, in red) of Acetylsalicylic Acid PhEur covered in a special coating, white in colour.

**Uses** Aspirin has analgesic, antipyretic and anti-inflammatory actions. It also has an antithrombotic action, mediated through inhibition of platelet activation, which has been shown to be useful in secondary prophylaxis following myocardial infarction and in patients with unstable angina or cerebral transient ischaemic attacks.

Nu-Seals Aspirin is indicated wherever high or prolonged dosage of aspirin is required. The special coating resists dissolution in gastric juice, but will dissolve readily in the relatively less acid environment of the duodenum. Owing to the delay that the coating imposes on the release of the active ingredient, Nu-Seals Aspirin is unsuitable for the short-term relief of pain.

**Dosage and administration** Nu-Seals Aspirin is for oral administration to adults only.

*Analgesic, antipyretic and anti-inflammatory actions:* 300–900 mg repeated three to four times daily according to clinical needs. In acute rheumatic disorders the dose is in the range of 4–8 g daily, taken in divided doses.

*Antithrombotic action:* 150 mg at diagnosis and 75 mg daily thereafter. Tablets taken at diagnosis should be chewed in order to gain rapid absorption.

Doses of 300 mg daily have been used with a low incidence of side-effects.

*The elderly: Analgesic, antipyretic and anti-inflammatory actions:* As for adults. The elderly are more likely to experience gastric side-effects and tinnitus. *Antithrombotic action:* The risk-benefit ratio has not been fully established.

*Children:* Aspirin should not be given to children, particularly those under 12 years (see *Warnings*).

**Contra-indications, warnings, etc**
*Contra-indications:* Hypersensitivity to aspirin. Hypoprothrombinaemia, haemophilia and active peptic ulceration.

*Warnings:* Aspirin should not be given to children, particularly those under 12 years, unless the expected benefits outweigh the possible risks. Aspirin may be a contributory factor in the causation of Reye's syndrome in some children.

Salicylates should be used with caution in patients with a history of peptic ulceration or coagulation abnormalities. They may also induce gastro-intestinal haemorrhage, occasionally major.

Aspirin should be used with caution in patients with impaired renal function, hepatic function (avoid if severe), or in patients who are dehydrated.

In large doses, salicylates may also decrease insulin requirements.

*Usage in pregnancy:* Aspirin does not appear to have teratogenic effects. However, prolonged pregnancy and labour, with increased bleeding before and after delivery, decreased birth weight and increased rate of stillbirth were reported with high blood salicylate levels. Aspirin should be avoided during the last 3 months of pregnancy.

*Usage in nursing mothers:* As aspirin is excreted in breast milk, Nu-Seals should not be taken by patients who are breast-feeding.

*Precautions:* Salicylates may enhance the effect of anticoagulants, oral hypoglycaemic agents, phenytoin and sodium valproate. They inhibit the uricosuric effect of probenecid and may increase the toxicity of sulphonamides. They may also precipitate bronchospasm or induce attacks of asthma in susceptible subjects.

Patients using enteric-coated aspirin should be advised against ingesting antacids simultaneously, to avoid premature drug release.

Patients with hypertension should be carefully monitored.

*Side-effects:* Salicylates may induce hypersensitivity, asthma, urate kidney stones, chronic gastro-intestinal blood loss, tinnitus, nausea and vomiting. The special coating of Nu-Seals Aspirin helps to reduce the incidence of side-effects resulting from gastric irritation.

*Overdosage:* Overdosage produces dizziness, tinnitus, sweating, nausea and vomiting, confusion and hyperventilation. Gross overdosage may lead to CNS depression with coma, cardiovascular collapse and respiratory depression. If overdosage is suspected, the patient should be kept under observation for at least 24 hours, as symptoms and salicylate blood levels may not become apparent for several hours. Treatment of overdosage consists of gastric lavage and forced alkaline diuresis. Haemodialysis may be necessary in severe cases.

**Pharmaceutical precautions** Store below 25°C. Keep bottles tightly closed.

**Legal category** P.

**Package quantities** Tablets 75 mg: Blister packs of 56.

Tablets 300 mg: Bottles of 100.

**Further information** Nil.

**Product licence numbers**
Tablets 75 mg: 0006/0293
Tablets 300 mg: 0006/5093R

## NU-SEALS CARDIO 75* ASPIRIN

**Presentation** Enteric sealed tablets of aspirin. Nu-Seals Cardio 75 Aspirin is available as 75 mg tablets (coded 75, in red) of Acetylsalicylic Acid PhEur covered in a special coating, white in colour.

**Uses** Aspirin has an antithrombotic action, mediated through inhibition of platelet activation, which has been shown to be useful in secondary prophylaxis following myocardial infarction and in patients with unstable angina or cerebral transient ischaemic attacks.

Nu-Seals Cardio 75 Aspirin is indicated wherever prolonged dosage of aspirin is required. The special coating resists dissolution in gastric juice, but will dissolve readily in the relatively less acid environment of the duodenum. Owing to the delay that the coating imposes on the release of the active ingredient, Nu-Seals Cardio 75 Aspirin is unsuitable for the short-term relief of pain.

**Dosage and administration** Nu-Seals Cardio 75 Aspirin is for oral administration to adults only.

*Antithrombotic action:* 150 mg at diagnosis and 75 mg daily thereafter. Tablets taken at diagnosis should be chewed in order to gain rapid absorption.

*The elderly: Antithrombotic action:* The risk-benefit ratio has not been fully established.

*Children:* Aspirin should not be given to children, particularly those under 12 years (see *Warnings*).

**Contra-indications, warnings, etc**

*Contra-indications:* Hypersensitivity to aspirin. Hypoprothrombinaemia, haemophilia and active peptic ulceration.

*Warnings:* Aspirin should not be given to children, particularly those under 12 years, unless the expected benefits outweigh the possible risks. Aspirin may be a contributory factor in the causation of Reye's syndrome in some children.

Salicylates should be used with caution in patients with a history of peptic ulceration or coagulation abnormalities. They may also induce gastro-intestinal haemorrhage, occasionally major.

Aspirin should be used with caution in patients with impaired renal function, hepatic function (avoid if severe), or in patients who are dehydrated.

In large doses, salicylates may also decrease insulin requirements.

*Usage in pregnancy:* Aspirin does not appear to have teratogenic effects. However, prolonged pregnancy and labour, with increased bleeding before and after delivery, decreased birth weight and increased rate of stillbirth were reported with high blood salicylate levels. Aspirin should be avoided during the last 3 months of pregnancy.

*Usage in nursing mothers:* As aspirin is excreted in breast milk, Nu-Seals Cardio 75 should not be taken by patients who are breast-feeding.

*Precautions:* Salicylates may enhance the effect of anticoagulants, oral hypoglycaemic agents, phenytoin and sodium valproate. They inhibit the uricosuric effect of probenecid and may increase the toxicity of sulphonamides. They may also precipitate bronchospasm or induce attacks of asthma in susceptible subjects.

Patients using enteric-coated aspirin should be advised against ingesting antacids simultaneously, to avoid premature drug release.

Patients with hypertension should be carefully monitored.

*Side-effects:* Salicylates may induce hypersensitivity, asthma, urate kidney stones, chronic gastro-intestinal blood loss, tinnitus, nausea and vomiting. The special coating of Nu-Seals Cardio 75 Aspirin helps to reduce the incidence of side-effects resulting from gastric irritation.

*Overdosage:* Overdosage produces dizziness, tinnitus, sweating, nausea and vomiting, confusion and hyperventilation. Gross overdosage may lead to CNS depression with coma, cardiovascular collapse and respiratory depression. If overdosage is suspected, the patient should be kept under observation for at least 24 hours, as symptoms and salicylate blood levels may not become apparent for several hours. Treatment of overdosage consists of gastric lavage and forced alkaline diuresis. Haemodialysis may be necessary in severe cases.

**Pharmaceutical precautions** Store below 25°C.

**Legal category** P

**Package quantities** Blister packs of 28 tablets.

**Further information** Nil.

**Product licence number** 0006/0293

## ONCOVIN*

WARNING
THIS PRODUCT IS **NOT**
FOR INTRATHECAL USE

**Presentation**

*Oncovin Solution:* 1 ml vials containing 1 mg Oncovin (Vincristine Sulphate BP) and 100 mg Mannitol BP.

2 ml vials containing 2 mg Oncovin (Vincristine Sulphate BP) and 200 mg Mannitol BP.

The vials also contain 1.8 mg per 1 ml Methyl Hydroxybenzoate PhEur and 0.2 mg per 1 ml Propyl Hydroxybenzoate PhEur as preservatives. Acetic acid and sodium acetate have been added for pH control.

**Uses** Oncovin is an anti–neoplastic drug for intravenous use.

Information available at present suggests that Oncovin may be useful either alone or in conjunction with other oncolytic drugs for the treatment of:

1. Leukaemias, including acute lymphocytic leukaemia, chronic lymphocytic leukaemia, acute myelogenous leukaemia and blastic crisis of chronic myelogenous leukaemia.
2. Malignant lymphomas, including Hodgkin's disease and non–Hodgkin's lymphomas.
3. Multiple myeloma.
4. Solid tumours, including breast carcinoma, small cell bronchogenic carcinoma, head and neck carcinoma and soft tissue sarcomas.
5. Paediatric solid tumours, including Ewing's sarcoma, embryonal rhabdomyosarcoma, neuroblastoma, Wilms' tumour, retinoblastoma and medulloblastoma.
6. Idiopathic thrombocytopenic purpura. Patients with true ITP refractory to splenectomy and short-term treatment with adrenocortical steroids may respond to vincristine but the drug is not recommended as primary treatment of this disorder. Recommended weekly doses of vincristine given for 3 to 4 weeks have produced permanent remissions in some patients. If patients fail to respond after 3 to 6 doses, it is unlikely that there will be any beneficial results with additional doses.

**Dosage and administration** *This preparation is for intravenous use only. It should be administered only by individuals experienced in vincristine administration.*

Intrathecal administration
usually results in death
(see 'Warnings' for treatment).

Extreme care must be used in calculating and administering the dose of vincristine since overdosage may have a very serious or fatal outcome.

The drug is administered intravenously *at weekly intervals.* The recommended dose is 1.4 to 1.5 mg/m², up to a maximum weekly dose of 2 mg.

The dosage must always be adjusted individually because of the narrow range between therapeutic and toxic levels, and individual variations in response.

*The elderly:* As for adults.

*Children:* The usual dose is 2 mg/m². For children weighing 10 kg or less, the starting dose should be 0.05 mg/kg, administered once a week.

An increase in the severity of side-effects may be experienced by patients with liver disease sufficient to decrease biliary excretion. A 50 per cent reduction in the dose of vincristine is recommended for patients having a direct serum bilirubin value above 3 mg/100 ml (51 micromol/l).

The metabolism of vinca alkaloids has been shown to be mediated by hepatic cytochrome P450 isoenzymes in the CYP 3A subfamily. This metabolic pathway may be impaired in patients with hepatic dysfunction or who are taking concomitant potent inhibitors of these isoenzymes (see *Precautions*).

*Oncovin solution:* The concentration of vincristine is 1 mg/ml. Do not add extra fluid to the vial prior to removal of the dose. Withdraw the solution of Oncovin into an accurate dry syringe, measuring the dose carefully. Do not add extra fluid to the vial in an attempt to empty it completely.

The calculated dose of the solution for injection is drawn up into a syringe and injected either directly into a vein or into the tubing of a running intravenous infusion of normal saline or glucose in water, whichever is more suitable for the patient.

Care should be taken to avoid infiltration of subcutaneous tissues. Injection may be completed in about one minute.

*Caution:* If leakage into surrounding tissue should occur during intravenous administration of vincristine, it may cause considerable irritation. The injection should be discontinued immediately and any remaining portion of the dose should then be introduced into another vein. Local injection of hyaluronidase and the application of moderate heat to the area of leakage help to disperse the drug and are thought to minimise discomfort and the possibility of cellulitis.

**Contra-indications, warnings, etc**

*Contra-indications*

Intrathecal administration
usually results in death
(see 'Warnings' for treatment).

Patients with the demyelinating form of Charcot-Marie–Tooth syndrome should not be given vincristine.

*Warnings:* Syringes containing this product should be labelled 'FATAL IF GIVEN INTRATHECALLY. FOR INTRAVENOUS USE ONLY'. An auxiliary sticker is provided in the pack with this warning.

Extemporaneously prepared syringes containing this product must be packaged in an overwrap which is labelled 'DO NOT REMOVE COVERING UNTIL MOMENT OF INJECTION. FATAL IF GIVEN INTRATHECALLY. FOR INTRAVENOUS USE ONLY'.

After intrathecal administration, removal of cerebrospinal fluid, and flushing with Lactated Ringer's and other solutions, has not prevented ascending paralysis leading to death. In one adult paralysis was arrested, with some recovery, by the following treatment initiated immediately after the intrathecal injection:

1. Removal of as much CSF as is safely possible.
2. Flushing with Lactated Ringer's solution by continuous infusion at 150 ml/h, through a catheter in a cerebral lateral ventricle and removed through lumbar access, until fresh frozen plasma became available.
3. Fresh frozen plasma, 25 ml, diluted with 1 l of Lactated Ringer's was then infused similarly at

75 ml/h. The rate of infusion was adjusted to maintain a spinal fluid protein level of 150 mg/dl.

4. Glutamic acid, 10 gm, was given i.v. over 24 hours, followed by 500 mg tds by mouth for 1 month. Glutamic acid may not be essential.

*Usage in pregnancy:* Caution is necessary with the use of all oncolytic drugs during pregnancy.

Vincristine can cause foetal harm when administered to a pregnant woman, although there are no adequate and well controlled studies. In several animal species, vincristine can induce teratogenic effects as well as embryolethality with doses that are non-toxic to the pregnant animal. Women of child-bearing potential should be advised to avoid becoming pregnant while receiving vincristine. If vincristine is used during pregnancy or if the patient becomes pregnant while receiving this drug she should be informed of the potential hazard to the foetus.

*Usage in nursing mothers:* It is not known whether Oncovin is excreted in human breast milk. Because of the potential for serious adverse reactions due to Oncovin in nursing infants, a decision should be made whether to discontinue nursing or the drug, taking into account the importance of the drug to the mother.

*Precautions:* Effective therapy with Oncovin is less likely to be followed by leucopenia than is the case with Velbe (vinblastine sulphate) and other oncolytic agents. A study of the side–effects of Oncovin in all age groups reveals that it is usually neuromuscular rather than bone marrow toxicity that limits dosage. However, because of the possibility of leucopenia, both clinician and patient should remain alert for signs of any complicating infection. Although pre-existing leucopenia does not necessarily contra-indicate the administration of Oncovin, the appearance of leucopenia during treatment warrants careful consideration before giving the next dose.

Acute uric acid nephropathy, which may occur after the administration of oncolytic agents, has also been reported with Oncovin.

If central-nervous-system leukaemia is diagnosed, additional agents may be required, since vincristine does not appear to cross the blood-brain barrier in adequate amounts.

Particular attention should be given to dosage and neurological side effects if Oncovin is administered to patients with pre-existing neuromuscular disease and also when other drugs with neurotoxic potential are being used.

Acute shortness of breath and severe bronchospasm have been reported following the administration of vinca alkaloids. These reactions have been encountered most frequently when the vinca alkaloid was used in combination with mitomycin-C and may be serious when there is pre-existing pulmonary dysfunction. The onset may be within minutes or several hours after the vinca is injected and may occur up to 2 weeks following the dose of mitomycin. Progressive dyspnoea, requiring chronic therapy, may occur. Vincristine should not be readministered.

The simultaneous oral or intravenous administration of phenytoin and antineoplastic chemotherapy combinations, that included vincristine sulphate, have been reported to reduce blood levels of the anticonvulsant and to increase seizure activity. Although the contribution of the vinca alkaloids has not been established, dosage adjustment of phenytoin, based on serial blood level monitoring, may need to be made when it is used in combination with vincristine.

Caution should be exercised in patients concurrently taking drugs known to inhibit drug metabolism by hepatic cytochrome P450 isoenzymes in the CYP 3A subfamily, or in patients with hepatic dysfunction. Concurrent administration of vincristine sulphate with itraconazole (a known inhibitor of the metabolic pathway) has been reported to cause an earlier onset and/or an increased severity of neuromuscular side-effects (see 'Adverse reactions'). This interaction is presumed to be related to inhibition of the metabolism of vincristine.

When Oncovin is used in combination with L-asparaginase, it should be given 12 to 24 hours before administration of the enzyme in order to minimise toxicity, since administering L-asparaginase first may reduce hepatic clearance of vincristine.

When chemotherapy is being given in conjunction with radiation therapy through portals which include the liver, the use of vincristine should be delayed until radiation therapy has been completed.

Both *in vivo* and *in vitro* laboratory tests have failed to demonstrate conclusively that this product is mutagenic. Fertility following treatment with vincristine alone for malignant disease has not been studied in humans. Clinical reports of both male and female patients who received multiple-agent chemotherapy that included vincristine indicate that azoospermia and amenorrhoea can occur in postpubertal patients. Recovery occurred many months after completion of chemotherapy in some but not all patients. When the same treatment is administered to prepubertal patients, it is much less likely to cause permanent azoospermia and amenorrhoea.

Patients who received vincristine chemotherapy in combination with anticancer drugs known to be carcinogenic have developed second malignancies. The contributing role of vincristine in this development has not been determined. No evidence of carcinogenicity was found following intraperitoneal administration in rats and mice, although this study was limited.

Care must be taken to avoid contamination of the eye with concentrations of Oncovin used clinically. If accidental contamination occurs, severe irritation (or, if the drug was delivered under pressure, even corneal ulceration) may result. The eye should be washed immediately and thoroughly.

*Adverse reactions:* Prior to the use of this drug, patients and/or their parents/guardians should be advised of the possibility of untoward symptoms.

In general, adverse reactions are reversible and are related to dosage size and cumulative dosage. The use of small amounts of vincristine daily for long periods is not advised. The most common adverse reaction is alopecia; the most troublesome adverse reactions are neuromuscular in origin.

When single weekly doses of the drug are employed, the adverse reactions of leucopenia, neuritic pain, and constipation are usually of short duration (i.e. less than 7 days). When the dosage is reduced, these reactions may lessen or disappear. They seem to be increased when the calculated amount of drug is given in divided doses. Other adverse reactions, such as alopecia, sensory loss, paraesthesia, difficulty in walking, slapping gait, loss of deep-tendon reflexes and muscle wasting may persist for at least as long as therapy is continued. Generalised sensorimotor dysfunction may become progressively more severe with continued treatment. In most instances, they have disappeared by about the sixth week after discontinuance of treatment, but the neuromuscular difficulties may persist for prolonged periods in some patients. Regrowth of hair may occur while maintenance therapy continues.

The following adverse reactions have been reported:

*Neuromuscular (often dose limiting):* Neuritic pain, sensory loss, paraesthesiae, difficulty in walking, slapping gait, loss of deep tendon reflexes, muscle wasting, ataxia, paresis, foot drop and cranial nerve palsies, especially ocular palsies and laryngeal nerve paralysis. Jaw pain, pharyngeal pain, parotid gland pain, bone pain, back pain, limb pain, and myalgias have been reported; pain in these areas may be severe. Convulsions, frequently with hypertension, have been reported in a few patients receiving vincristine. Several instances of convulsions followed by coma have been reported in children. Transient cortical blindness and optic atrophy with blindness have been reported. Treatment with vinca alkaloids has resulted rarely in both vestibular and auditory damage to the eighth cranial nerve. Manifestations include partial or total deafness, which may be temporary or permanent, and difficulties with balance, including dizziness, nystagmus and vertigo. Particular caution is warranted when vincristine sulphate is used in combination with other agents known to be ototoxic, such as the platinum-containing oncolytics.

Frequently, there appears to be a sequence in the development of neuromuscular side-effects. Initially, one may encounter only sensory impairment and paraesthesiae. With continued treatment, neuritic pain may appear and later, motor difficulties. No reports have yet been made of any agent that can reverse the neuromuscular manifestations of Oncovin.

*Haematological:* Leucopenia; vincristine does not appear to have any constant or significant effect upon the platelets or the red blood cells, however, anaemia and thrombocytopenia have been reported. If thrombocytopenia is present when treatment with Oncovin is begun, it may actually improve before the appearance of marrow remission.

*Gastro-intestinal:* Constipation, abdominal cramps, paralytic ileus, diarrhoea, weight loss, nausea, vomiting, oral ulceration, intestinal necrosis and/or perforation, and anorexia have occurred. The constipation which may be encountered responds well to such usual measures as enemas and laxatives. Constipation may take the form of upper colon impaction and the rectum may be found to be empty on physical examination. Colicky abdominal pain, coupled with an empty rectum, may mislead the clinician. A flat film of the abdomen is useful in demonstrating this condition. A routine prophylactic regimen against constipation is recommended for all patients receiving Oncovin. Paralytic ileus may occur, particularly in young children. The ileus will reverse itself upon temporary discontinuance of vincristine and with symptomatic care.

*Pulmonary:* See under *Precautions.*

*Endocrine:* Rare occurrences of a syndrome attributable to inappropriate anti-diuretic hormone secretion have been observed in patients treated with vincristine. There is a high urinary sodium excretion in the presence of hyponatraemia; renal or adrenal disease, hypotension, dehydration, azotaemia and clinical oedema are absent. With fluid deprivation, improvement occurs in the hyponatraemia and in the renal loss of sodium.

*Genitourinary:* Polyuria, dysuria and urinary retention due to bladder atony have occurred. Other drugs known to cause urinary retention (particularly in the elderly) should, if possible, be discontinued for the first few days following administration of vincristine.

*Cardiovascular:* Hypertension and hypotension have occurred. Chemotherapy combinations which have included vincristine, when given to patients previously treated with mediastinal radiation, have been associated with coronary artery disease and myocardial infarction. Causality has not been established.

*Hypersensitivity:* Rare cases of allergic-type reactions, such as anaphylaxis, rash and oedema, temporally related to vincristine therapy have been reported in patients receiving vincristine as a part of multi-drug chemotherapy regimens.

*Cutaneous:* Alopecia, rash.

*Other:* Fever, headache, injection site reaction (see *Dosage and administration—Caution).*

*Overdosage:* Side–effects following the use of vincristine are dose related. In children under 13 years of age, death has occurred following doses of vincristine that were 10 times those recommended for therapy. Severe symptoms may occur in this patient group following dosages of 3 to 4 mg/m$^2$. Adults can be expected to experience severe symptoms after single doses of 3 mg/m$^2$ or more. Therefore, following administration of doses higher than those recommended, patients can be expected to experience side-effects in an exaggerated fashion. Supportive care should include the following: (a) prevention of side-effects resulting from the syndrome of inappropriate antidiuretic hormone secretion (this would include restriction of fluid intake and perhaps the administration of a diuretic affecting the function of Henle's loop and the distal tubule); (b) administration of anticonvulsants; (c) use of enemas or cathartics to prevent ileus (in some instances, decompression of the gastro-intestinal tract may be necessary); (d) monitoring the cardiovascular system; (e) determining daily blood counts for guidance in transfusion requirements.

Folinic acid has been observed to have a protective effect in normal mice which were administered lethal doses of vincristine. Isolated case reports suggest that folinic acid may be helpful in treating humans who have received an overdose. A suggested schedule is to administer 100 mg of folinic acid intravenously every 3 hours for 24 hours and then every 6 hours for at least 48 hours. Theoretical tissue levels of vincristine derived from pharmacokinetic data are predicted to remain significantly elevated for at least 72 hours. Treatment with folinic acid does not eliminate the need for the above-mentioned supportive measures.

Most of an intravenous dose of vincristine is excreted into the bile after rapid tissue binding. Because only very small amounts of the drug appear in dialysate, haemodialysis is not likely to be helpful in cases of overdosage.

Enhanced faecal excretion of parenterally administered vincristine has been demonstrated in dogs pretreated with cholestyramine. There are no published clinical data on the use of cholestyramine as an antidote in humans.

There are no published clinical data on the consequences of oral ingestion of vincristine. Should oral ingestion occur, the stomach should be evacuated followed by oral administration of activated charcoal and a cathartic.

**Pharmaceutical precautions**

*Special dispensing information:* When dispensing vincristine sulphate in other than the original container, it is imperative that it be packaged in a overwrap bearing the statement 'DO NOT REMOVE COVERING UNTIL MOMENT OF INJECTION. FATAL IF GIVEN INTRATHECALLY. FOR INTRAVENOUS USE ONLY'. A syringe containing a specific dose must be labelled, using the auxiliary sticker provided in the pack, with this warning.

*Guidelines for the safe handling of antineoplastic agents:* Cytotoxic preparations should not be handled by pregnant staff.

Trained personnel should reconstitute the drug. This should be performed in a designated area. The work surface should be covered with disposable plastic-backed absorbent paper.

Adequate protective gloves, masks and clothing should be worn. Precautions should be taken to avoid the drug accidentally coming into contact with the eyes. If accidental contamination occurs, the eye should be washed with water thoroughly and immediately.

Use Luer-lock fittings on all syringes and sets. Large

bore needles are recommended to minimise pressure and the possible formation of aerosols. The latter may also be reduced by the use of a venting needle.

Adequate care and precaution should be taken in the disposal of items (syringes, needles, etc.) used to reconstitute cytotoxic drugs.

*Oncovin Solution:* Store in a refrigerator between 2° and 8°C. Protect from light.

Oncovin should never be mixed with any other drug and should not be diluted in solutions that raise or lower the pH outside the range of 3.5 to 5.5. It should not be mixed with anything other than normal saline or glucose in water.

Whenever solution and container permit, parenteral drug products should be inspected visually for particulate matter and discolouration prior to administration.

**Legal category** POM.

**Package quantities**
Vials 1 mg/1 ml: Single vials
Vials 2 mg/2 ml: Single vials

**Further information** Nil.

**Product licence numbers**
Vials 1 mg/1 ml: 0006/0169
Vials 2 mg/2 ml: 0006/0169

# REOPRO* ▼

**Qualitative and quantitative composition** Abciximab 2 mg/ml (10 mg/5 ml vial; 40 mg/20 ml vial).

**Pharmaceutical form** Solution for injection.

## Clinical particulars

*Therapeutic indications:* ReoPro is indicated as an adjunct to heparin and aspirin for the prevention of ischaemic cardiac complications in high risk patients undergoing percutaneous transluminal coronary angioplasty (PTCA). Because administration of ReoPro is associated with an increased frequency of bleeding, use by experienced physicians with adequate diagnostic and treatment facilities is required and should be limited to patients with a high risk of acute coronary thrombosis. These patients will have at least one of the following criteria:

1. Angina of the following characteristics:
- angina at rest with ischaemic ST changes refractory to medical therapy
- recurrent angina with ischaemic ST changes refractory to medical therapy
- postinfarction angina with ischaemic ST changes within 7 days of myocardial infarction refractory to medical therapy
2. Acute Q-wave myocardial infarction within 12 hours of onset that necessitates:
- direct intervention
- rescue for failed thrombolytic therapy
3. Angiographically-defined obstructions of the coronary circulation (based on the American Heart Association (AHA) and American College of Cardiology (ACC) classification – Ryan *et al, Circulation,* 1988, **78**, 486–502 and Ryan *et al, J Am Coll Cardiol,* 1993, **22**, 2033–54).
- 2 type B lesion characteristics
- 1 type C lesion characteristic
- 1 type B lesion characteristic and female ≥ 65 years of age and/or diabetes mellitus

Prior to treating with ReoPro on the basis of angiographically defined coronary lesion morphology, review of cine-angiograms should be performed to verify the severity of the lesions to be treated.

*Posology and method of administration:* ReoPro is for single use intravenous (IV) administration in adults.

*Adults:* The recommended dose of ReoPro is a 0.25 mg/kg intravenous bolus **10 minutes prior to PTCA** immediately followed by a 10µg/min continuous intravenous infusion for 12 hours.

*Administration instructions:*

1. Parenteral drug products should be inspected visually for particulate matter prior to administration. Preparations of ReoPro containing visibly opaque particles should NOT be used.
2. Hypersensitivity reactions should be anticipated whenever protein solutions such as ReoPro are administered. Adrenaline, dopamine, theophylline, antihistamines and corticosteroids should be available for immediate use. If symptoms of an allergic reaction or anaphylaxis appear, the infusion should be stopped immediately. Subcutaneous administration of 0.3 to 0.5 ml of aqueous adrenaline (1:1000 dilution), and use of corticosteroids, respiratory assistance and other resuscitative measures are essential.
3. As with all parenteral drug products, aseptic procedures should be used during the administration of ReoPro.
4. Withdraw the necessary amount of ReoPro for bolus injection through a sterile, non–pyrogenic, low protein–binding 0.2 or 0.22µm filter into a syringe. The

bolus should be administered 10 minutes before the procedure over one (1) minute.
5. Withdraw the necessary amount of ReoPro for the infusion through a sterile, non–pyrogenic, low protein–binding 0.2 or 0.22µm filter into a syringe. Inject into sterile 0.9% saline or 5% dextrose and infuse at a rate of 10µg/min for 12 hours via a continuous infusion pump equipped with an in–line sterile, non–pyrogenic, low protein–binding 0.2 or 0.22µm filter. (For example, withdraw 4.5 ml ReoPro and inject into 250 ml of 0.9% saline or 5% dextrose and infuse at 17 ml/hour for 12 hours.) Discard the unused portion at the end of the 12–hour infusion.
6. Although incompatibilities have not been shown with intravenous infusion fluids or commonly used cardiovascular drugs, it is recommended that ReoPro be administered in a separate intravenous line whenever possible and not mixed with other medications.
7. No incompatibilities have been observed with glass bottles or polyvinyl chloride bags or administration sets.

*Contra-indications:* ReoPro should not be administered to patients with known sensitivity to abciximab, to any component of the product or to murine monoclonal antibodies.

Because inhibition of platelet aggregation increases the risk of bleeding, ReoPro is contra–indicated in the following clinical situations: active internal bleeding; history of cerebrovascular accident within two years; recent (within two months) intracranial or intraspinal surgery or trauma; recent (within two months) major surgery; intracranial neoplasm, arteriovenous malformation or aneurysm; known bleeding diathesis or severe uncontrolled hypertension; pre–existing thrombocytopenia; vasculitis; hypertensive or diabetic retinopathy; severe hepatic or severe renal failure.

*Special warnings and special precautions for use:* ReoPro has been shown to be of benefit in patients who have high risk of ischaemic complications in relation to PTCA. However, due to the increased risk of bleeding, careful assessment of risk:benefit should be made in individual patients before commencing therapy with ReoPro.

*Requirement for specialist facilities:* ReoPro should only be administered in conjunction with extensive specialist medical and nursing care. In addition, there must be availability of laboratory tests of haematology function and facilities for administration of blood products.

*Concomitant aspirin and heparin therapy:* ReoPro should be used as an adjunct to aspirin and heparin therapy.

*Aspirin:* Aspirin should be administered orally at a daily dose of approximately but not less than 300 mg.

*Heparin: Heparin bolus pre-PTCA:* If a patient's activated clotting time (ACT) is less than 200 seconds prior to the start of the PTCA procedure, an initial bolus of heparin should be given upon gaining arterial access according to the following algorithm:

ACT <150 seconds: administer 70U/kg
ACT 150–199 seconds: administer 50U/kg

The initial heparin bolus dose should not exceed 7,000U.

ACT should be checked a minimum of 2 minutes after the heparin bolus. If the ACT is <200 seconds, additional heparin boluses of 20U/kg may be administered. Should the ACT remain <200 seconds, additional 20U/kg boluses are to be given until an ACT ≥200 seconds is achieved.

Should a situation arise where higher doses of heparin are considered clinically necessary in spite of the possibility of a greater bleeding risk, it is recommended that heparin be carefully titrated using weight–adjusted boluses and that the target ACT not exceed 300 seconds.

*Heparin bolus during PTCA:* During the PTCA procedure, ACT should be checked every 30 minutes. If ACT is <200 seconds, additional heparin boluses of 20U/kg may be administered. Should the ACT remain <200 seconds, additional 20U/kg boluses may be given until an ACT ≥200 seconds is achieved. ACT should be checked prior to and a minimum of 2 minutes after each heparin bolus.

As an alternative to giving additional boluses as described above, a continuous heparin infusion may be initiated after the initial heparin bolus doses achieve the ACT target ≥200 seconds at a rate of 7U/kg/hour and continued for the duration of the procedure.

*Heparin infusion after PTCA :* Discontinuation of heparin immediately following completion of the procedure, with removal of the arterial sheath within 6 hours, is *strongly recommended.* In individual patients, if prolonged heparin therapy after PTCA or later sheath removal is used, then an initial infusion rate of 7U/kg/hr is recommended (see Bleeding Precautions: Femoral Artery Sheath Removal).

*Bleeding precautions:*

*Femoral artery access site:* ReoPro is associated with an increase in bleeding rate particularly at the site of

arterial access for femoral artery sheath placement. The following are specific recommendations for access site care:

*Femoral artery sheath insertion:* When appropriate, place only an arterial sheath for vascular access (avoid venous sheath placement)

Puncture only the anterior wall of the artery or vein when establishing vascular access

The use of a through and through technique to identify the vascular structure is *strongly discouraged*

*While femoral artery sheath is in place:* Check sheath insertion site and distal pulses of affected leg(s) every 15 minutes for 1 hour, then hourly for 6 hours

Maintain complete bed rest with head of bed ≤30°

Maintain affected leg(s) straight via sheet tuck method or soft restraint

Medicate for back/groin pain as necessary

Educate patient on post-PTCA care via verbal instructions

*Femoral artery sheath removal:* Heparin should be discontinued at least 4 hours prior to arterial sheath removal

Check APTT or ACT prior to arterial sheath removal: do not remove sheath unless APTT ≤50 seconds or ACT ≤175 seconds

Apply pressure to access site for at least 30 min following sheath removal, using either manual compression or a mechanical device

Apply pressure dressing after haemostasis has been achieved

*After femoral artery sheath removal:* Check groin for bleeding/haematoma and distal pulses every 15 minutes for the first hour or until stable, then hourly for 6 hours following sheath removal

Continue complete bed rest with head of bed ≤30° and affected leg(s) straight for 6–8 hours following femoral artery sheath removal, 6–8 hours following discontinuation of ReoPro or 4 hours following discontinuation of heparin, whichever is later

Remove pressure dressing prior to ambulation

Continue to medicate for discomfort.

*Management of femoral access site bleeding/haematoma formation:* In the event of groin bleeding with or without haematoma formation, the following procedures are recommended:

Lower head of bed to 0°

Apply manual pressure/compression device until haemostasis has been achieved

Any haematoma should be measured and monitored for enlargement

Change pressure dressing as needed

If heparin is being given, obtain APTT and adjust heparin as needed

Maintain intravenous access if sheath has been removed

If groin bleed continues or the haematoma expands during ReoPro infusion despite the above measures, the ReoPro infusion should be immediately discontinued and the arterial sheath removed according to the guidelines listed above. After sheath removal intravenous access should be maintained until bleeding is controlled (see Overdose, *Uncontrolled Bleeding*).

*Potential bleeding sites:* Careful attention should be paid to all potential bleeding sites, including arterial and venous puncture sites, catheter insertion sites, cutdown sites, and needle puncture sites.

*Retroperitoneal bleeding:* ReoPro is associated with an increased risk of retroperitoneal bleeding in association with femoral vascular puncture. The use of venous sheaths should be minimised and only the anterior wall of the artery or vein should be punctured when establishing vascular access (see Bleeding Precautions, *Femoral Artery Access Site*).

*GI Bleeding prophylaxis:* In order to prevent spontaneous GI bleeding it is recommended that patients are pretreated with H₂–histamine receptor antagonists or liquid antacids. Antiemetics should be given as needed to prevent vomiting.

*General nursing care:* Unnecessary arterial and venous punctures, intramuscular injections, routine use of urinary catheters, nasotracheal intubation, nasogastric tubes and automatic blood pressure cuffs should be avoided. When obtaining intravenous access, non–compressible sites (eg, subclavian or jugular veins) should be avoided. Saline or heparin locks should be considered for blood drawing. Vascular puncture sites should be documented and monitored. Gentle care should be provided when removing dressings.

*Patient monitoring:* Before administration of ReoPro, platelet count, ACT, prothrombin time (PT) and APTT should be measured to identify pre-existing coagulation abnormalities. Haemoglobin and haematocrit measurements should be obtained prior to the ReoPro administration, at 12 hours following the ReoPro bolus injection, and again at 24 hours following the bolus injection. Twelve lead electrocardiograms (ECG) should be obtained prior to the bolus injection of ReoPro, and repeated once the patient has returned to the hospital ward from the catheterisation laboratory, and at 24 hours after the bolus injection of ReoPro. Vital signs (including blood pressure and pulse) should be obtained hourly for the first 4 hours following the ReoPro bolus injection, and then at 6, 12, 18 and 24 hours following the ReoPro bolus injection.

*Restoration of platelet function:* Transfusion of donor platelets has been shown to restore platelet function following ReoPro administration in animal studies and transfusions of fresh random donor platelets have been given empirically to restore platelet function in humans. In the event of serious uncontrolled bleeding or the need for surgery, a bleeding time should be determined by the Ivy method (see below). If the bleeding time is greater than 12 minutes, 10 units of platelets may be given. ReoPro may be displaced from endogenous platelet receptors and subsequently bind to platelets which have been transfused. Nevertheless, a single transfusion may be sufficient to reduce receptor blockade to 60% to 70% at which level platelet function is restored. Repeat platelet transfusions may be required to maintain the bleeding time at or below 12 minutes.

*Ivy method for determination of bleeding time:* Using an automated incision template, make a small incision on the lateral volar surface of the forearm while maintaining 40 mmHg pressure on the arm with a sphygmomanometer cuff. Determine the time for bleeding to stop with a stopwatch. Every 15 to 30 seconds a filter paper should be used to capture the blood from the incision but should not come in contact with the incision.

*Use of thrombolytics, anticoagulants and other anti-platelet agents:* Because ReoPro inhibits platelet aggregation, caution should be employed when used with other drugs affecting haemostasis such as heparin, oral anticoagulants such as warfarin, thrombolytics and antiplatelet agents other than aspirin, such as dipyridamole, ticlopidine or low molecular weight dextrans (see *Interactions with other medicaments and other forms of interaction*).

There are limited data on the use of ReoPro in patients receiving thrombolytic agents. However these data suggest an increase in the risk of bleeding when ReoPro is administered to patients treated with thrombolytics at doses sufficient to produce a systemic fibrinolytic state. If urgent intervention is required for refractory symptoms in a patient receiving ReoPro (or who has received the drug in the previous 48 hours), it is recommended that PTCA be attempted first to salvage the situation. Prior to further surgical interventions, the bleeding time should be determined by the Ivy method (see above) and should be 12 minutes or less. Should PTCA and any other appropriate procedures fail, and should the angiographic appearance suggest that the aetiology is due to thrombosis, consideration may be given to the administration of adjunctive thrombolytic therapy via the intracoronary route. A systemic fibrinolytic state should be avoided.

*Thrombocytopenia:* To reduce the possibility of thrombocytopenia, platelet counts should be monitored prior to treatment, 2 to 4 hours following the bolus dose of ReoPro and at 24 hours. If a patient experiences an acute platelet decrease, additional platelet counts should be determined. These platelet counts should be drawn in separate tubes containing ethylenediaminetetraacetic acid (EDTA), citrate and heparin to exclude pseudothrombocytopenia due to *in vitro* anticoagulant interaction. If true thrombocytopenia is verified, ReoPro should be immediately discontinued and the condition appropriately monitored and treated. A daily platelet count should be obtained until it returns to normal. If a patient's platelet count drops to 60,000 cells/μl, heparin and aspirin should be discontinued. If a patient's platelet count drops below 50,000 cells/μl, platelets should be transfused.

*Readministration:* There are no data concerning readministration of ReoPro. Therefore, readministration of ReoPro is not recommended. Human antichimeric antibodies (HACA) but not human anti-mouse antibodies (HAMA) have been observed after single administrations of ReoPro (see *Undesirable effects*). Available evidence suggests that human antibodies to other monoclonal antibodies do not cross–react with ReoPro. Nevertheless, the possibility of allergic or hypersensitivity reactions or diminished benefit cannot be excluded when ReoPro is administered to patients who have previously received monoclonal antibody therapy.

*Renal disease and peripheral vascular disease:* Benefits may be reduced in patients with renal disease or peripheral vascular disease.

*Children or age over 80 years:* Children or patients older than 80 years have not been studied.

*Interactions with other medicaments and other forms of interaction:* ReoPro has been formally studied as

an adjunct to heparin and aspirin treatment. In the presence of ReoPro, heparin is associated with an increase in the incidence of bleeding. Although there have been no formal studies of ReoPro with other commonly used cardiovascular drugs, in clinical studies there have been no adverse drug reactions associated with concomitant use of other medications used in the treatment of angina, myocardial infarction or hypertension nor with common intravenous infusion fluids. These medications have included warfarin (before and following but not during PTCA), beta–adrenergic receptor blockers, calcium channel antagonists, angiotensin converting enzyme (ACE) inhibitors, and intravenous and oral nitrates.

*Pregnancy and lactation:* Animal reproduction studies have not been conducted with ReoPro. It is also not known whether ReoPro can cause foetal harm when administered to a pregnant woman or can affect reproduction capacity. ReoPro should be given to a pregnant woman only if clearly needed.

Breast feeding of infants should be discontinued in nursing mothers since the secretion of abciximab in animal or human breast milk has not been studied.

*Effects on ability to drive and use machines:* Not applicable.

*Undesirable effects:* In the EPIC trial, the pivotal efficacy and safety trial of ReoPro, a non–weight-adjusted, standard heparin regimen was used. In the EPIC trial, the most common complication during ReoPro therapy was bleeding during the first 36 hours. The incidences of major bleeding (decrease in haemoglobin >5g/dL), minor bleeding (spontaneous gross haematuria or haematemesis, or observed blood loss with a haemoglobin decrease >3g/dL or with a decrease in haemoglobin ≥4g/dL with no observed blood loss) and transfusion of blood products were approximately doubled to 14%, 17% and 17%, respectively. However, the incidence of blood loss related to the performance of coronary artery bypass graft (CABG) surgery did not change. In patients who had major bleeding, 67% had bleeding associated with the arterial access site in the groin. Major, non-spontaneous retroperitoneal bleeding that was associated with the arterial access site occurred in 1.8% of ReoPro-patients compared to 0.3% of placebo-patients. There is no increase in the incidence of intracranial haemorrhage. Other major organ bleeding sites occurring in approximately 2% of patients treated with ReoPro were gastro-intestinal (spontaneous gross haematemesis) and genitourinary (spontaneous gross haematuria). Women over 65 years of age and low weight patients had the highest risk of bleeding events.

In a subsequent clinical trial, EPILOG, using the heparin regimen, sheath removal and femoral access care guidelines outlined in the section *Special warnings and special precautions for use*, the incidence of major bleeding in patients treated with ReoPro (1.8%) was not significantly different from patients receiving placebo (3.1%) and there was no significant increase in the incidence of intracranial haemorrhage. The reduction in major bleeding observed in the EPILOG trial was achieved without loss of efficacy.

Based on the EPIC trial experience, the most frequent adverse events are hypotension, nausea, vomiting, thrombocytopenia, haematoma, bradycardia, fever and vascular disorders. Human antichimeric antibody (HACA) appears, generally as a low titre, in approximately 6.5% of patients after 2 to 4 weeks. No hypersensitivity or allergic reactions have been observed following single treatments with ReoPro. Nevertheless, anaphylaxis may potentially occur at any time during administration (see Administration Instructions).

*Overdose:* There has been no experience of adverse events associated with overdosage. However, in the event of acute allergic reactions, thrombocytopenia or uncontrolled bleeding the administration of ReoPro should be immediately discontinued. In the event of thrombocytopenia or uncontrolled bleeding, platelet transfusion is recommended.

*Allergic reactions:* See Administration Instructions.

*Thrombocytopenia:* To reduce the possibility of thrombocytopenia, platelet counts should be monitored prior to treatment, 2 to 4 hours following the bolus dose of ReoPro and at 24 hours. If a patient experiences an acute platelet decrease, additional platelet counts should be determined. These platelet counts should be drawn in separate tubes containing ethylenediaminetetraacetic acid (EDTA), citrate and heparin to exclude pseudothrombocytopenia due to *in vitro* anticoagulant interaction. If true thrombocytopenia is verified, ReoPro should be immediately discontinued and the condition appropriately monitored and treated. A daily platelet count should be obtained until it returns to normal. If a patient's platelet count drops to 60,000 cells/μl, heparin and aspirin should be discontinued. If a patient's platelet count drops below 50,000 cells/μl, platelets should be transfused.

*Uncontrolled bleeding:* (Specific guidelines for access site bleeding are given above under *Bleeding Precautions, Femoral Artery Access Site*.) When considering the need to transfuse patients, the patient's intravascular volume should be assessed. If hypovolaemic, intravascular volume should be adequately restored with crystalloids. In asymptomatic patients, normovolaemic anaemia (haemoglobin 7–10 g/dL) can be well tolerated; transfusion is not indicated unless a deterioration in vital signs is seen or unless the patient develops signs and symptoms. In symptomatic patients (eg, syncope, dyspnoea, postural hypotension, tachycardia), crystalloids should be used to replace intravascular volume. If symptoms persist, the patient should receive transfusions with packed red blood cells or whole blood on a unit–by–unit basis to relieve symptoms; one unit may be sufficient. Transfusion of donor platelets has been shown to restore platelet function following ReoPro administration in animal studies and transfusions of fresh random donor platelets have been given empirically to restore platelet function in humans. In the event of serious uncontrolled bleeding or the need for surgery, a bleeding time should be determined by the Ivy method. If the bleeding time is greater than 12 minutes, 10 units of platelets may be given. ReoPro may be displaced from endogenous platelet receptors and subsequently bind to platelets which have been transfused. Nevertheless, a single transfusion may be sufficient to reduce receptor blockade to 60% to 70% at which level platelet function is restored. Repeat platelet transfusions may be required to maintain the bleeding time at or below 12 minutes.

## Pharmacological properties

*Pharmacodynamic properties:* ReoPro is the Fab fragment of the chimeric monoclonal antibody 7E3. It is directed against the glycoprotein IIb/IIIa (GPIIb/IIIa) receptor located on the surface of human platelets. ReoPro inhibits platelet aggregation by preventing the binding of fibrinogen, von Willebrand factor and other adhesive molecules to GPIIb/IIIa receptor sites on activated platelets.

Intravenous administration in humans of single bolus doses of ReoPro from 0.15 mg/kg to 0.30 mg/kg produced rapid dose-dependent inhibition of platelet function as measured by *ex vivo* platelet aggregation in response to adenosine diphosphate (ADP) or by prolongation of bleeding time. At the two highest doses (0.25 and 0.30 mg/kg) at 2 hours post injection, over 80% of the GPIIb/IIIa receptors were blocked and platelet aggregation in response to 20μM ADP was almost abolished. The median bleeding time increased to over 30 minutes at both doses compared with a baseline value of approximately 5 minutes. The 80% level of receptor blockade was selected as a target for pharmacological efficacy because animal models of severe coronary stenosis have shown that platelet inhibition associated with this degree of blockade prevents platelet thrombosis.

Intravenous administration in humans of a single bolus dose of 0.25 mg/kg followed by a continuous infusion of 10μg/min for periods of 12 to 96 hours produced sustained high–grade GPIIb/IIIa receptor blockade (≥80%) and inhibition of platelet function (*ex vivo* platelet aggregation in response to 20μm ADP less than 20% of baseline and bleeding time greater than 30 minutes) for the duration of the infusion in most patients. Results in patients who received the 0.25 mg/kg bolus followed by a 5μg/min infusion for 24 hours showed a similar initial receptor blockade and inhibition of platelet aggregation, but the response was not maintained throughout the infusion period. Although low levels of GPIIb/IIIa receptor blockade are present for up to 10 days following cessation of the infusion, platelet function typically returned to normal over a period of 24 to 48 hours.

*Pharmacokinetic properties:* Following intravenous bolus administration of ReoPro, free plasma concentrations decrease very rapidly with an initial half–life of less than 10 minutes and a second phase half-life of about 30 minutes, probably related to rapid binding to the platelet GPIIb/IIIa receptors. Platelet function generally recovers over the course of 48 hours, although ReoPro remains in the circulation for several days in a platelet-bound state. Intravenous administration of a 0.25 mg/kg bolus dose of ReoPro followed by continuous infusion of 10μg/min produces relatively constant free plasma concentrations throughout the infusion. At the termination of the infusion period, free plasma concentrations fall rapidly for approximately 6 hours then decline at a slower rate.

*Preclinical safety data:* No remarkable findings.

## Pharmaceutical particulars

*List of excipients:* ReoPro is formulated in a buffered aqueous solution (pH 7.2) containing sodium phosphate, dibasic, dihydrate; sodium phosphate, monobasic, monohydrate; sodium chloride and polysorbate 80. The total sodium content is approximately

3.45 mg/ml. Trace amounts of papain resulting from the production process may be present.

*Incompatibilities:* No incompatibilities have been shown with intravenous infusion fluids or commonly used cardiovascular drugs. Nevertheless, it is recommended that ReoPro be administered in a separate intravenous line whenever possible and not mixed with other medications.

No incompatibilities have been observed with polyvinyl chloride bags or administration sets.

*Shelf life:* Three (3) years at the recommended storage temperature.

ReoPro does not contain a preservative and is for single use only. Unused portions should be discarded. When intended for use by intravenous infusion, ReoPro should be used promptly after dilution.

*Special precautions for storage:* ReoPro should be stored at 2°C to 8°C. Do not freeze.

*Nature and contents of container:* ReoPro is supplied in either 5 ml (10 mg) or 20 ml (40 mg) glass vials with rubber stoppers and aluminium crimps protected by a plastic cap.

*Instructions for use/handling:* Do not shake vials. For administration instructions see *Posology and method of administration* section above.

*Marketing authorisation holder:* Centocor BV, Einsteinweg 101, 2333 CB Leiden, The Netherlands.

**Marketing authorisation number**   8563/0015

**Legal category**   POM

**Package quantities**   5 ml glass vials – single vials.

## VANCOCIN* CP INJECTION

**Presentation**   Rubber-stoppered 10 ml vials each containing chromatographically purified vancomycin hydrochloride, 250,000 iu or 500,000 iu, equivalent to 250 mg or 500 mg vancomycin, respectively, as an off-white lyophilised plug. Rubber-stoppered 20 ml vials containing chromatographically purified vancomycin hydrochloride, 1,000,000 iu, equivalent to 1 g vancomycin, as an off–white lyophilised plug. When reconstituted in water, it forms a clear solution with a pH range of 2.8 to 4.5.

**Uses**   Vancomycin is a glycopeptide antibiotic derived from *Nocardia orientalis* (formerly *Streptomyces orientalis*), and is active against many Gram-positive bacteria including *Staphylococcus aureus*, *Staph. epidermidis*, alpha and beta haemolytic streptococci, group D streptococci, corynebacteria and clostridia.

Vancomycin is indicated in potentially life-threatening infections which cannot be treated with other effective, less toxic antimicrobial drugs, including the penicillins and cephalosporins.

Vancomycin is useful in the therapy of severe staphylococcal infections in patients who cannot receive or who have failed to respond to the penicillins and cephalosporins, or who have infections with staphylococci resistant to other antibiotics.

Vancomycin is used in the treatment of endocarditis and as prophylaxis against endocarditis in patients at risk from dental or surgical procedures.

Its effectiveness has been documented in other infections due to staphylococci, including osteomyelitis, pneumonia, septicaemia and soft tissue infections.

Vancomycin may be used orally for the treatment of staphylococcal enterocolitis and pseudomembranous colitis due to *Clostridium difficile*. Parenteral administration of vancomycin is not effective for these indications.

Vancomycin is not significantly absorbed from the normal gastro–intestinal tract and is therefore not effective by the oral route for other types of infection. Intravenous administration may be used concomitantly if required.

**Dosage and administration**   For intravenous infusion and oral use only and not for intramuscular administration.

Infusion-related adverse events are related to both concentration and rate of administration of vancomycin. Concentrations of no more than 5 mg/ml are recommended. In selected patients in need of fluid restriction, a concentration up to 10 mg/ml may be used; use of such higher concentrations may increase the risk of infusion–related events. Infusions should be given over at least 60 minutes. In adults, if doses exceeding 500 mg are used, a rate of infusion of no more than 10 mg/min is recommended. Infusion-related events may occur, however, at any rate or concentration.

*Intravenous Infusion in patients with normal renal function*
*Adults:* The usual intravenous dose is 500 mg every six hours or 1 g every 12 hours, in Sodium Chloride Intravenous Infusion BP or 5% Dextrose Intravenous Infusion BP. Each dose should be administered at no

more than 10 mg/min. Other patient factors, such as age, obesity or pregnancy, may call for modification of the usual daily dose. The majority of patients with infections caused by organisms sensitive to the antibiotic show a therapeutic response within 48–72 hours. The total duration of therapy is determined by the type and severity of the infection and the clinical response of the patient. In staphylococcal endocarditis, treatment for three weeks or longer is recommended.

*Pregnancy:* It has been reported that significantly increased doses may be required to achieve therapeutic serum concentrations in pregnant patients, but see *Warnings*.

*The elderly:* Dosage reduction may be necessary to a greater extent than expected because of decreasing renal function (see below). Monitor auditory function – see *Warnings* and *Precautions*.

*Children:* The usual intravenous dosage is 10 mg/kg per dose given every 6 hours (total daily dosage 40 mg/kg of body weight). Each dose should be administered over a period of at least 60 minutes.

In neonates and young infants, the total daily dosage may be lower. An initial dose of 15 mg/kg is suggested, followed by 10 mg/kg every 12 hours in the first week of life and every 8 hours thereafter until one month of age. Each dose should be administered over 60 minutes. Close monitoring of serum vancomycin concentrations may be warranted in these patients.

*Patients with impaired renal function:* Dosage adjustments must be made to avoid toxic serum levels. In premature infants and the elderly, greater dosage reductions than expected may be necessary because of decreased renal function. Regular monitoring of serum levels is advised in such patients, as accumulation has been reported, especially after prolonged therapy. Vancomycin serum concentrations may be determined by use of a microbiological assay, radioimmunoassay, fluorescence polarisation immunoassay, fluorescence immunoassay or high-pressure liquid chromatography. The following nomogram, based on creatinine clearance values, is provided.

The nomogram is not valid for functionally anephric patients on dialysis. For such patients, a loading dose of 15 mg/kg body weight should be given to achieve therapeutic serum levels promptly, and the dose required to maintain stable levels is 1.9 mg/kg/24 hours. Since individual maintenance doses of 250 mg to 1 g are convenient, in patients with marked renal impairment a dose may be given every several days rather than on a daily basis. In anuria a dose of 1 g every 7 to 10 days has been recommended.

*Measurement of serum concentrations:* Following multiple intravenous doses, peak serum concentrations, measured 2 hours after infusion is complete, range from 18–26 mg/l. Trough levels measured immediately prior to the next dose should be 5–10 mg/l. Ototoxicity has been associated with serum drug levels of 80–100 mg/l, but this is rarely seen when serum levels are kept at or below 30 mg/l.

*Preparation of solution:* At the time of use, add 5 ml of Water for Injections PhEur to the 250 mg vial, 10 ml of Water for Injections PhEur to the 500 mg vial, or 20 ml Water for Injections PhEur to the 1 g vial. Vials reconstituted in this manner will give a solution of 50 mg/ml.

FURTHER DILUTION IS REQUIRED. Read instructions which follow:

1. *Intermittent infusion* is the preferred method of administration. Reconstituted solutions containing 250 mg vancomycin must be diluted with at least 50 ml of diluent. Reconstituted solutions containing 500 mg vancomycin must be diluted with at least 100 ml diluent. Reconstituted solutions containing 1 g vancomycin must be diluted with at least 200 ml diluent. Sodium Chloride Intravenous Infusion BP or 5% Dextrose Intravenous Infusion BP are suitable diluents. The desired dose should be given by intravenous infusion over a period of at least 60 minutes. If administered over a shorter period of time or

in higher concentrations, there is the possibility of inducing marked hypotension in addition to thrombophlebitis. Rapid administration may also produce flushing and a transient rash over the neck and shoulders.

2. *Continuous infusion* (should be used only when intermittent infusion is not feasible). 1–2 g can be added to a sufficiently large volume of Sodium Chloride Intravenous Infusion BP or 5% Dextrose Intravenous Infusion BP to permit the desired daily dose to be administered slowly by intravenous drip over a 24–hour period.

*Oral administration:* The contents of vials for parenteral administration may be used.

*Adults and the elderly:* The usual daily dose given is 500 mg in divided doses for 7 to 10 days, although up to 2 g/day have been used in severe cases. The total daily dosage should not exceed 2 g. Each dose may be reconstituted in 30 ml water and either given to the patient to drink, or administered by nasogastric tube.

*Children:* The usual daily dose is 40 mg/kg in three or four divided doses for 7 to 10 days. The total daily dosage should not exceed 2 g.

Common flavouring syrups may be added to the solution at the time of administration to improve the taste.

Capsules are also available.

**Contra-indications, warnings, etc**
*Contra-indication:* Hypersensitivity to vancomycin.

*Warnings:* Rapid bolus administration (e.g. over several minutes) may be associated with exaggerated hypotension, including shock, and, rarely, cardiac arrest. Vancomycin should be infused in a dilute solution over a period of not less than 60 minutes to avoid rapid infusion–related reactions. Stopping the infusion usually results in a prompt cessation of these reactions (see *Dosage and administration* and *Side-effects* sections).

Some patients with inflammatory disorders of the intestinal mucosa may have significant systemic absorbtion of oral vancomycin and, therefore, may be at risk for the development of adverse reactions associated with the parenteral administration of vancomycin. The risk is greater in patients with renal impairment. It should be noted that the total systemic and renal clearances of vancomycin are reduced in the elderly.

Due to its potential ototoxicity and nephrotoxicity, vancomycin should be used with care in patients with renal insufficiency and the dose should be reduced according to the degree of renal impairment. The risk of toxicity is appreciably increased by high blood concentrations or prolonged therapy. Blood levels should be monitored and renal function tests should be performed regularly.

Vancomycin should also be avoided in patients with previous hearing loss. If it is used in such patients, the dose should be regulated, if possible, by periodic determination of the drug level in the blood. Deafness may be preceded by tinnitus. The elderly are more susceptible to auditory damage. Experience with other antibiotics suggests that deafness may be progressive despite cessation of treatment.

There have been reports that the frequency of infusion–related events increases with the concomitant administration of anaesthetic agents. Infusion-related events may be minimised by the administration of vancomycin as a 60-minute infusion prior to anaesthetic induction.

Concurrent or sequential systemic or topical use of other potentially neurotoxic or nephrotoxic drugs, such as amphotericin B, aminoglycosides, bacitracin, polymixin B, colistin, viomycin or cisplatin, when indicated, requires careful monitoring.

*Drug interaction:* Concomitant administration of vancomycin and anaesthetic agents has been associated with erythema, histamine–like flushing and anaphylactoid reactions.

Vancomycin solution has a low pH that may cause chemical or physical instability when it is mixed with other compounds.

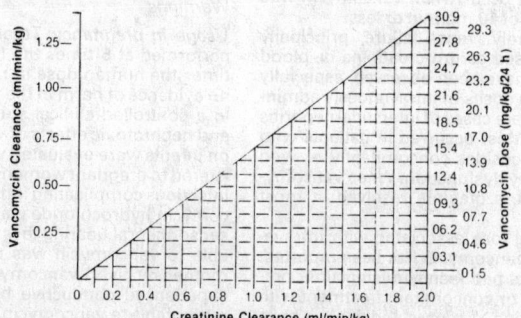

Dosage Nomogram for Vancomycin in Patients with Impaired Renal Function

*Usage in pregnancy:* Teratology studies have been performed at 5 times the human dose in rats and 3 times the human dose in rabbits, and have revealed no evidence of harm to the foetus due to vancomycin. In a controlled clinical study, the potential ototoxic and nephrotoxic effects of vancomycin hydrochloride on infants were evaluated when the drug was administered to pregnant women for serious staphylococcal infections complicating intravenous drug abuse. Vancomycin hydrochloride was found in cord blood. No sensorineural hearing loss or nephrotoxicity attributable to vancomycin was noted. One infant, whose mother received vancomycin in the third trimester, experienced conductive hearing loss that was not attributable to vancomycin. Because vancomycin was administered only in the second and third trimesters, it is not known whether it causes foetal harm. Vancomycin should be given in pregnancy only if clearly needed and blood levels should be monitored carefully to minimise the risk of foetal toxicity. It has been reported, however, that pregnant patients may require significantly increased doses of vancomycin to achieve therapeutic serum concentrations.

*Usage in nursing mothers:* Vancomycin hydrochloride is excreted in human milk. Caution should be exercised when vancomycin is administered to a nursing woman. It is unlikely that a nursing infant can absorb a significant amount of vancomycin from its gastrointestinal tract.

*Usage in paediatrics:* In premature neonates and young infants, it may be appropriate to confirm desired vancomycin serum concentrations. Concomitant administration of vancomycin and anaesthetic agents has been associated with erythema and histamine-like flushing in children.

*Usage in the elderly:* The natural decrement of glomerular filtration with increasing age may lead to elevated vancomycin serum concentrations if dosage is not adjusted (see *Dosage and administration*).

*Precautions:* Clinically significant serum concentrations have been reported in some patients being treated for active *C. difficile*-induced pseudomembranous colitis after multiple oral doses of vancomycin. Therefore, monitoring of serum concentrations may be appropriate in these patients.

Patients with borderline renal function and individuals over the age of 60 should be given serial tests of auditory function and of vancomycin blood levels. All patients receiving the drug should have periodic haematological studies, urine analysis and renal function tests.

Vancomycin is very irritating to tissue, and causes necrosis when injected intramuscularly; it must be infused intravenously. Pain and thrombophlebitis occur in many patients receiving vancomycin and are occasionally severe.

The frequency and severity of thrombophlebitis can be minimised by administering the drug slowly as a dilute solution (2.5 to 5.0 g/l) and by rotating the sites of infusion.

Prolonged use of vancomycin may result in the overgrowth of non-susceptible organisms. Careful observation of the patient is essential. If superinfection occurs during therapy, appropriate measures should be taken. In rare instances, there have been reports of pseudomembranous colitis, due to *C. difficile*, developing in patients who received intravenous vancomycin.

*Side-effects*

*Infusion-related events:* During or soon after rapid infusion of vancomycin, patients may develop anaphylactoid reactions including hypotension, wheezing, dyspnoea, urticaria or pruritus. Rapid infusion may also cause flushing of the upper–body ('red-neck syndrome') or pain and muscle spasm of the chest and back. These reactions usually resolve within 20 minutes but may persist for several hours. In animal studies, hypotension and bradycardia occurred in animals given large doses of vancomycin at high concentrations and rates. Such events are infrequent if vancomycin is given by slow infusion over 60 minutes. In studies of normal volunteers, infusion-related events did not occur when vancomycin was administered at a rate of 10 mg/min or less.

*Nephrotoxicity:* Rarely, renal failure, principally manifested by increased serum creatinine or blood urea concentrations, have been observed, especially in patients given large doses of intravenously administered vancomycin. Rare cases of interstitial nephritis have been reported. Most occurred in patients who were given aminoglycosides concomitantly or who had pre-existing kidney dysfunction. When vancomycin was discontinued, azotaemia resolved in most patients.

*Ototoxicity:* Hearing loss associated with intravenously administered vancomycin has been reported. Most of these patients had kidney dysfunction, pre-existing hearing loss, or concomitant treatment with an ototoxic drug. Vertigo, dizziness and tinnitus have been reported rarely.

*Haematological:* Reversible neutropenia, usually starting one week or more after onset of intravenous therapy or after a total dose of more than 25 g. Neutropenia appears to be promptly reversible when vancomycin is discontinued. Thrombocytopenia has rarely been reported. Reversible agranulocytosis (less than 500 granulocytes per mm³) has been reported rarely, although causality has not been established.

*Miscellaneous:* Phlebitis, hypersensitivity reactions, anaphylaxis, nausea, chills, drug fever, eosinophilia, rashes (including exfoliative dermatitis), Stevens-Johnson syndrome, toxic epidermal necrolysis and rare cases of vasculitis.

*Overdosage:* Supportive care is advised, with maintenance of glomerular filtration.

Vancomycin is poorly removed from the blood by haemodialysis or peritoneal dialysis. Haemoperfusion with Amberlite resin XAD–4 has been reported to be of limited benefit.

**Pharmaceutical precautions** Store below 25°C.

*After reconstitution:* May be stored in a refrigerator (2°–8°C) for 24 hours.

Prior to administration, parenteral drug products should be inspected visually for particulate matter and discolouration whenever solution or container permits.

Solutions of the parenteral powder intended for oral administration may be stored in a refrigerator (2°–8°C) for 96 hours.

**Legal category** POM.

**Package quantities**
Vials 250 mg (250,000 iu vancomycin): Single vials
Vials 500 mg (500,000 iu vancomycin): Single vials
Vials 1 g (1,000,000 iu vancomycin): Single vials

**Further information** Nil.

**Product licence number** 0006/5076.

# VANCOCIN* MATRIGEL CAPSULES

**Presentation** Matrigel capsules (dark blue and grey, coded Lilly 3126) containing chromatographically purified vancomycin hydrochloride, equivalent to 250 mg vancomycin base. Matrigel capsules (dark blue and peach, coded Lilly 3125) containing chromatographically purified vancomycin hydrochloride, equivalent to 125 mg vancomycin base.

This preparation is for oral use only. If parenteral vancomycin therapy is desired, use Vancocin CP Injection (Sterile Vancomycin Hydrochloride BP) and consult literature accompanying that preparation.

**Uses** Vancomycin may be used orally for the treatment of staphylococcal enterocolitis and pseudomembranous colitis due to *Clostridium difficile*.

Vancomycin is not significantly absorbed from the normal gastro–intestinal tract and is therefore not effective by the oral route for other types of infection. Intravenous administration may be used concomitantly if required.

**Dosage and administration** For oral administration. Either the Matrigel capsules or the contents of the 500 mg vial for parenteral administration may be used.

*Adults and the elderly:* The usual daily dose is 500 mg in divided doses for 7 to 10 days, although up to 2 g/day, in three or four divided doses, have been used in severe cases. The total daily dosage should not exceed 2 g.

*Children:* The usual daily dose is 40 mg/kg in three or four divided doses for 7 to 10 days. The total daily dosage should not exceed 2 g.

*Oral solution:* The contents of the 500 mg vial for parenteral administration may be used and either given to the patient to drink, or administered by nasogastric tube. Mix thoroughly to dissolve. Common flavouring syrups may be added to the solution at the time of administration to improve the taste.

**Contra-indications, warnings, etc**
*Contra-indication:* Hypersensitivity to vancomycin.

*Warnings*

*Usage in pregnancy:* Teratology studies have been performed at 5 times the human dose in rats and 3 times the human dose in rabbits, and have revealed no evidence of harm to the foetus due to vancomycin. In a controlled clinical study, the potential ototoxic and nephrotoxic effects of vancomycin hydrochloride on infants were evaluated when the drug was administered to pregnant women for serious staphylococcal infections complicating intravenous drug abuse. Vancomycin hydrochloride was found in cord blood. No sensorineural hearing loss or nephrotoxicity attributable to vancomycin was noted. One infant, whose mother received vancomycin in the third trimester, experienced conductive hearing loss that was not attributable to vancomycin. Because vancomycin was administered only in the second and third trimesters,

it is not known whether it causes foetal harm. Therefore vancomycin should be given to a pregnant woman only if clearly needed.

*Usage in nursing mothers:* Vancomycin hydrochloride is excreted in human milk. Caution should be exercised when vancomycin is administered to a nursing woman.

*Precautions:* Clinically significant serum concentrations have been reported in some patients who have taken multiple oral doses of vancomycin for active *C. difficile*-induced pseudomembranous colitis. Therefore, monitoring of serum concentrations may be appropriate in these patients.

Some patients with inflammatory disorders of the intestinal mucosa may have significant systemic absorption of vancomycin and, therefore, may be at risk for the development of adverse reactions associated with the parenteral administration of vancomycin (see package insert accompanying the intravenous preparation). The risk is greater in patients with renal impairment. It should be noted that the total systemic and renal clearances of vancomycin are reduced in the elderly.

Ototoxicity has occurred in patients receiving vancomycin. It may be transient or permanent. It has been reported mostly in patients who have been given excessive intravenous doses, have an underlying hearing loss, or are receiving concomitant therapy with an ototoxic agent such as an aminoglycoside. Serial tests of auditory function may be helpful in order to minimise the risk of ototoxicity.

When treating patients with underlying renal dysfunction or patients receiving concomitant therapy with an aminoglycoside, serial monitoring of renal function should be performed.

Prolonged use of vancomycin may result in the overgrowth of non-susceptible organisms. Careful observation of the patient is essential. If superinfection occurs during therapy, appropriate measures should be taken.

*Side-effects:* Since vancomycin is not usually significantly absorbed from the gastro-intestinal tract, the toxicity encountered with parenteral therapy is unlikely to occur after oral administration (but see 'Precautions').

*Nephrotoxicity:* Rarely, renal failure, principally manifested by increased serum creatinine or blood urea concentrations, have been observed, especially in patients given large doses of intravenously administered vancomycin. Rare cases of interstitial nephritis have been reported. Most occurred in patients who were given aminoglycosides concomitantly or who had pre-existing kidney dysfunction. When vancomycin was discontinued, azotaemia resolved in most patients.

*Ototoxicity:* Hearing loss associated with *intravenously* administered vancomycin has been reported. Most of these patients had kidney dysfunction, pre-existing hearing loss, or concomitant treatment with an ototoxic drug. Vertigo, dizziness and tinnitus have been reported rarely.

*Haematological:* Reversible neutropenia, usually starting one week or more after onset of *intravenous* therapy or after a total dose of more than 25 g. Neutropenia appears to be promptly reversible when vancomycin is discontinued. Thrombocytopenia and reversible agranulocytosis (granulocyte count less than 500/mm³) have been reported rarely.

*Miscellaneous:* Hypersensitivity reactions, anaphylaxis, chills, drug fever, eosinophilia, hypotension, wheezing, dyspnoea, urticaria, pruritus, flushing of the upper body ('red-neck syndrome'), pain, muscle spasm of the chest and back, nausea and rashes, including exfoliative dermatitis, Stevens-Johnson syndrome, toxic epidermal necrolysis and rare cases of vasculitis.

*Treatment of overdosage:* Supportive care is advised, with maintenance of glomerular filtration. Vancomycin is poorly removed by dialysis. Haemofiltration and haemoperfusion with Amberlite resin XAD–4 have been reported to be of limited benefit.

**Pharmaceutical precautions** Protect from moisture. Store below 25°C.

After reconstitution, solutions of the parenteral powder intended for oral administration may be stored in a refrigerator (2°–8°C) for 96 hours.

**Legal category** POM.

**Package quantity** Blister packs of 20 (2 strips of 10 capsules).

**Further information** The bitter taste of vancomycin can be avoided by the use of the Matrigel capsules. Vancomycin powder should be used when the patient is unable to swallow the capsules.

**Product licence numbers**
Matrigel Capsules 125 mg: 0006/0193
Matrigel Capsules 250 mg: 0006/0194

## VELBE*

WARNING
THIS PRODUCT IS **NOT**
FOR INTRATHECAL USE

**Presentation** Vials containing 10 mg Velbe (Vinblastine Sulphate BP) in the form of a lyophilised plug.

Velbe is supplied in a combination package with an accompanying vial of diluting solution, 10 ml containing 90 mg Sodium Chloride PhEur, with 2% Benzyl Alcohol BP as a preservative.

**Uses** Velbe is an anti-neoplastic drug for intravenous use.

Information available at present suggests that Velbe may be useful, either alone or in combination with other oncolytic drugs for the treatment of: Hodgkin's disease; non-Hodgkin's lymphoma; carcinoma of the breast; methotrexate-resistant choriocarcinoma; renal cell carcinoma; testicular teratoma and seminoma; histiocytosis X.

Other neoplasms occasionally show a marked response to Velbe, but less frequently than the more susceptible conditions listed above.

**Dosage and administration** This preparation is for intravenous use only. It should be administered only by individuals experienced in vinblastine administration.

Fatal if given intrathecally (see 'Warnings' for treatment).

The recommended dose for adults, the elderly and children is 6 mg/m² usually administered no more frequently than once every seven days. For testicular tumours, the dosage may be increased to 0.2 mg/kg administered on each of two consecutive days every three weeks.

As vinblastine is excreted principally by the liver, toxicity may be increased when there is hepatic insufficiency and it may be necessary to reduce initial doses in the presence of significantly impaired hepatic or biliary function. A reduction of 50% in the dose is recommended for patients having a direct serum bilirubin value above 3 mg/100 ml. Since metabolism and excretion are primarily hepatic, no modification is recommended for patients with impaired renal function.

The metabolism of vinca alkaloids has been shown to be mediated by hepatic cytochrome P450 isoenzymes in the CYP 3A subfamily. This metabolic pathway may be impaired in patients with hepatic dysfunction or who are taking concomitant potent inhibitors of these isoenzymes. (See *Precautions*.)

To prepare a solution containing 1 mg/ml, add 10 ml of the accompanying diluting solution to the 10 mg vial. The drug dissolves rapidly to give a clear solution.

The dose of Velbe solution may be injected either into the tubing of a running intravenous infusion of sodium chloride 0.9% or directly into a vein. In either case, the injection should be completed in about one minute. If care is taken to ensure that the needle is securely within the vein and that no solution containing vinblastine is spilled extravascularly, cellulitis and/or phlebitis will not occur.

To minimise further the possibility of extravascular spillage, it is suggested that the syringe and needle be rinsed with venous blood before withdrawal. The dose should not be diluted in large volumes of diluent (i.e. 100 to 250 ml) or given intravenously for prolonged periods (ranging from 30 to 60 minutes or more), since this frequently results in irritation of the vein and increases the chance of extravasation.

Because of the enhanced possibility of thrombosis, it is considered inadvisable to inject a solution of Velbe into an extremity in which the circulation is impaired, or potentially impaired, by such conditions as compressing or invading neoplasm, phlebitis or varicosity.

*Caution:* If leakage into surrounding tissue should occur during intravenous administration of vinblastine, it may cause considerable irritation. The injection should be discontinued immediately, and any remaining portion of the dose should then be introduced into another vein. Local injection of hyaluronidase and the application of moderate heat to the area of leakage help disperse the drug and are thought to minimise discomfort and the possibility of cellulitis.

**Contra-indications, warnings, etc**
*Contra-indications*

Intrathecal administration has resulted in death
(see 'Warnings' for treatment).

Vinblastine is contra-indicated in patients who are leucopenic unless this is the result of the disease being treated. It should not be used in the presence of bacterial infection. Such infections must be brought under control with antiseptics or antibiotics before using vinblastine.

*Warnings:* Syringes containing this product should be labelled 'FATAL IF GIVEN INTRATHECALLY. FOR INTRAVENOUS USE ONLY'. An auxiliary sticker is provided in the pack with this warning.

Extemporaneously prepared syringes containing this product must be packaged in an overwrap which is labelled 'DO NOT REMOVE COVERING UNTIL MOMENT OF INJECTION. FATAL IF GIVEN INTRATHECALLY. FOR INTRAVENOUS USE ONLY'.

The following treatment successfully arrested progressive paralysis in a single patient mistakenly given the related vinca alkaloid, vincristine sulphate, intrathecally. This treatment should be initiated immediately after the intrathecal injection:

1. Removal of as much CSF as is safely possible.
2. Flushing with Lactated Ringer's solution by continuous infusion at 150 ml/h, through a catheter in a cerebral lateral ventricle and removed through lumbar access, until fresh frozen plasma became available.
3. Fresh frozen plasma, 25 ml, diluted with 1l of Lactated Ringer's was then infused similarly at 75 ml/h. The rate of infusion should be adjusted to maintain a spinal fluid protein level of 150 mg/dl.
4. Glutamic acid, 10 gm, was given i.v. over 24 hours, followed by 500 mg t.d.s. by mouth for 1 month. Glutamic acid may not be essential.

*Usage in pregnancy:* Caution is necessary with the use of all oncolytic drugs during pregnancy. Information on the use of vinblastine during human pregnancy is very limited but vinblastine can cause foetal harm when administered to a pregnant woman. There are no adequate and well-controlled studies in pregnant women. Animal studies with vinblastine suggest that teratogenic effects may occur. Laboratory animals given this drug early in pregnancy suffer resorption of the conceptus; surviving foetuses demonstrate gross deformities.

Women of childbearing potential should be advised to avoid becoming pregnant while receiving vinblastine. If Velbe is used during pregnancy or if the patient becomes pregnant while receiving this drug she should be informed of the potential hazard to the foetus.

*Usage in nursing mothers:* It is not known whether vinblastine is excreted in human milk. Because of the potential for serious adverse reactions due to Velbe in nursing infants, a decision should be made whether to discontinue nursing or the drug taking into account the importance of the drug to the mother.

Aspermia has been reported in men. Animal studies show metaphase arrest and degenerative changes in germ cells. Amenorrhoea has occurred in some patients treated with vinblastine in combination with other drugs. Recovery of menses was frequent.

Stomatitis and neurological toxicity, although not common or permanent, can be disabling.

*Precautions:* The dose–limiting factor is myelosuppression. Effective therapy with vinblastine is more likely to be followed by leucopenia than is the case with Oncovin (vincristine sulphate).

In general, the larger the dose employed, the more profound and longer lasting the leucopenia will be. The fact that the granulocyte count returns to normal levels after drug-induced leucopenia is an indication that the granulocyte–producing mechanism is not permanently depressed.

Following therapy with vinblastine, the nadir in the granulocyte count may be expected to occur five to ten days after the last day of drug administration. Recovery of the granulocyte count is fairly rapid thereafter and is usually complete within another seven to fourteen days.

If granulocytopenia with less than 1,000 granulocytes/mm³ occurs following a dose of vinblastine, the patient should be watched carefully for evidence of infection until the granulocyte count has returned to a safe level. Any infection must be brought under control immediately.

When cachexia or ulcerated areas of the skin surface are present, there may be a more profound granulocytopenic response to the drug; therefore, its use should be avoided in older persons suffering from either of these conditions.

Although the thrombocyte count is not usually significantly lowered by therapy with vinblastine, patients whose bone marrow has been recently impaired by prior therapy with radiation or with other oncolytic drugs may show thrombocytopenia (less than 150,000 platelets/mm³). When other chemotherapy or radiation has not been employed previously, thrombocyte reduction below the level of 150,000/mm³ is rarely encountered, even when vinblastine may be causing significant granulocytopenia. Rapid recovery from thrombocytopenia within a few days is the rule.

The effect of vinblastine upon the red blood cell count and haemoglobin is usually insignificant when other treatment does not complicate the picture.

In patients with malignant-cell infiltration of the bone marrow, the granulocyte and platelet counts have sometimes fallen drastically after moderate doses of vinblastine. Further use of the drug in such patients is inadvisable.

When chemotherapy is being given in conjunction with radiation therapy through portals which include the liver, the use of vinblastine should be delayed until radiation therapy has been completed.

Acute shortness of breath and severe bronchospasm have been reported following the administration of the vinca alkaloids. These reactions have been encountered most frequently when the vinca alkaloid was used in combination with mitomycin-C and may be serious when there is pre-existing pulmonary dysfunction. The onset may be within minutes, or several hours after the vinca is injected, and may occur up to 2 weeks following a dose of mitomycin. Progressive dyspnoea, requiring chronic therapy, may occur. Vinblastine should not be readministered.

The simultaneous oral or intravenous administration of phenytoin and anti-neoplastic chemotherapy combinations, that included vinblastine sulphate, have been reported to reduce blood levels of the anticonvulsant and to increase seizure activity. Although the contribution of the vinca alkaloids has not been established, dosage adjustment of phenytoin, based on serial blood level monitoring, may need to be made when it is used in combination with vinblastine.

Caution should be exercised in patients concurrently taking drugs known to inhibit drug metabolism by hepatic cytochrome P450 isoenzymes in the CYP 3A subfamily, or in patients with hepatic dysfunction. Concurrent administration of vinblastine sulphate with an inhibitor of this metabolic pathway may cause an earlier onset and/or an increased severity of side-effects.

Care must be taken to avoid contamination of the eye with concentrations of Velbe used clinically. If accidental contamination occurs, severe irritation (or, if the drug was delivered under pressure, even corneal ulceration) may result. The eye should be washed with water immediately and thoroughly.

Sperm abnormalities have been noted in mice. Additional studies in mice demonstrated no reduction in fertility of males. Breaks and aberrations were not observed on chromosome analysis of marrow cells from patients treated with vinblastine although chromosomal changes have been noted in some hamster lung cell *in vitro* tests.

There is no currently available evidence to indicate that vinblastine itself has been carcinogenic in humans although some patients have developed leukaemia following radiation therapy and the administration of vinblastine in combination with alkylating agents.

*Adverse reactions:* Leucopenia is the most common adverse reaction and is usually the dose-limiting factor.

In general, the incidence of side-effects attending the use of Velbe appears to be related to the size of dosage employed. Symptoms commonly encountered when high doses are employed include constipation, abdominal pain, ileus and myalgia.

The use of small amounts of vinblastine daily for long periods is not advisable, even though the resulting total dosage may be similar to the recommended dosage. Little or no therapeutic advantage has been demonstrated when such regimens have been used and side-effects are increased.

The constipation which may be encountered responds well to such usual measures as enemas and laxatives. Constipation may take the form of upper colon impaction and the rectum may be found to be empty on physical examination. A flat film of the abdomen is useful in demonstrating this condition. A routine prophylactic regimen against constipation is recommended for patients receiving high doses of vinblastine.

The following symptoms may occur after usual doses of vinblastine:

*Haematological:* Leucopenia, thrombocytopenia, anaemia.

*Gastro-intestinal:* Nausea, vomiting, constipation, ileus, diarrhoea, anorexia, abdominal pain, rectal bleeding, pharyngitis, haemorrhagic enterocolitis, bleeding from an old peptic ulcer.

*Neurological:* Numbness, paraesthesiae, peripheral neuritis, mental depression, loss of deep tendon reflexes, headache, convulsions. Treatment with vinca alkaloids has resulted rarely in both vestibular and auditory damage to the eighth cranial nerve. Manifestations include partial or total deafness, which may be temporary or permanent, and difficulties with balance, including dizziness, nystagmus and vertigo. Particular caution is warranted when vinblastine sulphate is used in combination with other agents known to be ototoxic, such as the platinum-containing oncolytics.

*Pulmonary:* See under 'Precautions'.

*Cutaneous:* Stomatitis, ulceration of the skin and

alopecia. When alopecia develops it is frequently not total and, in some cases, hair regrows while maintenance therapy continues.

*Cardiovascular:* Hypertension. Cases of unexpected myocardial infarction and cerebrovascular accidents have occurred in patients undergoing combination chemotherapy with vinblastine, bleomycin and cisplatin.

*Miscellaneous:* Malaise, weakness, dizziness, bone pain, jaw pain, and pain in tumour-containing tissue. Injection site reaction (see *Dosage and administration – Caution*). Syndrome of inappropriate ADH secretion has been reported with higher than recommended doses. Raynaud's phenomenon has occurred when patients are being treated with vinblastine in combination with bleomycin and cisplatin for testicular cancer.

*Overdosage:* Side-effects following the use of vinblastine are dose related. Therefore, following administration of more than the recommended dose, patients can be expected to experience these effects in an exaggerated fashion. Any dose that results in elimination of platelets and neutrophils from blood and marrow and their precursors from marrow is life-threatening.

Overdoses occurring during prolonged, consecutive day infusions may be more toxic than the same total dose given by rapid i.v. injection.

In addition, neurotoxicity similar to that seen with Oncovin (vincristine sulphate) may be observed.

Supportive care should include: (a) prevention of the side-effects that result from the syndrome of inappropriate secretion of antidiuretic hormone. This includes restriction of fluid intake and perhaps the use of a diuretic acting on the loop of Henle and distal tubule function; (b) administration of an anticonvulsant; (c) prevention and treatment of ileus; (d) monitoring the patient's cardiovascular system; (e) daily blood counts for guidance in transfusion requirement and assessing the risk of infection.

The major effect of excessive doses of vinblastine will be on granulocytopoiesis, and this may be life-threatening.

There is no specific antidote. The use of folinic acid in addition to the other supportive measures recommended may be considered although, unlike vincristine, studies have not been conducted to confirm its protective action.

There is no information regarding the effectiveness of dialysis nor of cholestyramine for the treatment of overdosage.

Vinblastine in the dry state is irregularly and unpredictably absorbed from the gastro-intestinal tract following oral administration. Absorption of the solution has not been studied. If vinblastine is swallowed, activated charcoal in a water slurry may be given by mouth along with a cathartic. The use of cholestyramine in this situation has not been reported.

**Pharmaceutical precautions**

*Special dispensing information:* When dispensing vinblastine sulphate in other than the original container, it is imperative that it be packaged in an overwrap bearing the statement 'DO NOT REMOVE COVERING UNTIL MOMENT OF INJECTION. FATAL IF GIVEN INTRATHECALLY. FOR INTRAVENOUS USE ONLY'. A syringe containing a specific dose must be labelled, using the auxiliary sticker provided in the pack, with this warning.

*Guidelines for the safe handling of antineoplastic agents:* Cytotoxic preparations should not be handled by pregnant staff.

Trained personnel should reconstitute and administer the drug. This should be performed in a designated area. The work surface should be covered with disposable plastic-backed absorbent paper.

Adequate protective gloves, masks and clothing should be worn. Precautions should be taken to avoid the drug accidentally coming into contact with the eyes. If accidental contamination occurs, the eye should be washed with water thoroughly and immediately.

Use Luer-lock fittings on all syringes and sets. Large bore needles are recommended to minimise pressure and the possible formation of aerosols. The latter may also be reduced by the use of a venting needle.

Adequate care and precaution should be taken in the disposal of items (syringes, needles, etc) used to reconstitute cytotoxic drugs.

Vials of Velbe should be stored in a refrigerator between 2° and 8°C.

*After reconstitution:* After a portion of the solution has been removed from a vial, the remainder of the contents of the vial may be stored in a refrigerator for further use for 30 days without significant loss of potency. When the reconstituted vial of Velbe is to be stored for more than 48 hours, it is essential to use the accompanying diluting solution or a diluent which contains a preservative.

Velbe should never be mixed with any other drug and should not be diluted with solvents that raise or lower the pH from between 3.5 and 5.

Whenever solution and container permit, parenteral drug products should be inspected visually for particulate matter and discolouration prior to administration.

**Legal category** POM.

**Package quantity** Vials 10 mg: Single vials.

**Further information** The presence of this drug or its metabolites in blood or body tissues is not known to interfere with clinical laboratory tests.

**Product licence numbers**
Vials 10 mg: 0006/5073
Diluent: 0006/5174

## ZYPREXA* ▼

**Qualitative and quantitative composition**

Each Zyprexa 5 mg tablet contains 5 mg olanzapine.

Each Zyprexa 7.5 mg tablet contains 7.5 mg olanzapine.

Each Zyprexa 10 mg tablet contains 10 mg olanzapine.

**Pharmaceutical form** Coated tablets for oral administration.

Zyprexa 5 mg tablets are white, coated tablets imprinted with 'LILLY 4115'.

Zyprexa 7.5 mg tablets are white, coated tablets imprinted with 'LILLY 4116'.

Zyprexa 10 mg tablets are white, coated tablets imprinted with 'LILLY 4117'.

**Clinical particulars**

*Therapeutic indications:* Olanzapine is indicated for the treatment of schizophrenia.

Olanzapine is effective in maintaining the clinical improvement during continuation therapy in patients who have shown an initial treatment response.

*Further information on clinical trials:* In a multinational, double-blind, comparative study of schizophrenia, schizoaffective and related disorders, which included 1481 patients with varying degrees of associated depressive symptoms (baseline mean of 16.6 on the Montgomery-Asberg Depression Rating Scale), a prospective secondary analysis of baseline to endpoint mood score change demonstrated a statistically significant improvement ($P = 0.001$) favouring olanzapine (-6.0) versus haloperidol (-3.1).

*Posology and method of administration:* The recommended starting dose for olanzapine is 10 mg/day, administered as a single daily dose without regard to meals. Daily dosage may subsequently be adjusted on the basis of individual clinical status within the range of 5-20 mg daily. An increase to a dose greater than the routine therapeutic dose of 10 mg/day, ie, to a dose of 15 mg/day or greater, is recommended only after appropriate clinical reassessment.

*Children:* Olanzapine has not been studied in subjects under 18 years of age.

*Elderly patients:* A lower starting dose (5 mg/day) is not routinely indicated but should be considered for those 65 and over when clinical factors warrant.

*Patients with hepatic and/or renal impairment:* A lower starting dose (5 mg) may be considered for such patients.

*Female compared with male patients:* The starting dose and dose range need not be routinely altered for female patients relative to male patients.

*Non-smoking patients compared with smoking patients:* The starting dose and dose range need not be routinely altered for non-smoking patients relative to smoking patients.

When more than one factor is present which might result in slower metabolism (female gender, geriatric age, non-smoking status), consideration should be given to decreasing the starting dose. Dose escalation, when indicated, should be conservative in such patients.

(See also *Interaction with other medicaments and other forms of interaction* and *Pharmacokinetic properties.*)

*Contra-indications:* Olanzapine is contra-indicated in those patients with a known hypersensitivity to any ingredient of the product. Olanzapine is contra-indicated in patients with known risk for narrow-angle glaucoma.

*Special warnings and special precautions for use:*
*Concomitant illnesses:* While olanzapine demonstrated anticholinergic activity *in vitro*, experience during the clinical trials revealed a low incidence of related events. However, as clinical experience with olanzapine in patients with concomitant illness is limited, caution is advised when prescribing for patients with prostatic hypertrophy, or paralytic ileus and related conditions.

*Lactose:* Olanzapine tablets contain lactose.

Transient, asymptomatic elevations of hepatic transaminases, ALT, AST have been seen occasionally, especially in early treatment. Caution should be exercised in patients with elevated ALT and/or AST, in patients with signs and symptoms of hepatic impairment, in patients with pre-existing conditions associated with limited hepatic functional reserve, and in patients who are being treated with potentially hepatotoxic drugs. In the event of elevated ALT and/or AST during treatment, follow-up should be organised and dose reduction should be considered.

As with other neuroleptic drugs, caution should be exercised in patients with low leucocyte and/or neutrophil counts for any reason, in patients with a history of drug-induced bone marrow depression/toxicity, in patients with bone marrow depression caused by concomitant illness, radiation therapy or chemotherapy and in patients with hypereosinophilic conditions or with myeloproliferative disease. Thirty-two patients with clozapine-related neutropenia or agranulocytosis histories received olanzapine without decreases in baseline neutrophil counts.

*Neuroleptic malignant syndrome (NMS):* In clinical trials there were no reported cases of NMS in patients receiving olanzapine. NMS, a potentially fatal symptom complex, has been reported in association with other antipsychotic drugs. Clinical manifestations of NMS are hyperpyrexia, muscle rigidity, altered mental status, and evidence of autonomic instability (irregular pulse or blood pressure, tachycardia, diaphoresis, and cardiac dysrhythmia). Additional signs may include elevated creatinine phosphokinase, myoglobinuria (rhabdomyolysis), and acute renal failure. In such an event, or with unexplained high fever without additional clinical manifestations of NMS, all antipsychotic drugs, including olanzapine, must be discontinued.

Olanzapine should be used cautiously in patients who have a history of seizures or have conditions associated with seizures.

*Tardive dyskinesia:* In comparator studies of one year or less duration, olanzapine was associated with a statistically significant lower incidence of treatment emergent dyskinesia. However, the risk of tardive dyskinesia increases with long-term exposure, and therefore if signs or symptoms of tardive dyskinesia appear in a patient on olanzapine, a dose reduction or drug discontinuation should be considered. These symptoms can temporally deteriorate or even arise after discontinuation of treatment.

Given the primary CNS effects of olanzapine, caution should be used when it is taken in combination with other centrally acting drugs and alcohol. As it exhibits *in vitro* dopamine antagonism, olanzapine may antagonise the effects of direct and indirect dopamine agonists.

Postural hypotension was infrequently observed in the elderly in olanzapine clinical trials. As with other antipsychotics, it is recommended that blood pressure is measured periodically in patients over 65 years.

In clinical trials, olanzapine was not associated with a persistent increase in absolute QT intervals. Only 8 of 1685 subjects had increased QTc interval on multiple occasions. However, as with other antipsychotics, caution should be exercised when olanzapine is prescribed with drugs known to increase QTc interval, especially in the elderly.

*Interaction with other medicaments and other forms of interaction:*
*Potential for other drugs to affect olanzapine:* Single-doses of antacid (aluminium, magnesium) or cimetidine did not affect the oral bioavailability of olanzapine. However, the concomitant administration of activated charcoal reduced the oral bioavailability of olanzapine by 50 to 60%. The metabolism of olanzapine may be induced by concomitant smoking (the clearance of olanzapine is 33% lower and the terminal elimination half-life is 21% longer in non-smokers compared to smokers) or carbamazepine therapy (clearance is increased 44% and the terminal elimination half-life is reduced by 20% when administered with carbamazepine). Smoking and carbamazepine therapy induce P450-1A2 activity. The pharmacokinetics of theophylline, which is metabolised by P450-1A2, is not altered by olanzapine. The effect of potent inhibitors of P450-1A2 activity on olanzapine pharmacokinetics has not been studied.

*Potential for olanzapine to affect other drugs:* In clinical trials with single doses of olanzapine, no inhibition of the metabolism of imipramine/desipramine (P450-2D6 or P450-3A1/A2), warfarin (P450-2C9), theophylline (P450-1A2), or diazepam (P450-3A4 and P450-2C19) was evident. Olanzapine showed no interaction when co-administered with lithium or biperiden. The *in vitro* ability of olanzapine to inhibit metabolism by five principal cytochromes has been examined. These studies found inhibitory constants for 3A4 (491μM), 2C9 (751μM), 1A2 (36μM), 2C19 (920μM), 2D6 (89μM), that compared to olanzapine plasma concentrations of approximately 0.2μM, would mean maximum inhibition of these P450 systems by olanzapine would be less than 0.7%. The clinical relevance of these findings is unknown.

*Pregnancy and lactation:*

*Pregnancy:* There are no adequate and well-controlled studies in pregnant women. Patients should be advised to notify their physician if they become pregnant or intend to become pregnant during treatment with olanzapine. Nevertheless, because human experience is limited, this drug should be used in pregnancy only if the potential benefit justifies the potential risk to the fetus.

*Lactation:* Olanzapine was excreted in milk of treated rats during lactation. It is not known if olanzapine is excreted in human milk. Patients should be advised not to breast-feed an infant if they are taking olanzapine.

*Effects on ability to drive and use machines:* Because olanzapine may cause somnolence, patients should be cautioned about operating hazardous machinery, including motor vehicles.

*Undesirable effects:*

*Frequent (>10%):* The only frequent undesirable effects associated with the use of olanzapine in clinical trials were somnolence and weight gain. Weight gain was related to a lower pre-treatment body mass index (BMI) and initial starting dose of 15 mg or greater.

*Occasional (1-10%):* Occasional undesirable effects associated with the use of olanzapine in clinical trials included dizziness, increased appetite, peripheral oedema, orthostatic hypotension, and mild, transient anticholinergic effects, including constipation and dry mouth.

Transient, asymptomatic elevations of hepatic transaminases, ALT, AST have been seen occasionally, especially in early treatment (see *Special warnings and special precautions for use*).

In active-controlled studies, olanzapine-treated patients had a lower incidence of parkinsonism, akathisia and dystonia compared with titrated doses of haloperidol. In the absence of detailed information on the pre-existing history of individual acute and tardive extrapyramidal movement disorders, it can not be concluded at present that olanzapine produces less tardive dyskinesia and/or other tardive extrapyramidal syndromes.

*Rare (<1%):* Photosensitivity reaction was reported rarely.

*Other findings:* Plasma prolactin levels were sometimes elevated, but associated clinical manifestations (eg, gynaecomastia, galactorrhoea and breast enlargement) were rare. In most patients, levels returned to normal ranges without cessation of treatment.

High creatine phosphokinase levels have been observed in rare cases.

As with other neuroleptic drugs, asymptomatic haematologic variations were occasionally seen.

*Overdose:* Experience with olanzapine in overdosage is limited. In clinical trials, accidental or intentional acute overdosage of olanzapine was identified in 67 patients. In the patient taking the largest identified amount, 300 mg, the only symptoms reported were drowsiness and slurred speech. In the limited number of patients who were evaluated in hospitals, including the patient taking 300 mg, there were no observations indicating an adverse change in laboratory analytes or ECGs. Vital signs were usually within normal limits following overdoses.

Based on animal data, the predicted symptoms would reflect an exaggeration of the drug's known pharmacological actions. Symptoms may include somnolence, mydriasis, blurred vision, respiratory depression, hypotension and possible extrapyramidal disturbances.

There is no specific antidote to olanzapine; therefore, appropriate supportive measures should be initiated. The possibility of multiple drug involvement should be considered.

In case of acute overdosage, establish and maintain an airway and ensure adequate oxygenation and ventilation. The use of activated charcoal for overdose should be considered because the concomitant administration of activated charcoal was shown to reduce the oral bioavailability of olanzapine by 50 to 60%. Gastric lavage (after intubation, if patient is unconscious) may also be considered.

Hypotension and circulatory collapse should be treated with appropriate measures, such as intravenous fluids and/or sympathomimetic agents such as norepinephrine (do not use epinephrine, dopamine or other sympathomimetic agents with beta-agonist activity since beta stimulation may worsen hypotension in the setting of alpha blockade induced by olanzapine). Cardiovascular monitoring should be considered to detect possible arrhythmias. Close medical supervision and monitoring should continue until the patient recovers.

## Pharmacological properties

*Pharmacodynamic properties:* Pharmaco--therapeutic group: Olanzapine is an antipsychotic, ATC code N05A H03 (Diazepines and oxazepines).

Olanzapine is an antipsychotic agent that demonstrates a broad pharmacologic profile across a number of receptor systems.

In preclinical studies, olanzapine exhibited a range of receptor affinities (Ki; <100nmol) for serotonin 5HT2A/2C, 5HT3, 5HT6; dopamine D1, D2, D3, D4, D5; cholinergic muscarinic receptors m1-m5; a1 adrenergic; and histamine H1 receptors. Animal behavioural studies with olanzapine indicated 5HT, dopamine, and cholinergic antagonism, consistent with the receptor-binding profile. Olanzapine demonstrated a greater *in vitro* affinity for serotonin 5HT2 than dopamine D2 receptors and greater 5HT2 than D2 activity *in vivo*, models. Electrophysiological studies demonstrated that olanzapine selectively reduced the firing of mesolimbic (A10) dopaminergic neurons, while having little effect on the striatal (A9) pathways involved in motor function. Olanzapine reduced a conditioned avoidance response, a test indicative of antipsychotic activity, at doses below those producing catalepsy, an effect indicative of motor side-effects. Unlike some other antipsychotic agents, olanzapine increases responding in an 'anxiolytic' test.

In a single oral dose (10 mg) Positron Emission tomography (PET) study in healthy volunteers, olanzapine produced a higher 5HT2A than dopamine D2 receptor occupancy. In addition, a SPECT imaging study in schizophrenic patients revealed that olanzapine-responsive patients had lower striatal D2 occupancy than some other antipsychotic- and risperidone-responsive patients, while being comparable to clozapine-responsive patients.

In two of two placebo and two of three comparator controlled trials with over 2,900 schizophrenic patients presenting with both positive and negative symptoms, olanzapine was associated with statistically significantly greater improvements in negative as well as positive symptoms.

*Pharmacokinetic properties:* Olanzapine is well absorbed after oral administration, reaching peak plasma concentrations within 5 to 8 hours. The absorption is not affected by food. Absolute oral bioavailability relative to intravenous administration has not been determined.

Olanzapine is metabolised in the liver by conjugative and oxidative pathways. The major circulating metabolite is the 10-N-glucuronide, which does not pass the blood brain barrier. Cytochromes P450-CYP1A2 and P450-CYP2D6 contribute to the formation of the N-desmethyl and 2-hydroxymethyl metabolites, both exhibited significantly less *in vivo* pharmacological activity than olanzapine in animal studies. The predominant pharmacologic activity is from the parent olanzapine. After oral administration, the mean terminal elimination half-life of olanzapine in healthy subjects varied on the basis of age and gender.

In healthy elderly (65 and over) versus non-elderly subjects, the mean elimination half-life was prolonged (51.8 versus 33.8 hr) and the clearance was reduced (17.5 versus 18.2L/hr). The pharmacokinetic variability observed in the elderly is within the range for the non-elderly. In 44 patients with schizophrenia >65 years of age, dosing from 5 to 20 mg/day was not associated with any distinguishing profile of adverse events.

In female versus male subjects the mean elimination half-life was somewhat prolonged (36.7 versus 32.3 hrs) and the clearance was reduced (18.9 versus 27.3L/hr). However, olanzapine (5-20 mg) demonstrated a comparable safety profile in female (n = 467) as in male patients (n = 869).

In renally impaired patients (creatinine clearance <10 ml/min) versus healthy subjects, there was no significant difference in mean elimination half-life (37.7 versus 32.4 hr) or drug clearance (21.2 versus 25.0L/hr). A mass balance study showed that approximately 57% of radiolabeled olanzapine appeared in urine, principally as metabolites.

In smoking subjects with mild hepatic dysfunction, mean elimination half-life (39.3 hr) was prolonged and clearance (18.0L/hr) was reduced analogous to non-smoking healthy subjects (48.8hr and 14.1L/hr, respectively).

In non-smoking versus smoking subjects (males and females) the mean elimination half-life was prolonged (38.6 versus 30.4 hr) and the clearance was reduced (18.6 versus 27.7L/hr).

The plasma clearance of olanzapine is lower in elderly versus young subjects, in females versus males, and in non-smokers versus smokers. However, the magnitude of the impact of age, gender, or smoking on olanzapine clearance and half-life is small in comparison to the overall variability between individuals.

In a study of Caucasians, Japanese and Chinese subjects, there were no differences in the pharmacokinetic parameters among the three populations.

The plasma protein binding of olanzapine was about 93% over the concentration range of about 7 to about 1000ng/ml. Olanzapine is bound predominantly to albumin and a₁-acid--glycoprotein.

*Preclinical safety data:*

*Acute (single-dose) toxicity:* Signs of oral toxicity in rodents were characteristic of potent neuroleptic compounds: hypoactivity, coma, tremors, clonic convulsions, salivation, and depressed weight gain. The median lethal doses were approximately 210 (mice) and 175 (rats) mg/kg. Dogs tolerated single oral doses up to 100 mg/kg without mortality. Clinical signs included sedation, ataxia, tremors, increased heart rate, laboured respiration, miosis and anorexia. In monkeys, single oral doses up to 100 mg/kg resulted in prostration and, at higher doses, semi-consciousness.

*Repeated-dose toxicity:* In studies up to 3 months duration in mice and up to 1 year in rats and dogs, the predominant effects were CNS depression, anticholinergic effects and peripheral haematological disorders. Tolerance developed to the CNS depression. Growth parameters were decreased at high doses. Reversible effects consistent with elevated prolactin in rats included decreased weights of ovaries and uterus and morphologic changes in vaginal epithelium and in mammary gland.

*Haematologic toxicity:* Effects on haematology parameters were found in each species, including dose-related reductions in circulating leucocytes in mice and non-specific reductions of circulating leucocytes in rats; however, no evidence of bone marrow cytotoxicity was found. Reversible neutropenia, thrombocytopenia, or anaemia developed in a few dogs treated with 8 or 10 mg/kg/day (total olanzapine exposure [AUC] is 12- to 15-fold greater than that of a man given a 12 mg dose). In cytopenic dogs, there were no adverse effects on progenitor and proliferating cells in the bone marrow.

*Reproductive toxicity:* Olanzapine had no teratogenic effects. Sedation affected mating performance of male rats. Estrous cycles were affected at doses of 1.1 mg/kg (3 times the maximum human dose) and reproduction parameters were influenced in rats given 3 mg/kg (9 times the maximum human dose). In the offspring of rats given olanzapine, delays in fetal development and transient decreases in offspring activity levels were seen.

*Mutagenicity:* Olanzapine was not mutagenic or clastogenic in a full range of standard tests, which included bacterial mutation tests and *in vitro* and *in vivo* mammalian tests.

*Carcinogenicity:* Based on the results of studies in mice and rats, it was concluded that olanzapine is not carcinogenic.

## Pharmaceutical particulars

*List of excipients:* Inactive ingredients are carnauba wax (PhEur), colour mixture white (titanium dioxide E171, macrogol, polysorbate 80), crospovidone (PhEur), edible blue ink (contains indigo carmine colour E132), hydroxypropyl cellulose (PhEur), lactose monohydrate (PhEur), magnesium stearate (PhEur), methylhydroxypropylcellulose (PhEur), microcrystalline cellulose (PhEur).

*Incompatibilities:* None.

*Shelf life:* Two years when stored under appropriate conditions.

*Special precautions for storage:* Store at 15°-30°C. Sensitive to light. Keep tablets in the original package, in a dry place.

*Nature and contents of container:* Blister strips.

Zyprexa 5 mg tablets are available in cold-formed aluminium blister strips in cartons of 28 tablets per carton.

Zyprexa 7.5 mg tablets are available in cold-formed aluminium blister strips in cartons of 56 tablets per carton.

Zyprexa 10 mg tablets are available in cold-formed aluminium blister strips in cartons of 7, 28 or 56 tablets per carton.

*Marketing authorisation holder:* Eli Lilly Nederland BV, Kritjwal 17-23, 3432 ZT Nieuwegein, Netherlands

**Marketing authorisation numbers**
| | |
|---|---|
| 5 mg x 28 tablets: | EU/1/96/022/004 |
| 7.5 mg x 56 tablets: | EU/1/96/022/006 |
| 10 mg x 7 tablets: | EU/1/96/022/008 |
| 10 mg x 28 tablets: | EU/1/96/022/009 |
| 10 mg x 56 tablets: | EU/1/96/022/010 |

**Date of approval/revision of SPC** September 1996

**Legal category** POM

*\*Trade Mark*

## Link Pharmaceuticals Ltd
7/8 Sterling Buildings
Carfax
Horsham
West Sussex RH12 1DR

### COBALIN-H*

**Presentation** 1 ml ampoules containing a sterile, clear, red solution providing 1000 micrograms hydroxocobalamin per millilitre for injection. Cobalin-H complies with the specification for Hydroxocobalamin Injection BP.

**Uses** Addisonian pernicious anaemia. Prophylaxis and treatment of other macrocytic anaemias due to $B_{12}$ deficiency. Tobacco amblyopia and Leber's atrophy.

**Dosage and administration** The following dosages are suitable for children and adults.

*Addisonian pernicious anaemia and other macrocytic anaemias without neurological involvement:* Initially – 250 micrograms to 1000 micrograms intramuscularly on alternate days for one or two weeks then 250 micrograms weekly until blood count is normal. Maintenance – 1000 micrograms every two or three months.

*Addisonian pernicious anaemia and other macrocytic anaemias with neurological involvement:* Initially – 1000 micrograms on alternate days as long as improvement continues. Maintenance – 1000 micrograms every two months.

*Prophylaxis of macrocytic anaemias associated with Vitamin $B_{12}$ deficiency resulting from gastrectomy, ileal resection, certain malabsorption states and vegetarianism:* 1000 micrograms every two or three months.

*Tobacco amblyopia and Leber's optic atrophy:* Initially – 1000 micrograms daily by intramuscular injection for two weeks then twice weekly as long as improvement is maintained. Maintenance – 1000 micrograms every three months or as required.

**Contra-indications, warnings, etc**

*Contra-indications:* Sensitivity to hydroxocobalamin.

*Interactions:* The serum concentration of hydroxocobalamin may be reduced by concurrent administration of oral contraceptives. Chloramphenicol treated patients may respond poorly to hydroxocobalamin. Vitamin $B_{12}$ assays by microbiological techniques are invalidated by antimetabolites and most antibiotics.

*Effects on ability to drive and use machines:* None stated.

*Other undesirable effects:* Allergic hypersensitivity reactions have occurred rarely following the administration of hydroxocobalamin.

*Use in pregnancy and lactation:* Hydroxocobalamin should not be used to treat megaloblastic anaemia of pregnancy.

*Other special warnings and precautions:* Should not be given before a megaloblastic marrow has been demonstrated. Regular monitoring of the blood is advisable. Doses of hydroxocobalamin greater than 10 micrograms daily may produce a haematological response in patients with a folate deficiency. Indiscriminate use may mask the exact diagnosis. Cardiac arrhythmias secondary to hypokalaemia have been reported during initial therapy and plasma potassium should therefore be monitored during this period.

*Overdose:* Treatment is unlikely to be needed in cases of overdosage.

*Incompatibilities:* None stated.

**Pharmaceutical precautions** Protect from light. Store below 25°C.

**Legal category** POM.

**Package quantities** Boxes of 5 ampoules.

**Further information** Hydroxocobalamin injection has completely replaced Cyanocobalamin injection and is now the form of Vitamin $B_{12}$ therapy of choice.

**Product licence number** 12406/0001.

### NOZINAN*

**Presentation**

*Injection:* Colourless isotonic solution containing 2.5% w/v methotrimeprazine hydrochloride in ampoules of 1 ml. The injection also contains ascorbic acid, sodium sulphite and sodium chloride.

*Tablets:* Greyish white or cream tablets containing 25 mg methotrimeprazine maleate impressed NOZINAN '25' on one face, with a break line on the reverse.

**Uses** Methotrimeprazine resembles chlorpromazine and promethazine in the pattern of its pharmacology. It possesses anti-emetic, anti-histamine and anti-adrenaline activity and exhibits a strong sedative effect. Nozinan potentiates the action of other central nervous system depressants but may be given in conjunction with appropriately modified doses of narcotic analgesics in the management of severe pain. Nozinan does not significantly depress respiration and is particularly useful where pulmonary reserve is low.

Nozinan is indicated in the management of severe pain and accompanying anxiety and distress. Nozinan is also indicated in psychiatry as an alternative to Largactil in schizophrenia especially when it is desirable to reduce psychomotor activity.

*Kinetics:* Maximum serum concentrations are achieved in 2–3 hours depending on route of administration. Excretion is slow, with a half-life of about 30 hours. It is eliminated via urine and faeces.

**Dosage and administration** Dosage varies with the condition and individual response of the patient.

*1. Terminal illness:* The usual dose for adults and the elderly is 12.5–25 mg (0.5–1 ml) by intramuscular injection, or by the intravenous route after dilution with an equal volume of normal saline immediately before use. In cases of severe agitation up to 50 mg (2 ml) may be used, repeated every six to eight hours.

*Continuous subcutaneous infusion:* Nozinan may be administered over a 24 hour period via a syringe driver. The required dose of Nozinan (25–200 mg per day) should be diluted with the calculated volume of normal saline. Diamorphine hydrochloride is compatible with this solution and may be added if greater analgesia is required.

Nozinan tablets 25 mg may be substituted for the injection if oral therapy is more convenient the dosage being 12.5–50 mg 4–8 hourly.

*Children:* Clinical experience with parenteral methotrimeprazine in children is limited. Where indicated doses of 0.35 mg to 3.0 mg/kg/day are recommended.

*2. Psychiatric conditions: Adults:* Ambulant patients: initially the total daily oral dose should not exceed 25–50 mg, usually divided into 3 doses; a larger portion of the dosage may be taken at bedtime to minimise diurnal sedation. The dosage is then gradually increased to the most effective level compatible with sedation and other side-effects.

*Bed patients:* Initially the total daily oral dosage may be 100–200 mg, usually divided into 3 doses, gradually increased to 1 g daily if necessary. When the patient is stable attempts should be made to reduce the dosage to an adequate maintenance level.

*Children:* Children are very susceptible to the hypotensive and soporific effects of methotrimeprazine. It is advised that a total daily oral dosage of $1\frac{1}{2}$ tablets should not be exceeded. The average effective daily intake for a 10-year-old is $\frac{1}{2}$ to 1 tablet.

*Elderly patients:* It is not advised to give methotrimeprazine to ambulant patients over 50 years of age unless the risk of a hypotensive reaction has been assessed.

**Contra-indications, warnings, etc** Safety in pregnancy has not been established.

There are no absolute contra-indications to the use of Nozinan in terminal care.

The drug should be avoided or used with caution in patients with liver dysfunction or cardiac disease.

*Precautions:* The hypotensive effects of Nozinan should be taken into account when it is administered to patients with cardiac disease and the elderly or debilitated. Patients receiving large initial doses should be kept in bed.

Nozinan may cause drowsiness, disorientation, confusion or excessive hypotension, which may affect patient's ability to drive or operate machinery. Avoid alcoholic drinks.

*Side-effects:* Somnolence and asthenia are frequent side effects. Dry mouth is encountered occasionally. Hypotension may occur, especially in elderly patients. A raised ESR may occasionally be encountered. Agranulocytosis has been reported, as have photosensivity and allergic skin reactions. Parkinsonian-like reactions may occur in patients receiving prolonged high dosage. Jaundice is a rare side effect. Other adverse effects common to phenothiazine neuroleptics may be seen.

*Interactions:* Simultaneous administration of desferrioxamine and prochlorperazine has been observed to induce a transient metabolic encephalopathy characterised by loss of consciousness for 48–72 hours. It is possible that this may occur with Nozinan since it shares many of the pharmacological activities of prochlorperazine. Adrenaline must not be used in patients overdosed with neuroleptics.

*Toxicity and treatment of overdosage:* Symptoms of methotrimeprazine overdosage include drowsiness or loss of consciousness, hypotension, tachycardia, ECG changes, ventricular arrhythmias and hypothermia. Severe extra-pyramidal dyskinesias may occur.

If the patient is seen sufficiently soon (up to 6 hours) after ingestion of a toxic dose, gastric lavage may be attempted. Pharmacological induction of emesis is unlikely to be of any use. Activated charcoal should be given. There is no specific antidote. Treatment is supportive.

Generalised vasodilatation may result in circulatory collapse; raising the patient's legs may suffice, in severe cases, volume expansion by intravenous fluids may be needed; infusion fluids should be warmed before administration in order not to aggravate hypothermia.

Positive inotropic agents such as dopamine may be tried if fluid replacement is insufficient to correct the circulatory collapse. Peripheral vasoconstrictor agents are not generally recommended; avoid the use of adrenaline.

Ventricular or supraventricular tachy-arrhythmias usually respond to restoration of normal body temperature and correction of circulatory or metabolic disturbances. If persistent or life threatening, appropriate anti-arrhythmic therapy may be considered. Avoid lignocaine and, as far as possible, long acting anti-arrhythmic drugs.

Pronounced central nervous depression requires airway maintenance or, in extreme circumstances, assisted respiration. Severe dystonic reactions usually respond to procyclidine (5–10 mg) or orphenadrine (20–40 mg) administered intramuscularly or intravenously. Convulsions should be treated with intravenous diazepam.

Neuroleptic malignant syndrome should be treated with cooling. Dantrolene sodium may be tried.

**Pharmaceutical precautions** Protect from light. Nozinan Injection Solution, on exposure to light, rapidly develops a pink or yellow colouration and any such solution should be discarded. Nozinan Injection Solution is incompatible with alkaline solutions.

**Legal category** POM.

**Package quantities** Injection Solution 2.5% Box of 10×1 ml ampoules. Tablets container of 500×25 mg.

**Further information** Dilutions of Nozinan injection in normal saline, with or without the addition of diamorphine hydrochloride, are stable for 24 hours and may be used in syringe drivers.

**Product licence numbers**

| | |
|---|---|
| Nozinan Injection Solution 2.5% | 12406/0006 |
| Nozinan Tablets 25 mg | 12406/0007 |

### PABRINEX* INTRAVENOUS HIGH POTENCY
### PABRINEX* INTRAMUSCULAR HIGH POTENCY

**Presentation** Pairs of amber glass ampoules of Vitamins B and C Injection BPC for intravenous and intramuscular injection:
I.V. High Potency – 5 ml No. 1+5 ml No. 2 Blue Carton
I.M. High Potency – 5 ml No. 1+2 ml No. 2 Red Carton

Ingredients:

| Active ingredient | Intravenous High Potency Blue carton No. 1 | No. 2 | Intramuscular High Potency Red carton No. 1 | No. 2 |
|---|---|---|---|---|
| Thiamine Hydrochloride BP (Vitamin B₁) | 250 mg | | 250 mg | |
| Riboflavin (as Phosphate Sodium BP) (Vitamin B₂) | 4 mg | | 4 mg | |
| Pyridoxine Hydrochloride BP (Vitamin B₆) | 50 mg | | 50 mg | |
| Nicotinamide BP | | 160 mg | | 160 mg |
| Ascorbic Acid BP (Vitamin C) | | 500 mg | | 500 mg |
| Anhydrous Glucose BP | | 1 gm¹ | | |
| Benzyl Alcohol BP | | | | 140 mg² |
| Volume per ampoule | 5 ml | 5 ml | 5 ml | 2 ml |
| Dose volume | | 10 ml | | 7 ml |

¹ provides 10% w/v in mixed ampoules
² provides 2% w/v in mixed ampoules

Pabrinex Injections are aqueous solutions for intravenous and intramuscular injection and also contain edetic acid and sodium hydroxide as excipients.

**Uses** Rapid therapy of severe depletion or malabsorption of the water soluble Vitamins B and C, particularly in alcoholism, after acute infections, post operatively and in psychiatric states.

Also used to maintain levels of Vitamins B and C in patients on chronic intermittent haemodialysis.

**Dosage and administration**
*INTRAVENOUS:* The preferred method of administration is by drip infusion. The contents of each pair of ampoules should be diluted with 50–100 ml physiological saline or 5% glucose and infused over 15–30 minutes (see *Storage* section for further information).

Alternatively the contents of each pair of ampoules (total 10 ml) are drawn up into a syringe to mix them just before use, then injected slowly, over a period of 10 minutes, into a vein.

NOT FOR INTRAMUSCULAR USE.

*INTRAMUSCULAR* – The contents of each pair of ampoules (total 7 ml) are drawn up into a syringe to mix them just before use, then injected slowly high into the gluteal muscle, 5 cm below the iliac crest.

NOT FOR INTRAVENOUS USE.

*Adult dose (including the elderly):* Pabrinex is indicated for rapid therapy of severe vitamin depletion or malabsorption encountered in the following conditions:

| | |
|---|---|
| Coma or delirium from alcohol, narcotics or barbiturates; collapse following narcosis: | The contents of 2–3 pairs of ampoules INTRAVENOUS HIGH POTENCY (Blue No. 1 and No. 2) injected at intervals of 8 hours or at the discretion of the physician. |
| Psychosis following narcosis or ECT; toxicity from acute infections: | The contents of one pair of ampoules INTRAVENOUS HIGH POTENCY (Blue No. 1 and No. 2) or INTRAMUSCULAR HIGH POTENCY (Red No. 1 and No. 2) twice daily for up to 7 days. |
| Haemodialysis: | The contents of one pair of ampoules INTRAVENOUS HIGH POTENCY (Blue No. 1 and No. 2) every two weeks diluted with saline and given at the end of the dialysis. |

*Children's dose:* Pabrinex is rarely indicated for administration to children, but suitable doses are:

| | |
|---|---|
| Under 6 years | 0.25 adult dose |
| 6–10 years | 0.33 adult dose |
| 10–14 years | 0.50–0.66 adult dose |
| 14 years and over | adult dose |

**Contra-indications, warnings, etc**
*Contra-indications:* Known hypersensitivity to any of the active constituents.

*Interactions:* The content of pyridoxine may interfere with the effects of concurrent levodopa therapy.

*Effects on ability to drive and use machinery:* None known.

*Other undesirable effects:* Occasionally, hypotension and mild paraesthesia from continued high doses of thiamine; occasionally mild ache at local site of injection.

*Use in pregnancy and lactation:* No adverse effects at recommended doses when clinically indicated.

*Other special warnings and precautions:* Repeated injections of preparations containing high concentrations of Vitamin B₁ (thiamine) may give rise to anaphylactic shock. Mild allergic reactions such as sneezing or mild asthma are warning signs that further injections may give rise to anaphylactic shock. Facilities for treating anaphylactic reactions should be available whenever Pabrinex is administered.

*Overdosage:* Unlikely to occur but if it does, treatment is symptomatic and supportive.

*Incompatibilities:* If it is necessary to administer Pabrinex I.V. in infusion fluids it is recommended that it be given in Glucose 5% or Sodium Chloride 0.9% by intermittent infusion (i.e. over a short time in a relatively small volume) or by adding via drip tubing.

**Pharmaceutical precautions** Store blow 25°C protected from light. Do not freeze.

*Storage of diluted Pabrinex IVHP:* The stability of IVHP Vitamins B and C Injection BPC in intravenous infusion fluids, at room temperature, is as follows:

Intravenous infusion fluid: In the light.
Glucose 5%: 7 hours.
Sodium chloride 0.9%: 7 hours.
Glucose 4.3% with sodium chloride 0.18%: 4 hours.
Glucose 5% with potassium chloride 0.3%: 4 hours.
Sodium lactate M/6: 7 hours.

Although no further specific data are available, the solutions are expected to be stable for longer periods when protected from light. Store diluted solutions at 2–8°C if not used immediately. Do not freeze.

**Legal category** POM.

**Package quantities** Packs of 10 pairs of ampoules.

**Further information** Nil.

**Product licence numbers**
I.V. High Potency    12406/0003
I.M. High Potency    12406/0004

# SYTRON*

**Presentation** A clear red mixture with a cherry taste.

*Composition:* Each 5 ml contains: Sodium ironedetate 190 mg (equivalent to 27.5 mg of iron).

**Uses**
*Action:* Sodium ironedetate is not an iron salt as it contains iron in an un-ionised form. In this compound the iron is 'insulated' or 'sequestered' with the sodium salt of ethylenediamine tetra-acetic acid to form a chelate. This accounts for the fact that Sytron is not astringent and does not discolour teeth. Studies using radioactive tracers have shown that iron chelate is split within the gastro-intestinal tract, releasing elemental iron which is absorbed and rendered available for haemoglobin regeneration.

*Indications:* Iron deficiency anaemia, in paediatrics, and anaemias complicating rheumatoid arthritis. It is especially suitable in pregnancy when other forms of oral iron are not well tolerated.

**Dosage and administration** Oral.
*Adults:* 5 ml increasing gradually to 10 ml three times daily.

*Elderly (over 65 years):* As for adults.

*Children (including premature infants) up to 1 year:* 2.5 ml twice daily; somewhat smaller doses should be used initially.

*1 to 5 years:* 2.5 ml three times daily.
*6 to 12 years:* 5 ml three times daily.

**Contra-indications, warnings, etc**
*Contra-indications:* None known.

*Precautions:* None known.

*Pregnancy:* No adverse effects have been reported.

*Side effects:* Patients have occasionally complained of nausea or mild diarrhoea in the early stages of treatment. In such cases it has been found that if treatment is withdrawn for a short time these symptoms quickly disappear and subsequently the patient will tolerate further doses, which should be on a somewhat reduced scale. Normal individuals have taken Sytron in twice the recommended dosage and some of these have experienced mild diarrhoea. This should be taken into account if dosage is increased much higher than the recommended scale.

*Interactions:* None known.

*Overdose:* Initial symptoms of iron overdosage include nausea, vomiting, diarrhoea, abdominal pain, haematemesis, rectal bleeding, lethargy and circulatory collapse. Hyperglycaemia and metabolic acidosis may occur.

*Treatment of overdosage:*
1. Administer an emetic.
2. Emesis should be followed by gastric lavage with desferrioxamine solution (2 g/l). Desferrioxamine 5 g in 50–100 ml water should be introduced into the stomach following gastric emptying.
3. Keep the patient under constant surveillance to detect possible aspiration of vomitus. Maintain suction apparatus and standby emergency oxygen in case of need.
4. In adults, a drink of mannitol or sorbitol should be given to induce small bowel emptying. Inducing diarrhoea in children may be dangerous and should not be undertaken in young children.
5. Severe poisoning: In the presence of shock and/or coma with high serum iron levels (adults>142 µmol/l, children>90 µmol/l), immediate supportive measures should be introduced. Desferrioxamine should be given by slow I.V. infusion (adults 5 mg/kg/H, children 15 mg/kg/H). The maximum dose is 80 mg/kg/24 H.
*Warning:* Hypotension may occur if the infusion rate is too rapid.
6. Less severe poisoning: I.M. desferrioxamine should be administered (adults 50 mg/kg to a maximum of 4 g, children 1 g 4–6 hourly).
7. Serum iron levels should be monitored throughout.

**Pharmaceutical precautions** Store below 30°C. Recommended diluent: Water. When diluted use within 14 days of preparation.

**Legal category** P.

**Package quantities** Bottles of 500 ml.

**Further information** Nil.

**Product licence number** 12406/0005.

*Trade Mark

# Lipha Pharmaceuticals Limited
## Harrier House, High Street
## West Drayton
## Middlesex UB7 7QG

## CAMPRAL EC*

**Qualitative and quantitative composition** Each tablet contains acamprosate (I.N.N.) calcium 333.0 mg as the active ingredient.

**Pharmaceutical form** Enteric coated tablets.

**Clinical particulars**

*Therapeutic indications:* Campral EC is indicated as therapy to maintain abstinence in alcohol dependent patients. It should be combined with counselling.

*Posology and method of administration*
*Adults:* Within the age range 18-65 years:
Subjects weighing 60 kg or more: 2 tablets three times daily with meals (2 tablets morning, noon and night).
Subjects weighing less than 60 kg: 4 tablets divided into three daily doses with meals (2 tablets in the morning, 1 at noon, 1 at night).
The recommended treatment period is one year. Treatment with acamprosate should be initiated as soon as possible after the withdrawal period and should be maintained if the patient relapses.

*Children and the elderly:* Campral EC should not be administered to children and the elderly.

*Contra-indications:*
–in patients with a known hypersensitivity to the drug
–in pregnant women and lactating women
–in cases of renal insufficiency (serum creatinine >120 micromol/L)
–in cases with severe hepatic failure (Childs- Pugh Classification C)

*Special warnings and precautions for use:* Campral EC does not constitute treatment for the withdrawal period. Campral EC does not prevent harmful effects of continuous alcohol abuse. Continued alcohol abuse negates the therapeutic benefit, therefore Campral EC treatment should only be initiated after weaning therapy, once the patient is abstinent from alcohol.

*Interactions with other medicaments and other forms of interaction:* The concomitant intake of alcohol and Campral EC does not affect the pharmacokinetics of either alcohol or Campral EC. Administering Campral EC with food diminishes the bioavailability of the drug compared with its administration in the fasting state. Pharmacokinetic studies have been completed and show no interaction between acamprosate and diazepam, disulfiram or imipramine. There is no information available on the concomitant administration of Campral EC with diuretics.

*Pregnancy and lactation:* Although animal studies have not shown any evidence of foetotoxicity or teratogenicity, the safety of Campral EC has not been established in pregnancy women. Acamprosate is excreted in the milk of lactating animals and safe use of Campral EC has not been demonstrated in lactating women. Campral EC therefore should not be administered to pregnant or to breast feeding women.

*Effects on ability to drive and use machines:* Campral EC should not impair the patient's ability to drive or operate machinery.

*Undesirable effects:* Adverse events associated with Campral EC tend to be mild and transient in nature. They are predominantly gastrointestinal or dermatological. Diarrhoea, and less frequently nausea, vomiting and abdominal pain are the gastrointestinal adverse events. Pruritus is the predominant dermatological adverse event. An occasional maculopapular rash and rare cases of bullous skin reactions have been reported. Fluctuation in libido has been reported by patients receiving Campral EC as well as by patients receiving the placebo.

*Overdose:* Five cases of overdose associated with Campral EC therapy have been reported in humans, including one patient who ingested 43 g. After gastric lavage all patients had an uneventful recovery. Diarrhoea was observed in two cases. No case of hypercalaemia was reported in the course of these overdoses. However, should this occur, the patients should be treated for acute hypercalcaemia.

**Pharmacological properties**

*Pharmacodynamic properties:* Acamprosate calcium (calcium acetylhomotaurinate) has a chemical structure similar to that of amino acid neurotransmitters, such as taurine or gamma-amino-butyric acid (GABA), including an acetylation to permit passage across the blood brain barrier. Acamprosate may act by stimulating GABAergic inhibitory neurotransmission and antagonising excitatory amino-acids, particularly glutamic acid. Animal experimental studies have demonstrated that acamprosate affects alcohol dependence in rats, decreasing the voluntary intake of alcohol without affecting food and total fluid intake.

*Pharmacokinetic properties:* Acamprosate absorption across the gastrointestinal tract is moderate, slow and sustained and varies substantially from person to person. Oral absorption shows considerable variability and is usually less than 10% of the ingested drug in the first 24 hours. Food reduces the oral absorption of acamprosate. Steady state levels of acamprosate are achieved by the seventh day of dosing. Acamprosate is not protein bound. The drug is excreted in the urine and is not significantly metabolised. There is a linear relationship between creatinine clearance values and total apparent plasma clearance, renal clearance and plasma half-life of acamprosate. The pharmacokinetics of acamprosate are not altered by hepatic dysfunction.

*Preclinical safety data:* In preclinical studies, signs of toxicity are related to the excessive intake of calcium and not acetylhomotaurine. Disorders of phosphorus/calcium metabolism have been observed including diarrhoea, soft tissue calcification, renal and cardiac lesions. There were no mutagenic or carcinogenic effects, nor any teratogenic or adverse affects on the male or female reproductive systems of animals. Detailed *in vitro* and *in vivo* research on acamprosate to detect genetic and chromosomal mutations has not produced any evidence of potential genetic toxicity.

**Pharmaceutical particulars**

*List of excipients:* Crospovidone (Kollidon CL); microcrystalline cellulose (Avicel PH 101); magnesium silicate (Compressil); sodium starch glycolate (Explotab); anhydrous colloidal silica (Aerosil 200); magnesium stearate; anionic copolymer of methacrylic and acrylic acid ethyl ester (Eudragit L30 D); talc; propylene glycol.

*Incompatibilities:* None known.

*Shelf life:* 3 years.

*Special precautions:* None.

*Nature and contents of container:* Aluminium/PVC sheets of blisters containing 12 tablets. Sheets of blisters are presented in cartons of 84 tablets.

*Instructions for use / handling:* Not applicable.

*Marketing authorisation holder:* Lipha S.A., 34 rue Saint Romain, 69379 Lyon Cedex 08,France.

**Marketing authorisation number** 13466/0001

**Date of approval/revision of SPC** December 1995.

**Legal category** POM

## GLUCOPHAGE*

**Presentation** White, film-coated tablets containing Metformin Hydrochloride BP. 500 mg marked GL500; 850 mg marked GL850.

**Uses** *Indications:* Non-insulin dependent diabetes when diet has failed and especially if the patient is overweight. Glucophage can be given alone as initial therapy, or can be administered in combination with a sulphonylurea.
In insulin-dependent diabetes, Glucophage may be given as an adjuvant to patients whose symptoms are poorly controlled.

*Pharmacology:* Glucophage is a biguanide oral antihyperglycaemic agent. Its mode of action is thought to be multifactorial and includes delayed uptake of glucose from the gastro-intestinal tract, increased peripheral glucose utilisation mediated by increased insulin sensitivity and inhibition of increased hepatic and renal gluconeogenesis.

**Dosage and administration**

*Adults:* Initially, one 850 mg tablet twice a day or one 500 mg tablet three times a day, with or after food. Good diabetic control may be achieved within a few days, but it is not unusual for the full effect to be delayed for up to two weeks. If control is incomplete a cautious increase in dosage to a maximum of 3 g daily is justified. Once control has been obtained it may be possible to reduce the dosage of Glucophage.

*Children:* Glucophage is not recommended for use.

*Elderly:* Glucophage is indicated in the elderly, but not when renal function is impaired.

**Contra-indications, warnings, etc**

*Contra-indications:* Hypersensitivity to the drug. Diabetic coma and ketoacidosis, impairment of renal function, chronic liver disease, cardiac failure and recent myocardial infarction. History of, or states associated with, lactic acidosis such as shock or pulmonary insufficiency, alcoholism (acute or chronic), and conditions associated with hypoxaemia.

*Precautions:* Glucophage is excreted by the kidney and regular monitoring of renal function is advised in all diabetics. Glucophage therapy should be stopped 2–3 days before surgery and clinical investigations such as intravenous urography and intravenous angiography, and reinstated only after control of renal function has been regained. The use of Glucophage is not advised in conditions which may cause dehydration or in patients suffering from serious infections or trauma.
Patients receiving continuous Glucophage therapy should have an annual estimation of Vitamin $B_{12}$ levels because of reports of decreased Vitamin $B_{12}$ absorption.
During concomitant therapy with a sulphonylurea, blood glucose should be monitored because combined therapy may cause hypoglycaemia. Stabilisation of diabetic patients with Glucophage and insulin should be carried out in hospital because of the possibility of hypoglycaemia until the correct ratio of the two drugs has been obtained.
Reduced renal clearance of Glucophage has been reported during cimetidine therapy, so a dose reduction should be considered. As with a number of drugs, an interaction between Glucophage and anticoagulants is a possibility and dosage of the latter may need adjustment.

*Use in pregnancy and lactation:* Pregnancy: The use of Glucophage is not advised. Lactation: No information is available.

*Adverse reactions:* Glucophage is normally well tolerated but gastro-intestinal disturbances sometimes occur. These are usually minor and can often be avoided by taking Glucophage with or after food. Occasionally a temporary lowering of the dose may be needed. It is important that Glucophage treatment is not abandoned at the first sign of intolerance, since this has been found to resolve spontaneously.
Lactic acidosis has been associated with Glucophage but, in the few cases reported, has occurred in patients with contra-indications to therapy. In patients with a metabolic acidosis lacking evidence of ketoacidosis (ketonuria and ketonaemia), lactic acidosis should be suspected and Glucophage therapy stopped. Lactic acidosis is a medical emergency which must be treated in hospital.

*Overdosage – Signs and Symptoms:* Hypoglycaemia does not occur with Glucophage monotherapy (fifty tablets have been ingested with no untoward effects on blood glucose levels). However, it can occur when Glucophage is given concomitantly with a sulphonylurea, insulin or alcohol.
In excessive dosage, and particularly if there is a possibility of accumulation, lactic acidosis may develop.

*Overdosage – Treatment:* Intensive supportive therapy is recommended which should be particularly directed at correcting fluid loss and metabolic disturbance.

**Pharmaceutical precautions** Store below 25°C in a dry place. The shelf-life is 5 years.

**Legal category** POM.

**Package quantities** 500 mg: Blister packs of 84 tablets (OP); containers of 500 tablets. 850 mg: Blister packs of 56 tablets (OP); containers of 300 tablets.

**Further information** Glucophage does not lower blood glucose levels in non-diabetics, and does not cause hypoglycaemia in diabetics when used as monotherapy. Weight loss often occurs during therapy and levels of plasma cholesterol, triglycerides and prebeta-lipoproteins may be lowered. Glucophage has been shown to improve peripheral glucose metabolism.

**Product licence numbers**
Glucophage 500 mg   3759/0012
Glucophage 850 mg   3759/0013

## NITROLINGUAL* PUMP SPRAY

**Qualitative and quantitative composition** Each metered dose contains 400 micrograms glyceryl trinitrate.

**Pharmaceutical form** Oromucosal spray.

**Clinical particulars**

*Therapeutic indications:* For the treatment and prophylaxis of angina pectoris and the treatment of variant angina.

*Posology and method of administration*
*Adults and the elderly:* At the onset of an attack or prior to a precipitating event: one or two 400 microgram metered-doses sprayed under the tongue. It is recommended that no more than three metered-doses are taken at any one time and that there should be a minimum interval of 15 minutes between consecutive treatments.

For the prevention of exercise induced angina or in other precipitating conditions: one or two 400 microgram metered doses sprayed under the tongue immediately prior to the event.

*Children:* Nitrolingual Pump spray is not recommended for use.

*Administration:*The bottle should be held vertically with the valve head uppermost. If the pump is new, or has not been used for a week or more, the first actuation should be released into the air. The spray orifice should then be placed as close to the mouth as possible. The dose should be sprayed under the tongue and the mouth should be closed immediately after each dose. The spray should not be inhaled. Patients should be instructed to familiarise themselves with the position of the spray orifice, which can be identified by the finger rest on the top of the valve, in order to facilitate orientation for administration at night. During application the patient should rest, ideally in the sitting position.

*Contra-indications:*Hypersensitivity to nitrates or any constituent of the formulation. Hypotension, hypovolaemia, cerebral haemorrhage and brain trauma, mitral stenosis and angina caused by hypertrophic obstructive cardiomyopathy.

*Special warnings and special precautions for use:* Any lack of effect may be an indicator of early myocardial infarction.

As with all glyceryl trinitrate preparations, use in patients with incipient glaucoma should be avoided.

*Interaction with other medicaments and other forms of interaction:* Tolerance to this drug and cross tolerance to other nitrates may occur. Alcohol may potentiate any hypotensive effect.

*Pregnancy and lactation:* Nitrolingual Pump spray is not generally recommended and should be used only if its potential benefit justifies any potential risk to the foetus or neonate.

*Effects on ability to drive and use machines:* Only as a result of hypotension.

*Undesirable effects:* Headache, dizziness, postural hypotension, flushing, tachycardia and paradoxical bradycardia have been reported.

*Overdose*
*Signs and symptoms:* Flushing, severe headache, a feeling of suffocation, hypotension, fainting, restlessness, blurred vision, impairment of respiration, bradycardia and rarely, cyanosis and methaemoglobinaemia may occur. In a few patients there may be a reaction comparable to shock with nausea, vomiting, weakness, sweating and syncope.

*Treatment:* Recovery often occurs without special treatment. Hypotension may be corrected by elevation of the legs to promote venous return. Methaemoglobinaemia should be treated by intravenous methylene blue.

Symptomatic treatment should be given for respiratory and circulatory defects in more serious cases.

**Pharmacological properties**

*Pharmacodynamic properties:* Glyceryl trinitrate relieves angina pectoris by reduction of cardiac work and dilation of the coronary arteries. In this way, not only is there a lessening in arterial oxygen requirement but the amount of oxygenated blood reaching the ischaemic heart is increased.

*Pharmacokinetics properties:* The pharmacokinetics of glyceryl trinitrate are complex; venous plasma levels of the drug show wide and variable fluctuations and are not predictive of clinical effect. In a human pharmacodynamic study, pharmacological activity had commenced one minute after dosing and was obvious by two minutes.

**Pharmaceutical particulars**

*List of excipients:* Fractionated coconut oil, ethanol, medium chain partial glycerides, peppermint oil.

*Incompatibilities:* None known.

*Shelf life:* 3 years.

*Special precautions for storage:* Store below 25°C.

*Nature and contents of container:* Red plastic coated glass bottle fitted with metering pump. Each bottle contains 4.9, 11.2 or 14.1 g solution (equivalent to about 75, 200 or 250 doses).

*Instructions for use/handling:* See 'Administration' section.

**Marketing authorisation number**   03759/0042.

**Date of approval/revision of SPC**   April 1995.

**Legal category** P

## NITRONAL*

**Presentation** Amber glass 5 ml ampoules and clear glass 50 ml vials filled with a colourless isotonic solution containing 1 mg/ml glyceryl trinitrate.

Excipients: Dextrose, polyethylene glycol 400, water for injections.

**Uses**
*Indications:*

1. Unresponsive congestive heart failure, including that secondary to acute myocardial infarction.
2. Refractory unstable angina pectoris and coronary insufficiency, including Prinzmetal's angina.
3. Control of hypertensive episodes and/or myocardial ischaemia during and after cardiac surgery. For the induction of controlled hypotension for surgery.

*Pharmacology:* Glyceryl trinitrate exerts a spasmolytic action on smooth muscle, particularly in the vascular system. The predominant effect is an increase in venous capacitance resulting in marked diminution of both the left ventricular filling pressure and volume (preload). There is also a reduction in afterload due to moderate dilation of the arteriolar resistance vessels. These haemodynamic changes lower the myocardial oxygen demand. By direct action and through the reduction of myocardial wall tension, glyceryl trinitrate also lowers the resistance to flow in the coronary collateral channels and allows re-distribution of blood flow to ischaemic areas of the myocardium.

Administration of Nitronal by intravenous infusion to patients with congestive heart failure results in a marked improvement in haemodynamics, reduction of elevated left ventricular filling pressure and systolic wall tension, and an increase in the depressed cardiac output. It reduces the imbalance that exists between myocardial oxygen demand and delivery, thereby diminishing myocardial ischaemia and controlling ischaemia-induced ventricular arrhythmias.

**Dosage and administration**
*Dosage: Adults and the Elderly* – The dose should be titrated against the individual clinical response.

1. Unresponsive congestive heart failure. The normal dose range is 10–100 micrograms/minute administered as a continuous intravenous infusion with frequent monitoring of blood pressure and heart rate. The infusion should be started at the lower rate and increased cautiously until the desired clinical response is achieved. Other haemodynamic measurements are extremely important in monitoring response to the drug: these may include pulmonary capillary wedge pressure, cardiac output and precordial electrocardiogram depending on the clinical picture.
2. Refractory unstable angina pectoris. An initial infusion rate of 10–15 micrograms/minute is recommended; this may be increased cautiously in increments of 5–10 micrograms until either relief of angina is achieved, headache prevents further increase in dose, or the mean arterial pressure falls by more than 20 mm Hg.
3. Use in surgery. An initial infusion rate of 25 micrograms/minute is recommended; this should be increased gradually until the desired systolic arterial pressure is attained. The usual dose is 25–200 micrograms/minute.

*Children:* There is no recommended dose for children.

*Administration:* Nitronal need not be diluted before use but can be diluted with Dextrose Injection BP, Sodium Chloride and Dextrose Injection BP, 0.9% Sodium Chloride Injection BP or other protein-free infusion solution, if required.

The solution, whether or not diluted, should be infused *slowly* (see dosage section) and *not* given by bolus injection.

To ensure a constant infusion rate of glyceryl trinitrate, it is recommended that Nitronal be administered by means of a syringe pump or polyethylene infusion bag with a counter, with a glass or rigid polyethylene syringe and polyethylene tubing. Systems made of polyvinylchloride may adsorb up to 50% of the glyceryl trinitrate from the solution, thus reducing the efficacy of the infusion. If the recommended type of system is unavailable, a 1:10 dilution of Nitronal should be used and the infusion rate modified according to the haemodynamic response of the patient, until the required parameters are attained.

**Contra-indications, warnings, etc** These are common to all nitrates.

*Contra-indications:* Hypersensitivity to nitrates. Hypotensive shock, severe anaemia, cerebral haemorrhage, arterial hypoxaemia, uncorrected hypovolaemia and angina caused by hypertrophic obstructive cardiomyopathy.

*Precautions:* Caution should be exercised in patients with severe liver or renal disease, hypothermia or hypothyroidism. Glyceryl trinitrate may potentiate the action of other hypotensive drugs and the hypotensive and anticholinergic effects of tricyclic anti-depressants; it may also slow the metabolism of morphine-like analgesics.

*Pregnancy and lactation:* No information is available.

*Adverse reactions:* Nitronal is generally well tolerated because a minimum dose is administered in unit time. Headache, dizziness, flushing, hypotension and tachycardia may be encountered, particularly if the infusion is administered too rapidly. Nausea, diaphoresis, restlessness, retrosternal discomfort, abdominal pain and paradoxical bradycardia have been reported. These symptoms should be readily reversible on reducing the rate of infusion or, if necessary, discontinuing treatment.

*Overdosage – Signs and Symptoms:* Vomiting, restlessness, hypotension, syncope, cyanosis, coldness of the skin, impairment of respiration, bradycardia, psychosis and methaemoglobinaemia may occur.

*Overdosage – Treatment:* The symptoms may be readily reversed by discontinuing treatment; if hypotension persists, raising the foot of the bed and the use of vasoconstrictors such as intravenous methoxamine or phenylephrine is recommended. Methaemaglobinaemia should be treated by intravenous methylene blue. Oxygen and assisted respiration may be required.

**Pharmaceutical precautions** Store in a cool place away from light. The vial is for single dose use only, and should be stored in the carton until ready for use. The shelf life is 2 years.

The diluted solution should be administered as soon as possible; it is stable for up to 24 hours in the recommended infusion system.

**Legal category** POM.

**Package quantities** 10 ampoules; single vials.

**Further information** Nitronal is free of alcohol, propylene glycol and potassium. Glyceryl trinitrate is also known as nitroglycerin.

**Product licence number** 3759/0025.

## PRAXILENE*

**Presentation** Pale pink capsules marked PRAXILENE and LIPHA, each containing 100 mg of naftidrofuryl oxalate.

**Uses** *Indications:* Peripheral vascular disorders – intermittent claudication, night cramps, rest pain, incipient gangrene, trophic ulcers, Raynaud's syndrome, diabetic arteriopathy and acrocyanosis.

Cerebral vascular disorders – cerebral insufficiency and cerebral atherosclerosis, particularly where these manifest themselves as mental deterioration and confusion in the elderly.

*Pharmacology:* Praxilene has been shown to exert a direct effect on intracellular metabolism. Thus it has been demonstrated in man and animals that it produces an increase of ATP levels and a decrease of lactic acid levels in ischaemic conditions, evidence for an enhancement of cellular oxidative capacity. Furthermore Praxilene is a powerful spasmolytic agent.

**Dosage and administration**
*Adults and the Elderly:* Peripheral vascular disorders: one or two 100 mg capsules three times daily for a minimum of three months, or at the discretion of the Physician.

Cerebral vascular disorders: one 100 mg capsule three times daily for a minimum of three months, or at the discretion of the Physician.

*Children:* There is no recommended dose.

**Contra-indications, warnings, etc**
*Contra-indications:* Hypersensitivity to the drug.

*Use in pregnancy and lactation:* Pregnancy: There is no, or inadequate, evidence of safety of Praxilene in human pregnancy, but it has been in wide use for many years without apparent ill consequence, animal studies having shown no hazard. If drug therapy is needed in pregnancy, this drug can be used if there is no safer alternative.
Lactation: No information is available.

*Adverse reactions:* Praxilene is normally well tolerated in the dosage recommended. Occasionally nausea, epigastric pain and rashes have been noted. Rarely, hepatitis has been reported.

*Overdosage – Signs and symptoms:* Depression of cardiac conduction and convulsions may occur.

*Overdosage – Treatment:* The stomach should be emptied by gastric lavage and emesis. Activated charcoal may be employed if necessary. Cardiovascular function and respiration should be monitored and, in severe cases, electrical pacemaking or the use of isoprenaline should be considered. Convulsions may be managed by diazepam.

**Pharmaceutical precautions** Store below 20°C in a dry place away from light. The shelf-life is 3 years.

**Legal category** POM.

**Package quantities** Blister pack of 84 capsules (OP); containers of 100 and 500 capsules.

**Further information** Nil.

**Product licence number** 3759/0002.

## SLO-PHYLLIN*

**Presentation** Capsules marked SLO-PHYLLIN, LIPHA and with the capsule strength, containing Theophylline BP in a timed release formulation which provides a prolonged therapeutic effect over 12 hours.

*60 mg:* Opaque white capsule with a clear colourless cap, filled with white pellets.

*125 mg:* Opaque dark brown capsule with a clear colourless cap, filled with white pellets.

*250 mg:* Opaque blue capsule with a clear colourless cap, filled with white pellets.
Slo-Phyllin also contains sucrose.

**Uses** As a bronchodilator in the symptomatic and prophylactic treatment of asthma and for reversible bronchoconstriction associated with chronic bronchitis and bronchial asthma.

**Dosage and administration**
*Children:*

| | |
|---|---|
| 2–6 years (10–20 kg) | 60–120 mg twice daily |
| 6–12 years (20–35 kg) | 125–250 mg twice daily |
| Over 12 years | 250–500 mg twice daily |

*Adults:* 250–500 mg twice daily.

*Elderly:* There is a tendency for theophylline clearance to decrease with age leading to higher serum levels. A reduction of the adult dosage may therefore be necessary, and close monitoring is advised.

Each patient should be titrated to a suitable dosage regimen by clinical assessment. It may also be necessary to measure plasma theophylline levels.

Initially the lowest dosage for each group is recommended. This may be increased gradually if optimal bronchodilator effects are not achieved. The total dosage should not normally exceed 24 mg/kg bodyweight for children and 13 mg/kg for adults. However the plasma theophylline level measured 4–8 hours after dosing and at least 3 days after any dosage adjustment, provides a more accurate assessment of the patient's dosage need, especially as significant variations in the rate of drug elimination can occur between individuals. The following table provides a guide:

| *Plasma level (microgram/ml)* | *Result* | *Directions (if clinically indicated)* |
|---|---|---|
| Below 10 | Too low | Increase dose by 25% |
| 10–20 | Correct | Maintain dose |
| 20–25 | Too high | Decrease dose by 10% |
| 25–30 | | Miss next dose and decrease subsequent doses by 25% |
| Over 30 | | Miss next 2 doses and decrease subsequent doses by 50% |

It is advisable to recheck the plasma level after dose adjustment and every 6–12 months.

It is not possible to ensure bioequivalence between different sustained release theophylline products. Once titrated to an effective dose, patients should not be changed from Slo-Phyllin to another sustained release xanthine preparation without re-titration and clinical assessment.

Patients should be instructed not to chew or suck the capsules or pellets as this destroys the timed release properties. However, for those who experience difficulty in swallowing capsules, the contents of a capsule may be sprinkled on to a spoonful of soft food, e.g. yoghurt.

**Contra-indications, warnings, etc**
*Contra-indications:* Hypersensitivity to theophylline or other xanthines. Concomitant use with ephedrine in children.

*Precautions:* Smoking and alcohol consumption can increase the clearance of theophylline and a higher dosage may be necessary.

Careful monitoring is recommended for patients with congestive heart failure, chronic alcoholism, hepatic dysfunction or viral infections as they may have lower total clearance of theophylline which could lead to higher than normal plasma levels.

Caution should be exercised in patients with peptic ulcers, cardiac arrhythmias, other cardiovascular diseases, hyperthyroidism or hypertension.

Slo-Phyllin should not be used concurrently with other preparations containing xanthine derivatives. If it is necessary to administer aminophylline to a patient who is already receiving Slo-Phyllin, plasma theophylline concentrations should be monitored.

The use of alternative treatment is advised in patients with a history of seizures as these may be exacerbated by theophylline.

*Use in pregnancy and lactation:* Pregnancy: Slo-Phyllin is not recommended since theophylline is known to cross the placenta and its safety in pregnancy has not been established.

Lactation: Theophylline is distributed in breast milk and therefore Slo-Phyllin should be used with caution in nursing mothers.

*Adverse reactions:* These usually occur when theophylline blood levels exceed 20 micrograms/ml and include gastric irritation, nausea, vomiting, abdominal discomfort, palpitations, a fall in blood pressure, headache, occasional diarrhoea and insomnia. CNS stimulation and diuresis may also occur, especially in children.

*Overdosage – Signs and Symptoms:* Headache, nausea, vomiting, restlessness, hypotension, tachycardia, arrhythmias (usually supraventricular tachyarrhythmias), hypokalaemia, CNS depression, convulsions, dehydration and coma may occur. Massive overdosage may result in cardiac inhibition, circulatory and respiratory failure.

*Overdosage – Treatment:* The stomach should be emptied by gastric lavage and emesis. Repeated doses of activated charcoal should be considered. Blood glucose, electrolytes, arterial gases and pH should be monitored. Serum theophylline should be measured 4 h after ingestion and at 4 to 12 hourly intervals thereafter if symptoms are severe.

Intensive supportive therapy may be required to maintain respiration and cardiovascular function. Convulsions may be controlled by diazepam. Haemoperfusion may be necessary.

Slo-Phyllin is a timed-release capsule and effects may be slow in onset and prolonged.

*Drug interactions:* Theophylline has been reported to interact with a number of drugs.

The following increase clearance and it may therefore be necessary to increase dosage to ensure a therapeutic effect: barbiturates, carbamazepine, lithium, phenytoin, rifampicin, and sulphinpyrazone.

The following reduce clearance and a reduced dosage may therefore be necessary to avoid side-effects: allopurinol, cimetidine, ciprofloxacin, corticosteroids, diltiazem, erythromycin, frusemide, isoprenaline, oral contraceptives, thiabendazole, and verapamil.

There is some evidence of an interaction between theophylline and influenza vaccine.

Xanthines can potentiate hypokalaemia resulting from $beta_2$ agonist therapy, steroids, diuretics and hypoxia. Particular caution is advised in severe asthma. It is recommended that serum potassium levels are monitored in such situations.

The concomitant use of theophylline and fluvoxamine should usually be avoided. Where this is not possible, patients should have their theophylline dose halved and plasma theophylline should be monitored closely.

**Pharmaceutical precautions** Store below 25°C in a dry place. The shelf-life is 3 years.

**Legal category** P.

**Package quantities** Blister pack of 56 capsules (OP). Container of 100 capsules (250 mg strength only).

**Further information** The active pellets in each strength of Slo-Phyllin capsule are identical and the three presentations are therefore equally bioavailable. The three strengths thus allow optimum dose titration.

**Product licence numbers**

| | |
|---|---|
| Slo-Phyllin 60 mg | 0161/0021 |
| Slo-Phyllin 125 mg | 0161/0019 |
| Slo-Phyllin 250 mg | 0161/0020 |

## SLOZEM*

**Presentation** Hard gelatin capsules containing 120 mg, 180 mg and 240 mg diltiazem hydrochloride in sustained release pellet form. Each capsule is marked with the product name and strength. Each strength also has a unique colour coding:

120 mg natural transparent/pink transparent
180 mg natural transparent/pink opaque
240 mg natural transparent/scarlet opaque

Inactive ingredients in Slozem capsules include maize starch, sucrose, povidone, shellac, ethylcellulose, talc and the colourants E127, E132 and E172 (all strengths) and E171 (180 and 240 mg strengths).

**Uses**
*Mode of action:* Diltiazem hydrochloride is a calcium antagonist. It selectively reduces calcium entry through voltage-dependent calcium channels into vascular smooth muscle cells and myocardial cells. This lowers the concentration of intracellular calcium which is available to activate contractile proteins. In vascular tissue, diltiazem relaxes arterial smooth muscle, reducing systemic peripheral resistance and dilating the coronary arteries. In cardiac muscle diltiazem reduces contractility and slows the heart rate through its negative chronotropic and inotropic actions. Cardiac work and oxygen demand can therefore be reduced and high blood pressure lowered without reflex tachycardia.

The sustained release pellets in this presentation usually achieve maximum plasma diltiazem levels six to eight hours after dosing and have an apparent plasma elimination half-life of approximately 7 hours, allowing once daily dosing.

*Indications:* Mild to moderate hypertension. Angina pectoris.

**Dosage and administration** One dose should be given every 24 hours. There is no apparent food interaction with Slozem and the capsule(s) may, therefore, be taken with a meal or swallowed whole with a little water on an empty stomach.

*Adults:* Angina and hypertension: The recommended starting dose is one 240 mg capsule once daily. Patient responses may vary and dosage requirements can differ significantly between individual patients.

Dosage titration in 60 mg to 120 mg steps at 2-weekly intervals may be required to obtain satisfactory clinical response (usually 240 mg to 360 mg daily will suffice).

Dosage should be reduced in the presence of adverse reactions or if the pulse rate falls below 50 per minute.

*Elderly and patients with impaired hepatic or renal function:* Angina and hypertension: Dosage should be reduced, using a 120 mg starting dose, and 60 mg titration steps every two weeks until clinical response is satisfactorily achieved. Dosage should be reduced in the presence of adverse reactions or a pulse rate below 50 per minute. For co-prescription with other antihypertensive or antianginal agents see *interactions* below.

*Children:* Safety and efficacy in children have not been established.

**Contra-indications, warnings, etc**
*Contra-indications:* Slozem is contra-indicated in pregnancy and in women of childbearing potential. Slozem depresses atrioventricular node conduction and is therefore contraindicated in patients with marked bradycardia, sick sinus syndrome, uncontrolled heart failure or second or third degree AV block.

Hypersensitivity to diltiazem or any of the inactive ingredients is also a contra-indication.

*Warning and precautions:* Slozem should be used with caution in patients with reduced left ventricular function. Patients with mild bradycardia, and/or having a prolonged PR interval, should be observed closely.

*Interactions:* In common with other calcium antagonists, when Slozem is used with drugs which may induce bradycardia (e.g. amiodarone and beta-blockers) or with other antihypertensive drugs the possibility of an additive effect should be borne in mind.

Diltiazem has been used safely in combination with beta-blockers, diuretics, ACE inhibitors and other antihypertensive agents. It is recommended that patients receiving these combinations should be regularly monitored. Concomitant use of Slozem with alpha blockers such as prazosin should be strictly monitored because of the possible marked synergistic hypotensive effect of this combination.

Case reports have suggested that blood levels of carbamazepine, cyclosporin, and theophylline may be increased when given concurrently with diltiazem hydrochloride. Care should be exercised in patients taking these drugs. In common with other calcium antagonists diltiazem may cause small increases in plasma levels of digoxin.

In patients taking $H_2$ receptor antagonists concurrently with diltiazem, increased levels of diltiazem may be produced.

Diltiazem hydrochloride treatment has been continued without problem during anaesthesia, but the anaesthetist should be informed that the patient is receiving a calcium antagonist.

*Pregnancy:* Diltiazem hydrochloride is teratogenic in some animal species. In the absence of adequate evidence of safety in human pregnancy Slozem should not be used in pregnancy or in women of child bearing potential.

*Nursing mothers:* Diltiazem hydrochloride is excreted in breast milk. One report suggests that concentrations in breast milk reach similar levels to those in serum. If use of Slozem is considered essential, an alternative method of infant feeding should be instituted.

*Adverse effects:* The following have been reported: ankle oedema, malaise, headache, hot flushes, gastrointestinal disturbances and very rarely symptomatic bradycardia, sino-atrial block and atrio-ventricular block. Rash has been reported in association with diltiazem. These reactions are generally mild and resolve on cessation of therapy; however, severe

vascular skin reactions have been reported occasionally. Isolated cases of moderate and transient elevation of liver transaminases have been observed at the start of treatment. Isolated cases of clinical hepatitis have been reported which resolved on cessation of therapy.

The current literature suggests that the effects of vasodilation, particularly ankle oedema, are dose dependent and are more frequent in the elderly.

*Overdose – Signs and symptoms:* Acute intoxication can lead to severe hypotension, bradycardia, first to third degree atrioventricular block and, on occasion, to cardiac arrest. Hyperglycaemia may require treatment. Onset of symptoms may be delayed for several hours after ingestion and have been described after as little as 900 mg diltiazem.

*Treatment:* Observation in a coronary or intensive care unit is advisable if a substantial overdose has been ingested. Soon after ingestion, gastric lavage followed by 50–100 mg activated charcoal may reduce absorption. Profound hypotension requires plasma expanders, IV calcium gluconate and inotropic agents (e.g. dopamine, dobutamine or isoprenaline). Symptomatic bradycardia and heart block may respond to atropine, isoprenaline or, if necessary, cardiac pacing.

Slozem capsules are extended release capsules and effects may be slow in onset and prolonged.

**Pharmaceutical precautions**  Store below 30°C in a dry place. The shelf life is 3 years.

**Legal category**  POM.

**Package quantities**  Blister packs of 28 and 56 capsules.

**Further information**  Diltiazem is well absorbed from

the gastrointestinal tract and is subject to an extensive first-pass effect, giving an absolute bioavailability (compared to intravenous administration) of about 40%.

Diltiazem in plasma is 80–85% protein bound. Plasma levels above 40–50 ng/ml are associated with pharmaceutical activity.

Diltiazem is extensively metabolised by the liver, the apparent plasma half-life being on average 3–4.5 hours.

The two major active circulating metabolites, desacetyl-diltiazem and N-monodesmethyl diltiazem possess coronary artery vasodilatory activity equivalent to about 50% of that of diltiazem. Only 0.2 to 4% diltiazem is found unchanged in the urine.

The bioavailability of diltiazem from the Slozem formulation given once a day is equivalent to that obtained from a conventional release tablet given three times a day, when the same total daily dose is administered.

Data from studies in patients and healthy volunteers have also demonstrated that trough plasma levels (i.e. 24 hours post dosing) can be maintained within the minimum therapeutic range by appropriate dose titration.

Plasma concentrations in elderly patients and in hepatic failure are in general higher than in young subjects, due to an increase in apparent bioavailability. In renal failure, a reduction in dosage is only necessary as a function of the clinical response.

**Product licence numbers**
120 mg   03759/0043
180 mg   03759/0044
240 mg   03759/0045

*Trade Mark

# The Liposome Company Ltd
## 3 Shortlands
## Hammersmith International Centre
## London W6 8EH

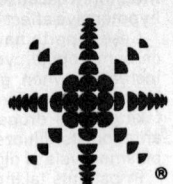

## ABELCET* ▼

**Qualitative and quantitative composition** Abelcet is supplied as a sterile, pyrogen-free suspension in isotonic saline. Each ml of the suspension contains 5.0 mg (5000 IU) of Amphotericin B USP. The full composition is presented in the following table:

| | |
|---|---|
| Amphotericin B USP | 5.0 mg |
| L-α-Dimyristoylphosphatidylcholine (DMPC) | 3.4 mg |
| L-α-Dimyristoylphosphatidylglycerol (DMPG) (as sodium and ammonium salts) | 1.5 mg |
| Sodium Chloride | 9.0 mg |
| Water for Injection, q.s. ad | 1.0 ml |

**Pharmaceutical form** Abelcet is supplied as a suspension containing 5.0 mg amphotericin B per ml, in vials containing 20 ml (100 mg, 100 000 IU of amphotericin B) which must be diluted before intravenous infusion, according to Posology and method of administration section.

### Clinical particulars

*Clinical indications:* Abelcet is indicated for the treatment of severe invasive candidiasis.

Abelcet is also indicated as second line therapy for the treatment of severe systemic fungal infections in patients who have not responded to conventional amphotericin B or other systemic antifungal agents, in those who have renal impairment or other contra-indications to conventional amphotericin B, or in patients who have developed amphotericin B nephrotoxicity. Abelcet treatment is indicated as second line treatment for invasive aspergillosis, cryptococcal meningitis and disseminated cryptococcosis in HIV patients, fusariosis, coccidioidomycosis, zygomycosis and blastomycosis.

*Posology and method of administration:* Abelcet is a sterile, pyrogen-free suspension to be diluted for intravenous infusion only.

For severe systemic infections treatment is generally recommended at 5.0 mg/kg for at least 14 days. Abelcet should be administered by intravenous infusion at a rate of 2.5 mg/kg/hr. An initial test dose of 1.0 mg should be infused intravenously over 15 minutes. As for use with all amphotericin B products, facilities for cardiopulmonary resuscitation should be readily at hand when administering Abelcet, due to the possible occurrence of anaphylactoid reactions. Abelcet has been administered for as long as 11 months, and cumulative doses have been as high as 56.6 g without significant toxicity.

An in-line filter may be used for intravenous infusion of Abelcet. The mean pore diameter of the filter should be no less than 5.0 microns.

*Paediatric use:* Systemic fungal infections in children have been treated successfully with Abelcet at doses comparable to the recommended adult dose on a body weight basis.

Adverse events seen in paediatric patients are similar to those seen in adults.

*Use in elderly patients:* Systemic fungal infections in elderly patients have been treated successfully with Abelcet at doses comparable to the recommended dose on a body weight basis.

*Use in neutropenic patients:* Abelcet has been used successfully to treat systemic fungal infections in patients who are severely neutropenic as a consequence of haematological malignancy or the use of cytotoxic or immunosuppressive drugs.

*Contra-indications:* Abelcet is contra-indicated in patients with known hypersensitivity to any of its constituents, unless in the opinion of the physician the advantages of using Abelcet outweigh the risks of hypersensitivity.

*Special warnings and special precautions for use*

*Systemic fungal infections:* Abelcet should not be used for treating common or superficial, clinically inapparent fungal infections that are detectable only by positive skin or serologic tests.

*Renal disease:* Since Abelcet is a potentially nephrotoxic drug, monitoring of renal function should be performed before initiating treatment in patients with pre-existing renal disease, and at least once weekly during therapy. Abelcet should be administered to renal dialysis patients only after the completion of dialysis. Serum potassium and magnesium levels should be monitored regularly.

*Liver disease:* Patients with concurrent hepatic impairment due to infection, graft-versus-host disease, other liver disease or administration of hepatotoxic drugs have been successfully treated with Abelcet. In cases where serum bilirubin, alkaline phosphatase or serum transaminases increased, factors other than Abelcet were present and possibly accounted for the abnormalities. These factors included infection, hyperalimentation, concomitant hepatotoxic drugs and graft-versus-host disease.

*Interactions with other medicaments and other forms of interactions:*

*Nephrotoxic drugs:* Abelcet is a potentially nephrotoxic drug, and particularly close monitoring of renal function is required in patients receiving nephrotoxic drugs concomitantly.

*Zidovudine:* In dogs, exacerbated myelotoxicity and nephrotoxicity were observed when Abelcet was administered concomitantly with zidovudine. If concomitant treatment with zidovudine is required, renal and haematologic function should be closely monitored.

*Cyclosporin:* Preliminary data suggest that patients receiving Abelcet concomitantly with high dose cyclosporin experience an increase in serum creatinine. The data also suggest that the increase in serum creatinine is caused by cyclosporin and not Abelcet.

The interaction of Abelcet with other drugs has not been studied to date. Conventional amphotericin B has been reported to interact with antineoplastic agents, corticosteroids and corticotrophin (ACTH), digitalis glycosides and skeletal muscle relaxants.

*Leukocyte transfusions:* Acute pulmonary toxicity has been reported in patients receiving intravenous amphotericin B and leukocyte transfusions.

*Pregnancy and lactation:* Conventional amphotericin B has been used successfully to treat systemic fungal infections in pregnant women with no obvious effects on the foetus, but only a small number of cases have been reported. Reproductive toxicity studies of Abelcet in rats and rabbits showed no evidence of embryotoxicity, foetotoxicity or teratogenicity. However, safety for use in pregnant or lactating women has not been established for Abelcet. Therefore, Abelcet should be administered to pregnant or lactating women only for life-threatening disease when the likely benefit exceeds the risk to the mother and foetus.

*Effect on ability to drive and use machines:* Abelcet is unlikely to affect the ability of an individual to drive or use machines, since adverse reactions are usually infusion-related. However, the clinical condition of patients who require Abelcet generally precludes driving or operating machinery.

*Undesirable effects:* Patients in whom significant renal toxicity was observed following conventional amphotericin B frequently did not experience similar effects when Abelcet was substituted. Adverse reactions related to the administration of Abelcet have generally been mild or moderate, and have been most prevalent during the first 2 days of dosing.

Premedication (e.g. paracetamol) may be administered for the prevention of infusion related adverse events. The most common clinical adverse events have been chills, fever, nausea and vomiting, which may occur during the first 2 days of treatment.

Declines in renal function, shown by increased serum creatinine, azotaemia and hypokalaemia, have not typically required discontinuation of treatment. Abelcet has not been reported to directly cause changes in hepatic or haemotologic function.

Adverse reactions that have been reported to occur with conventional amphotericin B may occur with Abelcet. In general, the physician should monitor the patient for any type of adverse event associated with conventional amphotericin B.

*Overdose:* No instance of toxicity due to overdose with Abelcet has been reported. One paediatric patient received a single dose of 13.1 mg/kg on one occasion, without adverse effects. Should an overdose occur, the patient should be treated as deemed appropriate by the physician.

**Pharmacological properties** Abelcet consists of the antifungal agent, amphotericin B, complexed to two phospholipids. Amphotericin B is a macrocyclic, polyene, broad-spectrum antifungal antibiotic produced by *Streptomyces nodosus*. The lipophilic moiety of amphotericin B allows molecules of the drug to be complexed in a ribbon-like structure with the phospholipids.

*Pharmacodynamic properties*

*Mechanism of action:* Amphotericin B, the active antifungal agent in Abelcet, may be fungistatic or fungicidal, depending on its concentration and on fungal susceptibility. The drug probably acts by binding to ergosterol in the fungal cell membrane causing subsequent membrane damage. As a result, cell contents leak from the fungal cell, and, ultimately, cell death occurs. Binding of the drug to sterols in human cell membranes may result in toxicity, although amphotericin B has greater affinity for fungal ergosterol than for the cholesterol of human cells.

*Microbiological activity:* Amphotericin B is active against many fungal pathogens *in vitro*, including *Candida* spp., *Cryptococcus neoformans*, *Aspergillus* spp., *Mucor* spp., *Sporothrix schenckii*, *Blastomyces dermatitidis*, *Coccidioides immitis* and *Histoplasma capsulatum*. Most strains are inhibited by amphotericin B concentrations of 0.03–1.0 mcg/ml. Amphotericin B has little or no activity against bacteria or viruses. The activity of Abelcet against fungal pathogens *in vitro* is comparable to that of amphotericin B. However, activity of Abelcet *in vitro* may not predict activity in the infected host.

*Pharmacokinetic properties:* Amphotericin B is complexed to phospholipids in Abelcet. The pharmacokinetic properties of Abelcet and conventional amphotericin B are different. Pharmacokinetic studies in animals showed that, after administration of Abelcet, amphotericin B levels were highest in the liver, spleen and lung. Amphotericin B in Abelcet was rapidly distributed to tissues. The ratio of drug concentrations in tissues to those in blood increased disproportionately with increasing dose, suggesting that elimination of the drug from the tissues was delayed. Peak blood levels of amphotericin B were lower after administration of Abelcet than after administration of equivalent amounts of conventional drug. Administration of conventional amphotericin B resulted in much lower tissue levels than did dosing with Abelcet. However, in dogs, conventional amphotericin B produced 20-fold higher kidney concentrations than did Abelcet given at comparable doses.

The pharmacokinetics of Abelcet in whole blood were determined in patients with mucocutaneous leishmaniasis. Results for mean pharmacokinetic parameters at 5.0 mg/kg/day were as follows:

| | Abelcet |
|---|---|
| Dose: (mg/kg/day) | 5.0 |
| Peak blood level $C_{max}$: (mcg/ml) | 1.7 |
| Area under time-concentration curve | |
| $AUC_{0-24}$: (mcg•hr/ml) | 9.5 |
| Clearance: (ml/hr•kg) | 211.0 |
| Volume of distribution Vd: (l) | 2286.0 |
| Half-life $T_{1/2}$: (hr) | 173.4 |

The rapid clearance and large volume of distribution of Abelcet result in a relatively low AUC and are consistent with preclinical data showing high tissue concentrations. The kinetics of Abelcet are linear and the AUC increases proportionately with dose.

Details of the tissue distribution and metabolism of Abelcet in humans, and the mechanisms responsible for reduced toxicity, are not well understood. The following data are available from necropsy in a heart transplant patient who received Abelcet at a dose of 5.3 mg/kg for 3 consecutive days immediately before death:

| Organ | Abelcet tissue concentration expressed as Amphotericin B content (mg/kg) |
|---|---|
| Spleen | 290.0 |
| Lung | 222.0 |
| Liver | 196.0 |
| Kidney | 6.9 |
| Lymph node | 7.6 |
| Heart | 5.0 |
| Brain | 1.6 |

*Preclinical safety data:* Acute toxicity studies in rodents showed that Abelcet was 10-fold to 20-fold less toxic than conventional amphotericin B. Multiple-dose toxicity studies in dogs lasting 2–4 weeks showed that on a mg/kg basis, Abelcet was 8-fold to 10-fold less nephrotoxic than conventional amphotericin B.

This decreased nephrotoxicity was presumably a result of lower drug concentrations in the kidney.

*Carcinogenesis, mutagenesis and impairment of fertility:* Since conventional amphotericin B first became available, there have been no reports of drug-related carcinogenicity, mutagenicity, teratogenicity or adverse effect on fertility. Abelcet has been shown not to be mutagenic by the *in vivo* mouse micronucleus assay, *in vitro* bacterial and lymphoma mutation assays, and an *in vivo* cytogenetic assay. It has been shown not to be teratogenic in mice and rabbits.

Phospholipids are essential constituents of human cell membranes. The average diet provides several grams of phospholipids each day. There is no evidence that phospholipids, including DMPC and DMPG, are carcinogenic, mutagenic or teratogenic.

## Pharmaceutical particulars

*List of excipients:* Each ml of Abelcet contains 3.4 mg L-α-dimyristoylphosphatidylcholine (DMPC), 1.5 mg L-α-dimyristoylphosphatidylglycerol (sodium and ammonium salts) (DMPG), 9.0 mg sodium chloride, and Water for Injection, q.s. ad 1.0 ml.

*Incompatibilities:* Abelcet should not be mixed with other drugs or electrolytes.

*Shelf life:* Results of stability studies substantiate a shelf life of 24 months at 5°C.

*Special precautions for storage:* Abelcet should be stored under refrigeration at +2 to +8°C. Do not freeze. Protect from light.

*Nature and contents of container:* Abelcet is a sterile, pyrogen-free yellow suspension in a single use vial containing 20 ml (100 mg amphotericin B). The vial is sealed with a rubber stopper and aluminium seal. Vials are packaged in cartons of 10 vials.

*Instructions for use/handling:* Abelcet is a sterile, pyrogen-free suspension to be diluted for intravenous infusion only.

*Preparation of the suspension for infusion:* Aseptic technique must be strictly observed throughout handling of Abelcet, since no bacteriostatic agent or preservative is present. Allow the suspension to come to room temperature. Shake gently until there is no evidence of any yellow settlement at the bottom of the vial. Withdraw the appropriate dose of Abelcet from the required number of vials into one or more sterile 20 ml syringes using a 17 to 19 gauge needle. Remove the needle from each syringe filled with Abelcet and replace with the 5 micron filter needle (supplied by B. Braun Medical, Inc.) provided with

each vial. Insert the filter needle of the syringe into an IV bag containing 5.0% Dextrose for Injection and empty the content of the syringe into the bag using either manual pressure or an infusion pump. The final infusion concentration should be 1 mg/ml. Do not use the agent after dilution with 5.0% Dextrose for Injection if there is any evidence of foreign matter. Vials are single use. Unused material should be discarded. The infusion is best administered by means of an infusion pump.

DO NOT DILUTE WITH SALINE SOLUTIONS OR MIX WITH OTHER DRUGS OR ELECTROLYTES. The compatibility of Abelcet with these materials has not been established. An existing intravenous line should be flushed with 5.0% Dextrose for Injection before infusion of Abelcet or a separate infusion line should be used.

The diluted ready for use suspension is stable for up to 15 hours at +2 to +8°C, and may be stable for a further 6 hours at room temperature. Do not store for later use.

**Marketing authorisation number** 14188/0001.

**Date of approval/revision of SPC** 12 March 1996.

**Legal catetgory** POM.

*\*Trade Mark*

# Lorex Synthélabo Ltd
Foundation Park
Roxborough Way
Maidenhead
Berkshire SL6 3UD

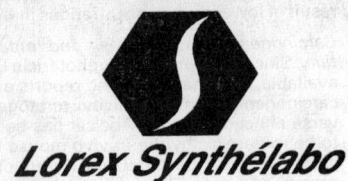

## TILDIEM*

**Presentation** Off-white biconvex tablets, engraved Tildiem 60. Each tablet contains 60 mg of diltiazem hydrochloride in a modified release formulation.

### Uses
*Mode of action:* Tildiem (diltiazem hydrochloride) is a calcium antagonist. It selectively reduces calcium entry through voltage-dependent calcium channels into vascular smooth muscle cells and myocardial cells. This lowers the concentration of intracellular calcium which is available to activate contractile proteins. This action of diltiazem results in dilation of coronary arteries causing an increase in myocardial oxygen supply. It reduces cardiac work by moderating the heart rate and reducing systemic vascular resistance thus reducing oxygen demand.

When Tildiem is given alone or with a beta-blocking agent only slight negative inotropic effects have been reported in patients with preserved ventricular function.

*Indication:* Angina pectoris.

### Dosage and administration
*Adults:* The usual dose is one tablet (60 mg) three times daily. However, patient responses may vary and dosage requirements can differ significantly between individual patients. If necessary the dosage may be increased to 360 mg/day. Higher doses up to 480 mg/day have been used with benefit in some patients especially in unstable angina. There is no evidence of any decrease in efficacy at these high doses.

*Elderly and patients with impaired hepatic or renal function:* The recommended starting dose is one tablet (60 mg) twice daily. The heart rate should be measured regularly in these groups of patients and the dose should not be increased if the heart rate falls below 50 beats per minute.

*Children:* Safety and efficacy in children have not been established.

### Contra-indications, warnings, etc
*Contra-indications:* Tildiem is contra-indicated in pregnancy and in women of child-bearing potential.

Tildiem depresses atrioventricular node conduction and is therefore contra-indicated in patients with marked bradycardia, sick sinus syndrome, left ventricular failure with stasis, or second or third degree AV block except in the presence of a functioning pacemaker.

Tildiem, like any calcium antagonist, should not be administered concurrently with dantrolene infusion because of the risk of ventricular fibrillation.

*Warnings and precautions:* Tildiem should be used with caution in patients with reduced left ventricular function. Patients with mild bradycardia, first degree AV block or prolonged PR interval should be observed closely.

*Drug interactions:* In common with other calcium antagonists, when Tildiem is used with drugs which may induce bradycardia or with antiarrhythmic or other antihypertensive drugs the possibility of an additive effect should be borne in mind.

Case reports have suggested that blood levels of carbamazepine, cyclosporin, and theophylline may be increased when given concurrently with diltiazem hydrochloride. Care should be exercised in patients taking these drugs. In common with other calcium antagonists Tildiem may cause small increases in plasma levels of digoxin.

In patients taking $H_2$ antagonists concurrently with Tildiem there may be increased levels of diltiazem.

Tildiem has been used safely in combination with beta-blockers, diuretics, ACE inhibitors and other antihypertensive agents. It is recommended that patients receiving these combinations should be regularly monitored. Concomitant use of Tildiem with alpha blockers such as prazosin should be strictly monitored because of the possible synergistic hypotensive effect of this combination.

Diltiazem hydrochloride treatment has been continued without problem during anaesthesia, but the anaesthetist should be informed that the patient is receiving a calcium antagonist.

*Pregnancy:* Diltiazem hydrochloride is teratogenic in some animal species. In the absence of adequate evidence of safety in human pregnancy, Tildiem should not be used in pregnancy or in women of child bearing potential.

*Nursing mothers:* Diltiazem hydrochloride is excreted in breast milk. One report suggests that concentrations in breast milk reach similar levels to those in serum. If use of Tildiem is considered essential, an alternative method of infant feeding should be instituted.

*Adverse effects:* Adverse effects are generally mild and transient and are most commonly vasodilatory related events. The following have been described: lower limb oedema, headache, hot flushes/flushing, asthenia/fatigue, palpitations, malaise, minor gastro-intestinal disorders (dyspepsia, abdominal pain, dry mouth) and skin rash. Vasodilatory related events (in particular, oedema) are dose-dependent and appear to be more frequent in elderly subjects.

Rare cases of symptomatic bradycardia, sino-atrial block and atrioventricular block were also recorded.

Experience with diltiazem has shown that skin rashes such as cases of simple erythema, urticaria or occasionally desquamative erythema with or without fever are usually localised and regress when treatment is discontinued. However, erythema multiforme and vasculitis have been reported occasionally.

Isolated cases of moderate and transient elevation of liver transaminases have been observed at the start of treatment. Isolated cases of clinical hepatitis have been reported which resolved on cessation of therapy.

*Overdosage:* The clinical consequences of overdose can be severe hypotension leading to collapse, and sinus bradycardia which may be accompanied by isorhythmic dissociation and atrioventricular conduction disturbances. Observation in a coronary care unit is advisable. Vasopressors such as adrenaline may be indicated in patients exhibiting profound hypotension. Calcium gluconate may help reverse the effects of calcium entry blockade. Atropine administration and temporary cardiac pacing may be required to manage bradycardia and/or conduction disturbances.

**Pharmaceutical precautions** Store in a dry place below 30°C (86°F).

**Legal category** POM.

**Package quantities** Packs of 100 tablets containing blister strips of 10 tablets.

**Further information** Diltiazem hydrochloride is effective in angina, protecting the heart against ischaemia, vasodilating coronary arteries and reducing myocardial oxygen requirements. It is well tolerated and does not generally give rise to side effects associated with peripheral vasodilators, nor cause significant myocardial depression.

In pharmacokinetic studies in healthy volunteers, diltiazem was well absorbed. Peak plasma concentrations were reached 3 to 4 hours after dosing. Due to a first pass effect the bioavailability of the Tildiem tablet is about 50%. Mean apparent plasma half life is 5 hours. Diltiazem in plasma is 80–85% protein bound and is poorly dialysed. Diltiazem is extensively metabolised by the liver. The two major active circulating metabolites, desacetyl-diltiazem and N-monodemethyl diltiazem possess pharmacological activity equivalent to about 50% of that of diltiazem. Only 0.2 to 4% of diltiazem is found unchanged in the urine.

There is a linear relationship between dose and plasma concentration. During long-term administration in any one patient plasma concentrations of diltiazem remained constant.

**Product licence number** 4969/0005.

## TILDIEM* LA 200
## TILDIEM* LA 300

**Qualitative and quantitative composition** Each capsule contains a combination of immediate-release and sustained-release pellets with 200 mg or 300 mg diltiazem hydrochloride as the active ingredient.

**Pharmaceutical form** Opaque capsules for oral administration with a grey body and pink cap (Tildiem LA 200) or white body and yellow cap (Tildiem LA 300).

### Clinical particulars
*Therapeutic indications:* Mild to moderate hypertension and angina pectoris.

*Posology and method of administration:* Tildiem LA 200 and Tildiem LA 300 are sustained release products for once daily dosing. The capsules should not be chewed but swallowed whole with water, ideally before or during a meal. The dosage requirements may differ in patients with angina or hypertension.

Tildiem (diltiazem hydrochloride) is available in a range of presentations to enable dosage to be adjusted to meet the individual requirements of the patient. Careful titration of the dose should be considered where appropriate, as individual patient response may vary. When changing from one type of Tildiem formulation to another it may be necessary to adjust the dosage until a satisfactory response is obtained. To ensure consistency of response once established, particularly in the sustained release formulations, Tildiem LA 200 and 300 should continue to be prescribed by brand name.

*Adults:*

*Angina and hypertension:* the usual starting dose is Tildiem LA 300 once daily. This dose may be increased to 2 capsules of Tildiem LA 200 daily (400 mg), and if clinically indicated a higher dose of one Tildiem LA 300 plus one Tildiem LA 200 capsule (total 500 mg) may be considered.

*Elderly and patients with impaired hepatic or renal function:* Heart rate should be monitored and if it falls below 50 beats per minute the dose should not be increased. Plasma levels of diltiazem can be increased in this group of patients.

*Angina and hypertension:* the initial dose should be one Tildiem LA 200 capsule daily. This dose may be increased to one capsule of Tildiem LA 300 daily if clinically indicated.

*Children:* Safety and efficacy in children have not been established.

*Contra-indications:* Sick sinus syndrome, 2nd or 3rd degree AV block in patients not fitted with a pacemaker.

Severe bradycardia (less than 50 beats per minute).

Left ventricular failure with pulmonary stasis.

Pregnancy, women of childbearing potential and lactation.

Concurrent use with dantrolene infusion.

*Special warnings and special precautions for use:* Close observation is necessary in patients with reduced left ventricular function, mild bradycardia (risk of exacerbation) or with a 1st degree AV block or prolonged PR interval detected on the electrocardiogram (risk of exacerbation and rarely, of complete block). Plasma diltiazem concentrations can be increased in the elderly and patients with renal and hepatic insufficiency. The contraindications and precautions should be carefully observed and close monitoring, particularly of heart rate and the electrocardiogram, should be carried out at the beginning of treatment.

In the case of general anaesthesia, the anaesthetist must be informed that the patient is taking diltiazem.

*Interaction with other medicaments and other forms of interaction:* Combination contra-indicated for safety reasons: *Dantrolene* (infusion): The combination of a calcium antagonist and dantrolene is potentially dangerous because of the risk of ventricular fibrillation and this combination should not be used.

*Combinations requiring caution:*

*Alpha₁-antagonists:* Increased hypotensive effect. Concomitant treatment with alpha₁ antagonists should be considered only with strict monitoring of blood pressure.

*Beta-blockers:* Possibility of rhythm disturbances (pronounced bradycardia, sinus arrest), sino-atrial and atrioventricular conduction disturbances and heart failure (synergistic effect). Such a combination must only be used under close clinical and ECG monitoring, particularly at the beginning of treatment.

*Digoxin:* Increased risk of bradycardia; caution is required when digoxin is combined with diltiazem, particularly in elderly subjects and when high doses are used.

*Antiarrhythmic agents:* Since diltiazem has antiarrhythmic properties, its concomitant prescription with other antiarrhythmic agents is not recommended due to the risk of increased adverse effects on the heart due to an additive effect. This combination is not without problems and should only be used under close clinical and ECG monitoring.

*Nitrate derivatives:* Increased hypotensive effects and faintness (additive vasodilating effects). In all patients treated with calcium antagonists, the prescription of nitrate derivatives should only be carried out at gradually increasing doses.

*Cyclosporin:* Increase in circulating cyclosporin levels. It is recommended that the cyclosporin dose be reduced, renal function be monitored, circulating cyclosporin levels be assayed and that the dose should be adjusted during combined therapy and after its discontinuation.

*Carbamazepine:* Increase in circulating carbamazepine levels.

*Theophylline:* Increase in circulating theophylline levels.

*$H_2$ antagonists (cimetidine and ranitidine):* Increase in plasma diltiazem concentrations.

*Use during pregnancy and lactation:* Pregnancy: this drug has been shown to be teratogenic in certain animal species and is therefore contraindicated in pregnancy and in women of child-bearing potential.

Breast feeding: as this drug is excreted in breast milk, breast feeding whilst taking diltiazem should be avoided.

*Effects on ability to drive and use machines:* No effect reported to date.

*Undesirable effects:* Adverse effects are generally mild and transient and are most commonly vasodilatory related events. The following have been described: lower limb oedema, headache, hot flushes/flushing, asthenia/fatigue, palpitations, malaise, minor gastrointestinal disorders (dyspepsia, abdominal pain, dry mouth) and skin rash. Vasodilatory related events (in particular, oedema) are dose-dependent and appear to be more frequent in the elderly.

Rare cases of symptomatic bradycardia and exceptionally sino-atrial block and atrioventricular block were also recorded.

Experience with use in other indications and with other formulations, has shown that skin rashes are usually localised and are limited to cases of erythema, urticaria or occasionally desquamative erythema, with or without fever, which regress when treatment is discontinued. Isolated cases of moderate and transient elevation of liver transaminases have been observed at the start of treatment. Isolated cases of clinical hepatitis have been reported which resolved on cessation of therapy.

*Overdose:* The clinical effects of acute overdose can involve pronounced hypotension leading to collapse, sinus bradycardia with or without isorhythmic dissociation, and atrioventricular conduction disturbances.

Treatment, under hospital supervision, will include gastric lavage, osmotic diuresis. Conduction disturbances may be managed by temporary pacing.

Proposed antidotes: atropine, adrenaline, glucagon or calcium gluconate.

**Pharmacological properties** Calcium antagonist, antihypertensive agent.

*Pharmacodynamic properties:* Diltiazem restricts calcium entry into the slow calcium channel of vascular smooth muscle and myocardial muscle fibres in a voltage-dependent manner. By this mechanism, diltiazem reduces the concentration of intracellular calcium in contractile protein.

*In animals* diltiazem increases coronary blood flow without inducing any coronary steal phenomena. It acts both on small, large and collateral arteries. This vasodilator effect, which is moderate on peripheral systemic arterial territories, can be seen at doses that are not negatively inotropic.

The two major active circulating metabolites, i.e. deacetyl diltiazem and N-monodemethyl diltiazem, possess pharmacological activity in angina corresponding to 10 and 20% respectively of that of the parent compound.

*In humans* diltiazem increases coronary blood flow by reducing coronary resistance.

Due to its moderate bradycardia-inducing activity and the reduction in systemic arterial resistance, diltiazem reduces cardiac workload.

Tildiem LA does not have a significant myocardial depressant action in man.

*Pharmacokinetic particulars:* Diltiazem is well absorbed (90%) in healthy volunteers following chronic oral administration. The sustained release capsule provides prolonged absorption of the active constituent, producing steady state plasma concentrations

between 2 and 14 hours post-dose, during which time peak plasma levels occur.

Bioavailability of Tildiem LA relative to the Tildiem 60 mg formulation is approximately 80%. The mean apparent plasma half-life is 8 hours.

Diltiazem in plasma is 80 to 85% protein bound and is poorly dialysed. It is extensively metabolised by the liver.

The major circulating metabolites, deacetyldiltiazem and N-monodemethyl diltiazem, possess pharmacological activity equivalent to about 50% that of diltiazem.

Only 0.7 to 5% of diltiazem is found unchanged in the urine.

There is a linear relationship between dose and plasma concentration. During long term administration in any one patient, plasma concentrations of diltiazem remained constant. Mean plasma concentrations in the elderly and patients with renal and hepatic insufficiency are higher than in young subjects.

*Preclinical safety data:* No data of therapeutic relevance.

**Pharmaceutical particulars**

*List of excipients*

*Tildiem LA 200:* microcrystalline cellulose, acrylic and methacrylic esters copolymer, ethylcellulose, sodium carboxymethylcellulose, diacetylated monoglycerides, magnesium stearate. *In the capsule:* gelatin, black iron oxide (E172), red iron oxide (E172), titanium dioxide (E171).

*Tildiem LA 300:* microcrystalline cellulose, acrylic and methacrylic esters copolymer, ethylcellulose, sodium carboxymethylcellulose, diacetylated monoglycerides, magnesium stearate. *In the capsule:* gelatin, titanium dioxide (E171), yellow iron oxide (E172).

*Incompatibilities:* Not applicable.

*Shelf life:* Three years (Tildiem LA 200). Two years (Tildiem LA 300).

*Special precautions for storage:* To be stored below 25°C.

*Nature and contents of container:* 7 or 28 capsules, in a PVC/foil blister strip.

*Instructions for use:* Please consult the package insert before use. Do not use after the stated expiry date on the carton and blister strip. Keep out of the reach of children.

**Marketing authorisation numbers**
Tildiem LA 200    4969/0016
Tildiem LA 300    4969/0014.

**Date of approval/revision of SPC**    18 March 1996.

**Legal category**   POM.

# TILDIEM RETARD* 90 mg
# TILDIEM RETARD* 120 mg

**Qualitative and quantitative composition**   Each tablet contains 90 mg or 120 mg diltiazem hydrochloride as the active ingredient.

**Pharmaceutical form**   Off white biconvex sustained release tablet for oral administration.

**Clinical particulars**

*Therapeutic indications:* Mild to moderate hypertension and angina pectoris.

*Posology and method of administration:* Tildiem Retard tablets should be swallowed with a little water and not chewed.

Patients should be advised that the tablet membrane may pass through the gastro-intestinal tract unchanged.

Tildiem (diltiazem hydrochloride) is available in a range of presentations to enable dosage to be adjusted to meet the individual requirements of the patient. Careful titration of the dose should be considered where appropriate, as individual patient response may vary. When changing from one type of Tildiem formulation to another it may be necessary to adjust the dosage until a satisfactory response is obtained. To ensure consistency of response once established, particularly in the sustained release formulations, Tildiem Retard 90 mg and 120 mg should continue to be prescribed by brand name.

*Adults: Angina and hypertension:* The usual starting dose is one tablet (90 mg or 120 mg) twice daily. Patient responses may vary and dosage requirements can differ significantly between individual patients. Higher divided doses up to 480 mg/day have been used with benefit in some angina patients especially in unstable angina. Doses of 360 mg/day may be required to provide adequate BP control in hypertensive patients.

*Elderly and patients with impaired hepatic or renal function:* Heart rate should be monitored in these patients and if it falls below 50 beats per minute the dose should not be increased.

*Angina:* The recommended starting dose is one

Tildiem 60 mg tablet twice daily. This dose may be increased to one 90 mg or 120 mg Tildiem Retard tablet twice daily.

*Hypertension:* The starting dose should be one 120 mg Tildiem Retard tablet daily. Dose adjustment to one 90 mg or one 120 mg Tildiem Retard tablet twice daily may be required.

*Children:* Safety and efficacy in children have not been established.

*Contra-indications:* Tildiem Retard is contra-indicated in pregnancy and in women of child bearing potential.

Tildiem Retard depresses atrioventricular node conduction and is therefore contraindicated in patients with marked bradycardia, sick sinus syndrome, left ventricular failure with stasis or second or third degree AV block except in the presence of a functioning pacemaker.

Tildiem Retard, like any calcium antagonist, should not be administered concurrently with Dantrolene infusion because of the risk of ventricular fibrillation.

*Special warnings and special precautions for use:* Tildiem Retard should be used with caution in patients with reduced left ventricular function. Patients with mild bradycardia, first degree AV block or a prolonged PR interval should be observed closely. Diltiazem does not affect the glucose or endogenous insulin responses to hypoglycaemia.

*Interaction with other medicaments and other forms of interaction:* In common with other calcium antagonists, when Tildiem Retard is used with drugs which may induce bradycardia or with other antiarrhythmic or antihypertensive drugs, the possibility of an additive effect should be borne in mind.

Tildiem Retard has been used safely in combination with beta-blockers, diuretics, ace inhibitors and other antihypertensive agents. It is recommended that patients receiving these combinations should be regularly monitored. Particular care should be taken with the combination diltiazem and a beta-blocker. Concomitant use of Tildiem Retard with alpha blockers such as prazosin should be strictly monitored because of the possible synergistic hypotensive effect of this combination.

Case reports have suggested that blood levels of carbamazepine, cyclosporin, and theophylline may be increased when given concurrently with diltiazem hydrochloride. Care should be exercised in patients taking these drugs. In common with other calcium antagonists Tildiem Retard may cause small increases in plasma levels of digoxin.

In patients taking $H_2$ antagonists concurrently with Tildiem Retard there may be increased levels of diltiazem.

Diltiazem hydrochloride treatment has been continued without problem during anaesthesia, but the anaesthetist should be informed that the patient is receiving a calcium antagonist.

*Use during pregnancy and lactation:* Diltiazem hydrochloride is teratogenic in some animal species. In the absence of adequate evidence of safety in human pregnancy, Tildiem Retard should not be used in pregnancy or in women of child bearing potential.

Diltiazem hydrochloride is excreted in breast milk. One report suggests that concentrations in breast milk reach similar levels to those in serum. If use of Tildiem Retard is considered essential, an alternative method of infant feeding should be instituted.

*Effects on ability to drive and use machines:* No effect reported to date.

*Undesirable effects:* Adverse effects are generally mild and transient and are most commonly vasodilatory related events. The following have been described: lower limb oedema, headache, hot flushes/flushing, asthenia/fatigue, palpitations, malaise, minor gastro-intestinal disorders (dyspepsia, abdominal pain, dry mouth) and skin rash. Vasodilatory related events (in particular oedema) are dose-dependent and appear to be more frequent in elderly subjects.

Rare cases of symptomatic bradycardia, sino-atrial block and atrioventricular block were also recorded.

Experience with diltiazem has shown that skin rashes such as cases of simple erythema, urticaria, or occasionally desquamative erythema, with or without fever are usually localised and regress when treatment is discontinued. However, erythema multiforme and vasculitis have been reported occasionally.

Isolated cases of moderate and transient elevation of liver transaminases have been observed at the start of treatment. Isolated cases of clinical hepatitis have been reported which resolved on cessation of therapy.

*Overdose:* The clinical consequences of overdose can be severe hypotension leading to collapse, and sinus bradycardia which may be accompanied by isorhythmic dissociation and atrioventricular conduction disturbances. Observation in a coronary care unit is advisable. Vasopressors such as adrenaline may be indicated in patients exhibiting profound hypotension. Calcium gluconate may help reverse the effects of calcium entry blockade. Atropine administration and temporary cardiac pacing may be required to manage bradycardia and/or conduction disturbances.

## Pharmacological properties

*Pharmacodynamic properties:* Tildiem is a calcium antagonist. It restricts the slow channel entry of calcium into the cell and so reduces the liberation of calcium from stores in the sarcoplasmic reticulum. This results in a reduction of the amount of available intracellular calcium reducing myocardial oxygen consumption. It increases exercise capacity and improves all indices of myocardial ischaemia in the angina patient. Tildiem relaxes large and small coronary arteries and relieves the spasm of vasospastic (prinzmetals) angina and the response to catecholamines but has little effect on the peripheral vasculature. There is therefore no possibility of reflex tachycardia. A small reduction in heart rate occurs which is accompanied by an increase in cardiac output, improved myocardial perfusion and reduction of ventricular work. In animal studies, Tildiem protects the myocardium against the effects of ischaemia and reduces the damage produced by excessive entry of calcium into the myocardial cell during reperfusion.

*Pharmacokinetic particulars:* In pharmacokinetic studies in healthy volunteers, diltiazem was well absorbed. Peak plasma concentrations were reached approximately 4 to 8 hours after dosing. Diltiazem in plasma is 80–85% protein bound and is poorly dialysed. Diltiazem is extensively metabolised by the liver. The two major active circulating metabolites, deacetyldiltiazem and N-monodemethyl diltiazem possess pharmacological activity in angina equivalent to about 50% of that of diltiazem. Only 0.2–4% of diltiazem is found unchanged in the urine.

*Preclinical safety data:* No data of therapeutic relevance.

## Pharmaceutical particulars

*List of excipients:* Tablet core: Sodium dihydrogen citrate, sucrose powdered, povidone, magnesium stearate, polyethylene glycol 6000 powder. Coating: Sucrose powdered, coating polymer, acetate tributyl citrate, castor oil polymerised, sodium bicarbonate, ethyl vanillin, titanium dioxide (E171).

*Incompatibilities:* Not applicable.

*Shelf-life:* Two years.

*Special precautions for storage:* Store in a dry place below 30°C (86°F). Tildiem Retard tablets are coated with a porous polymer membrane which enables the diltiazem to diffuse out of the tablet at a gradual rate. This membrane may pass through the gastro-intestinal tract unchanged. This has no bearing on the efficacy of the product.

*Nature and contents of container:* 14 or 56 tablets in PVC/foil strips.

*Instructions for use/handling:* Please consult the package insert before use. Do not use after the stated expiry date on the carton and blister strip. Keep out of the reach of children.

**Marketing authorisation numbers**
Tildiem Retard 90 mg      4969/0012
Tildiem Retard 120 mg    4969/0013

**Date of approval/revision of SPC**   November 1996.

**Legal category**   POM.

*Trade Mark

# Lorex Synthélabo UK & Ireland Ltd
Foundation Park
Roxborough Way
Maidenhead
Berkshire SL6 3UD

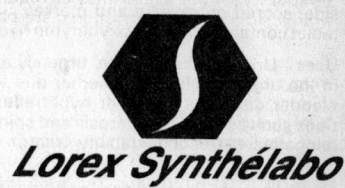

## DICYNENE* 500 TABLETS

**Presentation** Dicynene 500 Tablets. Each white, scored, capsule-shaped tablet contains 500 mg ethamsylate and is engraved 'D500' one side, with a breakmark on the other.

*Mode of action:* Dicynene is a non-hormonal agent which reduces capillary exudation and blood loss. Dicynene does not affect the normal coagulation mechanism since administration is without effect on prothrombin time, fibrinolysis, platelet count or function.

Dicynene is thought to act by increasing capillary vascular wall resistance and platelet adhesiveness in the presence of a vascular lesion, by inhibiting the biosynthesis and actions of those prostaglandins which cause platelet disaggregation, vasodilation and increased capillary permeability and does not have a vasoconstricting action.

**Uses** Dicynene is used clinically for the short term treatment of blood loss in primary and IUCD-induced menorrhagia.

**Dosage and administration** The normal dosage is 500 mg four times daily from the start of bleeding until menstruation ceases.

**Contra-indications, warnings, etc** Treatment should only be undertaken following exclusion of other pelvic pathology, in particular the presence of fibroids.

*Precautions:* In patients receiving Dicynene for menorrhagia the use of the product before onset of bleeding is not recommended.

*Use in pregnancy and lactation:* Studies in animals have revealed no teratogenic effect of Dicynene, but since there is inadequate evidence of safety in human pregnancy, clinical use in pregnancy is not recommended.

Dicynene is secreted in breast milk and administration to nursing mothers is not recommended.

*Side-effects:* Occasional headaches or skin rashes may occur which usually disappear on reduced dosage. A few patients may experience nausea, however this may be overcome by administering the dose after food.

**Pharmaceutical precautions** Dicynene tablets should be stored in a cool, dry place. Dispense in airtight containers offering adequate protection from light and moisture.

**Legal category** POM.

**Package quantities** Securitainers of 28 or 100 tablets.

**Further information** Dicynene is fully absorbed when given orally and is excreted unchanged, largely by the urinary route.

**Product licence number** 15819/0013.

## DICYNENE* INJECTION

**Presentation** Each clear glass 2 ml ampoule, printed DICYNENE, contains 250 mg ethamsylate.

*Mode of action:* Dicynene is a non-hormonal agent which reduces capillary exudation and blood loss. Dicynene does not affect the normal coagulation mechanism since administration is without effect on prothrombin time, fibrinolysis, platelet count or function.

Dicynene is thought to act by increasing capillary vascular wall resistance and platelet adhesiveness in the presence of a vascular lesion, by inhibiting the biosynthesis and actions of those prostaglandins which cause platelet disaggregation, vasodilation and increased capillary permeability and does not have a vasoconstricting action.

**Uses** Dicynene injection is used for the prophylaxis and treatment of periventricular haemorrhage in low birth weight infants.

**Dosage and administration** The normal dosage is 12.5 mg/kg given by intravenous or intramuscular route every six hours.

### Contra-indications, warnings, etc
*Precautions:* Dicynene Injection is intended for neonatal use only.

*Side-effects:* Dicynene is well tolerated. However, occasional headaches, nausea or skin rashes may occur which usually disappear on reduced dosage.

**Pharmaceutical precautions** Dicynene Injection should be stored in a cool place, protected from light. If the contents of the ampoules become coloured they should not be administered.

Dicynene Injection is incompatible with solutions of sodium bicarbonate and compound sodium lactate. When Dicynene Injection is mixed with saline it should be used immediately.

**Legal category** POM.

**Package quantities** Boxes containing 10×2 ml ampoules.

**Further information** Following intravenous administration maximum blood levels of ethamsylate are achieved in 2–3 minutes, while after intramuscular injection, maximum blood levels of ethamsylate are achieved after about one hour. Ethamsylate is excreted unchanged, largely by the urinary route.

**Product licence number** 15819/0014.

## DITROPAN* ELIXIR

**Presentation** Clear, colourless elixir. Each 5 ml contains 2.5 mg oxybutynin hydrochloride.

**Uses** Urinary incontinence, urgency and frequency in the unstable bladder, whether due to neurogenic bladder disorders (detrusor hyperreflexia) in conditions such as multiple sclerosis and spina bifida, or to idiopathic detrusor instability (motor urge incontinence).

*Children over 5 years of age:* In addition to neurogenic bladder disorders, Ditropan may also be used in nocturnal enuresis in conjunction with non-drug therapy where this alone, or in conjunction with other drug treatment, has failed.

### Dosage and administration
*Adult:* The usual dose is 5 mg (10 ml) two or three times a day. This may be increased to a maximum of 5 mg (10 ml) four times a day to obtain a clinical response provided the side effects are tolerated.

*Elderly (including frail elderly):* The elimination half-life is increased in the elderly. Therefore, a dose of 2.5 mg (5 ml) twice a day, particularly if the patient is frail, is likely to be adequate. This dose may be titrated upwards to 5 mg (10 ml) two times a day to obtain a clinical response provided the side effects are well tolerated.

*Children (under 5 years of age):* Not recommended.

*Children (over 5 years of age):* Neurogenic bladder: the usual dose is 2.5 mg (5 ml) twice a day. This dose may be titrated upwards to 5 mg (10 ml) two or three times a day to obtain a clinical response provided the side effects are tolerated. Nocturnal enuresis: the usual dose is 2.5 mg (5 ml) twice a day. This dose may be titrated upwards to 5 mg (10 ml) two or three times a day to obtain a clinical response provided the side effects are tolerated. The last dose should be given before bedtime.

### Contra-indications, warnings, etc
*Contra-indications:* Ditropan is contra-indicated in patients with obstruction of the bowel and in patients with a significant degree of bladder outflow obstruction where urinary retention may be precipitated.

It is also contra-indicated in patients with intestinal atony, severe ulcerative colitis, toxic megacolon, myasthenia gravis or glaucoma.

*Precautions:* Ditropan should be used with caution in the frail elderly and in patients with autonomic neuropathy, hepatic or renal disease.

The symptoms of hyperthyroidism, coronary artery disease, congestive cardiac failure, cardiac arrhythmias, tachycardias and prostatic hypertrophy may be aggravated following administration of Ditropan.

Special care should be taken in patients with hiatus hernia associated with reflux oesophagitis, as anticholinergic drugs may aggravate this condition.

As Ditropan may produce drowsiness or blurred vision, the patient should be cautioned regarding activities requiring mental alertness such as driving, operating machinery or performing hazardous work while taking this drug.

*Pregnancy:* There is no evidence as to the safety of Ditropan in human pregnancy nor is there evidence from animal work that it is totally free from hazard. Avoid in pregnancy unless there is no safer alternative.

*Lactation:* Ditropan has been detected in breast milk and should therefore not be taken by breastfeeding mothers.

*Side-effects:* The most frequently reported side effects (>1%) to oxybutynin are: dry mouth (about 22%), constipation, blurred vision, nausea, abdominal discomfort, facial flushing and difficulty in micturition. The incidence of facial flushing is more marked in children than adults. The occurrence of these effects may be reduced by lowering the dose. Those side effects reported less frequently include: headache, urinary retention, dizziness, dry skin, diarrhoea and cardiac arrhythmias.

*Drug interaction:* Care should be taken if other anticholinergic agents are administered together with Ditropan, as potentiation of anticholinergic effects could occur.

Occasional cases of interaction between anticholinergics and phenothiazines, amantidine, butyrophenones, L-dopa, digitalis and tricyclic antidepressants have been reported and care should be taken if Ditropan is administered concurrently with such drugs.

*Overdosage:* The symptoms of overdosage with Ditropan progress from an intensification of the usual side effects of CNS disturbances (from restlessness and excitement to psychotic behaviour), circulatory changes (flushing, fall in blood pressure, circulatory failure etc), respiratory failure, paralysis and coma.

Measures to be taken are: (1) Immediate gastric lavage, and (2) slow intravenous injection of 1.0 to 2.0 mg of physostigmine, repeated as necessary up to a total of 5 mg.

Fever should be treated symptomatically with tepid sponging or ice packs.

In pronounced restlessness or excitation, diazepam 10 mg may be given by intravenous injections, tachycardia may be treated with intravenous injection of propranolol, and urinary retention can be managed by catheterisation.

In the event of progression of the curare-like effect to the paralysis of the respiratory muscles, mechanical ventilation will be required.

**Pharmaceutical precautions** Store below 25°C. Protect from light. Discard any remaining medicine 28 days after opening.

**Legal category** POM.

**Package quantities** 150 ml bottle contained within a carton with a patient information leaflet.

**Further information** Oxybutynin has both direct antispasmodic action on the smooth muscle of the bladder detrusor as well as anticholinergic action in blocking the muscarinic effects of acetylcholine on smooth muscle.

These properties cause relaxation of the detrusor muscle of the bladder and in patients with an unstable bladder, Ditropan increases bladder capacity and reduces the incidence of spontaneous contractions of the detrusor muscle.

Ditropan elixir contains 1.3 g sucrose per 5 ml dose.

**Product licence number** 15819/0010.

## DITROPAN* TABLETS
**Presentation**
*Ditropan tablets 5 mg:* Pale blue bi-convex circular tablets, 8 mm in diameter, marked Ditropan on one side, scored on reverse and marked S&N 5. Each tablet containing 5 mg oxybutynin hydrochloride.

*Ditropan tablets 2.5 mg:* Pale blue bi-convex oval

tablets, 8.5 mm×5.8 mm marked Ditropan on one side, scored on reverse and marked S&N 2.5. Each tablet containing 2.5 mg oxybutynin hydrochloride.

**Uses** Urinary incontinence, urgency and frequency in the unstable bladder, whether due to neurogenic bladder disorders (detrusor hyperreflexia) in conditions such as multiple sclerosis and spina bifida, or to idiopathic detrusor instability (motor urge incontinence).

*Children over 5 years of age:* In addition to neurogenic bladder disorders, Ditopan may also be used in nocturnal enuresis in conjunction with non-drug therapy where this alone, or in conjunction with other drug therapy, has failed.

**Dosage and administration**
*Adult:* The usual dose is 5 mg two or three times a day. This may be increased to a maximum of 5 mg four times a day to obtain a clinical response provided the side effects are tolerated.

*Elderly (including frail elderly):* The elimination half-life is increased in the elderly. Therefore, a dose of 2.5 mg twice a day, particularly if the patient is frail, is likely to be adequate. This dose may be titrated upwards to 5 mg two times a day to obtain a clinical response provided the side effects are well tolerated.

*Children (under 5 years of age):* Not recommended.

*Children (over 5 years of age):* Neurogenic bladder: the usual dose is 2.5 mg twice a day. This dose may be titrated upwards to 5 mg two or three times a day to obtain a clinical response provided the side effects are tolerated. Noctural enuresis: the usual dose is 2.5 mg twice a day. This dose may be titrated upwards to 5 mg two or three times a day to obtain a clinical response provided the side effects are tolerated. The last dose should be given before bedtime.

**Contra-indications, warnings, etc**
*Contra-indications:* Ditropan is contra-indicated in patients with obstruction of the bowel and in patients with a significant degree of bladder outflow obstruction where urinary retention may be precipitated.

It is also contra-indicated in patients with intestinal atony, severe ulcerative colitis or toxic megacolon, myasthenia gravis or glaucoma.

*Precautions:* Ditropan should be used with caution in the frail elderly and in patients with autonomic neuropathy, hepatic or renal disease.

The symptoms of hyperthyroidism, coronary artery disease, congestive cardiac failure, cardiac arrhythmias, tachycardias and prostatic hypertrophy may be aggravated following administration of Ditropan.

Special care should be taken in patients with hiatus hernia associated with reflux oesophagitis, as anticholinergic drugs may aggravate this condition.

As Ditropan may produce drowsiness or blurred vision, the patient should be cautioned regarding activities requiring mental alertness such as driving, operating machinery or performing hazardous work while taking this drug.

*Pregnancy:* There is no evidence as to the safety of Ditropan in human pregnancy nor is there evidence from animal work that it is totally free from hazard. Avoid in pregnancy unless there is no safer alternative.

*Lactation:* Ditropan has been detected in breast milk and should therefore not be taken by breastfeeding mothers.

*Side-effects:* The most frequently reported side effects (>1%) to oxybutynin are: dry mouth (about 22%), constipation, blurred vision, nausea, abdominal discomfort, facial flushing and difficulty in micturition. The incidence of facial flushing is more marked in children than adults. The occurrence of these effects may be reduced by lowering the dose. Those side effects reported less frequently include: headache, urinary retention, dizziness, dry skin, diarrhoea and cardiac arrhythmias.

*Drug interactions:* Care should be taken if other anticholinergic agents are administered together with Ditropan, as potentiation of anticholinergic effects could occur.

Occasional cases of interaction between anticholinergics and phenothiazines, amantidine, butyrophenones, L-dopa, digitalis and tricyclic antidepressants have been reported and care should be taken if Ditropan is administered concurrently with such drugs.

*Overdosage:* The symptoms of overdosage with Ditropan progress from an intensification of the usual side effects of CNS disturbances (from restlessness and excitement to psychotic behaviour), circulatory changes (flushing, fall in blood pressure, circulatory failure etc), respiratory failure, paralysis and coma.

Measures to be taken are: (1) Immediate gastric lavage, and (2) slow intravenous injection of 1.0 to 2.0 mg of physostigmine, repeated as necessary up to a total of 5 mg.

Fever should be treated symptomatically with tepid sponging or ice packs.

In pronounced restlessness or excitation, diazepam 10 mg may be given by intravenous injections, tachycardia may be treated with intravenous injection of propranolol, and urinary retention can be managed by catheterisation.

In the event of progression of the curare-like effect to the paralysis of the respiratory muscles, mechanical ventilation will be required.

**Pharmaceutical precautions** Store under dry ambient conditions.

**Legal category** POM.

**Package quantities** Original packs containing 21 or 84 tablets in blister strips of 21 tablets each.

**Further information** Oxybutynin has both direct antispasmodic action on the smooth muscle of the bladder detrusor as well as anticholinergic action in blocking the muscarinic effects of acetylcholine on smooth muscle.

These properties cause relaxation of the detrusor muscle of the bladder and in patients with an unstable bladder, Ditropan increases bladder capacity and reduces the incidence of spontaneous contractions of the detrusor muscle.

**Product licence numbers**

| | |
|---|---|
| 2.5 mg tablets | 15819/0008 |
| 5 mg tablets | 15819/0009. |

## KERLONE*

**Presentation** White, biconvex, film-coated tablets engraved KE20 on one side with breakline on reverse. Each tablet contains betaxolol hydrochloride 20 mg.

**Uses**
*Actions:* Kerlone (betaxolol hydrochloride) is a beta-adrenoceptor blocking agent which is cardioselective, i.e. acts preferentially on beta$_1$-adrenergic receptors in the heart. It has prolonged activity, permitting once-daily administration which aids patient compliance. Its principal effects are to lower heart rate, especially on exercise, and to lower systolic and diastolic blood pressure in hypertensive subjects. It is devoid of intrinsic sympathomimetic activity and has little membrane stabilising activity. As with other beta-blockers, its mechanism of action in the treatment of hypertension is unclear. Absorption from the gastrointestinal tract is complete and not affected by food. There is little first-pass extraction in the liver. This results in blood levels which vary little within and between subjects and a reproducible bioavailability of 80–90%.

Its long elimination half-life of 16–20 hours results in protection from excessive or inappropriate sympathetic activity throughout the 24 hours after administration of a once daily dose.

*Indications:* Management of hypertension.

**Dosage and administration**
*Adults:* The usual adult dose is one tablet (20 mg) daily. The single daily dose may be increased to two tablets (40 mg) if response is inadequate.

*Elderly patients or those with a history of bronchospasm:* A starting dose of half tablet (10 mg) daily is recommended.

*Impaired renal function:* An adjustment of dose is usually unnecessary in patients with renal insufficiency where creatinine clearance is greater than 20 ml/min. However, clinical surveillance is recommended at the start of treatment until steady state blood levels are attained (4 days on average).

For patients on haemo- or peritoneal dialysis the initial recommended dose is 10 mg daily independent of the dialysis schedule.

*Hepatic insufficiency:* Adjustment of dosage is usually unnecessary in patients with hepatic insufficiency. However, clinical surveillance is recommended at the start of treatment.

*Children:* Paediatric experience with Kerlone is limited and for this reason it is not currently recommended for use in children.

Most of the reduction of blood pressure is seen during the first 3 hours following the initial dose, permitting an early evaluation of the antihypertensive effect. Little further reduction is seen after seven days of treatment and the response is undiminished in subsequent months. Should an inadequate response be obtained, a further decrease may be achieved by combining Kerlone with another antihypertensive agent such as a diuretic. However, in a large series of controlled clinical trials, 70–80% of patients responded to betaxolol alone.

Patients can be transferred to Kerlone from other anti-hypertensive treatments with the exception of clonidine (see precautions below).

**Contra-indications, warnings, etc**
*Contra-indications:* Kerlone is contra-indicated in cardiogenic shock, in patients with uncontrolled congestive cardiac failure and in second or third degree AV block if no pacemaker is present and in patients with marked bradycardia (heart rate less than 50 beats per minute).

*Warnings:* Concomitant administration of Kerlone and a myocardial depressant or inhibitor of AV conduction, such as the calcium antagonists of the verapamil type, should be carried out only under close supervision, especially in the case of intravenous administration.

Although cardio-selective beta-blockers may have less effect on lung function than non-selective beta-blockers, as with all beta-blockers these should be avoided in patients with wheezing or reversible obstructive airways disease unless there are compelling clinical reasons for their use.

It is recommended that Kerlone treatment is started at the dose of 10 mg daily in such patients. If any increase in airway resistance is provoked, it can be relieved by beta$_2$-mimetics whose effect is not inhibited.

*Precautions:* Secondary sympathetic hyperactivity has sometimes been reported following discontinuation of treatment with other beta-blockers. Even though Kerlone blood levels decrease slowly, care should be exercised if treatment is withdrawn, especially in patients with ischaemic heart disease.

Patients with a history of cardiac failure, cardiomyopathy, or cardiomegaly should be monitored carefully during treatment with a beta-blocker as sympathetic stimulation may be essential to their circulatory function.

Use with caution where the PR conduction interval is prolonged.

Studies in normal subjects have shown that, unlike non-selective beta-blockers, Kerlone does not inhibit the recovery from insulin-induced hypoglycaemia, nor does it mask the cardiovascular response. Due to its beta$_1$ selectivity, Kerlone is unlikely to interfere with glucose metabolism in insulin-treated diabetics. However, caution is advised when treating such patients.

*Anaesthesia:* In the event of surgical intervention, the anaesthetist should be advised in advance that the patient is receiving Kerlone. In patients with severe ischaemic heart disease the risk/benefits of continuation of treatment have to be evaluated. If treatment is continued care should be taken when using anaesthetic agents such as ether, cyclopropane and trichloroethylene.

*Drug interactions:* As with other beta-blockers, use with care in combination with myocardial depressants or drugs which depress AV conduction. If Kerlone and clonidine are given concurrently, clonidine should not be discontinued until several days after withdrawal of the beta-blocker.

*Pregnancy:* No teratogenic effects have been demonstrated in animal studies but the safety of Kerlone during human pregnancy has not been established. Like other beta-blockers, Kerlone crosses the placental barrier and its use in pregnant women requires that the anticipated benefit be weighed against the possible hazards to the mother and foetus.

*Nursing mothers:* Kerlone is excreted in human breast milk and the possibility of bradycardic and hypotensive effects on the newborn should therefore be considered if Kerlone is given to nursing mothers.

*Side effects:* Kerlone is generally well tolerated. The side effects are usually those due to its pharmacological actions and rarely require discontinuation of treatment. Minor side effects include lassitude at the start of treatment, exacerbation of Raynaud's disease or intermittent claudication, and paraesthesia of the extremities. Possible side effects include marked bradycardia and hypotension, AV block, cardiac insufficiency and bronchospasm. There have been reports of rashes and dry eyes associated with the use of all beta-blockers but in most cases the signs and symptoms have cleared when treatment was withdrawn. Nevertheless, the drug should be discontinued if any such reaction is suspected.

*Overdosage:* Excessive bradycardia can usually be corrected with atropine. If there is no response isoprenaline may be administered with caution. Cardiac failure should be managed with digitalisation and diuretics. Hypotension may be managed with vasopressors such as adrenaline.

**Pharmaceutical precautions** Store in a dry place below 30°C.

**Legal category** POM.

**Package quantities** Pack of 28 tablets (2×14).

**Further information** Kerlone is unique in having high bioavailability, long blood half-life and high selectivity for cardiac beta$_1$-receptors. Unlike most other cardio-selective beta-blockers it has high lipid solubility. This may facilitate rapid arrival of the drug at the receptor, but does not induce an increased incidence of side effects.

These characteristics and the rapidity of response

increase patient compliance by virtue of the drug's acceptability, the simple dose regimen and narrow dose range.

The only active metabolite is cardioselective and does not contribute to the clinical effect. Kerlone does not modify the hypoglycaemic response to insulin nor mask the cardiovascular response. It can be used in patients with respiratory disease, and is compatible with most other hypotensive agents.

**Product licence number** 15819/0011.

## MONIT* TABLETS
## MONIT* LS TABLETS

**Qualitative and quantitative composition** Each tablet of Monit contains isosorbide mononitrate 20 mg.

Each tablet of Monit LS contains isosorbide mononitrate 10 mg.

**Pharmaceutical form** Tablet.

### Clinical particulars

*Therapeutic indications:* Monit and Monit LS are indicated in the prophylaxis of angina pectoris.

Monit is indicated as adjunctive therapy in congestive heart failure which does not respond adequately to cardiac glycosides and/or diuretics.

*Posology and method of administration:* The tablets should be swallowed whole with a little fluid.

*Adults:* Angina pectoris: Usually one tablet twice or three times daily. Patients already accustomed to prophylactic nitrate therapy (for example with isosorbide dinitrate) may normally be transferred directly to a therapeutic dose of Monit or Monit LS. For patients not receiving prophylactic nitrate therapy, it is recommended that the initial dose should be one Monit LS tablet twice daily. Maintenance dose in individual patients will be between 20 and 120 mg daily. Congestive heart failure: In severe congestive cardiac failure Monit tablets may be taken in doses of 20 mg two to three times daily depending on patients requirements. In this situation optimal individual dose is best determined by continuous haemodynamic monitoring. The use of Monit in severe congestive cardiac failure should be considered adjunctive therapy to more conventional treatment (e.g. cardiac glycosides, diuretics etc).

*Elderly:* There is no evidence to suggest an adjustment of dosage is necessary. However, caution may be required in elderly patients who are known to be susceptible to the effects of hypotensive medication.

*Children:* The safety and efficacy of Monit and Monit LS in children has not been established.

*Patients with renal or hepatic impairment:* No dosage reduction is necessary in patients with renal or hepatic impairment.

*Contra-indications:* Monit and Monit LS are contra-indicated in patients with a known sensitivity to the drug or to isosorbide dinitrate and in cases of marked low blood pressure, shock and acute myocardial infarction with low left ventricular filling pressure.

*Special warnings and special precautions for use:* Monit and Monit LS are not indicated for relief of acute anginal attacks. In the event of an acute attack, sublingual or buccal glyceryl trinitrate tablets or spray should be used.

*Interaction with other medicaments and other forms of interaction:* The hypotensive effects of other drugs may be potentiated.

Beta-adrenoceptor blocking drugs have a different pharmacological action in angina and may have a complementary effect when co-administered with Monit or Monit LS.

*Pregnancy and lactation:* Animal studies have shown no adverse effects on the foetus, however, since its safety and efficacy during pregnancy and lactation have not been established, Monit, like other drugs should not be administered to pregnant women and nursing mothers unless considered essential. No data are available on the presence of isosorbide-5-mononitrate in breast milk.

*Effects on ability to drive and use machines:* The effect of isosorbide mononitrate upon an individual's performance of skilled and potentially dangerous tasks such as car driving and the operation of machinery has not been evaluated. However, there have been no published reports of impaired performance of such tasks.

*Undesirable effects:* A number of nitrate-related adverse effects may occur during treatment, including flushing, headache, dizziness and weakness. The incidence of such effects is normally highest at the commencement of treatment and tends to decline with time. If headache is a problem, a temporary lowering of the dose may be necessary. Nausea and vomiting may occur occasionally. Postural hypotension may occur, especially with high doses. Dry rash and/or exfoliative dermatitis have been described

rarely with isosorbide dinitrate and similar reactions might be expected.

*Overdose:* Overdosage should be treated symptomatically. The stomach should be aspirated to remove any remaining tablets. The main symptom is likely to be hypotension and this may be treated by elevation of the legs to promote venous return. Symptomatic and supportive treatment e.g. plasma expanders and if necessary the careful use of vasopressor agents to counterbalance the hypotensive effects may be necessary.

Methaemoglobinaemia will normally respond to methylene blue infusion.

### Pharmacological properties

*Pharmacodynamic properties:* Isosorbide mononitrate is an active metabolite of isosorbide dinitrate. The predominant action is that of a vasodilator with effects on both veins and arteries.

*Pharmacokinetic properties:* Isosorbide-5-mononitrate is completely absorbed after oral administration.

The elimination half-life is approximately 5 hours. The volume of distribution is about 0.62 l/kg. The time to maximum plasma level is approximately 1 hour and peak plasma concentration is approximately 500 ng/ml for Monit and 250 ng/ml for Monit LS. In patients with renal failure, the half-life is unchanged, remaining at approximately 5 hours.

*Preclinical safety data:* Not applicable.

### Pharmaceutical particulars

*List of excipients:* Lactose, microcrystalline cellulose, sodium starch glycollate, povidone 25000, colloidal silicon dioxide, magnesium stearate.

*Incompatibilities:* None known.

*Shelf life:* 5 years.

*Special precautions for storage:* Store below 25°C. Protect from moisture.

*Nature and contents of container:* Monit: PVC (250 micron), aluminium foil (20 micron) blister pack. 56 tablets. Plastic (white HDPE) bottle 100 or 500 tablets.

Monit LS: PVC (250 micron), aluminium foil (20 micron) blister pack. 14, 56 or 100 tablets.

*Instructions for use/handling:* None.

**Marketing authorisation numbers**
Monit 15819/0005
Monit LS 15819/0006

**Date of approval/revision of SPC** May 1997

**Legal category** P.

## MONIT* SR TABLETS

**Qualitative and quantitative composition** Isosorbide mononitrate 40 mg.

**Pharmaceutical form** Slow release, sugar coated tablet.

### Clinical particulars

*Therapeutic indications:* Monit SR is indicated in the prophylaxis of angina pectoris.

*Posology and method of administration:* The tablets should be swallowed whole without chewing.

*Adults:* One tablet daily to be taken in the morning.

*Elderly:* There is no evidence to suggest that an adjustment of dosage is necessary. However, caution may be required in elderly patients who are known to be susceptible to the effects of hypotensive medication.

*Children:* The safety and efficacy of Monit SR in children has not been established.

*Patients with renal or hepatic impairment:* No dosage reduction is necessary in patients with renal or hepatic impairment.

Patients who have not previously received nitrates may be started with a low dose which should be increased gradually before introducing Monit SR.

*Contra-indications:* Monit SR is contra-indicated in patients with a known hypersensitivity to isosorbide mononitrate or isosorbide dinitrate and in cases of marked low blood pressure, shock and acute myocardial infarction with low left ventricular filling pressure.

*Special warnings and special precautions for use:* Monit SR is not indicated for relief of acute anginal attacks. In the event of an acute attack, sublingual or buccal glyceryl trinitrate tablets or spray should be used.

*Interaction with other medicaments and other forms of interaction:* The hypotensive effects of other drugs may be potentiated.

Beta-adrenoceptor blocking drugs have a different pharmacological action in angina and may have a complementary effect when co-administered with Monit SR.

*Pregnancy and lactation:* Animal studies have shown no adverse effects on the foetus, however, since its

safety and efficacy during pregnancy and lactation have not been established, Monit SR, like other drugs should not be administered to pregnant women and nursing mothers unless considered essential. No data are available on the presence of isosorbide-5-mononitrate in breast milk.

*Effects on ability to drive and use machines:* The effect of isosorbide mononitrate upon an individual's performance of skilled and potentially dangerous tasks such as car driving and the operation of machinery has not been evaluated. However, there have been no published reports of impaired performance of such tasks.

*Undesirable effects:* A number of nitrate-related adverse effects may occur during treatment, including flushing, headache, dizziness and weakness. The incidence of such effects is normally highest at the commencement of treatment and tends to decline with time. If headache is a problem, a temporary reduced dose of isosorbide-5-mononitrate may be necessary. Nausea and vomiting may occur occasionally. Postural hypotension may occur, especially with high doses. Dry rash and/or exfoliative dermatitis have been described rarely with isosorbide dinitrate and similar reactions might be expected.

*Overdose:* In the event of overdosage with Monit SR the main sign is likely to be hypotension. The stomach should be aspirated to remove any remaining tablets. The patient should be placed in a supine position with the legs elevated to promote venous return. Symptomatic and supportive treatment, e.g. plasma expanders and if necessary the careful use of vasopressor agents to counterbalance the hypotensive effects may be necessary.

Methaemoglobinaemia will normally respond to methylene blue infusion.

### Pharmacological properties

*Pharmacodynamic properties:* Isosorbide-5-mononitrate is an active metabolite of isosorbide dinitrate. The predominant action is that of a vasodilator with effects on both veins and arteries.

*Pharmacokinetic properties:* Monit SR has been developed to provide a convenient, once daily dosage form of isosorbide-5-mononitrate. It is designed to achieve therapeutic blood concentrations within 30 minutes which persist up to 17 hours. A nitrate free interval of up to 7 hours makes the development of anti-anginal tolerance during chronic therapy unlikely.

*Preclinical safety data:* Not applicable.

### Pharmaceutical particulars

*List of excipients:* Anhydrous lactose; Hoechst Wax E; povidone 25000; colloidal silicon dioxide; magnesium stearate; Eudragit E12.5; talc; sucrose; kaolin; macrogol; titanium dioxide; liquid glucose.

*Incompatibilities:* None known.

*Shelf life:* 36 months.

*Special precautions for storage:* Store below 25°C. Protect from moisture.

*Nature and contents of container:* Blister pack 250 micron PVC and 20 micron aluminium foil. 28 tablet pack size.

*Instructions for use/handling:* None.

**Marketing authorisation number** 15819/0007

**Date of approval/revision of SPC** May 1997

**Legal category** P.

## PARAMAX* SACHETS
## PARAMAX* TABLETS

**Presentation** *Paramax Tablets:* White, round scored tablets, engraved 'Paramax' on one side.

*Paramax Sachets:* Sachets containing effervescent powder.

Each tablet or sachet contains 500 mg Paracetamol BP with 5 mg Metoclopramide Hydrochloride BP.

Paramax presentations do not contain sucrose, tartrazine or any other azo dyes.

**Uses** *Indications:* Paramax is indicated for the symptomatic treatment of migraine.

*Action:* Paracetamol relieves pain. More rapid absorption is promoted by the action of metoclopramide which also relieves gastric stasis and overcomes nausea and vomiting.

**Dosage and administration** For oral administration only.

Paramax should be taken at the first warning of an attack. If symptoms persist, further doses may be taken at four-hourly intervals. Total dosage in any 24-hour period should not exceed the quantity stated.

The dosage recommendations given below should be strictly adhered to if side-effects of the dystonic type are to be avoided. It should be noted that total daily dosage of metoclopramide, especially for adolescents and young adults, should not normally exceed 0.5 mg/kg body weight.

*Usual Recommended Dosage (Tablets or Sachets)*

|  | Initial dose at first warning of attack | Maximum dosage in any 24-hour period |
|---|---|---|
| Adults (including elderly patients) | 2 | 6 |
| Young Adults (12–19 years) | 1 | 3 |

*Young adults and adolescents:* Paramax should only be used after careful examination to avoid masking an underlying disorder, e.g. cerebral irritation. In the treatment of this group attention should be given primarily to bodyweight.

*Children:* A presentation of Paramax suitable for the treatment of children under 12 years of age is not available.

*Paramax Sachets:* Empty a sachet into about ¼ of a glass of water and stir before taking.

### Contra-indications, warnings, etc

*Use in pregnancy and lactation:* There is no evidence that metoclopramide or paracetamol by themselves have teratogenic effects. Nevertheless, Paramax should only be used when there are compelling reasons and is not advised during the first trimester.

During lactation, metoclopramide and paracetamol may be found in breast milk.

*Precautions:* If vomiting persists the patient should be reassessed to exclude the possibility of an underlying disorder, e.g. cerebral irritation.

Care should be exercised in patients being treated with other centrally active drugs e.g. in epilepsy.

Care should be exercised in the event of Paramax being prescribed concurrently with a phenothiazine since extrapyramidal symptoms may occur with both products. The action of metoclopramide on the gastrointestinal tract is antagonised by anticholinergics.

Metoclopramide may induce an acute hypertensive response in patients with phaeochromocytoma.

*Side-effects:* Various extrapyramidal reactions to metoclopramide, usually of the dystonic type, have been reported. The incidence of these reactions may be increased if the metoclopramide dosage exceeds 0.5 mg/kg body weight/day. Reactions include: spasm of the facial muscles, trismus, rhythmic protrusion of the tongue, a bulbar type of speech, spasm of extraocular muscles, including oculogyric crises, unnatural positioning of the head and shoulders and opisthotonos. The majority of reactions occur within 36 hours of starting treatment and the effects usually disappear within 24 hours of withdrawal of the drug. Should treatment of a dystonic reaction be required, a benzodiazepine or an anticholinergic anti-parkinsonian drug may be used.

Rarely, drowsiness, restlessness and diarrhoea have been reported in patients receiving metoclopramide therapy.

Raised serum prolactin levels have been observed during metoclopramide therapy; this effect is similar to that noted with many other compounds.

*Overdosage:* As with other paracetamol-containing products, an overdose of Paramax can be toxic to the liver. Overdosage should be treated by gastric lavage with appropriate supportive measures. Intravenous N-acetylcysteine or oral methionine if administered within 10 hours of paracetamol overdosage appears to exert a protective effect on the liver.

**Pharmaceutical precautions**    Protect tablets from light. Store sachets in a dry place.

**Legal category**    POM.

**Package quantities**    *Paramax tablets:* Original Pack of 42 with Patient Information Leaflet.
*Paramax sachets:* Original Pack of 42. Each sachet carries instructions for preparation and each pack contains a Patient Information Leaflet.

**Further information**    An acute attack of migraine is frequently characterised by impaired absorption of analgesics even when abdominal symptoms are absent. The beneficial effect of Paramax on delayed gastric emptying, nausea and vomiting contrasts with the gastric stasis which may occur following administration of phenothiazine or antihistamine antiemetics.

**Product licence numbers**
Paramax Tablets  15819/0015
Paramax Sachets  15819/0016

## STILNOCT*
## STILNOCT* 10 mg

**Qualitative and quantitative composition**
*Stilnoct:* Round white film coated tablets containing 5 mg zolpidem hemitartrate.

*Stilnoct 10 mg:* Oblong, white, scored, film-coated tablets, engraved SN 10, containing 10 mg zolpidem hemitartrate.

**Pharmaceutical form**    Coated tablets for oral administration.

**Clinical particulars**
*Therapeutic indications:* The short-term treatment of insomnia in situations where the insomnia is debilitating or is causing severe distress for the patient.

*Posology and method of administration:* Zolpidem acts rapidly and therefore should be taken immediately before retiring, or in bed. The recommended daily dose for adults is 10 mg. Elderly or debilitated patients may be especially sensitive to the effects of zolpidem therefore a 5 mg dose is recommended. These recommended doses should not be exceeded.

As clearance and metabolism of zolpidem is reduced in hepatic impairment, dosage should begin at 5 mg with particular caution being exercised in elderly patients. In adults (under 65 years) dosage may be increased to 10 mg only where the clinical response is inadequate and the drug is well tolerated.

The duration of treatment should usually vary from a few days to two weeks with a maximum of four weeks including tapering off where clinically appropriate.

As with all hypnotics, long-term use is not recommended and a course of treatment should not exceed four weeks.

Zolpidem should not be used in children.

*Contra-indications:* Zolpidem is contra-indicated in patients with a hypersensitivity to zolpidem, obstructive sleep apnoea, myasthenia gravis, severe hepatic insufficiency, acute pulmonary insufficiency or respiratory depression. Zolpidem should not be prescribed for children or patients with psychotic illness.

*Special warnings and special precautions for use:* The cause of insomnia should be identified wherever possible and the underlying factors treated before a hypnotic is prescribed. The failure of insomnia to remit after a 7–14 day course of treatment may indicate the presence of a primary psychiatric or physical disorder which should be evaluated.

*Use in depression:* As with other sedative/hypnotic drugs, zolpidem should be administered with caution in patients exhibiting symptoms of depression. Suicidal tendencies may be present therefore the least amount of drug that is feasible should be supplied to these patients because of the possibility of intentional overdosage by the patient.

*Use in patients with a history of drug or alcohol abuse:* Extreme caution should be exercised when prescribing for patients with a history of drug or alcohol abuse. These patients should be under careful surveillance when receiving zolpidem or any other hypnotic, since they are at risk of habituation and psychological dependence.

General information relating to effects seen following administration of benzodiazepines and other hypnotic agents which should be taken into account by the prescribing physician are described below.

*Tolerance:* Some loss of efficacy to the hypnotic effects of short-acting benzodiazepines and benzodiazepine-like agents may develop after repeated use for a few weeks.

*Dependence:* Use of benzodiazepines or benzodiazepine-like agents may lead to the development of physical and psychological dependence of these products. The risk of dependence increases with dose and duration of treatment; it is also greater in patients with a history of alcohol or drug abuse. Once physical dependence has developed, abrupt termination of treatment will be accompanied by withdrawal symptoms. These may consist of headaches or muscle pain, extreme anxiety and tension, restlessness, confusion and irritability. In severe cases the following symptoms may occur: derealisation, depersonalisation, hyperacusis, numbness and tingling of the extremities, hypersensitivity to light, noise and physical contact, hallucinations or epileptic seizures.

*Rebound insomnia:* A transient syndrome whereby the symptoms that led to treatment with a benzodiazepine or benzodiazepine-like agent recur in an enhanced form, may occur on withdrawal of hypnotic treatment. It may be accompanied by other reactions including mood changes, anxiety and restlessness.

It is important that the patient should be aware of the possibility of rebound phenomena, thereby minimising anxiety over such symptoms should they occur when the medicinal product is discontinued. Since the risk of withdrawal phenomena or rebound has been shown to be greater after abrupt discontin-

uation of treatment, it is recommended that the dosage is decreased gradually where clinically appropriate.

There are indications that, in the case of benzodiazepines and benzodiazepine-like agents with a short duration of action, withdrawal phenomena can become manifest within the dosage interval, especially when the dosage is high.

*Amnesia:* Benzodiazepines and benzodiazepine-like agents may induce anterograde amnesia. The condition occurs most often several hours after ingesting the product and therefore to reduce the risk patients should ensure that they will be able to have an uninterrupted sleep of 7–8 hours.

*Psychiatric and 'paradoxical' reactions:* Reactions like restlessness, agitation, irritability, aggressiveness, delusion, rages, nightmares, hallucinations, psychoses, inappropriate behaviour and other adverse behavioural effects are known to occur when using benzodiazepines or benzodiazepine-like agents. Should this occur, use of the product should be discontinued. These reactions are more likely to occur in the elderly.

*Interactions with other medicaments and other forms of interaction:*
*Not recommended:* Concomitant intake with alcohol. The sedative effect may be enhanced when the product is used in combination with alcohol. This affects the ability to drive or use machines.

*Combination requiring caution:* Combination with CNS depressants. Enhancement of the central depressive effect may occur in cases of concomitant use with antipsychotics (neuroleptics), hypnotics, anxiolytics/sedatives, antidepressant agents, narcotic analgesics, antiepileptic drugs, anaesthetics and sedative antihistamines.

In the case of narcotic analgesics enhancement of euphoria may also occur leading to an increase in psychological dependence.

Compounds which inhibit certain hepatic enzymes (particularly cytochrome P450) may enhance the activity of benzodiazepines and benzodiazepine-like agents.

*Pregnancy and lactation:* Although animal studies have shown no teratogenic or embryotoxic effects, safety in pregnancy has not been established. As with all drugs zolpidem should be avoided in pregnancy particularly during the first trimester.

If the product is prescribed to a woman of child-bearing potential, she should be warned to contact her physician about stopping the product if she intends to become or suspects that she is pregnant. If, for compelling medical reasons, zolpidem is administered during the late phase of pregnancy, or during labour, effects of the neonate, such as hypothermia, hypotonia and moderate respiratory depression, can be expected due to the pharmacological action of the product. Infants born to mothers who took benzodiazepines or benzodiazepine-like agents chronically during the latter stages of pregnancy may have developed physical dependence and may be at some risk of developing withdrawal symptoms in the postnatal period.

Small quantities of zolpidem appear in breast milk. The use of zolpidem in nursing mothers is, therefore, not recommended.

*Effects on ability to drive and use machines:* Although studies have shown that during the day following medication with zolpidem, simulated vehicle driving is unaffected, vehicle drivers and machine operators should be warned that, as with other hypnotics, there may be a possible risk of drowsiness the morning after therapy.

*Undesirable effects:* There is evidence of a dose-relationship for adverse effects associated with zolpidem use, particularly for certain CNS and gastrointestinal events. These occur most frequently in elderly patients.

In clinical trials side effects observed during treatment at doses up to 10 mg included drowsiness, dizziness, diarrhoea, headache, nausea and vertigo.

Daytime drowsiness, dizziness, headache, asthenia, nausea and vomiting occasionally led to withdrawal of treatment in clinical trials of zolpidem.

Memory disturbance (anterograde amnesia), nightmares, nocturnal restlessness, depressive syndrome, episodes of confusion, perceptual disturbances or diplopia, tremor, unsteady gait and falls have been observed very rarely in long-term clinical trials.

*Overdose:* In reports of overdose with zolpidem alone, impairment of consciousness has ranged from somnolence to light coma. Individuals have fully recovered from zolpidem overdoses up to 400 mg, 40 times the recommended dose.

General symptomatic and supportive measures should be used, along with immediate gastric lavage where appropriate; intravenous fluids should be administered as needed. If there is no advantage in emptying the stomach, activated charcoal should be given to reduce absorption. Sedating drugs should be withheld even if excitation occurs. Use of flumazenil may be considered where serious symptoms are observed.

In the management of overdose with any medicinal product, it should be borne in mind that multiple agents may have been taken.

### Pharmacological properties

*Pharmacodynamic properties:* (GABA-A receptor agonist selective for omega-1-type sub-unit hypnotic agent). Zolpidem is an imidazopyridine which selectively binds the omega-1 receptor subtype (also known as the benzodiazepine-1 subtype) which is the alpha unit of the GABA-A receptor complex. Whereas benzodiazepines non-selectively bind all three omega receptor subtypes, zolpidem preferentially binds the omega-1 subtype. The modulation of the chloride anion channel via this receptor leads to the specific sedative effects demonstrated by zolpidem. These effects are reversed by the benzodiazepine antagonist flumazenil.

*In animals:* The selective binding of zolpidem to omega-1 receptors may explain the virtual absence at hypnotic doses of myorelaxant and anti-convulsant effects in animals which are normally exhibited by benzodiazepines which are not selective for omega-1 sites.

*In humans:* The preservation of deep sleep (stages 3 and 4 – slow-wave sleep) may be explained by the selective omega-1 binding by zolpidem. All identified effects of zolpidem are reversed by the benzodiazepine antagonist flumazenil.

*Pharmacokinetic properties:* Zolpidem has both a rapid absorption and onset of hypnotic action. Bioavailability is 70% following oral administration and demonstrates linear kinetics in the therapeutic dose range. Peak plasma concentration is reached at between 0.5 and 3 hours.

The elimination half-life is short, with a mean of 2.4 hours (0.7–3.5) and a duration of action of up to 6 hours.

Protein binding amounts to 92.5%±0.1%. First pass metabolism by the liver amounts to approximately 35%. Repeated administration has been shown not to modify protein binding indicating a lack of competition between zolpidem and its metabolites for binding sites. The distribution volume in adults is 0.54±0.02 L/kg and decreases to 0.34±0.05 L/kg in the very elderly.

All metabolites are pharmacologically inactive and are eliminated in the urine (56%) and in the faeces (37%).

Zolpidem has been shown in trials to be non-dialysable.

Plasma concentrations in elderly subjects and those with hepatic impairment are increased. In patients with renal insufficiency, whether dialysed or not, there is a moderate reduction in clearance. The other pharmacokinetic parameters are unaffected.

*Preclinical safety data:* No data of therapeutic relevance.

### Pharmaceutical particulars

*List of excipients:* Tablet core: lactose, microcrystalline cellulose, methylhydroxypropylcellulose, sodium starch glycollate, magnesium stearate. Film coating: methylhydroxypropylcellulose, titanium dioxide (E171), polyoxyethyleneglycol 400.

*Incompatibilities:* None known.

*Shelf life:* 3 years.

*Special precautions for storage:* Store in a dry place below 30˚C.

*Nature and contents of container:* Stilnoct: Cartons of 28 tablets in PVC/foil blister strips. Stilnoct 10 mg: Cartons of 4 or 28 tablets in PVC/foil blister strips.

*Instructions for use/handling:* Please consult the package insert before use. Do not use after the stated expiry date on the carton and blister. Keep out of the reach of children.

### Marketing authorisation numbers

Stilnoct          15819/0017
Stilnoct 10 mg    15819/0018.

### Date of first authorisation/renewal of authorisation

Stilnoct:          16.12.93
Stilnoct: 10 mg    16.09.96.

### Date of approval/revision of SPC   21 January 1997.

### Legal category   POM.

## XATRAL* SR   ▼
## XATRAL*   ▼

**Qualitative and quantitative composition**   Each Xatral SR tablet contains 5 mg alfuzosin hydrochloride.

Each Xatral tablet contains 2.5 mg alfuzosin hydrochloride.

**Pharmaceutical form**   Xatral SR is a pale yellow, biconvex, film coated sustained release tablet for oral administration.

Xatral is a white round, film coated tablet for oral administration.

### Clinical particulars

*Therapeutic indications:* Alleviation of the functional symptoms of benign prostatic hypertrophy, particularly if surgery has to be delayed for some reason.

*Posology and method of administration:* Xatral SR and Xatral tablets should be swallowed whole. The first dose should be given just before bedtime.

*Adults:*

*Xatral SR:* The usual dose is one tablet Xatral SR 5 mg twice daily (morning and evening).

*Xatral:* The usual dose is one tablet Xatral 2.5 mg three times daily. The dose may be increased to a maximum of 4 tablets (10 mg) per day depending on the clinical response.

*Elderly (over 65 years), treated hypertensive patients, patients with renal insufficiency:* The initial dose should be one tablet Xatral SR 5 mg in the evening. If additional efficacy is required and Xatral SR is well tolerated the patient may be given Xatral SR 5 mg one tablet twice daily.

*Patients with hepatic insufficiency:* In patients with mild to moderate hepatic insufficiency, it is recommended that therapy should commence with a single dose of Xatral 2.5 mg once daily to be increased to Xatral 2.5 mg twice daily according to clinical response.

*Contra-indications:* Hypersensitivity to the product. History of orthostatic hypotension. Combination with other α-blockers. Severe hepatic insufficiency.

*Special warnings and special precautions for use:*

*Warnings:* In some subjects, in particular patients receiving antihypertensive medications, postural hypotension with or without symptoms (dizziness, fatigue, sweating) may develop within a few hours following administration. In such cases, the patient should lie down until the symptoms have completely disappeared.

These effects are transient and do not usually prevent the continuation of treatment after adjustment of the dose. The patient should be warned of the possible occurrence of such events.

*Precautions:* Treatment should be initiated gradually in patients with hypersensitivity to α-1-blockers. Xatral SR or Xatral should be administered carefully to patients being treated with antihypertensives. Blood pressure should be monitored regularly, especially at the beginning of treatment. In patients with coronary insufficiency specific anti-anginal therapy should be continued, but if the angina reappears or worsens Xatral SR or Xatral should be discontinued.

*Interaction with other medicaments and other forms of interaction:* Concomitant use with other α-1-receptor blockers should be avoided and antihypertensive agents should be used with caution because of the risk of a hypotensive effect.

The administration of general anaesthetics to patients receiving Xatral SR or Xatral could cause profound hypotension. It is recommended that Xatral SR or Xatral be withdrawn 24 hours before surgery.

No pharmacodynamic or pharmacokinetic interaction has been observed in healthy volunteers between alfuzosin and the following drugs: warfarin, digoxin, hydrochlorothiazide and atenolol.

*Use during pregnancy and lactation:* Due to the type of indication this section is not applicable.

*Effects on ability to drive and use machines:* There are no data available on the effect on driving vehicles. Adverse reactions such as vertigo, dizziness and asthenia may occur. This has to be taken into account when driving vehicles and operating machinery.

*Undesirable effects:* The following side-effects have been observed: faintness, vertigo, dizziness or malaise, headache, gastrointestinal disorders (nausea, gastralgia, diarrhoea, vomiting). The following occurred less frequently: hypotension (postural), syncope, tachycardia, palpitations, chest pain, fatigue, drowsiness, rash, pruritus, flushes and oedema.

*Overdosage:* No cases of accidental or deliberate overdosage have been reported. Should an overdose occur, the patient should be hospitalised, kept in a supine position, and cardiovascular support should be given. The most appropriate antidote is probably a vasoconstrictor that acts directly on vascular muscle fibres. Particular care should be exercised in patients

with cardiac or cerebrovascular complications. As alfuzosin is protein bound it is not easily dialysed. Activated charcoal may be administered after gastric lavage.

### Pharmacological properties

*Pharmacodynamic properties:* Alfuzosin is an orally active quinazoline derivative. It is a selective antagonist of postsynaptic α-adrenoceptors.

*In vitro* pharmacology studies have documented the specificity of alfuzosin for the α-receptors located in the trigone of the urinary bladder, urethra and prostate.

*In vivo* animal studies have shown that alfuzosin decreases urethral pressures and therefore resistance to the urine flow during micturition.

In benign prostatic hyperplasia, the development and severity of urinary functional symptoms are related not only to the size of the prostate but also to the tone of the sympathic nerve system. An α-adrenergic influence has been shown in smooth muscle fibres of the prostatic stroma. Blockade of post-synaptic α-1-receptors by alfuzosin results in relaxation of smooth muscle fibres. Alfuzosin may cause moderate antihypertensive effects.

*Pharmacokinetic particulars:* Xatral is well absorbed with a mean bioavailability of 64%, peak plasma levels are generally reached in 0.5–3 hours. The elimination half-life is 3–5 hours. For Xatral SR the peak plasma level is achieved approximately 3 hours post dose. The elimination half-life of alfuzosin is 8 hours. Bioavailability is decreased by approximately 15% as compared with Xatral. Alfuzosin is well absorbed. Alfuzosin is 90% protein bound in plasma, 68.2% to human serum albumin and 52.5% to human serum alpha-glycoprotein. It is partially metabolised and excreted mainly in the bile and faeces.

None of the metabolites found in man has any pharmacodynamic activity. The pharmacokinetic profile is not affected by taking Xatral with food.

In subjects over 75 years, absorption is more rapid and peak plasma levels are higher. Bioavailability may be increased and in some patients the volume of distribution is reduced. The elimination half-life does not change.

The volume of distribution and clearance of alfuzosin are increased in renal insufficiency, with or without dialysis, owing to an increase in the free fraction. Chronic renal insufficiency even when severe (creatinine clearance between 25 and 40 mls/min) is not adversely affected by alfuzosin. In patients with severe hepatic insufficiency, the elimination half-life is prolonged. A two-fold increase in Cmax values and a three-fold increase in the AUC is observed. Bioavailability is increased compared with healthy volunteers.

The pharmacokinetic profile of alfuzosin is not affected by chronic cardiac insufficiency.

*Preclinical safety data:* No data of therapeutic relevance.

### Pharmaceutical particulars

*List of excipients:*

*Xatral SR:* Tablet core – microcrystalline cellulose, polyvinyl pyrrolidone, dicalcium phosphate dihydrate, magnesium stearate, hydrogenated castor oil. Coating – methylhydroxypropylcellulose, polyethylene glycol, titanium dioxide (E171), iron oxide (E172).

*Xatral:* Tablet core – microcrystalline cellulose, lactose, povidone, sodium starch glycollate, magnesium stearate, purified water. Coating – methylhydroxypropylcellulose, polyethylene glycol 400, titanium dioxide suspension (E171), purified water.

*Incompatibilities:* Not known.

*Shelf life:* 3 years.

*Special precautions for storage:* Xatral SR: Store at room temperature (15–25˚C). Xatral: Store in a dry place at or below 30˚C.

*Nature and contents of containers:* Xatral SR: Boxes with 60 tablets in pvc/foil blister strips. Xatral: Boxes with 60 or 90 tablets in pvc/foil blister strips.

*Instructions for use/handling:* Please consult insert text before use. Do not use after the stated expiry date on packaging and blisters. Keep out of the reach of children.

### Marketing authorisation numbers
Xatral SR   15819/0024
Xatral      15819/0023.

### Date of approval/revision of SPC   September 1996.

### Legal category   POM.

*Trade Mark

# LRC Products Limited
London International House
Turnford Place
Broxbourne
Herts EN10 6LN

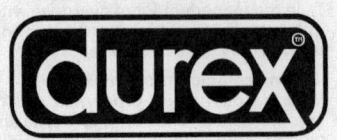

## DURAGEL*

**Presentation** *Duragel:* A colourless unscented gel containing Nonoxynol 9 USP, 2% w/w.

*Other constituents:* Docusate Sodium BP, Isopropyl Alcohol BP, Propylene Glycol EP, Sodium Hydroxide BP, Carbomer 934P USP, Benzoic Acid EP, Purified Water EP.

**Uses** Duragel is for use as a spermicidal contraceptive in conjunction with barrier methods of contraception.

**Dosage and administration** For use only by adult females of child bearing age.

*Vaginal diaphragm*
At insertion: Two strips (5 cm each) on each side of the diaphragm.At topping up: 1 applicator full (approximately 22 cm strip).

*Cervical Cap*
At insertion: One 5 ml teaspoonful inside the cap.At topping up: 1 applicator full (approximately 22 cm strip).

*All uses:* Apply or top up not more than 3 hours before intercourse. Top up between repeated acts of intercourse. Leave in place for at least 6 hours after last intercourse. Do not leave in place for longer than 24 hours.

**Contra-indications, warnings, etc**
*Contra-indications:* Hypersensitivity to Nonoxynol 9 or to any component of the preparation. Patients with absent vaginal sensation e.g. paraplegics and quadriplegics.

*Undesirable effects:* May cause irritation of the vagina or penis.

*Use in pregnancy and lactation:* There is no evidence from animal and human studies that Nonoxynol 9 is teratogenic. Human epidemiological studies have not shown any firm evidence of adverse effects on the foetus, however some studies have shown that Nonoxynol 9 may be embryotoxic in animals. This product should not be used if pregnancy is suspected or confirmed. Animal studies have detected Nonoxynol 9 in milk after intravaginal administration. Use by lactating women has not been studied.

*Other special warnings and precautions:* Spermicidal intravaginal preparations are intended for use in conjunction with barrier methods of contraception such as condoms, diaphragms and caps.

Where avoidance of pregnancy is important the choice of contraceptive method should be made in consultation with a doctor or a family planning clinic.

If vaginal or penile irritation occurs discontinue use. If symptoms worsen or continue for more than 48 hours medical advice should be sought.

*Overdose:* If taken orally the surfactant properties of this preparation may cause gastric irritation. General supportive therapy should be carried out. Hepatic and renal function should be monitored if medically indicated.

**Pharmaceutical precautions** Store below 30°C. Do not freeze.

**Legal category** GSL.

**Package quantities** The product is presented in a collapsible tube containing 100 g. The tubes are supplied in packs of four.

**Further information** Duragel is suitable for patients requiring extra lubrication in addition to spermicidal action.

**Product licence number** 2156/5001R

*Trade Mark

# Lundbeck Limited
## Sunningdale House
## Caldecotte Lake Business Park
## Caldecotte, Milton Keynes, MK7 8LF

*Lundbeck*

## BLEOMYCIN INJECTION

**Presentation** Bleomycin Lundbeck Injection is a whitish-yellow freeze-dried plug of bleomycin sulphate equivalent to 15 000 I.U ($15 \times 10^3$ I.U.) bleomycin in a clear glass ampoule.

*Active ingredients:* 15 000 I.U ($15 \times 10^3$ I.U.) bleomycin per ampoule, as the sulphate.

**Uses** *Pharmacology:* Bleomycin is a basic water-soluble glycopeptide with cytotoxic activity. The mechanism of action of bleomycin is believed to involve single-strand scission of DNA, leading to inhibition of cell division, of growth and of DNA synthesis in tumour cells.

Apart from its antibacterial and antitumour properties, bleomycin is relatively free from biological activity. When injected intravenously it may have a histamine-like effect on blood pressure and may cause a rise in body temperature. Blood concentrations of bleomycin in patients indicate that the drug is excreted more rapidly after intravenous than after intramuscular injection and that up to one third of the dose is excreted unchanged in the urine within 24 hours.

*Indications:*

1. Squamous cell carcinoma affecting the mouth, nasopharynx and paranasal sinuses, larynx, oesophagus, external genitalia, cervix or skin. Well-differentiated tumours usually respond better than anaplastic ones.
2. Hodgkin's disease and other malignant lymphomas, including mycosis fungoides.
3. Testicular teratoma.
4. Malignant effusions of serous cavities.
5. Secondary indications in which bleomycin has been shown to be of some value (alone or in combination with other drugs) include metastatic malignant melanoma, carcinoma of the thyroid, lung and bladder.

**Dosage and administration** *Adults:* Bleomycin is usually administered intramuscularly but may be given intravenously (bolus or drip), intra-arterially, intrapleurally or intraperitoneally as a solution in physiological saline. Local injection directly into the tumour may occasionally be indicated.

1. *Squamous cell carcinoma and testicular teratoma:* Used alone the normal dosage is $15 \times 10^3$ I.U. (1 ampoule) three times a week or $30 \times 10^3$ I.U. (2 ampoules) twice a week, either intramuscularly or intravenously. Treatment may continue on consecutive weeks, or more usually at intervals of 3–4 weeks, up to a total cumulative dose of $500 \times 10^3$ I.U. although young men with testicular tumours have frequently tolerated twice this amount. Continuous intravenous infusion at a rate of $15 \times 10^3$ I.U. (1 ampoule) per 24 hours for up to 10 days, or $30 \times 10^3$ I.U. (2 ampoules) per 24 hours for up to 5 days may produce a therapeutic effect more rapidly. The development of stomatitis is the most useful guide to the determination of individual tolerance of maximum therapeutic response. The dose may need to be adjusted when bleomycin is used in combination chemotherapy. Use in elderly or children – see below.

2. *Malignant lymphomas:* Used alone the recommended dosage regimen is $15 \times 10^3$ I.U. (1 ampoule) once or twice a week, intramuscularly, to a total dose of $225 \times 10^3$ I.U. (15 ampoules). Dosage should be reduced in the elderly. The dose may need to be adjusted when bleomycin is used in combination chemotherapy. Use in children – see below.

3. *Malignant effusions:* After drainage of the affected serous cavity, $60 \times 10^3$ I.U. (4 ampoules) bleomycin dissolved in 100 ml physiological saline is introduced via the drainage needle or cannula. After instillation, the drainage needle or cannula may be withdrawn. Administration may be repeated if necessary subject to a total cumulative dose of $500 \times 10^3$ I.U. (about 33 ampoules). Use in elderly or childen – see below.

*Combination therapy:* Bleomycin is commonly used in conjunction with radiotherapy, particularly in treatment of cancer of the head and neck region. Such a combination may enhance mucosal reactions if full doses of both forms of treatment are used and bleomycin dosage may require reduction, e.g. to $5 \times 10^3$ I.U. at the time of each radiotherapy fraction five days a week. Bleomycin is frequently used as one of the drugs in multiple chemotherapy regimens (e.g.

in squamous cell carcinoma, testicular teratoma, lymphoma). The mucosal toxicity of bleomycin should be borne in mind in the selection and dosage of drugs with similar toxic potential used in such combinations.

*Elderly patients:* The total dose of bleomycin used in the treatment of squamous cell carcinoma, testicular teratoma or malignant effusions should be reduced as indicated below.

| Age in years | Total dose (I.U.) | Dose per week (I.U.) |
|---|---|---|
| 80 and over | $100 \times 10^3$ | $15 \times 10^3$ |
| 70–79 | $150–200 \times 10^3$ | $30 \times 10^3$ |
| 60–69 | $200–300 \times 10^3$ | $30–60 \times 10^3$ |
| Under 60 | $500 \times 10^3$ | $30–60 \times 10^3$ |

*Children:* Until further data are available, administration of bleomycin to children should take place only under exceptional circumstances and in special centres. The dosage should be based on that recommended for adults and adjusted to body surface area or body weight.

*Reduced kidney function:* With serum creatinine values of 2–4 mg%, half the above individual dosage is recommended. With serum creatinine above 4 mg%, a further reduction in dose is indicated.

*Preparation of solutions:* For intramuscular injections the required dose is dissolved in up to 5 ml of a suitable solvent such as physiological saline. If pain occurs at the site of injection a 1% solution of lignocaine may be used as a solvent.

For intravenous injections the dose required is dissolved in 5–200 ml of physiological saline and injected slowly or added to the reservoir of a running intravenous infusion. For intra-arterial administration a slow infusion in physiological saline is used. For intra-cavitary injection $60 \times 10^3$ I.U. is dissolved in 100 ml normal saline.

For local injections bleomycin is dissolved in physiological saline to make a $1–3 \times 10^3$ I.U./ml solution.

**Contra-indications, warnings, etc** Bleomycin is contra-indicated in patients with acute pulmonary infection or greatly reduced lung function. It should not normally be administered to patients who are pregnant or to mothers who are breast feeding.

*Adverse reactions:* Like most cytotoxic agents bleomycin can give rise both to immediate and to delayed toxic effects. The most immediate effect is fever on the day of injection. Anorexia, tiredness or nausea may also occur.

Local pain may occur after intravenous or intra-cavitary injection and other rare adverse effects are hypotension and local thrombophlebitis after intravenous administration.

The majority of patients who receive a full course of bleomycin develop lesions of the skin or oral mucosa. Induration, hyperkeratosis, reddening, tenderness, and swelling of the tips of the fingers, ridging of the nails, bulla formation over pressure points such as elbows, loss of hair and stomatitis are rarely serious and usually disappear soon after completion of the course.

The most serious delayed effect is interstitial pneumonia, which may develop during, or occasionally after, a course of treatment. This condition may sometimes develop into fatal pulmonary fibrosis, although such an occurrence is rare at recommended doses. Previous or concurrent radiotherapy to the chest is an important factor in increasing the incidence and severity of lung toxicity. It has been suggested that those patients who have received bleomycin preoperatively are at a greater risk of developing pulmonary toxicity, and a reduction in inspired oxygen concentration during the operation and post-operatively is recommended.

Acute fulminant reactions with hyperpyrexia and cardiorespiratory collapse have been reported after intravenous injections of doses higher than those recommended. Hypotension, hyperpyrexia and drug-related deaths have been reported rarely following intra-cavitary instillation of bleomycin.

When bleomycin is used as one of the drugs in multiple chemotherapy regimens the toxicity of bleomycin should be borne in mind in the selection and dosage of drugs with similar toxic potential. The

addition of other cytotoxic drugs can necessitate changes and dose alterations.

In patients treated for testicular cancer with a combination of bleomycin and vinca alkaloids a syndrome has been reported corresponding to morbus Raynaud, ischaemia which can lead to necrosis of peripheral parts of the body (fingers, toes, nose tip).

*Precautions:* Patients undergoing treatment with bleomycin should have chest X-rays weekly. These should continue to be taken for up to four weeks after completion of the course. If breathlessness or infiltrates, not obviously attributable to tumour or to co-existent lung disease, appear, administration of the drug must be stopped immediately and patients should be treated with a corticosteroid (e.g. hydrocortisone 100 mg i.m. as the sodium succinate daily for five days, followed by oral prednisolone 10 mg twice daily) and a broad-spectrum antibiotic. No specific clinical incompatibilities with other drugs or food have been encountered.

This product should not normally be administered to patients who are pregnant or mothers who are breast feeding. Animal experiences have revealed that bleomycin, like most cytotoxics, may have teratogenic and carcinogenic potential.

*Overdosage:* No specific antidote. The acute reaction to an overdosage with bleomycin would probably include hypotension, fever, rapid pulse and general symptoms of shock. Treatment is purely symptomatic. In the event of respiratory complications, the patient should be treated with a corticosteroid and a broad-spectrum antibiotic.

**Pharmaceutical precautions** Bleomycin should be stored at room temperature and protected from light. It should be administered as a freshly prepared solution.

Because of possible skin changes, direct contact of bleomycin with the skin should be avoided.

*Pharmaceutical incompatibilities:* Bleomycin solutions should not be mixed with solutions of essential amino acids, riboflavine, ascorbic acid, dexamethasone, aminophylline or frusemide.

**Legal category** POM.
The supply of bleomycin is restricted to centres with special experience in the chemotherapy of malignant diseases and it is available on prescription only.

**Package quantities** Boxes of 10 ampoules, each ampoule containing 15 000 I.U. ($15 \times 10^3$ I.U.).

**Further information** Bleomycin has little or no toxic effect on the bone marrow, and has no immuno-suppressive action.

**Product licence number** 0458/0009.

## CIPRAMIL* TABLETS ▼

**Qualitative and quantitative composition** Tablets of 10 or 20 mg (12.49 or 24.98 mg citalopram hydrobromide corresponding to 10 or 20 mg citalopram base).

**Pharmaceutical form** Tablet.

**Clinical particulars**
*Therapeutic indications:* Treatment of depressive illness in the initial phase and as maintenance against potential relapse/recurrence. Cipramil is also indicated in the treatment of panic disorder with or without agoraphobia.

*Posology and method of administration*
*Posology – Treating depression:*

*Adults:* Citalopram should be administered as a single oral dose of 20 mg daily. Dependent on individual patient reponse this may be increased to a maximum of 60 mg daily. The dose may be taken in the morning or evening without regard for food.

*Elderly patients:* The recommended daily dose is 20 mg. Dependent on individual patient response this may be increased to a maximum of 40 mg daily.

*Children:* Not recommended, as safety and efficacy have not been established in this population.

*Reduced hepatic function:* Dosage should be restricted to the lower end of the dose range.

*Reduced renal function:* Dosage adjustment is not necessary in cases of mild or moderate renal impairment. No information is available in cases of severe renal impairment (creatinine clearance <20 mL/min).

*Duration of treatment:* A treatment period of at least six months is usually necessary to provide adequate maintenance against the potential for relapse.

*Treating panic disorder:* In common with other pharmacotherapy used in this patient group, a low starting dose is advised to reduce the likelihood of a paradoxical initial anxiogenic effect. A single oral dose of 10 mg daily is recommended for the first week before increasing the dose to 20 mg daily. The dose may be further increased up to a maximum of 60 mg daily dependent on individual patient response; however an optimum dose of 20–30 mg daily was indicated in a clinical study.

Maximum effectiveness of citalopram in treating panic disorder is reached after about 3 months and the response is maintained during continued treatment. Dependent on individual patient response it may be necessary to continue treatment for several months.

*Method of administration:* Citalopram tablets are administered as a single daily dose. Citalopram tablets can be taken any time of the day without regard to food intake.

*Contra-indications:* Hypersensitivity to citalopram. Sumatriptan's serotonergic effects are suspected to be enhanced by SSRIs. Until further evidence is available it is advised not to use citalopram simultaneously with 5-HT agonists e.g. sumatriptan.

*Special warnings and special precautions for use:* As with other SSRIs, citalopram should not be given to patients receiving Monoamine Oxidase Inhibitors (MAOIs), or for 14 days after their discontinuation. MAOIs should not be introduced for seven days after discontinuation of citalopram. Rarely, the occurrence of 'serotonin syndrome' has been reported in patients receiving SSRIs. A combination of symptoms, possibly including agitation, tremor, myoclonus and hyperthermia, may indicate the development of this condition.

Experience with citalopram has not revealed any clinically relevant interactions with neuroleptics. However, as with other SSRIs, the possibility of a pharmacodynamic interaction cannot be excluded.

Consideration should be given to factors which may affect the disposition of a minor metabolite of citalopram (didemethylcitalopram) since increased levels of this metabolite could theoretically prolong the QTc interval in susceptible individuals. However, in ECG monitoring of 2500 patients in clinical trials, including 277 patients with pre-existing cardiac conditions, no clincally significant changes were noted.

As with most antidepressants, citalopram should be discontinued if the patient enters a manic phase. There is little clinical experience of concurrent use of citalopram and ECT.

*Interactions with other medicaments and other forms of interaction:* Monoamine Oxidase Inhibitors (MAOIs) should not be used in combination with SSRIs (see above).

The metabolism of citalopram is only partly dependent on the hepatic cytochrome P450 isozyme CYP2 D6 and, unlike some other SSRIs, citalopram is only a weak inhibitor of this important enzyme system which is involved in the metabolism of many drugs (including antiarrhythmics, neuroleptics, beta-blockers, TCAs and some SSRIs). Protein binding is relatively low (<80%). These properties give citalopram a low potential for clinically significant drug interactions.

There is no pharmacokinetic interaction between lithium and citalopram. However, there have been reports of enhanced serotonergic effects when SSRIs have been given with lithium or tryptophan and therefore the concomitant use of citalopram with these drugs should be undertaken with caution. Routine monitoring of lithium levels need not be adjusted. In a pharmacokinetic study no effect was demonstrated on either citalopram or imipramine levels, although the level of desipramine, the primary metabolite of imipramine, was increased. In animal studies cimetidine has little or no influence on citalopram kinetics.

No pharmacodynamic interactions have been noted in clinical studies in which citalopram has been given concomitantly with benzodiazepines, neuroleptics, analgesics, lithium, alcohol, antihistamines, antihypertensive drugs, beta-blockers and other cardiovascular drugs.

*Pregnancy and lactation:* Category B1. Animal studies have not shown any evidence of teratogenic potential and citalopram does not affect reproduction or perinatal conditions. Citalopram appears in milk in very low concentrations.

Due to limited human data citalopram should only be used in pregnancy if considered necessary and under the close supervision of a physician. In nursing mothers, caution is recommended as it is not known whether citalopram excreted in milk may affect the infant.

*Effects on ability to drive and use machines:* Citalopram does not impair intellectual function and psychomotor performance. However, patients who are prescribed psychotropic medication may be expected to have some impairment of general attention and concentration either due to the illness itself, the medication or both and should be cautioned about their ability to drive a car and operate machinery.

*Undesirable effects:* Adverse effects observed with citalopram are in general mild and transient. They are most prominent during the first one or two weeks of treatment and usually attenuate as the depressive state improves.

The most commonly observed adverse events associated with the use of citalopram and not seen at an equal incidence among placebo-treated patients were: nausea, somnolence, mouth dry, sweating increased and tremor. The incidence of each in excess over placebo is low (<10%).

In comparative clinical trials with tricyclic antidepressants the incidence of adverse events occurring with citalopram was found to be lower in all cases.

Treatment emergent adverse events reported in clinical trials (N=2985):

*Frequent:* (≥5–20%) Sweating increased, headache, tremor, dizziness, accommodation abnormal, somnolence, insomnia, agitation, nervousness, nausea, mouth dry, constipation, diarrhoea, palpitation, asthenia.

*Less frequent:* (1–<5%) Rash, pruritus, paraesthesia, migraine, vision abnormal, taste perversion, sleep disorder, libido decreased, concentration impaired, dreaming abnormal, amnesia, anxiety, appetite increased, anorexia, apathy, impotence, suicide attempt, confusion, yawning, dyspepsia, vomiting, abdominal pain, flatulence, saliva increased, weight decrease, weight increase, hypotension postural, tachycardia, rhinitis, micturition disorder, polyuria, ejaculation failure, anorgasmia female, fatigue.

*Rare:* (<1%) Myalgia, exrapyramidal disorder, convulsion, tinnitus, euphoria, libido increased, coughing, malaise.

*Overdose:* Citalopram is given to patients at potential risk of suicide and some reports of attempted suicide have been received. Detail is often lacking regarding precise dose or combination with other drugs and/or alcohol.

*Symptoms:* Experience from 8 cases considered due to citalopram alone has recorded the following symptoms/signs: somnolence, coma, stiffened expression, episode of grand mal convulsion, sinus tachycardia, occasional nodal rhythm, sweating, nausea, vomiting, cyanosis, hyperventilation. No case was fatal. The clinical picture was inconsistent, no observation being made in more than two individuals.

Six fatalities have been reported. In one overdose was suspected; high post mortem plasma levels were seen although it is not technically possible to interpret these with confidence.

In the remaining five a combination with other drugs had been taken. The clinical syndrome observed prior to death in three of these cases where citalopram was taken with moclobemide was interpreted as that of serotonin syndrome. No clinical details are available on the other two.

*Treatment:* There is no specific antidote. Treatment is symptomatic and supportive. Gastric lavage should be carried out as soon as possible after oral ingestion. Medical surveillance is advisable.

**Pharmacological properties**

*Pharmacodynamic properties:* ATC-code: N 06 AB 04. Biochemical and behavioural studies have shown that citalopram is a potent inhibitor of serotonin (5-HT)-uptake. Tolerance to the inhibition of 5-HT-uptake is not induced by long-term treatment with citalopram.

Citalopram is the most Selective Serotonin Reuptake Inhibitor (SSRI) yet described, with no, or minimal, effect on noradrenaline (NA), dopamine (DA) and gamma aminobutyric acid (GABA) uptake.

In contrast to many tricyclic antidepressants and some of the newer SSRI's, citalopram has no or very low affinity for a series of receptors including 5-HT$_{1A}$, 5-HT$_2$, dopamine D$_1$ and D$_2$ receptors, alpha1-, alpha2- and beta-adrenoceptors, histamine H$_1$, muscarine cholinergic, benzodiazepine, and opioid receptors. A series of functional *in vitro* tests in isolated organs as well as functional *in vivo* tests have confirmed the lack of receptor affinity. This absence of effects on receptors could explain why citalopram produces fewer of the traditional side effects such as dry mouth, bladder and gut disturbance, blurred vision, sedation, cardiotoxicity and orthostatic hypotension. Although citalopram does not bind to opioid receptors it potentiates the anti-nociceptive effect of commonly used opioid analgesics. There was potentiation of d-amphetamine-induced hyperactivity following administration of citalopram.

Suppression of rapid eye movement (REM) sleep is considered a predictor of antidepressant activity. Like tricyclic antidepressants, other SSRI's and MAO inhibitors, citalopram suppresses REM-sleep and increases deep slow-wave sleep.

The main metabolites of citalopram are all SSRIs although their potency and selectivity ratios are lower than those of citalopram. However, the selectivity ratios of the metabolites are higher than those of many of the newer SSRIs. The metabolites do not contribute to the overall antidepressant effect.

In humans citalopram does not impair cognitive (intellectual function) and psychomotor performance and has no or minimal sedative properties, either alone or in combination with alcohol.

Citalopram did not reduce saliva flow in a single dose study in human volunteers and in none of the studies in healthy volunteers did citalopram have significant influence on cardiovascular parameters. Citalopram has no effect on the serum levels of prolactin and growth hormone.

*Pharmacokinetic properties*

*Absorption:* Absorption is almost complete and independent of food intake (T$_{max}$ average/mean 3.8 hours). Oral bioavailability is about 80%.

*Distribution:* The apparent volume of distribution (V$_d$)$_\beta$ is about 12.3 L/kg. The plasma protein binding is below 80% for citalopram and its main metabolites.

*Biotransformation:* Citalopram is metabolised to the active demethylcitalopram, didemethylcitalopram, citalopram-N-oxide and an inactive deaminated propionic acid derivative. All the active metabolites are also SSRIs, although weaker than the parent compound. Unchanged citalopram is the predominant compound in plasma.

*Elimination:* The elimination half-life (T$_{1/2\beta}$) is about 1½ days and the systemic citalopram plasma clearance (Cl$_S$) is about 0.33 L/min, and oral plasma clearance (Cl$_{oral}$) is about 0.41 L/min.

Citalopram is excreted mainly via the liver (85%) and the remainder (15%) via the kidneys. About 12% of the daily dose is excreted in urine as unchanged citalopram. Hepatic (residual) clearance is about 0.35 L/min and renal clearance about 0.068 L/min.

The kinetics is linear. Steady state plasma levels are achieved in 1–2 weeks. Average concentrations of 250 nmol/L (100–500 nmol/L) are achieved at a daily dose of 40 mg. There is no clear relationship between citalopram plasma levels and therapeutic response or side effects.

*Elderly patients* (≥65 years): Longer half-lives and decreased clearance values due to a reduced rate of metabolism have been demonstrated in elderly patients.

*Reduced hepatic function:* Citalopram is eliminated more slowly in patients with reduced hepatic function. The half-life of citalopram is about twice as long and steady state citalopram concentrations at a given dose will be about twice as high as in patients with normal liver function.

*Reduced renal function:* Citalopram is eliminated more slowly in patients with mild to moderate reduction of renal function, without any major impact on the pharmacokinetics of citalopram. At present no information is available for treatment of patients with severely reduced renal function (creatinine clearance <20 mL/min).

*Preclinical safety data:* Citalopram has low acute toxicity. In chronic toxicity studies there were no findings of concern for the therapeutic use of citalopram. Based on data from reproduction toxicity studies (segment I, II and III) there is no reason to have special concern for the use of citalopram in women of child-bearing potential. Citalopram has no mutagenic or carcinogenic potential.

**Pharmaceutical particulars**

*List of excipients:* Maize starch, lactose, microcrystalline-cellulose, copolyvidone, glycerol, croscarmellose sodium type A, magnesium stearate, methylhydroxypropyl-cellulose, macrogol, titanium dioxide.

*Incompatibilities:* Nil.

*Shelf life:* 5 years. Each pack has an expiry date.

*Special precautions for storage:* Store at room temperature (at or below 25˚C).

*Nature and contents of container:* Press through packs (UPVC/PVdC with aluminium closure) containing 28 tablets.

*Instructions for use/handling:* Nil.

**Marketing authorisation numbers**
10 mg  0458/0057
20 mg  0458/0058

**Date of approval/revision of SPC**  19 February 1997.

**Legal category**  POM.

## CLOPIXOL* ACUPHASE* INJECTION

**Qualitative and quantitative composition**  Zuclopenthixol acetate 5.0% w/v equivalent to 4.526% w/v of zuclopenthixol base.

**Pharmaceutical form** Oily solution for deep intramuscular injection.

**Clinical particulars**

*Therapeutic indications:* For the initial treatment of acute psychoses including mania and exacerbation of chronic psychoses, particularly where a rapid onset of action, and a duration of effect of 2–3 days is desirable.

*Posology and method of administration*
*Dosage*

*Adults:* Dosage should be adjusted according to the severity of the patient's illness. Clopixol Acuphase is administered by deep intramuscular injection, into the upper outer buttock or lateral thigh.

The usual dosage is 50–150 mg (1–3 mL), repeated if necessary after 2 or 3 days. Some patients may need an additional injection between 1 and 2 days after the first injection.

Clopixol Acuphase is not intended for long-term use and duration of treatment should not be more than two weeks. The maximum accumulated dosage in a course should not exceed 400 mg and the number of injections should not exceed four.

Patients with compromised hepatic function should receive half the recommended dosages for normal patients. Where there is reduced renal function, it is not necessary to reduce the dosage but where there is renal failure dosage should be reduced to half the normal dosage.

*Elderly:* The dosage may need to be reduced in the elderly owing to reduced rates of metabolism and elimination. Maximum dosage per injection should be 100 mg.

*Children:* Not recommended for children.

*Maintenance therapy:* Clopixol Acuphase is not intended for long-term use.

A single injection of Clopixol Acuphase has an onset of sedative action shortly after injection and an antipsychotic action persisting for 2 to 3 days. In this period, maintenance treatment with tablets or a longer acting depot neuroleptic can be initiated. The possible side-effects of long-term maintenance treatment with a neuroleptic, including tardive dyskinesia, should be considered.

Maintenance treatment where required can be continued with Clopixol tablets, Clopixol injection or Clopixol Conc. injection, according to the following guidelines:

1. Introduce Clopixol tablets at a dosage of 20–60 mg/day in divided doses, 2 to 3 days after the last injection of Clopixol Acuphase. If necessary increase the tablet dosage by 10–20 mg each day up to a maximum of 150 mg/day.
or

2. Concomitantly with the last injection of Clopixol Acuphase, administer 200–500 mg of Clopixol injection or Clopixol Conc injection by deep intramuscular injection and repeat the Clopixol injection or Clopixol Conc injection at intervals of 2 to 4 weeks. Higher dosages or a shorter interval may be necessary.

*Route of administration:* Deep intramuscular injection, into the upper outer buttock or lateral thigh.

*Contra-indications:* Comatose states, including acute alcohol, barbiturate, and opiate intoxication.

*Special warnings and special precautions for use:* Like other neuroleptics zuclopenthixol acetate should be used with caution in patients with convulsive disorders or advanced hepatic, renal or cardiovascular disease.

Zuclopenthixol is not suitable for patients who do not tolerate oral neuroleptic drugs or for patients suffering from Parkinson's disease.

*Interactions with other medicaments and other forms of interaction:* Zuclopenthixol enhances the response to alcohol and the effects of barbiturates and other CNS depressants. Potentiation of the effects of general anaesthetics may occur. Zuclopenthixol acetate should not be given concomitantly with guanethidine or similarly acting compounds, since neuroleptics may block the antihypertensive effect of these compounds. Tricyclic antidepressants and neuroleptics mutually inhibit the metabolism of each other. Zuclopenthixol may reduce the effect of levodopa and the effect of adrenergic drugs. Concomitant use of metoclopramide and piperazine increases the risk of extrapyramidal symptoms.

The possibility of interaction with lithium salts should be borne in mind.

*Pregnancy and lactation:* Animal tests have not revealed any evidence that zuclopenthixol causes an increased incidence of foetal damage. Nevertheless, zuclopenthixol acetate should not be administered during pregnancy or to women of childbearing potential, unless they are taking adequate contraceptive precautions or unless the expected benefit to the patient outweighs the potential risk to the foetus.

Zuclopenthixol is found in very low concentrations in the breast milk of mothers receiving Clopixol treatment. It is recommended that mothers treated with Clopixol Acuphase should not breast feed.

*Effects on ability to drive and use machines:* The ability to drive a car or operate machinery may be affected and patients should be warned of this risk.

*Undesirable effects:* The frequency of unwanted effects is in general low and the severity of the symptoms is most often mild. The frequency and severity are most pronounced the day after the first injection and then decrease rapidly.

Extrapyramidal symptoms, including dystonia, rigidity, motor akathisia, hypokinesia and tremor, have been reported. These side effects can be satisfactorily controlled by antiparkinson drugs.

Orthostatic dizziness occurs rarely and only occasionally to a severe degree.

Reduced salivation of a mild degree has been observed.

*Overdose:* Symptoms: somnolence, coma, extrapyramidal symptoms, convulsions, hypotension, shock, hyper or hypothermia.

Treatment is symptomatic and supportive. Measures aimed at supporting the respiratory and cardiovascular systems should be instituted. Adrenaline (epinephrine) must not be used in these patients. There is no specific antidote.

**Pharmacological properties**

*Pharmacodynamic properties:* Zuclopenthixol is a potent neuroleptic of the thioxanthene series with a piperazine side-chain. The antipsychotic effect of neuroleptics is related to their dopamine receptor blocking effect. The thioxanthenes have a high affinity for both the adenylate cyclase coupled dopamine $D_1$ receptors and for the dopamine $D_2$ receptors; in the phenothiazine group the affinity for $D_1$ receptors is much lower than that for $D_2$ receptors, whereas butyrophenones, diphenylbutylpiperidines and benzamides only have affinity for $D_2$ receptors.

In the traditional tests for antipsychotic effect, e.g. antagonism of stereotypic behaviour induced by dopamine agonists, the chemical groups of neuroleptics mentioned reveal equal but dosage dependent activity. However, the antistereotypic effect of phenothiazines, butyrophenones, diphenylbutylpiperidines, and benzamindes is strongly counteracted by the anticholinergic drug, scopolamine, while the antisteriotype effect of the thioxanthenes, e.g. zuclopenthixol, is not, or only very slightly, influenced by concomitant treatment with anticholinergics.

*Pharmacokinetic properties:* By esterification of zuclopenthixol with acetic acid, zuclopenthixol has been converted to a more lipophilic substance, zuclopenthixol acetate. When dissolved in oil and injected intramuscularly this substance diffuses slowly into the surrounding body water, where enzymatic breakdown occurs releasing the active component zuclopenthixol.

Maximum serum concentrations of zuclopenthixol are usually reached 36 hours after an injection, after which the serum levels decline slowly. The average maximum serum level corresponding to the 100 mg dose is 41 ng/mL. Three days after the injection the serum level is about one third of the maximum.

Zuclopenthixol is distrubuted in the body in a similar way to other neuroleptics; with the higher concentrations of drug and metabolites in liver, lungs, intestines and kidneys and lower concentrations in heart, spleen, brain and blood. The apparent volume of distribution is about 20 L/kg and the protein binding about 98%.

Zuclopenthixol crosses the placental barrier in small amounts. Zuclopenthixol is excreted in small amounts with the milk – the ratio milk concentration/serum concentration in women is on average 0.3.

The metabolism of zuclopenthixol proceeds via three main routes – sulphoxidation, side chain N-dealkylation and glucuronic acid conjugation. The metabolites are devoid of psychopharmacolical activity. The excretion proceeds mainly with the faeces but also to some degree with the urine. The systemic clearance is about 0.9 L/min.

The kinetics seem to be linear, since highly significant correlation exist between the dose and the area under the serum concentration curve.

*Preclinical safety data:* Zuclopenthixol has low acute toxicity and was not mutagenic or carcinogenic in appropriate tests. Local muscle damage is less pronounced with oily solutions of zuclopenthixol (including Clopixol Acuphase) than with aqueous solutions of zuclopenthixol and other neuroleptics.

**Pharmaceutical particulars**

*List of excipients:* Thin vegetable oil (derived from coconuts).

*Incompatibilities:* Zuclopenthixol acetate should not be mixed with other injection fluids.

*Shelf life:* 2 years was packaged for sale.

*Special precautions for storage:* Protect from light.

*Nature and contents of container:* Clear glass ampoules containing either 1 or 2 mL of zuclopenthixol acetate 5% w/v in thin vegetable oil.

The ampoules are packed in boxes of 5.

*Instructions for use/handling:* Nil.

**Marketing authorisation number** 0458/0063.

**Date of approval/revision of SPC** 12 September 1995.

**Legal category** POM.

# CLOPIXOL* INJECTION
# CLOPIXOL*-CONC. INJECTION

**Presentation** *Clopixol Injection* is a sterile, straw-coloured solution of 200 mg/ml (20%) zuclopenthixol decanoate in thin vegetable oil. It is presented in glass ampoules (1 ml).

*Clopixol-Conc. Injection* is a sterile, straw-coloured solution of 500 mg/ml (50%) zuclopenthixol decanoate in thin vegetable oil. It is presented in glass ampoules (1 ml).

**Uses** The maintenance treatment of schizophrenia and paranoid psychoses.

**Dosage and administration**

*Note:* As with all oil based injections it is important to ensure, by aspiration before injection, that inadvertent intravascular entry does not occur.

*Adults:* Clopixol Injection and Clopixol-Conc. Injection are administered by deep intramuscular injection into the upper outer buttock or lateral thigh.

Dosage and dosage interval should be adjusted according to the patients' symptoms and response to treatment.

The usual dosage range of zuclopenthixol decanoate is 200–500 mg every one to four weeks, depending on response, but some patients may require up to 600 mg per week. In patients who have not previously received depot neuroleptics, treatment is usually started with a small dose (e.g. 100 mg) to assess tolerability. An interval of at least one week should be allowed before the second injection is given at a dose consistent with the patients' condition.

Adequate control of severe psychotic symptoms may take up to 4 to 6 months at high enough dosage. Once stabilised lower maintenance doses may be considered, but must be sufficient to prevent relapse.

Injection volumes of greater than 2 ml should be distributed between two injection sites.

When transferring patients from oral to depot neuroleptic treatment, the oral medication should not be discontinued immediately, but gradually withdrawn over a period of several days after administering the first injection.

*Elderly:* In accordance with standard medical practice initial dosage may need to be reduced to a quarter or half the normal starting dose in the frail or elderly.

*Children:* Clopixol Injection and Clopixol-Conc. Injection are not indicated for children.

**Contra-indications, warnings, etc**

*Contra-indications:* Comatose states, including acute alcohol, barbiturates or opiate intoxication.

*Warnings and precautions for use:* Caution should be exercised in patients having: liver disease; cardiac disease, or arrhythmias; severe respiratory disease; renal failure; epilepsy (and conditions predisposing to epilepsy, e.g. alcohol withdrawal or brain damage); Parkinson's disease; narrow angle glaucoma; prostatic hypertrophy; hypothyroidism; hyperthyroidism; myasthenia gravis; phaeochromocytoma and patients who have shown hypersensitivity to thioxanthenes or other neuroleptics.

The elderly require close supervision because they are especially prone to experience such adverse effects as sedation, hypotension, confusion and temperature changes.

*Interactions:* In common with other neuroleptics, zuclopenthixol enhances the response to alcohol, and the effects of barbiturates and other CNS depressants, and may potentiate the effects of general anaesthetics. Neuroleptics may antagonise the effects of adrenaline and other sympathomimetic agents, and reverse the antihypertensive effects of guanethidine and similar adrenergic-blocking agents. Neuroleptics may impair the effect of levodopa, adrenergic drugs and anticonvulsants. The metabolism of tricyclic antidepressants may be inhibited and the control of diabetes may be impaired. The effect of anticoagulants may be increased. The anticholinergic effects of atropine may be increased. Anticholinergic effects may be enhanced by antiparkinson drugs and tardive dyskinesia precipitated. Concomitant use of metoclopramide and piperazine increases the risk of extrapyramidal symptoms. Neuroleptics may enhance the cardiac depressant effects of quinidine; the absorption of corticosteroids and digoxin; the hypotensive effect of vasodilator antihypertensive agents such as hydralazine and prolong the action of neuromuscular blocking agents. The possibility of interaction with lithium salts should be borne in mind.

*Pregnancy and lactation:* As the safety of this drug during pregnancy has not been established, use during pregnancy, especially the first and last trimesters, should be avoided, unless the expected benefit to the patient outweighs the potential risk to the foetus.

Zuclopenthixol is excreted into breast milk. If the use of Clopixol is considered essential, nursing mothers should be advised to stop breast feeding.

The newborn of mothers treated with neuroleptics in late pregnancy, or labour, may show signs of intoxication such as lethargy, tremor and hyperexcitability, and have a low apgar score.

*Effects on ability to drive and use machines:* Alertness may be impaired, especially at the start of treatment, or following the consumption of alcohol; patients should be warned of this risk and advised not to drive or operate machinery until their susceptibility is known.

*Undesirable effects:* Drowsiness and sedation may occur but are more often seen with high dosage and at the start of treatment, particularly in the elderly. Other adverse effects include blurring of vision, tachycardia and urinary incontinence and frequency. Dose-related postural hypotension may occur, particularly in the elderly.

Because Clopixol may impair alertness, especially at the start of treatment or following the consumption of alcohol, patients should be warned of this risk and advised not to drive or operate machinery, until their susceptibility is known.

Extrapyramidal reactions in the form of acute dystonias (including oculogyric crisis), parkinsonian rigidity, tremor, akinesia and akathisia have been reported and may occur even at lower dosage in susceptible patients. Such effects would usually be encountered early in treatment, but delayed reactions may also occur. Antiparkinson agents should not be prescribed routinely because of the possible risk of precipitating toxic-confusional states, impairing therapeutic efficacy or causing anticholinergic side-effects. They should only be given if required and their requirement reassessed at regular intervals.

Tardive dyskinesia can occur with neuroleptic treatment. It is more common at high doses for prolonged periods and has been reported at lower dosage for short periods. The risk seems to be greater in the elderly, especially females. It has been reported that fine vermicular movements of the tongue are an early sign. It has been observed occasionally in patients receiving Clopixol. The concurrent use of anticholinergic antiparkinson drugs may exacerbate this effect. The potential irreversibility and seriousness, as well as the unpredictability of the syndrome, requires especially careful assessment of the risk versus benefit, and the lowest possible dosage and duration of treatment consistent with therapeutic efficacy. Short-lived dyskinesia may occur after abrupt withdrawal of the drug.

The neuroleptic malignant syndrome has rarely been reported in patients receiving neuroleptics including zuclopenthixol. This potentially fatal syndrome is characterised by hyperthermia, a fluctuating level of consciousness, muscular rigidity and autonomic dysfunction with pallor, tachycardia, labile blood pressure, sweating and urinary incontinence. Neuroleptic therapy should be discontinued immediately and vigorous symptomatic treatment implemented.

Epileptic fits have occasionally been reported. Confusional states can occur.

The hormonal effects of antipsychotic neuroleptic drugs include hyperprolactinaemia, which may be associated with galactorrhoea, gynaecomastia, oligomenorrhoea or amenorrhoea. Sexual function, including erection and ejaculation may be impaired; but increased libido has also been reported.

ECG changes with prolongation of the QT interval and T-wave changes may occur with moderate to high doses; they are reversible on reducing the dose.

Zuclopenthixol may impair body temperature control, and cases of hyperthermia have occurred rarely. The possible development of hypothermia, particularly in the elderly and hypothyroid, should be borne in mind.

Blood dyscrasias have occasionally been reported. Blood counts should be carried out if a patient develops signs of persistent infection. Jaundice and other liver abnormalities have been reported rarely.

Weight gain and less commonly weight loss have been reported; oedema has occasionally been reported and has been considered to be allergic in origin. Rashes have occurred rarely. Although less likely than with phenothiazines, zuclopenthixol can rarely cause increased susceptibility to sunburn.

Occasional local reactions, such as erythema, swelling or tender fibrous nodules have been reported.

Zuclopenthixol, even in low doses, in susceptible (especially non-psychotic) individuals may unusually cause nausea, dizziness or headache, excitement, agitation, insomnia, or unpleasant subjective feelings of being mentally dulled or slowed down.

Because acute withdrawal symptoms, including nausea, vomiting and insomnia have rarely been described after abrupt cessation of high doses of neuroleptics, gradual withdrawal of Clopixol is advisable. If drugs are withdrawn, recurrence of psychotic symptoms may not become apparent for several weeks or months.

*Overdosage:* Overdosage may cause somnolence, or even coma, extrapyramidal symptoms, convulsions, hypotension, shock, hyper- or hypothermia. Treatment is symptomatic and supportive, with measures aimed at supporting the respiratory and cardiovascular systems. The following specific measures may be employed if required:

- anticholinergic antiparkinson drugs if extrapyramidal symptoms occur.
- sedation (with benzodiazepines) in the unlikely event of agitation or excitement or convulsions.
- noradrenaline in saline intravenous drip if the patient is in shock. Adrenaline must not be given.

**Pharmaceutical precautions** The products should be stored at room temperature protected from light.

The products may be mixed in the same syringe with other products in the Clopixol Injection range including Clopixol Acuphase Injection (zuclopenthixol acetate 50 mg/ml).

They should not be mixed with any other injection fluids.

**Legal category** POM.

**Package quantities**
*Clopixol Injection:* Boxes of 10 × 200 mg (1 ml) ampoules
*Clopixol Conc. Injection:* Boxes of 5 × 500 mg (1 ml) ampoules.

**Further information** Clopixol Injection and Clopixol Conc. Injection contain the decanoic ester of zuclopenthixol in a thin vegetable oil (Viscoleo). The decanoic ester is slowly released from the oil depot and rapidly hydrolysed to release zuclopenthixol. Whereas zuclopenthixol itself is relatively short acting, the decanoic ester in oil provides a predictable slow-release depot preparation.

**Product licence numbers**
Clopixol Injection: 0458/0017
Clopixol-Conc. Injection: 0458/0060

## CLOPIXOL* TABLETS

**Qualitative and quantitative composition** Tablets of 2, 10 or 25 mg (2.36, 11.9 or 29.7 mg zuclopenthixol dihydrochloride corresponding to 2, 10 or 25 mg zuclopenthixol base respectively).

**Pharmaceutical form** Round, biconvex, film-coated tablets (2 mg tablets are pale-red, 10 mg tablets are light red-brown and 25 mg tablets are red-brown).

**Clinical particulars**
*Therapeutic indications:* The treatment of psychoses, especially schizophrenia.

*Posology and method of administration:*
*Route of administration:* Oral.

*Adults:* The dosage range is 4–150 mg/day in divided doses. The usual initial dose is 20–30 mg/day (sometimes with higher dosage requirements in acute cases), increasing as necessary. The usual maintenance dose is 20–50 mg/day.

*Elderly:* In accordance with standard medical practice, initial dosage may need to be reduced to a quarter or half the normal starting dose in the frail or elderly.

*Children:* Not indicated for children.

*Contra-indications:* Comatose states, including acute alcohol, barbiturate, or opiate intoxication.

*Special warnings and special precautions for use:* Caution should be exercised in patients having: liver disease; cardiac disease or arrhythmias; severe respiratory disease; renal failure; epilepsy (and conditions predisposing to epilepsy e.g. alcohol withdrawal or brain damage); Parkinson's disease; narrow angle glaucoma; prostatic hypertrophy; hypothyroidism; hyperthyroidism; mayasthenia gravis; phaeochromocytoma and patients who have shown hypersensitivity to thioxanthenes or other neuroleptics.

The elderly require close supervision because they are specially prone to experience such adverse effects as sedation, hypotension, confusion and temperature changes.

*Interactions with other medicaments and other forms of interaction:* In common with other neuroleptics, zuclopenthixol enhances the response to alcohol, and the effects of barbiturates and other CNS depressants, and may potentiate the effects of general anaesthetics. Neuroleptics may antagonise the effects of adrenaline and other sympathomimetic agents, and reverse the antihypertensive effects of guanethidine and similar adrenergic-blocking agents. Neuroleptics may impair the effect of levodopa, adrenergic drugs and anticonvulsants. The metabolism of tricyclic antidepressants may be inhibited and the control of diabetes may be impaired. The effect of anticoagulants may be increased. The anticholinergic effects of atropine may be increased. Anticholinergic effects may be enhanced by antiparkinson drugs and tardive dyskinesia precipitated. Concomitant use of metoclopramide and piperazine increases the risk of extrapyramidal symptoms. Neuroleptics may enhance the cardiac depressant effects of quinidine; the absorption of corticosteroids and digoxin; the hypotensive effect of vasodilator antihypertensive agents such as hydralazine and prolong the action of neuromuscular blocking agents. The possibility of interaction with lithium salts should be borne in mind.

*Pregnancy and lactation:* As the safety of this drug during pregnancy has not been established, use during pregnancy, especially the first and last trimesters, should be avoided, unless the expected benefit to the patient outweighs the potential risk to the foetus.

Zuclopenthixol is excreted into the breast milk. If the use of Clopixol is considered essential, nursing mothers should be advised to stop breast feeding.

The newborn of mothers treated with neuroleptics in late pregnancy, or labour, may show signs of intoxication such as lethargy, tremor and hyperexcitability, and have a low apgar score.

*Effects on ability to drive and use machines:* Alertness may be impaired, especially at the start of treatment, or following the consumption of alcohol; patients should be warned of this risk and advised not to drive or operate machinery until their susceptibility is known.

*Undesirable effects:* Drowsiness and sedation may occur but are more often seen with high dosage and at the start of treatment, particularly in the elderly. Other adverse effects include blurring of vision, tachycardia and urinary incontinence and frequency. Dose-related postural hypotension may occur, particularly in the elderly.

Because Clopixol may impair alertness, especially at the start of treatment or following the consumption of alcohol, patients should be warned of the risk and advised not to drive or operate machinery, until their susceptibility is known.

Extrapyramidal reactions in the form of acute dystonias (including oculogyric crisis), parkinsonian rigidity, tremor, akinesia and akathisia have been reported and may occur even at lower dosage in susceptible patients. Such effects would usually be encountered early in treatment, but delayed reactions may also occur. Antiparkinson agents should not be prescribed routinely because of the possible risk of precipitating toxic-confusional states, impairing therapeutic efficacy or causing anticholinergic side-effects. They should only be given if required and their requirement reassessed at regular intervals.

Tardive dyskinesia can occur with neuroleptic treatment. It is more common at high doses for prolonged periods but has been reported at lower dosage for short periods. The risk seems to be greater in the elderly, especially females. It has been reported that fine vermicular movements of the tongue are an early sign. It has been observed occasionally in patients receiving Clopixol. The concurrent use of anticholinergic antiparkinson drugs may exacerbate this effect. The potential irreversibility and seriousness, as well as the unpredictability of the syndrome, requires especially careful assessment of the risk versus benefit, and the lowest possible dosage and duration of treatment consistent with therapeutic efficacy. Short-lived dyskinesia may occur after abrupt withdrawal of the drug.

The neuroleptic malignant syndrome has rarely been reported in patients receiving neuroleptics, including zuclopenthixol. This potentially fatal syndrome is characterised by hyperthermia, a fluctuating level of consciousness, muscular rigidity and autonomic dysfunction with pallor, tachycardia, labile blood pressure, sweating and urinary incontinence. Neuroleptic therapy should be discontinued immediately and vigorous symptomatic treatment implemented.

Epileptic fits have occasionally been reported. Confusional states can occur.

The hormonal effects of antipsychotic neuroleptic drugs include hyperprolactinaemia, which may be associated with galactorrhoea, gynaecomastia, oligomenorrhoea or amenorrhoea. Sexual function, including erection and ejaculation may be impaired; but increased libido has also been reported.

ECG changes with prolongation of the QT interval and T-wave changes may occur with moderate to high doses; they are reversible on reducing the dose.

Zuclopenthixol may impair body temperature control, and cases of hyperthermia have occurred rarely. The possible development of hypothermia, particularly in the elderly and hypothyroid, should be borne in mind.

Blood dyscrasias have occasionally been reported. Blood counts should be carried out if a patient develops signs of persistent infection. Jaundice and other liver abnormalities have been reported rarely.

Weight gain and less commonly weight loss have been reported; oedema has occasionally been reported and has been considered to be allergic in origin. Rashes have occurred rarely. Although less likely than with phenothiazines, zuclopenthixol can rarely cause increased susceptibility to sunburn.

Zuclopenthixol, even in low doses, in susceptible (especially non-psychotic) individuals may unusually cause nausea, dizziness or headache, excitement, agitation, insomnia, or unpleasant subjective feelings of being mentally dulled or slowed down.

Because acute withdrawal symptoms, including nausea, vomiting and insomnia have rarely been described after abrupt cessation of high doses of neuroleptics, gradual withdrawal of Clopixol is advisable. If drugs are withdrawn, recurrence of psychotic symptoms may not become apparent for several weeks or months.

*Overdose:* Overdose may cause somnolence, or even coma, extrapyramidal symptoms, convulsions, hypotension, shock, hyper- or hypothermia. Treatment is symptomatic and supportive, with measures aimed at supporting the respiratory and cardiovascular systems. The following specific measures may be employed if required.

– Anitcholinergic antiparkinson drugs if extrapyramidal symptoms occur.
– Sedation (with benzodiazepines) in the unlikely event of agitation or excitement or convulsions.
– Noradrenaline in saline intravenous drip if the patient is in shock. Adrenaline must not be given.
– Gastric lavage should be considered.

**Pharmacological properties**
*Pharmacodynamic properties:* The action of zuclopenthixol as with other neuroleptics is mediated through dopamine receptor blockage. Zuclopenthixol has a high affinity for $D_1$ and $D_2$ receptors and activity has been demonstrated in standard animal models used to assess neuroleptic action. Serotonergic blocking properties, a high affinity for alpha-adrenoreceptors and slight antihistaminergic properties have been observed.

*Pharmacokinetic particulars:* Zuclopenthixol given orally in man is relatively quickly absorbed and maximum serum concentrations are reached in 3–6 hours. There is good correlation between the dose of zuclopenthixol and the concentrations achieved in serum. The biological half-life in man is about one day. Zuclopenthixol is distributed in the liver, lungs, intestines and kidney, with somewhat lower concentration in the brain. Small amounts of drug or metabolites cross the placenta and are excreted in milk.

Zuclopenthixol is metabolised by sulphoxidation, N-Dealkylation and glucuronic acid conjugation.

The faecal route of excretion predominates and mostly unchanged zuclopenthixol and N-dealkylated metabolite are excreted in this way.

*Preclinical safety data:* Nil of relevance.

**Pharmaceutical particulars**
*List of excipients:* Potato starch, lactose, microcrystalline cellulose, polyvidone acetate, glycerol, talc, hydrogenated caster oil, magnesium stearate, methylhydroxypropyl cellulose, macrogol, titanium dioxide (E171) and red iron oxide (E172).

*Incompatibilities:* None known.

*Shelf life:* Clopixol Tablets 2 mg are stable for two years. Clopixol Tablets 10 mg and 25 mg are stable for 5 years. Each container has an expiry date.

*Special precautions for storage:* Store in original container, protected from light and moisture, below 25°C.

*Nature and contents of container:* Grey polypropylene container (with desiccant capsule in 2 mg). Contents: 100 tablets.

*Instructions for use handling:* Nil.

**Marketing authorisation numbers**
2 mg tablets    0458/0027
10 mg tablets   0458/0028
25 mg tablets   0458/0029

**Date of approval/revison of SPC**   15 April 1997.

**Legal category**   POM.

# DEPIXOL* INJECTION
# DEPIXOL*-CONC. INJECTION
# DEPIXOL* LOW VOLUME INJECTION

**Presentation**   *Depixol Injection* is a sterile, straw-coloured solution of *20 mg/ml* (2%) cis(Z)-flupenthixol decanoate in thin vegetable oil. It is presented in glass ampoules (1 ml and 2 ml).

*Depixol-Conc. Injection* is a sterile, straw-coloured solution of *100 mg/ml* (10%) cis(Z)-flupenthixol decanoate in thin vegetable oil. It is presented in glass ampoules (0.5 ml and 1 ml).

*Depixol Low Volume Injection* is a sterile, straw coloured solution of *200 mg/ml* (20%) cis(Z)-flupenthixol decanoate in thin vegetable oil. It is presented in glass ampoules (1 ml).

**Uses**   The treatment of schizophrenia and other psychoses.

**Dosage and administration**
*Note:* As with all oil based injections it is important to ensure, by aspiration before injection, that inadvertent intravascular entry does not occur.

*Adults:* Depixol Injection, Depixol-Conc. Injection and Depixol Low Volume Injection are administered by deep intramuscular injection into the upper, outer buttock or lateral thigh.

Dosage and dosage interval should be adjusted according to the patients' symptoms and response to treatment.

The usual dosage of flupenthixol decanoate lies between 50 mg every 4 weeks and 300 mg every 2 weeks, but some patients may require up to 400 mg weekly. Other patients may be adequately maintained on dosages of 20–40 mg flupenthixol decanoate every 2–4 weeks. In patients who have not previously received depot neuroleptics, treatment is usually started with a small dose (e.g. 20 mg) to assess tolerability. An interval of at least one week should be allowed before the second injection is given at a dose consistent with the patients' condition.

Adequate control of severe psychotic symptoms may take up to 4 to 6 months at high enough dosage. Once stabilised lower maintenance doses may be considered, but must be sufficient to prevent relapse.

The appropriate presentation of Depixol should be selected to achieve an injection volume which does not exceed 2 ml. Volumes greater than 2 ml should be distributed between two injection sites.

When transferring patients from oral to depot neuroleptic treatment, the oral medication should not be discontinued immediately, but gradually withdrawn over a period of several days after administering the first injection.

*Elderly:* In accordance with standard medical practice, initial dosage may need to be reduced to a quarter or half the normal starting dose in the frail or elderly.

*Children:* Depixol Injection, Depixol-Conc. Injection and Depixol Low Volume Injection are not indicated for children.

**Contra-indications, warnings, etc**
*Contra-indications:* Comatose states, including alcohol, barbiturates or opiate intoxication. Not recommended for excitable or agitated patients.

*Warnings and precautions for use:* Caution should be exercised in patients having: liver disease; cardiac disease, or arrhythmias; severe respiratory disease; renal failure; epilepsy (and conditions predisposing to epilepsy, e.g. alcohol withdrawal or brain damage); Parkinson's disease; narrow angle glaucoma; prostatic hypertrophy; hypothyroidism; hyperthyroidism; myasthenia gravis; phaeochromocytoma and patients who have shown hypersensitivity to thioxanthenes or other neuroleptics.

The elderly require close supervision because they are especially prone to experience such adverse effects as sedation, hypotension, confusion and temperature changes.

*Interactions:* In common with other neuroleptics, flupenthixol enhances the response to alcohol, and the effects of barbiturates and other CNS depressants, and may potentiate the effects of general anaesthetics. Neuroleptics may antagonise the affects of adrenaline and other sympathomimetic agents, and reverse the antihypertensive effects of guanethidine and similar adrenergic-blocking agents. Neuroleptics may impair the effect of levodopa, adrenergic drugs and anticonvulsants. The metabolism of tricyclic antidepressants may be inhibited and the control of diabetes may be impaired. The effect of anticoagulants may be increased. The anticholinergic effects of atropine may be increased. Anticholinergic effects may be enhanced by antiparkinson drugs and tardive dyskinesia precipitated. Concomitant use of metoclopramide and piperazine increases the risk of extrapyramidal symptoms. Neuroleptics may enhance the cardiac depressant effects of quinidine; the absorption of corticosteroids and digoxin; the hypotensive effect of vasodilator antihypertensive agents such as hydralazine and prolong the action of neuromuscular blocking agents. The possibility of interaction with lithium salts should be borne in mind.

*Pregnancy and lactation:* As the safety of this drug during pregnancy has not been established, use during pregnancy, especially the first and last trimes-

ters, should be avoided, unless the expected benefit to the patient outweighs the potential risk to the foetus.

Flupenthixol is excreted into breast milk. If the use of Depixol is considered essential, nursing mothers should be advised to stop breast feeding.

The newborn of mothers treated with neuroleptics in late pregnancy, or labour, may show signs of intoxication such as lethargy, tremor and hyperexcitability, and have a low apgar score.

*Effects on ability to drive and use machines:* Alertness may be impaired, especially at the start of treatment, or following the consumption of alcohol; patients should be warned of this risk and advised not to drive or operate machinery until their susceptibility is known.

*Undesirable effects:* Drowsiness and sedation are unusual. Sedation, if it occurs, is more often seen with high dosage and at the start of treatment, particularly in the elderly. Other adverse effects include blurring of vision, tachycardia and urinary incontinence and frequency. Dose-related postural hypotension may occur, particularly in the elderly.

Because Depixol may impair alertness, especially at the start of treatment or following the consumption of alcohol, patients should be warned of this risk and advised not to drive or operate machinery, until their susceptibility is known.

Extrapyramidal reactions in the form of acute dystonias (including oculogyric crisis), parkinsonian rigidity, tremor, akinesia and akathisia have been reported and may occur even at lower dosage in susceptible patients. Such effects would usually be encountered early in treatment, but delayed reactions may also occur. Antiparkinson agents should not be prescribed routinely because of the possible risk of precipitating toxic-confusional states, impairing therapeutic efficacy or causing anticholinergic side-effects. They should only be given if required and their requirement reassessed at regular intervals.

Tardive dyskinesia can occur with neuroleptic treatment. It is more common at high doses for prolonged periods but has been reported at lower dosage for short periods. The risk seems to be greater in the elderly, especially females. It has been reported that fine vermicular movements of the tongue are an early sign. It has been observed occasionally in patients receiving Depixol. The concurrent use of anticholinergic antiparkinson drugs may exacerbate this effect. The potential irreversibility and seriousness, as well as the unpredictability of the syndrome, requires especially careful assessment of the risk versus benefit, and the lowest possible dosage and duration of treatment consistent with therapeutic efficacy. Short-lived dyskinesia may occur after abrupt withdrawal of the drug.

The neuroleptic malignant syndrome has rarely been reported in patients receiving neuroleptics, including flupenthixol. This potentially fatal syndrome is characterised by hyperthermia, a fluctuating level of consciousness, muscular rigidity and autonomic dysfunction with pallor, tachycardia, labile blood pressure, sweating and urinary incontinence. Neuroleptic therapy should be discontinued immediately and vigorous symptomatic treatment implemented.

Epileptic fits have occasionally been reported. Confusional states can occur.

The hormonal effects of antipsychotic neuroleptic drugs include hyperprolactinaemia, which may be associated with galactorrhoea, gynaecomastia, oligomenorrhoea or amenorrhoea. Sexual function, including erection and ejaculation may be impaired; but increased libido has also been reported.

ECG changes with prolongation of the QT interval and T-wave changes may occur with moderate to high doses; they are reversible on reducing the dose.

Flupenthixol may impair body temperature control, and cases of hyperthermia have occurred rarely. The possible development of hypothermia, particularly in the elderly and hypothyroid, should be borne in mind.

Blood dyscrasias have occasionally been reported. Blood counts should be carried out if a patient develops signs of persistent infection. Jaundice and other liver abnormalities have been reported rarely.

Weight gain and less commonly weight loss have been reported; oedema has occasionally been reported and has been considered to be allergic in origin. Rashes have occurred rarely. Although less likely than with phenothiazines, flupenthixol can rarely cause increased susceptibility to sunburn.

Occasional local reactions, such as erythema, swelling or tender fibrous nodules have been reported.

Flupenthixol, even in low doses, in susceptible (especially non-psychotic) individuals may unusually cause nausea, dizziness or headache, excitement, agitation, insomnia, or unpleasant subjective feelings of being mentally dulled or slowed down.

Because acute withdrawal symptoms, including nausea, vomiting and insomnia have rarely been described after abrupt cessation of high doses of neuroleptics, gradual withdrawal of Depixol is advisable. If drugs are withdrawn, recurrence of psychotic symptoms may not become apparent for several weeks or months.

*Overdosage:* Overdosage may cause somnolence, or even coma, extrapyramidal symptoms, convulsions, hypotension, shock, hyper- or hypothermia. Treatment is symptomatic and supportive, with measures aimed at supporting the respiratory and cardiovascular systems. The following specific measures may be employed if required:
- anticholinergic antiparkinson drugs if extrapyramidal symptoms occur.
- sedation (with benzodiazepines) in the unlikely event of agitation or excitement or convulsions.
- noradrenaline in saline intravenous drip if the patient is in shock. Adrenaline must not be given.

**Pharmaceutical precautions** The products should be stored at room temperature protected from light.

Whereas it is acceptable to mix these products together in the same syringe, they should not be mixed with any other injection fluids.

**Legal category** POM.

**Package quantities** *Depixol Injection:*
Boxes of 10 × 20 mg (1 ml) ampoules
Boxes of 10 × 40 mg (2 ml) ampoules

*Depixol-Conc. Injection:*
Boxes of 10 × 50 mg (0.5 ml) ampoules
Boxes of 10 × 100 mg (1 ml) ampoules

*Depixol Low Volume Injection:*
Boxes of 5 × 200 mg (1 ml) ampoules.

**Further information** Depixol Injection, Depixol Conc. Injection, and Depixol Low Volume Injection contain the decanoic ester of flupenthixol in a thin vegetable oil (Viscoleo). The decanoic ester is slowly released from the oil depot and is rapidly hydrolysed to release flupenthixol. Whereas flupenthixol itself is relatively short acting, the decanoic ester in oil provides a predictable slow-release depot preparation.

**Product licence numbers**

| | |
|---|---|
| Depixol Injection | 0458/0007 |
| Depixol-Conc. Injection | 0458/0015 |
| Depixol Low Volume Injection | 0458/0065 |

## DEPIXOL* TABLETS 3 mg

**Qualitative and quantitative composition** 3.504 mg flupenthixol dihydrochloride corresponding to 3 mg flupenthixol base.

**Pharmaceutical form** Round, biconvex, yellow, sugar-coated tablets.

**Clinical particulars**
*Therapeutic indications:* The treatment of schizophrenia and other psychoses.

*Posology and method of administration:*
*Route of administration:* Oral

*Adults:* 1–3 tablets twice daily, to a maximum of 18 mg (6 tablets) per day. It is recommended that commencement of treatment and increase in dosage should be carried out under close supervision. As with all neuroleptic drugs, the dose of Depixol should be titrated to the needs of each patient.

*Elderly:* In accordance with standard medical practice, initial dosage may need to be reduced to a quarter or half the normal starting dose in the frail or elderly.

*Children:* Not indicated for children.

*Contra-indications:* Comatose states, including alcohol, barbiturate, or opiate poisoning. Not recommended for excitable or agitated patients.

*Special warnings and special precautions for use:* Caution should be exercised in patients having: liver disease; cardiac disease or arrhythmias; severe respiratory disease; renal failure; epilepsy (and conditions predisposing to epilepsy, e.g. alcohol withdrawal or brain damage); Parkinson's disease; narrow angle glaucoma; prostatic hypertrophy; hypothyroidism; hyperthyroidism; myasthenia gravis; phaeochromocytoma and patients who have shown hypersensitivity to thioxanthenes or other neuroleptics.

The elderly require close supervision because they are specially prone to experience such adverse effects as sedation, hypotension, confusion and temperature changes.

*Interactions with other medicaments and other forms of interaction:* In common with other neuroleptics, flupenthixol enhances the response to alcohol, and the effects of barbiturates and other CNS depressants, and may potentiate the effects of general anaesthetics. Neuroleptics may antagonise the effects of adrenaline and other sympathomimetic agents, and reverse the antihypertensive effects of guanethidine and similar adrenergic-blocking agents. Neuroleptics may impair the effect of levodopa, adrenergic drugs and anticonvulsants. The metabolism of tricyclic antidepressants may be inhibited and the control of diabetes may be impaired. The effect of anticoagulants may be increased. The anticholinergic effects of atropine may be increased. Anticholinergic effects may be enhanced by antiparkinson drugs and tardive dyskinesia precipitated. Concomitant use of metoclopramide and piperazine increases the risk of extrapyramidal symptoms. Neuroleptics may enhance the cardiac depressant effects of quinidine; the absorption of corticosteroids and digoxin; the hypotensive effect of vasodilator antihypertensive agents such as hydralazine and prolong the action of neuromuscular blocking agents. The possibility of interaction with lithium salts should be borne in mind. Antacids may impair absorption, as may tea and coffee.

*Pregnancy and lactation:* As the safety of this drug during pregnancy has not been established, use during pregnancy, especially the first and last trimesters, should be avoided, unless the expected benefit to the patient outweighs the potential risk to the foetus.

Flupenthixol is excreted into the breast milk. If the use of Depixol is considered essential, nursing mothers should be advised to stop breast feeding.

The newborn of mothers treated with neuroleptics in late pregnancy, or labour, may show signs of intoxication such as lethargy, tremor and hyperexcitability, and have a low apgar score.

*Effects on ability to drive and use machines:* Alertness may be impaired, especially at the start of treatment, or following the consumption of alcohol; patients should be warned of this risk and advised not to drive or operate machinery until their susceptibility is known.

*Undesirable effects:* Drowsiness and sedation are unusual. Sedation, if it occurs, is more often seen with high dosage and at the start of treatment, particularly in the elderly. Other adverse effects include blurring of vision, tachycardia and urinary incontinence and frequency. Dose-related postural hypotension may occur, particularly in the elderly.

Because Depixol may impair alertness, especially at the start of treatment or following the consumption of alcohol, patients should be warned of this risk and advised not to drive or operate machinery, until their susceptibility is known.

Extrapyramidal reactions in the form of acute dystonias (including oculogyric crisis), parkinsonian rigidity, tremor, akinesia and akathisia have been reported and may occur even at lower dosage in susceptible patients. Such effects would usually be encountered early in treatment, but delayed reactions may also occur. Antiparkinson agents should not be prescribed routinely because of the possible risk of precipitating toxic-confusional states, impairing therapeutic efficacy or causing anticholinergic side-effects. They should only be given if required and their requirement reassessed at regular intervals.

Tardive dyskinesia can occur with neuroleptic treatment. It is more common at high doses for prolonged periods but has been reported at lower dosage for short periods. The risk seems to be greater in the elderly, especially females. It has been reported that fine vermicular movements of the tongue are an early sign. It has been observed occasionally in patients receiving Depixol. The concurrent use of anticholinergic antiparkinson drugs may exacerbate this effect. The potential irreversibility and seriousness, as well as the unpredictability of the syndrome, requires especially careful assessment of the risk versus benefit, and the lowest possible dosage and duration of treatment consistent with therapeutic efficacy. Short-lived dyskinesia may occur after abrupt withdrawal of the drug.

The neuroleptic malignant syndrome has rarely been reported in patients receiving neuroleptics, including flupenthixol. This potentially fatal syndrome is characterised by hyperthermia, a fluctuating level of consciousness, muscular rigidity and autonomic dysfunction with pallor, tachycardia, labile blood pressure, sweating and urinary incontinence. Neuroleptic therapy should be discontinued immediately and vigorous symptomatic treatment implemented.

Epileptic fits have occasionally been reported. Confusional states can occur.

The hormonal effects of antipsychotic neuroleptic drugs include hyperprolactinaemia, which may be associated with galactorrhoea, gynaecomastia, oligomenorrhoea or amenorrhoea. Sexual function, including erection and ejaculation may be impaired; but increased libido has also been reported.

ECG changes with prolongation of the QT interval and T-wave changes may occur with moderate to high doses; they are reversible on reducing the dose.

Flupenthixol may impair body temperature control, and cases of hyperthermia have occurred rarely. The possible development of hypothermia, particularly in the elderly and hypothyroid, should be borne in mind.

Blood dyscrasias have occasionally been reported. Blood counts should be carried out if a patient develops signs of persistent infection. Jaundice and other liver abnormalities have been reported rarely.

Weight gain and less commonly weight loss have been reported; oedema has occasionally been reported and has been considered to be allergic in origin. Rashes have occurred rarely. Although less likely than with phenothiazines, flupenthixol can rarely cause increased susceptibility to sunburn.

Flupenthixol, even in low doses, in susceptible (especially non-psychotic) individuals may unusually cause nausea, dizziness or headache, excitement, agitation, insomnia, or unpleasant subjective feelings of being mentally dulled or slowed down.

Because acute withdrawal symptoms, including nausea, vomiting and insomnia have rarely been described after abrupt cessation of high doses of neuroleptics, gradual withdrawal of Depixol is advisable. If drugs are withdrawn, recurrence of psychotic symptoms may not become apparent for several weeks or months.

*Overdose:* Overdosage may cause somnolence, or even coma, extrapyramidal symptoms, convulsions, hypotension, shock, hyper- or hypothermia. Treatment is symptomatic and supportive, with measures aimed at supporting the respiratory and cardiovascular systems. The following specific measures may be employed if required:
- Anticholinergic antiparkinson drugs if extrapyramidal symptoms occur.
- Sedation (with benzodiazepines) in the unlikely event of agitation or excitement or convulsions.
- Noradrenaline in saline intravenous drip if the patient is in shock. Adrenaline must not be given.
- Gastric lavage should be considered.

**Pharmacological properties**
*Pharmacodynamic properties:* Flupenthixol is a neuroleptic of the thioxanthene series.

The antipsychotic effect of neuroleptics is believed to be related to their dopamine receptor blocking effect. The thioxanthenes have high affinity for $D_1$ and $D_2$ receptors.

**Pharmacokinetic particulars:** Oral administration to volunteers (8 mg single dose and 1.5 mg/day) and patients (5–60 mg/d) resulted in serum drug concentration curves with a maximum around four hours after administration. Mean biological half-title was about 35 hours in patients. No difference was seen in patients between half-lives estimated after single-dose administration and those estimated after repeated administration. Mean oral bioavailability of flupenthixol varied between 40% and 55%.

*Preclinical safety data:* Nil of relevance.

**Pharmaceutical particulars**
*List of excipients:* Potato starch, lactose, gelatin, talc, magnesium stearate, sucrose and yellow iron oxide (E172).

*Incompatibilities:* Not applicable.

*Shelf-life:* Depixol tablets are stable for 5 years. Each container has an expiry date.

*Special precautions for storage:* Store in original container, protected from light and moisture, below 25°C.

*Nature and contents of container:* Glass bottles with white plastic stoppers or polypropylene container and screw cap. Contents 100 tablets.

*Instructions for use/handling:* Nil.

**Marketing authorisation number** 0458/0013.

**Date of approval/revision of SPC** 3 December 1996.

**Legal category** POM.

## FLUANXOL* TABLETS

**Presentation** Fluanxol tablets contain flupenthixol as the dihydrochloride. The tablets are red, round, biconvex and sugar-coated. The 0.5 mg tablet has a diameter of 6 mm and the 1 mg tablet has a diameter of 8 mm.

**Uses** Fluanxol tablets are indicated in the short-term symptomatic treatment of depression of mild to moderate severity (with or without anxiety) or where treatment with other antidepressants has failed.

**Dosage and administration** *Adults:* Standard initial dosage is 1 mg as a single morning dose. After one week the dose may be increased to 2 mg if there is inadequate clinical response. Daily dosage of more than 2 mg should be in divided doses up to a maximum 3 mg. In view of the activating properties of Fluanxol it is advisable to give the last dose of the day no later than 4.00 p.m.

Patients often respond to Fluanxol within two or three days. If no effect has been observed within one week at maximum dosage the drug should be withdrawn.

*Elderly:* Standard initial dosage is 0.5 mg as a single morning dose. After one week, if response is inadequate, dosage may be increased to 1 mg once a day. Caution should be exercised in further increasing the dosage but occasional patients may require up to a maximum of 2 mg a day which should be given in divided doses (1 mg at breakfast time and 1 mg at about 4.00 pm).

*Children:* Not recommended for children.

**Contra-indications, warnings, etc** Fluanxol is not recommended for the treatment of severe depression requiring ECT and/or hospitalisation. It is not recommended in states of excitement or overactivity (including mania).

*Precautions:* Fluanxol should be used with caution in patients with Parkinson's disease, severe arteriosclerosis, senile confusional state or severe hepatic, renal or cardiovascular disease.

*Warnings and adverse effects:* precipitation of hypomania has been occasionally reported. Restlessness or insomnia are occasional side-effects. Others more rarely reported include, dizziness, tremor, visual disturbances, headache, migraine and hyperprolactinaemia. Extrapyramidal symptoms, such as akinesia, may occur rarely at the recommended dose and if they do occur treatment with Fluanxol should be withdrawn. Late onset movement disorders, including tardive dyskinesia, have occasionally been reported in patients receiving flupenthixol. Fluanxol may initially cause drowsiness. Patients should be warned of this possibility if driving or operating machinery. Alcohol may potentiate this effect.

Recurrence of depressive symptoms on abrupt withdrawal is rare. However gradual reduction of dosage is advisable. Dependence has not been reported.

The central depressant effect of alcohol may be increased. The anticholinergic effects of atropine and tricyclic antidepressants may be increased and undesirable anticholinergic effects can be enhanced by antiparkinson drugs. Flupenthixol weakly antagonizes the action of adrenaline and other sympathomimetic agents and may reverse the blood pressure lowering effects of adrenergic blocking agents such as guanethidine, possibly also clonidine. It may also affect the control of diabetes or the action of anticoagulants.

*Pregnancy and lactation:* As there is no unequivocal evidence as to the safety of Fluanxol in human pregnancy, use during pregnancy, especially the first and last trimesters, should be avoided. Flupenthixol is excreted in small amounts in breast milk. It is recommended that mothers receiving flupenthixol should not breast feed.

*Treatment of overdose:* Overdosage should be treated by gastric lavage and parenteral antiparkinson drugs administered if extrapyramidal symptoms occur.

**Further information** Clinical trials have shown that symptoms of apathy, lowered mood, asthenia, despondency, lack of initiative, or inertia are likely to respond well to Fluanxol. Its high therapeutic index is an advantage in view of the suicide risk associated with depressive illness.

No adverse interactions have been reported between Fluanxol and benzodiazepines or tricyclic antidepressants.

Flupenthixol is available in higher doses as Depixol tablets. These are indicated only in the treatment of functional psychotic disorders.

**Pharmaceutical precautions** The tablets should be stored in their original container, protected from light and moisture.

**Legal category** POM.

**Package quantities** 0.5 mg tablets and 1.0 mg tablets in packs of 60, as 6×10 blister strips.

**Product licence numbers**
Fluanxol 0.5 mg, 0458/0011
Fluanxol 1.0 mg, 0458/0037

# SERDOLECT*  ▼

**Qualitative and quantitative composition**
Serdolect  4 mg: Sertindole  4 mg
Serdolect 12 mg: Sertindole 12 mg
Serdolect 16 mg: Sertindole 16 mg
Serdolect 20 mg: Sertindole 20 mg

**Pharmaceutical form** Coated tablets intended for oral administration.

**Clinical particulars**
*Therapeutic indications:* Serdolect is indicated for the treatment of schizophrenia.

Serdolect should not be used in emergency situations for urgent relief of symptoms in acutely disturbed patients.

*Posology and method of administration:* Serdolect is administered orally once daily with or without meals. In patients where sedation is required, a benzodiazepine may be co-administered.

*Adults:* All patients should be started on Serdolect 4 mg/day. The dose should be increased by 4 mg

increments after 4–5 days on each dose to the optimal daily maintenance dosage range of 12–20 mg. Dependent upon individual patient response the dose may be increased to a maximum of 24 mg/day. During maintenance treatment further dose adjustments should be made on the basis of an assessment of the clinical response and should preferably be performed after at least five days of administration of that dose.

Patients' blood pressure should be monitored during the period of dose titration and early follow up on maintenance dose.

A starting dose of 8 mg or a rapid increase in dose carries a significantly increased risk of severe hypotension.

*Elderly:* A pharmacokinetic study showed no difference between young and elderly subjects, however until further clinical experience is available the product should be used with care.

Slower titration and lower maintenance doses may be appropriate in elderly patients, who potentially have greater sensitivity to cardiovascular effects of sertindole.

*Children:* The safety and efficacy of Serdolect in children have not been established.

*Reduced renal function:* Serdolect can be given in usual dosage even to patients with severe renal impairment. The pharmacokinetics of sertindole were not affected by haemodialysis.

*Reduced hepatic function:* Patients with mild/moderate hepatic impairment require slower titration and a lower maintenance dose.

*Retitration of Serdolect in patients previously discontinued:* When restarting patients who have had an interval of less than one week without Serdolect, retitration of Serdolect is not required and their maintenance dose can be reintroduced. Otherwise the recommended titration schedule should be followed.

*Switching from other antipsychotics:* Treatment with Serdolect can be initiated according to the recommended titration schedule concomitantly with either a gradual withdrawal or immediate cessation of other oral antipsychotics. For patients on depot antipsychotics Serdolect is initiated in place of the next depot injection.

*Contra-indications:* Serdolect is contra-indicated in patients with known prolongation of the QT interval and in patients receiving drugs known to prolong QT interval (e.g. terfenadine and astemizole; thioridazine; a number of antiarrhythmic agents; some antidepressants) and in patients with clinically significant cardiac disease or uncorrected hypokalaemia.

If diuretic treatment is needed, concomitant treatment with a potassium-sparing diuretic is required in order not to affect the potassium balance. Other drugs that may induce hypokalaemia are contra-indicated.

*Severe hepatic impairment:* Administration of Serdolect is contra-indicated in patients with severe hepatic impairment.

Co-administration of Serdolect with systemic treatment with ketoconazole or itraconazole is contra-indicated (see *Interactions* section).

Known hypersensitivity to sertindole or any of the ingredients in the product.

Serdolect should not be used during pregnancy and lactation (see *Pregnancy and lactation* and *Preclinical safety data*).

*Special warnings and precautions*
*Cardiovascular:* Due to the $\alpha_1$-blocking activity of Serdolect, symptoms of orthostatic hypotension may occur during the initial dose-titration period.

Serdolect lengthens the QT interval in some patients. The risk of QT prolongation is increased in patients receiving concomitant treatment with drugs that prolong the QT interval (see section 4.3) or drugs that inhibit sertindole metabolism. Other risk factors are cardiovascular disease, hypokalaemia, hypomagnesaemia and bradycardia.

Serdolect should be used with caution in patients with known cardiovascular disease, or other conditions that would predispose patients to hypotension.

An ECG should be performed before commencing treatment with Serdolect to establish prospective patients' baseline QT interval.

In clinical trials, $QT_{c2}$ interval (cube root correction of the observed QT interval) prolongation to ≥500 msec was observed in 24 of the 1,446 patients (1.66%). For these 24 patients, the mean (±SD) increase was 26.5 (±7)% to values ranging from 500 msec to 581 msec. This effect did not correlate with plasma concentrations of sertindole and/or its metabolites. Although the effect was observed most often during the first 3–6 weeks of treatment, patients should be monitored by periodic ECGs while receiving Serdolect. If the $QT_{c2}$ interval exceeds 520 msec, the treatment with Serdolect should be discontinued.

Hypokalaemia and hypomagnesaemia should be corrected and maintained within normal range during treatment.

Antipsychotic drugs may inhibit the effects of

dopamine agonists. Serdolect should be used cautiously in patients with Parkinson's disease.

*Reduced hepatic function:* Patients with mild/moderate hepatic dysfunction should be closely observed. Slower titration and a lower maintenance dose are more appropriate.

*Diabetic patients:* Serdolect may modify insulin and glucose responses in diabetic patients calling for adjustment of antidiabetic therapy.

*Tardive dyskinesia:* Tardive dyskinesia is thought to be caused by dopamine receptor hypersensitivity in the basal ganglia as a result of chronic receptor blockade by antipsychotics. A low incidence of Extrapyramidal Symptoms on Serdolect (comparable to that of placebo) has been seen in clinical studies. However, long-term treatment with antipsychotic compounds (especially at high dosages) is associated with the risk of tardive dyskinesia. If signs of tardive dyskinesia appear dosage reduction or drug discontinuation should be considered.

*Seizures:* Serdolect should be used with caution in patients with a history of seizures.

*Neuroleptic Malignant Syndrome:* A potentially fatal symptom complex sometimes referred to as Neuroleptic Malignant Syndrome (NMS) has been reported in association with antipsychotic drugs. The management of NMS should include immediate discontinuation of antipsychotic drugs.

*Interactions with other medicaments and other forms of interaction:* Serdolect is extensively metabolised by the CYP2D6 and CYP3A isozymes of the cytochrome P450 system. CYP2D6 is polymorphic in the population and both isozymes can be inhibited by a variety of psychotropic and other drugs.

CYP2D6: The plasma concentration of sertindole is increased by a factor of 2–3 in patients concurrently taking fluoxetine or paroxetine (potent CYP2D6 inhibitors) and a lower maintenance dose of sertindole may be required. Although not investigated, comparable effects are expected for quinidine (potent CYP2D6 inhibitor), which in addition is known to prolong the QT interval (see *Contra-indications*). Other potential CYP2D6 inhibitors (such as sertraline, tricyclic antidepressants, and propranolol) appear not to influence the plasma concentration of sertindole. *In vitro* studies have shown that high concentrations of sertindole and its major metabolites inhibit the activity of CYP2D6. Sertindole is proposed to be a weak inhibitor of CYP2D6 substrates since the dextromethorphan metabolic ratio was only slightly affected during Serdolect treatment.

Substrates of CYP2D6 isozyme include β-blockers, antiarrhythmic agents, some antihypertensives and a large number of neuroleptics and antidepressants. CYP2D6 is markedly inhibited by quinidine, fluoxetine and paroxetine.

CYP3A: Of the interactions detected for CYP3A substrates, none are of sufficient magnitude to be clinically significant. Minor increases (<25%) in sertindole plasma concentrations have been noted for macrolide antibiotics (e.g. erythromycin, CYP3A inhibitor) and calcium channel antagonists (weak CYP3A inhibitors). Ketoconazole and itraconazole are both very strong inhibitors of CYP3A (see *Contra-indications*); however with CYP2D6 poor metabolisers the inhibitory effect could be much larger, since elimination of sertindole by both CYP2D6 and CYP3A would be affected.

Substrates of CYP3A isozyme include immunomodulators, calcium channel blockers and class III antiarrhythmic agents. The most well known inhibitors of CYP3A are cimetidine, many imidazole antifungal agents and macrolide antibiotics.

The metabolism of sertindole is significantly enhanced by agents known to induce CYP isozymes, notably carbamazepine and phenytoin, which can decrease the plasma concentrations of sertindole by a factor of 2 to 3. Reduced antipsychotic efficacy in patients receiving these drugs or other inducing agents may require the dose of Serdolect to be adjusted to the upper dosage range.

Other potent inhibitors of CYP2D6 and CYP3A may increase the AUC and the $C_{max}$ of sertindole. A reduction in the Serdolect dose should be considered for patients taking such drugs.

*Pregnancy and lactation:* The safety of Serdolect for use during pregnancy has not been established and therefore, Serdolect should not be used during pregnancy. Sertindole was not teratogenic in animal reproduction studies. A peri/postnatal study in rats showed a decrease in offspring fertility at a dose within the therapeutic range for humans (0.2 mg/kg/day) and at higher dosages a decreased pup survival in early lactation period, reduced weight gain and delayed development of pups in doses not clearly free of producing maternal toxicity.

Sertindole is excreted in the milk in rats, however it is not known whether it is excreted in human milk. Therefore, Serdolect should not be used duration lactation. Nursing mothers should not breast feed if they are under treatment with Serdolect.

*Effects on ability to drive and use machines:* Sertindole is not sedative, however patients should be advised not to drive or operate machinery until their individual susceptibility is known.

### Undesirable effects

*Side-effects:* In clinical trials, adverse events with an incidence greater than 1% associated with the use of Serdolect and significantly different from placebo were (listed in order of decreasing frequency): Rhinitis/nasal congestion, abnormal ejaculation (decreased ejaculatory volume), dizziness, dry mouth, postural hypotension, weight gain, peripheral oedema, dyspnoea, paraesthesia and prolonged QT interval.

*Extrapyramidal symptoms (EPS):* The incidences of patients treated with Serdolect reporting EPS-related adverse events, were similar to the frequencies occurring in patients receiving placebo. In addition, in placebo-controlled clinical trials, the percentage of Serdolect patients requiring anti-EPS medication was indistinguishable from those receiving placebo.

*Decreased ejaculatory volume:* Male patients may experience decreased ejaculatory volume. This symptom, which usually occurs within two months of treatment, is generally not associated with decreased libido, erection and orgasm. Patients do produce sperm and should be advised to use appropriate contraceptive measures to avoid unwanted pregnancy. Normal ejaculatory volume generally returns upon discontinuation.

*Body weight:* As with the use of other antipsychotic drugs, patients should be advised of the potential for weight gain when taking Serdolect.

Convulsions, hyperglycaemia and syncope have been reported rarely. An ECG is desirable to check the QT interval in patients who experience syncope and seizure on Serdolect.

In comparison with control groups, patients on sertindole had a higher frequency of red and white blood cells on microscopy of urine but the clinical significance of this finding is not clear at present.

After long-term treatment (months to years) movement disorders (in particular tardive dyskinesia) may arise either during or after treatment (see *Special warnings and precautions for use*).

*Overdose:* Experience with Serdolect in acute overdose is limited. Patients taking estimated dosages up to 240 mg have recovered without sequelae. In general, reported signs and symptoms of overdose were somnolence, slurred speech, tachycardia, hypotension and transient prolongation of the QT interval.

*Treatment:* In case of acute overdose, establishment of an airway and maintenance of adequate oxygenation should be ensured. Cardiovascular monitoring should commence immediately and monitoring of cardiac conduction should be considered to detect possible arrhythmias. Intravenous access should be established, and the administration of activated charcoal with laxative should be considered. The possibility of multiple drug involvement should be considered.

There is no specific antidote to sertindole, and it is not dialysable, therefore appropriate supportive measures should be instituted. Hypotension and circulatory collapse should be treated with appropriate measures such as intravenous fluids. If sympathomimetic agents are used for vascular support, epinephrine and dopamine should not be used, since $\beta$-stimulation combined with $\alpha_1$ antagonism associated with sertindole may worsen hypotension.

If antiarrhythmic therapy is administered, agents such as quinidine, disopyramide, and procainamide carry a theoretical hazard of QT interval-prolonging effects that might be additive to those of sertindole.

In cases of severe extrapyramidal symptoms, anticholinergic medication should be administered. Close medical supervision and monitoring should continue until the patient recovers.

### Pharmacological properties

*Pharmacodynamic properties:* ATC-code: N05A

Serdolect is a novel, limbic selective antipsychotic drug.

It has been proposed that the unique neuropharmacological profile of sertindole is derived from its selective inhibitory effect on mesolimbic dopaminergic neurons and is due to balanced inhibitory effects on central dopamine $D_2$ and serotonin 5HT$_2$ receptors as well as on $\alpha_1$-andrenergic receptors.

In animal pharmacology studies, sertindole inhibited spontaneously active dopamine neurons in the mesolimbic ventral tegmental area (VTA) of the brain without affecting dopamine neurons in substantia nigra pars compacta (SNC). Inhibition of SNC activity is thought to be involved in movement side effects associated with many antipsychotic drugs.

Antipsychotic drugs are known to increase serum prolactin levels through dopamine blockade. Patients receiving Serdolect remained within normal limits both in short-term studies and during long-term treatment (one year).

Sertindole has no effect on muscarinic and histaminic H$_1$ receptors. This is confirmed by the absence of anticholinergic and sedative effects related to those receptors.

*Pharmacokinetic properties:* Elimination of sertindole is via hepatic metabolism, with a mean terminal half-life of approximately three days. The clearance of sertindole decreases with multiple dosing to a mean around 14 L/h (females have approximately 20% lower apparent clearance than males, although lean-mass corrected clearances are comparable). Therefore upon multiple dosing, accumulation is greater than predicted from a single dose, due to an increase in the systemic bioavailability. However, at steady state, clearance is dose-independent and concentrations are proportional to dose. There is a moderate intersubject variability in sertindole pharmacokinetics which is due to the polymorphism in the cytochrome P450 2D6 (CYP2D6). Patients who are deficient in this hepatic enzyme have sertindole clearances that are $\frac{1}{2}$ to $\frac{1}{3}$ of those who are CYP2D6 extensive metabolisers. These poor metaboliser patients (up to 10% of the population) will therefore have plasma levels 2–3 times the normal. Sertindole concentration is not predictive of therapeutic effect for an individual patient; thus, dosing individualisation is best achieved by assessment of therapeutic effect and tolerability.

*Absorption:* Serdolect is well absorbed with a T$_{max}$ of sertindole after oral administration of approximately 10 hours. Different dose strengths are bioequivalent. Food and aluminium-magnesium antacids have no clinically significant effect on the rate or the extent of sertindole absorption.

*Distribution:* The apparent volume of distribution ($V_\beta$/F) of sertindole after multiple dosing is approximately 20 L/kg. Sertindole is about 99.5% bound to plasma proteins, primarily to albumin and $\alpha_1$-acid glycoprotein. In patients treated with recommended doses, 90% of the measured concentrations are below

140 ng/ml ($\sim$320 nmol/L). Sertindole penetrates into red blood cells with a blood/plasma ratio of 1.0. Sertindole readily penetrates the blood-brain and placental barriers.

*Metabolism:* Two metabolites have been identified in human plasma; dehydrosertindole (oxidation of the imidazolidinone ring) and norsertindole (N-dealkylation). Concentrations of dehydrosertindole and norsertindole are approximately 80% and 40% respectively, of the parent compound at steady state. Sertindole activity is primarily due to the parent drug and the metabolites do not appear to have significant pharmacological effects in humans.

*Excretion:* Sertindole and its metabolites are eliminated very slowly, with a total recovery of 50–60% of a radiolabelled oral dose, 14 days after administration. Approximately 4% of the dose is excreted into the urine as parent drug plus metabolites of which less than 1% of the dose is parent drug. Faecal excretion is the major route of excretion and accounts for the rest of the parent drug and metabolites.

*Preclinical safety data:* The acute toxicity of sertindole is low. In chronic toxicity studies in the rat and dog (3–5 times clinical exposure) several effects were observed. These effects are in line with the pharmacological properties of the drug.

Animal reproduction studies have not given evidence of teratogenic effects. Exposure of rats during the last third of pregnancy and during lactation resulted in a decrease in offspring fertility at a dose within the therapeutic range for humans (0.2 mg/kg/day). Mating and fertility were affected in adult male rats at dosages above 0.04 mg/kg/day. The adult fertility impairment, which was reversible, was ascribed to the pharmacological profile of sertindole.

Sertindole was not toxic in a battery of in vitro and in vivo genotoxicity studies. Carcinogenicity studies conducted in the mouse and rat did not indicate any development of tumours relevant to the clinical use of sertindole.

### Pharmaceutical particulars

*List of excipients:* Tablets: Maize starch, lactose, hydroxypropylcellulose, microcrystalline-cellulose, croscarmellose sodium, magnesium stearate, macrogol 400 and titanium dioxide (E171).

*Incompatibilities:* None known.

*Shelf life:* Serdolect tablets have a shelf-life of 24 months.

*Special precautions for storage:* Store tablets in original pack to protect from light.

*Nature and contents of container:* Serdolect tablets 4 mg, 12 mg, 16 mg and 20 mg are provided in PVC/PVdC laminate (clear or white) with aluminium foil, inside a carton blackened on the inside, containing 28 or 30 tablets.

*Instructions for use/handling:* No special precautions.

*Marketing authorisation holder:* H. Lundbeck A/S, Ottiliavej 9, DK-2500 Copenhagen-Valby, Denmark.

**Marketing authorisation numbers**

| | |
|---|---|
| 4 mg tablets | 13761/0001 |
| 12 mg tablets | 13761/0003 |
| 16 mg tablets | 13761/0004 |
| 20 mg tablets | 13761/0005 |

**Date of approval/revision of SPC** 25 October 1996.

**Legal category** POM.

*Trade Mark

# 3M Health Care Limited
Morley Street
Loughborough
Leics LE11 1EP

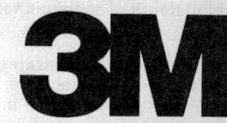

## ACUPAN*

**Presentation**   Acupan Tablets: White, film-coated, circular, biconvex tablets, 7 mm in diameter, marked APN on one side. Each tablet contains nefopam hydrochloride 30 mg.

Acupan Injection: Each 2 ml ampoule contains 1 ml of a solution of nefopam hydrochloride 20 mg/ml.

It also contains the following inactive ingredients: Sodium Acid Phosphate BP; Sodium Phosphate PhEur.

**Uses**   Acupan is indicated for the relief of acute and chronic pain, including: post-operative pain; dental pain; musculo-skeletal pain; acute traumatic pain and cancer pain.

Acupan is a potent and rapidly-acting analgesic. It is totally distinct from other centrally-acting analgesics such as morphine, codeine, pentazocine and pro-poxyphene.

Unlike the narcotic agents, Acupan has been shown not to cause respiratory depression. There is no evidence from pre-clinical research of habituation occurring with Acupan.

**Dosage and administration**   *Adults: Acupan Tablets:* Dosage may range from 1 to 3 tablets three times daily depending on response. The recommended starting dosage is 2 tablets three times daily.

*Acupan Injection:* 20 mg (1 ml) intramuscularly repeated if necessary every six hours (see instructions for administration). Onset of effect after intramuscular injection is within 15–20 minutes and peak effect is reached at one to one-and-a-half hours after administration.

Treatment started with Acupan injection may be continued with Acupan Tablets. 60 mg Acupan (2 tablets) is approximately bioequivalent to 20 mg (1 ampoule) given by injection.

Instructions for administration of Acupan Injection: Acupan Injection should always be given with the patient lying down and after injection the patient should remain lying down for 15–20 minutes. The patient should then get up slowly.

*Elderly:* Elderly patients may require reduced dosage due to slower metabolism. It is strongly recommended that the starting dose does not exceed one tablet three times daily as the elderly appear more susceptible to, in particular, the CNS side-effects of Acupan and some cases of hallucination and confusion have been reported in this age group.

*Children:* Since Acupan has not been evaluated in children no dosage recommendation can be given for patients under 12 years.

**Contra-indications, warnings, etc**   *Side-effects:* Nausea, nervousness, dry mouth, lightheadedness and urinary retention may occur. Less frequently, vomiting, blurred vision, drowsiness, sweating, insomnia, headache and tachycardia have been reported.

*Caution:* The side-effects of Acupan may be additive to those of other agents with anticholinergic or sympathomimetic activity.

It should not be used in the treatment of myocardial infarction since there is no clinical experience in this indication.

Hepatic and renal insufficiency may interfere with the metabolism and excretion of nefopam.

Caution should be exercised when nefopam is administered concurrently with tricyclic anti-depressants.

Acupan should be used with caution in patients with, or at risk of, urinary retention. Rarely a temporary, harmless pink discolouration has occurred.

*Use in pregnancy:* There is no evidence as to the drug safety in human pregnancy nor is there evidence from animal work that it is free from hazard. Avoid in pregnancy unless there is no safer treatment.

*Contra-indications:* Acupan is contra-indicated in patients with a history of convulsive disorders and should not be given to patients taking mono-amine-oxidase (MAO) inhibitors.

*Overdosage:* The clinical pattern of nefopam toxicity in overdose is on the neurological (convulsions, hallucinations and agitation) and cardiovascular systems (tachycardia with a hyperdynamic circulation). Routine supportive measures should be taken and prompt removal of ingested drug by gastric lavage or

induced vomiting with Syrup of Ipecacuanha should be carried out. Oral administration of activated charcoal may help prevent absorption. Convulsions and hallucinations should be controlled (e.g. with intravenously or rectally administered diazepam). Beta-adrenergic blockers may help control the cardiovascular complications.

**Pharmaceutical precautions**
Acupan tablets: Store below 30°C.
Acupan Injection: Store between 5°C and 30°C. Do not freeze.

**Package quantities**   Acupan Tablets; Packs of 90 tablets (OP).
Acupan Injection; Boxes containing 5×2 ml ampoules filled with 1 ml of solution.

**Legal category**   POM.

**Further information**   Nil.

**Product licence numbers**
Acupan Tablets        0068/0061
Acupan Injection      0068/0069

## AEROBEC* 50 AUTOHALER*
## AEROBEC* 100 AUTOHALER*

**Presentation**   AeroBec 50 Autohaler is a breath-actuated pressurised aerosol for inhalation therapy. Each actuation delivers 50 micrograms beclomethasone dipropionate (as propellant solvate) into the mouthpiece of a breath-actuated adapter. It also delivers the following inactive ingredients: sorbitan trioleate; propellants 11, 12 and 114.

AeroBec 100 Autohaler is a breath-actuated pressurised aerosol for inhalation therapy. Each actuation delivers 100 micrograms beclomethasone diproprionate (as propellant solvate) into the mouthpiece of a breath-actuated adapter. It also delivers the same inactive ingredients as AeroBec 50 Autohaler.

**Uses**   AeroBec 50 and AeroBec 100 Autohaler are indicated for the prophylactic treatment of chronic reversible obstructive airways disease.

**Dosage and administration**
*Adults:* for maintenance: 200 micrograms, twice daily or 100 micrograms, three or four times daily. In more severe cases a dose of 600–800 micrograms daily is recommended with subsequent reductions. The maximum recommended daily dose of this preparation is 1 mg. In patients receiving doses of 1500 micrograms or more daily, adrenal suppression may occur.

*Children:* 50–100 micrograms, two to four times daily.

*Elderly:* No special dosage recommendations are made for elderly patients.

**Contra-indications, warnings, etc**
*Contra-indications:* Hypersensitivity to beclomethasone is a contra-indication. Caution should be observed in patients with pulmonary tuberculosis.

*Side-effects:* Candidiasis of the throat and mouth may develop in some patients, but this can be treated without discontinuation of beclomethasone therapy. Hoarseness may also occur.

*Precautions:* Patients should be instructed on the proper use of the inhaler. They should be made aware of the prophylactic nature of AeroBec Autohaler therapy and that it should be used regularly at the intervals recommended and not when immediate relief is required.

In patients who have been transferred to inhalation therapy, systemic steroid therapy may need to be re-instated rapidly during periods of stress or where airways obstruction or mucus prevents absorption from the inhalation.

Patients who have received systemic steroids for long periods of time or at high doses, or both, need special care and subsequent management when being transferred to beclomethasone therapy. Recovery from impaired adrenocortical function, caused by prolonged systemic steroid therapy, is slow. The patient should be in a reasonably stable state before being given AeroBec Autohaler in addition to his usual maintenance dose of systemic steroid. Withdrawal of the systemic steroid should be gradual, starting after about seven days by reducing the daily oral dose by 1 mg prednisolone, or equivalent, at

intervals not less than one week. Adrenocortical function should be monitored regularly.

Most patients can be successfully transferred to AeroBec Autohaler with maintenance of good respiratory function, but special care is necessary for the first months after the transfer until the hypothalamic-pituitary-adrenal (HPA) system has sufficiently recovered to enable the patient to cope with emergencies such as trauma, surgery or infections.

Patients who have been transferred to inhalation therapy should carry a warning card indicating that systemic steroid therapy may need to be re-instated without delay during periods of stress. It may be advisable to provide such patients with a supply of oral steroid to use in emergency, for example when the asthma worsens as a result of a chest infection. The dose of AeroBec Autohaler should be increased at this time and then gradually reduced to the maintenance level after the systemic steroid has been discontinued.

Discontinuation of systemic steroids may cause exacerbation of allergic diseases such as atopic eczema and rhinitis. These should be treated as required with antihistamine and topical therapy.

*Overdosage:* Acute overdosage is unlikely to cause problems. The only harmful effect that follows inhalation of large amounts of the drug over a short time period is suppression of HPA function. Specific emergency action need not be taken. Treatment with AeroBec Autohaler should be continued at the recommended dose to control the asthma; HPA function recovers in a day or two.

If grossly excessive doses of beclomethasone dipropionate were taken over a prolonged period a degree of atrophy of the adrenal cortex could occur in addition to HPA suppression. In this event the patient should be treated as steroid-dependent and transferred to a suitable maintenance dose of a systemic steroid such as prednisolone. Once the condition is stabilised the patient should be returned to AeroBec Autohaler by the method recommended above.

*Pregnancy:* There is inadequate evidence of safety in human pregnancy. In animals, systemic administration of relatively high doses can cause abnormalities of foetal development including growth retardation and cleft palate. There may therefore be a very small risk of such effects in the human foetus. However, inhalation of beclomethasone dipropionate into the lungs avoids the high level of exposure that occurs with administration by systemic routes.

The use of beclomethasone dipropionate in pregnancy requires that the possible benefits of the drug be weighed against the possible hazards. The drug has been in widespread use for many years without apparent ill consequence.

*Lactation:* It is probable that beclomethasone is excreted in milk. However, given the relatively low doses used by the inhalation route, the levels are likely to be low. In mothers breast feeding their baby the therapeutic benefits of the drug should be weighed against the potential hazards to mother and baby.

**Pharmaceutical precautions**   Store below 30°C, protected from frost and direct sunlight. As the vial is pressurised, no attempt should be made to puncture or dispose of it by burning.

**Legal category**   POM.

**Package quantities**   Each canister provides 200 inhalations (OP).

**Further information**   Nil.

**Product licence numbers**
AeroBec 50 Autohaler      0068/0143
AeroBec 100 Autohaler     0068/0145

## AEROBEC* FORTE AUTOHALER*

**Presentation**   AeroBec Forte Autohaler is a breath-actuated pressurised aerosol for inhalation therapy. Each actuation delivers 250 micrograms beclomethasone dipropionate (as propellant solvate) into the mouthpiece of a breath-actuated adapter. It also delivers the following inactive ingredients: sorbitan trioleate, propellants 11, 12 and 114.

**Uses**   AeroBec Forte Autohaler is indicated for the prophylactic treatment of chronic reversible obstructive airways disease in those patients who require high doses of beclomethasone to control their symptoms.

## Dosage and administration

*Adults:* for maintenance: 2 inhalations (500 micrograms), twice daily or 1 inhalation (250 micrograms), four times daily; may be increased to 2 inhalations four times daily if necessary. In patients receiving doses of 1500 micrograms or more daily, adrenal suppression may occur. The degree of suppression may not always be clinically significant but it is advisable to provide such patients with a supply of oral steroid to use in stressful situations. The risk of adrenal suppression occurring should be balanced against the therapeutic advantages.

*Children:* AeroBec Forte Autohaler is not recommended for use in children.

*Elderly:* No special dosage recommendations are made for elderly patients.

## Contra-indications, warnings, etc

*Contra-indication:* Hypersensitivity to beclomethasone is a contra-indication. Caution should be observed in patients with pulmonary tuberculosis.

*Side-effects:* Candidiasis of the throat and mouth may develop in some patients, but this can be treated without discontinuation of beclomethasone therapy. Hoarseness may also occur.

*Precautions:* Patients should be instructed on the proper use of the inhaler. They should be made aware of the prophylactic nature of AeroBec Forte Autohaler therapy and that it should be used regularly at the intervals recommended and not when immediate relief is required.

In patients who have been transferred to inhalation therapy, systemic steroid therapy may need to be re-instated rapidly during periods of stress or where airways obstruction or mucus prevents absorption from the inhalation.

Patients who have received systemic steroids for long periods of time or at high doses, or both, need special care and subsequent management when being transferred to beclomethasone therapy.

Recovery from impaired adrenocortical function, caused by prolonged systemic steroid therapy, is slow. The patient should be in a reasonably stable state before being given AeroBec Forte Autohaler in addition to his usual maintenance dose of systemic steroid. Withdrawal of the systemic steroid should be gradual, starting after about seven days by reducing the daily oral dose by 1 mg prednisolone, or equivalent, at intervals not less than one week. Adrenocortical function should be monitored regularly.

Most patients can be successfully transferred to AeroBec Forte Autohaler with maintenance of good respiratory function, but special care is necessary for the first months after the transfer until the hypothalamic-pituitary-adrenal (HPA) system has sufficiently recovered to enable the patient to cope with emergencies such as trauma, surgery or infections.

Patients who have been transferred to inhalation therapy should carry a warning card indicating that systemic steroid therapy may need to be re-instated without delay during periods of stress. It may be advisable to provide such patients with a supply of oral steroid to use in an emergency, for example when the asthma worsens as a result of a chest infection. The dose of AeroBec Forte Autohaler should be increased at this time and then gradually reduced to the maintenance level after the systemic steroid has been discontinued.

Discontinuation of systemic steroids may cause exacerbation of allergic diseases such as atopic eczema and rhinitis. These should be treated as required with antihistamine and topical therapy.

*Overdosage:* If grossly excessive doses of beclomethasone dipropionate were taken over a prolonged period a degree of atrophy of the adrenal cortex could occur in addition to HPA suppression. In this event the patient should be treated as steroid-dependent and transferred to a suitable maintenance dose of a systemic steroid such as prednisolone. Once the condition is stabilised the patient should be returned to AeroBec Forte Autohaler by the method recommended above. To guard against the unexpected occurrence of adrenal suppression regular tests of adrenal function are advised.

*Pregnancy:* There is inadequate evidence of safety in human pregnancy. In animals, systemic administration of relatively high doses can cause abnormalities of foetal development including growth retardation and cleft palate. There may therefore be a very small risk of such effects in the human foetus. However, inhalation of beclomethasone dipropionate into the lungs avoids the high level of exposure that occurs with administration by systemic routes.

The use of beclomethasone dipropionate in pregnancy requires that the possible benefits of the drug be weighed against the possible hazards. The drug has been in widespread use for many years without apparent ill consequence.

*Lactation:* It is probable that beclomethasone is excreted in milk. However, given the relatively low doses used by the inhalation route, the levels are likely to be low. In mothers breast feeding their baby the therapeutic benefits of the drug should be weighed against the potential hazards to mother and baby.

**Pharmaceutical precautions** Store below 30°C, protected from frost and direct sunlight. As the vial is pressurised, no attempt should be made to puncture or dispose of it by burning.

**Legal category** POM.

**Package quantities** Each canister provides 200 inhalations.

**Further information** Nil.

**Product licence number** 0068/0140.

# AEROLIN* AUTOHALER*

**Qualitative and quantitative composition** Each actuation of Aerolin Autohaler delivers Salbutamol Sulphate PhEur equivalent to salbutamol 100 micrograms into the mouthpiece of a breath-actuated adapter.

**Pharmaceutical form** Aerolin Autohaler is a pressurised aerosol for bronchodilator inhalation therapy.

## Clinical particulars

*Therapeutic indications:* Aerolin Autohaler is indicated in the management of bronchial asthma, for the relief of wheezing and shortness of breath used on an as required basis. Aerolin Autohaler may be used as necessary to relieve attacks of acute dyspnoea and may be used prophylactically before exertion or to prevent exercise-induced asthma.

Aerolin Autohaler may also be used in the treatment of reversible airways obstruction associated with chronic bronchitis and emphysema.

*Posology and method of administration:*

*Adults:* For the relief of wheezing, shortness of breath and attacks of acute dyspnoea in patients with asthma, or reversible airways obstruction associated with chronic bronchitis and emphysema, one or two inhalations may be administered as a single dose.

For prophylaxis of exercise-induced asthma, two inhalations before exercise.

*Children:* For the relief of wheezing, shortness of breath and attacks of acute dyspnoea in children with asthma, one inhalation increasing to two if necessary may be administered as a single dose.

For prophylaxis of exercise-induced asthma, one inhalation increasing to two if necessary before exercise.

*Elderly:* No special dosage recommendations are made for elderly patients.

For all patients, the maximum recommended dose should not exceed eight inhalations in 24 hours. With repetitive dosing, inhalations should not usually be repeated more often than every 4 hours.

*Contra-indications:* Hypersensitivity to salbutamol or any of the inactive ingredients in Aerolin Autohaler.

Aerolin Autohaler is contra-indicated for use in the management of premature labour and threatened abortion.

*Special warnings and special precautions for use:*

*Special warnings:* Potentially serious hypokalaemia has been reported in patients taking beta-2-agonist therapy. Particular caution is advised in patients with severe asthma. Hypokalaemia may also occur in hypoxic patients and those treated with xanthine derivatives, steroids, diuretics and long-term laxatives. Extra care should therefore be taken if beta-2-agonists are used in these groups of patients and serum potassium levels should be monitored.

Unwanted stimulation of cardiac adrenergic receptors can occur in patients taking beta-2-agonist therapy.

*Special precautions for use:* The patient should be advised to seek medical advice if the treatment ceases to be effective and/or their asthma seems to be worsening, and not to increase the dose without medical advice.

Administer cautiously to patients with thyrotoxicosis.

*Interaction with other medicaments and other forms of interaction:* Salbutamol and beta-blockers should not usually be prescribed together.

Hypokalaemia occurring with beta-2-agonist therapy may be exacerbated by treatment with xanthines, steroids, diuretics and long-term laxatives.

*Pregnancy and lactation:* Aerolin should not be used in pregnancy and lactation unless the expected benefit to the mother is thought to outweigh any risk to the foetus or neonate.

The safe use of inhaled salbutamol during pregnancy has not been established but it has been in widespread use for many years in human beings without apparent ill consequence. In mice and rabbits large doses of salbutamol have been shown to be teratogenic.

It is not known whether salbutamol is distributed into breast milk.

*Effects on ability to drive and use machines:* None.

*Undesirable effects:* Mild tremor, headache, palpitations, tachycardia and transient muscle cramps may rarely occur. Potentially serious hypokalaemia has been reported in patients taking beta-2-agonist therapy.

Hypersensitivity reactions and hyperactivity in children have been reported rarely.

As with other inhalation therapy, paradoxical bronchospasm may occur immediately after dosing. In this instance, Aerolin Autohaler should be discontinued immediately and alternative therapy instituted if necessary.

*Overdose:* Treatment: Asthmatic patients: Monitor biochemical abnormalities, particularly hypokalaemia which should be treated with potassium replacement where necessary. Beta-adrenoceptor antagonists, even beta-1-selective antagonists, are potentially life-threatening and should be avoided.

Non-asthmatic patients: Monitor and correct biochemical abnormalities, particularly hypokalaemia. A non-selective beta-adrenoceptor antagonist (e.g. nadolol, propranolol) will competitively reverse both hypokalaemia and tachycardia (beta-1-selective drugs will be largely ineffective).

## Pharmacological properties

*Pharmacodynamic properties:* Salbutamol is a sympathomimetic agent which has a selective action on beta-2-adrenergic receptors in bronchial smooth muscle.

*Pharmacokinetic properties:* Salbutamol is readily absorbed from the gastro-intestinal tract, but the systemic absorption of the inhaled drug substance is low. The action of inhaled salbutamol depends on direct stimulation of receptors in the lung. Onset of action is usually within 10 minutes of inhalation and lasts 4–6 hours in most patients.

Salbutamol is subject to first-pass metabolism in the liver; about half is excreted in the urine as an inactive sulphate conjugate. It does not appear to be metabolised in the lung and therefore its fate following inhalation therapy depends on the delivery method used, which determines the proportion of salbutamol inhaled relative to the proportion inadvertently swallowed. It has been suggested that the slightly extended half-life following inhalation may reflect slow removal of active drug from the lungs.

*Preclinical safety data:* Salbutamol has been in widespread use for many years; there have been no adverse clinical findings with Aerolin Autohaler which might reflect pre-clinical safety issues (see *Pregnancy and lactation*).

## Pharmacuetical particulars

*List of excipients:* The excipients in Aerolin Autohaler are sorbitan trioleate, propellants 11, 12 and 114.

*Incompatibilities:* None known.

*Shelf life:* The shelf life expiry date for this product shall not exceed 3 years from the date of its manufacture.

*Special precautions for storage:* Aerolin Autohaler should be stored below 30°C. Avoid storage in direct sunlight or heat. Protect from frost.

*Nature and contents of container:* Aerolin Autohaler contains 200 metered doses.

*Instructions for use/handling:* The patient should read the patient leaflet before use.

As the canister is pressurised, no attempt should be made to puncture it or dispose of it by burning.

**Marketing authorisation number** 0068/0117

**Date of approval/revision of SPC** July 1996.

**Legal category** POM.

# AIROMIR* INHALER

**Qualitative and quantitative composition** Each actuation of Airomir Inhaler delivers Salbutamol Sulphate PhEur equivalent to salbutamol 100 micrograms into the mouthpiece of the adapter.

**Pharmaceutical form** Airomir Inhaler is a pressurised aerosol for bronchodilator inhalation therapy.

Airomir Inhaler contains a new propellant and does not contain chlorofluorocarbons (CFCs).

## Clinical particulars

*Therapeutic indications:* Airomir Inhaler is indicated in the management of bronchial asthma, for the relief of wheezing and shortness of breath used on an as required basis. Airomir Inhaler may be used as necessary to relieve attacks of acute dyspnoea and may be used prophylactically before exertion or to prevent exercise-induced asthma.

Airomir Inhaler may also be used in the treatment of reversible airways obstruction associated with chronic bronchitis and emphysema.

*Posology and method of administration*

*Adults:* For the relief of wheezing, shortness of breath and attacks of acute dyspnoea in patients with asthma, or reversible airways obstruction associated with chronic bronchitis and emphysema, one or two inhalations may be administered as a single dose.

For prophylaxis of exercise-induced asthma, two inhalations before exercise.

*Children:* For the relief of wheezing, shortness of breath and attacks of acute dyspnoea in children with asthma, one inhalation increasing to two if necessary may be administered as a single dose.

For prophylaxis of exercise-induced asthma, one inhalation increasing to two if necessary before exercise.

*Elderly:* No special dosage recommendations are made for elderly patients.

For all patients, the maximum recommended dose should not exceed eight inhalations in 24 hours. With repetitive dosing, inhalations should not usually be repeated more often than every 4 hours.

*Contra-indications:* Hypersensitivity to salbutamol or any of the inactive ingredients in Airomir Inhaler.

Airomir Inhaler is contra-indicated for use in the management of premature labour and threatened abortion.

*Special warnings and special precautions for use*

*Special warnings:* Potentially serious hypokalaemia has been reported in patients taking beta-2-agonist therapy. Particular caution is advised in patients with severe asthma. Hypokalaemia may also occur in hypoxic patients and those treated with xanthine derivatives, steroids, diuretics and long-term laxatives. Extra care should therefore be taken if beta-2-agonists are used in these groups of patients and serum potassium levels should be monitored.

Unwanted stimulation of cardiac adrenergic receptors can occur in patients taking beta-2-agonist therapy.

*Special precautions for use:* The patient should be advised to seek medical advice if the treatment ceases to be effective and/or their asthma seems to be worsening, and not to increase the dose without medical advice.

Administer cautiously to patients with thyrotoxicosis.

*Interaction with other medicaments and other forms of interaction:* Salbutamol and beta-blockers should not usually be prescribed together.

Hypokalaemia occurring with beta-2-agonist therapy may be exacerbated by treatment with xanthines, steroids, diuretics and long-term laxatives.

Because Airomir contains ethanol there is a theoretical potential for interaction in patients taking disulfiram or metronidazole. The amount of ethanol in Airomir is small but it may be enough to precipitate a reaction in some sensitive patients.

*Pregnancy and lactation*

*Airomir:* There is no experience of this product in pregnancy and lactation in humans. An inhalation reproductive study with Airomir Inhaler in rats did not exhibit any teratogenic effects. It should not be used in pregnancy and lactation unless the expected benefit to the mother is thought to outweigh any risk to the foetus or neonate.

*Propellant 134A:* Studies of propellant 134a administered to pregnant and lactating rats and rabbits have not revealed any special hazard.

*Salbutamol:* The safe use of inhaled salbutamol during pregnancy has not been established but it has been in widespread use for many years in human beings without apparent ill consequence. In mice and rabbits large doses of salbutamol have been shown to be teratogenic.

It is not known whether salbutamol is distributed into breast milk.

*Effects on ability to drive and use machines:* None.

*Undesirable effects:* Mild tremor, headache, palpitations, tachycardia and transient muscle cramps may rarely occur. Potentially serious hypokalaemia has been reported in patients taking beta-2-agonist therapy.

Hypersensitivity reactions and hyperactivity in children have been reported rarely.

No additional adverse effects have been seen with Airomir Inhaler.

As with other inhalation therapy, paradoxical bronchospasm may occur immediately after dosing. In this instance, Airomir Inhaler should be discontinued immediately and alternative therapy instituted if necessary.

*Overdose*

*Treatment:* Asthmatic patients: Monitor biochemical abnormalities, particularly hypokalaemia which should be treated with potassium replacement where necessary. Beta-adrenoceptor antagonists, even beta-1-selective antagonists, are potentially life-threatening and should be avoided.

Non-asthmatic patients: Monitor and correct biochemical abnormalities, particularly hypokalaemia. A non-selective beta-adrenoceptor antagonist (e.g. nadolol, propranolol) will competitively reverse both hypokalaemia and tachycardia (beta-1-selective drugs will be largely ineffective).

**Pharmacological properties**

*Pharmacodynamic properties:* Salbutamol is a sympathomimetic agent which has a selective action on beta-2-adrenergic receptors in bronchial smooth muscle.

*Pharmacokinetic properties:* Salbutamol is readily absorbed from the gastro-intestinal tract, but the systemic absorption of the inhaled drug substance is low. The action of inhaled salbutamol depends on direct stimulation of receptors in the lung. Onset of action is usually within 10 minutes of inhalation and lasts 4–6 hours in most patients.

Salbutamol is subject to first-pass metabolism in the liver; about half is excreted in the urine as an inactive sulphate conjugate. It does not appear to be metabolised in the lung and therefore its fate following inhalation therapy depends on the delivery method used, which determines the proportion of salbutamol inhaled relative to the proportion inadvertently swallowed. It has been suggested that the slightly extended half-life following inhalation may reflect slow removal of active drug from the lungs.

*Preclinical safety data*

*Propellant 134a:* In animal studies propellant 134a has been shown to have no significant pharmacological effects other than at very high exposure concentrations, when narcosis and a relatively weak cardiac sensitising effect were found. The potency of the cardiac sensitisation was less than that of CFC-11 (trichlorofluoromethane).

In studies to detect toxicity, repeated high dose levels of propellant 134a indicated that safety margins based on systemic exposure would be of the order 2200, 1314 and 381 for mouse, rat and dog with respect to humans.

There are no reasons to consider propellant 134a as a potential mutagen, clastogen or carcinogen judged from *in vitro* and *in vivo* studies including long-term administration by inhalation in rodents.

*Airomir:* Safety studies with Airomir in rate and dog showed few adverse effects. These occurred at high doses and were consistent with the known effects of salbutamol inhalation.

**Pharmaceutical particulars**

*List of excipients:* The excipients in Airomir Inhaler are Oleic Acid PhEur, Ethanol BP and Propellant 134a.

Airomir Inhaler contains a new propellant and does not contain chlorofluorocarbons (CFCs).

*Incompatibilities:* None known.

*Shelf life:* The shelf life expiry date for this product shall not exceed 2 years from the date of its manufacture.

*Special precautions for storage:* Airomir Inhaler should be stored below 30°C; storage in direct sunlight or heat should be avoided. Protect from frost.

*Nature and contents of container:* Airomir Inhaler contains either 100 or 200 metered doses.

*Instructions for use/handling:* For patients requiring a spacer device, the Aerochamber has been shown to be compatible with Airomir Inhaler.

The patient should read the instruction leaflet before use.

As the canister is pressurised, no attempt should be made to puncture or dispose of it by burning.

**Marketing authorisation number** 0068/0165.

**Date of approval/revision of SPC** February 1995.

**Legal category** POM.

## ALU-CAP* CAPSULES

**Presentation** Opaque green/red hard gelatin capsule, size 0, marked 3M. Each capsule contains 475 mg Dried Aluminium Hydroxide Gel BP as a white powder.

It also contains the following inactive ingredients: E104; E110; E127; E131.

**Uses** Alu-Cap is recommended for use as a phosphate-binding agent in the management of renal failure. It may also be used as an antacid.

In the gut, aluminium hydroxide adsorbs phosphate ions. This reduces absorption of phosphate into the body, and thereby reduces serum phosphate levels. In patients with renal failure, the problem of high serum phosphate levels may be partially solved by a diet low in phosphorus. However, a more liberal diet is feasible when a phosphate-binding agent, such as aluminium hydroxide, is used.

Aluminium hydroxide gel is a slow-acting antacid. It is used to provide symptomatic relief in gastric hyperacidity. In addition, the antipeptic and demulcent activity of aluminium hydroxide helps to protect inflamed gastric mucosa against further irritation by gastric secretions.

**Dosage and administration** *For phosphate-binding: Adults and children:* The dosage must be selected in accordance with individual patient requirements, and may range from 4 to 20 capsules of Alu-Cap daily (approximately 2–10 g dried aluminium hydroxide gel), taken with meals.

*As an antacid: Adults:* One Alu-Cap four times daily and on retiring. Alu-Cap is not suitable for antacid therapy in children.

*Elderly:* No special dosage recommendations are made for elderly patients.

**Contra-indications, warnings, etc**

*Side-effects:* Aluminium hydroxide is astringent and may cause constipation.

*Precautions:* Serum phosphate levels should be monitored in all patients receiving phosphate binders, to prevent the development of a phosphate depletion syndrome.

Aluminium hydroxide may form complexes with certain antibiotics (tetracyclines); concomitant administration may result in reduced absorption of the antibiotic.

*Pregnancy:* There is no evidence of safety of the drug in human pregnancy but it has been in wide use for many years without apparent ill consequence – animal studies having shown no hazard.

*Contra-indications:* Patients with hypophosphataemia and acute porphyria.

*Overdosage: Symptoms and treatment:* A single massive dose of aluminium hydroxide is unlikely to have harmful sequelae, as aluminium is not absorbed systemically to any great extent. Gastric lavage should be administered, followed by a mild aperient if required.

**Pharmaceutical precautions** Store below 30°C.

**Legal category** P.

**Package quantities** Bottles of 120 capsules (OP).

**Further information** Nil.

**Product licence number** 0068/0052.

## CALCISORB* SACHETS

**Qualitative and quantitative composition** Each sachet of Calcisorb contains 5 g of sodium cellulose phosphate.

**Pharmaceutical form** Calcisorb is a creamy-white to beige fibrous powder.

**Clinical particulars**

*Therapeutic indications:* Calcisorb is used to diminish calcium absorption from the diet in:

(1) the treatment of hypercalciuria and recurrent formation of renal stones;

(2) in osteopetrosis.

It can also be used in:

(3) the treatment of idiopathic hypercalcaemia of infancy;

(4) the treatment of hypercalcaemia in sarcoidosis;

(5) the treatment of vitamin D intoxication.

Calcisorb can also be used as a basis for a test for calcium absorption.

Each 5 g dose will bind approximately 350 mg calcium.

*Posology and method of administration*

*Adults:* 15 g daily, divided as three 5 g doses with meals.

*Children:* 10 g daily, divided as three doses with meals. Growing children should be prescribed Calcisorb only at the discretion of a senior physician and under his direct supervision.

*Elderly:* No special dosage instructions are required for the elderly.

The required dose should be dispersed in water and taken orally. Alternatively the powder may be sprinkled onto food.

*Contra-indications:* Renal failure. Congestive heart failure and other conditions in which a low sodium intake is essential.

*Special warnings and special precautions for use:* Calcisorb should be used in conjunction with a low calcium diet in which dairy products in particular are severely restricted.

During treatment with Calcisorb, restriction of oxalate-rich foods, such as spinach, rhubarb, peanuts, beetroot and chololate may be beneficial. An oral magnesium supplement of 58–87 mg elemental magnesium, twice daily, in patients receiving 10 and 15 g sodium cellulose phosphate daily, respectively, is also recommended. This supplement should be administered at least 1 hour before or 1 hour after Calcisorb.

*Interaction with other medicaments and other forms of interaction:* Interactions may occur with oral preparations containing calcium or magnesium salts, such as some antacids and laxatives.

*Pregnancy and lactation:* In view of the absence of data on the effect of cellulose phosphate on calcium levels in pregnant women it is recommended that treatment is discontinued during pregnancy and lactation. No signs of calcium deficiency have been reported during the continuous use of cellulose phosphate for up to 11 years. Therefore, this theoretical hazard in pregnancy is unlikely.

*Effects on ability to drive and use machines:* None.

*Undesirable effects:* Side-effects are rare. Isolated cases of diarrhoea have been reported. One patient with mild renal disease developed a moderate magnesium deficiency. This was readily corrected by halving the dose.

*Overdose:* An overdose of Calcisorb would potentially cause hypocalcaemia. The dose should be reduced. Complete withdrawal of treatment and supplementary calcium may be necessary.

**Pharmacological properties**
*Pharmacodynamic properties:* Sodium cellulose phosphate is an ion-exchange compound with a particular affinity for divalent cations. The product binds calcium ions in the lumen of the stomach and intestine and thus prevents hyperabsorption of dietary calcium. Calcium bound by cellulose phosphate is no longer available for absorption and is therefore excreted in the faeces. Each dose of Calcisorb will bind approximately 350 mg calcium.

*Pharmacokinetic properties:* Calcisorb is not absorbed.

**Pharmaceutical particulars**
*List of excipients:* None.

*Incompatibilities:* None known.

*Shelf life:* The shelf life expiry date for this product shall not exceed 3 years from the date of its manufacture.

*Special precautions for storage:* Since cellulose phosphate is an ester, some hydrolysis occurs on storage, the rate increasing with temperature. Calcisorb should therefore be kept in a refrigerator between 2°C and 8°C for long term storage. For short term storage by the patient, i.e. of the order of one month, refrigeration is unnecessary.

*Nature and contents of container:* Calcisorb is supplied in parchment, foil and polythene sachets. The 5 g sachets are packed in boxes of 90.

*Instructions for use/handling:* Not applicable.

**Marketing authorisation number**   0068/5900R.

**Date of approval/revision of SPC**   March 1996.

**Legal category**   P.

## DIFFLAM* CREAM

**Presentation**   Difflam is a white, pleasant-smelling cream, containing benzydamine hydrochloride 3% w/w.

It also contains the following inactive ingredients: Cutina* MD; Cetyl Alcohol USNF; Cetiol* V; Eumulgin* B1; Propylene Glycol PhEur; Perfume, Crematest*; Methyl Hydroxybenzoate PhEur; Propyl Hydroxybenzoate PhEur.

**Uses**   Difflam cream is a topical analgesic and non-steroidal anti-inflammatory agent. It is recommended as a short-term treatment for the relief of symptoms associated with painful inflammatory conditions of the musculo-skeletal system, including:

Acute inflammatory disorders such as myalgia and bursitis.

Traumatic conditions such as sprains, strains, contusions and the after-effects of fractures.

Difflam cream is well absorbed through the skin and it has been shown to have anti-inflammatory and local anaesthetic actions.

**Dosage and administration**   Difflam cream should be massaged lightly into the affected area. Depending on the size of the site to be treated, 35–85 mm (1–2.5 g) should be applied three times daily and at the discretion of the doctor, up to six times daily in more severe conditions. It is recommended that treatment be limited to not more than 10 days.

*Elderly:* No special dosage recommendations are made for elderly patients.

**Contra-indications, warnings, etc**   *Side-effects:* Photosensitivity reactions have been reported and local skin reactions which have varied from erythema to papular eruption. The skin returned to normal on stopping treatment.

*Use in pregnancy:* There is inadequate evidence of safety of the drug in human pregnancy but it has been in wide use for many years without apparent ill consequence.

*Caution:* To avoid possible irritation, Difflam cream should be kept away from eyes and mucosal surfaces.

*Overdosage:* Difflam is unlikely to cause adverse systemic effects, even if accidental ingestion should occur. No special measures are required.

**Pharmaceutical precautions**   Store between 5 and 30°C. Do not freeze.

**Legal category**   P.

**Package quantities**   Tubes containing 100 g (OP).

**Further information**   Nil.

**Product licence number**   0068/0088.

## DIFFLAM* ORAL RINSE

**Presentation**   Difflam Oral Rinse is a pleasant tasting, clear green solution, containing benzydamine hydrochloride 0.15% w/v. It also contains the following inactive ingredients: Ethanol BP; Methylhydroxybenzoate PhEur; E104; E131.

**Uses**   Difflam Oral Rinse is a locally acting analgesic and anti-inflammatory treatment for the relief of painful inflammatory conditions of the mouth and throat including:
*Traumatic conditions:* Pharyngitis following tonsillectomy or the use of a naso-gastric tube.
*Inflammatory conditions:* Pharyngitis, aphthous ulcers and oral ulceration due to radiation therapy.
*Dentistry:* For use after dental operations.

Benzydamine exerts an anti-inflammatory and analgesic action by stabilising the cellular membrane and inhibiting prostaglandin synthesis.

**Dosage and administration**   Rinse or gargle with 15 ml (approximately 1 tablespoonful) every 1½ to 3 hours as required for pain relief. Not suitable for children aged 12 years or under. The solution should be expelled from the mouth after use. Difflam Oral Rinse should generally be used undiluted, but if 'stinging' occurs the rinse may be diluted with water. Uninterrupted treatment should not exceed seven days, unless under medical supervision.

*Elderly:* No special dosage recommendations are made for elderly patients.

**Contra-indications, warnings, etc**
*Precautions:* Avoid contact with eyes.

*Side-effects:* Side-effects are minor. Occasionally, oral tissue numbness or 'stinging' sensations may occur.

*Overdosage:* Difflam is unlikely to cause adverse systemic effects, even if accidental ingestion should occur. No special measures are required.

*Use in pregnancy:* There is inadequate evidence of safety of the drug in human pregnancy, but it has been in wide use for many years without apparent ill consequence.

**Pharmaceutical precautions**   Do not leave the uncartonned bottle in direct sunlight. Store between 5°C and 30°C. Do not freeze.

**Legal category**   P.

**Package quantities**   Bottle containing 300 ml (OP).

**Further information**   Nil.

**Product licence number**   0068/0096.

## DIFFLAM* SPRAY

**Qualitative and quantitative composition**   Each metered dose pump spray delivers benzydamine hydrochloride 0.15% w/v, approximately 175 microlitres per puff.

**Pharmaceutical form**   Difflam Spray is a metered dose pump throat spray.

**Clinical particulars**
*Therapeutic indications:* Difflam Spray is a locally acting analgesic and anti-inflammatory treatment for the throat and mouth.

It is especially useful for the relief of pain in traumatic conditions such as following tonsillectomy or the use of a naso-gastric tube; dental surgery.

*Posology and method of administration:* For oral administration.

*Adults and elderly:* 4 to 8 puffs, 1½–3 hourly.

*Children (6 to 12):* 4 puffs, 1½–3 hourly.

*Children under 6:* One puff to be administered per 4 kg body weight, up to a maximum of 4 puffs, 1½–3 hourly.

Because of the small amount of drug applied, elderly patients can receive the same dose as adults.

*Contra-indications:* None.

*Special warnings and special precautions for use:* Avoid contact with the eyes.

*Interaction with other medicaments and other forms of interaction:* None known.

*Pregnancy and lactation:* There is inadequate evidence of safety of the drug in human pregnancy, but it has been in wide use for many years without apparent ill consequence.

*Effects on ability to drive and use machines:* None.

*Undesirable effects:* Side-effects are minor. Occasionally, oral tissue numbness or 'stinging' sensations may occur. The stinging has been reported to disappear upon continuation of the treatment, however if it persists it is recommended that treatment be discontinued.

*Overdose:* Difflam is unlikely to cause adverse systemic effects, even if accidental ingestion should occur. No special measures are required.

**Pharmacological properties**
*Pharmacodynamic properties:* Benzydamine exerts an anti-inflammatory and analgesic action by stabilising the cellular membrane and inhibiting prostaglandin synthesis.

*Pharmacokinetic properties:* Following oral administration, Benzydamine is rapidly absorbed from the gastrointestinal tract and maximum plasma levels reached after 2–4 hours. The most important aspect of the tissue distribution of benzydamine is its tendency to concentrate at the site of inflammation.

About half of the Benzydamine is excreted unchanged via the kidney at a rate of 10% of the dose within the first 24 hours. The remainder is metabolised, mostly to N-Oxide.

**Pharmaceutcal particulars**
*List of excipients:* The excipients in Difflam Spray include: Glycerol PhEur, Saccharin FU, Sodium Bicarbonate PhEur, Ethanol FU, Methylhydroxybenzoate PhEur, Mouthwash Flavour, Polysorbate 20 PhEur, Purified Water PhEur.

*Incompatibilities:* None.

*Shelf life:* The shelf life expiry date for this product shall not exceed 3 years from the date of its manufacture.

*Special precautions for storage:* Difflam Spray should be stored between 5°C and 30°C, do not freeze.

*Nature and contents of container:* Difflam Spray is presented in a 30 ml glass bottle with 170 µl valve pump spray and an outer coating of green coloured PVC.

*Instructions for use/handling:* The patient should read the instruction leaflet before use.

**Marketing authorisation number**   0068/0112.

**Date of approval/revision of SPC**   February 1990.

**Legal category**   P.

## DUROMINE* 15 mg CAPSULES

**Qualitative and quantitative composition**   Phentermine resin complex equivalent to 15 mg phentermine.

**Pharmaceutical form**   Capsules.

**Clinical particulars**
*Therapeutic indications:* Adjunctive therapy to diet, in patients with obesity and a body mass index (BMI) of 30 kg/m² or higher who have not responded to an appropriate weight-reducing regimen alone.

Note: short-term efficacy only has been demonstrated with regard to weight reduction. No significant data on changes in morbidity or mortality are yet available.

*Posology and method of administration:* For oral administration.

*Adults:* One 15 mg capsule daily at breakfast time.

Evening dosing should be avoided, as this agent may induce nervousness and insomnia.

It is recommended that treatment should be conducted under the care of physicians experienced in the treatment of obesity.

Secondary organic causes of obesity must be excluded by diagnosis before prescribing this agent.

The management of obesity should be undertaken using a global approach which should include dietary, medical and psychotherapeutic methods.

*Duration of treatment:* The duration of treatment is 4–6 weeks and should not exceed three months.

*Children:* Duromine is not recommended for children.

*Elderly:* Duromine is not recommended for the elderly.

*Contra-indications:*
– Patients sensitive to sympathomimetic agents.
– Pulmonary artery hypertension.
– Severe arterial hypertension.

– Current or past medical history of cardio-vascular or cerebro-vascular disease.
– Current or past medical history of psychiatric disorders including anorexia nervosa and depression.
– Propensity towards drug abuse, known alcoholism.
– Thyrotoxicosis.
– Children below 12 years.
– Women during lactation.

*Combination drug therapy* with any other centrally acting anorectic agent is contraindicated due to the increased risk of potentially fatal pulmonary artery hypertension.

*Special warnings and special precautions for use:*
*Special warnings:* Cases of severe, often fatal pulmonary artery hypertension, have been reported in patients who have received anorectics of the type in this product. An epidemiological study has shown that anorectic intake is a risk factor involved in the development of pulmonary artery hypertension and that use of anorectics is strongly associated with an increased risk for this adverse drug reaction. In view of this rare but serious risk, it must be emphasised that:
– careful compliance with the indication and the duration of treatment is required;
– duration of treatment greater than 3 months and a BMI ≥ 30 kg/m² increase the risk of pulmonary artery hypertension;
– the onset or aggravation of exertional dyspnoea suggests the possibility of occurrence of pulmonary artery hypertension. Under these circumstances, treatment should be immediately discontinued and the patient referred to a specialist unit for investigation.

*Special precautions for use:* Prolonged treatment may give rise to pharmacological tolerance and drug dependence, and more rarely to severe psychotic disorders in predisposed patients.

Rarely, cases of cardiac and cerebro-vascular accidents have been reported, often following rapid weight loss. Special care should be taken to ensure gradual and controlled weight loss in obese patients, who are subject to a risk of vascular disease. This anorectic agent should not be prescribed in patients with current or a past medical history of cardio-vascular or cerebro-vascular disease.

Duromine should be used with caution in patients under treatment with anti-hypertensive agents, since it may cause some loss of blood pressure control, and in patients receiving psychotrophic drugs, including sedatives and sympathomimetic agents.

This anorectic agent should be used with caution in epileptic patients.

*Interaction with other medicaments and other forms of interaction:* Duromine should not be given to patients under treatment with monoamine-oxidase (MAO) inhibitors, within 2 weeks of stopping such treatment. There may be an interaction with alcohol.

*Pregnancy and lactation:* Do not use in pregnancy or lactation. There is inadequate evidence of safety in pregnancy and there is no information from animal studies.

*Effects on ability to drive and use machines:* Patients may be at risk whilst driving or operating machinery.

*Undesirable effects:* An epidemiological study has shown that anorectic intake is a risk factor involved in the development of pulmonary artery hypertension and that the use of anorectics is strongly associated with an increased risk for this adverse drug reaction. Cases of pulmonary artery hypertension have been reported in patients treated with this agent. Pulmonary artery hypertension is a severe and often fatal disease. The occurrence or aggravation of exertional dyspnoea is usually the first clinical sign and requires treatment discontinuation and investigation in a specialised unit (see *Special warnings*).

*CNS effects:* The prolonged use of this agent is associated with a risk of pharmocological tolerance, dependence and withdrawal syndrome. The most common adverse reactions which have been described are: psychotic reactions or psychosis, depression, nervousness, agitation, sleep disorders and vertigo. Hallucinations and dizziness may also occur. Convulsions have been reported.

*Cardio-vascular effects:* The most common reported reactions are tachycardia, palpitations, hypertension, precordial pain. Rarely cases of cardiovascular or cerebro-vascular accidents have been described in patients treated with anorectic agents. In particular stroke, angina, myocardial infarction, cardiac failure and cardiac arrest have been reported. Other side-effects reported are vomiting, dry mouth, facial oedema, rash, headache and urinary frequency.

*Overdose: Symptoms:* Initially irritability, agitation, disorientation and tremor may occur, followed by cardiac arrhythmias, convulsions, hallucinations and coma.
*Treatment:* The stomach should be emptied by emesis or stomach tube and washed out with water if

the preparation has been ingested within the last three or four hours. Diazepam, preferably by mouth (cautiously by intravenous injection) should be used to control marked excitement and convulsions. Provided renal function is adequate, elimination of phentermine may be assisted by acidification of the urine by agents such as lysine hydrochloride or arginine hydrochloride.

**Pharmacological properties**
*Pharmacodynamic properties:* Phentermine is a weak sympathomimetic amine having marked anorexigenic activity. Its appetite suppressant effect is generally considered to be exerted through the hypothalamus, but it is not certain that this is the only effect related to weight loss. In vitro, it has been shown to inhibit phospholipase activity. It may also increase glucose uptake into skeletal muscle, as has been shown with fenfluramine. Phentermine has major effects on the dopaminergic and noradrenergic nervous systems.

Hence in addition to effects upon appetite suppression in the CNS, phentermine may also have peripheral metabolic effects which can help weight loss. The exact mechanisms are not clear.

*Pharmacokinetic properties:* Phentermine is readily absorbed from the gastro-intestinal tract and approximately 70–80% of all oral dose is excreted unchanged in the urine; the remainder is metabolised in the liver.

*Preclinical safety data:* Not applicable.

**Pharmaceutical particulars**
*List of excipients:* Lactose PhEur, Magnesium Stearate PhEur.

*Incompatibilities:* None known.

*Shelf life:* 5 years.

*Special precautions for storage:* Store below 30°C.

*Nature and contents of container:* Amber glass bottle with pilfer-proof screw cap.

*Instructions for use/handling:* Not applicable.

**Marketing authorisation number** 00068/5055R

**Date of approval/revision of SPC** January 1997.

**Legal category** CD(Sch 3), POM.

## DUROMINE* 30 mg CAPSULES

**Qualitative and quantitative composition** Phentermine resin complex equivalent to 30 mg phentermine.

**Pharmaceutical form** Capsules.

**Clinical particulars**
*Therapeutic indications:* Adjunctive therapy to diet, in patients with obesity and a body mass index (BMI) of 30 kg/m² or higher who have not responded to an appropriate weight-reducing regimen alone.
Note: short-term efficacy only has been demonstrated with regard to weight reduction. No significant data on changes in morbidity or mortality are yet available.

*Posology and method of administration:* For oral administration.

*Adults:* One 30 mg capsule daily at breakfast time.
Evening dosing should be avoided, as this agent may induce nervousness and insomnia.

It is recommended that treatment should be conducted under the care of physicians experienced in the treatment of obesity.

Secondary organic causes of obesity must be excluded by diagnosis before prescribing this agent.

The management of obesity should be undertaken using a global approach which should include dietary, medical and psychotherapeutic methods.

*Duration of treatment:* The duration of treatment is 4–6 weeks and should not exceed three months.

*Children:* Duromine is not recommended for children.

*Elderly:* Duromine is not recommended for the elderly.

*Contra-indications:*
– Patients sensitive to sympathomimetic agents.
– Pulmonary artery hypertension.
– Severe arterial hypertension.
– Current or past medical history of cardio-vascular or cerebro-vascular disease.
– Current or past medical history of psychiatric disorders including anorexia nervosa and depression.
– Propensity towards drug abuse, known alcoholism.
– Thyrotoxicosis.
– Children below 12 years.
– Women during lactation.

*Combination drug therapy* with any other centrally acting anorectic agent is contraindicated due to the increased risk of potentially fatal pulmonary artery hypertension.

*Special warnings and special precautions for use:*
*Special warnings:* Cases of severe, often fatal pulmonary artery hypertension, have been reported in patients who have received anorectics of the type in this product. An epidemiological study has shown

that anorectic intake is a risk factor involved in the development of pulmonary artery hypertension and that use of anorectics is strongly associated with an increased risk for this adverse drug reaction. In view of this rare but serious risk, it must be emphasised that:
– careful compliance with the indication and the duration of treatment is required;
– duration of treatment greater than 3 months and a BMI ≥ 30 kg/m² increase the risk of pulmonary artery hypertension;
– the onset or aggravation of exertional dyspnoea suggests the possibility of occurrence of pulmonary artery hypertension. Under these circumstances, treatment should be immediately discontinued and the patient referred to a specialist unit for investigation.

*Special precautions for use:* Prolonged treatment may give rise to pharmacological tolerance and drug dependence, and more rarely to severe psychotic disorders in predisposed patients.

Rarely, cases of cardiac and cerebro-vascular accidents have been reported, often following rapid weight loss. Special care should be taken to ensure gradual and controlled weight loss in obese patients, who are subject to a risk of vascular disease. This anorectic agent should not be prescribed in patients with current or a past medical history of cardio-vascular or cerebro-vascular disease.

Duromine should be used with caution in patients under treatment with anti-hypertensive agents, since it may cause some loss of blood pressure control, and in patients receiving psychotrophic drugs, including sedatives and sympathomimetic agents.

This anorectic agent should be used with caution in epileptic patients.

*Interaction with other medicaments and other forms of interaction:* Duromine should not be given to patients under treatment with monoamine-oxidase (MAO) inhibitors, within 2 weeks of stopping such treatment. There may be an interaction with alcohol.

*Pregnancy and lactation:* Do not use in pregnancy or lactation. There is inadequate evidence of safety in pregnancy and there is no information from animal studies.

*Effects on ability to drive and use machines:* Patients may be at risk whilst driving or operating machinery.

*Undesirable effects:* An epidemiological study has shown that anorectic intake is a risk factor involved in the development of pulmonary artery hypertension and that the use of anorectics is strongly associated with an increased risk for this adverse drug reaction. Cases of pulmonary artery hypertension have been reported in patients treated with this agent. Pulmonary artery hypertension is a severe and often fatal disease. The occurrence or aggravation of exertional dyspnoea is usually the first clinical sign and requires treatment discontinuation and investigation in a specialised unit (see *Special warnings*).

*CNS effects:* The prolonged use of this agent is associated with a risk of pharmocological tolerance, dependence and withdrawal syndrome. The most common adverse reactions which have been described are: psychotic reactions or psychosis, depression, nervousness, agitation, sleep disorders and vertigo. Hallucinations and dizziness may also occur. Convulsions have been reported.

*Cardio-vascular effects:* The most common reported reactions are tachycardia, palpitations, hypertension, precordial pain. Rarely cases of cardiovascular or cerebro-vascular accidents have been described in patients treated with anorectic agents. In particular stroke, angina, myocardial infarction, cardiac failure and cardiac arrest have been reported. Other side-effects reported are vomiting, dry mouth, facial oedema, rash, headache and urinary frequency.

*Overdose: Symptoms:* Initially irritability, agitation, disorientation and tremor may occur, followed by cardiac arrhythmias, convulsions, hallucinations and coma.
*Treatment:* The stomach should be emptied by emesis or stomach tube and washed out with water if the preparation has been ingested within the last three or four hours. Diazepam, preferably by mouth (cautiously by intravenous injection) should be used to control marked excitement and convulsions. Provided renal function is adequate, elimination of phentermine may be assisted by acidification of the urine by agents such as lysine hydrochloride or arginine hydrochloride.

**Pharmacological properties**
*Pharmacodynamic properties:* Phentermine is a weak sympathomimetic amine having marked anorexigenic activity. Its appetite suppressant effect is generally considered to be exerted through the hypothalamus, but it is not certain that this is the only effect related to weight loss. In vitro, it has been shown to inhibit phospholipase activity. It may also increase glucose uptake into skeletal muscle, as has been shown with

fenfluramine. Phentermine has major effects on the dopaminergic and noradrenergic nervous systems.

Hence in addition to effects upon appetite suppression in the CNS, phentermine may also have peripheral metabolic effects which can help weight loss. The exact mechanisms are not clear.

*Pharmacokinetic properties:* Phentermine is readily absorbed from the gastro-intestinal tract and approximately 70–80% of all oral dose is excreted unchanged in the urine; the remainder is metabolised in the liver.

*Preclinical safety data:* Not applicable.

**Pharmaceutical particulars**
*List of excipients:* Lactose PhEur, Magnesium Stearate PhEur.

*Incompatibilities:* None known.

*Shelf life:* 5 years.

*Special precautions for storage:* Store below 30°C.

*Nature and contents of container:* Amber glass bottle with pilfer-proof screw cap.

*Instructions for use/handling:* Not applicable.

**Marketing authorisation number** 00068/5056R

**Date of approval/revision of SPC** January 1997.

**Legal category** CD(Sch 3), POM.

## EXIREL* INHALER

**Presentation** Exirel is a pressurised aerosol for inhalation therapy. Each actuation delivers pirbuterol acetate equivalent to pirbuterol 200 microgramms into the mouthpiece of the adapter. It also delivers the following inactive ingredients: sorbitan trioleate, propellant 11 and propellant 12. Pirbuterol acetate is a white crystalline powder which is very soluble in water.

**Uses** *Actions:* Exirel is a beta-adrenergic receptor agonist, which has been shown *in vitro* and in *in vivo* animal studies to exert a more selective action on beta$_2$-adrenergic receptors located in the lung than on beta$_1$-receptors in the heart muscle. No data exist to confirm this in man. Onset of action is usually within 5–10 minutes of inhalation and lasts 5 hours in most patients.

*Indications:* Exirel inhaler is indicated for the treatment of acute attacks or exacerbations of bronchial asthma and for the treatment of reversible airways obstruction.

**Dosage and administration**
*Adults and children over 12 years:* One inhalation (200 micrograms) increasing to two inhalations (400 micrograms) if necessary.

*Elderly:* No special dosage recommendations are made for eldelry patients.

*Use in children:* Exirel inhaler is not presently recommended for children below the age of 12 due to lack of clinical data in this age group.

For all patients, the maximum recommended dose should not exceed 8 inhalations in 24 hours. With repetitive dosing, inhalation should usually not be repeated more often than every 4 hours.

**Contra-indications, warnings, etc**
*Contra-indications:* Exirel inhaler is contra-indicated in patients known to be sensitive to sympathomimetic agents, and in patients who are receiving non-selective beta-adrenergic blocking agents.

*Warnings:* Excessive use of sympathomimetic inhalants has been associated with an increased incidence of adverse reactions including life-threatening dysrhythmias.

Potentially serious hypokalaemia has been reported in patients taking B$_2$-agonist therapy. Hypokalaemia may also occur in hypoxic patients and those treated with xanthine derivatives, steroids, diuretics and long-term laxatives. Extra care should therefore be taken if B$_2$-agonists are used in these groups of patients and serum potassium levels should be monitored.

*Use in pregnancy:* Animal tests show no teratogenic effects, but the safety of Exirel inhaler during pregnancy or lactation has not yet been established. The expected therapeutic effects of the drug should be weighed against the possible hazard to the mother or child in these situations.

*Precautions:* As with other sympathomimetic agents, Exirel inhaler should be used with caution in patients with thyrotoxicosis. The patient should be advised to seek medical advice if the treatment ceases to be effective and/or their asthma seems to be worsening and not to increase the dose without medical advice.

*Side-effects:* Side-effects such as tremors, headache, nervousness, insomnia, palpitations have been reported infrequently and are similar to those reactions recorded with other beta$_2$-agonists. Potentially serious hypokalaemia has been reported in patients taking B$_2$-agonist therapy. As with other inhalation therapy, paradoxical bronchospasm may occur immediately after dosing. In this instance, Exirel should be discontinued immediately and alternative therapy instituted if necessary.

*Overdosage:* In the event of overdosage with Exirel inhaler, supportive and symptomatic treatment is indicated. Cardioselective beta-blocking drugs may be useful but should be used with caution in patients with a history of bronchospasm.

**Pharmaceutical precautions** Store below 30°C and protect from frost and direct sunlight. As the vial is pressurised, no attempt should be made to puncture or dispose of it by burning.

**Legal category** POM.

**Package quantities** Each canister provides 200 inhalations (OP).

**Further information** Nil.

**Product licence number** 0068/0135.

## FILAIR* 50 INHALER
## FILAIR* 100 INHALER

**Presentation** Filair 50 Inhaler is a pressurised aerosol for inhalation therapy. Each actuation delivers 50 micrograms beclomethasone dipropionate (as propellant solvate) into the mouthpiece of the adapter. It also delivers the following inactive ingredients: sorbitan trioleate; propellants 11, 12 and 114.

Filair 100 Inhaler is a pressurised aerosol for inhalation therapy. Each actuation delivers 100 micrograms beclomethasone dipropionate (as propellant solvate) into the mouthpiece of the adapter. It also delivers the same inactive ingredients as Filair 50 Inhaler.

**Uses** Filair 50 and Filair 100 Inhaler are indicated for the prophylactic treatment of chronic reversible obstructive airways disease.

**Dosage and administration**
*Adults:* for maintenance: 200 micrograms, twice daily or 100 micrograms, three or four times daily. In more severe cases a dose of 600–800 micrograms daily is recommended, with subsequent reductions. The maximum recommended daily dose of this preparation is 1 mg. In patients receiving doses of 1500 micrograms or more daily adrenal suppression may occur.

*Children:* 50–100 micrograms, two to four times daily.

*Elderly:* No special dosage recommendations are made for elderly patients.

**Contra-indications, warnings, etc**
*Contra-indication:* Hypersensitivity to beclomethasone is a contra-indication. Caution should be observed in patients with pulmonary tuberculosis.

*Side-effects:* Candidiasis of the throat and mouth may develop in some patients, but this can be treated without discontinuation of beclomethasone therapy. Hoarseness may also occur.

*Precautions:* Patients should be instructed on the proper use of the inhaler. They should be made aware of the prophylactic nature of Filair Inhaler therapy and that it should be used regularly at the intervals recommended and not when immediate relief is required.

In patients who have been transferred to inhalation therapy, systemic steroid therapy may need to be re-instated rapidly during periods of stress or where airways obstruction or mucus prevents absorption from the inhalation.

Patients who have received systemic steroids for long periods of time or at high doses, or both, need special care and subsequent management when being transferred to beclomethasone therapy.

Recovery from impaired adrenocortical function, caused by prolonged systemic steroid therapy, is slow. The patient should be in a reasonably stable state before being given Filair Inhaler in addition to his usual maintenance dose of systemic steroid. Withdrawal of the systemic steroid should be gradual, starting after about seven days by reducing the daily oral dose by 1 mg prednisolone, or equivalent, at intervals not less than one week. Adrenocortical function should be monitored regularly.

Most patients can be successfully transferred to Filair Inhaler with maintenance of good respiratory function, but special care is necessary for the first months after the transfer until the hypothalamic-pituitary-adrenal (HPA) system has sufficiently recovered to enable the patient to cope with emergencies such as trauma, surgery or infections.

Patients who have been transferred to inhalation therapy should carry a warning card indicating that systemic steroid therapy may need to be re-instated without delay during periods of stress. It may be advisable to provide such patients with a supply of oral steroid to use in an emergency, for example when the asthma worsens as a result of a chest infection. The dose of Filair Inhaler should be increased at this time and then gradually reduced to the maintenance level after the systemic steroid has been discontinued.

Discontinuation of systemic steroids may cause exacerbation of allergic diseases such as atopic eczema and rhinitis. These should be treated as required with antihistamine and topical therapy.

*Overdosage:* Acute overdosage is unlikely to cause problems. The only harmful effect that follows inhalation of large amounts of the drug over a short time period is suppression of HPA function. Specific emergency action need not be taken. Treatment with Filair Inhaler should be continued at the recommended dose to control the asthma; HPA function recovers in a day or two.

If grossly excessive doses of beclomethasone dipropionate were taken over a prolonged period a degree of atrophy of the adrenal cortex could occur in addition to HPA suppression. In this event the patient should be treated as steroid-dependent and transferred to a suitable maintenance dose of a systemic steroid such as prednisolone. Once the condition is stabilised the patient should be returned to Filair Inhaler by the method recommended above.

*Pregnancy:* There is inadequate evidence of safety in human pregnancy. In animals, systemic administration of relatively high doses can cause abnormalities of foetal development including growth retardation and cleft palate. There may therefore be a very small risk of such effects in the human foetus.

However, inhalation of beclomethasone dipropionate into the lungs avoids the high level of exposure that occurs with administration by systemic routes.

The use of beclomethasone dipropionate in pregnancy requires that the possible benefits of the drug be weighed against the possible hazards. The drug has been in widespread use for many years without apparent ill consequence.

*Lactation:* It is probable that beclomethasone is excreted in milk. However, given the relatively low doses used by the inhalation route, the levels are likely to be low. In mothers breast feeding their baby the therapeutic benefits of the drug should be weighed against the potential hazards to mother and baby.

**Pharmaceutical precautions** Store below 30°C, protected from frost and direct sunlight. As the vial is pressurised, no attempt should be made to puncture or dispose of it by burning.

**Legal category** POM.

**Package quantities** Each canister provides 200 inhalations

**Further information** Nil.

**Product licence numbers**
Filair 50 Inhaler 68/0121
Filair 100 Inhaler 68/0144

## FILAIR* FORTE INHALER

**Presentation** Filair Forte Inhaler is a pressurised aerosol for inhalation therapy. Each actuation delivers 250 micrograms beclomethasone dipropionate (as propellant solvate) into the mouthpiece of the adapter. It also delivers the following inactive ingredients: sorbitan trioleate; propellants 11, 12 and 114.

**Uses** Filair Forte Inhaler is indicated for the prophylactic treatment of chronic reversible obstructive airways disease in those patients who require high doses of beclomethasone to control their symptoms.

**Dosage and administration**
*Adults:* for maintenance: 2 inhalations (500 micrograms), twice daily or 1 inhalation (250 micrograms), four times daily; may be increased to 2 inhalations four times daily if necessary. In patients receiving doses of 1500 micrograms or more daily, adrenal suppression may occur. The degree of suppression may not always be clinically significant but it is advisable to provide such patients with a supply of oral steroid to use in stressful situations. The risk of adrenal suppression occurring should be balanced against the therapeutic advantages.

*Children:* Filair Forte Inhaler is not recommended for use in children.

*Elderly:* No special dosage recommendations are made for elderly patients.

**Contra-indications, warnings, etc**
*Contra-indication:* Hypersensitivity to beclomethasone is a contra-indication. Caution should be observed in patients with pulmonary tuberculosis.

*Side-effects:* Candidiasis of the throat and mouth may develop in some patients, but this can be treated without discontinuation of beclomethasone therapy. Hoarseness may also occur.

*Precautions:* Patients should be instructed on the proper use of the inhaler. They should be made aware of the prophylactic nature of Filair Forte Inhaler therapy and that it should be used regularly at the intervals recommended and not when immediate relief is required.

In patients who have been transferred to inhalation therapy, systemic steroid therapy may need to be re-instated rapidly during periods of stress or where airways obstruction or mucus prevents absorption from the inhalation.

Patients who have received systemic steroids for long periods of time or at high doses, or both, need special care and subsequent management when being transferred to beclomethasone therapy.

Recovery from impaired adrenocortical function, caused by prolonged systemic steroid therapy, is slow. The patient should be in a reasonably stable state before being given Filair Forte Inhaler in addition to his usual maintenance dose of systemic steroid. Withdrawal of the systemic steroid should be gradual, starting after about seven days by reducing the daily oral dose by 1 mg prednisolone, or equivalent, at intervals not less than one week. Adrenocortical function should be monitored regularly.

Most patients can be successfully transferred to Filair Forte Inhaler with maintenance of good respiratory function, but special care is necessary for the first months after the transfer until the hypothalamic-pituitary-adrenal (HPA) system has sufficiently recovered to enable the patient to cope with emergencies such as trauma, surgery or infections.

Patients who have been transferred to inhalation therapy should carry a warning card indicating that systemic steroid therapy may need to be re-instated without delay during periods of stress. It may be advisable to provide such patients with a supply of oral steroid to use in an emergency, for example when the asthma worsens as a result of a chest infection. The dose of Filair Forte Inhaler should be increased at this time and then gradually reduced to the maintenance level after the systemic steroid has been discontinued.

Discontinuation of systemic steroids may cause exacerbation of allergic diseases such as atopic eczema and rhinitis. These should be treated as required with antihistamine and topical therapy.

*Overdosage:* If grossly excessive doses of beclomethasone dipropionate were taken over a prolonged period a degree of atrophy of the adrenal cortex could occur in addition to HPA suppression. In this event the patient should be treated as steroid-dependent and transferred to a suitable maintenance dose of a systemic steroid such as prednisolone. Once the condition is stabilised the patient should be returned to Filair Forte Inhaler by the method recommended above. To guard against the unexpected occurrence of adrenal suppression regular tests of adrenal function are advised.

*Pregnancy:* There is inadequate evidence of safety in human pregnancy. In animals, systemic administration of relatively high doses can cause abnormalities of foetal development including growth retardation and cleft palate. There may therefore be a very small risk of such effects in the himan foetus. However, inhalation of beclomethasone dipropionate into the lungs avoids the high level of exposure that occurs with administration by systemic routes.

The use of beclomethasone dipropionate in pregnancy requires that the possible benefits of the drug be weighed against the possible hazards. The drug has been in widespread use for many years without apparent ill consequence.

*Lactation:* It is probable that beclomethasone is excreted in milk. However, given the relatively low doses used by the inhalation route, the levels are likely to be low. In mothers breast feeding their baby the therapeutic benefits of the drug should be weighed against the potential hazards to mother and baby.

**Pharmaceutical precautions** Store below 30°C, protected from frost and direct sunlight. As the vial is pressurised, no attempt should be made to puncture or dispose of it by burning.

**Legal category** POM.

**Package quantities** Each canister provides 200 inhalations

**Further information** Nil.

**Product licence number** *0068/0139*

## HIPREX* TABLETS

**Presentation** White, oblong tablet with breakline, marked HX on one side and 3M on the other. Each Hiprex tablet contains hexamine hippurate 1 g.

**Uses**
Hiprex is indicated in the prophylaxis and treatment of urinary tract infections:

1. As maintenance therapy after successful initial treatment of acute infections with antibiotics.

2. As long-term therapy in the prevention of recurrent cystitis.

3. To suppress urinary infection in patients with indwelling catheters and to reduce the incidence of catheter blockage.

4. To provide prophylaxis against the introduction of infection into the urinary tract during instrumental procedures.

5. Asymptomatic bacteriuria.

Hexamine hippurate is readily absorbed from the gastro-intestinal tract and excreted via the kidney.

With Hiprex, as with other specific urinary antibacterial agents of this type, antibacterial activity is confined to the urinary tract.

The antibacterial action is achieved by the slow release of the bactericidal formaldehyde, from the hexamine part, in the urine; acid pH less than pH 5.5 is necessary for this reaction to occur. It is obtained and maintained there by the presence of hippuric acid.

Hiprex has a wide antibacterial spectrum covering both gram-positive and gram-negative organisms. It is active against the bacteria which most commonly cause urinary tract infection – *Escherichia coli, Aerobacter aerogenes,* Pseudomonas and some strains of Proteus. Urinary antibacterial activity can be shown within 30 minutes of administration.

Hiprex is particularly useful for long-term treatment because neither tolerance to its effect nor bacterial resistance occurs. The incidence of side-effects is extremely low.

**Dosage and administration** *Adults:* 1 g twice daily.

In patients with catheters the dosage may be increased to 1 g three times daily.

*Children under 6 years:* Not recommended.

*Children: 6–12 years:* 500 mg twice daily.

The tablets may be halved, or they can be crushed and taken with a drink of milk or fruit juice if the patient prefers.

**Contra-indications, warnings, etc** *Side-effects:* Occasionally rashes, gastric irritation or irritation of the bladder may occur.

All side-effects are reversible on withdrawal of the drug.

*Contra-indications:* Severe dehydration, metabolic acidosis, or severe renal failure (creatinine clearance or GFR<10 ml/min.). Hiprex may be used where mild (20–50 ml/min.) to moderate (10–20 ml/min.) renal insufficiency is present. (If the GFR is not available, the serum creatinine concentration can be used as a guide).

Hiprex should not be administered concurrently with sulphonamides because of the possibility of crystalluria, or with alkalising agents, such as mixture of potassium citrate.

*Use in pregnancy:* There is inadequate evidence of safety of the drug in human pregnancy but it has been in wide use for many years without apparent ill consequence, animal studies having shown no hazard.

Hexamine is excreted in breast milk but the quantities will be insignificant to the infant. Mothers can therefore breast feed their infants.

*Overdosage:* Vomiting and haematuria may occur. These can be treated by the use of an anti-emetic and drinking copious quantities of water respectively. Bladder symptoms can be treated by the consumption of copious quantities of water and 2–3 teaspoonfuls of bicarbonate of soda.

**Pharmaceutical precautions** The container should be kept tightly closed.

**Legal category** P.

**Package quantities** Bottles of 60 tablets (OP).

**Further information** Nil.

**Product licence number** 0068/5003R.

## INTRALGIN* GEL

**Presentation** Intralgin contains Benzocaine BP 2 per cent w/w and salicylamide 5 per cent w/w in an alcoholic vehicle. It contains the following inactive ingredients: Carbopol*; Brij*; Isopropyl Alcohol BP; Strong Ammonia Solution BP. Intralgin is a clear, pleasant-smelling preparation – non-greasy and non-staining.

**Uses** Intralgin is indicated for the relief of muscle pain from strains, sprains and injuries, and pain associated with fibrositis, lumbago and non-articular rheumatism.

The use of isopropyl alcohol as a vehicle for the medicaments contributes significantly to the action of Intralgin. Isopropyl alcohol because of its penetrative properties facilitates the percutaneous absorption of benzocaine and salicylamide. Vigorous massage is not needed with Intralgin, unlike traditional rubs which rely for effect on erythema or counter-irritation.

**Dosage and administration** Intralgin Gel should be applied liberally and rubbed gently into the skin until penetration is complete. Vigorous massage is unnecessary.

For more rapid absorption the painful area should be warmed before applying Intralgin.

*Children and the elderly:* There are no special dosage recommendations for children and elderly patients.

**Contra-indications, warnings, etc**
*Contra-indications:* None.

*Precautions:* If irritation or itching occurs due to hypersensitivity, Intralgin should be discontinued and a soothing cream applied.

*Interactions:* There are no known interactions with Intralgin therapy.

*Side-effects:* Local sensitivity reactions to the benzocaine constituent have occasionally been reported.

*Overdosage:* Not applicable.

*Use in pregnancy:* There is inadequate evidence of the safety of Intralgin in human pregnancy but it has been in wide use for many years without apparent ill consequence. Excretion in breast milk, if any, is expected to be too low to affect the infant.

**Pharmaceutical precautions** Store in a cool dry place. Avoid extremes of temperature.

**Legal category** P.

**Package quantities** Tubes containing 50 g (OP).

**Further information** Nil.

**Product licence number** 0068/5076R.

## MEDIHALER-EPI*

**Presentation** Medihaler-Epi is a pressurised aerosol for inhalation therapy. The vial contains a creamy-white suspension of Adrenaline Acid Tartrate BP 14 mg/ml in aerosol propellent, and delivers 400 measured doses, each containing 280 micrograms Adrenaline Acid Tartrate BP. The vial contains the following inactive ingredients: sorbitan trioleate; propellants 11, 12 and 114.

**Uses** Medihaler-Epi may be used as an adjunct to the standard therapy in anaphylactic reactions due to drug sensitivity or insect stings.

Adrenaline is a sympathomimetic amine which activates both alpha- and beta-adrenergic receptors. As a result, it causes vasoconstriction, bronchodilatation, relieves mucosal congestion and is a cardiac stimulant.

By inhalation, adrenaline relaxes bronchial smooth muscle and constricts bronchial mucosal vessels, relieving congestion and oedema. However, tolerance to adrenaline can develop after repeated use and the action of adrenaline in reducing bronchial secretion may make mucus more viscid.

**Dosage and administration** Each puff from Medihaler-epi delivers a measured dose of 280 micrograms adrenaline acid tartrate.

Correct technique is essential if the patient is to obtain full benefit from each treatment. It is important that the doctor shows the patient how to use Medihaler-epi by personal demonstration, as patients may not be familiar with the use of inhalers. A Demonstration Unit containing no active medicament can be obtained for this purpose, on request.

*Adults:* In the adjunctive treatment of anaphylactic reactions, a minimum dose of 20 puffs is recommended.

*Children:* Medihaler-epi has not been evaluated in children but, should the need arise, it may be used as an adjunct to standard anaphylactic therapy. A dose of 10 to 15 puffs is recommended. Medihaler-epi should be administered to children only under the supervision of a responsible adult.

*Elderly:* No special dosage recommendations are made for elderly patients.

**Contra-indications, warnings, etc**
*Side-effects:* Gastric pain has been reported, probably as a result of swallowed adrenaline. Overdosage may cause dry mouth, palpitations or nervousness.

*Contra-indications:* Medihaler-epi should be used with caution in the presence of cardiac disease, hypertension and hyperthyroidism.

Prolonged use of adrenaline may lead to the development of tolerance (adrenaline 'fastness'). When this occurs, isoprenaline is a most effective alternative.

Theoretically, no interaction with monoamine oxidase inhibitors (MAOI) would be expected, but some enhancement of the cardiovascular effects of adrenaline is seen especially if the MAOI induces hypotension.

*Pregnancy:* There is inadequate evidence of safety of the drug in human pregnancy but it has been in wide use for many years without apparent ill consequence, animal studies having shown no hazard. If drug therapy is needed in pregnancy, this drug can be used if there is no safer alternative.

*Overdosage*

*Acute poisoning:* No cases have been reported. The following guidance is based on acute adrenaline poisoning following parenteral administration.

*Symptoms:* Restlessness, palpitations, rapid pulse, tremor, weakness, dizziness, headache, coldness of extremities, elevated blood pressure, tachycardia. The symptoms are rapid in onset and of short duration.

*Treatment:* It is essential to administer immediately intravenous injections of quick-acting sympatholytics, e.g. phentolamine or piperoxan.

*Chronic poisoning:* Some cases have been reported, but no details of treatment have been given, other than withdrawal of the aerosol.

**Pharmaceutical precautions** Medihaler-epi shold be stored in a cool place, protected from frost and sunlight.

As the Medihaler vial is pressurised, no attempt should be made to puncture it or to dispose of it by burning.

**Legal category** POM.

**Package quantities** Each canister provides 400 inhalations (OP).

**Further information** Nil.

**Product licence number** 0068/5060R.

## MEDIHALER-ERGOTAMINE*

**Qualitative and quantitative composition** Ergotamine Tartrate BP 9 mg/ml.

**Pharmaceutical form** Pressurised aerosol for inhalation therapy.

**Clinical particulars**
*Therapeutic indications:* Medihaler-ergotamine is indicated for the rapid relief of migraine.

*Posology and method of administration:*
*Adults and children aged 10 or over:* One inhalation should be taken at the first sign of attack and should be repeated if necessary after five minutes.

Caution: no more than 6 inhalations should be taken in any 24 hour period. There should be an interval of at least four treatment free days between treatment days.

*Children:* Medihaler ergotamine is not recommended for children younger than 10 years of age.

*Elderly:* No special dosage recommendations are made for elderly patients.

*Contra-indications:* Sepsis, coronary artery disease, peripheral vascular disease, renal or hepatic dysfunction, hypertension.

*Special warnings and special precautions for use:* Maximum dosage in one week should not exceed 12 inhalations.

*Interaction with other medicaments and other forms of interaction:* None reported.

*Pregnancy and lactation:* Ergotamine tartrate should not be used during pregnancy. Avoid during breast feeding.

*Effects on ability to drive and use machines:* None.

*Undesirable effects:* Ergotamine tartrate may cause nausea and vomiting in some patients. As these symptoms can occur in migraine attacks, it may be difficult to determine whether the illness or the medication is responsible. Muscle pain or cramps may occasionally be experienced.

Ergotamine may cause precordial pain, myocardial ischemia or infarction in patients with no history of coronary heart disease.

*Overdose:* Acute poisoning is rare. Symptoms are nausea, vomiting, diarrhoea, thirst, coolness of the skin, pruritus, rapid and weak pulse, numbness and tingling of the extremities, confusion and unconsciousness.

Treatment of poisoning is symptomatic. Vasodilators such as sodium nitroprusside may be used, together with mechanical procedures to restore the circulation. Nausea and vomiting may be relieved by atropine.

**Pharmacological properties**
*Pharmacodynamic properties:* One or two inhalations from Medihaler-Ergotamine can abort the migraine attack before cephalic vasodilatation becomes fixed and before oedema of the vascular wall and perivascular tissues has developed. In the majority of patients, full therapeutic effect is achieved within 15 minutes.

*Pharmacokinetic properties:* Micronised ergotamine tartrate taken by inhalation is rapidly absorbed from

the highly vascular epithelium of the respiratory tract into the systemic circulation. Two factors make this route of administration particularly effective: speed of absorption and lack of interference with the drug's action by either the digestive tract or the liver. Another advantage is that the dose is retained in spite of vomiting.

**Pharmaceutical particulars**
*List of excipients:* Sorbitan trioleate; Trichlorofluoromethane (Propellant 11) BP; Dichlorotetrafluoroethane (Propellant 114) BP; Dichlorodifluoromethane (Propellant 12) BP.

*Incompatibilities:* None.

*Shelf life:* 2 years. 6 months after dispensed.

*Special precautions for staorage:* Wholesaler/pharmacist: Store at 5°C until dispensed.

Patient: The inhaler should be stored for up to 6 months; no special storage conditions are required.

*Nature and contents of container:* Aluminium canister closed with a 50 µl metering valve containing 75 doses.

*Instructions for use/handling:* Pressurised canister. Do not puncture. Do not burn, even when empty.

**Marketing authorisation number** 0068/5014R

**Date of approval/revision of SPC** August 1996.

**Legal category** POM.

## MEDIHALER-ISO*

**Qualitative and quantitative composition** Each Medihaler-iso inhaler contains Isoprenaline Sulphate BP 0.4% w/v.

**Pharmaceutical form** Pressurised aerosol for inhalation therapy.

**Clinical particulars**
*Therapeutic indications:* Medihaler-iso is indicated for the relief of bronchospasm in bronchial asthma and chronic bronchitis.

*Posology and method of administration:*
*Adults:* Each puff from Medihaler-iso delivers a measured dose of 80 µg isoprenaline sulphate. One, two or at the most three puffs should be sufficient to provide relief in most cases. Before each puff, the patient should wait at least one minute to allow the full effect of the previous puff to become apparent. It should not be necessary for the patient to take further treatment for at least 30 minutes, or more than eight treatments in any 24 hour period.

*Children:* Medihaler-iso should be administered only under the supervision of a responsible adult to children who are responsive to bronchodilators.

*Elderly:* No special dosage recommendations are made for elderly patients.

*Contra-indications:* Medihaler-iso should not be used in the presence of severe cardiac disease, pre-existing ventricular arrhythmia, severe hypertension and hyperthyroidism.

*Special warnings and special precautions for use:* Use with care in patients with heart disease and hypertension and those taking other sympathomimetic agents. There is a theoretical possibility that isoprenaline could trigger or aggravate cardiac arrhythmias. Theoretically no interaction with monoamine oxidase inhibitors (MAOI) would be expected but some enhancement of the cardiovascular effects of isoprenaline is seen, particularly if the MAOI induces hypotension.

*Interaction with other medicaments and other forms of interactions:* Concurrent administration of cardiac glycosides, antidepressants, xanthine derivatives, thyroxine and anaesthetics may result in the myocardium being sensitised. This is also seen in patients with abnormalities of electrolytes and blood gases.

*Pregnancy and lactation:* There is inadequate evidence of the safety of the drug in human pregnancy but it has been in wide use for many years without apparent ill consequence, animal studies having shown no hazard. If drug therapy is needed in pregnancy, this drug can be used if there is no safer alternative.

*Effects on ability to drive and use machines:* None.

*Undesirable effects:* Overdosage may cause dry mouth, palpitations or nervousness. Rebound bronchospasm has been reported but this is rare. Elderly patients are more susceptible to side-effects.

*Overdose:* Acute poisoning in non-asthmatics: No cases have been reported. In the absence of details of such practical experience, the following guidance is based on theoretical considerations.

Symptoms of acute isoprenaline poisoning are likely to be mainly cardiovascular effects, e.g. tachycardia, palpitations, peripheral vasodilation and fall in blood pressure.

Treatment: General symptomatic therapy.

Chronic poisoning in asthmatics: Some cases have

been reported, but no details of treatment have been given, other than withdrawal of the aerosol.

Excessive use during an attack of asthma indicates lack of response. This is a grave sign suggestive of status asthmaticus, or that the patient is ill. Patients should therefore be advised to seek urgent medical attention. It is recommended that 100 mg hydrocortisone be given immediately by intravenous injection, and the patient admitted to hospital without delay. Beta-blocking drugs should not be used.

**Pharmacological properties**
*Pharmacodynamic properties:* Isoprenaline is a bronchodilator which also produces vasodilatation in all blood vessels, including those of the pulmonary system. Pulse rate and cardiac output are increased, the degree of cardiac stimulation being proportional to the blood level. Isoprenaline inhibits histamine release in the lungs and has a beneficial effect on cilia and mucus flow. Cardiac stimulation does not usually occur and the maximum possible bronchodilatation is produced at doses below those which result in significant tachycardia. Appreciable cardiac stimulation occurs only at the upper end of the therapeutic dose range.

*Pharmacokinetic properties:* By inhalation isoprenaline has a rapid onset of bronchodilatation. Isoprenaline is quickly eliminated from the blood and therefore has no cumulative effect.

**Pharmaceutical particulars**
*List of excipients:* Sorbitan trioleate; Dichlorodifluoromethane (Propellant 12) BP; Trichlorofluoromethane (Propellant 11) BP; Dichlorotetrafluoroethane (Propellant 114) BP.

*Incompatbilities:* None.

*Shelf-life:* 3 years.

*Special precautions for storage:* Store below 30°C. Avoid storage in direct sunlight or heat.

*Nature and contents of container:* Aluminium vial closed with 25 µl metering valve containing 400 doses.

*Instructions for use/handling:* Pressurised vial. Do not puncture, do not burn, even when empty.

**Marketing authorisation number** 0068/5082R.

**Date of approval/revision of SPC** September 1995.

**Legal category** POM.

## MEDIHALER-ISO* FORTE

**Qualitative and quantitative composition** Each Medihaler-iso Forte inhaler contains Isoprenaline Sulphate BP 2.0% w/v.

**Pharmaceutical form** Pressurised aerosol for inhalation therapy.

**Clinical particulars**
*Therapeutic indications:* Medihaler-iso Forte is indicated for the relief of bronchospasm in bronchial asthma and chronic bronchitis.

*Posology and method of administration:*
*Adults:* Each puff from Medihaler-iso Forte delivers a measured dose of 400 µg isoprenaline sulphate. One, two or at the most three puffs should be sufficient to provide relief in most cases. Before each puff, the patient should wait at least one minute to allow the full effect of the previous puff to become apparent. It should not be necessary for the patient to take further treatment for at least 30 minutes, or more than eight treatments in any 24 hour period.

*Children:* Medihaler-iso Forte is not recommended for children.

*Elderly:* No special dosage recommendations are made for elderly patients.

*Contra-indications:* Medihaler-iso Forte should not be used in the presence of severe cardiac disease, pre-existing ventricular arrhythmia, severe hypertension and hyperthyroidism.

*Special warnings and special precautions for use:* Use with care in patients with heart disease and hypertension and those taking other sympathomimetic agents. There is a theoretical possibility that isoprenaline could trigger or aggravate cardiac arrhythmias. Theoretically no interaction with monoamine oxidase inhibitors (MAOI) would be expected but some enhancement of the cardiovascular effects of isoprenaline is seen, particularly if the MAOI induces hypotension.

*Interaction with other medicaments and other forms of interactions:* Concurrent administration of cardiac glycosides, antidepressants, xanthine derivatives, thyroxine and anaesthetics may result in the myocardium being sensitised. This is also seen in patients with abnormalities of electrolytes and blood gases.

*Pregnancy and lactation:* There is inadequate evidence of the safety of the drug in human pregnancy but it has been in wide use for many years without apparent ill consequence, animal studies having shown no hazard. If drug therapy is needed in pregnancy, this drug can be used if there is no safer alternative. It is recognised that even following topical use, significant systemic absorption of isoprenaline could occur following the use of Medihaler-iso Forte, and give rise to systemic effects. Excessive use near the term could delay the onset of labour. There is no information on the excretion of this drug in breast milk.

*Effects on ability to drive and use machines:* None.

*Undesirable effects:* Overdosage may cause dry mouth, palpitations or nervousness. Rebound bronchospasm has been reported but this is rare. Elderly patients are more susceptible to side-effects.

*Overdose:* Acute poisoning in non-asthmatics: No cases have been reported. In the absence of details of such practical experience, the following guidance is based on theoretical considerations.

Symptoms of acute isoprenaline poisoning are likely to be mainly cardiovascular effects, e.g. tachycardia, palpitations, peripheral vasodilation and fall in blood pressure.

Treatment: General symptomatic therapy.

Chronic poisoning in asthmatics: Some cases have been reported, but no details of treatment have been given, other than withdrawal of the aerosol.

Excessive use during an attack of asthma indicates lack of response. This is a grave sign suggestive of status asthmaticus, or that the patient is ill. Patients should therefore be advised to seek urgent medical attention. It is recommended that 100 mg hydrocortisone be given immediately by intravenous injection, and the patient admitted to hospital without delay. Beta-blocking drugs should not be used.

### Pharmacological properties

*Pharmacodynamic properties:* Isoprenaline is a bronchodilator which also produces vasodilatation in all blood vessels, including those of the pulmonary system. Pulse rate and cardiac output are increased, the degree of cardiac stimulation being proportional to the blood level. Isoprenaline inhibits histamine release in the lungs and has a beneficial effect on cilia and mucus flow. Cardiac stimulation does not usually occur and the maximum possible bronchodilatation is produced at doses below those which result in significant tachycardia. Appreciable cardiac stimulation occurs only at the upper end of the therapeutic dose range.

*Pharmacokinetic properties:* By inhalation isoprenaline has a rapid onset of bronchodilatation. Isoprenaline is quickly eliminated from the blood and therefore has no cumulative effect.

### Pharmaceutical particulars

*List of excipients:* Sorbitan trioleate; Dichlorodifluoromethane (Propellant 12) BP; Trichlorofluoromethane (Propellant 11) BP; Dichlorotetrafluoroethane (Propellant 114) BP.

*Incompatbilities:* None.

*Shelf-life:* 3 years.

*Special precautions for storage:* Store below 30°C. Avoid storage in direct sunlight or heat.

*Nature and contents of container:* Aluminium vial closed with 25 µl metering valve containing 400 doses.

*Instructions for use/handling:* Shake before use. Pressurised vial. Do not puncture, do not burn even when empty.

**Marketing authorisation number**  0068/5072R.

**Date of approval/revision of SPC**  September 1995.

**Legal category**  POM.

## NUELIN* TABLETS

**Qualitative and quantitative composition**  Each Nuelin tablet contains Theophylline PhEur 125 mg.

**Pharmaceutical form**  Tablet.

### Clinical particulars

*Therapeutic indications:* Nuelin is indicated for the prophylaxis and treatment of reversible bronchospasm associated with asthma and chronic obstructive pulmonary disease.

*Posology and method of administration:*
*Adults:* One tablet three or four times daily, preferably after food; this can be increased to two tablets three or four times daily depending on response.

*Elderly:* Elderly patients may require lower doses due to reduced theophylline clearance.

*Children: 7–12 years (20–35 kg):* Half or 1 tablet three or four times daily, preferably after food.

The difficulty of dividing the tablet accurately makes Nuelin unsuitable for use in children under the age of seven.

Nuelin tablets are soluble in water.

*Contra-indications:* Hypersensitivity to theophylline or other xanthines.

*Special warnings and special precautions for use:* Use with caution in patients with cardiac arrythmias, peptic ulcer, hyperthyroidism and severe hypertension.

Smoking and alcohol consumption may increase theophylline clearance and increased doses of theophylline are therefore required. In patients with cardiac failure, hepatic dysfunction/disease and fever the reverse is true and these patients may require a reduced dosage.

Alternative bronchodilator therapy should be used in patients with epilepsy.

It is not recommended that the product be used concurrently with other preparations containing xanthine derivatives.

Xanthines can potentiate hypokalaemia resulting from beta-2-agonist therapy, steroids, diuretics and hypoxia. Particular caution is advised in severe asthma. It is recommended that serum potassium levels are monitored in such situations.

*Interaction with other medicaments and other forms of interaction:* Cimetidine, allopurinol, corticosteroids, frusemide, isoprenaline, oral contraceptives, thiobendazole, ciprofloxacin, erythromycin or other macrolide antibiotics and the calcium channel blockers, diltiazem and verapamil delay the elimination of theophylline. A reduction of the theophylline dosage is recommended. Phenytoin, carbamazepine, barbiturates, lithium, rifampicin, sulphinpyrazone increase theophylline clearance and therefore the theophylline dosage may need to be increased.

The concomitant use of theophylline and fluvoxamine should usually be avoided. Where this is not possible, patients should have their theophylline dose halved and plasma theophylline should be monitored closely.

*Pregnancy and lactation:* There is inadequate evidence of safety of the drug in human pregnancy but it has been in wide use for many years without apparent ill consequences; there is evidence of harmful effects in pregnancy in animals. Use in pregnancy only when there is no safer alternative and when the condition itself carries risks for the mother.

Theophylline is excreted in breast milk and has been shown to cause irritability in infants. It is therefore recommended that the mother nurse her infant just prior to taking her next dose, when plasma theophylline levels are expected to be low.

*Effects on ability to drive and use machines:* No effect.

*Undesirable effects:* Nausea and other gastric disturbances may occur rarely. Palpitations, headache, CNS stimulation and insomnia have been reported occasionally.

*Overdose: Symptoms:* Characterised by nausea, vomiting, electrolyte imbalance and gastro-intestinal irritation. Tachycardia and convulsions may also occur.

*Treatment:* Gastric lavage and general supportive measures (e.g. to maintain circulation, respiration and fluid and electrolyte balance) are recommended. Oral activated charcoal may reduce serum theophylline levels, whilst in severe cases charcoal haemoperfusion may be required.

### Pharmacological properties

*Pharmacodynamic properties:* Theophylline directly relaxes smooth muscle thus acting mainly as a bronchodilator and vasodilator. The drug also possesses other actions typical of the xanthine derivatives; coronary vasodilator, diuretic, cardiac stimulant, cerebral stimulant and skeletal muscle stimulant.

*Pharmacokinetic properties:* It has been established that the xanthines, which include theophylline, are readily absorbed after oral, rectal or parenteral administration and this fact is well documented in published literature.

Theophylline is excreted in the urine as metabolites, mainly 1,3-dimethyluric acid and 3-methylxanthine and about 10% is excreted unchanged.

Plasma half-lives ranging from 3–9 hours and therapeutic plasma concentrations from about 5–20 µg per ml have been reported.

### Pharmaceutical particulars

*List of excipients:* Lactose Monohydrate PhEur, sodium carboxymethylcellulose, Magnesium Stearate PhEur.

*Incompatibilities:* None known.

*Shelf life:* 3 years.

*Special precautions for storage:* Store in a cool, dry place.

*Nature and contents of container:* Bottle or blister packs of 90 tablets.

*Instructions for use/handling:* None.

**Marketing authorisation number**  0068/0064R

**Date of approval/revision of SPC**  January 1997.

**Legal category**  P.

## NUELIN* LIQUID

**Presentation**  Clear, light brown, pleasantly flavoured liquid. Each 5 ml dose of Nuelin Liquid contains 60 mg Theophylline Hydrate BP as the sodium glycinate salt. It also contains the following inactive ingredients: sucrose; Sodium Butyl Hydroxybenzoate BP.

**Uses**  Nuelin Liquid is indicated for the prophylaxis and treatment of reversible bronchospasm in asthma, bronchitis and emphysema. Nuelin in tablet form (microcrystalline theophylline 125 mg) is established as a highly effective bronchodilator. Nuelin Liquid is designed to offer comparable relief of bronchospasm with the same low incidence of side-effects, for patients who prefer a liquid presentation. Each 10 ml of Nuelin Liquid approximates to one 125 mg Nuelin tablet.

**Dosage and administration**  *Adults:* 10–20 ml (two to four 5 ml spoonfuls) three or four times daily, preferably after food.

*Children: 7–12 years:* One-and-a-half or two 5 ml spoonfuls three or four times daily, preferably after food.

*2–6 years:* One or one-and-a-half 5 ml spoonfuls three or four times daily, preferably after food.

*Under 2 years:* Nuelin liquid is not recommended for children under 2 years of age.

*Elderly:* Elderly patients may require lower doses due to reduced theophylline clearance.

**Contra-indications, warnings, etc**

*Contra-indications:* Hypersensitivity to theophylline or other xanthines.

*Warnings:* Xanthines can potentiate hypokalaemia resulting from $B_2$-agonist therapy, steroids, diuretics and hypoxia. Particular caution is advised in severe asthma. It is recommended that serum potassium levels are monitored in such situations.

*Precautions:* Use with caution in patients with cardiac arrhythmias, peptic ulcer, hyperthyroidism and severe hypertension.

Smoking and alcohol consumption may increase theophylline clearance and increased doses of theophylline are therefore required. In patients with cardiac failure, hepatic dysfunction/disease and fever the reverse is true and these patients may require a reduced dosage.

Epilepsy may become uncontrolled.

It is not recommended that the product be used concurrently with other preparations containing xanthine derivatives.

*Interactions:* Cimetidine, allopurinol, corticosteroids, frusemide, isoprenaline, oral contraceptives, thiobendazole, ciprofloxacin, erythromycin or other macrolide antibiotics delay the elimination of theophylline. A reduction of the theophylline dosage is recommended. Phenytoin, carbamazepine, barbiturates, lithium, rifampicin, sulphin pyrazone increase theophylline clearance and therefore the theophylline dosage may need to be increased. The concomitant use of theophylline and fluvoxamine should usually be avoided. Where this is not possible, patients should have their theophylline dose halved and plasma theophylline should be monitored closely.

Also see 'Warnings'.

*Side-effects:* Nausea or other gastric disturbances may occur rarely. Palpitations, headache, CNS stimulation and insomnia have been reported occasionally.

*Overdosage*

*Symptoms:* Characterised by nausea, vomiting electrolyte imbalance and gastro-intestinal irritation. Tachycardia, convulsions and hypotension may also occur.

*Treatment:* Gastric lavage and general supportive measures (e.g. to maintain circulation, respiration and fluid and electrolyte balance) are recommended. Oral activated charcoal may reduce serum theophylline levels, whilst in severe cases charcoal haemoperfusion may be required.

*Use in pregnancy:* There is inadequate evidence of safety of the drug in human pregnancy but it has been in wide use for many years without apparent ill consequences; there is evidence of harmful effects in pregnancy in animals. Use in pregnancy only when there is no safer alternative and when the condition itself carries risks for the mother.

Theophylline is excreted in breast milk and has been shown to cause irritability in infants. It is therefore recommended that the mother nurse her infant just prior to taking her next dose, when plasma theophylline levels are expected to be low.

**Pharmaceutical precautions**  Store between 5°C and 30°C. Do not freeze.

**Legal category**  P.

**Package quantities**  Bottles of 300 ml (OP).

**Further information** Each 5 ml spoonful of Nuelin Liquid contains 0.38 mEq sodium (8.7 mg Na).

**Product licence number** 0068/0084.

## NUELIN* SA TABLETS

**Presentation** Nuelin SA: White, biconvex, round tablets, 9 mm in diameter and marked NLS 175 on one side and 3M on the other.

Each Nuelin SA tablet contains 175 mg anhydrous theophylline in a slow release formulation which gives a particularly smooth release of medicament over a prolonged period. It also contains the following inactive ingredient: lactose.

Nuelin SA-250: White, biconvex, round tablets with breakline, 11 mm in diameter and marked NLS 250 on one side and 3M on the other. Each Nuelin SA-250 tablet contains 250 mg anhydrous theophylline in a slow release formulation. It contains the same inactive ingredients as Nuelin SA.

**Uses** Nuelin SA and Nuelin SA-250 tablets are indicated for the prophylaxis and treatment of reversible bronchospasm in asthma, bronchitis and emphysema.

Because effective plasma levels are maintained for up to twelve hours from a single dose, less frequent dosing is required than with conventional theophylline preparations.

**Dosage and administration** *Nuelin SA: Adults:* One tablet twice daily, preferably after food, increasing to two tablets twice daily if necessary.

*Children:* 6 to 12 years: one tablet twice daily, preferably after food.

*Nuelin SA-250: Adults:* One tablet twice daily, preferably after food, increasing to two tablets twice daily if necessary.

*Children:* 6 to 12 years: Half or one tablet twice daily, preferably after food.

Nuelin SA and Nuelin SA-250 tablets are not recommended for children under six years.

*Elderly:* Elderly patients may require lower dosage due to reduced theophylline clearance.

*Nuelin* SA tablets should be swallowed whole and not crushed or chewed.

*Nuelin* SA-250 tablets are scored and may be halved but should not be crushed or chewed.

**Contra-indications, warnings, etc**
*Contra-indications:* Hypersensitivity to theophylline or other xanthines.

*Warnings:* Xanthines can potentiate hypokalaemia resulting from $B_2$-agonist therapy, steroids, diuretics and hypoxia. Particular caution is advised in severe asthma. It is recommended that serum potassium levels are monitored in such situations.

*Precautions:* In the case of an acute asthmatic attack in a patient receiving a sustained action theophylline preparation, great caution should be taken when administering intravenous aminophylline. Half the recommended loading dose of aminophylline (generally 6 mg/kg) should be given, i.e. 3 mg/kg, cautiously.

Use with caution in patients with cardiac arrhythmias, peptic ulcer, hyperthyroidism, severe hypertension, acute porphyria, hepatic dysfunction, chronic alcoholism, acute febrile illness and chronic lung disease.

Smoking and alcohol consumption may increase theophylline clearance and increased doses of theophylline are therefore required. In patients with cardiac failure, hepatic dysfunction/disease and fever the reverse is true and these patients may require a reduced dosage.

Epilepsy may become uncontrolled.

It is not recommended that the product be used concurrently with other preparations containing xanthine derivatives.

*Interactions:* Cimetidine, allopurinol, corticosteroids, frusemide, isoprenaline, oral contraceptives, thiobendazole, ciprofloxacin, erythromycin or other macrolide antibiotics delay the elimination of theophylline. A reduction of the theophylline dosage is recommended. Phenytoin, carbamazepine, barbiturates, lithium, rifampicin, sulphin pyrazone increase theophylline clearance and therefore the theophylline dosage may need to be increased. The concomitant use of theophylline and fluvoxamine should usually be avoided. Where this is not possible, patients should have their theophylline dose halved and plasma theophylline should be monitored closely.

Also see 'Warnings'.

*Side-effects:* The side-effects commonly associated with xanthine derivatives such as nausea, gastric irritation, palpitations, headache, CNS stimulation and insomnia are much diminished when a sustained action preparation such as Nuelin SA is used. These side-effects are mild and infrequent when the plasma

concentration is maintained at less than 20 microgrammes/ml.

*Overdosage*
  *Symptoms:* Characterised by nausea, vomiting, electrolyte imbalance and gastro-intestinal irritation. Tachycardia, convulsions and hypotension may also occur.

  *Treatment:* Gastric lavage and general supportive measures (e.g. to maintain circulation, respiration and fluid and electrolyte balance) are recommended. Oral activated charcoal may reduce serum theophylline levels, whilst in severe cases charcoal haemoperfusion may be required.

*Use in pregnancy:* There is inadequate evidence of safety of the drug in human pregnancy but it has been in wide use for many years without apparent ill consequence; there is evidence of harmful effects in animals. Use in pregnancy only when there is no safer alternative and when the condition itself carries risks for the mother.

Theophylline is excreted in breast milk and has been shown to cause irritability in infants. As it is recommended that the mother nurse her infant just prior to taking her next dose when plasma theophylline levels are expected to be low, a non-sustained release form such as Nuelin is therefore preferable for nursing mothers.

**Pharmaceutical precautions** Store below 30°C.

**Legal category** P.

**Package quantities** Nuelin SA: Packs of 60 tablets (OP).
Nuelin SA-250: Packs of 60 tablets (OP).

**Further information** Nil.

**Product licence numbers**
Nuelin SA          0068/0092
Nuelin SA-250    0068/0093

## PULMADIL* INHALER

**Qualitative and quantitative composition** Each Pulmadil Inhaler contains rimiterol hydrobromide 10 mg/ml. Each inhalation delivers to the patient rimiterol hydrobromide 200 μg.

**Pharmaceutical form** Aerosol for inhalation use.

**Clinical particulars**
*Therapeutic indications:* Pulmadil is indicated for the relief of bronchospasm in bronchial asthma and chronic bronchitis.

*Posology and method of administration:* For oral administration by inhalation.

  *Adults:* One to three puffs should provide relief in most cases. This treatment dose should not be repeated in less than thirty minutes. No more than eight treatments should be taken in any 24 hour period.

  *Children:* Pulmadil Inhaler should be administered to childen only under the supervision of a responsible adult.

  *Elderly:* No special dosage recommendations are made for elderly patients.

*Contra-indications:* There are no contra-indications to inhaled Pulmadil therapy.

*Special warnings and special precautions for use:* Administer cautiously to patients with thyrotoxicosis. The patient should be advised to seek medical advice if the treatment ceases to be effective.

*Excessive use in asthmatics:* Excessive use of any bronchodilator aerosol can indicate lack of response. This is a grave sign suggestive of status asthmaticus. It is recommended that 100 mg of hydrocortisone be given intravenously immediately and the patient admitted to hospital without delay.

Potentially serious hypokalaemia has been reported in patients taking $\beta_2$-agonist therapy. Hypokalaemia may also occur in hypoxic patients and those treated with xanthine derivatives, steroids, diuretics and long-term laxatives. Extra care should therefore be taken if $\beta_2$-agonists are used in these groups of patients and serum potassium levels should be monitored.

*Interactions with other medicaments and other forms of interaction:* See *Warnings.*

*Pregnancy and lactation:* There is inadequate evidence of safety of the drug in human pregnancy but it has been in wide use for many years without apparent ill consequence, animal studies having shown no hazard.

It is unlikely that sufficient drug will be excreted in the breast milk to affect the infant.

*Effects on ability to drive and use machines:* No effects.

*Undesirable effects:* Side-effects such as headache and rash have been reported infrequently and are similar to those reactions recorded with other $\beta_2$-agonists. Potentially serious hypokalaemia has been reported in patients taking $\beta_2$-agonist therapy.

*Overdose:* As rimiterol is rapidly eliminated from the blood, it carries little risk of accumulation even if used excessively. No cases of overdosage have been reported and the following guidance is based on theoretical considerations.

  *Symptoms:* The blood pressure may fall and cause dizziness and fainting. Anxiety, tremor and tachycardia may be present.

  *Treatment:* A cardioselective beta-blocking agent should be administered, but these should be used with caution in patients with a history of bronchospasm.

**Pharmacological properties**
*Pharmacodynamic properties:* Rimiterol hydrobromide is a direct-acting sympathomimetic agent with predominantly beta-adrenergic activity. It is used as a bronchodilator and has a similar duration of action to isoprenaline but has been reported to have a more selective action than isoprenaline, its bronchodilating action being relatively more predominant than its effect on the heart.

*Pharmacokinetic properties:* Rimiterol hydrobromide is readily absorbed from inhalations and has a plasma half-life of less than 5 minutes. It is metabolised by catechol 0-methyltransferase.

**Pharmaceutical particulars**
*List of excipients:* Sorbitan trioleate; Trichlorofluoromethane BP (Propellant 11); Dichlorotetrafluoroethane BP (Propellant 114); Dichlorodifluoromethane BP (Propellant 12).

*Incompatibilities:* None known.

*Shelf-life:* 3 years.

*Special precautions for storage:* Store in a cool, dry place. Protect from frost. Avoid storage in direct sunlight or heat.

*Nature and contents of container:* Aluminium vial closed with 25 μl metering valve and containing 300 doses.

*Instructions for use/handling:* Not applicable.

**Marketing authorisation number** 0068/0030R.

**Date of approval/revision of SPC** December 1995.

**Legal category** POM.

## SALBULIN* INHALER

**Qualitative and quantitative composition** Each actuation of Salbulin inhaler delivers Salbutamol PhEur 100 micrograms into the mouthpiece of the adapter.

**Pharmaceutical form** Salbulin inhaler is a pressurised aerosol for bronchodilator inhalation therapy.

**Clinical particulars**
*Therapeutic indications:* Salbulin inhaler is indicated in the management of bronchial asthma, for the relief of wheezing and shortness of breath used on an as required basis. Salbulin inhaler may be used as necessary to relieve attacks of acute dyspnoea and may be used prophylactically before exertion or to prevent exercise-induced asthma.

Salbulin inhaler may also be used in the treatment of reversible airways obstruction associated with chronic bronchitis and emphysema.

*Posology and method of administration:*
*Adults:* For the relief of wheezing, shortness of breath and attacks of acute dyspnoea in patients with asthma, or reversible airways obstruction associated with chronic bronchitis and emphysema, one or two inhalations may be administered as a single dose.

For prophylaxis of exercise-induced asthma, two inhalations before exercise.

*Children:* For the relief of wheezing, shortness of breath and attacks of acute dyspnoea in children with asthma, one inhalation increasing to two if necessary may be administered as a single dose.

For prophylaxis of exercise-induced asthma, one inhalation increasing to two if necessary before exercise.

*Elderly:* No special dosage recommendations are made for elderly patients.

For all patients, the maximum recommended dose should not exceed eight inhalations in 24 hours. With repetitive dosing, inhalations should not usually be repeated more often than every 4 hours.

*Contra-indications:* Hypersensitivity to salbutamol or any of the inactive ingredients in Salbulin inhaler.

Salbulin inhaler is contra-indicated for use in the management of premature labour and threatened abortion.

*Special warnings and special precautions for use:*
*Special warnings:* Potentially serious hypokalaemia has been reported in patients taking beta-2-agonist therapy. Particular caution is advised in patients with severe asthma. Hypokalaemia may also occur in hypoxic patients and those treated with xanthine

derivatives, steroids, diuretics and long-term laxatives. Extra care should therefore be taken if beta-2-agonists are used in these groups of patients and serum potassium levels should be monitored.

Unwanted stimulation of cardiac adrenergic receptors can occur in patients taking beta-2-agonist therapy.

*Special precautions for use:* The patient should be advised to seek medical advice if the treatment ceases to be effective and/or their asthma seems to be worsening, and not to increase the dose without medical advice.

Administer cautiously to patients with thyrotoxicosis.

**Interaction with other medicaments and other forms of interaction:** Salbutamol and beta-blockers should not usually be prescribed together.

Hypokalaemia occurring with beta-2-agonist therapy may be exacerbated by treatment with xanthines, steroids, diuretics and long-term laxatives.

*Pregnancy and lactation:* Salbulin should not be used in pregnancy and lactation unless the expected benefit to the mother is thought to outweigh any risk to the foetus or neonate. The safe used of inhaled salbutamol during pregnancy has not been established but it has been in widespread use for many years in human beings without apparent ill consequence. In mice and rabbits large doses of salbutamol have been shown to be teratogenic.

It is not known whether salbutamol is distributed into breast milk.

*Effects on ability to drive and use machines:* None.

*Undesirable effects:* Mild tremor, headache, palpitations, tachycardia, and transient muscle cramps may rarely occur. Potentially serious hypokalaemia has been reported in patients taking beta-2-agonist therapy.

Hypersensitivity reactions and hyperactivity in children have been reported rarely.

As with other inhalation therapy, paradoxical bronchospasm may occur immediately after dosing. In this instance, Salbulin inhaler should be discontinued immediately and alternative therapy instituted if necessary.

*Overdose: Treatment: Asthmatic patients:* Monitor biochemical abnormalities, particularly hypokalaemia which should be treated with potassium replacement where necessary. Beta-adrenoceptor antagonists, even beta-1-selective antagonists, are potentially life-threatening and should be avoided.

*Non-asthmatic patients:* Monitor and correct biochemical abnormalities, particularly hypokalaemia. A non-selective beta-adrenoceptor antagonist (e.g. nadolol, propranolol) will competitively reverse both hypokalaemia and tachycardia (beta-1-selective drugs will be largely ineffective).

**Pharmacological properties**
*Pharmacodynamic properties:* Salbutamol is a sympathomimetic agent which has a selective action on beta-2-adrenergic receptors in bronchial smooth muscle.

*Pharmacokinetic properties:* Salbutamol is readily absorbed from the gastro-intestinal tract, but the systemic absorption of the inhaled drug substance is low. The action of inhaled salbutamol depends on direct stimulation of receptors in the lung. Onset of action is usually within 10 minutes of inhalation and lasts 4–6 hours in most patients.

Salbutamol is subject to first-pass metabolism in the liver; about half is excreted in the urine as an inactive sulphate conjugate. It does not appear to be metabolised in the lung and therefore its fate following inhalation therapy depends on the delivery method used, which determines the proportion of salbutamol. inhaled relative to the proportion inadvertently swallowed. It has been suggested that the slightly extended half-life following inhalation may reflect slow removal of active drug from the lungs.

*Preclinical safety data:* Salbutamol has been in widespread use for many years; there have been no adverse clinical findings with Salbulin inhaler which might reflect pre-clinical safety issues (see *Pregnancy and lactation*).

**Pharmaceutical particulars**
*List of excipients:* The excipients in Salbulin inhaler are sorbitan trioleate, propellants 11, 12 and 114.

*Incompatibilities:* None known.

*Shelf life:* The shelf life expiry date for this product shall not exceed 3 years from the date of its manufacture.

*Special precautions for storage:* Salbulin inhaler should be stored below 30°C. Avoid storage in direct sunlight or heat. Protect from frost.

*Nature and contents of container:* Salbulin inhaler contains 200 metered doses.

*Instructions for use/handling:* The patient should read the patient leaflet before use.

As the canister is pressurised, no atempt should be made to puncture it or dispose of it by burning.

**Marketing authorisation number** 0068/0108

**Date of approval/revision of SPC** July 1996.

**Legal category** POM.

## TAMBOCOR* (Flecainide)
**Presentation**
Tambocor 50 mg tablets: White, circular, biconvex tablets, 6.35 mm in diameter marked 3M on one side and TR50 on the other. Each tablet contains flecainide acetate 50 mg.

Tambocor 100 mg tablets: White, circular, biconvex tablets, 8.5 mm in diameter marked 3M on one side and TR 100 with a break-line on the other. Each tablet contains flecainide acetate 100 mg.

Tambocor injection: Each ampoule contains 15 ml of a solution of flecainide acetate 10 mg/ml, for intravenous use only. It also contains the following inactive ingredients: Sodium Acetate PhEur; Glacial Acetic Acid BP.

**Uses** Tambocor (Flecainide) is a potent sodium channel blocking agent for the treatment of the conditions listed below. It is recommended that treatment with Tambocor (Flecainide) should be initiated in hospitals.

Tambocor (Flecainide) slows conduction through the heart. Its actions may be reflected in the ECG by prolongation of the PR interval and widening of the QRS complex. The effect on the JT interval is insignificant at therapeutic plasma levels.

*Indications*
*Tablets:* Tambocor tablets are indicated for:

(a) AV nodal reciprocating tachycardia; arrhythmias associated with Wolff-Parkinson-White Syndrome and similar conditions with accessory pathways.

(b) Paroxysmal atrial fibrillation in patients with disabling symptoms, arrhythmias of recent onset will respond more readily.

(c) Symptomatic sustained ventricular tachycardia.

(d) Premature ventricular contractions and/or non-sustained ventricular tachycardia which are causing disabling symptoms, where these are resistant to other therapy or when other treatment has not been tolerated.

Tambocor tablets can be used for the maintenance of normal rhythm following conversion by other means.

*Injection:* Tambocor injection is indicated when rapid control of the following arrhythmias is the main clinical requirement:

(a) Ventricular tachyarrhythmias where these are resistant to other treatment.

(b) AV nodal reciprocating tachycardia; Arrhythmias associated with Wolff-Parkinson-White Syndrome and similar conditions with accessory pathways.

(c) Paroxysmal atrial fibrillation in patients with disabling symptoms. Arrhythmias of recent onset will respond more readily.

**Dosage and administration**
*Tablets: Adults:*
*Supraventricular arrhythmias:* The recommended starting dosage is 50 mg twice daily and most patients will be controlled at this dose. If required the dose may be increased to a maximum of 300 mg daily.
*Ventricular arrhythmias:* The recommended starting dosage is 100 mg twice daily. The maximum daily dose is 400 mg and this is normally reserved for patients of large build or where rapid control of the arrhythmia is required.

After 3–5 days it is recommended that the dosage be progressively adjusted to the lowest level which maintains control of the arrhythmia. It may be possible to reduce dosage during long-term treatment.

*Children:* Flecainide is not recommended in children under 12, as there is insufficient evidence of its use in this age group.

*Elderly patients:* The rate of flecainide elimination from plasma may be reduced in elderly people. This should be taken into consideration when making dose adjustments.

*Injection:*
a) *Bolus injection:* Tambocor injection can be given in an emergency or for rapid effect by a slow injection of 2 mg/kg over not less than ten minutes, or in divided doses. If preferred the dose may be diluted with 5% glucose and given as a mini-infusion.

Continuous ECG monitoring is recommended in all patients receiving the bolus dose. The injection should be stopped when there is control of the arrythmia.

It is recommended that Tambocor injection should be administered more slowly to patients in sustained ventricular tachycardia, with careful monitoring of the electrocardiogram. Similar caution should apply to patients with a history of cardiac failure, who may become decompensated during the administration. For such patients it is recommended that the initial dose is given over 30 minutes.

The maximum recommended bolus dose is 150 mg.

b) *Intravenous infusion:* When prolonged parenteral administration is required, it is recommended that therapy is initiated by slow injection of 2 mg/kg over 30 minutes as above and continued by intravenous infusion at the following rates:
*First hour:* 1.5 mg/kg per hour. *Second and later hours:* 0.1–0.25 mg/kg per hour.

It is recommended that the infusion duration should not exceed 24 hours. However, where this is considered necessary, or for patients receiving the upper end of the dose range, plasma level monitoring is strongly recommended. The maximum cumulative dose given in the first 24 hours should not exceed 600 mg.

In patients with severe renal impairment (creatinine clearance of less than 35 ml/min/1.73 sq m), each of the above dosage recommendations should be reduced by half.

Transition to oral dosing should be accomplished as soon as possible by stopping the infusion and administering the first required oral dose.

Oral maintenance is then continued as indicated in the relevant oral dosage instructions.

*Plasma levels:* Based on PVC suppression, it appears that plasma levels of 200–1000 ng/ml may be needed to obtain the maximum therapeutic effect. Plasma levels above 700–1000 ng/ml are associated with increased likelihood of adverse experiences.

*Dosage in impaired renal function:* In patients with significant renal impairment (creatinine clearance of 35 ml/min/1.73 sq. m. or less) the maximum initial dosage should be 100 mg daily (or 50 mg twice daily). When used in such patients, frequent plasma level monitoring is strongly recommended.

**Contra-indications, warnings, etc**
*Contra-indications:* Flecainide is contra-indicated in cardiac failure, and in patients with a history of myocardial infarction who have either asymptomatic ventricular ectopics or asymptomatic non-sustained ventricular tachycardia.

It is also contraindicated in patients with long standing atrial fibrillation in whom there has been no attempt to convert to sinus rhythm, and in patients with haemodynamically significant valvular heart disease.

Unless pacing rescue is available, flecainide should not be given to patients with sinus node dysfunction, atrial conduction defects, second degree or greater atrio-ventricular block, bundle branch block or distal block.

*Precautions:* Electrolyte disturbances should be corrected before using flecainide.

Since flecainide elimination from the plasma can be markedly slower in patients with significant hepatic impairment, flecainide should not be used in such patients unless the potential benefits clearly outweigh the risks. Plasma level monitoring is strongly recommended in these circumstances.

Flecainide is known to increase endocardial pacing thresholds – ie. to decrease endocardial pacing sensitivity. This effect is reversible and is more marked on the acute pacing threshold than on the chronic. Flecainide should thus be used with caution in all patients with permanent pacemakers or temporary pacing electrodes, and should not be administered to patients with existing poor thresholds or non-programmable pacemakers unless suitable pacing rescue is available.

Generally, a doubling of either pulse width or voltage is sufficient to regain capture, but it may be difficult to obtain ventricular thresholds less than 1 Volt at initial implantation in the presence of flecainide.

The minor negative inotropic effect of flecainide may assume importance in patients predisposed to cardiac failure. Difficulty has been experienced in defibrillating some patients. Most of the cases reported had pre-existing heart disease with cardiac enlargement, a history of myocardial infarction, arterio-sclerotic heart disease and cardiac failure.

Tambocor should be used with caution in patients with acute onset of atrial fibrillation following cardiac surgery.

In a large scale, placebo-controlled clinical trial in post-myocardial infarction patients with asymptomatic ventricular arrhythmia, oral flecainide was associated with a 2.2 fold higher incidence of mortality or non-fatal cardiac arrest as compared with its matching placebo. In that same study, an even higher incidence of mortality was observed in flecainide-treated patients with more than one myocardial infarction. Comparable placebo-controlled clinical trials have not been done to determine if flecainide is associated with higher risk of mortality in other patient groups.

*Use in Pregnancy and Lactation:* There is no evidence as to drug safety in human pregnancy.

In New Zealand White rabbits high doses of flecainide caused some foetal abnormalities, but these effects were not seen in Dutch Belted rabbits or rats. The relevance of these findings to humans has not been established. Data have shown that flecainide crosses the placenta to the foetus in patients taking flecainide during pregnancy.

Flecainide is excreted in human milk and appears in concentrations which reflect those in maternal blood. The case of adverse effects to the nursing infant is very small.

*Drug interactions:* Use of flecainide with other Sodium Channel blockers is not recommended. Treatment with flecainide is compatible with use of oral anticoagulants. Flecainide can cause the plasma digoxin level to rise by about 15%, which is unlikely to be of clinical significance for patients with plasma levels in the therapeutic range. It is recommended that the digoxin plasma level in digitalised patients should be measured not less than six hours after any digoxin dose, before or after administration of flecainide. The possibility of additive negative inotropic effects of beta-blockers and other cardiac depressants with flecainide should be recognised.

Limited data in patients receiving known enzyme inducers (phenytoin, phenobarbital, carbamazepine) indicate only a 30% increase in the rate of flecainide elimination. In healthy subjects receiving cimetidine (1 g daily) for one week, plasma flecainide levels increased by about 30% and the half-life by about 10%.

When flecainide is given in the presence of amiodarone, the usual flecainide dosage should be reduced by 50% and the patient monitored closely for adverse effects. Plasma level monitoring is strongly recommended in these circumstances.

*Side-effects:*
*Cardiac:* Pro-arrhythmic effects occur but are most likely in patients with structural heart disease and/or significant left ventricular impairment.

In patients with atrial flutter the use of flecainide has been associated with 1:1 AV conduction following initial atrial slowing with resultant ventricular acceleration. This has been seen most commonly following the use of the injection for acute conversion. This effect is usually short lived and abates quickly following cessation of therapy.

*Dermatological:* There have been isolated cases of photosensitivity.

*Gastrointestinal:* Occasionally nausea and vomiting.

*Hepatic:* A number of cases of elevated liver enzymes and jaundice have been reported in association with flecainide treatment. So far this has always been reversible on stopping treatment.

*Neurological:* Most commonly giddiness, dizziness, and light-headedness which are usually transient.

*Opthalmological:* Visual disturbances, such as double vision and blurring of vision may occur but these are usually transient and disappear upon continuing or reducing the dosage.

During long term therapy a few cases of peripheral neuropathy, paraesthesia and ataxia have been reported. Extremely rare cases of corneal deposits and pneumonitis have also been reported.

*Overdosage:* No specific antidote is known. There is no known way of rapidly removing flecainide from the system, but forced acid diuresis may theoretically be helpful. Neither dialysis nor haemoperfusion are helpful and injections of anticholinergics are not recommended. Treatment may include therapy with an inotropic agent, intravenous calcium, giving circulatory assistance (e.g. balloon pumping) mechanically assisting respiration, or temporarily inserting a transvenous pacemaker if there are severe conduction disturbances or the patient's left ventricular function is otherwise compromised.

**Pharmaceutical precautions**
*Storage:* Tambocor tablets should be stored below 30°C. Tambocor injection should be stored between 5-30°C. Do not freeze.

*Dilution:* When necessary Tambocor injection should be diluted with, or injected into, sterile solutions of 5% glucose. If chloride containing solutions, such as sodium chloride or Ringer's lactate are used, the injection should be added to a volume of not less than 500 ml, otherwise a precipitate will form.

**Legal category**   POM.

**Package quantities**
   Tambocor 50 mg: Packs of 60 tablets (OP).
   Tambocor 100 mg: Packs of 60 tablets (OP).
   Tambocor Injection: Boxes containing 5×15 ml ampoules.

**Further information**   Nil.

**Product licence numbers**
Tambocor 50 mg tablets        0068/0152
Tambocor 100 mg tablets       0068/0102
Tambocor Injection            0068/0101

## TITRALAC* TABLETS

**Presentation**   White, circular, bi-convex tablets, 11.2 mm in diameter, marked TC on one side and 3M on the other. Each tablet contains Calcium Carbonate BP 420 mg and Glycine BP 180 mg.

**Uses**   Titralac is indicated as a calcium supplement or phosphate binding agent in the management of renal failure.

**Dosage and administration**
*As a calcium supplement:* 1 to 4 tablets a day according to patient requirements. The maximum dose should not exceed 12 tablets per day. Each Titralac tablet contains 4.2 mmol (168 mg) calcium.

*As a phosphate binder:* Starting dose of 6 tablets a day and then titrated up to a maximum of 40 tablets a day by the physician according to the needs of the patient or until undesirable effects are observed such as hypercalcaemia, hypophosphataemia or hypophosphataemic red cell dysfunction. The total daily dose is to be divided between the meals of the day in order to ensure that the tablet is available as a

phosphate binder. Each Titralac tablet binds, in vitro, about 340 mg phosphate.

These dosage instructions apply to adults, elderly and children.

Titralac tablets may be chewed, allowed to dissolve in the mouth or swallowed whole as desired.

**Contra-indications, warnings, etc**
*Side-effects:* Hypercalcaemia and hypophosphataemia are possible complications of vigorous therapy.

Symptoms of hypercalcaemia include anorexia, nausea, vomiting, constipation, abdominal pain, muscle weakness, thirst, polyuria, drowsiness, confusion, and cardiac arrhythmias leading to cardiac arrest.

Symptoms of hypophosphataemia include weakness, paraesthesia, seizures and coma.

Hypophosphataemic red cell dysfunction impairs effective oxygen delivery to the periphery.

*Precautions:* Serum phosphate levels should be monitored in all patients receiving phosphate binders, to prevent the development of a phosphate depletion syndrome.

In long-term treatment, serum and urinary calcium levels should be monitored to prevent hypercalcaemia occurring. Serum albumin, magnesium and potassium levels should also be monitored to ensure Ca++/PO4--- homeostasis, particularly following dialysis.

Sarcoidosis may increase the risk of hypercalcaemia.

*Pregnancy and lactation:* Epidemiological studies have shown no increase in the teratogenic hazard to the foetus if used in the usual doses recommended for calcium supplementation. The safety of high doses of calcium, however, is not established.

Although some supplemental calcium may be excreted in breast milk, the concentration is not sufficient to produce an adverse effect on the neonate and problems in humans have not been documented.

*Contra-indications:* Patients with hypophosphataemia, hypercalcaemia or hypercalciuria.

*Interactions:* Concurrent administration of 1,25-dihydroxycholecalciferol or thiazides increases the risk of hypercalcaemia. There is a risk of digoxin toxicity if hypercalcaemia develops in well-digitalised patients. Corticosteroids may interfere with calcium absorption while calcium interferes with absorption of tetracyclines.

*Overdosage:* Acute hypercalcaemia may result and this may be aggravated by dehydration. Management of acute hypercalcaemia should be along standard recommendations and should include full hydration, monitoring of other electrolytes, judicious use of frusemide and other symptomatic and supportive measures. ECG monitoring of cardiac rhythm is particularly advisable in patients with renal failure.

**Pharmaceutical precautions**   Store in a cool, dry place.

**Legal category**   GSL.

**Package quantities**   Bottles of 180 tablets (OP).

**Further information**   Nil.

**Product licence number**   0068/5004R.

*Trade Mark

# Martindale Pharmaceuticals
Bampton Road
Harold Hill
Romford, Essex RM3 8UG

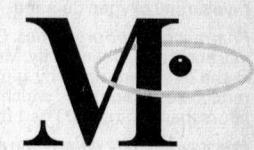

## FENTANYL CITRATE INJECTION
### 50 micrograms/ml

**Qualitative and quantitative composition** each 2 ml of solution contains 100 micrograms of fentanyl as Fentanyl Citrate BP. Each 10 ml of solution contains 500 micrograms of fentanyl as Fentanyl Citrate BP.

**Pharmaceutical form** Clear, colourless, sterile solution for injection intended for parenteral administration to human beings.

### Clinical particulars
*Therapeutic indications:* Fentanyl citrate is a narcotic analgesic. In low doses, it is used to provide analgesia during short surgical procedures and as a premedicant. In higher doses it is employed as an analgesic/respiratory depressant in patients who need assisted ventilation. In combination with a neuroleptic drug, fentanyl is employed as part of the technique of neuroleptanalgesia.

*Posology and method of administration:* Intravenous and Intramuscular routes. Fentanyl Citrate Injection can be administered to both adults and children via the intravenous route according to the following dosage regimen:

|  | Adults Initial μg | Supplemental μg | Children Initial μg/kg | Supplemental μg/kg |
|---|---|---|---|---|
| Spontaneous respiration | 50-200 | 50 | 3-5 | 1 |
| Assisted ventilation | 300-3500 | 100-200 | 15 | 1-3 |

Doses greater than 200 microgram are solely for use in anaesthesia.

As a premedicant, 1–2 ml may be administered intramuscularly before induction of anaesthesia.

Following intravenous administration in the non-premedicated adult patient, 2 ml fentanyl may be anticipated to provide adequate analgesia for 10–20 minutes in surgical procedures involving low pain intensity. A bolus of 10 ml fentanyl can be expected to provide analgesia for about 1 hour. The analgesia produced is generally adequate for surgery involving moderate pain intensity. Administration of 50 micrograms/kg will provide intense analgesia for some 4 to 6 hours for surgery associated with intense stimulation.

It is important when estimating the required dose to assess the likely degree of surgical stimulation, the effect of premedicant drugs, and the duration of the procedure.

Use in elderly: It is important to reduce the dosage in the elderly.

*Contra-indications:* Known hypersensitivity to fentanyl citrate; respiratory depression; obstructive airways disease, concurrent administration with monoamine oxidase inhibitors or within 2 weeks of their discontinuation.

*Special warnings and precautions for use:* In common with other narcotic analgesics, the most common serious adverse reactions with fentanyl are respiratory depression, bradycardia and skeletal muscle rigidity.

As with all narcotic analgesics, care should be observed when administering Fentanyl Citrate Injection to patients with myasthenia gravis.

It is desirable to reduce dosage in the elderly, in hypothyroidism and chronic hepatic disease.

Administration in labour may cause respiratory depression in the new-born infant.

As with all potent opioids, profound analgesia is accompanied by marked respiratory depression, which may persist into or recur in the early post-operative period. It is imperative to ensure that adequate spontaneous breathing has been established and maintained before discharge from the recovery area whenever large doses of infusions of Fentanyl Citrate Injection have been administered. Hyperventilation during anaesthesia may alter the patient's response to $CO_2$, thus affecting respiration post-operatively. Opioid pre-medication may potentiate or prolong depressant effects of fentanyl citrate.

Repeated use of fentanyl may result in the development of tolerance and dependence.

*Interaction with other medicaments and other forms of interaction:* If other narcotic or CNS-depressant drugs are used concurrently with fentanyl, the effects of the drugs may be expected to be additive. The pharmacological effects of fentanyl citrate can be reversed by Naloxone.

*Pregnancy and lactation:* Placental transfer of fentanyl occurs. There has been little usage in human pregnancy but no evidence of teratogenic effects in animals. Administration in labour may cause respiratory depression in the new-born infant. Fentanyl should be used during pregnancy only if the potential benefit justifies the potential risk to the foetus. It is not known whether fentanyl is excreted in human milk. Because many drugs are excreted in human milk, caution should be exercised when administering fentanyl to a nursing mother.

*Effects on ability to drive and use machines:* Where early discharge (from clinical care) is envisaged, patients should be advised not to drive or to operate machinery.

*Undesirable effects:* A transient fall in blood pressure may occur following intravenous administration of Fentanyl Citrate Injection.

Significant respiratory depression will occur following administration of fentanyl in doses in excess of 200 micrograms. This and other pharmacological effects of fentanyl can be reversed by naloxone.

Bradycardia may occur due to increased cardiac vagal stimulation; it can be reversed by atropine or glycopyrrolate. Skeletal muscle rigidity (morphine-like effect) may occur and muscle relaxants have been found helpful in such cases. Nausea and vomiting may be troublesome.

*Overdose:* As with other narcotic analgesics, the possible manifestations of fentanyl overdosage include respiratory depression and hypotension, with circulatory failure and deepening coma.

Intensive supporting therapy may be required to correct respiratory failure and shock. A patent airway must be maintained and assisted respiration may be required. The specific narcotic antagonist naloxone hydrochloride is used to counteract respiratory depression and coma. A dose of 0.4 to 2 mg is given intravenously and may be repeated at intervals of 2 to 3 minutes if necessary, up to 10 mg. The duration of respiratory depression following overdosage with fentanyl may exceed the duration of narcotic antagonist action.

### Pharmacological properties
*Pharmacodynamic properties:* Fentanyl citrate is a potent narcotic analgesic. The principal actions of therapeutic value are analgesia and sedation. When used with a neuroleptic agent it can induce a state of neuroleptanalgesia. As with other narcotic analgesics, fentanyl depresses respiration and this effect increases as the dose is increased.

Following intravenous injection fentanyl has rapid onset of action, although the maximal analgesic and respiratory depressant effect may not occur for several minutes.

Fentanyl Citrate Injection is usually given by the intravenous route, but it may be given intramuscularly as a premedicant.

*Pharmacokinetic properties:* Fentanyl is a lipid-soluble drug and its pharmacokinetics can be described in terms of a 3 compartment model. following intravenous injection, there is a short distribution phase during which high concentrations of fentanyl are achieved quickly in well perfused tissues such as the lungs, kidneys and brain. The drug is redistributed to other tissues, it accumulates more slowly in skeletal muscle and yet more slowly in fat, from which it is gradually released into the blood. Up to 80% of fentanyl is bound to plasma proteins.

Fentanyl is primarily metabolised in the liver, probably by N-dealkylation, and is excreted mainly in the urine with less than 10% representing the unchanged drug. The terminal half life of fentanyl is 3.7 hours.

*Preclinical safety data:* No further relevant information other than that which is included in other sections of the Summary of Product Characteristics.

### Pharmaceutical particulars
*List of excipients:* Sodium Chloride BP, Sodium Hydroxide BP, Water for Injections BP

*Incompatibilities:* Fentanyl citrate is incompatible with thiopentone and methohexitone

*Shelf life:* Unopened: 3 years (36 months) If only part of an ampoule is used, discard the remaining solution

*Special precautions for storage:* Store below 25°C. Protect from light.

*Nature and contents of container:* 2 ml or 10 ml clear glass ampoules, glass type I Ph Eur borosilicate glass, packed in cardboard cartons and contain 10 x 2 ml/10 ml ampoules.

*Instructions for use/handling:* CD(2), For IV or IM injection. If only part used, discard the remaining solution.

**Marketing authorisation number** 0156/0038

*Marketing authorisation holder:* Martindale Pharmaceuticals Limited, Bampton Road, Romford RM3 8UG.

**Date of approval/revision of SPC** 15 May 1997

**Legal category** CD (2), POM

## GTN 300 mcg

**Qualitative and quantitative composition** Glyceryl Trinitrate 300 micrograms per tablet + 6.67% overage.

**Pharmaceutical form** Sublingual tablet.

### Clinical particulars

*Therapeutic indications:* A short acting vasodilator for the prophylaxis and treatment of attacks of angina pectoris.

*Posology and method of administration.*
Adults and the elderly: One tablet to be allowed to dissolve slowly under the tongue. The treatment may be repeated as necessary.
  Children Not recommended for children

*Contra-indications:* Marked anaemia, closed angle glaucoma, head trauma, cerebral haemorrhage, hypersensitivity to nitrates, hypotensive conditions and hypovolaemia, hypertrophic obstructive cardiomyopathy, aortic stenosis, cardiac tamponade, constrictive pericarditis, mitral stenosis,

*Special warnings and special precautions for use:* Caution should be exercised in cases of severe hepatic or renal impairment; hypothyroidism, malnutrition, hypothermia or a recent history of myocardial infarction.

*Interactions with other medicaments and other forms of interaction:* When used with anti-muscarinic, anti-arrhythmic or cyclic antidepressant drugs the effect of Glyceryl Trinitrate may be lost. (due to failure to dissolve under the tongue)

*Use in pregnancy and lactation:* There is some evidence of hazard in animals when nitrates have been given in pregnancy. Avoid in pregnancy unless there is no safer alternative. Problems in breast feeding have not been documented.

*Effect on the ability to drive or operate machines:* Dizziness is a known side effect, if affected, patients should not drive or operate machinery.

*Undesirable effects:* The following side effects have been reported: Throbbing headache, facial flushing, dizziness, postural hypotension and tachycardia.

*Overdose:*
Symptoms: Vomiting, restlessness, hypotension, cyanosis, methaemoglobinaemia. Severe poisoning may result in bradycardia, respiratory depression and psychosis.

  Treatment: Remove any tablet from the mouth and place the patient in a recumbent position with the head down. If recovery is not rapid or in the case of known severe poisoning, the stomach should be emptied to prevent further absorption and general supportive measures, such as oxygen, assisted respiration and plasma expanders employed as necessary.

If methaglobinaemia has occurred it can be treated with Methylene Blue. Intravenous injection of 1–4 mg per kg body weight.

### Pharmacological properties

*Pharmacodynamic properties:* Glyceryl Trinitrate relaxes smooth muscle, including vascular muscle. The precise mechanism of action is not fully understood but it is thought that the cause is a reduction of myocardial oxygen demand.

*Pharmacokinetic properties:* Glyceryl Trinitrate is rapidly absorbed sublingually. Metabolism occurs mainly in the liver and blood by glutathione-organic nitrate reductase to dinitrates which are less potent vasodilators than trinitrates. T$\frac{1}{2}$ is 1 to 4 minutes.

*Preclinical safety data:* None stated

**Pharmaceutical particulars**

*List of excipients:* Mannitol, Lactose, Talc, Magnesium Stearate and Stearic Acid.

*Incompatibilities:* Not applicable.

*Shelf life:* 24 months. After first opening the product should be used within 8 weeks.

*Special precautions for storage and transport:* Storage in a dry place below 25°C. Protect from light.

*Nature and contents of container:* 100 tablets . Glass bottle with aluminium wadded cap.

*Instructions for use/handling:* After removing a tablet close the cap tightly. Do not transfer the tablets to another bottle. Use within 8 weeks of first opening.

*Marketing authorisation holder:* Macarthys Laboratories Limited, Bampton Road, Romford RM3 8UG.

**Marketing authorisation number**   1883/5958R

**Date of approval/revision of SPC**   25 August 1995

**Legal category**   P.

## METHADONE INJECTION BP 1%

**Presentation**   Clear, colourless, glass ampoules of 1 ml, 2 ml, 3.5 ml and 5 ml containing a colourless solution of Methadone Hydrochloride BP 10 mg per ml.

**Uses**   In the treatment of opioid drug addiction (as a narcotic abstinence syndrome suppressant). As an analgesic where the sedative effects of morphine are contra-indicated.

**Dosage and route of administration**

*Adults:* In the treatment of opioid drug addiction, by intramuscular or subcutaneous injection. Initially 10–20 mg per day, increasing by 10–20 mg per day until there are no signs of withdrawal or intoxication. The usual dose is 40–60 mg per day. If repeated doses are required the intramuscular route should be used.

The dose is adjusted according to the degree of dependence with the aim of gradual reduction.

As an analgesic, by intramuscular or subcutaneous injection. The dosage is 5–10 mg every 6–8 hours as needed. In prolonged use it should not be administered more than twice daily. If repeated doses are required the intramuscular route should be used.

*Elderly:* In the case of the elderly or ill patients repeated doses should only be given with extreme caution.

*Children:* Not recommended for children.

**Contra-indications, warnings, etc**
*Contra-indications:* Respiratory depression, obstructive airways disease, concurrent administration with M.A.O. inhibitors or within 2 weeks of discontinuation of treatment with them. Use during an acute asthma attack is not advisable.

Obstetric use not recommended, because in labour the prolonged duration of action increases the risk of neonatal depression.

Methadone is not suitable for children.

*Drug interactions:*
*Alcohol:* May induce serious respiratory depression and hypotension.

*Cimetidine:* Potentiation of opiate action due to displacement of Methadone from protein binding sites.

*Rifampicin:* Reduced opiate effect due to increased metabolism.

*Phenytoin:* Potentiation of opiate action due to displacement of Methadone from protein binding sites.

*MAOIs:* Possible CNS excitation or depression.

*Urinary acidifiers:* Increases rate of excretion of drug thus decreasing plasma concentration.

*CNS depressants:* Major and minor tranquillisers, sedatives and tricyclic antidepressants may result in increased CNS depression, respiratory depression and hypotension.

*Opioid agonist analgesics:* Additive CNS depression, respiratory depression and hypotension.

*Naloxone:* Antagonizes the analgesic, CNS and respiratory depressant effects of Methadone.

*Naltrexone:* Administration of Naltrexone to a patient addicted to Methadone will rapidly precipitate long term withdrawal symptoms.

*Buprenorphine/Pentazocine:* Administration to a patient addicted to Methadone may precipitate withdrawal symptoms.

*Effects on the ability to drive or operate machines:* This may be severely affected during and after treatment with Methadone. The time after which such activities may be safely resumed is extremely patient dependent and must be decided by the physician.

*Other undesirable effects:* Nausea, vomiting and dizziness. Methadone has the potential to increase intracranial pressure, particularly in circumstances where it is already raised. It causes pain at the injection site; subcutaneous injection causes local tissue irritation and induration.

In prolonged use as an analgesic it should not be administered more than twice daily to avoid the risk of accumulation and overdosage.

*Use in pregnancy and lactation:* There is no, or inadequate, evidence of safety in human pregnancy but the drug has been widely used for many years without apparent ill-consequence and animal studies have not shown any hazard.

It should not be used in labour, see *Contra-indications.*

Methadone is excreted in breast milk. This may be permissible during maintenance dosage.

*Other special warnings and precautions:* In the case of elderly or ill patients, repeated doses should only be given with extreme caution.

The formulation does not contain preservatives or antioxidants and therefore could be administered via the intravenous or intraspinal route. However, this should only be attempted by those with appropriate skill and experience in such administration and is therefore at the discretion of the physician.

Methadone is a drug of addiction and is controlled under the Misuse of Drugs Act 1971 (Schedule 2).

*Overdose:* Symptoms: Serious overdosage is characterised by respiratory depression, extreme somnolence progressing to stupor or coma, maximally constricted pupils, skeletal muscle flaccidity, cold and clammy skin and sometimes bradycardia and hypotension. In severe overdosage, particularly by the intravenous route, apnea, circulatory collapse, cardiac arrest and death may occur.

Treatment: A patent airway and assisted or controlled ventilation must be assured. Narcotic antagonists may be required, but it should be remembered that Methadone is a long-acting depressant (36 to 48 hours), whereas antagonists act for 1 to 3 hours, so that treatment with the latter must be repeated as needed. An antagonist should not be administered, however, in the absence of clinically significant respiratory or cardiovascular depression. Nalorphine (0.1 mg per kg) or Levallorphan (0.02 mg per kg) should be given intravenously as soon as possible and repeated, if necessary, every 15 minutes. Oxygen, intravenous fluids, vasopressors and other supportive measures should be employed as indicated. In a person physically dependent on narcotics, administration of the usual dose of a narcotic antagonist will precipitate an acute withdrawal syndrome; use of the antagonist in such a person should be avoided if possible but if it must be used to treat serious respiratory depression it should be administered with great care.

*Incompatibilities:* No major incompatibilities known.

**Pharmaceutical precautions**   Sterile until opened. Protect from light.

**Legal category**   CD (Sch. 2), POM.

**Package quantities**   Boxes of 10.

**Further information**   Nil.

**Product licence number**   1883/0058.

*Product licence holder:* Macarthys Laboratories Limited, Bampton Road, Romford RM3 8UG.

## METHADONE MIXTURE DTF
## 1 mg per ml

**Presentation**   A clear, yellow-green mixture containing methadone hydrochloride 1 mg per ml.

The mixture contains sodium methylparaben 0.1%, and sodium propylparaben 0.025% as preservatives.

Contains tartrazine (E102), Green S (E142) and Sunset Yellow (E110).

**Uses**   In the treatment of opioid drug addiction (as a narcotic abstinence syndrome suppressant).

**Dosage and administration**   For oral administration.

*Adults:* Initially 10–20 mg per day, increasing by 10–20 mg per day until there are no signs of withdrawal or intoxication. The usual dose is 40–60 mg per day.

The dose is adjusted according to the degree of dependence with the aim of gradual reduction.

*Elderly:* In the case of the elderly or ill patients repeated doses should only be given with extreme caution.

*Children:* Not recommended for children.

**Contra-indications, warnings, etc**
*Contra-indications:* Respiratory depression, obstructive airways disease, concurrent administration with MAO inhibitors or within 2 weeks of discontinuation of treatment with them. Use during an acute asthma attack is not advisable.

Use during labour is not recommended, the prolonged duration of action increases the risk of neonatal depression.

Methadone is not suitable for children.

*Drug interactions:*
*Alcohol:* May induce serious respiratory depression and hypotension.

*Cimetidine:* Potentiation of opiate action due to displacement of methadone from protein binding sites.

*Rifampicin:* Reduced opiate effect due to increased metabolism.

*Phenytoin:* Potentiation of opiate action due to displacement of methadone from protein binding sites.

*MAOIs:* Possible CNS excitation or depression.

*Urinary acidifiers:* Increases rate of excretion of drug thus decreasing plasma concentration.

*CNS depressants:* Major and minor tranquillisers, sedatives and tricyclic antidepressants may result in increased CNS depression, respiratory depression and hypotension.

*Opioid agonist analgesics:* Additive CNS depression, respiratory depression and hypotension.

*Naloxone:* Antagonises the analgesic, CNS and respiratory depressant effects of methadone.

*Naltrexone:* Administration of naltrexone to a patient addicted to methadone will rapidly precipitate long term withdrawal symptoms.

*Buprenorphine/pentazocine:* Administration to a patient addicted to methadone may precipitate withdrawal symptoms.

*Effects on the ability to drive or operate machines:* This may be severely affected during and after treatment with methadone. The time after which such activities may be safely resumed is extremely patient dependent and must be decided by the physician.

*Other undesirable effects:* Methadone has the potential to increase intracranial pressure, particularly in circumstances where it is already raised.

*Use in pregnancy and lactation:* There is no, or inadequate, evidence of safety in human pregnancy but the drug has been widely used for many years without apparent ill-consequence and animal studies have not shown any hazard.

It should not be used during labour, see 'Contra-indications'. Methadone is excreted in breast milk. This may be permissible during maintenance dosage.

*Other special warnings and precautions:* In the case of elderly or ill patients repeated doses should only be given with extreme caution. Methadone is a drug of addiction and is controlled under the Misuse of Drugs Act 1971 (Schedule 2).

*Overdose:* Symptoms: Serious overdosage is characterised by respiratory depression, extreme somnolence progressing to stupor or coma, maximally constricted pupils, skeletal muscle flaccidity, cold and clammy skin and sometimes bradycardia and hypotension. In severe overdosage, particularly by the intravenous route, apnea, circulatory collapse, cardiac arrest and death may occur.

Treatment: A patent airway and assisted or controlled ventilation must be assured. Narcotic antagonists may be required, but it should be remembered that Methadone is a long-acting depressant (36 to 48 hours), whereas antagonists act for 1 to 3 hours, so that treatment with the latter must be repeated as needed. An antagonist should not be administered, however, in the absence of clinically significant respiratory or cardiovascular depression. Nalorphine (0.1 mg per kg) or Levallorphan (0.02 mg per kg) should be given intravenously as soon as possible and repeated, if necessary, every 15 minutes. Oxygen, intravenous fluids, vasopressors and other supportive measures should be employed as indicated. In a person physically dependent on narcotics, administration of the usual dose of a narcotic antagonist will precipitate an acute withdrawal syndrome; use of the antagonist in such a person should be avoided if possible but if it must be used to treat serious respiratory depression it should be administered with great care.

*Incompatibilities:* No major incompatibilities known.

**Pharmaceutical precautions**   None.

**Legal category**   CD (Sch. 2), POM.

**Package quantities**   Amber glass bottles of 30 ml, 50 ml, 100 ml and 500 ml.

**Further information**   Nil.

**Product licence number**   1883/0018.

*Product licence holder:* Macarthys Laboratories Limited, Bampton Road, Romford RM3 8UG.

# METHADONE MIXTURE DTF (SUGAR FREE) 1 mg in 1 ml

**Qualitative and quantitative composition** Methadone Hydrochloride BP 0.1% w/v.

**Pharmaceutical form** Oral solution.

## Clinical particulars

*Therapeutic indications:* In the treatment of Opioid addiction as an abstinence syndrome suppressant.

*Posology and method of administration:* For oral use only. The dose is adjusted according to the degree of dependence with the aim of gradual reduction.

*Adults:* Initially 10–20 mg per day, increasing by 10–20 mg daily until there are no signs of withdrawal or intoxication.

*The elderly:* In the case of the elderly or ill patients, repeated doses should only be given with extreme caution.

*Children:* Not recommended for use in children.

*Contra-indications:* Contra-indications are: Respiratory depression, obstructive airways disease, concurrent administration with MAO inhibitors or within 2 weeks of discontinuation of treatment with them. Hypersensitivity to any of the product ingredients. Use during an acute asthma attack is not advisable.

Obstetric use not recommended during labour, as the prolonged duration of action increases the risk of neonatal depression.

Methadone is not suitable for children.

*Special warnings and precautions for use:* In the case of the elderly or ill patients repeated doses should only be given with extreme caution.

Methadone is a drug of addiction controlled under Schedule 2 of The Misuse of Drugs Act 1971.

*Interactions with other medicaments and other forms of interaction:*

*Alcohol:* This may induce serious respiratory depression and hypotension.

*Cimetidine:* Potentiation of opiate action due to displacement of methadone from protein binding sites.

*Rifampicin:* Reduced opiate effect due to increased metabolism.

*Phenytoin:* Potentiation of opiate action due to displacement of Methadone from protein binding sites.

*MAOIs:* Possible CNS excitation or depression.

*Urinary acidifiers:* Increases rate of excretion of drug thus decreasing plasma concentration.

*CNS depressants:* Major and minor tranquillisers, sedatives and tricyclic antidepressants may result in increased CNS depression, respiratory depression and hypotension.

*Opioid agonist analgesics:* Additive CNS depression, respiratory depression and hypotension.

*Naloxone:* Antagonises the analgesic, CNS and respiratory depressant effects of Methadone.

*Naltrexone:* Administration of Naltrexone to a patient addicted to Methadone will rapidly precipitate long term withdrawal symptoms.

*Buprenorphine pentazocine:* Administration to a patient addicted to Methadone may precipitate withdrawal symptoms.

*Pregnancy and lactation:* There is no, or inadequate evidence of safety of the drug in human pregnancy but it has been in wide use for a considerable number of years without apparent ill-consequence. Animal studies have not shown any evidence of hazard. It should not be used in labour as the prolonged duration of action increases the risk of neonatal depression. Methadone is excreted in breast milk. This may be permissible during maintenance therapy.

*Effects on ability to drive and use machines:* The ability to drive or operate machinery may be severely effected during and after treatment with Methadone. The time after which such activity may be safely resumed is extremely patient dependent and must be decided by the physician.

*Undesirable effects:* Nausea, vomiting and dizziness. Methadone has the potential to increase intracranial pressure, particularly in circumstances where it is already raised.

In prolonged use it should not be administered more than twice daily to avoid the risk of accumulation and overdosage.

*Overdose: Symptoms:* Serious overdosage is characterised by respiratory depression, extreme somnolence progressing to stupor or coma, maximally constricted pupils, skeletal muscle flaccidity, cold and clammy skin and sometimes bradycardia and hypotension. In severe overdosage, particularly by the intravenous route, apnea, circulatory collapse, cardiac arrest and death may occur.

*Treatment:* A patent airway and assisted or controlled ventilation must be assured. Narcotic antagonists may be required, but it should be remembered that Methadone is a long-acting depressant (36 to 48 hours), whereas antagonists act for 1 to 3 hours, so

that treatment with the latter must be repeated as needed. An antagonist should not be administered, however, in the absence of clinically significant respiratory or cardiovascular depression. Nalorphine (0.1 mg per kg) or levallorphan (0.02 mg per kg) should be given intravenously as soon as possible and repeated, if necessary, every 15 minutes. Oxygen, intravenous fluids, vasopressors and other supportive measures should be employed as indicated. In a person physically dependent on narcotics, administration of the usual dose of a narcotic antagonist will precipitate an acute withdrawal syndrome; use of the antagonist in such a person should be avoided if possible but if it must be used to treat serious respiratory depression it should be administered with great care.

## Pharmacological properties

*Pharmacodynamic properties:* Methadone is a narcotic analgesic in the manner of Morphine but has a less sedative effect.

It acts on the CNS system and smooth muscle. This action is caused by the response of structurally and sterically specific opiate receptor sites in the brain, spinal cord and nervous system.

Methadone depresses the cough and respiratory centres.

In the treatment of opioid addiction the drug of abuse is replaced by methadone. In some situations the use of methadone can reduce or eliminate the effects of other opioids taken during the treatment period. This process is referred to as "narcotic blockade".

*Pharmacokinetic properties:* Methadone is rapidly absorbed after oral administration.

Protein binding: up to 90% but considerable inter-subject variation. About 15% is bound to immuno-globulin the remainder to albumin.

Distribution in blood: Plasma: Whole blood ratio, about 1:3.

Clearance: Plasma clearance about 2 ml/min/kg.

Volume of distribution: approx. 5L/kg.

Half-life: a) single dose=10–25 hours
b) repeated doses=13–55 hours.

Therapeutic concentration: In plasma, usually in the range 0.05–1.0 μg/ml. During methadone maintenance treatment considerable fluctuations occur day to day.

*Dispositions in the body:* Widely distributed in the tissues, with higher concentrations in the liver, lungs, and kidneys than in the blood. The main metabolic reaction is N-demethylation resulting in a substance which spontaneously cyclises to form the major metabolites, 2-ethylene-1,5-dimethyl-3,3-diphenyl-pyrrolidine (EDDP) and 2-ethyl-5-methyl-3,3-diphenyl-1-pyrroline (EMDP), neither of which are active. Hydroxylation to Methadol followed by N-demethylation to Normethadol also occurs to some extent.

Other metabolic reactions occur and there are at least eight known metabolites. In subjects on Methadone maintenance, about 20–60% of a dose is excreted in the urine in 24 hours, with up to about 33% of the dose as unchanged drug and up to about 43% as EDDP; EMDP accounts for about 5 to 10% of the dose. The ratio of EDDP to unchanged Methadone is usually very much higher in the urine of patients on methadone maintenance treatment than in simple overdose cases. Urinary excretion of unchanged drug is pH-dependent, being increased in acid urine. Up to 30% of a dose may be eliminated in the faeces, but this appears to decrease with increasing dosage. About 75% of the total excreted material is unconjugated.

*Preclinical safety data:* None stated.

## Pharmaceutical particulars

*List of excipients:* Lycasin* 80/55, Potassium Sorbate, Green S, Sunset Yellow, Quinoline Yellow, Hydrochloric Acid and Purified Water.

*Incompatibilities:* No major incompatibilities known.

*Shelf life:* 12 months. Use within 28 days of opening.

*Special precautions for storage:* Store below 25°C.

*Nature and contents of container:* 30 ml, 50 ml, 100 ml and 500 ml of the oral solution in Amber glass bottles fitted with child-resistant closures. Contact material: Polypropylene.

*Instructions for use/handling:* None stated.

**Marketing authorisation number:** 00156/0030.

*Marketing authorisation holder:* Martindale Pharmaceuticals Limited, Bampton Road, Romford RM3 8UG.

**Date of approval/revision of SPC** 27 March 1996.

**Legal category** CD(Sch. 2), POM.

# PAMERGAN* P100

**Qualitative and quantitative composition**
Pethidine Hydrochloride BP 5% w/v

Promethazine Hydrochloride BP 2% w/v

**Pharmaceutical form** Injection.

## Clinical particulars

*Therapeutic indications:*
a. Pre-anaesthetic medication.
b. Obstetric analgesia and amnesia.
c. The management of severe pain.

*Posology and method of administration*

*a. Pre-anaesthetic medication:*

*Adults and the elderly:* 2 ml administered 60–90 minutes before anaesthesia by intramuscular or, if diluted to 10 ml with Water for Injections, by intravenous injection.

*Children 12–16 years:* 1 ml
8–12 years: 0.75 ml
Under 8 years: Not recommended.
Administered 60–90 minutes before anaesthesia by intramuscular or, if diluted to 10 ml with Water for Injections, by intravenous injection.

*b. Obstetric analgesia and amnesia:* 1–2 ml when labour is well established, repeated at 4 hourly intervals as required by intramuscular or, if diluted to 10 ml with Water for Injections, by intravenous injection.

*c. The management of severe pain:* Adults and the elderly: 1–2 ml every 4–6 hours as necessary by intramuscular or, if diluted to 10 ml with Water for Injections, by intravenous injection.

*Children:* Not recommended.

*Contra-indications:* Not to be used on patients with severe liver disease, cholecystectomy, biliary colic, increased intracranial pressure, respiratory depression, obstructive airways disease or those taking (or within 2 weeks of taking) any MAOI antidepressant.

*Special warnings and special precautions for use:* Repeated use may result in dependence of the morphine type.

Administration during labour may cause respiratory depression in the new-born infant.

Pamergan P100 should be given with caution and in reduced doses to patients who are elderly or debilitated or those with head injuries, severe hepatic or renal impairment, biliary tract disorders, hypothyroidism, adreno-cortical insufficiency, shock, prostatic hypertrophy, and supra-ventricular tachycardia.

Caution is also required in patients with acute alcoholism, raised intracranial pressure or convulsive disorders.

Pethidine neurotoxicity may be seen in patients with renal failure, cancer or sickle cell anaemia, during concomitant administration with anticholinergics or during prolonged administration of increasing pethidine doses.

*Interactions with other medicaments and other form of interaction:* Concurrent use of pethidine with CNS depressants or anaesthetics may potentiate the action of pethidine.

Alcohol potentiates the action of both promethazine and pethidine.

MAOI antidepressants may cause severe CNS excitation and hypertension.

Cimetidine increases the plasma concentration of pethidine.

Hypnotics and anxiolytics are potentiated by both pethidine and promethazine.

The absorption of mexiletine is delayed by pethidine.

Domperidone and metaclopramide have an opposing effect to pethidine on gastro-intestinal activity.

*Use in pregnancy and lactation:* There is inadequate evidence of safety in human pregnancy, but Pamergan P100 has been widely used for many years without apparent ill consequence. Animal studies have not shown any hazard associated with Pethidine or Promethazine. As with all drugs during pregnancy care should be taken in assessing the risk to benefit ratio.

Pethidine crosses the placental barrier and is excreted in breast milk. This should be taken into account when considering its use in patients during pregnancy or breast feeding.

Administration during labour may cause respiratory depression in the new-born infant.

Problems relating to the use of promethazine during lactation have not been reported however risk/benefit might be considered because of the higher risk of adverse effects of antihistamines on infants especially new born and premature.

*Effect on the ability to drive or operate machines:* This product will cause drowsiness: patients should not drive or operate machinery.

*Undesirable effects:* Dizziness, nausea, vomiting, hypertension and respiratory depression. Mild euphoria may occur and CNS excitation has been reported in certain patient groups.

Other side-effects include dryness of the mouth and blurred vision. Occasionally patients may develop a feeling of weakness or syncope accompanied by profuse perspiration.

*Overdosage:*
*Symptoms:* Accidental overdose may give rise to respiratory depression, hypotension, convulsions and circulatory collapse.

*Treatment:* Establish and maintain a patent airway, assisting respiration if necessary. If respiration is severely depressed give a small intravenous dose of Naloxone ( Adults: 0.4 mg, Children: 0.005–0.01 mg per kg. Neonates: 0.01 mg per kg. ) repeated if necessary at intervals of 2–3 minutes. Hypotension may improve with improved oxygenation but may require treatment with an infusion of plasma or suitable electrolyte solution. Convulsions may need to be treated with a short acting muscle relaxant, intubation and controlled respiration.

**Pharmacological properties**

*Pharmacodynamic properties:* Pethidine binds with stereospecific receptors at many sites within the central nervous system ( CNS ) to alter processes affecting the perception of pain and the emotional response to pain. Although the precise sites and mechanisms of action have not been fully determined, alterations in release of various neurotransmitters from afferent nerves sensitive to painful stimuli may be partially responsible for the analgesic effects. When these medications are used as adjuncts to anaesthesia, analgesic actions may provide dose related protection against haemodynamic responses to surgical stress

Promethazine acts as a CNS depressant possibly by indirect reduction of stimuli to the brain stem reticular system. It may also act as a anti-emetic by inhibition of the medullary chem-receptor trigger zone of the mid brain. In Pamergan P100 the promethazine is present for its ability to prolong the activity of and lower the maintenance requirement of pethidine. It is possible that this is achieved by promethazine stabilising the endoplastic reticulum which will prevent both access of pethidine to and egress of metabolites from the receptor sites.

*Pharmacokinetic properties: Pethidine* distribution: Rapidly thoughout tissues. Volume of distribution 200–300 Litres.

Crosses placenta and secreted in milk.

Protein binding: High. Half life: 2.4–4 hours.

Metabolism: Hepatic; also intestines. The processes involved are N- Demethylation, hydrolysis, glucuronic acid conjugation and N- Oxidation. The rate of metabolism is decreased in pregnancy and increased in the elderly.

Route of elimination: Renal.

Pethidine is principally metabolised to Norpethidine and only about 5% is eliminated unchanged. Norpethidine is active and toxic ( having CNS excitatory activity ) and accumulates in patients with impaired renal function.

*Promethazine* distribution: Volume of distribution about 170 Litres.

Crosses the placenta.

Protein binding: Very high.

Half life: 4 hours.

Metabolism: Subject to extensive first pass metabolism; major reactions appear to be sulphoxidation and glucuronic acid conjugation.

Route of elimination: Renal. Promethazine is principally excreted as the sulphoxide with only about 2% eliminated unchanged.

*Pre-clinical safety data:* None stated.

**Pharmaceutic particulars**

*List of excipients:* Sodium Metabisulphite BP, Sodium Sulphite, Anhydrous BP, Sodium Chloride BP and Water for Injection BP. pH adjustment may be made using either Hydrochloric acid BP or Sodium Hydroxide BP

*Incompatibilities:* Pamergan P100 has a pH of 5–6 and is incompatible with alkaline products including Thiopentone Sodium.

*Shelf life:* 36 months.

*Special precautions for storage:* Protect from light

*Nature and contents of container:* 2 ml in type 1 colourless neutral glass ampoules. Fusion sealed.

**Marketing authorisation number** 0156/0020R

*Marketing authorisation holder:* Martindale Pharmaceuticals Limited, Bampton Road, Romford RM3 8UG.

**Date of approval/revision of SPC** 27 March 1995

**Legal category** CD(Sch 2) POM.

## TIMOLOL EYE DROPS BP 0.25% w/v and 0.5% w/v

**Qualitative and quantitative composition** Timolol Maleate PhEur equivalent to 2.5 mg/ml Timolol, Timolol Maleate Ph Eur equivalent to 5.0 mg/ml Timolol.

**Pharmaceutical form** Ophthalmic solution.

**Clinical particulars**

*Therapeutic indications:* Timolol maleate ophthalmic solution is a beta-adrenergic receptor antagonist used topically for the reduction of elevated intra-ocular pressure in various conditions including patients with ocular hypertension; patients with chronic open-angle glaucoma including patients with aphakia; and some patients with secondary glaucoma.

**Posology and method of administration**

*Dosage schedule:* Recommended therapy is one drop Timolol Eye Drops 0.25%w/v in the affected eye(s) twice a day. If clinical response is not adequate, dosage may be increased to one drop Timolol Eye Drops 0.5% w/v in the affected eye(s) twice daily. If required, timolol maleate ophthalmic solution may be used with miotics, adrenaline or systemically administered carbonic anhydrous inhibitors.

Intra-ocular pressure should be reassessed approximately four weeks after starting treatment because response to Timolol Eye Drops may take a few weeks to stabilise. Provided that the intra-ocular pressure is maintained at satisfactory levels, many patients can then be placed on once-a-day therapy.

*Transfer from other agents:* If transferring from another topical beta-blocking agent, its use should be discontinued after a full day of treatment and treatment with Timolol Eye Drops 0.25% w/v started the next day with one drop twice daily in the affected eye(s). As above, if the clinical response is not adequate, the dosage may be increased to one drop of Timolol Eye Drops 0.5% w/v twice daily.

If transferring from a single anti-glaucoma agent which is not a beta-blocker, the agent should be continued and one drop added of the Timolol Eye Drops 0.25% w/v in the affected eye(s) twice daily. On the following day the previous agent should be discontinued and Timolol Eye Drops continued. The dosage may be increased to Timolol Eye Drops 0.5% w/v twice daily if the clinical response is inadequate.

*Use in children:* Paediatric use is not currently recommended.

*Use in the elderly:* There has been wide experience with the use of timolol maleate in elderly patients. The dosage recommendations above reflect the clinical data derived from this experience.

*Contra-indications:* Bronchial asthma, history of bronchial asthma or severe chronic obstructive pulmonary disease, sinus bradycardia, second and third degree AV block, overt cardiac failure, cardiogenic shock, and hypersensitivity to timolol maleate or other beta-blocking agents.

*Special warnings and precautions for use:* Like other topically applied ophthalmic drugs, timolol maleate ophthalmic solution may be absorbed systemically and adverse reactions seen with systemically administered beta-blockers may occur.

Cardiac failure should be adequately controlled before beginning therapy with timolol maleate ophthalmic solution. Patients with a history of severe cardiac disease should be closely observed for signs of cardiac failure and have their pulse rates checked.

Respiratory and cardiac reactions, including death due to bronchospasm in patients with asthma and, rarely, death associated with cardiac failure, have been reported.

The effect on intra-ocular pressure or the known effects of systemic beta-blockade may be exaggerated when timolol maleate ophthalmic solution is given to patients already receiving an oral beta-blocking agent. The response of these patients should be closely watched.

If timolol maleate ophthalmic solution is used to reduce elevated intra-ocular pressure in angle closure glaucoma it should be used with a miotic and not alone.

There have been reports of skin rashes and/or dry eyes associated with the use of beta-adrenergic receptor blocking drugs. The reported incidence is small and in most cases the symptoms have cleared when treatment was withdrawn. Discontinuation of the drug should be considered if any such reaction is not otherwise explicable. Cessation of therapy involving beta-blockade should be gradual.

Timolol Eye Drops contain benzalkonium chloride as a preservative which may be deposited in soft contact lenses. Therefore, timolol eye drops should not be used while wearing these lenses. The lenses should be removed before application of the drops and not reinserted earlier than 15 minutes after use.

Timolol Eye Drops have generally been well tolerated in glaucoma patients wearing conventional hard contact lenses. Timolol maleate ophthalmic solution has not been studied in patients wearing lenses made of material other than polymethylmethacrylate (PMMA) which is used to make hard contact lenses.

*Interaction with other medicaments and other forms of interaction:* Although timolol maleate ophthalmic solution alone has little or no effect on pupil size, mydriasis has occasionally been reported when timolol maleate ophthalmic solution is given with adrenaline.

*Pregnancy and lactation:* Timolol maleate ophthalmic solution has not been studied in human pregnancy. The use of timolol maleate ophthalmic solution requires that the anticipated benefit be weighed against possible hazards. Timolol maleate ophthalmic solution is detectable in human milk. A decision for breast-feeding mothers either to stop taking timolol or stop nursing should be based on the importance of the drug to the mother.

*Effects on ability to drive and use machines:* Instillation of Timolol Eye Drops may cause transient blurring of vision. Patients should be warned not to drive or operate moving machinery until any blurring of vision after instillation has totally regressed.

*Undesirable effects:* Timolol maleate ophthalmic solution is usually well tolerated.

*Special senses:* Signs and symptoms of ocular irritation, including conjunctivitis, blepharitis, keratitis and decreased corneal sensitivity, have been reported. Visual disturbances, including refractive changes (due to withdrawal of miotic therapy in some cases), diplopia and ptosis, can occur.

*Cardiovascular:* Bradycardia, arrhythmia, hypotension, syncope, heart block, cerebrovascular accident, cerebral ischaemia, congestive heart failure, palpitation and cardiac arrest may occur and are probably the result of systemic absorption.

*Respiratory:* Bronchospasm (predominantly in patients with pre-existing bronchospastic disease), respiratory failure and dyspnoea have been reported.

*Generally:* Headache, asthenia, nausea, dizziness, depression and hypersensitivity reactions including localised and generalised rash and urticaria may occasionally occur.

*Causal relationship unknown:* The following adverse effects have been reported, but a causal relationship to timolol maleate ophthalmic solution has not been established: Aphakic cystoid macular oedema, dry mouth, nasal congestion, anorexia, dyspepsia, CNS effects (eg behavioural change including confusion, hallucinations, anxiety, disorientation, nervousness, somnolence and other psychiatric disturbances), hypertension and retroperitoneal fibrosis.

The adverse reactions seen with oral timolol maleate may occur with timolol maleate ophthalmic solution due to systemic absorption.

*Overdose:* Overdosage reactions are more likely to follow oral ingestion of timolol maleate than by systemic absorption through its topical use. No specific data on overdosage in humans by either route are available. A study in patients with renal failure suggests that timolol does not readily dialyse. The most common signs and symptoms to be expected following overdosage with a beta-blocker are symptomatic bradycardia, hypotension, bronchospasm and acute cardiac failure. The standard measures to overcome beta-blockade should be undertaken.

**Pharmacological properties**

*Pharmacodynamic properties:* Timolol maleate is a non-selective beta-adrenergic antagonist used as an ophthalmic solution for the topical treatment of increased intra-ocular pressure. Timolol maleate has no intrinsic sympathomimetic activity nor membrane-stabilising activity. It is thought that the mode of action is by markedly reducing the production of aqueous humor, probably without any effect on the outflow tract. Timolol maleate ophthalmic solution is effective in a range of concentrations but the usual recommendation is for 0.25% w/v and 0.5% w/v strengths.

*Pharmacokinetic properties:* Timolol maleate ophthalmic solution lowers intra-ocular pressure within 30-60 minutes of being administered topically, has a maximum IOP-lowering effect 4-5 hours after administration, and the effect persists for 12-14 hours after a single dose. Minute amounts are absorbed systemically; plasma concentrations of up to 1 ng/ml can be detected after single eye drop administration.

*Preclinical safety data:* None presented

**Pharmaceutical particulars**

*List of excipients:* Potassium Dihydrogen Phosphate PhEur, Disodium Hydrogen Phosphate Dodecahydrate PhEur, Sodium Chloride PhEur, Benzalkonium Chloride, Purified Water PhEur.

*Incompatibilities:* None known

*Shelf life:*

Shelf life of the product as packaged for sale: 2 years (24 months).

Shelf life after first opening the container: 28 days.

*Special precautions for storage:* Store below 30°C. Protect from light.

*Nature and contents of container:* A 5 ml low density polyethylene bottle. The dropper insert is made from low density polyethylene and the bottle is closed by a screw cap manufactured from high density polyethylene. The cap is secured by a tamper evident closure.

*Instructions for use/handling:* Unscrew the cap from the bottle. Pull down the bottom lid of the eye to form a pocket. Place the tip close to the lower eye lid and squeeze the container gently. One drop of solution should fall into the eye.

### Marketing authorisation numbers

Timolol Eye Drops 0.25% w/v 0156/0032
Timolol Eye Drops 0.5% w/v 0156/0033

*Marketing authorisation holder:* Martindale Pharmaceuticals Limited, Bampton Road, Romford RM3 8UG.

**Date of approval/revision of SPC** August 1995

**Legal category** POM

*\* Trade Mark*

**medac GmbH**
Fehlandtstrasse 3
20354 Hamburg
Germany

## ACLARUBICIN medac* INJECTION

**Qualitative and quantitative composition** Aclarubicin hydrochloride equivalent to aclarubicin 20 mg.

**Pharmaceutical form** Freeze-dried powder for reconstitution and parenteral administration by injection or infusion.

**Clinical particulars**
*Therapeutic indications:* For the treatment of acute non-lymphocytic leukaemia in patients who have relapsed or are resistant or refractory to first line chemotherapy.

*Posology and method of administration:* Aclarubicin should be administered by intravenous infusion over 30 to 60 minutes.

*Dosage in adults including the elderly:* The usual initial dosage is 175–300 mg/m² of body surface over 3 to 7 consecutive days, e.g. 80–100 mg/m² on 3 consecutive days or 25 mg/m² daily for 7 consecutive days. Repetition of treatment schedules will be dependent on the patient's haematological profile and the response of the primary disease.

Maintenance dosage should be treatments of 25–100 mg/m² of body surface given as a single infusion every 3 to 4 weeks.

This is a guide to dosage using the drug alone. In combination with other cytotoxic drugs dosage may need to be reduced.

The maximum total dosage given to any individual patient should be decided according to their cardiological status. Most patients treated have received a maximum of 400 mg/m², however, larger doses in some patients have been used without ill consequence.

*Dosage in children:* Experience suggests that aclarubicin is well tolerated by children at the standard dosage level.

*Administration:* By parenteral infusion either (i) in a freely flowing iv peripheral line or (ii) in a patent central venous line.

*Contra-indications:* Severe bone marrow depression.

*Special warnings and special precautions for use:* Patients receiving aclarubicin require close observation and frequent laboratory monitoring therefore treatment should be carried out by doctors experienced in the use of cytotoxic drugs. Treatment should be carried out at centres where there are adequate laboratory facilities, supportive treatment and facilities for monitoring heart disease readily available.

Therapy should be initiated cautiously in patients with compromised hepatic, renal or cardiac function.

The patient's haematological profile should be taken into account when instituting therapy and monitored during the recovery phase post treatment. Anaemia and thrombocytopenia should be treated with appropriate blood product replacement.

Hyperuricaemia should be avoided (fluid and xanthine oxidase inhibitors) and infections should be treated.

Cardiac function should be monitored by ECG.

*Interactions with other medicaments and other forms of interaction:* Aclarubicin is a powerful myelosuppressive agent. The concurrent use of other chemotherapeutic drugs with similar actions may be expected to lead to additive myelosuppression and dosage reduction should be considered.

Aclarubicin has been used in combination chemotherapy without signs of interaction with the following drugs: cyclophosphamide, cytarabine, behenoyl cytarabine, 5-fluorouracil, 6-mercaptopurine, methotrexate, 6-thioguanine, prednisolone and vincristine.

Aclarubicin has caused higher myelosuppression in patients previously treated with nitrosourea or mitomycin.

There have been reports of increased toxicity consequent upon irradiation treatment shortly before the administration of anthracyclines. No such reactions have been observed following treatment with aclarubicin but the theoretical risk should be borne in mind.

*Pregnancy and lactation:* There is no evidence of the drug's safety in human pregnancy. There is evidence from animal work that it is foetotoxic but not teratogenic. Avoid in pregnancy unless there is no safer alternative. If used in pregnancy patients should be warned of the potential risk to the foetus.

Women of childbearing age should take adequate contraceptive precautions.

If the use of aclarubicin is considered essential, nursing mothers should be advised to stop breast feeding.

*Effects on ability to drive and use machines:* The patient's general condition is likely to be more significant in this consideration than any drug-induced effects.

*Undesirable effects:*
*Haematological:* The dose-limiting toxicity of aclarubicin is haematological with myelosuppression seen as leucopenia and thrombocytopenia. The platelet nadir precedes the leucocyte nadir. Myelosuppression is severe at total dosages greater than 300 mg/m². Higher total dosages should be administered in a cyclic schedule including rest periods for recovery of the bone marrow. Myelosuppression is not reduced by dividing a single dose over 2 to 5 days. Thrombocytopenia is at a maximum 1 to 2 weeks after the start of the drug administration with recovery within 2 to 4 weeks. Leucopenia is greatest 2 to 3 weeks after drug administration with recovery within 3 to 4 weeks.

*Gastro-intestinal:* Nausea and vomiting have been observed in 20–100% (average 60%) of patients depending on dosage and dose schedule used. Single dosages greater than 120 mg/m² given by iv infusion caused nausea and vomiting in all patients.

The same dosage divided over 5 days is better tolerated. A daily dose of up to 30 mg/m² for 7 consecutive days caused nausea and vomiting, (controllable with antiemetics) in about 50% of patients. Bolus injections of more than 50 mg/m² should not be given due to severe gastrointestinal side-effects. Diarrhoea, occasionally haemorrhagic, has been observed in 10–35% (average 26%) of patients. Diarrhoea has been most pronounced after high single dosages or consecutive use of low dosages for more than 10 days. Mucositis/stomatitis has been observed in 15–55% (average 30%) of patients and is also more pronounced at high dosages.

*Cardiac:* Acute cardiotoxicity during and after drug administration has been associated with ECG changes (including arrhythmia, atrial flutter, flattening or inversion of T waves, sinus tachycardia, ST depression and premature beats) in 10–40% (average 17%) of patients. The frequency of ECG changes is greater with high single doses of aclarubicin. The ECG changes are generally reversible, transient and frequently without clinical signs of cardiotoxocity. ECG QTc prolongation may herald a clinical risk of ventricular fibrillation.

Chronic cardiotoxicity has been observed rarely: in a follow up study of about 1,600 patients congestive heart failure occurred in 5 patients and in 2 patients clinical signs of cardiomyopathy were seen. The risk of cardiotoxicity may be increased in patients previously treated with other cytotoxic agents or irradiation to the thorax.

*Alopecia:* Mild alopecia has been observed in 1–5% of patients.

*Hepatic:* Transient and reversible serum transaminase elevation and hepatic dysfunction have been reported in 4–6% of patients.

*Other:* Phlebitis is rare, occurring in up to 7% of patients. It may be eliminated by dilution of infusion solutions. Allergic reactions (angioedema, urticaria, skin rash, conjunctivitis) have occurred in isolated cases.

After accidental extravasation, aclarubicin caused inflammation and induration, but no tissue necrosis.

Results from some mutagenicity studies with aclarubicin were positive and it showed the capacity to induce chromosomal aberrations. The carcinogenic potential of aclarubicin in man is unknown. The possibility of a carcinogenic effect should be kept in mind when planning long-term therapy.

*Overdose:* The haematologic profile should be monitored and, in the event of dangerously low haemoglobin, white cell or platelet counts, treatment with appropriate blood products should be carried out as clinically required. Fevers should be investigated and treated properly.

Cardiac function should be monitored and arrhythmias or congestive cardiac failure treated as they appear.

**Pharmacological properties**
*Pharmacodynamic properties:* Aclarubicin is a cytotoxic anthracycline antibiotic isolated from a strain of *Streptomyces galileaus*. Like other anthracyclines, aclarubicin is a glycoside but differs from daunorubicin and doxorubicin in having aklavinone as aglycone and in being a trisaccharide.

The cellular uptake is much more rapid and the cellular drug accumulation is significantly higher for aclarubicin than for daunorubicin and doxorubicin. Aclarubicin belongs to Class II anthracyclines which preferentially inhibit RNA synthesis, whereas Class I anthracyclines, daunorubicin and doxorubicin, inhibit RNA and DNA synthesis almost equally. Aclarubicin inhibition of cell progession is greatest for cells in mid $G_1$ followed by cells in late S and finally by cells in $G_2$. In contrast to daunorubicin and doxorubicin the cytotoxicity of aclarubicin in vitro is reversible at lower concentrations or after brief exposure to the drug. In vivo antineoplastic activity studies have shown that aclarubicin is more active in repeated daily or intermittent doses than in single dose, i.e. the effect seems to depend more on exposure to aclarubicin over longer periods of time than to high intracellular peak concentration. Aclarubicin induces maturation of human non-lymphocytic leukaemia blasts, unlike doxorubicin, which does not.

*Pharmacokinetic properties:* After a single iv injection the plasma drug concentration declines rapidly due to the rapid uptake of aclarubicin in the tissues. The initial disposition phases are short ($t_{1/2}$ α=2.6 (range 1.3–5.3) min, $t_{1/2}$ β=23 (range 11–75) min) and are followed by a terminal phase with an elimination half-life $t_{1/2}$ γ=3 (range 1.4–8.5) hours. (The corresponding figures for doxorubicin are: $t_{1/2}$ α=12 (±8) min, $t_{1/2}$ β=3.3 (±2.2) hours and $t_{1/2}$ γ=29.6 (±13.5) hours. Terminal half-lives for daunorubicin and its metabolite daunorubicinol were 18.5 (±4.9) and 26.7 (±12.8) hours.) The disposition half-lives are shorter and aclarubicin is removed more rapidly from plasma than daunorubicin and doxorubicin. Aclarubicin and the principal active metabolite M1 are highly bound to blood cells. The large apparent volume of distribution VD α=1249 (±648) L/m² (mean±sd) indicates that aclarubicin is highly bound to the tissues. The mean plasma total body clearance is 4.03±1.48 L/min/m² (range 1.61–8.83 L/min/m²). No accumulation is seen after repeated daily dosing of 20–40 mg/m² iv over 4–7 days.

An autoradiographic study in rats showed that small amounts of aclarubicin cross the placental barrier, distribution within the foetus is similar to that seen in the dam.

Aclarubicin is rapidly and highly metabolised before excretion. Only 1% or less of the total dose appears unchanged in the urine within 24 hours and only trace amounts are detected in the bile. The metabolic pathway for aclarubicin involves ketoreduction and hydrolysis of the terminal-sugars, reductive glycoside cleavage and glucuronide conjugation to form biologically active glycosides (M1, N1, S1, L1, T1) and inactive aglycones (AKN, C1, E, F1, F1-acid). M1, N1, S1 and F1 are found in plasma and urine. The other metabolites are found only in urine. M1 and, to a lesser extent, F1 are also found in bile.

In animal experiments active metabolites were found in high concentrations in the lung, spleen and lymph nodes; inactive metabolites were mainly found in the liver, kidneys and intestine.

Following aclarubicin injection the principal active glycoside metabolite M1 appears in plasma within 2–3 minutes and is the major metabolite during the first 2 hours. M1 plasma levels peak at 191±129 minutes after dosing, reaching concentrations of 130±43.8 ng/ml, with a terminal half-life of 13.4 (range 9.6–20.6) hours. The principal inactive aglycone metabolite F1 is detectable from 60 minutes and becomes the major metabolite from 3 hours after dosing. Peak plasma levels of F1, six times those of M1, occurred 18–23 hours after injection and declined slowly with a terminal half-life of 36.1±3 hours, suggesting that it is formed from tissue bound glycosides.

The rate of metabolism is independent of dose in the range 60–150 mg/m² and is unaffected by the rate of administration. There is correlation between plasma concentration of aclarubicin and the side-effects nausea and vomiting. Administration of the drug over a longer period of time by infusion or in divided doses may reduce the frequency of occurrence.

*Preclinical safety data:* Aclarubicin was non-mutagenic in the Ames test in contrast to daunorubicin and doxorubicin. No immunosuppressive effects were demonstrated for aclarubicin.

### Pharmaceutical particulars
*List of excipients:* Lactose, hydrochloric acid.

*Incompatibilities:* Aclarubicin is not stable at pH of less than 4.

Aclarubicin should only be reconstituted using 0.9% Sodium Chloride Injection or Water for Injections. Reconstituted aclarubicin should only be added to 0.9% intravenous sodium chloride infusion or to glucose infusion solutions having pH values between 5 and 6.

Exposure of very dilute solutions to light promotes degradation.

*Shelf life:* Aclarubicin medac injection, in the dry state, has a shelf-life of 3 years when stored at room temperature and protected from light.

Water and saline solutions (reconstituted aclarubicin) should be stored protected from light and should be used within 24 hours if stored below 4°C or within 6 hours if stored at room temperature.

Infusion solutions should be used immediately and protected from sunlight during administration.

*Special precautions for storage:* Aclarubicin medac injection, dry powder and reconstituted solution, should be stored protected from light.

*Nature and contents of container:* 10 ml colourless glass vial with butyl rubber stopper and cap of aluminium/polypropylene.

Each vial contains a quantity of freeze dried powder equivalent to 20 mg aclarubicin for reconstitution.

The vials are packed in boxes of 2.

*Instructions for use/handling:* Preparation of solutions: The vial contents should be reconstituted with 10 ml of 0.9% Sodium Chloride Injection or Water for Injection. The concentration of this reconstituted solution is 2 mg/ml.

To prepare an infusion solution dilute the required volume of reconstituted solution with 200 to 500 ml 0.9% sodium chloride intravenous infusion or, if necessary, 5% glucose intravenous infusion (of pH value between 5 and 6). The final concentration should be 0.2–0.5 mg/ml.

**Marketing authorisation number** 11587/0004

**Date of approval/revison of SPC** November 1996.

**Legal category** POM.

## CCNU* CAPSULES

**Presentation** Blue/colourless gelatin capsules containing 40 mg lomustine.

*Active ingredient:* 40 mg lomustine (CCNU: 1-(2-chloroethyl)-3-cyclohexyl-1-nitrosourea).

**Uses** The mechanism of action is believed to be partly as an alkylating agent and partly by inhibition of several other vital enzymatic processes. Cross-resistance with other nitrosoureas is usual but cross-resistance with conventional alkylating agents is unusual.

*Indications:* As palliative or supplementary treatment, usually in combination with radiotherapy and/or surgery or as part of multiple drug regimens in:

– brain tumours (primary or metastatic);
– lung tumours (especially oat-cell carcinoma);
– Hodgkin's disease (resistant to conventional combination chemotherapy);
– malignant melanoma (metastatic).

CCNU may also be of value as second-line treatment in non-Hodgkin's lymphoma, myelomatosis, gastrointestinal tumours, carcinoma of the kidney, the testis, the ovary, the cervix uteri and the breast.

### Dosage and administration
*Adults:* CCNU is given by mouth. The recommended dose in patients with normally functioning bone marrow receiving CCNU as their only chemotherapy is 120–130 mg/m² as a single dose every six to eight weeks (or as a divided dose over three days, e.g. 40 mg/m²/day). Dosage is reduced if:

(a) CCNU is being given as part of a drug regimen which includes other marrow-depressant drugs, and
(b) in the presence of leucopenia below 3,000/mm³ or thrombocytopenia below 75,000/mm³.

Marrow depression after CCNU is longer sustained than after nitrogen mustards and recover of white cell and platelet counts may not occur for six weeks or more. Blood elements depressed below the above levels should be allowed to recover to 4,000/mm³ (WBC) and 100,000/mm³ (platelets) before repeating CCNU dosage.

*Administration to children:* Until further data are available administration of CCNU to children with malignancies other than brain tumours should be restricted to specialised centres and exceptional situations. Dosage in children, like that in adults, is based on body surface area (120–130 mg/m² every six to eight weeks, with the same qualifications as apply to adults).

**Contra-indications, warnings, etc** This product should not normally be administered to patients who are pregnant or to mothers who are breast feeding. Other contra-indications are:

– Previous hypersensitivity to nitrosoureas;
– Previous failure of the tumour to respond to other nitrosoureas;
– Severe bone marrow depression.

*Precautions:* Patients receiving CCNU chemotherapy should be under the care of doctors experienced in cancer treatment. Blood counts should be carried out before starting the drug and at frequent intervals (preferably weekly) during treatment. Treatment and dosage is governed principally by the haemoglobin, white cell count and platelet count. Liver function should also be assessed periodically.

*Interactions:* CCNU used in combination with theophylline may potentiate bone marrow toxicity. Cross-resistance with other nitrosoureas is usual, but cross-resistance with conventional alkylating agents is unusual.

*Adverse effects:*
*Haematological:* The principal adverse effect is marrow toxicity of a delayed or prolonged nature. Thrombocytopenia appears about four weeks after a dose of CCNU and lasts one to two weeks at a level around 80–100,000/mm³; leucopenia appears after six weeks and persists for one to two weeks at about 4–5,000/mm³. The haematological toxicity may be cumulative, leading to successively lower white cell and platelet counts with successive doses of the drug.

*Gastro-intestinal:* Nausea and vomiting usually occur four to six hours after a full single dose of CCNU and last for 24–28 hours, followed by anorexia for two to three days. The effects are less troublesome if the six-weekly dose is divided into three doses and given on each of the first three days of the six-week period. Gastrointestinal tolerance is usually good, however, if prophylactic antinauseants are given (e.g. metoclopramide or chlorpromazine). Transient elevation of liver enzymes (SGOT, SGPT, LDH or alkaline phosphatase) are occasionally observed. More rarely patients are troubled by stomatitis.

*Other side-effects:* Loss of scalp hair has been reported infrequently.

*Overdosage:* Symptoms of overdosage with CCNU will probably include bone marrow toxicity, haematological toxicity, nausea and vomiting. Overdosage should be treated immediately by gastric lavage. There is no specific antidote. In the event of dangerously low red cell, white cell or platelet counts, cross-matched whole blood should be given as necessary.

**Pharmaceutical precautions** The capsules should be stored in the original container and protected from light and moisture.

**Legal category** POM.

The supply of CCNU capsules is restricted to centres with special experience in the chemotherapy of malignant disease. CCNU capsules are available on prescription only.

**Package quantities** Plastic bottles of 20 capsules each containing 40 mg lomustine.

**Further information** Nil.

**Product licence number** 11587/0003.

## TREOSULFAN* CAPSULES
## TREOSULFAN* INJECTION

**Presentation** *Capsules:* White opaque capsules each containing 250 mg Treosulfan.

*Injection;* Infusion bottles containing 1 g or 5 g Treosulfan, a white crystalline powder.

**Uses** Treosulfan is a bifunctional alkylating agent which has been shown to possess antineoplastic activity in the animal tumour screen and in clinical trials. The activity of Treosulfan is due to the formation of epoxide compounds in vivo.

*Indications:* For the treatment of all types of ovarian cancer, either supplementary to surgery or palliatively. Some uncontrolled studies have suggested activity in a wider range of neoplasms.

Because of a lack of cross-resistance reported between Treosulfan and other cytotoxic agents Treosulfan may be useful in any neoplasm refractive to conventional therapy.

Treosulfan has been used in combination regimens in conjunction with vincristine, methotrexate, 5-FU and procarbazine.

**Dosage and administration** *Capsules:* The following dosage regimens have been indicated. All regimens indicate that a total dose of 21–28 g of Treosulfan should be given in the initial 8 weeks of treatment.

*Regimen A:* 1 g daily, given in four divided doses for four weeks followed by four weeks off therapy.

*Regimen B:* 1 g daily, given in four divided doses for two weeks, followed by two weeks off therapy.

*Regimen C:* 1.5 g daily, given in three divided doses for one week only, followed by three weeks off therapy. If no evidence of haematological toxicity at this dose in Regimen C, increase to 2 g daily in four divided doses for one week for the second and subsequent courses.

These cycles should be repeated with the dose being adjusted if necessary, as outlined below, according to the effect on the peripheral blood counts.

The capsules should be swallowed whole and not allowed to disintegrate within the mouth.

*Dose modification (All regimens):* For excessive haematological toxicity (white blood cell count less than 3,000/microlitre or thrombocyte count less than 100,000/microlitre) a repeat blood count should be made after 1–2 weeks interval and treatment restarted if haematological parameters are satisfactory, reducing dose as follows:

*Regimen A:* 1 g daily×28 to 0.75 g daily×28 (and to 0.5 g daily×28 if necessary).

*Regimen B:* 1 g daily×14 to 0.75 g daily×14 (and to 0.5 g daily×14 if necessary).

*Regimen C:* 2 g daily×7 to 1.5 g daily×7 (and to 1 g daily×7 if necessary).

Present evidence, while not definitive, suggests that Regimens B and C are less myelosuppressive than Regimen A, whilst retaining maximum cytotoxic efficacy.

*Injection:* 3–8 g/m² i.v. every 1–3 weeks depending on blood count and concurrent chemotherapy. Single injections of up to 8 g/m² have been given with no serious adverse effects. Doses up to 1.5 g/m² have been given intraperitoneally. Doses up to 3 g/m² treosulfan may be given as a bolus injection. Larger doses should be administered as an i.v. infusion at a rate of 3 g/m² every 5–10 minutes (8 g/m² as a 30 minutes infusion).

Treosulfan Injection 1 g or 5 g is used for intravenous infusion after being dissolved in 20 or 100 ml of water for injection. Once brought into solution the injection should be used immediately.

Treatment should not be given if the white blood cell count is less than 3,000/microlitre or the thrombocyte count less than 100,000/microlitre. A repeat blood count should be made after a weeks interval, when treatment may be restarted if haematological parameters are satisfactory. Lower doses of Treosulfan should be used if other cytotoxic drugs or radiotherapy are being given concurrently. Treatment is initiated as soon as possible after diagnosis.

Care should be taken in administration of the injection to avoid extravasation into tissues since this will cause local pain and tissue damage. If extravasation occurs, the injection should be discontinued immediately and any remaining portion of the dose should be introduced into another vein.

*Dosage in the elderly:* Treosulfan is renally excreted. Blood counts should be carefully monitored in the elderly and dosage adjusted accordingly.

*Children:* Not recommended.

**Contra-indications, warnings, etc**
*Contra-indication:* Severe and lasting bone marrow depression.

*Warning:* This product should not normally be administered to patients who are pregnant or to mothers who are breast feeding.

Women of child-bearing age should take adequate contraceptive precautions.

*Adverse reactions:* The dose-limiting side-effect of treosulfan is a myelosuppression, which is usually reversible. It is manifested by a reduction in leukocytes and platelets and a decrease in haemoglobin.

The leukocytes and platelets usually reach their baseline level after 28 days.

Because the inhibition of bone marrow function is cumulative, the blood count should be monitored at shorter intervals starting with the third course of treatment.

This is especially important if combined with other forms of therapy that suppress bone marrow function such as radiotherapy.

During long-term therapy with oral treosulfan doses eight patients (1.4% of 553 patients) developed an acute non-lymphatic leukaemia.

*Skin:* Mild alopecia is observed in 16% of the patients and a skin pigmentation in the form of a bronze discoloration in up to 30% of the cases.

The occurrence of urticaria, erythemas, a sclero-derma and triggering of a psoriasis have been reported.

*Respiratory:* In rare cases allergic alveolitis, pneumonia and pulmonary fibrosis have developed.

*Gastro-intestinal:* Nausea with or without vomiting is observed in approx. 50% of the patients.

*Other adverse reactions:* In rare cases flu-like complaints, a. paraesthesia, haemorrhagic cystitis, Addison's disease and hypoglycaemia have been observed. It cannot be totally ruled out that one case of cardiomyopathy was related to treosulfan.

Due to the possible development of a haemorrhagic cystitis patients are advised to drink more fluids for up to 24 hours after infusion.

During infusion, care must be taken to use a flawless technique, since painful inflammatory reactions may occur as a result of extravasation of treosulfan solution into surrounding tissue.

*Overdosage:* Although there is no experience of acute overdosage with Treosulfan, nausea, vomiting and gastritis may occur.

Prolonged or excessive therapeutic doses may result in bone marrow depression which has occasionally been irreversible. The drug should be withdrawn, a blood transfusion given and general supportive measures given.

**Pharmaceutical precautions**  As with all cytotoxic substances appropriate precautions should be taken when handling treosulfan.

*Guidelines for the safe handling of antineoplastic agents:*
1. Trained personnel should reconstitute the drug.
2. This should be performed in a designated area.
3. Adequate protective gloves, masks and clothing should be worn.
4. Precautions should be taken to avoid the drug accidentally coming into contact with the eyes.
5. Cytotoxic preparations should not be handled by staff who may be pregnant.
6. Adequate care and precautions should be taken in the disposal of items (syringes, needles, etc.) used to reconstitute cytotoxic drugs.
7. The work surface should be covered with disposable plastic-backed absorbent paper.

8. Use Luer-lock fittings on all syringes and sets. Large bore needles are recommended to minimize pressure and the possible formation of aerosols. The latter may also be reduced by the use of a venting needle.

**Legal category**  POM.

**Package quantities**  *Capsules:* Amber glass bottles of 100 capsules.
*Injection:* Boxes of 5×100 ml infusion bottles, each containing 1 g or 5 g Treosulfan, complete with 5 plastic bottle holders.

**Further information**  All centres using Treosulfan have reported noteworthy improvements in the general condition of patients responding to treatment, particularly in regard to reduction or disappearance of ascites. Treosulfan is remarkably well tolerated allowing many patients to become fully ambulatory and return to their normal day to day work.

**Product licence numbers**
Capsules          11587/0001
Injection          11587/0002

*\*Trade Mark*

# E. Merck Pharmaceuticals

(A Division of Merck Ltd)
Harrier House
High Street
West Drayton
Middlesex UB7 7QG

# MERCK

## AKNEMIN*
## AKNEMIN* 50

### Presentation
*Capsules 100 mg:* Red capsule containing minocycline hydrochloride equivalent to 100 mg minocycline base.

*Capsules 50 mg:* Red/caramel capsule containing minocycline hydrochloride equivalent to 50 mg minocycline base.

**Uses** Minocycline is an antibiotic with a spectrum of activity similar to other tetracyclines but is more active against *Staphylococcus aureus* and Nocardia.

It is indicated for the treatment of organisms sensitive to tetracycline such as acne, respiratory infections, gonorrhoea, urinary tract infections, nocardiosis, staphylococcal infections; the chemoprophylaxis of meningococcal infections.

### Dosage and administration
*Adults:*
1. Routine antibiotic use: 200 mg daily in divided doses.
2. Acne: 50 mg twice daily or 100 mg once daily.
3. Gonorrhoea: In adult males – 200 mg initially followed by 100 mg every 12 hours for a minimum of 4 days with post-therapy cultures within 2–3 days. Adult females may require more prolonged therapy.
4. Prophylaxis of meningococcal infections: 100 mg twice daily for 5 days, usually followed by a course of rifampicin.

*Children:* Aknemin is not recommended for children under 12 years old. For children above 12 years old the recommended dose is 50 mg every 12 hours or 100 mg once daily.

*Elderly:* Aknemin may be used at the normal recommended dosage in elderly patients but caution is advised in patients with severe renal impairment.

Unlike earlier tetracyclines, absorption of Aknemin is not impaired significantly by the intake of food or moderate amounts of milk.

The treatment of acne should be continued for a minimum of 6 weeks. If after 6 months there is no satisfactory response, Aknemin should be discontinued and other therapies considered. If Aknemin is to be continued for longer than 6 months, patients should be monitored at least 3 monthly thereafter for signs and symptoms of hepatitis or SLE (see *Warnings and precautions*).

### Contra-indications, warnings, etc
*Contra-indications:* Hypersensitivity to tetracyclines, systemic lupus erythematosus, complete renal failure, children under 12 years old, pregnancy, lactation.

*Warnings and precautions:* Aknemin should be used with caution in patients with hepatic dysfunction and in conjunction with alcohol and other hepatotoxic drugs. Although clinical studies have shown that at the recommended doses there is not significant drug accumulation in renally impaired patients, in cases of severe renal insufficiency a reduction in the dose and monitoring of renal function may be required.

Cross-resistance between tetracyclines may develop in micro-organisms and cross-sensitisation in patients. Aknemin should be discontinued if there are signs/symptoms of overgrowth of resistant organisms, e.g. enteritis, glossitis, stomatitis, vaginitis, pruritis ani or staphyloccal enteritis.

Patients taking oral contraceptives should be warned that if diarrhoea or breakthrough bleeding occur there is a possibility of contraceptive failure.

Rare case of autoimmune hepatotoxicity and isolated cases of systemic lupus erythematosus (SLE) and also exacerbation of pre-existing SLE have been reported. If patients develop signs or symptoms of SLE, or hepatoxicity, or suffer exacerbation of existing SLE, minocycline should be discontinued.

*Interactions:* Tetracyclines decrease plasma prothrombin activity; reduced doses of concomitant anticoagulants may therefore be required. Aknemin should not be used with penicillins. The absorption of Aknemin is impaired by concomitant administration of antacids and preparations containing iron, calcium, aluminium, magnesium or zinc salts.

*Use in pregnancy:* Aknemin should not be used in pregnancy unless essential. Animal studies have indicated that tetracyclines cross the placenta, are found in foetal tissues, and can cause toxicity in the foetus usually related to a retardation of skeletal development. Yellow/brown discolouration of the teeth and enamel hypoplasia can occur when drugs of the tetracycline group are administered after the first trimester of pregnancy.

*Lactation:* Aknemin should not be given to lactating women. Tetracyclines have been found in the milk of lactating women who are taking drugs of this class. Permanent tooth discolouration may occur in the nursing infant and enamel hypoplasia has been reported.

*Side-effects:* Headache, dizziness, vertigo, ataxia and tinnitus may occur. Patients should therefore be warned of the hazards of driving and operating machinery until the effect of treatment is known. These disturbances are reversible within 3–48 hours of discontinuing therapy and occur less frequently when a low dose is given. Gastrointestinal disturbances may occur. Dermatological reactions are rare but erythema multiforme, Stevens-Johnson syndrome, exfoliative dermatitis and photosensitivity have been reported.

Hypersensitivity reactions can include urticaria, fever, arthralgia, angioneurotic oedema, anaphylaxis and anaphylactoid purpura. Rarely pericarditis, pulmonary infiltration have been reported.

Isolated cases of systemic lupus erythematosus (SLE) and also exacerbation of existing SLE have been reported. As with other tetracyclines, bulging fontanelles in infants and benign intracranial hypertension in adults have been reported. Treatment should be stopped if evidence of raised intracranial pressure develops.

Haemolytic anaemia, thrombocytopenia, neutropenia and eosinophilia have been reported with tetracyclines.

In common with other tetracyclines, transient increases in liver function test values and, rarely, hepatitis have been reported. There have been isolated incidences of pancreatitis.

Some hepatic reactions have an autoimmune basis, and may occur after several months of minocycline treatment (see *Dosage and administration*).

When given over long periods, tetracyclines have been reported to produce brownish black microscopic discolouration of thyroid tissue. No abnormalities of function are known to occur.

Hyperpigmentation of skin or discolouration of teeth and buccal mucosa has been reported occasionally. These are generally reversible on cessation of therapy. There are isolated cases of discolouration of the conjunctiva, lacrimal secretions, breast secretions and perspiration. See also Uses in Pregnancy and Lactation.

*Overdosage:* There is no specific antidote. Treatment is gastric lavage with appropriate supportive treatment.

**Pharmaceutical precautions** The product should be stored at room temperature (below 25°C) in the original pack.

**Legal category** POM.

**Package quantities** 50 mg capsules: Blister packs of 56 OP. 100 mg capsules: Blister packs of 28 OP.

**Further information** Nil.

**Product licence numbers**
50 mg capsules   10669/0002
100 mg capsules  10669/0003

## BALNEUM*

**Presentation** A liquid preparation for external use.

*Active ingredient:* Soya oil 84.75% w/w.

*Inactive ingredients:* Laureth 4, oleic acid diethanolamide, perfume oil, antioxidant (containing propylene glycol and butylated hydroxytoluene).

**Uses** Balneum has emollient properties and is recommended for the treatment of dry skin conditions including those associated with dermatitis and eczema.

**Dosage and administration** For full bath (~100 L)–20 ml = 1 measure.
For bath for children (~25 L)–5 ml = ¼ measure.
For partial bath (~5L)–2.5 ml = ⅛ measure.
For particularly dry skin, 2–3 times the above quantities can be used.
Add Balneum to the bath water and mix well. The frequency and duration of bathing will depend on the type and severity of the condition. Generally 2–3 baths should be taken weekly. For babies and infants a daily bath is recommended.

**Contra-indications, warnings, etc** Balneum is contraindicated in patients with a known hypersensitivity to any of the ingredients.
No side-effects have been observed.

**Pharmaceutical precautions** None.

**Legal category** GSL.

**Package quantities** Bottles of 200 ml, 500 ml and 1000 ml.

**Further information** Balneum contains vegetable oil well tolerated by the skin. Since the product contains no wool alcohols or lanolin it can be safely used by patients sensitive to these materials. The bath can easily be cleaned after use.

**Product licence number** 0493/0064.

## BALNEUM PLUS*

**Presentation** An oily liquid for external use.

*Active ingredients:* soya oil 82.95% w/w and mixed lauromacrogols 15% w/w.

*Inactive ingredients:* liquid paraffin, stabiliser, perfume oil, antioxidant (containing butylated hydroxytoluene and propylene glycol)

**Uses** Balneum Plus is a bath oil which has emollient and local anaesthetic properties and provides relief of pruritus. It is recommended for the treatment of dry skin conditions including those associated with dermatitis and eczema where pruritus is also experienced.

**Dosage and administration** After shaking the bottle Balneum Plus is added to the bath water and mixed well. Frequency and duration of the application depends on the type and severity of the condition. Balneum Plus should be used when bathing.
For babies and infants a daily application is recommended.
For full bath (~100 L)–20 ml = 1 measure.
For bath for children (~25 L)–5 ml = ¼ measure.
For partial bath (~5 L)–2.5 ml = ⅛ measure.
A partial bath may be required when the condition is localised eg the arm.
Balneum Plus can also be used in the shower. In this case the preparation should first be evenly applied over the body without dilution. Subsequently the excess is removed under the shower. Soap, which would remove the desired oil film on the skin, should not be used.
If the skin requires considerable moisturising, 2–3 times the above quantities can be used.
Excessive rinsing with water after the bath counteracts the therapeutic action of Balneum Plus.
After the bath the skin should only be lightly dabbed with a towel. Strong wiping and rubbing decreases the therapeutic effect.
The bath can be easily cleaned after use.

**Contra-indications, warnings, etc** Balneum Plus should not be used for the treatment of patients sensitive to any of the ingredients.
As Balneum Plus deposits a film of oil over the skin, care should be taken to guard against slipping, especially in the bath or shower.

**Legal category** GSL.

**Package quantities** Bottles of 500 ml.

**Further information** Balneum Plus contains a vegetable oil that is well tolerated by the skin. Since the product contains no wool alcohols or lanolin it can be used safely by patients sensitive to these materials. Cooler bath temperatures (circa 30°C) will enhance the anti-pruritic effect of the lauromacrogols.

The lauromacrogols contained in the product exert their local anaesthetic action directly to the skin surface, where it is required, thus optimising their efficacy.

**Product licence number** 0493/0137.

## BALNEUM* WITH TAR

**Presentation** Balneum with Tar is a clear, brownish-black medicinal bath oil.

*Active ingredients:* Soya oil 55% w/w, coal tar distillate 30% w/w.

*Inactive ingredient:* Laureth 4.

**Uses** Balneum with Tar is particularly recommended in the treatment of eczema, psoriasis, pruritic dermatoses and ichthyosis.

**Dosage and administration** Balneum with Tar is added to the bath water and well mixed. Frequency and duration of bathing depends on the type and severity of the condition. Unless otherwise prescribed by a physician, 2 to 3 baths weekly for up to 20 minutes each are recommended.

*Adults:* One measure (20 ml) of Balneum with Tar should be added to the usual bath of ~100 litres.

*Babies and children:* In small baths (~50 litres), up to half a measure (10 ml) will be sufficient.

**Contra-indications, warnings, etc**
*Contra-indications:* Do not apply the preparation to moist and weeping dermatoses, or severely broken skin.

*Warnings:* Avoid contact with the eyes and prolonged exposure to sunlight after bathing.

*Side-effects:* Very rarely sensitisation of normal skin may occur.

**Pharmaceutical precautions** No special requirements.

**Legal category** P.

**Package quantities** Bottles of 200 ml.

**Further information** Balneum with Tar combines the emollient properties of the medicinal bath oil Balneum with the therapeutic properties of coal tar distillate.

**Product licence number** 0493/0113.

## BALTAR* SHAMPOO

**Presentation** Baltar Shampoo is a clear, light brown liquid for scalp application.

*Active ingredient:* Coal tar distillate 1.5% w/w.

*Inactive ingredients:* Coconut fatty acid derivatives, sodium laureth sulphate, perfume oil, sodium chloride, purified water.

**Uses** For the treatment of scalp disorders such as psoriasis, eczema, dandruff, seborrhoeic and pruritic dermatoses.

**Dosage and administration** Wet hair and scalp. Apply sufficient Baltar shampoo to make a rich lather and massage well into the scalp. Wait one minute. Rinse and repeat. Finally rinse hair thoroughly.

Baltar shampoo should be used as above once to three times weekly, depending on the severity of the condition, or as directed by the physician.

**Contra-indications, warnings, etc**
*Contra-indications:* Do not apply the preparation to moist and weeping dermatoses, or severely broken skin.

Not recommended for use in children under 2 years old.

*Warnings:* Avoid contact with the eyes.

*Side-effects:* Very rarely, sensitisation of normal skin may occur.

**Pharmaceutical precautions** No special requirements.

**Legal category** GSL.

**Package quantities** Bottles of 200 ml.

**Further information** Baltar Shampoo combines the properties of a soap-free skin cleansing agent with the therapeutic effects of tar in a formulation designed to encourage patient compliance.

**Product licence number** 0493/0123.

## CURATODERM* OINTMENT 4µg/g ▼

**Qualitative and quantitative composition** Tacalcitol monohydrate 4.17 µg/g (tacalcitol 4µg/g)

**Pharmaceutical form** Ointment.

**Clinical particulars**
*Therapeutic indication:* Psoriasis vulgaris.

*Posology and method of administration:*
*Adults and the elderly:* Apply sparingly, once daily to the affected areas, preferably at bedtime. The amount applied should not exceed 5 g of ointment/day. Normally duration of treatment depends on the severity of the lesions and should be decided by the physician. Experience shows that treatment will not usually need to exceed 2 periods of 12 weeks each year.

*Children:* Not recommended. There is no clinical experience in children.

*Contra-indications:* Hypersensitivity to constituents; in patients with hypercalcaemia or other known disorders of calcium metabolism.

*Special warnings and precautions for use:* In patients at risk of hypercalcaemia, albumin corrected serum calcium levels should be closely monitored. Treatment should be stopped if hypercalcaemia occurs. Serum calcium levels should also be monitored in patients with renal impairment. Curatoderm is not recommended for use on the scalp.

Care should be exercised in patients with generalised pustular or erythrodermic exfoliative psoriasis as the risk of hypercalcaemia may be enhanced.

When applying to the face avoid contact with the eyes. Patients should be advised to wash their hands after applying the ointment to avoid inadvertent transfer to other parts of the body.

*Interaction with other medicaments and other forms of interaction:* No interactions are likely in patients using multivitamin preparations with up to 500 IU vitamin D.

Ultraviolet light including sunlight may degrade tacalcitol. When combining UV-treatment with tacalcitol topical therapy, UV-light should be given in the morning and tacalcitol at bedtime.

When patients are likely to be exposed to sunlight, tacalcitol should be applied at bedtime.

*Pregnancy and lactation:* The safety of this medicinal product for use in human pregnancy has not been established. Evaluation of experimental animal studies does not indicate direct or indirect harmful effects with respect to the development of the embryo or foetus, the course of gestation or peri- or postnatal development.

Avoid use in pregnancy unless there are no safer alternatives.

During lactation the breast area should not be treated. It is not known whether tacalcitol is excreted in breast milk.

*Effects on ability to drive and use machines:* Curatoderm is unlikely to produce any effect on the ability to drive and use machines.

*Undesirable effects:* Local skin reactions (itching, erythema, burning, paraesthesia) have been reported. When they do appear, they are usually mild and transient and seldom lead to treatment interruption. Other local reactions may occur.

*Overdose:* Overdosing by ingestion of an ointment is very unlikely. It cannot be excluded that topical application of excessive amounts may lead to hypercalcaemia. In this case Curatoderm treatment and other vitamin D or calcium supplements must be stopped until serum calcium returns to normal.

**Pharmacological properties**
*Pharmacodynamic properties:* Pharmacotherapeutic group: D05AX02.

Tacalcitol is a vitamin D₃ derivative, which inhibits keratinocyte hyper-proliferation and induces differentiation of these cells. The normalisation of these mechanisms is the basis for the efficacy in the treatment of psoriasis.

In biopsies from patients treated with tacalcitol specific indicators for inflammation were improved.

Tacalcitol binds to the keratinocyte vitamin D receptor to the same extent as natural active vitamin D3.

*Pharmacokinetic properties:* Single or repeated application of tacalcitol ointment in humans results in less than 0.5% of the drug being systemically absorbed through psoriatic skin.

Tacalcitol is completely bound to plasma proteins (vitamin D binding protein). The main metabolite is 1α, 24, 25 (OH) 3 vitamin D₃, a metabolite shared with the natural active vitamin, with 5-10 times less vitamin D activity. Tacalcitol and metabolites are excreted mainly in the faeces in rat and dog studies with excretion in urine in man. It cannot therefore be excluded that if there is sufficient systemic absorption accumulation may occur in patients with renal failure.

*Preclinical safety data:* Tacalcitol is effective in very low concentrations. The no-effect-level following cutaneous application for 12 months in rats was 4 ng/kg daily. Toxicity is typically that of the calciferols.

Tacalcitol showed no teratogenic effects in mice and rats.

The results of mutagenicity studies (Ames test, chromosomal aberration test and micronucleus test), indicate no genotoxic potential.

**Pharmaceutical particulars**
*List of excipients:* White petrolatum, liquid paraffin, diisopropyl adipate.

*Incompatibilities:* None known.

*Shelf life:* 36 months at up to 30°C. 6 months after first opening the tube.

*Special precautions for storage:* None.

*Nature and contents of container:* Aluminium tubes containing 20 g, 30 g, or 60 g.

*Instructions for use/handling:* External use only.

**Marketing authorisation number** 11648/0019

**Date of approval/revision of SPC** January 1996

Legal category POM

## EMCOR*
## EMCOR LS

**Presentation** Emcor LS tablets, containing 5 mg bisoprolol fumarate (2:1) are heart-shaped, pale yellow and film-coated. Emcor tablets, containing 10 mg bisoprolol fumarate (2:1) are heart-shaped, pale orange and film-coated. Both tablets are scored.

**Uses**
(i)  Management of hypertension
(ii) Management of angina pectoris

*Mode of action:* Bisoprolol is a potent, highly β₁-selective-adrenoreceptor blocking agent devoid of intrinsic sympathomimetic activity and without relevant membrane stabilising activity.

As with other β₁-blocking agents, the mode of action in hypertension is not clear but it is known that bisoprolol markedly depresses plasma renin activity.

In patients with angina, the blockade of β₁-receptors reduces heart action and thus reduces oxygen demand. Hence bisoprolol is effective in eliminating or reducing the symptoms.

*Pharmacokinetics:* Bisoprolol is absorbed almost completely from the gastrointestinal tract. Together with the very small first pass effect in the liver, this results in a high bioavailability of approximately 90%. The drug is cleared equally by the liver and kidney.

The plasma elimination half-life (10–12 hours) provides 24 hours efficacy following a once daily dosage. About 95% of the drug substance is excreted through the kidney, half of this is as unchanged bisoprolol. There are no active metabolites in man.

**Dosage and administration**
*Adults:* The usual dose is 10 mg once daily with a maximum recommended dose of 20 mg per day. In some patients 5 mg per day may be adequate. In patients with final stage impairment of renal (creatinine clearance <20 ml/min) or liver function, the dose should not exceed 10 mg bisoprolol once daily.

Experience of the use of bisoprolol in renal dialysis patients is limited, however, there is no evidence that the dosage regimen needs to be altered.

*Elderly:* No dosage adjustment is normally required but 5 mg per day may be adequate in some patients; as for other adults, dosage may have to be reduced in cases of severe renal or hepatic dysfunction.

*Children:* There is no paediatric experience with bisoprolol, therefore its use cannot be recommended for children.

**Contra-indications, warnings, etc**
*Contra-indications:* As with other β₁-adrenoceptor antagonists, bisoprolol should not be used in cases of untreated cardiac failure, cardiogenic shock, sinoatrial block, second or third degree AV block, marked bradycardia (heart rate less than 50 beats/min), extreme hypotension, or severe asthma.

*Precautions:* Use with care in patients with a prolonged PR conduction interval, poor cardiac reserve and peripheral circulatory disturbances, such as Raynaud's phenomenon.

In patients with ischaemic heart disease, treatment should not be withdrawn abruptly.

Although bisoprolol is a highly selective β₁-adrenoceptor blocking agent, it should be used with caution in patients with chronic obstructive airways diseases or a family history of asthma. In some asthmatic patients some increase in airways resistance may occur, this may be regarded as a signal to discontinue therapy. This bronchospasm can usually be reversed by commonly used bronchodilators such as salbutamol.

Due to the low affinity of bisoprolol for $\beta_2$-receptors, the drug does not appear to have a hypoglycaemic effect. However, it should be used with caution in diabetic patients since the symptoms of hypoglycaemia (in particular, tachycardia) may be masked.

*Pregnancy:* No teratogenic effects have been demonstrated in animal studies, but the safety of bisoprolol during human pregnancy has not been established. Like other β-blockers, the benefits of use during pregnancy should be weighed against the possible hazard to mother and foetus. β-blockers administered in late pregnancy may cause bradycardia or hypotension in the foetus/neonate. Studies in animals suggest that no clinically relevant levels of bisoprolol reach the milk. However, as in pregnancy, caution should be exercised for use during lactation.

*Drug interactions:* Bisoprolol may potentiate the effect of other concurrently administered antihypertensive drugs. Concomitant treatment with reserpine, α-methyldopa and clonidine may cause an exaggerated decrease in heart rate. In particular, if clonidine is to be discontinued, this should not be done until bisoprolol treatment has been discontinued for several days.

Bisoprolol should also be used with care when myocardial depressants, inhibitors of AV conduction such as calcium antagonists of the verapamil and diltiazem type, or class I antidysrhythmic agents such as disopyramide are used concurrently.

The intravenous administration of calcium antagonists and antiarrythmic agents is not recommended during bisoprolol therapy.

The concurrent use of rifampicin can reduce the elimination half-life of bisoprolol, although an increase in dose is generally not necessary. The effects of insulin or oral hypoglycaemic agents may be potentiated when used concurrently with bisoprolol.

*Anaesthesia:* Prior to anaesthesia, the anaesthetist should be informed if the patient is taking bisoprolol. In cases of severe ischaemic heart disease the risk/benefit of continuing treatment should be evaluated. Care should be taken when using either cyclopropane or trichloroethylene.

*Side-effects:* Bisoprolol is usually well tolerated. The reported side effects are generally attributable to its pharmacological actions and include lassitude, fatigue, dizziness, mild headache, muscle and joint ache, perspiration, aggravation of intermittent claudication or Raynaud's disease and parasthaesia and coldness of the extremities, bronchospasm, oedema and occasional GI side-effects such as nausea, vomiting and diarrhoea. Occasionally a marked decrease in blood pressure, and pulse rate or a disturbance of AV conduction, skin rashes and dry eyes may be observed. Sleep disturbances including vivid dreams of the type noted with other β-blockers have rarely been reported.

*Overdosage:* In the case of overdosage or a precipitous drop in pulse rate and/or blood pressure, treatment with bisoprolol must be discontinued. If necessary, the following antidotes should be administered alone or consecutively: intravenous atropine 0.5–2.0 mg, intravenous orciprenaline 0.5 mg by slow intravenous injection; also glucagon may be given at a dose level of 1 to 5 mg.

**Pharmaceutical precautions** No special requirement.

**Legal category** POM.

**Package quantities** Calendar blister packs of 28 tablets OP. Strips of 14 tablets, two strips in each carton.

**Further information** Bisoprolol is effective in hypertension and angina pectoris for at least 24 hours following a single oral dose. The high bioavailability and the dual pathway of clearance lead to predictable blood levels. Patient compliance is increased by the reliable and simple administration regimen.

**Product licence numbers**
Emcor LS    0493/0126
Emcor       0493/0127

## EMFLEX* CAPSULES

**Qualitative and quantitative composition** Each capsule contains Acemetacin 60 mg.

**Pharmaceutical form** Gelatine capsule.

**Clinical particulars**
*Therapeutic indications:* Rheumatoid arthritis, osteoarthritis, low back pain, and post-operative pain and inflammation.

*Posology and method of administration:* The recommended starting dose is 120 mg/day in divided doses, increasing to 180 mg/day in divided doses, depending on patient response.

For the treatment of elderly patients, adjustment of dosage is not normally required. However, non-steroidal anti-inflammatory drugs should be used with particular care in older patients who may be more prone to adverse reactions.

Emflex should be taken with food, milk or an antacid to reduce the possibility of gastro-intestinal disturbance.

*Contra-indications:* Active peptic ulcer; history of recurrent ulceration; known hypersensitivity to acemetacin or indomethacin. Patients who have experienced asthma attacks, urticaria or acute rhinitis resulting from treatment with aspirin or non-steroidal anti-inflammatory drugs. Patients with nasal polyps associated with angioneurotic oedema. Safety in children is not established.

*Special warnings and special precautions for use:* As rare instances of peptic ulceration have been reported administration should be closely supervised in patients with a history of upper gastrointestinal disease. Treatment should be discontinued if peptic ulceration or gastrointestinal bleeding occurs.

Inhibition of platelet aggregation may occur.

Aggravation of psychiatric disorders, epilepsy or parkinsonism may occur.

Signs and symptoms of infection may be masked.

Emflex should be used with caution in patients with reduced renal blood flow where renal perfusion may be maintained by prostaglandins. In patients at particular risk – renal or hepatic dysfunction, congestive heart failure, electrolyte or fluid imbalance, sepsis, concomitant use of nephrotoxic drugs – the dose should be kept as low as possible and renal function should be monitored.

Patients receiving long-term treatment should be periodically screened for renal and hepatic function and blood counts. Borderline elevation of renal and hepatic function test parameters may occur. If this persists or worsens, treatment should be stopped.

Eye changes may occur in chronic rheumatoid disease and patients should receive periodic ophthalmological examinations and therapy discontinued if changes occur.

Hyperkalaemia has been reported with use of indomethacin and this should be considered when administration with potassium sparing diuretics is proposed.

*Interactions with other medicaments and other forms of interaction:* Emflex is highly protein bound and it may therefore be necessary to modify the dosage of other highly protein bound drugs e.g. anti-coagulants. As there is a possibility of either a pharmacokinetic or pharmacodynamic interaction with aspirin or other salicylates, diflusinal, probenecid, lithium, triamterene, ACE inhibitors, haloperidol and methotrexate, patients receiving such combinations should be carefully monitored and dosages adjusted as necessary. Non-steroidal anti-inflammatory drugs may reduce the anti-hypertensive effects of beta-blockers, although clinical studies showed no propensity for Emflex to antagonise the effects of propranolol. Likewise the reduction of diuretic effects of thiazides and frusemide may occur with non-steroidal anti-inflammatory drugs and this should be borne in mind when treating patients with compromised cardiac function or hypertension.

*Pregnancy and lactation:* The safety of this product for use in human pregnancy and lactation has not been established. Animal reproduction studies do not provide reassurance regarding the lack of reproductive toxicity/teratogenicity. Due to maternal toxicity, the studies were conducted at doses below the therapeutic dose or a very low multiple of the therapeutic dose. It should not therefore be used in pregnancy or lactation in women of childbearing age unless they are taking adequate contraceptive precautions.

*Effects on ability to drive and use machines:* The ability to drive a car or operate machinery may be affected.

*Undesirable effects:* The following side effects have been either reported with Emflex or could possibly occur as they are common to a number of NSAIDs:
*Gastro-intestinal:* Gastro-intestinal discomfort/pain, anorexia, nausea, vomiting, indigestion, diarrhoea and constipation, peptic ulceration, gastrointestinal perforation and haemorrhage.
*Central nervous system:* Symptoms most frequently encountered are headache, dizziness, vertigo and insomnia. Rarely, confusion, depressed mood, irritability.
*Hepatic:* Occasional elevation of liver function test parameters without overt clinical symptomology. Very rarely, symptoms of cholestasis.
*Cardiovascular/renal:* Rarely, oedema, chest pain, palpitations, blood urea elevation. NSAIDs have been reported to cause nephrotoxicity in various forms and their use can lead to interstitial nephritis, nephrotic syndrome and renal failure.
*Dermatological/hypersensitivity:* Pruritus, urticaria, erythema, skin rash, alopecia, angio-neurotic oedema and excessive sweating have been reported.
*Haematological:* Rarely, thrombocytopenia, leucopenia and reduced haemoglobin levels. Very rarely, reversible agranulocytosis, bone marrow depression.
*Ocular/auditory:* Infrequently, tinnitus, blurred vision and rarely, eye pain.

*Overdose:* Symptomatic and supportive therapy is indicated. If ingestion is recent, vomiting should be induced or gastric lavage should be performed. Progress should be followed for several days as gastrointestinal ulceration and haemorrhage have been reported with overdosage of other NSAIDs. Antacids may be helpful.

**Pharmacological properties**
*Pharmacodynamic properties:* Acemetacin is a glycolic acid ester of indomethacin and the pharmacological activity resulting from acemetacin administration in man is derived from the presence of both acemetacin and indomethacin. The precise pharmacological mode of action of acemetacin is not known. However, unlike other NSAIDs, acemetacin is only a relatively weak inhibitor of prostaglandin synthetase. Prostaglandins are known to have an antisecretory and cytoprotective effect on the gastric mucosa. Acemetacin shows activity in many of the established in vitro tests of anti-inflammatory activity, including inhibition of the release of a number of mediators of inflammation.

*Pharmacokinetic properties:* Acemetacin is well absorbed after oral administration. Its major metabolite is indomethacin which, after repeated administration, is present at levels in excess of those of acemetacin. Acemetacin is bound to plasma protein to a slightly lesser extent than indomethacin and has a relatively short plasma elimination half-life. It is eliminated by both hepatic and renal mechanisms. The pharmacokinetics appear to be linear at recommended therapeutic doses, unaffected by moderate renal or hepatic impairment, and unchanged in the elderly.

*Preclinical safety data:* Emflex Capsules show similar toxicity to other non-steroidal anti-inflammatory drugs.

**Pharmaceutical particulars**
*List of excipients:* Gelatine capsule (colourings: erythrosine red E127, quinoline yellow E104 and titanium dioxide E171), lactose, magnesium stearate, silicon dioxide, talc.

*Incompatibilities:* None known.

*Shelf life:* Thirty six months.

*Special warnings and precautions:* Store below 25°C.

*Nature and contents of container:* White polypropylene bottles with polypropylene screw caps containing 90 capsules. PVC/PVDC foil blister packs in cartons: Four different pack sizes of 90, 30, 10, and 6 capsules

*Instructions for use/handling:* To be taken with food.

**Marketing authorisation number** 0493/0141

**Date of approval/revision of SPC** March 1996.

**Legal category** POM

## FEMSEVEN*

**Quantitative and qualitative composition** Estradiol hemihydrate 1.5 mg (corresponding to a release rate of 50 micrograms in 24 hours)

**Pharmaceutical form** Transdermal patch (patch size 15 cm² active surface area)

**Clinical particulars**
*Therapeutic indications:* Hormone replacement therapy for the symptomatic relief of menopausal symptoms including:
Vasomotor symptoms such as sweating and flushing,
Other symptoms related to oestrogen deficiency, e.g. urogenital atrophy, urinary urgency, sleeping disorders and mood swings.
Hormone replacement therapy is also indicated for the:
Prevention of postmenopausal bone loss in women considered at risk of developing fractures. Epidemiological studies have suggested that there are a number of risk factors associated with accelerated post menopausal bone loss such as early menopause, a family history of osteoporosis, prolonged exposure to corticosteroid therapy, small and thin skeletal frame and excessive cigarette smoking.

**Posology and method of administration**
*Adults and the elderly:* FemSeven should be applied once each week on a continuous basis, i.e. each patch is replaced with a new one after 7 days.
Therapy should be started with one FemSeven patch (delivering 50 micrograms of estradiol in 24 hours). If the prescribed dose does not eliminate the menopausal symptoms the dose should be adjusted

to two patches after the first few months. A maximum of two patches per week should not be exceeded. If there are persistent signs of overdose, such as breast tenderness, the dose should be reduced accordingly. In women with an intact uterus the addition of a progestogen for at least 10 days per cycle is essential.

Consecutive new patches should be applied to different sites. It is recommended that sites are chosen below the waist where little wrinkling of the skin occurs e.g., buttock, hip or abdomen. FemSeven must not be applied on or near the breasts. The patch should be applied to clean, dry, healthy and intact skin. The patch should be applied to the skin as soon as it is removed from its wrapping. The patch is applied by removing both parts of the protective liner and then holding it in contact with the skin for at least 30 seconds (warmth is essential to ensure maximal adhesive strength). Should part or all of a patch detach prematurely (before 7 days) it should be removed and a new patch applied. (To aid compliance it is recommended the patient then continues to change the patch on their usual day).

*Children:* Not indicated

*Contra-indications:* FemSeven is contra-indicated in:

Known or suspected pregnancy or lactation.

History of, known or suspected cancer of the breast.

Known or suspected oestrogen-dependent neoplasia.

Severe forms of endometriosis.

Undiagnosed abnormal genital bleeding.

Acute or chronic liver disease, severe liver disease or history of liver disease where the liver function tests have failed to return to normal. Rotor syndrome or Dubin-Johnson syndrome.

Active thrombophlebitis or thromboembolic disease.

Severe renal disease.

Known hypersensitivity to components of this product.

*Special warnings and special precautions for use:* Prior to commencing oestrogen replacement therapy, it is recommended that the patient should have a complete medical which includes a gynaecological examination and a family history taken. Periodically they should be given a thorough physical and gynaecological examination.

At the present time there is suggestive evidence of an overall change in the relative risk of breast cancer in post menopausal women receiving hormone replacement therapy. A careful appraisal of the risk/benefit ratio should be undertaken before treating for longer than 5 years. Regular breast examinations should be carried out.

There is no indication from published studies that the risk of myocardial infarction and stroke is increased with oestrogen replacement therapy at the current recommended low dosage in apparently normal women.

Several observational studies have suggested that the incidence of deep vein thrombosis and thromboembolism may be increased from a spontaneous incidence of 1/10,000 women/year to 2–3/10,000 women/year, especially during the first year of treatment.

Patients with a history or a known risk of thromboembolic diseases (e.g. blood coagulation disorders, immobilisation, severe varicose veins, certain malignant diseases, certain cardiac diseases) should not be treated with oestrogens unless the benefit of the treatment outweighs the increased risk for thromboses.

Similar caution should be exercised in patients with a history of endometriosis.

Close monitoring of patients with epilepsy, diabetes, hypertension, mild to moderate liver or renal disease, benign breast diseases, porphyria, otosclerosis, uterine fibroids and hypophyseal tumours or a significant family history of breast cancer is recommended.

If jaundice, migraine-like headaches, visual disturbances or a significant increase in blood pressure develop after initiating therapy, the medication should be discontinued while the cause is investigated. Discontinuation of treatment should also be considered 2–3 weeks before impending surgery entailed with a risk of thrombosis or in cases of extended immobilisation.

Hormone replacement therapy for 5 or more years has been shown in epidemiological studies to reduce fracture frequency by up to 50%, however, data showing benefit extending beyond 10 years is limited at present. A careful review of benefit versus risk is necessary in patients treated longer than 5 to 10 years.

FemSeven is not a contraceptive nor will it restore fertility. If FemSeven is administered together with a progestogen to women with an intact uterus of child bearing potential they should be advised to adhere to non-hormonal contraceptive methods. Repeated breakthrough bleeding should be investigated, including an endometrial biopsy.

*Interaction with other medicaments and other forms of interaction:* Liver enzyme inducing drugs, e.g. barbiturates, carbamazepine, rifampicin, phenylbutazone, meprobamate, and hydantoins, may impair the activity of oestrogens. Whether this is as relevant with transdermally applied oestrogens which are not subject to first pass metabolism is unknown.

*Pregnancy and lactation:* Accidental use during pregnancy or lactation is unlikely to have adverse effects, because only physiological levels of estradiol are achieved with the transdermal patch. There are no reports of risk for embryonic or foetal malformation.

*Effects on ability to drive and use of machinery:* There is no evidence from the clinical data available on oestrogen therapy to suggest that FemSeven should have any effect on a patient's ability to drive or operate machinery.

*Undesirable effects:* The following side effects have been reported:

*Skin:* Transient erythema and irritation at the site of application with or without pruritus. This usually disappears 2-3 days after patch removal and is similar to the effect sometimes observed after occlusion of the skin with sticking plasters.

*Urogenital tract:* Breakthrough bleeding. Unopposed oestrogen treatment may cause hyperplasia of the endometrium, when given to women with an intact uterus, unless regular therapy with a progestogen takes place.

*Endocrine system:* Breast tenderness.

*Gastro-intestinal tract:* Nausea, abdominal cramps, bloating.

*Central nervous system:* Headache, migraine. Rarely: dizziness.

*Cardiovascular system:* Rarely: thrombophlebitis, exacerbation of varicose veins, and increase in blood pressure.

*Miscellaneous:* Leg cramps (not related to thromboembolic disease and usually transient lasting 3-6 weeks, if symptoms persist the dose of oestrogen should be reduced). Rarely: Oedema and/or weight changes.

*Overdose:* The mode of administration makes significant overdose unlikely; removal of the patches is all that is required should it occur.

## Pharmacological properties

*Pharmacodynamic properties:* Estradiol, produced by the female from the menarche through to the menopause predominantly by the ovarian follicle, is the most active oestrogen at receptor level. After the menopause, when the functions of the ovaries cease, only a small amount of estradiol continues to be produced in the body, by the liver and adipose tissue from oestrone.

In many women, the loss of ovarian estradiol leads to vasomotor and thermoregulatory instability (hot flushes), sleep disturbances, as well as increasing atrophy of mucosa and other tissues of the urogenital system. In a large proportion of women, osteoporosis especially of the spinal column develops after the menopause as a result of the oestrogen deficiency. These disorders can be largely avoided by oestrogen substitution.

Administration of exogenous oestrogens to post menopausal women has been shown to decrease the potentially atherogenic low density lipoproteins (LDLs) and increase the cholesterol scavenging high density lipoproteins (HDLs). This produces an improvement in the HDL to LDL ratio and as seen in observational studies, an improvement of the lipid profile can be a factor contributing to the beneficial effect of oestrogens on the risk of coronary heart disease in post-menopausal women. In addition oestrogens have been shown to favourably affect the relative activity of osteoblasts and osteoclasts. This has been demonstrated in epidemiological studies to reduce the amount of bone loss in post-menopausal women. A number of factors are believed to be related to post-menopausal osteoporosis including early menopause, family history of osteoporosis, recent prolonged corticosteroid therapy, excessive cigarette consumption and a small, thin frame.

If a patient is at risk of osteoporosis consideration should be given to oestrogen replacement therapy. Therapy may be commenced at any convenient time, but for maximal effect therapy should be started as soon as possible after the menopause.

*Pharmacokinetic properties:* FemSeven delivers therapeutic estradiol levels within 3 hours of application and maintains these throughout the application interval (7 days). After removal of the patch, estradiol levels return to baseline values within 24 hours.

By transdermal administration of FemSeven, there is no hepatic first-pass effect and the estradiol reaches the bloodstream directly in unchanged form and in physiological amounts. With the use of FemSeven the estradiol concentrations are raised to values similar to those of the early to middle follicular phase.

*Preclinical safety data* No adverse effects can be predicted from animal toxicology studies other than those documented from human use of estradiol.

## Pharmaceutical particulars

*List of excipients:* Backing layer: Transparent polyethylene terephthalate (PET) foil. Adhesive matrix: Styrene-isoprene-styrene block copolymer, glycerine esters of completely hydrogenated resins.

*Incompatibilities:* None known.

*Shelf life:* 2 years.

*Special precautions for storage:* Store below 30°C.

*Nature and contents of the container:* The container (primary packaging) consists of a sealed laminated sachet. This comprises layers of food grade paper/polyethylene/aluminium/ethylene copolymer. Package sizes: Carton of 4 and 12 patches.

*Instructions for use/handling:* After removal from the laminated sachet, peel off the two part protective liner. Try to avoid touching the adhesive. Stick the adhesive side down to the upper left or right buttock on a clean and dry area of skin. Hold the applied patch to the skin with the palm of the hand for at least 30 seconds, in order to ensure optimal adhesion to the skin.

Recommended application sites are clean, dry and intact areas of skin on the trunk below the waistline. FemSeven should not be applied on or near the breasts. After removal the used patch should be folded and disposed of with the normal household solid waste.

**Marketing authorisation number** 11648/0021

**Date of approval/revision of SPC** 8 May 1997.

**Legal category** POM.


## GAMANIL*

**Presentation** Round, film-coated, brownish violet tablets with a spindle shaped scoring on one side, containing lofepramine hydrochloride equivalent to 70 mg lofepramine base.

**Use** The treatment of symptoms of depressive illness.

### Dosage and administration

*Adults:* The usual dose 70 mg twice daily (140 mg) or three times daily (210 mg) depending upon patient response.

*Elderly:* Elderly patients may respond to lower doses in some cases.

*Children:* Not recommended.

### Contra-indications, warnings, etc

*Contra-indications:* Lofepramine should not be used in patients hypersensitive to dibenzazepines, in mania, severe liver impairment and/or severe renal impairment, heart block, cardiac arrythmias, or during the recovery phase following a myocardial infarction.

*Precautions and warnings:* Lofepramine should be used with caution in patients with cardiovascular disease, impaired liver or renal function, narrow angle glaucoma, symptoms suggestive of prostatic hypertrophy, a history of epilepsy or recent convulsions, hyperthyroidism, blood dyscrasias or porphyria.

Ability to drive a car and operate machinery may be affected. Therefore caution should be exercised initially until the individual reaction to treatment is known.

*Use in pregnancy:* The safety of lofepramine for use during pregnancy has not been established and there is evidence of harmful effects in pregnancy in animals when high doses are given. Lofepramine has been shown to be excreted in breast milk. The administraton of lofepramine in pregnancy and during breast feeding therefore, is not advised unless there are compelling medical reasons.

*Side-effects:* Lofepramine has been shown to be well tolerated and side-effects when they occur tend to be mild.

Comparative clinical trials have shown that lofepramine is associated with a low incidence of anticholinergic side-effects.

The following side-effects have been reported with lofepramine:

*Cardiovascular:* hypotension, tachycardia.

*CNS and neuromuscular:* dizziness, drowsiness, agitation, confusion, headache, malaise, paraesthesia and rarely hypomania and convulsions.

*Anticholinergic:* dryness of mouth, constipation, disturbances of accommodation, urinary hesitancy, urinary retention, sweating and tremor.

*Allergic:* skin rash, allergic skin reactions, photosensitivity reactions.

*Gastrointestinal:* nausea, vomiting.

*Endocrine:* rarely, inappropriate secretion of antidiuretic hormone, interference with sexual function.

*Haematological/biochemical:* rarely, bone marrow depression including isolated reports of: agranulocytosis, eosinophilia, granulocytopenia, leucopenia, pancytopenia, thrombocytopenia.

Increases in liver enzymes, sometimes progressing to clinical hepatitis and jaundice, have been reported in some patients, usually occurring within the first 3 months of starting therapy.

The following adverse effects have been encountered in patients under treatment with tricyclic antidepressants and should therefore be considered as theoretical hazards of lofepramine even in the absence of substantiation: psychotic manifestations, including mania and paranoid delusions may be exacerbated during treatment with tricyclic antidepressants; withdrawal symptoms may occur on abrupt cessation of therapy and include insomnia, irritability and excessive perspiration; adverse effects such as withdrawal symptoms, respiratory depression and agitation have been reported in neonates whose mothers have taken tricyclic antidepressants during the last trimester of pregnancy.

*Drug interactions:* Lofepramine should not be administered concurrently with or within 2 weeks of cessation of therapy with monoamine oxidase inhibitors. It should then be introduced cautiously using a low initial dosage.

Lofepramine should not be given with sympathomimetic agents, central nervous depressants including alcohol or thyroid hormone therapy since its effects may be potentiated.

Lofepramine may decrease the antihypertensive effect of adrenergic neurone-blocking drugs; it is therefore advisable to review this form of antihypertensive therapy during treatment.

Anaesthetics given during tricyclic antidepressant therapy may increase the risk of arrhythmias and hypotension. If surgery is necessary, the anaesthetist should be informed that a patient is being so treated. Barbiturates may increase the rate of metabolism.

*Overdosage:* Treatment of overdosage is symptomatic and supportive. It should include immediate gastric lavage and routine close monitoring of cardiac function.

Reports of overdosage with lofepramine, with quantities ranging from 0.7 g up to 6.72 g, have shown no serious sequelae directly attributable to the drug.

**Pharmaceutical precautions** The tablets should be stored at room temperature, in their original container, protected from light and moisture.

**Legal category** POM.

**Package quantities** Containers of 250 tablets 70 mg. Blister calendar packs of 4 × 14 tablets 70 mg(OP).

**Further information** Nil.

**Product licence number** 0493/0060.

## GASTROMIRO*

**Qualitative and quantitative composition** Active component Iopamidol (INN) 612.4 mg per ml (61.24% w/v).

**Pharmaceutical form** Gastromiro is an aqueous solution for oral or rectal administration (enema)

**Clinical particulars**

*Therapeutic indications:* All forms of radiological investigations of gastrointestinal tract, in particular:

*Paediatric radiology of the gastro-intestinal tract* (GIT) where there is the possibility of:
-spill into the respiratory tract, for example in:
swallowing disorders
oesophageal obstruction with a foreign body, atresia or stricture
tracheo-oesophageal fistula.
-spill into the mediastinum, pleura, peritoneum or retroperitoneal tissues, for example due to perforation of the GIT.
- Inspissation of fluid, for example in:
Meconium ileus equivalent.
Intussusception.
Colonic obstruction.
Hirschsprung's disease.

*Adult radiology of the gastro-intestinal tract, such as:*
- Suspected upper gastro-intestinal perforation for example in:
Oesophagogastrectomy, endoscopy, partial gastrectomy, pneumonectomy, ingestion of foreign body, duodenal ulceration, small bowel resection, Whipples procedure and blunt abdominal trauma.
-Computer Tomography (CT) of the abdominal and pelvic regions, for example:
Suspicion of expanding lesions of pancreas, liver and gall bladder.
Space occupying metastatic lesions originating from prostate or recto-sigmoidal region in postsurgical staging of cancer.

*Posology and method of administration*
Adults:

*Radiology of gastro-intestinal tract*
*Oral:* 40-100 ml undiluted
*Rectal:* 200 ml of a 50% dilution, up to 1000 ml of a 2% dilution

*Computer tomography*
*Oral:* Abdominal CT: 100 ml of a 17% dilution, up to 600 ml of a 3% dilution.
*Rectal–Pelvic CT:* 500-700 ml of a 3% dilution

*Infants and children:*

*Radiology of gastro-intestinal tract*
*Oral:*10-100 ml undiluted or, for use in infants 20-200 ml of up to a 50% dilution to provide isotonic contrast medium
*Rectal:* 200 ml of 50-60% dilution

*Elderly:* Dosage as for adults.

Dilution of Gastromiro should be carried out using sterile water. Any unused solution should be discarded after 6 hours.

*Contra-indications:* Proven or suspected hypersensitivity to iodine containing preparations of this type. It must not be used for parenteral administration.

*Special warnings and precautions for use:* Disturbances in water or electrolyte balance must first be corrected. This product is formulated for gastrointestinal use only and should not be used parenterally.

Care should also be exercise in patients with severe functional impairment of the liver, kidney or myocardium, severe systemic disease and in myelomatosis. In such patients adequate hydration should be maintained and parameters of hepatic and renal function, especially urinary output should be monitored after the procedure.

Patients with hepato-renal insufficiency should not be examined unless benefits clearly outweigh risks and re-examination should be delayed for 5-7 days.

In patients with a history of adverse reactions during similar investigations additional caution should be exercised and the procedure should only be carried out if benefits clearly outweigh any risks.

X-ray examination of women should be conducted as far as possible during the pre-ovulation phase of the menstrual cycle. This product may interfere with tests of thyroid function.

*Interactions with other medicaments and other forms of interaction:* None known.

*Pregnancy and lactation:* The safety of iopamidol during pregnancy and lactation has not been demonstrated clinically. Due, however, to the extremely low absorption of iopamidol from the gastro-intestinal tract it is unlikely that a foetus could be exposed to significant levels. In animal experiments iopamidol is neither teratogenic nor foetotoxic. Similarly, during lactation breast fed infants are unlikely to be exposed to significant levels of iopamidol. However, the product should not be used during pregnancy or when breast feeding unless considered essential.

*Effects on ability to drive and use machines:* None known.

*Undesirable effects:* Systemic effects are rare since Gastromiro is only poorly absorbed from the alimentary tract. Owing to slight hypertonicity Gastromiro may occasionally cause diarrhoea in infants and children.

*Overdose:* The contrast agent is not absorbed from the gastrointestinal tract, therefore any systemic accumulation of the contrast medium following overdosage will not occur. Any treatment should be symptomatic.

**Pharmacological properties**

*Pharmacodynamic properties:* Iopamidol is a contrast medium belonging to the new generation of non-ionic compounds whose solubility is due to the presence of hydrophilic substituents in the molecule. This results in a solution of low osmolality when compared with ionic media.

Iopamidol has been shown to be effective as an X-ray contrast medium in neuroradiology, angiography, venography, arthrography, urography, cerebral angiography, and left ventriculography, coronary arteriography, and investigations of the gastrointestinal tract. Its toxicity, particularly cardiac and CNS toxicity are less than those of non-ionic contrast media.

*Pharmacokinetic properties:* Serum iopamidol concentration curves conform to an open two compartment pharmacokinetic model with first order elimination. Iopamidol is very poorly absorbed (about 1-2%) after oral or rectal administration.

Distribution volume is equivalent to extracellular fluid.

Following parenteral administration elimination is almost completely through the kidneys. Less than 1% of the administered dose has been recovered in the faeces up to seventy two hours after dosing. Renal elimination is rapid and up to half the administered

dose may be recovered in the urine within the first two hours of dosing.

There is no evidence of biotransformation.

Serum protein binding is negligible.

*Preclinical safety data:* In animals, Gastromiro was well tolerated after repeated oral administration. After 4 weeks adminstration of Gastromiro equivalent to 9 gl/kg day, i.e. about 20 times higher than the recommended clinical dose, no severe symptoms of sub-acute intoxication were observed in rats. Following intraperitoneal injection of Gastromiro in rats, iopamidol was rapidly cleared and almost totally eliminated by the renal route within the first 24 hours.

The intraperitoneal acute toxicity was relatively low. Necroscopic examination revealed no irritant effects on the peritoneal membrane. Gastromiro also showed good local tolerability after both local intratracheal installation and systemic administration . It therefore offers a good margin of safety for examination in which there is the risk of an accidental inspiration of the diagnostic medium.

**Pharmaceutical particulars**

*List of Excipients Quantity per ml*
Orange flavour 2.2 mg
Sodium cyclamate 1.5 mg
Red Curaçao flavour 1.1 mg
Disodium edetate dihydrate 0.3 mg
Sodium saccharinate 0.176 mg
Citric acid monohydrate 0.055 mg
Water for injections

*Incompatibilities:* No incompatibility studies have been performed: other drugs should not be mixed with Gastromiro.

*Shelf life:* Three years.

*Special warnings and precautions:* Protect from light.

*Nature and contents of container:* The containers are amber glass bottles (Type III) with aluminium screw caps, guarantee seals, and elastomer inserts.
Boxes of 1 bottle 20 ml
Boxes of 1 bottle 50 ml
Boxes of 1 bottle 100 ml

*Instructions for use / handling:* Gastromiro is formulated for gastro-intestinal use only and should not be administered parenterally.

The dosage of Gastromiro should be adjusted according to age, total weight, the segment of the digestive tract to be examined and the X-ray procedure.

The bottle once opened has to be used immediately. Solutions not used in one examination session must be discarded.

Gastromiro formulation is a colourless to pale yellow solution containing undissolved solids. Discard in case of discolouration.

**Marketing authorisation number** 0493/01139

**Date of approval/revision of SPC** 9 January 1996.

**Legal category** POM

## IOMERON ▼

**Qualitative and quantitative composition**
Iomeron 150 contains 30.62% w/v iomeprol equivalent to 15% iodine or 150 mg iodine/ml.
Iomeron 200 contains 40.82% w/v iomeprol equivalent to 20% iodine or 200 mg iodine/ml.
Iomeron 250 contains 51.03% w/v iomeprol equivalent to 25% iodine or 250 mg iodine/ml.
Iomeron 300 contains 61.24% w/v iomeprol equivalent to 30% iodine or 300 mg iodine/ml.
Iomeron 350 contains 71.44% w/v iomeprol equivalent to 35% iodine or 350 mg iodine/ml.
Iomeron 400 contains 81.65% w/v iomeprol equivalent to 40% iodine or 400 mg iodine/ml.

**Pharmaceutical form** Solution for parenteral administration.

**Clinical particulars**
*Therapeutic indications:* X-ray contrast medium. For indications see table overleaf.

*Posology and method of administration:*
† repeat as necessary
‡ according to body size and age
Peripheral arteriography: adults 10–90 ml†; children ‡
Venography: adults 10–100 ml†, max 250 ml
– 10–50 ml upper extremity
– 50–100 ml lower extremity
Aortography: adults 50–80 ml; children ‡
Angiocardiography and left ventriculography: adults 30–80 ml max 250 ml; children ‡
Cerebral arteriography: adults 5–12 ml†; children 3–7 ml or ‡
Coronary arteriography: adults 4-10 ml per artery†
Visceral arteriography: adults 5–50 ml† or according to type of examination; max 250 ml; children ‡
Digital subtraction angiography:
*Intra arterial:*
cerebral: adults 6–10 ml per artery†

## Iomeron: Indications for use

| Indication | Iomeron 150 | 200 | 250 | 300 | 350 | 400 |
|---|---|---|---|---|---|---|
| peripheral arteriography | | | | ✓ | ✓ | ✓ |
| venography | | | ✓ | ✓ | ✓ | ✓ |
| aortography | | | | ✓ | ✓ | ✓ |
| angiocardiography and left ventriculography | | | | ✓ | ✓ | ✓ |
| cerebral arteriography | | | ✓ | ✓ | | |
| coronary arteriography | | | | | ✓ | ✓ |
| visceral arteriography | | | | ✓ | ✓ | ✓ |
| digital subtraction angiography | | | | | | |
| *Intra-arterial* | | | | | | |
| cerebral | ✓ | ✓ | | | | |
| visceral | ✓ | ✓ | ✓ | ✓ | | |
| peripheral | ✓ | ✓ | ✓ | ✓ | | |
| *Intravenous* | | | | | | |
| computed tomography enhancement | | | | | | |
| brain | | | ✓ | ✓ | ✓ | ✓ |
| body | | | ✓ | ✓ | ✓ | ✓ |
| urography | | | | | | |
| infusion | ✓ | | | | | |
| intravenous | | | ✓ | ✓ | ✓ | ✓ |
| ERCP (endoscopic retrograde cholangiopancreatography) | | | ✓ | ✓ | ✓ | ✓ |
| arthrography | | | ✓ | ✓ | | |
| dacryocystography | | | | ✓ | ✓ | ✓ |
| sialography | | | | ✓ | ✓ | ✓ |
| fistulography | | | | ✓ | ✓ | ✓ |
| galactography | | | | ✓ | ✓ | ✓ |
| hysterosalpingography | | ✓ | ✓ | | | |
| cavernosography | ✓ | ✓ | ✓ | | | |

visceral: adults 2–20 ml per artery†
  aorta 25–50 ml†
  both 250 ml max
peripheral: adults 5–10 ml per artery†, max 250 ml
*Intravenous:* adults 30–60 ml†, max 250 ml
Computed tomography:
brain: adults 50–150 ml; children‡
body: adults 40–150 ml, max 250 ml; children‡
Urography:
*Infusion:* adults 250 ml
*Intravenous:* adults 50–150 ml
  neonates 3–4.8 ml/kg
  babies 2.5–4 ml/kg
  children 1–2.5 ml/kg or †
Arthrography: adults 1–10 ml
ERCP: adults 12–30 ml
Dacryocystography: adults 3–8 ml
Sialography: adults 1–3 ml
Fistulography: adults 1–50 ml
Galactography: adults 0.2–1.5 ml
Hysterosalpingography: adults 8–20 ml
Cavernosography: adults 40–250 ml
In elderly patients the lowest effective dose should be used.

*Contra-indications:* Proven or suspected hypersensitivity to iodine containing preparations of this type.

*Special warnings and precautions for use:* A positive history of allergy, asthma or untoward reaction during previous similar investigations indicates a need for extra caution since, as with other contrast media, this product may provoke anaphylaxis or other manifestations of allergy with nausea, vomiting, dyspnoea, erythema, urticaria and hypotension. The benefits should clearly outweigh the risks in such patients and appropriate resuscitative measures should be immediately available. The primary treatments are as follows:

| Effect | Major Symptoms | Primary Treatment |
|---|---|---|
| Vasomotor effect | warmth | reassurance |
| | nausea/ vomiting | |
| Cutaneous | scattered hives severe urticaria | H₁ -antihistamines H₂ -antihistamines |
| Bronchospastic | wheezing | oxygen β₂ agonist inhalers |
| Anaphylactoid reaction | angioedema urticaria bronchospasm hypotension | oxygen iv fluids adrenergics (iv epinephrine) β₂ agonist inhalers antihistamines (H₁ and H₂ antagonist) corticosteroids |
| Hypotensive | hypotension | iv fluids |
| vagal reaction | bradycardia | iv atropine |

From Bush WH The Contrast Media Manual
Katzburg RW Ed. Williams and Wilkins
Baltimore 1992 Chapter 2 p23

Any severe disorders of water and electrolyte balance must be corrected prior to administration. Adequate hydration must be ensured particularly in patients with multiple myeloma, diabetes mellitus, polyuria, oliguria and hyperuricaemia; also in babies, small children and the elderly. Rehydration prior to use of iomeprol is recommended in patients with sickle cell disease.

Care should be taken in severe cardiac disease particularly heart failure and coronary artery disease. Reactions may include pulmonary oedema, haemodynamic changes, ischaemic ECG changes and arrhythmias.

In severe, chronic hypertension the risk of renal damage following administration of a contrast medium is increased. In these cases the risks associated with the catheterization procedure are increased. Care should be taken in renal impairment and diabetes. In these patients it is important to maintain hydration in order to minimise deterioration in renal function.

A combination of severe hepatic and renal impairment delays excretion of the contrast medium therefore such patients should not be examined unless absolutely necessary.

The product should be used with caution in patients with hyperthyroidism or goitre. Use may interfere with thyroid function tests.

Particular care is needed in patients with acute cerebral infarction, acute intracranial haemorrhage and any conditions involving damage to the blood brain barrier, brain oedema or acute demyelination. Convulsive seizures are more likely in patients with intracranial tumours or metastases or with a history of epilepsy.

Neurological symptoms related to cerebrovascular diseases, intracranial tumours/metastases or degenerative or inflammatory pathologies may be exacerbated.

There is an increased risk of transient neurological complications in patients with symptomatic cerebrovascular disease eg stroke, transient ischaemic attacks. Cerebral ischaemic phenomena may be caused by intravascular injection.

In acute and chronic alcoholism the increase in blood brain barrier permeability facilitates the passage of the contrast medium into cerebral tissue possibly leading to CNS disorders. There is a possibility of a reduced seizure threshold in alcoholics. In patients with a drug addiction there is also the possibility of a reduced seizure threshold.

Patients with phaeochromocytoma may develop severe, occasionally uncontrollable hypertensive crises during intravascular administration. Premedication with an alpha blocker is recommended in these patients. Pronounced excitement, anxiety and pain can cause side effects or intensify reaction to the contrast medium. A sedative may be given.

Since, on rare occasions, delayed reactions can occur, driving or operating machinery is not advisable for the first 24 hours after the procedure. Anticonvulsant therapy should not be discontinued. A normal diet should be maintained until the patient refrains from eating 2 hours before the procedure.

Non ionic contrast media have less anticoagulant activity in vitro than ionic media. Meticulous attention should therefore be paid to angiographic technique. Non ionic media should not be allowed to remain in contact with blood in a syringe, and intravascular catheters should be flushed frequently to minimise the risk of clotting which, rarely, has led to serious thromboembolic complications.

The presence of renal damage in diabetic patients is one of the factors predisposing to renal impairment following contrast media administration. This may precipitate lactic acidosis in patients who are taking metformin. As a precaution, metformin should be stopped 48 hours prior to examination and reinstated only after control of renal function has been regained.

Intravascular administration should be performed if possible with the patient lying down. The patient should be kept in this position and closely observed for at least 30 minutes after the procedure since the majority of severe incidents occur within this time.

*Children:* Infants up to 1 year, especially the newborn, are particularly susceptible to electrolyte imbalance and haemodynamic alterations. Care should be taken regarding the dosage used.

*Elderly:* There is special risk of reactions involving the circulatory system such that myocardial ischaemia, major arrhythmias and extrasystoles are more likely to occur. A combination of neurological disturbances and vascular pathologies present a serious complication. The probability of acute renal insufficiencies is higher in these people.

*Interaction with other medicaments and other forms of interaction:* Use of the product may interfere with tests for thyroid function. Vasopressor agents should not be administered prior to iomeprol.

*Pregnancy and lactation:* Animal studies have not indicated any harmful effects with respect to the course of pregnancy or on the health of the unborn or neonate. The safety of iomeprol in human pregnancy however has not been established. Therefore avoid in pregnancy unless there is no safer alternative.

No human data exist concerning the excretion of iomeprol in breast milk. Animal studies have demonstrated that the excretion of iomeprol in breast milk is similar to that of other contrast agents and that these compounds are only minimally absorbed by the gastrointestinal tract of the young. Adverse effects on the nursing infant are therefore unlikely to occur.

*Effects on ability to drive and use machines:* Driving or operating machinery is not advisable for the first 24 hours following the procedure in case of delayed reaction.

*Undesirable effects:* Common reactions are pain at the site of injection, sensations of heat and a disturbance of the taste sensation.

The product may occasionally provoke the following mild to moderate effects: generalised transient pain sensation, chills, fever, asthenia, dizziness, fainting, nausea, vomiting, sweating, pallor, dyspnoea, moderate hypotension, generalised and localised flushing, widespread erythema, oedema, agitation, headache, laryngeal oedema and nasal congestion, rashes ac1369companied by itching. Symptoms related to CNS disturbances are usually mild and short lived.

More severe effects involve the cardiovascular system. These are peripheral vasodilation with pronounced hypotension, hypertension, tachycardia or bradycardia, cyanosis, dyspnoea and circulatory collapse. More severe neurological effects can occur but only as a result of pre-existing pathologies.

A transient renal failure may arise, particularly in patients with a pre existing impairment of renal function. Haemorrhage and oedema may arise at the site of injection.

*Overdose:* The effects of overdose on the pulmonary and cardiovascular systems may become life-threatening. Treatment consists of support of the vital functions and prompt use of symptomatic therapy. Iomeprol does not bind to plasma or serum proteins and is therefore dialyzable.

### Pharmacological properties

*Pharmacodynamic properties:* Iomeprol is a low osmolality, non-ionic organic molecule with radioopacity conferred by an iodine content of 49% of the molecular weight. It is formulated for use as an intravascular/intracavitary contrast medium in concentrations of up to 400 mg iodine per ml. Even at this concentration the low viscosity allows delivery of high doses through thin catheters.

*Pharmacokinetic properties:* The pharmacokinetics of intravascularly administered iomeprol are similar to those of other iodinated contrast media and conform to a two-compartment model with a rapid distribution and a slower elimination phase. In healthy subjects, the mean distribution and elimination half-lives of iomeprol were 0.5 hours and 1.9 hours respectively.

Distribution volume is similar to that of extra cellular fluid. There is no significant serum protein binding and iomeprol is not metabolized.

Elimination is almost exclusively through the kid-

| | Iomeron 150 | Iomeron 200 | Iomeron 250 | Iomeron 300 | Iomeron 350 | Iomeron 400 |
|---|---|---|---|---|---|---|
| 50 ml | | | ✓ | ✓ | ✓ | ✓ |
| 75 ml | | ✓ | | ✓ | ✓ | ✓ |
| 100 ml | ✓ | | | ✓ | ✓ | ✓ |
| 150 ml | | | ✓ | | | |
| 200 ml | | | | ✓ | ✓ | ✓ |
| 250 ml | | | | | | ✓ |

neys (90% of the dose recovered in the urine within 96 hours of its administration) and is rapid (50% of an intravascularly administered dose within 2 hours).

**Pharmaceutical particulars**

*List of excipients:* trometamol, hydrochloric acid, water for injection.

*Incompatibilities:* No other drug should be mixed with the contrast medium.

*Shelf life:* Five years. Solutions not used in one examination session must be discarded.

*Special precautions for storage:* Store below 30°C. Protect from light.

*Nature and contents of container:* Colourless Type 1 glass bottles with rubber/aluminium cap (see table above).

*Instructions for use/handling:* Not relevant.

**Marketing authorisation number** 11648/0005-0010

**Date of approval/revision of SPC 7** July 1997

**Legal category** POM

## MULTIBIONTA* for INFUSION

**Presentation** A 10 ml ampoule of an aqueous solution containing:

*Active ingredients:*

| | |
|---|---|
| Vitamin A as palmitate PhEur | 10,000 iu |
| Thiamine hydrochloride PhEur | 50 mg |
| Riboflavin sodium phosphate BP | 10 mg |
| Nicotinamide BP | 100 mg |
| Pantothenol INN | 25 mg |
| Pyridoxine hydrochloride PhEur | 15 mg |
| Vitamin C | 500 mg |
| Alpha tocopheryl acetate PhEur | 5 mg |

*Inactive ingredients:* Polysorbate 80, propylene glycol, glycerol 85%, benzyl alcohol, DL-α-tocopherol, trometamol.

**Uses** Intravenous infusions of vitamins should only be considered when oral intake is impossible or inadequate.

*Infants:* Multibionta for infusion is indicated as part of a total parenteral feeding regimen in young children in the following conditions.

1. Protracted diarrhoea unresponsive to dietary treatment.
2. Renal failure.

*In older children and adults:*

1. Obstructing lesions of the gastro-intestinal tract.
2. Massive bowel resection.
3. Extensive burns.
4. Major trauma and severe infections.
5. Acute states of inflammatory bowel disease.
6. Severe uncontrolled malabsorptive states with undernutrition.
7. Disorders of swallowing as might occur in poliomyelitis, tetanus or following severe trauma.
8. Prolonged coma.

**Dosage and administration** The exact requirements of intravenously administered vitamins (particularly in sick infants) are not known. For adults 10 ml of Multibionta in an average daily dose should be added to a full infusion bottle containing not less than 250 ml of the infusion. For small children 2 ml per litre of the infusion fluid is adequate; alternatively the dose can be calculated as 0.15 ml/kilogram/24 hours. However, if preferred, the adult dose may be used with complete safety.

There is no preparation which contains all the essential vitamins in recommended amounts. It is, therefore, suggested that the following are given during prolonged intravenous nutrition in the dosage indicated.

| | |
|---|---|
| Folic acid | 0.1–0.5 mg/day |
| Vitamin B₁₂ | 100 micrograms/month |
| Vitamin D | 300 Units/day (administered IM as calciferol. 1 ml contains 300,000 Units) |
| Vitamin K | 3 mg twice weekly |
| Choline chloride | 500 mg/day (normally present in adequate amounts as cholinephosphatides in fat emulsions) |

Their compatibility with the carrier intravenous infusion should always be checked with the pharmacy before addition.

*Additional information:* The miscibility of 10 ml of Multibionta has been tested and it was found to be compatible with amino-acid solutions, carbohydrate solutions such as glucose at various concentrations, and fat solutions.

Although Multibionta is compatible with many infusion fluids, it is best introduced into separate normal saline or dextrose-saline mixtures.

**Contra-indications, warnings, etc** Rarely, intravenous thiamine may act as an allergen.

Multibionta must not be used in neonates, especially in immature preterm babies, because of the benzyl alcohol content.

Multibionta should only be given in pregnancy if there are compelling reasons because of the possible embryotoxic effect of propylene glycol.

In order to minimise possible loss of active substance in a mixture (masked incompatibility), it is recommended that solutions to which Multibionta is added should not be kept for longer than six hours. Amino-acid solutions or dextran solutions containing Multibionta should not be kept longer than one hour.

A mixture should be discarded if visible turbidity or crystallisation appear in the infusion solution.

Especial care should be taken to avoid exposure of a plastic bag or giving set containing Multibionta to direct sunlight.

**Pharmaceutical precautions** Should be stored at a temperature not exceeding 8°C.

**Legal category** POM.

**Package quantities** 10 ml ampoules in packs of 3.

**Further information** Nil.

**Product licence number** 0493/0076.

## NIOPAM*

**Presentation** Ampoules or bottles containing sterile aqueous solutions of varying strengths of iopamidol.

*Niopam 150:* contains a 30.62% w/v concentration of the active constituent equivalent to 15% iodine or 150 mg iodine/ml.

*Niopam 200:* contains a 40.8% w/v concentration of the active constituent equivalent to 20% iodine or 200 mg iodine/ml.

*Niopam 300:* contains a 61.2% w/v concentration of the active constituent equivalent to 30% iodine or 300 mg iodine/ml.

*Niopam 340:* contains a 69.4% w/v concentration of the active constituent equivalent to 34% iodine or 340 mg iodine/ml.

*Niopam 370:* contains a 75.5% w/v concentration of the active constituent equivalent to 37% iodine or 370 mg iodine/ml.

**Uses** X-ray contrast media for lumbar and thoracocervical myelography, cerebral angiography, peripheral arteriography and venography, angiocardiography, digital subtraction angiography, left ventriculography and coronary arteriography, aortography, selective visceral angiography, computer tomography enhancement, urography, arthrography.

**Dosage and administration** See table following.

*Elderly:* There are no special dosage requirements for elderly patients, but as with all medicines, the lowest effective dose should be used.

**Contra-indications, warnings, etc**

*Contra-indications:* Proven or suspected hypersensitivity to iodine containing preparations of this type.

*Warnings:* As with all other contrast media this product may provoke anaphylaxis or other manifestations of allergy with nausea, vomiting, dyspnoea, erythema, urticaria and hypotension. A positive history of allergy, asthma or untoward reaction during previous similar investigations indicates a need for extra caution; the benefit should clearly outweigh the risk in such patients. Appropriate resuscitative measures should be immediately available.

Care should be exercised in carrying out radiographic procedures with contrast media in patients with severe functional impairment of the liver or myocardium, severe systemic disease and in myelo-

matosis. In the latter condition patients should not be exposed to dehydration; similarly abnormalities of fluid or electrolyte balance should be corrected prior to use.

Care should also be exercised in patients with moderate to severe impairment of renal function (as reflected by a raised blood urea) or in diabetes. Substantial deterioration in renal function is minimised if the patient is well hydrated. Renal function parameters should be monitored after the procedure in these patients.

The presence of renal damage in diabetic patients is one of the factors predisposing to renal impairment following contrast media administration. This may precipitate lactic acidosis in patients who are taking metformin. As a precaution, metformin should be stopped 48 hours prior to examination and reinstated only after control of renal function has been regained.

Patients with severe hepato-renal insufficiency should not be examined unless absolutely indicated. Re-examination should be delayed for 5–7 days.

Special care should be exercised when this product is injected into the right heart or pulmonary artery in patients with pulmonary hypertension. Right heart angiography should be carried out only when absolutely indicated.

During intracardiac and/or coronary arteriography, ventricular arrhythmias may infrequently occur.

In patients who are known epileptics or have a history of epilepsy, anticonvulsant therapy should be maintained before and following myelographic procedures. In some instances, anticonvulsant therapy may be increased for 48 hours before the examination.

Use of this product may interfere with tests for thyroid function.

Niopam should be used with caution in patients with hyperthyroidism. It is possible that hyperthyroidism may recur in patients previously treated for Graves' disease.

Non-ionic contrast media have less anti-coagulant activity in-vitro than ionic media. Meticulous attention should therefore be paid to angiographic technique. Non-ionic media should not be allowed to remain in contact with blood in the syringe and intravascular catheters should be flushed frequently, to minimise the risk of clotting, which rarely has led to serious thromboembolic complications after procedures.

X-ray examination of women should if possible be conducted during the pre-ovulation phase of the menstrual cycle and should be avoided during pregnancy; also since it has not been demonstrated that Niopam is safe for use in pregnant women, it should be administered only if the procedure is considered essential by the physician.

No other drugs should be mixed with the contrast media.

*Side Effects:* Side effects are infrequent and normally mild and may consist of headache, nausea, vomiting, heat sensation, dyspnoea and hypotension. Skin rashes may occur in some patients.

Following use in myelography, water soluble nonionic contrast media have been reported to cause neurological side effects. These include rare cases of seizures, transient confusion or transient motor or sensory dysfunction. Meningism or meningitis have also been reported. The possibility of an infective meningitis should be considered. Headaches, dizziness, nausea and vomiting may also occasionally occur.

More severe reactions involving the cardiovascular system may call for emergency treatment; appropriate resuscitative measures should be immediately available.

**Pharmaceutical precautions** Protect the solution from light. Store at room temperature.

Discard if solution is not clear of particulate matter.

**Legal category** POM.

**Package quantities**

*Niopam 150:* Box containing 10×50 ml bottles
Box containing 10×100 ml bottles
Box containing 10×200 ml bottles

*Niopam 200:* Box containing 5×10 ml ampoules
Box containing 5×20 ml ampoules
Box containing 10×50 ml bottles

*Niopam 300:* Box containing 5×10 ml ampoules
Box containing 5×20 ml ampoules
Box containing 10×50 ml bottles
Box containing 10×70 ml bottles
Box containing 10×100 ml bottles
Box containing 10×200 ml bottles

*Niopam 340:* Box containing 10×50 ml bottles
Box containing 10×100 ml bottles

*Niopam 370:* Box containing 5×10 ml ampoules
Box containing 5×20 ml ampoules
Box containing 10×50 ml bottles
Box containing 10×70 ml bottles
Box containing 10×100 ml bottles
Box containing 10×200 ml bottles

**Further information** Niopam is a water soluble nonionic contrast media. The development of this compound has led to considerable reduction in general

*NIOPAM – Recommended Dosage Schedule*

| Procedure | Niopam product and dosage | |
|---|---|---|
| Lumbar Myelography | Niopam 200 | Adults 10–15 ml |
| | Niopam 300 | Adults 5–10 ml |
| Thoraco-Cervical Myelography | Niopam 200 | Adults 5–15 ml |
| | Niopam 300 | Adults 5–10 ml |
| Cerebral Angiography | Niopam 300 | Adults 5–10 ml† Children 5–7 ml‡ |
| Peripheral Arteriography | Niopam 300 Niopam 340 Niopam 370 | Adults 20–50 ml† Children ‡ |
| Venography | Niopam 300 | Adults 20–50 ml Children ‡ |
| Angiocardiography & Left Ventriculography | Niopam 340 Niopam 370 | Adults 30–80 ml Children ‡ |
| Coronary Arteriography | Niopam 340 Niopam 370 | Adults 4–8 ml per artery† |
| Aortography —retrograde | Niopam 340 Niopam 370 | Adults 30–80 ml |
| Selective Renal Arteriography | Niopam 340 Niopam 370 | Adults 5–10 ml Children ‡ |
| Selective Visceral Angiography: Hepatic Coeliac Superior Mesenteric Inferior Mesenteric | Niopam 340 Niopam 370 | Adults 30–70 ml 40–70 ml 25–70 ml 5–30 ml |
| Digital Subtraction Angiography Intra-arterial injection | Niopam 150 | Adults 1–40 ml Children 0.5–0.75 ml/kg |
| Intra-venous injection | Niopam 340 Niopam 370 | Adults 30–50 ml Children 0.5–0.75 ml/kg‡ |
| Left ventriculography | Niopam 340 Niopam 370 Niopam 150 | Adults 25 ml Children 1.0–1.5 ml/kg |
| Selective coronary arteriography by intra-arterial DSA | Niopam 340 Niopam 370 | Adults 2–5 ml |
| Computer Tomography Enhancement | Niopam 200 Niopam 300 Niopam 340 | Adults *Brain Scanning* 50–100 ml *Whole Body Scanning* 40–100 ml |
| Intravenous Urography | Niopam 300 Niopam 340 Niopam 370 | Adults 40–80 ml In severe renal failure the usual high dose methods should be employed (up to 1.5 ml/kg) Children 1–2.5 ml/kg or ‡ |
| Arthrography | Niopam 300 Niopam 340 | Adults 1–10 ml According to joint being examined. |

† Repeat as necessary.
‡ According to body size and age.

toxicity particularly with regard to vascular endothelium and nervous tissues.

**Product licence numbers**
Niopam 150  0493/0119
Niopam 200  0493/0065
Niopam 300  0493/0066
Niopam 340  0493/0131
Niopam 370  0493/0067

## NUTRIZYM* GR

**Presentation** Hard gelatin capsules with opaque olive green cap and orange body each containing Pancreatin BP 300 mg with not less than the following activities:
Lipase   10,000 BP-U
Protease  650 BP-U
Amylase  10,000 BP-U

**Uses** Fibrocystic disease of the pancreas, chronic pancreatitis, steatorrhoea and other pancreatic deficiency states.

**Dosage and administration**
*Adults:* 1–2 capsules with meals. In severe cases dosage may be increased.

*Children:* 1–2 capsules to be taken with meals and further capsules may be taken according to the degree of exocrine sufficiency.

Colonic damage has been reported in patients with cystic fibrosis taking in excess of 10,000 units of lipase/kg/day. The dose of Nutrizym GR should usually not exceed this dose.

Capsules should be swallowed whole with water. Where swallowing of capsules proves to be difficult,

the capsule may be opened and the pellets sprinkled on soft foods which do not require chewing. When Nutrizym GR is mixed with foods in this way, the resulting mixture should not be allowed to stand for more than one hour prior to use.

**Contra-indications, warnings, etc**
*Contra-indications:* Known hypersensitivity to active ingredient (porcine pancreatin).

*Precautions:* Hyperuricaemia and hyperuricosuria have been reported to occur in cystic fibrosis patients; pancreatin extracts contain a very small amount of purine which might, in high doses, contribute to this condition.

Patients who are taking or have been given in excess of 10,000 units of lipase/kg/day are at risk of developing colon damage. Abdominal symptoms (not usually experienced by the patient) or changes in abdominal symptoms should be reviewed to exclude the possibility of colonic damage – especially if the patient is taking in excess of 10,000 units of lipase/kg/day.

*Use in pregnancy:* Safety in pregnancy has not been established.

*Side-effects:* Very rarely hypersensitivity reactions may occur. As with any pancreatin extract, high doses may cause buccal and perianal irritation, in rare cases amounting to inflammation.

Stricture of the ileo-caecum and large bowel and colitis have been reported in children with cystic fibrosis taking pancreatic enzymes.

**Pharmaceutical precautions** Store below 25°C in tightly closed containers.

**Legal category** P.

**Package quantities** Containers of 100 capsules.

**Further information** Each Nutrizym GR capsule contains enteric coated pellets of pancreatin extract thus giving maximum enzymatic activity in the gastrointestinal tract.

**Product licence number** 0493/0121.

## NUTRIZYM* 10

**Presentation** Hard gelatin capsules with opaque red cap and yellow body each containing enteric coated minitablets of Pancreatin BP 155 mg with not less than the following activities:
Lipase   10,000 BP-Units
Amylase  9,000 BP-Units
Protease  500 BP-Units

**Uses** Pancreatic exocrine insufficiency as in fibrocystic disease of the pancreas and chronic pancreatitis.

**Dosage and administration**
*Adults and children:* 1–2 capsules with meals and 1 capsule with snacks.

Since the individual response to pancreatin supplements is variable, the number of capsules taken may need to be titrated to the individual according to symptoms at the discretion of the physician.

Dose increases, if required, should be added slowly with careful monitoring of response and symptomatology.

Colonic damage has been reported in patients with cystic fibrosis taking in excess of 10,000 units of lipase/kg/day. The dose of Nutrizym 10 should usually not exceed this dose.

Capsules should be swallowed whole with water. Where swallowing of capsules proves to be difficult, the minitablets may be removed and taken with water or mixed with a small amount of soft food and swallowed immediately without chewing.

It is important to ensure adequate hydration of patients at all times whilst treating with Nutrizym 10.

**Contra-indications, warnings, etc**
*Contra-indications:* Known hypersensitivity to porcine pancreatin or any of the excipients.

Safety in pregnancy and during lactation has not been established, therefore use of Nutrizym 10 during pregnancy and lactation is not recommended.

*Precautions:* Hyperuricaemia and hyperuricosuria have been reported to occur in cystic fibrosis patients; pancreatin extracts contain a small amount of purine which might, in high doses, contribute to this condition.

Patients who are taking or who have been given in excess of 10,000 units of lipase/kg/day are at risk of developing colon damage.

Abdominal symptoms (not usually experienced by the patient) or changes in abdominal symptoms should be reviewed to exclude the possibility of colonic damage – especially if the patient is taking in excess of 10,000 units of lipase/kg/day.

*Side-effects:* Stricture of the ileo-caecum and large bowel, and colitis have been reported in children with cystic fibrosis taking pancreatic enzymes. Hypersensitivity reactions may occur. As with any pancreatin extract, high doses may cause buccal and perianal irritation, in some cases resulting in inflammation.

*Overdose:* Inappropriately large doses could result in abdominal discomfort, nausea, vomiting and perianal irritation or inflammation.

**Pharmaceutical precautions** Store below 25°C in tightly closed containers.

**Legal category** P.

**Package quantities** Containers of 100 capsules.

**Further information** Each Nutrizym 10 capsule contains enteric coated minitablets of pancreatin extract with identical potency of enzymes in each coated minitablet as in Nutrizym 22, which resist gastric inactivation thus giving maximal enzymatic activity in the upper small intestine.

Inactive ingredients: castor oil, silicon dioxide, magnesium stearate, sodium carboxymethylcellulose, microcrystalline cellulose, simethicone emulsion, methacrylic acid copolymer, talc and triethyl citrate. The gelatin capsules contain titanium dioxide, iron oxide red and iron oxide yellow.

**Product licence number** 0493/0157.

## NUTRIZYM* 22

**Presentation** Hard gelatin capsules with opaque red cap and yellow body each containing enteric coated minitablets of Pancreatin BP 340 mg with not less than the following activities:
Lipase   22,000 BP-Units
Amylase  19,800 BP-Units
Protease  1,100 BP-Units

This activity is higher than that of standard preparations.

**Uses** Pancreatic exocrine insufficiency as in fibrocystic disease of the pancreas and chronic pancreatitis.

**Dosage and administration**
*Adults and children:* 1–2 capsules with meals and 1 capsule with snacks. Nutrizym 22 should not be used in children aged 15 years and under with cystic fibrosis.

Since the individual response to pancreatin supplements is variable, the number of capsules taken may need to be titrated to the individual according to symptoms. Colonic damage has been reported in children with cystic fibrosis taking in excess of 10,000 units of lipase/kg/day. The dose of Nutrizym 22 should usually not exceed this dose.

Where a patient is already receiving a lower unit dose enteric coated pancreatin supplement, i.e. a product containing 10,000 BP units lipase, then Nutrizym 22 may be substituted at $\frac{1}{2}$ of the number of capsules normally consumed with the previous preparation. Further dose increases, if required, should be added slowly with careful monitoring of response and symptomatology.

Capsules should be swallowed whole with water. Where swallowing of capsules proves to be difficult, the minitablets may be removed and taken with water or mixed with a small amount of soft food and swallowed immediately without chewing.

It is important to ensure adequate hydration of patients at all times whilst treating with Nutrizym 22.

**Contra-indications, warnings, etc**
*Contra-indications:* Children aged 15 years and under with cystic fibrosis. Known hypersensitivity to porcine pancreatin or any of the excipients.

*Precautions and warnings:* Safety in pregnancy and during lactation has not been established, therefore use of Nutrizym 22 during pregnancy and lactation is not recommended.

Hyperuricaemia and hyperuricosuria have been reported to occur in cystic fibrosis patients. Pancreatin extracts contain a small amount of purine which might, in high doses, contribute to this condition.

Abdominal symptoms (not usually experienced by the patient) or changes in abdominal symptoms should be reviewed to exclude the possibility of colonic damage – especially if the patient is taking in excess of 10,000 units of lipase/kg/day. All patients should be reviewed regularly.

Until the risk of bowel stricture has been fully investigated patients with cystic fibrosis should not be prescribed this product unless there are special reasons for doing so. Patients who continue to use it should be reviewed regularly.

*Side-effects:* Hypersensitivity reactions may occur. Stricture of the ileo-caecum and large bowel, and colitis have been reported in children with cystic fibrosis taking pancreatic enzymes. As with any pancreatin extract, high doses may cause buccal and perianal irritation, in some cases resulting in inflammation.

*Overdose:* Inappropriately large doses could result in abdominal discomfort, nausea, vomiting and perianal irritation or inflammation.

**Pharmaceutical precautions** Store below 25°C in tightly closed containers.

**Legal category** POM.

**Package quantities** Containers of 100 capsules.

**Further information** Each Nutrizym 22 capsule contains enteric coated minitablets of pancreatin extract which resist gastric inactivation thus giving maximal enzymatic activity in the upper small intestine.

**Product licence number** 0493/0158.

## OPTIMAX* ▼

**Presentation** Optimax Tablets: White capsule shaped tablets, Optimax engraved on one side with a break line on the reverse. Each tablet contains 500 mg L-tryptophan.

**Uses** Optimax should only be used by hospital specialists in patients who have had severe and disabling depressive illness continuously for more than 2 years, only after an adequate trial of standard antidepressant drug treatments, and only as an adjunct to other antidepressant medication.

Prior to supply of Optimax, the prescriber and patient must be registered with the Optimax Information and Clinical Support (OPTICS) Unit, E Merck Pharmaceuticals (see Further Information).

**Dosage and administration**
*Adults:* The usual dose is two tablets, three times daily; for some patients up to 6 g L-tryptophan may be required. A lower dose may be appropriate in the elderly, especially where there is evidence of renal or hepatic impairment.

*Children:* Not recommended.

**Contra-indications, warnings, etc**
*Contra-indications:* Patients with a previous history of eosinophilia myalgia syndrome (EMS) following the use of L-tryptophan. This syndrome which is a multisystem disorder, is characterised by raised eosinophils ($>1.0\times10^9$/1), and severe myalgia in the absence of either an infectious or neoplastic cause.

*Warnings:* Eosinophilia Myalgia Syndrome (EMS) has been reported in association with the use of oral L-tryptophan – containing products. It is a multisystem disorder which is usually reversible but rarely, fatal. Various investigations have not as yet identified the aetiological factors precisely.

It is recommended therefore, that patients who are receiving L-tryptophan should be kept under close and regular surveillance with particular attention to monitoring eosinophil levels, haematological changes and muscle symptomatology. If the patient develops any of the symptoms of EMS, treatment with L-tryptophan should be stopped and the symptoms investigated further.

The possible interaction between L-tryptophan and 5HT reuptake inhibitors could lead to the 'serotonin syndrome' characterised by a combination of agitation, restlessness and gastro-intestinal symptoms including diarrhoea. Combinations with 5HT reuptake inhibitors should only be used with care (see Interactions).

Safety in pregnancy or lactation has not been established.

*Precautions:* Caution should be exercised with patients who may have experienced some, but not all of the symptoms of EMS after taking L-tryptophan. Treatment with L-tryptophan should be withheld and the symptoms investigated until the possibility of EMS can be excluded. These symptoms have been reported to include eosinophilia, arthralgia or myalgia, fever, dyspnoea, neuropathy, peripheral oedema, and skin lesions which can include sclerosis or papular and urticarial lesions.

*Drug interactions:* Where L-tryptophan is combined with an MAO Inhibitor the side effects of the latter may be enhanced. Use of L-tryptophan in combination with a 5-HT reuptake inhibitor has the potential for increasing the severity of the adverse effects of the latter and could lead to serotonin syndrome (see Warnings).

In patients taking L-tryptophan in conjunction with phenothiazines or benzodiazepines there have been isolated reports of sexual disinhibition.

*Adverse effects:* L-tryptophan may produce drowsiness. Patients who drive or operate machinery should be warned of the possible hazard.

In some patients, L-tryptophan may cause a slight feeling of nausea which usually disappears within 2 or 3 days. Such nausea can be minimised by giving L-tryptophan after food. Other adverse reactions include headache and lightheadedness.

*Overdosage:* Drowsiness and vomiting may occur; supportive measures should be employed.

**Pharmaceutical precautions** Store in a cool dry place.

**Legal category** POM.

**Package quantities** Containers of 84 (OP).

**Further information** Optimax can only be supplied once the prescriber and patient have been registered with the Optimax Information and Clinical Support (OPTICS) Unit. Following supply of the product, the prescriber will be contacted and asked to provide particular information relating to therapy. Further contact will be made at 3 months, and 6 monthly thereafter. All orders for Optimax will be dealt with through the OPTICS Unit. Ordering and other information is available from the OPTICS Unit, E Merck Pharmaceuticals, Harrier House, High Street, West Drayton, Middlesex UB7 7QC. Tel: 0345 626902. Fax: 01895 452297.

**Product licence number** 0493/5900

## OSTRAM* 1.2 g

**Presentation:** Ostram sachets contain a powder for the preparation of a lime flavoured drink containing 3.3 g tricalcium phosphate equivalent to 1.2 g calcium.
*Inactive ingredients:* sodium saccharin, sodium carboxymethylcellulose, natural lime flavouring.

**Uses** Calcium supplement for the treatment of osteoporosis (post-menopausal, senile and under corticosteroid therapy), and for the treatment of calcium deficiencies during growth, pregnancy or lactation.

**Dosage and administration**
*Adults and elderly:* One sachet to be taken daily, dispersed in water.

**Contra-indications, warnings, etc**
*Contra-indications:* Hypercalciuria, calcium lithiasis, tissue calcification, chronic renal insufficiency, prolonged immobilisation accompanied by hypercalciuria and/or hypercalcaemia.

*Precautions:* Patients having prolonged treatment should undergo regular checks of urinary calcium; if this exceeds 200 mg per 24 hours, treatment must be reduced or stopped. Patients treated concomitantly with high doses of vitamin D should undergo weekly checks on blood and urinary calcium.

*Interactions:* In cases of treatment with oral tetracyclines, the dose of Ostram should be taken at least 3 hours later, in order to avoid possible interference with the absorption of tetracycline. Thiazide diuretics reduce urinary calcium excretion so the risk of hypercalcaemia should be considered.

*Use in pregnancy and lactation:* Epidemiological studies have shown no evidence of hazard to the foetus; however, the likelihood of hypercalcaemia is increased in pregnant women in whom calcium and vitamin D are co-administered. Although supplemental calcium may be excreted in the breast milk, the concentration is unlikely to be sufficient to produce any adverse effects in the neonate.

*Side-effects:* Mild gastrointestinal disturbance; if thirst, polyuria, nausea, vomiting, dehydration, arterial hypertension, vascular disorders or constipation are experienced this might indicate hypercalcaemia.

*Overdose:* This is manifested by thirst, polyuria, nausea, vomiting, dehydration, arterial hypertension, vascular disorders, constipation. Administration of calcium, and vitamin D, should cease and the patient should be hydrated. Depending on the extent of the hypercalcaemia, loop diuretics, corticosteroids, calcitonin and peritoneal dialysis (alone or in association), should be administered.

**Pharmaceutical precautions** None.

**Legal category** P

**Package quantities** Boxes of 30 sachets.

**Further information** Nil

**Product licence number** 10144/0002

## SEPTOPAL* CHAINS

**Presentation** Methylmethacrylate-methylacrylate copolymer (PMMA) beads (7 mm in diameter) each containing gentamicin sulphate 7.5 mg (corresponding to 4.5 mg of gentamicin base) and 20 mg of zirconium dioxide as X-ray medium.

Chains consisting of 10 or 30 beads threaded on multiple-thread surgical wire.

**Uses** Gentamicin is a proven broad spectrum antibiotic active against both gram-positive and gram-negative organisms. Following insertion of the Chains, gentamicin is released gradually from the PMMA beads over a prolonged period and the high bactericidal concentrations of the antibiotic reached at the site of infection enable the infection to be controlled, or provide protection against infection when used prophylactically.

Septopal Chains are indicated for:

Short term and longer term therapy in bone infection, e.g. osteomyelitis, infected pseudoarthroses, infected osteosyntheses.

Short term preventive treatment of potentially infected bone injuries.

Short term prevention and therapy of soft tissue infections associated with abdominoperineal resections; operations on the small or large bowel. Other therapeutic indications for use include bacterial peritonitis, infection associated with cholecystectomies, infective fistulae, infected vascular grafts, soft tissue abscesses.

**Dosage and administration**
*Administration:* Septopal Chains are implanted in the cavity resulting from thorough surgical removal of infected tissue and/or sequestrated bone or that remaining after operation in the sacral cavity. The chains are laid in the cavity in such a way as to facilitate easy removal.

Septopal Chains may be used as follows:

*1. Bone Infection*
(a) *Short term application:* For the implantation of Chains, it is recommended to take into account the direction in which the Chain will later be pulled out and to let the last bead anchored by a loose suture, project above skin level through a separate stab incision in order that the Chain may be removed by careful, steady traction a few beads at a time daily. The Chains are in general removed within 10–14 days

following insertion and preferably not more than 10 days after the operation.

Where there is evidence of persisting local infection beyond 5 days post-operatively, it is recommended that the Chain be removed and the cause of infection determined prior to recommending further antibacterial therapy.

The less the Chains are fixed to connective tissue, the easier it is to remove them; this procedure is thus also less painful and more comfortable for the patient.

If the beads become fixed to connective tissue to an advanced extent, or if the traction on the beads is not adapted to the tissue conditions, one or several beads may rarely detach themselves from the multistranded wire or, in exceptional circumstances the wire may break on the removal of the Chain. In such an event one should generally try to remove the single beads (together with the remaining wire). Should, however, extensive surgical procedures be necessary, the single beads may be left in the body, taking into consideration the comparative risk of reoperation. For the above reasons the surgeons should count the beads on their removal as a check.

*(b) Longer Term Application:* This may be as above or if circumstances require it, the Chains may be implanted completely, and removed by reoperation up to 3 months later. The length of time the Chains are left in situ prior to secondary intervention will depend on the orthopaedic procedure. Inserted Chains will be completely enclosed by primary wound closure. Control of local infection allows subsequent surgical procedures, e.g. cancellous bone grafting.

*2. Soft tissue infections (Short term applications only):* The insertion of chains is carried out as described under 1a above. In this indication, the chains are best removed by the sixth and the very latest by the tenth day after the operation. In most cases it is advised that the chains are withdrawn gradually a few beads at a time daily from about the second post insertion day.

In considering wound closure/drainage it should be remembered that excess drainage will dilute the gentamicin concentration at the site of infection so, if possible, primary wound closure should always be employed. Local circumstances and degree of inflammation however should be considered.

An overflow drain may be employed only when considered necessary. Suction drainage is not employed but may be temporarily used in cases of obstructed wound secretion flow.

Toxic effects due to the antibiotics are not anticipated since after use of Septopal Chains, barely detectable systemic gentamicin concentrations (no more than 0.5 micrograms/ml) are found in the serum for up to 4 days postoperatively following insertion of the Chains.

*Dosage:* The number of Chains used will depend upon the size of the cavity. Usually 1–3 Chains are inserted but up to 5 have been used.

**Contra-indications, warnings, etc** There is no absolute contra-indication other than established intolerance of gentamicin.

Septopal Chains should not be used concurrently in apposition to metal-containing implants because of the theoretical possibility of surgical wire and implant corrosion. Septopal Chains should be removed prior to implant of a metal prosthesis.

Since the beads are strung on surgical wire containing chrome and nickel, there is a potential for local sensitivity reactions to these metals.

Gentamicin crosses the placenta barrier and may cause ototoxicity in the foetus although no problems in clinical use have been positively identified. Implantation of Septopal Chains results in only a transient, barely detectable plasma concentration of gentamicin which is well below toxic levels therefore, no ototoxic effects on the foetus are to be expected. Nevertheless, it is recommended that the product should not be used in pregnancy.

Septopal Chains should not be used alone in those situations where culture of wound secretion reveals the presence of anaerobic bacteria, or organisms which could be insensitive to gentamicin therapy. In these instances, additional systemic therapy with an appropriate antibiotic should be used.

Septopal may be used in all orthopaedic surgical procedures where gentamicin sensitive organisms are found to be present from routine bacteriological screening. Where resistant organisms are encountered to the standard 10 microgram disc test, a MIC determination is recommended. In view of the high bactericidal gentamicin concentration at the infection site, organisms found resistant to the standard 10 microgram sensitivity disc screen may in fact be sensitive and therefore results of such screening may not give a true reflection of clinical effectiveness.

In soft tissue, the chains should not be implanted intra-peritoneally.

*Young and elderly:* There is no evidence to suggest that use of Septopal Chains is either nephrotoxic or ototoxic. Nevertheless, for those patients who have moderate to severe impairment of renal function and when Septopal therapy is desirable, monitoring of renal state is advised.

**Pharmaceutical precautions** Store at room temperature – do not freeze.

Resterilisation of Septopal Chains should not be attempted under any circumstances.

**Legal category** POM.

**Package quantities** One Chain consists of 10 or 30 beads threaded on surgical wire in a sterile inner sachet (peel-off pack). Packs of 1 chain of 10 beads. Packs of 1 Chain of 30 beads. Packs of 5 Chains of 30 beads.

**Further information** Septopal Chains have been sterilised in ethylene oxide. They are contained in a triple sachet. The two outer sachets are opened (aluminium covering followed by the non-sterile peel-off pack) and the chain in the inner, sterile sachet is then removed under aseptic conditions.

Gentamicin is released in bactericidal concentrations at the site of infection with negligible systemic spread. Granulation tissue grows into the hollow spaces between the beads during the healing process, the flow of secretion is not inhibited and the biomechanics of the bone are not changed. Local control of infection lessens the risk of secondary infection developing with subsequent bone grafting.

**Product licence number** 0493/0091.

## SEPTOPAL* MINICHAINS

**Presentation** Methylmethacrylate-methylacrylate copolymer (PMMA) oval beads (approximately 3×5 mm) each containing gentamicin sulphate BP 2.8 mg (corresponding to 1.7 mg of gentamicin base) and 3.9 mg of zirconium dioxide as X-ray contrast medium.

Chains consisting of 10 beads threaded on multiple-thread surgical wire. The chain is approximately 10 cm long.

**Uses** Gentamicin is a proven broad spectrum antibiotic active against both gram-positive and gram-negative organisms. Following insertion of the chains, gentamicin is released gradually from the PMMA beads over a prolonged period and the high bactericidal concentrations of the antibiotic reached at the site of infection enable the infection to be controlled, or provide protection against infection when used prophylactically.

Septopal Minichains are used in bone infections together with conventional surgical methods, where Septopal Chains are too large for the anatomical conditions. They are indicated for:

Short and longer term therapy in bone infection, e.g. osteomyelitis, infected pseudoarthroses, infected osteosyntheses.

Short term preventative treatment of potentially infected bone injuries.

Surgical fields for which Septopal Minichains have been expressly developed are hand and foot surgery, face and jaw surgery and paediatrics.

**Dosage and administration**
*Administration:* Septopal Minichains are designed exclusively for temporary application. They are implanted in the cavity resulting from thorough surgical removal of sequestrated bone and infected tissue. The chains are laid in the cavity in such a way as to facilitate easy removal.

Septopal Minichains may be used as follows:

*(a) Short term:* For the implantation of chians, it is recommended that account should be taken of the direction in which the chain will later be pulled out and that the last bead, anchored by a loose suture, is allowed to project above skin level through a separate stab incision in order that the chain may be removed by careful, steady, traction a few beads at a time daily.

The chains are in general totally removed by 10–14 days following insertion and preferably no more than 10 days after the operation. Where there is evidence of persisting local infection beyond 4 days post operatively, it is recommended that the chain be removed and the cause of infection determined prior to recommending further anti-bacterial therapy.

The less the chains are fixed to connective tissue, the easier it is to remove them and the more comfortable the procedure is for the patient.

If the beads become fixed to connective tissue to a great extent, or if the traction of the beads is not adapted to the tissue conditions, then there is a small possibility that one or several beads may become detached from the wire or, inexceptional circumstances, the wire may break on removal of the chain. In such an event one should generally try to remove the single beads (together with the remaining wire). Should, however, extensive surgery be necessary then the risk of reoperation should be considered carefully. In high risk patients, it may be preferable to leave the beads in situ permanently. For the above reasons, the surgeon should count the beads on their removal as a check.

*(b) Longer term application:* This may be as above or if circumstances require it, the chains may be implanted completely, and removed by reoperation up to 3 months later. The latter applies particularly to oral surgery.

The length of time the chains are left in situ prior to secondary intervention will depend on the orthopaedic procedure.

Inserted chains will be completely enclosed by primary wound closure. Control of local infection allows subsequent surgical procedure, e.g. cancellous bone grafting.

In considering wound closure/drainage it should be remembered that excess drainage will dilute gentamicin concentration at the site of infection so, if possible, primary would closure should always be employed. Local circumstances and degree of inflammation however should be considered.

An overflow drain may be employed only when considered necessary. Suction drainage should not be employed but may be temporarily used in cases of obstructed wound secretion flow.

Toxic effects due to the antibiotic are not anticipated since after use of Septopal Minichains, barely detectable plasma gentamicin concentrations (no more than 0.42 micrograms/ml) are found in systemic circulation for up to 4 days postoperatively.

There is no distinguishing factor between doses for the young, adults and elderly since the number of chains used depends on the size of the cavity in individual cases and on the clinical conditions at the site of infection.

*Dosage:* The number of chains used will depend upon the size of the cavity.

**Contra-indications, warnings, etc** There is no absolute contra-indication other than established intolerance of gentamicin and hypersensitivity to chrome and nickel.

Septopal Minichains should not be used concurrently in apposition to metal-containing implants because of the theoretical possibility of surgical wire and implant corrosion. Septopal Minichains should be removed prior to implant of a metal prosthesis.

Because the beads are strung on surgical wire containing chrome and nickel, there is a potential for local sensitivity to these metals.

Granulation tissue grows into the hollow spaces between the beads during the healing process. This may cause difficulties at the time of removal.

Gentamicin crosses the placenta barrier and may cause ototoxicity in the foetus although no problems in clinical use have been positively identified. Implantation of Septopal Minichains results in only a transient, barely detectable plasma concentration of gentamicin (no more than 0.42 micrograms/ml) which is well below toxic levels therefore, no ototoxic effects on the foetus are to be expected. Nevertheless, it is recommended that the product should not be used in pregnancy.

Septopal Minichains should not be used alone in those situations where culture of wound secretion reveals the presence of anaerobic bacteria, or organisms which could be insensitive to gentamicin therapy. In these instances, additional systemic therapy with an appropriate antibiotic should be used.

Septopal Minichains may be used in all orthopaedic surgical procedures where gentamicin sensitive organisms are found to be present from routine bacteriological screening. Where resistant organisms are encountered to the standard 10 microgram disc test, a MIC determination is recommended. In view of the high bactericidal gentamicin concentration at the infection site, organisms found resistant to the standard 10 microgram sensitivity disc screen may in fact be sensitive and therefore results of such screening may not give a true reflection of clinical effectiveness.

*Young and elderly:* There is no evidence to suggest that use of Septopal Minichains is either nephrotoxic or ototoxic. Nevertheless, for those patients who have moderate to severe impairment of renal function and when Septopal therapy is desirable, monitoring of renal state and plasma gentamicin levels is advised.

**Pharmaceutical precautions** Store at room temperature—do not freeze.

Resterilisation of the chains should not be attempted under any circumstances.

**Legal category** POM.

**Package quantities** One chain consisting of 10 threaded on surgical wire in a sterile inner sachet (peel-off pack).

Packs of 1 Chain of 10 beads.

**Further information** Septopal Minichains have been sterilised in ethylene oxide. They are contained in a triple sachet. The two outer sachets are opened (aluminium covering followed by the non-sterile peel-off pack) and the chain in the inner, sterile sachet is then removed under aseptic conditions.

Gentamicin is released locally in bactericidal concentrations at the site of infection with negligible systemic spread. Granulation tissue grows into the hollow spaces between the beads during the healing process, the flow of secretion is not inhibited and the biomechanics of the bone are not changed. Local control of infection lessens the risk of secondary infection developing with subsequent bone grafting.

**Product licence number** 0493/0138.

# UNGUENTUM MERCK*

**Presentation** Unguentum Merck is a stable emulsion system with a uniform distribution of fat and water (ambiphilic); thus it combines the properties of a) an oil in water emulsion (cream) and b) a water in oil emulsion (ointment), for use on dry or weeping conditions of the skin.

*Composition:* Dispersed silicic acid; liquid paraffin; white soft paraffin; cetostearyl alcohol; polysorbate-40; glyceryl monostearate; saturated neutral oils; sorbic acid; propylene glycol; purified water, sodium hydroxide. Fat content: about 60%. Water content: about 40%.

**Uses** Unguentum Merck is to be used as a diluent for various topical corticosteroid formulations in those instances where a lower strength preparation is considered desirable by the physician and as a general base for extemporaneous dispensing.

Unguentum Merck has emollient properties and is recommended for the symptomatic treatment of dermatitis, nappy rash, ichthyosis, eczema, protection of raw and abraded skin areas, pruritus and related conditions where dry scaly skin is a problem, and as a pre-bathing emollient for dry/eczematous skin, to alleviate drying effects.

**Dosage and administration** *Administration:* A thin application of the cream should be gently massaged into the skin three times daily or at appropriate intervals.

When used as a protective cream Unguentum Merck should be applied sparingly to the affected areas of the skin before, or immediately after, exposure to a potentially harmful factor.

**Contra-indications, warnings, etc** Unguentum Merck should not be used for the treatment of patients sensitive to any of the ingredients.

**Pharmaceutical precautions** No special requirements.

**Legal category** GSL.

**Package quantities** Tubes of 50 g, 100 g. Jar of 500 g. 200 ml dispenser.

**Further information** Unguentum Merck contains no common allergens such as lanolin or parabens.

**Product licence number** 0493/0013.

*Trade Mark

# Merck Sharp & Dohme Limited
Hertford Road
Hoddesdon
Hertfordshire EN11 9BU

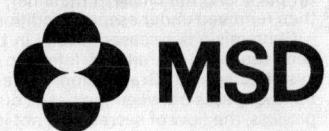

## ALDOMET*

**Presentation** Yellow, film-coated tablets containing Methyldopa PhEur equivalent to the following amounts of anhydrous methyldopa: 125 mg (marked 'ALDOMET MSD 135'), 250 mg (marked 'ALDOMET MSD 401'), or 500 mg (marked 'ALDOMET MSD 516').

Fruit-flavoured, oral suspension containing 250 mg of methyldopa per 5 ml. The oral suspension contains sodium metabisulphite as preservative

Injection, ampoules containing 50 mg Methyldopate Hydrochloride BP per millilitre, as a colourless solution. The injection contains sodium metabisulphite as preservative.

**Uses** Hypertension. Aldomet Injection is indicated for hypertension when parenteral medication is required. Treatment of acute hypertensive crises may be initiated with Aldomet Injection when an immediate effect is not necessary.

*Mode of action:* The antihypertensive effect of methyldopa is probably due to its metabolism to alphamethylnoradrenaline, which lowers arterial pressure by stimulation of central inhibitory alpha-adrenergic receptors, false neurotransmission, and/or reduction of plasma renin activity.

**Dosage and administration** *Oral therapy – Adults: Initial dosage:* Usually 250 mg two or three times a day, for two days.

*Adjustment:* Usually adjusted at intervals of not less than two days, until an adequate response is obtained. The maximum recommended daily dosage is 3 g.

Many patients experience sedation for two or three days when therapy with Aldomet is started or when the dose is increased. When increasing the dosage, therefore, it may be desirable to increase the evening dose first.

*General considerations:* Methyldopa is largely excreted by the kidney, and patients with impaired renal function may respond to smaller doses.

Withdrawal of Aldomet is followed by return of hypertension, usually within 48 hours. This is not complicated generally by an overshoot of blood pressure.

Therapy with Aldomet may be initiated in most patients already on treatment with other antihypertensive agents by terminating these antihypertensive medications gradually if required (see manufacturer's recommendations on stopping these drugs). Following such previous antihypertensive therapy, Aldomet should be limited to an initial dose of not more than 500 mg daily and increased as required at intervals of not less than two days.

A thiazide may be added at any time during methyldopa therapy and is recommended if therapy has not been started with a thiazide or if effective control of blood pressure cannot be maintained on 2.0 g of methyldopa daily.

Aldomet may also be used concomitantly with the combination of amiloride hydrochloride and hydrochlorothiazide (such as Moduretic*) or beta-blocking agents, such as timolol maleate (Blocadren*).

When methyldopa is given to patients on other antihypertensives the dose of these agents may need to be adjusted to effect a smooth transition.

*Oral therapy – Children:* Initial dosage is based on 10 mg/kg of body weight daily in 2–4 oral doses. The daily dosage then is increased or decreased until an adequate response is achieved. The maximum dosage is 65 mg/kg or 3.0 g daily, whichever is less.

*Intravenous therapy:* Aldomet Injection is for intravenous use only, it must not be given intramuscularly or subcutaneously. An effective dose will produce a fall in blood pressure that may begin in 4 to 6 hours and be maintained for 10 to 16 hours.

The required dose of Aldomet Injection should be added to 100 ml of 5% Dextrose Injection BP. Alternatively, Aldomet may be given with 5% dextrose infusion solution BP at a concentration of 100 mg to each 10 ml solution. This intravenous infusion should be given slowly over a period of 30 to 60 minutes.

When practicable, oral therapy with Aldomet may be substituted, starting with the same dosage as that being used by the parenteral route.

*Usual adult dosage:* 250–500 mg (5–10 ml) six-hourly. In severe cases, up to 1 g (20 ml) six-hourly may be needed, and this is the maximum recommended dosage. If there is renal impairment, lower dosages should suffice.

*Children's dosage:* The recommended intravenous dosage for children is 20–40 mg/kg of body weight daily in divided doses every six hours. The maximum dosage is 65 mg/kg or 3.0 g daily, whichever is less. If there is renal impairment, lower dosages should suffice.

*Use in the elderly:* The initial dose in elderly patients should be kept as low as possible, not exceeding 250 mg daily; an appropriate starting dose in the elderly would be 125 mg b.d. increasing slowly as required, but not to exceed a maximum daily dosage of 2 g.

**Contra-indications, warnings, etc**
*Contra-indications:* Active hepatic disease, such as acute hepatitis and active cirrhosis; hypersensitivity (including hepatic disorders associated with previous methyldopa therapy), depression.

Aldomet is not recommended for the treatment of phaeochromocytoma (see 'Precautions').

*Precautions:* Acquired haemolytic anaemia has occurred rarely; should symptoms suggest anaemia, haemoglobin and/or haematocrit determinations should be made. If anaemia is confirmed, tests should be done for haemolysis. If haemolytic anaemia is present, Aldomet should be discontinued. Stopping therapy, with or without giving a corticosteroid, has usually brought prompt remission. Rarely, however, deaths have occurred.

Some patients on continued therapy with methyldopa develop a positive direct Coombs test. From the reports of different investigators, the incidence averages between 10% and 20%. A positive Coombs test rarely develops in the first six months of therapy, and if it has not developed within 12 months, it is unlikely to do so later on continuing therapy. Development is also dose-related, the lowest incidence occurring in patients receiving 1 g or less of methyldopa per day. The test becomes negative usually within weeks or months of stopping methyldopa.

Prior knowledge of a positive Coombs reaction will aid in evaluating a cross-match for transfusion. If a patient with a positive Coombs reaction shows an incompatible minor cross-match, an indirect Coombs test should be performed. If this is negative, transfusion with blood compatible in the major cross-match may be carried out. If positive, the advisability of transfusion should be determined by a haematologist.

Reversible leucopenia, with primary effect on granulocytes has been reported rarely. The granulocyte count returned to normal on discontinuing therapy. Reversible thrombocytopenia has occurred rarely.

Occasionally, fever has occurred within the first three weeks of therapy, sometimes associated with eosinophilia or abnormalities in liver function tests. Jaundice, with or without fever, also may occur. Its onset is usually within the first two or three months of therapy. In some patients the findings are consistent with those of cholestasis. Rare cases of fatal hepatic necrosis have been reported. Liver biopsy, performed in several patients with liver dysfunction, showed a microscopic focal necrosis compatible with drug hypersensitivity. Liver function tests and a total and differential white blood cell count are advisable before therapy and at intervals during the first six weeks to twelve weeks of therapy, or whenever an unexplained fever occurs. Should fever, abnormality in liver function, or jaundice occur, therapy should be withdrawn. If related to methyldopa, the temperature and abnormalities in liver function will then return to normal. Methyldopa should not be used again in these patients. Methyldopa should be used with caution in patients with a history of previous liver disease or dysfunction.

The antihypertensive effect of Aldomet may be diminished by sympathomimetics, phenothiazines, tricyclic antidepressants and MAOIs.

A paradoxical pressor response has been reported with Aldomet Injection.

Patients may require reduced doses of anaesthetics when on methyldopa. If hypotension does occur during anaesthesia, it can usually be controlled by vasopressors. The adrenergic receptors remain sensitive during treatment with methyldopa.

Dialysis removes methyldopa; therefore, hypertension may recur after this procedure.

Rarely, involuntary choreoathetotic movements have been observed during therapy with methyldopa in patients with severe bilateral cerebrovascular disease. Should these movements occur, therapy should be discontinued.

Aldomet should be used with extreme caution in patients, or in near relatives of patients, with hepatic porphyria.

The preservatives in both Aldomet Injection and Suspension have been reported to cause hypersensitivity. Sodium metabisulphite in particular is associated with circulatory collapse, and depression of the central nervous system in certain susceptible individuals with allergic tendencies.

*Interference with laboratory tests:* Methyldopa may interfere with the measurement of urinary uric acid by the phosphotungstate method, serum creatinine by the alkaline picrate method, and AST (SGOT) by colorimetric method. Interference with spectrophotometric methods for AST (SGOT) analysis has not been reported.

As methyldopa fluoresces at the same wavelengths as catecholamines, spuriously high amounts of urinary catecholamines may be reported interfering with a diagnosis of phaeochromocytoma.

It is important to recognise this phenomenon before a patient with a possible phaeochromocytoma is subjected to surgery. Methyldopa does not interfere with measurements of VMA (vanillylmandelic acid) by those methods which convert VMA to vanillin.

Rarely, when urine is exposed to air after voiding, it may darken because of breakdown of methyldopa or its metabolites.

*Pregnancy and breast-feeding mothers:* Aldomet has been used under close medical supervision for the treatment of hypertension during pregnancy. There was no clinical evidence that Aldomet caused fetal abnormalities or affected the neonate.

Methyldopa crosses the placental barrier and appears in cord blood and breast milk.

Although no obvious teratogenic effects have been reported, the possibility of fetal injury cannot be excluded and the use of the drug in women who are, or may become, pregnant or who are breast-feeding their newborn infant requires that anticipated benefits be weighed against possible risks.

*Drug interactions:* When methyldopa and lithium are given concomitantly the patient should be monitored carefully for symptoms of lithium toxicity.

When methyldopa is used with other antihypertensive drugs, potentiation of antihypertensive action may occur. The progress of patients should be carefully followed to detect side reactions or manifestations of drug idiosyncrasy.

*Side-effects:* Sedation, usually transient, may occur during the initial period of therapy or whenever the dose is increased. If affected, patients should not attempt to drive, or operate machinery. Headache, asthenia or weakness may be noted as early and transient symptoms.

The following reactions have been reported:

*Central nervous system:* Sedation (usually transient), headache, asthenia or weakness, paraesthesiae, parkinsonism, Bell's palsy, involuntary choreoathetotic movements. Psychic disturbances including nightmares, impaired mental acuity and reversible mild psychoses or depression. Dizziness, light-headedness, and symptoms of cerebrovascular insufficiency (may be due to lowering of blood pressure).

*Cardiovascular:* Bradycardia, prolonged carotid sinus hypersensitivity, aggravation of angina pectoris. Orthostatic hypotension (decrease daily dosage). Oedema (and weight gain) usually relieved by use of a diuretic. (Discontinue methyldopa if oedema progresses or signs of heart failure appear.)

*Gastro-intestinal:* Nausea, vomiting, distension, constipation, flatus, diarrhoea, colitis, mild dryness of mouth, sore or 'black' tongue, pancreatitis, sialadenitis.

*Hepatic:* Liver disorders including hepatitis, jaundice, abnormal liver function tests.

*Haematological:* Positive Coombs test, haemolytic anaemia, bone marrow depression, leucopenia, granulocytopenia, thrombocytopenia. Positive tests for antinuclear antibody, LE cells, and rheumatoid factor.

*Allergic:* Drug-related fever and lupus-like syndrome, myocarditis, pericarditis.

*Dermatological:* Rash as in eczema or lichenoid eruption, toxic epidermal necrolysis.

*Other:* Nasal stuffiness, rise in blood urea, breast enlargement, gynaecomastia, hyperprolactinaemia, amenorrhoea, lactation, impotence, decreased libido, failure of ejaculation, mild arthralgia with or without joint swelling, myalgia.

*Overdosage:* Acute overdosage may produce acute hypotension with other responses attributable to brain and gastro-intestinal malfunction (excessive sedation, weakness, bradycardia, dizziness, light-headedness, constipation, distension, flatus, diarrhoea, nausea, and vomiting). If ingestion is recent, emesis may be induced or gastric lavage performed. There is no specific antidote. Methyldopa is dialysable. Treatment is symptomatic. Infusions may be helpful to promote urinary excretion. Special attention should be directed towards cardiac rate and output, blood volume, electrolyte balance, paralytic ileus, urinary function and cerebral activity. Administration of sympathomimetic agents may be indicated. When chronic overdosage is suspected, Aldomet should be discontinued.

The plasma half-life of methyldopa is 105 minutes. Peak plasma levels were reached about two hours after oral ingestion.

**Pharmaceutical precautions** Keep containers well closed and store the tablets and suspension below 25°C, protected from light. The injection should also be protected from freezing. Only 5% dextrose should be used as diluent for the injection.

Aldomet Suspension should not be diluted.

**Legal category** POM.

**Package quantities** *Tablets 125 mg:* Packs of 60. *Tablets 250 mg:* Packs of 60 and 90. *Tablets 500 mg:* Packs of 30. *Oral Suspension 250 mg/5 ml:* Bottles of 200 ml. *Injection:* Ampoules of 5 ml.

**Further information** Aldomet reduces both supine and standing blood pressure. Symptomatic postural hypotension, exercise hypotension and diurnal blood pressure variations rarely occur. By adjustment of dosage, morning hypotension can be prevented without sacrificing control of afternoon blood pressure.

Methyldopa has no direct effect on cardiac function and usually does not reduce glomerular filtration rate, renal blood flow or filtration fraction. Cardiac output usually is maintained without cardiac acceleration. In some patients, the heart rate is slowed.

Because of its relative freedom from adverse effects on kidney function, methyldopa can be of benefit in the control of high blood pressure, even in the presence of renal impairment. It may help arrest or retard the progression of renal function impairment and damage due to sustained elevation of blood pressure.

Normal or elevated plasma renin activity may decrease in course of methyldopa therapy.

**Product licence numbers**

| | |
|---|---|
| Tablets 125 mg | 0025/0098 |
| Tablets 250 mg | 0025/0099 |
| Tablets 500 mg | 0025/0100 |
| Oral Suspension 250 mg/5 ml | 0025/0154 |
| Injection | 0025/5003 |

## ARAMINE*

**Presentation** A clear, colourless solution containing, in each millilitre, Metaraminol Tartrate BP equivalent to 10 mg metaraminol. Aramine also contains methylhydroxybenzoate, propylhydroxybenzoate and sodium bisulphite as preservatives; with the solution made isotonic by the inclusion of sodium chloride.

**Uses** Sympathomimetic amine (vasopressor agent). For the treatment of acute hypotension due to loss of vasoconstrictor tone as may occur during spinal anaesthesia, and as an adjunct to accepted remedial procedures (e.g. tilting of patient and attention to fluid volumes). (See 'Precautions'.)

The pressor effect of a single dose of Aramine lasts from about twenty minutes up to one hour. Its onset is around one or two minutes after direct intravenous injection.

**Dosage and administration** Aramine Injection may be given intravenously either directly or by infusion. Because the maximum effect is not immediately apparent, allow at least ten minutes before increasing the dose. Since the vasopressor effect tapers off when therapy is stopped, be prepared to restart promptly if the blood pressure falls too rapidly. Patients with coexistent shock and acidosis may show poor response.

Direct intravenous injection is recommended only in grave emergencies. *Particular care should be taken to use the correct dose.*

*Intravenous infusion (for adjunctive treatment of hypotension):* 15–100 mg (1.5–10 ml) in 500 ml of Sodium Chloride Injection BP or 5% Dextrose Injection BP, adjusting the rate of infusion to maintain the blood pressure at the desired level. Higher concentrations of Aramine 150–500 mg per 500 ml of infusion fluid, have been used. If the patient needs additional saline or dextrose at a rate of flow that would provide an excessive dose of Aramine when used as recommended, the volume of infusion fluid should be increased accordingly. Aramine may also be added to *less* than 500 ml of infusion fluid if a smaller volume is desired.

Aramine is physically and chemically compatible with Injection Sodium Chloride BP, 5% Injection Dextrose BP, Ringer's Injection USP, Lactated Ringer's Injection USP, Dextran 70 Injection.

When Aramine is mixed with an infusion solution, sterile precautions should be observed. Mixtures should be used within 24 hours since infusion solutions do not contain preservatives.

*Direct intravenous injection (to be employed only in grave emergencies, when immediate action is necessary to save life):* 0.5–5 mg (0.05–0.5 ml), followed by an infusion of 15–100 mg (1.5–10 ml) in 500 ml of infusion liquid. *Particular care should be taken to use the correct dose when injecting undiluted Aramine.*

*Children:* Aramine should not be used in children.

*Use in the elderly:* The dosage may not require modification for elderly patients; however geriatric patients may be more sensitive to sympathomimetic agents, therefore particular caution should be taken in this age group.

**Contra-indications, warnings, etc**

*Contra-indications:* Concurrent use with cyclopropane or halothane anaesthesia, unless clinical circumstances demand it. Hypersensitivity to any component of Aramine including sulphites. Children.

*Precautions:* Each preservative in Aramine has been reported to cause hypersensitivity. Sodium bisulphite in particular is associated with circulatory or respiratory collapse, and depression of the CNS in certain susceptible individuals, particularly in those with asthma.

Caution should be exercised to avoid excessive blood pressure changes since response to treatment with Aramine is very variable and the ensuing control of the blood pressure may prove difficult.

Rapidly induced hypertensive responses have been reported to cause acute pulmonary oedema, cardiac arrhythmias and arrest. Aramine should be used with caution in patients with cirrhosis; electrolyte levels should be adequately restored if a diuresis ensues. A fatal ventricular arrhythmia was reported in a patient with Laënnec's cirrhosis while receiving metaraminol tartrate. In several instances, ventricular extrasystoles that appeared during infusion of Aramine promptly subsided when the rate of flow was reduced.

With the prolonged action of Aramine, a cumulative effect is possible. An excessive vasopressor response may cause a prolonged elevation of blood pressure, even after discontinuation of therapy.

Aramine should be used with caution in cases of heart disease, hypertension, thyroid disease or diabetes mellitus because of its vasoconstrictor action.

Sympathomimetic amines may provoke a relapse in patients with a history of malaria.

When vasopressor amines are used for long periods, the resulting vasoconstriction may prevent adequate expansion of circulating volume and may cause perpetuation of the shock state. There is evidence that plasma volume may be reduced in all types of shock, and that the measurement of central venous pressure is useful in assessing the adequacy of the circulating blood volume. Blood, or plasma-volume expanders, should therefore be employed when the principal reason for hypotension or shock is decreased circulating volume.

In choosing the site for injection, it is important to avoid those areas generally recognised as being unsuitable for the use of any pressor agent and to discontinue the infusion immediately if infiltration or thrombosis occurs. Although the urgent nature of the patient's condition may force the choice of an unsuitable injection site, the preferred areas of injection should be used when possible. The larger veins of the antecubital fossa or thigh are preferred to the veins in the ankle or dorsum of the hand, particularly in patients with peripheral vascular disease, diabetes mellitus, Buerger's disease or conditions with coexistent hypercoagulability.

Accidental spillage of Aramine on the skin can cause dermatitic reactions linked to the presence of the agent's preservatives.

*Pregnancy:* There are no well-controlled studies in pregnant women. Aramine should be used during pregnancy only if the potential benefit justifies the potential risk to the fetus.

*Breast-feeding mothers:* It is not known whether Aramine is secreted in human milk. Because many drugs are secreted in human milk, caution should be exercised if Aramine is given to a breast-feeding mother.

*Drug interactions:* Aramine should be used with caution in digitalised patients since the combination of digitalis and sympathomimetic amines is capable of causing ectopic arrhythmic activity.

Monoamine oxidase inhibitors have been reported to potentiate the action of sympathomimetic amines. The pressor effect of Aramine is decreased but not reversed by alpha-adrenergic blocking agents.

*Side effects:* Sympathomimetic amines, including Aramine, may cause sinus or ventricular tachycardia, or other arrhythmias, especially in patients with myocardial infarction.

Abscess formation, tissue necrosis, and sloughing rarely may follow the use of Aramine.

*Overdosage:* Aramine acts rapidly. Its major therapeutic effects are complete within an hour of parenteral administration. Overdosage may result in severe hypertension accompanied by headache, constricting sensation in the chest, nausea, vomiting, euphoria, diaphoresis, pulmonary oedema, tachycardia, bradycardia, sinus arrhythmia, atrial or ventricular arrhythmias, myocardial infarction, cardiac arrest or convulsions.

If the drug has been ingested, induce emesis or perform gastric lavage. If Aramine has been administered by subcutaneous or intramuscular injection, local ice packs may be applied to delay absorption. Intravenous infusion should be stopped immediately, but reinstated if hypotension occurs. If needed, an alpha-adrenergic blocking agent such as phenoxybenzamine may be used to reduce hypertension. Intravenous beta-adrenergic blocking agents may also be useful for reducing hypertension and may have a beneficial effect on cardiac arrhythmia, if present. Parenteral diazepam may be given for convulsions.

**Pharmaceutical precautions** Store below 25°C, protected from light and from freezing. Aramine is physically and chemically compatible with Injection Sodium Chloride BP, 5% Injection Dextrose BP, Ringer's Injection USP, Lactated Ringer's Injection USP, Dextran 70 Injection. The ampoule may be autoclaved.

**Legal category** POM.

**Package quantities** Ampoules of 1 ml.

**Further information** Aramine is a potent sympathomimetic amine which increases the force of myocardial contractions as well as having a peripheral vasoconstrictor action. It increases both systolic and diastolic blood pressures.

Renal, coronary, and cerebral blood flow are a function of perfusion pressure and regional resistance. In most instances of cardiogenic shock, the beneficial effect of sympathomimetic amines is attributable to their positive inotropic effect. In patients with insufficient or failing vasoconstriction, there is additional advantage to the peripheral action of Aramine, but in most patients with shock, vasoconstriction is adequate and any further increase is unnecessary. Therefore, blood flow to vital organs may decrease with Aramine if the regional resistance increases excessively.

The pressor effect of Aramine is decreased but not reversed by alpha-adrenergic blocking agents. Primary or secondary fall in blood pressure and tachyphylactic response to repeated use are uncommon.

**Product licence number** 10 mg/ml injection 0025/5020.

## BENEMID* TABLETS 500 mg

**Qualitative and quantitative composition** Benemid contains 500 mg of the active ingredient, Probenecid PhEur.

**Pharmaceutical form** Benemid is supplied as white, half-scored tablets marked 'MSD 501'.

**Clinical particulars**

*Therapeutic indications:* Probenecid is a uricosuric and renal tubular blocking agent designed for maintenance treatment of gout and gouty arthritis. It inhibits the reabsorption of urate ions in the renal tubules, thus increasing urinary excretion of uric acid and decreasing serum uric acid levels. This action is reversible upon withdrawal of the drug and is demonstrable in normal individuals as well as in patients under treatment. Effective uricosuria reduces the miscible urate pool, retards the deposition of urates, and promotes reabsorption of urate deposits. Also selectively inhibits the urinary excretion of β-lactam antibiotics (other than cephaloridine) and p-amino-salicylic acid.

*Gout and other forms of hyperuricaemia:* Benemid is an effective uricosuric agent for the treatment of hyperuricaemia in gout and gouty arthritis. Time is required to achieve clinical results with Benemid despite the marked uricosuric activity of Benemid. Although acute attacks may occur in the early stages of therapy, as therapy is continued these attacks should become less frequent and less intense. Benemid may also be given prophylactically, to treat the asymptomatic hyperuricaemia that often occurs in 'gouty' families, in an attempt to forestall the development of acute gouty attacks and urate deposition in tissues.

Benemid may be used to control the hyperuricaemia induced or aggravated by diuretics employed in oedema and hypertension.

*Beta-lactam antibiotic therapy:* Benemid is indicated as an adjunctive therapy with β-lactam antibiotics (other than cephaloridine) and p-aminosalicylic acid. Benemid interferes with the renal tubular excretion of these substances and thus elevates and prolongs the plasma levels by whatever route the antibiotics are given. A twofold to fourfold increase in plasma concentration has been demonstrated for: penicillin G or V; the synthetic penicillins, ampicillin, methicillin, oxacillin, cloxacillin, carbenicillin, and nafcillin; the cephamycin, cefoxitin sodium; and the cephalosporins, cephalothin, cephalexin, and cephaloglycin.

Adjunctive therapy of this type is particularly useful when treating severe or resistant infections, such as gonorrhoea, subacute bacterial endocarditis, staphylococcal osteomyelitis, staphylococcal septicaemia, and meningitis due to Gram-positive organisms.

*Posology and method of administration*

*Uricosuric therapy:* The usual adult dosage is ½ tablet (250 mg) twice a day for one week, followed thereafter by 1 tablet (500 mg) twice a day.

Some degree of renal impairment is common in patients with gout; therefore, a daily dosage of 2 tablets (1 g) may be adequate in many patients. If, however, symptoms of gouty arthritis remain uncontrolled or the 24-hour urate excretion is not above 700 mg, the daily dosage may be increased by 1 tablet (500 mg) every four weeks within tolerance [usually not more than 4 tablets (2 g) a day]. Benemid may not be effective in chronic renal insufficiency, particularly when the glomerular filtration rate is 30 ml/min or less.

Gastric intolerance may be indicative of overdosage, and may be corrected by reducing the dosage without losing the therapeutic response.

Benemid should be continued at a dosage that will maintain a normal serum uric acid level. When acute attacks have been absent for at least six months and serum uric acid levels remain within normal limits, dosage of Benemid may be reduced by 1 tablet (500 mg) every six months to the minimum effective dosage. The maintenance dosage should not be reduced to the point where serum uric acid levels tend to rise.

*Gonorrhoea:* For uncomplicated gonorrhoea in men or women, a single dose of 2 tablets (1 g) with adequate doses of either oral ampicillin or intramuscular aqueous procaine penicillin G, or cefoxitin. If oral ampicillin is used, Benemid should be given simultaneously; if a parenteral antibiotic is administered, Benemid should be given at least 30 minutes before the injection.

*β-lactam antibiotic therapy (general): Adults:* 4 tablets (2 g) a day in divided doses. Elderly patients with suspected renal impairment should be given a reduced dosage. Benemid should not be given concurrently with a β-lactam antibiotic in known cases of renal impairment.

*Children over 2 years:* 25 mg per kg bodyweight (or 0.7 g/m² body surface) initially, followed by 40 mg per kg (or 1.2 g/m²) a day in divided doses every six hours. For children weighing more than 50 kg, the adult dosage is recommended.

*Use in the elderly:* As with all drugs which are primarily renally excreted, care should be taken in the elderly whose renal function may be impaired.

*Contra-indications:* Known hypersensitivity to any component of this product. History of blood dyscrasias. Uric acid kidney stones. Children under 2 years old. Therapy with Benemid should not be started until an acute gouty attack has subsided. Salicylates are contra-indicated in patients taking Benemid.

*Special warnings and precautions for use:* Benemid should be used with caution in patients with a history of peptic ulcer.

If hypersensitivity reactions appear during therapy, the drug should be withdrawn.

Haematuria, renal colic, costovertebral pain and the formation of urate stones associated with the use of probenecid in gouty patients may be prevented by a liberal fluid intake and enough sodium bicarbonate (3–7.5 g daily) or potassium citrate (7.5 g daily) to keep the urine alkaline. When alkali is given, the acid-base balance of the patient should be carefully monitored.

Alkalisation of urine is recommended until the serum uric acid level returns to normal tophaceous deposits disappear, i.e. during the period when urinary excretion of urates is at a high level. After the miscible pool of uric acid decreases to normal (about 1 g) and deposited urates are reabsorbed and eliminated, alkalisation of the urine probably is unnecessary, since the urinary urate concentration is lower and less likely to cause crystallisation.

Exacerbation of gout during therapy with Benemid may occur; if so, a full therapeutic dosage of colchicine, indomethacin, or other appropriate therapy should be given.

*Interaction with other medicaments and other forms of interaction:* The use of acetylsalicylic acid is contra-indicated because it antagonises the uricosuric action of probenecid. If patients on Benemid require a mild analgesic, paracetamol is preferred.

Since probenecid decreases the renal excretion of conjugated sulphonamides, plasma concentrations of the latter should be determined from time to time when a sulphonamide and probenecid are given together for prolonged periods. Probenecid may prolong or enhance the action of oral sulphonylureas and thereby increase the risk of hypoglycaemia.

Benemid increases the mean plasma elimination half-life of a number of other drugs which can lead to increased peak plasma concentrations. These drugs include paracetamol, naproxen, indomethacin, ketoprofen, meclofenamate, lorazepam, and rifampicin acyclovir, ganciclovir and zidovudine. The clinical significance of this effect is not known; however, adjustment in the usual dosage of these drugs may be required.

Caution should be used if Benemid is administered simultaneously with methotrexate, as Benemid has been reported to decrease the tubular secretion of methotrexate and potentiate toxicity. If Benemid is given with methotrexate, the dosage of methotrexate should be reduced and serum levels may need to be monitored.

The uricosuric action of Benemid is antagonised by pyrazinamide.

Because of the mechanism of action, Benemid is not recommended in conjunction with a beta-lactam antibiotic in the presence of known renal impairment.

In addition to the effect of Benemid on the excretion of uric acid and β-lactam antibiotics (other than cephaloridine), Benemid decreases the urinary excretion of ρ-aminosalicylic acid (PAS), ρ-aminohippuric acid (PAH), phenolsulphonylphthalein (PSP), pantothenic acid, 17-ketosteroids, indomethacin, and sodium iodomethamate and related iodinated organic acids. Benemid decreases both hepatic and renal excretion of sulphobromophthalein (BSP). The renal tubular reabsorption of phosphorus is inhibited in hypoparathyroid, but not in euparathyroid, individuals.

Benemid does not affect the excretion of streptomycin, chloramphenicol, chlortetracycline, oxytetracycline, or neomycin. The effects on the excretion of cephaloridine are not clinically significant.

*Pregnancy and lactation*

*Use in pregnancy:* Probenecid crosses the placental barrier and appears in cord blood. Its use in women of childbearing age requires that the anticipated benefit be weighed against possible hazards.

*Use in breast-feeding:* It is not known whether this drug is excreted in human milk. Because many drugs are excreted in human milk, caution should be exercised when Benemid is administered to a breast-feeding mother.

*Effects on ability to drive and use machines:* Benemid may cause dizziness in some patients. If patients experience dizziness, they should be instructed not to drive and to avoid operating machinery or performing other hazardous activities requiring alertness.

*Undesirable effects:* Headache, gastro-intestinal symptoms (e.g. anorexia, nausea, vomiting), frequency of micturition, hypersensitivity reactions (including anaphylaxis, dermatitis, pruritus, urticaria, and fever and Stevens Johnson syndrome), sore gums, flushing, alopecia, dizziness, anaemia and haemolytic anaemia (in some cases associated with genetic deficiency of glucose-6-phosphate dehydrogenase in red blood cells) have occurred. Toxic epidermal necrolysis has been reported rarely after combination therapy of colchicine and probenecid. The nephrotic syndrome, leucopenia, hepatic necrosis, and aplastic anaemia occur rarely. In gouty patients, exacerbation of gout, and uric acid stones with or without haematuria, renal colic, or costovertebral pain, have been seen.

*Laboratory tests:* A reducing substance may appear in the urine of patients receiving Benemid. This may give a false-positive Benedict's test, but the substance disappears when therapy is discontinued.

Falsely high readings for theophylline have been reported in an *in vitro* study using the Schack and Waxler technique, when therapeutic concentrations of theophylline and Benemid were added to human plasma.

*Overdosage:* No specific antidote is available. The usual measures to remove unabsorbed material from the gastro-intestinal tract, clinical monitoring, and supportive therapy should be employed. If signs of CNS excitation are present, a short-acting barbiturate or intravenous diazepam should be given parenterally. Adrenaline should be given for anaphylactoid reactions. For less severe hypersensitivity reactions, antihistamines or corticosteroids may be given.

The plasma half-life of probenecid is between six to twelve hours; between 85 to 95% of the drug is bound to plasma proteins.

**Pharmacological properties**

*Pharmacodynamic properties:* Probenecid increases the excretion of urate in the urine by inhibiting its reabsorption in the renal tubule. It also decreases the excretion of penicillin and other beta-lactam antibiotics (therapy raising and prolonging plasma levels) by inhibiting their secretion in the renal tubule.

*Pharmacokinetic properties:* Probenecid is completely absorbed on oral administration. Peak plasma levels are reached in two to four hours. Plasma half life varies from less than five hours to more than eight hours, depending on the dose. Between 85% and 95% is bound to plasma albumin. It is partially metabolised to the glucuronide and hydroxylated, carboxylated, and N-depropylated metabolites. Unchanged drug and its metabolites are excreted in the urine.

*Preclinical safety data:* No evidence of mutagenicity was observed in a microbial mutagenicity test using mutant strains of salmonella typhimurium with or without rat or hamster liver metabolic activation. No genetic damage was noted in a chromosome aberration study in CHO cells. Variable results were obtained in a sister chromatid exchange (SCE) text in CHO cells. One trial caused a dose-related increase in SCEs; a second trial was negative, and a third trial had significant increases at the lowest and highest doses tested (but not the intermediate doses).

In a 23 month carcinogenic study in mice, a significant increase in the incidence of heptocellular carcinomas and adenomas was observed at a dose of 400 mg/kg/day (10 times the maximum recommended human dose) in the females. These changes were not observed in male mice or rats of either sex that received the same dose, or in mice of either sex at a dose of 100 mg/kg/day (2.5 times the maximum recommended human dose).

The oral $LD_{50}$ of probenecid is 1.7 g/kg and 1.6 g/kg in the mouse and rat respectively.

**Pharmaceutical particulars**

*List of excipients:* Calcium Stearate PhEur, Gelatin PhEur, Magnesium Carbonate, Heavy PhEur, Maize Starch PhEur.

*Incompatibilities:* None.

*Shelf life:* Blister pack: 36 months.

*Special precautions for storage:* Store below 25°C.

*Nature and contents of container:* PVC/Al blister pack containing 60 tablets.

*Instruction for use/handling:* None.

**Marketing authorisation number** 0025/5021R.

**Date of approval/revision of SPC** December 1996.

**Legal category** POM.

## BLOCADREN*

**Presentation** Light blue, half-scored tablets, marked 'MSD 136' on one side and scored on the other, containing 10 mg Timolol Maleate BP.

**Uses** Beta-adrenergic-receptor blocking agent. For the treatment of essential hypertension and in angina pectoris due to ischaemic heart disease.

Blocadren is also indicated for the long-term prevention of myocardial infarction and cardiac death (including sudden death) in those who have survived the acute phase of a myocardial infarction.

Prophylactic treatment of common and classic migraine.

**Dosage and administration**

*Hypertension:* The initial dosage is 10 mg a day in a single or divided dosage. Depending on the response of the patient, increases in dosage may be made gradually to a maximum of 60 mg daily. Daily dosages above 20 mg should be given on a divided dose schedule.

*Use with Moduretic* (amiloride hydrochloride and hydrochlorothiazide, MSD):* Studies have shown that Blocadren can be administered once daily when used concomitantly with Moduretic. The majority of patients will respond to a regimen of 10 or 20 mg of Blocadren once a day and 1 tablet of Moduretic.

*Use with other antihypertensives:* Blocadren may be used with thiazides, hydralazine, or methyldopa. Dosage adjustments are usually required.

For concomitant use with catecholamine-depleting

drugs such as reserpine or guanethidine, see 'Precautions'.

*Angina:* Therapy should be initiated with 5 mg two or three times a day. Dosage increases may be necessary, depending on the symptomatic response, pulse rate, and blood pressure. The first increase should not exceed 10 mg a day in divided doses, and subsequent increases should not exceed 15 mg a day in divided doses. There should be an interval of at least three days between increases in dosage.

The usual dosage range is 15 to 45 mg a day. The majority of patients respond to a dosage in the range of 35 to 45 mg a day.

*Preventive use in ischaemic heart disease:* For long-term preventive use in patients who have survived the acute phase of myocardial infarction, the maintenance dose is 10 mg twice daily. Therapy should be initiated with 5 mg twice daily and the patient observed carefully. If no adverse reaction occurs, the dosage should then be increased after 2 days to 10 mg twice daily. In the studies evaluating Blocadren following myocardial infarction, treatment was begun 7 to 28 days after the acute phase.

*Migraine:* The recommended dosage in the prophylactic treatment of common and classic migraine is 10 to 20 mg administered once-a-day.

*Paediatric use:* not established (see 'Precautions').

*Use in the elderly:* Initial dosage should be 5 mg b.d. Dosage may be increased cautiously depending on clinical response. *For the preventive use in ischaemic heart disease:* The dosage should be increased to 10 mg b.d. after the second day of treatment.

**Contra-indications, warnings, etc**

*Contra-indications:* Bronchospasm (including bronchial asthma), history of bronchospasm, severe chronic obstructive pulmonary disease; sinus bradycardia; atrioventricular block; overt heart failure (see 'Precautions'); right ventricular failure secondary to pulmonary hypertension; significant cardiomegaly; cardiogenic shock; hypersensitivity to this product.

See also 'Use in pregnancy and breast-feeding mothers', under 'Precautions'.

*Precautions: Congestive heart failure:* Blocadren may be given cautiously to patients with a history of cardiac failure who are well compensated, usually with digitalis or diuretics. Both digitalis and timolol maleate slow AV conduction. If cardiac failure persists, Blocadren should be withdrawn.

*In patients without history of cardiac failure:* At the first sign or symptom of cardiac failure, patients receiving Blocadren should be digitalised and/or given a diuretic, and the response closely observed. If cardiac failure still continues, Blocadren should be withdrawn.

*Thyrotoxicosis:* Beta-adrenergic blockade may mask certain clinical signs (e.g. tachycardia) of hyperthyroidism. Patients suspected of developing thyrotoxicosis should be managed carefully to avoid abrupt withdrawal of Blocadren which might precipitate a thyroid storm.

*Exacerbation of ischaemic heart disease following abrupt withdrawal:* Hypersensitivity to catecholamines has been seen in patients withdrawn from beta-blocker therapy; exacerbation of angina and, in some cases, myocardial infarction has occurred after *abrupt* withdrawal of such therapy. When discontinuing chronically administered Blocadren, particularly in patients with ischaemic heart disease, the dosage should be gradually reduced over one to two weeks and the patient carefully monitored. If angina markedly worsens or acute coronary insufficiency develops, Blocadren should be reinstated promptly, at least temporarily, and other appropriate measures taken. Patients should be warned against interruption or discontinuation of Blocadren without the physician's advice. Because coronary artery disease is both common and may be unrecognised, it may be prudent not to discontinue Blocadren abruptly, even when only treating hypertension.

*Major surgery:* Because beta-adrenergic-receptor blockade impairs the heart's response to beta-adrenergic mediated reflex stimuli, some patients on beta-adrenergic receptor blocking agents have shown protracted severe hypotension during anaesthesia. Difficulty in restarting and maintaining the heartbeat has also been reported.

Some authorities now recommend gradual withdrawal of beta-adrenergic-receptor blocking agents from anginal patients before elective surgery. If necessary during surgery, the effects of Blocadren may be reversed by sufficient doses of such agonists as isoprenaline, dopamine, dobutamine or noradrenaline (see 'Overdosage').

*Diabetes mellitus:* Blocadren should be administered with caution to patients liable to spontaneous hypoglycaemia, or to diabetic patients (especially those with labile diabetes) who are receiving insulin or oral hypoglycaemic agents. Beta-adrenergic receptor blocking agents may mask the premonitory signs and symptoms of acute hypoglycaemia.

*Impaired hepatic or renal function:* Since Blocadren is partially metabolised in the liver and excreted mainly by the kidney, dosage reduction may be necessary when hepatic and/or renal insufficiency is present.

*In the presence of marked renal failure:* Although the pharmacokinetics of Blocadren are not greatly altered by renal impairment, marked hypotensive responses have been seen in patients with marked renal impairment undergoing dialysis after 20 mg doses. Dosing in such patients should, therefore, be especially cautious.

*Musculoskeletal:* Beta-blockers have been reported to induce myasthenic symptoms such as diplopia, ptosis and generalised weakness. Timolol has been reported rarely to increase muscle weakness in some patients with myasthenic symptoms.

*Cerebrovascular insufficiency:* As an agent affecting both pulse and blood pressure, Blocadren should be used cautiously in patients with cerebrovascular insufficiency. Signs or symptoms suggesting reduced cerebral blood flow should prompt consideration of withdrawing therapy with Blocadren.

*General:* There have been reports of skin rashes and/or dry eyes associated with the use of beta-adrenoceptor-blocking drugs. The reported incidence is small and in most cases the symptoms have cleared when treatment was withdrawn. Discontinuation of the drug should be considered if any such reaction is not otherwise explicable. Cessation of therapy involving beta-blockade should be gradual.

*Paediatric use:* Safety and efficacy in children has not been established.

*Use in pregnancy and breast-feeding mothers:* There are no adequate and well-controlled studies in pregnant women. Blocadren should only be used if the potential benefit justifies the risk to the fetus.

Timolol is detectable in human milk. Because of the potential for serious adverse reactions in breast-feeding babies, a decision to discontinue breast-feeding, or Blocadren, should be made taking into account the importance of the drug to the mother.

*Risk from anaphylactic reaction:* While taking beta-blockers, patients with a history of atopy or a history of severe anaphylactic reaction to a variety of allergens, may be more reactive to repeated challenge with such allergens, either accidental, diagnostic or therapeutic. Such patients may be unresponsive to the usual doses of adrenaline used to treat anaphylactic reactions.

*Drug interactions:* Close observation of the patient is recommended when Blocadren is administered to patients on catecholamine-depleting drugs such as reserpine, because of possible additive effects and the production of hypotension and/or marked bradycardia, which may produce vertigo, syncope, or postural hypotension.

Attenuation of the antihypertensive effect of beta-blockers by NSAIDs has been reported. Patients treated with both agents should be monitored to confirm that the desired therapeutic effect has been obtained.

Oral calcium antagonists may be combined with Blocadren only when heart function is normal. The potential exists for hypotension, AV conduction disturbances, and left ventricular failure to occur in patients receiving a beta-blocking agent when an oral calcium antagonist is added to the treatment regimen. The nature of any cardiovascular adverse effect tends to depend on the type of calcium antagonist used. Dihydropyridine derivatives, such as nifedipine, may lead to hypotension, whereas verapamil or diltiazem have a greater propensity to lead to AV conduction disturbances or left ventricular failure when used with a beta-blocker. Intravenous calcium antagonists and Blocadren should only be used together with caution.

Concomitant use of beta-blockers and digitalis with either diltiazem or verapamil may further prolong the AV conduction time.

*Side-effects:* Blocadren is usually well tolerated. Most adverse reactions have been mild and transient. *General:* Asthenia, fatigue, headache, chest pain, extremity pain, decreased exercise tolerance, weight loss. *Cardiovascular:* Bradycardia, cardiac arrest, cerebral vascular accident, palpitation, arrhythmia, sinoatrial block, AV block (2nd or 3rd degree), syncope, hypotension, oedema, pulmonary oedema, cardiac failure, Raynaud's phenomenon, cold extremities, claudication, worsening of arterial insufficiency or angina pectoris, vasodilatation. *Digestive:* Dyspepsia, nausea, vomiting, diarrhoea, hepatomegaly. *Endocrine:* Hyperglycaemia, hypoglycaemia. *Integumentary:* Rash, pruritus, skin irritation, increased pigmentation, sweating, exfoliative dermatitis (one case). *Musculoskeletal:* Arthralgia. *Nervous system:* Dizziness, vertigo, paraesthesiae, local weakness. *Psychiatric:* Nervousness, diminished concentration, hallucinations, nightmares, increased dreaming, insomnia, depression, somnolence, decreased libido. *Haematological:* Non-thrombocytopenic purpura. *Respiratory:* Dyspnoea, bronchial spasm, rales, cough. *Special senses:* Tinnitus, visual disturbances, diplopia, ptosis, eye irritation, dry eyes. *Urogenital:* Impotence, micturition difficulties. *Clinical laboratory tests:* Changes in clinical laboratory tests are rare. Slight increases in blood urea, serum potassium and serum uric acid, and slight decreases in haemoglobin and haematocrit occurred, but were not progressive or associated with clinical manifestations.

*Overdosage:* No specific data are available in humans. A study in patients with renal failure suggests that Blocadren does not readily dialyse.

The most common signs and symptoms to be expected following overdosage with a beta-adrenergic-receptor blocking agent are symptomatic bradycardia, hypotension, bronchospasm, acute cardiac failure, and heart block. If overdosage occurs, the following measures are suggested. In all cases therapy with Blocadren should be stopped, and the patient closely observed.

1. Gastric lavage.
2. Symptomatic bradycardia: atropine sulphate, 0.25 to 2 mg intravenously, should be used to induce vagal blockade. If bradycardia persists, intravenous isoprenaline hydrochloride should be administered cautiously. In refractory cases, the use of a cardiac pacemaker may be considered.
3. Hypotension: a sympathomimetic pressor agent such as dopamine, dobutamine or noradrenaline should be used. In refractory cases, the use of glucagon has been reported to be useful.
4. Bronchospasm: isoprenaline hydrochloride should be used. Additional therapy with aminophylline may be considered.
5. Acute cardiac failure: conventional therapy with digitalis, diuretics, and oxygen should be instituted immediately. In refractory cases, the use of intravenous aminophylline is suggested. This may be followed, if necessary, by glucagon which has been reported useful.
6. Heart block: isoprenaline hydrochloride or a pacemaker should be used.

Timolol is rapidly and nearly completely absorbed following ingestion. Plasma half-life is approximately four hours.

**Pharmaceutical precautions** Keep container well closed; store in a cool place, protected from light.

**Legal category** POM.

**Package quantities** Packs of 60.

**Further information** Blocadren reduces blood pressure without acute hypotensive episodes in most patients with essential hypertension. The exact mechanism of action is still unknown. Blocadren does not usually affect normal blood pressure.

Blocadren effectively delays or prevents the development of anginal pain in most patients. It acts by modifying the cardiac response to stress or exercise.

Blocadren has been shown to be highly effective in reducing the incidence of cardiac death, including sudden death, and of reinfarction in patients who have survived the acute phase of a myocardial infarction.

**Product licence number** 0025/0091.

## CLINORIL*
## CLINORIL* 200

**Presentation** Brilliant yellow, scored, hexagonal tablets, biconvex in shape, containing 200 mg and 100 mg Sulindac PhEur. The 200 mg tablets are marked 'MSD 942' and the 100 mg tablets are marked 'MSD 943'.

**Uses** Non-steroidal, analgesic/anti-inflammatory agent with antipyretic properties.

Indicated in osteoarthritis, rheumatoid arthritis, ankylosing spondylitis, acute gouty arthritis, periarticular disorders such as bursitis, tendinitis, and tenosynovitis.

*Mode of action:* Prostglandin synthetase inhibition is hypothesised as the basis by which non-steroidal anti-inflammatory agents act. Following absorption, sulindac undergoes two major biotransformations: reversible reduction to the sulphide metabolite, and irreversible oxidation to the inactive sulphone metabolite. The sulphide metabolite is a potent inhibitor of prostaglandin synthesis and accounts for the activity of sulindac (Clinoril). Sulindac is thus a prodrug.

**Dosage and administration** The dosage should be taken twice a day and adjusted to the severity of the disease.

The usual dose is 400 mg a day. However, the dosage may be lowered depending on the response. Doses above 400 mg per day are not recommended.

In the treatment of acute gouty arthritis, therapy for seven days is usually adequate.

In peri-articular disorders, treatment should be limited to seven to ten days.

Clinoril should be adminstered with fluids or food.

*Children:* The use of Clinoril in children is contra-indicated.

*Use in the elderly:* The dosage does not require modification for the elderly patient.

**Contra-indications, warnings, etc**
*Contra-indications:* Hypersensitivity to any component of this product.

Clinoril should not be used in patients in whom acute asthmatic attacks, urticaria, or rhinitis have been precipitated by aspirin or other non-steroidal anti-inflammatory agents.

The drug should not be administered to patients with active gastro-intestinal bleeding.

The use of Clinoril should be avoided in patients with active peptic ulcer.

Since paediatric indications and dosage have not yet been established, Clinoril should not be given to children.

*Use in pregnancy:* Clinoril should be used during the first two trimesters of pregnancy only if the potential benefit justifies the potential risk to the fetus.

The known effects of drugs of this class on the human fetus during the third trimester of pregnancy include: constriction of the ductus arteriosus prenatally, tricuspid incompetence, and pulmonary hypertension; non-closure of the ductus arteriosus postnatally which may be resistant to medical management; myocardial degenerative changes, platelet dysfunction with resultant bleeding, intracranial bleeding, renal dysfunction or failure, renal injury/dysgenesis which may result in prolonged or permanent renal failure, oligohydramnios, gastro-intestinal bleeding or perforation and increased risk of necrotising enterocolitis. Use of Clinoril during the third trimester of pregnancy is not recommended.

*Precautions: Use in breast-feeding:* It is not known whether sulindac is excreted in human milk. Because other drugs of this class are excreted in human milk, a decision should be made whether to discontinue breast-feeding or discontinue the drug, taking into account the importance of the drug to the mother.

*Gastro-intestinal effects:* Clinoril should be used with caution in patients having a history of gastro-intestinal haemorrhage or ulcers.

*Platelet aggregation:* Clinoril has less effect on platelet function and bleeding time than aspirin; however, since Clinoril is an inhibitor of platelet function, patients who may be adversely affected should be carefully observed when 'Clinoril' is administered.

*Hypersensitivity syndrome:* A potentially life-threatening, apparent hypersensitivity syndrome has been reported. In cases where the syndrome is suspected, therapy should be discontinued immediately, and not recontinued. This syndrome may include constitutional symptoms (fever, chills, diaphoresis, flushing), cutaneous findings (rash or other dermatological reactions, see 'side effects'), conjunctivitis, involvement of major organs (changes in liver-function tests, hepatic failure, jaundice, pancreatitis, pneumonitis with or without pleural effusion, leucopenia, leucocytosis, eosinophilia, disseminated intravascular coagulation, anaemia, renal impairment, including renal failure), and other less specific findings (adenitis, arthralgia, arthritis, myalgia, fatigue, malaise, hypotension, chest pain, tachycardia).

*Infections:* Non-steroidal anti-inflammatory drugs, including Clinoril, may mask the usual signs and symptoms of infection. Therefore, the physician must be continually on the alert for this and should use the drug with extra care in the presence of existing infection.

*Ocular effects:* Because of reports of adverse eye findings with agents of this class it is recommended that patients who develop eye complaints during treatment with Clinoril have ophthalmological evaluations.

*Cardiovascular effects:* Peripheral oedema has been observed in some patients taking Clinoril. Therefore, as with other drugs in this class, Clinoril should be used with caution in patients with compromised cardiac function, hypertension, or other conditions predisposed to fluid retention.

*Hepatic effects:* A patient with signs and/or symptoms suggesting liver dysfunction, or in whom an abnormal liver-function test has occurred, should be evaluated for evidence of a more severe hepatic reaction while on therapy. Significant elevations of AST(SGOT) and ALT(SGPT) (three times higher than normal) were seen in less than 1% of patients in controlled clinical trials.

Poor liver function may alter the blood levels of circulating metabolites of Clinoril. Patients with liver dysfunction on Clinoril should be monitored closely; daily dosage reduction may be required.

Cases of hepatitis, jaundice, or both, with or without

fever, may occur within the first three months of therapy. In some patients, the findings are consistent with those of cholestatic hepatitis.

Fever or other evidence of hypersensitivity, including abnormalities in one or more liver function tests and skin reactions, have occurred during therapy. Some fatalities have occurred.

Whenever a patient develops unexplained fever, rash or other dermatological reactions, or constitutional symptoms, Clinoril should be permanently stopped and liver function investigated. Fever and abnormal liver function are reversible.

*Renal effects:* As with other non-steroidal anti-inflammatory drugs, there have been reports of acute interstitial nephritis with haematuria, proteinuria, and occasionally nephrotic syndrome in patients receiving sulindac.

In patients with reduced renal blood flow where renal prostaglandins play a major role in maintaining renal perfusion, administration of a non-steroidal anti-inflammatory agent may precipitate overt renal decomposition. Patients at greatest risk of this reaction are those with renal or hepatic dysfunction, diabetes mellitus, advanced age, extracellular volume depletion, congestive heart failure, sepsis, or concomitant use of any nephrotoxic drug. A non-steroidal anti-inflammatory drug should be given with caution and renal function should be monitored in any patient who may have reduced renal reserve. Discontinuation of non-steroidal anti-inflammatory therapy is usually followed by recovery to the pre-treatment state.

Since Clinoril is eliminated primarily by the kidneys, patients with significantly impaired renal function should be closely monitored; a lower daily dosage should be used to avoid excessive drug accumulation.

Sulindac metabolites have been reported rarely as the major, or a minor, component in renal stones in association with other calculus components. Clinoril should be used with caution in patients with a history of renal lithiasis and they should be kept well hydrated while receiving Clinoril. In patients with renal functional impairment, since the major route of excretion of the drug is via the kidney, the dosage may need to be reduced.

*Drug interactions: Dimethylsulphoxide:* Dimethyl sulphoxide should not be used with Clinoril. Concomitant use has been reported to reduce plasma levels of the active metabolite of Clinoril, and also cause peripheral neuropathy.

*Methotrexate:* Caution should be used if Clinoril is administered concomitantly with methotrexate. Non-steroidal anti-inflammatory drugs have been reported to decrease the tubular secretion of methotrexate and potentiate the toxicity.

*Cyclosporin:* Administration of non-steroidal anti-inflammatory drugs concomitantly with cyclosporin has been associated with an increase in cyclosporin-induced toxicity, possibly due to decreased synthesis of renal prostacyclin. NSAID's should be used with caution in patients taking cyclosporin, and renal function should be monitored carefully.

*Oral anticoagulants and hypoglycaemic agents:* Although sulindac and its sulphide metabolite are highly bound to protein, studies (in which Clinoril was given at a dose of 400 mg daily) have shown no clinically significant interaction with oral anticoagulants or oral hypoglycaemic agents. However, patients should be monitored carefully until it is certain that no change in their anticoagulant or hypoglycaemic dose is required.

*Aspirin:* Concomitant administration with aspirin in normal volunteers significantly depressed plasma levels of the active sulphide metabolite. Clinical study of the combination showed an increase in GI side effects with no improvement in the therapeutic response to Clinoril. The combination is not recommended.

*Diflunisal:* Concomitant administration with diflunisal in normal volunteers reduced the plasma level of active sulphide metabolite by approximately one-third.

*Other NSAIDs:* The concomitant use of Clinoril with other NSAIDs is not recommended due to the increased possibility of gastro-intestinal toxicity, with little or no increase in efficacy.

*Probenecid:* Probenecid given concomitantly with sulindac had only a slight effect on plasma sulphide levels, while plasma levels of sulindac and sulphone were increased. Sulindac was shown to produce a modest reduction in the uricosuric action of probenecid which probably is not usually significant.

*Dextropropoxyphene hydrochloride/paracetamol:* Neither dextropropoxyphene hydrochloride nor paracetamol had any effect on the plasma levels of sulindac or its sulphide metabolite.

*Antacids:* In a drug interaction study, an antacid (magnesium and aluminium hydroxides in suspension) was administered with Clinoril with no significant difference in absorption.

*Anti-hypertensive agents:* In contrast to most other non-steroidal anti-inflammatory drugs, Clinoril does

not reduce the antihypertensive effect of thiazides and a variety of other agents used to treat mild-to-moderate hypertension. However, the blood pressure of patients taking Clinoril with antihypertensive agents should be closely monitored.

*Side-effects:* Clinoril is generally well tolerated. Those side-effects experienced are usually mild and may often respond to a reduction in dosage.

*Side effects reported frequently:*
*Gastro-intestinal:* The most frequent types of side-effects occurring with Clinoril are gastro-intestinal; these include gastro-intestinal pain, dyspepsia, nausea with or without vomiting, diarrhoea, constipation, flatulence, anorexia, and gastro-intestinal cramps.

*Dermatological:* Rash, pruritus.

*Central nervous system:* Dizziness, headache, nervousness.

*Special senses:* Tinnitus.

*Miscellaneous:* Oedema.

*Side effects reported less frequently:*
The following side-effects were reported less frequently. The probability exists of a causal relationship between Clinoril and these side-effects:

*Gastro-intestinal:* Stomatitis, gastritis or gastro-enteritis. Peptic ulcer, colitis, as well as gastro-intestinal bleeding and perforations have been reported rarely. Fatalities have occurred. Liver-function test abnormalities, jaundice sometimes with fever, cholestasis, hepatitis, hepatic failure, pancreatitis, ageusia and glossitis, and intestinal strictures (diaphragm). It has also been reported that a probable sulindac metabolite has been found in biliary sludge in patients with symptoms of cholecystitis who underwent a cholecystectomy.

*Dermatological:* Sore or dry mucous membranes, alopecia, photosensitivity. Erythema multiforme, toxic epidermal necrolysis, Stevens-Johnson syndrome, exfoliative dermatitis.

*Cardiovascular:* Congestive heart failure, especially in patients with marginal cardiac function; palpitation, hypertension.

*Haematological:* Thrombocytopenia; ecchymosis; purpura; leucopenia; agranulocytosis; neutropenia; bone-marrow depression, including aplastic anaemia; haemolytic anaemia, increased prothrombin time in patients on oral anticoagulants.

*Genito-urinary:* Urine discoloration, dysuria, vaginal bleeding, haematuria, proteinuria, crystalluria, renal impairment including renal failure, interstitial nephritis, nephrotic syndrome.

*Nervous system:* Vertigo, somnolence, insomnia, sweating, asthenia, paraesthesia, convulsions, syncope, depression, psychic disturbances including acute psychosis, aseptic meningitis.

*Metabolic:* hyperkalaemia.

*Musculoskeletal:* Muscle weakness.

*Special senses:* Visual disturbances including blurred vision, decreased hearing, metallic or bitter taste.

*Respiratory:* Epistaxis.

*Hypersensitivity reactions:* Anaphylaxis and angioneurotic oedema. Bronchial spasm, dyspnoea, hypersensitivity vasculitis, hypersensitivity syndrome (see Precautions).

*Causal relationship unknown:* Other reactions have been reported in clinical trials or since the drug was marketed, but occurred under circumstances where a causal relationship could not be established. However, in these rarely reported events, that possibility cannot be excluded. Therefore, these observations are listed to serve as alerting information to physicians.

*Nervous system:* Neuritis.

*Special senses:* Disturbances of the retina and its vasculature.

*Cardiovascular:* Arrhythmia.

*Metabolic:* Hyperglycaemia.

*Miscellaneous:* Gynaecomastia.

Rarely, occurrences of fulminant necrotising fasciitis, particularly in association with Group A β-haemolytic streptococcus, has been described in persons treated with non-steroidal anti-inflammatory agents, sometimes with fatal outcome (see also Precautions).

*Overdosage:* Cases of overdosage have been reported and, rarely, fatalities have occurred. The following signs and symptoms may be observed following overdosage: stupor, coma, diminished urine output, and hypotension. In isolated cases, patients have received up to 600 mg a day without adverse consequences being reported.

In the event of acute overdosage, if ingestion is recent, the stomach should be emptied by inducing vomiting or by gastric lavage, and the patient carefully observed and given symptomatic and supportive treatment.

Animal studies show that absorption is decreased by the prompt administration of activated charcoal, and excretion is enhanced by alkalinisation of the urine.

The readiness of sulindac and its metabolites to dialyse is unknown at present. But because they are highly bound to plasma proteins, dialysis is not likely to be effective.

The mean half-life of sulindac is 7.8 hours while the mean half-life of the active sulphide metabolite is 16.4 hours.

**Pharmaceutical precautions**  Keep container well closed; store in a cool place, protected from light.

**Legal category**  POM.

**Package quantities**  *200 mg:* Packs of 60. *100 mg:* Packs of 60.

**Further information**  Clinoril usually provides symptomatic relief of inflammation, pain and tenderness, and promotes early improvement in joint mobility. Clinoril has a prolonged duration of activity, which permits a twice-a-day dose schedule. Based on extensive studies, Clinoril has been shown to be suitable for the long-term relief of pain and inflammation.

**Product licence numbers**
100 mg  0025/0121
200 mg  0025/0122

# COGENTIN* TABLETS
# COGENTIN* INJECTION

**Qualitative and quantitative composition**  Each tablet of Cogentin contains 2 mg of Benztropine Mesylate BP.

Each sterile injection of Cogentin contains 0.1% w/v Benztropine Mesylate BP.

**Pharmaceutical form**  Cogentin Tablets are supplied as white, quarter-scored tablets, marked 'MSD 60'.

Cogentin Injection is supplied as a colourless, sterile solution for injection.

## Clinical particulars

*Therapeutic indications:* Cogentin is an anti-parkinsonian agent with powerful anticholinergic effects.

It is indicated for symptomatic treatment of all types of 'classical' parkinsonism including arteriosclerotic, post-encephalitic, and idiopathic parkinsonism, and of extrapyramidal reactions induced by phenothiazines or reserpine.

Cogentin is particularly effective in the relief of rigidity and tremor. Among other symptoms which it can ameliorate are: sialorrhoea, drooling, mask-like facies, oculogyric crises, speech and writing difficulties, gait disturbances, dysphagia, and pain and insomnia due to muscle spasm and cramps.

Cogentin often is helpful in patients who have become unresponsive to other agents. Therapy is directed toward control of disturbing symptoms to permit the patient maximum integration of function with minimum discomfort. In non-drug-induced parkinsonism, partial control of symptoms is usually achieved.

Cogentin Injection is only to be used in an emergency or when a patient is unable to swallow tablets.

*Posology and method of administration:* As Cogentin is cumulative in action, treatment should begin with a low dosage, which can be increased by amounts of 0.5 mg at intervals of five to six days, to the smallest dosage necessary for optimal relief without excessive side-effects. Maximum dosage, 6 mg a day.

For Cogentin Tablets, the route of administration is oral.

Cogentin Injection may be used intramuscularly or intravenously in emergencies, or for patients unable to swallow tablets. (As there is no significant difference in time of onset of effect between intramuscular and intravenous administration, the intravenous route is not usually necessary.)

In emergencies, 1–2 ml (1–2 mg) of Cogentin Injection will normally provide quick relief. If signs of parkinsonism begin to return, the dose can be repeated.

*'Classical' parkinsonism: Usual dosage:* 1–2 mg a day. with a range of 0.5–6 mg a day. Dosage must be adjusted on an individual basis, taking into consideration the age and weight of the patient, and the type of parkinsonism. Older patients, thin patients and those with arteriosclerotic parkinsonism usually cannot tolerate large dosages. Most patients with post-encephalitic parkinsonism need and indeed tolerate fairly large dosages. Patients with a poor mental outlook may respond poorly. In arteriosclerotic and idiopathic parkinsonism, therapy may be initiated with a single daily dose of 0.5–1 mg at bedtime. This dosage will be adequate in some patients, whereas 4–6 mg a day may be required by others. In post-encephalitic parkinsonism, therapy may be initiated in most patients with 2 mg a day in one or more doses. In highly sensitive individuals, therapy may be initiated with 0.5 mg at bedtime, and increased as necessary.

Some patients obtain greatest relief by taking the entire dose at bedtime; others react more favourably to divided dosage, two to four times a day. One dose a day frequently is sufficient; divided doses may be unnecessary or even undesirable.

*Drug-induced parkinsonism:* Usual dosage range: 1–4 mg once or twice a day.

*Acute dystonic reactions:* 1–2 ml (1–2 mg) by intravenous injection followed usually by 1–2 mg orally twice a day.

Extrapyramidal reactions appearing soon after starting phenothiazine or reserpine therapy are likely to be temporary, and are usually controlled in one or two days by 1–2 mg of Cogentin orally two or three times a day. Cogentin should be withdrawn after one or two weeks to determine if it is still needed. It can be reinstated if necessary.

Certain extrapyramidal reactions which develop slowly (e.g. tardive dyskinesia) do not usually respond to Cogentin.

*Paediatric use:* Use with caution in children over 3 years old (see *Contra-indications*).

*Use in the elderly:* As with younger patients, dosage should be the smallest possible for optimum relief of symptoms. Initial dosage should be 0.5–1 mg preferably at night, increasing until optimum effect is seen. Older patients usually cannot tolerate large doses.

*Contra-indications:* Because of the atropine-like side effects, Cogentin is contra-indicated in children under 3 years old and should be used with caution in older children. Cogentin is contra-indicated in patients who are hypersensitive to this product.

*Special warnings and special precautions for use:* Continued supervision of patients is recommended as Cogentin has a cumulative action. Patients with a tendency towards tachycardia and those with prostatic hypertrophy, should be closely observed.

Patients with mental disorders should be carefully supervised when Cogentin is used to control drug-induced extrapyramidal reactions, especially when therapy is started or the dosage of Cogentin is increased. Intensification of mental symptoms may occasionally occur. Cogentin should be temporarily withdrawn if the reactions are severe.

Cogentin has anticholinergic effects, and glaucoma is a possibility. Although Cogentin does not appear to have any adverse effect on simple glaucoma, its use is probably not advisable in narrow-angle glaucoma. It may cause anhidrosis; this should be borne in mind, particularly in hot weather, especially when given concomitantly with other atropine-like drugs to the chronically ill, alcoholics, or patients with a central nervous system disease and those who do manual labour in a hot environment. Cogentin should be used cautiously in patients with or prone to abnormalities of sweating. If there is evidence of anhidrosis, the possibility of hyperthermia should be considered. Dosage should be decreased as necessary to maintain body heat equilibrium by the action of perspiration. Severe anhidrosis and fatal hyperthermia have occurred.

*Interaction with other medicaments and other forms of interaction:* Extra care should be taken when Cogentin is given concomitantly with phenothiazines, haloperidol or other drugs with anticholinergic or antidopaminergic activity. Patients should be advised to report gastro-intestinal complaints, fever or heat intolerance promptly. Paralytic ileus, sometimes fatal, has occurred to patients taking anticholinergic-type anti-parkinsonian drugs, including Cogentin, in combination with phenothiazines and/or tricyclic antidepressants.

Tardive dyskinesia may appear in some patients on long-term therapy with phenothiazines or related agents, or after discontinuation of such therapy. Anti-parkinsonian agents do not usually alleviate symptoms of tardive dyskinesia, and in some cases may aggravate or unmask them. Cogentin is not recommended in tardive dyskinesia.

*Pregnancy and lactation:* It is not known whether Cogentin can cause fetal harm when administered to a pregnant woman or can affect reproductive capacity. Cogentin should be given to a pregnant woman only if clearly needed.

*Breast-feeding mothers:* it is not known whether this drug is excreted in human milk. Because many drugs are excreted in human milk, caution should be exercised when Cogentin is administered to a breast-feeding mother.

*Effects on ability to drive and use machines:* Cogentin may impair the mental alertness and physical ability required for the performance of such hazardous tasks as driving a car or operating machinery.

*Undesirable effects:* Side-effects, most of which are anticholinergic or antihistaminic in nature are listed below by body system in order of decreasing severity.

*Cardiovascular:* Tachycardia.

*Digestive:* Constipation, dry mouth, nausea, vomiting.

If dry mouth is so severe that there is difficulty in swallowing or speaking, or loss of appetite and weight occur, reduce dosage, or discontinue the drug temporarily.

Slight reduction in dosage may control nausea and still give sufficient relief of symptoms. Vomiting may be controlled by temporary discontinuation, followed by resumption at a lower dosage.

*Nervous system:* Toxic psychosis, including confusion, disorientation, memory impairment, visual hallucinations; exacerbation of pre-existing psychotic symptoms; nervousness; depression; listlessness; numbness of fingers.

*Special senses:* Blurred vision, dilated pupils.

*Urogenital:* Urinary retention, dysuria.

*Metabolic/immune and skin:* Occasionally, an allergic reaction, e.g., skin rash, develops. If this cannot be controlled by dosage reduction, the medication should be discontinued.

*Other:* Heat stroke, hyperthermia, fever.

*Overdosage:* Symptoms may be any of those seen in atropine poisoning or antihistamine overdosage: CNS depression, preceded or followed by stimulation; confusion; nervousness; listlessness; intensification of mental symptoms or toxic psychosis in patients with mental illness being treated with neuroleptic drugs (e.g. phenothiazines); hallucinations (especially visual); dizziness; muscle weakness; ataxia; dry mouth; mydriasis; blurred vision; palpitations; tachycardia; nausea; vomiting; dysuria; numbness of fingers; dysphagia, allergic reactions, e.g. skin rash; headache; hot, dry, flushed skin; delirium; coma; shock; convulsions; respiratory arrest; anhidrosis; hyperthermia; glaucoma; constipation.

Physostigmine salicylate (1–2 mg, subcutaneously or intravenously) is reported to reverse symptoms of anticholinergic intoxication. A second injection may be given after two hours if needed. Otherwise, treatment is symptomatic and supportive.

If ingestion is recent, emesis should be induced or gastric lavage performed. A short-acting barbiturate may be used for CNS excitement, but with caution to avoid subsequent depression. Supportive care for CNS depression may be required (such convulsant stimulants as picrotoxin, leptazol or bemegride should be avoided). In severe respiratory depression, artificial respiration may be required. Also needed may be a local miotic for mydriasis and cycloplegia, ice bags or other cold applications and alcohol sponges for hyperpyrexia, a vasopressor and fluids for circulatory collapse, and a darkened room for photophobia.

Data on the metabolism of benztropine maleate are not available at present; but a death was recorded 1½ hours after ingestion.

## Pharmacological properties

*Pharmacodynamic properties:* Anticholinergic drugs exert their anti-parkinsonian effect by correcting the relating cholinergic excess which is thought to occur in parkinsonism as a result of dopamine deficiency.

The deficiency of dopamine in the striatum of patients with parkinsonism intensifies the excitatory effects of the cholinergic system within the striatum. Anticholinergics aid such patients by blunting this component of the nigrostriated pathway.

*Pharmacokinetic properties:* Following i.m. injection, the clinical effects of benztropine are apparent within 10 minutes and the maximal effect is seen within 30 minutes.

Benztropine has a cumulative effect and a prolonged duration of action when compared with other anticholinergic agents used in the treatment of Parkinson's disease such as trihexyphenidyl. In patients on long-term maintenance therapy, it may take up to seven days before all evidence of drug-related effects have ceased.

*Preclinical safety data:* No relevant information.

## Pharmaceutical particulars

*List of excipients:*

*Tablet:* Calcium hydrogen phosphate PhEur, cellulose powder PhEur, lactose PhEur, magnesium stearate PhEur E572, and maize starch PhEur.

*Injection:* Sodium chloride PhEur, and water for injection PhEur.

*Incompatibilities:* None known.

*Shelf life:* 60 months.

*Special precautions for storage: Tablet:* Store below 25°C. *Injection:* Store below 25°C, protected from light and freezing.

*Nature and contents of container: Tablet:* Amber glass, HDPE, or polypropylene bottles of 500.

*Injection:* Type I glass ampoules of 2 ml.

*Instructions for use/handling:* None.

**Marketing authorisation numbers**  Cogentin tablet 0025/5023R
Cogentin injection 0025/5024R.

**Date of approval/revision of SPL**  March 1996.

**Legal category**  POM.

# CONCORDIN*

**Presentation** Concordin-5, salmon-red, film-coated tablets, marked 'MSD 26', containing 5 mg Protriptyline Hydrochloride BP.

Concordin-10, white, film-coated tablets, marked 'MSD 47', containing 10 mg Protriptyline Hydrochloride BP.

**Uses** Symptoms of depressive illness.

Concordin may be used successfully in depression that is a manifestation of psychosis or neurosis, whether endogenous or reactive. Endogenous depression is more likely to respond. Concordin is especially recommended in apathetic, withdrawn patients, because it promptly relieves anergia, and it lacks sedative activity.

The following 'target' symptoms of depression may be expected to respond well to Concordin: depressed mood; excessive crying; apathy; withdrawal; psychomotor retardation; loss of interest; fatigue; lassitude; feelings of guilt; anorexia; headache; functional somatic complaints (e.g. gastro-intestinal symptoms).

**Dosage and administration** Dosage should be adjusted for each patient, bearing in mind the cyclic nature and variable severity of depression, the danger of relapse, and the possibility of spontaneous remission.

*Adults:* Dosage range, 15–60 mg. Usual starting dosage, 30–40 mg a day, divided into 3 or 4 doses. Any increase in dosage should be made gradually, and added to the morning dose first. If insomnia is present, the last dose should be given no later than mid-afternoon. When a satisfactory response is noted, the dosage should be reduced to the smallest amount necessary to maintain relief. Maintenance therapy should be continued for at least three months after satisfactory improvement. If relapse occurs, Concordin may be reinstated.

If the dosage required for adequate antidepressant effect produces overstimulation, concurrent use of a tranquilliser will provide effective control. Overstimulation is unlikely if the dosage of Concordin is kept below 20 mg a day.

Therapy may be usefully initiated with a tranquilliser and preventive supervision in suicidal patients, because these patients usually have a high level of anxiety, and Concordin may relieve anergia before recovery from depression is complete.

*Children:* Concordin is not recommended for children under 16 years old.

*Elderly patients:* Initially 5 mg three times a day. These patients may not tolerate higher doses as well as other patients. If the elderly receive more than 20 mg a day, they should be observed for effects on the cardiovascular system.

**Contra-indications, warnings, etc**
*Contra-indications:* Hypersensitivity to any component of this product. Concurrent use with a monoamine oxidase inhibitor. Hyperpyretic crises, severe convulsions, and deaths have occurred when tricyclic antidepressants and MAOIs have been given simultaneously (see also 'Precautions'); the acute recovery phase after recent myocardial infarction; known sensitivity to protriptyline. Any degree of heart block or other cardiac arrhythmias, mania, marked agitation, severe liver disease, during breast feeding. For 'Use in pregnancy', see 'Precautions'.

*Precautions:* Protriptyline should be used with caution in patients with a history of epilepsy, impaired liver function, a tendency to urinary retention, prostatic hypertrophy, or increased intra-ocular pressure.

Concordin should be used cautiously in elderly patients and patients with cardiovascular disorders. Such patients should be closely observed because of the tendency of protriptyline to produce tachycardia, hypotension, arrhythmias, and prolongation of the conduction time. The elderly are particularly liable to experience agitation and confusion. Myocardial infarction and stroke have occurred with drugs of this class.

Protriptyline may impair abilities needed for performing hazardous tasks, such as driving a vehicle or operating machinery.

In patients who may use alcohol excessively, potentiation may increase the danger inherent in any suicide attempt or overdosage.

Psychotic symtoms may be aggravated when Concodin is used in schizophrenic patients. Manic depressive patients may shift towards the manic phase. Paranoid delusions, with or without hostility, may be exaggerated. In any of these circumstances, it may be advisable to reduce the dosage, or to use a major tranquilliser concurrently.

Concordin may aggravate anxiety or agitation in over-active or agitated patients.

The possibility of suicide in depressed patients remains during treatment until significant remission has occurred; suicidal patients should not have access to large quantities of Concordin tablets and should be carefully supervised.

The natural course of depression often is of many months' duration. It is appropriate, therefore, to continue maintenance therapy for three months or longer to lessen the possibility of relapse.

Discontinue the drug several days before elective surgery if possible.

*Drug interactions:* A minimum of 14 days should elapse between discontinuing a monoamine oxidase inhibitor and introducing Concordin, which should then be started cautiously, with gradual increases in dosage until optimum response is achieved.

Protriptyline may block the antihypertensive effect of guanethidine, debrisoquine, bethanidine, and possibly clonidine or similar compounds. Review all antihypertensive therapy during treatment.

Protriptyline should not be given with sympathomimetic agents such as ephedrine, isoprenaline, noradrenaline, phenylephrine, and phenylpropanolamine.

Protriptyline may enhance the response to alcohol and the effects of barbiturates and other CNS depressants.

Cimetidine is reported to reduce hepatic metabolism of certain tricyclic antidepressants.

Concurrent administration of Concordin may increase the hazards of electroconvulsive therapy. Such combined treatment should be limited to those for whom it is essential.

Anaesthetics given during tricyclic antidepressant therapy may increase the risk of arrhythmias and hypotension. If surgery is necessary, the anaesthetist should be informed that the patient is receiving protriptyline.

On rare occasions, hyperthyroid patients or those receiving thyroid medication may develop arrhythmias when protriptyline is given.

*Use in pregnancy and lactation:* Safe use in pregnancy and lactation has not been established. Avoid during pregnancy, especially during the first and last trimesters. Use in pregnant women, breast-feeding mothers or women who may become pregnant requires that possible benefits be weighed against possible hazards to the mother and child.

There is no evidence as to drug safety in human pregnancy, nor is there evidence from animal work that it is free from hazard.

*Side-effects:* Some of the adverse reactions below have not been specifically reported for Concordin, but are included because of the similar pharmacological properties of the tricyclic group of antidepressants. Concordin is more likely to aggravate anxiety and agitation and to produce such cardiovascular reactions as tachycardia and hypotension.

As improvement may not occur during the first two to four weeks of treatment, patients should be closely monitored during this period.

*Cardiovascular:* Hypotension (particularly orthostatic hypotension), hypertension, tachycardia, palpitation, myocardial infarction, arrhythmias, heart block, stroke.

*Psychiatric:* Confusional states (especially in the elderly) with hallucinations, disorientation, delusions, anxiety, restlessness, agitation; insomnia, panic, and nightmares; hypomania; exacerbation of psychosis.

*Neurological:* Numbness, tingling and paraesthesiae of extremities; incoordination, ataxia, tremors, peripheral neuropathy; extrapyramidal symptoms; seizures; alteration in EEG patterns, tinnitus, drowsiness, dizziness, weakness and fatigue; headache.

*Anticholinergic:* Dry mouth and rarely associated sublingual adenitis; blurred vision, disturbance of accommodation, mydriasis; constipation, paralytic ileus; hyperpyrexia; urinary retention, delayed micturition, dilatation of the urinary tract.

*Allergic:* Skin rash, petechiae, urticaria, itching, oedema (generally, or of face and tongue), drug fever. Some rashes have been associated with photosensitisation. In view of this, patients should avoid excessive exposure to sunlight, including sunbathing.

*Haematological:* Bone-marrow depression; agranulocytosis; leucopenia; eosinophilia; purpura; thrombocytopenia.

*Gastro-intestinal:* Nausea and vomiting, anorexia, epigastric distress, diarrhoea, peculiar taste, stomatitis, abdominal cramps, black tongue.

*Endocrine:* Gynaecomastia in the male; breast enlargement and galactorrhoea in the female; increased or decreased libido, impotence; testicular swelling; elevation or depression of blood sugar levels; syndrome of inappropriate ADH secretion.

*Other:* Jaundice (simulating obstructive); altered liver function; weight gain or loss; perspiration; flushing; urinary frequency; nocturia; parotid swelling; alopecia.

*Withdrawal symptoms:* Though not indicative of addiction, abrupt cessation of treatment after prolonged therapy may produce nausea, insomnia, irritability, excessive perspiration, headache and malaise.

Gradual dosage reduction has been reported to produce, within two weeks, transient symptoms including irritability, restlessness, and dream and sleep disturbance. These symptoms are not indicative of addiction. Rare instances have been reported of mania or hypomania occurring within 2–7 days following cessation of chronic therapy with tricyclic antidepressants.

Withdrawal symptoms in neonates whose mothers receive tricyclic antidepressants during the third trimester have also been reported.

*Overdosage:* High doses may cause temporary confusion, disturbed concentration, or transient visual hallucinations. Overdosage may cause drowsiness; hypothermia; tachycardia and other arrhythmic abnormalities, for example bundle branch block; ECG evidence of impaired conduction; congestive heart failure; dilated pupils; convulsions; severe hypotension; stupor; and coma. Other symptoms may be agitation, hyperactive reflexes, muscle rigidity, vomiting, and hyperpyrexia, or any of those listed under 'Side-effects'.

Experience in the management of overdosage with protriptyline is limited. All patients suspected of having taken an overdosage should be admitted to a hospital as soon as possible. Treatment is symptomatic and supportive. If ingestion is recent, empty the stomach as quickly as possible by emesis followed by gastric lavage upon arrival at the hospital. Following gastric lavage, activated charcoal may be administered; 20 to 30 g of activated charcoal may be given every four to six hours during the first 24 to 48 hours after ingestion. An ECG should be taken and close monitoring of cardiac function instituted if there is any sign of abnormality. Maintain an open airway and adequate fluid intake; regulate body temperature.

Anticonvulsants may be given to control convulsions.

Dialysis is of no value because of low plasma concentrations of the drug.

The intravenous administration of 1–3 mg of physostigmine salicylate is reported to reverse the symptoms of tricyclic antidepressant poisoning in humans. Because physostigmine is rapidly metabolised, the dosage of physostigmine should be repeated as required, particularly if life-threatening signs such as arrhythmias, convulsions, and deep coma recur or persist after the initial dosage of physostigmine. Because physostigmine itself may be toxic, it is not recommended for routine use.

Standard measures should be used to manage circulatory shock and metabolic acidosis. Cardiac arrhythmias may be treated with neostigmine, pyridostigmine, or propranolol. Should cardiac failure occur, the use of digitalis should be considered. Close monitoring of cardiac function for not less than five days is advisable.

Protriptyline has been estimated to have a very prolonged half-life ranging from 55 to 198 hours, which may be further prolonged in overdosage.

**Pharmaceutical precautions** Store below 25°C, protected from light.

**Legal category** POM.

**Package quantities**
5 mg: Blister packs of 30.
10 mg: Blister packs of 30.

**Further information** Concordin is a member of the tricyclic group of antidepressants. Concordin is not a monoamine oxidase inhibitor, and dietary restrictions are not necessary. Concordin has not produced addiction or habituation.

Concordin has a rapid onset of effect, which can be of particular importance where there is a risk of suicide. It is advisable, however, to administer a tranquilliser and to ensure preventative supervision when starting Concordin in suicidal patients since they usually have a high level of anxiety, and especially because Concordin may relieve the anergia before there is complete recovery from the depressed state.

When Concordin has to be used in conjunction with ECT, the total number of shock treatments required may be reduced.

**Product licence numbers**
5 mg    0025/5004
10 mg   0025/5005

# COSMEGEN* LYOVAC*

**Qualitative and quantitative composition** Cosmegen Lyovac is supplied as a yellow, lyophilised powder, in a vial containing 500 micrograms dactinomycin with 20 mg of mannitol.

**Pharmaceutical form** Lyophilised powder for reconstitution and injection.

**Clinical particulars**
*Therapeutic indications:* Dactinomycin is a cytotoxic, antineoplastic antibiotic with immunosuppressant properties.

Recommended only in the treatment, under appropriate supervision, of hospitalised patients with Wilms' tumour, rhabdomyosarcoma, and carcinoma of the testis or uterus. All other indications for dactinomycin are as yet experimental (e.g. Ewing's sarcoma, osteogenic sarcoma).

*Wilms' tumour:* The neoplasm responding most frequently to Cosmegen is Wilms' tumour. With low doses of both dactinomycin and radiotherapy, temporary objective improvement may be as good as, and may last longer than, that obtained with higher doses of each given alone.

*Rhabdomyosarcoma:* Temporary regression of the tumour and beneficial subjective results have occurred with dactinomycin in rhabdomyosarcoma, which, like most soft-tissue sarcomas, is comparatively radioresistant.

*Carcinoma of the testis and uterus:* The sequential use of dactinomycin and methotrexate, along with meticulous monitoring of human chorionic gonadotrophin levels until normal, has resulted in survival in the majority of women with metastatic choriocarcinoma.

Sequential therapy is used if there is:
(1) stability in gonadotrophin titres following two successive courses of an agent.
(2) rising gonadotrophin titres during treatment.
(3) severe toxicity preventing adequate therapy.

In patients with non-metastatic choriocarcinoma, dactinomycin or methotrexate or both have been used successfully with or without surgery.

Cosmegen has been beneficial as a single agent in the treatment of metastatic non-seminomatous testicular carcinoma.

*Other neoplasms:* Dactinomycin has been given intravenously or by regional perfusion, alone or with other antineoplastic compounds or with X-ray therapy, in the palliative treatment of Ewing's sarcoma and sarcoma botryoides. For non-metastatic Ewing's sarcoma, promising results were obtained when dactinomycin (45 micrograms/m$^2$) and cyclophosphamide (1,200 mg/m$^2$) were given sequentially and with radiotherapy over an 18-month period. Those with metastatic disease remain the subject of continued investigation with a more aggressive chemotherapeutic regimen employed initially.

Temporary objective improvement and relief of pain and discomfort have followed the use of dactinomycin, usually in conjunction with radiotherapy for sarcoma botryoides. This palliative effect ranges from transitory inhibition of tumour growth to a considerable but temporary regression in tumour size.

*Cosmegen and radiation therapy:* Much evidence suggests that Cosmegen potentiates the effects of X-ray therapy. The converse also appears likely: that Cosmegen may be more effective when radiation therapy is given concurrently.

With combined Cosmegen and radiation therapy, the normal skin, as well as the buccal and pharyngeal mucosa, shows early erythema. When given with dactinomycin, a smaller than usual X-ray dose causes erythema and vesiculation, which progresses more rapidly through the stages of tanning and desquamation.

Healing may occur in four to six weeks rather than in two to three months. Erythema from previous X-ray therapy may be reactivated by the administration of Cosmegen alone, especially when the interval between the two forms of therapy is brief. This potentiation of radiation effects represents a special problem when the irradiation treatment area includes the mucous membrane. When irradiation is directed towards the nasopharynx, the combination may produce severe oropharyngeal mucositis.

*Severe reactions may ensue if high doses of both Cosmegen and radiation therapy are used, or if the patient is particularly sensitive to such combined therapy.*

Because of this potentiating effect, Cosmegen may be tried in radiosensitive tumours not responding to doses of X-ray therapy that can be tolerated. Objective improvement in tumour size and activity may be observed when lower, better tolerated doses of both types of therapy are employed.

*Isolation-perfusion technique:* Cosmegen, alone or with other antineoplastic agents, has also been given by the isolation-perfusion technique, either as palliative treatment or as an adjunct to resection of a tumour. Some tumours that are considered resistant to chemotherapy and radiation therapy may respond when the drug is given by the perfusion technique. Neoplasms in which dactinomycin has been tried by this technique include various types of sarcoma, carcinoma and adenocarcinoma.

In some instances, tumours regressed, pain was relieved for variable periods, and surgery made possible. On other occasions, however, the outcome has been less favourable. Nevertheless, in selected cases, Cosmegen given by the perfusion technique may provide more effective palliation than when given systemically.

*Posology and method of administration:* Toxic reactions due to Cosmegen are frequent and may be severe, thus limiting the amount that may be given in many cases. However, the severity of toxicity varies markedly and is only partly dependent on the dosage used.

Cosmegen must be given only in short courses.

*Intravenous use:* The dosage of Cosmegen will vary with the tolerance of the patient, the size and location of the neoplasm, and the use of other forms of therapy. It may be necessary to reduce the usual dosage suggested below when other chemotherapy or X-ray therapy is used concurrently or has been employed previously.

The dosage of Cosmegen is calculated in micrograms. The dosage for adults or children should not exceed 15 micrograms per kg or 400–600 micrograms per square metre of body surface daily, intravenously, for five days. Calculation of the dosage for obese or oedematous patients should be on the basis of surface area in an effort to relate dosage to lean body mass.

*Adults:* Usually 500 micrograms a day for a maximum of five days, given intravenously.

*Children:* 15 micrograms per kg bodyweight a day for a maximum of five days, given intravenously. Alternatively, a total dosage of 2,500 micrograms per square metre of body surface is given intravenously over a one-week period.

Cosmegen should not normally be given to infants under the age of 12 months.

In both adults and children, a second course may be given, but not until at least three weeks have elapsed, and all evidence of toxicity has disappeared.

*Isolation-perfusion technique:* Administration by the isolation-perfusion technique offers certain advantages, provided leakage of the drug through the general circulation into other areas of the body is minimal. By this technique, dactinomycin is in continuous contact with the tumour for the duration of treatment. The dose may be increased well above that used by the systemic route, usually without adding to the danger of toxic effects. If the agent is confined to an isolated part, it should not interfere with the patient's defence mechanisms. Systemic absorption of toxic products from neoplastic tissue can be minimised by removing the perfusate when the procedure is finished.

The dosage schedules and the technique itself vary from one investigator to another, and the published literature should, therefore, be consulted for details. In general the following doses are suggested:

For a lower extremity or pelvis – 50 micrograms per kg bodyweight.

For an upper extremity – 35 micrograms per kg bodyweight.

It may be advisable to use lower doses in obese patients, or when previous chemotherapy or radiation therapy has been employed.

*Use in the elderly:* The general considerations already outlined also apply to elderly patients.

When reconstituted, the solution of dactinomycin can be added to an infusion solution of 5% dextrose injection or sodium chloride injection, either directly or into the tubing of a running intravenous infusion.

Since dactinomycin is extremely corrosive to soft tissue, precautions for materials of this nature should be observed. To avoid extravasation, the calculated dose of Cosmegen should be given through the tubing of a running intravenous infusion, so that when administration is completed, the tubing can be flushed immediately to avoid damage to the vein.

If extravasation occurs, stop the infusion and disconnect the i.v. administration set, but leave the cannula or needle *in situ.* Attempt to aspirate the extravasated drug via the cannula or needle, inject antidote if desired, and remvoe the cannula or needle. Elevate the limb and apply a cold compress for 45 minutes. There is no generally accepted antidote for local use, but the following have been used with some success:

Sodium thiosulphate 25% (1.6 ml+3 ml of Water for Injection)
Sodium thiosulphate 10% (4 ml+6 ml of Water for Injection)
Ascorbic acid injection (50 mg/ml) (1 ml).

In severe cases, debridement may become necessary.

Partial removal of dactinomycin from intravenous solutions by cellulose ester membrane filters used in some intravenous in-line filters has been reported.

If Cosmegen is to be injected directly into the vein without the use of an infusion, the 'two-needle' technique should be used. The calculated dose should be reconstituted and withdrawn from the vial with one sterile needle; direct injection into the vein should then be performed with another sterile needle.

Although reconstituted Cosmegen is chemically stable, the product does not contain a preservative and accidental microbial contamination might result. Any unused portion of the solution should be discarded.

*Contra-indications:* If Cosmegen is given at or about the time of infection with chickenpox or herpes zoster, a severe generalised disease, which may be fatal, can occur.

*Special warnings and precautions for use:* Cosmegen should be administered only under the supervision of a physician who is experienced in the use of a cancer chemotherapeutic agent.

Cosmegen is highly toxic and both powder and solution must be handled and administered with care. This drug is extremely corrosive to soft tissue. If extravasation occurs during intravenous use, severe damage to soft tissue will occur.

Cosmegen, like all antineoplastic agents, is a toxic drug, and very careful and frequent observation of the patient for adverse reactions is necessary. These reactions may involve any tissue of the body. The possibility of an anaphylactic reaction should be borne in mind.

An increased incidence of gastro-intestinal toxicity and bone marrow depression has been reported when dactinomycin was given with X-ray therapy.

Particular caution is necessary when administering dactinomycin within two months of irradiation for the treatment of right-sided Wilms' tumour, since hepatomegaly and elevated AST (SGOT) levels have been seen.

Nausea and vomiting due to dactinomycin make it necessary to give Cosmegen intermittently. It is extremely important to observe the patient daily for toxic side effects when combined therapy is employed, since a full course of therapy is occasionally not tolerated. If stomatitis, diarrhoea or severe haemopoietic depression appear during therapy, these drugs should be discontinued until the patient has recovered.

Recent reports indicate an increased incidence of secondary primary tumours following treatment with radiation and antineoplastic agents, such as dactinomycin. Multi-modal therapy creates the need for careful, long-term observation of cancer survivors.

Dactinomycin can affect male fertility adversely.

*Laboratory tests:* A variety of abnormalities of renal, hepatic and bone-marrow function have been reported in patients with neoplastic disease receiving dactinomycin. It is advisable to make frequent checks of renal, hepatic and bone-marrow functions.

*Interaction with other medicaments and other forms of interaction:* Much evidence suggests that Cosmegen potentiates the effects of X-ray therapy. The converse also appears likely: that Cosmegen may be more effective when radiation therapy is given concurrently. See *Cosmegen and radiation therapy.*

It has been reported that dactinomycin may interfere with bio-assay procedures for the determination of antibacterial drug levels.

*Pregnancy and lactation:* Dactinomycin has been shown to be teratogenic in animals and should not normally be given to pregnant women.

Dactinomycin should not be administered to mothers who are breast-feeding.

*Use in children:* As there is a greater frequency of toxic effects of dactinomycin in infants, Cosmegen should not normally be given to children less than 12 months old.

*Effects on ability to drive and use machines:* There are no data available. The potential side effects, fatigue and lethargy, should be taken into account.

*Side-effects:* Toxic effects (except nausea and vomiting) do not usually become apparent until two to four days after a course of therapy is stopped, and may not reach a maximum before one to two weeks have elapsed. Deaths have been reported. However, side effects are usually reversible on discontinuing therapy, they include the following:

*General:* malaise, fatigue, lethargy, fever, myalgia, proctitis, hypocalcaemia.

*Oral:* cheilitis, dysphagia, oesophagitis, ulcerative stomatitis, pharyngitis.

*Gastro-intestinal:* anorexia, nausea, vomiting, abdominal pain, diarrhoea, gastro-intestinal ulceration, liver toxicity including ascites, hepatomegaly, hepatitis and liver-function test abnormalities. Nausea and vomiting, which occur early during the first few hours after administration, may be alleviated by giving anti-emetics.

*Haematological:* anaemia (even to the point of aplastic anaemia, agranulocytosis, leucopenia, thrombocytopenia, pancytopenia, reticulocytopenia). Platelet and white blood-cell counts should be done daily to detect severe haemopoietic depression. If either count shows a marked decrease, dactinomycin should be withheld to allow marrow recovery. This often takes up to three weeks.

*Dermatological:* alopecia, skin eruptions, acne,

flare-up of erythema or increased pigmentation of previously irradiated skin.

*Soft tissues:* dactinomycin is extremely corrosive to soft tissues. If extravasation occurs during intravenous use, severe damage to soft tissues will occur. In at least one instance this has led to contracture of the arms.

*Side-effects relating especially to the isolation-perfusion technique:* Complications of the perfusion technique are related mainly to the amount of drug that escapes into the systemic circulation and may consist of haemopoietic depression, increased susceptibility of infection, absorption of toxic products from massive destruction of neoplastic tissue, impaired wound healing and superficial ulceration of the gastric mucosa. Other side effects may include oedema of the extremity involved, damage to the soft tissues of the perfused area, and potentially venous thrombosis.

*Overdose:* In the event of overdosage, dactinomycin therapy should be withdrawn immediately. Limited information is available on overdosage in humans. Manifestations of overdose have included nausea, vomiting, diarrhoea, stomatitis, gastro-intestinal ulceration, severe haemopoietic depression, acute renal failure and death. Treatment should be symptomatic and supportive. There is no known antidote. It is advisable to check renal, hepatic and bone-marrow functions frequently.

**Pharmacological properties**

*Pharmacodynamic properties: Mode of action:* Cosmegen inhibits the proliferation of cells by forming a stable complex with DNA and interfering with DNA-dependent RNA synthesis.

Generally, the actinomycins exert an inhibitory effect on Gram-positive and Gram-negative bacteria and on some fungi. However, the toxic properties of the actinomycins (including dactinomycin) in relation to antibacterial activity are such as to preclude their use as antibiotics in the treatment of infectious diseases.

Because the actinomycins are cytotoxic, they have an antineoplastic effect which has been demonstrated in experimental animals with various types of tumour implant. This cytotoxic action is the basis for their use in the palliative treatment of certain types of cancer.

*Pharmacokinetic properties:* Results of a study in patients with malignant melanoma indicate that dactinomycin ($^3$H actinomycin D) is minimally metabolised, is concentrated in nucleated cells and does not penetrate the blood brain barrier. Approximately 30% of the dose was recovered in urine and faeces in one week. The terminal plasma half-life for radioactivity was approximately 36 hours.

*Preclinical safety data:* The international Agency on Research on Cancer has judged that dactinomycin is a positive carcinogen in animals. Local sarcomas were produced in mice and rats after repeated subcutaneous or intraperitoneal injection. Mesenchymal tumours occurred in male F344 rats given intraperitoneal injections of 0.05 mg/kg, two to five times per week for 18 weeks. The first tumour appeared at 23 weeks.

Dactinomycin has been shown to be mutagenic in a number of test systems *in vitro* and *in vivo*, including human fibroblasts and leucocytes, and HELA cells. DNA damage and cytogenetic effects have been demonstrated in the mouse and the rat.

Adequate fertility studies have not been reported.

*Impairment of fertility:* Cosmegen has been shown to cause malformations and embryotoxicity in the rat, rabbit and hamster when given in doses of 50–100 mcg/kg intravenously (three to seven times the maximum recommended human dose).

**Pharmaceutical particulars**

*List of excipients:* Mannitol PhEur.

*Incompatibilities:* Use of water containing preservatives (benzyl alcohol or parabens) to reconstitute Cosmegen for injection results in the formation of a precipitate.

*Shelf life:* The shelf life is 60 months.

*Special precautions for storage:* Cosmegen Lyovac should be stored below 25°C, protected from light. Avoid freezing.

*Nature and contents of container:* Glass vials containing 500 micrograms dactinomycin with 20 mg mannitol.

*Instructions for use/handling:*

*Reconstitution and administration:* Cosmegen is reconstituted by adding 1.1 ml of Water for Injections BP without preservative to the vial. For injection, 1.0 ml of the reconstituted solution, which will contain 500 micrograms of dactinomycin, is withdrawn into the syringe. Only Water for Injections BP (which does not contain preservatives) should be used. Other injection fluids may cause precipitation. Cosmegen should be inspected for particulate matter and discolouration, whenever possible. The reconstituted solution is clear and gold-coloured.

It is recommended that Cosmegen is reconstituted

only by trained personnel wearing protective gloves. A designated area should be set aside for this purpose and the work surface covered with disposable plastic-backed absorbent paper.

Luer-lock fittings on all syringes and sets are recommended, and use of large-bore needles or a venting needle will help to minimise back pressure and the possible formation of aerosols. Accidental splashing on to the skin or eye should be treated immediately with copious irrigation of isotonic saline or water. Pregnant staff should not handle Cosmegen.

Adequate care should be taken in the disposal of equipment after contact with Cosmegen.

*Disposal of unwanted Cosmegen:*

*(a) Unwanted made-up solution and open empty vials:* Treatment with a solution of 5% trisodium phosphate for 30 minutes has been shown to destroy dactinomycin. Approximately twice the volume of trisodium phosphate solution as made-up dactinomycin solution is considered adequate. After such treatment, vials and solution are safe for disposal by normal laboratory procedures.

*(b) Unopened vials:* Incinerate at high temperature (982°–1204°C [1800°–2200°F]). Allow incinerator to cool. Scrape off the residue and re-incinerate it.

**Marketing authorisation number** 0025/5075R.

**Date of approval/revision of SPC** March 1996.

**Legal category** POM.

## COZAAR* TABLETS 50 mg ▼
## COZAAR* HALF STRENGTH TABLETS 25 mg ▼

**Qualitative and quantitative composition** Cozaar contains 50 mg of the active ingredient, losartan potassium.

Cozaar Half Strength contains 25 mg of losartan potassium.

**Pharmaceutical form** Cozaar is supplied as white, film-coated tablets with a single score line on one side and '952' on the other.

Cozaar Half Strength is supplied as white, film-coated tablets marked '951' on one side and plain on the other.

**Clinical particulars**

*Therapeutic indications:* Cozaar is indicated for the treatment of hypertension.

*Posology and method of administration:* The starting and maintenance dose is 50 mg once daily for most patients. The maximal antihypertensive effect is attained 3–6 weeks after initiation of therapy. Some patients may receive an additional benefit by increasing the dose to 100 mg once daily.

*Use in the elderly: Patients up to 75 years:* No initial dosage adjustment is necessary for this group of patients.

*Patients over 75 years:* Presently there is limited clinical experience in this group; a lower starting dose of 25 mg once daily is recommended.

*Use in renal impairment:* No initial dosage adjustment is necessary in patients with mild renal impairment (i.e. creatinine clearance 20–50 ml/min). For patients with moderate to severe renal impairment (i.e. creatinine clearance <20 ml/min) or patients on dialysis, a lower starting dose of 25 mg once daily is recommended.

*Use in patients with intravascular volume depletion:* For the very small proportion of patients who have intravascular volume depletion (e.g. those treated with high-dose diuretics), a starting dose of 25 mg once daily is recommended (see *Special warnings and special precautions for use*).

*Use in hepatic impairment:* A lower dose should be considered for patients with a history of hepatic impairment (see *Special warnings and special precautions for use*).

Cozaar may be administered with other antihypertensive agents.

Cozaar may be administered with or without food.

*Contra-indications:* Cozaar is contra-indicated in pregnancy (see *Pregnancy and lactation*) and in patients who are hypersensitive to any component of this product.

*Special warnings and special precautions for use:* In patients who are intravascularly volume depleted (e.g. those treated with high-dose diuretics), symptomatic hypotension may occur. These conditions should be corrected prior to administration of Cozaar, or a lower starting dose should be used (see *Posology and method of administration*).

Based on pharmacokinetic data which demonstrate significantly increased plasma concentrations of losartan in cirrhotic patients, a lower dose should be considered for patients with a history of hepatic impairment (see *Posology and method of administration* and *Pharmacological properties, Pharmacokinetic properties*).

As a consequence of inhibiting the renin-angiotensin-aldosterone system, changes in renal function including renal failure have been reported in susceptible individuals; these changes in renal function may be reversible upon discontinuation of therapy.

Other drugs that affect the renin-angiotensin-aldosterone system may increase blood urea and serum creatinine in patients with bilateral renal artery stenosis or stenosis of the artery to a solitary kidney. Similar effects have been reported with Cozaar; these changes in renal function may be reversible upon discontinuation of therapy.

Cozaar should not be used with potassium-sparing diuretics.

*Interaction with other medicaments and other forms of interaction:* No drug interactions of clinical significance have been identified. Compounds which have been studied in clinical pharmacokinetic trials include hydrochlorothiazide, digoxin, warfarin, cimetidine, ketoconazole and and phenobarbital.

*Pregnancy and lactation*

*Use in pregnancy:* Although there is no experience with the use of Cozaar in pregnant women, animal studies with losartan potassium have demonstrated fetal and neonatal injury and death, the mechanism of which is believed to be pharmacologically mediated through effects on the renin-angiotensin-aldosterone system.

In humans, fetal renal perfusion, which is dependent upon the development of the renin-angiotensin-aldosterone system, begins in the second trimester; thus risk to the fetus increases if Cozaar is administered during the second or third trimesters of pregnancy.

**When used in pregnancy during the second and third trimesters, drugs that act directly on the renin-angiotensin-aldosterone system can cause injury and even death in the developing fetus. Cozaar should not be used in pregnancy, and if pregnancy is detected Cozaar should be discontinued as soon as possible.**

*Use during lactation:* It is not known whether losartan is excreted in human milk. However, significant levels of losartan and the active metabolite were shown to be present in rat milk. Because of the potential for adverse effects on the nursing infant, a decision should be made whether to discontinue breast-feeding or discontinue the drug, taking into account the importance of the drug to the mother.

*Effects on ability to drive and use machines:* There are no data to suggest that Cozaar affects the ability to drive and use machines.

*Undesirable effects:* Side effects have usually been mild and transient in nature and have not required discontinuation of therapy. The overall incidence of side effects reported with Cozaar was comparable to placebo.

In controlled clinical trials for essential hypertension, dizziness was the only side effect reported as drug related that occurred with an incidence greater than placebo in 1% or more of patients treated with Cozaar. In addition, dose-related orthostatic effects were seen in less than 1% of patients. Rarely, rash was reported, although the incidence in controlled clinical trials was less than placebo.

The following adverse reactions have been reported in post-marketing experience:

*Hypersensitivity:* Angioedema (involving swelling of the face, lips, pharynx and/or tongue) has been reported rarely in patients treated with losartan.

*Gastro-intestinal:* Diarrhoea, liver function abnormalities.

*Musculoskeletal:* Myalgia.

*Nervous system/psychiatric:* Migraine.

*Skin:* Urticaria, pruritus.

*Laboratory test findings:* In controlled clinical trials, clinically important changes in standard laboratory parameters were rarely associated with administration of Cozaar. Hyperkalaemia (serum potassium >5.5 mmol/l) occurred in 1.5% of patients. Serum potassium should be monitored, particularly in the elderly and patients with renal impairment. Elevations of ALT occurred rarely and usually resolved upon discontinuation of therapy.

*Overdose:* Significant lethality was observed in mice and rats after oral administration of 1000 mg/kg (3000 mg/m²) and 2000 mg/kg (11,800 mg/m²) (500 and 1000 times† the maximum recommended daily human dose), respectively.

Limited data are available in regard to overdosage in humans. The most likely manifestation of overdosage would be hypotension and tachycardia; bradycardia could occur from parasympathetic (vagal) stimulation. If symptomatic hypotension should occur, supportive treatment should be instituted.

Neither losartan nor the active metabolite can be removed by haemodialysis.

† Based on a patient weight of 50 kg.

**Pharmacological properties**

*Pharmacodynamic properties:* Losartan is an oral, specific angiotensin-II receptor (type AT₁) antagonist. Angiotensin II binds to the AT₁ receptor found in many tissues (e.g. vascular smooth muscle, adrenal gland, kidneys, and the heart) and elicits several important biological actions, including vasoconstriction and the release of aldosterone. Angiotensin II also stimulates smooth-muscle proliferation. Based on binding and pharmacological bioassays, it binds selectively to the $AT_1$ receptor. In vitro and in vivo, both losartan and its pharmacologically active carboxylic acid metabolite (E-3174) block all physiologically relevant actions of angiotensin II, regardless of the source or route of synthesis.

During losartan administration, removal of angiotensin-II negative feedback on renin secretion leads to increased plasma renin activity. Increases in plasma renin activity lead to increases in angiotensin II in plasma. Even with these increases, antihypertensive activity and suppression of plasma aldosterone concentration are maintained, indicating effective angiotensin-II receptor blockade.

Losartan binds selectively to the $AT_1$ receptor and does not bind to or block other hormone receptors or ion channels important in cardiovascular regulation. Furthermore, losartan does not inhibit ACE (kininase II), the enzyme that degrades bradykinin. Consequently, effects not directly related to blocking the $AT_1$ receptor, such as the potentiation of bradykinin-mediated effects, the generation of oedema (losartan 1.7%, placebo 1.9%) or fatigue (losartan 3.8%, placebo 3.9%), are not associated with losartan.

Losartan has been shown to block responses to angiotensin I and angiotensin II without affecting responses to bradykinin, a finding which is consistent with the specific mechanism of action of Losartan. In contrast, ACE inhibitors have been shown to block responses to angiotensin I and enhance responses to bradykinin without altering the response to angiotensin II, thus providing a pharmacodynamic distinction between losartan and ACE inhibitors.

A study was carried out which was specifically designed to assess the incidence of cough in patients treated with Cozaar as compared to patients treated with ACE inhibitors. In this study and in the controlled clinical trials for hypertension, the incidence of cough reported by patients receiving Cozaar or an agent not associated with ACE-inhibitor-induced cough (hydrochlorothiazide or placebo) was similar and was significantly less than in patients treated with an ACE inhibitor. In addition, in an overall analysis of 16 double-blind clinical trials in 4,131 patients, the incidence of spontaneously reported cough in patients treated with Cozaar was similar (3.1%) to that of patients treated with placebo (2.6%) or hydrochlorothiazide (4.1%), whereas the incidence with ACE inhibitors was 8.8%.

In non-diabetic hypertensive patients with proteinuria, the administration of losartan potassium significantly reduces proteinuria, fractional excretion of albumin and IgG. Losartan maintains glomerular filtration rate and reduces filtration fraction. Generally, losartan causes a decrease in serum uric acid (usually <24 µmol) which was persistent in chronic therapy.

Losartan has no effect on autonomic reflexes and no sustained effect on plasma noradrenaline.

Losartan potassium administered in doses of up to 150 mg once daily did not cause clinically important changes in fasting triglycerides, total cholesterol or HDL cholesterol in patients with hypertension. The same doses of losartan had no effect on fasting glucose levels.

In clinical studies, once-daily administration of 50 mg Cozaar to patients with mild to moderate essential hypertension produced statistically significant reductions in systolic and diastolic blood pressure; the antihypertensive effect was maintained in clinical studies for up to one year. Measurement of blood pressure at trough (24 hours post-dose) relative to peak (5–6 hours post-dose) demonstrated relatively smooth blood pressure reduction over 24 hours. The antihypertensive effect paralleled the natural diurnal rhythms. Blood pressure reduction at the end of the dosing interval was approximately 70–80% of the effect seen 5–6 hours post-dose. Discontinuation of losartan in hypertensive patients did not result in an abrupt rebound of blood pressure. Despite the significant decrease in blood pressure, administration of Cozaar had no clinically significant effect on heart rate.

The antihypertensive effect of Cozaar 50 mg is similar to once-daily administration of enalapril 20 mg. The antihypertensive effect of once-daily administration of Cozaar 50–100 mg is comparable to once-daily administration of atenolol 50–100 mg. The effect of administration of Cozaar 50–100 mg once daily also is equivalent to felodipine extended-release 5–10 mg in older hypertensives (≥65 years) after 12 weeks of therapy.

Although Cozaar is antihypertensive in all races, as with other drugs that affect the renin-angiotensin-aldosterone system, black hypertensive patients have a smaller average response to losartan monotherapy than non-black patients.

If Cozaar is given together with thiazide-type diuretics, the blood-pressure-lowering effects are approximately additive.

### Pharmacokinetic properties

*Absorption:* Following oral administration, losartan is well absorbed and undergoes first-pass metabolism, forming an active carboxylic acid metabolite and other inactive metabolites. The systemic bioavailability of losartan tablets is approximately 33%. Mean peak concentrations of losartan and its active metabolite are reached in 1 hour and in 3–4 hours, respectively. There was no clinically significant effect on the plasma concentration profile of losartan when the drug was administered with a standardised meal.

*Distribution:* Both losartan and its active metabolite are ≥99% bound to plasma proteins, primarily albumin. The volume of distribution of losartan is 34 litres. Studies in rats indicate that losartan crosses the blood-brain barrier poorly, if at all.

*Biotransformation:* About 14% of an intravenously or orally-administered dose of losartan is converted to its active metabolite. Following oral and intravenous administration of $^{14}$C-labelled losartan potassium, circulating plasma radioactivity primarily is attributed to losartan and its active metabolite.

In addition to the active metabolite, inactive metabolites are formed, including two major metabolites formed by hydroxylation of the butyl side chain and a minor metabolite, an N-2 tetrazole glucuronide.

*Elimination:* Plasma clearance of losartan and its active metabolite is about 600 ml/min and 50 ml/min, respectively. Renal clearance of losartan and its active metabolite is about 74 ml/min and 26 ml/min, respectively. When losartan is administered orally, about 4% of the dose is excreted unchanged in the urine, and about 6% of the dose is excreted in the urine as active metabolite. The pharmacokinetics of losartan and its active metabolite are linear with oral losartan potassium doses up to 200 mg.

Following oral administration, plasma concentrations of losartan and its active metabolite decline polyexponentially with a terminal half-life of about 2 hours and 6–9 hours, respectively. During once-daily dosing with 100 mg, neither losartan nor its active metabolite accumulates significantly in plasma.

Both biliary and urinary excretion contribute to the elimination of losartan and its metabolites. Following an oral dose of $^{14}$C-labelled losartan in man, about 35% of radioactivity is recovered in the urine and 58% in the faeces.

*Characteristics in patients:* Following oral administration in patients with mild to moderate alcoholic cirrhosis of the liver, plasma concentrations of losartan and its active metabolite were, respectively, 5-fold and 1.7-fold greater than those seen in young male volunteers.

Plasma concentrations of losartan are not altered in patients with creatinine clearance above 10 ml/min. Compared to patients with normal renal function, the AUC for losartan is approximately 2-fold greater in haemodialysis patients. Plasma concentrations of the active metabolite are not altered in patients with renal impairment or in haemodialysis patients. Neither losartan nor the active metabolite can be removed by haemodialysis.

*Preclinical safety data:* The toxic potential of losartan potassium was evaluated in a series of repeated dose oral toxicity studies of up to three months in monkeys and up to one year in rats and dogs. There were no findings that would preclude administration at the therapeutic dosage level.

Losartan potassium was not carcinogenic when administered at maximum tolerated dosage levels to rats and mice for 105 and 92 weeks, respectively. These maximum tolerated dosage levels provided respective margins of systemic exposure for losartan and its pharmacologically active metabolite over that achieved in humans treated with 50 mg of losartan of approximately 270- and 150-fold in rats and 45- and 27-fold in mice.

There was no evidence of direct genotoxicity in studies conducted with losartan potassium or its primary pharmacologically active metabolite (E-3174).

Fertility and reproductive performance were not affected in studies with male and female rats given oral doses of losartan potassium up to approximately 150 and 300 mg/kg/day, respectively. These dosages provide respective margins of systemic exposure for losartan and its pharmacologically active metabolite of approximately 150/125-fold in male rats and 300/170-fold in female rats over that achieved in man at the recommended daily dose.

Losartan potassium has been shown to produce adverse effects in rat fetuses and neonates. The effects include decreased bodyweight, mortality and/or renal toxicity. In addition, significant levels of losartan and its active metabolite were shown to be present in rat milk. Based on pharmacokinetic assessments, these findings are attributed to drug exposure in late gestation and during lactation.

### Pharmaceutical particulars
*List of excipients:* Cozaar and Cozaar Half Strength Tablets contain the following inactive ingredients: Hydroxypropyl Cellulose PhEur; Hydroxypropyl Methylcellulose PhEur; Lactose PhEur; Magnesium Stearate PhEur; Microcrystalline Cellulose PhEur; Pregelatinised Starch BP; Titanium Dioxide PhEur.

Cozaar 50 mg also contains Carnauba Wax PhEur.

Cozaar 50 mg also contains 4.24 mg (0.108 mmol) of potassium.

Cozaar Half Strength 25 mg also contains 2.12 mg (0.054 mmol) of potassium.

*Incompatibilities:* None.

*Shelf life:* 24 months.

*Special precautions for storage:* Store in a dry place at temperatures below 30°C (86°F).

*Nature and contents of container:* White, opaque PVC/PE/PVDC blisters with aluminium foil lidding. 50 mg tablets: Pack of 28 tablets. 25 mg tablets: Pack of 7 tablets.

*Instructions for use/handling:* None.

### Marketing authorisation numbers
50 mg tablet     0025/0324
25 mg tablet     0025/0336

**Date of approval/revision of SPC**   January 1997.

**Legal category**   POM.

## COZAAR*-COMP ▼
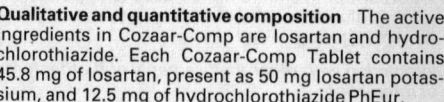

**Qualitative and quantitative composition**   The active ingredients in Cozaar-Comp are losartan and hydrochlorothiazide. Each Cozaar-Comp Tablet contains 45.8 mg of losartan, present as 50 mg losartan potassium, and 12.5 mg of hydrochlorothiazide PhEur.

**Pharmaceutical form**   Cozaar-Comp is supplied as oval, yellow, film-coated tablets '717' on one side and plain on the other.

### Clinical particulars
*Therapeutic indications:* For the treatment of hypertension in patients whose blood pressure has been stabilised on losartan and hydrochlorothiazide given separately in the same proportion.

*Posology and method of administration:* The usual starting and maintenance dose is 1 tablet once daily for most patients. For patients who do not respond adequately, the dosage may be increased to 2 tablets once daily. The maximum dose is 2 tablets once daily. In general, the antihypertensive effect is attained within three weeks after initiation of therapy.

*Use in the elderly: Patients up to 75 years:* No initial dosage adjustment is necessary for elderly patients.

*Patients over 75 years:* Presently there is limited clinical experience in this group. Cozaar-Comp can be initiated if the patient has already been stabilised on Cozaar. (In this age group initiation with Cozaar Half Strength is recommended.)

*Use in renal impairment:* No initial dosage adjustment is necessary in patients with mild renal impairment (i.e. creatinine clearance 20–50 ml/min). Cozaar-Comp is not recommended for patients with moderate to severe renal impairment (i.e. creatinine clearance <20 ml/min) or patients on dialysis.

*Use in patients with intravascular volume depletion:* Cozaar-Comp should not be initiated in patients who are intravascularly volume depleted (e.g. those treated with high-dose diuretics).

*Use in hepatic impairment:* Cozaar-Comp is not recommended for patients with hepatic impairment.

*Comcomitant therapy:* Cozaar-Comp may be administered with other antihypertensive agents.

Cozaar-Comp may be administered with or without food.

*Use in children:* Safety and efficacy in children have not been established.

*Contra-indications:* Cozaar-Comp is contra-indicated in pregnancy (see *Pregnancy and lactation*), in patients who are hypersensitive to any component of this product, in patients with anuria, and in patients who are hypersensitive to other sulphonamide-derived drugs.

*Special warnings and special precautions for use:*
*Losartan and hydrochlorothiazide combination tablet:*
*Hepatic and renal impairment:* Cozaar-Comp is not recommended for patients with hepatic impairment or moderate to severe renal impairment (creatinine clearance <20 ml/min) (see *Posology and method of administration*).

*Losartan:*
*Renal function impairment:* Other drugs that affect the renin-angiotensin system may increase serum urea and creatinine in patients with bilateral renal artery stenosis or stenosis of the artery to a solitary kidney. While not confirmed, this potentially may occur with angiotensin-II receptor antagonists.

*Hydrochlorothiazide:*

*Hypotension and electrolyte/fluid imbalance:* As with all antihypertensive therapy, symptomatic hypotension may occur in some patients. This was rarely seen in uncomplicated hypertensive patients, but was more likely in the presence of fluid or electrolyte imbalance. Periodic determination of serum electrolytes should be performed at appropriate intervals, as in any patients receiving diuretics.

*Metabolic and endocrine effects:* Thiazide therapy may impair glucose tolerance. Dosage adjustment of antidiabetic agents, including insulin, may be required (see *Interaction with other medicaments and other forms of interaction*).

Thiazides may decrease urinary calcium excretion and may cause intermittent and slight elevation of serum calcium. Marked hypercalcaemia may be evidence of hidden hyperparathyroidism. Thiazides should be discontinued before carrying out tests for parathyroid function.

Increases in cholesterol and triglyceride levels may be associated with thiazide diuretic therapy.

Thiazide therapy may precipitate hyperuricaemia and/or gout in certain patients. Because losartan decreases uric acid, losartan in combination with hydrochlorothiazide attenuates the diuretic-induced hyperuricaemia.

*Other:* In patients receiving thiazides, hypersensitivity reactions may occur with or without a history of allergy or bronchial asthma. Exacerbation or activation of systemic lupus erythematosus has been reported with the use of thiazides.

Cozaar-Comp should not be used with potassium-sparing diuretics, without appropriate serum potassium monitoring.

*Interaction with other medicaments and other forms of interaction:*

*Losartan:* No drug interactions of clinical significance have been identified. Compounds which have been studied in clinical pharmacokinetic trials include hydrochlorothiazide, digoxin, warfarin, cimetidine, and phenobarbitone (see *Hydrochlorothiazide: alcohol, barbiturates, or narcotics* below).

*Hydrochlorothiazide:* When given concurrently, the following drugs may interact with thiazide diuretics:

*Alcohol, barbiturates, or narcotics* – potentiation of orthostatic hypotension may occur.

*Antidiabetic drugs* (oral agents and insulin) – dosage adjustment of the antidiabetic drug may be required.

*Other antihypertensive drugs* – there may be an additive effect.

*Cholestyramine and colestipol resins* – absorption of hydrochlorothiazide is impaired in the presence of anionic exchange resins. Single doses of either cholestyramine or colestipol resins bind the hydrochlorothiazide and reduce its absorption from the gastro-intestinal tract by up to 85% and 43%, respectively.

*Corticosteroids, ACTH* – there may be intensified electrolyte depletion, particularly hypokalaemia.

*Pressor amines (e.g. adrenaline)* – possible decreased response to pressor amines, but not sufficient to preclude their use.

*Skeletal muscle relaxants, non-depolarising (e.g. tubocurarine)* – possible increased responsiveness to the muscle relaxant.

*Lithium* – diuretic agents reduce the renal clearance of lithium and add a high risk of lithium toxicity. Therefore, concomitant use is not recommended. Refer to the prescribing information for lithium preparations before use of such preparations.

*Non-steroidal anti-inflammatory drugs* – in some patients, the administration of a non-steroidal anti-inflammatory agent can reduce the diuretic, natriuretic, and antihypertensive effects of diuretics.

*Drug/laboratory test interactions:* Because of their effects on calcium metabolism, thiazides may interfere with tests for parathyroid function (see *Special warnings and special precautions for use*).

*Pregnancy and lactation:*

*Use during pregnancy:* Although there is no experience with the use of Cozaar-Comp in pregnant women, animal studies with losartan potassium have demonstrated fetal and neonatal injury and death, the mechanism of which is believed to be pharmacologically mediated through effects on the renin-angiotensin system.

In humans, fetal renal perfusion, which is dependent upon the development of the renin-angiotensin system, begins in the second trimester; thus, risk to the fetus increases if Cozaar-Comp is administered during the second or third trimesters of pregnancy.

Thiazides cross the placental barrier and appear in cord blood. The routine use of diuretics in otherwise healthy pregnant women is not recommended and exposes mother and fetus to unnecessary hazard, including fetal or neonatal jaundice, thrombocytopenia and possibly other adverse reactions which have occurred in the adult. Diuretics do not prevent development of toxaemia of pregnancy and there is no satisfactory evidence that they are useful in the treatment of toxaemia.

**When used in pregnancy during the second and third trimesters, drugs that act directly on the renin-angiotensin system can cause injury and even death to the developing fetus. When pregnancy is detected, Cozaar-Comp should be discontinued as soon as possible.**

*Use during lactation:* It is not known whether losartan is excreted in human milk. Significant levels of losartan and the active metabolite were shown to be present in rat milk. Thiazides appear in human milk. Because of the potential for adverse effects on the breast-feeding infant, a decision should be made whether to discontinue breast-feeding or discontinue the drug, taking into account the importance of the drug to the mother.

*Effects on ability to drive and use machines:* There are no data to suggest that Cozaar-Comp affects the ability to drive and use machines.

*Undesirable effects:* In clinical trials with the combination tablet of losartan and hydrochlorothiazide, no adverse experiences peculiar to this combination drug have been observed. Adverse experiences have been limited to those that were reported previously with losartan potassium and/or hydrochlorothiazide. The overall incidence of adverse experiences reported with the combination was comparable to placebo. The percentage of discontinuations of therapy was also comparable to placebo. For the most part, adverse experiences have been mild and transient in nature and have not required discontinuation of therapy.

In controlled clinical trials for essential hypertension, dizziness was the only adverse experience reported as drug related that occurred with an incidence greater than placebo in 1% or more of patients treated with losartan potassium-hydrochlorothiazide.

The following adverse reactions have been reported in post-marketing experience:

*Hypersensitivity:* Angioedema (involving swelling of the face, lips, and/or tongue) has been reported rarely in patients treated with losartan.

Additional side-effects that have been seen with one of the individual components and may be potential side effects with Cozaar-Comp are the following:

*Losartan:* Rash, dose-related orthostatic effects.

*Hydrochlorothiazide:* Anorexia, gastric irritation, nausea, vomiting, cramping, diarrhoea, constipation, jaundice (intrahepatic cholestatic jaundice), pancreatitis, sialadenitis, vertigo, paraesthesiae, headache, xanthopsia, leucopenia, agranulocytosis, thrombocytopenia, aplastic anaemia, haemolytic anaemia, purpura, photosensitivity, fever, urticaria, necrotising angiitis (vasculitis, cutaneous vasculitis), respiratory distress (including pneumonitis and pulmonary oedema), anaphylactic reactions, toxic epidermal necrolysis, hyperglycaemia, glycosuria, hyperuricaemia, electrolyte imbalance (including hyponatraemia and hypokalaemia), renal dysfunction, interstitial nephritis, renal failure, muscle spasm, weakness, restlessness, transient blurred vision.

*Laboratory test findings:* In controlled clinical trials, clinically important changes in standard laboratory parameters were rarely associated with administration of Cozaar-Comp. Hyperkalaemia (serum potassium >5.5 mmol/l) occurred in 0.7% of patients, but in these trials discontinuation of Cozaar-Comp due to hyperkalaemia was not necessary. Serum potassium should be monitored, particularly in the elderly and patients with renal impairment. Elevations of ALT occurred rarely and usually resolved upon discontinuation of therapy.

*Overdosage:* No specific information is available on the treatment of overdosage with Cozaar-Comp. Treatment is symptomatic and supportive. Therapy with Cozaar-Comp should be discontinued and the patient observed closely. Suggested measures include induction of emesis if ingestion is recent, and correction of dehydration, electrolyte imbalance, hepatic coma, and hypotension by established procedures.

*Losartan:* Limited data are available in regard to overdosage in humans. The most likely manifestation of overdosage would be hypotension and tachycardia; bradycardia could occur from parasympathetic (vagal) stimulation. If symptomatic hypotension should occur, supportive treatment should be instituted.

Neither losartan nor the active metabolite can be removed by haemodialysis.

*Hydrochlorothiazide:* The most common signs and symptoms observed are those caused by electrolyte depletion (hypokalaemia, hypochloraemia, hyponatraemia) and dehydration resulting from excessive diuresis. If digitalis has also been administered, hypokalaemia may accentuate cardiac arrhythmias.

The degree to which hydrochlorothiazide is removed by haemodialysis has not been established.

**Pharmacological properties**

*Pharmacodynamic properties:*

*Losartan and hydrochlorothiazide combination tablet:* The components of Cozaar-Comp have been shown to have an additive effect on blood-pressure reduction, reducing blood pressure to a greater degree than either component alone. This effect is thought to be a result of the complimentary actions of both components. Further, as a result of its diuretic effect, hydrochlorothiazide increases plasma-renin activity, increases aldosterone secretion, decreases serum potassium, and increases the levels of angiotensin II. Administration of losartan blocks all the physiologically relevant actions of angiotensin II and through inhibition of aldosterone could tend to attenuate the potassium loss associated with the diuretic.

Losartan has been shown to have a mild and transient uricosuric effect. Hydrochlorothiazide has been shown to cause modest increases in uric acid; the combination of losartan and hydrochlorothiazide tends to attenuate the diuretic-induced hyperuricaemia.

The antihypertensive effect of Cozaar-Comp is sustained for a 24-hour period. In clinical studies of at least one year's duration, the antihypertensive effect was maintained with continued therapy. Despite the significant decrease in blood pressure, administration of Cozaar-Comp had no clinically significant effect on heart rate. In clinical trials, after 12 weeks of therapy with losartan 50 mg/hydrochlorothiazide 12.5 mg, trough sitting diastolic blood pressure was reduced by an average of up to 13.2 mm Hg.

Cozaar-Comp is effective in reducing blood pressure in males and females, blacks and non-blacks, and in younger (<65 years) and older (≥65 years) patients and is effective in all degrees of hypertension.

*Losartan:* Losartan is an oral, specific angiotensin-II receptor (type $AT_1$) antagonist. Angiotensin II binds to the $AT_1$ receptor found in many tissues (e.g. vascular smooth muscle, adrenal gland, kidneys, and the heart) and elicits several important biological actions, including vasoconstriction and the release of aldosterone. Angiotensin II also stimulates smooth-muscle proliferation. Based on binding and pharmacological bioassays, angiotensin II binds selectively to the $AT_1$ receptor. *In vitro* and *in vivo*, both losartan and its pharmacologically active carboxylic acid metabolite (E-3174) block all physiologically relevant actions of angiotensin II, regardless of the source or route of synthesis.

During losartan administration, removal of angiotensin-II negative feedback on renin secretion leads to increased plasma-renin activity. Increases in plasma-renin activity lead to increases in angiotensin II in plasma. Even with these increases, antihypertensive activity and suppression of plasma-aldosterone concentration are maintained, indicating effective angiotensin-II receptor blockade.

Losartan binds selectively to the $AT_1$ receptor and does not bind to or block other hormone receptors or ion channels important in cardiovascular regulation. Furthermore, losartan does not inhibit ACE (kininase II), the enzyme that degrades bradykinin. Consequently, effects not directly related to blocking the $AT_1$ receptor, such as the potentiation of bradykinin-mediated effects or the generation of oedema (losartan 1.7%, placebo 1.9%), are not associated with losartan.

Losartan has been shown to block responses to angiotensin I and angiotensin II without affecting responses to bradykinin, a finding which is consistent with the specific mechanism of action of losartan. In contrast, ACE inhibitors have been shown to block responses to angiotensin I and enhance responses to bradykinin without altering the response to angiotensin II, thus providing a pharmacodynamic distinction between losartan and ACE inhibitors.

A study was carried out which was specifically designed to assess the incidence of cough in patients treated with losartan as compared to patients treated with ACE inhibitors. In this study, the incidence of cough reported by patients receiving losartan or hydrochlorothiazide was similar and was significantly less than in patients treated with an ACE inhibitor. In addition, in an overall analysis of 16 double-blind clinical trials in 4,131 patients, the incidence of spontaneously reported cough in patients treated with losartan was similar (3.1%) to that of patients treated with placebo (2.6%) or hydrochlorothiazide (4.1%), whereas the incidence with ACE inhibitors was 8.8%.

In non-diabetic hypertensive patients with proteinuria, the administration of losartan potassium significantly reduces proteinuria, fractional excretion of albumin and IgG. Losartan maintains glomerular filtration rate and reduces filtration fraction. Generally, losartan causes a decrease in serum uric acid (usually <24 µmol/l) which was persistent in chronic therapy.

Losartan has no effect on autonomic reflexes and no sustained effect on plasma noradrenaline.

In clinical studies, once-daily administration of losartan to patients with mild to moderate essential hypertension produced statistically significant reductions in systolic and diastolic blood pressure; in clinical studies of up to one year the antihypertensive effect was maintained. Measurement of blood pressure at trough (24 hours post-dose) relative to peak (5–6 hours post-dose) demonstrated relatively smooth blood pressure reduction over 24 hours. The antihypertensive effect paralleled the natural diurnal rhythms. Blood-pressure reduction at the end of the dosing interval was approximately 70–80% of the effect seen 5–6 hours post-dose. Discontinuation of losartan in hypertensive patients did not result in an abrupt rebound of blood pressure. Despite the significant decrease in blood pressure, administration of losartan had no clinically significant effect on heart rate.

The antihypertensive effect of losartan 50 mg is similar to once-daily administration of enalapril 20 mg. The antihypertensive effect of once-daily administration of losartan 50–100 mg is comparable to once-daily administration of atenolol 50–100 mg. The effect of administration of losartan 50–100 mg once daily also is equivalent to felodipine extended-release 5–10 mg in older hypertensives (≥65 years) after 12 weeks of therapy.

Losartan is equally effective in males and females and in younger (<65 years) and older (≥65 years) hypertensives. Although losartan is antihypertensive in all races, as with other drugs that affect the renin-angiotensin system, black hypertensive patients have a smaller average response to losartan monotherapy than non-black patients.

When given together with thiazide-type diuretics, the blood-pressure lowering effects of losartan are approximately additive.

*Hydrochlorothiazide:* The mechanism of the antihypertensive effect of thiazides is unknown. Thiazides do not usually affect normal blood pressure.

Hydrochlorothiazide is a diuretic and antihypertensive. It affects the distal renal tubular mechanism of electrolyte reabsorption. Hydrochlorothiazide increases excretion of sodium and chloride in approximately equivalent amounts. Natriuresis may be accompanied by some loss of potassium and bicarbonate.

After oral use, diuresis begins within 2 hours, peaks in about 4 hours and lasts about 6 to 12 hours.

*Pharmacokinetic properties:*
*Absorption – Losartan:* Following oral administration, losartan is well absorbed and undergoes first-pass metabolism, forming an active carboxylic acid metabolite and other inactive metabolites. The systemic bioavailability of losartan tablets is approximately 33%. Mean peak concentrations of losartan and its active metabolite are reached in 1 hour and in 3–4 hours, respectively. There was no clinically significant effect on the plasma-concentration profile of losartan when the drug was administered with a standardised meal.

*Distribution – Losartan:* Both losartan and its active metabolite are ≥99% bound to plasma proteins, primarily albumin. The volume of distribution of losartan is 34 litres. Studies in rats indicate that losartan crosses the blood-brain barrier poorly, if at all.

*Hydrochlorothiazide:* Hydrochlorothiazide crosses the placental but not the blood-brain barrier and is excreted in breast milk.

*Biotransformation – Losartan:* About 14% of an intravenously or orally administered dose of losartan is converted to its active metabolite. Following oral and intravenous administration of $^{14}$C-labelled losartan potassium, circulating plasma radioactivity primarily is attributed to losartan and its active metabolite. Minimal conversion of losartan to its active metabolite was seen in about 1% of individuals studied.

In addition to the active metabolite, inactive metabolites are formed, including two major metabolites formed by hydroxylation of the butyl side chain and a minor metabolite, an N-2 tetrazole glucuronide.

*Elimination – Losartan:* Plasma clearance of losartan and its active metabolite is about 600 ml/min and 50 ml/min, respectively. Renal clearance of losartan and its active metabolite is abot 74 ml/min and 26 ml/min, respectively. When losartan is administered orally, about 4% of the dose is excreted unchanged in the urine, and about 6% of the dose is excreted in the urine as active metabolite. The pharmacokinetics of losartan and its active metabolite are linear with oral losartan potassium doses up to 200 mg.

Following oral administration, plasma concentrations of losartan and its active metabolite decline polyexponentially with a terminal half-life of about 2 hours and 6–9 hours, respectively. During once-daily dosing with 100 mg, neither losartan nor its active metabolite accumulates significantly in plasma.

Both biliary and urinary excretion contribute to the elimination of losartan and its metabolites. Following an oral dose of $^{14}$C-labelled losartan in man, about 35% of radioactivity is recovered in the urine and 58% in the faeces.

*Hydrochlorothiazide:* Hydrochlorothiazide is not metabolised but is eliminated rapidly by the kidney. When plasma levels have been followed for at least 24 hours, the plasma half-life has been observed to vary between 5.6 and 14.8 hours. At least 61% of the oral dose is eliminated unchanged within 24 hours.

*Characteristics in patients – Losartan and hydrochlorothiazide combination tablet:* The plasma concentrations of losartan and its active metabolite and the absorption of hydrochlorothiazide in elderly hypertensives are not significantly different from those in young hypertensives.

*Losartan:* Following oral administration in patients with mild to moderate alcoholic cirrhosis of the liver, plasma concentrations of losartan and its active metabolite were, respectively, fivefold and 1.7-fold greater than those seen in young male volunteers.

Neither losartan nor the active metabolite can be removed by haemodialysis.

*Preclinical safety data:* The toxic potential of losartan potassium and hydrochlorothiazide was evaluated in repeated-dose oral toxicity studies for up to six months in rats and dogs. There were no findings that would preclude administration to man at the therapeutic dosage level.

There was no evidence of direct genotoxicity in studies conducted with the losartan and hydrochlorothiazide combination.

Losartan potassium and hydrochlorothiazide administration had no effect on the reproductive performance or fertility in male rats at dosage levels of up to 135 mg/kg/day losartan in combination with 33.75 mg/kg/day hydrochlorothiazide. These dosage levels provided respective plasma concentrations (AUC) for losartan, the active metabolite and hydrochlorothiazide that were approximately 260-, 120-, and 50-fold greater than those achieved in man with 50 mg losartan potassium in combination with 12.5 mg hydrochlorothiazide. In female rats, however, the co-administration of losartan potassium and hydrochlorothiazide (10/2.5 mg/kg/day) induced a slight but statistically significant decrease in fecundity and fertility indices. Compared to plasma concentrations in man (see above) these dosage levels provided respective increases in plasma concentration (AUC) for losartan, the active metabolite, and hydrochlorothiazide of approximately 15-, 4-, and 5-fold.

There was no evidence of teratogenicity in rats or rabbits treated with losartan potassium and hydrochlorothiazide combination. Fetal toxicity in rats, as evidenced by a slight increase in supernumerary ribs in the $F_1$ generation, was observed when females were treated prior to and throughout gestation. As observed in studies with losartan alone, adverse fetal and neonatal effects, including decreased body-weight, mortality and/or renal toxicity, also occurred when pregnant rats were treated with losartan potassium and hydrochlorothiazide combination during late gestation and/or lactation.

**Pharmaceutical particulars**
*List of excipients:* Each Cozaar-Comp Tablet contains the following inactive ingredients: Hydroxypropylcellulose PhEur; Methylhydroxypropylcellulose PhEur; Lactose Monohydrate PhEur; Magnesium Stearate PhEur; Microcrystalline Cellulose PhEur; Pregelatinised Maize Starch BP; Titanium Dioxide PhEur; Quinoline yellow aluminium lake E104; Carnauba Wax PhEur.

Cozaar-Comp also contains 4.24 mg (0.108 mmol) of potassium.

*Incompatibilities:* None.

*Shelf life:* 24 months.

*Special precautions for storage:* Store in a dry place at temperatures below 30°C (86°F).

*Nature and contents of container:* White, opaque PVC/PE/PVDC blisters with aluminium foil lidding. Available in blister calendar packs of 28 tablets.

*Instructions for use/handling:* None.

**Marketing authorisation number** 0025/0338.

**Date of approval/revision of SPC** April 1997.

**Legal category** POM.

# CRIXIVAN* ▼

**Qualitative and quantitative composition** Crixivan 200 mg Capsules contain 250 mg of indinavir sulphate corresponding to 200 mg of indinavir.

Crixivan 400 mg Capsules contain 500 mg of indinavir sulphate corresponding to 400 mg of indinavir.

**Pharmaceutical form** Capsules.

**Clinical particulars**
*Therapeutic indications:* Crixivan is indicated in combination with antiretroviral nucleoside analogues for the treatment of HIV-1 infected adult patients with advanced or progressive immunodeficiency.

The combinations with zidovudine, zidovudine/

didanosine and zidovudine/lamivudine reduce viral load in serum and increase CD4 cell counts. A preliminary analysis from early and ongoing studies indicates that indinavir slows progression of disease. Clinical studies are underway to confirm the clinical benefits of indinavir.

See *Pharmacodynamic properties.*

*Posology and method of administration:* The recommended dosage of Crixivan is 800 mg orally every 8 hours.

Crixivan should be used in combination with other antiretroviral agents (i.e. nucleoside analogues).

The capsules should be swallowed whole.

Since Crixivan must be taken at intervals of 8 hours, a schedule convenient for the patient should be developed. For optimal absorption, Crixivan should be administered without food but with water 1 hour before or 2 hours after a meal. Alternatively, Crixivan may be administered with a low-fat, light meal.

To ensure adequate hydration, it is recommended that the patient drinks at least 1.5 litres of liquids during the course of 24 hours.

Due to an increase in the plasma concentrations of rifabutin and a decrease in the plasma concentrations of indinavir, a dosage reduction of rifabutin to half the standard dose (consult manufacturer's package circular for rifabutin) and a dosage increase of Crixivan to 1000–1200 mg every 8 hours are suggested when rifabutin is co-administered with Crixivan. This dose regimen has not been confirmed in clinical studies and could result in a clinically significant increase in the plasma concentrations of rifabutin.

Due to an increase in the plasma concentrations of indinavir, a dosage reduction of Crixivan to 600 mg every 8 hours should be considered when administering ketoconazole concurrently.

In patients with mild-to-moderate hepatic insufficiency due to cirrhosis, the dosage of Crixivan should be reduced to 600 mg every 8 hours.

Medical management in patients with one or more episodes of nephrolithiasis must include adequate hydration and may include temporary interruption of therapy (e.g. 1–3 days) during the acute episode of nephrolithiasis or discontinuation of therapy.

*Contra-indications:* Clinically significant hypersensitivity to any component of this product.

Indinavir should not be administered concurrently with drugs with narrow therapeutic windows and which are substrates of CYP3A4. Co-administration may result in competitive inhibition of the metabolism of these drugs and create the potential for serious and/or life-threatening adverse events such as cardiac arrhythmias (e.g. terfenadine, astemizole, cisapride) prolonged sedation or respiratory depression (e.g. alprazolam, triazolam, midazolam).

Indinavir should not be administered concurrently with rifampicin because co-administration results in 90% reduction in indinavir plasma concentrations.

*Special warnings and special precautions for use:* Manifestations of nephrolithiasis, including flank pain with or without haematuria (including microscopic haematuria), have been reported infrequently (see *Undesirable effects, Post-marketed experience*). Adequate hydration is recommended in all patients on Crixivan (see *Posology and method of administration*).

Patients with mild to moderate hepatic insufficiency due to cirrhosis will require a dosage reduction of Crixivan due to decreased metabolism of indinavir (see *Posology and method of administration*). Patients with severe hepatic impairment have not been studied. In the absence of such studies, caution should be exercised as increased levels of indinavir may occur.

Safety in patients with impaired renal function has not been studied; however, less than 20% of indinavir is excreted in the urine as unchanged drug or metabolites.

In clinical trials, the majority of investigated patients were Caucasian males.

Safety and effectiveness in children have not been established.

Indinavir should be used cautiously with other drugs that are potent inducers of CYP3A4. Co-administration may result in decreased plasma concentrations of indinavir and as a consequence an increased risk for suboptimal treatment and facilitation of development of resistance (see *Interaction with other medicinal products and other forms of interaction*).

In clinical trials, patients treated with rifampicin, rifabutin, or chronically with acyclovir were excluded. However, patients treated intermittently with acyclovir were not excluded from the clinical trials.

Each 200 mg capsule contains 74 mg lactose (anhydrous). Each 400 mg capsule contains 149 mg lactose (anhydrous). These quantities are probably not sufficient to induce specific symptoms of intolerance.

There have been reports of increased bleeding, including spontaneous skin haematomas and haemarthroses, in haemophiliac patients type A and B treated with protease inhibitors. In some patients additional factor VIII was given. In more than a half of the reported cases, treatment with protease inhibitors was continued or reintroduced if treatment had been discontinued. A causal relationship has been evoked, although the mechanism of action has not been elucidated. Haemophiliac patients should therefore be made aware of the possibility of increased bleeding.

**Acute haemolytic anaemia has been reported which in some cases was severe and progressed rapidly. Once diagnosis is apparent, appropriate measures for the treatment of haemolytic anaemia should be instituted which may include discontinuation of Crixivan.**

*Interaction with other medicinal products and other forms of interaction:* Specific drug interaction studies were performed with indinavir and the following drugs: zidovudine, zidovudine/lamivudine, stavudine, trimethoprim/sulphamethoxazole, fluconazole, isoniazid, clarithromycin, quinidine, cimetidine, and an oral contraceptive (norethindrone/ethinyl oestradiol 1/35). No clinically significant interactions were observed with these drugs. Clinically significant interactions with other drugs are described below.

*Rifabutin:* The co-administration of indinavir 800 mg q8h with rifabutin either 300 mg once daily or 150 mg once daily was evaluated in two separate clinical studies. The results of these studies showed a decrease in indinavir AUC (34% and 33%, respectively, vs indinavir 800 mg q8h alone) and an increase in rifabutin AUC (173% and 55%, respectively, vs rifabutin 300 mg once daily alone). This increase in rifabutin plasma concentrations is likely related to inhibition of CYP3A4-mediated metabolism of rifabutin by indinavir. A dosage increase of idinavir and a dosage reduction of rifabutin are necessary when indinavir and rifabutin are co-administered (see *Posology and method of administration*).

*Ketoconazole:* Administration of a 400 mg dose of ketoconazole, a potent inhibitor of CYP3A4, with a 400 mg dose of indinavir, resulted in a 62% increase in the AUC of indinavir, which is clinically significant, and a 14% increase in the $C_{max}$ of indinavir. A dosage reduction of indinavir to 600 mg every 8 hours should be considered when indinavir and ketoconazole are co-administered.

*Other:* A formal drug-interaction study between indinavir and methadone has not been performed. Concomitant use may result in increased plasma concentrations of methadone. The clinical relevance of this is unknown.

A formal drug-interaction study between indinavir and itraconazole has not been performed. Because itraconazole is a potent inhibitor of CYP3A4, concomitant use could result in clinically significant increases in plasma concentrations of indinavir and such combinations should be avoided.

Concomitant use of other drugs that are inducers of CYP3A4, such as phenobarbital, phenytoin, dexamethasone and carbamazepine, may reduce indinavir plasma concentrations.

The efficacy and safety of indinavir in combination with other protease inhibitors have not been established. Co-administration with ritonavir is likely to result in significant increases in plasma concentrations of indinavir.

A formal drug-interaction study between indinavir and didanosine has not been performed. However, a normal (acidic) gastric pH may be necessary for optimum absorption of indinavir whereas acid rapidly degrades didanosine which is formulated with buffering agents to increase pH. Indinavir and didanosine should be administered at least one hour apart on an empty stomach (consult the manufacturer's prescribing information for didanosine). Antiretroviral activity was unaltered when didanosine was administered three hours after treatment with indinavir in one clinical study.

For optimal absorption, indinavir should be administered with water 1 hour before or 2 hours after a meal. Alternatively, indinavir may be taken with a low-fat light meal. Ingestion of indinavir with a meal high in calories, fat and protein reduces the absorption of indinavir.

*Use during pregnancy and lactation:*

*Use during pregnancy:* Crixivan has not been studied in pregnant women. Until additional data become available, Crixivan should be used during pregnancy only if the potential benefit justifies the potential risk to the fetus.

Hyperbilirubinaemia, reported predominantly as elevated indirect bilirubin, has occurred in 10% of patients during treatment with Crixivan. Because it is unknown whether indinavir will exacerbate physiological hyperbilirubinaemia in neonates, careful consideration must be given to the use of Crixivan in pregnant women at the time of delivery (see *Undesirable effects*).

Developmental toxicity studies performed in rats and rabbits at doses comparable to or slightly greater than human exposure revealed no evidence of teratogenicity. No treatment-related external or visceral changes were observed in rats. Treatment-related increases in the incidence of supernumerary ribs (at or below human exposure) and of cervical ribs (doses comparable to or slightly greater than human exposure) were seen in rats. No treatment-related external, visceral, or skeletal changes were observed in rabbits. In both species, no treatment-related abortions or effects on embryonic/fetal survival or fetal weights were observed.

*Use during lactation:* Health experts recommend that HIV-infected women should not breast-feed their infants under any circumstances in order to avoid transmission of HIV. It is not known whether indinavir is excreted in human milk. However, indinavir was shown to be present in rat milk and excretion in rat milk was also manifested as decreased pup weight gain during lactation. Until more data become available, mothers should be instructed to discontinue breast-feeding during treatment.

*Effects on ability to drive and use machines:* There are no data to suggest that indinavir affects the ability to drive and use machines. However, patients should be informed that dizziness and blurred vision have been reported during treatment with indinavir.

*Undesirable effects:* In controlled clinical trials conducted worldwide, indinavir was administered alone or in combination with other antiretroviral agents (zidovudine, didanosine, stavudine, and/or lamivudine) to approximately 2,000 patients, the majority of whom were Caucasian males (15% females).

Indinavir did not alter the type, frequency, or severity of known major adverse effects associated with the use of zidovudine, didanosine, or lamivudine.

Clinical adverse experiences reported by the investigators as possibly, probably, or definitely drug related in ≥5% of patients treated with Crixivan alone or in combination (n=309) for 24 weeks are listed below. Many of these adverse experiences were also identified as common pre-existing or frequently occurring medical conditions in this population. These adverse experiences were: nausea (35.3%), headache (25.2%), diarrhoea (24.6%), asthenia/fatigue (24.3%), rash (19.1%), taste perversion (19.1%), dry skin (16.2%), abdominal pain (14.6%), vomiting (11.0%), dizziness (10.7%), dyspepsia (10.7%), flatulence (7.8%), insomnia (7.4%), pruritus (7.4%), hypaesthesia (7.1%), dry mouth (6.8%), dysuria (6.5%), acid regurgitation (6.5%), paraesthesia (5.2%), and myalgia (5.2%). With the exception of dry skin, rash, and taste perversion, the incidence of clinical adverse experiences was similar or higher among patients treated with antiretroviral nucleoside analogue controls than among patients treated with Crixivan alone or in combination. This overall safety profile remained similar for 107 patients treated with Crixivan alone or in combination for up to 48 weeks.

Nephrolithiasis, including flank pain with or without haematuria (including microscopic haematuria), has been reported in approximately 4% (79/2205) of patients receiving Crixivan in clinical trials. In general, these events were not associated with renal dysfunction and resolved with hydration and temporary interruption of therapy (e.g. 1–3 days).

*Laboratory test findings:* The laboratory abnormalities reported by the investigators as possibly, probably, or definitely drug related in ≥10% of patients treated with Crixivan alone or in combination were: increases in MCV, ALT, AST, indirect bilirubin, total serum bilirubin; a decrease in neutrophils; haematuria, proteinuria, crystalluria.

Isolated asymptomatic hyperbilirubinaemia (total bilirubin ≥2.5 mg/dl, 43 mcmol/l), reported predominantly as elevated indirect bilirubin and rarely associated with elevations in ALT, AST, or alkaline phosphatase, has occurred in approximately 10% of patients treated with Crixivan alone or in combination with other antiretroviral agents. Most patients continued treatment with Crixivan without dosage reduction and bilirubin values gradually declined toward baseline. Hyperbilirubinaemia occurred more frequently at doses exceeding 2.4 g/day compared to doses less than 2.4 g/day.

*Post-marketed experience:* The following additional adverse reactions have been reported in post-marketed experience:

*Body as a whole/site unspecified:* abdominal distension.

*Digestive system:* liver-function abnormalities; hepatitis including rare reports of hepatic failure.

*Haematological:* increased spontaneous bleeding in patients with haemophilia; acute haemolytic anaemia (see *Special warnings and special precautions for use*).

*Skin and skin appendage:* hyperpigmentation.

*Urogenital system:* nephrolithiasis, in some cases with renal dysfunction including acute renal failure.

*Overdose:* It is not known whether indinavir is dialysable by peritoneal or haemodialysis.

**Pharmacological properties**

*Pharmacodynamic properties:* Pharmacotherapeutic group: protease inhibitor, ATC code JO5AE02.

*Mechanism of action:* Indinavir inhibits recombinant HIV-1 and HIV-2 protease with an approximate tenfold selectivity for HIV-1 over HIV-2 proteinase. Indinavir binds reversibly to the protease active site and inhibits competitively the enzyme, thereby preventing cleavage of the viral precursor polyproteins that occurs during maturation of the newly formed viral particle. The resulting immature particles are non-infectious and are incapable of establishing new cycles of infection. Indinavir did not significantly inhibit the eukaryotic proteases human renin, human cathepsin D, human elastase, and human factor Xa.

*Microbiology:* Indinavir at concentrations of 50 to 100 nM mediated 95% inhibition ($IC_{95}$) of viral spread (relative to an untreated virus-infected control) in human T-lymphoid cell cultures and primary human monocytes/macrophages infected with HIV-1 variants LAI, MN, RF, and a macrophage-tropic variant SF-162, respectively. Indinavir at concentrations of 25 to 100 nM mediated 95% inhibition of viral spread in cultures of mitogen-activated human peripheral blood mononuclear cells infected with diverse, primary clinical isolates of HIV-1, including isolates resistant to zidovudine and non-nucleoside reverse transcriptase inhibitors. Synergistic antiretroviral activity was observed when human T-lymphoid cells infected with the LAI variant of HIV-1 were incubated with indinavir and either zidovudine, didanosine, or a non-nucleoside reverse transcriptase inhibitor.

*Drug resistance:* Loss of suppression of viral RNA levels occurred in some patients; however, CD4 cell counts were often sustained above pretreatment levels. When loss of viral RNA suppression occurred, it was typically associated with replacement of circulating susceptible virus with resistant viral variants. Resistance was correlated with the accumulation of mutations in the viral genome that resulted in the expression of amino-acid substitutions in the viral protease.

At least eleven HIV-1 protease amino-acid residue positions, at which substitutions are associated with resistance, have been identified. No single substitution was capable of engendering measurable resistance to the inhibitor. In general, higher levels of resistance result from the co-expression of greater numbers of substitutions at the eleven identified positions. Substitutions at these positions appeared to accumulate sequentially, probably as the result of ongoing viral replication.

It should be noted that the decrease in suppression of viral RNA levels was seen more frequently when therapy with Crixivan was initiated at doses lower than the recommended oral dose of 2.4 g/day. **Therefore, therapy with Crixivan should be initiated at the recommended dose to increase suppression of viral replication and therefore inhibit the emergence of resistant virus.**

The concomitant use of indinavir with nucleoside analogues (to which the patient is naive) may lessen the risk of the development of resistance to both indinavir and the nucleoside analogues. In one comparative trial, combination therapy with nucleoside analogues (triple therapy with zidovudine plus didanosine) conferred protection against the selection of virus expressing at least one resistance-associated amino-acid substitution to both indinavir (from 13/24 to 2/20 at therapy week 24) and to the nucleoside analogues (from 10/16 to 0/20 at therapy week 24).

Combination treatment with Crixivan is preferred because of the concern about the emergence of resistance.

*Cross-resistance:* HIV-1 patient isolates with reduced susceptibility to indinavir expressed varying patterns and degrees of cross-resistance to a series of diverse HIV protease inhibitors, including ritonavir and saquinavir. Complete cross-resistance was noted between indinavir and ritonavir; however, cross-resistance to saquinavir varied among isolates. Many of the protease amino-acid substitutions reported to be associated with resistance to ritonavir and saquinavir were also associated with resistance to indinavir.

*Pharmacodynamic effects:* Treatment with indinavir alone or in combination with other antiretroviral agents (i.e. nucleoside analogues) has so far been documented to reduce viral load and increase CD4 lymphocytes in patients with CD4 cell counts below 500 cells/$mm^3$.

The effects of indinavir (alone or combined with other antiretroviral agents) on the biological markers of disease activity, CD4 cell counts and serum viral RNA, were evaluated in several studies involving HIV-1 seropositive patients with CD4 cell counts <500 cells/$mm^3$. These studies have documented that indinavir, 2.4 g/day was consistently associated with increases in median CD4 cell counts of 90–100 cells/$mm^3$ and median declines in serum viral RNA in excess of 1 $log_{10}$ copies/ml which were sustained to at least 24 weeks. Approximately 40% of these patients had serum viral RNA levels decrease to below 500 copies/ml, the limit of detection of the assay.

In one study at 24 weeks, the median declines in serum viral RNA for the group treated with indinavir alone, the group treated with indinavir in combination with zidovudine and lamivudine, and the group treated with zidovudine plus lamivudine were 0.67 $\log_{10}$ (79%), 1.88 $\log_{10}$ (98%), and 0.66 $\log_{10}$ (78%), respectively. At 24 weeks, the percentage of patients whose serum viral RNA levels had decreased to below the limit of detection of the assay (<500 copies/ml) were 35% and 91%, for the groups treated with indinavir alone or in combination, respectively. A total of 0% of the patients in the zidovudine plus lamivudine group experienced this level of serum viral RNA decline at the 24-week time-point. Median CD4 cell counts at 24 weeks were increased for all treatment groups.

*Pharmacokinetic properties:*

*Absorption:* Indinavir is rapidly absorbed in the fasted state with a time to peak plasma concentration of 0.8 hours±0.3 hours (mean±S.D.). A greater than dose-proportional increase in indinavir plasma concentrations was observed over the 200–800 mg dose range. Between 800-mg and 1000-mg dose levels, the deviation from dose-proportionality is less pronounced. As a result of the short half-life, 1.8±0.4 hours, only a minimal increase in plasma concentrations occurred after multiple dosing.

Administration of indinavir with a meal high in calories, fat, and protein resulted in a blunted and reduced absorption with an approximate 80% reduction in AUC and an 86% reduction in $C_{max}$. Administration with light meals (e.g. dry toast with jam or fruit conserve, apple juice, and coffee with skimmed or fat-free milk and sugar or corn flakes, skimmed or fat-free milk and sugar) resulted in plasma concentrations comparable to the corresponding fasted values.

*Distribution:* Indinavir was not highly bound to human plasma proteins (39% unbound).

There are no data concerning the penetration of indinavir into the central nervous system in humans.

*Biotransformation:* Seven major metabolites were identified and the metabolic pathways were identified as glucuronidation at the pyridine nitrogen, pyridine-N-oxidation with and without 3'-hydroxylation on the indane ring, 3'-hydroxylation of indane, p-hydroxylation of phenylmethyl moiety, and N-depyridomethylation with and without the 3'-hydroxylation. *In vitro* studies with human liver microsomes indicated that CYP3A4 is the only P450 isozyme that plays a major role in the oxidative metabolism of indinavir. Analysis of plasma and urine samples from subjects who received indinavir indicated that indinavir metabolites had little proteinase inhibitory activity.

*Elimination:* Over the 200–1000 mg dose range administered in both volunteers and HIV-infected patients, there was a slightly greater than dose-proportional increase in urinary recovery of indinavir. Renal clearance (116 ml/min) of indinavir is concentration-independent over the clinical dose range. Less than 20% of indinavir is excreted renally. Mean urinary excretion of unchanged drug following single dose administration in the fasted state was 10.4% following a 700-mg dose, and 12.0% following a 1000-mg dose. Indinavir was rapidly eliminated with a half-life of 1.8 hours.

*Characteristics in patients:* Pharmacokinetics of indinavir do not appear to be affected by gender or by race.

Patients with mild-to-moderate hepatic insufficiency and clinical evidence of cirrhosis had evidence of decreased metabolism of indinavir resulting in approximately 60% higher mean AUC following a 400-mg dose. The mean half-life of indinavir increased to approximately 2.8 hours.

At steady state following a dosage regimen of 800 mg every 8 hours, HIV-seropositive patients in one study achieved AUC values of 28,713 nM h, peak plasma concentrations of 11,144 nM and plasma concentrations at 8 hours post dose of 211 nM.

*Preclinical safety data:* Crystals have been seen in the urine of rats, one monkey, and one dog. The crystals have not been associated with drug-induced renal injury. An increase in thyroidal weight and thyroidal follicular-cell hyperplasia, due to an increase in thyroxine clearance, was seen in rats treated with indinavir at doses ≥160 mg/kg/day. An increase in hepatic weight occurred in rats treated with indinavir at doses ≥40 mg/kg/day and was accompanied by hepatocellular hypertrophy at doses ≥320 mg/kg/day.

The maximum non-lethal oral dose of indinavir was at least 5000 mg/kg in rats and mice, the highest dose tested in acute toxicity studies.

Studies in rats indicated that uptake into brain tissue was limited, distribution into and out of the lymphatic system was rapid, and excretion into the milk of lactating rats was extensive. Distribution of indinavir across the placental barrier was significant in rats, but limited in rabbits.

*Mutagenicity:* Indinavir did not have any mutagenic

or genotoxic activity in studies with or without metabolic activation.

*Carcinogenicity:* Carcinogenicity studies of indinavir are ongoing.

**Pharmaceutical particulars**

*List of excipients:* each capsule contains the inactive ingredients anhydrous lactose and magnesium stearate. The capsule shell contains the excipients gelatine, titanium dioxide, silicon dioxide, and sodium lauryl sulphate. The 200-mg capsules are printed with printing ink containing titanium dioxide (E 171) and indigo carmine (E 132). The 400-mg capsules are printed with printing ink containing titanium dioxide (E 171), indigo carmine (E 132) and iron oxide (E 172).

The 200 mg capsules are white opaque and coded 'Crixivan 200 mg' in blue.

The 400 mg capsules are white opaque and coded 'Crixivan 400 mg' in green.

*Incompatibilities:* Not applicable.

*Shelf life:* The shelf life is 18 months.

*Special precautions for storage:* Sensitive to moisture. Store in a well-closed container.

*Nature and contents of container:* Crixivan 200 mg is supplied in HDPE bottles with a polypropylene cap and a foil induction cap containing 360 capsules.

Crixivan 400 mg is supplied in HDPE bottles with a polypropylene cap and a foil induction cap containing 180 capsules or 90 capsules.

The containers contain desiccant canisters that should remain in the bottle. Patients should be advised not to swallow desiccant.

**Marketing authorisation numbers**

Crixivan 200 mg, 180 capsules EU/1/96/024/001
Crixivan 200 mg, 270 capsules EU/1/96/024/002
Crixivan 200 mg, 360 capsules EU/1/96/024/003
Crixivan 400 mg, 90 capsules EU/1/96/024/004
Crixivan 400 mg, 180 capsules EU/1/96/024/005

**Date of approval/revision of SPC** May 1997.

**Legal category** POM.

## DECADRON* INJECTION

**Presentation** A clear, colourless solution containing, in each millilitre, Dexamethasone Sodium Phosphate BP equivalent to 4 mg dexamethasone phosphate or approximately 3.33 mg dexamethasone.

**Uses** Corticosteroid.

For use in certain endocrine and non-endocrine disorders responsive to corticosteroid therapy.

*Systemic administration:* Decadron Injection is recommended for systemic administration by intravenous or intramuscular injection when oral therapy is not feasible or desirable in the following conditions.

*Endocrine disorders: Primary or secondary adrenocortical insufficiency* (hydrocortisone or cortisone is the first choice, but synthetic analogues may be used with mineralocorticoids where applicable and, in infancy, mineralocorticoid supplementation is particularly important.)

*Non-endocrine disorders:* Decadron Injection may be used in the treatment of non-endocrine corticosteroid responsive conditions including:

*Allergy and anaphylaxis:* Angioneurotic oedema and anaphylaxis.

*Gastro-intestinal:* Crohn's disease and ulcerative colitis.

*Infection (with appropriate chemotherapy):* Miliary tuberculosis and endotoxic shock.

*Neurological disorders:* Raised intracranial pressure secondary to cerebral tumours and infantile spasms.

*Respiratory:* Bronchial asthma and aspiration pneumonitis.

*Skin disorders:* Toxic epidermal necrolysis.

*Shock:* Adjunctive treatment where high pharmacological doses are needed. Treatment is an adjunct to, and not a substitute for, specific and supportive measures the patient may require. Dexamethasone has been shown to be beneficial when used in the early treatment of shock, but it may not influence overall survival.

*Local administration*

Decadron Injection is suitable for intra-articular or soft-tissue injection as adjunctive therapy for short-term administration in:

*Soft-tissue disorders* such as carpal tunnel syndrome and tenosynovitis.

*Intra-articular disorders* such as rheumatoid arthritis and osteoarthritis with an inflammatory component.

Decadron Injection may be injected intralesionally in selected skin disorders such as cystic acne vulgaris, localised lichen simplex, and keloids.

**Dosage and administration** Decadron Injection can be given without mixing or dilution, but if preferred,

can be added without loss of potency to sodium chloride injection or dextrose injection and given by intravenous drip. The infusion mixture must be used within 24 hours, and the usual aseptic techniques for injections should be observed.

Solutions used for intravenous administration or further dilution of this product should be preservative-free when used in the neonate, especially the premature infant.

*All dosage recommendations are given in units of dexamethasone phosphate.*

*Intravenous and intramuscular injection:*

*General considerations:* Dosage must be individualised on the basis of the disease and the reponse of the patient. In order to minimise side effects, the lowest possible dosage adequate to control the disease process should be used (see 'Side effects').

Usually the parenteral dosage ranges are one-third to one-half the oral dose, given every 12 hours.

The usual initial dosage is 0.5–20 mg (0.125–5 ml) a day. In situations of less severity, lower doses will generally suffice. However, in certain overwhelming, acute, life-threatening situations, administration in dosages exceeding the usual dosages may be justified. In these circumstances, the slower rate of absorption by intramuscular administration should be recognised.

Both the dose in the evening, which is useful in alleviating morning stiffness, and the divided dosage regimen are associated with greater suppression of the hypothalamo-pituitary-adrenal axis. After a favourable response is noted, the proper maintenance dosage should be determined by decreasing the initial dosage by small amounts at appropriate intervals to the lowest dosage which will maintain an adequate clinical response. Chronic dosage should preferably not exceed 500 micrograms dexamethasone daily. Close monitoring of drug dosage is needed.

If Decadron is to be stopped after it has been given for more than a few days, the drug should be withdrawn gradually rather than stopped abruptly.

Whenever possible, the intravenous route should be used for the initial dose and for as many subsequent doses as are given while the patient is in shock (because of the irregular rate of absorption of any medicament administered by any other route in such patients). When the blood pressure responds, use the intramuscular route until oral therapy can be substituted. For the comfort of the patient, not more than 2 ml should be injected intramuscularly at any one site.

In emergencies, the usual dose of Decadron Injection by intravenous or intramuscular injection is 4 mg–20 mg (1 ml–5 ml) (in shock use only the i.v. route). This dose may be repeated until adequate response is noted.

After initial improvement, single doses of 2 mg–4 mg (0.5 ml–1 ml) repeated as necessary, should be sufficient. The total daily dosage usually need not exceed 80 mg (20 ml), even in severe conditions.

When constant maximal effect is desired, dosage must be repeated at three-hour or four-hour intervals, or maintained by slow intravenous drip.

Intravenous and intramuscular injections are advised in acute illness. When the acute stage has passed, oral steroid therapy should be substituted as soon as feasible.

*Shock (of haemorrhagic, traumatic or surgical origin):* Usually 2 mg–6 mg/kg body weight as a single intravenous injection. This may be repeated in two to six hours if shock persists. Alternatively, this may be followed immediately by the same dose in an intravenous infusion. Therapy with Decadron Injection is an adjunct to, and not a replacement for conventional therapy.

Administration of these high doses should be continued only until the patient's condition has stabilised and usually no longer than 48–72 hours.

*Cerebral oedema:* Associated with primary or metastatic brain tumour, pre-operative preparation of patients with increased intracranial pressure secondary to brain tumour: initially 10 mg (2.5 ml) intravenously, followed by 4 mg (1 ml) intramuscularly every six hours until symptoms of cerebral oedema subside. Response is usually noted within 12–24 hours; dosage may be reduced after two to four days and gradually discontinued over five to seven days.

High doses of Decadron Injection are recommended for initiating short-term intensive therapy for acute life-threatening cerebral oedema. Following the high loading dose schedule of the first day of therapy, the dose is scaled down over the seven- to ten-day period of intensive therapy and subsequently reduced to zero over the next seven to ten days. When maintenance therapy is required, substitute oral Decadron as soon as possible (see table below).

*Palliative management of recurrent or inoperable brain tumours:* Maintenance therapy should be determined for each patient; 2 mg (0.5 ml) two or three times a day may be effective.

The smallest dosage necessary to control cerebral oedema should be used.

*Suggested high dose schedule in cerebral oedema:*

*Adults:*

| | |
|---|---|
| Initial Dose | 50 mg IV |
| 1st day | 8 mg IV every 2 hours |
| 2nd day | 8 mg IV every 2 hours |
| 3rd day | 8 mg IV every 2 hours |
| 4th day | 4 mg IV every 2 hours |
| 5th–8th days | 4 mg IV every 4 hours |
| Thereafter | decrease by daily reduction of 4 mg |

*Children (35 kg and over):*

| | |
|---|---|
| Initial Dose | 25 mg IV |
| 1st day | 4 mg IV every 2 hours |
| 2nd day | 4 mg IV every 2 hours |
| 3rd day | 4 mg IV every 2 hours |
| 4th day | 4 mg IV every 4 hours |
| 5th–8th days | 4 mg IV every 6 hours |
| Thereafter | decrease by daily reduction of 2 mg |

*Children (below 35 kg):*

| | |
|---|---|
| Initial Dose | 20 mg IV |
| 1st day | 4 mg IV every 3 hours |
| 2nd day | 4 mg IV every 3 hours |
| 3rd day | 4 mg IV every 3 hours |
| 4th day | 4 mg IV every 6 hours |
| 5th–8th days | 2 mg IV every 6 hours |
| Thereafter | decrease by daily reduction of 1 mg |

*Dual therapy:* In acute self-limiting allergic disorders or acute exacerbations of chronic allergic disorders, the following schedule combining oral and parenteral therapy is suggested:

| | |
|---|---|
| First day | Decadron Injection, 4 mg–8 mg (1 ml–2 ml) intramuscularly |
| Second day | Two 500 microgram Decadron Tablets twice a day |
| Third day | Two 500 microgram Decadron Tablets twice a day |
| Fourth day | One 500 microgram Decadron Tablet twice a day |
| Fifth day | One 500 microgram Decadron Tablet twice a day |
| Sixth day | One 500 microgram Decadron Tablet |
| Seventh day | One 500 microgram Decadron Tablet |
| Eighth day | Reassessment day |

(For information on Decadron Tablets, see separate entry.)

*Intrasynovial, intralesional, and soft-tissue injection:* In general, these injections are employed when only one or two joints or areas are affected.

Some of the usual single doses are:

| Site of injection | Amount of dexamethasone phosphate |
|---|---|
| Large joints (e.g. knee) | 2–4 mg (0.5–1 ml) |
| Small joints (e.g. interphalangeal, temporomandibular) | 0.8–1 mg (0.2–0.25 ml) |
| Bursae | 2–3 mg (0.5–0.75 ml) |
| Tendon sheaths* | 0.4–1 mg (0.1–0.25 ml) |
| Soft-tissue infiltration | 2–6 mg (0.5–1.5 ml) |
| Ganglia | 1–2 mg (0.25–0.5 ml) |

* Injection should be made into the tendon sheath, and not directly into the tendon.

Frequency of injection: once every three to five days to once every two to three weeks, depending on response.

*Use in children:* Dosage should be limited to a single dose on alternate days to lessen retardation of growth and minimise suppression of the hypothalamo-pituitary-adrenal axis.

*Use in the elderly:* Treatment of elderly patients, particularly if long term, should be planned bearing in mind the more serious consequences of the common side effects of corticosteroids in old age, especially osteoporosis, diabetes, hypertension, susceptibility to infection and thinning of the skin.

Close clinical supervision is required to avoid life-threatening reactions (see 'Side-effects').

**Contra-indications, warnings, etc**
*Contra-indications:* Systemic fungal infection; systemic infection unless specific anti-infective therapy is employed; hypersensitivity to sulphites or any other component of this medication. Administration of live virus vaccines (see 'Precautions').

*Warnings:* Frequent intra-articular injections over a prolonged period may lead to joint destruction with bone necrosis. Intra-articular injection of corticosteroid may produce systemic adverse reactions including adrenal suppression.

*Precautions:* Undesirable effects may be minimised by using the lowest effective dose for the minimum period. Frequent patient review is required to appropriately titrate the dose against disease activity. Where

reduction in dosage is possible, the reduction should be gradual (see 'Dosage and administration').

Decadron Injection contains sodium bisulphite, a sulphite that may cause allergic-type reactions, including anaphylactic symptoms and life-threatening or less severe asthmatic episodes in certain susceptible people. The overall prevalence of sulphite sensitivity in the general population is unknown and probably low. Sulphite sensitivity is seen more frequently in asthmatic than in non-asthmatic people.

Corticosteroids may exacerbate systemic fungal infections and, therefore, should not be used in the presence of such infections unless they are needed to control drug reactions due to amphotericin. Moreover, there have been cases reported in which concomitant use of amphotericin and hydrocortisone was followed by cardiac enlargement and congestive failure.

Average and large doses of hydrocortisone or cortisone can cause elevation of blood pressure, retention of salt and water, and increased excretion of potassium, but these effects are less likely to occur with synthetic derivatives, except when used in large doses. Dietary salt restriction and potassium supplementation may be necessary. All corticosteroids increase calcium excretion.

The slower rate of absorption by intramuscular administration should be recognised.

In patients on corticosteroid therapy subjected to unusual stress (e.g. intercurrent illness, trauma, or surgical procedures), dosage should be increased before, during and after the stressful situation.

Drug-induced secondary adrenocortical insufficiency may result from too rapid withdrawal of corticosteroids and may be minimised by gradual dosage reduction, being tapered off over weeks and months depending on the dose and duration of treatment, but may persist for up to a year after discontinuation of therapy. In any stressful situation during that period, therefore, corticosteroid therapy should be reinstated. If the patient is already receiving corticosteroids, the dosage may have to be increased. Salt and/or a mineralocorticoid should be given concurrently, since mineralocorticoid secretion may be impaired.

Stopping corticosteroids after prolonged therapy may cause withdrawal symptoms including fever, myalgia, arthralgia, and malaise. This may occur in patients even without evidence of adrenal insufficiency. **Patients should carry 'steroid treatment' cards, which give clear guidance on the precautions to be taken to minimise risk and which provide details of prescriber, drug, dosage and the duration of treatment.**

Because anaphylactoid reactions have occurred, rarely, in patients receiving parenteral corticosteroid therapy, appropriate precautions should be taken prior to administration, especially when the patient has a history of allergy to any drug.

Administration of live virus vaccines is contra-indicated in individuals receiving immunosuppressive doses of corticosteroids. If inactivated viral or bacterial vaccines are administered to individuals receiving immunosuppressive doses of corticosteroids, the expected serum antibody response may not be obtained. However, immunisation procedures may be undertaken in patients who are receiving corticosteroids as replacement therapy, e.g. for Addison's disease.

Literature reports suggest an apparent association between use of corticosteroids and left ventricular free wall rupture after a recent myocardial infarction; therefore, therapy with corticosteroids should be used with great caution in these patients.

The use of Decadron Injection in active tuberculosis should be restricted to those cases of fulminating or disseminated tuberculosis in which the corticosteroid is used for the management of the disease in conjunction with an appropriate antituberculosis regimen. If the corticosteroids are indicated in patients with latent tuberculosis or tuberculin reactivity, close observation is necessary as reactivation may occur. During prolonged corticosteroid therapy, these patients should receive prophylactic chemotherapy.

Corticosteroids may mask some signs of infection, and new infections may appear during their use. Suppression of the inflammatory response and immune function increases the susceptibility to infections and their severity. The clinical presentation may often be atypical, and serious infections such as septicaemia and tuberculosis may be masked and reach an advanced stage before being recognised. There may be decreased resistance, and inability to localise infection.

A report shows that the use of corticosteroids in cerebral malaria is associated with a prolonged coma and an increased incidence of pneumonia and gastro-intestinal bleeding.

**Chickenpox is of particular concern, since this normally minor illness may be fatal in immunosuppressed patients.** Patients (or parents of children) without a definite history of chickenpox should be advised to avoid close personal contact with chicken-

pox or herpes zoster, and if exposed they should seek urgent medical attention. Passive immunisation with varicella/zoster immunoglobulin (VZIG) is needed by exposed non-immune patients who are receiving systemic corticosteroids or who have used them within the previous three months; this should be given within ten days of exposure to chickenpox. **If a diagnosis of chickenpox is confirmed, the illness warrants specialist care and urgent treatment. Corticosteroids should not be stopped and the dose may need to be increased.**

Measles can have a more serious or even fatal course in immunosuppressed patients. In such children or adults particular care should be taken to avoid exposure to measles. If exposed, prophylaxis with intramuscular pooled immunoglobulin (IG) may be indicated. Exposed patients should be advised to seek medical advice without delay.

Corticosteroids may activate latent amoebiasis or strongyloidiasis or exacerbate active disease. Therefore, it is recommended that latent or active amoebiasis and strongyloidiasis be ruled out before initiating corticosteroid therapy in any patient at risk of or with symptoms of either condition.

Prolonged use of corticosteroids may produce posterior subcapsular cataracts, glaucoma with possible damage to the optic nerves, and may enhance the establishment of secondary ocular infections due to fungi or viruses. Corticosteroids may increase or decrease motility and number of spermatozoa.

*Special precautions:* Particular care is required when considering the use of systemic corticosteroids in patients with the following conditions, and frequent patient monitoring is necessary: renal insufficiency, hypertension, diabetes or in those with a family history of diabetes, congestive heart failure, osteoporosis, previous steroid myopathy, glaucoma (or family history of glaucoma), myasthenia gravis, non-specific ulcerative colitis, diverticulitis, fresh intestinal anastomoses, active or latent peptic ulcer, existing or previous history of severe affective disorders (especially previous steroid psychosis), liver failure, and epilepsy. Signs of peritoneal irritation following gastro-intestinal perforation in patients receiving large doses of corticosteroids may be minimal or absent. Fat embolism has been reported as a possible complication of hypercortisonism.

There is an enhanced effect of corticosteroids in patients with hypothyroidism and in those with cirrhosis.

Corticosteroids should be used cautiously in patients with ocular herpes simplex because of possible corneal perforation.

Local steroid injection should be undertaken in an aseptic environment to reduce the particular risk of bacterial infection. Injection of a steroid into an infected site should be avoided.

Appropriate examination of joint fluid is necessary to exclude a septic process.

A marked increase in pain accompanied by local swelling, further restriction of joint motion, fever, and malaise are suggestive of septic arthritis. If this complication occurs and the diagnosis of sepsis is confirmed, appropriate antimicrobial therapy should be instituted.

Patients should understand the great importance of not over-using joints that are still diseased, despite symptomatic improvement.

Corticosteroids should not be injected into unstable joints.

Frequent intra-articular injections have been reported to cause development of Charcot-like arthropathies.

*Children:* Corticosteroids cause growth retardation in infancy, childhood and adolescence, which may be irreversible. Treatment should be limited to the minimum dosage for the shortest possible time. In order to minimise suppression of the hypothalamo-pituitary-adrenal axis and growth retardation, treatment should be limited, where possible, to a single dose on alternate days.

Growth and development of infants and children on prolonged corticosteroid therapy should be carefully monitored.

*Use in pregnancy and lactation:* There is inadequate evidence of safety in human pregnancy and there may be a very small risk of cleft palate and intra-uterine growth retardation in the fetus; there is evidence of harmful effects on pregnancy in animals. Infants born of mothers who have received substantial doses of corticosteroids during pregnancy should be carefully observed for signs of hypoadrenalism.

When corticosteroids are essential, however, patients with normal pregnancies may be treated as though they were in the non-gravid state. Patients with pre-eclampsia or fluid retention require close monitoring.

Corticosteroids appear in breast milk and could suppress growth, interfere with endogenous corticosteroid production, or cause other unwanted effects.

Mothers taking pharmacological doses of corticosteroids should be advised not to breast-feed.

*Drug interactions:* Aspirin should be used cautiously in conjunction with corticosteroids in hypoprothrombinaemia.

The renal clearance of salicylates is increased by corticosteroids and therefore salicylate dosage should be reduced along with steroid withdrawal.

As phenytoin, barbiturates, ephedrine, rifabutin, carbamazepine, rifampicin, and aminoglutethimide may enhance the metabolic clearance of corticosteroids, resulting in decreased blood levels and reduced physiological activity, the dosage may have to be adjusted. These interactions may interfere with dexamethasone suppression tests, which should be interpreted with caution during administration of these drugs.

False-negative results in the dexamethasone suppression test in patients being treated with indomethacin have been reported.

The efficacy of coumarin anticoagulants may be changed by concurrent corticosteroid treatment. The prothrombin time should be checked frequently in patients who are receiving corticosteroids and coumarin anticoagulants at the same time, in order to avoid spontaneous bleeding.

The desired effects of hypoglycaemic agents (including insulin), are antagonised by corticosteroids.

When corticosteroids are administered concomitantly with potassium-depleting diuretics, patients should be observed closely for development of hypokalaemia.

Corticosteroids may affect the nitrobluetetrazolium test for bacterial infection and produce false-negative results.

*Side-effects:* The incidence of predictable undesirable effects, including hypothalamic-pituitary-adrenal suppression, correlates with the relative potency of the drug, dosage, timing of administration and the duration of treatment (see 'Precautions').

*Fluid and electrolyte disturbances:* Sodium retention, fluid retention, congestive heart failure in susceptible patients, potassium loss, hypokalaemic alkalosis, hypertension, increased calcium excretion (see 'Precautions').

*Musculoskeletal:* Muscle weakness, steroid myopathy, loss of muscle mass, osteoporosis (especially in post-menopausal females), vertebral compression fractures, aseptic necrosis of femoral and humeral heads, pathological fracture of long bones, tendon rupture, and post-injection flare (following intra-articular use).

*Gastro-intestinal:* Peptic ulcer with possible perforation and haemorrhage, perforation of the small and large bowel, particularly in patients with inflammatory bowel disease, pancreatitis, abdominal distension, ulcerative oesophagitis, dyspepsia, oesophageal candidiasis.

*Dermatological:* Impaired wound healing, thin fragile skin, petechiae and ecchymoses, erythema, striae, telangiectasia, acne, increased sweating, possible suppression of skin tests, burning or tingling especially in the perineal area (after intravenous injection), other cutaneous reactions such as allergic dermatitis, urticaria, angioneurotic oedema, and hypo- or hyperpigmentation.

*Neurological:* Convulsions, increased intracranial pressure with papilloedema (pseudotumour cerebri) usually after treatment, vertigo, headache, psychic disturbances (e.g. euphoria, psychological dependence, depression, insomnia).

*Endocrine:* Menstrual irregularities, amenorrhoea, development of Cushingoid state, suppression of growth in children and adolescents, secondary adrenocortical and pituitary unresponsiveness (particularly in times of stress, as in trauma, surgery or illness), decreased carbohydrate tolerance, manifestations of latent diabetes mellitus, increased requirements for insulin or oral hypoglycaemic agents in diabetes, hirsutism.

*Anti-inflammatory and immunosuppressive effects:* Increased susceptibility and severity of infections with suppression of clinical symptoms and signs. Opportunistic infections, recurrence of dormant tuberculosis (see 'Precautions').

*Ophthalmic:* Posterior subcapsular cataracts, increased intra-ocular pressure, papilloedema, corneal or scleral thinning, exacerbation of ophthalmic viral disease, glaucoma, exophthalmos, rare instances of blindness associated with intra-lesional therapy around the face and head, retinopathy of prematurity.

*Metabolic:* Negative nitrogen balance due to protein catabolism. Negative calcium balance.

*Cardiovascular:* Myocardial rupture following recent myocardial infarction (see 'Precautions'). Hypertrophic cardiomyopathy in low birth-weight infants.

*Other:* Hypersensitivity, including anaphylaxis has been reported, leucocytosis, thrombo-embolism, weight gain, increased appetite, nausea, malaise, hiccups, and sterile abscess.

*Withdrawal symptoms and signs:* Too rapid a reduction of corticosteroid dosage following prolonged treatment can lead to acute adrenal insufficiency, hypotension, and death (see 'Precautions').

In some instances, withdrawal symptoms may simulate a clinical relapse of the disease for which the patient has been undergoing treatment.

*Overdosage:* Reports of acute toxicity and/or deaths following overdosage with glucocorticoids are rare. No antidote is available. Treatment is probably not indicated for reactions due to chronic poisoning unless the patient has a condition that would render a patient unusually susceptible to ill effects from corticosteroids. In this case, symptomatic treatment should be instituted as necessary.

Anaphylactic and hypersensitivity reactions may be treated with adrenaline, positive-pressure artificial respiration and aminophylline. The patient should be kept warm and quiet.

The biological half-life of dexamethasone in plasma is about 190 minutes.

**Pharmaceutical precautions** Decadron Injection is sensitive to heat and should not be autoclaved to sterilise the outside of the vial. Store below 25°C, protected from light and freezing. Only sodium chloride injection or dextrose injection should be used as diluent. Any infusion mixture must be used within 24 hours.

**Legal category** POM.

**Package quantities** Vials of 2 ml.

**Further information** Also available is Injection Decadron Shock-Pak containing, per millilitre, dexamethasone sodium phosphate equivalent to 20 mg dexamethasone, indicated exclusively for intravenous use as adjunctive therapy in severe shock. For information about this special high-dose form of Decadron Injection, see separate entry.

Decadron Injection is ready for immediate use. An adequate dose is contained in a small volume of vehicle, and small-bore needles can be used wherever appropriate.

**Product licence number** 0025/5045.

# INJECTION DECADRON* SHOCK-PAK

**Presentation** An injection containing, per millilitre, dexamethasone sodium phosphate equivalent to 20 mg dexamethasone, as a colourless solution.

**Uses** Corticosteroid.

Only for the adjunctive treatment of shock where massive doses of corticosteroids are needed: Severe shock of haemorrhagic, traumatic or surgical origin. It is an adjunct to, and not a substitute for, specific or supportive measures that the patient may require, e.g. restoration of circulating blood volume, correction of fluid and electrolyte balance, oxygen, surgical measures.

**Dosage and administration** Injection Decadron Shock-Pak is for administration by the intravenous route only.

*Intravenous injection in shock:* Injection Decadron Shock-Pak can be used without mixing or diluting. Injection should be made slowly.

The usual dosage by intravenous injection is 2–6 mg/kg body weight given as a single intravenous injection. This may be repeated in two to six hours, if shock persists. As an alternative, the initial intravenous injection may be followed immediately by an intravenous infusion containing the same dose. (Although Injection Decadron Shock-Pak was not primarily designed for intravenous infusion, it can be added to sodium chloride injection, or to dextrose injection, and administered by intravenous drip without loss of potency. When the Shock-Pak is added to an infusion solution, the mixture must be used within 24 hours as infusion solutions do not contain preservatives.)

Solutions used for intravenous administration or further dilution of this product should be preservative-free when used in the neonate, especially the premature infant.

These dosages are large in comparison with the usual recommended dosages of dexamethasone sodium phosphate. They are, however, for emergency use in acute conditions needing massive doses of corticosteroid, and reflect the tendency in current medical practice to use such high doses in the treatment of shock.

Therapy with Injection Decadron Shock-Pak is an adjunct to, and not a replacement for, conventional therapy. Administration of high doses of corticosteroids should be continued only until the patient's condition has stabilised, and usually no longer than 48–72 hours. Prolonged therapy at such high doses should be avoided to prevent possible complications, such as adrenal suppression or gastro-intestinal ulceration.

*Use in the elderly:* These dosage recommendations apply to all adults, including the elderly.

**Contra-indications, warnings, etc**
*Contra-indications:* Systemic fungal infections; hypersensitivity to sulphites or to any other component of this product. Administration of live virus vaccines.

*Precautions:* Decadron Injection Shock-Pak contains sodium bisulphite, a sulphite that may cause allergic-type reactions, including anaphylactic symptoms and life-threatening or less severe asthmatic episodes in certain susceptible people. The overall prevalence of sulphite sensitivity in the general population is unknown and probably low. Sulphite sensitivity is seen more frequently in asthmatic than in non-asthmatic people.

Decadron Injection Shock-Pak is for adjunctive use in the treatment of shock, and therapy must be accompanied by the usual standard measures employed in its management.

The pronounced hormonal effects associated with prolonged corticosteroid therapy will probably not be seen when this injection is used for short-term adjunctive therapy in shock.

Because rare instances of anaphylactic reactions have occurred in patients receiving parenteral corticosteroid therapy, appropriate precautionary measures should be taken prior to administration, especially when the patient has a history of allergy to any drug.

Administration of live virus vaccines is contra-indicated in individuals receiving immunosuppressive doses of corticosteroids. If inactivated viral or bacterial vaccines are administered to individuals receiving immunosuppressive doses of corticosteroids, the expected serum antibody response may not be obtained.

Literature reports suggest an apparent association between use of corticosteroids and left ventricular free wall rupture after a recent myocardial infarction; therefore, therapy with corticosteroids should be used with great caution in these patients.

**Chickenpox is of particular concern, since this normally minor illness may be fatal in immunosuppressed patients.** Patients (or parents of children) without a definite history of chickenpox should be advised to avoid close personal contact with chickenpox or herpes zoster, and if exposed they should seek urgent medical attention. Passive immunisation with varicella/zoster immunoglobulin (VZIG) is needed by exposed non-immune patients who are receiving systemic corticosteroids or who have used them within the previous three months; this should be given within 10 days of exposure to chickenpox. **If a diagnosis of chickenpox is confirmed, the illness warrants specialist care and urgent treatment. Corticosteroids should not be stopped and the dose may need to be increased.**

Measles can have a more serious or even fatal course in immunosuppressed patients. In such children or adults, particular care should be taken to avoid exposure to measles. If exposed, prophylaxis with intramuscular pooled immunoglobulin (IG) may be indicated. Exposed patients should be advised to seek medical advice without delay.

*Precautions for prolonged corticosteroid therapy:* The following precautions are listed for Decadron Injection and should be considered for any dexamethasone preparation.

Undesirable effects may be minimised by using the lowest effective dose for the minimum period. Frequent patient review is required to appropriately titrate the dose against disease activity. When reduction in dosage is possible, the reduction should be gradual.

Corticosteroids may exacerbate systemic fungal infections and, therefore, should not be used in the presence of such infections unless they are needed to control drug reactions due to amphotericin. Moreover, there have been cases reported in which concomitant use of amphotericin and hydrocortisone was followed by cardiac enlargement and congestive failure.

Average and large doses of hydrocortisone or cortisone can cause elevation of blood pressure, retention of salt and water, and increased excretion of potassium, but these effects are less likely to occur with synthetic derivatives, except when used in large doses. Dietary salt restriction and potassium supplementation may be necessary. All corticosteroids increase calcium excretion.

In patients on corticosteroid therapy subjected to unusual stress (e.g. intercurrent illness, trauma, or surgical procedures), dosage should be increased before, during and after the stressful situation. Drug-induced secondary adrenocortical insufficiency may result from too rapid withdrawal of corticosteroids and may be minimised by gradual dosage reduction, being tapered off over weeks and months depending on the dose and duration of treatment, but may persist for up to a year after discontinuation of therapy. In any stressful situation during that period, therefore, corticosteroid therapy should be reinstated. If the patient is already receiving corticosteroids, the current dosage may have to be temporarily increased. Salt and/or a mineralocorticoid should be given concurrently, since mineralocorticoid secretion may be impaired.

Stopping corticosteroids after prolonged therapy may cause withdrawal symptoms, including fever, myalgia, arthralgia, and malaise. This may occur in patients even without evidence of adrenal insufficiency.

**Patients should carry 'steroid treatment' cards, which give clear guidance on the precautions to be taken to minimise risk and which provide details of prescriber, drug, dosage and the duration of treatment.**

The use of Decadron Injection in active tuberculosis should be restricted to those cases of fulminating or disseminated tuberculosis in which the corticosteroid is used for the management of the disease in conjunction with an appropriate antituberculosis regimen. If the corticosteroids are indicated in patients with latent tuberculosis or tuberculin reactivity, close observation is necessary as reactivation may occur. During prolonged corticosteroid therapy, these patients should receive prophylactic chemotherapy.

Corticosteroids may mask some signs of infection, and new infections may appear during their use. Suppression of the inflammatory response and immune function increases the susceptibility to infections and their severity. The clinical presentation may often be atypical, and serious infections such as septicaemia and tuberculosis may be masked and reach an advanced stage before being recognised. There may be decreased resistance, and inability to localise infection.

A report shows that the use of corticosteroids in cerebral malaria is associated with a prolonged coma and an increased incidence of pneumonia and gastrointestinal bleeding.

Corticosteroids may activate latent amoebiasis or strongyloidiasis or exacerbate active disease. Therefore, it is recommended that latent or active amoebiasis and strongyloidiasis be ruled out before initiating corticosteroid therapy in any patient at risk of or with symptoms of either condition.

Prolonged use of corticosteroids may produce posterior subcapsular cataracts, glaucoma with possible damage to the optic nerves, and may enhance the establishment of secondary ocular infections due to fungi or viruses. Corticosteroids may increase or decrease motility and number of spermatozoa.

*Special precautions:* Particular care is required when considering the use of systemic corticosteroids in patients with the following conditions, and frequent patient monitoring is necessary: renal insufficiency, hypertension, diabetes or in those with a family history of diabetes, congestive heart failure, osteoporosis, previous steroid myopathy, glaucoma (or family history of glaucoma), myasthenia gravis, non-specific ulcerative colitis, diverticulitis, fresh intestinal anastomoses, active or latent peptic ulcer, existing or previous history of severe affective disorders (especially previous steroid psychosis), liver failure, and epilepsy. Signs of peritoneal irritation following gastro-intestinal perforation in patients receiving large doses of corticosteroids may be minimal or absent. Fat embolism has been reported as a possible complication of hypercortisonism.

There is an enhanced effect of corticosteroids in patients with hypothyroidism and in those with cirrhosis.

Corticosteroids should be used cautiously in patients with ocular herpes simplex because of possible corneal perforation.

*Children:* Corticosteroids cause growth retardation in infancy, childhood and adolescence, which may be irreversible. Treatment should be limited to the minimum dosage for the shortest possible time. In order to minimise suppression of the hypothalamo-pituitary-adrenal axis and growth retardation, treatment should be limited, where possible, to a single dose on alternate days.

Growth and development of infants and children on prolonged corticosteroid therapy should be carefully monitored.

*Use in pregnancy:* There is inadequate evidence of safety in human pregnancy and there may be a very small risk of cleft palate and intra-uterine growth retardation in the fetus; there is evidence of harmful effects on pregnancy in animals. Infants born of mothers who have received substantial doses of corticosteroids during pregnancy should be carefully observed for signs of hypoadrenalism.

Corticosteroids appear in breast milk and could suppress growth, interfere with endogenous corticosteroid production, or cause other untoward effects. Mothers taking pharmacological doses of corticosteroids should be advised not to breast-feed.

*Drug interactions:* Aspirin should be used cautiously in conjunction with corticosteroids in hypoprothrombinaemia.

As phenytoin, barbiturates, ephedrine, rifabutin, carbamazepine, rifampicin, and aminoglutethimide may enhance the metabolic clearance of corticosteroids, resulting in decreased blood levels and reduced physiological activity, the dosage may have to be adjusted. These interactions may interfere with dexamethasone suppression tests, which should be interpreted with caution during administration of these drugs.

False-negative results in the dexamethasone suppression test in patients being treated with indomethacin have been reported.

The efficacy of coumarin anticoagulants may be changed by concurrent corticosteroid treatment. The prothrombin time should be checked frequently in patients who are receiving corticosteroids and coumarin anticoagulants at the same time, in order to avoid spontaneous bleeding.

When corticosteroids are administered concomitantly with potassium-depleting diuretics, patients should be observed closely for development of hypokalaemia.

Corticosteroids may affect the nitrobluetetrazolium test for bacterial infection and produce false-negative results.

*Side-effects:* Although adverse reactions associated with short-term corticosteroid therapy in high doses are uncommon, peptic ulceration may occur. Some patients have reported transitory burning or tingling sensations, often in the perineal area, when intravenous injections of large doses of dexamethasone sodium phosphate were given. The usual aseptic techniques governing injections should be observed.

The following side-effects reported with Decadron Injection should be regarded as potential side effects for any dexamethasone preparation.

*Fluid and electrolyte disturbances:* Sodium retention, fluid retention, congestive heart failure in susceptible patients, potassium loss, hypokalaemic alkalosis, hypertension, increased calcium excretion (see 'Precautions').

*Musculoskeletal:* Muscle weakness, steroid myopathy, loss of muscle mass, osteoporosis (especially in post-menopausal females), vertebral compression fractures, aseptic necrosis of femoral and humeral heads, pathological fracture of long bones, tendon rupture, and post-injection flare (following intra-articular use).

*Gastro-intestinal:* Peptic ulcer with possible perforation and haemorrhage, perforation of the small and large bowel, particularly in patients with inflammatory bowel disease, pancreatitis, abdominal distension, ulcerative oesophagitis, dyspepsia, oesophageal candidiasis.

*Dermatological:* Impaired wound healing, thin fragile skin, petechiae and ecchymoses, erythema, striae, telangiectasia, acne, increased sweating, possible suppression of skin tests, burning or tingling especially in the perineal area (after intravenous injection), other cutaneous reactions such as allergic dermatitis, urticaria, angioneurotic oedema, and hypo- or hyperpigmentation.

*Neurological:* Convulsions, increased intracranial pressure with papilloedema (pseudotumour cerebri) usually after treatment, vertigo, headache, psychic disturbances (e.g. euphoria, psychological dependence, depression, insomnia).

*Endocrine:* Menstrual irregularities, amenorrhoea, development of Cushingoid state, suppression of growth in children and adolescents, secondary adrenocortical and pituitary unresponsiveness (particularly in times of stress, as in trauma, surgery or illness), decreased carbohydrate tolerance, manifestations of latent diabetes mellitus, increased requirements for insulin or oral hypoglycaemic agents in diabetes, hirsutism.

*Anti-inflammatory and immunosuppressive effects:* Increased susceptibility and severity of infections with suppression of clinical symptoms and signs. Opportunistic infections, recurrence of dormant tuberculosis (see 'Precautions').

*Ophthalmic:* Posterior subcapsular cataracts, increased intra-ocular pressure, papilloedema, corneal or scleral thinning, exacerbation of ophthalmic viral disease, glaucoma, exophthalmos, rare instances of blindness associated with intra-lesional therapy around the face and head, retinopathy of prematurity.

*Metabolic:* Negative nitrogen balance due to protein catabolism. Negative calcium balance.

*Cardiovascular:* Myocardial rupture following recent myocardial infarction (see 'Precautions'). Hypertrophic cardiomyopathy in low birth-weight infants.

*Other:* Hypersensitivity, including anaphylaxis has been reported, leucocytosis, thrombo-embolism, weight gain, increased appetite, nausea, malaise, hiccups, and sterile abscess.

*Overdosage:* Reports of acute toxicity and/or deaths following overdosage with glucocorticoids are rare. No antidote is available. Treatment is probably not indicated for reactions due to chronic poisoning unless the patient has a condition that would render a patient unusually susceptible to ill effects from corticosteroids. In this case, symptomatic treatment should be instituted as necessary.

Anaphylactic and hypersensitivity reactions may be treated with adrenaline, positive-pressure artificial respiration and aminophylline. The patient should be kept warm and quiet.

The biological half-life of dexamethasone in plasma is about 190 minutes.

**Pharmaceutical precautions**    Injection Decadron Shock-Pak is sensitive to heat, and should not be autoclaved to sterilise the outside of the vial. It should be stored in a cool place and protected from freezing.

Only sodium chloride injection or dextrose injection should be used as diluents for infusion. Any infusion mixture must be used within 24 hours.

**Legal category**   POM.

**Package quantities**   Vials of 5 ml.

**Further information**    Injection Decadron Shock-Pak is a special dosage form of dexamethasone sodium phosphate designed exclusively for intravenous use as adjunctive therapy in the treatment of severe shock. For other indications requiring an injectable steroid, Decadron Injection, a formulation containing, per millilitre, dexamethasone sodium phosphate equivalent to 4 mg dexamethasone phosphate (approximately 3.33 mg dexamethasone), is available.

**Product licence number**   0025/0077.

# DECADRON* TABLETS

**Presentation**   White, half-scored tablets, marked 'MSD 41', containing 500 micrograms Dexamethasone BP.

**Uses**   Corticosteroid.

For use in certain endocrine and non-endocrine disorders, in certain cases of cerebral oedema, and for diagnostic testing of adrenocortical hyperfunction.

*Endocrine disorders:* Primary or secondary adrenocortical insufficiency (the first choice is hydrocortisone or cortisone, but synthetic analogues may be used with mineralocorticoids where applicable; in infancy, mineralocorticoid supplementation is particularly important), congenital adrenal hyperplasia.

*Non-endocrine disorders:* Dexamethasone may be used in the treatment of non-endocrine corticosteroid responsive conditions including:

*Allergy and anaphylaxis:* Angioneurotic oedema, anaphylaxis.

*Arteritis collagenosis:* Polymyalgia rheumatica, polyarteritis nodosa.

*Blood disorders:* Haemolytic anaemia, leukaemia, myeloma.

*Cardiovascular disorders:* Post-myocardial infarction syndrome.

*Gastro-intestinal:* Crohn's disease, ulcerative colitis.

*Hypercalcaemia:* Sarcoidosis.

*Infections (with appropriate chemotherapy):* Miliary tuberculosis.

*Muscular disorders:* Polymyositis.

*Neurological disorders:* Raised intra-cranial pressure secondary to cerebral tumours.

*Ocular disorders:* Anterior and posterior uveitis, optic neuritis.

*Renal disorders:* Lupus nephritis.

*Respiratory disease:* Bronchial asthma, aspiration pneumonitis.

*Rheumatic disorders:* Rheumatoid arthritis.

*Skin disorders:* Pemphigus vulgaris.

**Dosage and administration**   *General considerations:* Dosage must be individualised on the basis of the disease and the response of the patient. In order to minimise side-effects, the lowest possible dosage adequate to control the disease process should be used (see 'Side-effects').

The initial dosage varies from 0.5–9 mg a day depending on the disease being treated. In more severe diseases, doses higher than 9 mg may be required. The initial dosage should be maintained or adjusted until the patient's response is satisfactory. Both the dose in the evening, which is useful in alleviating morning stiffness, and the divided dosage regimen are associated with greater suppression of the hypothalamo-pituitary-adrenal axis. If satisfactory clinical response does not occur after a reasonable period of time, discontinue Decadron Tablets and transfer the patient to other therapy.

After a favourable initial response, the proper maintenance dosage should be determined by decreasing the initial dosage in small amounts to the lowest dosage that maintains an adequate clinical response. Chronic dosage should preferably not exceed 1.5 mg dexamethasone daily.

Patients should be monitored for signs that might require dosage adjustment, including changes in clinical status resulting from remissions or exacerbations of the disease, individual drug responsiveness, and the effect of stress (e.g. surgery, infection, trauma). During stress it may be necessary to increase dosage temporarily.

If the drug is to be stopped after more than a few days of treatment, it should be withdrawn gradually.

The following equivalents facilitate changing to Decadron from other glucocorticoids.

Milligram for milligram, dexamethasone is approximately equivalent to betamethasone, 4 to 6 times more potent than methylprednisolone and triamcinolone, 6 to 8 times more potent than prednisone and prednisolone, 25 to 30 times more potent than hydrocortisone, and about 35 times more potent than cortisone.

*In acute, self-limiting allergic disorders or acute exacerbations of chronic allergic disorders,* the following dosage schedule combining parenteral and oral therapy is suggested.

| | |
|---|---|
| First day | Decadron Injection, 4 mg or 8 mg (1 ml or 2 ml) intramuscularly |
| Second day | Two 500 microgram Decadron Tablets twice a day |
| Third day | Two 500 microgram Decadron Tablets twice a day |
| Fourth day | One 500 microgram Decadron Tablet twice a day |
| Fifth day | One 500 microgram Decadron Tablet twice a day |
| Sixth day | One 500 microgram Decadron Tablet |
| Seventh day | One 500 microgram Decadron Tablet |
| Eighth day | Reassessment day |

This schedule is designed to ensure adequate therapy during acute episodes while minimising the risk of overdosage in chronic cases.

*Dexamethasone suppression tests:*

1. *Tests for Cushing's syndrome:* Two milligrams of Decadron is given orally at 11 p.m., then blood is drawn for plasma cortisol determination at 8 a.m. the following morning.

For greater accuracy, 500 microgram Decadron is given orally every 6 hours for 48 hours. Plasma cortisol is measured at 8 a.m. on the third morning. Twenty-four-hour urine collections are made for determination of 17-hydroxycorticosteroid excretion.

2. *Test to distinguish Cushing's syndrome caused by pituitary ACTH excess from the syndrome induced by other causes:* Two milligrams of Decadron is given orally every 6 hours for 48 hours. Plasma cortisol is measured at 8 a.m. on the morning following the last dose. Twenty-four-hour urine collections are made for determination of 17-hydroxycorticosteroid excretion.

*Use in children:* Dosage should be limited to a single dose on alternate days to lessen retardation of growth and minimise suppression of hypothalamo-pituitary-adrenal axis.

*Use in the elderly:* Treatment of elderly patients, particularly if long term, should be planned bearing in mind the more serious consequences of the common side effects of corticosteroids in old age, especially osteoporosis, diabetes, hypertension, hypokalaemia, susceptibility to infection and thinning of the skin. Close clinical supervision is required to avoid life-threatening reactions (see 'Side-effects').

**Contra-indications, warnings, etc**
*Contra-indications:* Systemic fungal infections; systemic infection unless specific anti-infective therapy is employed; hypersensitivity to any component of the drug. Administration of live virus vaccines (see 'Precautions').

*Precautions:* Undesirable effects may be minimised by using the lowest effective dose for the minimum period and when appropriate by administering the daily requirement as a single morning dose or whenever possible as a single morning dose on alternative days. Frequent patient review is required to appropriately titrate the dose against disease activity. When reduction in dosage is possible, the reduction should be gradual (see 'Dosage and administration').

Corticosteroids may exacerbate systemic fungal infections and should not be used unless they are needed to control drug reactions due to amphotericin.

Moreover, there have been cases reported in which concomitant use of amphotericin and hydrocortisone was followed by cardiac enlargement and heart failure.

Reports in the literature suggest an apparent association between use of corticosteroids and left ventricular free wall rupture after a recent myocardial infarction; therefore corticosteroids should be used with great caution in these patients.

A report shows that the use of corticosteroids in cerebral malaria is associated with a prolonged coma and an increased incidence of pneumonia and gastrointestinal bleeding.

Average and large doses of hydrocortisone or cortisone can cause elevation of blood pressure, retention of salt and water, and increased excretion of potassium, but these effects are less likely to occur with synthetic derivatives, except when used in large doses. Dietary salt restriction and potassium supplementation may be necessary. All corticosteroids increase calcium excretion.

In patients on corticosteroid therapy subjected to unusual stress, e.g. intercurrent illness, trauma, or surgical procedure, dosage should be increased before, during and after the stressful situation. Drug-induced secondary adrenocortical insufficiency may result from too rapid withdrawal of corticosteroids and may be minimised by gradual dosage reduction, being tapered off over weeks and/or months depending on the dose and duration of treatment, but may persist for up to a year after discontinuation of therapy. In any stressful situation during that period, therefore, corticosteroid therapy should be reinstated. If the patient is already receiving corticosteroids, the current dosage may have to be temporarily increased. Salt and/or a mineralocorticoid should be given concurrently, since mineralocorticoid secretion may be impaired.

Stopping corticosteroids after prolonged therapy may cause withdrawal symptoms including fever, myalgia, arthralgia, and malaise. This may occur in patients even without evidence of adrenal insufficiency.

**Patients should carry 'steroid treatment' cards, which give clear guidance on the precautions to be taken to minimise risk, and which provide details of prescriber, drug, dosage and the duration of treatment.**

Administration of live virus vaccines is contra-indicated in individuals receiving immunosuppressive doses of corticosteroids. If inactivated viral or bacterial vaccines are administered to individuals receiving immunosuppressive doses of corticosteroids, the expected serum antibody response may not be obtained. However, immunisation procedures may be undertaken in patients who are receiving corticosteroids as replacement therapy, e.g. for Addison's disease.

The use of Decadron Tablets in active tuberculosis should be restricted to those cases of fulminating or disseminated tuberculosis in which the corticosteroid is used for the management of the disease in conjunction with an appropriate antituberculous regimen. If corticosteroids are indicated in patients with latent tuberculosis or tuberculin reactivity, close observation of the disease is necessary as reactivation may occur. During prolonged corticosteroid therapy, these patients should receive prophylactic chemotherapy.

There is an enhanced effect of corticosteroids in patients with hypothyroidism and in those with cirrhosis.

Corticosteroids may mask some signs of infection, and new infections may appear during their use. Suppression of the inflammatory response and immune function increases the susceptibility to infections and their severity. The clinical presentation may often be atypical, and serious infections such as septicaemia and tuberculosis may be masked and reach an advanced stage before being recognised. There may be decreased resistance and inability to localise infection in patients on corticosteroids.

**Chickenpox is of particular concern, since this normally minor illness may be fatal in immunosuppressed patients.** Patients (or parents of children) without a definite history of chickenpox should be advised to avoid close personal contact with chickenpox or herpes zoster, and if exposed they should seek urgent medical attention. Passive immunisation with varicella/zoster immunoglobulin (VZIG) is needed by exposed non-immune patients who are receiving systemic corticosteroids or who have used them within the previous three months; this should be given within ten days of exposure to chickenpox. **If a diagnosis of chickenpox is confirmed, the illness warrants specialist care and urgent treatment. Corticosteroids should not be stopped and the dose may need to be increased.**

Measles can have a more serious or even fatal course in immunosuppressed patients. In such children or adults particular care should be taken to avoid exposure to measles. If exposed, prophylaxis with intramuscular pooled immunoglobulin (IG) may be indicated. Exposed patients should be advised to seek medical advice without delay.

Corticosteroids may activate latent amoebiasis or strongyloidiasis or exacerbate active disease. Therefore, it is recommended that latent or active amoebiasis and strongyloidiasis be ruled out before initiating corticosteroid therapy in any patient at risk of or with symptoms suggestive of either condition.

Prolonged use of corticosteroids may produce subcapsular cataracts, glaucoma with possible damage to the optic nerves, and may enhance the establishment of secondary ocular infections due to fungi or viruses. Steroids may increase or decrease the motility and number of spermatozoa.

*Special precautions:* Particular care is required when considering the use of systemic corticosteroids in patients with the following conditions, and frequent patient monitoring is necessary: renal insufficiency, hypertension, diabetes or in those with a family history of diabetes, congestive heart failure, osteoporosis, previous steroid myopathy, glaucoma (or family history of glaucoma), myasthenia gravis, non-specific ulcerative colitis, diverticulitis, fresh intestinal anastomosis, active or latent peptic ulcer, existing or previous history of severe effective disorders (especially previous steroid psychosis), liver failure, and epilepsy. Signs of peritoneal irritation following gastro-intestinal perforation in patients receiving large doses of corticosteroids may be minimal or absent. Fat embolism has been reported as a possible complication of hypercortisonism.

Corticosteroids should be used cautiously in patients with ocular herpes simplex, because of possible corneal perforation.

*Children:* Corticosteroids cause growth retardation in infancy, childhood and adolescence which may be irreversible. Treatment should be limited to the minimum dosage for the shortest possible time. In order to minimise suppression of the hypothalamo-pituitary-adrenal axis and growth retardation, treatment should be limited, where possible, to a single dose on alternate days.

Growth and development of infants and children on prolonged corticosteroid therapy should be carefully monitored.

*Use in pregnancy and lactation:* There is inadequate evidence of safety in human pregnancy and there may be a very small risk of cleft palate and intra-uterine growth retardation in the fetus; there is evidence of harmful effects on pregnancy in animals. Infants born of mothers who have received substantial doses of corticosteroids during pregnancy should be carefully observed for signs of hypoadrenalism.

When corticosteroids are essential however, patients with normal pregnancies may be treated as though they were in the non-gravid state. Patients with pre-eclampsia or fluid retention require close monitoring.

Corticosteroids appear in breast milk and could suppress growth, interfere with endogenous corticosteroid production, or cause other unwanted effects. Mothers taking pharmacological doses of corticosteroids should be advised not to breastfeed.

*Drug interactions:* Aspirin should be used cautiously in conjunction with corticosteroids in hypoprothrombinaemia.

The renal clearance of salicylates is increased by corticosteroids and, therefore, salicylate dosage should be reduced along with steroid withdrawal.

As phenytoin, barbiturates, ephedrine, rifabutin, carbamazepine, rifampicin and aminoglutethimide may enhance the metabolic clearance of corticosteroids, resulting in decreased blood levels and reduced physiological activity, the dosage of Decadron may have to be adjusted. These interactions may interfere with dexamethasone suppression tests which should be interpreted with caution during administration of these drugs.

False-negative results in the dexamethasone suppression test in patients being treated with indomethacin have been reported.

The efficacy of coumarin anticoagulants may be changed by concurrent corticosteroid treatment. The prothrombin time should be checked frequently in patients who are receiving corticosteroids and coumarin anticoagulants at the same time, in order to avoid spontaneous bleeding.

The desired effects of hypoglycaemic agents (including insulin) are antagonised by corticosteroids.

When corticosteroids are administered concomitantly with potassium-depleting diuretics, patients should be observed closely for development of hypokalaemia.

Corticosteroids may affect the nitrobuletetrazolium test for bacterial infection and produce false-negative results.

*Side-effects:* The incidence of predictable undesirable effects, including hypothalamic-pituitary-adrenal suppression, correlates with the relative potency of the drug, dosage, timing of administration and the duration of treatment (see *Precautions*).

*Fluid and electrolyte disturbances:* Sodium retention, fluid retention, congestive heart failure in susceptible patients, potassium loss, hypokalaemic alkalosis, hypertension, increased calcium excretion (see 'Precautions').

*Musculoskeletal effects:* Muscle weakness, steroid myopathy, loss of muscle mass, osteoporosis (especially in post-menopausal females), vertebral compression fractures, aseptic necrosis of femoral and humeral heads, pathological fracture of long bones, tendon rupture.

*Gastro-intestinal:* Peptic ulcer with possible perforation and haemorrhage, perforation of the small and large bowel particularly in patients with inflammatory bowel disease, pancreatitis, abdominal distension, ulcerative oesophagitis, dyspepsia, oesophageal candidiasis.

*Dermatological:* Impaired wound healing, thin fragile skin, petechiae and ecchymoses, erythema, striae, telangiectasia, acne, increased sweating, suppressed reaction to skin tests, other cutaneous reactions such as allergic dermatitis, urticaria, angioneurotic oedema.

*Neurological:* Convulsions, vertigo, headache. Increased intracranial pressure with papilloedema (pseudotumour cerebri) may occur usually after treatment. Psychic disturbances, (e.g. euphoria, psychological dependence, depression, insomnia).

*Endocrine:* Menstrual irregularities, amenorrhoea, development of Cushingoid state, suppression of growth in children and adolescents, secondary adrenocortical and pituitary unresponsiveness (particularly in times of stress as in trauma, surgery or illness), decreased carbohydrate tolerance, manifestations of latent diabetes mellitus, increased requirements for insulin or oral hypoglycaemic agents in diabetics, hirsutism.

*Anti-inflammatory and immunosuppressive effects:* Increased susceptibility and severity of infections with suppression of clinical symptoms and signs. Opportunistic infections, recurrence of dormant tuberculosis (see 'Precautions').

*Ophthalmic:* Posterior subcapsular cataracts, increased intra-ocular pressure, papilloedema, corneal or scleral thinning, exacerbation of ophthalmic viral disease, glaucoma, exophthalmos.

*Metabolic:* Negative nitrogen balance due to protein catabolism. Negative calcium balance.

*Cardiovascular:* Myocardial rupture following recent myocardial infarction (see *Precautions*).

*Other:* Hypersensitivity including anaphylaxis has been reported, leucocytosis, thrombo-embolism, weight gain, increased appetite, nausea, malaise, hiccups.

*Withdrawal symptoms and signs:* Too rapid a reduction of corticosteroid dosage following prolonged treatment can lead to acute adrenal insufficiency, hypotension, and death (see *Precautions*).

In some instances, withdrawal symptoms may simulate a clinical relapse of the disease for which the patient has been undergoing treatment.

*Overdosage:* Reports of acute toxicity and/or deaths following overdosage with glucocorticoids are rare. No antidote is available. Treatment is probably not indicated for reactions due to chronic poisoning unless the patient has a condition that would render him unusually susceptible to ill effects from corticosteroids. In this case, the stomach should be emptied and symptomatic treatment should be instituted as necessary.

Anaphylactic and hypersensitivity reactions may be treated with adrenaline, positive-pressure artificial respiration and aminophylline. The patient should be kept warm and quiet.

The biological half-life of dexamethasone in plasma is about 190 minutes.

**Pharmaceutical precautions** Keep container well closed; store in a cool place, protected from light.

**Legal category** POM.

**Package quantities** *0.5 mg:* Packs of 30 tablets.

**Further information** Decadron is a potent glucocorticoid with little mineralocorticoid activity. It has considerable anti-inflammatory properties, but its effect on electrolyte metabolism is slight, and thus, electrolyte imbalance is not normally a problem with Decadron. In low or average doses, Decadron does not usually cause elevation of blood pressure, salt and water retention, or excessive potassium excretion.

**Product licence number**
500 microgram tablet    0025/5046

## DEMSER*

**Presentation** Available as, two-tone blue, opaque capsules, marked 'MSD 690', and 'DEMSER', containing 250 mg metirosine.

**Uses** The treatment of phaeochromocytoma during: pre-operative preparation of patients for surgery; management of patients when surgery is contra-indicated; prolonged treatment of patients with phaeochromocytoma.

Demser is not recommended for the control of essential hypertension.

**Dosage and administration** *Adults and children over*

*12 years of age:* Initially, 1 capsule (250 mg) four times a day. This may be increased by 1 or 2 capsules (250 or 500 mg) daily to a maximum of 4 g daily in divided doses. When used pre-operatively, the optimum dosage should be given for at least five to seven days before surgery.

The optimum dosage range is usually between 8 and 12 capsules (2 to 3 g) a day, titrated by monitoring clinical symptoms and catecholamine excretion. In patients who are hypertensive, dosage should be adjusted to lower blood pressure and control symptoms; in patients whose blood pressure is normal, adjust dosage until the urinary excretion of catecholamines and/or vanillylmandelic acid is reduced by 50% or more.

It is recommended that an alpha-adrenergic blocking agent such as phenoxybenzamine be added if control with Demser is not adequate.

The use of Demser in children under twelve years of age has been limited, and a dosage recommendation cannot be made.

*Use in the elderly:* These dosage recommendations apply to all adults, including the elderly.

**Contra-indications, warnings, etc**
*Contra-indications:* Hypersensitivity.

*Warnings:* When Demser is used pre-operatively, especially in combination with alpha-adrenoceptor blocking agents, blood volume must be maintained during and after surgery to avoid hypotension and decreased perfusion of vital organs. During surgery, life-threatening arrhythmias may occur requiring treatment with a beta-blocker or lignocaine. Blood pressure and ECG should be monitored continuously throughout surgery.

Demser does not eliminate the danger of arrhythmias or hypertensive crises occurring during manipulation of the tumour and additional alpha-blockade may be necessary.

*Precautions:* Crystalluria and urolithiasis have occurred in dogs; and crystalluria has been seen in a few patients. To minimise the risk, fluid intake should be sufficient to maintain a urine volume of 2,000 ml or more daily. Urine should be examined routinely, and if metirosine crystals (needles or rods) are seen, fluid intake should be increased. If crystalluria persists, the dosage of Demser should be reduced or discontinued.

Caution should be observed in administering Demser to patients receiving phenothiazines or haloperidol because the extrapyramidal effects of these drugs can be expected to be potentiated by inhibition of catecholamine synthesis; this has been documented to date only for haloperidol.

No evidence of adverse effects on hepatic, haematological or other functions (except for a few instances of increased AST) has been seen during clinical trials. However, total experience in man is limited to approximately 300 patients, and few patients have been studied long-term. Therefore, suitable laboratory tests should be carried out periodically in patients on prolonged therapy, particularly those with impaired hepatic or renal function.

Demser may cause spurious increases in urinary catecholamine measurements.

*Breast-feeding mothers:* It is not known whether Demser is excreted in human milk. Mothers who need Demser should stop breast-feeding.

*Pregnancy:* Demser is not recommended for use in pregnant patients. Complete reproduction studies have not been performed in animals to determine whether Demser affects fertility in males or females, has teratogenic potential, or has other adverse effects on the fetus. There are no well-controlled studies of Demser in pregnant women. The use of Demser in pregnant women should be avoided, if possible, but may be appropriate when anticipated benefits outweigh the potential risks.

*Adverse reactions:* The most common adverse reaction to Demser is moderate to severe sedation, which has been observed in almost all patients. It occurs at both low and high dosages. Sedative effects begin within the first 24 hours of therapy, are maximal after two to three days, and tend to wane during the next few days. Sedation usually is not obvious after one week unless the dosage is increased, but at dosages greater than 2,000 mg/day some degree of sedation or fatigue may persist.

When receiving Demser, patients should be warned about engaging in activities requiring mental alertness and motor co-ordination, such as driving a motor vehicle or operating machinery. Demser may have additive effects with alcohol and other CNS depressants, e.g. hypnotics, sedatives, tranquillisers, anti-anxiety agents.

In most patients who experience sedation, temporary changes in sleep pattern occur following withdrawal of the drug. Changes consist of insomnia that may last for two or three days and feelings of increased alertness and ambition. Even patients who do not

experience sedation while on Demser may report symptoms of psychic stimulation when the drug is discontinued.

Extrapyramidal signs such as drooling, speech difficulty and tremor have been reported in approximately 10% of patients, occasionally with trismus and frank parkinsonism.

Anxiety, depression, hallucinations, disorientation and confusion have occurred but may disappear on reduction of the dosage.

Diarrhoea occurs in about 10% of patients, and may be severe. Infrequently, slight swelling of the breast, galactorrhoea, nasal stuffiness, decreased salivation, dry mouth, headache, nausea, vomiting, abdominal pain, and impotence or failure of ejaculation may occur. Crystalluria transient dysuria and haematuria have been seen in a few patients. Eosinophilia, increased AST levels, peripheral oedema, and hypersensitivity such as urticaria and pharyngeal oedema has been reported rarely.

*Overdosage:* Signs of metirosine overdosage include the CNS effects seen at therapeutic dosages such as fatigue, anxiety or agitated depression, neuromuscular effects, diarrhoea, and decreased salivation. At therapeutic levels, reduction of dose or cessation of treatment usually results in the disappearance of these symptoms.

Since there is little clinical experience, the treatment of overdosage has not been identified. There is no antidote.

Metirosine is well-absorbed from the gastro-intestinal tract. Maximal biochemical effect is usually seen within two or three days.

**Pharmaceutical precautions** Store in a cool place, protected from light.

**Legal category** POM.

**Package quantities** Bottles of 100.

**Further information** Nil.

**Product licence number** 0025/0132.

## DOLOBID*
## DOLOBID* 500

**Presentation** Peach-coloured, capsule-shaped, film-coated tablets, marked 'MSD 675', containing 250 mg Diflunisal BP; and orange-coloured, film-coated tablets, marked 'MSD 697', containing 500 mg Diflunisal BP.

**Uses** Dolobid is indicated for the relief of pain.

Dolobid is also indicated in the relief of pain and inflammation associated with osteoarthritis and rheumatoid arthritis.

Dolobid is also indicated in the relief of pain and associated symptoms of primary dysmenorrhoea.

**Dosage and administration** Tablets should be swallowed whole, not crushed or chewed.

It is prudent to start at the bottom end of the dose range. In certain cases, it will be necessary to start with a high initial dose as described in the dosage recommendations below.

*For relief of pain:* An initial dose of 1000 mg, followed by 500 mg every 12 hours, is recommended for most patients. Following the initial dose some patients may require 500 mg every eight hours. Maintenance doses higher than 1500 mg a day are not recommended.

*For osteoarthritis and rheumatoid arthritis:* The recommended dosage range is 500 mg to 1000 mg per day. Dolobid may be administered once or twice a day.

Dosage should be adjusted to the nature and intensity of the pain being treated.

*For dysmenorrhoea:* The recommended dosage is 1000 mg at the onset of cramps or bleeding, followed by 500 mg every 12 hours for as long as symptoms last, usually a maximum of five days.

*Use in children:* Dolobid is not recommended for children.

*Use in the elderly:* The dosage does not require modification for elderly patients.

**Contra-indications, warnings, etc**
*Contra-indications:* Hypersensitivity to any component of this product.

In patients who have previously experienced acute asthmatic attacks, urticaria, or rhinitis precipitated by aspirin or non-steroidal anti-inflammatory agents.

The drug should not be administered to patients with active gastro-intestinal bleeding.

NSAIDs including Dolobid should not be given to patients with active peptic ulceration.

Dolobid should not be given to pregnant women, since the safety for this use has not been established. Breast-feeding mothers should not take Dolobid, or should stop breast-feeding.

*Precautions:* Although Dolobid has less effect on platelet function and bleeding time than aspirin, it does inhibit platelet function at higher doses; patients who may be adversely affected should be carefully observed.

Because of reports of adverse eye findings with agents of this class, if eye complaints develop during treatment with Dolobid they should be fully examined.

Dolobid should be used with caution in patients having a history of gastro-intestinal haemorrhage or ulcers. Fatalities have occurred, rarely.

In patients with a history of peptic-ulcer disease and in the elderly, NSAIDS should be given only after other forms of treatment have been carefully considered.

Although there have been no known reports associated with the use of Dolobid to date, acetylsalicylic acid has been associated with Reye's syndrome. Because diflunisal is a compound related to salicylic acid, the possibility of an association with Reye's syndrome cannot be excluded.

As with other NSAIDs, Dolobid should be used with caution in patients with reduced renal blood flow since renal prostaglandins play a supportive role in the maintenance of renal perfusion.

The dosage of Dolobid may need to be reduced in patients with renal functional impairment since the major route of excretion is via the kidney. In patients with severe renal impairment, the drug should not be used.

In rats and dogs, high oral doses of diflunisal (50–200 mg/kg/day) as with aspirin, produced similar pathological changes (gastro-intestinal ulceration and renal papillary oedema). These dosages are approximately 3 to 12 times the maximum dosages recommended in man.

Peripheral oedema has been observed in some patients taking Dolobid. Therefore, as with other drugs in this class, Dolobid should be used with caution in patients with compromised cardiac function, hypertension, or other conditions predisposing to fluid retention.

A potentially life-threatening apparent hypersensitivity syndrome has been reported. This multisystem syndrome includes constitutional symptoms, (fever, chills), and cutaneous findings (see Dermatological under 'Side-effects'). It may also include involvement of major organs (changes in liver function), jaundice, leucopenia, thrombocytopenia, eosinophilia, disseminated intravascular coagulation, renal impairment (including renal failure); and less specific findings (adenitis, arthralgia, myalgia, arthritis, malaise, anorexia, disorientation).

*Laboratory tests:* AST (SGOT) and ALT (SGPT) levels rose significantly by three times the upper limit of normal in less than 1% of patients in controlled clinical trials of non-steroidal anti-inflammatory drugs.

A patient on Dolobid with signs or symptoms suggesting liver disease or in whom abnormal liver function tests have occurred should be evaluated for evidence of a more severe hepatic reaction. If abnormal liver tests persist or worsen, if signs or symptoms of liver disease develop or if systemic manifestations such as eosinophilia or rash occur, Dolobid should be discontinued.

*Drug interactions: Indomethacin:* The combined use of indomethacin and Dolobid has been associated with fatal gastro-intestinal haemorrhage. The combination should not be used. Co-administration of Dolobid with indomethacin increases the plasma level of indomethacin by about 30 to 35% with a concomitant decrease in renal clearance of indomethacin and its conjugate. *Aspirin:* Co-administration of aspirin causes approximately a 15% decrease in plasma levels of Dolobid. *Codeine:* Co-administration with Dolobid improves the analgesic efficacy of either drug taken alone. *Methotrexate:* Caution should be used if Dolobid is administered concomitantly with methotrexate. Non-steroidal anti-inflammatory drugs have been reported to decrease the tubular secretion of methotrexate and potentiate the toxicity. *Cyclosporin:* Administration of NSAIDs concomitantly with cyclosporin has been associated with an increase in cyclosporin-induced toxicity, possibly due to decreased synthesis of renal prostacyclin. NSAIDs should be used with caution in patients taking cyclosporin, and renal function should be monitored carefully. *Oral anticoagulant drugs:* The concomitant administration of Dolobid and warfarin or nicoumalone resulted in prolongation of prothrombin time in normal volunteers. This may occur because diflunisal competitively displaces coumarins from protein binding sites. Accordingly, prothrombin time should be monitored during, and for several days after, the concomitant drug administration of Dolobid and oral anticoagulants. The dosage of oral anticoagulants may require adjustment. *Tolbutamide:* No significant changes occurred in the plasma levels of tolbutamide or in the fasting blood sugar levels of diabetic patients who also took Dolobid. *Hydrochlorothiazide:* Co-administration increases the plasma levels of hydrochlorothiazide by 25 to 35% with a concomitant decrease in renal clearance of the diuretic. This change is not clinically important. Dolobid counteracts the hyperuricaemic effect of hydrochlorothiazide. *Frusemide:* Co-administration did not affect the diuretic activity of frusemide in normal volunteers, but its hyperuricaemic activity was decreased by Dolobid. *Antacids:* The clinical effect of occasional doses of antacid is insignificant, but this becomes significant when antacids are used continuously. Co-administration of aluminium hydroxide suspension significantly decreases the absorption of Dolobid by approximately 40%. *Paracetamol:* Co-administration significantly increased the plasma levels of paracetamol by 50%, but the plasma levels of Dolobid were unaffected. *Other non-steroidal, anti-inflammatory agents:* No clinical data on the safety and efficacy of concomitant administration are available. No recommendations can be made. However, normal volunteers given sulindac and Dolobid showed substantial but no statistically significant lower levels of the active sulphide metabolite of sulindac. Normal volunteers given naproxen and Dolobid showed no changes in plasma levels of either drug, but a significant decrease in urinary excretion of naproxen and its glucuronide metabolite. *Gold salts:* In clinical studies of patients with rheumatoid arthritis, Dolobid added to the regimen of gold salts usually resulted in additional symptomatic relief.

*Drug/laboratory test interactions:* Serum Salicylate Assays: caution should be used in interpreting the results of serum salicylate assays when diflunisal is present. Because of the cross-reactivity between the two compounds, salicylate levels have been found to be falsely elevated with some assay methods.

*Side effects: 3% to 9% incidence: Gastro-intestinal:* gastro-intestinal pain, dyspepsia, diarrhoea, nausea. *Dermatological:* rash. *Central nervous system:* headache.

*1% to 3% incidence: Gastro-intestinal:* vomiting, constipation, flatulence. *Central nervous system/Psychiatric:* dizziness, somnolence, insomnia. *Special senses:* tinnitus. *Miscellaneous:* fatigue.

*Less than 1% incidence: Gastro-intestinal:* peptic ulcer, gastro-intestinal perforation and bleeding, anorexia, jaundice, cholestasis, liver function abnormality, hepatitis, gastritis. *Dermatological:* pruritus, sweating, dry mucous membranes, stomatitis, photosensitivity, urticaria, erythema multiforme and Stevens-Johnson syndrome, toxic epidermal necrolysis, exfoliative dermatitis. *Genito-urinary:* dysuria, renal impairment including renal failure, interstitial nephritis, haematuria. *Central nervous system/Psychiatric:* vertigo, lightheadedness, paraesthesiae, nervousness, depression, hallucinations, confusion. *Haematological:* thrombocytopenia, agranulocytosis, haemolytic anaemia. *Special senses:* transient visual disturbances including blurred vision. *Miscellaneous:* asthenia, oedema. *Hypersensitivity reactions:* acute anaphylactic reaction with bronchospasm, angioedema, hypersensitivity vasculitis, hypersensitivity syndrome (see 'Precautions').

*Side-effects—causal relationship unknown:* Other reactions have been reported in clinical trials or since the drug was marketed, but occurred under circumstances where a causal relationship could not be established. However, in these rarely reported events, that possibility cannot be excluded. Therefore, the following observations are listed to serve as alerting information to physicians.

*Respiratory:* Dyspnoea. *Cardiovascular:* Palpitation, syncope. *Musculoskeletal:* Muscle cramps. *Miscellaneous:* Chest pain. *Genitourinary:* Nephrotic syndrome.

*Treatment of overdosage:*

Cases of overdosage have occurred and fatalities have been reported. The most common signs and symptoms observed with overdosage were drowsiness, vomiting, nausea, diarrhoea, hyperventilation, tachycardia, sweating, tinnitus, disorientation, stupor, and coma. Diminished urine output and cardiorespiratory arrest have also been reported. The lowest dose of Dolobid alone at which death was reported was 15 g; death has been reported from a mixed drug overdose that included 7.5 g Dolobid.

In the event of recent overdosage, the stomach should be emptied by inducing vomiting or gastric lavage, and the patient observed carefully and given symptomatic and supportive treatment.

To facilitate urinary elimination of the drug, attempt to maintain renal function. Because of the high degree of protein binding, haemodialysis is not recommended.

The initial plasma half-life following single oral doses of diflunisal seems to be dose dependent, ranging from approximately 7.5 hours for a 250 mg dose to 11 hours for a 500 mg dose.

**Pharmaceutical precautions** Store below 25°C, protected from light.

**Legal category** POM.

**Package quantities** Dolobid 250 mg tablets and Dolobid 500 mg tablets are supplied in packs of 60.

**Further information** Following a single therapeutic dose, significant relief of pain usually occurs within the first hour, reaches a maximum in 2–3 hours and lasts for up to 12 hours or more.

Dolobid has a dose-related effect on platelet function. In normal volunteers given Dolobid over eight days, 250 mg twice daily had no effect on platelet function and 500 mg twice daily affected platelet function only slightly. However, at 1,000 mg twice daily, which exceeds the maximum recommended dose, platelet function was inhibited. In contrast to aspirin, these effects were reversible.

Bleeding time was unaffected by 250 mg twice daily, slightly increased at 500 mg twice daily, and the greater increase at 1,000 mg twice daily was not statistically significant from placebo.

When Dolobid was given to normal volunteers at the usual recommended dose of 500 mg twice daily, faecal blood loss was significantly different from placebo. Dolobid at 1000 mg twice daily (Note: exceeds the recommended dosage) caused a statistically significant increase in faecal blood loss, but this increase was only one-half as large as that associated with aspirin 1300 mg twice daily.

**Product licence numbers**

250 mg tablet 0025/0128
500 mg tablet 0025/0146

## EDECRIN*

**Presentation** Injection, vials containing sodium ethacrynate equivalent to 50 mg ethacrynic acid, as a dry, lyophilised powder.

**Uses** Diuretic. Edecrin is indicated when urgent and potent diuresis is essential. It is particularly recommended in oedema associated with: Congestive heart failure; pulmonary oedema; renal oedema; hepatic cirrhosis with ascites; ascites due to malignancy; oedema due to other causes, including idiopathic oedema and lymphoedema.

**Dosage and administration** Dosage should be carefully regulated to prevent a more rapid or substantial diuresis than necessary. Daily weighing of the patient and, where possible, serum electrolyte determinations will greatly contribute to the success of treatment.

Edecrin Injection is intended for intravenous injection when oral treatment is impractical or when urgent diuresis is essential, as in acute pulmonary oedema.

*Usual adult intravenous dose:* 0.5–1 mg/kg of bodyweight. The dosage for an average-sized adult is 50 mg. Usually only one dose is necessary; however, if a second dose is required, it should be given at a new injection site to avoid thrombophlebitis.

Single intravenous doses of up to 100 mg have been used in critical situations.

The solution may be given slowly through the tubing of a running infusion, or by direct intravenous injection over several minutes.

Edecrin Injection should not be mixed with whole blood or blood derivatives. If it is desired to administer it at the same time as a blood transfusion, it should be given independently.

*Children:* As paediatric experience with Edecrin Injection is limited, it is not recommended for children.

*Use in the elderly:* The general considerations on adjustment of dosage to meet individual needs apply equally to elderly patients (see 'Precautions').

**Contra-indications, warnings, etc**

*Contra-indications:* Anuria, infants (under 2 years). For 'Use in pregnancy' and 'Use in breast-feeding mothers', see 'Precautions'. Hypersensitivity to this product.

*Precautions:* The effects of Edecrin on electrolytes are based on its renal pharmacology and are usually dose related.

To minimise the possibility of profound electrolyte and water loss, therapy should be initiated with a low dosage and this carefully adjusted as necessary; intermittent dosage should be used where possible and the patient weighed regularly throughout treatment. If diuresis is excessive, Edecrin should be withdrawn until homeostasis is restored.

Frequent serum electrolyte, alkali reserve and blood urea determinations should be made early in therapy, and periodically thereafter while active diuresis is taking place. Any electrolyte abnormality should be corrected or the drug temporarily withdrawn. If increasing electrolyte imbalance, azotaemia and/or oliguria occur during treatment of severe progressive renal disease, the diuretic should be discontinued.

Inclusion of potassium supplements or potassium-sparing agents is often advisable, especially during the treatment of cirrhotic or nephrotic patients and patients receiving digitalis.

Although treatment with Edecrin generally allows patients greater freedom with their salt intake, cirrhotic patients should usually have their salt moderately restricted while on therapy.

Edecrin should be given with caution to patients with advanced cirrhosis of the liver, particularly those with a history of episodes of electrolyte imbalance or hepatic encephalopathy. Edecrin may precipitate hepatic coma and death.

When metabolic alkalosis may be anticipated (e.g. in cirrhosis with ascites), a potassium-conserving agent or potassium chloride may mitigate or prevent hypokalaemia.

Loop diuretics may cause hypomagnesaemia.

Too vigorous a diuresis may induce an acute hypotensive episode. In elderly cardiac patients, severe diuresis may cause a rapid contraction of plasma volume, which should be avoided to prevent possible thrombo-embolic episodes.

Weakness, muscle cramps, paraesthesiae, thirst, anorexia, and signs of hyponatraemia, hypokalaemia and/or hypochloraemic alkalosis may follow vigorous or excessive diuresis or be accentuated by rigid salt restriction. Rarely, tetany has been reported following vigorous diuresis. Adequate salt intake and potassium chloride supplements are often necessary.

A few patients have had a sudden onset of profuse watery diarrhoea. If this occurs and other causes are eliminated, Edecrin should be discontinued and not re-administered.

Edecrin should be used cautiously in critically ill patients, particularly (1) those patients with severe myocardial disease who have been receiving digitalis; they may develop acute hypokalaemia with fatal arrhythmias. (2) Patients with severely decompensated hepatic cirrhosis with ascites (with or without accompanying encephalopathy) who are in electrolyte imbalance may undergo further deterioration of the electrolyte defect. A number of possible drug-related deaths have occurred among such patients.

Edecrin has little or no effect on glomerular filtration rate or renal blood flow, except immediately after a pronounced reduction in plasma volume following rapid diuresis. An increase in blood urea may occur, although transient it may usually be readily reversed by discontinuing Edecrin.

Edecrin may potentiate the effect of carbonic anhydrase inhibitors, increasing sodium and potassium excretion. If Edecrin is given to patients already receiving a carbonic anhydrase inhibitor, the initial dose and increments should be only 25 mg (½ tablet).

*Drug interactions*
*Antihypertensive agents* may require adjustment of dosage with concurrent use. Orthostatic hypotension may occur in patients on antihypertensive agents when given Edecrin.

*Antibiotics:* The concurrent use of such drugs as aminoglycosides with Edecrin should be avoided because of the risk of increasing their ototoxic potential.

*Warfarin:* Several drugs, including Edecrin, have been shown to displace warfarin from plasma protein. In patients receiving both types of drug, a reduction in the dosage of the anticoagulant may therefore be required.

*Lithium:* Lithium should generally not be given to patients receiving diuretics, since the risk of lithium toxicity is very high in such patients.

*Corticosteroids:* Edecrin may increase the risk of gastric haemorrhage associated with corticosteroid treatment.

*Use in pregnancy:* As clinical experience is limited, Edecrin is not recommended in pregnant patients. The routine use of diuretics in otherwise healthy pregnant women with or without mild oedema is not indicated because they may be associated with hypovolaemia, increased blood viscosity and decreased placental perfusion. If administration in confirmed or suspected pregnancy is considered, the benefits of therapy should be weighed against the possible hazard to the fetus.

*Use in breast-feeding mothers:* Edecrin is contraindicated in breast-feeding mothers. If its use is deemed essential, the patient should stop breast-feeding.

*Side-effects*
*Gastro-intestinal:* Anorexia, malaise, abdominal discomfort or pain, dysphagia, nausea, vomiting and diarrhoea. A few patients have had profuse, watery diarrhoea, gastro-intestinal bleeding, and acute pancreatitis.

*Metabolic:* Reversible hyperuricaemia, decreased urinary urate excretion and hyperglycaemia may occur. Acute gout may be precipitated. Rarely, acute symptomatic hypoglycaemia with convulsions, jaundice and abnormal liver-function tests have been reported.

*Haematological:* Agranulocytosis, severe neutropenia, thrombocytopenia and Henoch-Schönlein purpura have been reported rarely.

*Special senses:* Deafness, tinnitus and vertigo with a sense of fullness in the ears, and blurred vision have occurred.

*Central nervous system:* Fatigue, apprehension and confusion.

*Other:* Skin rash, headache, fever, rigors, and haematuria. Edecrin Injection has occasionally caused local irritation and pain due to extravasation of injected fluid.

*Overdosage:* Treatment should be symptomatic and supportive; no specific antidote is available. Dehydration, electrolyte imbalance, hepatic coma and hypotension should be corrected by standard methods. If respiration is impaired, oxygen or artificial respiration should be given.

**Pharmaceutical precautions**   Injection: to reconstitute the lyophilised material, add 50 ml of 5% dextrose injection or of isotonic saline to the vial. (Some 5% dextrose injection solutions have a pH below 5. If such a preparation is used as diluent, the resulting solution may be cloudy. The use of such a solution is not recommended.) After reconstitution, can be stored up to 24 hours at 2–8°C.

**Legal category**   POM.

**Package quantities**   Vials containing sodium ethacrynate equivalent to 50 mg ethacrynic acid.

**Further information**   Nil.

**Product licence number**   0025/5007

## FOSAMAX*   ▼

**Qualitative and quantitative composition**   Each tablet of Fosamax contains 13.05 mg of alendronate sodium, which is the molar equivalent to 10 mg of alendronic acid.

**Pharmaceutical form**   Fosamax is supplied as round white tablets, with convex faces, marked with an embossed bone symbol and Fosamax on one side, and an embossed bone symbol and 'MSD 936' on the other.

**Clinical particulars**
*Therapeutic indications:* Fosamax is indicated for the treatment of osteoporosis in post-menopausal women.

*Posology and method of administration:* The recommended dosage is 10 mg once a day.

*To permit adequate absorption of Fosamax:* Fosamax must be taken at least 30 minutes before the first food, beverage, or medication of the day with plain water only. Other beverages (including mineral water), food and some medications are likely to reduce the absorption of Fosamax (see 'Interaction with other medicaments and other forms of interaction').

*To facilitate delivery to the stomach and thus reduce the potential for local and oesophageal irritation/adverse experiences* (see 'Special warnings and special precautions for use'): Fosamax should only be swallowed upon rising for the day with a full glass of water (not less than 200 ml or 7 fl. oz.).

Patients should not chew or suck the tablets.

Patients should not lie down for at least 30 minutes after taking Fosamax.

Patients should not lie down until after their first food of the day, which should be at least 30 minutes after taking the tablet.

Fosamax should not be taken at bedtime or before rising for the day.

All patients with osteoporosis should have adequate dietary calcium (see 'Special warnings and special precautions for use').

*Use in the elderly:* In clinical studies there was no age-related difference in the efficacy or safety profiles of Fosamax. Therefore no dosage adjustment is necessary for the elderly.

*Use in renal impairment:* No dosage adjustment is necessary for patients with mild renal impairment where GFR is greater than 35 ml/min. Fosamax is not recommended for patients with mild renal impairment where GFR is 20–35 ml/min, or for patients with moderate to severe renal impairment (GFR <20 ml/min).

*Use in children:* Fosamax has not been studied in children and should not be given to them.

*Contra-indications:* Abnormalities of the oesophagus and other factors which delay oesophageal emptying, such as stricture or achalasia.

Inability to stand or sit upright for at least 30 minutes.

Hypersensitivity to any component of this product.

Hypocalcaemia (see 'Special warnings and special precautions for use').

*Special warnings and special precautions for use:* Fosamax can cause local irritation of the upper gastro-intestinal mucosa. Because there is a potential for worsening of the underlying disease, caution should be used when Fosamax is given to patients with active

upper gastro-intestinal problems, such as dysphagia, oesophageal disease, gastritis, duodenitis, or ulcers (see 'Contra-indications').

Oesophageal reactions (sometimes severe and requiring hospitalisation), such as oesophagitis, oesophageal ulcers and oesophageal erosions, have been reported in patients receiving Fosamax. Physicians should therefore be alert to any signs or symptoms signalling a possible oesophageal reaction, and patients should be instructed to discontinue Fosamax and seek medical attention if they develop symptoms of oesophageal irritation such as dysphagia, pain on swallowing, retrosternal pain, or new or worsening heartburn.

In order to reduce potential for oesophageal adverse reactions, and to facilitate delivery to the stomach, patients should be instructed to swallow Fosamax with a full glass of water and not lie down for at least 30 minutes and until after their first food of the day (see 'Posology and method of administration'). Patients should be specifically instructed not to take the tablets at bedtime or before rising for the day. Patients should not chew or suck the tablets because of a potential for oropharyngeal ulceration.

While no increased risk was observed in extensive clinical trials, there have been rare (post-marketing) reports of gastric and duodenal ulcers, some severe and with complications. However, a causal relationship has not been established.

Fosamax is not recommended for patients with mild renal impairment where GFR is 20–35 ml/min, or for patients with moderate to severe renal impairment (see 'Posology and method of administration').

*Interaction with other medicaments and other forms of interaction:* If taken at the same time, it is likely that calcium supplements, antacids, and some oral medications will interfere with absorption of Fosamax. Therefore, patients must wait at least 30 minutes after taking Fosamax before taking any other oral medication.

No other drug interations of clinical significance are anticipated. A small number of patients in the clinical trials received oestrogen (intravaginal, transdermal, or oral) while taking Fosamax. No adverse experiences attributable to their concomitant use were identified.

Although specific interaction studies were not performed, Fosamax was used concomitantly in postmenopausal osteoporosis studies with a wide range of commonly prescribed drugs without evidence of clinical adverse interactions. However, the incidence of upper gastro-intestinal adverse events associated with non-steroidal anti-inflammatory drugs and aspirin appears to be greater with concomitant administration of Fosamax.

*Pregnancy and lactation*
*Use during pregnancy:* Fosamax has not been studied in pregnant women and should not be given to them.

In developmental toxicity studies in animals, there were no adverse effects at doses up to 25 mg/kg/day in rats and 35 mg/kg/day in rabbits.

*Use during lactation:* Fosamax has not been studied in breast-feeding women and should not be given to them.

*Effects on ability to drive and use machines:* There are no data to suggest that Fosamax affects the ability to drive or use machines.

*Undesirable effects:*
*Clinical studies:* Side-effects, which usually were mild, generally did not require discontinuation of therapy.

In two large, three-year studies of virtually identical design, with a total of 994 post-menopausal women (Fosamax: N=597, placebo: N=397) the overall safety profiles of Fosamax 10 mg/day and placebo were similar. Adverse experiences reported by the investigators as possibly, probably or definitely drug related in ≥1% of patients treated with 'Fosamax' 10 mg/day and at a greater incidence than in patients given placebo are presented in the following table:

| | FOSAMAX 10 mg/day (n=196) | Placebo (n=397) |
|---|---|---|
| | % | % |
| *Gastro-intestinal* | | |
| abdominal pain | 6.6 | 4.8 |
| dyspepsia | 3.6 | 3.5 |
| constipation | 3.1 | 1.8 |
| diarrhoea | 3.1 | 1.8 |
| flatulence | 2.6 | 0.5 |
| oesophageal ulcer | 1.5 | 0.0 |
| dysphagia | 1.0 | 0.0 |
| abdominal distension | 1.0 | 0.8 |
| *Musculoskeletal* | | |
| musculoskeletal (bone, muscle or joint) pain | 4.1 | 2.5 |
| *Neurological* | | |
| headache | 2.6 | 1.5 |

Rarely, rash and erythema have occurred.

*Post-marketing experience:* In addition to the adverse experiences reported during clinical studies and listed above under *Clinical studies,* the following adverse experiences have been reported during post-marketing use.

*Uncommon (>0.1% and <1%) – Gastro-intestinal:* nausea, vomiting, oesophagitis, oesophageal erosions, and as previously noted in clinical trials, oesophageal ulcers (see *Special warnings and special precautions for use* and *Posology and method of administration*).

*Rare (≥0.01% and <0.1%) – Body as a whole:* hypersensitivity reactions including urticaria and rarely angioedema. *Gastro-intestinal:* oropharyngeal ulceration; gastric or duodenal ulcers, some severe and with complications although a causal relationship has not been established (see *Special warnings and special precautions for use* and *Posology and method of administration*).

*Laboratory test findings:* In clinical studies, asymptomatic, mild and transient decreases in serum calcium and phosphate were observed in approximately 18% and 10%, respectively, of patients taking Fosamax versus approximately 12% and 3% of those taking placebo. However, the incidences of decreases in serum calcium to <2.0 mmol/l and serum phosphate to ≤0.65 mmol/l were similar in both treatment groups.

*Overdose:* Significant lethality after single oral doses was seen in female rats and mice at 552 mg/kg (3256 mg/m²) and 966 mg/kg (2898 mg/m²) (equivalent to human oral doses* of 27,600 and 48,300 mg), respectively. In males, these values were slightly higher, 626 and 1280 mg/kg, respectively. There was no lethality in dogs at oral doses up to 200 mg/kg (4000 mg/m²) (equivalent to human oral dose* of 10,000 mg).

* Based on a patient weight of 50 kg.

No specific information is available on the treatment of overdosage with Fosamax. Hypocalcaemia, hypophosphataemia and upper gastro-intestinal adverse events, such as upset stomach, heartburn, oesophagitis, gastritis, or ulcer, may result from oral overdosage. Milk or antacids should be given to bind alendronate. Owing to the risk of oesophageal irritation, vomiting should not be induced and the patient should remain fully upright.

**Pharmacological properties**
*Pharmacodynamic properties:* Osteoporosis is characterised by low bone mass and a consequent increased risk of fracture, most commonly of the spine, hip, and wrist. It occurs in both males and females but is most common among women following the menopause, when bone turnover increases and the rate of bone resorption exceeds that of bone formation, leading to loss of bone mass.

Alendronate is an aminobisphosphonate. In animal studies, alendronate localises preferentially to sites of bone resorption, specifically under osteoclasts. The localisation under osteoclasts is about tenfold higher than under osteoblasts. Alendronate does not interfere with osteoclast recruitment or attachment, but it does inhibit osteoclast activity. Following exposure to alendronate, normal bone is formed that incorporates alendronate into its matrix where it is pharmacologically inactive. Therefore, alendronate must be continuously administered to suppress osteoclasts on newly formed resorption surfaces. Alendronate reduces bone resorption with no direct effect on bone formation and thus reduces the elevated rate of bone turnover in post-menopausal women to approximate more closely that in pre-menopausal women. However, because bone formation and resorption are coupled, bone formation is also reduced. Nevertheless, bone formation exceeds bone resorption, leading to progressive gains in bone mass.

Evidence from animal models confirms the selective nature of alendronate's activity. In growing rats, the doses causing inhibition of bone resorption were significantly lower than those leading to inhibition of mineralisation.

Daily oral doses of alendronate in post-menopausal women produced biochemical changes indicative of dose-dependent inhibition of bone resorption, including suppression of urinary calcium and urinary markers of bone collagen degradation (such as hydroxyproline, deoxypyridinoline, and cross-linked N-telopeptides of type I collagen). These biochemical changes returned towards baseline values as early as three weeks following the discontinuation of alendronate, despite the long retention of alendronate in the skeleton.

Alendronate 10 mg once daily reduced urinary excretion of a specific marker of bone collagen breakdown, deoxypyridinoline, by approximately 50%. The suppression of bone resorption, as indicated by this measurement, was evident by as early as one month, and at three months reached a plateau that in two-year studies was maintained for their duration. Other markers of bone turnover, such as serum osteocalcin and alkaline phosphatase, were also reduced, by approximately 50% and 25–30%, respectively, and reached a plateau after 6 to 12 months. These data indicate that the rate of bone turnover reached a new steady-state, despite the progressive increase in the total amount of alendronate deposited within bone.

The efficacy of Fosamax 10 mg once daily in post-menopausal women with osteoporosis was demonstrated in four clinical studies of two years' duration. In patients receiving Fosamax 10 mg/day, the mean increases in bone-mineral density (BMD) of the spine, femoral neck, and trochanter at two years for the pooled data from the virtually identically designed two largest studies were 7.7%, 4.3%, and 6.4%, respectively, relative to placebo.

These increases were highly significant relative both to baseline and placebo at each measurement site in each study. Total body BMD also increased significantly in both studies, suggesting that the increases in bone mass of the spine and hip did not occur at the expense of the other skeletal sites. Increases in BMD were evident as early as three months and continued throughout the entire two years of treatment with no evidence of a plateau. Fosamax is equally effective in older (≥65 years) and younger (≤65 years) patients.

Bone histology in 130 post-menopausal patients with osteoporosis treated with Fosamax at doses ranging from 1 to 20 mg/day for either one or two years revealed normal mineralisation and structure, as well as the expected decrease in bone turnover. These data, together with the normal bone histology and increased bone strength observed in ovariectomised rats and baboons exposed to long-term alendronate treatment, indicate that bone formed during therapy with Fosamax is of normal quality and should translate into increased bone strength and reduced risk of fracture. That such a risk reduction occurs is supported by the findings of a significant decrease in the rate of loss of height in osteoporotic women treated with Fosamax relative to placebo-treated controls.

*Pharmacokinetic properties*
*Absorption:* Relative to an intravenous (IV) reference dose, the oral bioavailability of alendronate was 0.7% for doses ranging from 5 to 40 mg when administered after an overnight fast and two hours before a standardised breakfast. Bioavailability was decreased similarly to an estimated 0.46% and 0.39% when alendronate was administered one hour or half an hour before a standardised breakfast. However, in the two largest controlled studies (see 'Pharmacodynamic properties') that demonstrated efficacy, Fosamax 10 mg/day was administered one hour before the first food or beverage of the day. Therefore, bioavailability and therapeutic response should be similar to that seen in the studies if Fosamax is taken as directed (see 'Posology and method of administration').

Bioavailability was negligible whether alendronate was administered with, or up to two hours after, a standardised breakfast. Concomitant administration of alendronate with coffee or orange juice reduced bioavailability by approximately 60%.

*Distribution:* Preclinical studies show that alendronate transiently distributes to soft tissues following administration but is then rapidly redistributed to bone or excreted in the urine. The mean steady-state volume of distribution, exclusive of bone, is at least 28 litres in humans. Concentrations of drug in plasma following therapeutic oral doses are too low for analytical detection (<5 ng/ml). Protein binding in human plasma is approximately 78%.

*Biotransformation:* There is no evidence that alendronate is metabolised in animals or humans.

*Elimination:* Following a single i.v. dose of [¹⁴C]alendronate, approximately 50% of the radioactivity was excreted in the urine within 72 hours and little or no radioactivity was recovered in the faeces. Following a single 10 mg i.v. dose, the renal clearance of alendronate was 71 ml/min, and systemic clearance did not exceed 200 ml/min. Plasma concentrations fell by more than 95% within 6 hours following i.v. administration. The terminal half-life in humans is estimated to exceed 10 years, reflecting release of alendronate from the skeleton. Alendronate is not excreted through the acidic or basic transport systems of the kidney in rats, and thus it is not anticipated to interfere with the excretion of other drugs by those systems in humans.

*Characteristics in patients:* Preclinical studies show that the drug that is not deposited in bone is rapidly excreted in the urine. No evidence of saturation of bone uptake was found after chronic dosing with cumulative i.v. doses up to 35 mg/kg in animals. Although no clinical information is available, it is likely that, as in animals, elimination of alendronate via the kidney will be reduced in patients with impaired renal function. Therefore, somewhat greater accumulation of alendronate in bone might be expected in patients with impaired renal function (see 'Posology and method of administration').

*Preclinical safety data:* In test animal species the main target organs for toxicity were kidneys and gastrointestinal tract. Renal toxicity was seen only at doses >2 mg/kg/day orally (ten times the recommended dose) and was evident only on histological examination as small widely scattered foci or nephritis, with no evidence of effect on renal function. The gastrointestinal toxicity, seen in rodents only, occurred at doses >2.5 mg/kg/day and appears to be due to a direct effect on the mucosa. There is no additional relevant information.

**Pharmaceutical particulars**
*List of excipients:* Microcrystalline Cellulose PhEur, Anhydrous Lactose USNF, Croscarmellose Sodium USNF, and Magnesium Stearate PhEur.

*Incompatibilities:* None known.

*Shelf life:* 24 months.

*Special precautions for storage:* Store at temperatures below 30°C.

*Nature and contents of container:* Blister packs of opaque PVC lidded with aluminium foil. Pack size: 28 tablets.

*Instructions for use/handling:* None.

**Marketing authorisation number** 0025/0326.

**Date of approval/revision of SPC** March 1997.

**Legal category** POM.

# HYDROCORTONE* TABLETS

**Presentation** White, quarter-scored tablets, marked 'MSD 619', containing 10 mg hydrocortisone. White, half-scored tablets, marked 'MSD 625', containing 20 mg hydrocortisone.

**Uses** Corticosteroid.

For use as replacement therapy in primary, secondary, or acute adrenocortical insufficiency.

Pre-operatively, and during serious trauma or illness in patients with known adrenal insufficiency or doubtful adrenocortical reserve.

**Dosage and administration** Dosage must be individualised according to the response of the individual patient. The lowest possible dosage should be used.

Patients should be observed closely for signs that might require dosage adjustment, including changes in clinical status resulting from remissions or exacerbations of the disease, individual drug responsiveness, and the effect of stress (e.g. surgery, infection, trauma). During stress it may be necessary to increase the dosage temporarily.

If the drug is to be stopped after more than a few days of treatment, it should be withdrawn gradually.

In chronic adrenocortical insufficiency, a dosage of 10–20 mg a day or occasionally more is recommended, together with 4–6 g of sodium chloride or 1–3 mg of deoxycorticosterone acetate. When immediate support is mandatory, one of the soluble adrenocortical hormone preparations (e.g. Decadron* Injection, dexamethasone sodium phosphate, MSD), which may be effective within minutes after parenteral administration, can be life-saving.

*Use in children:* In chronic adrenocortical insufficiency, the dosage should be approximately 0.4 to 0.8 mg/kg/day in two or three divided doses, adjusted to the needs of the individual child.

*Use in the elderly:* Treatment of elderly patients, particularly if long term, should be planned bearing in mind the more serious consequences of the common side effects of corticosteroids in old age, especially osteoporosis, diabetes, hypertension, susceptibility to infection and thinning of the skin.

**Contra-indications, warnings, etc**
*Contra-indications:* Systemic fungal infections. Hypersensitivity to any component of this product.

*Precautions:* The lowest possible dosage of corticosteroid should be used and when reduction in dosage is possible, the reduction should be gradual.

Corticosteroids may exacerbate systemic fungal infections and therefore should not be used in the presence of such infections unless they are needed to control drug reactions due to amphotericin. Moreover, there have been cases reported in which concomitant use of amphotericin and hydrocortisone was followed by cardiac enlargement and congestive heart failure.

Literature reports suggest an apparent association between use of corticosteroids and left ventricular free wall rupture after a recent myocardial infarction; therefore, therapy with corticosteroids should be used with great caution in these patients.

Average and large dosages of hydrocortisone or cortisone can cause elevation of blood pressure, salt and water retention, and increase excretion of potassium. These effects are less likely to occur with the synthetic derivatives except when used in large doses. Dietary salt restriction and potassium supplementation may be necessary. All corticosteroids increase calcium excretion.

A report shows that the use of corticosteroids in cerebral malaria is associated with a prolonged coma and an increased incidence of pneumonia and gastro-intestinal bleeding.

Drug-induced secondary adrenocortical insufficiency may result from too rapid a withdrawal of corticosteroids and may be minimised by gradual reduction of dosage. This type of relative insufficiency may persist for months after discontinuation of therapy; therefore, in any situation of stress occurring during that period, corticosteroid therapy should be reinstated. If the patient is receiving steroids already, the dosage may have to be increased. Since mineralocorticoid secretion may be impaired, salt and/or a mineralocorticoid should be administered concurrently.

Stopping corticosteroids after prolonged therapy may cause withdrawal symptoms including fever, myalgia, arthralgia, and malaise. This may occur in patients even without evidence of adrenal insufficiency.

If corticosteroids are indicated in patients with latent tuberculosis or tuberculin reactivity, close observation is necessary as reactivation may occur. During prolonged corticosteroid therapy, these patients should receive prophylactic chemotherapy.

The use of Hydrocortone Tablets in active tuberculosis should be restricted to those cases of fulminating or disseminated tuberculosis.

Corticosteroids should be used with caution in renal insufficiency, hypertension, diabetes or in those with a family history of diabetes, congestive heart failure, osteoporosis, previous steroid myopathy, glaucoma (or family history), myasthenia gravis, non-specific ulcerative colitis, diverticulitis, fresh intestinal anastomoses, active or latent peptic ulcer. Signs of peritoneal irritation following gastro-intestinal perforation in patients receiving large doses of corticosteroids may be minimal or absent. Fat embolism has been reported as a possible complication of hypercortisonism.

There is an enhanced effect of corticosteroids in patients with hypothyroidism and in those with cirrhosis.

Corticosteroids may mask some signs of infection, and new infections may appear during their use. There may be decreased resistance and inability to localise infection in patients on corticosteroids. Corticosteroids may affect the nitrobluetetrazolium test for bacterial infection and produce false negative results.

Corticosteroids may activate latent amoebiasis. Therefore, it is recommended that latent or active amoebiasis be excluded before initiating corticosteroid therapy in any patient who has either spent time in the tropics, or has unexplained diarrhoea.

Prolonged use of corticosteroids may produce posterior subcapsular cataracts, glaucoma with possible damage to the optic nerves, and may enhance the establishment of secondary ocular infections due to fungi and viruses.

Corticosteroids should be used cautiously in patients with ocular herpes simplex because of possible corneal perforation.

Corticosteroids may increase or decrease motility and number of spermatozoa.

*Drug interactions:* Aspirin should be used cautiously in conjunction with corticosteroids in hypoprothrombinaemia.

Phenytoin, ephedrine, rifabutin, carbamazepine, barbiturates, rifampicin and aminoglutethimide may enhance the metabolic clearance of corticosteroids, resulting in decreased blood levels and lessened physiological activity, thus requiring adjustment in corticosteroid dosage.

The prothrombin time should be checked frequently in patients who are receiving corticosteroids and coumarin anticoagulants at the same time because of reports of altered response to these anticoagulants. Studies have shown that the usual effect produced by adding corticosteroids is inhibition of reponse to coumarins, although there have been some conflicting reports of potentiation not substantiated by studies.

When corticosteroids are administered concomitantly with potassium-depleting diuretics, patients should be observed closely for development of hypokalaemia.

*Children:* Corticosteroids cause growth retardation in infancy, childhood and adolescence. Treatment should be limited to the minimum dosage in order to minimise suppression of the hypothalamo-pituitary-adrenal axis and growth retardation.

Growth and development of infants and children on prolonged corticosteroid therapy should be carefully monitored.

*Use in pregnancy and lactation:* There is inadequate evidence of safety in human pregnancy. Use of these drugs in pregnancy or in women of childbearing potential requires that the anticipated benefits be weighed against the possible hazards to the mother and embryo or fetus. There may be a very small risk of cleft palate and intra-uterine growth retardation in the fetus; there is evidence of harmful effects on pregnancy in animals. Infants born of mothers who have received substantial doses of corticosteroids during pregnancy should be carefully observed for signs of hypoadrenalism.

Corticosteroids appear in breast milk and could suppress growth, interfere with endogenous corticosteroid production, or cause other unwanted effects. Mothers taking pharmacological doses of corticosteroids should be advised not to breast feed.

*Side-effects: Fluid and electrolyte disturbances:* Sodium retention, fluid retention, congestive heart failure in susceptible patients, potassium loss, hypokalaemic alkalosis, hypertension, increased calcium excretion.

*Musculoskeletal effects:* Muscle weakness, steroid myopathy, loss of muscle mass, osteoporosis (especially in post-menopausal females), vertebral compression fractures, aseptic necrosis of femoral and humeral heads, pathological fracture of long bones, tendon rupture.

*Gastro-intestinal:* Peptic ulcer with possible perforation and haemorrhage, perforation of the small and large bowel particularly in patients with inflammatory bowel disease, pancreatitis, abdominal distension, ulcerative oesophagitis, dyspepsia, oesophageal candidiasis.

*Dermatological:* Impaired wound healing, thin fragile skin, petechiae, and ecchymoses, erythema, striae, telangiectasia, acne, increased sweating, may suppress reactions to skin tests, other cutaneous reactions such as allergic dermatitis, urticaria, angioneurotic oedema.

*Neurological:* Convulsions, increased intracranial pressure with papilloedema (pseudotumour cerebri) usually after treatment, vertigo, headache. Psychic disturbances.

*Endocrine:* Menstrual irregularities, amenorrhoea, development of Cushingoid state, suppression of growth in children, secondary adrenocortical and pituitary unresponsiveness (particularly in times of stress, as in trauma, surgery, or illness), decreased carbohydrate tolerance, manifestations of latent diabetes mellitus, increased requirements for insulin or oral hypoglycaemic agents in diabetics, hirsutism.

*Ophthalmic:* Posterior subcapsular cataracts, increased intra-ocular pressure, papilloedema, corneal or scleral thinning, exacerbation of ophthalmic viral disease, glaucoma, exophthalmos.

*Metabolic:* Negative nitrogen balance due to protein catabolism.

*Cardiovascular:* Myocardial rupture following recent myocardial infarction (see 'Precautions').

*Other:* Hypersensitivity, leucocytosis, thrombo-embolism, weight gain, increased appetite, nausea, malaise.

*Overdosage:* Reports of acute toxicity and/or deaths following overdosage with glucocorticoids are rare. No antidote is available. Treatment is probably not indicated for reactions due to chronic poisoning unless the patient has a condition that would render him unusually susceptible to ill effects from corticosteroids. In this case, symptomatic treatment should be instituted as necessary.

Anaphylactic and hypersensitivity reactions may be treated with adrenaline, positive-pressure artificial respiration and aminophylline. The patient should be kept warm and quiet.

The biological half-life of hydrocortisone is about 100 minutes.

**Pharmaceutical precautions**   Keep container well closed, store in a cool place, below 25°C, protected from light.

**Legal category**   POM.

**Package quantities**   *10 mg:* Packs of 30. *20 mg:* Packs of 30.

**Further information**   Nil.

**Product licence numbers**
10 mg   0025/5053
20 mg   0025/5054

# HYDROSALURIC*

**Presentation**   White, half-scored tablets, marked 'MSD 42', containing 25 mg Hydrochlorothiazide BP.

White, half-scored tablets, marked 'MSD 105', containing 50 mg Hydrochlorothiazide BP.

**Uses**   Thiazide diuretic and antihypertensive.

Oedema associated with congestive heart failure, hepatic cirrhosis, premenstrual tension and oedema due to various forms of renal dysfunction (i.e. the nephrotic syndrome, acute glomerulonephritis, chronic renal failure). Hypertension, either alone or as an adjunct to other antihypertensive drugs.

**Dosage and administration**   Dosage should be determined on an individual basis, and the lowest dosage necessary to achieve the desired result should be used.

*Adults – for oedema:* Usually 25–100 mg a day given in a single dose or in two divided doses. Many patients respond to intermittent therapy; for example, every other day, or three to five days a week. Intermittent therapy is less likely to produce excessive diuretic response with resulting undesirable electrolyte imbalance. The maximum recommended daily dose is 100 mg.

*In oedema accompanying premenstrual tension:* 25–50 mg once or twice a day, from the first morning of symptoms until the onset of the menses.

*Adults – for control of hypertension:* Usual starting dosage, 25 mg a day as a single or divided dose. In some patients, a starting dose of 12.5 mg, alone or with another antihypertensive, may be sufficient. Dosage should be adjusted to response, but should not exceed 50 mg a day.

Thiazides may add to the action of other antihypertensives. If HydroSaluric is used with other antihypertensive agents, it may be necessary to reduce the dosage of such agents so as to prevent an excessive drop in blood pressure.

*Infants and children:* Usually 2.5 mg per kg bodyweight a day, given in two doses. Infants under 6 months may need up to 3.5 mg per kg a day, in two doses. Infants up to 2 years of age may be given 12.5–37.5 mg of HydroSaluric a day in two doses. Children from 2 to 12 years of age may be given 37.5–100 mg a day in two doses. Dosage should be based on bodyweight.

*Uses in the elderly:* Particular caution is needed in the elderly because of their susceptibility to electrolyte imbalance; the dosage should be carefully adjusted according to renal function and clinical response. If lower dosage is required, 25 mg tablets are available.

**Contra-indications, warnings, etc**

*Contra-indications:* Anuria, hypersensitivity to any component of this product or to other sulphonamide-derived drugs, severe renal or hepatic failure, Addison's disease, hypercalcaemia, concurrent lithium therapy. See 'Use in pregnancy' and 'Use in breast-feeding mothers', under 'Precautions'.

*Precautions:* Patients should be carefully monitored for signs of fluid and electrolyte imbalance (hyponatraemia, hypochloraemic alkalosis, hypokalaemia and hypomagnesaemia). It is particularly important to make serum and urine electrolyte determinations when the patient is vomiting excessively or receiving parenteral fluids. Warning signs or symptoms of fluid and electrolyte imbalance include: dryness of mouth, thirst, weakness, lethargy, drowsiness, restlessness, seizures, confusion, muscle pains or cramps, muscle fatigue, hypotension, oliguria, tachycardia, and gastro-intestinal disturbances such as nausea and vomiting.

Hypokalaemia may develop, especially with brisk diuresis, when severe cirrhosis is present, or after prolonged therapy. Hypokalaemia can sensitise or exaggerate the response of the heart to the toxic effects of digitalis (e.g. increased ventricular irritability).

Sensitivity reactions may occur in patients with or without history of allergy or bronchial asthma.

Hypokalaemia may be avoided or treated in the adult by concurrent use of amiloride hydrochloride (Midamor*), a potassium-conserving agent. It may also be avoided by giving potassium chloride or foods with a high potassium content. (Note that symptoms and signs which might indicate ulceration or obstruction of the small bowel in patients taking tablets or capsules containing potassium salts are indications for stopping treatment with such preparations immediately.)

Diuretic-induced hyponatraemia is usually mild and asymptomatic. Dilutional hyponatraemia may occur in oedematous patients in hot weather; and, except in rare instances when hyponatraemia is life-threatening, appropriate therapy is water restriction rather than administration of salt.

Thiazides may decrease serum Protein Bound Iodine levels without signs of thyroid disturbances.

Thiazides may decrease urinary calcium excretion, and may also cause intermittent and slight elevation of serum calcium in the absence of known disorders of calcium metabolism. Thiazides should be discontinued before carrying out tests for parathyroid function.

When creatinine clearance falls below 30 ml/min, thiazide diuretics become ineffective.

Uraemia may be precipitated or increased by chlorothiazide. Cumulative effects of the drug may develop in patients with impaired renal function. If increasing uraemia and oliguria occur during treatment of renal disease, HydroSaluric should be discontinued.

Thiazides should be used with caution in patients with impaired hepatic function or progressive liver disease, since minor alterations of fluid and electrolyte balance may precipitate hepatic coma.

Hyperuricaemia may occur, or gout may be precipitated, in certain patients receiving thiazide therapy.

Thiazide therapy may impair glucose tolerance.

Increases in cholesterol and triglyceride levels may be associated with thiazide diuretic therapy.

The possibility of exacerbation or activation of systemic lupus erythematosus has been reported.

Latent diabetes may become manifest during thiazide administration.

*Use in pregnancy:* Thiazides cross the placental barrier and appear in cord blood. The use of HydroSaluric when pregnancy is present or suspected requires, therefore, that the benefits of the drug be weighed against possible hazards to the fetus. These hazards include fetal or neonatal jaundice, thrombocytopenia, and possibly other adverse reactions which have occurred in the adult. The routine use of diuretics in otherwise healthy pregnant women with or without mild oedema is not recommended, because their use may be associated with hypovolaemia, increased blood viscosity and decreased placental perfusion.

*Use in breast-feeding mothers:* Thiazides appear in breast milk. If use of the drug is deemed essential, the patient should stop breast-feeding.

*Drug interactions: Alcohol, barbiturates or narcotics:* Co-administration may potentiate orthostatic hypotension. *Oral and parenteral antidiabetic drugs* may require adjustment of dosage with concurrent use. *Other antihypertensive drugs* may have an additive effect. Discontinuation of diuretic therapy 2–3 days before the initiation of treatment with an ACE inhibitor may reduce the likelihood of first-dose hypotension. The antihypertensive effect of the drug may be enhanced in the post-sympathectomy patient. *Cholestyramine and colestipol resin:* Absorption of hydrochlorothiazide is impaired in the presence of anionic exchange resins. Single doses of either cholestyramine or colestipol resins bind hydrochlorothiazide and reduce its absorption from the gastro-intestinal tract by up to 85% and 43%, respectively. *Corticosteroids or ACTH* may intensify any thiazide-induced electrolyte depletion, particularly hypokalaemia. *Pressor amines such as adrenaline* may show decreased arterial responsiveness when used with HydroSaluric, but this reaction is not enough to preclude their therapeutic usefulness. *Non-depolarising muscle relaxants such as tubocurarine* may possibly interact with HydroSaluric to increase muscle relaxation. *Non-steroidal anti-inflammatory drugs* may attenuate the diuretic and antihypertensive effect of diuretics.

*Drug/laboratory tests:* Because thiazides may affect calcium metabolism, HydroSaluric may interfere with tests for parathyroid function.

*Side-effects*

*Gastro-intestinal system:* Anorexia, gastric irritation, nausea, vomiting, cramps, diarrhoea, constipation, jaundice (intrahepatic cholestatic jaundice), pancreatitis, salivary gland inflammation.

*Central nervous system:* Dizziness, vertigo, paraesthesiae, headache, yellow vision.

*Haematological:* Leucopenia, agranulocytosis, thrombocytopenia, aplastic anaemia, haemolytic anaemia.

*Cardiovascular:* Hypotension, including orthostatic hypotension.

*Hypersensitivity:* Purpura, photosensitivity, rash, urticaria, necrotising angiitis (vasculitis, cutaneous vasculitis), fever, respiratory distress including pneumonitis and pulmonary oedema, anaphylactic reactions, toxic epidermal necrolysis.

*Metabolic:* Hyperglycaemia, glycosuria, hyperuricaemia, electrolyte imbalance including hyponatraemia and hypokalaemia.

*Renal:* Renal dysfunction, interstitial nephritis, renal failure.

*Other:* Muscle spasm, weakness, restlessness, transient blurred vision, impotence.

Whenever side-effects are moderate to severe, thiazide dosage should be reduced or therapy withdrawn.

*Overdosage:* The most common signs and symptoms observed are those caused by electrolyte depletion (hypokalaemia, hypochloraemia, hyponatraemia) and dehydration resulting from excessive diuresis. If digitalis has also been administered, hypokalaemia may accentuate cardiac arrhythmias.

In the event of overdosage, symptomatic and supportive measures should be employed. If ingestion is recent, emesis should be induced or gastric lavage performed. Dehydration, electrolyte imbalance, hepatic coma and hypotension should be corrected by established methods. If required, give oxygen or artificial respiration for respiratory impairment.

**Pharmaceutical precautions** Keep container tightly closed; store in a cool place, protected from light.

**Legal category** POM.

**Package quantities** 25 mg: Packs of 30. 50 mg: Packs of 30.

**Further information** Diuresis begins within two hours following administration, is at a peak after four hours and persists for six to twelve hours. No rigid dietary salt restriction required.

The plasma half-life of hydrochlorothiazide is 5.6 hours with a subsequently longer terminal phase. The biological half-life is 14.8 hours when the plasma level can be followed for at least 24 hours.

**Product licence numbers**
25 mg tablet   0025/5009
50 mg tablet   0025/5010

# INDOCID*

**Presentation** Ivory, opaque capsules containing 25 mg or 50 mg Indomethacin PhEur, marked 'MSD 25' and 'MSD 50' respectively.

Opaque ivory headed, transparent blue based, sustained release capsules carrying white and blue pellets containing 75 mg indomethacin, marked 'INDOCID R 693'. The 75 mg of indomethacin provides 25 mg of free indomethacin for immediate dissolution, and 50 mg of time-release coated pellets.

A fruit-flavoured suspension containing in each 5 ml, 25 mg Indomethacin PhEur.

Polyethylene glycol suppositories containing 100 mg Indomethacin PhEur.

**Uses** Non-steroidal anti-inflammatory agent indicated for the active stages of rheumatoid arthritis, osteoarthritis, ankylosing spondylitis, degenerative joint disease of the hip, acute musculoskeletal disorders, low-back pain, and acute gouty arthritis.

Also indicated in inflammation, pain and oedema following orthopaedic procedures; and the treatment of pain and associated symptoms of primary dysmenorrhoea.

Indocid Suppositories may be used where night pain and morning stiffness are prominent. One suppository at bedtime will frequently give relief from pain and stiffness for 13 to 16 hours after administration.

*Indocid-R:* Indocid-R may be substituted for all the indications of Indocid except acute gouty arthritis, as clinical evidence is not currently available for this dosage form in this condition.

**Dosage and administration** The dosage of Indocid should be carefully adjusted to suit the needs of the individual patient.

*Oral therapy:* In order to reduce the possibility of gastro-intestinal disturbances, *Indocid/Indocid-R Capsules and Suspension should always be taken with food or an antacid.* (Note, however, that Indocid Suspension should not be mixed with an antacid, but should be taken separately, because indomethacin is unstable in an alkaline medium.) Indocid Suspension should not be diluted.

In chronic conditions, starting therapy with a low dosage, increasing this gradually as necessary, and continuing a trial of therapy for an adequate period (in some cases, up to one month) will give the best results with a minimum of unwanted reactions. The recommended oral dosage range is 50–200 mg daily in divided doses. Paediatric dosage not established.

*Dosage in dysmenorrhoea:* Up to 75 mg a day, starting with onset of cramps or bleeding, and continuing for as long as the symptoms usually last.

*Dosage in acute gouty arthritis:* 150–200 mg daily in divided doses until all symptoms and signs subside.

*Adult dosage for suppositories:* 1 suppository to be inserted once or twice a day. One should be used at bedtime. If another is necessary, it should be used in the morning.

*Dosage for Indocid-R:* The sustained-release capsule may be given once or, where necessary, twice a day depending on patient needs and response.

*Use in the elderly:* Indocid should be used with particular care in older patients who are more prone to adverse reactions.

**Contra-indications, warnings, etc**
*Contra-indications:* Active peptic ulcer; a recurrent history of gastro-intestinal lesions; in patients who have nasal polyps associated with angioneurotic oedema, who show sensitivity to Indocid, or who have experienced acute asthmatic attacks, urticaria or rhinitis as a result of therapy with aspirin or other non-steroidal anti-inflammatory drugs. Safety for use in children has not been established. Indocid Suppositories are contra-indicated in patients with a history of proctitis or recent rectal bleeding.

*Use in pregnancy:* Indocid should be used during the first two trimesters of pregnancy only if the potential benefit justifies the potential risk to the fetus.

The known effects of indomethacin and other drugs of this class on the human fetus during the third trimester of pregnancy include: constriction of the ductus arteriosus prenatally, tricuspid incompetence, and pulmonary hypertension; non-closure of the ductus arteriosus postnatally which may be resistant to medical management; myocardial degenerative changes, platelet dysfunction with resultant bleeding, intracranial bleeding, renal dysfunction or failure, renal injury/dysgenesis which may result in prolonged or permanent renal failure, oligohydramnios, gastro-intestinal bleeding or perforation and increased risk of necrotising enterocolitis. Use of Indocid during the third trimester of pregnancy is not recommended.

*Use in breast-feeding mothers*
Administration of Indocid is not recommended in breast-feeding mothers. Indomethacin is excreted in breast milk.

*Precautions:* Headache, sometimes accompanied by dizziness and lightheadedness, may occur, usually early in treatment. Starting therapy with a low dosage and increasing it gradually will usually minimise the incidence of headache. These symptoms frequently disappear on continuing therapy or reducing the dosage, but if headache persists despite dosage reduction, Indocid should be withdrawn. Patients should be warned that they may experience dizziness and, if they do, should not drive a car or undertake potentially dangerous activities needing alertness.

Indocid should be used cautiously in patients with psychiatric disorders, epilepsy, or parkinsonism, as it may tend to aggravate these disorders.

Gastro-intestinal disturbances may be minimised by giving Indocid orally with food or an antacid. They usually disappear on reducing the dosage; if not, the risks of continuing therapy should be weighed against the possible benefits. If gastro-intestinal bleeding does occur, Indocid should immediately be discontinued.

Single or multiple ulcerations, including perforation and haemorrhage of the oesophagus, stomach, duodenum or small or large intestine have been reported to occur with Indocid. Fatalities have been reported in some instances. Rarely, intestinal ulceration has been associated with stenosis and obstruction.

Gastro-intestinal bleeding without obvious ulcer formation and perforation of pre-existing sigmoid lesions (diverticulum, carcinoma, etc.) have occurred. Increased abdominal pain in ulcerative colitis patients or the development of ulcerative colitis and regional ileitis have been reported to occur rarely.

Fluid retention and peripheral oedema have been observed in some patients taking Indocid. It should therefore be used with caution in patients with cardiac dysfunction, hypertension or other conditions predisposing to fluid retention.

Tenesmus and irritation of the rectal mucosa have been reported occasionally with Indocid Suppositories.

Indocid may mask the signs and symptoms of infection. Indocid should be used with caution in patients with existing, but controlled infection.

In patients with rheumatoid arthritis, eye changes may occur which may be related to the underlying disease or to the therapy. Therefore, in chronic rheumatoid disease, ophthalmological examinations at periodic intervals are recommended. Discontinue therapy if eye changes are observed.

Patients should be periodically observed to allow early detection of any unwanted effects on peripheral blood (anaemia), liver function or gastro-intestinal tract.

Indocid can inhibit platelet aggregation. This effect usually disappears within 24 hours of discontinuing Indocid. Bleeding time is prolonged (but within normal range) in normal adults. Because this effect may be exaggerated in patients with underlying haemostatic defects, Indocid should be used cautiously in patients with coagulation defects.

As with other non-steroidal anti-inflammatory drugs, there have been reports of acute interstitial nephritis with haematuria, proteinuria, and occasionally nephrotic syndrome, in patients receiving long-term administration of indomethacin.

In patients with reduced renal blood flow where renal prostaglandins play a major role in maintaining renal perfusion, administration of a non-steroidal anti-inflammatory agent may precipitate overt renal decompensation. Patients at greatest risk of this reaction are those with renal or hepatic dysfunction, diabetes mellitus, advanced age, extracellular volume depletion, congestive heart failure, sepsis, or concomitant use of any nephrotoxic drug. A non-steroidal anti-inflammatory drug should be given with caution and renal function should be monitored in any patient who may have reduced renal reserve. Discontinuation of non-steroidal anti-inflammatory therapy is usually followed by recovery to the pretreatment state.

Increases in plasma potassium concentration, including hyperkalaemia, have been reported, even in some patients without renal impairment. In patients with normal renal function, these effects have been attributed to a hyporeninaemic-hypoaldosteronism state (see 'Drug interactions').

Since Indocid is eliminated primarily by the kidneys, patients with significantly impaired renal function should be closely monitored; a lower daily dosage should be used to avoid excessive drug accumulation.

*Laboratory tests:* Borderline elevations of one or more liver tests may occur, and significant elevations of ALT (SGPT) or AST (SGOT) have been seen in less than 1% of patients receiving therapy with non-steroidal anti-inflammatory drugs in controlled clinical trials. If abnormal liver tests persist or worsen, if clinical signs and symptoms consistent with liver disease develop or if systemic manifestations such as rash or eosinophilia occur, Indocid should be stopped.

False negative results in the dexamethasone suppression test (DST) in patients being treated with Indocid have been reported. Thus, results of this test should be used with caution in these patients.

*Drug interactions:* Aspirin: The use of Indocid with aspirin or other salicylates is not recommended. Controlled clinical studies have shown no enhanced therapeutic effect, and one study showed a significant increase in the incidence of gastro-intestinal side effects. A study in normal volunteers showed that chronic administration of 3.6 g aspirin with indomethacin lowered the indomethacin blood levels by approximately 20%.

Diflunisal: Co-administration of diflunisal with Indocid increases the plasma level of indomethacin by about a third with a concomitant decrease in renal clearance. Fatal gastro-intestinal haemorrhage has occurred. The combination should not be used.

*Other NSAIDs:* the concomitant use of Indocid with other NSAIDs is not recommended due to the increased possibility of gastro-intestinal toxicity, with little or no increase in efficacy.

Anticoagulants: Although clinical studies suggest that Indocid does not influence the hypoprothrombinaemia induced by anticoagulants, patients also receiving anticoagulants should be closely observed for alterations of the prothrombin time.

Probenecid: Co-administration of probenecid may increase plasma levels of indomethacin.

Methotrexate: Caution should be exercised with simultaneous use of Indocid with methotrexate. Indocid has been reported to decrease the tubular secretion of methotrexate and to potentiate toxicity.

Cyclosporin: Administration of non-steroidal anti-inflammatory drugs concomitantly with cyclosporin has been associated with an increase in cyclosporin-induced toxicity, possibly due to decreased synthesis of renal prostacyclin. NSAIDs should be used with caution in patients taking cyclosporin and renal function should be monitored carefully.

Lithium: Indomethacin 50 mg three times a day produced a clinically relevant elevation of plasma lithium and reduction in renal lithium clearance in psychiatric patients and normal subjects with steady state plasma lithium concentrations. This effect has been attributed to inhibition of prostaglandin synthesis. As a consequence, when indomethacin and lithium are given concomitantly, the patient should be observed carefully for signs of lithium toxicity.

In addition, the frequency of monitoring serum lithium concentrations should be increased at the outset of such combination drug treatment.

Diuretics: In some patients, the administration of Indocid can reduce the diuretic and antihypertensive effects of loop, potassium-sparing, and thiazide diuretics. Therefore, when Indocid and diuretics are used concomitantly, the patient shoud be observed closely to determine if the desired effect of the diuretic is obtained.

Indocid reduces basal plasma renin activity (PRA), as well as those elevations of PRA induced by frusemide administration, or salt or volume depletion. These facts should be considered when evaluating plasma renin activity in hypertensive patients.

It has been reported that the addition of triamterene to a maintenance schedule of Indocid resulted in reversible acute renal failure in two of four healthy volunteers. Indocid and triamterene should not be administered together.

Indocid and potassium-sparing diuretics each may be associated with increased plasma potassium levels. The potential effects of Indocid and potassium-sparing diuretics on potassium kinetics and renal function should be considered when these agents are administered concurrently.

Most of the above effects concerning diuretics have been attributed, at least in part, to mechanisms involving inhibition of prostaglandin synthesis by Indocid.

Digoxin: Indocid given concomitantly with digoxin has been reported to increase the serum concentration and prolong the half life of digoxin. Therefore when 'Indocid' and digoxin are used concomitantly serum digoxin levels should be closely monitored.

Antihypertensive medications: Coadministration of Indocid and some antihypertensive agents may atten-

uate acutely the hypotensive effect of the latter, due partly to indomethacin's inhibition of prostaglandin synthesis. Therefore caution should be exercised when considering the addition of Indocid to the regimen of a patient taking any of the following antihypertensive agents: alpha-adrenergic blocking agents, ACE inhibitors, beta-adrenergic blocking agents, diuretics or hydralazine.

Phenylpropanolamine: Hypertensive crises have been reported due to oral phenylpropanolamine alone and rarely to phenylpropanolamine given with Indocid. This additive effect is probably due partly to indomethacin's inhibition of prostaglandin synthesis. Caution should be exercised when Indocid and phenylpropanolamine are administered concomitantly.

*Warnings and adverse reactions: CNS reactions –* headaches, dizziness, lightheadedness, depression, vertigo, and fatigue (including malaise and listlessness). Reactions reported infrequently include mental confusion, anxiety, syncope, drowsiness, convulsions, coma, peripheral neuropathy, muscle weakness, involuntary muscle movements, insomnia, psychiatric disturbances such as depersonalisation; and, rarely, paraesthesiae, dysarthria, aggravation of epilepsy and parkinsonism. These are often transient and disappear frequently with continued or with reduced dosage. However, occasionally, severe reactions require stopping therapy.

*Gastro-intestinal –* the more frequent reactions are nausea, anorexia, vomiting, epigastric distress, abdominal pain, constipation, and diarrhoea. Others which may develop are ulceration (single or multiple) of oesophagus, stomach, duodenum or small or large intestine including perforation and haemorrhage with a few fatalities having been reported; gastro-intestinal tract bleeding without obvious ulcer formation; increased abdominal pain when used in patients with pre-existing ulcerative colitis. Reactions occurring infrequently are stomatitis; gastritis; flatulence; bleeding from the sigmoid colon (occult or from a diverticulum); perforation of pre-existing sigmoid lesions (diverticulae and carcinoma).

Rarely, intestinal strictures (diaphragms) and intestinal ulceration followed by stenosis and obstruction have been reported. With suppositories, tenesmus and irritation of the rectal mucosa have occasionally been reported. Other gastro-intestinal side effects which may or may not be caused by indomethacin include ulcerative colitis and regional ileitis.

*Hepatic –* rarely, hepatitis and jaundice (some fatalities reported).

*Cardiovascular/renal –* oedema, increased blood pressure, tachycardia, chest pain, arrhythmia, palpitation, hypotension, congestive heart failure, blood urea elevation, and haematuria (all infrequent).

*Dermatological/hypersensitivity –* pruritus, urticaria, angioneurotic oedema, angiitis, erythema nodosum, skin rash, exfoliative dermatitis, Stevens-Johnson syndrome, erythema multiforme, toxic epidermal necrolysis, loss of hair, rapid fall in blood pressure resembling a shock-like state, acute anaphylaxis, acute respiratory distress including sudden dyspnoea, asthma and pulmonary oedema (all infrequent). Bronchospasm may be precipitated in patients suffering from, or with a history of, bronchial asthma or allergic disease.

*Haematological –* infrequently, blood dyscrasias may occur, including leucopenia, petechiae or ecchymosis, purpura, aplastic or haemolytic anaemia, agranulocytosis, bone-marrow depression, disseminated intravascular coagulation, and particularly thrombocytopenia. Because some patients may develop anaemia secondary to obvious or occult gastro-intestinal bleeding, appropriate blood determinations are recommended.

*Ocular –* infrequently, blurred vision, diplopia, and orbital and peri-orbital pain. Corneal deposits and retinal disturbances, including those of the macula, have been reported in patients with rheumatoid arthritis on prolonged therapy, but similar changes may also be expected in patients with rheumatoid arthritis who have not received indomethacin.

*Aural –* tinnitus, hearing disturbances (rarely deafness).

*Genito-urinary –* proteinuria, nephrotic syndrome, interstitial nephritis, and renal insufficiency including renal failure (all rare).

*Miscellaneous –* vaginal bleeding, hyperglycaemia, glycosuria, hyperkalaemia, flushing and sweating, epistaxis, breast changes including enlargement and tenderness, gynaecomastia, and ulcerative stomatitis (all rare).

*The following adverse reactions have been associated with use of Indocid Suppositories:* tenesmus; proctitis; rectal bleeding, burning, pain, discomfort, and itching.

*Overdosage:* The following symptoms may be ob-

served following overdosage: nausea, vomiting, intense headache, dizziness, mental confusion, disorientation, or lethargy. There have been reports of paraesthesiae, numbness, and convulsions.

Treatment is symptomatic and supportive. The stomach should be emptied as quickly as possible if the ingestion is recent.

If vomiting has not occurred spontaneously, the patient should be induced to vomit with syrup of ipecac. If the patient is unable to vomit, gastric lavage should be performed. Once the stomach has been emptied, 25 or 50 g of activated charcoal may be given. Depending on the condition of the patient, close medical observation and nursing care may be required. The patient should be followed for several days because gastro-intestinal ulceration and haemorrhage have been reported as adverse reactions of indomethacin. Use of antacids may be helpful.

The plasma elimination of indomethacin is biphasic with the half-life of the terminal plasma half-life phase between 2.6 and 11.2 hours.

**Pharmaceutical precautions**   Store in a dry place below 25°C, protected from light.

*Indocid/Indocid-R Capsules and Suspension should always be taken with food or an antacid.* (Note, however, that Indocid Suspension should not be mixed with an antacid but should be taken separately because indomethacin is unstable in an alkaline medium.) Indocid Suspension should not be diluted.

**Legal category**   POM.

**Package quantities**   *Capsules:* 25 mg, packs of 90; 50 mg, packs of 90; 75 mg, packs of 30.
*Suppositories:* Boxes of 10.
*Suspension:* Bottles of 200 ml.

**Further information**   Nil.

**Product licence numbers**
| | |
|---|---|
| 25 mg | 0025/0111 |
| 50 mg | 0025/0112 |
| 75 mg | 0025/0125 |
| Suppositories | 0025/0062 |
| Suspension | 0025/0120 |

# INDOCID* PDA

**Qualitative and quantitative composition**   Indocid PDA contains indomethacin sodium trihydrate equivalent to 1.0 mg indomethacin PhEur.

**Pharmaceutical form**   Indocid PDA is available in vials containing a sterile, off-white to yellow lyophilised mass of indomethacin sodium trihydrate.

**Clinical particulars**
*Therapeutic indications:* Indocid PDA is indicated for the closure of patent ductus arteriosus in premature babies.

*Posology and method of administration: For intravenous use only.*

A course of therapy is defined as three intravenous doses of Indocid PDA given at 12- to 24-hour intervals, with careful attention to urinary output.

If anuria or marked oliguria (urinary output of 0.6 ml/kg/hour) is evident at the time of the scheduled second or third dose, Indocid PDA must not be given until laboratory studies indicate that renal function has returned to normal.

Dosage recommendations depend closely on the age of the infant:

| | Dosage (mg/kg) | | |
|---|---|---|---|
| Age at 1st dose | 1st | 2nd | 3rd |
| Less than 48 hours | 0.2 | 0.1 | 0.1 |
| 2–7 days | 0.2 | 0.2 | 0.2 |
| Over 7 days | 0.2 | 0.25 | 0.25 |

If the ductus arteriosus is closed or significantly reduced in size 48 hours after the first course of therapy, no further treatment is necessary. If the ductus arteriosus reopens, a second course of therapy may be given.

If the condition is unchanged after the second course of therapy, surgery may then be necessary. If severe adverse reactions occur, stop the treatment.

*Contra-indications:* Indocid PDA is contra-indicated in infants with established or suspected untreated infection; infants who are bleeding, especially with active intracranial haemorrhage or gastro-intestinal bleeding; infants with congenital heart disease in whom patency of the ductus arteriosus is necessary for satisfactory pulmonary or systemic blood flow (e.g. pulmonary atresia, severe tetralogy of Fallot, severe coarctation of the aorta); infants with thrombocytopenia; infants with coagulation defects; infants with known or suspected necrotising enterocolitis; infants with significant impairment of renal function.

*Special warnings and special precautions for use:*
*General:* Indocid may mask the usual signs and symptoms of infection. The drug must therefore be used cautiously in the presence of existing controlled infection.

Because severe hepatic reactions have been reported in adults on prolonged therapy with oral indomethacin, Indocid PDA should be discontinued if signs and symptoms consistent with liver disease develop in the neonate.

Indocid PDA may inhibit platelet aggregation. Premature babies should be observed for signs of bleeding.

Indocid PDA should be administered carefully to avoid extravasation and resultant irritation to tissues.

*Gastro-intestinal effects:* Clinical results indicate that major gastro-intestinal bleeding was no more common in those babies receiving indomethacin than those receiving placebo. However, minor gastro-intestinal bleeding (i.e. chemical detection of blood in the stool) was more common in infants treated with indomethacin. Severe gastro-intestinal effects have been reported in adults treated for prolonged periods with oral indomethacin.

*CNS reactions:* Prematurity *per se* is associated with an increased incidence of spontaneous intraventricular haemorrhage. Because indomethacin may inhibit platelet aggregation, the potential for intraventricular bleeding may be increased.

*Renal effects:* Indocid PDA may cause significant reduction in urine output (50% or more) with elevated blood urea and creatinine, and reduced GFR and creatinine clearance. In most babies, these effects are transient and disappear when therapy with Indocid PDA is stopped. However, because adequate renal function can depend on renal prostaglandin synthesis, Indocid PDA may precipitate renal insufficiency including acute renal failure. This is most likely in babies with conditions such as extracellular volume depletion from any cause, CHF, sepsis, or hepatic dysfunction or who are undergoing therapy with nephrotoxic drugs which may affect renal function.

Whenever a significant suppression of urine volume occurs with treatment, treatment with Indocid PDA must stop until urine output returns to normal.

Indocid PDA may suppress water excretion in premature babies to a greater extent than the excretion of sodium. This may result in hyponatraemia. Renal function and plasma electrolytes should be monitored.

*Interaction with other medicaments and other forms of interaction:* The half-life of digitalis in premature babies with patent ductus arteriosus and with cardiac failure is often prolonged by indomethacin. When both drugs are used concomitantly, frequent monitoring of ECG and serum digitalis may help prevention or early detection of digitalis toxicity.

In a study of premature infants treated with Indocid PDA and also receiving gentamicin or amikacin, both peak and trough levels of these aminoglycosides were significantly elevated.

Indocid may reduce the diuretic effect of frusemide.

*Pregnancy and lactation:* Not applicable.

*Effects on ability to drive and use machines:* Not applicable.

*Undesirable effects:*

*Haemorrhagic:* gross or microscopic bleeding into the gastro-intestinal tract; oozing from the skin after needle puncture; pulmonary haemorrhage; and disseminated intravascular coagulopathy.

*Renal:* renal dysfunction including one or more of the following: reduced urinary output; reduced urine sodium, chloride or potassium, urine osmolality, free water clearance, or glomerular filtration rate; uraemia; transient oliguria; and hypercreatinaemia.

*Gastro-intestinal:* vomiting; abdominal distension; melaena; transient ileus; and localised perforations of the small and/or large intestine.

*Metabolic:* hypersensitivity; hyponatraemia; elevated plasma potassium; elevated blood urea; hypoglycaemia.

*Cardiovascular:* pulmonary hypertension, intracranial bleeding.

*Coagulation:* decreased platelet aggregation.

*General:* weight gain (fluid retention); and exacerbation of infection.

See Summary of Product Characteristics for Indocid (indomethacin) for additional information concerning side-effects reported in the treatment of inflammatory and other conditions in patients of two years of age and older.

*Causal relationship unknown:* Although the following reactions have been reported in babies, a definite causal relationship has not been established.

*Cardiovascular:* bradycardia.

*Respiratory:* apnoea; exacerbation of pre-existing pulmonary infection.

*Haematological:* disseminated intravascular coagulation.

*Metabolic:* acidosis, alkalosis.

*Gastro-intestinal:* necrotising enterocolitis.

*Ophthalmic:* retrolental fibroplasia.

*Overdosage:* It is recommended that Indocid PDA should be administered only in a neonatal intensive-care unit.

Dosage is critical. The following signs and symptoms have occurred in individuals (not necessarily in premature infants) following an overdose of oral indomethacin: nausea, vomiting, intense headache, dizziness, mental confusion, disorientation, lethargy, paraesthesiae, numbness, and convulsions. There are no specific measures to treat acute overdosage with Indocid PDA. The patient should be monitored for several days because gastro-intestinal ulceration and haemorrhage have been reported as adverse reactions of indomethacin. Any complications occurring in the gastro-intestinal, renal and central nervous systems should be treated symptomatically and supportively.

Plasma half-life of intravenous indomethacin was inversely variable to the post-natal age and weight of the baby. In one study, a mean plasma half-life in babies less than a week old averaged 20 hours, while older babies showed a 12-hour average. Grouping the same babies by weight, the mean plasma half-life seen in babies under 1,000 g was 21 hours, in heavier babies the half-life was reduced to an average of 15 hours.

**Pharmacological properties**

*Pharmacodynamic properties:* Although the exact mechanism of action through which indomethacin causes closure of patent ductus arteriosus is not known, it is believed to be through inhibition of prostaglandin synthesis. Indomethacin has been shown to be a potent inhibitor of prostaglandin synthesis, both *in vitro* and *in vivo.* In human newborns with certain congenital heart malformations, PGE 1 dilates the ductus arteriosus. In fetal and newborn lambs, E type prostaglandins have also been shown to maintain the patency of the ductus; as in human newborns, indomethacin causes its conjunction.

*Pharmacokinetic properties:* The disposition of indomethacin following intravenous administration in preterm neonates with patent ductus arteriosus has not been extensively evaluated. Even though the plasma half-life of indomethacin was variable among premature infants, it was shown to vary inversely with post-natal age and weight. In one study of 28 evaluable infants, the plasma half-life in those infants less than 7 days old averaged 20 hours, and in infants older than 7 days, the mean plasma half-life was 12 hours. Grouping the infants by weight, the mean plasma half-life in those weighing less than 1,000 g was 21 hours, and in those weighing more than 1,000 g was 15 hours.

*Preclinical safety data:* No relevant information.

**Pharmaceutical particulars**

*List of excipients:* Water for injection PhEur.

*Incompatibilities:* None reported.

*Shelf life:* 36 months.

*Special precautions for storage:* The vial may be shipped and stored below 25°C. Intravenous solution should be prepared just prior to use and any unused portion remaining in the opened vial should be discarded.

When reconstituted, Indocid PDA is acceptable for use only when clear and free from particulate matter.

Further dilution with intravenous infusion solutions is not recommended. Indocid PDA is not buffered, and reconstitution at pH levels below 6 may cause precipitation of insoluble indomethacin.

*Nature and contents of container:* Available in cartons of three Type I glass vials each containing 1 ml.

*Instructions for use/handling:* The solution should be prepared only with 1 to 2 ml 0.9% Sodium Chloride Injection BP or Water for Injections PhEur. Preparations containing dextrose must not be used.

Preservatives should be carefully avoided at every stage because of the risk of toxicity in the newborn; any unused portion remaining in the opened vial should be discarded.

A fresh solution should be prepared just prior to each administration according to the dilution table below:

| *Amount of diluent used for each vial* | *Concentration achieved* |
|---|---|
| 1 ml | 0.1 mg/0.1 ml |
| 2 ml | 0.05 mg/0.1 ml |

The indomethacin solution may be injected intravenously over 5 to 10 seconds.

Further dilution with intravenous infusion solutions is not recommended.

**Marketing authorisation number** 0025/0201

**Date of approval/revision of SPC** February 1996.

**Legal category** POM.

# INNOVACE*

**Qualitative and quantitative composition** There are four strengths of Innovace Tablets available, each containing 2.5 mg, 5 mg, 10 mg and 20 mg of the active ingredient enalapril maleate.

**Pharmaceutical form**

2.5 mg–White, round tablets, marked 'INNOVACE'.

5 mg–White, half-scored, triangular tablets, marked 'INNOVACE'.

10 mg–Red, triangular tablets, marked 'INNOVACE'.

20 mg–Peach-coloured, triangular tablets, marked 'INNOVACE'.

**Clinical particulars**

*Therapeutic indications:*

*Treatment of hypertension:* All grades of essential hypertension and renovascular hypertension.

*Treatment of heart failure:* In heart failure, Innovace should be used as an adjunctive therapy with non-potassium-sparing diuretics and, where appropriate, digitalis. Innovace has been shown to improve symptoms, retard the progression of the disease, and reduce mortality and hospitalisation.

*Prevention of symptomatic heart failure:* When used in asymptomatic patients with left ventricular dysfunction, Innovace retards the development of symptomatic heart failure, and reduces hospitalisation for heart failure.

*Prevention of coronary ischaemic events in patients with left ventricular dysfunction:* Innovace reduces the incidence of myocardial infarction and reduces hospitalisation for unstable angina pectoris.

*Posology and method of administration:* The maximum daily dose is 40 mg.

The absorption of Innovace is not affected by food.

*Essential and renovascular hypertension:* Treatment should be initiated with 5 mg once a day. Where concomitant therapy is a diuretic, the recommended initial dose of Innovace is 2.5 mg (see *With concomitant diuretic therapy*). The dose should be titrated to give optimum control of blood pressure. The usual maintenance dose is 10–20 mg given once daily. In severe hypertension, the dosage may be increased incrementally to a maximum of 40 mg once daily.

The dosage of other antihypertensive agents being used together with Innovace may need to be adjusted. Where Innovace replaces a beta-blocking drug in the therapeutic regime, the beta-blocking agent should not be discontinued abruptly; the dosage should be titrated down after commencing therapy with Innovace.

*With concomitant diuretic therapy:* The recommended initial dose of Innovace is 2.5 mg. Symptomatic hypotension can occur following the initial dose of Innovace; this is more likely when Innovace is added to previous diuretic therapy. Caution is recommended, therefore, since these patients may be volume- or salt-depleted. If possible, the diuretic therapy should be discontinued for 2–3 days prior to initiation of therapy with Innovace.

Innovace minimises the development of thiazide-induced hypokalaemia and hyperuricaemia.

*Use in the elderly (over 65 years):* The starting dose should be 2.5 mg. Innovace is effective in the treatment of hypertension in the elderly. Some elderly patients may be more responsive to Innovace than younger patients.

The dose should be titrated according to need for the control of blood pressure.

*Heart failure/Asymptomatic left ventricular dysfunction:* The recommended starting dose in patients with symptomatic heart failure or asymptomatic left ventricular dysfunction is 2.5 mg once daily initiated under close medical supervision. For patients with severe heart failure, therapy should be initiated in hospital. Evidence of systolic left ventricular dysfunction should be obtained by relevant techniques (e.g. radionuclide ventriculography or echocardiography or equivalent) prior to initiation of preventive treatment; however, a repeated measurement may not be necessary in patients with one or more myocardial infarctions and documented reduction in cardiac function.

Following initiation of therapy, the dose should be titrated gradually to the usual maintenance dose of 20 mg, given as a single dose or two divided doses, according to the tolerability of the patient. In patients with symptomatic heart failure, this dosage schedule has been shown to improve survival.

The dose titration of Innovace may be performed over a two- to four-week period or more rapidly if indicated by the presence of residual signs and symptoms of heart failure. Blood pressure and renal function should be monitored closely both before and during treatment with Innovace. Serum potassium should also be monitored.

Some patients, other than those with severe heart failure, are considered to be at higher risk when started on an ACE inhibitor and are recommended for initiation of therapy in hospital. Research data have shown such patients to be: those on multiple or high-dose diuretics (e.g. >80 mg frusemide); patients with hypovolaemia; hyponatraemia (serum sodium <130 mmol/l); pre-existing hypotension (systolic blood pressure <90 mm Hg); patients with unstable cardiac failure; renal impairment (serum creatinine >150 μ mol/l); those on high-dose vasodilator therapy; patients aged 70 years or over (see *Special warnings and special precautions for use*).

In order to decrease the possibility of symptomatic hypotension, patients on previous high-dose diuretics should have the diuretic dose reduced before introducing Innovace. The appearance of hypotension after the initial dose of Innovace does not preclude subsequent careful dose titration with the drug, following effective treatment of the hypotension.

*Use in impaired renal function:* (see *Special warnings and special precautions for use*) Innovace is excreted by the kidney. It should be used with caution in patients with renal impairment. The recommended starting dose is 2.5 mg. The dose should be titrated against the response, and should be kept as low as possible to maintain adequate control of blood pressure or heart failure.

Innovace is dialysable. Dialysis patients may be given the usual dose of Innovace on dialysis days (see *Haemodialysis patients*). On the days when patients are not on dialysis the dosage should be tailored to the blood-pressure response.

*Children:* The paediatric use of Innovace has not been studied.

*Contra-indications:*
*Pregnancy:* (see *Pregnancy and lactation*).

*Hypersensitivity* to the product or any of the components, and in patients with a history of angioneurotic oedema relating to previous treatment with an ACE inhibitor.

*Special warnings and special precautions for use:*
*Pretreatment assessment of renal function:* Evaluation of the patient should include assessment of renal function prior to initiation of therapy, and during treatment where appropriate.

*Symptomatic hypotension* was seen rarely in uncomplicated hypertensive patients. In hypertensive patients receiving Innovace, hypotension is more likely to occur if the patient has been volume-depleted, e.g. by diuretic therapy, dietary salt restriction, dialysis, diarrhoea or vomiting. In patients with heart failure, with or without associated renal insufficiency, symptomatic hypotension has been observed. This is most likely to occur in those patients with more severe degrees of heart failure, as reflected by the use of high doses of loop diuretics, hyponatraemia or functional renal impairment (see *Posology and method of administration* for management of these patients).

Similar considerations may apply to patients with ischaemic heart or cerebrovascular disease in whom an excessive fall in blood pressure could result in a myocardial infarction or cerebrovascular accident.

If hypotension develops, the patient should be placed in a supine position. Volume repletion with oral fluids or intravenous normal saline may be required. Intravenous atropine may be necessary if there is associated bradycardia. A transient hypotensive response is not a contra-indication to further doses, which can usually be given without difficulty once the blood pressure has increased after volume expansion.

In some patients with heart failure who have normal or low blood pressure, additional lowering of systemic blood pressure may occur with Innovace. This effect is anticipated, and usually is not a reason to discontinue treatment. If such hypotension becomes symptomatic, a reduction of dose and/or discontinuation of the diuretic and/or Innovace may become necessary.

*Impaired renal function:* Innovace should be used with caution in patients with renal insufficiency as they may require reduced or less frequent doses (see *Posology and method of administration*).

Close monitoring of renal function before and during therapy should be performed as deemed appropriate in those with renal insufficiency. In the majority, renal function will not alter, or may improve.

Renal failure has been reported in association with Innovace and has been mainly in patients with severe heart failure or underlying renal disease, including renal artery stenosis. If recognised promptly and treated appropriately, renal failure when associated with therapy with Innovace is usually reversible.

Some hypertensive patients, with no apparent pre-existing renal disease, have developed increases in blood urea and creatinine when Innovace has been given concurrently with a diuretic. Dosage reduction of Innovace and/or discontinuation of the diuretic may be required. This situation should raise the possibility of underlying renal artery stenosis (see comment below).

*Renovascular hypertension:* Innovace can be used when surgery is not indicated, or prior to surgery. In some patients with bilateral renal artery stenosis or stenosis of the artery to a solitary kidney, increases of blood urea and creatinine, reversible upon discontinuation of therapy, have been seen. This is especially likely in patients treated with diuretics and/or those with renal insufficiency.

Angioneurotic oedema has been reported with angiotensin-converting enzyme inhibitors, including Innovace. This may occur at any time during treatment. In such cases, Innovace should be discontinued immediately and appropriate monitoring should be instituted to ensure complete resolution of symptoms prior to dismissing the patient. Where swelling is confined to the face, lips and mouth the condition will usually resolve without further treatment, although antihistamines may be useful in relieving symptoms. These patients should be monitored carefully until the swelling has resolved. However, where there is involvement of the tongue, glottis or larynx, likely to cause airways obstruction, appropriate therapy such as subcutaneous adrenaline (0.5 ml, 1:1000) should be administered promptly.

Patients with a history of angioedema unrelated to ACE-inhibitor therapy may be at increased risk of angioedema while receiving an ACE inhibitor (see also *Contra-indications*).

Other hypersensitivity reactions including urticaria have been reported.

*Anaphylactic reactions during hymenoptera desensitisation:* Rarely, patients receiving ACE inhibitors during desensitisation with hymenoptera venom (e.g. Bee or Wasp venom) have experienced life-threatening anaphylactoid reactions. These reactions were avoided by temporarily withholding ACE-inhibitor therapy prior to each desensitisation.

*Haemodialysis patients:* A high incidence of anaphylactoid reactions have been reported in patients dialysed with high-flux membranes and treated concomitantly with an ACE inhibitor. This combination should therefore be avoided.

*Anaphylactoid reactions during LDL apheresis:* Rarely, patients receiving ACE inhibitors during low-density lipoprotein (LDL) apheresis with dextran sulphate have experienced life-threatening anaphylactoid reactions. These reactions were avoided by temporarily withholding ACE-inhibitor therapy prior to each apheresis.

*Cough:* Cough has been reported with the use of ACE inhibitors. Characteristically, the cough is non-productive, persistent and resolves after discontinuation of therapy. ACE-inhibitor-induced cough should be considered as part of the differential diagnosis of cough.

*Surgery/anesthesia:* In patients undergoing major surgery or during anesthesia with agents that produce hypotension, Innovace blocks angiotensin-II formation secondary to compensatory renin release. This may lead to hypotension which can be corrected by volume expansion.

*General:* Where Innovace has been used as a single agent in hypertension, Afro-Caribbean patients may show a reduced therapeutic response.

Innovace should not be used in patients with aortic stenosis or outflow tract obstruction.

*Interaction with other medicaments and other forms of interaction:*
*Drug interactions:* Combination with other antihypertensive agents such as beta-blockers, methyldopa, calcium antagonists, and diuretics may increase the antihypertensive efficacy. Adrenergic-blocking drugs should only be combined with Innovace under careful supervision. Concomitant propranolol may reduce the bioavailability of Innovace, but this does not appear to be of any clinical significance.

Concomitant therapy with lithium may increase the serum lithium concentration.

*Plasma potassium* usually remains within normal limits, although cases of hyperkalaemia have been reported. If Innovace is given with a potassium-losing diuretic, the likelihood of diuretic-induced hypokalaemia may be lessened. Innovace may elevate plasma potassium levels in patients with renal failure. Potassium supplements, potassium-sparing diuretics and potassium-containing salt substitutes are not recommended, particularly in patients with impaired renal function, since they may lead to significant increases in plasma potassium. However, if the concomitant use of these agents is deemed appropriate, they should be used with caution and with frequent monitoring of plasma potassium.

Epidemiological studies have suggested that concomitant administration of ACE inhibitors and antidiabetic medicines (insulins, oral hypoglycaemic agents) may cause an increased blood-glucose-lowering effect with risk of hypoglycaemia. This phenomenon appeared to be more likely to occur during the first weeks of combined treatment and in patients with renal impairment. Long-term controlled clinical trials with enalapril have not confirmed these findings, and do not preclude the use of enalapril in diabetic patients. It is advised however, that caution should be exercised in this patient population.

*Narcotic drugs/antipsychotics:* Postural hypotension may occur with ACE inhibitors.

*Allopurinol, cytostatic or immunosuppressive agents, systemic corticosteroids or procainamide:* Concomitant administration with ACE inhibitors may lead to an increased risk for leucopenia.

*Non-steroidal anti-inflammatory drugs:* The administration of a non-steroidal anti-inflammatory agent may reduce the antihypertensive effect of an ACE inhibitor. However, in a clinical pharmacology study indomethacin or sulindac was administered to hypertensive patients receiving Innovace and there was no evidence of a blunting of the antihypertensive action of Innovace. Furthermore, it has been described that NSAIDs and ACE inhibitors exert an additive effect on the increase in serum potassium, whereas renal function may decrease. These effects are in principle reversible, and occur especially in patients with compromised renal function.

*Antacids:* induce decreased bioavailability of ACE inhibitors.

*Sympathomimetics:* may reduce the antihypertensive effects of ACE inhibitors; patients should be carefully monitored to confirm that the desired effect is being obtained.

*Alcohol:* enhances the hypotensive effect with ACE inhibitors.

*Cyclosporin:* increase in the risk of hyperkalaemia with ACE inhibitors.

*Pregnancy and lactation:*
*Use in pregnancy:* Innovace has been shown to be fetotoxic in rabbits during middle and late pregnancy.

Fetal exposure in humans during the second and third trimesters of pregnancy has been associated with fetal and neonatal morbidity and mortality.

ACE inhibitors in human pregnancy have been associated with oligohydramnios which may result in limb contractures, craniofacial deformations and hypoplastic lung development. Hypotension, renal failure, hyperkalaemia and skull hypoplasia have occurred in the newborn. These adverse effects to the embryo and fetus do not appear to have resulted from intra-uterine ACE-inhibitor exposure limited to the first trimester.

Because of these findings, Innovace is contraindicated in pregnancy. When pregnancy is detected, treatment with Innovace should be discontinued as soon as possible.

*Use during lactation:* Enalapril and enalaprilat are secreted in human milk; caution should be exercised if Innovace is given to breast-feeding mothers.

*Effects on ability to drive and use machines:* There are no data to suggest that Innovace affects the ability to drive and use machines.

*Undesirable effects:* Severe hypotension and renal failure have occurred in association with therapy with Innovace. These appear to occur in certain specific sub-groups (see *Special warnings and special precautions for use*).

*Other adverse reactions:* Dizziness and headaches are the most commonly reported side effects. Less frequently, fatigue, asthenia, hypotension, orthostatic hypotension, syncope, nausea, diarrhoea, muscle cramps, rash, and cough have been reported. Even less frequently, renal dysfunction, renal failure, and oliguria have been reported.

Rarely reported side effects include:
*Cardiovascular:* myocardial infarction or cerebrovascular accident, possibly secondary to severe hypotension in high-risk patients (see *Special warnings and special precautions for use*), chest pain, palpitations, rhythm disturbances, angina pectoris.

*Gastr-intestinal:* ileus, pancreatitis, hepatic failure, hepatitis–either hepatocellular or cholestatic, jaundice, abdominal pain, vomiting, dyspepsia, constipation, anorexia, stomatitis.

*Nervous system/psychiatric:* depression, confusion, somnolence, insomnia, nervousness, paraesthesiae, vertigo.

*Respiratory:* pulmonary infiltrates, bronchospasm, asthma, dyspnoea, rhinorrhoea, sore throat, and hoarseness.

*Skin:* diaphoresis, erythema multiforme, exfoliative dermatitis, Stevens-Johnson syndrome, toxic epidermal necrolysis, pemphigus, pruritus, urticaria, alopecia.

*Other:* impotence, flushing, taste alteration, tinnitus, glossitis, blurred vision.

A complex of symptoms has been reported which may include fever, serositis, vasculitis, myalgia/myositis, arthralgia/arthritis, a positive ANA, elevated ESR, eosinophilia, and leucocytosis. Rash, photosensitivity or other dermatological manifestations may occur.

*Hypersensitivity/angioneurotic oedema:* angioneurotic oedema of the face, extremities, lips, tongue, glottis and/or larynx has been reported rarely (see *Special warnings and special precautions for use*).

*Laboratory test findings:* Increases in blood urea and plasma creatinine, reversible on discontinuation of Innovace, are most likely in the presence of severe heart failure or bilateral renal artery stenosis, especially in patients with renal insufficiency (see *Special warnings and special precautions for use*). However, increases in blood urea and plasma creatinine may occur without evidence of pre-existing renal impairment, especially in patients taking diuretics. In this event, undiagnosed renal artery stenosis should be suspected. Dosage reduction of Innovace and/or discontinuation of the diuretic should be considered.

Hyperkalaemia and hyponatraemia have also been reported in a few cases (for further information see *Interaction with other medicaments and other forms of interaction, Plasma potassium*).

Decreases in haemoglobin and haematocrit as well as elevation of liver enzymes and/or serum bilirubin have been reported in a few patients, and are usually reversible upon discontinuation of Innovace.

Decreases in platelets and white cell count, and rare cases of neutropenia, thrombocytopenia, bone-marrow depression, and agranulocytosis have been reported, but a causal relationship to Innovace has not been established.

*Overdose:* Limited data are available for overdosage in humans. The most prominent features of overdosage reported to date are marked hypotension, beginning some six hours after ingestion of tablets, concomitant with blockade of the renin-angiotensin-aldosterone system, and stupor. Serum enalaprilat levels 100 times and 200 times higher than usually seen after therapeutic doses have been reported after ingestion of 300 mg and 440 mg of enalapril, respectively.

The recommended treatment of overdosage is intravenous infusion of normal saline solution. If ingestion is recent, induce emesis. Innovace can be removed from the general circulation by haemodialysis.

### Pharmacological properties

*Pharmacodynamic properties:* Innovace is the maleate salt of enalapril, a derivative of two amino acids; L-alanine and L-proline. Angiotensin-converting enzyme (ACE) is a peptidyl dipeptidase which catalyses the conversion of angiotensin I to the pressor substance angiotensin II. After absorption Innovace is hydrolysed to enalaprilat which inhibits ACE. Inhibition of ACE results in decreased plasma renin activity (due to removal of negative feedback of renin release) and decreased aldosterone secretion.

ACE is identical to kinase II, and may therefore block the degradation of bradykinin. The possible role of this mechanism in the therapeutic effects of enalapril has not yet been elucidated.

While the mechanism through which Innovace lowers blood pressure is believed to be primarily suppression of the renin-angiotensin-aldosterone system, which plays a major role in the regulation of blood pressure, Innovace is anthypertensive even in patients with low-renin hypertension.

*Pharmacokinetic properties:* Innovace is rapidly absorbed, with peak serum concentrations of enalapril occurring within one hour. Based on urinary recovery, the extent of absorption of enalapril from Innovace is approximately 60%.

Following absorption, Innovace is rapidly and extensively hydrolysed to enalaprilat. Peak serum concentrations of enalaprilat occur 3 to 4 hours after an oral dose of Innovace. Excretion of Innovace is primarily renal. The principal components in urine are enalaprilat, accounting for about 40% of the dose and intact enalapril. In subjects with normal renal function, steady state serum concentrations of enalaprilat were achieved by the fourth day of administration. The effective half-life for accumulation of enalaprilat following multiple doses of Innovace is 11 hours. Accumulation may occur, however in patients with severely impaired renal function, and the dosage of enalapril should be adjusted accordingly. The absorption of Innovace is not influenced by the presence of food in the gastro-intestinal tract. The extent of absorption and hydrolysis of enalapril are similar for the various doses in the recommended therapeutic range.

*Preclinical safety data:* No relevant information.

### Pharmaceutical particulars

*List of excipients:* All Innovace Tablets contain the following inactive ingredients: Lactose PhEur; Magnesium Stearate PhEur; Maize Starch PhEur; Pregelatinised Maize Starch BP; Sodium Bicarbonate PhEur. In addition the red 10 mg tablets contain red iron oxide E172 and the peach-coloured 20 mg tablets containing red iron oxide E172 and yellow iron oxide E172.

*Incompatibilities:* None.

*Shelf life:* 36 months.

*Special precautions for storage:* Store in a dry place below 25°C.

*Nature and contents of container:* Innovace Tablets are available in calendar packs of 28

*Instructions for use/handling:* None.

**Marketing authorisation numbers**

| | |
|---|---|
| 2.5 mg tablet | 0025/0220 |
| 5 mg tablet | 0025/0194 |
| 10 mg tablet | 0025/0195 |
| 20 mg tablet | 0025/0196 |

**Date of approval/revision of SPC** April 1997

**Legal category** POM

## INNOZIDE*

**Presentation** Round, fluted, yellow tablets with MSD 718 on one side and scored. Each tablet contains 20 mg enalapril maleate and 12.5 mg hydrochlorothiazide.

**Uses** For the treatment of mild to moderate hypertension in patients who have been stabilised on the individual components given in the same proportions.

*Mode of action:* Innozide is a combination of an angiotensin-converting enzyme inhibitor (enalapril maleate) and a diuretic (hydrochlorothiazide).

Innozide is highly effective in the treatment of hypertension. The antihypertensive effects of the two components are additive and are sustained for at least 24 hours. A higher percentage of patients with hypertension respond satisfactorily to Innozide than to either component administered alone.

Enalaprilat, the active metabolite of enalapril maleate, is a highly specific, long-acting, non-sulphydryl angiotensin-converting enzyme inhibitor. Enalapril maleate modulates a specific physiological mechanism, the renin-angiotensin-aldosterone system, which plays a major role in the regulation of blood pressure.

Hydrochlorothiazide is a diuretic and antihypertensive agent. Use of this agent alone results in increased renin secretion. Although enalapril maleate alone is antihypertensive, concomitant administration with hydrochlorothiazide results in a greater reduction in blood pressure. Enalapril maleate attenuates the potassium loss associated with hydrochlorothiazide.

**Dosage and administration** The dosage of Innozide should be determined primarily by the experience with the enalapril maleate component.

*Adults*

*Essential hypertension:* The usual dosage is one tablet, taken once daily. If necessary, the dosage may be increased to two tablets, taken once daily.

*Prior diuretic therapy:* Symptomatic hypotension may occur following the initial dose of Innozide; this is more likely in patients who are volume and/or salt depleted as a result of prior diuretic therapy. The diuretic therapy should be discontinued for 2–3 days prior to initiation of therapy with Innozide.

*Dosage in renal insufficiency:* Thiazides may not be appropriate diuretics for use in patients with renal impairment and are ineffective at creatinine clearance values of 30 ml/min or below (i.e. moderate or severe renal insufficiency).

In patients with creatinine clearance of >30 and <80 ml/min, Innozide should be used only after titration of the individual components.

*Use in the elderly:* In clinical studies the efficacy and tolerability of enalapril maleate and hydrochlorothiazide, administered concomitantly, were similar in both elderly and younger hypertensive patients.

*Paediatric use:* Safety and effectiveness in children have not been established.

### Contra-indications, warnings, etc

*Contra-indications:* Innozide is contra-indicated in patients with anuria.

Innozide is contra-indicated in patients who are hypersensitive to any component of the product and in patients with a history of angioneurotic oedema relating to previous treatment with an angiotensin-converting enzyme inhibitor.

Innozide is contra-indicated in patients who are hypersensitive to other sulphonamide-derived drugs.

Innozide is contra-indicated in pregnancy. ACE inhibitors have been shown to be fetotoxic in rabbits during middle and late pregnancy. Effects of exposure of the fetus to ACE inhibitors during the first trimester of human pregnancy are unknown. Fetal exposure during the second and third trimesters of pregnancy has been associated with fetal and neonatal morbidity and mortality. ACE inhibitors in human pregnancy have been associated with oligohydramnios. Hypotension and renal failure have occurred in the newborn.

See also 'Breast-feeding mothers' under 'Precautions'.

*Precautions*

*Hypotension and electrolyte/fluid imbalance:* As with all antihypertensive therapy, symptomatic hypoten-

sion may occur in some patients. This was rarely seen in uncomplicated hypertensive patients but is more likely in the presence of fluid or electrolyte imbalance, e.g. volume depletion, hyponatraemia, hypochloraemic alkalosis, hypomagnesaemia or hypokalaemia which may occur from prior diuretic therapy, dietary salt restriction, dialysis, or during intercurrent diarrhoea or vomiting. Periodic determination of serum electrolytes should be performed at appropriate intervals in such patients.

Particular consideration should be given when therapy is administered to patients with ischaemic heart or cerebrovascular disease because an excessive fall in blood pressure could result in a myocardial infarction or cerebrovascular accident.

If hypotension occurs, the patient should be placed in the supine position and, if necessary, should receive an intravenous infusion of normal saline. A transient hypotensive response is not a contra-indication to further doses. Following restoration of effective blood volume and pressure, reinstitution of therapy at reduced dosage may be possible; or either of the components may be used appropriately alone.

*Renal function impairment:* Thiazides may not be appropriate diuretics for use in patients with renal impairment and are ineffective at creatinine clearance values of 30 ml/min or below (i.e. moderate or severe renal insufficiency).

Innozide should not be administered to patients with renal insufficiency (creatinine clearance ≤80 ml/min) until titration of the individual components has shown the need for the doses present in the combination tablet.

Some hypertensive patients with no apparent pre-existing renal disease have developed usually minor and transient increases in blood urea and serum creatinine when enalapril maleate has been given concomitantly with a diuretic. If this occurs during therapy with Innozide, the combination should be discontinued. Reinstitution of therapy at reduced dosage may be possible, or either of the components may be used appropriately alone.

In some patients, with bilateral renal artery stenosis or stenosis in the artery to a solitary kidney, increases in blood urea and serum creatinine, reversible upon discontinuation of therapy, have been seen with angiotensin-converting enzyme (ACE) inhibitors.

*Haemodialysis patients:* A high incidence of anaphylactoid reactions has been reported in patients dialysed with high-flux membranes and treated concomitantly with an ACE inhibitor. This combination should therefore be avoided.

*Anaphylactic reactions during LDL apheresis:* Rarely, patients receiving ACE inhibitors during low-density lipoprotein (LDL) apheresis with dextran sulphate have experienced life-threatening anaphylactoid reactions. These reactions were avoided by temporarily withholding ACE-inhibitor therapy prior to each apheresis.

*Hepatic disease:* Thiazides should be used with caution in patients with impaired hepatic function or progressive liver disease, since minor alterations of fluid and electrolyte balance may precipitate hepatic coma.

*Surgery/anaesthesia:* In patients undergoing major surgery or during anaesthesia with agents that produce hypotension, enalaprilat blocks angiotensin-II formation secondary to compensatory renin release. If hypotension occurs and is considered to be due to this mechanism, it can be corrected by volume expansion.

*Metabolic and endocrine effects:* Thiazide therapy may impair glucose tolerance. Dosage adjustment of antidiabetic agents, including insulin, may be required.

Thiazides may decrease urinary calcium excretion and may cause intermittent and slight elevation of serum calcium. Marked hypercalcaemia may be evidence of hidden hyperparathyroidism. Thiazides should be discontinued before carrying out tests for parathyroid function.

Increases in cholesterol and triglyceride levels may be associated with thiazide diuretic therapy; however, at the 12.5 mg dose contained in Innozide, minimal or no effect was reported.

Thiazide therapy may precipitate hyperuricaemia and/or gout in certain patients. However, enalapril may increase urinary uric acid and thus may attenuate the hyperuricaemic effect of hydrochlorothiazide.

*Hypersensitivity/angioneurotic oedema:* Angioneurotic oedema of the face, extremities, lips, tongue, glottis and/or larynx has been reported rarely in patients treated with angiotensin-converting enzyme inhibitors, including enalapril maleate. This may occur any time during treatment. In such cases, enalapril maleate should be discontinued promptly and appropriate monitoring should be carried out to ensure complete resolution of symptoms before dismissing the patient.

In those instances where swelling has been confined

to the face and lips the condition generally resolved without treatment, although antihistamines have been useful in relieving symptoms.

Angioneurotic oedema associated with laryngeal oedema may be fatal. Where there is involvement of the tongue, glottis or larynx, likely to cause airway obstruction, appropriate therapy such as subcutaneous adrenaline solution 1:1000 (0.3 ml to 0.5 ml) should be administered promptly.

Patients with a history of angioedema unrelated to ACE-inhibitor therapy may be at increased risk of angioedema while receiving an ACE inhibitor. (See also: 'Contra-indications').

In patients receiving thiazides, sensitivity reactions may occur with or without a history of allergy or bronchial asthma. Exacerbation or activation of systemic lupus erythematosus has been reported with the use of thiazides.

*Anaphylactoid reactions during Hymenoptera desensitisation:* Rarely, patients receiving ACE inhibitors during desensitisation with hymenoptera venom (e.g. Bee or Wasp venom) have experienced life-threatening anaphylactoid reactions. These reactions were avoided by temporarily withholding ACE-inhibitor therapy prior to each desensitisation.

*Cough:* Cough has been reported with the use of ACE inhibitors. Characteristically, the cough is non-productive, persistent and resolves after discontinuation of therapy. ACE inhibitor-induced cough should be considered as part of the differential diagnosis of cough.

*Breast-feeding mothers:* Enalapril, enalaprilat and thiazides appear in human milk. If use of Innozide is deemed essential, breast-feeding should stop.

*Drug Interactions*
*Serum potassium:* The potassium-losing effect of thiazide diuretics is usually attenuated by the effect of enalapril maleate. Serum potassium usually remains within normal limits, although in clinical trials with enalapril maleate hyperkalaemia did occur in a few cases.

The use of potassium supplements, potassium-sparing agents or potassium-containing salt substitutes, particularly in patients with impaired renal function, may lead to a significant increase in serum potassium. If concomitant use of 'Innozide' and any of these agents is deemed appropriate, they should be used with caution and with frequent monitoring of serum potassium.

*Lithium:* Lithium generally should not be given with diuretics or ACE inhibitors (ACE-I). Diuretic agents and ACE-I reduce the renal clearance of lithium and add a high risk of lithium toxicity. Refer to the prescribing information for lithium preparations before use of such preparations.

*Non-depolarising muscle relaxants:* Thiazides may increase the responsiveness to tubocurarine.

*Other agents:* The combination of enalapril maleate with beta-adrenergic blocking agents, methyldopa, or calcium entry blockers has been shown to improve the efficacy of lowering the blood pressure.

Ganglionic-blocking agents or adrenergic-blocking agents, combined with enalapril, should only be administered under careful observation of the patient.

When administered concurrently, the following drugs may interact with thiazide diuretics:

*Alcohol, barbiturates, narcotics or phenothiazines:* Potentiation of orthostatic hypotension may occur.

*Antidiabetic drugs* (oral agents and insulin): Dosage adjustment of the antidiabetic drug may be required.

*Corticosteroids, ACTH:* Intensified electrolyte depletion, particularly hypokalaemia.

*Pressor amines (e.g. adrenaline):* Possible decreased response to pressor amines but not sufficient to preclude their use.

*Non-steroidal anti-inflammatory drugs:* In some patients, the administration of non-steroidal anti-inflammatory agent can reduce the diuretic, natriuretic, and antihypertensive effects of diuretics.

*Side-effects:* Innozide is usually well tolerated. In clinical studies, side effects have usually been mild and transient, and in most instances have not required interruption of therapy.

The most common clinical side-effects were dizziness and fatigue, which generally responded to dosage reduction and seldom required discontinuation of therapy.

Other side-effects (1–2%) were: Muscle cramps, nausea, asthenia, orthostatic effects including hypotension, headache, cough, and impotence.

Less common side-effects which occurred either during controlled trials or during marketed use include:

*Cardiovascular:* Syncope, non-orthostatic hypotension, palpitation, tachycardia, chest pain.

*Gastro-intestinal:* Pancreatitis, diarrhoea, vomiting, dyspepsia, abdominal pain, flatulence, constipation. Pancreatitis has been reported rarely with enalapril

and with hydrochlorothiazide and, therefore, is a potential side-effect of Innozide.

*Nervous system/psychiatric:* Insomnia, somnolence, paraesthesia, vertigo, nervousness.

*Respiratory:* Dyspnoea.

*Skin:* Stevens–Johnson syndrome, rash, pruritis, diaphoresis.

*Other:* Renal dysfunction, renal failure, decreased libido, dry mouth, gout, tinnitus, arthralgia.

A symptom complex has been reported which may include fever, serositis, vasculitis, myalgia/myositis, arthralgia/arthritis, a positive ANA, elevated ESR, eosinophilia and leucocytosis. Rash, photosensitivity or other dermatological manifestations may occur.

*Hypersensitivity/angioneurotic oedema:* Angioneurotic oedema of the face, extremities, lips, tongue, glottis and/or larynx has been reported rarely (see 'Precautions').

*Side-effects due to individual components:* Additional side-effects that have been seen with one of the individual components and may be potential side-effects with Innozide are the following:

*Enalapril maleate:* Ileus, hepatic failure, hepatitis – either hepatocellular or cholestatic jaundice, depression, confusion, pulmonary infiltrates, bronchospasm/asthma, rhythm disturbances, angina pectoris, myocardial infarction or cerebrovascular accident, rhinorrhoea, photosensitivity, alopecia, flushing, taste alteration, anorexia, blurred vision, urticaria, stomatitis, glossitis, oliguria, toxic epidermal necrolysis, erythema multiforme, exfoliative dermatitis, pemphigus.

*Hydrochlorothiazide:* Anorexia, gastric irritation, constipation, jaundice (intrahepatic cholestatic jaundice), sialoadenitis, vertigo, xanthopsia, leucopenia, agranulocytosis, thrombocytopenia, aplastic anaemia, haemolytic anaemia, purpura, photosensitivity, fever, urticaria, necrotising angiitis (vasculitis), respiratory distress (including pneumonitis and pulmonary oedema), anaphylactic reaction, glycosuria, electrolyte imbalance including hyponatraemia, restlessness, muscle spasm, transient blurred vision.

*Laboratory test findings:* Clinically important changes in standard laboratory parameters were rarely associated with administration of 'Innozide'. Occasional hyperglycaemia, hyperuricaemia and hyper- or hypokalaemia have been noted. Increases in blood urea and serum creatinine, and elevations of liver enzymes and/or serum bilirubin have been seen. Decreases in haemoglobin and haematocrit have been reported in hypertensive patients treated with Innozide. These are usually reversible upon discontinuation of Innozide.

Decreases in platelets and white cell count, and rare cases of neutropenia, thrombocytopenia and bone marrow depression have been reported, but a causal relationship to 'Innozide' has not been established.

Hyponatraemia has occurred with enalapril and may be a potential finding with 'Innozide'.

*Overdosage:* No specific information is available on the treatment of overdosage with 'Innozide'. Treatment is symptomatic and supportive. Therapy with 'Innozide' should be discontinued and the patient observed closely. Suggested measures include induction of emesis and/or gastric lavage, and correction of dehydration, electrolyte imbalance and hypotension by established procedures.

*Enalapril maleate:* The most prominent feature of overdosage reported to date is marked hypotension, beginning some six hours after ingestion of tablets, concomitant with blockade of the renin-angiotensin system, and stupor. Serum enelaprilat levels 100 times and 200 times higher than usually seen after therapeutic doses have been reported after ingestion of 300 mg and 440 mg of enalapril maleate respectively.

Enalaprilat may be removed from the general circulation by haemodialysis.

*Hydrochlorothiazide:* The most common signs and symptoms observed are those caused by electrolyte depletion (hypokalaemia, hypochloraemia, hyponatraemia) and dehydration resulting from excessive diuresis. If digitalis has also been administered, hypokalaemia may accentuate cardiac arrhythmias.

**Pharmaceutical precautions** Store in a dry place below 25°C.

**Legal category** POM.

**Package quantities** Calendar pack of 28 tablets.

**Further information** Nil.

**Product licence number** 0025/0249.

## MEFOXIN* INJECTION

**Presentation** In vials containing 1 g or 2 g of cefoxitin as the sodium salt. Each gram of cefoxitin contains approximately 2.3 mEq sodium.

**Uses** Mefoxin is indicated for the treatment of the following infections caused by sensitive bacteria: peritonitis and other intra-abdominal and intrapelvic infections; gonorrhoea; female genital tract infections; septicaemia; urinary tract infections; respiratory tract infections; bone and joint infections; and skin and soft-tissue infections.

Mefoxin is a broad-spectrum bactericidal antibiotic indicated for the treatment of infections caused by susceptible strains of Gram-positive and Gram-negative pathogens both aerobic and anaerobic.

Mefoxin has been clinically effective not only in infections due to antibiotic-sensitive organisms, but also in infections due to organisms resistant to one or more of the following antibacterial agents: penicillin, ampicillin, carbenicillin, tetracyclines, erythromycin, chloramphenicol, cephalosporins, kanamycin, gentamicin, tobramycin, and sulphamethoxazole-trimethoprim.

Many Gram-negative pathogens are resistant to penicillins and cephalosporins through the action of the beta-lactamases which are produced by these pathogens. Mefoxin is remarkably stable in the presence of these bacterial beta-lactamases, both penicillinases and cephalosporinases. Hence, the clinical efficacy of Mefoxin extends to many infections caused by such pathogens.

Mefoxin is indicated for the treatment of mixed infections caused by susceptible strains of aerobic and anaerobic bacteria. The majority of these mixed infections are associated with contamination by faecal flora as well as flora originating from the vagina, skin, and mouth. In these mixed infections, *Bacteroides fragilis* is the most commonly encountered anaerobic pathogen and is usually resistant to aminoglycosides, cephalosporins, and virtually all penicillins. However, *Bacteroides fragilis* is usually susceptible to Mefoxin.

Mefoxin is indicated for adjunctive therapy in the surgical treatment of infections, including abscesses, infection complicating hollow visceral perforations, cutaneous infections, and infections of serous surfaces, whether caused by aerobes, mixed aerobes and anaerobes, or anaerobes.

Clinical experience has demonstrated that Mefoxin can be administered to patients who are also receiving carbenicillin, kanamycin, gentamicin, tobramycin, or amikacin (see 'Precautions' and 'Dosage and administration').

*Prophylaxis:* Mefoxin is indicated for the prevention of certain post-operative infections in patients undergoing contaminated or potentially contaminated surgical procedures or where the occurrence of post-operative infection could be especially serious.

*Microbiology:* Mefoxin is active *in vitro* against: Aerobic bacteria: *Gram-positive cocci* including: *Staphylococci:* (including coagulase-positive, coagulase-negative, and penicillinase-producing strains); Group A beta-haemolytic streptococci (*Streptococcus pyogenes*); Group B beta-haemolytic streptococci (*Streptococcus agalactiae*); *Streptococcus pneumoniae* (*Diplococcus pneumoniae*); other streptococci (except group D streptococci including enterococci, most strains of which are resistant, e.g. *Streptococcus faecalis*), *Gram-negative cocci* including: *Neisseria gonorrhoeae* (including penicillinase-producing strains); *Neisseria meningitidis. Gram-negative rods* (facultative anaerobes) including: *Escherichia coli; Klebsiella pneumoniae; Klebsiella* spp.; *Proteus mirabilis. Proteus* (indole-positive): *Morganella morganii* (formerly *Proteus morganii*); *Proteus vulgaris; Haemophilus influenzae; Serratia marcescens; Providencia* spp.; *Providencia rettgeri* (formerly *Proteus rettgeri*); *Salmonella* and *Shigella* spp.

Anaerobic bacteria: *Gram-positive cocci* including: *Peptococcus* spp.; *Peptostreptococcus* spp.; Micro-aerophilic *streptococcus. Gram-positive rods* including: *Clostridium perfringens; Clostridium* spp.; *Eubacterium* spp.; *Propionibacterium acnes. Gram-negative cocci* including: *Veillonella* spp. *Gram-negative rods* including: *Bacteroides fragilis; Bacteroides melaninogenicus; Bacteroides* spp. (including both penicillin-susceptible and penicillin-resistant strains); *Fusobacterium* spp.

Mefoxin is active against some strains of the following bacteria: *Acinetobacter calcoaceticus var. anitratum* (*Herellea vaginicola*); *Acinetobacter calcoaceticus var. lwoffi* (*Mima polymorpha*); *Alcaligenes faecalis; Citrobacter* spp. and *Flavo-bacterium* spp.; *Enterobacter* spp.

Mefoxin is not active against *Pseudomonas* spp., most strains of enterococci, many strains of *Enterobacter cloacae*, and methicillin-resistant staphylococci, and *Listeria monocytogenes.*

*Human pharmacology:* Mefoxin administered parenterally, produces high serum and urine concentrations. It is excreted virtually unchanged as active Mefoxin by the kidneys, and has a mean terminal serum half-life of approximately one hour. Mefoxin passes rapidly into body fluids such as pleural, bile, and ascitic fluids. Probenecid slows tubular excretion and increases and prolongs blood levels.

*Intravenous:* Peak serum concentrations of Mefoxin following 1 g infused intravenously over 3 minutes was 125 micrograms/ml, infused over 30 minutes was 72 micrograms/ml, and infused over 120 minutes was 25 micrograms/ml. Following 2 g infused intravenously over 3 minutes, peak serum concentration was 221 micrograms/ml. In a number of studies using 0.5 g, 1 g, or 2 g intravenous doses of Mefoxin mean total urinary recovery ranged from 77% to 99% of the cefoxitin dose.

*Intramuscular:* When Mefoxin was reconstituted for intramuscular injection with 0.5% or 1% lidocaine (lignocaine) hydrochloride, the lidocaine (lignocaine) had no effect on the absorption or elimination of Mefoxin.

Intramuscular injections of 1 g of Mefoxin in 0.5% lidocaine (lignocaine) hydrochloride solution produced a peak serum concentration of 30 micrograms/ml at 20 minutes. Approximately 85% of an intramuscular dose is excreted by the kidneys in the first six hours; this results in high urine levels (e.g. >3,000 micrograms/ml between one and two hours after a 1 g dose).

**Dosage and administration** Mefoxin may be administered intravenously or intramuscularly. (See reconstitution directions for each route below.) Dosage and route of administration should be determined by severity of infection, susceptibility of the causative organisms, and condition of the patient.

Therapy may be started while awaiting the results of susceptibility testing.

Usual adult dosage

| *Type of infection* | *Dose (g)* | *Frequency (hrs)* | *Total daily dosage* |
|---|---|---|---|
| Uncomplicated | 1 | Every 8 (occasionally every 6) | 3 g (4 g) |
| Moderately severe or severe | 2 | Every 8 (occasionally every 6) | 6 g (8 g) |
| Infections generally needing antibiotics in higher dosage | 3 (2) | Every 6 (every 4) | 12 g |

Maintenance dosage of Mefoxin in adults with reduced renal function

| Renal function | Creatinine clearance (ml/min) | Dose (g) | Frequency (hrs) |
|---|---|---|---|
| Mild impairment | 50–30 | 1–2 | Every 8–12 |
| Moderate impairment | 29–10 | 1–2 | Every 12–24 |
| Severe impairment | 9–5 | 0.5–1 | Every 12–24 |
| Essentially no function | <5 | 0.5–1 | Every 24–48 |

*Adults Dosage:* The usual dosage is 1 g or 2 g of Mefoxin every eight hours. (See 'Usual adult dosage' chart.)

In adults with renal insufficiency, an initial loading dose of 1 g to 2 g may be given. After a loading dose, the following recommendations for *maintenance dosage* may be used as a guide.

In the patients undergoing haemodialysis, the loading dose of 1–2 g should be given after each haemodialysis, and the maintenance dose should be given as indicated in the chart giving 'Maintenance dosage of Mefoxin in adults with reduced renal function'.

*Uncomplicated urinary tract infections:* In uncomplicated urinary tract infections due to susceptible organisms, 1 g intramuscularly twice a day for ten days has been shown to be effective.

*Uncomplicated gonorrhoea:* For single dose therapy of uncomplicated gonorrhoea, including that caused by penicillinase-producing strains, the recommended dose is 2 g of Mefoxin intramuscularly given with 1 g of probenecid by mouth (at the same time or up to one hour before).

*Neonates, infants and children:*

| | |
|---|---|
| *Neonates** | |
| 0–1 week of age | 20–40 mg/kg every 12 hours |
| 1–4 weeks of age | 20–40 mg/kg every 8 hours |
| *Infants** | 20–40 mg/kg every 6 hours or every 8 hours |
| *Children* | 20–40 mg/kg every 6 hours or every 8 hours |

*Clinical data are insufficient to recommend use of the intramuscular formulation in infants less than 3 months of age.

In severe infections, the total daily dosage may be increased to 200 mg/kg, but not to exceed 12 g per day.

Mefoxin is not recommended for the therapy of meningitis. If meningitis is suspected an appropriate antibiotic should be used.

In children with renal insufficiency dosage frequency should be reduced as indicated for adults.

*Prophylactic administration to adults:* 2 g administered intramuscularly or intravenously just prior to surgery (½–1 hour before initial incision), then 2 g every 6 hours. Prophylactic therapy should not usually be given for more than 24 hours.

*Prophylactic administration for neonates, infants and children:* In infants and children, 30–40 mg/kg doses may be given at the same times as designated for adults. However, in neonates, 30–40 mg/kg doses may be given ½ to 1 hour before initial incision and the second and third dose may be given every 8–12 hours.

Clinical data are insufficient to recommend use of the intramuscular formulation in infants less than 3 months of age.

*Obstetric and gynaecological surgery:* For patients undergoing caesarean section, a single 2 g dose is administered intravenously as soon as the cord is clamped. If necessary, a second and third dose of 2 g may be administered intravenously 4 hours and 8 hours after the first dose.

In gynaecological surgical procedures, a single prophylactic dose of 2 g intravenously or intramuscularly has been effective given ½ to 1 hour before surgery.

In prolonged or heavily contaminated cases, additional 2 g doses may be given at 6-hour intervals. Prophylactic therapy does not ordinarily extend beyond 24 hours.

*Intravenous administration:* Reconstitute Mefoxin with Water for Injections BP: 1 g is soluble in 2 ml. Although Mefoxin is very soluble, for intravenous use it is preferable to add 10 ml of Water for Injections BP to the 1 g vial or to the 2 g vial. Shake to dissolve and then withdraw entire contents of vial into syringe.

Solutions of Mefoxin range from clear to light amber in colour. The pH of freshly reconstituted solutions usually ranges from 4.2 to 7.0.

For direct intravenous injection, Mefoxin may be slowly injected into the vein over a period of three to five minutes or may be given through the tubing when the patient is receiving parenteral solutions.

An intermittent intravenous infusion of Mefoxin may be employed when large amounts of fluid are to be given. However, during infusion of the solution containing Mefoxin, it may be advisable temporarily to discontinue administration of any other infusion solution at the same site (by using an appropriate IV infusion set).

A solution of Mefoxin may also be given by continuous intravenous infusion (see below for compatibility and stability).

*Intramuscular administration ONLY:* Reconstitute Mefoxin 1 g with 2 ml of Water for Injections BP, or 0.5% or 1% lidocaine (lignocaine) hydrochloride (without adrenaline) solution. Mefoxin is given by deep injection into a large muscle mass. Avoid injection into a blood vessel.

*Note:* Some patients may be hypersensitive to lidocaine (lignocaine).

*Preparation of solution:* The following table is provided for convenience in reconstituting Mefoxin for both intravenous and intramuscular administration.

| *Strength* | *Amount of diluent to be added (ml*)* | *Approximate final volume (ml)* | *Approximate average concentration (mg/ml)* |
|---|---|---|---|
| 1 gram vial | 2 (Intramuscular) | 2.5 | 400 |
| 1 gram vial | 10 (IV) | 10.5 | 95 |
| 2 gram vial | 10 or 20 (IV) | 11 or 21 | 180 or 95 |

* Shake to dissolve and let stand until clear.

*Compatibility and stability:* A solution of Mefoxin in Water for Injections BP may be added to the following solutions: 0.9% Sodium Chloride Injection BP, 5% or 10% Dextrose Injection BP, Dextrose and Sodium Chloride Injection BP (5%/0.9%, 5%/0.45%, or 5%/0.2%). Lactated Ringer's Injection USP, 5% Dextrose Injection in 0.02% sodium bicarbonate solution, 5% Dextrose in Lactated Ringer's Injection, 5% or 10% invert sugar in water, 10% invert sugar in saline solution, 5% Sodium Bicarbonate Injection BP, M/6 Sodium Lactate Injection BP, insulin (in normal saline or 10% invert sugar), heparin (100 units/ml and 0.1 units/ml), mannitol (2.5%, 5% and 10%).

Mefoxin has been shown to be chemically and visually compatible with aminoglycosides such as amikacin, gentamicin, kanamycin, and tobramycin mixed in 200 ml of 0.9% sodium chloride or 5% dextrose in water.

*Use in the elderly:* The dosage should be determined by the severity of the infection, the susceptibility of the causative organisms, the patient's clinical condition and renal function.

**Contra-indications, warnings, etc**

*Contra-indications:* Mefoxin is contra-indicated in persons who have shown hypersensitivity to cefoxitin. In the absence of clinical experience, Mefoxin should not be administered to patients who have shown hypersensitivity to cephalosporins.

*Precautions:* There is some clinical and laboratory evidence of partial cross-allergenicity between cephamycins and other beta-lactam antibiotics, penicillins, and cephalosporins. Severe reactions (including anaphylaxis) have been reported with most beta-lactam antibiotics.

Before therapy with Mefoxin, careful inquiry should be made concerning previous hypersensitivity reactions to beta-lactam antibiotics. Mefoxin should be given cautiously to penicillin-allergic patients.

Any patient who has demonstrated some form of allergy, particularly to drugs, should receive antibiotics cautiously. If an allergic reaction to Mefoxin occurs, the drug should be discontinued.

Pseudomembranous colitis, reported with virtually all antibiotics, can range from mild to life threatening in severity. Antibiotics should be prescribed with caution in patients with a history of gastro-intestinal disease, particularly colitis. Treatment-related diarrhoea should always be considered as a pointer to this diagnosis. While studies indicate that a toxin of *Clostridium difficile* is one of the primary causes of antibiotic-related colitis, other causes should be considered.

The total daily dosage should be reduced when Mefoxin is administered to patients with transient or persistent reduction of urinary output due to renal insufficiency (see 'Dosage and administration') because high and prolonged serum antibiotic concentrations can occur from usual doses.

*Interference with laboratory tests:* A false-positive reaction to glucose in the urine may occur with reducing substances but not with the use of specific glucose oxidase methods.

Using the Jaffe technique, falsely high creatinine values in serum may occur if Mefoxin serum concentrations exceed 100 mcg/ml. Serum samples from patients treated with Mefoxin should not be analysed for creatinine if withdrawn within two hours of drug administration.

High concentration of cefoxitin in the urine may interfere with the measurement of 17-hydroxy-corticosteroids by the Porter-Silber reaction to give slight, falsely increased results.

*Use in pregnancy:* Use of the drug in women of childbearing potential requires that the anticipated benefits be weighed against possible hazards. Reproductive and teratogenic studies have been performed in mice and rats and have revealed no evidence of impaired fertility or harm to the fetus due to Mefoxin. There are no controlled studies with Mefoxin in pregnant women.

*Nursing mothers:* Mefoxin is excreted in human milk. Caution should be exercised if use is indicated.

*Side-effects:* Mefoxin is generally well tolerated. Side-effects have usually been mild and transient and treatment rarely needs to be stopped. The most common side effects have been local reactions following intravenous or intramuscular injection.

*Local reactions:* Thrombophlebitis has occurred with intravenous administration. Pain, induration and tenderness after intramuscular injections have been reported.

*Allergic:* Rash (including exfoliative dermatitis and toxic epidermal necrolysis), urticaria, pruritus, eosinophilia, fever and other allergic reactions (including anaphylaxis, interstitial nephritis and angioedema) have been reported.

*Cardiovascular:* Hypotension.

*Gastro-intestinal:* Diarrhoea, including pseudomembraneous colitis can appear during or after antibiotic treatment. Nausea and vomiting have been reported rarely.

*Blood:* Eosinophilia, leucopenia including granulocytopenia, neutropenia, anaemia including haemolytic anaemia, thrombocytopenia and bone-marrow depression have been reported. Some individuals, particularly those with azotaemia, may develop positive direct Coombs tests during therapy with Mefoxin.

*Musculoskeletal:* Worsening myasthenia gravis (single case).

*Liver function:* Transient elevations in AST (SGOT), ALT (SGPT), serum LDH, serum alkaline phosphatase and jaundice have been reported.

*Kidney function:* Elevations in serum creatinine and/or blood urea levels have been observed. Acute renal failure has been reported rarely. The role of Mefoxin in changes in renal function tests is difficult to assess, since factors predisposing to pre-renal azotaemia or to impaired renal function usually have been present.

*Overdosage:* No specific information is available on the treatment of overdose with Mefoxin.

After injection, cefoxitin has a half-life between 45 and 60 minutes with a 70% binding to plasma proteins.

The parenteral dose of Mefoxin is carefully controlled by the physician and no case of overdosage has been recorded. No known antidote is available.

**Pharmaceutical precautions** Mefoxin may be reconstituted with Water for Injections BP, Water for Injections BP preserved with parabens or benzyl alcohol, 0.9% Sodium Chloride Injection BP, 5% Dextrose Injection BP, or 0.5% and 1.0% lidocaine (lignocaine) hydrochloride (preserved in parabens). When reconstituting Mefoxin for neonates, Water for Injections must be preservative free.

Mefoxin, as reconstituted above, maintains satisfactory potency for 24 hours at room temperature, for one week under refrigeration (below 5°C) and for at least 30 weeks in the frozen state and will maintain potency after thawing for at least 24 hours at room temperature.

In keeping with good clinical and pharmaceutical practice, 'Mefoxin' should be administered as a freshly prepared solution. If circumstances make this impracticable, reconstituted material, should be used on the same day and stored at 2°C to 8°C before use.

*Note:* Mefoxin in the dry state should be stored below 30°C. The dry material as well as solutions tend to darken, depending on storage conditions; product potency, however, is not adversely affected.

**Legal category** POM.

**Package quantities** Sterile Mefoxin is supplied in vials containing 1 g or 2 g of cefoxitin as the sodium salt, both strengths available in packs of 5 vials.

**Further information** Nil.

**Product licence numbers**
1 g   0025/0130
2 g   0025/0131

## MINTEZOL*

**Presentation** Orange-coloured chewable tablets, marked 'MSD 907', containing 500 mg Thiabendazole BP.

**Uses** Anthelmintic.

Mintezol is indicated as primary treatment against Strongyloidiasis; Cutaneous larva migrans (creeping eruption); Dracunculiasis (guinea worm); Visceral larva migrans.

Mintezol is indicated as secondary treatment against Enterobiasis (threadworm) when the infestation is mixed with a primary indication.

Mintezol can relieve the symptoms and fever of trichinosis during the invasion stage.

Mintezol is indicated (a) when specific therapy is unavailable, (b) when other therapy cannot be used or (c) as additive therapy against *Necator americanus* and *Ancylostoma duodenale* (hookworm); *Trichuriasis* (whipworm); *Ascariasis* (large roundworm).

**Dosage and administration** Dosage depends on the body weight of the patient and is independent of the condition being treated. Usually, 2 doses are given each day. For patients weighing less than 60 kg (132 lb), each dose is based on 25 mg thiabendazole per kg body weight. For patients weighing 60 kg or more, each dose is 1.5 g thiabendazole. The maximum daily dosage for adults weighing 60 kg or more is 3 g.

Mintezol should be taken with meals and chewed before swallowing. Dietary restrictions, complementary medications and cleansing enemas are not necessary.

The table below relates dosage to body weight:

| Patient's weight | | Dose (twice daily) |
|---|---|---|
| kg | lb | Tablets (500 mg thiabendazole) |
| 10 | 22 | ½ |
| 20 | 44 | 1 |
| 30 | 66 | 1½ |
| 40 | 88 | 2 |
| 50 | 110 | 2½ |
| 60 (or more) | 132 (or more) | 3 |

Clinical experience, as well as safety experience in children weighing less than 15 kg has been limited. Duration of therapy depends on the particular nematode infestation, and is as follows:

*Strongyloidiasis, ascariasis, uncinariasis and trichuriasis:* 2 doses a day for two successive days. Alternatively, a single dose of 50 mg/kg may be given, but a higher incidence of side-effects would be expected.

*Cutaneous larva migrans:* 2 doses a day for two successive days. If active lesions are still present two days after completion of this therapy, a second similar course is recommended.

*Visceral larva migrans:* 2 doses a day for 7 successive days. (Safety and efficacy data on this duration of treatment are limited.)

*Trichinosis:* 2 doses a day for two to four successive days, according to the response of the patient. The optimum dosage in trichinosis has not yet been established.

*Dracunculiasis:* 50–100 mg/kg in two equally divided doses for one day. The lower dosage for patients with 1 or 2 visible worms; the higher dosage for patients with multiple infection (3 or more worms). In massive infections (10 worms or more), a second dose of 50 mg/kg can be given five to eight days after treatment, if required.

*Further considerations:* In certain patients, 2 doses a day may lead to a higher incidence of side-effects. In these circumstances, 25 mg per kg body weight may be given after the largest meal on the first day and repeated 24 hours later after a similar meal on the second day.

For mass treatment, a single dose of 50 mg/kg after the evening meal is highly effective and most convenient, though a higher incidence of side-effects may be expected.

*Use in the elderly:* Since CNS and hepatic side effects have been reported to occur and since excretion is primarily renal, use with caution in elderly patients who have renal, hepatic or CNS dysfunction. As with younger patients, the dosage should be calculated on the basis of body weight.

*Use in children:* Clinical experience, as well as safety experience with thiabendazole treatment in children weighing less than 15 kg has been limited.

**Contra-indications, warnings, etc**
*Contra-indication:* Hypersensitivity to any component of this product.

*Precautions:* If any hypersensitivity reactions occur, therapy should be discontinued immediately and not resumed. Erythema multiforme, including fatal cases of Stevens-Johnson syndrome, has been associated with thiabendazole therapy.

Mintezol may impair alertness in some patients, who should avoid driving, operating machinery, or other activities made hazardous by diminished alertness.

Ideally, anaemic, dehydrated or malnourished patients should be given supportive therapy before starting treatment with Mintezol. Liver and renal function should be carefully monitored in patients with disorders of these organs.

Mintezol is not suitable for the treatment of mixed infections with ascaris because it may cause these worms to migrate.

Mintezol should not be used prophylactically.

*Pregnancy and the nursing mother:* Mintezol should not be used during pregnancy or lactation. Reports have suggested that thiabendazole is teratogenic in mice, although reproduction studies in generations of rabbits, rats, sheep, cattle and pigs have shown no fetal abnormalities attributable to the drug. Nevertheless, Mintezol should not be used in women of childbearing potential unless pregnancy has been excluded.

*Drug interactions:* Thiabendazole may compete with other drugs, such as theophylline, for sites of metabolism in the liver and thus elevate the serum levels of such drugs to potentially toxic levels. Therefore, when the concomitant use of thiabendazole and xanthine derivatives is anticipated, it may be necessary to monitor blood levels and/or reduce the dosage of such compounds. Such concomitant use should only be made under careful medical supervision.

*Side-effects:* The most common are anorexia, nausea, vomiting and dizziness. Diarrhoea, epigastric distress, pruritus, weariness, giddiness, headache and drowsiness occur less often.

Rare side-effects are tinnitus, collapse, abnormal sensation in the eyes, blurring of vision, reduced vision, hyperirritability, numbness, hyperglycaemia, yellow vision (in isolated cases these ocular effects persisted for prolonged intervals), enuresis, hypotension, jaundice, transient leucopenia, perianal rash, crystalluria, haematuria, convulsions, psychic disturbances, drying of mucous membranes (mouth, eyes etc.), intrahepatic cholestasis and parenchymal liver damage (in isolated cases liver damage has been severe and irreversible). The appearance of live ascaris in the mouth and nose has been reported on rare occasions.

Hypersensitivity reactions include fever, facial flush, chills, conjunctival injection, angioneurotic oedema, anaphylaxis, skin rashes, erythema multiforme including Stevens-Johnson syndrome, and lymphadenopathy.

Some patients excrete a metabolite which imparts a characteristic odour to their urine, similar to that which occurs after eating asparagus.

*Laboratory test findings:* Rarely a transient rise in cephalin flocculation and aspartate transferase (AST) has occurred in patients receiving Mintezol.

*Overdosage:* The stomach should be emptied promptly either by inducing emesis, if necessary, or by gastric lavage. Toxic disturbances of the GI and CNS systems can be expected and these should be treated symptomatically and supportively. There is no known antidote.

Thiabendazole is readily absorbed from the GI tract with a peak plasma level reached in 1 to 2 hours.

**Pharmaceutical precautions** Store in a dry place below 25°C. Protect from light.

**Legal category** POM.

**Package quantities** *Tablets:* Packs of 6.

**Further information** Nil.

**Product licence number** 0025/5031.

## MODUCREN*

**Presentation** Blue, square, half-scored tablets, marked 'MSD 17', containing 25 mg hydrochlorothiazide, 2.5 mg amiloride hydrochloride, and 10 mg timolol maleate.

**Uses** Mild to moderate hypertension.

**Dosage and administration** 1 to 2 tablets once a day.

*Use in the elderly:* Moducren has been shown to be as well tolerated in the elderly as in younger patients. The recommended starting dose is one tablet daily.

*Children:* Because the safety and efficacy of Moducren has not been established in children, it is not recommended for paediatric use.

**Contra-indications, warnings, etc**
*Contra-indications:* Patients with bronchial asthma or with a history of bronchial asthma, severe chronic obstructive pulmonary disease, sinus bradycardia, second- or third-degree AV block, overt cardiac failure, right ventricular failure secondary to pulmonary hypertension, significant cardiomegaly, and cardiogenic shock. Hyperkalaemia (plasma potassium over 5.5 mmol/l). Anuria, acute and chronic renal insufficiency, severe progressive renal disease and diabetic nephropathy. Patients with blood urea over 10 mmol/l or serum creatinine over 130 mmol/l or diabetes mellitus should not receive Moducren without careful and frequent serum urea and serum electrolyte monitoring.

Anaesthetic agents causing myocardial depression, hypersensitivity to any component of Moducren or other sulphonamide-derived drugs. Use with other potassium-conserving agents. Use with potassium supplements or potassium-rich food except in severe and/or refractory cases of hypokalaemia when careful monitoring of the serum potassium level is necessary.

See also 'Pregnancy', 'Breast-feeding mothers' and 'Children', under 'precautions'.

*Precautions:*
*Congestive cardiac failure:* care should be exercised before and during treatment of patients with cardiomegaly or history of cardiac failure. *Cardiac arrhythmias:* patients at risk of congestive heart failure should be carefully observed for bradycardia, AV block and respiratory distress. If congestive cardiac failure persists, Moducren should be withdrawn. Beta-adrenergic blocking agents should be used with caution in patients with cerebrovascular insufficiency. If signs or symptoms suggesting reduced cerebral blood flow are observed, consideration should be given to discontinuing these agents. *Exacerbation of ischaemic heart disease following abrupt withdrawal:* Exacerbation of angina and, in some cases, myocardial infarction have occurred after abrupt withdrawal of beta-blocker therapy. Therefore, it is recommended that if Moducren is to be withdrawn, dosage should be gradually reduced. *Elective or emergency surgery:* Moducren should also be gradually withdrawn prior to elective surgery of anginal patients. Agonists such as isoprenaline, dopamine, dobutamine or noradrenaline may be used to counter the effects of beta-blockade in emergency surgery. *Renal and hepatic disease and electrolyte disturbances:* Moducren should be used with caution in patients with renal or hepatic disease and in those patients in whom fluid and electrolyte balance is critical. When creatinine clearance falls below 30 ml/min, thiazide diuretics are ineffective. Azotaemia may be precipitated or increased by hydrochlorothiazide. Cumulative effects of the drug may develop in patients with impaired renal function. If increasing azotaemia and oliguria occur during treatment of renal disease, the diuretic should be discontinued. *Metabolic or respiratory acidosis:* acid-base balance should be monitored frequently in severely ill patients at risk of respiratory or metabolic acidosis. *Electrolyte and fluid balance:* serum and urine electrolyte determinations should be made in patients vomiting excessively or receiving parenteral fluids. Dilutional hyponatraemia may occur in oedematous patients in hot weather which calls for appropriate therapy; hypochloraemia requires specific treatment only under exceptional circumstances.

Hyponatraemia, hypochloraemic alkalosis, hypokalaemia, hyperkalaemia or hypomagnesaemia may occur. If hyperkalaemia occurs, Moducren should be discontinued immediately and, if necessary, active measures taken to reduce the plasma potassium level. The degree of thiazide-induced hypomagnesaemia is reduced. *Diabetes mellitus, hypoglycaemia:* Moducren should be given with caution to diabetic patients and to patients subject to spontaneous hypoglycaemia as the symptoms and signs of acute hypoglycaemia may be masked. To minimise the risk of hyperkalaemia in diabetic or suspected diabetic patients, the status of renal function should be known before initiating therapy with Moducren. Therapy should be discontinued for at least three days prior to glucose tolerance testing. Thiazide therapy may impair glucose tolerance. Dosage adjustment of antidiabetic agents, including insulin, may be required. *Skin and sensitivity reactions:* there have been reports of skin rashes and/or dry eyes associated with the use of beta-adrenergic blocking drugs. The reported incidence is small and in most cases the symptoms have cleared when treatment was withdrawn. Discontinuation of the drug should be considered if any such reaction is not otherwise explicable. Withdrawal should be gradual. Sensitivity reactions to Moducren may occur with or without a history of allergy or bronchial asthma. Possible exacerbation or activation of systemic lupus erythematosus reactions have been reported with thiazide diuretics. *Metabolic and endocrine:* beta-adrenergic blocking agents may mask the signs of hyperthyroidism. Patients suspected of developing thyrotoxicosis should be managed carefully to avoid abrupt withdrawal of beta blockade which might precipitate a thyroid storm. Hypercalcaemia and hypophosphataemia have also been reported with thiazide diuretics. Moducren should be discontinued in patients prior to testing for parathyroid function. Increases in cholesterol and triglyceride levels may be associated with thiazide diuretic therapy. Hyperuricaemia or acute gout may be precipitated in some patients. *Musculoskeletal:* beta-blockers have been reported to induce myasthenic symptoms such as diplopia, ptosis, and generalised weakness.

*Drug interactions:* Moducren may potentiate other antihypertensive agents, such as reserpine or guanethidine. The antihypertensive effect of beta-blockers may be reduced by NSAIDs. NSAIDs may reduce the diuretic, natriuretic and antihypertensive effects of diuretics. Its effect may be enhanced in the post-sympathectomy patient.

Oral calcium antagonists may be combined with Moducren only when heart function is normal. When the heart function is impaired, combination of beta-blockers with dihydropyridine derivatives such as nifedipine may lead to hypotension; and combination with verapamil or diltiazem may cause AV conduction disturbances or left ventricular failure. Intravenous calcium antagonists and Moducren should only be used together with caution. Concomitant beta-blockers and digitalis with either diltiazem or verapamil may further prolong the AV conduction time.

When Moducren (which contains amiloride HCl) is administered concomitantly with an angiotensin-converting enzyme inhibitor, the risk of hyperkalaemia may be increased. Therefore, if concomitant use of these agents is indicated because of demonstrated hypokalaemia, they should be used with caution and with frequent monitoring of serum potassium.

When given concomitantly, the following drugs may interact with thiazide diuretics.

*Alcohol, barbiturates, or narcotics:* Co-administration may potentiate orthostatic hypotension. *Oral and parenteral antidiabetic drugs* may require adjustment of dosage with concurrent use.

*Corticosteroids or ACTH* may intensify any thiazide-induced electrolyte depletion, particularly hypokalaemia. *Pressor amines such as adrenaline* may show decreased arterial responsiveness when used with Moducren, but this reaction is not enough to preclude their therapeutic usefulness. *Non-depolarising muscle relaxants such as tubocurarine* may possibly interact with Moducren to increase muscle relaxation. *Lithium* should not generally be given with diuretics, because they reduce its renal clearance and add a high risk of lithium toxicity. *Drug/laboratory test interactions:* because thiazides may affect calcium metabolism, Moducren may interfere with tests for parathyroid function (see *Precautions*).

*Breast-feeding mothers:* Thiazides appear in breast milk, but it is not known whether timolol maleate or amiloride are also excreted. If the use of Moducren is deemed essential, the mother should stop breast-feeding.

*Pregnancy:* Moducren is not recommended for use during pregnancy. The use of any drug in women of child-bearing age requires that the anticipated benefit be weighed against possible hazards, which include fetal or neonatal jaundice, thrombocytopenia, and possibly other adverse reactions which have occurred in the adult.

*Side effects:* Moducren is usually well tolerated with significant side effects only infrequently reported.

Most common side-effects are dizziness, asthenia, fatigue, and bradycardia. Other clinical adverse reactions are: *Body as a whole:* Asthenia, fatigue, headache. *Cardiovascular:* Bradycardia, peripheral vascular disorder (cold extremities), hypotension, syncope, arrhythmia, angina pectoris. *Respiratory:* Dyspnoea, wheezing. *Digestive:* Nausea, dyspepsia, constipation, diarrhoea, vomiting, GI pain, anorexia, thirst, dry mouth, stomatitis. *Urogenital:* Impotence. *Nervous:* Dizziness, vertigo, paraesthesiae, tremors. *Integumentary:* Sweating. *Musculoskeletal:* Muscle cramps. *Psychiatric:* Insomnia, nervousness, depression, somnolence, abnormal dreaming, sleep disturbance. *Special senses:* Visual disturbances.

Side-effects that have been reported with the individual components may be considered as potential adverse effects of Moducren.

*Amiloride-related effects*
*Digestive:* abnormal liver function, activation of probable pre-existing peptic ulcer, jaundice. *Integumentary:* dry mouth, alopecia. *Haematological:* aplastic anaemia, neutropenia. *Cardiovascular:* one patient with partial heart block developed complete heart block, palpitation. *Psychiatric:* decreased libido. *Respiratory:* cough. *Special senses:* tinnitus, increased intra-ocular pressure. *Urogenital:* polyuria, urinary frequency, bladder spasm.

*Hydrochlorothiazide-related effects*
*Body as a whole:* Anaphylactic reaction, fever. *Cardiovascular:* Necrotising angiitis (vasculitis, cutaneous vasculitis). *Digestive:* Jaundice (intrahepatic cholestatic jaundice), pancreatitis, cramping, gastric irritation. *Integumentary:* Photosensitivity. *Endocrine/metabolic:* Glycosuria, hypoglycaemia, hyperglycaemia, hyperuricaemia, sialadenitis, urticaria. *Psychiatric:* Restlessness. *Renal:* Renal dysfunction, interstitial nephritis, renal failure. *Respiratory:* Respiratory distresses including pneumonitis, pulmonary oedema. *Special senses:* Transient blurred vision, xanthopsia. *Haematological:* Agranulocytosis, aplastic anaemia, haemolytic anaemia, leucopenia, purpura, thrombocytopenia.

*Timolol maleate-related effects.*
*Body as a whole:* chest pain, extremity pain, decreased exercise tolerance, weight loss. *Cardiovascular:* cardiac arrest, cerebral vascular accident, palpitation, second- or third-degree AV block, sino-atrial block, oedema and pulmonary oedema, cardiac failure, Raynaud's phenomenon, claudication, worsening of arterial insufficiency and angina pectoris, vasodilatation. *Digestive:* diarrhoea, hepatomegaly. *Endocrine:* hypoglycaemia, hyperglycaemia. *Integumentary:* rash, pruritus, skin irritation, increased pigmentation, exfoliative dermatitis (one case). *Musculoskeletal:* arthralgia. *Nervous system:* local weakness. *Psychiatric:* diminished concentration, hallucinations, decreased libido. *Haematological:* non-thrombocytopenic purpura. *Respiratory:* bronchial spasm, rales, cough. *Special senses:* tinnitus, visual disturbances, diplopia, ptosis, eye irritation, dry eyes. *Urogenital:* micturition difficulties.

*Clinical laboratory tests:* Clinically important changes in standard laboratory tests associated with timolol maleate are rare. Slight increases in blood urea, serum potassium and serum uric acid, and slight decreases in haemoglobin and haematocrit occurred but were not progressive or associated with clinical manifestations.

*Overdosage:* No specific data are available regarding symptoms or the treatment of overdosage with Moducren and no antidote is available. Little is known about dialysability of its components; a study of patients with renal failure showed that timolol did not readily dialyse. Treatment is symptomatic and supportive.

Therapy with Moducren should be stopped and emesis and/or gastric lavage induced.

*Hydrochlorothiazide and amiloride hydrochloride:* The signs and symptoms most likely are dehydration and electrolyte imbalance. If hyperkalaemia occurs, active measures should be taken to reduce plasma potassium levels.

*Timolol maleate:* The most common signs and symptoms to be expected following overdosage with a beta-blocker are symptomatic bradycardia, hypotension, bronchospasm, acute cardiac failure, and heart block.

If overdosage occurs, the following measures are recommended:

1. *Gastric lavage*

2. *For symptomatic bradycardia:* Atropine sulphate, 0.25 to 2 mg intravenously, should be used to induce vagal blockade. If bradycardia persists, intravenous isoprenaline hydrochloride should be administered cautiously. In refractory cases, the use of a transvenous cardiac pacemaker may be considered.

3. *For hypotension:* A sympathomimetic pressor agent such as dopamine, dobutamine or noradrenaline should be used. In refractory cases, the use of glucagon has been reported useful.

4. *For bronchospasm:* Isoprenaline hydrochloride should be used. Additional therapy with aminophylline may be considered.

5. *For acute cardiac failure:* Conventional therapy with digitalis, diuretics, and oxygen should be instituted immediately. In refractory cases, the use of intravenous aminophylline is suggested. This may be followed, if necessary, by glucagon which has been reported useful.

6. *For heart block:* Isoprenaline hydrochloride or a transvenous cardiac pacemaker should be used.

The components of Moducren have, respectively, plasma half-lives of: Hydrochlorothiazide at 5.6 hours with a longer terminal phase; amiloride at about 6–9.5 hours; and timolol at about four hours.

**Pharmaceutical precautions** Store in a dry place below 25°C, protected from light.

**Legal category** POM.

**Package quantities** Calendar packs of 28 tablets.

**Further information** The combination of amiloride with hydrochlorothiazide has been shown to cause less magnesium excretion than either the thiazides or loop diuretics alone.

Similar dosage schedules and similar bioavailability rationalise the combination of hydrochlorothiazide (a saluretic), timolol maleate (a beta-adrenergic receptor blocking agent), and amiloride hydrochloride (a potassium-conserving agent) for the treatment of hypertension.

**Product licence number** 0025/0141.

## PEPCID*

**Presentation** Brown, round-cornered square tablets, marked 'PEPCID' on one face with '40' on the other, containing 40 mg famotidine.

Beige, round-cornered square tablets, marked 'PEPCID' on one face with '20' on the other, containing 20 mg famotidine.

**Uses**

*Indications:* Duodenal ulcer.
Prevention of relapses of duodenal ulceration.
Benign gastric ulcer.
Hypersecretory conditions such as Zollinger-Ellison syndrome.
Treatment of gastro-oesophageal reflux disease.
Prevention of relapse of symptoms and erosions or ulcerations associated with gastro-oesophageal reflux disease.

*Mode of action:* Pepcid is a highly specific and potent competitive $H_2$-receptor antagonist. It has a rapid onset of action. Although the plasma half-life of famotidine in patients is approximately 3.0 hours, Pepcid has a long duration of action, and a single 40 mg dose has been shown to reduce gastric acid secretion for at least 10 hours.

Pepcid reduces the acid and pepsin content, as well as the volume of basal, nocturnal and stimulated gastric secretion.

**Dosage and administration** It is unnecessary to time the dose in relation to meals; bioavailability is not clinically affected by food in the stomach. In all cases the clinical response of the patient should be taken into consideration

In benign gastric and duodenal ulceration, the dose of Pepcid is one 40 mg tablet at night.

*Duodenal ulcer:* The recommended initial dose is one 40 mg tablet of Pepcid at night. Treatment should continue for four to eight weeks. In most patients, healing occurs on this regimen within four weeks. In those patients whose ulcers have not healed completely after four weeks, a further four-week period of treatment is recommended.

*Maintenance therapy:* For preventing the recurrence of duodenal ulceration, the reduced dose of 20 mg of Pepcid at night is recommended. This 20 mg maintenance dose has been continued effectively in clinical studies of 12 months duration.

*Benign gastric ulcer:* The recommended dose is one 40 mg tablet of Pepcid at night. Treatment should continue for four to eight weeks unless endoscopy reveals earlier healing.

*Zollinger-Ellison syndrome:* Patients without prior antisecretory therapy should be started on 20 mg of Pepcid every six hours. Dosage should then be adjusted to individual response: doses up to 800 mg daily have been used up to one year without the development of significant adverse effects or tachyphylaxis. Patients who have been receiving another $H_2$ antagonist may be switched directly to Pepcid at a dose higher than that recommended for new cases. This starting dose will depend on the severity of the condition and the last dose of $H_2$ antagonist previously used.

*Gastro-oesophageal reflux disease:* The recommended dosage for the symptomatic relief of gastro-oesophageal reflux disease is 20 mg of famotidine twice daily, which may be given for six to twelve weeks. Most patients experience improvement after two weeks.

Where gastro-oesophageal reflux disease is associated with the presence of oesophageal erosion or ulceration, the recommended dosage is 40 mg of famotidine, twice daily, which may be given for six to twelve weeks.

*Maintenance therapy:* For the prevention of recurrence of symptoms and erosions or ulcerations associated with gastro-oesophageal reflux disease, the recommended dosage is 20 mg of famotidine twice daily.

*Use in the elderly:* The recommended dosage in most elderly patients is the same as in younger patients for all indications (see above). No change in the incidence or type of drug-related side-effects were seen in treated elderly patients.

*Use in impaired renal function:* Since Pepcid is excreted primarily by the kidney, caution should be observed in patients with impaired renal function. The dose should be reduced to 20 mg *nocte* if creatinine clearance falls below 10 ml/min.

*Paediatric use:* The efficacy and safety of Pepcid in children have not been established.

### Contra-indications, warnings, etc

*Contra-indications:* Hypersensitivity to any component of this product.

*Precautions*

*Gastric carcinoma:* Gastric malignancy should be excluded prior to initiation of therapy of gastric ulcer with Pepcid. Symptomatic response of gastric ulcer to therapy with Pepcid does not preclude the presence of gastric malignancy.

*Impaired renal function:* Since Pepcid is primarily excreted via the kidney, caution should be exercised when treating patients with impaired renal function.

The dose should be reduced to 20 mg *nocte* when creatinine clearance falls below 10 ml/min.

*Pregnancy:* Pepcid is not recommended for use in pregnancy, and should be prescribed only if clearly needed. Before a decision is made to use Pepcid during pregnancy, the physician should weigh the potential benefits from the drug against the possible risks involved.

*Breast-feeding mothers:* Pepcid is secreted in human milk, therefore breast-feeding mothers should either stop breast-feeding or stop taking the drug.

*Drug interactions:* No clinically important drug interactions have been identified. Pepcid does not interact with the cytochrome P450-linked drug metabolising enzyme system. Compounds metabolised by this system which have been tested in man have included warfarin, theophylline, phenytoin, diazepam, propranolol, aminopyrine and phenazone. Indocyanine green as an index of hepatic blood flow and/or hepatic drug extraction has been tested and no significant effects have been found.

*Side-effects:* In controlled studies, Pepcid has been shown to be generally well tolerated.

Headache, dizziness, constipation, and diarrhoea have been reported rarely. Other side effects reported even less frequently included dry mouth, nausea and/or vomiting, abdominal discomfort or distension, anorexia, fatigue, rash, pruritus and urticaria, liver enzyme abnormalities, cholestatic jaundice, anaphylaxis, angioedema, arthralgia, muscle cramps, reversible psychic disturbances including depression, anxiety disorders, agitation, confusion and hallucinations. Toxic epidermal necrolysis has been reported very rarely with $H_2$-receptor antagonists. Pancytopenia, leucopenia, and isolated cases of worsening of existing hepatic disease have been reported; however, a causal relationship to therapy with Pepcid has not been established. No clinically significant increase in endocrine or gonadal function has been reported.

Gynaecomastia has been reported rarely. In most cases that were followed up, it was reversible on discontinuing treatment.

*Overdosage:* There is no experience to date with overdosage.

The usual measures to remove unabsorbed material from the gastro-intestinal tract, clinical monitoring, and supportive therapy only should be employed.

Patients with Zollinger-Ellison syndrome have tolerated a dosage of 800 mg daily for more than a year without the development of significant adverse effects.

**Pharmaceutical precautions** Store in a dry place below 25°C.

**Legal category** POM.

**Package quantities** Calendar packs of 28 tablets.

**Further information** Pepcid is a chemically novel competitive $H_2$-receptor antagonist with a guanidino-thiazole ring. Pepcid is rapidly absorbed, with dose-related peak plasma concentrations reached in one to three hours. When used as recommended, there was no accumulation effect with repeated doses.

In clinical studies, a single dose of Pepcid at night relieved the pain associated with peptic ulcer, usually within a week, and suppressed gastric secretion.

Studies in animals and human volunteers have not shown anti-androgenic effects.

**Product licence numbers**
20 mg tablets   0025/0215
40 mg tablets   0025/0216

## PERIACTIN*

**Presentation** White, half-scored tablets, marked 'MSD 62', containing Cyproheptadine Hydrochloride PhEur equivalent to 4 mg anhydrous cyproheptadine hydrochloride.

**Uses** Periactin is a serotonin and histamine antagonist with anticholinergic and sedative properties.

*In allergy and pruritus:* Periactin has a wide range of anti-allergic and antipruritic activity, and can be used successfully in treatment of acute and chronic allergic and pruritic conditions, such as: dermatitis, including neurodermatitis and neurodermatitis circumscripta; eczema; eczematoid dermatitis; dermatographism; mild, local allergic reactions to insect bites; hay fever and other seasonal rhinitis; perennial allergic and vasomotor rhinitis; allergic conjunctivitis due to inhalant allergens and foods; urticaria; angioneurotic oedema; drug and serum reactions; anogenital pruritus; pruritus of chickenpox.

Periactin is indicated as adjunctive therapy to adrenaline and other standard measures for the relief of anaphylactic reactions after the acute manifestations have been controlled.

*In migraine headache:* Periactin has been reported to have beneficial effects in a significant number of patients having vascular types of headache. Many patients who have responded inadequately to all other agents have reported amelioration of symptoms with Periactin. The characteristic headache and feeling of malaise may disappear within an hour or two of the first dose.

**Dosage and administration** There is no recommended dosage for children under 2 years old. Periactin is not recommended for elderly debilitated patients.

*In allergy and pruritus:* Dosage must be determined on an individual basis. The effect of a single dose usually lasts for four to six hours. For continuous effective relief, the daily requirement should be given in divided doses, usually three times a day, or as often as necessary, to provide continuous relief.

*Adults:* The therapeutic range is 4–20 mg a day, most patients requiring 12–16 mg a day. It is recommended that dosage be initiated with 4 mg three times a day and then adjusted according to the weight and response of the patient.

*Maximum:* 32 mg a day.

*Children aged 7–14 years:* Usually 4 mg two or three times a day, according to the patient's weight and response. If an additional dose is required it should be given at bedtime. Maximum 16 mg a day.

*Children aged 2–6 years:* Initially 2 mg two or three times a day, adjusted according to the patient's weight and response. If an additional dose is required it should be given at bedtime. Maximum 12 mg a day.

*In vascular headache and migraine:* For both prophylactic and therapeutic use at an initial dose of 4 mg repeated if necessary after half an hour. Patients who respond usually obtain relief with 8 mg, and this dose should not be exceeded within a 4- to 6-hour period.

*Maintenance:* 4 mg every four to six hours.

*Use in the elderly:* Periactin should not be used in elderly, debilitated patients. Elderly patients are more likely to experience dizziness, sedation, and hypotension.

### Contra-indications, warnings, etc

*Contra-indications:* Therapy of an acute asthmatic attack; newborn or premature infants; breast-feeding mothers; known sensitivity to cyproheptadine hydrochloride or drugs with similar chemical structure; concurrent use with monoamine oxidase inhibitors; glaucoma; stenosing peptic ulcer; symptomatic prostatic hypertrophy; bladder neck obstruction; pyloroduodenal obstruction; elderly, debilitated patients; predisposition to urinary retention.

*Precautions:* Antihistamines should not be used to treat lower respiratory tract symptoms including those of acute asthma.

The safety and efficacy of Periactin is not established in children under 2 years old.

Antihistamines may diminish mental alertness; conversely, particularly in the young child, they may occasionally produce excitation.

Patients should be warned against engaging in activities requiring motor co-ordination and mental alertness such as driving a car or operating machinery.

Rarely, prolonged therapy with antihistamines may cause blood dyscrasias.

Because Periactin has an atropine-like action, it should be used cautiously in patients with a history of bronchial asthma, increased intra-ocular pressure, hyperthyroidism, cardiovascular disease, or hypertension.

*Drug interactions:* MAO inhibitors prolong and intensify the anticholinergic effects of antihistamines.

Antihistamines may have additive effects with alcohol and other CNS depressants, e.g. hypnotics, sedatives, tranquillisers and anti-anxiety agents.

*Pregnancy and breast-feeding mothers:* The use of any drug in pregnancy or in women of child-bearing age requires that the potential benefit of the drug should be weighed against possible hazards to the embryo or fetus. It is not known whether Periactin is excreted in human milk, and because of the potential for serious adverse reactions in breast-feeding infants from Periactin, a decision should be made whether to discontinue breast-feeding or to discontinue the drug, taking into account the importance of the drug to the mother (see 'Contra-indications').

*Side-effects:* The side-effects that appear frequently are drowsiness and somnolence. Many patients who initially complain of drowsiness may no longer do so after the first three to four days of continuous administration. Side-effects reported with antihistamines are:

*Central nervous system:* Sedation, sleepiness (often transient), dizziness, disturbed co-ordination, confusion, restlessness, excitation, nervousness, tremor, irritability, insomnia, parasthesiae, neuritis, convulsions, euphoria, hallucinations, hysteria, faintness.

*Integumentary:* Allergic manifestations of rash and oedema, excessive perspiration, urticaria, photosensitivity.

*Special senses:* Acute labyrinthitis, blurred vision, diplopia, vertigo, tinnitus.

*Cardiovascular:* Hypotension, palpitation, tachycardia, extrasystoles, anaphylactic shock.

*Haematological:* Haemolytic anaemia, leucopenia, agranulocytosis, thrombocytopenia.

*Digestive system:* Dryness of mouth, epigastric distress, anorexia, nausea, vomiting, diarrhoea, constipation, jaundice.

*Genito-urinary:* Frequency and difficulty of micturition, urinary retention, early menses.

*Respiratory:* Dryness of the nose and throat, thickening of bronchial secretions, tightness of chest and wheezing, nasal stuffiness.

*Miscellaneous:* Fatigue, rigors, headache.

*Overdosage:* Antihistamine overdosage may vary from CNS depression or stimulation to convulsions and death, especially in infants and children. Atropine-like and GI symptoms may occur.

If vomiting has not occurred spontaneously, it should be induced in the conscious patient with syrup of ipecac. If the patient cannot vomit, gastric lavage with isotonic or half isotonic saline is indicated followed by activated charcoal. Precautions against aspiration must be taken, especially in infants and children.

Life-threatening CNS signs and symptoms should be treated appropriately.

Saline cathartics usefully draw water into the bowel by osmosis to dilute bowel content rapidly.

Central stimulants must not be used, but vasopressors may be used to counteract hypotension.

**Pharmaceutical precautions** Periactin should be stored below 25°C, protected from light.

**Legal category** P.

**Package quantities** Packs of 30 tablets.

**Further information** Nil.

**Product licence number** 0025/5017.

## PRIMAXIN*

### Presentation

*For intravenous infusion:* Vials containing sterile powders of:

250 mg imipenem (as the monohydrate) with 250 mg cilastatin (as the sodium salt) named Primaxin IV 250 mg.

500 mg imipenem (as the monohydrate) with 500 mg cilastatin (as the sodium salt) named Primaxin IV 500 mg.

Monovial presentation: A monovial of 500 mg imipenem (as the monohydrate) with 500 mg cilastatin (as the sodium salt), named 'Primaxin' IV 500 mg Monovial. The monovial has a built-in transfer needle to allow constitution of the product directly into an infusion bag.

*For intramuscular administration:* Vials containing sterile powders of:

500 mg imipenem (as the monohydrate) with 500 mg cilastatin (as the sodium salt), named Primaxin IM 500 mg.

**Uses** Broad-spectrum beta-lactam antibiotic.

Primaxin contains imipenem, a member of a new class of beta-lactam antibiotics – the thienamycins; and cilastatin sodium, a specific enzyme-inhibitor, that blocks the metabolism of imipenem in the kidney and substantially increases the concentration of unchanged imipenem in the urinary tract.

Primaxin is bactericidal against an unusually wide-spectrum of Gram-positive, Gram-negative, aerobic and anaerobic pathogens. Primaxin is useful for treating single, and polymicrobic infections, and initiating therapy prior to identification of the causative organisms.

Primaxin is indicated for the treatment of the following infections due to susceptible organisms:

| *Primaxin IV* | *Primaxin IM* |
|---|---|
| Lower respiratory tract infections | Lower respiratory tract infections (except those caused by *Pseudomonas aeruginosa)* |
| Intra-abdominal infections | Intra-abdominal infections |
| Genito-urinary infections | Genito-urinary infections |
| Gynaecological infections | Gynaecological infections |
| Septicaemia | Not indicated |
| Bone and joint infections | Bone and joint infections (there is limited experience in patients with these infections) |
| Skin and soft tissue infections | Skin and soft tissue infections |

*Note:* Primaxin is not indicated against central nervous system infections.

Primaxin is indicated against mixed infections caused by susceptible aerobic and anaerobic bacteria. The majority of these infections are associated with contamination by faecal flora, or flora originating from the vagina, skin, and mouth. In these mixed infections, Primaxin is usually effective against *Bacteroides fragilis* sp., the most commonly encountered anaerobic pathogen, that is usually resistant to the aminoglycosides, cephalosporins and penicillins.

*Prophylaxis:* Primaxin IV is also indicated for the prevention of certain post-operative infections in patients undergoing contaminated or potentially contaminated surgical procedures or where the occurrence of post-operative infection could be especially serious.

*Mode of action:* Imipenem is a potent inhibitor of bacterial cell wall synthesis and is highly reactive towards penicillin-binding protein. Imipenem is more potent in its bactericidal effect than other antibiotics studied. Imipenem also provides excellent stability to degradative bacterial beta-lactamases. Imipenem is therefore active against a high percentage of organisms resistant to other beta-lactam antibiotics.

Cilastatin sodium is a competitive, reversible, and specific inhibitor of dehydropeptidase-I, the renal enzyme which metabolises and inactivates imipenem. Cilastatin sodium is devoid of intrinsic antibacterial activity itself and does not affect the antibacterial activity of imipenem.

*Bacteriology:* Primaxin has a unique anti-bacterial spectrum. Against Gram-negative species, it shares the spectrum of the newer cephalosporins and penicillins; against Gram-positive species Primaxin exerts the high bacterial potency previously only associated with narrow-spectrum beta-lactam antibiotics and the first-generation cephalosporins.

The antibiotic spectrum of Primaxin is broader than other antibiotics studied and includes virtually all clinically significant pathogenic genera.

Organisms against which Primaxin is usually active *in vitro* include:

Gram-negative aerobes: *Escherichia coli; Proteus mirabilis; Proteus vulgaris; Proteus* spp.; *Morganella morganii* (formerly *Proteus morganii*); *Providencia rettgeri* (formerly *Proteus rettgeri*); *Providencia stuartii; Providencia* spp; *Hafnia alvei; Serratia marcescens; Serratia liquefaciens; Serratia* spp.; *Klebsiella oxytoca; Klebsiella pneumoniae; Klebsiella* spp.; *Enterobacter aerogenes; Enterobacter agglomerans; Enterobacter cloacae; Enterobacter* spp.; *Citrobacter freundii; Citrobacter diversus; Citrobacter* spp.; *Campylobacter* spp.; *Salmonella typhi; Salmonella* spp.; *Shigella* spp.; *Pseudomonas aeruginosa; Pseudomonas fluorescens; Pseudomonas* spp.†; *Acinetobacter* spp. (formerly *Mima-Herellea*); *Haemophilus influenzae* (including beta-lactamase-producing strains); *Haemophilus parainfluenzae; Neisseria gonorrhoeae* (including penicillinase-producing strains); *Moraxella* spp.; *Pasteurella multocida; Aeromonas hydrophila; Yersinia* spp. (formerly *Pasteurella*); *Yersinia enterocolitica; Achromobacter* spp.; *Gardnerella* spp.

†*Xanthomonas maltophilia* and some strains of *Pseudomonas cepacia* are generally not sensitive to Primaxin.

Gram-positive aerobes: Streptococcus Group A (*S. pyogenes*); Streptococcus Group B (*S. agalactiae*); Streptococcus Group C; Enterococcus including *Enterococcus faecalis;* Streptococcus Group D; Streptococcus Group G; *Streptococcus pneumoniae; Viridans streptococci* (including alpha and gamma haemolytic strains); *Staphylococcus aureus* (including penicillinase-producing strains); *Staphylococcus epidermidis* (including penicillinase-producing strains); *Erysipelothrix rhusiopathiae.*

Some methicillin-resistant staphylococci and some group D streptococci are not sensitive to Primaxin.

Microaerophilic streptococcus

Gram-negative anaerobes: *Bacteroides fragilis; Bacteroides vulgatus; Bacteroides melaninogenicus; Bacteroides asaccharolyticus; Bacteroides distasonis; Bacteroides ovatus; Bacteroides thetaiotaomicron; Bacteroides* spp.; *Fusobacterium nucleatum; Fusobacterium necrophorum; Fusobacterium* spp.; *Veillonella* spp.

Gram-positive anaerobes: *Actinomyces* spp.; *Clostridium perfringens; Clostridium* spp.; *Eubacterium* spp.; *Peptococcus* spp.; *Peptostreptococcus* spp.; *Propionibacterium* spp. including *P. acnes.*

*In vitro* tests show that imipenem acts synergistically with aminoglycoside antibiotics against some isolates of *Pseudomonas aeruginosa.*

**Dosage and administration** The total daily dosage and route of administration of Primaxin should be based on the type or severity of infection, consideration of degree of susceptibility of the pathogen(s), renal function and bodyweight. Doses cited are based on a bodyweight of 70 kg. The total daily requirement should be given in equally divided doses.

The dosage recommendations that follow specify the amounts of imipenem to be given. An equivalent amount of cilastatin is provided with this. One vial of Primaxin IV 250 mg therefore provides the equivalents of 250 mg anhydrous imipenem and 250 mg cilastatin; similarly one vial of Primaxin IV or IM 500 mg, provides the equivalents of 500 mg anhydrous imipenem and 500 mg cilastatin.

*Use in the elderly:* Age does not usually affect the tolerability and efficacy of Primaxin. The dosage should be determined by the severity of the infection, the susceptibility of the causative organism(s), the patient's clinical condition, and renal function.

*INTRAVENOUS ADMINISTRATION:* This formulation should not be used intramuscularly. The dosage of Primaxin IV should be determined by the severity of the infection, the antibiotic susceptibility of the causative organism(s) and the condition of the patient.

*Note:* All recommended doses refer to the imipenem fraction of Primaxin.

*Adults (based on 70 kg bodyweight):* The usual adult daily dosage is 1–2 g of Primaxin administered in 3–4 equally divided doses (see chart below). In infections due to less sensitive organisms, the daily dose of Primaxin may be increased to a maximum dose of 50 mg/kg/day (or not exceeding 4 g daily).

*Usual adult intravenous dosage*

Each 250 mg or 500 mg dose should be given by intravenous infusion over 20–30 minutes. Each 1000 mg dose should be infused over 40–60 minutes. In patients who develop nausea during infusion, the infusion rate may be slowed.

| | *I.V. administration* | | |
|---|---|---|---|
| *Severity of infection* | *Dose* | *Dosage interval* | *Total daily dose* |
| Mild | 250 mg | 6 hours | 1.0 g |
| Moderate | 500 mg | 8 hours | 1.5 g |
| Severe – fully susceptible | 500 mg | 6 hours | 2.0 g |
| Severe and/or life-threatening infections due to less sensitive organisms (primarily some strains of *P. aeruginosa*) | 1000 mg<br>1000 mg | 8 hours<br>6 hours | 3.0 g<br>4.0 g |

Primaxin has been used successfully as monotherapy in immunocompromised cancer patients for confirmed or suspected infections such as sepsis.

*Prophylactic use:* For prophylaxis against post-surgical infections in adults, 1 g of Primaxin should be given intravenously on induction of anaesthesia and 1 g three hours later. For high-risk (i.e. colorectal) surgery, two additional 0.5 g doses can be given at 8 and 16 hours after induction.

*In patients with renal insufficiency:* As in patients with normal renal function, dosing is based on the severity of the infection. The maximum dosage for patients with various degrees of renal functional impairment is shown in the following Table. Doses cited are based on a bodyweight of 70 kg. Proportionate reduction in dose administered should be made for patients with lower bodyweight.

*Maximum dosage in relation to renal function*

| *Renal function* | *Creatinine clearance (ml/min)* | *Dose (mg)* | *Dosage interval (hrs)* | *Maximum total daily dose† (g)* |
|---|---|---|---|---|
| Mild impairment | 31–70 | 500 | 6–8 | 1.5–2 |
| Moderate impairment | 21–30 | 500 | 8–12 | 1–1.5 |
| Severe‡ impairment | 0–20 | 250–500 | 12 | 0.5–1.0 |

†The higher dose should be reserved for infections caused by less susceptible organisms.

‡Patients with creatinine clearance of 6–20 ml/min should be treated with 250 mg (or 3.5 mg/kg, whichever is lower) every 12 hours for most pathogens. When the 500 mg dose is used in these patients, there may be an increased risk of convulsions.

Patients with a creatinine clearance of ≤5 ml/min should not receive Primaxin IV unless haemodialysis is started within 48 hours.

Primaxin is cleared by haemodialysis. The patient should receive Primaxin IV immediately after haemodialysis and at 12-hourly intervals thereafter. Dialysis patients, especially those with background CNS disease, should be carefully monitored; patients on haemodialysis should only receive Primaxin IV when the benefit outweighs the potential risk of convulsions (see 'Precautions').

There are currently inadequate data to recommend the use of Primaxin IV for patients on peritoneal dialysis.

*Paediatric dosage*

| *Age* | *Dose* | *Dosage interval* | *Total daily dose* |
|---|---|---|---|
| 3 months of age and older (less than 40 kg bodyweight) | 15 mg/kg | 6 hours | 60 mg/kg |

Children over 40 kg bodyweight should receive adult doses.

The maximum daily dose should not exceed 2 g.

Clinical data are insufficient to recommend an optimal dose for children under 3 months of age or infants and children with impaired renal function.

Primaxin IV is not recommended for the therapy of meningitis. If meningitis is suspected an appropriate antibiotic should be used.

Primaxin IV may be used in children with sepsis as long as they are not suspected of having meningitis.

*Preparation of solution:* The following table is provided for convenience in reconstituting Primaxin IV for intravenous infusion.

| *Amount of Primaxin (mg)* | *Volume of diluent added (ml)†* | *Approximate concentration of imipenem (mg/ml)* |
|---|---|---|
| Primaxin IV 500 mg | 100 | 5 |
| Primaxin IV 250 mg | 50 | 5 |

†Shake to dissolve to a colourless or yellow solution. Variation of colour within this range does not affect potency.

*Compatibility and stability:* In keeping with good clinical and pharmaceutical practice, Primaxin IV should be administered as a freshly prepared solution. On the few occasions where changing circumstances make this impracticable, reconstituted Primaxin IV retains satisfactory potency for 3 hours at room temperature (up to 25°C) or 24 hours in a refrigerator (below 4°C) when prepared in any of the following diluents: 0.9% Sodium Chloride Injection; 5% Dextrose and 0.9% Sodium Chloride; 5% Dextrose and 0.225% Sodium Chloride; 5% Mannitol; 2.5% Mannitol.

Primaxin IV is chemically incompatible with lactate and should not be reconstituted with diluents containing lactate. Primaxin IV can, however, be administered into an IV tubing through which a lactate solution is being infused.

Primaxin IV should not be mixed with, or physically added to, other antibiotics.

*Addition of Primaxin IV Injection in a Monovial to an infusion solution*

### Step 1   EXAMINE

Examine the vial for any foreign material in the powder and make sure the tamper-evident seal between the cap and the vial is intact.

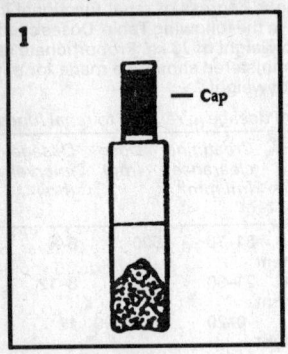

### Step 2   REMOVE CAP

Remove the cap by first twisting it and pulling it up to break the tamper-evident seal.

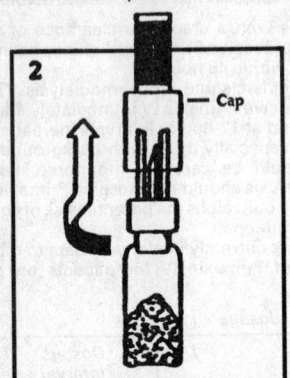

### Step 3   CONNECT

*Insert* the needle into the infusion-bag connector. *Push* the needle-holder and vial together until they 'click' into place.

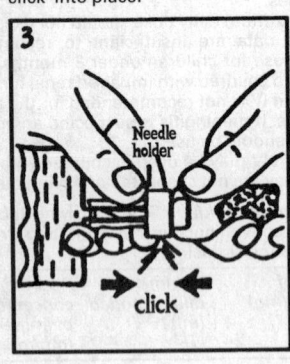

### Step 4   MIX

Hold the vial in an upright position. *Squeeze* the infusion bag several times to transfer the diluent into the vial. Shake the vial to reconstitute the substance.

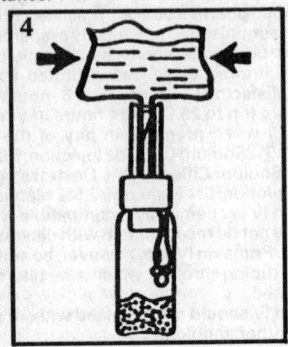

### Step 5   TRANSFER

Now reverse the connected IV assembly, holding the vial upside down. Squeeze the infusion bag several times. This will create an over-pressure in the vial, allowing the contents of the vial to be transferred back into the infusion bag. Repeat steps 4 and 5 until the vial is completely empty.

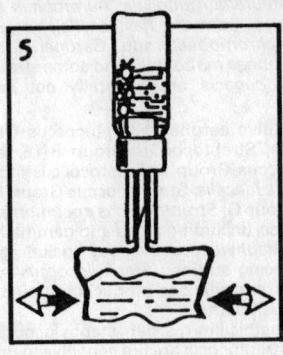

### Step 6   IDENTIFY

Fill out the peel-off label on the vial and *affix* it to the infusion bag for proper identification.

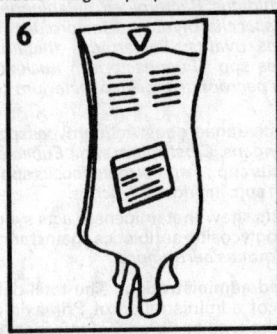

**INTRAMUSCULAR ADMINISTRATION:** This formulation is for intramuscular use only and should not be administered intravenously.

*Note:* All recommended doses refer to the imipenem fraction of Primaxin.

*Adults:* A single 500 mg dose of the intramuscular formulation may be used for the treatment of urethritis or cervicitis due to non-penicillinase-producing *Neisseria gonorrhoeae.*

The intramuscular formulation may be used as an alternative to the intravenous formulation in the treatment of mild and moderate infections.

Primaxin IM should be given by deep intramuscular injection into a large muscle mass (such as the gluteal muscle or lateral part of the thigh).

*Usual adult intramuscular dose*

| Type or severity of infection | IM administration | | |
|---|---|---|---|
| | Dose of imipenem | Dosage interval | Total daily dose |
| Gonococcal urethritis/cervicitis | 500 mg | single dose | 0.5 g |
| Mild infections | 500 mg | 12 hours | 1.0 g |
| Moderate infections | 750 mg | 12 hours | 1.5 g |

*In infants and children:* The safety and efficacy of the intramuscular formulation have not been studied in the paediatric group.

*In patients with renal insufficiency:* The safety and efficacy of the intramuscular formulation have not been studied in patients with renal insufficiency.

*Preparation of intramuscular suspension:* The following table is provided for convenience in reconstituting Primaxin IM with 1% lidocaine (lignocaine) solution for intramuscular use.

| Strength | Volume of 1% lidocaine (lignocaine) solution to be added (ml†) | Final volume (ml) |
|---|---|---|
| Primaxin IM 500 mg | 2 | 2.8 |

†Shake to prepare a white to light-tan-coloured suspension. Variation of colour within this range does not affect potency. Use immediately after making up. Lidocaine (Lignocaine) should not be used if patients are known or suspected to be hypersensitive to local anaesthetics of the amide type or in patients with severe shock or heart block.

### Contra-indications, warnings, etc

*Contra-indication:* Hypersensitivity to this product.

*Warning:* There is some clinical and laboratory evidence of partial cross-allergenicity between Primaxin and the other beta-lactam antibiotics, penicillins and cephalosporins. Severe reactions (including anaphylaxis) have been reported with most beta-lactam antibiotics. Before initiating therapy with Primaxin, careful inquiry should be made concerning previous hypersensitivity reactions to beta-lactam antibiotics. If an allergic reaction to Primaxin occurs, the drug should be discontinued and appropriate measures undertaken.

*Precautions:* Pseudomembranous colitis, reported with virtually all antibiotics, can range from mild to life-threatening in severity. Primaxin should be prescribed with caution in patients with a history of gastro-intestinal disease, particularly colitis. Treatment-related diarrhoea should always be considered as a pointer to this diagnosis. While studies indicate that a toxin of *Clostridium difficile* is one of the primary causes of antibiotic-associated colitis, other causes should be considered.

*Use in pregnancy and lactation:* Pregnant monkeys showed evidence of maternal and fetal toxicity with bolus injections at doses equivalent to twice the human dose.

The use of Primaxin in pregnant women has not been studied and Primaxin should therefore not be given in pregnancy unless the anticipated benefit to the mother outweighs the possible risk to the fetus.

It is not known whether Primaxin is excreted in human milk. Because many drugs are excreted by this route, the breast feeding mother should not receive Primaxin. If the use of Primaxin is deemed essential, the mother should stop breast feeding.

*Paediatric use:* Primaxin IV: Efficacy and tolerability in infants under three months of age have yet to be established; therefore, Primaxin is not recommended for use below this age.

Primaxin IM: Tolerability and efficacy of 'Primaxin' IM have not yet been studied in the paediatric group; therefore, at present, Primaxin IM is not recommended for use in this group.

*Drug interactions:* There are no data on adverse drug interactions. However, concomitant probenecid has been shown to double the plasma level and half-life of cilastatin, but with no effect on its urinary recovery.

Concomitant probenecid showed only minimal increases in plasma level and half-life of imipenem, with urinary recovery of active imipenem decreased to approximately 60% of the administered dose.

*Central nervous system:* Patients with CNS disorders and/or compromised renal function (accumulation of Primaxin may occur) have shown CNS side-effects, especially when recommended dosages based on body weight and renal function were exceeded. Hence it is recommended that the dosage schedules of Primaxin should be strictly adhered to, and established anticonvulsant therapy continued.

If focal tremors, myoclonus or convulsions occur, the patient should be evaluated neurologically and placed on anticonvulsant therapy if not already instituted. If these symptoms still continue, the dosage should be reduced, or Primaxin withdrawn completely.

*Use in patients with renal insufficiency:* Primaxin IV: Patients with creatinine clearances of ≤5 ml/min should not receive Primaxin IV unless haemodialysis is instituted within 48 hours. For patients on haemodialysis, Primaxin IV is only recommended when the benefit outweighs the potential risk of convulsions.

Primaxin IM: Safety and efficacy of Primaxin IM have not yet been studied in patients with renal insufficiency, therefore, at present, Primaxin IM is not recommended for use in this group.

*Side-effects:* Primaxin is generally well tolerated. Side-effects rarely require cessation of therapy and are generally mild and transient; serious side-effects are rare.

*Local reactions:* Erythema, local pain and induration, thrombophlebitis.

*Allergic:* Rash, pruritus, urticaria, toxic epidermal necrolysis (rarely), fever, anaphylactic reactions.

*Gastro-intestinal:* Nausea, vomiting, diarrhoea. Pseudomembranous colitis has been reported.

*Blood:* Eosinophilia, leucopenia, neutropenia including agranulocytosis, thrombocytopenia, thrombocytosis decreased haemoglobin, and hepatitis (rarely). A positive direct Coombs test may develop.

*Liver function:* Mild increases in serum transaminases, bilirubin and/or serum alkaline phosphatase have been reported.

*Renal function:* Oliguria/anuria, polyuria, acute renal failure (rarely). The role of Primaxin in changes in renal function is difficult to assess, since factors predisposing to pre-renal azotemia or to impaired renal function usually have been present. Elevated serum creatinine and blood urea have been seen. A harmless reddish urine discoloration, not to be confused with haematuria, has been seen in children.

*Central nervous system:* Myoclonic activity, psychic disturbances, confusional states or convulsions have been reported.

*Special senses:* Taste perversion.

*Other reported reactions with an unknown causal relationship*

*Gastro-intestinal:* Haemorrhagic colitis, gastro-enteritis, abdominal pain, glossitis, tongue papillar hypertrophy, heartburn, pharyngeal pain, increased salivation.

*Central nervous system:* Dizziness, somnolence, encephalopathy, paraesthesiae, vertigo, headache.

*Special senses:* Transient hearing loss in patients with impaired hearing, tinnitus.

*Respiratory:* Chest discomfort, dyspnoea, hyperventilation, thoracic spine pain.

*Cardiovascular:* Hypotension, palpitations, tachycardia.

*Skin:* Erythema multiforme, facial oedema, flushing, cyanosis hyperhidrosis, skin texture changes, candidiasis, pruritus vulvae.

*Body as a whole:* Polyarthralgia, asthenia/weakness.

*Treatment of overdosage:* No information is available at present.

**Pharmaceutical precautions** Vials of dry Primaxin should be stored below 25°C protected from light until immediately before use. They should not be frozen, or exposed to temperatures above 50°C.

**Legal category** POM.

**Package quantities** *For intravenous use:* Single 50-ml vial containing sterile powders of 250 mg imipenem (as the monohydrate) with 250 mg cilastatin (as the sodium salt).

Single 100-ml vial containing sterile powders of 500 mg imipenem (as the monohydrate) with 500 mg cilastatin (as the sodium salt).

Monovial presentation: Single 20-ml vial with transfer needle containing 500 mg imipenem (as the monohydrate) with 500 mg cilastatin (as the sodium salt).

*For intramuscular use:* Single 13-ml vial containing sterile powders of 500 mg imipenem (as the monohydrate) with 500 mg cilastatin (as the sodium salt).

**Further information** *The differences between intramuscular and intravenous administration should be recognised.*

Intramuscular use has a 75% bioavailability of intravenous infusion. Effective absorption from the intramuscular site is longer; plasma levels of a single 500 mg or 750 mg dose of imipenem remained above 2 mcg/ml for at least six to eight hours. This is above the $MIC_{90}$ of such pathogens as *Serratia* spp., *Acinetobacter* spp., *Bacteroides fragilis* and all Gram-positive cocci except enterococci. Alternatively, intravenous infusion offers peak plasma levels from single 250, 500 and 1000 mg doses of 17, 39 and 66 mcg/ml, respectively. The plasma levels of these doses decline below 1 microgram/ml or less in four to six hours.

Approximately 70% of the antibiotic administered intravenously was recovered intact from the urine in 10 hours. Concentrations exceeded 10 micrograms/ml for up to eight hours after a single intravenous dose of 500 mg Primaxin. However, intramuscular administration of a single dose of 500 mg or 750 mg of the antibiotic gave urine levels above 10 micrograms/ml for 12 hours with a total urinary recovery of 50% of the dose.

No accumulation of imipenem is seen in patients with normal kidney function in either plasma or urine at any of the dosage regimens recommended.

**Product licence numbers**

*Primaxin for intravenous administration:*

250 mg 0025/0228

500 mg 0025/0229

*Primaxin for intramuscular administration:* 500 mg 0025/0230.

## PROSCAR*

**Qualitative and quantitative composition** Active constituent finasteride 5.0 mg per dose unit.

**Pharmaceutical form** Film-coated tablets.

**Clinical particulars**

*Therapeutic indications:* Proscar is indicated for the treatment and control of benign prostatic hyperplasia (BPH) to cause regression of the enlarged prostate, improve urinary flow, and improve the symptoms associated with BPH.

*Posology and method of administration:* The recommended adult dose is one 5 mg tablet daily, with or without food.

Although early improvement may be seen, treatment for at least six months may be necessary to assess whether a beneficial response has been achieved. Thereafter treatment should be continued long term.

No dosage adjustment is required in the elderly or in patients with varying degrees of renal insufficiency (creatinine clearances as low as 9 ml/min).

There are no data available in patients with hepatic insufficiency.

Proscar is contra-indicated in children.

*Contra-indications:* Hypersensitivity to any component of this product; women who are or may become pregnant; children.

*Special warnings and special precautions for use*

*General:* Since the beneficial response to Proscar may not be manifested immediately, patients with large residual urine volume and/or severely diminished urinary flow should be carefully monitored for obstructive uropathy.

*Prostate cancer:* Digital rectal examination, as well as other evaluations for prostate cancer, should be performed on patients with BPH prior to initiating therapy with Proscar and periodically thereafter. Serum prostate specific antigen (PSA) is being increasingly used for prostate cancer detection. Generally, a baseline PSA >10 ng/ml (Hybritech) prompts further evaluation and consideration of biopsy; for PSA levels between 4 and 10 ng/ml, further evaluation is advisable. The physician should be aware that a baseline PSA <4 ng/ml does not exclude prostate cancer.

Finasteride causes a decrease in serum concentrations of markers of prostatic cancer such as PSA even in the presence of prostate cancer; therefore, reduction of serum levels of these markers in patients with BPH treated with Proscar should be considered when evaluating PSA data and does not rule out concomitant prostate cancer.

Any sustained increase in PSA levels of patients treated with finasteride should be carefully evaluated, including consideration of non-compliance to therapy with Proscar.

No clinical benefit has yet been demonstrated in patients with prostate cancer treated with finasteride. In controlled clinical trials in patients with BPH, finasteride did not appear to alter the rate of prostate cancer detection.

*Interaction with other medicaments and other forms of interaction:* No clinically important drug interactions have been identified. Proscar does not appear to significantly affect the cytochrome P450-linked drug metabolising enzyme system. Compounds which have been tested in man include propranolol, digoxin, glibenclamide, warfarin, theophylline, and antipyrine.

*Other concomitant therapy:* Although specific interaction studies were not performed in clinical studies, Proscar was used concomitantly with ACE inhibitors, alpha-blockers, beta-blockers, calcium channel blockers, cardiac nitrates, diuretics, $H_2$ antagonists, HMG-CoA reductase inhibitors, non-steroidal anti-inflammatory drugs (NSAIDs), quinolones and benzodiazepines without evidence of clinically significant adverse interactions.

*Pregnancy and lactation*

*Pregnancy:* Proscar is contra-indicated in women who are or may become pregnant.

Because of the ability of 5 alpha-reductase inhibitors to inhibit conversion of testosterone to dihydrotestosterone, these drugs, including finasteride, may cause abnormalities of the external genitalia of a male fetus when administered to a pregnant woman.

In animal developmental studies, hypospadias were observed in the male offspring of pregnant rats given finasteride at doses ranging from 100 μg/kg/day to 100 mg/kg/day, at an incidence of 3.6% to 100%. Additionally, pregnant rats produced male offspring with decreased prostatic and seminal vesicular weights, delayed preputial separation, transient nipple development and decreased anogenital distance, when given finasteride at doses below the recommended human dose. The critical period during which these effects can be induced has been defined in rats as days 16–17 of gestation.

The changes described above are expected pharmacological effects of 5 alpha-reductase inhibitors. Many of the changes, such as hypospadias, observed in male rats exposed *in utero* to finasteride are similar to those reported in male infants with a genetic deficiency of 5 alpha reductase. It is for these reasons that Proscar is contra-indicated in women who are or may become pregnant.

No effects were seen in female offspring exposed *in utero* to any dose of finasteride.

*Exposure to finasteride – risk to male fetus:* Crushed or broken Proscar Tablets should not be handled by women who are or may become pregnant because of the possibility of absorption of finasteride and the subsequent potential risk to a male fetus.

Similarly, small amounts of finasteride have been recovered from the semen in subjects receiving Proscar 5 mg/day. It is not known whether a male fetus may be adversely affected if his mother is exposed to the semen of a patient being treated with finasteride. Therefore, when the patient's sexual partner is or may become pregnant, the patient should either avoid exposure of his partner to semen (e.g. by use of a condom) or discontinue Proscar.

*Lactation:* Proscar is not indicated for use in women. It is not known whether finasteride is excreted in human milk.

*Effects on ability to drive and use machines:* None reported.

*Undesirable effects:* Proscar is well tolerated. The most frequently reported side-effects have been related to sexual function. In clinical studies, the following adverse experiences have been reported as possibly, probably or definitely drug related in ≥1% of patients treated for 12 months with Proscar 5 mg/day: impotence (3.7% on Proscar, 1.1% on placebo), decreased libido (3.3%, 1.6%), and decreased volume of ejaculate (2.8%, 0.9%).

The adverse experience profile for approximately 1,100 patients treated with 5 mg Proscar for up to 24 months, 400 patients treated for 36 months and 50 patients treated for 48 months (controlled studies of 6 to 12 months' duration and their extensions) was similar to that observed in the 12-month studies. There is no evidence of increased adverse experiences with increased duration of treatment with Proscar. The incidence of new drug-related sexual adverse experiences decreases with duration of treatment with Proscar, and in over 60% of patients who develop sexual adverse experiences they resolve with continued treatment.

The following adverse experiences have been reported in post-marketing experience: breast tenderness and enlargement; hypersensitivity reactions, including lip swelling and skin rash.

*Laboratory test findings:* When laboratory determinations of markers of prostate cancer such as PSA are evaluated, consideration should be given to the fact that levels are decreased in patients treated with Proscar.

Serum PSA concentration is correlated with patient age and prostatic volume, and prostatic volume is correlated with patient age. When PSA laboratory determinations are evaluated, consideration should be given to the fact that PSA levels generally decrease in patients treated with Proscar (see 'Special warnings and special precautions for use', Prostate cancer). In most patients, a rapid decrease in PSA is seen within the first months of therapy, after which time PSA levels stabilise to a new baseline. The post-treatment baseline approximates half of the pre-treatment value. This decrease is predictable over the entire range of PSA values, although it may vary in individual patients. Therefore, in typical patients treated with Proscar for six months or more, PSA values should be doubled for comparison to normal ranges in untreated men. There is considerable overlap in PSA levels among men with and without prostate cancer. Therefore, in men with BPH, PSA values within the normal reference range do not rule out prostate cancer, regardless of finasteride treatment.

Based on a comparison of PSA levels between men diagnosed with prostate cancer while taking Proscar (n = 10) and men not diagnosed with prostate cancer while taking Proscar, any ability of PSA to distinguish between BPH and cancer was not adversely affected by treatment with Proscar.

No other difference was observed in patients treated with placebo or Proscar in standard laboratory tests.

*Overdose:* No specific treatment of overdosage with Proscar is recommended. Patients have received single doses of Proscar up to 400 mg and multiple doses of Proscar up to 80 mg/day for up to three months without any adverse effects.

**Pharmacological properties**

*Pharmacodynamic properties:* Finasteride is a competitive inhibitor of human 5 alpha reductase, an intracellular enzyme which metabolises testosterone into the more potent androgen, dihydrotestosterone (DHT). Finasteride has no affinity for the androgen receptor.

Benign prostatic hyperplasia (BPH) is a common disease in men over the age of 50 years. The development of the prostate gland and subsequent BPH is dependent upon the potent androgen, dihydrotestosterone (DHT). Testosterone, secreted by the testes and adrenal glands, is rapidly converted to DHT by 5 alpha reductase predominantly in the prostate gland, liver and skin, where it is then preferentially bound to the cell nucleus in these tissues.

*Pharmacokinetic properties:* After an oral dose of $^{14}C$-finasteride in man, 39% of the dose was excreted in the urine in the form of metabolites (virtually no unchanged drug was excreted in the urine), and 57% of total dose was excreted in the faeces. Two metabolites have been identified which possess only a small fraction of the 5 alpha-reductase activity of finasteride.

The oral bioavailability of finasteride is approximately 80%, relative to an intravenous reference dose, and is unaffected by food. Maximum plasma concentrations are reached approximately two hours after dosing and the absorption is complete within 6–8 hours. Protein binding is approximately 93%. Plasma clearance and the volume of distribution are approximately 165 ml/min and 76 l, respectively.

In the elderly, the elimination rate of finasteride is somewhat decreased. Half-life is prolonged from a mean half-life of approximately 6 hours in men aged 18–60 years to 8 hours in men aged more than 70 years. This is of no clinical significance and does not warrant a reduction in dosage.

In patients with chronic renal impairment, whose creatinine clearance ranged from 9–55 ml/min, the disposition of a single dose of $^{14}$C-finasteride was not different from that in healthy volunteers. Protein binding also did not differ in patients with renal impairment. A portion of the metabolites which normally is excreted renally was excreted in the faeces. It therefore appears that faecal excretion increases commensurate to the decrease in urinary excretion of metabolites. Dosage adjustment in non-dialysed patients with renal impairment is not necessary.

There are not data available in patients with hepatic insufficiency.

Finasteride has been found to cross the blood-brain barrier. Small amounts of finasteride have been recovered in the seminal fluid of treated patients.

*Preclinical safety data:* No further information provided.

**Pharmaceutical particulars**

*List of excipients:* Cellulose, Microcrystalline PhEur; Docusate Sodium BP; Lactose PhEur; Magnesium Stearate PhEur; Pregelatinised Maize Starch BP; Sodium Starch Glycollate BP; Yellow Iron Oxide EEC; Hydroxypropylcellulose PhEur; Indigo Carmine Aluminium Lake EEC; Methylhydroxypropylcellulose PhEur; Talc PhEur; Titanium Dioxide PhEur.

*Incompatibilities:* None reported.

*Shelf life:* Two years.

*Special precautions for storage:* Protect from light. Keep container closed. Store below 25°C.

*Nature and contents of container:* Opaque PVC/PE/PVDC blisters lidded with aluminium foil; packs of 28 tablets.

*Instructions for use/handling:* Crushed or broken Proscar Tablets should not be handled by women who are or may become pregnant.

**Marketing authorisation number** 0025/0279.

**Date of approval/revision of SPC** April 1994.

**Legal category** POM.

## SALURIC*

**Presentation** White, half-scored tablets, marked 'MSD 432', containing 500 mg Chlorothiazide BP.

**Uses** Thiazide diuretic and antihypertensive.

Oedema associated with congestive heart failure, hepatic cirrhosis, premenstrual tension, and in oedema due to various forms of renal dysfunction (i.e. nephrotic syndrome, acute glomerulonephritis and chronic renal failure). Hypertension, either alone or as an adjunct to other antihypertensive drugs.

**Dosage and administration** Dosage should be determined on an individual basis, and the lowest dosage necessary to achieve the desired result should be used.

*Adults – for oedema:* Usually ½–2 tablets (250–1,000 mg) a day given in a single dose or in two divided doses. Many patients respond to intermittent therapy: every other day, or three to five consecutive days a week. Intermittent therapy is less likely to produce excessive diuretic response with resulting electrolyte imbalance. The maximum recommended daily dose is 2 tablets (1000 mg).

*In oedema accompanying premenstrual tension:* ½–1 tablet (250–500 mg) once or twice a day, from the first morning of symptoms until the onset of the menses.

*Adults – for control of hypertension:* The usual starting dose is ½ tablet (250 mg) a day as a single or divided dose.

In some patients, a ¼ tablet (125 mg), alone or with another antihypertensive, may be sufficient to initiate therapy. Dosage should be adjusted to response, but should not exceed 1 tablet (500 mg) a day.

Thiazides may add to the action of other antihypertensives. If Saluric is added to therapy with other antihypertensive agents, dosage reduction of such agents may be necessary to prevent an excessive drop in blood pressure.

*Infants and children:* Usually 25 mg per kg bodyweight a day, given in two doses. Infants under six months may need up to 35 mg per kg a day, in two doses.

On this basis, infants up to two years of age may be given 125–375 mg of Saluric daily in two doses. Children from 2 to 12 years of age may be given 375 mg to 1.0 g daily in two doses. Dosage in both age groups should be based on bodyweight.

*Use in the elderly:* Particular caution is needed in the elderly because of their susceptibility to electrolyte imbalance; the dosage should be carefully adjusted according to renal function and clinical response.

**Contra-indications, warnings, etc**

*Contra-indications:* Anuria, known hypersensitivity to this product or to other sulphonamide-derived drugs, severe renal or hepatic failure, Addison's disease, hypercalcaemia, concurrent lithium therapy. See 'Use in pregnancy' and 'Use in breast-feeding mothers', under 'Precautions'.

*Precautions:* Patients should be carefully monitored for signs of fluid and electrolyte imbalance (hyponatraemia, hypochloraemic alkalosis, hypokalaemia and hypomagnesaemia). It is particularly important to make serum and urine electrolyte determinations when the patient is vomiting excessively or receiving parenteral fluids. Warning signs or symptoms of fluid and electrolyte imbalance include: dryness of mouth, thirst, weakness, lethargy, drowsiness, restlessness, seizures, confusion, muscle pains or cramps, muscular fatigue, hypotension, oliguria, tachycardia, and gastro-intestinal disturbances such as nausea and vomiting.

Hypokalaemia may develop, especially with brisk diuresis, when severe cirrhosis is present, or after prolonged therapy. Hypokalaemia can sensitise or exaggerate the response of the heart to the toxic effects of digitalis (e.g. increased ventricular irritability).

Sensitivity reactions may occur in patients with or without history of allergy or bronchial asthma.

Hypokalaemia may be avoided or treated in the adult by concurrent use of amiloride hydrochloride (Midamor*), a potassium-conserving agent. It may also be avoided by giving potassium chloride or foods with a high potassium content. (Note that symptoms and signs which might indicate ulceration or obstruction of the small bowel in patients taking tablets or capsules containing potassium salts are indications for stopping treatment with such preparations immediately.)

Diuretic-induced hyponatraemia is usually mild and asymptomatic. Dilutional hyponatraemia may occur in oedematous patients in hot weather; and, except in rare instances when hyponatraemia is life-threatening, appropriate therapy is water restriction rather than administration of salt.

Thiazides may decrease serum Protein Bound Iodine levels without signs of thyroid disturbances.

Thiazides may decrease urinary calcium excretion, and may also cause intermittent and slight elevation of serum calcium in the absence of known disorders of calcium metabolism. Thiazides should be discontinued before carrying out tests for parathyroid function.

When creatinine clearance falls below 30 ml/min, thiazide diuretics become ineffective.

Uraemia may be precipitated or increased by Saluric. Cumulative effects of chlorothiazide may develop in patients with impaired renal function. If increasing uraemia and oliguria occur during treatment of renal disease, Saluric should be discontinued.

Thiazides should be used with caution in patients with impaired hepatic function or progressive liver disease, since minor alterations of fluid and electrolyte balance may precipitate hepatic coma.

Hyperuricaemia may occur, or gout may be precipitated, in certain patients receiving thiazide therapy.

Thiazide therapy may impair glucose tolerance.

Increases in cholesterol and triglyceride levels may be associated with thiazide diuretic therapy.

The possibility of exacerbation or activation of systemic lupus erythematosus has been reported.

Latent diabetes may become manifest during thiazide administration.

*Use in pregnancy:* Thiazides cross the placental barrier and appear in the cord blood. The use of Saluric when pregnancy is present or suspected, requires that the benefits of the drug be weighed against the possible hazards to the fetus. These hazards include fetal or neonatal jaundice, thrombocytopenia, and possibly other adverse reactions which have occurred in the adult. The routine use of diuretics in otherwise healthy, pregnant women with or without mild oedema is not recommended, because their use may be associated with hypovolaemia, increased blood viscosity and decreased placental perfusion.

*Use in breast-feeding mothers:* Thiazides appear in breast milk. If use of the drug is deemed essential, the patient should stop breast-feeding.

*Drug interactions: Alcohol, barbiturates or narcotics:* Co-administration may potentiate orthostatic hypotension. *Oral and parenteral antidiabetic drugs* may require adjustment of dosage with concurrent use. *Other antihypertensive drugs* may have an additive effect. Discontinuation of diuretic therapy 2–3 days before the initiation of treatment with an ACE-inhibitor may reduce the likelihood of first-dose hypotension. The antihypertensive effect of the drug may be enhanced in the post-sympathectomy patient. *Cholestyramine and colestipol resins:* Both cholestyramine and colestipol resins have the potential of binding thiazide diuretics and reducing diuretic absorption from the gastro-intestinal tract. *Corticosteroids or ACTH* may intensify any thiazide-induced electrolyte depletion, particularly hypokalaemia. *Pressor amines such as adrenaline* may show decreased arterial responsiveness when used with Saluric, but this reaction is not enough to preclude their therapeutic usefulness. *Non-depolarising muscle relaxants such as tubocurarine* may possibly interact with Saluric to increase muscle relaxation. *Non-steroidal anti-inflammatory drugs* may attenuate the diuretic and antihypertensive effect of diuretics.

*Drug/laboratory tests:* Because thiazides may affect calcium metabolism, Saluric may interfere with tests for parathyroid function.

*Side-effects:* The following side-effects have been reported with chlorothiazide or other thiazide diuretics:

*Gastro-intestinal system:* Anorexia, gastric irritation, nausea, vomiting, cramps, diarrhoea, constipation, jaundice (intrahepatic cholestatic jaundice), pancreatitis, salivary gland inflammation.

*Central nervous system:* Dizziness, vertigo, paraesthesiae, headache, yellow vision.

*Haematological:* Leucopenia, agranulocytosis, thrombocytopenia, aplastic anaemia, haemolytic anaemia.

*Cardiovascular:* Hypotension, including orthostatic hypotension.

*Hypersensitivity:* Purpura, photosensitivity, rash, urticaria, necrotising angiitis (vasculitis, cutaneous vasculitis), fever, respiratory distress including pneumonitis and pulmonary oedema, anaphylactic reactions, toxic epidermal necrolysis.

*Metabolic:* Hyperglycaemia, glycosuria, hyperuricaemia, electrolyte imbalance including hyponatraemia and hypokalaemia.

*Renal:* renal dysfunction, interstitial nephritis, renal failure.

*Other:* Muscle spasm, weakness, restlessness, transient blurred vision, impotence.

*Overdosage:* The most common signs and symptoms observed are those caused by electrolyte depletion (hypokalaemia, hypochloraemia, hyponatraemia) and dehydration resulting from excessive diuresis. If digitalis has also been administered, hypokalaemia may accentuate cardiac arrhythmias.

In the event of overdosage, symptomatic and supportive measures should be employed. If ingestion is recent, emesis should be induced or gastric lavage performed. Dehydration, electrolyte imbalance, hepatic coma, and hypotension should be corrected by established procedures. If required, give oxygen or artificial respiration for respiratory impairment.

**Pharmaceutical precautions** Keep container tightly closed; store in a cool place, protected from light.

**Legal category** POM.

**Package quantities** Bottles of 100. Packs of 30.

**Further information** Diuresis usually begins within two hours, is at a peak after four hours and persists for six to twelve hours. No rigid dietary salt restriction required.

The plasma half-life of chlorothiazide is 45–120 minutes.

**Product licence number** 0025/5019.

## SODIUM PARA-AMINOHIPPURATE

**Presentation** A clear, colourless to slightly yellow solution for intravenous injection, containing in each 10 ml of sterile solution 2 g sodium para-aminohippurate. Inactive ingredient: Sodium Hydroxide BP.

**Uses** As a diagnostic agent for the estimation of effective renal plasma flow (RPF). In research procedures, for the measurement of the functional capacity of the renal tubular secretory mechanism ($Tm_{PAH}$).

**Dosage and administration** For intravenous use only.

For the measurement of RPF, the concentration of sodium para-aminohippurate in the plasma is maintained at 2 mg per 100 ml. As a research procedure for the measurement of $Tm_{PAH}$, the plasma level of sodium para-aminohippurate must be sufficient to saturate the capacity of the tubular secretory cells. Concentrations of from 40 to 60 mg per 100 ml are necessary.

**Contra-indications, warnings, etc**

*Contra-indication*

Hypersensitivity to this product or its components.

*Precautions:* Intravenous solutions must be administered with caution in patients with low cardiac reserve, since a rapid increase in plasma volume can precipitate congestive heart failure.

For measurement of RPF, small doses of sodium

para-aminohippurate are used. However, in research procedures for Tm_PAH determinations high plasma levels are required to saturate the capacity of the tubular cells. During these procedures the intravenous administration of sodium para-aminohippurate solutions should be carried out slowly and with caution. The patient should be continuously observed for any adverse reactions.

Renal clearance measurement of sodium para-aminohippurate cannot be made with any significant accuracy in patients receiving sulphonamides, procaine or thiazolesulphone. These compounds interfere with chemical colour development essential to the analytical procedures.

Probenecid depresses tubular secretion of certain weak acids such as sodium para-aminohippurate; therefore, patients receiving probenecid will have erroneously low RPF and Tm_PAH values. Clearance is also affected by penicillins and salicylates.

*Pregnancy and lactation:* Animal reproduction studies have not been conducted with sodium para-aminohippurate. It is also not known whether sodium para-aminohippurate can cause fetal harm when administered to a pregnant woman or can affect reproduction capacity. Sodium Para-aminohippurate should be given to a pregnant woman only if clearly needed.

It is not known whether this drug is excreted in human milk. Because many drugs are excreted in human milk, caution should be exercised when Sodium Para-aminohippurate is administered to a breast-feeding woman.

*Side-effects:* Vasomotor disturbances, flushing, tingling, nausea, vomiting, cramps. Patients may have a sensation of warmth or the desire to defaecate or urinate during or shortly after the administration of a primary dose.

*Overdosage:* The dose is carefully controlled by experiment; no data are available on the symptoms of overdosage. No antidote is available.

The biological half-life of sodium para-aminohippurate is 10.2 minutes.

**Pharmaceutical precautions** No special requirements.

**Legal category** POM.

**Package quantities** Vials of 10 ml.

**Further information** Methods of calculating renal function are to be found in the package leaflet.

**Product licence number** 0025/5080.

# TIMOPTOL*

**Presentation** Clear, colourless to light yellow, sterile eye drops containing Timolol Maleate BP equivalent to 0.25% and 0.5% w/v solution of timolol. Each concentration is presented in:
Metered-dose Ocumeter* Dispensers containing 5 ml Ophthalmic Solution Timoptol with preservative;
Unit-dose dispensers containing 0.20 ml Ophthalmic Solution Timoptol without preservative.

**Uses** Timoptol Ophthalmic Solution is a beta-adrenoreceptor blocking agent used topically in the reduction of elevated intra-ocular pressure in various conditions including the following: patients with ocular hypertension; patients with chronic open-angle glaucoma including aphakic patients; some patients with secondary glaucoma.

**Dosage and administration** Recommended therapy is one drop 0.25% solution in the affected eye twice a day.

If clinical response is not adequate, dosage may be changed to one drop 0.5% solution in each affected eye twice a day. If needed, Timoptol may be used with miotics, adrenaline or systemically-administered carbonic anhydrase inhibitors.

Intra-ocular pressure should be reassessed approximately four weeks after starting treatment because response to Timoptol may take a few weeks to stabilise.

Provided that the intra-ocular pressure is maintained at satisfactory levels, many patients can then be placed on once-a-day therapy.

*Transfer from other agents:* When another topical beta-blocking agent is being used, discontinue its use after a full day of therapy and start treatment with Timoptol the next day with one drop of 0.25% Timoptol in each affected eye twice a day. The dosage may be increased to one drop of 0.5% solution in each affected eye twice a day if the response is not adequate.

When transferring a patient from a single anti-glaucoma agent other than a topical beta-blocking agent, continue the agent and add one drop of 0.25% Timoptol in each affected eye twice a day. On the following day, discontinue the previous agent completely, and continue with Timoptol. If a higher dosage of Timoptol is required, substitute one drop of 0.5%

solution in each affected eye twice a day (see 'Further information').

*Timoptol Unit-dose:* The Unit-dose Dispenser of Timoptol is free from preservative and should be used for patients who may be sensitive to the preservative benzalkonium chloride, or when use of a preservative-free topical medication is advisable.

Timoptol Unit-dose is a sterile solution. The solution from one individual unit is to be used immediately after opening for administration to one or both eyes. Since sterility cannot be maintained after the individual unit is opened, the remaining contents should be discarded immediately after administration.

*Paediatric use* is not currently recommended.

*Use in the elderly:* There has been wide experience with the use of timolol maleate in elderly patients. The dosage recommendations above reflect the clinical data derived from this experience.

**Contra-indications, warnings, etc**
*Contra-indications:* Bronchial asthma, history of bronchial asthma, or severe chronic obstructive pulmonary disease; sinus bradycardia, second and third degree AV block, overt cardiac failure, cardiogenic shock; and hypersensitivity to this product or other beta-blocking agents.

*Precautions:* Like other topically applied ophthalmic drugs, Timoptol may be absorbed systemically and adverse reactions seen with oral beta-blockers may occur.

Cardiac failure should be adequately controlled before beginning therapy with Timoptol. Patients with a history of severe cardiac disease should be watched for signs of cardiac failure and have their pulse rates checked.

Respiratory and cardiac reactions, including death due to bronchospasm in patients with asthma and, rarely, death associated with cardiac failure have been reported.

The effect on intra-ocular pressure or the known effects of systemic beta-blockade may be exaggerated when Timoptol is given to patients already receiving an oral beta-blocking agent. The response of these patients should be closely observed.

There have been reports of skin rashes and/or dry eyes associated with the use of beta-adrenoreceptor blocking drugs. The reported incidence is small and in most cases the symptoms have cleared when treatment was withdrawn. Discontinuation of the drug should be considered if any such reaction is not otherwise explicable. Cessation of therapy involving beta-blockade should be gradual.

The Ocumeter Dispenser of Timoptol contains benzalkonium chloride as a preservative which may be deposited in soft contact lenses; therefore, Timoptol should not be used while wearing these lenses. The lenses should be removed before application of the drops and not reinserted earlier than 15 minutes after use.

Timoptol has been generally well tolerated in glaucoma patients wearing conventional hard contact lenses. Timoptol has not been studied in patients wearing lenses made with material other than poly-methylmethacrylate (PMMA), which is used to make hard contact lenses.

The Unit-dose Dispenser of Timoptol is free from preservative and should, therefore, be discarded after single use to one or both eyes.

In patients with angle-closure glaucoma, the immediate objective of treatment is to reopen the angle. This requires constricting the pupil with a miotic. Timoptol has little or no effect on the pupil. When Timoptol is used to reduce elevated intraocular pressure in angle closure glaucoma it should be used with a miotic and not alone.

*Risk from anaphylactic reaction:* While taking beta-blockers, patients with a history of atopy or a history of severe anaphylactic reaction to a variety of allergens may be more reactive to repeated challenge with such allergens, either accidental, diagnostic or therapeutic. Such patients may be unresponsive to the usual doses of adrenaline used to treat anaphylactic reactions.

*Drug interactions:* Although Timoptol alone has little or no effect on pupil size, mydriasis has occasionally been reported when Timoptol is given with adrenaline.

Timoptol may potentially add to the effects of oral calcium antagonists, rauwolfia alkaloids or beta-blockers to induce hypotension and/or marked bradycardia.

*Breast-feeding mothers:* Timoptol is detectable in human milk. A decision for breast-feeding mothers either to stop taking Timoptol or stop nursing should be based on the importance of the drug to the mother.

*Use in pregnancy:* Timoptol has not been studied in human pregnancy. The use of Timoptol requires that the anticipated benefit be weighed against possible hazards.

*Side-effects:* Timoptol is usually well tolerated.

*Special senses:* Signs and symptoms of ocular irritation, including conjunctivitis, blepharitis, kerati-

tis, and decreased corneal sensitivity. Visual disturbances, including refractive changes (due to withdrawal of miotic therapy in some cases), diplopia, and ptosis.

*Cardiovascular:* Bradycardia, arrhythmia, hypotension, syncope, heart block, cerebrovascular accident, cerebral ischaemia, congestive heart failure, palpitation, cardiac arrest.

*Respiratory:* Bronchospasm (predominantly in patients with pre-existing bronchospastic disease), respiratory failure, dyspnoea.

*Body as a whole:* Headache, asthenia, fatigue, chest pain.

*Integumentary:* Hypersensitivity reactions including localised and generalised rash and urticaria, alopecia.

*Nervous system/psychiatric:* Dizziness, depression, increase in signs and symptoms of myasthenia gravis.

*Digestive:* Nausea.

*Causal relationship unknown:* The following adverse effects have been reported, but a causal relationship to Timoptol has not been established; aphakic cystoid macular oedema, dry mouth, nasal congestion, anorexia, dyspepsia, CNS effects (e.g. behavioural changes including confusion, hallucinations, anxiety, disorientation, nervousness, somnolence, and other psychiatric disturbances), hypertension, and retroperitoneal fibrosis. The adverse reactions seen with oral timolol maleate may occur with Timoptol.

*Overdosage:* No specific data are available. The most common signs and symptoms to be expected following overdosage with a beta-adrenoreceptor blocking agent are symptomatic bradycardia, hypotension, bronchospasm, and acute cardiac failure. If overdosage occurs, the following measures should be considered:

1. Gastric lavage, if ingested. Studies have shown that timolol does not dialyse readily.

2. Symptomatic bradycardia: Atropine sulphate, 0.25 to 2 mg intravenously, should be used to induce vagal blockade. If bradycardia persists, intravenous isoprenaline hydrochloride should be administered cautiously. In refractory cases, the use of a cardiac pacemaker may be considered.

3. Hypotension: A sympathomimetic pressor agent such as dopamine, dobutamine or noradrenaline should be used. In refractory cases, the use of glucagon has been reported to be useful.

4. Bronchospasm: Isoprenaline hydrochloride should be used. Additional therapy with aminophylline may be considered.

5. Acute cardiac failure: Conventional therapy with digitalis, diuretics, and oxygen should be instituted immediately. In refractory cases, the use of intravenous aminophylline is suggested. This may be followed, if necessary, by glucagon which has been reported useful.

6. Heart block (second or third degree): Isoprenaline hydrochloride or a pacemaker should be used.

**Pharmaceutical precautions** Timoptol is stable at room temperature. Protect from light.

**Legal category** POM.

**Package quantities** Both the 0.25% and 0.5% w/v solution are presented in:
Special metered-dose Ocumeter* Dispensers, each containing 5 ml;
Unit-dose Dispensers, available in cartons of 30 unit doses.

**Further information** Unlike miotics, Timoptol reduces IOP with little or no effect on accommodation or pupil size. In patients with cataracts, the inability to see around lenticular opacities when the pupil is constricted is avoided. When changing patients from miotics to Timoptol a refraction might be necessary when these effects of the miotic have passed.

Diminished response after prolonged therapy with Timoptol has been reported in some patients.

**Product licence numbers**
0.25% Ophthalmic Solution 5 ml
| | |
|---|---|
| Ocumeter | 0025/0134 |
| 0.20 ml Unit-dose | 0025/0210 |

0.5% Ophthalmic Solution 5 ml
| | |
|---|---|
| Ocumeter | 0025/0135 |
| 0.20 ml Unit-dose | 0025/0211 |

# TIMOPTOL*-LA ▼

**Qualitative and quantitative composition** Each millilitre of 0.25% w/v solution contains an amount of Timolol Maleate PhEur equivalent to 2.5 mg timolol.
Each millilitre of 0.5% w/v solution contains an amount of Timolol Maleate PhEur equivalent to 5 mg timolol.

**Pharmaceutical form** Sterile ophthalmic gel-forming solution.

**Clinical particulars**
*Therapeutic indications:* A beta-adrenoreceptor

blocker used topically in the reduction of elevated intra-ocular pressure in various conditions including the following: patients with ocular hypertension; patients with chronic open-angle glaucoma including aphakic patients; some patients with secondary glaucoma.

*Posology and method of administration:* Invert the closed container and shake once before each use. It is not necessary to shake the container more than once.

Recommended therapy is one drop 0.25% solution in each affected eye once a day.

If clinical response is not adequate, dosage may be changed to one drop 0.5% solution in each affected eye once a day.

If needed, Timoptol-LA may be used with miotics, adrenaline or systemically-administered carbonic anhydrase inhibitors. Other topically applied medication should be administered no less than 10 minutes before Timoptol-LA.

Intra-ocular pressure should be reassessed approximately four weeks after starting treatment because response to Timoptol-LA may take a few weeks to stabilise.

*Transfer from other agents:* When transferring a patient from Timoptol to Timoptol-LA, discontinue Timoptol after a full day of therapy, starting treatment with the same concentration of Timoptol-LA on the following day.

When another topical beta-blocking agent is being used, discontinue its use after a full day of therapy and start treatment with Timoptol-LA the next day with one drop of 0.25% Timoptol-LA in each affected eye once a day. The dosage may be increased to one drop of 0.5% solution in each affected eye once a day if the response is not adequate.

When transferring a patient from a single anti-glaucoma agent other than a topical beta-blocking agent, continue the agent and add one drop of 0.25% Timoptol-LA in each affected eye once a day. On the following day, discontinue the previous agent completely, and continue with Timoptol-LA. If a higher dosage of Timoptol-LA is required, substitute one drop of 0.5% solution in each affected eye once a day (see 'Pharmacodynamic properties').

*Paediatric use* is not currently indicated.

*Use in the elderly:* There has been wide-experience with the use of timolol maleate in elderly patients. The dosage recommendations given above reflect the clinical data derived from this experience.

*Contra-indications:* Bronchial asthma, history of bronchial asthma or severe chronic obstructive pulmonary disease; sinus bradycardia, second- or third-degree AV block, overt cardiac failure, cardiogenic shock; and hypersensitivity to any component of this product or other beta-blocking agents. Timoptol-LA should not be used in patients wearing contact lenses as it has not been studied in these patients.

*Special warnings and special precautions for use:* Like other topically applied ophthalmic drugs, this drug may be absorbed systemically and adverse reactions seen with oral beta-blockers may occur.

Cardiac failure should be adequately controlled before beginning therapy with Timoptol LA. Patients with a history of severe cardiac disease should be watched for signs of cardiac failure and have their pulse rates monitored.

Respiratory and cardiac reactions, including death due to bronchospasm in patients with asthma and, rarely, death associated with cardiac failure, are potential complications of therapy with Timoptol-LA.

The effect on intra-ocular pressure or the known effects of systemic beta-blockade may be exaggerated when Timoptol-LA is given to patients already receiving an oral beta-blocking agent. The response of these patients should be closely observed.

There have been reports of skin rashes and/or dry eyes associated with the use of beta-adrenoreceptor blocking drugs. The reported incidence is small and in most cases the symptoms have cleared when treatment was withdrawn. Discontinuation of the drug should be considered if any such reaction is not otherwise explicable. Cessation of therapy involving beta-blockade should be gradual.

The dispenser of Timoptol-LA contains benzododecinium bromide as a preservative. In a clinical study, the time required to eliminate 50% of the gellan solution from the eye was up to 30 minutes.

In patients with angle-closure glaucoma, the immediate objective of treatment is to reopen the angle. This requires constricting the pupil with a miotic. Timoptol-LA has little or no effect on the pupil. When Timoptol-LA is used to reduce elevated intra-ocular pressure in angle-closure glaucoma it should be used with a miotic and not alone.

Transient blurred vision following instillation may occur, generally lasting from 30 seconds to 5 minutes, and in rare cases up to 30 minutes or longer. Blurred vision and potenial visual disturbances may impair the ability to perform hazardous tasks such as operating machinery or driving a motor vehicle.

*Risk from anaphylactic reactions:* While taking beta-blockers, patients with a history of atopy or a history of severe anaphylactic reaction to a variety of allergens may be more reactive to repeated challenge with such allergens, either accidental, diagnostic, or therapeutic. Such patients may be unresponsive to the usual doses of adrenaline used to treat anaphylactic reactions.

*Interactions with other medicaments and other forms of interaction:* Although Timoptol alone has little or no effect on pupil size, mydriasis has occasionally been reported when Timoptol is given with adrenaline. The potential for mydriasis exists from concomitant therapy with Timoptol-LA and adrenaline.

Close observation of the patient is recommended when a beta-blocker is administered to patients receiving catecholamine-depleting drugs such as reserpine, because of possible additive effects and the production of hypotension and/or marked bradycardia, which may produce vertigo, syncope, or postural hypotension.

The potential exists for hypotension, atrioventricular (AV) conduction disturbances and left ventricular failure to occur in patients receiving a beta-blocking agent when an oral calcium-channel blocker is added to the treatment regimen. The nature of any cardiovascular adverse effect tends to depend on the type of calcium-channel blocker used. Dihydropyridine derivatives, such as nifedipine, may lead to hypotension, whereas verapamil or diltiazem have a greater propensity to lead to AV conduction disturbances or left ventricular failure when used with a beta-blocker.

The concomitant use of beta-adrenergic blocking agents and digitalis with either diltiazem or verapamil may have additive effects in prolonging AV conduction time.

Oral calcium-channel antagonists may be used in combination with beta-adrenergic blocking agents when heart function is normal, but should be avoided in patients with impaired cardiac function.

Intravenous calcium-channel blockers should be used with caution in patients receiving beta-adrenergic blocking agents.

*Pregnancy and lactation*

*Use in pregnancy:* Timoptol-LA has not been studied in human pregnancy. The use of Timoptol-LA requires that the anticipated benefit be weighed against possible hazards.

*Breast-feeding mothers:* Timolol is detectable in human milk. Because of the potential for adverse reactions to Timoptol-LA in infants, a decison should be made whether to discontinue nursing or to discontinue the drug, taking into account the importance of the drug to the mother.

*Effects on the ability to drive and use machines:* Transient blurred vision following instillation may occur, generally lasting from 30 seconds to 5 minutes, and in rare cases, up to 30 minutes or longer. Blurred vision and potential visual disturbances may impair the ability to perform hazardous tasks such as operating machinery or driving a motor vehicle.

*Undesirable effects*

*Side-effects:* Timopotol-LA is usually well tolerated. The most frequent drug-related complaint in clinical studies was transient blurred vision (6.0%), lasting from 30 seconds to 5 minutes following instillation.

The following possibly, probably, or definitely drug-related adverse reactions occurred with frequency of at least 1% in parallel active treatment controlled clinical trials:

*Ocular:* Burning and stinging, discharge, foreign body sensation, itching.

The following side-effects reported with Timoptol, either in clinical trials or since the drug has been marketed, are potential side effects of Timoptol-LA.

*Special senses:* Signs and symptoms of ocular irritation, including conjunctivitis, blepharitis, keratitis, and decreased corneal sensitivity. Visual disturbances, including refractive changes (due to withdrawal of miotic therapy in some cases), diplopia, and ptosis.

*Cardiovascular:* Bradycardia, arrhythmia, hypotension, syncope, heart block, cerebrovascular accident, cerebral ischaemia, congestive heart failure, palpitation, cardiac arrest.

*Respiratory:* Bronchospasm (predominantly in patients with pre-existing bronchospastic disease), respiratory failure, dyspnoea.

*Body as a whole:* Headache, asthenia, fatigue, chest pain.

*Integumentary:* Hypersensitivity reactions including localised and generalised rash and urticaria; alopecia.

*Nervous system/psychiatric:* Dizziness, depression.

*Neuromuscular:* Increase in signs and symptoms of myasthenia gravis.

*Digestive:* Nausea.

*Causal relationship unknown:* The following adverse effects have been reported but a causal relationship to therapy with timolol maleate has not been established: aphakic cystoid macular oedema, dry mouth, nasal congestion, anorexia, dyspepsia, CNS effects (e.g. behavioural changes including confusion, hallucinations, anxiety, disorientation, nervousness, somnolence, and other psychic disturbances), hypertension, and retroperitoneal fibrosis.

*Potential side-effects associated with oral administration of timolol:* The following additional side effects have been reported in clinical experiences with oral timolol maleate, and may be considered potential effects of ophthalmic timolol maleate:

*Body as a whole:* Extremity pain, decreased exercise tolerance.

*Cardiovascular:* AV block (second- or third-degree), sino-atrial block, oedema, pulmonary oedema, Raynaud's phenomenon, cold hands and feet, claudication, worsening of arterial insufficiency, worsening of angina pectoris, vasodilatation.

*Digestive:* Dyspepsia, vomiting, diarrhoea.

*Endocrine:* Hyperglycaemia, hypoglycaemia.

*Integumentary:* Pruritus, sweating, exfoliative dermatitis (one case).

*Musculoskeletal:* Arthralgia.

*Nervous system:* Vertigo, paraesthesia, local weakness.

*Psychiatric:* Nervousness, diminished concentration, hallucinations, nightmares, increased dreaming, insomnia, somnolence, decreased libido.

*Haematological:* Non-thrombocytopenic purpura.

*Respiratory:* Rales, cough.

*Special senses:* Tinnitus, dry eyes.

*Urogenital:* Impotence, micturition difficulties.

*Overdosage:* No specific data are available.

The most common signs and symptoms to be expected following overdosage with a beta-adrenoreceptor blocking agent are symptomatic bradycardia, hypotension, bronchospasm, and acute cardiac failure. If overdosage occurs, the following measures should be considered:

1. Symptomatic bradycardia: atropine sulphate, 0.25 to 2 mg intravenously, should be used to induce vagal blockade. If bradycardia persists, intravenous isoprenaline hydrochloride should be administered cautiously. In refractory cases, the use of a cardiac pacemaker may be considered.

2. Hypotension: a sympathomimetic pressor agent such as dopamine, dobutamine or noradrenaline should be used. In refractory cases, the use of glucagon has been reported to be useful.

3. Bronchospasm: isoprenaline hydrochloride should be used. Additional therapy with aminophylline may be considered.

4. Acute cardiac failure: conventional therapy with digitalis, diuretics, and oxygen should be instituted immediately. In refractory cases, the use of intravenous aminophylline is suggested. This may be followed, if necessary, by glucagon, which has been reported useful.

5. Heart block (second- or third-degree): isoprenaline hydrochloride or a pacemaker should be used.

Timolol does not dialyse readily.

**Pharmacological properties**

*Pharmacodynamic properties*

*Pharmacotherapeutic group:* Beta-adrenergic receptor blocking agent.

*Mechanism of action:* The precise mechanism of action of timolol maleate in lowering intra-ocular pressure is not clearly established. A fluorescein study and tonography studies indicate that the predominant action may be related to reduced aqueous formation. However, in some studies a slight increase in outflow facility was also observed.

Timoptol-LA is a new ophthalmic formulation comprising timolol maleate and a new delivery vehicle. Gellan solution contains a highly purified anionic heteropolysaccharide derived from gellan gum. Aqueous solutions of gellan gum form a clear transparent gel at low polymer concentrations in the presence of cations. When Timoptol-LA contacts the precorneal tear film, it becomes a gel. Gellan gum increases the contact time of the drug with the eye.

*Pharmacodynamics:* In parallel active treatment controlled, double-masked, multiclinic studies in patients with untreated elevated intra-ocular pressure of greater than 22 mm Hg in one or both eyes, 0.25% and 0.5% Timoptol-LA administered once daily had an intra-ocular pressure-lowering effect equivalent to the same concentration of Timoptol administered twice daily (see table below).

For the five independent comparative studies listed in the table below, the entrance criterion was an intraocular pressure of greater than 22 mm Hg in one or both eyes after a washout period of one week for most antiglaucoma medications and up to three weeks for ophthalmic beta-adrenergic antagonists. The dosage used was one drop of Timoptol-LA in each affected eye once daily versus one drop of Timoptol in each affected eye twice daily.

*Mean change in intra-ocular pressure (mm Hg) from baseline at trough (immediately before the morning dose) for the final week of the double-masked study*

| *Concentration* | *Timoptol-LA (n)* | *Timoptol (n)* | *Week* |
|---|---|---|---|
| 0.25% | −5.8 (94) | −5.9 (96) | 12 |
| 0.25% | −6.0 (74) | −5.9 (73) | 12 |
| 0.50% | −8.3 (110)* | −8.2 (111)* | 12 |
| 0.50% | −5.6 (189) | −6.3 (94) | 24 |
| 0.50% | −6.4 (212) | −6.1 (109) | 24 |

* The baseline intra-ocular pressure was elevated in comparison to the other studies due to the higher intra-ocular pressure of patients with pseudoexfoliative glaucoma.

Onset of action of timolol maleate is usually rapid, occurring approximately 20 minutes after topical application to the eye.

Maximum reduction of intra-ocular pressure occurs in two to four hours with Timoptol-LA. Significant lowering of intra-ocular pressure has been maintained for 24 hours with both 0.25% and 0.5% Timoptol-LA.

As compared with 0.5% Timoptol administered twice daily, in three clinical studies 0.5% Timoptol-LA administered once daily reduced mean heart rate less and produced bradycardia less frequently (see 'Special warnings and special precautions for use'). At trough (24 hours post-dose Timoptol-LA, 12 hours post-dose Timoptol), the mean reduction in heart rate was 0.8 beats/minute for Timoptol-LA and 3.6 beats/minute for Timoptol, whereas at two hours post-dose, the mean reduction was comparable (3.8 beats/minute for Timoptol-LA and 5 beats/minute for Timoptol).

Timolol maleate is a non-selective beta-adrenergic receptor blocking agent that does not have significant intrinsic sympathomimetic, direct myocardial depressant, or local anaesthetic (membrane-stabilising) activity.

Unlike miotics, timolol maleate reduces intra-ocular pressure with little or no effect on accommodation or pupil size. Thus, changes in visual acuity due to increased accommodation are uncommon, and the dim or blurred vision and night blindness produced by miotics are not evident. In addition, in patients with cataracts the inability to see around lenticular opacities when the pupil is constricted by miotics is avoided. When changing patients from miotics to Timoptol-LA, refraction may be necessary after the effects of the miotic have passed.

As with other antiglaucoma drugs, diminished responsiveness to timolol maleate after prolonged therapy has been reported in some patients. However, in clinical studies of Timoptol in which 164 patients were followed for at least three years, no significant difference in mean intra-ocular pressure was observed after initial stabilisation. This indicates that the intra-ocular pressure-lowering effects of timolol maleate is well maintained.

*Pharmacokinetic properties:* Onset of action of timolol maleate is usually rapid, occurring approximately 20 minutes after topical application to the eye.

Maximum reduction of intra-ocular pressure occurs in two to four hours with Timoptol-LA. Significant lowering of intra-ocular pressure has been maintained for 24 hours with both 0.25% and 0.5% Timoptol-LA. In a study of plasma timolol concentrations, the systemic exposure to timolol was less when normal healthy volunteers received 0.5% Timoptol-LA once daily than when they received 0.5% Timoptol twice daily.

*Preclinical safety data:* No adverse ocular effects were observed in monkeys and rabbits administered Timoptol-LA topically in studies lasting 12 months and one month, respectively. The oral $LD_{50}$ of timolol is 1,190 and 900 mg/kg in female mice and female rats, respectively. The oral $LD_{50}$ of gellan gum is greater than 5,000 mg/kg in rats.

In a two-year oral study of timolol maleate in rats there was a statistically significant ($p \leq 0.05$) increase in the incidence of adrenal phaeochromocytomas in male rats administered 300 mg/kg/day (300 times the maximum recommended human oral dose*). Similar differences were not observed in rats administered oral doses equivalent to 25 or 100 times the maximum recommended human oral dose.

* The maximum recommended daily oral dose of timolol is 60 mg. One drop of 0.5% Timoptol-LA contains about 1/300 of this dose, which is about 0.2 mg.

In a lifetime oral study in mice, there were statistically significant ($p \leq 0.05$) increases in the incidence of benign and malignant pulmonary tumours, benign uterine polyps and mammary adenocarcinoma in female mice at 500 mg/kg/day (500 times the maximum recommended human dose), but not at 5 or 50 mg/kg/day. In a subsequent study in female mice, in which post-mortem examinations were limited to uterus and lungs, a statistically significant increase in the incidence of pulmonary tumours was again observed at 500 mg/kg/day.

The increased occurrence of mammary adenocarcinoma was associated with elevations in serum prolactin which occurred in female mice administered timolol at 500 mg/kg, but not at doses of 5 or 50 mg/kg/day. An increased incidence of mammary adenocarcinomas in rodents has been associated with administration of several other therapeutic agents which elevate serum prolactin, but no correlation between serum prolactin levels and mammary tumours has been established in man. Furthermore, in adult human female subjects who received oral dosages of up to 60 mg of timolol maleate, the maximum recommended human oral dosage, there were no clinically meaningful changes in serum prolactin.

In oral studies of gellan gum administered to rats for up to 105 weeks at concentrations up to 5% of their diet and to mice for 96–98 weeks at concentrations up to 3% of their diet, no overt signs of toxicity and no increase in the incidence of tumours was observed.

Timolol maleate was devoid of mutagenic potential when evaluated *in vivo* (mouse) in the micronucleus test and cytogenetic assay (doses up to 800 mg/kg) and *in vitro* in a neoplastic cell-transformation assay (up to 100 mcg/ml). In Ames tests the highest concentrations of timolol employed, 5,000 or 10,000 mcg/plate, were associated with statistically significant elevations ($p \leq 0.05$) of revertants observed with tester strain TAIOO (in seven replicate assays), but not in the remaining three strains. In the assays with tester strain TAIOO, no consistent dose-response relationship was observed, nor did the ratio of test to control revertants reach 2. A ratio of 2 is usually considered the criterion for a positive Ames test.

Gellan gum was devoid of mutagenic potential when evaluated *in vivo* (mouse) in micronucleus assay using doses up to 450 mg/kg. In addition, gellan gum in concentrations up to 20 mg/ml was not detectably mutagenic in the following *in-vitro* assays: (1) unscheduled DNA synthesis in rat hepatocytes assay, (2) V-79 mammalian cell mutagenesis assay, and (3) chromosomal aberrations in Chinese hamster ovary cells assay.

In Ames tests, gellan gum (in concentrations up to 1,000 mcg/plate, which is its limit of solubility) did not induce a twofold or greater increase in revertants relative to the solvent control. It is therefore not detectably mutagenic.

**Pharmaceutical particulars**

*List of excipients:* Gellan gum, Trometamol PhEur, Mannitol PhEur, and Purified Water PhEur. Benzododecinium bromide (0.012%) is added as preservative.

*Incompatibilities:* None known.

*Shelf life:* 'Use not later than' date is printed on the package. The shelf life is 24 months.

*Special precautions for storage:* Store at or below 25°C. Avoid freezing. Protect from light.

*Nature and contents of the container:* Flexible-walled vials with controlled drop-size tips made from translucent low-density polyethylene contained in an outer sleeve, activated by pressing once on the bottom, closed by light-blue polypropylene caps (0.25%) or dark-blue polypropylene caps (0.5%).

Each metered-dose dispenser contains 2.5 ml Timoptol-LA-Ophthalmic gel-forming solution 0.25% or 0.5%.

*Instructions for use/handling:* Invert the container and shake once energetically before instillation.

**Marketing authorisation numbers**

| | |
|---|---|
| 0.25% | 0025/0310 |
| 0.5% | 0025/0311 |

**Date of approval/revision of SPC** 3 April 1996.

**Legal category** POM.

## TRUSOPT* ▼

**Qualitative and quantitative composition** Trusopt Sterile Ophthalmic Solution is supplied as an isotonic, buffered, slightly viscous, aqueous solution of dorzolamide hydrochloride. Each ml of Trusopt 2% contains 20 mg dorzolamide (22.3 mg of dorzolamide hydrochloride).

**Pharmaceutical form** Ophthalmic solution.

**Clinical particulars**

*Therapeutic indications:* Trusopt Ophthalmic Solution is indicated:

- as adjunctive therapy to beta-blockers
- as monotherapy in patients unresponsive to beta-blockers or in patients in whom beta-blockers are contra-indicated in the treatment of elevated intra-ocular pressure in:
  - ocular hypertension
  - open-angle glaucoma
  - pseudo-exfoliative glaucoma.

*Posology and method of administration:* When used as monotherapy, the dose is one drop of Trusopt Ophthalmic Solution in the conjunctival sac of the affected eye(s) three times daily.

When used as adjunctive therapy with an ophthalmic beta-blocker, the dose is one drop of Trusopt in the affected eye(s) twice daily.

When substituting Trusopt for another ophthalmic antiglaucoma agent, discontinue the other agent after proper dosing on one day, and start Trusopt on the next day.

If more than one topical ophthalmic drug is being used, the drugs should be administered at least 10 minutes apart.

*Contra-indications:* Trusopt is contra-indicated in patients who are hypersensitive to any component of this product.

Trusopt has not been studied in patients with severe renal impairment (CrCl <30 ml/min) or in patients with hyperchloraemic acidosis. Because Trusopt and its metabolite are excreted predominantly by the kidney, Trusopt is therefore contra-indicated in such patients.

*Special warnings and special precautions for use:* Trusopt has not been studied in patients with hepatic impairment and should therefore be used with caution in such patients.

The management of patients with acute angle-closure glaucoma requires therapeutic interventions in addition to ocular hypotensive agents. Trusopt has not been studied in patients with acute angle-closure glaucoma.

Trusopt is a sulphonamide and, although administered topically, is absorbed systemically. Therefore, the same types of adverse reactions that are attributable to sulphonamides may occur with topical administration. If signs of serious reactions or hypersensitivity occur, discontinue the use of this preparation.

In clinical studies, local ocular adverse effects, primarily conjunctivitis and lid reactions, were reported with chronic administration of Trusopt. Some of these reactions had the clinical appearance and course of an allergic-type reaction that resolved upon discontinuation of drug therapy. If such reactions are observed, discontinuation of treatment with Trusopt should be considered.

There is a potential for an additive effect on the known systemic effects of carbonic anhydrase inhibition in patients receiving an oral carbonic anhydrase inhibitor and Trusopt. The concomitant administration of Trusopt and oral carbonic anhydrase inhibitors has not been studied and is not recommended.

Safety and effectiveness in children has not been established.

Trusopt has not been studied in patients wearing contact lenses. The preservative in Trusopt Ophthalmic Solution, benzalkonium chloride, may be absorbed by soft contact lenses. Trusopt should not be administered while wearing soft contact lenses.

*Interaction with other medicaments and other forms of interaction:* Specific drug interaction studies have not been performed with Trusopt Ophthalmic Solution. In clinical studies, Trusopt was used concomitantly with the following medications without evidence of adverse interactions: timolol ophthalmic solution, betaxolol ophthalmic solution, and systemic medications including ACE inhibitors, calcium-channel blockers, diuretics, non-steroidal anti-inflammatory drugs including aspirin, and hormones (e.g. oestrogen, insulin, thyroxine). Association between Trusopt and miotics and adrenergic agonists has not been fully evaluated during glaucoma therapy.

Trusopt is a carbonic anhydrase inhibitor and, although administered topically, is absorbed systemically. In clinical studies, Trusopt was not associated with acid-base disturbances. However, these disturbances have been reported with oral carbonic anhydrase inhibitors and have, in some instances, resulted in drug interactions (e.g. toxicity associated with high-dose salicylate therapy). Therefore, the potential for such drug interactions should be considered in patients receiving Trusopt.

*Pregnancy and lactation*

*Pregnancy:* No studies were performed in pregnant women. Trusopt should not be used during pregnancy. In rabbits given maternotoxic doses associated with metabolic acidosis, malformations of the vertebral bodies were observed.

*Breast-feeding:* There are no data showing whether the drug is excreted in human milk. Trusopt should not be used during lactation. In lactating rats, decreases in the body weight gain of offspring were observed.

*Effects on ability to drive and operate machinery:* Possible side-effects such as dizziness and visual disturbances may affect the ability to drive and use machines.

*Undesirable effects:* The following adverse events have been reported either during clinical trials or during post-marketing experience:

*Ocular:* Burning and stinging, blurred vision, eye itching, tearing, conjunctivitis, eyelid inflammation, eyelid irritation, irritation including redness, pain, superficial punctate keratitis, iridocyclitis, transient myopia (which resolved upon discontinuation of therapy).

*Nervous system:* Headache, asthenia/fatigue, dizziness, paraesthesia.

*Hypersensitivity:* Signs and symptoms of systemic allergic reactions including angioedema, urticaria, pruritus, shortness of breath, rarely bronchospasm.

*Body as whole:* Rash, nausea, bitter taste, urolithiasis.

*Laboratory findings:* Trusopt was not associated with clinically meaningful electrolyte disturbances.

*Overdose:* No data are available in humans in regard to overdosage by accidental or deliberate ingestion.

Treatment should be symptomatic and supportive. Electrolyte imbalance, development of an acidotic state, and possible central nervous system effects may occur. Serum electrolyte levels (particularly potassium) and blood pH levels should be monitored.

The oral $LD_{50}$ of the drug is 1,320 mg/kg (3,960 mg/$m^2$) in mice and 1,927 mg/kg (11,369 mg/$m^2$) in female rats.

## Pharmacological properties
### Pharmacodynamic properties

*Mechanism of action:* Carbonic anhydrase (CA) is an enzyme found in many tissues of the body, including the eye. In humans, carbonic anhydrase exists as a number of isoenzymes, the most active being carbonic anhydrase II (CA-II) found primarily in red blood cells (RBCs) but also in other tissues. Inhibition of carbonic anhydrase in the ciliary processes of the eye decreases aqueous humour secretion. The result is a reduction in intra-ocular pressure (IOP).

Trusopt Ophthalmic Solution contains dorzolamide hydrochloride, a potent inhibitor of human carbonic anhydrase II. Following topical ocular administration, Trusopt reduces elevated intra-ocular pressure, whether or not associated with glaucoma. Elevated intra-ocular pressure is a major risk factor in the pathogenesis of optic-nerve damage and glaucomatous visual-field loss. Trusopt does not cause pupillary constriction and reduces intra-ocular pressure without side effects such as night blindness and accommodative spasm. Trusopt has minimal or no effect on pulse rate or blood pressure.

Topically applied beta-adrenergic blocking agents also reduce IOP by decreasing aqueous humour secretion but by a different mechanism of action. Studies have shown that when Trusopt is added to a topical beta-blocker additional reduction in IOP is observed; this finding is consistent with the reported additive effects of beta-blockers and oral carbonic anhydrase inhibitors.

*Pharmacodynamic effects: Clinical effects:* In patients with glaucoma or ocular hypertension, the efficacy of Trusopt given t.d.s. as monotherapy (baseline IOP ≥23 mm Hg) or given b.d. as adjunctive therapy while receiving ophthalmic beta-blockers (baseline IOP ≥22 mm Hg) was demonstrated in large-scale clinical studies of up to one-year duration. The IOP-lowering effect of Trusopt as monotherapy and as adjunctive therapy was demonstrated throughout the day and this effect was maintained during long-term administration. Efficacy during long-term monotherapy was similar to betaxolol and slightly less than timolol. When used as adjunctive therapy to ophthalmic beta-blockers, Trusopt demonstrated additional IOP lowering similar to pilocarpine 2% q.d.s.

*Pharmacokinetic properties:* Unlike oral carbonic anhydrase inhibitors, topical administration of dorzolamide hydrochloride allows for the drug to exert its effects directly in the eye at substantially lower doses and therefore with less systemic exposure. In clinical trials, this resulted in a reduction in IOP without the acid-base disturbances or alterations in electrolytes characteristic of oral carbonic anhydrase inhibitors.

When topically applied, dorzolamide reaches the systemic circulation. To assess the potential for systemic carbonic anhydrase inhibition following topical administration, drug and metabolite concentrations in RBCs and plasma and carbonic anhydrase inhibitions in RBCs were measured. Dorzolamide accumulates in RBCs during chronic dosing as a result of selective binding to CA-II while extremely low concentrations of free drug in plasma are maintained. The parent drug forms a single N-desethyl metabolite that inhibits CA-II less potently than the parent drug but also inhibits a less active isoenzyme (CA-I). The metabolite also accumulates in RBCs where it binds primarily to CA-I. Dorzolamide binds moderately to plasma proteins (approximately 33%). Dorzolamide is primarily excreted unchanged in the urine; the metabolite is also excreted in urine. After dosing ends, dorzolamide washes out of RBCs non-linearly, resulting in a rapid decline of drug concentration initially, followed by a slower elimination phase with a half-life of about 4 months.

When dorzolamide was given orally to simulate the maximum systemic exposure after long-term topical occular administration, steady state was reached within 13 weeks. At steady state, there was virtually no free drug or metabolite in plasma; CA inhibition in RBCs was less than that anticipated to be necessary for a pharmacological effect on renal function or respiration. Similar pharmacokinetic results were observed after chronic, topical administration of Trusopt. However, some elderly patients with renal impairment (estimated CrCl 30–60 ml/min) had higher metabolite concentrations in RBCs but no meaningful differences in carbonic anhydrase inhibition, and no clinically significant systemic side effects were directly attributable to this finding.

*Preclinical safety data:* The main findings in animal studies with dorzolamide hydrochloride administered orally were related to the pharmacological effects of systemic carbonic anhydrase inhibition. Some of these findings were species-specific and/or were a result of metabolic acidosis.

In clinical studies, patients did not develop signs of metabolic acidosis or serum electrolyte changes which are indicative to systemic CA inhibition. Therefore, it is not expected that the effects noted in animal studies would be observed in patients receiving therapeutic doses of Trusopt.

## Pharmaceutical particulars
*List of excipients:* Hydroxyethylcellulose, mannitol, sodium citrate, sodium hydroxide (to adjust pH), and water for injection. Benzalkonium chloride 0.0075% is added as preservative.

*Incompatibilities:* None known.

*Shelf life:* The shelf life is 24 months.

Trusopt should be used no longer than 4 weeks after first opening the container.

*Special precautions for storage:* Store Trusopt Ophthalmic Solution below 30°C. Protect from light.

*Nature and contents of container:* The 5 ml ALP vial consists of an oval, translucent, low-density polyethylene container with a metered dropper tip and an orange-coloured polypropylene cap. The tip and orange cap are covered with a translucent tamper-evident, disposable overcap.

*Instructions for use/handling:* Patients should be instructed to avoid allowing the tip of the dispensing container to contact the eye or surrounding structures.

Patients should also be instructed that ocular solutions, if handled improperly, can become contaminated by common bacteria known to cause ocular infections. Serious damage to the eye and subsequent loss of vision may result from using contaminated solutions.

**Marketing authorisation number** 0025/0323.

**Date of approval/revision of SPC** March 1996.

**Legal category** POM.

# TRYPTIZOL*

**Presentation** Blue, film-coated tablets, marked 'MSD 23', containing 10 mg Amitriptyline Hydrochloride BP; yellow, film-coated tablets, marked 'MSD 45', containing 25 mg; and brown, film-coated tablets, marked 'MSD 102', containing 50 mg.

Injection, a colourless solution containing per ml 10 mg amitriptyline hydrochloride.

Syrup, a pink suspension containing, in each 5 ml, Amitriptyline Embonate BP equivalent to 10 mg amitriptyline.

**Uses** Symptoms of depression (especially where sedation is required); also effective in nocturnal enuresis where organic pathology is excluded.

## Dosage and administration *Depression.*

*Oral therapy:* Therapy should be started with a low dosage and increased gradually, according to the clinical response and any evidence of intolerance.

*Adults – initial dosage:* Usually 75 mg a day in divided doses (or a single dose at night). If necessary, this may be increased to a total of 150 mg a day, the additional doses being given in the late afternoon and/or at bedtime.

The sedative effect is usually rapidly apparent. The antidepressant activity may be seen within three or four days or may take up to 30 days to develop adequately.

*Adults – maintenance dosage:* Usually 50–100 mg a day. For maintenance therapy, the total dosage may be given in a single dose preferably in the evening or at bedtime. When satisfactory improvement has been reached, dosage should be reduced to the lowest amount that will maintain relief of symptoms. Maintenance therapy should be continued for three months or longer to lessen the chances of relapse.

*Parenteral therapy:* Parenteral use of amitriptyline should be restricted to patients for whom oral therapy is inappropriate or difficult. Substitute oral therapy as soon as possible: 10–20 mg (1–2 ml) four times a day. The dosage should not exceed that for oral therapy

and should always be given in divided doses, intramuscularly or intravenously.

*Children:* Due to lack of clinical experience, Tryptizol is not recommended for the treatment of *depression* in children under 16 years of age.

*Enuresis:* Children aged 6–10 years may receive 10–20 mg a day, while those aged 11–16 years may need 25–50 mg a day. The recommended dosage must not be exceeded. Treatment should not exceed three months.

Most patients who respond, do so in the first few days of therapy.

This medication should be kept out of the reach of children. Tryptizol Syrup can be diluted with Syrup BP.

*Plasma levels:* Because of the wide variation in the absorption and distribution of tricyclic antidepressants in body fluids, dosage should be adjusted to clinical response and not based on plasma levels. However, plasma levels may be used as a guide to toxicity or to non-compliance.

*Elderly patients:* In general, lower dosages are recommended for these patients and an initial dosage of 10–25 mg t.d.s. is recommended, which should be increased slowly. A daily dosage of 50 mg may be satisfactory in elderly patients who may not tolerate higher dosages. The required dosage may be administered either as divided doses or as a single dose preferably in the evening or at bedtime.

## Contra-indications, warnings, etc
*Contra-indications:* Co-administration with monoamine oxidase inhibitors; prior sensitisation to amitriptyline; during the recovery phase after myocardial infarction; arrhythmias, particularly heartblock of any degree; mania; severe liver disease; lactation; children under 6 years of age. See also 'Use in pregnancy' under 'Precautions'.

*Precautions:* General: Tryptizol should be used with caution in patients with a history of epilepsy, in patients with impaired liver function and, because of its atropine-like action, in patients with a history of urinary retention, prostatic hypertrophy, narrow-angle glaucoma, or increased intra-ocular pressure. In patients with narrow-angle glaucoma, even average doses may precipitate an attack of glaucoma.

There has been a report of fatal dysarrhythmia occurring as late as 56 hours after amytriptyline overdose.

If possible, discontinue Tryptizol several days before surgery. But if emergency surgery is unavoidable, the anaesthetist should be informed that the patient is being treated with Tryptizol, because anaesthesia may increase the risk of hypotension and arrhythmias.

Hyperpyrexia has been reported when tricyclic antidepressants are administered with anticholinergic agents or with neuroleptic drugs, particularly during hot weather.

Tryptizol may impair alertness in some patients and activities made hazardous by diminished alertness (e.g. driving a car) should be avoided.

Elderly patients are particularly liable to experience adverse reactions: especially agitation, confusion, and postural hypotension.

Cardiovascular/endocrine disorders: Patients with cardiovascular disorders, hyperthyroid patients, and those receiving thyroid medication or anticholinergic agents should be closely supervised and the dosage of all medications carefully adjusted.

Central nervous system disorders: When Tryptizol is used for the depressive component of schizophrenia, psychotic symptoms may be aggravated. In manic-depressives, a shift towards the manic phase may occur; paranoid delusions, with or without associated hostility, may be aggravated. In such cases, a major tranquilliser should be given concurrently, or the dosage of Tryptizol reduced.

The risk of suicide remains during treatment of depressed patients and until significant remission occurs. Such patients require careful supervision.

Use in Children: Behavioural changes have been observed in children receiving tricyclics for the treatment of enuresis.

*Use in pregnancy:* The safety of Tryptizol for use during pregnancy has not been established. Tryptizol is not recommended during pregnancy, especially during the first and third trimesters unless there are compelling reasons, and in these patients the benefits should be weighed against possible hazards to the fetus, child, or mother. Clinical experience of the use of Tryptizol in pregnancy has been limited. Animal studies have shown harmful effects at exceptionally high doses.

*Breast-feeding mothers:* Amitriptyline is detectable in breast milk. Because of the potential for serious adverse reactions in infants from amitriptyline, a decision should be made whether to discontinue breast-feeding or discontinue the drug.

*Drug interactions:* Other antidepressant drugs: The concurrent use of antidepressants having varying modes of action should be made only with due recognition of their possible potentiation and with a thorough knowledge of their respective pharmacologies. Monoamine oxidase inhibitors can potentiate the effects of tricyclic antidepressants such as Tryptizol, and hyperpyretic crises, severe convulsions, and fatalities have occurred. A minimum of 14 days should elapse between discontinuing an MAOI and starting Tryptizol, which should be introduced cautiously and dosage increased gradually.

Guanethidine: Tryptizol may block the antihypertensive action of guanethidine, debrisoquine, bethanidine, and possibly clonidine. It would be advisable to review all antihypertensive therapy during treatment with tricyclic antidepressants.

Anticholinergic agents/sympathomimetic drugs: Amitriptyline should not be given with sympathomimetic agents such as adrenaline, ephedrine, isoprenaline, noradrenaline, phenylephrine, and phenylpropanolamine.

Paralytic ileus may occur in patients taking tricyclic antidepressants in combination with drugs having an anticholinergic action.

Central nervous system depressants: Tryptizol may enhance the response to alcohol, barbiturates, and other CNS depressants. In turn, barbiturates may decrease, and methylphenidate may increase, the antidepressant action of amitriptyline. Caution is advised if patients receive large doses of ethchlorvynol concurrently. Transient delirium has been reported in patients treated with 1 g ethchlorvynol and 75 mg to 150 mg of Tryptizol.

Disulfiram: Delirium has been reported in patients taking amitriptyline with disulfiram.

Cimetidine: Cimetidine is reported to reduce hepatic metabolism of certain tricyclic antidepressants.

Electroconvulsive therapy: Concurrent administration with ECT may increase the hazards of treatment, and should be limited to patients for whom it is deemed essential.

*Warnings and adverse effects:* In general, Tryptizol is well tolerated. The side effects given below are essentially a combined list of all those of the tricyclic group of antidepressants. Some of them have not been reported with Tryptizol, but are included because of the similar pharmacologies of the group members. As the antidepressant effects of Tryptizol may not become apparent for the first 2–4 weeks of therapy, patients should be closely monitored during this period.

*Cardiovascular reactions:* hypotension, syncope, postural hypotension, hypertension, tachycardia, palpitations, myocardial infarction, arrhythmias, heart block, stroke, non-specific ECG changes and changes in AV conduction. Arrhythmias and severe hypotension are likely to occur with high dosage or overdosage.

*CNS and neuromuscular:* confusional states, disturbed concentration, disorientation, delusions, hallucinations, hypomania, excitement, anxiety, restlessness, drowsiness, insomnia, nightmares, numbness, tingling, and paraesthesiae of the extremities, peripheral neuropathy, incoordination, ataxia, tremors, coma, convulsions, alteration of the EEG, extrapyramidal symptoms, including abnormal involuntary movements and tardive dyskinesia, dysarthria, tinnitus.

*Anticholinergic:* dry mouth, blurred vision, mydriasis, disturbance of accommodation, increased intraocular pressure, constipation, paralytic ileus, hyperpyrexia, urinary retention, urinary tract dilatation.

*Allergic:* skin rash, urticaria, photosensitisation, oedema of face and tongue.

*Haematological:* bone-marrow depression including agranulocytosis, leucopenia, eosinophilia, purpura, thrombocytopenia.

*Gastro-intestinal:* nausea, epigastric distress, vomiting, anorexia, stomatitis, unpleasant taste, diarrhoea, parotid swelling, black tongue, rarely hepatitis (including altered liver function and jaundice).

*Endocrine:* testicular swelling, gynaecomastia, breast enlargement, galactorrhoea, increased or decreased libido, impotence, interference with sexual function, elevation or lowering of blood sugar levels, syndrome of inappropriate ADH (antidiuretic hormone) secretion.

*Other reactions:* dizziness, weakness, fatigue, headache, weight loss, oedema, increased perspiration, urinary frequency, alopecia, increased appetite and weight gain (may be a drug reaction or due to relief of the depression). Abrupt withdrawal after prolonged administration has caused nausea, headache and malaise. Reports have associated gradual withdrawal with transient symptoms including irritability, restlessness, as well as dream and sleep disturbances during the first two weeks of dosage reduction. These symptoms are not indicative of addiction.

Adverse reactions such as withdrawal symptoms, respiratory depression and agitation have been reported in neonates whose mothers had taken tricyclic anti-depressants in the last trimester of pregnancy.

Mania or hypomania has been reported rarely within 2–7 days of stopping chronic therapy with tricyclic antidepressants.

*Side effects in enuresis:* Dosages used in enuresis are low compared with those used in depression, and side effects are therefore less frequent. The most common are drowsiness and anticholinergic effects. The only other side effects, reported infrequently at these dosages, have been mild sweating and itching.

The recommended dosage must not be exceeded.

*Side effects—causal relationship unknown:* The following additional side-effects have been reported; however, a causal relationship to therapy with amitriptyline has not been established: lupus-like syndrome (migratory arthritis, positive ANA and rheumatoid factor).

*Overdosage:* High dosage may cause temporary confusion, disturbed concentration, or transient visual hallucinations. Overdosage may cause drowsiness; hypothermia; tachycardia and other arrhythmic abnormalities such as bundle branch block; ECG evidence of impaired conduction; congestive heart failure; dilated pupils; disorders of ocular motility, convulsions; severe hypotension; stupor, coma and polyradiculoneuropathy, constipation. Other symptoms may be agitation, hyperactive reflexes, muscle rigidity, vomiting, hyperpyrexia, or any of those listed as adverse effects.

All persons suspected of having taken an overdosage should be admitted to hospital as soon as possible. Treatment is symptomatic and supportive. The stomach should be emptied as quickly as possible by emesis, followed by gastric lavage upon arrival at hospital. Following lavage, activated charcoal may be given during the first 24–48 hours at a dosage of 20–30 g every four to six hours. An ECG should be taken and close monitoring of cardiac function instituted if there is any sign of abnormality. An open airway and an adequate fluid intake should be maintained, and body temperature regulated.

Intravenous physostigmine salicylate, 1–3 mg, has been reported to reverse the symptoms of tricyclic antidepressant poisoning. Because physostigmine is rapidly metabolised, the dosage of physostigmine should be repeated as required, particularly if life-threatening signs such as arrhythmias, convulsions, and deep coma recur or persist after the initial dose of physostigmine. Because physostigmine itself may be toxic, it is not recommended for routine use.

Standard measures should be used to manage circulatory shock and metabolic acidosis. Cardiac arrhythmias may be treated with neostigmine, pyridostigmine or propranolol. Should cardiac failure occur, use of digitalis should be considered. Close monitoring of cardiac function for not less than five days is advisable.

If convulsions occur, they should be treated with paraldehyde, diazepam or an inhalation anaesthetic. Barbiturates should not be used because Tryptizol increases their CNS-depressant action.

Dialysis is of no value because of low plasma concentrations of amitriptyline. Since overdosage is often deliberate, patients may attempt suicide by other means during the recovery phase. Deaths by deliberate or accidental overdosage have occurred with this class of medicament.

**Pharmaceutical precautions** Keep containers well closed and store below 25°C, protected from light. The injection and the syrup should also be protected from freezing. Tryptizol Syrup may be diluted with Syrup BP; the mixture should be used within 14 days.

**Legal category** POM.

**Package quantities**
*Tablets 10 mg:* Blister packs of 30.
*Tablets 25 mg:* Blister packs of 30.
*Tablets 50 mg:* Blister packs of 30.
*Injection:* Vials of 10 ml.
*Syrup:* Bottles of 200 ml.

**Further information** Tryptizol is a member of the tricyclic group of antidepressants. Its mode of action in man is not known, but it is not a monoamine oxidase inhibitor (special dietary restrictions are not necessary), and it does not act primarily by stimulating the CNS.

**Product licence numbers**
Tablets 10 mg    0025/0093
Tablets 25 mg    0025/0094
Tablets 50 mg    0025/0095
Injection         0025/5036
Syrup             0025/5037

# UTINOR* TABLETS

**Qualitative and quantitative composition** Utinor contains 400 mg of the active ingredient, norfloxacin USP.

**Pharmaceutical form** Utinor is supplied as white, oval tablets marked 'MSD 705'.

**Clinical particulars**
*Therapeutic indications:* Broad-spectrum, bactericidal agent indicated for the treatment of:

Upper and lower, complicated and uncomplicated, acute and chronic urinary tract infections. These infections include cystitis, pyelitis, pyelonephritis, chronic prostatitis and those urinary infections associated with urological surgery, neurogenic bladder or nephrolithiasis caused by bacteria susceptible to Utinor.

*Posology and method of administration:* Susceptibility of the causative organism to Utinor should be tested. However, therapy may be initiated before obtaining the results of these tests.

| Diagnosis | Dosage | Therapy duration |
|---|---|---|
| Uncomplicated lower urinary tract infections (e.g. cystitis)† | 400 mg twice daily | 3 days |
| Urinary tract infections | 400 mg twice daily | 7–10 days |
| Chronic relapsing urinary tract infection‡ | 400 mg twice daily | up to 12 weeks |

†Trials in over 600 patients have demonstrated the efficacy and tolerability of Utinor in the three-day treatment of uncomplicated urinary tract infections.
‡If adequate suppression is obtained within the first four weeks of therapy, the dose of Utinor may be reduced to 400 mg daily.

*Patients with renal impairment:* Utinor is suitable for the treatment of patients with renal impairment. In studies involving patients whose creatinine clearance was less than 30 ml/min, but who did not require haemodialysis, the plasma half-life of norfloxacin was approximately eight hours. Clinical studies showed there was no difference in the mean half-life of norfloxacin in patients with a creatinine clearance of less than 10 ml/min, compared to patients with creatinine clearance of 10–30 ml/min. Hence, for these patients, the recommended dose is one 400 mg tablet once daily. At this dosage, concentrations in appropriate body tissues or fluids exceed the MICs for most pathogens sensitive to norfloxacin.

*Use in the elderly:* Pharmacokinetic studies have shown no appreciable changes when compared to younger patients, apart from a slight prolongation of half-life. In the absence of renal impairment, no adjustment of dosage is necessary. Limited clinical studies have shown Utinor to be well tolerated.

*Contra-indications:* Hypersensitivity to any component of this product or any chemically related quinolone antibacterials.

Utinor is contra-indicated in prepubertal children and growing adolescents.

*Special warnings and precautions for use:*
*Precautions:* Convulsions have been reported rarely with norfloxacin, although a causal relationship has not been established.

As with other drugs in this class, Utinor should not be used in patients with a history of convulsions or known factors that predispose to seizures unless there is an overwhelming clinical need.

Tendinitis and/or tendon rupture, particularly affecting the Achilles tendon, may occur with quinolone antibiotics. Such reactions have been observed, particularly in older patients and in those treated concurrently with corticosteroids. At the first sign of pain or inflammation, patients should discontinue Utinor and rest the affected limbs.

Photosensitivity reactions have been observed in patients who are exposed to excessive sunlight while receiving some members of this drug class. Excessive sunlight should be avoided. Therapy should be discontinued if photosensitivity occurs.

Rarely, haemolytic reactions have been reported in patients with latent or actual defects in glucose-6-phosphate dehydrogenase activity who take quinolone antibacterial agents, including norfloxacin (see *Side effects*).

*Use in children:* As with other quinolones, Utinor has been shown to cause arthropathy in immature animals. The safety of Utinor in children has not been adequately explored and therefore the use of Utinor in prepubertal children or growing adolescents is contra-indicated.

*Interaction with other medicaments and other forms of interaction:* Co-administration of probenecid does not affect serum concentrations of norfloxacin, but urinary excretion of the drug diminishes.

As with other organic acid antibacterials, antagonism has been demonstrated *in vitro* between Utinor and nitrofurantoin.

Elevated plasma levels of theophylline have been reported with concomitant quinolone use. There have been rare reports of theophylline-related side effects in patients on concomitant therapy with norfloxacin and theophylline. Therefore, monitoring of theophylline plasma levels should be considered and dosage of theophylline adjusted as required.

Elevated serum levels of cyclosporin have been reported with concomitant use of norfloxacin. Cyclosporin serum levels should be monitored and appropriate cyclosporin dosage adjustments made when these drugs are used concomitantly.

Quinolones, including norfloxacin, may enhance the effects of the anticoagulant warfarin, or its derivatives, by displacing significant amounts from serum albumin-binding sites. When concomitant administration of these products cannot be avoided, measurements of prothrombin time or other suitable coagulation tests should be carried out.

Multivitamins, products containing iron or zinc, antacids or sucralfate should not be administered concomitantly with, or within two hours of, the administration of norfloxacin because they may interfere with absorption, resulting in lower serum and urine levels of norfloxacin.

Some quinolones, including norfloxacin, have also been shown to interfere with the metabolism of caffeine. This may lead to reduced clearance of caffeine and a prolongation of its plasma half-life.

Animal data have shown that quinolones in combination with fenbufen can lead to convulsions. Therefore, concomitant administration of quinolones and fenbufen should be avoided.

*Pregnancy and lactation:* There is no evidence from animal studies that norfloxacin has any teratogenic or mutagenic effects. Embryotoxicity secondary to maternotoxicity was observed after large doses in rabbits. Embryonic losses were observed in cynomolgus monkeys without any teratogenic effects. The relevance of these findings for humans is uncertain.

The safe use of Utinor in pregnant women has not been established; however, as with other quinolones, norfloxacin has been shown to cause arthropathy in immature animals and therefore its use during pregnancy is not recommended.

It is not known whether Utinor is excreted in human milk; administration to breast-feeding mothers is thus not recommended.

*Effects on ability to drive and use machines:* There are no specific data. However, dizziness has been reported as a side effect in some patients. Patients should know how they react to Utinor before driving or operating machines.

*Undesirable effects:* The overall incidence of drug-related side effects reported during clinical trials was approximately 3%.

The most common side effects have been gastrointestinal, neuropsychiatric and skin reactions, and include nausea, headache, dizziness, rash, heartburn, abdominal pain/cramps, and diarrhoea.

Less commonly, other side effects such as anorexia, sleep disturbances, depression, anxiety/nervousness, irritability, euphoria, disorientation, hallucination, tinnitus, and epiphora have been reported.

Abnormal laboratory side effects observed during clinical trials included: leucopenia, elevation of ALAT (SGPT), ASAT (SGOT), eosinophilia, neutropenia, thrombocytopenia.

With more widespread use the following additional side effects have been reported:

*Hypersensitivity reactions:* Hypersensitivity reactions including anaphylaxis, interstitial nephritis, angioedema, vasculitis, urticaria, arthritis, myalgia, arthralgia.

*Skin:* Photosensitivity: Stevens-Johnson syndrome, toxic epidermal necrolysis, exfoliative dermatitis, erythema multiforme, pruritus.

*Gastro-intestinal:* Pseudomembranous colitis, pancreatitis (rare), hepatitis, including elevated liver-function tests.

*Nervous system/psychiatric:* Confusion, paraesthesia.

*Haematological:* Haemolytic anaemia, sometimes associated with glucose-6-phosphate dehydrogenase deficiency.

*Overdose:* No information is available at present.

In the event of recent acute overdosage, the stomach should be emptied by induced vomiting or by gastric lavage and the patient carefully observed and given symptomatic and supportive treatment. Adequate hydration must be maintained.

**Pharmacological properties**
*Pharmacodynamic properties:* Norfloxacin inhibits bacterial deoxyribonucleic acid synthesis and is bactericidal. At the molecular level, three specific events were attributed to norfloxacin in *Escherichia coli* cells:
1. Inhibition of the ATP-dependent DNA supercoiling reaction catalysed by DNA gyrase.
2. Inhibition of the relaxation of supercoiled DNA
3. Promotion of double-stranded DNA breakage.

Spontaneous mutation resistance to norfloxacin has occurred rarely, and resistance of the organism

during therapy has developed in less than 1% of patients treated.

*Bacteriology:* Utinor has a broad spectrum of antibacterial activity against Gram-positive and Gram-negative aerobic pathogens. The fluorine atom of the 6 position provides increased potency against Gram-negative organisms and the piperazine moiety at the 7 position is responsible for the anti-pseudomonal activity.

Utinor is active *in vitro* against the following bacteria:

*Bacteria found in urinary tract infections:*
*Enterobacteriaceae* – *Citrobacter* spp, *Citrobacter diversus, Citrobacter freundii, Edwardsiella tarda, Enterobacter* spp, *Enterobacter agglomerans, Enterobacter aerogenes, Enterobacter cloacae, Escherichia coli, Hafnia* spp, *Klebsiella* spp, *Klebsiella oxytoca, Klebsiella pneumoniae, Morganella morganii, Proteus* spp. (indole positive), *Proteus mirabilis, Proteus vulgaris, Providencia* spp, *Providencia rettgeri, Providencia stuartii, Serratia* spp, *Serratia marcescens.*
*Pseudomonadaceae* – *Pseudomonas aeruginosa, Pseudomonas cepacia, Pseudomonas fluorescens.*
*Other* – *Alcaligenes* spp, *Flavobacterium* spp.
*Gram-positive cocci* – *Enterococci, Staphylococcus* spp, *Staphylococcus* Coag. negative, *Staphylococcus aureus* (including penicillinase-producing and most methicillin-resistant strains), *Staphylococcus epidermidis, Staphylococcus saprophyticus, Streptococcus* Group B, Group D (including *Enterococcus faecalis*), Group G, *Streptococcus viridans.*

In addition, Utinor is active against *Bacillus cereus, Neiserria gonorrhoea, Ureaplasma urealyticum,* and *Haemophilus influenzae.*

Utinor is not active against anaerobes, including *Actinomyces* spp, *Fusobacterium* spp, *Bacteroides* spp, and *Clostridium* spp, other than *C. perfringens.*

There is no cross-resistance between norfloxacin and structurally unrelated antibacterial agents such as penicillins, cephalosporins, tetracyclines, macrolides, aminocyclitols and sulphonamides, 2,4 diaminopyrimidines, or combinations thereof (e.g. co-trimoxazole).

*Pharmacokinetic properties:* Norfloxacin is rapidly absorbed following oral administration. In healthy volunteers, at least 30–40% of an oral dose of norfloxacin is absorbed. This results in a serum concentration of 1.5 mcg/ml being attained approximately 1 hour after administration of a 400 mg dose. Mean serum half-life is 3 to 4 hours, and is independent of dose.

The following are mean concentrations of norfloxacin in various fluids and tissues measured 1 to 4 hours post-dose after the two 400 mg doses, unless otherwise indicated:

| | |
|---|---|
| Renal parenchyma | 7.3 mcg/g |
| Prostate | 2.5 mcg/g |
| Seminal fluid | 2.7 mcg/ml |
| Testicle | 1.6 mcg/g |
| Uterus/cervix | 3.0 mcg/g |
| Vagina | 4.3 mcg/g |
| Fallopian tube | 1.9 mcg/g |
| Bile | 6.9 mcg/ml |
| | (after 2×200 mg doses). |

Norfloxacin is eliminated through metabolism, biliary excretion and renal excretion. After a single 400 mg dose of norfloxacin, mean antimicrobial activities equivalent to 278,773 and 82 mcg of norfloxacin/g of faeces were obtained at 12, 24 and 48 hours, respectively.

Renal excretion occurs by both glomerular filtration and net tubular secretion, as evidenced by the high rate of renal clearance (approximately 275 ml/min). After a single 400 mg dose, urinary concentrations reach a value of 200 or more mcg/ml in healthy volunteers and remain above 30 mcg/ml for at least 12 hours. In the first 24 hours, 33–48% of the drug is recovered in the urine.

Norfloxacin exists in the urine as norfloxacin and six active metabolites of lesser antimicrobial potency. The parent compound accounts for over 70% of total excretion. The bactericidal potency of norfloxacin is not affected by the pH of urine.

Protein binding is less than 15%.

*Preclinical safety data:* Norfloxacin, when administered to 3- to 5-month-old dogs at doses four or more times the usual human dose, produced blister formation and eventual erosion of the articular cartilage of the weight-bearing joints. Similar changes have been produced by other structurally related drugs. Dogs six months or older were not susceptible to these changes.

Teratology studies in mice and rats and fertility studies in mice at oral doses of 30 to 50 times the usual dose for humans did not reveal teratogenic or fetal toxic effects. Embryotoxicity was observed in rabbits at does of 100 mg/kg/day. This was secondary to maternal toxicity and it is a non-specific antimicrobial effect in the rabbit due to an unusual sensitivity to antibiotic-induced changes in the gut microflora.

Although the drug was not teratogenic in cynomolgus monkeys at several times the therapeutic human dosage, an increased percentage of embryonic losses was observed.

**Pharmaceutical particulars**
*List of excipients:* Utinor contains the following inactive ingredients: Croscarmellose Sodium USNF; Magnesium Stearate PhEur; Microcrystalline Cellulose PhEur; Hydroxypropylcellulose PhEur; Hypromellose BP; Titanium Dioxide PhEur; Carnauba Wax PhEur.

*Incompatibilities:* None.

*Shelf life:* 36 months shelf life for blister packs.

*Special precautions for storage:* Store in a cool, dry place protected from light.

*Nature and contents of container:* Utinor is available as blister packs of 6 and 14 tablets.

*Instruction for use/handling:* None.

**Marketing authorisation number**  0025/0254

**Date of approval/revision of SPC**  April 1996.

**Legal category**  POM.

## ZINAMIDE*

**Qualitative and quantitative composition**  Each tablet of Zinamide contains 500 mg of pyrazinamide PhEur.

**Pharmaceutical form**  White tablets, with one side scored and the other side marked 'MSD 504'.

**Clinical particulars**
*Therapeutic indications:* Zinamide is indicated in patients with active tuberculosis caused by *Mycobacterium tuberculosis.* Zinamide is not active against the atypical mycobacteria. Zinamide should only be given in combination with other antituberculous agents.

*Posology and method of administration:*
*Usual adult dosage:* 20–35 mg/kg a day divided into three or four doses; the maximum daily dosage is 3 g regardless of body weight. Zinamide should be administered with at least one other effective antituberculous drug. The use of Zinamide in combination therapy does not modify the accepted dosages of other antituberculous agents.

*Paediatric use* has not been established (see *Special warnings and special precautions for use*).

*Use in the elderly:* The general considerations outlined above should also apply to elderly patients.

*Contra-indications:* Zinamide is contra-indicated in patients hypersensitive to any component of this product; in patients with hepatic disease; and in those with hyperuricaemia and/or gouty arthritis.

Zinamide is contra-indicated in breast-feeding mothers (see *Pregnancy and lactation*).

*Special warnings and special precautions for use:* Zinamide should only be used when close daily observation of the patient is possible, and when laboratory facilities are available for performing frequent liver-function tests and blood uric acid determinations. Pre-treatment examinations should include *in vitro* sensitivity tests of recent cultures of *M. tuberculosis* from the patient as measured against the usual antituberculous drugs.

Liver-function tests, especially aspartate transferase (AST) and alanine transferase (ALT) determinations, should be carried out prior to therapy, and then every two to four weeks during therapy. Therapy with Zinamide should be withdrawn and not reinstated if signs of hepatocellular damage occur.

Reduction in the size and/or frequency of dose is recommended for patients with renal insufficiency.

If hyperuricaemia accompanied by an acute gouty arthritis occurs, therapy should be discontinued and not reinstated. Close monitoring is advised to detect any increasing difficulty in the management of patients with a history of gout or diabetes mellitus.

*Children:* The safety of Zinamide for use in children has not been established. Because of its potential toxicity, the use of Zinamide in children should be avoided unless it is considered crucial.

*Interaction with other medicaments and other forms of interaction:* None known.

*Pregnancy and lactation:*
*Use during pregnancy:* There have been no well-controlled studies in pregnant women. Zinamide should only be used if the potential benefit justifies the risk to the fetus.

*Use during lactation:* Zinamide is contra-indicated in breast-feeding mothers. If its use is deemed essential, the patient should stop breast-feeding.

*Effects on ability to drive and use machines:* There are no data to suggest that Zinamide affects the ability to drive or use machines.

*Undesirable effects:* A hepatic reaction is the most

common side-effect of Zinamide. This varies from a symptomless abnormality of hepatic cell function, detectable only by laboratory tests, through a mild syndrome of fever, anorexia, malaise, liver tenderness, hepatomegaly and spleenomegaly, to more serious reactions such as clinical jaundice, and rare cases of progressive fulminating acute yellow atrophy and death.

Other side-effects – active gout, sideroblastic anaemia, arthralgias, anorexia, nausea and vomiting, dysuria, malaise, fever, urticaria, aggravation of peptic ulcer.

*Overdose:* Liver toxicity and hyperuricaemia may occur with overdosage.

The stomach should be emptied by gastric lavage if necessary.

There is no specific antidote. General supportive measures should be employed. Liver function should be monitored closely, and a high-carbohydrate, low-fat diet employed. Care should be taken to avoid exposure of the patient to other potential hepatotoxic agents, including alcohol. Benzodiazepines may be given if there is evidence of central nervous system stimulation.

Probenecid may be given for hyperuricaemia.

The plasma half-life of pyrazinamide is about nine to ten hours.

**Pharmacological properties**

*Pharmacodynamic properties:* Pyrazinamide exhibits tuberculostatic activity *in vitro* only at slightly acidic pH. The growth of tubercle bacilli within monocytes *in vitro* is completely inhibited by pyrazinamide at a concentration of 12.5 mcg/ml.

Pyrazinamide is active only at an acid pH, and it is therefore active mainly on the tubercle bacilli located within the cell. It is these bacteria which are probably responsible for microbial persistence and thus for relapses after chemotherapy has stopped.

Pyrazinamide has low bacterial activity compared with isoniazide. It is thought that when these are used in combination, isoniazide is the key bactericidal drug, whilst pyrazinamide has a sterilising role, acting on a special bacterial population inhibited by the acid environment inside the macrophage or the walls of tuberculous cavities.

*Pharmacokinetic properties:* Pyrazinamide is readily absorbed from the gastrointestinal tract. Peak concentrations occur about 2 hours after an oral dose and have been reported to be 33 mcg per ml after 1.5 g and 59 mcg per ml after 3 g.

Serum concentrations then decline, with a plasma half-life of about 9–10 hours.

About 30% of the dose is excreted in the urine as pyrazinoic acid and 4% as unchanged pyrazinamide within 24 hours.

*Preclinical safety data:* No relevant information.

**Pharmaceutical particulars**

*List of excipients:* Lactose PhEur, maize starch PhEur, magnesium stearate PhEur, silicon dioxide USNF, and purified water PhEur.

*Incompatibilities:* None known.

*Shelf life:* 60 months.

*Special precautions for storage:* Store at temperatures below 25°C.

*Nature and contents of container:* Amber glass bottles or HDPE bottles containing 100 tablets.

*Instructions for use/handling:* None.

**Marketing authorisation number** 0025/5038R

**Date of approval/revision of SPC** January 1996.

**Legal category** POM.

# ZOCOR*

**Qualitative and quantitative composition** Simvastatin 10 mg/20 mg/40 mg.

**Pharmaceutical form** Zocor is supplied as oval-shaped, film-coated tablets. The peach coloured tablets marked 'Zocor 10' contain 10 mg simvastatin, MSD. The tan coloured tablets marked 'Zocor 20' contain 20 mg simvastatin, MSD. The brick-red coloured tablets marked 'MSD 749' contain 40 mg simvastatin, MSD.

**Clinical particulars**

*Therapeutic indications*

*Hypercholesterolaemia:* For use in patients with primary hypercholesterolaemia, in whom response to diet and other non-pharmacological measures has been inadequate.

*Coronary heart disease:* In patients with coronary heart disease with a plasma cholesterol level of 5.5 mmol/l or greater, Zocor is indicated to:

- reduce the risk of mortality;
- reduce the risk of coronary death and non-fatal myocardial infarction;
- reduce the risk of undergoing myocardial revascularisation procedures (coronary artery bypass grafting and percutaneous transluminal coronary angioplasty); and
- slow the progression of coronary atherosclerosis, including reducing the development of new lesions and new total occlusions.

*Posology and method of administration:* Route of administration is oral.

The patient should be placed on a standard cholesterol-lowering diet before receiving Zocor and should continue on this diet during treatment with Zocor.

*Hypercholesterolaemia:* The recommended starting dose is 10 mg once daily taken in the evening. The dose range is 10 to 40 mg a day in single doses taken at night. A marked response to Zocor is seen within two weeks and the maximum therapeutic response occurs within four to six weeks. The response is maintained during continuation of therapy. When therapy with Zocor is stopped, total cholesterol has been shown to return to pretreatment levels. Adjustment of dosage, if required, should be made at intervals of not less than four weeks, depending on the patient's individual response.

If LDL-cholesterol levels fall below 1.94 mmol/l or total serum cholesterol levels fall below 3.6 mmol/l, consideration should be given to reducing the dose of Zocor.

*Coronary heart disease:* Patients with coronary heart disease can be treated with a starting dose of 20 mg/day given as a single dose in the evening. Adjustment of dosage, if required, should be made as specified above (see 'Posology and method of administation', *'Hypercholesterolaemia'*).

*Concomitant therapy:* Zocor is effective alone or in combination with bile-acid sequestrants. In patients taking immunosuppressive drugs concomitantly with Zocor, the maximum recommended dosage is 10 mg/day (see 'Special warnings and special precautions for use', *'Muscle effects'*).

*Dosage in renal insufficiency:* Because Zocor does not undergo significant renal excretion, modification of dosage should not be necessary in patients with moderate renal insufficiency.

In patients with severe renal insufficiency (creatinine clearance <30 ml/min), dosages above 10 mg/day should be carefully considered and, if deemed necessary, implemented cautiously.

*Use in the elderly:* Although experience in elderly patients is limited, efficacy using standard doses appears similar to that seen in the population as a whole. There is no apparent increase in the frequency of clinical or laboratory adverse findings.

*Children:* Studies to show safety and effectiveness in children have not been carried out.

*Contra-indications:* Hypersensitivity to this product; active liver disease or unexplained persistent elevations of serum transaminases; porphyria; pregnancy and breast-feeding (see also 'Special warnings and special precautions for use'); women of childbearing potential unless adequately protected by non-hormonal methods.

*Special warnings and special precautions for use*

*Homozygous familial hypercholesterolaemia:* In patients with the homozygous form of familial hypercholesterolaemia, in whom there is a complete absence of LDL receptors, therapy with Zocor is unlikely to result in clinical benefit.

*Hypertriglyceridaemia:* Zocor has only a moderate triglyceride-lowering effect and is not indicated where hypertriglyceridaemia is the abnormality of most concern (i.e. hyperlipidaemia types I, IV and V).

*Hepatic effects:* Minor asymptomatic transient rises in serum transaminase may occur soon after initiation of therapy with simvastatin which do not require the drug to be discontinued. There is no evidence that these changes are due to hypersensitivity to Zocor.

In the Scandinavian Simvastatin Survival Study (see *Pharmacodynamic properties*) the number of patients with one or more transaminase elevation to >3 times the upper limit of normal, over the course of the study, was not significantly different between the simvastatin and placebo groups (14 [0.7%] vs 12 [0.6%]), the number of patients with single elevations of SGPT (ALT) to 3 times the upper limit of normal was significantly higher in the simvastatin group in the first year of the study (20 vs 8, p=0.023), but not thereafter. Elevated transaminases resulted in the discontinuation of 8 patients from therapy in the simvastatin group (n=2,221) and 5 in the placebo group (n=2,223). All of the patients in this study received a starting dose of 20 mg of simvastatin; 37% were titrated to 40 mg.

It is recommended that liver-function tests be performed before treatment begins, and periodically thereafter (e.g. twice a year) for the first year of treatment or until one year after the last elevation in dose in all patients.

Special attention should be paid to patients who develop elevated serum transaminase levels, and in these patients measurements should be repeated promptly and then performed more frequently. If the transaminase levels show evidence of progression, particularly if they rise to three times the upper limit of normal and are persistent, the drug should be discontinued.

The drug should be used with caution in patients who consume substantial quantities of alcohol and/or have a past history of liver disease. Active liver diseases or unexplained transaminase elevations are contra-indications to the use of simvastatin.

*Muscle effects:* Transient mild elevations of creatinine phosphokinase (CPK) levels (from skeletal muscle) have been seen commonly in patients receiving Zocor, but these have been usually of no clinical significance. Therapy with HMG-CoA reductase inhibitors has rarely been associated with myopathy (0.1%). Myopathy should be considered in any patient with marked elevations of CPK levels (≥10 times the upper limit of normal), or with diffuse myalgias, muscle tenderness and such marked elevations of CPK levels. The patient should be asked to report promptly unexplained muscle pain, tenderness or weakness. Therapy with Zocor should be discontinued if markedly elevated CPK levels occur or if myopathy is diagnosed. These CPK elevations should be considered in the differential diagnosis of chest pain in a patient on therapy with Zocor.

The risk of myopathy with HMG-CoA reductase inhibitors is known to be increased by concomitant immunosuppressive therapy, including cyclosporins, and by concomitant therapy with a fibric acid derivative or lipid-lowering doses of nicotinic acid. There have been rare reports of severe rhabdomyolysis with secondary acute renal failure. Therefore, the benefits and risks of using simvastatin concomitantly with immunosuppressive or fibrate drugs or lipid-lowering doses of nicotinic acid should be carefully considered.

Myopathy or rhabdomyolysis has occurred in transplant and non-transplant patients receiving Zocor or another HMG-CoA reductase inhibitor following the initiation of treatment with the antifungal agent itraconazole. In a study in normal volunteers, plasma levels of another HMG-CoA reductase inhibitor were increased about 20 fold when administered concomitantly with itraconazole. This is probably related to metabolism of both drugs by the same P-450 isoform. Based on this data, therapy with Zocor should be temporarily interrupted if systemic azole derivative antifungal therapy is required.

Therapy with Zocor should be temporarily withheld or discontinued in any patient with an acute, serious condition suggestive of a myopathy or having a risk factor predisposing to the development of renal failure secondary to rhabdomyolysis.

*Ophthalmic examination:* In the absence of any drug therapy, an increase in the prevalence of lens opacities with time is expected as a result of ageing. Current long-term data from clinical trials do not indicate an adverse effect of simvastatin on the human lens.

*Paediatric use:* Safety and effectiveness in children have not been established. Zocor is not recommended for paediatric use at this time.

*Interactions with other medicaments and other forms of interaction:*

*Phenazone* is a model for drugs metabolised by the microsomal hepatic enzyme system (cytochrome P450 system). Zocor had little or no detectable effect on the pharmacokinetics of phenazone in hypercholesterolaemic patients. However since Zocor is metabolised by the cytochrome P-450 isoform 3A4, this does not preclude an interaction with other drugs metabolised by the same form.

*Propranolol:* In normal volunteers, there was no clinically significant pharmacokinetic or pharmacodynamic interaction with concomitant administration of single doses of Zocor and propranolol.

*Digoxin:* Concomitant administration of Zocor and digoxin resulted in a slight elevation (less than 0.3 ng/ml) in drug concentrations (as measured by a digoxin radio-immuno-assay) in plasma compared to concomitant administration of placebo and digoxin.

*Coumarin derivatives:* In two clinical studies, one in normal volunteers and the other in hypercholesterolaemic patients, simvastatin 20–40 mg/day modestly potentiated the effect of coumarin anticoagulants: the prothrombin time, reported as International Normalised Ratio (INR), increased from a baseline of 1.7 to 1.8 and from 2.6 to 3.4 in the volunteer and patient studies, respectively. In patients taking coumarin anticoagulants, prothrombin time should be determined before starting simvastatin and frequently enough during early therapy to ensure that no significant alteration of prothrombin time occurs. Once a stable prothrombin time has been documented, prothrombin times can be monitored at the intervals usually recommended for patients on coumarin anticoagulants. If the dose of simvastatin is changed, the same procedure should be repeated. Simvastatin therapy has not been associated with bleeding or with changes in prothrombin time in patients not taking anticoagulants.

*Fibric acid derivatives:* (see 'Special warnings and special precautions for use', 'Muscle effects').

*Other concomitant therapy:* In clinical studies, Zocor was used concomitantly with ACE inhibitors, beta-blockers, calcium antagonists, diuretics, and non-steroidal anti-inflammatory drugs (NSAIDs) without evidence of clinically significant adverse interactions.

Caution should be exercised in the concomitant use of Zocor with immunosuppressant therapy, itraconazole or nicotinic acid (see 'Special warnings and special precautions for use', 'Muscle effects').

*Pregnancy and lactation*

*Pregnancy:* Zocor is contra-indicated in pregnancy.

Atherosclerosis is a chronic process and the discontinuation of lipid-lowering drugs during pregnancy should have little impact on the outcome of long-term therapy of primary hypercholesterolaemia. Moreover, cholesterol and other products of the cholesterol biosynthesis pathway are essential components for fetal development, including synthesis of steroids and cell membranes. Because of the ability of inhibitors of HMG-CoA reductase such as Zocor to decrease the synthesis of cholesterol and possibly other products of the cholesterol biosynthesis pathway, Zocor is contra-indicated for use in pregnancy and women of child bearing potential unless such patients are highly unlikely to conceive or such patients are adequately protected by non-hormonal methods. An interval of one months should elapse between the end of therapy with Zocor and planned conception. If the patient becomes pregnant while taking this drug Zocor should be discontinued immediately and the patient apprised of the potential hazard to the foetus.

The active metabolite of simvastatin was shown to produce fetal malformations in the offspring of pregnant rats. A few reports have been received of congenital anomalies in infants whose mothers were treated during pregnancy with HMG-CoA reductase inhibitors.

In a review of approximately 100 prospectively followed pregnancies in women exposed to Zocor or another structurally related HMG-CoA reductase inhibitor, the incidences of congenital anomalies, spontaneous abortions and fetal death/stillbirths did not exceed what would be expected in the general population. As safety in pregnant women has not been established and there is no apparent benefit to therapy with Zocor during pregnancy, treatment should be immediately discontinued as soon as pregnancy is recognised.

*Breast-feeding mothers:* It is not known whether simvastatin or its metabolites are excreted in human milk. Zocor should be avoided during lactation.

*Effects on the ability to drive and use machines:* Not applicable.

*Undesirable effects:* Zocor is generally well tolerated; for the most part, side-effects have been usually mild and transient in nature. Less than 2% of patients on Zocor were discontinued from controlled clinical studies due to side-effects attributable to Zocor.

In the pre-marketing controlled clinical studies, adverse effects occurring with a frequency of 1% or more and considered by the investigator as possibly, probably or definitely drug related were: abdominal pain, constipation, and flatulence. Other side-effects occurring in 0.5–0.9% of patients were asthenia and headache. Myopathy has been reported rarely.

In the Scandinavian Simvastatin Survival Study (4S) involving 4,444 patients treated with Zocor 20–40 mg/day (n=2,221) or placebo (n=2,223), the safety and tolerability profiles were comparable between groups over the median 5.4 years of the study.

The following additional side-effects were reported either in long-term extension studies or in marketed use: nausea, diarrhoea, rash, dyspepsia, pruritus, alopecia, dizziness, muscle cramps, myalgia, pancreatitis, paraesthesia, peripheral neuropathy, vomiting, and anaemia. Rarely, rhabdomyolysis and hepatitis/jaundice occurred. An apparent hypersensitivity syndrome has been reported rarely which has included some of the following features: angioedema, lupus-like syndrome, polymyalgia rheumatica, vasculitis, thrombocytopenia, eosinophilia, ESR increased, arthritis, arthralgia, urticaria, photosensitivity, fever, flushing, dyspnoea, and malaise.

*Laboratory test findings:* Marked and persistent increases of serum transaminases have been reported infrequently. Elevated alkaline phosphatase and γ-glutamyl transpeptidase have been reported.

Liver-function test abnormalities have generally been mild and transient. Increases in serum creatinine phosphokinase (CPK) levels derived from skeletal muscle have been reported (see 'Special warnings and special precautions for use').

*Side-effects – causal relationship unknown:* The following side-effects have been reported; however, a causal relationship to therapy with Zocor has not been established: depression, erythema multiforme, including Stevens-Johnson syndrome, leucopenia, and purpura.

*Overdosage:* A few cases of overdosage have been reported; no patient had any specific symptoms, and all patients recovered without sequelae. The maximum dosage taken was 450 mg. General measures should be adopted.

The maximum plasma concentration of inhibitors occurred within 1.3 to 2.4 hours of administration.

**Pharmacological properties**

*Pharmacodynamic properties:* The involvement of LDL cholesterol in atherogenesis has been well documented in clinical and pathological studies, as well as in many animal experiments. Epidemiological studies have established that high LDL cholesterol and low HDL (high-density lipoprotein) cholesterol are both risk factors for coronary heart disease.

The value of drug- and/or diet-induced reduction in plasma cholesterol levels has long been controversial, but recently the beneficial effect of reduction of LDL cholesterol on morbidity and mortality due to coronary heart disease has been established. The Lipid Research Clinics – Coronary Primary Prevention Trial (LRC–CPPT) demonstrated in a seven-year, double-blind, placebo-controlled study that lowering LDL cholesterol with diet and cholestyramine decreased the combined rate of coronary heart disease death plus non-fatal myocardial infarction.

Zocor has been shown to reduce both normal and elevated LDL-cholesterol concentrations. LDL is formed from VLDL and is catabolised predominantly by the high affinity LDL receptor. The mechanism of the LDL-lowering effect of Zocor may involve both reduction of VLDL-cholesterol concentration and induction of the LDL receptor, leading to reduced production and increased catabolism of LDL cholesterol. Apolipoprotein B also falls substantially during treatment with Zocor. Since each LDL particle contains one molecule of apolipoprotein B, and since little apolipoprotein B is found in other lipoproteins, this strongly suggests that Zocor does not merely cause cholesterol to be lost from LDL but also reduces the concentration of circulating LDL particles. In addition, Zocor moderately increases HDL cholesterol and reduces plasma triglycerides. As a result of these changes the ratios of total to HDL cholesterol and LDL to HDL cholesterol are reduced.

In the Scandinavian Simvastatin Survival Study (4S), the effect on total mortality of therapy with Zocor for a median of 5.4 years was assessed in 4,444 patients with coronary heart disease (CHD) and baseline total cholesterol 5.5 to 8.0 mmol/l. In this multicentre, randomised, double-blind, placebo-controlled study, Zocor reduced the risk of death by 30%, of CHD death by 42%, and of having a hospital-verified non-fatal myocardial infarction by 37%. Furthermore, Zocor reduced the risk for undergoing myocardial revascularisation procedures (coronary artery by-pass grafting or percutaneous transluminal coronary angioplasty) by 37%.

In a post hoc analysis performed on fatal plus non-fatal cerebrovascular events (stroke and transient ischaemic attacks), there were 75 patients with such events in the Zocor group and 102 in the placebo group (risk reduction 28%, p=0.033). Prospective trials are needed to confirm this result.

In a multicentre, placebo-controlled clinical trial in 404 patients using quantitative coronary angiography, Zocor slowed the progression of coronary atherosclerosis and reduced the development of both new lesions and new total occlusions, whereas coronary atherosclerosis lesions steadily worsened over four years in patients receiving standard care.

Zocor is a specific inhibitor of HMG-CoA reductase, the enzyme which catalyses the conversion of HMG CoA to mevalonate. However, at therapeutic doses, the enzyme is not completely blocked, thereby allowing biologically necessary amounts of mevalonate to be available. Because the conversion of HMG CoA to mevalonate is an early step in the biosynthetic pathway of cholesterol, therapy with Zocor would not be expected to cause an accumulation of potentially toxic sterols. In addition, HMG CoA is metabolised readily back to acetyl CoA, which participates in many biosynthetic processes in the body.

*Pharmacokinetic properties:* Simvastatin is an inactive lactone which is readily hydrolysed *in vivo* to the corresponding β-hydroxyacid, L-654,969, a potent inhibitor of HMG-CoA reductase. Inhibition of HMG-CoA reductase is the basis for an assay in pharmacokinetic studies of the β-hydroxyacid metabolites (active inhibitors) and, following base hydrolysis, active plus latent inhibitors (total inhibitors). Both are measured in plasma following administration of simvastatin.

In a disposition study with $^{14}C$-labelled simvastatin, 100 mg (20 uCi) of drug was administered as capsules (5×20 mg), and blood, urine, and faeces collected. Thirteen per cent of the radioactivity was recovered in the urine and 60% in faeces. The latter represents absorbed drug equivalents excreted in bile as well as any unabsorbed drug. Less than 0.5% of the dose was recovered in urine as HMG-CoA reductase inhibitors. In plasma, the inhibitors account for 14% and 28% (active and total inhibitors) of the AUC of total radioactivity, indicating that the majority of chemical species present were inactive or weak inhibitors.

Both simvastatin and L-654,969 are highly bound to human plasma proteins (>94%). The major metabolites of simvastatin present in human plasma are L-654,969 and four additional active metabolites. The availability of L-654,969 to the systemic circulation following an oral dose of simvastatin was estimated using an i.v. reference dose of L-654,969; the value was found to be less than 5% of the dose. By analogy to the dog model, simvastatin is well absorbed and undergoes extensive first-pass extraction in the liver, its primary site of action, with subsequent excretion of drug equivalents in the bile. Consequently, availability of active drug to the general circulation is low.

In dose-proportionality studies, utilising doses of simvastatin of 5, 10, 20, 60, 90 and 120 mg, there was no substantial deviation from linearity of AUC of inhibitors in the general circulation with an increase in dose. Relative to the fasting state, the plasma profile of inhibitors was not affected when simvastatin was administered immediately before a test meal.

The pharmacokinetics of single and multiple doses of simvastatin showed that no accumulation of drug occurred after multiple dosing. In all of the above pharmacokinetic studies, the maximum plasma concentration of inhibitors occurred 1.3 to 2.4 hours post-dose.

*Preclinical safety data:* The oral $LD_{50}$ of simvastatin in mice is approximately 3.8 g/kg and in rats approximately 5 g/kg.

Administration of high dosage levels of simvastatin and related analogues to a variety of animal species has revealed a spectrum of changes in several tissues. These changes were not unexpected in view of the large doses used, the potency of these drugs in inhibiting mevalonate synthesis, and the essential role of the target enzyme in maintenance of cellular homeostasis. Extensive data generated on several of these changes indicate that they represent an exaggeration of the biochemical effect of these drugs at the high end of the dose-response curve. Thus, morphological changes in the livers of rats, squamous epithelial hyperplasia of the forestomach of rats and mice, and hepatotoxicity in rabbits have all been shown to be directly related to inhibition of HMG-CoA reductase.

Cataracts have been detected at high dosage levels in dog studies with simvastatin, although at a very low incidence. While there is no clear correlation between the magnitude of serum lipid-lowering and the development of cataracts, a consistent relationship has been observed between high serum levels of drug and cataract development with simvastatin and related HMG-CoA reductase inhibitors.

Serum levels (expressed as total inhibitors) in dogs receiving the minimally cataractogenic dose of simvastatin of 50 mg/kg/day are 21 times higher than those in man receiving the maximally anticipated therapeutic dose of 0.8 mg/kg (based on a 50 kg man).

Elevated serum transaminases have been observed in dogs receiving simvastatin. These occur either as chronic low-level elevations or as transient enzyme spikes in approximately 10–40% of the dogs receiving this drug. None of the dogs experiencing these transaminase elevations demonstrated any symptoms of illness; and none of the transaminase elevations have progressed to levels associated with frank hepatic necrosis, despite continued drug administration. No histopathological changes have been identified in the liver of any dogs receiving simvastatin.

Testicular degeneration has been seen in two dog safety studies with simvastatin. Special studies designed to further define the nature of these changes have not met with success, since the effects are poorly reproducible and unrelated to dose, serum cholesterol levels, or duration of treatment. Simvastatin has been administered for up to 2 years to dogs at a dose of 50 mg/kg/day without any testicular effects.

Skeletal muscle necrosis was seen in one study in rats given 90 mg/kg b.d., but this was a lethal dosage in rats.

*Genetic toxicology and carcinogenicity:* An extensive battery of *in vitro* and *in vivo* genetic toxicity tests have been conducted on both simvastatin and the corresponding open acid L-654,969. These include assays for microbial mutagenesis, mammalian cell mutagenesis, single stranded DNA breakage, and tests for chromosome aberrations. The results of these studies provided no evidence of an interaction between simvastatin or L-654,969 with genetic material at the highest soluble non-cytotoxic concentration tests in *in vitro* assay systems or at maximally tolerated doses tested *in vivo*.

Initial carcinogenicity studies conducted in rats and mice with simvastatin employed doses ranging from

1 mg/kg/day to 25 mg/kg/day. No evidence of a treatment-related incidence of tumour types was found in mice in any tissue. A statistically significant (p≤0.05) increase in the incidence of thyroid follicular cell adenomas was observed in female rats receiving 25 mg/kg of simvastatin per day (31 times the maximum recommended human dose). This benign tumour type was limited to female rats; no similar changes were seen in male rats or in female rats at lower dosages (up to 5 mg/kg/day). These tumours are a secondary effect reflective of a simvastatin-mediated enhancement of thyroid hormone clearance in the female rat. No other statistically significant increased incidence of tumour types was identified in any tissues in rats receiving simvastatin.

Data from both of these studies indicated that squamous epithelial hyperplasia of the forestomach occurred at all dosage levels. These gastric changes are confined to an anatomical structure which is not found in man. Moreover, identical cells found in other locations (e.g. oesophagus and anorectal junction of the rat, mouse and dog) are unaffected.

Results of a 73-week carcinogenicity study in mice receiving simvastatin doses up to 400 mg/kg/day (500 times the maximum recommended human dose, based on a 50 kg person) exhibited increased incidences of hepatocellular adenomas and carcinomas, pulmonary adenomas and Harderian gland adenomas. A no-effect dose of 25 mg/kg/day (31 times the maximum recommended human dose) was established in this study and from the results of the initial 92-week carcinogenicity study in mice.

Results of an additional 106-week carcinogenicity study in rats receiving simvastatin doses ranging from 50 mg/kg/day to 100 mg/kg/day (62.5 to 125 times the maximum recommended human dose) exhibited a treatment-related increase in the incidence of hepatocellular neoplasms. The no-effect dose remains at 25 mg/kg/day (31 times the maximum recommended human dose) as established in the initial carcinogenicity study. An increase in the incidence of thyroid hyperplastic lesions was also observed; however, this is consistent with the previous finding that this is a species-specific response and has no implications for man.

**Pharmaceutical particulars**

*List of excipients:* Each simvastatin tablet strength contains the following excipients: Ascorbic Acid PhEur, Butylated Hydroxyanisole BP, Citric Acid Monohydrate PhEur, Lactose PhEur, Magnesium Stearate PhEur, Microcrystalline Cellulose PhEur, Pregelatinised Maize Starch BP, Hydroxypropylcellulose PhEur, Methylhydroxypropylcellulose PhEur, Talc PhEur, Titanium Dioxide PhEur.

The 10 mg and 20 mg simvastatin tablets contain yellow iron oxide E172 and red iron oxide E172.

The 40 mg simvastatin tablet contains red iron oxide E172.

*Incompatibilities:* None known.

*Shelf life:* The shelf life is 24 months.

*Special precautions for storage:* Tablets should be stored below 25°C in a dry place.

*Nature and contents of container:* Blister packs of opacified PVC lidded with aluminium foil containing 28 tablets.

*Instructions for use/handling:* Not applicable.

**Marketing authorisation numbers**
| | |
|---|---|
| 10 mg Tablet | 0025/0241 |
| 20 mg Tablet | 0025/0242 |
| 40 mg Tablet | 0025/0243 |

**Date of approval/revision of SPC** December 1996

**Legal category** POM.

*\*Trade Mark*

# Monmouth Pharmaceuticals Limited
3 & 4 Huxley Road
The Surrey Research Park
Guildford GU2 5RE

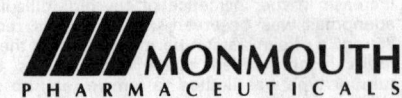

## BARATOL* TABLETS

**Presentation** Baratol tablets are round, convex, film coated tablets containing indoramin hydrochloride equivalent to 25 or 50 mg indoramin base. The 25 mg tablets are blue, 8.00 mm in diameter and marked MPL 020 on one face and '25' on the other. The 50 mg tablets are green, 9.5 mm in diameter, marked MPL 021 on one face and '50' on the other face which is also scored.

**Uses** *Actions:* Baratol is an alpha adrenoceptor blocking agent which acts selectively and competitively on post-synaptic alpha-1 receptors, causing a decrease in peripheral resistance.

*Indications:* Baratol tablets are indicated for the treatment of all grades of essential hypertension.

### Dosage and administration
*Adults: Initial dose:* 25 mg twice daily for all patients.

*Dose titration:* The dosage of Baratol should be titrated as necessary to control blood pressure to a maximum of 200 mg daily in two or three divided doses. The daily dosage may be increased by the progressive addition of 25 mg or 50 mg, made at intervals of two weeks. When unequal doses are used, the largest dose should be given at night in order to avoid daytime sedation.

*Elderly:* Clearance of indoramin may be affected in the elderly. A reduced dose and/or reduced frequency of dosing may be sufficient for effective control of blood pressure in some elderly patients.

*Children:* Not recommended for children.

*Combination with other anti-hypertensive agents:* Baratol is effective in lowering blood pressure in all grades of hypertension, either used alone or when combined with other anti-hypertensive agents. The anti-hypertensive effect of Baratol is enhanced by concomitant administration of a thiazide diuretic or a beta-adrenoceptor blocking drug. Control of most cases of mild and moderate hypertension should be achieved by using Baratol alone or by adding Baratol to the regimen of a patient already under treatment with a thiazide diuretic. In severe hypertension, a combination of Baratol, a thiazide diuretic and a beta-adrenoceptor blocking drug is effective in many such patients.

When Baratol is used in combination with other anti-hypertensive agents, the dose of Baratol should be titrated in the same way as when it is used alone.

### Contra-indications, warnings, etc
*Contra-indications:* Baratol tablets should not be prescribed for:

1. Patients with established heart failure.
2. Patients already under treatment with MAOIs.

*Precautions and warnings:*

1. Drowsiness is sometimes seen in the initial stages of treatment with Baratol or when dosage is increased too rapidly. Patients should be warned not to drive or operate machinery until it is established that they do not become drowsy while taking Baratol, and further cautioned to avoid the ingestion of alcohol or other central nervous system depressants.
2. The ingestion of ethanol has been shown to increase both the rate and extent of absorption of Baratol, and patients should be cautioned to avoid ingestion of alcohol.
3. Incipient cardiac failure should be controlled with diuretics and digitalis before treatment with Baratol.
4. Caution should be observed in prescribing Baratol for patients with hepatic or renal insufficiency.
5. A few cases of extrapyramidal disorders have been reported in patients treated with Baratol. Caution should be observed in prescribing Baratol in patients with Parkinson's disease.
6. In animals and in the one reported case of overdose in humans, convulsions have occurred. Due consideration should be given and great caution exercised in the use of Baratol in patients with epilepsy.
7. Caution should be observed in prescribing Baratol for patients with a history of depression.
8. Animal experiments indicate no teratogenic effects but Baratol tablets should not be prescribed for pregnant women unless considered essential by the physician.
9. There are no data available on the excretion of Baratol in human milk but the drug should not be administered during lactation unless in the judgement of the physician such administration is clinically justifiable.
10. Clearance of indoramin may be affected in the elderly. A reduced dose, and/or reduced frequency of dosing may be sufficient for effective control of blood pressure in some elderly patients.

*Side-effects:* Sedation occurs in some patients but is rarely intolerable and is usually overcome by a modest reduction in dosage. Less commonly, dry mouth, nasal congestion, weight gain, dizziness, failure of ejaculation and depression have also been noted.

*Treatment of overdosage:* The information available at present of the effects of acute overdosage in humans with Baratol is limited to one case. Effects seen in this case included deep sedation leading to coma, hypotension and fits. Results of animal work suggest that hypothermia may also occur.

Suggested therapy is along the following lines:
1. Recent ingestion of large numbers of tablets would require gastric lavage or a dose of ipecacuanha to remove any of the product still in the stomach of the conscious patient.
2. Ventilation should be monitored and assisted if necessary.
3. Circulatory support and control of hypotension should be maintained.
4. If convulsions occur diazepam may be tried.
5. Temperature should be closely monitored. If hypothermia occurs, rewarming should be carried out very slowly to avoid possible convulsions.

**Legal category** POM.

**Pharmaceutical precautions** Store below 25°C and protect from light.

**Package quantities** Bottles of 100.

**Further information** Baratol may be especially suitable for patients for whom beta-adrenoceptor blockade is contra-indicated, for example, in patients with a history of obstructive airways disease.

Reflex tachycardia is not associated with treatment with Baratol.

Postural hypotension is not a problem.

In one study, patients on Baratol who were treated with a tricyclic antidepressant showed no adverse effect on their blood pressure control.

Baratol has been used concomitantly with cardiac glycosides and other anti-hypertensive drugs with no interaction.

Rebound hypertension has not been observed after withdrawal of Baratol.

Selective alpha-1-blockade has been shown to be useful in the treatment of congestive heart failure. As yet, there is insufficient data to determine whether Baratol can also be indicated in this disorder.

Inactive ingredients include lactose.

**Product licence numbers**
25 mg tablets    10536/0015
50 mg tablets    10536/0016

## CELEVAC* TABLETS

**Presentation** Pink tablets, with breakline on one face and Celevac on the other, containing 500 mg Methylcellulose BP.

**Uses** *Action:* Methylcellulose is a hydrophilic colloid which absorbs water to swell to a soft gel of uniform consistency.

*Indications:*
1. In the control of colostomy, ileostomy and diarrhoea.
2. In the management of diverticular disease.
3. In the management of simple constipation.
4. As an aid to appetite control and as an aid in the management of obesity.

### Dosage and administration
1. *Colostomy and ileostomy control and for diarrhoea:* 3–6 tablets twice daily with the minimum of liquid. Liquids should be avoided for 30 minutes before and after each dose. Dosage should be adjusted to give stools the required consistency.

2. *Diverticular disease:* 3–6 tablets twice daily, adjusted according to the degree of constipation, diarrhoea or spastic pain.

3. *Simple constipation:* 3–6 tablets twice daily, to be taken with at least 300 ml of liquid. The dose may be reduced as normal bowel function is restored.

4. *Appetite control and obesity:* 3 tablets, with at least 300 ml of warm liquid, half an hour before each meal, and between meals when hunger pangs are severe.

No specific information on the use of this product in the elderly is available. Clinical trials have included patients over 65 years and no adverse reactions specific to this age group have been reported.

**Contra-indications, warnings, etc** Celevac should not be used in cases where the physician believes there is a pathological cause for the diarrhoea which would render the condition unsuitable for symptomatic medical treatment, e.g. infective bowel disease and imminent or threatened bowel obstruction. Bowel obstruction is a rare complication of treatment with any bulk-forming hydrophilic colloid.

Although Celevac has been in wide general use for many years there is no evidence of ill-consequence during human pregnancy.

Medicines should not be used in pregnancy, especially the first trimester, unless the expected benefit is thought to outweigh any possible risk to the foetus.

*Overdosage:* Methylcellulose is not absorbed. The features to be expected would be abdominal distension which may be followed by intestinal obstruction.

Gastric lavage should be employed where appropriate. The patient should be observed and fluids given. If obstruction develops, appropriate measures such as rectal washout must be taken.

**Pharmaceutical precautions** Protect from heat and moisture.

**Legal category** GSL.

**Package quantities** Tablet pack of 112 (OP).

**Further information** Methylcellulose is a hydrophilic colloid which bonds loosely with $H_2O$ and with $H_2S$, thus acting as a bulking agent and a deodorising agent. In diverticular disease its use has been associated with a fall in intracolonic pressures as well as relief of symptoms.

Inactive ingredients include lactose.

**Product licence number** 10536/0017.

## EMINASE*

**Presentation** Eminase is presented as a white to off-white sterile, freeze-dried solid in vials containing 30 Units of anistreplase.

Its chemical name is p-anisoylated (human) lys-plasminogen-streptokinase activator complex (APSAC). The approved name is anistreplase.

The potency of Eminase is measured using a reference standard which is specific for Eminase and is not comparable with units used for other thrombolytic agents.

Eminase includes the following inactive ingredients as solubilisers and stabilisers: aminocaproic acid, human albumin, lysine hydrochloride, mannitol, p-amidinophenyl-p'-anisate hydrochloride.

**Uses**
*Indication:* Eminase is indicated in the treatment of acute myocardial infarction to establish reperfusion, to preserve left ventricular function, to limit infarct size and to reduce mortality.

Clinical studies have shown that Eminase significantly reduces 30 day and 1 year mortality, limits infarct size and preserves left ventricular function.

*Action:* Eminase is a thrombolytic enzyme complex in which the catalytic centre of the activator complex is temporarily masked by an anisoyl group.

Eminase binds to fibrin strongly: this assists both its initial uptake and retention within the thrombus.

After intravenous injection, deacylation proceeds immediately with formation of the enzymatically active lys-plasminogen-streptokinase activator complex. Deacylation of Eminase proceeds in a controlled and sustained manner, resulting in a long plasma half-life which allows progressive clot uptake. This ensures sustained activation which may be useful in facilitating a low rate of early reocclusion.

The generation of lys-plasminogen-streptokinase activator complex within the thrombus converts fibrin-bound plasminogen to plasmin. The plasmin then dissolves the fibrin of the thrombus. The enzymatic efficiency of lys-plasminogen-streptokinase activator complex is enhanced by clot fibrin, ensuring efficient thrombolysis.

### Dosage and administration

*Dosage*
*Adults:* Eminase is given as a single 30 Unit dose as a 4 to 5 minute intravenous injection.
*Elderly:* As above. See *Precautions*.

Thrombolytic therapy should be administered as soon as possible after the onset of symptoms and preferably within 6 hours. The ease of administration of Eminase should facilitate early treatment of the patient with acute myocardial infarction, for whom time is critical.

*Preparation:* Eminase should be reconstituted by dissolving the contents of a 30 Unit vial in 5 ml Water for Injections BP. (5 ml Sodium Chloride Injection BP [0.9% w/v] is a suitable alternative.) To avoid foaming, the diluent should be directed against the wall of the vial and the powder dissolved by gently swirling. AVOID SHAKING. Eminase dissolves immediately to give a clear or slightly turbid, colourless to pale yellow solution.

NO OTHER MEDICATION SHOULD BE ADDED TO THE VIAL OR SYRINGE CONTAINING EMINASE.

*Administration:* Eminase should be given by slow intravenous injection over 4 to 5 minutes.

The reconstituted solution should be administered as soon as possible. If unused after 30 minutes the solution must be discarded.

Discoloured solutions should not be used.

RECONSTITUTED SOLUTION MUST NOT BE ADMINISTERED BY INTRAMUSCULAR INJECTION OR ADDED TO INFUSION FLUIDS.

*Anticoagulation:* The use of anticoagulants or anti-platelet drugs following administration of Eminase has not been shown to be of unequivocal benefit. In clinical studies a majority of patients treated with Eminase received heparin therapy 4 to 6 hours after Eminase during their hospital stay, followed by oral anticoagulation as appropriate.

Following Eminase, there is a decrease in plasma fibrinogen and plasminogen concentrations and an increase in fibrin degradation products. Values have generally returned to normal within 24 to 48 hours of therapy.

### Contra-indications, warnings, etc

*Contra-indications:* Since all thrombolytic therapies increase the risk of bleeding, Eminase is contra-indicated in the following situations:
– After surgery or major trauma within the previous 10 days.
– Recent neurosurgical procedure (previous 2 months).
– Recent traumatic cardio-pulmonary resuscitation.
– In patients with active gastro-intestinal bleeding or other internal bleeding (within the previous 6 months), e.g. active peptic ulcer.
– History of cerebrovascular accident.
– In patients with known bleeding diathesis.
– In patients with severe, uncontrolled hypertension.
– In patients with known intracranial neoplasm, or aneurysm.
– In women with heavy vaginal bleeding.

Eminase should not be administered to patients who have experienced severe allergic reactions to this product or streptokinase.

*Precautions:* The most common complication associated with Eminase therapy is bleeding.

Patients with any condition in which bleeding constitutes a significant hazard, or which would be particularly difficult to manage because of its location, should be monitored carefully. The risks of Eminase therapy may be increased in such patients and should be weighed against the anticipated benefits.

Venepuncture and other invasive procedures should be kept to a minimum in order to reduce the risk of bleeding. In patients undergoing cardiac catheterisation the sheath should not be removed until 24 hours after dosing.

In the following conditions the risks associated with thrombolytic therapy may be increased and should be weighed against the anticipated benefits: haemorrhagic retinopathy, coagulation defects and treatment with anticoagulants.

Patients with evidence of intramural ventricular thrombus or thrombus within abdominal aneurysms should be treated with caution as there is a risk of dissolution of clot with subsequent embolisation. This risk should be considered against the benefits of Eminase therapy.

Accelerated idioventricular rhythm may be associated with reperfusion of the coronary artery. Other arrhythmias (such as sinus bradycardia, ventricular tachycardia and ventricular fibrillation) may occur. These are not different from those often seen in the course of acute myocardial infarction and should be managed with standard measures.

Experience is limited in patients over 70 years of age and the benefits of Eminase should be balanced against risk in this group.

Because of the increased likelihood of resistance due to anti-streptokinase antibody, Eminase may not be effective if administered more than 5 days after prior Eminase or streptokinase therapy, particularly between 5 days and 12 months. Furthermore, increased anti-streptokinase antibody levels after Eminase or streptokinase may also increase the risk of allergic reactions following readministration.

Rapid injection of Eminase has been followed, in some patients, by a precipitate but transient fall in blood pressure. Eminase should be given by slow intravenous injection over 4 to 5 minutes.

*Use in pregnancy and lactation:* There is no evidence as to the drug safety in human pregnancy nor is there evidence from animal work that it is free from hazard. Avoid in pregnancy unless there is no safer alternative.

There is no information regarding the use of Eminase in lactating mothers.

*Drug interactions:* The interaction of Eminase and other drugs has not been formally studied.

*Side-effects*
*Early reactions:* Bradycardia and/or occasionally ventricular arrhythmias (including ventricular fibrillation) can occur, as in the course of acute myocardial infarction. Flushing and transient hypotension (usually within the first hour) as well as fever and nausea/vomiting (usually within 6 to 24 hours) have been reported but such reactions are generally not severe.

Allergic reactions including bronchoconstriction and anaphylaxis have been reported but are uncommon and usually reversible. Vasculitis generally manifest as a purpuric rash has occasionally been reported. All patients recovered spontaneously without sequelae.

Transient back pain immediately following administration of Eminase has been reported rarely.

*Other reactions:* The most common complication associated with thrombolytic therapy is bleeding, most frequently from arterial and venous puncture sites. Haemoptysis, haematuria, haematemesis and melaena have been reported occasionally. Cerebrovascular accidents have been reported but the incidence is low and there has usually been a predisposing factor.

Careful patient selection with due regard to risk factors and contra-indications can reduce the likelihood of haemorrhage.

Guillain-Barré syndrome has been rarely reported after streptokinase treatment.

*Treatment of reactions:* Local bleeding can be controlled with pressure. In cases of severe uncontrolled bleeding, if the haematocrit has fallen significantly, transfusion with packed cells or whole blood may be necessary. Cryoprecipitate or purified clotting factor concentrates may also be used to correct the haemostatic deficiency. Tranexamic acid (10 mg/kg body weight given by slow intravenous injection) or aprotinin (see manufacturer's literature) will competitively inhibit the fibrinolytic action of Eminase.

Mild to moderate allergic reactions may be treated, if required, with an antihistamine. Severe anaphylactic reactions should be treated with adrenaline, corticosteroids and antihistamines as appropriate. Corticosteroids may be given prophylactically, if desired.

*Treatment of overdosage:* see under *Treatment of reactions.*

### Pharmaceutical precautions

*Stability and storage:* Eminase must be stored at 2–8°C (not frozen) and must not be used after the expiry date printed on the pack and vial. The IV Injection Pack, which includes Water for Injections, must not be frozen. Eminase vials must not be stored at room temperature. If a vial of Eminase is removed from the refrigerator in anticipation of being used, but is then not used, the vial can be returned to the refrigerator provided the material has not been reconstituted and is returned within 2 to 3 hours.

Reconstituted solution should be administered as soon as possible. If unused after 30 minutes the solution must be discarded.

*Compatibility:* No other medication should be added to the vial or syringe containing Eminase.

### Legal category POM.

### Package quantities

Vials of Eminase 30 Units, boxed singly.
IV Injection Pack: 1 vial Eminase 30 Units, a 5 ml ampoule of Water for Injections BP, a 5 ml disposable syringe and needle.
Each pack contains instructions for use.

### Further information

Eminase belongs to a new class of thrombolytic agents designed for use in the treatment of acute myocardial infarction. Eminase can be given as a single, slow intravenous injection, over 4 to 5 minutes, unlike other thrombolytic agents which require intravenous infusions of various degrees of complexity. The ease of administration of Eminase facilitates early treatment of the patient with acute myocardial infarction, for whom time is critical.

The fibrinolytic mean half-life of Eminase is 94 minutes (range of 70 to 120 minutes).

At the recommended dose of 30 Units injected intravenously in patients with acute myocardial infarction of less than 6 hours' duration, patency of coronary arteries has occurred in 70–80% of patients.

The incidence of early reocclusion with Eminase is low and is less than 10% in reported studies.

Clinical studies have shown that reperfusion with Eminase preserves myocardial function and improves patient survival.

Randomised controlled studies have demonstrated that treatment with Eminase reduces mortality for at least 1 year when administered within 6 hours after the onset of symptoms of acute myocardial infarction.

It is recommended that antiarrhythmic therapy for bradycardia, ventricular tachycardia and ventricular fibrillation be available when infusions of Eminase are administered as would normally be required in the early phase of acute myocardial infarction.

### Product licence numbers

| | |
|---|---|
| Eminase 30 Unit vial | 0038/0353. |
| Water for Injections BP | 0038/0118. |

## ETHMOZINE* ▼ TABLETS 200 mg, 250 mg and 300 mg

**Qualitative and quantitative composition** Each tablet contains moracizine hydrochloride (200 mg, 250 mg or 300 mg).

**Pharmaceutical form** White film-coated tablets: 200 mg tablets are round, 250 mg tablets are oval and 300 mg tablets capsule shaped. The tablets are marked 'ROBERTS' on one face and 'ETHMOZINE' and an indication of the tablet strength on the other face.

### Clinical particulars

*Therapeutic indications:* Ethmozine is indicated for the treatment of ventricular arrhythmias in patients with underlying cardiac disease and a history of:
- ventricular fibrillation or sustained ventricular tachycardia
- symptomatic non-sustained ventricular tachycardia
- disabling symptoms due to premature ventricular contractions.

*Posology and method of administration:* The usual adult dosage is between 600 mg and 900 mg per day, given every 8 hours in three equally divided doses. Within this range, the dose can be adjusted as tolerated, in increments of 150 mg/day at 3-day intervals, until the desired effect is obtained.

When rapid control of life-threatening ventricular arrhythmias is essential, an initial dose of 400 mg to 500 mg should be administered followed by 200 mg every 8 hours. Patients who exhibit a beneficial response can be maintained on chronic Ethmozine therapy.

Patients who are well-controlled on an 8-hour regimen may be given the same total daily dose in a 12-hour regimen.

A maximum daily dosage of 900 mg is recommended.

It is recommended that treatment with Ethmozine should be initiated in hospitals.

Patients with hepatic disease have reduced plasma clearance and increased half life of moracizine. Consequently, the Ethmozine dose required for these patients should be lower and the dosing interval should possibly be less frequent than in patients with normal liver function.

In patients with renal disease, clearance and plasma protein binding are reduced and AUC is increased. Consequently, the Ethmozine dose may be lower and the dosing interval may be less frequent than in patients with normal renal function.

*Use in children:* The safety and effectiveness of Ethmozine use in children has not been established.

*Use in the elderly:* Clearance of moracizine in elderly patients is reduced and a lower effective dose can be expected. The dose should be individualised on the basis of antiarrhythmic response and tolerance.

*Contra-indications:* As with other antiarrhythmics, Ethmozine is contra-indicated in patients with pre-existing second or third degree heart block unless a pacemaker is present, or in the presence of cardiogenic shock or known hyper-sensitivity to the drug.

*Special warnings and precautions for use:*
*Warnings:* In controlled studies with antiarrhythmic

drugs, an improvement in survival has not been demonstrated. Ethmozine has not been shown to be of benefit to patients who have had recent (4-90 days) myocardial infarction together with left ventricular ejection fractions less than 40%.

*Proarrhythmia:* Ethmozine, like other antiarrhythmic agents, can cause a new onset of a higher grade of ventricular arrhythmia, an increase in frequency of a previously documented arrhythmia, or a change in severity of symptoms. A spontaneous variation in the patient's underlying rhythm disorder may be difficult to distinguish from drug-induced worsening. The incidence of proarrhythmia measured using Holter monitoring is generally less than 4%, however, some risk factors are known and include poor ventricular function, previous MI, CHF and previous proarrhythmia.

*Sick sinus syndrome:* Ethmozine, like other antiarrhythmic drugs, should be used only with extreme caution in patients with sick sinus syndrome, since it may cause sinus bradycardia, sinus pause or sinus arrest.

*Electrocardiographic changes:* In patients who have pre-existing conduction abnormalities, Ethmozine therapy should be initiated cautiously. If second or third degree AV block occurs, Ethmozine therapy should be discontinued unless a temporary or permanent ventricular pacemaker is in place. When changing the dose of Ethmozine or adding concomitant medications which may also affect cardiac conduction, patients, especially those who have conduction abnormalities, should be closely monitored with electrocardiograms.

*Electrolyte disturbance:* Hypokalaemia, hyperkalaemia or hypomagnesaemia may alter the effects of class I antiarrhythmic drugs. Pre-existing hypokalaemia, hyperkalaemia or hypomagnesaemia should be corrected before administration of Ethmozine.

*Use in children:* The safety and effectiveness of Ethmozine use in children has not been established.

*Use in the elderly:* Clearance of moracizine and two of its metabolites is reduced in elderly patients and a lower effective dose can be expected. The dose should be individualised on the basis of antiarrhythmic response and tolerance.

*Precautions:* Patients with cardiovascular diseases, including coronary artery disease, congestive heart failure and cardiomegaly should be carefully monitored.

Pharmacokinetic studies have demonstrated that patients with significant liver disease have reduced plasma clearance and increased half-life of moracizine. Consequently, the Ethmozine dose required for these patients should be lower and the dosing interval should possibly be less frequent than in patients with normal liver function.

In patients with renal disease, clearance and plasma protein binding are reduced and AUC is increased. Consequently, the Ethmozine dose may be lower and the dosing interval may be less frequent than in patients with normal renal function.

Clearance of moracizine and two of its metabolites is reduced in elderly patients and a lower effective dose can be expected. The dose should be individualised on the basis of antiarrhythmic reponse and tolerance.

Caution is advised in patients who develop unexplained signs of hepatic dysfunction, and consideration should be given to discontinuing Ethmozine therapy.

Dizziness may occur in a small number of patients, particularly at higher doses. Patients should be advised not to drive or operate machinery during treatment with Ethmozine until their susceptibility is known.

*Interaction with other medicaments and other forms of interaction:* Significant changes in serum digoxin levels have not been observed in patients and healthy volunteers receiving concomitant Ethmozine therapy. Concomitant administration of Ethmozine and digoxin is associated with additive prolongation of the PR interval, but is not associated with a significant increase in the risk of development of second or third degree AV block.

Ethmozine plasma levels are increased (mean 1.6 fold) and oral clearance decreased in healthy subjects receiving a single dose of Ethmozine concomitantly with multiple doses of cimetidine. Patients should be carefully monitored when concomitant cimetidine therapy is instituted or discontinued or when the Ethmozine dose is changed.

In healthy subjects, Ethmozine increases the oral clearance (>43%) and decreases the half-life of both conventional and sustained-release theophylline, (33% and 20%, respectively). Ethmozine has similar effects on the clearance and the half-life of antipyrine, after multiple doses. Ethmozine has minimal effect on the plasma warfarin levels, but no effect on prothrombin time.

Experience has not indicated any obvious problems with the concomitant use of Ethmozine and diuretics,

vasodilators, antihypertensives, warfarin, calcium channel blockers, beta blockers or ACE inhibitors. However, because of possible additive pharmacological effects, caution is indicated when Ethmozine is used with other drugs that affect cardiac electrophysiology.

*Pregnancy and lactation:* Animal studies have not shown any teratogenic effects, but as there is no experience with the use of Ethmozine in human pregnancy, Ethmozine should not be used during pregnancy unless the benefits outweigh the risks. Since moracizine is secreted in the milk of laboratory animals and has been reported to be present in human milk, it should not be administered to nursing women.

*Effects on ability to drive and use machines:* Dizziness may occur in a small number of cases, particularly at higher doses. Patients should be advised not to drive or operate machinery while taking Ethmozine therapy until their susceptibility is known.

*Undesirable effects:* The most frequently reported adverse reactions were dizziness, nausea, headache, fatigue, palpitations and dyspnoea. Proarrhythmic effects have been observed in a small number of patients, none of whom were treated for benign ventricular arrhythmia.

Less frequently reported adverse reactions were nervousness, hypoaesthesia, paraesthesia, dry mouth, dyspepsia, vomiting, diarrhoea, constipation, sweating, chest pain, musculoskeletal pain, sleep disorders and blurred vision.

Very infrequently reported events included congestive heart failure, fever, elevations in liver function tests, jaundice and thrombocytopaenia.

*Overdose:* Deaths have occurred after accidental or intentional overdoses of 2,250 and 10,000 mg of moracizine.

*Signs, symptoms and laboratory findings associated with an overdose of drug:* Overdose with Ethmozine may produce emesis, lethargy, coma, syncope, hypotension, conduction disturbances, exacerbation of congestive heart failure, myocardial infarction, sinus arrest, arrhythmias (including junctional bradycardia, ventricular tachycardia, ventricular fibrillation and asystole), and respiratory failure.

*Recommended general treatment procedures:* A specific antidote for Ethmozine has not been identified. In the event of overdose, treatment should be supportive. Patients should be hospitalised and monitored for cardiac, respiratory and CNS changes. Appropriate resuscitation equipment should be provided as necessary. Acute overdose should be treated with appropriate gastric evacuation, with special care to avoid aspiration and rapid absorption of the drug.

**Pharmacological properties**

*Pharmacodynamic properties:* Ethmozine has potent local anaesthetic activity and is included among the membrane stabilising (Class I) antiarrhythmic agents. Ethmozine does not clearly belong to a currently existing electrophysiological subclass. Although structurally related to neuroleptic phenothiazines, Ethmozine has not demonstrated central or peripheral dopaminergic antagonist activity in animals. Serum prolactin concentrations do not increase in patients receiving multiple doses of Ethmozine, indicating that Ethmozine lacks dopaminergic antagonist activity in man. Haemodynamic studies have shown that moracizine has a minimal negative inotropic effect. Clinical experience indicates that Ethmozine can be administered to patients with significant left ventricular dysfunction without further deterioration of their condition.

*Pharmacokinetic properties:* Following oral administration, Ethmozine undergoes significant first-pass metabolism. Less than 0.1% of the administered dose is excreted unchanged in the urine of healthy subjects. Analysis of urine extracts from healthy subjects revealed in excess of 26 putative metabolites, and no single urinary metabolite has been found to represent as much as 1% of the administered dose. Two metabolites, moracizine sulphoxide and phenothiazine-2-carbamic acid ethyl ester sulphoxide (P2CAEES) have been shown to be effective against ventricular arrhythmias in the rat. Each of these metabolites represents a small percentage (<0.6%) of the administered dose, and is present in lower concentrations in the plasma than the parent drug, and has a plasma elimination half-life of approximately 3 hours.

Approximately 56% of an orally administered radioactive dose is excreted in the faeces and 39% is excreted in the urine.

Peak plasma concentrations are usually reached within 0.5 to 2.0 hours following oral administration.

The apparent mean plasma elimination half-life is 2-6 hours following multiple oral doses. Average plasma concentrations are observed to decrease with multiple dosing, suggesting that Ethmozine may induce its own metabolism. The data suggest that

plasma levels are approximately proportional to dose over the recommended therapeutic dose range.

Patients with hepatic disease had an increased Cmax (59%), t1/2 (141%) and AUC (229%) when given moracizine hydrochloride compared to healthy volunteers. For P2CAEES, an increase in AUC (192%), t1/2 (164%) but no change in Cmax from healthy volunteers was observed. Although there was an increase in the t1/2 (148%) for the moracizine sulfoxide metabolite, there was a reduction of Cmax (57%) with no change in AUC.

For patients with renal disease, the AUC for moracizine hydrochloride and P2CAEES increased by 85% and 145%, respectively, as compared to healthy volunteers. A small increase in t1/2 was found for moracizine hydrochloride (2.1 to 3.2 hr.), moracizine sulfoxide (1.3 to 2.4 hr.) and P2CAEES (1.5 to 4.3 hr.).

For elderly subjects the increases in AUC were up to 115% for moracizine hydrochloride, 50% for moracizine sulphoxide, and 39% for P2CAEES, while the t1/2 for moracizine increased 136%, for moracizine sulphoxide 92%, and for P2CAEES 62%, compared to younger subjects. There was no effect of age on the plasma binding of moracizine hydrochloride.

Based on these pharmacokinetic results, the ETHMOZINE dose required for arrhythmia patients with hepatic disease, renal disease and for elderly patients may be lower and the dosing interval may need to be less frequent.

*Preclinical safety data:* All preclinical data, relevant to the prescriber, are mentioned in the appropriate section of the SPC.

**Pharmaceutical particulars**

*List of excipients:* Lactose; microcrystalline cellulose; sodium starch glycollate; magnesium stearate; purified water; hydroxypropyl methylcellulose; titanium dioxide; polyethylene glycol 400; polysorbate 80.

*Incompatibilities:* Not applicable

*Shelf life:* The tablets have a shelf-life of 60 months when stored at or below 25 degrees Centigrade.

*Special precautions for storage:* Store at or below 25 degrees Centigrade.

*Nature and contents of container:* All pack sizes are packed in PVC blisters with aluminium foil* or aluminium foil with paper backing* High density polyethylene bottles of 100 tablets.
*Not available.

*Instructions for use/handling:* None

**Marketing authorisation numbers**
(200 mg)   10536/0027
(250 mg)   10536/0028
(300 mg)   10536/0029

**Date of approval/revision of SPC**   28 May 1996

**Legal category** POM.

# HRF*

**Presentation**   HRF (gonadorelin hydrochloride) is a synthetic decapeptide that has a chemical composition and structure identical to the naturally-occurring luteinizing hormone-releasing hormone (LH-RH) isolated from porcine or ovine hypothalami, in a freeze-dried form. HRF is available in 2 strengths, 100 micrograms and 500 micrograms with 100 mg lactose. An ampoule of sterile diluent is supplied which contains 2% benzyl alcohol and water for injection.

**Uses**   HRF as a single injection is indicated for evaluating the functional capacity and response of the gonadotropes of the anterior pituitary. The LH response is used in testing patients with suspected gonadotropin deficiency, whether due to the hypothalamus alone or in combination with anterior pituitary failure. HRF is also indicated for evaluating residual gonadotropic function of the pituitary following removal of a pituitary tumour or surgery and/or irradiation.

**Dosage and administration**   *Adults:* 100 micrograms dose, subcutaneously or intravenously. In females for whom the phase of the menstrual cycle can be established, the test should be performed in early follicular phase (days 1–7).

*Test methodology:* To determine the status of the gonadotropin secretory capacity of the anterior pituitary, a test procedure requiring seven venous blood samples for LH is recommended.

*Procedure*
1. Venous blood samples should be drawn at −15 minutes and immediately prior to HRF administration. The LH baseline is obtained by averaging the LH values of the two samples.
2. Administer a bolus of HRF subcutaneously or intravenously.
3. Draw venous blood samples at 15, 30, 45, 60 and 120 minutes after administration.
4. Blood samples should be handled as recommended

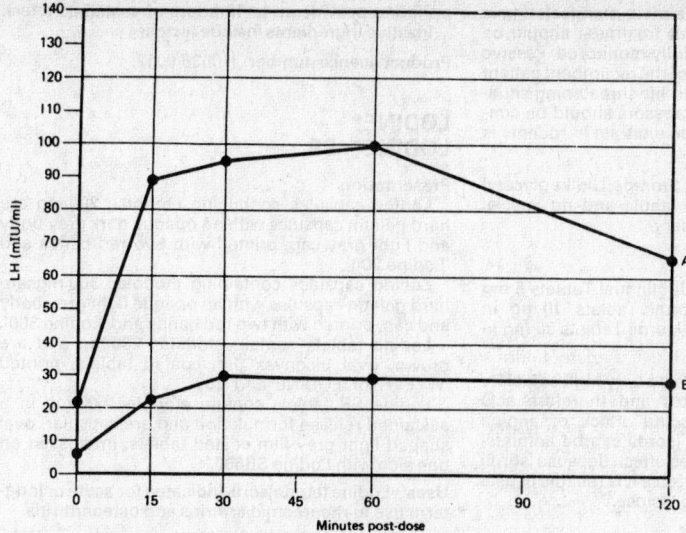

*Figure 1.* Normal male LH response after HRF 100 micrograms subcutaneous administration 10th and 90th percentiles.

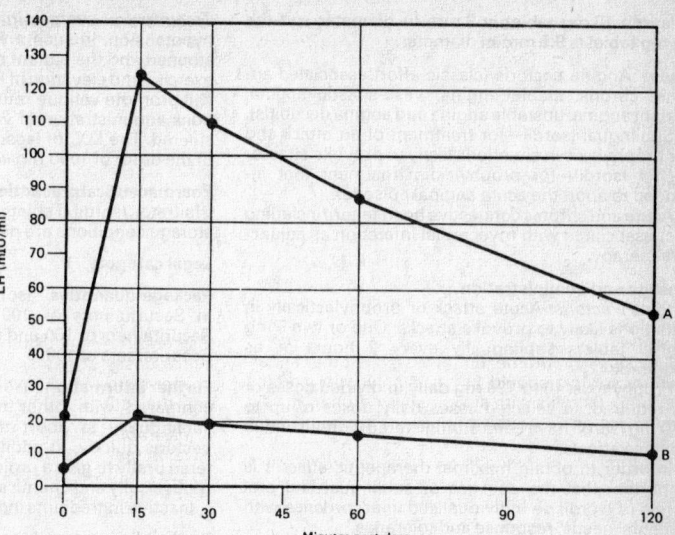

*Figure 2.* Normal male LH response after HRF 100 micrograms intravenous administration 10th and 90th percentiles.

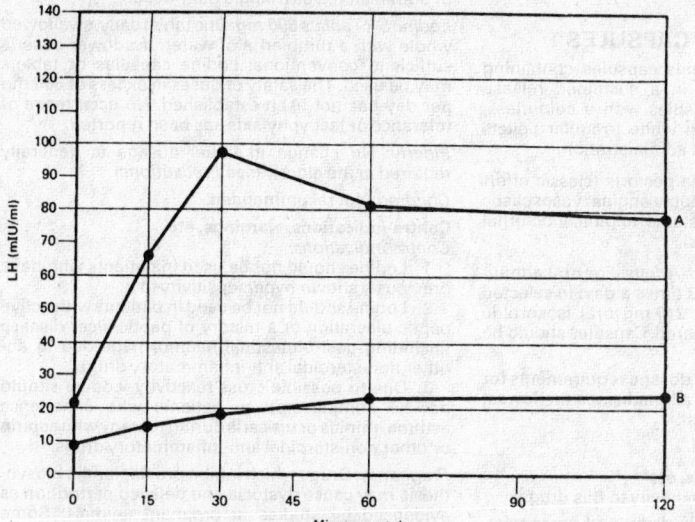

*Figure 3.* Normal female LH response after HRF 100 micrograms subcutaneous administration 10th and 90th percentiles.

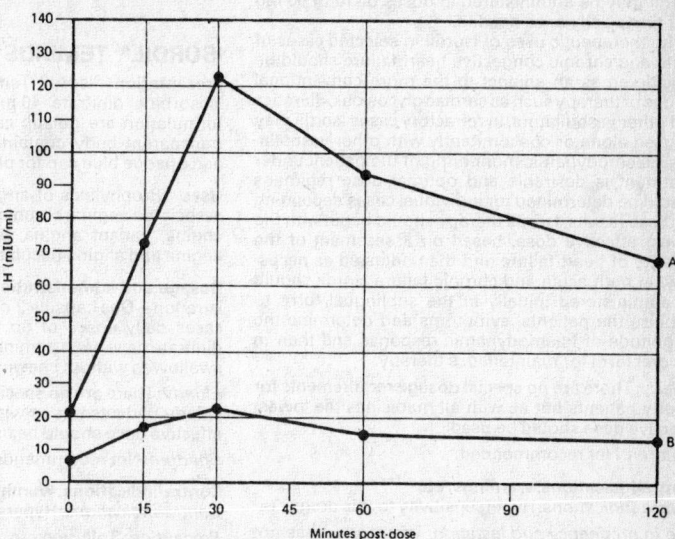

*Figure 4.* Normal female LH response after HRF 100 micrograms intravenous administration 10th and 90th percentiles.

by the laboratory that will determine the LH content. It must be emphasised that the reliability of the test is directly related to the inter-assay and intra-assay reliability of the laboratory performing the assay.

*Interpretation of test results:* Interpretation of the LH response to HRF requires an understanding of the hypothalamic-pituitary physiology, knowledge of the clinical status of the individual patient, and familiarity with the normal ranges and the standards used in the laboratory performing the LH assays.

Figures 1–4 represent the LH response curves after HRF administration in normal subjects. The normal LH response curves were established between the 10th percentile (B line) and 90th percentile (A line) of all LH responses in normal subjects analysed from the results of clinical studies. Individual patient responses should be plotted on the appropriate curve. A subnormal response in patients is defined as three or more LH values which fall below the B line of the normal LH response curve.

In cases where there is a blunted or borderline response, the HRF test should be repeated.

The HRF test complements the clinical assessment of patients with a variety of endocrine disorders involving the hypothalamic-pituitary axis. In cases where there is a normal response, it indicates the presence of functional pituitary gonadotropes. The single injection test does not determine the pathophysiological cause for the subnormal response and does not measure pituitary gonadotropic reserve.

**Contra-indications, warnings, etc**

*Contra-indications:* Hypersensitivity to HRF or any of the components. Known or suspected pregnancy. Do not use in children under one year of age as diluent contains 2% benzyl alcohol.

*Precautions:* Although allergic and hypersensitivity reactions have been observed with other polypeptide hormones, to date no such reactions have been

encountered following the administration of a single 100 micrograms dose of HRF used for diagnostic purposes. Rare instances of hypersensitivity reactions have been reported (see Side Effects). Therefore, patients treated by intermittent pulsatile therapy in whom re-administration is considered, particularly by the intravenous route, should be carefully observed. Administration during the follicular phase of a normal cycle may result in premature ovulation and appropriate measures are advised to prevent an unwanted pregnancy in these circumstances.

*Drug interactions:* The HRF test should be conducted in the absence of other drugs which directly affect the pituitary secretion of the gonadotrophins. These would include a variety of preparations which contain androgens, oestrogens, progestins, or glucocorticoids. The gonadotropin levels may be transiently elevated by spironolactone, minimally elevated by levodopa, and suppressed by oral contraceptives and digoxin. The response to HRF may be blunted by phenothiazines and dopamine antagonists which cause a rise in prolactin.

*Side-effects:* Systemic complaints such as headaches, nausea, lightheadedness, abdominal discomfort and flushing have been reported rarely following administration of HRF. Local swelling, occasionally with pain and pruritus at the injection site may occur if HRF is administered subcutaneously. Local and generalised skin rash have been noted after chronic subcutaneous administration.

Thrombophlebitis with septicaemia, mild and severe, has been reported in isolated cases at the site of intravenous injection. Rare instances of hypersensitivity reaction (bronchospasm, tachycardia, flushing, urticaria, swelling, itching and redness of face, eyelids and lips, induration at injection site) have been reported following multiple-dose administration of large doses. Antibody formation has also been reported rarely after chronic administration of large doses.

*Overdosage:* HRF has been administered parenterally in doses up to 3 mg bd for 28 days without any signs or symptoms of overdosage. In case of overdosage or idiosyncrasy, symptomatic treatment should be administered as required.

**Pharmaceutical precautions** Both the lyophilised powder vials and diluent ampoules have a shelf life of 3 years. Store at room temperature (approximately 25°C). Preparation for single injection administration: Reconstitute 100 micrograms vial with 1.0 ml of the accompanying sterile diluent of 2% benzyl alcohol. Reconstitute 500 micrograms vial with 2.0 ml of the accompanying sterile diluent of 2% benzyl alcohol. Prepare solution immediately before use. After reconstitution, refrigerate and use within 1 day. Discard unused reconstituted solution and diluent.

**Legal category** POM.

**Package quantities** Packs comprise a vial containing 100 micrograms or 500 micrograms freeze-dried material and a 2 ml ampoule of sterile diluent (OP).

**Further information** Nil.

**Product licence numbers**
HRF 100 micrograms   10536/0013
HRF 500 micrograms   10536/0014

## ISORDIL* TABLETS

**Presentation** Isordil Sublingual Tablets, containing isosorbide dinitrate 5 mg, are small, round, flat, bevelled pink tablets specially formulated for sublingual administration.

Isordil Tablets, containing isosorbide dinitrate 10 mg, are white, round, bi-convex tablets, scored on one side and engraved 'Isordil 10' on the other.

Isordil Tablets, containing isosorbide dinitrate 30 mg, are white, round, bi-convex tablets, scored on one side and engraved 'Isordil 30' on the other.

Isordil 10 mg tablet is 8 mm in diameter and the 30 mg tablet is 9.5 mm in diameter.

**Uses** Angina pectoris (classic effort associated angina, chronic stable angina, vaso-spastic angina, variant angina, unstable angina and angina decubitis).

Sublingual Isordil—for treatment of an attack and for prophylaxis in situations likely to provoke attacks.

Oral Isordil—for prophylactic treatment (not intended to abort the acute anginal episode).

Acute and chronic congestive heart failure including that associated with myocardial infarction as adjunctive therapy.

**Dosage and administration**
*Angina Pectoris:* Acute attack or prophylactically in situations likely to provoke attacks: One or two 5 mg Isordil tablets sublingually every 2 hours or as required.

Prophylaxis: 40 to 120 mg daily in divided doses or as required. In selected cases daily doses of up to 240 mg Isordil have been administered without undue adverse effects.

In order to obtain maximal therapeutic effect it is important that the dosages of sublingual and oral forms of Isordil be individualised in accordance with patients' needs, response and tolerance.

*Congestive heart failure:* Acute and chronic, including after myocardial infarction: Sublingual Isordil 5 to 15 mg every 2–3 hours or as needed. The oral form of Isordil may be administered in doses of 10 to 60 mg four times daily or as needed.

The therapeutic uses of Isordil in selected cases of acute and chronic congestive heart failure should be considered as an adjunct to the more conventional modes of therapy such as cardiac glycosides, diuretics and other vasodilators. In refractory cases Isordil may be used alone or concomitantly with other vasodilators. Haemodynamic monitoring of the patient under treatment is desirable and optimal dose regimens should be determined for individual cases depending on these results. Isordil therapy should begin with the lowest effective dose, based on assessment of the severity of heart failure and then adjusted as necessary. In both acute and chronic failure Isordil should be administered initially in the sublingual form to stabilise the patients' symptoms and determine the magnitude of haemodynamic response and then in the oral form for maintenance therapy.

*Elderly:* There are no special dosage requirements for elderly patients but as with all medicines the lowest effective dose should be used.

*Children:* Not recommended.

**Contra-indications, warnings, etc**
*Contra-indications:* Hypersensitivity to this drug.

*Use in pregnancy and lactation:* The product has not been studied in human pregnancy. The use of Isordil requires that the anticipated benefit be weighed against possible hazard. It is not known whether isosorbide dinitrate is excreted in human milk. It is unlikely that a nursing woman would require Isordil but the decision depends on the condition of the patient and caution should be exercised.

*Precautions:*
1. Tolerance to this drug and cross tolerance to other nitrates and nitrites, may occur; withdrawal restores the original sensitivity.
2. In congestive heart failure, as a rule, pulmonary capillary pressure should not be allowed to fall below 15 mm Hg or systolic blood pressure below physiological range in normal or hypertensive patients. In patients with hypotension in the range of 90–100 mm Hg of systolic pressure there should be no fall at all. As with other vasodilators in sensitive patients Isordil may cause paradoxical side-effects which may increase ischaemia and may even lead to extension of myocardial damage and advanced congestive heart failure. Treatment should therefore be discontinued.

*Side-effects:* Side effects due to Isordil are common to all nitrates used for the treatment of angina pectoris.
1. Cutaneous vasodilation with flushing.
2. Headache is common and in some patients may be severe and persistent. Analgesics have been useful in some cases.
3. Transient episodes of dizziness and weakness and other signs of cerebral ischaemia associated with postural hypotension may occur.
4. This drug can act as a physiological antagonist to noradrenaline, acetylcholine, histamine and many other agents.
5. An occasional individual exhibits a marked sensitivity to the hypotensive effects of nitrate and severe responses (nausea, vomiting, weakness, restlessness, pallor, perspiration and collapse) can occur even with the usual therapeutic dose. Appropriate treatment should be given. Alcohol may enhance this effect.
6. Drug rash and/or exfoliative dermatitis may occasionally occur.

*Treatment of overdosage:* The main manifestation is hypotension. In such an event treatment should be stopped and the patient carefully monitored. Passive exercise and elevation of legs of the recumbent patient will promote venous return. In life threatening situations administration of vasopressors should be considered. The $LD_{50}$ of isosorbide dinitrate in rodents is of the order of 1000 mg/kg.

**Pharmaceutical precautions** *Storage:* Unlike glyceryl trinitrate, Isordil Tablets are stable and no special storage conditions are necessary.

**Legal category** P.

**Package quantities** Isordil Sublingual Tablets 5 mg in Securitainers of 100. Isordil Tablets 10 mg in Securitainers of 100 and 500. Isordil Tablets 30 mg in Securitainers of 100.

**Further information** Isordil has a very high solubility compared with other nitrates and therefore acts sublingually to abort the acute attack of angina pectoris quickly. In addition, Isordil can be administered orally to give a prolonged effect. Because Isordil is physically and chemically stable it is reliable in use.

Inactive ingredients include lactose.

**Product licence numbers**
Isordil Tablets 5 mg    10536/0009
Isordil Tablets 10 mg    10536/0010
Isordil Tablets 30 mg    10536/0011

## ISORDIL* TEMBIDS* CAPSULES

**Presentation** Isordil Tembids capsules containing isosorbide dinitrate 40 mg in a sustained release formulation are gelatin capsules with a colourless, transparent body containing white irregular pellets and opaque blue cap for oral administration.

**Uses** Prophylaxis of angina pectoris (classic effort associated angina, chronic stable angina, vasospastic angina, variant angina, unstable angina, nocturnal angina and angina decubitus).

**Dosage and administration** *Adults:* For oral administration—One capsule 2 or 3 times a day. In selected cases daily doses of up to 240 mg oral isosorbide dinitrate have been administered. Capsules should be swallowed without chewing.

*Elderly:* There are no special dosage requirements for elderly patients but as with all medicines the lowest effective dose should be used.

*Children:* Not recommended.

**Contra-indications, warnings, etc**
*Contra-indications:* Hypersensitivity to this drug.

*Precaution:* Tolerance to this drug, and cross-tolerance to other nitrates and nitrites may occur; withdrawal restores the original sensitivity.

*Use in pregnancy:* The product has not been studied in human pregnancy. The use of Isordil Tembids requires that the anticipated benefit be weighed against possible hazard.

*Side-effects:* Side effects due to Isordil are common to all nitrates used for the treatment of angina pectoris:
1. Cutaneous vasodilation with flushing.
2. Headache is common and in some patients may be severe and persistent. Analgesics have been useful in some cases.
3. Transient episodes of dizziness and weakness and other signs of cerebral ischaemia associated with postural hypotension may occur.
4. This drug can act as a physiological antagonist to noradrenaline, acetylcholine, histamine and many other agents.
5. An occasional individual exhibits a marked sensitivity to the hypotensive effects of nitrate and severe responses (nausea, vomiting, weakness, restlessness, pallor, perspiration and collapse) can occur even with the usual therapeutic dose. Alcohol may enhance this effect.
6. Drug rash and/or exfoliative dermatitis may occasionally occur.

*Treatment of overdosage:* The main manifestation is hypotension. In such event the drug should be withheld and the patient carefully monitored. Passive exercise and elevation of legs of the recumbent patient will promote venous return. In life threatening situations administration of vasopressors should be considered. The $LD_{50}$ of isosorbide dinitrate in rodents is of the order of 1000 mg/kg.

**Pharmaceutical precautions** *Storage:* Unlike glyceryl trinitrate, Isordil Tembids are stable and no special storage conditions are necessary.

**Legal category** P.

**Package quantities** Securitainers of 100.

**Further information** Isosorbide dinitrate is released from the slow release formulation over a 6 hour period to provide up to 12 hours of sustained effect.

Inactive ingredients include lactose.

**Product licence number** 10536/0012.

## LODINE*
## LODINE* SR

**Presentation**
Lodine capsules containing etodolac 200 mg are hard gelatin capsules with an opaque dark grey body and light grey cap, printed with two red bands and 'Lodine 200'.

Lodine capsules containing etodolac 300 mg are hard gelatin capsules with an opaque light grey body and cap, printed with two red bands and 'Lodine 300'.

Lodine tablets contain etodolac 200 mg and are brown, oval biconvex film coated tablets, printed 'WYETH' or 'LODINE' and '200'.

Lodine SR tablets contain etodolac 600 mg in a sustained release formulation and are capsular, oval shaped light grey film coated tablets, impressed on one side with Lodine SR600.

**Uses** Lodine (etodolac) is indicated for acute or long-term use in rheumatoid arthritis and osteoarthritis.

**Dosage and administration**
*Adults: Lodine Capsules 200 mg, 300 mg and Lodine Tablets 200 mg* – The recommended dosage for Lodine is 400 mg to 600 mg daily in two divided doses or administered as a single daily dose.

*Lodine SR Tablets 600 mg:* One tablet daily, swallowed whole with a tumblerful of water. If a lower dose is sufficient, conventional Lodine capsules or tablets may be used. The safety of doses in excess of 600 mg per day has not been established. No occurrence of tolerance or tachyphylaxis has been reported.

*Elderly:* No change in initial dosage is generally required in the elderly (see *Precautions*).

*Children:* Not recommended.

**Contra-indications, warnings, etc**
*Contra-indications:*
1. Lodine should not be used in patients who have previously shown hypersensitivity to it.
2. Lodine should not be used in patients with active peptic ulceration or a history of peptic ulcer disease (including gastrointestinal haemorrhage due to another non-steroidal anti-inflammatory drug).
3. Due to possible cross-reactivity, Lodine should not be administered to patients who experience asthma, rhinitis or urticaria during therapy with aspirin or other non-steroidal anti-inflammatory drugs.

*Pregnancy:* Drugs which inhibit prostaglandin biosynthesis may cause dystocia and delayed parturition as evidenced by studies in pregnant animals. Some inhibitors of prostaglandin biosynthesis have been shown to interfere with the closure of the ductus arteriosus. Safety in human pregnancy has not been established and Lodine should not be used during pregnancy. Safety of Lodine use during lactation has not been established and as such its use in nursing mothers should be avoided.

*Precautions:*
1. Although non-steroidal anti-inflammatory drugs do not have the same direct effects on platelets as does aspirin, all drugs which inhibit the biosynthesis of prostaglandins may interfere, to some extent, with platelet function. Patients receiving Lodine who may be adversely affected by such actions should be carefully observed.
2. In patients with renal, cardiac or hepatic impairment especially those taking diuretics, caution is required since the use of NSAIDs may result in deterioration of renal function. The dose should be kept as low as possible and renal function should be monitored. However, impairment of renal or hepatic functions due to other causes may alter drug metabolism; patients receiving concomitant long term therapy, especially the elderly, should be observed for potential side effects and their drug doses adjusted as needed, or the drug discontinued.
3. Serious gastrointestinal adverse effects such as bleeding, ulceration and perforation can occur at any time with or without warning symptoms in patients treated with NSAIDs. If any sign of gastrointestinal bleeding occurs, Lodine should be stopped immediately.
4. Patients on long-term treatment with Lodine should be regularly reviewed as a precautionary measure e.g. for changes in renal function, haematological parameters, or hepatic function.
5. Lodine should be used with caution in patients with fluid retention, hypertension or heart failure.

*Drug interactions:*
1. Since Lodine is extensively protein-bound, it may be necessary to modify the dosage of other highly protein-bound drugs.

The concomitant administration of warfarin and Lodine should not require a dosage adjustment of either drug, however it has rarely led to prolonged prothrombin times, therefore caution should be exercised when Lodine is administered with warfarin.

2. Concomitant use of clyclosporin, digoxin, or lithium with NSAIDs may cause an increase in serum levels of these compounds and associated toxicities.

3. Bilirubin tests can give a false positive result due to the presence of phenolic metabolites of Lodine in the urine.

*Side-effects:*

1. Reported side effects include nausea, epigastric pain, diarrhoea, indigestion, heartburn, flatulence, abdominal pain, constipation, vomiting, ulcerative stomatitis, dyspepsia, gastritis, haematemesis, melaena, rectal bleeding, colitis, vasculitis, headaches, dizziness, abnormal vision, pyrexia, drowsiness, tinnitus, rash, pruritus, fatigue, depression, insomnia, confusion, paraesthesia, tremor, weakness/malaise, dyspnoea, oedema, palpitations, bilirubinuria, hepatic function abnormalities and jaundice, urinary frequency, dysuria, angioedema, anaphylactoid reaction, photosensitivity, urticaria and Stevens-Johnson syndrome.

2. More serious adverse reactions which may occasionally occur are gastro-intestinal ulceration and peptic ulceration.

3. NSAIDs have been reported to cause nephrotoxicity in various forms and their use can lead to interstitial nephritis, nephrotic syndrome and renal failure. There have been reports of nephritis and renal failure with etodolac.

4. Occasionally blood disorders have been reported including: thrombocytopenia, neutropenia, agranulocytosis and anaemia.

*Overdosage:* The standard practices of gastric lavage, activated charcoal administration and general supportive therapy should be undertaken.

**Pharmaceutical precautions** Store at room temperature – below 25°C.

**Legal category** POM

**Package quantities**
Lodine 200 mg capsules: Securitainers of 60.
Lodine 300 mg capsules: Cartons containing 60 capsules, (blisters of 10).
Lodine 200 mg tablets: White HDPE bottles of 60.
Lodine SR 600 mg tablets: Cartons containing 30 tablets, (blisters of 10).

**Further information** All non-steroidal anti-inflammatory drugs (NSAIDs) have been shown to inhibit the formation of prostaglandins. It is this action which is primarily responsible both for their therapeutic effects and some of their side-effects. The inhibition of prostaglandin synthesis observed with etodolac differs from that of other NSAIDs. In an animal model at an established anti-inflammatory dose, cytoprotective PGE concentrations in the gastric mucosa have been shown to be reduced to a lesser degree and for a shorter period with eotdolac than with other NSAIDs

This finding is consistent with subsequent in-vitro studies which have found etodolac to be selective for induced cyclo-oxygenase 2 (COX-2, associated with inflammation) over COX-1 (cytoprotective). Furthermore, studies in human cell models have confirmed that etodolac is selective for the inhibition of COX-2. The clinical benefit of preferential COX-2 inhibition over COX-1 has yet to be proven.

**Product licence numbers**

| | |
|---|---|
| Lodine Capsules 200 mg | 0011/0144 |
| Lodine Capsules 300 mg | 0011/0145 |
| Lodine Tablets 200 mg | 0011/0148 |
| Lodine SR Tablets 600 mg | 0011/0197 |

*Product licence holder:* Wyeth Laboratories, Huntercombe Lane South, Taplow, Maidenhead.

# MAXOLON*

## Qualitative and quantitative composition

*Maxolon Tablets 5 mg:* Each tablet contains Metoclopramide Hydrochloride BP equivalent to 5 mg of the anhydrous substance.

*Maxolon Tablets 10 mg:* Each tablet contains Metoclopramide Hydrochloride BP equivalent to 10 mg of the anhydrous substance.

*Maxolon Syrup:* The syrup contains Metoclopramide Hydrochloride BP equivalent to 1 mg/ml of the anhydrous substance.

*Maxolon Paediatric Liquid:* The liquid contains Metoclopramide Hydrochloride BP equivalent to 1 mg/ml of the anhydrous substance.

*Maxolon Injection:* Each 2 ml ampoule contains Metoclopramide Hydrochloride BP equivalent to 10 mg of the anhydrous substance.

## Pharmaceutical form

*Maxolon Tablets 5 mg:* White to ivory-white circular tablets.

*Maxolon Tablets 10 mg:* White uncoated tablets scored and engraved Maxolon.

*Maxolon Syrup and Paediatric Liquid:* Clear colourless lemon-lime solution for oral administration.

*Maxolon Injection:* Clear colourless solution for intramuscular or intravenous administration.

## Clinical particulars

*Therapeutic indications. Adults (20 years and over): Digestive disorders:* Maxolon restores normal coordination and tone to the upper digestive tract. Maxolon relieves the symptoms of gastro-duodenal dysfunction including: dyspepsia, heartburn, flatulence, sickness, regurgitation of bile, pain. These symptoms may be associated with such conditions as: peptic ulcer, duodenitis, reflux oesophagitis, hiatus hernia, gastritis, cholelithiasis and post-cholecystectomy dyspepsia.

*Nausea and vomiting:* Maxolon is indicated for the treatment of the nausea and vomiting associated with: gastro-intestinal disorders, cyclical vomiting, intolerance to cytotoxic drugs, congestive heart failure, deep x-ray or cobalt therapy, post-anaesthetic vomiting.

*Migraine:* Maxolon relieves symptoms of nausea and vomiting, and overcomes gastric stasis associated with attacks of migraine. This improvement in gastric emptying assists the absorption of concurrently administered oral anti-migraine therapy (e.g. paracetamol) which may otherwise be impaired in such patients.

*Post-operative conditions:* Post-operative gastric hypotonia, post-vagotomy syndrome. Maxolon promotes normal gastric emptying and restores motility in vagotomised patients, and where post-operative symptoms suggest gastro-duodenal dysfunction.

Diagnostic procedures: Radiology, Duodenal intubation. Maxolon speeds up the passage of a barium meal by decreasing gastric emptying time, co-ordinating peristalsis and dilating the duodenal bulb. Maxolon also facilitates duodenal intubation procedures.

*Young adults and children:* The use of Maxolon in patients under 20 years should be restricted to the following:

Severe intractable vomiting of known cause, vomiting associated with radiotherapy and intolerance to cytotoxic drugs, as an aid to gastro-intestinal intubation, and as part of the premedication before surgical procedures.

*Posology and method of administration:*

*Route of administration*
*Oral:* The dosage recommendations given below should be strictly adhered to if side effects of the dystonic type are to be avoided. It should be noted that total daily dosage of Maxolon, especially for children and young adults, should not normally exceed 0.5 mg/kg body weight.

In patients with clinically significant degrees of renal or hepatic impairment, therapy should be at reduced dosage. Metoclopramide is metabolised in the liver and the predominant route of elimination of metoclopramide and its metabolites is via the kidney.

*Injection:* Maxolon injection may be administered either intramuscularly or by slow intravenous injection (1-2 minutes).

Otherwise as for oral dosage.

*Medical indications:*
*Adults 20 years and over:* 10 mg three times daily. For patients of less than 60 kg see below.

*Elderly patients:* As for adults. To avoid adverse reactions adhere strictly to dosage recommendations and where prolonged therapy is considered necessary, patients should be regularly reviewed.

Young adults and children: Maxolon should only be used after careful examination to avoid masking an underlying disorder, e.g. cerebral irritation. In the treatment of this group attention should be given primarily to body weight and treatment should commence at the lower dosage where stated.

| | | |
|---|---|---|
| Young adults: | 15-19 years, 60 kg and over | 10 mg three times daily |
| | 30-59 kg | 5 mg three times daily |
| Children: | 9-14 years, 30 kg and over | 5 mg three times daily |
| | 5-9 years, 20-29 kg | 2½ mg two to three times daily |
| | 3-5 years, 15-19 kg | 2 mg two to three times daily |
| | 1-3 years, 10-14 kg | 1 mg two to three times daily |
| | Under 1 year, up to 10 kg | 1 mg twice daily |

Tablets should not be used in children under the age of 15. Maxolon Injection or an oral liquid presentation should be used in the younger age groups; more accurate dosage is facilitated by the use of the Paediatric Liquid.

*Diagnostic indications:* A single dose of Maxolon may be given 5-10 minutes before the examination subject to body weight consideration,(see above); the following dosages are recommended:

| | | |
|---|---|---|
| Adults: | 20 years and over | 10-20 mg |
| Young adults: | 15-19 years | 10 mg |
| Children: | 9-14 years | 5 mg |
| | 5-9 years | 2½ mg |
| | 3-5 years | 2 mg |
| | Under 3 years | 1 mg |

Maxolon Injection or an oral liquid presentation should be used in the younger age groups; more accurate dosage is facilitated by the use of the Paediatric liquid.

*Contra-indications:* No absolute contra-indications to the use of Maxolon.

*Special warnings and special precautions for use:* Precautions: If vomiting persists the patient should be reassessed to exclude the possibility of an underlying disorder e.g. cerebral irritation.

Care should be exercised in patients being treated with other centrally active drugs e.g. in epilepsy.

Since extrapyramidal symptoms may occur with both metoclopramide and neuroleptics such as the phenothiazines, particular care should be exercised in the event of these drugs being prescribed concurrently.

The neuroleptic malignant syndrome has been reported with metoclopramide in combination with neuroleptics as well as with metoclopramide monotherapy (see side effects).

Special care should be taken in cases of severe renal insufficiency (see also under dosage and administration).

Following operations such as pyloroplasty or gut anastomosis metoclopramide therapy should be withheld for three or four days as vigorous muscular contractions may not help healing.

Metoclopramide may induce an acute hypertensive response in patients with phaeochromocytoma.

*Interaction with other medicaments and other forms of interaction:* The action of Maxolon on the gastrointestinal tract is antagonised by anticholinergics. The absorption of any concurrently administered oral medication may be modified by the effect of Maxolon on gastric motility.

*Pregnancy and lactation:* Animal tests in several mammalian species and clinical experience have not indicated a teratogenic effect. Nevertheless Maxolon should only be used when there are compelling reasons and is not advised during the first trimester.

During lactation metoclopramide is found in breast milk.

*Effects on ability to drive and use machines:* None but see below.

*Undesirable effects:* Various extrapyramidal reactions to Maxolon, usually of the dystonic type, have been reported. The incidence of dystonic reactions, particularly in children and young adults, is increased if daily dosages higher than 0.5 mg per kg body weight are administered. Dystonic reactions include: spasm of the facial muscles, trismus, rhythmic protrusion of the tongue, a bulbar type of speech, spasm of extraocular muscles including oculogyric crises, unnatural positioning of the head and shoulders and opisthotonos. There may be a generalised increase in muscle tone. The majority of reactions occur within 36 hours of starting treatment and the effects usually disappear within 24 hours of withdrawal of the drug. Should treatment of a dystonic reaction be required an anticholinergic anti-Parkinsonian drug, or a benzodiazepine may be used.

Very rare occurrences of the neuroleptic malignant syndrome have been reported. This syndrome is potentially fatal and comprises hyperpyrexia, altered consciousness, muscle rigidity, autonomic instability and elevated levels of creatine phosphokinase (CPK) and must be treated urgently (recognised treatments include dantrolene and bromocriptine). Metoclopramide should be stopped immediately if this syndrome occurs.

Tardive dyskinesia has been reported during prolonged treatment in a small number of mainly elderly patients. Patients on prolonged treatment should be regularly reviewed.

Rarely, drowsiness, restlessness and diarrhoea have been reported in patients receiving metoclopramide therapy. Depression has been reported extremely rarely.

Raised serum prolactin levels have been observed during metoclopramide therapy: this effect is similar to that noted with many other compounds.

Extremely rarely cases of red cell disorders such as methaemoglobinaemia and sulphaemoglobinaemia have been reported, particularly at high doses of metoclopramide. If this occurs the drug should be withdrawn. Methaemoglobinaemia may be treated using methylene blue.

For intravenous use: There have been very rare reports of abnormalities of cardiac conduction (such as bradycardia and heart block) in association with intravenous metoclopramide.

*Overdose:* In cases of overdosage, acute dystonic reactions have occurred. Overdosage should be treated by gastric lavage with appropriate supportive measures. For treatment of a dystonic reaction see *Side effects.* Very rarely AV block has been observed with Maxolon Injection.

**Pharmacological properties**

*Pharmacodynamic properties:* The action of metoclopramide is closely associated with parasympathetic nervous control of the upper gastro-intestinal tract, where it has the effect of encouraging normal peristaltic action. This provides for a fundamental approach to the control of those conditions where disturbed gastro-intestinal motility is a common underlying factor.

*Pharmacokinetic properties:* Metoclopramide is metabolised in the liver and the predominant route of elimination of metoclopramide and its metabolites is via the kidney.

*Preclinical safety data:* No additional data available.

**Pharmaceutical particulars**

*List of excipients:* Maxolon Tablets 5 mg and 10 mg: Maize starch (dried), colloidal silicon dioxide, magnesium stearate, pregelatinised maize starch, lactose.

Maxolon Syrup and Paediatric Liquid: Hydroxyethylcellulose, methyl parahydroxybenzoate, propyl parahydroxybenzoate, saccharin sodium, citric acid monohydrate, soluble lemon oil, No.1 lime flavour, purified water.

Maxolon Injection: Sodium chloride, sodium metabisulphite, water for injection.

*Incompatibilities:* Not applicable.

*Shelf life:* Maxolon Tablets 10 mg and Injection: Sixty months.

Maxolon Tablets 5 mg and Syrup: Thirtysix months.

Maxolon Paediatric Liquid: Thirtysix months. The liquid should be used within 14 days of opening.

*Special precautions for storage:* Maxolon Tablets 5 mg: Store at or below 25°C.

Maxolon Tablets 10 mg: None. Maxolon Syrup and Paediatric Liquid: Protect from light. Maxolon Injection: If ampoules are removed from their carton, they should be stored away from light. If inadvertent exposure occurs, ampoules showing discolouration must be discarded.

*Nature and contents of container:*
*Maxolon Tablets 5 mg:* PVC (250 microns)/PVDC (60 gsm) blister (6 tablets) backed with aluminium foil (20 microns). The underside of the foil is coated with vinyl based lacquer.
*Maxolon Tablets 10 mg:* Plastic recloseable containers packed into carton of 100 or 500 tablets. PVC blister (300 microns) of 84 tablets backed with aluminium foil (20 microns). The underside of the foil is coated with vinyl based lacquer.
*Maxolon Syrup:* Amber glass bottles of 100 ml, 200 ml or 1000 ml.
*Maxolon Paediatric Liquid:* Amber glass bottles with pipette administration device of 15 ml liquid.
*Maxolon Injection:* Clear glass 2 ml ampoules (PhEur, Type I neutral glass) in packs of 12 ampoules.

*Instructions for use/handling:*
*Maxolon Tablets 5 mg, 10 mg, Syrup, Paediatric Liquid:* None.
*Maxolon Injection:* Protect from light.

**Marketing authorisation numbers**
Maxolon Tablets 10 mg: 10536/0031
Maxolon Syrup: 10536/0032
Maxolon Paediatric Liquid: 10536/0033
Maxolon Injection: 10536/0034
Maxolon Tablets 5 mg: 10536/0037

**Date of approval/revision of SPC** January 1997

**Legal category** POM.

## MAXOLON* HIGH DOSE

**Qualitative and quantitative composition** Each 20 ml ampoule contains Metoclopramide Hydrochloride BP equivalent to 100 mg of the anhydrous substance.

**Pharmaceutical form** Clear colourless solution for intravenous infusion.

**Clinical particulars**

*Therapeutic indications:* Maxolon High Dose is indicated for the treatment of nausea and vomiting associated with intolerance to cytotoxic drugs.

*Posology and method of administration:* Maxolon High Dose is administered by IV infusion, suitably diluted. The recommended method of administration is by continuous infusion which allows steady serum levels of metaclopramide to be maintained.

*Continuous infusion (recommended method):* Maxolon High Dose is given by IV infusion as a loading dose followed by a continuous infusion to maintain a metoclopramide serum concentration of 0.85 microgram–1.0 microgram/ml. The loading dose should be given before starting cytotoxic chemotherapy.

| | *Maxolon High Dose* | *Volume of Diluent* | *IV Infusion Time* |
|---|---|---|---|
| Loading dose | 2-4 mg/kg body weight | 50-100 ml | 15-20 minutes |
| Maintenance dose | 3-5 mg/kg body weight | 500 ml | 8-12 hours |

Total dosage in any 24 hour period should not normally exceed 10 mg/kg body weight. Where cisplatin is to be used the loading dose of Maxolon High Dose should be at least 3 mg/kg body weight and the maintenance dose at least 4 mg/kg body weight.

*Intermittent Infusion (alternative regimen):* Maxolon High Dose can be given by intermittent IV infusion suitably diluted. The initial dose should be given before starting cytotoxic chemotherapy.

| | *Maxolon High Dose* | *Volume of Diluent* | *IV Infusion Time* |
|---|---|---|---|
| Initial dose | Up to 2 mg/kg body weight | at least 50 ml | at least 15 minutes |
| Repeat doses at 2 hourly intervals | Up to 2 mg/kg body weight | at least 50 ml | at least 15 minutes |

Total dosage in any 24 hour period should not normally exceed 10 mg/kg body weight.

*Abnormal renal or liver function:* In patients with clinically significant degrees of renal or hepatic impairment, therapy should be at reduced dosage. Metoclopramide is metabolised in the liver and the predominant route of elimination of metoclopramide and its metabolites is via the kidney.

*Compatibility with cytotoxic agents:* Maxolon High Dose is compatible with a number of cytotoxic drugs; however it should not be mixed in solution with therapeutic agents other than those stated. Maxolon High Dose is compatible with cisplatin, cyclophosphamide and doxorubicin hydrochloride and is stable over the concentration ranges listed below for 24 hours at room temperature when protected from light.

40-200 ml cisplatin (1 mg/ml) per 100 mg/20 ml of Maxolon High Dose in 1 litre of sodium chloride 0.9%.

Up to 40 mg doxorubicin hydrochloride (powder) per 100 mg/20 ml of Maxolon High Dose.

Up to 4 g cyclophosphamide (1 g/50 ml) per 100 mg/20 ml of Maxolon High Dose.

*Compatibility with morphine/diamorphine:* Maxolon High Dose is compatible with morphine hydrochloride and diamorphine hydrochloride and is stable over the concentration ranges listed below for 48 hours at room temperature under normal fluorescent lighting. Up to 100 mg of morphine hydrochloride per 100 mg/20 ml of Maxolon High Dose. Up to 50 mg of diamorphine hydrochloride per 100 mg/20 ml of Maxolon High Dose. Maxolon High Dose 100 mg/20 ml also remains stable for 48 hours at room temperature with 100 mg of morphine hydrochloride, or 50 mg diamorphine hydrochloride, when diluted 1 in 10 with sodium chloride 0.9%.

*Stability in intravenous fluids:* Ideally intravenous solutions should be prepared at the time of infusion.

However, Maxolon High Dose has been shown to be stable for at least 48 hours at room temperature in the following solutions when administered in a PVC infusion bag (e.g. Viaflex[R] Travenol).

Sodium chloride intravenous infusion BP (0.9% w/v), Glucose intravenous infusion BP (5% w/v), Sodium chloride and glucose intravenous infusion BP (sodium chloride 0.18% w/v; glucose 4% w/v), Compound sodium lactate intravenous infusion BP (ringer-lactate solution; Hartmann's solution).

Note: preparation must be under appropriate aseptic conditions if the above extended storage periods are required. The high dose ampoule presentation is not suitable for multidose use.

*Contra-indications:* No absolute contraindications to the use of Maxolon.

*Special warnings and special precautions for use: Other special warnings and precautions:* Precautions: Care should be exercised in patients being treated with other centrally active drugs e.g. in epilepsy.

Since extrapyramidal symptoms may occur with both metoclopramide and neuroleptics such as the phenothiazines, particular care should be exercised in the event of these drugs being prescribed concurrently.

The neuroleptic malignant syndrome has been reported with metoclopramide in combination with neuroleptics as well as with metoclopramide monotherapy (see undesirable side effects).

Following operations such as pyloroplasty or gut anastomosis metoclopramide therapy should be withheld for three or four days as vigorous muscular contractions may not help healing.

Metoclopramide may induce an acute hypertensive response in patients with phaeochromocytoma.

*Interaction with other medicaments and other forms of interaction:* The action of Maxolon on the gastro-intestinal tract is antagonised by anticholinergics. The absorption of any concurrently administered oral medication may be modified by the effect of Maxolon on gastric motility.

*Pregnancy and lactation:* Animal tests in several mammalian species and clinical experience have not indicated a teratogenic effect. Nevertheless Maxolon should only be used when there are compelling reasons and is not advised during the first trimester.

During lactation metoclopramide is found in breast milk.

*Effects on ability to drive and use machines:* None but see *'Undesirable effects'.*

*Undesirable effects:* When given at high dose in association with cancer chemotherapy, Maxolon has been found to be well tolerated with few adverse events. Various extrapyramidal reactions to Maxolon, usually of the dystonic type, have been reported. Studies of Maxolon given in doses up to 10 mg/kg body weight/day by IV infusion report an incidence of extrapyramidal reactions of less than 10%. The incidence of such reactions may be increased in the younger patient. Reactions to Maxolon have included spasm of the facial muscles, trismus, rhythmic protrusion of the tongue, a bulbar type of speech, spasm of extra-ocular muscles including oculogyric crises, unnatural positioning of the head and shoulders and opisthotonos. There may be a generalised increase in muscle tone. The majority of reactions occur within 36 hours of starting treatment and the effects usually disappear within 24 hours of withdrawal of the drug. Should treatment of a dystonic reaction be required an anticholinergic anti-Parkinsonian drug, or a benzodiazepine may be used.

Very rare occurrences of the neuroleptic malignant syndrome have been reported. This syndrome is potentially fatal and comprises hyperpyrexia, altered consciousness, muscle rigidity, autonomic instability and elevated levels of creatine phosphokinase (CPK) and must be treated urgently (recognised treatments include dantrolene and bromocriptine). Metoclopramide should be stopped immediately if these syndrome occurs.

There have been very rare reports of abnormalities of cardiac conduction (such as bradycardia and heart block) in association with intravenous metoclopramide.

Mild drowsiness and diarrhoea have been noted. Depression has been reported extremely rarely.

Raised serum prolactin levels have been observed during metoclopramide therapy: this effect is similar to that noted with many other compounds.

Extremely rarely cases of red cell disorders such as methaemoglobinaemia and sulphaemoglobinaemia have been reported, particularly at high doses of metoclopramide. If this occurs the drug should be withdrawn. Methaemoglobinaemia may be treated using methylene blue.

*Overdose:* In cases of overdosage, acute dystonic reactions have occurred. Very rarely AV block has been observed. For treatment of a dystonic reaction see *'Undesirable effects'.*

**Pharmacological properties**

*Pharmacodynamic properties:* Maxolon High Dose is indicated for the treatment of nausea and vomiting associated with intolerance to cytotoxic drugs. It is specially formulated to ensure compatibility in solution with cisplatin.

Maxolon exerts a three-fold anti-emetic action: by inhibiting central dopamine receptors Maxolon raises the threshold of the chemoreceptor trigger zone, and reduces the reaction of the adjacent vomiting centre to centrally-acting emetics. Maxolon decreases the sensitivity of the visceral afferent nerves to the vomiting centre, reducing the effect of locally-acting emetics and irritant substances. In the upper gastro-intestinal tract Maxolon promotes normal gastric emptying and it may thus abolish gastric stasis which is part of the vomiting reflex.

Maxolon High Dose is not intended for use in the wider range of indications for which Maxolon at standard dose is indicated.

*Pharmacokinetic properties:* Based on current literature, a metoclopramide concentration range of about 0.85 microgram/ml would appear desirable for the control of cytotoxic drug induced emesis. Such plasma concentrations may be achieved by the administration of a loading dose of 2-4 mg/kg infused over 15-30 minutes prior to cytotoxic drug therapy followed by a maintenance continuous infusion of 3-5 mg/kg over 8-12 hours.

Metoclopramide is metabolised in the liver and the predominant route of elimination of metoclopramide and its metabolites is via the kidney. In patients with clinically significant degrees of renal or hepatic impairment, therapy should be at reduced dosage.

*Preclinical safety data:* No additional data available.

**Pharmaceutical particulars**

*List of excipients:* Sodium chloride, water for injections.

*Incompatibilities:* Not applicable.

*Shelf life:* Thirty six months.

*Special precautions for storage:* If ampoules are removed from their carton, they should be stored away from light. If inadvertent exposure occurs, ampoules showing discolouration must be discarded.

*Nature and contents of container:* Clear glass 20 ml ampoules (PhEur Type I neutral glass) packed in boxes of 10.

*Instructions for use/handling:* Protect from light.

**Marketing authorisation number** 10536/0035

**Date of approval/revision of SPC** May 1996

**Legal category** POM.

# MAXOLON* SR

**Qualitative and quantitative composition** Each capsule contains Metoclopramide Hydrochloride BP equivalent to 15 mg of the anhydrous substance.

**Pharmaceutical form** Colourless, transparent capsules, overprinted 'Maxolon SR 15', containing white sustained release microgranules.

Maxolon SR does not contain tartrazine or any other azo dyes.

**Clinical particulars**

*Therapeutic indications:* Digestive disorders: Maxolon SR restores normal co-ordination and tone to the upper digestive tract. Maxolon SR relieves symptoms of gastro-duodenal dysfunction. Including: dyspepsia, heartburn, flatulence, sickness, pain, regurgitation of bile. These symptoms may be associated with such conditions as: reflux oesophagitis, hiatus hernia, gastritis, duodenitis, peptic ulcer, cholelithiasis and post-cholecystectomy dyspepsia.

Nausea and vomiting: Maxolon SR is indicated for the treatment of the nausea and vomiting associated with gastro-intestinal disorders and intolerance to cytotoxic drugs.

*Posology and method of administration:* Adults: In adults 20 years and over: 1 capsule (15 mg) twice daily, swallowed whole. Total daily dosage of Maxolon SR should not normally exceed 0.5 mg/kg body weight.

Elderly: As for adults. To avoid adverse reactions adhere strictly to dosage recommendations and where prolonged therapy is considered necessary, patients should be regularly reviewed.

The interval between doses many need to be extended in patients with clinically significant degrees of renal or hepatic impairment. The predominant route of elimination is via the kidney.

Children and young adults: A presentation of Maxolon SR suitable for patients under 20 years of age is not available.

Note: Presentations suitable for patients of low body weight are described on the separate Maxolon data sheet.

*Contra-indications:* Maxolon SR is contra-indicated in patients under 20 years since the dose level cannot be reduced.

*Special warnings and special precautions for use:* Precautions: If vomiting persists the patient should be reassessed to exclude the possibility of an underlying disorder e.g. cerebral irritation.

Care should be exercised in patients being treated with other centrally active drugs e.g. epilepsy.

Since extrapyramidal symptoms may occur with both metoclopramide and neuroleptics such as the phenothiazines, particular care should be exercised in the event of these drugs being prescribed concurrently.

The neuroleptic malignant syndrome has been reported with metoclopramide in combination with neuroleptics as well as with metoclopramide monotherapy (see side effects).

Special care should be taken in cases of severe renal insufficiency (see Posology).

Following operations such as pyloroplasty or gut anastomosis metoclopramide therapy should be withheld for three or four days as vigorous muscular contractions may not help healing.

Metoclopramide may induce an acute hypertensive response in patients with phaeochromocytoma.

*Interaction with other medicaments and other forms of interaction:* The action of metoclopramide on gastro-intestinal tract is antagonised by anticholinergics. The absorption of any concurrently administered oral medication may be modified by the effect of metoclopramide on motility. See also under *Special warnings.*

*Pregnancy and lactation:* Animal tests in several mammalian species and clinical experience have not indicated a teratogenic effect. Nevertheless Maxolon SR should only be used when there are compelling reasons and is not advised during the first trimester.

During lactation metoclopramide is found in breast milk.

*Effects on ability to drive and use machines:* None but see *Undesirable effects.*

*Undesirable effects:* Various extrapyramidal reactions to metoclopramide, usually of the dystonic type, have been reported. The incidence of these reactions may be increased if daily dosages higher than 0.5 mg per kg body weight are administered. Dystonic reactions include: spasm of the facial muscles, trismus, rhythmic protrusion of the tongue, a bulbar type of speech, spasm of extra-ocular muscles including oculogyric crises, unnatural positioning of the head and shoulders and opisthotonos. There may be a generalised increase in muscle tone. The majority of reactions occur within 36 hours of starting treatment and the effects usually disappear within 24 hours of withdrawal of the drug. Should treatment of a dystonic reaction be required an anticholinergic anti-Parkinsonian drug, or a benzodiazepine may be used.

Very rare occurrences of the neuroleptic malignant syndrome have been reported. This syndrome is potentially fatal and comprises hyperpyrexia, altered consciousness, muscle rigidity, autonomic instability and elevated levels of creatine phosphokinase (CPK) and must be treated urgently (recognised treatments include dantrolene and bromocriptine).

Tardive dyskinesia has been reported during prolonged treatment in a small number of mainly elderly patients. Patients on prolonged treatment should be regularly reviewed.

Rarely, drowsiness, restlessness and diarrhoea have been reported in patients receiving metoclopramide therapy. Depression has been reported extremely rarely.

Raised serum prolactin levels have been observed during metoclopramide therapy: this effect is similar to that noted with many other compounds.

Extremely rarely cases of red cell disorders such as methaemoglobinaemia and sulphaemoglobinaemia have been reported, particularly at high doses of metoclopramide. If this occurs the drug should be withdrawn. Methaemoglobinaemia may be treated using methylene blue.

*Overdose:* In cases of overdosage, acute dystonic reactions have occurred. Overdosage should be treated by gastric lavage with appropriate supportive measures. For treatment of a dystonic reaction see Undesirable effects.

**Pharmacological properties**

*Pharmacodynamic properties:* The action of metoclopramide is closely associated with parasympathetic nervous control of the upper gastro-intestinal tract, where it has the effect of encouraging normal peristaltic action. This provides for a fundamental approach to the control of those conditions where disturbed gastro-intestinal motility is a common underlying factor.

*Pharmacokinetic properties:* The following pharmacokinetic parameters for Maxolon SR after a single administration have been established.

$C_{max}$ 102.5 nmol/litre; $T_{max}$ 4.5 hours; AUC 1514.25 nmol.hr/litre; t $_{1/2}$ (elim) 7.04 hours; C12 hrs 54.75 nmol/litre

On repeated administration the following parameters have been established.

$C_{max}$ 188 nmol/l; $C_{min}$ 109 nmol/l

*Preclinical safety data:* No relevant information available.

**Pharmaceutical particulars**

*List of excipients:* Sucrose; maize starch; stearic acid, dibutyl phthalate; talc; polymethacrylates; gelatin; black iron oxide.

*Incompatibilities:* Not applicable.

*Shelf life:* 24 months.

*Special precautions for storage:* Protect from direct light.

*Nature and contents of container:* All pack sizes (8*,14* or 56 capsules) are available in the following packaging:

PVC blister (300 microns) backed with aluminium foil (20 microns)*. The underside of the foil is coated with vinyl based lacquer.

PVC (200 microns)/PVDC (60 gsm) blister*.

Polypropylene containers with polyethylene caps.
*Not available.

*Instructions for use/handling:* None.

**Marketing authorisation number** 10536/0030

**Date of approval/revision of SPC** July 1996

**Legal category** POM.

# MEPTID* INJECTION

**Presentation** Meptid injection is a clear solution, containing meptazinol hydrochloride at a concentration equivalent to 100 mg meptazinol base per ml, supplied in 1 ml quantities in clear glass ampoules.

**Uses** Meptid injection is indicated for the treatment of moderate to severe pain, including post-operative pain, obstetric pain and the pain of renal colic.

**Dosage and administration** *Adults: Intramuscular dosage:* 75–100 mg Meptid. The injection may be repeated 2–4 hourly as required. For obstetric pain a dose of 100–150 mg should be used according to weight. This dose should approximate 2 mg/kg.

*Intravenous dosage:* 50–100 mg Meptid by slow intravenous injection. The injection may be repeated 2–4 hourly as required. If vomiting occurs, a suitable antiemetic should be given.

*Epidural/Intrathecal use:* This formulation is *not* suitable for these routes.

*Elderly:* The adult dosage schedule may be used in the elderly.

*Children:* Meptid Injection has not been evaluated for use in children.

**Contra-indications, warnings, etc**
*Contra-indications:* None known, except for individuals with known sensitivity to the product.

*Precautions:*
1. Caution should be observed in treating patients with hepatic or renal insufficiency.
2. Clinical studies have indicated absence of clinically significant respiratory depression but caution should be exercised in patients already severely compromised.
3. Safety for use in myocardial infarction has not been established.
4. Meptid injection is a useful analgesic in labour but in accordance with general medical principles it should not be given in other stages of pregnancy unless considered essential by the physician. There is no evidence from animal reproductive studies to anticipate a teratogenic risk.
5. Meptid should be used cautiously in patients with head injuries, as other drugs of this class have the potential to elevate cerebrospinal fluid pressure and to obscure the clinical course of such patients.

*Warnings:* Since dizziness and occasionally drowsiness have been reported, patients should be cautioned against driving or operating machinery until it is established that they do not become dizzy or drowsy while taking meptazinol. Other central nervous system depressants should be used with caution in patients receiving Meptid.

*Treatment of overdosage:* Overdosage with Meptid injection has not been reported. Large doses, including seven times the recommended therapeutic dose, have been given in balanced and total intravenous anaesthesia, without significant respiratory depressant effects.

In the event of cardiovascular and respiratory collapse, normal resuscitative procedures should be employed. Respiratory depression caused by overdosage with meptazinol may be reversed in part with therapeutic doses of naloxone.

*Side-effects:* The most commonly reported adverse reactions after treatment with meptazinol are nausea, vomiting, dizziness, diarrhoea, increased sweating, abdominal pain, rash, vertigo, headache, somnolence and dyspepsia.

**Pharmaceutical precautions** Store below 25°C.

Meptid injection should *not* be mixed with other drugs in the same infusion solution or in the same syringe. Meptid injection is an acidic solution of the hydrochloride salt of meptazinol and is therefore pharmaceutically incompatible with injection solutions known to be strongly basic (for example thiopentone) as precipitation of the meptazinol base may occur.

Meptid at concentrations of 200 mg in 500 ml and

500 mg in 500 ml has been shown to be compatible with the following intravenous infusion fluids when added immediately prior to use:

Dextrose 5% w/v
Dextrose 10% w/v
Sodium chloride 0.9% w/v
Ringers solution
Hartmanns solution
Sodium chloride 0.9% w/v and dextrose 5% w/v

If Meptid is administered through an intravenous cannula, it is essential to flush the system with saline before and after administration.

**Legal category** POM.

**Package quantities** Cartons of 10 ampoules (OP).

**Further information** Nil.

**Product licence number** 10536/0008.

## MEPTID* TABLETS

**Presentation** Meptid tablets are oval orange film coated tablets marked MPL 023 on one side, 14.5 mm in length and containing 200 mg meptazinol.

**Uses** Meptid tablets are indicated for the short term treatment of moderate pain.

**Dosage and administration** For oral administration only.

*Adults:* 200 mg 3–6 hourly as required. Usually one tablet four hourly.

*Elderly:* The adult dosage schedule may be used in the elderly.

*Children:* Meptid tablets have not been evaluated for use in children.

**Contra-indications, warnings, etc**

*Contra-indications:* None known, except for individuals with known sensitivity to the product.

*Precautions:*

1. Caution should be observed in treating patients with hepatic or renal insufficiency.

2. Clinical studies have indicated absence of clinically significant respiratory depression but caution should be exercised in patients already severely compromised.

3. In accordance with general medical principles Meptid tablets should not be given to pregnant or lactating women unless considered essential by the physician. There is no evidence from animal reproductive studies to anticipate a teratogenic risk.

4. Meptid should be used cautiously in patients with head injuries, as other drugs of this class have the potential to elevate cerebrospinal fluid pressure and to obscure the clinical course of such patients.

5. Safety for use in myocardial infarction has not yet been established.

*Warnings:* Since dizziness and occasionally drowsiness have been reported, patients should be cautioned against driving or operating machinery until it is established that they do not become dizzy or drowsy while taking meptazinol. Other central nervous system depressants should be used with caution in patients receiving Meptid.

*Treatment of overdosage:* Meptid tablets are subject to a hepatic first pass metabolism which prevents systemic concentrations of the drug reaching levels achieved by parenteral administration. In the unlikely event of overdose producing respiratory depression naloxone is the treatment of choice.

Recommended treatment includes gastric lavage, supportive therapy and naloxone if required.

*Side-effects:* The most commonly reported adverse reactions after treatment with meptazinol are nausea, vomiting, dizziness, diarrhoea, increased sweating, abdominal pain, rash, vertigo, headache, somnolence and dyspepsia.

**Pharmaceutical precautions** None.

**Legal category** POM.

**Package quantities** Cartons of 100 tablets (5 blister packs of 20 tablets).

**Further information** Meptazinol is eliminated rapidly via the kidney. The main metabolite is a glucuronide conjugate and there is no accumulation of the drug or of active metabolites.

**Product licence number** 10536/0007.

## MINTEC*

**Qualitative and quantitative composition** Each capsule contains 0.2 ml Peppermint Oil BP

**Pharmaceutical form** Enteric coated, soft gelatin capsule. Oral, size no. 4, one half green, the other half ivory.

**Clinical particulars**

*Therapeutic indications:* Symptomatic relief of irritable bowel or spastic colon syndrome.

*Posology and method of administration:* Adults and elderly: one capsule orally three times a day, preferably before meals with a small quantity of water, but not immediately after food. The capsules must not be broken or chewed. When symptoms are more severe, the dose may be increased to two capsules three times a day. Mintec should be taken until symptoms resolve, but may be continued for up to 2 to 3 months.

Children: Not recommended for children.

*Contra-indications:* None known.

*Special warnings and special precautions for use:* In patients with pre-existing heartburn, symptoms may be exacerbated.

*Interaction with other medicaments and other forms of interaction:* None known.

*Pregnancy and lactation:* The usual precautions concerning the administration of any drug during pregnancy should be observed.

*Effects on ability to drive and use machines:* None known.

*Undesirable effects:* Heartburn, and rarely allergic reactions including erythematous skin rash, bradycardia, muscle tremor and ataxia.

*Overdose:* Treatment consists of gastric lavage, together with symptomatic and supportive measures.

**Pharmacological properties**

*Pharmacodynamic properties:* Mintec (peppermint oil) is an aromatic carminative which acts locally to relax gastro-intestinal smooth muscle and relieve gastro-intestinal flatulence and colic. The enteric coating of the capsules is designed to delay release of the peppermint oil beyond the stomach and upper small bowel.

*Pharmacokinetic properties:* An open cross-over study was conducted in eight healthy volunteers, to compare the excretion pattern of menthol (the major constituent of peppermint oil) from peppermint oil contained in enteric coated soft gelatin capsules ('Mintec'), and similar, uncoated capsules. In each leg of the study, each volunteer received 0.4 ml of peppermint oil as two capsules of one of the preparations. The excretion of the oil in the urine (as the glucuronide) was followed over a 24 hour period. 'Mintec' capsules significantly delayed the rate of excretion of menthol compared with the non-coated capsules. The maximum amounts of menthol were excreted within 0 to 2 hours following administration of uncoated capsules and between 2 to 4 hours following 'Mintec' administration. There were no significant differences between treatments in terms of the maximum or total amounts of menthol excreted over the 24 hour post-dose period.

*Preclinical safety data:* No additional data available.

**Pharmaceutical particulars**

*List of excipients:* Capsule shell: Gelatin, glycerol, titanium dioxide (E171), chlorophyll KK (E141). Enteric coat: Hydroxypropylmethyl cellulose phthalate, dibutyl phthalate.

*Incompatibilities:* Not applicable.

*Shelf life:* Thirty months.

*Special precautions for storage:* Store at a temperature not exceeding 25°. Protect from light.

*Nature and contents of container:* Aluminium/PVC/PVDC blister strips in packs of 3 (sample), 12, 25 and 84.

*Instructions for use/handling:* None.

**Marketing authorisation number** 10536/0036

**Date of approval/revision of SPC** March 1996

**Legal category** GSL.

## TOPICYCLINE*

**Qualitative and quantitative composition** One bottle of powder containing 154 mg of Tetracycline Hydrochloride PhEur.

One bottle containing 70 ml of diluent for use only with Topicycline Powder (PL 10536/0025). Once reconstituted, Topicycline contains tetracycline hydrochloride 2.2 mg per ml.

**Pharmaceutical form** Topicycline is presented in two separate bottles as a yellow powder and as a diluent which must be combined prior to topical application.

**Clinical particulars**

*Therapeutic indications:* For the treatment of acne vulgaris

*Posology and method of administration:* Topicycline is first prepared by the Pharmacist according to the manufacturer's instructions.

Once reconstituted, Topicycline is applied topically, twice daily. It should be applied generously to the entire affected area, not just to the individual lesions, until the skin is thoroughly wet.

The average amount of Topicycline delivered to the skin by application to the face and neck twice a day is approximately 1.3 ml/day. This quantity of the medication contains approximately 2.9 mg of tetracycline hydrochloride. Twice-daily use of Topicycline on other acne-involved areas, in addition to the face and neck, has resulted in an average application of about 2.2 ml/day, or 4.8 mg of tetracycline hydrochloride.

*Contra-indications:* In patients who have shown hypersensitivity to any of its ingredients or to any of the other tetracyclines.

*Special warnings and special precautions for use:* Topicycline is for external use only, and care should be taken to keep it out of eyes, nose and other mucosal surfaces. Liver damage from Topicycline is highly unlikely because of the low levels of systemic absorption, however the warnings and precautions associated with the use of oral tetracyclines should be considered before prescribing to patients with renal impairment.

*Interaction with other medicaments and other forms of interaction:* None.

*Pregnancy and lactation:* Reproduction studies in rats and rabbits have revealed no evidence of impaired fertility or harm to the foetus from Topicycline. There are no data on the use of this product in pregnant women. It is not known whether tetracycline or any other component of Topicycline, administered in this topical form, is secreted in human milk. Because many drugs are secreted in human milk, caution should be exercised if Topicycline is administered to nursing mothers.

*Effects on ability to drive and use machines:* None.

*Undesirable effects:* Some patients may experience stinging or tingling sensations, skin rashes and skin discolouration at the site of application. The stinging or tingling reaction normally occurs for no more than a few minutes, does not occur on every application and often diminishes with continued use.

Topicycline may leave a faint yellow colour on the skin which could result in the staining of clothing and bed linen. This can be avoided by advising the patient to wash lightly the affected area one hour *after* applying Topicycline.

*Overdose:* Not applicable.

**Pharmacological properties**

*Pharmacodynamic properties:* Topicycline is a topical antibiotic preparation containing the active ingredient tetracycline hydrochloride. It has a broad spectrum of antimicrobial activity against both gram positive and gram negative pathogenic bacteria and it is mainly bacteriostatic.

In this topical preparation, Topicycline delivers tetracycline hydrochloride to the pilosebaceous apparatus and the adjacent tissues. Topicycline reduces the inflammatory acne lesions but its mode of action is not fully understood.

*Pharmacokinetic properties:* Very small amounts of tetracycline hydrochloride are absorbed systemically after application of Topicycline to the skin, compared with oral dosing. The serum level of tetracycline resulting from the use of Topicycline is less than 0.1 microgram/ml which is less than 7% of the level associated with an oral therapeutic dose of 500 mg/day.

*Preclinical safety data:* Not applicable.

**Pharmaceutical particulars**

*List of excipients:* The powder also contains 4-epitetracycline hydrochloride and sodium bisulphite (E223). The diluent contains n-decyl methyl sulphoxide and citric acid (E330) in 70 ml of a 40% ethanol solution.

*Incompatibilities:* None.

*Shelf life:* Shelf life of unreconstituted product is 24 months. Shelf life of reconstituted product is 8 weeks.

*Special precautions for storage:* Store at or below 25°.

*Nature and contents of container:* A single carton containing a plastic bottle and cap with an applicator and overcap supplied for the reconstituted product. On reconstitution of active powder (PL 10536/0025) and diluent (PL 10536/0026), the pack size is 70 ml.

*Instructions for use/handling:* At the time of dispensing the entire contents of the diluent–containing bottle are poured into the bottle containing the powder. The resultant mixture is then shaken well. Any unused material should be discarded.

**Marketing authorisation numbers**
Topicycline Powder 10536/0025
Diluent for Topicycline Powder 10536/0026

**Date of approval/revision of SPC** 9 December, 1995

**Legal category** POM.

*Trade Mark

# Napp Laboratories Limited
## Cambridge Science Park
## Milton Road
## Cambridge CB4 4GW

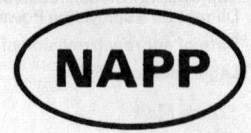

## ADIZEM*-60 TABLETS

**Presentation** White, film coated, capsule shaped tablets marked with 60/DL on one side. Each tablet contains 60 mg of diltiazem hydrochloride in a modified release formulation.

### Uses
*Actions:* Diltiazem is a calcium antagonist. It restricts the slow channel entry of calcium ions into the cell and so reduces the liberation of calcium from stores in the sarcoplasmic reticulum. This results in a reduction in the amount of available intracellular calcium and consequently a (1) reduction of myocardial oxygen consumption (2) dilation of small and large coronary arteries (3) mild peripheral vasodilation (4) negative dromotropic effects (5) a slight reduction or no change in heart rate due to the negative chronotropic effects of diltiazem counteracting the reflex increase in heart rate that occurs as a result of peripheral vasodilation.

The antihypertensive effect is due to the reduction in peripheral vascular resistance.

The antianginal effect is due to reduction in peripheral resistance, thereby decreasing the after-load, whilst a reduction in the vasomotor tone of the coronary circulation maintains the coronary blood flow. Cardiac contractility and ventricular ejection fraction are unchanged. Diltiazem increases exercise capacity and improves indices of myocardial ischaemia in the angina patient. Diltiazem relieves the spasm of vasospastic (Prinzmetal's) angina.

*Indications:* Management of angina pectoris and treatment of mild to moderate hypertension.

**Dosage and administration** Dosage requirements may differ between patients with angina and patients with hypertension. The tablets should be swallowed whole and not chewed.

*Adults:* The usual dose is one tablet (60 mg) three times a day, however, patients' responses may vary and dosage requirements can differ significantly between individual patients. There is no evidence of any decrease in efficacy at high doses. If necessary the dose may be increased to 480 mg/day.

*Elderly (over 65 years) and patients with renal or hepatic impairment:* The recommended starting dose is one tablet (60 mg) twice daily. The heart rate should be measured regularly in these groups of patients and the dosage should not be increased if the heart rate falls below 50 beats per minute.

*Children:* Adizem-60 Tablets are not recommended for children.

### Contra-indications, warnings, etc
*Contra-indications:* Pregnancy and in women of childbearing capacity. Patients with bradycardia (less than 50 bpm), second or third degree heart block, sick sinus syndrome, decompensated cardiac failure, patients with left ventricular dysfunction following myocardial infarction. Concurrent use with dantrolene infusion is contra-indicated because of the risk of ventricular fibrillation.

*Warnings and precautions:* The product should be used with caution in patients with reduced left ventricular function. Patients with mild bradycardia, first degree atrioventricular block or prolonged PR interval should be observed closely. Diltiazem is considered unsafe in patients with acute porphyria.

*Drug interactions:* Due consideration should be given to the possibility of an additive effect when diltiazem is prescribed with drugs which may induce bradycardia or other anti-arrhythmic drugs.

Diltiazem hydrochloride has been used safely in combination with beta-blockers, diuretics, ACE-inhibitors and other antihypertensive agents. It is recommended that patients receiving these combinations should be regularly monitored and the doses adjusted as required. Concomitant use with alpha-blockers such as prazosin should be strictly monitored because of the possible synergistic hypotensive effect of this combination. Patients with pre-existing conduction defects should not receive the combination of diltiazem and beta-blockers.

Case reports have suggested that blood levels of carbamazepine, cyclosporin and theophylline may be increased when given concurrently with diltiazem hydrochloride. Care should be exercised in patients

taking these drugs. In common with other calcium antagonists, diltiazem hydrochloride may cause small increases in plasma levels of digoxin.

Concurrent use with $H_2$-antagonists may increase serum levels of diltiazem.

Treatment with diltiazem has been continued without problem during anaesthesia, but the anaesthetist should be made aware of the treatment regimen.

*Use in pregnancy and lactation:* Diltiazem hydrochloride is contra-indicated in pregnant women or women of child-bearing potential, and is not recommended in nursing mothers.

*Side-effects:* Diltiazem is generally well tolerated. Occasional undesirable effects are nausea, headache, skin rashes, oedema of the legs, flushing, hypotension and fatigue which disappear on cessation of treatment. Diltiazem may cause depression of atrioventricular nodal conduction and bradycardia. Changes in liver function tests and renal function have been reported in a few cases.

*Overdosage:* The clinical symptoms of acute intoxication may include pronounced hypotension or even collapse, and sinus bradycardia with or without atrioventricular conduction defects.

The patient should be closely monitored in hospital to exclude arrhythmias or atrioventricular conduction defects. Gastric lavage and osmotic diuresis should be undertaken when considered appropriate. Symptomatic bradycardia and high grade atrioventricular block may respond to atropine, isoprenaline or occasionally temporary cardiac pacing. Hypotension may require correction with plasma volume expanders, intravenous calcium gluconate and positive inotropic agents.

The release of diltiazem from Adizem-60 Tablets is retarded and this should be considered in the event of an overdose.

**Pharmaceutical precautions** Store in a dry place at less than 30°C.

**Legal category** POM.

**Package quantities** Securitainers of 100 tablets.

**Further information** Diltiazem is well tolerated and does not normally give rise to the side-effects associated with peripheral vasodilators, nor cause significant myocardial depression. It protects against excessive catecholamine stimulation but is free of the side-effects seen with beta-blockade. Adizem-60 Tablets do not interfere with glucose metabolism.

**Product licence number** 0337/0163.

## ADIZEM*-SR CAPSULES 90, 120, 180 mg
## ADIZEM-SR TABLETS 120 mg

### Presentation
*Adizem-SR Capsules 90 mg* are size 3 capsules with opaque white caps and bodies with "90 mg" printed in black on the caps and bodies. Each capsule contains 90 mg of Diltiazem Hydrochloride USP in a controlled release formulation.

*Adizem-SR Capsules 120 mg* are size 3 capsules with opaque brown caps and opaque white bodies with "120 mg" printed in black on the caps and bodies. Each capsule contains 120 mg of Diltiazem Hydrochloride USP in a controlled release formulation.

*Adizem-SR Capsules 180 mg* are size 2 capsules with opaque pale brown caps and opaque white bodies with "180 mg" printed in black on the caps and bodies. Each capsule contains 180 mg of Diltiazem Hydrochloride USP in a controlled release formulation.

*Adizem-SR Tablets 120 mg* are white, film coated, capsule shaped tablets marked with DL/120 on one side, scoreline on the other. Each tablet contains 120 mg of Diltiazem Hydrochloride USP in a controlled release formulation.

### Uses
*Actions:* Diltiazem is a calcium antagonist. It restricts the slow channel entry of calcium ions into the cell and so reduces the liberation of calcium from stores in the sarcoplasmic reticulum. This results in a reduction in the amount of available intracellular calcium and consequently a (1) reduction of myocar-

dial oxygen consumption (2) dilation of small and large coronary arteries (3) mild peripheral vasodilation (4) negative dromotropic effects (5) a slight reduction or no change in heart rate due to the negative chronotropic effects of diltiazem counteracting the reflex increase in heart rate that occurs as a result of peripheral vasodilation.

The antihypertensive effect is due to the reduction in peripheral vascular resistance.

The antianginal effect is due to a reduction in peripheral resistance, thereby decreasing the afterload, whilst a reduction in the vasomotor tone of the coronary circulation maintains the coronary blood flow. Cardiac contractility and ventricular ejection fraction are unchanged. Diltiazem increases exercise capacity and improves indices of myocardial ischaemia in the angina patient. Diltiazem relieves the spasm of vasospastic (Prinzmetal's) angina.

*Indications:* For the management of angina pectoris and treatment of mild to moderate hypertension.

**Dosage and administration** Dosage may be taken with or without food, and should be swallowed whole and not chewed.

*Angina*
*Adults:* The usual initial dose is 90 mg, 12-hourly. Dosage may be increased gradually to 120 mg, 12-hourly or 180 mg, 12-hourly if required. Patients' responses may vary and dosage requirements can differ significantly between individual patients.

*Elderly and patients with renal and hepatic dysfunction:* In the elderly, dosage should commence at one Adizem-60 Tablet 12-hourly and the dose carefully titrated as required.

*Hypertension*
*Adults:* The usual dose is one Adizem-SR 120 mg Tablet or Capsule 12-hourly. Patients may benefit by titrating from a lower total daily dose.

*Elderly and patients with renal and hepatic dysfunction:* The starting dose should be one Adizem-60 Tablet 12-hourly, increasing to one Adizem-SR 90 mg Capsule 12-hourly and then to one Adizem-SR 120 mg Tablet or Capsule 12-hourly if clinically indicated.

*Children:* The Adizem preparations are not recommended for children. Safety and efficacy in children have not been established.

### Contra-indications, warnings, etc
*Contra-indications:* Pregnancy and in women of child bearing capacity. Patients with bradycardia (less than 50 bpm), second or third degree heart block, sick sinus syndrome, decompensated cardiac failure, patients with left ventricular dysfunction following myocardial infarction. Concurrent use with dantrolene infusion is contra-indicated because of the risk of ventricular fibrillation.

*Warnings and precautions:* The product should be used with caution in patients with reduced left ventricular function. Patients with mild bradycardia, first-degree atrioventricular block or prolonged PR interval should be observed closely.

*Drug interactions:* Due consideration should be given to the possibility of an additive effect when diltiazem is prescribed with drugs which may induce bradycardia or other anti-arrhythmic drugs.

Diltiazem hydrochloride has been used safely in combination with beta-blockers, diuretics, ACE-inhibitors and other anti-hypertensive agents. It is recommended that patients receiving these combinations should be regularly monitored. Concomitant use with alpha-blockers such as prazosin should be strictly monitored because of the possible synergistic hypotensive effect of this combination. Patients with pre-existing conduction defects should not receive the combination of diltiazem and beta-blockers.

Case reports have suggested that blood levels of carbamazepine, cyclosporin and theophylline may be increased when given concurrently with diltiazem hydrochloride. Care should be exercised in patients taking these drugs. In common with other calcium antagonists diltiazem hydrochloride may cause small increases in plasma levels of digoxin.

Concurrent use with $H_2$-antagonists may increase serum levels of diltiazem.

Treatment with diltiazem has been continued without problem during anaesthesia, but the anaesthetist should be made aware of the treatment regimen.

*Use in pregnancy and lactation:* Diltiazem hydrochloride is contra-indicated in pregnant women or women of child bearing capacity, and is not recommended in nursing mothers.

*Side-effects:* Diltiazem is generally well tolerated. Occasional undesirable effects are nausea, headache, skin rashes, oedema of the legs, flushing, hypotension and fatigue which disappear on cessation of treatment. Diltiazem may cause depression of atrioventricular nodal conduction and bradycardia. Isolated cases of moderate and transient increased liver transaminases have been observed at the start of treatment. Isolated cases of clinical hepatitis have been reported, which resolved when diltiazem was withdrawn. Changes in renal function have been reported in a few cases.

*Overdosage:* The clinical symptoms of acute intoxication may include pronounced hypotension or even collapse, sinus bradycardia with or without atrioventricular conduction defects.

The patient should be closely monitored in hospital to exclude arrhythmias or atrioventricular conduction defects. Gastric lavage and osmotic diuresis should be undertaken when considered appropriate. Symptomatic bradycardia and high grade atrioventricular block may respond to atropine, isoprenaline or occasionally temporary cardiac pacing.

Hypotension may require correction with plasma volume expanders, intravenous calcium gluconate and positive inotropic agents.

The formulations are controlled release systems which will continue to release diltiazem for some hours.

**Pharmaceutical precautions** Store in a dry place at less than 30°C.

**Legal category** POM.

**Package quantities**
*Capsules 90, 120, 180 mg:* Blister packs containing 56 capsules.
*Tablets 120 mg:* Blister packs containing 56 tablets.

**Further information**
*Transferability:* In order to avoid confusion it is suggested that patients once titrated to an effective dose using any of the ADIZEM preparations should remain on this treatment and should not be changed between different presentations.

**Product licence numbers**
Adizem-SR Capsules 90 mg 0337/0221
Adizem-SR Capsules 120 mg 0337/0222
Adizem-SR Tablets 120 mg 0337/0137
Adizem-SR Capsules 180 mg 0337/0223

## ADIZEM*-XL CAPSULES 120, 180, 240 and 300 mg

**Presentation**
*Adizem-XL Capsules 120 mg* are size 3 hard gelatin capsules with pale pink bodies and navy blue caps, marked "DCR 120". Each capsule contains 120 mg Diltiazem Hydrochloride USP in a controlled release formulation.

*Adizem-XL Capsules 180 mg* are size 2 hard gelatin capsules with dark pink bodies and royal blue caps, marked "DCR 180". Each capsule contains 180 mg Diltiazem Hydrochloride USP in a controlled release formulation.

*Adizem-XL Capsules 240 mg* are size 1 hard gelatin capsules with dark red bodies and blue caps, marked "DCR 240". Each capsule contains 240 mg Diltiazem Hydrochloride USP in a controlled release formulation.

*Adizem-XL Capsules 300 mg* are size 0 hard gelatin capsules with maroon bodies and pale blue caps, marked "DCR 300". Each capsule contains 300 mg Diltiazem Hydrochloride USP in a controlled release formulation.

**Uses**
*Actions:* Diltiazem is a calcium antagonist. It restricts the slow channel entry of calcium ions into the cell and so reduces the liberation of calcium from stores in the sarcoplasmic reticulum. This results in a reduction in the amount of available intracellular calcium and consequently a (1) reduction of myocardial oxygen consumption (2) dilation of small and large coronary arteries (3) mild peripheral vasodilation (4) negative dromotropic effects (5) a slight reduction or no change in heart rate due to the negative chronotropic effects of diltiazem counteracting the reflex increase in heart rate that occurs as a result of peripheral vasodilation.

The antihypertensive effect is due to the reduction in peripheral vascular resistance.

The antianginal effect is due to reduction in the peripheral resistance, thereby decreasing the afterload, whilst a reduction in the vasomotor tone of the coronary circulation maintains the coronary blood flow. Cardiac contractility and ventricular ejection fraction are unchanged. Diltiazem increases exercise capacity and improves indices of myocardial ischaemia in the angina patient. Diltiazem relieves the spasm of vasospastic (Prinzmetal's) angina.

*Indications:* Management of angina pectoris and treatment of mild to moderate hypertension.

**Dosage and administration** Dosage requirements may differ between patients with angina and patients with hypertension. In addition, individual patients' responses may vary, necessitating careful titration. This range of capsule strengths facilitates titration to the optimal dose.

The capsules should be swallowed whole and not chewed.

*Adults:* For patients new to diltiazem therapy, the usual starting dose is one 240 mg capsule daily.

Patients currently receiving a total daily dose of 180 mg diltiazem (as 90 mg bd or 60 mg tid) and transferring to Adizem-XL Capsules, should be given the 240 mg capsule (od). A patient receiving 240 mg/day of diltiazem (as 120 mg bd) should commence treatment on the 240 mg capsule (od), titrating to the 300 mg capsule (od) if required.

*Elderly and patients with impaired hepatic and renal function:* For patients new to diltiazem therapy, the usual starting dose is one 120 mg capsule daily. If necessary the dose may be gradually increased, but careful monitoring of this group of patients is advised.

Elderly patients transferring to Adizem-XL Capsules should receive the same total daily dose, titrating upwards as required.

*Children:* Adizem-XL Capsules are not recommended for children. Safety and efficacy in children have not been established.

In order to avoid confusion it is suggested that patients once titrated to an effective dose using Adizem-XL Capsules, should remain on this treatment and should not be changed between different presentations.

**Contra-indications, warnings, etc**
*Contra-indications:* Pregnancy and in women of child bearing capacity. Patients with bradycardia (less than 50 bpm), second or third degree heart block, sick sinus syndrome, decompensated cardiac failure, patients with left ventricular dysfunction following myocardial infarction. Concurrent use with dantrolene infusion is contra-indicated because of the risk of ventricular fibrillation.

*Warnings and precautions:* The product should be used with caution in patients with reduced left ventricular function. Patients with mild bradycardia, first degree atrioventricular block or prolonged PR interval should be observed closely. Diltiazem is considered unsafe in patients with acute porphyria.

*Drug interactions:* Due consideration should be given to the possibility of an additive effect when diltiazem is prescribed with drugs which may induce bradycardia or other anti-arrhythmic drugs.

Diltiazem hydrochloride has been used safely in combination with beta-blockers, diuretics, ACE-inhibitors and other anti-hypertensive agents. It is recommended that patients receiving these combinations should be regularly monitored. Concomitant use with alpha-blockers such as prazosin should be strictly monitored because of the possible synergistic hypotensive effect of this combination. Patients with pre-existing conduction defects should not receive the combination of diltiazem and beta-blockers.

Case reports have suggested that blood levels of carbamazepine, cyclosporin and theophylline may be increased when given concurrently with diltiazem hydrochloride. Care should be exercised in patients taking these drugs. In common with other calcium antagonists diltiazem hydrochloride may cause small increases in plasma levels of digoxin.

Concurrent use with $H_2$-antagonists may increase serum levels of diltiazem.

Treatment with diltiazem has been continued without problem during anaesthesia, but the anaesthetist should be made aware of the treatment regimen.

*Use in pregnancy and lactation:* Diltiazem hydrochloride is contra-indicated in pregnant women or women of child bearing potential, and is not recommended in nursing mothers.

*Side-effects:* Diltiazem is generally well tolerated. Occasional undesirable effects are nausea, headache, oedema of the legs, flushing, hypotension and fatigue which disappear on cessation of treatment. Allergic skin reactions including erythema multiforme and vasculitis have been reported. Diltiazem may cause depression of atrioventricular nodal conduction and bradycardia. Isolated cases of moderate and transient increased liver transaminases have been observed at the start of treatment. Isolated cases of clinical hepatitis have been reported, which resolved when diltiazem was withdrawn.

*Overdosage:* The clinical symptoms of acute intoxication may include pronounced hypotension or even collapse and sinus bradycardia with or without atrioventricular conduction defects.

The patient should be closely monitored in hospital to exclude arrhythmias or atrioventricular conduction defects. Gastric lavage and osmotic diuresis should be undertaken when considered appropriate. Symptomatic bradycardia and high grade atrioventricular block may respond to atropine, isoprenaline or occasionally temporary cardiac pacing.

Hypotension may require correction with plasma volume expanders, intravenous calcium gluconate and positive inotropic agents. The formulations employ a controlled release system which will continue to release diltiazem for some hours.

**Pharmaceutical precautions** Store at or below 25°C.

**Legal category** POM.

**Package quantities** Blister packs containing 30 capsules.

**Further information** An oral dose of diltiazem is almost completely absorbed. Despite this, diltiazem has a low bioavailability owing to extensive first pass metabolism. This process is saturable at higher doses of the drug, resulting in a non-linear accumulation and higher blood concentrations at steady state than would be anticipated from those following a single dose. Adizem-XL Capsules reduce the degree of saturation by presenting diltiazem in a retarded fashion therefore eliminating the high peak concentrations of the absorption phase. This allows the capsule to be administered once daily.

In pharmacokinetic studies in healthy volunteers, diltiazem was well absorbed. The controlled release capsules provided prolonged absorption of the drug, producing peak steady state plasma concentrations between 4 and 14 hours post-dose. The availability of diltiazem from Adizem-XL Capsules 120 mg (od) relative to a modified release 60 mg diltiazem preparation (bd) was approximately 79% at steady state. Similarly, the availability of diltiazem from the 240 mg capsule (od) relative to Adizem-SR Tablets 120 mg (bd) was approximately 78%. The extent of absorption of diltiazem was not affected when Adizem-XL Capsules were co-administered with a high-fat meal.

**Product licence numbers**
Adizem-XL Capsules 120 mg 0337/0217
Adizem-XL Capsules 180 mg 0337/0218
Adizem-XL Capsules 240 mg 0337/0219
Adizem-XL Capsules 300 mg 0337/0220

## ADIZEM*-XL PLUS CAPSULES

**Qualitative and quantitative composition**
Diltiazem Hydrochloride USP 150.0 mg
Hydrochlorothiazide PhEur 12.5 mg

**Pharmaceutical form** Controlled release capsules.

**Clinical particulars**
*Therapeutic indications:* For the treatment of mild to moderate hypertension in patients who have been stabilised on the individual components given in the same proportions where monotherapy was found inadequate.

*Posology and method of administration*
*Route of administration:* Oral.
*Dosage and administration:* The capsules should be swallowed whole and not chewed and should be taken in the morning.
*Adults:* The usual dose is two capsules daily.
*Elderly:* As for adults. Care should be taken to exclude electrolyte imbalance and/or impaired renal function (GFR less than 30 $ml.min^{-1}$).
*Children:* Not recommended for children.

*Contra-indications:* Known hypersensitivity to hydrochlorothiazide or other sulphonamide derived drugs. Anuria, Addison's disease, severe renal or hepatic failure, hypercalcaemia and in patients taking concurrent lithium therapy. Pregnant women or those of child bearing capacity. Patients with bradycardia (less than 50 bpm), second or third degree heart block, sick sinus syndrome, decompensated cardiac failure, patients with left ventricular dysfunction following myocardial infarction. Concurrent use with dantrolene infusion because of the risk of ventricular fibrillation.

*Special warnings and special precautions for use:* The product should be used with caution in patients with reduced left ventricular function. Patients with mild bradycardia, first degree AV block or prolonged PR interval should be observed closely.

Use with care in patients who have fluid or electrolyte imbalance. Use with caution in patients with impaired hepatic function or progressive liver disease, since minor alterations of fluid and electrolyte balance may precipitate hepatic coma.

Hypokalaemia may develop after prolonged therapy, or in patients with severe cirrhosis. Dehydration in oedematous patients leads to increased sensitivity to the effects of thiazides causing hyponatraemia.

Thiazides may decrease serum plasma bound iodine levels without signs of thyroid disturbance. Thiazides may interefere with tests for parathyroid function. Thiazide therapy may impair glucose tolerance. Dose adjustment of antidiabetic agents, including insulin, may be required. The product may decrease urinary calcium excretion and may cause intermittent and slight elevation of serum calcium. Increases in cholesterol and triglyceride levels may be associated with thiazide therapy. Gout may be exacerbated in patients with a previous family history of the condition. The possibility of exacerbation or activation of systemic lupus erythematous has been reported.

*Interaction with other medicaments and other forms of interaction:* The product may have an additive effect when prescribed with drugs that induce bradycardia, or other anti-arrhythmic drugs.

Concomitant use with alpha-blockers such as prazosin should be strictly monitored becuse of the possible synergistic hypotensive effect of this combination. Patients with pre-existing conduction defects should not receive this product in combination with beta-blockers.

Case reports have suggested that blood levels of carbamazepine, cyclosporin and theophylline may be increased when given concurrently with diltiazem hydrochloride. Concurrent use with $H_2$-antagonists may increase serum levels of diltiazem. Treatment with diltiazem has been continued without problem during anaesthesia, but the anaesthetist should be made aware of the treatment regimen.

The action of tricyclic antidepressants and monoamine oxidase inhibitors may be potentiated by the product. Concomitant use with lithium may increase the risk of neurotoxicity. Co-administration of alcohol, barbiturates or narcotics may potentiate orthostatic hypotension.

Oral and parenteral antidiabetic drugs may require dose adjustment with concurrent use. Corticosteroids or ACTH may intensify any thiazide-induced electrolyte depletion, particularly hypokalaemia. Non-steroidal anti-inflammatory drugs may decrease the diuretic and antihypertensive effect of diuretics.

*Pregnancy and lactation:* The product is contra-indicated in pregnant women or women of child bearing potential, and is not recommended for use in breast-feeding mothers.

*Effects on ability to drive and use machines:* None known.

*Undesirable effects:* Side-effects may include anorexia, nausea, constipation, diarrhoea, headache, skin rashes, oedema of the legs, flushing, hypotension, fatigue and photo-sensitivity. Diliazem may cause depression of atrioventricular nodal conduction and bradycardia. Changes in liver function tests and renal function have been reported in a few patients treated with diltiazem. Electrolyte imbalance, especially hypokalaemia can occur.

There have been reports of blood dyscrasias, including thrombocytopenia following thiazide therapy, but these are rare.

*Overdose:* An overdose of diltiazem may lead to hypotension or even collapse and sinus bradycardia with or without atrioventricular conduction defects.

The most prominent feature of poisoning due to hydrochlorothiazide is acute loss of fluid and electrolytes. The following symptoms may also be observed: dizziness, sedation/impairment of consciousness, hypotension, cardiac arrhythmias and muscle cramps.

Treatment should include close monitoring of cardiovascular, respiratory and renal functions, and blood glucose and electrolytes. Gastric lavage should be undertaken when considered appropriate. Cardiovascular complications should be treated symptomatically, which may require the use of atropine, isoprenaline or occasional temporary cardiac pacing. Hypotension may require correction with plasma volume expanders, intravenous calcium gluconate and positive inotropic agents.

**Pharmacological properties**

*Pharmacodynamic properties:* Diltiazem is a calcium antagonist. It restricts the slow channel entry of calcium ions into the cell and so reduces the liberation of calcium from stores in the sarcoplasmic reticulum. This results in a reduction in the amount of available intra-cellular calcium and consequently, (1) a reduction of myocardial oxygen consumption, (2) dilation of small and large coronary arteries, (3) mild peripheral vasodilation, (4) negative dromotropic effects, (5) reflex positive chronotropic and inotropic effects due to reflex sympathetic activity are partially inhibited and result in a slight reduction or no change in heart rate. The antihypertensive effect is due to the reduction in peripheral vascular resistance. The exact mechanism for reduction of arterial blood pressure by diuretics is not certain. The drugs first decrease extracellular volume and cardiac output. However, the hypotensive effect is maintained during long-term therapy because of reduced vascular resistance. Several potential mechanisms for this reduction in vascular resistance have been postulated.

*Pharmacokinetic properties:* In Adizem-XL Plus capsules, hydrochlorothiazide is available for immediate absorption whereas the diltiazem release is controlled to provide a prolonged, therapeutically effective plasma concentration over 24 hours.

Hydrochlorothiazide is fairly rapidly absorbed from the gastrointestinal tract and is reported to have a bioavailability of about 55 to 70%. It has been estimated to have a plasma half-life of about 5 hours with a subsequent longer terminal phase; its biological half-life is up to about 15 hours. It is excreted unchanged in the urine.

A pharmacokinetic study has demonstrated a mean increase of 11% in the bioavailability of hydrochlorothiazide from Adizem-XL Plus capsules when compared to hydrochlorothiazide administered alone. This may be due to an increase in the gastrointestinal transit time of the diuretic. There is no evidence that this small increase has any pharmacodynamic consequences.

An oral dose of diltiazem is almost completely absorbed. Despite this, diltiazem has a low bioavailability owing to extensive first pass metabolism. This process is saturable at higher doses of the drug resulting in a non-linear accumulation and higher blood concentrations at steady state than would be anticipated from those following a single dose. The degree of saturation is reduced with this product since diltiazem is presented in a retarded fashion, therefore eliminating the high peak concentrations of the absorption phase. This allows the capsules to be administered once-daily.

*Pre-clinical data:* Not applicable.

**Pharmaceutical particulars**

*List of excipients:* Microcrystalline Cellulose PhEur; Ethylcellulose N10 USNF; Colloidal Anhydrous Silica PhEur; Polysorbate 80 PhEur; Dibutyl Sebacate USNF; Methylhydroxypropylcellulose 5 cps PhEur; Magnesium Stearate PhEur. *Capsule shell:* Sodium dodecylsulphate DAB; Gelatin PhEur; titanium dioxide (E171); erythrosine (E127); indigo carmine (E132).

*Incompatibilities:* None known.

*Shelf life:* Two years.

*Special precautions for storage:* Store at or below 25°C in a dry place.

*Nature and contents of container:*

1. PVC/PVdC blister backed with aluminium foil containing 4, 28 or 30 capsules. Blister strips are contained in a boxboard carton.
2. Polypropylene container fitted with a polyethylene lid.

*Instructions for use/handling:* None stated.

**Marketing authorisation number** 0337/0250

**Date of approval/revision of SPC** 9 May 1996

**Legal category** POM.

## CODAFEN CONTINUS* TABLETS

**Presentation** Codafen Continus Tablets are capsule shaped, bilayer tablets consisting of pink and white layers of approximately equal thickness marked IBC3 on the white layer. They contain 300 mg of Ibuprofen BP in the pink controlled release layer and 20 mg of Codeine Phosphate BP in the white normal release layer.

**Uses** The combination of ibuprofen and codeine in Codafen Continus Tablets provides optimum pain relief, with a clinically demonstrated synergistic effect between the two ingredients. Codafen Continus Tablets are indicated for the relief of pain in rheumatoid arthritis, osteoarthritis, ankylosing spondylitis and sero-negative arthropathies. It is also indicated in inflammatory disorders such as bursitis, capsulitis of the shoulder, tendinitis, tenosynovitis and for the relief of severe pain in such clinical conditions as post-episiotomy pain, dental extraction pain, post-operative pain, dysmenorrhoea, migraine, sprains, strains and low back pain.

**Dosage and administration** Codafen Continus Tablets must be swallowed whole and not chewed, and taken after food.

*Adults and children over 12 years:* The starting dose is two tablets taken twelve hourly. This may be increased to three tablets twelve hourly. The maintenance dose is one to three tablets taken twelve hourly.

*Elderly:* No special dosage modifications are required for elderly patients unless renal or hepatic function is impaired, in which case dosage should be assessed individually.

*Children under 12 years:* Not recommended.

**Contra-indications, warnings, etc**

*Contra-indications:* Respiratory depression, hypersensitivity to ibuprofen or codeine, a history of peptic ulceration, chronic constipation. Not recommended in children under 12 years of age.

*Precautions:* Bronchospasm may be precipitated in patients suffering from or with a history of bronchial asthma or allergic disease. The possibility of cross-sensitivity with aspirin and other non-steroidal anti-inflammatory agents should be considered.

Codafen Continus Tablets should be used with caution in patients with gastro-intestinal disease.

NSAIDs have been reported to cause nephrotoxicity in various forms: interstitial nephritis, nephrotic syndrome and renal failure. In patients with renal, cardiac or hepatic impairment, caution is required since the use of NSAIDs may result in deterioration of renal function. The dose should be kept as low as possible and renal function should be monitored in these patients.

Codafen Continus Tablets should be used with caution in patients with hypotension, hypothyroidism, hepatic and/or renal impairment (GFR <20 ml per minute).

Caution is also advised when administering Codafen Continus Tablets to those patients taking monoamine oxidase inhibitors, thiazide diuretics or oral anticoagulants.

If given to patients receiving anti-coagulant therapy, prothrombin time should be monitored daily for the first few days of combined treatment.

Codafen Continus Tablets should be used with caution in patients with raised intracranial pressure or head injury.

It should be noted that tolerance to codeine may develop with large doses of Codafen Continus Tablets.

*Warnings:* Patients should be advised not to drive or operate machinery if affected by dizziness or sedation. The effects of CNS depressants (including alcohol) may be potentiated.

*Use in pregnancy and lactation:* Based on animal studies and clinical experience, there is no evidence to suggest foetal abnormalities associated with the use of ibuprofen and codeine. However, as with all drugs Codafen Continus Tablets should be avoided during pregnancy unless essential. Ibuprofen and codeine are both excreted in breast milk.

*Adverse effects:* The most frequent adverse effect occurring with ibuprofen is gastro-intestinal disturbance. Peptic ulceration and gastro-intestinal bleeding have been reported. Other adverse effects to ibuprofen include headache, dizziness, nervousness, skin rash, pruritus, tinnitus, oedema, depression, drowsiness, insomnia, blurred vision and other ocular reactions. Hypersensitivity reactions, abnormalities of liver function tests, impairment of renal function, agranulocytosis and thrombocytopenia have occasionally been observed.

Side-effects to codeine include constipation, respiratory depression, cough suppression, nausea and drowsiness.

*Overdosage:* Symptoms of overdose with ibuprofen could be expected to include the following: headache, vomiting, drowsiness and gastrointestinal irritation or bleeding. Nausea and vomiting are prominent features of codeine overdose. Respiratory depression, excitability, convulsions, hypotension and loss of consciousness may also occur with a large codeine overdose.

The stomach should be emptied.

Symptoms should be treated on appearance and any imbalance in electrolyte levels should be corrected. Monitoring of potassium levels should be considered.

If severe CNS depression has occurred, artificial respiration, oxygen and parenteral naloxone may be needed.

The physician should bear in mind that the tablets in the intestine may release ibuprofen for a number of hours.

**Pharmaceutical precautions** Store at or below 20°C.

**Legal category** CD (Sch 5), POM.

**Package quantities** Securitainers of 112 tablets.

**Further information** By incorporating ibuprofen in a controlled release system and combining it with codeine in immediate release form, long acting anti-inflammatory activity and rapid pain relief can be achieved simultaneously.

**Product licence number** 0337/0146.

## CO-DANTHRAMER SUSPENSIONS (Codalax) AND CAPSULES STRONG CO-DANTHRAMER SUSPENSIONS (Codalax Forte) AND CAPSULES

**Presentation** Co-danthramer Suspension and Strong Co-danthramer Suspension are peach flavoured, orange liquids. Each 5 ml spoonful of Co-danthramer Suspension contains: Poloxamer 188 BP, 200 mg and Danthron BP, 25 mg. Each 5 ml spoonful of Strong Co-danthramer Suspension contains: Poloxamer 188 BP, 1000 mg and Danthron BP, 75 mg.

Co-danthramer Capsules have light brown bodies, opaque orange caps and are marked CX. Each capsule contains: Poloxamer 188 BP, 200 mg and Danthron BP, 25 mg. Strong Co-danthramer Capsules have light brown bodies, opaque green caps and are marked CXF. Each capsule contains: Poloxamer 188 BP, 500 mg and Danthron BP, 37.5 mg.

**Uses**
*Action:* As a lubricant, faecal softener and laxative for oral administration. Danthron is a hydroquinone compound that acts on the nerve endings of the myenteric plexus to stimulate the muscle of the large intestine. It acts between 6 and 12 hours after administration.

Poloxamer 188 increases the penetration of water into faecal material thus preventing the faecal mass from drying and hardening excessively. The surface activity of poloxamer improves the penetration of water and thereby lubricates the contents of the distal colon.

*Indications:* The use of these products is strictly limited to:

Constipation in geriatric practice.

The prophylaxis of analgesic-induced constipation in terminally ill cancer patients.

Analgesic-induced constipation in the terminally ill, in all age groups.

Constipation in cardiac failure and coronary thrombosis, conditions in which defaecation must be free of strain.

**Dosage and administration**
*Co-danthramer Suspension and Capsules:*
*Adults:* One or two 5 ml spoonfuls *or* one or two capsules at bedtime.
*Children:* Half to one 5 ml spoonful *or* one capsule at bedtime.
*Strong Co-danthramer Suspension and Capsules:*
*Adults:* One 5 ml spoonful *or* one or two capsules at bedtime.
*Children:* Not recommended for children under 12 years.

Please note that *one* 5 ml spoonful of Strong Co-danthramer Suspension is equivalent to *two* Strong Co-danthramer Capsules.

**Contra-indications, warnings, etc**
*Contra-indications:* In common with other gastrointestinal evacuants Co-Danthramer preparations should not be given when acute or painful conditions of the abdomen are present, or the cause of constipation is suspected to be intestinal inflammation or obstruction. Pregnancy and lactation.

*Caution:* Co-Danthramer preparations may cause staining of the buttocks in incontinent and/or bedridden patients. This may lead to superficial sloughing of the skin. Therefore, these products should not be given to infants in nappies and should be used with caution in all incontinent patients.

*Use in pregnancy and lactation:* As there is inadequate evidence of the safety of these products in pregnancy and lactation, Co-danthramer preparations are contra-indicated.

*Special warning:* Oral administration of danthron has been reported to cause liver or intestinal tumours in rats and mice. There is no sound evidence to conclude a no-effect dose and therefore there may be a risk of such effects in humans. The use of Co-danthramer preparations should be restricted to the licensed indications.

*Side-effects:* Danthron may cause temporary harmless pink or red colouring of the urine and perianal skin. With prolonged high dosage the mucosa of the large intestine may become coloured.

*Overdosage:* Patients should be given plenty of fluids. An anticholinergic preparation such as atropine sulphate may be given to offset the excessive intestinal motility.

**Pharmaceutical precautions** Suspensions: Store in a cool place, away from stong light. Capsules: Store at or below 30°C.

*Suspension diluents:* Tragacanth Mucilage BP or Syrup BP should be used if diluents are required.

N.B. It is not possible to dilute Strong Co-Danthramer Suspension to obtain Co-Danthramer Suspension since the proportions of the two active ingredients are different.

**Legal category** POM.

**Package quantities**
Co-danthramer Suspension: Bottles of 300 ml and 1 litre.
Strong Co-danthramer Suspension: Bottles of 300 ml.
Co-danthramer Capsules: Blister packs of 60 capsules.
Strong Co-danthramer Capsules: Blister packs of 60 capsules.

**Further information** Nil.

**Product licence numbers**

| | |
|---|---|
| Co-Danthramer Suspension | 12724/0001 |
| Strong Co-Danthramer Suspension | 12724/0002 |
| Co-danthramer Capsules | 0337/0248 |
| Strong Co-danthramer Capsules | 0337/0249. |

## DF 118 FORTE* TABLETS 40 mg

**Presentation** DF 118 Forte Tablets are white tablets engraved DF 118 on one side and Forte on the other. Each tablet contains Dihydrocodeine Tartrate BP 40 mg.

**Uses** Relief of severe and chronic severe pain.

**Dosage and administration** DF 118 Forte Tablets should be administered with or after food.

*Adults, elderly and children over 12 years of age:* One or two tablets, three times daily. The maximum daily dose is 240 mg. DF 118 Forte Tablets are not recommended for children under 12 years of age.

**Contra-indications, warnings, etc**
*Contra-indications:* Respiratory depression; obstructive airways disease.

*Precautions:* As dihydrocodeine may bring about histamine-release, DF 118 Forte Tablets should not be given during an attack of asthma and should be administered with due care to persons liable to such attacks.

Dosage should be reduced in hypothyroidism, in chronic hepatic disease and in renal insufficiency. Alcohol should be avoided whilst under treatment with DF 118 Forte Tablets. Opioid analgesics should be avoided in those patients with raised intracranial pressure.

*Pregnancy:* There is no, or inadequate evidence of safety in human pregnancy but the drug has been used for many years without apparent ill consequence.

*Side-effects:* Constipation, nausea, vomiting, headache and vertigo may occur. If constipation occurs, it can be treated with a gentle laxative.

*Effects on ability to drive and to use machinery:* Dihydrocodeine may cause drowsiness, and, if affected, patients should not drive or operate machinery.

*Overdosage:* Administer naloxone 0.8 mg intravenously. Repeat at 2–3 minute intervals as necessary, or by an infusion of 2 mg in 500 ml of normal saline or 5% dextrose (0.004 mg/ml). The infusion should be run at a rate related to the previous bolus doses administered and should be in accordance with the patient's response. Empty the stomach. Assist respiration if necessary. Maintain fluid and electrolyte levels.

**Pharmaceutical precautions** Store at or below 25°C. Store in a dry place and protect from light.

**Legal category** CD (Sch 5), POM.

**Package quantities** Polypropylene containers of 100 tablets.

**Further information** In patients already habituated to a drug such as pethidine, the substitution of dihydrocodeine in equi-analgesic doses has led to the appearance of abstinence symptoms. This suggests that dihyrodocodeine, despite its effectiveness as an analgesic, has a low addiction potential. Nevertheless, when dihydrocodeine is prescribed for chronic use the physician should take care to avoid any unnecessary increase in dosage especially where there is a previous history of drug dependence or abuse.

**Product licence number** 0337/0230.

## DHC CONTINUS* TABLETS

**Qualitative and quantitative composition** Dihydrocodeine Tartrate BP 60 mg, 90 mg, 120 mg.

**Pharmaceutical form** Controlled release tablet.

**Clinical particulars**
*Therapeutic indications:* For the relief of severe pain in cancer and other chronic conditions.

*Posology and method of administration:*
*Route of administration:* Oral.
*Adults and children over 12 years:* 60 mg–120 mg every 12 hours.
*Elderly:* Dosage should be reduced.
*Children 12 years or under:* Not recommended.

*Contra-indications:* Respiratory depression, obstructive airways disease. As dihydrocodeine may cause the release of histamine, it should not be given during an asthma attack and should be given with caution to asthmatics.

*Special warnings and special precautions for use:* Dosage should be reduced in the elderly, in hypothyroidism, chronic hepatic disease and renal insufficiency. Opioid analgesics should be avoided in those patients with raised intracranial pressure or head injury.

*Interaction with other medicaments and other forms of interaction:* Alcohol should be avoided whilst under treatment with dihydrocodeine. Dihydrocodeine should be used with caution in patients taking monoamine oxidase inhibitors.

*Pregnancy and lactation:* There is little published evidence on safety in human pregnancy but dihydrocodeine has been used for many years without apparent ill effects. Dihydrocodeine has not been reported to be excreted in breast milk. However, it is advisable that dihydrocodeine only be administered to breast-feeding mothers if considered essential.

*Effects on ability to drive and use machines:* Dihydrocodeine may cause drowsiness and, if affected, patients should not drive or operate machinery.

*Undesirable effects:* Constipation, nausea, vomiting, headache, vertigo and urinary retention can occur.

*Overdose:* Conservative management is recommended and should include gastric lavage. Severe respiratory depression can be treated with naloxone hydrochloride 0.8 mg intravenously, repeated as required at 2–3 minute intervals.

**Pharmacological properties**
*Pharmacodynamic properties:* Dihydrocodeine is a semisynthetic narcotic analgesic with a potency between morphine and codeine. It acts on opioid receptors in the brain to reduce the patient's perception of pain and improve the psychological reaction to pain by reducing the associated anxiety.

*Pharmacokinetic properties:* Dihydrocodeine is well absorbed from the gastrointestinal tract following administration of DHC Continus tablets and plasma levels are maintained throughout the twelve hour dosing interval.

Like other phenanthrene derivatives, dihydrocodeine is mainly metabolised in the liver with the resultant metabolites being excreted mainly in the urine. Metabolism of dihydrocodeine includes o-demethylation, n-demethylation and 6-keto reduction.

*Preclinical safety data:* There are no preclinical data of relevance to the prescriber which are additional to that already included in other sections of the SPC.

**Pharmaceutical particulars**
*List of excipients:* Lactose (anhydrous) USNF; Hydroxyethylcellulose PhEur; Cetostearyl Alcohol BP; Magnesium Stearate BP; Purified Talc BP; Purified Water PhEur.

*Incompatibilities:* None known.

*Shelf life:* Three years.

*Special precautions for storage:* Store at or below 25°C.

*Nature and contents of container:* Polypropylene containers with polyethylene lids containing 56 tablets.

*Instructions for use/handling:* None stated.

**Marketing authorisation numbers**

| | |
|---|---|
| 60 mg | 0337/0115 |
| 90 mg | 0337/0140 |
| 120 mg | 0337/0141 |

**Date of approval/revision of SPC** November 1996

**Legal category** POM.

## DIHYDROCODEINE ELIXIR BP

**Presentation** A brown syrup. Each 5 ml contains Dihydrocodeine Tartrate BP 10 mg.

**Uses** For the relief of moderate to severe pain in all painful conditions where an alert patient is required, e.g. sciatica, osteoarthritis, chronic rheumatoid arthritis, arthritis of the spine, peripheral vascular disease, post-herpetic neuralgia, Paget's disease, malignant disease and post-operative pain. Dihydrocodeine Elixir is also indicated as an anti-tussive.

**Dosage and administration** Dihydrocodeine Elixir BP is best administered with or after food.

*Analgesia:*
*Adults:* One to three 5 ml spoonfuls (10 to 30 mg) every four to six hours or at the discretion of the physician.
*Elderly:* A reduced dose should be given.
*Children aged 4 to 12 years:* 0.5 to 1.0 mg/kg body weight every 4 to 6 hours. Not recommended for children under 4 years of age.
*Anti-tussive:*
*Adults:* One 5 ml spoonful (10 mg) every four to six hours or at the discretion of the physician.
*Children aged 4 to 12 years:* 200 micrograms/kg body weight every 4 to 6 hours. Not recommended for children under 4 years of age.

**Contra-indications, warnings, etc**

*Contra-indications:* Respiratory depression, obstructive airways disease.

*Precautions:* As dihydrocodeine may bring about histamine-release, Dihydrocodeine Elixir BP should not be given during an attack of asthma and should be administered with due care to persons liable to such attacks.

Dosage should be reduced in the elderly, in hypothyroidism, in chronic hepatic disease and in renal insufficiency. Opioid analgesics should be avoided in those patients with raised intra-cranial pressure or head injury.

*Pregnancy:* There is no, or inadequate evidence of safety in human pregnancy but the drug has been used for many years without apparent ill consequence. Dihydrocodeine should only be administered to nursing mothers if considered essential.

*Side-effects:* Constipation, nausea, vomiting, headache, vertigo and urinary retention may occur. Constipation can be treated with a gentle laxative.

*Overdosage:* Conservative management is recommended; gastric lavage should be carried out. Severe respiratory depression can be treated with naloxone 0.8 mg intravenously, repeated as required at 2-3 minute intervals.

**Pharmaceutical precautions** The recommended diluent of the elixir is Unpreserved Syrup BP or syrup preserved with p-hydroxybenzoic acid. The resulting dilution will keep for 14 days at room temperature.

**Legal category** POM.

**Package quantities** 1 litre amber glass bottles. 150 ml amber glass bottles.

**Further information** Nil.

**Product licence number** 0337/0197.

## FLEXIN* CONTINUS* TABLETS 75 mg FLEXIN*-LS TABLETS and FLEXIN*-25 TABLETS

**Presentation**

*Flexin Continus Tablets 75 mg* are yellow, capsule-shaped tablets with 75 IC on one side and a plain reverse. Each tablet contains 75 mg Indomethacin BP in a controlled release system.

*Flexin-LS Tablets* are red, capsule-shaped tablets with 50 IC on one side and a plain reverse. Each tablet contains 50 mg Indomethacin BP in a controlled release system.

*Flexin-25 Tablets* are green, capsule-shaped tablets with 25 IC on one side and a plain reverse. Each tablet contains 25 mg Indomethacin BP in a controlled release system.

**Uses** Non-steroidal anti-inflammatory agent indicated in rheumatoid arthritis; osteoarthritis; ankylosing spondylitis; gout; degenerative joint disease of the hip; painful musculoskeletal disorders; low-back pain and any periarticular disorders such as bursitis, tendinitis, synovitis, tenosynovitis and capsulitis. Also indicated in inflammation, in pain and oedema following orthopaedic procedures and treatment of dysmenorrhoea.

**Dosage and administration** In order to reduce the possibility of gastro-intestinal disturbance, the Flexin range of tablets should always be given with food, milk or an antacid.

*Adults:* The recommended total daily dosage of indomethacin is 25 mg–200 mg taken in one or two divided doses depending on patient needs and response.

In dysmenorrhoea up to 75 mg daily may be taken, starting with the onset of cramps or bleeding and continuing for as long as the symptoms last.

*Elderly:* Indomethacin should be used with particular care in older patients who are more prone to adverse reactions.

*Children:* A paediatric dose has not been established.

**Contra-indications, warnings, etc**

*Contra-indications:* Since safety of indomethacin has not been established in children, pregnant or lactating women, the Flexin range of tablets should not be given to such patients.

Also contra-indicated in active peptic ulcer, a history of recurrent gastro-intestinal lesions, sensitivity to indomethacin, aspirin or other non-steroidal anti-inflammatory drugs.

*Precautions:* The Flexin range of tablets should be used with caution in patients with hepatic or renal dysfunction. Hepatitis and jaundice have been reported rarely with indomethacin treatment.

Patients should be warned not to drive or operate machinery if they become dizzy or light-headed.

In common with other anti-inflammatory analgesic anti-pyretic agents, indomethacin may mask the signs and symptoms of infections.

The Flexin range of tablets should be used with caution in patients with psychiatric disorders, epilepsy or Parkinsonism as indomethacin may tend to aggravate these disorders.

The Flexin range of tablets should be used with caution in patients with coagulation defects. Indomethacin can inhibit platelet aggregation. The effect usually diappears within 24 hours of discontinuing therapy.

In patients with renal, cardiac or hepatic impairment caution is required since the use of NSAIDs may result in deterioration of renal function. The dose should be kept as low as possible and renal function should be monitored.

The patient should be periodically monitored to allow early detection of any unwanted effects on peripheral blood (anaemia), liver function and gastro-intestinal tract.

*Drug interactions:* Co-administration of aspirin may decrease blood levels of indomethacin. Diflunisal and probenecid may increase plasma levels of indomethacin.

Indomethacin and triamterene should not be administered together.

The Flexin range of tablets may reduce the antihypertensive effect of beta-blockers and the diuretic and antihypertensive effect of thiazides and frusemide in some patients.

When the Flexin range of tablets are used in patients receiving anticoagulant therapy, they should be closely observed for changes in prothrombin time.

The Flexin range of tablets may reduce the tubular secretion and therefore potentiate the toxicity of methotrexate.

If the patient is receiving corticosteroids concomitantly, a reduction in dosage of these may be possible but should only be effected slowly under supervision.

Co-administration to patients with steady state lithium concentrations may reduce clearance of lithium and raise plasma lithium levels.

*Warnings and adverse effects:* Treatment should be started with one 75 mg tablet per day. Dosage increases or decreases can be made in 25 mg or 50 mg steps to achieve the desired symptomatic relief. This procedure will minimise the incidence of side-effects.

Headache, dizziness and dyspepsia may occur. If headache persists, even after dosage reduction, indomethacin should be withdrawn.

Other CNS side-effects which may occur include mental confusion, depression, convulsions, depersonalisation and tinnitus. These are often transient and disappear with time or on reduction of dosage. Coma has also been reported.

Gastro-intestinal side-effects which may occur with indomethacin therapy are anorexia, nausea, vomiting, epigastric distress, abdominal pain and diarrhoea. Giving indomethacin with food, milk or antacids lowers the incidence of these side-effects. Ulceration of the oesophagus, stomach or duodenum, which may be accompanied by either haemorrhage or perforation has been reported with indomethacin preparations. Use of the Flexin range of tablets will minimise these gastro-intestinal effects. Gastro-intestinal bleeding without obvious ulceration may also occur. If this happens indomethacin treatment should be discontinued.

Blood dyscrasias, particularly thrombocytopenia, have been reported with indomethacin therapy.

Blurred vision and orbital and peri-orbital pain are seen infrequently with indomethacin therapy. Corneal deposits and retinal disturbances have been reported in some patients with rheumatoid arthritis on prolonged therapy with indomethacin, and ophthalmic examinations are desirable in patients given prolonged treatment.

Oedema and increased blood pressure and haematuria have been reported with indomethacin therapy.

Reported hypersensitivity reactions to indomethacin include pruritus, urticaria, angiitis, erythema nodosum. Hair loss may also occur.

Acute respiratory distress including sudden dyspnoea and asthma, have been reported on rare occasions with indomethacin therapy. Bronchospasm may be precipitated in patients suffering from, or with a previous history of bronchial asthma or allergic disease.

NSAIDs have been reported to cause nephrotoxicity in various forms and their use can lead to interstitial nephritis, nephrotic syndrome and renal failure.

*Treatment of overdosage:* Empty stomach contents. Supportive therapy should be initiated and a watch should be kept for gastro-intestinal bleeding for several days. Antacids may be useful.

**Pharmaceutical precautions** Store at or below 20°C.

**Legal category** POM.

**Package quantities** Flexin Continus Tablets 75 mg: Containers of 28 tablets.
Flexin-LS Tablets: Containers of 28 tablets.
Flexin-25 Tablets: Containers of 56 tablets.

**Further information** Nil.

**Product licence numbers**
Flexin Continus Tablets 75 mg 0337/0128
Flexin-LS Tablets 0337/0145
Flexin-25 Tablets 0337/0144.

## GASTROBID* CONTINUS* TABLETS

**Presentation** White biconvex tablets with (NAPP) on one side and 15 mg on the other. Each tablet contains Metoclopramide Hydrochloride BP equivalent to 15 mg of the anhydrous substance in a controlled release system.

**Uses** Gastrobid Continus Tablets restore normal co-ordination and tone to the upper digestive tract and relieve symptoms of gastro-duodenal dysfunction including heartburn, dyspepsia, nausea and vomiting associated with such conditions as reflux oesophagitis, gastritis, duodenitis and hiatus hernia.

Gastrobid Continus Tablets are also indicated as an anti-emetic for the treatment of nausea and vomiting associated with cytostatic and cytotoxic drugs.

**Dosage and administration**

*Adults (over 20 years) and elderly:* 1 tablet (15 mg) 12-hourly. In patients with significant degrees of renal impairment, therapy should be at a reduced dosage.

*Adults under 20 years and children:* Contra-indicated.

**Contra-indications, warnings, etc**

*Contra-indications:* Gastrobid Continus Tablets are contra-indicated in patients under 20 years, since dosage titration is not possible; patients with phaeochromocytoma, and epileptic patients since the frequency and severity of seizures may be increased.

*Precautions:* Gastrobid Continus Tablets should not be given during, or within 15 days of completing, treatment with monoamine oxidase inhibitors, nor with tricyclic antidepressants or sympathomimetic drugs. It is also recommended that combination with neuroleptics (synergy of central effect) and derivatives of anticholinergic drugs (neutralisation of effect) be avoided.

Special care should be taken if Gastrobid Continus Tablets are administered concomitantly with other medicines. For example, the presence of metoclopramide may decrease gastric absorption of digoxin and increase the intestinal absorption of paracetamol.

Use with caution in patients with renal impairment.

Following operations such as pyloroplasty or gut anastomosis, therapy with Gastrobid Continus Tablets should be withheld for three or four days as vigorous muscular contractions may impair healing.

Metoclopramide may cause drowsiness and if affected patients should not drive or operate machinery.

*Use in pregnancy and lactation:* Although animal tests in several mammalian species have shown no teratogenic effects, treatment with Gastrobid Continus Tablets is not advised during the first trimester of pregnancy. Metoclopramide is excreted in breast milk and should not be given to nursing mothers.

*Side-effects:* The following side-effects have occasionally been reported with metoclopramide therapy: drowsiness, lethargy, dizziness and headache. More rarely, various extrapyramidal reactions, usually of the dystonic type, have been reported. These include spasm of the facial muscles, trismus, rhythmic protrusion of the tongue, a bulbar type of speech, spasm of extra-ocular muscles including oculogyric crises, unnatural positioning of the head and shoulders and opisthotonos. These have been shown to be more common in young adults, particularly females aged 12–19. Parkinsonian reactions are significantly more common in the elderly. Tardive dyskinesia has been reported during prolonged treatment with metoclopramide in a small number of mainly elderly patients. Insomnia, diarrhoea and flatulence have also been reported.

Cases of neuroleptic malignant syndrome or idiosyncratic response characterised by hyperthermia, muscle rigidity, altered consciousness including coma and elevated creatine phosphokinase have been reported with metoclopramide.

The majority of reactions occur within 36 hours of starting treatment and the effects are reversible, usually disappearing within 24 hours of stopping treatment.

Raised serum prolactin levels have been observed during metoclopramide therapy; this effect is similar to that noted with many other compounds.

To avoid adverse reactions adhere strictly to dosage recommendations and where prolonged therapy is considered necessary patients should be regularly reviewed.

*Overdosage:* Gastric lavage and intensive supportive therapy should be initiated. Should treatment of a dystonic reaction be required, an anticholinergic antiparkinsonian drug, or a benzodiazepine may be used. The physician should be aware that tablets remaining in the intestine will continue to release metoclopramide hydrochloride for a period of hours.

**Pharmaceutical precautions** Store at or below 25°C.

**Legal category** POM.

**Package quantities** Blister packs of 56 tablets.

**Further information** The action of Gastrobid Continus Tablets is closely associated with parasympathetic nervous control of the upper gastro-intestinal tract, where it has the effect of encouraging normal peristaltic action. This provides a fundamental approach to the treatment of those conditions where disturbed gastro-intestinal motility is a common underlying factor. The controlled release formulation allows Gastrobid Continus Tablets to be administered 12-hourly.

**Product licence number** 0337/0106.

# MST* CONTINUS* TABLETS

## Presentation

*MST Continus Tablets:* Film coated bi-convex tablets marked with the NAPP logo on one side and the strength of the preparation on the other. Each tablet contains Morphine Sulphate BP in a controlled release system.

MST Continus Tablets 10 mg are golden brown
MST Continus Tablets 15 mg are green
MST Continus Tablets 30 mg are dark purple
MST Continus Tablets 60 mg are orange
MST Continus Tablets 100 mg are grey
MST Continus Tablets 200 mg are teal green.

**Uses** MST Continus Tablets are indicated for the prolonged relief of severe and intractable pain.

**Dosage and administration** MST Continus Tablets should be swallowed whole and not chewed.

*For the prolonged relief of severe and intractable pain Adults:* MST Continus Tablets should be used at 12-hourly intervals. The dosage is dependent upon the severity of the pain, the patient's age and previous history of analgesic requirements.

Increasing severity of pain will require an increased dosage of MST Continus Tablets. The tablets can be used alone or in combination to achieve pain relief.

Patients presenting with severe pain uncontrolled by weaker opioids should normally be started on a 30 mg preparation, 12-hourly increasing to 60 mg, 12-hourly when required. If higher doses are necessary increases should be made, where possible, in 30%–50% increments. The correct dosage for any individual patient is that which controls the pain with no or tolerable side-effects, for a full 12 hours.

In debilitated and underweight patients a reduction in starting dose is advisable.

Patients previously on normal release oral morphine or diamorphine should be given the same total daily dose as MST Continus Tablets but in divided doses at 12-hourly intervals. Occasionally dose adjustment may be necessary.

Patients receiving MST Continus Tablets in place of parenteral morphine should be given an increased dosage to compensate for any reduction in analgesic effects associated with oral administration. In such patients, individual dose adjustments are required but are usually of the order of 100% increase.

*Children:* For severe and intractable pain in cancer a starting dose in the range of 0.2 to 0.8 mg/kg 12-hourly is recommended. Doses should be titrated in the normal way as for adults.

*Elderly:* As with all narcotics, a reduction in dosage may be advisable in the elderly.

*Post-operative pain Adults and elderly:* MST Continus Tablets are not recommended in the first 24 hours post-operatively; thereafter it is suggested that the following dosage schedule be observed at the physician's discretion:

(a) MST Continus Tablets 20 mg 12-hourly to patients under 70 kilograms.

(b) MST Continus Tablets 30 mg 12-hourly to patients over 70 kilograms.

Supplemental parenteral morphine may be given if required but with careful attention to the total dosage of morphine, and bearing in mind the prolonged effects of morphine in the MST Continus formulation.

As with all oral morphine preparations, MST Continus Tablets should be used with caution post-operatively, and particularly following abdominal surgery.

*Children:* MST Continus Tablets are not recommended for treatment of post-operative pain in children.

## Contra-indications, warnings, etc

*Contra-indications:* Respiratory depression, head injury, paralytic ileus, acute abdomen, delayed gastric emptying, obstructive airways disease, known morphine sensitivity, acute hepatic disease, concurrent administration of monoamine oxidase inhibitors (MAOIs) or within two weeks of discontinuation of their use. Children under one year of age.

MST Continus Tablets are not recommended for use in pregnancy or lactation, or for the treatment of post-operative pain in children.

Pre-operative administration of MST Continus Tablets is not recommended and is not an approved indication.

*Precautions:* As with all narcotics a reduction in dosage may be advisable in the elderly, in hypothyroidism, and in patients with significantly impaired renal or hepatic function.

Use with caution in opiate dependent patients and patients with raised intracranial pressure, hypotension with hypovolaemia, diseases of the biliary tract, pancreatitis, inflammatory bowel disorders, prostatic hypertrophy and adrenocortical insufficiency.

*Warnings and adverse effects:* MST Continus Tablets should not be used where there is a possibility of paralytic ileus occurring. Should paralytic ileus be suspected or occur during use, MST Continus Tablets should be discontinued immediately. As with all morphine preparations, patients who are to undergo cordotomy or other pain relieving surgical procedures should not receive MST Continus Tablets for 24 hours prior to surgery. If further treatment with MST Continus Tablets is then indicated the dosage should be adjusted to the new post-operative requirement.

As with all oral morphine preparations, MST Continus tablets should be used with caution post-operatively, and following abdominal surgery as morphine impairs intestinal motility and should not be used until the physician is assured of normal bowel function.

It is not possible to ensure bio-equivalence between different brands of controlled release morphine products. Therefore, it should be emphasised that patients, once titrated to an effective dose, should not be changed from MST Continus preparations to other slow, sustained or controlled release morphine or other potent narcotic analgesic preparations without retitration and clinical assessment.

Morphine potentiates the effects of tranquillisers, anaesthetics, hypnotics, sedatives, alcohol, muscle relaxants and antihypertensives. Cimetidine inhibits the metabolism of morphine. Monoamine oxidase inhibitors are known to interact with narcotic analgesics producing CNS excitation or depression with hyper- or hypotensive crisis.

In normal doses, the commonest side effects of morphine are nausea, vomiting, constipation and drowsiness. With chronic therapy, nausea and vomiting are unusual with MST Continus tablets but should they occur the tablets can be readily combined with an anti-emetic if required. Constipation may be treated with appropriate laxatives. Dry mouth, sweating, vertigo, headache, disorientation, facial flushing, mood changes, palpitations, hallucinations, bronchospasm and colic may occur in a few patients. Micturition may be difficult and there may be biliary or ureteric spasm. Overdose may produce respiratory depression. Rarely, clinically relevant reductions in blood pressure and heart rate have been observed. Morphine has histamine releasing effects which may be responsible in part for reactions such as urticaria and pruritus.

The effects of morphine have led to its abuse and dependence may develop with regular, inappropriate use. This is not a major concern in the treatment of patients with severe pain.

Morphine may modify the patient's reactions to a varying extent depending on the dosage and susceptibility. If affected, patients should not drive or operate machinery.

*Use in pregnancy:* MST Continus Tablets are not recommended during pregnancy or labour due to the risk of neonatal respiratory depression. Administration to nursing mothers is not recommended as morphine is excreted in breast milk. Withdrawal symptoms may be observed in the newborn of mothers undergoing chronic treatment.

*Overdosage:* Signs of morphine toxicity and overdosage are pin-point pupils, respiratory depression and hypotension. Circulatory failure and deepening coma may occur in more severe cases.

*Treatment of morphine overdosage:* Primary attention should be given to the establishment of a patent airway and institution of assisted or controlled ventilation.

In the case of massive overdosage, administer naloxone 0.8 mg intravenously. Repeat at 2–3 minute intervals as necessary, or by an infusion of 2 mg in 500 ml of normal saline or 5% dextrose (0.004 mg/ml).

The infusion should be run at a rate related to the previous bolus doses administered and should be in accordance with the patient's response. However, because the duration of action of naloxone is relatively short, the patient must be carefully monitored until spontaneous respiration is reliably re-established. MST Continus tablets will continue to release and add to the morphine load for up to 12 hours after administration and the management of morphine overdosage should be modified accordingly.

For less severe overdosage, administer naloxone 0.2 mg intravenously followed by increments of 0.1 mg every 2 minutes if required.

Naloxone should not be administered in the absence of clinically significant respiratory or circulatory depression secondary to morphine overdosage. Naloxone should be administered cautiously to persons who are known or suspected, to be physically dependent on morphine. In such cases, an abrupt or complete reversal of opioid effects may precipitate an acute withdrawal syndrome.

Gastric contents may need to be emptied as this can be useful in removing unabsorbed drug, particularly when a modified release formulation has been taken.

**Pharmaceutical precautions** Store at or below 25°C.

**Legal category** CD (Sch 2), POM.

**Package quantities** MST Continus Tablets: Blister packs of 60 tablets.

**Further information** Nil.

**Product licence numbers**
*MST Continus Tablets*

| | |
|---|---|
| 10 mg | 0337/0055 |
| 15 mg | 0337/0180 |
| 30 mg | 0337/0059 |
| 60 mg | 0337/0087 |
| 100 mg | 0337/0088 |
| 200 mg | 0337/0149 |

# MST* CONTINUS* SUSPENSION

**Qualitative and quantitative composition** Morphine equivalent to Morphine Sulphate BP 20, 30, 60, 100 and 200 mg.

**Pharmaceutical form** Modified release granules for oral suspension.

**Clinical particulars**
*Therapeutic indications:* For the prolonged relief of severe and intractable pain.

*Posology and method of administration*
*Route of administration:* Oral.

*20, 30 & 60 mg strengths:* The contents of one sachet should be mixed with at least 10 ml water or sprinkled on to soft food, for example yogurt.

*100 mg strength:* The contents of one sachet should be mixed with at least 20 ml water or sprinkled on to soft food, for example yogurt.

*200 mg strength:* The contents of one sachet should be mixed with at least 30 ml water or sprinkled on to soft food, for example yogurt.

MST Continus suspension should be used at 12-hourly intervals. The dosage is dependent upon the severity of the pain, the patient's age and previous history of analgesic requirements.

*Adults:* A patient presenting with severe pain, uncontrolled by weaker opioids (eg dihydrocodeine) should normally be started on 30 mg 12 hourly. Patients previously on normal release oral morphine should be given the same total daily dose as MST Continus suspension but in divided doses at 12-hourly intervals.

Increasing severity of pain will require an increased dosage of the suspension. Higher doses should be made, where possible in 30–50% increments as required. The correct dosage for any individual patient is that which is sufficient to control pain with no, or tolerable, side effects for a full 12 hours. It is recommended that the 200 mg strength is reserved for patients who have already been titrated to a stable analgesic dose using lower strengths of morphine or other opioid preparations.

Patients receiving MST Continus Suspension in place of parenteral morphine should be given a sufficiently increased dosage to compensate for any reduction in analgesic effects associated with oral administration. Usually such increased requirement is of the order of 100%. In such patients individual dose adjustments are required.

*Children:* The use of MST Continus suspension in children has not been extensively evaluated. For children with severe cancer pain, a starting dose in the range of 0.2 to 0.8 mg morphine per kg bodyweight 12 hourly is recommended. Doses should then be titrated as for adults.

*Post-operative pain:* MST Continus suspension is not recommended in the first 24 hours post-operatively or until normal bowel function has returned; thereafter it is suggested that the following dosage schedule be observed at the physician's discretion:

(a) MST Continus suspension 20 mg 12 hourly to patients under 70 kg.
(b) MST Continus suspension 30 mg 12 hourly to patients over 70 kg.
(c) Elderly – a reduction in dosage may be advisable in the elderly
(d) Children – not recommended

Supplemental parenteral morphine may be given if required but with careful attention to the total dosage of morphine, and bearing in mind the prolonged effects of morphine in this controlled release formulation.

*Contra-indications:* Respiratory depression, head injury, paralytic ileus, 'acute abdomen', delayed gastric emptying, obstructive airways disease, known morphine sensitivity, acute hepatic disease, concurrent administration of monoamine oxidase inhibitors or within two weeks of discontinuation of their use. Children under one year of age. Pre-operative administration of MST Continus suspension is not recommended.

*Special warnings and special precautions for use:* As with all narcotics a reduction in dosage may be advisable in the elderly, in hypothyroidism and in patients with significantly impaired renal or hepatic function. Use with caution in opiate dependent patients and in patients with raised intracranial pressure, hypotension with hypovolaemia, diseases of the biliary tract, pancreatitis, inflammatory bowel disorders, prostatic hypertrophy and adrenocortical insufficiency.

Should paralytic ileus be suspected or occur during use, MST Continus suspension should be discontinued immediately. As with all morphine preparations, patients who are to undergo cordotomy or other pain relieving surgical procedures should not receive MST Continus suspension for 24 hours prior to surgery. If further treatment with MST Continus suspension is then indicated, the dosage should be adjusted to the new post-operative requirement.

As with all oral morphine preparations, MST Continus suspension should be used with caution post-operatively, and following abdominal surgery as morphine impairs intestinal motility and should not be used until the physician is assured of normal bowel function.

It is not possible to ensure bio-equivalence between different brands of controlled release morphine products. Therefore, it should be emphasised that patients, once titrated to an effective dose, should not be changed from MST Continus preparations to other slow, sustained or controlled release morphine or other potent narcotic analgesic preparations without retitration and clinical assessment.

*Interactions with other medicament and other forms of interaction:* Morphine potentiates the effects of tranquillisers, anaesthetics, hypnotics, sedatives, alcohol, muscle relaxants and antihypertensives. Concurrent administration of antacids may result in a more rapid release of morphine than otherwise expected; dosing should therefore be separated by a minimum of two hours. Cimetidine inhibits the metabolism of morphine. Monoamine oxidase inhibitors are known to interact with narcotic analgesics producing CNS excitation or depression with hyper- or hypotensive crisis.

*Pregnancy and lactation:* MST Continus Suspension is not recommended during pregnancy and labour due to the risk of neonatal respiratory depression. Administration to nursing mothers is not recommended as morphine is excreted in breast milk. Withdrawal symptoms may be observed in the newborn of mothers undergoing chronic treatment.

*Effects on ability to drive and use machines:* Morphine may modify the patient's reactions to a varying extent depending on the dosage and susceptibility. If affected, patients should not drive or operate machinery.

*Undesirable effects:* In normal doses, the commonest side effects of morphine are nausea, vomiting, constipation and drowsiness. With chronic therapy, nausea and vomiting are unusual with MST Continus suspensions but should they occur the suspensions can be readily combined with an anti-emetic if required. Constipation may be treated with appropriate laxatives. Dry mouth, sweating, vertigo, headache, disorientation, facial flushing, mood changes, palpitations, hallucinations, bronchospasm and colic may occur in a few patients. Micturition may be difficult and there may be biliary or ureteric spasm. Overdose may produce respiratory depression. Rarely, clinically relevant reductions in blood pressure and heart rate have been observed. Morphine has histamine releasing effects which may be responsible in part for reactions such as urticaria and pruritus.

The effects of morphine have led to its abuse and dependence may develop with regular, inappropriate use. This is not a major concern in the treatment of patients with severe pain.

*Overdosage:* Signs of morphine toxicity and overdosage are pin-point pupils, respiratory depression and hypotension. Circulatory failure and deepening coma may occur in more severe cases.

*Treatment of morphine overdosage:* Primary attention should be given to the establishment of a patent airway and institution of assisted or controlled ventilation.

In the case of massive overdosage, administer naloxone 0.8 mg intravenously. Repeat at 2–3 minute intervals as necessary, or by an infusion of 2 mg in 500 ml of normal saline or 5% dextrose (0.004 mg/ml).

The infusion should be run at a rate related to the previous bolus doses administered and should be in accordance with the patient's response. However, because the duration of action of naloxone is relatively short, the patient must be careflly monitored until spontaneous respiration is reliably re-established. MST Continus suspension will continue to release and add to the morphine load for up to 12 hours after administration and the management of morphine overdosage should be modified accordingly.

For less severe overdosage, administer naloxone 0.2 mg intravenously followed by increments of 0.1 mg every 2 minutes if required.

Naloxone should not be administered in the absence of clinical significant respiratory or circulatory depression secondary to morphine overdosage. Naloxone should be administered cautiously to persons who are known, or suspected, to be physically dependent on morphine. In such cases, an abrupt or complete reversal of opioid effects may precipitate an acute withdrawal syndrome.

Gastric contents may need to be emptied as this can be useful in removing unabsorbed drug, particularly when a modified release formulation has been taken.

**Pharmacological properties**
*Pharmacodynamic properties:* Morphine acts as an agonist at opiate receptors in the CNS particularly Mu and to a lesser extent Kappa receptors. Mu receptors are thought to mediate supraspinal analgesia, respiratory depression and euphoria, and Kappa receptors, spinal analgesia, miosis and sedation. Morphine also has a direct action on the bowel wall nerve plexuses causing constipation.

*Pharmacokinetic properties:* Morphine is bound to a cationic exchange resin and drug release is effected when morphine is displaced by ions in the gastrointestinal tract. Morphine is well absorbed and adequate plasma morphine levels are achieved following the recommended dosage regimen. However, first pass metabolism occurs in the liver. In a single dose study in healthy volunteers, the systemic availability of morphine from MST Continus suspension 30 mg was equivalent to that from an immediate release solution 30 mg (mean 91%, 95% CI 81–102%) and from MST Continus tablet 30 mg (mean 101%, 95% CI 93–109%). The suspension provided a retarded plasma profile which was comparable to that of the MST Continus tablet.

*Preclinical data:* There are no pre-clinical data of relevance to the prescriber which are additional to that already included in other sections of the SPC.

**Pharmaceutical particulars**
*List of excipients:* Dowex 50WX8 100–200 mesh cationic exchange resin; xylitol; xanthan gum; raspberry flavour; Ponceau 4R (E 124).

*Incompatibilities:* None known.

*Shelf life:* Two years.

*Special precautions for storage:* Store at or below 25°C.

*Nature and contents of container:* Pack type: Surlyn lined, laminated aluminium foil sachets coated with polyethylene and clay coated Kraft paper.

Pack size: Boxboard cartons of 10, 20, 30, 60 sachets or medical sample packs of up to 14 sachets.

*Instructions for use/handling:* The contents of the sachet should be added to water or sprinkled onto soft food, e.g. yogurt (see *Posology and method of administration*).

**Marketing authorisation numbers** 0337/0165, 0166, 0225–0227.

**Date of approval/revision of SPC** February 1997.

**Legal category** CD (Sch 2) POM.

## MXL* CAPSULES

**Qualitative and quantitative composition** Capsules containing Morphine Sulphate BP 30 mg, 60 mg, 90 mg, 120 mg, 150 mg, 200 mg.

**Pharmaceutical form** Modified release capsules containing white to off white multiparticulates.

MXL capsules 30 mg are size 4, light blue capsules marked MS OD30.

MXL capsules 60 mg are size 3, brown capsules marked MS OD60.

MXL capsules 90 mg are size 2, pink capsules marked MS OD90.

MXL capsules 120 mg are size 1, olive capsules marked MS OD120.

MXL capsules 150 mg are size 1, blue capsules marked MS OD150.

MXL capsules 200 mg are size 0, rust capsules marked MS OD200.

**Clinical particulars**
*Therapeutic indications:* The prolonged relief of severe and intractable pain.

*Posology and method of administration:*
*Route of administration:* Oral.

The capsules may be swallowed whole or opened and the contents sprinkled on to soft cold food. MXL capsules should be used at 24-hourly intervals. The dosage is dependent upon the severity of the pain, the patient's age and previous history of analgesic requirements.

*Adults and elderly:* Patients presenting with severe uncontrolled pain, who are not currently receiving opioids, should have their dose requirements calculated through the use of immediate release morphine, where possible, before conversion to MXL capsules.

Patients presenting in pain, who are currently receiving weaker opioids should be started on:

(a) 60 mg MXL capsule once-daily if they weigh over 70 kg.

(b) 30 mg MXL capsule once-daily if they weigh under 70 kg, are frail or elderly.

Increasing severity of pain will require an increased dosage of MXL capsules using 30 mg, 60 mg, 90 mg, 120 mg, 150 mg or 200 mg alone or in combination to achieve pain relief. Higher doses should be made, where appropriate in 30%–50% increments as required. The correct dosage for any individual patient is that which controls the pain with no or tolerable side effects for a full 24 hours.

Patients receiving MXL capsules in place of parenteral morphine should be given a sufficiently increased dosage to compensate for any reduction in analgesic effects associated with oral administration. Usually such increased requirement is of the order of 100%. In such patients individual dose adjustments are required.

*Children aged 1 year and above:* The use of MXL capsules in children has not been extensively evaluated. For severe and intractable pain in cancer a starting dose in the range of 0.4 to 1.6 mg morphine per kg bodyweight daily is recommended. Doses should be titrated in the normal way as for adults.

*Contra-indications:* Respiratory depression, head injury, paralytic ileus, acute abdomen, delayed gastric emptying, obstructive airways disease, known morphine sensitivity, acute hepatic disease, concurrent administration of monoamine oxidase inhibitors (MAOIs) or within two weeks of discontinuation of their use. Not recommended during pregnancy or for pre-operative use or for the first 24 hours post-operatively. Children under one year of age.

*Special warnings and special precautions for use:* As with all narcotics, a reduction in dosage may be advisable in the elderly, in hypothyroidism, in renal and chronic hepatic disease. Use with caution in patients with raised intracranial pressure, hypotension with hypovolaemia, opioid dependent patients, diseases of the biliary tract, pancreatitis, inflammatory bowel disorders, prostatic hypertrophy and adrenocortical insufficiency. MXL capsules should not be used where there is a possibility of paralytic ileus occurring. Should paralytic ileus be suspected or occur during use, MXL capsules should be discontinued immediately. As with all morphine preparations, patients who are to undergo cordotomy or other pain relieving surgical procedures should not receive MXL capsules for 24 hours prior to surgery. If further treatment with MXL capsules is then indicated the dosage should be adjusted to the new post-operative requirement.

It is not possible to ensure bio-equivalence between different brands of controlled release morphine products. Therefore, it should be emphasised that patients, once titrated to an effective dose should not be changed from MXL capsules to other slow, sustained or controlled release morphine or other potent narcotic analgesic preparations without retitration and clinical assessment.

*Interaction with other medicaments and other forms of interaction:* Monoamine oxidase inhibitors have been reported to react with narcotic analgesics, producing CNS excitation or depression with hyper- or hypotensive crisis. Morphine potentiates the effects of tranquillisers, anaesthetics, hypnotics and sedatives, alcohol, muscle relaxants and antihypertensives. Cimetidine inhibits the metabolism of morphine.

*Pregnancy and lactation:* MXL capsules are not recommended for use in pregnancy and labour due to the risk of neonatal respiratory depression. Administration to nursing mothers is not recommended as morphine is excreted in breast milk. Withdrawal symptoms may be observed in the newborn of mothers undergoing chronic treatment.

*Effects on ability to drive and use machines:* Morphine may modify the patient's reactions to a varying extent depending on the dosage and individual susceptibility. If affected, patients should not drive or operate machinery.

*Undesirable effects:* In normal doses, the commonest side effects of morphine are nausea, vomiting, constipation and drowsiness. With chronic therapy, nausea and vomiting are unusual with MXL capsules but should they occur the capsules can be readily combined with an anti-emetic if required. Constipation may be treated with appropriate laxatives. Dry mouth, sweating, vertigo, headache, disorientation, facial flushing, mood changes, palpitations, hallucinations, bronchospasm and colic may occur in a few patients. Micturition may be difficult and there may be biliary or ureteric spasm. Overdose may produce respiratory depression. Rarely, clinically relevant reductions in blood pressure and heart rate have been observed. Morphine has histamine releasing effects which may be responsible in part for reactions such as urticaria and pruritus.

The effects of morphine have led to its abuse and dependence may develop with regular, inappropriate use. This is not a major concern in the treatment of patients with severe pain.

*Overdose:* Signs of morphine toxicity and overdosage are pin-point pupils, respiratory depression and hypotension. Circulatory failure and deepening coma may occur in more severe cases.

*Treatment of morphine overdosage:* Primary attention should be given to the establishment of a patent airway and institution of assisted or controlled ventilation.

In the case of massive overdosage, administer naloxone 0.8 mg intravenously. Repeat at 2–3 minute intervals as necessary, or by an infusion of 2 mg in 500 ml of normal saline or 5% dextrose (0.004 mg/ml). The infusion should be run at a rate related to the previous bolus doses administered and should be in accordance with the patient's response. However, because the duration of action of naloxone is relatively short, the patient must be carefully monitored until spontaneous respiration is reliably re-established. MXL capsules will continue to release and add to the morphine load for up to 24 hours after administration and the management of morphine overdosage should be modified accordingly.

For less severe overdosage, administer naloxone 0.2 mg intravenously followed by increments of 0.1 mg every 2 minutes if required.

Naloxone should not be administered in the absence of clinically significant respiratory or circulatory depression secondary to morphine overdosage. Naloxone should be administered cautiously to persons who are known, or suspected, to be physically dependent on morphine. In such cases, an abrupt or complete reversal of opioid effects may precipitate an acute withdrawal syndrome.

Gastric contents may need to be emptied as this can be useful in removing unabsorbed drug, particularly when a modified release formulation has been taken.

**Pharmacological properties**

*Pharmacodynamic properties:* Morphine acts as an agonist at opiate receptors in the CNS particularly mu and to a lesser extent kappa receptors. mu receptors are thought to mediate supraspinal analgesia, respiratory depression and euphoria and kappa receptors, spinal analgesia, miosis and sedation. Morphine has also a direct action on the bowel wall nerve plexuses causing constipation.

*Pharmacokinetic properties:* Morphine is well absorbed from the capsules and, in general, peak plasma concentrations are achieved 2–6 hours following administration. The availability is complete when compared to an immediate release oral solution or MST Continus tablets. The pharmacokinetics of morphine are linear across a very wide dose range. Morphine is subject to a significant first-pass effect which results

in a lower bioavailability when compared to an equivalent intravenous or intramuscular dose.

The major metabolic transformation of morphine is glucuronidation to morphine-3-glucuronide and morphine-6-glucuronide which then undergo renal excretion. These metabolites are excreted in bile and may be subject to hydrolysis and subsequent reabsorption.

Because of the high inter-patient variation in morphine pharmacokinetics, and in analgesic requirements, the daily dosage in individual patients must be titrated to achieve appropriate pain control. Daily doses of up to 11.2 g have been recorded from twelve-hourly MST Continus tablets. For this reason the capsules have been formulated in strengths of 30 mg, 60 mg, 90 mg, 120 mg, 150 mg and 200 mg.

*Pre-clinical safety data:* There are no pre-clinical data of relevance to the prescriber which are additional to that already included in other sections of the SPC.

**Pharmaceutical particulars**

*List of excipients:* Hydrogenated Vegetable Oil BP; Macrogol 6000 PhEur; Talc PhEur; Magnesium Stearate PhEur.

*Capsule shells:* Gelatin (containing sodium dodecylsulphate). The following colours are also present:

30 mg: indigo carmine (E132); titanium dioxide (E171)
60 mg: indigo carmine (E132); titanium dioxide (E171); iron oxide (E172)
90 mg: erythrosine (E127); titanium dioxide (E171); iron oxide (E172)
120 mg: indigo carmine (E132); titanium dioxide (E171); iron oxide (E172)
150 mg: erythrosine (E127); indigo carmine (E132); titanium dioxide (E171); iron oxide (E172)
200 mg: titanium dioxide (E171); iron oxide (E172)

*Printing ink:* IMS 74 OP, Shellac DAB 10, iron oxide, black (E172), soya lecithin, dimethylpolysiloxane.

*Incompatibilities:* None known.

*Shelf life:* 3 years.

*Special precautions for storage:* Store at or below 25°C.

*Nature and contents of container:* Polypropylene containers with polyethylene caps, containing 28 or 30 capsules.

PVDC (≥40 gsm) coated PVC (250 µm) blister strip with aluminium backing foil. The blister strips will be enclosed in a cardboard box. Each box will contain 28 or 30 capsules.

*Instructions for use/handling:* None.

**Marketing authorisation numbers**   0337/0259–0264

**Date of approval/revision of SPC**   7 October 1996

**Legal category**   CD (Sch 2), POM.

# NARPHEN* TABLETS

**Qualitative and quantitative composition**   Phenazocine Hydrobromide BP 5 mg.

**Pharmaceutical form**   White, round, biconvex tablets marked with N on one side and 5 on the other.

**Clinical particulars**

*Therapeutic indications:* Narphen is a powerful analgesic for the relief of severe pain. Pain relief usually occurs within 20 minutes and lasts for five to six hours. Narphen is indicated for acute and chronic pain, including pre- and post-operative pain, and for obstetric analgesia. Narphen is particularly suitable for the treatment of intractable pain such as that of carcinoma as it produces minimal sedation.

In treating biliary or pancreatic pain, constriction of the Sphincter of Oddi is undesirable and the low spasmogenic activity of Narphen may be advantageous.

*Posology and method of administration:*
*Route of administration:* Orally/sublingually.

*Adults and elderly:* One tablet every four to six hours; up to 20 mg may be given in a single dose if necessary.

*Children:* A paediatric dosage has not been established.

*Contra-indications:* Narphen is contra-indicated in coma, convulsive disorders, delirium tremens, myxoedema, alcoholism, respiratory depression and obstructive airways disease.

*Special warnings and special precautions for use:* It is wise to reduce dosage in the elderly and in hypothyroidism or chronic hepatic disease.

Care is required in the presence of renal insufficiency.

*Interaction with other medicaments and other forms of interaction:* Narphen should not be given concurrently with monoamine oxidase inhibitors, nor within two weeks of discontinuation of treatment with them.

Care is required with concurrent administration of other narcotic analgesics, sedatives/hypnotics or anaesthetics.

*Pregnancy and lactation:* Although there is insufficient evidence of the safety of this drug in human pregnancy, animal studies have not shown any hazard. Nevertheless the use of phenazocine during pregnancy is not recommended.

Administration in labour may cause respiratory depression in the new-born infant.

*Effects on ability to drive and use machines:* Initially some patients may experience a feeling of light-headedness or dizziness, which soon passes, but if affected the patient should not attempt to drive or operate machinery.

*Undesirable effects:* Nausea and vomiting may be troublesome although emetic symptoms and constipation are less than with other narcotic analgesics. If nausea and vomiting occur phenazocine can be readily combined with an anti-emetic. Pruritus and occasionally dryness of the mouth and sweating have occurred. Hypotension is rare. As with other narcotics respiratory depression, tolerance and dependence may occur.

*Overdose:* Naloxone may be used as an antidote to overdosage or to antagonise any respiratory depression that may occur.

**Pharmacological properties**

*Pharmacodynamic properties:* Phenazocine is a synthetic morphine-like compound with agonist activity on mu opioid receptors. There is speculation that phenazocine may also possess some antagonist activity.

The knowledge of the pharmacological similarities between phenazocine and morphine has permitted the long and safe clinical use of Narphen.

Phenazocine produces only minimal sedation, and euphoria, and low spasmogenic activity on the Sphincter of Oddi.

Naloxone may be used as an antidote to overdosage or to antagonise any respiratory depression that may occur.

*Pharmacokinetic properties:* There are no data on the pharmacokinetics of phenazocine. It is considered unnecessary to provide such data as phenazocine is used in the treatment of severe pain, particularly in patients who are terminally ill. The interpretation of pain relief is subjective and therefore cannot be clearly related to specific blood levels.

*Preclinical safety data:* There are no preclinical data of relevance to the prescriber which are additional to that already included in other sections of the SPC.

**Pharmaceutical particulars**

*List of excipients:* Lactose PhEur, Maize Starch PhEur, Magnesium Stearate PhEur.

*Incompatibilities:* None known.

*Shelf life:* 42 months.

*Special precautions for storage:* Store at or below 25°C.

*Nature and contents of container:* Polypropylene securitainer with polyethylene lid (pack sizes 25, 28, 100, 112 tablets).

*Instructions for use/handling:* None stated.

**Marketing authorisation number**   0337/0198

**Date of approval/revision of SPC**   November 1996

**Legal category**   CD (Sch 2), POM.

# PALLADONE* CAPSULES

**Qualitative and quantitative composition**   Palladone capsules contain Hydromorphone Hydrochloride USP 1.3 mg or 2.6 mg.

**Pharmaceutical form**   Palladone capsules 1.3 mg are orange/clear capsules marked HNR 1.3.

Palladone capsules 2.6 mg are red/clear capsules marked HNR 2.6.

**Clinical particulars**

*Therapeutic indications:* For the relief of severe pain in cancer.

*Posology and method of administration*
*Route of administration:* The capsules can be swallowed whole or opened and their contents sprinkled on to cold soft food.

*Dosage*
*Adults and children over 12 years:* Palladone capsules should be used at 4-hourly intervals. The dosage is dependent upon the severity of the pain and the patient's previous history of analgesic requirements. 1.3 mg of hydromorphone has an efficacy approximately equivalent to 10 mg of morphine given orally. A patient presenting with severe pain should normally be started on a dosage of one Palladone capsule 4-hourly. Increasing severity of pain will require increased dosage of hydromorphone to achieve the desired relief.

*Elderly and patients with renal impairment:* The elderly and patients with renal impairment should be dose titrated with Palladone capsules in order to achieve adequate analgesia. It should be noted, however, that these patients may require a lower dosage to achieve adequate analgesia.

*Patients with hepatic impairment:* Contra-indicated.

*Children under 12 years:* Not recommended.

*Contra-indications:* Respiratory depression, pregnancy, coma, acute abdomen, hepatic impairment, known hydromorphone sensitivity, concurrent administration of monoamine oxidase inhibitors or within 2 weeks of discontinuation of their use. Hydromorphone should be avoided in patients with raised intracranial pressure or head injury, and also in patients with convulsive disorders or acute alcoholism.

*Special warnings and special precautions for use:* As with all narcotics, a reduction in dosage may be advised in the elderly, in hypothyroidism, in chronic obstructive airways disease, in renal or adrenocortical insufficiency, prostatic hypertrophy, shock or reduced respiratory reserve. Palladone capsules are not recommended in the first 24 hours post-operatively. After this time they should be used with caution, particularly following abdominal surgery.

Palladone capsules should not be used where there is the possibility of paralytic ileus occurring. Should paralytic ileus be suspected or occur during use, Palladone capsules should be discontinued immediately.

Patients about to undergo cordotomy or other pain-relieving surgical procedures should not receive Palladone capsules for 4 hours prior to surgery. If further treatment with Palladone capsules is indicated, the dosage should be adjusted to the new post-operative requirement.

*Interaction with other medicaments and other forms of interaction:* Hydromorphone potentiates the effects of tranquillisers, anaesthetics, hypnotics and sedatives.

*Pregnancy and lactation:* Palladone capsules are not recommended in pregnancy or in the breast-feeding mother as there are insufficient animal or human data to justify such use.

*Effects on ability to drive and use machines:* Hydromorphone may cause drowsiness and patients should not drive or operate machinery if affected.

*Undesirable effects:* Hydromorphone may cause constipation, nausea and vomiting. Constipation may be treated with appropriate laxatives. When nausea and vomiting are troublesome, Palladone capsules can be readily combined with anti-emetics. Tolerance and dependence may occur.

*Overdose:* Signs of hydromorphone toxicity and overdosage are pin-point pupils, respiratory depression and hypotension. Circulatory failure and deepening coma may occur in more severe cases.

*Treatment of overdosage:* Primary attention should be given to the establishment of a patent airway and institution of assisted or controlled ventilation.

In the case of massive overdosage, administer naloxone 0.8 mg intravenously. Repeat at 2–3 minute intervals as necessary, or by an infusion of 2 mg in 500 ml of normal saline or 5% dextrose (0.004 mg/ml).

The infusion should be run at a rate related to the previous bolus doses administered and should be in accordance with the patient's response. However, because the duration of action of naloxone is relatively short, the patient must be carefully monitored until spontaneous respiration is reliably re-established.

For less severe overdosage, administer naloxone 0.2 mg intravenously followed by increments of 0.1 mg every 2 minutes if required.

Naloxone should not be administered in the absence of clinically significant respiratory or circulatory depression secondary to hydromorphone overdosage. Naloxone should be administered cautiously to persons who are known, or suspected, to be physically dependent on hydromorphone. In such cases, an abrupt or complete reversal of opioid effects may precipitate an acute withdrawal syndrome.

Gastric contents may need to be emptied as this can be useful in removing unabsorbed drug.

**Pharmacological properties**
*Pharmacodynamic properties:* Like morphine, hydromorphone is an agonist of mu receptors. The pharmacological actions of hydromorphone and morphine do not differ significantly. The oral analgesic potency ratio of hydromorphone to morphine is approximately 5–10:1. Hydromorphone and related opioids produce their major effects on the central nervous system and bowel. The effects are diverse and include analgesia, drowsiness, changes in mood, respiratory depression, decreased gastrointestinal motility, nausea, vomiting, and alteration of the endocrine and autonomic nervous system.

*Pharmacokinetic properties:* Hydromorphone is absorbed from the gastrointestinal tract and undergoes pre-systemic elimination resulting in an oral bioavailability of about 50%. It is metabolised and excreted in the urine mainly as conjugated hydromorphone, dihydroisomorphine and dihydromorphine.

*Preclinical safety data:* There are no preclinical data of

relevance to the prescriber which are additional to that already included in other sections of the SPC.

**Pharmaceutical particulars**
*List of excipients:* Microcrystalline Cellulose PhEur, Lactose (anhydrous) USNF.

*Capsule shells:* Gelatin PhEur, erythrosine (E127), iron oxide (E172), titanium dioxide (E171), sodium dodecylsulphate DAB.

*Incompatibilities:* None known.

*Shelf life:* Two years.

*Special precautions for storage:* Store at or below 25°C. Protect from moisture.

*Nature and contents of container:* PVdC coated PVC blisters with aluminium backing foil containing 30, 56 or 60 capsules.

*Instructions for use/handling:* None stated.

**Marketing authorisation numbers**
Palladone capsules 1.3 mg     0337/0238
Palladone capsules 2.6 mg     0337/0239

**Date of approval/revision of SPC**     January 1997

**Legal category**     CD (Sch 2), POM.

## PALLADONE-SR* CAPSULES

**Qualitative and quantitative composition**     The capsules contain Hydromorphone Hydrochloride USP 2 mg, 4 mg, 8 mg, 16 mg, 24 mg.

**Pharmaceutical form**     Hard gelatin capsule containing spherical controlled release pellets.

Palladone-SR capsules 2 mg are yellow/clear capsules marked HCR 2.

Palladone-SR capsules 4 mg are pale blue/clear capsules marked HCR 4.

Palladone-SR capsules 8 mg are pink/clear capsules marked HCR 8.

Palladone-SR capsules 16 mg are brown/clear capsules marked HCR 16.

Palladone-SR capsules 24 mg are dark blue/clear capsules marked HCR 24.

**Clinical particulars**
*Therapeutic indications:* For the relief of severe pain in cancer.

*Posology and method of administration*
*Route of administration:* The capsules can be swallowed whole or opened and their contents sprinkled on to cold soft food.

*Dosage*
*Adults and children over 12 years:* Palladone-SR capsules should be used at 12-hourly intervals. The dosage is dependent upon the severity of the pain and the patient's previous history of analgesic requirements. 4 mg of hydromorphone has an efficacy approximately equivalent to 30 mg of morphine sulphate given orally. A patient presenting with severe pain should normally be started on a dosage of 4 mg Palladone-SR capsules 12-hourly. Increasing severity of pain will require increased dosage of hydromorphone to achieve the desired relief.

*Elderly and patients with renal impairment:* The elderly and patients with renal impairment should be dose titrated with Palladone-SR capsules in order to achieve adequate analgesia. It should be noted, however, that these patients may require a lower dosage to achieve adequate analgesia.

*Patients with hepatic impairment:* Contra-indicated.

*Children under 12 years:* Not recommended.

*Contra-indications:* Respiratory depression, pregnancy, coma, acute abdomen, hepatic impairment, known hydromorphone sensitivity, concurrent administration of monoamine oxidase inhibitors or within 2 weeks of discontinuation of their use. Use of Palladone-SR capsules should be avoided in patients with raised intracranial pressure or head injury, and also in patients with convulsive disorders or acute alcoholism.

Pre-operative administration of Palladone-SR capsules is not recommended and is not an approved indication.

*Special warnings and special precautions for use:* As with all narcotics, a reduction in dosage may be advised in the elderly, in hypothyroidism, in chronic obstructive airways disease, in renal or adrenocortical insufficiency, prostatic hypertrophy, shock or reduced respiratory reserve. Palladone-SR capsules are not recommended in the first 24 hours post-operatively. After this time they should be used with caution, particularly following abdominal surgery.

Palladone-SR capsules should not be used where there is the possibility of paralytic ileus occurring. Should paralytic ileus be suspected or occur during use, Palladone-SR capsules should be discontinued.

Patients about to undergo cordotomy or other pain relieving surgical procedures should not receive Palladone-SR capsules for 24 hours prior to surgery. If further treatment with Palladone-SR capsules is

indicated, then the dosage should be adjusted to the new post-operative requirement.

*Interaction with other medicaments and other forms of interaction:* Hydromorphone potentiates the effects of tranquillisers, anaesthetics, hypnotics and sedatives.

*Pregnancy and lactation:* Palladone-SR capsules are not recommended in pregnancy or in the breast-feeding mother as there are insufficient animal or human data to justify such use.

*Effects on ability to drive and use machines:* Hydromorphone may cause drowsiness and patients should not drive or operate machinery if affected.

*Undesirable effects:* Hydromorphone may cause constipation, nausea and vomiting. Constipation may be treated with appropriate laxatives. When nausea and vomiting are troublesome, Palladone-SR capsules can be readily combined with antiemetics. Tolerance and dependence may occur.

*Overdose:* Signs of hydromorphone toxicity and overdosage are pin-point pupils, respiratory depression and hypotension. Circulatory failure and deepening coma may occur in more severe cases.

*Treatment of overdosage:* Primary attention should be given to the establishment of a patent airway and institution of assisted or controlled ventilation.

In the case of massive overdosage, administer naloxone 0.8 mg intravenously. Repeat at 2–3 minute intervals as necessary, or by an infusion of 2 mg in 500 ml or normal saline or 5% dextrose (0.004 mg/ml).

The infusion should be run at a rate related to the previous bolus doses administered and should be in accordance with the patient's response. However, because the duration of action of naloxone is relatively short, the patient must be carefully monitored until spontaneous respiration is reliably re-established. Palladone-SR capsules will continue to release and add to the hydromorphone load for up to 12 hours after administration, and the management of the overdosage should be modified accordingly.

For less severe overdosage, administer naloxone 0.2 mg intravenously followed by increments of 0.1 mg every 2 minutes if required.

Naloxone should not be administered in the absence of clinically significant respiratory or circulatory depression secondary to hydromorphone overdosage. Naloxone should be administered cautiously to persons who are known, or suspected, to be physically dependent on hydromorphone. In such cases, an abrupt or complete reversal of opioid effects may precipitate an acute withdrawal syndrome.

Gastric contents may need to be emptied as this can be useful in removing unabsorbed drug, particularly when a modified release formulation has been taken.

**Pharmacological properties**
*Pharmacodynamic properties:* Like morphine, hydromorphone is an agonist of mu receptors. The pharmacological actions of hydromorphone and morphine do not differ significantly. The oral analgesic potency ratio of hydromorphone to morphine is approximately 5–10:1. Hydromorphone and related opioids produce their major effects on the central nervous system and bowel. The effects are diverse and include analgesia, drowsiness, changes in mood, respiratory depression, decreased gastrointestinal motility, nausea, vomiting and alteration of the endocrine and autonomic nervous system.

*Pharmacokinetic properties:* Hydromorphone is absorbed from the gastrointestinal tract and undergoes pre-systemic elimination resulting in an oral bioavailability of about 50%. It is metabolised and excreted in the urine mainly as conjugated hydromorphone and with smaller amounts of unchanged hydromorphone, dihydroisomorphine and dihydromorphine. Palladone-SR capsules have been formulated to produce therapeutic plasma levels following 12-hourly dosing.

*Preclinical safety data:* There are no preclinical data of relevance to the prescriber which are additional to that already included in other sections of the SPC.

**Pharmaceutical particulars**
*List of excipients:* Microcrystalline Cellulose PhEur; Hydroxypropylmethylcellulose (15 cps) PhEur; Purified Water PhEur; Ethylcellulose (N10) USNF; Colloidal Anhydrous Silica PhEur; Dibutyl Sebacate USNF; Methanol BP (1973), Dichloromethane.

*Capsule shells:* Gelatin PhEur; Sodium Dodecylsulphate DAB.

The following colours are included in the capsule shells: 2 mg (E104, E171), 4 mg (E127, E132, E171), 8 mg (E127, E171), 16 mg (E171, E172), 24 mg (E132, E171).

*Incompatibilities:* None known.

*Shelf life:* Two years.

*Special precautions for storage:* Store at or below 25°C.

*Nature and contents of container:*

(a) PCdC/PVC blister packs with aluminium backing foil.

(b) Polypropylene containers with polyethylene lids.

The capsules will be sold in packs of 30, 56 or 60 capsules.

*Instructions for use/handling:* None stated.

### Marketing authorisation numbers
| | |
|---|---|
| Palladone-SR capsules 2 mg | 0337/0246 |
| Palladone-SR capsules 4 mg | 0337/0242 |
| Palladone-SR capsules 8 mg | 0337/0243 |
| Palladone-SR capsules 16 mg | 0337/0244 |
| Palladone-SR capsules 24 mg | 0337/0245 |

**Date of approval/revision of SPC** January 1997

**Legal category** CD (Sch 2), POM.

## PHYLLOCONTIN* CONTINUS* TABLETS 225 mg
## PHYLLOCONTIN FORTE CONTINUS TABLETS 350 mg
## PHYLLOCONTIN PAEDIATRIC CONTINUS TABLETS 100 mg

### Presentation
*Phyllocontin Continus Tablets* are pale yellow, film-coated tablets with the logo (NAPP) on one side and SA on the other. Each tablet contains Aminophylline Hydrate BP 225 mg in a controlled release system.

*Phyllocontin Forte Continus Tablets* are pale yellow, film-coated, capsule-shaped tablets with the logo (NAPP) on one side and $\frac{SA}{350}$ on the other. Each tablet contains Aminophylline Hydrate BP 350 mg in a controlled release system.

*Phyllocontin Paediatric Continus Tablets* are pale mottled peach, bi-convex tablets with the logo (NAPP) on one side and $\frac{SA}{2}$ on the other. Each tablet contains Aminophylline Hydrate BP 100 mg in a controlled release system.

**Uses** Aminophylline is a bronchodilator. In addition it affects the function of a number of cells involved in the inflammatory processes associated with asthma and chronic obstructive airways disease. Of most importance may be enhanced suppressor T-lymphocyte activity and reduction of eosinophil and neutrophil function. These actions may contribute to anti-inflammatory prophylactic activity in asthma and chronic obstructive airways disease.

*Indications:* For the treatment and prophylaxis of bronchospasm associated with asthma, emphysema and chronic bronchitis. Also indicated in adults for the treatment of cardiac asthma and left ventricular or congestive cardiac failure.

### Dosage and administration
*N.B.* Tablets should be swallowed whole and not chewed.

*Children:* Not recommended for children under 3 years of age. The maintenance dose (expressed as mg aminophylline) is 12 mg/kg, 12-hourly adjusted to the nearest 125 mg. It is recommended that half the maintenance dose be given for the first week of therapy if the patient has not previously been receiving xanthine preparations.

Some children with chronic asthma require and tolerate much higher doses (13–20 mg/kg, 12-hourly). Lower doses (based on the usual adult dose) may be required by adolescents.

*Adults:* The usual daily dose is two Phyllocontin Continus Tablets 225 mg, 12-hourly following an initial week of therapy on one Phyllocontin Continus Tablet 225 mg 12-hourly.

*The elderly:* The dose should be adjusted following the response to the initial week of therapy on one tablet 12-hourly.

*Dose titration:* Patients vary in their response to xanthines and it may be necessary to titrate dosage individually. Steady state theophylline levels are generally attained 3–4 days after dose adjustment. If a satisfactory clinical response is not achieved, serum theophylline level should be measured 4–6 hours after the last dose. Based on serum theophylline assay results dosage should be titrated using the following as a guide:

| Peak serum theophylline level | Dosage adjustment to nearest 125 mg |
|---|---|
| <10 micrograms/ml | Increase total daily dose by half. |
| 10–15 micrograms/ml | Increase total daily dose by one quarter if symptoms persist. |
| 16–20 micrograms/ml | No adjustment required. |
| 21–25 micrograms/ml | Decrease dose by one quarter. |
| 26–30 micrograms/ml | Miss next dose and decrease maintenance dose by one half. |

It is advisable to re-check serum theophylline concentration after dose adjustment, when steady state is attained.

*Pharmacokinetics: In vivo* and *in vitro* bioavailability/dissolution studies have shown that the three strengths of Phyllocontin Continus Tablets are equally bioavailable. It has also been demonstrated that 12-hourly dosing produces minimal peak to trough variation and with appropriate dose titration plasma theophylline levels can be maintained within the therapeutic range of 10–20 micrograms/ml throughout the 12-hour dosing interval.

*Transferability:* It is not possible to ensure bioequivalence between different sustained release theophylline products. Therefore, it should be emphasised that patients, once titrated to an effective dose, should not be changed from Phyllocontin Continus Tablets to other slow or sustained release xanthine preparations without re-titration and clinical assessment.

### Contra-indications, warnings, etc
*Contra-indications:* Should not be given concomitantly with ephedrine in children.

*Warnings:* Theophylline has been reported to interact with a number of drugs.

The following increase clearance and it may therefore be necessary to increase dosage to ensure a therapeutic effect: aminoglutethimide, carbamazepine, moracizine, phenytoin, rifampicin, sulphinpyrazone and barbiturates. Smoking and alcohol consumption can also increase clearance of theophylline.

The following reduce clearance and a reduced dosage may therefore be necessary to avoid side-effects: allopurinol, carbimazole, cimetidine, ciprofloxacin, clarithromycin, diltiazem, disulfiram, erythromycin, fluconazole, interferon, isoniazid, isoprenaline, methotrexate, mexiletine, nizatidine, norfloxacin, oxpentifylline, propafenone, propranolol, ofloxacin, thiabendazole, verapamil, viloxazine hydrochloride and oral contraceptives. The concomitant use of theophylline and fluvoxamine should usually be avoided. When this is not possible, patients should have their theophylline dose halved and plasma theophylline should be monitored closely.

Factors such as viral infections, liver disease and heart failure also reduce theophylline clearance. Thyroid disease or associated treatment may alter theophylline plasma levels. There are conflicting reports concerning the potentiation of theophylline by influenza vaccine and physicians should be aware that interaction may occur. A reduction of dosage may also be necessary in the elderly patient. There is also a pharmacological interaction with adenosine, benzodiazepines, halothane, lomustine, and lithium and these drugs should be used with caution.

Theophylline may decrease steady state phenytoin levels.

The hypokalaemia resulting from beta$_2$ agonist therapy, steroids, diuretics and hypoxia may be potentiated by xanthines. Particular care is advised in patients suffering from severe asthma who require hospitalisation. It is recommended that serum potassium levels are monitored in such situations.

Safety in human pregnancy has not been established but it has been in use for many years without apparent ill consequence. Theophylline crosses the placental barrier and is secreted in breast milk. Use of theophylline during the third trimester or during breast feeding, may be associated with irritability in the infant. Use in pregnancy only when there is no safe alternative, or when the disease itself carries risk for the mother or child.

*Side-effects:* Side-effects usually associated with aminophylline and xanthine derivatives such as nausea, gastric irritation, headache, palpitations and CNS stimulation are only frequent above 20 micrograms/ml theophylline plasma concentrations. Phyllocontin Continus Tablets reduce the risk of such effects by minimising peak/trough variations in plasma levels.

*Overdosage:* Empty stomach contents. Monitor electrocardiogram and maintain fluid balance. Oral activated medical charcoal has been found to reduce high theophylline blood levels. In severe poisoning employ charcoal-column haemoperfusion. Treat symptoms

on appearance. The physician should be aware that tablets in the intestine will continue to release aminophylline for a period of hours.

In the event of hypokalaemia, potassium chloride should be given by slow intravenous infusion. Repeated measurements of plasma potassium should be made.

**Pharmaceutical precautions** Store at or below 25°C.

**Legal category** P.

### Package quantities
Phyllocontin Continus Tablets 225 mg: Blister packs of 60 tablets, containers of 250 and 1000 tablets. Phyllocontin Forte Continus Tablets 350 mg: Containers of 60 tablets. Blister packs of 60 tablets. Phyllocontin Paediatric Continus Tablets 100 mg: Containers of 50 and 250 tablets.

**Further information** By incorporating aminophylline in the Continus controlled release system, therapeutic blood levels of theophylline between 10 and 20 micrograms/ml can be maintained over a full 24-hour period on a simple 12-hourly dosage. The availability of three strengths of Phyllocontin Continus Tablets permits dosage flexibility. The Continus tablet formulation shows minimal tablet to tablet variation in aminophylline release.

### Product licence numbers
| | |
|---|---|
| Phyllocontin Continus Tablets 225 mg | 0337/0026 |
| Phyllocontin Forte Continus Tablets 350 mg | 0337/0090 |
| Phyllocontin Paediatric Continus Tablets 100 mg | 0337/0040 |

## REMEDEINE* EFFERVESCENT and REMEDEINE FORTE* EFFERVESCENT TABLETS

**Qualitative and quantitative composition** Remedeine Effervescent Tablets contain Dihydrocodeine Tartrate BP 20 mg, Paracetamol PhEur 250 mg, Paracetamol (direct compression containing gelatin) 260 mg.

Remedeine Forte Effervescent Tablets contain Dihydrocodeine Tartrate BP 30 mg, Paracetamol PhEur 250 mg, Paracetamol (direct compression containing gelatin) 260 mg.

**Pharmaceutical form** Effervescent tablet

### Clinical particulars
*Therapeutic indications:* For the treatment of severe pain. Remedeine Forte Effervescent Tablets are for the treatment of severe pain, where there is a higher analgesic requirement (higher than Remedeine Effervescent Tablets 500/20 mg).

*Posology and method of administration:*
*Route of administration:* Oral.

*Dosage and administration:* The tablets should be taken during or after meals. The tablets should be dissolved in water.

*Adults and children over 12 years:* One or two tablets every four to six hours. Do not exceed eight tablets in any 24 hour period.

*Children under 12 years:* Not recommended.

*Elderly:* One tablet every four to six hours increasing to two tablets every four to six hours if required and tolerated. Do not exceed eight tablets in any 24 hour period.

*Contra-indications:* Respiratory depression, obstructive airways disease.

*Special warnings and special precautions for use:* The tablets should be given with caution to patients with allergic disorders and should not be given during an attack of asthma.

Caution should also be observed if there is marked impairment of liver function or advanced kidney disease.

Dosage should be reduced in the elderly, in hypothyroidism and in chronic hepatic disease. An overdose can cause hepatic necrosis.

Dihydrocodeine should be used with caution in patients taking monoamine oxidase inhibitors and should be avoided in those patients with raised intracranial pressure or head injury.

Remedeine Effervescent Tablets and Remedeine Forte Effervescent Tablets contain approximate 350 mg sodium. This should be taken into account in patients requiring sodium restriction.

*Interaction with other medicaments and other forms of interaction:* Additive CNS depression may occur with alcohol.

*Pregnancy and lactation:* There is no, or inadequate evidence of safety in human pregnancy but the drugs have been used for many years without apparent ill consequence.

*Effects on ability to drive and use machines:* Dihydrocodeine may cause drowsiness and, if affected, patients should not drive or operate machinery.

*Undesirable effects:* Constipation, if it occurs, is readily treated with a mild laxative. Nausea, headache, vertigo, giddiness and urinary retention may occur in a few patients.

*Overdose:* Conservative management is recommended; gastric lavage should be carried out. Severe respiratory depression can be treated with naloxone hydrochloride 0.8 to 2 mg subcutaneously, repeated as required at two or three minute intervals. An overdose of paracetamol may cause hepatic necrosis, treatment should be commenced as soon as possible after ingestion using preferably acetylcysteine or cysteamine or methionine.

### Pharmacological properties

*Pharmacodynamic properties:* Paracetamol is an effective analgesic possessing a remarkably low level of side effects. Its broad clinical utility has been extensively reported, and it now largely replaces aspirin for routine use. Paracetamol is well tolerated; having a bland effect on gastric mucosa, unlike aspirin, it neither exacerbates symptoms of peptic ulcer nor precipitates bleeding. Dihydrocodeine tartrate has been widely used for a number of years as a powerful analgesic.

In addition the compound exhibits well-defined anti-tussive activity.

Fortifying paracetamol with dihydrocodeine tartrate provides an effective combination of drugs for the treatment of severe pain.

*Pharmacokinetic properties:* Dihydrocodeine is well absorbed from the gastrointestinal tract. Like other phenanthrene derivatives, dihydrocodeine is mainly metabolised in the liver with the resultant metabolites being excreted mainly in the urine. Metabolism of dihydrocodeine includes o-demethylation, n-demethylation and 6-keto reduction.

Paracetamol is readily absorbed from the gastrointestinal tract with peak plasma concentrations occurring 30 minutes to 2 hours after ingestion. It is metabolised in the liver and excreted in the urine mainly as the glucuronide and sulphate conjugates.

*Pre-clinical data:* There are no pre-clinical data of relevance to the prescriber which are additional to that already included in other sections of the SPC.

### Pharmaceutical particulars

*List of excipients:* Citric Acid PhEur (anhydrous, added as Citric Acid Monohydrate); Sodium Hydrogen Carbonate PhEur; Sodium Carbonate (anhydrous) PhEur; Sodium Benzoate PhEur; Sucrose PhEur; Saccharin Sodium PhEur; Gelatin PhEur.

*Incompatibilities:* None known.

*Shelf life:* 24 months.

*Special precautions for storage:* Store at or below 25°C.

*Nature and contents of container:*
1. Blister packs: 43 µm soft tempered aluminium foil coated with 25 µm nylon on the outside and 25 µm polyethylene on the inside.
2. Aluminium foil strip packs: 30 µm soft tempered aluminium foil and 38 µm polyethylene on the inside.
   Pack sizes: 2, 4, 12, 24, 56, 60, 100, 112 tablets.

*Instructions for use/handling:* None stated.

### Marketing authorisation numbers
Remedeine Effervescent tablets          0337/0257
Remedeine Forte Effervescent tablets    0337/0258

**Date of approval/revision of SPC**  20 March 1996

**Legal category**  POM.

## REMEDEINE* and REMEDEINE FORTE* TABLETS

### Presentation
*Remedeine Tablets* are white to off-white, circular, flat-faced tablets impressed PD/20 on one side. Each tablet contains:
  Paracetamol BP 500 mg
  Dihydrocodeine Tartrate BP 20 mg.

*Remedeine Forte Tablets* are white to off-white, circular, flat-faced tablets impressed PD/30 on one side. Each tablet contains:
  Paracetamol BP 500 mg
  Dihydrocodeine Tartrate BP 30 mg.

**Uses**  Paracetamol is an effective analgesic possessing a remarkably low level of side effects. Its broad clinical utility has been extensively reported, and it now largely replaces aspirin for routine use. Paracetamol is well tolerated; having a bland effect on gastric mucosa, unlike aspirin, it neither exacerbates symptoms of peptic ulcer nor precipitates bleeding. Dihydrocodeine tartrate has been widely used for a number of years as a powerful analgesic.

The addition of paracetamol to dihydrocodeine provides an effective combination of drugs for the treatment of severe pain.

**Dosage and administration**  Tablets should, if possible, be taken during or after meals. Do not exceed eight tablets in any 24-hour period.

*Adults and children aged 12 years and over:* One or two tablets every four to six hours.

*Children under 12 years:* Not recommended.

*Elderly:* One tablet every four to six hours increasing to two tablets every four to six hours if required and tolerated.

### Contra-indications, warnings, etc
*Contra-indications:* Respiratory depression, obstructive airways disease.

*Precautions:* Dihydrocodeine may cause drowsiness and, if affected, patients should not drive or operate machinery. Additive CNS depression may occur with alcohol.

Caution should be observed in patients with allergic disorders and tablets should not be given during an attack of asthma. Caution should also be observed if there is marked impairment of liver function or advanced kidney disease.

Dihydrocodeine should be used with caution in patients taking monoamine oxidase inhibitors (MAOIs) and should be avoided in those patients with raised intracranial pressure or head injury.

Dosage should be reduced in the elderly, hypothyroidism and in chronic hepatic disease. An overdose can cause hepatic necrosis.

*Use in pregnancy and lactation:* There is no or inadequate evidence of safety in human pregnancy but the drugs have been used for many years without apparent ill consequence.

*Side-effects:* Constipation, if it occurs, is readily treated with a mild laxative. Nausea, vomiting, headache, vertigo, giddiness and urinary retention may occur in a few patients.

*Overdosage:* Overdosage with Remedeine Tablets may result in initial acute opioid induced coma, respiratory depression, pinpoint pupils and circulatory collapse. Conservative management is recommended; gastric lavage should be carried out. Severe respiratory depression can be treated with naloxone hydrochloride 0.8 to 2 mg intravenously, repeated as required at 2 or 3 minute intervals as advised by experts. An overdose of paracetamol (as little as 20 tablets) may cause hepatic necrosis. Treatment should be commenced as soon as possible after ingestion using acetylcysteine, cysteamine or methionine.

**Pharmaceutical precautions**  No special requirements or precautions.

**Legal category**  CD (Sch 5), POM.

**Package quantities**  Remedeine Tablets are available in plastic tamper evident containers of 112 tablets.

Remedeine Forte Tablets are available in plastic tamper evident containers of 56 tablets.

**Further information**  Nil.

**Product licence numbers**
Remedeine Tablets        0337/0192
Remedeine Forte Tablets  0337/0193.

## SEVREDOL* TABLETS 10 mg, 20 mg, 50 mg

**Qualitative and quantitative composition**  Morphine Sulphate BP 10 mg, 20 mg, 50 mg.

### Pharmaceutical form
*10 mg:* Blue film-coated capsule shaped, biconvex tablet with a score line on one side. 'IR' is marked on the left side and '10' on the right.

*20 mg:* Pink film-coated capsule shaped, biconvex tablet, with a score line on one side. 'IR' is marked on the left side and '20' on the right.

*50 mg:* Pale green film-coated capsule shaped, biconvex tablet, with a score line on one side. 'IR' is marked on the left side and '50' on the right.

### Clinical particulars
*Therapeutic indications:* Sevredol tablets are indicated for the relief of severe pain.

*Posology and method of administration*
  *Route of administration:* Oral.
  *Adults and children over 12 years:* The dosage of Sevredol tablets is dependent on the severity of pain and the patient's previous history of analgesic requirements. One tablet to be taken every four hours or as directed by a physician. Increasing severity of pain or tolerance to morphine will require increased dosage of Sevredol tablets using 10 mg, 20 mg or 50 mg alone or in combination to achieve the desired relief.

Patients receiving Sevredol tablets in place of parenteral morphine should be given a sufficiently increased dosage to compensate for any reduction in analgesic effects associated with oral administration. Usually such increased requirement is of the order of

100 per cent. In such patients individual dose adjustments are required.

*Elderly:* A reduction in adult dosage may be advisable.

*Children 3–12 years of age:* Only Sevredol 10 mg tablets are suitable for children.
  3–5 years – 5 mg, 4-hourly.
  6–12 years – 5–10 mg, 4-hourly.

*Contra-indications:* Respiratory depression, head injury, obstructive airways disease, paralytic ileus, acute abdomen, delayed gastric emptying, known morphine sensitivity, acute hepatic disease, concurrent administration of monoamine oxidase inhibitors or within two weeks of discontinuation of their use. Not recommended during pregnancy.

Not recommended for children below 3 years of age.

*Special warnings and special precautions for use:* Sevredol tablets should not be used where there is a possibility of paralytic ileus occurring. Should paralytic ileus be suspected or occur during use, Sevredol tablets should be discontinued immediately. Patients who are about to undergo cordotomy or other pain relieving procedures should not receive Sevredol tablets 4 hours prior to surgery. A reduction in dosage may be advisable in hypothyroidism, and in renal and chronic hepatic disease. Sevredol tablets should be used with caution post-operatively particularly following abdominal surgery.

Use with caution in opiate dependent patients and in patients with raised intracranial pressure, hypotension with hypovolaemia, diseases of the biliary tract, pancreatitis, inflammatory bowel disorders, prostatic hypertrophy and adrenocortical insufficiency, acute alcoholism, and in patients with convulsive disorders.

*Interaction with other medicaments and other forms of interaction:* Monoamine oxidase inhibitors are known to interact with narcotic analgesics producing CNS excitation or depression with hyper- or hypotensive crisis. Morphine potentiates the effects of tranquilisers, anaesthetics, hypnotics, sedatives, alcohol, muscle relaxants and antihypertensives. Cimetidine inhibits the metabolism of morphine.

*Pregnancy and lactation:* Not recommended.

*Effects on ability to drive and use machines:* Treatment with Sevredol tablets may cause sedation and it is not recommended that patients drive or use machines if they experience drowsiness.

*Undesirable effects:* In normal doses, the commonest side effects of morphine are nausea, vomiting, constipation and drowsiness. With chronic therapy, nausea and vomiting are unusual with Sevredol tablets but should they occur the tablets can be readily combined with an anti-emetic if required. Constipation may be treated with appropriate laxatives. Dry mouth, sweating, vertigo, headache, disorientation, facial flushing, mood changes, palpitations, hallucinaitons, bronchospasm and colic may occur in a few patients. Micturition may be difficult and there may be biliary or ureteric spasm. Overdosage may produce respiratory depression. Rarely, clinically relevant reductions in blood pressure and heart rate have been observed. Morphine has histamine releasing effects which may be responsible in part for reactions such as urticaria and pruritus.

The effects of morphine have led to its abuse and dependence may develop with regular, inappropriate use. This is not a major concern in the treatment of patients with severe pain.

*Overdose:* Signs of morphine toxicity and overdosage are pin-point pupils, respiratory depression and hypotension. Circulatory failure and deepening coma may occur in more severe cases.

*Treatment of morphine overdosage:* Primary attention should be given to the establishment of a patent airway and institution of assisted or controlled ventilation.

In the case of massive overdosage, administer naloxone 0.8 mg intravenously. Repeat at 2–3 minute intervals as necessary, or by an infusion of 2 mg in 500 ml of normal saline or 5% dextrose (0.004 mg/ml).

The infusion should be run at a rate related to the previous bolus doses administered and should be in accordance with the patient's response. However, because the duration of action of naloxone is relatively short, the patient must be carefully monitored until spontaneous respiration is reliably re-established.

For less severe overdosage, administer naloxone 0.2 mg intravenously followed by increments of 0.1 mg every 2 minutes if required.

Naloxone should not be administered in the absence of clinically significant respiratory or circulatory depression secondary to morphine overdosage. Naloxone should be administered cautiously to persons who are known, or suspected, to be physically dependent on morphine. In such cases, an abrupt or complete reversal of opioid effects may precipitate an acute withdrawal syndrome.

Gastric contents may need to be emptied as this can be useful in removing unabsorbed drug.

## Pharmacological properties

*Pharmacodynamic properties:* Morphine acts as an agonist at opiate receptors in the CNS particularly mu and to a lesser extent kappa receptors. mu receptors are thought to mediate supraspinal analgesia, respiratory depression, and euphoria, and kappa receptors, spinal analgesia, miosis and sedation. Morphine also has a direct action on the bowel wall nerve causing constipation.

*Pharmacokinetic properties:* Morphine is well absorbed from Sevredol tablets, however first pass metabolism does occur. Apart from the liver, metabolism also occurs in the kidney and intestinal mucosa. The major urinary metabolite is morphine-3-glucuronide but morphine 6-glucuronide is also formed. The half life for morphine in the plasma is approximately 2.5–3.0 hours.

*Pre-clinical safety data:* There are no pre-clinical data of relevance to the prescriber which are additional to that already included in other sections of the SPC.

## Pharmaceutical particulars

*List of excipients:*
*Tablet core:* Lactose (anhydrous) NF; Pregelatinised Maize Starch BP; Povidone K25 BP; Purified Water PhEur; Magnesium Stearate BP; Purified Talc BP.

*Film coat*
*10 mg tablet:* Opaspray M-1F-4448 blue containing hydroxypropylmethylcellulose E464, titanium dioxide E171, polyethylene glycol 400, Patent Blue V E131, industrial methylated spirit.

*20 mg tablet:* Opaspray M-1-15503 pink containing hydroxypropylmethylcellulose E464, titanium dioxide E171, erythrosine E127, Sunset yellow E110, industrial methylated spirit.

*50 mg tablet:* Opadry 0Y-21037 green containing hydroxypropylmethylcellulose E464, titanium dioxide E171, quinoline yellow E104, indigo carmine E132, iron oxide E172, polyethylene glycol 400.

*Incompatibilities:* None stated.

*Shelf life:* 3 years.

*Special precautions for storage:* Store at or below 30°C.

*Nature and contents of container:* PVdC coated PVC blister packs and polypropylene containers with polyethylene lids containing 56 and 112 tablets.

Medical sample packs containing up to 24 tablets are also available.

*Instructions for use/handling:* None.

## Marketing authorisation numbers

| | |
|---|---|
| Sevredol tablets 10 mg | 0337/0142 |
| Sevredol tablets 20 mg | 0337/0143 |
| Sevredol tablets 50 mg | 0337/0265 |

**Date of approval/revision of SPC** June 1997.

**Legal category** CD (Sch 2), POM.

# UNIPHYLLIN* CONTINUS* TABLETS 400 mg
# UNIPHYLLIN* CONTINUS* TABLETS 300 mg
# UNIPHYLLIN* CONTINUS* TABLETS 200 mg

**Presentation** *Uniphyllin Continus Tablets 400 mg* are white, capsule-shaped scored tablets with the logo (NAPP) U400 embossed on one side and 'UNIPHYLLIN' on the other. Each tablet contains Theophylline BP 400 mg in a controlled release system.

*Uniphyllin Continus Tablets 300 mg* are white, capsule-shaped, scored tablets with U300 embossed on one side. Each tablet contains Theophylline BP 300 mg in a controlled release system.

*Uniphyllin Continus Tablets 200 mg* are white, capsule-shaped, scored tablets with U200 embossed on one side. Each tablet contains Theophylline BP 200 mg in a controlled release system.

**Uses** Theophylline is a bronchodilator. In addition it affects the function of a number of cells involved in the inflammatory processes associated with asthma and chronic obstructive airways disease. Of most importance may be enhanced suppressor T-lymphocyte activity and reduction of eosinophil and neutrophil function. These actions may contribute to anti-inflammatory prophylactic activity in asthma and chronic obstructive airways disease.

For the treatment and prophylaxis of bronchospasm associated with asthma, emphysema and chronic bronchitis. Also indicated in adults for the treatment of cardiac asthma and left ventricular or congestive cardiac failure.

## Dosage and administration

*N.B.* Tablets should be swallowed whole and not chewed.

*Children:* Not recommended for children under 7 years of age. The maintenance dose is 9 mg/kg, 12-hourly. Some children with chronic asthma require and tolerate much higher doses (10–16 mg/kg, 12-hourly). Lower dosages (based on usual adult dose) may be required by adolescents.

*Adults:* The usual maintenance dose for elderly patients or those less than 70 kg body weight is 300 mg, 12-hourly following an initial week of therapy on 200 mg, 12-hourly.

The usual maintenance dose for patients of 70 kg body weight or over is 400 mg 12-hourly following an initial week of therapy on 200 mg or 300 mg 12-hourly.

It may be appropriate to administer a larger evening or morning dose in some patients, in order to achieve optimum therapeutic effect when symptoms are most severe, e.g. at the time of the 'morning dip' in lung function.

In patients whose night time or day time symptoms persist despite other therapy and who are not currently receiving theophylline, then the total daily requirement of Uniphyllin Continus Tablets (as specified above) may be added to their treatment regimen as either a single evening or morning dose.

*Elderly:* The initial dose should be 200 mg 12-hourly increasing to 300 mg 12-hourly.

*Dose titration:* Patients vary in their response to xanthines and it may be necessary to titrate dosage individually. Steady state theophylline levels with 12-hourly dosing are generally attained 3–4 days after dose adjustment. If a satisfactory clinical response is not achieved, serum theophylline should be measured 6–8 hours after the last dose. Based on serum theophylline assay results, dosage should be titrated using the following as a guide:

| Peak serum theophylline level | Dosage adjustment to nearest 100 mg |
|---|---|
| <10 micrograms/ml | Increase total daily dose by half. |
| 10–15 micrograms/ml | Increase total daily dose by one quarter if symptoms persist. |
| 16–20 micrograms/ml | No adjustment required. |
| 21–25 micrograms/ml | Decrease dose by one quarter. |
| 26–30 micrograms/ml | Miss next dose and decrease maintenance dose by one half. |

It is advisable to re-check serum theophylline concentration after dose adjustment, when steady state is attained.

*Pharmacokinetics: In-vivo* bioavailability studies have shown that the three strengths of Uniphyllin Continus Tablets are equally bioavailable. It has also been demonstrated that twice-daily dosing produces minimal peak to trough variation and plasma theophylline levels can be maintained within the therapeutic range of 10–20 micrograms/ml throughout the 12-hour dosing interval.

*Transferability:* It is not possible to ensure bioequivalence between different sustained release theophylline products. Therefore, it should be emphasised that patients, once titrated to an effective dose, should not be changed from Uniphyllin Continus Tablet preparations to other slow or sustained release xanthine preparations without re-titration and clinical assessment.

After an effective therapeutic regimen is attained, it is important that practitioners, pharmacists and patients be aware of the possible dangers of inefficacy or toxicity if an alternative sustained release theophylline preparation is substituted. This may be a particular hazard because the products are available without prescription. Likewise there may be a hazard if the doctor prescribes 'generically' or if the preparation used in hospital is unknown by the general practitioner.

## Contra-indications, warnings, etc

*Contra-indications:* Should not be given concomitantly with ephedrine in children.

*Warnings:* Theophylline has been reported to interact with a number of drugs.

The following increase clearance and it may therefore be necessary to increase dosage to ensure a therapeutic effect: aminoglutethimide, carbamazepine, moracizine, phenytoin, rifampicin, sulphinpyrazone and barbiturates. Smoking and alcohol consumption can also increase clearance of theophylline.

The following reduce clearance and a reduced dosage may therefore be necessary to avoid side-effects: allopurinol, carbimazole, cimetidine, ciprofloxacin, clarithromycin, diltiazem, disulfiram, erythromycin, fluconazole, interferon, isoniazid, isoprenaline, methotrexate, mexiletine, nizatidine, norfloxacin, oxpentifylline, propafenone, propranolol, ofloxacin, thiabendazole, verapamil, viloxazine hydrochloride and oral contraceptives. The concomitant use of theophylline and fluvoxamine should usually be avoided. Where this is not possible, patients should have their theophylline dose halved and plasma theophylline should be monitored closely.

Factors such as viral infections, liver disease and heart failure also reduce theophylline clearance. Thyroid disease or associated treatment may alter theophylline plasma levels. There are conflicting reports concerning the potentiation of theophylline by influenza vaccine and physicians should be aware that interaction may occur. A reduction of dosage may also be necessary in the elderly patient. There is also a pharmacological interaction with adenosine, benzodiazepines, halothane, lomustine, and lithium and these drugs should be used with caution.

Theophylline may decrease steady state phenytoin levels.

The hypokalaemia resulting from beta$_2$ agonist therapy, steroids, diuretics and hypoxia may be potentiated by xanthines. Particular care is advised in patients suffering from severe asthma who require hospitalisation. It is recommended that serum potassium levels are monitored in such circumstances.

Safety in human pregnancy has not been established but it has been in use for many years without apparent ill consequence. Theophylline crosses the placental barrier and is secreted in breast milk. Use of theophylline during the third trimester, or during breast feeding, may be associated with irritability in the infant. Use in pregnancy only when there is no safe alternative, or when the disease itself carries risk for the mother or child.

*Side-effects:* The risk of side-effects usually associated with theophylline and xanthine derivatives such as nausea, gastric irritation, headache and CNS stimulation is significantly reduced when Uniphyllin Continus Tablet preparations are given. Furthermore, the side-effects can be minimised by dose titration downwards.

*Overdosage:* Empty stomach contents. Monitor electrocardiogram and maintain fluid balance. Oral activated medical charcoal has been found to reduce high theophylline blood levels. In severe poisoning employ charcoal-column haemoperfusion. Treat symptoms on appearance. The physician should be aware that tablets in the intestine will continue to release theophylline for a period of hours.

In the event of hypokalaemia, potassium chloride should be given by slow intravenous infusion. Repeated measurements of plasma potassium should be made.

**Pharmaceutical precautions** Store at room temperature in a dry place protected from light.

**Legal category** P.

**Package quantities** Uniphyllin Continus Tablets 400 mg: Blister packs of 56 tablets, containers of 250 and 1000 tablets.

Uniphyllin Continus Tablets 300 mg: Blister packs of 56 tablets and containers of 250 tablets.

Uniphyllin Continus Tablets 200 mg: Blister packs of 56 tablets.

**Further information** By incorporating theophylline in the Continus controlled release system, therapeutic blood levels of theophylline between 10 and 20 micrograms/ml can be maintained over a full 24 hour period on a simple twice daily dosage. The availability of 3 strengths of Uniphyllin Continus tablets permits dosage flexibility. The Continus tablet formulation shows minimal tablet to tablet variation in theophylline release.

**Product licence numbers**

| | |
|---|---|
| Uniphyllin Continus Tablets 400 mg | 0337/0074 |
| Uniphyllin Continus Tablets 300 mg | 0337/0129 |
| Uniphyllin Continus Tablets 200 mg | 0337/0057 |

*Trade Mark

# Newport Synthesis Ltd
Baldoyle Industrial Estate
Dublin 13
Ireland

## IMUNOVIR*

**Presentation** White, ovoid tablets with the number 148 on one side and the letters IMV on the other. Each tablet contains 500 mg inosine pranobex.

**Uses** Imunovir is an agent demonstrating anti-viral activity and possessing immunopotentiating action in viral diseases.

*Indications:* Imunovir is indicated in the management of:
(a) Mucocutaneous infections due to herpes simplex virus (type I and/or type II).
(b) Genital warts as adjunctive therapy to podophyllin or carbon dioxide laser.
(c) Subacute sclerosing panencephalitis.

**Dosage and administration**
*Mucocutaneous herpes simplex:* 1 g q.d.s. (4 g daily) for 7–14 days.
*Genital warts:* 1 g t.d.s. (3 g daily) for 14–28 days as adjunctive therapy to podophyllin or carbon dioxide laser.

*Subacute sclerosing panencephalitis:* 50–100 mg/kg daily in divided doses every 4 hours.

*Dosage in the elderly:* No dosage alterations are necessary in the elderly.

*Children:* No information is available in children.

**Contra-indications, warnings, etc**
*Contra-indications:* None known.

*Warnings:* As the inosine component of Imunovir is metabolised to uric acid, it should be used with caution in patients with renal impairment, a history of gout or hyperuricaemia.

*Pregnancy:* Although animal tests have shown no teratogenic effect, the use of Imunovir in women where pregnancy is suspected or confirmed, should be avoided.

*Adverse reactions:* Side-effects are rare and usually of a mild and transitory nature. The only commonly associated adverse effects occurring during treatment with Imunovir are elevated serum and urinary concentrations of uric acid. These return to normal once treatment is withdrawn.

*Symptoms and treatment of overdosage:* There has been no experience of overdosage with Imunovir. However, serious adverse effects, apart from increased levels of uric acid in the body, seem unlikely in view of the animal toxicity studies. Treatment should be restricted to symptomatic and supportive measures.

**Pharmaceutical precautions** Store below 25°C.

**Legal category** POM.

**Package quantities** Available in bottles of 100 tablets.

**Further information** Nil.

**Product licence number** 14806/0001.

# Nexstar Pharmaceuticals Ltd
## The Quorum
## Barnwell Road
## Cambridge CB5 8RE

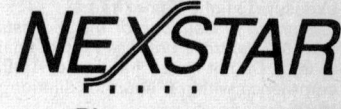

**NEXSTAR**
*Pharmaceuticals Ltd.*

## AMBISOME*

### Qualitative and quantitative composition

AmBisome is a sterile lyophilized product for intravenous infusion. Each vial contains 50 mg of Amphotericin BP (50,000 units) encapsulated in liposomes consisting of approximately 213 mg hydrogenated soy phosphatidylcholine, 52 mg Cholesterol USNF, 84 mg distearoylphosphatidylglycerol, 0.64 mg alpha tocopherol, PhEur, together with 900 mg Sucrose BP, PhEur and 27 mg disodium succinate hexahydrate.

Amphotericin B has a molecular weight of 924.10 and is represented by the formula and structure shown below:

$$C_{47} H_{73} NO_{17}$$

**Pharmaceutical form** AmBisome is a sterile, lyophilized product for intravenous infusion. After reconstitution, the product is an injectable intended to be administered by intravenous infusion.

### Clinical particulars

*Therapeutic indications:* AmBisome is indicated in the treatment of severe *systemic and/or deep mycoses* where toxicity (particularly nephrotoxicity) precludes the use of conventional systemic amphotericin B in effective dosages.

AmBisome is indicated in the treatment of *visceral leishmaniasis* in immunocompetent patients including both adults and children.

Infections successfully treated with AmBisome include: disseminated candidiasis, aspergillosis, mucormycosis, chronic mycetoma, cryptococcal meningitis and visceral leishmaniasis.

This drug should not be used to treat the common clinically inapparent forms of fungal disease which show only positive skin or serologic tests.

*Posology and method of administration:* AmBisome should be administered by intravenous infusion over a 30–60 minute period. The recommended concentration for intravenous infusion is 0.20 mg/ml to 2.00 mg/ml amphotericin as AmBisome. Dosage of amphotericin as AmBisome must be adjusted to the specific requirements of each patient. AmBisome therapy has been administered for as long as three months, with a cumulative dose of 16.8 g of amphotericin as AmBisome without significant toxicity.

Therapy is usually instituted at a daily dose of 1.0 mg/kg of body weight, and increased stepwise to 3.0 mg/kg, as required. Data are presently insufficient to define total dosage requirements and duration of treatment necessary for resolution of *mycoses*. However, a cumulative dose of 1.0–3.0 g of amphotericin as AmBisome over 3–4 weeks has been typical.

A total dose of 21.0–30.0 mg/kg given over 10–21 days may be used in *visceral leishmaniasis*. Particulars as to the optimal dosage and the eventual development of resistance are as yet incomplete. The product should be administered under strict medical supervision.

*Paediatric patients:* Systemic fungal infections have been successfully treated with AmBisome in paediatric patients, without reports of unusual adverse events. Paediatric patients have received AmBisome at doses comparable to those used in adults on a per kilogram body weight basis.

*Elderly patients:* No specific dosage recommendations or precautions.

*Contra-indications:* AmBisome is contra-indicated in those patients who have shown hypersensitivity to any of its constituents unless, in the opinion of the physician, the condition requiring treatment is life-threatening and amenable only to AmBisome therapy.

*Special warnings and special precautions for use:* AmBisome has been shown to be substantially less toxic than conventional amphotericin; however, adverse events may still occur. In particular, caution should be exercised when prolonged therapy is required. Laboratory evaluation of renal, hepatic and haematopoietic function should be performed regularly, and at least once weekly. Particular attention should be paid to patients receiving concomitant therapy with nephrotoxic drugs. Renal function should be closely monitored in these patients.

Although the frequencies of severe allergic or anaphylactic reactions after AmBisome are rare, administration of a test dose is still advisable before a new course of treatment. For this purpose a small amount of an AmBisome infusion (e.g. 1 mg) can be administered for about 10 minutes, the infusion stopped and the patient observed carefully for the next 30 minutes. If there have been no severe allergic or anaphylactic reactions the infusion of AmBisome dose can be continued.

*In the treatment of diabetic patients:* It should be noted that AmBisome contains approximately 900 mg of sucrose in each vial.

*In the treatment of renal dialysis patients:* The administration of AmBisome should commence *only* when dialysis is completed.

Levels of serum potassium and magnesium should be monitored regularly.

*Drug interactions with other medicaments and other forms of interaction:* Although interactions of AmBisome with other drugs have not been observed to date, patients requiring concomitant drug therapy should be monitored closely. Conventional amphotericin has been reported to interact with the following drugs: antineoplastic agents, corticosteroids and corticotropin (ACTH), digitalis glycosides and skeletal muscle relaxants.

No evidence of benefit from the use of flucytosine with AmBisome has been observed. Whilst synergy between amphotericin and flucytosine has been reported, amphotericin may enhance the toxicity of flucytosine by increasing its cellular uptake and impeding its renal excretion.

*Pregnancy and lactation:* No reproductive toxicity studies have been conducted with AmBisome in pregnant women. Systemic fungal infections have been successfully treated in pregnant women with conventional amphotericin without obvious effect on the foetus, but the number of cases reported have been small. Safety for use in pregnant women has not been established with AmBisome. Therefore, AmBisome should only be used during pregnancy if the possible benefits to be derived outweigh the potential risks involved. Breast feeding should be discontinued during treatment.

*Effects on ability to drive and use machines:* The effects of AmBisome on the ability to drive and/or use machines has not been investigated.

*Undesirable effects:* Generally, patients who experienced significant acute toxicity with conventional amphotericin did not experience acute toxicity when AmBisome was substituted.

Patients who developed renal dysfunction, while receiving conventional amphotericin, improved or stabilised when AmBisome was substituted, even when doses were increased. Transient decreases in renal function (hypokalaemia, azotaemia, increased serum creatinine, and renal tubular acidosis) were reported, but did not require discontinuation of AmBisome treatment.

No significant changes in hepatic or haematopoietic function have been observed. However, the possibility of haemolysis must be considered, as it has been associated with the use of conventional amphotericin B. In general, the clinician should monitor the patient for any type of adverse event associated with the use of amphotericin.

Mild headache, nausea, vomiting and lumbar pain have been rarely reported.

Reduction of the infusion rate may lessen the infusion related toxicity.

Phlebitis and thrombophlebitis at infusion sites have not been observed.

Rash and anaphylactic reactions have been reported rarely.

*Overdose:* If overdosage should occur, cease administration immediately. Carefully monitor renal function.

### Pharmacological properties

*Pharmacodynamic properties:* Amphotericin is a macrocyclic, polyene antifungal antibiotic produced by *Streptomyces nodosus*.

Liposomes are closed, spherical vesicles formed from a variety of amphiphilic substances such as phospholipids. Phospholipids arrange themselves into membrane bilayers when exposed to aqueous solutions. The lipophilic moiety of amphotericin allows the drug to be integrated into the lipid bilayer of the liposomes.

Amphotericin is fungistatic or fungicidal depending on the concentration attained in body fluids and the susceptibility of the fungus. The drug probably acts by binding to sterols in the fungal cell membrane, with a resultant change in membrane permeability, allowing leakage of a variety of small molecules. Mammalian cell membranes also contain sterols, and it has been suggested that the damage to human cells and fungal cells caused by amphotericin B may share common mechanisms.

*Microbiology:* Amphotericin, the antifungal component of AmBisome, shows a high order of *in vitro* activity against many species of fungi. Most strains of *Histoplasma capsulatum, Coccidioides immitis, Candida* spp., *Blastomyces dermatitidis, Rhodotorula, Cryptococcus neoformans, Sporothrix schenkii, Mucor mucedo* and *Aspergillus fumigatus*, are inhibited by concentrations of amphotericin ranging from 0.03 to 1.0 mcg/ml *in vitro*. Amphotericin has minimal or no effect on bacteria and viruses.

*Pharmacokinetic properties:* Pharmacokinetic data from animal studies demonstrated that higher peak plasma levels and greater total area under the curve values for amphotericin were achieved after AmBisome administration, as compared to conventional amphotericin. Higher levels of amphotericin were achieved in hepatic and splenic tissues with AmBisome in biodistribution studies in mice and rats. However, in rats amphotericin levels in renal tissue were 5 to 6 fold lower for a given dose of AmBisome, compared to conventional drug after repeated administration for 28 days. For other organs, tissue levels of amphotericin were similar, following dosing with AmBisome or with the conventional drug.

The following table shows the results of human studies with AmBisome at doses of 2.0, 3.0 and 4.0 mg/kg/day. Some variability of the data in patients has been observed.

|  | 2.0 mg/kg | 3.0 mg/kg | 4.0 mg/kg |
|---|---|---|---|
| Distribution half-life (hrs) | 1.70 | 1.82 | 1.30 |
| Elimination half-life (hrs) | 8.33 | 6.76 | 8.57 |
| AUC (mcg-hr/ml) | 84.80 | 158.00 | 283.30 |
| Clearance (L/hr) | 1.30 | 1.27 | 0.97 |
| Volume of Distribution (L) | 15.70 | 12.40 | 11.90 |

These values were determined by pooling serum data at each dose level, generating a curve fit and calculating the pharmacokinetic parameters from that curve.

Detailed human tissue distribution and possible metabolic pathways of conventional amphotericin are not fully understood, and have not been established for AmBisome.

### Pharmaceutical particulars

*List of excipients:* 213 mg hydrogenated soy phosphatidylcholine, 52 mg cholesterol USNF, 84 mg distearoylphosphatidylglycerol, 0.64 mg alpha tocopherol PhEur, 900 mg sucrose PhEur, 27 mg disodium succinate hexahydrate.

*Incompatibilities:* AmBisome is incompatible with saline solutions and may not be mixed with other drugs or electrolytes.

*Shelf life:* A shelf life of 30 months when stored at 2°–8°C and protected from light is recommended. The reconstituted product concentrate may be stored for up to 24 hours at 2°–8°C following reconstitution with water. When diluted with 5% dextrose, AmBisome may be stored for up to 6 hours.

*Special precautions for storage:*

*Storage:* Unopened vials of lyophilized material must be stored under refrigeration at 2°–8°C (36°–46°F). Protect against exposure to light. Do not freeze.

*Storage precautions of reconstituted product concentrate:* The reconstituted product concentrate may be stored for up to 24 hours at 2°–8°C (36°–46°F) following reconstitution with water. Protect against exposure to light. Do not freeze.

*Storage precautions of the reconstituted, diluted with 5% dextrose product:* Protect against exposure to light. Do not freeze. Infusion of AmBisome should commence within 6 hours of dilution with 5% Dextrose.

DO NOT STORE partially used vials for future patient use.

*Nature and contents of container:* AmBisome is presented in 30 ml, sterile, Type I glass vials. The closure consists of West 4416/50 gray butyl rubber stoppers and aluminium ring seals fitted with removable plastic caps. Single-dose vials are packed in ten per carton with 10 filters.

*Instructions for use/handling:* READ THIS ENTIRE SECTION CAREFULLY BEFORE BEGINNING RECONSTITUTION.

**AmBisome must be reconstituted by suitably trained staff.**

AmBisome must be reconstituted using Sterile Water for Injection (**without a bacteriostatic agent**).

**Vials of AmBisome containing 50 mg of Amphotericin are prepared as follows:**

1. Add 12 ml of Sterile Water for Injection to each AmBisome vial, to yield a preparation containing 4 mg/ml amphotericin.

2. SHAKE VIALS VIGOROUSLY for at least 15 seconds to completely disperse the AmBisome.

3. Calculate the amount of reconstituted (4 mg/ml) AmBisome to be further diluted.

4. The infusion solution is obtained by dilution of the reconstituted AmBisome with between one (1) and nineteen (19) parts 5% Dextrose Injection by volume, to give a final concentration in the recommended range of 2.00 mg/ml to 0.20 mg/ml amphotericin as AmBisome.

5. Withdraw the calculated volume of reconstituted AmBisome into a sterile syringe. Using the 5-micron filter provided, instill the AmBisome preparation into a sterile container with the correct amount of 5% Dextrose Injection.

**Do not reconstitute the lyophilized powder/cake with saline or add saline to the reconstituted concentrate, or mix with other drugs. Use only Water for Injection to reconstitute the powder/cake. Use only 5% Dextrose Injection to dilute the reconstituted product to the appropriate concentration for infusion.**

Aseptic technique must be strictly observed in all handling, since no preservative or bacteriostatic agent is present in AmBisome, or in the materials specified for reconstitution and dilution. The use of any solution other than those recommended, or the presence of a bacteriostatic agent (e.g. benzyl alcohol) in the solution, may cause precipitation of AmBisome. Do not use material if there is any evidence of precipitation of foreign matter.

An in-line membrane filter may be used for intravenous infusion of AmBisome. However, **the mean pore diameter of the filter should not be less than 1.0 micron.**

*Note:* AmBisome is not physically compatible with saline solutions and should not be mixed with other drugs or electrolytes. An existing intravenous line must be flushed with 5% Dextrose Injection prior to infusion of AmBisome. If this is not feasible, AmBisome should be administered through a separate line.

Marketing authorisation number  11972/0001.

Date of approval/revision of SPC  7 February 1996.

Legal category  POM.

## DAUNOXOME* ▼

**Qualitative and quantitative composition**  Each 50 ml vial contains 50 mg Daunorubicin PhEur, encapsulated in liposomes consisting of approximately 753 mg distearoylphosphatidylcholine and 180 mg cholesterol USNF and 7 mg citric acid PhEur, suspended in a buffer of 2,125 mg sucrose PhEur, 94 mg glycine BP, and 7 mg calcium chloride PhEur, q.s. to approximately 25 ml with Water for Injection PhEur. The liposomes are small unilamellar vesicles with mean diameter of about 45 nm. The active ingredient is daunorubicin, an anthracycline antibiotic with antineoplastic activity originally obtained from *Streptomyces peucetius*. Daunorubicin has a four-ring anthracycline moiety linked by a glycosidic bond to daunosamin, an amino sugar. Daunorubicin is currently isolated from *Streptomyces coeruleorubidus* and is described by the following chemical name:

(8S, 10S)-8-acetyl-10-[(3-amino-2, 3, 6-trideoxy-α-L-lyxo-hexopyranosyl)oxy]-6, 8, 11-trihydroxy-1-methoxy-7, 8, 9, 10-tetrahydronaphthacene-5, 12-dione

Daunorubicin has a molecular weight of 527.5 and is represented by the formula $C_{27}H_{29}NO_{10}$.

**Pharmaceutical form**  Each vial contains a sterile, pyrogen-free, preservative-free liposomal emulsion. This emulsion is red and clear to slightly opalescent in appearance. The product is an injectable intended to be administered by intravenous infusion.

## Clinical particulars

*Therapeutic indications:* DaunoXome is indicated for the treatment of advanced HIV-related Kaposi's sarcoma.

*Posology and method of administration:* Dosage of DaunoXome must be adjusted for each patient. Therapy should be instituted at 40 mg/m² every two weeks. Therapy should be continued as long as disease control can be maintained.

DaunoXome should be diluted with 5% Dextrose Injection (D5W) before administration. The recommended concentration after dilution is between 0.2 mg and 1 mg daunorubicin/ml of solution. DaunoXome should be administered intravenously over a 30–60 minute period and within six hours of dilution with D5W.

Myelosuppression is a known reaction to DaunoXome therapy. The colony stimulating factor G-CSF has been used to manage patients whose absolute neutrophil count (ANC) fell below 1000/mm³.

Safety and effectiveness in children and the elderly has not been established.

*Contra-indications:* DaunoXome is a bone marrow suppressant. Suppression may occur in patients given therapeutic doses of this drug. Combination of DaunoXome with other cancer chemotherapeutic agents which suppress blood counts is contra-indicated. Therapy with DaunoXome is contra-indicated in patients who have had a serious hypersensitivity reaction to previous doses of DaunoXome or to any of its constituents unless the benefit from such treatment warrants the risk.

*Special warnings and precautions for use:* Conventional daunorubicin has been associated with cardiomyopathy and congestive heart failure. Although no such side-effects have been observed in the clinical use of DaunoXome, there must be a presumption that this is possible. As such, cardiac function should be evaluated in each patient, by means of history, physical examination and appropriate measurements of cardiac ejection fraction as indicated.

Also, it is recommended to give special attention to patients who received cumulative doses of daunorubicin equal to or in excess of 400 mg/m². These patients should undergo four weekly monitoring of the cardiac function by echo cardiography. Conventional daunorubicin has also been associated with local tissue necrosis at the site of drug infiltrations. No such local necrosis has been observed with DaunoXome. Nonetheless, care should be taken to ensure that there is no extravasation of drug when DaunoXome is administered.

Aseptic technique must be strictly observed in all handling, since no preservative or bacteriostatic agent is present in DaunoXome or in the materials recommended for dilution.

**Caution: The only fluid which may be mixed with DaunoXome is D5W; DaunoXome should not be mixed with saline, bacteriostatic agents such as benzyl alcohol, or any other solution.**

An in-line filter is not recommended for the intravenous infusion of DaunoXome. However, if such a filter is used, the mean pore diameter of the filter should not be less than 5 µm.

All parenteral drug products should be inspected visually for particulate matter prior to administration, wherever solution and container permit.

Procedures for proper handling and disposal of anticancer drugs should be followed.

*Interactions with other medicaments and other forms of interaction:* No interactions between DaunoXome and other drugs have been observed to date. DaunoXome has been safely administered during antiretroviral therapy with zidovudine (AZT), dideoxycytidene (ddC, zalcitabine), and dideoxyinosine (ddI, didanosine) and with the colony stimulating factor G-CSF. Although interaction of DaunoXome with other drugs has not been observed, patients requiring concomitant drug therapy should be monitored closely. During preparation and administration DaunoXome should not be mixed with saline; aggregation of the liposomes may result.

So far no safety information is available on the combination of DaunoXome with other cancer chemotherapeutic agents which suppress blood counts. Concomitant use of DaunoXome and parenteral nutritional lipid solutions or other liposomal products should be avoided.

*Pregnancy and lactation:* Safety for use of DaunoXome in pregnant and lactating women has not been established. Since it is not known if the administration of DaunoXome during pregnancy can cause fetal harm, DaunoXome should only be used during pregnancy if the possible benefits to be derived outweigh the potential risks involved. Breast feeding should be discontinued during treatment.

Daunorubicin, the active component of DaunoXome, has been shown to impair fertility and to have teratogenic effects in experimental animals, and there is also positive evidence of human fetal risk. Daunorubicin is also mutagenic both *in vitro* and *in vivo*, and carcinogenic *in vivo*. A high incidence of mammary tumours was observed in rats treated with daunorubicin. Although no such studies have been conducted with DaunoXome, it is most likely that DaunoXome will have a similar profile for carcinogenesis, teratogenesis, mutagenesis, and impairment of fertility as that of daunorubicin.

*Effects on ability to drive and use machines:* Since DaunoXome is being administered to sick patients and may induce delayed nausea and vomiting, administration prior to driving or the use of heavy machinery is contra-indicated.

*Undesirable effects:* Conventional daunorubicin has been associated with cardiomyopathy and congestive heart failure. Although no such side-effects have been observed in the clinical use of DaunoXome, there must be a presumption that this is possible. As such, cardiac function should be evaluated in each patient, including history, physical examination, and appropriate measures of cardiac ejection fraction as indicated.

Conventional daunorubicin has also been associated with local tissue necrosis at the site of drug infiltrations. No such local necrosis has been observed with DaunoXome. Nonetheless, care should be taken to ensure that there is no infiltration of drug when DaunoXome is administered intravenously.

The primary toxicity of DaunoXome is myelosuppresion and, as such, close patient observation and frequent monitoring of the blood cell counts is mandated. In patients with malignancies or with HIV infection, the immune system is already compromised, and the use of a cytotoxic agent decreasing the white blood cell count may cause further immunosuppression and make the patient more susceptible to intercurrent or opportunistic infections.

Back pain, flushing, and chest tightness were occasionally reported during the clinical trials. This syndrome may occur during a patient's initial infusion and may also occur in patients who have previously been exposed to DaunoXome without incident. This combination of symptoms does not always appear to be dose related, and generally occurs during the first ten minutes of the infusion. The etiology is unclear. The symptoms usually subside when the infusion is slowed or halted, and acetaminophen (paracetamol) may be used for analgesia. Other allergic or immune reactions may also be seen, and have been reported to be associated with hypotension. Anaphylactic reactions have been reported in rare cases.

Various other minor reactions, such as headache, fatigue, chills, mucositis, lightheadedness, nausea and vomiting, have also been reported.

*Overdose:* No experience exists for an overdose with this medication. The primary anticipated toxicity from such an overdose would be myelosuppression, and under these circumstances bone marrow function should be carefully monitored with appropriate therapy for any severe side-effects.

**Pharmacological properties**

*Pharmacodynamic properties:* DaunoXome is a liposomal preparation of daunorubicin formulated to maximise the selectivity of daunorubicin for solid tumours *in situ*. This tumour selectivity has been demonstrated for transplanted tumours in animal models. While in the circulation, the DaunoXome formulation protects the entrapped daunorubicin from chemical and enzymatic degradation, minimises protein binding, and generally decreases uptake by normal tissues, as well as by the non-reticuloendothelial system. The specific mechanism by which DaunoXome is able to deliver daunorubicin to solid tumours *in situ* is not known. However, it is believed to be a function of increased permeability of the tumour neovasculature to some particulates in the size range of DaunoXome. Thus, by a decrease in distribution and uptake of normal tissues and binding to plasma proteins and by selective extravasation in tumour neovasculature, the pharmacokinetics of daunorubicin are favourably shifted towards an accumulation of DaunoXome in tumour tissue. Once within the tumour environment, DaunoXome vesicles enter the tumour cells intact. Daunorubicin is then released over time in the cytoplasm, where it is able to exert its antineoplastic activity over a longer period.

*Pharmacokinetic properties:* DaunoXome has a pharmacokinetic profile significantly different from that of conventional daunorubicin. DaunoXome was administered intravenously over approximately 30 minutes as a single dose of 10, 20, 40, 60 or 80 mg/m². Plasma pharmacokinetic profiles for most patients demonstrated monoexponential declines, although biexponential or Michaelis-Menton (saturation) kinetics occurred in some instances. Peak plasma levels at 40 mg/m² ranged from 14.8 to 22.0 micrograms/ml with a mean peak plasma level of 18.0 micrograms/ml. The mean terminal half-life at this dose was 4.0 hours and mean total body clearance was 10.5 ml/minute. This resulted in a mean area under the plasma curve of 120 micrograms.hr/ml. Metabolism of DaunoXome appeared not to be significant at lower doses. At 60 mg/m² and above, three metabolites were observed, although they have not yet been identified.

DaunoXome's pharmacokinetic parameters were also compared to published values for conventional daunorubicin. At 80 mg/m², peak plasma levels ranged from 33.4 to 52.3 micrograms/ml for DaunoXome compared to 0.40 micrograms/ml for conventional drug. At this dose, DaunoXome plasma levels decline monoexponentially with a terminal half-life of 5.2 hours versus an initial half-life of 0.77 hours and a final half-life of 55.4 hours for conventional daunorubicin. Mean clearance for DaunoXome is 6.6 ml/min versus 223 ml/minute for daunorubicin. When combined, these parameters indicate that DaunoXome produces a 36-fold increase in mean area under the plasma curve compared to conventional drug (375.3 versus 10.33 micrograms.hr/ml).

*Preclinical safety data:* Animal studies with tumour models in mice have demonstrated that DaunoXome can increase daunorubicin tumour exposure ten-fold (in terms of area under the tumour concentration vs. time curve, AUC) when compared with equivalent doses of conventional (free) drug. The rate of drug accumulation in tumour tissues, however, appears to be slower for DaunoXome than for conventional daunorubicin. This difference is thought to be due to a slow diffusion process by which DaunoXome extravasates through the tumour neovasculature into the extracellular space while free drug, in contrast, is able to rapidly equilibrate from the circulation to both normal and neoplastic tissues. Since tumour accumulation of DaunoXome-delivered daunorubicin is a gradual process, it is important that DaunoXome

remains in the circulation at high levels for prolonged periods. This has been shown to occur in animal studies where plasma AUC values for daunorubicin were approximately 200-fold greater for DaunoXome than for conventional drug. In contrast to tumour tissue, however, AUC values for normal tissues were only moderately elevated in DaunoXome-treated animals, relative to conventional daunorubicin. Exclusive of reticuloendothelial tissues (liver and spleen, AUC values increased by 110% and 60%, respectively) and brain tissue (AUC value increased by 3.5 fold) AUC increases ranged from 10% for heart and lungs to 30% for kidney and small intestines.

## Pharmaceutical particulars

*List of excipients: Liposome:* 753 mg distearoylphosphatidylcholine; 180 mg cholesterol USNF; 7 mg citric acid PhEur. *Buffer:* 2,125 mg sucrose PhEur; 94 mg glycine BP; 7 mg calcium chloride PhEur, q.s. to approximately 25 ml with Water for Injection PhEur.

*Incompatibilities:* To date, no incompatibilities of DaunoXome with other drugs have been reported. However, it is known that the active component daunorubicin is physically incompatible with heparin sodium and with dexamethasone phosphate when directly admixed. A precipitate is produced with either drug. Additionally, because of the chemical instability of the glycosidic bond of daunorubicin, admixture into a highly alkaline media (pH >8.0) is not recommended.

DaunoXome should not be mixed with saline; aggregation of the liposomes may result.

Admixtures containing bacteriostatic agents such as benzyl alcohol or other detergent-like molecules should be avoided as well because such compounds can rupture the bilayer wall of the liposomes causing premature leakage of the active drug.

*Shelf life:* An expiry period of 40 weeks, when stored at 2°–8°C, is recommended. The product should be used within six hours of dilution in 5% dextrose as DaunoXome does not contain a preservative or bacteriostatic agent.

*Special precautions for storage:* Store at 2°–8°C. Do not freeze. Protect against exposure to light. Do not store partially used vials for future patient use. Vials are for single use only.

*Nature and contents of container:* DaunoXome is presented in 50-ml, sterile, Type I glass vials. The closure consists of West 4416/50 gray butyl rubber and aluminium ring seals fitted with removable plastic caps. Each single-dose vial is packed in a white chipboard carton. Included in each carton are directions for use.

## Instruction for use/handling

**Use aseptic technique:** Aseptic technique must be strictly observed in all handling, since no preservative or bacteriostatic agent is present in DaunoXome or in the materials recommended for dilution.

Withdraw the calculated volume of DaunoXome into a sterile syringe. Instil the DaunoXome preparation into a sterile container with the correct amount of 5% Dextrose Injection (D5W) and administer within six hours. The recommended concentration after dilution is between 0.2 mg and 1 mg daunorubicin/ml of solution. Infuse over a 30–60 minute period. As with all parenteral drug products, inspect the solution visually for particulate matter prior to administration.

**Caution: The only fluid which may be mixed with DaunoXome is D5W; DaunoXome should not be mixed with saline, bacteriostatic agents such as benzyl alcohol, or any other solution.**

An in-line filter is not recommended for the intravenous infusion of DaunoXome. However, if such a filter is used, the mean pore diameter of the filter should not be less than 5 μm.

Procedures for proper handling and disposal of anticancer drugs should be followed.

**Marketing authorisation number** 11972/0002.

**Date of approval/revision of SPC** February 1997.

**Legal category** POM.

*\*Trade Mark*

# Norgine Limited

Chaplin House
Widewater Place
Moorhall Road
Harefield
Middlesex UB9 6NS

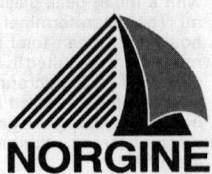

**NORGINE**

## ALVERCOL*

**Qualitative and quantitative composition** The active ingredients are 62% Sterculia BP and 0.5% alverine citrate.

**Pharmaceutical form** Beige granules for oral administration.

**Clinical particulars**

*Therapeutic indications:* The treatment of hypertonic disorders of the colon and irritable bowel syndrome.

*Posology and method of administration*
Adults (including the elderly): 1-2 heaped 5 ml spoonfuls, once or twice daily after meals.

*Children:* (6-12 years): a reduced amount may be given at the discretion of the doctor.

The granules should be placed dry on the tongue and, without chewing or crushing, swallowed immediately with plenty of water or a cool drink.

*Contra-indications:* Intestinal obstruction, faecal impaction, and total atony of the colon.

*Special warnings and special precautions for use:* Patients should be advised to maintain an adequate fluid intake and to avoid taking Alvercol immediately before going to bed (especially if they are elderly).

*Interaction with other medicaments and other forms of interaction:* None known.

*Pregnancy and lactation*
*Pregnancy:* No teratogenic effects have been reported, but caution should be exercised during the first trimester.

*Lactation:* There is no evidence to suggest that Alvercol is unsuitable for use.

*Effects on the ability to drive and use machines:* None known.

*Undesirable effects:* Occasionally mild abdominal distension may occur. Oesophageal obstruction is possible if the product is not adequately washed down with fluid.

*Overdose:* Intestinal obstruction is possible in overdosage, particularly in combination with inadequate fluid intake. Management is as for intestinal obstruction from other causes. Alverine in overdosage can produce hypotension and atropine-like toxic effects, which should be treated as for atropine poisoning.

**Pharmacological properties**
*Pharmacodynamic properties:* Sterculia is insoluble in water and has no known pharmacological actions. Its pharmacodynamic properties are attributable entirely to the mechanical consequences of the expansion of the bulk and water content, and softening of the consistency of the colonic contents. Alverine citrate is a spasmolytic which acts selectively on the smooth muscle of the alimentary tract and uterus.

*Pharmacokinetic properties:* Sterculia is pharmacokinetically inert, having no significant absorption, metabolism or excretion. With only a change in physical state, resulting from the absorption or adsorption of water, it is evacuated in the faeces. Alverine is a prodrug and is rapidly converted *in vivo* to metabolites which are excreted by the kidney.

*Preclinical safety data:* There are no preclinical data of relevance to the prescriber.

**Pharmaceutical particulars**
*List of excipients:* Sucrose BP; Talc USP; Sodium Bicarbonate PhEur; Paraffin Wax; Titanium Dioxide BP; Flavourings: Anethole; Caramel (E150).

The sugar provides 7.5 calories (1.9 g carbohydrate) per heaped 5 ml spoonful, and the sodium content is 0.8 mmol. Alvercol is gluten free.

*Incompatibilities:* None known.

*Shelf life:* The shelf life is 4 years.

*Special precautions for storage:* Store in a dry place below 25°C.

*Nature and contents of container:* Lined box of 200 g and 500 g containing beige granules.

*Instructions for use/handling:* None.

Marketing authorisation number    00322/5009
Date of approval/revision of SPC    December 1994.
Legal category    P

## CAMCOLIT* 400

**Qualitative and quantitative composition** The active ingredient is Lithium Carbonate BP; 400 mg/tablet.

**Pharmaceutical form** White film, coated tablets, engraved 'CAMCOLIT-S' around one face and having a breakline on the reverse. For oral administration.

**Clinical particulars**
*Therapeutic indications:* The treatment and prophylaxis of mania, manic-depressive illness and recurrent depression, and the treatment of aggressive or self mutilating behaviour.

*Posology and method of administration*
*Acute mania:*
*Adults:* Sufficient to produce a serum lithium level of between 0.6 and 1.2 mmol/l 12 hours after the last dose.
*Elderly:* As above but with a recommended upper serum lithium limit of 1.0 mmol/l.
*Children:* Not recommended.

*Prophylaxis of recurrent affective disorders:*
*Adults:* Sufficient to produce a serum lithium level of between 0.5 and 1.2 mmol/l 12 hours after the last dose.
*Elderly:* As above but with a recommended upper serum lithium limit of 1.0 mmol/l.
*Children:* Not recommended.

*Contra-indications:* Patients with renal disease, cardiovascular disease, Addison's disease or those breast feeding.

*Special warnings and special precautions for use:* Pretreatment and periodic routine clinical monitoring is essential. This should include assessment of renal function, urine analysis, assessment of thyroid function and cardiac function, especially in patients with cardiovascular disease.

Patients should be euthyroid before initiation of lithium therapy.

Clear instructions regarding the symptoms of impending toxicity should be given by the doctor to all patients receiving long-term lithium therapy.

Patients should also be warned to report if polyuria or polydipsia develop. Episodes of nausea and vomiting or other conditions leading to salt/water depletion (including severe dieting) should also be reported. Patients should be advised to maintain their usual salt and fluid intake.

Elderly patients are particularly liable to lithium toxicity.

*Interactions with other medicaments and other forms of interaction:* Lower doses of lithium may be required during diuretic therapy as lithium clearance is reduced.

Serum lithium concentrations may increase during concomitant therapy with non-steroidal anti-inflammatory drugs or tetracycline, possibly resulting in lithium toxicity. Serum lithium concentrations therefore should be monitored more frequently if NSAID or tetracycline therapy is initiated or discontinued.

Raised plasma levels of ADH may occur during treatment.

Symptoms of nephrogenic diabetes insipidus are particularly prevalent in patients receiving concurrent treatment with tricyclic or tetracyclic anti-depressants.

*Pregnancy and lactation*
*Pregnancy:* There is epidemiological evidence to suggest that the drug may be harmful during human pregnancy. Should the use of lithium be unavoidable, close monitoring of serum concentrations should be made throughout pregnancy and parturition.

*Lactation:* Infants of mothers on lithium should be bottle fed as lithium is present in the breast milk.

*Effects on the ability to drive and use machines:* None known.

*Undesirable effects:* Long term treatment with lithium may result in permanent changes in the kidney and impairment of renal function. High serum concentrations of lithium, including episodes of acute lithium toxicity may enhance these changes. The minimum clinically effective dose of lithium should always be used. Patients should only be maintained on lithium after 3-5 years if, on assessment, benefit persists.

Renal function should be routinely monitored in patients with polyuria and polydipsia.

Side effects are usually related to serum lithium concentrations and are infrequent at levels below 1.0 mmol/l.

Mild gastro-intestinal effects, nausea, vertigo, muscle weakness and a dazed feeling may occur, but frequently disappear after stabilisation. Fine hand tremors, polyuria and mild thirst may persist. Some studies suggest that the tremor can be controlled by relatively small doses of propranolol.

Long term treatment with lithium is frequently associated with disturbances of thyroid function including goitre and hypothyroidism. These can be controlled by administration of small doses of thyroxine (0.05-0.2 mg daily) concomitantly with lithium. Thyrotoxicosis has also been reported.

Mild cognitive impairment may occur during long term use.

Hypercalcaemia, hypermagnesaemia, hyperparathyroidism and an increase in antinuclear antibodies have also been reported.

Exacerbation of psoriasis may occur.

*Overdose:* Appearance or aggravation of gasto-intestinal symptoms, muscle weakness, lack of co-ordination, drowsiness or lethargy may be early signs of intoxication. With increasing toxicity, ataxia, giddiness, tinnitus, blurred vision, coarse tremor, muscle twitching and a large output of dilute urine may be seen. At blood levels above 2-3 mmol/l, increasing disorientation, seizures, coma and death may occur.

There is no antidote to lithium poisoning. In the event, lithium treatment should be stopped immediately and serum lithium levels estimated every 6 hours. When ingestion is recent, gastric lavage should be carried out, together with general supportive measures. Special attention must be given to the maintenance of fluid and electroylyte balance, and also adequate renal function. Sodium-depleting diuretics should not be used in any circumstances. Forced alkaline diuresis may be used. If the serum lithium level is above 4.0 mmol/l, or if there is a deterioration in the patient's condition, or if the serum lithium concentration is not falling at a rate equivalent to a half-life of less than 30 hours, peritoneal dialysis or haemodialysis should be instituted promptly. This should be continued until the serum and dialysis fluid are free of lithium. Serum lithium levels should be monitored for at least another 7 days thereafter, as a rebound rise is possible due to delayed diffusion from the tissues.

**Pharmacological properties**
*Pharmacodynamic properties:* The precise mechanism of action of lithium as a mood-stabilising agent remains unknown, although many cellular actions of lithium have been characterised.

*Pharmacokinetic properties:* The pharmacokinetics of lithium are extremely well documented. A single oral dose of Camcolit 400 gives a peak plasma level approximately 3-4 hours later, with the level at 24 hours being approximately 40% of peak levels.

*Preclinical safety data:* There is no preclinical data of relevance to the prescriber.

**Pharmaceutical particulars**
*List of excipients:* Maize Starch PhEur; Acacia PhEur; Magnesium Stearate PhEur; Sodium Lauryl Sulphate PhEur; Hydroxypropylmethyl Cellulose 2910 USP; Polyethylene Glycol 400 USNF; Opaspray M-1-7111B.

*Incompatibilities:* See *Interactions* and *Undesirable effects* above.

*Shelf life:* The shelf life is 3 years.

*Special precautions for storage:* Store in a cool dry place below 25°C.

*Nature and contents of container:* Polypropylene containers of 100 or 500 tablet capacity, and for hospital use only, screw-cap amber glass bottles of 50 or 100 tablet capacity.

*Instructions for use/handling:* None.

**Marketing authorisation number** 00322/0015

**Date of approval/revision of SPC** June 1997

**Legal category** POM

## CAMCOLIT* 250

**Qualitative and quantitative composition** The active ingredient is Lithium Carbonate BP; 250 mg/tablet.

**Pharmaceutical form** White film, coated tablets, engraved 'CAMCOLIT' around one face and having a breakline on the reverse. For oral administration.

**Clinical particulars**
*Therapeutic indications:* The treatment and prophylaxis of mania, manic-depressive illness and
recurrent depression, and the treatment of aggressive or self mutilating behaviour.

*Posology and method of administration*
*Acute mania:*
*Adults:* Sufficient to produce a serum lithium level of between 0.6 and 1.2 mmol/l 12 hours after the last dose.
*Elderly:* As above but with a recommended upper serum lithium limit
of 1.0 mmol/l.
*Children:* Not recommended.

*Prophylaxis of recurrent affective disorders:*
*Adults:* Sufficient to produce a serum lithium level of between 0.5 and 1.2 mmol/l 12 hours after the last dose.
*Elderly:* As above but with a recommended upper serum lithium limit of 1.0 mmol/l.
*Children:* Not recommended.

*Contra-indications:* Patients with renal disease, cardiovascular disease, Addison's disease or those breast feeding.

*Special warnings and special precautions for use:* Pretreatment and periodic routine clinical monitoring is essential. This should include assessment of renal function, urine analysis, assessment of thyroid function and cardiac function, especially in patients with cardiovascular disease.
Patients should be euthyroid before initiation of lithium therapy.
Clear instructions regarding the symptoms of impending toxicity should
be given by the doctor to all patients receiving long-term lithium therapy.
Patients should also be warned to report if polyuria or polydipsia develop. Episodes of nausea and vomiting or other conditions leading to salt/water depletion (including severe dieting) should also be reported. Patients should be advised to maintain their usual salt and fluid intake.
Elderly patients are particularly liable to lithium toxicity.

*Interactions with other medicaments and other forms of interaction:* Lower doses of lithium may be required during diuretic therapy as lithium clearance is reduced.
Serum lithium concentrations may increase during concomitant therapy with non-steroidal anti-inflammatory drugs or tetracycline, possibly resulting in lithium toxicity. Serum lithium concentrations therefore should be monitored more frequently if NSAID or tetracycline therapy is initiated or discontinued.
Raised plasma levels of ADH may occur during treatment.
Symptoms of nephrogenic diabetes insipidus are particularly prevalent
in patients receiving concurrent treatment with tricyclic or tetracyclic antidepressants.

*Pregnancy and lactation*
*Pregnancy:* There is epidemiological evidence to suggest that the drug may be harmful during human pregnancy. Should the use of lithium be unavoidable, close monitoring of serum concentrations should be made throughout pregnancy and parturition.
*Lactation:* Infants of mothers on lithium should be bottle fed as lithium is present in the breast milk.

*Effects on the ability to drive and use machines:* None known.

*Undesirable effects:* Long term treatment with lithium may result in permanent changes in the kidney and impairment of renal function. High serum concentrations of lithium, including episodes of acute lithium toxicity may enhance these changes. The minimum clinically effective dose of lithium should always be

used. Patients should only be maintained on lithium after 3-5 years if, on assessment, benefit persists.
Renal function should be routinely monitored in patients with polyuria and polydipsia.
Side effects are usually related to serum lithium concentrations and are infrequent at levels below 1.0 mmol/l.
Mild gastro-intestinal effects, nausea, vertigo, muscle weakness and a dazed feeling may occur, but frequently disappear after stabilisation.
Fine hand tremors, polyuria and mild thirst may persist. Some studies suggest that the tremor can be controlled by relatively small doses of propranolol.
Long term treatment with lithium is frequently associated with disturbances of thyroid function including goitre and hypothyroidism. These can be controlled by administration of small doses of thyroxine (0.05-0.2 mg daily) concomitantly with lithium. Thyrotoxicosis has also been reported.
Mild cognitive impairment may occur during long term use.
Hypercalcaemia, hypermagnesaemia, hyperparathyroidism and an increase in antinuclear antibodies have also been reported.
Exacerbation of psoriasis may occur.

*Overdose:* Appearance or aggravation of gasto-intestinal symptoms, muscle weakness, lack of co-ordination, drowsiness or lethargy may be early signs of intoxication. With increasing toxicity, ataxia, giddiness, tinnitus, blurred vision, coarse tremor, muscle twitching and a large output of dilute urine may be seen. At blood levels above 2-3 mmol/l, increasing disorientation, seizures, coma and death may occur.
There is no antidote to lithium poisoning. In the event, lithium treatment should be stopped immediately and serum lithium levels estimated every 6 hours. When ingestion is recent, gastric lavage should be carried out, together with general supportive measures. Special attention must be given to the maintenance of fluid and electrolyte balance, and also adequate renal function. Sodium-depleting diuretics should not be used in any circumstances. Forced alkaline diuresis may be used. If the serum lithium level is above 4.0 mmol/l, or if there is a deterioration in the patient's condition, or if the serum lithium concentration is not falling at a rate equivalent to a half-life of less than 30 hours, peritoneal dialysis or haemodialysis should be instituted promptly. This should be continued until the serum and dialysis fluid are free of lithium. Serum lithium levels should be monitored for at least another 7 days thereafter, as a rebound rise is possible due to delayed diffusion from the tissues.

**Pharmacological properties**
*Pharmacodynamic properties:* The precise mechanism of action of lithium as a mood-stabilising agent remains unknown, although many cellular actions of lithium have been characterised.

*Pharmacokinetic properties:* The pharmacokinetics of lithium are extremely well documented. A single oral dose of Camcolit 250 gives a peak plasma level approximately 2-3 hours later, with the level at 24 hours being approximately 40% of peak levels.

*Preclinical safety data:* There is no preclinical data of relevance to the prescriber.

**Pharmaceutical particulars**
*List of excipients:* Maize Starch PhEur; Magnesium Stearate PhEur; Pregelatinised Maize Starch BP; Hydroxypropylmethyl Cellulose 2910 USP; Polyethylene Glycol 400 USNF

*Incompatibilities:* See *Interactions* and *Undersirable effects* above.

*Shelf life:* The shelf life is 5 years.

*Special precautions for storage:* Store below 25°C.

*Nature and contents of container:* Polypropylene containers of 100 or 1000 tablet capacity, and for hospital use only, screw-cap amber glass bottles of 50 or 100 tablet capacity.

*Instructions for use/handling:* None.

**Marketing authorisation number** 00322/5900R

**Date of approval/revision of SPC** May 1997

**Legal category** POM

## DESTOLIT*

**Presentation** White half-scored tablet containing 150 mg ursodeoxycholic acid marked Destolit.

**Uses** Destolit is indicated for the dissolution of radiolucent (i.e. non-radio opaque) cholesterol gallstones in patients with a functioning gallbladder.

**Dosage and administration** The daily dose for most patients is 3 or 4 tablets of 150 mg according to body weight. This dose should be divided into 2 administrations after meals, with one administration always to be taken after the evening meal.

A daily dose of about 8 to 10 mg/kg will produce cholesterol desaturation of bile in the majority of cases. The measurement of the lithogenic index on bile-rich duodenal drainage fluid after 4–6 weeks of therapy may be useful for determining the minimal effective dose. The lowest effective dose has been found to be 4 mg/kg.
The duration of treatment required to achieve gallstone dissolution will usually not be extended beyond 2 years and should be monitored by regular cholecystograms. Treatment should be continued for 3–4 months after the radiological disappearance of the gallstones.
Any temporary discontinuation of treatment, if prolonged for 3–4 weeks, will allow the bile to return to a state of supersaturation and will extend the total time required for litholysis. In some cases stones may recur after successful treatment.

**Contra-indications, warnings, etc**
*Use in pregnancy and lactation:* In common with all drugs, it is advised that ursodeoxycholic acid should not be given during the first trimester of pregnancy. (In the rabbit, embryotoxicity has been observed, but this has not been seen in the rat.) Treatment in women of child-bearing age should only be undertaken if measures to prevent pregnancy are used. Non-hormonal contraceptive measures are recommended. In cases of conception during treatment, therapy should be discontinued.

*Contra-indications:* Active gastric or duodenal ulcers are contra-indications, as are hepatic and intestinal conditions interfering with the enterohepatic circulation of bile acids (ileal resection and stoma, regional ileitis, extra and intra-hepatic cholestasis, severe, acute, and chronic liver diseases). A product of this class has been found to be carcogenic in animals. The relevance of these findings to the clinical use of ursodeoxycholic acid has not been established.

*Precautions:* Excessive dietary intake of calories and cholesterol should be avoided; a low cholesterol diet will probably improve the effectiveness of Destolit tablets.

*Drug interactions:* It is also recommended that drugs known to increase cholesterol elimination in bile, such as oestrogenic hormones, oral contraceptive agents and certain blood cholesterol lowering agents should also not be prescribed concomitantly.

*Side-effects:* Destolit is normally well tolerated. Diarrhoea has been found to occur only occasionally. No significant alterations have so far been observed in liver function.

*Overdosage:* It is unlikely that overdosage will cause serious adverse effects. Diarrhoea may occur and it is recommended that liver function tests be monitored. Ion-exchange resins may be useful to bind bile acids in the intestines.

**Pharmaceutical precautions** None.

**Legal category** POM.

**Package quantities** Blister packs of 60 tablets.

**Further information** Nil.

**Product licence number** 4425/0045.

*Product licence holder:* Marion Merrell Limited, Broadwater Park, Denham, Uxbridge, Middlesex UB9 5HP.

## KAMILLOSAN*

**Presentation** Light brown ointment containing Chamomile extracts 10.5% (standardised to provide 0.01% L-α bisabolol) in a base containing lanolin. Kamillosan also contains beeswax, maize oil and mixed esters of p-hydroxy-benzoic acid.

**Uses** Prophylaxis and treatment of sore nipples in nursing mothers, nappy rash, nappy chafe and chapped hands.

**Dosage and administration** Ointment for topical application.
*Sore nipples:* Apply after breastfeeding.
*Nappy chafe and nappy rash:* Apply at every nappy change.
*Other conditions:* Apply twice daily as necessary.

**Contra-indications, warnings, etc**
*Contra-indications:* None known.
*Precautions:* None known.
*Use in pregnancy:* There is no evidence to suggest that Kamillosan should not be used during pregnancy or lactation.
*Side-effects:* None reported.
*Overdosage:* There are no known symptoms of overdosage.

**Pharmaceutical precautions** Store in a cool, dry place below 25°C.

**Legal category** GSL.

**Package quantities** Tubes of 30 g.

**Further information** Breast pads may be worn to prevent staining of clothing by the ointment.

**Product licence number** 0322/5914

## KLEAN-PREP*

**Qualitative and quantitative composition** Each sachet of Klean-Prep contains the following active ingredients:

| | |
|---|---|
| Polyethylene Glycol 3350 USNF | 59.000 g |
| Anhydrous Sodium Sulphate PhEur | 5.685 g |
| Sodium Bicarbonate PhEur | 1.685 g |
| Sodium Chloride PhEur | 1.465 g |
| Potassium Chloride PhEur | 0.7425 g |

The content of electrolyte ions per sachet when made up to one litre of water is as follows:

| | |
|---|---|
| Sodium | 125 mM |
| Sulphate | 40 mM |
| Chloride | 35 mM |
| Bicarbonate | 20 mM |
| Potassium | 10 mM |

**Pharmaceutical form** A whitish powder which, when dissolved in water, gives a clear, colourless solution for oral administration.

**Clinical particulars**

*Therapeutic indications:* For colonic lavage prior to diagnostic examination or surgical procedures requiring a clean colon, e.g. colonoscopy, barium enema or colonic resection.

*Posology and method of administration*
*Adults:* Each sachet should be dissolved in 1 litre of water. The usual dose is up to 4 sachets taken at a rate of 250 ml every 10 to 15 minutes until the total volume is consumed or rectal effluent is clear, or as directed by the physician.

The solutions from all 4 sachets should be drunk within 4 to 6 hours. Alternatively, administration may be divided, for example, taking 2 sachets during the evening before the examination, and the remaining 2 sachets on the morning of the examination.

If administration is by nasogastric tube, the usual rate should be 20 to 30 ml/minute.

*Children:* There is no recommended dosage for children.

*Renal patients:* No dosage adjustment need be made.

*Contra-indications:* Use in patients with known or suspected gastrointestinal obstruction or perforation, ileus, gastric retention, acute intestinal or gastric ulceration, toxic colitis or toxic megacolon.

*Special warnings and special precautions for use:* No solid food should be eaten for at least 2 hours before taking Klean-Prep. The product should only be administered with caution to patients with impaired gag reflex, reflux oesophagitis or those with diminished levels of consciousness and patients with ulcerative colitis.

Unconscious, semi-conscious patients or patients prone to aspiration or regurgitation should be observed during administration especially if this is via the nasogastric route.

*Interaction with other medicaments and other forms of interaction:* Oral medication taken within one hour of administration of Klean-Prep may be flushed from the gastro-intestinal tract and not absorbed.

*Pregnancy and lactation:* The preparation should only be used during pregnancy and lactation if considered essential by the physician. There is no experience of use during pregnancy. The purpose and mechanisms of use should be borne in mind if the physician is considering administration.

*Effects on the ability to drive and use machines:* There is no known effect on the ability to drive and use machines.

*Undesirable effects:* Nausea, abdominal fullness and bloating may be experienced. Should distension or pain arise, the rate of administration should be slowed down or temporarily stopped until symptoms subside. Abdominal cramps, vomiting and anal irritation occur less frequently.

These effects normally subside rapidly. Urticaria and allergic reactions have been reported rarely.

*Overdose:* In case of gross accidental overdosage, where diarrhoea is severe, conservative measures are usually sufficient; generous amounts of fluid, especially fruit juices, should be given.

**Pharmacological properties**
*Pharmacodynamic properties:* Polyethylene glycol 3350 exerts its effects by virtue of its osmotic effect in the gut, which induces a laxative effect. The electrolytes also present in the formulation ensure that there is virtually no net gain or loss of sodium, potassium or water, and thus no dehydration.

*Pharmacokinetic properties:* Polyethylene glycol 3350 is unchanged along the gut. It is virtually unabsorbed from the gastro-intestinal tract and has no known pharmacological activity. Any polyethylene glycol 3350 that is absorbed is excreted via the urine.

*Preclinical safety data:* Preclinical studies provide evidence that polyethylene glycol 3350 has no significant systemic toxicity potential.

**Pharmaceutical particulars**
*List of excipients:* Vanilla flavour; aspartame.

*Incompatibilities:* None are known.

*Shelf life:* Sachets: 2 years. Solution: 24 hours.

*Special precautions for storage:* Sachets: Store in a dry place below 25°C.

*Nature and contents of container:* Sachets containing 69 gm white powder, in boxes of 4 sachets.

*Instructions of use/handling:* The solution should be used within 24 hours.

**Marketing authorisation number** 00322/0068

**Date of approval/revision of SPC** March 1997

**Legal category** P

## MOVICOL*

**Qualitative and quantitative composition** Each sachet of Movicol contains the following active ingredients:

| | |
|---|---|
| Polyethylene Glycol 3350 USP | 13.125 g |
| Sodium Bicarbonate PhEur | 178.5 mg |
| Sodium Chloride PhEur | 350.7 mg |
| Potassium Chloride PhEur | 46.6 mg |

The content of electrolyte ions per sachet when made up to 125 ml of solution is as follows:

| | |
|---|---|
| Sodium | 65 mM |
| Potassium | 5.4 mM |
| Chloride | 53 mM |
| Bicarbonate | 17 mM |

**Pharmaceutical form** Powder for oral solution.

**Clinical particulars**
*Therapeutic indications:* For the treatment of chronic constipation.

*Posology and method of administration*
*Adults:* 2 or 3 sachets daily in divided doses each reconstituted in 125 ml water and taken orally.
*Elderly:* Initially 1 sachet per day is recommended.
*Children:* Not recommended.

No dosage change need be made for patients with renal insufficiency. As for all laxatives, prolonged use of Movicol is not recommended. A course of treatment with Movicol does not normally exceed two weeks, although this can be repeated if required.

*Contra-indications:* Intestinal perforation or obstruction due to structural or functional disorder of the gut wall, ileus and severe inflammatory conditions of the intestinal tract, such as Crohn's disease, ulcerative colitis and toxic megacolon. Known hypersensitivity to polyethylene glycol.

*Special warnings and special precautions for use:* Mild adverse drug reactions are possible as indicated in *Undesirable effects* below.

*Interaction with other medicaments and other forms of interaction:* No clinical interactions with other medicaments have been reported. Polyethylene glycol raises the solubility of drugs that are soluble in alcohol and relatively insoluble in water. There is therefore a theoretical possibility that the absorption of such drugs could be transiently reduced.

*Pregnancy and lactation:* There is no experience of the use of Movicol during pregnancy and lactation and it should only be used if considered essential by the physician.

*Effects on the ability to drive and use machines:* There is no effect on the ability to drive and use machines.

*Undesirable effects:* Abdominal distension and pain, borborygmi and nausea, attributable to the expansion of the contents of the intestinal tract can occur. Allergic reactions are a possibility.

*Overdose:* Severe pain or distension can be treated by nasogastric aspiration. Extensive fluid loss by diarrhoea or vomiting may require correction of electrolyte disturbances.

**Pharmacological properties**
*Pharmacodynamic properties:* Polyethylene glycol exerts its effects by virtue of its osmotic effect in the gut, which induces a laxative effect. The electrolytes also present in the formulation ensure that there is virtually no net gain or loss of sodium, potassium or water. The laxative action of polyethylene glycol has a time course which will vary according to the severity of the constipation being treated.

*Pharmacokinetic properties:* Polyethylene glycol is unchanged along the gut. It is virtually unabsorbed from the gastro-intestinal tract and has no known pharmacological activity. Any polyethylene glycol that is absorbed is excreted via the urine.

*Preclinical safety data:* Preclinical studies provide evidence that polyethylene glycol 3350 has no significant systemic toxicity potential, although no tests of its effects on reproduction or genotoxicity have been conducted.

**Pharmaceutical particulars**
*List of excipients:* Acesulfame K (E950), lime and lemon flavour.

*Incompatibilities:* None are known.

*Shelf life:* The shelf life is 3 years.

*Special precautions for storage:* Store below 25°C.

*Nature and contents of container:* Sachets containing white powder.

*Instructions for use/handling:* Before administration, the contents of each sachet must be dissolved in 125 ml of water. The reconstituted liquid should not be stored.

**Marketing authorisation number** 0332/0070.

**Date of approval/revision of SPC** September 1996.

**Legal category** P.

## NORGALAX*

**Presentation** Ready-to-use, disposable micro-enema of 10 g liquid containing Docusate Sodium USP 120 mg.

**Uses** Norgalax is indicated for symptomatic treatment of constipation, whenever an enema is required, and for the preparation of the colon and rectum for endoscopic examination. Norgalax is usually effective in 5 to 20 minutes.

**Dosage and administration** For rectal administration. *Adults, elderly and children over 12:* One enema is usually sufficient.
*Children under 12:* Not recommended.

Remove the protective cap, insert the nozzle into the rectum, squeezing gently until the tube is empty. No additional lubricant is needed as a drop of the mixture is sufficient.

**Contra-indications, warnings, etc**
*Contra-indications:* Haemorrhoids, anal fissures, rectocolitis bleeding, abdominal pain, intestinal obstruction, nausea, vomiting and inflammatory bowel disease.

*Use in pregnancy and lactation:* Norgalax may be used in pregnancy and lactation.

*Interactions:* Norgalax may increase the resorption of medicines and is not be used in combination with hepatotoxic agents.

*Side-effects:* Anal or rectal burning and pain, usually short lasting, diarrhoea, congestion of the rectal mucosa, rectal bleeding may occur occasionally. Hepatotoxicity has been described, especially when used in association with other laxatives. As with all laxatives, Norgalax should not be administered chronically. Prolonged use can precipitate the onset of an atonic non-functioning colon and hypokalaemia.

*Overdosage:* Excessive use will lead to excessive purgation, which should be treated symptomatically.

**Pharmaceutical precautions** Store in a cool place, below 25°C.

**Legal category** P.

**Package quantities** Boxes of 6.

**Further information** Norgalax utilises docusate sodium as a faecal softening agent. It is an anionic surfactant which acts by increasing the penetration of fluid into the faeces.

**Product licence number** 0322/0065.

## NORMACOL*

**Presentation** White, coated granules containing Sterculia BP 62%. The coating of the granules also contains sucrose. The product is gluten-free.

**Uses** Treatment of constipation, particularly simple or idiopathic constipation, and constipation arising in pregnancy.
Management of colostomies and ileostomies.
The 'high residue diet' management of diverticular disease of the colon and other conditions requiring a high fibre regime.
The initiation and maintenance of bowel action after rectal and anal surgery.
Administration after ingestion of sharp foreign bodies to provide a coating and reduce the possibility of intestinal damage during transit.

**Dosage and administration** Granules for oral administration.

*Adults:* (including the elderly): 1 or 2 sachets or 1–2 heaped 5 ml spoonfuls, once or twice daily after meals.

*Children (6–12 years):* One half of the above amount.
*Children (under 6 years):* Only at the discretion of the physician.

The granules should be placed dry on the tongue and, without chewing or crushing, swallowed immediately with plenty of liquid (water or a cool drink).

**Contra-indications, warnings, etc**
*Contra-indications:* Intestinal obstruction, faecal impaction, and total atony of the colon.

*Precautions:* Not to be taken immediately before retiring to bed, especially in the elderly. Adequate fluid intake should be maintained. Caution should be exercised in cases of ulcerative colitis.

*Use in pregnancy and lactation:* Normacol is recommended for use during pregnancy or lactation.

*Side-effects:* Occasionally, mild abdominal distension. Oesophageal obstruction is possible if the product is taken in overdosage or if it is not adequately washed down with fluid.

*Overdosage:* Intestinal obstruction is possible in overdosage particularly in combination with inadequate fluid intake. Management is as for intestinal obstruction from other causes.

**Pharmaceutical precautions** Store in a dry place below 25°C.

**Legal category** GSL.

**Package quantities** Packs of 60 sachets, each sachet containing 7 g of granules, or packs of 500 g.

**Further information** Each 7 g sachet of granules contains 1.72 g of available carbohydrate, equivalent to 6.75 kcal.

**Product licence number** 0322/5010.

## NORMACOL* PLUS

**Presentation** Brown, coated granules containing:
Sterculia BP 62%
Frangula BPC 1949 8%

The coating of the granules also contains sucrose and colouring including azo dye. The product is gluten-free.

**Uses** Treatment of constipation, particularly hypotonic or slow transit constipation resistant to bulk alone.

The initiation and maintenance of bowel action after rectal surgery and after haemorrhoidectomy.

**Dosage and administration** Granules for oral administration.

*Adults (including the elderly):* 1 or 2 sachets or 1–2 heaped 5 ml spoonfuls once or twice daily after meals.

*Children (6–12 years):* A reduced amount may be given at the discretion of the physician.

The granules should be placed dry on the tongue and, without chewing or crushing, swallowed immediately with plenty of liquid (water or a cool drink). Prior to drinking they may also be sprinkled onto and taken with soft foods such as yoghurt.

**Contra-indications, warnings, etc**
*Contra-indications:* Intestinal obstruction, faecal impaction, and total atony of the colon.

*Precautions:* Not to be taken immediately before retiring to bed, especially in the elderly. Adequate fluid intake should be maintained. Caution should be exercised in cases of ulcerative colitis. Not to be taken for more than 4 days if there has been no movement of the bowels.

*Use in pregnancy:* No teratogenic effects have been reported, but caution should be exercised during the first trimester of pregnancy.

*Use during lactation:* There is no evidence to suggest that Normacol Plus is unsuitable for use during lactation, though Normacol (sterculia alone) is available, if preferred.

*Side-effects:* Abdominal distension. Intestinal obstruction is possible if the product is taken in overdosage or is not adequately washed down with fluid.

*Overdosage:* Intestinal obstruction is possible in overdosage particularly in combination with inadequate fluid intake. Management is as for intestinal obstruction from other causes.

**Pharmaceutical precautions** Store in a dry place below 25°C.

**Legal category** GSL.

**Package quantities** Packs of 60 sachets, each sachet containing 7 g of granules, or packs of 500 g.

**Further information** Normacol Plus is likely to take about 12 hours to exert its effect. Each 7 g sachet of granules contains 1.72 g of available carbohydrate, equivalent to 6.75 kcal.

**Product licence number** 0322/5011.

## POSALFILIN* OINTMENT

**Qualitative and quantitative composition** Each 10 g tube of Posalfilin Ointment contains 20% w/w Podophyllum Resin BP and 25% w/w Salicylic Acid BP.

**Pharmaceutical form** Dark brown ointment.

**Clinical particulars**
*Therapeutic indications:* For the treatment of plantar warts.

*Posology and method of administration*
*Adults (including the elderly) and Children:* A corn ring should be placed around the wart, cutting the ring to fit if necessary. A minimal amount of ointment should be applied to the exposed wart, taking care to avoid normal skin. The wart and corn ring should be covered with a plaster and the treatment repeated daily. When the wart appears soft and spongy, it should be left exposed and allowed to drop off. If the wart remains, the procedure should be repeated.

*Contra-indications:* Use in pregnancy and breastfeeding mothers. Patients with peripheral neuropathy, diabetes mellitus or peripheral vascular insufficiency.

*Special warnings and special precautions for use:* Misapplication of Posalfilin Ointment to healthy skin may cause inflammation, desquamation or necrosis. Treatment should be suspended if such inflammation occurs. If applied to delicate areas of skin such as in the ano-genital area, the skin may be seriously damaged, depending on the amount applied.

*Interaction with other medicaments and other forms of interaction:* None known.

*Pregnancy and lactation:* Contra-indicated in pregnancy and breastfeeding mothers.

*Effects on the ability to drive and use machines:* There is no effect on the ability to drive and use machines.

*Undesirable effects:* Posalfilin Ointment does not normally cause side effects when used as directed.

*Overdose:* Over-application can cause cutaneous necrosis and should be treated as a caustic burn.

**Pharmacological properties**
*Pharmacodynamic properties:* The salicylic acid macerates the horny layer covering the wart and allows the podophyllum to penetrate the wart where it has a specific cytotoxic effect on the nuclei of the hyperplastic cells.

*Pharmacokinetic properties:* Not applicable, as Posalfilin Ointment applied topically directly to the wart.

*Preclinical safety data:* There are no preclinical data of relevance to the prescriber which are additional to that already included in other sections of the SPC.

**Pharmaceutical particulars**
*List of excipients:* Yellow Soft Paraffin BP; Liquid Paraffin BP.

*Incompatibilities:* None known.

*Shelf life:* The shelf life is 4 years.

*Special precautions for storage:* Store below 25°C.

*Nature and contents of container:* Aluminium tube containing 10 g of ointment.

*Instruction of use/handling:* None.

**Marketing authorisation number** 00322/5901R

**Date of approval/revision of SPC** July 1996.

**Legal category** P

## PYRALVEX*

**Qualitative and quantitative composition** Pyralvex contains the following active ingredients in each 1 ml of solution: Rhubarb extract 50 mg (equivalent to 5 mg anthraquinone glycosides) and Salicylic Acid BP 10 mg.

**Pharmaceutical form** Oromucosal solution.

**Clinical particulars**
*Therapeutic indications:* For the symptomatic relief of pain associated with recurrent mouth ulcers and denture irritation.

*Posology and method of administration*
*Adults (including the elderly):* To be applied to the inflamed oral mucosa (after removing any dentures) three or four times daily using the brush provided.
*Children:* Not recommended below the age of 12 years.

*Contra-indications:* None known.

*Special warnings and special precautions for use:* Each bottle of Pyralvex should be used by only one person.

*Interaction with other medicaments and other forms of interaction:* None known.

*Pregnancy and lactation:* There is no evidence to suggest that Pyralvex should not be used during pregnancy or lactation.

*Effects on the ability to drive and use machines:* None.

*Undesirable effects:* None known.

*Overdose:* Not applicable.

**Pharmacological properties**
*Pharmacodynamic properties:* Pharmacological studies have shown that the active ingredients of Pyralvex display anti-inflammatory, analgesic and anti-microbial properties, which are the basis of its clinical efficacy.

*Pharmacokinetic properties:* Systemic availability of Pyralvex is unlikely to be significant, owing to the low levels of ingredients administered.

*Preclinical safety data:* Preclinical studies indicate that at clinically effective doses, the ingredients in Pyralvex are unlikely to have any potential for toxic effects.

**Pharmaceutical particulars**
*List of excipients:* Ethanol BP; Water.

*Incompatibilities:* None known.

*Shelf life:* The shelf life is 3 years.

*Special precautions for storage:* Store below 25°C.

*Nature and contents of container:* An amber glass bottle with brush applicator containing 10 ml of solution.

*Instructions of use/handling:* Avoid rinsing of the mouth or eating for 15 minutes after application. Any discolouration which may occur will disappear during normal cleaning of the teeth.

**Marketing authorisation number** 00322/5013

**Date of approval/revision of SPC** October 1996.

**Legal category** P

## SOMNITE* SUSPENSION
(Nitrazepam Mixture)

**Presentation** An off-white, translucent, thixotropic suspension with a cherry flavour. Each 5 ml spoonful contains Nitrazepam BP 2.5 mg. The suspension also contains sucrose and mixed esters of p-hydroxybenzoic acid.

**Uses** Short term treatment of insomnia where daytime sedation is acceptable. Benzodiazepines should be used to treat insomnia only when it is severe, disabling, or subjecting the individual to extreme distress. An underlying cause for insomnia should be sought before deciding upon the use of benzodiazepines for symptomatic relief.

**Dosage and administration** Suspension for oral administration. *Adults:* 5 mg (two 5 ml spoonfuls) before retiring. This dose may, if necessary, be increased to 10 mg (four 5 ml spoonfuls).

*Elderly patients:* 2.5 mg (one 5 ml spoonful) before retiring. This dose may, if necessary, be increased to 5 mg (two 5 ml spoonfuls).

*Children:* Not recommended.

The lowest dose which can control the symptoms should be used. It should not be continued beyond four weeks. Long term chronic use is not recommended. Treatment should always be tapered off gradually. Patients who have taken benzodiazepines for a long time may require a longer period during which doses are reduced. When a benzodiazepine is used as a hypnotic, treatment should, if possible, be intermittent.

**Contra-indications, warnings, etc**
*Contra-indications:* Known sensitivity to benzodiazepines. Acute pulmonary insufficiency.

*Precautions:* Chronic pulmonary insufficiency. In chronic renal or hepatic disease. In labour. High single doses or repeated low doses have been reported to produce hypotonia, poor sucking and hypothermia in the neonate and irregularities in the foetal heart. Avoid if possible in lactation. The concurrent use of other CNS depressant drugs should be avoided. Benzodiazepines should not be used alone to treat depression or anxiety associated with depression. Suicide may be precipitated in such patients. They should not be used for phobic or obsessional states. They should not be used for the treatment of chronic psychosis. In cases of loss or bereavement, psychological adjustment may be inhibited by benzodiazepines. Disinhibiting effects may be manifested in various ways. Suicide may be precipitated in patients who are depressed, and aggressive behaviour towards self and others may be precipitated. Extreme caution should therefore be used in prescribing benzodiazepines in patients with personality disorders.

*Pregnancy and lactation:* If the product is prescribed to a woman of childbearing potential, she should be warned to contact her physician regarding discontinuance of the product if she intends to become or suspects that she is pregnant.

If, for compelling medical reasons, the product is administered during the late phase of pregnancy, or during labour at high doses, effects on the neonate, such as hypothermia, hypotonia and moderate respiratory depression, can be expected, due to the pharmacological action of the compound.

Moreover, infants born to mothers who took benzodiazepines chronically during the latter stages of pregnancy may have developed physical dependence and may be at some risk for developing withdrawal symptoms in the postnatal period.

Since benzodiazepines are found in the breast milk, benzodiazepines should not be given to breast feeding mothers.

*Side-effects:* Common adverse effects include drowsiness, sedation, blurring of vision, unsteadiness and ataxia. These effects occur following single as well as repeated dosage and may persist well into the following day. Performance at skilled tasks and alertness may be impaired. Patients should be warned of this hazard and advised not to drive or operate machinery during treatment. These effects are potentiated by alcohol. The elderly are particularly liable to experience these symptoms together with confusion especially if organic brain symptoms are present. See also Dependence Potential and Withdrawal Symptoms below.

Abnormal psychological reactions to benzodiazepines have been reported. Behavioural adverse effects include paradoxical aggressive outbursts, excitement, confusion, and the uncovering of depression with suicidal tendencies.

Other rare adverse effects including hypotension, gastrointestinal and visual disturbances, skin rashes, urinary retention, headache, vertigo, changes in libido; blood dyscrasias and jaundice have also been reported.

*Dependence potential and withdrawal symptoms:* In general the dependence potential of benzodiazepines is low but this increases when high dosages are attained, especially when given over long periods. This is particularly so in patients with a history of alcoholism, drug abuse or in patients with marked personality disorders. Regular monitoring of treatment in such patients is essential and routine repeat prescriptions should be avoided.

Treatment in all patients should be withdrawn gradually. Withdrawal from benzodiazepines may be associated with physiological and psychological symptoms of withdrawal including depression, nervousness, rebound insomnia, irritability, sweating and diarrhoea. Withdrawal symptoms occur with benzodiazepines following normal therapeutic doses given for short periods of time.

Abrupt withdrawal following excessive dosage may produce confusion, toxic psychosis, convulsions or a condition resembling delirium tremens.

*Overdosage:* The primary symptoms of overdosage are drowsiness, dizziness, ataxia and slurred speech.

Treatment is symptomatic but gastric lavage may be useful if performed soon after ingestion.

**Pharmaceutical precautions** Somnite suspension should be stored in a cool place, protected from light. Avoid freezing.

**Legal category** CD (Sch 4) POM.

**Package quantities** Bottles of 150 ml

**Further information** Nil.

**Product licence number** 0322/0039.

## SPASMONAL*

**Presentation** Blue/grey, opaque, hard gelatin capsules, marked '78' on one half and with a sailing boat design on the other. Each capsule contains 60 mg Alverine Citrate.

**Uses** Smooth muscle spasmolytic effective on smooth muscle of the alimentary tract and uterus. Spasmonal is indicated for use in the relief of smooth muscle spasm, in conditions such as irritable bowel syndrome, painful diverticular disease of the colon, primary dysmenorrhoea.

**Dosage and administration** Capsules for oral administration.

*Adults (including the elderly):* 1 or 2 capsules one to three times daily.

*Children (below the age of 12 years):* Not recommended.

### Contra-indications, warnings, etc
*Contra-indications:* Paralytic ileus or known hypersensitivity to any of the ingredients.

*Precautions:* None known.

*Use in pregnancy:* Not recommended during pregnancy and lactation.

*Side-effects:* Possible side-effects may include nausea, headache, itching, rash, dizziness and allergic reaction.

*Overdosage:* Can produce hypotension and atropine-like toxic effects. Management is as for atropine poisoning with supportive therapy for hypotension.

**Pharmaceutical precautions** Store in a cool, dry place below 25°C.

**Legal category** P.

**Package quantities** Packs of 100 capsules.

**Further information** Alverine citrate is a synthetic, non-narcotic, non-habit-forming spasmolytic of a low order of toxicity in comparison with other antispasmodics. It is selectively active on the smooth muscle of the intestine and uterus, but not on those of the respiratory or cardiovascular system.

**Product licence number** 0322/5014.

## WAXSOL* EAR DROPS

**Qualitative and quantitative composition** Waxsol Ear Drops contain the following active ingredient: Docusate Sodium BP 0.5% w/v.

**Pharmaceutical form** Ear drops.

### Clinical particulars
*Therapeutic indications:* Waxsol Ear Drops are indicated as an aid in the removal of ear wax.

*Posology and method of administration:* Recommended dose and dosage schedules:

*Adults (including the elderly):* The application of ear drops sufficient to fill the affected ear on not more than two consecutive nights, prior to attending syringing if this is necessary.

*Children:* As for adult dose.

*Contra-indications:* Perforation of the ear drum or inflammation of the ear.

*Special warnings and special precautions for use:* If pain or inflammation is experienced, treatment should be discontinued.

*Interaction with other medicaments and other forms of interaction:* None known.

*Pregnancy and lactation:* There is no evidence to suggest that Waxsol Ear Drops should not be used during pregnancy and lactation.

*Effects on ability to drive and use machines:* None known.

*Undesirable effects:* Rarely, transient stinging or irritation may occur.

*Overdose:* None known.

**Pharmacological properties** The so-called 'wax' which often obstructs the external auditory meatus of the ear contains less than 50% of fatty matter derived from secretions of the sebaceous ceruminous glands. The majority of the wax consists of desquamated epithelium, foreign matter and shed hairs. This non-fatty material forms a matrix holding together the granules of fatty matter to form the ceruminous mass.

The addition of oils or solvents binds the mass more firmly together, but aqueous solutions, if they are able to penetrate the matrix, cause a disintegration of the ceruminous mass.

Waxsol Ear Drops, because of their low surface tension and miscibility, rapidly penetrate the dry matrix of the ceruminous mass, reducing the solid material to a semi-solid debris. This can be syringed away readily, or in less severe or chronic cases, is ejected by normal physiological processes.

### Pharmaceutical particulars
*List of excipients:* Glycerine BP; Phenonip (solution of esters of 4-hydroxybenzoic acid in phenoxetol); water.

*Incompatibilities:* None known.

*Shelf life:* The shelf life is 3 years.

*Special precautions for storage:* Store below 25°C.

*Nature and contents of container:* Amber glass bottle of 10 ml capacity with a dropper applicator.

*Instructions for use/handling:* The dropper applicator must be filled before dripping Waxsol Ear Drops into the affected ear.

**Marketing authorisation number** 00322/5016.

**Date of approval/revision of SPC** June 1995.

**Legal category** P.

*Trade Mark

**Novartis Consumer Health**
Wimblehurst Road
Horsham
West Sussex RH12 4AB

⊍ NOVARTIS

## EURAX* CREAM

**Qualitative and quantitative composition** Crotamiton BP 10%.

**Pharmaceutical form** Topical cream.

**Clinical particulars**

*Therapeutic indications:* (1) For the relief of itching and skin irritation caused by, for example sunburn, dry eczema, itchy dermatitis, allergic rashes, hives, nettle rash, chickenpox, insect bites and stings, heat rashes and personal itching.
(2) The treatment of scabies.

*Posology and method of administration:* For cutaneous use.

*Recommended dose and dosage schedules*
PRURITUS: *Adults (including the elderly) and children:* Apply to the affected area 2–3 times daily. Eurax will provide relief from irritation for 6–10 hours after each application. Eurax can be used in children. There are no special dosage recommendations in the elderly.

SCABIES: *Adults (including the elderly):* After the patient has taken a warm bath, the skin should be well dried and Eurax rubbed into the entire body surface (excluding the face and scalp) until no traces of the preparation remain visible on the surface. The application should be repeated once daily, preferably in the evening, for a total of 3–5 days. Depending on the response, special attention should be paid to sites that are particularly susceptible to infestation by the mites (e.g. interdigital spaces, wrists, axillae and genitalia). Areas where there is pus formation should be covered with a dressing impregnated with Eurax. While the treatment is in progress the patient may take a bath shortly before the next application. After completion of the treatment, a cleansing bath should be taken followed by a change of bed linen and underclothing.

*Children:* Application as described for adults but in children under 3 years of age Eurax should not be applied more than once a day.

*Contra-indications:* Acute exudative dermatoses. Hypersensitivity to any of the ingredients. Eurax should not be used in or around the eyes since contact with the eyelids may give rise to conjunctival inflammation.

*Special warnings and special precautions for use:* Eurax can be used for children; consult your doctor before use on children under 3 years of age.
  For external use only.
  Do not use in or around the eyes, on broken skin, for weeping skin conditions or if you are sensitive to any of the ingredients.
  Keep all medicines out of the reach of children.
  Consult your doctor or pharmacist before using Eurax if you are pregnant or breast feeding, or suffering from genital itching.
  If symptoms persist consult your doctor.

*Interactions with other medicaments and other forms of interaction:* None.

*Pregnancy and lactation:* There is no experience to judge the safety of Eurax in pregnancy, therefore Eurax is not recommended during pregnancy, especially in the first three months. It is not known whether the active substance passes into breast milk. Nursing mothers should avoid applying Eurax in the area of the nipples.

*Effect on ability to drive and use machines:* None.

*Undesirable effects:* Occasionally irritation of the skin or contact allergy may occur. In such cases the preparation should be discontinued.

*Overdose:* Eurax is for application to the skin only. Following accidental ingestion, nausea, vomiting and irritation of the buccal, oesophageal and gastric mucosa have been reported. If accidental ingestion of large quantities occurs, there is no specific antidote and general measures to eliminate the drug and reduce its absorption should be undertaken. Symptomatic treatment should be administered as appropriate. A risk of methaemoglobinaemia exists, which may be treated with methylene blue.

**Pharmacological properties**

*Pharmacodynamic properties:* Eurax has a symptomatic action on pruritus and is an acaricide.

*Pharmacokinetic properties:* Eurax penetrates rapidly into human skin. Low but measurable concentrations of crotamiton are found in plasma, with a maximum level after 4–10 hours, declining rapidly thereafter.

*Preclinical safety data:* Eurax cream administered dermally once daily under occlusive dressing for 3 months to rabbits was tolerated at doses of up to 250 mg/kg without signs of toxicity, apart from transient skin irritation. No sensitising or photo-sensitising potential has been observed in animal studies. Crotamiton does not induce mutations in bacteria nor chromosomal damage in mammalian cells. Studies to detect a possible effect on fertility and reproductive behaviour also gave negative results.

**Pharmaceutical particulars**

*List of excipients:* Methyl hydroxybenzoate, phenylethyl alcohol, glycerol, triethanolamine, sodium lauryl sulphate, ethylene glycol monostearate, stearyl alcohol, strong ammonia solution, stearic acid, hard paraffin, white beeswax, perfume, purified water.

*Incompatibilities:* None.

*Shelf life:* 5 years.

*Special precautions for storage:* Protect from heat.

*Nature and contents of container:* Internally lacquered aluminium tube, with a screw cap, in a cardboard carton.

*Instructions for use/handling:* Medicines should be kept out of the reach of children.

*Marketing authorisation holder:* Ciba-Geigy PLC, Macclesfield SK10 2NX.

**Marketing authorisation number** 0001/5008R.

**Date of approval/revision of SPC** March 1997.

**Legal category** GSL.

## EURAX* LOTION

**Qualitative and quantitative composition** Crotamiton BP 10%.

**Pharmaceutical form** Topical lotion.

**Clinical particulars**

*Therapeutic indications:* (1) For the relief of itching and skin irritation caused by, for example sunburn, dry eczema, itchy dermatitis, allergic rashes, hives, nettle rash, chickenpox, insect bites and stings, heat rashes and personal itching.
(2) The treatment of scabies.

*Posology and method of administration:* For cutaneous use.

*Recommended dose and dosage schedules*
PRURITUS: *Adults (including the elderly) and children:* Apply to the affected area 2–3 times daily. Eurax will provide relief from irritation for 6–10 hours after each application. Eurax can be used in children. There are no special dosage recommendations in the elderly.

SCABIES: *Adults (including the elderly):* After the patient has taken a warm bath, the skin should be well dried and Eurax rubbed into the entire body surface (excluding the face and scalp) until no traces of the preparation remain visible on the surface. The application should be repeated once daily, preferably in the evening, for a total of 3–5 days. Depending on the response, special attention should be paid to sites that are particularly susceptible to infestation by the mites (e.g. interdigital spaces, wrists, axillae and genitalia). Areas where there is pus formation should be covered with a dressing impregnated with Eurax. While the treatment is in progress the patient may take a bath shortly before the next application. After completion of the treatment, a cleansing bath should be taken followed by a change of bed linen and underclothing.

*Children:* Application as described for adults but in children under 3 years of age Eurax should not be applied more than once a day.

*Contra-indications:* Acute exudative dermatoses. Hypersensitivity to any of the ingredients. Eurax should not be used in or around the eyes since contact with the eyelids may give rise to conjunctival inflammation.

*Special warnings and special precautions for use:* Eurax can be used for children; consult your doctor before use on children under 3 years of age.
  For external use only.
  Do not use in or around the eyes, on broken skin, for weeping skin conditions or if you are sensitive to any of the ingredients.
  Keep all medicines out of the reach of children.
  Consult your doctor or pharmacist before using Eurax if you are pregnant or breast feeding, or suffering from genital itching.
  If symptoms persist consult your doctor.

*Interactions with other medicaments and other forms of interaction:* None.

*Pregnancy and lactation:* There is no experience to judge the safety of Eurax in pregnancy, therefore Eurax is not recommended during pregnancy, especially in the first three months. It is not known whether the active substance passes into breast milk. Nursing mothers should avoid applying Eurax in the area of the nipples.

*Effect on ability to drive and use machines:* None.

*Undesirable effects:* Occasionally irritation of the skin or contact allergy may occur. In such cases the preparation should be discontinued.

*Overdose:* Eurax is for application to the skin only. Following accidental ingestion, nausea, vomiting and irritation of the buccal, oesophageal and gastric mucosa have been reported. If accidental ingestion of large quantities occurs, there is no specific antidote and general measures to eliminate the drug and reduce its absorption should be undertaken. Symptomatic treatment should be administered as appropriate. A risk of methaemoglobinaemia exists, which may be treated with methylene blue.

**Pharmacological properties**

*Pharmacodynamic properties:* Eurax has a symptomatic action on pruritus and is an acaricide.

*Pharmacokinetic properties:* Eurax penetrates rapidly into human skin. Low but measurable concentrations of crotamiton are found in plasma, with a maximum level after 4–10 hours, declining rapidly thereafter.

*Preclinical safety data:* Eurax cream administered dermally once daily under occlusive dressing for 3 months to rabbits was tolerated at doses of up to 250 mg/kg without signs of toxicity, apart from transient skin irritation. No sensitising or photo-sensitising potential has been observed in animal studies. Crotamiton does not induce mutations in bacteria nor chromosomal damage in mammalian cells. Studies to detect a possible effect on fertility and reproductive behaviour also gave negative results.

**Pharmaceutical particulars**

*List of excipients:* Glyceryl monostearate, cetomacrogol, cetyl alcohol, stearyl alcohol, sodium cetearyl sulphate, 2-octyl dodecanol, sorbic acid, citric acid, phenylethyl alcohol, propylene glycol, perfume, purified water.

*Incompatibilities:* None.

*Shelf life:* 5 years.

*Special precautions for storage:* Protect from heat.

*Nature and contents of container:* Amber glass bottle with cap-to-cap closure in cardboard carton. Pack sizes 100, 150 and 1000 ml.
  Amber glass bottle with wadless polypropylene cap in cardboard carton. Pack sizes 100 and 150 ml.

*Instructions for use/handling:* Medicines should be kept out of the reach of children.

*Marketing authorisation holder:* Ciba-Geigy PLC, Macclesfield SK10 2NX.

**Marketing authorisation number** 0001/5009R.

**Date of approval/revision of SPC** March 1997.

**Legal category** GSL.

## EURAX*-HYDROCORTISONE

**Presentation** White to cream coloured soft cream with a faint odour of perfume, containing Crotamiton BP 10% and Hydrocortisone BP 0.25%.
  Also contains: methyl hydroxybenzoate, propyl hydroxybenzoate, polyoxyl 40 stearate, propylene glycol, stearyl alcohol, white soft paraffin, and perfume.

**Uses**

*Mode of action:* Eurax-Hydrocortisone combines the

antipruritic action of crotamiton with the anti-inflammatory and anti-allergic properties of hydrocortisone.

*Indications:* Eczema and dermatitis of all types including atopic eczema, photodermatitis, otitis externa, primary irritant and allergic dermatitis, intertrigo, prurigo nodularis, seborrhoeic dermatitis and insect bite reactions.

**Dosage and administration** Eurax-Hydrocortisone is indicated for external application only.

*Method of application:* A thin layer of Eurax-Hydrocortisone cream should be applied to the affected area 2–3 times a day. Occlusive dressings should not be used. Treatment should be limited to 10–14 days or up to 7 days if applied to the face.

*Use in the elderly:* Clinical evidence would indicate that no special dosage regime is necessary.

*Use in children:* Eurax-Hydrocortisone should be used with caution in infants and for not more than 7 days. Eurax-Hydrocortisone should not be applied more than once a day to large areas of the body surface in young children.

**Contra-indications, warnings, etc**

*Contra-indications:* Hypersensitivity to any component of the formulation. Bacterial, viral or fungal infections of the skin. Acute exudative dermatoses. Application to ulcerated areas.

*Precautions:* Eurax-Hydrocortisone should be used with caution in infants and for not more than 7 days; long-term continuous topical therapy should be avoided since this can lead to adrenal suppression even without occlusion.

Eurax-Hydrocortisone should not be allowed to come into contact with the conjunctiva and mucous membranes.

*Side-effects:* Occasionally at the site of application signs of irritation such as a burning sensation, itching, contact dermatitis/contact allergy may occur. Treatment should be discontinued if patients experience severe irritation or sensitisation.

*Use in pregnancy and lactation:* There is inadequate evidence of safety in human pregnancy. Topical administration of corticosteroids to pregnant animals can cause abnormalities of foetal development, including cleft palate and intra-uterine growth retardation. There may therefore be a very small risk of such effects in the human foetus.

It is not known whether the active substances of Eurax-Hydrocortisone and/or their metabolite(s) pass into the breast milk after topical administration. Use in lactating mothers should only be at the doctor's discretion.

*Overdosage:* Eurax-Hydrocortisone cream is for application to the skin only. If accidental ingestion of large quantities occurs, there is no specific antidote and general measures to eliminate the drug and reduce its absorption should be undertaken. Symptomatic treatment should be administered as appropriate.

**Pharmaceutical precautions** Protect from heat. Dilution of or addition to this formulation is not recommended.

**Legal category** POM.

**Package quantities** Tubes of 30 g (OP).

**Further information** Nil.

**Product licence number** 0001/0158.

## LACTITOL*

**Presentation** Lactitol is a white, crystalline, slightly sweet tasting powder composed of lactitol monohydrate. There are no other ingredients.

**Uses**

*Mode of action:* Lactitol is a disaccharide derivative consisting of galactose and sorbitol which is only minimally absorbed and is not hydrolysed by the disaccharidases of the gastrointestinal tract and thus reaches the colon unchanged. In the colon it is broken down to short chain organic acids, mainly acetic, propionic and butyric acid, by the intestinal flora, in particular by the bacteroides and lactobacilli, thus acidifying the contents of the colon. The effect of this acidification is to reduce the absorption of ammonia. It also seems that the above-mentioned bacteria prefer Lactitol to amino acids: an in-vitro faecal incubation study has shown that the presence of Lactitol reduces the production of ammonia by bacteria.

The transformation of Lactitol into low molecular weight organic acids results in an increase in osmotic pressure in the colon, thereby causing an increase in the stool water content and stool volume, which explains the laxative effect.

Lactitol produces its effect in the lumen of the colon, where it is virtually 100% bioavailable. It is absorbed only in minimal amounts. Up to 2% can be found unchanged in the urine.

*Indications:* Constipation. Acute and chronic portal systemic encephalopathy.

**Dosage and administration** For oral administration. It can be mixed with hot or cold beverages, cereals, puddings, etc. Due to variations in individual patient response the dosage will require adjustment to obtain one daily bowel movement in constipated patients and two daily bowel movements in patients with portal systemic encephalopathy.

*Constipation:* Lactitol should be given in a single daily dose, in the morning or in the evening, at meal times, mixed with food or drink. The choice between morning or evening intake should be left to the patient, according to the individual response: the laxative effect has been found mostly to occur within a few hours after intake.

Patients should be informed that in some cases the first laxative response may be delayed until the second or third day of administration. Patients should be advised to maintain an adequate daily fluid intake.

*Adults (including the elderly):* The initial daily dosage should be 20 g (two 10 g sachets) taken in a single dose with the morning or evening meal. After a few days, a daily dose of 10 g (one sachet) may be sufficient for many patients.

*Children:* The mean dosage is 0.25 g/kg body weight daily, e.g.:

| | | |
|---|---|---|
| 1 to 6 years old: | $\frac{1}{4}$ to $\frac{1}{2}$ sachet daily | (2.5 to 5 g). |
| 6 to 12 years old: | $\frac{1}{2}$ to 1 sachet daily | (5 to 10 g). |
| 12 to 16 years old: | 1 to 2 sachets daily | (10 to 20 g). |

In all cases dosage should be individually adjusted to obtain one daily bowel movement.

*Portal systemic encephalopathy:* The dosage should be adjusted according to the severity of the patient's disease and their individual response. The initial recommended dose is 0.5 to 0.7 g/kg body weight daily, divided into three daily doses with meals. The dosage should then be adjusted to produce two soft bowel movements daily.

To obtain a 40% solution for administration by nasogastric tube if required, in patients with acute portal systemic encephalopathy proceed as follows: add 200 g of lactitol monohydrate to 200 ml of hot distilled water, stirring continuously. When dissolved, complete to a final volume of 500 ml with cold distilled water. This solution can be given by nasogastric tube at a dosage of 1 to 2 ml/kg body weight daily (corresponding to 0.4 to 0.8 g/kg). Unused solution should be disposed of in the normal manner.

**Contra-indications, warnings, etc**

*Contra-indications:* In common with other laxatives, Lactitol should not be used in patients with intestinal obstruction, where an underlying organic lesion of the gastrointestinal tract is suspected, or in cases of unexplained abdominal pain or bleeding. Faecal impaction should be treated by alternative methods prior to using Lactitol.

Lactitol is not recommended for use in patients with galactosaemia.

*Precautions:* To avoid disturbances of electrolyte balance which may occur as a result of overdose-induced diarrhoea, the doctor should try, from the beginning of the treatment, to determine the optimal dosage (see 'Dosage and Administration') to achieve one daily bowel movement in constipated patients and two daily bowel movements in cirrhotic patients.

Elderly or debilitated patients receiving long-term treatment with Lactitol should have their serum electrolytes monitored regularly.

As for all laxatives, pre-existing fluid or electrolyte imbalance should be corrected before starting treatment with Lactitol.

Following treatment with Lactitol, hydrogen may accumulate in the bowel. Patients who need to undergo electrocauterisation procedures should therefore have a thorough bowel cleansing with a non-fermentable solution.

Patients who complain of nausea should be advised to take Lactitol with a meal.

Lactitol is not recommended in cases of ileostomy or colostomy.

Prolonged use of laxatives without interruption should be avoided.

All cases of chronic constipation should first be treated by a fibre-rich diet, intake of liquids or physical activity.

*Interactions:* Antacids and neomycin, as they can neutralise the stool acidifying effect of Lactitol, should not be given simultaneously with Lactitol to cirrhotic patients with portal systemic encephalopathy. Antacids and neomycin do not alter the laxative effect in constipated patients.

Like all laxatives, Lactitol may increase the potassium loss caused by other drugs e.g. thiazide diuretics, corticosteroids, carbenoxolone, amphotericin B. Potassium deficiency may enhance the risk of toxic effects of glycosides in patients receiving concomitant therapy.

Lactitol monohydrate has a calorific value of 2 kcal/g (8.5 KJ/g) and has no effect on blood glucose levels. It can therefore be given to diabetic patients.

*Use in pregnancy and lactation:* At present there is inadequate evidence of safety in human pregnancy. Therefore, it is recommended that, during the first trimester of pregnancy, Lactitol should only be used if there is no safer alternative.

Although the passage of Lactitol into breast milk has not been studied, it appears unlikely to have any clinical relevance since it is only minimally absorbed.

*Side-effects:* At the start of treatment Lactitol may produce abdominal discomfort such as meteorism and flatulence, pain, cramps or sensation of fullness. In clinical trials these untoward effects were observed in about 25% of adult patients and 35% of elderly patients. Such effects tend to diminish or disappear after a few days of regular intake of Lactitol. Occasionally, nausea, borborygmi or anal pruritus have been reported as well as vomiting in rare cases. Because of inter-individual variation, some patients may experience diarrhoea at the recommended dosage. A reduction in dosage will overcome this.

*Overdosage:* Doses of up to 72 g/day in portal systemic encephalopathy and up to 40 g/day in constipation have been tolerated in some patients. The sign of overdosage is diarrhoea, which can be stopped by decreasing the dosage. It may also result in an alteration of serum electrolytes which may need correcting.

**Pharmaceutical precautions** No special precautions.

**Legal category** P.

**Package quantities** Sachets: packs of 10 sachets, each sachet containing 10 g of lactitol monohydrate powder.

**Further information** Nil.

**Product licence number** 0030/0062.

## LOCORTEN*-VIOFORM* EAR DROPS

**Presentation** A clear, yellowish solution containing 1% w/v Clioquinol BP and 0.02% w/v flumethasone pivalate. Also contains: polyethylene glycol.

**Uses**

*Mode of action:* Locorten-Vioform Ear Drops combine the anti-bacterial and anti-fungal properties of clioquinol with the anti-inflammatory activity of flumethasone pivalate.

*Indications:* Inflammatory conditions of the external ear where a secondary infection is suspected. Otorrhoea.

**Dosage and administration**

*Method of application:* Instil 2 or 3 drops twice daily directly into the auditory canal of the affected ear. Treatment should be limited to 7–10 days.

If there is little improvement after 7 days treatment with Locorten-Vioform, appropriate microbiological investigations should be carried out and local or systemic antibiotic treatment given.

*Use in the elderly:* There is no evidence to suggest that dosage should be different in the elderly.

*Use in children:* Locorten-Vioform Ear Drops are contra-indicated in children below the age of two years.

**Contra-indications, warnings, etc**

*Contra-indications:* Hypersensitivity to any component of the formulation, or iodine. Primary bacterial, viral or fungal infections of the outer ear. Perforation of the tympanic membrane. Use in children below the age of two years.

*Precautions:* Long-term continuous topical therapy should be avoided since this can lead to adrenal suppression.

Topical application of clioquinol-containing preparations may lead to a marked increase in protein-bound iodine (PBI). The results of thyroid function tests, such as PBI, radioactive iodine and butanol extractable iodine may be affected. However, other thyroid function tests, such as the $T_3$ resin sponge test or $T_4$ determination, are unaffected.

The ferric chloride test for phenylketonuria may yield a false-positive result when clioquinol is present in the urine.

Locorten-Vioform should not be allowed to come into contact with the conjunctiva.

*Side-effects:* Locorten-Vioform is generally well tolerated, but occasionally, at the site of application, there may be signs of irritation such as a burning sensation, itching, or skin rash. Hypersensitivity reactions may also occasionally occur. Treatment should be discontinued if patients experience severe irritation or sensitisation.

Locorten-Vioform may cause hair discolouration.

*Use in pregnancy and lactation:* There is inadequate evidence of safety in human pregnancy. Topical administration of corticosteroids to pregnant animals can cause abnormalities of foetal development, including cleft palate and intra-uterine growth retardation. There may therefore be a very small risk of such effects in the human foetus.

It is not known whether the active substances of Locorten-Vioform and/or their metabolite(s) pass into breast milk after topical administration. Use in lactating mothers should only be at the doctor's discretion.

*Overdosage:* Locorten-Vioform is for topical (external) use only. If accidental ingestion of large quantities occurs, there is no specific antidote and general measures to eliminate the drug and reduce its absorption should be undertaken. Symptomatic treatment should be administered as appropriate.

**Pharmaceutical precautions**  No special precautions.

**Legal category**  POM.

**Package quantities**  7.5 ml dropper bottles (OP).

**Further information**  Clothing stained with Locorten-Vioform should be washed immediately or soaked overnight.

**Product licence number**  0030/0049.

## NICOTINELL* ORIGINAL CHEWING GUM 2 mg

**Qualitative and quantitative composition**  Nicotine 2 mg per gum in a resin complex.

**Pharmaceutical form**  Chewing gum.

### Clinical particulars

*Therapeutic indications:* Nicotinell treatment is indicated for the relief of nicotine withdrawal symptoms, in nicotine dependency as an aid to smoking cessation.

*Posology and method of administration*

*Adults and elderly:* Users should stop smoking completely during treatment with Nicotinell gum. One piece of Nicotinell gum to be chewed when the user feels the urge to smoke.

Normally, 8–12 pieces per day, up to a maximum of 25 pieces per day.

*Directions for use:* 1.  One piece of gum should be chewed until the taste becomes strong.

2.  The chewing gum should be rested between the gum and cheek.

3.  When the taste fades, chewing should commence again.

4.  The chewing routine should be repeated for 30 minutes.

After three months, the user should gradually cut down the number of pieces chewed each day until they have stopped using the product.

*Children:* Not to be used by children.

Concomitant use of acidic beverages such as coffee or soda may interfere with the buccal absorption of nicotine. Acidic beverages should be avoided for 15 minutes prior to chewing the gum.

*Contra-indications:* Nicotinell gum should not be used by non-smokers or people under 18 years of age. Furthermore, people should not use the gum and smoke concomitantly.

Use is contra-indicated during pregnancy and lactation, acute myocardial infarction, unstable or worsening angina pectoris, severe cardiac arrhythmias, and recent cerebrovascular accident.

*Special warnings and precautions for use:* Swallowed nicotine may exacerbate symptoms in subjects suffering from active oesophagitis, oral or pharyngeal inflammation, gastritis or peptic ulcer.

Use with caution in patients with hypertension, stable angina pectoris, cerebrovascular disease, occlusive peripheral arterial disease, heart failure, hyperthyroidism, diabetes mellitus, and renal or hepatic impairment.

Counselling may help smokers to quit.

Doses of nicotine that are tolerated by adult smokers during treatment may produce severe symptoms of poisoning in small children and may prove fatal (please see *Overdose*).

*Interactions with other medicaments and other forms of interaction:*

*Drug interactions:* No information is available on interactions between Nicotinell gum and other drugs.

*Smoking cessation:* This is different in the case of smoking where interactions with other medications may occur due to a multitude of other substances contained in the smoke. Presumably due to the polycyclic aromatic hydrocarbons contained in the smoke, the metabolism of different medicinal products may be speeded up by enzyme induction: e.g. caffeine, theophylline, paracetamol, phenazone, phenylbutazone, pentazocine, lidocaine, benzodiazepines, imipramine, warfarin, oestrogen and vitamin B12.

Upon smoking cessation it may be expected that the hitherto increased metabolism of these medicinal products is slowed down or normalised. Unaltered dosage of the products may result in an increase in their blood concentration.

Therefore when prescribing Nicotinell a possible dose adjustment should be considered in patients treated with the above mentioned medicinal products.

Other reported effects of smoking include a reduction of the analgesic effects of propoxyphene, reduced diuretic response to frusemide, change in the pharmacological effect of propranolol and altered responder rates in ulcer hearing with $H_2$-antagonists.

Smoking and nicotine may raise the blood levels of cortisol and catecholamines. Dose adjustment of nifedipine, adrenergic agonists or adrenergic antagonists may be necessary.

Increased subcutaneous absorption of insulin which occurs upon smoking cessation may necessitate a reduction in insulin dose.

*Pregnancy and lactation:* In common with medical advice on stopping smoking in these situations, Nicotinell gum is contra-indicated in pregnant women and during breast feeding.

Reproductive toxicity studies with nicotine in several animal studies have demonstrated non-specific retardation of foetal growth. Studies in rats produced evidence of decreased fertility, prolonged pregnancy, and behavioural disorders in the offspring. In mice the offspring of animals exposed to very high doses of nicotine showed skeletal defects in the peripheral parts of the limbs.

Overall, there are no clear cut grounds for believing that nicotine at the concentrations reached by treatment with nicotine gum has any teratogenic potential and/or inhibitory effects on fertility.

*Effects on ability to drive and use machines:* Smoking cessation can cause behavioural changes. There is no evidence of any risks associated with driving or operating machinery when the gum is used following the recommended use.

*Undesirable effects:* In principle, Nicotinell gum can cause adverse reactions similar to those associated with nicotine administered by smoking.

Nicotine from gum may sometimes cause a slight irritation of the throat and increase salivation at the start of treatment. Excessive swallowing of dissolved nicotine may, at first, cause hiccuping. Those with a tendency to indigestion may suffer initially from minor indigestion or heartburn. Slower chewing will usually overcome this problem. Excessive consumption of gum by subjects who have not been in the habit of inhaling tobacco smoke could possibly lead to nausea, faintness or headaches.

*Overdose:* In overdose, symptoms corresponding to heavy smoking may be seen.

The acute lethal oral dose of nicotine is about 0.5–0.75 mg per kg body weight, corresponding in an adult to 40–60 mg. Even small quantities of nicotine are dangerous in children, and may result in severe symptoms of poisoning which may prove fatal. If poisoning in suspected in a child, a doctor must be consulted immediately.

Overdose with Nicotinell gum may only occur if many pieces are chewed simultaneously. Risk of overdose is small as nausea or vomiting usually occurs at an early stage. Risk of poisoning by swallowing the gum is small. Since the release of nicotine from the gum is slow, very little nicotine is absorbed from the stomach and intestine, and if any is, it will be inactivated in the liver.

General symptoms of nicotine poisoning include: weakness, perspiration, salivation, throat burn, nausea, vomiting, diarrhoea, abdominal pain, hearing and visual disturbances, headache, tachycardia and cardiac arrhythmia, dyspnoea, prostration, circulatory collapse, coma and terminal convulsions.

*Treatment of overdosage:* In the event of overdosage, vomiting should be induced with syrup of ipecacuanha or gastric lavage carried out (wide bore tube). A suspension of activated charcoal should then be passed through the tube and left in the stomach. Artificial respiration with oxygen should be instituted if needed and continued for as long as necessary. Other therapy, including treatment of shock, is purely symptomatic.

### Pharmacological properties

*Pharmacodynamic properties:* Nicotine gum mimics the pharmacological effects of nicotine from smoking, and may therefore be used to help provide relief from nicotine withdrawal symptoms. In addition to effects on the central nervous system, nicotine produces haemodynamic effects such as increased heart rate and systolic blood pressure.

*Pharmacokinetic properties:* When the gum is chewed, nicotine is steadily released into the mouth and is rapidly absorbed through the buccal mucosa. A proportion, by the swallowing of nicotine containing saliva, reaches the stomach and intestine where it is inactivated.

The peak plasma concentration of the 2 mg gum after a single dose is approximately 4.8 nanograms per ml and following steady state administration is approximately 14 nanograms per ml (average plasma concentration of nicotine when smoking a cigarette is 15–30 nanograms per ml). Following chewing of a single 4 mg gum, peak plasma concentration of approximately 10 nanograms per ml is reached after about 30 minutes.

Nicotine is eliminated mainly via hepatic metabolism; small amounts of nicotine are eliminated in unchanged form via the kidneys. The plasma half-life is approximately three hours. Nicotine crosses the blood-brain barrier, the placenta and is detectable in breast milk.

*Pre-clinical safety data:* No animal studies have been undertaken on Nicotinell Chewing Gum.

The toxicity of nicotine as a constituent of tobacco has been well documented. Acute toxic effects include convulsions, cardiac insufficiency, and paralysis of the respiratory system.

At high doses in cats and dogs, nicotine has been shown to potentiate histamine-induced peptic ulcer.

All excipients used in Nicotinell Chewing Gum are of food grade.

### Pharmaceutical particulars

*List of excipients:* Gum base, calcium carbonate, sorbitol, glycerin, sodium carbonate, sodium bicarbonate, amberlite, menthol, fruit flavour, butylated hydroxytoluene, acesulfame potassium, saccharin, sodium saccharin, talc, carnauba wax.

Nicotinell gum is sugar-free.

*Incompatibilities:* Not applicable.

*Shelf life:* 2 years.

*Special precautions for storage:* Store below 25˚C.

*Nature and contents of container:* The chewing gum is packed in PVC/aluminium blister packs each containing 12 pieces of gum. The blisters are packed in boxes of 12, 24 and 96 pieces of gum.

*Instructions for use/handling:* Medicines should be kept out of the reach of children.

*Marketing authorisation holder:* Ciba-Geigy plc, Hulley Road, Macclesfield, Cheshire SK10 2NX.

**Marketing authorisation number**  0001/0195.

**Date of approval/revision of SPC**  25 September 1996.

**Legal category**  P.

## NICOTINELL* MINT CHEWING GUM 2 mg

**Qualitative and quantitative composition**  Nicotine 2 mg per gum, in a resin complex.

**Pharmaceutical form**  Chewing gum.

### Clinical particulars

*Therapeutic indications:* Nicotinell treatment is indicated for the relief of nicotine withdrawal symptoms, in nicotine dependency as an aid to smoking cessation.

*Posology and method of administration*

*Adults and elderly:* Users should stop smoking completely during treatment with Nicotinell gum. One piece of Nicotinell gum to be chewed when the user feels the urge to smoke.

Normally, 8–12 pieces per day, up to a maximum of 25 pieces per day.

*Directions for use:* 1.  One piece of gum should be chewed until the taste becomes strong.

2.  The chewing gum should be rested between the gum and cheek.

3.  When the taste fades, chewing should commence again.

4.  The chewing routine should be repeated for 30 minutes.

After three months, the user should gradually cut down the number of pieces chewed each day until they have stopped using the product.

*Children:* Not to be used by children.

Concomitant use of acidic beverages such as coffee or soda may interfere with the buccal absorption of nicotine. Acidic beverages should be avoided for 15 minutes prior to chewing gum.

*Contra-indications:* Nicotinell gum should not be used by non-smokers or people under 18 years of age.

Use is contra-indicated during pregnancy and lactation, acute myocardial infarction, unstable or worsening angina pectoris, severe cardiac arrhythmias, and recent cerebrovascular accident.

*Special warnings and precautions for use:* Swallowed nicotine may exacerbate symptoms in subjects suffering from active oesophagitis, oral or pharyngeal inflammation, gastritis or peptic ulcer.

Use with caution in patients with hypertension, stable angina pectoris, cerebrovascular disease, occlusive peripheral arterial disease, heart failure, hyperthyroidism, diabetes mellitus, and renal or hepatic impairment.

Counselling may help smokers to quit.

Doses of nicotine that are tolerated by adult smokers during treatment may produce severe symptoms of poisoning in small children and may prove fatal (please see *Overdose*).

*Interactions with other medicaments and other forms of interaction:*

*Drug interactions:* No information is available on interactions between Nicotinell gum and other drugs.

*Smoking cessation:* This is different in the case of smoking where interactions with other medications may occur due to a multitude of other substances contained in the smoke. Presumably due to the polycyclic aromatic hydrocarbons contained in the smoke, the metabolism of different medicinal products may be speeded up by enzyme induction: e.g. caffeine, theophylline, paracetamol, phenazone, phenylbutazone, pentazocine, lidocaine, benzodiazepines, imipramine, warfarin, oestrogen and vitamin B12.

Upon smoking cessation it may be expected that the hitherto increased metabolism of these medicinal products is slowed down or normalised. Unaltered dosage of the products may result in an increase in their blood concentration.

Therefore when prescribing Nicotinell a possible dose adjustment should be considered in patients treated with the above mentioned medicinal products.

Other reported effects of smoking include a reduction of the analgesic effects of propoxyphene, reduced diuretic response to frusemide, change in the pharmacological effect of propranolol and altered responder rates in ulcer healing with $H_2$-antagonists.

Smoking and nicotine may raise the blood levels of cortisol and catecholamines. Dose adjustment of nifedipine, adrenergic agonists or adrenergic antagonists may be necessary.

Increased subcutaneous absorption or insulin which occur under smoking cessation may necessitate a reduction in insulin doses.

*Pregnancy and lactation:* In common with medical advice on stopping smoking in these situations, Nicotinell gum is contra-indicated in pregnant women and during breast feeding.

Reproductive toxicity studies with nicotine in several animal studies have demonstrated non-specific retardation of foetal growth. Studies in rats produced evidence of decreased fertility, prolonged pregnancy, and behavioural disorders in the offspring. In mice the offspring of animals exposed to very high doses of nicotine showed skeletal defects in the peripheral parts of the limbs.

Overall, there are no clear cut grounds for believing that nicotine at the concentrations reached by treatment with nicotine gum has any teratogenic potential and/or inhibitory effects on fertility.

*Effects on ability to drive and use machines:* Smoking cessation can cause behavioural changes. There is no evidence of any risks associated with driving or operating machinery when the gum is used following the recommended dose.

*Undesirable effects:* In principle, Nicotinell gum can cause adverse reactions similar to those associated with nicotine administered by smoking.

Nicotine from gum may sometimes cause a slight irritation of the throat and increase salivation at the start of treatment. Excessive swallowing of dissolved nicotine may, at first, cause hiccuping. Those with a tendency to indigestion may suffer initially from minor indigestion or heartburn. Slower chewing will usually overcome this problem. Excessive consumption of gum by subjects who have not been in the habit of inhaling tobacco smoke could possibly lead to nausea, faintness or headaches.

*Overdose:* In overdose, symptoms corresponding to heavy smoking may be seen.

The acute lethal oral dose of nicotine is about 0.5–0.75 mg per kg bodyweight, corresponding in an adult of 40–60 mg. Even small quantities of nicotine are dangerous in children, and may result in severe symptoms of poisoning which may prove fatal. If poisoning is suspected in a child, a doctor must be consulted immediately.

Overdose with Nicotinell gum may only occur if many pieces are chewed simultaneously. Risk of overdose is small as nausea or vomiting usually occurs at an early stage. Risk of poisoning by swallowing the gum is small. Since the release of nicotine from the gum is slow, very little nicotine is absorbed from the stomach and intestine, and if any is, it will be inactivated in the liver.

General symptoms of nicotine poisoning include: weakness, perspiration, salivation, throat burn, nausea, vomiting, diarrhoea, abdominal pain, hearing and visual disturbances, headache, tachycardia and cardiac arrhythmia, dyspnoea, prostration, circulatory collapse, coma and terminal convulsions.

*Treatment of overdosage:* In the event of overdosage, vomiting should be induced with syrup of ipecacuanha or gastric lavage carried out (wide bore tube). A suspension of activated charcoal should then be passed through the tube and left in the stomach. Artificial respiration with oxygen should be instituted if needed and continued for as long as necessary. Other therapy, including treatment of shock, is purely symptomatic.

## Pharmacological properties

*Pharmacodynamic properties:* Nicotine gum mimics the pharmacological effects of nicotine from smoking, and may therefore be used to help provide relief from nicotine withdrawal symptoms. In addition to effects on the central nervous system, nicotine produces haemodynamic effects such as increased heart rate and systolic blood pressure.

*Pharmacokinetic properties:* When the gum is chewed, nicotine is steadily released into the mouth and is rapidly absorbed through the buccal mucosa. A proportion, by the swallowing of nicotine containing saliva, reaches the stomach and intestine where it is inactivated.

The peak plasma concentration of the 2 mg gum after a single dose is approximately 4.8 nanograms per ml and following steady state administration is approximately 14 nanograms per ml (average plasma concentration of nicotine when smoking a cigarette is 15–30 nanograms per ml). Following chewing of a single 4 mg gum, peak plasma concentration of approximately 10 nanograms per ml is reached after about 30 minutes.

Nicotine is eliminated mainly via hepatic metabolism; small amounts of nicotine are eliminated in unchanged form via the kidneys. The plasma half-life is approximately three hours. Nicotine crosses the blood-brain barrier, the placenta and is detectable in breast milk.

*Pre-clinical safety data:* No animal studies have been undertaken on Nicotinell Chewing Gum.

The toxicity of nicotine as a constituent of tobacco has been well documented. Acute toxic effects include convulsions, cardiac insufficiency, and paralysis of the respiratory system.

At high doses in cats and dogs, nicotine has been shown to potentiate histamine-induced peptic ulcer.

All excipients used in Nicotinell Chewing Gum are of food grade.

## Pharmaceutical particulars

*List of excipients:* Gum base, calcium carbonate, sorbitol, glycerin, sodium carbonate, sodium bicarbonate, amberlite, menthol, peppermint, eucalyptus, butylated hydroxytoluene, acesulfame potassium, saccharin, sodium saccharin, talc, carnauba wax.

Nicotinell gum is sugar-free.

*Incompatibilities:* Not applicable.

*Shelf life:* 2 years.

*Special precautions for storage:* Store below 25°C.

*Nature and contents of container:* The chewing gum is packed in PVC/aluminium blister packs each containing 12 pieces of gum. The blisters are packed in boxes of 12, 24 and 96 pieces of gum.

*Instructions for use/handling:* Medicines should be kept out of the reach of children.

*Marketing authorisation holder:* Ciba-Geigy plc, Hulley Road, Macclesfield, Cheshire SK10 2NX.

**Marketing authorisation number** 0001/0197.

**Date of approval/revision of SPC** 25 September 1996.

**Legal category** P.

# NICOTINELL TTS*

**Presentation** Nicotinell TTS is a transdermal therapeutic system, consisting of a round, flat, matrix-type self-adhesive, yellowish-ochre coloured patch. It is protected by a rectangular metallic release liner backing to be discarded before application.

Three sizes of patch are available: Nicotinell TTS 10, containing 17.5 mg S(-)-nicotine with a drug releasing area of 10cm² and printed CG CWC on the patch surface; Nicotinell TTS 20, containing 35 mg S(-)-nicotine with a drug releasing area of 20cm² and printed CG FEF on the patch surface; and Nicotinell TTS 30 containing 52.5 mg S(-)-nicotine with a drug releasing area of 30 cm² and printed CG EME on the patch surface.

Nicotinell Transdermal Therapeutic Systems also contain acrylate esters vinylacetate co-polymers, fractionated coconut oil and methacrylic acid esters co-polymers.

## Uses

*Indications:* The treatment of nicotine dependence, as an aid to smoking cessation.

*Mode of action:* S(-)-Nicotine is the most pharmacologically active form of nicotine, the major alkaloid of tobacco. S(-)-Nicotine acts primarily on cholinergic receptors of the nicotinic type in the peripheral and central nervous system. For many effects, low doses of S(-)-nicotine have a stimulant action, and high doses a depressant effect. Intermittent administration of S(-)-nicotine affects neurohormonal pathways, and results in the release of acetylcholine, noradrenaline, dopamine, serotonin, vasopressin, beta-endorphin, growth hormone, cortisol and ACTH. These neuroregulators may be involved in the reported behavioural and subjective effects of smoking.

Nicotine replacement is an established therapy as an aid to smoking cessation. Nicotinell TTS provides for a convenient once daily administration by exploiting the fact that S(-)-nicotine is readily absorbed through the skin into the systemic circulation. Placebo-controlled, double-blind studies have shown that nicotine replacement with Nicotinell TTS produces smoking abstinence rates statistically significantly better than placebo, with or without group support. There was also a strong trend towards reduction of withdrawal symptoms.

Application of Nicotinell TTS 20 to smokers abstinent overnight resulted in small increases in mean heart rate and systolic blood pressure and a decrease in stroke volume. The effects were smaller in magnitude than those produced by cigarette smoking.

*Pharmacokinetics:* Following single application of Nicotinell TTS to the skin of healthy abstinent smokers there is an initial 1–2 hours delay followed by a progressive rise in nicotine plasma concentrations, with a plateau attained at about 8–10 hours after application.

In the majority of subjects the area under the plasma concentration time curve (AUC 0–24 hours) varies approximately in proportion to the drug releasing area of the patch. Nicotinell TTS is designed to deliver approximately 0.7 mg/cm²/24 hours. In comparison with an i.v. infusion, 76.8% of the nicotine released from Nicotinell TTS is systemically available. Steady state plasma concentrations after repeated daily administration are within the range observed during moderate cigarette smoking.

Absorption of nicotine over 24 hours varies by a factor of two between different individuals; however within-individual variability is small indicating consistent performance of the transdermal system.

S(-)-Nicotine is distributed widely in the body with a volume of distribution of approximately 180 litres. It crosses the blood-brain barrier, placenta and is detectable in breast milk. Plasma protein binding is only 5%. Total plasma clearance of nicotine ranges from 0.92 to 2.43 litres/min. It is eliminated mainly via hepatic metabolism. Only small amounts of nicotine are eliminated in unchanged form via the kidneys, a process which is pH dependent, being negligible under alkaline conditions.

## Dosage and administration

*Adults:* Users should stop smoking completely during treatment with Nicotinell TTS.

For individuals smoking more than 20 cigarettes a day it is recommended that treatment be started with Nicotinell TTS 30 once daily, applied to a dry non-hairy area of the skin on the trunk or upper arm. Those smoking less than this are recommended to start with Nicotinell TTS 20. Sizes of 30 cm², 20 cm² and 10 cm² are available to permit gradual withdrawal of nicotine replacement, using treatment periods of 3–4 weeks for each size. The size of patch may be adjusted according to individual response, maintaining or increasing the dose if abstinence is not achieved or if withdrawal symptoms are experienced. Total treatment periods of more than 3 months and daily doses above 30 cm² have not been evaluated. The treatment is designed to be used continuously for 3 months but not beyond. However, if abstinence is not achieved at the end of the 3 month treatment period, further treatments may be recommended following a re-evaluation of the patient's motivation. The dosage must not be adjusted by cutting a patch.

Nicotinell TTS should be used as soon as it has been removed from the child-resistant pouch. Following removal of the metallic backing, the Nicotinell TTS patch should be applied to the skin and held in position for 10–20 seconds with the palm of the hand. Each patch should be removed after 24 hours and disposed of safely (see 'Warnings'). A different site of application should be chosen each day and several days should be allowed to elapse before a new patch is applied to the same area of skin.

*Children:* Safety and efficacy in individuals under 18 years of age have not been established. Nicotinell TTS is contra-indicated in children.

*Elderly:* Experience in the use of Nicotinell TTS in smokers over the age of 65 years is limited. Nicotinell TTS does not appear to pose safety problems in this age group.

*Potential for abuse and dependence:* Transdermal nicotine is likely to have a very low abuse potential because of its slow onset of action, low fluctuations in blood concentrations, inability to produce high blood concentrations of nicotine, and the infrequent (once daily) use. Moreover, gradual weaning from Nicotinell TTS is instituted within the treatment schedule, and the risk of dependence after therapy is minimal. The effects of abrupt withdrawal from Nicotinell TTS are likely to be similar to those observed with tobacco withdrawal from comparable nicotine concentrations.

### Contra-indications, warnings, etc

*Contra-indications:* Nicotinell TTS should not be administered to non-smokers, occasional smokers or children. The system is also contra-indicated during pregnancy and breast-feeding (see 'Use in Pregnancy and Lactation'), and in acute myocardial infarction, unstable or worsening angina pectoris, severe cardiac arrhythmias, recent cerebrovascular accident, diseases of the skin which may complicate patch therapy, and known hypersensitivity to nicotine or any of the components of the patch.

*Warnings:* Nicotine is a toxic drug and milligram doses are potentially fatal if rapidly absorbed. Treatment with Nicotinell TTS should be discontinued if symptoms of nicotine overdosage appear. Mild intoxication produces nausea, vomiting, abdominal pain, diarrhoea, headache, sweating and pallor (see 'Overdosage').

Doses of nicotine that are tolerated by adult smokers during treatment, can produce severe symptoms of poisoning in small children and may prove fatal. Both before and after use, Nicotinell TTS contains a significant amount of nicotine. Subjects must be cautioned that the patches must not be handled casually or left where they might be inadvertently misused or consumed by children. Used patches must be disposed of with care by folding them in half with the adhesive sides inwards, and ensuring that they do not fall into the hands of children under any circumstances.

*Precautions:* Users should stop smoking completely during therapy with Nicotinell TTS. They should be informed that if they continue to smoke while using Nicotinell TTS, they may experience increased adverse effects due to the hazards of smoking, including cardiovascular effects.

In subjects with the conditions listed below, Nicotinell TTS should only be used following a careful risk-benefit assessment, and only in cases where subjects have found it impossible to stop smoking without use of Nicotinell TTS: hypertension, stable angina pectoris, cerebrovascular disease, occlusive peripheral arterial disease, heart failure, hyperthyroidism, diabetes mellitus, renal or hepatic impairment and peptic ulcer.

Discontinuation of treatment may be advisable in cases of severe or persistent skin reactions.

Contact sensitisation was reported in a few patients using transdermal nicotine in clinical trials. Patients who develop contact sensitisation to nicotine should be cautioned that a severe reaction could occur from exposure to smoking or other nicotine containing products.

When Nicotinell TTS is used as recommended there are minimal risks for driving vehicles or operating machinery.

*Use in pregnancy and lactation:* In common with medical advice on stopping smoking in these situations, Nicotinell TTS is contra-indicated in pregnant women and during breast feeding.

Teratogenicity studies with nicotine in several animal species have demonstrated non-specific retardation of foetal growth. Studies in pregnant rats have indicated the presence of behavioural disorders in the offspring, and in the mouse the unborn offspring of animals treated with approximately 120 times the human transdermal dose showed skeletal defects in the peripheral parts of the limbs. Embryo implantation in rats and rabbits may be inhibited or delayed by nicotine. Overall, there are no clear cut grounds for believing that nicotine at the concentrations reached by treatment with Nicotinell TTS has any teratogenic potential and/or inhibitory effects on fertility.

*Drug interactions:* No information is available on interactions between Nicotinell TTS and other drugs.

Cessation of smoking, with or without nicotine replacement, may alter the individual's response to concomitant medication and may require adjustment of dose. Smoking is thought to increase the metabolism through enzyme induction and thus to lower the blood concentrations of drugs such as antipyrine, caffeine, oestrogens, desmethyldiazepam, imipramine, lignocaine, oxazepam, pentazocine, phenacetin, theophylline, and warfarin. Cessation of smoking may result in increased concentrations of these drugs.

Other reported effects of smoking include reduced analgesic efficacy of propoxyphene, reduced diuretic response to frusemide, and reduced pharmacological response to propranolol, as well as reduced rates of ulcer healing with H₂-antagonists.

Both smoking and nicotine can increase levels of circulating cortisol and catecholamines. Dosages of

nifedipine, adrenergic agonists, or adrenergic blocking agents may need to be adjusted.

*Side-effects:* In principle, Nicotinell TTS can cause adverse reactions similar to those associated with nicotine administered by smoking. Since the maximum plasma concentrations of nicotine that are produced by Nicotinell TTS are lower than those produced by smoking and fluctuate less, nicotine-related adverse reactions occurring during treatment with Nicotinell TTS can be expected to be less marked than during smoking.

Some of the symptoms listed below are hard to differentiate from recognised tobacco withdrawal symptoms when comparison with placebo is made. The placebo used contained about 13% of the nicotine of a matching Nicotinell TTS (to match colour and odour for blinding purposes).

The main unwanted effect of Nicotinell TTS is application site reaction. This led to premature discontinuation of Nicotinell TTS in about 6% of clinical trial participants. Skin reactions consisted of erythema or pruritus at the patch site. Oedema, burning sensation, blisters, rash, or pinching sensation at the application site were also noted. The majority of these reactions were mild. Most of the skin reactions resolved within 48 hours, but in more severe cases the erythema and infiltration lasted from 1 to 3 weeks. The time of onset of important skin reactions was between 3 and 8 weeks from the start of therapy. In isolated cases the skin reactions extended beyond the application sites. Isolated cases of urticaria, angioneurotic oedema and dyspnoea were reported.

The following are the adverse events/withdrawal symptoms, most commonly reported in three double-blind clinical trials *irrespective of causal association to study drug.*

|  | Nicotinell TTS (N=401) | Placebo (N=391) |
| --- | --- | --- |
| Application site reaction | 34.9% | 17.6% |
| Headache | 29.7% | 29.2% |
| Cold and Flu-like Symptoms | 12.0% | 8.4% |
| Dysmenorrhoea (% of female subjects) | 6.6% | 8.8% |
| Insomnia | 6.5% | 5.4% |
| Nausea | 6.2% | 4.6% |
| Myalgia | 6.0% | 4.1% |
| Dizziness | 6.0% | 5.9% |

Other unwanted experiences reported (irrespective of causal association with Nicotinell TTS) with an incidence of 1%–5.9% and more frequently than placebo, included: abdominal pain, vomiting, dyspepsia, allergy, motor dysfunction, chest pain, vivid dreams, blood pressure changes, generalised rash, somnolence, impaired concentration and fatigue.

*Overdosage:* The toxicity of nicotine cannot be directly compared with that of smoking, because tobacco smoke contains additional toxic substances (e.g. carbon monoxide and tar).

Chronic smokers can tolerate doses of nicotine that, in a non-smoker, would be more toxic, because of the development of tolerance.

Application of several Nicotinell TTS patches could result in serious overdosage. Slower absorption after cutaneous exposure to nicotine favours the development of tolerance to toxic effects.

Rapid systemic delivery of nicotine from Nicotinell TTS would not be expected on chewing and swallowing, owing to the slow release of nicotine from the patch and first-pass metabolism.

Acute toxic effects: Signs and symptoms of overdosage would be the same as those of acute nicotine poisoning. In non-smoking children and adults, these include pallor, sweating, nausea, salivation, vomiting, abdominal cramps, diarrhoea, headache, dizziness, hearing and vision disturbances, tremor, mental confusion, muscle weakness, convulsions, prostration, absence of neurological reaction, and respiratory failure. Lethal doses may produce convulsions, and death follows as a result of peripheral or central respiratory paralysis or, less frequently, cardiac failure.

The acute lethal oral dose of nicotine in non-smoking adults is approximately 60 mg.

Management: If the patient shows signs of overdosage, Nicotinell TTS should be removed immediately. The skin surface may be washed with water and dried (no soap should be used). The skin will continue to deliver nicotine into the blood stream for several hours after removal of the system, possibly because of a depot of nicotine in the skin.

Other treatment measures for acute nicotine poisoning include artificial respiration in the case of respiratory paralysis, maintaining normal body temperature and treatment for hypotension and cardiovascular collapse.

Each Nicotinell TTS patch is sealed in a child-resistant sachet and the product must be kept out of

the reach of children at all times (see 'Warnings'). Even doses of nicotine which are tolerated by adults during treatment with Nicotinell TTS could produce severe symptoms of poisoning in small children following accidental application, and may prove fatal.

**Pharmaceutical precautions** Store below 25°C.

**Legal category** P.

**Package quantities**
Nicotinell TTS 10: Packs of 7 patches.
Nicotinell TTS 20: Packs of 7 patches.
Nicotinell TTS 30: Packs of 7 patches.

**Further information** Smokers' support materials are included in 7 day packs of Nicotinell TTS 20 and 30.

**Product licence numbers**
Nicotinell TTS 10    0001/0173
Nicotinell TTS 20    0001/0174
Nicotinell TTS 30    0001/0175

## OTRIVINE*

**Presentation** Clear, colourless, odourless solutions, Otrivine Adult Formula Nasal Drops and Spray contain 0.1% w/v Xylometazoline Hydrochloride BP. Otrivine Children's Formula Nasal Drops contain 0.05% w/v Xylometazoline Hydrochloride BP. Otrivine also contains sodium acid phosphate, sodium phosphate, sodium chloride, disodium edetate and benzalkonium chloride.

### Uses

*Mode of action:* Otrivine is a sympathomimetic agent with marked alpha-adrenergic activity, and is intended for use in the nose. It constricts the nasal blood vessels, thereby decongesting the mucosa of the nose and neighbouring regions of the pharynx. This enables patients suffering from colds to breathe more easily through the nose. The effect of Otrivine begins within a few minutes and persists for several hours. Otrivine is generally well tolerated and does not impair the function of ciliated epithelium.

*Pharmacokinetics:* Systemic absorption may occur following nasal application of xylometazoline hydrochloride solutions. It is not used systemically.

*Indications:* For the symptomatic relief of nasal congestion, perennial and allergic rhinitis (including hay fever), sinusitis.

### Dosage and administration

*Adults:* 2 or 3 drops of Otrivine Adult Formula Nasal Drops or one application of Otrivine Formula Nasal Spray in each nostril, two or three times daily.

*N.B.* The Otrivine Adult Formula Nasal Drops and Spray should not be used for children under the age of 12 years.

*Children under 12:* 1 or 2 drops of the Otrivine Children's Formula Nasal Drops in each nostril once or twice daily. Not to be used in infants less than 3 months.

### Contra-indications, warnings, etc

*Contra-indications:* Patients with trans-sphenoidal hypophysectomy or surgery exposing the dura mater. Known hypersensitivity to Otrivine.

*Warnings:* Each Otrvine pack should be used by one person only to prevent any cross-infection.

*Precautions:* Patients are advised not to take decongestants for more than seven consecutive days. Otrivine, like other preparations belonging to the same class of active substances, should be used only with caution in patients showing a strong reaction to sympathomimetic agents as evidenced by signs of insomnia, dizziness, etc.

*Side-effects:* The following side-effects have occasionally been encountered: a burning sensation in the nose and throat, local irritation, nausea, headache, and dryness of the nasal mucosa. Systemic cardiovascular effects have occurred, and this should be kept in mind when giving Otrivine to people with cardiovascular disease.

*Pregnancy and lactation:* No foetal toxicity or fertility studies have been carried out in animals. In view of its potential systemic vasoconstrictor effect, it is advisable to take the precaution of not using Otrivine during pregnancy.

*Drug interactions:* No drug interactions have been reported.

*Overdosage:* No cases of overdosage in adults have yet been reported. In rare instances of accidental poisoning in children, the clinical picture has been marked chiefly by signs such as acceleration and irregularity of the pulse, elevated blood pressure, drowsiness, respiratory depression or irregularity. There is no specific treatment and appropriate supportive treatment should be initiated.

**Pharmaceutical precautions** Protect from heat. For

reasons of hygiene, do not use the bottle more than 28 days after opening it.

**Legal category** GSL.

**Package quantities**
Otrivine Adult Formula Nasal Drops 10 ml (OP).
Otrivine Adult Formula Nasal Spray 10 ml (OP).
Otrivine Children's Formula Nasal Drops 10 ml (OP).

**Further information** May be prescribed under the NHS Pharmaceutical Services as Xylometazoline Hydrochloride.

**Product licence numbers**
Otrivine Adult Formula Nasal Drops 0008/5023R
Otrivine Adult Formula Nasal Spray 0008/5024R
Otrivine Children's Formula Nasal
   Drops               0008/5022R.

## PAROVEN* CAPSULES

**Qualitative and quantitative composition** Oxerutins 250 mg.

**Pharmaceutical form** Capsules.

**Clinical particulars**
*Therapeutic indications:* Relief of symptoms of oedema associated with chronic venous insufficiency.

*Posology and method of administration:*
  *Adults and elderly:* 2 capsules (500 mg) twice daily.
  *Children:* not recommended for children under 12 years.

*Contra-indications:* Hypersensitivity to any of the ingredients.

*Special warnings and special precautions for use:* Treatment of leg oedema due to cardiac, renal or hepatic disease should be directed to the underlying cause; Paroven should not be used in these conditions. If leg pain and swelling do not improve, or get worse, the patient should consult their doctor.

*Interactions with other medicaments and other forms of interaction:* None reported. Oxerutins have been shown not to interact with warfarin anticoagulants.

*Pregnancy and lactation:* Clinical trials and animal studies have shown no increase in teratogenic (or other) hazard to the foetus if used in the recommended dosage during pregnancy. However, in keeping with current medical opinion, Paroven should not be used during the first trimester of pregnancy.

In animal studies traces of oxerutins and/or their metabolites have been found in breast milk, but the levels are not considered to be of clinical relevance. The use of Paroven in lactating women is therefore at the physician's discretion.

*Effect on ability to drive and use machines:* None known.

*Undesirable effects:* Occasionally, mild adverse reactions (skin allergies, minor gastrointestinal disturbances, headaches and flushes) have been reported. They disappear rapidly on stopping treatment.

*Overdose:* No cases of overdosage with symptoms have been reported. No specific antidotes are known.

**Pharmacological properties**
*Pharmacodynamic properties:* Oxerutins has uniquely useful therapeutic actions in the microcirculation and particularly in the post-capillary venous segment. Oxerutins reduces capillary leakage and hence oedema formation.

*Pharmacokinetic properties:* Not all conventional pharmacokinetic parameters are available due to technical difficulties. Oxerutins is absorbed from the gastrointestinal tract of mammals. Its metabolism is, in part, determined by the degree of hydroxyethylation of the aromatic ring systems of the constituent rutoside derivatives. Biliary excretion plays a major role in elimination in the animal species studied. It is, however, not clear if this route of elimination is equally important in man since quantitative data in humans are not available. The same applies to enterohepatic recycling.

*Preclinical safety data:* Not applicable.

**Pharmaceutical particulars**
*List of excipients:* Polyethylene glycol, gelatin, titanium dioxide E171, yellow iron oxide E172, black iron oxide E172.

*Incompatibilities:* None.

*Shelf life:* 36 months.

*Special precautions for storage:* Protect from moisture.

*Nature and contents of container:* Blister pack composed of PVC blisters sealed with aluminium foil. Pack sizes: 120 capsules.

*Instructions for use/handling:* Medicines should be kept out of the reach of children.

**Marketing authorisation number** 0030/5002R.

---

**Date of approval/revision of SPC** March 1997.

**Legal category** P.

## PECRAM*

**Presentation** Round, biconvex, pale yellow tablets imprinted on one face with the Zyma logo and on the other with the symbol SRA/225.
  Each tablet contains 225 mg Aminophylline Hydrate BP in a slow release formulation.

**Uses** For the treatment and prophylaxis of asthmatic bronchospasm and that associated with emphysema and chronic bronchitis. For the treatment of cardiac asthma and left ventricular or congestive heart failure.

**Dosage and administration** For oral administration. The tablets should be swallowed whole and not chewed.
*Standard dosing*
*Adults:* The recommended initial dose is one tablet twice daily (one tablet to be taken in the morning and one in the evening).
*The elderly:* Reduced dosages may be required in elderly patients. The dosage should be titrated to attain optimum clinical response.
*Children:* Pecram tablets have not been fully evaluated in children.
*Dose titration:* The response to xanthines may vary between patients so that dosage must be individually titrated by clinical assessment and serum theophylline monitoring to a suitable dosage regimen, and when necessary the dose can be increased up to two tablets twice daily.
  Steady state theophylline levels are generally reached with Pecram after 3–4 days. If satisfactory clinical response is not achieved, serum theophylline should be measured 4–6 hours after the last dose. Based on serum theophylline assay results, the dosage should be titrated using the following as a guide for twice daily administration.

| Peak serum theophylline level | Dosage adjustment |
|---|---|
| <10 micrograms/ml | Increase total daily dose by one tablet. |
| 10–15 micrograms/ml | If the patient's symptoms persist, increase the total daily dose to a maximum of 2 tablets twice daily. |
| 16–20 micrograms/ml | Do not adjust the dose unless side effects occur, in which case reduce the total daily dose by 1 tablet per day. |
| 21–25 micrograms/ml | Decrease the total daily dose by 1 tablet per day |
| 26–30 micrograms/ml | Miss the next dose and decrease the maintenance dose by one half. |

It is advisable to re-check serum theophylline concentration after dose adjustment, when steady state is attained.
*Pharmacokinetics:* It has been demonstrated that twice-daily dosing produces minimal peak to trough variations. A dose regimen of 1 tablet twice daily for 6 days resulted in a peak plasma theophylline concentration of 9.5 micrograms/ml ($C_{Max}$) at 4.0 hours ($T_{Max}$) and a minimum plasma concentration of 4.5 micrograms/ml ($C_{Min}$) at 12 hours.
  With appropriate dosage titration, plasma theophylline levels can be maintained in the range of 10–20 micrograms/ml for 12 hours.
  Smoking and alcohol consumption may increase theophylline clearance thus necessitating an increased dosage.
  Other factors such as viral infections, liver disease and heart failure may reduce theophylline clearance requiring a reduction in dosage.
*Transferability:* It is not possible to ensure bioequivalence between different sustained release xanthine products. Once an effective dose has been established, patients should not be changed from Pecram to another preparation without re-titration and clinical assessment.

**Contra-indications, warnings, etc**
*Contra-indications:* Patients with a known hypersensitivity to the xanthine group of drugs.

*Precautions:* Suspected interactions have been documented between theophylline and the following drugs: Allopurinol, thiabendazole, halothane, lithium, oral contraceptives, erythromycin, triacetyloleandomycin, lomustine, phenobarbitone, propranolol, cimetidine, ciprofloxin and hydrocortisone. Care should be taken on its concomitant use with β-adrenergic agonists, glucagon and other xanthine drugs, as these will potentiate the effects of theophylline. The incidence of toxic effects may be enhanced by the concomitant use of ephedrine. Physicians should be aware that interaction may occur with influenza vaccine. Some reports have suggested that this may

---

potentiate theophylline. The following drugs increase theophylline clearance and it may therefore be necessary to increase dosage to ensure a therapeutic effect: phenytoin, carbamazepine, rifampicin, sulphinpyrazone and barbiturates.
  The prolonged release characteristic of this product should be kept in mind if intravenous aminophylline is to be administered, lest unintended high serum levels lead to toxicity.
  Xanthines can potentiate hypokalaemia resulting from beta 2 agonist therapy, steroids, diuretics and hypoxia. Particular caution is advised in severe asthma. It is recommended that serum potassium levels are monitored in such situations.

*Side-effects:* Those associated with theophylline and xanthine derivatives such as nausea, gastric irritation, headache and CNS stimulation, are reduced when controlled release formulations such as Pecram are administered because the peak/trough variation is reduced.

*Use in pregnancy and lactation:* Theophylline crosses the placental barrier and is secreted in breast milk. It has been used during pregnancy without attributable adverse foetal effects. However, as with all drugs theophylline should only be used during pregnancy if considered essential by the physician.

*Overdosage:* In the event of overdosage, empty the stomach contents, monitor the patient's electrocardiogram and maintain fluid balance. Orally administer activated charcoal to reduce high theophylline plasma levels. With severe poisoning, charcoal column haemoperfusion should be used. Other treatment is symptomatic. Oxygen should be given as necessary.
  Convulsions may be controlled by intravenous administration of diazepam 5 or 10 mg, or if necessary thiopentone sodium. The physician should be aware that tablets in the intestine will continue to release the drug over several hours.
  In the event of blood monitoring showing low serum potassium levels it is recommended that potassium replacement therapy be instituted by mouth. Cases of acute hypokalaemia should be admitted to hospital.

**Pharmaceutical precautions** Protect from light. Store in a cool dry place.

**Legal category** P.

**Package quantities** Containers of 60 tablets (OP).

**Further information** Nil.

**Product licence number** 10013/0002.

## PROFLEX* CREAM

**Qualitative and quantitative composition** Ibuprofen BP 5% w/w.

**Pharmaceutical form** Cream.

**Clinical particulars**
*Therapeutic indications:* Topical analgesic and anti-inflammatory treatment for the fast relief of the symptoms of rheumatic pain, muscular aches and pains, backache, lumbago, fibrositis, pains or swellings such as strains, sprains, and sports injuries.

*Route of administration:* Topical.

*Posology and method of administration:*
  *Adults and elderly:* 4–10 cm (1½–4 inches) of cream (50–125 mg ibuprofen) 3–4 times daily, massaged into the skin over a large area at the affected site.
  A period of at least 4 hours should be left between each application.
  *Children:* Not recommended for children under 12 years.

*Contra-indications:* Hypersensitivity to any of the constituents. Hypersensitivity to aspirin or other non-steroidal anti-inflammatory drugs including provocation or exacerbation of asthma, rhinitis, or urticaria.

*Special warnings and precautions for use:* Keep away from inflamed or broken skin, lips and near the eyes. Discontinue if rash develops. Wash hands after use.

*Interactions with other medicaments and other forms of interaction:* Concurrent aspirin or other NSAIDs may result in an increased incidence of adverse reactions.

*Pregnancy and lactation:* Whilst no teratogenic effects have been demonstrated in animal experiments, ibuprofen should be avoided during pregnancy. The onset of labour may be delayed and duration of labour may be increased. Ibuprofen appears in breast milk in very low concentration and is unlikely to affect the breast-fed infant adversely.

*Effect on ability to drive and use machines:* Proflex Cream will not impair the ability to drive and the ability to use machines.

*Undesirable effects:* Skin reactions are most frequently reported.

*Skin:* Application site reactions, rashes, pruritus, urticaria.

*Gastro-intestinal:* Abdominal pain, dyspepsia.

*Respiratory:* Bronchospasm may be precipitated in patients suffering from or with a previous history of bronchial asthma or allergic disease.

*Overdose:* Overdosage with a topical presentation of ibuprofen is unlikely. Symptoms of ibuprofen overdose include headache, vomiting, drowsiness and hypotension. Correction of severe electrolyte abnormalities should be considered.

## Pharmacological properties

*Pharmacodynamic properties:* Ibuprofen is a phenylpropionic acid derivative which has analgesic anti-inflammatory and anti-pyretic actions.

*Pharmacokinetic properties:* Percutaneous absorption approximately 5% that of oral ibuprofen. $C_{max}$=0.64 mcg/ml (higher concentrations achieved locally) $T_{max}$=2.00 h

*Preclinical safety data:* Not applicable.

## Pharmaceutical particulars

*List of excipients:* Fractionated coconut oil; Arlacel 165 (glyceryl stearate); Arlatone 983S (polyoxyethylene fatty acid ester); propylene glycol; sodium methyl hydroxybenzoate; Keltrol F (xanthan gum); purified water.

*Incompatibilities:* None stated.

*Shelf life:* 36 months.

*Special precautions for storage:* Store in a cool place.

*Nature and contents of container:* Internally lacquered aluminium tube. Contents 100 g.

*Instructions for use/handling:* Keep all medicines out of the reach of children. For external use only. Wash hands after use.

**Marketing authorisation number** 0030/0052.

**Date of approval/revision of SPC** 18 March 1997.

**Legal category** P.

# VIOFORM*-HYDROCORTISONE

**Presentation** The active ingredients Clioquinol BP 3% w/w and Hydrocortisone BP 1% w/w are presented as a white, water miscible cream and a smooth, off-white ointment.

Ointment also contains: light liquid paraffin and white soft paraffin.

Cream also contains: cetostearyl alcohol, cetyl palmitate, glycerol, sodium lauryl sulphate, 2-phenoxyethanol, and white soft paraffin.

## Uses

*Mode of action:* Vioform-Hydrocortisone combines the anti-fungal and anti-bacterial properties of clioquinol with the anti-inflammatory, anti-allergic and antipruritic effects of hydrocortisone.

*Indications:* Exudative and secondarily infected eczema and dermatitis, including atopic eczema, primary irritant dermatitis, allergic and seborrhoeic dermatitis. Infected insect bite reactions. Genital or perianal intertrigo.

**Dosage and administration** Vioform-Hydrocortisone is indicated for external application only.

*Method of application:* The preparation should be applied sparingly to the affected area, 1–3 times daily. Treatment should be limited to 7 days. Occlusive dressings should not be used.

If there is little improvement after 7 days treatment with Vioform-Hydrocortisone cream or ointment, the appropriate microbiological investigations should be carried out and local or systemic antibiotic treatment given.

*Use in the elderly:* There is no evidence to suggest that dosage should be different in the elderly.

*Use in children:* Vioform-Hydrocortisone is contra-indicated in children below the age of two years.

**Contra-indications, warnings, etc**

*Contra-indications:* Hypersensitivity to any component of the formulation, or iodine. Primary bacterial, viral or fungal infections of the skin. Secondary infections due to yeasts. Application to ulcerated areas. Use in children below the age of two years.

*Precautions:* Long-term continuous topical therapy should be avoided since this can lead to adrenal suppression even without occlusion.

Application to relatively large and/or eroded areas of skin, use of occlusive dressings, and treatment for longer than one week, should be avoided, because this may lead to a marked increase in protein-bound iodine (PBI). Thyroid function tests such as PBI, radioactive iodine and butanol extractable iodine, may be affected, consequently it is advisable that such tests are not performed within one month of discontinuing treatment. However, other thyroid function tests, such as the $T_3$ resin sponge test or $T_4$ determination are unaffected.

The ferric chloride test for phenylketonuria may

yield a false-positive result when clioquinol is present in the urine.

Vioform-Hydrocortisone should be used with caution in patients suffering from hepatic and/or renal failure.

Vioform-Hydrocortisone should not be allowed to come into contact with the conjunctiva.

*Side-effects:* Vioform-Hydrocortisone is usually well tolerated but occasionally, at the site of application, there may be signs of irritation such as a burning sensation, itching or skin rash. Hypersensitivity reactions may also occasionally occur. Treatment should be discontinued if patients experience severe irritation or sensitisation.

Vioform-Hydrocortisone may cause hair discolouration.

*Use in pregnancy and lactation:* There is inadequate evidence of safety in human pregnancy. Topical administration of corticosteroids to pregnant animals can cause abnormalities of foetal development, including cleft palate and intra-uterine growth retardation. There may, therefore, be a very small risk of such effects in the human foetus.

It is not known whether the active substances of Vioform-Hydrocortisone and/or their metabolite(s) pass into the breast milk after topical administration. Use in lactating mothers should only be at the doctor's discretion.

*Overdosage:* Vioform-Hydrocortisone cream and ointment are for topical (external) use only. If accidental ingestion of large quantities occurs, there is no specific antidote and general measures to eliminate the drug and reduce its absorption should be undertaken. Symptomatic treatment should be administered as appropriate.

**Pharmaceutical precautions** Protect from heat. Dilution of or addition to these formulations is not recommended.

**Legal category** POM.

**Package quantities** Cream: Tubes of 30 g (OP). Ointment: Tubes of 30 g (OP).

**Further information** Clothing stained with Vioform-Hydrocortisone cream or ointment should be washed immediately or soaked overnight.

**Product licence numbers**

| | |
|---|---|
| Vioform-Hydrocortisone cream | 0030/0050 |
| Vioform-Hydrocortisone ointment | 0030/0051 |

*Trade Mark

## Novartis Pharmaceuticals UK Ltd
Frimley Business Park
Frimley
Camberley
Surrey GU16 5SG

**NOVARTIS**

## ANAFRANIL
## ANAFRANIL SR*

**Presentation** The active ingredient, Clomipramine Hydrochloride BP, is presented as:

Dull greyish red, film coated tablets, round, slightly convex with slightly bevelled edges, imprinted 'GEIGY' on one face and GD on the other, diameter approximately 8 mm, thickness approximately 4.3 mm, each containing 75 mg in a sustained release formulation.

SR tablets also contain: ethylacrylate methylmethacrylate copolymer, calcium hydrogen phosphate, silicon dioxide, calcium stearate, hydroxypropyl methylcellulose, red iron oxide, polyethoxylated castor oils, talc, titanium dioxide and water.

Two-tone light grey/caramel-coloured capsules, hard gelatin size no. 4, imprinted 'GEIGY', each containing 50 mg.

Two-tone brownish-orange/caramel-coloured capsules, hard gelatin size no. 4, imprinted 'GEIGY', each containing 25 mg.

Two-tone greyish-yellow/caramel coloured capsules, hard gelatin size no. 4, imprinted 'GEIGY', each containing 10 mg.

The capsules also contain: lactose, gelatin, magnesium stearate, titanium dioxide, black iron oxide, red iron oxide, yellow iron oxide and brown printing ink.

An off-white, pourable, viscous suspension with a characteristic citrus odour and taste containing the equivalent of 25 mg clomipramine hydrochloride in 5 ml.

The syrup also contains: powdered tragacanth, microcrystalline cellulose, methyl- and propyl-hydroxybenzoates, sorbitol, flavours (tetrarome orange and lemon) and water.

Ampoules of clear glass containing 25 mg Clomipramine Hydrochloride BP in 2 ml.

The ampoules also contain: glycerine, water and pressurised carbon dioxide.

## Uses

*Indications:* Symptoms of depressive illness especially where sedation is required. Obsessional and phobic states. Adjunctive treatment of cataplexy associated with narcolepsy.

*Mode of action:* Clomipramine is a tricyclic antidepressant and its pharmacological action includes alpha-adrenolytic, anticholinergic, anti-histaminic and 5-HT receptor blocking properties. The therapeutic activity of Anafranil is thought to be based on its ability to inhibit the neuronal re-uptake of noradrenaline and 5-HT. Inhibition of the latter is the dominant component.

*Pharmacokinetics:*
*Absorption:* The active substance is completely absorbed following oral administration and intramuscular injection.

The systemic bioavailability of unchanged clomipramine is reduced by 50% by 'first-pass' metabolism to desmethylclomipramine (an active metabolite). The bioavailability of clomipramine is not markedly affected by the ingestion of food but the onset of absorption and therefore the time to peak may be delayed. Coated tablets and sustained release tablets are bioequivalent with respect to amount absorbed.

During oral administration of constant daily doses of Anafranil the steady state plasma concentrations of clomipramine and desmethylclomipramine (active metabolite) and the ratio between these concentrations show a high variability between patients, e.g. 75 mg Anafranil daily produces steady state concentrations of clomipramine ranging from about 20 to 175ng/ml. Levels of desmethylclomipramine follow a similar pattern but are 40-85% higher.

Following repeated intravenous or intramuscular administration of 50-150 mg Anafranil daily, steady-state plasma concentrations are attained in the second week of treatment. These range from <15 to 447 ng/ml for clomipramine and from <15 to 669 ng/ml for desmethylclomipramine.

*Distribution:* Clomipramine is 97.6% bound to plasma proteins. The apparent volume of distribution is about 12-17 L/kg bodyweight. Concentrations in cerebrospinal fluid are about 2% of the plasma concentration.

*Biotransformation:* The major route of transformation of clomipramine is demethylation to desmethylclomipramine. In addition, clomipramine and desmethylclomipramine are hydroxylated to 8-hydroxyclomipramine and 8-hydroxy-desmethylclomipramine but little is known about their activity in vivo. The hydroxylation of clomipramine and desmethylclomipramine is under genetic control similar to that of debrisoquine. In poor metabolisers of debrisoquine this may lead to high concentrations of desmethylclomipramine; concentrations of clomipramine are less significantly influenced.

*Elimination:* Oral clomipramine is eliminated from the blood with a mean half-life of 21 hours (range 12-36 h), and desmethylclomipramine with a half-life of 36 hours.

After intramuscular and intravenous administration, clomipramine is eliminated from plasma with a mean terminal half-life of 25 hours (range 20-40h) and 18 hours respectively.

About two-thirds of a single dose of clomipramine is excreted in the form of water-soluble conjugates in the urine, and approximately one-third in the faeces. The quantity of unchanged clomipramine and desmethylclomipramine excreted in the urine amounts to about 2% and 0.5% of the administered dose respectively.

*Characteristics in patients:* In elderly patients, plasma clomipramine concentrations may be higher for a given dose than would be expected in younger patients because of reduced metabolic clearance.

The effects of hepatic and renal impairment on the pharmacokinetics of clomipramine have not been determined.

## Dosage and administration
*Depression:*

*Adults:* Oral–10 mg/day initially, increasing gradually to 30-150 mg/day, if required, in divided doses throughout the day or as a single dose at bedtime. Many patients will be adequately maintained on 30-50 mg/day. Higher doses may be needed in some patients. In severe cases this dosage can be increased up to a maximum of 250 mg per day. Once a distinct improvement has set in, the daily dosage may be adjusted to a maintenance level averaging either 2-4 capsules of 25 mg or 1 tablet of 75 mg. Where a higher dose is required, the 75 mg SR formulation may be preferable.

*Intramuscular/Intravenous*–see below.

*Elderly:* The initial dose should be 10 mg/day, which may be increased with caution under close supervision to an optimum level of 30-50 mg daily, which should be reached after about 10 days and then maintained until the end of treatment.

*Children:* Not recommended.

*Obsessional/phobic states (oral or parenteral treatment):* The maintenance dosage of Anafranil is generally higher than that used in depression. It is recommended that the dose be built up to 100-150 mg Anafranil daily, according to the severity of the condition. This should be attained gradually over a period of 2 weeks starting with 1 x 25 mg Anafranil daily. In elderly patients and those sensitive to tricyclic antidepressants a starting dose of 1 x 10 mg Anafranil daily is recommended. Again where a higher dosage is required, the SR 75 mg formulation may be preferable.

*Adjunctive treatment of cataplexy associated with narcolepsy (oral treatment):* 10-75 mg daily. It is suggested that treatment is commenced with 10 mg Anafranil daily and gradually increased until a satisfactory response occurs. Control of cataplexy should be achieved within 24 hours of reaching the optimal dose.

Where necessary, therapy may be combined with capsules and syrup up to the maximum dose of 75 mg per day.

*Intramuscular administration:* Commence with 1-2 ampoules of 25 mg daily, then increase the dosage by 1 ampoule daily until the patient is receiving 4-6 ampoules a day. Once improvement has occurred, the number of injections should be gradually reduced

while at the same time switching the patient to oral treatment (maintenance doses).

*Intravenous infusion: administration and dosage:* Any standard giving set may be used but a cannula or fine needle with a flange which can be strapped in position should be chosen. Anafranil ampoules may be diluted with either physiological saline or 5% Dextrose BP The required dose of Anafranil should be introduced into the infusion fluid with a sterile syringe and the contents should be agitated to ensure even distribution of the drug before infusion is commenced into a forearm vein.

In the first instance a small dose of Anafranil (25 mg or 50 mg) should be diluted in 250-500 ml of infusion fluid and infused over a period of 1.5-3 hours to assess tolerability. If satisfactory, the dose may be increased by 25 mg daily until an optimum therapeutic dose has been achieved. At the same time the volume of fluid may be reduced (to a minimum of 125 ml) and the duration of infusion decreased (to a minimum of 45 minutes). The normal therapeutic dose will be in the region of 100 mg but higher doses may be required in more severe depressions or in obsessional and phobic states.

*Length of treatment:* Infusions should be given only to patients who are unable to take the drug orally. Oral therapy should be substituted once therapy has started to be effective, usually after 7-10 days.

*Changeover to oral therapy:* it is advisable to give double the maximum intravenous dosage orally until the patient's response is assured. Thereafter, a suitable maintenance dose, if considered necessary, can be selected.

*Monitoring during treatment:* During the course of infusion, patients should be monitored carefully for adverse effects. Particular attention should be paid to blood pressure recording, especially if there are any changes of position after conclusion of the infusion, as hypotension may occur. Patients often feel drowsy during treatment and not infrequently fall asleep.

## Contra-indications, warnings, etc
*Contra-indications:* Known hypersensitivity to clomipramine, or any of the excipients or cross-sensitivity to tricyclic antidepressants of the dibenzazepine group. Recent myocardial infarction. Any degree of heart block or other cardiac arrhythmias. Mania, severe liver disease, narrow angle glaucoma. Retention of urine. Anafranil should not be given in combination or within 3 weeks before or after treatment with a MAO inhibitor (see Drug Interactions). The concomitant treatment with selective, reversible MAO-A inhibitors, such as moclobemide, is also contra-indicated.

*Warnings:* Patients receiving Anafranil should be warned that blurred vision, drowsiness and other CNS symptoms (see Side Effects) may occur in which case they should not drive, operate machinery or do anything else which may require alertness or quick actions. Patients should also be warned that consumption of alcohol or other drugs may potentiate these effects (see Drug Interactions).

As improvement in depression may not occur for the first two to four weeks treatment, patients should be closely monitored during this period.

Tricyclic antidepressants are known to lower the convulsion threshold and Anafranil should therefore be used with extreme caution in patients with epilepsy and other predisposing factors, e.g. brain damage of varying aetiology, concomitant use of neuroleptics, withdrawal from alcohol or drugs with anticonvulsive properties (e.g. benzodiazepines). It appears that the occurence of seizures is dose dependent, therefore the recommended total daily dose of Anafranil should not be exceeded.

Caution is called for when giving tricyclic antidepressants to patients with tumours of the adrenal medulla (e.g. phaeochromocytoma, neuroblastoma), in whom they may provoke hypertensive crises.

Concomitant treatment of Anafranil and electroconvulsive therapy should only be resorted to under careful supervision.

Elderly patients are particularly liable to experience adverse effects, especially agitation, confusion, and postural hypotension.

Many patients with panic disorders experience intensified anxiety symptoms at the start of the treatment with antidepressants. This paradoxical initial increase in anxiety is most pronounced during the first few days of treatment and generally subsides within two weeks.

Isolated cases of anaphylactic shock have been reported. Caution is called for when administering Anafranil intravenously.

*Precautions:* Before initiating treatment it is advisable to check the patient's blood pressure, because individuals with hypotension or a labile circulation may react to the drug with a fall in blood pressure.

Caution is indicated in patients with hyperthyroidism or during concomitant treatment with thyroid preparations since aggravation of unwanted cardiac effects may occur.

Although changes in the white blood cell count have been reported with Anafranil only in isolated cases, periodic blood cell counts and monitoring for symptoms such as fever and sore throat are called for, particularly during the first few months of therapy. They are also recommended during prolonged therapy.

It is advisable to monitor cardiac and hepatic function during long-term therapy with Anafranil. In patients with liver disease, periodic monitoring of hepatic enzyme levels is recommended.

Because of its anticholinergic properties, Anafranil should be used with caution in patients with a history of increased intra-ocular pressure, narrow angle glaucoma or urinary retention (e.g. diseases of the prostate).

Caution is called for in patients with chronic constipation. Tricyclic antidepressants may cause paralytic ileus, particularly in the elderly and in bedridden patients.

An increase in dental caries has been reported during long-term treatment with tricyclic antidepressants. Regular dental check-ups are therefore advisable during long-term treatment.

Decreased lacrimation and accumulation of mucoid secretions due to the anticholinergic properties of tricyclic antidepressants may cause damage to the corneal epithelium in patients with contact lenses.

Risk of suicide is inherent to severe depression and may persist until significant remission occurs. Patients posing a high suicide risk require close initial supervision.

Activation of psychosis has occasionally been observed in schizophrenic patients receiving tricyclic antidepressants. Hypomanic or manic episodes have also been reported during a depressive phase in patients with cyclic affective disorders receiving treatment with a tricyclic antidepressant. In such cases it may be necessary to reduce the dosage of Anafranil or to withdraw it and administer an antipsychotic agent. After such episodes have subsided, low dose therapy with Anafranil may be resumed if required.

Anafranil may cause anxiety, feelings of unrest, and hyperexcitation in agitated patients and patients with accompanying schizophrenic symptoms.

In predisposed and elderly patients, Anafranil may, particularly at night, provoke pharmacogenic (delirious) psychoses, which disappear without treatment within a few days of withdrawing the drug.

Before general or local anaesthesia, the anaesthetist should be aware that the patient has been receiving Anafranil and of the possible interactions (see Drug Interactions).

Abrupt withdrawal should be avoided because of possible adverse reactions (see Side-Effects).

*Use in pregnancy and lactation:* There is inadequate evidence of safety of Anafranil in human pregnancy. Do not use unless there are compelling reasons, especially during the first and last trimesters. Animal work has not shown clomipramine to be free from hazard.

Neonates whose mothers had taken tricyclic antidepressants up until delivery have developed dyspnoea, lethargy, colic, irritability, hypotension or hypertension, tremor or spasms, during the first few hours or days. Anafranil should–if this is at all justifiable–be withdrawn at least 7 weeks before the calculated date of confinement.

The active substance of Anafranil passes into the breast milk in small quantities. Therefore nursing mothers should be advised to withdraw the medication or cease breast-feeding.

*Drug interactions:*
*MAO inhibitors:* Do not give Anafranil for at least 3 weeks after discontinuation of treatment with MAO inhibitors (there is a risk of severe symptoms such as hypertensive crisis, hyperpyrexia, myoclonus, agitation, seizures, delirium and coma). The same applies when giving a MAO inhibitor after previous treatment with Anafranil. In both instances the treatment should initially be given in small gradually increasing doses and its effects monitored. There is evidence to suggest that Anafranil may be given as little as 24 hours after a reversible MAO-A inhibitor such as moclobemide, but the 3 week wash-out period must be observed if the MAO-A inhibitor is used after Anafranil.

*Selective serotonin reuptake inhibitors:* Co-medication may lead to additive effects on the serotonin system. Fluoxetine and fluvoxamine may also increase plasma concentrations of clomipramine, with corresponding effects.

*CNS depressants:* Tricyclic antidepressants may potentiate the effects of alcohol and other central depressant substances (e.g. barbiturates, benzodiazepines, or general anaesthetics).

*Neuroleptics:* Comedication may result in increased plasma levels of tricyclic antidepressants, a lowered convulsion threshold, and seizures. Combination with thioridazine may produce severe cardiac arrhythmias.

*Adrenergic neurone blockers:* Anafranil may diminish or abolish the antihypertensive effects of guanethidine, betanidine, reserpine, clonidine and alpha-methyldopa. Patients requiring comedication for hypertension should therefore be given antihypertensives of a different type (e.g. diuretics, vasodilators, or beta-blockers).

*Anticoagulants:* Tricyclic antidepressants may potentiate the anticoagulant effect of coumarin drugs by inhibiting their metabolism by the liver. Careful monitoring of plasma prothrombin is therefore advised.

*Anticholinergic agents:* Tricyclic antidepressants may potentiate the effects of these drugs (e.g. phenothiazine, antiparkinsonian agents, antihistamines, atropine, biperiden) on the eye, central nervous system, bowel and bladder.

*Sympathomimetic drugs:* Anafranil may potentiate the cardiovascular effects of adrenaline, ephedrine, isoprenaline, noradrenaline, phenylephrine, and phenylpropanolamine (e.g. as contained in local and general anaesthetic preparations and nasal decongestants).

*Quinidine:* Tricyclic antidepressants should not be employed in combination with antiarrhythmic agents of the quinidine type.

*Liver-enzyme inducers:* Drugs which activate the hepatic mono-oxygenase enzyme system (e.g. barbiturates, carbamazepine, phenytoin, nicotine and oral contraceptives) may accelerate the metabolism and lower the plasma concentrations of clomipramine, resulting in decreased efficacy. Plasma levels of phenytoin and carbamazepine may increase, with corresponding adverse effects. It may be necessary to adjust the dosage of these drugs.

*Cimetidine, methylphenidate and estrogens:* these drugs increase plasma concentrations of tricyclic antidepressants, whose dosage should therefore be reduced.

*Side-effects:* Unwanted effects are usually mild and transient, disappearing under continued treatment or with a reduction in the dosage. They do not always correlate with plasma drug levels or dose. It is often difficult to distinguish certain undesirable effects from symptoms of depression such as fatigue, sleep disturbances, agitation, anxiety, constipation and dry mouth.

If severe neurological or psychiatric reactions occur, Anafranil should be withdrawn.

Elderly patients are particularly sensitive to anticholinergic, neurological, psychiatric, or cardiovascular effects. Their ability to metabolise and eliminate drugs may be reduced, leading to a risk of elevated plasma concentrations at therapeutic doses.

The following side-effects, although not necessarily observed with Anafranil, have occured with tricyclic antidepressants.

Frequency estimate: frequent > 10%, occasional > 1-10%, rare > 0.001-1%, isolated cases < 0.001%.

*Anticholinergic effects:* Frequently: dryness of the mouth, sweating, constipation, disorders of visual accommodation and blurred vision, disturbances of micturition. Occasionally: hot flushes, mydriasis. Isolated cases: of glaucoma.

*Central nervous system: Psychiatric effects:* Frequently: drowsiness, transient fatigue, feelings of unrest, increased appetite. Occasionally: confusion accompanied by disorientation and hallucinations (particularly in geriatric patients and patients suffering from Parkinson's disease), anxiety states, agitation, sleep disturbances, mania, hypomania, aggressiveness, impaired memory, yawning, depersonalisation, insomnia, nightmares, aggravated depression, impaired concentration. Isolated cases of activation of psychotic symptoms.

*Neurological effects:* Frequently: dizziness, tremor, headache, myoclonus. Occasionally: delirium, speech disorders, paraesthesia, muscle weakness, muscle hypertonia. Rarely: convulsions, ataxia. Isolated cases: EEG changes, hyperpyrexia.

*Cardiovascular system:* Occasionally: postural hypotension, sinus tachycardia, and clinically irrelevant ECG changes in patients of normal cardiac status (e.g. T and ST changes), palpitations. Rarely: arrhythmias, increased blood pressure. Isolated cases: conduction disorders (e.g. widening of QRS complex, PQ changes, bundle-branch block).

*Gastro-intestinal tract:* Frequently: nausea. Occasionally: vomiting, abdominal disorders, diarrhoea, anorexia.

*Hepatic effects:* Rarely: elevated transaminases. Isolated cases: hepatitis with or without jaundice.

*Skin:* Occasionally: allergic skin reactions (skin rash, urticaria), photosensitivity, pruritus. Isolated cases: local reactions after intravenous injections (thrombophlebitis, lymphangitis, burning sensation, and allergic skin reactions), oedema (local or generalised), hair loss.

*Endocrine system and metabolism:* Frequently: weight gain, disturbances of libido and potency. Occasionally: galactorrhoea, breast enlargement. Isolated cases: SIADH (inappropriate antidiuretic hormone secretion syndrome).

*Hypersensitivity:* Isolated cases: allergic alveolitis (pneumonitis) with or without eosinophilia, systemic anaphylactic/anaphylactoid reactions including hypotension.

*Blood:* Isolated cases: leucopenia, agranulocytosis, thrombocytopenia, eosinophilia, and purpura.

*Sense organs:* Occasionally: taste disturbances, tinnitus.

*Others:* The following symptoms occasionally occur after abrupt withdrawal or reduction of the dose: nausea, vomiting, abdominal pain, diarrhoea, insomnia, headache, nervousness and anxiety.

*Overdose:* Overdose with ampoules has not been reported. The following information relates to overdosage with oral dosage forms.

The signs and symptoms of overdose with Anafranil are similar to those reported with other tricyclic antidepressants. Cardiac abnormalities and neurological disturbances are the main complications. In children accidental ingestion of any amount should be regarded as serious and potentially fatal.

*Signs and symptoms:* Symptoms generally appear within 4 hours of ingestion and reach maximum severity after 24 hours. Owing to delayed absorption (anticholinergic effect), long half-life, and enterohepatic recycling of the drug, the patient may be at risk for up to 4-6 days.

*The following signs and symptoms may be seen:*
Central nervous system: drowsiness, stupor, coma, ataxia, restlessness, agitation, enhanced reflexes, muscular rigidity and choreoathetoid movements, convulsions

Cardiovascular system: hypotension, tachycardia, arrhythmias, conduction disorders, shock, heart failure; in very rare cases cardiac arrest

Respiratory depression, cyanosis, vomiting, fever, mydriasis, sweating and oliguria or anuria may also occur.

*Treatment:* There is no specific antidote, and treatment is essentially symptomatic and supportive.

Anyone suspected of receiving an overdose of Anafranil, particularly children, should be hospitalised and kept under close surveillance for at least 72 hours.

Perform gastric lavage or induce vomiting as soon as possible if the patient is alert. If the patient has impaired consciousness, secure the airway with a cuffed endotracheal tube before beginning lavage, and do not induce vomiting. These measures are recommended for up to 12 hours or even longer after the overdose, since the anticholinergic effect of the drug may delay gastric emptying. Administration of activated charcoal may help to reduce drug absorption.

Treatment of symptoms is based on modern methods of intensive care, with continuous monitoring of cardiac function, blood gases, and electrolytes and, if necessary, emergency measures such as:
- anticonvulsive therapy
- artificial respiration,
- insertion of a temporary cardiac pacemaker,
- plasma expander, dopamine or dobutamine administered by intravenous drip,
- resuscitation.

Since it has been reported that physostigmine may cause severe bradycardia, asystole and seizures, its use is not recommended in cases of overdosage with Anafranil. Haemodialysis or peritoneal dialysis are ineffective because of the low plasma concentrations of clomipramine.

**Pharmaceutical precautions**
*Storage:* Capsules- protect from moisture. Store below 30°C.

Anafranil SR- protect from moisture.

Syrup- store below 25°C. Keep the container tightly closed.

Ampoules- protect from light. Discard any unused portion.

*Dilutions:* Syrup–dilutions down to 15 mg/5 ml can be prepared with boiled, distilled or de-ionised water. For dilutions below 15 mg/5 ml the recommended diluent is equal parts simple Syrup BP and freshly prepared Tragacanth Mucilage BPC 1973. After dilution the solution should be used within a few days.

**Legal category** POM

**Package quantities**
Tablets 75 mg SR:Blister packs of 28
Capsules 50 mg:Blister packs of 56
Capsules 25 mg:Blister packs of 84
Capsules 10 mg:Blister packs of 84
Syrup 25 mg/5 ml:Bottles of 150 ml
Ampoules 25 mg/2 ml:Boxes of 10

**Further information** Anafranil SR tablets should be swallowed whole.

**Product licence numbers**
Tablets 75 mg SR 00101/0436
Capsules 50 mg 00101/0440
Capsules 25 mg 00101/0439
Capsules 10 mg 00101/0438
Syrup 25 mg/5 ml 00101/0441
Ampoules 25 mg/2 ml 00101/0437

## ANTURAN*

**Presentation** The active ingredient, Sulphinpyrazone BP is presented as light yellow, sugar coated, round, biconvex, approximately 10.6 mm diameter, printed GEIGY on one side, each containing 200 mg.

Pale-yellow, sugar coated tablets, round, biconvex, approximately 8.5 mm diameter, printed GEIGY on one side, each containing 100 mg.

The tablets also contain lactose and sucrose.

**Uses**
*Indications:* Chronic, including tophaceous gout; recurrent gouty arthritis; hyperuricaemia.

*Mode of action:* Anturan lowers serum urate levels by blocking tubular reabsorption, thereby increasing renal excretion of uric acid. As a result of increased excretion, serum urate deposits are mobilised and tophi are no longer formed.

*Pharmacokinetics:* After oral administration the active substance is absorbed rapidly and almost completely (> 85%).

Following a single oral dose of 100 mg or 200 mg, sulphinpyrazone, peak plasma concentrations of 5-6µg/ml or 13-22µg/ml, respectively, are attained after 1-2 hours. Sulphinpyrazone has a half-life of 2-4 hours.

Following repeated administration of sulphinpyrazone in a dosage of 400 mg bid for 23 days, a significant decrease in the AUC values and an increase in the drug's clearance was observed as compared with the values recorded after a single dose. After multiple dosing with 400 mg bid, the mean steady-state concentration of sulphinpyrazone amounts to 5.1µg/ml, which corresponds to only half of the calculated value after a single dose (9.6µg/ml). The reason for this is an increase in total clearance brought about by the fact that the drug induces its own metabolism.

Sulphinpyrazone is metabolised by reduction to the sulphide and by oxidation to the sulphone and to hydroxy-compounds. The sulphide metabolite inhibits platelet aggregation *in vitro* about 12 times more strongly than sulphinpyrazone itself. In comparison with sulphinpyrazone the plasma concentrations of the sulphide metabolite are low. Peak sulphide concentrations are reached approx. 19 hours after administration of a single dose.

**Dosage and administration** Anturan is administered orally in tablet form with meals or milk.

*Hyperuricaemia*
*Adults:* 100-200 mg daily increasing gradually (over the first two or three weeks) to 600 mg daily (rarely 800 mg), and maintained until the serum urate level has fallen within the normal range. Subsequent dosage should be reduced, to the lowest level which maintains serum urate within the normal range. Maintenance dose may be as low as 200 mg daily. Reduced dose required in renal impairment. Not to be used in severe renal impairment.

*Children:* Paediatric usage not established.

**Contra-indications, warnings, etc**
*Contra-indications:* Acute attacks of gout. Treatment with Anturan should not be initiated during an acute attack of gout.

Gastric and duodenal ulcer (overt or case-history). Known hypersensitivity to sulphinpyrazone and other pyrazolone derivatives. Sulphinpyrazone is contra-indicated in patients in whom attacks of asthma, urticaria, or acute rhinitis are precipitated by acetylsalicylic acid or by other drugs with prostaglandin-synthetase inhibiting activity.

Severe parenchymal lesions of the liver or kidneys (also in the case history). Porphyria. Blood dyscrasias (also in the case history). Haemorrhagic diatheses (e.g. blood coagulation disorders).

In the treatment of chronic gout salicylates antagonise the action of Anturan and should not be given concurrently.

*Warnings:* During the early stages of treatment in patients with hyperuricaemia or gout, acute attacks of gout may be precipitated. To help prevent episodes of urolithiasis or renal colic, ensure adequate fluid intake and alkalinisation of the urine during initial stages of therapy.

Since Anturan may cause salt and water retention, caution is called for in patients with overt or latent heart failure.

For the early detection of a haematological abnormality, careful clinical supervision and full blood count should be done before and at regular intervals during treatment.

*Precautions:* Use with caution in patients with impaired renal function.

In patients with an elevated plasma uric acid level and/or with a history of nephrolithiasis or renal colic, and also when resuming treatment after interruption of the medication, a cautious incremental dosage schedule should be adopted. As with any form of long-term uricosuric medication, renal function tests should be performed regularly, particularly in cases where there is pre-existing evidence of renal failure.

*Use during pregnancy and lactation:* Anturan should be used with caution in pregnant women, weighing the potential risk against the possible benefits.

It is not known whether the active substance of Anturan and/or its metabolite(s) pass into breast milk. For safety reasons mothers should refrain from taking the drug.

*Drug interactions:* Since Anturan may potentiate the action of coumarin-type anticoagulants, frequent estimation of prothrombin time should be undertaken when these drugs are given concurrently, and the dosage of anticoagulant adjusted accordingly.

Anturan may also potentiate the action of other plasma protein binding drugs such as hypoglycaemic agents and sulphonamides, which may necessitate a modification in dosage.

Penicillins (e.g. penicillin G): Inhibition of tubular secretion may raise the plasma concentrations of penicillins.

Theophylline: Activation of microsomal liver enzymes and resultant acceleration of metabolism lowers the plasma concentration of theophylline.

Phenytoin: Displacement of phenytoin from its plasma protein-binding sites as well as inhibition of microsomal liver enzymes delays the metabolism of phenytoin, thus prolonging its half-life and raising its plasma concentration.

Substances affecting haemostasis: Such substances, e.g. non-steroidal antirheumatic drugs, may exert a synergistic effect on the blood coagulation system and thus increase the risk of haemorrhage.

*Side effects:*
*Gastro-intestinal tract:* Frequent: mild transient gastro-intestinal upsets, such as nausea, vomiting, diarrhoea. In isolated cases: gastro-intestinal bleeding and ulcers.

*Urogenital system:* Rare: acute renal failure (mostly reversible), especially with high initial dosages. In isolated cases: salt and water retention.

*Skin:* Rare: allergic skin reactions (e.g. drug rash, urticaria).

*Blood:* In isolated cases: leucopenia, thrombocytopenia, agranulocytosis, aplastic anaemia.

*Liver:* In isolated cases: hepatic dysfunction (increase in transaminases and alkaline phosphatase), jaundice, and hepatitis.

*Overdosage:* There is no antidote to Anturan.
*Signs and symptoms:* Nausea, vomiting, abdominal pains, diarrhoea, hypotension, cardiac arrhythmias, hyperventilation, respiratory disorders, impairment of consciousness, coma, epileptic seizures, oliguria or anuria, acute renal failure, renal colic.

*Treatment:* Immediate treatment consists of forced emesis to recover undigested tablets. This is followed by gastric lavage preferably with mild alkaline solution such as sodium bicarbonate solution and supportive therapy as indicated.

Note that forced diuresis is of no value.

**Pharmaceutical precautions**
*Storage:* Protect from moisture and store below 25°C.

**Legal category** POM.

**Package quantities**
Tablets 100 mg and 200 mg: Containers and blister packs of 84 tablets.

**Product licence numbers**
Tablets 100 mg 0001/5002R
Tablets 200 mg 0001/0080

*Product licence holder:* Ciba-Geigy plc, Hulley Road, Macclesfield, Cheshire SK10 2NX.

## APRESOLINE*

**Presentation** Tablets containing 25 mg Hydralazine Hydrochloride BP, circular, polished, sugar-coated, pale yellow in colour marked CIBA on one side and the letters GF on the other.

Ampoules for intravenous use containing 20 mg hydralazine hydrochloride, as a white or yellowish lyophilised powder (requiring reconstitution before use–see Dosage below).

The tablets also contain gluten (wheat starch) and sucrose.

The ampoules contain hydralazine hydrochloride active substance only.

**Uses**
*Indications:*
*Hypertension:* Oral: Moderate to severe hypertension as an adjunct to other anti-hypertensive agents.

Use in combination with long active nitrates in moderate to severe chronic congestive cardiac failure in patients in whom optimal doses of diuretics and cardiac glycosides have proved insufficient.

*Intravenous:* Hypertensive emergencies, particularly those associated with pre-eclampsia and toxaemia of pregnancy and in hypertension with renal complications

*Mode of action:* Hydralazine is a direct acting vasodilator which exerts its effects principally on the arterioles. Its precise mode of action is not known. Administration of hydralazine produces a fall in peripheral resistance and a decrease in arterial blood pressure, effects which induce reflex sympathetic cardiovascular responses. The concomitant use of a beta-blocker will reduce these reflex effects and enhance the anti-hypertensive effect. The use of hydralazine can result in sodium and fluid retention, producing oedema and reduced urinary volume. These effects can be prevented by concomitant administration of a diuretic.

*Pharmacokinetics:* Orally administered Apresoline is rapidly and completely absorbed but is subject to a dose-dependent first pass effect (systemic bioavailability: 26-55%) which is dependent upon the individuals acetylator status. Peak plasma concentrations are attained after 0.5 to 1.5 hours. Apresoline appears in the plasma chiefly in the form of a readily hydrolysable conjugate with pyruvic acid. Plasma half-life averages 2-3 hours but is prolonged up to 16 hours in severe renal failure (creatinine clearance less than 20 ml/min) and shortened to approximately 45 minutes in rapid acetylators. Apresoline is rapidly distributed in the body and displays a particular affinity for the blood-vessel walls. Plasma protein binding is of the order of 90%. Within 24 hours after an oral dose, the quantity recovered in the urine averages 80% of the dose.

The bulk of the dose is excreted as acetylated and hydroxylated metabolites, some of which are conjugated with glucuronic acid.

**Dosage and administration** SEE PRECAUTIONS BEFORE USE.

*Adults:*
*Hypertension:* The dose should be adjusted to the individual requirements of the patient. Treatment should begin with low doses of Apresoline which, depending on the patients response should be increased stepwise to achieve optimal therapeutic effect whilst keep unwanted effects to a minimum.

*Oral:* Initially 25 mg bid. This can be increased gradually to a dose not exceeding 200 mg daily. The dose should not be increased beyond 100 mg daily without first checking the patients acetylator status (see Warnings).

*Parenteral:* Initially 5 to 10 mg by slow intravenous injection, to avoid precipitous decreases in arterial pressure with a critical reduction in cerebral or utero-placental perfusion. If necessary a repeat injection can be given after an interval of 20-30 minutes, throughout which blood pressure and heart rate should be monitored. A satisfactory response can be defined as a decrease in diastolic blood pressure to 90/100 mmHg. The contents of the vial should be reconstituted by dissolving in 1 ml of Water for Injection BP. This should then be further diluted with 10 ml of Sodium Chloride injection BP 0.9% and be administered by slow intravenous injection. The injection must be given immediately and any remainder discarded. Apresoline may also be given by continuous intravenous infusion, beginning with a flow rate of 200-300µg/min. Maintenance flow rates must be determined individually and are usually within the range 50-150µg/min. The product reconstituted as for direct iv injection may be added via the infusion container to 500 ml of Sodium Chloride Injection BP 0.9% and given by continuous infusion. The addition should be made immediately before administration and the mixture should not be stored. Apresoline for infusion can also be used with 5% sorbitol solution or isotonic inorganic infusion solutions such as Ringer's solution.

*Incompatibility:* Dextrose infusion solutions are not compatible because contact between hydralazine and glucose causes hydralazine to be rapidly broken down.

*Chronic congestive heart failure.* Treatment with

Apresoline should always be initiated in hospital, where the patients' individual haemodynamic values can be reliably determined with the help of invasive monitoring. It should then be continued in hospital until the patient has become stabilised on the requisite maintenance dose. Doses vary greatly between individual patients and are generally higher than those used for treating hypertension. After progressive titration (initially 25 mg tid or qid increasing every second day) the maintenance dosage averages 50-75 mg qid.

*Children*: Not recommended.

*Elderly*: Clinical evidence would indicate that no special dosage regime is necessary. Advancing age does not affect either blood concentration or systemic clearance. Renal elimination may however be affected insofar as kidney function diminishes with age.

### Contra-indications, warnings, etc
*Contra-indications*: Known hypersensitivity to hydralazine or dihydralazine.

Idiopathic systemic lupus erythematosus (SLE) and related diseases.

Severe tachycardia and heart failure with a high cardiac output (e.g. in thyrotoxicosis).

Myocardial insufficiency due to mechanical obstruction (e.g. in the presence of aortic or mitral stenosis or constrictive pericarditis).

Isolated right ventricular failure due to pulmonary hypertension (cor pulmonale).

Dissecting aortic aneurysm.

*Warnings*: The overall 'hyperdynamic' state of the circulation induced by hydralazine may accentuate certain clinical conditions. Myocardial stimulation may provoke or aggravate angina pectoris. Patients with suspected or confirmed coronary artery disease should therefore be given Apresoline only under cover of beta-blocker or in combination with other suitable sympatholytic agents. It is important that the beta-blocker medication should be commenced a few days before the start of treatment with Apresoline.

Patients who have survived a myocardial infarction should not receive Apresoline until a post-infarction stabilisation phase has been achieved.

Prolonged treatment with hydralazine (i.e. usually for more than 6 months) may provoke a lupus erythematosus (LE) like syndrome, especially where doses exceed 100 mg daily. First symptoms are likely to be arthralgia, sometimes associated with fever and rash and are reversible after withdrawal of the drug. In its more severe form it resembles acute SLE, and in rare cases renal and ocular involvement have been reported. Long term treatment with corticosteroids may be required to reverse these changes. Since such reactions tend to occur more frequently the higher the dose and the longer its duration, and since they are also more common in slow acetylators, it is recommended that for maintenance therapy the lowest effective dose should be used. If 100 mg daily fails to elicit an adequate clinical effect, the patient's acetylator status should be evaluated. Slow acetylators and women run a greater risk of developing the LE-like syndrome and every effort should therefore be made to keep the dosage below 100 mg daily and a careful watch kept for signs and symptoms suggestive of this syndrome. If such symptoms do develop the drug should be gradually withdrawn. Rapid acetylators often respond inadequately even to doses of 100 mg daily and therefore the dose can be raised with only a slightly increased risk of an LE-like syndrome.

During long-term treatment with Apresoline it is advisable to determine the antinuclear factors and conduct urine analysis at intervals of approximately 6 months. Microhaematuria and/or proteinuria, in particular together with positive titres of ANF, may be initial signs of immune-complex glomerulonephritis associated with the SLE-like syndrome. If overt clinical signs or symptoms develop, the drug should be withdrawn immediately.

Skin rash, febrile reactions and change in blood count occur rarely and drug should be withdrawn. Peripheral neuritis in the form of paraesthesia has been reported, and may respond to pyridoxine administration or drug withdrawal.

In high (cyto-) toxic concentrations, Hydralazine induces gene mutations in single cell organisms and in mammalian cells *in-vitro*. No unequivocally mutagenic effects have been detected *in-vivo* in a great number of test systems.

Hydralazine, in lifetime carcinogenicity studies, caused, towards the end of the experiments, small but statistically significant increases in lung tumours in mice and in hepatic and testicular tumours in rats. These tumours also occur spontaneously with fairly high frequency in aged rodents.

With due consideration of these animal and *in-vitro* toxicological findings, hydralazine in therapeutic doses does not appear to bear a risk that would necessitate a limitation of its administration. Many

years of clinical experience have not suggested that human cancer is associated with hydralazine use.

Apresoline may impair the patient's reactions, especially at the start of treatment. The patient should be warned of the hazard when driving or operating machinery.

*Precautions*: In patients with renal impairment (creatinine clearance < 30 ml/min or serum creatinine concentrations > 2.5 mg/100 ml or 221µmol/l) and in patients with hepatic dysfunction the dose or interval between doses should be adjusted according to clinical response, in order to avoid accumulation of the 'apparent' active substance.

Apresoline should be used with caution in patients with coronary artery disease (since it may increase angina) or cerebrovascular disease.

When undergoing surgery, patients treated with Apresoline may show a fall in blood pressure, in which case one should not use adrenalin to correct the hypotension, since it enhances the cardiac-accelerating effects of hydralazine.

When initiating therapy in heart failure, particular caution should be exercised and the patient kept under surveillance and/or haemodynamic monitoring for early detection of postural hypotension or tachycardia. Where discontinuation of therapy in heart failure is indicated, Apresoline should be withdrawn gradually (except in serious situations, such as SLE-like syndrome or blood dyscrasias) in order to avoid precipitation and/or exacerbation of heart failure.

*Use in pregnancy and lactation*: Use of Apresoline in pregnancy, before the third trimester should be avoided but the drug may be employed in later pregnancy if there is no safer alternative or when the disease itself carries serious risks for the mother or child e.g. pre-eclampsia and/or eclampsia.

Hydralazine has been found to be teratogenic in mice producing a small incidence of cleft palate and certain other bony malformations, in oral doses ranging from 20-120 mg/kg i.e. 20-30 times the maximum human daily dose. It was not teratogenic in rats or rabbits.

No serious adverse effects in human pregnancy have been reported to date with Apresoline, although experience in the third trimester is extensive.

Hydralazine passes into breast milk but reports available so far have not shown adverse effects on the infant. Mothers in whom use of Apresoline proves unavoidable may breast feed their infant provided that the infant is observed for possible adverse effects.

*Drug interactions*: Potentiation of effects: Concurrent therapy with other antihypertensives (vasodilators, calcium antagonists, ACE inhibitors, diuretics), anaesthetics, tricyclic antidepressants, major tranquillisers or drugs exerting central depressant actions (including alcohol).

Administration of Apresoline shortly before or after diazoxide may give rise to marked hypotension.

MAO inhibitors should be used with caution in patients receiving Apresoline.

Concurrent administration of Apresoline with beta-blockers subject to a strong first-pass effect (e.g. propranolol) may increase their bioavailability. Downward adjustment of these drugs may be required when they are given concomitantly with Apresoline.

*Side-effects*: Some of the adverse effects listed below e.g. tachycardia, palpitation, anginal symptoms, flushing, headache, dizziness, nasal congestion and gastrointestinal disturbances are commonly seen at the start of treatment, especially if the dose is raised quickly. However such effects generally subside in the further course of treatment.
*Cardiovascular system:* Frequently: tachycardia, palpitation. Occasionally: flushing, hypotension, anginal symptoms. Rarely: oedema, heart failure. Isolated cases: paradoxical pressor responses.
*Central and peripheral nervous system:* Frequently: headache. Rarely: dizziness. Isolated cases: peripheral neuritis, polyneuritis, paraesthesiae (these unwanted effects may be reversed by administering pyridoxine).
*Musculo-skeletal system:* Occasionally: arthralgia, joint swelling, myalgia.
*Skin and appendages:* Rarely: rash.
*Urogenital system:* Rarely: proteinuria, increased plasma creatinine, haematuria sometimes in association with glomerulonephritis. Isolated cases: acute renal failure, urinary retention.
*Gastro-intestinal tract: Occasionally:* gastro-intestinal disturbances, diarrhoea, nausea, vomiting. Rarely: jaundice, liver enlargement, abnormal liver function sometimes in association with hepatitis. Isolated cases: paralytic ileus.
*Blood:* Rarely: anaemia, leucopenia, neutropenia, thrombocytopenia with or without purpura. Isolated cases: haemolytic anaemia, leucocytosis, lymphadenopathy, pancytopenia, splenomegaly, agranulocytosis.
*Psyche:* Rarely: agitation, anorexia, anxiety. Isolated cases: depression, hallucinations.

*Sense organs:* Rarely: increased lacrimation, conjunctivitis, nasal congestion.
*Hypersensitivity reactions:* Occasionally: SLE-like syndrome (see under Warnings). Rarely: hypersensitivity reactions such as pruritus, urticaria, vasculitis, eosinophilia, hepatitis.
*Respiratory tract:*Rarely: dyspnoea, pleural pain.
*Miscellaneous:*Rarely: fever, weight decrease, malaise. Isolated cases: exophthalmos.
*Overdosage:* Symptoms include hypotension, tachycardia, myocardial ischaemia, dysrrhythmias and coma.

Gastric lavage should be instituted as soon as possible. Supportive measures including intravenous fluids are also indicated. If hypotension is present, an attempt should be made to raise the blood pressure without increasing the tachycardia. Adrenaline should therefore be avoided.

**Pharmaceutical precautions** The tablets should be protected from moisture and heat and stored below 30°C.

The ampoules should be protected from light and stored below 30°C. The reconstituted solution should be stored below 25°C and used within 24 hours.

**Legal category** POM.

**Package quantities**
Apresoline tablets:Securitainers of 84 and 100
Apresoline ampoules:Boxes of 5

**Further information** Nil.

**Product licence numbers**
Apresoline tablets 25 mg 00101/0443
Apresoline ampoules 20 mg 00101/0442

## AREDIA* DRY POWDER

**Qualitative and quantitative composition** The active ingredient is disodium 3-amino-1-hydroxypropylidene-1, 1-bisphosphonate pentahydrate (pamidronate disodium).

One vial contains 15 mg, 30 mg or 90 mg of sterile, lyophilised pamidronate disodium. An ampoule containing 5 mL sterile water for injections is supplied with each 15 mg vial, and a 10 mL ampoule with each 30 mg or 90 mg vial.

**Pharmaceutical form** Powder in vials together with ampoules of water for reconstitution.

**Clinical particulars**
*Therapeutic indications:* Treatment of conditions associated with increased osteoclast activity:
– Tumour-induced hypercalcaemia
– Osteolytic lesions and bone pain in patients with bone metastases associated with breast cancer or multiple myeloma
– Paget's disease of bone.

*Posology and method of administration:* Aredia must never be given as a bolus injection (see 'Warnings'). The reconstituted solution of Aredia from powder in vials should be diluted in a calcium-free infusion solution (0.9% w/v Sodium Chloride Intravenous Infusion BP is recommended) and infused slowly.

The infusion rate should never exceed 60 mg/hour (1 mg/min), and the concentration of Aredia in the infusion solution should not exceed 60 mg/250 ml. In patients with established or suspected renal impairment (e.g. those with tumour-induced hypercalcaemia or multiple myeloma) it is recommended that the infusion rate does not exceed 20 mg/h (see also 'Renal Impairment'). In order to minimise local reactions at the infusion site, the cannula should be inserted carefully into a relatively large vein.

Until further experience is gained, Aredia is only recommended for use in adult patients.

*Tumour-induced hypercalcaemia:* It is recommended that patients be rehydrated with 0.9% w/v sodium chloride solution before or during treatment.

The total dose of Aredia to be used for a treatment course depends on the patient's initial serum calcium levels. The following guidelines are derived from clinical data on uncorrected calcium values. However, doses within the ranges given are also applicable for calcium values corrected for serum or albumin in rehydrated patients.

| Initial serum calcium (mmol/L) | (mg %) | Recommended total dose (mg) |
|---|---|---|
| up to 3.0 | up to 12.0 | 15–30 |
| 3.0–3.5 | 12.0–14.0 | 30–60 |
| 3.5–4.0 | 14.0–16.0 | 60–90 |
| > 4.0 | > 16.0 | 90 |

The total dose of Aredia may be administered either in a single infusion or in multiple infusions over 2–4 consecutive days. The maximum dose per treatment course is 90 mg for both initial and repeat courses.

A significant decrease in serum calcium is generally observed 24–48 hours after administration of Aredia, and normalisation is usually achieved within 3 to 7 days. If normocalcaemia is not achieved within this time, a further dose may be given. The duration of the response may vary from patient to patient, and treatment can be repeated whenever hypercalcaemia recurs. Clinical experience to date suggests that Aredia may become less effective as the number of treatments increases.

*Osteolytic lesions and bone pain in multiple myeloma:* The recommended dose is 90 mg every 4 weeks.

*Osteolytic lesions and bone pain in bone metastases associated with breast cancer.*

The recommended dose is 90 mg every 4 weeks. This dose may also be administered at 3 weekly intervals to coincide with chemotherapy if desired.

*Paget's disease of bone:* The recommended treatment course consists of a total dose of 180 mg administered in unit doses of either 30 mg once a week for 6 consecutive weeks, or 60 mg every other week over 6 weeks. Experience to date suggests that any mild and transient unwanted effects (see 'Side-effects') tend to occur after the first dose. For this reason if unit doses of 60 mg are used it is recommended that treatment be started with an initial additional dose of 30 mg (i.e. total dose 210 mg). Each dose of 30 or 60 mg should be diluted in 125 or 250 ml 0.9% w/v Sodium Chloride Intravenous Infusion BP respectively, and the infusion rate should not exceed 60 mg/hour (1 mg/min). This regimen or increased dose levels according to disease severity, up to a maximum total dose of 360 mg (in divided doses of 60 mg) can be repeated every 6 months until remission of disease is achieved, and if relapse occurs.

*Renal impairment:* Pharmacokinetic studies indicate that no dose adjustment is necessary in patients with any degree of renal impairment. However, until further experience is gained a maximum infusion rate of 20 mg/h is recommended in renally impaired patients.

*Contra-indications:* Known hypersensitivity to Aredia or to other bisphosphonates.

*Special warnings and precautions for use:*
*Warnings:* Aredia must not be given as a bolus injection, but should always be diluted and given as a slow intravenous infusion (see 'Posology and method of administration').

Aredia should not be given with other bisphosphonates because their combined effects have not been investigated.

Convulsions have been precipitated in some patients with tumour-induced hypercalcaemia due to the electrolyte changes associated with this condition and its effective treatment.

*Precautions:* Serum electrolytes, calcium and phosphate should be monitored following initiation of therapy with Aredia. Patients who have undergone thyroid surgery may be particularly susceptible to develop hypocalcaemia due to relative hypoparathyroidism.

Patients receiving frequent infusions of Aredia over a prolonged period of time, especially those with pre-existing renal disease or a predisposition to renal impairment (e.g. patients with multiple myeloma and/or tumour-induced hypercalcaemia), should have periodic evaluations of standard laboratory and clinical parameters of renal function as deterioration of renal function (including renal failure) has been reported following long-term treatment with Aredia in patients with multiple myeloma. However, underlying disease progression and/or concomitant complications were also present and therefore a causal relationship with Aredia is unproven.

There is very little experience of the use of Aredia in patients receiving haemodialysis.

In patients with cardiac disease, especially in the elderly, additional saline overload may precipitate cardiac failure (left ventricular failure or congestive heart failure). Fever (influenza-like symptoms) may also contribute to this deterioration.

Pagetic patients at risk of calcium or Vitamin D deficiency (e.g. through malabsorption or lack of exposure to sunlight) should take oral supplements of both during Aredia therapy to minimise the potential risk of hypocalcaemia.

*Interactions with other drugs and other types of interactions:* Aredia has been administered concomitantly with commonly used anticancer agents without interactions occurring.

Aredia has been used in combination with calcitonin in patients with severe hypercalcaemia, resulting in a synergistic effect producing a more rapid fall in serum calcium.

Since pamidronate binds to bone, it could in theory interfere with bone scintigraphy examinations.

*Pregnancy and lactation:* In animal experiments, pamidronate showed no teratogenic potential and did not affect general reproductive performance or fertility. In rats, prolonged parturition and reduced survival rate of pups were probably caused by a decrease in maternal serum calcium levels. In pregnant rats, pamidronate has been shown to cross the placental

barrier and accumulate in fetal bone in a manner similar to that observed in adult animals.

There is insufficient clinical experience to support the use of Aredia in pregnant women. Therefore, Aredia should not be administered during pregnancy except in cases of life-threatening hypercalcaemia.

A study in lactating rats has shown that pamidronate will pass into the milk. Mothers treated with Aredia should therefore not breast-feed their infants.

*Effects on ability to drive or use machines:* Patients should be warned that in rare cases somnolence and/or dizziness may occur following Aredia infusion, in which case they should not drive, operate potentially dangerous machinery, or engage in other activities that may be hazardous because of decreased alertness.

*Undesirable effects:* Adverse reactions to Aredia are usually mild and transient. The most common adverse reactions are asymptomatic hypocalcaemia and fever (an increase in body temperature of 1–2°C), typically occurring within the first 48 hours of infusion. Fever usually resolves spontaneously and does not require treatment. Symptomatic hypocalcaemia is rare.

Frequency estimate: frequent >10%, occasional >1–10%, rare >0.001–1%, isolated cases <0.001%.

*Body as a whole:* Frequent: fever and influenza-like symptoms sometimes accompanied by malaise, rigor, fatigue, and flushes.

*Local reactions:* Occasional: reactions at the infusion site: pain, redness, swelling, induration, phlebitis, thrombophlebitis.

*Musculoskeletal system:* Occasional: transient bone pain, arthralgia, myalgia, generalised pain. Rare: muscle cramps.

*Gastrointestinal tract:* Occasional: nausea, vomiting. Rare: anorexia, abdominal pain, diarrhoea, constipation, dyspepsia. Isolated cases: gastritis.

*Central nervous system:* Occasional: headache. Rare: symptomatic hypocalcaemia (paraesthesia, tetany), agitation, confusion, dizziness, insomnia, somnolence, lethargy. Isolated cases: seizures, visual hallucinations.

*Blood:* Occasional: lymphocytopenia. Rare: anaemia, leukopenia. Isolated cases: thrombocytopenia.

*Cardiovascular system:* Rare: hypotension, hypertension.

*Renal system:* Isolated cases: haematuria, acute renal failure, deterioration of pre-existing renal disease.

*Skin:* Rare: rash, pruritus.

*Special senses:* Isolated cases: conjunctivitis, uveitis (iritis, iridocyclitis), scleritis, episcleritis, xanthopsia.

*Others:* Isolated cases: reactivation of herpes simplex and herpes zoster.

*Biochemical changes:* Frequent: hypocalcaemia, hypophosphataemia. Occasional: hypomagnesaemia. Rare: hyperkalaemia, hypokalaemia, hypernatraemia. Isolated cases: abnormal liver function tests, increase in serum creatinine and urea.

Many of these undesirable effects may have been related to the underlying disease.

*Overdose:* Patients who have received doses higher than those recommended should be carefully monitored. In the event of clinically significant hypocalcaemia with paraesthesia, tetany and hypotension, reversal may be achieved with an infusion of calcium gluconate.

**Pharmacological properties**
*Pharmacodynamic properties:* Pamidronate disodium, the active substance of Aredia, is a potent inhibitor of osteoclastic bone resorption. It binds strongly to hydroxyapatite crystals and inhibits the formation and dissolution of these crystals in vitro. Inhibition of osteoclastic bone resorption in vivo may be at least partly due to binding of the drug to the bone mineral.

Pamidronate suppresses the accession of osteoclast precursors onto the bone. However, the local and direct antiresorptive effect of bone-bound bisphosphonate appears to be the predominant mode of action in vitro and in vivo.

Experimental studies have demonstrated that pamidronate inhibits tumour-induced osteolysis when given prior to or at the time of inoculation or transplantation with tumour cells. Biochemical changes reflecting the inhibitory effect of Aredia on tumour-induced hypercalcaemia, are characterised by a decrease in serum calcium and phosphate and secondarily by decreases in urinary excretion of calcium, phosphate, and hydroxyproline.

Hypercalcaemia can lead to a depletion in the volume of extracellular fluid and a reduction in the glomerular filtration rate (GFR). By controlling hypercalcaemia, Aredia improves GFR and lowers elevated serum creatinine levels in most patients.

Clinical trials in patients with breast cancer and predominantly lytic bone metastases or with multiple myeloma showed that Aredia prevented or delayed skeletal-related events (hypercalcaemia, fractures, radiation therapy, surgery to bone, spinal cord compression) and decreased bone pain.

Paget's disease of bone, which is characterised by local areas of increased bone resorption and formation with qualitative changes in bone remodelling, responds well to treatment with Aredia. Clinical and biochemical remission of the disease has been demonstrated by bone scintigraphy, decreases in urinary hydroxyproline and serum alkaline phosphatase, and by symptomatic improvement.

*Pharmacokinetic properties:*
*General characteristics:* Pamidronate has a strong affinity for calcified tissues, and total elimination of pamidronate from the body is not observed within the time-frame of experimental studies. Calcified tissues are therefore regarded as site of 'apparent elimination'.

*Absorption:* Pamidronate disodium is given by intravenous infusion. By definition, absorption is complete at the end of the infusion.

*Distribution:* Plasma concentrations of pamidronate rise rapidly after the start of an infusion and fall rapidly when the infusion is stopped. The apparent half-life in plasma is about 0.8 hours. Apparent steady-state concentrations are therefore achieved with infusions of more than about 2–3 hours' duration. Peak plasma pamidronate concentrations of about 10 nmol/mL are achieved after an intravenous infusion of 60 mg given over 1 hour, and the apparent plasma clearance is about 180 mL/min.

In animals and in man, a similar percentage of the dose is retained in the body after each dose of pamidronate disodium. Thus the accumulation of pamidronate in bone is not capacity-limited, and is dependent solely on the total cumulative dose administered.

The percentage of circulating pamidronate bound to plasma proteins is relatively low (about 54%), and increases when calcium concentrations are pathologically elevated.

*Elimination:* Pamidronate does not appear to be eliminated by biotransformation. After an intravenous infusion, about 20–55% of the dose is recovered in the urine within 72 hours as unchanged pamidronate. Within the time-frame of experimental studies the remaining fraction of the dose is retained in the body. The percentage of the dose retained in the body is independent of both the dose (range 15–180 mg) and the infusion rate (range 1.25–60 mg/h). From the urinary elimination of pamidronate, two decay phases, with apparent half-lives of about 1.6 and 27 hours, can be observed. The apparent renal clearance is about 54 mL/min, and there is a tendency for the renal clearance to correlate with creatinine clearance.

*Characteristics in patients:* Hepatic and metabolic clearance of pamidronate are insignificant. Impairment of liver function is therefore not expected to influence the pharmacokinetics of Aredia. Aredia thus displays little potential for drug-drug interactions both at the metabolic level and at the level of protein binding (see above).

*Preclinical safety data:* The toxicity of pamidronate is characterised by direct (cytotoxic) effects on organs with a copious blood supply, particularly the kidneys following i.v. exposure. The compound is not mutagenic and does not appear to have carcinogenic potential.

**Pharmaceutical particulars**
*List of excipients:* Mannitol, phosphoric acid.

*Incompatibilities:* Pamidronate will form complexes with divalent cations and should not be added to calcium-containing intravenous solutions.

*Shelf-life:* 3 years.

*Special precautions for storage:* Protect vials from heat (store below 30°C). Reconstituted solutions that have been further diluted with one of the recommended diluents for intravenous infusion should be used immediately. Discard the unused portion.

*Nature and contents of container:* Colourless glass vials of 10 mL, with closures made from a butyl rubber derivative.

*Instructions for use/handling:* Powder in vials should be first dissolved in sterile water for injection, i.e. 15 mg in 5 mL, and 30 mg or 90 mg in 10 mL. The sterile water for injection is available in ampoules which are supplied together with vials. The pH of the reconstituted solution is 6.0–7.4. The reconstituted solution should be further diluted with a calcium-free infusion solution (0.9% w/v Sodium Chloride Intravenous Infusion BP is recommended) before administration. It is important that the powder be completely dissolved before the reconstituted solution is withdrawn for dilution.

**Marketing authorisation numbers**
Aredia Dry Powder 15 mg 00101/0518
Aredia Dry Powder 30 mg 00101/0519
Aredia Dry Powder 90 mg 00101/0521
Water for Injections PhEur 00101/0479

**Date of approval/revision of SPC**  June 1996.

**Legal category**  POM.

# BUTACOTE*

**Presentation** The active ingredient, Phenylbutazone BP is presented as: sugar-coated, enteric tablets, bi-convex, approximately 7.8 mm diameter, pale blue coloured and imprinted GEIGY on one side and DM on the other, each tablet containing 100 mg.

*Excipients:* Silica aerogel, gelatin, maize starch, sodium carboxymethyl starch, magnesium stearate, stearic acid, microcrystalline cellulose, polyethylene glycol, sucrose, talc, polyvidone, titanium dioxide, cellulose acetate phthalate, diethyl phthalate, colourings – E132, E127, E171, E172.

**Uses** Ankylosing spondylitis. Butacote should only be used where other therapies have been found unsuitable.

*Pharmacokinetics:* Phenylbutazone, the active substance of Butacote is rapidly and completely absorbed from the gastrointestinal tract. At therapeutic plasma concentrations, phenylbutazone is 98–99% plasma bound, exclusively to albumin. It is extensively metabolised in the liver and less than 1% is excreted unchanged in the urine. It inhibits the metabolism of several drugs, but it can also act as an inducer of liver enzymes (see *Interactions*). The drug forms the active metabolite oxyphenbutazone. The mean plasma elimination half life of phenylbutazone is about 75 hours, with wide inter- and intra-individual variations.

**Dosage and administration** The dosage selected should be as low as possible, and duration of treatment should be as short as possible; when long term treatment is unavoidable, special precautions should be taken (see *Precautions*) and the dosage should be adjusted to the needs of each patient taking account of the patient's age and general condition.

Butacote tablets should be swallowed whole with a meal together with liquid.

*Adults:* For the initial 48 hours 400-600 mg daily in divided doses. Thereafter, reduce to the minimum amount necessary, usually 200-300 mg daily in divided doses.

*Elderly:* In the elderly, always use the minimum effective dose (see *Precautions*).

*Children:* Not recommenced for children under 14 years.

## Contra-indications, warnings, etc

*Contra-indications:* History, however remote, of peptic ulcer, gastro-intestinal haemorrhage, patients with symptoms or a history of inflammatory bowel disease with or without ulceration, blood dyscrasia. Haemorrhagic diathesis (thrombocytopenia, disorders of blood coagulation), severe cardiac, hepatic, renal or pulmonary insufficiency, oedema or hypertension where there is danger of cardiac decompensation, thyroid disease, salivary gland disorder, Sjögren's syndrome and previous adverse reactions to pyrazoles.

Like other non-steroidal anti-inflammatory agents, Butacote is also contra-indicated in asthmatic patients in whom attacks of asthma, urticaria, or acute rhinitis are precipitated by acetylsalicylic acid or by other drugs with prostaglandin synthetase inhibiting activity.

There is not enough experience with the use of Butacote in pregnant women. Butacote may appear in cord blood and should not be used during pregnancy. If other drugs have been tried and found ineffective, Butacote may be used, but only if the benefits to the mother justify the potential risk to the foetus (e.g. premature closure of ductus arteriosus). Since phenylbutazone passes into breast milk, albeit in small quantities, nursing mothers taking Butacote should not breast feed their infants.

*Precautions:* Like all potent drugs, Butacote should be used only under close medical supervision.

In elderly patients, who are generally more prone to side-effects, particular caution should be exercised.

Serious gastrointestinal reactions such as bleeding, ulceration and perforation can occur at any time, with or without warning symptoms, in patients treated with non-steroidal anti-inflammatory drugs. Although minor upper gastrointestinal symptoms such as dyspepsia are common, usually developing early in therapy, physicians should watch for ulceration and bleeding in patients treated with non-steroidal anti-inflammatory drugs, even in the absence of previous gastrointestinal tract symptoms. If any of the symptoms or signs suggestive of gastrointestinal toxicity occur, Butacote should be discontinued immediately.

As blood dyscrasias may occur suddenly after a small dose or insidiously after prolonged therapy, particularly in the elderly, blood counts should be monitored before and regularly during therapy, if it is anticipated that treatment may continue for more than one week. If significant changes occur, e.g. decrease in leucocyte and/or platelet count or in the haematocrit, the drug should be withdrawn. Therapy should also be stopped if symptoms suggestive of

these complications arise, (e.g. bruising, fever, sore throat, rash, mouth ulceration), and patients should be advised accordingly.

Sodium retention and oedema may occur, and this should be considered in patients with cardiovascular disease.

Severe hepatic reactions including jaundice and hepatitis have been reported with Butacote, as with other non-steroidal anti-inflammatory drugs. If abnormal liver tests persist or worsen, or clinical signs and symptoms consistent with liver disease develop, the drug should be discontinued.

Patients with impaired renal function should be closely monitored. Overt renal failure may be precipitated due to the inhibition of prostaglandin synthesis.

Granulocytopenia or aplastic anaemia have to be excluded in patients with stomatitis before treatment with Butacote is started, because stomatitis might be an indication of pre-existing haematological abnormality of this type.

If Butacote is given for more than one week, liver function tests, kidney function tests, and blood counts should be performed periodically. In case of significant changes, the drug should be withdrawn.

Use of acetylsalicylic acid and other NSAIDs should be avoided in patients receiving therapy with Butacote, since concomitant administration of these drugs may increase the risk of serious gastrointestinal adverse reactions.

Butacote should not be given to patients on oral anticoagulant therapy because of an increased risk of bleeding. Patients being treated with oral antidiabetics should not receive Butacote owing to possible occurrence of serious hypoglycaemia.

Patients receiving treatment with Butacote should be warned that drowsiness or dizziness may occur, in which case they should not drive, operate potentially dangerous machinery, or engage in other activities that may become hazardous because of decreased alertness. Concomitant ingestion of alcohol may potentiate these effects.

In a 2-year carcinogenicity study in mice and rats a small increase in the incidence of neoplasms in the liver or kidney was seen. The incidence of liver tumours in male mice might be a response to rodent-specific hepatotrophic effects, including liver-enzyme induction. The clinical significance of these findings is not clear.

*Side-effects:*

*Gastrointestinal tract:* Frequent: nausea, gastritis. Occasional: gastrointestinal discomfort, heartburn, epigastric pain, peptic ulcer, diarrhoea. Rare: Vomiting, gastrointestinal bleeding (haematemesis and/or melaena), bleeding or perforation of peptic ulcer. Isolated cases: Pancreatitis, oesophagitis, oesophageal ulcer, benign stricture of the oesophagus, exacerbation of inflammatory bowel disease, including Crohn's disease with bleeding, ulceration or perforation, small bowel obstruction, constipation.

*Body as a whole:* Frequent: oedema, water retention.

*Skin:* Occasional: rash. Rare: urticaria, pruritus, purpura, exfoliative dermatitis. Isolated cases: bullous eruptions, fixed drug eruptions, erythema multiforme, Steven's-Johnson syndrome, toxic epidermal necrolysis (Lyells's syndrome), photosensitivity, erythema nodosum, precipitation of generalised pustula psoriasis.

*Others:* Occasional: stomatitis. Rare: salivary gland enlargement, dry mouth.

*Endocrine system:* Occasional: goitre, lowering of plasma thyroid hormone concentration. Isolated cases: hypothyroidism.

*Nervous system:* Rare: dizziness, headache. Isolated cases: peripheral neuropathy, confusional states, excitation.

*Blood and lymph:* Rare: anaemia due to occult gastrointestinal blood loss, haemolytic anaemia, thrombocytopenia, agranulocytosis, leucopenia, pancytopenia, bone marrow depression, aplastic anaemia.

*Liver:* Rare: increase in serum transaminases, hepatitis with or without jaundice. Isolated cases: fulminant hepatitis.

*Kidneys:* Rare: impaired renal function, acute renal failure, haematuria, proteinuria. Isolated cases: acute tubular necrosis, acute interstitial nephritis, nephrotic syndrome, glomerulonephritis, papillary necrosis, ureteral obstruction with uric acid crystal formation.

*Cardiovascular system:* Rare: congestive heart failure, pulmonary oedema. Isolated cases: hypertension, myocarditis, pericarditis.

*Hypersensitivity:* Isolated cases: anaphylactic/anaphylactoid reactions with and without shock, angioedema, serum sickness, lymphadenopathy, vasculitis, systemic lupus erythematosus-like syndrome, eosinophilic pulmonary infiltrates, fever.

*Respiratory tract:* Isolated cases: exacerbation of bronchial asthma. Isolated occurrences of an 'acute pulmonary syndrome' marked by dyspnoea, fever, shadows in radiographs of the lungs and sometimes

also by eosinophilia – have been reported. Although a causal relationship has not been proven, the drug should be withdrawn at first signs of this potentially serious syndrome, for the treatment of which corticosteroids and supportive cardiotherapy may be necessary.

*Special senses:* Isolated cases: blurred vision, retinal haemorrhage, hearing loss.

*Drug interactions:* By competitively displacing them from their serum-protein binding sites, phenylbutazone may increase the activity and duration of effect of other drugs, e.g. other anti-inflammatory agents, oral anticoagulants, oral antidiabetic drugs, phenytoin, and sulphonamides. Phenylbutazone may also accelerate the metabolism of dicoumarol, digitoxin, and cortisone by inducing hepatic microsomal enzymes. Conversely, it may inhibit the metabolic degradation of phenytoin and potentiate the effect of insulin. In patients previously treated with drugs which activate the hepatic microsomal enzyme system, e.g. barbiturates, chlorpheniramine, rifampicin, promethazine, and corticosteroids (e.g. prednisone), the elimination half-life of phenylbutazone is shortened. When phenylbutazone is given together with methylphenidate, the serum concentration of the metabolite oxyphenbutazone rises and the elimination half-life of phenylbutazone is prolonged.

During concomitant administration of anabolic steroids and phenylbutazone, the serum concentration of the metabolite oxyphenbutazone rises.

Since phenylbutazone may potentiate the effect of methotrexate, caution is indicated in cases where the two drugs are given concomitantly. Concomitant administration of cholestyramine reduces the enteral absorption of phenylbutazone. Phenylbutazone displaces thyroid hormone from its serum protein-binding sites and may thus make it more difficult to interpret tests of thyroid function.

When given together with lithium preparations, phenylbutazone causes increased tubular reabsorption of lithium, thereby raising the latter's serum concentration.

Concomitant administration of Butacote with aspirin, other NSAID's or corticosteroids increases the risk of serious gastrointestinal adverse reactions.

When given concomitantly, Butacote and misoprostol may induce adverse symptoms related to the central nervous system, such as dizziness, headache and transient diplopia.

Butacote may potentiate the effects of alcohol on the central nervous system.

*Overdosage:* Where the recommended dosage has been appreciably exceeded, the following are the signs and symptoms liable to be encountered: Nausea, vomiting, abdominal pain, diarrhoea, gastrointestinal bleeding, peptic ulceration. Hyperpyrexia, restlessness, dizziness, somnolence, agitation, convulsions, coma.

Alkalosis, acidosis, electrolyte disturbances, oedema.

Tachycardia, hyperventilation, respiratory arrest, cyanosis, hypotension, electrocardiographic abnormalities, cardiac arrest.

Acute renal failure.

Abnormal liver function test, jaundice, hepatic failure.

Anaemia, leucopenia, thrombocytopenia, hypoprothrombinaemia.

*Treatment:* Evacuation of the stomach (induction of vomiting, gastric lavage), and activated charcoal. If necessary, saline purgatives, artificial respiration, measures to support the circulation, anticonvulsants (e.g. diazepam i.v.). Forced diuresis and haemodialysis are considered to be ineffective in removing the drug. Haemoperfusion may be useful.

**Pharmaceutical precautions** Protect tablets from moisture. Store below 25°C.

**Legal category** POM.

**Package quantities** Containers of 100 and 500

**Further information** Butacote tablets are available through hospitals only.

**Product licence number** 0001/0024R

*Product licence holder:* Ciba-Geigy plc, Hulley Road, Macclesfield, Cheshire SK10 2NX.

# CAFERGOT*

## Presentation

*Tablets:* Whitish, round, coated tablets, 9.5 to 10 mm diameter, 5.4 to 5.6 mm thick, weighing 370 mg. Each tablet contains 1 mg Ergotamine Tartrate PhEur and 100 mg Caffeine PhEur.

*Suppositories:* Off-white suppositories weighing 2.0 g. Each suppository contains 2 mg Ergotamine Tartrate PhEur and 100 mg Caffeine PhEur.

## Uses

*Principal actions:* Ergotamine aborts attacks of migraine and other vascular headaches by its specific vasoconstrictor effect on distended extracranial arteries. Concomitant administration of caffeine enhances the absorption of ergotamine.

Cafergot suppositories are especially valuable for patients who have nausea and vomiting early in the attack and cannot retain or absorb anything taken by mouth.

To be fully effective the tablets must be taken, or the suppositories used, as early as possible in the attack.

*Indications:* Acute attacks of migraine and migraine variants unresponsive to simple analgesics.

**Dosage and administration** There is considerable inter-individual variation in the sensitivity of patients to ergotamine. Care should therefore be exercised in selecting the optimum therapeutic dose for an individual patient which will not give rise to unwanted effects, either acutely or chronically. The maximum recommended dosages should not be exceeded and ergotamine treatment should not be administered at intervals of less than 4 days.

For maximum efficacy, the optimal dose (in the preferred galenical form) should be administered immediately prodromal symptoms are experienced.

*Tablets:* One or two tablets taken at the first warning of an attack are normally sufficient to obtain migraine relief. Some individuals may require higher dosages which should never exceed 4 tablets (4 mg ergotamine) in 24 hours. It is essential to use the minimum effective dose.

The maximum recommended weekly dose of 8 tablets (8 mg ergotamine) should not be exceeded and there should be an interval of at least 4 days between successive doses.

*Suppositories:* One suppository should be administered at the first warning of an attack. This dose is normally sufficient, although some individuals may require higher dosages which should never exceed 2 suppositories (4 mg ergotamine) in 24 hours. It is essential to use the minimum effective dose.

The maximum recommended weekly dosage of 4 suppositories (8 mg ergotamine) should never be exceeded and there should be an interval of at least 4 days between successive doses.

*Use in children under 12 years:* Not recommended.

*Use in the elderly:* Whilst there is no evidence to suggest that the elderly require different dosages of Cafergot, nevertheless, the contra-indications of this drug are common in the elderly, e.g. coronary heart disease, renal impairment, hepatic impairment and severe hypertension. Caution should therefore be exercised when prescribing for this age group.

**Contra-indications, warnings, etc**
*Contra-indications:* Cafergot should not be used for migraine prophylaxis, nor should the recommended dosages be exceeded. Frequent attacks of migraine may be an indication for the use of a suitable prophylactic agent.

Cafergot should not be used in patients with peripheral vascular disease, coronary heart disease, obliterative vascular disease and Raynaud's Syndrome in view of the increased risk of peripheral vasospasm secondary to ergotamine. Impaired hepatic or renal function, sepsis, and severe hypertension are all contra-indications for treatment with Cafergot.

*Use in pregnancy and lactation:* Ergotamine containing products are contra-indicated in pregnancy due to oxytocic effects on the pregnant uterus and in breast-feeding mothers due to the risk of the infant developing ergotism. Repeated doses of ergotamine may inhibit lactation.

*Precautions:* Concomitant use of erythromycin and ergotamine should be avoided, as this can result in an elevated concentration of ergotamine in the plasma.

If symptoms such as tingling in the fingers or toes occur, the drug should be discontinued at once and the physician consulted.

As vasospastic reactions have been reported with beta-blockers alone and in a few patients treated concomitantly with ergotamine and propranolol, caution is advised in the concomitant use of these agents with Cafergot.

The caffeine component of Cafergot may give rise to unwanted stimulant effects.

*Side-effects:* Side-effects of Cafergot are related in the main to the ergotamine component. Acutely, these may include nausea, vomiting and abdominal pain. Paraesthesia and peripheral vasoconstriction or pain and weakness in the extremities may develop after both acute and chronic dosing. Numbness and tingling of the extremities can be indicative of peripheral vasospasm and treatment must be stopped immediately if signs of circulatory impairment appear. Failure to observe this precaution can lead to the development of ergotism. Due to its vasoconstrictive properties, ergotamine may cause precordial pain, myocardial

ischaemia or, in rare cases, infarction, even in patients with no known history of coronary heart disease.

Excessive use of ergotamine containing products for prolonged periods may result in fibrotic changes, in particular of the pleura and retroperitoneum.

*Overdosage:* Symptoms of overdosage are: nausea, vomiting, drowsiness, confusion, tachycardia, dizziness, tingling and numbness in the extremities due to ischaemia, respiratory depression, coma.

Treatment should be directed to the elimination of ingested material by aspiration and gastric lavage.

Rarely, headache may be provoked either by chronic overdosage or by rapid withdrawal of the product. Caffeine is a weak stimulant and excessive use of Cafergot may lead to a state of arousal and anxiety.

If severe arteriospasms occur, vasodilators such as nitroprusside sodium should be administered. General supportive measures should be applied with particular reference to the respiratory and cardiovascular systems.

**Pharmaceutical precautions** Store suppositories below 25°C.

**Legal category** POM.

**Package quantities**
*Tablets:* Blister pack of 30.
*Suppositories:* Boxes of 30.

**Further information** Caffeine is not an active ingredient but enhances the action of ergotamine, probably by facilitating its absorption.

**Product licence numbers**
*Tablets* 0101/5023R
*Suppositories* 0101/5001R

# CLIMAGEST*

## Presentation
*1 mg tablets:* 16 tablets each containing 1 mg Oestradiol Valerate USP, grey-blue in colour. Biconvex, circular tablets, diameter 6.05–6.65 mm, weight 83.0–91.6 mg, thickness, 2.5–2.9 mm. Marked E1 on one side.

12 tablets each containing 1 mg Oestradiol Valerate USP and 1 mg Norethisterone BP, white in colour. Biconvex, circular tablets, diameter 6.05–6.65 mm, weight 83.0–91.6 mg, thickness 2.5–2.9 mm. Marked N1 on one side.

*2 mg tablets:* 16 tablets each containing 2 mg Oestradiol Valerate USP, blue in colour. Biconvex circular tablets, diameter 6.05–6.65 mm, weight 83.0–91.6 mg, thickness 2.5–2.9 mm. Marked E2 on one side.

12 tablets each containing 2 mg Oestradiol Valerate USP and 1 mg Norethisterone BP, pale yellow in colour. Biconvex, circular tablets diameter 6.05–6.65 mm, weight 83.0–91.6 mg thickness 2.5–2.9 mm. Marked N2 on one side.

**Use** Hormone replacement therapy for the treatment of menopausal symptoms.

**Dosage and administration** Treatment commences with one oestradiol valerate tablet daily for the first 16 days followed by one combination tablet containing oestradiol valerate and norethisterone daily for the next 12 days, as directed on the 28 day calendar pack. Therapy may start at any time during the cycle. However, if the patient is menstruating regularly it is advised that the patient starts therapy on the first day of bleeding. Menstrual bleeding during initial Climagest therapy may be irregular. Pregnancy should be excluded before starting therapy.

The lowest dose compatible with the control of symptoms should always be used.

Climagest may be taken continuously by women with an intact uterus as it provides both oestrogen and progestogen to reduce endometrial hyperstimulation.

*Use in children:* Climagest should not be used in children.

*Use in elderly:* Climagest should only be used in the elderly for the indications listed.

**Contra-indications, warnings, etc**
*Contra-indications:* Known or suspected pregnancy. History of, known or suspected cancer of the breast. Known or suspected oestrogen-dependent neoplasia. Undiagnosed abnormal genital bleeding or endometriosis. Active thrombophlebitis or thromboembolic disorders. Severe cardiac, hepatic or renal disease.

*Precautions:* If migrainous or frequent unusually severe headaches occur for the first time, or any other symptoms that are possible prodromata of vascular occlusion occur, treatment should be suspended pending further investigation.

If jaundice or a significant rise in blood-pressure occur treatment should be stopped immediately. Consider discontinuation of treatment when impending surgery, trauma or illness is considered to entail a risk of thrombosis.

Patients with a mild chronic liver disease should have their liver function checked every 8–12 weeks. Patients with cholelithiasis, Dubin-Johnson syndrome or Rotor syndrome should be closely monitored.

Some conditions can deteriorate on hormone replacement therapy and it is essential that patients with these conditions should be closely monitored, including otosclerosis, migraine, multiple sclerosis, epilepsy, diabetes, hypertension, porphyria, uterine fibroids and tetany.

At the present time there is suggestive evidence of a slight increase in the relative risk of carcinoma of the breast with hormone replacement therapy used for longer than five years. Regular breast examinations should be carried out in women on HRT and mammography where appropriate. Breast status should also be closely monitored in women with a history of, or known, breast nodules, or fibrocystic disease.

Caution should be exercised in patients with a history or increased risk of thromboembolic disorders including myocardial infarction, stroke, pulmonary embolism and thrombophlebitis.

A thorough gynaecological and physical examination is advised before and periodically during treatment with Climagest.

Irregular bleeding during tablet taking is common during the first few months of therapy. If this persists an endometrial assessment including biopsy should be carried out.

As Climagest is not an oral contraceptive adequate non-hormonal measures should be taken to exclude pregnancy.

*Use in pregnancy and lactation:* Climagest should not be used in pregnant or nursing women.

*Side-effects:* A number of side-effects have been reported during treatment. They are dyspepsia, flatulence, nausea, vomiting, abdominal pain and bloating, weight-gain, breast tension and pain, palpitations, cardiac symptoms, changes in libido, headaches, dizziness, vertigo, epistaxis, biliary stasis, hypertension, urticaria and other rashes, thrombophlebitis, mucous vaginal discharge.

*Overdosage:* No reports of ill-effects from overdosage have been reported. There are no specific antidotes for overdosage and if further treatment is required it should be symptomatic.

**Pharmaceutical precautions** Store the tablets below 25°C, in a dry place. Protect from light.

**Legal category** POM.

**Package quantities**
1 mg tablets: 1 calendar pack of 28 tablets
1 mg tablets: 3 calendar packs of 28 tablets
2 mg tablets: 1 calendar pack of 28 tablets
2 mg tablets: 3 calendar packs of 28 tablets

**Product licence numbers**
Climagest 1 mg Tablets 0101/0328.
Climagest 2 mg Tablets 0101/0366.

*Product licence holder:* Sandoz Pharmaceuticals (UK) Ltd, Frimley Business Park, Frimley, Camberley GU16 5SG.

# CLIMAVAL*

## Presentation
*1 mg Tablets:* Grey-blue, biconvex circular tablets, diameter 6.05–6.65 mm, weight 83.0–91.6 mg, thickness 2.5–2.9 mm. Marked E1 on one side. Each tablet contains 1 mg oestradiol valerate.

*2 mg Tablets:* Blue, biconvex, circular tablets, diameter 6.05–6.65 mm, weight 83.0–91.6 mg, thickness 2.5–2.9 mm. Marked E2 on one side. Each tablet contains 2 mg oestradiol valerate.

**Uses** Hormone Replacement Therapy for the treatment of menopausal symptoms in hysterectomised women.

**Dosage and administration** 1 mg to 2 mg to be taken daily. Dosage may be adjusted according to severity of symptoms or clinical response. Climaval may be taken continuously in hysterectomised patients. The lowest dose compatible with the control of symptoms should always be used.

*Use in children:* Climaval should not be used in children.

*Use in the elderly:* Climaval should not be used except for the control of postmenopausal symptoms.

**Contra-indications, warnings, etc**
*Contra-indications:* History of, known or suspected cancer of the breast. Known or suspected oestrogen-dependent neoplasia. Undiagnosed abnormal genital bleeding or endometriosis. Active thrombophlebitis or thromboembolic disorders. Severe cardiac, hepatic or renal disease.

*Precautions:* If migrainous or frequent unusually severe headaches occur for the first time, or any other symptoms that are possible prodromata of vascular occlusion occur, treatment should be suspended pending further investigation.

If jaundice or a significant rise in blood-pressure occur treatment should be stopped immediately. Consider discontinuation of treatment when trauma, illness or impending surgery is considered to entail a risk of thrombosis.

Patients with mild chronic liver disease should have their liver function checked every 8–12 weeks. Those patients with cholelithiasis, Dubin-Johnson syndrome or Rotor syndrome should be closely monitored.

Some conditions can deteriorate on hormone replacement therapy and it is essential that patients with these conditions should be closely monitored, including otosclerosis, migraine, multiple sclerosis, epilepsy, diabetes, hypertension, porphyria, uterine fibroids and tetany.

At the present time there is suggestive evidence of a slight increase in the relative risk of carcinoma of the breast with hormone replacement therapy used for longer than five years. Regular breast examinations should be carried out in women on HRT and mammography where appropriate. Breast status should also be closely monitored in women with a history of, or known, breast nodules, or fibrocystic disease.

Caution should be exercised in patients with a history or increased risk of thromboembolic disorders including myocardial infarction, stroke, pulmonary embolism and thrombophlebitis.

A thorough gynaecological and physical examination is advised before and periodically during treatment with Climaval.

As Climaval is not an oral contraceptive adequate non-hormonal measures should be taken to exclude pregnancy.

*Use in pregnancy and lactation:* Climaval should not be used in pregnant or nursing women.

*Side-effects:* A number of side-effects have been reported during treatment. They are dyspepsia, flatulence, nausea, vomiting, abdominal pain and bloating, weight gain, breast tension and pain, palpitations, cardiac symptoms, increased libido, headaches, dizziness, vertigo, epistaxis, biliary stasis, hypertension, urticaria and other rashes, thrombophlebitis, mucous vaginal discharge, general pruritus.

*Overdosage:* No reports of ill-effects from overdosage have been reported. There are no specific antidotes for overdosage and if further treatment is required it should be symptomatic.

**Pharmaceutical precautions** Store the tablets below 25˚C, in a dry place. Protect from light.

**Legal category** POM.

**Package quantities**
*1 mg Tablets:* 1 calendar pack of 28 tablets; 3 calendar packs of 28 tablets.
*2 mg Tablets:* 1 calendar pack of 28 tablets; 3 calendar packs of 28 tablets.

**Further information** After the menopause the protective effects which endogenous oestrogens appear to have on the female cardiovascular system are lost, therefore the risk of women developing cardiovascular disease rises to become similar to that of men. Studies have shown that the oral administration of oestradiol valerate to post-menopausal women decreases low density lipoprotein cholesterol (LDLC-C) and also increases high density lipoprotein cholesterol (HDLC-C). Such changes are recognised as potentially offering protection from the development of coronary artery disease.

**Product licence number**
1 mg Tablets     0101/0307
2 mg Tablets     0101/0308.

*Product licence holder:* Sandoz Pharmaceuticals (UK) Ltd, Frimley Business Park, Frimley, Camberley GU16 5SG.

## CLIMESSE*

**Presentation** 28 tablets each containing 2 mg Oestradiol Valerate USP and 0.7 mg Norethisterone BP. Pink in colour. Biconvex, circular tablets, diameter 5.7–6.3 mm, weight 95.9 mg, thickness 2.7–3.1 mm.

**Uses** Hormone Replacement Therapy for the treatment of menopausal symptoms.

Prophylaxis of post-menopausal osteoporosis in women at risk of developing fractures.

Climesse is effective in the prevention of progressive bone loss following the menopause. For maximum benefit treatment should begin as soon as permissible after the onset of the menopause (see Dosage and administration). Epidemiological studies indicate a number of risk factors which may contribute to post-menopausal osteoporosis. These include an early menopause, a family history of osteoporosis,

recent corticosteroid therapy, cigarette smoking and a thin small frame. Bone mineral density measurements can confirm the presence of low bone mass and may be a useful aid to diagnosis.

**Dosage and administration** One tablet to be taken daily, as directed on the 28 day calendar pack. Climesse should be taken continuously without a break between packs.

It is recommended that Climesse should not be taken by women until at least 12 months after their last natural menstrual bleed. Irregular bleeding during tablet taking may occur during the first few months of therapy but is usually transient, and amenorrhoea will develop in a majority of women. Amenorrhoea is most likely to occur in women who are more than 2 years post-menopausal but may also be achieved before that in a significant proportion of women.

Climesse is designed to prevent stimulation of the endometrium in postmenopausal women, usually resulting in amenorrhoea. Irregular bleeding may occur in the first few months of therapy but this will usually settle completely. A certain proportion of women, particularly those closer to the menopause, may fail to develop amenorrhoea and for these women an alternative form of Hormone Replacement Therapy may be more suitable.

If after 3–4 months treatment, continued unacceptable bleeding is still being experienced, Climesse should be discontinued. If bleeding subsides, no further investigation is necessary.

Bleeding after a period of amenorrhoea or heavy bleeding after a period of light bleeding may occur. Any doubt as to the cause of such bleeding should be investigated. Certain conditions may predispose to persistent irregular bleeding, such as uterine polyps and fibroids and this may warrant further investigation. As for all postmenopausal bleeding, appropriate investigations, including endometrial assessment should be carried out in all women who experience prolonged bleeding or who begin to bleed sometime after initiation of therapy.

Pregnancy should be excluded before starting therapy.

*Changing from sequential hormone replacement therapy:* Patients changing from sequential Hormone Replacement Therapy preparations to Climesse should do so at the end of the oestrogen plus progestogen phase of the sequential therapy, without a tablet free interval. Climesse should normally be used only in women more than 12 months postmenopause. When changing from sequential therapy menopausal status may not be known, and in some women endogenous oestrogens may still be being produced. This could result in unpredictable bleeding patterns.

*Use in children:* Climesse should not be used in children.

*Use in the elderly:* Climesse should only be used in the elderly for the indications listed.

**Contra-indications, warnings, etc**
*Contra-indications:* Known or suspected pregnancy. History of, known or suspected cancer of the breast. Known or suspected oestrogen-dependent neoplasia. Undiagnosed abnormal genital bleeding. Active thrombophlebitis or thromboembolic disorders. Severe cardiac, hepatic or renal disease. Allergy to one or more of the constituents.

*Precautions:* Premenopausal women should not receive Climesse therapy because it may inhibit ovulation, disturb cycle regularity and result in unpredictable bleeding patterns. Climesse is not intended to be an oral contraceptive and should not be used to prevent pregnancy.

At the present time there is suggestive evidence of a slight increase in the relative risk of carcinoma of the breast with hormone replacement therapy used for longer than five to ten years. Regular breast examinations should be carried out in women on HRT and mammography performed where appropriate and these women should be instructed in self breast examination. Breast status should also be closely monitored in women with a history of, or known, breast nodules, or fibrocystic disease.

A thorough gynaecological and physical examination is advised before and periodically during treatment with Climesse.

Patients should be carefully observed if they suffer with diseases which may be subject to deterioration during pregnancy or with oestrogen use. These include otosclerosis, migraine, multiple sclerosis, epilepsy, diabetes, porphyria, uterine fibroids and systemic lupus erythematosus. Patients with endometriosis should be closely monitored.

If jaundice, migrainous or frequent unusually severe headaches occur for the first time, or any other symptoms that are possible prodromata of vascular occlusion occur, treatment should be suspended pending further investigation.

Consider discontinuation of treatment when

trauma, illness or impending surgery is considered to entail a risk of thrombosis.

Rarely an idiosyncratic rise in blood pressure may occur and necessitate a suspension of treatment pending investigation. Although most studies indicate Hormone Replacement therapy has little effect on blood pressure, patients with pre-existing hypertension should be monitored at regular intervals.

Patients with mild chronic liver disease should have their liver function checked every 8–12 weeks. Patients with cholelithiasis, Dubin-Johnson syndrome or Rotor syndrome should be closely monitored.

*Use in pregnancy and lactation:* Climesse should not be used in pregnant or nursing women.

*Side-effects:* During the first few months of therapy irregular bleeding or spotting may occur; this is usually transient. Other side-effects that have been observed during treatment include: breast tenderness, acne, depression, weight gain and fatigue.

Other side effects that might be expected with this type of therapy include: abdominal cramps, nausea, leg cramps, irritability, fluid retention, palpitations, flatulence, bloating, headaches, dizziness, skin rashes, dysmenorrhoea, vomiting, change in libido, enlargement of breasts and vaginal discharge.

*Overdosage:* No reports of ill-effects from overdosage have been reported. There are no specific antidotes for overdosage and if further treatment is required it should be symptomatic.

**Pharmaceutical precautions** Store the tablets below 25˚C, in a dry place.

**Legal category** POM.

**Package quantities** 1 calendar pack of 28 tablets. 3 calendar packs of 28 tablets.

**Further information** Nil.

**Product licence number** 0101/0396.

*Product licence holder:* Sandoz Pharmaceuticals (UK) Ltd, Frimley Business Park, Frimley, Camberley GU16 5SG.

## CLOZARIL*

**Presentation**
*25 mg tablets:* Yellow, flat, circular tablets with a bevelled edge, of 6.3 mm diameter and weighing approximately 95 mg, coded CLOZ 25 on one side and with a breakline on the other. Each tablet contains 25 mg clozapine.

*100 mg tablets:* Yellow, flat, circular tablets with a bevelled edge, of 10 mm diameter and weighing approximately 380 mg, coded CLOZARIL 100 on one side and plain on the other. Each tablet contains 100 mg clozapine.

**Uses**
*Principal action:* Clozapine is an antipsychotic agent which differs from conventional neuroleptics. In animal experiments, it does not induce catalepsy or inhibit apomorphine- or amphetamine-induced stereotyped behaviour. It has weak dopamine receptor-blocking activity at both D1, D2, D3 and D5 receptors, but shows high potency for the D4 receptor, in addition to potent noradrenolytic, anticholinergic, antihistaminic and arousal reaction inhibiting effects. It has also been shown to possess antiserotoninergic properties.

Clinically, Clozaril produces rapid and marked sedation, and exerts strong antipsychotic effects. In particular, the antipsychotic effects have been demonstrated in schizophrenic patients resistant to other drug treatment. In such cases, Clozaril has proven effective in relieving both positive and negative schizophrenic symptoms, with more than half of patients showing clinically relevant improvement.

*Indications:* Clozaril is indicated in treatment-resistant schizophrenic patients, ie patients who are non-responsive to, or intolerant of, conventional neuroleptics.

*Non-responsiveness* is defined as lack of satisfactory clinical improvement despite the use of adequate doses of at least two marketed neuroleptics prescribed for adequate durations.

*Intolerance* is defined as the impossibility to achieve adequate benefit with conventional neuroleptic drugs because of severe and untreatable neurological adverse reactions (extrapyramidal symptoms or tardive dyskinesia).

**Dosage and administration** Initiation of Clozaril treatment must be in hospital in-patients and is restricted to those patients with a white blood cell count >3.5×10⁹/L and a normal differential blood count. *The use of Clozaril is restricted to patients who are registered with the Clozaril Patient Monitoring Service.*

The dosage must be adjusted individually. For each patient the lowest effective dose should be used.

*Adults*

*Initial dose:* 12.5 mg (one half of a 25 mg tablet) once or twice on the first day, followed by one or two 25 mg tablets on the second day. If well tolerated, the daily dose may then be increased slowly in increments of 25 to 50 mg in order to achieve a dose level of up to 300 mg/day within 2 to 3 weeks. Thereafter, if required, the daily dose may be further increased in increments of 50 to 100 mg at half-weekly or, preferably, weekly intervals.

*Therapeutic dose range:* In most patients, antipsychotic efficacy can be expected with 200 to 450 mg/day in divided doses. The total daily dose may be divided unevenly, with the larger portion at bedtime.

*Maximum dose:* A few patients may require larger doses to obtain maximum therapeutic benefit. Judicious increments (not exceeding 100 mg per increment) are permissible up to a maximum dose of 900 mg/day. Adverse reactions may increase at doses over 450 mg/day, in particular seizures.

*Maintenance dose:* After achieving maximum therapeutic benefit, many patients can be maintained on lower doses. Careful downward titration to the level of 150 to 300 mg/day given in divided doses is recommended. At daily doses not exceeding 200 mg, a single administration in the evening may be appropriate.

*Ending therapy:* If termination of Clozaril therapy is planned, a gradual reduction in dose is recommended over a 1 to 2 week period. If abrupt discontinuation is necessary the patient should be carefully observed for the recurrence of psychotic symptoms.

*Re-starting therapy (providing the patient has not ceased therapy due to a haematological abnormality – see Precautions):* In patients in whom the interval since the last dose of Clozaril exceeds 2 days, treatment should be re-initiated with 12.5 mg (one half of a 25 mg tablet) given once or twice on the first day. If this dose is well tolerated, it may be feasible to titrate the dose to the therapeutic level more quickly than is recommended for initial treatment. However, if patients have previously experienced respiratory or cardiac arrest with initial dosing, and were then able to be successfully titrated to a therapeutic dose, re-titration should be done with extreme caution.

*Switching from a conventional neuroleptic to Clozaril:* It is generally recommended that Clozaril should not be used in combination with conventional neuroleptics, including depot preparations, which may have a myelosuppressive effect. When Clozaril treatment is to be initiated in a patient who is on oral neuroleptic therapy, it is recommended that the conventional neuroleptic be discontinued by tapering the dosage downwards, before Clozaril therapy is initiated as described above.

*Children:* Not recommended.

*Use in the elderly:* In elderly patients it is recommended to initiate treatment at a particularly low dose (12.5 mg given once on the first day) and to restrict subsequent dose increments to 25 mg/day.

*Other special patient groups:* Patients with a history of epilepsy should be closely monitored during Clozaril therapy since dose-related convulsions have been reported. Therefore in patients with a history of seizures, as well as those suffering from cardiovascular, renal, or hepatic disorders, the initial dose should be 12.5 mg given once on the first day, and dosage increase should be slow and in small increments.

**Contra-indications, warnings, etc**

*Contra-indications:* Allergy to one or more of the constituents of the formulation. Patients with a history of drug-induced neutropenia/agranulocytosis, or with myeloproliferative disorders, must not be treated with Clozaril.

Other contra-indications are uncontrolled epilepsy, alcoholic and toxic psychoses, drug intoxication, comatose conditions, circulatory collapse and/or CNS depression of any cause and severe renal or cardiac failure.

Patients with active liver disease associated with nausea, anorexia or jaundice; progressive liver disease or hepatic failure are also contra-indicated.

*Warning: Clozaril can cause agranulocytosis.* A fatality rate of up to 1 in 300 has been estimated when Clozaril was used prior to recognition of the risk of agranulocytosis and the need for routine blood monitoring. Since that time careful monitoring of patients has been demonstrated to be effective in markedly reducing the risk of fatality.

Because of the risk associated with Clozaril therapy its use is limited to treatment-resistant schizophrenic patients (see 'indications'):

1. who have normal leucocyte findings (white blood cell count and differential blood count), and
2. in whom regular leucocyte counts can be performed weekly during the first 18 weeks and at least every two weeks for the first year of therapy. After the patient has been on treatment for 1 consecutive year with stable neutrophil counts over that period, then the frequency of monitoring may be changed to four-week intervals. Monitoring must continue throughout treatment and for four weeks after complete discontinuation of Clozaril.

The patient must be under the supervision of a specialist and supply of Clozaril is restricted to hospital and community pharmacies registered with the Clozaril Patient Monitoring Service.

Prescribing physicians must register themselves, their patients and a nominated pharmacist with the Clozaril Patient Monitoring Service. This service provides for the required leucocyte counts as well as a drug supply audit so that Clozaril treatment is promptly withdrawn from any patient who develops abnormal leucocyte findings.

Each time Clozaril is prescribed, patients should be reminded to contact the treating physician immediately if any kind of infection begins to develop. Particular attention should be paid to flu-like complaints or other symptoms which might suggest infection, such as fever or sore throat.

*Precautions: Clozaril can cause agranulocytosis.* The following precautionary measures are mandatory: Clozaril should not be used concurrently with drugs known to have a substantial potential to depress bone marrow function, such as co-trimoxazole, chloramphenicol, sulphonamides, pyrazolone analgesics, phenylbutazone, penicillamine, carbamazepine or cytotoxic agents. Concomitant use of long-acting depot antipsychotics (which have myelosuppressive potential) is not recommended because these medications cannot rapidly be removed from the body in situations where this may be required eg neutropenia.

Before starting Clozaril treatment, a white blood cell count and a differential count must be performed. Only patients with normal findings may receive the drug.

During Clozaril treatment the white blood cell count and differential count must be monitored weekly for the first 18 weeks and at least at two-week intervals for the first year of therapy. After the patient has been on treatment for 1 year with stable neutrophil counts over that period, then the frequency of monitoring may be changed to four week intervals. Monitoring must continue for as long as the patient is on the drug.

Particular attention should be paid to the white blood cell count and the differential count if any flu-like complaints or other symptoms develop which might suggest infection. Each time Clozaril is prescribed the patient should be reminded to contact the treating physician immediately if any kind of infection begins to develop. An immediate differential blood count must be obtained when any symptoms or signs of infection develop.

If the white blood cell count falls below $3.0\times10^9$/L and/or the absolute neutrophil count drops below $1.5\times10^9$/L, Clozaril must be withdrawn at once and the patient closely monitored. The patient must not be re-exposed to Clozaril.

In the event of an infection or a routine white blood cell count between 3.0 and $3.5\times10^9$/L and/or a neutrophil count between 1.5 and $2.0\times10^9$/L, the patient should be re-evaluated immediately with respect to the white blood cell count and the differential count. Should there be a decline in either, Clozaril must be withdrawn at once. If the blood cell count remains the same or increases, treatment with Clozaril may continue provided that the leucocytes and granulocytes are checked at least twice weekly until it is certain that the patient has a stable leucocyte count within the range 3.0 and $3.5\times10^9$/L or higher.

If Clozaril has been withdrawn and a further fall of white blood cell count below $1.0\times10^9$/L occurs and/or the neutrophils decrease below $0.5\times10^9$/L, the patient should be referred immediately to a unit experienced in the management of febrile neutropenia. If possible, the patient should be referred to a specialised haematological unit, where protective isolation and the administration of broad spectrum antibiotics and GM-CSF (granulocyte-macrophage colony stimulating factor) or G-CSF (granulocyte colony stimulating factor) should be considered. Due to the myelotoxic potential of some antibiotics, careful consideration should be given to the antibiotics chosen. It is recommended that the colony stimulating factor therapy be discontinued when the neutrophil count has returned to a level above $1.0\times10^9$/l.

Clozaril lowers the seizure threshold – see *'Dosage and administration – other special patient groups'*.

Orthostatic hypotension, with or without syncope, can occur with Clozaril treatment. Rarely, collapse can be profound and may be accompanied by cardiac and/or respiratory arrest. Such events are more likely to occur during initial titration in association with rapid dose escalation; on very rare occasions they have occurred even after the first dose. Therefore, patients commencing Clozaril treatment require close medical supervision.

Drowsiness may occur, especially at the beginning of therapy. Owing to its sedative action, Clozaril may impair the reactions of the patients e.g. when driving vehicles or operating machinery. Clozaril should be administered with caution to patients who participate in activities requiring complete mental alertness.

Clozaril exerts anticholinergic activity; therefore, careful supervision is indicated in the presence of prostatic enlargement, narrow-angle glaucoma and paralytic ileus.

Patients with stable pre-existing liver disorders may receive Clozaril but need regular liver function test monitoring. Patients who develop symptoms of possible liver dysfunction such as nausea, vomiting and/or anorexia during Clozaril treatment should have liver function tests performed immediately. If the elevation is clinically relevant or if the patient is jaundiced Clozaril should be immediately discontinued. It may be resumed (see *Re-starting therapy*) only when the liver function tests have returned to normal values. In such cases liver function should be closely monitored after the reintroduction of the drug (see *Side effects* section).

During Clozaril therapy patients may experience transient temperature elevations above 38°C, with a peak incidence within the first 3 weeks of treatment. This fever is generally benign. Occasionally, it may be associated with an increase or decrease in the WBC count. Patients with fever should be carefully evaluated to rule out the possibility of an underlying infection or the development of agranulocytosis. In the presence of high fever, the possibility of neuroleptic malignant syndrome (NMS) must be considered.

*Drug interactions:* Drugs known to have a substantial potential to depress bone marrow function should not be used concurrently with Clozaril (see *Precautions*, second paragraph).

Clozaril may enhance the central effects of alcohol, MAO inhibitors, CNS depressants including narcotics, benzodiazepines and antihistamines. Particular caution is advised when Clozaril therapy is initiated in patients who are receiving (or have recently received) a benzodiazepine or any other psychotropic drug, as these patients may have an increased risk of circulatory collapse, which, on rare occasions, can be profound and may lead to cardiac and/or respiratory arrest.

Because of the possibility of additive effects, caution in the concomitant administration of drugs with anticholinergic, hypotensive or respiratory depressant effects is essential.

Since clozapine is highly bound to plasma proteins, the administration of Clozaril to a patient taking another drug which is highly protein bound (e.g. warfarin) may cause an increase in plasma concentrations of this drug, potentially resulting in adverse effects. Conversely, adverse effects may result from displacement of protein-bound clozapine by other highly protein-bound drugs.

The metabolism of clozapine is mediated mainly by cytochrome P450 1A2 and probably to a minor extent by cytochrome P450 2D6. The concomitant administration of drugs which possess affinity to one or both of these enzymes may result in either a decrease or an increase in the plasma levels of clozapine and/or the co-administered drug.

However with tricyclic antidepressants, phenothiazines and type 1c antiarrhythmics, which are known to bind to cytochrome P450 2D6, no clinically relevant interactions with clozapine have been observed thus far. On theoretical grounds, however, it is possible that the plasma levels of such drugs are increased by clozapine, so that it may be appropriate to use them at doses lower than usually prescribed.

Administration of cimetidine concomitantly with high-dose Clozaril therapy was associated with increased plasma clozapine levels and the occurrence of adverse effects.

Elevated serum levels of clozapine have been reported in patients receiving drug in combination with fluoxetine (up to 2 fold) or fluvoxamine (up to 10 fold).

Drugs known to increase the activities of cytochrome P450 enzymes may decrease the plasma levels of clozapine. Discontinuation of the concomitant administration of carbamazepine resulted in an increase of the clozapine plasma levels. The concomitant use of phenytoin has been found to decrease the clozapine plasma concentration, resulting in reduced effectiveness of a previously effective Clozaril dose.

Concomitant use of lithium or other CNS-active agents may increase the risk of development of neuroleptic malignant syndrome (NMS).

Owing to its noradrenolytic action, Clozaril may reduce the blood pressure increasing effect of noradrenaline or other predominantly alpha-adrenergic agents and reverse the pressor effect of adrenaline.

*Use in pregnancy and lactation:* The safe use of Clozaril in pregnancy has not been established and its use is not recommended. A return to normal menstrual cycling may occur as a result of switching from conventional neuroleptics to Clozaril, therefore adequate contraceptive measures must be ensured in women of child bearing potential.

Animal studies suggest that Clozaril is excreted in breast milk; therefore, mothers receiving Clozaril must not breast-feed.

*Overdosage:* In cases of acute intentional or accidental Clozaril overdosage, for which information on the outcome is available, to date the mortality is about 12%. Most of the fatalities were associated with cardiac failure or pneumonia caused by aspiration and occurred at doses above 2000 mg. There have been reports of patients recovering from an overdose in excess of 10,000 mg. However, in a few adult individuals, primarily those not previously exposed to Clozaril the ingestion of doses as low as 400 mg led to life-threatening comatose conditions and, in one case, to death. In young children, the intake of 50 to 200 mg resulted in strong sedation or coma without being lethal.

*Signs and symptoms:* drowsiness, lethargy, coma, areflexia, confusion, hallucinations, extrapyramidal symptoms, agitation, delirium, hyperreflexia, convulsions, hypersalivation, mydriasis, blurred vision, thermolability, tachycardia, hypotension, collapse, cardiac arrhythmias, aspiration pneumonia, dyspnoea, respiratory depression or failure.

*Treatment:* gastric lavage and/or the administration of activated charcoal within the first 6 hours after the ingestion of the drug. (Peritoneal dialysis and haemodialysis are not very effective.) Symptomatic treatment under continuous cardiac monitoring, surveillance of respiration, monitoring of electrolytes and acid-base balance. The use of adrenaline and its derivatives should be avoided in the treatment of hypotension because of the possibility of a 'reverse adrenaline' effect. Close medical supervision is necessary for at least five days because of the possibility of delayed reactions.

*Side-effects: Neutropenia leading to agranulocytosis is a risk of Clozaril treatment.* This reaction, although generally reversible, can prove fatal. The majority of cases occur in the first 18 weeks of treatment. Because immediate withdrawal of the drug is required to prevent the development of life-threatening agranulocytosis, monitoring of the white blood cell count is mandatory (see *Warning* and *Precautions*).

Patients on Clozaril may develop unexplained leucocytosis, including eosinophilia, especially in the initial weeks of treatment. Isolated cases of various types of leukaemia have been reported in patients treated with Clozaril. However, there is no evidence to suggest a causal relationship between the drug and any type of leukaemia. The reported occurrence rate is in the range of the background incidence of these diseases in the general population. Isolated cases of thrombocytopenia have been reported but no causal relationship has been established.

*Central nervous system:* Fatigue, drowsiness and sedation are among the most common side-effects observed. Dizziness or headache may also occur.

Clozaril lowers the seizure threshold in a dose-dependent manner and may cause EEG changes, including the occurrence of spike and wave complexes. Myoclonic jerks or convulsions may, therefore, be precipitated in individuals who have epileptogenic potential but no previous history of epilepsy. In this case Clozaril treatment should be suspended for 24 hours and then resumed at a lower dose. It may be possible to control the problem by reducing the dosage and if necessary, raising it again very gradually. Anticonvulsant treatment may be considered but carbamazepine should be avoided because of its potential to depress bone marrow function, and with other anticonvulsant drugs the possibility of a pharmacokinetic interaction should be considered. Valproic acid was found to cause only non-significant increases in clozapine blood levels and to be well tolerated in the majority of patients receiving it in combination with clozapine.

In rare cases Clozaril may cause confusion, restlessness, agitation and delirium.

Extrapyramidal symptoms are limited mainly to tremor, akathisia and rigidity and if such effects occur, they tend to be mild and transient. Very rarely, tardive dyskinesia has been reported in patients on Clozaril. Some patients in whom tardive dyskinesia developed with other neuroleptics have improved on Clozaril.

There have been several reported cases of neuroleptic malignant syndrome (NMS) in patients receiving Clozaril either alone or in combination with lithium or other CNS-active agents.

*Autonomic nervous system:* dry mouth, disturbances of accommodation and disturbances in sweating and temperature regulation have been reported. Hypersalivation is a common side-effect.

*Cardiovascular system:* tachycardia and postural hypotension, with or without syncope, may occur,

especially in the initial weeks of treatment. Less commonly, hypertension may also occur. In rare cases profound circulatory collapse has been reported. ECG changes may occur and isolated cases of cardiac arrhythmias, pericarditis and myocarditis (with or without eosinophilia) have been reported, some of which have been fatal. Myocarditis can be difficult to diagnose as symptoms may be non-specific. Heart failure, arrhythmias or symptoms mimicking myocardial infarction or pericarditis may, however, be presenting features. Confirmation of diagnosis may not be possible but if suspicion is high, Clozaril medication should be stopped. Rare cases of thromboembolism have been reported.

*Respiratory system:* In isolated cases, with or without circulatory collapse, respiratory depression or arrest has occurred.

Rarely, aspiration of ingested food may occur in patients presenting with dysphagia or as a consequence of acute overdosage.

*Gastro-intestinal system:* Clozaril has been reported to cause nausea and vomiting. Constipation may occur, probably due to the anticholinergic properties of the drug. This is usually mild; however, on occasions more severe complications have been reported, including obstipation and paralytic ileus. The importance of recognising and treating constipation is emphasised.

Asymptomatic elevations in liver enzymes occur commonly particularly in the first three months of treatment. Rarely hepatitis and cholestatic jaundice may occur. Very rarely fulminant hepatic necrosis has been reported. If jaundice develops, Clozaril should be discontinued.

As a rare event, Clozaril treatment may be associated with dysphagia a possible cause of aspiration.

In rare cases, acute pancreatitis has been reported.

*Genito-urinary system:* both urinary incontinence and retention and, in a few cases, priapism have been reported. Isolated cases of acute interstitial nephritis have been reported in association with Clozaril.

*Miscellaneous:* benign hyperthermia may occur, especially in the initial weeks of treatment (see 'Precautions').

Isolated reports of skin reactions have been received.

On rare occasions, hyperglycaemia has been reported in patients on Clozaril treatment.

Rarely, increases in CPK values have occurred.

Clozaril has not been associated with elevated prolactin levels.

With prolonged treatment considerable weight gain has been observed in some patients.

Sudden unexplained deaths are known to occur among psychiatric patients who receive antipsychotic medication as well as those who do not. Isolated cases of such deaths have been reported in patients receiving Clozaril.

**Pharmaceutical precautions** Nil.

**Legal category** POM.

**Package quantities** Containers of 28 and 84 tablets.

**Further information**

*Clozaril Patient Monitoring Service:* The use of Clozaril is restricted to patients who are registered with the Clozaril Patient Monitoring Service (CPMS). This service provides for the required leucocyte counts as well as a drug supply audit to ensure that Clozaril is withdrawn from any patient with an abnormal leucocyte count. Full details of the service are available from the Clozaril Patient Monitoring Service Manager at Sandoz Pharmaceuticals, Sandoz Pharmaceuticals (UK) Limited, Frimley Business Park, Frimley, Camberley, Surrey GU16 5SG. Tel: 01276 692255.

Supply of Clozaril is restricted to hospital and community pharmacies registered within the Clozaril Patient Monitoring Service.

*Pharmacokinetics:* The absorption of orally administered Clozaril is 90 to 95%; the rate or extent of absorption is not influenced by food.

Clozapine is subject to a moderate first-pass metabolism, resulting in an absolute bioavailability of 50 to 60%. In steady-state conditions, when given twice daily, peak blood levels occur on an average at 2.1 hours (range: 0.4 to 4.2 hours) and the volume of distribution is 1.6 l/kg. Clozapine is approximately 95% bound to plasma proteins. Its elimination is biphasic with a mean terminal half-life of 12 hours (range: 6 to 26 hours).

After single doses of 75 mg the mean terminal half-life was 7.9 hours; it increased to 14.2 hours when steady-state conditions were reached by administering daily doses of 75 mg for at least 7 days. Dosage increases from 37.5 to 75 and 150 mg given twice daily were found to result during steady state in linearly dose-proportional increases in the area under the plasma concentration/time curve (AUC), as well as in the peak and minimum plasma concentrations.

Clozapine is almost completely metabolised prior

to excretion. Of the main metabolites only the desmethyl metabolite was found to be active. Its pharmacological actions resemble those of clozapine, but are considerably weaker and of short duration. Only trace amounts of unchanged drug are detected in the urine and faeces, approximately 50% of the administered dose being excreted as metabolites in the urine and 30% in the faeces.

**Product licence numbers**
25 mg tablets: 0101/0228
100 mg tablets: 0101/0229

## DESERIL*

**Presentation** White, sugar-coated, round, biconvex tablets weighing 100 mg, of 6 mm diameter and 3.4 to 3.9 mm thick, branded DSL on one side. Each tablet contains 1.33 mg Methysergide Maleate BP (equivalent to 1 mg methysergide base).

**Uses** *Principal action:* Deseril is a potent serotonin antagonist. In addition to inhibiting the pain-facilitating and permeability-increasing actions of serotonin, Deseril can potentiate the effects of vasoconstrictor stimuli.

*Indications:* Prophylactic treatment of migraine, cluster headache and other vascular headaches in patients who, despite other attempts at control, experience headaches of such severity or regularity that their social or economic life is seriously disrupted. (Note: Deseril is not recommended for treatment of the acute attack.)

Control of profuse diarrhoea associated with carcinoid disease.

**Dosage and administration** *Adults: Prophylactic treatment of headache:* 1 or 2 tablets two or three times a day, with meals.

Treatment should start with one tablet at bedtime and dosage should then be increased gradually over about two weeks until effective levels are reached. The minimum effective dose should be used – often that which will prevent 75% of attacks rather than all headaches.

From the outset, patients should understand that regular clinical supervision and periodic withdrawal of treatment are essential so that adverse effects can be recognised and minimised.

*Carcinoid syndrome:* High doses are usually necessary. In most reported cases dosage ranged between 12 and 20 tablets daily.

*Children:* Deseril is not recommended for the treatment of children.

*Use in the elderly:* No evidence exists that elderly patients require different dosages or show different side effects from younger patients.

**Contra-indications, warnings, etc**
*Contra-indications:* Hypersensitivity to the drug. Pregnancy, lactation, peripheral vascular disorders, progressive arteriosclerosis, severe hypertension, coronary heart disease, valvular heart disease, phlebitis or cellulitis of the lower extremities, pulmonary disease, collagen disease, impaired kidney or liver function, diseases of the urinary tract, cachectic or septic conditions.

*Warnings:* Continuous Deseril administration should not exceed six months without a drug-free interval of at least one month for reassessment; dosage should be reduced gradually over two to three weeks to avoid rebound headaches. In patients undergoing treatment with Deseril the dose of ergotamine required to control acute attacks may have to be reduced.

*Precautions:* Regular clinical supervision of patients treated with Deseril is essential. Particular attention should be paid to complaints of urinary dysfunction, pain in the loin, flank or chest, and pain, coldness or numbness in the limbs. Patients should be regularly examined for the presence of cardiac murmurs, vascular bruits, pleural or pericardial friction rubs and abdominal or flank masses or tenderness. Treatment with Deseril should be stopped should any of these symptoms or signs occur.

Caution is also advised during drug administration to patients with a past history of peptic ulceration.

In carcinoid syndrome the risk of adverse reactions due to the higher dosage must be weighed against the therapeutic benefit.

Concomitant use of Deseril and vasoconstrictors or vasopressors may result in enhanced vasoconstriction.

*Overdosage:* Symptoms of overdosage are: headache, agitation, hyperactivity, nausea, vomiting, abdominal pain, mydriasis, tachycardia, cyanosis, peripheral vasospasm with diminished pulses, coldness of the extremities. Treatment should be directed to elimination of the ingested material by aspiration and gastric lavage. General supportive measures should be applied. The patient should be carefully observed for peripheral vasospasm which may be treated by warmth, care being taken to protect ischaemic limbs. If there is evidence of impending tissue damage vasodilators may be used.

*Side-effects:*

*General:* The most commonly reported side-effects are nausea, heartburn, abdominal discomfort, vomiting, dizziness, lassitude and drowsiness. These side-effects can often be minimised by taking Deseril with food. Tissue oedema, insomnia, leg cramps and weight gain have occurred, and skin eruptions or loss of scalp hair have occasionally been reported. Mental and behavioural disturbances have occurred in isolated instances.

*Inflammatory fibrosis:* Retroperitoneal fibrosis: Continuous long-term Deseril administration has been associated with the development of retroperitoneal fibrosis. This is very rare when continuous treatment has not exceeded 6 months. Retroperitoneal fibrosis usually presents with symptoms of urinary tract obstruction such as persistent loin or flank pain, oliguria, dysuria, increased blood nitrogen and vascular insufficiency of the lower limbs. Deseril must be withdrawn if retroperitoneal fibrosis develops; drug withdrawal is often associated with clinical improvement over a few days to several weeks.

*Fibrosis in other areas:* Fibrotic processes involving lungs, pleura, heart valves and major vessels have been reported in a small number of patients. Presenting symptoms include chest pain, dyspnoea or pleural friction rub and pleural effusion. Cardiac murmurs or vascular bruits have also been reported. Appearance of these symptoms demands immediate withdrawal of Deseril. These fibrotic manifestations are often reversible although less readily so than retroperitoneal fibrosis.

*Vascular:* Vascular reactions, including arterial spasm, have been seen in some patients. The following have all been described: arterial spasm in a limb causing coldness, numbness, pain or intermittent claudication; renal artery spasm giving rise to transitory hypertension; mesenteric artery spasm causing abdominal pain; retinal artery spasm causing reversible loss of vision; coronary artery spasm causing angina and questionably resulting in myocardial infarction. Arterial spasm is rapidly reversible following drug withdrawal.

**Pharmaceutical precautions** Nil.

**Legal category** POM.

**Package quantities** Blister pack of 60 tablets.

**Further information** Deseril tablets no longer contain tartrazine.

**Product licence number** 0101/5026R.

## DESFERAL*

**Presentation** A sterile, lyophilised powder available in vials containing 500 mg of Desferrioxamine Mesylate BP.

**Uses**

*Indications:* Iron overload–Acute iron poisoning; primary and secondary haemochromatosis including thalassaemia and transfusional haemosiderosis; in patients in whom concomitant disorders (eg severe anaemia, hypoproteinaemia, renal or cardiac failure) preclude phlebotomy; and for the diagnosis of iron storage disease and certain anaemias.

Aluminium overload–in patients on maintenance dialysis for end stage renal failure where preventative measures (eg reverse osmosis) have failed and with proven aluminium-related bone disease and/or anaemia, dialysis encephalopathy; and for diagnosis of aluminium overload.

*Mode of action*: Desferal is a chelating agent for trivalent iron and aluminium ions; the resulting chelates (ferrioxamine and aluminoxamine) are stable and non-toxic. Neither chelate undergoes significant intestinal absorption, and any formed systemically as a result of parenteral administration is rapidly excreted via the kidneys without deleterious effects. Desferal takes up iron either free or bound to ferritin and haemosiderin. Similarly it mobilises and chelates tissue bound aluminium. It does not remove iron from haemin containing substances including haemoglobin and transferrin. Since both ferrioxamine and aluminoxamine are completely excreted, Desferal promotes the excretion of iron and aluminium in urine and faeces thus reducing pathological iron or aluminium deposits in the organs and tissues.

*Pharmacokinetics*: Desferrioxamine mesylate is rapidly absorbed following intramuscular or subcutaneous administration. In healthy volunteers peak plasma concentrations of desferrioxamine (15.5μmol/l/ 8.7μg/ml) and ferrioxamine (3.7μmol/l/ 2.3μg/ml) were observed at 30 minutes and 1 hour respectively, following an injection (10 mg/kg) of desferrioxamine. It is only poorly absorbed from the gastrointestinal tract in the presence of intact mucosa.

Serum protein binding of desferrioxamine is less than 10% *in vitro*.

In healthy subjects elimination is biphasic, first phase half-lives for desferrioxamine and ferrioxamine are 1 hour and 2.4 hours, respectively. In the second phase both compounds have a half-life of 6 hours. Of the injected dose 22% appears in the urine as desferrioxamine and 1% as ferrioxamine, after 6 hours.

In patients with haemochromatosis peak plasma levels of 7.0μmol/l (3.9μg/ml) were measured for desferrioxamine, and 15.7μmol/l (9.6μg/ml) for ferrioxamine, 1 hour after intramuscular injection of 10 mg/kg desferrioxamine. These patients eliminated desferrioxamine and ferrioxamine with half-lives of 5.6 and 4.6 hours, respectively. Six hours after the injection 17% of the dose was excreted in the urine as desferrioxamine and 12% as ferrioxamine.

In patients dialysed for renal failure who received 40 mg/kg desferrioxamine infused iv within 1 hour, the plasma concentration at the end of the infusion was 152μmol/l (85.2μg/ml) when the infusion was given between dialysis sessions. Plasma concentrations of desferrioxamine were between 13% and 27% lower when the infusion was administered during dialysis. Concentrations of ferrioxamine were in all cases approx. 7.0μmol/l (4.3μg/ml) with concomitant aluminoxamine levels of 2-3μmol/l (1.2-1.8μg/ml). After the infusion was discontinued, the plasma concentration of desferrioxamine decreased rapidly with a half-life of 20 minutes. A smaller fraction of the dose was eliminated with a longer half-life of 14 hours. Plasma concentrations of aluminoxamine continued to increase for up to 48 hours post-infusion and reached values of approx. 7μmol/l (4μg/ml). Following dialysis the plasma concentration of aluminoxamine fell to 2.2μmol/l (1.3μg/ml), indicating that the aluminoxamine complex is dialysable.

During peritoneal dialysis desferrioxamine is absorbed if administered in the dialysis fluid.

**Dosage and administration** Desferal may be administered parenterally or orally (for acute iron poisoning only).

*Preparation:* For parenteral administration: The drug should preferably be employed in the form of a 10% solution, eg by dissolving the contents of one vial (500 mg) in 5 ml of water for injection. When administered subcutaneously the needle should not be inserted too close to the dermis. The 10% Desferal solution can be diluted with routinely employed infusion solutions (saline, dextrose or dextrose-saline), although these should not be used as solvent for the dry substance. Dissolved Desferal can also be added to dialysis fluid and given intraperitoneally to patients on continuous ambulatory peritoneal dialysis (CAPD) or continuous cyclic peritoneal dialysis (CCPD).

Only clear pale yellow Desferal solutions should be used. Opaque, cloudy or discoloured solutions should be discarded. Heparin is pharmaceutically incompatible with Desferal solutions.

For oral administration: 5-10 g Desferal should be dissolved in 50-100 ml of water.

*Treatment: Acute iron poisoning:*

*Adults and children*: Desferal may be administered both orally and parenterally. It is important to initiate treatment as soon as possible.

Gastric lavage should be carried out as quickly as possible using, if readily available, 1% sodium bicarbonate solution. This should be followed by oral administration of Desferal which will chelate any iron remaining in the stomach and prevent any further absorption. Further measures, eg. sodium bicarbonate, sedatives, oxygen etc., may be given as necessary.

Patients with–

- serum iron levels >500 μg/dl (89.5 μmol/l), or
- serum iron levels >350 μg/dl (62.6μmol/l) with evidence of free iron, or
- with signs and symptoms of acute iron poisoning,

should be given Desferal either intramuscularly or intravenously to eliminate iron that has already been absorbed. The dosage and route of administration should be adapted to the severity of the poisoning.

*Dosage*: The normal dose is 2 g for an adult and 1 g for a child, administered as a single intramuscular dose.

If the patient is hypotensive or in shock, the intravenous route of administration is recommended. Initially the maximum rate of iv administration should be 15 mg/kg/h. It should be reduced after 4-6 hours so that the total dose does not exceed 80 mg/kg/24 hours. However, in the absence of adverse effects much larger doses may be tolerated.

Therapy should be continued until serum iron levels are less than the total iron binding capacity.

The effectiveness of treatment is dependent on an adequate urine output in order that the iron complex (ferrioxamine) is excreted from the body. Therefore, if oliguria or anuria develop, peritoneal dialysis or haemodialysis may become necessary to remove ferrioxamine.

It should be noted that the serum iron level may rise sharply when the iron is released from the tissues.

Theoretically 100 mg Desferal can chelate 8.5 mg of ferric iron.

*Primary and secondary haemochromatosis including thalassaemia, in patients in whom concomitant disorders (e.g. severe anaemia, hypoproteinaemia) preclude phlebotomy:* The main aim of therapy in younger patients is to achieve an iron balance and prevent haemosiderosis, whilst in the older patient a negative iron balance is desirable in order to slowly deplete the increased iron stores and to prevent the toxic effects of iron.

*Adults and children*: Desferal therapy should be commenced after the first 10–15 blood transfusions, or when serum ferritin levels reach 1,000ng/ml. The dose and mode of administration should be individually adapted according to the degree of iron overload.

*Dose*: The lowest effective dose should be used. The average daily dose will probably lie between 20 and 60 mg/kg. Patients with serum ferritin levels of <2,000ng/ml should require about 25 mg/kg/day, and those with levels between 2,000 and 3,000ng/ml about 35 mg/kg/day. Higher doses should only be employed if the benefit for the patient outweighs the risk of unwanted effects.

To assess the chelation therapy, 24 hour urinary iron excretion should initially be monitored daily. Starting with a dose of 500 mg daily the dose should be raised until a plateau of iron excretion is reached. Once the appropriate dose has been established, urinary iron excretion rates can be assessed at intervals of a few weeks.

*Mode of administration*: Slow subcutaneous infusions by means of a portable, light-weight, infusion pump over a period of 8-12 hours is effective and particularly convenient for ambulant patients. It may be possible to achieve a further increase in iron excretion by infusing the same daily dose over a 24 hour period. Patients should be treated 4-7 times a week depending on the degree of iron overload.

As intramuscular injections are less effective they should be given only when subcutaneous infusions are not appropriate.

Desferal can be administered by intravenous infusion during blood transfusion.

Continuous intravenous infusion is recommended for patients incapable of continuing subcutaneous infusions and in those who have cardiac problems secondary to iron overload. Implanted intravenous systems can be used when intensive chelation is carried out at home

*Diagnosis of iron storage disease and certain anaemias*: The Desferal test for iron overload is based on the principle that normal subjects do not excrete more than a fraction of a milligram of iron in their urine daily, and that a standard intramuscular injection of 500 mg of Desferal will not increase this above 1 mg (18μmol). In iron storage diseases, however, the increase may be well over 1.5 mg (27μmol). It should be borne in mind that the test only yields reliable results when renal function is normal.

Desferal is administered as a 500 mg intramuscular injection. Urine is then collected for a period of 6 hours and its iron content determined. Excretion of 1-1.5 mg (18-27μmol) of iron during this 6-hour period is suggestive of iron overload; values greater than 1.5 mg (27μmol) can be regarded as pathological.

*Use in the elderly*: No special dosage regime is necessary but concurrent renal insufficiency should be taken into account.

*Treatment for aluminium overload in patients with end-stage renal failure:* Patients should receive Desferal if:

- they have symptoms or evidence of organ impairment due to aluminium overload
- they are asymptomatic but their serum aluminium levels are consistently above 60ng/ml and associated with a positive Desferal test (see below), particularly if a bone biopsy provides evidence of aluminium-related bone disease

*Adults and children:* Patients on maintenance haemodialysis or haemofiltration: 5 mg/kg once a week administered during the last hour of a dialysis as a slow intravenous infusion (to reduce loss of free drug in the dialysate).

Four weeks after the completion of a 3 month course of Desferal treatment a Desferal infusion test should be performed, followed by a second test 1 month later. Serum aluminium increases above baseline of less than 75ng/ml measured in 2 successive infusion tests indicate that further Desferal treatment is not necessary.

*Patients on CAPD or CCPD*: 5 mg/kg once a week prior to the final exchange of the day. Desferal may be administered iv (by slow infusion), im, sc or intraperitoneally; the intraperitoneal route is recommended for these patients.

*Diagnosis of aluminium overload in patients with end-stage renal failure:* A Desferal infusion test is recommended in patients with serum aluminium levels > 60ng/ml associated with serum ferritin levels > 100ng/ml.

Serum aluminium values should be determined from blood samples taken:
- immediately before a haemodialysis session (baseline); 5 mg/kg should then be administered as a slow intravenous infusion during the last hour of the dialysis
- at the start of the next haemodialysis session

An increase in serum aluminium above baseline of more than 150ng/ml is suggestive of aluminium overload. It should be noted that a negative test does not completely exclude the possibility of aluminium overload.

Theoretically 100 mg Desferal can bind 4.1 mg Al+++.

### Contra-indications, warnings, etc
*Contra-indications:* Hypersensitivity to desferrioxamine mesylate unless the patient can be desensitised.

*Warnings and precautions:* Desferal should be used with caution in patients with renal impairment since the metal complexes are excreted via the kidneys. In these patients, dialysis will increase the elimination of chelated iron and aluminium.

Used alone Desferal may exacerbate neurological impairment in patients with aluminium-related encephalopathy. This deterioration (manifest as seizures) is probably related to an acute increase in brain aluminium secondary to elevated circulating levels. Pretreatment with clonazepam has been shown to afford protection against such impairment.

Treatment with Desferal by the intravenous route should only be administered in the form of *slow* infusions. If an intramuscular injection is accidentally given intravenously, this may lead to circulatory collapse.

Desferal should not be administered s.c. in concentrations and/or doses higher than those recommended as otherwise local irritation at the site of administration may occur more frequently.

Patients suffering from iron overload are particularly susceptible to infection. There have been reports of Desferal promoting some infections such as *Yersinia enterocolitica* and *Y.pseudotuberculosis*. If patients develop fever with pharyngitis, diffuse abdominal pain or enteritis/enterocolitis, Desferal therapy should be stopped, and appropriate treatment with antibiotics should be instituted. Desferal therapy may be resumed once the infection has cleared.

In patients undergoing haemodialysis while receiving Desferal, there have been rare reports of severe fungal infection (i.e. cases of mucormycosis). If any characteristic signs or symptoms occur Desferal treatment should be discontinued, mycological tests carried out and appropriate treatment immediately instituted. Mucormycosis has been reported to occur in dialysis patients not receiving Desferal, thus no causal link with the use of the drug has been established.

Disturbances of vision and hearing have been reported during prolonged Desferal therapy. In particular this has occurred in patients on higher than recommended therapy or in patients with low serum ferritin levels. Therefore, ophthalmological and audiological tests should be carried out both prior to the institution of long-term therapy with Desferal and at 3-monthly intervals during treatment. A detailed ophthalmological assessment is recommended (visual field measurements, funduscopy, colour vision testing using pseudoisochromatic plates and the Farnsworth D-15 colour test, slit lamp investigation, visual evoked potential studies).

If disturbances of vision or hearing do occur, treatment with Desferal should be stopped. Such disturbances may be reversible. If Desferal therapy is re-instituted later at a lower dosage, close monitoring of ophthalmological/ auditory function should be carried out with due regard to the risk-benefit ratio.

The use of inappropriately high doses of Desferal in patients with low ferritin levels has also been associated with growth retardation; dose reduction has been found to restore the growth rate to pretreatment levels in some cases. Three monthly checks on body weight and height are recommended in children.

Patients experiencing CNS effects such as dizziness or impaired vision or hearing should be warned against driving or operating machinery.

*Use in pregnancy and lactation:* Desferal has caused teratogenic effects in animals when given during pregnancy, particularly in the first trimester.

In rabbits, desferrioxamine caused skeletal malformations. However, these teratogenic effects in the foetuses were observed at doses which were toxic to the mother. In mice and rats desferrioxamine appears to be free of teratogenic activity.

Malformations have not occurred in children borne by patients reported to have received Desferal during pregnancy.

It is not known whether Desferal is excreted into the breast milk.

Desferal should not be given to pregnant or lactating women unless in the judgement of the physician, the expected benefits to the mother outweigh the potential risk to the child. This particularly applies to the first trimester.

*Drug interactions:* Oral administration of vitamin C (up to a maximum of 200 mg daily, given in divided doses) may serve to enhance excretion of the iron complex in response to Desferal; larger doses of vitamin C fail to produce an additional effect. Monitoring of cardiac function is indicated during such combined therapy. Vitamin C should be given only if the patient is receiving Desferal regularly, and should not be administered within the first month of Desferal therapy. In patients with severe chronic iron-storage disease undergoing combined treatment with Desferal and high doses of vitamin C (more than 500 mg daily) impairment of cardiac function has been encountered; this proved reversible when the vitamin C was withdrawn. Vitamin C supplements should not therefore be given to patients with cardiac failure.

Desferal should not be used in combination with prochlorperazine (a phenothiazine derivative) since prolonged unconsciousness may result.

Gallium[67] imaging results may be distorted because of the rapid urinary excretion of Desferal-bound radiolabel. Discontinuation of Desferal 48 hours prior to scintigraphy is advised.

There is evidence that aluminium intoxication causes reduced erythropoiesis. In dialysed patients with aluminium and/or iron overload treated with desferrioxamine and erythropoietin some dosage adjustment of the latter may be necessary. Regular monitoring of iron stores should also be carried out.

*Side-effects:* The following unwanted effects have been reported:
*Local reactions:* Frequent: pain, swelling, induration, erythema, burning, pruritus, wheals; rash at the injection/infusion site, occasionally accompanied by fever, chills and malaise
*Allergy:* Rare: anaphylactic/anaphylactoid reactions with or without shock, angioedema
*Special senses:* Rare: blurred vision, decreased visual acuity, loss of vision, impairment of colour vision, night blindness, visual field defects, scotoma, retinopathy (pigmentary degeneration of the retina), optic neuritis, cataracts, corneal opacities; tinnitus; hearing loss (including high-frequency sensorineural hearing loss).
*Skin:* Rare: generalised rash, pruritus, urticaria.
*Endocrine system:* Rare: growth retardation.
*Pulmonary system:* Isolated cases: adult respiratory distress syndrome (with dyspnoea, cyanosis and interstitial pulmonary infiltrates; following excessively high iv doses of Desferal).
*Central nervous system:* Rare: neurological disturbances, dizziness, convulsions, exacerbation of neurological impairment in aluminium-related encephalopathy. Isolated cases: precipitation of dialysis dementia, peripheral sensory neuropathy, paraesthesia
*Gastrointestinal system:* Rare: nausea, vomiting, diarrhoea, abdominal cramps.
*Renal system:* Isolated cases: impaired renal function.
*Liver:* Rare: impaired hepatic function.
*Cardiovascular system:* Rare: hypotension.
*Haematological system:* Isolated cases: blood dyscrasias (e.g. thrombocytopenia).
*Other:* Rare: leg cramps. Isolated cases: malaise, bone pain.

Some of the side-effects mentioned above must be considered as signs and symptoms of the underlying disease. Excretion of iron complex during treatment with Desferal causes reddish-brown discolouration of the urine.

*Overdosage:* Desferal is usually administered parenterally and acute poisoning is unlikely to occur.
*Signs and symptoms:* Tachycardia, hypotension and gastrointestinal symptoms have occasionally occurred in patients who received an overdose of Desferal. Accidental administration of Desferal by the iv route may be associated with acute but transient loss of vision, aphasia, agitation, headache, nausea, bradycardia and hypotension.
*Treatment:* There is no specific antidote to Desferal but signs and symptoms may be eliminated by reducing the dosage and Desferal is dialysable. Appropriate supportive therapy should be instituted.

### Pharmaceutical precautions
*Storage:* Desferal should be stored below 25°C.
*Dilution:* The reconstituted solution should be stored at room temperature (23°C or below) and used within 24 hours.

**Legal category** POM.

**Package quantities** Packs of 10 vials containing 500 mg Desferal.

**Further information** Nil.

**Product licence number** 00101/0523

## DIOVAN* ▼

**Qualitative and quantitative composition** Active substance: (S)-N-valeryl-N-{[2'-(1H-tetrazol-5-yl)biphenyl-4-yl]methyl}-valine (INN=valsartan). One capsule contains 40 mg, 80 mg or 160 mg valsartan.

**Pharmaceutical form** Capsules.

Appearance:
| | |
|---|---|
| 40 mg: | Light grey cap and body, marked CG HBH in black ink on the cap. |
| 80 mg: | Light grey cap and flesh opaque body, marked CG FZF in black ink on the cap. |
| 160 mg: | Dark grey cap and flesh opaque body, marked CG GOG in white ink on the cap. |

### Clinical particulars
*Therapeutic indications:* Treatment of hypertension.

*Posology and method of administration:* The recommended dose of Diovan is 80 mg once daily for most patients. The antihypertensive effect is substantially present within 2 weeks and maximal effects are seen after 4 weeks. In some patients whose blood pressure is not adequately controlled, the dose can either be increased to 160 mg, or a greater decrease in BP may be achieved by adding in a thiazide diuretic.

Diovan may also be administered with other antihypertensive agents.

*Use in patients over 75 years:* A lower starting dose of 40 mg once daily is recommended.

*Use in renal impairment:* No initial dose adjustment is required in patients with mild renal impairment (i.e. creatinine clearance 20–50 ml/min). For patients with moderate to severe renal impairment (i.e. creatinine less than 20 ml/min) or patients on dialysis, a lower starting dose of 40 mg once daily is recommended.

*Use in patients with intravascular volume depletion:* For those patients who have intravascular volume depletion (e.g. those treated with high dose diuretics who are unable to have their dose of diuretic reduced) a starting dose of 40 mg is recommended.

*Use in patients with mild to moderate hepatic impairment:* Treatment should commence at a dose of 40 mg once daily. A daily dose of 80 mg should not be exceeded. Patients with severe hepatic impairment, cirrhosis or biliary obstruction should not use Diovan (see *Contra-indications*).

*Use in children:* The safety and efficacy of Diovan have not been established in children.

*Contra-indications:* Hypersensitivity to any of the components of Diovan.
Pregnancy (see *Pregnancy and lactation*).
Severe hepatic impairment, cirrhosis, biliary obstruction.

*Special warnings and precautions for use:*
*Sodium and/or volume depleted patients*—In severely sodium-depleted and/or volume-depleted patients, such as those receiving high doses of diuretics, symptomatic hypotension may occur in rare cases after initiation of therapy with Diovan. For those patients whose diuretic dose cannot be reduced in order to correct their sodium and/or volume depletion a starting dose of 40 mg is recommended.
*Renal artery stenosis*—Short-term administration of Diovan to twelve patients with renovascular hypertension secondary to unilateral renal artery stenosis did not induce any significant changes in renal haemodynamics, serum creatinine, or blood urea nitrogen (BUN). However, since other drugs that affect the renin-angiotensin-aldosterone system may increase blood urea and serum creatinine in patients with bilateral or unilateral renal artery stenosis, monitoring is recommended as a safety measure.
*Hepatic impairment*—Based on pharmacokinetic data which demonstrate significantly increased plasma concentrations of valsartan in mild to moderately hepatically impaired patients, a lower dose is recommended (see *Posology and method of administration*). In these patients the dose of 80 mg should not be exceeded. Patients with severe hepatic impairment, cirrhosis or biliary obstruction are contra-indicated from using Diovan (see *Contra-indications*).

*Interaction with other medicaments and other forms of interaction:* Compounds which have been studied in clinical trials include cimetidine, warfarin, furosemide, digoxin, atenolol, indomethacin, hydrochlorothiazide, amlodipine, glibenclamide. Used together with cimetidine, the systemic exposure of valsartan may be marginally increased. A combination with glibenclamide may cause a decrease in the systemic exposure to valsartan.

As Diovan is not metabolised to a significant extent, clinically relevant drug-drug interactions in the form of metabolic induction or inhibition of the cytochrome P450 system are not expected with valsartan. Although valsartan is highly bound to plasma proteins, *in vitro* studies have not shown any interaction at this level with a range of molecules which are also highly protein-bound, such as diclofenac, furosemide, and warfarin.

Concomitant use of potassium-sparing diuretics (e.g. spironolactone, triamterene, amiloride), potassium supplements, or salt substitutes containing potassium may lead to increases in serum potassium. Comedication is not advisable.

*Pregnancy and lactation:* Although there is no experience with Diovan in pregnant women, in utero exposure to angiotensin converting enzyme (ACE) inhibitors given to pregnant women during the second and third trimesters has been reported to cause injury and death to the developing fetus. Thus, as for any drug that also acts directly on the renin-angiotensin-aldosterone system (RAAS), Diovan should not be used during pregnancy. If pregnancy is detected during therapy, Diovan should be discontinued as soon as possible.

It is not known whether valsartan is excreted in human milk. Valsartan was excreted in the milk of lactating rats. Thus, it is not advisable to use Diovan in lactating mothers.

*Effects in ability to drive and use machines:* As with other antihypertensive agents, it is advisable to exercise caution when driving or operating machinery.

*Undesirable effects:* In general, Diovan has a side-effect profile comparable to placebo; adverse experiences have been mild and transient in nature.

In placebo controlled clinical trials of essential hypertension in 3204 patients, side effects that were reported whether or not drug related with an incidence greater than placebo in patients treated with Diovan were:

*Body as a whole:* Occasionally: Fatigue.

*Respiratory system:* Rarely: Epistaxis. There was one isolated case of angioedema.

[Frequency estimates are as follows: frequently, >10%; occasionally, 1–10%; rarely, 0.001–1%].

*Laboratory findings:* In controlled clinical trials, clinically significant changes in laboratory parameters were rarely seen in patients taking Diovan.

In rare cases, Diovan was associated with decreases in haemoglobin and haematocrit; neutropoenia was observed occasionally.

Occasional elevations of liver function tests occurred in Diovan treated patients but no more frequently than in patients taking placebo.

Occasional elevation of serum potassium was seen but rarely was this of clinical significance and no patient discontinued for hyperkalaemia. Serum potassium should be monitored in renally impaired or elderly patients if they are also taking potassium supplements.

Occasional minor elevations of creatinine and bilirubin were also seen in controlled trials.

*Overdose:* Although there is no experience of overdosage with Diovan, the major sign that might be expected is marked hypotension. If the ingestion is recent, vomiting should be induced. Otherwise, the usual treatment would be intravenous infusion of normal saline solution.

Valsartan is unlikely to be removed by haemodialysis.

**Pharmacological properties**

*Pharmacodynamic properties:* The active hormone of the RAAS is angiotensin II, which is formed from angiotensin I through ACE. Angiotensin II binds to specific receptors located in the cell membranes of various tissues. It has a wide variety of physiological effects, including in particular both direct and indirect involvement in the regulation of blood pressure. As a potent vasoconstrictor, angiotensin II exerts a direct pressor response. In addition it promotes sodium retention and stimulation of aldosterone secretion.

Diovan (valsartan) is an orally active, potent, and specific angiotensin II (Ang II) receptor antagonist. It acts selectively on the $AT_1$ receptor subtype, which is responsible for the known actions of angiotensin II. The $AT_2$ subtype is unrelated to cardiovascular effects. Valsartan does not exhibit any partial agonist activity at the $AT_1$ receptor and has much (about 20,000 fold) greater affinity for the $AT_1$ receptor than for the $AT_2$ receptor.

Valsartan does not inhibit ACE, also known as kininase II, which converts Ang I to Ang II and degrades bradykinin. Since there is no effect on ACE and no potentiation of bradykinin or substance P, angiotensin II antagonists are unlikely to be associated with cough. In clinical trials where valsartan was compared with an ACE inhibitor, the incidence of dry cough was significantly (P<0.05) less in patients treated with valsartan than in those treated with an ACE inhibitor (2.6% versus 7.9% respectively). In a clinical trial of patients with a history of dry cough during ACE inhibitor therapy, 19.5% of trial subjects receiving valsartan and 19.0% of those receiving a thiazide diuretic experienced cough compared to 68.5% of those treated with an ACE inhibitor (P<0.05). Valsartan does not bind to or block other hormone receptors or ion channels known to be important in cardiovascular regulation.

Administration of Diovan to patients with hypertension results in reduction of blood pressure without affecting pulse rate.

In most patients, after administration of a single oral dose, onset of antihypertensive activity occurs within 2 hours, and the peak reduction of blood pressure is achieved within 4–6 hours. The antihypertensive effect persists over 24 hours after dosing. During repeated dosing, the maximum reduction in blood pressure with any dose is generally attained within 2–4 weeks and is sustained during long-term therapy. Combined with hydrochlorothiazide, a significant additional reduction in blood pressure is achieved.

Abrupt withdrawal of Diovan has not been associated with rebound hypertension or other adverse clinical events.

In multiple dose studies in hypertensive patients valsartan had no notable effects on total cholesterol, fasting triglycerides, fasting serum glucose, or uric acid.

*Pharmacokinetic properties:* Absorption of valsartan after oral administration is rapid, although the amount absorbed varies widely. Mean absolute bioavailability for Diovan is 23%. Valsartan shows multi-exponential decay kinetics ($t_{1/2}\,\alpha$<1 h and $t_{1/2}\,\beta$ about 9 h).

The pharmacokinetics of valsartan are linear in the dose range tested. There is no change in the kinetics of valsartan on repeated administration, and little accumulation when dosed once daily. Plasma concentrations were observed to be similar in males and females.

Valsartan is highly bound to serum protein (94–97%), mainly serum albumin. Steady-state volume of distribution is low (about 17 L). Plasma clearance is relatively slow (about 2 L/h) when compared with hepatic blood flow (about 30 L/h). After oral dosing, 83% is excreted in the faeces and 13% in the urine, mainly as unchanged compound.

When Diovan is given with food, the area under the plasma concentration curve (AUC) of valsartan is reduced by 48%, although from about 8 h post dosing plasma valsartan concentrations are similar for the fed and fasted group. This reduction in AUC, however, is not accompanied by a clinically significant reduction in the therapeutic effect, and Diovan can therefore be given either with or without food.

*Special populations:*

*Elderly:* A somewhat higher systemic exposure to valsartan was observed in some elderly subjects compared with young subjects; and a lower starting dose (40 mg) is recommended for the elderly.

*Impaired renal function:* As expected for a compound where renal clearance accounts for only 30% of total plasma clearance, no correlation was seen between renal function and systemic exposure to valsartan. Dose adjustment is therefore not required in patients with mild renal impairment (creatinine clearance 20–50 ml/min). Limited data are available in patients with moderate-severe impairment of renal function and a starting dose of 40 mg is recommended for these patients. No studies have been performed in patients undergoing dialysis. However, valsartan is highly bound to plasma protein and is unlikely to be removed by dialysis.

*Hepatic impairment:* In a pharmacokinetics trial in patients with mild to moderate hepatic dysfunction, exposure to valsartan was increased approximately 2-fold compared with healthy volunteers.

*Preclinical safety data:* In a variety of preclinical safety studies conducted in several animal species, there was no evidence of systemic or target organ toxicity, apart from fetotoxicity. Offspring from rats given 600 mg/kg during the last trimester and during lactation showed a slightly reduced survival rate and a slight developmental delay (see *Pregnancy and lactation*). The main preclinical safety findings are attributed to the pharmacological action of the compound, and have not been demonstrated to have any clinical significance.

There was no evidence of mutagenicity, clastogenicity or carcinogenicity.

**Pharmaceutical particulars**

*List of excipients:* Microcrystalline cellulose, polyvidone, sodium lauryl sulfate, crospovidone, magnesium stearate.

*Incompatibilities:* None known.

*Shelf life:* 3 years.

*Special precautions for storage:* Protect from moisture and heat, store below 30°C.

*Nature and contents of container:* PVC/PE/PVDC blister packs.

80 mg and 160 mg capsules are supplied in packs of 7 or 28.

40 mg capsules are supplied in packs of 7 capsules.

*Instructions for use/handling:* No specific instructions for use/handling.

**Marketing authorisation numbers**

40 mg 00101/0524
80 mg 00101/0525
160 mg 00101/0526

**Date of approval/revision of SPC** October 1996.

**Legal category** POM.

## ESTRACOMBI TTS*

**Presentation** Estracombi TTS is a transdermal therapy comprising:

(i) Estraderm TTS 50: Four self-adhesive, circular, transparent, transdermal therapeutic systems (patches) marked CG EFE, each containing a drug reservoir of 17β-oestradiol with an absorption rate of approximately 50 μg of oestradiol per day (drug releasing area 10cm², oestradiol content 4 mg).

(ii) Estragest TTS: Four self-adhesive, goggle-shaped, transparent, transdermal therapeutic systems marked CG FNF, each with two similar drug reservoirs containing 17β-oestradiol plus Norethisterone Acetate BP. The absorption rates from the system are approximately 50 μg of oestradiol per day and 250 μg of norethisterone acetate per day (drug releasing area 20cm², oestradiol content 10 mg, norethisterone acetate content 30 mg).

Patches contain: ethanol, hydroxypropylcellulose, polyethylene terephthalate, ethylenevinylacetate copolymer, liquid paraffin, polyisobutylene, silicone-coating (on the inner side of the protective release liner which is removed before patch application).

**Uses**

*Indications:* Hormone replacement therapy for patients with disorders due to natural or surgically induced menopause, e.g. vasomotor symptoms (hot flushes and nocturnal sweating), urogenital conditions such as atrophic vaginitis/vulvitis, and/or atrophic urethritis and trigonitis.

Prevention of postmenopausal osteoporosis in women considered at risk of developing fractures. Epidemiological studies suggest a number of risk factors may contribute to postmenopausal osteoporosis, including:

- early menopause (either natural or surgically induced)
- family history of osteoporosis
- recent prolonged corticosteroid therapy
- a small, thin frame
- excessive cigarette consumption.

If several risk factors are present consideration should be given to hormone replacement therapy. Bone mineral density measurements may help to confirm the presence of low bone mass. For maximum prophylactic benefit treatment should commence as soon as possible after the menopause.

*Mode of action:* Oestrogen substitution effectively prevents the symptomatic, metabolic and trophic changes due to loss of ovarian function associated with the menopause.

The patch formulation (transdermal therapeutic system, TTS) delivers hormone into the bloodstream via intact skin. Estraderm TTS and Estragest TTS are both designed to deliver 17β-oestradiol at a low rate over several days.

With Estragest TTS progestogen is added for the last 14 days in each cycle in order to prevent endometrial hyperstimulation. A regular cyclic bleed can be expected to start on day 24-26 of treatment.

Studies of bone mineral content have shown Estracombi TTS to be effective in the prevention of progressive bone loss following the menopause.

*Pharmacokinetics:* Within four hours of application of the first Estraderm TTS 50 patch plasma oestradiol levels reach the therapeutic range, and these are maintained throughout the dose interval (for up to four days).

After removal of the last patch plasma oestrogen levels return to baseline values in less than 24 hours, and urinary oestrogen conjugates within 2-3 days.

Mean plasma concentrations of oestradiol are similar during both phases of the treatment (i.e. transdermal oestradiol alone with Estraderm TTS 50, or transdermal oestradiol plus norethisterone acetate with Estragest TTS).

Norethisterone acetate is metabolised to the active progestogen, norethisterone, which reaches plasma levels of 0.5–1.0 ng/ml within 2 days after Estragest TTS application. These levels are maintained throughout the dose interval and are sufficient to prevent endometrial hyperstimulation. After removal of the system, levels of norethisterone return to baseline within 2 days.

Absorption rates may vary between individual patients.

## Dosage and administration

*Adults and elderly:* Estracombi TTS provides continuous oestrogen and sequential progestogen therapy.

One treatment cycle of Estracombi TTS consists of 4 patches of transdermal oestradiol followed by 4 patches of transdermal oestradiol and norethisterone acetate. Therapy is started with transdermal oestradiol (Estraderm TTS 50) which should be applied twice weekly for 2 weeks, i.e. the patch should be changed once every 3 to 4 days. For the following 2 weeks, one transdermal oestradiol plus norethisterone acetate patch (Estragest TTS) is applied twice weekly. The next treatment cycle should be started immediately after the removal of the last Estragest TTS patch.

Each fresh patch should be applied to a slightly different site. Recommended application sites are clean, dry and intact areas of skin on the trunk below the waistline. The site selected should be one at which little wrinkling of the skin occurs during movement of the body, e.g. buttock, hip, abdomen. Experience to date has shown that less irritation of the skin occurs on the buttocks than at other sites of application, and this site is preferred by patients. It is therefore recommended to apply Estracombi TTS to the buttock. Estracombi TTS should NOT be applied on or near the breasts.

In the woman with an intact uterus, combined oestrogen/progestogen hormone replacement therapy is required, as in Estracombi TTS.

Estracombi TTS incorporates a combined oestrogen and progestogen patch to induce withdrawal bleeding, thereby minimising the risk of endometrial hyperplasia and carcinoma which can occur with unopposed oestrogen therapy. Most patients will bleed towards the end of progestogen therapy. The first transdermal patch of the new cycle should be applied irrespective of the duration of bleeding. It is important that the patches be used in the correct sequence (i.e. 2 weeks Estraderm TTS 50 followed by 2 weeks Estragest TTS each cycle) to ensure regular cyclic bleeding.

For most postmenopausal women Estracombi TTS therapy may be started at any convenient time. However, if the patient is still menstruating commencement within 5 days of the onset of bleeding is recommended.

Some breakthrough bleeding or spotting may be seen until therapy has become established. Some effects, usually of oestrogenic origin, e.g. breast discomfort, water retention or bloating, are often observed at the start of treatment, especially in patients receiving hormone replacement therapy for the first time. However, if symptoms persist for more than 6 weeks, treatment should be reconsidered.

The system should not be exposed to sunlight.

The use of creams, oils or lotions should be avoided since these may reduce patch adhesion.

*Children:* Estracombi TTS is not indicated.

*Pregnancy and lactation:* Estracombi TTS is not indicated.

## Contra-indications, warnings, etc

*Contra-indications:* Cancer of the breast, genital tract or other oestrogen-dependent neoplasia; severe hepatic, renal or cardiac disease; undiagnosed vaginal bleeding; active thrombophlebitis and thromboembolic disorders; Dubin-Johnson syndrome; Rotor syndrome; endometriosis; known hypersensitivity to the components of the patch.

*Precautions and warnings:* Contact sensitisation is known to occur with all topical applications. Although it is extremely rare, patients who develop contact sensitisation to any of the components of the patch should be warned that a severe hypersensitivity reaction may occur with continuing exposure to the causative agent.

Before commencing any oestrogen replacement therapy it is recommended that the patient should have a thorough general medical and gynaecological examination to rule out endometrial abnormalities and breast cancer. In patients receiving prolonged treatment these examinations, including endometrial assessment where necessary, should be repeated at regular intervals (e.g. every 6 to 12 months). Persistent breakthrough bleeding is an indication for endometrial assessment, which may include biopsy. In patients experiencing recurrent early onset of bleeding (i.e. before day 24), treatment should be re-evaluated.

At the present time there is some evidence which suggests a slight increase in the relative risk of breast cancer in postmenopausal women receiving long-term hormone replacement therapy. A careful appraisal of the risk/benefit ratio should be undertaken before treating for longer than 5 years.

Women on this therapy, in particular those with fibrocystic disease of the breast, or with a family history of breast cancer (first degree relatives) should have regular breast examinations, including mam-

mography, and should be instructed in breast self examination.

Close monitoring of patients with conditions reportedly worsened by oestrogens is recommended: uterine fibroids; history of oestrogen-related hearing impairment, jaundice or thromboembolic disorders; cholelithiasis; diabetes

Oestrogen overdosage may cause water retention, therefore patients with heart failure, hypertension, disorders of renal or hepatic function, epilepsy or migraine should be kept under special surveillance. Regular monitoring of blood pressure should be carried out in hypertensive patients.

Estracombi TTS is not a contraceptive.

*Drug interactions:* Preparations inducing microsomal liver enzymes e.g. barbiturates, hydantoins, carbamazepine, meprobamate, phenylbutazone, antibiotics (including rifampicin) and activated charcoal, may impair the activity of oestrogens and progestogens (irregular bleeding and recurrence of symptoms may occur).

The extent of interference with transdermally administered oestradiol and norethisterone acetate is not known; these problems should be minimised by the transdermal route of administration which avoids any first pass hepatic metabolism.

*Side-effects:*
*Skin:* Frequently: Transient erythema and irritation at site of application with or without pruritus. This usually disappears 3-4 days after patch removal and is similar to the effect observed after occlusion of the skin with household medical adhesive plasters. Very infrequently: Local swelling, papules/vesicles and scaling have been reported, which also resolved spontaneously and did not result in permanent skin damage. Isolated cases: Allergic contact dermatitis, reversible post-inflammatory pigmentation; generalised pruritus and exanthema.

*Urogenital tract:* Frequently: Breakthrough bleeding, spotting. Occasionally: Heavy, sometimes prolonged bleeding, dysmenorrhoea, pre-menstrual syndrome-like symptoms; endometrial hyperplasia (incidence similar to that reported for other opposed HRT regimes). Amenorrhoea may occur during treatment.

*Endocrine system:* Frequently: Breast discomfort.

*Gastrointestinal tract:* Occasionally: Nausea, abdominal cramps, bloating. Isolated cases: Asymptomatic impaired liver function, cholestatic jaundice.

*Central nervous system:* Occasionally: Headache, migraine. Rarely: Dizziness.

*Cardiovascular system:* Isolated cases: Thromboembolic disorders, exacerbation of varicose veins, increase in blood pressure.

*Miscellaneous:* Rarely: Oedema and/or weight changes. Occasionally: Leg cramps (not related to thromboembolic disease and usually transient lasting 3-6 weeks; if symptoms persist treatment should be reviewed). Isolated cases: anaphylactoid reactions (history of previous allergy or allergic disorders in some cases)

*Overdosage:* Due to the mode of administration overdosage is unlikely .

Signs and symptoms: Signs of acute oestrogen overdosage may be either one of, or a combination of breast discomfort, fluid retention and bloating, or nausea.

Signs of progestogen overdosage may be nausea, vomiting, breast enlargement and vaginal bleeding.

Treatment: Overdosage can if necessary be reversed by removal of the patch.

**Pharmaceutical precautions** Store below 25°C.

**Legal category** POM.

**Package quantities** Cartons containing four transdermal oestradiol and four transdermal oestradiol and norethisterone acetate patches each individually sealed in a protective pouch (sufficient for one month's treatment). A three-monthly pack containing twelve transdermal oestradiol and twelve transdermal oestradiol and norethisterone acetate patches each individually sealed in a protective pouch is also available.

**Further information** Adverse effects on lipid and non-lipid mediated markers of cardiovascular disease may contribute to the increased incidence of cardiovascular disease seen in women post-menopause.

An improved lipid profile may be one factor contributing to the beneficial effect of oestrogen replacement therapy on the risk of coronary heart disease in postmenopausal women. Studies have indicated beneficial effects of Estraderm TTS with progestogen on serum total cholesterol, low density lipoprotein (LDL), triglyceride and high density lipoprotein (HDL) levels. There have been few long-term studies of the effect of Estraderm TTS alone on these measurements and the results are thus less conclusive although generally favourable. Studies of Estraderm TTS incorporating progestogen treatment have demonstrated effects on arterial tone which may have a beneficial effect on cardiovascular risk, and have not shown deleterious

effects on blood pressure, coagulation and insulin resistance.

Epidemiological studies indicate that a useful reduction in fracture frequency of approx. 50% is achieved with 5 to 6 years oestrogen therapy.

**Product licence number** 00101/0485

## ESTRADERM TTS*

**Presentation** Estraderm TTS is a self-adhesive, transparent, transdermal therapeutic system (patch), containing a drug reservoir of 17β-oestradiol. It is available in three sizes: Estraderm TTS 25, with an absorption rate of approx. 25 micrograms oestradiol/24 hours (active surface area 5cm², oestradiol content 2 mg); Estraderm TTS 50, with an absorption rate of approx. 50 micrograms oestradiol/24 hours (active surface area 10cm², oestradiol content 4 mg); Estraderm TTS 100, with an absorption rate of approx. 100 micrograms oestradiol/24 hours (active surface area 20cm², oestradiol content 8 mg).

Patches also contain: ethanol, hydroxypropylcellulose, polyethylene terephthalate, ethylenevinylacetate copolymer, liquid paraffin, polyisobutylene, silicone-coating (on the inner side of the protective release liner which is removed before patch application).

## Uses

*Indications:* Oestrogen replacement therapy for patients with disorders due to natural or surgically induced menopause e.g. vasomotor symptoms (hot flushes and nocturnal sweating), urogenital conditions such as atrophic vaginitis/vulvitis, and/or atrophic urethritis and trigonitis).

Prevention of postmenopausal osteoporosis in women considered at risk of developing fractures. Epidemiological studies suggest a number of risk factors may contribute to postmenopausal osteoporosis, including:

- early menopause (either natural or surgically induced)
- family history of osteoporosis
- recent prolonged corticosteroid therapy
- a small, thin frame
- excessive cigarette consumption

If several risk factors are present consideration should be given to hormone replacement therapy. Bone mineral density measurements may help to confirm the presence of low bone mass. For maximum prophylactic benefit treatment should commence as soon as possible after the menopause.

Oestrogen therapy must not be used in patients with an intact uterus unless an appropriate dose of progestogen is administered for twelve days per month.

*Mode of action:* Oestrogen substitution effectively prevents the characteristic symptomatic, metabolic and trophic changes associated with loss of ovarian function due to natural or surgical menopause.

The patch formulation (transdermal therapeutic system, TTS) delivers hormone into the bloodstream via intact skin. Estraderm TTS is designed to deliver 17β-oestradiol at a low rate over several days.

*Pharmacokinetics:* Within four hours after application of the first system, plasma oestradiol levels reach the therapeutic range and these are maintained throughout the dose interval (for up to four days).

After removal of the last system plasma oestrogen levels return to baseline values in less than 24 hours and urinary oestrogen conjugates within 2-3 days.

Absorption rate may vary between individual patients. However, the plasma oestradiol levels achieved with different sized systems have been shown to be proportional to the drug-releasing area of the dosage form.

## Dosage and administration

*Adults and elderly:* Menopausal symptoms–Therapy should be initiated with one Estraderm TTS 50 and the dose adjusted after the first treatment month depending on efficacy and signs of overdosage. Effects usually of oestrogenic origin eg breast discomfort, water retention or bloating are often observed at the start of treatment especially in patients receiving hormone replacement therapy for the first time, however, if symptoms persist for more than six weeks the dose should be reduced. For maintenance therapy the lowest effective dose should be used; a maximum dose of 100 micrograms per day should not be exceeded. Unopposed oestrogen therapy should not be used unless the patient has had a hysterectomy. *Postmenopausal osteoporosis:* Estraderm TTS 50 is recommended as an effective bone-sparing dose. Estraderm TTS 100 is not recommended as the risk/benefit of the higher dose in osteoporosis has not been assessed in clinical studies. However, it may be used if necessary to control concurrent menopausal symptoms. Estraderm TTS 25 is not recommended as it has been shown to slow down but not completely halt the rate of bone loss.

Where a progestogen is considered necessary, the

appropriate dose should be administered for 12 days per month. If the oestrogen is adequately combined with a progestogen withdrawal bleeding occurs, in a way similar to normal menstrual bleeding. Breakthrough bleeding or spotting may be seen until therapy has become established. Signs of breakthrough bleeding early in the cycle should be investigated.

Estraderm TTS should be applied twice weekly on a continuous basis, each used system being removed after 3-4 days and a fresh system applied to a slightly different site. Recommended application sites are clean, dry and intact areas of skin on the trunk below the waistline. The site selected should be one at which little wrinkling of the skin occurs during movement of the body, eg buttock, hip, abdomen. Experience to date has shown that less irritation of the skin occurs on the buttocks than on other sites of application. It is therefore advisable to apply Estraderm TTS to the buttock. Estraderm TTS should **NOT** be applied on or near the breasts.

The system should not be exposed to sunlight.

*Children:* Estraderm TTS is not indicated in children.

*Use in pregnancy and lactation:* Estraderm TTS is not indicated.

### Contra-indications, warnings, etc

*Contra-indications:* Cancer of the breast, genital tract or other oestrogen-dependent neoplasia. Severe hepatic, renal or cardiac disease. Undiagnosed vaginal bleeding. Active thrombophlebitis and thromboembolic disorders. Dubin-Johnson syndrome. Rotor syndrome. Endometriosis; known hypersensitivity to the components of the patch.

*Precautions and warnings:* Contact sensitisation is known to occur with all topical applications. Although it is extremely rare, patients who develop contact sensitisation to any of the components of the patch should be warned that a severe hypersensitivity reaction may occur with continuing exposure to the causative agent.

Before commencing any oestrogen therapy it is recommended that the patient should have a thorough physical and gynaecological examination. This should be repeated regularly, e.g. at 6 monthly intervals.

At the present time there is some evidence which suggests a slight increase in the relative risk of breast cancer in postmenopausal women receiving long-term hormone replacement therapy. A careful appraisal of the risk/benefit ratio should be undertaken before treating for longer than 5 years.

Women on this therapy, in particular those with fibrocystic disease of the breast, or with a family history of breast cancer (first degree relatives) should have regular breast examinations, including mammography, and should be instructed in breast self examination.

Close monitoring of patients with conditions reportedly worsened by oestrogens is also recommended: uterine fibroids; history of oestrogen-related hearing impairment, jaundice or thromboembolic disorders; cholelithiasis; diabetes.

Oestrogen overdosage may cause water retention, therefore patients with heart failure, hypertension, disorders of renal or hepatic function, epilepsy or migraine should be kept under special surveillance. Regular monitoring of blood pressure should be carried out in hypertensive patients.

*Drug interactions:* Preparations inducing microsomal liver enzymes, eg barbiturates, hydantoins, anticonvulsants (including carbamazepine), meprobamate, phenylbutazone; antibiotics (including rifampicin) and activated charcoal, may impair the activity of oestrogens (irregular bleeding and recurrence of symptoms may occur).

The extent of interference with transdermally administered oestradiol is not known; these problems should be minimised by the transdermal route of administration which avoids any first pass hepatic metabolism.

*Side-effects:*

*Skin:* Frequently: transient erythema and irritation at the site of application with or without pruritus. This usually disappears 3-4 days after patch removal and is similar to the effect sometimes observed after occlusion of the skin with household medical adhesive plasters. Very infrequently: local swelling, papules/vesicles and scaling have been reported, which also resolved spontaneously and did not result in permanent skin damage. Isolated cases: Allergic contact dermatitis, reversible post-inflammatory pigmentation; generalised pruritus and exanthema

*Urogenital tract:* Frequently: breakthrough bleeding (usually a sign of oestrogen overdosage, see 'Dosage and administration').

*Endocrine system:* Frequently: breast discomfort

*Gastrointestinal tract:* Occasionally: nausea, abdominal cramps, bloating. Isolated cases: asymptomatic impaired liver function, cholestatic jaundice.

*Central nervous system:* Occasionally: headache, migraine. Rarely: dizziness.

*Cardiovascular system:* Isolated cases: thromboembolic disorders, exacerbation of varicose veins, increase in blood pressure.

*Miscellaneous:* Occasionally: leg cramps (not related to thromboembolic disease and usually transient lasting 3-6 weeks, if symptoms persist the dose of oestrogen should be reduced). Rarely: Oedema and/or weight changes. Isolated cases: Anaphylactoid reactions (history of previous allergy or allergic disorders in some cases)

*Overdosage:* This is not likely due to the mode of administration.

*Signs and symptoms:* (see *Dosage and administration*).

*Treatment:* Overdosage can if necessary be reversed by removal of the patch(es).

**Pharmaceutical precautions** Store below 25°C.

**Legal category** POM.

**Package quantities** Cartons containing eight Estraderm TTS patches, each individually sealed in a protective pouch (sufficient for one month's treatment). A three-monthly pack containing twenty-four Estraderm TTS patches, each individually sealed in a protective pouch is also available.

**Further information** Adverse effects on lipid and non-lipid mediated markers of cardiovascular disease may contribute to the increased incidence of cardiovascular disease seen in women post-menopause.

An improved lipid profile may be one factor contributing to the beneficial effect of oestrogen replacement therapy on the risk of coronary heart disease in postmenopausal women. Studies have indicated beneficial effects of Estraderm TTS with progestogen on serum total cholesterol, low density lipoprotein (LDL), triglyceride and high density lipoprotein (HDL) levels. There have been few long-term studies of the effect of Estraderm TTS alone on these measurements and the results are thus less conclusive although generally favourable. Studies of Estraderm TTS incorporating progestogen treatment have demonstrated effects on arterial tone which may have a beneficial effect on cardiovascular risk, and have not shown deleterious effects on blood pressure, coagulation and insulin resistance.

Epidemiological studies indicate that a useful reduction in fracture frequency of approx. 50% is achieved with 5 to 6 years oestrogen therapy.

**Product licence numbers**
Estraderm TTS 25 00101/0489
Estraderm TTS 50 00101/0490
Estraderm TTS 100 00101/0491

## ESTRADERM* MX

**Qualitative and quantitative composition** The active ingredient is Estra-1, 3,5(10)-triene-3,17β-diol (17β-oestradiol).

Patches contain 0.75, 1.5 and 3.0 mg active substance corresponding to surface areas of 11, 22 and 44 cm² respectively.

**Pharmaceutical form** Estraderm MX is a square-shaped, self-adhesive, transparent, transdermal therapeutic system (patch) for application to the skin surface. Each patch comprises an impermeable polyester backing film, an adhesive matrix containing 17β-oestradiol and an oversized protective liner which is removed prior to application of the patch to the skin. Estraderm MX releases oestradiol into the circulation via intact skin at a low rate for up to 4 days.

Cross section:

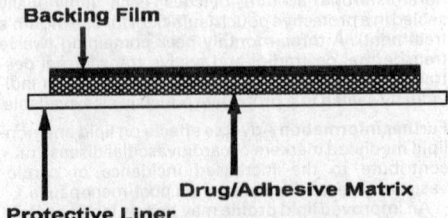

**Backing Film**

**Drug/Adhesive Matrix**

**Protective Liner**

| Dosage strength | Estraderm MX 25 |
|---|---|
| Nominal rate of oestradiol release | 25 µg/day |
| Oestradiol content | 0.75 mg |
| Drug-releasing area | 11 cm² |
| Imprint (on backing film) | CG GRG |

| Dosage strength | Estraderm MX 50 |
|---|---|
| Nominal rate of oestradiol release | 50 µg/day |
| Oestradiol content | 1.5 mg |
| Drug-releasing area | 22 cm² |

| Imprint (on backing film) | CG GSG |
|---|---|

| Dosage strength | Estraderm MX 100 |
|---|---|
| Nominal rate of oestradiol release | 100 µg/day |
| Oestradiol content | 3.0 mg |
| Drug-releasing area | 44 cm² |
| Imprint (on backing film) | CG GTG |

### Clinical particulars

*Therapeutic indications:* Oestrogen replacement therapy for patients with disorders due to natural or surgically induced menopause e.g. vasomotor symptoms (hot flushes and nocturnal sweating), urogenital conditions such as atrophic vaginitis/ vulvitis, and/or atrophic urethritis and trigonitis.

Prevention of postmenopausal osteoporosis in women considered at risk of developing fractures. Epidemiological studies suggest a number of risk factors may contribute to postmenopausal osteoporosis, including:
- early menopause (either natural or surgically induced)
- family history of osteoporosis
- recent prolonged corticosteroid therapy
- a small, thin frame
- excessive cigarette consumption

If several risk factors are present consideration should be given to hormone replacement therapy. Bone mineral density measurements may help to confirm the presence of low bone mass. For maximum prophylactic benefit treatment should commence as soon as possible after the menopause.

Oestrogen therapy must not be used in patients with an intact uterus unless an appropriate dose of progestogen is administered for twelve days per month.

*Posology and method of administration:*
*Dosage:*

*Menopausal symptoms:* Therapy should be initiated with one Estraderm MX 50 and the dose adjusted after the first treatment month depending on efficacy and signs of overdosage. Effects usually of oestrogenic origin e.g. breast discomfort, water retention or bloating are often observed at the start of treatment especially in patients receiving hormone replacement therapy for the first time, however, if symptoms persist for more than six weeks the dose should be reduced. For maintenance therapy the lowest effective dose should be used; a maximum dose of 100 micrograms per day should not be exceeded. Unopposed oestrogen therapy should not be used unless the patient has had a hysterectomy.

*Postmenopausal osteoporosis:* Estraderm MX 50 is recommended as an effective bone-sparing dose. Estraderm MX 100 is not recommended as the risk/benefit of the higher dose in osteoporosis has not been assessed in clinical studies. However, it may be used if necessary to control concurrent menopausal symptoms. Estraderm MX 25 Is not recommended as it has been shown to slow down but not completely halt the rate of bone loss.

Where a progestogen is considered necessary, the appropriate dose should be administered for 12 days per month. If the oestrogen is adequately combined with a progestogen withdrawal bleeding occurs, in a way similar to normal menstrual bleeding. Breakthrough bleeding or spotting may be seen until therapy has become established. Signs of breakthrough bleeding early in the cycle should be investigated.

Estraderm MX is not indicated in children

*Administration:* Estraderm MX should be applied immediately after removal of the protective liner (see Figs.), to an area of clean, dry, and intact skin on the trunk below the waistline. The site chosen should be one at which little wrinkling of skin occurs during movement of the body, e.g. buttock. Estraderm MX should NOT be applied on or near the breasts.

Estraderm MX should be applied twice weekly on a continuous basis, each used patch being removed after 3-4 days and a fresh system applied to a slightly different site. The patch should not be exposed to sunlight.

*Contra-indications:* Cancer of the breast, genital tract or other oestrogen-dependent neoplasia. Severe hepatic, renal or cardiac disease. Undiagnosed vaginal bleeding. Active thrombophlebitis and thromboembolic disorders. Dubin-Johnson syndrome. Rotor syndrome. Endometriosis; known hypersensitivity to the components of the patch.

*Special warnings and special precautions for use:* Contact sensitisation is known to occur with all topical applications. Although it is extremely rare, patients who develop contact sensitisation to any of the components of the patch should be warned that a severe hypersensitivity reaction may occur with continuing exposure to the causative agent.

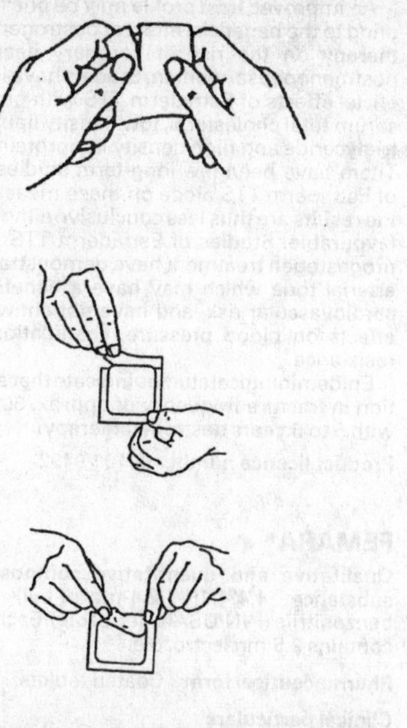

Before commencing any oestrogen therapy it is recommended that the patient should have a thorough physical and gynaecological examination. This should be repeated regularly, e.g. at 6 monthly intervals.

At the present time there is some evidence which suggests a slight increase in the relative risk of breast cancer in postmenopausal women receiving long-term hormone replacement therapy. A careful appraisal of the risk/benefit ratio should be undertaken before treating for longer than 5 years.

Women on this therapy, in particular those with fibrocystic disease of the breast, or with a family history of breast cancer (first degree relatives) should have regular breast examinations, including mammography, and should be instructed in breast self examination.

Close monitoring of patients with conditions reportedly worsened by oestrogens is also recommended: uterine fibroids; history of oestrogen-related hearing impairment, jaundice or thromboembolic disorders; cholelithiasis; diabetes.

Oestrogen overdosage may cause water retention, therefore patients with heart failure, hypertension, disorders of renal or hepatic function, epilepsy or migraine should be kept under special surveillance. Regular monitoring of blood pressure should be carried out in hypertensive patients.

*Interactions with other medicaments and other forms of interaction:* Preparations inducing microsomal liver enzymes, e.g. barbiturates, hydantoins, anticonvulsants, meprobamate, phenylbutazone; antibiotics and activated charcoal, may impair the activity of oestrogens (irregular bleeding and recurrence of symptoms may occur).

The extent of interference with transdermally administered oestradiol is not known; these problems should be minimised by the transdermal route of administration which avoids any first pass hepatic metabolism.

*Pregnancy and lactation:* Estraderm MX should not be used during pregnancy and lactation.

*Effects on ability to drive and use machines:* None known.

*Undesirable effects:* Frequency estimates are as follows: frequently >10%; occasionally 1-10%; rarely 0.001-1%; isolated cases <0.001%.

The following systemic effects have been reported for Estraderm TTS, which is bioequivalent to Estraderm MX:

*Urogenital tract:* Frequently: breakthrough bleeding (usually a sign of oestrogen overdosage).

*Endocrine system:* Frequently: breast discomfort.

*Gastrointestinal tract:* Occasionally: nausea, abdominal cramps, bloating. Isolated cases: asymptomatic impaired liver function, cholestatic jaundice.

*Central nervous system:* Occasionally: headache, migraine. Rarely: dizziness.

*Cardiovascular system:* Isolated cases: thromboembolic disorders, exacerbation of varicose veins, increase in blood pressure.

*Miscellaneous:* Rarely: oedema and/or weight changes, leg cramps (not related to thromboembolic disease and usually transient lasting 3-6 week; if symptoms persist the dose of oestrogen should be reduced).

*Skin:* The following have been reported in clinical trials performed with Estraderm MX:

Occasionally: transient erythema and irritation (observed in less than 6% of the cases) with pruritus (observed in less than 1%).

Isolated cases: generalized pruritus and rash.

*Overdose:* This is not likely due to the mode of administration.

*Signs and symptoms:* See *Dosage* section.

*Treatment:* Overdosage can if necessary be reversed by removal of the patch.

**Pharmacological properties**

*Pharmacodynamic properties:* Like all steroid hormones, oestrogens exert their metabolic effects intracellularly. In the cells of target organs oestrogens interact with specific receptors to form a complex which stimulates both DNA and protein synthesis. Such receptors have been identified in various organs, e.g. the hypothalamus, pituitary, vagina, urethra, breast, and liver, and in osteoblasts.

Oestradiol, which in women from the menarche to the menopause is produced mainly by the ovarian follicles, is the most active oestrogen at the receptor level. After the menopause, when the ovaries have ceased to function, only small amounts of oestradiol are still produced from aromatisation of androstenedione and to a lesser extent of testosterone by the aromatase enzyme, yielding oestrone and oestradiol, respectively. Oestrone is further transformed to oestradiol by the enzyme 17β–hydroxysteroid dehydrogenase. Both enzymes are found in fat, liver, and muscle tissue.

In many women, the cessation of ovarian oestradiol production results in vasomotor and thermoregulatory instability (hot flushes), sleep disturbances, and progressive atrophy of the urogenital system. These disorders can be largely eliminated by means of oestrogen replacement therapy. Owing to the accelerated loss of bone substance induced by postmenopausal oestrogen deficiency many women develop osteoporosis, particularly of the vertebral column, hip, and wrist. This can be prevented by oestrogen replacement therapy, preferably initiated early in the menopause. Epidemiological studies indicate that a useful reduction in fracture frequency of approx. 50% is achieved with 5 to 6 years oestrogen therapy.

Transdermal therapy with Estraderm MX delivers the physiological oestrogen oestradiol in unchanged form into the bloodstream via intact skin. Estraderm MX raises oestradiol concentrations to levels similar to those found in the early to mid–follicular phase and maintains them over the application period of 3-4 days. The oestradiol/oestrone ratio is restored to premenopausal levels.

The following pharmacodynamic effects have been reported for Estraderm TTS, which is bioequivalent to Estraderm MX:

Estraderm TTS treatment for 28 days did not result in changes in circulating levels of fibrinopeptide A, high molecular weight fibrinogen, or antithrombin III. There were no changes in concentrations either of circulating renin substrate or of the sex-hormone-binding, thyroxine-binding, and cortisol-binding globulins.

After only a few weeks treatment Estraderm TTS has been shown to elicit a dose-dependent reduction in urinary excretion of calcium and hydroxyproline which is indicative of a slowing down of the rate of bone loss.

Adverse effects on lipid and non-lipid mediated markers of cardiovascular disease may contribute to the increased incidence of cardiovascular disease seen in women post-menopause. An improved lipid profile may be one factor contributing to the beneficial effect of oestrogen replacement therapy on the risk of coronary heart disease in postmenopausal women. Studies have indicated beneficial effects of Estraderm TTS with progestogen on serum total cholesterol, low density lipoprotein (LDL), triglyceride and high density lipoprotein (HDL) levels. There have been few long-term studies of the effect of Estraderm TTS alone on these measurements and the results are thus less conclusive although generally favourable. Studies of Estraderm TTS incorporating progestogen treatment have demonstrated effects on arterial tone which may have a beneficial effect on cardiovascular risk, and have not shown deleterious effects on blood pressure, coagulation and insulin resistance.

Regardless of the route of administration, the oestrogen doses required to relieve menopausal symptoms and conserve bone mass are also a potent stimulus for endometrial mitosis and proliferation. Unopposed oestrogens increase the incidence of endometrial hyperplasia and the risk of endometrial carcinoma. Following 1 year of unopposed oestrogen therapy endometrial hyperplasia has been found in up to 57% of biopsies. Endometrial hyperplasia is also possible as a result of unopposed transdermal oestrogen therapy. A high rate of endometrial hyperplasia has been observed with the higher doses of Estraderm TTS.

*Pharmacokinetic properties:* Within 8 hours after application of Estraderm MX 25, 50, and 100 steady-state plasma oestradiol concentrations are reached and remain stable throughout the dose interval (up to 4 days). The average increase in oestradiol concentration over baseline reached with Estraderm MX 50 is 37 pg/ml. The oestradiol/oestrone ratio increases from a postmenopausal value of 0.3 to a value of 1.3, similar to the physiological ratio observed before menopause in women with normally functioning ovaries. Following 12 weeks treatment with Estraderm MX 50 the average increase in oestradiol concentration over baseline was 36 pg/ml, indicating an absence of oestradiol accumulation.

Absorption rates may vary between individual patients. However, the plasma oestradiol levels achieved with different sized systems have been shown to be proportional to the drug-releasing area of the dosage form.

After removal of the last system, plasma oestradiol levels return to baseline values in less than 24 hours.

*Oestradiol:* The plasma elimination half-life of oestradiol is approx. 1 hour. The metabolic plasma clearance ranges from 650 to 900 l/(day x m²). Oestradiol is mainly metabolised in the liver. Its most important metabolites are oestriol and oestrone and their conjugates (glucuronides, sulphates); these are far less active than oestradiol.

The bulk of the conjugates are excreted in urine. Oestrogen metabolites are also subject to enterohepatic circulation.

*Preclinical safety data:* At low physiological doses of oestradiol (similar to those delivered by Estraderm MX), the potential for neoplasia is negligible in experimental animals. Most of the documented effects of exogenously administered oestradiol in animal studies have been consequences of the administration of higher doses and are consistent with an exaggerated pharmacological response (most notably the promotion of tumours in oestrogen-responsive tissues). However, long term unopposed treatment with physiological doses of oestradiol may potentially lead to hyperplastic changes in oestrogen-dependent reproductive organs like the uterus.

Some dermal irritation associated with the patch has been observed in the rabbit.

**Pharmaceutical particulars**

*List of excipients:* Acrylate, methacrylate, isopropyl palmitate, polyethylene terephthalate, ethylenevinylacetate copolymer, silicone–coating (on the inner side of the protective release liner which is removed before patch application).

*Incompatibilities:* None known.

*Shelf life:* 2 years.

*Special precautions for storage:* Store below 25°C.

*Nature and contents of container:* Each system is individually heat sealed in a paper/aluminium/polyacrylonitrile pouch. Two, eight or twenty four Estraderm MX pouches are placed in an appropriately sized carton which comprises the finished product (a 'starter pack' of one month's treatment and a three month maintenance pack).

*Instructions for use/handling:* See administration section. Exposure of Estraderm MX patches to ultraviolet light results in degradation of oestradiol. Patches should not be exposed to sunlight. They should be applied immediately after removal from the pouch to skin sites covered by clothing.

*Marketing authorisation holder:* Ciba-Geigy plc, Hulley Road, Macclesfield, Cheshire SK10 2NX.

**Marketing authorisation numbers**

Estraderm MX 25 0001/0202
Estraderm MX 50 0001/0203
Estraderm MX 100 0001/0204

**Date of approval/revision of SPC** February 1996.

**Legal category** POM

## ESTRAPAK* 50

**Presentation** Estrapak 50 is a calendar pack comprising:

8 self-adhesive, transparent, transdermal therapeutic systems (patches), containing a drug reservoir of 17β-oestradiol with an absorption rate of approximately 50 micrograms of oestradiol per day (active surface area 10cm², oestradiol content 4 mg).

12 red tablets containing 1 mg Norethisterone Acetate BP. The tablets are round, have slightly convex faces, slightly bevelled edges, approximately 6.2 mm diameter, imprinted CG on one side and LK on the other.

Patches also contain: ethanol, hydroxypropylcellulose, polyethylene terephthalate, ethylenevinylacetate copolymer, liquid paraffin, polyisobutylene, silicone-coating (on the inner side of the protective release liner which is removed before patch application).

**Uses**

*Indications:* Hormone replacement therapy for patients with disorders due to natural or surgically induced menopause, e.g. vasomotor symptoms (hot flushes and nocturnal sweating), urogenital conditions such as atrophic vaginitis/ vulvitis, and/or atrophic urethritis and trigonitis.

Prevention of post menopausal osteoporosis in women considered at risk of developing fractures. Epidemiological studies suggest a number of risk factors may contribute to postmenopausal osteoporosis, including:

- early menopause (either natural or surgically induced)
- family history of osteoporosis
- recent prolonged corticosteroid therapy
- a small, thin frame
- excessive cigarette consumption.

If several risk factors are present consideration should be given to hormone replacement therapy. Bone mineral density measurements may help to confirm the presence of low bone mass. For maximum prophylactic benefit treatment should commence as soon as possible after the menopause.

*Mode of action:* Oestrogen substitution effectively prevents the characteristic symptomatic, metabolic and trophic changes associated with loss of ovarian function due to the menopause.

The patch formulation (transdermal therapeutic system, TTS) delivers hormone into the bloodstream via intact skin. Estraderm TTS is designed to deliver 17β-oestradiol at a low rate over several days.

An oral progestogen is included for 12 days in each cycle in order to prevent endometrial hyperstimulation. A withdrawal bleed can be expected to start on day 24-26 of treatment.

*Pharmacokinetics:* Within four hours after application of the first transdermal oestrogen patch, plasma oestradiol levels reach the therapeutic range and these are maintained throughout the dose interval (for up to four days).

After removal of the last patch, plasma oestradiol levels return to baseline values in less than 24 hours and urinary oestrogen conjugates within 2-3 days.

Absorption rates may vary between individual patients.

Norethisterone acetate is rapidly absorbed from the gastrointestinal tract and converted to norethisterone, which has a half-life of 7.5-8 hours.

**Dosage and administration**
*Adults and elderly:* Transdermal oestrogen administration is continued without a break in therapy; oral progestogen is included in the dosage regime for 12 days out of each month of oestrogen replacement.

The transdermal oestrogen patch should be applied twice weekly on a continuous basis, each used patch being removed after 3-4 days and a fresh patch applied to a slightly different site. Recommended application sites are clean, dry and intact areas of skin on the trunk below the waistline. The oestrogen patches should not be applied on or near the breasts. One norethisterone acetate tablet should be taken by mouth daily for days 15-26 of each 28 days of oestrogen replacement therapy.

In women with an intact uterus for whom hormone replacement is required, Estrapak 50 should be administered in preference to unopposed oestrogen therapy.

Estrapak 50 contains oestrogen and a progestogen to induce withdrawal bleeding, thereby avoiding endometrial hyperstimulation. Most patients will bleed towards the end of progestogen therapy.

For most postmenopausal women Estrapak 50 therapy may be started at any convenient time. However, if the patient is still menstruating commencement within 5 days of onset of bleeding is recommended. Some breakthrough bleeding or spotting may be seen until therapy has become established.

*Children:* Estrapak 50 is not indicated in children.
*Use in pregnancy and lactation:* Estrapak 50 is not indicated.

**Contra-indications, warnings, etc**
*Contra-indications:* Cancer of the breast, genital tract or other oestrogen-dependent neoplasia; severe hepatic, renal or cardiac disease; undiagnosed vaginal bleeding; active thrombophlebitis and thromboembolic disorders; Dubin-Johnson syndrome; Rotor syndrome; endometriosis; known hypersensitivity to the components of the patch.

*Precautions and warnings:* Contact sensitisation is known to occur with all topical applications. Although it is extremely rare, patients who develop contact sensitisation to any of the components of the patch should be warned that a severe hypersensitivity reaction may occur with continuing exposure to the causative agent.

Before commencing any oestrogen replacement therapy it is recommended that the patient should have a thorough physical and gynaecological examination. This should be repeated at regular intervals. Breakthrough bleeding is an indication for endometrial assessment, which may include biopsy.

At the present time there is some evidence which suggests a slight increase in the relative risk of breast cancer in postmenopausal women receiving long-term hormone replacement therapy. A careful appraisal of the risk/benefit ratio should be undertaken before treating for longer than 5 years.

Women on this therapy, in particular those with fibrocystic disease of the breast, or with a family history of breast cancer (first degree relatives) should have regular breast examinations, including mammography, and should be instructed in breast self examination.

Close monitoring of patients with conditions reportedly worsened by oestrogens is recommended: uterine fibroids; history of oestrogen-related hearing impairment, jaundice or thromboembolic disorders; cholelithiasis; diabetes.

Oestrogen overdosage may cause water retention, therefore patients with heart failure, hypertension, disorders of renal or hepatic function, epilepsy or migraine should be kept under special surveillance. Regular monitoring of blood pressure should be carried out in hypertensive patients.

Estrapak 50 is not an oral contraceptive.

Drug interactions: Preparations inducing microsomal liver enzymes, eg barbiturates, hydantoins, carbamazepine, meprobamate, phenylbutazone; antibiotics (including rifampicin) and activated charcoal, may impair the activity of oestrogens (irregular bleeding and recurrence of symptoms may occur).

The extent of interference with transdermally administered oestradiol is not known; these problems should be minimised by the transdermal route of administration which avoids any first pass hepatic metabolism.

*Side-effects:*
*Skin:* Frequently: Transient erythema and irritation at site of application with or without pruritus. This usually disappears 3-4 days after patch removal and is similar to the effect observed after occlusion of the skin with household medical adhesive plasters.

Very infrequently: Local swelling, papules/vesicles and scaling have been reported, which also resolved spontaneously and did not result in permanent skin damage.

Isolated cases: Allergic contact dermatitis, reversible post-inflammatory pigmentation; generalised pruritus and exanthema.

*Urogenital tract:* Frequently: Breakthrough bleeding, spotting. Occasionally: Heavy, sometimes prolonged bleeding, dysmenorrhoea, pre-menstrual syndrome-like symptoms; endometrial hyperplasia (incidence similar to that reported for other opposed HRT regimes). Amenorrhoea may occur during treatment.

*Endocrine system:* Frequently: Breast discomfort.

*Gastrointestinal tract:* Occasionally: Nausea, abdominal cramps, bloating. Isolated cases: asymptomatic impaired liver function, cholestatic jaundice.

*Central nervous system:* Occasionally: Headache, migraine. Rarely: Dizziness.

*Cardiovascular system:* Isolated cases: Thromboembolic disorders, exacerbation of varicose veins, increase in blood pressure.

*Miscellaneous:* Rarely: Oedema and/or weight changes. Occasionally: Leg cramps (not related to thromboembolic disease and usually transient lasting 3-6 weeks; if symptoms persist treatment should be reviewed). Isolated cases: Anaphylactoid reactions (history of previous allergy or allergic disorders in some cases).

*Overdosage:* This is not likely due to the mode of administration.

*Signs and symptoms:* Signs of acute oestrogen overdosage may be either one of, or a combination of, breast discomfort, fluid retention and bloating, or nausea.

Signs of progestogen overdosage may be nausea, vomiting, breast enlargement and vaginal bleeding.

*Treatment:* Oestrogen overdosage can if necessary be reversed by removal of the patch. There is no specific antidote for progestogen overdose and treatment should be symptomatic. Gastric lavage may be employed if the overdosage is large and the patient is seen sufficiently early (within 4 hours).

**Pharmaceutical precautions** Store below 25°C.

**Legal category** POM.

**Package quantities** Calendar pack containing 8 transdermal oestrogen patches (each individually sealed in a protective pouch) and 12 norethisterone acetate tablets (in a blister pack). A three-monthly pack containing 24 transdermal oestrogen patches (each individually sealed in a protective pouch) and 36 norethisterone acetate tablets (in a blister pack) is also available.

**Further information** Adverse effects on lipid and non-lipid mediated markers of cardiovascular disease may contribute to the increased incidence of cardiovascular disease seen in women post-menopause.

An improved lipid profile may be one factor contributing to the beneficial effect of oestrogen replacement therapy on the risk of coronary heart disease in postmenopausal women. Studies have indicated beneficial effects of Estraderm TTS with progestogen on serum total cholesterol, low density lipoprotein (LDL), triglyceride and high density lipoprotein (HDL) levels. There have been few long-term studies of the effect of Estraderm TTS alone on these measurements and the results are thus less conclusive although generally favourable. Studies of Estraderm TTS incorporating progestogen treatment have demonstrated effects on arterial tone which may have a beneficial effect on cardiovascular risk, and have not shown deleterious effects on blood pressure, coagulation and insulin resistance.

Epidemiological studies indicate that a useful reduction in fracture frequency of approx. 50% is achieved with 5 to 6 years oestrogen therapy.

**Product licence number** 00101/0492

## FEMARA*

**Qualitative and quantitative composition** Active substance: 4,4'-[(1H-1,2,4-triazol-l-yl)-methylene]bis-benzonitrile (INN/USAN=letrozole). Each coated tablet contains 2.5 mg lectrozole.

**Pharmaceutical form** Coated tablets.

**Clinical particulars**
*Therapeutic indications:* Treatment of advanced breast cancer in post-menopausal women in whom tamoxifen or other anti-oestrogen therapy has failed.

*Posology and method of administration:*
*Adult and elderly patients:* The recommended dose of Femara is 2.5 mg once daily. Treatment with Femara should continue until tumour progression is evident. No dose adjustment is required for elderly patients.

*Children:* Not recommended for use in children.

*Patients with hepatic and/or renal impairment:* No dosage adjustment is required for patients with mild to moderate hepatic impairment (Child-Pugh grade A and B) or renal impairment (creatinine clearance ≥10 mL/min) (see *Pharmacokinetic properties*).

*Contra-indications:* Hypersensitivity to the active substance or to any of the excipients. Pre-menopausal, pregnant or lactating women; patients with severe hepatic impairment (Child-Pugh grade C).

*Special warnings and special precautions for use:* Femara is not recommended for use in children as efficacy and safety in this patient group have not been assessed in clinical studies. There are no efficacy data to support the use of Femara in men with breast cancer.

Femara has not been investigated in patients with creatinine clearance <10 mL/min. As letrozole is weakly bound to plasma proteins (see *Pharmacokinetic properties*), it is anticipated that it could be removed from circulation by dialysis. The potential risk/benefit to such patients should be carefully considered before administration of Femara.

*Interaction with other medicaments and other forms of interaction:* Clinical interaction studies with cimetidine and warfarin indicated that the co-administration of Femara with these drugs does not result in clinically significant drug interactions, even though cimetidine is a known inhibitor of one of the cytochrome P450 isoenzymes capable of metabolising letrozole *in vitro* (see also *Metabolism and elimination*).

Additionally, in a large clinical trial there was no evidence of clinically relevant interaction in patients receiving other commonly prescribed drugs (e.g. benzodiazepines; barbiturates; NSAIDs such as diclofenac sodium, ibuprofen; paracetamol; furosemide; omeprazole).

There is no clinical experience to date on the use of Femara in combination with other anti-cancer agents.

*Pregnancy and lactation:* There is no experience of the use of Femara in human pregnancy or lactation. Femara is contra-indicated during pregnancy, lactation and in pre-menopausal women.

Embryotoxicity and foetotoxicity were seen in pregnant rats following oral administration of Femara, and there was an increase in the incidence of foetal malformation among the animals treated. However, it is not known whether this was an indirect consequence of the pharmcological activity of Femara (inhibition of oestrogen biosynthesis) or a direct drug effect.

*Ability to drive and use machines:* Femara is unlikely to impair the ability of patients to drive or to operate machinery. However, fatigue and dizziness have been observed with the use of Femara. Patients should be advised that their physical and/or mental abilities required for operating machinery or driving a car may be impaired.

*Undesirable effects:* In clinical trials, adverse experiences were generally mild to moderate and rarely severe enough to require discontinuation of treatment. Many can be attributed to either the underlying disease or the normal pharmacological consequences of oestrogen deprivation (e.g. hot flushes, hair thinning).

Most frequently reported (>5%) adverse events (% patients) irrespective of trial drug relationship

| | *Comparative clinical trial* | | *All trials* |
|---|---|---|---|
| | *Femara 2.5 mg* | *Megestrol acetate 160 mg* | *Femara 2.5 mg* |
| musculoskeletal pain | 27.0 | 30.2 | 19.3 |
| arthralgia | 13.2 | 7.9 | 8.4 |
| headache | 12.6 | 9.0 | 8.9 |
| fatigue | 10.9 | 11.1 | 6.6 |
| nausea | 10.9 | 9.0 | 12.4 |
| dyspnoea | 9.2 | 16.4 | 6.8 |
| peripheral oedema | 8.6 | 7.9 | — |
| coughing | 8.0 | 7.4 | 5.8 |
| constipation | 7.5 | 8.5 | 5.6 |
| vomiting | 7.5 | 5.3 | 7.1 |
| chest pain | 6.9 | 7.4 | 5.3 |
| viral infection | 6.9 | 6.3 | 6.1 |
| diarrhoea | 6.3 | 2.6 | 5.6 |
| hot flushes | 5.7 | 3.7 | 5.3 |
| rash | 5.7 | 3.2 | — |
| abdominal pain | 5.7 | 8.5 | 5.6 |
| dyspepsia | 5.2 | 5.8 | — |
| anorexia | 5.2 | 4.8 | — |
| dizziness | 3.4 | 6.9 | — |
| weight increase | 2.3 | 8.5 | — |
| pruritus | 1.7 | 5.3 | — |

*Overdose:* There is no clinical experience of overdosage. In animal studies, Femara exhibits only a slight degree of acute toxicity. In clinical trials, the highest single and multiple dose tested in healthy volunteers was 30 mg and 5 mg, respectively, the latter also being the highest dose tested in post-menopausal breast cancer patients. Each of these doses was well tolerated. There is no clinical evidence for a particular dose of Femara resulting in life-threatening symptoms.

There is no specific antidote to Femara. Since Femara is not highly protein bound, dialysis may be helpful. Emesis may be induced if the patient is alert. In general, supportive care and frequent monitoring of vital signs is appropriate.

**Pharmacological properties**

*Pharmacodynamic properties:*

*Pharmacotherapeutic group:* Non-steroidal aromatase inhibitor (inhibitor of oestrogen biosynthesis); anti-neoplastic agent.

*Pharmacodynamic effects:* The elimination of oestrogen-mediated stimulatory effects is a prerequisite for tumour response in cases where the growth of tumour tissue depends on the presence of oestrogens. In post-menopausal women, oestrogens are mainly derived from the action of the aromatase enzyme, which converts adrenal androgens – primarily androstenedione and testosterone – to oestrone (El) and oestradiol (E2). The suppression of oestrogen biosynthesis in peripheral tissues and the cancer tissue itself can therefore be achieved by specifically inhibiting the aromatase enzyme.

Letrozole is a non-steroidal aromatase inhibitor. It inhibits the aromatase enzyme by competitively binding to the haem of the cytochrome P450 subunit of the enzyme, resulting in a reduction of oestrogen biosynthesis in all tissues.

In healthy post-menopausal women, single doses of 0.1, 0.5, and 2.5 mg letrozole suppress serum oestrone and oestradiol by 75–78% and 78% from baseline respectively. Maximum suppression is achieved in 48–78 h.

In post-menopausal patients with advanced breast cancer, daily doses of 0.1 to 5 mg suppress plasma concentration of oestradiol, oestrone, and oestrone sulphate by 75–95% from baseline in all patients treated. With doses of 0.5 mg and higher, many values of oestrone and oestrone sulphate are below the limit of detection in the assays, indicating that higher oestrogen suppression is achieved with these doses. Oestrogen suppression was maintained throughout treatment in all these patients.

Letrozole is highly specific in inhibiting aromatase activity. Impairment of adrenal steroidogenesis has not been observed.

No clinically relevant changes were found in the plasma concentrations of cortisol, aldosterone, 11-deoxycortisol, 17-hydroxy-progesterone, and ACTH or in plasma renin activity among post-menopausal patients treated with a daily dose of letrozole 0.1 to 5 mg. The ACTH stimulation test performed after 6 and 12 weeks of treatment with daily doses of 0.1, 0.25, 0.5, 1, 2.5, and 5 mg did not indicate any attenuation of aldosterone or cortisol production. Thus, glucocorticoid and mineralocorticoid supplementation is not necessary.

No changes were noted in plasma concentrations of androgens (androstenedione and testosterone) among healthy post-menopausal women after 0.1, 0.5, and 2.5 mg single doses of letrozole or in plasma concentrations of and ostenedione among post-menopausal patients treated with daily doses of 0.1 to 5 mg, indicating that the blockade of oestrogen biosynthesis does not lead to accumulation of androgenic precursors. Plasma levels of LH and FSH are not affected by letrozole in patients, nor is thyroid function as evaluated by TSH, T4 and T3 uptake.

*Pharmacokinetic properties:*

*Absorption:* Letrozole is rapidly and completely absorbed from the gastrointestinal tract (mean absolute bioavailability: 99.9%). Food slightly decreases the rate of absorption (median $t_{max}$: 1 hour fasted versus 2 hours fed; and mean $C_{max}$: 129±20.3 nmol/L fasted versus 98.7±18.6 nmol/L fed) but the extent of absorption (AUC) is not changed. The minor effect on the absorption rate is not considered to be of clinical relevance and therefore letrozole may be taken without regard to mealtimes.

*Distribution:* Plasma protein binding of letrozole is approximately 60%, mainly to albumin (55%). The concentration of letrozole in erythrocytes is about 80% of that in plasma. After administration of 2.5 mg $^{14}C$-labelled letrozole, approximately 82% of the radioactivity in plasma was unchanged compound. Systemic exposure to metabolites is therefore low. Letrozole is rapidly and extensively distributed to tissues. Its apparent volume of distribution at steady state is about 1.87±0.47 L/kg.

*Metabolism and elimination:* Metabolic clearance to a pharmacologically inactive carbinol metabolite is the major elimination pathway of letrozole ($CL_m$=2.1 L/h) but is relatively slow when compared to hepatic blood flow (about 90 L/h). The cytochrome P450 isoenzymes 3A4 and 2A6 were found to be capable of converting letrozole to this metabolite *in vitro*, but their individual contributions to letrozole clearance *in vivo* have not been established. In an interaction study co-administration with cimetidine, which is known to inhibit only the 3A4 isoenzyme, did not result in a decrease in letrozole clearance suggesting that *in vivo* the 2A6 isoenzyme plays an important part in total clearance. In this study a slight decrease in AUC and increase in $C_{max}$ were observed. Formation of minor unidentified metabolites and direct renal and faecal excretion play only a minor role in the overall elimination of letrozole. Within 2 weeks after administration of 2.5 mg $^{14}C$-labelled letrozole to healthy post-menopausal volunteers, 88.2±7.6% of the radioactivity was recovered in urine and 3.8±0.9% in faeces. At least 75% of the radioactivity recovered in urine up to 216 hours (84.7±7.8% of the dose) was attributed to the glucuronide of the carbinol metabolite, about 9% to two unidentified metabolites, and 6% to unchanged letrozole.

The apparent terminal elimination half-life in plasma is about 2 days. After daily administration of 2.5 mg steady-state levels are reached within 2 to 6 weeks. Plasma concentrations at steady state are approximately 7 times higher than concentrations measured after a single dose of 2.5 mg while they are 1.5 to 2 times higher than the steady-state values predicted from the concentrations measured after a single dose, indicating a slight non-linearity in the pharmacokinetics of letrozole upon daily administration of 2.5 mg. Since steady-state levels are maintained over time, it can be concluded that no continuous accumulation of letrozole occurs.

Age had no effect on the pharmacokinetics of letrozole.

*Special populations:* In a study involving volunteers with varying degrees of renal function (24 hours creatinine clearance 9–116 mL/min) no effect on the pharmacokinetics of letrozole or the urinary excretion of the glucoronide of its carbinol metabolite was found after a single dose of 2.5 mg. The $C_{max}$, AUC and half-life of the metabolite have not been determined. In a similar study involving subjects with varying degrees of hepatic function, the mean AUC values of the volunteers with moderate hepatic impairment was 37% higher than in normal subjects, but still within the range seen in subjects without impaired function.

*Preclinical safety data:* Femara showed a low degree of acute toxicity in rodents exposed to up to 2000 mg/kg. In dogs Femara caused signs of moderate toxicity at 100 mg/kg.

In repeated-dose toxicity studies in rats and dogs up to 12 months, the main findings can be attributed to the pharmacological action of the compound. Effects on the liver (increased weight, hepatocellular hypertrophy, fatty changes) were observed, mainly at high dose levels. Increased incidences of hepatic vacuolation (both sexes, high dose) and necrosis (intermediate and high dose females) were also noted in rats treated for 104 weeks in a carcinogenicity study. They may have been associated with the endocrine effects and hepatic enzyme-inducing properties of Femara. However, a direct drug effect cannot be ruled out.

In a 104-weeks mouse carcinogenicity study, dermal and systemic inflammation occurred, particularly at the highest dose of 60 mg/kg, leading to increased mortality at this dose level. Again it is not known whether these findings were an indirect consequence of the pharmacological activity of Femara (i.e. linked to long-term oestrogen deprivation) or a direct drug effect.

Both *in vitro* and *in vivo* investigations on Femara's mutagenic potential revealed no indication of any genotoxicity.

In the carcinogenicity studies no treatment-related tumours were noted in male animals. In female animals, treatment-related changes in genital tract tumours (a reduced incidence of benign and malignant mammary tumours in rats, an increased incidence of benign ovarian stromal tumours in mice) were secondary to the pharmacological effect of the compound.

**Pharmaceutical particulars**

*List of excipients:* Silica aerogel, cellulose, lactose, magnesium stearate, maize starch, sodium carboxymethyl starch, hydroxypropyl methylcellulose, polyethylene glycol, talc, titanium dioxide, iron oxide yellow.

*Incompatibilities:* None known.

*Shelf life:* Two years.

*Special precautions for storage:* Protect from heat, store below 30°C.

*Nature and contents of container:* PVC/PE/PVDC blister packs of 14 or 28 tablets.

*Instructions for use/handling:* No specific instructions for use/handling.

*Marketing authorisation holder:* Ciba-Geigy plc, Hulley Road, Macclesfield, Cheshire SK10 2NX.

**Marketing authorisation number** 00001/0224.

**Date of approval/revision of SPC** November 1996.

**Legal category** POM.

## FORADIL* ▼

**Qualitative and quantitative composition** Active substance: (±)–2′–Hydroxy–5′–[(RS)–1–hydroxy–2–[[(RS)–p–methoxy-a methylphenethyl]–amino] ethyl] formanilide fumarate dihydrate (= eformoterol fumarate).

One capsule contains 12 micrograms eformoterol fumarate.

**Pharmaceutical form** Inhalation powder in capsules.

**Clinical particulars**

*Therapeutic indications:* The treatment of reversible airways obstruction (including nocturnal asthma and prevention of exercise induced bronchospasm) in patients requiring long-term regular bronchodilator therapy. Such patients should normally also be receiving regular and adequate doses of inhaled anti-inflammatory agents (eg corticosteroids and/or sodium cromoglycate) or oral corticosteroids.

*Posology and method of administration:*

*For use in adults (including the elderly):*

*Regular maintenance therapy:* One inhalation capsule (12 micrograms) to be inhaled twice daily. For more severe cases two inhalation capsules twice daily. This dosing regimen provides symptomatic relief throughout day and night.

Foradil should be taken twice daily. The maximum daily dose is 24 micrograms b.d. (4 capsules).

Although Foradil has a rapid onset of action, current asthma management guidelines recommend that long-acting inhaled bronchodilators should be used for maintenance bronchodilator therapy. They further recommend that in the event of an acute attack, a β-agonist with a short duration of action should be used.

In accordance with the current management Guidelines, long-acting β2-agonists may be added to the treatment regimen in patients experiencing problems with high dose inhaled steroids. Alternatively, where regular symptomatic treatment of asthma is required in addition to inhaled steroids, then long-acting β2-agonists can be used. Patients should be advised not to stop or change their steroid therapy when Foradil is introduced.

If the symptoms persist or worsen, or if the recommended dose of Foradil fails to control symptoms (maintain effective relief), this is usually an indication of a worsening of the underlying condition.

*Children under 18 years:* Foradil inhalation capsules are not recommended in children, because of the limited clinical experience with this patient group.

*Renal and hepatic impairment:* There is no theoretical reason to suggest that Foradil dosage requires adjustment in patients with renal or hepatic impairment, however no clinical data have been generated to support its use in these groups.

Contra-indications: Hypersensitivity to eformoterol fumarate or lactose.

Special warnings and special precautions for use:
Anti-inflammatory therapy: In general, asthmatic patients who require regular therapy with a β2-agonist should also receive regular and adequate doses of an inhaled anti-inflammatory agent (e.g. corticosteroids, and/or sodium cromoglycate) or oral corticosteroids. Whenever Foradil is prescribed, patients should be evaluated for the adequacy of the anti-inflammatory therapy they receive. Patients must be advised to continue taking anti-inflammatory therapy unchanged after the introduction of Foradil, even when the symptoms improve. Should symptoms persist, or should the number of doses of Foradil required to control symptoms increase, this usually indicates a worsening of the underlying condition and warrants a reassessment of asthma therapy by a physician.

Concomitant conditions: Special care and supervision, with particular emphasis on dosage limits, is required in patients receiving Foradil when the following conditions may exist:

Ischaemic heart disease, cardiac arrhythmias, especially third degree atrioventricular block, severe cardiac decompensation, idiopathic subvalvular aortic stenosis, hypertrophic obstructive cardiomyopathy, thyrotoxicosis, known or suspected prolongation of the QT interval (QTc > 0.44 sec.; see section 4.5).

Due to the hyperglycaemic effect of β2–stimulants, additional blood glucose controls are recommended in diabetic patients.

Hypokalaemia: Potentially serious hypokalaemia may result from β2-agonist therapy. Particular caution is advised in severe asthma as this effect may be potentiated by hypoxia and concomitant treatment (see section 4.5). It is recommended that serum potassium levels be monitored in such situations.

Paradoxical bronchospasm: As with other inhalation therapy, the potential for paradoxical bronchospasm should be kept in mind. If it occurs, the preparation should be discontinued immediately and alternative therapy substituted.

Interaction with other medicaments and other forms of interaction: There are no clinical data to support the advice given below, but from consideration of first principles one might expect the following interactions:

Drugs such as quinidine, disopyramide, procainamide, phenothiazines, antihistamines, and tricyclic antidepressants may be associated with QT-interval prolongation and an increased risk of ventricular arrhythmia (see section 4.3).

Concomitant administration of other sympathomimetic agents may potentiate the undesirable effects of Foradil.

Administration of Foradil to patients being treated with monoamine oxidase inhibitors or tricyclic antidepressants should be performed with caution, since the action of β2-adrenergic stimulants on the cardiovascular system may be potentiated.

Concomitant treatment with xanthine derivatives, steroids, or diuretics may potentiate a possible hypokalaemic effect of β2-agonists. Hypokalaemia may increase susceptibility to cardiac arrhythmias in patients treated with digitalis (see section 4.4).

β-adrenergic blockers may weaken or antagonise the effect of Foradil. Therefore Foradil should not be given together with β-adrenergic blockers (including eye drops) unless there are compelling reasons for their use.

Pregnancy and lactation: There were no teratogenic effects revealed in animal tests. However, until further experience is gained, Foradil is not recommended for use during pregnancy (particularly at the end of pregnancy or during labour) unless there is no more established alternative. As with any medicine, use during pregnancy should only be considered if the expected benefit to the mother is greater than any risk to the foetus. The substance has been detected in the milk of lactating rats, but it is not known whether eformoterol passes into human breast milk, therefore mothers using Foradil should refrain from breast feeding their infants.

Effects on ability to drive and use machines: Foradil is unlikely to have any effect on the ability to drive and operate machinery.

Undesirable effects: Frequency estimate: Frequent=>10%, occasional=>1%-10%, rare=>0.001%-1%, isolated cases=<0.001%

Musculoskeletal system: Occasional:tremor. Rare:muscle cramps, myalgia.

Cardiovascular system: Occasional:palpitations. Rare:tachycardia.

Central nervous system: Occasional:headache. Rare:agitation, dizziness, anxiety, nervousness, insomnia.

Respiratory tract: Rare:aggravated bronchospasm.
Local irritation: Rare:oropharyngeal irritation.

Others: Isolated cases:pruritus, conjunctival irritation and eyelid oedema, taste disturbance, exanthema, nausea

Overdose:
Symptoms: There is no clinical experience to date on the management of overdose, however, an overdosage of Foradil would be likely to lead to effects that are typical of β2-adrenergic agonists: nausea, vomiting, headache, tremor, somnolence, palpitations, tachycardia, ventricular arrhythmias, metabolic acidosis, hypokalaemia, hyperglycaemia.

Treatment: Supportive and symptomatic treatment is indicated. Serious cases should be hospitalised.

Use of cardioselective beta-blockers may be considered, but only subject to extreme caution since the use of β-adrenergic blocker medication may provoke bronchospasm.

Serum potassium should be monitored.

**Pharmacological properties**

Pharmacodynamic properties:Eformoterol is a potent selective β2-adrenergic stimulant. It exerts a bronchodilator effect in patients with reversible airways obstruction. The effect sets in rapidly (within 1-3 minutes) and is still significant 12 hours after inhalation.

In man, Foradil has been shown to be effective in preventing bronchospasm induced by exercise and methacholine.

Pharmacokinetic properties:
Absorption:As reported for other inhaled drugs, it is likely that about 90% of eformoterol administered from an inhaler will be swallowed and then absorbed from the gastrointestinal tract. This means that the pharmacokinetic characteristics of the oral formulation largely apply also to the inhalation powder.

Oral doses of up to 300 micrograms eformoterol fumarate are readily absorbed from the gastrointestinal tract. Peak plasma concentrations of the unchanged substance are reached 0.5–1 hour after administration. The absorption of an oral 80 micrograms dose is 65% or more.

The pharmacokinetics of eformoterol appear linear in the range of oral doses investigated, i.e. 20–300 micrograms. Repeated oral administration of 40–160 micrograms daily does not lead to significant accumulation of the drug.

Following inhalation of therapeutic doses, eformoterol cannot be detected in the plasma using current analytical methods. However, analysis of urinary excretion rates suggests that inhaled eformoterol is rapidly absorbed. The maximum excretion rate after administration of 12–96 micrograms is reached within 1–2 hours of inhalation.

Cumulative urinary excretion of eformoterol after administration of the inhalation powder (12–24 micrograms) and two different aerosol formulations (12–96 micrograms) showed the amount of eformoterol available in the circulation to increase in proportion to the dose.

Distribution: The plasma protein binding of eformoterol is 61-64% (34% primarily to albumin). There is no saturation of binding sites in the concentration range reached with therapeutic doses.

Biotransformation: Eformoterol is eliminated primarily by metabolism, direct glucuronidation being the major pathway of biotransformation. O-demethylation followed by glucuronidation is another pathway.

Elimination: Elimination of eformoterol from the circulation seems to be polyphasic; the apparent half-life depends on the time interval considered. On the basis of plasma or blood concentrations up to 6, 8 or 12 hours after oral administration, an elimination half-life of about 2-3 hours was determined. From urinary excretion rates between 3 and 16 hours after inhalation, a half-life of about 5 hours was calculated.

The drug and its metabolites are completely eliminated from the body; about two-thirds of an oral dose appear in the urine and one-third in the faeces. After inhalation about 6-9% of the dose on average is excreted unchanged in the urine. Renal clearance of eformoterol is 150 mL/min.

Preclinical safety data:
Mutagenicity: Mutagenicity tests covering a broad range of experimental endpoints have been conducted. No genotoxic effects were found in any of the in vitro or in vivo tests performed.

Carcinogenicity: Two-year studies in rats and mice did not show any carcinogenic potential.

Male mice treated at very high dose levels showed a slightly higher incidence of benign adrenal subcapsular cell tumours, which are considered to reflect alterations in the physiological ageing process.

Two studies in rats, covering different dose ranges, showed an increase in mesovarial leiomyomas. These benign neoplasms are typically associated with long-term treatment of rats at high doses of β2-adrenergic drugs. Increased incidences of ovarian cysts and benign granulosa/theca cell tumours were also seen; β-agonists are known to have effects on the ovary in

rats in which are very likely specific to rodents. A few other tumour types noted in the first study using the higher doses were within the incidences of the historical control population, and were not seen in the lower-dose experiment.

None of the tumour incidences were increased to a statistically significant extent at the lowest dose of the second study, a dose leading to a systemic exposure 10 times higher than that expected from the maximum recommended dose of eformoterol.

On the basis of these findings and the absence of a mutagenic potential, it is concluded that use of eformoterol at therapeutic doses not present a carcinogenic risk.

Reproduction toxicity: Animal tests showed no teratogenic effects; after oral administration, eformoterol was excreted in the milk of lactating rats.

**Pharmaceutical particulars**
List of excipients: Lactose EP/USP NF/JP (150 mesh).

Incompatibilities: None known.

Shelf life: 3 years in PVC/PE/PVDC blisters

Special precautions for storage: In PVC/PE/PVDC blisters: protect from heat and moisture (store below 25°C).

Nature and contents of container: Blister calendar packs of 14 or 56 capsules, with an inhaler device in each pack.

Instructions for use/handling: To ensure proper administration of the drug, the patient should be shown how to use the inhaler by a physician or other health professional.

It is important for the patient to understand that the gelatin capsule may very occasionally break up and small pieces of gelatin might reach the mouth or throat after inhalation. The patient may be reassured that gelatin is harmless and will soften in the mouth and can be swallowed. The tendency for the capsule to break up is minimised by not piercing the capsule more than once.

The capsules should be removed from the blister strip **only** immediately before use.

**Marketing authorisation number** 00101/0494

**Date of approval/revision of SPC** July 1996

**Legal category** POM

# HYDERGINE*

**Presentation** 1·5 mg Tablets: Hydergine 1.5 mg is available as white, flat, bevel-edged tablets, scored on one side, with HYDERGINE 1.5 engraved on the other, and of 240 mg weight, 9 mm diameter and 2.9 mm thickness. Each tablet contains 1.5 mg Co-dergocrine Mesylate BP.

4·5 mg Tablets: Hydergine 4.5 mg is available as white, round, biconvex tablets coded HYDERGINE on one side with 4.5 engraved on the other, and of 240 mg weight and 9 mm diameter. Each tablet contains 4.5 mg Co-dergocrine Mesylate BP.

**Uses** Indications: As an adjunct in the management of elderly patients with mild to moderate dementia.

**Dosage and administration** 1.5 mg three times a day or a once daily dosage of 4.5 mg.

Hydergine should be taken before meals.

The effect of Hydergine is not immediate: alleviation of symptoms is usually gradual and may not be apparent for two to three weeks. Continuing improvement may be expected for at least three months.

**Contra-indications, warnings, etc**
Contra-indications: Known hypersensitivity to the drug.

Precautions: Caution should be exercised in the administration of Hydergine to patients with severe bradycardia.

There are no known drug interactions involving Hydergine.

Overdosage: Symptoms might include nausea, vomiting, nasal stuffiness, flushing of the face, headache, hypotension and collapse. Treatment should be directed to the elimination of the drug from the gastrointestinal tract by gastric lavage, followed by the administration of activated charcoal. General supportive measures should be applied with particular reference to the cardiovascular system.

Side-effects: Side-effects are infrequent following administration of Hydergine and even relatively large doses are well tolerated. Minor side-effects including gastro-intestinal disturbances, flushes, rashes, nasal stuffiness, abdominal cramps, headaches, dizziness and postural hypotension in hypotensive patients have on occasion been reported.

**Pharmaceutical precautions** Protect from light.

**Legal category** POM.

**Package quantities** *1.5 mg Tablets:* Blister pack of 100.
*4.5 mg Tablets:* Calendar pack of 28.

**Further information** Double-blind studies have shown that improvement occurs with all the symptoms listed in the Sandoz Clinical Assessment-Geriatric (SCAG) scale except for hostility; significant improvement can be expected for nine of the symptoms, namely confusion, impairment of recent memory, disorientation, anxiety, depression, emotional lability, irritability, unsociability and the overall impression of the patient.

**Product licence numbers**

| | |
|---|---|
| 1.5 mg Tablets | 0101/0042R |
| 4.5 mg Tablets | 0101/0117 |

## HYGROTON*

**Presentation** Pale yellow compressed tablets, containing 50 mg Chlorthalidone BP, approximately 7 mm diameter, flat with bevelled edges and impressed GEIGY on one side, breakline and ZA on the other.

**Uses**
*Indications:* Hygroton is indicated for the treatment of mild to moderate hypertension. Hygroton is also indicated for the treatment of diabetes insipidus and oedema associated with cardiac failure, renal or hepatic disease.

*Mode of action*: Hygroton is a sulphonamide derivative. It exerts diuretic and antihypertensive effects by inhibiting the reabsorption of sodium, chloride and water, probably at the distal renal tubules. In renal diabetes insipidus, Hygroton paradoxically reduces polyuria.

*Pharmacokinetics*: Chlorthalidone is absorbed slowly with peak drug concentrations attained approximately 12 hours after ingestion. Chlorthalidone is extensively bound to carbonic anhydrase of erythrocytes, and the plasma and blood elimination half-life is approximately 50 hours. In response to repeated daily doses steady-state blood concentrations are achieved after 1-2 weeks. Chlorthalidone is excreted mainly in the urine in unchanged form.

After a single oral dose a marked salt and water diuresis is evident within 2 hours and a maximum effect reached within 12 hours. This natriuretic activity of Hygroton persists for 48-72 hours.

**Dosage and administration** The dosage of Hygroton should be individually titrated to give the lowest effective dose; this is particularly important in the elderly. Hygroton should be taken orally preferably as a single daily dose at breakfast time.

*Adults*: Hypertension: In mild to moderate hypertension, 25 mg daily increasing to 50 mg if necessary. If a further reduction in blood pressure is required, other antihypertensive therapy may be added to the dosage regime.

*Oedema:* Initially 100 mg-200 mg on alternate days or if preferred, 1 x 50 mg tablet daily; in severe cases, 100-200 mg daily may be given. A maintenance dose should be the minimum effective dose which may be as low as 50-100 mg three times a week.

*Diabetes insipidus:* Initially 100 mg twice daily but reducing where possible to a daily maintenance dose of 50 mg.

*Use in children*: A dosage of up to 2 mg/kg daily may be appropriate but is dependent on the diagnosis.

*Use in the elderly*: Chlorthalidone may be excreted more slowly in the elderly and therefore a reduction in the recommended adult dosage may be necessary. Particular caution should be exercised since the elderly are more susceptible to electrolyte imbalances (see Precautions).

**Contra-indications, warnings, etc**
*Contra-indications:* Anuria, severe renal or hepatic insufficiency, hypersensitivity to chlorthalidone and other sulphonamide derivatives, refractory hypokalaemia and hyponatraemia, hypercalcaemia, symptomatic hyperuricaemia, untreated Addison's disease and concomitant lithium therapy.

*Precautions*: As with the use of other thiazide diuretics, glucose intolerance may occur; this is manifest as hyperglycaemia and glycosuria. Hygroton may very seldom aggravate or precipitate diabetes mellitus; this is usually reversible on stopping therapy.

Chlorthalidone can cause hyperuricaemia and thus provoke attacks of gout in predisposed patients. In cases where prolonged elevation of serum uric acid occurs, the concurrent use of a uricosuric agent will reverse the hyperuricaemia without loss of therapeutic effect.

As with other thiazide diuretics, Hygroton may cause disturbances in the serum electrolyte balance during prolonged treatment. Since the excretion of electrolytes is increased, a very strict low-salt diet should be avoided.

Periodic serum electrolyte determinations should be carried out, particularly in digitalised patients. If signs of potassium depletion occur, such as muscular weakness or cardiac arrhythmias, oral potassium supplements (16-40 mEq/day) should be used. Supplementary potassium medication is also indicated in cases where additional potassium loss occurs, such as vomiting, diarrhoea, malnutrition, nephrosis, hepatic cirrhosis, hyperaldosteronism or in patients receiving concomitant treatment with digitalis, glucorticoids or ACTH. Alternatively a potassium-sparing diuretic may be appropriate.

As with all antihypertensive agents, a cautious dosage schedule is indicated in patients with severe coronary or cerebral arteriosclerosis.

Since chlorthalidone is excreted largely unchanged in the urine, the drug may accumulate in patients with impaired renal function. At creatinine clearance levels of less than 30 ml/min (or at serum creatinine levels of greater than 2.5 mg/100 ml which is greater than or equal to 220μmol/litre) chlorthalidone will not exert an adequate diuretic effect. In such cases, loop diuretics are indicated.

The elderly, in particular those suffering from chronic disease and patients with hepatic cirrhosis, are very susceptible to electrolyte and fluid imbalance. There have been isolated reports of hyponatraemia with neurological symptoms (e.g. nausea, debility, progressive disorientation and apathy) following thiazide treatment. Serum electrolyte levels should be monitored particularly in the elderly and those with hepatic cirrhosis.

In patients with hyperlipidaemia, serum lipids should be monitored regularly. Withdrawal of Hygroton should be considered if serum lipids rise further.

*Pregnancy and lactation*: Diuretics are best avoided for the management of oedema or hypertension in pregnancy as their use may be associated with hypovolaemia, increased blood viscosity and reduced placental perfusion. There have been reports of foetal bone marrow depression, thrombocytopenia, and foetal and neonatal jaundice associated with the use of thiazide diuretics.

Chlorthalidone passes into the breast milk and thus mothers taking Hygroton should refrain from breast-feeding their infants.

*Side-effects*: Hygroton is generally well tolerated in the recommended dosage. The following unwanted effects may occur with higher dosages:
*Electrolytes:* Hypokalaemia, hyponatraemia, hypomagnesaemia. In isolated cases, hypochloraemic alkalosis and hypercalcaemia.
*Skin:* Allergic urticaria and other forms of skin rash, photosensitisation.
*Liver:* Rarely intrahepatic cholestasis or jaundice.
*Cardiovascular system:* Postural hypotension and cardiac arrhythmias.
*Central nervous system:* Dizziness and rarely, paraesthesia.
*Gastro-intestinal tract:* Loss of appetite, mild nausea, vomiting, gastrospasm, diarrhoea or constipation, pancreatitis.
*Metabolism:* Hyperuricaemia, hyperglycaemia, glycosuria, worsening of glucose intolerance (see Precautions), elevated blood lipids.
*Blood:* Thrombocytopenia and rarely leucopenia, agranulocytosis and eosinophilia.
*Other effects:* Idiosyncratic effects (e.g. pulmonary oedema), and occasionally impotence and disturbances of vision.

*Interactions*: Diuretics potentiate the action of curare derivatives and antihypertensive drugs (e.g. guanethidine, methyldopa, beta-blockers, vasodilators, calcium antagonists and ACE inhibitors).

The hypokalaemic effect of diuretics may be potentiated by corticosteroids, ACTH, amphotericin and carbenoxolone.

It may prove necessary to adjust the dosage of insulin and oral anti-diabetic agents.

Hypokalaemia or hypomagnesaemia possibly occurring as unwanted effects may cause onset of digitalis-induced cardiac arrhythmias.

Concomitant administration of certain non-steroidal anti-inflammatory drugs (e.g. indomethacin) may reduce the diuretic and antihypertensive activity of Hygroton; there have been isolated reports of a deterioration in renal function in predisposed patients.

*Overdosage*: Symptoms: Dizziness, nausea, somnolence, hypovolaemia, hypotension and electrolyte disturbances associated with cardiac arrhythmias and muscle spasms.

Treatment: There is no specific antidote to Hygroton. Gastric lavage, emesis or activated charcoal should be employed to reduce absorption. Blood pressure and fluid and electrolyte balance should be monitored and appropriate corrective measures taken. Intravenous fluid and electrolyte replacement may be indicated.

**Pharmaceutical precautions** None.

**Legal category** POM

**Package quantities** Tablets 50 mg: Blister pack of 28 tablets

**Further information** Nil

**Product licence number** 00101/0495

## ISMELIN* AMPOULES

**Presentation** Ismelin ampoules each containing 10 mg/ml, colourless solution of Guanethidine Monosulphate PhEur in a clear glass 1 ml ampoule for intramuscular administration.

**Uses**
*Indications*: For control of hypertensive crises, and to obtain more rapid blood pressure control.

*Mode of action*: Ismelin is a peripheral sympathetic blocking drug which lowers blood pressure by depleting and inhibiting reformation of noradrenaline in postganglionic nerve endings. Ismelin active substance, guanethidine, being highly polar does not cross the blood-brain barrier and is unlikely therefore to exert any effect on the central nervous system. In addition, guanethidine has no effect on the parasympathetic nervous system.

*Pharmacokinetics*: Guanethidine may be excreted more slowly in those patients with moderate to severely compromised renal function. Therefore the potential for accumulation of the drug will be higher.

**Dosage and administration**
*Adults*: In the management of hypertensive crises including toxaemia of pregnancy, Ismelin should be given by intramuscular injection. One injection of 10-20 mg will generally cause a fall in blood pressure within 30 minutes which reaches a maximum in one to two hours and is maintained for four to six hours. If a further dose of 10-20 mg is deemed necessary, then three hours should be allowed to elapse between doses.

In hypertensive patients with moderate renal insufficiency, the intervals between dosing should be extended or the dosage reduced to avoid accumulation as the drug is renally excreted. (For patients with renal failure, see Contra-indications).

*Use in children*: Ismelin is not recommended for use in children.

*Use in the elderly*: Clinical evidence would indicate that no special dosage regime is necessary, but concurrent coronary or cerebral insufficiency should be taken into account.

**Contra-indications, warnings, etc**
*Contra-indications*: Ismelin is contra-indicated in cases of phaechromocytoma and in patients previously treated with monoamine oxidase inhibitors (see Drug Interactions); in such cases, Ismelin may lead to the release of large quantities of catecholamines which may cause a hypertensive crisis.

Ismelin is also contra-indicated in patients with known hypersensitivity to guanethidine and related derivatives, in heart failure due to causes other than hypertension, and in those patients with renal failure (creatinine clearance 10-40 ml/min).

*Warnings*: Heat and physical exertion may increase the antihypertensive effect of Ismelin.

Ismelin may cause drowsiness. If affected, the patient should not drive or operate machinery.

*Precautions*: Ismelin should be used with caution in patients with moderate renal insufficiency (creatinine clearance 41-65 ml/min), or with coronary and/or cerebral arteriosclerosis; abrupt lowering of blood pressure should be avoided. Caution should be exercised in asthmatic patients or in patients with a history of gastro-intestinal ulceration.

The concurrent administration of guanethidine and β-blockers may provoke severe bradycardia.

When patients have to undergo surgery, it is recommended that treatment with Ismelin be withdrawn a few days before the operation. To avoid excessive bradycardia during anaesthesia, it is advisable to premedicate with larger than usual doses of atropine.

After prolonged treatment with Ismelin, latent heart failure may develop. This is due to salt and water retention, and mild negative inotropic and chronotropic effects. Concomitant administration of diuretics can readily correct this condition.

If patients develop fever, the dose of Ismelin should be lowered.

*Use in pregnancy and lactation*: No foetal toxicity or fertility studies have been carried out in animals. Therefore the drug should only be used if there is no safer alternative. However, in particular, it should not be used during the first trimester of pregnancy nor within at least two weeks prior to the birth or during labour since it may induce paralytic ileus in the newborn infant.

In mothers receiving Ismelin in therapeutic doses, the active substance passes into the breast milk, but in quantities so small that no undesirable effects on the infant are to be expected.

*Side-effects*: Side-effects are often an indication of excessive dosage. The following effects may occur:
*Central nervous system:* Particularly at the start of treatment: dizziness, tiredness, lethargy, paraesthesia and headache. Occasionally: blurred vision and depression. Rarely: myalgia and muscular tremor.

*Cardiovascular system:* Postural hypotension (which may be associated with cerebral or myocardial ischaemia in severe cases) especially when getting up in the morning or after physical exertion, sick-sinus syndrome, oedema, exacerbation of intermittent claudication and bradycardia. Occasionally: heart failure. Rarely: angina pectoris.

*Gastro-intestinal tract:* Diarrhoea and gaseous distension. Occasionally: vomiting, nausea and dry mouth. Rarely: swelling of parotid glands.

*Respiratory tract:* Nasal congestion. Rarely: asthma.

*Urogenital system:* Raised BUN levels or uraemia in patients with latent or manifest renal failure, and ejaculation disturbances.

*Skin and hair:* Occasionally: dermatitis. Rarely: hair loss.

*Blood:* Isolated reports of anaemia, leucopenia, and/or thrombocytopenia.

*Drug interactions*: Monoamine oxidase inhibitors should be withdrawn at least fourteen days before starting treatment with Ismelin (See Contra-indications).

Concurrent administration of Ismelin with anti-arrhythmic agents and digitalis may lead to sinus bradycardia.

The anti-hypertensive action of Ismelin may be enhanced by other anti-hypertensive agents such as reserpine, methyldopa, vasodilators (especially minoxidil), calcium antagonists, β-blockers, ACE inhibitors and alcohol.

The anti-hypertensive action of Ismelin may be reduced by chlorpromazine, phenothiazine derivatives, tricyclic antidepressants and related anti-psychotic drugs, and oral contraceptives. Consequently if larger doses of Ismelin are prescribed, care must be taken upon the withdrawal of any of the drugs listed as severe hypotension may ensue if the dose of Ismelin is not adjusted in advance.

After prolonged treatment with Ismelin, it may be necessary to adjust the dosage of insulin or oral anti-diabetic drugs.

Patients on Ismelin may become hypersensitive to adrenaline, amphetamines or other sympathomimetic agents. Therefore caution should be exercised when taking or using preparations containing these drugs.

*Overdosage*: Symptoms may include postural hypotension which may cause syncope, sinus bradycardia although tachycardia has been observed, tiredness, dizziness, blurring of vision, muscular weakness, nausea, vomiting, severe diarrhoea and oliguria.

*Treatment*: Postural hypotension may be overcome by keeping the patient recumbent, or by instituting fluid and electrolyte replacement, and if necessary, by cautious administration of pressor agents (see Drug Interactions).

Sinus bradycardia can be treated with atropine, and diarrhoea with an anti-cholinergic agent.

**Pharmaceutical precautions** Protect from light.

**Legal category**POM

**Package quantities** Ampoules of 1 ml containing 10 mg: boxes of 5.

**Further information** Nil.

**Product licence number** 00101/0497

## LACTULOSE SOLUTION BP

**Presentation** Lactulose Solution BP is available as a clear, almost colourless to brownish-yellow syrup. Each 5 ml spoonful contains 3.35 g lactulose and 1.34 g of other sugars (lactose, galactose, tagatose and other keto-sugars).

**Uses** *Principal action:* Lactulose prevents the formation of hard stools and encourages normal bowel movement. Unlike traditional laxative preparations which act either on the innervation or musculature of the intestine or by bulk stimulus, lactulose provides a natural substrate for the saccharolytic bacterial flora in the colon.

Lactulose is a disaccharide which is not hydrolysed in the small intestine. Therefore it cannot be absorbed and is transported to the colon with water to retain the osmotic balance. In the colon, several species of bacteria can hydrolyse lactulose to the monosaccharides galactose and fructose.

By encouraging this normal metabolic activity of the bacteria, the osmotic pressure of the colonic contents is doubled and more water is drawn into the bowel.

Further metabolism of the monosaccharides leads to the production of acetic and lactic acids and the subsequent lowering of colonic pH. This acidification of the colonic contents is considered to be the main reason for the effectiveness of lactulose solution. In chronic portal-systemic encephalopathy it may be associated with the decrease in the relative concentration of free ammonia, the major agent involved in the cerebral disturbance.

*Indications:* Chronic constipation. Chronic portal-systemic encephalopathy.

**Dosage and administration**
*Chronic constipation:* Because lactulose acts naturally to encourage the normal activity of the bowel, it may be two or three days before the full benefit of the treatment is obtained. It is important, therefore, to follow the dosage regimen set out below.

*Adults:*
*Initially:* Three to six 5 ml spoonfuls for the first two to three days of treatment. (Nine spoonfuls may be given in obstinate cases).

*Maintenance:* Two to three 5 ml spoonfuls daily or according to the needs of the patient.

*Children:*
*Initially:* Two to five 5 ml spoonfuls for the first two or three days of treatment.

*Maintenance:* One to three 5 ml spoonfuls daily or according to the needs of the patient.

*Chronic portal-systemic encephalopathy:* Six to ten 5 ml spoonfuls three times daily according to the requirements of the patient, for adequate acidification of the colonic contents.

*Use in the elderly:* No evidence exists that elderly patients require different dosages or show different side-effects from younger patients.

**Contra-indications, warnings, etc**
*Contra-indications:* In common with other preparations used for the treatment of constipation, lactulose solution should not be used in patients with gastrointestinal obstruction. Lactulose solution should not be given to patients with galactosaemia or lactose intolerance.

*Precautions:* Lactulose solution should be used with caution during the first trimester of pregnancy.

There are no known drug interactions involving lactulose.

There is no evidence that lactulose affects driving ability.

*Overdosage:* No cases of intoxication due to deliberate or accidental overdosage with lactulose solution have been reported to the Company.

*Side-effects:* Side-effects rarely occur after the administration of lactulose solution. Mild transient effects such as abdominal distension or cramps and flatulence, which subside after the initial stages of treatment, have occasionally been reported.

High doses may provoke nausea in some patients. This can be minimised by administration with water, fruit juice, or with meals.

**Pharmaceutical precautions** Lactulose solution should be stored below 25°C.

Dilution is not recommended.

**Legal category** P.

**Package quantities** Bottles of 200 ml, 300 ml, 500 ml and 1 litre.

**Further information** Lactulose solution has an *absolute* calorific content of approximately 19 kcals/5 ml. However, as lactulose is almost completely unabsorbed from the gastrointestinal tract, the *available* calories will be much lower. Therefore, at the usual maintenance dose for constipation, lactulose solution is unlikely to adversely affect diabetic control.

**Product licence number** 0101/0076.

## LAMISIL* CREAM

**Qualitative and quantitative composition** Terbinafine hydrochloride 1.0% w/w.

**Pharmaceutical form** White, smooth or almost smooth glossy cream.

**Clinical particulars**
*Therapeutic indications:* Fungal infections of the skin caused by *Trichophyton* (e.g. *T. rubrum, T. mentagrophytes, T. verrucosum, T. violaceum*), *Microsporum canis* and *Epidermophyton floccosum.*

Yeast infections of the skin, principally those caused by the genus *Candida* (e.g. *C. albicans*).

Pityriasis (tinea) versicolor due to *Pityrosporum orbiculare* (also known as *Malassezia furfur*).

*Posology and method of administration:* Lamisil can be applied once or twice daily. Cleanse and dry the affected areas thoroughly before application of Lamisil. Apply the cream to the affected skin and surrounding area in a thin layer and rub in lightly. In the case of intertriginous infections (submammary, interdigital, intergluteal, inguinal) the application may be covered with a gauze strip, especially at night.

The likely durations of treatment are as follows:

| | |
|---|---|
| Tinea corporis, cruris: | 1 to 2 weeks |
| Tinea pedis: | 1 week |
| Cutaneous candidiasis: | 2 weeks |
| Pityriasis versicolor: | 2 weeks |

Relief of clinical symptoms usually occurs within a few days. Irregular use or premature discontinuation of treatment carries the risk of recurrence. If there are no signs of improvement after two weeks, the diagnosis should be verified.

*Children:* The experience with topical Lamisil in children in still limited and its use cannot therefore be recommended.

*Use in the elderly:* There is no evidence to suggest that elderly patients require different dosages or experience side-effects different to those of younger patients.

*Method of administration:* Via the topical route.

*Contra-indications:* Hypersensitivity to terbinafine or any of the excipients contained in the cream.

*Special warnings and precautions for use:* Lamisil Cream is for external use only. Contact with the eyes should be avoided.

*Interaction with other medicaments and other forms of interaction:* There are no known drug interactions with Lamisil Cream.

*Pregnancy and lactation:* Foetal toxicity and fertility studies in animals suggest no adverse effects.

There is no clinical experience with Lamisil Cream in pregnant women, therefore, unless the potential benefits outweigh any potential risks, Lamisil Cream should not be administered during pregnancy.

Terbinafine is excreted in breast milk and therefore mothers should not receive Lamisil whilst breast-feeding.

*Effects on ability to drive and to use machines:* None known.

*Undesirable effects:* Redness, itching or stinging occasionally occur at the site of application; however, treatment rarely has to be discontinued for this reason. This must be distinguished from allergic reactions which are rare but require discontinuation.

*Overdose:* No case of ingestion of Lamisil Cream has been reported to the company. However, if accidental ingestion of Lamisil Cream occurs, an appropriate method of gastric emptying may be used if considered appropriate.

**Pharmacological properties**
*Pharmacodynamic properties:* Terbinafine is an allylamine which has a broad spectrum of antifungal activity. At low concentrations terbinafine is fungicidal against dermatophytes, moulds and certain dimorphic fungi. The activity versus yeasts is fungicidal or fungistatic depending on the species.

Terbinafine interferes specifically with fungal sterol biosynthesis at an early step. This leads to a deficiency in ergosterol and to an intracellular accumulation of squalene, resulting in fungal cell death. Terbinafine acts by inhibition of squalene epoxidase in the fungal cell membrane.

The enzyme squalene epoxidase is not linked to the cytochrome P450 system. Terbinafine does not influence the metabolism of hormones or other drugs.

*Pharmacokinetic properties:* Less than 5% of the dose is absorbed after topical application to humans; systemic exposure is therefore very slight.

**Pharmaceutical particulars**
*List of excipients:* Sodium hydroxide, benzyl alcohol, sorbitan monostearate, cetyl palmitate, cetyl alcohol, stearyl alcohol, polysorbate 60, isopropyl myristate, demineralised water.

*Incompatibilities:* None known.

*Shelf life:* Aluminium tube: 5 years.

*Special precautions for storage:* None.

*Nature and contents of container:* Aluminium tube with membrane, with an interior coating of phenol-epoxy based lacquer, closed with a polypropylene cap, containing 15 g or 30 g Lamisil Cream.

*Instruction for use/handling:* Not applicable.

**Marketing authorisation number** 0101/0305.

**Date of approval/revision of SPC** 3 March 1997.

**Legal category** POM.

## LAMISIL* TABLETS 250 mg

**Qualitative and quantitative composition** Each tablet contains 281.25 mg terbinafine hydrochloride, equivalent to 250 mg terbinafine.

**Pharmaceutical form** Tablets for oral administration.

**Clinical particulars**
*Therapeutic indications:* Fungal infections of the skin and nails caused by *Trichophyton* (e.g. *T. rubrum, T. mentagrophytes, T. verrucosum, T. violaceum*), *Microsporum canis* and *Epidermophyton floccosum.*

1. Oral Lamisil is indicated in the treatment of ringworm (tinea corporis, tinea cruris and tinea pedis) where oral therapy is considered appropriate due to the site, severity or extent of the infection.
2. Oral Lamisil is indicated in the treatment of onychomycosis.

*Posology and method of administration:*
*Adults:* 125 mg b.d. or 250 mg o.d. The duration of treatment varies according to the indication and the severity of the infection.
*Skin infections:*
Likely durations of treatment are as follows:

| | |
|---|---|
| Tinea pedia (interdigital, plantar/ moccasin type): | 2 to 6 weeks |
| Tinea corporis: | 4 weeks |
| Tinea cruris: | 2 to 4 weeks |

*Onychomycosis:* The duration of treatment for most patients is between 6 weeks and 3 months. Treatment periods of less than 3 months can be anticipated in patients with fingernail infection, toenail infection other than of the big toe, or patients of younger age. In the treatment of toenail infections, 3 months is usually sufficient although a few patients may require treatment of 6 months or longer. Poor nail outgrowth during the first weeks of treatment may enable identification of those patients in whom longer therapy is required.

Complete resolution of the signs and symptoms of infection may not occur until several weeks after mycological cure.

*Children:* A review of safety experience with oral Lamisil in children, which includes 314 patients involved in the UK Lamisil Post Marketing Surveillance study, has shown that the adverse event profile in children is similar to that seen in adults. No evidence of any new, unusual or more severe reactions to those seen in the adult population have been noted. However, as data is still limited its use is not recommended.

*Use in the elderly:* There is no evidence to suggest that elderly patients require different dosages or experience side-effects different to those of younger patients. The possibility of impairment of liver or kidney function should be considered in this age group (see *Precautions*).

*Method of administration:* Via the oral route.

*Contra-indications:* Hypersensitivity to Lamisil.

*Special warnings and precautions for use:* Rarely, cases of cholestasis and hepatitis have been reported, these usually occur within two months of starting treatment. If patients develop symptoms of liver dysfunction such as pruritis, anorexia, nausea, vomiting, fatigue, abdominal pain or dark urine, treatment should be immediately discontinued.

Patients with a known history of liver disease or pre-existing stable chronic liver dysfunction are not known to be at greater risk but should be carefully monitored. Patients with pre-existing, stable, chronic liver dysfunction or impaired renal function (creatinine clearance less than 50 ml/minute or serum creatinine of more than 300 μmol/l) should receive half the normal dose (see also *Undesirable effects*).

*Interaction with other medicaments and other forms of interaction:* Based on studies undertaken in-vitro and in healthy volunteers, terbinafine shows negligible potential to inhibit or induce the clearance of drugs that are metabolised via the cytochrome P450 system (e.g. cyclosporin, tolbutamide, oral contraceptives). However, some cases of menstrual disturbance (breakthrough bleeding and irregular cycle) have been reported in patients taking Lamisil concomitantly with oral contraceptives. The plasma clearance of terbinafine may however be accelerated by drugs which induce metabolism (such as rifampicin) and may be inhibited by drugs which inhibit cytochrome P450 (such as cimetidine). Where coadministration of such agents is necessary the dosage of Lamisil may need to be adjusted accordingly.

*Pregnancy and lactation:* Foetal toxicity and fertility studies in animals suggest no adverse effects.

There is no clinical experience with Lamisil in pregnant women, therefore, unless the potential benefits outweigh any potential risks, Lamisil should not be administered during pregnancy.

Terbinafine is excreted in breast milk and therefore mothers should not receive Lamisil treatment whilst breast-feeding.

*Effects on ability to drive and to use machines:* None.

*Undesirable effects:* Side effects are generally mild to moderate, and transient. The most common are gastrointestinal symptoms (dyspepsia, fullness, loss of appetite, nausea, mild abdominal pain, diarrhoea), allergic skin reactions (rash, urticaria) and headache. Paraesthesia, hypoaesthesia, dizziness, malaise and fatigue have also been reported rarely.

Musculo-skeletal disorders including arthralgia and myalgia have been reported. These may occur as part of a hypersensitivity reaction in association with allergic skin reactions.

Rare cases of serious skin reactions (e.g. Stevens-Johnson syndrome, toxic epidermal necrolysis, photosensitivity and angioneurotic oedema) have been reported. If progressive skin rash occurs, Lamisil treatment should be discontinued.

Taste loss and taste disturbance have been reported in approximately 0.6% of patients treated with Lamisil. This usually resolves slowly on drug discontinuation.

Rare cases of serious hepatic dysfunction, including jaundice, cholestasis and hepatitis have been reported. If hepatic dysfunction develops, treatment with Lamisil should be discontinued (see also *Precautions*).

Haematological disorders such as neutropenia, thrombocytopenia and agranulocytosis have been reported very rarely.

*Overdose:* Based on the observed adverse effects in man, the main symptoms of an acute overdosage are likely to be gastrointestinal, e.g. nausea or vomiting.

**Pharmacological properties**
*Pharmacodynamic properties:* Terbinafine is an allylamine which has a broad spectrum of antifungal activity. At low concentrations terbinafine is fungicidal against dermatophytes, moulds and certain dimorphic fungi. The activity versus yeasts is fungicidal or fungistatic depending on the species.

Terbinafine interferes specificlaly with fungal sterol biosynthesis at an early step. This leads to a deficiency in ergosterol and to an intracellular accumulation of squalene, resulting in fungal cell death. Terbinafine acts by inhibition of squalene epoxidase in the fungal cell membrane.

The enzyme squalene epoxidate is not linked to the cytochrome P450 system. Terbinafine does not influence the metabolism of hormones or other drugs.

When given orally, the drug concentrates in skin at levels associated with fungicidal activity.

*Pharmacokinetic properties:* A single oral dose of 250 mg terbinafine results in mean peak plasma concentrations of 0.97 mcg/ml within 2 hours after administration. The absorption half-life is 0.8 hours and the distribution half life is 4.6 hours. Terbinafine binds strongly to plasma proteins. It rapidly diffuses through the dermis and concentrates in the lipophilic stratum corneum.

Terbinafine is also secreted in sebum, thus achieving high concentrations in hair follicles, hair and sebum rich skins. There is also evidence that terbinafine is distributed into the nail plate within the first few weeks of commencing therapy. Biotransformation results in metabolites with no antifungal activity, which are excreted predominantly in the urine. The elimination half-life is 17 hours. There is no evidence of accumulation.

No age-dependent changes in pharmacokinetics have been observed but the elimination rate may be reduced in patients with renal or hepatic impairment, resulting in higher blood levels of terbinafine.

The bioavailability of Lamisil is unaffected by food.

**Pharmaceutical particulars**
*List of excipients:* Magnesium stearate, colloidal anhydrous silica, hydroxy propyl methylcellulose, sodium carboxy methyl starch, microcystalline cellulose.

*Incompatibilities:* None known.

*Shelf life:* 5 years.

*Special precautions for storage:* Protect from light.

*Nature and contents of container:* PVC/PVDC blister pack, containing 14 or 28 tablets.

*Instructions for use/handling:* Not applicable.

**Marketing authorisation number** 0101/0304.

**Date of approval/revision of SPC** 18 April 1997.

**Legal category** POM.

## LAMPRENE*

**Presentation** Red-brown, soft gelatin capsules each containing 100 mg of the active substance, Clofazimine BP. Lamprene is presented as a microcrystalline suspension in an oil-wax base.

Lamprene capsules also contain:
Butylated hydroxytoluene (E 321); sodium salt of ethyl hydroxybenzoate (E215); sodium salt of propyl hydroxybenzoate (E 217); p-methoxy acetophenone; propylene glycol; rapeseed oil; soybean lecithin; hydrogenated soybean oil; partially hydrogenated vegetable oils; beeswax; gelatin; glycerol; citric acid; ethylvanillin; black iron oxide, red iron oxide (E172).

**Uses**
*Indications:* Lamprene, given in combination with dapsone and rifampicin, can be used to treat the multibacillary forms of leprosy. These include lepromatous, borderline lepromatous and mid-borderline leprosy. In addition, this combination of drugs may be used to treat the lepra reaction, erythema nodosum leprosum. Combined chemotherapy should be employed to prevent the emergence of resistant strains of *M. leprae.*

*Mode of action:* Clofazimine exerts in man a bacteriostatic and weakly bactericidal effect on *Mycobacterium leprae* (M. leprae, Hansen's bacillus). Its precise mechanism of action against mycobacteria remains to be elucidated. Clofazimine appears to bind preferentially to mycobacterial DNA and inhibit mycobacterial replication and growth.

No cross-resistance occurs with dapsone and rifampicin, probably because clofazimine has a different mode of action. *M. leprae* resistant to clofazimine have been reported only in isolated cases.

The minimum inhibitory concentration of clofazimine for *M. leprae* in mouse tissue has been estimated at between 0.1 and 1 μg per gram; uneven tissue distribution precludes a more accurate estimate. In patients with lepromatous leprosy, the overall antibacterial effect of Lamprene is comparable to that of dapsone. However, the onset of antimicrobial activity of Lamprene is slow and can only be demonstrated after about 50 days of therapy.

Clofazimine also displays an anti-inflammatory effect, which may contribute to the efficacy of Lamprene in controlling ENL reactions.

*Pharmacokinetics:*
*Absorption and plasma concentrations:* Clofazimine is absorbed relatively slowly. Bioavailability of the micronised suspension in an oil-wax base is up to 70% after a dose of 100 mg, and decreases with higher doses. Peak plasma concentrations of the unchanged active substance are reached 8-12 hours after a single oral dose. Administering the drug with food increases bioavailability in terms of AUC (area under the concentration-time curve) by about 60% and tends to accelerate the absorption rate. After administration of a single oral dose of 200 mg clofazimine at breakfast, mean peak plasma concentrations of 861 (±289) pmol/g were measured in healthy volunteers. When clofazimine is taken on an empty stomach, the peak plasma concentration is approximately 20% lower.

After repeated administration of clofazimine to leprosy patients in daily doses of 50 mg and 100 mg, mean morning trough concentrations of 580 pmol/g and 910 pmol/g, respectively, were measured after 42 consecutive days. Steady-state concentrations were not reached within this time period.

*Distribution:* Clofazimine is strongly lipophilic and accumulates mainly in fatty tissue and in macrophages of the reticuloendothelial system. After long-term treatment, clofazimine has been detected in the following organs and tissues and body fluids: subcutaneous fat, mesenteric lymph nodes, bile and gall bladder, adrenals, spleen, small intestine, liver, muscle tissue, bones, and skin, but never in the brain. Clofazimine does not appear to cross the intact blood-brain barrier. Clofazimine crosses the placenta and passes into the breast milk in sufficient quantities to colour the milk

*Biotransformation:* Information on the metabolism of clofazimine is limited. Three metabolites, two glucuronides, have been identified in urine.

*Elimination:* Clofazimine is eliminated slowly from the plasma. The mean elimination half-life of the unchanged substance following a single dose of 200 mg in healthy volunteers is 10.6 (±4.0) days. After repeated administration of 50 mg and 100 mg daily to leprosy patients, the elimination half-life as estimated from the concentration/time curve was about 25 days.

Unchanged clofazimine is excreted via the bile mainly in the faeces. Within 3 days on average 35% of the dose is recovered. No more than 0.4% of the dose is found in the urine as unchanged clofazimine after 24 hours. The urinary metabolites account for about 0.6% of the daily dose.

**Dosage and administration** Lamprene should be taken at meal-times or together with milk.

Lamprene should be used in combination with rifampicin and dapsone. The following dosage regimen is recommended by the World Health Organisation:

*Adults:* The dosage of Lamprene should be adjusted according to body weight, but for adults weighing approximately 60 kg, the following doses are recommended:

*For the treatment of multibacillary forms of leprosy:*
*Lamprene:* 300 mg once a month under surveillance and 100 mg once every 2 days.

*Rifampicin:* 600 mg once a month under surveillance.

*Dapsone:* 100 mg once a day.

This combined therapy should be given for at least 2 years, and whenever possible, until such time the skin smears become negative.

*For the treatment of erythema nodosum leprosum:*

*Lamprene:* a maximum of 300 mg once a day for not longer than 3 months.

*Rifampicin:* 600 mg once a month under surveillance.

*Dapsone:* 100 mg once a day.

*Elderly:* Clinical evidence would indicate that no special dosage regime is necessary but concurrent renal or hepatic insufficiency should be taken into account.

*Children:* Children should receive lower doses according to their body weight.

### Contra-indications, warnings, etc

*Contra-indications:* Hypersensitivity to clofazimine or to excipients of Lamprene.

*Warnings:* After prolonged administration in high doses, clofazimine may accumulate in tissue, e.g. the wall of the small bowel, and precipitate. Enteropathy may develop if crystals are deposited in the lamina propria of the jejunal mucosa and the mesenteric lymph nodes, sometimes leading to intestinal obstruction. If gastrointestinal symptoms develop during treatment, the dosage should be reduced or the interval between doses prolonged. Symptoms may slowly regress on withdrawal of the drug

In the event of persistent diarrhoea or vomiting, the patient should be confined to hospital.

Dimness of vision, tiredness and headache have been reported under Lamprene therapy. Patients experiencing such adverse reactions should not drive a vehicle or operate machines.

*Precautions:* Lamprene should not be used to treat leprosy patients suffering from repeated attacks of abdominal pain and diarrhoea, or in patients with renal or hepatic damage, unless absolutely necessary.

Patients should be kept under medical supervision when treated with daily doses of Lamprene exceeding 100 mg; this dosage should not be continued for longer than 3 months.

Physicians should be aware that skin discoloration due to Lamprene may result in depression (two cases of depression with suicide have been reported). Patients should be warned that Lamprene may cause discoloration of the conjunctiva, lacrimal fluid, sweat, sputum, urine, faeces, nasal secretions, semen, breast milk and reddish to brownish-black discoloration of the skin. Patients should be told that discoloration of the skin, although reversible, may take several months or years to disappear after the end of therapy with Lamprene.

*Use in pregnancy and lactation:* Experience with Lamprene in pregnancy is limited. Clofazimine crosses the placenta, and skin discoloration in neonates has been observed. Lamprene should be used during pregnancy only if the potential benefit justifies the risk to the fetus. Since leprosy is exacerbated during pregnancy, the WHO recommends that treatment with Lamprene should be continued during pregnancy.

No mutagenic activity was detected in the Ames test and in cytogenic tests in patients treated with Lamprene. No teratogenic effect was observed in rabbits or rats given clofazimine doses 8 and 25 times the usual human dose, respectively. However, with doses 12 to 25 times those given to humans, retardation of fetal skull ossification and fetotoxicity were observed in mice.

Clofazimine passes into the breast milk, and skin discoloration may occur in the infant. Lamprene should be administered to a breast-feeding woman only if clearly indicated.

*Drug interactions:* Lamprene seems to have no important effects on the pharmacokinetics of dapsone, although a transient increase in the urinary excretion of dapsone occurred in a few patients. Preliminary data suggesting that dapsone inhibits the anti-inflammatory activity of Lamprene have not been confirmed. If leprosy-associated inflammatory reactions develop in patients being treated with dapsone and Lamprene, it is still advisable to continue treatment with both drugs.

Clofazimine reduces rifampicin absorption in leprosy patients, increasing the time it takes for peak serum concentration to be reached and prolonging the half-life. Bioavailability was not affected, so this interaction is unlikely to be clinically significant.

In patients receiving high doses of clofazimine (300 mg daily) and isoniazid (300 mg daily), elevated concentrations of clofazimine were detected in plasma and urine, although skin concentrations were found to be lower.

*Side effects:* Frequency estimates: frequent >10%,

occasional 1-10%, rare 0.001%-1%, isolated cases <0.001%).

*Skin and appendages:* Frequent: reddish to brownish-black discoloration of the skin and leprous lesions, particularly in fair-skinned patients at sites exposed to light, and discoloration of the hair (in 75-100% of patients). This discoloration is reversible, although in the case of the skin it may take several months to disappear after the end of treatment. Ichthyosis and dry skin. Occasional: rash, pruritus. Rare: photosensitivity, acneiform eruptions.

*Gastrointestinal tract:* Frequent: nausea, vomiting, abdominal pain, diarrhoea (in 40-50% of patients). Rare: anorexia, eosinophilic enteropathy. Isolated cases: bowel obstruction.

*Eyes:* Frequent to occasional: discoloration of the conjunctiva, cornea and lacrimal fluid. Occasional: dry, irritated eyes. Dimness of vision. Rare: pigmentation of the macula. Subepithelial corneal brownish pigmented lines due to crystal deposits, reversible on discontinuation of Lamprene.

*Central nervous system:* Rare: headache, tiredness. Isolated cases: depression due to skin discoloration.

*Laboratory values:* Rare: elevated levels of blood sugar.

*Others:* Frequent: discoloration of body fluids and secretions e.g. sweat, sputum, urine, faeces. Occasional: weight loss. Isolated cases: splenic infarction, lymphadenopathy.

*Overdosage:* No specific data are available on the treatment of overdosage with Lamprene. In cases of acute overdose the stomach should be emptied by inducing vomiting or performing gastric lavage, and symptomatic treatment should be given as required.

**Pharmaceutical precautions** Protect from moisture, (store below 25°C).

**Legal category** POM

**Package quantities** Capsules: containers of 100.

**Further information** Nil.

**Product licence number** 0001/5041R

*Product licence holder:* Ciba-Geigy plc, Hulley Road, Macclesfield, Cheshire SK10 2NX.

## LENTARON* I.M. DEPOT ▼

**Presentation** Vials of clear glass containing formestane 250 mg as a white or slightly yellowish sterile lyophilised cake, together with ampoules of clear glass containing 2 ml of 0.9% Sodium Chloride PhEur sterile aqueous suspension medium.

Lentaron vials also contain polyethylene glycol, soybean lecithin, and vitamin E.

### Uses

*Indication:* Treatment of advanced breast cancer in women with natural or artificially induced post-menopausal status.

*Mode of action:* Lentaron is a potent and highly specific competitive inhibitor of the aromatase enzyme which is responsible for the conversion of androgens to oestrogens. The anti-tumour effects are mediated via the primary endocrine effect of oestrogen deprivation. Clinical studies indicate that the response rate, as with other endocrine therapies, is higher in patients in whom the receptor status of the tumour tissue is positive than in those patients in whom this parameter is negative.

Injection of 250 mg Lentaron i.m. depot results in a clinically significant reduction of oestrogen biosynthesis. Plasma oestradiol and oestrone are suppressed in parallel.

Lentaron does not affect the plasma levels of androstenedione, testosterone or dihydrotestosterone. Levels of sex-steroid hormone binding globulin (SHBG) were decreased slightly in clinical studies, but this effect was not of statistical significance. However, no clinical androgenic effects have been observed.

No clinically relevant changes in plasma levels of cortisol, 11-desoxycortisol, 17-hydroxy-progesterone or dehydroepiandrosterone sulphate have been observed during treatment. Glucocorticoid supplements are therefore not necessary.

*Pharmacokinetics:* Intramuscular injection of Lentaron gives rise to the formation of a depot characterised by slow release of formestane into the systemic circulation. After single i.m. doses of 250 mg in post-menopausal breast cancer patients, maximum plasma concentrations are reached within 30-48 hours. After a relatively rapid decline between 2-4 days, the active substance is eliminated from plasma with an apparent half-life of about 5-6 days. Levels of formestane are still measurable in the plasma at 14 days, but are undetectable after 2 months.

Steady-state plasma levels are reached after the fourth dose, and accumulation does not occur after repeated dosing.

Formestane has not been shown to influence its

own metabolism and 82-86% of the circulating formestane is bound to plasma protein.

An assessment of the extent of the systemic uptake (or of the absolute bioavailability) is not possible due to the poor solubility of formestane in aqueous media. Assuming that plasma is the sole carrier of systemically available formestane, a preliminary estimate of the systemic uptake, which is based on hepatic clearance, is about 20-25% of the i.m. dose in 14 days.

As shown in oral studies, the major circulating and urinary metabolite of formestane is its pharmacologically inactive glucuronide.

### Dosage and administration

*Dosage:* The recommended dosage is 250 mg i.m. fortnightly. Lentaron should be administered by deep i.m. intragluteal injection high into the upper outer quadrant. The alternate buttock should be chosen for each subsequent injection. Lentaron should be given until further tumour progression is evident.

The contents of the vial should be reconstituted under aseptic conditions into an aqueous microcrystalline suspension by injecting 2 ml of 0.9% Sodium Chloride PhEur sterile aqueous suspension medium provided. Gentle shaking facilitates dispersal of the drug. It is recommended that the suspension is prepared freshly before use and allowed to come to room temperature before injection.

*Hepatic and renal impairment:* No specific studies have been performed in such patients. Conjugation appears to be a major route of elimination for Lentaron and its metabolites, and less than 1% of the dose is excreted unchanged in the urine. Impairment of either hepatic or renal function is therefore not expected to require dose adjustment. Lentaron has been used without problem in patients with mild impairment of renal function (creatinine clearance not less than 20 ml/min).

*Elderly:* There is no evidence to suggest that dosage requirements are different in the elderly.

*Children:* Not applicable.

### Contra-Indications, warnings and precautions.

*Contra-indications:* Lentaron is contra-indicated in women with pre-menopausal endocrine status and during pregnancy and lactation. Lentaron should not be given to patients with known hypersensitivity to the active substance, polyethylene glycol, soybean lecithin or Vitamin E.

*Precautions:* Care should be taken to inject the drug deep intramuscularly; intravascular injection must be avoided. Rapid venous uptake of the drug following intravascular injection has led to symptoms of bitter taste, feeling hot, tachycardia, breathlessness or dizziness immediately after administration. Care should also be taken to avoid injection into or near the sciatic nerve. The risks associated with improper injection include pain and temporary nerve trauma. There is the theoretical risk of severe or permanent damage if the nerve is injured directly. No injection should be given in an area where resistance is felt or where there is inflammation from a previous injection.

As with all i.m. injections, caution should be observed in patients taking anticoagulants owing to the risk of haematoma or bleeding at the injection site.

As occasional lethargy, drowsiness or dizziness have been reported, caution should be observed when driving or using machinery.

No studies have been performed in diabetic patients. Blood glucose should therefore be monitored as a precautionary measure.

*Use in pregnancy and lactation:* There is no experience of the use of Lentaron in human pregnancy or lactation. Lentaron is contra-indicated during pregnancy, lactation and in women of pre-menopausal endocrine status (see 'Contra-indications').

*Drug interactions:* No information is available at present on the use of Lentaron in combination with other anti-cancer agents.

Increased growth of facial hair was observed in a single patient concomitantly treated with phenytoin.

*Side-effects:* In clinical trials, adverse events were generally mild or moderate. All reactions resolved without permanent consequence. Local intolerability was the most frequent adverse reaction. Many of the adverse events which have been observed can be classified as being due to the pharmacological consequences of oestrogen deprivation (e.g. hot flushes). The following adverse events have been observed:

*Local adverse events:*

*Skin and appendages:* Frequent: itching, pain, irritation, burning sensation, indolent or painful lump, granuloma at the injection site. Occasional: sterile abscess, inflammation at the injection site. Rare: haematoma at the injection site.

*General adverse events:*

*Skin and appendages:* Occasional: rash, pruritus, exanthema. Rare: facial hypertrichosis, alopecia.

*Nervous system:* Rare: lethargy, drowsiness, emotional lability, headache, dizziness.

*Vascular system:* Rare: oedema of the lower leg, thrombophlebitis.

*Endocrine system:* Occasional: hot flushes.

*Urogenital system:* Rare: vaginal spotting or bleeding, pelvic cramps, colpitis.

*Digestive system:* Occasional: nausea, vomiting. Rare: constipation, diarrhoea.

*Musculoskeletal system:* Rare: muscle cramps, arthralgia, exacerbation of bone pain.

*Respiratory system:* Rare: sore throat.

*Others:* Rare: faintness due to vasovagal reaction, giddiness immediately following injection, anaphylactoid reaction (rash, nausea, vertigo, chest pain and tachycardia, fatigue).

*Overdosage:* There is no experience of accidental overdosage with Lentaron. In clinical trials, doses up to 1000 mg per week led only to an increased frequency of local adverse reactions.

**Pharmaceutical precautions** Lentaron vials should be stored below 25°C. The reconstituted suspension is stable for 24 hours in the refrigerator; (2–8°); after this period the suspension should be discarded.

Lentaron should not be mixed with any other medication for injection.

**Legal category** POM.

**Package quantities** Packs containing one vial of Lentaron i.m. depot 250 mg and one ampoule of Sodium Chloride PhEur 0.9% w/v sterile aqueous suspension medium.

Packs containing six vials of Lentaron i.m. depot 250 mg and six ampoules of Sodium Chloride PhEur 0.9% w/v sterile aqueous suspension medium.

**Further information** Nil.

**Product licence numbers**
Lentaron i.m. depot 250 m 00101/0528
Sodium Chloride PhEur 0.9% w/v sterile aqueous suspension medium 2 ml 00101/0529

# LESCOL* ▼

**Qualitative and quantitative composition** One capsule containing 21.06 mg/42.12 mg fluvastatin sodium corresponding to 20 mg/40 mg fluvastatin free acid.

**Pharmaceutical form** Capsules for oral administration.

**Clinical particulars**
*Therapeutic indications:* The therapeutic indication for Lescol is in the treatment of primary hypercholesterolaemia (with a cholesterol level in excess of 6.5 mmol/l) in patients who do not adequately respond to dietary control.

Lescol is also indicated to slow the progression of coronary atherosclerosis in patients with primary hypercholesterolaemia and concomitant coronary heart disease who do not adequately respond to dietary control.

*Posology and method of administration:* Prior to initiating Lescol, secondary causes of hypercholesterolaemia should be excluded and the patient placed on a standard cholesterol-lowering diet. Dietary therapy should be continued during treatment.

An initial starting dose of 20–40 mg once daily in the evening should be used. Since the maximal reduction in LDL-C at a given dose can be seen within four weeks, this dose should be adjusted at monthly intervals to achieve the desired effect up to 40 mg twice daily. Most patients will however require a dose of 20 to 40 mg daily. In a study in patients with primary hypercholesterolaemia and concomitant coronary heart disease 40 mg daily slowed the progression of coronary atherosclerosis. The therapeutic effect of Lescol is maintained with prolonged administration.

For patients requiring a daily dose of 40 mg twice daily, a calendar pack of 56 Lescol Capsules 40 mg is available containing morning and evening doses in marked blister strips.

Lescol is efficacious in monotherapy or in combination with bile acid sequestrants. When Lescol is used in combination with cholestyramine or other resins, it should be administered at least four hours after the resin to avoid a significant interaction due to binding of the drug to the resin. Minimal data exist to support the efficacy and safety of Lescol in combination with nicotinic acid or fibrates.

Since Lescol is cleared by the liver, with less than 6% of the administered dose excreted into the urine, dose adjustments for mild or moderate renal impairment (creatinine <160 µmol/l) are not necessary.

*Use in the elderly:* There is no evidence of reduced tolerability or altered dosage requirements in elderly patients.

*Use in children:* As there is no experience with the use of Lescol in individuals less than 18 years of age, its use is contra-indicated in this group.

*Contra-indications:*
Known hypersensitivity to any component of Lescol.
Patients with severe renal impairment (creatinine ≥160 µmol/l).
Patients with active liver disease, hepatic impairment, or unexplained, persistent elevations in serum transaminases.
Individuals under 18 years of age.

*Special warnings and special precautions for use:* HMG-CoA reductase inhibitors, including Lescol, are unlikely to be of benefit in patients with rare homozygous familial hypercholesterolaemia.

Although no hypersensitivity reactions have been reported with Lescol during clinical trials, these have occurred rarely with other HMG-CoA reductase inhibitors.

As with other lipid-lowering drugs, it is recommended that liver function tests be performed before the initiation of treatment and periodically thereafter in all patients. Should an increase in aspartate aminotransferase (AST) or alanine aminotransferase (ALT) exceed 3 times the upper limit of normal and persist, therapy should be discontinued. In very rare cases, possibly drug-related hepatitis was observed that resolved upon discontinuation of treatment.

Caution should be exercised when Lescol is administered to patients with a history of liver disease or heavy alcohol ingestion.

Since fluvastatin is eliminated primarily via the biliary route and is subject to significant pre-systemic metabolism, the potential exists for drug accumulation in patients with hepatic insufficiency.

*Skeletal muscle:* Myopathy including myositis and rhabdomyolysis has been reported in patients receiving other HMG-CoA reductase inhibitors. With Lescol such cases have been reported very rarely. In patients with unexplained diffuse myalgias, muscle tenderness or weakness, and marked elevation of creatinine phosphokinase (CPK) values (greater than 10 times the upper limit of normal), myopathy should be considered. Patients should be advised to report promptly unexplained muscle pain, tenderness, or weakness, particularly if accompanied by malaise or fever. Lescol therapy should be discontinued if markedly elevated CPK levels occur or myopathy is diagnosed or suspected.

The risk of myopathy is known to be increased in patients receiving immunosuppressive drugs (including cyclosporin), gemfibrozil, nicotinic acid or erythromycin together with other HMG-CoA reductase inhibitors. However, myopathy has not been observed in clinical trials involving small numbers of patients who were treated with Lescol for short periods together with nicotinic acid, its derivatives, fibrates or cyclosporin. Minimal data exist to support the efficacy or safety of Lescol in combination with nicotinic acid, its derivatives, fibrates or cyclosporin. Lescol should be used with caution in patients receiving such concomitant medication.

*Interactions with other medicaments and other forms of interaction:*
*Food:* Although AUC and $C_{max}$ were lowered and $t_{max}$ prolonged when Lescol was taken with food, there was no apparent difference in the lipid-lowering effects whether Lescol was taken with food or not.

*Immunosuppressive drugs (including cyclosporin), gemfibrozil, nicotinic acid, erythromycin:* Lescol has been safely administered concomitantly with nicotinic acid, gemfibrozil, bezafibrate and cyclosproin (at doses up to 40 mg Lescol) in clinical trials involving small numbers of patients for short periods (see *Special warnings and special precautions for use*).

*Antipyrine:* Administration of Lescol does not influence the metabolism and excretion of antipyrine. As antipyrine is a model for drugs metabolised by the microsomal hepatic enzyme systems, interactions with other drugs metabolised by these systems are not expected.

*Nicotinic acid/propranolol:* Concomitant administration of Lescol with nicotinic acid or propranolol has no effect on the bioavailability of Lescol.

*Bile-acid Sequestering agents:* Administration of Lescol 4 hours after cholestyramine results in a clinically significant additive effect compared with that achieved with either drug alone. Lescol should be administered at least 4 hours after the resin (e.g. cholestyramine) to avoid a significant interaction due to drug binding to the resin.

*Digoxin:* Concomitant administration of Lescol with digoxin has no effect on digoxin plasma concentrations.

*Cimetidine/ranitidine/omeprazole:* Concomitant administration of Lescol with cimetidine, ranitidine or omeprazole results in an increase in the bioavailability of Lescol, which, however, is of no clinical relevance.

*Rifampicin:* Administration of Lescol to subjects pre-treated with rifampicin resulted in a reduction of the bioavailability of Lescol by about 50%.

*Warfarin/salicylic acid/glibenclamide:* In vitro protein binding studies demonstrated no interaction at therapeutic concentrations.

*In vitro* findings have shown a potential effect of fluvastatin on the activity of $P_{450}$ CYP2C subfamily, indicating the theoretical possibility of an interaction with drugs also metabolised by this sub-family such as warfarin, sulphonylureas, diclofenac and phenytoin if co-administered with fluvastatin, although the clinical significance of this is unknown. However, *in vivo* study with warfarin as representative of the drugs metabolised through this $P_{450}$ enzyme sub-family, has shown that fluvastatin had no effect on prothrombin times or warfarin blood levels.

Bleeding and/or increased prothrombin times have, however, been reported very rarely in patients on Lescol receiving concomitant coumarin derivatives.

*Other concomitant therapy:* In clinical studies in which Lescol was used concomitantly with angiotensin converting enzyme (ACE) inhibitors, beta-blockers, calcium channel blockers, oral sulphonylureas, salicylic acid, $H_2$-blockers and non-steroidal anti-inflammatory drugs (NSAIDS), no clinically significant adverse interactions occurred.

*Pregnancy and lactation:* Animal studies have indicated that fluvastatin is devoid of embryotoxic and teratogenic potential. However, since HMG-CoA reductase inhibitors decrease the synthesis of cholesterol and possibly of other biologically active substances derived from cholesterol, they may cause fetal harm when administered to pregnant women. Therefore, HMG-CoA reductase inhibitors are contra-indicated during pregnancy, and in women of child-bearing potential, not taking adequate contraceptive precautions. If a patient becomes pregnant while taking this class of drug, therapy should be discontinued. As small amounts of fluvastatin have been found in rat milk, Lescol is contra-indicated in nursing mothers.

*Effects on ability to drive and use machines:* No data exist on the effects of Lescol on the ability to drive and use machines.

*Undesirable effects:* Adverse events, both clinical and biochemical, are usually mild and transient. In placebo controlled trials, events occurring with a frequency of 1% or more (over that with placebo) were: dyspepsia, nausea, abdominal pain, headache and insomnia. The only adverse events with an incidence of ≥1% that can be clearly attributed to Lescol treatment are minor gastrointestinal symptoms.

For a discussion of the very rarely occurring myopathies see *Special warnings and special precautions for use – skeletal muscle*.

Biochemical abnormalities of liver function have been associated with HMG-CoA reductase inhibitors and other lipid lowering agents. Confirmed elevations of transaminase levels to more than 3 times the upper limit of normal developed in a small number of patients (less than or equal to 1%). The majority of these abnormal biochemical findings were asymptomatic and resolved or improved towards pre-treatment values after discontinuation of treatment.

*Overdosage:* The experience with overdoses of Lescol is very limited. Should an accidental overdosage occur, administration of activated charcoal is recommended. In the case of a very recent oral intake gastric lavage may be considered. Treatment should be symptomatic.

**Pharmacological properties**
*Pharmacodynamic properties:* Lescol, a hydrophilic, fully synthetic cholesterol-lowering agent, is a competitive inhibitor of HMG-CoA reductase, which is responsible for the conversion of HMG-CoA to mevalonate, a precursor of sterols, including cholesterol. Lescol exerts its main effect in the liver. The inhibition of cholesterol biosynthesis reduces the cholesterol in hepatic cells, which stimulates the synthesis of LDL receptors and thereby increases the uptake of LDL particles. The overall cholesterol profile is improved with the principal effects being the reduction of total – C, and LDL-C. Lescol also produces a moderate reduction in triglycerides and a moderate increase in HDL-C.

A variety of clinical studies has demonstrated that elevated levels of total cholesterol (total-C), LDL-C and apolipoprotein B (a membrane transport complex for LDL-C) promote human atherosclerosis. Similarly, decreased levels of high density lipoprotein cholesterol (HDL-C) and its transport complex, apolipoprotein A, are associated with the development of atherosclerosis. Epidemiologic investigations have established that cardiovascular morbidity and mortality vary directly with the level of total-C and LDL-C and inversely with the level of HDL-C. In multicentre clinical trials, those pharmacologic and/or non-pharmacologic interventions that simultaneously lowered LDL-C and increased HDL-C reduced the rate of cardiovascular events (both fatal and non-fatal myocardial infarctions). The overall cholesterol profile is improved with the principal effects being the reduction of total-C and LDL-C. Lescol also produces a moderate reduction in triglycerides and a moderate increase in HDL-C.

*Pharmacokinetic properties:* Lescol is a racemate of the two erythro enantiomers of which one exerts the pharmacological activity. Lescol is absorbed rapidly and completely (98%) following oral administration to fasted volunteers. In a fed state, the drug is absorbed at a reduced rate. Fluvastatin exerts its main effect in the liver, which is also the main organ for its metabolism. The absolute bioavailability assessed from systemic blood concentrations is 24%. The apparent volume of distribution $(V_zf)$ for the drug is 330 l. More than 98% of the circulating drug is bound to plasma proteins, and this binding is unaffected by drug concentration.

The major circulating blood components are fluvastatin and the pharmacologically inactive N-desisopropyl-propionic acid metabolite. The hydroxylated metabolites have pharmacological activity but do not circulate systemically.

Following administration of $^3$H-fluvastatin to healthy volunteers, excretion of radioactivity is about 6% in the urine and 93% in the faeces, and fluvastatin accounts for less than 2% of the total radioactivity excreted. The plasma clearance (CL/f) for fluvastatin in man is calculated to be 1.8±0.8 l/min. Steady-state plasma concentrations show no evidence of fluvastatin accumulation following administration of 40 mg daily. Following oral administration of 40 mg of Lescol, the terminal disposition half-life for fluvastatin is 2.3±0.9 hours.

*Food:* Although AUC and $C_{max}$ were lowered and $t_{max}$ prolonged when Lescol was taken with food, there was no apparent difference in the lipid-lowering effect whether Lescol was taken with food or not.

Plasma concentrations of fluvastatin do not vary as a function of either age or gender in the general population.

*Preclinical safety data:* The safety of fluvastatin was extensively investigated in toxicity studies in rats, dogs, monkeys, mice and hamsters. A variety of changes were identified that are common to HMG-CoA reductase inhibitors, viz. hyperplasia and hyperkeratosis of the rodent non-glandular stomach, cataracts in dogs, myopathy in rodents, mild liver changes in most laboratory animals with gall bladder changes in dog, monkey and hamster, thyroid weight increases in the rat and testicular degeneration in the hamster. Fluvastatin is devoid of the CNS vascular and degenerative changes recorded in dogs with other members of this class of compound.

A carcinogenicity study was performed in rats at dose levels of 6, 9 and 18 mg/kg a day (escalated to 24 mg/kg a day after 1 year) to establish a clear maximum tolerated dose. These treatment levels yielded plasma drug levels approximately 9, 13 and 26 to 35 times the mean human plasma drug concentration after a 40-mg oral dose. A low incidence of forestomach squamous papillomas and one carcinoma of the forestomach was observed at the 24 mg/kg a day dose level. In addition, an increased incidence of thyroid follicular cell adenomas and carcinomas was recorded in male rats treated with 18 to 24 mg/kg a day.

The forestomach neoplasms observed in rats and mice reflect chronic hyperplasia caused by direct contact exposure to fluvastatin rather than a genotoxic effect of the drug. The increased incidence of thyroid follicular cell neoplasms in male rats given fluvastatin appears to be consistent with species-specific findings with other HMG-CoA reductase inhibitors. In contrast to other HMG-CoA reductase inhibitors, no treatment-related increases in the incidences of hepatic adenomas or carcinomas were observed.

The carcinogenicity study conducted in mice at dose levels of 0.3, 15 and 30 mg/kg a day revealed, as in rats, a statistically significant increase in forestomach squamous cell papillomas in males and females at 30 mg/kg a day and in females at 15 mg/kg a day. These treatment levels yielded plasma drug levels approximately 0.2, 10 and 21 times the mean human plasma drug concentration after a 40-mg oral dose.

No evidence of mutagenicity was observed *in vitro*, with or without rat-liver metabolic activation, in the following studies: microbial mutagen tests using mutant strains of *Salmonella typhimurium* or *Escherichia coli*; malignant transformation assay in BALB/3T3 cells; unscheduled DNA synthesis in rat primary hepatocytes; chromosomal aberrations in V79 Chinese hamster cells; HGPRT V79 Chinese hamster cells. In addition, there was no evidence of mutagenicity *in vivo* in either a rat or mouse micronucleus test.

In a study in rats at dose levels in females of 0.6, 2 and 6 mg/kg a day and in males of 2, 10 and 20 mg/kg a day, fluvastatin had no adverse effects on the fertility or reproductive performance. Teratology studies in rats and rabbits showed maternal toxicity at high dose levels, but there was no evidence of embryotoxic or teratogenic potential. A study in which female rats were dosed at 12 and 24 mg/kg a day during late gestation until weaning of the pups resulted in

maternal mortality at or near term and post partum accompanied by fetal and neonatal lethality. No effects on the pregnant females or fetuses occurred at the low dose level of 2 mg/kg a day.

A second study at levels of 2, 6, 12 and 24 mg/kg a day during late gestation and early lactation showed similar effects at 6 mg/kg a day and above caused by cardiotoxicity. In a third study, pregnant rats were administered 12 or 24 mg/kg a day during late gestation until weaning of pups with or without the presence of concurrent supplementation with mevalonic acid, a derivative of HMG-CoA that is essential for cholesterol biosynthesis. The concurrent administration of mevalonic acid completely prevented the cardiotoxicity and the maternal and neonatal mortality. Therefore, the maternal and neonatal lethality observed with fluvastatin reflects its exaggerated pharmacologic effect during pregnancy.

**Pharmaceutical particulars**

*List of excipients:* Magnesium stearate; sodium hydrogen carbonate; talc; cellulose microcrystalline, fine powder; cellulose microcrystalline, granular powder; maize starch, physically modified; calcium carbonate.

*Incompatibilities:* None.

*Shelf life:* On the basis of the results obtained so far, a shelf life of 3 years in temperate, hot or tropical climate is proposed.

*Special precautions for storage:* Store below 25˚C.

*Nature and contents of container:* Alu/alu blister consisting of an aluminium coating foil and an aluminium covering foil.

HDPE bottle with a tight closure consisting of a polyethylene container (high density polyethylene, grey pigmented) and a closure.

For 20 mg capsules, capsules are No 3 size hard gelatine capsules with a strong reddish brown opaque cap with a Sandoz triangle imprinted in white, and a pale yellow opaque body with XU 20 mg imprinted in red.

For 40 mg capsules, capsules are No 1 size hard gelatine capsules with a strong reddish brown opaque cap with a Sandoz triangle imprinted in white, and a moderate orange yellow body with XU 40 mg imprinted in red.

Both the 20 mg and 40 mg capsules are contained in calendar packs of 28 capsules. The 40 mg capsules are also available in calendar packs of 56 capsules for 40 mg twice daily dosing.

*Instructions for use/handling:* None.

**Marketing authorisation numbers**
20 mg capsules    0101/0360
40 mg capsules    0101/0361

**Date of approval/revision of SPC**  July 1997.

**Legal category**  POM.

## LEUCOMAX* ▼

**Presentation**  Leucomax contains molgramostim, a recombinant human granulocyte macrophage-colony stimulating factor (rHuGM-GSF), non-glycosylated with isoleucine at position 100.

Molgramostim is a water-soluble, non-glycosylated protein produced by recombinant techniques. Its activity is expressed in International Units (IU) with 1 million IU corresponding to approximately 90 mcg of molgramostim protein. Each vial of Leucomax contains the labelled quantity of molgramostim in million IU.

**Uses**  Leucomax is indicated for reduction of risk of infection and to allow better adherence to the chemotherapeutic regimen, by decreasing the severity of cytotoxic chemotherapy-induced neutropenia (see *Precautions, Laboratory tests*).

Leucomax is also indicated for the acceleration of myeloid recovery in patients following autologous or syngeneic bone marrow transplantation. Leucomax has not been shown to improve overall survival or increase time to relapse.

Leucomax is also indicated as adjuvant therapy in ganciclovir (DHPG)-induced neutropenia in patients with AIDS-related cytomegalovirus (CMV) retinitis in order to maintain recommended DHPG dosage.

**Dosage and administration**  Leucomax must be reconstituted before administration (see under *Pharmaceutical Precautions*). Leucomax dosing regimens vary according to the indication for therapy. The maximum daily dose should not exceed $0.11 \times 10^6$ IU/kg/day (10 mcg/kg). The recommended dosage regimens are:

*Cancer chemotherapy:* $0.06–0.11 \times 10^6$ IU/kg/day (5 to 10 mcg/kg/day) administered subcutaneously. Treatment should be initiated 24 hours after the last dose of chemotherapy and continued for 7 to 10 days. Dosing may be initiated at $0.06 \times 10^6$ IU/kg/day (5 mcg/kg/day).

*Bone marrow transplantation (BMT):* $0.11 \times 10^6$ IU/kg/

day (10 mcg/kg/day) administered by intravenous infusion over 4 to 6 hours, beginning the day after BMT. Continue until the absolute neutrophil count (ANC) is $\geq 1 \times 10^9$/l. The maximum duration of treatment is 30 days.

*AIDS-related CMV retinitis as adjuvant therapy to ganciclovir (DHPG):* $0.06 \times 10^6$ IU/kg (5 mcg/kg) once daily by subcutaneous injection. After the fifth Leucomax dose has been administered the dose may be titrated to maintain the ANC and the WBC count at the desired levels, usually $\geq 1 \times 10^9$/l and $< 20 \times 10^9$/l respectively.

*Use in children:* The safety of Leucomax has been demonstrated in a limited number of patients below the age of 18 years.

*Use in the elderly:* There are no apparent differences in safety of Leucomax in elderly patients.

**Contra-indications, warnings, etc**
*Contra-indications:* Leucomax is contra-indicated in patients with a history of hypersensitivity to molgramostim or any component of the injectable formulation.

Leucomax should not be used in patients with myeloid malignancies.

*Precautions:* Leucomax should be used under the supervision of a physician experienced in the treatment of oncologic and haematopoietic disorders or infectious diseases.

The first dose of Leucomax should be administered under medical supervision.

Acute severe, life threatening hypersensitivity reactions, including anaphylaxis, angioedema or bronchoconstriction have occurred in patients receiving Leucomax. If such reactions occur Leucomax should be withdrawn immediately and not re-introduced.

Leucomax has been associated infrequently with pleurisy, or pleural effusion. Pericarditis occurred in 2% (21/1098) and pericardial effusion in <2% (16/1098). If such reactions occur Leucomax should be withdrawn. Patients with pre-existing pulmonary disease may be predisposed to decreased pulmonary function and dyspnoea, and should be monitored closely when being treated with Leucomax.

In clinical trials, adverse events reported with initiation of dosing were mostly mild to moderate in severity and included rigors, dyspnoea, fever, nausea, vomiting, non-specific chest pain, asthenia, hypotension or flushing. These symptoms, which infrequently required withdrawal of Leucomax, were managed symptomatically.

In a few isolated instances, autoimmune disease developed or was exacerbated during rHuGM-CSF therapy. Therefore when administering Leucomax to patients with a history of, or predisposition to autoimmune disease, this should be considered.

Laboratory tests–Standard haematologic tests (full blood count with differential white cell count and platelet count) should be performed and serum albumin levels monitored during therapy with Leucomax.

Because of the potential of receiving higher doses of chemotherapy (ie full doses on the prescribed schedule), the patients may be at greater risk of thrombocytopenia and anaemia as consequences of increased chemotherapy doses. Regular monitoring of the platelet count and haematocrit is recommended.

*Drug interactions:* Since dosing with Leucomax has been associated with a decrease in serum albumin, drugs that are highly bound to serum albumin may require dosage adjustment.

*Use in pregnancy and lactation:* Safety of Leucomax for use in human pregnancy has not been established. Animal studies have shown reproductive toxicity. In primate models, administration of molgramostim was associated with foetal death and spontaneous abortion at doses of 0.07 and $0.11 \times 10^6$ IU/kg/day (6 and 10 mcg/kg/day).

In the absence of clinical data in pregnancy, the therapeutic benefit to the patient must be weighed against potential risks to the progress of pregnancy.

It is not known whether Leucomax is excreted in human milk. However, because of the potential for adverse effects in infants, nursing is not recommended in women receiving Leucomax.

*Side-effects:* Since many of the undesirable events reported during Leucomax clinical trials are often associated with underlying or concurrent disease or their treatment, the causal relationship of many of these events to Leucomax cannot be definitively determined. Most adverse reactions were mild to moderate in severity. Rarely were they severe or life threatening.

The most frequently reported undesirable effects across all indications were fever, nausea, dyspnoea, diarrhoea, rash, rigors, injection site reaction (with s.c administration), vomiting, fatigue, anorexia, musculoskeletal pain and asthenia.

Less frequently reported events include: non-specific chest pain, stomatitis, headache, increased sweating, abdominal pain, pruritus, dizziness, peripheral oedema, paraesthesia and myalgia.

Serious reactions, which occurred rarely in clinical trials, include: anaphylaxis, bronchospasm, cardiac failure, capillary leak syndrome, cerebrovascular disorders, confusion, convulsions, hypotension, cardiac rhythm abnormalities, intracranial hypertension, pericardial effusion, percarditis, pleural effusion, pulmonary oedema and syncope.

Laboratory findings – in all patient groups the most frequently occurring changes in laboratory values were decreased platelet count, decreased haemoglobin level, decreased serum albumin level and an increase in eosinophils (absolute count and percent). The causal relationship of these changes to Leucomax cannot be determined definitively.

The frequency of antibodies that bind to molgramostim, measured by enzyme-linked immunosorbent assay (ELISA) and bioassay, was determined to be 1% post treatment. No loss of activity of Leucomax was evident in these patients.

*Overdosage:* Overdosing has not been reported with Leucomax. As for any pharmacologically active compound, symptomatic treatment with frequent monitoring of vital signs and close observation of the patient is indicated if severe reactions occur.

**Pharmaceutical precautions** Leucomax sterile powder should be stored at 2°C to 8°C and protected from light.

Following reconstitution with sterile water for injection Leucomax solution can be used for 24 hours when refrigerated at 2°C to 8°C. Unused Leucomax solution should be discarded.

*Technical instructions*

*Reconstitution of Leucomax:* Add 1.0 ml of diluent (sterile water for injection) to the vial of Leucomax. Agitate the vial gently to dissolve the powder completely. This provides the labelled amount of Leucomax as an isotonic solution, which may be used for subcutaneous administration. When diluted further in accordance with the instructions below, Leucomax may be administered intravenously.

*Dilution for i.v. administration:* **Dilution instructions must be followed carefully to avoid loss of molgramostim as a result of adsorption to the infusion system.**

Reconstitute each of the required number of vials of lyophilised powder to the appropriate strength of molgramostim with 1 ml of sterile water for injection. The reconstituted molgramostim solution may be further diluted in 25 ml, 50 ml or 100 ml infusion bags or bottles of either normal saline solution or 5% dextrose in water. The number and the strength of lyophilised powder vials required must be such that the above infusion admixture solution contains a final concentration of molgramostim of *not less than* $0.08 \times 10^6$ *IU (7 micrograms) per ml.* The resulting infusion solution is stable for 24 hours when stored in a refrigerator.

Leucomax infusion solution is compatible with the following infusion sets: Travenol 2C0001 and C0334, Intrafix air, Infusionsgerat R, 87 Plus, Souplix, Steriflex, Intrafix Air Euroklappe-ISO, Soluset and Linfosol sets. **Significant adsorption of Leucomax has been observed in a Port-A-Cath (Pharmacia) system, and its use is not recommended.**

For i.v. administration, the use of an in-line, low protein binding 0.2 or 0.22 micrometer filter is recommended. The reconstituted solution is colourless to light yellow and should be inspected visually for discolouration and particulate matter prior to administration.

**Legal category** POM.

**Package quantities** Leucomax sterile lyophilised powder is supplied in Type 1 glass vials with butyl or halobutyl rubber closures and aluminium seal in the following strengths:

$1.67 \times 10^6$ IU/vial (150 microgram/vial)
$3.33 \times 10^6$ IU/vial (300 microgram/vial)
$4.44 \times 10^6$ IU/vial (400 microgram/vial)

**Further information** The excipients contained in Leucomax are mannitol, citric acid, dibasic sodium phosphate, polyethylene glycol and human albumin.

Molgramostim has an elimination half-life of one to two hours following intravenous administration and two to three hours following subcutaneous administration.

**Product licence numbers**
$1.67 \times 10^6$ IU/vial (150 micrograms/vial) 0201/0150
$3.33 \times 10^6$ IU/vial (300 micrograms/vial) 0201/0181
$4.44 \times 10^6$ IU/vial (400 micrograms/vial) 0201/0151

*Product licence holder:* Schering-Plough Ltd, Schering-Plough House, Welwyn Garden City, Hertfordshire AL7 1TW.

## LIORESAL*

**Presentation** Lioresal tablets each containing 10 mg Baclofen PhEur; circular, flat, white to faintly yellowish tablets, uncoated, with bevelled edges, having the monogram CG on one side and the letters KJ and a break line on the other.

Lioresal liquid containing 5 mg/5 ml baclofen Ph.Eur; clear, very slightly yellow solution with a raspberry flavour.

**Uses**
*Indications:* Lioresal is indicated for the relief of spasticity of voluntary muscle resulting from such disorders as: multiple sclerosis, other spinal lesions, e.g. tumours of the spinal cord, syringomyelia, motor neurone disease, transverse myelitis, traumatic partial section of the cord.

Lioresal is also indicated in adults and children for the relief of spasticity of voluntary muscle arising from eg. cerebrovascular accidents, cerebral palsy, meningitis, traumatic head injury.

Patient selection is important when initiating Lioresal therapy; it is likely to be of most benefit in patients whose spasticity constitutes a handicap to activities and/or physiotherapy. Treatment should not be commenced until the spastic state has become stabilised.

*Mode of action:* Lioresal is an antispastic agent acting at the spinal level. A gamma-aminobutyric acid (GABA) derivative, Lioresal is chemically unrelated to other antispastic agents.

Lioresal depresses monosynaptic and polysynaptic reflex transmission, probably by stimulating the $GABA_B$-receptors, this stimulation in turn inhibiting the release of the excitatory amino acids glutamate and aspartate. Neuromuscular transmission is unaffected by Lioresal.

The major benefits of Lioresal stem from its ability to reduce painful flexor spasms and spontaneous clonus thereby facilitating the mobility of the patient, increasing his independence and helping rehabilitation.

Lioresal also exerts an antinociceptive effect. General well being is often improved and sedation is less often a problem than with centrally acting drugs.

*Pharmacokinetics:* Lioresal (baclofen) is rapidly and completely absorbed from the gastro-intestinal tract. Following oral administration of single doses (10-30 mg) peak plasma concentrations are recorded after 0.5 to 1.5 hours and areas under the serum concentration curves are proportional to the dose.

In cerebrospinal fluid active substance concentrations are approximately 8.5 times lower than in the plasma.

The plasma elimination half-life of baclofen averages 3 to 4 hours. The serum protein binding rate is approximately 30%.

Baclofen is eliminated largely in unchanged form. Within 72 hours, about 75% of the dose is excreted via the kidneys with about 5% of this amount as metabolites.

**Dosage and administration** Lioresal is given orally in either tablet or liquid form. These two formulations are bioequivalent. The liquid may be particularly suitable for children or those adults who are unable to take tablets. Dosage titration can be more precisely managed with the liquid.

Before starting treatment with Lioresal it is prudent to realistically assess the overall extent of clinical improvement that the patient may be expected to achieve. Careful titration of dosage is essential (particularly in the elderly) until the patient is stabilised. If too high a dose is initiated or if the dosage is increased too rapidly side effects may occur. This is particularly relevant if the patient is ambulant in order to minimise muscle weakness in the unaffected limbs or where spasticity is necessary for support.

*Adults:* The following gradually increasing dosage regimen is suggested, but should be adjusted to suit individual patient requirements.

5 mg three times a day for three days
10 mg three times a day for three days
15 mg three times a day for three days
20 mg three times a day for three days

Satisfactory control of symptoms is usually obtained with doses of up to 60 mg daily, but a careful adjustment is often necessary to meet the requirements of each individual patient. The dose may be increased slowly if required, but a maximum daily dose of more than 100 mg is not advised unless the patient is in hospital under careful medical supervision. Small frequent dosage may prove better in some cases than larger spaced doses. Also some patients benefit from the use of Lioresal only at night to counteract painful flexor spasm. Similarly a single dose given approximately 1 hour prior to performance of specific tasks such as washing, dressing, shaving, physiotherapy, will often improve mobility.

Once the maximum recommended dose has been reached, if the therapeutic effect is not apparent within 6 weeks a decision whether to continue with Lioresal should be taken.

*Elderly:* Elderly patients may be more susceptible to side effects, particularly in the early stages of introducing Lioresal. Small doses should therefore be used at the start of treatment, the dose being titrated gradually against the response, under careful supervision. There is no evidence that the eventual average maximum dose differs from that in younger patients.

*Children:* A dosage range of 0.75-2 mg/kg body weight should be used. In children over 10 years of age however, a maximum daily dosage of 2.5 mg/kg body weight may be given. Treatment is usually started with 2.5 mg given 4 times daily. The dosage should be cautiously raised at about 3 day intervals, until it becomes sufficient for the child's individual requirements. The recommended daily dosages for maintenance therapy are as follows:

Children aged, 12 months–2 years : 10-20 mg;
2 years–6 years : 20-30 mg;
6 years–10 years : 30-60 mg

*Patients with impaired renal function:* In patients with impaired renal function or undergoing chronic haemodialysis, a particularly low dosage of Lioresal should be selected ie. approx. 5 mg daily.

*Patients with spastic states of cerebral origin:* Unwanted effects are more likely to occur in these patients. It is therefore recommended that a very cautious dosage schedule be adopted and that patients be kept under appropriate surveillance.

**Contra-indications, warnings, etc**
*Contra-indications:* Hypersensitivity to baclofen, peptic ulceration.

*Precautions:* Psychotic disorders, schizophrenia or confusional states may be exacerbated by treatment with Lioresal. Patients suffering from these conditions should therefore be treated cautiously and kept under close surveillance.

Lioresal may also exacerbate epileptic manifestations but can be employed provided appropriate supervision and adequate anticonvulsive therapy are maintained. Lioresal should be used with extreme care in patients already receiving antihypertensive therapy, (see Interactions).

Lioresal should be used with caution in patients suffering from cerebrovascular accidents or from respiratory, hepatic or renal impairment.

Since under treatment with Lioresal neurogenic disturbances affecting emptying of the bladder may show an improvement, whereas in patients with preexisting sphincter hypertonia acute retention of urine may occur, the drug should be used with caution in such patients.

Anxiety and confusional states, hallucinations, psychotic, manic or paranoid states, convulsions (status epilepticus), tachycardia and as rebound phenomenon temporary aggravation of spasticity have been reported with abrupt withdrawal of Lioresal, especially after long term medication. Treatment should, always (unless serious adverse effects occur) therefore, be gradually discontinued by successively reducing the dosage over a period of about 1-2 weeks.

The patients reactions may be adversely affected by Lioresal induced sedation or decreased alertness, patients should therefore exercise due caution. Operating equipment or machinery may be hazardous.

Since in rare instances elevated SGOT, alkaline phosphatase and glucose levels in serum have been recorded, appropriate laboratory tests should be performed in patients with liver diseases or diabetes mellitus in order to ensure that no drug induced changes in these underlying diseases have occurred.

*Use in pregnancy and lactation:* Baclofen increases the incidence of omphaloceles (ventral hernias) in the foetuses of rats at high doses. No teratogenic effects have been noted in mice or rabbits.

A dose related increase in the incidence of ovarian cysts, and a less marked increase in enlarged and/or haemorrhagic adrenals have been observed in female rats treated for 2 years. The clinical relevance of these findings is not known.

During pregnancy, especially in the first 3 months, Lioresal should only be employed if its use is of vital necessity. The benefits of the treatment for the mother must be carefully weighed against the possible risks for the child. Baclofen crosses the placental barrier.

In mothers taking Lioresal in therapeutic doses, the active substance passes into the breast milk, but in quantities so small that no undesirable effects on the infant are to be expected.

*Interactions:* Where Lioresal is taken concomitantly with other drugs acting on the CNS or with alcohol, increased sedation may occur.

Lioresal may produce severe aggravation of hyperkinetic symptoms in patients receiving Lithium.

Pretreatment with Lioresal may prolong the duration of Fentanyl induced analgesia.

During concurrent treatment with tricyclic antidepressants, the effect of Lioresal may be potentiated, resulting in pronounced muscular hypotonia.

Since concomitant treatment with Lioresal and antihypertensives is likely to increase the fall in blood pressure, the dosage of antihypertensive medication should be adjusted accordingly.

Drugs which may produce renal insufficiency eg. ibuprofen, may reduce baclofen excretion leading to toxic effects.

In patients with Parkinson's disease receiving treatment with Lioresal and levodopa plus carbidopa, there have been reports of mental confusion, hallucinations and agitation.

*Side-effects:* Unwanted effects occur mainly at the start of treatment, if the dosage is raised too rapidly, if large doses are employed, or in elderly patients. They are often transitory and can be attenuated or eliminated by reducing the dosage; they are seldom severe enough to necessitate withdrawal of the medication.

*Central nervous system:* Particularly at the start of treatment, unwanted effects such as daytime sedation, drowsiness, and nausea may frequently occur. Also occasionally encountered are dryness of the mouth, respiratory depression, light-headedness, lassitude, exhaustion, mental confusion, dizziness, retching, vomiting, headache, and insomnia.

Should nausea persist following a reduction in dosage, it is recommended that Lioresal be ingested with food or a milk beverage.

Neurological and/or psychiatric manifestations which have occasionally or rarely been reported include: euphoria, depressive states, paraesthesiae, myalgia, muscular weakness, ataxia, tremor, nystagmus, accommodation disorders, hallucinations and nightmares. It is often difficult to distinguish between these manifestations and those of the disease under treatment. Lowering of the convulsion threshold and attacks of convulsions may possibly occur, particularly in epileptic patients.

*Gastro-intestinal tract:* Occasionally, mild gastrointestinal disturbances (constipation, diarrhoea).

*Cardiovascular system:* Occasionally, hypotension, respiratory or cardiovascular depression.

*Urogenital system:* Occasionally or rarely, dysuria, frequency of micturition, enuresis. It is often difficult to distinguish between these manifestations and those of the diseases under treatment.

*Miscellaneous unwanted effects:* In rare or isolated cases visual disturbances, alterations in the taste sensation, hyperhidrosis, skin rash, deterioration in liver function tests.

Certain patients have shown increased spasticity as a paradoxical reaction to the medication.

An undesirable degree of muscular hypotonia–making it more difficult for patients to walk or fend for themselves–may occur and can usually be relieved by re-adjusting the dosage (ie. by reducing the doses given during the day and possibly increasing the evening dose).

*Overdosage*
*Symptoms:* Prominent features are signs of central nervous depression: drowsiness, impairment of consciousness, respiratory depression, coma. Also liable to occur are: confusion, hallucinations, agitation, accommodation disorders, absent pupillary reflex; generalised muscular hypotonia, myoclonia, hyporeflexia or areflexia; convulsions; peripheral vasodilatation, hypotension, bradycardia; hypothermia; nausea, vomiting, diarrhoea, hypersalivation; elevated LDH, SGOT and AP values.

A deterioration in the condition may occur if various substances or drugs acting on the central nervous system (eg. alcohol, diazepam, tricyclic antidepressants) have been taken at the same time.

*Treatment:* No specific antidote is known.

Elimination of the drug from the gastro-intestinal tract (induction of vomiting, gastric lavage; comatose patients should be intubated prior to gastric lavage), administration of activated charcoal; if necessary, saline aperient; in respiratory depression, administration of artificial respiration, also measures in support of cardiovascular functions. Since the drug is excreted chiefly via the kidneys, generous quantities of fluid should be given, possibly together with a diuretic. In the event of convulsions diazepam should be administered cautiously i.v.

**Pharmaceutical precautions** Lioresal tablets should be protected from heat (store below 25°C) and moisture.

Lioresal liquid should be protected from light and heat (store below 25°C) and should not be refrigerated.

Dilution: Lioresal liquid may be diluted with Purified Water BP and stored at room temperature for up to 14 days.

**Legal category**   POM

**Package quantities**
Tablets 10 mg: Blister packs of 84 and 100
Tablets 10 mg: Securitainers of 84 and 200

Liquid 5 mg/5 ml: Bottles of 300 ml with child proof closures.

**Further information** Lioresal liquid contains no sucrose and is therefore suitable for diabetics and children.

**Product licence numbers**
Tablets 10 mg 00101/0504
Liquid 5 mg/5 ml 00101/0503

# LIORESAL* INTRATHECAL

**Presentation** Ampoules for intrathecal administration containing baclofen in a sterile 0.9% sodium chloride solution:
-1 ml ampoules containing 50 micrograms baclofen (50 micrograms/ml)
-20 ml ampoules containing 10 mg baclofen (500 micrograms/ml)
-5 ml ampoules containing 10 mg baclofen (2000 micrograms/ml)

**Uses**
*Indications:* Lioresal Intrathecal is indicated in patients with severe chronic spasticity associated with spinal injury and multiple sclerosis who are unresponsive to oral baclofen or other orally administered antispastic agents and/or those patients who experience unacceptable side-effects at effective oral doses.

Lioresal Intrathecal may be considered as an alternative to ablative neurosurgical procedures.

*Mode of action:* Baclofen does not readily cross the blood-brain barrier, but administration directly into the spinal subarachnoid space permits immediate access to the drug receptor sites in the dorsal horn of the spinal cord. Intrathecal use therefore permits effective treatment of spasticity with doses less than one-hundredth of those required orally.

The onset of action is generally half an hour to 1 hour after administration of a single intrathecal bolus injection. Peak spasmolytic effects are seen approximately 4 hours after dosing, these effects lasting 4 to 8 hours. Variations may occur depending on the dose, disease severity and the speed of administration. A slower onset of spasmolytic action is observed when the drug is administered by an infusion pump delivering a constant low dose over a prolonged period. Under these conditions antispastic activity may not be seen until 6-8 hours after commencement of the infusion, with maximal efficacy within 24-48 hours.

*Pharmacokinetics:* After single intrathecal bolus injections or short-term infusions the volume of distribution (calculated from CSF levels) ranges from 22 to 157 ml.

At steady state, lumbar CSF concentrations of 130 to 1240ng/ml have been achieved with doses of 50 to 1200 micrograms. Based on CSF half-life calculations, steady state concentrations will be reached within 1 to 2 days of the start of a continuous intrathecal infusion. Under steady state conditions a baclofen concentration gradient is established between lumbar and cisternal CSF of between 2:1 and 9:1 (mean 4:1). This means that spasticity in the lower extremities can be effectively treated with little effect on the upper limbs, and with fewer adverse central effects due to actions on the higher brain centres.

During intrathecal infusion plasma concentrations do not exceed 5ng/ml, confirming poor blood-brain barrier penetration.

The CSF elimination half-life of baclofen following single intrathecal bolus injections or short-term infusions of 50 to 136 micrograms ranges from 1 to 5 hours. The half-life under steady state conditions has not been determined.

The mean CSF clearance following both single bolus injections or chronic lumbar subarachnoid infusions has been found to be about 30 ml/h.

**Dosage and administration** Lioresal Intrathecal 50 micrograms/1 ml is intended for administration in single bolus test injections via a lumbar puncture or intrathecal catheter. Lioresal Intrathecal 10 mg/20 ml and 10 mg/5 ml have been developed specifically for use with implantable pumps.

Individual titration of dosage is essential due to a high interindividual variability in response. Each patient must undergo an initial screening phase to determine the response to test bolus doses followed by a dose-titration phase to determine the optimum dose schedule for maintenance therapy with an appropriate implanted delivery system.

Respiratory function should be monitored and appropriate resuscitation facilities should be available during the introduction of treatment with Lioresal Intrathecal. Intrathecal administration using an implanted delivery system should only be undertaken by physicians with appropriate knowledge and experience. Specific instructions for using the implantable pump should be obtained from the pump manufacturers. Only pumps constructed of material known to

be compatible with the product and incorporating an in-line bacterial retentive filter should be used.

*Adults:*
*Screening phase:* Prior to initiation of a chronic infusion, the patient's response to intrathecal bolus doses administered via a catheter or lumbar puncture must be assessed. Low concentration ampoules containing 50 micrograms baclofen in 1 ml are available for the purpose. Patients should be infection-free prior to screening, as the presence of a systemic infection may prevent an accurate assessment of the response.

The usual initial test dose is 25 or 50 micrograms, increasing step-wise by 25 microgram increments at intervals of not less than 24 hours until a response of approximately 4 to 8 hours duration is observed. Each dose should be given **slowly** (over at least one minute). In order to be considered a responder the patient must demonstrate a significant decrease in muscle tone and/or frequency and/or severity of muscle spasms.

The variability in sensitivity to intrathecal baclofen between patients is emphasised. Signs of severe overdose (coma) have been observed in an adult after a single test dose of 25 micrograms. It is recommended that the initial test dose is administered with resuscitative equipment on hand.

Patients who do not respond to a 100 micrograms test dose should not be given further dose increments or considered for continuous intrathecal infusion.

Monitoring of respiratory and cardiac function is essential during this phase, especially in patients with cardiopulmonary disease and respiratory muscle weakness or those being treated with benzodiazepine-type preparations or opiates, who are at higher risk of respiratory depression.

*Dose-titration phase:* Once the patient's responsiveness to Lioresal Intrathecal has been established, an intrathecal infusion may be introduced. Lioresal Intrathecal is most often administered using an infusion pump which is implanted in the chest wall or abdominal wall tissues. **Implantation of pumps should only be performed in experienced centres to minimise risks during the perioperative phase.**

Infection may increase the risk of surgical complications and complicate attempts to adjust the dose.

The initial total daily infused dose is determined by doubling the bolus dose which gave a significant response in the initial screening phase and administering it over a 24 hour period. However, if a prolonged effect (ie. lasting more than 12 hours) is observed during screening the starting dose should be the unchanged screening dose delivered over 24 hours. No dose increases should be attempted during the first 24 hours.

After the initial 24 hour period dosage should be adjusted slowly to achieve the desired effect. If a programmable pump is used the dose should be increased only once every 24 hours; for non-programmable multi-dose reservoir pumps intervals of 48 hours between dose adjustments are recommended. In either case increments should be limited to 10-20% of the previous daily dose to avoid possible overdosage. If the dose has been significantly increased without apparent clinical effect, pump function and catheter patency should be investigated.

There is limited clinical experience using doses greater than 1000 micrograms/day.

It is important that patients are monitored closely in an appropriately equipped and staffed environment during screening and immediately following pump implantation. Resuscitative equipment should be available for immediate use in case of life-threatening adverse reactions.

*Maintenance therapy:* The clinical goal is to maintain as normal a muscle tone as possible, and to minimise the frequency and severity of spasms without inducing intolerable side-effects. The lowest dose producing an adequate response should be used. The retention of some spasticity is desirable to avoid a sensation of 'paralysis' on the part of the patient. In addition, a degree of muscle tone and occasional spasms may help support circulatory function and possibly prevent the formation of deep vein thrombosis.

Maintenance dosing for long-term continuous infusions of intrathecal baclofen ranges from 10 to 1200 micrograms/day, with most patients being adequately maintained on 300 to 800 micrograms/day. Lioresal Intrathecal ampoules of 20 ml containing 500 micrograms/ml and 5 ml containing 2 mg (2000 micrograms)/ml are intended for use with infusion pumps. The concentration to be used depends on the dose requirements and size of pump reservoir. Use of the more concentrated solution obviates the need for frequent re-filling in patients with high dosage requirements.

Provided the pump allows it, the administration may be adjusted to optimise control of spasticity. For example, patients who have increased spasm whilst asleep may require an increased hourly infusion rate at night.

Most patients require gradual dose increases to maintain optimum response during chronic therapy due to decreased responsiveness or disease progression. The daily dose may be increased gradually by 10-30% to maintain adequate symptom control; the daily dose may also be reduced by 10-20% if patients suffer side-effects. A sudden requirement for substantial dose escalation is indicative of a catheter complication (i.e. a kink or dislodgement) or pump malfunction.

In order to prevent excessive weakness the dosage of Lioresal Intrathecal should be adjusted with caution whenever spasticity is required to maintain function.

During long-term treatment approximately 10% of patients become refractory to increasing doses. There is insufficient clinical experience on which to base firm recommendations for tolerance management. However, sensitivity to baclofen may be restored by switching for 10 to 14 days to intrathecal preservative-free morphine sulphate treatment. Lioresal Intrathecal should be resumed at the initial continuous infusion dose followed by re-titration to avoid overdose; this should be performed in a hospital unit. Caution should be exercised when switching from Lioresal Intrathecal to morphine and vice versa (see 'Interactions').

*Reservoir refilling:* Reservoir refilling must be performed by trained and qualified personnel in accordance with the instructions provided by the pump manufacturer. Refills should be timed to avoid excessive depletion of the reservoir.

When refilling the pump, care should be taken to avoid discharging the contents of the catheter into the intrathecal space.

Strict asepsis is required to avoid microbial contamination and infection.

Extreme caution must be taken when filling a pump equipped with an injection port that allows direct access to the intrathecal catheter as a direct injection into the catheter through the access port could cause a life-threatening overdose.

*Elderly:* Several patients over the age of 65 years have been treated with intrathecal baclofen without specific problems and as doses are individually titrated there is unlikely to be any specific problems in elderly patients.

*Children:* Lioresal Intrathecal is not recommended for use in patients under 18 years of age due to limited clinical experience in this age group.

### Contra-indications, warnings, etc
*Contra-indications:* Hypersensitivity to baclofen, administration by any route other than intrathecal.

*Warnings:* Intrathecal baclofen therapy is valuable but hazardous. Careful pre-operative assessment is mandatory.

The patient must be given adequate information regarding the risks of this mode of treatment, and be physically and psychologically able to cope with the pump. It is essential that the responsible physicians and all those involved in the care of the patient receive adequate instruction on the signs and symptoms of overdose, procedures to be followed in the event of an overdose and the proper home care of the pump and insertion site.

*Precautions:* In patients with abnormal CSF flow the circulation of drug and hence antispastic activity may be inadequate.

Psychotic disorders, schizophrenia or confusional states may be exacerbated by treatment with oral Lioresal. Patients suffering from these conditions should therefore be treated cautiously and kept under close surveillance.

Special attention should be given to patients suffering from epilepsy as seizures have been occasionally reported during overdose with and withdrawal from Lioresal Intrathecal, as well as in patients maintained on therapeutic doses.

Lioresal Intrathecal should be used with caution in patients suffering from cerebrovascular or respiratory insufficiency.

Lioresal Intrathecal should be used with caution in patients with a history of autonomic dysreflexia; the presence of nociceptive stimuli or abrupt withdrawal of Lioresal Intrathecal may precipitate an autonomic dysreflexic episode.

An effect of Lioresal Intrathecal on underlying, non-CNS related diseases is unlikely because its systemic availability is substantially lower than after oral administration. Observations after oral baclofen therapy suggest that caution should be exercised in patients with a history of peptic ulcer, pre-existing sphincter hypertonia and impaired renal function.

Drowsiness has been reported in some patients receiving intrathecal baclofen, and patients should be advised to exercise due caution. Operating equipment or machinery may be hazardous.

*Treatment withdrawal:* Except in overdose-related emergencies or where serious adverse effects occur, treatment should always be discontinued gradually with successive reductions in dosage. Sudden cessa-

tion of treatment, especially after doses exceeding the average, may result in a hyperactive state with rapid uncontrolled spasms and increased rigidity to intolerable levels lasting for several days.

Confusional states, hallucinations, psychotic, manic or paranoid states, convulsions (status epilepticus), and–as a rebound phenomenon–temporary aggravation of spasticity have been reported upon the abrupt withdrawal of oral Lioresal, especially after long-term treatment.

*Use in pregnancy and lactation:* There are no adequate and well-controlled studies in pregnant women. Oral baclofen increases the incidence of omphaloceles (ventral hernias) in the foetuses of rats at high doses. No teratogenic effects have been noted in mice or rabbits.

A dose related increase in the incidence of ovarian cysts, and a less marked increase in enlarged and/or haemorrhagic adrenals have been observed in female rats treated for 2 years. The clinical relevance of these findings is not known.

Lioresal Intrathecal should not be used during pregnancy unless the potential benefit is judged to outweigh the potential risk to the foetus. Baclofen crosses the placental barrier.

In mothers taking oral Lioresal in therapeutic doses the active substance passes into the breast milk, but in quantities so small that no undesirable effects on the infant are to be expected. It is not known whether detectable levels of drug are present in the breast milk of nursing mothers receiving Lioresal Intrathecal.

*Drug interactions:* The co-administration of other intrathecal agents with Lioresal Intrathecal is not recommended.

An attempt should be made to reduce or discontinue concomitant oral antispastic medications, preferably before initiating baclofen infusion. However, abrupt reduction or discontinuation during chronic intrathecal baclofen therapy should be avoided.

There is inadequate experience with Lioresal Intrathecal in combination with systemic medications to be able to predict specific drug-drug interactions, although it is suggested that the lower plasma baclofen levels produced by intrathecal administration should reduce the potential for interactions. Experience with oral baclofen would suggest that:

– There may be increased sedation where Lioresal is taken concomitantly with other drugs acting on the CNS or with alcohol.
– During concurrent treatment with tricyclic antidepressants, the effect of Lioresal may be potentiated, resulting in muscular hypotonia.
– Since concomitant treatment with Lioresal and antihypertensives is likely to increase the fall in blood pressure, it may be necessary to reduce the dosage of antihypertensive medication.

The combined use of morphine and intrathecal baclofen has been responsible for hypotension in one patient; the potential for this combination to cause dyspnoea or CNS symptoms cannot be excluded.

*Side-effects:* A causal link between reported adverse events and baclofen treatment cannot be reliably established in many cases since many unwanted effects occur in association with the underlying conditions under treatment.

Adverse events associated with the delivery system (eg. misuse or malfunction of the device, pocket infection, meningitis) are not included here.

*Central nervous system: Occasional:* sedation, drowsiness, dizziness/lightheadedness, seizures, headache, paraesthesiae, accommodation disorders/blurred vision/double vision, slurred speech, lethargy. *Rare:* respiratory depression, hypothermia, nystagmus, dysphagia, insomnia, somnolence, fatigue, decreased co-ordination, memory loss, confusion/disorientation, anxiety, depression, suicidal ideation and attempt, euphoria, dysphoria, hallucinations, paranoia

*Cardiovascular system: Occasional:* hypotension, hypertension, bradycardia. *Rare:* deep vein thrombosis, skin flushing, pallor.

*Gastro-intestinal tract:Occasional:* nausea/vomiting, constipation. *Rare:* dry mouth, diarrhoea, decreased appetite, dehydration, ileus, decreased taste sensation.

*Respiratory system:Occasional:* Dyspnoea, bradypnoea.

*Urogenital system: Rare:* Enuresis, atonic bladder, bladder spasm, sexual dysfunction.

*Miscellaneous unwanted effects: Rare:* urticaria, alopecia, facial oedema, hyperhidrosis.

*Overdosage*
*Symptoms:* Special attention should be given to recognising the signs and symptoms of overdosage at all times, but especially during the initial 'screening' and 'dose titration' phases and also during the reintroduction of Lioresal Intrathecal after an interruption of therapy.

Signs of overdose usually appear insidiously: ex-

cessive muscular hypotonia, drowsiness, lightheadedness, nausea, dizziness, somnolence, loss of consciousness, respiratory depression and apnoea result from serious overdosage. Seizures may occur with increasing dosage or, more commonly, during recovery from an overdose. Serious overdose may occur through the inadvertent delivery of the catheter contents, errors in pump programming, excessively rapid dose increases or concomitant treatment with oral baclofen. Possible pump malfunction should also be investigated.

*Treatment:* There is no specific antidote for intrathecal baclofen overdose. Any instructions provided by the pump manufacturer should be followed, and the following steps should generally be taken:-

– Where a programmable continuous infusion pump is used further delivery of baclofen should be halted immediately by removal of residual drug solution from the reservoir.
– If it is possible to do so without surgical intervention the intrathecal catheter should be disconnected from the pump as soon as possible, and infusion fluid allowed to drain back together with some CSF (up to 30-40 ml is suggested).
– Patients with respiratory depression should be intubated if necessary, and ventilated artificially if required.

Anecdotal reports suggest that intravenous physostigmine may assist in the reversal of central side-effects (notably drowsiness and respiratory depression), but its use has been associated with the induction of seizures, bradycardia and cardiac conduction disturbances, and it should not be used in cases of severe overdose. In such cases intubation and ventilation are essential. A total dose of 1-2 mg physostigmine may be tried intravenously over 5-10 minutes. Patients should be monitored closely during this time.

Repeated doses of 1 mg may be administered at 30-60 minute intervals in an attempt to maintain adequate respiration in the absence of facilities for respiratory support.

**Pharmaceutical precautions** Lioresal Intrathecal ampoules should be protected from heat (store below 30°C). Each ampoule is intended for single use only, and any unused solution should be discarded. Ampoules should **not** be autoclaved.

Dilution: If alternative baclofen concentrations are required Lioresal Intrathecal may be diluted under aseptic conditions with sterile preservative-free sodium chloride for injections. The ampoules should not be mixed with other solutions for injection or infusion.

The compatibility of Lioresal Intrathecal with the components of the infusion pump (including the chemical stability of baclofen in the reservoir) and the presence of an in-line bacterial retentive filter should be confirmed with the pump manufacturer prior to use.

**Legal category** POM

**Package quantities** Packs containing single ampoules.

**Further information** Nil

**Product licence numbers**
Lioresal Intrathecal 50 micrograms/1 ml 00101/0500
Lioresal Intrathecal 10 mg/20 ml 00101/0501
Lioresal Intrathecal 10 mg/5 ml 00101/0502

## LOPRESOR*

**Presentation** The active ingredient Metoprolol Tartrate PhEur is presented as: pale red, round, slightly biconvex, film-coated tablets with slightly bevelled edges, approximately 9 mm diameter, engraved GEIGY on one side and scored on the other side. Each tablet contains 50 mg.

Lopresor is also available as: light blue, round, slightly biconvex, film- coated tablets with slightly bevelled edges, approximately 10 mm diameter, engraved GEIGY on one side and scored on the other. Each tablet contains 100 mg.

The 100 mg tablets also contain indigocarmine E132.

**Uses**
*Indications:* Hypertension and angina pectoris, cardiac arrhythmias, especially supraventricular tachyarrhythmias.

Adjunct to treatment of thryotoxicosis.

Early intervention with Lopresor in acute myocardial infarction reduces infarct size and the incidence of ventricular fibrillation. Pain relief may also decrease the need for opiate analgesics.

Lopresor has been shown to reduce mortality when administered to patients with acute myocardial infarction.

Prophylaxis of migraine.

*Mode of action:* Lopresor is a cardioselective beta-adrenergic blocking agent. It has a relatively greater blocking effect on beta$_1$-receptors (i.e. those mediating adrenergic stimulation of heart rate and contractility and release of free fatty acids from fat stores) than on beta$_2$-receptors, which are chiefly involved in broncho- and vasodilation.

*Pharmacokinetics*: Metoprolol is well absorbed after oral administration, peak plasma concentrations occurring 1.5–2 hours after dosing. The bioavailability of a single dose is approximately 50%, increasing to approximately 70% during repeated administration. The bioavailability also increases if metoprolol is given with food.

Elimination is mainly by hepatic metabolism and the average elimination half-life is 3.5 hours (range 1 to 9 hours). Rates of metabolism vary between individuals, with poor metabolisers (approximately 10%) showing higher plasma concentrations and slower elimination than extensive metabolisers. Within individuals, however, plasma concentrations are stable and reproducible.

Because of variation in rates of metabolism, the dose of metoprolol should always be adjusted to the individual requirements of the patient. As the therapeutic response, adverse effects and relative cardioselectivity are related to plasma concentration, poor metabolisers may require lower than normal doses. Dosage adjustment is not routinely required in the elderly or in patients with renal failure, but dosage may need to be reduced in patients with significant hepatic dysfunction when metoprolol elimination may be impaired.

**Dosage and administration** Lopresor tablets should be administered orally and swallowed unchewed.

The dose must always be adjusted to the individual requirements of the patient but should not exceed 400 mg/day. The following are guidelines:

*Adults: Hypertension:* Initially a dose of 100 mg per day should be prescribed either as single or divided doses.

Depending upon the response the dosage may be increased by 100 mg per day at weekly intervals to 200 mg daily given in single or divided doses. Over the dosage range most patients may be expected to respond rapidly and satisfactorily. A further reduction in blood pressure may be achieved if Lopresor is used in conjunction with an antihypertensive diuretic or other hypotensive agent.

Lopresor may be administered with benefit both to previously untreated patients with hypertension and to those in whom the response to previous therapy is inadequate. In the latter type of patient the previous therapy may be continued and Lopresor added into the regime with adjustment of the previous therapy if necessary.

*Angina pectoris:* 50-100 mg twice or three times daily.

In general a significant improvement in exercise tolerance and reduction of anginal attacks may be expected with a dose of 50-100 mg twice daily.

*Cardiac arrhythmias:* A dosage of 50 mg two or three times daily is usually sufficient. If necessary the dose can be increased up to 300 mg per day administered in divided doses.

*Hyperthyroidism:* 50 mg four times daily. The dosage should be progressively reduced as euthyroid state is slowly achieved.

*Myocardial infarction:* Early intervention.

Therapy should commence with 50 mg every 6 hours for 48 hours, preferably within 12 hours of the onset of chest pain.

Maintenance: the usual maintenance dose is 200 mg daily given in divided doses. The treatment should be continued for at least 3 months.

*Prophylaxis of migraine:* 100-200 mg daily, given in divided doses (morning and evening).

*Elderly*: There is no evidence to suggest that dosage requirements are different in otherwise healthy elderly patients. However, caution is indicated in elderly patients as an excessive decrease in blood pressure or pulse rate may cause the blood supply to vital organs to fall to inadequate levels.

In patients with significant hepatic dysfunction the lower dosage recommendations will be more appropriate.

*Children*: Not recommended.

**Contra-indications, warnings, etc**

*Contra-indications*: Known sensitivity to metoprolol and related derivatives, severe asthma, atrioventricular block of second or third degree, uncontrolled heart failure, clinically relevant sinus bradycardia, sick-sinus syndrome, severe peripheral arterial disease, cardiogenic shock. Metoprolol is also contra-indicated when myocardial infarction is complicated by significant bradycardia, first degree heart block, systolic hypotension (less than 100 mmHg) and/or severe heart failure.

*Precautions*: Metoprolol may aggravate bradycardia, symptoms of peripheral arterial circulatory disorders and anaphylactic shock. If the patient develops increasing bradycardia, Lopresor should be given in lower doses or gradually withdrawn.

Abrupt cessation of therapy with a beta-blocker should be avoided. When possible, Lopresor should be withdrawn gradually over a period of 10 days, the doses diminishing to 25 mg for the last 6 days. During its withdrawal the patient should be kept under close surveillance.

Although cardioselective beta-blockers may have less effect on lung function than non-selective beta-blockers, as with all beta-blockers these should be avoided in patients with reversible obstructive airway disease unless there are compelling clinical reasons for their use. Therapy with a $\beta_2$-stimulant may become necessary or current therapy require adjustment.

Lopresor may be administered when heart failure has been controlled. Digitalisation and/or diuretic therapy should also be considered for patients with a history of heart failure or patients known to have a poor cardiac reserve.

Lopresor may mask some of the symptoms of thyrotoxicosis and of hypoglycaemia by inhibition of sympathetic nerve functions.

In labile and insulin-dependent diabetes it may be necessary to adjust the hypoglycaemic therapy.

In patients with a phaeochromocytoma, an alpha-blocker should be given concomitantly.

In patients with significant hepatic dysfunction it may be necessary to adjust the dosage because metoprolol undergoes biotransformation in the liver.

The administration of adrenaline to patients undergoing beta-blockade can result in an increase in blood pressure and bradycardia although this is less likely to occur with beta$_1$-selective drugs.

Lopresor should be given cautiously to patients with metabolic acidosis.

Lopresor therapy should be brought to the attention of the anaesthetist prior to general anaesthesia. In a patient under beta-blockade, the anaesthetic selected should be one exhibiting as little negative inotropic activity as possible (halothane/nitrous oxide).

*Warnings*: As with all beta-blockers, metoprolol may affect patient's ability to drive and operate machinery. Patients should be warned accordingly.

*Use in pregnancy and lactation*: Lopresor should not be used in pregnancy or lactation unless it is considered that the benefit outweighs the possible risk to the foetus/infant. Metoprolol has, however, been used in pregnancy associated hypertension under close supervision after 20 weeks gestation. Although the drug crosses the placental barrier and is present in cord blood no evidence of foetal abnormalities have been reported. Animal experiments have shown neither teratogenic potential nor other adverse events on the embryo and/or foetus relevant to the safety assessment of the product.

The amount of metoprolol ingested via breast milk seems to be negligible with regard to its beta-blocking effects if the mother is treated in doses within the therapeutic range.

If Lopresor is used during pregnancy and lactation special attention should be paid to the foetus, neonate and breast-fed infant for undesirable effects of the drug's beta-blocking action (e.g. bradycardia, hypoglycaemia).

*Drug interactions*: The effects of metoprolol and other antihypertensive drugs on blood pressure are usually additive, and care should be taken to avoid hypotension. As with all beta-blockers particular caution is called for when metoprolol is administered together with prazosin for the first time. However, combinations of antihypertensive drugs may often be used with benefit to improve control of hypertension.

Metoprolol can reduce myocardial contractility and impair intracardiac conduction. Care should be exercised when drugs with similar activity, e.g. antiarrhythmic agents, general anaesthetics, are given concurrently. Like all other beta-blockers, metoprolol should not be given in combination with verapamil since this may cause bradycardia, hypotension and asystole.

Care should also be exercised when beta-blockers are given in combination with sympathetic ganglion blocking agents, other beta-blockers (also in the form of eye drops) or MAO inhibitors.

If combination treatment with clonidine is to be discontinued, metoprolol should be withdrawn several days before clonidine.

As beta-blockers may affect the peripheral circulation, care should be exercised when drugs with similar activity, e.g. ergotamine, are given concurrently.

Metoprolol will antagonise the beta$_1$ effects of sympathomimetic agents but should have little influence on the bronchodilator effects of beta$_2$-agonists at normal therapeutic doses.

Enzyme inducing agents (e.g. rifampicin) may reduce plasma concentration of metoprolol, whereas enzyme inhibitors (e.g. cimetidine) may increase plasma concentrations.

During concomitant ingestion of alcohol and metoprolol the concentration of blood alcohol may reach higher levels and may decrease more slowly.

Metoprolol may impair the elimination of lignocaine.

Indomethacin may reduce the antihypertensive effect of beta-blockers.

Nitroglycerin may enhance the hypotensive effect of Lopresor.

*Side-effects:*

*Central and peripheral nervous system:* Occasionally: fatigue, dizziness, headache. Rarely: paraesthesiae, muscle cramps, depression, decreased mental alertness, somnolence or insomnia, nightmares. In isolated cases: personality disorder, hallucinations.

*Cardiovascular system:* Occasionally: bradycardia, postural disorders (occasionally with syncope). Rarely: heart failure, cardiac arrhythmias, oedema, palpitation, Raynaud's phenomenon. In isolated cases: disturbances of cardiac conduction, precordial pain, gangrene in patients with pre-existing severe peripheral circulatory disorders.

*Gastro-intestinal tract:* Occasionally: nausea and vomiting, abdominal pain. Rarely: diarrhoea or constipation. In isolated cases: dryness of the mouth, liver function test abnormalities, hepatitis.

*Skin and appendages:* Rarely: skin rash (in the form of urticaria, psoriasiform and dystrophic skin lesions), occurrence of antinuclear antibodies (not associated with SLE). In isolated cases: photosensitivity, increase sweating, loss of hair.

*Respiratory tract:* Occasionally: exertional dyspnoea. Rarely: bronchospasm, also in patients without a history of obstructive lung disease. In isolated cases: rhinitis.

*Endocrine system and metabolism:* In isolated cases: weight gain.

*Urogenital system:* There are isolated reports on disturbances of libido and potency.

*Sense organs:* In isolated cases: disturbances of vision, dry and/or irritated eyes, tinnitus, in doses exceeding those recommended loss of hearing.

*Blood:* In isolated cases: thrombocytopenia.

*Other organ systems:* In isolated cases: arthritis.

The reported incidence of skin rashes and/or dry eyes associated with the use of beta-blockers is small and in most cases the symptoms have cleared when treatment was withdrawn. Discontinuation of the drug should be considered if any such reaction is not otherwise explicable.

*Overdosage*: *Signs:* In more severe cases an overdosage of metoprolol may lead to severe hypotension, sinus bradycardia, atrioventricular block, heart failure, cardiogenic shock, cardiac arrest, bronchospasm, impairment of consciousness, coma, nausea, vomiting, cyanosis, hypoglycaemia and occasionally hyperkalaemia. The first manifestations usually appear 20 minutes to 2 hours after drug ingestion.

*Treatment*: Treatment should include close monitoring of cardiovascular, respiratory and renal functions, and blood glucose and electrolytes. Further absorption may be prevented by induction of vomiting, gastric lavage or administration of activated charcoal if ingestion is recent. Cardiovascular complications should be treated symptomatically which may require the use of sympathomimetic agents (e.g. noradrenaline, metaraminol), atropine or inotropic agents (e.g. dopamine, dobutamine). Temporary pacing may be required for AV block. Glucagon can reverse the effects of excessive beta- blockade given in a dose of 1-10 mg intravenously. Intravenous beta$_2$- stimulants may be required to relieve bronchospasm. Metoprolol cannot be effectively removed by haemodialysis.

**Pharmaceutical precautions** Protect from moisture.

**Legal category** POM

**Package quantities**

Lopresor 50 mg: Blister packs of 56 tablets.
Lopresor 100 mg: Blister packs of 56 tablets.

**Product licence numbers**

Tablets 50 mg 00101/0418
Tablets 100 mg 00101/0419

## LOPRESOR SR*

**Qualitative and quantitative composition** The active ingredient is Di-[(±)-1-(isopropylamino)-3-[p-(2-methoxyethyl)phenoxy]-2-propanol] L(+)-tartrate (metoprolol tartrate).

One coated slow release tablet contains 200 mg metoprolol tartrate.

**Pharmaceutical form** Film coated tablets.

**Clinical particulars**

*Therapeutic indications:* For the treatment of hypertension, angina pectoris, prophylaxis of migraine.

*Posology and method of administration:* Lopresor SR tablets should be swallowed unchewed.

The dose must always be adjusted to the individual requirements of the patient but should not exceed 400 mg/day. The following are guidelines:

*Adults:*
*Hypertension:* One Lopresor SR tablet should be given in the morning. Most patients may be expected to respond satisfactorily within 14 days. Further anti-hypertensive effect may be achieved by the addition of a diuretic or a vasodilator.

Lopresor SR may be administered with benefit to both previously untreated patients with hypertension and to those in whom the response to previous therapy is inadequate. In the latter type of patient therapy may be continued and Lopresor SR added into the regime with adjustment of previous therapy if necessary.

*Angina pectoris:* Initially, one Lopresor SR tablet daily. The dose may be increased to two tablets once daily if required. In general a significant improvement in exercise tolerance and a reduction of anginal attacks may be expected with a dose of one Lopresor SR tablet daily.

*Prophylaxis of migraine:* One tablet daily given in the morning.

*Elderly:* There is no evidence to suggest that dosage requirements are different in otherwise healthy elderly patients. However, caution is indicated in elderly patients as an excessive decrease in blood pressure or pulse rate may cause the blood supply to vital organs to fall to inadequate levels.

In patients with significant hepatic dysfunction the lower dosage recommendations will be more appropriate.

*Children:* Not recommended.

*Contra-indications:* Known sensitivity to metoprolol and related derivatives, severe asthma, atrioventricular block of second or third degree, uncontrolled heart failure, clinically relevant sinus bradycardia, sick-sinus syndrome, severe peripheral arterial disease, cardiogenic shock. Metoprolol is also contra-indicated when myocardial infarction is complicated by significant bradycardia, first degree heart block, systolic hypotension (less than 100 mmHg) and/or severe heart failure.

*Special warnings and precautions for use:*
*Warnings:* None.

*Precautions:* Metoprolol may aggravate bracycardia, symptoms of peripheral arterial circulatory disorders and anaphylactic shock. If the patient develops increasing bradycardia, Lopresor should be given in lower doses or gradually withdrawn.

Abrupt cessation of therapy with a beta-blocker should be avoided. When possible, Lopresor SR should be withdrawn gradually over a period of 10 days, the doses diminishing to 25 mg for the last 6 days. During its withdrawal the patient should be kept under close surveillance.

Although cardioselective beta-blockers may have less effect on lung function than non selective beta-blockers, as with all beta-blockers these should be avoided in patients with reversible obstructive airways disease unless there are compelling clinical reasons for their use. Therapy with a beta-2-stimulant may become necessary or current therapy require adjustment.

Lopresor SR may be administered when heart failure has been controlled. Digitalisation and/or diuretic therapy should also be considered for patients with a history of heart failure or patients known to have a poor cardiac reserve.

Lopresor SR may mask some of the symptoms of thyrotoxicosis and of hypoglycaemia by inhibition of sympathetic nerve functions.

In labile and insulin-dependent diabetes it may be necessary to adjust the hypoglycaemic therapy.

In patients with a phaeochromocytoma, an alpha-blocker should be given concomitantly.

In patients with significant hepatic dysfunction it may be necessary to adjust the dosage because metoprolol undergoes biotransformation in the liver.

The administration of adrenaline to patients undergoing beta-blockade can result in an increase in blood pressure and bradycardia although this is less likely to occur with $beta_1$-selective drugs.

Lopresor SR should be given cautiously to patients with metabolic acidosis.

Lopresor SR therapy should be brought to the attention of the anaesthetist prior to general anaesthesia. In a patient under beta-blockade, the anaesthetic selected should be one exhibiting as little negative inotropic activity as possible (halothane/nitrous oxide).

*Interactions with other drugs and other types of interactions:*
*Drug interactions:* The effects of metoprolol and other antihypertensive drugs on blood pressure are usually additive, and care should be taken to avoid hypotension. As with all beta-blockers particular caution is called for when metoprolol is administered together with prazosin for the first time. However, combinations of antihypertensive drugs may often be used with benefit to improve control of hypertension.

Metoprolol can reduce myocardial contractility and impair intracardiac conduction. Care should be exercised when drugs with similar activity e.g. antiarrhythmic agents, general anaesthetics, are given concurrently. Like all other beta-blockers, metoprolol should not be given in combination with verapamil since this may cause bradycardia, hypotension and asystole.

Care should also be exercised when beta-blockers are given in combination with sympathetic ganglion blocking agents, other beta-blockers (also in the form of eye drops) or MAO inhibitors.

If combination treatment with clonidine is to be discontinued metoprolol should be withdrawn several days before clonidine.

As beta-blockers may affect the peripheral circulation, care should be exercised when drugs with similar activity e.g. ergotamine are given concurrently.

Metoprolol will antagonise the $beta_1$ effects of sympathomimetic agents but should have little influence on the bronchodilator effects of $beta_2$-agonists at normal therapeutic doses.

Enzyme inducing agents (e.g. rifampicin) may reduce plasma concentration of metoprolol, whereas enzyme inhibitors (e.g. cimetidine) may increase plasma concentrations.

During concomitant ingestion of alcohol and metoprolol the concentration of blood alcohol may reach higher levels and may decrease more slowly.

Metoprolol may impair the elimination of lignocaine.

Indomethacin may reduce the antihypertensive effect of beta-blockers.

Nitroglycerin may enhance the hypotensive effect of Lopresor SR.

*Pregnancy and lactation:* Lopresor SR should not be used in pregnancy or lactation unless it is considered that the benefit outweighs the possible risk to the foetus/infant. Metoprolol has, however, been used in pregnancy associated hypertension under close supervision after 20 weeks gestation. Although the drug crosses the placental barrier and is present in cord blood no evidence of foetal abnormalities have been reported. The amount of metoprolol ingested via breast milk seems to be negligible with regard to its beta-blocking effects if the mother is treated in doses within the therapeutic range.

If Lopresor SR is used during pregnancy and lactation special attention should be paid to the foetus, neonate and breast-fed infant for undesirable effects of the drug's beta-blocking action (e.g. bradycardia, hypoglycaemia).

*Effects on ability to drive or use machines:* As with all beta-blockers, metoprolol may affect patients ability to drive and operate machinery. Patients should be warned accordingly.

*Undesirable effects:* Frequency estimate: frequent, 10%; occasional, 1–10%; rare, 0.001–1%; isolated cases, 0.001%.

*Central and peripheral nervous system:* Occasionally: fatigue, dizziness, headache. Rarely: paraesthesiae, muscle cramps, depression, decreased mental alertness, somnolence or insomnia, nightmares. In isolated cases: personality disorder, hallucinations.

*Cardiovascular system:* Occasionally: bradycardia, postural disorders (occasionally with syncope). Rarely: heart failure, cardiac arrhythmias, oedema, palpitation, Raynaud's phenomenon. In isolated cases: disturbances of cardiac conduction, precordial pain, gangrene in patients with pre-existing severe peripheral circulatory disorders.

*Gastro-intestinal tract:* Occasionally: nausea and vomiting, abdominal pain. Rarely: diarrhoea or constipation. In isolated cases: dryness of the mouth, liver function test abnormalities, hepatitis.

*Skin and appendages:* Rarely: skin rash (in the form of urticaria, psoriasiform and dystrophic skin lesions), occurrence of antinuclear antibodies (not associated with SLE). In isolated cases: photosensitivity, increase sweating, loss of hair.

*Respiratory tract:* Occasionally: exertional dyspnoea. Rarely: bronchospasm, also in patients without a history of obstructive lung disease. In isolated cases: rhinitis.

*Endocrine system and metabolism:* In isolated cases: weight gain.

*Urogenital system:* There are isolated reports on disturbances of libido and potency.

*Sense organs:* In isolated cases: disturbances of vision, dry and/or irritated eyes, tinnitus, in doses exceeding those recommended loss of hearing.

*Blood:* In isolated cases: thrombocytopenia.

*Other organ systems:* In isolated cases: arthritis.

The reported incidence of skin rashes and/or dry eyes associated with the use of beta-blockers is small and in most cases the symptoms have cleared when treatment was withdrawn. Discontinuation of the drug should be considered if any such reaction is not otherwise explicable.

*Overdose:*
*Signs:* In more severe cases an overdosage of metoprolol may lead to severe hypotension, sinus bradycardia, atrioventricular block, heart failure, cardiogenic shock, cardiac arrest, bronchospasm, impairment of consciousness, coma, nausea, vomiting, cyanosis, hypoglycaemia and occasionally hyperkalaemia. The first manifestations usually appear 20 minutes to 2 hours after drug ingestion.

*Treatment:* Treatment should include close monitoring of cardiovascular, respiratory and renal functions, and blood glucose and electrolytes. Further absorption may be prevented by induction of vomiting, gastric lavage or administration of activated charcoal if ingestion is recent. Cardiovascular complications should be treated symptomatically which may require the use of sympathomimetic agents (e.g. noradrenaline, metaraminol), atropine or inotropic agents (e.g. dopamine, dobutamine). Temporary pacing may be required for AV block. Glucagon can reverse the effects of excessive beta-blockage given in a dose of 1–10 mg intravenously. Intravenous $beta_2$-stimulants may be required to relieve bronchospam. Metoprolol cannot be effectively removed by haemodialysis.

**Pharmacological properties**
*Pharmacodynamic properties:*
*Pharmacotherapeutic group:* Lopresor SR is a cardioselective beta-adrenergic receptor blocking agent.

*Mechanism of action:* It has a relatively greater blocking effect on $beta_1$-receptors (i.e. those mediating adrenergic stimulation of heart rate and contractility and release of free fatty acids from fat stores) than on $beta_2$-receptors, which are chiefly involved in broncho- and vasodilation.

*Pharmacokinetic properties:*
*Absorption:* Lopresor SR is well absorbed after oral administration, peak plasma concentrations occurring 4–5 hours after dosing. The bioavailability of a single dose is approximately 50%, increasing to approximately 70% during repeated administration. The bioavailability also increases if metoprolol is given with food.

*Biotransformation:* Rates of metabolism vary between individuals, with poor metabolisers (approximately 10%) showing higher plasma concentrations and slower elimination than extensive metabolisers. Within individuals, however, plasma concentrations are stable and reproducible.

*Elimination:* Elimination is mainly by hepatic metabolism and the average elimination half-life is 3.5 hours (range 1 to 9 hours).

*Characteristics in patients:* Because of variation in rates of metabolism, the dose of metoprolol should always be adjusted to the individual requirements of the patient. As the therapeutic response, adverse effects and relative cardioselectivity are related to plasma concentration, poor metabolisers may require lower than normal doses. Dosage adjustment is not routinely required in the elderly or in patients with renal failure, but dosage may need to be reduced in patients with significant hepatic dysfunction when metoprolol elimination may be impaired.

*Preclinical safety data:* Animal experiments have shown neither teratogenic potential nor other adverse events on the embryo and/or foetus relevant to the safety assessment of the product.

**Pharmaceutical particulars**
*List of excipients:* The coated tablets contain silicon dioxide, microcystalline cellulose, calcium phosphate, polyacrylic/methacrylic copolymer, magnesium stearate, stearic acid, hydroxypropyl methylcellulose, glyceryl palmitostearate, talc, titanium dioxide, polysorbate, and yellow iron oxide.

*Incompatibilities:* None known.

*Shelf-life:* Five years.

*Special precautions for storage:* No special recommendations. Medicines should be kept out of reach of children.

*Nature and contents of container:* The tablets are pale yellow, capsule shaped, biconvex, film coated tablets, one face imprinted CG/CG, the other face with the letters CDC/CDC and packed in PVC/PVdC/foil bubble packs of 28 tablets.

*Instruction for use/handling:* None.

**Marketing authorisation number** 00101/0420.

**Date of approval/revision of SPC** 27 September 1995.

**Legal category** POM.

# LUDIOMIL*

**Qualitative and quantitative composition** The active ingredient is 1-(3-methylaminopropyl)-dibenzo[b,e] bicyclo[2.2.2]octadiene hydrochloride (maprotiline hydrochloride INN).

One coated tablet contains 10 mg, 25 mg, 50 mg, or 75 mg maprotiline hydrochloride.

**Pharmaceutical form** Coated tablets.

## Clinical particulars

*Therapeutic indications:* Symptoms of depressive illness, especially where sedation is required.

*Posology and method of administration:* Ludiomil tablets should be swallowed with sufficient liquid. The dose should be gradually increased to achieve a therapeutic effect with the lowest possible dose. This is particularly important for elderly patients with an unstable autonomic nervous system as these patients show a more marked response to Ludiomil than younger patients. A daily dosage of 150 mg should not be exceeded.

*Adults:* The usual dose range is 25–75 mg daily which may be given either in one dose or in three divided doses.

For moderate or severe depression, treatment should start with 75 mg daily, increasing step-wise, if necessary, to a maximum of 150 mg daily. Initially the patient should be closely monitored and dosage adjusted after 1 to 2 weeks according to response. Once a distinct improvement has set in the daily dosage may be adjusted to a maintenance level, i.e. the lowest dose that maintains the improvement.

*Use in the elderly:* It may be advisable in elderly patients, or those who may be sensitive to this type of drug, to start treatment with lower doses such as 30 mg once a day or 10 mg three times a day. This should then be adjusted in a stepwise fashion over one or two weeks up to 25 mg tid or 75 mg once a day, depending on the patient's response. In the majority of cases, half the normal dose should be sufficient.

*Use in children:* Not recommended.

*Contra-indications:* Ludiomil is contra-indicated in: patients who are known or suspected to have epilepsy or have a lowered convulsion threshold, recent myocardial infarction, the presence of defects in bundle-branch conduction, narrow angle glaucoma, retention of urine (e.g. prostatic disease), severe liver or renal disease, mania.

Concurrent use in patients receiving or within 14 days of cessation of therapy with monoamine oxidase inhibitors.

Known hypersensitivity to maprotiline or any of the excipients, or cross-sensitivity to tricyclic antidepressants.

Acute poisoning with alcohol, hypnotics, or psychotropic drugs.

*Special warnings and precautions for use:*
*Warnings:* In some patients, improvement may not occur for 2–3 weeks.

There have been rare reports of seizures occurring in patients without a history of seizures who were treated with therapeutic doses of Ludiomil. In some cases, other confounding factors were present such as concomitant medications known to lower the seizure threshold. The risk of seizures may be increased in comedication with phenothiazines (see Interactions), with benzodiazepines that are withdrawn abruptly, or when the recommended dosage of Ludiomil is rapidly exceeded.

While a causal relationship has not been established, the risk of seizures may be reduced by:

– initiating therapy at a low dosage,
– maintaining the initial dosage for two weeks and then raising it gradually in small increments,
– keeping the maintenance dosage at a minimally effective level,
– cautious alteration or avoidance of co-medication with drugs that lower the seizure threshold (e.g. phenothiazines),
– avoidance of rapid tapering of benzodiazepines.

Tricyclic and tetracyclic antidepressants have been reported to produce cardiac arrhythmias, sinus tachycardia and prolongation of conduction time. Caution is indicated in elderly patients and patients with cardiovascular disease, including a history of myocardial infarction, arrhythmias and/or ischaemic heart disease. Monitoring of cardiac function, including ECG, is indicated in such patients, especially during long-term treatment. Regular measurements of blood pressure are called for in patients susceptible to postural hypotension.

Activation of psychosis has occasionally been observed in schizophrenic patients receiving tricyclic antidepressants and must be considered a risk with Ludiomil. Similarly, hypomanic or manic episodes have been reported in patients with cyclic effective disorders while under treatment with a tricyclic antidepressant during a depressive phase. In such cases it may be necessary to reduce the dosage of Ludiomil or to withdraw the drug and administer an antipsychotic agent.

*Precautions:* The possibility of suicide in depressed patients is inherent in their illness and may persist until significant remission occurs. There are reports that antidepressants can, in rare instances, exacerbate suicidal tendencies. One study where Ludiomil was given as prophylactic treatment for unipolar depression suggested an increase in suicidal behaviour in the treated group. Therefore, patients must be carefully supervised during all phases of treatment with Ludiomil and prescriptions should be written for the smallest number of tablets consistent with good patient management.

In predisposed and elderly patients, tricyclic antidepressants may provoke pharmacogenic (delirious) psychoses, especially at night; these disappear without treatment within a few days of withdrawing the drug.

The elderly are particularly liable to experience side effects, especially agitation, confusion and postural hypotension. The initial dosage should therefore be increased with caution and the patients kept under close supervision (see *Dosage*).

Concomitant treatment with electroconvulsive therapy should be carried out only under careful supervision.

Abrupt withdrawal or dose reduction should be avoided because of possible adverse reactions (see *Side effects*).

Although reductions in the white blood cell count have been reported with Ludiomil only in isolated cases, periodic blood cell counts and monitoring for symptoms such as fever and sore throat are called for, particularly during the first few months of therapy.

During long-term treatment it is advisable to monitor hepatic and renal function.

Caution is also called for when treating patients with hyperthyroidism, or when administering thyroid hormone preparations, in view of the possibility of an increase in unwanted cardiac effects.

Because of its anticholinergic properties, Ludiomil should be used with caution in patients with a history of increased intra-ocular pressure, chronic severe constipation or a history of urinary retention (see *Contra-indications*).

Caution is called for in patients with chronic constipation. Tricyclic antidepressants may cause paralytic ileus, particularly in the elderly and bedridden patients.

An increase in dental caries has been reported in long-term treatment with antidepressants. Regular dental inspections are therefore advisable during long-term therapy.

Decreased lacrimation and relative accumulation of mucoid secretion associated with the anticholinergic properties of tricyclic antidepressants may cause damage to the corneal epithelium in patients who wear contact lenses.

Before general or local anaesthesia, inform the anaesthetist that the patient has been receiving Ludiomil. It is safer to continue treatment than to risk the potential disruption due to discontinuation of the drug before surgery.

*Interactions with other drugs and other types of interactions:* Concomitant treatment with Ludiomil and major tranquillisers may give rise to elevated concentrations of maprotiline in the serum, to lowering of the convulsion threshold and to seizures. Combination with thioridazine may produce severe cardiac arrythmia.

The following drug interactions, although not necessarily reported with Ludiomil, have been reported with tri/tetracyclic antidepressants.

*Monoamine oxidase inhibitors (MAO):* Do not give Ludiomil for at least 14 days after discontinuation of treatment with MAO inhibitors (there is a risk of severe interactions such as hyperpyrexia, tremor, delirium and possibly death). The same applies with giving a MAO inhibitor after previous treatment with Ludiomil. In both instances, the treatment should initially be given in small gradually increasing doses and its effects monitored.

*Selective serotonin reuptake inhibitors (SSRI):* Comedication may lead to additive effects on the serotonergic system. Fluvoxetine and fluvoxamine may also increase plasma concentrations of imipramine, with corresponding adverse effects.

*Central nervous system depressants:* Tricyclic antidepressants may potentiate the effects of alcohol and other central depressant substances (e.g. barbiturates, benzodiazepines or general anaesthetics).

*Neuroleptics:* concomitant use of these agents may cause an increase in plasma levels of maprotiline, a lowered convulsion threshold and seizures. Combination with thioridazine may produce severe cardiac arrhythmias.

*Anticoagulants:* Tricyclic antidepressants may potentiate the anticoagulant effect of coumarin drugs by inhibiting their metabolism by the liver. Careful monitoring of plasma prothrombin is therefore advised.

*Anticholinergic agents:* The effects of anticholinergic agents (e.g. phenothiazines, antiparkinsonian agents, atropine, biperiden, antihistamines) on the eye, central nervous system, bowel and bladder, may be potentiated.

*Adrenergic neuronblockers:* Diminution or abolition of the antihypertensive effects of drugs such as guanethidine, bethanidine, reserpine, clonidine and alpha-methyldopa, may occur. Patients requiring co-medication for hypertension should therefore be given antihypertensives of a different type (e.g. diuretics, vasodilators or β-blockers).

Plasma concentrations of maprotiline may rise when the drug is given concomitantly with β-blockers that undergo substantial biotransformation, e.g. propranolol. In such cases, monitor plasma levels and adjust the dosage accordingly. Sudden withdrawal of Ludiomil can also result in serious hypotension.

*Sympathomimetic drugs:* Ludiomil may potentiate the cardiovascular effects of adrenaline, ephedrine, isoprenaline, noradrenaline, phenylephrine and phenylpropanolamine (e.g. as contained in local and general anaesthetic preparations and nasal decongestants). Close supervision (blood pressure, cardiac rhythm) and careful dosage adjustment are therefore required.

*Quinidine:* Tricyclic antidepressants should not be employed in combination with anti-arrhythmic agents of the quinidine type.

*Liver-enzyme inducers:* Drugs which activate the hepatic mono-oxygenase enzyme system (e.g. carbamazepine, barbiturates, phenytoin, nicotine and oral contraceptives) may accelerate the metabolism and lower the plasma concentrations of maprotiline, resulting in decreased efficacy. Plasma levels of phenytoin and carbamazepine may increase, with corresponding adverse effects. It may be necessary to adjust the dosage of these drugs.

*Cimetidine:* It is known that administration of cimetidine together with tricyclic antidepressants may lead to a rise in the latter's serum concentration and may cause unwanted effects (e.g. very severe dryness of the mouth, disturbances of vision).

Neuroleptics and methylphenidate may also increase plasma levels of Ludiomil.

*Oral sulfonylureas or insulin:* Comedication with antidiabetic agents may potentiate their hypoglycaemic effect. Diabetic patients should monitor their blood glucose when treatment with Ludiomil is initiated or discontinued.

*Pregnancy and lactation:* Use of Ludiomil during pregnancy should be avoided unless it is essential and there is no safer alternative.

As a general rule no drugs should be taken during the first 3 months of pregnancy, and the benefits and risks of taking drugs should be carefully considered throughout the whole of pregnancy.

Experience with Ludiomil in pregnancy is limited. Isolated cases suggesting a possible association between Ludiomil and adverse effects on the foetus have been reported. There is no evidence as to drug safety in human pregnancy; nor is there evidence that it is free from hazard.

Withdrawal symptoms in neonates whose mothers received tri/tetracyclic antidepressants during the third trimester have been reported.

Should use of Ludiomil during pregnancy be unavoidable Ludiomil should be withdrawn at least 7 weeks before the expected date of delivery, provided the clinical status of the patient permits, to prevent possible symptoms such as dyspnoea, lethargy, irritability, tachycardia, hypotonia, convulsions, jitters and hypothermia in the new-born.

Maprotiline passes into breast milk. After repeated administration of 150 mg daily for 5 days, the concentration measured in the breast milk exceeds that in the blood by a factor of 1.3–1.5. Nursing mothers should be advised to cease breast-feeding, although reports available so far have shown no adverse effects on the infant.

*Effects on ability to drive or use machines:* Patients receiving Ludiomil should be warned that blurred vision, drowsiness and other CNS symptoms (see *Side-effects*) may occur, in which case they should not drive, operate machinery or do anything else which may require alertness or quick actions. Patients should also be warned that consumption of alcohol or other drugs may potentiate these effects (see *Interactions*).

*Undesirable effects:* Side-effects: Various unwanted effects of Ludiomil are of a mild and transient nature and usually disappear in the further course of treatment or following a decrease in the dosage. Convulsions have been reported as occurring in patients both with and without a history of epilepsy. The rare occurrence of convulsions may increase at higher doses. Skin rashes are not uncommon, an incidence of 3% has been reported.

Elderly patients are particularly sensitive to adverse anticholinergic, neurological, psychiatric or cardiovascular reactions. Their ability to metabolise and eliminate drugs may be reduced, leading to a risk of elevated plasma concentrations at therapeutic doses.

The following adverse effects, although not necessarily reported with Ludiomil, have occurred with tri/tetracyclic antidepressants.

Frequency estimate: frequent >10%, occasional >1–10%, rare >0.001–1%, isolated cases <0.001%.

*Central nervous system: Psychiatric:* Frequent: drowsiness, fatigue. Occasional: increased appetite, restlessness, daytime sedation, anxiety, agitation, mania, hypomania, aggressiveness, impaired memory, sleep disturbances, insomnia, nightmares, aggravated depression, impaired concentration. Rare: delirium, hallucinations (particularly in geriatric patients), nervousness. Isolated cases: activation of psychotic symptoms, depersonalisation, fine tremor, myoclonus.

*Neurological:* Frequent: light-headedness, headache. Occasional: dizziness, dysarthria, muscle weakness, paraesthesiae (numbness, tingling). Rare: convulsions, ataxia, akathisia. Isolated cases: EEG changes, dyskinesia, inco-ordination, falls.

*Anticholinergic effects:* Frequent: dryness of the mouth. Occasional: constipation, sweating, hot flushes, blurred vision, disorders of visual accommodation, disturbances of micturition. Isolated cases: stomatitis, dental caries.

*Cardiovascular system:* Occasional: sinus tachycardia, postural hypotension, clinically irrelevant ECG changes (e.g. ST and T changes) in patients of normal cardiac status. Rare: arrhythmias, increased blood pressure. Isolated cases: conduction disorders (e.g. widening of QRS complex, bundle-branch block, PQ changes), syncope.

*Gastro-intestinal tract:* Occasional: nausea, vomiting; abdominal disorders. Rare: diarrhoea, elevated liver enzymes (transaminases, alkaline phosphatase). Isolated cases: hepatitis with or without jaundice.

*Skin:* Occasional: allergic skin reactions (rash, urticaria), sometimes with fever; photosensitivity. Isolated cases: itching, purpura, oedema (local or generalised), cutaneous vasculitis, alopecia, erythema multiforme.

*Endocrine system and metabolism:* Occasional: weight gain, disturbances of libido and potency. Isolated cases: enlarged mammary glands, galactorrhoea, SIADH (inappropriate antidiuretic hormone secretion syndrome).

*Respiratory tract:* Isolated cases: allergic alveolitis with or without eosinophilia, bronchospasm.

*Blood:* Isolated cases: leucopenia, agranulocytosis, eosinophilia, thrombocytopenia.

*Sense organs:* Isolated cases of tinnitus, taste disturbances, nasal congestion.

*Miscellaneous:* Withdrawal symptoms: Although not indicative of addiction, the following symptoms occasionally occur after abrupt cessation of therapy or reduction of the dose: nausea, vomiting, abdominal pain, diarrhoea, insomnia, headache, nervousness, anxiety, worsening of underlying depression or recurrence of depressed mood.

*Overdose:* The signs and symptoms of overdose with Ludiomil are similar to those reported with tricyclic antidepressants. Cardiac abnormalities and neurological disturbances are the main complications. In children accidental ingestion of any amount should be regarded as serious and potentially fatal.

*Signs and symptoms:* Symptoms generally appear within 4 hours of ingestion and reach a maximum severity at 24 hours. Due to delayed absorption (anticholinergic effect), long half-life and enterohepatic recycling, the patient may remain at risk for up to 4–6 days.

The following signs and symptoms may be seen.

*Central nervous system:* Drowsiness, stupor, coma, ataxia, restlessness, agitation, enhanced reflexes, muscular rigidity, choreo-athetotic movements, convulsions.

*Cardiovascular system:* Hypotension, tachycardia, arrhythmias, conduction disorders, shock, heart failure, in very rare cases, cadiac arrest. In addition, respiratory depression, cyanosis, vomiting, fever, midriasis, sweating and oliguria or anuria may occur.

*Treatment:* There is no specific antidote and treatment is essentially symptomatic and supportive.

Anyone suspected of receiving an overdose of Ludiomil, particularly children, should be hospitalised and kept under close surveillance for at least 72 hours.

Perform gastric lavage or induce vomiting as soon as possible if the patient is alert. If the patient has impaired consciousness, secure the airway with a cuffed endotracheal tube before beginning lavage, and do not induce vomiting. These measures are recommended for up to 12 hours or even longer after the overdose, since the anticholinergic effect of the drug may delay gastric emptying. Administration of activated charcoal may help to reduce drug absorption.

Treatment of symptoms is based on modern methods of intensive care, with continuous monitoring of cardiac function, blood gases, and electrolytes, and if necessary emergency measures such as:
- anticonvulsive therapy
- artificial respiration
- insertion of a temporary cardiac pacemaker
- plasma expander, dopamine or dobutamine administered by intravenous drip
- resuscitation.

Since it has been reported that physostigmine may cause severe bradycardia, asystole, and seizures, its use is not recommended in cases of overdosage with Ludiomil. Haemodialysis or peritoneal dialysis are ineffective because of the low plasma concentrations of maprotiline.

## Pharmacological properties

*Pharmacodynamic properties:* Mode of action: Maprotiline is a tetracyclic antidepressant which shares basic therapeutic properties with the tricyclic antidepressants but differs from them structurally and pharmacologically. It has a potent and selective inhibitory effect on the re-uptake of noradrenalin. Maprotiline has a weak affinity for the central alpha₁-adrenoceptors but exerts little inhibitory effect on re-uptake of serotonin. It displays marked antihistaminic activity and a moderate anticholinergic effect.

*Pharmacokinetic properties:*

*Absorption:* Maprotiline is completely absorbed from Ludiomil film coated tablets, peak levels in the blood occurring within 8 hours. Steady state concentrations in the blood are attained during the second week of treatment and they are linearly proportional to dose but tend to be higher in elderly patients.

*Distribution:* The protein binding rate is 88–89%, independent of the patient's age or disease. The partition coefficient between blood and plasma is 1.7 and the apparent volume of distribution is 23–27 litres/kg. Concentrations in the cerebrospinal fluid are 2–13% of those in serum.

*Biotransformation:* Maprotiline hydrochloride is extensively metabolised; only 2–4% of the dose is excreted unchanged in the urine. The principal metabolite is the pharmacologically active desmethyl derivative. There are also several hydroxylated or methoxylated metabolites, which are excreted by the kidneys as conjugates.

*Elimination:* Maprotiline is eliminated from blood with a mean half-life of 43 hours. The mean systemic clearance ranges between 510 and 570 ml/min. Within 21 days, about two thirds of a single dose is excreted in the urine (predominantly as unchanged drug and conjugated metabolites) and 30% in the faeces.

Impairment of renal function does not affect maprotiline elimination half life provided that hepatic function is normal.

*Characteristics in patients:* In patients over 60 years of age: The steady-state concentrations for a given dose are higher and the elimination half-life longer than in younger patients. The dose should be halved.

*Preclinical safety data:* Animal experiments showed no teratogenic or mutagenic effects and no evidence of impaired fertility or harm to the foetus.

## Pharmaceutical particulars

*List of excipients:* All coated tablets contain lactose, wheat starch, calcium phosphate, magnesium stearate, stearic acid, talc, hydroxypropyl methylcellulose, titanium dioxide, polysorbate 80, aerosil 200, yellow iron oxide.

Coated tablets of 25 mg, 50 mg and 75 mg also contain red iron oxide.

*Incompatibilities:* None known.

*Shelf life:* Five years.

*Special precautions for storage:* No special recommendations. Medicines should be kept out of reach of children.

*Nature and contents of container:* Tablets 10 mg: Pale yellow, circular, film-coated tablets with 'CIBA' on one side and the letters 'CO' on the reverse.

Tablets 25 mg: Greyish-red, circular, film-coated tablets with 'CIBA' on one side and the letters 'DP' on the reverse.

Tablets 50 mg: Light orange, circular, film-coated tablets with 'CIBA' on one side and the letters 'ER' on the reverse.

Tablets 75 mg: Brownish-orange, circular, film-coated tablets with 'CIBA' on one side and the letters 'FS' and a break line on the reverse.

All tablets are packed in PVC/foil bubble packs of 28 tablets.

*Instructions for use/handling:* None.

**Marketing authorisation numbers**
10 mg 00101/0505
25 mg 00101/0506
50 mg 00101/0507
75 mg 00101/0508

**Date of approval/revision of SPL** December 14, 1995.

**Legal category** POM.

# MELLERIL* SUSPENSION

**Qualitative and quantitative composition**
Melleril Suspension 0.5%: Thioridazine base USP 25 mg/5 ml.
Melleril Suspension 2%: Thioridazine base USP 100 mg/5 ml.

**Pharmaceutical form** Opaque, grey/white viscous liquid.

**Clinical particulars**

*Therapeutic indications:*

*Adults:* Schizophrenia: treatment of symptoms and prevention of relapse.

Mania and hypomania.

As an adjunct to the short-term management of anxiety, moderate to severe psychomotor agitation, excitement, violent or dangerously impulsive behaviour. Agitation and restlessness in the elderly.

*Children:* Behaviour disorders and epilepsy – only where there are severe mental or behavioural problems such as senseless hyperactivity, aggressiveness, temper tantrums, self injury or mutilation, or agitation.

*Posology and method of administration:* Oral administration.

*Adults:* Daily dose range in terms of the hydrochloride†:

Schizophrenia, mania, hypomania: 150–600 mg.

For acute schizophrenia, an initial loading dose of 200 mg may be given. In hospitalised, resistant patients under specialist supervision, up to 800 mg daily may be administered for not more than 4 weeks.

Psychomotor agitation, excitement, violent or dangerously impulsive behaviour: 75–200 mg.

Anxiety, agitation and restlessness in the elderly: 30–100 mg.

There may be great variability in individual response and dosage requirements. In underweight patients, or in those suffering from kidney or liver disease, lower initial doses and more gradual increases are indicated.

*Use in the elderly:* In elderly patients lower initial doses and more gradual increases are indicated.

*Children:*

1 to 5 years of age: 1 mg/kg bodyweight.

5 years and over: Usually 75–150 mg/day. In severe cases up to 300 mg/day may be used.

† Melleril suspension contains Thioridazine base. To convert from hydrochloride to base, multiply by 0.91.

As might be expected the *in vitro* dissolution profiles of the suspension and tablets differ; bioequivalence of the liquid and solid dose formulations should not therefore be assumed.

*Contra-indications:* Comatose states, severe depression of the CNS or a history of blood dyscrasia or severe cardiovascular disease. Phenothiazines can cause sleep apnoea and because of a possible correlation with sudden infant death syndrome, Melleril should not be given to children below one year of age.

*Special warnings and precautions for use:* Melleril should be used with caution in patients with cardiac arrhythmias, cardiac disease, severe respiratory disease, renal failure, Parkinson's disease, a personal or family history of narrow angle glaucoma, in prostatic hypertrophy, myasthenia gravis, epilepsy, phaeochromocytoma and in patients who have shown hypersensitivity to other phenothiazines. In patients with liver disease, regular monitoring of liver function is essential. Regular blood counts should be carried out during the first three to four months of treatment or if any clinical signs of blood dyscrasias appear. Phenothiazines generally may affect temperature regulation and decrease serum thyroxine concentrations, although this is very unlikely with Melleril.

Acute withdrawal symptoms including nausea, vomiting and insomnia have rarely been described after abrupt cessation of high dose Melleril. Gradual withdrawal is advisable. Drug withdrawal in children may lead to rapid clinical relapse and neurological symptoms, although this is less common with Melleril than with other antipsychotics.

*Interaction with other medicaments and other forms of interaction:* Melleril may enhance the central nervous system depression produced by other CNS depressant drugs including alcohol, hypnotics, sedatives or narcotic analgesics. In common with other phenothiazines, Melleril antagonises the action of adrenaline and other sympathomimetic agents, and may reverse the blood pressure lowering effects of adrenergic-blocking agents such as guanethidine and clonidine. Phenylpropanolamine has been reported to interact with phenothiazines and cause ventricular arrythmias. Melleril may affect the metabolism of tricyclic antidepressants, phenytoin and other anticonvulsants. It may also impair the antiparkinsonian effects of levodopa; it may possibly affect the control of diabetes or the action of anticoagulants. It may enhance the cardiac depressant effects of quinidine. Antacids should not be used within two hours of taking phenothiazines. Undesirable anticholinergic effects can be enhanced by anticholinergic drugs. Neurotoxicity resulting from combination with lithium has been reported rarely.

*Pregnancy and lactation:* Do not use during pregnancy unless there are compelling reasons. There is inadequate evidence for safety of the drug in human pregnancy, and there is some evidence of harmful effects in a few, but not all, animal studies. The newborn of mothers treated with Melleril in late pregnancy may show signs of intoxication such as excessive sleepiness, tremor and hyperactivity.

Do not use during lactation. If the use of Melleril is considered essential, breast feeding should be discontinued.

*Effects on ability to drive and to use machines:* Phenothiazines should be administered with caution to patients who participate in activities requiring complete mental alertness. They may impair the reactions of the patient e.g. when driving vehicles or operating machinery.

*Undesirable effects:* Common side-effects, particularly with higher dosage and at the start of treatment, include drowsiness, sedation, dry mouth and nasal stuffiness. Dose-related postural hypotension may occur, particularly in the elderly. Other dose-related anticholinergic-type side-effects including blurring of vision, tachycardia, constipation and urinary hesitancy or retention.

Even in low dosage, in susceptible (especially non-psychotic) individuals, Melleril may cause feelings of being mentally dulled or slowed down, nausea, dizziness, headache or paradoxical effects of excitement, agitation or insomnia. Confusional states or epileptic fits can occur.

At higher dose levels, as with other phenothiazines, ECG changes such as prolongation of the Q-T interval, flattening of the T-wave and the appearance of U-waves have been reported. These changes are more likely to occur in the presence of a low potassium blood level. Like all phenothiazines, Melleril may induce arrhythmias.

Pigmentary retinopathy has been observed in a small number of patients receiving long-term therapy with daily doses above the recommended maximum of 600 mg and has been seen rarely in patients taking less. It is characterised by decreased visual acuity, chromatopsia (usually brown-tinted vision) and impairment of dark adaption; progressive loss of vision may occur. Fundoscopic examination discloses deposits of pigment. The patient should be told of the importance of reporting any change in vision. If prolonged high-dose treatment is envisaged full ophthalmic examinations should be carried out at appropriate intervals.

The possibility of pigmentary retinopathy, together with the possibility of cardiotoxic reactions, emphasises the need not to increase doses beyond the recommended maximum daily dose of 600 mg. Extrapyramidal reactions may occur but are uncommon within the recommended dosage range; antiparkinsonian agents are therefore rarely required and should be prescribed with caution.

Whenever an antipsychotic agent is used, the possible risk of development of tardive dyskinesia should be considered, and the patient monitored for early signs. With Melleril the risk is less than with other phenothiazines, and tardive dyskinesia tends to be seen particularly with prolonged treatment at high doses. The potential seriousness and unpredictability of tardive dyskinesia and the fact that it has occasionally been reported to occur when neuroleptic antipsychotic drugs have been prescribed for relatively short periods in low dosage means that the prescribing of such agents requires especially careful assessment of risks versus benefit. Tardive dyskinesia can be precipitated or aggravated by antiparkinsonian drugs. Short-lived dyskinesias may occur after abrupt drug withdrawal.

Antipsychotic drugs such as Melleril may cause hyperprolactinaemia resulting in galactorrhoea and oligo- and amenorrhoea. Sexual function, including erection and ejaculation may be impaired. Weight gain is occasionally seen with Melleril and oedema has been reported. These effects may be prevented by reduction in dosage.

Blood dyscrasias have been reported: transient leucopenia can occur and agranulocytosis has been reported very rarely, most commonly in the first three months of treatment, but occasionally later. Blood counts should be performed if a patient develops signs of persistent infection.

Melleril very rarely may cause a photosensitivity reaction. The critical dose for this to occur is 400 to 600 mg daily. Other rare side-effects include skin rashes, altered seizure control, jaundice, hepatitis and liver dysfunction.

Long-term usage at doses above the recommended maximum may rarely cause increased melanin pigmentation of the skin, which may be irreversible. Although not reported with Melleril, phenothiazines have been reported to cause raised serum cholesterol, rarely hyperglycaemia, faecal impaction, severe paralytic ileus or megacolon.

Sudden and unexplained death, apparently due to arrhythmia or cardiac arrest, has been reported in patients treated with tricyclic neuroleptic agents including Melleril.

In isolated cases, neuroleptic malignant syndrome (muscular rigidity, hyperthermia, altered mental status, autonomic instability) a condition necessitating immediate discontinuation of the drug and appropriate symptomatic treatment, has been observed.

*Overdose:* Acute overdosage of Melleril usually gives rise to coma with shallow breathing, hypotension and absence of reflexes. Motor restlessness, hyperflexia, cardiac arrhythmias and epileptiform convulsions may occur. Treatment should be directed to the elimination of the ingested material by emesis and gastric lavage. General supportive measures should be applied with particular reference to the cardiovascular and respiratory systems.

Acute hypotension should be treated with plasma expanders. If treatment with a vasopressor (*not* adrenaline) proves necessary (as it might in resistant cases) careful monitoring of the patient, particularly of cardiac function, is indicated. Attention should be paid to symptoms of metabolic acidosis and delayed cardiac effects.

**Pharmacological properties**
*Pharmacodynamic properties:* Melleril exhibits the same general pharmacological properties as the other members of the phenothiazine class of compounds. However, probably, as a result of more selective dopaminergic-blocking action in the limbic forebrain region rather than the nigrostriatal region Melleril has been shown to exhibit less extrapyramidal side-effects compared to the other major tranquillisers.

*Pharmacokinetic properties:* Melleril is rapidly and completely absorbed from the gastrointestinal tract. Maximum plasma concentrations are reached 2–4 hours after ingestion. The average systemic bioavailability is approximately 60%. The relative distribution volume is about 10 l/kg. Protein binding is high (more than 95%). Thioridazine is metabolised in the liver; some of the metabolites (e.g. thioridazine sulforidazine) possess pharmacodynamic properties similar to those of the parent compound. Excretion is mainly with the faeces (50%), but also via the kidney (less than 4% as unchanged drug, about 30% as metabolites). Plasma elimination half-life is approximately 10 hours. Thioridazine crosses the placenta, and passes into breast milk.

*Preclinical safety data:* Thioridazine was examined for genotoxicity in Ames tests and *in vivo* examinations such as the micronucleus test in mice, cytogenetic analysis in Chinese hamster bone marrow cells and the dominant lethal test in mice. The results of these tests gave no indications that thioridazine has mutagenic potential.

Fertility and carcinogenicity studies were not performed.

**Pharmaceutical particulars**
*List of excipients:* Buttermint, polysorbate 80, sodium hydroxide, carbomer, sugar granulated No 1, purified water.

*Incompatibilities:* None.

*Shelf life:* 48 months.

*Special precautions for storage:* Protect from light and heat.

*Nature and contents of container:* Amber glass bottle with a polyethylene closure (polythene wad faced with PP, PVDC or PET lining).

*Instruction for use/handling:* None.

**Marketing authorisation numbers**
*Suspension 0.5%* 0101/0052R
*Suspension 2.0%* 0101/0053R

**Date of approval/revision of SPC** May 1997

**Legal category** POM.

# MELLERIL* SYRUP
# MELLERIL* TABLETS

**Qualitative and quantitative composition**
*Syrup:* Thioridazine Hydrochloride PhEur 27.5 mg/5 ml

*Tablets*
Thioridazine Hydrochloride PhEur 10 mg.
Thioridazine Hydrochloride PhEur 25 mg.
Thioridazine Hydrochloride PhEur 50 mg.
Thioridazine Hydrochloride PhEur 100 mg.

**Pharmaceutical form**
*Syrup:* Clear, pale brown syrup with the odour of spearmint/anise.

*Tablets:* White film coated tablets with a bevel edge, embossed MEL on one side with the strength on the other. Dimensions are as follows:
10 mg Tablets: 6.3 mm in diameter, 2.7 mm thick and weigh 82 mg.
25 mg Tablets: 7.3 mm in diameter, 3.4 mm thick and weigh 143 mg.
50 mg Tablets: 8.3 mm in diameter, 3.7 mm thick and weigh 204 mg.

100 mg Tablets: 9.3 mm in diameter, 3.8 mm thick and weigh 245 mg.

**Clinical particulars**
*Therapeutic indications:*
*Adults:* Schizophrenia: treatment of symptoms and prevention of relapse.

Mania and hypomania.

As an adjunct to the short-term management of anxiety, moderate to severe psychomotor agitation, excitement, violent or dangerously impulsive behaviour.

Agitation and restlessness in the elderly.

*Children:* Behaviour disorders and epilepsy – only where there are severe mental or behavioural problems such as senseless hyperactivity, aggressiveness, temper trantrums, self injury or mutilation, or agitation.

*Posology and method of administration:* Oral administration.

*Adults: Daily dose range in terms of the hydrochloride.* Schizophrenia, mania, hypomania: 150–600 mg.

For acute schizophrenia, an initial loading dose of 200 mg may be given. In hospitalised, resistant patients under specialist supervision, up to 800 mg daily may be administered for not more than 4 weeks.

Psychomotor agitation, excitement, violent or dangerously impulsive behaviour: 75–200 mg.

Anxiety, agitation and restlessness in the elderly: 30–100 mg.

There may be great variability in individual response and dosage requirements. In underweight patients, or in those suffering from kidney or liver disease, lower initial doses and more gradual increases are indicated.

*Use in the elderly:* In elderly patients lower initial doses and more gradual increases are indicated.

*Children:*
*Syrup:*
1 to 5 years of age: 1 mg/kg bodyweight.
5 years and over. Usually 75–150 mg/day. In severe cases up to 300 mg/day may be used.

*Tablets:*
0 to 1 year of age: Not recommended, see *Contraindications*.
1 to 5 years of age: 10 mg tablet: 1 mg/kg/body weight. The 25 mg, 50 mg and 100 mg tablets are not suitable for children.
5 years and over: Usually 75–150 mg/day. In severe cases up to 300 mg/day may be used.

*Contra-indications:* Comatose states, severe depression of the CNS or a history of blood dyscrasia or severe cardiovascular disease. Phenothiazines can cause sleep apnoea and because of a possible correlation with sudden infant death syndrome, Melleril should not be given to children below one year of age.

*Special warnings and precautions for use:* Melleril should be used with caution in patients with cardiac arrhythmias, cardiac disease, severe respiratory disease, renal failure, Parkinson's disease, a personal or family history of narrow angle glaucoma, in prostatic hypertrophy, myasthenia gravis, epilepsy, phaeochromocytoma and in patients who have shown hypersensitivity to other phenothiazines. In patients with liver disease, regular monitoring of liver function is essential. Regular blood counts should be carried out during the first three to four months of treatment or if any clinical signs of blood dyscrasias appear. Phenothiazines generally may affect temperature regulation and decrease serum thyroxine concentrations, although this is very unlikely with Melleril.

Acute withdrawal symptoms including nausea, vomiting and insomnia have rarely been described after abrupt cessation of high dose Melleril. Gradual withdrawal is advisable. Drug withdrawal in children may lead to rapid clinical relapse and neurological symptoms, although this is less common with Melleril than with other antipsychotics.

*Interaction with other medicaments and other forms of interaction:* Melleril may enhance the central nervous system depression produced by other CNS depressant drugs including alcohol, hypnotics, sedatives or narcotic analgesics. In common with other phenothiazines. Melleril antagonists the action of adrenaline and other sympathomimetic agents, and may reverse the blood pressure lowering effects of adrenergic-blocking agents such as guanethidine and clonidine. Phenylpropanolamine has been reported to interact with phenothiazines and cause ventricular arrythmias. Melleril may affect the metabolism of tricyclic antidepressants, phenytoin and other anticonvulsants. It may also impair the antiparkinsonian effects of levodopa; it may possibly affect the control of diabetes or the action of anticoagulants. It may enhance the cardiac depressant effects of quinidine. Antacids should not be used within two hours of taking phenothiazines. Undesirable anticholinergic effects can be enhanced by anticholinergic drugs.

Neurotoxicity resulting from combination with lithium has been reported rarely.

*Pregnancy and lactation:* Do not use during pregnancy unless there are compelling reasons. There is inadequate evidence for safety of the drug in human pregnancy, and there is some evidence of harmful effects in a few, but not all, animal studies. The newborn of mothers treated with Melleril in late pregnancy may show signs of intoxication such as excessive sleepiness, tremor and hyperactivity.

Do not use during lactation. If the use of Melleril is considered essential, breast feeding should be discontinued.

*Effects on ability to drive and to use machines:* Phenothiazines should be administered with caution to patients who participate in activities requiring complete mental alertness. They may impair the reactions of the patient e.g. when driving vehicles or operating machinery.

*Undesirable effects:* Common side-effects, particularly with higher dosage and at the start of treatment, include drowsiness, sedation, dry mouth and nasal stuffiness. Dose-related postural hypotension may occur, particularly in the elderly. Other dose-related anticholinergic-type side-effects including blurring of vision, tachycardia, constipation and urinary hesitancy or retention.

Even in low dosage, in susceptible (especially nonpsychotic) individuals, Melleril may cause feelings of being mentally dulled or slowed down, nausea, dizziness, headache or paradoxical effects of excitement, agitation or insomnia. Confusional states or epileptic fits can occur.

At higher dose levels, as with other phenothiazines, ECG changes such as prolongation of the Q-T interval, flattening of the T-wave and the appearance of U-waves have been reported. These changes are more likely to occur in the presence of a low potassium blood level. Like all phenothiazines, Melleril may induce arrhythmias.

Pigmentary retinopathy has been observed in a small number of patients receiving long-term therapy with daily doses above the recommended maximum of 600 mg and has been seen rarely in patients taking less. It is characterised by decreased visual acuity, chromatopsia (usually brown-tinted vision) and impairment of dark adaption; progressive loss of vision may occur. Fundoscopic examination discloses deposits of pigment. The patient should be told of the importance of reporting any change in vision. If prolonged high-dose treatment is envisaged full ophthalmic examination should be carried out at appropriate intervals.

The possibility of pigmentary retinopathy, together with the possibility of cardiotoxic reactions, emphasises the need not to increase doses beyond the recommended maximum daily dose of 600 mg. Extrapyramidal reactions may occur but are uncommon within the recommended dosage range; antiparkinsonian agents are therefore rarely required and should be prescribed with caution.

Whenever an antipsychotic agent is used, the possible risk of development of tardive dyskinesia should be considered, and the patient monitored for early signs. With Melleril the risk is less than with other phenothiazines, and tardive dyskinesia tends to be seen particularly with prolonged treatment at high doses. The potential seriousness and unpredictability of tardive dyskinesia and the fact that it has occasionally been reported to occur when neuroleptic antipsychotic drugs have been prescribed for relatively short periods in low dosage means that the prescribing of such agents requires especially careful assessment of risks versus benefit. Tardive dyskinesia can be precipitated or aggravated by antiparkinsonian drugs. Short-lived dyskinesias may occur after abrupt drug withdrawal.

Antipsychotic drugs such as Melleril may cause hyperprolactinaemia resulting in galactorrhoea and oligo- and amenorrhoea. Sexual function, including erection and ejaculation may be impaired. Weight gain is occasionally seen with Melleril and oedema has been reported. These effects may be prevented by reduction in dosage.

Blood dyscrasias have been reported: transient leucopenia can occur and agranulocytosis has been reported very rarely, most commonly in the first three months of treatment, but occasionally later. Blood counts should be performed if a patient develops signs of persistent infection.

Melleril very rarely may cause a photosensitivity reaction. The critical dose for this to occur is 400 to 600 mg daily. Other rare side-effects include skin rashes, altered seizure control, jaundice, hepatitis and liver dysfunction.

Long-term usage at doses above the recommended maximum may rarely cause increased melanin pigmentation of the skin, which may be irreversible. Although not reported with Melleril, phenothiazines have been reported to cause raised serum cholesterol,

rarely hyperglycaemia, faecal impaction, severe paralytic ileus or megacolon.

Sudden and unexplained death, apparently due to arrhythmia or cardiac arrest, has been reported in patients treated with tricyclic neuroleptic agents including Melleril.

In isolated cases, neuroleptic malignant syndrome (muscular rigidity, hyperthermia, altered mental status, autonomic instability) a condition necessitating immediate discontinuation of the drug and appropriate symptomatic treatment, has been observed.

*Overdose:* Acute overdosage of Melleril usually gives rise to coma with shallow breathing, hypotension and absence of reflexes. Motor restlessness, hyperflexia, cardiac arrhythmias and epileptiform convulsions may occur. Treatment should be directed to the elimination of the ingested material by emesis and gastric lavage. General supportive measures should be applied with particular reference to the cardiovascular and respiratory systems.

Acute hypotension should be treated with plasma expanders. If treatment with a vasopressor (*not* adrenaline) proves necessary (as it might in resistant cases) careful monitoring of the patient, particularly of cardiac function, is indicated. Attention should be paid to symptoms of metabolic acidosis and delayed cardiac effects.

### Pharmacological properties

*Pharmacodynamic properties:* Melleril exhibits the same general pharmacological properties as the other members of the phenothiazine class of compounds. However, probably as a result of more selective dopaminergic-blocking action in the limbic forebrain region rather than the nigrostriatal region Melleril has been shown to exhibit less extrapyramidal side-effects compared to the other major tranquillisers.

*Pharmacokinetic properties:* Melleril is rapidly and completely absorbed from the gastrointestinal tract. Maximum plasma concentrations are reached 2–4 hours after ingestion. The average systemic bioavailability is approximately 60%. The relative distribution volume is about 10 l/kg. Protein binding is high (more than 95%). Thioridazine is metabolised in the liver; some of the metabolites (e.g. thioridazine sulforidazine) possess pharmacodynamic properties similar to those of the parent compound. Excretion is mainly with the faeces (50%), but also via the kidney (less than 4% as unchanged drug, about 30% as metabolites). Plasma elimination half-life is approximately 10 hours. Thioridazine crosses the placenta, and passes into breast milk.

*Preclinical safety data:* Thioridazine was examined for genotoxicity in Ames tests and *in vivo* examinations such as the micronucleus test in mice, cytogenetic analysis in Chinese hamster bone marrow cells and the dominant lethal test in mice. The results of these tests gave no indications that thioridazine has mutagenic potential.

Fertility and carcinogenicity studies were not performed.

### Pharmaceutical particulars

*List of excipients:*

*Syrup:* Caramel 16398, menthol, ascorbic acid, spearmint essence, essence of anise, monopropylene glycol, ethyl alcohol, glycerol, polyvinylpyrrolidone, liquid glucose, sorbitol syrup (70%), sugar granulated No. 1, purified water.

*Tablets:* Collidal anhydrous silica, magnesium stearate, talc, polyvinylpyrrolidone, maize starch, lactose. The film coating constituents are hydroxypropyl methylcellulose, polyethylene glycol, titanium dioxide, carnuba wax.

*Incompatibilities:* None.

*Shelf life: Syrup:* 36 months. *Tablets:* 36 months.

*Special precautions for storage: Syrup:* Protect from light; shake bottle before use. *Tablets:* Protect from direct light.

*Nature and contents of container: Syrup:* Amber glass bottle with a polyethylene closure (polythene wad faced with PP, PVDC or PET lining). *Tablets:* Opaque white PVC/PVDC blister strip or polypropylene securitainers.

*Instructions for use/handling:* None.

### Marketing authorisation numbers

| | |
|---|---|
| Syrup | 0101/5034R |
| Tablets | |
| 10 mg | 0101/5033R |
| 25 mg | 0101/5053R |
| 50 mg | 0101/5054R |
| 100 mg | 0101/5055R |

**Date of approval/revision of SPC** May 1997.

**Legal category** POM.

## METOPIRONE*

**Presentation** Metopirone capsules each containing 250 mg Metyrapone BP in a soft gelatin capsule, coloured white.

These capsules also contain sodium salt of ethyl parahydroxybenzoate, ethylvanillin, gelatin, glycerol, p-methoxy acetophenone, macrogol 400, macrogol 4000, sodium salt of propyl parahydroxybenzoate, titanium dioxide and water.

### Uses

*Indications:* As a diagnostic aid in the differential diagnosis of ACTH-dependent Cushing's syndrome.

For the management of patients with Cushing's syndrome.

In conjunction with glucocorticoids in the treatment of resistant oedema due to increased aldosterone secretion in patients suffering from cirrhosis, nephrosis and congestive heart failure.

*Mode of action:* Metopirone inhibits the enzyme responsible for the 11β-hydroxylation stage in the biosynthesis of cortisol and to a lesser extent, aldosterone. The fall in plasma concentration of circulating glucocorticoids stimulates ACTH secretion, via the feedback mechanism which accelerates steroid biosynthesis. As a result, 11-desoxycortisol, the precursor of cortisol, is released into the circulation, metabolised by the liver and excreted in the urine. Unlike cortisol, 11-desoxycortisol does not suppress ACTH secretion and its urinary metabolites may be measured.

These metabolites can easily be determined by measuring urinary 17-hydroxycorticosteroids (17-OHCS) or 17-ketogenic steroids (17-KGS). Metopirone is used as a diagnostic test on the basis of these properties, with plasma 11-desoxycortisol and urinary 17-OHCS measured as an index of pituitary ACTH responsiveness. Metopirone may also suppress biosynthesis of aldosterone, resulting in mild natriuresis.

*Pharmacokinetics:*
*Absorption:* Metyrapone, the active substance of Metopirone, is rapidly absorbed and eliminated from the plasma. Peak plasma levels usually occur one hour after ingestion of metopirone; after a dose of 750 mg Metopirone, plasma drug levels average 3.7 µg/ml. Plasma drug levels decrease to a mean value of 0.5 µg/ml 4 hours after dosing. The half-life of elimination of Metopirone from the plasma is 20-26 minutes.

*Metabolism:* Metyrapol, the reduced form of metyrapone, is the main active metabolite. Eight hours after a single oral dose, the ratio of metyrapone to metyrapol in the plasma is 1:1.5. Metyrapol takes about twice as long as metyrapone to be eliminated in the plasma.

*Excretion:* Seventy-two hours after a first daily dose of 4.5 g Metopirone (750 mg every 4 hours), 5.3% of the total dose was excreted in the urine as metyrapone (9.2% in free form and 90.8% conjugated with glucuronic acid), and 38.5% in the form of metyrapol, the principal active metabolite (8.1% in free form and 91.9% conjugated with glucuronic acid).

**Dosage and administration** The capsules should be taken with milk or after a meal to minimise nausea and vomiting which can lead to impaired absorption.

*For use as a diagnostic aid:* The patient must be hospitalised. Urinary 17-oxygenic steroid excretion is measured over 24 hours on each of 4 consecutive days. The first 2 days serve as a control period. On the third day, 750 mg Metopirone (3 capsules) must be given at four-hourly intervals to give a total of 6 doses (i.e. 4.5 g). Maximum urine steroid excretion may occur on the fourth day. If urinary steroid excretion increases in response to Metopirone, this suggests the high levels of circulatory cortisol are due to adrenocortical hyperplasia following excessive ACTH production rather than a cortisol-producing adrenal tumour.

*For therapeutic use:* For the management of Cushing's syndrome, the dosage must be adjusted to meet the patients requirements; a daily dose from 250 mg to 6 g may be required to restore normal cortisol levels.

For the treatment of resistant oedema, the usual daily dose of 3 g (12 capsules) should be given in divided doses in conjunction with a glucocorticoid.

*Use in children:* Children should be given a smaller amount based upon 6 four-hourly doses of 15 mg per kg, with a minimum dose of 250 mg every four hours.

*Use in the elderly:* Clinical evidence would indicate that no special dosage regimen is necessary.

**Contra-indications, warnings, etc**
*Contra-indications:* Primary adrenocortical insufficiency. Hypersensitivity to Metopirone or to any of the excipients.

*Warning:* Since Metopirone may cause dizziness and sedation, patients should exercise caution when driving or operating machinery.

## Precautions:

*In relation to use as a diagnostic aid:* Anticonvulsants (e.g. phenytoin, barbiturates), anti-depressants and neuroleptics (e.g. amitriptyline, chlorpromazine), hormones that affect the hypothalamo-pituitary axis and anti-thyroid agents may influence the results of the Metopirone test. If these drugs cannot be withdrawn, the necessity of carrying out the Metopirone test should be reviewed.

If adrenocortical or anterior pituitary function is more severely compromised than indicated by the results of the test, Metopirone may trigger transient adrenocortical insufficiency. This can be rapidly corrected by giving appropriate doses of corticosteroids.

Long-term treatment with Metopirone can cause hypertension as the result of excessive secretion of desoxycorticosterone.

The ability of the adrenal cortex to respond to exogenous ACTH should be demonstrated before Metopirone is employed as a test, because Metopirone may induce acute adrenal insufficiency in patients with reduced adrenal secretory capacity as well as in patients with gross hypopituitarism.

Patients with liver cirrhosis often show a delayed response to Metopirone due to liver damage delaying the metabolism of cortisol.

In cases of thyroid hypofunction, urinary steroid levels may rise very slowly, or not at all, in response to Metopirone.

*Pregnancy and lactation:* No data are available from animal reproduction studies. Metopirone should not be administered during pregnancy since the drug can impair the biosynthesis of foetal-placental steroids. It is not known whether metyrapone passes into the breast milk, therefore nursing mothers should refrain from breast-feeding their infants during treatment with Metopirone.

*Interactions:* It has been observed that in some cases concomitant medication may affect the results of the Metopirone test (see *Precautions*).

## Side-effects:

*Gastro-intestinal tract:* Occasional: nausea, vomiting. Rare: abdominal pain.

*Central nervous system:* Occasional: dizziness, sedation, headache.

*Cardiovascular system:* Occasional: hypotension.

*Skin:* Rare: allergic skin reactions.

*Endocrine system:* Rare: hypoadrenalism, hirsutism.

## Overdosage:

*Signs and symptoms:* The clinical picture of acute Metopirone poisoning is characterised by gastrointestinal symptoms and acute adreno-cortical insufficiency. Laboratory findings: hyponatraemia, hypochloraemia, hyperkalaemia. In patients under treatment with insulin or oral antidiabetics, the signs and symptoms of acute poisoning with Metopirone may be aggravated or modified.

*Treatment:* There is no specific antidote. Gastric lavage and forced emesis should be employed to reduce the absorption of the drug. In addition to general measures, a large dose of hydrocortisone should be administered at once, together with i.v. saline and glucose. This should be repeated as necessary in accordance with the patient's clinical condition. For a few days blood pressure and fluid and electrolyte balance should be monitored.

**Pharmaceutical precautions** Protect from moisture and heat (Store below 30°C).

**Legal category** POM

**Package quantities** 250 mg capsules of Metopirone in Securitainers of 100.

**Further information** Nil.

**Product licence number** 0008/5078R

*Product licence holder:* Ciba-Geigy plc, Hulley Road, Macclesfield, Cheshire SK10 2NX.

# METROGEL*

**Presentation** A clear pale yellow water based gel containing Metronidazole BP 0.75% w/w.

## Uses

*Action:* The mode of action of topical metronidazole in the treatment of rosacea is not known at present.

*Indication:* The treatment of acute inflammatory exacerbations of rosacea.

## Dosage and administration

*Adults:* Apply to the affected skin of the face in a thin film twice daily for a period of eight to nine weeks. Thereafter, further applications may be necessary depending on the severity of the condition.

*Use in the elderly:* As detailed for adults.

*Use in children:* Not recommended.

## Contra-indications, warnings, etc

*Contra-indication:* Known hypersensitivity to metronidazole or bronopol.

*Warnings:* Avoid contact with the eyes. If contact with the eyes occurs the gel should be washed out carefully with water.

*Precautions:* The following statement takes into account the possibility that metronidazole may be absorbed after topical application. However, there is evidence to suggest that the systemic absorption of metronidazole following the topical administration of Metrogel is slight. A disulfiram-like reaction has been reported in a small number of patients taking oral metronidazole and alcohol concomitantly.

*Use in pregnancy and lactation:* The safety of Metrogel in pregnancy and lactation has not been adequately established and Metrogel should not be used in these circumstances. Stop medication if pregnancy occurs.

*Side-effects:* Dryness or irritation of the skin may be experienced after application.

*Overdosage:* Overdosage is unlikely. If necessary remove the medication by washing with warm water. If accidental ingestion of Metrogel occurs, an appropriate method of gastric emptying may be used if considered appropriate.

**Pharmaceutical precautions** Store at room temperature (15–25°C) Protect from light.

**Legal category** POM.

**Package quantities** 40 g tubes.

**Further information** Gel excipients, hydroxybenzoic acid esters, bronopol, hydroxyethyl cellulose, propylene glycol.

**Product licence number** 0041/0008.

*Product licence holder:* Bioglan Laboratories Limited, Hitchin, Herts.

# MIACALCIC* AMPOULES
# MIACALCIC* MULTIDOSE VIALS

## Qualitative and quantitative composition

*Ampoules:* Salcatonin BP 50 IU/ml and 100 IU/ml.

*Multidose vials:* Salcatonin BP 200 IU/ml.

**Pharmaceutical form** Clear, colourless parenteral solution.

## Clinical particulars

*Therapeutic indications:*

*Hypercalcaemic crisis:* Due to tumoral osteolysis secondary to breast, lung, kidney and other malignancies.

Due to osteolysis induced by myeloma.

Due to primary hyperparathyroidism.

*Short term treatment of chronic hypercalcaemia:* Paget's disease of bone (osteitis deformans), particularly in cases with:

– bone pain;
– neurological complications;
– increased bone turnover reflected in elevated alkaline phosphatase and hydroxyproline excretion;
– progressive extension of bone lesions;
– incomplete or repeated fractures.

*Pain associated with advanced metastatic bone cancer:*

*Short term use in post menopausal osteoporosis:* Studies based on total blood calcium determinators have indicated that Miacalcic may be effective in the prevention of progressive loss of bone mass in the treatment of post-menopausal osteoporosis.

*Posology and method of administration:* Miacalcic may be administered subcutaneously, intramuscularly or by intravenous injection.

The solution provided in multidose vials contains phenol (5 mg/ml) as a preservative and is not suitable for intravenous bolus injection.

The 50 IU/ml or 100 IU/ml ampoules can be used for intravenous infusion, which is the most effective method of administration and should always be used in emergencies or severe cases. However, there is a loss of potency of approximately 20% when Miacalcic is diluted. This should be taken into account when calculating dosage 5–10 IU (0.50–0.1 ml) Miacalcic per kg body weight daily, by slow intravenous infusion in 500 ml physiological saline over at least six hours.

*Short term treatment of chronic hypercalcaemia:* 5–10 IU per kg body weight daily by subcutaneous or intramuscular injection as a single dose or in two divided doses. If the volume for injection exceeds 2 ml intramuscular injection is preferable and multiple sites of injection should be used.

Treatment should be adjusted according to the patient's response and should not exceed three months; the definitive treatment should be for the underlying cause.

*Paget's disease:* 100 IU (1 ml) daily by subcutaneous or intramuscular injection. In some cases the injections may be given only every second day. In particular after improvement of the objective and subjective symptoms, an injection of 50 IU per day may be sufficient. Clinical improvement is usually seen within 3 months, but may occasionally be delayed for as long as a year.

Treatment should be limited to one course of 6 months followed by a treatment free period. A new treatment course of 6 months can be resumed in the case of biochemical relapse.

*Pain associated with advanced metastatic bone cancer:* 200 IU, depending on tolerability, up to 4 times in 24 hours by either the subcutaneous or intramuscular route has been shown to be effective in some patients and to permit reduction in the dose of concomitantly administered analgesics. Relief of pain may last for one week or longer. Treatment may be repeated at the discretion of the physician.

*Postmenopausal osteoporosis:* 100 IU daily by subcutaneous or intramuscular injection. Patients should also receive supplementary calcium (equivalent to 600 mg elemental calcium daily) and if necessary, vitamin D (400 units daily). An adequate diet is also essential.

*Use in children:* There is very little experience with use in children. The recommended adult dose should be reduced according to the child's lower body weight.

Miacalcic should be given to children for periods not more than a few weeks, unless physicians conclude that longer treatment is indicated on compelling grounds. Careful surveillance of bone growth is recommended.

*Use in elderly:* There is no evidence to suggest that elderly patients require different dosages or show different side-effects from younger patients. However, elderly patients should be supervised as factors sometimes associated with ageing such as poor diet or impaired renal function, may affect tolerance and may required dosage reduction.

*Contra-indications:* Hypersensitivity see *Precautions*.

*Special warnings and precautions for use:* Treatment with Miacalcic markedly reduces serum alkaline phosphatase and urinary hydroxyproline excretion, often to normal levels. In rare cases alkaline phosphatase and hydroxyproline excretion levels may rise after an initial fall; the physician must then judge from the clinical picture whether treatment should be continued. Disorders of bone metabolism may recur one or several months after treatment has been discontinued, necessitating a new course of Miacalcic.

Miacalcic is excreted mainly via the kidneys, therefore dosage adjustment may be required in patients with impaired renal function. Antibodies to salmon calcitonin may develop in a few patients following prolonged therapy. Clinical efficacy, however, is usually not affected. Escape phenomena are sometimes observed following prolonged use, but this is not necessarily related to the development of antibodies. Therapeutic response to Miacalcic may be restored after an interruption of treatment.

*Interaction with other medicaments and other forms of interaction:* Following injections of calcitonin, serum calcium levels may be transiently lowered but usually stay within normal values. This effect is noted most frequently on initiation of therapy where bone turnover is abnormally high, but diminishes as osteoclastic activity is reduced with Miacalcic. This phenomenon does not usually give rise to complications. It is theoretically possible that dosage adjustments may be required in patients receiving concurrent cardiac glycosides as their effect might be modified by changes in cellular electrolyte concentrations.

*Pregnancy and lactation:* Salmon calcitonin has been shown to cause decrease in foetal birth weight in rabbits when given in doses of 14–56 times the dose recommended for human use. Since calcitonin does not cross the placental barrier, this finding may be due to metabolic effects of calcitonin on the pregnant animal. Studies have not been carried out in pregnant women. Whenever possible, treatment should be avoided in women of child-bearing potential. Calcitonin has been shown to inhibit lactation in animals and should not be administered to nursing mothers.

*Effects on ability to drive and to use machines:* None known.

*Other undesirable side-effects:* Nausea and occasional vomiting, slight facial flushing accompanied by a sensation of heat.

Occasional irritation at injection site, skin rash, diarrhoea and dizziness have occurred. Effects are usually dose dependent and occur more frequently after intravenous than after subcutaneous or intramuscular administration. They usually subside spontaneously and a temporary reduction in dosage is only necessary in exceptional cases.

Anti-emetics may be used if necessary during treatment.

Hypersensitivity reactions may occur (see *Precautions*).

As Miacalcic is a polypeptide, local or general hypersensitivity reactions are a possibility in rare cases. Symptoms may include local effects at the injection site or generalised skin reactions. Isolated anaphylactic-type reactions resulting in tachycardia, dyspnoea, hypotension and collapse have been reported. If any symptoms observed can definitely be ascribed to the drug, the treatment should be stopped.

In patients with a history of allergic reactions a skin sensitivity test is advisable before starting treatment. A 1:100 dilution in physiological saline may be used.

*Overdosage:* No serious consequences due to overdosage have yet been reported. Treatment would be symptomatic.

### Pharmacological properties
*Pharmacodynamic properties:* Calcitonin is a major regulating factor in mineral and skeletal metabolism; it interferes with the action of parathyroid hormone in the maintenance of skeletal mass, by acting both on bone and on calcium homeostasis. It markedly reduces the removal of calcium from bone in conditions with a greatly increased rate of resorption and formation such as Paget's disease and malignant osteolysis. Osteoclast activity is inhibited and osteoblast formation and activity seem to be stimulated. Calcitonin inhibits osteolysis, thus lowering the abnormally increased serum calcium. Additionally, it increases the urinary excretion of calcium, phosphorus and sodium by reducing their tubular re-uptake. Serum calcium is not reduced below the normal range.

Calcitonin reduces gastric and exocrine pancreatic secretion without influencing gastrointestinal motility. Clinical experience demonstrates that Miacalcic possesses analgesic activity. Investigations have shown specific salmon calcitonin binding sites in some areas of the central nervous system.

All calcitonin structures show 32 amino-acids in a single chain, the sequence of which differs from species to species. Due to its greater affinity to receptor binding sites than synthetic calcitonins from mammalian species, including the synthetic human calcitonin, Miacalcic is clinically more potent and longer acting.

*Pharmacokinetic properties:* Pharmacokinetic studies indicate the bioavailability after intramuscular or subcutaneous injection to be about 70%. Maximum plasma concentrations are obtained within one hour. Elimination half-life of 70 to 90 minutes. Miacalcic and its metabolites are excreted up to 95% by the kidney, percentage of parent drug being about 2%. The apparent volume of distribution is 0.15–0.3 litre/kg and the protein binding is 30–40%.

*Pre-clinical safety data:* No relevant pre-clinical safety data are available. Miacalcic has been marketed for many years.

### Pharmaceutical particulars
*List of excipients:*
*50 IU/ml and 100 IU/ml ampoules:* Glacial acetic acid, sodium acetate trihydrate, sodium chloride, water for injection.

*400 IU/2 ml multidose vials:* Glacial acetic acid, sodium acetate trihydrate, sodium chloride, phenol, water for injection.

*Incompatibilities:* None.

*Shelf life:* 50 IU/ml and 100 IU/ml ampoules – 60 months. 400 IU/2 ml multidose vials – 36 months, 1 month after initial use.

*Special precautions for storage:* Store in a refrigerator (2–8°C). Do not freeze. Allow to reach room temperature before subcutaneous or intramuscular use.

The multidose vial can be stored at room temperature once started. Its unused portion of contents must be discarded one month after initial use.

*Nature and contents of container:* Ampoules: glass ampoule – uncoloured.

Multidose vial: glass vial – uncoloured, with rubber stopper.

*Instructions for use/handling:* Allow to reach room temperature before intramuscular or subcutaneous use. Solutions for infusions should be prepared immediately before use and glass or hard plastic containers should not be used.

### Marketing authorisation numbers
50 IU ampoule     0101/0202
100 IU ampoule     0101/0095
400 IU multidose vial     0101/0203

**Date of approval/revision of SPC**   May 1996.

**Legal category**   POM.

## NAVIDREX*

**Presentation** Navidrex tablets containing 0.5 mg of Cyclopenthiazide BP as white, flat, circular tablets with bevelled edges, bearing the monogram 'CIBA' on one side, and the letters AO on each side of a breakline on the other.

### Uses
*Indications:* Navidrex is indicated for:

The treatment of mild to moderate hypertension, in more severe hypertension it may be used in conjunction with other antihypertensive agents.

Stable , chronic heart failure of mild to moderate degree (functional class II, III), as long as creatinine clearance is > 30 ml/min.

Oedema of specific origin:
- fluid retention in pre-menstrual syndrome only as short-term therapy and only if the gain in weight is the main symptom and is well documented.
- ascites due to cirrhosis of the liver in stable patients under close control.
- oedema associated with renal disease.

*Mode of action:* Cyclopenthiazide, the active substance of Navidrex, is a benzothiadiazine (thiazide) diuretic.

Thiazide diuretics act primarily on the distal renal tubule (early convoluted part), inhibiting NaCL reabsorption (by antagonising the Na$_+$ Cl$_-$ cotransporter), promoting Ca$_{++}$ reabsorption (by an unknown mechanism). The enhanced delivery of Na$_+$ and water to the cortical collecting tubule and/or the increased flow rate leads to increased secretion and excretion of K$_+$ and H$_+$.

In healthy volunteers or in patients with oedema, cyclopenthiazide administration results in a dose dependent increase in urinary excretion of sodium and chloride and a less prominent dose dependent increase in potassium excretion. The diuretic and natriuretic effect appears within 1-3 hours and subsides within 24 hours.

Thiazide-induced diuresis initially leads to a decrease in plasma volume, cardiac output and systemic blood pressure. The renin-angiotensin-aldosterone system may possibly become activated. On continued administration the hypotensive effect is maintained, probably due to the fall in peripheral resistance; cardiac output returns to pretreatment values, plasma volume remains somewhat reduced and plasma renin activity may be elevated.

During repeated administration of Navidrex the antihypertensive effect is dose dependent from 125-500µg/day. The maximum hypotensive effect is reached with 500µg in most patients. In chronic heart failure, daily doses of 1 mg may enhance the therapeutic benefit but at higher doses the expected benefit must be balanced by the increased risk of side-effects.

As with other diuretics, when Navidrex is given as monotherapy, blood pressure control is achieved in about half of patients with mild to moderate hypertension. In general the elderly and black patients are found to respond well to diuretics as primary therapy.

Combined treatment with other antihypertensives has an additive effect and in a large proportion of patients failing to respond to monotherapy, a further decrease in blood pressure can thus be achieved.

*Pharmacokinetics:* Based on limited pharmacokinetic data the variability of the amount of cyclopenthiazide absorbed appears to be low. After oral administration of single doses of 0.5 or 1.0 mg cyclopenthiazide peak plasma levels of about 3 and 7ng/ml respectively, were reached after an average of 3-4 hours. Twelve hours after the administration of 1 mg cyclopenthiazide, the plasma concentration decreases to about 25% of the peak concentration.

In rats cyclopenthiazide is excreted mainly by tubular excretion. In humans receiving cyclopenthiazide the drug can be detected in the urine. At 24 hours after the administration of a 0.5 mg dose, for instance, the concentration in the urine is about 400 ng/ml.

**Dosage and administration** The dosage of Navidrex should be individually titrated to give the lowest effective dose; this is particularly important in the elderly. Navidrex should be taken orally, a single dose of up to 1 mg given in the morning is recommended.

*Adults:* Hypertension: Initially 0.25 mg daily, if necessary the dosage may be raised to 0.5 mg daily. For a given dose, the full effect is reached after 4-6 weeks. If the decrease in blood pressure proves inadequate with 0.5 mg/day, combined treatment with other antihypertensive drugs such as a β-blocker (if necessary, a β-blocker and vasodilator), or an ACE inhibitor is recommended. It is recommended that diuretics (Navidrex) should be withdrawn for several days before starting the ACE inhibitor.

Stable, chronic heart failure (NYHA class II, III): Initially 0.25-0.5 mg daily. If necessary the dose may be titrated up to 1 mg/day; higher doses rarely achieve any further benefit. The lowest effective dose should be used for maintenance therapy. If the response proves inadequate, a positive inotropic drug (e.g. digitalis), possibly combined with an ACE inhibitor may be added. In the latter case a reduction in the dose of Navidrex may be necessary.

Oedema: The lowest effective dose should be determined by titration and administered over limited periods only. Doses should not exceed 0.5 mg/day.

*Children:* Adequate experience regarding the dosage in children is lacking.

*Use in the elderly:* Particular caution should be exercised since the elderly are more susceptible to electrolyte imbalances (see Precautions).

*Use in patients with renal impairment:* There is no evidence on the effect of renal impairment on the excretion of cyclopenthiazide but experience with other thiazide diuretics indicates that a 50% reduction of the normal adult dose may be appropriate.

### Contra-indications, warnings, etc
*Contra-indications:* Anuria, severe renal and hepatic failure. Hypersensitivity to cyclopenthiazide and other sulphonamide derivatives. Refractory hypokalaemia, hyponatraemia and hypercalcaemia. Symptomatic hyperuricaemia (history of gout or uric acid calculi). Hypertension during pregnancy. Creatinine clearance lower than 30 ml/min. Conditions involving enhanced potassium loss, e.g. salt-losing nephropathies and prerenal (cardiogenic) impairment of kidney function. Untreated Addison's disease. Concomitant lithium therapy.

*Warnings:* Navidrex should be used with caution in patients with renal disease or with impaired hepatic function (see 'Contra-indications' and 'Precautions').

Navidrex especially at the start of treatment, may impair the patient's reactions, e.g. when driving or operating machinery.

*Precautions:*
Electrolytes: As with all thiazide diuretics, potassium loss induced by Navidrex is dose dependent. With daily doses of 125 and 500µg, given for 8 weeks the decreases in serum potassium concentrations averaged 0.2 and 0.6 mmol/l, respectively. For chronic treatment serum potassium concentrations should be checked initially and then after 3-4 weeks. Thereafter–if the potassium balance is not disturbed by additional factors (e.g. vomiting, diarrhoea, change in renal function etc.,–checks should be carried out every 4-6 months.

Titrated co-administration of an oral potassium salt (e.g. KCl) may be considered in patients receiving digitalis; glucocorticoids or ACTH, in patients exhibiting signs of coronary heart disease, unless they are also receiving an ACE inhibitor; in patients on high doses of a β-adrenergic agonist; and in all cases where plasma concentrations are < 3.0 nmol/l. If oral potassium preparations are not tolerated, Navidrex may be combined with a potassium-sparing diuretic (e.g. amiloride).

In all cases of combined treatment, maintenance or normalisation of the potassium balance should be checked closely. If hypokalaemia is accompanied by clinical signs (e.g. muscular weakness, paresis and ECG alteration), Navidrex should be discontinued.

Combined treatment consisting of Navidrex and a potassium salt or a potassium-sparing diuretic must be avoided in patients also receiving ACE inhibitors.

There have been isolated reports of hyponatraemia with neurological symptoms (e.g. nausea, debility, progressive disorientation and apathy).

Serum electrolyte levels should be monitored particularly in the elderly, and in patients with ascites due to liver cirrhosis and in patients with oedema due to nephrotic syndrome. For the latter condition, Navidrex should be used only under close control in normokalaemic patients with no signs of volume depletion or severe hypoalbuminaemia.

As with other diuretics, Navidrex may cause disturbances in the electrolyte balance during prolonged treatment. Since the excretion of electrolytes is increased, a very strict low salt diet should be avoided.
Metabolic effects:
Navidrex may raise the serum uric acid level but attacks of gout are rarely observed during chronic treatment.

Glucose intolerance may occur (this may manifest as hypoglycaemia and glycouria) but diabetes mellitus very seldom occurs under treatment.

In patients with hyperlipidaemia, serum lipids should be monitored regularly. Small and partly reversible increases in plasma concentrations of total cholesterol, triglycerides or low density lipoprotein cholesterol have been reported in patients during long term treatments with thiazides and thiazide-like diuretics. The clinical relevance of these findings is not clear. Withdrawal of Navidrex should be considered if serum lipids rise further.

Navidrex should not be used as first line therapy for long-term treatment in patients with overt diabetes mellitus or in subjects receiving therapy for hypercholesterolaemia (diet or combined).

Other precautions: Navidrex may accumulate in patients with impaired renal function. At creatinine clearance levels of < 30 ml/min (or at serum creatinine levels of > 2.5 mg/100 ml), thiazide diuretics including cyclopenthiazide will not exert a diuretic effect. In such cases, loop diuretics are indicated.

The antihypertensive effect of ACE inhibitors is potentiated by diuretics that increase plasma renin activity. A cautious dosage schedule should therefore be adopted when an ACE inhibitor is added to a diuretic agent.

As with all antihypertensive agents, a cautious dosage schedule is indicated in patients with severe coronary or cerebral arteriosclerosis.

Lupus erythematosus may possibly become activated under treatment with thiazides.

*Use in pregnancy and lactation:* Diuretics are best avoided for the management of oedema or hypertension in pregnancy as their use may be associated with hypovolaemia, increased blood viscosity and reduced placental perfusion. Diuretics do not prevent or alter the course of oedema, proteinuria or hypertension during pregnancy (pre-eclampsia). Cyclopenthiazide must not be used to treat hypertension during pregnancy (see Contra-indications), and the use of Navidrex for other indications (e.g. heart disease) during pregnancy should be avoided unless there are no safer alternatives. There have been reports of foetal bone marrow depression, thrombocytopenia, and foetal and neonatal jaundice associated with the use of thiazide diuretics.

Cyclopenthiazide may be excreted into the breast milk and thus mothers taking Navidrex should refrain from breast-feeding their infants.

*Drug interactions:* Curare derivatives and antihypertensive drugs: Diuretics potentiate the action of these drugs (e.g. guanethidine, methyldopa, beta-blockers, vasodilators, calcium antagonists and ACE inhibitors).

Lithium: Diuretics raise the blood level of lithium. Where lithium has produced polyuria, diuretics may exert a paradoxical antidiuretic effect. (see 'Contraindications').

Corticosteroids, ACTH, amphotericin and carbenoxolone: These may increase the hypokalaemic effect of diuretics.

Anti-diabetic agents: It may prove necessary to adjust the dosage of insulin and oral anti-diabetic agents.

Digitalis: Hypokalaemia or hypomagnesaemia possibly occurring as unwanted effects may cause onset of digitalis-induced cardiac arrhythmias.

Non-steroidal anti-inflammatory agents: Concomitant administration of certain NSAIDs (e.g. indomethacin) may reduce the diuretic and antihypertensive activity of Navidrex; there have been isolated reports of a deterioration in renal function in predisposed patients.

Allopurinol: Co-administration of thiazide diuretics may increase the incidence of hypersensitivity reactions to allopurinol. (see 'contra-indications')

Amantadine: Co-administration of thiazide diuretics may increase the risk of adverse effects from amantadine.

Antineoplastic agents (e.g. cyclophosphamide, methotrexate): Concomitant use of thiazide diuretics may reduce renal excretion of cytotoxic agents and enhance the myelosuppresive effects.

Anticholinergic agents (e.g. atropine, biperiden): The bioavailability of thiazide type diuretics may be increased by anticholinergic agents, apparently due to a decrease in gastro-intestinal motility and stomach emptying rate.

Cholestyramine: Absorption of thiazide diuretics is decreased by cholestyramine. A decrease of the pharmacological effect may be expected.

Vitamin D: Concomitant use of thiazide diuretics may decrease urinary excretion of calcium and coadministration of Vitamin D may potentiate the increase in serum calcium.

Cyclosporin: Concomitant treatment with diuretics may increase the risk of hyperuricaemia and gout type complications.

Calcium salts: Concomitant use of thiazide type diuretics may cause hypercalcaemia by increasing tubular calcium resorption.

Diazoxide: Thiazide diuretics may enhance the hyperglycaemic effect of diazoxide.

Methyldopa: There have been reports in the literature of haemolytic anaemia occurring with concomitant use of a thiazide diuretic and methyldopa.

*Side-effects:*
*Electrolytes and metabolic disorders:* Frequently: mainly at higher doses, hypokalaemia, and rise in blood lipids (see Precautions). Occasionally: hyponatraemia, hypomagnesaemia and hyperuricaemia. Rarely: hypercalcaemia, hyperglycaemia, glycosuria, worsening of diabetic metabolic state. In isolated cases: hypochloraemic alkalosis.
*Skin:* Occasionally: urticaria and other forms of skin rash. Rarely: photosensitisation. Isolated cases: necrotising vasculitis and toxic epidermal necrolysis, cutaneous lupus erythematosus-like reactions, reactivation of cutaneous lupus erythematosus.

*Gastro-intestinal tract:* Occasionally: loss of appetite, mild nausea and vomiting. Rarely: abdominal distress, constipation, diarrhoea and gastro-intestinal discomfort. Isolated cases: pancreatitis:
*Liver:* Rarely: intrahepatic cholestasis.
*Cardiovascular system:* Occasionally: postural hypotension which may be aggravated by alcohol, anaesthetics or sedatives. Rarely: cardiac arrhythmias.
*Central nervous system:* Rarely: headache, dizziness or muzziness, sleep disturbance, depression and paraesthesia.
*Special senses:* Visual disturbances particularly in the first few weeks of treatment.
*Blood:* Rarely: thrombocytopenia sometimes with purpura. Isolated cases: leucopenia, agranulocytosis, bone marrow depression and haemolytic anaemia.
*Other effects:* Occasionally: impotence. Isolated cases: hypersensitivity reactions–respiratory distress including pneumonitis and pulmonary oedema. Gout may be precipitated or aggravated in susceptible patients or those with a history of the illness but there have been only isolated reports of attacks occurring during chronic therapy.

*Overdosage:*
*Symptoms:* Dizziness, nausea, somnolence, hypovolaemia, hypotension and electrolyte disturbances associated with cardiac arrhythmias and muscle spasms.
*Treatment:* There is no specific antidote to Navidrex. Gastric lavage, emesis or activated charcoal should be employed to reduce absorption. Blood pressure and fluid and electrolyte balance should be monitored and appropriate corrective measures taken. Intravenous fluid and electrolyte replacement may be indicated.

**Pharmaceutical precautions** Protect from heat and moisture. Store below 25˚C.

**Legal category** POM.

**Package quantities** Navidrex tablets are available in blister packs of 28.

**Further information** Nil

**Product licence number** 00101/0423

# NAVISPARE*

**Presentation** Navispare tablets containing 0.25 mg Cyclopenthiazide BP and 2.5 mg Amiloride Hydrochloride BP as orange yellow, round film-coated tablets marked CIBA on one face and 'RC' on the other.

The tablets also contain gluten (wheat starch), lactose and polyethoxylated caster oils.

**Uses**
*Indications:* Navispare contains a thiazide diuretic in combination with a potassium-conserving diuretic and is indicated for the treatment of mild to moderate hypertension.

*Mode of action:* Cyclopenthiazide is a thiazide diuretic which exerts its diuretic effect by inhibiting the reabsorption of sodium, chloride and water probably at the distal renal tubules.

Amiloride hydrochloride is a mild diuretic that acts mainly on the distal part of the renal tubule. It increases the excretion of sodium and chloride and reduces the excretion of potassium.

**Dosage and administration**
*Adults:* Usually 1 or 2 Navispare tablets taken once a day in the morning.

*Elderly:* Although no special dosage regime is necessary in the elderly, particular caution should be exercised in the elderly since they are more susceptible to electrolyte imbalances.

*Children:* Navispare is not suitable for use in children.

**Contra-indications, warnings, etc**
*Contra-indications:* Navispare is contra-indicated in patients hypersensitive to cyclopenthiazide or other sulphonamide derivatives; Addison's disease; hyperkalaemia; in the presence of other potassium conserving agents or potassium supplements; anuria; severe renal and hepatic failure; diabetic nephropathy; concurrent lithium therapy; refractory hypokalaemia and hyponatraemia; hypercalcaemia; symptomatic hyperuricaemia.

*Precautions:*
Diabetes mellitus: Hyperkalaemia has occurred in diabetic patients receiving amiloride hydrochloride, especially those with chronic renal disease or prerenal azotaemia. The status of renal function should therefore be determined before use in a known or suspected diabetic patient. Navispare should be discontinued for at least three days before a glucose tolerance test. Prolonged doses may bring about a decrease in glucose tolerance and precipitate a diabetic condition. In known diabetics the addition of a thiazide to the treatment regime may alter their antidiabetic requirement.

Metabolic or respiratory acidosis: Potassium conserving therapy should be initiated with caution in patients in whom metabolic or respiratory acidosis may occur eg: patients with cardiopulmonary disease or decompensated diabetes. Shifts in acid-base balance alter the balance of extracellular-intracellular potassium and the development of acidosis may be associated with rapid increases in plasma potassium.

Electrolyte considerations: In patients with renal impairment, a rise in blood urea can occur. In such cases, either the dose should be reduced or the treatment interrupted temporarily. Thiazides may precipitate an attack of gout in patients predisposed to this condition.

The elderly, especially those suffering from chronic disease and patients with hepatic cirrhosis are more susceptible to a lack of electrolyte and fluid balance homeostasis. During treatment with thiazides hyponatraemia accompanied by neurological symptoms has been observed in isolated cases. In the elderly and patients with hepatic cirrhosis, the serum electrolytes should be monitored at more frequent intervals.

Patients receiving relatively high doses of thiazides may develop hypomagnesaemia accompanied by signs and symptoms such as nervousness, muscle spasms and cardiac arrhythmias.

Miscellaneous: In patients with hyperlipidaemia, the serum lipids should be regularly monitored. In the event of a rise in the serum lipids, withdrawal of the thiazide medication should be considered.

Lupus erythematosus may possibly become activated under treatment with thiazides.

*Use in pregnancy and lactation:* Diuretics are best avoided for the management of hypertension in pregnancy as their use may be associated with hypovolaemia, increased blood viscosity and reduced placental perfusion. There is inadequate evidence of safety in human pregnancy and there have been reports of foetal bone marrow depression, thrombocytopenia, and foetal and neonatal jaundice reported with the use of thiazide diuretics.

As cyclopenthiazide passes into breast milk, Navispare should be avoided in mothers who wish to breast-feed. It is not known whether amiloride hydrochloride passes into breast milk.

*Drug interactions:* The concomitant administration of thiazides with other antihypertensive agents (e.g. beta-blockers, vasodilators, calcium antagonists, may necessitate adjustment of the dosage of those drugs. The concomitant administration of potassium sparing agents such as amiloride and ACE inhibitors may increase serum potassium levels and is not to be recommended. However, if the concomitant use of these agents is deemed appropriate, they should be used with caution and with frequent monitoring of plasma potassium.

NSAIDs may attenuate the antihypertensive effect of thiazide diuretics. Thiazide containing drugs may increase the responsiveness to tubocurarine.

Orthostatic hypotension may occur and may be potentiated by alcohol, barbiturates and narcotics.

*Side-effects:* Navispare is generally well tolerated. Reported side effects of the combination include dizziness, headache, lightheadedness, tiredness, nausea and vomiting, discomfort/pain in the chest. However, the following side effects of cyclopenthiazide and amiloride as single agents have been reported.
Cyclopenthiazide:
*Skin:* Allergic urticaria (nettle rash) and other forms of skin rash, photosensitisation. In very rare cases: necrotising vasculitis.
*Gastro-intestinal tract:* Loss of appetite, mild nausea, vomiting, gastrospasm, diarrhoea or possibly constipation, pancreatitis.
*Central nervous system:* Headache, muzziness, dizziness. Occasionally: sleep disturbances, depression, paraesthesiae.
*Blood:* Thrombocytopenia. In isolated cases: leucopenia, agranulocytosis, anaemia, purpura, and very rarely bone marrow depression.
*Electrolytes:* Hypokalaemia, hyponatraemia, hypomagnesaemia. In isolated cases: hypochloraemic alkalosis and hypercalcaemia. If hypercalcaemia occurs, further diagnostic clarification is necessary (e.g. possibility of hyperparathyroidism).
*Liver:* In rare cases: intrahepatic cholestasis or jaundice.
*Miscellaneous:* Occasionally impotence.
*Metabolic:* Hyperuricaemia, hyperglycaemia, glycosuria. Gout or diabetes may be precipitated or aggravated. Increased blood lipid levels in response to higher doses.
*Cardiovascular system:* Postural hypotension and cardiac arrhythmias; postural hypotension may be aggravated by alcohol, anaesthetics, or sedatives.
Amiloride:
*Gastro-intestinal tract:* Anorexia, nausea, vomiting, diarrhoea, constipation, abdominal pain, GI bleeding, jaundice, thirst, dyspepsia, heartburn, flatulence.
*Central nervous system:* Dizziness, vertigo, paraes-

thesiae, tremors, encephalopathy, nervousness, mental confusion, insomnia, decreased libido, depression, somnolence.

*Cardiovascular system:* Angina pectoris, orthostatic hypotension, arrhythmias, palpitation.

*Respiratory:* Cough, dyspnoea.

*Special senses:* Nasal congestion, visual disturbances, increased intra-ocular pressure, tinnitus.

*Urogenital:* Impotence, polyuria, dysuria, frequency of micturition.

*Musculoskeletal:* Muscle cramps, joint pain.

*Skin and appendages:* Pruritus, rash, dryness of mouth, alopecia.

*Overdosage:*

*Signs:* In cases of overdosage the following signs and symptoms may occur: dizziness, nausea, somnolence, hypovolaemia, hypotension and electrolyte disturbances associated with cardiac arrhythmias and muscle spasms.

*Treatment:* Emesis should be induced or gastric lavage performed. Intravenous fluid and electrolyte replacement may be indicated.

**Pharmaceutical precautions** Protect from moisture. Store below 25°C.

**Legal category** POM

**Package quantities** Blister packs of 28 tablets.

**Further information** Nil.

**Product licence number** 00101/0424

## NAVOBAN*

### Presentation
*Ampoules 5 mg/5 ml:* Clear, colourless or very faintly brown-yellow solution in a 5 ml, uncoloured glass ampoule. Each ampoule contains 5.64 mg tropisetron hydrochloride in 5 ml, equivalent to 5 mg tropisetron base in 5 ml.

*Capsules 5 mg:* Opaque, yellow and white, hard gelatin capsules, 16 mm in length and 6 mm in diameter. Each capsule contains 5.64 mg tropisetron hydrochloride, equivalent to 5 mg tropisetron base and is marked Navoban 5 mg in red print.

### Uses
*Principal actions:* Navoban is a highly potent and selective competitive antagonist of the 5-HT$_3$ receptor, a subclass of serotonin receptors located on peripheral neurons and within the CNS. Certain substances, including some chemotherapeutic agents, are believed to trigger the release of serotonin (5-HT) from enterochromaffin-like cells in the visceral mucosa and initiate the emesis reflex and its accompanying feeling of nausea. Navoban selectively blocks the excitation of the pre-synaptic 5-HT$_3$ receptors of the peripheral neurons in this reflex, and may exert additional direct actions within the CNS on 5-HT$_3$ receptors mediating the actions of vagal input to the area postrema. Navoban has a 24 hour duration of action which allows once-a-day administration. In studies where Navoban has been administered over multiple chemotherapy cycles, treatment has remained effective.

Navoban prevents nausea and vomiting induced by cancer chemotherapy without causing extrapyramidal side effects.

*Indications:* Prevention of cancer chemotherapy-induced nausea and vomiting.

### Dosage and administration
*Adults:* Six-day courses of Navoban 5 mg daily are recommended.

On day one, shortly before chemotherapy commences, 5 mg Navoban should be given by intravenous administration as a slow injection or an injection into a running infusion. For intravenous infusion, one Navoban ampoule should be diluted in 100 ml of sodium chloride 0.9% w/v (physiological saline). Alternative diluents are Ringers solution, glucose 5% or fructose 5%. Diluents other than those specified should not be used.

On days two to six, one 5 mg Navoban capsule should be taken with water each morning upon rising, at least one hour before food.

*Children:* Navoban is not recommended for use in children.

*Use in the elderly:* There is no evidence that elderly patients require different dosages or experience side effects different from those in younger patients.

*Use in poor metabolisers of sparteine/debrisoquine:* In patients belonging to this group (about 8% of the caucasian population) the elimination half-life of tropisetron is prolonged (4 to 5 times longer than in extensive metabolisers). However, studies indicate that for 6-day courses in patients with poor metabolism the recommended daily dose of 5 mg Navoban does not need to be reduced.

*Use in patients with impaired hepatic or renal function:* No change in the pharmacokinetics of tropisetron occurs in patients with acute hepatitis or fatty liver disease. In contrast, patients with liver cirrhosis or impaired kidney function may have plasma concentrations up to 50% higher than those found in healthy volunteers belonging to the group of extensive metabolisers of sparteine/debrisoquine. Nevertheless, no dosage reduction is necessary in such patients when the recommended 6-day courses of Navoban 5 mg daily are given.

*Use in patients with uncontrolled hypertension:* In patients with uncontrolled hypertension, it is important not to exceed the recommended daily dose since higher dosages, particularly when administered after intravenous prehydration therapy, have been reported to aggravate this condition.

### Contra-indications, warnings, etc
*Contra-indications:* Hypersensitivity to tropisetron or other 5-HT$_3$ receptor antagonists.

*Use in pregnancy and lactation:* Navoban must not be used during pregnancy.

There is no experience with Navoban in human pregnancy. In animal studies no teratogenic effects occurred at doses which were not toxic to the dams, but effects on reproductive capacity were observed. Therefore, women should not try to conceive when on Navoban therapy.

It is not known whether tropisetron is excreted into human milk. Patients taking Navoban should not, therefore, breast-feed.

*Precautions:* Concomitant administration of Navoban with therapeutic agents known to induce hepatic enzymes may result in lower tropisetron plasma concentrations, particularly in extensive metabolisers. Conversely, the effects of agents which characteristically inhibit these enzyme systems may lead to enhanced plasma concentrations. Such changes are unlikely to be of practical importance provided the recommended 6-day courses of Navoban 5 mg daily are adhered to.

In several in vitro and in vivo tests, Navoban has been shown to have no mutagenic potential, but in a long-term study in male mice, at doses of 30 mg/kg per day (300 times the human daily dose) an increased incidence of hepatocellular adenomas was observed.

Patients should be cautioned against driving or operating machinery until it is established that they do not become dizzy or drowsy whilst taking Navoban.

*Side-effects:* The most frequently reported adverse reactions are headache, constipation, dizziness, fatigue and gastrointestinal disorders such as abdominal pain and diarrhoea.

In very rare instances, collapse, syncope, bradycardia or cardiovascular arrest have been reported with Navoban. However, as with other 5-HT$_3$ receptor antagonists, the relationship to Navoban has not been established. Some may have been caused by the concomitant chemotherapy or the underlying disease.

As with other 5-HT$_3$ receptor antagonists, hypersensitivity reactions ('type I-reactions') with one or more of the following symptoms have been rarely reported: facial flushing and/or generalised urticaria, chest tightness, dyspnoea, acute bronchospasm, hypotension.

*Overdosage:* At very high repeated doses, visual hallucinations have been noted and, in patients with pre-existing hypertension, an increase in blood pressure has been observed. Seizure threshold may also be reduced in susceptible patients. Symptomatic treatment with frequent monitoring of vital signs and close observation of the patient is indicated.

### Pharmaceutical precautions
*Capsules:* Store in a dry place below 25°C.

*Ampoules:* Diluted solution should be used immediately or prepared under aseptic conditions and stored between 2°C and 8°C for no more than 24 hours.

### Legal category POM.

### Package quantities
*5 mg capsules:* Boxes of 1 blister strip containing 5×5 mg capsules; boxes of 10 blister strips each containing 5×5 mg capsules.

*5 mg in 5 ml ampoules:* Boxes of 1×5 ml ampoule; boxes of 10×5 ml ampoules.

**Further information** The absorption of Navoban from the gastrointestinal tract is rapid (mean half-life of about 20 minutes) and extensive (more than 95%). The peak plasma concentration is attained within 3 hours. Owing to a saturable metabolic capacity, the absolute bioavailability is dependent on the dose.

Tropisetron is 71% bound to plasma protein in a non-specific manner. The volume of distribution is 400 to 600 L. The metabolism of tropisetron is linked to the sparteine/debrisoquine polymorphism.

Ingestion of the capsule with food has no relevant influence on the bioavailability but may slightly delay the absorption of Navoban.

**Product licence numbers**
*5 mg in 5 ml ampoules*     0101/0344
*5 mg capsules*            0101/0345

## NEORAL*
**Qualitative and quantitative composition** Neoral Soft Gelatin Capsules containing 10, 25, 50, or 100 mg cyclosporin.

Neoral Oral Solution containing 100 mg cyclosporin/mL.

**Pharmaceutical form** Neoral Soft Gelatin Capsules and Neoral Oral Solution are for oral administration.

Neoral is an improved pharmaceutical form of the active ingredient cyclosporin. Neoral is a pre-concentrate formulation of cyclosporin which undergoes a microemulsification process in the presence of water, either in the form of a beverage or in the form of the gastrointestinal fluid. Neoral reduces the intra-patient variability of pharmacokinetic parameters, with a more consistent absorption profile and less influence of concomitant food intake and the presence of bile. In pharmacokinetic and clinical studies it has been demonstrated that the correlation between trough concentration ($C_{min}$) and total exposure (AUC) is significantly stronger when cyclosporin is given as Neoral than when it is given as Sandimmun*. Neoral therefore allows greater predictability and consistency of cyclosporin exposure.

**Clinical particulars**
*Therapeutic indications:*
*Transplantation indications: Organ transplantation:* Prevention of graft rejection following kidney, liver, heart, combined heart-lung, lung or pancreas transplants.

Treatment of transplant rejection in patients previously receiving other immunosuppressive agents.

*Bone marrow transplantation:* Prevention of graft rejection following bone marrow transplantation and prophylaxis of graft-versus-host disease (GVHD).

Treatment of established graft-versus-host disease (GVHD).

*Non-transplantation indications:*
*Psoriasis:* Neoral Soft Gelatin Capsules and Neoral Oral Solution are indicated in patients with severe psoriasis in whom conventional therapy is ineffective or inappropriate.

*Atopic dermatitis:* Neoral Soft Gelatin Capsules and Neoral Oral Solution are indicated for the short term treatment (8 weeks) of patients with severe atopic dermatitis in whom conventional therapy is ineffective or inappropriate.

*Rheumatoid arthritis:* Neoral Soft Gelatin Capsules and Neoral Oral Solution are indicated for the treatment of severe, active rheumatoid arthritis in patients in whom classical, slow-acting anti-rheumatic agents are inappropriate or ineffective.

*Nephrotic syndrome:* Neoral Soft Gelatin Capsules and Neoral Oral Solution are indicated for the treatment of steroid dependent or steroid resistant nephrotic syndrome (associated with adverse prognostic features) due to minimal change glomerulonephritis, focal segmental glomerulosclerosis or membranous glomerulonephritis in both adults and children.

*Posology and method of administration:* Following initiation of treatment with Neoral, due to the different bioavailabilities of the different oral cyclosporin formulations, patients should not be transferred to any other oral formulation of cyclosporin without appropriate monitoring of cyclosporin blood concentrations, serum creatinine levels and blood pressure. This does not apply to the conversion between Neoral Soft Gelatin Capsules and Neoral Oral Solution as these two forms are bioequivalent.

Due to the differences in bioavailability between different oral fomulations of cyclosporin, it is important that prescribers, pharmacists, and patients be aware that substitution of Neoral with any other oral formulation of cyclosporin is not recommended as this may lead to alterations in cyclosporin blood levels. For this reason it may be appropriate to prescribe by brand.

*Dosage:*
*Transplantation indications – Organ transplantation:* Treatment with Neoral Soft Gelatin Capsules or Neoral Oral Solution should be initiated within 12 hours before transplantation at a dose of 10 to 15 mg/kg body weight given in two divided doses.

As a general rule, treatment should continue at a dose of 10 to 15 mg/kg per day given in two divided doses for one to two weeks post-operatively. Dosage should then be gradually reduced until a maintenance dose of about 2 to 6 mg/kg per day is reached. This total daily dose should be given in two divided doses. Dosage should be adjusted by monitoring cyclosporin trough levels and kidney function (see *Precautions*).

When Neoral is given with other immunosuppressants (e.g. with corticosteroids or as part of a triple or quadruple drug therapy), lower doses (e.g. 3 to 6 mg/

kg per day given orally in two divided doses) may be used for the initial treatment. For trough level monitoring, whole blood is preferred, measured by a specific analytical method. Target trough concentration ranges depend on organ type, time after transplantation and immunosuppressive regimen.

The use of Sandimmun Concentrate for Intravenous Infusion is recommended in organ transplant patients who are unable to take Neoral Soft Gelatin Capsules or Neoral Oral Solution (e.g. shortly after surgery) or in whom the absorption of Neoral might be impaired during episodes of gastrointestinal disturbances. It is recommended, however, that patients be transferred to Neoral therapy as soon as the given circumstances allow (please refer to Sandimmun data sheet/SmPC for prescribing information on Sandimmun Concentrate for I.V. Infusion).

*Bone marrow transplantation/prevention and treatment of graft-versus-host-disease (GVHD):* Sandimmun Concentrate for Intravenous Infusion is usually preferred for initiation of therapy, although Neoral Soft Gelatin Capsules or Neoral Oral Solution may be used (please refer to Sandimmun data sheet/SmPC for prescribing information on Sandimmun Concentrate for I.V. Infusion).

Treatment should continue using Neoral Soft Gelatin Capsules or Neoral Oral Solution at a dosage of 12.5 mg/kg per day, given in two divided doses, for at least three and preferably six months before tailing off to zero. In some cases it may not be possible to withdraw Neoral until a year after bone marrow transplantation. Higher doses of Neoral or the use of Sandimmun Concentrate for Intravenous Infusion may be necessary in the presence of gastro-intestinal disturbances which might decrease absorption.

If Neoral Soft Gelatin Capsules or Neoral Oral Solution are used to initiate therapy, the recommended dose is 12.5 to 15 mg/kg per day, given in two divided doses, starting on the day before transplantation.

If GVHD develops after Neoral is withdrawn it should respond to reinstitution of therapy. Low doses of Neoral should be used for mild, chronic GVHD.

*Non-transplantation indications:*
*Psoriasis* (refer also to *Additional precautions in psoriasis and atopic dermatitis* section): Due to the variability of this condition, treatment must be individualised. To induce remission, the recommended initial dose of Neoral is 2.5 mg/kg a day given orally in two divided doses. If there is no improvement after 1 month, the daily dose may be gradually increased, but should not exceed 5 mg/kg. Treatment should be discontinued if sufficient response is not achieved within 6 weeks on a daily basis of 5 mg/kg per day, or if the effective dose is not compatible with the safety guidelines given below (see *Precautions*). Initial doses of 5 mg/kg per day of Neoral are justified in patients whose condition requires rapid improvement. For *maintenance treatment*, Neoral dosage must be individually titrated to the lowest effective level, and the dosage should not exceed 5 mg/kg a day, given orally in two divided doses.

Some clinical data are available which provide evidence that once satisfactory response is achieved, Neoral may be discontinued and subsequent relapse managed with re-introduction of Neoral at the previous effective dose. In some patients continuous maintenance therapy may be necessary.

*Atopic dermatitis* (refer also to *Additional precautions in atopic dermatitis* section): The recommended dose range for Neoral is 2.5–5 mg/kg per day given orally in two divided doses for a maximum of 8 weeks. If a starting dose of 2.5 mg/kg per day does not achieve a good initial response within 2 weeks the dose may be rapidly increased to a maximum of 5 mg/kg per day. In very severe cases rapid and adequate control of disease is more likely with a starting dose of 5 mg/kg per day, given orally in two divided doses.

*Rheumatoid arthritis* (refer also to *Additional precautions in rheumatoid arthritis* section): It is recommended that initiation of Neoral therapy should take place over a period of 12 weeks. For the first 6 weeks of treatment, the recommended dose is 2.5 mg/kg per day, given orally in two divided doses. If the clinical effect is considered insufficient, the daily dose may be increased gradually as tolerability permits, but should not exceed 4 mg/kg per day.

If, after 3 months of treatment at the maximum permitted or tolerable dose the response is considered inadequate, treatment should be discontinued.

For maintenance treatment the dose has to be titrated individually according to tolerability.

Neoral can be given in combination with low-dose corticosteroids. Pharmacodynamic interactions can occur between cyclosporin and NSAIDs and therefore this combination should be used with care (see *Additional precautions in rheumatoid arthritis* section and *Interactions* section).

Long-term data on the use of cyclosporin in the treatment of rheumatoid arthritis are still limited.

Therefore, it is recommended that patients are re-evaluated after 6 months of maintenance treatment and therapy only continued if the benefits of treatment outweigh the risks.

*Nephrotic syndrome* (refer also to *Additional precautions in nephrotic syndrome* section): To induce remission, the recommended dose is 5 mg/kg per day given orally in two divided doses for adults and 6 mg/kg per day given orally in two divided doses for children if, with the exception of proteinuria, renal function is normal. In patients with impaired renal function, the initial dose should not exceed 2.5 mg/kg per day orally.

In focal segmental glomerulosclerosis, the combination of Neoral and low dose corticosteroids may be of benefit.

In the absence of efficacy after 3 months treatment for minimal change glomerulonephritis and focal segmental glomerulosclerosis or 6 months treatment for membranous glomerulonephritis, Neoral therapy should be discontinued.

For maintenance treatment the maximum recommended dose is 5 mg/kg per day orally in adults or 6 mg/kg per day orally in children. The doses need to be slowly reduced individually according to efficacy (proteinuria) and safety (primarily serum creatinine), to the lowest effective level.

Long term data of cyclosporin in the treatment of nephrotic syndrome are limited. However, in clinical trials patients have received treatment for 1 to 2 years. Long term treatment may be considered if there has been a significant reduction in proteinuria with preservation of creatine clearance and provided adequate precautions are taken (see *Additional precautions in nephrotic syndrome* section).

*Conversion of transplant patients from Sandimmun Soft Gelatin Capsules or Oral Solution to Neoral:* Cyclosporin absorption from Sandimmun oral formulations is highly variable and the relationship between Sandimmun dose and cyclosporin exposure (AUC) is non-linear. In contrast, with Neoral the absorption of cyclosporin is less variable and the correlation between cyclosporin trough concentrations and exposure is much stronger than with Sandimmun.

For converting patients from Sandimmun to Neoral an initial mg for mg conversion from Sandimmun to Neoral is recommended with subsequent dose titration if required. Available data confirm that following this initial mg for mg conversion comparable trough concentrations of cyclosporin in whole blood are achieved, maintaining adequate immunosuppression. In many patients, higher peak concentrations ($C_{max}$) and an increased exposure to the drug (AUC) may occur. No additional adverse events, including renal dysfunction, however, were observed due to these changes in pharmacokinetic parameters during long term treatment. In a small percentage of patients, these changes may be more marked and of clinical significance. Their magnitude depends largely on the individual ability to absorb cyclosporin from the originally used Sandimmun. In these patients, dose reduction should be undertaken to achieve the appropriate trough concentration range.

Long term clinical data in renal transplant patients have demonstrated that a large proportion of patients previously on Sandimmun therapy can be maintained at the same dose of Neoral as with Sandimmun.

All patients should be monitored according to the following recommendations:

(a) Preconversion (i.e. on Sandimmun): Measure cyclosporin trough concentration, serum creatinine and blood pressure.
(b) Day 1: Convert the patient to the same daily dose of Neoral as was previously used with oral Sandimmun (i.e. on a mg to mg basis).
(c) Day 4–7 post conversion: Follow-up visit to measure cyclosporin trough concentration, serum creatinine and blood pressure.
(d) Subsequent follow-up: Depending on the findings on review at day 4–7, subsequent follow-up visits may need to be arranged (e.g. week 2 and week 4) in the first 2 month period after conversion to Neoral. During these visits, cyclosporin trough concentrations, serum creatinine and blood pressure should be measured and, dependent on these measurements, the dose of Neoral adjusted accordingly.

Further information on conversion can be obtained via the Neoral Helpline (01276 698494).

*Conversion of non-transplant (i.e. psoriasis, atopic dermatitis, rheumatoid arthritis, nephrotic syndrome) patients from Sandimmun Soft Gelatin Capsules or Oral Solution to Neoral:* Cyclosporin absorption from Sandimmun oral formulations is highly variable and the relationship between Sandimmun dose and cyclosporin exposure (AUC) is non-linear. In contrast, with Neoral the absorption of cyclosporin is less variable.

With equivalent doses following conversion from

Sandimmun to Neoral, higher peak concentrations ($C_{max}$) and an increased exposure to the drug may occur. In a small percentage of patients, these changes may be more marked and of clinical significance. Their magnitude depends largely on the individual ability to absorb cyclosporin from the originally used Sandimmun. Therefore, the clinical status of each patient should be assessed prior to initiating Neoral therapy.

It is recommended that where any potential loss of efficacy results in considerable risk to the patients (e.g. rheumatoid arthritis), conversion from Sandimmun to Neoral is on a mg for mg basis. In other patients, the lowest recommended starting dose of Neoral is recommended initially with appropriate dose titration according to clinical response, serum creatinine and blood pressure levels.

All patients converting on a mg for mg basis should be monitored according to the following recommendations:

(a) Preconversion (i.e. on Sandimmun): Measure serum creatinine and blood pressure.
(b) Day 1: Start the patient with the same daily dose of Neoral as was previously used with oral Sandimmun (i.e. on a mg for mg basis).
(c) Week 2: Measure serum creatinine and blood pressure and consider reducing the dose of Neoral if either parameter significantly exceeds the preconversion level.
(d) Week 4: Measure serum creatinine and blood pressure and consider reducing the dose of Neoral if either parameter significantly exceeds the preconversion level.
(e) Week 8: Measure serum creatinine blood pressure and consider reducing the dose of Neoral if either parameter significantly exceeds the preconversion level.

If on more than one measurement, the serum creatinine increases more than 30% above the pre-Sandimmun baseline the dose of Neoral should be decreased (see *Additional precautions for psoriasis, atopic dermatitis, rheumatoid arthritis* and *nephrotic syndrome* sections).

*Administration:* The total daily dosage of Neoral Soft Gelatin Capsules or Neoral Oral Solution should always be given in two divided doses. Neoral Soft Gelatin Capsules should be taken with a mouthful of water and should then be swallowed whole.

Neoral Oral Solution should be diluted immediately before being taken. For improved taste the solution can be diluted with orange juice or squash or apple juice. However, it may also be taken with water if preferred. It should be stirred well.

Neoral Oral Solution has a characteristic taste which is distinct to that of Sandimmun Oral Solution.

The measuring device should not come into contact with the diluent. The measuring device should not be rinsed with water, alcohol or any other liquid. If it is necessary to clean the measuring device, the outside should be wiped with a dry tissue.

Owing to its possible interference with the P450-dependent enzyme system, grapefruit or grapefruit juice should not be ingested for 1 hour prior to dose administration, and grapefruit juice should not be used as a diluent for the Oral Solution.

*Use in the elderly:* There is currently no experience with Neoral in the elderly. However, no particular problems have been reported following the use of cyclosporin at the recommended dose. However, factors sometimes associated with ageing, in particular impaired renal function, make careful supervision essential and may necessitate dosage adjustment.

*Use in children:* There is currently no experience with Neoral in young children. However, transplant recipients from three months of age have received cyclosporin at the recommended dosage with no particular problems although at dosages above the upper end of the recommended range children seem to be more susceptible to fluid retention, convulsions and hypertension. This responds to dosage reduction.

*Contra-indications:* Known hypersensitivity to cyclosporin. Neoral is contra-indicated in psoriatic and atopic dermatitis patients with abnormal renal function, uncontrolled hypertension, uncontrolled infections or any kind of malignancy other than of the skin (see *Precautions* section). Neoral is contra-indicated in rheumatoid arthritis patients with abnormal renal function, uncontrolled hypertension, uncontrolled infections or any kind of malignancy. Neoral should not be used to treat rheumatoid arthritis in patients under the age or 18 years. Neoral is contra-indicated in nephrotic syndrome patients with uncontrolled hypertension, uncontrolled infections, or any kind of malignancy.

*Special warnings and special precautions for use:*
*Precautions:* Cyclosporin can impair renal function. Close monitoring of serum creatinine and urea is required and dosage adjustment may be necessary. Increases in serum creatinine and urea occurring during the first few weeks of cyclosporin therapy are

generally dose-dependent and reversible and usually respond to dosage reduction. During long-term treatment, some patients may develop structural changes in the kidney (e.g. interstitial fibrosis) which, in renal transplant recipients, must be distinguished from chronic rejection.

Cyclosporin may also affect liver function and dosage adjustment, based on the results of bilirubin and liver enzyme monitoring, may be necessary.

Since cyclosporin occasionally causes hyperkalaemia or may aggravate pre-existing hyperkalaemia, monitoring of serum potassium is recommended, especially in patients with marked renal dysfunction. Patients receiving cyclosporin should avoid a high dietary potassium intake (see also *Interactions*).

Caution is required in treating patients with hyperuricaemia.

Cyclosporin should preferably not be administered with other immunosuppressive agents except corticosteroids. However, some transplant centres use cyclosporin together with azathioprine and corticosteroids, or other immunosuppressive agents (all in low doses) with the aim of reducing the risk of cyclosporin-induced renal dysfunction or renal structural changes. When cyclosporin is used with other immunosuppressive agents, there is a risk of over-immunosuppression, which can lead to increased susceptibility to infection and to possible development of lymphoma.

There are differences in bioavailability between different oral formulations of cyclosporin however, Neoral Soft Gelatin Capsules are bioequivalent to Neoral Oral Solution.

Regular monitoring of blood pressure is required during treatment with cyclosporin. If hypertension develops, appropriate anti-hypertensive treatment must be instituted.

Cyclosporin can induce a reversible increase in blood lipids. It is, therefore, advisable to perform lipid determinations before treatment and thereafter as appropriate.

*Additional precautions in psoriasis and atopic dermatitis:* Careful dermatological and physical examinations, including measurements of blood pressure and renal function on at least two occasions prior to starting therapy should be performed to establish an accurate baseline status.

Development of malignancies (particularly of the skin) have been reported in psoriatic patients treated with cyclosporin as well as during treatment with conventional therapy. A search for all forms of pre-existing tumours, including those of the skin and cervix should be carried out. Skin lesions which are not typical for psoriasis should be biopsied before starting Neoral treatment to exclude skin cancers, mycosis fungoides or other pre-malignant disorders. Patients with malignant or pre-malignant alterations of the skin should be treated with Neoral only after appropriate treatment of such lesions and only if no other option for successful therapy exists.

Because of the possibility of renal dysfunction or renal structural changes, serum creatinine should be measured at two weekly intervals during the first three months of therapy. Thereafter, if creatinine remains stable, measurements should be made at monthly intervals. If serum creatinine increases and remains increased to more than 30% above baseline at more than one measurement, Neoral dosage must be reduced by 25 to 50%. These recommendations apply even if the patient's values still lie within the laboratory's normal range. If dosage reduction is not successful within one month, Neoral treatment should be discontinued.

In atopic dermatitis patients serum creatinine should be measured at two weekly intervals throughout the treatment period.

If hypertension develops which cannot be controlled by Neoral dosage reduction or appropriate antihypertensive therapy, discontinuation of Neoral is recommended.

Neoral treatment and its monitoring should be carried out under the supervision of a dermatologist experienced in the management of severe skin diseases.

In view of the potential risk of skin malignancy, patients on Neoral should be warned to avoid excessive unprotected sun exposure and should not receive concomitant therapeutic ultraviolet B irradiation or PUVA photochemotherapy.

*Additional precautions in atopic dermatitis:* Active herpes simplex infections should be allowed to clear before initiating treatment with Neoral but are not necessarily a reason for drug withdrawal if they occur during treatment unless infection is severe.

Skin infections with *Staphylococcus aureus* are not an absolute contra-indication for Neoral therapy but should be controlled with appropriate antibacterial agents. Oral erythromycin, known to have the potential to increase the blood concentration of cyclosporin (see *Interactions*) should be avoided or, if there is no alternative, its concomitant use must be accompanied by close monitoring of the blood levels of cyclosporin.

There is currently no experience with Neoral in children with atopic dermatitis. Its use in patients under 16 years of age cannot, therefore, be recommended.

*Additional precautions in rheumatoid arthritis:* Since cyclosporin can impair renal function, a reliable baseline level of serum creatinine should be established by at least two measurements prior to treatment, and serum creatinine should be monitored at 2 weekly intervals during the first 3 months of therapy. Thereafter, measurements can be made every 4 weeks, but more frequent checks are necessary when the Neoral dose is increased or concomitant treatment with a non-steroidal anti-inflammatory drug is initiated or its dosage increased. Because the pharmacodynamic interaction between cyclosporin and NSAIDs may adversely affect renal function, caution should be exercised if NSAID therapy is to be continued.

If the serum creatinine remains increased by more than 30% above creatinine levels recorded before starting cyclosporin therapy at more than one measurement, the dosage of Neoral should be reduced. If the serum creatinine increases by more than 50%, a dosage reduction by 50% is mandatory. These recommendations apply even if the patient's values still lie within the laboratory normal range. If dosage reduction is not successful in reducing levels within one month, Neoral treatment should be discontinued.

Discontinuation of the drug may also become necessary if hypertension developing during Neoral therapy cannot be controlled by appropriate anti-hypertensive therapy.

The combination of non-steroidal anti-inflammatory drugs and cyclosporin should be used with caution in patients with rheumatoid arthritis and should be accompanied by particularly close monitoring of renal function as detailed above.

As hepatotoxicity is a potential side effect of non-steroidal anti-inflammatory drugs, regular monitoring of hepatic function is advised when Neoral is co-administered with these drugs in rheumatoid arthritis patients.

The use of cyclosporin therapy for the treatment of patients with rheumatoid arthritis requires careful monitoring and follow-up. Neoral should only be used provided that the necessary expertise and adequate equipment, laboratory and supportive medical resources are available.

Patients with rheumatoid arthiritis have an increased incidence of malignancies compared to the general population. Use of disease modifying drugs increases the risk of malignancy further. The use of cyclosporin in the treatment of rheumatoid arthritis has not been shown to increase the incidence of malignancies more than other disease-modifying drugs.

*Additional precautions in nephrotic syndrome:* Development of malignancies (including Hodgkin's lymphoma) has occasionally been reported in nephrotic syndrome patients treated with cyclosporin, as well as during treatment with other immunosuppressive agents. However, malignancy may be related to the pathogenesis of the disease.

Since cyclosporin can impair renal function, it is necessary to assess renal function frequently and if the serum creatinine remains increased by more than 30% above baseline at more than one measurement, to reduce the dosage of Neoral by 25–50%. Patients with abnormal baseline renal function are at higher risk. They should initially be treated with 2.5 mg/kg per day orally and must be monitored very carefully.

In some patients it may be difficult to detect Neoral-induced renal dysfunction because of changes in renal function related to the underlying renal disease. If Neoral is indicated for more than one year in the long-term management, then renal biopsies should be performed at 1 yearly intervals to assess the progression of the renal disease and the extent of any Neoral-associated changes in the renal morphology that may co-exist.

The use of Neoral therapy for the treatment of patients with nephrotic syndrome requires careful monitoring and follow-up. Neoral should only be used provided that the necessary expertise and adequate equipment, laboratory and supporting medical resources are available.

*Interactions with other medicaments and other forms of interactions:* Care should be taken when using cyclosporin in combination with systemic antibiotics or other compounds known to have nephrotoxic effects e.g. aminoglycosides, amphotericin B, ciprofloxacin, melphalan and trimethoprim.

Various agents are known to either increase or decrease the plasma or whole blood concentrations of cyclosporin by competitive inhibition or induction of hepatic enzymes involved in the metabolism and excretion of cyclosporin, in particular cytochrome P450. Agents known to increase plasma or whole blood concentrations of cyclosporin include ketoconazole, erythromycin, oral contraceptives and some calcium channel blockers including diltiazem, nicardipine and verapamil. Doxycycline, fluconazole, itraconazole, propafenone and lipid solutions are also suspected of having the same effect. Agents known to decrease plasma or whole blood cyclosporin concentrations include phenytoin, carbamazepine, barbiturates and rifampicin. Sulphadiazine is also suspected of having the same effect.

In transplant patients, frequent measurement of cyclosporin and, if necessary, cyclosporin dosage adjustment is required, particularly during the introduction or withdrawal of co-administered drug. In non-transplant patients, the relationship between blood level and clinical effect is less well established. If drugs known to increase cyclosporin levels are given concomitantly, frequent assessment of renal function and careful monitoring for cyclosporin related side-effects may be more appropriate than blood level measurement.

Intraveneous (but not oral) administration of sulphadimidine and trimethoprim has also resulted in a marked reduction of plasma or whole blood levels of cyclosporin. Concomitant administration of such drugs with cyclosporin should, therefore, be avoided. Where combined administration is unavoidable, careful monitoring of cyclosporin blood levels and appropriate adjustment of cyclosporin dosage are essential.

In addition, it has been noted that cyclosporin reduces the clearance of prednisolone and, conversely, high-dose therapy with methylprednisolone can increase the blood concentration of cyclosporin.

As non-steroidal anti-inflammatory drugs alone can have an adverse effect on renal function, addition of these drugs to cyclosporin therapy or an increase in their dosages, should initially be accompanied by particularly close monitoring of renal function.

Cyclosporin given in combination with diclofenac causes an increase in plasma concentration of diclofenac. Diclofenac dosages should, therefore, be reduced by approximately half when given with cyclosporin. There have been reports of pharmacokinetic interactions between cyclosporin with other non-steroidal anti-inflammatory drugs, but there are insufficient data available to clarify their significance. However, a lack of pharmacokinetic interaction has been demonstrated between aspirin and cyclosporin.

Some studies have shown that various NSAIDs interact pharmacodynamically with cyclosporin to affect renal function. An analysis of clinical trials of cyclosporin and non-steroidal anti-inflammatory drugs suggest that plasma creatinine is not higher in patients if they receive concomitant NSAID therapy. The combination of these drugs, however, should be used with care.

Administration of cyclosporin may enhance the potential of the HMG-CoA reductase inhibitor lovastatin to induce rhabdomyolysis. The potential for interaction with other drugs in this class should be considered.

Muscular toxicity, including muscle pains and weakness, have also been reported in patients receiving colchicine concurrently with cyclosporin.

The concurrent administration of nifedipine and cyclosporin has resulted in an increased rate of gingival hyperplasia when compared with that for cyclosporin alone. It is recommended that nifedipine should be avoided in patients who develop gingival hypertrophy during therapy with cyclosporin. Where there is a risk of hyperkalaemia, potassium-sparing diuretics should be avoided and care should be taken when prescribing potassium supplements or potassium containing medications.

Since cyclosporin occasionally causes hyperkalaemia or may aggravate pre-existing hyperkalaemia, monitoring of serum potassium is recommended, especially in patients with marked renal dysfunction. Patients receiving cyclosporin should avoid a high dietary potassium intake.

During treatment with cyclosporin, vaccination may be less effective, and the use of live attenuated vaccines should be avoided.

*Pregnancy and lactation:* Cyclosporin is not teratogenic in animals. There is currently no clinical experience with Neoral and experience with Sandimmun is still limited. However, data available from organ transplant recipients indicate that, compared with traditional therapy, cyclosporin treatment imposes no increased risk of adverse effects on the course and outcome of pregnancy. However, there are no adequate and well controlled studies in pregnant women, therefore cyclosporin should be used during pregnancy only if the potential benefit justifies the potential risk to the foetus.

Cyclosporin passes into breast milk. Mothers receiving treatment with cyclosporin should not, therefore, breast-feed their infants.

*Effects on ability to drive and use machines:* No data exists on the effects of Neoral on the ability to drive and use machines.

*Undesirable effects:* The following side-effects have

been observed with cyclosporin treatment. They are usually dose dependent and responsive to dose reduction.

A frequent and potentially serious complication is a dose-dependent and reversible increase in serum creatinine and urea during the first few weeks of therapy. Less frequently, renal structural changes (e.g. interstitial fibrosis) may develop during long-term treatment. Impairment of renal function may necessitate dosage reduction or, in patients treated for psoriasis, discontinuation of cyclosporin therapy (see Precautions).

Apart from impaired renal function, the most frequently observed side-effects include hypertrichosis, tremor, hypertension (particularly in heart transplant patients) hepatic dysfunction, fatigue, gingival hypertrophy, gastrointestinal disturbances (abdominal pain, anorexia, nausea, vomiting, diarrhoea) and burning sensations of the hands and feet (usually during the first week of treatment).

Occasionally, headaches, rashes of possible allergic origin, mild anaemia, hyperkalaemia, hyperuricaemia, gout, hypomagnesaemia, hypercholesterolaemia, weight increase, oedema, pancreatitis, neuropathy, confusion, paraesthesia, convulsions, reversible dysmenorrhoea or amenorrhoea may develop.

Muscle weakness, muscle cramps, or myopathy have been reported.

Especially in liver transplant patients, signs of encephalopathy, vision and movement disturbances, and impaired consciousness are described. Whether these alterations are caused by cyclosporin, or are a consequence of the underlying disease, or other conditions, remains to be established.

On rare occasions, a syndrome of thrombocytopenia, in some patients in combination with micro-angiopathic haemolytic anaemia and renal failure (haemolytic uraemic syndrome) has been observed.

Gynaecomastia has been rarely reported, occasionally in patients receiving concomitant spironolactone.

Malignancies and lymphoproliferative disorders have developed, but their incidence and distribution were found to be similar to those in patients on conventional immunosuppressive therapy. Where lymphoproliferative disorders have developed in patients with psoriasis, they have been responsive to prompt drug discontinuation.

In a few cases, colitis has developed after treatment with cyclosporin.

Overdose: No experience of acute overdosage with Neoral is available and little experience is available with regards to overdosage with Sandimmun. Symptomatic treatment and general supportive measures should be followed in all cases of overdosage. Forced emesis could be of value within the first few hours after intake. Signs of nephrotoxicity might occur which should be expected to resolve following drug withdrawal. Cyclosporin is not dialysable to any great extent nor is it well cleared by charcoal haemoperfusion. Hypertension and convulsions have been reported in some patients receiving cyclosporin therapy at doses above the recommended range and in others with high trough blood levels of cyclosporin. This might, therefore, be expected as a feature of overdosage.

Pharmacological properties

Pharmacodynamic properties: Cyclosporin is a cyclic polypeptide consisting of 11 amino acids. It is a potent immunosuppressive agent which prolongs survival of allogeneic transplants involving skin, heart, kidney, pancreas, cornea, bone marrow, small intestine and lung in animals.

Successful solid organ and bone marrow allogeneic transplants have been performed in man, using cyclosporin to prevent and treat rejection and GVHD. Marked beneficial effects of cyclosporin therapy have also been shown in partients with severe psoriasis, atopic dermatitis and rheumatoid arthritis, conditions that may be considered to have an immunological mechanism.

Studies in animals suggest that cyclosporin inhibits the development of cell mediated reactions. It appears to block the resting lymphocytes in the $G_0$ or early $G_1$ phase of the cell cycle, and also inhibits lymphokine production and release, including interleukin 2 (T cell growth factor, TCGF). The available evidence suggests that cyclosporin acts specifically and reversibly on lymphocytes. It does not depress haemopoiesis and has no effect on the function of phagocytic cells.

Pharmacokinetic properties: Neoral is an improved pharmaceutical form of the active ingredient cyclosporin. Neoral is a pre-concentrate formulation of cyclosporin which undergoes a microemulsification process in the presence of water, either in the form of a beverage or in the form of the gastrointestinal fluid. Neoral reduces the intra-patient variability of pharmacokinetic parameters, with a more consistent absorption profile and less influence of concomitant food intake and the presence of bile. In pharmacokinetic and clinical studies it has been demonstrated

that the correlation between trough concentration ($C_{min}$) and total exposure (AUC) is significantly stronger when cyclosporin is given as Neoral than when it is given as Sandimmun. Neoral, therefore, allows greater predictability and consistency of cyclosporin exposure.

The data available indicate that following a 1:1 conversion from Sandimmun Soft Gelatin Capsules and Sandimmun Oral Solution to Neoral, trough concentrations in whole blood are comparable, thereby remaining in the desired therapeutic trough level range. Compared to oral administration of Sandimmun (with which peak blood concentrations are achieved within 1 to 6 hours), Neoral is more quickly absorbed (resulting in a 1 hour earlier mean $t_{max}$ and a 59% higher mean $C_{max}$) and exhibits, on average, a 29% higher bioavailability. In a clinical trial involving maintained renal transplant patients the correlation ($r^2$) between trough concentration ($C_{min}$) and exposure (AUC) was good (0.8).

Cyclosporin is extensively biotransformed to approximately 15 metabolites. There is no single major metabolic pathway. Elimination is primarily biliary, with only 6% of the oral dose excreted in the urine, only 0.1% is excreted in the urine as unchanged drug.

There is a high variability in the data reported on the terminal half-life of cyclosporin depending on the assay applied and the target population. The terminal half-life ranged from 6.3 hours in healthy volunteers to 20.4 hours in patients with severe liver disease.

Preclinical safety data: Cyclosporin gave no evidence of mutagenic or teratogenic effects in appropriate test systems. Only at dose levels toxic to dams were adverse effects seen in reproduction studies in rats. At toxic doses (rats at 30 mg/kg and rabbits at 100 mg/kg a day orally), cyclosporin was embryo- and fetotoxic as indicated by increased pre-natal and post-natal mortality and reduced fetal weight together with related skeletal retardation. In the well-tolerated dose range (rats up to 17 mg/kg and rabbits up to 30 mg/kg a day orally), cyclosporin proved to be without any embryolethal or teratogenic effects.

Carcinogenicity studies were carried out in male and female rats and mice. In the 78-week mouse study, at doses of 1, 4, and 16 mg/kg a day, evidence of a statistically significant trend was found for lymphocytic lymphomas in females, and the incidence of hepatocellular carcinomas in mid-dose males significantly exceeded the control value. In the 24-month rat study conducted at 0.5, 2, and 8 mg/kg a day, pancreatic islet cell adenomas significantly exceeded the control rate at the low dose level. The hepatocellular carcinomas and pancreatic islet cell adenomas were not dose related. No impairment in fertility was demonstrated in studies in male and female rats.

Cyclosporin has not been found to be mutagenic/genotoxic in the Ames test, the V79-HGPRT test, the micronucleus test in mice and Chinese hamsters, the chromosome-aberration tests in Chinese hamster bone marrow, the mouse dominant lethal assay, and the DNA repair test in sperm from treated mice. A study analysing sister chromatid exchange (SCE) induction by cyclosporin using human lymphocytes in vitro gave indication of a positive effect (i.e. induction of SCE) at high concentrations in this system.

An increased incidence of malignancy is a recognised complication of immunosuppression in recipients of organ transplants. The most common forms of neoplasms are non-Hodgkin's lymphoma and carcinomas of the skin. The risk of malignancies during cyclosporin treatment is higher than in the normal, healthy population, but similar to that in patients receiving other immunosuppressive therapies. It has been reported that reduction or discontinuance of immunosuppression may cause lesions to regress.

Pharmaceutical particulars

List of excipients:

Soft gelatin capsules: DL-α-tocopherol, absolute ethanol, propylene glycol, corn oil mono-di-triglycerides, polyoxyl 40 hydrogenated castor oil.

Capsule shell: Iron oxide black (25 mg and 100 mg capsules), titanium dioxide, glycerol 85% propylene glycol, gelatin.

Solution: DL-α-tocopherol, absolute ethanol, propylene glycol, corn oil mono-di-triglycerides, polyoxyl 40 hydrogenated castor oil.

Incompatibilities: None known.

Shelf life: Soft gelatin capsules and solution 36 months.

Special precautions for storage: Neoral Soft Gelatin Capsules should be stored below 25°C.

Neoral Soft Gelatin Capsules should be left in the blister pack until required for use. When a blister is opened, a characteristic smell is noticeable.

Neoral Oral Solution should be stored below 30°C (preferably not below 15°C, as it contains oily compo-

nents of natural origin which tend to solidify at low temperatures). A jelly-like formation may occur below 20°C which is, however, reversible at temperatures up to 30°C. Minor flakes or a slight sediment may still be observed. These phenomena do not affect the efficacy and safety of the product, and the dosing by means of the measuring device remains accurate.

Nature and contents of container: Neoral Soft Gelatin Capsules are available in 6×5 blister packs of double-sided aluminium consisting of an aluminium bottom foil and an aluminium covering foil.

Neoral Oral Solution is available in 50 ml amber glass bottles with an aluminium cap and rubber stopper. A dispenser set is also provided.

Instructions for use/handling: Initial use of Neoral Oral Solution:

1. Flip off plastic cap and bend right back.
2. Tear off whole of cap and sealing ring.
3. Remove black stopper from bottle and dispose of carefully.
4. Push tube unit firmly into neck of bottle.
5. Insert syringe into stopper.
6. Draw up prescribed volume of solution.
7. Expel any large bubbles by depressing and withdrawing plunger a few times before removing syringe containing prescribed dose from bottle. The presence of a few tiny bubbles is of no importance and will not affect the dose in any way.
8. After use, wipe syringe on outside only with a dry tissue and replace in its case. Dispose of the tissue carefully. White stopper and tube should remain in bottle. Close bottle with cap provided.

Subsequent use: Commence at point 5.

Marketing authorisation numbers

| Neoral Soft Gelatin Capsules | 10 mg | 0101/0483 |
| | 25 mg | 0101/0387 |
| | 50 mg | 0101/0388 |
| | 100 mg | 0101/0389 |
| Neoral Oral Solution | | 0101/0390 |

Date of approval/revision of SPC   May 1997.

Legal category   POM.

# NORPROLAC*

Qualitative and quantitative composition  Quinagolide as the hydrochloride, 25 mcg, 50 mcg, 75 mcg or 150 mcg.

Pharmaceutical form  Tablet for oral administration.

Clinical particulars

Therapeutic indications: Hyperprolactinaemia (idiopathic or originating from a prolactin-secreting pituitary microadenoma or macroadenoma).

Posology and method of administration: Since dopaminergic stimulation may lead to symptoms of orthostatic hypotension, the dosage of Norprolac should be initiated gradually with the aid of the 'starter pack', and given only at bedtime.

Adults: The optimal dose must be titrated individually on the basis of the prolactin-lowering effect and tolerability.

With the 'starter pack', treatment begins with 25 mcg/day for the first 3 days, followed by 50 mcg/day for a further 3 days. From day 7 onwards, the recommended dose is 75 mcg/day.

If necessary, the daily dose may then be increased stepwise until the optimal individual response is attained. The usual maintenance dosage is 75 to 150 mcg/day.

Daily doses of 300 mcg or higher doses are required in less than one-third of the patients. In such cases, the daily dosage may be increased in steps of 75 to 150 mcg at intervals not shorter than 4 weeks until satisfactory therapeutic effectiveness is achieved or reduced tolerability, requiring the discontinuation of treatment, occurs.

Elderly: Experience with the use of Norprolac in elderly patients is not available.

Children: Experience with the use of Norprolac in children is not available.

Method of administration: Norprolac should be taken once a day with some food at bedtime.

Contra-indications: Hypersensitivity to the drug. Impaired hepatic or renal function. For procedure during pregnancy, see Pregnancy and lactation.

Special warnings and precautions for use: Fertility may be restored by the treatment with Norprolac. Women of child-bearing age who do not wish to conceive should therefore be advised to practice a reliable method of contraception.

Since orthostatic hypotension may result in syncope, it is recommended to check blood pressure both lying and standing during the first days of therapy and following dosage increases.

In a few cases, including patients with no previous history of mental illness, treatment with Norprolac has been associated with the occurrence of acute psychosis, usually reversible upon discontinuation. Particular caution is required in patients who have had psychotic episodes in their previous history.

To date no data is available with the use of Norprolac in patients with impaired renal or hepatic function (see *Contra-indications*).

Norprolac should be kept out of the reach of children.

*Interaction with other medicaments and other forms of interaction:* No interactions between Norprolac and other drugs have so far been reported. On theoretical grounds, a reduction of the prolactin-lowering effect could be expected when drugs (e.g. neuroleptic agents) with strong dopamine antagonistic properties are used concomitantly. As the potency of Norprolac for 5-$HT_1$ and 5-$HT_2$ receptors is some 100 times lower than that for $D_2$ receptors, an interaction between Norprolac and 5-$HT_{1a}$ receptors is unlikely. However, care should be taken when using these medicaments concomitantly.

The tolerability of Norprolac may be reduced by alcohol.

*Pregnancy and lactation*

*Pregnancy:* Animal data provide no evidence that Norprolac has any embryotoxic or teratogenic potential, but experience in pregnant women is still limited. In patients wishing to conceive, Norprolac should be discontinued when pregnancy is confirmed, unless there is a medical reason for continuing therapy. No increased incidence of abortion has been observed following withdrawal of the drug at this point.

If pregnancy occurs in the presence of a pituitary adenoma and Norprolac treatment has been stopped, close supervision throughout pregnancy is essential.

*Lactation:* Breast-feeding is usually not possible since Norprolac suppresses lactation. If lactation should continue during treatment, breast-feeding cannot be recommended because it is not known whether quinagolide passes into human breast milk.

*Effects on ability to drive and to use machines:* Since, especially during the first days of treatment, hypotensive reactions may occasionally occur and result in reduced alertness, patients should be cautious when driving a vehicle or operating machinery.

*Undesirable effects:* The adverse reactions reported with the use of Norprolac are characteristic for dopamine receptor agonist therapy. They are usually not sufficiently serious to require discontinuation of treatment and tend to disappear when treatment is continued.

The most frequent side effects (>10%) are nausea, vomiting, headache, dizziness and fatigue. They occur predominantly during the first few days of the initial treatment or, as a mostly transient event, following dosage increase. If necessary, nausea and vomiting may be prevented by the intake of a peripheral dopaminergic antagonist, such as domperidone, for a few days, at least 1 hour before the ingestion of Norprolac.

Less frequent side effects (1 to 10%) include anorexia, abdominal pain, constipation or diarrhoea, insomnia, oedema, flushing, nasal congestion and hypotension. Orthostatic hypotension may result in faintness or syncope (see *Special warnings and special precautions for use*).

In a few isolated cases, treatment with Norprolac has been associated with the occurrence of acute psychosis, reversible upon discontinuation.

*Overdose:*

*Symptoms:* Acute overdosage with Norprolac tablets has not been reported. It would be expected to cause severe nausea, vomiting, headache, dizziness, drowsiness, hypotension and possibly collapse. Hallucinations could also occur.

*Treatment:* Should be symptomatic.

**Pharmacological properties**

*Pharmacodynamic properties:* Quinagolide, the active ingredient of Norprolac, is a selective dopamine $D_2$-receptor agonist not belonging to the chemical classes of ergot or ergoline compounds. Owing to its dopaminergic action, the drug exerts a strong inhibitory effect on the secretion of the anterior pituitary hormone prolactin, but does not reduce normal levels of other pituitary hormones. In some patients the reduction of prolactin secretion may be accompanied by short-lasting, small increases in plasma growth hormone levels, the clinical significance of which is unknown.

As a specific inhibitor of prolactin secretion with a prolonged duration of action, Norprolac has been shown to be effective and suitable for once-a-day oral treatment of patients presenting with hyperprolactinaemia and its clinical manifestations such as galactorrhoea, oligomenorrhoea, amenorrhoea, infertility and reduced libido.

*Pharmacokinetic properties:* After oral administration of radiolabelled drug, quinagolide is rapidly and well absorbed. Plasma concentration values obtained by a non-selective radio-immunoassay (RIA), measuring quinagolide together with some of it metabolites, were close to the limit of quantification and gave no reliable information.

The apparent volume of distribution of quinagolide after single oral administration of radiolabelled compound was calculated to be approx 100 L. For the parent drug, a terminal half-life of 11.5 hours has been calculated under single dose conditions, and of 17 hours at steady state.

Quinagolide is extensively metabolised during its first pass. Studies performed with $^3$H-labelled quinagolide revealed that more than 95% of the drug is excreted as metabolites. About equal amounts of total radioactivity are found in faeces and urine.

In blood, quinagolide and its N-desethyl analogue are the biologically active but minor components. Their inactive sulphate or glucuronide conjugates represent the major circulating metabolites. In urine, the main metabolites are the glucuronide and sulphate conjugates of quinagolide and the N-desethyl, N,N-didesethyl analogues. In the faeces unconjugated forms of the three components are found.

The protein binding of quinagolide is approximately 90% and is non-specific.

The results, obtained in pharmacodynamic studies, indicate that with the recommended therapeutic dosage a clinically significant prolactin-lowering effect occurs within 2 hours after ingestion, reaches a maximum within 4 to 6 hours and is maintained for about 24 hours.

A definite dose-response relationship could be established for the duration, but not for the magnitude, of the prolactin-lowering effect which, with a single oral dose of 50 mcg was close to maximum. Higher doses did not result in a considerably greater effect but prolonged its duration.

*Preclinical safety data:*

*Acute toxicity:* The $LD_{50}$ of quinagolide was determined for several species after single oral administration: mice 357 to >500 mg/kg; rats >500 mg/kg; rabbits >150 mg/kg.

*Chronic toxicity:* Decreased cholesterol levels of treated female rats suggest that quinagolide influences lipid metabolism. Since similar observations have been made with other dopaminergic drugs, a causal relationship with low prolactin levels is assumed. In several chronic studies with rats, enlarged ovaries resulting from an increased number of corpora lutea and, additionally, hydrometra and endometritis were observed. These changes were reversible and reflect the pharmacodynamic effect of quinagolide: suppression of prolactin secretion inhibits luteolysis in rats and thus influences the normal sexual cycle. In humans, however, prolactin is not involved in luteolysis.

*Carcinogenic and mutagenic potential:* In comprehensive in vitro and in vivo mutagenic studies there was no evidence of a mutagenic effect.

The changes which were observed in carcinogenicity studies reflect the pharmacodynamic activity of quinagolide. The drug modulates the prolactin level as well as, specially in male rats, the level of luteinising hormone and, in female rodents, the ratio of progesterone to oestrogen.

Long-term studies with high doses of quinagolide revealed Leydig cell tumours in rats and mesenchymal uterine tumours in mice. The incidence of Leydig cell tumours in a carcinogenicity study in rats was increased even at low doses (0.01 mg/kg). These results were without relevance for the therapeutic application in humans since there are fundamental differences between humans and rodents in the regulation of the endocrine system.

*Reproductive toxicity:* Animals studies in rats and rabbits showed no evidence for embryotoxic or teratogenic effects. The prolactin inhibiting effect led to a decrease of milk production in rats, which was associated with an increased loss of rat pups. Possible post-natal effects of exposure during fetal development (2nd and 3rd trimester) and effects on female fertility are not sufficiently investigated.

**Pharmaceutical particulars**

*List of excipients:* Iron oxide, red; indigotin lake; silica, colloidal anhydrous; magnesium stearate; methylhydroxypropylcellulose; maize starch; cellulose, microcrystalline; lactose.

*Incompatibilities:* Not applicable.

*Shelf life:* The shelf life is 3 years. The expiry date is printed on the box. On the blister the expiry date is marked with the letters EXP.

*Special precautions for storage:* The expiry date refers to original unopened boxes, which were stored under the correct conditions, i.e. between 15 and 30°C. No special warning with respect to light sensitivity or humidity is necessary because the tablets are protected by the packaging.

*Nature and contents of container:* The 'starter pack' (Norprolac 25/50) consists of 3 tablets of 25 mcg and 3 tablets of 50 mcg. These tablets are packed in an aluminium PVC/PVDC blister which is sealed in a moisture-proof aluminium bag.

The 75 mcg and 150 mcg tablets are in packs of 30 tablets (3 times 10 tablets in aluminium blisters).

*Instructions for use/handling:* None.

**Marketing authorisation numbers**

| | |
|---|---|
| 25 mcg | 0101/0380 |
| 50 mcg | 0101/0381 |
| 75 mcg | 0101/0382 |
| 150 mcg | 0101/0383 |

**Date of approval/revision of SPC** May 1997.

**Legal category** POM.

## ORIMETEN*

**Presentation** Tablets containing 250 mg aminoglutethimide. White to yellowish white, round with slightly convex faces and slightly bevelled edges, printed 'CG' on one side and 'GG' with score on the other.

The tablets also contain silica aerogel, hydroxypropyl methylcellulose, magnesium stearate, maize starch and talc.

**Uses**

*Indications:* Advanced carcinoma of the breast in post-menopausal or oophorectomised women (especially where the tumours are oestrogen-sensitive), including in particular patients who have previously responded to endocrine therapy or have painful bony metastases.

Advanced carcinoma of the prostate as palliative treatment. Subjective improvement and pain relief have been noted in up to 50% of patients.

Cushing's syndrome due to malignant disease, e.g. adrenocortical carcinoma or ectopic ACTH syndrome, in place of or in conjunction with surgery.

*Mode of action:* Aminoglutethimide inhibits the enzyme aromatase which converts androgens to oestrogens, and thus effects a reduction in oestrogen biosynthesis. In post-menopausal (or oophorectomised) women, oestrogens are derived primarily from extra-glandular (non-ovarian) aromatisation of adrenal precursors. Oestrogens are important in maintaining the growth of hormone dependent breast cancer. Treatment designed to lower circulating levels of oestrogens, results in tumour regression in patients with oestrogen receptor-positive tumours. In many cases of carcinoma of the breast, metastases or recurring tumours diminish in size, or even disappear during treatment with Orimeten. Such remission may be maintained for several years. Patients with soft tissue and bone metastases show the highest response rates, and some patients experience marked subjective relief from bone pain.

Orimeten also inhibits several other Cytochrome P450 mediated hydroxylation steps in the adrenal cortex, including conversion of cholesterol to 5 pregnenolone. Orimeten thus reduces the production of glucocorticoids and mineralocorticoids from the adrenal cortex, and reduces excessive plasma cortisol in patients with adrenocortical hyperfunction, such as Cushing's syndrome.

A decrease in adrenal secretion of cortisol leads to a reflex rise in adrenocorticotrophic hormone (ACTH) which will overcome the cortisol-lowering effect of Orimeten. This compensatory increase in ACTH secretion can be suppressed by the simultaneous administration of glucocorticoid.

The mode of action of Orimeten in prostatic carcinoma is not fully understood. Patients may benefit from marked relief of bone pain. Objective tumour regression has also been seen in some patients.

*Pharmacokinetics:* Orimeten is well absorbed and has a systemic availability of 92-98%. Peak plasma concentrations are attained within 1-4 hours. Mean steady state plasma concentrations vary between patients, but are proportional over the dose range 125-1000 mg/day. The drug is 21-25% bound to plasma proteins and during long term therapy the steady state elimination half-life averages 9 hours. Approximately 50% of the dose at steady state is excreted unchanged in the urine, and up to 25% in the form of N-hydroxylamino-glutethimide. Between 90% and 97% of the total dose is recovered in the urine. No reports of impaired metabolism or excretion of aminoglutethimide due to renal or hepatic dysfunction have been reported.

**Dosage and administration** Orimeten tablets should be administered orally.

Administration of Orimeten in small, gradually increasing doses substantially improves tolerability.

*Adults:*

*Advanced carcinoma of the breast and of the prostate:* The initial dose of one tablet daily, should be increased each week by one tablet per day to the maximum tolerated dose, not exceeding 1000 mg daily e.g. Week 1–250 mg once daily, Week 2–250 mg twice daily, Week 3–250 mg three times daily, Week 4–250 mg four times daily.

In some patients with breast cancer a dose of 250 mg twice daily has proved sufficient.

In the majority of patients treated for carcinoma of the prostate the effective dose has not exceeded 750 mg daily.

*Supplementary therapy:* Orimeten should be employed in combination with glucocorticoid in order to offset the decrease in endogenous corticosteroid biosynthesis which Orimeten may provoke. Hydrocortisone, 30 mg daily (preferably 20 mg in the morning plus 10 mg in the afternoon or evening) or cortisone acetate in daily doses of 37.5 mg (25 mg in the morning and 12.5 mg in the afternoon) are suitable for supplementary therapy. Orimeten accelerates the metabolism of dexamethasone (or other synthetic corticosteroids) to a variable extent, therefore individual titration to a relatively high dose (up to 3 mg daily) may be required if this glucocorticoid is used.

*Cushing's syndrome:* Initially 250 mg daily, increasing gradually according to response up to 1 g daily in divided doses. In some cases, especially ectopic ACTH syndrome, higher dosages (of up to 1.5-2 g daily) may occasionally prove necessary to achieve adequate suppression.

*Supplementary therapy:* When treating Cushing's syndrome, the plasma cortisol levels should be determined regularly and the dosage of aminoglutethimide adjusted accordingly. Substitution therapy with corticosteroids occasionally proves necessary.

*Elderly:* There is no evidence to suggest that dosage should be different in the elderly.

*Children:* Safety and efficacy have not been established in children.

### Contra-indications, warnings, etc

*Contra-indications:* History of severe hypersensitivity reactions to aminoglutethimide or glutethimide. Pregnancy and lactation. Porphyria.

*Use in pregnancy and lactation:* Since foetal abnormalities and an increase in foetal deaths and resorption have been observed in animals and there have been cases of pseudohermaphroditism in newborn infants of women treated with Orimeten, the possible presence of a pregnancy must be excluded before prescribing Orimeten for women of child-bearing age (see *Contra-indications*). During treatment, such women should employ non-hormonal contraceptives.

No mutagenic potential was observed with Orimeten in standard in vitro and in vivo mutagenicity tests.

*Warning and precautions:* Orimeten may cause adrenal hypofunction, especially under conditions of stress, such as surgery, trauma, or acute illness. Patients should be carefully monitored and given hydrocortisone as recommended in the dosage section. If inhibition of aldosterone synthesis leads to hyponatraemia, hypotension, or dizziness, a mineralocorticoid, e.g. fludrocortisone (0.1–0.15 mg daily or every other day) should be given in addition. Patients should be warned of the possibility of hypotension and its symptoms.

The patients blood pressure, plasma electrolytes, blood counts and thyroid function should be checked during treatment with Orimeten. Particularly during the first 2–3 months of treatment when blood counts should be carried out once every 2–3 weeks. If blood dyscrasias develop, Orimeten should be withdrawn. In the event of hypothyroidism, substitution therapy with thyroxine must be instituted; such therapy, however, very seldom proves necessary because the decrease in thyroxine provoked by Orimeten is usually offset by a reactive rise in TSH.

Patients frequently develop a skin rash at the start of treatment; if this does not disappear within 10 days, Orimeten should be temporarily withdrawn and/or the corticosteroid dosage increased.

If, during treatment for cancer of the breast or prostate, the supplementary glucocorticoid medication gives rise to Cushing–like symptoms, the dosage of the glucocorticoid should be reduced

Patients should be warned that drowsiness may occur, in which case they should not drive, operate potentially dangerous machinery, or engage in other activities that may become hazardous because of decreased alertness.

In a long-term rat carcinogenicity study an increased incidence in benign and malignant neoplasms of the adrenal cortex and the thyroid gland was noted in both sexes in one or more of the treated groups. These findings are not unexpected in view of the known pharmacodynamic properties of aminoglutethimide. The relevance of these findings in humans is not known.

*Drug interactions:* By inducing hepatic enzymes, Orimeten increases its own metabolism and also that of several drugs including synthetic glucocorticoids such as dexamethasone, warfarin and other oral anticoagulants, theophylline, medroxyprogesterone and oral antidiabetics. If necessary, the dosage of these drugs may have to be raised.

Concomitant therapy with diuretics may lead to hyponatraemia.

The effects of Orimeten may be potentiated if it is taken in combination with alcohol.

*Side-effects:* Frequency estimate: frequent >10%, occasional >1%-<10%, rare >0.001%-<1%, isolated cases <0.001%.

*Central nervous system:* Frequent: drowsiness, lethargy. These are commonly observed at the beginning of treatment and generally abate after about 6 weeks. Occasional: dizziness (vertigo). Rare: ataxia, headache, depression. Isolated cases: insomnia, confusion.

*Skin and appendages:* Frequent: rash, sometimes accompanied by fever. This commonly occurs within the first 2 weeks of starting treatment and usually resolves spontaneously despite continued treatment. Rare: pruritus, urticaria. Isolated cases: exfoliative dermatitis, Stevens–Johnson syndrome

*Gastrointestinal system:* Occasional: nausea. Rare: diarrhoea, vomiting, constipation, anorexia.

*Systemic:* Rare: fever, sweating.

*Liver:* Isolated cases: hepatitis (cholestatic type, associated with itching and skin rash), jaundice.

*Endocrine system:* Rare: adrenal insufficiency (hyponatraemia, hypotension, dizziness, hypoglycaemia). Isolated cases: hypothyroidism, inappropriate ADH secretion, masculinisation and hirsutism in females.

*Kidney:* Isolated cases: renal function abnormalities.
*Cardiovascular system:* Rare: hypotension.

*Haematological system:* Rare: agranulocytosis, leukopenia, thrombocytopenia. Isolated cases: pancytopenia, anaemia.

*Allergy:* Isolated cases: allergic/anaphylactic reactions, allergic alveolitis (eosinophilic pulmonary infiltrates). Where such alveolitis is suspected, Orimeten should be withdrawn immediately.

*Laboratory abnormalities:* Rare: increased gamma-glutamyl transferase (gamma–GT). This is due to the enzyme–inducing effect of Orimeten and is usually not a sign of liver damage.

Hyponatraemia, hyperkalaemia, hypoglycaemia. Isolated cases: hypercholesterolaemia.

*Adverse reactions due to glucocorticoid replacement therapy:* Isolated cases: Cushingoid symptoms (moon face, weight gain, oedema), arterial hypertension, hyperglycaemia, muscle cramps.

*Overdosage:* Following an overdosage of Orimeten, signs and symptoms may appear which are caused by its effects both on the adrenal cortex and on the central nervous system, e.g. hypotension, drowsiness, lethargy, dizziness, ataxia, coma, electrolyte disturbances, respiratory depression and hypoventilation.

The signs and symptoms of acute overdosage with Orimeten may be aggravated or modified if alcohol, hypnotics, tranquillisers, or tricyclic antidepressants have been taken at the same time.

The following countermeasures should be taken:
Removal of the tablets ingested; intravenous administration of a glucocorticoid such as hydrocortisone; measures to increase plasma volume; administration of oxygen; intravenous treatment with vasoactive drugs, e.g. noradrenaline; if necessary, artificial respiration. Haemoperfusion may be considered.

**Pharmaceutical precautions** Store below 30°C and protect from light and moisture.

**Legal category** POM.

**Package quantities** Blister pack of 56 tablets.

**Product licence number** 00101/0531.

## PARLODEL*
### Presentation
*1 mg tablets:* White, round, flat, bevel-edged Bromocriptine Mesylate Tablets PhEur, impressed PARLODEL 1 on one side and scored on the reverse. The tablets are 8 mm in diameter, with a nominal weight of 180 mg, and provide the equivalent of 1 mg bromocriptine base.

*2.5 mg tablets:* White, round, flat, bevel-edged Bromocriptine Mesylate Tablets PhEur, impressed PARLODEL 2.5 on one side and scored on the reverse. The tablets are 7 mm in diameter, with a nominal weight of 140 mg, and provide the equivalent of 2.5 mg bromocriptine base.

*5 mg capsules:* Opaque, hard gelatin Bromocriptine Mesylate Capsules PhEur. The capsules are size 3, upper part powder blue, lower part white, printed PARLODEL 5 in red and provide the equivalent of 5 mg bromocriptine base.

*10 mg capsules:* Opaque, hard gelatin Bromocriptine Mesylate Capsules PhEur. The capsules are size 1, white, printed PARLODEL 10 in red and provide the equivalent of 10 mg bromocriptine base.

**Uses** *Principal action:* Parlodel is a dopaminergic-receptor stimulant or dopamine agonist. This pharmacological action is manifested in normal individuals

and those with hyperprolactinaemic states by an inhibition of the secretion of prolactin by the pituitary; in many acromegalic patients a lowering of elevated circulating growth hormone levels results.

In patients with prolactin secreting adenomas there is radiological evidence to indicate tumour regression in some cases.

Because of its dopaminergic activity Parlodel is also effective in idiopathic Parkinson's disease, which is characterised by a specific nigro-striatal dopamine deficiency.

*Indications:* The inhibition or suppression of puerperal lactation for medical reasons. Parlodel is not recommended for the routine suppression of lactation, or for the relief of symptoms of postpartum pain and engorgement, which can be adequately treated with simple analgesics and breast support.

The treatment of hyperprolactinaemia in men and women with hypogonadism and/or galactorrhoea.

The treatment of hyperprolactinaemic infertility. Parlodel has been used successfully in the treatment of a number of infertile women who do not have demonstrable hyperprolactinaemia.

In a number of specialized units, patients who have been shown to have prolactin secreting adenomas have been treated successfully with Parlodel. In particular Parlodel can be considered as a first choice of treatment in patients with macroadenomas and as an alternative to the surgical procedure, transsphenoidal hypophysectomy, in patients with microadenomas.

The treatment of cyclical benign breast disease/cyclical pronounced mastalgia.

Cyclical menstrual disorders have also responded to Parlodel, particularly breast symptomatology, but in the premenstrual syndrome there is also some evidence that other symptoms, such as headache, mood changes and bloatedness, may be alleviated.

Parlodel has been used in a number of specialized units, as an adjunct to surgery and/or radiotherapy, to reduce circulating growth hormone levels in the management of acromegalic patients.

In the treatment of idiopathic Parkinson's disease, Parlodel has been used both alone and in combination with levodopa in the management of previously untreated patients and those disabled by 'on-off' phenomena. Parlodel has been used with occasional benefit in patients who do not respond to, or are unable to tolerate, levodopa and those whose response to levodopa is declining.

**Dosage and administration** Parlodel should always be taken during a meal.

A number of disparate conditions are amenable to treatment with Parlodel and, for this reason, the recommended dosage regimens are variable. In most indications, irrespective of the final dosage, the optimum response with the minimum of side-effects is best achieved by gradual introduction of Parlodel. The following scheme is suggested:

Initially 1 mg to 1.25 mg at bedtime, increasing after 2 to 3 days to 2 mg to 2.5 mg at bedtime. Dosage may then be increased by 1 mg to 2.5 mg at 2 to 3 day intervals, until a dosage of 2.5 mg twice daily is achieved. Further dosage increments, if necessary, should be added in a similar manner.

*Prevention of lactation:* 2.5 mg on the day of delivery, followed by 2.5 mg twice daily for 14 days. Gradual introduction of Parlodel is not necessary in this indication.

*Suppression of lactation:* 2.5 mg on the first day, increasing after 2 to 3 days to 2.5 mg twice daily for 14 days. Gradual introduction of Parlodel is not necessary in this indication.

*Hypogonadism/galactorrhoea syndromes/infertility:* Introduce Parlodel gradually according to the suggested scheme. Most patients with hyperprolactinaemia have responded to 7.5 mg daily, in divided doses, but doses of up to 30 mg daily have been used. In infertile patients without demonstrably elevated serum prolactin levels, the usual dosage is 2.5 mg twice daily.

*Prolactinomas:* Introduce Parlodel gradually according to the suggested scheme. Dosage may then be increased by 2.5 mg daily at 2 to 3 day intervals as follows: 2.5 mg eight-hourly, 2.5 mg six-hourly, 5 mg six-hourly. Patients have responded to doses of up to 30 mg daily.

*Cyclical benign breast disease/cyclical pronounced mastalgia/cyclical menstrual disorders:* Introduce Parlodel gradually, according to the suggested scheme, until the recommended dosage of 2.5 mg twice daily is reached.

*Acromegaly:* Introduce Parlodel gradually, according to the suggested scheme. Dosage may then be increased by 2.5 mg daily at 2 to 3 day intervals as follows: 2.5 mg eight-hourly, 2.5 mg six-hourly, 5 mg six-hourly.

*Parkinson's disease:* Introduce Parlodel gradually, as follows: Week 1: 1 mg to 1.25 mg at bed time. Week

2: 2 mg to 2.5 mg at bed time. Week 3: 2.5 mg twice daily. Week 4: 2.5 mg three times daily. Thereafter, take three times a day increasing by 2.5 mg every 3 to 14 days depending on the patient's response. Continue until the optimum dose is reached. This will usually be between 10 and 40 mg daily. In patients already receiving levodopa the dosage of this drug may be gradually decreased, while the dosage of Parlodel is increased until the optimum balance is determined.

*Use in children:* Administration of Parlodel is not appropriate for children less than 15 years old.

*Use in the elderly:* There is no clinical evidence that Parlodel poses a special risk to the elderly.

### Contra-indications, warnings, etc

*Contra-indications:* Hypersensitivity to bromocriptine or other ergot alkaloids. Toxaemia of pregnancy, hypertension postpartum and in the puerperium. For procedure during pregnancy see *Use in pregnancy.*

*Precautions:* Parlodel should not be used in the postpartum or puerperium in women with high blood pressure, coronary artery disease or symptoms and/ or a history of serious mental disorders (see 'Side-effects'). In postpartum women receiving Parlodel, blood pressure should be carefully monitored, especially during the first days of therapy. Particular caution is required in patients who are on concomitant therapy with, or have recently been treated with, drugs that can alter blood pressure. Although there is no conclusive evidence of an interaction between Parlodel and other ergot alkaloids, a concomitant course of these medications during the puerperium is not recommended. If hypertension, unremitting headache, or any signs of CNS toxicity develop, treatment should be discontinued immediately.

Hyperprolactinaemia may be idiopathic, drug-induced, or due to hypothalamic or pituitary disease. The possibility that hyperprolactinaemic patients may have a pituitary tumour should be recognised and complete investigation at specialized units to identify such patients is advisable. Parlodel will effectively lower prolactin levels in patients with pituitary tumours but does not obviate the necessity for radiotherapy or surgical intervention where appropriate in acromegaly.

In women suffering from prolactin-related fertility disorders, treatment with Parlodel results in ovulation. Patients who do not wish to conceive should be advised to practice a reliable method of contraception. Oral contraceptives have, however, been reported to increase serum prolactin levels. When women of child-bearing age are treated with Parlodel for conditions not associated with hyperprolactinaemia the lowest effective dose should be used. This is in order to avoid suppression of prolactin to below normal levels, with consequent impairment of luteal function.

Gynaecological assessment, preferably including cervical and endometrial cytology, is recommended for women receiving Parlodel for extensive periods. Six-monthly assessment is suggested for post-menopausal women and annual assessment for women with regular menstruation.

Hypotensive reactions may be disturbing in some patients during the first few days of treatment and particular care should be exercised when driving vehicles or operating machinery.

Tolerance to Parlodel may be reduced by alcohol.

The concomitant use of erythromycin may increase bromocriptine plasma levels.

In acromegalic patients, whilst Parlodel may effectively lower growth hormone levels, treatment to limit expansion of the tumour is also indicated. Acromegalic patients should be carefully assessed for peptic ulceration prior to treatment with Parlodel and advised to report gastro-intestinal side-effects promptly, as gastro-intestinal bleeding has been reported, though the connection with treatment is not proven.

Caution is required where Parlodel is being given in high doses to patients with a history of psychotic disorders or severe cardiovascular disease.

Among parkinsonian patients on long-term, high-dose Parlodel treatment, pleural effusions have been observed. Patients with unexplained pleuro-pulmonary signs or symptoms should be examined thoroughly and discontinuation of Parlodel therapy should be contemplated.

In a few patients treated for more than a year, with daily doses greater than 30 mg, retroperitoneal fibrosis has been reported. Patients on long-term, high-dose therapy should therefore be observed for manifestations of retroperitoneal fibrosis (e.g. back pain, oedema of the lower limbs or impaired kidney function) so that retroperitoneal fibrosis may be detected at an early stage. Parlodel should be withdrawn if fibrotic changes in the retroperitoneum are diagnosed or suspected.

*Use in pregnancy:* If pregnancy occurs it is generally advisable to withdraw Parlodel after the first missed menstrual period.

Rapid expansion of pituitary tumours sometimes occurs during pregnancy and this may also occur in patients who have been able to conceive as a result of Parlodel therapy. As a precautionary measure, patients should be monitored to detect signs of pituitary enlargement so that Parlodel may be reintroduced if necessary. Based on the outcome of more than 2,000 pregnancies, the use of Parlodel to restore fertility has not been associated with an increased risk of abortion, premature delivery, multiple pregnancy or malformation in infants. Because this accumulated evidence suggests a lack of teratogenic or embryopathic effect in humans, maintenance of Parlodel treatment during pregnancy may be considered where there is a large tumour or evidence of expansion.

*Overdosage:* Overdosage with Parlodel is likely to result in vomiting and other symptoms which could be due to over-stimulation of dopaminergic receptors and might include confusion, hallucinations and hypotension. General supportive measures should be undertaken to remove any unabsorbed material and maintain blood pressure if necessary.

*Side-effects:* Nausea is the most commonly occurring side-effect. Postural hypotension, dizziness, headache, vomiting, and mild constipation have also occasionally been reported. The occurrence of side-effects is minimised by taking Parlodel during a meal and by gradual introduction of the dose. If side-effects do occur, a reduction of dosage, followed in a few days by a more gradual increase, will ameliorate the symptoms.

Episodes of reversible pallor of the fingers and toes induced by cold have occasionally been reported to occur during prolonged treatment, particularly in patients previously exhibiting Raynaud's phenomenon. Drowsiness, and less frequently, confusion, psychomotor excitation, hallucinations, dyskinesia, dry mouth and leg cramps have been reported during high-dose treatment of Parkinson's disease with Parlodel. All these side-effects are dose-dependent and can usually be controlled by a reduction in dosage and a more gradual implementation of dosage increments.

In extremely rare cases (in post partum women treated with Parlodel for the prevention of lactation) serious adverse events including hypertension, myocardial infarction, seizures, stroke, or mental disorders, have been reported although the causal relationship is uncertain. In some patients the occurrence of seizures or stroke was preceded by severe headache and/or transient visual disturbances.

**Pharmaceutical precautions** Protect from light.

**Legal category** POM.

**Package quantities** 1 mg Tablets: Containers of 100. 2.5 mg Tablets: Blister pack of 30 and containers of 100.
5 mg Capsules: Containers of 100.
10 mg Capsules: Containers of 100.

**Further information** Nil.

**Product licence numbers**
1 mg Tablets      0101/0176
2.5 mg Tablets    0101/0061
5 mg Capsules     0101/0131
10 mg Capsules    0101/0108

## PHOSPHATE-SANDOZ*

**Presentation** Flat, round, white, effervescent tablets with a rough surface, weight 3.7 g, 25.4 mm diameter and 4.4 to 4.9 mm thick. Citrus flavoured. Each effervescent tablet contains 1.936 g Anhydrous Sodium Acid Phosphate HSE, 350 mg Sodium Bicarbonate PhEur and 315 mg Potassium Bicarbonate USP. This provides the equivalent of 500 mg elemental phosphorus (16.1 mmol phosphate), 468.8 mg sodium (20.4 mmol: 20.4 mEq Na⁺), 123 mg potassium (3.1 mmol: 3.1 mEq K⁺), also 800 mg anhydrous citric acid (787.4 mg citrate ion).

**Uses**   *Principal action:* Oral administration of inorganic phosphates produces a fall in serum calcium in patients with hypercalcaemia. The main effect of oral phosphate in hypercalcaemia is to bind calcium in the gut thus reducing absorption.

High-dose phosphate supplement.

*Indications:* Hypercalcaemia associated with such conditions as hyperparathyroidism, multiple myelomatosis and malignancy. Hypophosphataemia associated with vitamin D resistant rickets and vitamin D resistant hypophosphataemic osteomalacia.

**Dosage and administration** Phosphate-Sandoz Effervescent Tablets should be dissolved in ⅓ to ½ a tumblerful of water.

Dosage should be adjusted to suit the requirements of individual patients. Excessive dosage has been reported to produce hypocalcaemia in isolated cases. Particular care should therefore be taken to ensure appropriate dosage in the elderly.

*Adults*
*Hypercalcaemia:* Up to 6 tablets daily (adjustment being made according to requirements).
*Vitamin D resistant hypophosphataemic osteomalacia:* 4 to 6 tablets daily.

*Children under 5 years*
*Hypercalcaemia:* Up to 3 tablets daily (adjustment being made according to requirements).
*Vitamin D resistant rickets:* 2 to 3 tablets daily.

### Contra-indications, warnings, etc

*Precautions:* In cases of impaired renal function associated with hypercalcaemia and in cases where restricted sodium intake is required, e.g. congestive cardiac failure, hypertension or pre-eclamptic toxaemia, the sodium (20.4 mmol per tablet) and potassium (3.1 mmol per tablet) content of Phosphate-Sandoz should be taken into consideration. In cases of hypercalcaemia associated with impaired renal function and hyperphosphataemia, the main effect of oral phosphate is to bind calcium in the gut and thus reduce calcium absorption. The effect of oral phosphate on serum phosphate is likely to be minimal, but close monitoring of serum levels is recommended.

Concurrent administration of antacids, containing agents such as aluminium hydroxide, may result in displacement of calcium from binding to oral phosphate, thus reducing efficacy.

Soft-tissue calcification and nephrocalcinosis have been reported in isolated cases following intravenous therapy with phosphate. This is thought to be a function of dosage and rapidity of phosphate administration. While such effects appear less likely to occur following treatment with oral phosphates, careful surveillance of patients is recommended, especially if on long-term therapy.

*Use in pregnancy:* The safety of Phosphate-Sandoz in human pregnancy has not been formally studied, the drug has been widely used for many years without ill consequences. Nevertheless, the benefit of treatment should be considered in relation to the risk before Phosphate-Sandoz is given to pregnant or nursing women.

*Side-effects:* Apart from gastro-intestinal upsets, nausea and diarrhoea, very few side-effects have been reported.

*Overdosage:* Excessive dosage has been reported to produce hypocalcaemia in isolated cases. This has proved reversible when dosage has been adjusted.

**Pharmaceutical precautions** Protect from heat and moisture. Since Phosphate-Sandoz Tablets are hygroscopic they should be dispensed in their original containers.

**Legal category** GSL.

**Package quantities** Boxes of 100 (5 tubes of 20 effervescent tablets).

**Further information** Phosphate-Sandoz Tablets each contain 136 mg sucrose. Approximate calorific value – 3 kcals per tablet.

**Product licence number** 0101/5038R.

## PRESCAL*

**Presentation** The active ingredient, isradipine, is presented as: 2.5 mg yellow, flat circular angled scored tablets (designed to be easily divided), 6 mm diameter, marked NM on one face and CIBA on the other.

**Uses**
*Indication:* Prescal is recommended for the treatment of essential hypertension.

*Mode of action:* Isradipine is a dihydropyridine calcium antagonist with a higher affinity for calcium channels in arterial smooth muscle than for those in the myocardium. Thus it produces vasodilation of peripheral, coronary, and cerebral arteries without notably depressing cardiac function. As a result of the vasodilation of peripheral arteries, the arterial blood pressure is lowered; the attending after-load reduction improves myocardial contractility and increases cardiac output, while myocardial oxygen consumption decreases. In animal studies isradipine has been observed to exert a cardioprotective effect against ischaemic injury without cardiodepression.

*Pharmacokinetics:* Following oral administration of Prescal, isradipine is almost completely absorbed (90-95%) from the gastrointestinal tract and undergoes extensive first pass metabolism resulting in a bioavailability of about 15-24%. Single oral doses are detectable in the plasma within 20 minutes and peak plasma concentrations are reached approximately 2 hours after intake. Isradipine is approximately 95% bound to plasma proteins.

No clear correlation between renal function and pharmacokinetic parameters has been found; both an increase and decrease in bioavailability has been observed in patients with impaired renal function. The bioavailability of isradipine was increased in elderly patients with impaired liver function.

**Dosage and administration** Prescal can be administered with or without food.

The recommended dosage is 2.5 mg twice a day (i.e about every 12 hours). Treatment for 3-4 weeks is required for the maximum effect to develop. If blood pressure is not adequately controlled after this period patients may require a dosage of 5 mg twice a day, or if more appropriate, the addition of a low dose of another antihypertensive agent ie thiazide diuretic or beta-blocker. Exceptionally, some patients may require up to 10 mg twice a day. Prescal can also be added to an ongoing regimen of other antihypertensive agents.

*Use in the elderly and patients with impaired hepatic or renal function:* In elderly patients, or where hepatic or renal function is impaired, a more suitable starting dose is 1.25 mg twice a day for hypertension. However, the dosage may be increased according to the requirements of the individual patient. Once daily maintenance treatment with 2.5 mg or 5 mg may be sufficient in some hypertensive patients.

*Use in children:* The efficacy and safety of Prescal has not been established in children and is therefore not recommended in these patients.

**Contra-indications, warnings, etc**
*Contra-indications:* Patients with a previous allergic reaction to isradipine and other dihydropyridines because of the theoretical risk of cross-reactivity.

Dihydropyridines, including Prescal tablets, should be discontinued in patients who develop cardiogenic shock. They should also not be used in patients with symptomatic or tight aortic stenosis, and during or within one month of myocardial infarction.

Dihydropyridines including Prescal tablets should not be used for the prevention of secondary myocardial infarctions and they have not been approved for the treatment of hypertensive crisis.

*Precautions:* As for other calcium antagonists Prescal does not give protection against the danger of abrupt beta-blocker withdrawal. Beta-blockers should therefore be withdrawn gradually, preferably over 8–10 days.

Caution should be taken when treating patients with documented or strongly suspected sick sinus syndrome who are not fitted with a pacemaker.

Prescal should be used with caution in patients with poor cardiac reserve.

Care is recommended when treating patients with a low systolic blood pressure.

There is no evidence that Prescal interferes with glucose metabolism, however, diabetic patients should be initially monitored in accord with good clinical practice.

*Use in pregnancy and lactation:* Although some dihydropyridine compounds have been found to be teratogenic in animals, animal data in the rat and rabbit on isradipine provide no evidence for a teratogenic or embryotoxic effect. There is insufficient experience of the drug in pregnant women to justify its use during pregnancy, unless the potential benefit to the mother is expected to outweigh any potential risk to the offspring. Pre-natal observations in animals suggest that high doses of isradipine may cause prolongation of labour.

Animal data indicate that small quantities of isradipine may be excreted in the breast milk. Therefore breast-feeding should not be undertaken by mothers treated with Prescal.

*Drug interactions:* The bioavailability of isradipine is not affected by co-administration of food, however the lag time to absorption and time to peak plasma concentration may be delayed by about one hour.

The pharmacokinetics of isradipine is not modified by the concomitant administration of digoxin, propranolol, or hydrochlorothiazide. Nor are the kinetics of digoxin or hydrochlorothiazide altered by the concomitant administration of Prescal. However, Prescal increases the bioavailability of propranolol, but this does not appear to be of any clinical significance. Isradipine is non-specifically bound to proteins. Enzyme inducing anticonvulsants may be associated with reduced levels of isradipine. As with other dihydropyridines, Prescal should not be taken with grapefruit juice because bioavailability may be increased.

Concurrent administration of cimetidine, an inhibitor of the cytochrome P450 system, results in an increase of about 50% in the bioavailability of Prescal whereas concomitant administration of rifampicin, an inducer of the cytochrome P450 system, greatly reduces the plasma concentrations of Prescal. Therefore, when Prescal is administered together with other drugs which alter the activity of the cytochrome P450 system, patients should be monitored carefully and doses of these drugs altered accordingly.

*Side-effects:* Clinical studies indicate that Prescal is

well tolerated with an overall incidence of adverse events similar to that of placebo when used in doses up to 2.5 mg twice a day. Generally side effects are mild, dose dependent and tend to disappear or decrease in intensity as treatment is continued. Discontinuation of therapy is generally not required. Those side effects mentioned most often are related to the vasodilating properties of Prescal: headache, flushing, dizziness, tachycardia and palpitation, and localised peripheral oedema of non-cardiac origin; hypotension is uncommon and there have been no reports of orthostatic hypotension.

Non-specific side-effects are rare and include: weight gain, fatigue, abdominal discomfort, and skin rash.

Elevations of serum transaminases have been observed on very rare occasions; these changes were reversible both spontaneously and on following Prescal withdrawal.

As with other dihydropyridines, aggravation of underlying angina has been reported in a small number of individuals especially after starting treatment. This is more likely to happen in patients with symptomatic ischaemic heart disease. Prescal should be discontinued under medical supervision in patients who develop unstable angina.

*Overdosage*
*Symptoms:* Available data on calcium antagonists suggest that overdosage would result in marked and prolonged systemic hypotension requiring cardiovascular support, with monitoring of cardiac and respiratory functions and attention to possible cerebral ischaemia (elevation of the lower extremities) and to circulating blood volume (intravenous fluid or plasma volume expanders).

*Management:* In cases of severe hypotension, vasoconstrictors could be beneficial provided there is no contra-indication to their use. Intravenous calcium may help to reverse the effect of calcium entry blockade. Animal data suggest the risk for cardiodepression with Prescal should be minimal, but depression of the sinus node may occur in which case temporary pacemaker treatment may be useful.

Since isradipine is bound to plasma proteins to a very large extent, dialysis cannot be expected to be of benefit.

**Pharmaceutical precautions** The tablets should be protected from light.

**Legal category** POM

**Package quantities** Boxes of 56 tablets consisting of 2 blister strips each containing 28 tablets.

**Further information** Prescal is effective in both Negroid and Caucasian hypertensive patients, requiring no alteration of dose. Additionally, no potential deleterious first dose effects have been observed.

In asthmatic patients a single dose of isradipine has been found to blunt the bronchospastic response to exercise.

In patients with congestive heart failure, single oral doses of Prescal improved cardiac performance in terms of increasing cardiac output and decreasing pulmonary capillary venous pressure.

Prescal has not been shown to be arrhythmogenic and does not depress the atrioventricular node.

**Product licence number** 0001/0132

*Product licence holder:* Ciba-Geigy plc, Hulley Road, Macclesfield, Cheshire SK10 2NX.

# REGULOSE*

**Presentation** Regulose is a clear, almost colourless to brownish-yellow plum flavoured syrup. Each 5 ml spoonful contains 3.33 g lactulose and 1.33 g of other sugars (lactose, galactose, tagatose and other ketosugars).

**Uses**
*Principal actions:* Lactulose prevents the formation of hard stools and encourages normal bowel movement. Unlike traditional laxative preparations which act either on the innervation or musculature of the intestine or by bulk stimulus, lactulose provides a natural substrate for the saccharolytic bacterial flora in the colon.

Lactulose is a disaccharide which is not hydrolysed in the small intestine. Therefore it cannot be absorbed and is transported to the colon with water to retain the osmotic balance. In the colon, several species of bacteria can hydrolyse lactulose to the monosaccharides galactose and fructose.

By encouraging this normal metabolic activity of the bacteria, the osmotic pressure of the colonic contents is doubled and more water is drawn into the bowel.

Further metabolism of the monosaccharides leads to the production of acetic and lactic acids and the subsequent lowering of colonic pH. This acidification of the colonic contents is considered to be the main reason for the effectiveness of lactulose solution. In

chronic portal-systemic encephalopathy it may be associated with the decrease in the relative concentration of free ammonia, the major agent involved in the cerebral disturbance.

*Indications:* Chronic constipation. Chronic portal-systemic encephalopathy.

**Dosage and administration**
*Chronic constipation:* Because lactulose acts naturally to encourage the normal activity of the bowel, it may be two or three days before the full benefit of the treatment is obtained. It is important, therefore, to follow the dosage regimen set out below.

*Adults*
*Initially:* Three to six 5 ml spoonfuls for the first two to three days of treatment. (Nine spoonfuls may be given in obstinate cases).
*Maintenance:* Two to three 5 ml spoonfuls daily or according to the needs of the patient.

*Children*
*Initially:* Two to five 5 ml spoonfuls for the first two to three days of treatment.
*Maintenance:* One to three 5 ml spoonfuls daily or according to the needs of the patient.

*Chronic portal-systemic encephalopathy:* Six to ten 5 ml spoonfuls three times daily according to the requirements of the patient, for adequate acidification of the colonic contents.

*Use in the elderly:* No evidence exists that elderly patients require different dosages or show different side-effects from younger patients.

**Contra-indications, warnings, etc**
*Contra-indications:* In common with other preparations used for the treatment of constipation, Regulose should not be used in patients with gastrointestinal obstruction. Regulose should not be given to patients with galactosaemia or lactose intolerance.

*Precautions:* Regulose should be used with caution during the first trimester of pregnancy. There are no known drug interactions involving Regulose. There is no evidence that Regulose affects driving ability.

*Overdosage:* No cases of intoxication due to deliberate or accidental overdosage with Regulose have been reported to the company.

*Side-effects:* Side-effects rarely occur after the administration of Regulose. Mild transient effects such as abdominal distension or cramps and flatulence, which subside after the initial stages of treatment, have occasionally been reported.

High doses may provoke nausea in some patients. This can be minimised by administration with water, fruit juice, or with meals.

**Pharmaceutical precautions** Regulose should be stored below 25°C. Dilution is not recommended.

**Legal category** P.

**Package quantities** Bottles of 200 ml, 300 ml and 500 ml.

**Further information** Nil.

**Product licence number** 0101/0363

# RIMACTANE*

**Qualitative and quantitative composition** The active ingredient is 3-(4-Methyl-1-piperazinyliminomethyl)rifamycin SV.

One capsule contains 150 mg or 300 mg Rifampicin PhEur.

The syrup contains 100 mg Rifampicin BP in every 5 mls.

**Pharmaceutical form** Capsules and syrup.

**Clinical particulars**
*Therapeutic indications:* Rimactane is a major drug in the management of tuberculosis (all forms) and certain opportunistic mycobacterial infections. It is effective in cases resistant to other anti-tuberculosis agents and shows no cross-resistance outside the rifampycin group of drugs. In the treatment of tuberculosis Rimactane must always be combined with other anti-tuberculosis agents. It is effective in combination with isoniazid, streptomycin, pyrazinamide, ethambutol and the majority of second line drugs.

Rimactane is also indicated for the chemoprophylaxis of meningococcal meningitis.

*Posology and method of administration*
*For the management of tuberculosis and certain opportunistic mycobacterial infections:* Rimactane must always be given in association with other anti-tuberculosis drugs, to prevent emergence of resistant strains.

*Use in adults:* 450–600 mg daily as a single dose (based on approximately 10 mg per kg body weight). Those patients 50 kg (8 stone) and over should take

600 mg rifampicin daily, whilst patients under 50 kg should take 450 mg).

The following chemotherapeutic agents are employed today as combined therapy for tuberculosis; rifampicin (Rimactane) (RMP), isoniazid (INH), pyrazinamide (PZA), ethambutol (EMB), streptomycin (STM).

The dosages recommended by the Centres for Disease Control and Prevention are given in the table.

For the treatment of sputum-positive pulmonary tuberculosis, preference is given to the following regimens: (for dosage information please refer to the text above for Rimactane and to the table for other components of the treatment).

*Continuous therapy:*
*Daily for a total of 9 months:*

| | |
|---|---|
| Initial phase for 2 months: | RMP + INH + PZA + EMB or STM |
| Continuation phase for 7 months: | RMP + INH |

A total duration of 9 months is recommended for tuberculosis with HIV infection and for tuberculous meningitis, disseminated tuberculosis, or spinal involvement with neurological complications.

*Daily for a total of 6 months:*

| | |
|---|---|
| Initial phase for 2 months: | RMP + INH + PZA + EMB or STM |
| Continuation phase for 4 months: | RMP + INH |

*Partially intermittent therapy:*
*Total duration 6 months:*

| | |
|---|---|
| Initial phase for 2 months: | RMP + INH + PZA + EMB or STM |
| Continuation phase for 4 months: | RMP + INH twice or 3 times a week |

*Fully intermittent therapy:*

| | |
|---|---|
| Total duration 6 months: | RMP + INH + PZA + EMB or STM 3 times a week |

In the case of all regimens administered twice or three times weekly, the patient should be monitored with directly observed therapy (i.e. administration of tablets under supervision). The same applies for relapses and treatment failures.

*Use in children:* Up to 20 mg per kg body weight daily to a maximum of 600 mg as a single dose.

*Use in premature and new-born infants:* 10 mg/kg once daily. Premature and new-born infants should be treated only in cases of emergency and with extreme caution since their liver enzyme system may not be fully developed.

*Use in elderly:* No special dosage regime is necessary but concurrent hepatic insufficiency should be taken into account (see *Pharmacokinetics*).

*For the chemoprophylaxis of meningococcal meningitis: Note:* Rimactane should not be used to treat overt meningococcal meningitis.

*Use in adults:* 600 mg twice daily (12 hourly) for 2 days.

*Use in children (aged 1-12 years):* 10 mg/kg twice daily (12 hourly) for 2 days. Children at the lower end of this age range may metabolise rifampicin more rapidly and produce significantly lower serum levels than new-borns or adults. In such cases doses up to 15 mg/kg 12 hourly may be required.

*Use in infants (up to 1 year):* 5 mg/kg twice daily (12 hourly) for 2 days.

*Use in the elderly:* There is no evidence to suggest that dose adjustments are necessary.

This prophylactic administration should be started as soon as possible. It is recommended that Rimactane is only given for 2 days in this indication since resistance to this class of antibacterial agent may develop.

*Contra-indications:* Hypersensitivity to rifamycins or other excipients of the capsules or syrup.

*Special warnings and precautions for use:*
*Warnings:* Patients receiving Rimactane for the chemoprophylaxis of meningococcal meningitis should be kept under close surveillance. Special attention should be paid to signs of overt infection.

Rimactane should not be used to treat an overt meningococcal infection.

To prevent the emergence of resistant bacteria, Rimactane must always be combined with other antibiotics/chemotherapeutic agents when used to treat infections.

*Intermittent therapy:* The 'flu syndrome' (see *Side effects*) is chiefly encountered during intermittent therapy and may be a prelude to serious complications such as thrombocytopenia, purpura, haemolytic anaemia, dyspnoea and asthma-like attacks, shock and renal failure. In the event of its onset, therefore, one should consider the possibility of switching to daily medication. Such a switch must always be made where the 'flu syndrome' assumes a relatively severe form and if the aforementioned serious complications occur, the medication must be withdrawn at once and never reinstituted.

When changing over from intermittent to daily therapy, an incremental dosage must be employed, starting with approx. 75–150 mg on the first day. The desired therapeutic dose should be reached within 3–4 days. During this time the patient's renal function should be closely monitored. Corticosteroids may prove useful in attenuating possible immunopathological reactions.

Resumption of therapy after its interruption: since severe reactions such as shock and renal failure may occur in rare cases upon resumption of therapy, incremental dosing under close surveillance is mandatory (see *Intermittent therapy*).

*Precautions:* In the treatment of tuberculosis rifampicin should be given under the supervision of a respiratory or other suitably qualified physician.

As Rimactane is excreted principally by the biliary tract, caution should be exercised in treating patients with hepatic disorders.

All tuberculosis patients should have pretreatment measurement of liver function.

If a patient has no evidence of pre-existing liver disease and normal pretreatment liver function, liver function tests need only be repeated if fever, vomiting, jaundice or other deterioration in the patients condition occurs.

In patients with or likely to have liver function abnormalities including those with chronic liver disease, chronic alcoholism, the elderly and the undernourished, the benefit of combined treatment with rifampicin must be weighed against the possible risks. This applies particularly to combination of isoniazid and/or pyrazinamide with rifampicin. In the presence of severely impaired liver function or jaundice the dosage may have to be reduced.

Regular monitoring of liver function is required in patients with chronic liver disease throughout treatment with rifampicin. Weekly testing for two weeks followed by tests every two weeks for the next six weeks is recommended initially. Blood counts and liver function tests should also be performed periodically during prolonged treatment.

Rifampicin should be withdrawn if clinically significant changes in hepatic function occur. The need for other forms of antituberculous therapy and a different regimen should be considered. Urgent advice should be obtained from a specialist in the management of tuberculosis. If rifampicin is reintroduced after liver function has returned to normal, liver function should be monitored daily until the maintenance dose has been established. This should be followed by weekly testing for two weeks and then testing every two weeks for the next six weeks. Liver function should be monitored periodically thereafter.

Owing to its enzyme-inducing effect, rifampicin must be employed with extreme caution in patients with porphyria, because activation of delta-aminolaevulinic acid synthetase may lead to an acute manifestation of the porphyria.

To preclude all possibility of pregnancy during treatment with Rimactane, non-hormonal means of contraception must be employed (see *Interactions*).

*Interactions with other medicaments and other types of interactions:* Antacids, opiates, and anticholinergic drugs and ketoconazole reduce the bioavailability of rifampicin when given concomitantly by mouth. The same applies to PAS preparations containing bentonite. To avoid this interaction, rifampicin must be administered a few hours before these preparations.

Rifampicin is a potent inducer of liver enzymes which may increase the metabolism of concomitantly administered drugs such as those listed below. The activity of the following drugs may be impaired and their dosage must be reassessed during and after treatment with Rifampicin.

Oral anticoagulants; oral antidiabetic agents, digitalis preparations, antiarrhythmic agents (disopyramide, quinidine, mexiletine, tocainide, lorcainide, propafenone), methadone (withdrawal signs may set in), hydantoins (phenyltoin); hexobarbital, nortriptyline, benzodiazepines, corticosteroids (Addison patients may develop a crisis; exacerbation of pemphigus may occur; treatment for corticoid-dependent asthma patients may become more difficult or impossible); sex hormones (menstrual disorders may appear); oral contraceptives (their effect can no longer be relied upon); theophyllines, dapsone, chloramphenicol, azole antifungal agents (ketoconazole; itraconazole), cyclosporin A; azathioprine (transplants may be rejected); beta blockers, calcium-channel blockers (nifedipine, verapamil); enalapril, cimetidine.

Although concurrent use of isoniazid, pyrazinamide and rifampicin is common and therapeutically valuable, hepatic toxicity may be increased.

Rifampicin can delay the biliary excretion of contrast media employed to X-ray the gall bladder.

Microbiological techniques for assaying folic acid and vitamin $B_{12}$ in the serum are unsuitable for use during treatment with Rimactane.

*Pregnancy and lactation:* In studies of over 300 women exposed to rifampicin during pregnancy, no significant increase in the rate of malformations in their offspring, over and above the background level was observed. Rimactane should not be given during pregnancy unless the potential benefit justifies the potential risk to the foetus.

Administration of Rimactane during the last few weeks of pregnancy can cause post-natal haemorrhage in the mother and new-born infant. This may necessitate treatment with vitamin K preparations.

Rifampicin passes into the breast milk but no adverse effects on breast-fed infants have been observed. Therefore nursing mothers may continue to breast-feed their infants.

*Effects on ability to drive or use machines:* None known.

*Undesirable effects:* Rifampicin may cause reddish discolouration of body fluids and occasionally other body secretions, e.g. urine, sputum, lacrimal fluid, faeces, saliva, sweat. It may permanently discolour soft contact-lenses.

Unwanted effects which may occur during continuous daily or intermittent therapy.

Frequency estimates: frequent>10%, occasional>1–10%, rare>0.001%–1%, isolated cases<0.001%.

*Skin and appendages:* Occasionally: flushing, itching with or without skin rash, and reddening of the eyes. Isolated cases: severe signs and symptoms, such as exudative conjunctivitis or generalised hypersensitivity reactions involving the skin, e.g. exfoliative dermatitis, Lyell's syndrome and pemphigoid reactions.

*Gastro-intestinal tract:* Occasionally: anorexia, nausea, abdominal pains, gaseous distension; rarely: vomiting or diarrhoea; isolated occurrences of erosive gastritis and pseudomembranous colitis.

*Hepatic:* Frequently: an asymptomatic increase in liver enzymes; rarely: hepatitis or jaundice; here account should also be taken of the liver toxicity of chemotherapeutic agents, e.g. isoniazid or pyrazinamide, employed in combination with rifampicin. Induction of porphyria in isolated cases.

*Central and peripheral nervous system:* Occasionally: tiredness, drowsiness, headache, light-headedness, dizziness; rarely: ataxia, mental confusion. Isolated cases: muscular weakness, visual disturbances.

*Blood:* Isolated occurrences of transient leucopenia; eosinophilia; thrombocytopenia and thrombocytopenic purpura are encountered more frequently under intermittent therapy than on continuous daily treatment, during which they occur only in isolated cases.

*Endocrine:* In rare instances disturbances in the menstrual cycle (in extreme cases amenorrhoea); induction of a crisis in Addison patients (see *Interactions*).

Unwanted effects chiefly occurring during intermittent therapy or upon resumption of treatment after temporary interruption: In patients taking rifampicin other than on a daily basis or in those resuming treatment with the drug after a temporary interruption, an influenza-like syndrome ('flu syndrome') may occur, this being very probably of immunopathological origin. It is characterised by fever, shivering, and possibly headache, dizziness and musculoskeletal pain. In rare cases the 'flu syndrome' may be followed by thrombocytopenia, purpura, dyspnoea, asthma-like attacks, haemolytic anaemia, shock and acute renal failure. These serious complications may, however, also set in suddenly with no preceding 'flu syndrome', chiefly when treatment is resumed after a temporary interruption or when rifampicin is given only once a week in high doses (25 mg/kg or more). When Rimactane is administered in lower doses (600 mg) 2–3 times a week, the syndrome is encountered less frequently, its incidence then being comparable to that observed during daily medication.

*Overdose:*

*Signs and symptoms:* Nausea, vomiting, abdominal pains; enlargement of the liver, jaundice, elevated liver enzyme levels, possibly acute pulmonary oedema, lethargy, clouding of consciousness, convulsions.

*Treatment:* Gastric lavage together with instillation of an activated charcoal suspension via a stomach tube; general supportive measures to maintain vital functions; forced diureses; haemodialysis; in the presence of severe liver damage, cholecystotomy if necessary. Bear in mind that other drugs used in combination with Rimactane may also have been taken in an overdosage and necessitate additional specific measures.

**Pharmacological properties**

*Pharmacodynamic properties:*

*Pharmacotherapeutic group:* Rifampicin is a rifamycin antibiotic.

*Mechanisms of action:* Rimactane exerts, both *in vitro* and *in vivo* bactericidal effects on *Mycobacterium tuberculosis*. It also exhibits variable activity against other atypical species of Mycobacterium.

Combined therapy for tuberculosis: Dosages recommended by the Centres for Disease Control and Prevention

| Drug | Daily mg/kg Children | Adults | max. mg | Twice a week mg/kg Children | Adults | max. mg | 3 times a week mg/kg Children | Adults | max. mg |
|---|---|---|---|---|---|---|---|---|---|
| RMP | 10–20 | 10 | 600 | 10–20 | 10 | 600 | 10–20 | 10 | 600 |
| INH | 10–20 | 5 | 300 | 20–40 | 15 | 900 | 20–40 | 15 | 900 |
| PZA | 15–30 | 15–30 | 2,000 | 50–70 | 50–70 | 4,000 | 50–70 | 50–70 | 3,000 |
| EMB | 15–25 | 5–25 | 2,500 | 50 | 50 | 2,500 | 25–30 | 25–30 | 2,500 |
| STM | 20–30 | 15 | 1,000 | 25–30 | 25–30 | 1,500 | 25–30 | 25–30 | 1,000 |

*In vivo* it exerts its bactericidal effect not only on micro-organisms in the extracellular spaces but also on those located intracellularly. Rifampicin has a potent sterilising effect.

Rifampicin inhibits the DNA-dependent RNA polymerase of sensitive bacterial strains, but without affecting the corresponding mammalian enzyme.

Since relatively rapid 'one-step' selection of resistant bacteria occurs with rifampicin, the drug must not be employed as monotherapy to treat overt infections. Bacteria resistant to rifampicin display no cross-resistance to other antibiotics with the exception of the rifamycins.

*Pharmacokinetic properties:*

*Absorption:* Rifampicin is rapidly and completely absorbed. Following a single dose taken on an empty stomach (600 mg) the peak serum concentrations (approx. 10 mcg/ml) are observed after about 2 hours. Ingestion with food may adversely affect the absorption of rifampicin.

*Distribution:* The apparent distribution volume is 1.6 L/kg in adults and 1.1 L/kg in children. Binding to serum proteins amounts to 84%–91%.

Rifampicin penetrates rapidly into various body fluids and tissues, including bone tissue. Rifampicin crosses the blood/brain barrier in the case of inflamed meninges only, but concentrations in the cerebrospinal fluid may remain above the MIC for *Mycobacterium tuberculosis* for up to two months with continuous therapy of 600 mg/day orally.

Rifampicin crosses the human placenta and is secreted in human breast milk. However, it is estimated that a breast-fed infant would receive no more than 1% of the usual therapeutic dose.

*Biotransformation:* Rifampicin is metabolised in the liver, the principal metabolite being 25-O-deacetyl-rifampicin, which is microbiologically active and, like rifampicin, subject to enterohepatic circulation. Rifampicin induces its own metabolism.

*Elimination:* The plasma elimination half-life of rifampicin increases with increasing doses and amounts to 2.5 h, 3–4 h and about 5 h after single doses of 300 mg, 600 mg and 900 mg respectively. After a few days of repeated daily administration, the bioavailability of rifampicin diminishes, and the half-life value following repeated doses of 600 mg falls to 1–2 hours.

Owing to its enzyme-inducing effect in the liver, rifampicin accelerates its own metabolism, with the result that its systemic clearance, which amounts to approx. 6 L/h after the first dose, rises to approx. 9 L/h after repeated dosing.

Although the bulk of the drug is eliminated in the bile, 80% of the quantity excreted being accounted for by the deacetylrifampicin metabolite, rifampicin also appears in the urine. In a dosage range of 150–900 mg, 4–18% of a dose is excreted dose-dependently in the urine in unchanged form.

*Characteristics in patients:* In elderly patients, renal clearance is reduced, but, owing to the large scale on which the drug is eliminated via the liver, the plasma concentrations are similar to those in young patients.

With impaired renal function, the elimination half-life becomes prolonged only at doses exceeding 600 mg daily. Provided that hepatic excretory function is normal, the dosage in patients with impaired renal function does not need to be reduced below 600 mg daily. Rifampicin is eliminated by peritoneal or haemodialysis. Dosage adjustment is not necessary during dialysis. Because rifampicin is dialysable it is recommended that the drug should not be administered until after the period of dialysis is complete.

In patients with severe hepatic dysfunction the dosage may have to be adjusted as plasma concentrations are raised and half-life prolonged.

*Preclinical safety data:* There is limited evidence as to the carcinogenic potential of rifampicin in animals. In female mice of a strain known to be susceptible to hepatomas, a significant increase in such tumours was observed after 1 year of treatment with rifampicin in quantities equivalent to 2–10 times the maximum clinical doses.

In mice of another strain treated for 1 year, and in rats treated for 2 years, no significant increase was noted in the incidence of any type of tumour. Studies with various mammalian models, as well as with bacteria, yielded no evidence that rifampicin has a mutagenic effect.

In daily doses of 150–250 mg/kg, rifampicin proved teratogenic in mice and rats, insofar as an increased occurrence of spina bifida and cleft palate was observed. In rabbits it had no teratogenic effect. In all three animal species, unspecific embryotoxic effects occurred after doses>150 mg/kg.

**Pharmaceutical particulars**

*List of excipients:* The capsules contain calcium stearate, lactose, titanium dioxide (E171), iron oxide red (E172) and gelatin.

The syrup contains zanthan gum, methyl hydroxybenzoate (E218), propyl hydroxybenzoate (E216), sucrose, potassium sorbate (E202), saccharin, sodium metabisulphite (E223), raspberry flavour, antifoam AF (dimethylpolysiloxane and silica).

*Incompatibilities:* None known.

*Shelf-life:* Capsules: Four years. Syrup: Three years.

*Special precautions for storage:* Capsules: Protect from moisture and heat (store below 30°C). Syrup: Store below 25°C.

Medicines should be kept out of reach of children.

*Nature and contents of container:* The capsules are opaque, two-piece, hard gelatine capsule size 2, reddish-brown in colour, marked with the monogram CG on each half and the code JZ 150, and come in securitainers of 100 and PVC/PVdC blister packs of 56.

The syrup is an opaque, red-coloured suspension having the odour and taste of raspberry and is contained in a glass bottle with a child resistant clic-loc cap.

*Instructions for use/handling:* None.

**Marketing authorisation numbers**

| | |
|---|---|
| Capsules 150 mg | 00101/0445 |
| Capsules 300 mg | 00101/0446 |
| Syrup | 00101/0448 |

**Date of approval/revision of SPC** 16 July 1996.

**Legal category** POM.

# RIMACTANE* INFUSION

**Qualitative and quantitative composition** The active ingredient is 3-[[(4-Methyl-1-piperazinyl)-imino]-methyl]-rifamycin SV natrium (=rifampicin sodium) equivalent to rifampicin 300 mg.

One vial contains 308.2 mg rifampicin sodium salt, equivalent to 300 mg Rifampicin BP.

**Pharmaceutical form** Vial.

**Clinical particulars**

*Therapeutic indications:* Rimactane is a major drug in the management of tuberculosis (all forms) and certain opportunistic mycobacterial infections. It is effective in cases resistant to other anti-tuberculous agents and shows no cross-resistance outside the rifampycin group of drugs. In the treatment of tuberculosis Rimactane must always be combined with other anti-tuberculosis agents. It is effective in combination with isoniazid, streptomycin, pyrazinamide, ethambutol and the majority of second line drugs.

Rimactane infusion is indicated in patients with all forms of tuberculosis who are unable to tolerate oral therapy, e.g. post-operative or comatose patients or patients in whom gastro-intestinal absorption is impaired.

*Posology and method of administration*

*For the management of tuberculosis and certain opportunistic mycobacterial infections:* Rimactane must always be given in association with other anti-tuberculosis drugs, to prevent emergence of resistant strains.

*Use in adults:* 450–600 mg daily as a single dose (based on approximately 10 mg per kg body weight). A daily dose of 600 mg given in an intravenous infusion over two to three hours has been found to be effective and well tolerated for the majority of adult patients. Serum levels following this regimen are similar to those obtained following oral administration. Lower doses are recommended for small or frail patients. (Patients 50 kg (8 stone) and over should take 600 mg rifampicin daily, whilst patients under 50 kg should take 450 mg).

The chemotherapeutic agents usually employed today as combined therapy for tuberculosis are rifampicin (Rimactane) (RMP), isoniazid (INH), pyrazinamide (PZA), ethambutol (EMB), streptomycin (STM).

The dosages recommended by the Centres for Disease Control and Prevention are as follows (see Table below):

For the treatment of sputum-positive pulmonary tuberculosis, preference is given to the following regimens: (for dosage information please refer to the text above for Rimactane and to the table for other components of the treatment).

*Continuous therapy:*

*Daily for a total of 9 months:*

| | |
|---|---|
| Initial phase for 2 months: | RMP + INH + PZA + EMB or STM |
| Continuation phase for 7 months: | RMP + INH |

A total duration of 9 months is recommended for tuberculosis with HIV infection and for tuberculous meningitis, disseminated tuberculosis, or spinal involvement with neurological complications.

*Daily for a total of 6 months:*

| | |
|---|---|
| Initial phase for 2 months: | RMP + INH + PZA + EMB or STM |
| Continuation phase for 4 months: | RMP + INH |

*Partially intermittent therapy:*

*Total duration 6 months:*

| | |
|---|---|
| Initial phase for 2 months: | RMP + INH + PZA + EMB or STM |
| Continuation phase for 4 months: | RMP + INH twice or 3 times a week |

*Fully intermittent therapy:*

| | |
|---|---|
| Total duration 6 months: | RMP + INH + PZA + EMB or STM 3 times a week |

In the case of all regimens administered twice or three times weekly, the patient should be monitored with directly observed therapy (i.e. administration of tablets under supervision). The same applies for relapses and treatment failures.

*Use in children:* Paediatric usage has not yet been established. However, the following regimen is suggested. In tuberculosis, a single daily dose of up to 20 mg/kg body weight daily is recommended, although total daily dose should not usually exceed 600 mg.

*Use in premature and new-born infants:* 10 mg/kg once daily. Premature and new-born infants should be treated only in cases of emergency and with extreme caution since their liver enzyme system may not be fully developed.

*Use in elderly:* No special dosage regime is necessary but concurrent hepatic insufficiency should be taken into account (see *Pharmacokinetics*).

*Transfer to oral therapy:* When patients are able to accept oral medication, they should be transferred to Rimactane capsules or syrup. Oral dosage would be expected to be the same as that used with the infusion (see oral Rimactane data sheet).

*Contra-indications:* Hypersensitivity to rifamycins or other excipients of the infusion.

*Special warnings and precautions for use:*

*Warning:* To prevent the emergence of resistant bacteria, Rimactane must always be combined with other antibiotics/chemotherapeutic agents when used to treat infections.

There have been isolated reports of hypersensitivity reactions affecting the face and hands of nursing staff preparing and applying infusions. Care should be taken to avoid contact with rifampicin.

*Intermittent therapy:* The 'flu syndrome' (see *Side effects*) is chiefly encountered during intermittent therapy and may be a prelude to serious complications such as thrombocytopenia, purpura, haemolytic anaemia, dyspnoea and asthma-like attacks, shock and renal failure. In the event of its onset, therefore, one should consider the possibility of switching to daily medication. Such a switch must always be made where the 'flu syndrome' assumes a relatively severe form and if the aforementioned serious complications occur, the medication must be withdrawn at once and never reinstituted.

When changing over from intermittent to daily therapy, an incremental dosage must be employed, starting with approx. 75–150 mg on the first day. The desired therapeutic dose should be reached within 3–4 days. During this time the patient's renal function should be closely monitored. Corticosteroids may prove useful in attenuating possible immunopathological reactions.

Resumption of therapy after its interruption: since severe reactions such as shock and renal failure may occur in rare cases upon resumption of therapy, incremental dosing under close surveillance is mandatory (see 'intermittent therapy').

*Precautions:* In the treatment of tuberculosis rifampicin should be given under the supervision of a respiratory or other suitably qualified physician.

| Drug | Daily mg/kg Children | Adults | max. mg | Twice a week mg/kg Children | Adults | max. mg | 3 times a week mg/kg Children | Adults | max. mg |
|------|------|------|------|------|------|------|------|------|------|
| RMP | 10–20 | 10 | 600 | 10–20 | 10 | 600 | 10–20 | 10 | 600 |
| INH | 10–20 | 5 | 300 | 20–40 | 15 | 900 | 20–40 | 15 | 900 |
| PZA | 15–30 | 15–30 | 2,000 | 50–70 | 50–70 | 4,000 | 50–70 | 50–70 | 3,000 |
| EMB | 15–25 | 5–25 | 2,500 | 50 | 50 | 2,500 | 25–30 | 25–30 | 2,500 |
| STM | 20–30 | 15 | 1,000 | 25–30 | 25–30 | 1,500 | 25–30 | 25–30 | 1,000 |

As Rimactane is excreted principally by the biliary tract, caution should be exercised in treating patients with hepatic disorders.

All tuberculosis patients should have pretreatment measurement of liver function.

If a patient has no evidence of pre-existing liver disease and normal pretreatment liver function, liver function tests need only be repeated if fever, vomiting, jaundice or other deterioration in the patients condition occurs.

In patients with or likely to have liver function abnormalities including those with chronic liver disease, chronic alcoholism, the elderly and the undernourished, the benefit of combined treatment with rifampicin must be weighed against the possible risks. This applies particularly to combination of isoniazid and/or pyrazinamide with rifampicin. In the presence of severely impaired liver function or jaundice the dosage may have to be reduced.

Regular monitoring of liver function is required in patients with chronic liver disease throughout treatment with rifampicin. Weekly testing for two weeks followed by tests every two weeks for the next six weeks is recommended initially. Blood counts and liver function tests should also be performed periodically during prolonged treatment.

Rifampicin should be withdrawn if clinically significant changes in hepatic function occur. The need for other forms of antituberculous therapy and a different regimen should be considered. Urgent advice should be obtained from a specialist in the management of tuberculosis. If rifampicin is reintroduced after liver function has returned to normal, liver function should be monitored daily until the maintenance dose has been established. This should be followed by weekly testing for two weeks and then testing every two weeks for the next six weeks. Liver function should be monitored periodically thereafter.

Owing to its enzyme-inducing effect, rifampicin must be employed with extreme caution in patients with porphyria, because activation of delta-aminolaevulinic acid synthetase may lead to an acute manifestation of the porphyria.

To preclude all possibility of pregnancy during treatment with Rimactane, non-hormonal means of contraception must be employed (see *Interactions*).

*Interactions with other drugs and other types of interactions:* Antacids, opiates, and anticholinergic drugs and ketoconazole reduce the bioavailability of rifampicin when given concomitantly by mouth. The same applies to PAS preparations containing bentonite. To avoid this interaction, rifampicin must be administered a few hours before these preparations.

Rifampicin is a potent inducer of liver enzymes which may increase the metabolism of concomitantly administered drugs such as those listed below. The activity of the following drugs may be impaired and their dosage must be reassessed during and after treatment with Rifampicin.

Oral anticoagulants; oral antidiabetic agents, digitalis preparations, antiarrhythmic agents (disopyramide, quinidine, mexiletine, tocainide, lorcainide, propafenone), methadone (withdrawal signs may set in), hydantoins (phenytoin); hexobarbital, nortriptyline, benzodiazepines, corticosteroids (Addison patients may develop a crisis; exacerbation of pemphigus may occur; treatment for corticoid-dependent asthma patients may become more difficult or impossible); sex hormones (menstrual disorders may appear); oral contraceptives (their effect can no longer be relied upon); theophyllines, dapsone, chloramphenicol, azole antifungal agents (ketoconazole, itraconazole), cyclosporin A; azathioprine (transplants may be rejected); beta blockers, calcium-channel blockers (nifedipine, verapamil); enalapril, cimetidine.

Although concurrent use of isoniazid, pyrazinamide and rifampicin is common and therapeutically valuable, hepatic toxicity may be increased.

Rifampicin can delay the biliary excretion of contrast media employed to X-ray the gall bladder.

Microbiological techniques for assaying folic acid and vitamin $B_{12}$ in the serum are unsuitable for use during treatment with Rimactane.

*Pregnancy and lactation:* In studies of over 300 women exposed to rifampicin during pregnancy, no significant increase in the rate of malformations in their offspring, over and above the background level was observed. Rimactane should not be given during pregnancy unless the potential benefit justifies the potential risk to the foetus.

Administration of Rimactane during the last few weeks of pregnancy can cause post-natal haemorrhage in the mother and new-born infant. This may necessitate treatment with vitamin K preparations.

Rifampicin passes into the breast milk but no adverse effects on breast-fed infants have been observed. Therefore nursing mothers may continue to breast-feed their infants.

*Effects on ability to drive or use machines:* None known.

*Undesirable effects:*
*Effects relating to intravenous administration:* During prolonged (more than 30 days) administration i.v., local thrombophlebitis occasionally occurs. Nursing staff preparing and applying infusions may develop hypersensitivity reactions to the hands and face.

Rifampicin may cause reddish discolouration of body fluids and occasionally other body secretions, e.g. urine, sputum, lacrimal fluid, faeces, saliva, sweat. It may permanently discolour soft contact-lenses.

Unwanted effects which may occur during continuous daily or intermittent therapy.

Frequency estimates: frequent >10%, occasional >1–10%, rare >0.001%–1%, isolated cases <0.001%.

*Skin and appendages:* Occasionally: flushing, itching with or without skin rash, and reddening of the eyes. Isolated cases: severe signs and symptoms, such as exudative conjunctivitis or generalised hypersensitivity reactions involving the skin, e.g. exfoliative dermatitis, Lyell's syndrome and pemphigoid reactions.

*Gastro-intestinal tract:* Occasionally: anorexia, nausea, abdominal pains, gaseous distension; rarely: vomiting or diarrhoea; isolated occurrences of erosive gastritis and pseudomembranous colitis.

*Hepatic:* Frequently: an asymptomatic increase in liver enzymes; rarely: hepatitis or jaundice; here account should also be taken of the liver toxicity of chemotherapeutic agents, e.g. isoniazid or pyrazinamide, employed in combination with rifampicin. Induction of porphyria in isolated cases.

*Central and peripheral nervous system:* Occasionally: tiredness, drowsiness, headache, light-headedness, dizziness; rarely: ataxia, mental confusion. Isolated cases: muscular weakness, visual disturbances.

*Blood:* Isolated occurrences of transient leucopenia; eosinophilia; thrombocytopenia and thrombocytopenic purpura are encountered more frequently under intermittent therapy than on continuous daily treatment, during which they occur only in isolated cases.

*Endocrine:* In rare instances disturbances in the menstrual cycle (in extreme cases amenorrhoea); induction of a crisis in Addison patients (see *Interactions*).

Unwanted effects chiefly occurring during intermittent therapy or upon resumption of treatment after temporary interruption: In patients taking rifampicin other than on a daily basis or in those resuming treatment with the drug after a temporary interruption, an influenza-like syndrome ('flu syndrome') may occur, this being very probably of immunopathological origin. It is characterised by fever, shivering, and possibly headache, dizziness and musculoskeletal pain. In rare cases the 'flu syndrome' may be followed by thrombocytopenia, purpura, dyspnoea, asthmalike attacks, haemolytic anaemia, shock and acute renal failure. These serious complications may, however, also set in suddenly with no preceding 'flu syndrome', chiefly when treatment is resumed after a temporary interruption or when rifampicin is given only once a week in high doses (25 mg/kg or more). When Rimactane is administered in lower doses (600 mg) 2–3 times a week, the syndrome is encountered less frequently, its incidence then being comparable to that observed during daily medication.

*Overdose:*
*Signs and symptoms:* Nausea, vomiting, abdominal pains; enlargement of the liver, jaundice, elevated liver enzyme levels, possibly acute pulmonary oedema, lethargy, clouding of consciousness, convulsions.

*Treatment:* General supportive measures to maintain vital functions; forced diureses; haemodialysis; in the presence of severe liver damage, cholecystotomy if necessary. Bear in mind that other drugs used in combination with Rimactane may also have been taken in an overdosage and necessitate additional specific measures.

**Pharmacological properties**
*Pharmacodynamic properties:*
*Pharmacotherapeutic group:* Rifampicin is a rifamycin antibiotic.

*Mechanisms of action:* Rimactane exerts, both *in vitro* and *in vivo* bactericidal effects on *Mycobacterium tuberculosis*. It also exhibits variable activity against other atypical species of Mycobacterium.

*In vivo* it exerts its bactericidal effect not only on micro-organisms in the extracellular spaces but also on those located intracellularly. Rifampicin has a potent sterilising effect.

Rifampicin inhibits the DNA-dependent RNA polymerase of sensitive bacterial strains, but without affecting the corresponding mammalian enzyme.

Since relatively rapid 'one-step' selection of resistant bacteria occurs with rifampicin, the drug must not be employed as monotherapy to treat overt infections. Bacteria resistant to rifampicin display no cross-resistance to other antibiotics with the exception of the rifamycins.

*Pharmacokinetic properties:*
*Absorption:* An intravenous drip infusion of rifampicin (600 mg) lasting 3 hours produces peak plasma concentrations of approx. 10 mcg/ml. The plasma profiles are similar to those obtained following the administration of the same dose in capsules.

*Distribution:* The apparent distribution volume is 1.6 L/kg in adults and 1.1 L/kg in children. Binding to serum proteins amounts to 84%–91%.

Rifampicin penetrates rapidly into various body fluids and tissues, including bone tissue. Rifampicin crosses the blood/brain barrier in the case of inflamed meninges only, but concentrations in the cerebrospinal fluid may remain above the MIC for *Mycobacterium tuberculosis* for up to two months with continuous therapy of 600 mg/day orally.

Rifampicin crosses the human placenta and is secreted in human breast milk. However, it is estimated that a breast-fed infant would receive no more than 1% of the usual therapeutic dose.

*Biotransformation:* Rifampicin is metabolised in the liver, the principal metabolite being 25-O-deacetylrifampicin, which is microbiologically active and, like rifampicin, subject to enterohepatic circulation.

Rifampicin induces its own metabolism.

*Elimination/excretion:* The plasma elimination half-life of rifampicin increases with increasing doses and amounts to 2.5 h, 3–4 h and about 5 h after single doses of 300 mg, 600 mg and 900 mg respectively.

After a few days of repeated daily administration, the bioavailability of rifampicin diminishes, and the half-life value following repeated doses of 600 mg falls to 1–2 hours.

Owing to its enzyme-inducing effect in the liver, rifampicin accelerates its own metabolism, with the result that its systemic clearance, which amounts to approx. 6 L/h after the first dose, rises to approx. 9 L/h after repeated dosing.

Although the bulk of the drug is eliminated in the bile, 80% of the quantity excreted being accounted for by the deacetylrifampicin metabolite, rifampicin also appears in the urine. In a dosage range of 150–900 mg, 4–18% of a dose is excreted dose-dependently in the urine in unchanged form.

*Characteristics in patients:* In elderly patients, renal clearance is reduced, but, owing to the large scale on which the drug is eliminated via the liver, the plasma concentrations are similar to those in young patients.

With impaired renal function, the elimination half-life becomes prolonged only at doses exceeding 600 mg daily. Provided that hepatic excretory function is normal, the dosage in patients with impaired renal function does not need to be reduced below 600 mg daily.

Rifampicin is eliminated by peritoneal or haemodialysis. Dosage adjustment is not necessary during dialysis. Because rifampicin is dialysable it is recommended that the drug should not be administered until after the period of dialysis is complete.

In patients with severe hepatic dysfunction the dosage may have to be adjusted as plasma concentrations are raised and half-life prolonged.

*Preclinical safety data:* There is limited evidence as to the carcinogenic potential of rifampicin in animals. In female mice of a strain known to be susceptible to hepatomas, a significant increase in such tumours was observed after 1 year of treatment with rifampicin in quantities equivalent to 2–10 times the maximum clinical doses.

In mice of another strain treated for 1 year, and in rats treated for 2 years, no significant increase was noted in the incidence of any type of tumour. Studies with various mammalian models, as well as with bacteria, yielded no evidence that rifampicin has a mutagenic effect.

In daily doses of 150–250 mg/kg, rifampicin proved

teratogenic in mice and rats, insofar as an increased occurrence of spina bifida and cleft palate was observed. In rabbits it had no teratogenic effect. In all three animal species, unspecific embryotoxic effects occurred after doses>150 mg/kg.

**Pharmaceutical particulars**

*List of excipients:* The vials also contain sodium formaldehyde sulphoxylate (pyrogen free).

*Incompatibilities:* Rimactane infusion is incompatible with the following infusion solutions: sodium bicarbonate 5%, Ringer's solution (acetate) plus glucose, Perfudex and sodium lactate 0.167M.

Rimactane infusion diluted in glucose or saline is not compatible with: cephamandole, tetracycline, rolitetracycline, doxycycline.

Rimactane infusion should not be mixed with other drugs if there is a possibility that precipitation may occur; concurrent intravenous therapy should be administered via a different site of injection.

*Shelf-life:* Three years.

*Special precautions for storage:* Protect from light and heat (store below 30°C).

The reconstituted solution should be stored in a refrigerator (2–8°C) and used within 24 hours.

Medicines should be kept out of reach of children.

*Nature and contents of containers:* Colourless glass vials of 300 mg.

*Instructions for use/handling:*
*Preparation of infusion:* (see *Warnings*). Rimactane infusion is prepared for use by aseptically adding 5 ml Water for Injections PhEur to the vial of dry rifampicin powder and shaking vigorously and continuously for 30–60 seconds.

When the powder has completely dissolved, the solution should be immediately diluted in 250 ml of 5% glucose solution or other suitable infusion fluid (see *Pharmaceutical Precautions*). Freshly prepared solutions must be used within 6 hours. It is recommended that the infusion be administered over a period of 2–3 hours.

Care should be taken to avoid contact with rifampicin.

*Compatibility:* Rimactane infusion is compatible with the following infusion solutions: NaCl 0.9%, Ringer's solution (lactate or acetate), dextrose 5% or 10%, mannitol 10% or 20%, sodium bicarbonate 1.4%, Macrodex with saline solution, Macrodex with glucose solution, Rheomacrodex and Fructose 5% and 10%.

**Marketing authorisation number**   00101/0447.

**Date of approval/revision of SPC**   16 July 1996.

**Legal category**   POM.

# RIMACTAZID*

**Qualitative and quantitative composition**   The active ingredient for rifampicin is 3-[[(4-Methyl-1-piperazinyl)-imino]-methyl]-rifamycin SV.

The active ingredient for isoniazid is isonicotonic acid hydrazide.

One tablet contains 150 mg or 300 mg rifampicin PhEur and 100 mg or 150 mg Isoniazid PhEur.

**Pharmaceutical form**   Coated tablets.

**Clinical particulars**

*Therapeutic indications:* Rimactane and isoniazid are both major drugs in the management of tuberculosis and in certain opportunist mycobacterial infections. Rifampicin is effective in cases resistant to other antituberculous agents and shows no cross-resistance outside the rifamycin group of drugs. Rimactazid must always be used in combination with other antituberculosis agents, e.g. streptomycin, pyrazinamide, ethambutol and the majority of second-line drugs.

*Posology and method of administration:* Rimactazid should be given as a single dose, preferably on an empty stomach, at least 30 minutes before breakfast to ensure a high peak serum concentration.

*Adults:*
*Continuous therapy*

| | |
|---|---|
| Body weight less than 50 kg: | 3 tablets Rimactazid 150 (=450 mg Rifampicin +300 mg INH) once daily |
| Body weight 50 kg or more: | 2 tablets Rimactazid 300 (=600 mg Rifampicin +300 mg INH) once daily |

*Intermittent therapy*

| | |
|---|---|
| Body weight less than 50 kg: | 3 tablets Rimactazid 150 (=450 mg Rifampicin +300 mg INH) twice or 3 times weekly |
| Body weight 50 kg or more: | 2 tablets Rimactazid 300 (=600 mg Rifampicin +300 mg INH) twice or 3 times weekly |

Rimactazid has to be supplemented with 150 mg isoniazid for every 10 kg body weight above 20 kg (i.e.

body weight 60 kg: 150×4=600 mg additional isoniazid needed). To a maximum of 900 mg daily.

The chemotherapeutic agents usually employed today as combined therapy for tuberculosis are rifampicin (Rimactane) (RMP), isoniazid (INH), pyrazinamide (PZA), ethambutol (EMB), streptomycin (STM).

The dosages recommended by the Centres for Disease Control and Prevention are as follows (see Table below):

For the treatment of sputum-positive pulmonary tuberculosis, preference is given to the following regimens: (for dosages information please refer to the text above for rifampicin and isoniazid, and to the table for advice on the other components of the treatment).

*Continuous therapy:*
*Daily for a total of 9 months:*

| | |
|---|---|
| Initial phase for 2 months: | RMP + INH + PZA + EMB or STM |
| Continuation phase for 7 months: | RMP + INH |

A total duration of 9 months is recommended for tuberculosis with HIV infection and for tuberculous meningitis, disseminated tuberculosis, or spinal involvement with neurological complications.

*Daily for a total of 6 months:*

| | |
|---|---|
| Initial phase for 2 months: | RMP + INH + PZA + EMB or STM |
| Continuation phase for 4 months: | RMP + INH |

*Partially intermittent therapy:*
*Total duration 6 months:*

| | |
|---|---|
| Initial phase for 2 months: | RMP + INH + PZA + EMB or STM daily |
| Continuation phase for 4 months: | RMP + INH twice or 3 times a week |

*Fully intermittent therapy:*
Total duration 6 months: RMP + INH + PZA + EMB or STM 3 times a week

In the case of all regimens administered twice or three times weekly, the patient should be monitored with directly observed therapy (i.e. administration of tablets under supervision). The same applies for relapses and treatment failures.

*Use in children:* The ratios of Rimactane and isoniazid present in Rimactazid 150 and 300 make it difficult for both components to be administered in a dosage suitable for children. Rimactazid tablets are therefore not recommended for paediatric use.

*Use in elderly:* No special dosage regime is necessary but concurrent hepatic insufficiency should be taken into account (see *Pharmacokinetics*).

*Contra-indications:* Known hypersensitivity to rifampicin and/or to isoniazid, a history of drug induced hepatitis, acute liver diseases regardless of their origin, peripheral neuritis.

*Special warnings and precautions for use:*
*Warnings:* Intermittent therapy, resumption of therapy after its interruption – The presence of rifampicin means that, if treatment with Rimactazid is withdrawn for a while and then resumed again, or if the medication is not taken regularly, potentially serious side effects can occur (see under rifampicin in *Undesirable effects*). For this reason, both temporary interruption of treatment and non-compliance should if possible be avoided. Where temporary withdrawal of the medication is unavoidable, the two components rifampicin and INH should be administered separately when resuming the treatment, because rifampicin should then be given in an incremental dosage. A start should be made with approx. 75–150 mg rifampicin on the first day, and the desired therapeutic dose should be reached within 3–4 days. During this time the patient's renal function should be close monitored. Corticosteroids may prove useful in attenuating possible immunopathological reactions. Isoniazid should be given in its normal dosage from the first day onwards.

If severe acute hypersensitivity reactions set in, such as thrombocytopenia, purpura, haemolytic anaemia, dyspnoea and asthmas-like attacks, shock, or renal failure (these being side effects which rifampicin may provoke in exceptional cases), Rimactazid should be withdrawn at once. Patients developing such complications should never again be treated with rifampicin.

If other signs of hypersensitivity appear, such as fever or skin reactions, Rimactazid should be with-

drawn. For safety reasons, treatment should not be continued with rifampicin. Where isoniazid is considered essential, treatment should be resumed in low doses and under strict surveillance.

*Precautions:* In the treatment of tuberculosis rifampicin should be given under the supervision of a respiratory or other suitably qualified physician.

As rifampicin and isoniazid are metabolised in the liver, patients with impaired liver function should be treated with caution.

All tuberculosis patients should have pretreatment measurement of liver function.

If a patient has no evidence of pre-existing liver disease and normal pretreatment liver function, liver function tests need only be repeated if fever, vomiting, jaundice or other deterioration in the patients condition occurs.

The occurrence of liver function abnormalities is more common when rifampicin and isoniazid are used in combination and special care is therefore required in patients with pre-existing liver impairment or malnourished patients.

In patients with chronic liver disease, as well as in chronic alcoholics and undernourished patients, the therapeutic benefits of treatment with Rimactazid must be weighed against the possible risks. If the treatment is considered necessary, the dosage of both components must be correspondingly reduced. In such cases it is only possible to adapt the dosage by administering rifampicin and isoniazid separately.

Regular monitoring of liver function is required in patients with chronic liver disease throughout treatment with Rimactazid. Weekly testing for two weeks followed by tests every two weeks for the next six weeks is recommended initially. Blood counts and liver function tests should also be performed periodically during prolonged treatment. Any deterioration in liver function in these patients is an indication for stopping treatment

Rimactazid should be withdrawn if clinically significant changes in hepatic function occur. The need for other forms of antituberculous therapy and a different regimen should be considered. Urgent advice should be obtained from a specialist in the management of tuberculosis. If rifampicin or isoniazid are reintroduced after liver function has returned to normal, liver function should be monitored daily until the maintenance dose has been established. This should be followed by weekly testing for two weeks and then testing every two weeks for the next six weeks. Liver function should be monitored periodically thereafter.

Owing to its enzyme-inducing effect, rifampicin must be employed with extreme caution in patients with porphyria, because activation of delta-aminolaevulinic acid synthetase may lead to an acute manifestation of the porphyria.

To preclude all possibility of pregnancy during treatment with rifampicin, additional non-hormonal means of contraception must be employed (see *Interactions*).

Owing to the neurotoxic action of isoniazid, patients suffering from convulsive disorders must be kept under special observation during treatment with Rimactazid.

Pyridoxine may be useful in preventing the occurrence of peripheral neuritis and should be given in a dose of 10 mg daily from the start of treatment with Rimactazid.

Patients should abstain from alcohol while under treatment with Rimactazid.

*Interactions with other drugs and other types of interactions:*
*Rifampicin:* Antacids, opiates, and anticholinergic drugs and ketoconazole reduce the bioavailability of rifampicin when given concomitantly by mouth. The same applies to PAS preparations containing bentonite. To avoid this interaction, rifampicin must be administered a few hours before these preparations.

Rifampicin is a potent inducer of liver enzymes which may increase the metabolism of concomitantly administered drugs such as those listed below. The activity of the following drugs may be impaired and their dosage must be reassessed during and after treatment with Rifampicin.

Oral anticoagulants; oral antidiabetic agents, digitalis preparations, antiarrhythmic agents (disopyramide, quinidine, mexiletine, tocainide, lorcainide, propafenone), methadone (withdrawal signs may set in), hydantoins (phenytoin); hexobarbital, nortriptyline, benzodiazepines, corticosteroids (Addison patients may develop a crisis; exacerbation of pem-

| | Daily | | Twice a week | | 3 times a week | |
|---|---|---|---|---|---|---|
| Drug | mg/kg | max. mg | mg/kg | max. mg | mg/kg | max. mg |
| RMP | 10 | 600 | 10 | 600 | 10 | 600 |
| INH | 5 | 300 | 15 | 900 | 15 | 900 |
| PZA | 15–30 | 2,000 | 50–70 | 4,000 | 50–70 | 3,000 |
| EMB | 5–25 | 2,500 | 50 | 2,500 | 25–30 | 2,500 |
| STM | 15 | 1,000 | 25–30 | 1,500 | 25–30 | 1,000 |

phigus may occur; treatment for corticoid-dependent asthma patients may become more difficult or impossible); sex hormones (menstrual disorders may appear); oral contraceptives (their effect can no longer be relied upon); theophyllines, dapsone, chloramphenicol, azole antifungal agents (ketoconazole; itraconazole), cyclosporin A; azathioprine (transplants may be rejected); beta blockers, calcium-channel blockers (nifedipine, verapamil); enalapril, cimetidine.

Although concurrent use of isoniazid, pyrazinamide and rifampicin is common and therapeutically valuable, hepatic toxicity may be increased.

Rifampicin can delay the biliary excretion of contrast media employed to X-ray the gall bladder.

Microbiological techniques for assaying folic acid and vitamin $B_{12}$ in the serum are unsuitable for use during treatment with Rimactane.

*Isoniazid:* The absorption of isoniazid is reduced by antacids. Isoniazid retards the metabolism of various concomitantly administered drugs, including hydantoins (phenytoin), carbamazepine, primidone, and valproic acid. The dosages of these drugs may have to be reduced. It is not advisable to administer disulfiram concomitantly with isoniazid as this may lead to mental disturbances, the mechanism of this interaction is not known.

Concomitant use of halothane and isoniazid (and possibly rifampicin) may increase the risk of hepatotoxic reactions.

As alcohol tolerance is decreased under isoniazid, the consumption of alcoholic beverages should be avoided. The metabolism of isoniazid is increased in chronic alcoholics.

*Pregnancy and lactation:*
*Rifampicin:* In studies of over 300 women exposed to rifampicin during pregnancy, no significant increase in the rate of malformations in their offspring, over and above the background level was observed. Rimactane should not be given during pregnancy unless the potential benefit justifies the potential risk to the foetus.

Administration of Rimactane during the last few weeks of pregnancy can cause post-natal haemorrhage in the mother and new-born infant. This may necessitate treatment with vitamin K preparations.

*Isoniazid:* Isoniazid, besides having weak direct genotoxic activity, is a promutagen in the sense that the formation of the toxic metabolites, hydrazine and acetylhydrazine, is the first step in metabolic activation. In lymphocytes of patients treated with isoniazid no chromosomal alterations could be detected whereas in a study comparing the effects of combination treatment an increased frequency of chromosomal alterations was observed.

Nevertheless isoniazid has been found to entail relatively little risk during pregnancy in humans. Congenital malformations have not been observed to be any greater than those expected for the normal population. Since it is theoretically possible that the drug might exert neurotoxic effects on the child, it is recommended that the mother should take pyridoxine during her pregnancy.

Rimactazid should not be given during pregnancy unless the potential benefit justifies the potential risk to the foetus.

Although rifampicin and isoniazid pass into the breast milk, no adverse effects on breast-fed infants have been observed. It is therefore not absolutely necessary to wean the infant. However, in view of the theoretical possibility of neurotoxic effects due to isoniazid, beast-fed infants should be kept under careful surveillance. Prophylactic administration of pyridoxine to mother and child is recommended.

*Effects on ability to drive or use machines:* Doses of 10 mg/kg or greater, of isoniazid may produce adverse reactions of the nervous system, e.g. peripheral neuropathy and thus impair the patients ability to drive or operate machinery.

*Undesirable effects:* Rifampicin may cause reddish discolouration of body fluids and occasionally other body secretions, e.g. urine, sputum, lacrimal fluid, faeces, saliva, sweat. It may permanently discolour soft contact-lenses.

Unwanted effects which may occur during continuous daily or intermittent therapy.

Frequency estimates: frequent>10%, occasional>1–10%, rare>0.001–1%, isolated cases<0.001%.

*Associated with Rifampicin:*
*Skin and appendages:* Occasionally: flushing, itching with or without skin rash, and reddening of the eyes. Isolated cases: severe signs and symptoms, such as exudative conjunctivitis or generalised hypersensitivity reactions involving the skin, e.g. exfoliative dermatitis, Lyell's syndrome and pemphigoid reactions.

*Gastro-intestinal tract:* Occasionally: anorexia, nausea, abdominal pains, gaseous distension; rarely: vomiting or diarrhoea; isolated occurrences of erosive gastritis and pseudomembranous colitis.

*Hepatic:* Frequently: an asymptomatic increase in liver enzymes; rarely: hepatitis or jaundice; here account should also be taken of the liver toxicity of chemotherapeutic agents, e.g. isoniazid or pyrazinamide, employed in combination with rifampicin. Induction of porphyria in isolated cases.

*Central and peripheral nervous system:* Occasionally: tiredness, drowsiness, headache, light-headedness, dizziness; rarely: ataxia, mental confusion. Isolated cases: muscular weakness, visual disturbances.

*Blood:* Isolated occurrences of transient leucopenia; eosinophilia; thrombocytopenia and thrombocytopenic purpura are encountered more frequently under intermittent therapy than on continuous daily treatment, during which they occur only in isolated cases.

*Endocrine:* Rarely: disturbances in the menstrual cycle (in extreme cases amenorrhoea); induction of a crisis in Addison patients (see *Interactions*).

*Unwanted effects chiefly occurring during intermittent therapy or upon resumption of treatment after temporary interruption:* In patients taking rifampicin other than on a daily basis or in those resuming treatment with the drug after a temporary interruption, an influenza-like syndrome ('flu syndrome') may occur, this being very probably of immunopathological origin. It is characterised by fever, shivering, and possibly headache, dizziness and musculoskeletal pain. In rare cases the 'flu syndrome' may be followed by thrombocytopenia, purpura, dyspnoea, asthma-like attacks, haemolytic anaemia, shock and acute renal failure. These serious complications may, however, also set in suddenly with no preceding 'flu syndrome', chiefly when treatment is resumed after a temporary interruption or when rifampicin is given only once a week in high doses (25 mg/kg or more). When Rimactane is administered in lower doses (600 mg) 2–3 times a week, the syndrome is encountered less frequently, its incidence then being comparable to that observed during daily medication.

*Associated with Isoniazid:*
*Central nervous system:* Frequently: peripheral neuropathy (dose dependent and more common in undernourished patients, alcoholics and diabetes). Rarely: damage to the optic nerve, convulsions, psychoses, dizziness, light-headedness, headache. Isolated cases: toxic encephalopathy. High doses may increase seizure frequency in epileptics.

*Gastro-intestinal:* Occasionally: nausea, vomiting, epigastric distress.

*Hepatic:* Frequently: disburbances of liver function (usually transient). Rarely: hepatitis. Isolated cases: severe hepatitis. The incidence of hepatitis increases with the patient's age.

*Blood:* Isolated cases: agranulocytosis, eosinophilia, thrombocytopenia, anaemia (haemolytic, hypoplastic).

*Allergic and miscellaneous reactions:* Occasional: drug rash, fever. Rarely: dryness of the mouth, heartburn, disorders of micturition, rheumatic syndrome, lupus erythematosus-like signs and symptoms, pellagra. Isolated cases: gynaecomastia, vasculitis.

*Overdose:*
*Signs and symptoms: Rifampicin:* Nausea, vomiting, abdominal pains; enlargement of the liver, jaundice, elevated liver enzyme levels, possibly acute pulmonary oedema, lethargy, clouding of consciousness, convulsions.

*Isoniazid:* In mild poisoning – ataxia, symptoms of polyneuritis, disturbed articulation, vertigo. In severe poisoning – hallucinations, epileptiform tonic-clonic attacks, respiratory depression, coma, severe metabolic acidosis, hyperglycaemia, acetonuria.

*Treatment:* : General supportive measures to maintain vital functions; intravenous administration of anticonvulsants and pyridoxine in large doses; control of metabolic acidosis; gastric lavage together with instillation of an activated charcoal suspension via a stomach tube; forced diuresis; haemodialysis, in the presence of severe liver damage, cholecystotomy if necessary.

**Pharmacological properties**
*Pharmacodynamic properties:*
*Pharmacotherapeutic group:* Rifampicin is a rifamycin antibiotic and isoniazid is a specific antituberculous agent.

*Mechanism of action:* Rifampicin exerts, both *in vitro* and *in vivo* bactericidal effects on *Mycobacterium tuberculosis*. It also exhibits variable activity against other atypical species of Mycobacterium.

*In vivo* it exerts its bactericidal effect not only on micro-organisms in the extracellular spaces but also on those located intracellularly. Rifampicin has a potent sterilising effect.

Rifampicin inhibits the DNA-dependent RNA polymerase of sensitive bacterial strains, but without affecting the corresponding mammalian enzyme.

*Isoniazid* exerts a strong bactericidal effect mainly on rapidly growing populations of *Mycobacterium tuberculosis*. Its mechanism of action is probably based chiefly on inhibition of mycolic acid synthesis, mycolic acid being an important constituent of the mycobacterial cell wall.

*Pharmacokinetic properties:*
*Absorption:* An oral administration of the fixed combination on an empty stomach, the two active substances are well absorbed.

*Rifampicin,* following a single dose of 600 mg, reaches mean peak plasma concentrations of 9.4 mcg/mL after 2–3 hours.

*Isoniazid,* following a single dose of 300 mg, reaches mean peak plasma concentrations of 6.1 mcg/mL after 0.5–2 hours. However, plasma concentrations vary interindividually, depending on the acetylator status of the patient.

Concomitant intake of food reduces the absorption of both active components.

*Distribution: Rifampicin:* The apparent distribution volume is 1.6 L/kg in adults and 1.1 L/kg in children. Binding to serum proteins amounts to 84%–91%.

*Isoniazid:* The apparent distribution volume is 0.61 L/kg. Isoniazid is not appreciably bound to serum proteins.

Rifampicin and isoniazid penetrate rapidly into various body fluids and tissues, including bone tissue (rifampicin) and cerebrospinal fluid, in therapeutically active concentrations.

*Rifampicin* crosses the blood/brain barrier in the case of inflamed meninges only, but concentrations in the cerebrospinal fluid may remain above the MIC for *Mycobacterium tuberculosis* for up to two months with continuous therapy of 600 mg/day orally.

Rifampicin and isoniazid cross the human placenta and are secreted in human breast milk.

*Isoniazid* attains the highest levels, but it is estimated that a breast-fed infant would receive no more than 20%, and in the case of *rifampicin* less than 1% of the usual therapeutic dose.

*Biotransformation: Rifampicin* is metabolised in the liver, the principal metabolite being 25-O-deacetyl-rifampicin, which is microbiologically active and, like rifampicin, subject to enterohepatic circulation. Rifampicin induces its own metabolism.

*Isoniazid* is acetylated and hydrolysed in the liver. Acetylation is the most important metabolic pathway and is subject to genetic predisposition (fast and slow acetylators).

*Elimination/excretion: Rifampicin:* The plasma elimination half-life of rifampicin increases with increasing doses and amounts to 2.5 h, 3–4 h and about 5 h after single doses of 300 mg, 600 mg and 900 mg respectively. After a few days of repeated daily administration, the bioavailabilty of rifampicin diminishes, and the half-life value following repeated doses of 600 mg falls to 1–2 hours.

Owing to its enzyme-inducing effect in the liver, rifampicin accelerates its own metabolism, with the result that its systemic clearance, which amounts to approx. 6 L/h after the first dose, rises to approx. 9 L/h after repeated dosing.

Although the bulk of the drug is eliminated in the bile, 80% of the quantity excreted being accounted for by the deacetylrifampicin metabolite, rifampicin also appears in the urine.

In a dosage range of 150–900 mg, 4–18% of a dose is excreted dose-dependently in the urine in unchanged form.

*Isoniazid:* The plasma elimination half-life is 0.6–1.8 hours in fast acetylators and 1.8–6.7 hours in slow acetylators.

Within 24 hours 75–95% of the dose administered is excreted in the urine, mainly as metabolites. N-cetylisoniazid is eliminated in the urine together with other metabolites. The quantity appearing in the urine as unchanged isoniazid is equivalent to 12% of the dose in fast acetylators and to 27% in slow acetylators.

*Characteristics in patients: Rifampicin:* In elderly patients, plasma concentrations are similar to those in young patients.

With impaired renal function, the elimination half-life becomes prolonged only at doses exceeding 600 mg daily. Provided that hepatic excretory function is normal, the dosage in patients with impaired renal function does not need to be reduced below 600 mg daily.

Rifampicin is eliminated by peritoneal or haemodialysis. Dosage adjustment is not necessary during dialysis. Because rifampicin is dialysable it is recommended that the drug should not be administered until after the period of dialysis is complete.

In patients with impaired liver function, the plasma concentrations are raised and the elimination half-life prolonged. In the presence of severe hepatic dysfunction the dosage may have to be adjusted accordingly.

*Isoniazid:* Elderly patients: In fast acetylators, old age has no significant influence on the rate at which the drug is eliminated. However, clearance and elimination half-life vary significantly in elderly slow acetylators, so that it might be necessary to adjust the dosage accordingly.

In slow acetylators with severely impaired renal

function, accumulation of isoniazid may occur. In such cases, the serum concentration of isoniazid should be monitored and, if necessary, the dosage reduced.

In the presence of impaired liver function the elimination half-life of isoniazid is prolonged. To avoid unwanted effects it may therefore be necessary to adapt the dosage accordingly.

*Preclinical safety data: Rifampicin:* There is limited evidence as to the carcinogenic potential of rifampicin in animals. In female mice of a strain known to be susceptible to hepatomas, a significant increase in such tumours was observed after 1 year of treatment with rifampicin in quantities equivalent to 2–10 times the maximum clinical doses.

In mice of another strain treated for 1 year, and in rats treated for 2 years, no significant increase was noted in the incidence of any type of tumour. Studies with various mammalian models, as well as with bacteria, yielded no evidence that rifampicin has a mutagenic effect.

In daily doses of 150–250 mg/kg, rifampicin proved teratogenic in mice and rats, insofar as an increased occurrence of spina bifida and cleft palate was observed. In rabbits it had no teratogenic effect. In all three animal species, unspecific embryotoxic effects occurred after doses >150 mg/kg.

*Isoniazid:* Teratogenic effects have been noted in animal models. Limited evidence shows that isoniazid produces lung tumours in mice after various modes of administration. Available evidence of human exposure has not suggested that isoniazid is carcinogenic in man at doses applicable to the treatment and prophylaxis of tuberculosis.

**Pharmaceutical particulars**

*List of excipients:* The tablets contain calcium stearate, sodium lauryl sulphate, maize starch, sodium carboxymethylcellulose, talc, hydroxypropyl, methylcellulose, povidone, titanium dioxide, microcrystalline cellulose, polyethylene glycol, polyvinylpyrrolidone, sugar (sucrose), red iron oxide (E172), yellow iron oxide (E172) (300 mg only) and water.

*Incompatibilities:* None known.

*Shelf life:* Three years.

*Special precautions for storage:* Protect from moisture and heat (store below 25°C).

Medicines should be kept out of reach of children.

*Nature and contents of containers:* Rimactazid 150 tablets are round, pale red, sugar-coated tablets, printed CG on one side and EI on the other side in brown ink, and are packed in PVC/PVdC blister packs of 84.

Rimactazid 300 tablets are round, reddish-orange, sugar-coated tablets, printed CG on one side and DH on the other side in brown ink, and are packed in PVC/PVdC blister packs of 56.

*Instructions for use/handling:* None.

**Marketing authorisation numbers**
150 mg tablet     00101/0449
300 mg tablet     00101/0450

**Date of approval/revision of SPC**   27 June 1996.

**Legal category**   POM.

# RITALIN*

**Qualitative and quantitative composition**   The active ingredient is α-Phenyl-2-piperidineacetic acid methyl ester hydrochloride.

One tablet contains 10 mg methylphenidate hydrochloride.

**Pharmaceutical form**   Tablets.

**Clinical particulars**

*Therapeutic indications:* Ritalin is indicated as a part of a comprehensive treatment programme for attention-deficit hyperactivity disorder (ADHD) when remedial measures alone prove insufficient. Treatment must be under the supervision of a specialist in childhood behavioural disorders.

*Additional information on the safe use of the product:* ADHD is also known as attention-deficit disorder (ADD). Other terms used to describe this behavioural syndrome include: hyperkinetic child syndrome, minimal brain damage, minimal brain dysfunction in children, minimal cerebral dysfunction and psychoorganic syndrome of children.

A part of a comprehensive treatment programme, typically includes psychological, educational and social measures to stablise children with a behavioural syndrome characterised by symptoms which may include chronic history of short attention span, distractibility, emotional lability, impulsivity, moderate to severe hyperactivity, minor neurological signs and abnormal EEG. Learning may or may not be impaired.

Ritalin treatment is not indicated in all children with this syndrome and the decision to use the drug must be based on the physician's evaluation of the child's history and the duration and severity of symptoms.

*Posology and method of administration:*
*Adults:* Not applicable.

*Elderly:* Not applicable.

*Children:* (over 6 years). Begin with 5 mg once or twice daily, increasing the dose and frequency of administration if necessary by weekly increments of 5–10 mg in the daily dose. Doses above 60 mg daily are not recommended. The total daily dose should be administered in divided doses. Ritalin is not indicated in children less than 6 years of age.

In some children a rebound hyperactivity may occur if the effect of the drug wears off in the evening. An additional dose of Ritalin at bedtime may eliminate this difficulty. A trial dose at bedtime may indicate whether this is necessary.

Note: If improvement of symptoms is not observed after appropriate dosage adjustment over a one-month period, the drug should be discontinued. Ritalin should be discontinued periodically to assess the child's condition. Drug treatment is usually discontinued during or after puberty.

*Contra-indications:* The presence of marked anxiety, agitation or tension is a contra-indication to the use of Ritalin as it may aggravate these symptoms. Ritalin is also contra-indicated in patients with tics, tics in siblings, or a family history or diagnosis of Tourette's syndrome. It is also contra-indicated in patients with severe angina pectoris, cardiac arrhythmia, glaucoma, thyrotoxicosis, or known sensitivity to methylphenidate.

*Special warnings and precautions for use:*
*Warnings:* Ritalin should not be used in children under 6 years of age, since safety and efficacy in this age group have not been established.

Ritalin should not be used as treatment for severe depression of either exogenous or endogenous origin.

Available clinical experience suggests that in psychotic children administration of Ritalin may exacerbate symptoms of behavioural disturbance and thought disorder.

Available clinical evidence indicates that treatment with Ritalin during childhood does not increase the likelihood of addiction. Chronic abuse of Ritalin can lead to marked tolerance and psychic dependence with varying degrees of abnormal behaviour. Frank psychotic episodes can occur, especially in response to parenteral abuse.

*Precautions:* Height and weight should be carefully monitored in children, as growth retardation may occur during prolonged therapy. The retardation of growth is usually followed by a catch up growth when medication is discontinued. To minimise such complications, drug-free periods, especially during long vacations, are advocated by some specialists.

Use cautiously in patients with hypertension. Blood pressure should be monitored at appropriate intervals.

Ritalin should be employed with caution in emotionally unstable patients, such as those with a history of drug dependence or alcoholism, because such patients may increase the dosage on their own initiative.

Ritalin should be used with caution in patients with epilepsy. Clinical experience has shown that a small number of such patients may experience an increase in seizure frequency when treated with Ritalin. If seizure frequency rises, Ritalin should be discontinued.

Data on safety and efficacy of long-term use of Ritalin are not complete. Therefore, patients requiring long-term therapy should be monitored carefully. Periodic complete and differential blood counts, and platelet counts are advisable during prolonged therapy.

Careful supervision is required during drug withdrawal, since depression as well as renewed overactivity can be unmasked. Long-term follow-up may be needed for some patients.

*Interactions with other medicaments and other forms of interactions:* Human pharmacological studies have shown that Ritalin may inhibit the metabolism of coumarin anticoagulants, anticonvulsants (phenobarbitone, phenytoin, primidone), phenylbutazone and tricyclic antidepressants. Pressor agents and MAOIs may augment its effect.

Ritalin may also decrease the antihypertensive effect of guanethidine.

Alcohol may exacerbate the CNS adverse reactions of psychoactive drugs, including Ritalin. It is therefore advisable for patients to abstain from alcohol during treatment.

*Pregnancy and lactation:* There is no evidence of risk to the foetus but experience during pregnancy is limited. In animal studies, Ritalin did not affect the reproductive performance or fertility and had no embryotoxic, foetotoxic or teratogenic effects at about 2–5 times the therapeutic dose in humans. Ritalin should not be given to pregnant women unless the potential benefit outweighs the risk to the foetus.

It is not known whether the active substance of

Ritalin and/or its metabolites passes into breast milk. For safety reasons mothers taking Ritalin should refrain from breast feeding their infants.

*Effects on ability to drive or use machines:* Ritalin may affect the patient's reactions and adversely influence his or her ability to drive and use machinery.

*Undesirable effects:* Nervousness and insomnia are the most common adverse reactions occurring at the beginning of treatment. They are usually controlled by reducing the dosage and omitting the drug in the afternoon or evening.

Decreased appetite is also a common but usually transient adverse effect of Ritalin.

*Central and peripheral nervous system: Occasional:* Headache, drowsiness, dizziness, dyskinesia. *Rare:* Difficulties in accommodation, and blurring of vision may occur. *Isolated cases:* convulsions, muscle cramps, choreo-athetoid movements, tics or exacerbation of pre-existing tics, and Tourette's syndrome have been reported. Isolated cases of toxic psychosis (some with visual and tactile hallucinations), transient depressed mood.

*Gastro-intestinal tract: Occasional:* Abdominal pain, nausea, and vomiting may occur at the beginning of treatment and may be alleviated by concomitant food intake. Dry mouth.

*Cardiovascular system: Occasional:* Tachycardia, palpitations, arrhythmias, changes in blood pressure and heart rate (usually an increase). *Rare:* Angina pectoris.

*Skin and/or hypersensitivity reactions: Occasional:* Rash, pruritus, urticaria, fever, arthralgia, alopecia. Isolated cases of thrombocytopenic purpura, exfoliative dermatitis, and erythema multiforme have been reported.

*Blood:* Isolated cases of leucopenia, thrombocytopenia and anaemia have been reported.

*Others:* Rare: Moderately reduced weight gain and minor retardation of growth during prolonged therapy in children.

*Overdose: Signs and symptoms:* Acute overdose may result in vomiting, agitation, tremors, hyperreflexia, muscle twitching, convulsions (may be followed by coma), euphoria, confusion, hallucinations, delirium, sweating, flushing, headache, hyperpyrexia, tachycardia, palpitations, cardiac arrhythmias, hypertension, mydriasis, and dryness of mucous membrane.

*Treatment:* There is no specific antidote to Ritalin overdosage. Management consists of appropriate supportive measures.

The patient must be protected against self-injury and against external stimuli that would aggravate over-stimulation already present. If the signs and symptoms are not too severe and the patient is conscious, gastric contents may be evacuated by induction of vomiting or gastric lavage. In the presence of severe intoxication, a carefully titrated dose of a short-acting barbiturate should be given before performing gastric lavage.

Intensive care must be provided to maintain adequate circulation and respiratory exchange; external cooling procedures may be required for hyperpyrexia.

Efficacy of peritoneal dialysis or extracorporeal haemodialysis for overdose of Ritalin has not been established.

**Pharmacological properties**

*Pharmacodynamic properties: Mode of action:* Ritalin has a stimulant effect on the central nervous system. Its mode of action is not completely understood but it is thought to exert its stimulant effect by activating the brainstem arousal system and cortex.

*Pharmacokinetic properties: Absorption:* The active substance methylphenidate hydrochloride is rapidly and almost completely absorbed from the tablets. Owing to extensive first-pass metabolism its systemic availability amounts to only 30% (11–51%) of the dose. Ingestion together with food accelerates its absorption, but has no influence on the amount absorbed. Peak plasma concentrations of approximately 40 nmol/litres (11 ng/ml) are attained, on average, 2 hours after administration of 0.30 mg/kg. The peak plasma concentrations, however, show considerable intersubject variability. The area under the plasma concentration curve (AUC), as well as the peak plasma concentration, are proportional to the size of the dose administered.

*Distribution:* In the blood, methylphenidate and its metabolites become distributed in the plasma (57%) and the erythrocytes (43%). Methylphenidate and its metabolites have a low plasma protein-building rate (10–33%). The apparent distribution volume has been calculated as 13.1 litres/kg.

*Elimination:* Methylphenidate is eliminated from the plasma with a mean half-life of 2 hours, and the calculated mean systemic clearance is 10 litres/h/kg. Within 48–96 hours 78–97% of the dose administered is excreted in the urine and 1–3% in the faeces in the form of metabolites. Unchanged methylphenidate appears in the urine only in small quantities (<1%). The bulk of the dose is excreted in the urine as

2-phenyl-2-piperidyl acetic acid (PPAA, 60–86%). Peak plasma concentrations of PPAA are attained approximately 2 hours after administration of methylphenidate and are 30–50 times higher than those of the unchanged substance. The half-life of PPAA is roughly twice as long as that of methylphenidate, and the mean systemic clearance is 0.17 litres/h/kg. Therapeutic activity seems to be principally due to the parent compound.

*Characteristics in patients:* There are no apparent differences in the pharmacokinetic behaviour of methylphenidate in hyperactive children and normal adults. Renal excretion of the unchanged methylphenidate is hardly diminished at all in the presence of impaired renal function; however, renal excretion of PPAA may be reduced.

*Preclinical safety data:* In a lifetime carcinogenicity study carried out in mice, methylphenidate caused an increase in hepatocellular adenomas and, in males only, an increase in hepatoblastomas, at a daily dose of approximately 60 mg/kg/day. This is considerably higher than the recommended human dose on a mg/kg basis. Hepatoblastoma is a relatively rare rodent malignant tumour type. There was no increase in total malignant hepatic tumours. The mouse strain used is sensitive to the development of hepatic tumours, and the significance of these results to humans is unknown.

Similar studies in rats showed no evidence of carcinogenicity.

Sister chromatid exchange and chromosome aberrations were elevated in an in vitro test on cultured ovary cells of Chinese hamster. In two further in vitro tests (Ames reverse mutation test, mouse lymphoma forward mutation test) no mutagenic effects were observed.

In an in vivo study of the effect of methylphenidate on mouse bone marrow cells (micronucleus test), in which doses up to 250 mg/kg were tested, there was no evidence of clastogenic or aneugenic effects.

In the general population, the risk of hepatoblastoma is greatest in children under 4 years of age, for whom Ritalin treatment is not recommended. The estimated incidence is 1 per 10 million in children aged 5 to 9 years, and falls thereafter. There is no indication that the incidence is higher in patients exposed to Ritalin.

**Pharmaceutical particulars**

*Life of excipients:* The tablets also contain calcium phosphate, lactose, wheat starch, gelatin, magnesium stearate and talc.

*Incompatibilities:* None known.

*Shelf life:* Three years.

*Special precautions for storage:* Protect from moisture and store below 30°C. Medicines should be kept out of reach of children.

*Nature and contents of container:* The tablets are available in blister packs of 30 tablets.

*Instruction for use/handling:* None.

*Marketing authorisation holder:* Ciba-Geigy plc trading as Ciba Laboratories, Wimblehurst Road, Horsham, West Sussex RH12 4AB.

**Marketing authorisation number** 0008/0205

**Date of approval/revision of SPC** 9 September 1996.

**Legal category** POM.

## ROGITINE*

**Presentation** Clear glass ampoules each containing 10 mg Phentolamine Mesylate BP. presented as a colourless to pale yellow solution in 1 ml Water for Injections PhEur.

The ampoules also contain water, sodium metabisulphite and glucose for injection.

**Uses**

*Indications:* Management of hypertensive episodes that may occur in patients with phaeochromocytoma, for example during pre-operative preparation and surgical manipulation.

Diagnosis of phaeochromocytoma by Rogitine blocking test if other more specific tests are not available.

*Mode of action:* Phentolamine, the active substance of Rogitine, is a competitive non-selective $\alpha_1$, and $\alpha_2$-adrenergic receptor blocker of relatively short duration. It causes vasodilation and a fall in blood pressure which is based upon the blockade of both postjunctional vascular $\alpha_1$, and $\alpha_2$-adrenoceptors. It also antagonises the vasoconstrictor response to noradrenaline and adrenaline infusions. Enhanced neural release of noradrenaline due to presynaptic $\alpha_2$-blockade may contribute to the positive inotropic and chronotropic effects of Rogitine on cardiac muscle.

The administration of Rogitine intravenously to man produces transient declines in mean systemic vascular resistance and mean systemic arterial pressure as a result of dilatation in the arterial as well as in the venous vascular bed. These effects of Rogitine are accompanied by tachycardia, triggered by the baroreceptor reflex system and the autonomic nervous system.

*Pharmacokinetics:* The elimination of phentolamine from blood is rapid and does not follow first order kinetics. After two to four hours the concentration has fallen to about 15% of the peak value.

At concentrations of 0.02 to 109 mcg/ml, 54% of phentolamine is bound to human serum proteins.

Phentolamine is extensively metabolised, on average about 13% of a dose given by intravenous infusion is excreted unchanged in the urine.

Phentolamine metabolism is more pronounced following oral administration than after intravenous administration.

**Dosage and administration**

*Adults*

*Management of hypertensive episodes in patients with phaeochromocytoma:* For the management of hypertensive crises that arise during pre-operative phase or during induction of anaesthesia, intubation, or surgical removal of tumour, 2-5 mg of Rogitine is injected intravenously and repeated if necessary, the blood pressure response should be monitored.

*Diagnosis of phaeochromocytoma–Rogitine blocking test:* The test is most reliable in detecting phaeochromocytoma in patients with sustained hypertension and least reliable in those with paroxysmal hypertension. False-positive tests may occur in patients with hypertension without phaeochromocytoma.

*Preparation for the test:* Sedatives, analgesics and all other medications except those that might be deemed essential (such as digitalis and insulin) are withheld for at least 24 hours, and preferably 48-72 hours, prior to the test. Antihypertensive drugs are withheld until blood pressure returns to the untreated, hypertensive level. This test is not performed on a patient who is normotensive.

*Procedure: (intravenous):* The patient is kept at rest in the supine position throughout the test, preferably in a quiet, darkened room. Injection of Rogitine is delayed until blood pressure is stabilised, as evidenced by blood pressure readings taken every 10 minutes for at least 30 minutes.

The dose for adults is 5 mg. The syringe needle is inserted into the vein and injection delayed until the pressor response to venepuncture has subsided.

Rogitine is injected rapidly. Blood pressure is recorded immediately after injection, at 30-second intervals for the first 3 minutes, and at 60-second intervals for the next 7 minutes.

*Interpretation:* A positive response, suggestive of phaeochromocytoma, is indicated when the blood pressure is reduced by more than 35 mmHg systolic and by 25 mmHg diastolic. A typical positive response is a reduction in pressure of 60 mmHg systolic and 25 mmHg diastolic. Usually, the maximal effect is evident within 2 minutes after injection. A return to preinjection pressure commonly occurs within 15-30 minutes but may occur more rapidly.

If blood pressure decreases to a dangerous level, the patient should be treated as outlined under Overdosage.

A negative response is indicated when the blood pressure is elevated, unchanged, or reduced by less than 35 mmHg systolic and 25 mmHg diastolic after injection of Rogitine. A negative response to this test does not exclude the diagnosis of phaeochromocytoma, especially in patients with paroxysmal hypertension in whom the incidence of false-negative responses is high.

*Procedure: (intramuscular):* A dose of 5 mg is administered intramuscularly.

*Interpretation:* Blood pressure is recorded every 5 minutes for 30-45 minutes following injection. A positive response is indicated when the blood pressure is reduced by 35 mmHg systolic and by 25 mmHg diastolic, or more, within 20 minutes following injection.

*Children:* Management of hypertensive episodes in patients with phaeochromocytoma.

The dosage is 1 mg given intravenously.

Diagnosis of phaeochromocytoma–Rogitine blocking test.

The dosage is 1 mg given intravenously or 3 mg given intramuscularly.

*Elderly:* In elderly patients, it is advisable to use the lower dose or a slow infusion rate in case of undiagnosed coronary insufficiency (see Contra-indications).

*Patients with renal impairment:* Since no pharmacokinetic studies with Rogitine have been performed in patients with renal impairment, use caution in administering Rogitine to these patients.

**Contra-indications, warnings, etc**

*Contra-indications:* Known hypersensitivity to phentolamine and related compounds. Known hypersensitivity to sulphites. Hypotension. Myocardial infarction, history of myocardial infarction, coronary insufficiency, angina, or other evidence of coronary artery disease.

*Warnings:* Monitoring of the blood pressure is necessary for appropriate selection of patient, dosage, and duration of therapy. Myocardial infarction, cerebrovascular spasm, and cerebrovascular occlusion have been reported to occur following the administration of Rogitine, usually in association with marked hypotensive episodes.

The presence of sulphites in Rogitine ampoules can, especially in patients with bronchial asthma, lead to isolated hypersensitivity reactions, which may become manifest as an acute asthma attack, or shock, or clouding of consciousness.

For screening tests in patients with hypertension, the generally available urinary assay of catecholamines or other biochemical assays have largely replaced the Rogitine blocking test and other pharmacological tests for reasons of accuracy and safety, therefore, the Rogitine blocking test is not the procedure of choice and should be used only when these other specific tests are not available.

Rogitine may cause central nervous symptoms (See 'Side-effects') which may impair the patient's reactions. Patients must therefore be warned against engaging in activities that require quick reactions, such as driving motor vehicles and operating machinery.

*Precautions:* Tachycardia and cardiac arrhythmias may occur with the use of Rogitine.

Due to its stimulatory effect on the gastro-intestinal tract, including gastric secretion, Rogitine should be used with caution in patients with gastritis and peptic ulcer.

Excessive cardiac stimulation and hypertensive crisis may occur during surgical removal of a tumour due to manipulation of the phaeochromocytoma, despite the fact that phentolamine had been given as premedication to prevent such an occurrence. In the event of this complication use a $\beta_1$-selective, β-adrenergic blocking agent in slow i.v. injection.

*Use in pregnancy and lactation:* As a general rule no drugs should be taken during the first three months of pregnancy, and the benefits and risks of taking drugs should be carefully considered throughout the whole pregnancy.

Experience with Rogitine in pregnant women is not available. Do not use in pregnancy unless treatment is considered essential.

No information is available as to whether phentolamine passes into breast milk. For safety reasons, it is not recommended to use Rogitine during lactation.

According to the experimental data available, phentolamine did not reveal either a mutagenic or a teratogenic potential. Long-term carcinogenicity studies have not been conducted with phentolamine.

*Interactions:* Rogitine may augment the hypotensive effect of other antihypertensive agents. Antipsychotics may enhance the hypotensive effect of α-adrenergic blocking agents.

*Side-effects:*

*Cardiovascular system:* Frequently: Orthostatic hypotension and tachycardia. Occasionally: Acute or prolonged hypotensive episodes (flushing, sweating and feelings of apprehension). Myocardial infarction, cerebrospasm, and cerebrovascular occlusion may occur under these circumstances. Rarely: Anginal pain and cardiac arrhythmias.

*Central nervous system:* Occasionally: Dizziness and weakness.

*Gastro-intestinal tract:* Occasionally: Nausea, vomiting and diarrhoea.

*Other organ systems:* Occasionally: Nasal stuffiness and flushing. Rarely: Chest pain

*Overdosage:*

*Symptoms:* The main clinical manifestations of overdosage with Rogitine are arterial hypotension, reflex tachycardia, cardiac stimulation, arrhythmia, increase of systemic venous capacity, and possibly shock. These effects may be accompanied by headache, hyperexcitability and disturbances of vision, sweating, increased gastric motility, vomiting and diarrhoea, hypoglycaemia.

*Treatment:* Hypotension, excessive peripheral vasodilation: Noradrenaline, in cautiously titrated continuous i.v. infusion, can be considered the physiological antagonist; the effect of Rogitine may wear off in a short time, and administration of noradrenaline may have to be adjusted accordingly. When a pressor agent is used, ECG should be monitored, because major arrhythmias may occur. Alternative measures such as keeping the patient's legs raised and administering a plasma expander should be implemented concomitantly. Do not use adrenaline since this may cause a further fall of blood pressure under the given conditions.

*Disturbances of cardiac rhythm*: Adjust treatment to the nature of the arrhythmia.

*Hypoglycaemia*: Provide glucose i.v. until reaction is compensated.

**Pharmaceutical precautions** Rogitine should not be mixed with alkaline solutions.

Protect from light and heat (store below 25°C)..

**Legal category** POM.

**Package quantitities** Ampoules each containing 10 mg Rogitine in 1 ml Water for Injection. Boxes of 5.

**Further information** Nil.

**Product licence number** 0008/5070R

*Product licence holder:* Ciba-Geigy plc, Hulley Road, Macclesfield, Cheshire SK10 2NX.

## SANDIMMUN*

**Presentation**

*Soft gelatin capsules*

*25 mg Capsules:* Pale-pink, oval capsules, approximately 7.4 mm in diameter and approximately 11.3 mm in length, containing 25 mg cyclosporin.

*50 mg Capsules:* Corn-yellow, oblong capsules, approximately 7.5 mm in diameter and approximately 19.8 mm in length, containing 50 mg cyclosporin.

*100 mg Capsules:* Dusky-pink, oblong capsules, approximately 8.7 mm in diameter and approximately 24.9 mm in length, containing 100 mg cyclosporin.

*Oral solution:* Yellow or brownish-yellow, oily solution, clear or with a small amount of fine sediment, containing 100 mg cyclosporin per ml.

*Concentrate for intravenous infusion:* Each ml of concentrate contains 50 mg cyclosporin in a clear, brown-yellow, oily solution containing 650 mg polyethoxylated castor oil and 33% ethanol by volume. Sandimmun concentrate is available in 1 ml (50 mg) and 5 ml (250 mg) ampoules.

**Uses** *Principal action:* Cyclosporin is a cyclic polypeptide consisting of 11 amino acids. It is a potent immunosuppressive agent which prolongs survival of allogeneic transplants involving skin, heart, kidney, pancreas, bone marrow, cornea, small intestine and lung in animals. Successful solid organ and bone marrow allogeneic transplants have been performed in man using Sandimmun to prevent and treat rejection and graft-versus-host disease. Marked beneficial effects of Sandimmun therapy have also been shown in patients with severe psoriasis, atopic dermatitis and rheumatoid arthritis, conditions that may be considered to have an immunological mechanism.

Studies in animals suggest that cyclosporin inhibits the development of cell-mediated reactions. It appears to block the resting lymphocytes in the $G_0$ or early $G_1$ phase of the cell cycle and also inhibits lymphokine production and release, including interleukin 2 (T cell growth factor, TCGF). The available evidence suggests that cyclosporin acts specifically and reversibly on lymphocytes. It does not depress haemopoiesis and has no effect on the function of phagocytic cells.

*Indications*

*Organ transplantation:* Prevention of graft rejection following kidney, liver, heart, combined heart-lung, lung or pancreas transplant.

Treatment of transplant rejection in patients previously receiving other immunosuppressive agents.

*Bone marrow transplantation:* Prevention of graft rejection following bone marrow transplantation and prophylaxis of graft-versus-host disease (GVHD).

Treatment of established graft-versus-host disease (GVHD).

*Psoriasis:* The oral forms of Sandimmun (but not the Concentrate for intravenous infusion) are indicated in patients with severe psoriasis in whom conventional therapy is ineffective or inappropriate.

*Atopic dermatitis:* The oral forms of Sandimmun (but not the Concentrate for intravenous infusion) are indicated for the short term treatment (8 weeks) of patients with severe atopic dermatitis in whom conventional therapy is ineffective or inappropriate.

*Rheumatoid arthritis:* The oral forms of Sandimmun (but not the Concentrate for intravenous infusion) are indicated for the treatment of severe, active rheumatoid arthritis in patients in whom classical slow-acting antirheumatic agents are inappropriate or ineffective.

**Dosage and administration**

*Dosage:*

*Organ transplantation:* Initially, a single oral dose of 10 to 15 mg/kg body weight, should be given 4 to 12 hours before transplantation. As a general rule, treatment should continue at a dose of 10 to 15 mg/kg/day for one to two weeks post-operatively. Dosage should then be gradually reduced until a maintenance dose of 2 to 6 mg/kg/day is reached. Dosage should be adjusted by monitoring cyclosporin blood levels and kidney function (see 'Further information' and 'Precautions'). When Sandimmun is given with other immunosuppressants (e.g. with corticosteroids or as part of a triple or quadruple drug therapy) lower doses (e.g. 3 to 6 mg/kg/day orally initially) may be used.

The use of the Concentrate for intravenous infusion is recommended in organ transplant patients who are unable to take Sandimmun orally (e.g. shortly after surgery) or in whom the absorption of the oral forms might be impaired during episodes of gastrointestinal disturbances. In such cases the intravenous dose is *one third* of the recommended oral dose. It is recommended, however, that patients be transferred to oral therapy as soon as the given circumstances allow.

*Bone marrow transplantation/Prevention and treatment of graft-versus-host disease (GVHD):* Sandimmun Concentrate for intravenous infusion is usually preferred for initiation of therapy, although the oral forms may be used. The recommended dosage by the intravenous route is 3 to 5 mg/kg/day, starting on the day before transplantation and continuing during the immediate post-transplant period of up to two weeks until oral maintenance therapy begins.

Treatment with Sandimmun should continue using the oral forms at a dosage of 12.5 mg/kg/day for at least three and preferably six months before tailing off to zero. In some cases it may not be possible to withdraw Sandimmun until a year after bone marrow transplantation. Higher oral doses or the use of I.V. therapy may be necessary in the presence of gastrointestinal disturbances which might decrease absorption. If oral treatment is used to initiate therapy the recommended dose is 12.5 to 15 mg/kg/day starting on the day before transplantation. If GVHD develops after Sandimmun is withdrawn it should respond to reinstitution of therapy. Low doses should be used for mild, chronic GVHD.

*Psoriasis:* Refer also to Additional Precautions in psoriasis and atopic dermatitis section. To induce remission, the recommended initial dose is 2.5 mg/kg/day given orally in two divided doses. If there is no improvement after one month, the daily dose may be gradually increased, but should not exceed 5 mg/kg/day orally. Treatment should be discontinued if sufficient response is not achieved within six weeks on 5 mg/kg/day orally, or if the effective dose is not compatible with the safety guidelines given below (see Precautions). Initial doses of 5 mg/kg/day orally are justified in patients whose condition requires rapid improvement. For maintenance treatment, dosage must be individually titrated to the lowest effective level, and should not exceed 5 mg/kg/day orally.

*Atopic dermatitis:* Refer also to Additional Precautions in Psoriasis and Atopic Dermatitis section.

The recommended dose range is 2.5–5 mg/kg per day orally in two divided doses for a maximum of eight weeks. If a starting dose of 2.5 mg/kg per day does not achieve a good initial response within two weeks the dose may be rapidly increased to a maximum of 5 mg/kg per day. In very severe cases rapid and adequate control of disease is more likely with a starting dose of 5 mg/kg per day.

*Rheumatoid arthritis:* Refer also to Additional Precautions in Rheumatoid Arthritis section.

It is recommended that initiation of Sandimmun therapy should take place over a period of 12 weeks. For the first 6 weeks of treatment, the recommended dose is 2.5 mg/kg per day given orally in two divided doses. If the clinical effect is considered insufficient, the daily dose may then be increased gradually as tolerability permits, but should not exceed 4 mg/kg per day orally.

If, after 3 months of treatment at the maximum permitted or tolerable dose the response is considered inadequate, treatment should be discontinued.

For maintenance treatment the dose has to be titrated individually according to tolerability.

Sandimmun can be given in combination with low-dose corticosteroids. Pharmacodynamic interactions can occur between Sandimmun and NSAIDs and therefore this combination should be used with care (see *Additional precautions in rheumatoid arthritis* and *Drug interactions*).

Long term data on the use of Sandimmun in the treatment of rheumatoid arthritis are still limited. Therefore, it is recommended that patients are re-evaluated after 6 months of maintenance treatment and therapy only continued if the benefits of treatment outweigh the risks.

*Administration*

*Oral administration:* The total daily dosage of Sandimmun Capsules or Oral Solution may be given as a single daily dose or in two divided doses but a single daily dose may be used if appropriate for transplant recipients.

The Oral Solution should be diluted in a glass (not plastic) container, with cold milk, cold chocolate drink, fruit juice (e.g. orange juice) or cola according to individual taste, immediately before being taken. It should be stirred well and drunk at once. The measuring device should not come into contact with the diluent. The glass should then be rinsed well with more diluent to ensure that the total dose is taken.

Owing to its possible interference with the P450 dependent enzyme system, grapefruit or grapefruit juice should not be ingested for 1 hour prior to dose administration and grapefruit juice should not be used as a diluent.

The measuring device should not be rinsed with water, alcohol or any other liquid.

*Intravenous administration:* When Sandimmun is administered by the intravenous route, the intravenous dose is *one third* of the recommended oral dose.

Sandimmun Concentrate should be diluted 1:20 to 1:100 with normal saline or 5% glucose before use and given by slow intravenous infusion over two to six hours (see 'Pharmaceutical precautions').

*Use in the elderly:* Experience in the elderly is limited but no particular problems have been reported following the use of the drug at the recommended dose. However, factors sometimes associated with ageing, in particular impaired renal function, make careful supervision essential and may necessitate dosage adjustment.

*Use in children:* Experience with Sandimmun in young children is still limited. Transplant recipients from three months of age have received the drug at the recommended dosage with no particular problems although at dosages above the upper end of the recommended range, children seem to be more susceptible to fluid retention, convulsions and hypertension. This responds to dosage reduction.

**Contra-indications, warnings, etc**

*Contra-indications:* Known hypersensitivity to cyclosporin. Sandimmun is also contra-indicated in psoriasis and atopic dermatitis patients with abnormal renal function, uncontrolled hypertension, uncontrolled infections or any kind of malignancy other than of the skin (see 'Precautions'). Sandimmun is contra-indicated in rheumatoid arthritis patients with abnormal renal function, uncontrolled hypertension, uncontrolled infections or any kind of malignancy. Sandimmum should not be used to treat rheumatoid arthritis in patients under the age of 18 years. Sandimmun Concentrate for intravenous infusion should not be used in patients known to be hypersensitive to polyethoxylated castor oils.

*Precautions:* Sandimmun can impair renal function. Close monitoring of serum creatinine and urea is required and dosage adjustment may be necessary. Increases in serum creatinine and urea occurring during the first few weeks of Sandimmun therapy are generally dose-dependent and reversible and usually respond to dosage reduction. During long-term treatment, some patients may develop structural changes in the kidney (e.g. interstitial fibrosis) which, in renal transplant recipients, must be distinguished from chronic rejection.

Sandimmun may also affect liver function and dosage adjustment, based on the results of bilirubin and liver enzyme monitoring, may be necessary. Regular monitoring of blood pressure is required during Sandimmun therapy. If hypertension develops, appropriate antihypertensive treatment must be instituted.

Since Sandimmun occasionally causes hyperkalaemia or may aggravate pre-existing hyperkalaemia, monitoring of serum potassium is recommended, especially in patients with marked renal dysfunction. Patients receiving Sandimmun should avoid a high dietary potassium intake. Refer also to *Drug interactions.*

Caution is required in treating patients with hyperuricaemia because Sandimmun can aggravate this condition (see *Side-effects*).

Sandimmun should preferably not be administered with other immunosuppressive agents except corticosteroids. However, some transplant centres use Sandimmun together with azathioprine and corticosteroids or other immunosuppressive agents (all in low doses) with the aim of reducing the risk of Sandimmun-induced renal dysfunction or renal structural changes. When Sandimmun is used with other immunosuppressive agents, there is a risk of over-immunosuppression, which can lead to increased susceptibility to infection and to possible development of lymphoma.

In Sandimmun treated renal transplant recipients, a machine perfusion time of more than 24 hours and a reanastomosis time of more than 45 minutes can have a significant effect on graft function. Both factors appear to increase the incidence of acute tubular necrosis.

The Concentrate for intravenous infusion contains polyethoxylated castor oil, which has been reported to cause anaphylactoid reactions. These reactions consist of flushing of the face and upper thorax, acute respiratory distress with dyspnoea and wheezing, blood pressure changes and tachycardia. Special caution is therefore necessary in patients who have previously received intravenous injections or intravenous infusions containing polyethoxylated castor oil, or in patients with an allergic predisposition. Thus patients receiving Sandimmun intravenously should be under continuous observation for at least the first 30 minutes following start of the infusion and at frequent intervals thereafter. If anaphylaxis occurs, the infusion should be discontinued and the patient managed in accordance with common clinical practice.

Sandimmun can induce a reversible increase in blood lipids. It is therefore advisable to perform lipid determinations before treatment and thereafter as appropriate. The oral forms of Sandimmun do not contain polyethoxylated castor oil.

*Drug interactions:* Care should be taken when using Sandimmun in combination with systemic antibiotics or other compounds known to have nephrotoxic effects, e.g. aminoglycosides, amphotericin B, ciprofloxacin, melphalan and trimethoprim.

Various agents are known to either increase or decrease the plasma or whole blood concentrations of cyclosporin by competitive inhibition or induction of hepatic enzymes involved in the metabolism and excretion of Sandimmun, in particular cytochrome P450. Agents known to increase plasma or whole blood cyclosporin concentrations include ketoconazole, erythromycin, oral contraceptives and some calcium-channel blockers including diltiazem, nicardipine and verapamil. Doxycycline, fluconazole, itraconazole, propafenone and lipid solutions are also suspected of having the same effect. Agents known to decrease plasma or whole blood cyclosporin concentrations include phenytoin, carbamazepine, barbiturates and rifampicin. Sulphadiazine is also suspected of having the same effect.

In transplant patients, frequent measurement of cyclosporin and, if necessary, Sandimmun dosage adjustment is required, particularly during the introduction or withdrawal of co-administered drug. In non-transplant patients the relationship between cyclosporin blood level and clinical effect is less well established. If drugs known to increase cyclosporin levels are given concomitantly, frequent assessment of renal function and careful monitoring for Sandimmun-related side-effects may be more appropriate than blood level measurement.

Intravenous (but not oral) administration of sulphadimidine and trimethoprim has also resulted in a marked reduction of plasma or whole blood levels. Concomitant administration of such drugs with Sandimmun should therefore be avoided. Where combined administration is unavoidable, careful monitoring of cyclosporin blood levels and adjustment of Sandimmun dosage are essential.

In addition, it has been noted that Sandimmun reduces the clearance of prednisolone and, conversely, high-dose therapy with methylprednisolone can increase the blood concentration of cyclosporin. As non-steroidal anti-inflammatory drugs alone can have an adverse effect on renal function, addition of these drugs to Sandimmun therapy or an increase in their dosages should initially be accompanied by particularly close monitoring of renal function. Sandimmun given in combination with diclofenac causes an increase in plasma concentration of diclofenac. Diclofenac dosages should, therefore, be reduced by approximately half when given with Sandimmun. There have been other reports of pharmacokinetic interactions with other non-steroidal anti-inflammatory drugs, but there are insufficient data available to clarify their significance. However, a lack of pharmacokinetic interaction has been demonstrated between aspirin and Sandimmun. Some studies have shown that various NSAIDs interact pharmacodynamically with Sandimmun to affect renal function. An analysis of clinical trials of Sandimmun and non-steroidal anti-inflammatory drugs suggests that plasma creatinine is not higher in patients if they receive concomitant NSAID therapy. The combination of these drugs, however, should be used with care.

Sandimmun may enhance the potential of the HMG-CoA reductase inhibitor lovastatin to induce rhabdomyolysis. The potential for interaction with other drugs in this class should be considered.

Muscular toxicity, including muscle pains and weakness, have also been reported in patients receiving colchicine concurrently with Sandimmun.

The concurrent administration of nifedipine and Sandimmun has resulted in an increased rate of gingival hyperplasia when compared with that for Sandimmun alone.

Where there is a risk of hyperkalaemia, potassium-sparing diuretics should be avoided and care should be taken when prescribing potassium supplements or potassium-containing medications.

During treatment with Sandimmun, vaccination may be less effective, and the use of live attenuated vaccines should be avoided.

*Use in pregnancy and lactation:* Cyclosporin is not teratogenic in animals. As the safety of Sandimmun in human pregnancy has not been fully established it should only be used in pregnancy if the benefit outweighs any potential risks.

Cyclosporin passes into the breast milk and mothers receiving treatment with Sandimmun should not, therefore, breast feed their infants.

*Additional precautions in psoriasis and atopic dermatitis:* Only the oral forms of Sandimmun are recommended for the treatment of patients with psoriasis or atopic dermatitis. Sandimmun Concentrate for intravenous infusion should not be used for the treatment of these patients. Careful dermatological and physical examinations, including measurements of blood pressure and renal function on at least two occasions prior to starting therapy should be performed to establish an accurate baseline status.

Development of malignancies (particularly of the skin) have been reported in psoriatic patients treated with Sandimmun as well as during treatment with conventional therapy. A search for all forms of pre-existing tumours, including those of the skin and cervix, should be carried out.

Skin lesions which are not typical for psoriasis should be biopsied before starting Sandimmun treatment to exclude skin cancers, mycosis fungoides or other pre-malignant disorders. Patients with malignant or pre-malignant alterations of the skin should be treated with Sandimmun only after appropriate treatment of such lesions and only if no other option for successful therapy exists.

Because of the possibility of renal dysfunction or renal structural changes, serum creatinine should be measured at two weekly intervals during the first three months of therapy. Thereafter, if creatinine remains stable, measurements should be repeated at two-month intervals in patients receiving doses of 2.5 mg/kg/day and at monthly intervals in patients who require higher doses. If serum creatinine increases to more than 30% above baseline, even if the values are still within the normal range, Sandimmun dosage must be reduced by 25 to 50%. If dosage reduction is not successful within one month, treatment should be discontinued. In atopic dermatitis patients serum creatinine should be measured at two weekly intervals throughout the treatment period.

If hypertension develops which cannot be controlled by Sandimmun dosage reduction or appropriate antihypertensive therapy, discontinuation of the drug is recommended.

Sandimmun treatment and its monitoring should be carried out under the supervision of a dermatologist experienced in the management of severe skin disease.

In view of the potential risk of skin malignancy, patients on Sandimmun should be warned to avoid excess unprotected sun exposure and should not receive concomitant therapeutic ultraviolet B irradiation or PUVA photochemotherapy.

*Additional precautions in atopic dermatitis:* Active herpes simplex infections should be allowed to clear before initiating treatment with Sandimmun but are not necessarily a reason for drug withdrawal if they occur during treatment unless infection is severe.

Skin infections with *Staphylococcus aureus* are not an absolute contra-indication for Sandimmun therapy but should be controlled with appropriate antibacterial agents. Oral erythromycin, known to have the potential to increase the blood concentration of Sandimmun (see *Drug interactions*) should be avoided or, if there is no alternative, its concomitant use must be accompanied by close monitoring of the blood levels of Sandimmun.

As the experience with Sandimmun in children with atopic dermatitis is still limited, its use in patients under 16 years of age cannot be recommended.

*Additional precautions in rheumatoid arthritis:* Only the oral forms of Sandimmun are recommended for the treatment of patients with rheumatoid arthritis. Sandimmun concentrate for intravenous infusion should not be used for the treatment of patients with rheumatoid arthritis.

Since Sandimmun can impair renal function, a reliable baseline level of serum creatinine should be established by at least two measurements prior to treatment, and serum creatinine should be monitored at 2 weekly intervals during the first 3 months of therapy. Thereafter, measurements can be made every 4 weeks, but more frequent checks are necessary when the Sandimmun dose is increased or concomitant treatment with a non-steroidal anti-inflammatory drug is initiated or its dosage increased. Because the pharmacodynamic interaction between Sandimmun and NSAIDs may adversely affect renal function, caution should be exercised if NSAID therapy is to be continued.

If the serum creatinine remains increased by more than 30% above baseline at more than one measurement, the dosage of Sandimmun should be reduced. If the serum creatinine increases by more than 50%, a dosage reduction by 50% is mandatory. These recommendations apply even if the patient's values still lie within the laboratory normal range. If dosage reduction is not successful in reducing levels within one month, Sandimmun treatment should be discontinued.

Discontinuation of the drug may also become necessary if hypertension developing during Sandimmun therapy cannot be controlled by appropriate antihypertensive therapy.

The combination of non-steroidal anti-inflammatory drugs and Sandimmun should be used with caution in patients with rheumatoid arthritis and should be accompanied by particularly close monitoring of renal function as detailed above (please also see *Drug interactions* section).

As hepatotoxicity is a potential side effect of non-steroidal anti-inflammatory drugs, regular monitoring of hepatic function is advised when Sandimmun is co-administered with these drugs in rheumatoid arthritis patients.

The use of Sandimmun therapy for the treatment of patients with rheumatoid arthritis requires careful monitoring and follow-up. Sandimmun should only be used provided that the necessary expertise and adequate equipment, laboratory and supportive medical resources are available.

Patients with rheumatoid arthritis have an increased incidence of malignancies compared to the general population. Use of disease modifying drugs increases the risk of malignancy further. The use of Sandimmun in the treatment of rheumatoid arthritis has not been shown to increase the incidence of malignancies more than other disease modifying drugs.

*Side-effects:* Side-effects are usually dose dependent and responsive to dose reduction.

A frequent and potentially serious complication is a dose-dependent and reversible increase in serum creatinine and urea during the first few weeks of Sandimmun therapy. Less frequently, renal structural changes (e.g. interstitial fibrosis) may develop during long-term treatment. In patients who have undergone transplantation other than kidney transplant, impairment of renal function may necessitate a dosage reduction. In kidney transplant patients, impairment of renal function may necessitate a dosage reduction provided that graft rejection has been excluded. In non-transplant patients, impairment of renal function may necessitate discontinuation of Sandimmun therapy (see *Precautions*).

Apart from impaired renal function, the most frequently observed side-effects include hypertrichosis, tremor, hypertension (particularly in heart transplant patients) hepatic dysfunction, fatigue, gingival hypertrophy, gastrointestinal disturbances (abdominal pain, anorexia, nausea, vomiting, diarrhoea) and burning sensations of the hands and feet (usually during the first week of treatment).

Occasionally headaches, rashes of possible allergic origin, mild anaemia, hyperkalaemia, hyperuricaemia, gout, hypomagnesaemia, hypercholesterolaemia, weight increase, oedema, pancreatitis, neuropathy, confusion, paraesthesia, convulsions, reversible dysmenorrhoea or amenorrhoea may develop.

Muscle weakness, muscle cramps, or myopathy have also been reported.

Especially in liver transplant patients, signs of encephalopathy, vision and movement disturbances, and impaired consciousness are described. Whether these alterations are caused by Sandimmun, or are a consequence of the underlying disease or other conditions, remains to be established.

On rare occasions, a syndrome of thrombocytopenia, in some patients in combination with microangiopathic haemolytic anaemia and renal failure (haemolytic uraemic syndrome) has been observed.

Gynaecomastia has been rarely reported, occasionally in patients receiving concomitant spironolactone.

Malignancies and lymphoproliferative disorders have developed, but their incidence and distribution were found to be similar to those in patients on conventional immunosuppressive therapy. Where lymphoproliferative disorders have developed in patients with psoriasis they have been responsive to prompt drug discontinuation.

In a few cases, colitis has developed after treatment with Sandimmun.

*Overdosage:* Little experience is available with overdosage. Symptomatic treatment and general supportive measures should be followed in all cases of overdosage. Forced emesis could be of value within the first few hours after intake. Signs of nephrotoxicity might occur which would be expected to resolve following drug withdrawal. Sandimmun is not dialysable to any great extent nor is it well cleared by charcoal haemoperfusion. Hypertension and convulsions have been reported in some patients receiving Sandimmun therapy at doses above the recommended range and in others with high trough blood levels of cyclosporin. This might, therefore, be expected as a feature of overdosage.

**Pharmaceutical precautions** All forms of Sandimmun (Capsules, Oral Solution, Concentrate for intravenous infusion) may be stored at room temperature not exceeding 30°C. Sandimmun Capsules should be left in the blister-pack until required for use. When a blister is opened, a characteristic smell is noticeable.

Sandimmun Oral Solution should be used within 2 months of opening the bottle. At temperatures between 5°C and 10°C a reversible precipitate may be observed. At temperatures below 5°C an intensive precipitate may form. This precipitate will not completely redissolve at room temperature. Therefore, the preparation should not be refrigerated and the use of Sandimmun Oral Solution which has been stored in a refrigerator cannot be recommended.

Sandimmun Concentrate for intravenous infusion contains polyethoxylated castor oil which can cause phthalate stripping from PVC. Once an ampoule is opened the contents should be used immediately.

Sandimmun Concentrate for intravenous infusion should be diluted 1:20 to 1:100 with physiological saline or 5% glucose immediately before use. As compatibility with other intravenous infusion fluids is not known, their use cannot be recommended.

**Legal category** POM.

**Package quantities**
Soft Gelatin Capsules (25 mg, 50 mg and 100 mg): Boxes of 30 (OP).
Oral Solution: Bottles of 50 ml (OP).
Concentrate for infusion: Boxes of 10×5 ml ampoules. Boxes of 10×1 ml ampoules.

**Further information** Sandimmun therapy requires careful monitoring and follow up and the drug should only be used in units with experience of immunosuppressive therapy where adequate equipment, laboratory and supportive medical resources are available.

Further information on cyclosporin blood level monitoring and drug interactions with Sandimmun (cyclosporin) is available on request.

**Product licence numbers**

| | |
|---|---|
| 25 mg Soft Gelatin Capsules | 0101/0207 |
| 50 mg Soft Gelatin Capsules | 0101/0310 |
| 100 mg Soft Gelatin Capsules | 0101/0208 |
| Oral Solution | 0101/0124 |
| Concentrate for infusion | 0101/0153 |

## SANDOCAL* CALCIUM-SANDOZ*

**Presentation**
*Sandocal 400:* White, round, flat-faced, effervescent tablets with a slightly rough surface, weighing 2.92 g, 25 mm diameter and 4.35 mm thick, citrus flavoured. Each effervescent tablet contains 930.8 mg calcium lactate gluconate and 700 mg calcium carbonate and provides 400 mg calcium (10 mmol: 20 mEq $Ca^{++}$), and 1.189 g anhydrous citric acid.
*Sandocal 1000:* White, round, flat-faced effervescent tablets with a slightly rough surface, weighing 7.30 g, 33 mm diameter and 6.4 mm thick, citrus flavoured. Each effervescent tablet contains 2.327 g calcium lactate gluconate, 1.75 g calcium carbonate and provides 1 g calcium (25 mmol: 50 mEq $Ca^{++}$), 2.973 g anhydrous citric acid.
*Calcium-Sandoz Syrup:* Colourless to pale straw coloured, fruit flavoured syrup. Each 15 ml contains 3.27 g calcium glubionate and 2.18 g calcium lactobionate. Three 5 ml spoonfuls provide 325 mg calcium (8.1 mmol: 16.2 mEq $Ca^{++}$).

**Uses**
*Principal action:* Calcium is an essential body electrolyte. It is involved in the maintenance of normal muscle and nerve function, is essential for normal cardiac function and is essential to blood coagulation. There is a dynamic equilibrium between the calcium in blood and that in the skeleton. Homeostasis is mainly regulated by parathyroid hormone, by calcitonin and by vitamin D.
*Indications*
1. As an adjunct to conventional therapy in the arrest or slowing down of bone demineralisation in osteoporosis.
2. In the arrest or slowing down of bone demineralisation in osteoporosis where other effective treatment is contra-indicated.
3. As a supplemental source of calcium in the correction of dietary deficiencies or when normal requirements are high.
4. Calcium-Sandoz syrup is indicated for the treatment of neonatal hypocalcaemia.

Signs of hypocalcaemia may occur when the serum calcium concentration falls below 2.25 mmol per litre (or 4.5 mEq per litre). Symptoms may include paraesthesia, laryngospasm, muscle cramps, increased muscle excitability leading to tetany, prolongation of the Q-T interval on the ECG, convulsions and mental changes (e.g. anxiety, depression, delusions). Also ectodermal changes including loss of hair, grooved and brittle fingernails, defects of dental enamel and fungal infections, typically generalised candidiasis.

**Dosage and administration** In health the concentration of calcium in serum is maintained close to 2.5 mmol per litre (normal range 2.25–2.75 mmol or 4.5–5.5 mEq per litre). Treatment or therapeutic supplementation should aim to restore or maintain this level.

Effervescent tablets must be dissolved in ⅓ to ½ a tumblerful of water.

| Indication | Daily Dose Tablets Sandocal 400 | Sandocal 1000 | Syrup (5 ml spoonfuls) |
|---|---|---|---|
| *Adults* | | | |
| Osteoporosis | 3–4 | 1–2 | 11–15 |
| Therapeutic supplement (dose dependent upon severity) | 1–4 | 1–2 | 3–15 |
| *Children* | | | |
| Calcium deficiency | 1–2 | 1 | 6–9 |
| Dietary supplementation | 1 | — | 2–6 |

Neonatal hypocalcaemia: Calcium-Sandoz syrup may be given at a dose of 1 mmol calcium/kg/24 hours in divided doses. Serum calcium levels should be monitored and the dosage adjusted if necessary. Doses may be mixed with the first (small) part of milk feeds. Note: 1 mmol of calcium is equivalent to 1.85 ml Calcium-Sandoz syrup.

*Use in the elderly:* No evidence exists that tolerance of Sandocal 400, Sandocal 1000 or Calcium-Sandoz is directly affected by advanced age; however, elderly patients should be supervised as factors sometimes associated with ageing, such as poor diet or impaired renal function, may indirectly affect tolerance and may require dosage reduction.

**Contra-indications, warnings, etc**
*Contra-indications:* Hypercalcaemia (e.g. in hyperparathyroidism, vitamin D overdosage, decalcifying tumours such as plasmocytoma, severe renal failure, bone metastases), severe hypercalciuria, and renal calculi.

Due to its galactose component Calcium-Sandoz syrup should not be given to patients with galactosaemia.

*Precautions:* In mild hypercalciuria (exceeding 300 mg (7.5 mmol)/24 hours) or renal failure, or where there is evidence of stone formation in the urinary tract, adequate checks must be kept on urinary calcium excretion; if necessary the dosage should be reduced or calcium therapy discontinued. High vitamin D intake should be avoided during calcium therapy, unless especially indicated.

Thiazide diuretics reduce urinary calcium excretion so the risk of hypercalcaemia should be considered.

Oral calcium supplementation is aimed at restoring normal serum calcium levels. Although it is extremely unlikely that high enough levels will be achieved to adversely affect digitalised patients, this theoretical possibility should be considered.

The sugar content of Calcium-Sandoz syrup should be taken into account in diabetic patients.

Oral calcium administration may reduce the absorption of oral tetracycline or fluoride preparations. An interval of 3 hours should be observed if the two are to be given.

*Use in pregnancy and lactation:* The likelihood of hypercalcaemia is increased in pregnant women in whom calcium and vitamin D are co-administered. Epidemiological studies with calcium have shown no increase in the teratogenic hazard to the foetus if used in the doses recommended. Although supplemental calcium may be excreted in breast milk, the concentration is unlikely to be sufficient to produce any adverse effect on the neonate.

*Side-effects:* Mild gastrointestinal disturbances have occurred rarely (e.g. constipation, diarrhoea). Although hypercalcaemia would not be expected in patients unless their renal function were impaired, the following symptoms could indicate the possibility of hypercalcaemia: nausea, vomiting, anorexia, constipation, abdominal pain, bone pain, thirst, polyuria, muscle weakness, drowsiness or confusion.

*Overdosage:* The amount of calcium absorbed following overdosage with Sandocal 400, Sandocal 1000 or Calcium-Sandoz Syrup will depend on the individual's calcium status. Deliberate overdosage is unlikely with effervescent preparations and acute overdosage has not been reported. It might cause gastrointestinal disturbances but would not be expected to cause hypercalcaemia except in patients treated with excessive doses of vitamin D. Treatment should be aimed at lowering serum calcium levels, e.g. administration of oral phosphates.

**Pharmaceutical precautions** Sandocal 400 and Sandocal 1000 tablets must be stored below 30°C. Protect from humidity.

Calcium-Sandoz Syrup may be diluted with Syrup BP; the diluted syrup should be used within 14 days.

**Legal category** P.

**Package quantities**
Sandocal 400 Effervescent Tablets: Boxes of 100 (5 tubes of 20).
Sandocal 1000 Effervescent Tablets: Boxes of 30 (3 tubes of 10).
Calcium-Sandoz Syrup: Bottles of 500 ml.

**Further information** Sandocal 400 and Sandocal 1000 contain aspartame as an artificial sweetener, so that the preparations are free from sucrose. There is no added sodium or potassium in the tablets.

Calcium-Sandoz Syrup contains 1.512 g sucrose per 5 ml (4.536 g sucrose per 15 ml dose). Approximate calorific value of 13 kcals per 5 ml (39 kcals per 15 ml dose).

**Product licence numbers**

| | |
|---|---|
| Calcium-Sandoz Syrup | 0101/5024R |
| Sandocal 400 | 0101/5043R |
| Sandocal 1000 | 0101/0205 |

## SANDOGLOBULIN*

**Presentation** Freeze-dried substance for preparation of an intravenous solution of human normal immunoglobulin. Sodium chloride 0.9% w/v (physiological saline) for reconstitution.

Sandoglobulin is a polyvalent antibody preparation containing, in concentrated form, all the antibodies normally occurring in the donor pool. The distribution of IgG subclasses in the preparation corresponds closely to that found in normal plasma.

Sandoglobulin is available in three pack sizes: one containing 1 g protein, 1.67 g sucrose as stabiliser and a 33 ml bottle of saline; one containing 3 g protein, 5 g sucrose and a 100 ml bottle of saline; and one containing 6 g protein, 10 g sucrose and a 200 ml bottle of saline. It does not contain any preservative.

**Uses** *Principal actions:* Sandoglobulin contains intact immunoglobulin which possesses unchanged Fab and Fc functional activity. The anticomplementary activity of the preparation is only detectable at very low levels, but in the presence of an appropriate antigen it activates complement by the classical pathway.

The exact mechanism of action in idiopathic thrombocytopenic purpura remains to be elucidated. Changes have been shown to occur in the function of Fc receptors in mononuclear phagocytes, leading to a decreased binding affinity and prolonged clearance rates within the reticulo-endothelial system. It would appear that Sandoglobulin may block platelet removal by temporary competitive inhibition.

*Indications:* Replacement therapy for congenital agammaglobulinaemia and hypogammaglobulinaemia.

Treatment of idiopathic thrombocytopenic purpura.

**Dosage and administration**
*Dosage: Replacement therapy for congenital agammaglobulinaemia and hypogammaglobulinaemia:* 0.1 to 0.3 g/kg body weight every 2 to 4 weeks according to severity of clinical signs and symptoms.

*Idiopathic thrombocytopenic purpura:* 0.4 g/kg body weight/day on 5 successive days. Maintenance doses of 0.4 g/kg body weight may be given as required in order to maintain platelet count.

*Reconstitution:* Prepare the solution immediately before use. Dissolve the contents of the bottle in sodium chloride 0.9% w/v (physiological saline) as follows:
1 g in 33 ml to produce a 3% solution.
3 g in 100 ml to produce a 3% solution.
6 g in 200 ml to produce a 3% solution.
1 g in 16.5 ml to produce a 6% solution.
3 g in 50 ml to produce a 6% solution.
6 g in 100 ml to produce a 6% solution.

After disinfecting the stoppers, use the transfer needle provided to connect the bottles of saline and Sandoglobulin. Invert the connected bottles to allow the saline to flow into the Sandoglobulin bottle. Discard the empty saline bottle and transfer needle. Turn the Sandoglobulin bottle to wet any undissolved substance. Avoid frothing and *do not shake the solution.* Sandoglobulin usually dissolves in a few minutes, but in exceptional cases may take up to 20 minutes. When reconstituted Sandoglobulin should appear as an opalescent solution devoid of any particulate matter.

*Administration:* Sandoglobulin is for intravenous use. Use only solutions at close to body temperature which contain no undissolved Sandoglobulin. The first infusion of Sandoglobulin should be of a 3% solution, infused at a rate not exceeding 10 to 20 drops per minute. This is because the first infusion of immunoglobulin, particularly in previously untreated agammaglobulinaemic patients, may lead to inflammatory side-effects as a result of the reaction between the antibodies administered and the free antigen in the blood and tissues of the recipient. After 15 minutes the rate of infusion may be increased to 20 to 30 drops per minute and, after 30 minutes, it may be further increased to 40 to 50 drops per minute. Subsequent infusions may be administered at a rate of 40 to 50 drops per minute. For repeated administration of high doses a 6% solution may be used. In this case the initial rate of infusion should again be 20 to 30 drops per minute, increasing after 15 minutes to a maximum of 50 drops per minute. Antihistamines may be administered to prevent inflammatory reactions in agammaglobulinaemic patients being treated for the first time.

*Note:* 20 drops = approximately 1 ml.

*Use in the elderly:* Since there is an increased susceptibility to left ventricular overload in the elderly, particular caution is required with infusion volumes and infusion rates.

**Contra-indications, warnings, etc**
*Contra-indications:* Like all blood products containing IgA, Sandoglobulin is contra-indicated in IgA deficient patients who have circulating antibodies to IgA as anaphylactoid reactions may occur.

*Precautions:* Live virus vaccines should not normally be given until three months after a dose of normal immunoglobulin injection. If a live virus vaccine has been given, Sandoglobulin should not be given for at least two weeks, except in special circumstances. The risk of transmission of infection, in particular non-A non-B hepatitis, by intravenous immunoglobulin preparations cannot be entirely excluded.

*Side-effects:* If the correct dosage and administration routine is followed (Dosage and Administration) severe adverse reactions rarely occur. Nevertheless, the patient should be closely monitored for signs of anaphylactoid reactions such as a sensation of pressure in the chest, hypotension and cyanosis. In such cases the infusion should be stopped until the symptoms have passed.

Delayed inflammatory reactions including headache, nausea, mild pyrexia, shivering and tachycardia are more likely to occur in agammaglobulinaemic and hypogammaglobulinaemic patients who have never received immunoglobulin substitution therapy before or who have not received therapy within the previous 8 weeks. These reactions usually occur 30 to 60 minutes after the start of the infusion and disappear after it has been completed.

*Overdosage:* An overdosage of Sandoglobulin has never been reported, but is unlikely to leave harmful effects either on blood circulation or on other body functions. The only consequence of an abnormally increased level of IgG is the accelerated catabolic rate of this protein.

High infusion rates may produce symptoms resembling shock.

**Pharmaceutical precautions** Sandoglobulin should be protected from light and stored at a temperature not exceeding 25°C.

Once the freeze-dried substance has been reconstituted it should be used without delay.

Do not shake the Sandoglobulin solution.

Any solution remaining after infusion must be discarded. Open bottles must not be used again because of the danger of bacterial contamination.

Infuse only solutions devoid of any undissolved particulate matter at close to body temperature.

Sodium chloride 0.9% w/v (physiological saline) should be used to reconstitute Sandoglobulin. No other compatibilities have yet been evaluated so due consideration should be given to the advisability of adding other intravenous fluids or medications to Sandoglobulin.

**Legal category** POM.

**Package quantities** 1 g pack including 33 ml saline and transfer needle. 3 g pack including 100 ml saline transfer needle and 6 g pack including 200 ml saline and transfer needle.

**Further information** Sandoglobulin is prepared by cold alcohol fractionation of pooled plasma from blood donors and contains at least 96% IgG.

Individual donor units of plasma are screened for hepatitis B surface antigen and for the presence of antibodies to human immunodeficiency virus (HIV) which, combined with careful donor selection, minimises the risk of viral transmission. To date, no new antigenic properties have been shown to be acquired during fractionation and sensitisation has not been recognised as a clinical problem even after repeated administration. At least 90% of the immunoglobulin is intact monomeric and dimeric (7S) IgG; the remainder consists of a small amount of polymeric IgG and traces of IgA, IgM and immunoglobulin fragments.

**Product licence numbers**
1 g pack    0101/0181
3 g pack    0101/0182
6 g pack    0101/0186

## SANDO-K*

**Presentation** Flat, round, white, effervescent tablets with a slightly rough surface, weighing 2.4 g and of 22 mm diameter and 4.2 mm thickness. Salty taste. Each tablet contains 600 mg Potassium Chloride PhEur, 400 mg Potassium Bicarbonate USP and 800 mg of anhydrous citric acid. This provides the equivalent of 470 mg potassium (12 mmol: 12 mEq K+) and 285 mg chloride (8 mmol: 8 mEq Cl–). Sodium content 2.6 mg (0.1 mmol: 0.1 mEq Na+).

**Uses** *Principal action:* Potassium is the major cation in intracellular fluid and is essential for carbohydrate metabolism, glycogen storage and protein synthesis. It is also involved in transmembrane potentials thereby having important effects on muscle.

The concentration of potassium in the plasma is usually maintained between 3.5–5 mmol/l. Signs of hypokalaemia may occur when the plasma concentration falls below 3.5 mmol/l. Signs of deficiency include vomiting, abdominal distention, paralytic ileus, muscular weakness, confusion, reduced reflexes, respiratory failure and cardiac arrythmias.

Administration of potassium salts may cause gastric irritancy, intestinal ulceration has been seen with enteric-coated and matrix-type solid dose form potassium supplements. Sando-K effervescent tablets when dissolved in water prevent such local concentration, thereby minimising irritation.

**Indications:** Prevention and treatment of hypokalaemic states such as those associated with:
(i) use of drugs which can induce potassium depletion, eg, frusemide, thiazide diuretics, corticosteroids, carbenoxolone and cardiac glycosides, especially in combination with diuretics;
(ii) potassium loss resulting from severe diarrhoea, vomiting or fistulas;
(iii) acid-base disturbances eg alkalosis, renal tubular acidosis, states in which there is aldosterone excess, Cushing's syndrome;
(iv) decreased intake of potassium eg malnutrition, alcoholism, some elderly patients with deficient diets;
(v) since Sando-K effervescent tablets contain Cl– they may be used in the treatment of hypokalaemia associated with hypochloraemic alkalosis.

**Dosage and administration** Sando-K Effervescent Tablets must be dissolved in ⅓ to ½ a tumblerful of water and may be taken with food if preferred.

*Use in adults and children:* Dosage is dependent upon the clinical conditions and diet of the patient, however the administration of 2 to 4 tablets daily (24 to 48 mmol K+) is likely to provide an adequate prophylactic or therapeutic dose in most patients. Large doses may be indicated in more severe hypokalaemic conditions when the dose should be regulated by the patient's response as determined by serum electrolyte levels and acid-base studies.

*Dosage guidelines:* A drop in serum potassium level of 1 mmol/l represents a loss of about 100–200 mmol of potassium from body stores. While serum potassium levels below 2 mmol/l may warrant intravenous replacement therapy, the following are approximate guidelines in less severe potassium depletion: For serum levels between 2–3 mmol/l, a maximum daily dose of 100–200 mmol K+ (8–16 tablets) and for serum levels between 3–4 mmol/l, a maximum daily dose of 50–100 mmol K+ (4–8 tablets) should be considered.

*Use in the elderly:* No evidence exists that elderly patients require different dosages or show different side-effects than younger patients. However, such patients should be carefully supervised as factors sometimes associated with ageing, such as poor diet or impaired renal function, may indirectly affect the dosage or tolerability.

**Contra-indications, warnings, etc**
*Contra-indications and precautions:* The use of Sando-K is contra-indicated in patients with severe renal impairment with oliguria, inadequately treated Addison's disease, hyperkalaemia from any cause, crush injuries and acute dehydration.

If co-administered with potassium-sparing diuretics and ACE-inhibitors, the risk of hyperkalaemia must be considered.

*Use in pregnancy and lactation:* No clinical problems have been encountered during pregnancy or lactation. Nevertheless, the benefit of treatment should be considered in relation to the risks before Sando-K is given to pregnant or nursing women.

*Warning:* Periodic evaluation of the patient's clinical status, serum electrolytes and the ECG should be carried out when replacement therapy is undertaken. This is particularly important in patients with cardiac disease and in those receiving digitalis. Care should

be taken to avoid dosage in excess of requirements for patients with impaired renal function. Caution is also necessary in patients receiving potassium-sparing diuretics and ACE-inhibitors and in patients with myotonia congenita or severe haemolysis. In patients with acidosis, the acid-base balance should be monitored. In patients with hypertension, it should be remembered that correction of hypokalaemia may lower blood pressure.

*Side-effects:* Abdominal discomfort, diarrhoea, nausea and vomiting may occur. If there are any signs of gastric irritancy, Sando-K, in common with all other potassium salts, should be given with or after food. Gastric irritancy has occurred but this is rare since the tablets dissolve in water and are taken in solution thus preventing high local concentrations. Moderate hyperkalaemia may be asymptomatic. If suspected, reference to the section on overdosage is recommended.

*Overdosage:* Hyperkalaemia. Poisoning is usually minimal below 6.5 mmol/l but may be severe above 8 mmol/l.

However, comparatively low doses may cause adverse effects when excretion is delayed as in renal insufficiency. The absolute toxicity is dependent on other electrolytes and acid-base levels.

Hyperkalaemic symptoms include paraesthesia of the extremities, listlessness, mental confusion, weakness, paralysis, hypotension, cardiac arrhythmias, heart block and cardiac arrest.

Hyperkalaemia is often asymptomatic. However, increasing serum potassium levels can be detected by changes in the ECG; initially the appearance of tall, peaked T waves, followed by a widening of the QRS complex blending into the abnormal T waves. P-wave voltage decreases and the PR interval is prolonged.

Severe cardiac toxicity may be treated with calcium gluconate (10–20 ml of a 10% injection given over 1–5 minutes with ECG monitoring). The effect may be transient and the injection may need to be repeated.

Raised serum potassium levels respond to administration of dextrose (300–500 ml/hr of 10 or 25% solution), dextrose and insulin (as for dextrose with 10 units of insulin per 20 g dextrose), or sodium bicarbonate solution.

Cation exchange resins may be used, or in severe cases peritoneal dialysis or haemodialysis may be necessary.

Caution should be exercised in patients who are digitalised and who may experience acute digitalis intoxication in the course of potassium removal.

**Pharmaceutical precautions** Store in a cool dry place. Sando-K Effervescent Tablets are hygroscopic and should be dispensed in their original containers.

**Legal category** P.

**Package quantities** Boxes of 100 (5×20 effervescent tablets).

**Further information** Sando-K Tablets each contain 521.5 mg sucrose. Approximate calorific value – 4 kcals per tablet.

**Product licence number** 0101/5044R.

## SANDOSTATIN*

**Presentation**
Clear, colourless solution of octreotide acetate, available as ampoules and multidose vials. Ampoules provide 50 micrograms octreotide per ml, 100 micrograms octreotide per ml and 500 micrograms octreotide per ml. Multidose vials provide 1 mg octreotide in 5 ml, phenol 0.5% w/v as preservative.

**Uses**

*Principal actions:* Sandostatin is a synthetic octapeptide analogue of naturally occurring somatostatin with similar pharmacological effects, but with a longer duration of action. It inhibits the secretion of peptides of the gastroenteropancreatic endocrine system and of growth hormone.

In animals, Sandostatin is a more potent inhibitor of growth hormone, glucagon and insulin release than somatostatin with greater selectivity for growth hormone and glucagon suppression.

In normal healthy subjects Sandostatin inhibits the release of growth hormone stimulated by arginine, exercise and insulin-induced hypoglycaemia; postprandial release of insulin, glucagon, gastrin, other peptides of the gastroenteropancreatic system; arginine-stimulated release of insulin and glucagon and thyrotropin releasing hormone-stimulated release of thyroid stimulating hormone.

Because of its diverse endocrine effects, Sandostatin modifies different clinical features in patients with tumours of the gastroenteropancreatic endocrine system. Its effects in the different tumour types are as follows:

*Carcinoid tumours:* Sandostatin may improve symptoms, particularly flush and diarrhoea. In some cases there is a fall in plasma serotonin and reduced urinary excretion of 5-hydroxyindole acetic acid.

*VIPomas:* In most cases, Sandostatin alleviates the severe secretory diarrhoea typical of the condition, with consequent improvement in quality of life. This is accompanied by an improvement in associated electrolyte abnormalities, e.g. hypokalaemia, enabling enteral and parenteral fluid and electrolyte supplementation to be withdrawn. A reduction in plasma VIP levels, often into the normal reference range, usually accompanies clinical improvement.

*Glucagonomas:* Sandostatin produces an improvement of the characteristic necrolytic migratory rash in most patients. Its effect on the mild diabetes mellitus which frequently occurs is variable. Sandostatin produces improvement of diarrhoea, and hence weight gain in those patients affected. Its administration often leads to an immediate reduction in plasma glucagon levels which is generally not maintained long-term, despite continued symptomatic improvement.

*Acromegaly:* Sandostatin lowers plasma levels of GH and/or somatomedin C. In most patients Sandostatin markedly reduces the clinical symptoms of the disease such as headache, skin and soft tissue swelling, hyperhidrosis, arthralgia and paraesthesia.

*Indications:* (i) For the relief of symptoms associated with the gastroenteropancreatic endocrine tumours, including carcinoid tumours with features of the carcinoid syndrome, VIPomas, and glucagonomas.

Sandostatin is not an antitumour therapy and is not curative in these patients.

(ii) For symptomatic control and reduction of GH and somatomedin C plasma levels in patients with acromegaly:
(a) In short-term treatment prior to pituitary surgery, or
(b) In long-term treatment in those who are inadequately controlled by pituitary surgery, dopamine agonist treatment, radiotherapy, or in the interim period until radiotherapy becomes fully effective.

Sandostatin is indicated for acromegalic patients for whom surgery is inappropriate. Evidence from short-term studies demonstrates that tumour size is reduced in some patients (prior to surgery); further tumour shrinkage, however, cannot be expected as a feature of continued long-term treatment.

### Dosage and administration

(i) *Carcinoid tumours, VIPomas, glucagonomas*

*Adults:* The initial dose is 50 micrograms once or twice daily by subcutaneous injection. Depending on response, dosage can be gradually increased to 200 micrograms three times daily. Under exceptional circumstances higher doses may be required. Maintenance doses are variable.

The recommended route of administration is subcutaneous. However, in instances where a rapid response is required eg carcinoid crises, the initial recommended dose of Sandostatin may be administered by the intravenous route diluted and given as a bolus, whilst monitoring the cardiac rhythm.

For intravenous use Sandostatin should be diluted with sodium chloride 0.9% w/v solution to a ratio of not less than 1:1 and not more than 1:9. Dilution of Sandostatin with glucose solution is not recommended.

In carcinoid tumours, if there is no beneficial effect within a week, continued therapy is not recommended.

(ii) *Acromegaly*

*Adults:* 100 to 200 micrograms three times daily by subcutaneous injection.

If no relevant reduction of GH levels and no improvement of clinical symptoms have been achieved within 3 months of starting treatment with Sandostatin, therapy should be discontinued.

*Children:* Experience with Sandostatin in children is very limited.

*Use in the elderly:* In elderly patients treated with Sandostatin there is no evidence of reduced tolerability or altered dosage requirements.

Note: To reduce local discomfort, let the solution reach room temperature before injection. Avoid multiple injections at short intervals at the same site. To prevent contamination, it is recommended that the cap of multidose vials should be punctured not more than 10 times.

### Contra-indications, warnings, etc

*Contra-indications:* Hypersensitivity to the drug.

*Precautions:* Sudden escape of gastroenteropancreatic endocrine tumours from symptomatic control by Sandostatin may occur infrequently, with rapid recurrence of severe symptoms.

Sandostatin may increase the depth and duration of hypoglycaemia in patients with insulinoma. This is because it is relatively more potent in inhibiting growth hormone and glucagon secretion than in inhibiting insulin and because its duration of insulin

inhibition is shorter. If Sandostatin is given to a patient with insulinoma, close observation is necessary on introduction of therapy and at each change of dosage. Marked fluctuations of blood glucose concentration may be reduced by more frequent administration of Sandostatin.

Sandostatin may reduce insulin or oral hypoglycaemic requirements in patients with diabetes mellitus.

Thyroid function should be monitored in patients receiving long-term Sandostatin therapy.

Sandostatin exerts an inhibitory effect on gallbladder motility, bile acid secretion and bile flow and there is an acknowledged association with the development of gallstones. In some studies, an incidence of up to 20% has been reported. Therefore ultrasound examination of the gallbladder is recommended before treatment is initiated and at 6 to 12 month intervals thereafter. If gallstones do occur, they are usually asymptomatic; symptomatic stones should be treated in the normal manner with due attention to abrupt withdrawal of the drug.

Sandostatin has been reported to reduce the intestinal absorption of cyclosporin and to delay that of cimetidine.

*Use in pregnancy and lactation:* Experience with Sandostatin in pregnant or nursing women is not available. Studies in animals showed transient growth retardation of offspring, possibly consequent upon the specific endocrine profiles of the species tested, but there was no evidence of foetotoxic, teratogenic or other reproduction effects. Nevertheless, Sandostatin should not be given during pregnancy except in compelling circumstances.

Women receiving treatment with Sandostatin should not breast feed their infants.

*Side-effects:* The main side-effects are local and gastrointestinal.

Local reactions after subcutaneous administration of Sandostatin include pain, a sensation of stinging, tingling or burning at the site of injection, with redness and swelling. They rarely last more than fifteen minutes. Local discomfort may be reduced by allowing the solution to reach room temperature before injection.

Gastrointestinal side-effects include anorexia, nausea, vomiting, abdominal pain, abdominal bloating, flatulence, loose stools, diarrhoea and steatorrhoea. Although measured faecal fat excretion may increase, there is no evidence to date that long-term treatment with Sandostatin has led to nutritional deficiency due to malabsorption. In rare instances, gastrointestinal side-effects may resemble acute intestinal obstruction with progressive abdominal distention, severe epigastric pain, abdominal tenderness and guarding. Occurrence of gastrointestinal side-effects may be reduced by avoiding meals around the time of Sandostatin administration, that is, by injecting between meals or on retiring to bed.

Formation of gallstones has been reported in patients on long-term Sandostatin treatment and there have been isolated reports of biliary colic following the abrupt withdrawal of the drug in acromegalic patients in whom biliary sludge or gallstones had developed.

Because of its inhibitory action on insulin release, Sandostatin may impair postprandial glucose tolerance. In rare instances, with chronic administration, a state of persistent hyperglycaemia may be induced. Hypoglycaemia has also been observed. Rarely, hair loss has been reported in patients receiving Sandostatin treatment.

There have been isolated reports of hepatic dysfunctions associated with Sandostatin administration. These consist of acute hepatitis, without cholestasis, where transaminase values have normalised on withdrawal of Sandostatin, or slow development of hyperbilirubinaemia in association with elevation of alkaline phosphatase, gamma-glutamyl transferase and, to a lesser extent, transaminases.

*Overdosage:* No life-threatening reactions have been reported after acute overdosage. The maximum single dose so far given to an adult has been 1 mg by intravenous bolus injection. The observed signs and symptoms were a brief drop in heart rate, facial flushing, abdominal cramps, diarrhoea, an empty feeling in the stomach and nausea, all of which resolved within twenty-four hours of drug administration.

One patient has been reported to have received an accidental overdosage of Sandostatin by continuous infusion (250 micrograms per hour for forty-eight hours instead of 25 micrograms per hour). He experienced no side-effects.

The management of overdosage is symptomatic.

**Pharmaceutical precautions** For prolonged storage Sandostatin ampoules and multidose vials should be stored between 2° and 8°C and protected from light. For day-to-day use they may be stored at room temperature for up to 2 weeks. Unused portion of

contents of multidose vials should be discarded after 2 weeks.

If Sandostatin Injection needs to be given by the intravenous route, it should be diluted with sodium chloride 0.9% w/v solution to a ratio of of not less than 1:1 and not more than 1:9. Dilution with glucose solution is not recommended. The prepared solution may be kept at room temperature but should be administered within 8 hours of preparation.

**Legal category** POM.

**Package quantities**
50 micrograms per ml: boxes of 5×1 ml ampoules.
100 micrograms per ml: boxes of 5×1 ml ampoules.
500 micrograms per ml: boxes of 5×1 ml ampoules.
1 mg per 5 ml: boxes of 1×5 ml multidose vial.

**Further information** After subcutaneous injection Sandostatin is rapidly and completely absorbed. Peak plasma concentrations are reached within 30 minutes. The elimination half-life after subcutaneous administration is 100 minutes. After intravenous injection the elimination is biphasic with half-lives of 10 and 90 minutes respectively. The volume of distribution is 0.27 l/kg and the total body clearance 160 ml/min. Plasma protein binding amounts to 65%. The amount of Sandostatin bound to blood cells is negligible.

**Product licence numbers**
50 micrograms per ml: 0101/0212.
100 micrograms per ml: 0101/0213.
500 micrograms per ml: 0101/0214.
1 mg per 5 ml: 0101/0300.

## SANOMIGRAN*

### Presentation

*0.5 mg Tablets:* Ivory/yellow, coated, bi-convex tablets of 5.5 to 5.6 mm diameter, weighing 90 mg. Printed SMG on one face. Each tablet contains 725 micrograms pizotifen hydrogen malate (equivalent to 500 micrograms pizotifen base).

*1.5 mg Tablets:* Ivory/yellow, coated, bi-convex tablets of 9.0 mm diameter, weighing 280 mg. Printed SMG 1.5 on one face. Each tablet contains 2.175 mg pizotifen hydrogen malate (equivalent to 1.5 mg pizotifen base).

*Elixir 0.25 mg in 5 ml:* Clear, colourless, fruit flavoured elixir. Each 5 ml spoonful contains 365 micrograms pizotifen hydrogen malate (equivalent to 250 micrograms pizotifen base).

**Uses** *Principal action:* Pharmacodynamic studies demonstrate pizotifen to have powerful antiserotonin and antitryptaminic properties, marked antihistaminic effects and some antagonistic activity against kinins. It also possesses weak anticholinergic effects and sedative properties.

Pizotifen also possesses appetite-stimulating properties.

The prophylactic effect of Sanomigran in migraine is associated with its ability to modify the humoral mechanisms of headache. It inhibits the permeability-increasing effect of serotonin and histamine on the affected cranial vessels, thereby checking the transudation of plasmakinin so that the pain threshold of the receptors is maintained at 'normal' levels. In the sequence of events leading to the migraine attack, depletion of plasma serotonin contributes to loss of tone in the extracranial vessels. Pizotifen inhibits serotonin re-uptake by the platelets, thus maintaining plasma serotonin and preventing the loss of tone and passive distension of the extracranial arteries.

*Indications:* Prophylactic treatment of recurrent vascular headaches, including classical migraine, common migraine and cluster headache (periodic migrainous neuralgia).

### Dosage and administration

*Adults:* Usually 1.5 mg daily. This may be taken as a single dose at night or in three divided doses, using 1.5 mg tablets, 0.5 mg tablets or elixir as appropriate. Dosage should be adjusted to individual patients' requirements up to a maximum of 4.5 mg daily. Up to 3 mg may be given as a single daily dose.

*Children:* Up to 1.5 mg daily, usually as a divided dose. Use of the 1.5 mg tablets is not recommended but up to 1 mg has been given as a single daily dose at night. 0.5 mg tablets or elixir may be used.

*Use in the elderly:* Clinical work with Sanomigran has not shown that elderly patients require different dosages from younger patients.

### Contra-indications, warnings, etc

*Contra-indications:* Hypersensitivity to the drug.

*Precautions:* Patients should be cautioned about the possibility of drowsiness and informed of its significance in the driving of vehicles and the operation of machinery. The central effects of sedatives, hypnotics, antihistamines (including certain common cold preparations) and alcohol may be enhanced by Sanomigran.

Although the anticholinergic activity of Sanomigran is relatively weak, caution is required in the presence of closed angle glaucoma and in patients with a predisposition to urinary retention. Dosage adjustment may be necessary in patients with kidney insufficiency.

*Use in pregnancy and lactation:* As clinical data with Sanomigran in pregnancy are very limited it should only be administered during pregnancy under compelling circumstances.

Although the concentrations of Sanomigran measured in the milk of treated mothers are not likely to affect the infant, its use in nursing mothers is not recommended.

*Side-effects:* The most commonly occurring side-effects are drowsiness and an increased appetite which may lead to an increase in body weight. Other side-effects such as dizziness, dry mouth, nausea and constipation have been reported infrequently. In children CNS stimulation may occur.

*Overdosage:* Symptoms of overdosage may include drowsiness, dizziness, hypotension, dryness of the mouth, confusion, excitatory states (in children), ataxia, nausea, vomiting, dyspnoea, cyanosis, tachycardia, convulsions (particularly in children), coma and respiratory paralysis. Treatment should be directed to the elimination of the drug by gastric lavage and diuresis. Severe hypotension must be corrected (*cave:* adrenaline may produce paradoxical effects). Convulsions may be treated with short-acting barbiturates or benzodiazepines. General surveillance measures are indicated.

**Pharmaceutical precautions** Protect tablets from direct light.

**Legal category** POM.

**Package quantities** 0.5 mg tablets: Blister pack of 84. 1.5 mg tablets: Calendar packs of 28. Elixir: Bottles of 300 ml.

**Further information** Sanomigran elixir does not contain sucrose and neither Sanomigran tablets nor elixir now contains tartrazine. The sweetening agent in Sanomigran elixir is Lycasin* 80/55 (hydrogenated glucose syrup) at a concentration of 4 g in 5 ml. Lycasin contains 45% readily absorbable carbohydrate. This should be considered if prescribing the drug for diabetic patients.

The absorption of pizotifen is fast (absorption half-life 0.5 to 0.8 hours) and nearly complete (80%). The substance is metabolised with a half-life of about one hour. The main metabolite (N-glucuronide) is eliminated with a half life of approximately 23 hours. Protein binding amounts to 91% and distribution volume to 485 litres. Less than 1% of the administered dose is excreted unchanged in the urine, whereas 55% is excreted as metabolites.

**Product licence numbers**
0.5 mg tablets    0101/0036
1.5 mg tablets    0101/0129
Elixir            0101/0163

## SCOPODERM* TTS

**Presentation** Scopoderm TTS is a transdermal drug delivery system consisting of a self-adhesive, pink-coloured system, containing a drug reservoir of hyoscine. The average amount of hyoscine absorbed from each system in 72 hours is 1 mg. Each system has a contact surface area measuring 2.5cm² and hyoscine content of 1.5 mg.

**Uses**

*Indications:* For the prevention of symptoms of motion sickness such as nausea, vomiting and vertigo.

*Mode of action:* The transdermal therapeutic system (TTS) is a novel form of drug delivery designed to achieve a continuous release of hyoscine through the intact skin to the systemic circulation for up to 72 hours.

Hyoscine has anticholinergic properties. It acts as a competitive antagonist to acetylcholine and other parasympathomimetic agents. Its mechanism of action in the central nervous system in preventing motion sickness has yet to be elucidated. Hyoscine produces classical symptoms of parasympathetic blockade.

*Pharmacokinetics:* Following Scopoderm TTS administration, measurement of the urinary excretion has shown the equilibrium between absorption and elimination to be reached within about 6 hours. Steady plasma concentrations of hyoscine in the range of 0.17-0.33nmol/litre are produced. Provided the system is not removed, this equilibrium is maintained and plasma hyoscine levels are within the therapeutic range for up to 72 hours.

After removal of Scopoderm TTS, the plasma concentration diminishes slowly to approximately one third over the following 24 hours because hyoscine in the skin continues to enter the blood stream.

**Dosage and administration**
*Adults:* To achieve the optimum protective effect, one system should be applied about 5-6 hours before embarking on a journey (or on the evening before). The system should be placed onto a clean, dry, hairless area of skin behind the ear, taking care to avoid any cuts or irritation. One system can provide protection for up to 72 hours. Should protection be required for longer periods of time, a fresh system should be placed behind the other ear after 72 hours. (No more than one system should be used at a time). Conversely, if protection is only required for shorter periods of time, the system should be removed at the end of the journey.

Patients should wash their hands thoroughly after handling the system. In addition, after removal of the system, the site of application should also be washed. These precautions are necessary to minimise any chance of hyoscine accidentally being transferred to the eyes (see *Side-effects*).

Limited contact with water (i.e. during bathing or swimming), should not affect the system, although it should be kept as dry as possible.

If the Scopoderm TTS becomes accidentally detached, it should be replaced by a fresh system.

*Use in elderly:* Scopoderm TTS may be used in the elderly (see dosage recommendations for adults) although the elderly may be more prone to suffer from the side-effects of hyoscine (see *Precautions*).

*Use in children:* Scopoderm TTS can be used in children aged 10 years or over (see dosage recommendations for adults). Insufficient data are available to recommend the use of Scopoderm TTS for younger children.

**Contra-indications, warnings, etc**
*Contra-indications:* Scopoderm TTS is contra-indicated in patients with glaucoma or with a history of the condition, and in patients with known hypersensitivity to hyoscine.

*Warnings:* Scopoderm TTS may cause drowsiness, dizziness, confusion or visual disturbance in certain individuals. Patients using the system must not drive, operate machinery, pilot an aircraft, dive or engage in any other activities in which such symptoms could be dangerous (see *Side-effects*).

Care should be taken after removal of the system as side-effects may persist for up to 24 hours or longer.

Patients should not consume alcohol whilst using Scopoderm TTS.

*Precautions:* Scopoderm TTS should be used with caution in patients with pyloric stenosis, those who have bladder outflow obstruction, or in patients with intestinal obstruction.

Scopoderm TTS should also be used with caution in elderly patients, and in patients with impaired hepatic or renal function.

In rare cases, confusional states and visual hallucinations may occur. In such cases, Scopoderm TTS should be removed immediately. If severe symptoms persist, appropriate therapeutic measures should be taken (see *Overdosage* section).

Idiosyncratic reactions may occur with ordinary therapeutic doses of hyoscine.

In isolated cases an increase in seizure frequency in epileptic patients has been reported.

*Use in pregnancy and lactation:* Teratogenic studies have been performed in pregnant rats and rabbits with hyoscine administered by daily intravenous injection. No adverse effects were noted in rats. In rabbits, the drug had a marginal embryotoxic effect at a high dose (at drug plasma levels approximately 100 times those observed in humans using Scopoderm TTS).

Scopoderm TTS should only be used during pregnancy if the expected benefits to the mother outweigh the potential risks to the foetus.

It is not known if hyoscine passes into the breast milk. Therefore nursing mothers should refrain from breast feeding their infants whilst using Scopoderm TTS.

*Drug interactions:* Scopoderm TTS should be used with caution in patients being treated with drugs that act on the central nervous system or drugs with anticholinergic properties.

*Side-effects:* The following side-effects may occur:
*Eyes:* In isolated cases pupillary dilatation may precipitate acute glaucoma, particularly narrow angle glaucoma (see *Contra-indications*). Occasional: irritation of the eyelids. If traces of hyoscine on the hands enter the eyes, transient cycloplegia and pupillary dilatation (occasionally unilateral) frequently occur.
*Mouth:* Frequent: transient dryness of the mouth.
*Central nervous system:* Occasional: drowsiness. Rare: impairment of memory and concentration, restlessness, dizziness, disorientation, confusion and visual hallucinations (see *Precautions*).

*Skin:* Occasional: local irritation. In isolated cases: a generalised skin rash.
*Urogenital system:* Rare: disturbances of micturition (i.e. urine retention).
*Side-effects after removal of Scopoderm TTS:* Rare: unwanted effects, including headache, nausea, vomiting and disturbance of balance, occurring after removal of the system. These symptoms have occurred most often in patients who have used the system for several days. In such cases, patients should not drive or engage in other activities requiring concentration (see *Warnings*).

*Overdosage:*
*Symptoms:* Initially, restlessness, excitation and confusion may be observed. In response to higher doses, delirium, hallucinations and convulsions set in. At very high doses, coma and respiratory paralysis may occur.

*Treatment:* If symptoms of overdosage occur, the system(s) should be removed immediately. Physostigmine is the most effective antidote. Depending on the severity of poisoning, physostigmine should be given by slow intravenous injection in doses of 1-4 mg (0.5 mg in children). Repeated injections may be necessary since physostigmine is rapidly metabolised. Diazepam may be used to counter excitation and convulsions although at higher doses it may cause respiratory depression. In severe cases, artificial respiration may be necessary.

If hyperthermia occurs, immediate action should be taken to dissipate heat.

**Pharmaceutical precautions** Store below 25°C. Do not freeze.

**Legal category** POM

**Package quantities** Cartons containing 2 Scopoderm TTS systems, each individually sealed in a protective pouch (OP).

**Further information** Scopoderm TTS contains hyoscine which is a potent anticholinergic agent.

*Instructions for use:* Tear open the pouch and remove the system. Peel off the transparent hexagonal protective foil taking care not to touch the silver adhesive side. Press the system (silver adhesive side downwards) firmly onto a clean, dry area of skin behind the ear. Undue pressure should not be applied to the system. Once the system has been fixed in place, it should not be touched again until it is necessary to remove it. Wash hands after applying or removing the system. The system should be disposed of carefully and out of the reach of children.

**Product licence number** 0001/0099

*Product licence holder:* Ciba-Geigy plc, Hulley Road, Macclesfield, Cheshire SK10 2NX.

## SINTHROME*

**Presentation** The active ingredient, Nicoumalone BP, is presented as:
White, round, flat, compressed tablets with slightly bevelled edges, approx. 5.1 mm diameter, imprinted 'CG' on one side and 'AA' on the other, containing 1 mg in each tablet.
The tablet also contain lactose.

**Uses**
*Indications:* Sinthrome is an oral anticoagulant for the treatment and prevention of thromboembolic diseases.

*Mode of action:* To initiate blood clotting, vitamin K causes -carboxylation of certain glutamic acid molecules on the coagulation factors II, VII, IX and X. Coumarin derivatives such as Sinthrome prevent -carboxylation of these proteins by vitamin K although the precise nature of this antagonism has yet to be established.

Depending on the initial dosage, Sinthrome prolongs the thromboplastin time within approximately 36-72 hours. Following withdrawal of Sinthrome, the thromboplastin time usually reverts to normal after a few days.

*Pharmacokinetics:* Following oral administration, Sinthrome is rapidly absorbed; at least 60% of the administered dose is systemically available. Peak plasma concentrations are achieved within 1-3 hours after a single dose of 10 mg and AUC values are proportional to the size of the dose over a dosage range of 8-16 mg.

No correlation between plasma concentrations of Sinthrome active substance (nicoumalone) and the apparent prothrombin levels can be established due to the variation of plasma drug concentrations between patients.

Plasma drug concentrations are generally higher in patients of 70 years or over when compared with younger patients, after the same dose.

Over 98% of nicoumalone is protein-bound, mainly to albumin. The calculated apparent volume of distribution is 0.16-0.18 l/kg for the R(+) enantiomer and 0.22-0.34 l/kg for the S(-) enantiomer.

Nicoumalone is extensively metabolised although the metabolites appear to be pharmacologically inactive in man.

The elimination half-life of nicoumalone from the plasma is 8-11 hours. Less than 0.2% of the dose is renally excreted unchanged with 60% being excreted in the urine and 29% in the faeces.

**Dosage and administration** Sensitivity to anticoagulants varies from patient to patient and may also fluctuate during the course of treatment. Therefore it is essential to perform regular coagulation tests and to adjust the patients dosage accordingly. If this is not possible, Sinthrome should not be used.

Sinthrome should be given in a single dose at the same time every day.

*Adults*: Initial dosage: If the thromboplastin time before starting treatment is within the normal range, the following dosage schedule is recommended:

First day : 8-12 mg
Second day : 4- 8 mg

If the initial thromboplastin time is abnormal, treatment should be instituted with caution.

Maintenance therapy: The maintenance dose of Sinthrome varies from patient to patient and must be determined on the basis of regular laboratory estimations of the patient's blood coagulation time.

Adjustment of the maintenance dose can only be made by monitoring the Quick value or International Normalised Ratio (INR) at regular intervals so that dosage remains within the therapeutic range. Depending on the individual, the maintenance dose generally lies between 1-8 mg daily.

Before the start of treatment, up to the time when the coagulation valency is stabilised within the optimum range, routine measurement of the thromboplastin time should be carried out daily in hospital. Blood samples for laboratory tests should always be taken at the same time of day.

The INR is the ratio of the patient's plasma thromboplastin time and the normal thromboplastin time raised to a power determined for a reference thromboplastin. As the Quick value decreases, the patient's thromboplastin time increases and the INR is greater. The therapeutic range generally lies between INR values of 2-4.5.

Generally after withdrawal of Sinthrome, there is usually no danger of reactive hypercoagulability and therefore it is not necessary to give gradually diminishing doses. However, in extremely rare cases in some high risk patients (e.g. after myocardial infarction) withdrawal should be gradual.

*Use in children*: Not recommended.

*Use in the elderly*: A dose lower than the recommended adult dose may be sufficient in elderly patients. (See 'Precautions').

**Contra-indications, warnings, etc**
*Contra-indications*: Sinthrome is contra-indicated in patients with a known hypersensitivity to nicoumalone and related coumarin derivatives, and in patients unable to co-operate (e.g. unsupervised and senile patients, alcoholics and patients with psychiatric disorders).

Sinthrome is also contra-indicated in all conditions where the risk of haemorrhage exceeds possible clinical benefit e.g. haemorrhagic diathesis and/or blood dyscrasia, immediately prior to, or after surgery on the central nervous system or eyes and traumatising surgery involving extensive exposure of the tissues, peptic ulceration or haemorrhage in the gastro-intestinal tract, urogenital tract or respiratory system, cerebrovascular haemorrhages, pericarditis, pericardial effusion, subacute bacterial endocarditis, severe hypertension (due to occult risks), severe hepatic or renal disease, and in cases of increased fibrinolytic activity following operations on the lung, prostate and uterus.

*Precautions*: Strict medical supervision should be given in cases where the disease or condition may reduce the protein binding of Sinthrome (e.g. thyrotoxicosis, tumours, renal diseases, infections and inflammation).

Particular care should be taken in patients with hepatic dysfunction since the synthesis of blood coagulation factors may be impaired. Disorders affecting gastro-intestinal absorption may alter the anticoagulant activity of Sinthrome. In severe heart failure, a very cautious dosage schedule must be adopted, since hepatic congestion may reduce the activation or -carboxylation of coagulation factors. However with reversal of the hepatic congestion, it may be necessary to raise the dosage.

In elderly patients, anticoagulant medication should be monitored with special care (see 'Pharmacokinetics' and 'Dosage' recommendations).

Since nicoumalone is extensively metabolised by the liver, impaired renal function will not greatly affect the elimination of the drug although care should be

taken due to the possibility of underlying platelet dysfunction.

During treatment with anticoagulants, intramuscular injections may cause haematomas and should be avoided. Subcutaneous and intravenous injections may be given without such complications.

Meticulous care should be taken where it is necessary to shorten the thromboplastin time for diagnostic or therapeutic procedures (e.g. angiography, lumbar puncture, minor surgery, tooth extractions, etc.).

*Use in pregnancy and lactation*: Sinthrome, like other coumarin derivatives may be associated with congenital malformations of the embryo. Therefore Sinthrome is contra-indicated for use in pregnancy. Women of child-bearing potential should take contraceptive measures during treatment with Sinthrome.

Sinthrome active substance passes into the breast milk of lactating mothers, but in quantities so small that no undesirable effects on the infant are to be expected. However, as a precaution, the infant should be given 1 mg vitamin $K_1$ per week as a prophylactic measure.

*Drug interactions*: There are many possible interactions between coumarins and other drugs; the interactions of clinical relevance are given below. The mechanisms of these interactions include disturbances of absorption, inhibition or induction of liver microsomal enzyme systems and reduced availability of vitamin K necessary for -carboxylation of coagulation factors. Every form of therapy may involve the risk of an interaction although not all will be significant. Thus careful surveillance is important and frequent coagulation tests (e.g. twice weekly) should be carried out when initially prescribing any drug in combination with Sinthrome or withdrawing a concomitantly administered drug.

The anticoagulant effect may be potentiated by concomitant administration of the following drugs:

allopurinol, anabolic steroids, androgens, anti-arrhythmic agents (e.g. amiodarone, quinidine), antibiotics (e.g. erythromycin, tetracyclines, neomycin, chloramphenicol), clofibric acid, its derivatives and structural analogues, disulfiram, ethacrynic acid, glucagon, histamine $H_2$-receptor antagonists, imidazole derivatives (e.g. metronidazole and, even when administered locally, miconazol), long-acting sulphonamides (including co-trimoxazoles), oral antidiabetics, thyroid hormones (incl. dextrothyroxine), sulphinpyrazone.

Drugs altering haemostasis may potentiate the anticoagulant activity of Sinthrome and thereby increase the risk of gastro-intestinal haemorrhage. Consequently, Sinthrome should not be prescribed with such drugs, which include heparin, salicylic acid and its derivatives.

When Sinthrome is prescribed in combination with NSAIDs, coagulation tests should be performed more frequently.

The anticoagulant effect may be diminished by concomitant administration of the following drugs:

aminoglutethimide, barbiturates, carbamazepine, cholestyramine (see below), griseofulvin, oral contraceptives, rifampicin, and thiazide diuretics.

During concomitant treatment with hydantoin derivatives, the serum hydantoin concentration may rise.

Sinthrome may potentiate the hypoglycaemic effect of sulphonylurea derivatives.

Patients being treated with Sinthrome (especially those suffering from hepatic dysfunction), should limit their alcohol intake since it is not possible to predict the severity of any drug interactions nor identify any early signs of such interactions.

*Side-effects*: Haemorrhage, in various organs, is the most common side-effect associated with Sinthrome; its occurrence is related to the dosage of the drug, the patient's age and the nature of the underlying disease (but not the duration of treatment).

Possible sites of haemorrhage include the gastrointestinal tract, brain, urogenital tract, uterus, liver, gall bladder and the eye.

If haemorrhage occurs in a patient with a thromboplastin time within the therapeutic range, diagnosis of their condition must be clarified.

Rare effects noted with similar coumarin derivatives include gastro-intestinal disorders (loss of appetite, nausea, vomiting), allergic reactions (urticaria, dermatitis and fever) and reversible alopecia.

Isolated cases of haemorrhagic skin necrosis (usually associated with congenital protein C deficiency) and liver damage have also been reported.

*Overdosage*: Clinical manifestations of overdosage are unlikely with large single doses but more likely following prolonged use of daily doses exceeding those required therapeutically.

*Symptoms*: The onset and severity of the symptoms are dependent on the individual's sensitivity to oral anticoagulants, the size of the overdose and the duration of treatment.

Haemorrhage is the prominent feature of an overdose and may occur within 1-5 days after ingestion.

Nose-bleeds, haematemesis, haemoptysis, gastrointestinal haemorrhage, vaginal bleeding, haematuria (with renal colic), cutaneous haemorrhages, bleeding into the joints or menorrhagia may be experienced.

Further symptoms include tachycardia, hypotension, peripheral circulatory disorders due to loss of blood, nausea, vomiting, diarrhoea, and abdominal pains.

Laboratory tests will show an extremely low Quick value (or high INR value) pronounced prolongation of the recalcification time or thromboplastin time and disturbed -carboxylation of factors II, VII, IX and X.

*Treatment*: If, at the time of overdosage, the patient's thromboplastin time was normal, drug absorption may be reduced by emesis or gastric lavage in combination with giving activated charcoal or a fast-acting laxative. Cholestyramine may markedly enhance the drug's elimination by inhibiting the enterohepatic circulation.

A temporary reduction of the dose of Sinthrome is often sufficient to control slight bleeding.

Vitamin $K_1$ may antagonise the effect of Sinthrome within 3-5 hours. In cases of moderate haemorrhage, 2-5 mg vitamin $K_1$ should be given orally; in severe haemorrhage, 1-10 mg vitamin $K_1$ should be injected very slowly (at a rate less than 1 mg/min) intravenously. Additional doses (up to a maximum dose of 40 mg daily) should be given at 4-hour intervals. Vitamin $K_1$ should not be given by intramuscular injection.

Doses of vitamin $K_1$ in excess of 5 mg can cause resistance to further anticoagulant therapy for several days. If an anticoagulant is required, heparin may be used temporarily, although oral anticoagulant therapy should be resumed at the same time and heparin withdrawn once the therapeutic range has been reached.

In the case of life-threatening haemorrhage, intravenous transfusions of fresh frozen plasma or whole blood can abolish the effects of Sinthrome.

**Pharmaceutical precautions** None.

**Legal category** POM

**Package quantities** Tablets 1 mg : Containers of 200 and blister packs of 100.

**Further information** Nil

**Product licence number** 00101/0427

## SLOW-FE*

**Presentation** A circular, biconvex, greenish-white tablet, impressed with the letters CG 503 on one side and plain on the other side. The tablets have a thin, transparent film coat and contain 160 mg of dried ferrous sulphate in a special slow-release wax core (equivalent to approx. 50 mg elemental iron). The tablets also contain lactose.

**Uses**
*Indication:* As a haematinic for the treatment of, or for the prophylaxis of iron deficiency anaemia, including that associated with post-gastrectomy and other malabsorption syndromes.

*Mode of action:* Slow-Fe (Ferrous Sulphate in a slow release preparation) provides a source of iron which is an essential constituent of the body. It is necessary for haemoglobin formation and for the oxidative processes of living tissues. Insufficient iron in the body results in iron deficiency anaemia which may be treatable with an iron supplement such as Slow-Fe.

*Pharmacokinetics:* Iron is a dietary requirement, about 5%–10% of the iron ingested with food is absorbed. Absorption is increased in conditions of deficiency and decreased when body stores are overloaded. Apart from haemorrhage iron is lost from the body in: urine, hair, nails, skin and sweat. In healthy men and non-menstruating women absorption of 1 mg/day is required, in menstruating women this rises to 2 mg/day and in pregnancy/lactation 3 mg/day is required.

In therapy haemoglobin levels return to normal after about 10 weeks. Three to six months are required to replenish body stores.

There is no significant difference between the absorption of iron from ferrous sulphate tablets and from Slow-Fe in healthy persons, in anaemia, following gastrectomy, or in coeliac disease.

**Dosage and administration**
*Adults:* For prophylaxis, one tablet daily. For the treatment of iron deficiency anaemia, two tablets daily.

*Children:* For treatment, one tablet daily for children over the age of six years.

The tablets should be swallowed whole with fluid and may be taken at any time of the day.

**Contra-indications, warnings, etc**
*Contra-indications:* Known hypersensitivity to ferrous sulphate.

Iron therapy is contra-indicated in the presence of

haemochromatosis, haemosiderosis and haemolytic anaemia.

*Precautions:* As with all iron preparations, Slow-Fe should be used with care in patients with known or suspected gastro-intestinal strictures or diverticulae.

*Pregnancy and lactation:* Slow-Fe can be used in the iron deficiency anaemia of pregnancy, with or without additional folic acid as appropriate.

*Drug interactions:* Concurrent administration of antacids may reduce absorption of iron preparations. Iron chelates with tetracyclines and absorption of both agents may be impaired. Iron may reduce the absorption of penicillamine and zinc salts.

*Side-effects:* As with all iron containing preparations gastro-intestinal side effects such as abdominal discomfort, nausea, vomiting, constipation, diarrhoea and dark stools may occur.

*Overdosage:*
   *Symptoms:* Include abdominal pain, nausea and vomiting, diarrhoea and haematemesis.
   *Treatment:* Gastric lavage or emesis should be carried out immediately. To chelate excess free iron in the gastro-intestinal tract, 5 g desferrioxamine dissolved in 50 ml water should be introduced into the stomach. To chelate excess free iron in the blood, desferrioxamine may be given parenterally; depending on the patients condition, 1 g desferrioxamine given every three hours intramuscularly may be appropriate.

**Pharmaceutical precautions** Tablets should be protected from moisture.

**Legal category** P

**Package quantities** The tablets are available form-packed in quantities of 28 and 150.

**Further information** The precision release principle of Slow-Fe ensures that the iron is released evenly over a period of 1 to 2 hours. Complete release therefore normally occurs before the tablet has left the duodenum or upper jejunum, and maximum iron absorption can take place.
   The incidence of side-effects would appear to be lower than with plain ferrous sulphate.

**Product licence number** 00101/0509

## SLOW-FE* FOLIC

**Presentation** A circular biconvex yellowish-white tablet impressed with the monogram CIBA on one side and the letters TP on the other. The tablets have a thin transparent film-coat and contain 160 mg dried ferrous sulphate U.S.P (equivalent to 50 mg elemental iron) in a special slow-release core and 0.4 mg Folic Acid BP. The tablets also contain lactose.

### Uses
*Indications:* Slow-Fe Folic is indicated throughout pregnancy for prophylaxis of iron and folic acid deficiency. Slow-Fe folic is designed to minimise the problems of gastro-intestinal disturbance associated with most oral iron preparations, and contains 0.4 mg of folic acid, a daily supplement which prevents the occurrence of megaloblastic anaemia due to folate deficiency.

*Mode of action:* Slow-Fe Folic incoporates iron (as ferrous sulphate) and folic acid in a slow release preparation. Both are essential constituents of the body. Iron is necessary for haemoglobin formation and for the oxidative processes of the tissues. Folic acid undergoes reduction in the body to tetrahydrofolate which is a co-enzyme for various metabolic processes including DNA synthesis. Deficiency of iron causes microcytic hypochromic anaemia; deficiency of folic acid leads to megaloblastic anaemia. Epidemiological work has shown that folic acid deficiency in pregnancy is associated with an increased risk of neural tube defect. A supplement of folic acid given from the time of conception to the 12th week of pregnancy may reduce this risk. In the absence of supplementation of dietary iron and folic acid during pregnancy anaemia is likely to occur. Slow-Fe Folic can be used for prophylaxis of anaemia of pregnancy.

*Pharmacokinetics:* Both iron and folic acid are obtained in the diet. Iron absorption is increased in conditions of deficiency and decreased when body stores are overloaded. In healthy men and non-menstruating women absorption of 1 mg/day is required. This rises to >3 mg/day in pregnancy. Folic acid is absorbed mainly from the proximal small intestine and circulates bound to plasma proteins. 4-5µg is excreted daily in urine. A high proportion is stored in the liver; folic acid undergoes enterohepatic circulation.
   A combination of iron and folic acid acts more effectively against the anaemia of pregnancy than either substance alone.

**Dosage and administration**
*Adults:* The product is intended for oral administration, one tablet to be taken daily throughout pregnancy. In the case of a multiple pregnancy the dosage should be increased to two tablets daily. The tablets should be swallowed whole and for preference taken after food.

*Use in children:* Not indicated.

*Use in the elderly:* Not indicated.

**Contra-indications,warnings, etc**
*Contra-indications:* Iron therapy is contra-indicated in the presence of haemochromatosis, haemosiderosis and haemolytic anaemia. Hypersensitivity to the active ingredient.

*Precautions:* In epileptic patients who have become folate deficient (for instance during phenytoin treatment) folic acid supplementation can result in decreased anticonvulsant serum concentrations, which (unless the anticonvulsant dosage is adjusted) can lead to loss of seizure control.

*Use in pregnancy and lactation:* Slow-Fe Folic is indicated throughout pregnancy for prophylaxis of iron and folic acid deficiency.

*Drug interactions:* Concurrent administration of antacids may reduce absorption of iron preparations. Iron chelates with tetracyclines and absorption of both agents may be impaired. Iron may reduce the absorption of penicillamine and zinc salts.

*Side-effects:* Slow-Fe Folic is particularly well tolerated although gastro-intestinal side effects such as nausea, vomiting, constipation or diarrhoea may occur infrequently. On very rare occasions, skin rashes have been reported.

*Overdosage:*
   *Symptoms:* Symptoms include abdominal pain, nausea and vomiting, diarrhoea and haematemesis.
   *Treatment:* Gastric lavage or emesis should be carried out immediately. To chelate excess free iron in the gastro-intestinal tract, 5 g desferrioxamine dissolved in 50 ml water should be introduced into the stomach. To chelate excess free iron in the blood, desferrioxamine may be given parenterally; depending on the patient's condition, 1 g desferrioxamine given every 3 hours intramuscularly may be appropriate.

**Pharmaceutical precautions** Tablets should be protected from moisture.

**Legal category** Slow-Fe folic is not subject to poisons regulations but it is recommended for use only under medical supervision.

**Package quantities** Slow-Fe folic tablets are available form-packed in quantities of 28.

**Further information** The precision-release principle of Slow-Fe folic ensures that the iron is released evenly over a period of 1½ to 2 hours. Complete release therefore occurs before the tablet has left the duodenum or upper jejunum, and maximum iron absorption can take place. This avoids wastage, and associated side effects, whilst producing an effective haematinic response from a relatively low dose of iron.
   The incidence of side effects is comparable with placebo levels and considerably lower than with plain ferrous sulphate.

**Product licence number** 00101/0510

## SLOW-K*

**Presentation** Pale orange, polished, sugar-coated tablets about 12 mm in diameter, printed with the name Slow-K, containing 600 mg (8.06 mmol) of Potassium Chloride BP. The tablets also contain sucrose.

### Uses
*Indications:* Slow-K is indicated for the correction and/or prevention of hypokalaemia in those patients who cannot tolerate and/or refuse to take liquid or effervescent potassium chloride, or when there is a problem of compliance with these preparations.

*Mode of action:* The potassium chloride in Slow-K is finely distributed in a neutral wax base, from which it is gradually released over a period of 3-6 hours during its passage through the digestive tract. This special form of potassium subtitution therapy is designed to avoid high localised concentrations of potassium chloride which might irritate or damage the mucosa. The potassium chloride in Slow-K is completely absorbed in the intestinal tract.

*Pharmacokinetics:* The potassium chloride in Slow-K has been shown to be completely absorbed, occasionally patients may notice 'ghost' tablet cores in the faeces, these have been shown not to contain any potassium.
   Following a single dose of Slow-K, potassium chloride is released over a period of approximately 4

hours. Renal excretion of potassium chloride following ingestion of Slow-K occurs 30-60 minutes later than when the same dose is given in the form of a solution. In the presence of a normal potassium balance 90% of the potassium supplied by Slow-K is excreted renally within 8 hours and more than 98% by 24 hours.

**Dosage and administration** It is important that the tablets should be swallowed whole, with fluid during meals, whilst the patient is sitting upright.

*Adults:* The dosage of Slow-K should be adapted to the cause, degree and duration of potassium depletion. 2-3 tablets daily are usually an adequate supplement. In states of severe potassium deficiency, a higher dose of 9-12 tablets daily may be needed. If the dosage exceeds 16 mmol K⁺ (2 tablets) it should be taken in divided doses. Where intermittent diuretic therapy is being used, it is advisable to give Slow-K on intervening days between administration of the diuretic. The response to treatment should preferably be monitored by repeat determination of plasma potassium and Slow-K continued until the hypokalaemia has been corrected.

*Children:* Not recommended.

*Use in the elderly:* No special dosage regime is usually necessary, but concurrent renal insufficiency should be taken into account (also see Precautions).

**Contra-indications, warnings, etc**
*Contra-indications:* Hypersensitivity to potassium administration e.g. hyperkalaemic periodic paralysis, congenital paramyotonia. Marked renal failure (even when not yet associated with manifest hyperkalaemia), untreated Addison's disease, hyporeninaemic hypoaldosteronism, acute dehydration, hyperkalaemia and conditions involving extensive cell destruction (e.g. severe burns).
   All solid forms of potassium medication are contra-indicated in the presence of obstructions in the digestive tract (e.g. resulting from compression of the oesophagus due to dilation of the left atrium or from stenosis of the gut).
   In cases of metabolic acidosis, the hypokalaemia should be treated not with potassium chloride but with an alkaline potassium salt (e.g. potassium bicarbonate).
   Concomitant treatment with potassium sparing diuretics (e.g. spironolactone, triamterene, amiloride).

*Precautions:* If a patient under treatment with Slow-K develops severe vomiting, severe abdominal pains or flatulence, or gastro-intestinal haemorrhage, the preparation should be withdrawn at once, because in the presence of an obstruction it could conceivably give rise to ulceration or perforation.
   Oral potassium preparations should be prescribed with particular caution in patients with a history of peptic ulcer.
   Caution should be exercised when prescribing solid oral potassium preparations, particularly in high dosage, in patients concurrently receiving anticholinergics because of their potential to slow gastro-intestinal motility.
   Patients with ostomies may have altered intestinal transit times and are better treated with other forms of potassium salts.
   In patients suffering from impaired renal function, special care should be exercised when prescribing potassium salts owing to the risk of their producing hyperkalaemia. Monitoring of the serum electrolytes is particularly necessary in patients with diseases of the heart or kidneys.
   In some patients diuretic induced magnesium deficiency will prevent restoration of intracellular deficits of potassium so that hypomagnesaemia should be corrected at the same time as hypokalaemia.

*Use in pregnancy:* As a general rule, no drugs should be taken during the first three months of pregnancy and the risks and benefits of taking drugs should be carefully considered throughout pregnancy.
   Because of gastro-intestinal hypomotility associated with pregnancy, solid forms of oral potassium preparations should be given to pregnant women only if clearly needed.
   The normal K⁺ content of human milk is about 13 mmol/litre. Since oral potassium becomes part of the body's potassium pool, provided this is not excessive, Slow K can be expected to have little or no effect on the potassium level in human milk.

*Drug interactions:* Combined treatment with the following increase the risk of hyperkalaemia:-
   Angiotensin-converting enzyme inhibitors, cyclosporin, NSAIDs, beta blockers, heparin, digoxin, potassium sparing diuretics (see Contra-indications).

*Side-effects:* Side-effects are rare with Slow-K, as any excess potassium is rapidly excreted in the urine.

*Gastro-intestinal tract:* In rare cases, oral potassium preparations may provoke gastro-intestinal disturbances (nausea, vomiting, abdominal pains, diarrhoea) necessitating either a reduction in dosage or withdrawal of medication (see Precautions).

In isolated cases; obstruction, bleeding and ulceration, with or without perforation of the upper or lower GIT, have been reported, usually associated with other factors known to predispose a patient to these effects (e.g. delayed GIT transit time, obstruction of GIT).

*Skin:* Rare: Pruritus and/or skin rash, urticaria.

*Electrolytes:* Hyperkalaemia may develop in patients having difficulty with either renal potassium excretion or potassium metabolism.

*Overdosage:*

*Signs and symptoms:* Mainly cardiovascular (hypotension, shock, ventricular arrhythmias, bundle-branch block, ventricular fibrillation leading possibly to cardiac arrest) and neuromuscular (paraesthesiae, convulsions, areflexia, flaccid paralysis of striated muscle leading possibly to respiratory paralysis). Beside elevation of serum potassium concentration, typical ECG changes are also encountered (increasing amplitude and peaking of T waves, disappearance of P wave, widening of QRS complex and S-T segment depression).

*Treatment:* Gastric lavage, administration of cation-exchange agents, infusion of glucose and insulin, forced diuresis and possibly peritoneal dialysis or haemodialysis.

**Pharmaceutical precautions** Slow-K tablets should be protected from heat and moisture. The tablets should be dispensed in moisture-proof containers.

**Legal category** P

**Package quantities** Slow-K tablets (600 mg Potassium Chloride BP in a special slow-release core, equivalent to 8.06 mmol K+) Securitainers of 500, and containers of 5000.

**Further information** Slow-K has been successfully used in those patients who cannot tolerate liquid potassium chloride preparations or who find their taste unacceptable.

**Product licence number** 00101/0542

## SLOW SODIUM*

**Qualitative and quantitative composition** The active ingredient is Sodium Chloride PhEur. Sodium Chloride contains not less than 99.0 per cent and not more than 100.5 per cent of NaCl. One coated tablet contains 600 mg sodium chloride.

**Pharmaceutical form** Coated tablets.

**Clinical particulars**

*Therapeutic indications:* For the treatment and prophylaxis of sodium chloride deficiency.

*Posology and method of administration:* It is important that the tablets should be swallowed whole with water (approx. 70 ml per tablet where kidney function is normal to avoid hypernatraemia), and not chewed.

*Adults:* For prophylaxis 4-8 tablets per day. For treatment dosage to be adjusted to individual needs up to a maximum of 20 tablets per day in cases of severe salt depletion.

For control of muscle cramps during routine maintenance haemodialysis usually 10-16 tablets per dialysis. In cases of chronic renal salt-wasting up to 20 tablets per day may be required with appropriate fluid intake.

*Children:* Dosage should be adjusted to individual needs.

*Elderly:* No special dosage adjustment.

*Contra-indications:* Slow Sodium is contra-indicated in any situation where salt retention is undesirable, such as oedema, heart disease, cardiac decompensation and primary or secondary aldosteronism; or where therapy is being given to produce salt and water loss.

*Special warnings and precautions for use:*

*Warnings:* None.

*Precautions:* Use of Slow Sodium without adequate water supplementation can produce hypernatraemia. The matrix (ghost) is often eliminated intact and owing to the risk of obstruction Slow Sodium should not be given to patients suffering from Crohn's disease or any other intestinal condition where strictures or diverticula may form.

*Interactions with other drugs and other types of interactions:* In hypertensive patients with chronic renal failure Slow Sodium may tend to impair the efficacy of antihypertensive drugs.

*Pregnancy and lactation:* No additional precautions required.

*Effects on ability to drive or use machines:* Nil.

*Undesirable-effects:* No side-effects have been reported with Slow Sodium at the recommended dosage.

*Overdosage:*

*Signs and symptoms:* Excessive intake of sodium

chloride can result in hypernatraemia. Symptoms of hypernatraemia include restlessness, weakness, thirst, reduced salivation and lachrymation, swollen tongue, flushing of the skin, pyrexia, dizziness, headache, oliguria, hypertension, tachycardia, delirium, hyperpnoea and respiratory arrest.

*Treatment:* Treatment requires the use of sodium-free liquids and the cessation of excessive sodium intake. In the event of a significant overdose serum sodium levels should be evaluated as soon as possible and appropriate steps taken to correct any abnormalities. The use of a loop diuretic e.g. frusemide (with potassium supplementation as required) may be appropriate in severe cases of hypernatraemia. Levels should be monitored until they return to normal.

**Pharmacological properties**

*Pharmacodynamic properties:*

*Mode of action:* Sodium chloride is the principal salt involved in maintaining the osmotic tension of blood and tissues, changes in osmotic tension influence the movement of fluids and diffusion of salts in cellular tissue.

Slow Sodium provides a source of sodium (in the form of sodium chloride) where a deficiency exists.

*Pharmacokinetic properties:* Sodium chloride is readily absorbed from the gastro-intestinal tract. It is present in all body fluids but especially in the extracellular fluid. The amount of sodium lost (as sweat) is normally small. Osmotic balance is maintained by excretion of surplus amounts in the urine.

*Preclinical safety data:* No information available.

**Pharmaceutical particulars**

*List of excipients:* The coated tablets contain ceto-stearyl alcohol, gelatin, magnesium stearate, acacia, talc, titanium dioxide and polyethylene glycol.

*Incompatibilities:* None known.

*Shelf life:* Five years.

*Special precautions for storage:* Protect from moisture and store below 30°C. The tablets should be dispensed in moisture proof containers. Medicines should be kept out of reach of children.

*Nature and contents of container:* The tablets are white, biconvex, polished, coated tablets about 11.4 mm in diameter, printed "CIBA" on one side and available in containers of 100 tablets.

*Instructions for use/handling:* None.

**Marketing authorisation number** 00101/0457.

**Date of approval/revision of SPC** 7 March 1996.

**Legal category** GSL.

## SLOW-TRASICOR*

**Presentation** Slow-Trasicor tablets each containing 160 mg Oxprenolol Hydrochloride PhEur in a special sustained release formulation. Circular, slightly biconvex, white film-coated tablets, having the monogram CIBA impressed on one side and Slow-Trasicor on the other.

The tablets also contain lactose, silicon dioxide, calcium stearate, methacrylic acid copolymer, glyceryl palmitostearate, hydroxypropylmethylcellulose, magnesium stearate, polysorbate, talc and titanium dioxide.

**Uses**

*Indications: Hypertension:* As monotherapy or for use in combination with other antihypertensives, e.g. with a diuretic, peripheral vasodilator, calcium channel blocker or ACE inhibitor.

*Angina pectoris:* For long-term prophylactic use (if necessary nitrates should be employed for alleviating acute attacks).

*Mode of action:* Oxyprenolol, the active substance of Trasicor, is a non-selective, lipophilic beta-blocker exerting a sympatholytic effect and displaying mild to modest partial agonistic activity (PAA), also known as intrinsic sympathomimetic activity (ISA).

Drugs like oxprenolol with PAA cause comparatively less slowing of the resting heart rate and a less marked negative-inotropic effect than those without PAA. The risk of substantial bradycardia at rest and heart failure is lessened.

The antiarrhythmic effect of oxprenolol is primarily due to suppression of the arrhythmogenic sympathetic influence of catecholamines. Evidence that increased sympathetic stimulation predisposes to many arrhythmias is strong. This is supported by the increased incidence of arrhythmias in man in situations associated with high sympathetic drive or myocardial sensitisation to catecholamines e.g. exercise, emotional stress, phaeochromocytoma, trauma, myocardial ischaemia, anaesthesia, hyperthyroidism.

Oxprenolol decreases cardiac impulse formation in the sinus node with resultant slowing of the sinus rate; it slightly prolongs the sino-atrial conduction

time; both the atrio-ventricular (AV) conduction time and the AV node refractory periods are lengthened.

Some β-blockers such as oxprenolol possess a membrane stabilising activity (MSA) on the cardiac action potential, also known as 'quinidine-like' or 'local anaesthetic' action, a property that tends to result in greater cardiac depression than is seen with β-blockers which do not have this pharmacological characteristic. However, at normal therapeutic doses, this property is probably clinically irrelevant and it only becomes manifest after overdose.

In coronary artery disease, oxprenolol is beneficial in increasing exercise tolerance and decreasing the frequency and severity of anginal attacks.

Emotional stress and anxiety states the symptoms of which are largely caused by increased sympathetic drive are alleviated by the sympatholytic effect of oxprenolol.

The exact way in which β-blockers exert their antihypertensive action is still not fully understood. Various modes of action have been postulated. During chronic therapy the antihypertensive effect of β-blockers is associated with a decline in peripheral resistance.

Oxprenolol is effective in lowering elevated supine, standing and exercise blood pressure; postural hypotension is unlikely to occur.

*Pharmacokinetics:*

*Absorption:* Oxprenolol is rapidly and completely absorbed from the sustained release tablets, regardless of whether or not they are taken together with food. Peak plasma concentrations are attained after an average of approximately 3 hours.

During treatment with the sustained release forms, prolongation of the absorption phase enables therapeutically active plasma concentrations to be maintained over a longer period than when the same doses are given in conventional dosage forms and avoids high peak drug concentrations in the plasma.

*Biotransformation:* Oxprenolol is subject to first-pass metabolism. Its systemic bioavailability is 20–70%.

*Distribution:* Oxprenolol has a plasma-protein binding rate of approx. 80% and a calculated distribution volume of 1.2 L/kg.

Oxprenolol crosses the placental barrier. The concentration in the breast milk is equivalent to approx. 30% of that in the plasma.

*Elimination:* Oxprenolol has an elimination half-life of 1–2 hours. Oxprenolol is extensively metabolised, direct O-glucuronidation being the major metabolic pathway and oxidative reactions minor ones. Oxprenolol is excreted chiefly in the urine (almost exclusively in the form of inactive metabolites). The drug is not likely to accumulate.

*Characteristics in patients:* Age has no effect on the pharmacokinetics of oxprenolol.

In patients with acute or chronic inflammatory diseases an increase in the plasma levels of oxprenolol has been observed. The plasma levels may also increase in the presence of severe hepatic insufficiency associated with a reduced metabolism.

Impaired renal function generally leads to an increase in the blood levels of oxprenolol, but the concentrations measured remain within – although at the upper limit of – the concentration range recorded in subjects with healthy kidneys. In addition, in patients with renal failure the apparent elimination half-life for unchanged, i.e. active, oxprenolol is comparable with the corresponding half-life values determined in subjects with no renal disease. Hence, there is no need to readjust the dosage in the presence of impaired renal function.

**Dosage and administration** The dosage should be individualised. Before raising the dosage, the heart rate at rest should always be checked. If it is 50–55 beats/min, the dosage should not be increased, see *Contra-indications.* The tablets should be swallowed with liquid.

If the maximum recommended dose is insufficient to produce the desired response, appropriate combined therapy should be considered.

When discontinuing prolonged treatment with a beta-blocker, the medication should not be interrupted abruptly, but withdrawn gradually.

The sustained-release formulation provides a longer pharmacological action from a given dose, thus allowing once daily administration. When the dose is raised to more than one Trasicor sustained-release tablet, it is usual for this to continue to be given once daily.

The sustained-release tablets should be swallowed whole with liquid. Oxprenolol is only gradually released from the sustained-release tablet, extending the duration of effect. The occurrence of high peak concentrations in the plasma is thus avoided.

*Elderly:* No special dosage regime is necessary but concurrent hepatic insufficiency should be taken into account.

*Children:* No adequate experience has been acquired on the use of Slow-Trasicor in children.

*Adults:*

*Hypertension:* 160 mg once daily. If necessary, the dosage can be raised to 320 mg.

*Angina pectoris:* 160 mg once daily. If necessary, the dosage can be raised to 320 mg.

**Contra-indications, warnings, etc**

*Contra-indications:* Slow-Trasicor is contra-indicated in patients with:

Hypersensitivity to oxprenolol and related derivatives, cross-sensitivity to other β-blockers or to any of the excipients
Cardiogenic shock
Second or third degree atrioventricular block
Uncontrolled heart failure
Sick-sinus syndrome
Bradycardia (<45–50 bpm)
Hypotension
Untreated phaeochromocytoma
Severe peripheral arterial circulatory disturbances
History of bronchospasms and broncial asthma
Prinzmetal's angina (variant angina pectoris)
Use of anaesthetics which are known to have a negative inotropic effect
Metabolic acidosis

*Warnings:* Patients receiving oxprenolol should be warned that dizziness, fatigue or visual disturbances (see *Side-effects*) may occur, in which case they should not drive, operate machinery or do anything else requiring alertness, particularly if they also consume alcohol.

*Precautions:* Owing to the risk of bronchoconstriction, non-selective beta-blockers such as Slow-Trasicor should be used with particular caution in patients with chronic obstructive lung disease (see *Contra-indications*).

As β-blockers increase the AV conduction time, beta-blockers should only be given with caution to patients with first degree AV block.

Beta-blockers should not be used in patients with untreated congestive heart failure. This condition should first be stabilised.

If the patient develops increasing bradycardia less than 50–55 beats per minute at rest and the patient experiences symptoms related to bradycardia, the dosage should be reduced or gradually withdrawn (see *Contra-indications*).

β-blockers are liable to affect carbohydrate metabolism. Diabetic patients, especially those dependent on insulin, should be warned that β-blockers can mask the symptoms of hypoglycaemia (e.g. tachycardia) (see *Interactions with other medicaments and other forms of interaction*). Hypoglycaemia, producing loss of consciousness in some cases, may occur in non-diabetic individuals who are taking β-blockers, particularly those who undergo prolonged fasting or severe exercise. The concurrent use of β-blockers and anti-diabetic medication should always be monitored to confirm that diabetic control is well maintained.

β-blockers may mask certain clinical signs (e.g. tachycardia) of hyperthyroidism and the patients should be carefully monitored.

Beta-blockers may reduce liver function and thus affect the metabolism of other drugs. Like many beta-blockers oxprenolol undergoes substantial first-pass hepatic metabolism. In the presence of liver cirrhosis the bioavailability of oxprenolol may be increased leading to higher plasma concentrations (see *Pharmacokinetics*). Patients with renal failure might be more susceptible to the effects of antihypertensive drugs due to haemodynamic effects. Careful monitoring is advisable (see *Pharmacokinetics*).

In patients with peripheral circulatory disorders (e.g. Raynaud's disease or syndrome, intermittent claudication), beta-blockers should be used with great caution as aggravation of these disorders may occur (see *Contra-indications*).

In patients with phaeochromocytoma a β-blocker should only be given together with an α-blocker (see *Contra-indications*).

Owing to the danger of cardiac arrest, a calcium antagonist of the verapamil type must not be administered intravenously to a patient already receiving treatment with a β-blocker. Furthermore, since β-blockers may potentiate the negative-inotropic and dromotropic effects of calcium antagonists, like verapamil or diltiazem, any oral comedication (e.g. in angina pectoris) requires close clinical control (see also *Drug interactions*).

Anaphylactic reactions precipitated by other agents may be particularly severe in patients taking beta-blockers, especially non-selective drugs, and may require higher than normal doses of adrenaline for treatment. Whenever possible, β-blockers should be discontinued in patients in patients who are at increased risk for anaphylaxis.

Especially in patients with ischaemic heart disease, treatment should not be discontinued suddenly. The dosage should gradually be reduced, i.e. over 1–3 weeks, if necessary, at the same time initiating alternative therapy, to prevent exacerbation of angina pectoris.

If a patient receiving oxprenolol requires anaesthesia, the anaesthetist should be informed of the use of the medication prior to the use of general anaesthetic to permit him to take the necessary precautions. The anaesthetic selected should be one exhibiting as little inotropic activity as possible, e.g. halothane/nitrous oxide. If, on the other hand, inhibition of sympathetic tone during the operation is regarded as undesirable, the β-blocker should be withdrawn gradually at least 48 hours prior to surgery.

The full development of the 'oculomucocutaneous syndrome', as previously described with practolol has not been reported with oxprenolol. However, some features of this syndrome have been noted such as dry eyes alone or occasionally associated with skin rash. In most cases the symptoms cleared after withdrawal of the treatment. Discontinuation of oxprenolol should be considered, and a switch to another antihypertensive drug might be advisable, see advice on discontinuation above.

*Use in pregnancy and lactation:* As in the case of any form of drug therapy, oxprenolol should be employed with caution during pregnancy, especially in the first 3 months.

β-blockers may reduce placental perfusion, which may result in intrauterine foetal death, immature and premature deliveries. Use the lowest possible dose. If possible, discontinue beta-blocker therapy at least 2 to 3 days prior to delivery to avoid the effects on uterine contractility and possible adverse effects, especially bradycardia and hypoglycaemia, in the foetus and neonate.

Oxprenolol is excreted into breast milk (see *Pharmacokinetic properties*) and although the estimated daily infant dose derived from breast-feeding is likely to be very low, breast feeding is not recommended.

*Drug interactions:*

*Calcium channel blockers:* e.g. verapamil, dilitiazem: potentiation of bradycardia, myocardial depression and hypotension; particularly after intravenous administration of verapamil in patients taking oral β-blockers, the possibility of hypotension and cardiac arrhythmia cannot be excluded (see *Warnings* and *Precautions*).

*Class I anti-arrhythmic drugs and amiodarone:* Drugs like disopyramide, quinidine and amiodarone may increase atrial-conduction time and induce negative inotropic effect when administered concomitantly with beta-blockers.

*Sympathomimetic drugs:* Non-cardioselective beta-blockers such as oxprenolol enhance the pressor response to sympathomimetic drugs such as adrenaline, noradrenaline, isoprenaline, ephedrine and phenylephrine (e.g. local anaesthetics in dentistry, nasal and ocular drops), resulting in hypertension and bradycardia.

*Clonidine:* When clonidine is used in conjunction with non-selective beta-blockers, such as oxprenolol, treatment with clonidine should be continued for some time after β-blocker has been discontinued to reduce the danger of rebound hypertension.

*Catecholamine-deleting drugs:* e.g. guanethidine, reserpine, may have an additive effect when administered concomitantly with beta-blockers. Patients should be closely observed for hypotension.

Beta-blockers may modify blood glucose concentrations in patients being treated with insulin and oral antidiabetic drugs and may alter the response to hypoglycaemia by prolonging the recovery (blood glucose rise) from hypoglycaemia, causing hypotension and blocking tachycardia. In diabetic patients receiving β-blockers hypoglycaemic episodes may not result in the expected tachycardia but hypoglycaemia-induced sweating will occur and may even be intensified and prolonged (see *Warnings* and *Precautions*).

*Non-steroidal anti-inflammatory drugs (NSAIDs):* Neosteroidal anti-inflammatory drugs (NSAIDs) can reduce the hypotensive effect of beta-blockade.

*Cimetidine:* Hepatic metabolism of beta-blockers may be reduced, resulting in increased plasma levels of β-blocker and prolonged serum half-life. Marked bradycardia may occur.

*Ergot alkaloids:* Concomitant administration with beta-blockers may enhance the vasoconstrictive action of ergot alkaloids.

*Anesthetic drugs:* β-blockers and certain anaesthetics (e.g. halothane) are additive in their cardiodepressant effect. However, continuation of beta-blockers reduces the risk of arrhythmia during anaesthesia (see *Warnings* and *Precautions*).

*Digitalis glycosides:* Beta-blockers and digitalis glycosides may be additive in their depressant effect on myocardial conduction, particularly through the atrioventricular node, resulting in bradycardia or heart block.

*Lidocaine:* Concomitant administration with beta-blockers may increase lidocaine blood concentrations and potential toxicity; patients should be closely monitored for increased lidocaine effects.

Alcohol and beta-blocker effects on the central nervous system have been observed to be additive and it is possible that symptoms such as dizziness may be exaggerated if alcohol and Trasicor are taken together (see also *Warnings*).

*Side-effects:* Frequency estimate: *very common* >10%, *common* >1%–<10%, *uncommon* >0.1%–<1%, *rare* >0.01%–<0.1%, *very rare* <0.01%.

*Central nervous system: Common:* fatigue, dizziness, headache, mental depression. *Uncommon:* sleep disturbances, nightmares. Rare: hallucinations, exertional tiredness.

*Cardiovascular system: Common:* hypotension, heart failure, peripheral vascular disorders (e.g. cold extremities, paraesthesia). *Uncommon:* bradycardia, disturbance of cardiac conduction. *Rare:* Raynaud-like symptoms.

*Gastro-intestinal tract: Very common:* dry mouth, constipation. *Common:* nausea. *Uncommon:* diarrhoea, vomiting, flatulence..

*Skin and appendages: Uncommon:* Allergic skin rash (e.g. urticarial, psoriasiform, ezcematous, lichenoid). *Rare:* worsening of psoriasis.

*Respiratory system: Common:* dyspnoea, bronchoconstriction (see *Precautions* and *Contra-indications*).

*Sense organs: Uncommon:* visual disturbances ('blurred vision', 'vision abnormal'). *Rare:* dry eyes, keratoconjunctivitis.

Others: disturbances of libido and potency. Very rare: thrombocytopenia.

*Overdosage:*

*Signs and symptoms:* Poisoning due to an overdosage of β-blocker may lead to pronounced hypotension, bradycardia, hypoglycaemia, heart failure, cardiogenic shock, conduction abnormalities (first or second degree block, complete heart block, asystole), or even cardiac arrest. In addition, dyspnoea, bronchospasm, vomiting, impairment of consciousness, and also generalised convulsions may occur.

The manifestations of poisoning with beta-blockers are dependent on the pharmacological properties of the ingested drug. Although the onset of action is rapid, effects of massive overdose may persist for several days despite declining plasma levels. Watch carefully for cardiovascular or respiratory deterioration in an intensive care setting, particularly in the early hours. Observe mild overdose cases for at least 4 hours for the development of signs of poisoning.

*Treatment:* Patients who are seen soon after potentially life-threatening overdosage (within 4 hours) should be treated by gastric lavage and activated charcoal.

Treatment of symptoms is based on modern methods of intensive care, with continuous monitoring of cardiac function, blood gases, and electrolytes, and if necessary, emergency measures such as artificial respiration, resuscitation or cardiac pacemaker.

Significant bradycardia should be treated initially with atropine. Large doses of isoprenaline may be necessary for control of heart rate and hypotension. Glucagon has positive chronotropic and inotropic effects on the heart rate that are independent of interactions with beta-adrenergic receptors and it represents a useful alternative treatment for hypotension and heart failure.

For seizures, diazepam has been effective and is the drug of choice.

For bronchospasms, aminophylline, salbutamol or terbutaline ($\beta_2$ agonist) are effective bronchodilator drugs. Monitor the patient for dysrhythmias during and after administration.

Patients who recover should be observed for signs of β-blocker withdrawal phenomenon (see *Warnings* and *Precautions*).

**Pharmaceutical precautions** No special storage requirements.

**Legal category** POM.

**Package quantities** Cartons of 28 Slow-Trasicor tablets consisting of two reminder calendar foils of 14 (each carton of 28 represents 2-4 weeks treatment, depending on whether the dosage is one or two tablets daily).

**Further information** Nil.

**Product licence number** 00101/0429.

## SYMMETREL*

**Qualitative and quantitative composition** The active ingredient is 1-Adamantanamine hydrochloride (=amantadine hydrochloride).

The capsules contain 100 mg Amantadine Hydrochloride PhEur.

The syrup contains 50 mg/5 ml Amantadine Hydrochloride PhEur.

**Pharmaceutical form** Capsules and syrup.

**Clinical particulars**

*Therapeutic indications:* Parkinson's disease.

Herpes zoster.

*Note:* Herpes zoster: It is recommended that the

drug be given to elderly or debilitated patients in whom the physician suspects that a severe and painful rash could occur. Symmetrel can significantly reduce the proportion of patients experiencing pain of long duration.

Prophylaxis and treatment of signs and symptoms of infection caused by influenza A virus.

Influenza A: It is suggested that Symmetrel be given to patients suffering from clinical influenza in whom complications might be expected to occur. In addition, Symmetrel is recommended prophylactically in cases particularly at risk, for example those with chronic respiratory disease or debilitating conditions, the elderly, those living in crowded conditions and for individuals in families where influenza has already been diagnosed, control of institutional outbreaks or those in essential services who are unvaccinated or when vaccination is unavailable or contra-indicated.

Symmetrel does not completely prevent the host immune response to influenza A infection so individuals who take this drug still develop immune responses to the natural disease or vaccination and may be protected when later exposed to antigenically related viruses. Symmetrel may also be used in post-exposure prophylaxis in conjunction with inactivated vaccine during an outbreak until protective antibodies develop or in patients who are not expected to have a substantial antibody response (immunosuppression).

*Posology and method of administration:*

*Parkinson's disease:* Initially 100 mg daily for the first week, increasing to 100 mg twice daily.

The dose can be titrated against signs and symptoms. In some cases amounts exceeding 200 mg daily may provide some additional relief but may also be associated with increasing toxicity. A dose of 400 mg/day should not be exceeded. The dose should be increased gradually, at intervals of not less than 1 week. Since patients over 65 years of age tend to show lower renal clearance and consequently higher plasma concentrations, the recommended dose for elderly patients with Parkinsonism is 100 mg daily.

Amantadine acts within a few days but sometimes appears to lose some of its efficacy within a few months of continuous treatment.

The effectiveness of amantadine may be prolonged by a temporary withdrawal of three to four weeks, which seems to restore activity. During this time existing concomitant antiparkinsonian therapy should be continued or low dose L-dopa treatment initiated if clinically necessary.

Treatment with Symmetrel must be reduced gradually, e.g. at a rate of half the dose at weekly intervals because abrupt discontinuation may exacerbate Parkinson's syndrome, regardless of the patient's response to therapy (see *Special warnings and special precautions for use*).

Combined treatment: any antiparkinson drug with which the patient is already being treated should be continued during the first stage of treatment with Symmetrel. In many cases it is then possible gradually to reduce the dosage of the other drug without prejudicing the treatment response. If increased side effects occur, however, its dosage should be reduced more quickly. In patients already receiving large doses of anticholinergic agents or L-dopa the initial low-dosage phase of treatment with Symmetrel should be extended to 15 days.

*Herpes zoster:* Treatment should be started as soon as possible after the diagnosis has been made. The dosage is 100 mg twice daily for 14 days. If post-herpetic pain persists after this period it is recommended that treatment be continued for a further 14 days.

*Treatment of influenza A:* It is advisable to start treating influenza as early as possible and to continue for 4–5 days. When amantadine is started within 48 hours of symptoms appearing the duration of fever and other effects is reduced by one or two days and the inflammatory reaction of the bronchial tree that usually accompanies influenza resolves more quickly.

*Prophylaxis of influenza A:* Treatment daily for as long as protection from influenza infection is required. In most instances this is expected to be for 6 weeks but when used with inactivated influenza A vaccine amantadine is continued for 2–3 weeks following inoculation.

*Adults:* 100 mg daily for the recommended period.

*Use in children aged 10–15 years:* 100 mg daily for the recommended period.

*Use in children under 10 years of age:* Dosage not established.

*Adults over 65 years of age:* Plasma amantadine concentrations are influenced by renal function. In elderly patients, the elimination half-life is longer and renal clearance of the compound is diminished in comparison to young people. Therefore a daily dose of less than 100 mg or 100 mg given at intervals of greater than one day may be appropriate.

*Use in patients with renal impairment:* in patients with compromised renal function, the dose of amantadine should be reduced accordingly. This can be achieved by reducing the daily dose or prolonging the dosage interval in accordance with the creatinine clearance. For example:

| *Creatinine clearance [ml/(min. 1.73 $m^2$)]* | *Dose* |
|---|---|
| <15 | Symmetrel contra-indicated |
| 15–35 | 100 mg/2–3 days |
| >35 | 100 mg/day |

The above recommendations are for guidance only and physicians should continue to monitor their patients for signs of unwanted effects.

*Contra-indications:* It is not recommended that Symmetrel be used to treat individuals who are subject to convulsions, or who have a history of gastric ulceration.

Symmetrel should not be used in patients with severe renal disease. Pregnancy.

Known hypersensitivity to amantadine, or any of the excipients of the capsules and syrup.

*Special warnings and precautions for use:* Symmetrel should be used with caution in patients with confusional or hallucinatory states or underlying psychiatric disorders.

Particular care is called for in patients suffering from, or who have a history of, cardiovascular disorders.

Symmetrel should be used cautiously in patients with liver or kidney disorders.

Discontinuation of treatment. Abrupt discontinuation of amantadine may result in worsening of symptoms.

There have been isolated reports of a possible association with the occurrence or aggravation of neuroleptic malignant syndrome or neuroleptic-induced catatonia in patients treated concurrently with neuroleptics and amantadine, following abrupt cessation of the latter. Treatment should not be stopped abruptly in such patients.

Because of the possibility of serious adverse effects, caution should be observed when prescribing Symmetrel to patients being treated with drugs having CNS effects, or for whom the potential risks outweigh the benefit of treatment. Because some patients have attempted suicide on amantadine, prescriptions should be written for the smallest quantity consistent with good patient management.

Peripheral oedema thought to be due to an alteration in the responsiveness of peripheral vessels may occur in some patients during treatment with Symmetrel. This should be considered when the drug is prescribed for those with congestive heart failure.

Resistance to amantadine occurs during serial passage of influenza virus strains *in vitro* or *in vivo* in the presence of the drug. Apparent transmission of drug-resistant viruses may have been the cause of failure of prophylaxis and treatment in household contacts and in nursing-home patients. However, there is no evidence to date that the resistant virus produces a diseases that is in any way different from that produced by sensitive viruses.

*Interactions with other drugs and other types of interactions:* Concurrent administration of amantadine and anticholinergic agents or levodopa may increase confusion, hallucinations, nightmares, gastro-intestinal disturbances, or other atropine-like side effects (see also *Overdose*).

In isolated cases psychotic decompensation has been reported in patients receiving amantadine and concomitant neuroleptic medication.

Psychotic reactions have been observed in patients receiving amantadine and levodopa.

Concurrent administration of amantadine and drugs or substances (e.g. alcohol) acting on the central nervous system may result in additive CNS toxicity. Close observation is recommended (see also *Overdose*).

There have been isolated reports of a suspected interaction between amantadine and combination diuretics (hydrochlorothiazide+potassium sparing diuretics. One or both of the components apparently reduce the clearance of amantadine, leading to higher plasma concentrations and toxic effects (confusion, hallucinations, ataxia, myoclonus).

*Pregnancy and lactation:* Reproductive toxicity studies were performed in rats and rabbits. In rat oral doses of 50 and 100 mg/kg proved to be teratogenic.

Amantadine-related complications during pregnancy have been reported. Symmetrel is contra-indicated during pregnancy and in women wishing to become pregnant.

Amantadine passes into breast milk. Undesirable effects have been reported in breast-fed infants. Nursing mothers should not take Symmetrel.

*Effects on ability to drive or use machines:* Patients who note central nervous system effects or blurring of vision should be advised to avoid situations where alertness is essential.

*Undesirable effects:*

*Side effects:* Amantadine's undesirable effects are often of mild and transient nature. They usually appear within the first 2–4 days of treatment and promptly disappear in 24–48 hours after discontinuation of amantadine.

A direct relationship between dose and incidence of side effects has not been demonstrated; however, there seems to be a tendency towards more frequent undesirable effects (particularly affecting the central nervous system) with increasing doses.

Frequency estimates: frequent>10%, occasional 1%–10%, rare 0.001%–1%, isolated cases<0.001%.

*Central nervous system:* Occasional: depression, anxiety, elevation of mood, agitation, nervousness, difficulty in concentrating, dizziness, lightheadedness, headache, insomnia, lethargy, hallucinations, nightmares, ataxia, slurred speech, blurred vision. Hallucinations, confusion, and nightmares are more common when amantadine is administered concurrently with anticholinergic agents or when the patient has an underlying psychiatric disorder. Rare: confusion, disorientation, psychosis, tremor, dyskinesia, convulsions. Delirium, hypomanic state, and mania, have been reported but their incidence cannot be readily deduced from the literature.

*Cardiovascular system:* Frequent: oedema of ankles, livedo reticularis. Occasional: palpitations, orthostatic hypotension. Isolated cases: heart insufficiency/failure.

*Blood:* Isolated cases: leucopenia, reversible elevation of liver enzymes.

*Gastrointestinal tract:* Occasional: dry mouth, anorexia, nausea, vomiting, constipation. Rare: diarrhoea.

*Skin and appendages:* Occasional: diaphoresis. Rare: exanthema. Isolated cases: photosensitisation.

*Sense organs:* Rare: corneal lesions, e.g. punctate subepithelial opacities which might be associated with superficial punctate keratitis, corneal epithelial oedema, and markedly reduced visual acuity.

*Urogenital tract:* Rare: urinary retention, urinary incontinence.

*Overdose: Signs and symptoms:* neuromuscular disturbances and symptoms of acute psychosis are prominent features of acute poisoning with amantadine.

Central nervous system: Hyperreflexia, motor restlessness; convulsions; extrapyramidal signs: torsion spasms, dystonic posturing: dilated pupils. Confusion, disorientation, delirium, visual hallucinations.

Respiratory system: hyperventilation, pulmonary oedema, respiratory distress, including adult respiratory distress syndrome.

Cardiovascular system: sinus tachycardia, arrhythmia.

Gastrointestinal system: nausea, vomiting, dry mouth.

Renal function: urine retention, renal dysfunction, including increase in BUN and decreased creatinine clearance.

Overdose from combined drug treatment: the peripheral and central adverse effects of anticholinergic drugs are increased by the concomitant use of amantadine, and acute psychotic reactions, which may be identical to those caused by atropine poisoning, may occur when large doses of anticholinergic agents are used. Where alcohol or central nervous stimulants have been taken at the same time, the signs and symptoms of acute poisoning with amantadine may be aggravated and/or modified.

*Management:* There is no specific antidote. Removal and/or activation of poisoning agent(s): induction of vomiting and/or gastric aspiration and lavage if patient is conscious, activated charcoal, saline cathartic, if judged appropriate. Since amantadine is excreted for a large part unchanged in the urine, maintenance of renal excretory function, copious diuresis, and forced diuresis if necessary, are effective ways to remove it from the blood stream. Acidification of the urine favours the excretion of amantadine in the urine. Haemodialysis does not remove significant amounts of amantadine.

Monitoring of blood pressure, heart rate, ECG, respiration, body temperature and treatment for possible hypotension and cardiac arrhythmias, as necessary.

Convulsions and excessive motor restlessness: administer anticonvulsants such as diazepam i.v., paraldehyde i.m. or per rectum, or phenobarbital i.m.

Acute psychotic symptoms, delerium, dystonic posturing, myoclonic manifestations: physostigmine by slow intravenous infusion (1 mg doses in adults, 0.5 mg in children) repeated administration according to the initial response and the subsequent need, has been reported.

Retention of urine: bladder should be catheterised; an indwelling catheter can be left in place for the time required.

**Pharmacological properties** Pharmacotherapeutic group: Antiparkinson agent and anti-influenza virostatic.

*Pharmacodynamic properties;*

*Parkinson's disease:* Symmetrel probably acts by enhancing the release of dopamine and delaying the reuptake into synaptic vesicles. It may also exert some anticholinergic activity. When administered either alone or in combination with other drugs, amantadine produces an improvement in the cardinal signs and symptoms of parkinsonism and improves functional capacity in about 60% of patients.

The effect generally sets in two to five days after the start of treatment. It exerts a positive effect particularly on akinesia, rigidity and tremor.

*Herpes zoster:* The mechanism of action of Symmetrel in herpes zoster has not been fully characterised.

*Influenza:* Amantadine specifically inhibits the replication of influenza A viruses at low concentrations. Using a sensitive plaque-reduction assay human influenza viruses including $H_1N_1$, $H_2N_2$, $H_3N_2$ subtypes, are inhibited by 0.4 mcg/ml of amantadine or less. The exact mechanism of action of amantadine is unclear but it appears to inhibit an early stage in viral replication. Effects on late replicative steps have been found for representative avian influenza viruses.

Data from tests with representative strains of influenza A virus indicate that Symmetrel is likely to be active against previously unknown strains and could be used in the early stages of an epidemic before a vaccine against the causative strain is generally available.

*Pharmacokinetic properties:*

*Absorption:* Amantadine is absorbed slowly but almost completely. Peak plasma concentrations of approximately 250 ng/ml and 500 ng/ml are attained within 3–4 hours after single oral administration of 100 mg and 200 mg amantadine, respectively.

Following repeated administration of 200 mg daily the steady-state plasma concentration settles at 300 ng/ml within 3 days.

*Distribution: In vitro,* 67% of amantadine is bound to plasma proteins. A substantial amount of amantadine is bound to red blood cells. The concentration of amantadine in erythrocytes in normal healthy volunteers is 2.66 times the plasma concentration.

The apparent volume of distribution of the drug is 5–10 L/kg, suggesting extensive tissue binding. It declines with increasing doses. The concentration of amantadine in the lung, heart, kidney, liver and spleen is higher than in the blood.

The drug accumulates after several hours in nasal secretions.

Amantadine passes the blood-brain barrier; it is, however, not possible to quantify this event.

*Biotransformation:* Amantadine is metabolised to a minor extent, principally by N-acetylation.

*Elimination:* The drug is eliminated in healthy young adults with a mean plasma elimination half-life of 15 hours (10–31 hours).

The total plasma clearance is about the same as renal clearance (250 ml/min). The renal amantadine clearance is much higher than the creatinine clearance, suggesting renal tubular secretion.

A single dose of amantadine is excreted over 72 hours as follows: 65–85% unchanged, 5–15% as acetyl metabolite in urine, and 1% in stools. After 4–5 days 90% of the dose appears unchanged in urine. The rate is considerably influenced by urinary pH. A rise in pH brings about a fall in excretion.

*Characteristics in special patient populations: Elderly patients:* compared with healthy young adults, the half-life may be doubled and renal clearance diminished. Tubular secretion diminishes more than glomerular filtration in the elderly. In elderly patients repeated administration of 100 mg daily may raise the plasma concentration into the toxic range.

*Renal impairment:* accumulation of amantadine may occur in renal failure causing severe adverse drug reactions. The rate of elimination of amantadine from plasma is correlated to creatinine clearance values divided by body surface area (1.73 m²) but total renal elimination exceeds this value, possibly due to tubular secretion. The effects of reduced kidney function on elimination are dramatic (a reduction in creatinine clearance to 40 ml/min/1.73 m² may result in a five-fold increase in elimination half-life). The urine remains the almost exclusive route of excretion even in cases of renal failure, where amantadine may persist in the plasma for several days.

*Haemodialysis:* little amantadine is removed by haemodialysis; this inefficiency may be related to extensive tissue binding. Less than 5% of a dose is eliminated in 4 hours and the mean dialysis time taken to remove half of the dose is 24 hours.

*Preclinical safety data:* There are no pre-clinical data of relevance to the prescriber which are additional to that already included in other sections of the SPC.

**Pharmaceutical particulars**

*List of excipients:* The capsules also contain lactose, polyvinylpyrrolidone, magnesium stearate, red iron oxide, titanium dioxide, gelatin and white printer's ink.

The syrup also contains methyl hydroxybenzoate, propyl hydroxybenzoate, sorbitol, disodium hydrogen citrate, lemon flavouring, strawberry flavouring and water.

*Incompatibilities:* None known.

*Shelf life:* Five years.

*Special precautions for storage:* Capsules: Protect from moisture. Syrup: Protect from heat and light. Keep container closed.

Medicines should be kept out of reach of children.

*Nature and contents of container:* The capsules of 100 mg (brownish-red, hard gelatin capsules, imprinted GEIGY in white on both cap and body) are packed in PVC/PVdC blister packs of 56 and 100.

The clear, citrus flavoured syrup is contained in 150 ml amber glass bottles with child proof closures.

*Instruction for use/handling:* There is no specific instruction for use/handling.

**Marketing authorisation numbers**

| | |
|---|---|
| Capsules | 00101/0452 |
| Syrup | 00101/0453 |

**Date of approval/revision of SPC** 24 June 1997.

**Legal category** POM.

## SYNACTHEN*

**Presentation** Tetracosactrin Acetate $\beta_{1\text{-}24}$ Corticotrophin BP (Tetracosactide INN) as a clear, colourless, sterile solution containing the equivalent of 250 micrograms of tetracosactrin per ml. This preparation is available in 1 ml ampoules.

The ampoules contain acetic acid, sodium acetate, sodium chloride and water.

**Uses**

*Indications:* As a diagnostic test for the investigation of adrenocortical insufficiency.

*Mode of action*: Tetracosactrin, the active substance of Synacthen, consists of the first 24 amino acids occurring in the natural corticotrophic hormone (ACTH) sequence and displays the same physiological properties as ACTH. Like ACTH, it stimulates adrenocortical production of glucocorticoids and mineralocorticoids, and to a lesser extent androgens.

The site of action of ACTH is the plasma membrane of the adrenocortical cells, where it binds to a specific receptor. The hormone-receptor complex activates adenylate cyclase, stimulating the production of cyclic AMP (adenosine monophosphate) and so promoting the synthesis of pregnenolone from cholesterol. From pregnenolone the various corticosteroids are produced via different enzymatic pathways.

*Pharmacokinetics*: Tetracosactrin has an apparent volume of distribution of approximately 0.4 litres/kg.

Following an intravenous injection, elimination of the compound from the plasma consists of 3 phases. The half-lives of these phases are approximately 7 minutes (0-1 hour), 37 minutes (1-2 hours) and 3 hours thereafter.

In the serum, tetracosactrin is broken down by serum endopeptidases into inactive oligopeptides and then by aminopeptidases into free amino acids. The rapid elimination from plasma is probably not attributable to this relatively slow cleavage process, but rather to the rapid concentration of the active substance in the adrenal glands and kidneys.

Following an intravenous dose of $^{131}$I-labelled tetracosactrin, 95-100% of the radioactivity is excreted in the urine within 24 hours.

**Dosage and administration** This preparation of Synacthen is intended for administration for diagnostic purposes only as a single intramuscular or intravenous dose; it is not to be used for repeated therapeutic administration.

The 30-minute Synacthen diagnostic test: This test is based on measurement of the plasma cortisol concentration immediately before and exactly 30 minutes after an intramuscular or intravenous injection of 250 mcg (1 ml) Synacthen. Adrenocortical function can be regarded as normal if the post-injection rise in plasma cortisol concentration amounts to at least 200nmol/litre (70 mcg/litre).

Where the 30-minute test has yielded inconclusive results, or where it is desired to determine the functional reserve of the adrenal cortex, a 5-hour test can be performed with Synacthen Depot (see separate data sheet). Furthermore, a 3-day test with Synacthen Depot may be used to differentiate between primary and secondary adrenocortical insufficiency.

*Use in the elderly*: There is no evidence to suggest that dosage should be different in the elderly.

*Use in children*: An intravenous dose of 250 mcg/ 1.73²m body surface area has been suggested. Thus for children aged 5-7 years, approximately half the adult dose will be adequate. For more accurate dosing of other ages, standard body surface area tables should be consulted.

**Contra-indications, warnings, etc**

*Contra-indications*: History of hypersensitivity to ACTH, Synacthen or Synacthen Depot. Synacthen is contra-indicated in patients with allergic disorders (e.g. asthma).

*Warnings*: Patients should be made aware that very occasionally they may suffer from side effects which could interfere with their ability to drive a car or operate machinery.

*Precautions*: Before using Synacthen, the doctor should make every effort to find out whether the patient is suffering from, or has a history of allergic disorders, (see contra-indications). In particular, he should enquire whether the patient has previously experienced adverse reactions to ACTH, Synacthen or other drugs.

Synacthen should only be administered under the supervision of appropriate senior hospital medical staff (e.g. consultants).

If local or systemic hypersensitivity reactions occur after the injection (for example, marked redness and pain at the injection site, urticaria, pruritus, flushing, faintness or dyspnoea), Synacthen or other ACTH preparations should be avoided in the future. Hypersensitivity reactions tend to occur within 30 minutes of an injection. The patient should therefore be kept under observation during this time.

Preparation should be made in advance to combat any anaphylactic reaction that may occur after an injection of Synacthen. In the event of a serious anaphylactic reaction occurring, the following measures must be taken immediately: administer adrenaline (0.4-1 ml of a 0.1% solution intramuscularly or 0.1-0.2 ml of a 0.1% solution in 10 ml physiological saline *slowly* intravenously) as well as a large intravenous dose of a corticosteroid (for example 100-500 mg hydrocortisone, three or four times in 24 hours), repeating the dose if necessary.

The hydrocortisone product information prepared by the manufacturer should also be consulted.

*Pregnancy and lactation*: The Synacthen test should not be utilised during pregnancy and lactation unless there are compelling reasons for doing so.

*Side-effects*: Hypersensitivity reactions:

Synacthen may provoke hypersensitivity reactions, which in patients suffering from, or susceptible to, allergic disorders (especially asthma) may take the form of anaphylactic shock (see Contra-indications).

Hypersensitivity may be manifested as skin reaction at the injection site, dizziness, nausea, vomiting, urticaria, pruritus, flushing, malaise, dyspnoea, angioneurotic oedema and Quincke's oedema.

Other side effects are unlikely to be observed with short-term use of Synacthen as a diagnostic tool. For an extended list of side effects reported with long-term use of tetracosactrin, see Synacthen Depot data sheet.

*Overdosage*: Overdosage is unlikely to be a problem when the product is used as a single dose for diagnostic purposes.

**Pharmaceutical precautions** Synacthen should be protected from light and stored in a refrigerator (2-8°C).

**Legal category** POM.

**Package quantities** Synacthen ampoules 250 micrograms per ml in boxes of 5.

**Further information** Nil

**Product licence number** 0008/0034R

*Product licence holder:* Ciba-Geigy plc, Hulley Road, Macclesfield, Cheshire SK10 2NX.

## SYNACTHEN* DEPOT

**Presentation** Tetracosactrin Acetate ($\beta^{1\text{-}24}$ corticotrophin) BP is absorbed on to zinc phosphate. A sterile, white suspension, which settles on standing, containing 1 mg of Synacthen per ml and 10 mg benzyl alcohol per ml. This preparation is available in 1 ml ampoules.

The ampoules contain zinc, sodium phosphate, benzyl alcohol, sodium chloride, sodium hydroxide and water.

**Uses**

*Indications:*

*Therapeutic use*: Synacthen Depot should normally only be used for short-term therapy in conditions for which glucocorticoids are indicated in principal, for example, in ulcerative colitis and Crohn's disease, juvenile rheumatoid arthritis, or as adjunct therapy in patients with rheumatoid arthritis and osteoarthrosis.

Synacthen Depot may be particularly useful in patients unable to tolerate oral glucocorticoid therapy or in patients where normal therapeutic doses of glucocorticoids have been ineffective.

*Diagnostic use*: As a diagnostic aid for the investigation of adrenocortical insufficiency.

*Mode of action*: Tetracosactrin, the active substance of Synacthen, consists of the first 24 amino acids occurring in the natural corticotrophic hormone (ACTH) sequence and displays the same physiological properties as ACTH. Like ACTH, it stimulates adrenocortical production of glucocorticoids and mineralocorticoids, and to a lesser extent androgens, which explains its therapeutic effect in conditions responsive to glucocorticoid treatment.

However, its pharmacological activity is not comparable to that of corticosteroids, because under ACTH treatment–in contrast to treatment with a single glucocorticoid–the tissues are exposed to a physiological spectrum of corticosteroids.

The site of action of ACTH is the plasma membrane of the adrenocortical cells, where it binds to a specific receptor. The hormone-receptor complex activates adenylate cyclase, stimulating the production of cyclic AMP (adenosine monophosphate) and so promoting the synthesis of pregnenolone from cholesterol. From pregnenolone the various corticosteroids are produced via different enzymatic pathways.

*Pharmacokinetics*: Tetracosactrin is absorbed on to a zinc phosphate complex which ensures the sustained release of the active substance from the intramuscular injection site. After an intramuscular injection of 1 mg Synacthen Depot, the radioimmunologically determined plasma concentrations of tetracosactrin range between 200-300 pg/ml and are maintained for 12 hours.

Tetracosactrin has an apparent volume of distribution of approximately 0.4 litres/kg.

In the serum, tetracosactrin is broken down by serum endopeptidases into inactive oligopeptides and then by aminopeptidases into free amino acids.

Following an intravenous dose of $^{131}$I-labelled tetracosactrin, 95-100% of the radioactivity is excreted in the urine within 24 hours.

**Dosage and administration** Synacthen Depot is intended for intramuscular injection. The ampoule should be shaken before use.

*Therapeutic use*: Initially, daily doses of Synacthen Depot should be given but after approximately 3 days, intermittent doses may be given.

*Adults*: Initially 1 mg intramuscularly daily or 1 mg every 12 hours in acute cases. After the acute symptoms of the disease have disappeared, treatment may be continued at a dose of 1 mg every 2-3 days; in patients who respond well, the dosage may be reduced to 0.5 mg every 2-3 days or 1 mg per week.

*Infants aged 1 month-2 years*: Initially 0.25 mg intramuscularly daily; the maintenance dose is 0.25 mg every 2-8 days.

*Children aged 2-5 years*: Initially 0.25-0.5 mg intramuscularly daily; the maintenance dose is 0.25-0.5 mg every 2-8 days.

*Children aged 5-12 years*: Initially 0.25-1 mg intramuscularly daily; the maintenance dose is 0.25-1 mg every 2-8 days.

*Elderly*: There is no evidence to suggest that dosage should be different in the elderly.

*Diagnostic use:* In cases of suspected adrenocortical insufficiency, where the 30-minute diagnostic test with Synacthen ampoules (see Synacthen data sheet) has yielded inconclusive results or where it is desired to determine the functional reserve of the adrenal cortex, a 5-hour test with Synacthen Depot may be performed.

*Adults:* This test is based on measurement of the plasma cortisol concentration before and exactly 30 minutes, 1, 2, 3, 4 and 5 hours after an intramuscular injection of 1 mg Synacthen Depot. Adrenocortical function can be regarded as normal if the post-injection rise in plasma cortisol concentration increases 2-fold in the first hour, and continues to rise steadily. The values expected would be 600-1,250 nmol/l in the first hour increasing slowly up to 1,000-1,800 nmol/l by the fifth hour. Lower concentrations of plasma cortisol may be attributable to Addison's disease, secondary adrenocortical insufficiency due to a disorder of hypothalamo-pituitary function or overdosage of corticosteroids.

A 3-day test with Synacthen Depot may be used to differentiate between primary and secondary adrenocortical insufficiency.

*Children:* No paediatric dosage has been established.

*Elderly:* There is no evidence to suggest that dosage should be different in the elderly.

**Contra-indications, warnings, etc**
*Contra-indications*: History of hypersensitivity to ACTH, Synacthen or Synacthen Depot. Synacthen Depot therapy is also contra-indicated in acute psychoses, in infectious diseases, in Cushings syndrome, in patients with peptic ulcer, refractory heart failure, adrenogenital syndrome and for therapeutic use in adrenocortical insufficiency.

In view of the increased risk of anaphylactic reactions, Synacthen Depot should not be used in patients known to have asthma and/or other forms of allergy.

Synacthen Depot is contra-indicated for use in neonates (especially premature infants) since it contains benzyl alcohol which can cause severe poisoning.

Synacthen Depot must not be administered intravenously.

*Warnings*: Patients should be made aware that very occasionally they may suffer from side effects which could interfere with their ability to drive a car or operate machinery.

*Precautions*: Before using Synacthen Depot, the doctor should make every effort to find out whether the patient is suffering from, or has a history of allergic disorders. In particular, he should enquire whether the patient has previously experienced adverse reactions to ACTH, Synacthen Depot or other drugs.

Synacthen Depot should only be administered under medical supervision.

If local or systemic hypersensitivity reactions occur during or after an injection (for example, marked redness and pain at the injection site, urticaria, pruritus, flushing, faintness or dyspnoea), Synacthen Depot or other ACTH preparations should be avoided in the future. Hypersensitivity reactions tend to occur within 30 minutes of the injection. The patient should therefore be kept under observation during this time.

In the event of a serious anaphylactic reaction occurring, despite these precautions, the following measures must be taken immediately: administer adrenaline (0.4-1 ml of a 0.1% solution intramuscularly or 0.1-0.2 ml of a 0.1% solution in 10 ml physiological saline *slowly* intravenously) as well as a large intravenous dose of a corticosteroid (for example 100-500 mg hydrocortisone, three or four times in 24 hours) repeating the dose if necessary.

The hydrocortisone product information prepared by the manufacturer should also be consulted.

Synacthen Depot should not be used in the presence of active infectious or systemic diseases, when the use of live vaccine is contemplated or in the presence of a reduced immune response, unless adequate disease specific therapy is being given.

Use with care in patients with non-specific ulcerative colitis, diverticulitis, recent intestinal anastomosis, renal insufficiency, hypertension, thromboembolic tendencies, osteoporosis and myasthenia gravis.

The increased production of adrenal steroids may result in corticosteroid type effects:

- Salt and water retention can occur and may respond to a low salt diet. Potassium supplementation may be necessary during long term treatment

- Psychological disturbances may be triggered or aggravated

- Latent infections (e.g. amoebiasis, tuberculosis) may become activated

- Ocular effects may be produced (e.g. glaucoma, cataracts)

- Provided the dose is chosen to meet the individual's needs, Synacthen Depot is unlikely to inhibit growth in children. Nevertheless, growth should be monitored in children undergoing long-term treatment. In infants and children aged up to 5 years, reversible myocardial hypertrophy may occur in rare cases following long-term treatment with high doses. Therefore echocardiographic recordings should be made regularly.

- Dosage adjustments may be necessary in patients being treated for diabetes or hypertension

An enhanced effect of tetracosactide therapy may occur in patients with hypothyroidism and in those with cirrhosis of the liver.

*Use in pregnancy*: Synacthen Depot is contra-indicated for therapeutic use during pregnancy and lactation and should not be used as a diagnostic tool unless there are compelling reasons for doing so.

*Drug interactions:* Interactions are likely with drugs whose actions are affected by adrenal steroids (See Precautions).

*Side-effects:* Since Synacthen Depot stimulates the adrenal cortex to increase the output of glucocorticoids and mineralocorticoids, side-effects associated with excessive adrenocorticotrophic activity may be encountered.

*Hypersensitivity reactions:* Synacthen Depot may provoke hypersensitivity reactions, which in patients suffering from, or susceptible to allergic disorders (especially asthma) may take the form of anaphylactic shock. (See Precautions). Hypersensitivity may be manifested as skin reaction at the injection site, dizziness, nausea, vomiting, urticaria, pruritus, flushing, malaise, dyspnoea, angioneurotic oedema and Quincke's oedema. In rare cases, the benzyl alcohol in Synacthen Depot may provoke hypersensitivity reactions.

The following side-effects have also been reported during corticotrophin/corticosteroid therapy, although not necessarily observed during tetracosactide therapy:

*Musculoskeletal system:* Osteoporosis, muscle weakness, steroid myopathy, loss of muscle mass, vertebral compression fractures, aseptic necrosis of femoral and humeral heads, pathologic fracture of long bones and tendon rupture.

*Gastro-intestinal tract:* Peptic ulceration with possible perforation and haemorrhage, pancreatitis, abdominal distension and ulcerative oesophagitis.

*Skin and appendages:* Impaired wound healing, thin fragile skin, petechia and ecchymosis, facial erythema, increased sweating, suppression of skin test reactions, acne and skin pigmentation.

*Central and peripheral nervous system:* Convulsions, increased intracranial pressure with papilloedema (pseudotumour cerebri) usually after treatment, vertigo, headache and psychic changes.

*Endocrine system:* Sodium retention, fluid retention, potassium loss, hypokalaemic alkalosis and calcium loss. Menstrual irregularities, Cushing's syndrome, suppression of growth in children, secondary adrenocortical and pituitary unresponsiveness, particularly in times of stress, as in trauma, surgery or illness; decreased carbohydrate tolerance, hyperglycaemia, manifestations of latent diabetes mellitus, hirsutism.

*Ophthalmic:* Posterior subcapsular cataracts, increased intraocular pressure, glaucoma and exophthalmos.

*Metabolism:* Negative nitrogen balance due to protein catabolism.

*Cardiovascular system:* A rise in blood pressure, necrotising angiitis and congestive heart failure. In infants and small children treated over a prolonged period with high doses, reversible myocardial hypertrophy may occur in isolated cases.

*Miscellaneous:* Increased susceptibility to infection, abscess, thromboembolism, weight gain, increased appetite, leucocytosis.

*Overdosage:*
*Relating to therapeutic usage of Synacthen Depot*: Overdosage may lead to fluid retention and signs of excessive adrenocorticotrophic activity (Cushing's Syndrome). In such cases, Synacthen Depot should either be withdrawn temporarily, given in lower doses or the interval between injections should be prolonged (e.g. 5-7 days).

*Treatment*: There is no known antidote. Treatment should be symptomatic.

**Pharmaceutical precautions** Synacthen Depot should be protected from light and stored in a refrigerator (2-8°C).

**Legal category** POM.

**Package quantities** Ampoules of 1 mg in 1 ml packed in boxes of 10.

**Further information** Nil.

**Product licence number** 00101/0544

# SYNTOCINON* PARENTERAL SOLUTION

**Presentation** Syntocinon is available in clear, glass ampoules as Oxytocin Injection BP containing 5 units in 1 ml and 10 units in 1 ml. The solution is clear, colourless and sterile.

**Uses** *Principal action:* The active principle of Syntocinon is a synthetic nonapeptide identical with oxytocin, a hormone released by the posterior lobe of the pituitary. It exerts a stimulatory effect on the smooth musculature of the uterus, particularly towards the end of pregnancy, during labour, after delivery, and in the puerperium, i.e. at times when the number of specific oxytocin receptors in the myometrium is increased.

When given by low-dose intravenous infusion, Syntocinon elicits rhythmic uterine contractions that are indistinguishable in frequency, force, and duration from those observed during spontaneous labour. At higher infusion dosages, or when given by single injection, the drug is capable of causing sustained uterine contractions.

Being synthetic, Syntocinon does not contain vasopressin, but even in its pure form oxytocin possesses some weak intrinsic vasopressin-like antidiuretic activity.

Another pharmacological effect observed with high doses of oxytocin, particularly when administered by rapid intravenous bolus injection, consists in a transient direct relaxing effect on vascular smooth muscle, resulting in brief hypotension, flushing, and reflex tachycardia.

*Indications:* Syntocinon Parenteral Solution may be used for: Induction of labour for medical reasons; stimulation of labour in hypotonic uterine inertia; during caesarian section following the delivery of the child; prevention and treatment of postpartum uterine atony and haemorrhage.

Syntocinon may also be indicated in early stages of pregnancy as an adjunctive therapy for the management of incomplete, inevitable or missed abortion.

**Dosage and administration**
*Induction or enhancement of labour:* Syntocinon should be administered as an intravenous drip infusion or, preferably, by means of a variable-speed infusion pump. For drip infusion it is recommended that 5 IU of Syntocinon be added to 500 ml of a physiologic electrolyte solution. For patients in whom infusion of sodium chloride must be avoided, 5% dextrose solution may be used as the diluent (see 'Precautions'). To ensure even mixing, the bottle or bag must be turned upside down several times before use.

The initial infusion rate should be set at 1–4 mU/min (2–8 drops/min). It may be gradually increased at intervals not shorter than 20 min, until a contraction pattern similar to that of normal labour is established. In pregnancy near term this can often be achieved with an infusion of less than 10 mU/min (20 drops/min), and the recommended maximum rate is 20 mU/min (40 drops/min). In the unusual event that higher rates are required, as may occur in the management of foetal death in utero or for induction of labour at an earlier stage of pregnancy, when the uterus is less sensitive to oxytocin, it is advisable to use a more concentrated Syntocinon solution, e.g. 10 IU in 500 ml.

When using a motor-driven infusion pump which delivers smaller volumes than those given by drip infusion, the concentration suitable for infusion within the recommended dosage range must be calculated according to the specifications of the pump.

The frequency, strength, and duration of contractions as well as the foetal heart rate must be carefully monitored throughout the infusion. Once an adequate level of uterine activity is attained, the infusion rate can often be reduced. In the event of uterine hyperactivity and/or foetal distress, the infusion must be discontinued immediately.

If, in women who are at term or near term, regular contractions are not established after the infusion of a total amount of 5 IU, it is recommended that the attempt to induce labour be ceased; it may be repeated on the following day, starting again from a rate of 1–4 mU/min.

*Caesarean section:* 5 IU by slow intravenous injection immediately after delivery.

*Prevention of postpartum uterine haemorrhage:* The usual dose is 5 IU slowly iv after delivery of the placenta. In women given Syntocinon for induction or enhancement of labour, the infusion should be continued at an increased rate during the third stage of labour and for the next few hours thereafter.

*Treatment of postpartum uterine haemorrhage:* 5 IU slowly iv, followed in severe cases by intravenous infusion of a solution containing 5–20 IU of oxytocin in 500 ml of a non-hydrating diluent, run at the rate necessary to control uterine atony.

*Incomplete, inevitable, or missed abortion:* 5 IU slowly iv, if necessary followed by intravenous infusion at a rate of 20–40 mU/min or higher.

**Contra-indications, warnings, etc**
*Contra-indications:* Hypersensitivity to the drug.

Hypertonic uterine contractions, mechanical obstruction to delivery, foetal distress. Any condition in which for foetal or maternal reasons spontaneous labour is inadvisable and/or vaginal delivery is contra-indicated: e.g. significant cephalopelvic disproportion, foetal malpresentation; placenta praevia and vasa praevia, placental abruption, cord presentation or prolapse, overdistension or impaired resistance of the uterus to rupture as in multiple pregnancy, polyhydramnios, grand multiparity and in the presence of a uterine scar resulting from major surgery including classical caesarean section.

Syntocinon should not be used for prolonged periods in patients with oxytocin-resistant uterine inertia, severe pre-eclamptic toxaemia or severe cardiovascular disorders.

*Precautions:* The induction of labour by means of oxytocin should be attempted only when strictly indicated for medical reasons. Administration should only be under hospital conditions and qualified medical supervision. When given for induction and enhancement of labour, Syntocinon must only be administered as an intravenous infusion and never by intravenous bolus injection. Careful monitoring of foetal heart rate and uterine motility (frequency, strength, and duration of contractions) is essential, so that the dosage may be adjusted to individual response.

When Syntocinon is given for induction or enhancement of labour, particular caution is required in the presence of borderline cephalopelvic disproportion, secondary uterine inertia, mild to moderate degrees of pregnancy-induced hypertension or cardiac disease, and in patients above 35 years of age or with a history of lower-uterine-segment caesarean section.

In the case of foetal death in utero, and/or in the presence of meconium-stained amniotic fluid, tumultuous labour must be avoided, as it may cause amniotic fluid embolism.

Because oxytocin possesses slight antidiuretic activity, its prolonged intravenous administration at high doses in conjunction with large volumes of fluid, as may be the case in the treatment of inevitable or missed abortion, or in the management of postpartum haemorrhage, may cause water intoxication associated with hyponatraemia. To avoid this rare complication, the following precautions must be observed whenever high doses of oxytocin are administered over a long time: an electrolyte-containing diluent must be used (not dextrose); the volume of infused fluid should be kept low (by infusing oxytocin at a higher concentration than recommended for the induction or enhancement of labour at term); fluid intake by mouth must be restricted; a fluid balance chart should be kept, and serum electrolytes should be measued when electrolyte imbalance is suspected.

When Syntocinon is used for prevention or treatment of uterine haemorrhage, rapid intravenous injection should be avoided, as it may cause an acute short-lasting drop in blood pressure.

Prostaglandins may potentiate the uterotonic effect of oxytocin and vice versa; therefore, concomitant administration requires very careful monitoring.

Some inhalation anaesthetics, e.g. cyclopropane or halothane, may enhance the hypotensive effect of oxytocin and reduce its oxytocic action. Their concurrent use with oxytocin has also been reported to cause cardiac rhythm disturbances.

When given during or after caudal block anaesthesia, oxytocin may potentiate the pressor effect of sympathomimetic vasoconstrictor agents.

*Overdosage:* The fatal dose of Syntocinon has not been established. Syntocinon is subject to inactivation by proteolytic enzymes of the alimentary tract. Hence it is not absorbed from the intestine and is not likely to have toxic effects when ingested.

The symptoms and consequences of overdosage are those mentioned under 'Side-effects'. In addition, as a result of uterine overstimulation, placental abruption and/or amniotic fluid embolism have been reported.

*Treatment:* When signs or symptoms of overdosage occur during continuous iv administration of Syntocinon, the infusion must be discontinued at once and oxygen should be given to the mother. In cases of water intoxication it is essential to restrict fluid intake, promote diuresis, correct electrolyte imbalance, and control convulsions that may eventually occur, by judicious use of diazepam. In the case of coma, a free airway should be maintained with routine measures normally employed in the nursing of the unconscious patient.

*Side-effects:* As there is a wide variation in uterine sensitivity, uterine spasm may be caused in some instances by what are normally considered to be low doses.

When oxytocin is used by iv infusion for the induction or enhancement of labour, its administration at too high doses results in uterine overstimulation which may cause foetal distress, asphyxia, and death, or may lead to hypertonicity, tetanic contractions, soft tissue damage or rupture of the uterus.

Water intoxication associated with maternal and neonatal hyponatraemia has been reported in cases where high doses of oxytocin together with large amounts of electrolyte-free fluid have been administered over a prolonged period of time (see 'Precautions'). Symptoms of water intoxication include:

1. Headache, anorexia, nausea, vomiting and abdominal pain.
2. Lethargy, drowsiness, unconsciousness and grand-mal type seizures.
3. Low blood electrolyte concentration.

Rapid intravenous bolus injection of oxytocin at doses amounting to several IU may result in acute short-lasting hypotension accompanied with flushing and reflex tachycardia.

Oxytocin may occasionally cause nausea, vomiting, or cardiac arrhythmias. In a few cases, skin rashes and anaphylactoid reactions associated with dyspnoea, hypotension, or shock have been reported.

**Pharmaceutical precautions** Protect from light. Store between 4° and 22°C.

Syntocinon should not be infused via the same apparatus as blood or plasma, because the peptide linkages are rapidly inactivated by oxytocin-inactivating enzymes. Syntocinon is incompatible with solutions containing sodium metabisulphite as a stabiliser.

Syntocinon is compatible with the following infusion fluids, but due attention should be paid to the advisability of using electrolyte fluids in individual patients: Dextrose 5%, Sodium/potassium chloride (103 mmol $Na^+$ and 51 mmol $K^+$), Laevulose 20%, Macrodex 6%, Sodium bicarbonate 1.39%, Sodium chloride 0.9%, Sodium lactate 1.72%, Rheomacrodex 10%, Ringer's solution.

**Legal category** POM.

**Package quantities**
5 Units/1 ml: Boxes of 10.
10 Units/1 ml: Boxes of 10.

**Further information** Snap ampoules: no file required.

Oxytocin (used as an intravenous infusion) has a short half life, values reported by various investigators range from 3 to 17 minutes. Plasma protein binding is very low. Removal of oxytocin from plasma is mainly via the liver and the kidneys. Less than 1% of a given dose is excreted unchanged in the urine.

**Product licence numbers**
5 Units/1 ml 0101/0069
10 Units/1 ml 0101/0070

## SYNTOMETRINE* AMPOULES

**Qualitative and quantitative composition** Each 1 ml ampoule contains 5.0 IU Oxytocin PhEur and 0.5 mg of Ergometrine Maleate PhEur.

**Pharmaceutical form** Injection.

**Clinical particulars**
*Therapeutic indications:* Syntometrine is indicated in the active management of the third stage of labour, or routinely, following the birth of the placenta, to prevent or treat postpartum haemorrhage.

*Posology and method of administration*
*Adults:*
*Active management of third stage of labour:* Intramuscular injection of 1 ml after delivery of the anterior shoulder, or at the latest, immediately after delivery of the child. Expulsion of the placenta, which is normally separated by the first strong uterine contraction, should be assisted by gentle suprapubic pressure and controlled cord traction.

*Prevention and treatment of postpartum haemorrhage:* Intramuscular injection of 1 ml following expulsion of the placenta, or when bleeding occurs.

*Third stage of labour and postpartum haemorrhage:* Syntometrine may also be administered by a slow intravenous injection in a dose of 0.5 to 1 ml. This route of administration is not generally recommended.

*Children:* Not applicable.

*Use in the elderly:* Not applicable.

*Method of administration:* Intramuscular, intravenous.

*Contra-indications:* Hypersensitivity to any of the components.

Pregnancy, first stage of labour, primary or secondary uterine inertia.

Second stage of labour before crowning of the head.

Severe disorders of cardiac, liver or kidney functions; occlusive vascular disease, sepsis, severe hypertension, pre-eclampsia, eclampsia.

*Special warnings and precautions for use:* When the intravenous route is employed, care should be exercised in patients of doubtful cardiac status.

In breech presentations and other abnormal presentations, Syntometrine should not be given until after delivery of the child, and in multiple births not until the last child has been delivered. In postpartum haemorrhage, if bleeding is not arrested by the injection of Syntometrine, the possibility of retained placental fragments, of soft tissue injury (cervical or vaginal laceration), or of a clotting defect, should be excluded before a further injection is given. Caution should be exercised in the presence of mild or moderate hypertension, or with mild or moderate degrees of cardiac, liver of kidney disease.

*Interaction with other medicaments and other forms of interaction:* Halothane anesthesia may diminish the uterotonic effect of Syntometrine. Syntometrine may enhance the effects of vasoconstrictors and of prostaglandins.

*Pregnancy and lactation:* See indications.

*Effects on ability to drive and to use machines:* Not applicable.

*Undesirable effects:* Nausea, vomiting, abdominal pain, headache, dizziness and skin rashes. On rare occasions hypertension, bradycardia, cardiac arrhythmias, chest pain or anaphylactoid reactions associated with dyspnoea, hypotension, collapse or shock.

*Overdose:* No case of maternal intoxication with Syntometrine has been reported to the company. If such a case were to occur the most likely symptoms would be those of ergometrine intoxication: nausea, vomiting, hypertension or hypotension, vasospastic reactions, respiratory depression, convulsions, coma. Treatment would have to be symptomatic.

Accidental administration to the newborn infant has been reported and has proved fatal. In these accidental neonatal overdosage cases, symptoms such as respiratory depression, convulsions, hypertonia, heart arrhythmia have been reported. Treatment has been symptomatic in most cases, respiratory and cardiovascular support have been required.

**Pharmacological properties**
*Pharmacodynamic properties:* Syntometrine combines the known sustained oxytotic action of ergometrine with the more rapid action of oxytocin on the uterus.

*Pharmacokinetic properties:* Ergometrine is reported to be rapidly and completely absorbed after an intramuscular injection. Uterine stimulation occurs within 7 minutes of i.m. injection and immediately after intravenous injection. Oxytocin is also rapidly absorbed and is rapidly metabolised by the liver and the kidneys.

*Preclinical safety data:* There are no pre-clinical data of relevance to the prescriber which are additional to that already included in other sections of the SPC.

**Pharmaceutical particulars**
*List of excipients:* Sodium Chloride PhEur, Maleic Acid PhEur, Water for Injection PhEur.

*Incompatibilities:* None.

*Shelf life:* 36 months.

*Special precautions for storage:* For prolonged periods store between 2° and 8°C. Protect from light. Syntometrine may be stored at temperatures up to 25°C for 2 months when protected from light.

*Nature and contents of container:* Uncoloured borosilicate glass Type I snap ampoule. Pack of 10 ampoules.

*Instructions for use/handling:* None.

**Marketing authorisation number** 0101/5046R.

**Date of approval/revision of SPC** 3 March 1997.

**Legal category** POM.

## SYNTOPRESSIN* NASAL SPRAY

**Presentation** Syntopressin is available as a solution containing lypressin 50 IU per ml for use as a nasal spray.

**Uses** *Principal action:* Syntopressin is synthetic 8-lysine-vasopressin (lypressin). It is completely free of oxytocin and extraneous animal protein. Syntopressin has a direct antidiuretic action. It is used for the control of polyuria in diabetes insipidus.

*Indications:* Diabetes insipidus, spontaneous or induced.

**Dosage and administration** Before the spray is used for the first time the pump must be primed by depressing the actuator several times until the spray is released.

Once the cap has been removed, the spray device should be held upright to the nostril and the actuator depressed. The patient should be in the sitting position and should be instructed to inhale gently through the nose. Each actuation delivers a metered dose of 5 IU.

The dosage should be individually adjusted to take account of the patient's specific hormone deficiency. On average, the dosage required amounts to 1 or 2 sprays (5 to 10 IU) 3 or 4 times a day. If two sprays per dose are required, one should be given into each nostril. For patients who need more than two actuations per dose it is recommended that the time interval between doses be shortened rather than increasing the number of actuations per dose.

If an excess volume of intranasally administered spray solution is swallowed vasopressin is quickly inactivated in the digestive track by trypsin.

The effectiveness of Syntopressin nasal spray may be reduced in patients with nasal congestion, allergic rhinitis and upper respiratory infections because these conditions may interfere with the absorption of drug from the nasal mucosa. In this event, larger doses or more frequent administration of the spray may be needed.

*Use in the elderly:* No evidence exists that elderly patients require different dosages, or show different side-effects from younger people.

**Contra-indications, warnings, etc**
*Contra-indications:* Hypersensitivity. Coronary heart disease, Chronic nephritis, anaesthesia with halothane or cyclopropane.

*Precautions:* As with other forms of vasopressin, caution is advised in the administration of this drug during pregnancy, particularly toxaemia, since vaso-

pressin can impair the blood supply to the uterus. Caution is indicated in all conditions in which an increase in blood pressure is undesirable, e.g. peripheral vascular disease, hypertension, as vasopressin can give rise to a temporary increase in blood pressure. Vasopressin should also be given with caution in the presence of cardiac dysfunction, advanced arteriosclerosis, bronchial asthma and epilepsy.

Syntopressin should not be inhaled through the mouth.

The antidiuretic effect of Syntopressin may be enhanced by carbamazepine, chlorpropamide or clofibrate and decreased by lithium.

*Overdosage:* Symptoms: as under *Side-effects*.
Treatment: temporary withdrawal of vasopressin medication, symptomatic measures. In case of water retention, restriction of fluid intake and if necessary correction of electrolyte imbalance may be required.

*Side-effects:* Nausea, abdominal pain or urge to defaecate may occur. On rare occasions nasal congestion with ulceration of the nasal mucosa has been reported.

Headache, dizziness, increase in blood pressure, cardiac arrhythmias or hyponatraemia with water retention may occur. Such reactions are seen in particular after overdosage.

**Pharmaceutical precautions** Store between 2° and 8°C, but do NOT freeze. Allow to reach room temperature before use.

Once in use the nasal spray should be stored at room temperature. Use within one month of opening.

**Legal category** POM.

**Package quantities** Spray glass bottles of 5 ml.

**Further information** Chlorbutol is added to Syntopressin Nasal Spray to prevent antimicrobial contamination during manufacture. For this reason, a low concentration of chlorbutol (approximately 2.5 mg/ml) is present in the finished product.

**Product licence number** 0101/5047R.

## TAVEGIL*

**Presentation**
*Tablets:* White, uncoated, round tablets, 7 mm in diameter, with bevelled edges, branded TAVEGIL on one side with a single break line on the other. Each tablet contains 1.34 mg clemastine hydrogen fumarate (equivalent to 1 mg clemastine base).

*Elixir:* A clear, colourless liquid with an odour of peaches. Each 5 ml spoonful contains 670 micrograms (0.67 mg) clemastine hydrogen fumarate (equivalent to 500 micrograms (0.5 mg) clemastine base).

**Uses** *Principal action:* Tavegil is a potent, specific antihistamine which is innately long-acting.

*Indications:* Allergic rhinitis, including hay fever and perennial rhinitis, vasomotor rhinitis. Allergic dermatoses, including pruritus, atopic eczema and contact dermatitis. Urticaria. Angioneurotic oedema. Drug allergy.

**Dosage and administration**
*Adults:* 1 mg clemastine base (one tablet or two 5 ml spoonfuls of elixir) night and morning.

In individual cases the dose may be increased to 6 mg clemastine base daily if necessary (six tablets or twelve 5 ml spoonfuls of elixir).

*Children:*
| | |
|---|---|
| 1 to 3 years: | 250 micrograms to 500 micrograms clemastine base night and morning. |
| 3 to 6 years: | 500 micrograms clemastine base night and morning. |
| 6 to 12 years: | 500 micrograms to 1000 micrograms (1 mg) clemastine base night and morning. |

For doses less than 500 micrograms Tavegil Elixir may be diluted. For dilution details see 'Pharmaceutical precautions'.

*Use in the elderly:* No evidence exists that elderly patients require different dosages or show different side-effects from younger patients.

**Contra-indications, warnings, etc**
*Contra-indications:* Tavegil is contra-indicated in patients with a known hypersensitivity to clemastine or other arylalkylamine antihistamines.

Tavegil should not be given to children below one year of age.

*Precautions:* Patients should be warned not to take charge of vehicles or machinery until the effect of Tavegil treatment on the individual is known. Tavegil may potentiate the effects of sedatives, hypnotics, monoamine-oxidase inhibitors and alcohol. Patients should be advised to avoid alcoholic drinks.

Antihistamines should be used with caution in patients with narrow-angle glaucoma, stenosing pep-

tic ulcer, pyloroduodenal obstruction, prostatic hypertrophy with urinary retention and bladder neck obstruction.

*Use in pregnancy and lactation:* Tavegil should not be given during pregnancy and breast feeding unless it is strictly indicated.

*Side-effects:* Drowsiness, fatigue, occasionally CNS stimulation has been reported, particularly in children. Very occasional miscellaneous side-effects such as weakness, dizziness, dry mouth, headache, palpitations, gastro-intestinal disturbance, heartburn and skin rash have occurred. In general, these adverse effects can be controlled by a diminution of dosage.

*Overdosage:* May give rise to confusion, nausea and vomiting. Treatment should be directed to the removal of ingested material by induced emesis or gastric lavage as appropriate. Routine supportive measures are indicated to combat respiratory depression and hypotension.

**Pharmaceutical precautions** Store both the tablets and elixir below 25°C. Tavegil Elixir may be diluted with Syrup BP or Sorbitol Syrup (70%). The diluted elixir should be used within 14 days.

**Legal category** P.

**Package quantities** *Tavegil Tablets:* Blister pack of 60 (OP).

*Tavegil Elixir:* Bottles of 150 ml.

**Further information** Tavegil Elixir is sucrose free and is suitable for diabetic patients. It has an approximate calorific value of 11 kcals per 5 ml spoonful.

**Product licence numbers**
Tavegil Tablets 0101/0033
Tavegil Elixir 0101/0058

## TEGRETOL*

**Presentation** The active ingredient, Carbamazepine PhEur, is presented as:

White suspension with a flavour of caramel, containing 100 mg/5 ml Carbamazepine PhEur,

100 mg white, scored, compressed tablets, 7 mm diameter, impressed TEGRETOL 100 on one side, breakline on the other.

200 mg white, scored, compressed tablets, 9 mm diameter impressed TEGRETOL 200 on one side, breakline on the other.

400 mg white, rod-shaped, flat faced tablets with bevelled edges, 17 mm long, 5.5 mm wide and 5.5 mm thick, impressed GEIGY/GEIGY on one face with breakline. Other face impressed TEGRETOL with breakline.

Retard divisible tablets containing 200 mg Carbamazepine PhEur, in a formulation to reduce peak plasma levels, beige-orange, capsule shaped, convex faces, with deep break-score on both sides, 13.2 mm long, 5.2 mm wide, 5.0 mm thick, impressed C/G on one side and H/C on the other side.

Retard divisible tablets containing 400 mg Carbamazepine PhEur, in a formulation to reduce peak plasma levels, brown-orange, capsule shaped, convex faces, with deep break-score on both sides, 17.2 mm long, 6.6 mm wide, 6.0 mm thick, impressed CG/CG score on one side and ENE/ENE on the other side.

Chewtabs containing 100 mg Carbamazepine PhEur, in a chewable formulation, pale orange, square-shaped, width 10 mm, height 4.0 mm, first side embossed with 'T', second side impressed with TEGRETOL 100.

Chewtabs containing 200 mg Carbamazepine PhEur, in a chewable formulation, pale orange, square-shaped, width 12.5 mm, height 5.1 mm, first side embossed with 'T', second side impressed with TEGRETOL 200.

Suppositories containing 125 mg Carbamazepine PhEur in a white to off-white, torpedo-shaped hard fat base weighing approximately 1 g.

Suppositories containing 250 mg carbamazepine Ph. Eur in a white to off-white, torpedo-shaped hard fat base weighing approximately 2 g.

Tegretol Liquid also contains polyethoxylated castor oils, methyl hydroxybenzoate and propyl hydroxybenzoate.

Tegretol Retard divisible tablets also contain polyethoxylated castor oils.

Tegretol chewtabs contain sorbitol.

Tegretol Suppositories also contain hydroxypropyl methylcellulose.

**Uses**
*Indications:* Epilepsy–generalised tonic-clonic and partial seizures.

Note: Tegretol is not usually effective in absences (petit mal). Moreover, anecdotal evidence suggests that seizure exacerbation may occur in patients with atypical absences.

The paroxysmal pain of trigeminal neuralgia.

For the prophylaxis of manic-depressive psychosis in patients unresponsive to lithium therapy.

Tegretol Retard is indicated in newly diagnosed patients with epilepsy and in those patients who are uncontrolled or unable to tolerate their current anticonvulsant therapy.

No clinical data are available on the use of Tegretol Suppositories in indications other than epilepsy.

*Mode of action:* Carbamazepine is a dibenzazepine derivative with anti-epileptic, neurotropic and psychotropic properties.

The mechanism of action of carbamazepine has only been partially elucidated. It is conceivable that blockade of voltage-sensitive sodium channels may be one or even the main primary effect of carbamazepine.

*Pharmacokinetics:*

*Absorption:* Carbamazepine is almost completely absorbed but the rate of absorption from the tablets is slow and may vary amongst the various formulations and between patients. Peak plasma concentrations of the unchanged active substance after administration of single doses of Tegretol conventional tablets, Retard divisible tablets, chewable tablets and syrup are attained at 12 hours, within 24 hours, 6 hours and 2 hours, respectively.

The retard formulation shows about 15% lower bioavailability than standard preparations due mainly to the considerable reduction in peak plasma levels occasioned by controlled release of the same dosage of carbamazepine. Plasma concentrations show less fluctuation. Auto-induction of carbamazepine occurs as with standard carbamazepine preparations.

The elimination half-life of unchanged drug in the plasma averages approximately 36 hours following a single dose, whereas after repeated administration, which leads to auto-induction of hepatic enzymes, it averages only 16-24 hours, depending on the duration of the medication. In patients receiving co-medication with other enzyme-inducing drugs (phenytoin, phenobarbitone) half-life values averaging 9-10 hours have been observed. The therapeutic plasma concentration range of carbamazepine at steady state is usually between 4-12 µg/ml (17-50µmol/l).

The bioavailability of Tegretol in various oral formulations has been shown to lie between 85-100%. Bioavailability is unaffected by food regardless of dosage form.

As measured by AUC calculations the total bioavailability of carbamazepine from Tegretol Suppositories is approximately 25% less than from oral formulations. For doses up to 300 mg approximately 75% of the total amount absorbed reaches the general circulation within 6 hours of application. For these reasons the maximum recommended daily dose is limited to 250 mg qid (1,000 mg per day), the equivalent of 800 mg per day orally. Clinical trials have shown that when Tegretol Suppositories are substituted for oral dosage forms plasma levels within the range 5-8µg/ml (19-34µmol/L) are reached. It should be possible, therefore, to maintain therapeutically effective plasma levels in most patients.

Serum protein binding: 70-80%

*Distribution:* The concentration of unchanged substance in the CSF and saliva represents the unbound portion in plasma i.e. 20-30% of total plasma concentration, breast milk 25-60% of total plasma concentration. Carbamazepine crosses the placental barrier. Apparent volume of distribution 0.8-1.5 L/kg.

*Metabolism:* Carbamazepine is extensively metabolised in the liver, mainly by oxidative pathways and the greater part is excreted as the inactive glucuronide with up to 40% as metabolites, of which only carbamazepine epoxide is pharmacologically active. This may constitute up to 30% of the circulating active material originating as carbamazepine; in particular polytherapy is an important factor in augmenting epoxide levels. The inactive 10, 11- diol represents the final stage of carbamazepine biotransformation. Only about 3% of pharmacologically active material (unchanged plus epoxide) is excreted.

In advanced hepatic disease carbamazepine metabolism may be impaired.

The pharmacokinetics of carbamazepine are unaltered in the elderly but its metabolism may be affected by hepatic dysfunction (see above). In children the relatively high rate of metabolism of the drug may require higher doses (in mg/kg b.w.) of carbamazepine to maintain therapeutic concentrations.

**Dosage and administration** Tegretol is given orally in either tablet or liquid form, usually in two or three divided doses. In the case of Retard tablets Tegretol is usually given in two divided doses. Tegretol is also available as suppositories for short-term use as replacement therapy (maximum period recommended: 7 days) in patients for whom oral treatment is temporarily not possible, for example in postoperative or unconscious subjects.

Tegretol tablets or liquid (the liquid should be shaken before use) may be taken during, after or between meals. The tablets should be taken with a little liquid e.g. a glass of water.

Tegretol Retard divisible tablets are given orally, generally in the same total daily dose as conventional Tegretol dosage forms. In a few patients when changing from other oral dosage forms of Tegretol to Tegretol Retard divisible tablets the total daily dose may need to be increased, particularly when it is used in polytherapy. When starting treatment with Tegretol Retard divisible tablets in monotherapy, 100-200 mg once or twice daily is recommended. This may be followed by a slow increase in dosage until the best response is obtained, often 800-1,200 mg daily. In some instances, 1,600 mg or even 2,000 mg daily may be necessary.

Tegretol Retard (either the whole or half divisible tablet as prescribed), should not be chewed but should be swallowed with a little liquid, before, during or between meals. The divisible tablet presentation enables flexibility of dosing to be achieved.

The chewtabs should be chewed before swallowing, preferably with a little liquid to wash down possible remnants of the tablets.

The chewtabs are particularly suitable for children and adults who have difficulty in swallowing tablets.

Since a given dose of Tegretol liquid will produce higher peak levels than the same dose in tablet form, it is advisable to start with low doses of the liquid and to increase them slowly so as to avoid adverse effects on the central nervous system such as dizziness and lethagy.

When switching a patient from tablets to liquid the same overall dose may be used but in smaller, more frequent, doses.

When switching from oral formulations to suppositories the dosage should be increased by approximately 25% (the 125 mg and 250 mg suppositories correspond to 100 mg and 200 mg tablets respectively). The final dose adjustment should always depend on the clinical response in the individual patient (plasma level monitoring is recommended). Tegretol Suppositories have been shown to provide plasma levels which are well within the therapeutic range (see pharmacokinetics).

*Epilepsy:*
*Adults:* It is advised that with all formulations of Tegretol, a gradually increasing dosage scheme is used and this should be adjusted to suit the needs of the individual patient. It may be helpful to monitor the plasma concentration of carbamazepine to establish the optimum dose (see pharmacokinetics, precautions and interactions).

Where suppositories are used the maximum daily dose is limited to 1,000 mg (250 mg qid at 6 hour intervals; see pharmacokinetics).

Tegretol should be taken in a number of divided doses although intially 100-200 mg once or twice daily is recommended. This may be followed by a slow increase until the best response is obtained, often 800-1,200 mg daily. In some instances, 1,600 mg or even 2,000 mg daily may be necessary.

*Elderly:* There is no evidence to suggest that dosage requirements are different in the elderly but it is recommended that the initial dose be small.

*Children:* It is advised that with all formulations of Tegretol, a gradually increasing dosage scheme is used and this should be adjusted to suit the needs of the individual patient. It may be helpful to monitor the plasma concentration of carbamazepine to establish the optimum dose, (see pharmacokinetics, precautions and interactions). Usual dosage 10-20 mg/kg bodyweight daily in several divided doses.

Tegretol conventional tablet formulations are not recommended for very young children and Tegretol Retard is not recommended for children under 5 years. Where suppositories are used the maximum daily dose is limited to 1,000 mg (250 mg qid at 6 hour intervals; see pharmacokinetics).

Age up to 1 year: for flexibility of dosage, use Tegretol liquid: 5-10 ml per day
1-5 years: 10-20 ml liquid per day, or 2-4 x 100 mg chewtabs per day,
where appropriate,
5-10 years: 400-600 mg as 2-3 x 200 mg tablets, or 20-30 ml liquid per day.
When conventional tablets or chewtabs are used Tegretol should be taken in divided doses. When Retard tablets are used the dose may be given twice daily.
10-15 years: 3-5 x 200 mg tablets or 30-50 ml liquid per day.
When conventional tablets or chewtabs are used Tegretol should be taken in divided doses. When Retard tablets are used the dose may be given twice daily.

Wherever possible, anti-epileptic agents should be prescribed as the sole anti-epileptic agent but if used in polytherapy the same incremental dosage pattern is advised.

*Trigeminal neuralgia:* The individual dosage require-

ments of Tegretol vary considerably. It is recommended that the initial dose be small but in some patients a high dose early in treatment may be required. In elderly patients, an initial dose of 100 mg twice daily is recommended.

The dose may be increased gradually until a satisfactory clinical response is obtained, which in some instances necessitates 1,600 mg Tegretol daily. It has been found that in the majority of patients a dosage of 200 mg three or four times a day is sufficient to maintain a pain-free state. When the pain goes into remission the dose may be gradually reduced and Tegretol discontinued in the absence of recurrence.

*For the prophylaxis of manic depressive psychosis in patients unresponsive to lithium therapy.* Initial starting dose of 400 mg daily, in divided doses, increasing gradually until symptoms are controlled or a total of 1,600 mg given in divided doses is reached. The usual dosage range is 400-600 mg daily, given in divided doses.

**Contra-indications, warnings, etc**
*Contra-indications:* Previous drug sensitivity to carbamazepine or structurally related drugs, e.g. tricyclic antidepressants. Because Tegretol depresses AV-conduction, it is inadvisable to administer this drug to patients with atrioventricular conduction abnormalities. Patients with a history of previous bone marrow depression or a history of intermittent porphyria. On theoretical grounds i.e. a structural relationship to tricyclic anti-depressants, the use of Tegretol is not recommended in combination with monoamine oxidase inhibitors (MAOIs); before administering Tegretol, MAOIs should be discontinued for a minimum of 2 weeks, or longer if the clinical situation permits.

*Warnings:* Agranulocytosis and aplastic anaemia have been associated with Tegretol; however, due to the very low incidence of these diseases, meaningful risk estimates for Tegretol are difficult to obtain. The overall risk in the general untreated population has been estimated at 4.7 persons per million per year for agranulocytosis and 2.0 persons per million per year for aplastic anaemia.

Blood counts, platelet count and serum biochemistry including electrolytes and indices of hepatic function should be checked before commencing treatment with Tegretol. Blood counts should be performed before and periodically during treatment. Clinical monitoring is of primary importance during the whole treatment.

Patients and their relatives should be informed on how to recognise early toxic signs and symptoms indicative of a potential haematological problem, or of dermatological or hepatic reactions. If reactions such as fever, sore throat, rash, ulcers in the mouth, easy bruising, petechial or purpuric haemorrhage appear, the patient should be advised to consult his physician immediately.

Non-progressive or fluctuating asymptomatic leucopenia, which occurs in about 10% of treated patients does not generally call for withdrawal of Tegretol. However, treatment with Tegretol should be discontinued if the patient develops leucopenia which is severe, progressive or accompanied by clinical manifestations, e.g. fever or sore throat. Tegretol should be discontinued if any evidence of significant bone marrow depression appears.

Liver function tests should also be performed before commencing treatment and periodically thereafter, particularly in patients with a history of liver disease and in elderly patients.

Some liver function tests in patients receiving carbamazepine may be found to be abnormal, particularly gamma glutamyl transferase. This is probably due to hepatic enzyme induction. Enzyme induction may also produce modest elevations in alkaline phosphatase. These enhancements of hepatic metabolising capacity are not an indication for the withdrawal of carbamazepine.

Severe hepatic reactions to carbamazepine occur very rarely. The development of signs and symptoms of liver dysfunction or active liver disease should be urgently evaluated and treatment with Tegretol suspended pending the outcome of the evaluation.

Mild skin reactions eg. isolated macular or maculopapular exanthemata, are mostly transient and not hazardous, and they usually disappear within a few days. However, the patient should be kept under close surveillance and a worsening rash or accompanying symptoms are an indication for the immediate withdrawal of Tegretol. Severe skin reactions e.g. Stevens-Johnson syndrome, Lyell's syndrome (toxic epidermal necrolysis), also necessitate immediate withdrawal.

If treatment with Tegretol has to be withdrawn abruptly, the changeover to another anti-epileptic drug should if necessary be effected under the cover of a suitable drug eg i.v. or rectal benzodiazepines, or i.v. phenytoin.

The patient's reactions, e.g. as a road user, may be impaired by Tegretol, especially in the early stages of treatment. Patients should be warned of the possible hazard when driving or operating machinery.

The induction of hepatic enzymes by carbamazepine may reduce the activity of the hormones contained in the combined oral contraceptive pill. This may appear clinically as breakthrough bleeding or spotting. Patients taking Tegretol and requiring oral contraception should receive a preparation containing not less than 50µg oestrogen or use of some alternative non-hormonal method of contraception should be considered.

Although correlations between dosages and plasma levels of carbamazepine, and between plasma levels and clinical efficacy or tolerability are rather tenuous, serum level monitoring of carbamazepine may prove useful during stabilisation, for optimum seizure control and in particular situations e.g. pregnancy, for verification of compliance, in suspected toxicity and when carbamazepine is used in polytherapy.

In rats treated with carbamazepine for two years, the incidence of tumours of the liver was found to be increased. There is, however, no evidence to indicate that this observation has any significant bearing on the therapeutic use of the drug.

*Precautions:* Tegretol should be prescribed only after a critical benefit-risk appraisal and under close monitoring in patients with a history of cardiac, hepatic, or renal damage, adverse haematological reactions to other drugs, or interrupted courses of therapy with Tegretol.

Baseline and periodic complete urinalysis and BUN determinations are recommended.

Tegretol has shown mild anticholinergic activity; patients with glaucoma should therefore be warned and advised regarding possible hazards.

The possibility of activation of a latent psychosis, and in elderly patients the possibility of agitation or confusion, especially when high doses of Tegretol are administered, should be borne in mind.

*Use in pregnancy and lactation:* If pregnancy occurs in a woman receiving Tegretol or if the use of Tegretol is considered necessary during pregnancy the need to control seizures in the mother should be carefully weighed against the possible risk to the foetus. This is particularly important during the first three months of pregnancy. Minimum effective doses should be given and monitoring of plasma levels is recommended.

In women of childbearing age Tegretol should be administered as monotherapy, whenever possible.

Cases of developmental disorders and malformations, including spina bifida, have been reported in association with carbamazepine. However, offspring of mothers with untreated epilepsy are known to be prone to an increased incidence of development disorders and conclusive evidence that carbamazepine given alone increases the risk further is not available. Patients should be counselled regarding the possibility of an increased risk of malformations and given the opportunity of antenatal screening.

In animals (mice, rats and rabbits) oral administration of carbamazepine during organogenesis led to increased embryo mortality at daily doses which caused maternal toxicity (above 200 mg/kg b.w. daily i.e. 20 times the usual human dosage). No evidence of a teratogenic effect was observed in the three species studied but in one study using mice carbamazepine (40-240 mg/kg b.w. daily orally) caused defects in 4.7% of exposed foetuses compared with 1.3% in controls.

Anti-epileptic drugs may contribute to folic acid deficiency, a possible contributory cause of foetal abnormality. Folic acid supplementation is recommended before and during pregnancy.

Bleeding disorders in the newborn caused by anti-epileptic agents have been reported. As a precaution, Vitamin $K_1$ should be administered as a preventive measure in the last weeks of pregnancy and to the newborn.

Carbamazepine passes into the breast milk in concentrations of about 25-60% of the plasma level. This is not believed to present a significant hazard to the infant, which is likely to receive at most 10% of an appropriate therapeutic dose of carbamazepine for an infant with epilepsy. As with all drugs, the benefits of breast-feeding should be weighed against the remote possibility of an adverse effect occurring in the infant. There is one report of a severe skin (hypersensitivity) reaction in a breast-fed baby.

*Drug interactions:* Induction of hepatic enzymes in response to Tegretol may increase the metabolism and reduce the effectiveness of certain other drugs that are metabolised in the liver including: clobazam, clonazepam, ethosuximide, primidone, valproic acid, alprazolam, corticosteroids, hormonal contraceptive agents, cyclosporin, digoxin, doxycycline, felodipine, haloperidol, imipramine, methadone, theophylline, warfarin. The concurrent administration of carbamazepine has been reported to both raise and lower phenytoin levels and in rare instances mephenytoin plasma levels have been reported to increase.

Certain drugs have been shown to increase carbamazepine serum levels: macrolide antibiotics (erythromycin), isoniazid, calcium antagonists (verapamil, diltiazem), dextropropoxyphene, viloxazine, fluoxetine, cimetidine, acetazolamide, danazol, possibly desipramine and nicotinamide (only in adults and at high doses). Since raised carbamazepine levels may produce signs of overdosage (e.g. dizziness, drowsiness, ataxia, diplopia), the dosage of Tegretol should be adjusted accordingly.

Concomitant use of carbamazepine and isoniazid has been reported to increase isoniazid hepatotoxicity.

The combination of lithium and carbamazepine may cause enhanced neurotoxicity in spite of lithium plasma concentrations being within the therapeutic range.

Combined use of carbamazepine with metoclopramide or major tranquillisers, e.g. haloperidol, thioridazine, may also result in an increase in neurological side-effects.

Plasma levels of carbamazepine may be reduced by phenobarbitone, phenytoin, primidone, theophylline, also possibly clonazepam, and valproic acid (the data on the latter two compounds are contradictory).

Valproic acid, valpromide and primidone have been reported to increase the degree of conversion of carbamazepine to the active metabolite carbamazepine-10, 11-epoxide.

Concomitant medication with Tegretol and some diuretics (hydrochlorothiazide, frusemide) may lead to symptomatic hyponatraemia.

Carbamazepine may antagonise the effects of non-depolarising muscle relaxants (e.g. pancuronium); their dosage may need to be raised and patients monitored closely for unexpectedly rapid recovery from neuromuscular blockade.

Isotretinoin has been reported to alter unpredictably the bioavailability and/or clearance of carbamazepine and carbamazepine-10, 11-epoxide; carbamazepine plasma concentrations should be monitored.

Alcohol may exacerbate the CNS side-effects of psychoactive drugs including Tegretol; it is therefore advised that patients abstain from alcohol during treatment.

*Side-effects:* Provided a gradually increasing dosage scheme is followed, Tegretol is generally well tolerated but side effects may occur particularly at the start of treatment, or if the initial dose is too high. Dizziness, headache, ataxia, drowsiness, fatigue, diplopia, nausea or vomiting may be symptoms of carbamazepine overdosage and usually abate within a few days either spontaneously or after a transient dosage reduction. It is advisable to monitor the plasma levels and divide the daily dosage into smaller (i.e. 3-4) fractional doses.

*Central nervous system: Neurological:* Frequent: dizziness, ataxia, drowsiness, fatigue. Occasional: headache, diplopia, accommodation disorders (blurred vision). Rare: abnormal involuntary movements (tremor, asterixis, orofacial dyskinesia, choreoathetotic disorders, dystonia, tics), nystagmus. Isolated cases: oculomotor disturbances, speech disorders (e.g. dysarthria or slurred speech), peripheral neuritis, paraesthesiae, muscle weakness, and paretic symptoms.

*Psychiatric:* Isolated cases: hallucinations (visual or acoustic), depression, loss of appetite, restlessness, aggressive behaviour, agitation, confusion, activation of psychosis.

*Skin and appendages:* Occasional or frequent: allergic skin reactions, urticaria, which may be severe. Rare: exfoliative dermatitis and erythroderma, Stevens-Johnson syndrome, systemic lupus erythematosus-like syndrome. Isolated cases: toxic epidermal necrolysis, photosensitivity, erythema multiforme and nodosum, alterations in skin pigmentation, purpura, pruritus, acne, sweating, hair loss, hirsutism.

*Blood:* Occasional or frequent: leucopenia. Occasional: eosinophilia, thrombocytopenia. Rare: leucocytosis. Isolated cases: agranulocytosis, aplastic anaemia, pure red cell aplasia, megaloblastic anaemia, acute intermittent porphyria, reticulocytosis, folic acid deficiency, and possibly haemolytic anaemia.

*Liver:* Frequent: elevated gamma-GT (due to hepatic enzyme induction), usually not clinically relevant. Occasional: elevated alkaline phosphatase, rarely transaminases. Rare: jaundice, hepatitis of cholestatic, parenchymal (hepatocellular), or mixed type. Isolated cases: granulomatous hepatitis.

*Gastro-intestinal tract:* Occasional or frequent: nausea, vomiting. Occasional: dryness of the mouth. Rare: diarrhoea or constipation. Isolated cases: abdominal pain, glossitis, stomatitis. With suppositories occasional rectal irritation may occur.

*Hypersensitivity reactions:* Rare: a delayed multi-organ hypersensitivity disorder (of serum sickness type) with fever, skin rashes, vasculitis, lymphadenopathy, disorders mimicking lymphoma, arthralgia, leucopenia, eosinophilia, hepato-splenomegaly and abnormal liver function tests, occurring in various combinations. Other organs may also be affected (e.g. lungs, kidneys, pancreas, myocardium). Isolated

cases: aseptic meningitis, with myoclonus and peripheral eosinophilia, anaphylactic reaction.

Treatment must be discontinued immediately if such hypersensitivity reactions occur.

*Cardiovascular system:* Rare: disturbances of cardiac conduction.

Isolated cases: bradycardia, arrhythmias, AV-block with syncope, collapse, congestive heart failure, hypertension or hypotension, aggravation of coronary artery disease, thrombophlebitis, thromboembolism.

*Endocrine system and metabolism:* Occasional: Hyponatraemia, fluid retention, oedema, weight gain, and reduced plasma osmolality due to an antidiuretic hormone (ADH)-like effect, leading in isolated cases to water intoxication accompanied by lethargy, vomiting, headache, mental confusion, neurological abnormalities.

Isolated cases: gynaecomastia or galactorrhoea. Impaired male fertility and/or abnormal spermatogenesis; loss of libido/impotence; abnormal thyroid function tests: decreased L-thyroxine ($FT_4$, $T_4$, $T_3$) and increased TSH, usually without clinical manifestations; disturbances of bone metabolism (decrease in plasma calcium and 25-OH-cholecalciferol), leading to osteomalacia; elevated levels of cholesterol, including HDL cholesterol, and triglycerides.

*Renal:* Isolated cases: interstitial nephritis and renal failure. Signs of renal dysfunction including albuminuria, haematuria, oliguria and elevated BUN/ azotaemia, urinary frequency, urinary retention.

*Sense organs:* Isolated cases: taste disturbances; lens opacities, conjunctivitis, tinnitus, hyperacusis.

*Musculoskeletal system:* Isolated cases: arthralgia, muscle pain or cramp.

*Respiratory tract:* Isolated cases: pulmonary hypersensitivity characterised by dyspnoea, pneumonitis or pneumonia.

*Overdosage:*
*Signs and symptoms:* The presenting signs and symptoms of overdosage involve the central nervous, cardiovascular or respiratory systems.

Central nervous system: CNS depression; disorientation, somnolence, agitation, hallucination, coma; blurred vision, slurred speech, dysarthria, nystagmus, ataxia, dyskinesia, initially hyperreflexia, later hyporeflexia; convulsions, psychomotor disturbances, myoclonus, hypothermia.

Respiratory system: Respiratory depression, pulmonary oedema.

Cardiovascular system: Tachycardia, changes in blood pressure (hypotension and at times hypertension), cardiac arrhythmias, conduction disturbance with widening of QRS complex; syncope.

Gastro-intestinal system: Vomiting, delayed gastric emptying, reduced bowel motility.

Renal function: Retention of urine, oliguria or anuria; fluid retention, water intoxication due to ADH-like effect of carbamazepine.

Laboratory findings: Hyponatraemia, possibly metabolic acidosis, possibly hyperglycaemia, increased muscle creatinine phosphokinase.

*Treatment:* There is no specific antidote.

Management according to the patient's clinical condition. Possible admission to hospital. Measurement of the plasma level to confirm carbamazepine poisoning and to ascertain the size of the overdose. Evacuation of the stomach, gastric lavage, and administration of activated charcoal. Supportive medical care in an intensive care unit with cardiac monitoring and careful correction of electrolyte imbalance, if required.

Special recommendations:
Hypotension: administer dopamine or dobutamine i.v.

Disturbances of cardiac rhythm: to be managed on an individual basis.

Convulsions: administer a benzodiazepine (e.g. diazepam) or another anticonvulsant, e.g. phenobarbitone (with caution because of increased respiratory depression) or paraldehyde.

Hyponatraemia (water intoxication): fluid restriction and slow careful NaCl 0.9% infusion i.v. These measures may be useful in preventing brain damage.

Charcoal haemoperfusion has been recommended. Forced diuresis, haemodialysis, and peritoneal dialysis have been reported not to be effective.

Relapse and aggravation of symptomatology on the 2nd and 3rd day after overdose, due to delayed absorption, should be anticipated.

**Pharmaceutical precautions**
*Storage:* Liquid- Protect from heat (store below 25°C), keep container tightly closed.
Tablets 400 mg–Protect from moisture.
Retard tablets- Store below 25°C and protect from moisture.
Chewtabs–Protect from heat (store below 30°C).
Suppositories- Protect from heat (store below 30°C).

*Dilutions:* Tragacanth Mucilage BPC 1973 is suitable when used in 1:1 ratio with Tegretol liquid. After dilution, the liquid should be used within 14 days.

**Legal category** POM.

**Package quantities**
Liquid 100 mg/5 ml: Bottles of 300 ml
Tablets 100 mg: Blister packs of 84 and 100 and containers of 500
Tablets 200 mg: Blister packs of 84 and 100 and containers of 500
Tablets 400 mg: Blister packs of 56
Retard divisible tablets 200 mg: Blister packs of 56 and 100
Retard divisible tablets 400 mg: Blister packs of 56 and 100
Chewtabs 100 mg: Blister packs of 56
Chewtabs 200 mg: Blister packs of 56
Suppositories 125 mg: Packs of 5
Suppositories 250 mg: Packs of 5

**Further information** Tegretol chewtabs and liquid contain no sucrose and are therefore suitable for diabetics and children.

No problems would be expected if chewtabs were allowed to disintegrate in the mouth, i.e. sucked.

Pharmacokinetic studies have shown that chewtabs also perform well if inadvertently swallowed whole.

**Product licence numbers**
Liquid 100 mg/5 ml 00101/0456
Tablets 100 mg 00101/0461
Tablets 200 mg 00101/0462
Tablets 400 mg 00101/0463
Retard divisible tablets 200 mg 00101/0457
Retard divisible tablets 400 mg 00101/0458
Chewtabs 100 mg 00101/0454
Chewtabs 200 mg 00101/0455
Suppositories 125 mg 00101/0459
Suppositories 250 mg 00101/0460

## TOFRANIL*

**Qualitative and quantitative composition** The active ingredient is N-(γ-dimethylaminopropyl)-iminodibenzyl hydrochloride (imipramine hydrochloride).

One coated tablet contains 10 mg or 25 mg imipramine hydrochloride.

The syrup contains 25 mg imipramine base (equivalent to 25 mg imipramine hydrochloride) in every 5 mls.

**Pharmaceutical form** Coated tablets. Syrup.

**Clinical particulars**
*Therapeutic indications:* Symptoms of depressive illness. Relief of nocturnal enuresis in children.

*Posology and method of administration*
*Depression: Adults:* 1 x 25 mg up to three times daily, increasing stepwise to 150-200 mg. This should be reached by the end of the first week and maintained until definite improvement has occurred. The subsequent maintenance dose should be individually determined by gradually reducing the dosage, usually to about 50-100 mg daily.

In patients in hospital, i.e. severe cases, the dose may be increased to 100 mg three times daily until a distinct improvement is seen. Again the subsequent maintenance dose should be determined individually by reducing the dosage, usually to about 100 mg daily.

*Elderly patients:* Patients over 60 years of age may respond to lower doses of Tofranil than those recommended above. Treatment should be initiated with 10 mg daily, gradually increasing to 30-50 mg daily. The optimum dose should be reached after about 10 days and then continued until the end of treatment.

*Children:* (for nocturnal enuresis only). Not for use in children under 6 years.

6–7 years (weight 20-25 kg or 44-55lbs) 25 mg
8–11 years (weight 25-35 kg or 55-77lbs) 25–50 mg
Over 11 years (weight 35-54 kg or 77-119lbs) 50–75 mg

A daily dosage of 2.5 mg/kg should not be exceeded in children. The dose should be taken just before bedtime. The maximum period of treatment should not exceed three months and withdrawal should be gradual. Should a relapse occur, a further course of treatment should not be started until a full physical examination has been made.

*Contra-indications:* Known hypersensitivity to imipramine, any of the excipients or cross-sensitivity to other tricyclic antidepressants of the dibenzazepine group. Recent myocardial infarction. Any degree of heart block or other cardiac arrhythmias, mania, severe liver disease, narrow angle glaucoma. Infants and children under 6 years old. Retention of urine. Concurrent use in patients receiving, or within 3 weeks of cessation of therapy with, monoamine oxidase inhibitors. Concomitant treatment with selective, reversible MAO-A inhibitors such as moclobemide, is also contra-indicated.

*Special warnings and precautions for use*
*Warnings:* As improvement in depression may not occur for the first two to four weeks treatment, patients should be closely monitored during this period.

*Precautions:* Tricyclic antidepressants are known to lower the convulsion threshold and Tofranil should therefore be used with extreme caution in patients with epilepsy and other predisposing factors, e.g. brain damage of varying aetiology, concomitant use of neuroleptics, withdrawal from alcohol or drugs with anticonvulsive properties (e.g. benzodiazepines). It appears that the occurrence of seizures is dose dependent.

Concomitant treatment of Tofranil and electroconvulsive therapy should only be resorted to under careful supervision.

Caution is called for when giving tricyclic antidepressants to patients with severe renal disease.

Caution is called for when giving tricyclic antidepressants to patients with tumours of the adrenal medulla (e.g. phaeochromocytoma, neuroblastoma), in whom they may provoke hypertensive crises.

Many patients with panic disorders experience intensified anxiety symptoms at the start of the treatment with antidepressants. This paradoxical initial increase in anxiety is most pronounced during the first few days of treatment and generally subsides within two weeks.

Caution is indicated in patients with hyperthyroidism or during concomitant treatment with thyroid preparations, since aggravation of unwanted cardiac effects may occur.

Before initiating treatment it is advisable to check the patient's blood pressure, because individuals with hypotension or a labile circulation may react to the drug with a fall in blood pressure.

Althought changes in the white blood cell count have been reported with Tofranil only in isolated cases, periodic blood cell counts and monitoring for symptoms such as fever and sore throat are called for, particularly during the first few months of therapy.

Periodic monitoring of hepatic enzyme levels is recommended in patients with liver disease.

In elderly patients monitoring of cardiac function is indicated.

Because of its anticholinergic properties, Tofranil should be used with caution in patients with a history of increased intra-ocular pressure, narrow angle glaucoma, or urinary retention (e.g. diseases of the prostate).

Caution is called for in patients with chronic constipation. Tricyclic antidepressants may cause paralytic ileus, particularly in the elderly and bedridden patients.

Before general or local anaesthesia, the anaesthetist should be aware that the patient has been receiving Tofranil. Anaesthetics given during tri/tetracyclic antidepressant therapy may increase the risk of arrhythmias and hypotension (see interactions).

An increase in dental caries has been reported during long-term treatment with tricyclic antidepressants. Regular dental check-ups are therefore advisable during long-term treatment.

Decreased lacrimation and accummulation of mucoid secretions due to the anticholinergic properties of tricyclic antidepressants may cause damage to the corneal epithelium in patients with contact lenses.

Risk of suicide is inherent to severe depression and may persist until significant remission occurs. Patients posing a high suicide risk require close supervision.

Tofranil may cause anxiety, feelings of unrest, and hyperexcitation in agitated patients and patients with accompanying schizophrenic symptoms.

Activation of psychosis has occasionally been observed in schizophrenic patients receiving tricyclic antidepressants. Hypomanic or manic episodes have also been reported during a depressive phase in patients with cyclic affective disorders receiving treatment with a tricyclic antidepressant. In such cases it may be necessary to reduce the dosage of Tofranil or to withdraw it and administer an antipsychotic agent. After such episodes have subsided, low dose therapy with Tofranil may be resumed if required.

In predisposed and elderly patients, Tofranil may, particularly at night, provoke pharmacogenic (delirious) psychoses, which disappear without treatment within a few days of withdrawing the drug. Agitation, confusion and postural hypotension may occur.

Abrupt withdrawal should be avoided because of possible adverse reactions (see side effects).

Behavioural changes may occur in children receiving Tofranil for treatment of nocturnal enuresis.

*Interactions with other drugs and other types of interactions*
MAO inhibitors: Do not give Tofranil for at least 3 weeks after discontinuation of treatment with MAO inhibitors (there is a risk of severe symptoms such as hypertensive crisis, hyperpyrexia, myoclonus, agitation, seizures, dilirium and coma). The same applies when giving a MAO inhibitor after previous treatment with Tofranil. In both instances Tofranil or the MAO inhibitor should initially be given in small, gradually increasing doses and its effects monitored. There is evidence to suggest that tricyclic antidepressants may be given as little as 24 hours after a reversible MAO inhibitor such as moclobemide, but the 3 week washout period must be observed if the MAO inhibitor is given after a tricyclic antidepressant has been used.

Selective serotonin reuptake inhibitors: Co-medication may lead to additive effects on the serotonergic system. Fluvoxetine and fluvoxamine may also increase plasma concentrations of imipramine, with corresponding adverse effects, resulting in increased plasma levels of tricyclic antidepressants, a lowered convulsion threshold and seizures.

CNS depressants: Tricyclic antidepressants may also increase the effect of alcohol and central depressant drugs (eg barbiturates, benzodiazepines or general anaesthetics).

Alprazolam and disulfiram: It may be necessary to reduce the dosage of imipramine if it is administered concomitantly with aprazolam or disulfiram.

Neuroleptics: Co-medication may result in increased plasma levels of tricyclic antidepressants, a lowered convulsion threshold and seizures. Combination with thioridazine may produce severe cardiac arrhythmias.

Adrenergic neurone blockers: Tofranil may diminish or abolish the antihypertensive effects of guanethidine, betanidine, reserpine, clonidine and α-methyldopa. Patients requiring co-medication for hypertension should therefore be given antihypertensives of a different type (e.g. diuretics, vasodilators, or β-blockers).

Anticoagulants: Tricyclic antidepressants may potentiate the anti-coagulant effect of coumarin drugs by inhibiting hepatic metabolism of these anticoagulants. Careful monitoring of plasma prothrombin is therefore advised.

Anticholinergic agents: Tricyclic antidepressants may potentiate the effects of these drugs (e.g. phenothiazine, antiparkinsonian agents, antihistamines, atropine, biperiden) on the eye, central nervous system, bowel and bladder.

Sympathomimetic drugs: Tofranil may potentiate the cardiovascular effects of adrenaline, ephedrine, isoprenaline, noradrenaline, phenylephrine and phenylpropanolamine (e.g. as contained in local anaesthetic preparations and nasal decongestants).

Quinidine: Tricyclic antidepressants should not be employed in combination with anti-arrhythmic agents of the quinidine type.

Liver enzyme inducers: Drugs which activate the hepatic mono-oxygenase enzyme system (e.g. barbiturates, carbamazepine, phenytoin, nicotine, and oral contraceptives) may accelerate the metabolism and lower plasma concentrations of imipramine, resulting in decreased efficacy. Plasma levels of phenytoin and carbamazepine may increase, with corresponding adverse effects. It may be necessary to adjust the dosage of these drugs.

Cimetidine, methylphenidate: These drugs may increase the plasma concentrations of tricyclic antidepressants, whose dosage should therefore be reduced.

Oestrogens: There is evidence that oestrogens can sometimes paradoxically reduce the effects of Tofranil yet at the same time cause Tofranil toxicity.

*Pregnancy and lactation:* There is no evidence of the safety of the drug in human pregnancy. There have been isolated reports of a possible connection between the use of tricyclic antidepressants and adverse effects (developmental disorders) on the foetus, treatment with Tofranil should be avoided during pregnancy, unless the anticipated benefits justify the potential risk to the foetus.

Neonates whose mothers had taken Tofranil up until delivery have developed dyspnoea, lethargy, colic, irritability, hypotension or hypertension, tremor or spasms, during the first few hours or days. Tofranil should if possible be gradually withdrawn at least 7 weeks before the calculated date of confinement.

The active substance of Tofranil and its metabolite, desmethylimipramine, pass into the breast milk in small quantities. Tofranil should be gradually withdrawn or the mother advised to cease breast-feeding.

*Effects on ability to drive or use machines:* Patients receiving Tofranil should be warned that blurred vision, drowsiness and other CNS symptoms (see side effects) may occur, in which case they should not drive, operate machinery, or do anything which may require alertness or quick actions. Patients should also be warned that alcohol or other drugs may potentiate these effects (see Interactions).

*Undesirable effects:* If severe neurological or psychiatric reactions occur, Tofranil should be withdrawn.

Elderly patients are particularly sensitive to anticholinergic, neurological, psychiatric, or cardiovascular effects. Their ability to metabolise and eliminate drugs may be reduced, leading to a risk of elevated plasma concentrations at therapeutic doses.

The following side-effects, although not necessarily observed with Tofranil, have occured with tricyclic antidepressants.

(The following frequency estimates are used: frequent > 10%, occasional >1-10%, rare >0.001-1%, isolated cases < 0.001%)

*Central nervous system:*

*Psychiatric effects:* Occasionally fatigue, drowsiness, restlessness, delirium confusion, disorientation and hallucinations (particularly in geriatric patients and those suffering from Parkinsons's disease), increased anxiety, agitation, sleep disturbances, swings from depression to hypomania or mania. Rare: activation of psychotic symptoms. Isolated cases: aggresiveness.

*Neurological effects:* Frequently: tremor. Occasionally: paraesthesiae, headache, dizziness. Rarely, epileptic seizures. Isolated cases of EEG changes, myoclonus, weakness, extrapyramidal symptoms, ataxia, speech disorders, drug fever.

*Cardiovascular system:* Frequently sinus tachycardia and clinically irrelevant ECG changes (T and ST changes) in patients of normal cardiac status, postural hypotension.

Occasionally arrhythmias, conduction disorders (widening of QRS complex and PR interval, bundle-branch block), palpitations.

Isolated cases of increased blood pressure, cardiac decompensation, peripheral vasospastic reactions.

*Anticholinergic effects:* Frequently: dry mouth, sweating, constipation, disorders of visual accomodation, blurred vision, hot flushes. Occasionally: disturbances of micturition. Isolated cases of mydriasis, glaucoma, paralytic ileus.

*Gastro-intestinal tract:* Occasionally nausea, vomiting, anorexia. Isolated cases of stomatitis, tongue lesions, abdominal disorders.

*Hepatic effects:* Occasionally: elevated transaminases. Isolated cases of hepatitis with or without jaundice.

*Skin:* Occasionally: allergic skin reactions (skin rash, urticaria). Isolated cases of oedema (local or generalised), photosensitivity, pruritus, petechiae, hair loss.

*Endocrine system and metabolism:* Frequently weight gain. Occasionally disturbances of libido and potency. Isolated cases of enlarged mammary glands, galactorrhoea, SIADH (syndrome of inappropriate antidiuretic hormone secretion), increase or decrease in blood sugar, weight loss.

*Hypersensitivity:* Isolated cases of allergic alveolitis (pneumonitis) with or without eosinophilia, systemic anaphylactic/anaphylactoid reactions including hypotension.

*Blood:* Isolated cases of eosinophilia, leucopenia, agranulocytosis, thrombocytopenia and purpura.

*Sense organs:* Tinnitus.

*Miscellaneous:* Occasional withdrawal symptoms following abrupt discontinuation of treatment : nausea, vomiting, abdominal pain, diarrhoea, insomnia, headache, nervousness and anxiety.

*Overdose:* The signs and symptoms of overdose with Tofranil are similar to those reported with other tricyclic antidepressants. Cardiac abnormalities and neurological disturbances are the main complications. In children accidental ingestion of any amount should be regarded as serious and potentially fatal.

*Signs and symptoms:* Symptoms generally appear within 4 hours of ingestion and reach a maximum severity after 24 hours. Owing to delayed absorption (increased anticholinergic effect due to overdose), long half-life and enterohepatic recycling of the drug, the patient may be at risk for up to 4-6 days.

The following may be encountered :

Central nervous system : drowsiness, stupor, coma, ataxia, restlessness, agitation, enhanced reflexes, muscular rigidity, athetoid and choreiform movements, convulsions.

Cardiovascular System: Hypotension, tachycardia, arrhythmia, conduction disorders, heart failure; in very rare cases, cardiac arrest.

In addition, respiratory depression, cyanosis, shock, vomiting, fever, hydriasis, sweating and oliguria or anuria may occur.

*Treatment:* There is no specific antidote and treatment is essentially symptomatic and supportive

Anyone suspected of receiving an overdose of Tofranil, particularly children, should be admitted to hospital and kept under close surveillance for at least 72 hours.

Perform gastric lavage or induce vomiting as soon as possible if the patient is fully conscious. If the patient has impaired consciousness, secure the airway with a cuffed endotracheal tube before beginning lavage, and do not induce vomiting. These measures are recommended for up to 12 hours or even longer after the overdose, since the anticholinergic effect of the drug may delay gastric emptying. Administration of activated charcoal may help reduce drug absorption.

Treatment of symptoms is based on modern methods of intensive care, with continuous monitoring of cardiac function, blood gases and electrolytes, and if necessary emergency measures such as:

- anticonvulsive therapy,
- artificial respiration,
- insertion of a temporary cardiac pacemaker,
- plasma expander, dopamine or dobutamine administered by intravenous drip,
- resuscitation.

Since it has been reported that physostigmine may cause severe bradycardia, asystole and seizures, its use is not recommended in cases of overdosage with Tofranil. Haemodialysis or peritoneal dialysis are ineffective because of the low plasma concentrations of Tofranil.

**Pharmacological properties**

*Pharmacodynamic properties:* Pharmacotherapeutic group: Tricyclic antidepressant. Noradrenaline (NA) and serotonin (5HT) re-uptake inhibitor.

*Mechanism of action:* Imipramine is a tricyclic antidepressant and has several pharmacological actions including alpha-adrenolytic, anti-histaminic, anticholinergic and 5HT-receptor blocking properties. However, the main therapeutic activity is believed to be inhibition of the neuronal re-uptake of noradrenaline and 5HT. Imipramine is a so-called 'mixed' re-uptake blocker, i.e.it inhibits the reuptake of NA and 5HT to about the same extent.

*Pharmacokinetic properties*

*Absorption:* Imipramine is absorbed quickly and completely following oral administration. The intake of food has no effect on its absorption and bioavailability. During its first passage through the liver, orally administered imipramine becomes partly converted to desmethylimipramine, a metabolite which also exhibits antidepressant activity.

During oral administration of 50 mg 3 times daily for 10 days, the mean steady-state plasma concentrations of imipramine and desmethylimipramine were 33-85ng/ml and 43-109ng/ml respectively. Owing to lower clearance in the plasma, resulting in increased systemic availability, elderly patients require lower doses of imipramine than patients in intermediate age groups. Renal impairment is not expected to have any influence on the kinetics of unchanged imipramine and its desmethyl metabolite since both are excreted only in small amounts by the kidneys.

*Distribution:* About 86% of imipramine binds to plasma proteins. Concentrations of imipramine in the cerebrospinal fluid and the plasma are highly correlated. The mean distribution volume is about 21L/kg.

Imipramine and its metabolite desmethylimipramine both pass into breast milk in concentrations similar to those found in the plasma.

*Biotransformation:* Imipramine is extensively metabolised in the liver. It is cleared mainly by demethylation and to a lesser extent by hydroxylation. Both metabolic pathways are under genetic control.

*Elimination:* Imipramine is eliminated from the blood with a mean half-life of about 19 hours. About 80% is excreted in the urine and about 20% in the faeces, mainly in the form of inactive metabolites. Urinary excretion of unchanged imipramine and of the active metabolite desmethylimipramine is about 5% and 6%, respectively. Only small quantities of these are excreted in the faeces.

*Characteristics in patients:* Owing to reduced metabolic clearance, plasma concentrations of imipramine are higher in elderly patients than in younger patients.

In children the mean clearance and elimination half-life does not differ significantly from adult controls but the between-patient variability is high.

In patients with severe renal impairment, no change occurs in renal excretion of imipramine and its biologically active unconjugated metabolites. However steady-state plasma concentrations of the conjugated metabolites, which are considered to be biologically inactive are elevated. The clinical significance of this finding is not known.

*Preclinical safety data:* Imipramine has no mutagenic or carcinogenic potential. Studies in four species (mouse, rat, rabbit and monkey) led to the conclusion that orally administered imipramine has no teratogenic potential. Experiments with high doses of parenterally administered imipramine resulted mainly in severe maternal and embryotoxic effects, they were thus inconclusive with regard to teratogenic effects.

**Pharmaceutical particulars**

*List of excipients:* Coated tablets of 10 mg and 25 mg contain glycerol, lactose, magnesium stearate, maize starch, stearic acid, silicon dioxide, hydroxypropyl methylcellulose, microcrystalline cellulose, titanium dioxide, red iron oxide, polyethylene glycol, povidone, sucrose, talc.

The syrup contains tragacanth, sucrose, methyl hydroxybenzoate, propyl hydroxybenzoate, sorbitol, titanium dioxide, cream flavour (Cornish C9014) and water.

*Incompatibilities:* None known.

*Shelf-life:* Coated tablets of 10 mg and 25 mg: Five years.

Syrup: Four years

*Special precautions for storage:* Coated tablets of 10 mg and 25 mg: Protect from moisture.

Syrup: Store below 25°C. Keep containers tightly closed.

Medicines should be kept out of reach of children.

*Nature and contents of container:* Tablets 10 mg: Red-brown, sugar coated, triangular shaped tablets, 5.8 mm in diameter, imprinted with GEIGY on one side–packed in PVC/foil bubble packs of 84 tablets.

Tablets 25 mg: Red-brown, sugar coated, round biconvex tablets, 5.5 mm in diameter imprinted GEIGY on one side–packed in PVC/foil bubble packs of 84 tablets.

Syrup 25 mg/5 ml: White, viscous syrup contained in a glass bottle with a child resistant clic-loc cap.

*Instruction for use/handling:* None.

*Marketing authorisation holder:* Ciba-Geigy plc, Hulley Road, Macclesfield, Cheshire SK10 2NX.

**Marketing authorisation numbers**

Tablets 10 mg 0001/5030R
Tablets 25 mg 0001/5029R
Syrup 25 mg/5 ml 0001/5032R

**Date of approval/revision of SPC** 15 January 1996

**Legal category** POM

## TRANSIDERM-NITRO* 5 and 10

**Presentation** Transiderm-Nitro is a transdermal drug delivery system, comprising a self-adhesive, pink coloured patch, containing a drug reservoir of glyceryl trinitrate.

For each Transiderm-Nitro 5, the average amount of glyceryl trinitrate absorbed per patch in 24 hours is 5 mg. Each patch has a contact surface measuring 10cm², and a glyceryl trinitrate content of 25 mg.

For Transiderm-Nitro 10, the average amount of glyceryl trinitrate absorbed per patch in 24 hours is 10 mg. Each patch has a contact surface measuring 20cm², and a glyceryl trinitrate content of 50 mg.

**Uses**

*Indications:* Prophylactic treatment of attacks of angina pectoris, as monotherapy or in combination with other anti-anginal agents.

Transiderm-Nitro 5 only: Prophylactic treatment of phlebitis and extravasation secondary to venous cannulation for intravenous fluid and drug administration when the duration of treatment is expected to last for 2 days or longer.

*Mode of action:* Nitroglycerin relaxes smooth muscle. It acts chiefly on systemic veins and large coronary arteries, with more predominant effects on the former. In angina pectoris the fundamental mechanism of action of nitroglycerin is based on an increase in venous capacitance leading to a decreased return of blood to the heart. Owing to this, preload and hence filling volume diminishes, resulting in a decreased myocardial oxygen requirement at rest and especially during exercise.

In the coronary arterial circulation nitroglycerin dilates extramural conductance and small resistance vessels. It appears to cause redistribution of coronary blood flow to the ischaemic subendocardium by selectively dilating large epicardial vessels and also relaxes vasospasm.

Nitroglycerin dilates the arteriolar vascular bed, as a result of which afterload and left ventricular systolic wall tension decrease, leading to a reduction in myocardial oxygen consumption.

*Pharmacokinetics:* Following single application, plasma concentrations of nitroglycerin reach a plateau within 2 hours, which is maintained throughout the day until patch removal. The height of this plateau is directly proportional to the size of the system's drug-releasing area.

The same plasma levels are attained regardless of whether the system is applied to the skin of the upper arm, pelvis or chest. Upon removal of Transiderm-Nitro the plasma level falls rapidly. After repeated application of Transiderm-Nitro no cumulation occurs.

**Dosage and administration**

*Adults:*

*Angina:* Treatment should be initiated with one Transiderm-Nitro 5 patch daily. If a higher dosage is required a Transiderm-Nitro 10 patch may be substituted. The dosage may be increased to a maximum of two Transiderm-Nitro 10 patches daily in resistant cases. Transiderm-Nitro may be given either continuously, or intermittently with a patch-off period of 8-12 hours, usually at night, during each 24 hour period. Development of tolerance or attenuation of therapeutic effect commonly occurs with prolonged or frequent administration of all long-acting nitrates. Recent evidence suggests that intermittent therapy with Transiderm-Nitro may reduce the incidence of tolerance.

Prior to the use of intermittent therapy, the clinical benefits to the patient should be weighed against the risks of angina in the patch-free interval. In patients considered to be at risk, concomitant anti-anginal therapy should be implemented (see 'Precautions').

It is recommended that the patch is applied to the lateral chest wall. The replacement patch should be applied to a new area of skin. Allow several days to elapse before applying a fresh patch to the same area of skin.

If acute attacks of angina pectoris occur, rapidly acting nitrates may be required.

*Phlebitis and extravasation:* One Transiderm-Nitro 5 patch is to be applied distal to the site of intravenous cannulation at the time of venepuncture. The patch should be removed after 3-4 days and a new replacement patch applied to a different area of skin. Treatment with Transiderm-Nitro should be discontinued once intravenous therapy has stopped.

*Use in the elderly:* No specific information on use in the elderly is available, however, no evidence exists to suggest that an alteration in dosage is required.

*Use in children:* There is insufficient knowledge of the effects of Transiderm-Nitro in children and therefore recommendations for its use cannot be made.

### Contra-indications, warnings, etc

*Contra-indications:* Transiderm-Nitro should not be prescribed to patients hypersensitive to nitrates. Severe hypotension. Increased intracranial pressure. Myocardial insufficiency due to obstruction (e.g. in the presence of aortic or mitral stenosis or of constrictive pericarditis).

*Precautions:* In recent myocardial infarction or acute heart failure, Transiderm-Nitro should be employed only under careful surveillance.

As with all anti-anginal nitrate preparations, withdrawal of long-term treatment should be gradual, by replacement with decreasing doses of long-acting oral nitrates.

The system should be removed before cardioversion or DC defibrillation is attempted. This is to avoid the possibility of arcing between the patch and the electrodes. Also the system should be removed before diathermy treatment.

Caution should be exercised in patients with arterial hypoxaemia due to severe anaemia because, in such patients the biotransformation of nitroglycerin is reduced. Similarly, caution is called for in patients with hypoxaemia and a ventilation/perfusion imbalance due to lung disease or ischaemic heart failure.

Postural hypotension has been reported rarely following initiation of treatment with Transiderm-Nitro and care is advised when driving or operating machinery.

Nitrate therapy may aggravate the angina caused by hypertrophic cardiomyopathy.

The possibility of increased frequency of angina during patch-off periods should be considered. In such cases, the use of concomitant anti-anginal therapy is desirable.

If tolerance to nitroglycerin patches develops, the effect of sublingual nitroglycerin on exercise tolerance may be partially diminished.

*Pregnancy and lactation:* As with all drugs, Transiderm-Nitro should not be prescribed during pregnancy, particularly during the first trimester, unless there are compelling reasons for doing so.

It is not known whether the active substance passes into the breast milk. The benefits for the mother must be weighed against the risks for the child.

*Drug interactions:* Concomitant treatment with other vasodilators, calcium antagonists, ACE inhibitors, beta-blockers, diuretics, antihypertensives, tricyclic antidepressants and major tranquillisers, as well as the consumption of alcohol, may potentiate the blood pressure lowering effects of Transiderm-Nitro.

Concurrent administration of Transiderm-Nitro with dihydroergotamine may increase the bioavailability of dihydroergotamine and lead to coronary vasoconstriction.

The possibility that the ingestion of acetylsalicylic acid and non-steroidal anti-inflammatory drugs might diminish the therapeutic response to Transiderm-Nitro cannot be excluded.

*Side effects:*
*Central nervous system:* Like other preparations, Transiderm-Nitro may give rise to headache, which is due to cerebral vasodilation and is dose-dependant. Such headaches, however, may regress after a few days despite continuation of the therapy. If they do not disappear, they should be treated with mild analgesics. In cases where headaches are unresponsive to treatment, the dosage of nitroglycerin should be reduced or use of the product discontinued.

*Skin:* Reddening of the skin, with or without local itching or burning sensation, as well as allergic contact dermatitis may occasionally occur. Upon removal of the patch, any slight reddening of the skin will usually disappear within a few hours. The application site

should be changed on patch replacement to prevent local irritation.

*Cardiovascular:* Facial flushing, faintness, dizziness or lightheadedness, and postural hypotension, which may be associated with reflex-induced tachycardia, have been reported rarely. Reflex tachycardia can be controlled by concomitant treatment with a beta-blocker.

*Gastro-intestinal:* Rarely nausea, vomiting.

*Treatment of overdosage:*
*Signs:* High doses of glyceryl trinitrate are known to cause pronounced systemic side effects, eg a marked fall in blood pressure and reflex tachycardia resulting in collapse and syncope. Methemoglobinaemia has also been reported following accidental overdosage of nitroglycerin. However, with Transiderm-Nitro, the release membrane will reduce the likelihood of overdosage occurring.

*Management:* In contrast to long acting oral nitrate preparations, the effect of Transiderm-Nitro can be rapidly terminated simply by removing the system. Any fall in blood pressure or signs of collapse that may occur, may be managed by general resuscitative measures.

**Pharmaceutical precautions** Store below 25°C.

**Legal category** P

**Package quantities** Boxes of 28 and 30 patches.

**Further information** Transiderm-Nitro gives a controlled release of glyceryl trinitrate over at least 24 hours, and thereby avoids high peaks of blood levels, minimising the incidence of side-effects.

Although glyceryl trinitrate is volatile, resulting, in the case of most products, in a loss of the drug after relatively short storage, the design of the Transiderm-Nitro patch ensures that the dosage to the patient is maintained even after 2 years storage.

**Product licence numbers**
Transiderm-Nitro 5   00101/0464
Transiderm-Nitro 10   00101/0465

*Product licence holder:* Ciba-Geigy plc, Hulley Road, Macclesfield, Cheshire SK10 2NX.

## TRASICOR*

**Presentation** Trasicor tablets each containing 20 mg oxprenolol hydrochloride PhEur. Circular, flat, white film-coated tablets with bevelled edges having the monogram CIBA impressed on one side and Trasicor 20 on the other.

Trasicor tablets each containing 40 mg oxprenolol hydrochloride PhEur. Circular, flat, white film-coated tablets with bevelled edges having the monogram CIBA impressed on one side and Trasicor 40 on the other.

Trasicor tablets each containing 80 mg oxprenolol hydrochloride PhEur. Circular, flat, pale-yellow film-coated tablets with bevelled edges having the monogram CIBA impressed on one side and Trasicor 80 on the other.

All strengths of Trasicor tablets contain: calcium phosphate hydroxypropyl-methylcellulose, magnesium stearate, talc, and titanium dioxide.

In addition: 20 mg and 40 mg tablets contain: polyvinylpyrrolidone, sucrose, wheat starch and vinylpyrrolidone-vinylacetate copolymer.

80 mg tablets contain: maize starch, polyvinylpyrrolidone, silicon dioxide, sodium starch glycollate (sodium carboxymethyl starch), polysorbate and yellow iron oxide.

### Uses

*Indications:* Angina pectoris: for long-term prophylactic use (if necessary nitrates should be employed for alleviating acute attacks).

Hypertension: as monotherapy or for use in combination with other antihypertensives, e.g. with a diuretic, peripheral vasodilator, calcium channel blocker or ace inhibitor.

Disburbances of cardiac rhythm: especially supraventricular tachycardia, atrial fibrillation and digitalis-induced arrhythmias, ventricular tachycardia.

Short-term relief of functional cardiovascular disorders due to adrenergic hyperactivity: such as cardiac neurosis, hyperkinetic heart syndrome and anxiety-induced cardiovascular disorders.

*Mode of action:* Oxprenolol, the active substance of Trasicor, is a non-selective, lipophilic beta-blocker exerting a sympatholytic effect and displaying mild to modest partial agonistic activity (PAA), also known as intrinsic sympathomimetic activity (ISA).

Drugs like oxprenolol with PAA cause comparatively less slowing of the resting heart rate and a less marked negative-inotropic effect than those without PAA. The risk of substantial bradycardia at rest and heart failure is lessened.

The antiarrhythmic effect of oxprenolol is primarily due to suppression of the arrhythmogenic sympathetic influence of catecholamines. Evidence that

increased sympathetic stimulation predisposes to many arrhythmias is strong. This is supported by the increased incidence of arrhythmias in man in situations associated with high sympathetic drive or myocardial sensitisation to catecholamines e.g. exercise, emotional stress, phaeochromocytoma, trauma, myocardial ischaemia, anaesthesia, hyperthyroidism.

Oxprenolol decreases cardiac impulse formation in the sinus node with resultant slowing of the sinus rate; it slightly prolongs the sino-atrial conduction time; both the atrio-ventricular (AV) conduction time and the AV node refractory periods are lengthened.

Some β-blockers such as oxprenolol possess a membrane stabilising activity (MSA) on the cardiac action potential, also known as 'quinidine-like' or 'local anaesthetic' action, a property that tends to result in greater cardiac depression than is seen with β-blockers which do not have this pharmacological characteristic. However, at normal therapeutic doses, this property is probably clinically irrelevant and it only becomes manifest after overdose.

In coronary artery disease, oxprenolol is beneficial in increasing exercise tolerance and decreasing the frequency and severity of anginal attacks.

Emotional stress and anxiety states, the symptoms of which are largely caused by increased sympathetic drive, are alleviated by the sympatholytic effect of oxprenolol.

The exact way in which β-blockers exert their antihypertensive action is still not fully understood. Various modes of action have been postulated. During chronic therapy the antihypertensive effect of β-blockers is associated with a decline in peripheral resistance.

Oxprenolol is effective in lowering elevated supine, standing and exercise blood pressure; postural hypotension is unlikely to occur.

*Pharmacokinetics:* Absorption: Oral oxprenolol is rapidly and completely absorbed. Food has no significant effect on absorption. Peak plasma concentrations are achieved approximately 1 hour after drug administration.

Biotransformation: Oxprenolol is subject to a first-pass metabolism. Its systemic bioavilability is 20–70%.

Distribution: Oxprenolol has a plasma protein binding rate of approximately 80% and a calculated distribution volume of 1.2 l/kg.

Oxprenolol crosses the placental barrier. The concentration in the breast milk is equivalent to approx. 30% of that in the plasma.

Elimination: Oxprenolol has an elimination half-life of 1-2 hours. Oxprenolol is extensively metabolised, direct O-glucuronidation being the major metabolic pathway and oxidative reactions minor ones. Oxprenolol is excreted chiefly in the urine (almost entirely in the form of inactive metabolites). The drug is not likely to accumulate.

Characteristics in patients: Age has no effect on the pharmacokinetics of oxprenolol.

In patients with acute or chronic inflammatory diseases, an increase in the plasma levels of oxprenolol has been observed. The plasma levels may also increase in the presence of severe hepatic insufficiency associated with a reduced metabolism.

Impaired renal function generally leads to an increase in the blood levels of oxprenolol, but the concentrations measured remain within – although at the upper limit of – the concentration range recorded in subjects with healthy kidneys. In addition, in patients with renal failure the apparent elimination half-life for unchanged, i.e. active, oxprenolol is comparable with the corresponding half-life values determined in subjects with no renal disease. Hence, there is no need to readjust the dosage in the presence of impaired renal function.

**Dosage and administration** The dosage should be individualised. Before raising the dosage, the heart rate at rest should always be checked. If it is 50-55 beats/min, the dosage should not be increased, see *Contra-indications.* The tablets should be swallowed with liquid.

If the maximum recommended dose is insufficient to produce the desired response appropriate combined therapy should be considered.

When discontinuing prolonged treatment with a beta-blocker, the medication should not be interrupted abruptly, but withdrawn gradually.

Higher doses using conventional Trasicor tablets may be administered in two or more divided doses.

*Elderly:* no special dosage regime is necessary but concurrent hepatic insufficiency should be taken into account.

*Children:* no adequate experience has been acquired on the use of Trasicor in children.

*Hypertension:* 80-160 mg total daily dose, given in 2 to 3 doses. If necessary the dosage can be raised to 320 mg.

*Angina pectoris:* 80–160 mg total daily dose, given in

2 to 3 doses. If necessary the dosage can be raised to 320 mg.

*Disturbances of cardiac rhythm:* 40–240 mg total daily dose given in 2 to 3 doses. The maximum dose recommended is 240 mg/day.

*Short-term relief of functional cardiovascular disorders due to adrenergic hyperactivity, e.g. short-term relief of sympathomimetic symptoms of anxiety:* 40–80 mg daily, given in 1 or 2 doses, is usually sufficient.

**Contra-indications, warnings, etc**

*Contra-indications:* Trasicor is contra-indicated in patients with:

- Hypersensitivity to oxprenolol and related derivatives, cross-sensitivity to other β-blockers or to any of the excipients
- Cardiogenic shock
- Second or third degree atrioventricular block
- Uncontrolled heart failure
- Sick-sinus syndrome
- Bradycardia (<45–50 bpm)
- Hypotension
- Untreated phaeochromocytoma
- Severe peripheral arterial circulatory disturbances
- History of bronchospasm and broncial asthma
- Prinzmetal's angina (variant angina pectoris)
- Use of anaesthetics which are known to have a negative inotropic effect
- Metabolic acidosis

*Warnings:* Patients receiving oxprenolol should be warned that dizziness, fatigue or visual disturbances (see *Side effects*) may occur, in which case they should not drive, operate machinery or do anything else requiring alertness, particularly if they also consume alcohol.

*Precautions:* Owing to the risk of bronchoconstriction, non-selective beta-blockers such as Trasicor should be used with particular caution in patients with chronic bronchitis or emphysema (see *Contra-indications*).

As β-blockers increase the AV conduction time, beta-blockers should only be given with caution to patients with first degree AV block.

Beta-blockers should not be used in patients with untreated congestive heart failure. This condition should first be stabilised.

If the patient develops increasing bradycardia less than 50–55 beats per minute at rest and the patient experiences symptoms related to bradycardia, the dosage should be reduced or gradually withdrawn (see *Contra-indications*).

β-blockers are liable to affect carbohydrate metabolism. Diabetic patients, especially those dependent on insulin, should be warned that β-blockers can mask the symptoms of hypoglycaemia (e.g. tachycardia) (see *Interactions with other medicaments and other forms of interaction*). Hypoglycaemia, producing loss of consciousness in some cases, may occur in non-diabetic individuals who are taking β-blockers, particularly those who undergo prolonged fasting or severe exercise. The concurrent use of β-blockers and anti-diabetic medication should always be monitored to confirm that diabetic control is well maintained.

β-blockers may mask certain clinical signs (e.g. tachycardia) of hyperthyroidism and the patients should be carefully monitored.

Beta-blockers may reduce liver function and thus affect the metabolism of other drugs. Like many beta-blockers, oxprenolol undergoes substantial first-pass hepatic metabolism. In the presence of liver cirrhosis the bioavailability of oxprenolol may be increased leading to higher plasma concentrations (see *Pharmacokinetic properties*). Patients with severe renal failure might be more susceptible to the effects of antihypertensive drugs due to haemodynamic effects. Careful monitoring is advisable (see *Pharmacokinetic properties*).

In patients with peripheral circulatory disorders (e.g. Raynaud's disease or syndrome, intermittent claudication), beta-blockers should be used with great caution as aggravation of these disorders may occur (see *Contra-indications*).

In patients with phaeochromocytoma a β-blocker should only be given with an α-blocker (see *Contra-indications*).

Owing to the danger of cardiac arrest, a calcium antagonist of the verapamil type must not be administered intravenously to a patient already receiving treatment with a β-blocker. Furthermore, since β-blockers may potentiate the negative-inotropic and dromotropic effects of ca-antagonists, like verapamil or diltiazem, any oral co-medication (e.g. in angina pectoris) requires close clinical control (see also *Drug interactions*).

Anaphylactic reactions precipitated by other agents may be particularly severe in patients taking beta-blockers, especially non-selective drugs, and may require higher than normal doses of adrenaline for treatment. Whenever possible, β-blockers should be discontinued in patients who are at increased risk for anaphylaxis.

Especially in patients with ischaemic heart disease, treatment should not be discontinued suddenly. The dosage should gradually be reduced, i.e. over 1–3 weeks, if necessary, at the same time initiating alternative therapy to prevent exacerbation of angina pectoris.

If a patient receiving oxprenolol requires anaesthesia, the anesthetist should be informed of the use of the medication prior to the use of a general anaesthetic to permit him to take the necessary precautions. The anaesthetic selected should be one exhibiting as little negative inotropic activity as possible, e.g. halothane/nitrous oxide. If, on the other hand, inhibition of sympathetic tone during the operation is regarded as undesirable, the β-blocker should be withdrawn gradually at least 48 hours prior to surgery.

The full development of the 'oculomucocutaneous syndrome', as previously described with practolol has not been reported with oxprenolol. However, some features of this syndrome has been noted, such as dry eyes alone or occasionally associated with skin rash. In most cases the symptoms cleared after withdrawal of the treatment. Discontinuation of oxprenolol should be considered, and a switch to another antihypertensive drug might be advisable, see advice on discontinuation above.

*Use in pregnancy and lactation:* As in the case of any form of drug therapy, oxprenolol should be employed with caution during pregnancy, especially in the first 3 months.

β-blockers may reduce placental perfusion, which may result in intrauterine foetal death, immature and premature deliveries. Use the lowest possible dose. If possible, discontinue beta-blocker therapy at least 2 to 3 days prior to delivery to avoid the effects on uterine contractility and possible adverse effects, especially bradycardia and hypoglycaemia, in the foetus and neonate.

Oxprenolol is excreted into breast milk (see *Pharmacokinetic properties*) and although the esimated daily infant dose derived from breast-feeding is likely to be very low, breast feeding is not recommended.

*Drug interactions:*

*Calcium channel blockers:* e.g. Verapamil, diltiazem: Potentiation of bradycardia, myocardial depression and hypotension; particularly after intravenous administration of verapamil in patients taking oral β-blockers, the possibility of hypotension and cardiac arrhythmia cannot be excluded (see *Warnings* and *Precautions*).

*Class 1 anti-arrhythmic drugs and amiodarone:* Drugs like disopyramide, quinidine and amiodarone may increase atrial-conduction time and induce negative isotropic effect when administered concomitantly with beta-blockers.

*Sympathomimetic drugs:* Non-cardioselective beta-blockers such as oxprenolol enhance the pressor response to sympathomimetic drugs such as adrenaline, noradrenaline, isoprenaline, ephedrine and phenylphrine (e.g. local anaesthetics in dentistry, nasal and ocular drops), resulting in hypertension and bradycardia.

*Clonidine:* When clonidine is used in conjunction with non-selective beta-blockers, such as oxprenolol, treatment with clonidine should be continued for some time after β-blocker has been discontinued to reduce the danger of rebound hypertension.

*Catecholamine-depleting drugs:* e.g. guanethidine, reserpine, may have an additive effect when administered concomitantly with beta-blockers. Patients should be closely observed for hypotension.

Beta-blockers may modify blood glucose concentrations in patients being treated with insulin and oral antidiabetic drugs and may alter the response to hypoglycaemia by prolonging the recovery (blood glucose rise) from hypoglycaemia, causing hypotension and blocking tachycardia. In diabetic patients receiving β-blockers hypoglycaemic episodes may not result in the expected tachycardia but hypoglycaemia-induced sweating will occur and may even be intensified and prolonged (see *Warnings* and *Precautions*).

*Non-steroidal anti-inflammatory drugs (NSAIDs):* Non-steroidal anti-inflammatory (NSAIDs) can reduce the hypotensive effect of beta-blockade.

*Cimetidine:* Hepatic metabolism of beta-blockers may be reduced resulting in increased plasma levels of β-blocker and prolonged serum half-life. Marked bradycardia may occur.

*Ergot alkaloids:* Concomitant administration with beta-blockers may enhance the vasoconstrictive action of ergot alkaloids.

*Anaesthetic drugs:* β-blockers and certain anaesthetics (e.g. halothane) are additive in their cardio-depressant effect. However, continuation of beta-blockers reduces the risk of arrhythmia during anaesthesia (see *Warnings* and *Precautions*).

*Digitalis glycosides:* Beta-blockers and digitalis glycosides may be additive in their depressant effect on myocardial conduction, particularly through the atrioventricular node, resulting in bradycardia or heart block.

*Lidocaine:* Concomitant administration with beta-blockers may increase lidocaine blood concentrations and potential toxicity; patients should be closely monitored for increased lidocaine effects.

Alcohol and beta-blocker effects on the central nervous system have been observed to be additive and it is possible that symptoms such as dizziness may be exaggerated if alcohol and Trasicor are taken together (see also *Warnings*).

*Side-effects:* Frequency estimate: Very common >10%, common >1%–10%, uncommon >0.1%–1%, rare >0.01%–0.1%, very rare <0.01%.

Central nervous system: Common: fatigue, dizziness, headache, mental depression. Uncommon: sleep disturbances, nightmares. Rare: hallucinations, exertional tiredness.

Cardiovascular system: Common: hypotension, heart failure, peripheral vascular disorders (e.g. cold extremities, paraesthesia). Uncommon: bradycardia, disturbance of cardiac conduction. Rare: Raynaud-like symptoms.

Gastro-intestinal tract: Very common: dry mouth, constipation. Common: nausea. Uncommon: diarrhoea, vomiting, flatulence.

Skin and appendages: Uncommon: allergic skin rash (e.g. urticarial, psoriasiform, eczematous, lichenoid). Rare: worsening of psoriasis.

Respiratory system: Common: dyspnoea, bronchoconstriction (see *Precautions* and *Contra-indications*).

Sense organs: Uncommon: visual disturbances ('blurred vision', 'vision abnormal'). Rare: dry eyes, keratoconjunctivitis.

Others: disturbances of libido and potency. Very rare: thrombocytopenia.

*Overdosage: Signs and symptoms:* Poisoning due to an overdosage of β-blocker may lead to pronounced hypotension, bradycardia, hypoglycaemia, heart failure, cardiogenic shock, conduction abnormalities (first or second degree block, complete heart block, asystole), or even cardiac arrest. In addition, dyspnoea, bronchospasm, vomiting, impairment of consciousness, and also generalised convulsions may occur.

The manifestations of poisoning with beta-blocker are dependent on the pharmacological properties of the ingested drug. Although the onset of action is rapid, effects of massive overdose may persist for several days despite declining plasma levels. Watch carefully for cardiovascular or respiratory deterioration in an intensive care setting, particularly in the early hours. Observe mild overdose cases for at least 4 hours for the development of signs of poisoning.

*Treatment:* Patients who are seen soon after potentially life-threatening overdosage (within 4 hours) should be treated by gastric lavage and activated charcoal.

Treatment of symptoms is based on modern methods of intensive care, with continuous monitoring of cardiac function, blood gases, and electrolytes, and if necessary, emergency measures such as artificial respiration, resuscitation or cardiac pacemaker.

Significant bradycardia should be treated initially with atropine. Large doses of isoprenaline may be necessary for control of heart rate and hypotension. Glucagon has positive chronotropic and inotropic effects on the heart that are independent of interactions with beta-adrenergic receptors and it represents a useful alternative treatment for hypotension and heart failure.

For seizures, diazepam has been effective and is the drug of choice.

For bronchospasm, aminophylline, salbutamol or terbutaline ($\beta_2$ agonist) are effective bronchodilator drugs. Monitor the patient for dysrhythmias during and after administration.

Patients who recover should be observed for signs of β-blocker withdrawal phenomenon (see *Special warnings and precautions*).

**Pharmaceutical precautions** The tablets should be protected from moisture.

**Legal category** POM.

**Package quantities**
Tablets 20 mg: Blister packs of 56 and 100.
Tablets 40 mg: Blister packs of 56 and 100.
Tablets 80 mg: Blister packs of 56.

**Further information** Nil.

**Product licence numbers**

| | |
|---|---|
| Tablets 20 mg | 00101/0430 |
| Tablets 40 mg | 00101/0431 |
| Tablets 80 mg | 00101/0432 |

## TRASIDREX*

**Presentation** Trasidrex tablets each contain 160 mg oxprenolol hydrochloride PhEur in a sustained release core and 0.25 mg cyclopenthiazide BP in the coat. The tablets are circular, with a pinkish-red sugar coat, and are printed CIBA on one side and TRASIDREX on the other, both words in black.

Trasidrex tablets also contain sucrose.

**Uses**

*Indications:* Hypertension.

*Mode of action:* Trasidrex contains two components which have different sites of action and whose antihypertensive effects are mutually complimentary.

*Oxprenolol* – Oxprenolol, one of the active substance of Trasidrex, is a non-selective, lipophilic β-blocker exerting a sympatholytic effect and displaying mild to moderate partial agonist activity (PAA), also known as intrinsic sympathomimetic activity (ISA).

The exact way in which β-blockers exert their antihypertensive action is still not fully understood. Various modes of action have been postulated. In the long run the antihypertensive effect of β-blockers always parallels a decline in peripheral vascular resistance.

Oxprenolol is effective in lowering elevated supine, standing and exertional blood pressure; substantial hypotensive reactions are less likely to occur. Emotional stress and anxiety states which are largely caused by increased sympathetic drive are alleviated by the sympatholytic effect of oxprenolol.

*Cyclopenthiazide*– Cyclopenthiazide, one of the two active substances of Trasidrex, is a benzothiadiazine (thiazide) diuretic.

Thiazide diuretics act primarily on the distal renal tubule (early convoluted part), inhibiting NaCl reabsorption (by antagonising the $Na^+Cl^-$ co-transporter), and promoting $Ca^{++}$ reabsorption (by an unknown mechanism). Increased delivery of $Na^+$ and water to the cortical collecting tubule and/or the higher flow rate lead to more secretion and excretion of $K^+$ and $H^+$.

In healthy volunteers or in patients with oedema, diuresis is already enhanced after administration of a single dose of 0.125 mg of cyclopenthiazide. The resulting increase in urinary excretion of sodium and chloride and the less marked increase in kaliuresis are dose dependent. The diuretic/natriuretic effect appears within 1–3 hours after oral administration of cyclopenthiazide, reaches its maximum after 6–9 hours, and subsides within 24 hours.

Thiazide-induced diuresis initially leads to decreases in plasma volume, cardiac output, and systemic blood pressure. The renin-angiotensin-aldosterone system may become activated. The hypotensive effect is maintained during continued administration, probably owing to a fall in total peripheral vascular resistance; cardiac output returns to pretreatment values, plasma volume remains slightly reduced, and plasma renin activity may be elevated.

During chronic administration, the antihypertensive effect of cyclopenthiazide is dose dependent.

Like other diuretics, cyclopenthiazide given as monotherapy achieves blood pressure control in about 40–50% of patients with mild to moderate hypertension.

Combination with oxprenolol potentiates the blood-pressure-lowering effect, making it possible to achieve a further decrease in blood pressure in a large proportion of patients who have failed to respond adequately to monotherapy.

*Pharmacokinetics:* The active substances of Trasidrex show the same pharmacokinetic behaviour in the fixed combination as following simultaneous administration of Slow-Trasicor and Navidrex.

*Oxprenolol – general characteristics:*

*Absorption:* In the gastrointestinal tract, oxprenolol is completely absorbed from the sustained-release tablets, regardless of whether or not they are taken together with food. Peak plasma concentrations are reached after an average of approx. 3 hours.

During treatment with sustained-release forms, prolongation of the absorption phase enables therapeutically active plasma concentrations to be maintained over a longer period of time than when the same doses are given in conventional dosage forms and avoids high peak drug concentrations in the plasma.

After the active substance has been absorbed, the insoluble matrix of the tablet is excreted in a softened form in the faeces.

Oxprenolol is subject to a first-pass effect. Its systemic bioavailability amounts to 20–70%.

*Distribution:* Oxprenolol has a plasma-protein binding rate of approx. 80% and a calculated distribution volume of 1.2 L/kg.

Oxprenolol crosses the placental barrier. The concentration in the breast milk is equivalent to approx. 30% of that in the plasma.

*Elimination (biotransformation and excretion):* Oxprenolol has an elimination half-life of 1–2 hours.

Oxprenolol is extensively metabolised, direct O-glucuronidation being the major metabolic pathway and oxidative reactions minor ones. Oxprenolol is excreted chiefly in the urine (almost exclusively in the form of inactive metabolites). Oxprenolol is not likely to accumulate.

*Characteristics in patients:* Age has no effect on the pharmacokinetics of oxyprenolol.

In patients with acute or chronic inflammatory diseases an increase in the plasma levels of oxprenolol has been observed.

The plasma levels may also increase in the presence of severe hepatic insufficiency associated with a reduced metabolic rate.

Impaired renal function generally leads to an increase in the blood levels of oxprenolol, but the concentrations measured remain within – although at the upper limit of – the concentration range recorded in subjects with healthy kidneys. In addition, in patients with renal failure the apparent elimination half-life for unchanged, i.e. active oxprenolol is comparable with the corresponding half-life values determined in subject with no renal disease. Hence there is no need to readjust the dosage in the presence of impaired renal function.

*Cyclopenthiazide – general characteristics:* After oral administration of single doses of 0.5 mg or 1 mg cyclopenthiazide, peak plasma levels of about 3 and 7 ng/mL respectively were reached after an average of 3–4 hours. Twelve hours after administration of 1 mg cyclopenthiazide, plasma concentrations fall to about 25% of the peak concentrations. Thiazide diuretics cross the placental barrier and also pass into the breast milk.

Lipophilic thiazides also have a higher protein-binding rate, that of cyclopenthiazide amounting to approx. 92%. They therefore exert a more prolonged action than the more hydrophilic thiazides.

In humans receiving cyclopenthiazide, the drug can be detected in the urine. 24 hours after administration of 0.5 mg, for instance, concentrations in the urine are about 400 ng/mL.

*Characteristics in patients:* In patients with impaired renal function thiazides accumulate and uraemia may become more marked. Thiazide diuretics (including cyclopenthiazide) lose their diuretic effect when creatinine clearance is <30 mL/min (or at serum creatinine levels of >2.5 mg/100 mL).

**Dosage and administration** The dosage should be individualised. The sustained release tablets should be swallowed whole with liquid. When discontinuing prolonged treatment with a β-blocker, the medication should not be stopped abruptly, but withdrawn gradually. The physician may wish to switch to products containing the individual components of Trasidrex, i.e. conventional oxprenolol and cyclopenthiazide tablets to facilitate a stepwise reduction in dose.

*Adults:* In mild to moderate hypertension the recommended dosage is 1 tablet daily in the morning. Depending on the response it may be necessary to raise the dosage to two tablets daily. This should be done after an interval of about 1 week, because the antihypertensive effect often only sets in slowly after 1–2 weeks. In resistant cases, treatment in combination with other antihypertensives can be given, e.g. with a peripheral vasodilator, calcium channel blocker, or ACE inhibitor (see *Interaction with other medicaments*).

*Children:* Adequate experience of the use of Trasidrex in children has not been acquired.

*Elderly:* No special dosage regime is necessary but concurrent hepatic insufficiency and susceptibility to electrolyte imbalances should be taken into account. The lowest effective dosage should be used.

**Contra-indications, warnings, etc.** Hypersensitivity to oxprenolol, cyclopenthiazide and related derivatives or to any of the excipients, or cross sensitivity to other β-blockers.

*Oxprenolol:*

- Cardiogenic shock.
- Heart failure refractory to treatment.
- Atrioventricular block of second or third degree.
- Sick sinus syndrome.
- Bradycardia (<45–50 beats/min).
- Hypotension.
- Severe peripheral arterial circulatory disturbances.
- Bronchial asthma and history of bronchospasm.
- Prinzmetal's angina (variant angina pectoris).
- Untreated phaeochromocytoma.
- Metabolic acidosis.
- Use of anaesthetics with a negative inotropic effect.

*Cyclopenthiazide:*

- Anuria.
- Renal failure.
- Hepatic failure.
- Refractory hyponatraemia and hypercalcaemia.
- Refractory hypokalaemia and conditions involving increased potassium loss, e.g. salt-losing nephropathies and prerenal (cardiogenic) impairment of kidney function.
- Untreated Addison's disease.
- Symptomatic hyperuricaemia (history of gout or uric acid calculi).
- Concomitant treatment with Lithium.
- Hypertension during pregnancy.

*Warnings:* Trasidrex should be used with caution in patients with renal disease or with impaired hepatic function (see *Contra-indications* and *Precautions*).

Patients receiving Trasidrex should be warned that dizziness, fatigue or visual disturbances (see *Side effects*) may occur, in which case they should not drive, operate machinery, or do anything else requiring alertness, particularly if they also consume alcohol.

*Precautions:*

*Oxprenolol:* Owing to the danger of cardiac arrest, a calcium antagonist of the verapamil type must not be administered intravenously to a patient already receiving treatment with a β-blocker (see *Drug interactions*).

Owing to the risk of bronchoconstriction, non-selective β-blockers such as oxprenolol should be used with caution in patients with chronic bronchitis or emphysema.

Due to the negative effect on AV conduction time, β-blockers should only be given with caution to patients with AV block of first degree (see *Contra-indications*).

β-blockers should not be used in patients with untreated congestive heart failure (see *Contra-indications*). This condition should first be stabilised.

If the patient develops increasing bradycardia (<50–55 beats/min at rest) and experiences related symptoms, the dosage should be reduced or gradually withdrawn (see *Contra-indications*).

β-blockers may mask certain clinical signs of hyperthyroidism (e.g. tachycardia), and the patients should be carefully monitored.

β-blockers may reduce liver function and thus affect the metabolism of other drugs. Like many β-blockers, oxprenolol undergoes substantial first-pass hepatic metabolism. In the presence of liver cirrhosis the bioavailability of oxprenolol may be increased leading to higher plasma concentrations (see *Pharmacokinetic properties*).

In patients with peripheral circulatory disorders (e.g. Raynaud's disease or syndrome, intermittent claudication), β-blockers should be used with great caution as aggravation of these disorders may occur (see *Contra-indications*).

In patients with phaeochromocytoma a β-blocker should only be given with an α-blocker, see *Contra-indications*.

Anaphylactic reactions precipitated by other agents may be particularly severe in patients taking β-blockers, require higher than normal doses of adrenaline. Whenever possible, β-blockers should be avoided (replaced by other antihypertensive drugs) in patients who are at increased risk for anaphylaxis.

In patients with ischaemic heart disease, treatment should not be discontinued suddenly. The dosage should be gradually reduced, i.e. over 1–3 weeks, if necessary at the same time initiating alternative therapy, to prevent exacerbation of angina pectoris.

If a patient receiving oxprenolol requires anaesthesia, the anesthetist should be informed of the use of the medication prior to the use of a general anaesthetic to permit him to take the necessary precautions. The anaesthetic selected should be one exhibiting as little negative inotropic activity as possible, e.g. halothane/nitrous oxide. If, on the other hand, inhibition of sympathetic tone during the operation is regarded as undesirable, the β-blocker should be withdrawn gradually at least 48 hours prior to surgery.

The full development of the 'oculomucocutaneous syndrome', as previously described with practolol, has not been reported with oxprenolol. However, some features of this syndrome have been noted, such as dry eyes alone or occasionally associated with skin rash. In most cases the symptoms cleared after withdrawal of the treatment. Discontinuation of oxprenolol should be considered and a switch to another antihypertensive drug might be advisable.

*Cyclopenthiazide: Electrolytes:* all patients receiving thiazide therapy should be observed for clinical signs of fluid or electrolyte unbalance, namely dose dependent hyponatraemia, hypochloremic alkalosis and hypokalaemia. Since the excretion of electrolytes is increased during thiazide treatment an excessively strict low-salt diet should be avoided.

Periodic serum electrolyte determinations should be carried out, especially in digitalised patients, in the elderly, especially in those suffering from chronic diseases, in patients with liver cirrhosis, who are more susceptible to regulatory disorders affecting the electrolytes and fluid balance, and in patients with oedema due to nephrotic syndrome.

Serum potassium concentrations should be checked initially and 3–4 weeks after the start of therapy. Unless the potassium balance is disturbed by other factors (e.g. vomiting, diarrhoea, change in renal function malnutrition, liver cirrhosis, hyperaldosteronism, treatment with ACTH or corticosteroids) controls should be carried out every 4–6 months.

Hypokalaemia may be avoided or treated by the use of potassium supplements and/or foods with a high potassium content.

Oral potassium supplementation (e.g. KCl) may be considered in patients receiving digitalis and diuretics, particularly if their plasma potassium concentrations are <3.0 mmol/L. If oral potassium supplementation is not well tolerated, Trasidrex may be combined with a potassium sparing diuretic e.g. amiloride.

Combined treatment consisting of Trasidrex and a potassium salt or a potassium-sparing diuretic must be avoided in patients also receiving ACE inhibitors.

If hypokalaemia is acocmpanied by clinical signs (e.g. muscular weakness, paresis, or ECG changes) Trasidrex should be discontinued.

During treatment with thiazides, hyponatraemia accompanied by neurological symptoms (nausea, asthenia, progressive disorientation, apathy) has been observed in isolated cases.

Patients receiving relatively high doses of thiazides may develop hypomagnesaemia accompanied by signs and symptoms such as irritability, muscle cramps, and cardiac arrhythmias.

*Metabolic effects:* Like other diuretics, thiazides may raise serum uric acid levels, but attacks of gout are rarely observed during chronic treatment.

Small and partly reversible increases in plasma concentrations of total cholesterol, triglycerides or low-density lipoprotein cholesterol were reported in patients during long-term treatment with thiazides and thiazide-like diuretics. The clinical relevance of these findings is not clear.

Calcium excretion is decreased by thiazides. Pathological changes in the parathyroid gland associated with hypercalcaemia and hypophosphataemia have been observed in a few patients on prolonged thiazide therapy. If hypercalcaemia occurs, further diagnostic clarification is necessary. The usual complications of hyperparathyroidism, e.g. renal lithiasis, bone resorption, and peptic ulceration, have not been observed.

*Others:* Lupus erythematosus may become activated under treatment with thiazides.

*Oxprenolol and cyclopenthiazide*

*Diabetes/glucose tolerance:* β-blockers as well as thiazide diuretics are liable to affect carbohydrate metabolism. Diabetic patients, especially those dependent on insulin, should be warned that β-blockers can mask the signs of hypoglycaemia (e.g. tachy-

cardia) (see *Drug interactions*). Hypoglycaemia, producing loss of consciousness in some cases, may occur in non-diabetic individuals who are taking β-blockers, particularly those who undergo prolonged fasting or strenuous exercise.

Although glucose tolerance may be adversely affected, diabetes mellitus very seldom occurs under treatment.

The concurrent use of β-blockers, thiazide diuretics and antidiabetic medication should always be monitored to confirm that glycaemic control is well maintained (see *Drug interactions*).

*Renal function:* In patients with renal impairment, the elimination half-life for unchanged oxprenolol is not expected to be significantly different from the subjects with normal renal function, but thiazides accumulate and uraemia may become more marked.

Creatinine clearance, urea and electrolytes should be monitored in patients with renal impairment since they might be more susceptible to the effects of antihypertensive drugs. At creatinine clearance levels of <30 mL/min (or at serum creatinine levels of greater than 2.5 mg/100 mL=221 mmol/l), thiazides no longer exert an adequate diuretic effect.

The antihypertensive effect of ACE inhibitors is potentiated by diuretics that increase plasma renin activity. A cautious dosage schedule should therefore be adopted when an ACE inhibitor is added to a diuretic agent.

As with all antihypertensive agents, a cautious dosage schedule is indicated in patients with severe coronary or cerebral arteriosclerosis.

*Use in pregnancy and lactation:* Trasidrex should not be given during pregnancy unless there are no safer alternatives. If used, as in the case of any form of drug therapy, Trasidrex should be employed with caution, especially in the first 3 months.

β-blockers may reduce placental perfusion, which may result in intrauterine foetal death, immature and premature deliveries. Use the lowest possible dose. If possible, discontinue β-blocker therapy at least 2–3 days prior to delivery to avoid the effects of uterine contractility and possible adverse effects, especially bradycardia and hypoglycaemia, in the foetus and neonate.

Cyclopenthiazide must not be used to treat hypertension during pregnancy (see *Contra-indications*). There have been reports of foetal bone marrow depression, thrombocytopenia, and foetal and neonatal jaundice associated with the use of thiazide diuretics. Other adverse reactions associated with use in adults may also occur.

Oxprenolol and cyclopenthiazide pass into breast milk (see *Pharmacokinetic properties*) and although the estimated daily infant dose derived from breast feeding is likely to be very low, breast feeding is not recommended.

Trasidrex may also suppress lactation.

*Drug interactions:* The antihypertensive effect of Trasidrex is enhanced by concomitant treatment with other antihypertensives.

In addition, the following interactions may occur with the individual components.

*Oxprenolol:* Alcohol and β-blocker effects on the central nervous system have been observed to be additive and it is possible that symptoms such as dizziness may be exaggerated if alcohol and Trasidrex are taken together (see also *Effects on ability to use machines*).

*Oxprenolol and cyclopenthiazide:*

*Antidiabetics:* Trasidrex may modify blood glucose concentrations in patients being treated with insulin and oral antidiabetic drugs, and may alter the response to hypoglycaemia by prolonging the recovery (blood glucose rise) from hypoglycaemia, reversing hypotension, and blocking tachycardia. In diabetic patients receiving Trasidrex hypoglycaemic episodes may not result in the expected tachycardia, but hypoglycaemia-induced sweating will occur, and may even be intensified and prolonged (see *Warnings* and *Precautions*).

Hyperglycaemia may also occur with thiazide diuretics. Thus latent diabetes mellitus may become manifest during Trasidrex therapy.

During concurrent therapy with antidiabetics a close watch should therefore be kept on carbohydrate metabolism, and the dosage of hypoglycaemic medication may have to be readjusted (see *Warnings* and *Precautions*).

*Non-steroidal anti-inflammatory drugs (NSAIDs):* NSAIDs such as indomethacin can reduce the hypotensive effect of Trasidrex and there have been isolated reports of a deterioration in renal function in predisposed patients.

*Calcium channel blockers:* Calcium channel blockers such as verapamil and diltiazem may protentiate bradycardia, myocardial depression, and hypotension induced by Trasidrex, particularly after intravenous administration of verapamil, the possibility of hypotension cardiac arrhythmia and cardiac arrest cannot be excluded (see *Warnings* and *Precautions*).

*Catecholamine-depleting drugs:* Catecholamine-depleting drugs, such as guanethidine or monoamine oxydase inhibitors may have an additive effect when administered concomitantly with β-blockers such as oxprenolol and with thiazide diuretics. Patients should be closely observed for hypotension.

*Digitalis glycosides:* β-blockers and digitalis glycosides may be additive in their depressant effect on myocardial conduction, particularly at the atrioventricular node, resulting in bradycardia or heart block.

Thiazide induced hypokalaemia or hypomagnesaemia may also favour the onset of digitalis-induced cardiac arrhythmias (see *Warnings* and *Precautions*).

In addition, the following interactions may occur with the individual components:

*Oxprenolol:* Class I anti-arrhythmic drugs and amiodarone.

Drugs such as disopyramide, quinidine and amiodarone may have a potentiating effect on atrial conduction time and induce negative isotropic effect when administered concomitantly with β-blockers.

*Sympathomimetic drugs:* Non-cardioselective β-blockers such as oxprenolol may enhance the pressor response to sympathomimetic drugs such as adrenaline, noradrenaline, isoprenaline, ephedrine, and phenylephrine (e.g. local anaesthetics in dentistry, nasal and ocular drops), resulting in hypertension and bradycardia.

*Clonidine:* When clonidine is used in conjunction with a non-selective β-blocker, such as oxprenolol, treatment with clonidine should be continued for some time after the β-blocker has been discontinued to reduce the danger of rebound hypertension.

*Cimetidine:* Hepatic metabolism of β-blockers may be reduced by cimetidine, resulting in increased plasma concentrations and prolonged serum half-life. Marked bradycardia may occur.

*Ergot alkaloids:* Concomitant administration with β-blockers may enhance the vasoconstrictive action of ergot alkaloids.

*Anaesthetic agents:* Beta-blockers and certain inhaled anaesthetics may be additive in their cardio-depressant effect. However, continued use of β-blockers during anaesthesia reduces the risk of cardiac arrhythmias and hypertension (see *Warnings* and *Precautions*).

*Lignocaine:* Concomitant administration with β-blockers may increase blood lidocaine concentrations and potential toxicity; patients should be closely monitored for increased lidocaine effects.

*Cyclopenthiazide:*

*Lithium:* Diuretics raise the blood level of lithium. Where lithium has produced polyuria, diuretics may exert a paradoxical antidiuretic effect (see *Contra-indications*)

*Curare derivatives and antihypertensive drugs:* Thiazides potentiate the action of curare derivatives and antihypertensive drugs (e.g. methyldopa, β-blockers, vasodilators, ACE inhibitors.

*Potassium lowering drugs* (such as corticosteroids, ACTH, amphotericin B, carbenoxolene): These drugs may increase the hypokalaemic effect of thiazides.

*Allopurinol:* Co-administration of thiazide diuretics may increase the incidence of hypersensitivity reactions to allopurinol.

*Amantadine:* Co-administration of thiazide diuretics may increase the risk of adverse effects caused by amantadine.

*Antineoplastic agents* (e.g. cyclophosphamide, methotrexate): Concomitant use of thiazide diuretics may reduce renal excretion of cytotoxic agents and potentiate their myelosuppressive effects.

*Anticholinergics* (e.g. atropine, biperiden): The bioavailability of thiazide-type diuretics may be increased by anticholinergic agents, apparently owing to a decrease in gastrointestinal motility and stomach-emptying rate.

*Cholestyramine:* Absorption of thiazide diuretics is decreased by cholestyramine. A decrease in the pharmacological effect of thiazides may be expected.

*Vitamin D:* Thiazide diuretics may reduce urinary calcium excretion caused by vitamin D, while vitamin D may potentiate the increase in serum calcium caused by thiazides.

*Cyclosporin:* Concomitant use of thiazide-type diuretics and cyclosporin may increase the risk of hyperuricemia and gout-type complications.

*Calcium salts:* Concomitant use of thiazide-type diuretics and calcium salts may cause hypercalcaemia by increasing tubular calcium reabsorption.

*Diazoxide:* Thiazide diuretics may enhance the hyperglycaemia effect of diazoxide.

*Methyldopa:* There have been reports in the literature of haemolytic anaemia occurring when a thiazide diuretic and methyldopa were administered concomitantly.

*Alcohol, barbiturates or narcotics:* may potentiate orthostatic hypotension induced by cyclopenthiazide.

*Side-effects:* Frequency estimate: very common 10%, common 1% to >10%, uncommon 0.1% to <1%, rare 0.01% to <0.1%, very rare <0.01%.

*Central nervous system* – Common: fatigue, dizziness, headache, mental depression, sleep disturbances, nightmares.

Rare: hallucinations, exertional tiredness.

Uncommon: paresthesias.

*Cardiovascular system* – Common: postural hypotension which can be aggravated by alcohol, anaesthetics or sedatives, heart failure, peripheral vascular disorders (peripheral coldness).

Uncommon: bradycardia, disturbances of cardiac conduction.

Rare: Raynaud-like symptoms, cardiac arrhythmia.

*Gastronintestinal tract* – Very common: dry mouth, constipation.

Common: nausea, vomiting, flatulence, loss of appetite.

Uncommon: diarrhoea.

Very rare: pancreatitis, abdominal distress.

*Skin and appendages* – Common: allergic skin rash, urticaria.

Rare: worsening of psoriasis, photosensitivity.

Very rare: necrotising vasculitis and toxic epidermal necrolysis, cutaneous lupus erythematosus like-lesions, and reactivation of cutaneous lupus erythematosus.

*Respiratory system* – Common: dyspnoea, bronchospasm.

*Sense organs* – Uncommon: visual disturbances.

Very rare: dry eyes, keratoconjunctivitis.

*Blood* – Very rare: thrombocytopenia sometimes with purpura, leucopenia, agranulocytosis, bone marrow depression and haemolytic anaemia.

*Liver* – Rare: intrahepatic cholestasis or jaundice.

*Electrolytes and metabolic disorders* – Very common: mainly with higher doses, hypokalaemia and rise in serum lipids.

Common: hyponatraemia, hypomagnesaemia, and hyperuricaemia.

Rare: hypercalcaemia, hyperglycaemia, glycosuria and worsening of diabetic metabolic status.

Very rare, hypocloraemic alkalosis.

*Other effects:* Common: disturbances of libido and potency.

Very rare: hypersensitivity reactions – respiratory distress including pneumonitis and pulmonary oedema.

*Overdosage:*

*Signs and symptoms:*

*Oxprenolol* – Poisoning due to an overdose of a β-blocker may lead to pronounced hypotension, bradycardia, conduction abnormalities (first or second degree block, complete heart block, asystole), or even cardiac arrest; heart failure, cardiogenic shock, hypoglycaemia, in addition, dyspnoea, bronchospasm, vomiting, impairment of consciousness, and also generalised convulsions may occur.

The manifestations of poisoning with β-blockers are dependent on the pharmacological properties of the ingested drug. Although the onset of action is rapid, effects of massive overdose may persist for several days despite declining plasma levels. Watch carefully for cardiovascular or respiratory deterioration in an intensive care setting, particularly in the early hours. Observe mild overdose cases for at least 4 hours for the development of signs of poisoning.

*Cyclopenthiazide* – Additional symptoms due to overdosage with cyclopenthiazide are nausea, dizziness, somnolence, hypovolaemia, electrolyte disturbances associated with cardiac arrhythmias and muscles spasms.

*Treatment:* Patients who are seen soon after potentially life-threatening overdosage (within 4 hours) should be treated by gastric lavage and activated charcoal.

Treatment of symptoms is based on modern methods of intensive care, with continuous monitoring of cardiac function, blood gases, electrolytes, and if necessary intravenous fluid and electrolytes replacement, and emergency measures such as artificial respiration, resuscitation or cardiac pacemaker.

Significant bradycardia should be treated initially with atropine. Large doses of isoprenaline may be necessary for control of heart rate and hypotension. Glucagon has positive chronotropic and inotropic effect on the heart that are independent of interactions with β-adrenergic receptors, and it represents a useful alternative treatment for hypotension and heart failure.

For the treatment of seizures, diazepam has been effective and is the drug of choice.

For the treatment of bronchospasm, $\beta_2$-agonists (such as salbutamol or terbutaline) or aminophylline are effective bronchodilator drugs. Monitor the patient for dysrhythmias during and after administration.

Patients who recover should be observed for signs of β-blocker withdrawal phenomenon (see *Warnings and Precautions*).

**Pharmaceutical precautions** Protect from heat, light and moisture. Store below 25°C.

**Legal category** POM.

**Package quantities** Cartons of 28 tablets consisting of two reminder calendar foils of 14 tablets (each carton of 28 represents 2–4 weeks' treatment depending on whether dosage is one or two tablets daily).

**Further information** Nil.

**Product licence number** 00101/0434.

## VISKALDIX* TABLETS

**Qualitative and quantitative composition** Each tablet contains 10 mg pindolol and 5 mg clopamide.

**Pharmaceutical form** Tablet.

**Clinical particulars**

*Therapeutic indications:* Mild to moderate hypertension.

*Posology and method of administration*

*Adults:* One tablet daily in the morning. If blood pressure is not satisfactorily lowered after 2 to 3 weeks then two tablets daily as a single dose in the morning. Maximum dose of three tablets daily, if required.

*Children:* There is no experience with Viskaldix in children.

*Use in the elderly:* There is no evidence that the dosage or tolerability of Viskaldix is directly affected by advanced age. However, because of the diuretic component, such patients should be carefully supervised as factors sometimes associated with aging, such as poor diet or impaired renal function may indirectly affect the dosage or tolerability.

*Method of administration:* Oral.

*Contra-indications:* Untreated cardiac failure, sick sinus syndrome (include sino-atrial block), second and third degree heart block, Prinzmetal's angina, history of bronchospasm and broncial asthma (a warning stating 'do not take this medicine if you have a history of wheezing or asthma' will appear on the label), untreated phaeochromocytoma, metabolic acidosis, pronounced bradycardia, obstructive pulmonary disease, cor pulmonale, prolonged fasting hypokalaemia, refractory hypokalaemia, hyponatraemia, hypercalcaemia, Addison's disease, severe renal or hepatic impairment and symptomatic hyperuricaemia. Viskaldix should not be used with agents which inhibit calcium transport e.g. verapamil.

*Special warnings and precautions for use:* Especially in patients with ischaemic heart disease, treatment should not be discontinued suddenly. The dosage should be gradually reduced, i.e. over 1–2 weeks, if necessary at the same time initiating replacement therapy, to prevent exacerbation of angina pectoris.

Patients with a poor cardiac reserve should be stabilised with digitalis before treatment with Viskaldix to prevent impairment of myocardial contractility.

As with all beta-blockers, Viskaldix should be used with caution in patients with a history of non-asthmatic chronic obstructive lung disease or recent myocardial infarction.

Patients with spontaneous hypoglycaemia or diabetes should be monitored closely as concomitant use of beta-blockers may intensify the blood sugar lowering effect of insulin and other antidiabetic drugs and also as thiazide diuretics can lower insulin tolerance. Use of beta-blockers may mask the symptoms of hypoglycaemia (tachycardia, tremor). Beta-blockers may also mask the symptoms of thyrotoxicosis.

During treatment with Viskaldix, patients should not undergo anaesthesia with agents causing myocardial depression (e.g. Halothane, cyclopropane, trichlorethylene, ether, chloroform). Viskaldix should be gradually withdrawn before elective surgery. In emergency surgery or cases where withdrawal of Viskaldix would cause deterioration in cardiac condition, atropine sulphate 1 to 2 mg intravenously should be given to prevent severe bradycardia.

If a beta-blocker is indicated in a patient with phaeochromocytoma it must always be given in conjunction with an alpha-blocker, Pre-existing peripheral vascular disorders may be aggravated by beta-blockers. Patients with known psoriasis should take beta-blockers only after careful consideration.

Beta-blockers may increase both the sensitivity towards allergens and the seriousness of anaphylactic reactions.

There have been reports of skin rashes and/or dry eyes associated with the use of beta-adrenoceptor blocking drugs. The reported incidence is small and in most cases the symptoms have cleared when treatment was withdrawn. Discontinuance of the drug should be considered if any such reaction is not otherwise explicable. Cessation of therapy with a beta-blocker should be gradual.

In severe renal failure a further impairment of renal function following beta blockade has been reported in a few cases. Potassium levels should be checked in patients with renal or hepatic failure and urate levels should be checked in patients with gout.

Dilutional hyponatraemia may occur in hot weather in oedematous patients on Viskaldix. The appropriate therapy is water restriction rather than the administration of salt, except in rare instances when the hyponatraemia is life-threatening. In true salt depletion, appropriate replacement is the treatment of choice.

*Interaction with other medicaments and other forms of interaction:* Viskaldix should not be used during concomitant administration of lithium, or by patients with known hypersensitivity to sulphonamides.

Calcium-channel blocking agents: Viskaldix should not be used with clacium-channel blockers with negative ionotropic effects e.g. verapamil and to a lesser extent diltiazem. The concomitant use of oral beta-blockers and calcium antagonists of the dihydropyridine type can be useful in hypertension or angina pectoris. However, because of their potential effect on the cardiac condution system and contractility, the I.V. Route must be avoided. The concomitant use with dihydropyridines e.g. nifedipine may increase the risk of hypotension. In patients with cardiac insufficiency, treatment with beta-blocking agents may lead to cardiac failure.

Use of digitalis glycosides in association with beta-blockers may increase atrio-ventricular conduction time.

Clonidine: when therapy is discontinued in patients receiving a beta-blocker and clonidine concurrently, the beta-blockers should be gradually discontinued several days before clonidine is discontinued, in order to reduce the potential risk of a clonidine withdrawal hypertensive crisis.

Mao inhibitors: concurrent use with beta-blockers is not recommended. Possibly significant hypertension may theoretically occur up to 14 days following discontinuation of the mao inhibitor.

Caution should be exercised in the concurrent use of beta-blocking agents with class 1 antiarrhythmics (e.g. disopyramide, quinidine) and amiodarone.

Concomitant use of beta-blockers may intensify the blood sugar lowering effect of insulin and other antidiabetic drugs.

Cimetidine, hydralazine and alcohol may induce increased plasma level of beta-blockers.

Prostaglandin synthetase inhibiting drugs may decrease the hypotensive effects of beta-blockers.

Sympathomimetics with beta-adrenergic stimulant activity and xanthines: concurrent use with beta-blockers may result in mutual inhibition of therapeutic effects; in addition, beta-blockers may decrease theophylline clearance.

Concomitant use of beta-blockers with tricyclic antidepressants, barbiturates and phenothiazines as well as other anti-hypertensive agents may increase the blood pressure lowering effect.

Reserpine: concurrent use may result in an additive and possibly excessive beta-adrenergic blockade.

*Pregnancy and lactation:* Viskaldix should not be given to pregnant or lactating women.

*Effects on ability to drive and to use machines:* Because dizziness or fatigue may occur during initiation of treatment with antihypertensive drugs, patients driving vehicles or operating machinery should exercise caution until their individual reaction to treatment has been determined.

*Undesirable effects:* Side-effects associated with beta-blockade: bradycardia, a slowed av-conduction or increase of an existing av-block, hypotension, heart failure, cold and cyanotic extremities, Raynaud's phenomenon, paraesthesia of the extremities, increase of an existing intermittent claudication. Fatigue, headaches, impaired vision, hallucinations, psychoses, confusion, impotence, dizziness, sleep disturbances, depression, nightmares. Gastro-intestinal problems, nausea, vomiting, diarrhoea. Bronchospasm in patients with bronchial asthma or a history of asthmatic complaints. Disorder of the skin, especially rash. Dry eyes. Beta-blockers may mask the symptoms of thyrotoxicosis or hypoglycaemia. An increase in ana (anti nuclear antibodies) has been seen; its clinical relevance is not clear.

Thiazide diuretics may cause postural hypotension and mild gastrointestinal effects; importence (reversible on withdrawal of treatment); hypokalaemia, hypomagnesaemia, hyponatraemia, hypercalcaemia, hypochloraemic alkalosis, hyperuricaemia, gout, hyperglycaemia, and increases in plasma cholesterol. Less commonly rashes, photosensitivity; blood disorders (including neutropenia and thrombocytopenia), pancreatitis; intrahepatic cholestatis and hypersensitivity reactions (including pneumonitis, pulmonary oedema, severe skin reactions) have also been reported.

*Overdose:* Overdosage may cause alterations in heart rate, nausea, vomiting, orthostatic disturbances, collapse, hypokalaemia and its accompanying disorders. Treatment by elimination of any unabsorbed drug and general supportive measures.

Plasma electrolytes should be closely monitored. Marked bradycardia, as a result of overdosage (or idiosyncrasy) should be treated with atropine sulphate 1–2 mg iv.

If necessary isoprenaline hydrochloride can be administered by slow iv under constant supervision beginning with 25 mcg (5 mcg/min) until desired effect is achieved. A cardiac pacemaker may be required. Glucagon (5 to 10 mg) iv has been reported to overcome some of the features of serious overdosage.

**Pharmacological properties**

*Pharmacodynamic properties:* Viskaldix is a combination of pindolol and clopamide, both acting to lower blood pressure, although by two separate mechanisms.

Pindolol is a non-selective Beta-adrenergic antagonist which blocks both B1 and B2 adrenoceptors for more than 24 hours following administration. It has negligible membrane stabilising activity. The intrinsic sympathomimetic activity (ISA) provides the heart with basal stimulation similar to that elicited by normal resting sympathetic activity. Thus resting cardiac output and heart rate are not unduly depressed, subsequently reducing the risk of bradycardia.

Clopamide enhances the elimination of sodium and chloride by inhibiting their reabsorption in the renal tubules which in turn leads to increased water excretion. The mechanistic relationship to the diuretic action and reduced blood pressure is not fully understood, however the diuretic effect is proportional to the dosage. Diuresis is initiated after about 2 hours and can last for up to 24 hours with maximal effect after 3 to 6 hours.

This combination can produce a clear antihypertensive effect after a few days, but in some cases, to achieve the full effect, two to three weeks treatment may be necessary.

*Pharmacokinetic properties:* The pharmacokinetics of the two active ingredients are very similar and are not influenced by their combination or by being taken with food. Both components are rapidly and almost completely absorbed. They show negligible hepatic first-pass metabolism. Thus the bioavailability of both is at least 85%. The maximum plasma concentration of pindolol is reached within one hour after ingestion, and that of clopamide, one or two hours after ingestion. Plasma protein binding is 40% for pindolol, and 46% for clopamide. The volume of distribution is about 2 L/kg for pindolol, and 1.5 L/kg for clopamide.

The total body clearance of pindolol is 400 ml/min, that of clopamide is 165 ml/min. The elimination half-life is 3–4 hours for pindolol, and 6 hours for clopamide. Approximately one third of the dose of both drugs is excreted unchanged in the urine. The excretion of clopamide occurs mainly via the kidneys, whereas pindolol shows a balanced excretion between the renal and hepatic routes.

*Preclinical safety data:* There are no pre-clinical data of relevance to the prescriber which are additional to that already included in other sections of the SPC.

## Pharmaceutical particulars

*List of excipients:* Magnesium stearate , maize starch and lactose.

*Incompatibilities:* None.

*Shelf life:* 5 years from date of manufacture.

*Special precautions for storage:* None.

*Nature and contents of container:* PVDC opaque blister pack containing 28 tablets.

*Instructions for use/handling:* None.

**Marketing authorisation number**    0101/0113

**Date of approval/revision of SPC**    23 April 1997

**Legal category**    POM.

# VISKEN*

**Presentation**    *5 mg Tablets:* Visken 5 mg is available as white, round, flat, bevel-edged tablets of 7 mm diameter, and weighing 120 mg. The tablets are marked VISKEN 5 on one side with a single break line on the reverse. Each tablet contains 5 mg Pindolol PhEur.

*15 mg Tablets:* Visken 15 mg is available as white, round, flat, bevel-edged tablets of 9 mm diameter and weighing 200 mg. The tablets are marked VISKEN 15 on one side, and scored on the reverse. Each tablet contains 15 mg Pindolol PhEur.

**Uses**    *Principal action:* Visken is a specific beta-adrenoceptor blocking agent with low cardiodepressant activity at therapeutic dose. Its beta-blocking activity prevents excessive sympathetic drive to the heart, resulting in a fall in heart rate, and a decrease in cardiac work and myocardial oxygen consumption. Visken possesses some intrinsic sympathomimetic activity even at low dosage which may prevent reduction of resting sympathetic tone to an undesirably low level and minimise myocardial depression.

*Indications: Hypertension:* For reduction of blood pressure in essential hypertension. Onset of action of Visken is usually rapid, most patients showing a response within the first one to two weeks of treatment. However, maximum response may take several weeks to develop.

*Angina pectoris:* Prophylactic treatment with Visken reduces the frequency and severity of anginal attacks and increases work capacity.

**Dosage and administration**    *Hypertension:* Initially one 15 mg tablet daily, with breakfast or 5 mg two or three times daily. Most patients respond to a once-daily dose of from 15 mg to 30 mg.

If necessary, dosage may be increased at weekly intervals up to a maximum of 45 mg daily in single or divided doses. Patients not responding after three to four weeks at this dosage level rarely benefit from further elevations in dosage. Addition of Visken to existing diuretic therapy increases the hypotensive effect and combination with other antihypertensives enables reduction in dosage of these agents.

*Angina pectoris:* Usually half to one 5 mg tablet up to three times a day according to response.

*Use in the elderly:* No evidence exists that elderly patients require different dosages or show different side-effects from younger patients.

*Use in children:* Experience with Visken in children is still limited. Its use in children cannot, therefore, be recommended.

## Contra-indications, warnings, etc

*Contra-indications:* Cardiac failure unless satisfactorily controlled by digitalis (see also 'Precautions'). Atrioventricular block, pronounced bradycardia, obstructive pulmonary disease, bronchial asthma, cor pulmonale, metabolic acidosis, prolonged fasting, severe renal failure.

Visken should not be taken in conjunction with agents which inhibit calcium transport, e.g. verapamil.

*Use in pregnancy and lactation:* Visken is contra-indicated in pregnancy and passes in small quantities into breast milk.

*Precautions:* Patients with a poor cardiac reserve should be stabilised with digitalis before treatment with Visken to prevent impairment of myocardial contractility.

As with all beta-blockers, Visken should be used with caution in patients with a history of non-asthmatic chronic obstructive lung disease or recent myocardial infarction. Caution must be exercised when beta-blocking agents are administered to patients with spontaneous hypoglycaemia or diabetics under treatment with insulin or oral hypoglycaemic agents, since hypoglycaemia may occur during prolonged fasting and some of its symptoms (tachycardia, tremor) may be masked.

During treatment with Visken, patients should not undergo anaesthesia with agents causing myocardial depression (e.g. halothane, cyclopropane, trichlorethylene, ether, chloroform). Visken should be gradually withdrawn before elective surgery. In emergency surgery or cases where withdrawal of Visken would cause deterioration in cardiac condition, atropine sulphate 1 to 2 mg intravenously should be given to prevent severe bradycardia.

If a beta-blocker is indicated in a patient with a phaeochromocytoma it must always be given in conjunction with an alpha-blocker. Pre-existing peripheral vascular disorders may be aggravated by beta-blockers.

In severe renal failure a further impairment of renal function following beta blockade has been reported in a few cases.

There have been reports of skin rashes and/or dry eyes associated with the use of beta-adrenoceptor blocking drugs. The reported incidence is small and in most cases the symptoms have cleared when treatment was withdrawn. Discontinuance of the drug should be considered if any such reaction is not otherwise explicable. Cessation of therapy with a beta-blocker should be gradual.

Because dizziness or fatigue may occur during the initial phase of treatment with antihypertensive drugs, patients driving vehicles or operating machinery should exercise caution until their individual response to treatment has been determined.

*Drug interactions:*

Calcium-channel blocking agents: experience has shown that the concomitant use of oral beta-blockers and calcium antagonists of the dihydropyridine type can be useful in hypertension or angina pectoris. However, because of their potential effect on the cardiac conduction system and contractility, the i.v. route must be avoided.

Cimetidine may increase the plasma level of beta-blockers, possibly by interference with hepatic metabolism.

Clonidine: when therapy is discontinued in patients receiving a beta-blocker and clonidine concurrently, the beta-blockers should be gradually discontinued several days before clonidine is discontinued, in order to reduce the potential risk of a clonidine withdrawal hypertensive crisis.

MAO inhibitors: concurrent use with beta-blockers is not recommended. Possibly significant hypertension may theoretically occur up to 14 days following discontinuation of the MAO inhibitor.

Non-steroidal anti-inflammatory drugs (NSAIDs): the effect of many antihypertensive agents, including beta-blockers, may be reduced when they are used concurrently with these drugs, possibly as a result of the inhibition of renal prostaglandin synthesis and sodium and fluid retention caused by NSAIDs.

Phenothiazines: concurrent use with beta-blockers may result in an increased plasma concentration of either drug.

Reserpine: concurrent use may result in an additive and possibly excessive beta-adrenergic blockade.

Sympathomimetics with beta-adrenergic stimulant activity and xanthines: concurrent use with beta-blockers may result in mutual inhibition of therapeutic effects; in addition, beta-blockers may decrease theophylline clearance.

*Side-effects:* Few serious side-effects have been reported. Depression gastrointestinal distubances (including diarrhoea, nausea and epigastric pain), muscle cramps, tremors, insomnia, headaches, sleep disturbance, fatigue, dizziness and hypotension have occurred but are usually transient and disappear if dosage is reduced. Allergic skin reactions have occasionally been reported.

*Overdosage:* Treat by elimination of any unabsorbed drug and general supportive measures. Marked bradycardia as a result of overdosage or idiosyncrasy should be treated with atropine sulphate 1 to 2 mg intravenously. If necessary, isoprenaline hydrochloride can be administered by a slow intravenous injection, under constant supervision, beginning with 25 micrograms (5 micrograms/min) until the desired effect is achieved. A cardiac pacemaker may be required; i.v. glucagon (5 to 10 mg) has been reported to overcome some of the features of serious overdosage and may be useful.

**Pharmaceutical precautions**    Nil.

**Legal category**    POM.

**Package quantities**    *5 mg tablets:* Blister pack of 100 (OP).

*15 mg tablets:* Blister pack of 30 (OP).

**Further information**    Nil.

**Product licence numbers**
Tablets 5 mg    0101/0065
Tablets 15 mg    0101/0110

# VOLTAROL* AMPOULES

**Qualitative and quantitative composition**    The active ingredient is sodium-[o-[(2,6-dichlorophenyl)-amino]-phenyl]-acetate) (diclofenac sodium).

Each 3 ml ampoule contains 75 mg diclofenac sodium.

**Pharmaceutical form**    Solution for injection in ampoules.

## Clinical particulars

*Therapeutic indications:*

*Ampoules for intramuscular use:* The ampoules are effective in acute forms of pain, including renal colic, exacerbations of osteo- and rheumatoid arthritis, acute back pain, acute gout, acute trauma and fractures, and post-operative pain.

*Ampoules used in intravenous infusion:* For treatment or prevention of post-operative pain in the hospital setting.

*Posology and method of administration:*

*Adults:* Voltarol Ampoules (given i.m. or i.v.) should not be given for more than two days; if necessary, treatment can be continued with Voltarol Tablets or Suppositories.

*Intramuscular injection:* The following directions for intramuscular injection must be adhered to in order to avoid damage to a nerve or other tissue at the injection site.

One ampoule once (or in severe cases twice) daily intramuscularly by deep intragluteal injection into the upper outer quadrant. If two injections daily are required it is advised that the alternative buttock be used for the second injection. Alternatively, one ampoule of 75 mg can be combined with other dosage forms of Voltarol (Tablets or Suppositories) up to the maximum daily dosage of 150 mg.

*Renal colic:* One 75 mg ampoule intramuscularly. A further ampoule may be administered after 30 minutes if necessary. The recommended maximum daily dose of Voltarol is 150 mg.

*Intravenous infusion:* Immediately before initiating an intravenous infusion, Voltarol must be diluted with 100–500 ml of either sodium chloride solution (0.9%) or glucose solution (5%). Both solutions should be buffered with sodium bicarbonate solution (0.5 ml 8.4% or 1 ml 4.2%). Only clear solutions should be used.

Voltarol must not be given as an intravenous bolus injection.

Two alternative regimens are recommended:

For the *treatment* of moderate to severe post-operative pain, 75 mg should be infused continuously over a period of 30 minutes to 2 hours. If necessary, treatment may be repeated after 4–6 hours, not exceeding 150 mg within any period of 24 hours.

For the *prevention* of post-operative pain, a loading dose of 25 mg–50 mg should be infused after surgery over 15 minutes to 1 hour, followed by a continuous infusion of approx. 5 mg per hour up to a maximum daily dosage of 150 mg.

*Children:* Voltarol Ampoules are not recommended for use in children.

*Elderly:* Although the pharmacokinetics of Voltarol are not impaired to any clinically relevant extent in elderly patients, non-steroidal anti-inflammatory drugs should be used with particular caution in such patients who, generally, are more prone to adverse reactions. In particular, it is recommended that the lowest effective dosage be used in frail elderly patients or those with a low body weight (see also *Precautions*).

The recommended maximum daily dose of Voltarol is 150 mg.

*Contra-indications:* Active or suspected gastro-intestinal ulcers or bleeding.

Previous sensitivity to diclofenac.

Patients in whom attacks of asthma, urticaria or acute rhinitis are precipitated by aspirin or other non-steroidal anti-inflammatory agents.

Hypersensitivity to the excipients sodium metabisulphite, benzyl alcohol, propylene glycol, mannitol.

*Specifically for iv use:* Concomitant NSAID or anti-coagulant use (including low dose heparin).

History of haemorrhagic diathesis, a history of confirmed or suspected cerebrovascular bleeding.

Operations associated with a high risk of haemorrhage.

A history of asthma.

Moderate or severe renal impairment (serum creatinine >160 µmol/l).

Hypovolaemia or dehydration from any cause.

*Special warnings and special precautions for use*
*Warnings: Gastro-intestinal:* Close medical surveillance is imperative in patients with symptoms indicative of gastro-intestinal disorders, with a history suggestive of gasto-intestinal ulceration, with ulcerative colitis or with Crohn's disease.

Gastro-intestinal bleeding or ulcerative/perforation, haematemesis and melaena have, in general, more serious consequences in the elderly. They can occur at any time during treatment, with or without warning symptoms or a previous history. In the rare instances where gastro-intestinal bleeding or ulceration occurs in patients receiving Voltarol, the drug should be withdrawn.

*Hepatic:* Close medical surveillance is also imperative in patients suffering from severe impairment of hepatic function.

*Hypersensitivity reactions:* As with other nonsteroidal anti-inflammatory drugs, allergic reactions, including anaphylactic/anaphylactoid reactions, can also occur without earlier exposure to the drug.

Like other NSAIDs, Voltarol may mask the signs and symptoms of infection due to its pharmacodynamic properties.

*Precautions: Renal:* Patients with renal, cardiac or hepatic impairment and the elderly should be kept under surveillance, since the use of NSAIDs may result in deterioration of renal function. The lowest effective dose should be used and renal function monitored.

The importance of prostaglandins in maintaining renal blood flow should be taken into account in patients with impaired cardiac or renal function, those being treated with diuretics or recovering from major surgery. Effects on renal function are usually reversible on withdrawal of Voltarol.

*Hepatic:* If abnormal liver function tests persist or worsen, clinical signs or symptoms consistent with liver disease develop or if other manifestations occur (eosinophilia, rash), Voltarol should be discontinued. Hepatitis may occur without prodromal symptoms.

Use of Voltarol in patients with hepatic porphyria may trigger an attack.

*Haematological:* Voltarol may reversibly inhibit platelet aggregation (see *Anticoagulants* in *Drug interactions*). Patients with defects of haemostasis, bleeding diathesis or haematological abnormalities should be carefully monitored.

*Long-term treatment:* All patients who are receiving non-steroidal anti-inflammatory agents should be monitored as a precautionary measure e.g. renal function, hepatic function (elevation of liver enzymes may occur) and blood counts. This is particularly important in the elderly.

*Interaction with other medicaments and other forms of interaction:*
*Lithium and digoxin:* Voltarol may increase plasma concentrations of lithium and digoxin.

*Anticoagulants:* Although clinical investigations do not appear to indicate that Voltarol has an influence on the effect of anticoagulants, there are isolated reports of an increased risk of haemorrhage with the combined use of diclofenac and anticoagulant therapy. Therefore, to be certain that no change in anticoagulant dosage is required, close monitoring of such patients is required. As with other non-steroidal anti-inflammatory agents, diclofenac in a high dose can reversibly inhibit platelet aggregation.

*Antidiabetic agents:* Clinical studies have shown that Voltarol can be given together with oral antidiabetic agents without influencing their clinical effect. However, there have been isolated reports of hypoglycaemic and hyperglycaemic effects which have required adjustment to the dosage of hypoglycaemic agents.

*Cyclosporin:* Cases of nephrotoxicity have been reported in patients receiving concomitant cyclosporin and NSAIDs, including Voltarol. This might be mediated through combined renal antiprostaglandin effects of both the NSAID and cyclosporin.

*Methotrexate:* Cases of serious toxicity have been reported when methotrexate and NSAIDs are given within 24 hours of each other. This interaction is mediated through accumulation of methotrexate resulting from impairment of renal excretion in the presence of the NSAID.

*Quinolone antimicrobials:* Convulsions may occur due to an interaction between quinolones and NSAIDs. This may occur in patients with or without a previous history of epilepsy or convulsions. Therefore, caution should be exercised when considering the use of a quinolone in patients who are already receiving an NSAID.

*Other NSAIDs and steroids:* Co-administration of Voltarol with other systemic NSAIDs and steroids may increase the frequency of side-effects. Concomitant therapy with aspirin lowers the plasma levels of each, although no clinical significance is known.

*Diuretics:* Various NSAIDs are liable to inhibit the activity of diuretics. Concomitant treatment with potassium-sparing diuretics may be associated with increased serum potassium levels, hence serum potassium should be monitored.

*Pregnancy and lactation:* Although animal studies have not demonstrated teratogenic effects, Voltarol should not be prescribed during pregnancy, unless there are compelling reasons for doing so. The lowest effective dosage should be used.

Use of prostaglandin synthetase inhibitors may result in premature closure of the ductus arteriosus or uterine inertia; such drugs are, therefore, not recommended during the last trimester of pregnancy.

Following doses of 50 mg enteric coated tablets every 8 hours, traces of active substance have been detected in breast milk, but in quantities so small that no undesirable effects on the infant are to be expected.

*Effects on ability to drive and use machines:* Patients who experience dizziness or other central nervous disturbances, while taking NSAIDs should refrain from driving or operating machinery.

*Undesirable effects:* If serious side-effects occur, Voltarol should be withdrawn.

Frequency estimate: *frequent:* >10%, *occasional:* >1–10%, *rare:* >0.001–1%, *isolated cases:* <0.001%.

*Gastro-intestinal tract: Occasional:* Epigastric pain, other gastro-intestinal disorders (e.g. nausea, vomiting, diarrhoea, abdominal cramps, dyspepsia, flatulence, anorexia). *Rare:* Gastro-intestinal bleeding (haematemesis, melaena, bloody diarrhoea), gastrointestinal ulcers with or without bleeding or perforation. *Isolated cases:* Aphthous stomatitis, glossitis, oesophageal lesions, lower gut disorders (e.g. nonspecific haemorrhagic colitis and exacerbations of ulcerative colitis or Crohn's proctocolitis, colonic damage and stricture formation), pancreatitis, constipation.

*Central nervous system: Occasional:* Headache, dizziness, or vertigo. *Rare:* drowsiness, tiredness. *Isolated cases:* Disturbances of sensation, paraesthesia, memory disturbance, disorientation, insomnia, irritability, convulsions, depression, anxiety, nightmares, tremor, psychotic reactions, aseptic meningitis.

*Special senses: Isolated cases:* Disturbances of vision (blurred vision, diplopia), impaired hearing, tinnitus, taste disturbances.

*Skin: Occasional:* Rashes or skin eruptions. *Rare:* Urticaria. *Isolated cases:* Bullous eruptions, eczema, erythema multiforme, Steven's-Johnson syndrome, Lyell's syndrome (acute toxic epidermolysis), erythroderma (exfoliative dermatitis), loss of hair, photosensitivity reactions, purpura including allergic purpura.

*Kidney: Rare:* Oedema. *Isolated cases:* Acute renal insufficiency, urinary abnormalities (e.g. haematuria, proteinuria), interstitial nephritis, nephrotic syndrome, papillary necrosis.

*Liver: Occasional:* Elevation of serum aminotransferase enzymes (ALT, AST). *Rare:* Liver function disorders including hepatitis (in isolated cases fulminant) with or without jaundice.

*Blood: Isolated cases:* Thrombocytopenia, leucopenia, agranulocytosis, haemolytic anaemia, aplastic anaemia.

*Hypersensitivity: Rare:* Hypersensitivity reactions (e.g. bronchospasm, anaphylactic/anaphylactoid systemic reactions including hypotension). *Isolated cases:* Vasculitis, pneumonitis.

*Cardiovascular system: Isolated cases:* palpitations, chest pain, hypertension, congestive heart failure.

*Reactions to the intramuscular injection: Occasional:* Reactions such as local pain and induration. *Isolated cases:* Abscesses and local necrosis at the intramuscular injection site.

*Overdose:* Management of acute poisoning with NSAIDs essentially consists of supportive and symptomatic measures. There is no typical clinical picture resulting from Voltarol overdosage. Supportive and symptomatic treatment should be given for complications such as hypotension, renal failure, convulsions, gastro-intestinal irritation, and respiratory depression; specific therapies such as forced diuresis, dialysis or haemoperfusion are probably of no help in eliminating NSAIDs due to their high rate of protein binding and extensive metabolism.

**Pharmacological properties**
*Pharmacodynamic properties:*
*Pharmacotherapeutic group:* Non-steroidal anti-inflammatory drugs (NSAIDs).
*Mechanism of action:* Voltarol is a non-steroidal agent with marked analgesic/anti-inflammatory properties. It is an inhibitor of prostaglandin synthetase (cyclo-oxygenase). Diclofenac sodium *in vitro* does not suppress proteoglycan biosynthesis in cartilage at concentrations equivalent to the concentrations reached in human beings. When used concomitantly with opioids for the management of post-operative pain, Voltarol often reduces the need for opioids.

*Pharmacokinetic properties:*
*Absorption:* After administration of 75 mg diclofenac by intramuscular injection, absorption sets in immediately, and mean peak plasma concentrations of about 2.558±0.968 mcg/ml (2.5 mcg/ml≡8 µmol/l) are reached after about 20 minutes. The amount absorbed is in linear proportion to the size of the dose.

Intravenous infusion: When 75 mg diclofenac is administered as an intravenous infusion over 2 hours, mean peak plasma concentrations are about 1.875±0.436 mcg/ml (1.9 mcg/ml≡5.9 µmol/l). Shorter infusions result in higher peak plasma concentrations, while longer infusions give plateau concentrations proportional to the infusion rate after 3 to 4 hours. This is in contrast to the rapid decline in plasma concentrations seen after peak levels have been achieved with oral, rectal or intramuscular administration.

*Bioavailability:* The area under the concentration curve (AUC) after intramuscular or intravenous administration is about twice as large as it is following oral or rectal administration as this route avoids 'firstpass' metabolism.

*Distribution:* The active substance is 99.7% protein bound, mainly to albumin (99.4%).

Diclofenac enters the synovial fluid, where maximum concentrations are measured 2–4 hours after the peak plasma values have been attained. The apparent half-life for elimination from the synovial fluid is 3–6 hours. Two hours after reaching the peak plasma values, concentrations of the active substance are already higher in the synovial fluid than they are in the plasma and remain higher for up to 12 hours.

*Metabolism:* Biotransformation of diclofenac takes place partly by glucuronidation of the intact molecule, but mainly by single and multiple hydroxylation and methoxylation, resulting in several phenolic metabolites, most of which are converted to glucuronide conjugates. Two phenolic metabolites are biologically active, but to a much lesser extent than diclofenac.

*Elimination:* Total systemic clearance of diclofenac in plasma is 263±56 ml/min (mean value±SD). The terminal half-life in plasma is 1–2 hours. Four of the metabolites, including the two active ones, also have short plasma half-lives of 1–3 hours.

About 60% of the administered dose is excreted in the urine in the form of the glucuronide conjugate of the intact molecule and as metabolites, most of which are also converted to glucuronide conjugates. Less than 1% is excreted as unchanged substance. The rest of the dose is eliminated as metabolites through the bile in the faeces.

*Characteristics in patients: Elderly:* No relevant agedependent differences in the drug's absorption, metabolism or excretion have been observed, other than the finding that in five elderly patients, a 15 minute iv infusion resulted in 50% higher plasma concentrations than expected with young healthy subjects.

*Patients with renal impairment:* In patients suffering from renal impairment, no accumulation of the unchanged active substance can be inferred from the single-dose kinetics when applying the usual dosage schedule. At a creatinine clearance of <10 ml/min, the calculated steady-state plasma levels of the hydroxy metabolites are about 4 times higher than in normal subjects. However, the metabolites are ultimately cleared through the bile.

*Patients with hepatic disease:* In patients with chronic hepatitis or non-decompensated cirrhosis, the kinetics and metabolism of diclofenac are the same as in patients without liver disease.

*Preclinical safety data:* None stated.

**Pharmaceutical particulars**
*List of excipients:* Voltarol ampoules also contain mannitol, sodium metabisulphite (E.223), benzyl alcohol, propylene glycol, sodium hydroxide and water.

*Incompatibilities:* The ampoules used im or iv as an infusion should not be mixed with other injection solutions.

*Shelf life:* Two years.

*Special precautions for storage:* Protect from light and heat (store below 30°C).

Medicines should be kept out of the reach of children.

The infusion solution should not be used if crystals or precipitates are observed.

*Nature and contents of container:* The glass ampoules (PhEur Type I) contain colourless to faintly yellow liquid and come in packs of 2 and 10.

*Instructions for use/handling:* Intravenous infusions should be freshly made up and used immediately. Once prepared, the infusion should not be stored.

**Marketing authorisation number** 00101/0466.

**Date of approval/revision of SPC** 11 July 1997.

**Legal category** POM.

## VOLTAROL* DISPERSIBLE TABLETS

**Qualitative and quantitative composition** The active ingredient is o-[(2,6-dichlorophenyl)amino]phenyl-acetic acid (diclofenac). Each tablet contains 46.5 mg diclofenac free acid, which is equivalent to 50 mg of diclofenac sodium.

**Pharmaceutical form** Tablet.

**Clinical particulars**
*Therapeutic indications:*
*Adults and elderly:* The rapid onset of absorption of diclofenac from Voltarol Dispersible makes this preparation more suitable for *short-term* use in acute conditions for which treatment is required for no more than 3 months including: acute episodes of arthritic conditions, acute musculo-skeletal disorders and acute pain resulting from trauma.

There is no information on the use of Voltarol Dispersible for more than 3 months.

*Posology and method of administration:*
*Adults:* 100–150 mg daily in two or three divided doses. The Voltarol Dispersible tablet should be dropped into a glass of water, and the liquid stirred to aid dispersion, before swallowing.

The recommended maximum daily dose of Voltarol is 150 mg.

*Children:* Not recommended.

*Elderly:* Although the pharmacokinetics of Voltarol are not impaired to any clinically relevant extent in elderly patients, non-steroidal anti-inflammatory drugs should be used with particular caution in such patients who, generally, are more prone to adverse reactions. In particular it is recommended that the lowest effective dosage be used in frail elderly patients or those with a low body weight (see also *Precautions*).

*Contra-indications:* Active or suspected gastro-intestinal ulcers or bleeding. Previous sensitivity to diclofenac. Patients in whom attacks of asthma, urticaria or acute rhinitis are precipitated by aspirin or other non-steroidal anti-inflammatory agents.

*Special warnings and special precautions for use*
*Warnings: Gastro-intestinal:* Close medical surveillance is imperative in patients with symptoms indicative of gastro-intestinal disorders, with a history suggestive of gastro-intestinal ulceration, with ulcerative colitis, or with Crohn's disease.

Gastro-intestinal bleeding or ulcerative/perforation, haematemesis and melaena have, in general, more serious consequences in the elderly. They can occur at any time during treatment, with or without warning symptoms or a previous history. In the rare instances when gastro-intestinal bleeding or ulceration occurs in patients receiving Voltarol, the drug should be withdrawn.

In choosing to prescribe Voltarol Dispersible it should be remembered that any liquid NSAID preparation does not have the advantages of an enteric-coated tablet in relation to gastric tolerability. In clinical trials of three months duration, a slight increase in the frequency and reported severity of G.I. side-effects and higher rates of withdrawal because of these have been noted in patients receiving dispersible tablets compared with those receiving enteric-coated tablets.

An endoscopy study also revealed Voltarol Dispersible to have a slightly higher mucosal injury score than enteric-coated tablets, although no ulcers occurred with either treatment.These observations must be taken into account and weighed against the advantages of the dispersible formulation.

*Hepatic:* Close medical surveillance is also imperative in patients suffering from severe impairment of hepatic function.

*Hypersensitivity reactions:* As with other non-steroidal anti-inflammatory drugs, allergic reactions, including anaphylactic/anaphylactoid reactions, can also occur without earlier exposure to the drug.

Like other NSAIDs, Voltarol may mask the signs and symptoms of infection due to its pharmacodynamic properties.

*Precautions:*
*Renal:* Patients with renal, cardiac or hepatic impairment and the elderly should be kept under surveillance, since the use of NSAIDs may result in deterioration of renal function. The lowest effective dose should be used and renal function monitored.

The importance of prostaglandins in maintaining renal blood flow should be taken into account in patients with impaired cardiac or renal function, those being treated with diuretics or recovering from major surgery. Effects on renal function are usually reversible on withdrawal of Voltarol.

*Hepatic:* If abnormal liver function tests persist or worsen, clinical signs or symptoms consistent with liver disease develop or if other manifestations occur (eosinophilia, rash), Voltarol should be discontinued. Hepatitis may occur without prodromal symptoms.

Use of Voltarol in patients with hepatic porphyria may trigger an attack.

*Haematological:* Voltarol may reversibly inhibit platelet aggregation (see *Anticoagulants* in *Drug interactions*). Patients with defects of haemostasis, bleeding diathesis or haematological abnormalities should be carefully monitored.

*Long-term treatment:* All patients who are receiving non-steroidal anti-inflammatory agents should be monitored as a precautionary measure e.g. renal function, hepatic function (elevation of liver enzymes may occur) and blood counts. This is particularly important in the elderly.

*Interaction with other medicaments and other forms of interaction:*
*Lithium and digoxin:* Voltarol may increase plasma concentrations of lithium and digoxin.

*Anticoagulants:* Although clinical investigations do not appear to indicate that Voltarol has an influence on the effect of anticoagulants, there are isolated reports of an increased risk of haemorrhage with the combined use of diclofenac and anticoagulant therapy. Therefore, to be certain that no change in anticoagulant dosage is required, close monitoring of such patients is required. As with other non-steroidal anti-inflammatory agents, diclofenac in high dose can reversibly inhibit platelet aggregation.

*Antidiabetic agents:* Clinical studies have shown that Voltarol can be given together with oral antidiabetic agents without influencing their clinical effect. However, there have been isolated reports of hypoglycaemic and hyperglycaemic effects which have required adjustment to the dosage of hypoglycaemic agents.

*Cyclosporin:* Cases of nephrotoxicity have been reported in patients receiving concomitant cyclosporin and NSAIDs, including Voltarol. This might be mediated through combined renal antiprostaglandin effects of both the NSAID and cyclosporin.

*Methotrexate:* Cases of serious toxicity have been reported when methotrexate and NSAIDs are given within 24 hours of each other. This interaction is mediated through accumulation of methotrexate resulting from impairment of renal excretion in the presence of the NSAID.

*Quinolone antimicrobials:* Convulsions may occur due to an interaction between quinolones and NSAIDs. This may occur in patients with or without a previous history of epilepsy or convulsions. Therefore, caution should be exercised when considering the use of a quinolone in patients who are already receiving an NSAID.

*Other NSAIDs and steroids:* Co-administration of Voltarol with other systemic NSAIDs and steroids may increase the frequency of unwanted effects. Concomitant therapy with aspirin lowers the plasma levels of each, although no clinical significance is known.

*Diuretics:* Various NSAIDs are liable to inhibit the activity of diuretics. Concomitant treatment with potassium-sparing diuretics may be associated with increased serum potassium levels, hence serum potassium should be monitored.

*Pregnancy and lactation:* Although animal studies have not demonstrated teratogenic effects, Voltarol should not be prescribed during pregnancy, unless there are compelling reasons for doing so. The lowest effective dosage should be used.

Use of prostaglandin synthetase inhibitors may result in premature closure of the ductus arteriosus or uterine inertia; such drugs are, therefore, not recommended during the last trimester of pregnancy.

Following doses of 50 mg enteric coated tablets every 8 hours, traces of active substance have been detected in breast milk, but in quantities so small that no undesirable effects on the infant are to be expected.

*Effects on ability to drive and use machines:* Patients who experience dizziness or other central nervous disturbances while taking NSAIDs should refrain from driving or operating machinery.

*Undesirable effects:* If serious side-effects occur, Voltarol should be withdrawn.

Frequency estimate: *frequent:* >10%, *occasional:* >1–10%, *rare:* >0.001–1%, *isolated cases:* <0.001%.

*Gastro-intestinal tract: Occasional:* Epigastric pain, other gastro-intestinal disorders (e.g. nausea, vomiting, diarrhoea, abdominal cramps, dyspepsia, flatulence, anorexia). *Rare:* Gastro-intestinal bleeding (haematemesis, melaena, bloody diarrhoea), gastro-intestinal ulcers with or without bleeding or perforation. *Isolated cases:* Aphthous stomatitis, glossitis, oesophageal lesions, lower gut disorders (e.g. non-specific haemorrhagic colitis and exacerbations of ulcerative colitis or Crohn's proctocolitis, colonic damage and stricture formation), pancreatitis, constipation.

*Central nervous system: Occasional:* Headache, dizziness, or vertigo. *Rare:* drowsiness, tiredness. *Isolated cases:* Disturbances of sensation, paraesthesia, memory disturbance, disorientation, insomnia, irritability, convulsions, depression, anxiety, nightmares, tremor, psychotic reactions, aseptic meningitis.

*Special senses: Isolated cases:* Disturbances of vision (blurred vision, diplopia), impaired hearing, tinnitus, taste disturbances.

*Skin: Occasional:* Rashes or skin eruptions. *Rare:* Urticaria. *Isolated cases:* Bullous eruptions, eczema, erythema multiforme, Steven's-Johnson syndrome, Lyell's syndrome (acute toxic epidermolysis), erythroderma (exfoliative dermatitis), loss of hair, photosensitivity reactions, purpura including allergic purpura.

*Kidney: Rare:* Oedema. *Isolated cases:* Acute renal insufficiency, urinary abnormalities (e.g. haematuria, proteinuria), interstitial nephritis, nephrotic syndrome, papillary necrosis.

*Liver: Occasional:* Elevation of serum aminotransferase enzymes (ALT, AST). *Rare:* Liver function disorders including hepatitis (in isolated cases fulminant) with or without jaundice.

*Blood: In isolated cases:* Thrombocytopenia, leucopenia, agranulocytosis, haemolytic anaemia, aplastic anaemia.

*Hypersensitivity: Rare:* Hypersensitivity reactions (e.g. bronchospasm, anaphylactic/anaphylactoid systemic reactions including hypotension). *Isolated cases:* Vasculitis, pneumonitis.

*Cardiovascular system: Isolated cases:* Palpitations, chest pain, hypertension, congestive heart failure.

*Overdose:* Management of acute poisoning with NSAIDs essentially consists of supportive and symptomatic measures. There is no typical clinical picture resulting from Voltarol overdosage. The therapeutic measures to be taken are: supportive and symptomatic treatment should be given for complications such as hypotension, renal failure, convulsions, gastro-intestinal irritation, and respiratory depression; specific therapies such as forced diuresis, dialysis or haemoperfusion are probably of no help in eliminating NSAIDs due to their high rate of protein binding and extensive metabolism.

**Pharmacological properties**
*Pharmacodynamic properties:*
*Pharmacotherapeutic group:* Non-steroidal anti-inflammatory drugs (NSAIDs).

*Mechanism of action:* Voltarol is a non-steroidal agent with marked analgesic/anti-inflammatory properties. It is an inhibitor of prostaglandin synthetase (cyclo-oxygenase).

Diclofenac sodium *in vitro* does not suppress proteoglycan biosynthesis in cartilage at concentrations equivalent to the concentrations reached in human beings.

*Pharmacokinetic properties:*
*Absorption:* Absorption begins immediately upon administration. Mean peak plasma concentrations of diclofenac are reached at about 1 hour 0.9±0.0.4 mcg/ml (1 mcg/ml≡3 µmol/l). Ingestion of dispersible tablets together with or immediately after a meal does not delay the onset of absorption but reduces the amount absorbed by on average of about 16% and the maximum concentrations by about 50%.

*Bioavailability:* The bioavailability is 82% of that of enteric-coated tablets. Ingestion with food affects the bioavailability (see above).

Pharmacokinetic behaviour does not change on repeated administration. Accumulation does not occur, provided the recommended dosage intervals are observed.

*Distribution:* The active substance is 99.7% protein bound, mainly to albumin (99.4%).

Diclofenac enters the synovial fluid, where maximum concentrations are measured 2–4 hours after the peak plasma values have been attained. The apparent half-life for elimination from the synovial fluid is 3–6 hours. Two hours after reaching the peak plasma values, concentrations of the active substance are already higher in the synovial fluid than they are in the plasma and they remain higher for up to 12 hours.

*Metabolism:* Biotransformation of diclofenac takes place partly by glucuronidation of the intact molecule, but mainly by single and multiple hydroxylation and methoxylation, resulting in several phenolic metabolites, most of which are converted to glucuronide conjugates. Two phenolic metabolites are biologically active, but to a much lesser extent than diclofenac.

*Elimination:* The total systemic clearance of diclofenac in plasma is 263±56 ml/min (mean value±SD). The terminal half-life in plasma is 1–2 hours. Four of the metabolites, including the two active ones, also have short plasma half-lives of 1–3 hours.

About 60% of the administered dose is excreted in the urine in the form of the glucuronide conjugate of the intact molecule and as metabolites, most of which are also converted to glucuronide conjugates. Less than 1% is excreted as unchanged substance. The rest of the dose is eliminated as metabolites through the bile in the faeces.

*Characteristics in patients: Elderly:* No relevant age-dependent differences in the drug's absorption, metabolism, or excretion have been observed, other than the finding that in five elderly patients, a 15 minute iv infusion resulted in 50% higher plasma concentrations than expected with young healthy subjects.

*Patients with renal impairmment:* In patients suffering from renal impairment, no accumulation of the unchanged active substance can be inferred from the single-dose kinetics when applying the usual dosage schedule. At a creatinine clearance of <10 ml/min, the calculated steady-state plasma levels of the hydroxy metabolites are about 4 times higher than in normal subjects. However, the metabolites are ultimately cleared through the bile.

*Patients with hepatic disease:* In patients with chronic hepatitis or non-decompensated cirrhosis, the kinetics and metabolism of diclofenac are the same as in patients without liver disease.

*Preclinical safety data:* None stated.

**Pharmaceutical particulars**

*List of excipients:* The dispersible tablets also contain microcrystalline cellulose, croscarmellose sodium type A, sodium starch glycollate, sodium saccharin, hydrogenated caster oil, purified talc special, colloidal anhydrous silica, blackcurrant and F.D. and C. red No. 3.

*Incompatibilities:* None known.

*Shelf life:* Five years.

*Special precautions for storage;* Protect from heat (store below 30°C) and moisture. Medicines should be kept out of the reach of children.

*Nature and contents of container:* The tablets are pink speckled with white, triangular shaped, uncoated tablets, impressed GEIGY on one side with an embossed 'V' on the other, with a blackcurrant odour and come in aluminium blister packs of 21.

*Instructions for use/handling:* The dispersible tablets should be dissolved in water.

**Marketing authorisation number** 00101/0467.

**Date of approval/revision of SPC** 11 July 1997.

**Legal category** POM.

## VOLTAROL* EMULGEL

**Qualitative and quantitative composition** Diethylammonium-{-o-[2,6-dichlorophenyl)-amino]-phenyl}-acetate. 100 g of Voltarol Emulgel contains 1.16 g of the active substance diclofenac diethylammonium, which corresponds to 1 g diclofenac sodium.

**Pharmaceutical form** Gel for topical administration.

**Clinical particulars**

*Therapeutic indications:*

For the local symptomatic relief of pain and inflammation in:

- trauma of the tendons, ligaments, muscles and joints, e.g. due to sprains, strains and bruises
- localised forms of soft tissue rheumatism

It is recommended that treatment be reviewed after 14 days in these indications.

For the treatment of osteoarthritis of superficial joints such as the knee.

In the treatment of osteoarthritis, therapy should be reviewed after 4 weeks.

*Posology and method of administration:*

*Adults:* Voltarol Emulgel should be rubbed gently into the skin. Depending on the size of the affected site to be treated 2–4 g (a circular shaped mass approximately 2.0–2.5 cm in diameter) should be applied 3–4 times a day. After application, the hands should be washed unless they are the site being treated.

*Use in the elderly:* The usual adult dosage may be used.

*Children:* Voltarol Emulgel is not recommended for use in children as dosage recommendations and indications for use in this group of patients have not been established.

Voltarol Emulgel is suitable for the transmission of ultrasound and may be used as a couplant in combination with ultrasound therapy. If large areas of the body are covered with gel, systemic absorption will be greater and the risk of side-effects increased, especially if the therapy is used frequently.

*Contra-indications:* Patients with or without chronic asthma in whom attacks of asthma, urticaria or acute rhinitis are precipitated by aspirin or other non-steroidal anti-inflammatory agents. Hypersensitivity to diclofenac, acetylsalicylic acid or other non-steroidal anti-inflammatory drugs. Hypersensitivity to propylene glycol, isopropanol or other components of the gel base.

*Special warnings and special precautions for use:*

*Warnings:* None stated.

*Precautions:* Concomitant use of oral NSAIDs should be cautioned as the incidence of untoward effects, particularly systemic side effects, may increase (see also *Interactions*).

Voltarol Emulgel should not be co-administered with other products containing diclofenac.

Voltarol Emulgel should be applied only to intact, non-diseased skin and not to skin wounds or open injuries. It should not be used with occlusion. It should not be allowed to come into contact with the eyes or mucous membranes, and should never be taken by mouth.

Some possibility of gastro-intestinal bleeding in those with a significant history of this condition has been reported in isolated cases.

*Interactions with other medicaments and other forms of interaction:* Systemic absorption of Voltarol Emulgel is low and hence the risk of an interaction is small. There are no known interactions with Volterol Emulgel but for a list of interactions known with oral diclofenac the SPC for oral dosage forms should be consulted.

*Pregnancy and lactation:* Since no experience has been acquired with Voltarol Emulgel in pregnancy or lactation, it is not recommended for use in these circumstances.

During the last trimester of pregnancy the use of prostaglandin synthetase inhibitors may result in premature closure of the ductus arteriosus, or in uterine inertia.

Animal data have shown an increased incidence of dystonia and delayed parturition when drug administration is continued into late pregnancy.

*Effects on ability to drive and use machines:* None known.

*Undesirable effects: Local reactions:* Voltarol Emulgel is usually well tolerated. *Occasional:* allergic or non-allergic contact dermatitis (with symptoms and signs such as itching, reddening, oedema, papules, vesicles, bullae or scaling of skin).

*Systemic reactions: Isolated cases:* generalised skin rash, hypersensitivity reactions (e.g. asthmatic attacks, angio-oedema), photosensitivity reactions.

Patients should be warned against excessive exposure to sunlight in order to reduce the incidence of photosensitivity.

*General:* Systemic absorption of Voltarol Emulgel is low compared with plasma levels obtained following administration of oral forms of Voltarol and the likelihood of systemic side-effects occurring with topical diclofenac is small compared with the frequency of side-effects associated with oral diclofenac. However, where Voltarol Emulgel is applied to a relatively large area of skin and over a prolonged period, the possibility of systemic side-effects cannot be completely excluded. If such usage is envisaged, the SPC on Voltarol oral dosage forms should be consulted.

Asthma has been rarely reported in patients using topical NSAID preparations.

*Overdose:*

*Signs and symptoms:* The low systemic absorption of Voltarol Emulgel renders overdosage extremely unlikely. In the event of accidental ingestion, resulting in significant systemic side-effects, general therapeutic measures normally adopted to treat poisoning with non-steroidal anti-inflammatory drugs should be used.

*Treatment:* Management of overdosage with NSAIDs essentially consists of supportive and symptomatic measures. There is no typical clinical picture resulting from Voltarol overdosage. Supportive and symptomatic treatment should be given for complications such as hypotension, renal failure, convulsions, gastro-intestinal irritation, and respiratory depression; specific therapies such as forced diuresis, dialysis or haemoperfusion are probably of no help in eliminating NSAIDs due to their high rate of protein binding and extensive metabolism.

**Pharmacological properties**

*Pharmacodynamic properties:* Voltarol Emulgel is a non-steroidal anti-inflammatory (NSAID) and analgesic preparation designed for external application. Due to an aqueous-alcoholic base the gel exerts a soothing and cooling effect.

*Pharmacokinetic properties:* When Voltarol Emulgel is applied locally, the active substance is absorbed through the skin. In healthy volunteers approximately 6% of the dose applied is absorbed, as determined by urinary excretion of diclofenac and its hydroxylated metabolites. Findings in patients confirm that diclofenac penetrates inflamed areas following local application of Voltarol Emulgel.

After topical administration of Voltarol Emulgel to hand and knee joints diclofenac can be measured in plasma, synovial tissue and synovial fluid. Maximum plasma concentrations of diclofenac are about 100 times lower than after oral administration of Voltarol.

*Preclinical safety data:* None known.

**Pharmaceutical particulars**

*List of excipients:* Diethylamine, carbopol 934P, cetomacrogol 1000, cetiol LC, isopropyl alcohol, liquid paraffin heavy, perfume creme 45, propylene glycol dist., and water.

*Incompatibilities:* None known.

*Shelf life:* Three years.

*Special precautions for storage:* Protect from heat (store below 30°C). Voltarol Emulgel should be kept out of the reach of children.

*Nature and contents of container:* Aluminium tubes with protective inner coating, available in packs of 100 g.

*Instructions for use/handling:* None.

**Marketing authorisation number** 00101/0468.

**Date of approval/revision of SPC** 11 July 1997.

**Legal category** POM.

## VOLTAROL* TABLETS

**Qualitative and quantitative composition** The active substance is sodium-[o-[(2,6-dichlorophenyl)-amino]-phenyl]-acetate (diclofenac sodium).

Each enteric-coated tablet contains 25 mg or 50 mg Diclofenac Sodium PhEur.

**Pharmaceutical form** Enteric coated tablet.

**Clinical particulars**

*Therapeutic indications:*

*Adults and elderly:* Relief of all grades of pain and inflammation in a wide range of conditions, including:

(i) arthritic conditions: rheumatoid arthritis, osteoarthritis, ankylosing spondylitis, acute gout,

(ii) acute musculo-skeletal disorders such as periarthritis (for example, frozen shoulder), tendinitis, tenosynovitis, bursitis,

(iii) other painful conditions resulting from trauma, including fracture, low back pain, sprains, strains, dislocations, orthopaedic, dental and other minor surgery.

*Children (aged 1–12 years):* Juvenile chronic arthritis (25 mg enteric-coated tablets only).

*Posology and method of administration*

*Adults:* 75–150 mg daily in two or three divided doses.

The recommended maximum daily dose of Voltarol is 150 mg.

*Children (aged 1–12 years)* 25 mg enteric-coated tablets only: 1–3 mg/kg per day individed doses.

*Elderly:* Although the pharmacokinetics of Voltarol are not impaired to any clinically relevant extent in elderly patients, non-steroidal anti-inflammatory drugs should be used with particular caution in such patients who, generally, are more prone to adverse reactions. In particular, it is recommended that the lowest effective dosage be used in frail, elderly patients or those with a low body weight (see also *Precautions*).

*Contra-indications:* Active or suspected gastro-intestinal ulcers or bleeding.

Previous sensitivity to diclofenac.

Patients in whom attacks of asthma, urticaria or acute rhinitis are precipitated by aspirin or other non-steroidal anti-inflammatory agents.

*Special warnings and special precautions for use:*

*Warnings:* Close medical surveillance is imperative in patients with symptoms indicative of gastro-intestinal disorders, with a history suggestive of gastric or intestinal ulceration, with ulcerative colitis, or with Crohn's disease.

Gastro-intestinal bleeding or ulceration/perforation, haematemesis and melaena have, in general, more serious consequences in the elderly. They can occur at any time during treatment, with or without warning symptoms or a previous history. In the rare instances when gastro-intestinal bleeding or ulceration occurs in patients receiving Voltarol, the drug should be withdrawn.

*Hepatic:* Close medical surveillance is also imperative in patients suffering from severe impairment of hepatic function.

*Hypersensitivity reactions:* As with other non-steroidal anti-inflammatory drugs, allergic reactions, including anaphylactic/anaphylactoid reactions, can also occur without earlier exposure to the drug.

Like other NSAIDs, Voltarol may mask the signs and symptoms of infection due to its pharmacodynamic properties.

*Precautions:*

*Renal:* Patients with renal, cardiac or hepatic impairment and the elderly should be kept under surveillance, since the use of NSAIDs may result in deterioration of renal function. The lowest effective dose should be used and renal function monitored.

The importance of prostaglandins in maintaining renal blood flow should be taken into account in patients with impaired cardiac or renal function, those being treated with diuretics or recovering from major surgery. Effects on renal function are usually reversible on withdrawal of Voltarol.

*Hepatic:* If abnormal liver function tests persist or worsen, clinical signs or symptoms consistent with liver disease develop or if other manifestations occur (eosinophilia, rash), Voltarol should be discontinued. Hepatitis may occur without prodromal symptoms.

Use of Voltarol in patients with hepatic porphyria may trigger an attack.

*Haematological:* Voltarol may reversibly inhibit platelet aggregation (see *Anticoagulants* in *Drug interactions*). Patients with defects of haemostasis, bleeding diathesis or haematological abnormalities should be carefully monitored.

*Long-term treatment:* All patients who are receiving non-steroidal anti-inflammatory agents should be monitored as a precautionary measure e.g. renal function, hepatic function (elevation of liver enzymes may occur) and blood counts. This is particularly important in the elderly.

*Interaction with other medicaments and other forms of interaction:*
*Lithium and digoxin:* Voltarol may increase plasma concentrations of lithium and digoxin.
*Anticoagulants:* Although clinical investigations do not appear to indicate that Voltarol has an influence on the effect of anticoagulants, there are isolated reports of an increased risk of haemorrhage with the combined use of diclofenac and anticoagulant therapy. Therefore, to be certain that no change in anticoagulant dosage is required, close monitoring of such patients is required. As with other non-steroidal anti-inflammatory agents, diclofenac in high dose can reversibly inhibit platelet aggregation.
*Antidiabetic agents:* Clinical studies have shown that Voltarol can be given together with oral antidiabetic agents without influencing their clinical effect. However there have been isolated reports of hypoglycaemic and hyperglycaemic effects which have required adjustment to the dosage of hypoglycaemic agents.
*Cyclosporin:* Cases of nephrotoxicity have been reported in patients receiving concomitant cyclosporin and NSAIDs, including Voltarol. This might be mediated through combined renal antiprostaglandin effects of both the NSAID and cyclosporin.
*Methotrexate:* Cases of serious toxicity have been reported when methotrexate and NSAIDs are given within 24 hours of each other. This interaction is mediated through accumulation of methotrexate resulting from impairment of renal excretion in the presence of the NSAID.
*Quinolone antimicrobials:* Convulsions may occur due to an interaction between quinolones and NSAIDs. This may occur in patients with or without a previous history of epilepsy or convulsions. Therefore, caution should be exercised when considering the use of a quinolone in patients who are already receiving an NSAID.
*Other NSAIDs and steroids:* Co-administration of Voltarol with other systemic NSAIDs and steroids may increase the frequency of unwanted effects. Concomitant therapy with aspirin lowers the plasma levels of each, although no clinical significance is known.
*Diuretics:* Various NSAIDs are liable to inhibit the activity of diuretics. Concomitant treatment with potassium-sparing diuretics may be associated with increased serum potassium levels, hence serum potassium should be monitored.

*Pregnancy and lactation:* Although animal studies have not demonstrated teratogenic effects, Voltarol should not be prescribed during pregnancy, unless there are compelling reasons for doing so. The lowest effective dosage should be used.

Use of prostaglandin synthetase inhibitors may result in premature closure of the ductus arteriosus or uterine inertia; such drugs are, therefore, not recommended during the last trimester of pregnancy.

Following doses of 50 mg enteric coated tablets every 8 hours, traces of active substance have been detected in breast milk, but in quantities so small that no undesirable effects on the infant are to be expected.

*Effects on ability to drive and use machines:* Patients who experience dizziness or other central nervous disturbances, while taking NSAIDs should refrain from driving or operating machinery.

*Undesirable effects:* If serious side-effects occur, Voltarol should be withdrawn.
Frequency estimate: *frequent:* >10%, *occasional:* >1–10%, *rare:* >0.001–1%, *isolated cases:* <0.001%.
*Gastro-intestinal tract:* Occasional: Epigastric pain, other gastro-intestinal disorders (e.g. nausea, vomiting, diarrhoea, abdominal cramps, dyspepsia, flatulence, anorexia). *Rare:* Gastro-intestinal bleeding (haematemesis, melaena, bloody diarrhoea), gastrointestinal ulcers with or without bleeding or perforation. *Isolated cases:* Aphthous stomatitis, glossitis, oesophageal lesions, lower gut disorders (e.g. nonspecific haemorrhagic colitis and exacerbations of ulcerative colitis or Crohn's proctocolitis, colonic damage and stricture formation), pancreatitis, constipation.

*Central nervous system: Occasional:* Headache, dizziness, or vertigo. *Rare:* drowsiness, tiredness. *Isolated cases:* Disturbances of sensation, paraesthesia, memory disturbance, disorientation, insomnia, irritability, convulsions, depression, anxiety, nightmares, tremor, psychotic reactions, aseptic meningitis.
*Special senses: Isolated cases:* Disturbances of vision (blurred vision, diplopia), impaired hearing, tinnitus, taste disturbances.
*Skin: Occasional:* Rashes or skin eruptions. *Rare:* Urticaria. *Isolated cases:* Bullous eruptions, eczema, erythema multiforme, Steven's-Johnson syndrome, Lyell's syndrome (acute toxic epidermolysis), erythroderma (exfoliative dermatitis), loss of hair, photosensitivity reactions, purpura including allergic purpura.
*Kidney: Rare:* Oedema. *Isolated cases:* Acute renal insufficiency, urinary abnormalities (e.g. haematuria, proteinuria), interstitial nephritis, nephrotic syndrome, papillary necrosis.
*Liver: Occasional:* Elevation of serum aminotransferase enzymes (ALT, AST). *Rare:* Liver function disorders including hepatitis (in isolated cases fulminant) with or without jaundice.
*Blood: Isolated cases:* Thrombocytopenia, leucopenia, agranulocytosis, haemolytic anaemia, aplastic anaemia.
*Hypersensitivity: Rare:* Hypersensitivity reactions (e.g. bronchospasm, anaphylactic/anaphylactoid systemic reactions including hypotension). *Isolated cases:* Vasculitis, pneumonitis.
*Cardiovascular system: Isolated cases:* Palpitations, chest pain, hypertension, congestive heart failure.

*Overdose:* Management of acute poisoning with NSAIDs essentially consists of supportive and symptomatic measures. There is no typical clinical picture resulting from Voltarol overdosage. The therapeutic measures to be taken are: Supportive and symptomatic treatment should be given for complications such as hypotension, renal failure, convulsions, gastro-intestinal irritation, and respiratory depression; special therapies such as forced diuresis, dialysis or haemoperfusion are probably of no help in eliminating NSAIDs due to their high rate of protein binding and extensive metabolism.

## Pharmacological properties
*Pharmacodynamic properties*
*Pharmacotherapeutic group:* Non-steroidal antiinflammatory drugs (NSAIDs).
*Mechanism of action:* Voltarol is a non-steroidal agent with marked analgesic/anti-inflammatory properties. It is an inhibitor of prostaglandin synthetase (cyclo-oxygenase).
Diclofenac sodium *in vitro* does not suppress proteoglycan biosynthesis in cartilage at concentrations equivalent to the concentrations reached in human beings.

*Pharmacokinetic properties:*
*Absorption:* Absorption is complete but onset is delayed until passage through the stomach, which may be affected by food, which delays stomach emptying. The mean peak plasma diclofenac concentration reached at about 2 hours (50 mg dose produces 1.48±0.65 mcg/ml (1.5 mcg/ml≡5 µmol/l)).
*Bioavailability:* About half of the administered diclofenac is metabolised during its first passage through the liver ('first-pass' effect), the area under the concentrations-curve (AUC) following oral administration is about half that following an equivalent parenteral dose.
Pharmacokinetic behaviour does not change on repeated administration. Accumulation does not occur, provided the recommended dosage intervals are observed.
*25 mg enteric-coated tablet only:* The plasms concentrations attained in children given equivalent doses (mg/kg, b.w.) are similar to those obtained in adults.
*Distribution:* The active substance is 99.7% protein bound, mainly to albumin (99.4%).
Diclofenac enters the synovial fluid, where maximum concentrations are measured 2–4 hours after the peak plasma values have been attained. The apparent half-life for elimination from the synovial fluid is 3–6 hours. Two hours after reaching the peak plasma values, concentrations of the active substance are already higher in the synovial fluid than they are in the plasma and remain higher for up to 12 hours.
*Metabolism:* Biotransformation of diclofenac takes place partly by glucuronidation of the intact molecule, but mainly by single and multiple hydroxylation and methoxylation, resulting in several phenolic metabolites, most of which are converted to glucuronide conjugates. Two phenolic metabolites are biologically active, but to a much lesser extent than diclofenac.
*Elimination:* Total systemic clearance of diclofenac in plasma is 263±56 ml/min (mean value±SD). The terminal half-life in plasma is 1–2 hours. Four of the metabolites, including the two active ones, also have short plasma half-lives of 1–3 hours.

About 60% of the administered dose is excreted in the urine in the form of the glucuronide conjugate of the intact molecule and as metabolites, most of which are also converted to glucuronide conjugates. Less than 1% is excreted as unchanged substance. The rest of the dose is eliminated as metabolites through the bile in the faeces.
*Characteristics in patients: Elderly:* No relevant agedependent differences in the drug's absorption, metabolism or excretion have been observed, other than the finding that in five elderly patients, a 15 minute iv infusion resulted in 50% higher plasma concentrations than expected with young healthy subjects.
*Patients with renal impairment:* In patients suffering from renal impairment, no accumulation of the unchanged active substance can be inferred from the single-dose kinetics when applying the usual dosage schedule. At a creatinine clearance of <10 ml/min, the calculated steady-state plasma levels of the hydroxy metabolites are about 4 times higher than in normal subjects. However, the metabolites are ultimately cleared through the bile.
*Patients with hepatic disease:* In patients with chronic hepatitis or non-decompensated cirrhosis, the kinetics and metabolism of diclofenac are the same as in patients without liver disease.

*Preclinical safety data:* None stated.

**Pharmaceutical particulars**
*List of excipients:* The enteric-coated tablets also contain colloidal anhydrous silica, lactose, maize starch, sodium starch glycollate, povidone (K30), microcrystalline cellulose, magnesium stearate, hydroxypropylmethylcellulose, Cremophor RH40, yellow iron oxide (E.172), red iron oxide (E.172). *50 mg tablet only:* purified talc special, titanium dioxide (E.171), eudragit L30D-55, polyethylene glycol 8000 flakes, silicone antifoam emulsion SE2, ammonia 25% and purified water.

*Incompatibilities:* None known.

*Shelf life:* 5 years.

*Special precautions for storage:* Protect from moisture. Store below 30°C. Medicines should be kept out of the reach of children.

*Nature and contents of container:* The 25 mg tablets are yellow, round, biconvex, film coated tablets, impressed GEIGY on one face and VOLTAROL 25 on the other, and come in PVC/PVdC blister packs of 84.

The 50 mg tablets are light brown, round, biconvex, film coated tablets, impressed GEIGY on one face and VOLTAROL 50 on the other, and come in PVC/PVdC blister packs of 14 and 84.

*Instructions for use/handling:* The enteric-coated tablets should be swallowed whole, preferably before meals.

**Marketing authorisation numbers**
25 mg     00101/0476
50 mg     00101/0477

**Date of approval/revision of SPC**   11 July 1997.

**Legal category**   POM.

## VOLTAROL* SR and RETARD TABLETS

**Qualitative and quantitative composition** The active substance is sodium-[o-[(2,6-dichlorophenyl)-amino]-phenyl]-acetate (diclofenac sodium).
Each slow release/retard tablet contains 75 mg or 100 mg Diclofenac Sodium PhEur.

**Pharmaceutical form** Slow/sustained release, film-coated tablet.

**Clinical particulars**
*Therapeutic indications:*
*Adults and elderly:* Relief of all grades of pain and inflammation in a wide range of conditions, including:
(i) arthritic conditions: rheumatoid arthritis, osteoarthritis, ankylosing spondylitis, acute gout,
(ii) acute musculo-skeletal disorders such as periarthritis (for example, frozen shoulder), tendonitis, tenosynovitis, bursitis,
(iii) other painful conditions resulting from trauma, including fracture, low back pain, sprains, strains, dislocations, orthopaedic, dental and other minor surgery.
*Children:* Voltarol 75 mg SR tablets and Retard tablets 100 mg are not suitable for children.

*Posology and method of administration:*
*Adults:* One tablet once or twice daily, taken whole with liquid, preferably at meal times.
The recommended maximum daily dose of Voltarol is 150 mg.

*Children:* Voltarol 75 mg SR tablets and Retard tablets 100 mg are not suitable for children.

*Elderly:* Although the pharmacokinetics of Voltarol are not impaired to any clinically relevant extent in elderly patients, non-steroidal anti-inflammatory drugs should be used with particular caution in such patients who, generally, are more prone to adverse reactions. In particular, it is recommended that the lowest effective dosage be used in frail, elderly patients or those with a low body weight (see also *Precautions*).

*Contra-indications:* Active or suspected gastro-intestinal ulcers or bleeding.

Previous sensitivity to diclofenac.

Patients in whom attacks of asthma, urticaria or acute rhinitis are precipitated by aspirin or other non-steroidal anti-inflammatory agents.

*Special warnings and special precautions for use:*
*Warnings:* Close medical surveillance is imperative in patients with symptoms indicative of gastro-intestinal disorders, with a history suggestive of gastric or intestinal ulceration, with ulcerative colitis, or with Crohn's disease.

Gastro-intestinal bleeding or ulceration/perforation, haematemesis and melaena have, in general, more serious consequences in the elderly. They can occur at any time during treatment, with or without warning symptoms or a previous history. In the rare instances when gastro-intestinal bleeding or ulceration occur in patients receiving Voltarol, the drug should be withdrawn.

*Hepatic:* Close medical surveillance is also imperative in patients suffering from severe impairment of hepatic function.

*Hypersensitivity reactions:* As with other non-steroidal anti-inflammatory drugs, allergic reactions, including anaphylactic/anaphylactoid reactions, can also occur without earlier exposure to the drug.

Like other NSAIDs, Voltarol may mask the signs and symptoms of infection due to its pharmacodynamic properties.

*Precautions: Renal:* Patients with renal, cardiac or hepatic impairment and the elderly should be kept under surveillance, since the use of NSAIDs may result in deterioration of renal function. The lowest effective dose should be used and renal function monitored.

The importance of prostaglandins in maintaining renal blood flow should be taken into account in patients with impaired cardiac or renal function, those being treated with diuretics or recovering from major surgery. Effects on renal function are usually reversible on withdrawal of Voltarol.

*Hepatic:* If abnormal liver function tests persist or worsen, clinical signs or symptoms consistent with liver disease develop or if other manifestations occur (eosinophilia, rash), Voltarol should be discontinued. Hepatitis may occur without prodromal symptoms.

Use of Voltarol in patients with hepatic porphyria may trigger an attack.

*Haematological:* Voltarol may reversibly inhibit platelet aggregation (see *Anticoagulants* in *Drug interactions*). Patients with defects of haemostasis, bleeding diathesis or haematological abnormalities should be carefully monitored.

*Long-term treatment:* All patients who are receiving non-steroidal anti-inflammatory agents should be monitored as a precautionary measure e.g. renal function, hepatic function (elevation of liver enzymes may occur) and blood counts. This is particularly important in the elderly.

*Interaction with other medicaments and other forms of interaction:*
*Lithium and digoxin:* Voltarol may increase plasma concentrations of lithium and digoxin.

*Anticoagulants:* Although clinical investigations do not appear to indicate that Voltarol has an influence on the effect of anticoagulants, there are isolated reports of an increased risk of haemorrhage with the combined use of diclofenac and anticoagulant therapy. Therefore, to be certain that no change in anticoagulant dosage is required, close monitoring of such patients is required. As with other non-steroidal anti-inflammatory agents, diclofenac in high dose can reversibly inhibit platelet aggregation.

*Antidiabetic agents:* Clinical studies have shown that Voltarol can be given together with oral antidiabetic agents without influencing their clinical effect. However, there have been isolated reports of hypoglycaemic and hyperglycaemic effects which have required adjustment to the dosage of hypoglycaemic agents.

*Cyclosporin:* Cases of nephrotoxicity have been reported in patients receiving concomitant cyclosporin and NSAIDs, including Voltarol. This might be mediated through combined renal antiprostaglandin effects of both the NSAID and cyclosporin.

*Methotrexate:* Cases of serious toxicity have been reported when methotrexate and NSAIDs are given within 24 hours of each other. This interaction is mediated through accumulation of methotrexate resulting from impairment of renal excretion in the presence of the NSAID.

*Quinolone antimicrobials:* Convulsions may occur due to an interaction between quinolones and NSAIDs. This may occur in patients with or without a previous history of epilepsy or convulsions. Therefore, caution should be exercised when considering the use of a quinolone in patients who are already receiving an NSAID.

*Other NSAIDs and steroids:* Co-administration of Voltarol with other systemic NSAIDs and steroids may increase the frequency of unwanted effects. Concomitant therapy with aspirin lowers the plasma levels of each, although no clinical significance is known.

*Diuretics:* Various NSAIDs are liable to inhibit the activity of diuretics. Concomitant treatment with potassium-sparing diuretics may be associated with increased serum potassium levels, hence serum potassium should be monitored.

*Pregnancy and lactation:* Although animal studies have not demonstrated teratogenic effects, Voltarol should not be prescribed during pregnancy, unless there are compelling reasons for doing so. The lowest effective dosage should be used.

Use of prostaglandin synthetase inhibitors may result in premature closure of the ductus arteriosus or uterine inertia; such drugs are therefore not recommended during the last trimester of pregnancy.

Following doses of 50 mg enteric coated tablets every 8 hours, traces of active substance have been detected in breast milk, but in quantities so small that no undesirable effects on the infant are to be expected.

*Effects on ability to drive and use machines:* Patients who experience dizziness or other central nervous disturbances, while taking NSAIDs should refrain from driving or operating machinery.

*Undesirable effects:* If serious side-effects occur, Voltarol should be withdrawn.

Frequency estimate: *frequent:* >10%, *occasional:* >1–10%, *rare:* >0.001–1%, *isolated cases:* <0.001%.

*Gastro-intestinal tract: Occasional:* Epigastric pain, other gastro-intestinal disorders (e.g. nausea, vomiting, diarrhoea, abdominal cramps, dyspepsia, flatulence, anorexia). *Rare:* Gastro-intestinal bleeding (haematemesis, melaena, bloody diarrhoea), gastrointestinal ulcers with or without bleeding or perforation. *Isolated cases:* Aphthous stomatitis, glossitis, oesophageal lesions, lower gut disorders (e.g. non-specific haemorrhagic colitis and exacerbations of ulcerative colitis or Crohn's proctocolitis, colonic damage and stricture formation), pancreatitis, constipation.

*Central nervous system: Occasional:* Headache, dizziness, or vertigo. *Rare:* drowsiness, tiredness. *Isolated cases:* Disturbances of sensation, paraesthesia, memory disturbance, disorientation, insomnia, irritability, convulsions, depression, anxiety, nightmares, tremor, psychotic reactions, aseptic meningitis.

*Special senses: Isolated cases:* Disturbances of vision (blurred vision, diplopia), impaired hearing, tinnitus, taste disturbances.

*Skin: Occasional:* Rashes or skin eruptions. *Rare:* Urticaria. *Isolated cases:* Bullous eruptions, eczema, erythema multiforme, Steven's-Johnson syndrome, Lyell's syndrome (acute toxic epidermolysis), erythroderma (exfoliative dermatitis), loss of hair, photosensitivity reactions, purpura including allergic purpura.

*Kidney: Rare:* Oedema. *Isolated cases:* Acute renal insufficiency, urinary abnormalities (e.g. haematuria, proteinuria), interstitial nephritis, nephrotic syndrome, papillary necrosis.

*Liver: Occasional:* Elevation of serum aminotransferase enzymes (ALT, AST). *Rare:* Liver function disorders including hepatitis (in isolated cases fulminant) with or without jaundice.

*Blood: Isolated cases:* Thrombocytopenia, leucopenia, agranulocytosis, haemolytic anaemia, aplastic anaemia.

*Hypersensitivity: Rare:* Hypersensitivity reactions (e.g. bronchospasm, anaphylactic/anaphylactoid systemic reactions including hypotension). *Isolated cases:* Vasculitis, pneumonitis.

*Cardiovascular system: Isolated cases:* Palpitations, chest pain, hypertension, congestive heart failure.

*Overdose:* Management of acute poisoning with NSAIDs essentially consists of supportive and symptomatic measures. There is no typical clinical picture resulting from Voltarol overdosage. The therapeutic measures to be taken are: supportive and symptomatic treatment should be given for complications such as hypotension, renal failure, convulsions, gastro-intestinal irritation, and respiratory depression; special therapies such as forced diuresis, dialysis or haemoperfusion are probably of no help in eliminating NSAIDs due to their high rate of protein binding and extensive metabolism.

**Pharmacological properties**
*Pharmacodynamic properties:*
*Pharmacotherapeutic group:* Non-steroidal anti-inflammatory drugs (NSAIDs).
*Mechanism of action:* Voltarol is a non-steroidal agent with marked analgesic/anti-inflammatory properties. It is an inhibitor of prostaglandin synthetase (cyclo-oxygenase).

Diclofenac sodium *in vitro* does not suppress proteoglycan biosynthesis in cartilage at concentrations equivalent to the concentrations reached in human beings.

*Pharmacokinetic properties:*
*Absorption:* The same amount of active substance is released and absorbed from SR and Retard tablets as from enteric-coated tablets. Mean peak plasma concentrations of diclofenac are reached at 4 hours, 0.508±0.185 mcg/ml (0.5 mcg/mL≡1.6 µmol/l) or 0.4±0.184 mcg/ml (0.4 mcg/mL≡1.25 µmol/l) after Retard 100 mg or 75 mg SR, respectively. 75 mg SR and Retard 100 mg are modified release preparations and plasma concentrations of diclofenac of 13 ng/ml (40 µmol/l) can be recorded at 24 hours (Retard 100 mg) and 16 hours (75 mg SR) after administration. Absorption is unaffected by food.

*Bioavailability:* The systemic availability of diclofenac from the SR formulations is on average 82% of that achieved with the same dose of enteric-coated tablets (possibly due to release rate dependent first-pass metabolism). As a result of the slower release of active substance, peak plasma concentrations are lower than for the equivalent enteric-coated tablets.

Pharmacokinetic behaviour does not change on repeated administration. Accumulation does not occur, provided the recommended dosage intervals are observed. Trough levels of diclofenac in the plasma after Retard 100 mg daily or 75 mg SR twice daily are around 22 ng/ml or 25 ng/ml (70 nmol/l or 80 nmol/l), respectively.

*Distribution:* The active substance is 99.7% protein bound, mainly to albumin (99.4%).

Diclofenac enters the synovial fluid, where maximum concentrations are measured 2–4 hours after the peak plasma values have been attained. The apparent half-life for elimination from the synovial fluid is 3–6 hours. Two hours after reaching the peak plasma values, concentrations of the active substance are already higher in the synovial fluid than they are in the plasma and remain higher for up to 12 hours.

*Metabolism:* Biotransformation of diclofenac takes place partly by glucuronidation of the intact molecule, but mainly by single and multiple hydroxylation and methoxylation, resulting in several phenolic metabolites, most of which are converted to glucuronide conjugates. Two phenolic metabolites are biologically active, but to a much lesser extent than diclofenac.

*Elimination:* The total systemic clearance of diclofenac in plasma is 263±56 ml/min (mean value±SD). The terminal half-life in plasma is 1–2 hours. Four of the metabolites, including the two active ones, also have short plasma half-lives of 1–3 hours.

About 60% of the administered dose is excreted in the urine in the form of the glucuronide conjugate of the intact molecule and as metabolites, most of which are also converted to glucuronide conjugates. Less than 1% is excreted as unchanged substance. The rest of the dose is eliminated as metabolites through the bile in the faeces.

*Characteristics in patients: Elderly:* No relevant age-dependent differences in the drug's absorption, metabolism or excretion have been observed, other than the finding that in five elderly patients, a 15 minute iv infusion resulted in 50% higher plasma concentrations than expected with young healthy subjects.

*Patients with renal impairment:* In patients suffering from renal impairment, no accumulation of the unchanged active substance can be inferred from the single-dose kinetics when applying the usual dosage schedule. At a creatinine clearance of <10 ml/min, the calculated steady-state plasma levels of the hydroxy metabolites are about 4 times higher than in normal subjects. However, the metabolites are ultimately cleared through the bile.

*Patients with hepatic disease:* In patients with chronic hepatitis or non-decompensated cirrhosis, the kinetics and metabolism of diclofenac are the same as in patients without liver disease.

*Preclinical safety data:* None stated.

**Pharmaceutical particulars**
*List of excipients:* 75 mg SR and Retard 100 mg tablets also contain colloidal anhydrous silica, cetyl alcohol, sucrose (powder), povidone, magnesium stearate, hydroxypropylmethylcellulose, polysorbate 80, purified talc, titanium dioxide (E.171), red iron oxide (E.172) and purified water.

*Incompatibilities:* None known.

*Shelf life:* 75 mg SR tablets: Three years. Retard 100 mg tablets: Five years.

*Special precautions for storage:* 75 mg SR tablets: Protect from moisture and heat (store below 30°C).
Retard 100 mg tablets: No special precautions for storage.

Medicines should be kept out of the reach of children.

*Nature and contents of container:* 75 mg SR tablets are pale pink, triangular film coated tablets embossed GEIGY on one face, V 75 SR on the other, and come in PVC/PVdC blister packs of 2, 7, 28, 56 and 70.

The Retard 100 mg tablets are pale red, round, slightly convex, film coated tablets, impressed GEIGY on one side and VOLTAROL R on the other, and come in PVC/PVdC blister packs of 7, 28 and 70.

*Instructions for use/handling:* The tablets should be swallowed whole with liquid, preferably with meals.

**Marketing authorisation numbers**
75 mg SR tablets      00101/0471
Retard 100 mg tablets   00101/0470

**Date of approval/revision of SPC**   11 July 1997.

**Legal category**   POM.

## VOLTAROL* SUPPOSITORIES

**Qualitative and quantitative composition**   The active substance is sodium-[o-[(2,6-dichlorophenyl)-amino]-phenyl]-acetate (diclofenac sodium).

Each suppository contains 12.5 mg, 25 mg, 50 mg and 100 mg diclofenac sodium.

**Pharmaceutical form**   Suppositories.

**Clinical particulars**
*Therapeutic indications:*
*Adults and elderly:* Relief of all grades of pain and inflammation in a wide range of conditions, including:

(i)   arthritic conditions: rheumatoid arthritis, osteo-arthritis, ankylosing spondylitis, acute gout,

(ii)   acute musculo-skeletal disorders such as peri-arthritis (for example, frozen shoulder), tendinitis, tenosynovitis, bursitis,

(iii)   other painful conditions resulting from trauma, including fracture, low back pain, sprains, strains, dislocations, orthopaedic, dental and other minor surgery.

*Children (aged 1–12 years):* Juvenile chronic arthritis (12.5 mg and 25 mg suppositories only).

*Posology and method of administration:*
*Adults:* 25 mg, 50 mg and 100 mg: 75–150 mg daily, in divided doses.

The recommended maximum daily dose of Voltarol is 150 mg. This may be administered using a combination of dosage forms, e.g. tablets and suppositories.

*Children (aged 1–12 years) 12.5 mg and 25 mg suppositories only:* 1–3 mg/kg per day in divided doses.

*Elderly:* Although the pharmacokinetics of Voltarol are not impaired to any clinically relevant extent in elderly patients, non-steroidal anti-inflammatory drugs should be used with particular caution in such patients who, generally, are more prone to adverse reactions. In particular it is recommended that the lowest effective dosage be used in frail, elderly patients or those with a low body weight (see also *Precautions*).

*Contra-indications:* Active or suspected gastro-intestinal ulcers or bleeding.

Previous sensitivity to diclofenac.

Patients in whom attacks of asthma, urticaria or acute rhinitis are precipitated by aspirin or other non-steroidal anti-inflammatory agents.

In ulcerative or acute inflammatory conditions of the anus, rectum (proctitis) and sigmoid colon.

*Special warnings and special precautions for use:*
*Warnings:* Close medical surveillance is imperative in patients with symptoms indicative of gastro-intestinal disorders, with a history suggestive of gastric or intestinal ulceration, with ulcerative colitis, or with Crohn's disease.

Gastro-intestinal bleeding or ulceration/perforation, haematemesis and melaena have, in general, more serious consequences in the elderly. They can occur at any time during treatment, with or without warning symptoms or a previous history. In the rare instances when gastro-intestinal bleeding or ulceration occur in patients receiving Voltarol, the drug should be withdrawn.

*Hepatic:* Close medical surveillance is also imperative in patients suffering from severe impairment of hepatic function.

*Hypersensitivity reactions:* As with other non-steroidal anti-inflammatory drugs, allergic reactions, including anaphylactic/anaphylactoid reactions, can also occur without earlier exposure to the drug.

Like other NSAIDs, Voltarol may mask the signs and symptoms of infection due to its pharmacodynamic properties.

*Precautions: Renal:* Patients with renal, cardiac or hepatic impairment and the elderly should be kept under surveillance, since the use of NSAIDs may result in deterioration of renal function. The lowest effective dose should be used and renal function monitored.

The importance of prostaglandins in maintaining renal blood flow should be taken into account in patients with impaired cardiac or renal function, those being treated with diuretics or recovering from major surgery. Effects on renal function are usually reversible on withdrawal of Voltarol.

*Hepatic:* If abnormal liver function tests persist or worsen, clinical signs or symptoms consistent with liver disease develop or if other manifestations occur (eosinophilia, rash), Voltarol should be discontinued. Hepatitis may occur without prodromal symptoms.

Use of Voltarol in patients with hepatic porphyria may trigger an attack.

*Haematological:* Voltarol may reversibly inhibit platelet aggregation (see *Anticoagulants* in *Drug interactions*). Patients with defects of haemostasis, bleeding diathesis or haematological abnormalities should be carefully monitored.

*Long-term treatment:* All patients who are receiving non-steroidal anti-inflammatory agents should be monitored as a precautionary measure e.g. renal function, hepatic function (elevation of liver enzymes may occur) and blood counts. This is particularly important in the elderly.

*Interaction with other medicaments and other forms of interaction:*
*Lithium and digoxin:* Voltarol may increase plasma concentrations of lithium and digoxin.

*Anticoagulants:* Although clinical investigations do not appear to indicate that Voltarol has an influence on the effect of anticoagulants, there are isolated reports of an increased risk of haemorrhage with the combined use of diclofenac and anticoagulant therapy. Therefore, to be certain that no change in anticoagulant dosage is required, close monitoring of such patients is required. As with other non-steroidal anti-inflammatory agents, diclofenac in high dose can reversibly inhibit platelet aggregation.

*Antidiabetic agents:* Clinical studies have shown that Voltarol can be given together with oral anti-diabetic agents without influencing their clinical effect. However, there have been isolated reports of hypo-glycaemic and hyperglycaemic effects which have required adjustment to the dosage of hypoglycaemic agents.

*Cyclosporin:* Cases of nephrotoxicity have been reported in patients receiving concomitant cyclo-sporin and NSAIDs, including Voltarol. This might be mediated through combined renal antiprostaglandin effects of both the NSAID and cyclosporin.

*Methotrexate:* Cases of serious toxicity have been reported when methotrexate and NSAIDs are given within 24 hours of each other. This interaction is mediated through accumulation of methotrexate resulting from impairment of renal excretion in the presence of the NSAID.

*Quinolone antimicrobials:* Convulsions may occur due to an interaction between quinolones and NSAIDs. This may occur in patients with or without a previous history of epilepsy or convulsions. Therefore, caution should be exercised when considering the use of a quinolone in patients who are already receiving an NSAID.

*Other NSAIDs and steroids:* Co-administration of Voltarol with other systemic NSAIDs and steroids may increase the frequency of unwanted effects. Concomitant therapy with aspirin lowers the plasma levels of each, although no clinical significance is known.

*Diuretics:* Various NSAIDs are liable to inhibit the activity of diuretics. Concomitant treatment with potassium-sparing diuretics may be associated with increased serum potassium levels, hence serum potassium should be monitored.

*Pregnancy and lactation:* Although animal studies have not demonstrated teratogenic effects, Voltarol should not be prescribed during pregnancy, unless there are compelling reasons for doing so. The lowest effective dosage should be used.

Use of prostaglandin synthetase inhibitors may result in premature closure of the ductus arteriosus or uterine inertia; such drugs are, therefore, not recommended during the last trimester of pregnancy.

Following doses of 50 mg enteric coated tablets every 8 hours, traces of active substance have been detected in breast milk, but in quantities so small that no undesirable effects on the infant are to be expected.

*Effects on ability to drive and use machines:* Patients who experience dizziness or other central nervous disturbances, while taking NSAIDs should refrain from driving or operating machinery.

*Undesirable effects:* If serious side-effects occur, Voltarol should be withdrawn.

Frequency estimate: *frequent:* >10%, *occasional:* >1–10%, *rare:* >0.001–1%, *isolated cases:* <0.001%.

*Gastro-intestinal tract:* Occasional: Epigastric pain, other gastro-intestinal disorders (e.g. nausea, vomiting, diarrhoea, abdominal cramps, dyspepsia, flatulence, anorexia). *Rare:* Gastro-intestinal bleeding (haematemesis, melaena, bloody diarrhoea), gastro-intestinal ulcers with or without bleeding or perforation. *Isolated cases:* Aphthous stomatitis, glossitis, oesophageal lesions, lower gut disorders (e.g. non-specific haemorrhagic colitis and exacerbations of ulcerative colitis or Crohn's proctocolitis, colonic damage and stricture formation), pancreatitis, constipation.

*Suppositories only: Occasional:* Local reactions (e.g. itching, burning and increased bowel movement). *Isolated cases:* exacerbation of haemorrhoids.

*Central nervous system: Occasional:* Headache, dizziness, or vertigo. *Rare:* drowsiness, tiredness. *Isolated cases:* Disturbances of sensation, paraesthesia, memory disturbance, disorientation, insomnia, irritability, convulsions, depression, anxiety, nightmares, tremor, psychotic reactions, aseptic meningitis.

*Special senses: Isolated cases:* Disturbances of vision (blurred vision, diplopia), impaired hearing, tinnitus, taste disturbances.

*Skin: Occasional:* Rashes or skin eruptions. *Rare:* Urticaria. *Isolated cases:* Bullous eruptions, eczema, erythema multiforme, Steven's-Johnson syndrome, Lyell's syndrome (acute toxic epidermolysis), erythroderma (exfoliative dermatitis), loss of hair, photosensitivity reactions, purpura including allergic purpura.

*Kidney: Rare:* Oedema. In isolated cases: Acute renal insufficiency, urinary abnormalities (e.g. haematuria, proteinuria), interstitial nephritis, nephrotic syndrome, papillary necrosis.

*Liver: Occasional:* Elevation of serum aminotransferase enzymes (ALT, AST). *Rare:* Liver function disorders including hepatitis (in isolated cases fulminant) with or without jaundice.

*Blood: Isolated cases:* Thrombocytopenia, leucopenia, agranulocytosis, haemolytic anaemia, aplastic anaemia.

*Hypersensitivity: Rare:* Hypersensitivity reactions (e.g. bronchospasm, anaphylactic/anaphylactoid systemic reactions including hypotension). *Isolated cases:* Vasculitis, pneumonitis.

*Cardiovascular system: Isolated cases:* Palpitations, chest pain, hypertension, congestive heart failure.

*Overdose:* Management of acute poisoning with NSAIDs essentially consists of supportive and symptomatic measures. There is no typical clinical picture resulting from Voltarol overdosage. The therapeutic measures to be taken are: Supportive and symptomatic treatment should be given for complications such as hypotension, renal failure, convulsions, gastro-intestinal irritation, and respiratory depression; specific therapies such as forced diuresis, dialysis or haemoperfusion are probably of no help in eliminating NSAIDs due to the high rate of protein binding and extensive metabolism.

**Pharmacological properties**
*Pharmacodynamic properties:*
*Pharmacotherapeutic group:* Non-steroidal anti-inflammatory drugs (NSAIDs).

*Mechanism of action:* Voltarol is a non-steroidal agent with marked analgesic/anti-inflammatory properties. It is an inhibitor of prostaglandin synthetase (cyclo-oxygenase).

Diclofenac sodium *in vitro* does not suppress proteoglycan biosynthesis in cartilage at concentrations equivalent to the concentrations reached in human beings.

*Pharmacokinetic properties:*
*Absorption:* Absorption is rapid; although the rate of absorption is slower than from enteric-coated tablets administered orally. After the administration of 50 mg suppositories, peak plasma concentrations are attained on average within 1 hour, but maximum concentrations per dose unit are about two thirds of those reached after administration of enteric-coated tablets (1.95±0.8 mcg/ml (1.9 mcg/ml≡5.9 µmol/l)).

*Bioavailability:* As with oral preparations, the AUC is approximately a half of the value obtained from a parenteral dose.

Pharmacokinetic behaviour does not change on repeated administration. Accumulation does not occur, provided the recommended dosage intervals are observed. The plasma concentrations attained in children given equivalent doses (mg/kb, b.w.) are similar to those obtained in adults.

*Distribution:* The active substance is 99.7% protein bound, mainly to albumin (99.4%).

Diclofenac enters the synovial fluid, where maximum concentrations are measured 2–4 hours after the peak plasma values have been attained. The apparent half-life for elimination from the synovial fluid is 3–6 hours. Two hours after reaching the peak plasma values, concentrations of the active substance are already higher in the synovial fluid than they are in the plasma and remain higher for up to 12 hours.

*Metabolism:* Biotransformation of diclofenac takes place partly by glucuronidation of the intact molecule, but mainly by single and multiple hydroxylation and methoxylation, resulting in several phenolic metabolites, most of which are converted to glucuronide conjugates. Two phenolic metabolites are biologically active, but to a much lesser extent than diclofenac.

*Elimination:* The total systemic clearance of diclofenac in plasma is 263±56 ml/min (mean value±SD). The terminal half-life in plasma is 1–2 hours. Four of the metabolites, including the two active ones, also have short plasma half-lives of 1–3 hours.

About 60% of the administered dose is excreted in the urine in the form of the glucuronide conjugate of the intact molecule and as metabolites, most of which are also converted to glucuronide conjugates. Less than 1% is excreted as unchanged substance. The rest of the dose is eliminated as metabolites through the bile in the faeces.

*Characteristics in patients:* No relevant age-dependent differences in the drug's absorption, metabolism or excretion have been observed, other than the finding that in five elderly patients, a 15 minute iv infusion resulted in 50% higher plasma concentrations than expected with young healthy subjects.

*Patients with renal impairment:* In patients suffering from renal impairment, no accumulation of the unchanged active substance can be inferred from the single-dose kinetics when applying the usual dosage schedule. At a creatinine clearance of <10 ml/min, the calculated steady-state plasma levels of the hydroxy metabolites are about 4 times higher than in normal subjects. However, the metabolites are ultimately cleared through the bile.

*Patients with hepatic disease:* In patients with chronic hepatitis or non-decompensated cirrhosis, the kinetics and metabolism of diclofenac are the same as in patients without liver disease.

*Preclinical safety data:* None stated.

**Pharmaceutical particulars**

*List of excipients:* Voltarol suppositories also contain suppository mass 5 (a waxy base composed of hard fat).

*Incompatibilities:* None known.

*Shelf life:* Three years.

*Special precautions for storage:* Protect from heat (store below 30°C). Medicines should be kept out of the reach of children.

*Nature and contents of container:* The suppositories are white to yellowish, torpedo-shaped, with smooth surfaces and a slightly fatty odour and are sealed in polyethylene laminated aluminium foil. They come in packs of 10.

*Instructions for use/handling:* For rectal use only.

**Marketing authorisation numbers**

| | |
|---|---|
| 12.5 mg | 00101/0472 |
| 25 mg | 00101/0473 |
| 50 mg | 00101/0474 |
| 100 mg | 00101/0475 |

**Date of approval/revision of SPC** 11 July 1997.

**Legal category** POM.

## ZADITEN*

**Presentation** *1 mg capsules:* White, opaque, oblong, gelatin capsules, size 4, weighing 182 mg. Each capsule contains 1.38 mg ketotifen hydrogen fumarate (equivalent to 1 mg ketotifen base). Coded CS in red.

*1 mg tablets:* White, uncoated, round, flat, bevel-edged tablets weighing 130 mg, 7 mm diameter. The tablets are marked ZADITEN 1 on one side and scored on the other. Each tablet contains 1.38 mg ketotifen hydrogen fumarate (equivalent to 1 mg ketotifen base).

*Elixir:* Clear, colourless, strawberry flavoured elixir.

Each 5 ml spoonful contains 1.38 mg ketotifen hydrogen fumarate (equivalent to 1 mg ketotifen base).

For information on excipients, refer to *Further information.*

**Uses** *Principal action:* Ketotifen is a non-bronchodilator anti-asthmatic drug which inhibits the effect of certain endogenous substances known to be inflammatory mediators, and thereby exerts anti-allergic activity.

Laboratory experiments indicate that this anti-asthmatic activity may be due to the inhibition of release of allergic mediators such as histamine and leukotrienes and the inhibition of the development of airway hyperactivity associated with activation of platelets by PAF (platelet activating factor) or caused by neural activation following the use of sympathomimetic drugs or the exposure to allergen. In addition, ketotifen exerts a non-competitive blocking effect on histamine (H1) receptors.

Experimental investigations in asthmatic subjects have shown that Zaditen is as effective orally as a selective mast cell stabiliser administered by inhalation: antihistamines are ineffective in these tests.

The effectiveness of Zaditen in the prevention of bronchial asthma has been studied in long term clinical trials. Asthma attacks were reduced in number, severity and duration and in some cases the patients were completely freed from attacks. Progressive reduction of corticosteroids and/or bronchodilators was also possible.

The prophylactic activity of Zaditen may take several weeks to become fully established.

Zaditen will not abort established attacks of asthma.

*Indications:* Prophylactic treatment of bronchial asthma. Symptomatic treatment of allergic conditions including rhinitis and conjunctivitis.

**Dosage and administration** *Adults:* 1 mg twice daily with food. If necessary the dose may be increased to 2 mg twice daily.

Patients known to be easily sedated should begin treatment with 0.5 to 1 mg at night for the first few days.

*Children from two years:* 1 mg twice daily with food.

*Use in the elderly:* No evidence exists that elderly patients require different dosages or show different side effects from younger patients.

**Contra-indications, warnings, etc**

*Contra-indications:* Hypersensitivity to ketotifen or any of the excipients (see *Further information*). A reversible fall in the thrombocyte count in patients receiving Zaditen concomitantly with oral antidiabetic agents has been observed in a few cases. This combination of drugs should therefore be avoided until this phenomenon has been satisfactorily explained.

*Use in pregnancy and lactation:* Although there is no evidence of any teratogenic effect, recommendations for Zaditen in pregnancy cannot be given. Ketotifen is excreted in breast milk, therefore mothers receiving Zaditen should not breast feed.

*Precautions:* Post-marketing surveillance has shown exacerbation of asthma in approximately 2 per 1000 patients. Since some of these asthmatic attacks might have been related to stopping existing treatment, it is important to continue such treatment for a minimum of two weeks after starting Zaditen. Symptomatic and prophylactic anti-asthmatic drugs already in use should never be withdrawn abruptly when long-term treatment with Zaditen is begun. This applies especially to systemic corticosteroids and ACTH because of the possible existence of adrenocortical insufficiency in steroid-dependent patients; in such cases

recovery of a normal pituitary-adrenal response to stress may take up to one year. If it is necessary to withdraw Zaditen, this should be done progressively over a period of 2 to 4 weeks. Symptoms of asthma may recur.

If intercurrent infection occurs Zaditen treatment must be supplemented by specific antimicrobial therapy.

During the first days of treatment with Zaditen reactions may be impaired. Patients should be warned not to take charge of vehicles or machinery until the effect of Zaditen treatment on the individual is known. Patients should be advised to avoid alcoholic drinks.

Zaditen may potentiate the effects of sedatives, hypnotics, antihistamines and alcohol.

*Side-effects:* Drowsiness and, in isolated cases, dry mouth and slight dizziness may occur at the beginning of treatment, but usually disappear spontaneously after a few days. Occasionally symptoms of CNS stimulation have been observed. Weight gain has also been reported. Cystitis has been rarely described in association with Zaditen. Isolated cases of severe skin reactions (erythema multiforme, Stephen's-Johnson Syndrome) have been reported.

*Overdosage:* The reported features of overdosage include confusion, drowsiness, nystagmus, headache, disorientation, tachycardia, hypotension, reversible coma; especially in children, hyperexcitability or convulsions. Bradycardia and respiratory depression should be watched for. Elimination of the drug with gastric lavage or emesis is recommended. Otherwise general supportive treatment is all that is required.

**Pharmaceutical precautions** Nil.

**Legal category** POM.

**Package quantities** *1 mg capsules:* Blister pack of 60 capsules (OP).
*1 mg tablets:* Blister pack of 60 tablets (OP).
*Elixir 1 mg/5 ml:* Bottles of 150 ml. Bottles of 300 ml.

**Further information** Zaditen capsules: the excipients are colloidal anhydrous silica, magnesium stearate, maize starch and mannitol. The capsule shell is made of gelatin and contains titanium dioxide.

Zaditen tablets: the excipients are magnesium stearate, maize starch, lactose and pre-gel corn starch.

Zaditen elixir: the excipients are propyl hydroxybenzoate, methyl hydroxybenzoate, strawberry flavour, citric acid, disodium phosphate, ethyl alcohol, Lycasin* 80/55 (hydrogenated glucose syrup) and purified water.

Zaditen elixir is sugar free. It contains the sweetening agent Lycasin* 80/55 (hydrogenated glucose syrup) at a concentration of 4 g in 5 ml. Lycasin* 80/55 contains 45% readily absorbable carbohydrate. This should be considered if prescribing the drug for diabetic patients.

The bioavailability of Zaditen is not influenced by food. After oral administration, the absorption of Zaditen is almost complete. Bioavailability amounts to approximately 50% owing to a first-pass effect of about 50% in the liver. Maximal plasma concentrations are reached within 2 to 4 hours. Protein binding is 75%. Ketotifen is eliminated biphasically, with a short half-life of 3 to 5 hours and a longer one of 21 hours. About 1% of the substance is excreted unchanged in the urine within 48 hours and 60 to 70% is excreted as metabolites. The main metabolite is ketotifen-N-glucuronide. This is practically inactive.

**Product licence numbers**

| | |
|---|---|
| 1 mg capsules | 0101/0105 |
| 1 mg tablets | 0101/0125 |
| Elixir 1 mg/5 ml | 0101/0137 |

*Trade Mark

# Novex Pharma Ltd

Innovex House
Marlow Park
Marlow
Bucks., SL7 1TB

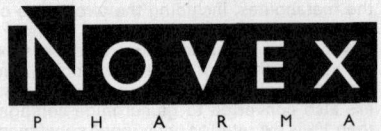

## ALVEDON* SUPPOSITORIES

**Qualitative and quantitive composition** Paracetamol 125 mg

**Pharmaceutical form** Suppositories

**Clinical particulars**

*Therapeutic indications:* For treatment of mild to moderate pain and pyrexia in children. Alvedon suppositories may be especially useful in patients unable to take oral forms of paracetamol eg post-operatively or with nausea or vomiting.

*Posology and method of administration:*
Children: 1-5 years, 1-2 suppositories. The dosage should be based on age and weight i.e.
  1 year (10 kg) 1 suppository
  5 years (20 kg) 2 suppositories.
These doses may be repeated up to 4 times daily.

*Contra-indications:* Hypersensivity to paracetamol

*Special warnings and special precautions for use:* Paracetamol should be given with care to patients with impaired kidney or liver function

*Interaction with other medicaments and other forms of interaction:* Drugs which induce hepatic microsomal enzymes such as alcohol, barbiturates and other anticonvulsants may increase the hepatotoxicity of paracetamol particularly after overdosage

*Using during pregnancy.* Not applicable

*Effects on ability to drive and use machines:* None known.

*Undesirable effects.* Side-effects at therapeutic doses are rare. Isolated cases of liver damage and allergic reactions such as skin rash have been reported.

Redness of the mucous membrane of the rectum and minor local vascular changes have been reported after the use of Alvedon Suppositories. Hepatic necrosis may occur after overdosage.

*Overdosage:* Clinical symptoms of liver damage are manifested usually after 48 hours.

Overdosage results in saturation of the conjugation capacity of the liver and irreversible binding of a reactive intermediate metabolite in the hepatocytes. N-acetylcysteine intravenously or L-methionine orally protects the liver if administered within 10-12 hours of ingesting an overdose.

**Pharmacological properties**

*Pharmacodynamic properties.* Paracetamol is an aniline derivative with analgesic and antipyretic actions similar to those of aspirin but with no demonstrable anti-inflammatory activity.

Paracetamol is less irritant to the stomach than aspirin. It does not affect thrombocyte aggregation or bleeding time. Paracetamol is generally well tolerated by patients hypersensitive to acetylsalicyclic acid.

*Pharmacokinetic properties:* Paracetamol is well absorbed by both oral and rectal routes.

Peak plasma concentrations occur about 2 to 3 hours after rectal administration. The plasma half life is about 2 hours.

Paracetamol is primarily metabolised in the liver by conjugation to glucuronide and sulphate. A small amount (about 3-10% of a therapeutic dose) is metabolised by oxidation and the reactive intermediate metabolite thus formed is bound preferentially to the liver glutathione and excreted as cystein and mercapturic acid conjugates. Excretion occurs via the kidneys. 2-3% of a therapeutic dose is excreted unchanged: 80-90% as glucuronide and sulphate and a smaller amount as cystein and mercapturic acid derivatives.

**Pharmaceutical particulars**

*List of excipients.* Hard fat (Witepsol H12).

*Incompatibilities.* None.

*Shelf-life.* 3 years.

*Special precautions for storage:* Store below 25°C.

*Nature and contents of container:* PVC/Polyethylene strips each containing 5 suppositories. Packs of 5, 10 or 50 suppositories.

PVC/Polyethylene strips each containing 1 suppository. Packs of 10 suppositories.

*Instructions for use/handling.* Not applicable.

*Marketing authorisation holder:* Astra Pharmaceuticals Ltd, Home Park, Kings Langley, Hertfordshire WD4 8DH.

**Marketing authorisation number** 0017/0250

**Date of approval/revision of SPC** October 1995

**Legal category** P

## FENOPRON* 300

**Qualitative and quantitative composition** Each tablet contains as active ingredient, fenoprofen calcium equivalent to 300 mg of fenoprofen.

**Pharmaceutical form** Tablet

**Clinical particulars**

*Therapeutic indications:* For the treatment of osteoarthritis, rheumatoid arthritis and ankylosing spondylitis. For the relief of mild/moderate pain.

*Posology and method of administration:* For oral administration to adults only and not recommended for administration to children.
*Dosage:* 300-600 mg three or four times a day.
*Fenopron 300:* Recommended initial dosage is 2 tablets three times per day, then adjusted to the needs of the patient.
*Fenopron 600:* Recommended initial dosage is one tablet three times per day plus one at night if necessitated by a more severe condition. The dosage may then be adjusted to the needs of the patient.
The maximum daily dose should not exceed 3 g.
If fenoprofen is administered with meals the total amount absorbed is not affected, although peak blood levels are delayed and diminished.
The elderly: There is no difference in the metabolism or pharmacokinetics of fenoprofen in the elderly. However, it may be advisable to start therapy with a low dose, as side-effects of non-steroidal anti-inflammatory drugs are more pronounced in this patient population.

*Contra-indications:* Hypersensitivity to the drug. Active or a history of, peptic or intestinal ulceration. Fenoprofen should not be given to patients in whom aspirin and other non-steroidal anti-inflammatory drugs induce the symptoms of asthma, rhinitis or urticaria because cross-sensitivity to these drugs occurs in a high proportion of patients. Patients with a history of significantly impaired renal function.

*Special warnings and special precautions:*
*Gastro-intestinal.* Serious toxicity, such as bleeding, ulceration and perforation, can occur at any time, without warning symptoms, in patients treated chronically. Elderly or debilitated patients tolerate ulceration or bleeding less well than other individuals and most spontaneous reports of fatal gastro-intestinal events are in this population. Minor upper gastro-intestinal problems, such as dyspepsia are common, usually developing early in therapy.

Fenoprofen should only be given under close supervision to patients with a history of upper gastro-intestinal disease or peptic ulcer risk factors.

*Genito-urinary:* The most frequently reported problems have been episodes of dysuria, cystitis, haernaturia, interstitial nephritis and nephrotic syndrome. This syndrome may be preceded by the appearance of fever, rash, arthralgia, oliguria and uraemia, and may progress to anuria. Early recognition of the syndrome and withdrawal of the drug have been followed by rapid recovery. Patients who have had similar reactions with other non-steroidal anti-inflammatory drugs should not be given fenoprofen. Patients likely to have compromised renal function should be monitored periodically.

Bronchospasm may be precipitated in patients suffering from, or with a previous history of, bronchial asthma or allergic disease.

In patients with conditions leading to reduction in renal blood flow or blood volume, administration of non-steroidal anti-inflammatory drugs may precipitate overt renal decompensation. Patients at greatest risk of this reaction are those with impaired renal function, heart failure, liver dysfunction, those taking diuretics and the elderly. Discontinuation of therapy is typically followed by recovery to the pre-treatment state.

Since fenoprofen is eliminated primarily by the kidneys, patients with possibly compromised renal function (such as the elderly) should be closely monitored, especially during long term therapy: a lower daily dosage should be anticipated to avoid excessive drug accumulation.

Some patients have developed elevation of serum transaminase, LDH and alkaline phosphatase and it is recommended that fenoprofen be discontinued if any significant liver abnormalities occur. Borderline elevations of one or more liver function tests may occur in up to 15% of patients. Severe hepatic reactions, including jaundice and cases of fatal hepatitis, have been reported. Patients in whom an abnormal liver test has occurred should be evaluated for evidence of more severe hepatic reactions. During long-term therapy, liver function tests should be monitored periodically. If fenoprofen is used in the presence of impaired liver function, it must be done under strict observation.

Patients with initial low haemoglobin values who are receiving long-term therapy with fenoprofen should have a haemoglobin determination at reasonable intervals.

Peripheral oedema has been observed in some patients taking fenoprofen, therefore, it should be used with caution in patients with compromised cardiac function or hypertension. The possibility of renal involvement should be considered.

Studies to date have not shown changes in the eyes attributable to the administration of fenoprofen. However, adverse ocular effects have been observed with other anti-inflammatory drugs, so eye examinations should be performed if visual disturbances occur in patients taking fenoprofen.

Since the safety of fenoprofen has not been established in patients with impaired hearing, these patients should have periodic tests of auditory function during chronic therapy

Fenoprofen decreases platelet aggregation and may prolong bleeding time.

*Interaction with other medicaments and other forms of interaction:*
*Laboratory test interactions:* Values of total and free triiodothyronine in patients receiving fenoprofen have been reported as falsely elevated. Thyroid stimulating hormones, total thyroxine and thyrotropin releasing hormone response are not affected.

*Drug interactions:* The concurrent use of fenoprofen and salicylates is not recommended.

Chronic administration of phenobarbitone may be associated with a decrease in the plasma half life of fenoprofen. Dosage adjustment of fenoprofen may be required

Patients treated with fenoprofen may be resistant to the effects of loop diuretics.

In-vitro studies have shown that fenoprofen may displace other drugs, for example hydantoins, sulphonamides, or sulphonylureas, from their binding sites and this may lead to drug interaction. Theoretically, fenoprofen could likewise be displaced. In patients receiving coumarin-type anti-coagulants, the addition of fenoprofen could prolong the prothrombin time.

*Pregnancy and lactation:* Usage in pregnancy: The safety of fenoprofen for use during pregnancy has not be established; therefore it should not be used during pregnancy unless considered essential by the physician. Animal studies showed prolongation of parturition, but no evidence of teratogenicity.

Usage in nursing mothers: Safety has not been established, therefore, administration to nursing mothers is not recommended.

*Effects on the ability to drive and use machines:* Caution should be exercised by patients whose activities require alertness if they experience central nervous system side-effects.

*Undesirable effects:*
*Gastro-intestinal:* These are the most commonly observed side-effects and include dyspepsia, constipation, diarrhoea, nausea, vomiting, anorexia, ulcer-

ation of the buccal mucosa, abdominal pain, flatulence, dry mouth, gastritis, metallic taste, pancreatitis and occult blood in the stool. Cases of peptic ulceration, including some complicated by bleeding or perforation have occurred.

*Renal:* Cases of acute renal insufficiency, in association with interstitial nephritis, nephrotic syndrome or papillary necrosis, have been reported. Episodes of dysuria, cystitis and haematuria, oliguria, azotaemia and anuria have occurred.

*Hepatic:* Severe hepatic reactions, including jaundice and fatal hepatitis, have been reported rarely. Increases in alkaline phosphatase, LDH and AST have been observed.

*Haematological:* Various syndromes involving the bone marrow have been reported rarely: thrombocytopenia, pancytopenia and aplastic anaemia have occurred. Purpura, bruising, haemorrhage, haemolytic anaemia and agranulocytosis have also been reported.

*Allergic skin:* Pruritus, rash, urticaria, anaphylaxis, Stevens-Johnson syndrome, angioneurotic oedema, increased sweating, exfoliative dermatitis, toxic epidermal necrolysis and alopecia have been reported

*Neurological:* Reactions reported include headache, somnolence, dizziness, tremor, confusion and insomnia, depression, disorientation, seizures and trigeminal neuralgia.

*Cardiovascular:* Palpitations, tachycardia, atrial fibrillation, pulmonary oedema, ECG changes and supraventricular tachycardia have been reported.

*Miscellaneous:* Tinnitus, hearing decrease, amblyopia, blurred vision, diplopia, optic neuritis, nervousness, peripheral oedema, asthenia, dyspnoea, fatigue, malaise, burning tongue, personality change, lymphadenopathy, mastodynia, fever, upper respiratory infection and nasopharyngitis have been reported.

*Overdose:* Symptoms of overdose appear within several hours and generally involve the gastrointestinal and central nervous systems. They include dyspepsia, nausea, vomiting, abdominal pain, dizziness, headache, ataxia, tinnitus, tremor, drowsiness and confusion. Hyperpyrexia, tachycardia, hypotension and acute renal failure may occur rarely following overdose. Respiratory depression and metabolic acidosis have also been reported following overdose with certain non-steroidal anti-inflammatory drugs.

*Treatment:* Standard therapy to evacuate gastric contents and to support vital functions should be employed. Alkalinisation of the urine, forced diuresis, peritoneal dialysis, haemodialysis and charcoal haemoperfusion do not enhance systemic drug elimination.

## Pharmacological properties

*Pharmacodynamic properties:* Fenoprofen calcium is a nonsteroidal, anti-inflammatory, antiarthritic drug that also possess analgesic and antipyretic activities. Its exact mode of action is unknown, but it is thought that prostaglandin synthetase inhibition is involved.

*Pharmacokinetic properties:* Under fasting conditions, fenoprofen is rapidly absorbed, and peak plasma levels of 50 mgc/L are achieved within 2 hours after oral administration of 600 mg doses. Good dose proportionality was observed between 200 mg and 600 mg doses in fasting male volunteers. The plasma half-life is approximately 3 hours. About 90% of a single oral dose is eliminated within 24 hours as fenoprofen glucuronide and 4-hydroxyfenoprofen glucuronide, the major urinary metabolites of fenoprofen. Fenoprofen is highly bound (99%) to albumin. The concomitant administration of antacid (containing both aluminium and magnesium hydroxide) does not interfere with absorption of fenoprofen.

*Preclinical safety data:* Reproduction studies in rats have shown fenoprofen calcium to be associated with prolonged labour and difficult parturition when given during late pregnancy, but no evidence of teratogenicity has been seen.

Fenoprofen shows anti-inflammatory effects in rodents by inhibiting the development of redness and oedema in acute inflammatory conditions by reducing soft tissue swelling and bone damage associated with chronic inflammation. It exhibits analgesic activity in rodents by inhibiting the writhing response caused by the introduction of an irritant into the peritoneal cavities of mice and by elevating pain thresholds that are related to pressure in edematous hindpaws of rats. In rats made febrile by the subcutaneous administration of brewer's yeast, fenoprofen produces antipyretic action.

In chronic studies in rats, high doses of fenoprofen calcium caused elevation of serum transaminase and hepatocellular hypertrophy.

## Pharmaceutical particulars

*List of excipients:* Calcium hydrogen phosphate; maize starch; polacrilin potassium; magnesium stearate; stearic acid powder; methylhydroxypropylcellulose;

polyethylene glycol 8000; propylene glycol; titanium dioxide; sunset yellow (E110).

*Incompatibilities:* Not applicable

*Shelf life:* Two years, when stored appropriately

*Special precautions for storage:* Store at room temperature (15°-25°C)

*Nature and contents of container:* Screw capped, high density polyethylene bottles of 100 tablets

*Instruction for use/handling:* No special instructions

**Marketing authorisation number** 11157/0005

**Date of approval/ revision of SPC** October 1996

**Legal category** POM

# FENOPRON* 600

**Presentation** Fenoprofen Calcium Tablets BP, each containing fenoprofen calcium equivalent to 600 mg fenoprofen.

Fenopron 600 tablets are orange, para-capsule, 20 mm long and marked 4021.

**Uses** For the treatment of osteoarthritis, rheumatoid arthritis and ankylosing spondylitis.

For the relief of mild/moderate pain.

**Dosage and administration** For oral administration to adults only, and not recommended for administration to children.

*Dosage:* 300 to 600 mg three or four times per day.

*Fenopron 600:* Recommended initial dosage is 1 tablet three times per day, plus one at night if necessitated by a more severe condition. The dosage may then be adjusted to the needs of the patient.

The maximum daily dose should not exceed 3 g.

If fenoprofen is administered with meals the total amount absorbed is not affected, although peak blood levels are delayed and diminished.

*The elderly:* There is no difference in the metabolism or pharmacokinetics of fenoprofen in the elderly. However, it may be advisable to start therapy with a low dose, as side-effects of non-steroidal anti-inflammatory drugs are more pronounced in this patient population.

**Contra-indications, warnings, etc**
*Contra-indications:* Hypersensitivity to the drug. Active, or a history of, peptic or intestinal ulceration.

Fenoprofen should not be given to patients in whom aspirin and other non-steroidal anti-inflammatory drugs induce the symptoms of asthma, rhinitis, or urticaria, because cross-sensitivity to these drugs occurs in a high proportion of patients.

Patients with a history of significantly impaired renal function.

*Warnings*

*Gastro-intestinal:* Serious toxicity, such as bleeding, ulceration and perforation, can occur at any time, without warning symptoms, in patients treated chronically. Elderly or debilitated patients tolerate ulceration or bleeding less well than other individuals and most spontaneous reports of fatal gastro-intestinal events are in this population. Minor upper gastro-intestinal problems, such as dyspepsia, are common, usually developing early in therapy.

Fenoprofen should only be given under close supervision to patients with a history of upper gastro-intestinal disease or peptic ulcer risk factors.

*Genito-urinary:* The most frequently reported problems have been episodes of dysuria, cystitis, haematuria, interstitial nephritis and nephrotic syndrome. This syndrome may be preceded by the appearance of fever, rash, arthralgia, oliguria and uraemia, and may progress to anuria. Early recognition of the syndrome and withdrawal of the drug have been followed by rapid recovery. Patients who have had similar reactions with other non-steroidal anti-inflammatory drugs should not be given fenoprofen. Patients likely to have compromised renal function should be monitored periodically.

Bronchospasm may be precipitated in patients suffering from, or with a previous history of, bronchial asthma or allergic disease.

*Usage in pregnancy:* The safety of fenoprofen for use during pregnancy has not been established; therefore it should not be used during pregnancy unless considered essential by the physician. Animal studies showed prolongation of parturition, but no evidence of teratogenicity.

*Usage in nursing mothers:* Safety has not been established, therefore administration to nursing mothers is not recommended.

*Precautions:* In patients with conditions leading to reduction in renal blood flow or blood volume, administration of non-steroidal anti-inflammatory drugs may precipitate overt renal decompensation. Patients at greatest risk of this reaction are those with

impaired renal function, heart failure, liver dysfunction, those taking diuretics, and the elderly. Discontinuation of therapy is typically followed by recovery to the pre-treatment state.

Since fenoprofen is eliminated primarily by the kidneys, patients with possibly compromised renal function (such as the elderly) should be closely monitored, especially during long-term therapy; a lower daily dosage should be anticipated to avoid excessive drug accumulation.

Some patients have developed elevation of serum transaminase, LDH and alkaline phosphatase and it is recommended that fenoprofen be discontinued if any significant liver abnormalities occur. Borderline elevations of one or more liver function tests may occur in up to 15% of patients. Severe hepatic reactions, including jaundice and cases of fatal hepatitis, have been reported. Patients in whom an abnormal liver test has occurred should be evaluated for evidence of more severe hepatic reactions. During long-term therapy, liver function tests should be monitored periodically. If fenoprofen is used in the presence of impaired liver function, it must be done under strict observation.

Patients with initial low haemoglobin values who are receiving long-term therapy with fenoprofen should have a haemoglobin determination at reasonable intervals.

Peripheral oedema has been observed in some patients taking fenoprofen, therefore it should be used with caution in patients with compromised cardiac function or hypertension. The possibility of renal involvement should be considered.

Studies to date have not shown changes in the eyes attributable to the administration of fenoprofen. However, adverse ocular effects have been observed with other anti-inflammatory drugs, so eye examinations should be performed if visual disturbances occur in patients taking fenoprofen.

Caution should be exercised by patients whose activities require alertness if they experience central nervous system side-effects.

Since the safety of fenoprofen has not been established in patients with impaired hearing, these patients should have periodic tests of auditory function during chronic therapy.

Fenoprofen decreases platelet aggregation and may prolong bleeding time.

*Laboratory test interactions:* Values of total and free triiodothyronine in patients receiving fenoprofen have been reported as falsely elevated. Thyroid stimulating hormones, total thyroxine and thyrotropin releasing hormone response are not affected.

*Drug interactions:* The concurrent use of fenoprofen and salicylates is not recommended.

Chronic administration of phenobarbitone may be associated with a decrease in the plasma half-life of fenoprofen. Dosage adjustment of fenoprofen may be required.

Patients treated with fenoprofen may be resistant to the effects of loop diuretics.

*In vitro* studies have shown that fenoprofen may displace other drugs, for example hydantoins, sulphonamides, or sulphonylureas, from their binding sites and this may lead to drug interaction. Theoretically, fenoprofen could likewise be displaced. In patients receiving coumarin-type anti-coagulants, the addition of fenoprofen could prolong the prothrombin time.

*Side-effects*
*Gastro-intestinal:* These are the most commonly observed side-effects and include dyspepsia, constipation, diarrhoea, nausea, vomiting, anorexia, ulceration of the buccal mucosa, abdominal pain, flatulence, dry mouth, gastritis, metallic taste, pancreatitis and occult blood in the stool. Cases of peptic ulceration, including some complicated by bleeding or perforation have occurred.

*Renal:* Cases of acute renal insufficiency, in association with interstitial nephritis, nephrotic syndrome or papillary necrosis, have been reported. Episodes of dysuria, cystitis and haematuria, oliguria, azotaemia and anuria have occurred.

*Hepatic:* Severe hepatic reactions, including jaundice and fatal hepatitis, have been reported rarely. Increases in alkaline phosphatase, LDH and AST have been observed.

*Haematological:* Various syndromes involving the bone marrow have been reported rarely; thrombocytopenia, pancytopenia and aplastic anaemia have occurred. Purpura, bruising, haemorrhage, haemolytic anaemia and agranulocytosis have also been reported.

*Allergic/skin:* Pruritus, rash, urticaria, anaphylaxis, Stevens-Johnson syndrome, angioneurotic oedema, increased sweating, exfoliative dermatitis, toxic epidermal necrolysis and alopecia have been reported.

*Neurological:* Reactions reported include headache, somnolence, dizziness, tremor, confusion and insomnia, depression, disorientation, seizures and trigeminal neuralgia.

*Cardiovascular:* Palpitations, tachycardia, atrial fibrillation, pulmonary oedema, ECG changes and supraventricular tachycardia have been reported.

*Miscellaneous:* Tinnitus, hearing decrease, amblyopia, blurred vision, diplopia, optic neuritis, nervousness, peripheral oedema, asthenia, dyspnoea, fatigue, malaise, burning tongue, personality change, lymphadenopathy, mastodynia, fever, upper respiratory infection and nasopharyngitis have been reported.

*Overdosage:* Symptoms of overdose appear within several hours and generally involve the gastrointestinal and central nervous systems. They include dyspepsia, nausea, vomiting, abdominal pain, dizziness, headache, ataxia, tinnitus, tremor, drowsiness and confusion. Hyperpyrexia, tachycardia, hypotension and acute renal failure may occur rarely following overdose. Respiratory depression and metabolic acidosis have also been reported following overdose with certain non-steroidal anti-inflammatory drugs.

*Treatment:* Standard therapy to evacuate gastric contents and to support vital functions should be employed. Alkalinisation of the urine, forced diuresis, peritoneal dialysis, haemodialysis and charcoal haemoperfusion do not enhance systemic drug elimination.

**Pharmaceutical precautions** Nil.

**Legal category** POM.

**Package quantities**
Bottles of 100 tablets

**Further information** Nil.

**Product licence number** 11157/0006

## HAELAN CREAM

**Qualitative and quantitative composition** Flurandrenolone (Fludroxycortide) 0.0125% w/w.

**Pharmaceutical form** Cream for topical administration.

**Clinical particulars**

*Therapeutic indications: Adults and children:* Eczema and dermatitis of all types including childhood and adult atopic eczema, photodermatitis, primary irritant and allergic dermatitis, lichen planus, lichen simplex, prurigo nodularis, discoid lupus erythematosus, necrobiosis lipoidica, pretibial myxoedema and erythroderma.

*Posology and method of administration:* For moist, weeping lesions, the cream should be applied gently to the affected area two or three times daily.
*The elderly:* As the skin is likely to be thin, apply sparingly to avoid development of atrophy.
    Dilution is not recommended, but if considered necessary, aqueous cream BP may be used.

*Contra-indications:* Tuberculosis of the skin, facial rosacea, acne vulgaris, perioral dermatitis, perianal and genital pruritus, dermatoses in infancy including eczema, dermatitic napkin eruption, bacterial (impetigo), viral (herpes simplex) and fungal (candida or dermatophyte) infections. Use in patients with a history of hypersensitivity to any of the components in the preparation.

*Special warnings and special precautions for use:* Preparations of Haelan are not intended for ophthalmic use.

    Local and systemic toxicity is common especially following long-term continuous use, continued use on large areas of damaged skin, flexures and with polythene occlusion.

    Systemic absorption of topical corticosteroids has produced reversible hypothalamic-pituitary-adrenal (HPA) axis suppression (see *Undesirable effects*). Therefore, patients receiving a large dose of a potent topical steroid applied to a large surface area or under an occlusive dressing should be evaluated periodically for evidence of HPA axis suppression by using urinary-free cortisol and ACTH stimulation tests. If HPA axis suppression is noted, an attempt should be made to withdraw the drug, to reduce the frequency of application or to substitute a less potent steroid. Recovery of HPA axis function is generally prompt and complete on discontinuation of the drug. Infrequently, signs and symptoms of steroid withdrawal may occur, so that supplemental systemic corticosteroids are required.

    Long-term continuous therapy should be avoided in all patients irrespective of age.

    Application under occlusion should be restricted to dermatoses in very limited areas.

    If used on the face, courses should be limited to five days and occlusion should not be used.

    In the presence of skin infections, the use of an appropriate antifungal or antibacterial agent should be instituted. If a favourable response does not occur promptly, flurandrenolone should be discontinued until the infection has been adequately controlled.

    *Usage in children:* If used in childhood courses should be limited to five days and occlusion should not be used.

    Children may absorb proportionally larger amounts of topical corticosteroids and thus may be more susceptible to systemic toxicity. Children may also demonstrate greater susceptibility to topical corticosteroid induced HPA axis suppression and Cushing's Syndrome than do mature patients because of a large skin surface to body weight ratio. Administration of topical corticosteroids to children should be limited to the least amount compatible with an effective therapeutic regimen. Chronic corticosteroid therapy may interfere with the growth and development of children.

    As with all topical steroids, the activity can be enhanced by the use of occlusive dressings. Preparations of Haelan are recommended only as a supplement to, and not as a substitute for, preparations (lotions, wet dressings, etc.) used in the conventional management of skin lesions. Haelan Cream does not contain parahydroxybenzoates or lanolin.

*Interaction with other medicaments and other forms of interaction:* Not known.

*Pregnancy and lactation: Usage in pregnancy:* There is inadequate evidence of safety in human pregnancy. There may be a very small risk of cleft palate and intra-uterine growth retardation as well as suppression of the neonatal HPA axis. There is evidence of harmful effects in animals.

    Use in pregnancy only when there is no safer alternative and when the disease itself carries risks for mother and child.

    Usage in nursing mothers: It is not known whether topical administration of corticosteroids could result in sufficient systemic absorption to produce detectable quantities in the breast milk of nursing mothers. Systemically administered corticosteroids are secreted into breast milk in quantities not likely to have a deleterious effect on the infant. Nevertheless, caution should be exercised when topical corticosteroids are administered to nursing mothers.

*Effects on ability to drive and to use machines:* Not applicable.

*Undesirable effects:* The following local adverse reactions are reported infrequently with topical corticosteroids but may occur more frequently with the use of occlusive dressings. These reactions are listed in approximate decreasing order of occurrence; burning, itching, irritation, dryness, folliculitis, hypertrichosis, acneform eruptions, hypopigmentation, perioral dermatitis, allergic contact dermatitis, maceration of the skin, secondary infection, skin atrophy, miliaria, striae and thinning and dilatations of the superficial blood vessels producing telangiectasia.

    Prolonged use of large doses to extensive areas can result in sufficient systemic absorption to produce generalised manifestations of steroid toxicity and may result in depression of HPA function on discontinuing treatment.

    Manifestations of Cushing's syndrome, hyperglycaemia and glycosuria have occurred in some patients.

    Manifestations of adrenal suppression in children include linear growth retardation, delayed weight gain, low plasma cortisol levels and absence of response to ACTH stimulation. Intracranial hypertension including bulging fontanelles, headaches and bilateral papilloedema have also been reported in children receiving topical corticosteroids.

    Infected skin lesions, viral, bacterial or fungal may be substantially exacerbated by topical steroid therapy. Wound healing is significantly retarded.

    Hypersensitivity reactions may occur.

*Overdose:* Topically applied corticosteroids can be absorbed in sufficient amounts to produce systemic effects (see *Special warnings and special precautions for use*).

**Pharmacological properties**

*Pharmacodynamic properties:* Flurandrenolone is a fluorinated, synthetic, moderately potent corticosteroid.

    As with other topical steroids, the therapeutic effect is primarily the result of its anti-inflammatory, anti-mitotic and anti-synthetic activities.

*Pharmacokinetic properties:* Flurandrenolone applied under occlusive dressing has shown therapeutic improvement without disturbance of electrolyte, liver or renal function or suppression of adrenal function.

*Preclinical safety data:* There are no preclinical data of relevance to the prescriber in addition to that summarised in other sections of the Summary of Product Characteristics.

**Pharmaceutical particulars**

*List of excipients:* Stearic acid, cetyl alcohol, polyoxyl 40 stearate, liquid paraffin, propylene glycol, sodium citrate, citric acid anhydrous, water purified

*Incompatibilities:* None known.

*Shelf life:* 24 months.

*Special precautions for storage:* None.

*Nature and contents of container:* 60 g aluminium tubes with screw cap.

*Instructions for use/handling:* No special instructions for handling.

**Marketing authorisation number** 11157/0008.

**Date of approval/revision of SPC** December 1996

**Legal category** POM

## HAELAN* OINTMENT

**Presentation** Collapsible tubes containing 0.0125% flurandrenolone in an ointment base. The ointment is translucent in colour.

**Uses** *Adults and children:* Eczema and dermatitis of all types including childhood and adult atopic eczema, photodermatitis, primary irritant and allergic dermatitis, lichen planus, lichen simplex, prurigo nodularis, discoid lupus erythematosus, necrobiosis lipoidica, pretibial myxoedema and erythroderma.

**Dosage and administration** For topical administration.

    For dry, scaly lesions, the ointment should be applied as a thin film to the affected area two or three times daily.

*The elderly:* As the skin is likely to be thin, apply sparingly to avoid development of atrophy.

    Dilution is not recommended, but if considered necessary White Soft Paraffin BP may be used.

**Contra-indications, warnings, etc**
*Contra-indications:* Tuberculosis of the skin. Facial rosacea. Acne vulgaris. Perioral dermatitis. Perianal and genital pruritus. Dermatoses in infancy including eczema, dermatitic napkin eruption, bacterial (impetigo), viral (herpes simplex) and fungal (candida or dermatophyte) infections. Use in patients with a history of hypersensitivity to any of the components in the preparation.

*Warnings and precautions:* Preparations of Haelan are not intended for ophthalmic use.

    Local and systemic toxicity is common especially following long-term continuous use, continued use on large areas of damaged skin, flexures and with polythene occlusion.

    Systemic absorption of topical corticosteroids has produced reversible hypothalamic-pituitary-adrenal (HPA) axis suppression (see 'Side-effects'). Therefore, patients receiving a large dose of a potent topical steroid applied to a large surface area or under an occlusive dressing should be evaluated periodically for evidence of HPA axis suppression by using urinary-free cortisol and ACTH stimulation tests. If HPA axis suppression is noted, an attempt should be made to withdraw the drug, to reduce the frequency of application or to substitute a less potent steroid. Recovery of HPA axis function is generally prompt and complete on discontinuation of the drug. Infrequently, signs and symptoms of steroid withdrawal may occur, so that supplemental systemic corticosteroids are required.

    Long-term continuous therapy should be avoided in all patients irrespective of age.

    Application under occlusion should be restricted to dermatoses in very limited areas.

    If used on the face, courses should be limited to five days and occlusion should not be used.

    In the presence of skin infections, the use of an appropriate antifungal or antibacterial agent should be instituted. If a favourable response does not occur promptly, flurandrenolone should be discontinued until the infection has been adequately controlled.

*Usage in children:* If used in childhood, courses should be limited to five days and occlusion should not be used.

    Children may absorb proportionally larger amounts of topical corticosteroids and thus may be more susceptible to systemic toxicity. Children may also demonstrate greater susceptibility to topical corticosteroid induced HPA axis suppression and Cushing's syndrome than do mature patients because of a larger skin surface to body weight ratio. Administration of topical corticosteroids to children should be limited to the least amount compatible with an effective therapeutic regimen. Chronic corticosteroid therapy may interfere with the growth and development of children.

*Usage in pregnancy:* There is inadequate evidence of safety in human pregnancy. There may be a very small risk of cleft palate and intra-uterine growth retardation as well as suppression of the neonatal HPA axis. There is evidence of harmful effects in animals.

    Use in pregnancy only when there is no safer

alternative and when the disease itself carries risks for mother and child.

*Usage in nursing mothers:* It is not known whether topical administration of corticosteroids could result in sufficient systemic absorption to produce detectable quantities in the breast milk of nursing mothers. Systemically administered corticosteroids are secreted into breast milk in quantities not likely to have a deleterious effect on the infant. Nevertheless, caution should be exercised when topical corticosteroids are administered to nursing mothers.

*Side-effects:* The following local adverse reactions are reported infrequently with topical corticosteroids but may occur more frequently with the use of occlusive dressings. These reactions are listed in an approximate decreasing order of occurrence: burning, itching, irritation, dryness, folliculitis, hypertrichosis, acneform eruptions, hypopigmentation, perioral dermatitis, allergic contact dermatitis, maceration of the skin, secondary infection, skin atrophy, miliaria, striae and thinning and dilatations of superficial blood vessels producing telangiectasia.

Prolonged use of large doses to extensive areas can result in sufficient systemic absorption to produce generalised manifestations of steroid toxicity and may result in depression of HPA function on discontinuing treatment.

Manifestations of Cushing's syndrome, hyperglycaemia and glycosuria have occurred in some patients.

Manifestations of adrenal suppression in children include linear growth retardation, delayed weight gain, low plasma cortisol levels and absence of response to ACTH stimulation. Intracranial hypertension including bulging fontanelles, headaches and bilateral papilloedema have also been reported in children receiving topical corticosteroids.

Infected skin lesions, viral, bacterial or fungal may be substantially exacerbated by topical steroid therapy. Wound healing is significantly retarded.

Hypersensitivity reactions may occur.

*Overdosage:* Topically applied corticosteroids can be absorbed in sufficient amounts to produce systemic effects (see 'Warnings and precautions').

**Pharmaceutical precautions** Do not store above 25°C.

See *Administration* for diluents.

**Legal category** POM.

**Package quantities**
Haelan Ointment (0.0125% flurandrenolone): Tubes of 60 g

**Further information** As with all topical steroids, the activity can be enhanced by the use of occlusive dressings. Preparations of Haelan are recommended only as a supplement to, and not as a substitute for, preparations (lotions, wet dressings, etc.) used in the conventional management of skin lesions. Haelan preparations do not contain parahydroxybenzoates or lanolin.

**Product licence number** 11157/009

# HAELAN* TAPE

**Qualitative and quantitative composition** The tape is impregnated with 4 micrograms flurandrenolone per square centimetre.

**Pharmaceutical form** Occlusive tape

**Clinical particulars**

*Therapeutic indications:* Occlusive topical steroid. Adjunctive therapy for chronic, localised, recalcitrant dermatoses that may respond to topical corticosteroids and particularly dry, scaling lesions.

*Posology and method of administration:*
*Adults and the elderly:* For application to the skin, which should be clean, dry and shorn of hair. In most instances the tape need only remain in place for 12 out of 24 hours. Cosmetics may be applied over the tape.

*Application:* The tape is cut so as to cover the lesion and a quarter inch margin of normal skin. Corners should be rounded off. After removing the lining paper, the tape is applied to the centre of the lesion with gentle pressure and worked to the edges, avoiding excessive tension of the skin. If longer strips of tape are to be applied, the lining paper should be removed progressively.

If irritation or infection develops, remove tape and consult a physician.

*Children:* If used in childhood, courses should be limited to five days and occlusion should not be used (see *Special warnings and special precautions for use*).

*Contra-indications:* Chicken pox. Vaccinia. Tuberculosis of the skin. Hypersensitivity to any of the components. Facial rosacea. Acne vulgaris. Perioral dermatitis. Perianal and genital pruritus. Dermatoses in infancy including eczema, dermatitic napkin eruption, bacterial (impetigo), viral (herpes simplex) and fungal (candida or dermatophyte) infections.

*Special warnings and special precautions for use:* Not advocated for acute and weeping dermatoses.

Local and systemic toxicity of medium and high potency topical corticosteroids is common, especially following long-term continuous use, continued use on large areas of damaged skin, flexures and with polythene occlusion.

Systemic absorption of topical corticosteroids has produced reversible hypothalamic-pituitary-adrenal (HPA) axis suppression (see *Undesirable effects*). Therefore, patients receiving a large dose of a potent topical steroid applied to a large surface area or under an occlusive dressing should be evaluated periodically for evidence of HPA axis suppression by using urinary-free cortisol and ACTH stimulation tests. If HPA axis suppression is noted, an attempt should be made to withdraw the drug, to reduce the frequency of application or to substitute a less potent steroid. Recovery of HPA axis function is generally prompt and complete on discontinuation of the drug. Infrequently, signs and symptoms of steroid withdrawal may occur, so that supplemental systemic corticosteroids are required.

Long-term continuous therapy should be avoided in all patients irrespective of age.

Application under occlusion should be restricted to dermatoses in very limited areas.

If used on the face, courses should be limited to five days and occlusion should not be used.

In the presence of skin infections, the use of an appropriate antifungal or antibacterial agent should be instituted. If a favourable response does not occur promptly, flurandrenolone should be discontinued until the infection has been adequately controlled.

Children may absorb proportionally larger amounts of topical corticosteroids and thus may be more susceptible to systemic toxicity. Children may also demonstrate greater susceptibility to topical corticosteroid induced HPA axis suppression and Cushing's syndrome than do mature patients because of a larger skin surface to bodyweight ratio. Administration of topical corticosteroids to children should be limited to the least amount compatible with an effective therapeutic regimen. Chronic corticosteroid therapy may interfere with the growth and development of children.

*Interaction with other medicaments and other forms of interaction:* None known.

*Pregnancy and lactation:* Usage in pregnancy: There is inadequate evidence of safety in human pregnancy. There may be a very small risk of cleft palate and intra-uterine growth retardation as well as suppression of the neonatal HPA axis. There is evidence of harmful effects in animals.

Use in pregnancy only when there is no safer alternative and when the disease itself carries risks for mother and child.

Usage in nursing mothers: It is not known whether topical administration of corticosteroids could result in sufficient systemic absorption to produce detectable quantities in the breast milk of nursing mothers. Systemically administered corticosteroids are secreted into breast milk in quantities not likely to have a deleterious effect on the infant. Nevertheless, caution should be exercised when topical corticosteroids are administered to nursing mothers.

*Effects on the ability to drive and use machines:* Not applicable.

*Undesirable effects:* The following local adverse reactions are reported infrequently with topical corticosteroids but may occur more frequently with the use of occlusive dressings. These reactions are listed in an approximate decreasing order of occurrence: burning, itching, irritation, dryness, folliculitis, hypertrichosis, acneform eruptions, hypopigmentation, perioral dermatitis, allergic contact dermatitis, maceration of the skin, secondary infection, skin atrophy, miliaria, striae and thinning and dilatations of superficial blood vessels producing telangiectasia.

Prolonged use of large doses to extensive areas can result in sufficient systemic absorption to produce generalised manifestations of steroid toxicity and may result in depression of HPA function on discontinuing treatment.

Manifestations of Cushing's syndrome, hyperglycaemia and glycosuria have occurred in some patients.

Manifestations of adrenal suppression in children include linear growth retardation, delayed weight gain, low plasma cortisol levels and absence of response to ACTH stimulation. Intracranial hypertension including bulging fontanelles, headaches and bilateral papilloedema have also been reported in children receiving topical corticosteroids. Infected skin lesions, viral, bacterial or fungal, may be substantially exacerbated by topical steroid therapy. Wound healing is significantly retarded.

Hypersensitivity reactions may occur.

*Overdose:* Topically applied corticosteroids can be absorbed in sufficient amounts to produce systemic affects (see *Special warnings and special precautions for use*).

**Pharmacological properties**

*Pharmacodynamic properties:* Flurandrenolone is a fluorinated, synthetic, moderately potent, topical corticosteroid. As with other topical steroids, the therapeutic effect is primarily the result of its anti-inflammatory, antimitotic and antisynthetic activities.

*Pharmacokinetic properties:* When applied topically, particularly to large areas, when skin is broken, or under occlusive dressings, corticosteroids may be absorbed in sufficient amounts to cause systemic effects.

*Preclinical safety data:* There are no preclinical data of relevance to the prescriber in addition to that summarised in other sections of the Summary of Product Characteristics.

**Pharmaceutical particulars**

*List of excipients:* Blenderm brand surgical tape.

*Incompatibilities:* None known.

*Shelf life:* 3 years.

*Special precautions for storage:* Store in a dry place, below 25°C.

*Nature and contents of container:* Polypropylene dispenser, in a cardboard box, containing 50cm or 200cm of translucent, polythene adhesive film, 7.5cm wide, protected by a removable paper liner.

*Instructions for use/handling:* Not applicable.

**Marketing authorisation number** 11157 / 0007

**Date of approval/revision of SPC** January 1997

**Legal category** POM

# TOPAL*

**Presentation** Round, pale cream tablets with a fragrant odour and sweet, slightly gelatinous taste containing dried aluminium hydroxide gel 30 mg, light magnesium carbonate 40 mg, alginic acid 200 mg, plus excipients to 1.65 g. The inactive ingredients are citric acid, flavour agents, lactose, magnesium stearate, polyvinylpyrrolidone, silica, sodium bicarbonate, sugar and water.

**Uses** Relief of discomfort due to gastric reflux or mucosal irritation in conditions such as: heartburn, reflux oesophagitis, hiatus hernia, gastritis, acid dyspepsia.

**Dosage and administration**
*Adults including the elderly:* One to three tablets chewed four times a day after meals and at bedtime.

*Children:* Half the adult dose.

**Contra-indications, warnings, etc** No specific contra-indications, but care should be observed if used by diabetics because of the sugar content (see 'Further information').

Topal is not recommended in patients who are severely debilitated or on low phosphorus diets and in patients with severe renal insufficiency, alkalosis or hypermagnesaemia.

Antacids may interfere with the absorption of some drugs, especially tetracyclines.

*Pregnancy:* It is probably wise to avoid any drug during first trimester of pregnancy unless there are compelling reasons for its use.

*Side-effects:* Topal is well tolerated and any side effects which occur are likely to be mild and transient.

*Overdosage:* Treatment should be symptomatic.

**Pharmaceutical precautions** Store below 30°C protected from moisture.

**Legal category** GSL.

**Package quantities** Blister packs of 42 tablets (OP).

**Further information** Each tablet also contains 40 mg sodium bicarbonate, 880 mg of sucrose and 220 mg lactose, but no added colouring.

**Product licence number** 0603/0021

*Product licence holder:* Pierre Fabre Limited, Hyde Abbey House, 23 Hyde Street, Winchester, Hants SO23 7DR.

*\*Trade Mark*

# Novo Nordisk Pharmaceuticals Limited
Novo Nordisk House, Broadfield Park
Brighton Road, Pease Pottage
Crawley, West Sussex, RH11 9RT

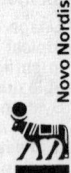

**ACTRAPID\* PENFILL\* 3 ml**
**INSULATARD\* PENFILL\* 3 ml**
**MIXTARD\* 10 PENFILL\* 3 ml**
**MIXTARD\* 20 PENFILL\* 3 ml**
**MIXTARD\* 30 PENFILL\* 3 ml**
**MIXTARD\* 40 PENFILL\* 3 ml**
**MIXTARD\* 50 PENFILL\* 3 ml**

### Qualitative and quantitative composition
Actrapid Penfill 3 ml: Insulin Injection.
Insulatard Penfill 3 ml: Isophane Insulin Injection.
Mixtard 10 Penfill 3 ml: Biphasic Isophane Insulin Injection 10/90.
Mixtard 20 Penfill 3 ml: Biphasic Isophane Insulin Injection 20/80.
Mixtard 30 Penfill 3 ml: Biphasic Isophane Insulin Injection 30/70.
Mixtard 40 Penfill 3 ml: Biphasic Isophane Insulin Injection 40/60.
Mixtard 50 Penfill 3 ml: Biphasic Isophane Insulin Injection 50/50.

*Active ingredient:* Human insulin (pyr) 100 iu/ml.

### Pharmaceutical form
Actrapid Penfill 3 ml: Sterile solution for injection.
Insulatard Penfill 3 ml and Mixtard Penfill 3 ml range: Sterile suspension for injection.

### Clinical particulars
*Therapeutic indications:* The treatment of insulin-requiring diabetics.

*Posology and method of administration:* The dosage is determined by the physician according to the needs of the patient.

The Penfill preparations are usually administered subcutaneously but may also be given intramuscularly. When injected subcutaneously, injection of Actrapid Penfill 3 ml into the abdominal wall ensures a faster absorption than from other regions of the body. The thigh is the recommended site for injection of Insulatard Penfill 3 ml, the abdominal wall or thigh for subcutaneous injection of Mixtard Penfill 3 ml preparations. Injection into a lifted skin fold minimises the risk of intramuscular injection.

When used alone Actrapid Penfill 3 ml is usually given three or more times daily; it is more commonly used in regimens where an intermediate or long-acting insulin is given in addition.

Insulatard Penfill 3 ml and the Mixtard Penfill 3 ml preparations may be given once or, more commonly, twice daily. Insulatard Penfill 3 ml may also be supplemented with shorter-acting insulin.

Penfill insulin cartridges are designed to be used with NovoPen insulin pens and NovoFine needles. The Penfill preparations are intended for use by one person only. The Penfill cartridges must not be used with conventional syringes or refilled.

*Use in the elderly:* There are no precautions concerning the use of insulin which are specific to the elderly diabetic. However, injection procedures may be difficult for the infirm or the confused patient, and the simplest regimen consistent with keeping the patient symptom-free should be considered.

*Contra-indications:* Insulin is contra-indicated in hypoglycaemia.

*Special warnings and special precautions for use:* Injection of Actrapid Penfill 3 ml or the Mixtard Penfill 3 ml preparations should be followed by a meal within approximately 30 minutes of administration.

The use of dosages which are inadequate, or discontinuation of treatment, especially in insulin-dependent diabetics, may lead to hyperglycaemia and diabetic ketoacidosis; conditions which are potentially lethal.

When patients are transferred from other insulins to highly purified human insulin the change should be made according to the following general guidelines:

For patients currently controlled on highly purified human or porcine insulin preparations no dosage change is anticipated other than the routine adjustments made in order to maintain stable diabetic control. Patients currently stabilised on mixed species or bovine insulin may require a dosage adjustment dependent upon dosage, purity, species and formulation of the insulin preparation(s) currently administered. Variations in glycaemic control may occur and

adjustments in therapy should be made under the guidance of a physician. A few patients have reported that after being transferred to human insulin the early warning symptoms for hypoglycaemia were less pronounced than they were with animal-source insulin.

Patients whose blood glucose is greatly improved, e.g. by intensified insulin therapy, may experience a change in their usual warning symptoms of hypoglycaemia and possibly lose some or all of the symptoms, and should be advised accordingly.

*Interaction with other medicaments and other forms of interaction:* Concomitant use of other drugs may influence insulin requirements. The following substances may enhance the hypoglycaemic effect of insulin: alcohol, non-selective beta adrenergic blocking agents, monoamine oxidase inhibitors (MAOI), ACE inhibitors, salicylate, anabolic steroids.

Other drugs may increase insulin requirements: oral contraceptives, thyroid hormones, corticosteroids, thiazides and sympathomimetics. Beta adrenergic blocking agents may blur the symptoms of hypoglycaemia. Alcohol may intensify and prolong the hypoglycaemic effect of insulin.

Diabetic patients treated with drugs other than insulin should discuss possible interactions with the prescribing physician.

*Pregnancy and lactation:* Intensified control in the treatment of pregnant insulin-dependent diabetics is recommended. Insulin requirements usually fall in the first trimester and increase during the second and third trimester. Insulin does not pass the placental barrier.

*Effects on ability to drive and use machines:* The ability to drive or use machinery may be impaired during hypoglycaemia or severe hyperglycaemia.

*Undesirable effects:* At initiation of insulin therapy, oedema and refraction anomalies may occur; these are usually transitory. The same applies to local hypersensitivity reactions (swelling and itching at the injection site) which usually disappear during continued treatment.

Persistent allergies to human insulin are very rare and are mostly due to cross-reacting antibodies to animal insulins. Lipodystrophy at injection sites is also rare and should be prevented by constantly changing injection sites.

*Overdose:* Overdosage causes hypoglycaemia; symptoms are variable but may include confusion, palpitations, sweating, malaise and loss of consciousness. In the event of an overdose, glucose should be given if the patient is conscious. Where the patient is unconscious an intramuscular, subcutaneous or intravenous injection of glucagon should be given and oral carbohydrate administered when the patient responds. Alternatively intravenous glucose may be administered; it must be given if there is no response to glucagon. If severe hypoglycaemia is not treated it can cause temporary or permanent brain damage and death.

### Pharmacological properties
*Pharmacodynamic properties:* Human insulin (pyr) is identical to pancreatic human insulin. It has hypoglycaemic actions in man, promotes uptake of glucose into liver, muscle and adipose tissue, inhibits gluconeognesis and promotes lipogenesis.

*Pharmacokinetic properties:* Actrapid Penfill 3 ml is a neutral solution of human insulin (pyr). When injected subcutaneously it has a duration of action of some $\frac{1}{2}$ to 8 hours and its maximum effect is exerted between 1 and 3 hours after injection. Insulatard Penfill 3 ml is an isophane insulin preparation. When injected subcutaneously it has a duration of action of some $1\frac{1}{2}$ up to 24 hours and its maximum effect is exerted between 4 and 12 hours after injection.

The Mixtard Penfill 3 ml preparations consist of soluble human insulin and isophane human insulin in the ratios:

Mixtard 10 Penfill 3 ml – 10/90
Mixtard 20 Penfill 3 ml – 20/80
Mixtard 30 Penfill 3 ml – 30/70
Mixtard 40 Penfill 3 ml – 40/60
Mixtard 50 Penfill 3 ml – 50/50

They are intermediate acting insulins with a pronounced initial effect. When injected subcutaneously

they have a duration of action of some $\frac{1}{2}$ up to 24 hours and their maximum effect is exerted between 2 and 8 hours after injection.

### Pharmaceutical particulars
*List of excipients:* Glycerol (E422), m-cresol, zinc oxide, sodium hydroxide, hydrochloric acid, water for injections.

Plus, Insulatard Penfill 3 ml and Mixtard Penfill 3 ml preparations: sodium phosphate dihydrate, phenol, protamine sulphate.

*Incompatibilities:* Not applicable.

*Shelf life:* 30 months. Cartridges in use or carried as a spare may be kept at ambient temperature (e.g. in the pocket or handbag) for up to one month but should not be exposed to excessive heat or sunlight.

*Special precautions for storage:* Store between 2 and 8˚C. Avoid freezing. Cartridges in use must not be stored in a refrigerator.

*Nature and contents of container:* 3 ml glass cartridges closed at one end with an aluminium cap and natural rubber/bromobutyl rubber laminate disc, and at the other end with a bromobutyl piston. A threaded colour-coded plastic cap is placed over the aluminium cap. Pack size: 5×3 ml cartridges.

*Instructions for use/handling:* Each carton contains a patient information leaflet with instructions for use; the leaflet includes a reference to the instruction manual accompanying the NovoPen 3 device.

### Marketing authorisation numbers
| | |
|---|---|
| Actrapid Penfill 3 ml | 03132/0105 |
| Insulatard Penfill 3 ml | 03132/0091 |
| Mixtard 10 Penfill 3 ml | 03132/0092 |
| Mixtard 20 Penfill 3 ml | 03132/0093 |
| Mixtard 30 Penfill 3 ml | 03132/0094 |
| Mixtard 40 Penfill 3 ml | 03132/0095 |
| Mixtard 50 Penfill 3 ml | 03132/0096 |

**Date of approval/revision of SPC** July 1996.

**Legal category** P.

**ACTRAPID\* PEN**
**HUMAN INSULATARD\* PEN**
**HUMAN MIXTARD\* 10 PEN**
**HUMAN MIXTARD\* 20 PEN**
**HUMAN MIXTARD\* 30 PEN**
**HUMAN MIXTARD\* 40 PEN**
**HUMAN MIXTARD\* 50 PEN**

*Human Mixtard 10 Pen, Human Mixtard 20 Pen, Human Mixtard 30 Pen, Human Mixtard 40 Pen and Human Mixtard 50 Pen were formerly named PenMix 10/90, PenMix 20/80, PenMix 30/70, PenMix 40/60 and PenMix 50/50 respectively.*

### Qualitative and quantitative composition
Actrapid Pen: Insulin Injection
Human Insulatard Pen: Isophane Insulin Injection
Human Mixtard 10 Pen: Biphasic Isophane Insulin Injection 10/90
Human Mixtard 20 Pen: Biphasic Isophane Insulin Injection 20/80
Human Mixtard 30 Pen: Biphasic Isophane Insulin Injection 30/70
Human Mixtard 40 Pen: Biphasic Isophane Insulin Injection 40/60
Human Mixtard 50 Pen: Biphasic Isophane Insulin Injection 50/50

*Active ingredient:* Human insulin (pyr) 100 iu/ml.

### Pharmaceutical form
Actrapid Pen: Sterile solution for injection.
Human Insulatard Pen and Human Mixtard Pen range: Sterile suspension for injection.

### Clinical particulars
*Therapeutic indications:* The treatment of insulin requiring diabetics.

*Posology and method of administration:* The dosage is determined by the physician according to the needs of the patient.

The Pen preparations are usually administered subcutaneously but may also be given intramuscularly. When injected subcutaneously, injection of Actrapid Pen into the abdominal wall ensures a faster absorption than from other regions of the body. The thigh is the recommended site for injection of Human Insulatard Pen, the abdominal wall or thigh for subcutaneous injection of Human Mixtard Pen preparations. Injection into a lifted skin fold minimises the risk of intramuscular injection.

When used alone Actrapid Pen is usually given three or more times daily; it is more commonly used in regimens where an intermediate or long-acting insulin is given in addition.

Human Insulatard Pen and the Human Mixtard Pen preparations may be given once or, more commonly, twice daily. Human Insulatard Pen may also be supplemented with shorter-acting insulin.

NovaFine needles are designed to be used with the Pen prefilled insulin syringes. The Pen preparations are for single-patient use only.

*Use in the elderly:* There are no precautions concerning the use of insulin which are specific to the elderly diabetic. However, injection procedures may be difficult for the infirm or the confused patient, and the simplest regimen consistent with keeping the patient symptom-free should be considered.

*Contra-indications:* Insulin is contra-indicated in hypoglycaemia.

*Special warnings and special precautions for use:* Injection of Actrapid Pen or the Human Mixtard Pen preparations should be followed by a meal within approximately 30 minutes of administration.

The use of dosages which are inadequate, or discontinuation of treatment, especially in insulin-dependent diabetics, may lead to hyperglycaemia and diabetic ketoacidosis; conditions which are potentially lethal.

When patients are transferred from other insulins to highly purified human insulin the change should be made according to the following general guidelines:

For patients currently controlled on highly purified human or porcine insulin preparations no dosage change is anticipated other than the routine adjustments made in order to maintain stable diabetic control. Patients currently stabilised on mixed species or bovine insulin may require a dosage adjustment dependent upon dosage, purity, species and formulation of the insulin preparation(s) currently administered. Variations in glycaemic control may occur and adjustments in therapy should be made under the guidance of a physician. A few patients have reported that after being transferred to human insulin the early warning symptoms for hypoglycaemia were less pronounced than they were with animal-source insulin.

Patients whose blood glucose is greatly improved, e.g. by intensified insulin therapy, may experience a change in their usual warning symptoms of hypoglycaemia and possibly lose some or all of the symptoms, and should be advised accordingly.

*Interaction with other medicaments and other forms of interaction:* Concomitant use of other drugs may influence insulin requirements. The following substances may enhance the hypoglycaemic effect of insulin: alcohol, non-selective beta adrenergic blocking agents, monoamine oxidase inhibitors (MAOI), ACE inhibitors, salicylate, anabolic steroids.

Other drugs may increase insulin requirements: oral contraceptives, thyroid hormones, corticosteroids, thiazides and sympathomimetics. Beta adrenergic blocking agents may blur the symptoms of hypoglycaemia. Alcohol may intensify and prolong the hypoglycaemic effect of insulin.

Diabetic patients treated with drugs other than insulin should discuss possible interactions with the prescribing physician.

*Pregnancy and lactation:* Instensified control in the treatment of pregnant insulin-dependent diabetics is recommended. Insulin requirements usually fall in the first trimester and increase during the second and third trimester. Insulin does not pass the placental barrier.

*Effects on ability to drive and use machines:* The ability to drive or use machinery may be impaired during hypoglycaemia or severe hyperglycaemia.

*Undesirable effects:* At initiation of insulin therapy, oedema and refraction anomalies may occur; these are usually transitory. The same applies to local hypersensitivity reactions (swelling and itching at the injection site) which usually disappear during continued treatment.

Persistent allergies to human insulin are very rare and are mostly due to cross-reacting antibodies to animal insulins. Lipodystrophy at injection sites is also rare and should be prevented by constantly changing injection sites.

*Overdose:* Overdosage causes hypoglycaemia; symptoms are variable but may include confusion, palpitations, sweating, malaise and loss of consciousness. In the event of an overdose, glucose should be given if the patient is conscious. Where the patient is unconscious an intramuscular, subcutaneous or intravenous injection of glucagon should be given and oral carbohydrate administered when the patient responds. Alternatively intravenous glucose may be administered; it must be given if there is no response to glucagon. If severe hypoglycaemia is not treated it can cause temporary or permanent brain damage and death.

**Pharmacological properties**

*Pharmacodynamic properties:* Human insulin (pyr) is identical to pancreatic human insulin. It has hypoglycaemic actions in man, promotes uptake of glucose into liver, muscle and adipose tissue, inhibits gluconeogenesis and promotes lipogenesis.

*Pharmacokinetic properties:* Actrapid Pen is a neutral solution of human insulin (pyr). When injected subcutaneously it has a duration of action of some ½ to 8 hours and its maximum effect is exerted between 1 and 3 hours after injection. Human Insulatard Pen is an isophane insulin preparation. When injected subcutaneously it has a duration of action of some 1½ up to 24 hours and its maximum effect is exerted between 4 and 12 hours after injection.

The Human Mixtard Pen preparations consist of soluble human insulin and isophane human insulin in the ratios:

Human Mixtard 10 Pen – 10/90
Human Mixtard 20 Pen – 20/80
Human Mixtard 30 Pen – 30/70
Human Mixtard 40 Pen – 40/60
Human Mixtard 50 Pen – 50/50

They are intermediate acting insulins with a pronounced initial effect. When injected subcutaneously they have a duration of action of some ½ up to 24 hours and their maximum effect is exerted between 2 and 8 hours after injection.

**Pharmaceutical particulars**

*List of excipients:* Glycerol (E422), m-cresol, zinc oxide, sodium hydroxide, hydrochloric acid, water for injections.

Plus, Human Insulatard Pen and Human Mixtard Pen preparations: sodium phosphate dihydrate, phenol, protamine sulphate.

*Incompatibilities:* Not applicable.

*Shelf life:* 30 months.

*Special precautions for storage:* Store between 2 and 8°C. Avoid freezing. Pens in use or carried as a spare may be kept at ambient temperature (maximum 25°C) for up to one month but should not be exposed to excessive heat or sunlight. Pens in use must not be refrigerated.

*Nature and contents of container:* 3 ml glass cartridges closed at one end with an aluminium cap and natural rubber/bromobutyl rubber laminate disc, and at the other end with a bromobutyl piston, and which is contained within a disposable injection device.

*Pack size:* 5×3 ml prefilled, disposable injection device.

*Instructions for use/handling:* Each carton contains a patient information leaflet with instructions for use.

**Marketing authorisation numbers**

| | |
|---|---|
| Actrapid Pen | 03132/0104 |
| Human Insulatard Pen | 03132/0067 |
| Human Mixtard 10 Pen | 03132/0068 |
| Human Mixtard 20 Pen | 03132/0069 |
| Human Mixtard 30 Pen | 03132/0070 |
| Human Mixtard 40 Pen | 03132/0071 |
| Human Mixtard 50 Pen | 03132/0072 |

**Date of approval/revision of SPC** 21 April 1997.

**Legal category** P.

## HUMAN ACTRAPID* PENFILL*
## HUMAN INSULATARD* PENFILL*
## HUMAN MIXTARD* 10 PENFILL*
## HUMAN MIXTARD* 20 PENFILL*
## HUMAN MIXTARD* 30 PENFILL*
## HUMAN MIXTARD* 40 PENFILL*
## HUMAN MIXTARD* 50 PENFILL*

*Human Insulatard Penfill was formerly named Human Protaphane Penfill. Human Mixtard 10 Penfill, Human Mixtard 20 Penfill, Human Mixtard 30 Penfill, Human Mixtard 40 Penfill and Human Mixtard 50 Penfill were formerly named PenMix 10/90 Penfill, PenMix 20/80 Penfill, PenMix 30/70 Penfill, PenMix 40/60 Penfill and PenMix 50/50 Penfill respectively.*

**Presentation** *Human Actrapid Penfill* (Insulin Injection) is a clear neutral solution of human insulin (pyr), containing glycerol and m-cresol as added preservative.

*Human Insulatard Penfill* (Isophane Insulin Injection) is a neutral suspension of isophane human insulin (pyr).

The Human Mixtard Penfill preparations are neutral suspensions of human insulin (pyr) consisting of soluble human insulin and isophane human insulin in the ratios:

| | | |
|---|---|---|
| Human Mixtard 10 Penfill | – | 10/90 |
| Human Mixtard 20 Penfill | – | 20/80 |
| Human Mixtard 30 Penfill | – | 30/70 |
| Human Mixtard 40 Penfill | – | 40/60 |
| Human Mixtard 50 Penfill | – | 50/50 |

Human Insulatard Penfill and the Human Mixtard Penfill preparations also contain glycerol, sodium phosphate, protamine sulphate as retarding agent, and m-cresol and phenol as added preservatives.

The Penfill preparations are contained in 1.5 ml cartridges; when agitated up and down the suspensions appear white and cloudy. Each preparation is available in a strength of 100 iu/ml.

**Uses** The treatment of insulin-requiring diabetics.

**Dosage and administration**

*Adults and children:* The dosage is determined by the physician according to the needs of the patient.

Penfill insulin cartridges are designed to be used with the NovoPen insulin pens and NovoFine needles. When used in these devices they are given by subcutaneous injection. Instructions for use of these preparations in NovoPen insulin pens are included with the devices and must be carefully followed. Prior to injection the suspensions should be agitated up and down until the insulin is white and cloudy; a glass ball is included in the cartridge to facilitate resuspension.

When injected subcutaneously, Human Actrapid Penfill has a duration of action of some ½ to 8 hours and its maximum effect is exerted between 1 and 3 hours after injection. When used alone it is usually given three or more times daily; it is most commonly used in regimens where an intermediate or long acting insulin is given in addition.

When injected subcutaneously, Human Insulatard Penfill has a duration of action of some 1½ up to 24 hours and its maximum effect is exerted between 4 and 12 hours after injection, and the Human Mixtard Penfill preparations have a duration of action of some ½ to 24 hours and their maximum effect is exerted between 2 and 8 hours after injection. Human Insulatard Penfill and the Human Mixtard Penfill preparations may be given once, or more commonly, twice daily. The Human Mixtard Penfill preparations are used especially when a strong initial effect is desired. Human Insulatard Penfill may also be supplemented with shorter-acting insulin.

When injected subcutaneously, injection of Human Actrapid Penfill into the abdominal wall ensures a faster absorption than from other regions of the body. The thigh is the recommended site for subcutaneous injection of Human Insulatard Penfill, the abdominal wall or thigh for subcutaneous injection of Human Mixtard Penfill preparations. Injection into a lifted skin fold minimises the risk of intramuscular injection.

The Penfill preparations must not be used with conventional syringes, or refilled.

*Use in the elderly:* There are no precautions concerning the use of insulin which are specific to the elderly diabetic. However, injection procedures may be difficult for the infirm, the poorly sighted, or the confused patient, and the simplest regimen consistent with keeping the patient symptom-free should be considered.

**Contra-indications, warnings, etc**

*Contra-indications:* Insulin is contra-indicated in hypoglycaemia.

*Precautions:* Owing to their strong early effect, injections of Human Actrapid Penfill or the Human Mixtard Penfill preparations should be followed by a meal within 30 minutes of administration.

The use of dosages which are inadequate or discontinuation of treatment, especially in insulin-dependent diabetics, may lead to hyperglycaemia and diabetic ketacidosis; conditions which are potentially lethal.

When patients are transferred from other insulins to Human Monocomponent insulin the change should be made according to the following general guidelines:

For patients currently controlled on Human Monocomponent, porcine monocomponent or other highly purified human or porcine insulin preparations, no dosage change is anticipated other than the routine adjustments made in order to maintain stable diabetic control.

Patients currently stabilised on mixed species or bovine insulin may require a dosage adjustment dependent upon dosage, purity, species and formulation of the insulin preparation(s) currently administered. Variations in glycaemic control may occur and adjustments in therapy should be made under the guidance of a physician.

A few patients have reported that after being transferred to human insulin, the early warning symptoms for hypoglycaemia were less pronounced than they were with animal source insulin.

Patients whose blood glucose control is greatly improved, e.g. by intensified insulin therapy, may experience a change in their usual warning symptoms of hypoglycaemia, and possibly lose some or all of the symptoms, and should be advised accordingly.

*Use in pregnancy:* Intensified control in the treatment of pregnant insulin-dependent diabetics is recommended. Insulin requirements usually fall in the first trimester and increase during the second and third trimester. Insulin does not pass the placental barrier.

Concomitant use of other drugs may influence insulin requirements. The following substances may enhance the hypoglycaemic effect of insulin: alcohol, non-selective beta-adrenergic blocking agents, monoamine oxidase inhibitors (MAOI), ACE inhibitors, salicylate, anabolic steroids. Other drugs may increase insulin requirements: oral contraceptives, thyroid hormones, corticosteroids, thiazides and sympathomimetics. Beta-adrenergic blocking agents may blur the symptoms of hypoglycaemia. Alcohol may intensify and prolong the hypoglycaemic effect of insulin. Diabetic patients treated with other drugs than insulin should discuss possible interactions with the prescribing physician.

*Side-effects:* At initiation of insulin therapy, oedema and refraction anomalies may occur; these are usually transitory. The same applies to local hypersensitivity reactions (swelling and itching at the injection site) which usually disappear during continued treatment.

Persistent allergies to human insulin are very rare and are mostly due to cross-reacting antibodies to animal insulins. Lipo-dystrophy at injection sites is also rare and should be prevented by constantly changing injection sites.

*Overdosage:* Overdosage causes hypoglycaemia, symptoms are variable but may include confusion, palpitations, sweating, malaise, and loss of consciousness.

In the event of an overdose, glucose should be given orally if the patient is conscious. Where the patient is unconscious an intra-muscular, subcutaneous or intravenous injection of glucagon should be given and oral carbohydrate administered when the patient responds. Alternatively intravenous glucose may be administered; it must be given if there is no response to glucagon.

If severe hypoglycaemia is not treated it can cause temporary or permanent brain damage and death.

**Pharmaceutical precautions** The Penfill cartridge preparations should be stored between 2 and 8°C, and should not be allowed to freeze. Cartridges in use or carried as a spare may be kept at ambient temperature (e.g. in the pocket or handbag) for up to one month, but should not be exposed to excessive heat or sunlight. Cartridges in use must not be stored in a refrigerator.

**Legal category** P.

**Package quantities** Pack of 5×1.5 ml cartridges.

**Further information** Nil.

**Product licence numbers**

| | |
|---|---|
| Human Actrapid Penfill | 4668/0024 |
| Human Insulatard Penfill | 4668/0019 |
| Human Mixtard 10 Penfill | 4668/0032 |
| Human Mixtard 20 Penfill | 4668/0033 |
| Human Mixtard 30 Penfill | 4668/0020 |
| Human Mixtard 40 Penfill | 4668/0034 |
| Human Mixtard 50 Penfill | 4668/0035 |

*Product licence holder:* Novo Nordisk A/S.

# HUMAN ACTRAPID*
# HUMAN MONOTARD*
# HUMAN INSULATARD* GE
# HUMAN MIXTARD* 30 GE
# HUMAN ULTRATARD*

*Human Insulatard ge and Human Mixtard 30 ge were formerly named Human Protaphane and Human Actraphane 30/70; they are not identical to the products Human Insulatard and Human Mixtard 30/70 which contained human insulin (emp) and which were discontinued in April 1995.*

**Presentation** Human Actrapid (Insulin Injection) is a clear neutral solution of human insulin (pyr), containing glycerol, and m-cresol as added preservative.

*Human Monotard* (Insulin Zinc Suspension) is a neutral suspension of amorphous (30%) and crystalline (70%) human insulin (pyr).

*Human Insulatard ge* (Isophane Insulin Injection) is a neutral suspension of isophane human insulin (pyr).

*Human Mixtard 30 ge* (Biphasic Isophane Insulin Injection) is a neutral suspension of human insulin (pyr), consisting of soluble human insulin and isophane human insulin in the ratio 3:7.

*Human Ultratard* (Insulin Zinc Suspension Crystalline) is a neutral suspension of crystalline human insulin (pyr).

Human Monotard and Human Ultratard contain sodium chloride, sodium acetate, zinc as retarding agent and methyl parahydroxybenzoate as added preservative. Human Insulatard ge and Human Mixtard 30 ge contain glycerol, sodium phosphate, protamine sulphate as retarding agent, and m-cresol and phenol as added preservative. When shaken, the suspensions appear white and cloudy.

Each preparation is available in a strength of 100 iu/ml.

**Uses** The treatment of insulin-requiring diabetics.

**Dosage and administration**
*Adults and children:* The dosage is determined by the physician according to the needs of the patient.

Human Actrapid may be given by subcutaneous, intramuscular or intravenous injection. When injected subcutaneously it has a duration of action of some ½ to 8 hours and its maximum effect is exerted between 1 and 3 hours after injection.

The suspensions may be given by subcutaneous or intramuscular injection. The vial should be gently shaken before use to ensure that the insulin is uniformly distributed throughout the liquid. The dose should then be immediately drawn into the syringe and injected.

Human Monotard and Human Insulatard ge may be used in once, or more commonly, twice daily injection regimens. When injected subcutaneously, Human Monotard has a duration of action of some 2½ to 24 hours and its maximum effect is exerted between 7 and 15 hours after injection, and Human Insulatard ge has a duration of action of some 1½ to 24 hours and its maximum effect is exerted between 4 and 12 hours after injection.

Human Mixtard 30 ge may be given once, or more commonly, twice daily, especially when a strong initial effect is desired. When injected subcutaneously it has a duration of action of some ½ to 24 hours and its maximum effect is exerted between 2 and 8 hours after injection.

Human Ultratard is usually given as a once daily insulin but may also be given twice daily if required. It is often used as a basal insulin in multiple injection regimens. Human Ultratard may be used as a once daily injection (if necessary with the addition of rapid acting insulin) in maturity onset diabetes when diet or oral hypoglycaemic drugs fail to produce good control. When injected subcutaneously Human Ultratard has a duration of action of some 4 to 28 hours and its maximum effect is exerted between 8 and 24 hours after injection.

The suspensions may be mixed in the syringe with Human Actrapid to intensify the initial effect. The Human Actrapid should be drawn into the syringe first and the injection given immediately after mixing. When injected subcutaneously, injection of Human Actrapid into the abdominal wall ensures a faster absorption than from other regions of the body. The thigh is the recommended site for subcutaneous injection of Human Insulatard ge, Human Monotard, or Human Ultratard, the abdominal wall or thigh for subcutaneous injection of Human Mixtard 30 ge. Injection into a lifted skin fold minimises the risk of intramuscular injection.

*Infusion pumps:* Due to the risk of precipitation in some pump catheters, Human Actrapid is not recommended for use in ambulatory insulin infusion pumps.

The suspensions must not be used in insulin infusion pumps.

*Use in the elderly:* There are no precautions concerning the use of insulin which are specific to the elderly diabetic. However the injection procedure may be difficult for the infirm, the poorly sighted, or the confused patient, and the simplest regimen consistent with keeping the patient symptom-free should be considered.

**Contra-indications, warnings, etc**
*Contra-indications:* Insulin is contra-indicated in hypoglycaemia.

*Precautions:* Owing to their strong early effect, injections of Human Actrapid or Human Mixtard 30 ge should be followed by a meal within 30 minutes of administration.

The use of dosages which are inadequate or discontinuation of treatment, especially in insulin-dependent diabetics, may lead to hyperglycaemia and diabetic ketoacidosis; conditions which are potentially lethal.

When patients are transferred from other insulins to Human Monocomponent insulin the change should be made according to the following general guidelines:

For patients currently controlled on Human Monocomponent, porcine monocomponent, or other highly purified human or porcine insulin preparation, no dosage change is anticipated other than the routine

adjustments made in order to maintain stable diabetic control.

Patients currently stabilised on mixed species or bovine insulin may require a dosage adjustment dependent upon dosage, purity, species, and formulation of the insulin preparation(s) currently administered. Variations in glycaemic control may occur and adjustment in therapy should be made under the guidance of a physician.

A few patients have reported that after being transferred to human insulin, the early warning symptoms for hypoglycaemia were less pronounced than they were with animal source insulin.

Patients whose blood glucose control is greatly improved, e.g. by intensified insulin therapy, may experience a change in their usual warning symptoms of hypoglycaemia, and possibly lose some or all of the symptoms, and should be advised accordingly.

*Use in pregnancy:* Intensified control in the treatment of pregnant insulin dependent diabetics is recommended. Insulin requirements usually fall in the first trimester and increase during the second and third trimester. Insulin does not pass the placental barrier.

Concomitant use of other drugs may influence insulin requirements. The following substances may enhance the hypoglycaemic effect of insulin: alcohol, non-selective beta-adrenergic blocking agents, monoamine oxidase inhibitors (MAOI), ACE inhibitors, salicylate, anabolic steroids. Other drugs may increase insulin requirements: oral contraceptives, thyroid hormones, corticosteroids, thiazides and sympathomimetics. Beta-adrenergic blocking agents may blur the symptoms of hypoglycaemia. Alcohol may intensify and prolong the hypoglycaemic effect of insulin. Diabetic patients treated with other drugs than insulin should discuss possible interactions with the prescribing physician.

*Side-effects:* At initiation of insulin therapy, oedema and refraction anomalies may occur; these are usually transitory. The same applies to local hypersensitivity reactions (swelling and itching at the injection site) which usually disappear during continued treatment.

Persistent allergies to human insulin are very rare and are mostly due to cross-reacting antibodies to animal insulins. Lipo-dystrophy at injection sites is also rare and should be prevented by constantly changing injection sites.

*Overdosage:* Overdosage causes hypoglycaemia, symptoms are variable but may include confusion, palpitations, sweating, malaise, and loss of consciousness.

In the event of an overdose, glucose should be given orally if the patient is conscious. Where the patient is unconscious an intra-muscular, subcutaneous or intravenous injection of glucagon should be given and oral carbohydrate administered when the patient responds. Alternatively intravenous glucose may be administered; it must be given if there is no response to glucagon.

If severe hypoglycaemia is not treated it can cause temporary or permanent brain damage and death.

**Pharmaceutical precautions** The human insulin preparations should be stored between 2° and 8°C. They should not be exposed to excessive heat or sunlight and should not be allowed to freeze. The vial in use may be kept at room temperature (max. 25°C) for up to four weeks.

**Legal category** P.

**Package quantities** 10 ml glass vials.

**Further information** Nil.

**Product licence numbers**

| | |
|---|---|
| Human Actrapid | 4668/0025 |
| Human Monotard | 4668/0021 |
| Human Insulatard ge | 4668/0018 |
| Human Mixtard 30 ge | 4668/0023 |
| Human Ultratard | 4668/0022 |

*Product licence holder:* Novo Nordisk A/S.

# HUMAN MIXTARD* 50

**Qualitative and quantitative composition** Biphasic Isophane Insulin Injection 50/50. *Active ingredient:* Insulin Human, Biosynthetic (pyr); 50% as soluble insulin, 50% as isophane insulin, 100 iu/ml.

**Pharmaceutical form** Sterile suspension for injection (subcutaneously).

**Clinical particulars**
*Therapeutic indications:* Treatment of diabetes mellitus.

*Posology and method of administration:* Dosage is individual and determined by the physician in accordance with the needs of the patient. Concomitant disease, especially if the patient is febrile, usually increases insulin requirements. Blood glucose monitoring is recommended.

The preparation is administered subcutaneously

into the abdominal wall or the thigh. Each injection should be followed within 30 minutes by a meal containing carbohydrate. The physician determines whether one or several daily injections are necessary. Injection into a lifted skin fold minimises the risk of intramuscular injection.

*Contra-indications:* Insulin should never be given to patients with hypoglycaemia. Hypersensitivity to human insulin or to one of the excipients. Insulin suspensions must not be administered intravenously.

*Special warnings and special precautions for use:* The use of too low doses or discontinuation of treatment may lead to hyperglycaemia and diabetic keto-acidosis. These conditions are potentially lethal. For diabetic ketoacidosis treatment soluble insulin should be used. Transfer of patients to this human insulin may lead to change in glycaemic control; adjustments in therapy should be made under the guidance of a physician. The following general guidelines apply:

For patients currently controlled on human or porcine highly purified insulin, no dosage change is anticipated other than routine adjustments to maintain stable diabetic control.

Patients currently controlled on mixed species or bovine insulin may require adjustment of their insulin dosage dependent upon purity, species and formulation of their current insulin preparation(s).

A few patients have reported that after being transferred to human insulin the early warning symptoms for hypoglycaemia were less pronounced than experienced with animal source insulin.

Patients whose blood glucose control is greatly improved, e.g. by intensified insulin therapy, may experience a change in their usual warning symptoms of hypoglycaemia, and should be advised accordingly.

*Interaction with other medicaments and other forms of interaction:* Omission of a meal or unplanned, vigorous physical exercise may lead to hypoglycaemia, see *Overdose.*

Concomitant use of other drugs may influence insulin requirements.

The following substances may enhance the hypoglycaemic effect of insulin: monoamine oxidase inhibitors (MAOI), non-selective beta-blocking agents, ACE inhibitors, salicylate, alcohol, anabolic steroids.

Other drugs may decrease the effect: oral contraceptives, thiazides, corticosteroids, thyroid hormones and sympathomimetics.

Beta-blocking agents may mask the symptoms of hypoglycaemia. Alcohol may intensify and prolong the hypoglycaemic effect of insulin.

Diabetic patients treated with other drugs than insulin should discuss possible interactions with their prescribing physician.

*Pregnancy and lactation:* Insulin does not pass the placental barrier. Breast-feeding involves no risk for the baby.

Intensified control of pregnant insulin-dependent diabetic patients is recommended. Insulin requirements usually fall in the first trimester and increase during the second and third trimester.

*Effects on ability to drive and use machines:* The ability to drive or use machines can be impaired depending on the tendency to experience hypoglycaemia.

*Undesirable effects:* Oedema and refraction anomalies may occur at initiation of insulin therapy. These conditions are usually of transitory nature. The same applies to local hypersensitivity reactions (redness, swelling and itching at the injection site), which usually disappear during continued treatment. Persistent allergic reactions and lipoatrophy rarely occur when using this human insulin. Lipohypertrophy may occur as a consequence of too frequent injections into the same small area.

*Overdose:* Hypoglycaemia, accompanied by a variety of symptoms, is a common phenomenon with insulin treatment. Hypoglycaemia is potentially lethal. In the event of an overdose causing hypoglycaemia, sugar or food rich in carbohydrate should be given immediately if the patient is conscious. If the patient is unconscious, a subcutaneous, intramuscular or intravenous injection of glucagon (0.5–1 mg) may be given, followed by oral carbohydrate when the patient regains consciousness. An alternative to glucagon is intravenous glucose; it must be given if there is no response to glucagon within 10–15 minutes.

### Pharmacological properties
*Pharmacodynamic properties:* The blood glucose lowering effect of insulin occurs when the molecules facilitate the uptake of glucose by binding to insulin receptors on muscle and fat cells – and simultaneously inhibit the output of glucose from the liver.

*Pharmacokinetic properties:* Insulin in the blood stream has a half-life of only a few minutes. Consequently, the time-action profile of an insulin preparation is determined solely by its absorption characteristics. This process is influenced by several factors, which is why considerable intra- and inter-

patient variations are seen. An approximate action profile following s.c. administration indicates:

Onset: ½ hour
Maximum: 2–8 hours
Duration: up to 24 hours

*Preclinical safety data:* Not applicable.

### Pharmaceutical particulars
*List of excipients:* Zinc chloride; protamine sulphate; glycerol; disodium phosphate dihydrate; m-cresol; phenol; water for injection; stabilising agent; protracting principle; isotonic agent; buffering agent; preservative; preservative.

*Incompatibilities:* Insulin is compatible with simple infusion fluids, however, other drugs added to the fluid together with insulin may cause degradation of the insulin, e.g. if the drugs contain substances such as thiols or sulphites.

It is therefore recommended not to mix insulin with other drugs. Only soluble insulin (i.e. not insulin suspensions) should be added to infusion fluids. An unpredictable amount of insulin will be absorbed to the infusion material. Monitoring of the patient's blood glucose during infusion is therefore recommended.

*Shelf life:* 30 months at 2°C to 8°C

*Special precautions for storage:* Insulin preparations should be stored between 2°C and 8°C, not near a freezing compartment. Insulin which has been frozen must not be used. Insulin should be protected from excessive heat or sunlight. Insulin vials can be kept at room temperature for up to 6 weeks (max. 25°C).

*Nature and contents of container:* 10 ml vial made of glass, closed with a rubber disc. Packed in a carton.

*Instructions for use/handling:* Immediately before use, the vial should be turned upside down several times in order to resuspend the insulin crystals. The liquid should appear uniformly white and cloudy. Each carton contains a patient insert with instructions for use.

**Marketing authorisation number** 3132/0120.

**Date of approval/revision of SPC** August 1996.

**Legal category** P.

## HUMAN VELOSULIN*
### Presentation
*Human Velosulin* (Insulin Injection) is a clear neutral solution of highly purified human insulin (emp).

Human Velosulin is available in 10 ml vials containing 100 iu/ml. It is buffered with Sodium Phosphate PhEur 2.4 mg/ml and is preserved with m-cresol 3.0 mg/ml.

The vials are fitted with tamper evident disposable plastic caps as a security safeguard. No attempt should be made to refit the caps after removal.

**Uses** For the treatment of insulin-requiring diabetic patients.

Human Velosulin has a rapid onset and a short duration of action, making it particularly suitable for the treatment of diabetic coma and pre-coma.

**Dosage and administration** The dosage of insulin is determined by the physician according to the needs of the patient.

Human Velosulin may be given by subcutaneous, intramuscular or intravenous injection or infusion.

Human Velosulin may be mixed with Human Mixtard 30 ge and Human Insulatard ge in all proportions without changing the characteristic effect of any of the types of insulin.

Human Velosulin should not be mixed with insulin zinc suspensions, since the phosphate buffer can interact with the zinc in the suspensions and alter the timing of action of the mixture in an unpredictable way.

The injection site should be changed regularly according to a set routine.

*Subcutaneous injection:* Human Velosulin has an onset of action of approximately half an hour after subcutaneous injection with a duration of about 8 hours, the maximum effect being exerted between 1 and 3 hours after injection.

*Intramuscular injection:* Following intramuscular injection, the onset of action is more rapid, while the overall duration of action is shorter, provided the injection site is well perfused muscle.

*Use in pregnancy and lactation:* It is important to maintain continuous good glycaemic control during conception and throughout pregnancy. In insulin-requiring pregnant diabetic patients, insulin requirements generally fall during the first trimester and increase during the second and third trimesters.

*Use in the elderly:* Clearance rates may be reduced in the elderly due to declining renal function. Insulin may therefore have a more prolonged action. Dose requirements should be regularly reviewed.

### Contra-indications, warnings, etc
*Contra-indications:* Insulin is contra-indicated in hypoglycaemia.

*Precautions:* Variations in lifestyle and other factors, e.g. infection and pregnancy, can affect insulin requirements.

The use of dosages which are inadequate or discontinuation of treatment, especially in insulin-dependent diabetics, may lead to hyperglycaemia and diabetic ketoacidosis; conditions which are potentially lethal.

Some patients previously treated with insulin of beef or pork origin may require a dosage adjustment on transfer to highly purified human insulin (emp). This is more likely in patients previously treated with beef or mixed beef/pork insulin.

Hypoglycaemia may be precipitated by some drugs including the following: aspirin; sulphonylureas and agents affecting them; and certain steroids. Hypoglycaemia may also occur following excessive physical activity, alcohol intake or reduced food intake.

Hyperglycaemia can be enhanced by drugs including the following: triiodothyronine; thyroxine; various natural and synthetic steroids, including some oral contraceptives; diuretics including thiazides; and cyclophosphamide.

Certain beta-blockers, especially propranolol, may affect insulin requirements and mask the signs of hypoglycaemia, mediated by the sympathetic nervous system. Monoamine oxidase inhibitors (MAOI) may potentiate the action of insulin.

A few patients have reported that after being transferred to human insulin, their early warning symptoms for hypoglycaemia were less pronounced than they had been with beef or porcine insulin. Patients should be alerted to this possibility on being transferred to human insulin.

Patients whose blood glucose control is greatly improved, e.g. by intensified insulin therapy, may experience a change in their usual warning symptoms of hypoglycaemia, and possibly lose some or all of the symptoms, and should be advised accordingly.

*Side- and adverse effects:* The most important side-effect is hypoglycaemia. Reduction of hyperglycaemia in newly diagnosed diabetic patients may alter visual refraction.

Insulin, like any other injected protein is potentially immunogenic. This may or may not have clinical implications. Local reactions at the injection site may include transient erythema, induration, urticaria and oedema. The incidence is minimal with highly purified human insulin (emp) and these usually resolve with continuing insulin usage. True generalised hypersensitivity reactions approaching anaphylaxis are very rare.

Clinical evidence suggests that highly purified human insulin (emp) is unlikely to cause localised lipodystrophy. However, at present, this possibility cannot be totally excluded.

*Toxicity and treatment of overdosage:* The symptoms and signs of hypoglycaemia depend on the patient's clinical state and on the rate and extent of the fall in blood glucose levels.

If possible, glucose, sucrose, or rapidly absorbable carbohydrate should be taken by mouth. Failing this, hypoglycaemia should be reversed as rapidly as possible by intravenous injection of glucose 50% solution. Alternative emergency treatments include the subcutaneous injection of up to 1 ml of adrenaline solution 1:1000 or the subcutaneous, intramuscular or intravenous injection of lyophilised glucagon 0.5–1.0 mg (1 unit = 1.0 mg). Both adrenaline and glucagon injections mobilise hepatic glycogen, but this effect is short lived and must be supplemented by freely available carbohydrate as soon as possible.

If severe hypoglycaemia is not treated it can cause temporary or permanent brain damage and death.

**Pharmaceutical precautions** Store at a temperature between 2 and 8°C, protected from sunlight. The shelf life is 3 years from the date of manufacture. Insulin which has been frozen should not be used.

**Legal category** P.

**Package quantities** 10 ml glass vials in individual cartons.

**Further information** Nil.

**Product licence number** 3132/0031.

## PORK VELOSULIN*
## PORK INSULATARD*
## PORK MIXTARD* 30

**Presentation** Pork Velosulin (Insulin Injection) is a clear neutral solution of highly purified pork insulin.

Pork Insulatard (Isophane Insulin Injection [NPH]) is a cloudy neutral suspension of highly purified microcrystalline pork insulin.

Pork Mixtard 30 (Biphasic Isophane Insulin Injection)

is a cloudy neutral suspension of highly purified pork insulin comprising 30% Neutral Insulin in solution and 70% Isophane Insulin in microcrystalline form.

All the above insulins are available in 100 units/ml strength and are buffered with Sodium Phosphate PhEur 2.4 mg/ml. Pork Velosulin is preserved with m-Cresol 3 mg/ml and Pork Insulatard and Pork Mixtard 30 are preserved with m-Cresol 1.5 mg/ml and Phenol 0.6 mg/ml.

The vials are fitted with tamper-evident disposable plastic caps as a security safeguard. No attempt should be made to refit the caps after removal.

**Uses** The treatment of insulin-requiring diabetic patients. Pork Velosulin has a rapid onset and a short duration of action making it particularly suitable for the treatment of diabetic coma and pre-coma.

**Dosage and administration** The dosage of insulin is determined by the physician according to the needs of the patient. Pork Velosulin, Pork Insulatard and Pork Mixtard 30 may be mixed in all proportions without changing the characteristic effect of any of the types of insulin.

Pork Velosulin may be given by subcutaneous, intramuscular or intravenous injection or infusion. It has an onset of action of approximately 30 minutes after subcutaneous injection with duration of about 8 hours, the maximum effect being 1 to 3 hours after injection.

Pork Insulatard and Pork Mixtard 30 should be well mixed by gently inverting the vial several times before being given by subcutaneous or intramuscular injection. Pork Insulatard and Pork Mixtard 30 should not be given intravenously.

Pork Insulatard has an onset of action of approximately 1½ hours after subcutaneous injection with an overall duration of action which may extend to 24 hours, the maximum effect occurring 4 to 12 hours after injection.

Pork Mixtard 30 has a duration of action of some ½ to 24 hours after subcutaneous injection, the maximum effect occurring 4 to 8 hours after injection.

Onset of action is more rapid and overall duration of action shorter following intramuscular injection than with the subcutaneous route assuming adequate vascular perfusion.

*Use in pregnancy and lactation:* It is essential to maintain continuous good glycaemic control throughout pregnancy. In the insulin-treated (gestational or insulin-dependent) pregnant diabetic patient, the insulin requirements fall during the first trimester and increase during the second and third trimesters.

*Use in the elderly:* Clearance rates may be reduced in the elderly due to falling renal function. Insulin may therefore have a more prolonged action. Dose requirements should be regularly reviewed.

**Contra-indications, warnings, etc**
*Contra-indications:* Insulin is contra-indicated in hypoglycaemia.
*Precautions:* Variations in lifestyle and other factors, eg. infection and pregnancy, can affect insulin requirements.

The use of dosages which are inadequate or discontinuation of treatment, especially in insulin-dependent diabetics, may lead to hyperglycaemia and diabetic ketoacidosis; conditions which are potentially lethal.

Some patients previously treated with insulin of beef or mixed beef/pork origin may require a dosage adjustment on transfer to highly purified pork insulin.

Hypoglycaemia can be enhanced by drugs including the following: aspirin; sulphonylureas and agents affecting them; certain steroids.

Hyperglycaemia can be enhanced by drugs including the following: triiodothyronine; thyroxine; various natural and synthetic steroids, including some oral contraceptives; diuretics, including thiazides; cyclophosphamide.

Certain beta-blockers, especially propranolol, may affect insulin requirements and mask the signs of hypoglycaemia mediated by the sympathetic nervous system.

Monoamine oxidase inhibitors (MAOI) may potentiate the action of insulin.

Patients whose blood glucose control is greatly improved, e.g. by intensified insulin therapy, may experience a change in their usual warning symptoms of hypoglycaemia, and possibly lose some or all of the symptoms, and should be advised accordingly.

*Side-and adverse effects:* The most important side-effect is hypoglycaemia. Reduction of hyperglycaemia in newly diagnosed diabetics may alter visual refraction.

Insulin and protamine, like any other injected proteins, are potentially immunogenic. This may or may not have clinical implications. Local reactions at the injection site may include transient erythema, induration, urticaria and oedema. The incidence is minimal with highly purified pork insulin. These usually resolve with continuing usage of insulin. True

generalised hypersensitivity reactions approaching anaphylaxis are very rare.

Clinical evidence suggests that highly purified pork insulins are unlikely to cause localised lipodystrophies, however, at present, this possibility cannot be totally excluded.

*Toxicity and treatment of overdosage:* The symptoms and signs of hypoglycaemia depend on the patient's clinical state and on the rate and extent of the fall in blood glucose levels.

If possible, glucose, sucrose, or rapidly absorbable carbohydrate should be taken by mouth. Failing this, hypoglycaemia should be reversed as rapidly as possible by intravenous injection of glucose 50% solution. Alternative emergency treatments include the subcutaneous injection of up to 1 ml of adrenaline solution 1:1000 or the subcutaneous, intramuscular or intravenous injection of lyophilised glucagon 0.5–1.0 mg (1 unit=1.0 mg). Both adrenaline and glucagon injections mobilise hepatic glycogen, but the effect is short lived and must be supplemented by freely available carbohydrate as soon as possible.

If severe hypoglycaemia is not treated it can cause temporary or permanent brain damage and death.

**Pharmaceutical precautions** The highly purified pork insulin preparations should be stored between 2 and 8°C, protected from sunlight. Under these storage conditions they have a shelf life of 3 years from date of manufacture. Insulin which has been frozen should not be used.

**Legal category** P.

**Package quantities** 10 ml glass vials.

**Further information** Nil.

**Product licence numbers**

| | |
|---|---|
| Pork Velosulin | 3132/0019 |
| Pork Insulatard | 3132/0018 |
| Pork Mixtard 30 | 3132/0021 |

## LENTARD* MC

**Presentation** Lentard MC (Insulin Zinc Suspension BP) is a neutral suspension of amorphous porcine MC insulin (30%) and crystalline bovine MC insulin (70%), containing sodium chloride, sodium acetate, zinc as retarding agent, and methyl parahydroxybenzoate as added preservative.

When shaken Lentard MC appears white and cloudy. It is available in a strength of 100 iu/ml.

**Uses** The treatment of insulin-requiring diabetic patients.

**Dosage and administration** *Adults and children:* The dosage of insulin is determined by the physician according to the needs of the patient.

Lentard MC may be given by subcutaneous or intramuscular injection. The vial should be gently shaken before use to ensure that the insulin is uniformly distributed throughout the liquid. The dose should then be immediately drawn into the syringe and injected.

Lentard MC has a duration of action of some 2½ to 24 hours and its maximum effect is exerted between 7 and 15 hours after injection. It may be given once or twice daily.

Lentard MC may be mixed in the syringe with Human Actrapid to intensify the initial effect. The insulin mixture should be injected immediately. When longer acting insulins are mixed with short acting soluble insulins, the short acting insulin should be drawn into the syringe first.

*Infusion pumps:* Insulin suspensions must not be used in insulin infusion pumps.

*Use in pregnancy:* It is essential to maintain continuous good control of the insulin requiring diabetic patient throughout pregnancy. In the insulin treated (gestational or insulin dependent) pregnant diabetic patient the insulin requirements usually fall in the first trimester and increase during the second and third trimester.

*Use in the elderly:* There are no precautions concerning the use of insulin which are specific to the elderly diabetic. However the injection procedure may be difficult for the infirm, the poorly sighted, or the confused patient, and the simplest regimen consistent with keeping the patient symptom-free should be considered.

**Contra-indications, warnings, etc**
*Contra-indications:* Insulin is contra-indicated in hypoglycaemia.

*Precautions:* The use of dosages which are inadequate or discontinuation of treatment, especially in insulin-dependent diabetics, may lead to hyperglycaemia and diabetic ketoacidosis; conditions which are potentially lethal.

Patients transferred from conventional (predominantly bovine) insulins may require a smaller dosage.

The dosage reduction may occur immediately after transfer or gradually over a period of weeks or months. In order to reduce the risk of hypoglycaemia, the patient and the physician should be aware of the possibility that the insulin requirement may be reduced.

If the daily insulin dosage is below 40 iu the risk is considered minimal. However, when higher dosages are required, stricter supervision of the patient is necessary and possibly a dosage reduction should be made initially on transfer. Insulin resistant patients receiving over 100 units daily should be referred to hospital for transfer.

Patients whose blood glucose control is greatly improved, e.g. by intensified insulin therapy, may experience a change in their usual warning symptoms of hypoglycaemia, and possibly lose some or all of the symptoms, and should be advised accordingly.

The addition of corticosteroids, oral contraceptives or thyroid hormone replacement therapy may lead to an increase in insulin requirements. The addition of a beta-adrenergic blocking agent or a monoamine oxidase inhibitor (MAOI), may also necessitate an adjustment of insulin dosage.

*Side-effects:* Lipodystrophy, insulin resistance and hypersensitivity reactions have been associated with insulin therapy, but the incidence and severity of these unwanted effects is minimal with the MC insulins.

Severe local or generalised allergic reactions require immediate treatment and, in some cases, desensitisation may be necessary.

*Overdosage:* Overdosage causes hypoglycaemia, symptoms are variable but may include confusion, palpitations, sweating, malaise and loss of consciousness. In the event of an overdose, glucose should be given orally if the patient is conscious. Where the patient is unconscious, an intramuscular, subcutaneous or intravenous injection of glucagon should be given and oral carbohydrate administered when the patient responds. Alternatively, intravenous glucose may be administered; it must be given if there is no response to glucagon.

If severe hypoglycaemia is not treated it can cause temporary or permanent brain damage and death.

**Pharmaceutical precautions** Lentard MC should be stored between 2°C and 8°C. It should not be exposed to excessive heat or sunlight, neither should they be frozen. The vial in use may be kept at room temperature (max. 25°C) for one month.

**Legal category** P.

**Package quantities** 10 ml glass vials.

**Further information** Nil.

**Product licence numbers** Lentard MC 3132/0090.

## GLUCAGEN* KIT 1 mg ▼
## GLUCAGEN* 1 mg ▼

**Qualitative and quantitative composition** GlucaGen Kit 1 mg consists of a vial containing 1 mg (1 iu) glucagon (rys) and a pre-filled syringe containing 1 ml Water for Injections.

GlucaGen 1 mg consists of a vial containing 1 mg (1 iu) glucagon (rys) and a vial containing 1 ml Water for Injections.

**Pharmaceutical form** Powder for injection with accompanying diluent for reconstitution.

**Clinical particulars**
*Therapeutic indications:*

(i) The treatment of acute hypoglycaemic reactions which may occur in the management of diabetic patients receiving insulin or oral hypoglycaemic agents.

(ii) As a motility inhibitor in examinations of the gastro-intestinal tract by radiography or endoscopy.

*Posology and method of administration:* The freeze-dried glucagon must be dissolved in the accompanying diluent before use. The reconstituted solution may be administered by intravenous, intramuscular or subcutaneous injection.

*Adults and children:*

(i) Treatment of acute hypoglycaemic reactions: Give 0.5 to 1 mg (20 micrograms/kg) by subcutaneous, intramuscular or intravenous injection. If the patient does not respond within 10 minutes, intravenous glucose must be given. When the patient responds, administer oral carbohydrate to restore the liver glycogen and prevent secondary hypoglycaemia.

(ii) Radiography and endoscopy of the gastro-intestinal tract: Doses range from 0.2 mg–2 mg depending on the diagnostic technique used and the rate of administration. The usual diagnostic dose for relaxation of the stomach, duodenal bulb, duodenum and small bowel is 0.2–0.5 mg given intravenously or 1 mg given intramuscularly; the usual dose to relax the colon is 0.5–0.75 mg intravenously or 1–2 mg intramuscularly.

*Contra-indications:* Hypersensitivity to glucagon or one of the excipients.

Glucagon is contra-indicated in patients with known or suspected phaeochromocytoma, insulinoma or glucagonoma.

The presence of fibril formation (viscous appearance) or solid particles in the solution is a contra-indication to its use at any time.

*Special warnings and special precautions for use:* Caution should be observed if GlucaGen is used in diabetic patients as an adjunct in radiography or endoscopy of the gastro-intestinal tract.

*Interaction with other medicaments and other forms of interaction:* Interactions of clinical significance between GlucaGen and drugs other than insulin have not been reported in the literature when GlucaGen is used in the approved indications.

It should be borne in mind that glucagon reacts antagonistically towards insulin.

*Pregnancy and lactation:* Glucagon does not cross the placental barrier. Experience of the use of glucagon during pregnancy is limited to the treatment of hypoglycaemia in a small number of pregnant diabetics; in this group all pregnancies were completed successfully and there was no evidence of harmful effects on the infants.

*Effects on ability to drive and use machines:* GlucaGen is not known to produce any effect on the ability to drive and to operate machines.

*Undesirable effects:* Glucagon has only few and minimal side effects consisting mainly of nausea and vomiting, especially when the dose is more than 1 mg.

Since glucagon is a protein there is a theoretical possibility of hypersensitivity.

*Overdose:* Adverse effects of overdose have not been reported.

### Pharmacological properties

*Pharmacodynamic properties:* Glucagon is a hyperglycaemic agent that rapidly mobilises hepatic glycogen which is released into the bloodstream as glucose.

Independent of its hyperglycaemic effect glucagon also has an inhibitory action on the tone and motility of the smooth muscles in the gastro-intestinal tract.

*Pharmacokinetic properties:* The metabolic clearance rate (MCR) of glucagon in humans is approximately 10 ml/kg/min. The MCR is independent of plasma glucagon concentrations over a wide concentration range. The liver and kidney are major sites of glucagon clearance, each organ contributing about 30% to the overall MCR. The plasma half-life of glucagon is approximately 5 minutes.

### Pharmaceutical particulars

*List of excipients:* Lactose, hydrochloric acid, water for injections.

*Incompatibilities:* Not applicable.

*Shelf life:* Prior to reconstitution, the shelf life is 36 months when stored at 2 to 8°C.

The reconstituted solution should be prepared immediately prior to use and any portion of the solution remaining after use should be discarded.

*Special precautions for storage:* Store in a refrigerator (2 to 8°C). Packs carried for use may be kept at ambient temperature (max 25°C) for up to 18 months, provided the expiry date is not exceeded.

*Nature and contents of container:* Freeze dried powder: 2 ml glass vial closed with bromobutyl rubber plug-in and aluminium cap.

Diluent: Pre-filled syringe (GlucaGen Kit 1 mg) or vial (GlucaGen 1 mg) containing 1 ml Water for Injections.

The vial closures are covered with a tamper-evident plastic snap-off cap.

*Instructions for use/handling:* The freeze-dried powder must be reconstituted with the accompanying diluent (Water for Injections) before use; a solution containing 1 mg/ml glucagon is produced. Each carton contains a patient information leaflet with instructions for reconstitution.

GlucaGen 1 mg is suitable for hospital use only.

**Marketing authorisation numbers**
GlucaGen 1 mg | 4668/0027
Diluent for GlucaGen 1 mg | 4668/0028
Water for Injections PhEur | 3132/0082

**Date of approval/revision of SPC** January 1997.

**Legal category** POM.

## KLIOFEM*

### Qualitative and quantitative composition
*Active ingredients:* Estradiol 2 mg and Norethisterone acetate 1 mg.

The tablets also contain lactose and maize starch, but do not contain clinically significant amounts of gluten.

**Pharmaceutical form** Film-coated tablet for oral administration.

### Clinical particulars
*Therapeutic indications:*
1. The treatment of symptoms due to oestrogen deficiency.
2. The prophylaxis of postmenopausal osteoporosis in women at risk of developing fractures.

At present there is no established screening programme for determining women at risk of developing osteoporotic fractures. Epidemiological studies suggest a number of individual risk factors which contribute to the development of postmenopausal osteoporosis. These include: early menopause, family history of osteoporosis, thin, small frame; cigarette use; recent prolonged systemic cortico-steroid use.

If several of these risk factors are present in a patient, consideration should be given to oestrogen replacement therapy.

Kliofem is for use in postmenopausal women with an intact uterus. In perimenopausal women treated with Kliofem the incidence of vaginal bleeding is unacceptably high and therefore therapy should not be initiated earlier than one year after the last natural menstrual period.

*Posology and method of administration*
*Dosage: Adults:* Menopausal symptoms and prophylaxis of osteoporosis.

Kliofem is administered orally, without chewing, one tablet daily without interruption, preferably at the same time each day.

*Prophylaxis of osteoporosis:* Hormone replacement therapy (HRT) has been found to be effective in the prevention of osteoporosis especially when started soon after the menopause and used for 5 years and probably up to 10 years or more. Treatment should ideally start as soon as possible after the onset of the menopause and certainly within 2 to 3 years, but benefit may also be obtained even if treatment is started at a later date. Protection appears to be effective for as long as treatment is continued. However, data beyond 10 years are limited. A careful re-appraisal of the risk-benefit ratio should be undertaken before treating for longer than 5 to 10 years.

Not intended for children or males.

*Use in the elderly:* There are no special dosage requirements.

*Administration:* In women not previously treated with HRT, treatment may be started on any convenient day. In women transferred from sequential HRT, treatment should probably be started at the end of the scheduled bleed.

During the first few months of Kliofem therapy, a high proportion of patients will experience bleeding or spotting. About half of women will become amenorrhoeic after 3–4 months' treatment with Kliofem. In a further group, bleeding or spotting may still occur infrequently but will remain acceptable. This means that after 3 months treatment the majority of women will derive benefit from Kliofem in terms of either having no bleeding at all or only light spotting. Some women may experience continued unacceptable bleeding and in these cases Kliofem should be discontinued. All patients on Kliofem require the routine follow up examinations which are recommended every 6 to 12 months (see below).

If, at any time, bleeding or spotting is unacceptable, Kliofem should be discontinued; if all bleeding subsides completely within 3 weeks of stopping Kliofem, then no further investigation is needed.

Bleeding after a period of amenorrhoea or heavy bleeding after a period of light bleeding may indicate poor compliance or concurrent antibiotics use. However, any doubt as to the cause of the bleeding is a reason for endometrial evaluation including some form of endometrial biopsy.

Before initiation of therapy it is recommended that the patient is fully informed of all likely benefits and potential risks. She should have a full physical and gynaecological examination, with special emphasis on blood pressure, breasts, abdominal and pelvic organs. Endometrial assessment should be carried out if indicated; this may be particularly relevant in patients who are, or who have been, previously treated with oestrogens unopposed by a progestogen. The patient should be asked to keep a diary of any spotting or bleeding that occurs during treatment with Kliofem. After the first 6 months, follow-up examinations are recommended every 6 to 12 months and should include examination of the diary.

Since progestogens are only administered to protect against hyperplastic changes of the endometrium patients without a uterus should be treated with an oestrogen-only preparation.

*Contra-indications:*
1. Known, suspected, or past history of cancer of the breast.

2. Known or suspected oestrogen-dependent neoplasia. Vaginal bleeding of unknown aetiology.
3. Known or suspected pregnancy.
4. Active thrombophlebitis or thromboembolic disorders. See also Warnings and precautions, number 4.
5. Acute or chronic liver disease or history of liver disease where the liver function tests have failed to return to normal.
6. Rotor's syndrome or Dubin-Johnson syndrome.
7. Severe cardiac or renal disease.
8. Allergy to one or more of the constituents.

*Special warnings and special precautions for use:*
1. In the female there is an increased risk of endometrial hyperplasia and carcinoma associated with unopposed oestrogen administered long term (for more than one year). However, the appropriate addition of a progestogen to an oestrogen regimen lowers this additional risk.
2. There has been concern about the possible risk of breast cancer in oestrogen-treated women. Although many studies have failed to disclose an increased incidence of breast cancer, some have shown a small increase upon prolonged therapy (e.g. 5 years or longer). It is not known whether concurrent progestogen use influences the risk of breast cancer in post-menopausal women taking HRT. Women on long-term therapy should have regular breast examinations, and should be instructed in self breast examination. Regular mammographic investigations should be conducted where considered appropriate.

There is a need for caution when prescribing oestrogens in women who have a history of, or known breast nodules or fibrocystic disease. Breast status should be closely monitored, supported by regular mammography.
3. Certain diseases may be made worse by hormone replacement therapy and patients with these conditions should be closely monitored. These include otosclerosis, multiple sclerosis, systemic lupus erythematosus, porphyria, melanoma, epilepsy, migraine and asthma. In addition, pre-existing uterine fibroids may increase in size during oestrogen therapy and symptoms associated with endometriosis may be exacerbated.
4. Studies to date do not indicate that there is an increased risk of thromboembolic disease, including stroke, myocardial infarction and thrombophlebitis, with oestrogen replacement therapy, at the current recommended low dosages in apparently normal women.

If an acute vascular thromboembolic event occurs coincidentally during therapy, current opinion suggests that treatment should be discontinued. However, there is no evidence that a past history of deep vein thrombosis, pulmonary embolism, stroke, or myocardial infarction, not associated with recognised risk factors such as prolonged immobilisation or surgery (particularly pelvic), should be a contra-indication to hormone replacement therapy, but in the absence of sufficient data, Kliofem should be used with caution in these patients.
5. Consideration should be given to discontinuing treatment at least four weeks prior to surgery or during periods of prolonged immobilisation.
6. Oestrogens may cause fluid retention and, therefore, patients with cadiac or renal dysfunction should be carefully observed.
7. If jaundice, migraine-like headaches, visual disturbance, or a significant increase in blood pressure develop after initiating therapy, the medication should be discontinued while the cause is investigated.
8. Kliofem is not a contraceptive, neither will it restore fertility.
9. Most studies indicate that oestrogen replacement therapy has little effect on blood pressure and some indicate that oestrogen use may be associated with a small decrease in B.P. In addition, most studies on combined therapy, including Kliofem, indicate that the addition of a progestogen also has little effect on blood pressure. Rarely, idiosyncratic hypertension may occur.

However, when oestrogens are administered to hypertensive women, supervision is necessary and blood pressure should be monitored at regular intervals.
10. Diabetic patients should be carefully observed when initiating hormone replacement therapy, as worsening glucose tolerance may occur.
11. Changed oestrogen levels may affect certain endocrine and liver function tests.
12. It has been reported that there is an increase in the risk of surgically confirmed gall bladder disease in women receiving postmenopausal oestrogens.

*Interactions with other medicaments and other forms of interaction:* Drugs such as barbiturates, phenytoin, rifampicin and carbamazepine which induce the activity of microsomal drug metabolising enzymes may decrease the effectiveness of Kliofem.

*Pregnancy and lactation:* Kliofem is contra-indicated during pregnancy and lactation.

*Effects on ability to drive and use machinery:* No effects known.

*Undesirable effects:* The following side-effects have been reported with oestrogen/progestogen therapy:

1. Genitourinary system – breakthrough bleeding, spotting, change in menstrual flow, dysmenorrhoea, premenstrual-like syndrome, increase in size of uterine fibromyomata, vaginal candidiasis, change in cervical erosion and in degree of cervical secretion, cystitis-like syndrome.
2. Breasts – tenderness, enlargement, secretion.
3. Gastrointestinal – nausea, vomiting, abdominal cramps, bloating, cholestatic jaundice.
4. Skin – chloasma or melasma which may persist when drug is discontinued, erythema multiforme, erythema nodosum, haemorrhagic eruption, loss of scalp hair, hirsutism.
5. Eyes – steepening of corneal curvature, intolerance to contact lenses.
6. CNS – headaches, migraine, dizziness, mental depression, chorea.
7. Miscellaneous – increase or decrease in weight, reduced carbohydrate tolerance, aggravation of porphyria, oedema, change in libido, leg cramps.

*Overdose:* Overdosage may be manifested by nausea and vomiting. There is no specific antidote and treatment should be symptomatic.

**Pharmacological properties**

*Pharmacodynamic properties:* The oestrogen component of Kliofem substitutes for the loss of endogenous oestrogen production in postmenopausal women, whilst the progestogen component counteracts hyperstimulation of the endometrium. A regular shedding of the endometrium is not induced by Kliofem. Studies based on measurement of bone mineral content have shown that Kliofem is effective in the prevention of progressive bone loss following the menopause.

*Pharmacokinetic properties:* The micronised oestradiol in Kliofem is rapidly and efficiently absorbed from the gastrointestinal tract, maximum plasma concentration being reached after 2–4 hours. Oestrogens are partly bound to plasma proteins. Oestradiol is oxidised to oestrone which, in turn, is hydrated to oestriol; both transformations take place mainly in the liver. Oestrogens are excreted into the bile and then undergo reabsorption from the intestine. During this entero-hepatic circulation, degradation of the oestrogens occur. They are excreted in the urine (90–95%) as biologically inactive glucuronide and sulphate conjugates or in the faeces (5–10%) most conjugated.

Norethisterone acetate is rapidly absorbed and transformed to norethisterone, then metabolised and excreted as glucuronide and sulphate conjugates. About half the dose is recovered in the urine within 24 hours, the remainder being reduced to less than 1% of the dose within 5–6 days. Mean plasma half-life is 3–6 hours.

**Pharmaceutical particulars**

*List of excipients:* Lactose; maize starch; gelatin; talc; magnesium stearate; methyl hydroxypropyl cellulose (E464); titanium dioxide (E171); iron oxide (E172); propylene glycol; purified water.

*Incompatibilities:* None known.

*Shelf life:* 24 months.

*Special precautions for storage:* Store at room temperature; protect from light and moisture.

*Nature and contents of container:* Polypropylene/polystyrene calendar dial pack containing 28 tablets. Calendar dial packs (3×28 tablets) are contained within outer carton.

*Instructions for use/handling:* Each carton contains a patient information leaflet with instructions for use of the calendar dial pack.

**Marketing authorisation number** 3132/0080.

**Date of revision/approval of SPC** February 1995.

**Legal category** POM.

# NORDITROPIN*

**Qualitative and quantitative composition**

*Norditropin Vials and PenSet:* Active ingredient Somatropin 12 IU (4 mg) and 24 IU (8 mg) (biosynthetic human growth hormone).

Solvent contains 0.9% benzyl alcohol.

Inactive ingredients: Mannitol, glycine, sodium hydrogen carbonate.

**Pharmaceutical form** Powder for injection supplied with diluent.

Route of administration: Subcutaneous injection.

**Clinical particulars**

*Therapeutic indications*

*Children:* Growth failure due to growth hormone insufficiency. Turner syndrome. Growth retardation in prepubertal children due to chronic renal disease.

*Adults:* Growth hormone insufficiency with known hypothalamic-pituitary disease where there is evidence of deficiency in at least one other axis (prolactin excepted) or pronounced growth hormone deficiency demonstrated by two different dynamic growth hormone stimulation tests. Tests for growth hormone deficiency should be undertaken only after adequate replacement therapy has been instituted for deficiencies in any other axis. Patients with childhood onset growth hormone deficiency should be retested as adults and the deficiency should be confirmed by two dynamic tests.

*Posology and method of administration:* The dosage is individual, based on body weight or body surface area and must always be adjusted in accordance with the individual's response to therapy. Generally, daily subcutaneous administration in the evening is recommended. The injection site should be varied to prevent lipoatrophy.

*Generally recommended dosages:*

*Children*

*Growth hormone insufficiency:*
0.07–0.1 IU/kg (2–3 IU/m²/day)
Equal to: 0.02–0.03 mg/kg/day or 0.7–1.0 mg/m²/day

*Turner syndrome:*
0.14 IU/kg/day (4.3 IU/m²/day)
Equal to: 0.05 mg/kg/day or 1.4 mg/m²/day

*Chronic renal disease:*
0.14 IU/kg/day (4.3 IU/m²/day)
Equal to: 0.05 mg/kg/day or 1.4 mg/m²/day

*Replacement therapy in adults:* The dosage must be adjusted to the need of the individual patient. It is recommended to start treatment with a very low dose like 0.5 IU (0.17 mg) per day or not more than 0.02 IU/kg/day, equal to 0.007 mg/kg/day. The starting dosage may be increased step-wise up to 0.04 IU/kg/day, equal to 0.013/mg/kg/day over a period of one or two months, depending on the obtained treatment results. Insulin-like Growth Factor 1 (IGF-1) in serum should be used as guidance. Dose requirements decline with age.

| Daily dosage | IU/kg | mg/kg |
|---|---|---|
| Starting dose 0.5 IU (0.17 mg) not more than | 0.02 | 0.007 |
| Maximum maintenance dosage | 0.04 | 0.013 |

*Administration:* Patients should be reminded to wash their hands thoroughly with soap and water and/or disinfectant prior to mixing the dry powder and solvent. The solution should not be shaken vigorously at any time.

*Norditropin PenSet:* Norditropin PenSet 12 and 24 should be prescribed only for use with Nordiject 12 and Nordiject 24 pen injection devices respectively. Instructions for preparing the cartridge for use and for using Nordiject are provided within the respective packs. Patients should be advised to read these instructions very carefully.

*Norditropin 12 IU:* Norditropin 12 IU is reconstituted by adding 3 ml solvent to the dry powder for injection. Prior to administration the rubber seals of the vials should be wiped with antiseptic solution. The solvent is then drawn into a syringe and injected into the vial containing the dry powder whilst directing the stream against the glass wall of the vial. The powder is dissolved by inverting the vial several times, avoiding vigorous shaking.

*Contra-indications:* Norditropin should not be used where there is evidence of active tumour. Anti-tumour therapy should be completed prior to the institution of therapy. Norditropin should be discontinued if there is any evidence of recurrent tumour growth.

In children with chronic renal disease treatment with Norditropin should be discontinued at renal transplantation.

Treatment during pregnancy and lactation is not recommended (see *Pregnancy and lactation* section).

Hypersensitivity to Norditropin preparations.

*Special warnings and special precautions for use:* Patients treated with Norditropin should be regularly assessed by a specialist in child growth. Norditropin treatment should always be instigated by a physician with special knowledge of growth hormone insufficiency and its treatment. This is also true for the management of Turner syndrome and chronic renal disease.

The stimulation of skeletal growth in children can only be expected until the epiphysial discs are closed.

Data on final adult height following the use of Norditropin in children with Turner syndrome and chronic renal disease are not available.

The dosage in children with chronic renal disease is individual and must be adjusted according to the individual response to therapy. The growth disturbance should be clearly established before treatment by following the growth on optimal conservative treatment for a minimum of 1 year. Conservative management of uraemia should be maintained during therapy. Patients with chronic renal disease normally experience a decline in renal function. During Norditropin treatment renal function should be observed for an excessive decline or an increase in the glomerular filtration rate (which could be attributed to hyper filtration).

Somatropin has been found to influence carbohydrate metabolism and, therefore, patients should be observed for evidence of glucose intolerance.

A state of hypothyroidism may develop during growth hormone treatment. Since untreated hypothyroidism may interfere with the response to Norditropin, patients should have a periodic thyroid function test and should be treated with thyroid hormone when indicated.

Patients with growth hormone deficiency secondary to an intracranial lesion should be examined frequently for progression or recurrence of the underlying disease process.

Leukaemia has been reported in a small number of growth hormone deficient patients, some of whom have been treated with somatropin. Based on current evidence, it is unlikely that somatropin is associated with this risk.

Slipped capital femoral epiphysis may occur more frequently in patients with endocrine disorders. This may result in the development of a limp or complaints of hip or knee pain in patients treated with somatropin and parents should be alerted to this possibility.

In the event of severe or recurrent headache, visual problems, nausea and/or vomiting, a funduscopy for papilloedema is recommended. If papilloedema is confirmed, a diagnosis of benign intracranial hypertension should be considered and if appropriate the growth hormone treatment should be discontinued. At present there is insufficient evidence to guide clinical decision making in patients with resolved intracranial hypertension. If growth hormone treatment is restarted, careful monitoring for symptoms of intracranial hypertension is necessary.

Experience in patients above 60 years of age is lacking. Experience with prolonged treatment in adults is limited.

*Interaction with other medicaments and other forms of interaction:* Concomitant glucocorticoid therapy may inhibit the growth promoting effect of Norditropin.

*Pregnancy and lactation:* There is currently insufficient evidence of safety of human growth hormone therapy during pregnancy. Norditropin is, therefore, contraindicated during pregnancy. In the event of pregnancy occurring during treatment, Norditropin therapy should be discontinued.

The possibility that human growth hormone is secreted in breast milk cannot be discounted.

*Effect of ability to drive and use machines:* No effects.

*Undesirable effects:* Fluid retention with peripheral oedema may occur. It is normally transient and dependent on the dosage.

Formation of antibodies directed against somatropin has rarely been observed during Norditropin therapy. The titres and binding capacities of these antibodies have been very low and have not interfered with the growth response to Norditropin.

During treatment with Norditropin a few children developed transient local skin reactions. General reactions are very rarely seen.

Some rare cases of benign intracranial hypertension have been reported.

Rare cases of hypersensitivity to the preservative benzyl alcohol may occur.

*Overdose:* Acute overdosage could lead initially to hypoglycaemia and subsequently to hyperglycaemia. Long-term overdosage could result in signs and symptoms consistent with the known effects of human growth hormone excess.

**Pharmacological properties**

*Pharmacodynamic properties:* Norditropin contains somatropin, which is human growth hormone produced by recombinant DNA-technology. It is an anabolic peptide of 191 amino acids stabilised by two disulphide bridges with a molecular weight of approximately 22.000 Daltons. The major effect is stimulation of skeletal and somatic growth and in addition to Norditropin's growth promoting effect, it has also other metabolic effects. When growth hormone deficiency is treated a normalisation of body composition takes place resulting in an increase in lean body mass and a decrease in fat mass.

The lipolytic and protein sparing effects become particularly important during stress. Somatropin exerts most of its actions through insulin-like growth factors (IGF). IGF is produced in tissues throughout the body, the most important contribution coming from hepatic synthesis. More than 90% of IGF is bound to binding proteins (IGF-BP) of which IGF-BP-3 is the most important.

*Pharmacokinetic properties:* Following i.v. infusion of Norditropin (33 ng/kg/min for 3 hours) in nine growth hormone deficient patients, the following results were found. Serum half-life was 21.1±1.7 min, metabolic clearance rate was 2.33±0.58 ml/kg/min and the distribution space was 67.6±14.6 ml/kg.

*Preclinical safety data:* The toxicity of Norditropin has been tested in mice, rats and monkeys and no findings of toxicological relevance were revealed. Norditropin has also been tested for mutagenic potential and none of the tests showed any mutagenic properties of the product.

### Pharmaceutical particulars

*List of excipients:* Lyophilised powder contains Glycine BP, Sodium Hydrogen Carbonate PhEur and Mannitol PhEur. Solvent contains Benzyl Alcohol PhEur 9 mg/ml as preservative in Water for Injections PhEur.

*Incompatibilities:* None.

*Shelf life:*
*Norditropin 12 IU in vials:* Powder for injection: 2 years (2–8°C). Reconstituted powder for injection: 14 days (2–8°C).

*Norditropin PenSet 12 IU and 24 IU:* Powder for injection: 3 years (2–8°C). Reconstituted powder for injection: 14 days (2–8°C).

*Special precautions for storage:* Avoid freezing. Protect from light. Storage between 2°C and 8°C.

*Nature and contents of container*
*Norditropin vials and PenSet:*
(a) Powder for injection: Colourless vials of glass.
(b) Solvent: Colourless vials or cartridge vials of glass.

Vials with powder for injection and its respective solvent are packed together in a light cardboard carton.

The PenSet package contains mixing devices packed in a carton.

### Marketing authorisation numbers

| | |
|---|---|
| Norditropin PenSet 12 | 3132/0060 |
| Norditropin PenSet 24 | 3132/0061 |
| Norditropin 12 IU | 3132/0046 |
| Diluent for Norditropin PenSet | 3132/0062 |
| Norditropin Diluent | 3132/0065 |

**Dat of approval/revision of SPC** July 1997.

**Legal category** CD (Sch 4), POM.

## NOVOSEVEN* ▼

**Qualitative and quantitative composition** Recombinant Coagulation Factor VIIa. Human Factor VII was cloned and expressed in baby hamster kidney cells (BHK cells). Recombinant Factor VII is secreted from the BHK cells and is activated during the purification procedure. NovoSeven Recombinant Coagulation Factor VIIa is structurally very similar to plasma-derived activated Factor VII (Human).

Proposed INN: eptacog alfa (activated).
Solvent: Water for injections PhEur.

*Quantitative composition:* Recombinant Coagulation Factor VIIa (rFVIIa) 60 KIU/bottle (corresponds to 1.2 mg/bottle). Water for injections PhEur 2.2 ml.

Recombinant Coagulation Factor VIIa 120 KIU/bottle (corresponds to 2.4 mg/bottle). Water for injections PhEur 4.3 ml.

Recombinant Coagulation Factor VIIa 240 KIU/bottle (corresponds to 4.8 mg/bottle). Water for injections PhEur 8.5 ml.

Please note that the above units are international units, measured with reference to the first international standard of FVIIa 89/688. Thus, these units should not be mistaken for units of other coagulation factors including FVII. 1 KIU equals 1000 IU (International Units). After reconstitution with the appropriate volume of diluent each vial contains 30 KIU/ml (0.6 mg/ml).

**Pharmaceutical form** Recombinant Coagulation Factor VIIa is supplied as a powder for injections. After reconstitution with the supplied diluent (Water for injections PhEur 2.2 ml, 4.3 ml or 8.5 ml) NovoSeven is administered intravenously as a bolus injection.

### Clinical particulars

*Therapeutic indications:* Serious bleeding events and surgery in patients with inhibitors to coagulation factors (FVIII or FIX).

*Posology and method of administration*
*Dosage:*
*Serious bleeding episodes and surgery:* From 3–6 KIU (60–120 µg) per kg body weight per single dose given by intravenous bolus injection. Administration time is 2–5 minutes.

Dose intervals: 2–3 hours initially, then 4–12 hours.

*Serious bleeding episodes:* The dosage varies according to the type and severity of the haemorrhages. As a guideline, an initial dosage of 4.5 KIU (90 µg) per kg body weight is recommended. Dosing frequency should initially be every second hour until clinical improvement is observed. If continued therapy is indicated the dosage interval can then be increased to 3 hours for 1–2 days. Thereafter, the dosage interval can be increased successively to every 4, 6, 8 or 12 hours for the period of time treatment is judged as being indicated. A major bleeding episode may be treated for 2–3 weeks but can be extended beyond this if clinically warranted.

*Surgery:* An initial dose of 4.5 KIU (90 µg) per kg body weight should be given immediately before the procedure. The dose should be repeated after 2 hours and then at 2–3 hour intervals for the first 24–48 hours depending on the surgery performed and the clinical status of the patient. In major surgery the dosage should be continued at 2–4 hour intervals for 6–7 days. The dosage interval may then be increased to 6–8 hours for another 2 weeks of treatment. Patients undergoing major surgery may be treated for up to 2–3 weeks until healing has occurred.

Anti-fibrinolytics have been reported to reduce blood loss in association with surgery in haemophilia patients, especially in regions rich in fibrinolytic activity, such as the oral cavity.

Preliminary experience indicates that concomitant use of anti-fibrinolytic therapy in minor and major surgery is clinically safe.

For patients with Factor IX inhibitors or acquired antibodies to Factor VIII, only experience of the use of NovoSeven in minor surgery exists.

*Other bleeding episodes:* In one study investigating joint and muscle bleeds using doses of 35 and 70 mg/kg body weight (1.75 and 3.5 KIU/kg b.w.) there was no clear difference in efficacy and safety between the two dosages.

*Administration:* Dissolve the preparation as described under Instructions for use/handling and administer as an intravenous bolus injection.

NovoSeven should not be mixed with infusion solutions or be given in a drip.

*Contra-indications:* Known hypersensitivity to mouse, hamster or bovine protein may be a contra-indication to the use of NovoSeven.

*Special warnings and special precautions for use:* In pathological conditions in which tissue factor can be expected in circulating blood there is a possibility of a thrombogenic potential or induction of DIC in association with NovoSeven treatment. Such situations may include patients with advanced atherosclerotic disease, crush injury, septicaemia or DIC.

As Recombinant Coagulation Factor VIIa Novo-Seven contains trace amounts of mouse IgG (maximum of 1.2 ng/mg rFVIIa), bovine IgG (maximum of 45 ng/ml rFVIIa) and hamster and other bovine proteins (maximum of 23 ng BHK protein/mg rFVIIa) the remote possibility exists that patients treated with this product may develop hypersensitivity to these proteins.

The product should only be administered in centres specialising in the treatment of patients with coagulation factor VIII or IX inhibitors.

*Interaction with other medicaments and other forms of interaction:* The risk of a potential interaction between NovoSeven and coagulation factor concentrates is unknown. Simultaneous use of prothrombin complex concentrates, activated or not, should be avoided.

*Laboratory tests:* The relationship between the prothrombin time (PT), activated partial thromboplastin time (aPTT) and levels of the plasma FVII clotting activity FVII:C has been investigated in one core laboratory.

*The therapeutic range has not been identified for any of the assays.*

FVII:C was measured in a one step coagulation system containing FVII-deficient plasma (immunodepleted, Novo Nordisk A/S) and rabbit brain thromboplastin (type C, Manchester Comparative Reagents Ltd., UK). Coagulation was started by adding thromboplastin and Ca++. Pooled citrated plasma from healthy normal subjects was used as calibrator and was assigned an arbitrary potency of 1 U/ml.

PT shortens to 7 seconds and seems to reach a plateau at plasma FVII:C levels of approximately 5 U/ml. Preliminary data indicate that a clinical improvement is associated with a shortening of the PT to 3–4 seconds from baseline and that this shortening is maintained throughout the treatment with therapeutic doses. The PT cannot be used to differentiate plasma FVII:C levels >5 U/ml. The PT assay is performed according to the instructions given in the kit 'IL TEST (TM) PT-Fibrinogen: Calcium thromboplastin for the simultaneous *in vitro* determination of Prothrombin Time (PT) and Fibrinogen in plasma' from Instrumentation Laboratory. CAVE: Penicillins cause a reduction in prothrombin time.

Although administration of NovoSeven shortens the aPTT, normalisation is usually not observed in doses shown to induce clinical improvement. Experience so far indicates that a shortening of 15–20 seconds was associated with clinical improvement. It is not known if aPTT is helpful in the monitoring of treatment. The aPTT assay is performed according to the instructions given in the kit 'IL TEST (TM) APTT-Micronised Silica: Cephalin with Micronised silica for the *in vitro* determination of activated partial thromboplastin time (APTT) in plasma' from Instrumentation Laboratory.

For all the assay different thromboplastins may give different results.

*Pregnancy and lactation:* From an animal reproduction study it was concluded that intravenous administration of NovoSeven to male and female rats at dose levels up to 3.0 mg/kg b.w./day (150 KIU/kg b.w./day had no effect upon mating performance, fertility and litter responses. It is not known whether NovoSeven can cause foetal harm when administered to a pregnant woman or can affect reproduction capacity. NovoSeven should only be given to a pregnant woman if clearly needed.

*Use during lactation:* It is now known whether this drug is excreted in human milk but, since many drugs are, caution should be exercised when NovoSeven is administered to nursing women.

*Effects on ability to drive and use machines:* None known.

*Undesirable effects:* During the clinical studies conducted there were 7 minor adverse reactions related to the skin (e.g. rash, itching) and 19 systemic complaints (nausea, fever, headache, malaise, diaphoresis and changes in blood pressure) reported out of more than 8,000 injections. Major adverse events possibly related to treatment were reported in 7 cases (e.g. renal failure, ataxia, cerebrovascular disorder, angina pectoris, atrial arrythmia, circulatory shock).

One FVII deficient patient has developed antibodies against FVII after treatment with NovoSeven.

*Overdose:* From human use no thrombotic complications to overdose have been reported, even after accidental administration of 800 µg/kg b.w. (40 KIU/kg b.w.).

### Pharmacological properties

*Pharmacodynamic properties:* Pharmacotherapeutic Group: Coagulation factors, ATC code B02B D05.

NovoSeven contains activated Recombinant Coagulation Factor VII. The working mechanism of FVIIa in the induction of haemostasis includes a direct activation of FX into FXa which then initiates the conversion of prothrombin into thrombin leading to the formation of the haemostatic plug by converting fibrinogen into fibrin. In addition, FVIIa activates FIX into FIXa. Accordingly, a pharmacodynamic effect of FVIa should give rise to an increased formation of FIXa and FXa as well as thrombin. However, the activity of FVIIa increases tremendously when it forms a complex with tissue factor/phospholipid which are exposed locally following an injury to the vessel wall. Therefore, the activity of rFVIIa will induce local haemostatsis only.

Systemic activation of the coagulation system may occur in patients suffering from underlying diseases predisposing for DIC.

*Pharmacokinetic properties:* Using a FVII clot assay, the pharmacokinetic properties of NovoSeven were investigated in 25 non-bleeding and in 5 bleeding study episodes. NovoSeven was given as a single dose of 17.5 mcg (0.875 KIU), 35 mcg (1.75 KIU) and 70 mcg (3.5 KIU) per kilo b.w.

Single dose pharmacokinetics of NovoSeven, 17.5, 35 and 70 mcg/kg (0.875, 1.75 and 3.5 KIU/kg) exhibited linear behaviour. FVII clotting activities measured in plasma drawn prior to and during a 24-hour period after NovoSeven administration were analysed. In non-bleeding episodes the median apparent volume of distribution at steady state and at elimination were 106 and 122 ml/kg and in bleeding episodes the figures were 107 and 121 ml/kg respectively. Median clearance was 31.0 ml/h×kg non-bleeding episodes and 32.6 ml/h×kg in bleeding episodes. The elimination of the drug was described also by mean residence time and half-time. In non-bleeding episodes mean residence time was 3.44 h and half-time was 2.89 h (median values). In bleeding episodes the elimination seemed faster, mean residence time being 2.97 h and half-time being 2.30 h (median values).

The median *in vivo* plasma recovery was 45.6% in non-bleeding episodes and 43.5% in bleeding episodes. A significantly lower plasma recovery was found in bleeding episodes than in non-bleeding episodes, indicating a consumption of rFVIIa in connection with tissue damage.

*Preclinical safety data:* All findings in the pre-clinical safety programme were related to the pharmacological effect of Recombinant Coagulation Factor VIIa.

### Pharmaceutical particulars

*List of excipients:* Sodium chloride, calcium chloride, glyclyglycine, polysorbate 80, mannitol.

After reconstitution with the appropriate volume of diluent (water for injections, PhEur) each bottle contains NovoSeven 30 KIU/ml (0.6 mg/ml). Sodium chloride 3 mg/ml, calcium chloride dihydrate 1.5 mg/ml, glycylglycine 1.3 mg/ml, polysorbate 80 0.1 mg/ml and mannitol 30 mg/ml are present in the preparation.

*Incompatibilities:* NovoSeven should not be mixed with infusion solutions or be given in a drip.

*Shelf life:* The shelf life for the product packed for sale is 2 years. The reconstituted product should be administered within 3 hours.

*Special precautions for storage:* NovoSeven should be stored under refrigeration (2°–8°C). Do not use after the expiry date.

Freezing should be avoided to prevent damage to the diluent bottle.

Avoid exposure to direct sunlight.

*Nature and contents of container*

*Vials for NovoSeven:* Glass type 1 PhEur, closed with a bromobutyl rubber plug, covered with an aluminium cap. The closed vials are equipped with a snap-off cap made of polypropylene for sealing.

*Vials for diluent:* Glass type 1 PhEur, closed with a bromobutyl rubber disc with teflon, covered with an aluminium cap. The closed vials are equipped with a snap-off cap made of polypropylene for sealing.

*Syringe for reconstitution and administration:* The disposable syringe is made of polypropylene and the size is 3 ml, 6 ml and 12 ml for 60 KIU/vial, 120 KIU/vial and 240 KIU/vial respectively.

*Instructions for use/handling*

*Reconstitution – Always use aseptic technique:*

1. Bring NovoSeven (powder) and water for injections, PhEur (diluent) to room temperature (but not above 37°C).
2. Remove caps from powder and diluent bottles to expose central portion of rubber stoppers.
3. Cleanse stoppers with alcohol swab and allow to dry prior to use.
4. To take the needle out of the package, press the needle end. Remove protective covering from the needle and attach the disposable syringe supplied in the package.
5. Draw back the plunger to admit air into the syringe.
6. Insert needle through the diluent bottle stopper at its centre and inject air into the bottle. Hold the bottle upside down, then withdraw the total content of the bottle into the syringe.
7. Inject the diluent from the syringe into the bottle containing the powder through the centre of the stopper (the powder bottle does not contain vacuum).
8. Gently swirl until all material is dissolved.

The enclosed disposable syringe should be used for reconstitution and administration of the preparation.

NovoSeven is for intravenous bolus injection only and should not be mixed with infusion solutions or be given in a drip.

Administration should preferably take place immediately or at least within 3 hours after reconstitution.

The enclosed disposable syringe is compatible with the reconstituted preparation, but **do not** store reconstituted NovoSeven in plastic syringes.

Parental drug products should be inspected visually for particulate matter and discolouration prior to administration whenever solution and container permit.

*Marketing authorisation holder:* Novo Nordisk A/S, Novo Alle, DK-2880 Bagsvaerd, Denmark.

**Marketing authorisation numbers**

| | |
|---|---|
| NovoSeven 60 KIU | EU/1/96/006/001 |
| NovoSeven 120 KIU | EU/1/96/006/002 |
| NovoSeven 240 KIU | EU/1/96/006/003 |

**Date of approval/revision of SPC** February 1996.

**Legal category** POM.

## TRISEQUENS*

**Presentation** Trisequens is supplied in a calendar dial-pack of 28 sequential tablets:

12 blue biconvex tablets marked 'NOVO 270' on one side, blank on the other side, each containing 2 mg oestradiol and 1 mg oestriol.

10 white biconvex tablets marked 'NOVO 271' on one side, blank on the other side, each containing 2 mg oestradiol, 1 mg oestriol and 1 mg Norethisterone Acetate BP.

6 red biconvex tablets marked 'NOVO 272' on one side, blank on the other side, each containing 1 mg oestradiol, and 0.5 mg oestriol.

**Uses** Trisequens is indicated for the treatment of symptoms due to oestrogenic deficiency and for the prophylaxis of postmenopausal osteoporosis in women at risk of developing fractures.

The oestrogen components of Trisequens counteract falling oestrogen levels during the menopause, whilst the progestogen component counteracts hyperstimulation of the endometrium. A regular shedding of the endometrium is normally induced by Trisequens during the red tablet phase or at the end of the white tablet phase.

Studies based on measurement of bone mineral content have shown that Trisequens is effective in the prevention of progressive bone loss following the menopause.

**Dosage and administration** Trisequens is administered orally without chewing, one tablet daily without interruption, starting with the blue tablets. In menstruating women the first tablet should be taken on the fifth day of menstrual bleeding. If menstruation has stopped altogether or is infrequent and sporadic (2–4 monthly intervals) the first tablet can be taken at any time.

*Menopausal symptoms:* Treatment may be stopped at approximately 6–12 monthly intervals to establish whether continued therapy for relief of menopausal symptoms is still required.

*Postmenopausal oesteoporosis:* Epidemiological studies which have examined risk factors for osteoporotic fractures (hip, lower forearm and spine) indicate that a useful reduction in fracture frequency is achieved with continuous long-term oestrogen therapy. In these studies, treatment for 5–6 years gave a reduction in fracture frequency of about 50%. Ideally, prophylactic therapy should commence during the perimenopausal period or as soon as possible thereafter. At present there is no diagnostic test for determining women at risk of developing osteoporotic fractures. Epidemiological studies give some indication of those women at risk. White women are more at risk than black women; other risk factors for fracture include: low body weight, tallness, early menopause, surgical menopause, cigarette smoking and high alcohol intake. A dietary intake of calcium ≥1000 mg/day is probably also important in maintaining bone mass and supplementation should be considered if the diet is deficient.

Not intended for children or males.

**Contra-indications, warnings, etc**

*Contra-indications:* Known or suspected mammary or genital carcinoma. Known or suspected oestrogen-dependent tumours. Thrombophlebitis, thromboembolic disorders or patients with a past history of these conditions.

Undiagnosed irregular vaginal bleeding. Acute or chronic liver disease or history of liver disease where the liver function tests have failed to return to normal. Jaundice or history of jaundice in pregnancy. Rotor syndrome or Dubin-Johnson syndrome. Hyperlipoproteinaemia, especially in the presence of other risk factors which may indicate a predisposition to cardiovascular or cerebrovascular disorders. Patients with existing cerebrovascular or cardiovascular disease. A history during pregnancy of severe pruritus, herpes gestationis, or a deterioration of otosclerosis. Pregnancy or suspected pregnancy.

*Precautions and warnings:* Before initiation of therapy with Trisequens it is advisable to undertake a thorough examination to exclude any possibility of genital or mammary tumours. Women receiving long-term therapy with Trisequens should be given a similar examination every 6 months. Special attention should be paid to body weight, blood pressure, heart, breasts, pelvic organs, legs and skin.

It has been established that treatment of women with an intact uterus with oestrogens unopposed by progestogens increases the risk of endometrial cancer. Endometrial hyperplasia (atypical or adenomatous) often precedes endometrial cancer. Recent prospective studies, however, suggest that endometrial hyperplasia can virtually be avoided if the endometrium is protected by administration of a sufficient dose of progestogen for at least 10 days each cycle.

Long-term use of oestrogen replacement therapy in high doses shows an increase in breast cancer risk. Use of small doses for short periods show no measurable increase in risk. The effects of smaller doses of oestrogens for long periods are not adequately studied but appear unlikely to be associated with any substantially increased risk of breast cancer.

Patients with epilepsy, migraine, diabetes, asthma or cardiac dysfunction should be carefully controlled, as oestrogens may worsen these conditions.

Thromboembolism has been reported in connection with oestrogen replacement therapy but there is no background to believe that the overall incidence is increased.

The indications for immediate withdrawal of therapy are as follows: thrombophlebitis; thromboembolic disorders; the appearance of jaundice; the occurrence of migraine-like headaches; sudden visual disturbances or a significant increase in blood pressure.

It is also advisable to withdraw treatment 6 weeks before elective surgery and during prolonged periods of immobilisation.

Trisequens may potentiate the side-effects of phenothiazines. Drugs such as barbiturates, phenytoin, and rifampicin, which induce the activity of hepatic microsomal drug-metabolizing enzymes, may decrease the effectiveness of Trisequens. Mineral oil may decrease the intestinal absorption of Trisequens.

Trisequens has no contraceptive effect.

Pre-existing uterine fibromyomata may increase in size under the influence of oestrogens and if this is observed administration of the preparation should be discontinued.

*Side-effects:* During the first few months of treatment, tension in the breasts, spotting or break-through bleeding can occur. These side-effects are usually of a temporary character and normally disappear after continued treatment. Other side-effects such as headache, oedema or nausea seldom occur.

**Pharmaceutical precautions** Protect from light.

**Legal category** POM.

**Package quantities** Trisequens is supplied in a calendar dial-pack of 28 tablets. Available in cartons containing three calendar dial packs.

**Further information** Nil.

**Product licence number** 4668/0015.

*Product licence holder:* Novo Nordisk A/S.

## TRISEQUENS FORTE*

**Qualitative and quantitative composition** 28 sequential tablets: 12 yellow, 10 white, 6 red.

*Active ingredients:*

Yellow tablets: estradiol 4 mg, oestriol 2 mg.

White tablets: estradiol 4 mg, oestriol 2 mg, norethisterone acetate 1 mg.

Red tablets: estradiol 1 mg, oestriol 0.5 mg.

The tablets also contain lactose and maize starch, but do not contain significant amounts of gluten.

**Pharmaceutical form** Film-coated tablets for oral administration.

**Clinical particulars**

*Therapeutic indications:* The treatment of symptoms due to oestrogen deficiency.

*Posology and method of administration:* Trisequens Forte is administered orally, without chewing, one tablet daily without interruption, starting with the yellow tablets. In menstruating women the first tablet should be taken on the fifth day of menstrual bleeding. If menstruation has stopped altogether or is infrequent and sporadic (2–4 monthly intervals) the first tablet can be taken at any time.

Treatment may be stopped at approximately 6–12 monthly intervals to establish whether contined therapy for relief of menopausal symptoms is still required.

Not intended for children or males.

*Contra-indications:* Known or suspected, mammary or genital carcinoma. Known or suspected oestrogen-dependent tumours. Thrombophlebitis, thromboembolic disorders or patients with a past history of these conditions. Undiagnosed irregular vaginal bleeding. Acute or chronic liver disease or history of liver disease where the liver function tests have failed to return to normal. Jaundice or history of jaundice in pregnancy. Rotor syndrome or Dubin-Johnson syndrome. Hyperlipoproteinaemia, especially in the presence of other risk factors which may indicate a predisposition to cardiovascular or cerebrovascular disorders. Patients with existing cerebrovascular or cardiovascular disease. A history during pregnancy of severe pruritus, herpes gestationis or a deterioration of otosclerosis. Pregnancy or suspected pregnancy.

*Special warnings and special precautions for use:* Before initiation of therapy with Trisequens Forte it is advisable to undertake a thorough examination to exclude any possibility of genital or mammary tumours. Women receiving long-term therapy with Trisequens Forte should be given a similar examination every 6 months. Special attention should be paid to body weight, blood pressure, heart, breasts, pelvic organs, legs and skin.

It has been established that treatment of women with an intact uterus with oestrogens unopposed by progestogens increases the risk of endometrial cancer. Endometrial hyperplasia (atypical or adenomatous) often precedes endometrial cancer. Recent prospective studies, however, suggest that endometrial hyperplasia can virtually be avoided if the endometrium is protected by administration of a sufficient dose of progestogen for at least 10 days each cycle.

Long-term use of oestrogen replacement therapy in

high doses shows an increase in breast cancer risk. Use of small doses for short periods show no measurable increase in risk. The effects of smaller doses of oestrogen for long periods are not adequately studied, but appear unlikely to be associated with any substantially increased risk of breast cancer.

Patients with epilepsy, migraine, diabetes, asthma or cardiac dysfunction should be carefully controlled as oestrogens may worsen these conditions. Thromboembolism has been reported in connection with oestrogen replacement therapy but there is no background to believe that the overall incidence is increased.

The indications for immediate withdrawal of therapy are as follows: thrombophlebitis, thromboembolic disorders, the appearance of jaundice, the occurrence of migraine-like headaches, sudden visual disturbances or a significant increase in blood pressure. It is also advisable to withdraw treatment 6 weeks before elective surgery and during prolonged periods of immobilisation.

*Interaction with other medicaments and other forms of interaction:* May potentiate side effects of phenothiazines. Drugs such as barbiturates, phenytoin and rifampicin, which induce the activity of hepatic microsomal drug metabolising enzymes, may decrease the effectiveness of Trisequens Forte. Mineral oil may decrease the intestinal absorption of Trisequens Forte.

*Pregnancy and lactation:* Trisequens Forte is contra-indicated during pregnancy.

*Effects on ability to drive and use machinery:* No effects known.

*Undesirable effects:* During the first few months of treatment, tension in the breasts, spotting or breakthrough bleeding may occur. These side effects are usually of a temporary character and normally disappear after continued treatment. Other side effects such as headache, oedema or nausea seldom occur. Pre-existing uterine fibromyomata may increase in size under the influence of oestrogens and if this is observed administration of the preparation should be discontinued.

*Overdose:* Overdosage may be manifested by nausea and vomiting. There is no specific antidote and treatment should be symptomatic.

### Pharmacological properties
*Pharmacodynamic properties:* Oestradiol and oestriol components have oestrogenic activity in man. Norethisterone acetate has protestagenic activity in man.

*Pharmacokinetic properties:* Oestradiol and oestriol are rapidly absorbed after oral administration. A large part of the oestradiol becomes interconvertible with oestrone, which is rapidly conjugated as the sulphate and is bound to albumin.

Noresthisterone acetate is rapidly absorbed after oral administration; it is also rapidly excreted.

### Pharmaceutical particulars
*List of excipients:* Lactose, maize starch, gelatin, talc, magnesium stearate, hydroxypropyl methylcellulose (E464), iron oxide (E172), propylene glycol, titanium dioxide (E171), triacetin, purified water.

*Incompatibilities:* None known.

*Shelf life:* 48 months.

*Special precautions for storage:* Store at room temperature, below 25°C. Protect tablets from light.

*Nature and contents of container:* Polypropylene/polystyrene calendar dial pack containing 28 tablets.

Calendar dial packs (3×28 tablets) are contained within outer carton.

*Instructions for use/handling:* Each carton contains a patient information leaflet with instructions for use of the calendar dial pack.

**Marketing authorisation number** 3132/0087.

**Date of approval/revision of SPC** November 1996.

**Legal category** P.

## VAGIFEM*

**Qualitative and quantitative composition** Active ingredient, Oestradiol 25 micrograms.

**Pharmaceutical form** Film-coated vaginal tablet inset in disposable applicator.

### Clinical particulars
*Therapeutic indications:* The treatment of atrophic vaginitis due to oestrogen deficiency.

*Posology and method of administration*
*Dosage:* Vagifem is administered intravaginally using the applicator. An initial dose of 1 tablet daily for two weeks will usually improve vaginal atrophy and associated symptoms; a maintenance dose of 2 tablets per week may then be instituted. Treatment should be discontinued after about 3 months to assess whether further therapy is necessary.
Not intended for childen or males.
Use in the elderly: there are no special dosage requirements.

*Administration:* The applicator is inserted into the vagina up to the end of the smooth part of the applicator (approximately 9 cms). The tablet is released by pressing the plunger. The applicator is then withdrawn and disposed of.

*Contra-indications:*
1. Known, suspected, or past history of carcinoma of the breast.
2. Known or suspected oestrogen-dependent neoplasia, e.g. endometrial carcinoma or other hormone-dependent tumours.
3. Abnormal genital bleeding of unknown aetiology.
4. Acute thrombophlebitis or thromboembolic disorders, or a past history of these conditions associated with previous oestrogen use.

*Special warnings and special precautions for use:* Although the dose of oestradiol is low and the treatment is local, a minor degree of systemic absorption may occur. Because of this, the increased risk of endometrial cancer after treatment with unopposed oestrogens should be kept in mind. Endometrial hyperplasia (atypical or adenomatous) often precedes endometrial cancer.
Patients with the following conditions who are treated with Vagifem should be monitored more frequently and if any of the conditions worsen Vagifem treatment should be withdrawn:

– Acute or chronic liver disease or history of liver disease where the liver function tests have failed to return to normal.
– Thrombophlebitis, thromboembolic disorders or cerebro vascular accident, or a past history of these disorders.
– Haemoglobinopathies or sickle cell anaemia.
– Porphyria.
– Epilepsy.

– Migraine.
– Diabetes.
– Asthma.
– Cardiac dysfunction.
– Hypertension requiring treatment.

Before initiation of therapy with Vagifem, it is advisable to undertake a thorough examination to exclude any possibility of genital or mammary tumours. Vaginal infections should be treated before initiation of Vagifem therapy.
Persistent or recurring vaginal bleeding should be investigated.
The present bulk of evidence shows that oestrogens given to post-menopausal women do not increase the risk of breast cancer.

*Interactions with other medicaments and othere forms of interaction:* Not applicable due to the low systemic absorption.

*Pregnancy and lactation:* Vagifem is contra-indicated in pregnant women.

*Effects on ability to drive and to use machines:* No effects known.

*Undesirable effects:* Few side-effects have been observed. Slight vaginal bleeding, vaginal discharge and skin rash have rarely been reported.

*Overdose:* Vagifem is intended for intravaginal use. The dose of oestradiol is so low that a considerable number of tablets would have to be ingested to approach a significant dose.

### Pharmacological properties
*Pharmacodynamic properties:* 17-β oestradiol is the principal and most active of the naturally occurring human oestrogens. It has pharmacological actions in common with all oestrogenic compounds. The action on the vagina is to increase maturation of vaginal epithelial cells and increase cervical secretory activity.

*Pharmacokinetic properties:* Oestrogens are well absorbed from the vagina. After treatment with Vagifem, marginal elevations of plasma oestradiol and conjugated oestrogens as well as suppression of pituitary gonadotrophins have been observed. This indicates that there is an absorption of the oestradiol. This absorption is, however, low and no other systemic oestrogen effect could be determined.

### Pharmaceutical particulars
*List of excipients:* Methyl hydroxypropyl cellulose (E464), lactose, maize starch, magnesium stearate, polyethylene glycol 6000, purified water.

*Incompatibilities:* None known.

*Shelf life:* 36 months.

*Special precautions for storage:* Store in a dry place, protect from light. Store below 25°C. Do not refrigerate.

*Nature and contents of container:* Laminated bubble strips containing 5 applicators with inset tablet. Packed in cartons containing 3 strips (15 tablets and applicators).

*Instructions for use/handling:* Each carton contains a patient information leaflet with instructions for use.

*Marketing authorisation holder:* Novo Nordisk A/S, Novo Alle, DK-2880 Bagsvaerd, Denmark.

**Marketing authorisation number** 4668/0026.

**Date of approval/revision of SPC** August 1995.

**Legal category** POM.

*Trade Mark

# Nycomed UK Limited

Nycomed House
2111 Coventry Road
Sheldon
Birmingham B26 3EA

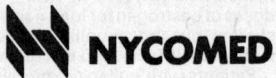

## CONDYLINE*

**Presentation** Condyline is presented as a clear colourless alcoholic solution containing 0.5% podophyllotoxin in vials of 3.5 ml, with a suitable quantity of special applicators.

**Uses** For the topical treatment of condylomata acuminata affecting the penis or the female external genitalia.

**Dosage and administration** By topical administration.

*Adults and the elderly:* Apply twice daily for three days directly to the warts. Allow to dry after treatment. Use the applicator provided, applying not more than 50 applicators-full for each application. This three-day treatment may be repeated, if necessary, at weekly intervals, for a total of five weeks of treatment.

Lesions in the female, and lesions greater than 4 cm² in the male, should be treated under direct medical supervision.

*Children:* Not recommended.

**Contra-indications, warnings, etc**
*Contra-indications:* Hypersensitivity to podophyllotoxin.

*Use in pregnancy and lactation:* Condyline is not recommended for use during pregnancy or during breast feeding.

*Special precautions:* Avoid contact with healthy skin; lesions in the female, and lesions greater than 4 cm² in the male, should be treated under direct medical supervision. Do not use on open wounds following surgical procedures.

*Side-effects:* Local irritation, usually mild, may occur.

*Overdosage:* In topical overdosage, wash well with soap and water; if the eyes are involved bathe thoroughly with water. If accidentally ingested give stomach washout and monitor electrolyte balance, blood gases, liver function and blood picture.

**Pharmaceutical precautions** Normal pharmaceutical storage and handling are indicated.

**Legal category** POM.

**Package quantities** 3.5 ml in an amber glass vial fitted with a child-resistant cap, together with a suitable quantity of special applicators (OP).

**Further information** The product should be discarded six weeks after first opening the vial. Keep away from naked flames.

**Product licence number** 04517/0020.

## FORTIPINE* LA40 TABLETS

**Qualitative and quantitative composition**
*Active Ingredient:* Nifedipine (international non-proprietary name): 40 mg.

Chemical name: Dimethyl 1,4.dihydro-2,6-dimethyl-4-(2-nitrophenyl) pyridine -3,5- dicarboxylate.

**Pharmaceutical form** Modified release tablets (matrix tablets) for oral administration.

**Clinical particulars**
*Therapeutic indications:* Treatment of all degrees of hypertension.

*Posology and method of administration:* Patients should be treated individually depending on the severity of the disease and the therapeutic response. The following recommendations for dosing in adults and adolescents over 14 years are applicable:

In general, one modified release tablet of Fortipine LA40 (40 mg) once daily should be adequate. If necessary this dose can be increased to 80 mg given once daily, or 40 mg twice daily.

The modified release tablets are to be taken after meals, e.g. breakfast. The modified release tablets should be swallowed whole with half a glass of water, and must not be broken or chewed.

In patients with renal dysfunction, a slight alteration of the pharmacokinetics of nifedipine may be seen. However, dose adjustment in these patients is not usually required.

In patients with hepatic dysfunction, significant alteration of the pharmacokinetics of nifedipine has usually been seen. These patients should be carefully monitored when initiating therapy and during dose titration.

*Elderly patients:* In elderly patients, a slight alteration of the pharmacokinetics of nifedipine may be seen. However, dose adjustment in these patients is not usually required.

*Children:* Not recommended for children under 14 years of age.

*Contra-indications:* Fortipine LA40 should not be administered to patients with an allergy to nifedipine or other tablet constituents, nor to patients with cardiogenic shock. It is contra-indicated in women with child-bearing potential and those breast-feeding their babies. Fortipine LA40 is contra-indicated in patients with advanced aortic stenosis, low cardiac reserve, severe hypotension or porphyria.

*Special warnings and precautions for use:* Patients at risk of hypotensive crisis should begin any therapy under close medical supervision. In patients on haemodialysis with malignant hypertension and irreversible renal failure with hypovolaemia, nifedipine should be given with caution. An exaggerated fall in blood pressure due to vasodilation may occur.

Ischaemic pain has been reported in a small proportion of patients following the introduction of nifedipine therapy. Although a 'steal' effect has not been demonstrated, patients experiencing this effect should discontinue nifedipine therapy.

*Interactions with other medicaments and other forms of interaction:* Fortipine LA40 can be administered concomitantly with other antihypertensives including beta-receptor blockers. These may have additive antihypertensive or potentiating effects and postural hypotension may therefore occur. Concomitant treatment of nifedipine with a beta-blocker occasionally results in the occurrence of heart failure. For this reason a combination with a beta-blocker is only recommended in patients with a sufficient ventricular function. After discontinuation of the beta-blocker a deterioration with regard to the symptoms of angina pectoris may occasionally occur, due to the abrupt withdrawal of the beta-blocker. Therefore, is it not recommended to switch abruptly from a beta-blocker to nifedipine.

Fortipine LA40 will not prevent the possibility that there might be a rebound effect when other antihypertensive treatment is stopped.

Concomitant therapy with cimetidine (and to a smaller extent with ranitidine) may potentiate the antihypertensive action of nifedipine. Nifedipine administration may suppress serum levels of quinidine and may increase plasma digoxin levels due to reduced drug clearance. Therefore, on combination therapy monitoring of quinidine levels as well as digoxin levels is recommended.

Fortipine LA40 may modify insulin and glucose responses, requiring adjustment in therapy of treated diabetics.

Grapefruit juice inhibits the oxidative metabolism of nifedipine; this may be potentially significant in some patients.

*Pregnancy and lactation:* Fortipine LA40 is contra-indicated in pregnant women and women of child-bearing potential because foetal risks, observed in animal experiments and during human use, far outweigh the potential benefits. Pregnancy category: B3.

Nifedipine is secreted into breast milk. Fortipine LA40 should not be administered during lactation.

*Effects on ability to drive and use machines:* Nifedipine may cause headache, dizziness, nausea and tiredness to such a degree that reaction time is affected. These effects can be aggravated by concurrent alcohol. If this occurs, the patient should be advised not to drive or operate machines.

*Undesirable effects:* Undesirable effects, usually mild and transient in nature, may occur and are more frequent at the beginning of therapy. Frequently, headache, flush (facial reddening), dizziness, as well as oedema, due to vasodilatation, may occur. Less common side effects include rash, nausea, lethargy and urinary frequency. In rare cases, in acute studies, a transient increase in glucose has been observed. This should be considered particularly in patients with diabetes mellitus. Nifedipine has no diabetogenic effect. Rarely gingival hyperplasia has been observed which was reversible after discontinuation of therapy. In elderly patients, very rarely gynaecomastia has been observed which was reversible after discontinuation of therapy. Chest pain due to myocardial ischemia may occur 1–4 hours after ingestion of nifedipine. Cases of hypersensitivity to nifedipine resulting in jaundice have been reported.

List of undesirable effects according to body system.
*Cardiovascular system:* Tachycardia, hypotension. As with other vasodilators coronary ischaemia (steal phenomenon) resulting in retrosternal pain, may occur.

*Central nervous system:* Dizziness, tiredness, paresthesia, tremor.

*Eyes:* Transient change in optical perception.
*Gastro-intestinal tract:* Nausea, disturbances.
*Skin:* Redness, itching, urticaria, exanthema and exceptionally exfoliative dermatitis.
*Urinary tract:* An increase in the daily amount of urine so that nocturia may occur.
*Legs:* Myalgia.
*Liver:* Very rarely liver function distiurbances (intrahepatic cholestasis, or increases in transaminases) have occurred which were reversible after discontinuation of therapy.
*Miscellaneous:* Gingival hyperplasia, gynaecomastia, increase in glucose in particular in patients with diabetes mellitus.

*Overdose:* Toxic effects arise from the three main actions of nifedipine in overdose: dilation of vascular smooth muscles (predominant effect); decreased myocardial contractility; and depression of AV nodal conduction. Hypotension and tachycardia or bradycardia are the most likely manifestations of overdose. Other toxic effects include nausea, vomiting, drowsiness, dizziness, confusion, lethargy, flushing, coma and convulsions. Cardiac effects may include heart block, AV dissociation and asystole; metabolic disturbances include hyperglycaemia, acidosis, hypo- or hyperkalaemia and hypocalcaemia; pulmonary oedema has been reported.

Primary treatment involves removal of nifedipine by gastric lavage or ipecacuanha and administration of activated charcoal (50 g adults; 10–15 g children). Fortipine LA40 is a modified release matrix tablet, therefore activated charcoal should be repeated at 4-hourly intervals (25 g adults; 10 g children). The patient should be closely monitored and treated according to predominating signs:

*for hypotension:* the feet should be raised and plasma expanders given. If this is not effective, 10% calcium gluconate or chloride can be given intravenously (calcium chloride should not be given to acidotic patients). If this fails, dopamine may be tried (large doses may be needed). Glucagon may be also of value;

*for bradycardia:* treatment with atropine, isoprenaline and cardiac pacing should be given as required.

The value of extracorporeal methods of removal of nifedipine have not been established.

**Pharmacological properties**
*Pharmacodynamic properties:* Nifedipine ia a Ca-antagonist of the 1,4-dihydropyridine type. Ca-antagonists inhibit the slow Ca-channel flux into the myocardial cells, the smooth muscle cells of the coronary arteries and the peripheral capillaries. Nifedipine brings about a substantial improvement in the oxygen supply of the myocardium while reducing oxygen demand. It has been shown to exhibit anti-anginal properties. High blood pressure is normalised due to a reduction in the peripheral resistance (vasodilatation).

In therapeutic doses nifedipine has almost no effect on the myocardium. Nifedipine dilates mainly the large coronary arteries and reduces the muscle tone of the coronary arteries, thereby increasing the oxygen supply. Simultaneously, the reduction in peripheral resistance (afterload reduction) leads to less work for the myocardium with the result of a decrease in oxygen demand.

In particular at the beginning of therapy heart rate

and cardiac output may increase due to baroreceptor reflex activation. After chronic therapy with nifedipine, heart rate and cardiac output return to pre-treatment values. A pronounced blood pressure lowering effect is observed in patients with hypertension.

*Pharmacokinetic properties*

*Absorption:* Fortipine LA40 is absorbed rapidly and almost completely following oral administration. Fortipine LA40 reaches maximal concentrations (29.4±12.0 (x±SD) ng/ml) 5.0±2.7 hours after drug intake at steady state.

The release of nifeipine from the Fortipine LA40 modified release tablet is almost linear, this means that the drug is delivered at a constant rate. The relative bioavailability of the modified release form compared to the slow release forms of nifedipine is not statistically different in steady state.

Trough levels after Fortipine LA40 (24 h post-dose) in steady state (12.0±6,5 ng/ml) are achieved already after the first dose.

Based on its pharmacokinetic profile, an effect due to Fortipine LA40 is expected over 24 hours.

Concomitant intake of food results in higher maximum plasma concentrations of nifedipine, which occurs earlier compared to administration in fasted state, but the concentrations at the end of the dose interval are similar.

*Distribution:* The protein binding of nifedipine amounts to 94–99%. Animal studies with labelled nifedipine have shown that distribution of the fraction not protein bound is throughout all organs and tissues, with higher concentrations in myocardium than in skeletal muscle. Neither nifedipine nor its metabolites are stored selectively in any tissue.

*Metabolism:* Nifedipine is almost completely metabolised to inactive matabolites.

*Elimination:* An apparent half-life of 14.9±6.0 hours was found. The apparent half-life of Fortipine LA40 did not change after repeated dosing. Only <1% of the dose is excreted in the urine as the parent compound. 70–80% of the dose is excreted in the urine as metabolites. The remainder is excreted as metabolites in the faeces. Elimination may be regarded by renal failure or insufficiency.

*Preclinical safety data:* Different animals were investigated. Studies in mice, rats and rabbits demonstrated a low intraperitoneal, subcutaneous and oral acute toxicity. No significant susceptibility was detected: $LD_{50}$ in mice p.o. was found to be 421–572 mg/kg, in rats p.o. 950–1087 mg/kg, in rabbits p.o. 250–500 mg/kg, in cats p.o. 100 mg/kg. Toxic symptoms were rapidly and completely reversible in surviving animals. No major differences have been observed between male and female animals.

*Subacute, subchronic* and *chronic* oral *toxicity* studies in rats demonstrated a low toxicity of high doses of nifedipine. With the exception of a dose-dependent increase in heart and liver phospholipids in the subchronic study, a no-effect dose has been evaluated to be equivalent to 75 times the human therapeutic dose. Only doses of 800 (1200 HTD) and to some extent 400 mg/kg/day were found to be clearly toxic.

*Teratogenicity* studies of nifedipine in rats and rabbits demonstrated a teratogenic potential which justify it to be contra-indicated in women who are, or may become pregnant.

Extensive *mutagenicity* studies in Ames Salmonella mutagenicity testing systems were all negative.

No *carcinogenic* potential has occurred during the long clinical experience with the compound and in the negative Ames.

Nifedipine seems to have a low *interaction* profile toward other drugs. The possible interaction between ethanol and nifedipine, causing increased plasma levels of nifedipine, should however, be noted.

The *pharmacokinetics* of nifedipine are well documented, especially in rats, with a fast absorption, dose independence and a low accumulation potential by repeated dosing. The ability to cross the blood-brain and placental barriers should be noted.

**Pharmaceutical particulars**

*List of excipients:* Microcrystalline cellulose; cellulose; methylhydroxypropylcellulose; lactose; magnesium stearate; Colloidal anhydrous silica; Macrogol 400 (polyethyleneglycol 400); Macrogol 6000 (polyethyleneglycol 6000); ferric oxide red (E172); titanium dioxide [E171]; talc.

*Incompatibilities:* None known.

*Shelf life:* Three years.

*Special precautions for storage:* Fortipine LA40 should be stored in the original pack below 25°C, in a dry place and protected from light.

Nifedipine is highly sensitive to light and is therefore protected both by materials in the tablet and in the packaging. Nonetheless tablets should not be exposed to direct sunlight and should only be removed from the blister pack when about to be taken.

*Nature and contents of container:* Thermoformed blister packs of red transparent, light protective PVC/PVDC-film/aluminum in boxes of 28, 30, 56, 60 and 100 tablets.

*Instruction for use/handling:* None.

**Marketing authorisation number** 04517/0024.

**Date of approval/revision of SPC** August 1996.

**Legal cateogry** POM.

## IMUNOVIR*

**Presentation** White, avoid tablets with the number '148' on one side and the letters 'IMV' on the other. Each tablet contains 500 mg inosine pranobex.

**Uses** Imunovir is an agent demonstrating anti-viral activity and possessing immunopotentiating action in viral diseases.

*Indications:* Imunovir is indicated in the mangement of:

(a) Mucocutaneous infections due to herpes simplex virus (type I and/or type II).
(b) Genital warts as adjunctive therapy to podophyllin or carbon dioxide laser.
(c) Subacute sclerosing panencephalitis.

**Dosage and administration**

*Adults:* Mucocutaneous herpes simplex: 1 g four times a day (4 g daily) for 7–14 days.

Genital warts: 1 g three times a day (3 g daily) for 14–28 days as adjunctive therapy to podophyllin or carbon dioxide laser.

Subacute sclerosing panencephalitis: 50–100 mg/kg daily in divided doses every 4 hours.

*Elderly:* No dosage alterations are necessary in the elderly.

*Children:* No information is available in children.

**Contra-indications, warnings, etc**

*Contra-indications:* None known.

*Warnings:* As the inosine component of Imunovir is metabolised to uric acid, it should be used with caution in patients with renal impairment, a history of gout or hyperuricaemia.

*Use in pregnancy:* Although animal tests have shown no teratogenic effect, the use of Imunovir in women where pregnancy is suspected or confirmed, should be avoided.

*Adverse reactions:* Side-effects are rare and usually of a mild and transitory nature. The only commonly associated adverse effects occurring during treatment are elevated serum and urinary concentrations of uric acid. These return to normal once treatment is withdrawn.

*Symptoms and treatment of overdosage:* There has been no experience of overdosage with Imunovir. However, serious adverse effects apart from increased levels of uric acid in the body, seem unlikely in view of the animal toxicity studies. Treatment should be restricted to symptomatic and supportive measures.

**Pharmaceutical precautions** Store below 25°C.

**Legal category** POM.

**Package quantities** Available in bottles of 100 tablets.

**Further information** Nil.

**Product licence number** 14806/0001.

*Product licence holder:* Newport Synthesis Ltd., Baldoyle Industrial Estate, Dublin 13, Republic of Ireland.

## NYCOPREN

**Qualitative and quantitative composition**

*Active constituent:* Naproxen BP 250 mg and 500 mg.

**Pharmaceutical form** Enteric coated tablets for oral administration.

**Clinical particulars**

*Therapeutic indications:* Rheumatoid arthritis, juvenile rheumatoid arthritis, osteoarthrosis (degenerative arthritis), ankylosing spondylitis, acute gout and acute inflammatory musculoskeletal disorders.

*Posology and method of administration:*
*Adult dosage:*

(a) Rheumatoid arthritis, osteoarthrosis, ankylosing spondylitis: 500 mg to 1 g per day taken in 2 doses at 12 hour intervals.
(b) In severe night-time pain and/or morning stiffness, in patients being switched to Nycopren from a high dose of another NSAID, or in osteoarthrosis where pain is the predominant symptom:
Loading dose of 750 mg–1 g per day during the acute phase.
(c) Acute gout: 750 mg at once then 250 mg every 8 hours until the attack has passed.
(d) Acute inflammatory musculoskeletal disorders: 500 mg initially, followed by 250 mg at 8 hour intervals as needed. Maximum daily dose is 1250 mg.

*Use in children over 50 kg:* In juvenile rheumatoid arthritis, the dosage is as the adult dose in rheumatoid arthritis.

*Use in the elderly:* Use adult doses, but with caution when high doses are required. A reduction in dosage may be necessary if there is impaired renal function.

*Dosage in patients with renal impairment:* Use with caution if renal impairment is significant. Do not use if creatinine clearance is less than 20 ml/minute.

*Contra-indications:* Active peptic ulceration. Hypersensitivity to naproxen or naproxen sodium formulations. Since the potential exists for cross-sensitivity reactions, naproxen should not be given to patients in whom aspirin or other non-steroidal anti-inflammatory/analgesic drugs induce asthma, rhinitis, or urticaria.

*Special warnings and special precautions for use:* Give under closee supervision to patients with a history of gastrointestinal disease. GI bleeding may occur.

Bronchospasm may be precipitated in patients with, or with a history of, bronchial asthma or allergic disease. Naproxen decreases platelet aggregation and prolongs bleeding time. Mild peripheral oedema may occur.

Patients with compromised cardiac function may be at greater risk of sodium retention. Use with great caution in patients with significantly impaired renal function and monitor renal function if given. Use with caution in patients with impaired hepatic function.

*Interactions with other medicaments and other forms of interaction:* Patients receiving hydantoin, anticoagulants or highly protein bound sulphonamides should be observed for signs of overdosage due to naproxen protein binding.

The natriuretic action of frusemide may be inhibited, as may the renal clearance of lithium.

The antihypertensive effect of propranolol and other beta blockers may also be reduced.

Probenecid given concurrently increases naproxen plasma levels and extends its half life.

Tubular secretion of methotrexate has been reported to be reduced in animal models, so increasing methotrexate toxicity; therefore caution is advised.

Naproxen may interfere with some tests for 17-ketogenic steroids or assays for urinary 5-hydroxyindoleacetic acid.

*Pregnancy and lactation:* Teratology studies in rats and rabbits, at high doses, have not produced evidence of fetal damage with naproxen. As with other drugs of this type, naproxen delays parturition in animals (the relevance of this finding to human patients is unknown) and also affects the human fetal cardiovascular system (closure of the ductus arteriosus). Balance possible risks against benefit to the mother and fetus especially in the first and third trimesters.

Should be avoided in patients who are breast feeding.

*Effects on ability to drive and use machines:* If CNS side effects such as headache and insomnia should occur (most likely at high doses), patients should be warned to assess their ability to drive or operate machinery.

*Undesirable effects:*

*Gastrointestinal:* The more frequent reactions are nausea, vomiting, abdominal discomfort and epigastric distress. More serious reactions which may occur occasionally are gastrointestinal bleeding and peptic ulceration (sometimes with haemorrhage and perforation).

*Dermatological hypersensitivity:* Skin rashes, urticaria, angio-oedema. Anaphylactic reactions to naproxen and naproxen sodium formulations and eosinophilic pneumonitis may occur rarely.

*CNS:* Headache, insomnia, inability to concentrate and cognitive dysfunction have been reported.

*Haematological:* Thrombocytopenia, granulocytopenia, aplastic anaemia and haemolytic anaemia may occur rarely.

*Other:* Tinnitus, hearing impairment, vertigo, mild peripheral oedema. Jaundice, fatal hepatitis, renal effects (glomerular nephritis, interstitial nephritis, nephrotic syndrome, haematuria, renal papillary necrosis, and renal failure) and ulcerative stomatitis have been reported rarely.

*Overdose:*

*Signficant overdosage may be characterised by:* Headache, tinnitus, drowsiness, indigestion, nausea, vomiting, tachycardia, hypoprothrombinaemia, and renal dysfunction.

*Emergency procedure: supportive and symptomatic:* The stomach should be emptied by lavage or inducing emesis. Activated charcoal may be given. Further treatment is symptomatic.

## Pharmacological properties

*Pharmacodynamic properties:* Naproxen is a non-steroidal anti-inflammatory agent (NSAID) with analgesic and antipyretic properties. It inhibits prostaglandin synthesis, as do other non-steroidal anti-inflammatory agents. As with other agents, however, the exact mechanism of its anti-inflammatory action is not known.

*Pharmacokinetic properties:* Nycopren is an enteric-coated tablet with an acid resistant film, and will pass through the stomach without disintergrating. In the intestine, the coating dissolves and naproxen is absorbed.

Complete absorption of Nycopren occurs, commencing 1–2 hours after ingestion. The peak plasma level occurs after 4–6 hours depending upon food intake. More than 99% of the drug is protein-bound, with only a small amount being distributed to the tissues.

The half-life is between 10–17 hours, and averages 13 hours; this being virtually independent of dose. Nycopren is metabolised mainly by demethylation and conjugation, and is excreted in the urine (95%), mostly as inactive metabolites, with 10% being unchanged naproxen. 1–2% is excreted in the faeces.

*Preclinical safety data:* The toxicological profile of naproxen is well known and documented, and no additional toxicity studies have been performed with Nycopren.

## Pharmaceutical particulars

*List of excipients:* Lactose, potato starch, povidone K-90, glycerolum, sodium starch glycolate, magnesium stearate, silicone antifoam 1510.

*The film coating contains:* Eudragit L12.5, Eudragit L30 D, Triacetin, Talc, Polyethylene glycol 600, Silicone antifoam 1510.

*Incompatibilities:* Not applicable.

*Shelf life:* 4 years, polypropylene container and blister pack.

*Special precautions for storage:* None. Should be kept in a well closed container.

*Nature and contents of container:* Aluminium foil and PVC blister pack – pack size 20, 56.

Polypropylene container and polyethylene cap – pack size 8, 56, 60, 84, 100 and 250.

*Instructions for use/handling:* Enteric coated tablets should be swallowed whole preferably with sufficient to drink.

## Marketing authorisation numbers
250 mg    4517/0009
500 mg    4517/0010

**Date of approval/revision of SPC**    January 1997.

**Legal category**    POM.

*\*Trade Mark*

# Organon Laboratories Limited
Cambridge Science Park
Milton Road
Cambridge CB4 4FL

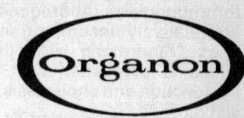

## DECA-DURABOLIN*

**Presentation** Deca Durabolin is a clear, sterile, oily, solution for injection containing Nandrolone Decanoate PhEur, 25 mg or 50 mg per ml.

Other constituents: Benzyl Alcohol PhEur, 0.1 ml and Arachis Oil PhEur, to 1.0 ml.

**Uses** For use in osteoporosis in post-menopausal women.

Established osteoporosis should have been diagnosed by the following parameters:

(i) crush or wedge fractures of the vertebrae
(ii) other osteoporotic fractures
(iii) established reduction in bone mineral content as measured by accepted BMC measurements.

**Dosage and administration**
*Dosage:* Post-menopausal women–50 mg every three weeks.

*Children:* There are no recommendations for use in children.

*Administration:* The duration of treatment depends on the clinical response and the possible occurrence of side-effects.

We would recommend that the effectiveness of therapy be monitored with the appropriate methods for osteoporosis on a 6-12 monthly basis.

Deca-Durabolin should be administered by deep intramuscular injection.

**Contra-indications, warnings, etc.** *Contra-indications:* Pregnancy. Known or suspected carcinoma of prostate or mammary carcinoma in the male.

*Use in pregnancy and lactation:* This medicine is contraindicated during pregnancy because of possible masculinization of the foetus. There are insufficient data on the use of this medicine during breast-feeding to assess potential harm to the infant or a possible influence on milk production.

*Warnings and precautions:* If signs of virilisation develop, discontinuation of the treatment should be considered.

Patients, especially the elderly, with the following conditions should be monitored: Latent or overt cardiac failure, renal dysfunction, hypertension, epilepsy or migraine (or a history of these conditions), since anabolic steroids may occasionally induce sodium and water retention;

Incomplete statural growth, since anabolic steroids in high dosages may accelerate epiphyseal closure;

Skeletal metastases, since anabolic steroids may induce hypercalcaemia and hypercalciuria in these patients;

Liver dysfunction.

*Effects on ability drive and use machines:* None known.

*Interactions:* Anabolic steroids may improve the glucose tolerance and decrease the need for insulin or other antidiabetic drugs in diabetics.

*Overdosage:* The acute toxicity of nandrolone decanoate in animals is very low. There are no reports of acute overdosage with Deca-Durabolin in the human.

*Adverse reactions:* Deca-Durabolin at the *recommended* dosages is unlikely to produce virilising effects.

High dosages, prolonged treatment and/or too frequent administration may cause:

Virilisation which appears in sensitive women as hoarseness, acne, hirsutism and increase of libido; in prepubertal boys as an increased frequency of erections and phallic enlargement, and in girls as an increase of pubic hair and clitoral hypertrophy. Hoarseness may be the first symptom of vocal change which may end in long-lasting, sometimes irreversible deepening of the voice;

Amenorrhoea and inhibition of spermatogenesis; Premature epiphyseal closure;

Sodium and water retention.

Abnormal liver function tests have been reported in patients treated with (high doses) of Deca-Durabolin. Liver tumours have been reported.

Liver tumours have been reported occasionally on prolonged treatment with orally active C17-alpha alkylated anabolic steroids. A relationship between liver tumours and non-C17-alkylated injectable ster-

oids, such as nandrolone esters, appears to be highly unlikely, but cannot be absolutely excluded.

**Pharmaceutical precautions** Protect from light. Store below 25°C.

**Legal category** POM.

**Package quantities** *25 mg per ml:* 1 ml ampoules in carton of 1 and 1 ml ampoules in cartons of 3. *50 mg per ml:* 1 ml ampoules in carton of 1 and 1 ml ampoules in cartons of 3

**Further information** Nandrolone is chemically related to testosterone and shows enhanced anabolic and a reduced androgenic activity.

In humans Deca-Durabolin has been shown to positively influence calcium metabolism and to increase bone mass in osteoporosis.

Androgenic effects (e.g. virilisation) are relatively uncommon at the recommended dosages. Nandrolone lacks the C17 alpha-alkyl group which is associated with the occurrence of liver dysfunction and cholestasis.

Nandrolone decanoate is slowly released from the injection site into the blood with a half-life of 6 days. The ester is rapidly hydrolysed to nandrolone in the blood with a half-life of one hour or less. The half-life for the combined process of hydrolysis of nandrolone decanoate and of distribution and elimination of nandrolone is 4.3 hours.

Nandrolone is metabolised by the liver. 19-norandrosterone, 19-noretiocholanolone and 19-norepiandrosterone have been identified as metabolites in the urine. It is not known whether these metabolites display a pharmacological action.

**Product licence numbers**
25 mg/ml    0065/5005R
50 mg/ml    0065/5063R.

## DECA-DURABOLIN 100*

**Qualitative and quantitative composition** Each ml of Deca-Durabolin 100 contains 100 mg nandrolone decanoate BP.

**Pharmaceutical form** 1 ml clear PhEur I type ampoules containing a sterile pale yellow oily liquid intended for intramuscular injection in human beings.

**Clinical particulars**

*Therapeutic indications:* Anaemia of chronic renal failure. Aplastic anaemia. Anaemia due to cytotoxic therapy

*Posology and method of administration:*
*Dosage: Adults:*
Anaemia of chronic renal failure. Males: 200 mg weekly. Females: 100 mg weekly.
Aplastic anaemia. The usual dose is 50 to 150 mg weekly.
Anaemia due to cytotoxic therapy.
The usual dose is 200 mg weekly commencing 2 weeks prior to the course of cytotoxic therapy. This treatment should be continued throughout cytotoxic therapy and thereafter during the recovery period until the blood count has returned to normal.
**NB:** Treatment with Deca-Durabolin 100 does not substitute for other therapeutic measures.
The onset of a therapeutic effect may vary widely among patients. If no satisfactory response occurs after 3-6 months of treatment, administration should be discontinued.
After a satisfactory improvement or a normalisation of the red blood picture has been obtained, treatment should be withdrawn gradually on the basis of regular monitoring of the haematological parameters. Should a relapse occur at any time whilst the dose is being reduced or after stopping the treatment, re-institution of therapy should be considered.
*Children:* There is insufficient clinical experience to permit specific recommendations
*Administration:* Deep Intramuscular injection

*Contra-indications:* Pregnancy. Known or suspected carcinoma of prostate or mammary carcinoma in males.

*Special warnings and special precautions for use:* The recommended doses should not be exceeded. If signs of virilisation develop, discontinuation of the treat-

ment should be considered, preferably in consultation with the patient.

It is recommended that patients with any of the following conditions should be monitored:

latent or overt cardiac failure, renal dysfunction, hypertension or migraine (or a history of these conditions), since anabolic steroids may occasionally induce fluid retention;

incomplete statural growth, since anabolic steroids in high dosages may accelerate epiphyseal closure; skeletal metastases of breast carcinoma. In these patients hypercalcaemia may develop both spontaneously and as a result of anabolic steroid therapy. The latter can be indicative of a positive tumour response to the treatment. Nevertheless, the hypercalcaemia should first be treated appropriately and after restoration of normal calcium levels the therapy can be resumed;

liver dysfunction.

The use of anabolic steroids to enhance athletic ability may carry severe risks to the user's health and should be discouraged.

*Interaction with other medicaments and other forms of interaction:* Anabolic steroids may improve glucose tolerance and decrease the need for insulin or other antidiabetic medicines in diabetes.

Although only one possible case of interaction with an oral anticoagulant has been observed, it is advisable to check the prothrombin time regularly when Deca-Durabolin 100 is used in conjunction with such an agent.

*Pregnancy and lactation:* This medicine is contraindicated during pregnancy because of possible masculinisation of the foetus. There are insufficient data on the use of this medicine during breast-feeding to assess potential harm to the infant or a possible influence on milk production.

*Effects on ability to drive and use of machines:* As far as is known Deca-Durabolin 100 has no effect on alertness and concentration.

*Undesirable effects:* The high dosages which are required to obtain a therapeutic effect in the indications mentioned may cause:
- Virilisation which appears in sensitive women as hoarseness, acne, hirsutism and increase of libido; in prepubertal boys as an increased frequency of erections and phallic enlargement, and in girls as an increase of pubic hair and clitoral hypertrophy. Hoarseness may be the first symptom of vocal change which may end in a long-lasting, sometimes irreversible deepening of the voice
- Amenorrhoea
- Inhibition of spermatogenesis
- Premature epiphyseal closure
- Fluid retention
- Occasionally, abnormal values in some liver function tests. These changes appear to be reversible after completion of the treatment course.

*Overdosage:* The acute toxicity of nandrolone decanoate in animals is very low. There are no reports of acute overdosage with Deca-Durabolin 100 in man.

**Pharmacological properties**

*Pharmacodynamic properties:* Deca-Durabolin 100 is a high dosage form of nandrolone decanoate designed especially for adjuvant therapy in the treatment of certain blood disorders. Nandrolone, the pharmacologically active substance of the preparation, is chemically related to testosterone. Compared to testosterone, it has an enhanced anabolic and a reduced androgenic activity. This has been demonstrated in animal bioassays and explained by receptor binding studies. The low androgenicity of nandrolone is confirmed in clinical use.

In animals, nandrolone decanoate possesses an erythropoiesis-stimulating effect probably by directly stimulating the haematopoietic stem cells in the bone marrow and by increasing the release of erythropoietin. It also affords protection against the bone marrow depression caused by cytotoxic agents.

In the human, Deca-Durabolin 100 stimulates erythropoiesis as demonstrated by rises in the red blood cell mass, and in the haemoglobin and haematocrit values. This effect is utilised therapeutically in the treatment of anaemia due to a decreased production of erythropoietin, bone marrow depression induced by chemotherapy, or hypoplasia of the stem cells in the bone marrow. In the latter condition (e.g. aplastic anaemia) the erythropoiesis response is frequently accompanied by a positive effect on leucopoiesis and thrombopoiesis. Androgenic effects (e.g. virilisation) are relatively uncommon at the recommended dosages. Nandrolone lacks the C17alpha-alkyl group which is associated with the occurrence of liver dysfunction and cholestasis.

*Pharmacokinetic properties:* Nandrolone decanoate is slowly released from the injection site into the blood with a half-life of 6 days. In the blood, the ester is rapidly hydrolysed to nandrolone with a half-life of one hour or less. The half-life for the combined process of hydrolysis of nandrolone decanoate and of distribution and elimination of nandrolone is 4.3 hours. Nandrolone is metabolised by the liver. 19-norandrosterone, 19-noretiocholanolone and 19-norepiandrosterone have been identified as metabolites in the urine. It is not known whether these metabolites display a pharmacological action

Preclinical safety data: Not applicable

**Pharmaceutical particulars**

*List of excipients:* Benzyl Alcohol PhEur, Arachis Oil PhEur.

*Incompatibilities:* None known

*Shelf life:* 5 years

*Special precautions for storage:* Protect from light. Store at room temperature 15-25˚C.

*Nature and contents of containers:* 1 ml clear glass ampoule with ring snap neck.

*Instructions for use/handling:* Not applicable.

**Marketing authorisation number**    0065/0036

**Date of approval/revision**    June 1995

**Legal category**    POM

## DEXAMETHASONE INJECTION

**Presentation** Each ml aqueous solution contains 5 mg Dexamethasone Sodium Phosphate BP, equivalent to approximately 4 mg dexamethasone.
*Other ingredients: 1 ml ampoule*–Glycerol PhEur, Disodium Edetate PhEur, Water for Injections PhEur.
*2 ml vials*–Glycerol PhEur, Disodium Edetate PhEur, Methylparaben BP, Propylparaben BP and Water for injections PhEur.

**Uses** Dexamethasone injection can be used for all forms of general and local glucocorticoid injection therapy and all acute conditions in which intravenous glucocorticoids may be life-saving.

**Dosage and administration** *Dosage: N.B.* All dosages are expressed as mg dexamethasone sodium phosphate.

In general, glucocorticoid dosage depends on the severity of the condition and response of the patient. Under certain circumstances, for instance in stress, extra dosage adjustments may be necessary. If no favourable response is noted within a couple of days, glucocorticoid therapy should be discontinued.

*Adults:* Once the disease is under control the dosage should be reduced or tapered off to the lowest suitable level under continuous monitoring and observation of the patient. This should be done by administering one early morning dose, daily (or preferably every other morning), of an oral glucocorticoid with a shorter biological half-life than dexamethasone e.g. prednisolone.

For acute life-threatening situations (e.g. anaphylaxis, acute severe asthma) substantially higher dosages may be needed. Cerebral oedema (adults): initial dose 10–20 mg i.v. followed by 6 mg i.v. or i.m. every 6 hours, until a satisfactory result has been obtained. In brain surgery these dosages may be necessary until several days after the operation. Thereafter, the dosage has to be tapered off gradually. Increase of intracranial pressure associated with brain tumours can be counteracted by continuous treatment.

For local treatment, the following dosages can be recommended:

intra-articularly: 2-4 mg large joints; 0.8–1 mg small joints; intrabursally: 2-4 mg; in tendon sheaths: 0.4–1 mg.

The frequency of these injections may vary from every 3-5 days to every 2-3 weeks.

For rectal drip in cases of ulcerative colitis: 5 mg diluted in 120 ml saline.

*Suggested doses for children:* Dosage requirements are variable and may have to be changed according to individual needs. Usually 0.25 mg/kg to 0.50 mg/kg of body weight daily.

*Administration:* Dexamethasone may be administered intravenously, subcutaneously, intramuscularly, by local injection or as a rectal drip. For administration by intravenous infusion: see section on compatibility with infusion fluids. With intravenous administration high plasma levels can be obtained rapidly.

Rapid intravenous injection of massive doses of glucocorticoids may sometimes cause cardiovascular collapse; the injection should therefore be given slowly over a period of several minutes.

Intra-articular injections should be given under strictly aseptic conditions.

Discontinuation of prolonged therapy should be carried out by gradual reduction of dosage and under strict medical supervision, since withdrawal may result in acute exacerbation of the disease and acute adrenocortical insufficiency.

*Use with infusion fluids:* Dexamethasone has been shown to retain its potency for at least 24 hours at room temperature, and in daylight conditions, when diluted with one of the following infusion fluids: sodium chloride 0.9%; anhydrous glucose 5%; invert sugar 10%; sorbitol 5%; Ringer's solution; Hartmann's solution (Ringer-lactate); Rheomacrodex; Haemaccel.

Using these infusion fluids, Dexamethasone can also be injected directly into the infusion line without causing precipitation of the ingredients. Direct injection into the infusion line is also possible with the following infusion fluids: mannitol 10%; Vamin N. See also *Precautions and warnings.*

**Contra-indications, warings, etc**
*Contra-indications:* Systemic infection unless specific anti-infective therapy is employed.

Hypersensitivity to any ingredient. Local injection of a glucocorticoid is contraindicated in bacteraemia and systemic fungal infections, unstable joints, infection at the injection site e.g. septic arthritis resulting from gonorrhoea or tuberculosis.

*Use during pregnancy and breast-feeding:* Intrauterine growth retardation in the foetus and a small increased risk of cleft palate have been reported. Hypoadrenalism may occur in the neonate.

When corticosteroids are essential however, patients with normal pregnancies may be treated as though they were in the non-gravid state. Patients with pre-eclampsia or fluid retention require close monitoring

Corticosteroids are excreted in small amounts in breast milk and infants of mothers taking pharmacological doses of steroids should be monitored carefully for signs of adrenal suppression.

*Precautions and warnings:* **A patient information leaflet should be supplied with this product.** Undesirable effects may be minimised by using the lowest effective dose for the minimum period, and by administering the daily requirement as a single morning dose or whenever possible as a single morning dose on alternative days. Frequent patient review is required to appropriately titrate the dose against disease activity.

After parenteral administration of glucocorticoids serious anaphylactoid reactions, such as glottis oedema, urticaria and bronchospasm, have occasionally occurred, particularly in patients with a history of allergy. If such an anaphylactoid reaction occurs, the following measures are recommended: immediate slow intravenous injection of 0.1–0.5 ml of adrenaline (solution of 1:1000: 0.1–0.5 mg adrenaline dependent on body weight), intravenous administration of aminophylline and artificial respiration if necessary.

*Adrenal suppression:* Adrenal cortical atrophy develops during prolonged therapy and may persist for years after stopping treatment. Withdrawal of corticosteroids after prolonged therapy must therefore always be gradual to avoid acute adrenal insufficiency, being tapered off over weeks or months according to the dose and duration of treatment. During prolonged therapy any intercurrent illness, trauma or surgical procedure will require a temporary increase in dosage; if corticosteroids have been stopped following prolonged therapy they may need to be temporarily reintroduced.

**Patients should carry 'Steroid treatment' cards which give clear guidance on the precautions to be taken to minimise risk and which provide details of prescriber, drug, dosage and the duration of treatment.**

*Anti-inflammatory/immunosuppressive effects and infection:* Suppression of the inflammatory response and immune function increases the susceptibility to infections and their severity. The clinical presentation may often be atypical, and serious infections such as septicaemia and tuberculosis may be masked and may reach an advanced stage before being recognised.

Appropriate antimicrobial therapy should accompany glucocorticoid therapy when necessary e.g. in tuberculosis and viral and fungal infections of the eye.

*Chickenpox is of particular concern since this normally minor illness may be fatal in immunosuppressed patients.* Patients (or parents of children) without a definite history of chickenpox should be advised to avoid close personal contact with chickenpox or herpes zoster and if exposed they should seek urgent medical attention. Passive immunisation with varicella zoster immunoglobulin (VZIG) is needed by

exposed non-immune patients who are receiving systemic corticosteroids or who have used them within the previous 3 months; this should be given within 10 days of exposure to chickenpox. If a diagnosis of chickenpox is confirmed, the illness warrants specialist care and urgent treatment. Corticosteroids should not be stopped and the dose may need to be increased.

Live vaccines should not be given to individuals with impaired immune responsiveness. The antibody response to other vaccines may be diminished.

*Special precautions:* Particular care is required when considering the use of systemic corticosteroids in patients with the following conditions and frequent patient monitoring is necessary.

a.  Osteoporosis (post-menopausal females are particularly at risk).
b.  Hypertension or congestive heart failure.
c.  Existing or previous history of severe affective disorders (especially previous steroid psychosis).
d.  Diabetes mellitus (or a family history of diabetes).
e.  History of tuberculosis since glucocorticoids may induce reactivation.
f.  Glaucoma (or a family history of glaucoma).
g.  Previous corticosteroid-induced myopathy.
h.  Liver failure.
i.  Renal insufficiency.
j.  Epilepsy.
k.  Gastrio-intestinal ulceration.
l.  Migraine
m.  Certain parasitic infestations in particular amoebiasis.
n.  Incomplete statural growth since glucocorticoids on prolonged administration may accelerate epiphyseal closure
o.  Patients with Cushing's syndrome

*Use in children:* Corticosteroids cause dose-related growth retardation in infancy, childhood and adolescence, which may be irreversible.

*Use in the elderly:* The common adverse effects of systemic corticosteroids may be associated with more serious consequences in old age, especially osteoporosis, hypertension, hypokalaemia, diabetes, susceptibility to infection and thinning of the skin. Close clinical supervision is required to avoid life-threatening reactions.

In the treatment of conditions such as tendinitis or tenosynovitis care should be taken to inject into the space between the tendon sheath and the tendon as cases of ruptured tendon have been reported.

*Adverse reactions:* Local adverse reactions include post-injection flare, and a painless destruction of the joint reminiscent of Charcots arthropathy especially with repeated intra-articular injection. The incidence of predictable undesirable effects, including hypothalamic-pituitary-adrenal suppression correlates with the relative potency of the drug, dosage, timing of administration and the duration of treatment. Cases of ruptured tendon have been reported. (see *Precautions and warnings*).

Local injections of glucocorticoid may produce systemic effects.

*Endocrine/metabolic:* Suppression of the hypothalamic-pituitary-adrenal axis, premature epiphyseal closure, growth suppression in infancy, childhood and adolescence, menstrual irregularity and amenorrhoea. Cushiongoid faces, hirsutism, weight gain, impaired carbohydrate tolerance with increased requirement for anti-diabetic therapy. Negative protein and calcium balance. Increased appetite.

*Anti-inflammatory and Immunosuppressive effects:* Increased susceptibility and severity of infections with suppression of clinical symptoms and signs. Diminished lymphoid tissue and immune response. Opportunistic infections, recurrence of dormant tuberculosis and decreased responsiveness to vaccination and skin tests (see *Precautions and warnings*).

*Musculoskeletal:* Osteoporosis, vertebral and long bone fractures, avascular osteonecrosis, tendon rupture. Proximal myopathy.

*Fluid and electrolyte disturbance:* Sodium and water retention, hypertension, potassium loss, hypokalaemic alkalosis.

*Neuropsychiatric:* Psychological dependence, depression, insomnia, and aggravation of schizophrenia. Increased intra-cranial pressure with papilloedema in children (pseudotumour cerebri), usually after treatment withdrawal. Aggravation of epilepsy. Psychic disturbances ranging from euphoria to frank psychotic manifestations.

*Ophthalmic:* Increased intra-ocular pressure, glaucoma, papilloedema, posterior subcapsular cataracts, corneal or scleral thinning, exacerbation of opthalmic viral or fungal diseases.

*Gastrointestinal:* Dyspepsia, peptic ulceration with perforation and haemorrhage, acute pancreatitis, candidiasis.

*Dermatological:* Impaired healing, skin atrophy, bruising, telangiectasia, striae, increased sweating and acne.

*General:* Hypersensitivity including anaphylaxis, has been reported. Leucocytosis. Thromboembolism.

A transient burning or tingling sensation mainly in the perineal area following intravenous injection of large doses of corticosteroid phosphates.

*Withdrawal symptoms and signs:* Too rapid a reduction of corticosteroid dosage following prolonged treatment can lead to acute adrenal insufficiency, hypotension and death. (see *Precautions and warnings*)

A 'withdrawal syndrome' may also occur including, fever, myalgia, arthralgia, rhinitis, conjunctivitis, painful itchy skin nodules and loss of weight.

*Interactions:* Rifampicin, rifabutin, ephedrine, carbamazepine, phenylbutazone, phenobarbitone, phenytoin, primidone, and aminoglutethimide enhance the metabolism of corticosteroids and its therapeutic effects may be reduced.

The desired effects of hypoglycaemic agents (including insulin), anti-hypertensives, cardiac glycosides and diuretics are antagonised by corticosteroids, and the hypokalaemic effects of acetazolamide, loop diuretics, thiazide diuretics and carbenoxolone are enhanced.

The efficacy of coumarin anticoagulants may be enhanced by concurrent corticosteroid therapy and close monitoring of the INR or prothrombin time is required to avoid spontaneous bleeding.

The renal clearance of salicylates is increased by corticosteroids and steroid withdrawal may result in salicylate intoxication.

There may be interaction with salicylates in patients with hypoprothrombinaemia.

*Overdosage:* It is difficult to define an excessive dose of a corticosteroid as the therapeutic dose will vary according to the indication and patient requirements. Massive i.v. corticosteroid doses given as a pulse in emergencies are relatively free from hazardous effects.

Exaggeration of corticosteroid related adverse effects may occur. Treatment should be asymptomatic and supportive as necessary.

**Pharmaceutical precautions** Store below 25°C, protected from light. Do not freeze ampoules.

**Legal category** POM

**Package quantities** Boxes of 10 x 2 ml vials containing Dexamethasone Sodium Phosphate BP 5 mg/ml equivalent to Dexamethasone (4 mg/ml).

Boxes of 10 x 1 ml ampoules. Each ampoule containing 5 mg/ml Dexamethasone Sodium Phosphate BP.

**Further information** Dexamethasone is a synthetic adrenocorticoid with approximately a 7 times higher anti-inflammatory potency than prednisolone and 30 times that of hydrocortisone. Adrenocorticoids act on the HPA at specific receptors on the plasma membrane. On other tissues the adrenocorticoids diffuse across cell membranes and complex with specific cytoplasmic receptors which enter the cell nucleus and stimulate protein synthesis. Adrenocorticoids have anti-inflammatory and immunosuppressive properties. Dexamethasone has only minor mineralocorticoid activities and does therefore, not induce water and sodium retention.

After administration of dexamethasone injection, dexamethasone sodium phosphate is rapidly hydrolysed to dexamethasone. After an iv dose of 20 mg dexamethasone plasma levels peak within 5 minutes. Dexamethasone is bound (up to 77%) by plasma proteins, mainly albumin. There is a high uptake of dexamethasone by the liver, kidney and adrenal glands. Metabolism in the liver is slow and excretion is mainly in the urine, largely as unconjugated steroids. The plasma half life is 3.5-4.5 hours but as the effects outlast the significant plasma concentrations of steroids the plasma half-life is of little relevance and the use of biological half life is more applicable. The biological half life of dexamethasone is 36-54 hours, therefore dexamethasone is especially suitable in conditions where continuous glucocorticoid action is desirable.

**Product licence numbers**
2 ml/vial          0065/5013R
1 ml ampoule          0065/0106R

# DEXAMETHASONE TABLETS BP

**Qualitative and quantitative composition** 500 microgram tablet contains 500 micrograms Dexamethasone PhEur. 2.0 mg tablet contains 2.0 mg Dexamethasone PhEur.

**Pharmaceutical form** Tablet

**Clinical particulars**

*Therapeutic indications:* Indicated in a wide variety of disorders amenable to glucocorticoid therapy, as well as an adjunct in the control of cerebral oedema.

*Posology and method of administration:* In general, glucocorticoid dosage depends on the severity of the condition and response of the patient. Under certain circumstances, for instance in stress, and changed clinical picture, extra dosage adjustments may be necessary. If no favourable response is noted within a couple of days, glucocorticoid therapy should be discontinued.

*Adults:* Usually, daily oral dosages of 0.5–10 mg are sufficient. In some patients higher dosages may be temporarily required to control the disease. Once the disease is under control the dosage should be reduced or tapered off to the lowest suitable level under continuous monitoring and observation of the patient. This should be done by administering one early morning dose, daily (or preferably every other morning), of an oral glucocorticoid with a shorter biological half-life than dexamethasone e.g. prednisolone.

For a short dexamethasone suppression test, 1 mg dexamethasone is given at 11 p.m. and plasma cortisol measured the next morning. Patients who do not show a decrease in cortisol can be exposed to a longer test: 500 micrograms dexamethasone is given at 6 hourly intervals for 48 hours followed by 2 mg every 6 hours for a further 48 hours. 24 hour-urine collections are made before, during and at the end of the test for determination of 17-hydroxycorticosteroids.

Discontinuation of prolonged therapy should be carried out by gradual reduction of dosage and under strict medical supervision, since withdrawal may result in acute exacerbation of the disease and acute adrenocortical insufficiency.

*Children:* 0.01-0.1 mg/kg of body weight daily.

Dosage of glucocorticoids should be adjusted on the basis of the individual patient's response.

*Contra-indications:* Systemic infection unless specific anti-infective therapy is employed. Hypersensitivity to any ingredient. In general no contra-indications apply in conditions where the use of glucocorticoids may be life saving.

*Special warnings and special precautions for use:* **A patient information leaflet should be supplied with this product.** Undesirable effects may be minimised by using the lowest effective dose for the minimum period, and by administering the daily requirement as a single morning dose or whenever possible as a single morning dose on alternative days. Frequent patient review is required to appropriately titrate the dose against disease activity. (see dosage section).

*Adrenal suppression:* Adrenal cortical atrophy develops during prolonged therapy and may persist for years after stopping treatment. Withdrawal of corticosteroids after prolonged therapy must therefore always be gradual to avoid acute adrenal insufficiency, being tapered off over weeks or months according to the dose and duration of treatment. During prolonged therapy any intercurrent illness, trauma or surgical procedure will require a temporary increase in dosage; if corticosteroids have been stopped following prolonged therapy they may need to be temporarily reintroduced.

**Patients should carry 'Steroid treatment' cards which give clear guidance on the precautions to be taken to minimise risk and which provide details of prescriber, drug, dosage and the duration of treatment.**

*Anti-inflammatory/Immunosuppressive effects and Infection:* Suppression of the inflammatory response and immune function increases the susceptibility to infections and their severity. The clinical presentation may often be atypical, and serious infections such as septicaemia and tuberculosis may be masked and may reach an advanced stage before being recognised.

Appropriate anti-microbial therapy should accompany glucocorticoid therapy when necessary e.g. in tuberculosis and viral and fungal infections of the eye.

*Chickenpox* is of particular concern since this normally minor illness may be fatal in immunosuppressed patients. Patients (or parents of children) without a definite history of chickenpox should be advised to avoid close personal contact with chickenpox or herpes zoster and if exposed they should seek urgent medical attention. Passive immunisation with varicella zoster immunoglobulin (VZIG) is needed by exposed non-immune patients who are receiving systemic corticosteroids or who have used them within the previous 3 months; this should be given within 10 days of exposure to chickenpox. *If a diagnosis of chickenpox is confirmed, the illness warrants specialist care and urgent treatment. Corticosteroids should not be stopped and the dose may need to be increased.*

Live vaccines should not be given to individuals with impaired immune responsiveness. The antibody response to other vaccines may be diminished.

Particular care is required when considering the use of systemic corticosteroids in patients with the following conditions and frequent patient monitoring is necessary.

a. Osteoporosis (post-menopausal females are particularly at risk).
b. Hypertension or congestive heart failure.
c. Existing or previous history of severe affective disorders (especially previous steroid psychosis).
d. Diabetes mellitus (or a family history of diabetes).
e. History of tuberculosis.
f. Glaucoma (or a family history of glaucoma).
g. Previous corticosteroid-induced myopathy.
h. Liver failure.
i. Renal insufficiency.
j. Epilepsy.
k. Peptic ulceration.
l. Migraine
m. Certain parasitic infestations in particular amoebiasis
n. Incomplete natural growth since glucocorticoids on prolonged administration may accelerate epiphyseal closure.

*Use in children:* Corticosteroids cause dose-related growth retardation in infancy, childhood and adolescence, which may be irreversible.

*Use in the elderly:* The common adverse effects of systemic corticosteroids may be associated with more serious consequences in old age, especially osteoporosis, hypertension, hypokalaemia, diabetes, susceptibility to infection and thinning of the skin. Close clinical supervision is required to avoid life-threatening reactions.

After administration of glucocorticoids serious anaphylactoid reactions such as glottis oedema, urticaria and bronchospasm have occasionally occurred particularly in patients with a history of allergy.

If such an anaphylactoid reaction occurs, the following measures are recommended: immediate slow intravenous injection of 0.1-0.5 ml of adrenaline (solution of 1:1000: 0.1-0.5 mg adrenaline dependent on body weight), intravenous administration of aminophylline and artificial respiration if necessary.

*Interaction with other medicaments and other forms of interaction:* Rifampicin, rifabutin, carbamazepine, phenobarbitone, phenytoin, primidone, and aminoglutethimide enhance the metabolism of corticosteroids and its therapeutic effects may be reduced.

The desired effects of hypoglycaemic agents (including insulin), anti-hypertensives and diuretics are antagonised by corticosteroids, and the hypokalaemic effects of acetazolamide, loop diuretics, thiazide diuretics and carbenoxolone are enhanced.

The efficacy of coumarin anticoagulants may be enhanced by concurrent corticosteroid therapy and close monitoring of the INR or prothrombin time is required to avoid spontaneous bleeding.

The renal clearance of salicylates is increased by corticosteroids and steroid withdrawal may result in salicylate intoxication.

Patients taking NSAIDs should be monitored since the incidence and/or severity of gastro-intestinal ulceration may increase.

Antacids, especially those containing magnesium trisilicate have been reported to impair the gastrointestinal absorption of glucocorticoid steroids. Therefore, doses of one agent should be spaced as far as possible from the other.

*Pregnancy and lactation:* There is evidence of harmful effects on pregnancy in animals. Intra-uterine growth retardation in the foetus and a small increased risk of cleft palate have been reported. Hypoadrenalism may occur in the neonate.

When corticosteroids are essential however, patients with normal pregnancies may be treated as though they were in the non-gravid state. Patients with pre-eclampsia or fluid retention require close monitoring

Corticosteroids are excreted in small amounts in breast milk and infants of mothers taking pharmacological doses of steroids should be monitored carefully for signs of adrenal suppression.

Mothers taking high doses of glucocorticoids should be advised not to breast feed.

*Effects on ability to drive and use machines:* None known

*Undesirable effects:* The incidence of predictable undesirable effects, including hypothalamic-pituitary-adrenal suppression correlates with the relative potency of the drug, dosage, timing of administration and the duration of treatment. (see *Special warnings and precautions for use*).

*Endocrine/metabolic:* Suppression of the hypothalamic-pituitary-adrenal axis, growth suppression in infancy, childhood and adolescence, menstrual irregularity and amenorrhoea. Cushingoid faces, hirsutism, weight gain, premature epiphyseal closure, impaired carbohydrate tolerance with increased requirement for anti-diabetic therapy. Negative protein and calcium balance. Increased appetite.

*Anti-inflammatory and immunosuppressive effects:* Increased susceptibility and severity of infections with suppression of clinical symptoms and signs, opportunistic infections, recurrence of dormant tuberculosis. Decreased responsiveness to vaccination and skin tests (see *Special warnings and precautions for use*).

*Musculoskeletal:* Osteoporosis, vertebral and long bone fractures, avascular osteonecrosis, tendon rupture. Proximal myopathy.

*Fluid and electrolyte disturbance:* Sodium and water retention, hypertension, potassium loss, hypokalaemic alkalosis.

*Neuropsychiatric:* Psychological dependence, depression, insomnia, and aggravation of schizophrenia. Increased intra-cranial pressure with papilloedema in children (pseudotumour cerebri), usually after treatment withdrawal. Aggravation of epilepsy. Psychic disturbances ranging from euphoria to frank psychotic manifestations.

*Ophthalmic:* Increased intra-ocular pressure, glaucoma, papilloedema, posterior subcapsular cataracts, corneal or scleral thinning, exacerbation of opthalmic viral or fungal diseases.

*Gastrointestinal:* Dyspepsia, peptic ulceration with perforation and haemorrhage, acute pancreatitis, candidiasis. Abdominal distension and vomiting.

*Dermatological:* Impaired healing, skin atrophy, bruising, telangiectasia, striae, acne.

*General:* Hypersensitivity including anaphylaxis, has been reported. Leucocytosis. Thromboembolism.

*Withdrawal symptoms and signs:* Too rapid a reduction of corticosteroid dosage following prolonged treatment can lead to acute adrenal insufficiency, hypotension and death. (see 'Special warnings and precautions for use').

A 'withdrawal syndrome' may also occur including, fever, myalgia, arthralgia, rhinitis, conjunctivitis, painful itchy skin nodules and loss of weight.

*Overdosage:* It is difficult to define an excessive dose of a corticosteroid as the therapeutic dose will vary according to indication and patient requirements. Exaggeration of corticosteroid related adverse effects may occur. Treatment should be asymptomatic and supportive as necessary.

### Pharmacological properties

*Pharmacodynamic properties:* Dexamethasone is a synthetic glucocorticoid whose anti-inflammatory potency is 7 times greater than prednisolone. Like other glucocorticoids, dexamethasone also has anti-allergic, antipyretic and immunosuppressive properties.

Dexamethasone has practically no water and salt-retaining properties and is, therefore, particularly suitable for the use in patients with cardiac failure or hypertension. Because of its long biological half-life (36-54 hours), dexamethasone is especially suitable in conditions where continuous glucocorticoid action is desired.

*Pharmacokinetic properties:* Corticosteroids, are, in general, readily absorbed from the gastro-intestinal tract. They are also well absorbed from sites of local application. Water-soluble forms of corticosteroids are given by intravenous injection for a rapid response; more prolonged effects are achieved using lipid-soluble forms of corticosteroids by intramuscular injection.

Corticosteroids are rapidly distributed to all body tissues. They cross the placenta and may be excreted in small amounts in breast milk.

Most corticosteroids in the circulation are extensively bound to plasma proteins, mainly to globulin and less so to albumin. The corticosteroid-binding globulin has high affinity but low binding capacity, while the albumin has low affinity but large binding capacity. The synthetic corticosteroids are less extensively protein bound than hydrocortisone (cortisol). They also tend to have longer half-lives.

Corticosteroids are metabolised mainly in the liver but also in the kidney, and are excreted in the urine. The slower metabolism of the synthetic corticosteroids with their lower protein-binding affinity may account for their increased potency compared with the natural corticosteroids.

*Preclinical safety data:* Not applicable

**Pharmaceutical particulars** *List of excipients:* 0.5 mg tablet Glycerol PhEur, Potato Starch PhEur, Magnesium Stearate PhEur, Talc PhEur and Lactose PhEur.

2 mg tablets Potato Starch PhEur, Propylene Glycol PhEur, Magnesium Stearate PhEur, and Lactose PhEur.

*Incompatibilities:* None known

*Shelf-life:* 5 years -when stored in polyethylene tampertainers. 3 years-when stored in polystyrene bottle

*Special precautions for storage:* Store below 25˚C protected from light

*Nature and contents of containers:* Polyethylene tampertainers with child resistant closures. Polystyrene bottles.

*Instructions for use/handling:* Not applicable

**Marketing authorisation numbers:** 0065/5044R and 0065/45R

**Date of approval/revision of SPC** May 1995

**Legal category** POM

## LIVIAL*

**Qualitative and quantitative composition** Each Livial tablet contains as active substance 2.5 mg of the steroid tibolone.

**Pharmaceutical form** Tablets for oral use.

### Clinical particulars

*Therapeutic indications:* In oestrogen deficiency states for the treatment of vasomotor symptoms (such as hot flushes and sweating), depressed mood, decreased libido and prevention of osteoporosis in women at risk of developing fractures.

However at present there is no established screening programme for determining women at risk of developing osteoporosis and osteoporotic fractures. Epidemiological studies suggest a number of individual risk factors which contribute to the development of postmenopausal osteoporosis. These include early menopause, family history of osteoporosis, thinness, small frame, cigarette use and recent prolonged systemic corticosteroid use. If several of these risk factors are present in a patient, consideration should be given to hormone replacement therapy.

*Posology and method of administration:* Adults and the elderly: Livial tablets should be swallowed without chewing, preferably at the same time of day.

The dosage is one tablet per day. Improvement of symptoms generally occurs within a few weeks, but optimal results are obtained when therapy is continued for at least 3 months. At the recommended dosage, Livial may be used uninterrupted for longer periods. For prevention of osteoporosis in postmenopausal women long term therapy (5-10 years) is required.

*Starting Livial:* For the treatment of vasomotor symptoms and the prevention of osteoporosis.

Women experiencing a natural menopause should commence treatment with Livial 12 months after their last natural bleed. If Livial is taken sooner than this irregular menstrual bleeding may occur.
Women experiencing a surgical menopause may commence treatment with Livial immediately
Women being treated with gonadotrophin releasing hormone (GnRH) analogues, for example, for endometriosis, may commence treatment with Livial immediately.

*Switching from another HRT preparation:* If changing from another HRT preparation the endometrium may already be stimulated, so induction of a withdrawal bleed with a progestogen is advisable.

*Missed pills:* A missed dose should be taken as soon as remembered, unless it is more than 12 hours overdue. In the latter case, the missed dose should be skipped and the next dose should be taken at the normal time.

*Children:* Not applicable.

*Contra-indications:*

– Hypersensitivity to the active ingredient or any of the constituents of the product.
– Pregnancy or lactation.
– Known or suspected hormone-dependent tumours.
– Cardiovascular or cerebrovascular disorders e.g. thrombophlebitis, thrombo-embolic processes, or a history of these conditions.
– Undiagnosed vaginal bleeding.
– Severe liver disorders.

*Special warnings and precautions for use:*

– Livial is not intended for contraceptive use.
– Risk-benefit should be considered when any of the following medical conditions exist:

liver disease or a history of this condition; hypercholesterolaemia

– Treatment should be discontinued if signs of thrombo-embolic processes occur, if results of liver function tests become abnormal, or if cholestatic jaundice appears.
– During prolonged treatment with steroids with hormonal activity, periodic medical examination is advisable.
– In women experiencing a natural menopause Livial should not be prescribed in the premenopause because, in view of the ovulation inhibition, cycle regularity may be disturbed.
– In postmenopausal women Livial does not stimulate the endometrium; the incidence of vaginal bleeding is no higher than that with placebo use. In women in whom some endogenous oestrogen is still produced, vaginal bleeding may occur during Livial therapy because of an apparently stimulated endometrium. Normally such a bleeding is of short duration. Bleeding commencing after three months of treatment or recurrent or persistent bleeding

should be appropriately investigated, however in most cases no apparent cause of the bleeding is found.
– In women changing from another form of hormonal substitution therapy to Livial therapy, it is always advisable to induce a withdrawal bleed with a progestogen, because also in these women the endometrium may be stimulated.
– Patients with any of the following conditions should be monitored:
– renal dysfunction, liver disease, epilepsy or migraine or a history of these conditions, since the use of steroids with hormonal activity may occasionally induce fluid retention;
– hypercholesterolaemia, since during Livial treatment changes in the serum lipid profile have been observed.
– impaired carbohydrate metabolism, since Livial may diminish glucose tolerance and increase the need for insulin or other antidiabetic drugs.

*Interaction with other medicaments and other forms of interaction:* No examples of interactions between Livial and other medicines have been reported in clinical practice. However, the following potential interactions should be considered on a theoretical basis:

Enzyme inducing compounds such as barbiturates, carbamazepine, hydantoins and rifampicin may enhance the metabolism of tibolone and thus decrease its therapeutic effect.

Since tibolone may increase blood fibrinolytic activity (lower fibrinogen levels, higher antithrombin III, plasminogen and fibrinolytic activity values) it may enhance the effect of anticoagulants.

*Pregnancy and lactation:* There is no clinical experience with Livial in pregnancy but animal studies have indicated that tibolone is fetotoxic. Livial is contraindicated in pregnancy and lactation.

*Effects on ability to drive and use machines:* Livial is not known to have any effects on alertness and concentration.

*Undesirable effects:* Occasionally, vaginal bleeding or spotting may occur, mainly during the first months of treatment. Other adverse events that have been observed occasionally include: change of body weight, dizziness, rash, pruritus, seborrhoeic dermatosis, increased facial hair growth, headache, migraine, visual disturbances (including blurred vision), gastrointestinal upset, abdominal pain, depression, oedema, effects on the musculoskeletal system such as arthralgia or myalgia and changes in liver function parameters. There have been reports of endometrial hyperplasia and endometrial cancer in patients treated with tibolone although a causal relationship has not been established.

*Overdosage:* The acute toxicity of tibolone in animals is very low. Therefore toxic symptoms are not expected to occur even when several tablets are taken simultaneously. In cases of acute overdose, nausea, vomiting and withdrawal bleeding in females may develop. No specific antidote is known. Symptomatic treatment can be given if necessary.

### Pharmacological properties

*Pharmacodynamic properties:* After oral administration tibolone is rapidly metabolised into three compounds which contribute to the pharmacological effects of Livial. Two of these metabolites have predominantly oestrogenic activity, a third metabolite and the parent compound have predominantly progestagenic activity.

Livial has an oestrogen-like effect on hot flushes and other climacteric complaints. In addition, oestrogen-like effects are exerted on the vagina and bone. Due to its progestagenic effects Livial does not stimulate the endometrium. Therefore, if bleeding occurs, this usually results from an atrophic endometrium. Finally, Livial has effects on certain metabolic and haematological parameters such as a decrease in plasma high density lipoprotein cholesterol, triglycerides, lipoprotein (a) and an increase in blood fibrinolytic activity.

*Pharmacokinetic properties:* After oral administration tibolone is rapidly and extensively absorbed. Due to rapid metabolism the plasma levels of tibolone are very low. Pharmacokinetic data indicate linear kinetics. Peak plasma levels are reached after 1–4 hours and accumulation does not occur.

Excretion of tibolone is mainly in the form of polar and very polar metabolites. A small amount of the administered compound is excreted in the urine, but most is eliminated via the bile and the faeces.

*Preclinical safety data:* Livial is not genotoxic. Although a carcinogenic effect was seen in certain strains of rat (hepatic tumours) and mouse (bladder tumours), the relevance of this evidence to man is uncertain.

**Pharmaceutical particulars**

*List of excipients*: Potato starch, magnesium stearate, ascorbyl palmitate and lactose.

*Incompatibilities*: None known

*Shelf-life*: When stored as indicated the tablets can be stored for up to two years.

*Special precautions for storage*: Livial tablets should be stored at room temperature (below 25°C), protected from moisture and light.

*Nature and contents of container:* Press-through strips of 28 or 30 tablets each containing 2.5 mg of tibolone. Cartons containing 1 strip or 3 strips.

*Instructions for use/handling*: Not applicable

**Marketing authorisation number** 0065/0086

**Date of approval/revision of SPC** April 1997

**Legal category** POM

## MARVELON*

**Presentation** White, round, biconvex tablets, diameter 6 mm, coded TR5 on one side and ORGANON* on the reverse side.

Each tablet contains 150 micrograms of Desogestrel and 30 micrograms Ethinyloestradiol BP.

Other ingredients: dl-alpha-tocopherol, potato starch, povidone, stearic acid, aerosil and lactose.

**Uses** Oral contraception.

**Dosage and administration** It is preferable that tablet intake from the first pack is started on the first day of menstruation in which case no extra contraceptive precautions are necessary.

If menstruation has already begun, (that is 2, 3, or 4 days previously), tablet taking should commence on day 5 of the menstrual period. In this case additional contraceptive precautions must be taken for the first 7 days of tablet taking.

If menstruation began more than 5 days previously then the patient should be advised to wait until her next menstrual period before starting to take Marvelon.

*How to take Marvelon:* One tablet is taken daily at the same time, (preferably in the evening) without interruption for 21 days, followed by a break of 7 tablet-free days. Each subsequent pack is started after the 7 tablet-free days have elapsed. Additional contraceptive precautions are not then required.

*Use during pregnancy and breast feeding:* Marvelon is contraindicated for use during pregnancy or suspected pregnancy and in mothers who are breast-feeding.

*Post-partum administration:* Following childbirth oral contraceptive administration to non-breast feeding mothers should be started 21 days post-partum in which case no additional contraceptive precautions are required.

If intercourse has taken place post-partum, oral contraceptive use should be delayed until the first day of the first menstrual period.

If post-partum administration of Marvelon begins more than 21 days after delivery then additional contraceptive precautions are required for the first 7 days.

N.B. Mothers who are breast feeding should be advised not to use the combined pill since this may reduce the amount of breast-milk, but may be advised instead to use a progestogen-only pill (POP).

After miscarriage or abortion administration should start immediately in which case no additional contraceptive precautions are required.

*Changing from a 21 day pill or a 22 day pill to Marvelon:* All tablets in the old pack should be finished. The first Marvelon tablet is taken the next day i.e. no gap is left between taking tablets nor does the patient need to wait for her period to begin. Tablets should be taken as instructed in 'How to take Marvelon'. The patient will not have a period until the end of the first Marvelon pack, but this is not harmful, nor does it matter if she experiences some bleeding on tablet-taking days.

*Changing from a combined Every Day Pill (28 day tablets) to Marvelon:* Marvelon should be started after taking the last **active** tablet from the 'Every Day Pill' pack (i.e. after taking 21 or 22 tablets). The first Marvelon tablet is taken the next day i.e. no gap is left between taking tablets nor does the patient need to wait for her period to begin. Tablets should be taken as instructed in 'How to take Marvelon'. Remaining tablets from the Every Day (ED) pack should be discarded. The patient will not have a period until the end of the first Marvelon pack, but this is not harmful, nor does it matter if she experiences some bleeding on tablet-taking days.

*Changing from a Progestogen-only Pill (POP or Mini Pill) to Marvelon:* The first Marvelon tablet should be taken on the first day of the period, even if the patient has already taken a mini pill on that day. Tablets should be taken as instructed in 'How to take Marvelon'. All the remaining progestogen-only pills in the mini pill pack should be discarded.

If the patient is taking a (mini) pill, then she may not always have a period, especially when she is breast feeding. The first Marvelon tablet should be taken on the day *after* stopping the mini pill. All remaining pills in the mini pill packet must be discarded. Additional contraceptive precautions must be taken for the first 7 days.

*Additional contraceptive precautions:* When additional contraceptive precautions are required the patient should be advised either not to have sex, or to use a cap plus spermicide, or for her partner to use a condom. Rhythm methods should not be advised as the pill disrupts the usual cyclical changes associated with the natural menstrual cycle e.g. changes in temperature and cervical mucus.

*To skip a period:* To skip a period, a new pack of Marvelon should be started on the day after finishing the current pack (the patient skips the tablet-free days). Tablet-taking should be continued in the usual way. During the use of the second pack she may experience slight spotting or break-through bleeding but contraceptive protection will not be diminished provided there are no tablet omissions. The next pack of Marvelon is started after the usual 7 tablet-free days, regardless of whether the period has completely finished or not.

*Reduced reliability:* The reliability of Marvelon may be reduced under the following circumstances:

*Forgotten tablets:* If the forgotten tablet is taken **within 12 hours,** no further precautions are necessary, further tablets should be taken at the usual time.

If one or more tablets are forgotten for **more than 12 hours,** contraceptive protection will be reduced. The patient should take the last forgotten tablet, even if this means taking two tablets in one day, and then continue to take tablets at the normal time. Additional contraceptive precautions should be taken for the next seven days, and the patient should follow the 'seven day rule'. (See *Precautions and Warnings* for further advice.)

*Vomiting or diarrhoea:* If symptoms persist for more than 12 hours the patient should follow the '7-day rule'. (See *Precautions and Warnings* for further advice.)

*Interactions:* The doctor should consider the possibility of interactions between oral contraceptives and other drugs commonly prescribed such as antibiotics, anticonvulsants and barbiturates. (See *Interactions* for further advice.)

*Surgery, varicose veins or immobilisation:* It is advisable to discontinue oral contraceptive use at least 4 to 6 weeks prior to these procedures, and to (re)start not less than 2 weeks after full ambulation. (See *Precautions and Warnings* for further advice.)

**Contra-indications, warnings, etc**

*Absolute contra-indications:*

- Pregnancy or suspected pregnancy (that cannot yet be excluded) or breast feeding.
- Circulatory disorders (cardiovascular or cerebrovascular) such as thrombophlebitis and thromboembolic processes (or a history of these conditions), moderate to severe hypertension, hyperlipoproteinaemia.
- In addition the presence of more than one of the risk factors for arterial disease which are discussed under *Serious adverse reactions*
- Severe liver disease, cholestatic jaundice or hepatitis (viral or non-viral), or a history of these conditions if the results of liver function tests have failed to return to normal, and for 3 months after liver function tests have been found to be normal; a history of jaundice of pregnancy or jaundice due to the use of steroids, Rotor syndrome and Dubin-Johnson syndrome, hepatic cell tumours and porphyria.
- Cholelithiasis
- Known or suspected oestrogen-dependent tumours, (see *Serious adverse reactions*); endometrial hyperplasia; undiagnosed vaginal bleeding.
- Systemic lupus erythematosus or a history of this condition.
- A history during pregnancy or previous use of steroids of: severe pruritus; herpes gestationis; a manifestation or deterioration of otosclerosis

*Relative contra-indications:* If any of the relative contra-indications listed below is present, the benefits of oestrogen/progestogen-containing preparations must be weighed against the possible risks for each individual case and the patient kept under close supervision. In case of aggravation or appearance of any of these conditions whilst the patient is taking the pill, its use should be discontinued.

Conditions implicating an increasing risk of developing venous thrombo-embolic complications, e.g. severe varicose veins or prolonged immobilisation or major surgery (see *Precautions and Warnings*). Disorders of coagulation.

Presence of any risk factor for arterial disease e.g. smoking, hyperlipidaemia or hypertension (see *Serious adverse reactions*).

Other conditions associated with an increased risk of circulatory disease such as latent or overt cardiac failure, renal dysfunction, or a history of these conditions.

Epilepsy or a history of this condition; Migraine or a history of this condition; A history of cholelithiasis; Presence of any risk factor for oestrogen-dependent tumours; oestrogen-sensitive gynaecological disorders such as uterine fibromyomata and endometriosis (see also under *Serious adverse reactions*); Diabetes mellitus.

Severe depression or a history of this condition. If this is accompanied by a disturbance in tryptophan metabolism, administration of vitamin $B_6$ might be of therapeutic value.

Sickle cell haemoglobinopathy, since under certain circumstances, e.g. during infections or anoxia, oestrogen-containing preparations may induce thromboembolic processes in patients with this condition.

If the results of liver function tests become abnormal, use should be discontinued.

*Precautions and warnings:*

*Reduced reliability:* When Marvelon is taken according to the directions for use the occurrence of pregnancy is highly unlikely. However, the reliability of oral contraceptives may be reduced under the following circumstances:

*Forgotten tablets:*

- Provided she is **less than 12 hours late** in taking her tablet the patient should take it as soon as she remembers, further tablets should be taken at the usual time. Marvelon will still give contraceptive protection during this cycle.
- If she is **more than 12 hours late** in taking one or more tablets then she will *not* be protected for the next 7 days.
- If one or more tablets are forgotten for **more than 12 hours**, contraceptive protection will be reduced. The patient should take the last forgotten tablet, even if this means taking two tablets in one day, and then continue to take tablets at the normal time. Additional contraceptive precautions should be taken for the next 7 days, and the patient should follow the '7-day rule'.

*Vomiting or diarrhoea:* If after tablet intake vomiting or diarrhoea occurs, a tablet may not be absorbed properly by the body. If the symptoms disappear within 12 hours of tablet-taking, the patient should take an extra tablet from a spare pack and continue with the rest of the pack as usual. However, if the symptoms continue beyond those 12 hours, additional contraceptive precautions are necessary for any sexual intercourse during the stomach or bowel upset and for the following 7 days (the patient must be advised to follow '7-day rule').

*If the patient is taking certain other medicines:* If the patient is taking any of the medicines given in the *Interactions* section she should be advised to follow the '7-day rule':

**THE 7-DAY RULE**

*If any **one** tablet is forgotten for more than 12 hours:*

*If the patient has vomiting or diarrhoea for more than 12 hours:*

*If the patient is taking any of the drugs listed under Interactions:*

The patient should continue to take her tablets as usual and:

– Additional contraceptive precautions must be taken for the next 7 days

**– BUT – if these 7 days run beyond the end of the current pack,** the next pack must be started as soon as the current one is finished, i.e. no gap should be left between packs. (This prevents an extended break in tablet taking which may increase the risk of the ovaries releasing an egg and thus reducing contraceptive protection). The patient will not have a period until the end of 2 packs but this is not harmful nor does it matter if she experiences some bleeding on tablet taking days.

If after taking Marvelon for several months there is a sudden occurrence of spotting or breakthrough bleeding (not observed in previous cycles) or the absence of withdrawal bleeding, contraceptive effectiveness may be reduced. If withdrawal bleeding fails to occur and none of the above mentioned events has taken place, pregnancy is highly unlikely and oral contraceptive use can be continued until the end of the next pack. If withdrawal bleeding fails to occur at the end of the second cycle, tablet intake should be discontinued and pregnancy excluded before oral contraceptive use can be resumed.) However, if withdrawal bleeding is absent and any of the above mentioned events has occurred, tablet intake should be discontinued and pregnancy excluded before oral contraceptive use can be resumed.

*Medical examination/consultation:* A complete medical history and physical examination should be taken prior to the initiation or reinstitution of oral contraceptives and should be repeated periodically.

These physical examinations should include special reference to blood pressure, breasts, abdomen and pelvic organs, including cervical cytology and, where indicated by the medical or family history, relevant laboratory tests.

Caution should be observed when prescribing oral contraceptives to young women whose cycles are not yet stabilised.

*Surgery, Varicose Veins or immobilisation:* In patients using oestrogen-containing preparations, the risk of deep-vein thrombosis may be temporarily increased when undergoing a major operation (e.g. abdominal, orthopaedic), any surgery to the legs, medical treatment for varicose veins or prolonged immobilisation. Therefore, it is advisable to discontinue oral contraceptive use at least 4 to 6 weeks prior to these procedures if performed electively and to (re)start not less than 2 weeks after full ambulation. The latter is also valid with regard to immobilisation after an accident or emergency surgery. In case of emergency surgery, thrombotic prophylaxis is usually indicated e.g. with subcutaneous heparin.

*Chloasma:* Chloasma may occasionally occur, especially in women with a history of chloasma gravidarum. Women with a tendency to chloasma should avoid exposure to the sun or ultraviolet radiation whilst taking this preparation.

*Laboratory tests:* The use of steroids may influence the results of certain laboratory tests. In the literature, at least a hundred different parameters have been reported to possibly be influenced by oral contraceptive use, predominantly by the oestrogenic component. Among these are: biochemical parameters of the liver, thyroid, adrenal and renal function, plasma levels of (carrier) proteins and lipid/lipoprotein fractions and parameters of coagulation and fibrinolysis.

*Adverse reactions:* Various adverse reactions have been associated with oral contraceptive use. The serious reactions are dealt with in more detail. The first appearance of symptoms indicative of any one of these reactions necessitates immediate cessation of oral contraceptive use while appropriate diagnostic and therapeutic measures are undertaken.

*Serious adverse reactions:* Various reports have associated oral contraceptive use with the occurrence of deep venous thrombosis, pulmonary embolism and other embolisms.

Other investigations involving oral contraceptives have suggested an increased risk of oestrogen and/or progestogen dose-dependent coronary and cerebrovascular accidents, predominantly in heavy smokers. Thrombosis has very rarely been reported to occur in other veins or arteries, e.g. hepatic, mesenteric, renal or retinal. It should be noted that there is no consensus about the often contradictory findings obtained in early studies. The physician should bear in mind, the possibility of vascular events occurring and take into account the presence of risk factors for arterial disease and deep venous thrombosis when prescribing oral contraceptives. Risk factors for arterial disease include smoking, the presence of hyperlipidaemia, hypertension, or diabetes. Signs and symptoms of a thromboembolic event may include: sudden severe pain in the chest, whether or not reaching to the left arm; sudden breathlessness; any unusual severe, prolonged headache, especially if it occurs for the first time or gets progressively worse, or is associated with any of the following symptoms: sudden partial or complete loss of vision or diplopia, aphasia, vertigo, a bad fainting attack or collapse with or without focal epilepsy, weakness or very marked numbness suddenly affecting one side or one part of the body, motor disturbances; severe pain in the calf of one leg; acute abdomen.

Cigarette smoking increases the risk of serious cardiovascular adverse reactions to oral contraceptive use. This risk increases with age and with heavy smoking and is more marked in women over 35 years of age. Women who use oral contraceptives should be strongly advised not to smoke.

The use of oestrogen-containing oral contraceptives may promote growth of existing sex steroid dependent tumours. For this reason, the use of these oral contraceptives in patients with such tumours is contraindicated.

Numerous epidemiological studies have been reported on the risks of ovarian, endometrial, cervical and breast cancer in women using combined oral contraceptives. The evidence is clear that combined oral contraceptives offer substantial protection against both ovarian and endometrial cancer.

An increased risk of cervical cancer in long term users of combined oral contraceptives has been reported in some studies, but there continues to be controversy about the extent to which this is attributable to the confounding effects of sexual behaviour and other factors.

The evidence linking combined oral contraceptive use and breast cancer remains inconclusive. The results of some studies suggest an increased risk of breast cancer presenting below the age of about 35, the risk rising with duration of use. Any possible increased risk of breast cancer with combined oral contraceptives is however likely to be small, and may be expected to be less with low dose pills. This possible risk should be weighed against the many benefits of combined oral contraceptives, including their protective effects against ovarian and endometrial cancers.

Malignant hepatic tumours have been reported on rare occasions in long-term users of oral contraceptives. Benign hepatic tumours have also been associated with oral contraceptive usage. A hepatic tumour should be considered in the differential diagnosis when upper abdominal pain, enlarged liver or signs of intra-abdominal haemorrhage occur.

The use of oral contraceptives may sometimes lead to the development of cholestatic jaundice or cholelithiasis.

On rare occasions the use of oral contraceptives may trigger or reactivate systemic lupus erythematosus.

A further rare complication of oral contraceptive use is the occurrence of Sydenhams' chorea which can be reversed by discontinuing the pill. The majority of cases of oral-contraceptive-induced chorea show a pre-existing predisposition which may relate to previous rheumatic fever.

*Other adverse reactions:*
*Cardiovascular system:* rise of blood pressure. If hypertension develops, treatment should be discontinued.

*Genital tract:* intermenstrual bleeding, post-medication amenorrhoea, changes in cervical secretion, increase in size of uterine fibromyomata, aggravation of endometriosis and certain vaginal infections, e.g. candidiasis.

*Breast:* tenderness, pain, enlargement, secretion.
*Gastro-intestinal tract:* nausea, vomiting, cholelithiasis, cholestatic jaundice.

*Skin:* erythema nodosum, rash, chloasma.
*Eyes:* discomfort of the cornea if contact lenses are used.

*CNS:* headache, migraine, mood changes, depression.

*Metabolic:* fluid retention, change in body weight, reduced glucose tolerance.

*Effects on ability to drive and to use machines:* None stated

*Interactions:* Irregular cycles and reduced reliability of oral contraceptives may occur when these preparations are used concomitantly with drugs such as anticonvulsants, barbiturates, antibiotics, (e.g. tetracyclines, ampicillin, rifampicin, etc.), griseofulvin, activated charcoal and certain laxatives.

Special consideration should be given to patients being treated with antibiotics for acne.

They should be advised to use a non-hormonal method of contraception, or to use an oral contraceptive containing a progestogen showing minimal androgenicity, which have been reported as helping to improve acne without using an antibiotic.

Oral contraceptives may diminish glucose tolerance and increase the need for insulin or other anti-diabetic drugs in diabetics.

*Overdosage:* There have been no reports of serious ill-effects from overdosage even when a considerable number of tablets have been taken by a small child. In general, it is therefore unnecessary to treat overdosage. However, if overdosage is discovered within two or three hours and is large, then gastric lavage can be safely used. There are no antidotes and further treatment should be symptomatic.

**Pharmaceutical precautions** Store below 25°C in a dry place. Protect from light.

**Legal category** POM.

**Package quantities** Plastic/aluminium foil blister strips containing 21 tablets, overwrapped with a sealed aluminium laminated sachet. Pack of 3 strips.

**Product licence number** 0065/0071.

# MERCILON*

**Presentation** White, round, biconvex tablets, 6 mm in diameter, engraved with Organon* motif on one side and T₄R on the other. Each pack of Mercilon consists of 21 tablets.

Each tablet contains: Desogestrel (a progestogen) 150 micrograms

Ethinyloestradiol (an oestrogen) PhEur 20 micrograms.

Other ingredients: dl-alpha-tocopherol, potato starch, povidone, stearic acid, aerosil and lactose.

**Uses** Oral contraception.

**Dosage and administration** It is preferable that tablet intake from the first pack is started on the first day of menstruation in which case no extra contraceptive precautions are necessary.

If menstruation has already begun, (that is 2, 3, or 4 days previously), tablet taking should commence on day 5 of the menstrual period. In this case additional contraceptive precautions must be taken for the first 7 days of tablet taking.

If menstruation began more than 5 days previously then the patient should be advised to wait until her next menstrual period before starting to take Mercilon.

*How to take Mercilon:* One tablet is taken daily at the same time, (preferably in the evening) without interruption for 21 days, followed by a break of 7 tablet-free days. Each subsequent pack is started after the 7 tablet-free days have elapsed. Additional contraceptive precautions are not then required.

*Use during pregnancy and breast feeding:* Mercilon is contraindicated for use during pregnancy or suspected pregnancy and in mothers who are breast-feeding.

*Post-partum administration:* Following childbirth oral contraceptive administration to non-breast feeding mothers should be started 21 days post-partum in which case no additional contraceptive precautions are required.

If intercourse has taken place post-partum, oral contraceptive use should be delayed until the first day of the first menstrual period.

If post-partum administration of Mercilon begins more than 21 days after delivery then additional contraceptive precautions are required for the first 7 days.

N.B. Mothers who are breast feeding should be advised not to use the combined pill since this may reduce the amount of breast-milk, but may be advised instead to use a progestogen-only pill (POP).

After miscarriage or abortion administration should start immediately in which case no additional contraceptive precautions are required.

*Changing from a 21 day pill or 22 day pill to Mercilon:* All tablets in the old pack should be finished. The first Mercilon tablet is taken the next day i.e. no gap is left between taking tablets nor does the patient need to wait for her period to begin. Tablets should be taken as instructed in 'How to take Mercilon'. The patient will not have a period until the end of the first Mercilon pack, but this is not harmful, nor does it matter if she experiences some bleeding on tablet-taking days.

*Changing from a combined Every Day Pill (28 day tablets) to Mercilon:* Mercilon should be started after taking the last **active** tablet from the 'Every Day Pill' pack (i.e. after taking 21 or 22 tablets). The first Mercilon tablet is taken the next day i.e. no gap is left between taking tablets nor does the patient need to wait for her period to begin. Tablets should be taken as instructed in 'How to take Mercilon'. Remaining tablets from the Every Day (ED) pack should be discarded. The patient will not have a period until the end of the first Mercilon pack, but this is not harmful, nor does it matter if she experiences some bleeding on tablet-taking days.

*Changing from a Progestogen-only Pill (POP or Mini Pill) to Mercilon:* The first Mercilon tablet should be taken on the first day of the period, even if the patient has already taken a mini pill on that day. Tablets should be taken as instructed in 'How to take Mercilon'. All the remaining progestogen-only pills in the mini pill pack should be discarded.

If the patient is taking a (mini) pill, then she may not always have a period, especially when she is breast feeding. The first Mercilon tablet should be taken on the day *after* stopping the mini pill. All remaining pills in the mini pill packet must be discarded. Additional contraceptive precautions must be taken for the first 7 days.

*Additional contraceptive precautions:* When additional contraceptive precautions are required the patient should be advised either not to have sex, or to use a cap plus spermicide, or for her partner to use a condom. Rhythm methods should not be advised as the pill disrupts the usual cyclical changes associated with the natural menstrual cycle e.g. changes in temperature and cervical mucus.

*To skip a period:* To skip a period, a new pack of Mercilon should be started on the day after finishing the current pack (the patient skips the tablet-free days). Tablet-taking should be continued in the usual way. During the use of the second pack she may experience slight spotting or break-through bleeding but contraceptive protection will not be diminished provided there are no tablet omissions. The next pack of Mercilon is started after the usual 7 tablet-free days, regardless of whether the period has completely finished or not.

*Reduced reliability:* The reliability of Mercilon may be reduced under the following circumstances:

*Forgotten tablets:* If the forgotten tablet is taken **within 12 hours,** no further precautions are necessary, further tablets should be taken at the usual time.

If one or more tablets are forgotten for **more than 12 hours,** contraceptive protection will be reduced. The patient should take the last forgotten tablet, even if this means taking two tablets in one day, and then continue to take tablets at the normal time. Additional contraceptive precautions should be taken for the next seven days, and the patient should follow the 'seven day rule'. (See *Precautions and Warnings* for further advice.)

*Vomiting or Diarrhoea:* If symptoms persist for more than 12 hours the patient should follow the '7-day rule'. (See *Precautions and Warnings* for further advice.)

*Interactions:* The doctor should consider the possibility of interactions between oral contraceptives and other drugs commonly prescribed such as antibiotics, anticonvulsants and barbiturates. (See *Interactions* for further advice.)

*Surgery, varicose veins or immobilisation:* It is advisable to discontinue oral contraceptive use at least 4 to 6 weeks prior to these procedures, and to (re)start not less than 2 weeks after full ambulation. (See *Precautions and Warnings* for further advice.)

**Contra-indications, warnings, etc**

*Absolute contra-indications:*

– Pregnancy or suspected pregnancy (that cannot yet be excluded) or breast feeding.
– Circulatory disorders (cardiovascular or cerebrovascular) such as thrombophlebitis and thromboembolic processes (or a history of these conditions), moderate to severe hypertension, hyperlipoproteinaemia.
  In addition the presence of more than one of the risk factors for arterial disease which are discussed under *Serious adverse reactions.*
– Severe liver disease, cholestatic jaundice or hepatitis (viral or non-viral), or a history of these conditions if the results of liver function tests have failed to return to normal, and for 3 months after liver function tests have been found to be normal; a history of jaundice of pregnancy or jaundice due to the use of steroids, Rotor syndrome and Dubin-Johnson syndrome, hepatic cell tumours and porphyria.
– Cholelithiasis
– Known or suspected oestrogen-dependent tumours, (see *Serious adverse reactions*); endometrial hyperplasia; undiagnosed vaginal bleeding.
– Systemic lupus erythematosus or a history of this condition.
– A history during pregnancy or previous use of steroids of: severe pruritis; herpes gestationis; a manifestation or deterioration of otosclerosis

*Relative contra-indications:* If any of the relative contra-indications listed below is present, the benefits of oestrogen/progestogen-containing preparations must be weighed against the possible risks for each individual case and the patient kept under close supervision. In case of aggravation or appearance of any of these conditions whilst the patient is taking the pill, its use should be discontinued.

– Conditions implicating an increasing risk of developing venous thrombo-embolic complications, e.g. severe varicose veins or prolonged immobilisation or major surgery (see *Precautions and warnings*). Disorders of coagulation.
– Presence of any risk factor for arterial disease e.g. smoking, hyperlipidaemia or hypertension (see *Serious adverse reactions*).
– Other conditions associated with an increased risk of circulatory disease such as latent or overt cardiac failure, renal dysfunction, or a history of these conditions.
– Epilepsy or a history of this condition.
– Migraine or a history of this condition.
– A history of cholelithiasis.
– Presence of any risk factor for oestrogen-dependent tumours; oestrogen-sensitive gynaecological disorders such as uterine fibromyomata and endometriosis (see also under *Serious adverse reactions*).
– Diabetes mellitus.
– Severe depression or a history of this condition. If this is accompanied by a disturbance in tryptophan

metabolism, administration of vitamin $B_6$ might be of therapeutic value.
– Sickle cell haemoglobinopathy, since under certain circumstances, e.g. during infections or anoxia, oestrogen-containing preparations may induce thromboembolic processes in patients with this condition.
– If the results of liver function tests become abnormal, use should be discontinued.

*Precautions and warnings:*
*Reduced reliability:* When Mercilon is taken according to the directions for use the occurrence of pregnancy is highly unlikely. However, the reliability of oral contraceptives may be reduced under the following circumstances:

*Forgotten tablets:* Provided she is **less than 12 hours late** in taking her tablet the patient should take it as soon as she remembers, further tablets should be taken at the usual time. Mercilon will still give contraceptive protection during this cycle.

– If she is **more than 12 hours late** in taking one or more tablets then she will *not* be protected for the next 7 days.
– If one or more tablets are forgotten for **more than 12 hours,** contraceptive protection will be reduced. The patient should take the last forgotten tablet, even if this means taking two tablets in one day, and then continue to take tablets at the normal time. Additional contraceptive precautions should be taken for the next 7 days, and the patient should follow the '7-day rule'.

*Vomiting or diarrhoea:* If after tablet intake vomiting or diarrhoea occurs, a tablet may not be absorbed properly by the body. If the symptoms disappear within 12 hours of tablet-taking, the patient should take an extra tablet from a spare pack and continue with the rest of the pack as usual. However, if the symptoms continue beyond those 12 hours, additional contraceptive precautions are necessary for any sexual intercourse during the stomach or bowel upset and for the following 7 days (the patient must be advised to follow '7-day rule').

*If the patient is taking certain other medicines:* If the patient is taking any of the medicines given in the *Interactions* section she should be advised to follow the '7-day rule':

**THE 7-DAY RULE**
*If any **one** tablet is forgotten for more than 12 hours:*
*If the patient has vomiting or diarrhoea for more than 12 hours:*
*If the patient is taking any of the drugs listed under Interactions:*
The patient should continue to take her tablets as usual and:
Additional contraceptive precautions must be taken for the next 7 days
BUT – if these 7 days run beyond the end of the current pack, the next pack must be started as soon as the current one is finished, i.e. no gap should be left between packs. (This prevents an extended break in tablet taking which may increase the risk of the ovaries releasing an egg and thus reducing contraceptive protection). The patient will not have a period until the end of 2 packs but this is not harmful nor does it matter if she experiences some bleeding on tablet taking days.

If after taking Mercilon for several months there is a sudden occurrence of spotting or breakthrough bleeding (not observed in previous cycles) or the absence of withdrawal bleeding, contraceptive effectiveness may be reduced. If withdrawal bleeding fails to occur and none of the above mentioned events has taken place, pregnancy is highly unlikely and oral contraceptive use can be continued until the end of the next pack. (If withdrawal bleeding fails to occur at the end of the second cycle, tablet intake should be discontinued and pregnancy excluded before oral contraceptive use can be resumed.) However, if withdrawal bleeding is absent and any of the above mentioned events has occurred, tablet intake should be discontinued and pregnancy excluded before oral contraceptive use can be resumed.

*Medical examination/consultation:* A complete medical history and physical examination should be taken prior to the initiation or reinstitution of oral contraceptives and should be repeated periodically.

These physical examinations should include special reference to blood pressure, breasts, abdomen and pelvic organs, including cervical cytology and, where indicated by the medical or family history, relevant laboratory tests.

Caution should be observed when prescribing oral contraceptives to young women whose cycles are not yet stabilised.

*Surgery, varicose veins or immobilisation:* In patients using oestrogen-containing preparations, the risk of deep-vein thrombosis may be temporarily increased when undergoing a major operation (e.g. abdominal,

orthopaedic), any surgery to the legs, medical treatment for varicose veins or prolonged immobilisation. Therefore, it is advisable to discontinue oral contraceptive use at least 4 to 6 weeks prior to these procedures if performed electively and to (re)start not less than 2 weeks after full ambulation. The latter is also valid with regard to immobilisation after an accident or emergency surgery. In case of emergency surgery, thrombotic prophylaxis is usually indicated e.g. with subcutaneous heparin.

*Chloasma:* Chloasma may occasionally occur, especially in women with a history of chloasma gravidarum. Women with a tendency to chloasma should avoid exposure to the sun or ultraviolet radiation whilst taking this preparation.

*Laboratory tests:* The use of steroids may influence the results of certain laboratory tests. In the literature, at least a hundred different parameters have been reported to possibly be influenced by oral contraceptive use, predominantly by the oestrogenic component. Among these are: biochemical parameters of the liver, thyroid, adrenal and renal function, plasma levels of (carrier) proteins and lipid/lipoprotein fractions and parameters of coagulation and fibrinolysis.

*Adverse reactions:* Various adverse reactions have been associated with oral contraceptive use. The serious reactions are dealt with in more detail. The first appearance of symptoms indicative of any one of these reactions necessitates immediate cessation of oral contraceptive use while appropriate diagnostic and therapeutic measures are undertaken.

*Serious adverse reactions:* Various reports have associated oral contraceptive use with the occurrence of deep venous thrombosis, pulmonary embolism and other embolisms.

Other investigations involving oral contraceptives have suggested an increased risk of oestrogen and/or progestogen dose-dependent coronary thromboses and cerebrovascular accidents, predominantly in heavy smokers. Thrombosis has very rarely been reported to occur in other veins or arteries, e.g. hepatic, mesenteric, renal or retinal. It should be noted that there is no consensus about the often contradictory findings obtained in early studies. The physician should bear in mind, the possibility of vascular events occurring and take into account the presence of risk factors for arterial disease and deep venous thrombosis when prescribing oral contraceptives. Risk factors for arterial disease include smoking, the presence of hyperlipidaemia, hypertension, or diabetes. Signs and symptoms of a thromboembolic event may include: sudden severe pain in the chest, whether or not reaching to the left arm; sudden breathlessness; any unusual severe, prolonged headache, especially if it occurs for the first time or gets progressively worse, or is associated with any of the following symptoms: sudden partial or complete loss of vision or diplopia, aphasia, vertigo, a bad fainting attack or collapse with or without focal epilepsy, weakness or very marked numbness suddenly affecting one side or one part of the body, motor disturbances; severe pain in the calf of one leg; acute abdomen.

Cigarette smoking increases the risk of serious cardiovascular adverse reactions to oral contraceptive use. This risk increases with age and with heavy smoking and is more marked in women over 35 years of age. Women who use oral contraceptives should be strongly advised not to smoke.

The use of oestrogen-containing oral contraceptives may promote growth of existing sex steroid dependent tumours. For this reason, the use of these oral contraceptives in patients with such tumours is contraindicated.

Numerous epidemiological studies have been reported on the risks of ovarian, endometrial, cervical and breast cancer in women using combined oral contraceptives. The evidence is clear that combined oral contraceptives offer substantial protection against both ovarian and endometrial cancer.

An increased risk of cervical cancer in long term users of combined oral contraceptives has been reported in some studies, but there continues to be controversy about the extent to which this is attributable to the confounding effects of sexual behaviour and other factors.

The evidence linking combined oral contraceptive use and breast cancer remains inconclusive. The results of some studies suggest an increased risk of breast cancer presenting below the age of about 35, the risk rising with duration of use. Any possible increased risk of breast cancer with combined oral contraceptives is however likely to be small, and may be expected to be less with low dose pills. This possible risk should be weighed against the many benefits of combined oral contraceptives, including their protective effects against ovarian and endometrial cancers.

– Malignant hepatic tumours have been reported on rare occasions in long-term users of oral contraceptives. Benign hepatic tumours have also been associated with oral contraceptive usage. A hepatic tumour should be considered in the differential diagnosis when upper abdominal pain, enlarged liver or signs of intra-abdominal haemorrhage occur.

- The use of oral contraceptives may sometimes lead to the development of cholestatic jaundice or cholelithiasis.
- On rare occasions the use of oral contraceptives may trigger or reactivate systemic lupus erythematosus.
- A further rare complication of oral contraceptive use is the occurrence of Sydenhams' chorea which can be reversed by discontinuing the pill. The majority of cases of oral-contraceptive-induced chorea show a pre-existing predisposition which often relates to acute rheumatism.

*Other adverse reactions:*
*Cardiovascular system:* rise of blood pressure. If hypertension develops, treatment should be discontinued.
*Genital tract:* intermenstrual bleeding, post-medication amenorrhoea, changes in cervical secretion, increase in size of uterine fibromyomata, aggravation of endometriosis and certain vaginal infections, e.g. candidiasis.
*Breast:* tenderness, pain, enlargement, secretion.
*Gastro-intestinal tract:* nausea, vomiting, cholelithiasis, cholestatic jaundice.
*Skin:* erythema nodosum, rash, chloasma.
*Eyes:* discomfort of the corneal if contact lenses are used.
*CNS:* headache, migraine, mood changes, depression.
*Metabolic:* fluid retention, change in body weight, reduced glucose tolerance.

*Effects on ability to drive and to use machines:* None stated

*Interactions:* Irregular cycles and reduced reliability of oral contraceptives may occur when these preparations are used concomitantly with drugs such as anticonvulsants, barbiturates, antibiotics, (e.g. tetracyclines, ampicillin, rifampicin, etc.), griseofulvin, activated charcoal and certain laxatives.

Special consideration should be given to patients being treated with antibiotics for acne.

They should be advised to use a non-hormonal method of contraception, or to use an oral contraceptive containing a progestogen showing minimal androgenicity, which have been reported as helping to improve acne without using an antibiotic.

Oral contraceptives may diminish glucose tolerance and increase the need for insulin or other anti-diabetic drugs in diabetics.

*Overdosage:* There have been no reports of serious ill-effects from overdosage even when a considerable number of tablets have been taken by a small child. In general, it is therefore unnecessary to treat overdosage. However, if overdosage is discovered within two or three hours and is large, then gastric lavage can be safely used. There are no antidotes and further treatment should be symptomatic.

**Pharmaceutical precautions**  Store below 25˚C. Protect from light and moisture.

**Legal category**  POM

**Package quantities**  Plastic/aluminium foil blister strips containing 21 tablets, overwrapped with a sealed aluminium laminated sachet. Pack of 3 strips.

**Product licence number** 0065/0085.

## OESTRADIOL IMPLANTS

**Presentation** Pellets of fused, crystalline oestradiol for implantation. Each pellet contains either 25 mg, 50 mg, or 100 mg of Oestradiol. The 25 mg weight has a diameter of 2.2 mm and the 50 mg and 100 mg weights have a diameter of 4.5 mm.

**Uses** Indicated in females for: Major post-menopausal symptoms due to oestrogen deficiency, including prevention of post-menopausal osteoporosis in hysterectomised patients.

Should women with an intact uterus be prescribed Oestradiol implants then the lowest effective dose should be used and it must be co-administered with a progestogen for 10-13 days in each cycle.

**Dosage and administration**  25-100 mg. Frequency of replacement depends on the duration of activity of the implants administered and the severity of the symptoms. Patients require a further implant when symptoms return, usually every 4 to 8 months.

Because of the sustained absorption of oestradiol, the endometrium of post-menopausal or ovariectomised women is liable to progressive hypertrophy. Therefore, in women with an intact uterus, additional administration of a progestogen is essential, for 10-13 days in each cycle, to prevent endometrial hyperplasia.

When the patient no longer requires or seeks reimplantation with oestradiol pellets, it is recommended that, in those women with an intact uterus, cyclical administration of an oral progestogen should be continued until there is a cessation of withdrawal bleeding, in order to prevent the possibility of continued endometrial stimulation.

Oestradiol Implants should be inserted subcutaneously, (either by means of a trocar and cannula or in the wound at the time of laparotomy), into an area where there is relatively little movement or blood supply, such as the lower abdominal wall or the buttock. Insertion is made under local anaesthesia and the wound is closed either with an adhesive dressing or a fine suture.

Full aseptic 'no touch' technique should be adopted.

**Contra-indications, warnings, etc**
*Contra-indications:* Pregnancy. Cardiovascular or cerebrovascular disorders, e.g. thrombophlebitis, thrombo-embolic processes or a history of these conditions. Moderate to severe hypertension. Severe liver disease or history of this condition if results of liver function tests have failed to return to normal; cholestatic jaundice, a history of jaundice in pregnancy or jaundice due to the use of steroids; Rotor syndrome and Dubin-Johnson syndrome. Known or suspected oestrogen-dependent tumours: Endometrial hyperplasia. Undiagnosed vaginal bleeding. Porphyria. Hyperlipoproteinaemia, especially in the presence of other risk factors predisposing to cardiovascular disorders. A history during pregnancy or previous steroid use of severe pruritus or herpes gestationis.

*Use in pregnancy and lactation:* Oestradiol implants are contraindicated during pregnancy. This is based on epidemiological evidence that use during pregnancy is harmful to the foetus.

Oestradiol implants are not recommended in lactating women.

*Precautions and warnings:* Chloasma is occasionally seen during the use of oestrogen and/or progestogen-containing preparations, especially in women with a history of chloasma gravidarum. Women with a tendency to chloasma should avoid exposure to the sun while taking this preparation.

Pain in the breasts or excessive production of cervical mucus may be indicative of too high a dosage.

The use of steroids may influence the results of certain laboratory tests e.g. thyroid function tests.

During prolonged treatment with oestrogen-containing preparations periodical medical examinations are advisable. Patients, especially the elderly, with the following conditions should be monitored:

- latent or overt cardiac failure, renal dysfunction, epilepsy or migraine (or a history of these conditions), since the use of steroids may occasionally induce fluid retention.
- hypertension (or a history of this condition); if hypertension develops, the implant should be removed.
- sickle cell haemoglobinopathy, since under certain circumstances, e.g. during infections or anoxia, oestrogen-containing preparations may induce thromboembolic processes in patients with this condition.
- oestrogen-sensitive gynaecological disorders, e.g. uterine fibromyomata which may increase in size and endometriosis which may become aggravated during oestrogen treatment.

*Effects on ability to drive and to use machines:* None stated

*Interactions:* Oestrogen and/or progestogen-containing preparations may diminish glucose tolerance and increase the need for insulin or other antidiabetic drugs in diabetics.

*Other undesirable effects (frequency and seriousness):* The following adverse reactions have been associated with oestrogen therapy:
*Genito-urinary tract:* Intermenstrual bleeding, increase in the size of the uterine fibromyomata, endometrial proliferation, excessive production of cervical mucus, aggravation of endometriosis, premenstrual like syndrome.
*Breast:* Tenderness, pain, enlargement, secretion.
*Gastro-intestinal tract:* Nausea, vomiting, cholelithiasis, cholestatic jaundice.
*Cardiovascular system:* Thrombosis, rise of blood pressure.
*Skin:* Chloasma, erythema nodosum, rash.
*Eyes:* Discomfort of the cornea if contact lenses are used.
*CNS:* Headache, migraine, mood changes.
*Metabolic:* Sodium and water retention, reduced glucose tolerance, and change in body weight.

Prolonged exposure to unopposed oestrogens may increase risk of development of cardiac and renal disease, melanoma, otosclerosis, multiple sclerosis and systemic lupus erythematous. If there is a history of breast nodules or fibrocystic disease then closely monitor breast status.

Changes in liver function.

High dosages and/or prolonged use of oestrogens may cause psychotic disturbances.

*Overdosage:* Acute overdose with oestradiol implants is not known to occur.

With chronic use supraphysiological levels of oestradiol can be found, however these do not generally result in adverse symptoms, signs or metabolic effects. None the less it would seem prudent in the circumstances to withhold further implantation or other administration of exogenous oestrogens until oestradiol levels have fallen to within the pre-menopausal physiological range.

**Pharmaceutical precautions** Store below 25˚C. Protect from light

**Legal category** POM

**Package quantities** Each sterile implant is supplied singly, in a sealed glass tube, available in the following weights: 25 mg, 50 mg, and 100 mg.

**Further information**

*Pharmacodynamic:* 17β Oestradiol is the main, naturally occurring female sex hormone. Among numerous effects Oestradiol is largely responsible for the development and maintenance of the reproductive system and secondary sexual characteristics in women.

Oestradiol implants are effective in relieving the major symptoms of the menopause due to oestrogen deficiency, whether naturally occurring or due to oophorectomy.

Oestradiol implants have also been shown to be effective in reducing the bone loss associated with oestrogen deficiency after the menopause.

*Pharmacokinetic:* After insertion of an implant into the subcutaneous fat the oestradiol plasma levels gradually increase and generally reach their maximum within approximately two months. Thereafter the concentrations remain nearly stationary until the 4th–6th month after insertion. As with other progestogens and oestrogens, there are large interindividual differences in oestradiol levels, but intraindividual variability appears to be small. Unlike oral oestrogen therapy, subcutaneous administration bypasses the gastrointestinal tract, where oestradiol is converted to oestrone and avoids the first-pass effect of the liver. Therefore more unconjugated oestradiol is observed and the liver is less burdened.

The transport, metabolism, and excretion of oestradiol released from the implants are comparable to those of endogenous oestradiol. Thus, about 38 per cent of circulatory oestradiol will be bound to SHBG, 60 per cent is bound to albumin, and only 2–3 per cent is free. The main metabolic end products are oestriol and 2-hydroxyestrone, which are synthesized after conversion of oestradiol to oestrone. Most of the oestradiol is excreted by the kidneys, mainly after conjugation with glucuronic and sulphuric acid. There is a significant enterohepatic circulation of oestradiol and its metabolites. Most of the conjugated biliary oestrogens undergo hydrolysis in the intestines after which they are reabsorbed. Therefore, only a small part of the administered oestradiol will ultimately be lost in the faeces.

After long-term treatment, accumulation may occur (with doses of 50 mg or more, especially when reimplantation is performed after periods of less than 6 months), but in most cases there is only a moderate increase and levels remain well within the normal premenopausal range. However, in rare cases (mainly with implantation intervals of only 3 or 4 months) plasma levels may rise above 1750 pmol/l. There are some indications that supraphysiological levels occur most frequently in women with a history of depression or surgical castration.

**Product licence numbers**

| | |
|---|---|
| 25 mg | 0065/5074R |
| 50 mg | 0065/5075R |
| 100 mg | 0065/5076R |

## OVESTIN* CREAM

**Presentation** An intravaginal cream containing 1 mg oestriol in 1 g of cream.
*Other ingredients:* 2 octyl-dodecanol (eutanol G); cetyl palmitate; glycerin; cetyl alcohol; stearyl alcohol; Polysorbate 60; sorbitan monostearate; chlorhexidine hydrochloride; lactic acid; sodium hydroxide to pH 4, purified water.

**Uses** Vulvo-vaginal complaints due to oestrogen deficiency associated with the climacteric and the post-menopause or after oophorectomy: atrophic vaginitis, kraurosis vulvae, pruritus vulvae, dyspareunia due to an atrophic vaginal mucosa and as pre-surgery therapy for vaginal operations and during subsequent convalescence.

**Dosage and administration** Ovestin Cream is administered intravaginally by means of a calibrated applicator. Ovestin Cream should be given at the lowest dose to control the symptoms and for as short a time as is found necessary. One applicator-dose (applicator filled to the ring mark) is 0.5 grams Ovestin Cream containing 0.5 mg oestriol. Usual dose for vulvo-vaginal complaints associated with the menopause: One application per day for 2 to 3 weeks.

As maintenance dosage, one application twice a week is recommended. Medication should be discontinued every 2 to 3 months for a period of 4 weeks to assess the necessity for further treatment. Pre-surgery therapy (one application per day) should begin 2 weeks before the operation. Following surgery a period of at least 2 weeks should be allowed before resuming therapy.

*Children:* There are no clinical trials to support use in children.

The following 'Instructions for Use' should be given to the patient and are included in the package interior leaflet:

*How to apply the cream:* Use the applicator to apply the cream in the vagina. It is a good idea to do this before going to bed. 1 application (applicator filled to the ring mark) contains 0.5 grams Ovestin cream, which has 0.5 mg of oestriol in it.

1. Remove cap from the tube, invert it, and use the sharp point to open the tube.
2. Screw the end of the applicator onto the tube.
3. Squeeze tube to fill the applicator with the cream until the plunger stops (at the ring mark).
4. Unscrew applicator from tube and replace cap on tube.
5. To apply the cream, lie down, insert the end of the applicator deep into the vagina and slowly push plunger all the way in.

After use, pull plunger out of barrel and wash both in warm, soapy water. Do not use detergents. Rinse well afterwards.

*DO NOT PUT THE APPLICATOR IN HOT OR BOILING WATER.*

**Contra-indications, warnings etc**
*Contra-indications:* Pregnancy or suspected pregnancy and during lactation. Thrombophlebitis, thrombo-embolic processes, or a history of these conditions. Known or suspected oestrogen-dependent tumours, e.g. mammary, genital carcinoma. Undiagnosed vaginal bleeding. Acute or chronic liver disease or history of liver disease where the liver function tests have failed to return to normal. Jaundice or history of jaundice in pregnancy. Rotor syndrome or Dubin-Johnson syndrome. Porphyria. Cerebrovascular or cardiovascular disease.

Hyperlipoproteinaemia, especially in the presence of other risk factors which may indicate a predisposition to cerebrovascular or cardiovascular disorders.

A history during pregnancy or previous use of steroids of severe pruritus, herpes gestationis or a deterioration of otosclerosis.

*Precautions and warnings:* Medication should be discontinued every 2-3 months for a period of 4 weeks to assess the necessity for further treatment.

In the event of persistent or recurring vaginal bleeding, appropriate diagnostic measures should be taken to rule out malignancy. In case of vaginal infections these should be treated before therapy with Ovestin Cream is started.

Prolonged exposure to unopposed oestrogens may increase the risk of the development of endometrial carcinoma.

Pain in the breasts or excessive production of cervical mucus may be indicative of too high a dosage.

During prolonged treatment with oestrogens, periodic medical examinations are advisable.

A cervical smear should be taken at regular intervals.

Oestrogen preparations may increase the risk of thrombosis and this should be taken into account when surgery is to be performed in patients using these preparations. Where possible, oestrogens should be discontinued approximately six weeks prior to elective surgery and not recommenced until the patient has recovered and is mobile.

Patients, especially the elderly, with any of the following conditions should be monitored: latent or overt cardiac failure; renal or hepatic dysfunction; hypertension; epilepsy or migraine or a history of these conditions; a history of thromboembolic disorders (since oestrogens may cause sodium and water retention and exacerbate the above conditions); endometriosis; fibrocystic mastopathy; diabetes mellitus.

*Adverse reactions:* As with any preparation that is to be applied to mucosal surfaces, Ovestin Cream may cause local irritation or itching at the beginning of treatment. During the first weeks of therapy, occasional mastodynia may occur. In general, these complaints are transient in nature.

*Interactions:* There is insufficient evidence to support the occurrence of clinically relevant interactions.

*Overdosage:* The acute toxicity of oestriol in animals is very low. Symptoms that may occur in the case of an acute oral overdosage are nausea, vomiting and possibly withdrawal bleeding in females. No specific antidote is known. If necessary a symptomatic treatment should be instituted.

**Pharmaceutical precautions** The preparation should be stored at room temperature (15–25°C)

**Legal category** POM

**Package quantities** Tube (+applicator) containing 15 g cream.

**Further information**
*Pharmacological particulars:* Oestriol, along with oestradiol and oestrone, is one of the three most important oestrogens found in the body.

Morphological and clinical investigations have shown that oestriol has a specific effect upon the cervix and upon the epithelium of the vagina and vulva, with only a mild proliferative effect upon the endometrium.

The local application of oestriol makes therapeutic use of its stimulating effect upon the epithelium of the vulva and vagina.

The vaginal mucosa reacts with a loosening up and hyperaemia of the sub epithelial tissue, and an increase in the desquamation of superficial and intermediate cells containing glycogen. Histological examination shows the vaginal smear exhibiting regular layering once again, which corresponds to the picture of oestrogen-stimulated tissue.

Oestriol is absorbed from the vagina into the general circulation as evidenced by a rise in plasma oestriol. There is no effect on plasma levels of oestradiol, oestrone and prolactin, nor on sex hormone binding globulin and corticosteroid binding globulin synthesis in the liver.

There is no clinically significant suppression of the FSH/LH release. Oestriol administered at therapeutically effective dosages as Ovestin Cream, does not induce a general oestrogenic effect in the body.

In particular no effect on the endometrium is found.

No other pharmacological effects are observed.

*Pharmacokinetic particulars:* Intravaginal application of oestriol ensures optimal availability of the product at the site of action. After administration of Ovestin Cream, oestriol is also absorbed from the vagina into the general circulation, shown by a sharp rise in plasma oestriol, followed by a gradual decline.

After 3 weeks of administration of a single daily dose, a similar absorption pattern to that seen for a single application was observed.

Daily treatment with 0.5 mg of oestriol (in 0.5 g of cream) leads to a sharp rise in unconjugated plasma oestriol levels to 110 pg/ml at one hour from previously undetectable levels (<12 pg/ml). This was followed by a gradual decline during the next 5 hours to around 60 pg/ml.

On day 21 of treatment mean baseline oestriol levels of about 26 pg/ml rose to a mean peak value of 95 pg/ml at 1 hour. A decline similar to that seen on day 1 was observed during the next 5 hours.

Vaginal administration permits the absorption of the active (unconjugated, or free) form of oestriol into the blood for transport to the target tissues, prior to its inactivation via conjugation by enterohepatic enzymes.

**Product licence number** 0065/0074

## OVESTIN TABLETS (1 mg)

**Presentation** Round, flat, white tablets, diameter 6 mm, code-marked 'DG7' on one side, with 'Organon' and a star on the reverse side. Each tablet contains 1 mg of Oestriol.

Other constituents: amylopectin, lactose, potato starch and magnesium stearate.

**Uses** In genito-urinary complaints due to oestrogen deficiency such as vaginal atrophy, atrophic vaginitis and recurrent urogenital infections.

**Dosage and administration** *Adults and the elderly:* The tablets should be swallowed without chewing. It is important that the total daily dose is taken at one time.

*Genito-urinary complaints:* 0.5–3 mg daily for up to 1 month. Maintenance dose 0.5–1 mg daily until restoration of the epithelial integrity and normal balance of vaginal flora is established.

***NB.*** Oestrogen therapy should be reviewed according to the individual patient's requirements and clinical picture. Long-term therapy requires regular monitoring procedures.

*Children:* There is no recommended dose for children.

*Use in pregnancy and lactation:* Ovestin tablets are contraindicated during pregnancy. This is based on observations in the human which have indicated that the use of oestrogens may be harmful in pregnancy.

There is insufficient data on the use of Ovestin tablets at recommended dosages during breast-feeding to assess potential harm to the child. It is known, however, that oestriol is excreted in breast milk and may inhibit lactation.

**Contra-indications, warnings etc**
*Contra-indications:* Pregnancy; thrombosis; known or suspected oestrogen-dependent tumours; undiagnosed vaginal bleeding; porphyria; severe hypertension; hepatic diseases

*Precautions and warnings:* Prolonged exposure to unopposed oestrogens may increase the risk of the development of endometrial carcinoma.

Pain in the breasts or excessive production of cervical mucus may be indicative of too high a dosage.

During prolonged treatment with oestrogens, periodical medical examinations are advisable.

With vaginal infections, a concomitant specific treatment is recommended.

Patients, with the following conditions should be monitored: a history of thromboembolic disorders; latent or overt cardiac failure; fluid retention due to renal dysfunction; hypertension; epilepsy or migraine (or a history of these conditions); endometriosis; fibrocystic mastopathy; hyperlipoproteinaemia; diabetes mellitus; a history during pregnancy or previous use of steroids of severe pruritus or herpes gestationis.

*Effects on ability to drive and to use machines:* None stated

*Interactions:* There is insufficient evidence to support the potential occurrence of clinically relevant interactions.

*Other undesirable effects (frequency and seriousness):* The following adverse reactions, associated with oestrogen treatment may occur during oestriol therapy: Nausea and vomiting, breast tenderness or pain in the breasts, spotting during or on withdrawal of therapy, excessive production of cervical mucus, headache.

*Overdosage:* The acute toxicity of the natural hormone oestriol is very low. Symptoms that may possibly occur in the case of an acute overdosage are nausea and vomiting. No specific antidote is known. If necessary a symptomatic treatment will probably be sufficient.

**Pharmaceutical precautions** Store between 2° and 30°C. Protect from light

**Legal category** POM

**Package quantities** Push through strips of 30 tablets

**Further information** Ovestin tablets contain the natural hormone oestriol. In the years just before and after the menopause (whether naturally or surgically induced) oestriol can be used in the treatment of symptoms and complaints related to oestrogen deficiency. In cases of vaginal atrophy oestriol induces normalisation of the vaginal epithelium and thus helps to restore the normal microflora and a physiological pH in the vagina. As a result it increases the resistance of the vaginal epithelial cells to infection and inflammation. Oestriol is a relatively short-acting oestrogen due to its short nuclear retention time in endometrial cells, its low affinity for plasma proteins and partly as a result of this, its rapid metabolic clearance. Endometrial proliferation is not expected when oestriol is given in a single daily dose, since this requires sustained occupancy of the nuclear oestrogen receptor. As a consequence, undesired vaginal bleeding rarely occurs during treatment with oestriol and an increased risk of endometrial carcinoma is unlikely.

**Product licence number** 0065/0130

## PREGNYL*

**Presentation** Pregnyl contains purified human chorionic gonadotrophin (hCG) prepared from the urine of pregnant women. Ampoules containing a white, freeze-dried powder, with 1 ml ampoules of solvent. Active ingredient: Chorionic Gonadotrophin BP 1,500 IU or 5,000 IU.

Other ingredients: sodium carboxymethylcellulose, mannitol, anhydrous disodium hydrogen phosphate, anhydrous sodium dihydrogen phosphate

**Uses** *In the male:* Hypogonadotrophic hypogonadism. Delayed puberty associated with insufficient gonadotrophic pituitary function. Sterility in selected cases of deficient spermatogenesis.

*In the female:* Sterility due to the absence of follicle-ripening or ovulation. In conjunction with human menopausal gonadotrophins (HMG), in the promotion of controlled superovulation in medically assisted reproduction programmes.

**Dosage and administration** *In the male: Hypogonadotrophic hypogonadism.* 500-1,000 IU 2-3 times weekly.

*Delayed puberty associated with insufficient gonad-*

*otrophic pituitary function.* 1,500 IU twice weekly for at least 6 months.

*Sterility in selected cases of deficient spermatogenesis.* Usually, 3,000 IU per week in combination with a HMG preparation.

*In the female: Sterility due to the absence of follicle-ripening or ovulation.* Usually 5,000-10,000 IU hCG to induce ovulation, following treatment with an HMG preparation. Up to 3 repeat injections of up to 5,000 IU hCG may then be given within the following 9 days to prevent insufficiency of the corpus luteum.

*In conjunction with HMG, in the promotion of controlled superovulation in medically assisted reproduction programmes.* 5,000-10,000 IU hCG 30-40 hours after the last HMG injection.

Pregnyl should not be administered if the following criteria have not been met: It is recommended that at least 3 follicles greater than 17 mm in diameter are present with 17β oestradiol levels of at least 3,500 pmol/L (920 picogram/ml).

Oocyte collection is carried out 32-36 hours after the hCG injection.

After addition of the solvent to the freeze-dried substance, the solution should be used immediately by intramuscular injection.

### Contra-indications, warnings, etc
*Contra-indications:* Known or suspected androgen-dependent tumours, carcinoma of the prostate or mammary carcinoma in males.

*Use in pregnancy and lactation:* Not applicable.

*Warnings and precautions:* Treatment of male patients with Pregnyl leads to increased androgen production. Therefore Pregnyl should be used cautiously in prepubertal boys to avoid premature epiphyseal closure or precocious sexual development.

Patients with latent or overt cardiac failure, renal dysfunction, hypertension, epilepsy or migraine (or a history of these conditions) should be monitored, since sodium and fluid retention have been observed after administration of high dosages of hCG.

Prior to treating patients for inadequate endogenous stimulation of the gonads, an examination should be performed to exclude anatomical abnormalities of the genital organs or nongonadal endocrinopathies (e.g. thyroid or adrenal disorders, diabetes). Primary ovarian failure should be excluded by the determination of gonadotrophin levels.

In the pregnancies occurring after induction of ovulation with gonadotrophic preparations, there is an increased risk of abortion and multiplets.

*Unwanted hyperstimulation:* During treatment of female patients, determinations of oestrogen levels and assessment of ovarian size and if possible, ultrasonography should be performed prior to treatment and at regular intervals during treatment. High dosages may cause oestrogen levels to rise excessively rapidly, e.g. more than doubling on 2 or 3 consecutive days, and possibly reaching excessively high pre-ovulatory values.

If unwanted hyperstimulation occurs (i.e. not as part of a treatment preparing for IVF/ET or GIFT or other assisted reproduction techniques), the administration of HMG should be discontinued immediately. hCG must not be given, because the administration of an hLH–active gonadotrophin at this stage may induce, in addition to multiple ovulations, the ovarian hyperstimulation syndrome. This warning is particularly important with respect to patients with polycystic ovarian disease.

The severe form of ovarian hyperstimulation syndrome may be life-threatening and is characterised by large ovarian cysts (prone to rupture), acute abdominal pain, ascites, very often hydrothorax and occasionally thrombo-embolic phenomena.

*Effects on ability to drive and use machines:* Not applicable.

*Interactions:* None known

*Adverse reactions:* Skin rashes have occasionally been reported.

Sodium and water retention is occasionally seen in males after administration of high dosages; this is regarded as a result of excessive androgen production.

*Overdosage:* The toxicity of human chorionic gonadotrophic hormone is very low. However, too high a dose may lead to hyperstimulation of the ovaries (see *Unwanted Hyperstimulation*)

**Pharmaceutical precautions** Protect from light and store at a temperature between 2 and 15°C. In the dry state, in sealed containers, Pregnyl will retain its full activity for three years from the date of manufacture. Solutions are unstable and should be used freshly prepared.

**Legal category** POM

**Package quantities** Single ampoules of Pregnyl 1500 IU or 5,000 IU with solvent. Boxes of 10 ampoules of Pregnyl 5,000 IU with solvent.

**Further information** Pregnyl stimulates the steroidogenesis in the gonads by virtue of a biological effect similar to that of LH (luteinizing hormone, which is the same as interstitial cell stimulating hormone). In the male it promotes the production of testosterone and in the female the production of oestrogens and particularly of progesterone after ovulation. In certain cases, this preparation is used in combination with human menopausal gonadotrophin (HMG). Because hCG is of human origin, no antibody formation is to be expected.

**Product licence numbers**
Pregnyl 1500 IU    0065/5078
Pregnyl 5000 IU    0065/5079
Solvent               0065/0114 (Sodium Chloride solution for injection 0.9%w/v)

## PUREGON* ▼

**Qualitative and quantitative composition** Puregon consists of a freeze-dried powder and a solvent for reconstitution. The powder for injection contains the active ingredient recombinant follicle-stimulating hormone (FSH) (Follitropin beta).

One container of Puregon contains 50 or 100 I.U. FSH activity corresponding to 5 or 10 micrograms of protein (specific in vivo bioactivity equal to approximately 10 000 I.U. FSH/ mg protein[1] ). Puregon is in the form of a lyophilised sphere or lyosphere.

[1] as determined by the PhEur test for FSH in vivo bioactivity and on the basis of the molar extinction coefficient at 277 nm (εs ; mg-1cm-1 ) = 1.066.

**Pharmaceutical form** Powder for injection. Prior to use, Puregon is reconstituted with the solvent for parenteral use provided.

**Clinical particulars**

*Therapeutic indications:* Puregon is indicated for the treatment of female infertility in the following clinical situations:
– Anovulation (including polycystic ovarian disease, PCOD) in women who have been unresponsive to treatment with clomiphene citrate.
– Controlled ovarian hyperstimulation to induce the development of multiple follicles in medically assisted reproduction programs [e.g. in vitro fertilisation/embryo transfer (IVF/ET), gamete intra-fallopian transfer (GIFT) and intracytoplasmic sperm injection (ICSI)].

*Posology and method of administration:*
*General:* The dosage recommendations given below are in line with those usually applied for urinary FSH. These dosages were also applied in comparative clinical studies with Puregon and urinary FSH. In these studies it was shown that Puregon is more effective than urinary FSH in terms of a lower total dose and a shorter treatment period needed to achieve pre-ovulatory conditions. Therefore, it may be appropriate to give a lower dosage of Puregon than for urinary FSH. This advice is not only relevant in order to optimise follicular development but also to minimise the risk of unwanted ovarian hyperstimulation. For this purpose the dosage range of Puregon includes the strengths of 50 I.U. and 100 I.U.

*Posology:* There are great inter- and intra-individual variations in the response of the ovaries to exogenous gonadotropins. This makes it impossible to set a uniform dosage scheme. The dosage should, therefore, be adjusted individually depending on the ovarian response. This requires ultrasonography and monitoring of oestradiol levels.

After pituitary desensitisation induced by a GnRH agonist a higher dose of Puregon may be necessary to achieve an adequate follicular response.

Clinical experience with Puregon is based on up to three treatment cycles in both indications. Overall experience with IVF indicates that in general the treatment success rate remains stable during the first four attempts and gradually declines thereafter.

*Anovulation:* In general, a sequential treatment scheme is recommended. This usually starts with daily administration of 75 I.U. FSH activity. The starting dose is maintained for at least seven days. If there is no ovarian response, the daily dose is then gradually increased until follicle growth and/or plasma oestradiol levels indicate an adequate pharmacodynamic response. A daily increase of oestradiol levels of 40-100 per cent is considered to be optimal. The daily dose is then maintained until pre-ovulatory conditions are reached. Pre-ovulatory conditions are reached when there is ultrasonographic evidence of a dominant follicle of at least 18 mm in diameter and/or when plasma oestradiol levels of 300-900 picograms/ml (1000-3000 pmol/L) are attained. Usually, 7 to 14 days of treatment is sufficient to reach this state. The administration of Puregon is then discontinued and ovulation can be induced by administering human chorionic gonadotropin (hCG). If the number of responding follicles is too high or oestradiol levels increase too rapidly, i.e. more than a daily doubling

for oestradiol for two or three consecutive days, the daily dose should be decreased.

Since follicles of over 14 mm may lead to pregnancies, multiple pre-ovulatory follicles exceeding 14 mm carry the risk of multiple gestations. In that case hCG should be withheld and pregnancy should be avoided in order to prevent multiple gestations.

*Controlled ovarian hyperstimulation in medically assisted reproduction programmes:* Various stimulation protocols are applied. A starting dose of 150-225 I.U. is recommended for at least the first four days. Thereafter, the dose may be adjusted individually, based upon ovarian response. In clinical studies it was shown that maintenance dosages ranging from 75-375 I.U. for six to twelve days are sufficient, although longer treatment may be necessary.

Puregon can be given either alone, or in combination with a GnRH agonist to prevent premature luteinisation. In the latter case a higher total treatment dose of Puregon may be required.

Ovarian response is monitored by ultrasonography and measurement of plasma oestradiol levels. When ultrasonographic evaluation indicates the presence of at least three follicles of 16-20 mm, and there is evidence of a good oestradiol response (plasma levels of about 300-400 picogram/ml (1000-1300 pmol/l) for each follicle with a diameter greater than 18 mm), the final phase of maturation of the follicles is induced by administration of hCG. Oocyte retrieval is performed 34-35 hours later.

*Method of administration:* Puregon should be reconstituted with the solvent provided. The reconstituted solution should be administered immediately

To prevent painful injections and minimise leakage from the injection site the Puregon* solution should be slowly administered intramuscularly or subcutaneously. The subcutaneous injection site should be alternated to prevent lipoatrophy. Any unused solution should be discarded.

Subcutaneous injection of Puregon may be carried out by patient or partner, provided that proper instructions are given by the physician. Self administration of Puregon should only be performed by patients who are well-motivated, adequately trained and with access to expert advice.

*Contra-indications:* Tumours of the ovary, breast, uterus, pituitary or hypothalamus. Pregnancy or lactation. Undiagnosed vaginal bleeding. Hypersensitivity to any of the substances in Puregon. Primary ovarian failure. Ovarian cysts or enlarged ovaries, not related to polycystic ovarian disease (PCOD). Malformations of the sexual organs incompatible with pregnancy. Fibroid tumours of the uterus incompatible with pregnancy.

*Special warnings and special precautions for use:* The presence of uncontrolled non-gonadal endocrinopathies (e.g. thyroid, adrenal or pituitary disorders) should be excluded.

In pregnancies occurring after induction of ovulation with gonadotropic preparations, there is an increased risk of multiple gestations.

There have been no reports of hypersensitivity to Puregon, but there remains the possibility of anaphylactic responses. The first injection of Puregon should only be performed under direct medical supervision.

Since infertile women undergoing assisted reproduction, and particularly IVF, often have tubal abnormalities the incidence of ectopic pregnancies might be increased. Early ultrasound confirmation that a pregnancy is intrauterine is therefore important.

Rates of pregnancy loss in women undergoing ART are higher than in the normal population.

*Unwanted ovarian hyperstimulation:* In the treatment of female patients, ultrasonographic assessment of follicular development, and determination of oestradiol levels should be performed prior to treatment and at regular intervals during treatment. Apart from the development of a high number of follicles, oestradiol levels may rise very rapidly, e.g. more than a daily doubling for two or three consecutive days, and possibly reaching excessively high values. The diagnosis of ovarian hyperstimulation may be confirmed by ultrasound examination. If this unwanted ovarian hyperstimulation occurs (i.e. not as part of controlled ovarian hyperstimulation in medically assisted reproduction programs), the administration of Puregon* should be discontinued. In that case pregnancy should be avoided and hCG must be withheld, because it may induce, in addition to multiple ovulation, the ovarian hyperstimulation syndrome. Clinical symptoms and signs of mild ovarian hyperstimulation syndrome are abdominal pain, nausea, diarrhoea, and mild to moderate enlargement of ovaries and ovarian cysts. In rare cases severe ovarian hyperstimulation syndrome occurs, which may be life-threatening. This is characterised by large ovarian cysts (prone to rupture), ascites, often hydrothorax and weight gain. In rare instances, arterio-thromboembolic processes have been associated with other gonadotropin therapy. This may also occur with Puregon/hCG.

*Interaction with other medicaments and other forms of interaction:* Concomitant use of Puregon* and clomiphene citrate may enhance the follicular response. After pituitary desensitisation induced by a GnRH agonist, a higher dose of Puregon may be necessary to achieve an adequate follicular response.

*Pregnancy and lactation:* Puregon must not be used during pregnancy and lactation.

*Effects on ability to drive and use machines:* As far as known this medicine has no influence on alertness and concentration.

*Undesirable effects:* Unwanted ovarian hyperstimulation has been observed in 5% of subjects treated with Puregon. Characteristic symptoms of these conditions have been described (see *Special warnings and special precautions for use*).

Clinical use of Puregon by the i.m. or s.c. routes may lead to reactions at the site of injection such as bruising, pain, redness, swelling and itching, the majority of which are mild. Generalised reactions have not been observed.

Formation of antibodies against follitropin beta or host cell-derived proteins have not been observed during therapy.

A slightly increased risk of ectopic pregnancy and multiple pregnancies has been seen.

In rare instances, arterio-thromboembolisms have been associated with menotrophin/human chorionic gonadotrophin therapy. This may also occur with Puregon/hCG therapy.

*Overdosage:* No data on acute toxicity of Puregon in humans is available, but the acute toxicity of Puregon and of urinary gonadotropin preparations in animal studies has been shown to be very low. Too high a dosage of FSH may lead to hyperstimulation of the ovaries (see *Unwanted ovarian hyperstimulation*).

**Pharmacological properties**

*Pharmacodynamic properties:* (ATC classification: gonadotrophins, GO3G)

Puregon contains a recombinant FSH. This is produced by recombinant DNA technology, using a Chinese hamster ovary cell line transfected with the human FSH subunit genes. The primary amino acid sequence is identical to that of natural human FSH. Small differences in the carbohydrate chain structure are known to exist. FSH is indispensable in normal follicular growth and maturation, and gonadal steroid production. In the female the level of FSH is critical for the onset and duration of follicular development, and consequently for the timing and number of follicles reaching maturity. Puregon can thus be used to stimulate follicular development and steroid production in selected cases of disturbed gonadal function. Furthermore Puregon can be used to promote multiple follicular development in medically assisted reproduction programs [e.g. in vitro fertilisation/embryo transfer (IVF/ET), gamete intra-fallopian transfer (GIFT) and intracytoplasmic sperm injection (ICSI)]. Treatment with Puregon is generally followed by administration of hCG to induce the final phase of follicle maturation, resumption of meiosis and rupture of the follicle.

*Pharmacokinetic properties:* After intramuscular or subcutaneous administration of Puregon, maximum concentrations of FSH are reached within about 12 hours. Due to the sustained release from the injection site and the elimination half-life of about 40 hours (ranging from 12 to 70 hours), FSH levels remain increased for 24-48 hours. Due to the relatively long elimination half-life, repeated administration of the same dose will lead to plasma concentrations of FSH that are approximately 1.5-2.5 times higher than after single dose administration. This increase enables therapeutic FSH concentrations to be reached.

There are no significant pharmacokinetic differences between intramuscular and subcutaneous administration of Puregon. Both have an absolute bioavailability of approximately 77 per cent. Recombinant FSH is biochemically very similar to urinary human FSH and is distributed, metabolised, and excreted in the same way.

*Preclinical safety data:* Single-dose administration of Puregon to rats induced no toxicologically significant effects. In repeated-dose studies in rats (two weeks) and dogs (13 weeks) up to 100-fold the maximal human dose, Puregon induced no toxicologically significant effects. Puregon showed no mutagenic potential in the Ames test or in the in vitro chromosome aberration test with human lymphocytes.

**Pharmaceutical particulars**

*List of excipients:* The powder for injection contains sucrose, sodium citrate, and polysorbate 20. The pH may have been adjusted with sodium hydroxide and/or hydrochloric acid. The ampoule of solvent contains sodium chloride (4.5 mg) and water for injections (1.0 ml). The quality of all excipients is in accordance with the specifications of the European Pharmacopoeia (PhEur.)

*Incompatibilities:* Incompatibilities with other medication have not been investigated and mixing with other medication should therefore be avoided.

*Shelf-life:* The shelf-life of Puregon is two years under the conditions specified below in *Special precautions for storage* Puregon may be used until the expiration date indicated on the package.

*Special precautions for storage:* Store below 30°C. Protect from light. Do not freeze. Store Puregon out of reach of children

*Nature and contents of containers:* Boxes of Puregon contain:

1 ampoule of follitropin beta plus 1 ampoule solvent or

5 ampoules of follitropin beta plus 5 ampoules solvent.

Ampoules of Puregon* contain a sterile lyophilised sphere (called lyosphere) corresponding to 50 or 100 I.U. FSH activity. Ampoules solvent contain 1 ml saline 0.45%.

*Instructions for use/handling:* Puregon should be reconstituted with the solvent provided using a gentle, swirling motion. Vigorous shaking should be avoided. Do not use if the solution contains particles or if the solution is not clear.

Since an opened ampoule cannot be resealed in such a way to further guarantee the sterility of the contents, the solution should be used immediately after reconstitution. Discard any remaining solution after single use.

*Marketing authorisation holder:* N.V. Organon, P O Box 20, 5340 BH Oss, The Netherlands

**Marketing authorisation numbers**

| | |
|---|---|
| 50 IU | 1 ampoule–EU/1/96/008/001, 5 ampoules–EU/1/96/008/003 |
| 100 IU | 1 ampoule–EU/1/96/008/009, 5 ampoules–EU/1/96/008/011 |

**Date of approval/revision of SPC** 9 August 1996

**Legal category** POM

## RESTANDOL*

**Qualitative and quantitative composition** Each capsule contains Testosterone Undecanoate 40.0 mg HSE

**Pharmaceutical form** Red/Brown soft gelatin capsule printed Org $D_3V$

**Clinical particulars**

*Therapeutic indications:* Testosterone replacement therapy in male hypogonadal disorders, for example: after castration; eunuchoidism; hypopituitarism; endocrine impotence; male climacteric symptoms like decreased libido and decreased mental and physical activity; certain types of infertility due to disorders of spermatogenesis

Testosterone therapy may also be indicated in osteoporosis due to androgenic deficiency.

*Posology and method of administration:*
*Dosage:*

*Adults:* The initial dosage required will usually be 120-160 mg daily for 2-3 weeks. Subsequent dosage (40-120 mg daily) should be based on the clinical effect obtained during the first weeks of therapy.

*Elderly patients:* It should be noted that smaller and less frequent doses may achieve the same response.

*Children:* Not applicable.

*Administration:* Oral. The capsules should be taken after meals, if necessary with a little water, and be swallowed whole without chewing. It is preferable that half of the daily dose be taken in the morning and the other half in the evening. If an uneven number of capsules is taken daily, the greater part should be taken in the morning.

*Contra-indications:* Known or suspected prostatic or mammary carcinoma; hypercalciuria, hypercalcaemia, nephrotic syndrome, ischaemic heart disease or untreated congestive heart failure.

*Special warnings and special precautions for use:* Patients, especially the elderly, with the following conditions should be monitored: latent or overt cardiac failure, renal or hepatic dysfunction, hypertension, epilepsy or migraine (or a history of these conditions), since androgens may occasionally induce sodium and water retention. Mammary carcinoma, hypernephroma, bronchial carcinoma, and skeletal metastases, since these conditions may produce hypercalcaemia or hypercalciuria which may in turn be exacerbated by androgen therapy. If hypercalcaemia or hypercalciuria develops treatment should be discontinued.

A decrease in protein-bound iodine (PBI) may occur, but this has no clinical significance.

Androgens should be used cautiously in prepubertal boys to avoid premature epiphyseal closure or precocious sexual development.

Androgen therapy should only be used in male hypogonadism in which testosterone levels have been demonstrated to be low.

In treating males, stimulation to the point of increasing nervous, mental and physical activities beyond the patient's cardiovascular capacity should be avoided.

Tumours and other histological abnormalities and disturbances of liver function have been reported in patients subjected to prolonged treatment with some testosterone derivatives. Most of these compounds were 17-alpha alkyl derivatives but a smaller number of cases has occurred with certain 17-beta esters of testosterone. The possibility that such changes result from the use of Restandol has not been excluded.

*Interaction with other medicaments and other forms of interaction:* Concurrent administration of liver enzyme inducing drugs such as rifampicin, barbiturates, carbamazepine, dichloralphenazone, phenylbutazone, phenytoin or primidone may decrease the effect of Restandol.

*Pregnancy and lactation:* Not applicable (only male indications).

*Effects on ability to drive and use of machines:* Restandol will not effect ability to drive or use machines.

*Undesirable effects:* Restandol, like any other androgen therapy, may give rise to the following adverse reactions: priapism and other signs of excessive sexual stimulation. Precocious sexual development, an increased frequency of erections, phallic enlargement and premature epiphyseal closure in pre-pubertal males. Sodium and water retention. Oligospermia and a decreased ejaculatory volume.

Treatment should be interrupted until these symptoms have disappeared, after which it should be continued at a lower dosage.

Hoarseness of the voice may be the first symptom of vocal change which may lead to irreversible lowering of the voice. If signs of virilisation, particularly lowering of the voice, develop, treatment should be discontinued.

*Overdosage:* Treatment of overdosage is by gastric lavage with appropriate supportive therapy. Standard resuscitative measures should be given as required.

**Pharmacological properties**

*Pharmacodynamic properties:* The pharmacological action of testosterone undecanoate can be attributed to the testosterone content, an androgenic hormone which controls the development and maintenance of the male sex organs and male secondary sex characteristics

*Pharmacokinetic properties:* Testosterone undecanoate, a fatty acid ester of the natural androgen testosterone, is an orally effective testosterone preparation. Testosterone is inactive on oral administration because it is prematurely inactivated by the liver. Testosterone undecanoate is able to by-pass the liver via the lymphatic system and is therefore orally active.

*Preclinical safety data:* Not applicable

**Pharmaceutical particulars**

*List of excipients:* Oleic Acid PhEur. Capsule shell: Glycerol (85%) PhEur, sorbitol concentrate (Karion 83) HSE, sodium ethylhydroxybenzoate FRP, sodium propylhydroxybenzoate BP, titanium dioxide PhEur, iron oxide (Red) NF, gelatin PhEur.

*Incompatibilities:* None stated.

*Shelf life:* 3 years

*Special precautions for storage:* Wholesaler/pharmacy: Store in the refrigerator (2-8°C). Protect from light and moisture. *Patient:* Store at room temperature (up to 30°C). Protect from light and moisture.

*Nature and contents of containers:* Polyethylene tampertainers 28. Polyethylene tampertainers 56

*Instructions for use/handling:* Not applicable

**Marketing authorisation number** 0065/0059

**Date of approval/revision of SPC** October 1995

**Legal category** POM

## SANDRENA

**Qualitative and quantitative composition** Estradiol hemihydrate corresponding to: 0.5 mg estradiol/dose (in single dose units containing 0.5 g gel).

Estradiol hemihydrate corresponding to: 1.0 mg estradiol/dose (in single dose units containing 1.0 g gel).

**Pharmaceutical form** Gel

**Clinical particulars**

*Therapeutic indications*: Treatment of the climacteric syndrome associated with natural or artificial menopause (oestrogenic deficiency, e.g. hot flushes, night sweats, urogenital atrophy).

*Posology and method of administration*: Sandrena can be used for continuous or cyclical treatment.

The dose can be adjusted individually from 0.5 g to 1.5 g per day, corresponding to 0.5 to 1.5 mg estradiol per day. The usual starting dose is 1.0 mg estradiol (1.0 g gel) daily and can be readjusted after 2-3 cycles.

In patients with an intact uterus, it is recommended to combine Sandrena treatment with an adequate dose of progestogen, for adequate duration e.g. for 10-12 consecutive days per month.

The Sandrena dose is applied once daily on the skin of the lower trunk of the right or left thigh, on alternate days. The application surface should be 1-2 times the size of the hand. Sandrena should not be applied on the breasts, on the face or on irritated skin. After application the gel should be allowed to dry for a few minutes and the application site should not be washed within 1 hour. Accidental contact of the gel with the eyes should be avoided. Hands should be washed after application.

If the patient forgets to apply a dose, it should be applied as soon as possible, unless the dose is more than 12 hours late. If the dose is more than 12 hours late, it should be skipped. Missed doses may induce breakthrough bleeding.

*Contra-indications:*

- Undiagnosed vaginal bleeding,
- Active or recent thromboembolic disease or thrombophlebitis,
- Severe hepatic disease (including Dubin-Johnson and Rotor's syndrome),
- Oestrogen dependent cancer (e.g. of the breast or endometrium),
- Hypersensitivity to the constituents of the preparation.

*Special warnings and special precautions for use:* Before therapy is initiated, a thorough medical history should be taken. A complete gynaecological examination should be performed and repeated at least once a year during therapy.

Prolonged use without addition of a progestogen may cause endometrial hyperplasia. Therefore, in women with an intact uterus, Sandrena treatment should be combined with cyclic progestogen administration. Withdrawal bleeding resembling normal menstruation will usually occur after each course of progestogen. The cause of unexpected or prolonged uterine bleeding during therapy should be clarified. A typical adenomatous hyperplasia of the endometrium must be treated before commencing oestrogen therapy.

Consider discontinuation prior to surgery or prolonged immobilisation. Development of de novo frequent severe headaches or migraine should be investigated and possible prodromal symptoms of vascular occlusion should be clarified.

The risks and benefits of treatment should be evaluated and close monitoring performed for patients with:

- endometriosis
- uterine leiomyoma
- endometrial hyperplasia (simple glandular hyperplasia or hyperplasia glandularis cystica)
- diseases of the cardiovascular system including cerebrovascular disorders,
- a history of thromboembolic disease,
- severe hypertension,
- history of (or close family history of) breast cancer,
- severe disturbances of lipid metabolism,
- renal dysfunction
- systemic lupus erythematosus
- porphyria

At present there is suggestive evidence of a slight increase in the relative risk of carcinoma of the breast with long-term hormone replacement therapy, however, the results are contradictory. Regular breast examinations and mammography, where appropriate, should be carried out in women on hormone replacement therapy.

Some conditions may be aggravated during oestrogen therapy or pregnancy. Women on Sandrena treatment with one of the following conditions (or with a history thereof during previous pregnancy or hormone use) should therefore be closely monitored. These conditions include:

- mild hypertension,
- migraine or severe headache,
- benign breast disease,
- liver function disturbances,
- cholestasis,
- cholelithiasis,
- diabetes mellitus,
- asthma,
- otosclerosis,
- multiple sclerosis,
- galactorrhea, elevated prolactin levels,
- history of herpes gestationis,
- epilepsy.

*Interaction with other medicaments and other forms of interaction:* No interactions between Sandrena and other medicines have been reported. There are some indications that oestrogens may reduce the effects of antihypertensive, anticoagulant and antidiabetic drugs. Concomitant treatment with potent inducers of liver enzymes (e.g. barbiturates, carbamazepine, griseofulvin and rifampicin) may reduce the plasma levels of estradiol. The significance of these interactions in transdermal application has not been elucidated.

*Pregnancy and lactation*: Sandrena is not indicated in women of child-bearing capacity. It has no contraceptive efficacy. Sandrena should not be used during pregnancy or lactation.

*Effects on ability to drive and use machines*: Oestrogens such as Sandrena do not affect the ability to drive or use machines.

*Undesirable effects:* Adverse drug reactions are usually mild and only seldom lead to discontinuation of treatment. If they do occur, it will usually be during the first months of treatment.

Occasionally for oestrogens in general: Breast tenderness, headache, oedema, weight increase, unscheduled vaginal bleeding or spotting.

Rarely for oestrogens in general: Migraine, changes in libido and mood, gastrointestinal discomfort (e.g. nausea, vomiting, stomach cramps), hypertension, alterations in liver function and biliary flow.

In clinical trials dermal irritation has been very infrequent with Sandrena.

*Overdosage:* Generally, oestrogens are well tolerated even in massive doses. Possible symptoms of overdose include those listed under undesirable effects. Treatment is symptomatic.

**Pharmacological properties** Therapeutic classification: G03 CA 03, Oestrogen preparation for hormone replacement therapy.

*Pharmacodynamic properties:* The pharmacodynamics of Sandrena are similar to those of oral oestrogens, but the major difference to oral administration lies in the pharmacokinetic profile.

The clinical efficacy of Sandrena in the treatment of menopausal symptoms is comparable to that of peroral oestrogen. Combined with medroxyprogesterone acetate, percutaneous oestradiol lowers total cholesterol without reducing the HDL cholesterol level.

*Pharmacokinetic properties:* Sandrena is an alcohol-based estradiol gel. When applied to the skin the alcohol evaporates rapidly and oestradiol is absorbed through the skin into the circulation. To some extent, however, the estradiol is stored in the subcutaneous tissue from where it is released gradually into circulation. Percutaneous administration circumvents the hepatic first-pass metabolism. For these reasons, the fluctuations in the plasma oestrogen concentrations with Sandrena are less pronounced than peroral oestrogen.

A 1.5 mg percutaneous dose of estradiol (1.5 g Sandrena) results in a plasma concentration of about 340 pmol/l, which corresponds to the level of early follicular stage in premenopausal women. During Sandrena treatment the estradiol/oestrone ratio remains at 0.7, while during peroral oestrogen treatment it usually drops to less than 0.2.

The mean estradiol exposure at steady state of Sandrena is 82 per cent compared with an equivalent oral dose of estradiol valerate. Otherwise the metabolism and excretion of transdermal oestradiol follow the fate of natural oestrogens.

*Preclinical safety data:* Estradiol is a natural female hormone with an established clinical use, therefore no toxicological studies have been performed with Sandrena. The necessary studies on the irritant effects of the gel have been studied in rabbits and skin sensitisation in guinea pig. Based on the results from these studies it can be concluded that Sandrena could very infrequently cause mild skin irritation. The frequency of the occurrence of dermal irritation can be reduced by daily change of the application site.

**Pharmaceutical particulars**

*List of excipients:* Carbomer 934 BP, sodium hydroxide, propylene glycol PhEur., Spir. fort.–Ethanol 96% BP, Aq. purif.–Purified water PhEur.

*Incompatibilities:* No incompatibilities have been found.

*Shelf life*: 3 years.

*Special precautions for storage*: At room temperature (below 25°C).

*Nature and contents of container*: Single dose aluminium foil sachets supplied in packages containing 28 of either dose or 91 sachets of 1 mg dose.

*Instructions for use/handling*: None

*Marketing authorisation holder:* Orion Corporation, Orioninite 1, P.O. Box 65, FIN-02101, Espoo, Finland.

**Marketing authorisation number** 13911/0004-0005

**Date of approval/revision of SPC** October 1996

**Legal category** POM

## SUSTANON* 100

**Qualitative and quantitative composition**

| | |
|---|---|
| Testosterone propionate PhEur | 20 mg |
| Testosterone phenylpriopionate BP | 40 mg |
| Testosterone isocaproate BP | 40 mg |

(equivalent to a total of 74 mg of testosterone)

**Pharmaceutical form** Sustanon 100 is a clear, sterile, oily solution for deep intramuscular injection.

**Clinical particulars**

*Therapeutic indications:* Testosterone replacement therapy in male hypogonadal disorders, for example: after castration; eunuchoidism; hypopituitarism; endocrine impotence; male climacteric symptoms like decreased libido; certain types of infertility due to disorders of spermatogenesis.

Testosterone therapy may also be indicated for the prevention and treatment of osteoporosis in hypogonadal males

*Posology and method of administration:* Dosage: In general, dosage should be adjusted to the individual response of the patient.

*Adults:* Usually, one injection of 1 ml per two weeks is adequate.

*Elderly:* It should be noted that smaller and less frequent doses may achieve the same response.

*Children:* It should be noted that smaller and less frequent doses may achieve the same response.

*Administration:* Deep intramuscular injection

*Contra-indications:* Known or suspected prostatic or mammary carcinoma. Pregnancy. Breast-feeding. Hypersensitivity to one of the excipients.

*Special warnings and special precautions for use:* Patients, especially the elderly, with the following conditions should be monitored: ischaemic heart disease, since androgens may produce hypercholesterolaemia. Latent or overt cardiac failure, renal dysfunction, hypertension, epilepsy or migraine (or a history of these conditions), since androgens may occasionally induce fluid and sodium retention. Skeletal metastases, since androgens may induce hypercalcaemia or hypercalciuria in these patients.

The use of steroids may influence the results of certain laboratory tests.

Androgens should be used cautiously in prepubertal boys to avoid premature epiphyseal closure or precocious sexual development.

If androgen-associated adverse reactions occur, Sustanon 100 treatment should be interrupted and, after disappearance of the symptoms, be resumed at a lower dosage.

*Interaction with other medicaments and other forms of interaction:* Enzyme-inducing agents may exert increasing or decreasing effects on testosterone levels. Therefore adjustment of the dose, and/or intervals between injections may be required.

*Pregnancy and lactation:* On the basis of its pharmacological effect, Sustanon 100 is suspected to cause birth defects and/or other irreversible adverse effects on pregnancy outcome. Therefore, Sustanon 100 is contraindicated during pregnancy and lactation.

*Effects on ability to drive and use of machines:* As far as is known Sustanon 100 has no influence on alertness and concentration

*Undesirable effects:* The following adverse reactions have been associated with androgen therapy in general: In prepubertal boys, precocious sexual development, an increased frequency of erections, phallic enlargement and premature epiphyseal closure; priapism and other signs of excessive sexual stimulation; water and sodium retention; oligospermia and a decreased ejaculatory volume.

Treatment should be interrupted until these symptoms have disappeared, after which it should be continued at a lower dosage.

Hoarseness of the voice may be the first symptom of vocal change which may lead to irreversible lowering of the voice. If signs of virilisation, particularly lowering of the voice, develop, treatment should be discontinued.

*Overdosage:* The acute intramuscular toxicity of Sustanon 100 is very low. Therefore toxic symptoms are not expected to occur.

### Pharmacological properties

*Pharmacodynamic properties:* Testosterone is the principal endogenous hormone essential for normal growth and development of the male sex organs and male secondary sex characteristics. During adult life testosterone is essential for the functioning of the testes and accessory structures, and for the maintenance of libido, sense of well-being, erectile potency, prostate and seminal vesicle function.

Treatment of hypogonadal males with Sustanon 100 results in a clinically significant rise of plasma concentrations of testosterone, dihydrotestosterone and androstenedione, as well as a decrease of SHBG (sex hormone binding globulin). In the males with primary (hypergonadotropic) hypogonadism treatment with Sustanon results in a normalisation of pituitary function.

*Pharmacokinetic properties:* Sustanon 100 contains a number of esters of testosterone with different durations of action. The esters are hydrolysed into the natural hormone testosterone, as soon as they enter the general circulation.

A single dose of Sustanon 100 leads to an increase of total plasma testosterone, with peak level reached approximately 24-48hrs ($t_{max}$) after administration. Plasma testosterone levels return to the lower limit of the normal range in males after approximately 21 days.

Testosterone is metabolised via the normal pathways. Excretion mainly takes place via the urine as conjugates of etiocholanolone and androsterone.

*Preclinical safety data:* Not applicable

### Pharmaceutical particulars

*List of excipients:*
Benzyl Alcohol PhEur 0.1 ml
Arachis Oil PhEur to 1.0 ml

*Incompatibilities:* No relevant incompatibilities are known.

*Shelf-life:* 5 years.

*Special precautions for storage:* Store between 15-25°C, protect from light.

*Nature and contents of containers:* 1 ml ampoules in boxes of 3.

*Instructions for use/handling:* not applicable.

**Marketing authorisation number** 0065/5019

**Date of approval/revision of SPC** March 1995

**Legal category** POM

## SUSTANON* 250

### Qualitative and quantitative composition

| | |
|---|---|
| Testosterone propionate PhEur | 30 mg |
| Testosterone phenylpriopionate BP | 60 mg |
| Testosterone isocaproate BP | 60 mg |
| Testosterone decanoate BP | 100 mg |

(equivalent to a total of 176 mg of Testosterone)

**Pharmaceutical form** Sustanon 250 is a clear, sterile, oily solution for deep intramuscular injection.

### Clinical particulars

*Therapeutic indications:* Testosterone replacement therapy in male hypogonadal disorders, for example: after castration; eunuchoidism; hypopituitarism; endocrine impotence; male climacteric symptoms like decreased libido; certain types of infertility due to disorders of spermatogenesis.

Testosterone therapy may also be indicated for the prevention and treatment of osteoporosis in hypogonadal males

*Posology and method of administration:* Dosage: In general, dosage should be adjusted to the individual response of the patient.
*Adults:* Usually, one injection of 1 ml per three weeks is adequate.
*Elderly:* It should be noted that smaller and less frequent doses may achieve the same response.
*Children:* It should be noted that smaller and less frequent doses may achieve the same response.

*Administration:* Deep intramuscular injection

*Contra-indications:* Known or suspected prostatic or mammary carcinoma. Pregnancy. Breast-feeding. Hypersensitivity to one of the excipients.

*Special warnings and special precautions for use:* Patients, especially the elderly, with the following conditions should be monitored: ischaemic heart disease, since androgens may produce hypercholesterolaemia. Latent or overt cardiac failure, renal dysfunction, hypertension, epilepsy or migraine (or a

history of these conditions), since androgens may occasionally induce fluid and sodium retention. Skeletal metastases, since androgens may induce hypercalcaemia or hypercalciuria in these patients.

The use of steroids may influence the results of certain laboratory tests.

Androgens should be used cautiously in prepubertal boys to avoid premature epiphyseal closure or precocious sexual development.

If androgen-associated adverse reactions occur, Sustanon 250 treatment should be interrupted and, after disappearance of the symptoms, be resumed at a lower dosage.

*Interaction with other medicaments and other forms of interaction:* Enzyme-inducing agents may exert increasing or decreasing effects on testosterone levels. Therefore adjustment of the dose, and/or intervals between injections may be required.

*Pregnancy and lactation:* On the basis of its pharmacological effect, Sustanon 250 is suspected to cause birth defects and/or other irreversible adverse effects on pregnancy outcome. Therefore, Sustanon 250 is contraindicated during pregnancy and lactation.

*Effects on ability to drive and use of machines:* As far as is known Sustanon 250 has no influence on alertness and concentration.

*Undesirable effects:* The following adverse reactions have been associated with androgen therapy in general:

In prepubertal boys, precocious sexual development, an increased frequency of erections, phallic enlargement and premature epiphyseal closure; priapism and other signs of excessive sexual stimulation; water and sodium retention; oligospermia and a decreased ejaculatory volume.

Treatment should be interrupted until these symptoms have disappeared, after which it should be continued at a lower dosage.

Hoarseness of the voice may be the first symptom of vocal change which may lead to irreversible lowering of the voice. If signs of virilisation, particularly lowering of the voice, develop, treatment should be discontinued.

*Overdosage:* The acute intramuscular toxicity of Sustanon 250 is very low. Therefore toxic symptoms are not expected to occur.

### Pharmacological properties

*Pharmacodynamic properties:* Testosterone is the principal endogenous hormone essential for normal growth and development of the male sex organs and male secondary sex characteristics. During adult life testosterone is essential for the functioning of the testes and accessory structures, and for the maintenance of libido, sense of well-being, erectile potency, prostate and seminal vesicle function.

Treatment of hypogonadal males with Sustanon 250 results in a clinically significant rise of plasma concentrations of testosterone, dihydrotestosterone and androstenedione, as well as a decrease of SHBG (sex hormone binding globulin). In the males with primary (hypergonadotropic) hypogonadism treatment with Sustanon results in a normalisation of pituitary function.

*Pharmacokinetic properties:* Sustanon 250 contains a number of esters of testosterone with different durations of action. The esters are hydrolysed into the natural hormone testosterone as soon as they enter the general circulation.

A single dose of Sustanon 250 leads to an increase of total plasma testosterone with peak-levels of approximately 70 nmol/1 ($C_{max}$), which are reached approximately 24-48h ($t_{max}$) after administration. Plasma testosterone levels return to the lower limit of the normal range in males in approximately 21 days.

Testosterone is metabolised via the normal pathways. Excretion mainly takes place via the urine as conjugates of etiocholanolone and androsterone.

*Preclinical safety data:* Not applicable

### Pharmaceutical particulars

*List of excipients:* Benzyl Alcohol PhEur 0.1 ml; Arachis Oil PhEur to 1.0 ml.

*Incompatibilities:* No relevant incompatibilities are known.

*Shelf-life:* 5 years

*Special precautions for storage:* Store between 15-25°C, protect from light

*Nature and contents of containers:* 1 ml ampoules in boxes of 3

*Instructions for use/handling:* not applicable.

**Marketing authorisation number** 0065/5086

**Date of approval/revision of SPC** March 1995

**Legal category** POM

## TESTOSTERONE IMPLANT

**Presentation** Testosterone implants are pellets containing 50, 100 or 200 mg testosterone in glass ampoules.

**Uses** In the male: testosterone replacement therapy in primary or secondary hypogonadal disorders, for example:

- after castration,
- eunuchoidism,
- hypopituitarism,
- endocrine impotence,
- infertility due to spermatogenic disorders,
- male climacteric symptoms such as decreased libido and decreased mental and physical activity.

Moreover, testosterone therapy may be indicated in osteoporosis in the male due to androgen deficiency.

In the female as an adjunct to oestrogen replacement therapy in postmenopausal women to alleviate symptoms, such as decreased libido and/or loss of energy.

### Dosage and administration

*In males:* 100-600 mg depending on individual requirements. A dosage of 600 mg (6 x 100 mg) usually maintains plasma testosterone levels within the normal physiological range for 4-5 months.

*In females:* 50-100 mg as an adjunct to oestradiol implants.

*Method of implantation:* Testosterone implants should be inserted subcutaneously into an area where there is relatively little movement or blood supply, such as the lower abdominal wall or the buttock. Insertion is made under local anaesthesia using a trocar and a cannula. The wound is closed either with an adhesive dressing or a fine suture. The implants must be placed subcutaneously to facilitate removal if necessary. Full aseptic 'no touch' technique should be adopted.

**Contra-indications, warnings, etc** *Contra-indications:* Known or suspected prostatic carcinoma or breast carcinoma in the male. Pregnancy. Breast-feeding.

*Use in pregnancy and lactation:* Testosterone implants are contra-indicated during pregnancy and lactation.

*Warnings and precautions:*

Androgens should be used with caution in women to avoid unacceptable and irreversible virilization. Female patients should therefore be counselled to report any deepening or hoarsening of the voice without delay.

Androgens should be used with caution in prepubertal boys to avoid premature epiphyseal closure or precocious sexual development. Skeletal maturation should be monitored regularly.

Due to the long-lasting action and the difficulty of removal, Testosterone implants should be used with extra caution. Therefore, it may be advisable to establish the beneficial effect and tolerance for androgen therapy by prior treatment with a shorter-acting testosterone preparation. This applies in particular to (pre)pubertal boys, women and elderly men.

Patients with latent or overt cardiac failure, renal or hepatic dysfunction, hypertension, epilepsy or migraine (or a history of these conditions) should be kept under close medical supervision, since aggravation of recurrence may occasionally be induced.

If androgen-associated adverse reactions occur the implant should be removed if possible.

The use of steroids may influence the results of certain laboratory tests.

*Effects on ability to drive and to use machines:* As far as is known Testosterone implants have no effects on alertness and concentration.

*Interactions:* Enzyme-inducing drugs may influence plasma testosterone levels.

*Other undesirable effects (frequency and seriousness):* The following adverse reactions have been associated with androgen therapy:
*in general:* water and sodium retention, hypercalcaemia;
*in women:* symptoms of virilization, such as voice changes (deepening, hoarsening) and hirsutism;
*in prepubertal boys:* precocious sexual development, increased frequency of erections, phallic enlargement and premature epiphyseal closure;
*in men:* priapism and other signs of excessive sexual stimulation, oligospermia and decreased ejaculatory volume

*Overdosage:* The acute toxicity of testosterone is low. Priapism in men and undesired deepening of the voice in women are symptoms of chronic overdosage. In this case the implant(s) should be removed.

**Pharmaceutical precautions:** Store below 25°C and protect from light

*Incompatibilities:* None

**Legal category** POM.

**Package quantities** Each sterile implant is supplied singly, in a sealed glass tube.

**Further information** Testosterone is a naturally-occurring hormone formed in the interstitial cells of the testes under the control of the anterior lobe of the pituitary gland which controls the development and maintenance of the male sex organs and male secondary sex characteristics. Testosterone also produces systemic effects, such as increasing the retention of nitrogen, calcium, sodium, potassium, chloride and phosphate leading to an increase in skeletal weight, water retention and an increase in the growth of bone.

Testosterone implants, when inserted subcutaneously release testosterone into the bloodstream at a relatively even rate supplying near physiological plasma testosterone levels.

Surface area of the implants is the most important factor influencing the rate of absorption. In general the absorption rate estimated by removal of implants at intervals and weighing appears to be appreciably more rapid than when the rate is assessed upon the clinical requirement. In addition to clinical evidence individual variation in the rate of absorption of implants must be taken into account.

The average daily absorption of testosterone has been estimated at 0.5 mg for a 100 mg implant with an approximate duration of 30 weeks.

**Product licence numbers**

| | |
|---|---|
| 50 mg | 0065/5082R |
| 100 mg | 0065/5083R |
| 200 mg | 0065/5084R |

## ZISPIN* ▼

**Qualitative and quantitative composition** Each tablet contains 15 mg or 30 mg of mirtazapine.

**Pharmaceutical form** Tablet.

**Clinical particulars**

*Therapeutic indications:* Treatment of depressive illness.

*Posology and method of administration:* The tablets should be taken orally, if necessary with fluid, and swallowed without chewing.

*Adults:* Treatment should begin with 15 mg daily. The dosage generally needs to be increased to obtain an optimal clinical response. The effective daily dose is usually between 15 and 45 mg.

*Elderly:* The recommended dose is the same as that for adults. In elderly patients an increase in dosing should be done under close supervision to elicit a satisfactory and safe response.

*Children:* Since safety and efficacy of Zispin has not been established in children, it is not recommended to treat children with Zispin.

The clearance of mirtazapine may be decreased in patients with renal or hepatic insufficiency. This should be taken into account when prescribing Zispin to this category of patients.

Mirtazapine has a half-life of 20-40 hours and therefore Zispin is suitable for once-a-day administration. It should be taken preferably as a single nighttime dose before going to bed. Zispin may also be given in sub-doses equally divided over the day (once in the morning and once at night-time).

Treatment should preferably be continued until the patient has been completely symptom-free for 4-6 months. After this, treatment can be gradually discontinued. Treatment with an adequate dose should result in a positive response within 2-4 weeks. With an insufficient response, the dose can be increased up to the maximum dose. If there is no response within a further 2-4 weeks, then treatment should be stopped.

*Contra-indications:* Hypersensitivity to mirtazapine or any of the other ingredients of Zispin.

*Special warnings and special precautions for use:* Reversible white blood cell disorders including agranulocytosis, leukopenia and granulocytopenia have been reported with Zispin. With respect to agranulocytosis the physician should be alert to symptoms such as fever, sore throat, stomatitis or other signs of infection; when such symptoms occur, treatment should be stopped and blood counts taken. Patients should also be advised of the importance of these symptoms.

Careful dosing as well as regular and close monitoring is necessary in patients with:

- epilepsy and organic brain syndrome; from clinical experience it appears that insults occur rarely in patients treated with Zispin
- hepatic or renal insufficiency
- cardiac diseases like conduction disturbances, angina pectoris and recent myocardial infarct, where normal precautions should be taken and concomitant medicines carefully administered

- low blood pressure.

As with other antidepressants care should be taken in patients with:

- micturation disturbances like prostate hypertrophy (although problems are not to be expected because Zispin possesses only very weak anticholinergic activity)
- acute narrow-angle glaucoma and increased intra-ocular pressure (also here little chance of problems with Zispin because of its very weak anticholinergic activity)
- diabetes mellitus.

Treatment should be discontinued if jaundice occurs.

Moreover, as with other antidepressants, the following should be taken into account:

- worsening of psychotic symptoms can occur when antidepressants are administered to patients with schizophrenia or other psychotic disturbances; paranoid thoughts can be intensified
- when the depressive phase of manic-depressive psychosis is being treated, it can transform into the manic phase
- with regard to the chance of suicide, in particular at the beginning of treatment, only a limited number of Zispin tablets should be given to the patient
- although antidepressants are not addictive, the abrupt termination of treatment after long-term administration may result in nausea, headache and malaise
- elderly patients are often more sensitive, especially with regard to the side-effects of antidepressants. During clinical research with Zispin, side-effects have not been reported more often in elderly patients than in other age groups; however experience until now is limited.

*Interaction with other medicaments and other forms of interaction:*

- Mirtazapine may potentiate the central nervous dampening action of alcohol; patients should therefore be advised to avoid alcohol during treatment with Zispin.
- Zispin should not be administered concomitantly with MAO inhibitors or within two weeks of cessation of therapy with these agents.
- Mirtazapine may potentiate the sedative effects of benzodiazepines; caution should be taken when these drugs are prescribed together with Zispin.
- No data are available from formal clinical studies on interactions with neuroleptics.
- In vitro data suggest that mirtazapine is a very weak competitive inhibitor of the cytochrome P450 enzymes CYP1A2, CYP2D6 and CYP3A and clinically significant interactions are unlikely with mirtazapine.

*Pregnancy and lactation:* The safety of Zispin in human pregnancy has not been established.

Reproduction studies in pregnant rats and rabbits at doses up to 100 mg/kg and 40 mg/kg (approx. 3 and 5 times respectively the maximum recommended human dose on the basis of exposure) have revealed no evidence of teratogenic effects. There was, however, in rats an increase in post-implantation loss; there was also an increase in pup deaths during the first three days of lactation (cause of death unknown) and a decrease in pup birth weights. These findings are common with CNS-active drugs at high dose levels in animals.

As the relevance of these findings to humans is not certain the use of Zispin during pregnancy is not recommended. Women of child bearing potential should employ an adequate method of contraception if taking Zispin.

Although animal experiments show that mirtazapine is excreted only in very small amounts in the milk, the use of Zispin in nursing mothers is not recommended since no human data in breast milk are available.

*Effects on ability to drive and use machines:* Zispin has sedative properties and may impair concentration and alertness. Patients treated with Zispin should avoid the performance of potentially dangerous tasks, which require alertness and good concentration, such as driving a motor vehicle or operating machinery.

*Undesirable effects:* Depressed patients display a number of symptoms that are associated with the illness itself. It is therefore sometimes difficult to ascertain which symptoms are a result of the illness itself and which are a result of treatment with Zispin.

The following adverse effects have been reported:

*Common* (>1/100): Increase in appetite and weight gain.

Drowsiness/sedation, generally occurring during the first few weeks of treatment. (N.B. dose reduction generally does not lead to less sedation but can jeopardize antidepressant efficacy.)

*Less common:* Increases in liver enzyme levels.

*Rare* (<1/1000): Oedema and accompanying weight gain. Reversible agranulocytosis has been reported

as a rare occurrence with Zispin. (see also *Special warnings and special precautions for use*). (Orthostatic) hypotension. Exanthema. Mania, convulsions (insults), tremor, myoclonus.

*Overdose:* Toxicity studies in animals suggest that clinically relevant cardiotoxic effects will not occur after overdosing with Zispin. Experience in clinical trials and from the market has shown that no serious adverse effects have been associated with Zispin in overdose. Symptoms of acute overdosage are confined to prolonged sedation.

Cases of overdose should be treated by gastric lavage with appropriate symptomatic and supportive therapy for vital functions.

**Pharmacological properties** Zispin (mirtazapine) is an antidepressant, which can be given as treatment for episodes of major depression. The presence of symptoms such as anhedonia, psychomotor inhibition, sleep disturbances (early wakening) and weight loss, increase the chance of a positive response. Other symptoms are: loss of interest, suicidal thoughts and changes in mood (better in the evening than in the morning). Zispin begins to exert its effect in general after 1-2 weeks of treatment.

*Pharmacodynamic properties:* Mirtazapine is a centrally active presynaptic $\alpha_2$-antagonist, which increases central noradrenergic and serotonergic neurotransmission. The enhancement of serotonergic neurotransmission is specifically mediated via 5-HT$_1$ receptors, because 5-HT$_2$ and 5-HT$_3$ receptors are blocked by mirtazapine. Both enantiomers of mirtazapine are presumed to contribute to the antidepressant activity, the S(+) enantiomer by blocking $\alpha_2$ and 5-HT$_2$ receptors and the R(-) enantiomer by blocking 5-HT$_3$ receptors.

The histamine H$_1$-antagonistic activity of mirtazapine is responsible for its sedative properties. Mirtazapine is generally well tolerated. It has practically no anticholinergic activity and, at therapeutic doses, has practically no effect on the cardiovascular system.

*Pharmacokinetic properties:* After oral administration of Zispin tablets, the active constituent mirtazapine is rapidly and well absorbed (bioavailability ≈ 50%), reaching peak plasma levels after about 2 hours. Binding of mirtazapine to plasma proteins is approx. 85%. The mean half-life of elimination is 20-40 hours; longer half-lives, up to 65 hours, have occasionally been recorded and shorter half-lives have been seen in young men. The half-life of elimination is sufficient to justify once-a-day dosing. Steady state is reached after 3-4 days, after which there is no further accumulation. Mirtazapine displays linear pharmacokinetics within the recommended dose range. Food intake has no influence on the pharmacokinetics of mirtazapine. Mirtazapine is extensively metabolized and eliminated via the urine and faeces within a few days. Major pathways of biotransformation are demethylation and oxidation, followed by conjugation. In vitro data from human liver microsomes indicate that cytochrome P450 enzymes CYP2D6 and CYP1A2 are involved in the formation of the 8-hydroxy metabolite of mirtazapine, whereas CYP3A4 is considered to be responsible for the formation of the N-demethyl and N-oxide metabolites. The demethyl metabolite is pharmacologically active and appears to have the same pharmacokinetic profile as the parent compound. There are no differences in the pharmacokinetic parameters of racemic mirtazapine or its demethyl metabolite in extensive and poor metabolisers. Plasma metabolite profiles for the individual enantiomers are qualitatively similar in extensive and poor metabolisers.

The clearance of mirtazapine may be decreased as a result of renal or hepatic insufficiency.

*Preclinical safety data:* No special particulars

**Pharmaceutical particulars**

*List of excipients:* Zispin 15 mg and 30 mg tablets contain:

Core: maize starch, hydroxypropyl cellulose, magnesium stearate, colloidal silicon dioxide, lactose

Coating layer: hydroxypropyl methylcellulose, polyethylene glycol 8000, titanium dioxide (E171).

Zispin 15 mg tablets also contain yellow iron oxide (E172). The 30 mg tablets yellow iron oxide (E172) and red iron oxide (E172).

*Incompatibilities:* Not applicable

*Shelf life:* The shelf life for Zispin tablets is 3 years, if stored in the dark and dry at 2-30 ˚C. Zispin tablets should not be used after the expiry date on the package.

*Special precautions for storage:* Zispin should be stored in the dark and dry.

*Nature and contents of containers:* Zispin tablets are oval, biconvex, scored and marked with 'Organon' on one side-and a code on the other side.

Zispin tablets are packed in child-safe, push-through strips made of opaque white polyvinyl chloride film and aluminium foil containing a heat-seal coating on the side in contact with the tablets.

The following packages are available:

3, 6 or 9 push-through strips with 10 yellow tablets each containing 15 mg mirtazapine (code TZ/3)

4 push-through strips with 7 red-brown tablets each containing 30 mg mirtazapine (code TZ/5).

*Instructions for use/handling:* Not applicable

**Marketing authorization number**   0065/0144-5

**Date of approval/revision of SPC** May 1997

**Legal category** POM

*Trade Mark

# Organon Teknika Limited
Science Park
Milton Road
Cambridge CB4 4FL

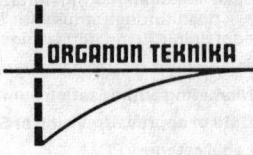

## ESMERON*

**Qualitative and quantitative composition** Each ml Esmeron contains 10 mg rocuronium bromide.

**Pharmaceutical form** Esmeron is supplied as a solution for intravenous injection.

### Clinical particulars

*Therapeutic indications:* Esmeron is indicated as an adjunct to general anaesthesia to facilitate endotracheal intubation, to provide skeletal muscle relaxation, and to facilitate mechanical ventilation.

*Posology and method of administration: Dosage:* As with other neuromuscular blocking agents, the dosage of Esmeron should be individualized in each patient. The anaesthetic method used, the expected duration of surgery, the possible interaction with other drugs that are administered before and/or during anaesthesia and the condition of the patient should be taken into account when determining the dose. The routine use of an appropriate neuromuscular monitoring technique is recommended for the evaluation of neuromuscular block and recovery.

Inhalational anaesthetics do potentiate the neuromuscular blocking effects of Esmeron. This potentiation, however, only becomes clinically relevant in the course of anaesthesia when the volatile agents have reached the tissue concentrations required for this interaction. Consequently, adjustments with Esmeron should be made by administering smaller maintenance doses at less frequent intervals or by using lower infusion rates of Esmeron during long lasting procedures (longer than 1 hour) under inhalational anaesthesia (see Interaction with other medicaments and other forms of interaction).

In adult patients the following dosage recommendations may serve as a general guideline for endotracheal intubation and muscle relaxation for short to long lasting surgical procedures.

*Endotracheal intubation:* The intubating dose is 0.6 mg Esmeron per kg body weight.

*Maintenance dosing:* The recommended maintenance dose is 0.15 mg Esmeron per kg body weight. The maintenance doses should best be given when twitch height has recovered to 25% of control twitch height.

*Continuous infusion:* If Esmeron is administered by continuous infusion, it is recommended to give a loading dose of 0.6 mg Esmeron per kg body weight and, when neuromuscular block starts to recover, to start administration by infusion. The infusion rate should be adjusted to maintain twitch response at 10% of control twitch height. In adults, the infusion rate required to maintain neuromuscular block at this level ranges from 0.3-0.6 mg.kg⁻¹.hour⁻¹ (300-600 micrograms.kg⁻¹.hour⁻¹). Continuous monitoring of neuromuscular block is essential since infusion rate requirements vary from patient to patient and with the anaesthetic method used.

*Dosing in paediatric patients:* Children (1-14 years) and infants (1-12 months) under halothane anaesthesia manifest similar sensitivity to Esmeron as adults. Onset of action is faster in infants and children than in adults. Clinical duration is shorter in children than in adults. There are no data to support recommendations for the use of Esmeron in neonates (0-1 month).

*Dosing in geriatric patients:* Geriatric patients manifest similar sensitivity to Esmeron as younger adults, however the duration of action might be somewhat longer.

*Dosing in overweight and obese patients:* When used in overweight or obese patients (defined as patients with a body weight of 30% or more above ideal body weight) doses should be reduced taking into account a lean body mass.

*Hepatic and/or biliary tract disease and renal failure:* Because rocuronium is excreted in urine (up to approximately 30% within 12-24 hours) and it is expected that it is also partly excreted in bile, Esmeron should be used with caution in patients with clinically significant hepatic and/or biliary diseases and/or renal failure. In these patient groups prolongation of action has been observed with doses of 0.6 mg Esmeron per kg body weight.

*Administration:* Esmeron is administered intravenously either as a bolus injection or as a continuous infusion (see also Instructions for use/handling).

*Contra-indications:* Former anaphylactic reactions to rocuronium or to the bromide ion.

*Special warnings and precautions for use:* Since Esmeron causes paralysis of the respiratory muscles, ventilatory support is mandatory for patients treated with this drug until adequate spontaneous respiration is restored.

Anaphylactic reactions to neuromuscular blocking agents in general have been reported. Although these are very rarely seen with Esmeron, precautions for treating such reactions if they would occur should always be taken (see also Undesirable effects).

Dose levels greater than 0.9 mg Esmeron per kg body weight may increase the heart rate; this effect could counteract the bradycardia produced by other anaesthetic agents or by vagal stimulation.

Presently there are insufficient data to give recommendations for use of Esmeron in the Intensive Care Unit or for rapid sequence intubation. However during continuous neuromuscular block it is essential that patients receive adequate analgesia and sedation and that neuromuscular transmission is monitored throughout; furthermore, muscle relaxants should be administered in carefully adjusted doses, sufficient for the maintenance of less than complete block by or under the supervision of experienced clinicians who are familiar with its actions and with appropriate neuromuscular monitoring techniques.

Because Esmeron is always used with other agents and because the occurrence of malignant hyperthermia during anaesthesia is possible, even in the absence of known triggering agents, clinicians should be familiar with early signs, confirmatory diagnosis and treatment of malignant hyperthermia prior to the start of any anaesthesia. In animal studies Esmeron was shown not to be a triggering factor for malignant hyperthermia. The following conditions may influence the pharmacokinetics and/or pharmacodynamics of Esmeron:

*Prolonged circulation time:* Conditions associated with prolonged circulation time such as cardiovascular disease, old age and oedematous state resulting in an increased volume of distribution, may contribute to a slower onset of action.

*Neuromuscular disease:* Like other neuromuscular blocking agents, Esmeron should be used with extreme caution in patients with a neuromuscular disease or after poliomyelitis since the response to neuromuscular blocking agents may be considerably altered in these cases. The magnitude and direction of this alteration may vary widely. In patients with myasthenia gravis or with the myasthenic (Eaton-Lambert) syndrome, small doses of Esmeron may have profound effects and Esmeron should be titrated to the response.

*Hypothermia:* In surgery under hypothermic conditions, the neuromuscular blocking effect of Esmeron is increased and the duration prolonged.

*Obesity:* Like other neuromuscular blocking agents, Esmeron may exhibit a prolonged duration and a prolonged spontaneous recovery in obese patients.

*Conditions which may increase the effects of Esmeron:* Hypokalaemia (e.g. after severe vomiting, diarrhoea and diuretic therapy), hypermagnesaemia, hypocalcaemia (after massive transfusions), hypoproteinaemia, dehydration, acidosis, hypercapnia, cachexia.

Severe electrolyte disturbances, altered blood pH or dehydration should therefore be corrected when possible.

*Interaction with other medicaments and other forms of interaction:* The following drugs have been shown to influence the magnitude and/or duration of action of non-depolarizing neuromuscular blocking agents.

*Increased effect:*

Anaesthetics:

– halothane, ether, enflurane, isoflurane, methoxyflurane, cyclopropane.
– high doses of thiopentone, methohexitone, ketamine, fentanyl, gammahydroxybutyrate, etomidate and propofol.
Other non-depolarising neuromuscular blocking agents.
Prior administration of suxamethonium.

Other drugs:

– antibiotics: aminoglycoside and polypeptide antibiotics, acylamino-penicillin antibiotics, high doses of metronidazole.
– diuretics, β-adrenergic blocking agents, thiamine, MAO inhibiting agents, quinidine, protamine, α-adrenergic blocking agents, magnesium salts.

*Decreased effect:*

– neostigmine, edrophonium, pyridostigmine, aminopyridine derivatives.
– prior chronic administration of corticosteroids, phenytoin or carbamazepine.
– noradrenaline, azathioprine (only transient and limited effect), theophylline, calcium chloride.

Note: Single doses of the antibiotics netilmicin, cefuroxime, metronidazole and the combination of cefuroxime and metronidazole do not potentiate the effect of Esmeron.

*Pregnancy and lactation:* In animal studies neither embryotoxicity nor teratogenicity was observed that could be attributed to treatment with rocuronium bromide.

There are no data on the use of Esmeron during human pregnancy to assess potential harm to the foetus. Esmeron should be given to pregnant women only when the attending physician decides that the benefits outweigh the risks. In patients receiving magnesium sulphate, the dose of Esmeron should be reduced and be carefully titrated to twitch response.

Insignificant levels of rocuronium bromide were found in the milk of lactating rats. There are no human data on the use of Esmeron during lactation. Esmeron should be given to lactating women only when the attending physician decided that the benefits outweigh the risks.

*Effects on ability to drive and use of machines:* It is not recommended to use potentially dangerous machinery or drive a car within 24 hours after the full recovery from the neuromuscular blocking action of Esmeron.

*Undesirable effects: Anaphylactic reactions:* Anaphylactic reactions to neuromuscular blocking agents in general have been reported. Although these are very rarely seen with Esmeron, precautions for treating such reactions if they would occur should always be taken. Particularly in the case of former anaphylactic reactions to neuromuscular blocking agents, special caution should be taken since allergic cross-reactivity between neuromuscular blocking agents has been reported.

*Histamine release and histaminoid reactions:* Since neuromuscular blocking agents are known to be capable of inducing histamine release both locally and systemically, the possible occurrence of itching and erythematous reaction at the site of injection and/or generalised histaminoid (anaphylactoid) reactions such as bronchospasm and cardiovascular changes should always be taken into consideration when administering these drugs.

Although slight increases in mean plasma histamine levels have been observed following rapid bolus administration of 0.3-0.9 mg Esmeron per kg body weight, no clinically significant tachycardia, hypotension or other clinical signs of histamine release associated with the administration of Esmeron, have been reported.

*Overdosage:* In the event of overdosage and prolonged neuromuscular block, the patient should continue to receive ventilatory support and upon start of spontaneous recovery an acetylcholinesterase inhibitor (e.g. neostigmine, edrophonium, pyridostigmine) should be administered in adequate doses. When administration of an acetylcholinesterase inhibiting agent fails to reverse the neuromuscular effects of Esmeron, ventilation must be continued until spontaneous breathing is restored. Repeated dosage of an acetylcholinesterase inhibitor can be dangerous.

In animal studies, severe depression of cardiovascular function, ultimately leading to cardiac collapse did not occur until a cumulative dose of 750 x ED₉₀ (135 mg per kg body weight) was administered.

### Pharmacological properties

*Pharmacodynamic properties:* Esmeron is a fast onset, intermediate acting non-depolarizing neuromuscular blocking agent, possessing all of the characteristic pharmacological actions of this class of drugs (curariform). It acts by competing for nicotinic cholinoceptors at the motor end-plate. This action is antagonised by acetylcholinesterase inhibitors such as neostigmine, edrophonium and pyridostigmine.

The $ED_{90}$ (dose required to produce 90% depression of the twitch response of the thumb to stimulation of the ulnar nerve) during balanced anaesthesia is approximately 0.3 mg per kg body weight.

Within 60 seconds following intravenous administration of a dose of 0.6 mg Esmeron per kg body weight (2 x $ED_{90}$ under balanced anaesthesia), adequate intubation conditions can be achieved in nearly all patients of which in 80% intubation conditions are rated excellent; within 2 minutes general muscle paralysis adequate for any type of surgery is established. The clinical duration (the duration until spontaneous recovery to 25% of control twitch height) with this dose is 30-40 minutes. The total duration (time until spontaneous recovery to 90% of control twitch height) is 50 minutes. The mean time of spontaneous recovery of twitch response from 25 to 75% (recovery index) after a bolus dose of 0.6 mg Esmeron per kg body weight is 14 minutes.

With lower dosages of 0.3-0.45 mg Esmeron per kg body weight (1-1½ x $ED_{90}$), onset of action is slower and duration of action is shorter (13-26 mins). After administration of 0.45 mg Esmeron per kg body weight, acceptable intubation conditions are present after 90 seconds.

With doses higher than 3 x $ED_{90}$ the intubation conditions will not improve appreciably; the duration of action, however, will be prolonged. Doses higher than 4 x $ED_{90}$ have not been studied.

The duration of action of maintenance doses of 0.15 mg Esmeron per kg body weight might be somewhat longer under enflurane and isoflurane anaesthesia in geriatric patients and in patients with hepatic or renal disease (approximately 20 minutes) than in patients without impairment of excretory organ functions under intravenous anaesthesia (approximately 13 minutes). No cumulation of effect (progressive increase in duration of action) with repetitive maintenance dosing at the recommended level has been observed.

In patients scheduled for cardiovascular surgery the most common cardiovascular changes during the onset of maximum block following 0.6-0.9 mg Esmeron per kg body weight are a slight and clinically insignificant increase in heart rate up to 9% and an increase in mean arterial blood pressure up to 16% from the control values.

Administration of acetylcholinesterase inhibitors, such as neostigmine, pyridostigmine or edrophonium, antagonises the action of Esmeron.

*Pharmacokinetic properties:* The Pharmacokinetics properties of Esmeron have been determined in adult patients with normal renal and hepatic function, in adults with renal dysfunction, with hepatic cirrhosis, and in geriatric and paediatric patients. Mean values are summarised in the following table.

In animal studies, biliary excretion is the main elimination route. Within a few hours 30-40% of the dose administered is excreted in the bile as unchanged rocuronium.

In humans, the amount of rocuronium excreted in the urine in the first 12 hours following Esmeron administration varied from 13.0 to 30.8% of the total dose administered. It is expected also that hepatic excretion is of importance in humans.

No metabolites of rocuronium could be detected in plasma or urine after administration of Esmeron.

*Preclinical safety data: Acute toxicity:* In acute toxicity studies rocuronium bromide was intravenously administered to cats and dogs up to a dose of 350 x $ED_{90}$ and 750 x $ED_{90}$ respectively. This last dose was administered in 4 consecutive doses at intervals of 30 minutes (9, 18, 36 and 72 mg per kg body weight) and resulted in death due to cardiac collapse.

*Subacute toxicity:* In subacute toxicity studies rocuronium bromide was intravenously administered to cats and dogs up to a dose of 37 x $ED_{90}$ and 60 x $ED_{90}$ respectively two times per week for a period of 4 weeks. Unforeseen mortalities occurred in three out of seven dogs at the dose of 60 x $ED_{90}$ (10.8 mg per kg body weight). The cause of death could not be established, but was considered to be related to interactions between rocuronium treatment and experimental procedures and/or instrumentation and anaesthesia.

*Chronic toxicity:* Chronic toxicity studies have not been performed with rocuronium bromide.

*Mutagenicity and carcinogenicity:* In vivo and in vitro mutagenicity studies revealed no mutagenic potential of rocuronium bromide.

Carcinogenicity studies have not been performed with rocuronium bromide.

*Reproductive toxicity:* Studies in rats with administration of rocuronium bromide during organogenesis using subpharmacological intravenous doses revealed no evidence of embryolethality, teratological changes or suppression of growth of the foetuses.

**Pharmaceutical particulars**

*List of excipients:* Esmeron contains the following excipients: sodium acetate, sodium chloride, acetic acid and water for injections.

*Incompatibilities:* Physical incompatibility has been documented for Esmeron when added to solutions containing the following drugs: amphotericin, amoxycillin, azathioprine, cefazolin, cloxacillin, dexamethasone, diazepam, enoximone, erythromycin, famotidine, frusemide, hydrocortisone sodium succinate, insulin, intralipid, methohexitone, methylprednisolone, prednisolone sodium succinate, thiopentone, trimethoprim and vancomycin.

*Shelf life:* Esmeron can be stored for three years provided it is stored under the prescribed conditions (see Special precautions for storage). The date mentioned behind 'exp.:' on the label of the vial is the expiry date; this is the date up to which Esmeron may be used. Since Esmeron does not contain a preservative, it is recommended to discard any unused solution.

*Special precautions for storage:* Esmeron should be stored at 2°C to 8°C in the dark.

Esmeron can be stored at 8°C to 30°C for 3 months prior to the expiry date. After any storage at 8°C to 30°C Esmeron should not be returned to the refrigerator and should be discarded.

*Nature and contents of containers:*
Esmeron 50 mg in 5 ml (10 mg/ml): Packaging of 12 vials each containing 50 mg rocuronium bromide.
Esmeron 100 mg in 10 ml (10 mg/ml): Packaging of 10 vials each containing 100 mg rocuronium bromide.
Esmeron 250 mg in 25 ml (10 mg/ml): Packaging of 4 vials each containing 250 mg rocuronium bromide.

*Instructions for use/handling:* Compatibility studies with the following infusion fluids have been performed. Esmeron has been shown to be compatible with: 0.9% NaCl, 5% dextrose, 5% dextrose in saline, sterile water for injections, Lactated Ringers and Haemaccel 35. Solutions should be used within 24 hours after mixing. Unused solutions should be discarded.

Esmeron can be injected into the intravenous line of a running infusion containing most of the commonly used intravenous drugs, except those mentioned under Incompatibilities.

**Marketing authorisation number** 3524/0025

**Date of approval/revision of SPC** 15 October 1996

**Legal category** POM

# NORCURON*

**Qualitative and quantitative composition** Norcuron 10 mg, 1 vial contains: Vecuronium bromide 10 mg

**Pharmaceutical form** Powder for injection.

**Clinical particulars**

*Therapeutic indications:* Norcuron is indicated as an adjunct to general anaesthesia to facilitate endotracheal intubation and to provide skeletal muscle relaxation during surgery.

*Posology and method of administration: Dosage:* As with all other neuromuscular blocking agents, the dosage of Norcuron should be individualised in each patient. The anaesthetic method used, the expected duration of surgery, the possible interaction with other drugs that are administered before or during anaesthesia and the condition of the patient should be taken into account when determining the dose. The use of a peripheral nerve stimulator is recommended to monitor neuromuscular blockade and recovery.

The following dosages may serve as general guidelines for initial and maintenance intravenous bolus dose requirements of Norcuron to assure appropriate muscle relaxation throughout short, medium and long lasting surgical procedures under balanced anaesthesia, with and without the use of Norcuron for facilitation of endotracheal intubation.

*Adults and children (see also Use in paediatrics):*
Intubating dose: 80 to 100 micrograms vecuronium bromide per kg body weight.

Dosages of Norcuron for surgical procedures after intubation with succinylcholine: 30 to 50 micrograms vecuronium bromide per kg body weight.

If succinylcholine is used for intubation, the administration of Norcuron should be delayed until the patient has clinically recovered from the neuromuscular block induced by succinylcholine.

Maintenance dose: 20 to 30 micrograms vecuronium bromide per kg body weight.

These maintenance doses should best be given when twitch height has recovered to 25% of control twitch height.

*Notes:* In obese patients, these doses should be reduced taking into account a lean body mass.

Since inhalational anaesthetics potentiate the action of Norcuron (see interactions), doses of Norcuron in general should be reduced during surgical procedures where these anaesthetics are used.

Should there be reason for selection of larger doses in individual patients, initial doses ranging from 150 micrograms up to 300 micrograms vecuronium bromide per kg body weight have been administered during surgery both under halothane and neurolept anaesthesia without adverse cardiovascular effects being noted as long as ventilation is properly maintained. The use of these high dosages of Norcuron pharmacodynamically decreases the onset time and increases the duration of action.

In caesarean section and neonatal surgery the dose should not exceed 100 micrograms/kg.

*Neonates and infants up to one year of age:* Because of the possible variations of the sensitivity of the neuromuscular junction, especially in neonates (up to 4 weeks) and probably in infants (up to 4 months of age), it is recommended that an initial test dose of 10 to 20 micrograms vecuronium bromide per kg body weight followed by incremental doses until 90 to 95% depression of twitch response is achieved is recommended. Dose requirements in infants of 5 months to 1 year of age are the same as in adults. However, since the onset time of Norcuron in these patients is considerably shorter than in adults and children, the

| Esmeron Pharmacokinetics | Adult patients | | Geriatric patients | Paediatric patients | | |
|---|---|---|---|---|---|---|
| | | | | Infants | children | |
| | Normal renal & hepatic function | Renal dys-function | Hepatic disease | | 3-12 months | 1-3 years | 3-8 years |
| Clearance (ml.kg⁻¹.min⁻¹) | 3.90 | 2.76 | 2.30 | 4 | 5.75 | 5.27 | 7.39 |
| Volume of central compartment (ml.kg⁻¹) | 60.5 | 57.5 | 92.2 | 29 | 79.2 | 83.4 | 75.7 |
| Volume of distribution at steady state (ml.kg⁻¹) | 228 | 274 | 378 | 221 | 298 | 238 | 213 |
| $T_{1/2}\pi$ rapid distribution half life (min) | 1.94 | 1.55 | N.D. | 1.5 | 1.71 | 2.38 | 2.05 |
| $T_{1/2}\alpha$ (slow) distribution half life (min) | 16.1 | 24.3 | 12.2 | 16 | 18.8 | 14.9 | 11.2 |
| $T_{1/2}\beta$ elimination half life (min) | 96.8 | 123.2 | 169.7 | 91 | 79.4 | 64.7 | 48.0 |
| Mean residence time (min) | 60.9 | 97.1 | 87.7 | N.D. | 53.3 | 45.5 | 30.6 |

N.D. = not determined

use of high intubating doses in general is not required for early development of good intubating conditions.

Since the duration of action and recovery time with Norcuron is longer in neonates and infants than in children and adults, maintenance doses could be lower and are required less frequently (see also *Use in paediatrics* in the section *Special warnings and precautions for use*).

*Dose requirements for administration of Norcuron by continuous infusion:* If Norcuron is administered by continuous infusion, it is recommended that a bolus dose of $ED_{90}$ or $2xED_{90}$ (40-100 micrograms per kg) is administered first and, when neuromuscular block starts to recover, administration of Norcuron by infusion is commenced. The infusion rate should be adjusted to maintain twitch response at 10% of control twitch height. In adults, the infusion rate required to maintain neuromuscular block at this level, ranges from 0.8 to 1.4 micrograms vecuronium bromide/kg/min. For neonates and infants see above. Repeated monitoring of neuromuscular block is essential since infusion rate requirements vary from patient to patient and with the anaesthetic method used.

*Administration:* Norcuron should be administered intravenously.

*Contra-indications:* Former anaphylactic reactions to vecuronium or the bromide ion.

*Special warnings and precautions for use:* As with other neuromuscular blocking agents, Norcuron should only be administered by, or under supervision of experienced clinicians who are familiar with the action and use of these drugs.

Since Norcuron causes relaxation of the respiratory muscles, mechanical ventilation until spontaneous respiration is restored, is necessary for patients treated with this drug.

Anaphylactic reactions to neuromuscular blocking agents in general have been reported. Although these are very rarely seen with Norcuron, precautions for treating such reactions if they would occur should always be taken (see also Undesirable effects).

Since Norcuron has no cardiovascular effects within the clinical dosage range, it does not attenuate bradycardia that may occur due to the use of some types of anaesthetics and opiates or due to vagal reflexes during surgery. Therefore, reassessment of the use and/or dosage of vagolytic drugs such as atropine for premedication or at induction of anaesthesia, may be of value for surgical procedures during which vagal reactions are more likely to occur (e.g. surgical procedures where anaesthetic drugs with known vagal stimulatory effects are used, opthalmic abdominal or anorectal surgery, etc.).

Presently there are insufficient data to give recommendations for the use of Norcuron in the Intensive Care Unit. As with other muscle relaxants prolonged neuromuscular block following long term use of Norcuron in seriously ill patients in the Intensive Care Unit has been reported. It is essential that during continuous neuromuscular block patients receive adequate analgesia and sedation and that neuromuscular transmission is monitored throughout; furthermore, muscle relaxants should be administered in carefully adjusted doses, sufficient for the maintenance of less than complete block by or under the supervision of experienced clinicians who are familiar with its actions with appropriate neuromuscular monitoring techniques.

The following disease states may influence the pharmacokinetics and/or pharmacodynamics of Norcuron:

*Hepatic and/or biliary tract disease:* Despite the fact that Norcuron is excreted mainly via the bile, in general only moderate changes of the course of neuromuscular block induced by Norcuron are found in patients with hepatic and/or biliary tract diseases. In addition, these changes are dose dependent. With a dose of 100 micrograms vecuronium bromide per kg body weight, a slight, statistically not significant prologation of the onset time and decrease of the duration of action were found as compared to normal patients. At doses of 150 and 200 micrograms vecuronium bromide per kg body weight, the prolongation of the onset time was even less pronounced (150 micrograms/kg) or absent (200 micrograms/kg), and no alterations of the duration of action were found in the 150 micrograms/kg group, while significant increases in the duration of action and in the recovery time were observed in the 200 micrograms/kg group.

*Renal failure:* Only limited changes of pharmacodynamic parameters were reported with Norcuron when administered to patients with renal failure.

As with other non-depolarising neuromuscular blocking agents, a limited degree of resistance to the action of Norcuron may occur in patients with renal failure. A slight, clinically not relevant, prolongation of onset time and recovery time may occur when Norcuron is administered to patients with renal failure.

*Prolonged circulation time:* Conditions associated with prolonged circulation time such as cardiovascular disease, old age, oedematous state resulting in an increased volume of distribution, may contribute to an increase in the onset time of neuromuscular block.

*Neuromuscular disease:* As with other neuromuscular blocking agents, Norcuron should be used with extreme caution in cases of neuromuscular disease or after poliomyelitis since the response to neuromuscular blocking agents may be considerably altered in these patients. The magnitude and direction of this alteration may vary widely. In patients with myasthenia gravis or the myasthenic (Eaton Lambert) syndrome, small doses of Norcuron may have profound effects and Norcuron should be titrated to the response.

*Hypothermia:* In operations under hypothermia, the neuromuscular blocking effect of Norcuron is prolonged.

*Other conditions which may increase the effects of Norcuron are:* hypokalaemia (e.g. after severe vomiting, diarrhoea, and diuretic therapy), hypermagnesaemia, hypocalcaemia (after massive transfusions), hypoproteinaemia, dehydration, acidosis, hypercapnoea, cachexia.

Severe electrolyte disturbances, altered blood pH or dehydration should therefore be corrected when possible.

Like pancuronium bromide, d-tubocurarine or other non-depolarising neuromuscular blocking agents, Norcuron may cause a reduction in the partial thromboplastin time and the prothrombin time.

*Interaction with other medicaments and other forms of interaction:* The following drugs have shown to influence the magnitude and/or duration of action of non-depolarising neuromuscular blocking agents:

*Increased effect:*

Anaesthetics:

– halothane, ether, enflurane, isoflurane, methoxyflurane,cycloproprane, propofol

– High doses of thiopentone, methohexitone, ketamine, fentanyl, gammahydroxybutyrate, etomidate.

Other non-depolarising neuromuscular blocking agents.

Prior administration of succinylcholine (1 mg/kg).

Other drugs:

– antibiotics: aminoglycoside and polypeptide antibiotics, acylaminopenicillin antibiotics, high doses of metronidazole

– diuretics, β-adrenergic blocking agents, thiamine, MAO inhibiting agents, quinidine, protamine, α-adrenergic blocking agents, magnesium salts.

*Decreased effect:*

– neostigmine, edrophonium, pyridostigmine, aminopyridine derivatives.

– prior chronic administration of corticosteroids, phenytoin or carbamazepine

– noradrenaline, azathioprine (only transient and limited effect), theophylline, $CaCl_2$.

Variable effect:

– depolarising muscle relaxants, e.g. succinylcholine, given after the administration of Norcuron may produce potentiation or attenuation of the neuromuscular blocking effect of Norcuron.

*Pregnancy and lactation:* There are insufficient data on the use of Norcuron during animal or human pregnancy to assess potential harm to the foetus. Norcuron should be given to a pregnant woman only when the attending physician decides that the benefits outweigh the risks.

*Caesarean section:* Studies with Norcuron, administered in doses up to 100 micrograms/kg, have shown its safety for use in Caesarean section. Norcuron does not affect Apgar score, foetal muscle tonus nor cardiorespiratory adaptation. From umbilical cord blood sampling it is apparent that only very little placental transfer of Norcuron does occur which did not lead to the observation of any clinical adverse effect in the newborn.

*Remark:* Reversal of Norcuron-induced neuromuscular block may be unsatisfactory in patients receiving magnesium sulphate for toxaemia of pregnancy because magnesium salts enhance neuromuscular blockade.

Therefore, in patients receiving magnesium sulphate, the dosage of Norcuron should be reduced and be carefully titrated to twitch response.

*Effects on ability to drive and use machines:* It is not recommended to use potentially dangerous machinery or drive a car within 24 hours after the full recovery from the neuromuscular blocking action of Norcuron.

*Undesirable effects:*

Anaphylactic and histaminoid reactions

Anaphylactic reactions

Anaphylactic reactions to neuromuscular blocking agents in general have been reported. Although these are very rarely seen with Norcuron, precautions for treating such reactions if they would occur should always be taken.

Particularly in the case of former anaphylactic reactions to neuromuscular blocking agents, special caution should be taken since allergic cross-reactivity between neuromuscular blocking agents has been reported.

*Histamine release and histaminoid reactions:* Since neuromuscular blocking agents are known to be capable of inducing histamine release both locally and systematically, the possible occurrence of itching and erythematous reactions at the site of injection and/or generalised histaminoid (anaphylactoid) reactions such as bronchospasm and cardiovascular changes should always be taken into consideration when administering these drugs.

Experimental studies with intradermal injection of Norcuron have demonstrated that this drug has only a weak capacity for inducing local histamine release. Controlled studies in man failed to demonstrate any significant rise in plasma histamine levels after intravenous administration of Norcuron. Nevertheless, such cases have rarely been reported during large scale use of Norcuron.

*Overdose:* In the event of overdosage and prolonged neuromuscular block, the patient should remain under mechanical ventilation and a cholinesterase inhibitor (e.g. neostigmine, pyridostigmine, edrophonium) in adequate doses should be administered as an antidote. When administration of a cholinesterase inhibiting agent fails to reverse the neuromuscular effects of Norcuron, ventilation must be continued until spontaneous breathing is restored. Repeated dosage of a cholinesterase inhibitor can be dangerous.

**Pharmacological properties**

*Pharmacodynamic properties:* Norcuron (vecuronium bromide) is a non-depolarising neuromuscular blocking agent, chemically designated as the aminosteroid 1-(3α, 17β-diacetoxy-2β piperidino-5α-androstan-16β-yl)-1 methylpiperidinium bromide. Norcuron blocks the transmission process between the motor nerve-ending and striated muscle by binding competitively with acetylcholine to the nicotinic receptors located in the motor end-plate region of striated muscle.

Unlike depolarising neuromuscular blocking agents, such as succinylcholine, Norcuron does not cause muscle fasciculations. Within 90 to 120 seconds following intravenous administration of a dose of 80 to 100 micrograms vecuronium bromide per kg body weight (approximately $2xED_{90}$ under neurolept anaesthesia), good to excellent conditions for endotracheal intubation occur and within 3 to 4 minutes following administration of these dosages, general muscle paralysis adequate for any type of surgery is established.

The duration of action to 25% recovery of control twitch height (clinical duration) with this dose is 20 to 30 minutes. The time to 95% recovery of control twitch height following this dose is approximately 40 to 50 minutes.

With higher dosages of Norcuron, onset time to maximal block is shortened and duration of action is prolonged. At dosages of 150, 200, 250 and 300 micrograms vecuronium bromide per kg body weight, the mean onset time under neurolept anaesthesia amounts to 146, 110, 92 and 77 seconds respectively. The mean clinical duration of action with these is 41, 55, 70 and 86 minutes respectively. With these high dosages, also a gradual, but relatively slight increase of the recovery rate from neuromuscular block occurs.

When Norcuron is administered by continuous intravenous infusion, a steady state neuromuscular blockade of 90% can be maintained at a constant rate of drug delivery and without clinically significant prolongation of the recovery time from neuromuscular block at termination of the infusion. Norcuron has no cumulative effects if maintenance doses are administered at 25% recovery of control twitch height. Several maintenance doses can therefore be give in succession.

These properties allow the use of Norcuron in short, medium and long lasting surgical procedures.

Within the clinical dosage range, Norcuron exerts no vagolytic no ganglion blocking activity.

Administration of acetylcholinesterase inhibitors, such as neostigmine, pyridostigmine or edrophonium, antagonises the action of Norcuron.

*Pharmacokinetic properties:* After intravenous administration of Norcuron, the distribution half-life of vecuronium amounts to approx. 2.2 (± 1.4) minutes. Vecuronium is mainly distributed in the extracellular fluid compartment. At steady state, the volume of distribution averages 0.27 $l.kg^{-1}$ and its plasma elimination half-life averages 71 (± 20) minutes.

The extent of metabolism of vecuronium is relatively low. In humans, a 3-hydroxy derivative having approximately 50% less neuromuscular blocking potency than vecuronium could be demonstrated in the urine and bile as metabolite of Norcuron. In patients not suffering from renal or hepatic failure, the plasma concentration of this derivative is below detection limit, and does not contribute to the neuromuscular block occurring after administration of Norcuron.

Biliary excretion is the main elimination route. It is

estimated that within 24 hours after intravenous administration of Norcuron, 40 to 80% of the dose administered is excreted into the bile as monoquaternary compounds. Approximately 95% of these monoquaternary compounds is unchanged vecuronium and 5% is 3-hydroxy vecuronium.

Renal elimination is relatively low. The amount of monoquaternary compounds excreted in the urine collected by intravesical catheter for 24 hours following Norcuron administration averages 30% of the dose administered.

*Use in paediatrics: Neonates and infants:* In neonates and infants the $ED_{90}$ dose of vecuronium bromide under halothane anaesthesia was found to be approximately the same (approx. 28 micrograms/kg body weight) as in adults.

The onset time of Norcuron in neonates and infants is considerably shorter as compared to children and adults, probably due to the shorter circulation time and larger cardiac output. Also, a greater sensitivity of the neuromuscular junction to the action of neuromuscular blocking agents in these patients may account for a more rapid onset of action. The duration of action and recovery time with Norcuron is longer in neonates and infants than in adults. Maintenance doses of Norcuron should therefore be less frequently administered.

*Children:* In children the $ED_{90}$ dose of vecuronium bromide under halothane anaesthesia was found to be somewhat higher (approx. 32 micrograms/kg body weight), although statistically not significant, than in adults. In comparison to adults, the duration of action and recovery time with Norcuron in children are in general approximately 30% and 20-30% shorter respectively.

Similar to adults, cumulative effects with repeat maintenance doses of approximately one quarter of the initial dose and administered at 25% recovery of control twitch height are not observed in paediatric patients. The longer recovery time of Norcuron in neonates and infants is not of a magnitude which would require routine use of reversal agents. If used, these reversal agents are as efficacious for antagonising the neuromuscular block in neonates and infants as they are in children and adults.

*Preclinical safety data:* In animal studies, at high doses, a toxicity related to the pharmacological activity of vecuronium bromide was seen.

**Pharmaceutical particulars**

*List of excipients:* Norcuron is supplied as a freeze dried powder containing citric acid monohydrate, disodium hydrogen phosphate dihydrate, mannitol, sodium hydroxide (for pH correction) and phosphoric acid (for pH correction). No preservative has been added.

*Incompatibilities:* As is the case for many other drugs, incompatibility has been documented for Norcuron when added to thiopentone or thiopentone containing solutions.

Except for those solutions with which Norcuron has been shown to be compatible, it is not recommended that Norcuron should be mixed with other solutions or drugs in the same syringe or bag (see *Compatibility*).

*Shelf life:* Norcuron can be kept until the expiry date indicated on the packaging, provided it is stored under the prescribed conditions.

The shelf life is as follows: Norcuron 10 mg–2 years

When reconstituted as indicated under *Reconstitution* or diluted as described under *Compatibility*, the solution obtained can be kept for 24 hours at room temperature and in daylight. However, in order to avoid microbiological contamination it is recommended to discard any unused solution.

*Special precautions for storage:* Norcuron should be stored at a temperature below 25°C, protected from light.

*Nature and contents of container:* Packaging of 20 vials each containing 10 mg vecuronium bromide, and 20 ampoules each containing 5 ml water for injections (solvent).

It is possible that one or more of the above mentioned presentations is not available in this country.

*Instructions for use/handling:*
*Reconstitution:* Norcuron 10 mg: Addition of 5 ml water for injections results in an isotonic solution of pH 4 containing 2 mg vecuronium bromide per ml. (2 mg/ml).

Alternatively, in order to obtain a solution with a lower concentration Norcuron 10 mg may be reconstituted with a volume up to 10 ml of the following infusion fluids:
5% glucose injection fluid
0.9% sodium chloride injection fluid
Lactated Ringer's solution
Lactated Ringer's injection and 5% glucose
Glucose 5% and 0,9% sodium chloride injection
Water for injections

*Compatibilities:* Norcuron can be injected into the line of a running infusion containing the following drugs: fentanyl, droperidol, nicomorphinehydrochloride and pancuronium bromide.

Compatibility studies with other drugs have not been performed.

When Norcuron is reconstituted with water for injections, the resultant solution can be mixed with the following infusion fluids, packed in PVC or glass, to a dilution up to 40 mg/litre:
0.9% NaCl solution
5% glucose solution
Ringer's solution
Ringer's glucose

The above-mentioned reconstituted solution can also be injected in to the line of a running infusion of the following fluids:
Lactated Ringer's solution
Lactated Ringer's solution and 5% glucose
Glucose 5% and 0.9% NaCl solution
Haemaccel
Dextran-40 5% in 0.9% NaCl solution
Water for injections

Compatibility studies with other infusion fluids have not been performed.

**Marketing authorisation number** 3524/0019

**Date of approval/revision of SPC** June 1996

**Legal Category** POM

## OncoTICE* ▼

**Qualitative and quantitative composition** BCG 12.5 mg equivalent to 2-8 x $10^8$ cfu

**Pharmaceutical form** Freeze dried powder for intravesical instillation fluid

**Clinical particulars**

*Therapeutic indications:* OncoTICE is indicated for treatment of primary or concurrent carcinoma-in-situ of the urinary bladder and for the prevention of recurrence of high grade and/or relapsing superficial papillary transitional cell carcinoma of the urinary bladder (Stage Ta or T1) after transurethral resection.

*Posology and method of administration:*
*Reconstitution:* Add 1 ml of a sterile physiological saline solution to the freeze dried powder by means of a sterile syringe and allow to stand for a few minutes. Then gently swirl the ampoule until a homogenous suspension is obtained, forceful agitation should be avoided.

*Intravesical instillation:* Insert a catheter via the urethra into the bladder and drain the bladder completely. Connect the 50 ml syringe containing the prepared OncoTICE suspension to the catheter, and instil the suspension into the bladder. After instillation, remove the catheter. The instilled OncoTICE suspension must remain in the bladder for a period of 2 hours. During this period care should be taken that the instilled OncoTICE suspension has sufficient contact with the whole mucosal surface of the bladder. Therefore the patient should not be immobilised or, in case of a bed-ridden patient, should be turned over from back to prone and vice versa every 15 minutes. After two hours, have the patient void the instilled suspension in a sitting position.

NOTE: The patient is not allowed any fluid for a period of 4 hours prior to instillation, nor during the time that the OncoTICE suspension remains in the bladder (2 hours).

*Dosage:* Adults and the elderly The contents of one ampoule of OncoTICE, reconstituted and diluted as indicated, are instilled into the urinary bladder.

*Initiation of treatment:* OncoTICE should be administered ten to fourteen days after TUR, biopsy or traumatic catheterisation. Treatment should be delayed in cases of gross haematuria or major bladder irritability.

*Carcinoma in situ with or without papillary carcinoma of the bladder:* A standard treatment schedule consists of one intravesical instillation of OncoTICE per week for six consecutive weeks. This schedule may be repeated if tumour remission has not been achieved and if the clinical circumstances warrant. After a treatment-free interval of 2 weeks intravesical OncoTICE administration should continue at monthly intervals for at least 6 months. Maintenance treatment for up to 24 months may be required in some patients. The duration of treatment should be determined by clinical response.

*Prophylaxis of papillary tumour after transurethral resection:*

A weekly instillation for six consecutive weeks, followed by a treatment free period of 2 weeks. Subsequent treatments to be given monthly for the next 11 months.

*Children:* Not recommended.

*Contra-indications:* Impaired immune response irrespective of whether this impairment is congenital or caused by disease, drugs or other therapy.

Positive HIV serology.

Pregnancy and lactation.

In patients with a positive Mantoux test, OncoTICE instillations are contra-indicated only if there is supplementary medical evidence for an active tuberculous infection.

Urinary tract infections. Therapy with OncoTICE should be interrupted until the bacterial culture from urine becomes negative and therapy with antibiotics and/or urinary antiseptics is stopped.

*Special warnings and special precautions for use:* Before the first intravesical instillation of OncoTICE, a Mantoux test (PPD) should be performed. If the test is positive, OncoTICE instillations are contraindicated only if there is supplementary medical evidence for an active tuberculous infection.

OncoTICE should not be administered intravenously, subcutaneously or intramuscularly.

Reconstitution and preparation of the OncoTICE suspension for instillation and administration should be performed under aseptic conditions.

Spillage of OncoTICE solution should be treated with a disinfectant such as strong hypochlorite. Spillage on the skin should be treated with dilute hypochlorite.

Traumatic catheterization can promote systemic BCG infection. Administration of OncoTICE should be delayed in such patients until mucosal damage has healed.

In patients with known risk factors for HIV infection, it is recommended that adequate HIV assays are performed prior to therapy.

*Interaction with other medicaments and other forms of interaction:* Tice BCG is sensitive to the routinely used tuberculostatic chemotherapeutic agents such as streptomycin, para-amino salicylic acid (PAS), isoniazid (INH), rifampicin and ethambutol.

Studies on interactions with other drugs have not been performed.

*Pregnancy and lactation:* OncoTICE instillation for carcinoma of the bladder is contraindicated during pregnancy and lactation.

*Effects on ability to drive and use machines:* Not applicable

*Undesirable effects:*
*Common side effects:* The intravesical administration of BCG frequently produces symptoms of cystitis or bladder irritation such as dysuria, urinary frequency and haematuria. The cystitis and inflammatory reaction (granulomata) may be an essential part of the antitumour activity. In most cases the symptoms disappear within two days after instillation and the cystitis does not require treatment. Where necessary the irritative bladder effects can be managed symptomatically.

Severe or prolonged (greater than 48 hours) frequency and dysuria may be treated with isoniazid (300 mg daily) and analgesics until the symptoms resolve. BCG treatment should be withheld until symptoms have resolved completely.

Malaise, low grade fever and/or a flu-like syndrome. These symptoms usually appear within 4 hours of administration and last for 24–48 hours and should be managed by standard symptomatic treatment.

*Less frequent complications:* BCG infection: Systemic BCG infection is a serious side effect of OncoTICE administration, and fatalities have occurred.

BCG infection may be more common after traumatic bladder catheterisation or bladder perforation. BCG treatment should be delayed in such patients until mucosal damage has healed.

Treatment should be delayed for 10–14 days after TUR or biopsy of bladder lesions.

All patients receiving the product should be carefullly monitored and advised to report all incidences of fever and other events outside the urinary tract. Fever lasting over 24 hours and any unusual event should be investigated to exclude another cause and to try and isolate organisms. Blood cultures and samples from affected sites should be cultured for BCG.

The infection may manifest as pneumonitis, hepatitis and/or cytopenia after a period of fever and malaise.

Fever lasting more than 48 hours for which there is no other explanation and any other unexplained reactions should be treated with antituberculous therapy, following the regular treatment schedules for tuberculosis.

OncoTICE is sensitive to Isoniazid, Rifampicin and Ethambutol.

No further treatment with BCG should be given.

*In rare cases,* arthritis/arthralgias, major haematuria, skin rash, transient urethral obstruction, orchitis or bladder contracture may occur. If these rare complications of OncoTICE instillation occur, it is almost exclusively during the maintenance treatment regimen. In most cases of arthritis, arthralgias and skin rash, these can be attributed to hypersensitivity reactions of the patient to BCG.

*Overdose:* Patients with manifest symptoms of therapy-induced BCG infections should be adequately treated with antituberculosis chemotherapeutics, following the normal treatment schedules used for tuberculosis infections.

**Pharmacological properties**

*Pharmacodynamic properties:* The precise mode of action of intravesical BCG instillation in the treatment and/or recurrence prophylaxis of superficial bladder cancer is still largely unknown. The primary mode of action is thought to involve local and systemic immunological mechanisms.

*Pharmacokinetic properties:* For the treatment and recurrence prophylaxis of bladder cancer, the attachment of BCG to the bladder wall after voiding has been shown to be important. This allows a targeted pharmacological effect at the site of application.

*Preclinical safety data:* As a result of the wide clinical application of BCG vaccination in the preceding decades the risks of BCG in human subjects are well-characterised. Intra-vesical administration to dogs has been found to be safe and without significant toxicity. No evidence of birth defects, genetic damage or carcinogenecity in humans are available from the extensive adverse reaction literature of BCG used as a vaccine.

**Pharmaceutical particulars**

*List of excipients:* Lactose PhEur, Asparagine USP, Citric Acid PhEur, Dibasic potassium phosphate USP, Magnesium sulphate PhEur, Ferric Ammonium Citrate USP, Glycerol PhEur, Zinc Formate and Ammonium Hydroxide PhEur.

*Incompatibilities:*OncoTICE is incompatible with hypo and hypertonic solutions.

*Shelf life:* 12 months. Once reconstituted the solution should be used within 1 hour.

*Special precautions for storage:* Store at 2-8°C, protect from light.

*Nature and contents of containers:* 2 ml glass ampoules in packs of 1, 3 and 6.

*Instructions for use/handling:* See *Posology and method of administration.*

**Marketing authorisation number** 03524/0016

**Date of approval/revision of SPC** April 1997

# PAVULON*

**Presentation** Each 2 ml ampoule contains pancuronium bromide BP 4 mg. Other ingredients: sodium chloride, sodium acetate, acetic acid to pH 4 and water for injection.

**Uses:** Pavulon is a non-depolarising neuromuscular blocking agent with a medium duration of action. It is used as an adjuvant in surgical anaesthesia to obtain relaxation of the skeletal muscles in a wide range of surgical procedures. Pavulon is also used for neuromuscular blockade during intensive care therapy for a variety of pathologies, including intractable status asthmaticus and tetanus.

**Dosage and administration** Pavulon is administered intravenously.

When determining the dose, the method of anaesthesia, expected duration of surgery, potential interaction with other drugs that are administered before or during anaesthesia and the condition of the patient should be taken into account. The use of a peripheral nerve stimulator is recommended for monitoring neuromuscular block and recovery.

The following may be used as a general guide to dosage:

*Adult surgery:* Initial dose: 50–80 micrograms/kg (intubation accomplished within 120 -150 seconds) or 80–100 micrograms/kg (intubation accomplished within 90–120 seconds).

Incremental doses: 10–20 micrograms/kg

*Child surgery:* Initial dose: 60–100 micrograms/kg Incremental doses: 10–20 micrograms/kg

*Neonatal surgery:* 30–40 micrograms/kg. Incremental doses: As neonates are sensitive this dose should be adjusted according to the initial response but generally incremental doses lie in the range 10–20 micrograms/kg body weight.

If succinylcholine is used for intubation the administration of Pavulon should be delayed until the patient has clinically recovered from the neuromuscular block induced by succinylcholine.

Following the administration of suxamethonium the dosage of Pavulon may be considerably reduced:

*Adults:* Initial dose 20–60 micrograms/kg. Incremental doses 10–20 micrograms/kg

*Children:* Initial dose: 20–60 micrograms/kg. Incremental doses 10–20 micrograms/kg

In obese patients all of these doses should be reduced.

The duration of action depends upon the clinical condition of the patient and the dose administered, but in normal subjects receiving perioperative muscle relaxant doses the duration of action is usually 45–60 minutes.

Pavulon is longer-acting in the intensive-care patient, and an intravenous dose of 60 micrograms/kg every one to one and a half hours, or even less frequently, is usually adequate.

The neuromuscular blocking activity of Pavulon is prolonged in the elderly.

In the control of tetanus, duration of Pavulon relaxation probably depends on the severity of the spasm: duration of effect can therefore be variable.

Pavulon should not be mixed with other agents in the same syringe, or with solutions for intravenous infusion, as a change in pH may induce precipitation.

Any unused solution should be discarded.

**Contra-indications, warnings, etc**

*Contra-indications:* Patients with a known hypersensitivity to Pavulon injection.

*Use in pregnancy and lactation:* There are insufficient data on the use of Pavulon during animal or human pregnancy to assess potential harm to the foetus. The drug should only be administered to a pregnant woman when the attending physician decides that the benefits outweigh the risks.

*Lactation:* There is no available evidence that breast-feeding, after a mother has been given Pavulon, has any adverse effects on the baby.

*Caesarean section:* Studies with Pavulon have shown its safety for use in Caesarean section. Pavulon does not affect Apgar score, foetal muscle tonus nor cardiorespiratory adaptation of the new-born. From assays of the Pavulon concentration in umbilical blood samples it is apparent that only very limited placental transfer of Pavulon occurs.

*Warning:* Reversal of neuromuscular block induced by Pavulon may be unsatisfactory in patients receiving magnesium sulphate for toxaemia of pregnancy because magnesium salts enhance neuromuscular blockade. Dosages should be reduced in such cases.

*Warnings and precautions:* Pavulon should be administered only by anaesthetists familiar with its use, and only when facilities for controlled ventilation insufflation with oxygen and endotracheal intubation are available for immediate use.

Since Pavulon causes relaxation of the respiratory muscles, respiration must be assisted in all patients. It is essential to ensure that the patient is breathing spontaneously, deeply and regularly before leaving the theatre after anaesthesia. The neuromuscular blockade achieved with Pavulon can be reversed with a cholinesterase inhibiting agent (e.g. neostigmine) in an adequate dose, together with atropine as an anticholinergic agent.

Care should be exercised if there is a danger of regurgitation when intubating the patient, for example during crash induction.

Pavulon (like d-tubocurarine) causes a reduction in the partial thromboplastin time and the prothrombin time.

The following disease states may influence the pharmacokinetics and/or pharmacodynamics of Pavulon:

*Renal failure:* Since renal excretion is the major elimination route of Pavulon, the elimination half-life is prolonged and the plasma clearance is reduced in patients with renal failure. Pavulon should be used with caution in patients with severe renal impairment as the duration of action can be prolonged.

The prolongation of half-life in patients with renal failure is often but not always associated with an extended duration of neuromuscular blockade. In these patients the recovery from neuromuscular block may also be prolonged.

Hyperdiuresis may result in a decreased neuromuscular blocking effect.

*Hepatic and/or biliary tract disease:* Despite the modest role of the liver in the elimination of Pavulon, major pharmacokinetic changes have been observed in patients with liver disease.

Resistance to the neuromuscular blocking activity of Pavulon may occur, because these conditions are characterised by a considerable increase (up to 50%) in the volume of distribution of the drug.

At the same time hepatic and/or biliary tract disease can prolong the elimination half-life of Pavulon and prolong the recovery from neuromuscular block.

The possibility of slower onset, higher total dosage requirements and prolongation of neuromuscular blockade and recovery time must be taken into consideration when Pavulon is used in these patients.

*Altered circulation time:* Conditions associated with slower circulation time, such as cardiovascular disease, old age, oedematous states resulting in an increased volume of distribution, may contribute to an increase of onset time.

*Neuromuscular disease:* As is the case with other curariform agents, in cases of neuromuscular disease or after poliomyelitis, Pavulon should be used with extreme caution since the response to neuromuscular blocking agents may be considerably altered in these patients. The magnitude and direction of this alteration may vary widely. In patients with myasthenia gravis or the myasthenic (Eaton Lambert) syndrome, small doses of Pavulon may have profound effects and only very small doses of Pavulon should be used initially.

*Hypothermia:* In operations requiring hypothermia the neuromuscular blockade of non-depolarising drugs is decreased and increases when re-warming the patient. Hypothermia in neonates therefore, requires a reduced dosage of Pavulon.

*Other conditions which may increase the effect of Pavulon are:* hypokalaemia (e.g. after severe vomiting, diarrhoea, digitalisation and diuretic therapy), hypermagnesaemia, hypocalcaemia (after massive transfusions), hypoproteinaemia, dehydration, acidosis, hypercapnoea, cachexia.

Severe electrolyte disturbances, altered blood pH or dehydration should therefore be corrected when possible.

Patients with carcinomatosis especially when associated with bronchial carcinoma, may exhibit a marked sensitivity to this agent, and the neuromuscular block produced may respond poorly to neostigmine.

*Effects on ability to drive and to use machines:* It is not recommended to use potentially dangerous machinery or drive a car within 24 hours after the full recovery from the neuromuscular blocking action of Pavulon.

*Interactions:* The following drugs have been shown to influence the magnitude and/or duration of action of non-depolarising neuromuscular blocking agents:

*Increased effect:* Anaesthetics: halothane, ether, enflurane, isoflurane, methoxyflurane, cyclopropane, thiopentone, methohexital, ketamine, fentanyl, gammahydroxybutyrate, etomidate.

Other drugs: other non-depolarising muscle relaxants, prior administration of succinylcholine, aminoglycoside and polypeptide antibiotics, diuretics, beta-adrenergic blocking agents, thiamine, M.A.O. inhibiting agents, quinidine, protamine, phenytoin, alpha-adrenergic blocking agents, imidazoles, metronidazole, nitroglycerin, diazepam, magnesium sulphate, narcotic analgesics.

*Decreased effect:* Anaesthetics: Neurolept analgesia, propanidid.

Other drugs: neostigmine, edrophonium, pyridostigmine, prior chronic administration of corticosteroids, noradrenaline, adrenaline, azathioprine, theophylline, KCl, $CaCl_2$, heparin (temporary decrease).

*Variable effect:* depolarising muscle relaxants given after the administration of Pavulon may produce potentiation or attenuation of the neuromuscular blocking effect.

The non-depolarising drug increases resistance towards the neuromuscular blocking effect of the depolarising drug. Therefore high doses of a depolarising drug are necessary before muscular relaxation can be obtained. These high doses of a depolarising drug may cause endplate desensitisation and prolong post-operative apnoea.

Unlike a non-depolarising block, a depolarising block cannot be overcome by, and may even be worsened by an anticholinesterase agent.

*Influence on the cardiovascular system:* Pavulon does not intensify the hypotension induced by halothane; in addition the cardiac depression is partly restored. The excessive bradycardia induced by neurolept analgesia and some of the cholinergic effects of morphine derivatives are counteracted by Pavulon.

Pavulon should be given with caution to a patient receiving chronic tricyclic antidepressant therapy who is anaesthetised with halothane or any inhalation anaesthetic, since this enhances the predisposition to the development of cardiac arrhythmias associated with tricyclic antidepressants.

Recent evidence suggests that alkylating drugs (nitrogen mustards) should be considered a possible hazard when given to patients during anaesthesia involving the use of muscle relaxants.

*Other undesirable effects (frequency and seriousness):* After Pavulon a slight to moderate rise in arterial pressure may occur. Increased pulse rate and cardiac output are frequently reported, showing Pavulon to have weak vagolytic activity. In general this is considered to be a favourable effect. Pavulon decreases intra-ocular pressure and induces miosis, both effects being favourable in ophthalmic surgery. A few cases of localised reactions at the site of injection have been reported. Although rare instances of bronchospasm have been reported, Pavulon has in general a lack of associated bronchospasm.

*Overdosage:* In the event of an overdosage i.e. a failure of neostigmine to reverse the neuromuscular block, the patient must continue to be ventilated. When administration of a cholinesterase inhibiting agent fails to reverse the neuromuscular blocking effects of Pavulon, ventilation must be continued until spontaneous breathing is restored. Repeated dosage of a cholinesterase inhibitor can be dangerous.

**Pharmaceutical precautions** Pavulon should be stored at 2–8°C and protected from light. Any unused solution should be discarded.

**Legal category** POM

**Package quantities** Boxes of 25 x 2 ml ampoules.

**Further information**

*Pharmacological particulars:* Pavulon (pancuronium bromide) is a non-depolarising neuromuscular blocking agent chemically designated as the amino-steroid 1,1'-(3α, 17β-diacetoxy-5α-androstan-2β, 16β-ylene) bis (1-methylpiperidinium) dibromide.

Pavulon blocks the transmission process between the motor nerve-ending and the striated muscle by binding competitively with acetylcholine to the nicotinic receptors located in the motor end-plate region of striated muscle.

Unlike depolarising neuromuscular blocking agents such as succinylcholine, Pavulon does not cause muscle fasciculations.

Pavulon has no hormonal activity. Pavulon exerts a slight and dose dependent vagolytic action. Within the clinical dose range it has no ganglion blocking action

Acetylcholinesterase inhibitors such as neostigmine, pyridostigmine or edrophonium antagonise the action of Pavulon.

The $ED_{95}$ (dose required to produce 95% suppression of twitch height) is approximately 0.06 mg pancuronium bromide per kilogram of bodyweight under neurolept anaesthesia .

The time from administration to occurrence of the maximal effect (onset time) and the duration of action largely depend on the dose administered. With a dose of 0.06 mg pancuronium bromide per kg body-weight ($ED_{95}$ under neurolept anaesthesia), the onset time is approximately 5 minutes and the time from administration to 25% recovery of control twitch height (duration of action) is approximately 35 minutes. The time from administration to 90% recovery of control twitch height with this dose averages 73 minutes . Higher doses up to 0.1 mg pancuronium bromide per kg bodyweight as used to facilitate endotracheal intubation, will reduce the onset time and prolong the duration of action.

*Pharmacokinetic particulars:* Following intravenous injection, the plasma half-life of the drug during the distribution phase ($T_{1/2}\alpha$) is less than 5 minutes. This rapid initial disappearance from the plasma is compatible with the assumption that a stable distribution of pancuronium between plasma and extracellular fluid is attained within 5 minutes of drug administration in man .

The plasma elimination half-life ($T_{1/2}\beta$) of pancuronium bromide averages 110 to 120 minutes. Renal excretion is the major route of elimination. Approximately 40 to 50% of the initial dose of pancuronium is excreted unchanged in the urine. 11% is excreted in the bile as unchanged pancuronium or its metabolites.

The metabolites of pancuronium are 3-OH, 17-OH 3,17 di-OH derivatives. These derivatives do not significantly contribute to the neuromuscular block occurring after the administration of Pavulon.

**Product licence number** 0065/5014R

*\*Trade Mark*

# Orion Pharma (UK) Limited
1st Floor, Leat House,
Overbridge Square,
Hambridge Lane
Newbury Berkshire RG14 5UX

## ELDEPRYL*

### Presentation
*Tablets:* White uncoated tablets scored on one side, 6 mm diameter, containing 5 mg selegiline hydrochloride.

White uncoated tablets scored on one side, 8 mm diameter, containing 10 mg selegiline hydrochloride.

*Syrup:* Oral liquid, each 5 ml containing 10 mg of selegiline hydrochloride.

### Uses
Eldepryl is a selective monoamine oxidase-B (MAO-B) inhibitor which prevents dopamine breakdown in the brain. The inhibitory effect of a single 10 mg dose lasts for 24 hours. It also inhibits the re-uptake of dopamine at the pre-synaptic dopamine receptor. These effects potentiate dopaminergic function in the brain and help to even out and prolong the effect of exogenous and endogenous dopamine. Thus Eldepryl potentiates and prolongs the effect of levodopa in the treatment of parkinsonism.

Double-blind studies on patients with early phase parkinsonism showed that patients receiving selegiline monotherapy manage significantly longer without levodopa therapy than controls on placebo. These patients could also maintain their ability to work longer.

The addition of Eldepryl to levodopa (with or without decarboxylase inhibitor) therapy helps to alleviate dose related fluctuations and end of dose deterioration. When Eldepryl is added to such a regimen it is possible to reduce the levodopa dosage by an average of 30%. Unlike conventional MAO-inhibitors, which inhibit both the MAO-A and MAO-B enzyme, Eldepryl is a specific MAO-B inhibitor and can be given safely with levodopa.

Eldepryl does not cause the so called "cheese effect" either when used alone as monotherapy or when used with other drugs, except for moclobemide or nonselective MAO-inhibitors.

*Indications:* Eldepryl is indicated for the treatment of Parkinson's disease and symptomatic parkinsonism. It may be used alone to delay the need for levodopa (with or without decarboxylase inhibitor) or as an adjunct to levodopa (with or without decarboxylase inhibitor).

### Dosage and administration
10 mg daily, either alone or as an adjunct to levodopa or levodopa/peripheral decarboxylase inhibitor. Eldepryl may be administered either as a single dose in the morning or in two divided doses of 5 mg, taken at breakfast and lunch.

### Contra-indications, warnings, etc
*Contra-indications:* Known hypersensitivity to selegiline or other components of the formulation.

*Drug interactions:* Foods containing tyramine have not been reported to induce hypertensive reactions during selegiline treatment at doses used in the treatment of Parkinson's disease. Concomitant use of non-selective monoamine oxidase inhibitors may cause severe hypotension.

No tolerability problems have been reported when a combination of selegiline and moclobemide, an inhibitor of MAO-A, has been used. However, when they are used together, the tyramine sensitivity factor may increase up to 8-9 (being 1 for selegiline alone and 2-3 for moclobemide alone). Although tyramine induced hypersensitive reactions are unlikely when selegiline and moclobemide are used together, dietary restrictions (e.g. excluding foods with a large amount of tyramine such as aged cheese and yeast products) are recommended when prescribing this combination.

Interactions between nonselective MAO-inhibitors and pethidine, as well as selegiline and pethidine have been described. The mechanism of this interaction is not fully understood and, therefore, use of pethidine concomitantly with selegiline should be avoided. Serious reactions with signs and symptoms that may include diaphoresis, flushing, ataxia, tremor, hyperthermia, hyper/hypotension, seizures, palpitation, dizziness and mental changes that include agitation, confusion and hallucinations progressing to delirium and coma have been reported in some patients receiving a combination of selegiline and fluoxetine. Similar experiences have been reported in patients receiving selegiline and either of two other serotonin re-uptake inhibitors, sertraline and paroxetine. Since the mechanisms of these reactions are not fully understood, it is recommended to avoid the combinations of selegiline and fluoxetine, sertraline or paroxetine. A minimum period of five weeks should be allowed between discontinuation of fluoxetine and initiation of selegiline treatment, due to the long half-lives of fluoxetine and its active metabolite. As the half-lives of selegiline and its metabolites are short, a wash-out period of 14 days after selegiline treatment should be sufficient before starting fluoxetine.

Severe CNS toxicity has been reported in patients with the combination of tricyclic antidepressants and selegiline. In one patient receiving amitriptyline and selegiline this included hyperpyrexia and death, and another patient receiving protriptyline and selegiline experienced tremor, agitation, and restlessness followed by unresponsiveness and death two weeks after selegiline was added.

Other adverse reactions occasionally reported in patients receiving a combination of selegiline with various tricyclic antidepressants include hyper/hypotension, dizziness, diaphoresis, tremor, seizures, and changes in behavioural and mental status. Since the mechanisms of these reactions are not fully understood, caution is recommended when using selegiline together with tricyclic antidepressants.

*Pregnancy and lactation:* The available safety data concerning the use of selegiline during pregnancy and lactation is insufficient to justify its use in these patient groups.

*Precautions:* Eldepryl should be administered with caution to patients with peptic or duodenal ulcer, labile hypertension, cardiac arrhythmias, severe angina pectoris or psychosis.

In higher doses (more than 30 mg daily) the selectivity of selegiline begins to diminish resulting in increased inhibition of MAO-A. Thus in higher doses there is a risk of hypertension after ingestion of food rich in tyramine.

*Adverse reactions:* In monotherapy, selegiline has been found to be well tolerated. Dry mouth, transient rise of serum alanine aminotransferase (ALAT) values and sleep disorders have been reported more frequently than in patients receiving placebo.

Because selegiline potentiates the effects of levodopa, the adverse reactions of levodopa, e.g. abnormal movements, nausea, agitation, confusion, hallucinations, headache, postural hypotension, cardiac arrhythmias and vertigo, may be emphasised, particularly if the dose of levodopa is too high. Such adverse reactions usually disappear when the levodopa dosage is decreased. Levodopa dosage can be reduced by an average of 30% when selegiline is added to the treatment.

Micturition difficulties and skin reactions have also been reported during selegiline treatment.

Following up of these possible adverse reactions is important.

*Overdosage:* No cases of overdosage are known.

However, experience gained during Eldepryl's development reveals that some individuals exposed to doses of 600 mg/day selegiline suffered severe hypotension and psychomotor agitation.

Theoretically, overdosage causes significant inhibition of both MAO-A and MAO-B and thus, symptoms of overdosage may resemble those observed with non-selective MAO-inhibitors, such as central nervous and cardiovascular system disorders (e.g. drowsiness, dizziness, faintness, irritability, hyperactivity, agitation, severe headache, hallucination, hypertension/hypotension, vascular collapse, rapid and irregular pulse, precordial pain, respiratory depression and failure, hyperpyrexia and diaphoresis).

There is no specific antidote and treatment should be symptomatic.

### Pharmaceutical precautions
*Syrup:* Store at room temperature (not exceeding 25°C), do not store in a refrigerator. Shake bottle before use and secure cap after use.

*Tablets:* Protect from heat, moisture and light.

### Legal category  POM

### Package quantities

| | |
|---|---|
| Syrup: | Bottles containing 200 ml. |
| 5 mg Tablets: | Blister packs of 60. |
| 10 mg Tablets: | Blister packs of 30. |

### Further information  Nil.

### Product licence numbers

| | |
|---|---|
| Syrup: | 06043/0013. |
| 5 mg Tablets: | 06043/0011. |
| 10 mg Tablets: | 06043/0112. |

*Product licence holder:* Orion Corporation, Orionintie 1, FIN-02200 Espoo, Finland.

## FRUSENE* TABLETS

**Qualitative and quantitative composition**  Frusemide PhEur 40.0 mg, Triamterene PhEur 50.0 mg.

**Pharmaceutical form**  Frusene is presented as pale yellowish, scored tablets of 9 mm diameter. Each tablet contains 40 mg frusemide and 50 mg triamterene.

### Clinical particulars
*Therapeutic indications:* Frusene is indicated when a prompt diuresis is required and where potassium conservation is important:- congestive heart failure, cardiac oedema, hepatic oedema and ascites.

*Posology and method of administration:* The dosage will depend on individual requirements. The usual adult dose is 1/2–2 tablets, taken in the morning. Maximum daily dose: 6 tablets.

*Contra-indications:* Frusene is contra-indicated in severe renal or hepatic failure or if the serum potassium level is elevated. Known sensitivity to frusemide, triamterene or any of the other ingredients.

*Special warnings and precautions for use:* In patients with mild renal failure, serum creatinine and electrolytes should be monitored regularly.

Frusemide may affect metabolic control in diabetes. Insulin requirements could increase, or latent diabetes become manifest. Triamterene may cause a blue fluorescence of the urine under certain light conditions.

*Interactions with other medicaments and other forms of interaction:* Hyperkalaemia may occur if Frusene is used in combination with other drugs which raise plasma potassium levels, including ACE-inhibitors, potassium sparing diuretics or potassium supplements. Concomitant administration of potent diuretics may increase the toxic effects of antibiotics known to exhibit nephrotoxicity. Plasma lithium levels may rise when frusemide is given with lithium. The effects of curariform muscle relaxants may be increased by frusemide. The dosage of concurrently administered cardiac glycosides or antihypertensive agents may require adjustment. The effects of theophylline may be potentiated.

Salicylates and certain other non-steroidal anti-inflammatory agents may antagonise the action of diuretics such as frusemide and may cause renal failure in pre-existing hypovolaemia. Rare cases of renal failure have been reported due to an interaction between triamterene and indomethacin.

*Pregnancy and lactation:* Frusene should be used with caution during the first trimester of pregnancy. Frusemide and triamterene are known to pass into breast milk. Therefore, Frusene should be used with caution in breast-feeding women.

*Effects on ability to drive and use machines:* None known.

*Undesirable effects:* Frusene is a combination of frusemide and triamterene and side-effects due to either component are possible. Reported side effects are as follows:
*Frusemide:* Frusemide is generally well tolerated. Side effects of a minor nature such as nausea, malaise or gastric upset may occur, but are not usually severe enough to cause withdrawal of treatment. The incidence of allergic reactions such as skin rashes is very low, but when these occur, treatment should be withdrawn. In common with other sulphonamide-based diuretics, hyperuricaemia may occur and in rare cases, clinical gout may be precipitated. Bone

marrow depression has been reported as a rare complication and necessitates withdrawal of treatment. As with other diuretics, electrolytes and water balance may be disturbed as a result of diuresis after prolonged therapy. This may cause symptoms such as headache, hypotension and muscle cramps. Ototoxicity has been rarely reported with high doses.

*Triamterene:* Nausea, diarrhoea, fatigue, headache, dry mouth or rash have been reported. If renal function is impaired, triamterene has been reported to cause elevation of BUN and the uric acid level. Leucopenia or photosensitivity have been rarely reported in association with the use of triamterene. Hyperkalaemia or hypokalaemia have been observed in some patients. Megaloblastic anaemia may rarely be induced by triamterene in patients with depleted folic acid stores.

Triamterene may rarely result in adverse effects on renal function.

*Overdose:* Treatment of overdose consists of fluid replacement and correction of the electrolyte imbalance.

**Pharmacological properties**

*Pharmacodynamic properties:*

*Frusemide:* Frusemide is a potent diuretic with a rapid action. Its effects are evident within 1 hour after a dose by mouth and lasts for about 4 to 6 hours. It has been reported to exert inhibiting effects on electrolyte reabsorption in the proximal and distal renal tubules and in the ascending Loop of Henle.

Excretion of sodium, potassium and chloride ions is increased and water excretion enhanced.

Unlike thiazide diuretics where, owing to their flat dose response curve, very little is gained by increasing the dose, frusemide has a steep dose-response curve, which gives it a wide therapeutic range.

*Triamterene:* Triamterene is a mild diuretic which appears mainly to act on the distal renal tubules. It produces a diuresis in about 2 to 4 hours, reaching a maximum effect in about 6 hours. Triamterene adds to the natriuretic but diminishes the kaliuretic effects of other diuretics and is used as an adjunct to frusemide to conserve potassium, in the treatment of refractory oedema associated with hepatic cirrhosis, congestive heart failure and the nephrotic syndrome.

*Pharmacokinetic properties:*

*Frusemide:* Frusemide is incompletely but fairly rapidly absorbed from the gastro-intestinal tract. It has a biphasic half-life in the plasma with a terminal elimination phase that has been estimated to range up to about 1 1/2 hours. It is up to 99% bound to plasma proteins and is mainly excreted in the urine, largely unchanged, but also in the form of the glucuronide and free amine metabolites. Variable amounts are also excreted in the bile, non renal elimination being considerably increased in renal failure. Frusemide crosses the placental barrier and is excreted in the breast milk.

*Triamterene:* Triamterene is incompletely but fairly rapidly absorbed from the gastro-intestinal tract. It has been estimated to have a plasma half-life of about 2 hours. It is extensively metabolised and is excreted in the urine in the form of metabolites with some unchanged triamterene. Variable amounts are also excreted in the bile. Animal studies have indicated that triamterene crosses the placental barrier and is excreted in the breast milk.

*Preclinical safety data:* None stated.

**Pharmaceutical particulars**

*List of excipients:* Lactose, maize starch, STa-Rx 1500 = pre-gelatinised starch, sodium starch glycolate = Explotab, Prejel PA5, polysorbate 80, gelatin, magnesium stearate.

*Incompatibilities:* None known.

*Shelf life:* 60 months.

*Special precautions for storage:* Store below 30°C, in a dry place protected from sunlight.

*Nature and contents of container:* Either a white PVC/aluminium foil blister strip containing 56 tablets or a white polyethylene bottle with snap cap containing 100 tablets.

*Instructions for use/handling:* None stated.

*Marketing authorisation holder:* Orion Corporation, PO Box 65, FIN-02101 Espoo, Finland.

**Marketing authorisation number** 6043/0020

**Date of approval/revision of SPC** November 1996.

**Legal category** POM.

## FARESTON* TABLETS 60 mg

**Qualitative and quantitative composition**

*Active ingredient:* Toremifene 60 mg (as toremifene citrate).

*Inactive ingredients:* Maize starch, lactose, povidone, sodium starch glycolate, microcrystalline cellulose, colloidal anhydrous silica, magnesium stearate.

**Pharmaceutical form** Tablet for oral administration.

**Clinical particulars**

*Therapeutic indications:* First line hormone treatment of hormone-dependent metastatic breast cancer in postmenopausal patients. Fareston is not recommended for patients with oestrogen receptor negative tumours.

*Posology and method of administration:* The recommended dose is 60 mg, one tablet, daily.

No dose adjustment is needed in renal insufficiency. Toremifene should be used cautiously in patients with hepatic impairment (see also *Pharmacokinetic properties,* (b) *Characteristics in patients*).

*Contra-indications:* Pre-existing endometrial hyperplasia and severe hepatic failure are contra-indications in long-term use of toremifene.

*Special warnings and special precautions for use:* Experience of the long-term use (more than one year) of toremifene is limited.

Patients with non-compensated cardiac insufficiency or severe angina pectoris should be closely monitored.

Because hypercalcaemia may occur at the beginning of the treatment patients with bone metastases should also be closely monitored.

There is no data on the bone effect of toremifene.

Patients with history of severe thromboembolic disease should generally not be treated.

There is no clinical data available in patients with labile or poorly controlled diabetes, in patients with severely altered performance status or in patients with non-compensated cardiac insufficiency or serious angina pectoris.

*Interaction with other medicaments and other forms of interaction:* No specific interaction studies have been performed.

Drugs which decrease renal calcium excretion e.g. thiazide diuretics, may increase the risk of hypercalcaemia. Enzyme inducers, like phenobarbital, phenytoin and carbamazepine, may increase the rate of toremifene metabolism thus lowering the steady-state concentration in serum. In such cases doubling of the daily dose may be necessary.

There is a known interaction between anti-oestrogens and warfarin-type anticoagulants leading to a seriously increased bleeding time. Therefore, the concomitant use of toremifene with such drugs should be avoided.

Theoretically the metabolism of toremifene is inhibited by drugs known to inhibit the CYP 3A4-6 enzyme system which is reported to be responsible for its main metabolic pathways. Examples of such drugs are ketoconazole and similar antimycotics, erythromycin and troleandomycin. Concomitant use of those drugs with toremifene should be carefully considered.

*Pregnancy and lactation:* Toremifene is recommended for postmenopausal patents.

Owing to the lack of specific data in humans toremifene should not be used during pregnancy and lactation.

In the animal reproduction studies toremifene has shown to prevent implantation, to induce parturition failures, and to reduce perinatal survival. In addition, treatment during organogenesis induces changes in ossification, rib abnormalities, and oedematous foetuses.

In rats, decreased body weight gain of the offspring during lactation was observed.

*Effects on ability to drive and use machines:* None.

*Undesirable effects:* Adverse drug reactions are usually mild. They are mostly due to the hormonal action of toremifene.

In clinical studies, the most frequent adverse reaction is hot flushes (up to 20%). Other common adverse reactions include sweating (14%), nausea (8%), leucorrhea (8%), dizziness (4%), oedema (3%), pain (2%) and vomiting (2%). Less frequent adverse reactions (frequency <1%) include vaginal bleeding, chest pain, fatigue, back pain, headache, skin discoloration, weight increase, insomnia, constipation, dyspnea, paresis, tremor, vertigo, pruritus, anorexia, reversible cornea verticillata (reversible corneal opacity) and asthenia. Thromboembolic events have been reported, although the causal relationship to toremifene treatment remains conjectural.

Rare adverse reactions with unclear causal relationship to toremifene include dermatitis, alopecia, emotional lability, depression, jaundice and stiffness.

Treatment was discontinued due to adverse reactions in about 3% of patients. Most of the cases were due to nausea, vomiting, vertigo, hypercalcaemia and vaginal bleeding. Development of hypercalcaemia in the beginning of the treatment is possible especially in patients with bone metastases.

Endometrial hypertrophy may develop during the treatment due to the hormonal (partial oestrogenic) effect of toremifene. There is a risk of increased endometrial changes including hyperplasia, polyps and cancer. This may be due to the underlying mechanism/oestrogenic stimulation.

*Overdose:* No overdose cases are known.

Vertigo, headache and dizziness were observed in healthy volunteer studies at daily dose of 680 mg. There is no specific antidote and the treatment is symptomatic.

**Pharmacological properties**

*Pharmacodynamic properties:* Toremifene is a nonsteroidal triphenylethylene derivative. As other members of this class, e.g. tamoxifen and clomifene, toremifene binds to oestrogen receptors and may produce oestrogenic or anti-oestrogenic, or both, effects, depending upon the duration of treatment, animal species, gender, target organ and variable selected. In general, however, nonsteroidal triphenylethylene derivatives are predominantly anti-oestrogenic in rats and man and oestrogenic in mice.

In female rats the lowest dose of toremifene that produces an intrinsic oestrogenic effect on the uterus is about 40 times higher than that of tamoxifen. In the same model the minimum anti-oestrogenically effective dose is 10 times higher than that of tamoxifen suggesting a lower oestrogenic to anti-oestrogenic ratio for toremifene than for tamoxifen. No data is available on this ratio in humans. In post-menopausal volunteers receiving oestrogen by oral or transdermal routes, toremifene was shown to exert an anti-oestrogenic effect on vaginal mucosa, by reducing the cornification index. The latter effect was reproducibly found for toremifene doses ranging from 20 to 200 mg daily and could not be distinguished from that of 20 mg tamoxifen. Lower doses of toremifene did not oppose the oestrogenic stimulation of vaginal epithelium.

Toremifene binds specifically to oestrogen receptors, competitively with oestradiol, and inhibits oestrogen-induced stimulation of DNA synthesis and cell replication. In some experimental cancers and/or using high-dose, toremifene displays anti-tumour effects which are not oestrogen-dependent.

The anti-tumour effect of toremifene in breast cancer is mainly due to the anti-oestrogenic effect, although other mechanisms (changes in oncogene expression, growth factor secretion, induction of apoptosis and influence on cell cycle kinetics) may also be involved in the anti-tumour effect.

*Pharmacokinetic properties:*

*(a) General characteristics:* Toremifene is readily absorbed after oral administration. Peak concentrations in serum are obtained within 3 (range 2-5) hours. Food intake has no effect on the extent of absorption but may delay the peak concentrations by 1.5–2 hours. The changes due to food intake are not clinically significant.

The serum concentration curve can be described by a biexponential equation.

The half-life of the first (distribution) phase is 4 (range 2-12) hours, and of the second (elimination) phase 5 (range 2-10) days. The basal disposition parameters (CL and V) could not be estimated due to the lack of intravenous study. Toremifene binds extensively (>99.5%) to serum proteins, mainly to albumin. Toremifene obeys linear serum kinetics at oral daily doses between 11 and 680 mg. The mean concentration of toremifene at steady-state is 0.9 (range 0.6–1.3) $\mu$ g/ml at the recommended dose of 60 mg per day.

Toremifene is extensively metabolised. In human serum the main metabolite is N-demethyltoremifene with mean half-life of 11 (range 4-20) days. Its steady-state concentrations are about twice compared to those of the parent compound. It has similar anti-oestrogenic, albeit weaker anti-tumour activity than the parent compound. It is bound to plasma proteins even more extensively than toremifene, the protein bound fraction being > 99.9%. Three minor metabolites have been detected in human serum: (deaminohydroxy) toremifene, 4-hydroxytoremifene, and N,N-didemethyltoremifene. Although they have theoretically interesting hormonal effects, their concentrations during toremifene treatment are too low to have any major biological importance.

Toremifene is eliminated mainly as metabolites to the faeces. Enterohepatic circulation can be expected. About 10% of the administered dose is eliminated via urine as metabolites. Owing to the slow elimination, steady-state concentrations in serum are reached in 4 to 6 weeks.

*(b) Characteristics in patients:* Clinical anti-tumour efficacy and serum concentrations have no positive correlation at the recommended daily dose of 60 mg.

No information is available concerning polymorphic metabolism. Enzyme complex, known to be responsible for the metabolism of toremifene in humans, is cytochrome P450-dependent hepatic mixed function oxidase. The main metabolic pathway, N-demethylation, is mediated mainly by CYP 3A4/3A5.

Pharmacokinetics of toremifene were investigated in an open study with four parallel groups of ten subjects: normal subjects, patients with impaired ( mean AST 57 U/L–mean ALT 76 U/L–mean gamma GT 329 U/L) or activated liver function ( mean AST 25 U/L–mean ALT 30 U/L–mean gamma GT 91 U/L), patients treated with antiepileptics and patients with impaired renal function (creatinine: 176 µ mol/L). In this study the kinetics of toremifene in patients with impaired renal function were not significantly altered as compared to normal subjects. The elimination of toremifene and its metabolites was significantly increased in patients with activated liver function and decreased in patients with impaired liver function.

*Preclinical safety data:* The acute toxicity of toremifene is low with LD-50 in rats and mice of more than 2000 mg/ kg. In repeated toxicity studies the cause of death in rats is gastric dilatation. In the acute and chronic toxicity studies most of the findings are related to the hormonal effects of toremifene. The other findings are not toxicologically significant. Toremifene has not shown any genotoxicity and has not been found to be carcinogenic in rats. In mice, oestrogens induce ovarian and testicular tumours as well as hyperostosis and osteosarcomas. Toremifene has a species-specific oestrogen-like effect in mice and causes similar tumours. These findings are postulated to be of little relevance for the safety in man, where toremifene acts mainly as an anti-oestrogen.

## Pharmaceutical particulars

*List of excipients:* Maize starch; lactose; povidone; purified water; sodium starch glycolate; magnesium stearate; microcrystalline cellulose; colloidal anhydrous silica.

*Incompatibilities:* None.

*Shelf life:* 5 years between +15°C and +30°C.

*Special precautions for storage:* None.

*Nature and contents of container:* Green PVC foil and aluminium foil blister in a cardboard box. Package sizes: 30 and 100 tablets.

*Instructions for use/handling:* None.

*Marketing authorisation holder:* Orion Corporation, Orionintie 1, FIN-02200 Espoo, Finland.

**Marketing authorisation numbers**
Fareston 60 mg, 30 tablets     EU/1/96/004/001
Fareston 60 mg, 100 tablets    EU/1/96/004/002

**Date of approval/revision of SPC**   2 October 1996.

**Legal category**   POM.

*Trade Mark

# Paines & Byrne Limited
Yamanouchi House
Pyrford Road
West Byfleet
Surrey KT14 6RA

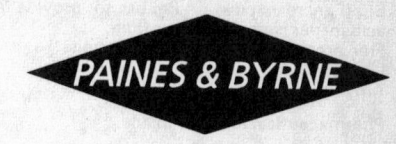

PAINES & BYRNE

## KETOVITE* LIQUID

**Presentation** A pink to yellow liquid containing the following active constituents in a formulation which does not include sucrose, glucose, fructose, lactose, starch, sodium or artificial colouring.

| | per 5 ml |
| --- | --- |
| Vitamin A | 2,500 Units |
| Ergocalciferol BP | 400 Units |
| Choline chloride | 150 mg |
| Cyanocobalamin BP | 12.5 micrograms |

**Uses** As a therapeutic supplement for the prevention of vitamin deficiency in conditions such as galactosaemia, disaccharide intolerance, phenylketonuria and other disorders of carbohydrate or amino acid metabolism, as well as in patients who are on restricted, specialised or synthetic diets.

**Dosage and administration** Ketovite Liquid should be administered orally. The dose for adults, children and the elderly is 5 ml daily.

**Contra-indications, warnings, etc**
*Contra-indications:* Hypersensitivity to the product. Hypercalcaemia.

*Interactions:* Absorption of some vitamins in the preparation may be reduced in conditions of fat malabsorption or with the concurrent use of neomycin, cholestyramine, liquid paraffin, aminoglycosides, aminosalicylic acid, anticonvulsants, biguanides, chloramphenicol, cimetidine, colchicine, potassium salts and methyl-dopa. Serum $B_{12}$ concentrations may be decreased by concurrent administration of oral contraceptives.

*Effects on ability to drive and to use machines:* None known.

*Other undesirable effects:* None in the absence of overdosage.

*Use in pregnancy and lactation:* Caution should be used in pregnancy as excessive doses of Vitamin A may be teratogenic, especially when taken in the first trimester. Large doses of Vitamin D in lactating mothers may cause hypercalcaemia in infants.

*Other special warnings and precautions:* The recommended dose should not be exceeded without medical advice. No other vitamin supplement containing Vitamins A and D should be taken with Ketovite Liquid except under medical supervision. *Warning:* do not exceed the stated dose.

*Overdose:* Symptoms of overdosage may include anorexia, nausea, vomiting, rough dry skin, polyuria, thirst, loss of hair, painful bones and joints as well as raised plasma and urine calcium and phosphate concentration.

No emergency procedure or antidote is applicable and symptoms are rapidly reduced upon withdrawal of the preparation.

*Incompatibilities (major):* None known.

**Pharmaceutical precautions** Store at a temperature between 5° and 15°C.

**Legal category** P.

**Package quantities** 150 ml.

**Further information** For complete vitamin supplementation, Ketovite Liquid should be used in conjunction with Ketovite Tablets. Ketovite Liquid is available on NHS prescription.

**Product licence number** 0051/5080R

## KETOVITE* TABLETS

**Presentation** Yellow biconvex tablets. Each tablet contains the following vitamins in a formulation which does not contain sucrose, glucose, fructose, lactose, starch, sodium, artificial colouring or preservatives:

| | |
| --- | --- |
| Thiamine Hydrochloride BP | 1.0 mg |
| Riboflavine BP | 1.0 mg |
| Pyridoxine Hydrochloride BP | 330 micrograms |
| Nicotinamide BP | 3.3 mg |
| Calcium Pantothenate PhEur | 1.16 mg |
| Ascorbic Acid BP | 16.6 mg |
| Alpha Tocopheryl Acetate BP | 5.0 mg |
| Inositol | 50.0 mg |
| Biotin | 170 micrograms |
| Folic Acid BP | 250 micrograms |
| Acetomenaphthone 1973 BP | 500 micrograms |

**Uses** As a therapeutic supplement for the prevention of vitamin deficiency in conditions such as galactosaemia, disaccharide intolerance, phenylketonuria and other disorders of carbohydrate or amino acid metabolism, as well as in patients who are on restricted, specialised or synthetic diets.

**Dosage and administration** Ketovite Tablets should be administered orally. The dose for adults, children and the elderly is one tablet three times a day.

**Contra-indications, warnings, etc**
*Contra-indications:* Hypersensitivity to the product.

*Interactions:* Pyridoxine may increase the peripheral metabolism of levodopa reducing therapeutic efficacy in patients with Parkinson's disease.

*Effects on ability to drive and to use machines:* None known.

*Other undesirable effects:* None known.

*Use in pregnancy and lactation:* The recommended dose should not be exceeded without medical advice.

*Overdose:* Large overdosages of water-soluble vitamins are readily excreted in the urine.

No emergency procedure or antidote is applicable and any symptoms are rapidly reduced upon withdrawal of the preparation.

*Incompatibilities (major):* None known.

**Pharmaceutical precautions** Store in a cool dry place.

**Legal category** POM.

**Package quantities** 100.

**Further information** For complete vitamin supplementation, Ketovite Tablets should be used in conjunction with Ketovite Liquid. Ketovite Tablets are available on NHS prescription.

**Product licence number** 0051/5079R.

## PANCREX* GRANULES

**Presentation** Pancrex Granules (Pancreatin Granules BP) – Coated granules of pancreatin with not less than the following BP Units of activity in each gram: Free protease 300, lipase 5,000, amylase 4,000.

**Uses** To compensate for reduced intestinal enzyme activity in pancreatic deficiency states.

*Indications:* Fibrocystic disease of the pancreas (cystic fibrosis), chronic pancreatitis and pancreatic steatorrhoea following pancreatectomy. May also be indicated following gastrectomy or vagotomy.

**Dosage and administration** Oral.
Dosage should be adjusted according to the needs of the individual patient and the amount and type of food consumed.
The following dosage range provides a suitable basis for adjustment.
*Adults and children:* 5–10 g swallowed dry or mixed with a little water or milk just before each meal.

**Contra-indications, warnings, etc**
*Contra-indications:* None stated.

*Interactions:* None stated.

*Effects on ability to drive and use machines:* None stated.

*Other undesirable effects:* Rare cases of hyperuricosuria and hyperuricaemia have been reported when extremely high doses of pancreatin have been taken.

*Use in pregnancy and lactation:* Safety in pregnancy has not been established. However no teratogenic effects have been observed in clinical cases.

*Other special warnings and precautions:* It is possible that some irritation of the skin of the mouth may occur if the granules are chewed and retained in the mouth. Irritation of the anus may also occur. A barrier cream may prevent this local irritation.

*Overdose:* None stated.

*Incompatibilities:* None stated.

**Pharmaceutical precautions** Store at a temperature not exceeding 15°C.

**Further information** Pancrex is prepared from Pancreatin of porcine origin. Three level 5 ml spoonfuls provide aproximately 10 g of Pancrex Granules. Palatability may be improved by mixing with fruit juice or puree.

**Legal category** P.

**Package quantities** 300 g.

**Product licence number** 0051/5003R.

## PANCREX* V CAPSULES 125

**Presentation** Clear hard gelatin capsules containing Pancreatin BP and providing not less than the following BP Units of activity: Free protease 160, lipase 2,950, amylase 3,300.

**Uses** To compensate for reduced intestinal enzyme activity in pancreatic deficiency states.

*Indications:* Fibrocystic disease of the pancreas (cystic fibrosis), chronic pancreatitis and pancreatic steatorrhoea following pancreatectomy. May also be indicated following gastrectomy or vagotomy.

**Dosage and administration** Oral. Dosage should be adjusted according to the needs of the individual patient and the amount and type of food consumed.
The following dosage range provides a suitable basis for adjustment.
These low dose capsules may be used when small amounts of Pancrex are required, for example for neonates.

*Neonates:* The contents of 1–2 capsules mixed with feeds.

**Contra-indications, warnings, etc**
*Contra-indications:* None stated.

*Interactions:* None stated.

*Effects on ability to drive and use machines:* None stated.

*Other undesirable effects:* Rare cases of hyperuricosuria and hyperuricaemia have been reported when extremely high doses of pancreatin have been taken.

*Use in pregnancy and lactation:* Safety in pregnancy has not been established. However no teratogenic effects have been observed in clinical cases.

*Other special warnings and precautions:* It is possible that some irritation of the skin of the mouth may occur if capsules are chewed or the contents retained in the mouth. Irritation of the anus may also occur. A barrier cream may prevent this local irritation.
Allergic/asthmatic reactions have occasionally occurred on handling the capsule contents.
If the capsule contents are mixed with liquids or feeds, the resulting mixture should not be allowed to stand for more than one hour prior to use.

*Overdose:* None stated.

*Incompatibilities:* None stated.

**Pharmaceutical precautions** Store at a temperature not exceeding 15°C.

**Further information** Pancrex is prepared from Pancreatin of porcine origin. Palatability of capsule contents may be improved by mixing with fruit juice or puree.
Some of the activity is destroyed by the activity of the stomach. Dosage recommendations reflect this. Cimetidine given 30–45 minutes before meals has been found to potentiate the enzyme activity by reducing gastric acid secretion.

**Legal category** P.

**Package quantities** 300 Pancrex V Capsules 125.

**Product licence number** 0051/5104R

# PANCREX* V CAPSULES

**Qualitative and quantitative composition** Pancreatin BP (Pancreas powder PhEur) to provide enzymic activity per capsule not less than:

| | |
|---|---|
| Free protease | 430 BP units |
| Lipase | 8000 BP units |
| Amylase | 9000 BP units |

**Pharmaceutical form** Capsule.

## Clinical particulars

*Therapeutic indications:* Pancrex is used to compensate for reduced intestinal enzyme activity in pancreatic deficiency states.

It is indicated for the treatment of fibrocystic disease of the pancreas (cystic fibrosis), chronic pancreatitis and pancreatic steatorrhoea following pancreatectomy. May also be indicated following gastrectomy as an aid to digestion.

*Posology and method of administration:* Dosage should be adjusted according to the needs of the individual patient and the amount and type of food consumed.

The following dosage ranges provide a suitable basis for adjustment.

*Infants:* The contents of 1–2 capsules mixed with feeds.

*Older children and adults:* The contents of 2–6 capsules with each snack or meal. The capsules may be swallowed.

The capsules may provide a suitable alternative to the enteric coated presentations in cases where the pH of the duodenum is not sufficiently alkaline to dissolve the enteric coat.

Capsules provide a simple and convenient method of dose measurement of pancreatin for administration to younger children requiring a low dose.

*Contra-indications:* None known.

*Special warnings and precautions for use:* It is possible that some irritation of the skin of the mouth may occur if capsules are chewed or the contents retained in the mouth. Irritation of the anus may also occur. A barrier cream may prevent this local irritation.

Allergic/asthmatic reactions have occasionally occurred on handling the capsule contents.

If the capsule contents are mixed with liquids or feeds the resulting mixture should not be allowed to stand for more than one hour prior to use.

*Interaction with other medicaments and other forms of interaction:* None known.

*Pregnancy and lactation:* Safety in pregnancy has not been established. However, no teratogenic effects have been observed in clinical use.

*Effects on ability to drive and use machines:* None.

*Undesirable effects:* Rare cases of hyperuricosuria and hyperuricaemia have been reported when extremely high doses of pancreatin have been taken.

*Overdose:* None stated.

## Pharmacological properties

*Pharmacodynamic properties:* Pancreatin is derived from mammalian pancreas and contains the enzymes, amylase, protease and lipase. The enzymes have the same actions as pancreatic juice and when administered to patients with pancreatic insufficiency improve the ability to metabolise starches, proteins and fats.

*Pharmacokinetic properties:* Pancreatin hydrolyses fats to glycerol and fatty acids, changes proteins into proteoses and derived substances, and converts starch into dextrins and sugars.

*Preclinical safety data:* No relevant pre-clinical safety data has been generated.

## Pharmaceutical particulars

*List of excipients:* Aluminium oxide, magnesium stearate, microcrystalline cellulose.

*Incompatibilities:* None known.

*Shelf life:* 2 years.

*Special precautions for storage:* Store at a temperature not exceeding 15˚C.

*Nature and contents of container:* Securitainer; 100, 300 and 500 capsules.

*Instructions for use/handling:* Not applicable.

**Marketing authorisation number** 0051/5043R

**Date of approval/revision of SPC** 10 October 1995.

**Legal category** P.

# PANCREX* V POWDER

**Presentation** Pancrex V Powder (Pancreatin BP): A white or buff coloured powder having not less than the following BP Units of activity in each gram: Free Protease 1,400, Lipase 25,000, Amylase 30,000.

**Uses** To compensate for reduced intestinal enzyme activity in pancreatic deficiency states.

*Indications:* Fibrocystic disease of the pancreas (cystic fibrosis), chronic pancreatitis and pancreatic steatorrhoea following pancreatectomy. May also be indicated following gastrectomy or vagotomy.

**Dosage and administration** Oral. Dosage should be adjusted according to the needs of the individual patient and the amount and type of food consumed.

The following dosage ranges provide a suitable basis for adjustment:

*Adults and children:* 0.5–2 g. Swallowed dry or mixed with a little water or milk with each meal.

*Newborn infants:* 0.25–0.5 g with each feed.

**Contra-indications, warnings, etc**
*Contra-indications:* None stated.

*Interactions:* None stated.

*Effects on ability to drive and use machines:* None stated.

*Other undesirable effects:* Rare cases of hyperuricosuria and hyperuricaemia have been reported when extremely high doses of pancreatin have been taken.

*Use in pregnancy and lactation:* Safety in pregnancy has not been established. However no teratogenic effects have been observed in clinical cases.

*Other special warnings and precautions:* It is possible that some irritation of the skin of the mouth may occur if the powder is retained in the mouth. Irritation of the anus may also occur. A barrier cream may prevent this local irritation.

Allergic/asthmatic reactions have occasionally occurred on handling the powder.

If Pancrex is mixed with liquids or feeds, the resulting mixture should not be allowed to stand for more than one hour prior to use.

*Overdose:* None stated.

*Incompatibilities:* None stated.

**Pharmaceutical precautions** Store at a temperature not exceeding 15˚C.

**Further information** Pancrex is prepared from Pancreatin of porcine origin. One level 5 ml spoonful will provide approximately 2 g of Pancrex V Powder. Palatability may be improved by mixing with fruit juice or puree.

Some of the activity is destroyed by the acidity of the stomach. Dosage recommendations reflect this.

Cimetidine given 30–45 minutes before meals has been found to potentiate the enzyme activity by reducing gastric acid secretion.

**Legal category** P.

**Package quantities** 300 g.

**Product licence number** 0051/5004R.

# PANCREX* V TABLETS
# PANCREX* V FORTE TABLETS

**Presentation**
*Pancrex V Tablets (Pancreatin Tablets BP)* (Pancreatin BP/Pancreas Powder EP 92.5 mg); White sugar and enteric coated tablets each containing not less than the following BP Units of activity: Free protease 110, lipase 1,900, amylase 1,700.

*Pancrex V Forte Tablets (Pancreatin Tablets BP)* (Pancreatin BP/Pancreas Powder EP 222 mg): White sugar and enteric coated tablets each containing not less than the following BP Units of activity: Free protease 330, lipase 5,600, amylase 5,000.

**Uses** To compensate for reduced intestinal enzyme activity in pancreatic deficiency states.

*Indications:* Fibrocystic disease of the pancreas (cystic fibrosis), chronic pancreatitis and pancreatic steatorrhoea following pancreatectomy. May also be indicated following gastrectomy or vagotomy.

**Dosage and administration** Oral. Dosage should be adjusted according to the needs of the individual patient and the amount and type of food consumed.

The following dosage range provides a suitable basis for adjustment.

*Adults and children:* 5–15 Pancrex V Tablets or 6–10 Pancrex V Forte Tablets before each meal swallowed whole.

**Contra-indications, warnings, etc**
*Contra-indications:* None stated.

*Interactions:* None stated.

*Effects on ability to drive and use machines:* None stated.

*Other undesirable effects:* Rare cases of hyperuricosuria and hyperuricaemia have been reported when extremely high doses of pancreatin have been taken.

*Use in pregnancy and lactation:* Safety in pregnancy has not been established. However no teratogenic effects have been observed in clinical cases.

*Other special warnings and precautions:* Variations in response to treatment may be due to enteric coating. It is possible that some irritation of the skin of the mouth may occur if tablets are chewed. Irritation of the anus may also occur. A barrier cream may prevent this local irritation.

*Overdose:* None stated.

*Incompatibilities:* None stated.

**Pharmaceutical precautions** Store at a temperature not exceeding 15˚C.

**Further information** Pancrex is prepared from Pancreatin of porcine origin.

**Legal category** P.

**Package quantities** 300.

**Product licence numbers**
| | |
|---|---|
| Pancrex V Tablets | 0051/5002R |
| Pancrex V Forte Tablets | 0051/5000R |

*Trade Mark

# Parke Davis
Lambert Court
Chestnut Avenue
Eastleigh
Hampshire SO53 3ZQ

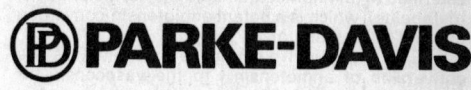 **PARKE-DAVIS**

## ACCUPRO*

**Qualitative and quantitative composition** Each Accupro 5 mg tablet contains: Quinapril hydrochloride 5.416 mg (equivalent to 5 mg quinapril base).

Each Accupro 10 mg tablet contains: Quinapril hydrochloride 10.832 mg (equivalent to 10 mg quinapril base).

Each Accupro 20 mg tablet contains: Quinapril hydrochloride 21.664 mg (equivalent to 20 mg quinapril base).

Each Accupro 40 mg tablet contains: Quinapril hydrochloride 43.328 mg (equivalent to 40 mg quinapril base).

**Pharmaceutical form** Accupro is supplied as brown film coated tablets imprinted with the dosage strength. The 5 mg tablet is elliptical. The 10 mg tablet is triangular. The 20 mg tablet is round. The 40 mg tablet is elliptical.

### Clinical particulars

*Therapeutic indications:* (1) For the treatment of all grades of essential hypertension. Accupro is effective as monotherapy or concomitantly with diuretics in patients with hypertension.

(2) For the treatment of congestive heart failure when given concomitantly with a diuretic and/or cardiac glycoside. Treatment of congestive heart failure with Accupro should always be initiated under close medical supervision.

*Posology and method of administration:* For oral use *Adults: Hypertension: Monotherapy:* The recommended initial dosage is 10 mg once daily in uncomplicated hypertension. Depending upon clinical response, patient's dosage may be titrated (by doubling the dose allowing adequate time for dosage adjustment) to a maintenance dosage of 20 to 40 mg/day given as a single dose or divided into 2 doses. Long-term control is maintained in most patients with a single daily dosage regimen. Patients have been treated with dosages up to 80 mg/day.
*Concomitant diuretics:* In order to determine if excess hypotension will occur, an initial dosage of 2.5 mg of Accupro is recommended in patients who are also being treated with a diuretic. After this the dosage of Accupro should be titrated (as described above) to the optimal response.
*Congestive heart failure:* In order to closely monitor patients for symptomatic hypotension, a single 2.5 mg initial dose is recommended. After this, patients should be titrated to an effective dose (up to 40 mg/day) given in 1 or 2 doses with concomitant diuretic and/or cardiac glycoside therapy. Patients are usually maintained effectively on doses of 10-20 mg/day given with concomitant therapy.

In the treatment of severe or unstable congestive heart failure, Accupro should always be initiated in hospital under close medical supervision.

Other patients who may also be considered to be at higher risk and should have treatment initiated in hospital include: patients who are on high dose loop diuretics (e.g. > 80 mg frusemide) or on multiple diuretic therapy, have hypovolaemia, hyponatraemia (serum sodium < 130 mgeq/l) or systolic blood pressure < 90 mm Hg, are on high dose vasodilator therapy, have a serum creatinine > 150 micromol/l or are aged 70 years or over.
*Elderly / Renal impairment:* In elderly patients and in patients with a creatinine clearance of less than 40 ml/min, an initial dosage in essential hypertension of 2.5 mg is recommended followed by titration to the optimal response.
*Children (6–12 years):* Not recommended. Safety and efficacy in children has not been established.
*Contra-indications:* Hypersensitivity to any of the ingredients.
Pregnancy: Accupro is contra-indicated throughout pregnancy. Accupro has been shown to be foetotoxic in rabbits. When ACE inhibitors have been used during the second and third trimesters of pregnancy, there have been reports of hypotension, renal failure, skull hypoplasia, and/or death in the newborn. Oligohydramnios has also been reported, presumably representing decreased renal function in the foetus; limb contractures, craniofacial deformities, hypoplastic lung development, and intrauterine growth retar-

dation have been reported in association with oligohydramnios. Should a woman become pregnant while receiving ACE inhibitors, the drug should be discontinued as soon as possible. Infants exposed *in utero* t o ACE inhibitors should be closely observed for hypotension, oliguria, and hyperkalaemia. If oliguria occurs, attention should be directed toward support of blood pressure and renal perfusion.

*Special warnings and special precautions for use:* Accupro should not be used in patients with aortic stenosis or outflow obstruction.

In patients with renal insufficiency, monitoring of renal function during therapy should be performed as deemed appropriate, although in the majority renal function will not alter or may improve.

As a consequence of inhibiting the renin-angiotensin-aldosterone system, changes in renal function may be anticipated in susceptible individuals. In patients with severe heart failure whose renal function may depend on the activity of the renin-angiotensin-aldosterone system, treatment with ACE inhibitors including quinapril, may be associated with oliguria and/or progressive azotemia and rarely acute renal failure and/or death.

Patients haemodialysed using high-flux polyacrylonitrile ('AN69') membranes are highly likely to experience anaphylactoid reactions if they are treated with ACE inhibitors. This combination should therefore be avoided, either by use of alternative antihypertensive drugs or alternative membranes for haemodialysis.

The half-life of quinaprilat is prolonged as creatinine clearance falls. Patients with a creatinine clearance of <40 ml/min require a lower initial dosage of quinapril. These patients' dosage should be titrated upwards based upon therapeutic response, and renal function should be closely monitored although initial studies do not indicate that quinapril produces further deterioration in renal function.

In clinical studies in hypertensive patients with unilateral or bilateral renal artery stenosis, increases in blood urea nitrogen and serum creatinine have been observed in some patients following ACE inhibitor therapy. These increases were almost always reversible upon discontinuation of the ACE inhibitor and/or diuretic therapy. In such patients, renal function should be monitored during the first few weeks of therapy.

Some patients with hypertension or heart failure with no apparent pre-existing renal vascular disease have developed increases (>1.25 times the upper limit of normal) in blood urea and serum creatinine, usually minor and transient, especially when quinapril has been given concomitantly with a diuretic and has been observed in 4% and 3% respectively of patients on monotherapy. This is more likely to occur in patients with pre-existing renal impairment. Dosage reduction and/or discontinuation of a diuretic and/or quinapril may be required.
*Angioedema:* Angioedema has been reported in patients treated with angiotensin- converting enzyme inhibitors. If laryngeal stridor or angioedema of the face, tongue, or glottis occur, treatment should be discontinued immediately, the patient treated appropriately in accordance with accepted medical care, and carefully observed until the swelling disappears. In instances where swelling is confined to the face and lips, the condition generally resolves without treatment; antihistamines may be useful in relieving symptoms. Angioedema associated with laryngeal involvement may be fatal. Where there is involvement of the tongue, glottis, or larynx likely to cause airway obstruction, appropriate therapy eg, subcutaneous adrenaline solution 1:1000 (0.3 to 0.5 ml) should be promptly administered.
*Hypotension:* Symptomatic hypotension was rarely seen in hypertensive patients treated with Accupro but is a possible consequence of ACE inhibition therapy particularly in salt/volume depleted patients such as those previously treated with diuretics, who have a dietary salt reduction, or who are on dialysis. If symptomatic hypotension occurs, the patient should be placed in the supine position and, if necessary, receive an intravenous infusion of normal saline. A transient hypotensive response is not a contraindication to further doses; however, lower doses of

quinapril or any concomitant diuretic therapy should be considered if this event occurs.
*Neutropenia/agranulocytosis:* ACE inhibitors have been rarely associated with agranulocytosis and bone marrow depression in patients with uncomplicated hypertension but more frequently in patients with renal impairment, especially if they also have collagen vascular disease. As with other ACE inhibitors, monitoring of white blood cell counts in patients with collagen vascular disease and/or renal diseases should be considered.

*Interactions with other medicaments and other forms of interaction: Tetracycline:* Because of the presence of magnesium carbonate in the formulation Accupro has been shown in healthy volunteers to reduce the absorption of tetracycline in concomitant administration by 28-37%. It is recommended that concomitant administration with tetracycline be avoided.
*Concomitant diuretic therapy:* Patients treated with diuretics may occasionally experience an excessive reduction of blood pressure after initiation of therapy with Accupro. This hypotensive effect may be effectively minimised by either discontinuing the diuretic or increasing the salt intake prior to the initial dose of Accupro. If discontinuation of the diuretic is not possible, medical supervision should be provided for up to two hours following administration of the initial dose.
*Surgery/anaesthesia:* Although no data are available to indicate there is an interaction between Accupro and anaesthetic agents that produces hypotension, caution should be exercised when patients undergo major surgery or anaesthesia since ACE inhibitors have been shown to block angiotensin II formation secondary to compensatory renin release. This may lead to hypotension which can be corrected by volume expansion.
*Agents increasing serum potassium:* Concomitant treatments with potassium sparing diuretics, potassium supplements or potassium containing salts should be used with caution and with appropriate monitoring of serum potassium. As with other ACE inhibitors, patients on quinapril alone may have increased serum potassium levels. When administered concomitantly, quinapril may reduce the hypokalaemia induced by thiazide diuretics.
*Lithium:* Increased serum lithium levels and symptoms of lithium toxicity have been reported in patients receiving concomitant lithium and ACE inhibitor therapy due to the sodium-losing effect of these agents. These drugs should be co-administered with caution and frequent monitoring of serum lithium levels is recommended. If a diuretic is also used, it may increase the risk of lithium toxicity.

*Pregnancy and lactation: Pregnancy*–see under *Contra-indications.*
*Lactation:* Since it is not known if this drug is secreted in human milk caution should be exercised when the product is given to nursing mothers.

*Effects on ability to drive or use machines:* None known

*Other undesirable effects:* The most frequent clinical adverse reactions in hypertension and congestive heart failure are headache, dizziness, rhinitis, coughing, upper respiratory tract infection, fatigue, and nausea and vomiting. Other less frequent side effects are dyspepsia, myalgia, chest pain, abdominal pain, diarrhoea, back pain, sinusitis, insomnia, paraesthesia, nervousness, asthenia, pharyngitis, hypotension, palpitations, flatulence, depression, pruritus, rash, impotence, oedema, arthralgia, amblyopia.

Renal dysfunction, angioedema, hypotension, hyperkalaemia, neutropenia, agranulocytosis. (see *special warnings and special precautions of use*).

Pancreatitis has been reported rarely in patients treated with ACE inhibitors; in some cases this has proved fatal.

*Overdose:* No data are available with respect to overdosage in humans. The most likely clinical manifestation would be symptoms attributable to severe hypotension, which should normally be treated by intravenous volume expansion.

Haemodialysis and peritoneal dialysis have little effect on the elimination of quinapril and quinaprilat.

**Pharmacological properties**

*Pharmacodynamic properties:* Quinapril is rapidly de-esterified to quinaprilat (quinapril diacid, the principal metabolite), which is a potent angiotensin-converting enzyme (ACE) inhibitor.

ACE is a peptidyl dipeptidase that catalyzes the conversion of angiotensin I to the vasoconstrictor angiotensin II which is involved in vascular control and function through many different mechanisms, including stimulation of aldosterone secretion by the adrenal cortex. The mode of action of quinapril in humans and animals is to inhibit circulating and tissue ACE activity, thereby decreasing vasopressor activity and aldosterone secretion.

In animal studies, the antihypertensive effect of quinapril outlasts its inhibitory effect on circulating ACE, whereas, tissue ACE inhibition more closely correlates with the duration of antihypertensive effects. Administration of 10-40 mg of quinapril to patients with mild to severe hypertension results in a reduction of both sitting and standing blood pressure with minimal effect on heart rate. Antihypertensive activity commences within one hour with peak effects usually achieved by two to four hours after dosing. Achievement of maximum blood pressure lowering effects may require two weeks of therapy in some patients. At the recommended doses, antihypertensive effects are maintained in most patients throughout the 24-hour dosing interval and continue during long-term therapy.

*Pharmacokinetic properties:* Peak plasma Accupro concentrations are observed within 1 hour of oral administration. The extent of absorption is approximately 60% and is not influenced by food. Following absorption, Accupro is deesterified to its major active metabolite, quinaprilat and to minor inactive metabolites. Accupro has an apparent half-life of approximately one hour. Peak plasma quinaprilat concentrations are observed approximately 2 hours following an oral dose of quinapril. Quinaprilat is eliminated primarily by renal excretion and has an effective accumulation half-life of 3 hours. In patients with renal insufficiency and creatinine clearance of ≤40 ml/min, peak and trough quinaprilat concentrations increase, time to peak concentration increases, apparent half-life increases and time to steady state may be delayed. The elimination of quinaprilat is also reduced in elderly patients (>65 years) and correlates well with the impaired renal function which frequently occurs in the elderly. Quinaprilat concentrations are reduced in patients with alcoholic cirrhosis due to impaired deesterification of Accupro. Studies in rats indicate that Accupro and its metabolites do not cross the blood-brain barrier.

*Pre-clinical safety data:* The results of the pre-clinical tests do not add anything of further significance to the prescriber

**Pharmaceutical particulars**

*List of excipients:* Accupro tablets contain the following excipients: Magnesium carbonate, lactose, gelatin, crospovidone, magnesium stearate, candelilla wax, colourings: red iron oxide (E172) and titanium dioxide (E171).

*Incompatibilities:* None known.

*Shelf-life:* Not less than 3 years when stored in the original packaging.

*Special precautions for storage:* Store below 25°C

*Nature and contents of container:* Polyamide / aluminium / PVC blister containing 28 tablets.

*Instructions for use/handling:* No special requirements.

*Marketing authorisation holder:* Parke, Davis & Company, Usk Road, Pontypool, NP4 0YH

**Marketing authorisation numbers**

Accupro 5 mg 0018/0148
Accurpo 10 mg 0018/0149
Accupro 20 mg 0018/0150
Accupro 40 mg 0018/0213

**Date of approval/revision of SPC** 1 May 1996

**Legal category** POM

## ACCURETIC*

**Presentation** Pink, scored, elliptical, biconvex film coated tablets.

*Composition:* Tablets containing 10 mg quinapril and 12.5 mg of hydrochlorothiazide.

**Uses**

*Indications:* Hydrochlorothiazide: For the treatment of essential hypertension.

Quinapril: For the treatment of all grades of essential hypertension where the standard therapy is ineffective or inappropriate because of adverse events.

Accuretic: For the treatment of hypertensive patients who have been stabilised on their individual components given in the same proportions.

**Dosage and administration** Oral

*Adults:* Effective blood pressure control is usually achieved with a daily dosage of 10/12.5 mg to a maximum of 20/25 mg.

*Renal Impairment:* Accuretic is not recommended for use in patients with creatinine clearance of less than 40 ml/min.

*Elderly:* The dose should be kept as low as possible commensurate with achievement of adequate blood pressure control.

*Children:* Not recommended. Safety and efficacy in children has not been established.

**Contra-indications, warnings, etc**

*Contra-indications:* Accuretic is contra-indicated in patients with anuria or hypersensitivity to quinapril, thiazides or any sulfonamide derived drug.

Pregnancy: Accuretic is contraindicated throughout pregnancy. Quinapril has been shown to be foetoxic in rabbits. Use of ACE inhibitors in the second and third trimesters have been associated with oligohydramnios. Hypotension and renal failure have occurred in the newborn.

Accuretic should not be used in nursing mothers.

*Precautions:* Sensitivity reactions may occur in patients with or without a history of allergy or bronchial asthma, eg. purpura, photosensitivity, urticaria, necrotising angiitis, respiratory distress including pneumonitis and pulmonary oedema.

Stevens-Johnson syndrome and exacerbations or activation of systemic lupus erythematosus have been reported with thiazides.

In patients with renal insufficiency, monitoring of renal function during therapy should be performed as deemed appropriate.

Renal failure has been reported in association with ACE inhibitors and has occurred mainly in patients with severe congestive heart failure or underlying renal disease, including renal artery stenosis. If recognised promptly and treated appropriately, renal failure is usually reversible.

Accuretic should be used cautiously in patients with impaired hepatic function or progressive liver disease because of the known risks associated with alterations in fluid and electrolyte balance resulting from thiazide treatment.

Patients receiving Accuretic should be observed for clinical signs of thiazide–induced fluid or electrolyte imbalance. In such patients periodic determination of serum electrolytes should be performed. Because quinapril reduces the production of aldosterone, its combination with hydrochlorothiazide may minimise diuretic induced hypokalaemia. However, some patients may still require potassium supplements.

Patients haemodialysed using high-flux polyacrylonitrile ('AN69') membranes are highly likely to experience anaphylactoid reactions if they are treated with ACE inhibitors. This combination should therefore be avoided, either by use of alternative antihypertensive drugs or alternative membranes for haemodialysis.

*Drug interactions: Tetracycline:* Because of the presence of magnesium carbonate in the formulation it is recommended that concomitant administration of Accuretic with tetracycline be avoided.

*Agents increasing serum potassium:* Accuretic contains a diuretic. The addition of a potassium sparing diuretic is not recommended since these may cause a significant increase in serum potassium.

*Surgery/anaesthesia:* Although no data are available to indicate there is an interaction between Accuretic and anaesthetic agents that produce hypotension, caution should be exercised when patients undergo major surgery or anaesthesia since ACE inhibitors have been shown to block angiotensin II formation secondary to compensatory renin release. This may lead to hypotension which can be corrected by volume expansion.

Thiazides may decrease the arterial response to noradrenaline. In emergency surgery pre-anaesthetic and anaesthetic agents should be administered in reduced doses. Thiazides may increase the response to tubocurarine.

*Lithium:* Increased serum lithium levels and symptoms of lithium toxicity have been reported in patients receiving concomitant lithium and ACE inhibitor therapy or lithium and thiazide therapy. Lithium should not generally be given with Accuretic since the risk of lithium toxicity may be increased.

*Corticosteroids, ACTH:* Intensified electrolyte depletion, particularly hypokalaemia has been observed.

*Non-steroidal anti-inflammatory drugs:* In some patients, the administration of a non-steroidal anti-inflammatory agent can reduce the diuretic, natriuretic, and antihypertensive effects of loop, potassium-sparing, and thiazide diuretics. Therefore, when Accuretic and non-steroidal anti-inflammatory agents are used concomitantly the patients should be observed closely to determine if the desired effect of Accuretic is obtained.

*Side-effects:* The most frequent clinical adverse reactions in hypertension are headache, dizziness, rhinitis, coughing and fatique. Other adverse experiences include myalgia, viral infection, nausea and vomiting, abdominal pains, back pain and upper respiratory infection. Less frequent side effects are dyspepsia, chest pain, diarrhoea, insomnia, bronchitis, somnolence, asthenia, pharyngitis, vasodilatation and vertigo.

Increases (>1.25 times the upper limit of normal) in serum creatinine and blood urea nitrogen were observed in 3% and 4% respectively of the patients treated with Accuretic. These increases were almost always reversible upon discontinuation of ACE inhibitor therapy. In such patients renal funtion should be monitored during the first few weeks of therapy.

Increases in cholesterol and triglyceride levels may be associated with thiazide diuretic therapy.

*Angioedema:* Angioedema has been reported in patients treated with ACE inhibitors. If laryngeal stridor or angioedema of the face, tongue, or glottis occur, treatment should be discontinued immediately, the patient treated appropriately in accordance with accepted medical care, and carefully observed until the swelling disappears. In instances where swelling is confined to the face and lips, the condition generally resolves without treatment; antihistamines may be useful in relieving symptoms. Angioedema associated with laryngeal involvement may be fatal. Where there is involvement of the tongue, glottis, or larynx likely to cause airway obstruction, appropriate therapy eg subcutaneous adrenaline solution 1:1000 (0.3 to 0.5 ml) should be promptly administered.

*Hypotension:* Symptomatic hypotension is a possible consequence of ACE inhibition therapy in volume depleted patients such as those previously treated with thiazides.

*Neutropenia/agranulocytosis:* ACE inhibitors have been rarely associated with agranulocytosis and bone marrow depression in patients with uncomplicated hypertension but more frequently in patients with renal impairment, especially if they also have collagen vascular disease. As with other ACE inhibitors, monitoring of white blood cell counts in patients with collagen vascular disease and/or renal diseases should be considered. With thiazides leucopenia, agranulocytosis thrombocytopenia and aplastic anaemia have been reported.

*Metabolic disorders:* Hyperuricaemia may occur or frank gout be precipitated by thiazides in certain patients. Insulin requirements in diabetic patients may be altered by thiazides and latent diabetes mellitus may occur.

Pancreatitis has been reported rarely in patients treated with ACE inhibitors; in some cases this has proved fatal.

*Overdosage:* No data are available with respect to overdosage in humans. The most likely clinical manifestation would be symptoms attributed to severe hypotension. Treatment is symptomatic and supportive. Therapy with Accuretic should be discontinued and the patient observed closely.

Haemodialysis and peritoneal dialysis have little effect on the elimination of quinapril and quinaprilat.

**Pharmaceutical precautions** Store at a temperature not exceeding 25°C.

**Legal category** POM.

**Package quantities** Blister strips of 7 tablets, 4 strips in a carton (28 tablets).

**Further information**

*Clinical chemistry:* Accuretic may cause a false positive urine test for Acetone.

Accuretic is designed to aid compliance by providing a convenient once daily preparation of quinapril combined with hydrochlorothiazide for the treatment of all grades of essential hypertension.

Significant antihypertensive activity is detectable throughout a 24 hour period following oral therapy. Quinaprilat is highly potent at binding to arterial and cardiac ACE.

By combining lower doses than might be required with each component used alone, side effects, especially the hypokalaemia associated with diuretics can be minimised.

**Product licence number** 0018/0196

## AMSIDINE* CONCENTRATE FOR INFUSION

**Presentation** Amsidine is formulated as two sterile liquids that are combined prior to use:

*Drug ampoule*–a 2 ml clear, neutral glass printed ampoule containing a clear bright orange/red coloured solution.

*Diluent vial*–a 20 ml amber glass vial containing a clear colourless solution.

*Composition:* Each 2 ml ampoule contains 1.5 ml of amsacrine solution in anhydrous N,N- dimethylacetamide in a strength of 50 mg amsacrine per ml. That is, each ampoule contains 75 mg amsacrine. Each 20 ml amber vial contains 13.5 ml of 0.0353M L- lactic acid. Exactly 1.5 ml of the solution from the ampoule is removed by the aid of a graduated glass syringe and immediately added to the vial with L-lactic acid, and the contents are mixed thoroughly by shaking. The resulting red solution contains 5 mg/ml Amsidine.

**Uses**
*Action:* Amsidine is a sterile antitumour chemotherapeutic agent for intravenous infusion. Although not completely clarified, the mode of action of amsacrine is related to its property of binding the DNA through intercalation and external (electrostatic) forces. Amsacrine inhibits the synthesis of DNA while the RNA may not be directly affected. An additional mode of action, involving modification of cell membrane function, has been suggested.

*(a) Properties:* Amsacrine is a synthetic aminocrine derivative. It acts by inhibiting DNA synthesis. It is 98% protein bound, has an elimination half-life of 5-8 hours, excretion occuring mainly through bile. Elimination is significantly slower in renal and hepatic insufficiency and in the elderly.

*(b) Indications:* Amsidine is indicated for the induction and maintenance of remission in acute leukaemia of adults. It is effective in patients refractory to the anthracycline antibiotics used singly or in combination with other chemotherapeutic agents, and in patients who were formerly treated with maximum cumulative doses of these antibiotics.

**Dosage and administration** Amsidine must be diluted in 500 ml 5% Dextrose Injection BP and infused over 60 to 90 minutes. Phlebitis or pain at the injection site may occur at doses greater than 70 mg/m². **(NOTE: DO NOT USE OTHER DILUENTS. AMSIDINE IS INCOMPATIBLE WITH SALINE).** Care must be taken that no extravasation occurs which might produce severe irritation or necrosis.

Caution in the handling and preparation of the solution should be exercised, and the use of polyethylene gloves is recommended. If the solution of Amsidine contacts the skin or mucosae, immediately wash thoroughly with soap and water. (See professional leaflet).

*Adults: Induction of remission phase:* The usual dosage of Amsidine in the induction phase is 90 mg/m² every day for five consecutive days (total dose 450 mg/m² per course of treatment). If bone marrow biopsy performed on day six displays over 50% cellularity and the blasts count is over 30%, the treatment may be extended for an additional three days, bringing the total dose per course of treatment to 720 mg/m².

More than one course of treatment may be required to achieve induction. Depending on the effectiveness of the first course in producing myelosuppression, the subsequent courses are given at two-week (if not effective) to four-week (if effective) intervals. In cases where a hypocellular marrow has not been achieved after the first course of treatment, the daily dose of Amsidine may be escalated to 120 mg/m² per day for the subsequent courses, provided that this is not contra-indicated for reasons of non-myelosuppressive toxicity.

For patients with impaired liver function or impaired renal function, the dose of Amsidine should be decreased by 20-30% (to 60-75 mg/m² per day).

*Maintenance phase:* The maintenance dose is about one third the induction dose, given either as a single I.V. infusion or divided in three daily doses; e.g. 150 mg/m² given once every 3-4 weeks or 50 mg/m² per day for three consecutive days, repeated every 3-4 weeks.

Each maintenance course should bring down the granulocyte count to 1,000- 1,500/μl and the platelet count to 50,000-100,000/μl. If this is not accomplished, the maintenance dose may be escalated by 20% every second course. The granulocyte and platelet counts should be allowed to recover between the courses to over 1,500/μl and 100,000/μl respectively; otherwise the subsequent course should be delayed.

*Elderly:* Elimination may be slower in this group. This should be considered when designing dose schedules for the elderly.

*Children under 12 years:* Not recommended.

**Contra-indications, warnings, etc**
*Contra-indications:* Amsidine treatment should not be started in patients who have pre-existing marked bone marrow suppression induced by other chemotherapeutic agents or radiotherapy.

*Precautions:* Patients should be hospitalised during the induction phase of treatment for close observation and extensive laboratory monitoring. Amsidine should be used only by physicians experienced in cancer chemotherapy. The drug may cause severe myelosuppression, and complete blood counts must be performed frequently. Leucocyte, red cell and platelet transfusions should be available.

With recommended dose schedules, leucopenia is usually transient, reaching its nadir at 10-13 days after treatment, with recovery usually following by the 17th to 25th day. White blood cell counts of 1000/μl or lower are to be expected during treatment with appropriate doses of Amsidine. Doses higher than recommended may produce more severe or more prolonged marrow suppression.

The potential for cardiotoxicity may be increased particularly by hypokalaemia, also concurrent use of diuretics, aminoglycosides or other nephrotoxic drugs and previous exposure to other anthracycline therapy.

Periodic monitoring of bone marrow, cardiac, liver, kidney and CNS functions should be carried out in patients receiving Amsidine and particularly in those with pre-existing disorders of these systems. In the case of an exceedingly large fall in white cell count and excessive depression of bone marrow, suspension of treatment or reduction of dosage may be necessary.

Studies have demonstrated a mutagenic potential. No carcinogenic studies have been carried out. As with other antineoplastic agents there is a possibility that prolonged use may lead to a carcinogenic effect. This should be borne in mind when undertaking long-term treatment.

*Use in pregnancy:* Animal studies have indicated that amsacrine has foetotoxic and teratogenic properties. In addition there may be an effect on fertility. There is no information on use in human pregnancy, therefore the benefit/risk considerations should be carefully weighed when administering Amsidine.

*Adverse reactions: Haematopoietic system:* The dose-limiting toxicity associated with Amsidine is myelosuppression and pancytopenia, requiring supportive treatment with white and red blood cells and platelets. Major complications during therapy were infections and haemorrhages treated, respectively, with antibiotics and platelet transfusions.

*Gastro-intestinal:* Nausea, with or without vomiting occurred frequently, but these symptoms were usually mild to moderate. Mucositis (stomatitis and oesophagitis) was almost as frequent and ranged in severity from mild to life-threatening; its frequency and severity were not strictly dose-related.

*Central nervous system:* A few cases of grand mal seizures in acute leukaemia patients have occurred during treatment with Amsidine. These patients were suffering, however, from a number of conditions related to far-advanced disease and were heavily pretreated; and it is unclear whether the seizures were attributable to Amsidine. The seizures generally were responsive to standard treatment, such as phenytoin.

*Hepatic:* Liver function tests showed occasional transient elevations of serum bilirubin and alkaline phosphatase, sometimes accompanied by jaundice, which required lowering the dose of Amsidine.

*Renal:* Occasional occurrence of haematuria, anuria, and rarely acute renal failure have been reported.

*Cardiac:* Cardiotoxicity occurred in several patients. It ranged from grand mal seizures followed by ventricular tachycardia to congestive heart failure or cardiac arrest.

*Cutaneous:* Local tissue irritation, necrosis and phlebitis have been reported. This problem is related to the concentration of drug infused per unit time; it is ameliorated by diluting the drug in a large volume of 5% Dextrose Injection BP and infusing over a longer period of time (1 to 2 hours).

Alopecia occurred in about 1 in 7 patients, sometimes precipitously. Since most patients were previously treated with other chemotherapeutic agents/or radiation, it is not clear whether this was a cumulative effect of all treatments.

*Treatment of overdosage:* Treatment of overdosage should be supportive and the blood picture should be closely monitored with appropriate blood transfusions being given if necessary.

**Pharmaceutical precautions** Store below 25°C. Protect from light.

Caution in handling and preparation of solution should be exercised, and the use of polyethylene gloves is recommended (see professional leaflet). If the solution of Amsidine contacts the skin or mucosae, immediately wash thoroughly with soap and water.

Amsidine must be diluted in 500 ml 5% Dextrose Injection BP and infused over 60 to 90 minutes. **(NOTE: DO NOT USE OTHER DILUENTS. AMSIDINE IS INCOMPATIBLE WITH SALINE).**

The solution when diluted for infusion is stable for eight hours at room temperature. It should be protected from exposure to sunlight, and any unused solution should be discarded (see professional leaflet).

**GLASS SYRINGES MUST BE USED. AMSIDINE IN SOLUTION REACTS WITH PLASTIC SYRINGES.**

**Legal category** POM.

**Package quantities** Each carton contains: six 2 ml ampoules containing amsacrine solution and six 20 ml vials of diluent.

**Further information** Nil

**Product licence number** 0018/0124

## ANUGESIC* HC CREAM

**Presentation** Buff coloured cream with the characteristic odour of Balsam Peru. Each 100 g of cream contains:

Pramoxine Hydrochloride USP 1.00 g
Hydrocortisone Acetate PhEur 0.50 g
Benzyl Benzoate PhEur 1.20 g
Bismuth Oxide 0.875 g
Balsam Peru PhEur 1.85 g
Zinc oxide Ph Eur 12.35 g

**Uses** Anugesic HC Cream provides antiseptic, astringent, emollient and decongestant properties. In addition hydrocortisone exerts an anti-inflammatory effect. Pramoxine is a rapidly acting local anaesthetic. The cream may be used to provide lubrication for suppositories.

Anugesic HC Cream is indicated for the comprehensive symptomatic treatment of severe and acute discomfort or pain associated with internal and external haemorrhoids, and pruritus ani.

**Dosage and administration** Topical

*Adults:* Apply cream to the affected area at night, in the morning and after each evacuation. Thoroughly cleanse the affected area, dry and apply cream by gently smoothing onto the affected area. For internal conditions use rectal nozzle provided and clean it after each use.

Not to be taken orally.

*Elderly (over 65 years):* As for adults.

*Children:* Not recommended.

**Contra-indications, warnings, etc**
*Contra-indications:* Tubercular, fungal and most viral lesions including herpes simplex, vaccinia and varicella.

History of sensitivity to any of the constituents.

*Warnings:* As with all products containing topical steroids the possibility of systemic absorption should be borne in mind.

Prolonged or excessive use may produce systemic corticosteroid effects, and use for periods longer than seven days is not recommended.

*Use in pregnancy:* There is inadequate evidence of safety in human pregnancy and there may be a very small risk of cleft palate and intrauterine growth retardation as well as suppression of the neonatal HPA axis. There is evidence of harmful effects in animals. Use in pregnancy only when there is no safer alternative and when the disease itself carries risks for the mother or child.

*Precautions:* Following symptomatic relief definite diagnosis should be established.

*Side-effects:* Rarely, sensitivity reactions. Patients may occasionally experience transient burning on application, especially if the anoderm is not intact.

*Overdosage:* If swallowed, fever, nausea, vomiting, stomach cramps and diarrhoea may develop 3-12 hours after ingestion.

Pramoxine is relatively non-toxic and less sensitising than other local anaesthetics.

Hydrocortisone does not normally produce toxic effects in an acute single overdose.

Treatment of a large acute overdosage should include gastric lavage, purgation with magnesium sulphate and complete bed rest. If necessary, give oxygen and general supportive measures. Methaemoglobinaemia should be treated by intravenous methylene blue.

**Pharmaceutical precautions** Store at a temperature not exceeding 25°C.

**Legal category** POM.

**Package quantities** Tubes containing 30 g

**Further information** Anugesic-HC Cream is prepared in a water miscible base which provides intimate contact with the area to be treated without having to cross an anhydrous barrier. A cream is also more convenient to use, being aesthetically more acceptable than ointments.

**Product licence numbers** 0018/0161

# ANUGESIC* HC SUPPOSITORIES

**Presentation** Buff coloured suppositories. Each 2.8 g suppository contains:
Pramoxine Hydrochloride USP 27 mg
Hydrocortisone Acetate PhEur 5 mg
Benzyl Benzoate PhEur 33 mg
Bismuth Oxide 24 mg
Bismuth Subgallate BP 59 mg
Balsam Peru PhEur 49 mg
Zinc Oxide PhEur 296 mg

**Uses** Anugesic HC suppositories provide antiseptic, astringent, emollient and decongestant properties. In addition hydrocortisone exerts an anti-inflammatory effect. Pramoxine is a rapidly acting local anaesthetic.

Anugesic HC Suppositories are indicated for the comprehensive symptomatic treatment of severe and acute discomfort or pain associated with internal haemorrhoids and pruritus ani.

**Dosage and administration**
*Adults:* Remove plastic cover and insert one suppository into the anus at night, in the morning and after each evacuation.
Not to be taken orally.

*Elderly (over 65 years):* As for adults.

*Children:* Not recommended.

**Contra-indications, warnings, etc**

*Contra-indications:* Tubercular, fungal and most viral lesions including herpes simplex, vaccinia and varicella. History of sensitivity to any of the constituents.

*Warnings:* As with all products containing topical steroids the possibility of systemic absorption should be borne in mind.

Prolonged or excessive use may produce systemic corticosteroid effects, and use for periods longer than seven days is not recommended.

*Use in pregnancy:* There is inadequate evidence of safety in human pregnancy and there may be a very small risk of cleft palate and intrauterine growth retardation as well as suppression of the neonatal HPA axis. There is evidence of harmful effects in animals. Use in pregnancy only when there is no safer alternative and when the disease itself carries risks for the mother or child.

*Precautions:* Following symptomatic relief definitive diagnosis should be established.

*Side-effects:* Rarely, sensitivity reactions.
Patients may occasionally experience transient burning on application, especially if the anoderm is not intact.

*Overdosage:* If swallowed, fever, nausea, vomiting, stomach cramps and diarrhoea may develop 3-12 hours after ingestion.

Pramoxine is relatively non-toxic and less sensitising than other local anaesthetics.

Hydrocortisone normally does not produce toxic effects in an acute single overdose.

Treatment of a large acute overdosage should include gastric lavage, purgation with magnesium sulphate and complete bed rest. If necessary, give oxygen and general supportive measures. Methaemoglobinaemia should be treated by intravenous methylene blue.

**Pharmaceutical precautions** Store in a dry place, at a temperature not exceeding 25°C.

**Legal category** POM.

**Package quantities** Box of 12 suppositories.

**Further information** Nil

**Product licence numbers** 0018/0162

# ANUSOL* HC OINTMENT

**Presentation** A buff coloured ointment having a characteristic odour of Balsam Peru. Each 100 mg of ointment contains:
Hydrocortisone Acetate PhEur 0.25 g
Benzyl Benzoate PhEur 1.25 g
Bismuth Subgallate BP 2.25 g
Bismuth Oxide 0.875 g
Balsam Peru PhEur 1.875 g
Zinc Oxide PhEur 10.75 g

**Uses** Anusol-HC Ointment provides antiseptic, astringent, emollient and decongestant properties. In addition hydrocortisone exerts an anti-inflammatory effect.

Indicated for the comprehensive symptomatic treatment of internal and external haemorrhoids and pruritus ani.

**Dosage and administration** Topical

*Adults:* Apply ointment to the affected area at night, in the morning and after each evacuation. Thoroughly cleanse the affected area, dry and apply ointment on a gauze dressing. For internal conditions use rectal nozzle provided and clean it after each use.
Not to be taken orally.

*Elderly (over 65 years):* As for adults.

*Children:* Not recommended.

**Contra-indications, warnings, etc**
*Contra-indications:* Tubercular, fungal and most viral lesions including herpes simplex, vaccinia and varicella. History of sensitivity to any of the constituents.

*Warnings:* As with all products containing topical steroids the possibility of systemic absorption should be borne in mind.

Prolonged or excessive use may produce systemic corticosteroid effects, and use for periods longer than seven days is not recommended.

*Use in pregnancy:* There is inadequate evidence of safety in human pregnancy and there may be a very small risk of cleft palate and intrauterine growth retardation as well as suppression of the neonatal HPA axis. There is evidence of harmful effects in animals. Use in pregnancy only when there is no safer alternative and when the disease itself carries risks for the mother or child.

*Precautions:* Following symptomatic relief, definitive diagnosis should be established.

*Side-effects:* Rarely, sensitivity reactions. Patients may occasionally experience transient burning on application, especially if the anoderm is not intact.

*Overdosage:* If swallowed, fever, nausea, vomiting, stomach cramps and diarrhoea may develop 3-l2 hours after ingestion.

Hydrocortisone normally does not produce toxic effects in an acute single overdose.

Treatment of a large acute overdose should include gastric lavage, purgation with magnesium sulphate and complete bed rest. If necessary give oxygen and general supportive measures. Methaemoglobinaemia should be treated by intravenous methylene blue.

**Pharmaceutical precautions** Store at a temperature not exceeding 25°C.

**Legal category** POM.

**Package quantities** Tubes containing 15, 25 or 30 g

**Further information** Nil

**Product licence number** 0018/0166

# ANUSOL* HC SUPPOSITORIES

**Presentation** Olive green suppositories. Each 2.8 g suppository contains:
Hydrocortisone Acetate PhEur 10 mg
Benzyl Benzoate PhEur 33 mg
Bismuth Subgallate BP 59 mg
Bismuth Oxide 24 mg
Balsam Peru PhEur 49 mg
Zinc Oxide PhEur 296 mg

**Uses** Anusol HC Suppositories provide antiseptic, astringent, emollient and decongestant properties which help to relieve discomforts associated with minor ano-rectal conditions. In addition hydrocortisone exerts an anti-inflammatory effect.

Anusol HC Suppositories are indicated for the symptomatic relief of internal haemorrhoids and pruritus ani.

**Dosage and administration**
*Adults:* Remove wrapper and insert one suppository into the anus at night, in the morning and after each evacuation.
Not to be taken orally.

*Elderly (over 65 years):* As for adults.

*Children:* Not recommended.

**Contra-indications, warnings, etc**
*Contra-indications:* Tubercular, fungal and most viral lesions including herpes simplex, vaccinia and varicella. History of sensitivity to any of the constituents.

*Warnings:* As with all products containing topical steroids the possibility of systemic absorption should be borne in mind.

Prolonged or excessive use may produce systemic corticosteroid effects, and use for periods longer than seven days is not recommended.

*Use in pregnancy:* There is inadequate evidence of safety in human pregnancy and there may be a very small risk of cleft palate and intrauterine growth retardation as well as suppression of the neonatal HPA axis. There is evidence of harmful effects in animals. Use in pregnancy only when there is no safer alternative and when the disease itself carries risks for the mother or child.

*Precautions:* Following symptomatic relief definitive diagnosis should be established.

*Side-effects:* Rarely, sensitivity reactions. Patients may occasionally experience transient burning on application, especially if the anoderm is not intact.

*Overdosage:* If swallowed, fever, nausea, vomiting, stomach cramps and diarrhoea may develop 3-12 hours after ingestion.

Hydrocortisone normally does not produce toxic effects in an acute single overdose. Treatment of a large acute overdose should include gastric lavage, purgation with magnesium sulphate and complete bed rest. If necessary, give oxygen and general supportive measures. Methaemoglobinaemia should be treated by intravenous methylene blue.

**Pharmaceutical precautions** Store at a temperature not exceeding 25°C.

**Legal category** POM.

**Package quantities** Box of 12 suppositories.

**Further information** Nil

**Product licence number** 0018/0167

# CHLOROMYCETIN* SUCCINATE

**Presentation** A plug of freeze-dried sterile powder which when reconstituted with Water for Injection makes a clear solution for injection.

*Composition:* Each 1.2 g vial contains: Chloramphenicol Sodium Succinate BP equivalent to Chloramphenicol PhEur 1.2 g.

Each 300 mg vial contains: Chloramphenicol Sodium Succinate BP equivalent to Chloramphenicol PhEur 300 mg.

**Uses**

*Action:* Chloramphenicol sodium succinate when administered intravenously is hydrolysed to the free antibiotic within the body. Part of the parenterally administered chloramphenicol sodium succinate is excreted by the kidneys prior to hydrolysis and although serum levels of free chloramphenicol are lower than when a comparable dose of chloramphenicol is given orally, they are clinically effective.

Chloramphenicol exerts mainly a bacteriostatic effect on a wide range of gram- positive and gram-negative bacteria including Vibrio cholerae and is also active against rickettsial organisms and, the lympho-granuloma psittacosis group. It is particularly active against Salmonella typhi and Haemophilus influenzae. The mode of action is through interference with or inhibition of protein synthesis in intact cells. Development of resistance to chloramphenicol, both experimentally and in man, appears to be low in contrast to other antibiotics.

The principal route of excretion of chloramphenicol is through the kidneys, total urinary excretion ranging from 68 to over 90 per cent. Small amounts of active drug are found in the bile and faeces. Chloramphenicol diffuses rapidly throughout the tissues and body fluids. Chloramphenicol enters cerebrospinal fluid even in the absence of meningeal inflammation. Measurable levels are also detectable in pleural and ascitic fluids, saliva and in milk. It diffuses readily into the aqueous and vitreous humours of the eye. Transport across the placental barrier occurs with somewhat lower concentration in cord blood than in maternal blood.

*Indications:* Chloramphenicol is a potent therapeutic agent and should not be used for trivial infections. It should be administered according to the instructions of a medical practitioner. It is recommended that chloramphenicol should be reserved for use in typhoid fever, Haemophilus influenzae meningitis, serious chest infections and situations where clinical assessment usually supplemented by laboratory studies indicates that no other antibiotic would suffice.

**Dosage and administration**
*Adults and children over 2 weeks old:* The conventional dosage of chloramphenicol of 50 mg/kg of bodyweight per day in divided doses at six-hour intervals is recommended for the average patient.

In exceptional cases, such as with patients having infections due to moderately resistant organisms or suffering from infections such as septicaemia or meningitis, dosage schedules up to 100 mg/kg/day may be prescribed. However, these high doses should be decreased as soon as clinically indicated. To prevent relapses treatment should be continued after the temperature has returned to normal for 4 days in rickettsial diseases and for 8-10 days in typhoid fever.

Chloramphenicol in the form of chloramphenicol succinate should be administered intravenously in seriously ill patients or under conditions in which the patient is not able to take the drug by mouth. In such instances, it is highly desirable that the physician change to orally administered chloramphenicol as soon as is practicable.

In instances of impaired hepatic or renal function, the ability to metabolise or excrete chloramphenicol may be reduced and the medical practitioner should adjust the dose accordingly.

*Elderly (over 65 years):* As for adults Chloramphenicol has been used successfully at normal dosage in elderly patients. The pattern and incidence of adverse effects does not appear to differ from younger adults.

*Premature and newborn infants and children with immature metabolic processes (see Gray syndrome under Adverse reactions):* 25 mg/kg/day divided into four doses at six-hour intervals usually produces and maintains a concentration of chloramphenicol in blood and tissues adequate to control most infections in premature and new born infants and children with immature metabolic processes. After the first two weeks of life, full term infants ordinarily may receive up to a total of 50 mg/kg/day equally divided into four doses at six-hour intervals. Caution should be used in therapy of premature and full term infants to avoid 'Gray Syndrome' toxicity. Serum levels should be carefully followed during therapy of the newborn infant.

*For administration to young children, infants, and neonates in particular:* Chloromycetin Succinate 300 mg vial is recommended for preparation of the solution. The Chloromycetin Succinate 1.2 g vial is more suitable for preparation of the solution for older children and adults. See above for actual dosage to be given.

*Method of preparation:*

*Chloromycetin 300 mg vial:* Prepare a solution of 25 mg/ml (2.5%) by the addition of 11.75 ml of aqueous diluent. This solution should be injected intravenously over at least a one minute period, the amount administered depending on the bodyweight of the patient.

*Chloromycetin 1.2 g vial:* Prepare a solution of 100 mg/ml (10%) by the addition of 11 ml of aqueous diluent. This solution should be injected intravenously over at least a one minute period, the amount administered depending on the bodyweight of the patient.

Further information is contained in the package insert which should be consulted before preparation and administration.

### Contra-indications, warnings, etc

*Contra-indications:* Chloramphenicol succinate is contra-indicated in persons with a history of previous hypersensitivity and/or toxic reaction to the drug. Lactation.

*Use in pregnancy and lactation:* Chloramphenicol succinate readily crosses the placental barrier. Chloramphenicol succinate should not be administered intravenously during labour and should be used with caution during pregnancy and at term because of the potential toxic effects on the foetus (Gray Syndrome). Chloramphenicol should not be used during pregnancy unless considered essential by the physician.

Chloramphenicol is excreted in breast milk and therefore mothers taking this drug should not breast-feed their infant.

*Warnings and precautions:* Blood dyscrasias including aplastic anaemia may be associated with the administration of chloramphenicol succinate. In addition, there have been reports of aplastic anaemia attributed to chloramphenicol which later resulted in leukaemia. Blood dyscrasias have occured after both short-term and prolonged therapy with this drug. If facilities are available, it is advisable to determine the routine blood profile before therapy, and blood studies should be repeated at appropriate intervals especially during prolonged or intermittent therapy. However, it should be noted that such determinations do not exclude the possible later appearance of the irreversible type of bone marrow depression. The intervals at which such studies should be performed depends on the circumstances of each individual case.

Consideration should be given to discontinuing the drug if evidence of depression of any of the blood elements appears attributable to chloramphenicol, after weighing these effects against the seriousness and course of the disease under treatment. Repeated courses of chloramphenicol succinate and concurrent therapy with other drugs known to cause bone marrow depression or even aplastic anaemia should be avoided. Chloramphenicol succinate should be administered according to the direction of a medical practitioner, and it should not be used for the treatment of trivial infections, because of the potential for these adverse effects.

As with other antibiotics, the use of chloramphenicol succinate may result in an overgrowth of non-susceptible organisms including fungi. Where this occurs, appropriate steps should be taken.

In patients with impaired liver or kidney function, including those with immature metabolic processes such as premature and full term infants, excessive blood levels may result from administration of the normal recommended dose. Dosage should be adjusted accordingly.

*Drug interactions:* Chloramphenicol has been shown to retard the biotransformation of warfarin, tolbutamide and phenytoin.

The metabolism of chloramphenicol is enhanced by phenobarbitone and rifampacin and the half life of chloramphenicol is considerably prolonged in patients receiving paracetamol (acetaminophen). Concurrent administration of these drugs should be avoided.

*Side effects:*

*Haematological reactions:* Blood dyscrasias including aplastic anaemia have been attributed to the administration of chloramphenicol. Two types of bone marrow depression have been observed.

One type may occur during therapy, is reversible on cessation of treatment and is dose related.

The second type which may occur weeks to months after therapy is rare, it may be genetically related, and is not dose related. In more than half of the cases it is irreversible. It may lead to aplastic anaemia which may be fatal. The reported incidence of aplastic anaemia varies throughout the world.

Hypoplastic anaemia, thrombocytopenia and agranulocytosis have all been described following administration of chloramphenicol.

Paroxysmal nocturnal haemoglobinuria has also been reported.

*Gastro-intestinal reactions:* Nausea, vomiting, glossitis and stomatitis, diarrhoea and enterocolitis may occur; the incidence is low.

*Neurological reactions:* Optic and peripheral neuritis have been reported usually following long-term dosage.

*Hypersensitivity reaction:* Sensitivity reactions are sometimes encountered.

*Gray syndrome:* Toxic reactions including fatalities have occurred in the premature and newborn infant, the signs and symptoms associated with these reactions are known as the 'Gray Syndrome'. Single reports have appeared in an infant as old as three months, and in an infant born of a mother receiving chloramphenicol intravenously during labour. The following points summarise the studies of the 'Gray Syndrome'.

1. In most instances therapy has been instituted within the first 48 hours of life.

2. Symptoms first appeared after 3 to 4 days of continued treatment with conventional adult dosage of chloramphenicol not tolerated by and incorrect for this age group.

3. The symptoms appeared in the following order:
   (a) Abdominal distension with or without vomiting.
   (b) Progressive pallid cyanosis.
   (c) Vasomotor collapse, frequently accompanied by irregular respiration.
   (d) Death within a few hours of onset of symptoms.

4. Progression of symptoms from onset to exitus were accelerated with higher dosage schedules.

5. In some cases upon early recognition of the associated symptomatology, termination of therapy frequently reversed the process with complete recovery.

*Treatment of overdosage:* Levels exceeding 25 mg/L are frequently considered toxic. In the case of serious overdosage, charcoal haemoperfusion may be effective in removing chloramphenicol from plasma. Exchange tranfusion is of questionable value following massive overdosage especially in neonates and infants. General supportive therapy should be undertaken to prevent cardiovascular collapse.

**Pharmaceutical precautions** Protect from light. Store at a temperature not exceeding 30°C.

To reduce the risk of microbial and particulate contamination the reconstituted solution should be used on one occasion only, immediately after preparation.

**Legal category** POM.

**Package quantities** Vials of 1.2 g and 300 mg.

**Further information** Chloramphenicol sodium succinate is generally compatible with infusion fluids when the pH range is 5.5 to 7.0. For further information contact the manufacturer.

**Product licence numbers**
Chloromycetin Succinate 1.2 g 0018/5078
Chloromycetin Succinate 300 mg 0018/5077

## CHOLEDYL*

**Presentation** An amber coloured, chocolate flavoured, clear syrup. Each 5 ml spoonful contains Choline Theophyllinate BP 62.5 mg.

**Uses** For the relief and prophylaxis of bronchospasm in chronic bronchitis and asthma.

**Dosage and administration** Oral administration

*Children (3 to 6 years):* One to two 5 ml spoonfuls three times daily. Use in children at more than six hourly intervals.

### Contra-indications, warnings, etc

*Contra-indications:* Use in patients with a known hypersensitivity to the xanthine group of drugs.

*Precautions and warnings:* Caution should be exercised in patients suffering from cardiac or liver disease as such individuals may show marked reductions in theophylline clearance, with consequent high serum levels at normal therapeutic doses. Great caution should especially be used in patients with congestive heart failure. It is particularly important that careful serum level monitoring is carried out in these patients and doses of choline theophyllinate adjusted accordingly. Half life may be prolonged in patients with chronic obstructive airways disease or cor pulmonale and in neonates. Care should be taken in its use in patients suffering from insomnia.

Xanthines can potentiate hypokalaemia resulting from beta$_2$ agonist therapy, steroids, diuretics and hypoxia. Particular caution is advised in severe asthma. It is recommended that serum potassium levels are monitored in such situations.

Theophylline clearance may be decreased in patients receiving trioleandomycin, erythromycin, cimetidine, high-dose allopurinol, propranolol, oral contraceptives, or influenza vaccine. Plasma concentrations of theophylline may be reduced when aminoglutethimide, carbamazepine, phenytoin, rifampicin and sulphinpyrazone are administered concurrently.

Smoking increases theophylline metabolism and this effect persists for 3–24 months after cessation of smoking. Care should be taken in its concomitant use with beta-adrenergic agonists, glucagon and the other xanthine drugs as these will potentiate the effect of theophylline. The incidence of toxic effects may be enhanced by the concomitant use of ephedrine. Choledyl syrup contains invert sugar syrup (3.7 ml/5 ml) and due care should be taken where it is prescribed for patients with diabetes mellitus.

*Use in pregnancy and lactation:* There is no conclusive evidence of safety in pregnancy, but choline theophyllinate has been widely used for many years and only one case of irritability and apnoea has been reported in a newborn infant exposed to theophylline during the third trimester of pregnancy. In view of this it is recommended that Choledyl should only be administered during the last trimester of pregnancy if no safer alternative is available. Methylxanthines are excreted in breast milk and irritability has been reported in breast-fed infants. It is therefore recommended that mothers taking choledyl should not breast feed.

*Side-effects:* Gastro-intestinal upsets, palpitations and CNS stimulation may occur occasionally.

*Overdosage:* Characterised by nausea, vomiting, gastro-intestinal irritation, hypokalaemia, unusual thirst, CNS stimulation including convulsions in severe cases, tachycardia, arrhythmias, fall in B.P. and collapse.

*Treatment:* Gastric lavage. For fall in blood pressure nurse in head-down position and treat with fluid replacement if necessary. Use general supportive measures and treat symptoms accordingly. Diazepam i.v. may be given to control convulsions. Charcoal haemoperfusion can be considered in severely intoxicated patients. Supportive treatment is indicated for hypokalaemia.

**Pharmaceutical precautions** Choledyl syrup should be stored in a dry place at a temperature not exceeding 25°C, and protected from light.

**Legal category** P

**Package quantities** Bottles containing 200 ml.

**Further information** Nil

**Product licence number** 0018/0169

## DICLOMAX RETARD*
## DICLOMAX SR*

**Qualitative and quantitative composition** Diclomax Retard is supplied in opaque white capsules containing 100 mg Diclofenac Sodium in a modified release formulation.

Diclomax SR is supplied in opaque yellow capsules containing 75 mg Diclofenac Sodium in a modified release formulation.

**Pharmaceutical form** Modified release capsules for oral use.

**Clinical particulars**

*Therapeutic indications:* Diclomax SR and Diclomax Retard are indicated for rheumatoid arthritis; osteoarthritis; low back pain; acute musculo-skeletal disorders and trauma such as periarthritis (especially frozen shoulder), tendinitis, tenosynovitis, bursitis, sprains, strains and dislocations; relief of pain in fractures; ankylosing spondylitis; acute gout; control in pain and inflammation in orthopaedic, dental and other minor surgery.

*Posology and method of administration:* For oral administration.

*Adults:* Diclomax Retard: One 100 mg capsule taken whole daily, preferably with food or after food.

Diclomax SR: One or two 75 mg capsules daily taken whole in single or divided doses preferably with or after food.

*Elderly:* Studies indicate the pharmacokinetics of diclofenac sodium are not impaired to any clinical extent in the elderly, however, as with all non-steroidal anti-inflammatory drugs, Diclomax should be used with caution in elderly patients and the lowest effective dose used. (See also precautions.)

*Children:* Not recommended.

*Contra-indications:* Diclomax is contra-indicated in patients with a known sensitivity to diclofenac sodium, patients with active peptic ulcer or gastrointestinal bleeding, asthmatic patients in whom attacks of asthma, urticaria or acute rhinitis are precipitated by aspirin or other non-steroidal anti-inflammatory agents.

*Special warnings and special precautions for use:* As with all non-steroidal anti-inflammatory drugs (NSAIDs) Diclomax should only be given to the elderly and to patients with a history of peptic ulcer after other forms of treatment have been carefully considered.

NSAIDs in general, have been reported to cause nephrotoxicity, interstitial nephritis, nephrotic syndrome and renal failure. In patients with renal, cardiac or hepatic impairment caution is required since the use of NSAIDs may result in deterioration of renal function. The dose should be kept as low as possible and renal function should be monitored in these patients.

Diclomax should be used with caution in patients with gastro-intestinal ulceration, haematemesis or melaena, ulcerative colitis, Crohn's disease, bleeding diathesis or haematological abnormalities.

Patients with severe hepatic, cardiac or renal insufficiency or the elderly should be kept under close surveillance.

All patients who are receiving long-term treatment with non-steroidal anti-inflammatory agents should be monitored as a precautionary measure, eg. renal, hepatic function (elevation of liver enzymes may occur) and blood counts.

If abnormal liver function tests persist or worsen, clinical signs or symptoms consistent with liver disease develop or if other manisfestations occur (eosinophilia, rash), Diclomax should be discontinued.

Use of Diclomax in patients with hepatic porpyhria may trigger an attack.

The importance of prostaglandins in maintaining renal blood flow should be taken into account in patients with impaired cardiac or renal function, those being treated with diuretics or recovering from major surgery. Effects on renal function are usually reversible on withdrawal of Diclomax.

Diclomax in common with other NSAIDs, can reversibly inhibit platelet aggregation.

*Interactions with other medicaments and other forms of interaction:* Drug interactions: Diclomax may increase plasma concentrations of lithium and digoxin.

Clinical investigations do not appear to indicate that Diclomax affects the activity of anticoagulants but there have been isolated reports of an increased risk of haemorrhage with the combined use of these agents. Close monitoring is therefore recommended. Clinical studies have shown that Diclomax can be given together with oral antidiabetic agents without influencing their clinical effect. However there have been isolated reports of hyperglycaemic effects which have required adjustments to the dosage of hypoglycaemic agents.

Cyclosporin nephrotoxicity may be increased by the effect of non-steroidal anti-inflammatory drugs on renal prostaglandins.

Caution should be exercised if NSAIDs and methotrexate are administered within 24 hours of each other, since NSAIDs may increase methotrexate plasma levels, resulting in increased toxicity.

Concomitant therapy with other systemic NSAIDs may increase the frequency of side-effects.

Various NSAIDs are liable to inhibit the activity of diuretics. Concomitant treatment with potassium-sparing diuretics may be associated with increased serum potassium levels, hence serum potassium should be monitored.

*Pregnancy and lactation:* Diclofenac sodium should not be prescribed during pregnancy unless the benefits outweigh the risk. Use of Diclomax in the last trimester of pregnancy is not recommended as regular use of NSAIDs may result in closure of the fetal ductus arteriosus in utero and possibly persistant pulmonary hypertension of the newborn, delay onset and increase duration of labour.

Traces of diclofenac sodium have been found in breast milk following oral doses of 50 mg every 8 hours.

*Effects on ability to drive or use machines:* None reported.

*Undesirable effects:* There have been occasional reports of epigastric pain, other gastrointestinal disorders, headache, dizziness, vertigo, rashes or skin eruptions and elevation of serum aminotransferase enzymes (SGOT, SGPT). Rare reports of gastrointestinal bleeding, peptic ulcer, bloody diarrhoea, drowsiness, tiredness, urticaria, liver function disorders including hepatitis with or without jaundice, oedema and hypersensitivity reactions have been reported.

*Overdose:* Symptomatology of overdose with diclofenac sodium is not well documented. The management of NSAID overdose should be supportive and the treatment symptomatic.

Should a patient ingest a large amount of Diclomax the stomach may be emptied, treatment with charcoal may reduce absorption. Haemodialysis is unlikely to decrease plasma protein concentration due to the high degree of protein binding.

**Pharmacological properties**

*Pharmacodynamic properties:* Diclofenac Sodium is a non-steroidal agent with marked analgesic/anti-inflammatory and anti-pyretic properties. It is an inhibitor of prostaglandin synthetase (cyclo-oxygenase).

*Pharmacokinetic properties:* Diclofenac Sodium is rapidly absorbed from the gut and is subject to first-pass metabolism. Capsules give peak plasma concentrations after approximately 2.5 hours. The active substance is 99.7% protein bound and plasma half-life for the terminal elimination phase is 1-2 hours. Approximately 60% of the administered dose is excreted via the kidneys in the form of metabolites and less than 1% in unchanged form. About 30% of the dose is excreted via the bile in metabolised form. The Diclomax modified release preparations:

(i) increase the duration of action of the drug,

(ii) maintain a relatively constant rate of absorption in the gastointestinal tract over a longer period of time,

(iii) increase the fraction of the ingested dose absorbed in the G.I. tract,

(iv) regulate the rate at which the drug is made available for absorption, thereby reducing the possibility of malabsorption and occurrence of side-effects.

**Pharmaceutical particulars**

*List of excipients:* Diclomax Retard capsules contain the following excipients: Sucrose PhEur, Maize Starch PhEur, purified stearic acid NF, polyethylene glycol 6000 NF, Ammonio methacrylate copolymer type A NF, Talc PhEur, Lactose PhEur and Polysorbate 80 PhEur.

Diclomax SR capsules contain the following excipients: Sucrose PhEur, Maize Starch PhEur, purified stearic acid NF, polyethylene glycol 6000 NF, ammonio methacrylate copolymer type A NF, Talc PhEur, Lactose PhEur, Polysorbate 80 PhEur, Gelatin PhEur, Titanium Dioxide (E171) PhEur, iron oxide yellow (E172), opacode S-1-8100HV Black 1007 HSE.

*Incompatibilities:* None known.

*Shelf life:* Diclomax Retard: Two years. Diclomax SR: 18 months.

*Special precautions for storage:* Diclomax SR: Protect from moisture and heat. Store below 25°C. Diclomax Retard: Protect from moisture. Store below 25°C.

*Nature and contents of container:* Diclomax Retard: Hard aluminium/PVC blister packs of 28 (OP).

Diclomax SR: White opaque PVC blister packs of 56 (OP) with hard tempered aluminium foil.

*Instructions for use/handling:* None.

*Marketing authorisation holder:* Parke, Davis & Company, Usk Road, Pontypool, NP4 0YH.

**Marketing authorisation numbers**
Diclomax Retard 0018/0208
Diclomax SR 0018/0228

**Date of approval/revision of SPC** Diclomax SR: September 1996. Diclomax Retard: June 1997

**Legal category** POM

## EPANUTIN* CAPSULES 25 mg, 50 mg and 100 mg

**Qualitative and quantitative composition** Epanutin Capsules containing 25 mg, 50 mg or 100 mg Phenytoin Sodium PhEur.

**Pharmaceutical form** *Epanutin Capsules 25 mg:* A white powder in a No 4 hard gelatin capsule with a white opaque body and purple cap, radially printed 'EPANUTIN 25'.

*Epanutin Capsules 50 mg:* A white powder in a No 4 hard gelatin capsule with a white opaque body and a pale pink opaque cap, radially printed 'EPANUTIN 50'.

*Epanutin Capsules 100 mg:* A white powder in a No 3 hard gelatin capsule with a white opaque body and orange cap, radially printed 'EPANUTIN 100'.

**Clinical particulars** *Therapeutic indications:* Control of tonic-clonic seizures (grand mal epilepsy), partial seizures (focal epilepsy including temporal lobe epilepsy) or a combination of these and the prevention and treatment of seizures occurring during or following neurosurgery and/or severe head injury. Epanutin has also been employed in the treatment of trigeminal neuralgia but it should only be used as second line therapy if carbamazepine is ineffective or patients are intolerant to carbamazepine.

*Posology and method of administration:* For oral administration only.

Dosage should be individualised as there may be wide interpatient variability in phenytoin serum levels with equivalent dosage. Epanutin should be introduced in small dosages with gradual increments until control is achieved or until toxic effects appear. In some cases serum level determinations may be necessary for optimal dosage adjustments–the clinically effective level is usually 10–20 mg/l (40–80 micromoles/l) although some cases of tonic-clonic seizures may be controlled with lower serum levels of phenytoin. With recommended dosage a period of seven to ten days may be required to achieve steady state serum levels with Epanutin and changes in dosage should not be carried out at intervals shorter than seven to ten days.

Maintenance of treatment should be the lowest dose of anticonvulsant consistent with control of seizures.

*Epanutin Capsules, Suspension and Infatabs:* Epanutin Capsules contain phenytoin sodium whereas Epanutin Suspension and Epanutin Infatabs contain phenytoin. Although 100 mg of phenytoin sodium is equivalent to 92 mg of phenytoin on a molecular weight basis, these molecular equivalents are not necessarily biologically equivalent. Physicians should therefore exercise care in those situations where it is necessary to change the dosage form and serum level monitoring is advised.

*Adults:* Initially 3 to 4 mg/kg/day with subsequent dosage adjustment if necessary. For most adults a satisfactory maintenance dose will be 200 to 500 mg daily in single or divided doses. Exceptionally, a daily dose outside this range may be indicated. Dosage should normally be adjusted according to serum levels where assay facilities exist.

*Elderly (over 65 years):* As with adults the dosage of Epanutin should be titrated to the patient's individual requirements using the same guidelines.

As elderly patients tend to receive multiple drug therapies, the possibility of drug interactions should be borne in mind.

*Infants and children:* Initially, 5 mg/kg/day in two divided doses, with subsequent dosage individualised to a maximum of 300 mg daily. A recommended daily maintenance dosage is usually 4-8 mg/kg.

Epanutin Infatabs may be chewed.

*Neonates:* The absorption of phenytoin following oral administration in neonates is unpredictable. Furthermore, the metabolism of phenytoin may be depressed. It is therefore especially important to monitor serum levels in the neonate.

*Contra-indications:* Hypersensitivity to hydantoins.

*Special warnings and special precautions for use:* Abrupt withdrawal of phenytoin in epileptic patients may precipitate status epilepticus. When, in the judgement of the clinician, the need for dosage reduction, discontinuation, or substitution of alternative anti-epileptic medication arises, this should be done gradually. However, in the event of an allergic or hypersensitivity reaction, rapid substitution of alternative therapy may be necessary. In this case, alternative therapy should be an anti-epileptic drug not belonging to the hydantoin chemical class.

Phenytoin is highly protein bound and extensively metabolised by the liver. Reduced dosage to prevent accumulation and toxicity may therefore be required in patients with impaired liver function. Where protein binding is reduced, as in uraemia, total serum phenytoin levels will be reduced accordingly. However, the pharmacologically active free drug concentration is unlikely to be altered. Therefore, under these circumstances therapeutic control may be achieved with total phenytoin levels below the normal range of 10–20 mg/l (40–80 micromoles/l). Patients with impaired liver function, elderly patients or those who are gravely ill may show early signs of toxicity.

Phenytoin should be discontinued if a skin rash appears. If the rash is exfoliative, purpuric, or bullous or if lupus erythematosus or Stevens-Johnson syndrome or toxic epidermal necrolysis is suspected, use of the drug should not be resumed (see *Adverse reactions*). If the rash is of a milder type (measles-like or scarlatiniform), therapy may be resumed after the rash has completely disappeared. If the rash recurs upon reinstitution of therapy, further phenytoin medication is contraindicated.

Phenytoin is not effective for absence (petit mal) seizures. If tonic-clonic (grand mal) and absence seizures are present together, combined drug therapy is needed.

Phenytoin may affect glucose metabolism and inhibit insulin release. Hyperglycaemia has been reported in association with toxic levels. Phenytoin is not indicated for seizures due to hypoglycaemia or other metabolic causes.

Serum levels of phenytoin sustained above the optimal range may produce confusional states referred to as 'delirium,' 'psychosis,' or 'encephalopathy,' or rarely irreversible cerebellar dysfunction. Accordingly, at the first sign of acute toxicity, serum drug level determinations are recommended. Dose reduction of phenytoin therapy is indicated if serum levels are excessive; if symptoms persist, termination of therapy with phenytoin is recommended.

Phenytoin therapy may interfere with Vitamin D metabolism. In the absence of an adequate dietary intake of Vitamin D or exposure to sunlight, osteomalacia, hypocalcemia or rickets may develop.

In view of isolated reports associating phenytoin with exacerbation of porphyria, caution should be exercised in using the medication in patients suffering from this disease.

*Interactions with other medicaments and other forms of interaction:* 1. Drugs which may *increase* phenytoin serum levels include: Amiodarone, antifungal agents, (such as, but not limited to, amphotericin B, fluconazole, ketoconazole, miconazole and itraconazole), chloramphenicol, chlordiazepoxide, diazepam, dicoumarol, disulfiram, H2-antagonists, halothane, isoniazid, methylphenidate, omeprazole, oestrogens, phenothiazines, phenylbutazone, salicylates, succinimides, sulphonamides, tolbutamide, trazodone and viloxazine.

2. Drugs which may *decrease* phenytoin serum levels include: carbamazepine, folic acid, reserpine, sucralfate and vigabatrin.

3. Drugs which may either *increase* or *decrease* phenytoin serum levels include: Phenobarbitone, valproic acid, sodium valproate, antineoplastic agents and certain antacids. Similarly, the effect of phenytoin on phenobarbitone and valproic acid and sodium valproate serum levels is unpredictable.

Acute alcohol intake may increase phenytoin serum levels while chronic alcoholism may decrease serum levels.

4. Although not a true pharmacokinetic interaction, tricylic antidepressants and phenothiazines may precipitate seizures in susceptible patients and phenytoin dosage may need to be adjusted.

5. Drugs whose effect is *impaired* by phenytoin include: antifungal agents, antineoplastic agents, clozapine, corticosteroids, dicoumarol, digitoxin, doxycycline, frusemide, oestrogens, oral contraceptives, quinidine, rifampicin, theophylline and vitamin D.

6. Drugs whose effect is *altered* by phenytoin include: warfarin. The effect of phenytoin on warfarin is variable and prothrombin times should be determined when these agents are combined.

Serum level determinations are especially helpful when possible drug interactions are suspected.

*Drug/laboratory test interactions:* Phenytoin may cause a slight decrease in serum levels of total and free thyroxine, possibly as a result of enhanced peripheral metabolism. These changes do not lead to clinical hypothyroidism and do not affect the levels of circulating TSH. The latter can therefore be used for diagnosing hypothyroidism in the patient on phenytoin. Phenytoin does not interfere with uptake and suppression tests used in the diagnosis of hypothyroidism. It may, however, produce lower than normal values for dexamethasone or metapyrone tests. Phenytoin may cause raised serum levels of glucose, alkaline phosphatase, and gamma glutamyl transpeptidase and lowered serum levels of calcium and folic acid. It is recommended that serum folate concentrations be measured at least once every 6 months, and folic acid supplements given if necessary. Phenytoin may affect blood sugar metabolism tests.

*Pregnancy and lactation:* There are intrinsic methodologic problems in obtaining adequate data on drug teratogenicity in humans. Genetic factors or the epileptic condition itself may be more important than drug therapy in leading to birth defects. The great majority of mothers on anticonvulsant medication deliver normal infants. It is important to note that anticonvulsant drugs should not be discontinued in patients in whom the drug is administered to prevent major seizures because of the strong possibility of precipitating status epilepticus with attendant hypoxia and threat to life. In individual cases where the severity and frequency of the seizure disorder are such that the removal of medication does not pose a serious threat to the patient, discontinuation of the drug may be considered prior to and during pregnancy although it cannot be said with any confidence that even minor seizures do not pose some hazard to the developing embryo or foetus.

Anticonvulsants including phenytoin may produce congenital abnormalities in the offspring of a small number of epileptic patients. The exact role of drug therapy in these abnormalities is unclear and genetic factors, in some studies, have also been shown to be important. Epanutin should only be used during pregnancy, especially early pregnancy, if in the judgement of the physician the potential benefits clearly outweigh the risk.

In addition to the reports of increased incidence of congenital malformations, such as cleft lip/palate and heart malformations in children of women receiving phenytoin and other antiepileptic drugs, there have more recently been reports of a foetal hydantoin syndrome. This consists of prenatal growth deficiency, micro-encephaly and mental deficiency in children born to mothers who have received phenytoin, barbiturates, alcohol or trimethadione. However, these features are all interrelated and are frequently associated with intrauterine growth retardation from other causes.

There have been isolated reports of malignancies, including neuroblastoma, in children whose mothers received phenytoin during pregnancy.

An increase in seizure frequency during pregnancy occurs in a proportion of patients, and this may be due to altered phenytoin absorption or metabolism. Periodic measurement of serum phenytoin levels is particularly valuable in the management of a pregnant epileptic patient as a guide to an appropriate adjustment of dosage. However, postpartum restoration of the original dosage will probably be indicated.

Neonatal coagulation defects have been reported within the first 24 hours in babies born to epileptic mothers receiving phenytoin. Vitamin K1 has been shown to prevent or correct this defect and may be given to the mother before delivery and to the neonate after birth.

Infant breast feeding is not recommended for women taking phenytoin because phenytoin appears to be secreted in low concentrations in human milk.

*Effects on ability to drive or use machines:* None known

*Undesirable effects:*
*Central nervous system:* The most common manifestations encountered with phenytoin therapy are referable to this system and are usually dose-related. These include nystagmus, ataxia, slurred speech, decreased coordination, mental confusion, paraesthesia, drowsiness and vertigo. Dizziness, insomnia, transient nervousness, motor twitchings, and headaches have also been observed. There have also been rare reports of phenytoin induced dyskinesias, including chorea, dystonia, tremor and asterixis, similar to those induced by phenothiazine and other neuroleptic drugs. There are occasional reports of irreversible cerebellar dysfunction associated with severe phenytoin overdosage. Peripheral neuropathy has been reported on rare occasions.

*Gastrointestinal:* Nausea, vomiting and constipation, toxic hepatitis, and liver damage.

*Dermatological:* Dermatological manifestations sometimes accompanied by fever have included scarlatiniform or morbilliform rashes. A morbilliform rash is the most common; dermatitis is seen more rarely. Other more serious and rare forms have included bullous, exfoliative or purpuric dermatitis, lupus erythematosus, Stevens-Johnson syndrome and toxic epidermal necrolysis (see *Special precautions and special warnings for use*).

*Connective tissue:* Coarsening of the facial features, enlargement of the lips, gingival hyperplasia, hirsutism, hypertrichosis, Peyronie's Disease and Dupuytren's contracture may occur rarely.

*Haemopoietic:* Haemopoietic complications, some fatal, have occasionally been reported in association with administration of phenytoin. These have included thrombocytopenia, leucopenia, granulocytopenia, agranulocytosis, pancytopenia with or without bone marrow suppression and aplastic anaemia. While macrocytosis and megaloblastic anaemia have occurred, these conditions usually respond to folic acid therapy.

There have been a number of reports suggesting a relationship between phenytoin and the development of lymphadenopathy (local and generalised) including benign lymph node hyperplasia, pseudolymphoma, lymphoma, and Hodgkin's Disease. Although a cause and effect relationship has not been established, the occurrence of lymphadenopathy indicates the need to differentiate such a condition from other types of lymph node pathology. Lymph node involvement may occur with or without symptoms and signs resembling serum sickness, eg fever, rash and liver involvement. In all cases of lymphadenopathy, follow-up observation for an extended period is indicated and every effort should be made to achieve seizure control using alternative antiepileptic drugs.

Frequent blood counts should be carried out during treatment with phenytoin.

*Immune system:* Hypersensitivity syndrome has been reported and may in rare cases be fatal (the syndrome may include, but is not limited to, symptoms such as arthralgias, eosinophilia, fever, liver dysfunction, lymphadenopathy or rash), systemic lupus erythematosus, polyarteritis nodosa, and immunoglobulin abnormalities may occur. Several individual case reports have suggested that there may be an increased, although still rare, incidence of hypersensitivity reactions, including skin rash and hepatotoxicity, in black patients.

*Other:* Polyarthropathy, interstitial nephritis, pneumonitis

*Overdose:* The lethal dose in children is not known. The mean lethal dose for adults is estimated to be 2 to 5 g. The initial symptoms are nystagmus, ataxia and dysarthria. The patient then becomes comatose, the pupils are unresponsive and hypotension occurs followed by respiratory depression and apnoea. Death is due to respiratory and circulatory depression.

There are marked variations among individuals with respect to phenytoin serum levels where toxicity may occur. Nystagmus on lateral gaze usually appears at 20 mg/l, and ataxia at 30 mg/l, dysarthria and lethargy appear when the serum concentration is greater than 40 mg/l, but a concentration as high as 50 mg/l has been reported without evidence of toxicity.

As much as 25 times therapeutic dose has been taken to result in serum concentration over 100 mg/l (400 micromoles/l) with complete recovery.

*Treatment:* Treatment is non-specific since there is no known antidote. If ingested within the previous 4 hours the stomach should be emptied. If the gag reflex is absent, the airway should be supported. Oxygen and assisted ventilation may be necessary for central nervous system, respiratory and cardiovascular depression. Haemodialysis can be considered since phenytoin is not completely bound to plasma proteins. Total exchange transfusion has been utilised in the treatment of severe intoxication in children.

**Pharmacological properties.**

*Pharmacodynamic properties:* Phenytoin is effective in various animal models of generalised convulsive disorders, reasonably effective in models of partial seizures but relatively ineffective in models of myoclonic seizures. It appears to stabilise rather than raise the seizure threshold and prevents spread of seizure activity rather than abolish the primary focus of seizure discharge. The mechanism by which phenytoin exerts its anticonvulsant action has not been fully elucidated however, possible contributory effects include: 1. Non-synaptic effects to reduce sodium conductance, enhance active sodium extrusion, block repetitive firing and reduce post-titanic potentiation. 2. Post-synaptic action to enhance gaba-mediated inhibition and reduce excitatory synaptic transmission. 3. Pre-synaptic actions to reduce calcium entry and block release of neurotransmitter.

*Pharmacokinetic properties:* Phenytoin is absorbed from the samll intestine after oral administration. Various formulation factors may affect the bioavailability of phenytoin, however, non-linear techniques have estimated absorption to be essentially complete. After absorption it is distributed into body fluids, including CSF. Its volume of distribution has been estimated to be between 0.52 and 1.19 litres/kg, and it is highly protein bound (usually 90% in adults). The plasma half-life of phenytoin in man averages 22 hours with a range of 7 to 42 hours. Steady state therapeutic drug levels are achieved at least 7 to 10 days after initiation of therapy. Phenytoin is hydroxylated in the liver by an enzyme system which is saturable. Small incremental doses may produce very substantial increases in serum levels when these are in the upper range of therapeutic concentrations. The parameters controlling elimination are also subject to wide interpatient variation. The serum level is achieved by a given dose is therefore also subject to wide variation.

*Preclinical safety data:* Pre-clinical safety data does not add anything of further significance to the prescriber.

**Pharmaceutical particulars**

*List of excipients: Epanutin Capsules 25 mg:* Each capsule contains lactose and magnesium stearate. The gelatin capsule shell also contains E127 (erythrosine), E131 (patent blue V) and E171 (titanium dioxide). *Epanutin Capsules 50 mg:* Each capsule contains lactose and magnesium stearate. The gelatin capsule shell also contains E127 (erythrosine), E104 (quinoline yellow) and E171 (titanium dioxide). *Epanutin Capsules 100 mg:* Each capsule contains lactose and magnesium stearate. The gelatin capsule shell also contains E127 (erythrosine), E104 (quinoline yellow) and E171 (titanium dioxide).

*Incompatibilities:* None known.

*Shelf life:* White HDPE container with white LDPE cap: 3 years.

*Special precautions for storage:* Store at a temperature not exceeding 30°C.

*Nature and contents of container:* White HDPE Bottle with white LDPE cap containing 500 capsules.

*Instructions for use/handling:* No special requirements.

*Marketing authorisation holder:* Parke, Davis & Company, Usk Road, Pontypool, NP4 0YH.

**Marketing authorisation numbers**
Epanutin Capsules 25 mg 0018/0112
Epanutin Capsules 50 mg 0018/5079
Epanutin Capsules 100 mg 0018/5080

**Date of approval/revision of SPC** April 1997

**Legal category** POM

## EPANUTIN* CAPSULES 300 mg, SUSPENSION AND INFATABS

**Presentation** *Epanutin Capsules 300 mg:* A white powder in a No 1 hard gelatin capsule with a white opaque body and dark green cap radially imprinted 'EPANUTIN 300'

*Epanutin Suspension:* Cherry red suspension.

*Epanutin Infatabs:* A yellow triangular flat chewable tablet with a breaking line on one side and with a spearmint flavour.

*Composition:* Epanutin Capsules 300 mg: Each Epanutin Capsule 300 mg contains 300 mg phenytoin sodium PhEur.

Epanutin Suspension (Phenytoin Mixture BP). Each 5 ml of Epauntin Suspension contains 30 mg phenytoin BP .

Epanutin Infatabs. Each Epauntin Infatab contains 50 mg Phenytoin BP.

**Uses**
*Pharmacology:* Anticonvulsant which appears to stabilise rather than raise the seizure threshold and prevent spread of seizure activity rather than abolish the primary focus of seizure discharge.

A small percentage of individuals who have been treated with phenytoin have been shown to metabolise the drug more slowly than normal and this appears to be genetically determined.

The plasma half-life of phenytoin in man averages 22 hours with a range of 7 to 42 hours. Steady state therapeutic drug levels are achieved at least 7 to 10 days after initiation of therapy.

Phenytoin is hydroxylated in the liver by an enzyme system which is saturable. Small incremental doses may produce very substantial increases in serum levels when these are in the upper range of therapeutic concentrations.

*Indications:* Control of tonic-clonic seizures (grand mal epilepsy), partial seizures (focal epilepsy including temporal lobe epilepsy) or a combination of these and the prevention and treatment of seizures occurring during or following neurosurgery and/or severe head injury. Epanutin has also been employed in the treatment of trigeminal neuralgia but it should only be used as second line therapy if carbamazepine is ineffective or patients are intolerant to carbamazepine.

**Dosage and administration** Dosage should be individualised as there may be wide interpatient variability in phenytoin serum levels with equivalent dosage. Epanutin should be introduced in small dosages with gradual increments until control is achieved or until toxic effects appear. In some cases serum level determinations may be necessary for optimal dosage adjustments – the clinically effective level is usually 10–20 mg/l (40–80 micromoles/l) although some cases of tonic-clonic seizures may be controlled with lower serum levels of phenytoin. With recommended dosage a period of seven to ten days may be required to achieve steady state serum levels with Epanutin and changes in dosage should not be carried out at intervals shorter than seven to ten days.

Maintenance of treatment should be the lowest dose of anticonvulsant consistent with control of seizures.

*Epanutin Capsules, Suspension and Infatabs:* Epanutin Capsules contain phenytoin sodium whereas Epanutin Suspension and Epanutin Infatabs contain phenytoin. Although 100 mg of phenytoin sodium is equivalent to 92 mg of phenytoin on a molecular weight basis, these molecular equivalents are not necessarily biologically equivalent. Physicians should therefore exercise care in those situations where it is necessary to change the dosage form and serum level monitoring is advised.

*Adults:* Initially 3 to 4 mg/kg/day with subsequent dosage adjustment if necessary. For most adults a satisfactory maintenance dose will be 200 to 500 mg daily in single or divided doses. Exceptionally, a daily dose outside this range may be indicated. Dosage should normally be adjusted according to serum levels where assay facilities exist.

*Elderly (over 65 years):* As with adults the dosage of Epanutin should be titrated to the patient's individual requirements using the same guidelines.

As elderly patients tend to receive multiple drug therapies, the possibility of drug interactions should be borne in mind.

*Infants and Children:* Initially, 5 mg/kg/day in two divided doses, with subsequent dosage individualised to a maximum of 300 mg daily. A recommended daily maintenance dosage is usually 4-8 mg/kg.

Epanutin Infatabs may be chewed.

*Neonates:* The absorption of phenytoin following oral administration in neonates is unpredictable. Furthermore, the metabolism of phenytoin may be depressed. It is therefore especially important to monitor serum levels in the neonate.

**Contra-indications, warnings, etc**
*Use in pregnancy:* There are intrinsic methodologic problems in obtaining adequate data on drug teratogenicity in humans. Genetic factors or the epileptic condition itself may be more important than drug therapy in leading to birth defects. The great majority of mothers on anticonvulsant medication deliver normal infants. It is important to note that anticonvulsant drugs should not be discontinued in patients in whom the drug is administered to prevent major seizures because of the strong possibility of precipitating status epilepticus with attendant hypoxia and threat to life. In individual cases where the severity and frequency of the seizure disorder are such that the removal of medication does not pose a serious threat to the patient, discontinuation of the drug may be considered prior to and during pregnancy although it cannot be said with any confidence that even minor seizures do not pose some hazard to the developing embryo or foetus.

Anticonvulsants including phenytoin may produce congenital abnormalities in the offspring of a small number of epileptic patients. The exact role of drug therapy in these abnormalities is unclear and genetic factors, in some studies, have also been shown to be important. Epanutin should only be used during pregnancy, especially early pregnancy, if in the judgement of the physician the potential benefits clearly outweigh the risk.

In addition to the reports of increased incidence of congenital malformations, such as cleft lip/palate and heart malformations in children of women receiving phenytoin and other antiepileptic drugs, there have more recently been reports of a foetal hydantoin syndrome. This consists of prenatal growth deficiency, micro-encephaly and mental deficiency in children born to mothers who have received phenytoin, barbiturates, alcohol, or trimethadione. However, these features are all interrelated and are frequently associated with intrauterine growth retardation from other causes.

There have been isolated reports of malignancies, including neuroblastoma, in children whose mothers received phenytoin during pregnancy.

An increase in seizure frequency during pregnancy occurs in a proportion of patients, and this may be due to altered phenytoin absorption or metabolism. Periodic measurement of serum phenytoin levels is particularly valuable in the management of a pregnant epileptic patient as a guide to an appropriate adjustment of dosage. However, postpartum restoration of the original dosage will probably be indicated.

Neonatal coagulation defects have been reported within the first 24 hours in babies born to epileptic mothers receiving phenytoin. Vitamin K1 has been shown to prevent or correct this defect and may be given to the mother before delivery and to the neonate after birth.

*Lactation:* Infant breast feeding is not recommended for women taking phenytoin because phenytoin appears to be secreted in low concentrations in human milk.

*Contra-indications:* Hypersensitivity to hydantoins.

*Precautions and warnings:* Abrupt withdrawal of phenytoin in epileptic patients may precipitate status epilepticus. When, in the judgement of the clinician, the need for dosage reduction, discontinuation, or substitution of alternative anti-epileptic medication arises, this should be done gradually. However, in the event of an allergic or hypersensitivity reaction, rapid substitution of alternative therapy may be necessary. In this case, alternative therapy should be an anti-epileptic drug not belonging to the hydantoin chemical class.

Phenytoin is highly protein bound and extensively metabolised by the liver. Reduced dosage to prevent accumulation and toxicity may therefore be required in patients with impaired liver function. Where protein binding is reduced, as in uraemia, total serum phenytoin levels will be reduced accordingly. However, the pharmacologically active free drug concentration is unlikely to be altered. Therefore, under these circumstances therapeutic control may be achieved with total phenytoin levels below the normal range of 10–20 mg/l (40–80 micromoles/l). Patients with impaired liver function, elderly patients or those who are gravely ill may show early signs of toxicity.

Phenytoin should be discontinued if a skin rash appears. If the rash is exfoliative, purpuric, or bullous or if lupus erythematosus or Stevens-Johnson syndrome or toxic epidermal necrolysis is suspected, use of the drug should not be resumed (see Adverse Reactions). If the rash is of a milder type (measles-like or scarlatiniform), therapy may be resumed after the rash has completely disappeared. If the rash recurs upon reinstitution of therapy, further phenytoin medication is contraindicated.

Phenytoin is not effective for absence (petit mal) seizures. If tonic-clonic (grand mal) and absence seizures are present together, combined drug therapy is needed.

Phenytoin may affect glucose metabolism and inhibit insulin release. Hyperglycaemia has been reported in association with toxic levels. Phenytoin is not indicated for seizures due to hypoglycaemia or other metabolic causes.

Serum levels of phenytoin sustained above the optimal range may produce confusional states referred to as 'delirium,' 'psychosis,' or 'encephalopathy,' or rarely irreversible cerebellar dysfunction. Accordingly, at the first sign of acute toxicity, serum drug level determinations are recommended. Dose reduction of phenytoin therapy is indicated if serum levels are excessive; if symptoms persist, termination of therapy with phenytoin is recommended.

Phenytoin therapy may interfere with Vitamin D metabolism. In the absence of an adequate dietary intake of Vitamin D or exposure to sunlight, osteomalacia, hypocalcemia or rickets may develop.

In view of isolated reports associating phenytoin with exacerbation of porphyria, caution should be exercised in using the medication in patients suffering from this disease.

Phenytoin may cause lowered serum levels of folic acid. It is recommended that serum folate concentrations be measured at least once every 6 months, and folic acid supplements given if necessary.

*Adverse reactions:*

*Central nervous system:* The most common manifestations encountered with phenytoin therapy are referable to this system and are usually dose-related. These include nystagmus, ataxia, slurred speech, decreased coordination, mental confusion, paraesthesia, drowsiness and vertigo. Dizziness, insomnia, transient nervousness, motor twitchings, and headaches have also been observed. There have also been rare reports of phenytoin induced dyskinesias, including chorea, dystonia, tremor and asterixis, similar to those induced by phenothiazine and other neuroleptic drugs. There are occasional reports of irreversible cerebellar dysfunction associated with severe phenytoin overdosage. Peripheral neuropathy has been reported on rare occasions.

*Gastrointestinal:* Nausea, vomiting and constipation, toxic hepatitis, and liver damage.

*Dermatological:* Dermatological manifestations sometimes accompanied by fever have included scarlatiniform or morbilliform rashes. A morbilliform rash is the most common; dermatitis is seen more rarely. Other more serious and rare forms have included bullous, exfoliative or purpuric dermatitis, lupus erythematosus, Stevens-Johnson syndrome and toxic epidermal necrolysis (see Precautions).

*Connective tissue:* Coarsening of the facial features, enlargement of the lips, gingival hyperplasia, hirsutism, hypertrichosis, Peyronie's Disease and Dupuytren's contracture may occur rarely.

*Haemopoietic:* Haemopoietic complications, some fatal, have occasionally been reported in association with administration of phenytoin. These have included thrombocytopenia, leucopenia, granulocytopenia, agranulocytosis, pancytopenia with or without bone marrow suppression, and aplastic anaemia. While macrocytosis and megaloblastic anaemia have occurred, these conditions usually respond to folic acid therapy.

There have been a number of reports suggesting a relationship between phenytoin and the development of lymphadenopathy (local and generalised) including benign lymph node hyperplasia, pseudolymphoma, lymphoma, and Hodgkin's Disease. Although a cause and effect relationship has not been established, the occurrence of lymphadenopathy indicates the need to differentiate such a condition from other types of lymph node pathology. Lymph node involvement may occur with or without symptoms and signs resembling serum sickness, eg fever, rash and liver involvement. In all cases of lymphadenopathy, follow-up observation for an extended period is indicated and every effort should be made to achieve seizure control using alternative antiepileptic drugs.

Frequent blood counts should be carried out during treatment with phenytoin.

*Immune system:* Hypersensitivity syndrome has been reported and may in rare cases be fatal (the syndrome may include, but is not limited to, symptoms such as arthralgias, eosinophilia, fever, liver dysfunction, lymphadenopathy or rash), systemic lupus erythematosus, polyarteritis nodosa, and immunoglobulin abnormalities may occur. Several individual case reports have suggested that there may be an increased, although still rare, incidence of hypersensitivity reactions, including skin rash and hepatotoxicity, in black patients.

*Other:* Polyarthropathy, interstitial nephritis , pneumonitis

*Drug interactions:* 1. Drugs which may *increase* phenytoin serum levels include: Amiodarone, antifungal agents, (such as, but not limited to, amphotericin B, fluconazole, ketoconazole, miconazole and itraconazole), chloramphenicol, chlordiazepoxide, diazepam, dicoumarol, disulfiram, H2-antagonists, halothane, isoniazid, methylphenidate, omeprazole, oestrogens, phenothiazines, phenylbutazone, salicylates, succinimides, sulphonamides, tolbutamide, trazodone and viloxazine.

2. Drugs which may *decrease* phenytoin serum levels include: carbamazepine, folic acid, reserpine, sucralfate and vigabatrin.

3. Drugs which may either *increase* or *decrease* phenytoin serum levels include: Phenobarbitone, valproic acid, sodium valproate antineoplastic agents and certain antacids. Similarly, the effect of phenytoin on phenobarbitone, valproic acid and sodium valproate serum levels is unpredictable.

Acute alcohol intake may increase phenytoin serum levels while chronic alcoholism may decrease serum levels.

4. Although not a true pharmacokinetic interaction, tricylic antidepressants and phenothiazines may precipitate seizures in susceptible patients and phenytoin dosage may need to be adjusted.

5. Drugs whose effect is *impaired* by phenytoin include: antifungal agents, antineoplastic agents, clozapine, corticosteroids, dicoumarol, digitoxin, doxycycline, frusemide, oestrogens, oral contraceptives, quinidine, rifampicin, theophylline and vitamin D.

6. Drugs whose effect is *altered* by phenytoin include: warfarin. The effect of phenytoin on warfarin is variable and prothrombin times should be determined when these agents are combined.

Serum level determinations are especially helpful when possible drug interactions are suspected.

*Drug/Laboratory test interactions:* Phenytoin may cause a slight decrease in serum levels of total and free thyroxine, possibly as a result of enhanced peripheral metabolism. These changes do not lead to clinical hypothyroidism and do not affect the levels of circulating TSH. The latter can therefore be used for diagnosing hypothyroidism in the patient on phenytoin. Phenytoin does not interfere with uptake and suppression tests used in the diagnosis of hypothyroidism. It may, however, produce lower than normal values for dexamethasone or metapyrone tests. Phenytoin may cause raised serum levels of glucose, alkaline phosphatase, and gamma glutamyl transpeptidase and lowered serum levels of calcium and folic acid. It is recommended that serum folate concentrations be measured at least once every 6 months, and folic acid supplements given if necessary. Phenytoin may affect blood sugar metabolism tests.

*Overdosage:* The lethal dose in children is not known. The mean lethal dose for adults is estimated to be 2 to 5 g. The initial symptoms are nystagmus, ataxia and dysarthria. The patient then becomes comatose, the pupils are unresponsive and hypotension occurs followed by respiratory depression and apnoea. Death is due to respiratory and circulatory depression.

There are marked variations among individuals with respect to phenytoin serum levels where toxicity may occur. Nystagmus on lateral gaze usually appears at 20 mg/l, and ataxia at 30 mg/l, dysarthria and lethargy appear when the serum concentration is greater than 40 mg/l, but a concentration as high as 50 mg/l has been reported without evidence of toxicity.

As much as 25 times therapeutic dose has been taken to result in serum concentration over 100 mg/l (400 micromoles/l) with complete recovery.

*Treatment:* Treatment is non-specific since there is no known antidote. If ingested within the previous 4 hours the stomach should be emptied. If the gag reflex is absent, the airway should be supported. Oxygen, and assisted ventilation may be necessary for central nervous system, respiratory and cardiovascular depression. Haemodialysis can be considered since phenytoin is not completely bound to plasma proteins.

Total exchange transfusion has been utilised in the treatment of severe intoxication in children.

**Pharmaceutical precautions** Epanutin Capsules 300 mg and Infatabs: Store at a temperature not exceeding 30°C.

Epanutin Suspension: Store at a temperature not exceeding 25°C.

**Legal category** POM.

**Package quantities**

Epanutin Capsules 300 mg are available in containers of 100 and 500.

Epanutin Suspension (30 mg per 5 ml) is available in bottles of 500 ml.

Epanutin Infatabs 50 mg are available in containers of 100

**Further information** The 25 mg Epanutin Capsule has been introduced because incremental doses of the drug should become progressively smaller as the serum concentration increases, since there is no linear relationship between dose and serum level–for example, an incremental dose of 50 mg may be enough to increase a serum level in a particular patient from 10 mg/l (40 micromoles/l) to a toxic level.

**Product licence numbers**
Epanutin Capsules 300 mg 0018/0158
Epanutin Suspension 0018/5106
Epanutin Infatabs 0018/0069

## EPANUTIN* READY-MIXED PARENTERAL

**Qualitative and quantitative composition** Each 5 ml ampoule of Epanutin Ready-Mixed Parenteral contains Phenytoin sodium PhEur 250 mg.

**Pharmaceutical form** Clear, sterile solution for injection

**Clinical particulars** *Therapeutic indications:* Parenteral Epanutin is indicated for the control of status epilepticus of the tonic-clonic (grand mal) type and prevention and treatment of seizures occurring during or following neurosurgery and/or severe head injury.

It is of use in the treatment of cardiac arrhythmias where first line therapy is not effective. It is of particular value when these are digitalis induced.

*Posology and method of administration:* For parenteral administration.

Parenteral drug products should be inspected visually for particulate matter and discolouration prior to administration, whenever solution and container permit. Parenteral Epanutin is suitable for use as long as it remains free of haziness and precipitate. Upon refrigeration or freezing a precipitate might form; this will dissolve again after the solution is allowed to stand at room temperature. The product is still suitable for use. Only a clear solution should be used. A faint yellow colouration may develop, however, this has no effect on the potency of this solution.

There is a relatively small margin between full therapeutic effect and minimally toxic doses of this drug. Optimum control without clinical signs of toxicity occurs most often with serum levels between 10 and 20 mg/l (40-80 micromoles/l).

Parenteral Epanutin should be injected **slowly** directly into a large vein through a large-gauge needle or intravenous catheter.

Each injection or infusion of intravenous Epanutin should be preceded and followed by an injection of sterile saline through the same needle or catheter to avoid local venous irritation due to alkalinity of the solution. (see warning section)

For infusion administration the parenteral phenytoin should be diluted in 50-100 ml of normal saline, with the final concentration of phenytoin in the solution not exceeding 10 mg/ml. Administration should commence immediately after the mixture has been prepared and must be completed within one hour (the infusion mixture should not be refrigerated). An in-line filter (0.22-0.50 microns) should be used. The diluted form is suitable for use as long as it remains free of haziness and precipitate.

Continuous monitoring of the electrocardiogram and blood pressure is essential. Cardiac resuscitative equipment should be available. The patient should be observed for signs of respiratory depression. If administration of intravenous Epanutin does not terminate seizures, the use of other measures, including general anaesthesia, should be considered.

Epanutin Ready Mixed Parenteral contains phenytoin sodium whereas Epanutin Suspension and Epanutin Infatabs contain phenytoin. Although 100 mg of phenytoin sodium is equivalent to 92 mg of phenytoin on a molecular weight basis; these molecular equivalents are not necessarily biologically equivalent. Physicians should therefore exercise care in those situations where it is necessary to change the dosage form and serum level monitoring is advised.

*Status epilepticus:* In a patient having continuous seizure activity, as compared to the more common rapidly recurring seizures, i.e. serial epilepsy, injection of intravenous diazepam or a short acting barbiturate is recommended because of their rapid onset of action, prior to administration of Epanutin.

Following the use of diazepam in patients having continuous seizures and in the initial management of serial epilepsy a loading dose of Epanutin 10-15 mg/kg should be injected **slowly** intravenously, at a rate not exceeding 50 mg per minute in adults (this will require approximately 20 minutes in a 70 kg patient). The loading dose should be followed by maintenance doses of 100 mg orally or intravenously every 6 to 8 hours.

Recent work in neonates has shown that absorption of phenytoin is unreliable after oral administration, but a loading dose of 15-20 mg/kg of Epanutin intravenously will usually produce serum concentrations of phenytoin within the generally accepted therapeutic range (10-20 mg/l). The drug should be injected slowly intravenously at a rate of 1-3 mg/kg/min.

Determination of phenytoin serum levels is advised when using Epanutin in the management of status epilepticus and in the subsequent establishing of maintenance dosage. The clinically effective level is usually 10-20 mg/l although some cases of tonic-clonic seizures may be controlled with lower serum levels of phenytoin.

Intramuscular administration should not be used in the treatment of status epilepticus because the attainment of peak plasma levels may require up to 24 hours.

*Use in cardiac arrhythmias:* 3.5-5 mg per kg of bodyweight intravenously initially, repeated once if necessary. The solution should be injected slowly, intravenously and at a uniform rate which should not exceed 1 ml (50 mg) per minute.

*Other clinical conditions:* It is not possible to set forth a universally applicable dosage schedule. **The intravenous route of administration is preferred.** Dosage and dosing interval will, of necessity, be determined by the needs of the individual patient. Factors such as previous antiepileptic therapy, seizure control, age and general medical condition must be considered. Notwithstanding the slow absorption of Epanutin when given intra-muscularly its use in certain conditions may be appropriate.

When short term intramuscular administration is necessary for a patient previously stabilised orally, compensating dosage adjustments are essential to maintain therapeutic serum levels. An intramuscular dose 50% greater than the oral dose is necessary to maintain these levels. When returned to oral administration, the dose should be reduced by 50% of the original oral dose, for the same period of time the patient received Epanutin intra-muscularly, to prevent excessive serum levels due to continued release from intramuscular tissue sites.

*Neurosurgery:* In a patient who has not previously received the drug, Parenteral Epanutin 100-200 mg (2-4 ml) may be given intramuscularly at approximately 4-hour intervals prophylactically during neurosurgery and continued during the postoperative period for 48–72 hrs. The dosage should then be reduced to a maintenance dose of 300 mg and adjusted according to serum level estimations.

If the patient requires more than a week of intramuscular Epanutin alternative routes should be explored such as gastric intubation. For time periods less than one week, the patient switched from intramuscular administration should receive one half the original oral dose for the same period of time the patient received Epanutin intra-muscularly. Measurement of serum levels is of value as a guide to an appropriate adjustment of dosage.

*Elderly (over 65 years):* As for adults. However, complications may occur more readily in elderly patients.

*Neonates:* Recent work in neonates has shown that absorption of phenytoin is unreliable after oral administration, but a loading dose of 15-20 mg/kg of Epanutin intravenously will usually produce serum concentrations of phenytoin within the generally accepted therapeutic range (10-20 mg/l). The drug should be injected slowly intravenously at a rate of 1-3 mg/kg/min.

*Infants and children:* As for adults. However, it has been shown that children tend to metabolise phenytoin more rapidly than adults. This should be borne in mind when determining dosage regimens. The use of serum level monitoring being particularly beneficial in such cases.

*Contra-indications:* Phenytoin is contraindicated in

patients who are hypersensitive to phenytoin or other hydantoins.

Intra-arterial administration must be avoided in view of the high pH of the preparation.

Because of its effect on ventricular automaticity, phenytoin is contraindicated in sinus bradycardia, sino-atrial block, and second and third degree A-V block, and patients with Adams-Stokes syndrome.

*Special warnings and special precautions for use:* In adults, intravenous administration should not exceed 50 mg per minute. In neonates, the drug should be administered at a rate of 1-3 mg/kg/min.

The most notable signs of toxicity associated with the intravenous use of this drug are cardiovascular collapse and/or central nervous system depression. Severe cardiotoxic reactions and fatalities due to depression of atrial and ventricular conduction and ventricular fibrillation, respiratory arrest and tonic seizures have been reported particularly in elderly or gravely ill patients, if the preparation is given too rapidly or in excess.

Hypotension usually occurs when the drug is administered rapidly by the intravenous route.

Soft tissue irritation and inflammation has occurred at the site of injection with and without extravasation of intravenous phenytoin. Soft tissue irritation may vary from slight tenderness to extensive necrosis, sloughing and in rare instances has led to amputation. Subcutaneous or perivascular injection should be avoided because of the highly alkaline nature of the solution.

The intramuscular route is not recommended for the treatment of status epilepticus because of slow absorption. Serum levels of phenytoin in the therapeutic range cannot be rapidly achieved by this method.

*General:* Intravenous Epanutin should be used with caution in patients with hypotension and severe myocardial insufficiency.

Phenytoin should be discontinued if a skin rash appears. If the rash is exfoliative, purpuric, or bullous or if lupus erythematosus, Stevens- Johnson syndrome, or toxic epidermal necrolysis is suspected, use of this drug should not be resumed and alternative therapy should be considered. If the rash is of a milder type (measles-like or scarlatiniform), therapy may be resumed after the rash has completely disappeared. If the rash recurs upon reinstitution of therapy, further phenytoin medication is contraindicated.

Phenytoin is not effective for absence (petit mal) seizures. If tonic-clonic (grand mal) and absence (petit mal) seizures are present together, combined drug therapy is needed.

Serum levels of phenytoin sustained above the optimal range may produce confusional states referred to as 'delirium,' 'psychosis,' or 'encephalopathy,' or rarely irreversible cerebellar dysfunction. Accordingly, at the first sign of acute toxicity, serum drug level determinations are recommended. Dose reduction of phenytoin therapy is indicated if serum levels are excessive; if symptoms persist, termination of therapy with phenytoin is recommended.

Phenytoin is highly protein bound and extensively metabolised by the liver.

Reduced maintenance dosage to prevent accumulation and toxicity may therefore be required in patients with impaired liver function. Where protein binding is reduced, as in uraemia, total serum phenytoin levels will be reduced accordingly. However, the pharmacologically active free drug concentration is unlikely to be altered. Therefore, under these circumstances therapeutic control may be achieved with total phenytoin levels below the normal range of 10-20 mg/l. Dosage should not exceed the minimum necessary to control convulsions.

The liver is the chief site of biotransformation of phenytoin. Patients with impaired liver function, elderly patients, or those who are gravely ill may show early signs of toxicity.

Phenytoin may affect glucose metabolism and inhibit insulin release. Hyperglycaemia has been reported. Phenytoin is not indicated for seizures due to hypoglycaemia or other metabolic causes. Caution is advised when treating diabetic patients.

In view of isolated reports associating phenytoin with exacerbation of porphyria, caution should be exercised in using this medication in patients suffering from this disease.

*Laboratory tests:* Phenytoin serum level determinations may be necessary to achieve optimal dosage adjustments.

*Interactions with other medicaments and other forms of interaction:* 1. Drugs which may *increase* phenytoin serum levels include: Amiodarone, antifungal agents, (such as, but not limited to, amphotericin B, fluconazole, ketoconazole, miconazole and itraconazole), chloramphenicol, chlordiazepoxide, diazepam, dicoumarol, disulfiram, H2-antagonists, halothane, isoniazid, methylphenidate, omeprazole, oestrogens, phenothiazines, phenylbutazone, salicylates, succinimides, sulphonamides, tolbutamide, trazodone and viloxazine.

2. Drugs which may *decrease* phenytoin serum levels include: carbamazepine, folic acid, reserpine, sucralfate and vigabatrin.

3. Drugs which may either *increase* or *decrease* phenytoin serum levels include: Phenobarbitone, valproic acid, sodium valproate, antineoplastic agents and certain antacids. Similarly, the effect of phenytoin on phenobarbitone and valproic acid and sodium valproate serum levels is unpredictable.

Acute alcohol intake may increase phenytoin serum levels while chronic alcoholism may decrease serum levels.

4. Although not a true pharmacokinetic interaction, tricylic antidepressants and phenothiazines may precipitate seizures in susceptible patients and phenytoin dosage may need to be adjusted.

5. Drugs whose effect is *impaired* by phenytoin include: antifungal agents, antineoplastic agents, clozapine, corticosteroids, dicoumarol, digitoxin, doxycycline, frusemide, oestrogens, oral contraceptives, quinidine, rifampicin, theophylline and vitamin D.

6. Drugs whose effect is *enhanced* by phenytoin include: warfarin.

Serum level determinations are especially helpful when possible drug interactions are suspected.

*Drug/Laboratory test interactions:* Phenytoin may cause decreased serum levels of protein-bound iodine (PBI). It may also produce lower than normal values for dexamethasone or metyrapone tests. Phenytoin may cause raised serum levels of glucose, alkaline phosphatase, gamma glutamyl transpeptidase and lowered serum levels of calcium and folic acid. Phenytoin may affect blood sugar metabolism tests.

*Pregnancy and lactation:* In considering the use of Epanutin intravenously in the management of status epilepticus in pregnancy, the following information should be weighed in assessing the risks and the benefits. The potential adverse effects upon the foetus of status epilepticus, specifically hypoxia, make it imperative to control the condition in the shortest possible time.

There are intrinsic methodologic problems in obtaining adequate data on drug teratogenicity in humans. Genetic factors or the epileptic condition itself may be more important than drug therapy in leading to birth defects.

The great majority of mothers on anticonvulsant medication deliver normal infants. It is important to note that anticonvulsant drugs should not be discontinued in patients in whom the drug is administered to prevent major seizures because of the strong possibility of precipitating status epilepticus and attendant hypoxia and threat to life. In individual cases where the severity and frequency of the seizure disorder are such that the removal of medication does not pose a serious threat to the patient, discontinuation of the drug may be considered prior to and during pregnancy although it cannot be said with any confidence that even minor seizures do not pose some hazard to the developing embryo or foetus.

There is some evidence that phenytoin may produce congenital abnormalities in the offspring of a small number of epileptic patients, therefore it should not be used as first drug during pregnancy, especially early pregnancy, unless in the judgement of the physician the potential benefits outweigh the risk.

In addition to the reports of increased incidence of congenital malformations, such as cleft lip/palate and heart malformations in children of women receiving phenytoin and other anti-epileptic drugs, there have more recently been reports of a foetal hydantoin syndrome. This consists of prenatal growth deficiency, microencephaly and mental deficiency in children born to mothers who have received phenytoin, barbiturates, alcohol, or trimethadione. However, these features are all interrelated and are frequently associated with intrauterine growth retardation from other causes.

There have been isolated reports of malignancies, including neuroblastoma, in children whose mothers received phenytoin during pregnancy.

An increase in seizure frequency during pregnancy occurs in a proportion of patients, because of altered phenytoin absorption or metabolism. Periodic measurement of serum phenytoin levels is particularly valuable in the management of a pregnant epileptic patient as a guide to an appropriate adjustment of dosage. However, post partum restoration of the original dosage will probably be indicated. Neonatal coagulation defects have been reported within the first 24 hours in babies born to epileptic mothers receiving phenytoin. Vitamin K has been shown to prevent or correct this defect and may be given to the mother before delivery and to the neonate after birth.

Infant breast feeding is not recommended for women taking this drug because phenytoin appears to be secreted in low concentrations in human milk.

*Effects on ability to drive or use Machines:* None known

*Undesirable effects:* Signs of toxicity are associated with cardiovascular and central nervous system depression.

*Central nervous system*: The most common manifestations encountered with phenytoin therapy are referable to this system and are usually dose-related. These include nystagmus, ataxia, slurred speech, decreased coordination, mental confusion, paraesthesia, drowsiness and vertigo. Dizziness, insomnia, transient nervousness, motor twitching, and headache have also been observed. There have also been rare reports of phenytoin-induced dyskinesia, including chorea, dystonia, tremor, and asterixis, similar to those induced by phenothiazine and other neuroleptic drugs. A predominantly sensory peripheral polyneuropathy has been observed in patients receiving long-term phenytoin therapy. Tonic seizures have also been reported.

*Cardiovascular:* Severe cardiotoxic reactions and fatalities have been reported with atrial and ventricular conduction depression and ventricular fibrillation. Severe complications are most commonly encountered in elderly or gravely ill patients.

*Respiratory:* Alterations in respiratory function including respiratory arrest may occur.

*Injection site:* Local irritation, inflammation and tenderness. Necrosis and sloughing have been reported after subcutaneous or perivascular injection. Subcutaneous or perivascular injection should be avoided. Soft tissue irritation and inflammation have occurred at the site of injection with and without extravasation of intravenous phenytoin.

*Dermatological system:* Dermatological manifestations sometimes accompanied by fever have included scarlatiniform or morbilliform rashes. A morbilliform rash (measles-like) is the most common. Other types of dermatitis are seen more rarely. Other more serious forms which may be fatal have included bullous, exfoliative or purpuric dermatitis, lupus erythematosus, Stevens-Johnson syndrome, and toxic epidermal necrolysis.

*Haemopoietic system:* Haemopoietic complications, some fatal, have occasionally been reported in association with administration of phenytoin. These have included thrombocytopenia, leucopenia, granulocytopenia, agranulocytosis, and pancytopenia with or without bone marrow suppression and aplastic anaemia. While macrocytosis and megaloblastic anaemia have occurred, these conditions usually respond to folic acid therapy. There have been a number of reports suggesting a relationship between phenytoin and the development of lymphadenopathy (local or generalised) including benign lymph node hyperplasia, pseudolymphoma, lymphoma, and Hodgkin's Disease. Although a cause and effect relationship has not been established, the occurrence of lymphadenopathy indicates the need to differentiate such a condition from other types of lymph node pathology. Lymph node involvement may occur with or without symptoms and signs resembling serum sickness, eg fever, rash and liver involvement.

In all cases of lymphadenopathy, follow-up observation for an extended period is indicated and every effort should be made to achieve seizure control using alternative antiepileptic drugs.

*Gastrointestinal system:* Nausea, vomiting, constipation, toxic hepatitis, and liver damage.

*Connective tissue system:* Coarsening of the facial features, enlargement of the lips, gingival hyperplasia, hirsutism, hypertrichosis, Peyronie's disease and Dupuytren's contracture may occur rarely.

*Immune system:* Hypersensitivity syndrome has been reported and may in rare cases be fatal (the syndrome may include, but is not limited to, symptoms such as arthralgias, eosinophilia, fever, liver dysfunction, lymphadenopathy or rash), systemic lupus erythematosus, periarteritis nodosa, and immunoglobulin abnormalities may occur. Several individual case reports have suggested that there may be an increased, although still rare, incidence of hypersensitivity reactions, including skin rash and hepatotoxicity, in black patients.

*Other:* Polyarthropathy, interstitial nephritis, pneumonitis.

*Overdose:* The lethal dose in children is not known. The mean lethal dose in adults is estimated to be 2 to 5 grams. The initial symptoms are nystagmus, ataxia, and dysarthria. Other signs are tremor, hyperflexia, lethargy, nausea, vomiting. The patient may become comatose and hypotensive. Death is due to respiratory and circulatory depression.

Attempts to relate serum levels of the drug to toxic effects have shown wide interpatient variation. Nystagmus on lateral gaze usually appears at 20 mg/l, and ataxia at 30 mg/l, dysarthria and lethargy appear when the serum concentration is >40 mg/l, but a concentration as high as 50 mg/l has been reported without evidence of toxicity.

As much as 25 times the therapeutic dose, which resulted in a serum concentration of 100 mg/l was taken with complete recovery.

*Treatment:* Treatment is non-specific since there is no known antidote. The adequacy of the respiratory and circulatory systems should be carefully observed and appropriate supportive measures employed. Haemodialysis can be considered since phenytoin is not completely bound to plasma proteins. Total exchange transfusion has been used in the treatment of severe intoxication in children.

In acute overdosage the possibility of other CNS depressants, including alcohol, should be borne in mind.

## Pharmacological properties.

*Pharmacodynamic properties:* Phenytoin is effective in various animal models of generalised convulsive disorders, reasonably effective in models of partial seizures but relatively ineffective in models of myoclonic seizures. It appears to stabilise rather than raise the seizure threshold and prevents spread of seizure activity rather than abolish the primary focus of seizure discharge. The mechanism by which phenytoin exerts its anticonvulsant action has not been fully elucidated however, possible contributory effects include: 1. Non-synaptic effects to reduce sodium conductance, enhance active sodium extrusion, block repetitive firing and reduce post-titanic potentiation. 2. Post-synaptic action to enhance gaba-meidated inhibition and reduce excitatory synaptic transmission. 3. Pre-synaptic actions to reduce calcium entry and block release of neurotransmitter.

*Pharmacokinetic properties:* After injection phneytoin is distributed into body fluids including CSF. Its volume of distribution has been estimated to be between 0.52 and 1.19 litres/kg, and it is highly protein bound (usually 90% in adults). In serum, phenytoin binds rapidly and reversibly to proteins. About 90% of phenytoin in plasma is bound to albumin. The plasma half-life of phenytoin in man averages 22 hours with a range of 7 to 42 hours. Phenytoin is hydroxylated in the liver by an enzyme system which is saturable. Small incremental doses may produce very substantial increases in serum levels when these are in the upper range of therapeutic concentrations. The parameters controlling elimination are also subject to wide interpatient variation. The serum level is achieved by a given dose is therefore also subject to wide variation.

*Pre-clinical safety data:* Pre-clinical safety data does not add anything of further significance to the prescriber.

## Pharmaceutical particulars

*List of excipients:* Each 5 ml contains: propylene glycol, ethanol 96%, water for injection, sodium hydroxide.

*Incompatibilities:* None stated.

*Shelf-life:* 36 months

*Special precautions for storage:* Store at room temperature not exceeding 25°C. Protect from light. The product should not be used if a precipitate or haziness develops in the solution in the ampoule. Epanutin Ready Mixed Parenteral should not be mixed with other drugs because of precipitation of phenytoin acid.

*Nature and contents of container:* Clear glass ampoules with red colour break band containing 5 ml of solution. Each pack contains 10 ampoules.

*Instructions for use/handling:* See *posology and method of administration* for further information.

*Marketing authorisation holder:* Parke Davis & Company, Usk Road, Pontypool, NP4 OYH

**Marketing authorisation number** 0018/0070R

**Date of approval/revision of SPC** February 1996

**Legal category** POM.

# KETALAR*

**Presentation** Parenteral general anaesthetic.

*Composition:* Ketalar, dl2-(o-chlorophenyl)-2-(methylamino) cyclohexanone hydrochloride, is a white crystalline solid, soluble in water to 20% clear and colourless solution.

The base component is 86.7% of the salt. It is supplied as a slightly acid (pH3.5- 5.5) solution for intravenous or intramuscular injection in concentrations containing the equivalent of either 10, 50 or 100 mg ketamine base per ml. All concentrations contain 1 : 10,000 Phemeride* (benzethonium chloride) as a preservative. The 10 mg per ml solution has been made isotonic with sodium chloride.

**Uses** Ketalar is recommended:

1. as the sole anaesthetic agent for diagnostic and surgical procedures. When used by intravenous or intramuscular injection, Ketalar is best suited for short procedures. With additional doses, or by intravenous infusion, Ketalar can be used for longer procedures. If skeletal muscle relaxation is desired, a muscle relaxant should be used and respiration should be supported.

2. for the induction of anaesthesia prior to the administration of other general anaesthetic agents.

3. to supplement other anaesthetic agents.

*Specific areas of application or types of procedures:*

1. when the intramuscular route of administration is preferred.

2. debridement, painful dressings, and skin grafting in burned patients, as well as other superficial surgical procedures.

3. neurodiagnostic procedures such as pneumoencephalograms, ventriculograms, myelograms, and lumbar punctures.

4. diagnostic and operative procedures of the eye, ear, nose, and mouth, including dental extractions.

**Note:** Eye movements may persist during ophthalmological procedures.

5. anaesthesia in poor-risk patients with depression of vital functions or where depression of vital functions must be avoided, if at all possible.

6. orthopaedic procedures such as closed reductions, manipulations, femoral pinning, amputations, and biopsies.

7. sigmoidoscopy and minor surgery of the anus and rectum, circumcision and pilonidal sinus.

8. cardiac catheterization procedures.

9. Caesarian section; as an induction agent in the absence of elevated blood pressure.

10. anaesthesia in the asthmatic patient, either to minimise the risks of an attack of bronchospasm developing, or in the presence of bronchospasm where anaesthesia cannot be delayed.

## Dosage and administration

*Adults, elderly(over 65 years) and children:* For surgery in elderly patients ketamine has been shown to be suitable either alone or supplemented with other anaesthetic agents.

*Preoperative preparations:* 1. Ketalar has been safely used alone when the stomach was not empty. However, since the need for supplemental agents and muscle relaxants cannot be predicted, when preparing for elective surgery it is advisable that nothing be given by mouth for at least six hours prior to anaesthesia.

2. Atropine, scopolamine, or another drying agent should be given at an appropriate interval prior to induction.

3. Midazolam, diazepam, lorazepam, or flunitrazepam used as a premedicant or as an adjunct to ketamine, have been effective in reducing the incidence of emergence reactions.

*Onset and duration:* As with other general anaesthetic agents, the individual response to Ketalar is somewhat varied depending on the dose, route of administration, age of patient, and concomitant use of other agents, so that dosage recommendation cannot be absolutely fixed. The dose should be titrated aginst the patient's requirements.

Because of rapid induction following intravenous injection, the patient should be in a supported position during administration. An intravenous dose of 2 mg/kg of body-weight usually produces surgical anaesthesia within 30 seconds after injection and the anaesthetic effect usually lasts 5 to 10 minutes. An intramuscular dose of 10 mg/kg of body-weight usually produces surgical anaesthesia within 3 to 4 minutes following injection and the anaesthetic effect usually lasts 12 to 25 minutes. Return to consciousness is gradual.

*A. Ketalar as the sole anaesthetic agent:*

*Intravenous Infusion:*

The use of Ketalar by continuous infusion enables the dose to be titrated more closely, thereby reducing the amount of drug administered compared with intermittent administration. This results in a shorter recovery time and better stability of vital signs.

A solution containing 1 mg/ml of ketamine in dextrose 5% or sodium chloride 0.9% is suitable for administration by infusion.

*Induction:* An infusion corresponding to 0.5–2 mg/kg** as total induction dose.

*Maintenance of anaesthesia:* Anaesthesia may be maintained using a microdrip infusion of 10–45 microgram/kg/min (1–3 mg/min)

The rate of infusion will depend on the patient's reaction and response to anaesthesia. The dosage required may be reduced when a long acting neuromuscular blocking agent is used.

*Intermittent Injection:*

*Induction:*

*Intravenous Route:* The initial dose of Ketalar administered intravenously may range from 1 mg/kg to 4.5 mg/kg**. The average amount required to produce 5 to 10 minutes of surgical anaesthesia has been 2.0 mg/kg. It is recommended that intravenous administration be accomplished slowly (over a period of 60 seconds). More rapid administration may result in respiratory depression.

*Intramuscular Route:* The initial dose of Ketalar administered intramuscularly may range from 6.5 to 13 mg/kg**. A low initial intramuscular dose of 4 mg/kg has been used in diagnostic manoeuvres and procedures not involving intensely painful stimuli. A dose of 10 mg/kg will usually produce 12 to 25 minutes of surgical anaesthesia. **In terms of ketamine base.

*Maintenance of anaesthesia:*

Lightening of anaesthesia may be indicated by nystagmus, movements in response to stimulation, and vocalization. Anaesthesia is maintained by the administration of additional doses of Ketalar by either the intravenous or intramuscular route.

Each additional dose is from ½ to the full induction dose recommended above for the route selected for maintenance, regardless of the route used for induction.

The larger the total amount of Ketalar administered, the longer will be the time to complete recovery.

Purposeless and tonic-clonic movements of extremities may occur during the course of anaesthesia. These movements do not imply a light plane and are not indicative of the need for additional doses of the anaesthetic.

*B. Ketalar as induction agent prior to the use of other general anaesthetics:*

Induction is accomplished by a full intravenous or intramuscular dose of Ketalar as defined above. If Ketalar has been administered intravenously and the principal anaesthetic is slow-acting, a second dose of Ketalar may be required 5 to 8 minutes following the initial dose. If Ketalar has been administered intramuscularly and the principal anaesthetic is rapid-acting, administration of the principal anaesthetic may be delayed up to 15 minutes following the injection of Ketalar.

*C. Ketalar as supplement to anaesthetic agents:*

Ketalar is clinically compatible with the commonly used general and local anaesthetic agents when an adequate respiratory exchange is maintained. The dose of Ketalar for use in conjunction with other anaesthetic agents is usually in the same range as the dosage stated above; however, the use of another anaesthetic agent may allow a reduction in the dose of Ketalar.

*Management of patients in recovery:*

Following the procedure the patient should be observed but left undisturbed. This does not preclude the monitoring of vital signs. If, during the recovery, the patient shows any indication of emergence delirium, consideration may be given to the use of diazepam (5 to 10 mg I.V. in an adult). A hypnotic dose of a thiobarbiturate (50 to 100 mg I.V.) may be used to terminate severe emergence reactions. If any one of these agents is employed, the patient may experience a longer recovery period.

## Contra-indications, warnings, etc

*Contra-indications:* Ketalar is contra-indicated in persons in whom an elevation of blood pressure would constitute a serious hazard (see Adverse Reactions section). Ketalar should not be used in patients with eclampsia or pre-eclampsia.

*Use in pregnancy and lactstion:* Ketalar crosses the placenta. This should be borne in mind during obstetric procedures.

With the exception of administration during surgery for abdominal delivery or vaginal delivery, no controlled studies in pregnancy have been conducted. The safe use in pregnancy has not been established and such use is not recommended.

*Precautions:* 1. To be used only in hospitals by or under the supervision of experienced medically qualified anaesthetists except under emergency conditions.

2. As with any general anaesthetic agent, resuscitative equipment should be available and ready for use.

3. Barbiturates and Ketalar, being chemically incompatible because of precipitate formation, should not be injected from the same syringe or infusion solution.

4. Prolonged recovery time may occur if barbiturates and/or narcotics are used concurrently with Ketalar.

5. Emergence delirium phenomena may occur during the recovery period. The incidence of these reactions may be reduced if verbal and tactile stimulation of the patient is minimised during the recovery period. This does not preclude the monitoring of vital signs.

6. Because pharyngeal and laryngeal reflexes usually remain active, mechanical stimulation of the pharynx should be avoided unless muscle relaxants, with proper attention to respiration, are used.

7. Although aspiration of contrast medium has been reported during Ketalar anaesthesia under experimental conditions (Taylor, P A and Towey, R M, Brit. Med.

J. 1971, 2: 688) in clinical practice aspiration is seldom a problem.

8. Cardiac function should be continually monitored during the procedure in patients found to have hypertension or cardiac decompensation.

9. Since an increase in cerebrospinal fluid pressure has been reported during Ketalar anaesthesia, Ketalar should be used with special caution in patients with preanaesthetic elevated cerebrospinal fluid pressure.

10. Respiratory depression may occur with overdosage of Ketalar, in which case supportive ventilation should be employed. Mechanical support of respiration is preferred to the administration of analeptics.

11. The intravenous dose should be administered over a period of 60 seconds. More rapid administration may result in transient respiratory depression or apnoea.

12. In surgical procedures involving visceral pain pathways, Ketalar should be supplemented with an agent which obtunds visceral pain.

13. Use with caution in the chronic alcoholic and the acutely alcohol- intoxicated patient.

14. When Ketalar is used on an outpatient basis, the patient should not be released until recovery from anaesthesia is complete and then should be accompanied by a responsible adult.

15. Patients should be cautioned that driving a car, operating hazardous machinery or engaging in hazardous activities should not be undertaken for 24 hours or more after anaesthesia.

*Adverse reactions:*
*Cardiovascular:* Temporary elevation of blood pressure and pulse rate is frequently observed following administration of ketamine hydrochloride. However, hypotension and bradycardia have been reported. Arrhythmia has also occurred. The medium peak rise of blood pressure has ranged from 20 to 25 per cent of preanaesthetic values. Depending on the condition of the patient, this elevation of blood pressure may be considered an adverse reaction or a beneficial effect.

*Respiratory:* Depression of respiration or apnoea may occur following too rapid intravenous administration or high doses of ketamine hydrochloride. Laryngospasm and other forms of airway obstruction have occurred during ketamine hydrochloride anaesthesia.

*Ocular:* Diplopia and nystagmus may occur following ketamine hydrochloride administration. A slight elevation in intraocular pressure may also occur.

*Psychological:* During recovery from anaesthesia the patient may experience emergence delirium, characterised by vivid dreams (pleasant or unpleasant), with or without psychomotor activity, manifested by confusion and irrational behaviour. The fact that these reactions are observed less often in the young (15 years of age or less) makes Ketalar especially useful in paediatric anaesthesia. These reactions are also less frequent in the elderly (over 65 years of age) patient. The incidence of emergence reactions is reduced as experience with the drug is gained. No residual psychological effects are known to have resulted from the use of Ketalar.

*Neurological:* In some patients, enhanced skeletal muscle tone may be manifested by tonic and clonic movements sometimes resembling seizures. These movements do not imply a light plane of anaesthesia and are not indicative of a need for additional doses of the anaesthetic.

*Gastro-intestinal:* Anorexia, nausea, and vomiting have been observed; however, these are minimal and are not usually severe. The great majority of patients are able to take liquids by mouth shortly after regaining consciousness.

*Other:* Local pain and exanthema at the injection site have infrequently been reported. Transient erythema and/or morbilliform rash have also been reported. Increased salivation leading to respiratory difficulties may occur unless an antisialogogue is used.

*Symptoms and treatment of overdosage:* Respiratory depression can result from an overdosage of ketamine hydrochloride. Supportive ventilation should be employed. Mechanical support of respiration that will maintain adequate blood oxygen saturation and carbon dioxide elimination is preferred to administration of analeptics.

Ketalar has a wide margin of safety; several instances of unintentional administration of overdoses of Ketalar (up to 10 times that usually required) have been followed by prolonged but complete recovery.

**Pharmaceutical precautions** Barbiturates and Ketalar, being chemically incompatible because of precipitate formation, should not be injected from the same syringe.

Protect from light. Do not freeze. Store at a temperature not exceeding 25°C.

A 1 mg/ml solution of ketamine in dextrose 5% or sodium chloride 0.9% is stable for 24 hours.

Discard any solution left after the end of each operating session

**Legal category** POM. Ketamine hydrochloride is to be used only in hospitals by or under the supervision of experienced medically qualified anaesthetists.

**Package quantities** Vials of 20 ml containing 10 mg ketamine base per ml.

Vials of 10 ml containing 50 mg ketamine base per ml.

Vials of 10 ml containing 100 mg ketamine base per ml.

**Further information** Nil

**Product licence numbers**
Ketalar 10 mg per ml 0018/5117
Ketalar 50 mg per ml 0018/5118
Ketalar 100 mg per ml 0018/0015

# LENTIZOL*

**Qualitative and quantitative composition** Lentizol 50 mg is supplied in white pellets in a size 2 capsule with a pink body and a red cap radially marked LENTIZOL 50, each capsule contains Amitriptyline Hydrochloride BP 50 mg.

Lentizol 25 mg is supplied in white pellets in a size 3 all-pink capsule radially marked LENTIZOL 25, each capsule contains Amitriptyline Hydrochloride BP 25 mg.

**Pharmaceutical form** Oral capsules

**Clinical particulars** *Therapeutic indications:* Symptoms of depressive illness especially where sedation is required.

*Posology and method of administration:* Oral administration.

*Adults and adolescents over 16 years old:* Initially 50-100 mg as a single dose at night, increasing to 200 mg/day according to clinical response. Once a satisfactory response has been obtained, the dosage should be reduced to the lowest dose that will maintain the symptomatic benefit. The usual maintenance dose is 50 -100 mg as a single dose at night.

*Elderly (over 65 years):* Initially 25-75 mg a day. Since the elderly are particularly prone to experience adverse effects such as agitation, confusion and postural hypotension; the initial dose should only be increased with caution under close medical supervision. Half the normal maintenance dose may be sufficient to produce a satisfactory clinical response.

*Children (under 16 years):* Not recommended.

*Contra-indications:* Recent cardiac infarction and patients with any degree of heart block or disorders of cardiac rhythm and those suffering from coronary artery insufficiency. Patients with mania, severe liver disease, or known hypersensitivity to dibenzazepines. Co-administration with monoamine oxidase inhibitors. Lactation. Porphyria.

*Special warnings and special precautions for use:* As improvement may not occur during the first 2-4 weeks of treatment, patients should be closely monitored during this period especially those posing a high suicidal risk.

Cardiac arrhythmias and severe hypotension are likely to occur with high dosage or in deliberate overdosage. They may also occur in patients with pre-existing heart disease taking normal dosage.

Unless essential it is inadvisable to combine Lentizol with ECT.

When Lentizol is used for the depressive component of schizophrenia, psychotic symptoms may be aggravated. In manic-depressives, a shift towards the manic phase may occur; paranoid delusions, with or without associated hostility, may be aggravated.

Avoid if possible in patients with a history of urinary retention, narrow angle glaucoma, impaired liver function, or increased ocular pressure, symptoms suggestive of prostatic hypertrophy and a history of epilepsy. Lentizol should be used with caution in hyperthyroid patients.

Anaesthetics given during tri/tetracyclic antidepressant therapy may increase the risk of arrhythmias and hypotension. If possible, discontinue Lentizol several days before surgery; if emergency surgery is unavoidable, the anaesthetist should be informed that the patient is being so treated.

Hyperpyrexia has been reported with tricyclic antidepressants when administered with anticholinergic or with neuroleptic medications.

Abrupt withdrawal of Lentizol should be avoided.

*Interactions with other medicaments and other forms of interaction:* Lentizol should not be administered concurrently, or within 14 days of termination of treatment with MAO inhibitors. It should not be given with sympathomimetic agents such as adrenaline, ephedrine, isoprenaline, noradrenaline, phenylephrine, and phenylpropanolamine, and should be used with caution when administered concurrently with anticholinergic drugs, or thyroid medications.

Lentizol may counteract the effect of adrenergic

neurone blocking agents, and possibly clonidine, and therefore it would be advisable to review all antihypertensive therapy during treatment.

The action of Lentizol may be decreased by barbiturates, and potentiated by methylphenidate. Lentizol may enhance the response to alcohol, barbiturates and other CNS depressants.

Cimetidine is reported to reduce hepatic metabolism of certain tricyclic antidepressants.

Delirium has been reported in patients taking amitriptyline with disulfiram.

*Pregnancy and lactation:* Do not use during pregnancy, especially during the first and last trimesters, unless there are compelling reasons. There is no, or inadequate, evidence of safety of the drug in human pregnancy. There is evidence of harmful effects in pregnancy in animals, when given in exceptionally high doses.

Adverse effects such as withdrawal symptoms, respiratory depression and agitation have been reported in neonates whose mothers had taken amitriptyline during the last trimester of pregnancy.

Amitriptyline is detectable in breast milk. Because of the potential for serious adverse reactions in infants from amitriptyline, Lentizol should not be given to mothers during breast feeding. A decision should be made whether to discontinue breast-feeding or discontinue the drug.

*Effects on ability to drive or use machines:* Amitriptyline may initially impair alertness and also potentiate the CNS depressant effects of alcohol. Patients should be warned of the possible hazard when driving or operating machinery. This can usually be controlled by reducing the dose. If necessary the dose can be subsequently increased gradually.

*Undesirable efects:* The following adverse effects, although not necessarily all reported with amitriptyline, have occurred with tricyclic antidepressants.

*Anticholinergic:* Excessive perspiration, dryness of mouth, blurred vision, mydriasis, disturbed accommodation, increased intraocular pressure, hyperpyrexia, urinary retention, and urinary tract dilatation. These symptoms are common but usually lessen on continuing therapy.

*Cardiovascular reactions:* hypotension, syncope, postural hypotension, hypertension, tachycardia, palpitations, myocardial infarction, arrhythmias, heart block, stroke, non-specific ECG and AV conduction changes.

*CNS and Neuromuscular:* confusional states, disturbed concentration, disorientation, delusions, hallucinations, hypomania, excitement, anxiety, restlessness, drowsiness, insomnia, nightmares, numbness, tingling, and paraesthesiae of the extremities, peripheral neuropathy, incoordination, ataxia, tremors, coma, convulsions, alteration of EEG, extrapyramidal symptoms, including abnormal involuntary movements and tardive dyskinesia, dysarthria, tinnitus, dizziness, weakness, fatigue, headache.

*Allergic:* Skin rash, urticaria, photosensitisation, oedema of face and tongue.

*Haematological:* bone-marrow depression including agranulocytosis, leucopenia, eosinophilia, purpura, thrombocytopenia.

*Gastrointestinal:* nausea, epigastric distress, vomiting, anorexia, stomatitis, unpleasant taste, diarrhoea, weight loss, increased appetite and weight gain (may be a drug reaction or due to relief of the depression), parotid swelling, black tongue, rarely hepatitis (including altered liver function and cholestatic jaundice) constipation, paralytic ileus.

*Endocrine:* testicular swelling, gynaecomastia, breast enlargement, galactorrhoea, increased or decreased libido, impotence, interference with sexual function, elevation or lowering of blood sugar levels, inappropriate ADH (antidiuretic hormone) secretion.

*Other:* oedema, urinary frequency, alopecia

Withdrawal symptoms may occur on abrupt cessation of therapy and include insomnia, irritability, nausea, headache and excessive perspiration.

Mania or hypomania has been reported rarely within 2-7 days of stopping chronic therapy with tricyclic antidepressants.

*Overdose:* Amitriptyline exerts an anticholinergic effect as well as antihistamine and adrenaline blocking actions. Large doses produce temporary confusion, disturbed concentration, transient visual hallucinations, drowsiness, hypothermia, convulsions, coma, apnoea, tachycardia and other rhythm dysfunctions such as bundle branch block, ECG evidence of impaired conduction, congestive heart failure, dilated pupils, disorders of ocular motility, severe hypotension, stupor, polyradiculoneuropathy, and intestinal stasis.

Other symptoms may be agitation, hyperactive reflexes, muscle rigidity, vomiting, hyperpyrexia, or any of those listed as adverse effects.

*Treatment:* Gastric lavage and emesis if appropriate. Following lavage, activated charcoal may be given during the first 24-48 hours at a dosage of 20-30 g every four to six hours. Vital signs should be continuously monitored and patients should be treated in hospital wherever possible. General supportive measures should be initiated with careful attention to electrolyte balance. An ECG should be taken and close monitoring of cardiac function instituted if there is any sign of abnormality. Cardiac irregularities may need controlling with antiarrhythmic drugs and physostigmine salicylate may be indicated. If convulsions occur, paraldelyde, diazepam or inhalation anaesthetics, but not barbiturates, may be indicated. Forced diuresis and haemodialysis have no place in treatment. An open airway and an adequate fluid intake should be maintained, and body temperature regulated.

**Pharmacological properties.**

*Pharmacodynamic properties:* Amitriptyline is a tricyclic antidepressant. It prevents re-uptake and hence inactivation of noradrenaline and serotonin at nerve terminals. The precise mechanism by which an antidepressant effect is achieved remains unclear.

*Pharmacokinetic properties:* After release from Lentizol capsules, amitriptyline is readily absorbed from the gastro-intestinal tract. Peak serum levels are reached between 6 and 12 hours after administration of Lentizol.

Amitriptyline is extensively demethylated in the liver to its primary active metabolite, nortriptyline. Paths of metabolism of both amitriptyline and nortriptyline include hydroxylation (possibly to active metabolites), n-oxidation, and conjugation with glucuronic acid. Amitriptyline is excreted in the urine, mainly in the form of its metabolites, either free or in conjugated form. Amitriptyline and nortriptyline are widely distributed throughout the body and are extensively bound to plasma and tissue protein. Amitriptyline has been estimated to have a half-life ranging from 9 to 25 hours, which may be considerably extended in overdosage. Plasma concentrations of amitriptyline and nortriptyline vary very widely between individuals and simple correlation with therapeutic reponse has been established. Amitriptyline and nortriptyline cross the placental barrier and are excreted in breast milk.

*Pre-clinical safety data:* Pre-clinical safety data does not add anything of further significance to the prescriber.

**Pharmaceutical particulars**

*List of excipients:* Lentizol 50 mg capsules contain the following excipients – Active pellets: Sucrose, maize starch, stearic acid, diffulac (shellac), povidone and talc. Neutral pellets: Sucrose, maize starch, stearic acid, talc and diffulac (shellac). Gelatin capsule shell: E127, E132, E122.

Lentizol 25 mg capsules contain the following excipients – Active pellets: Sucrose, maize starch, stearic acid, diffulac (shellac), povidone and talc. Neutral pellets: Sucrose, maize starch, stearic acid, talc and diffulac (shellac). Gelatin capsule shell: E127, E132.

*Incompatibilities:* Not applicable.

*Shelf-life:* Two years.

*Special precautions for storage:* Store in a dry place, at a temperature not exceeding 30°C

*Nature and contents of container:*

PVC/PVdC blister pack, containing 56 or 100 capsules.

*Instructions for use/handling:* No special requirements.

*Marketing authorisation holder:* Parke, Davis & Company, Usk Road, Pontypool, NP4 0YH

**Marketing authorisation numbers**
Lentizol 50 mg 0018/0174
Lentizol 25 mg 0018/0173

**Date of approval/revision of SPC** June 1995

**Legal category** POM

## LIPITOR* ▼

**Qualitative and quantitative composition** Lipitor Tablets contain atorvastatin calcium (trihydrate) equivalent to 10, 20 and 40 mg atorvastatin per tablet.

**Pharmaceutical form** Lipitor is supplied as 10, 20, and 40 mg film-coated tablets for oral administration.

**Clinical particulars** *Therapeutic indications:* Lipitor is indicated as an adjunct to diet for reduction of elevated total cholesterol, LDL-cholesterol, apolipoprotein B, and triglycerides in patients with primary hypercholesterolaemia, heterozygous familial hypercholesterolaemia or combined (mixed) hyperlipidaemia when response to diet and other nonpharmacological measures is inadequate.

Lipitor is also indicated as an adjunct to diet and other non-dietary measures in reducing elevated total cholesterol, LDL-cholesterol, and apolipoprotein B in patients with homozygous familial hypercholesterolaemia when response to these measures is inadequate.

*Posology and method of administration:* The patient should be placed on a standard cholesterol-lowering diet before receiving Lipitor and should continue on this diet during treatment with Lipitor. The usual starting dose is 10 mg once a day. Doses should be individualised according to baseline LDL-C levels, the goal of therapy, and patient response. Adjustment of dosage should be made at intervals of 4 weeks or more. The maximum dose is 80 mg once a day. Doses may be given at any time of day with or without food.

*Primary hypercholesterolaemia and combined (mixed) hyperlipidaemia:* The majority of patients are controlled with 10 mg Lipitor once a day. A therapeutic response is evident within 2 weeks, and the maximum response is usually achieved within 4 weeks. The response is maintained during chronic therapy.

The following treatment guidelines may be used to establish treatment goals (Table 1).

*TABLE 1. European Atherosclerosis Society Treatment Goals for Lipid Management*

| Patient Population | Treatment Goal | mg/dL | mmol/l |
|---|---|---|---|
| No risk factors and no CHD | LDL-C | 155-175 | 4-4.5 |
| One risk factor and no CHD | LDL-C | 135-155 | 3.5-4 |
| Two or more risk factors, CHD, PVD, or famililal hypercholesterolaemia | LDL-C | 115-135 | 3-3.5 |

CHD = Coronary heart disease; PVD = Peripheral vascular disease.

*Heterozygous familial hypercholesterolaemia:* Patients should be started with Lipitor 10 mg daily. Doses should be individualised and adjusted every 4 weeks to 40 mg daily. Thereafter, either the dose may be increased to a maximum of 80 mg daily or a bile acid sequestrant (eg, colestipol) may be combined with 40 mg Lipitor.

*Homozygous familial hypercholesterolaemia: Adults:* In a compassionate-use study of patients with homozygous familial hypercholesterolaemia, most patients responded to a dose of 80 mg of Lipitor (see *Pharmacodynamic properties*).

*Children:* Treatment experience in a paediatric population with doses of Lipitor up to 80 mg/day is limited.

*Dosage in patients with renal insufficiency:* Renal disease has no influence on the plasma concentrations nor lipid effects of Lipitor; thus, no adjustment of dose is required.

*Dosage in patients with hepatic dysfunction:* In patients with moderate to severe hepatic dysfunction, the therapeutic response to Lipitor is unaffected but exposure to the drug is greatly increased. Cmax increases by approximately 16 fold and AUC (0-24) by approximately 11 fold. Therefore, caution should be exercised in patients who consume substantial quantities of alcohol and/or have a history of liver disease.

*Geriatric use:* Adequate treatment experience in adults age 70 or older with doses of Lipitor up to 80 mg/day has been obtained. Efficacy and safety in older patients using recommended doses is similar to that seen in the general population.

*Contra-indications:* Lipitor is contra-indicated in patients with hypersensitivity to any component of this medication, active liver disease or unexplained persistent elevations of serum transaminases exceeding 3 times the upper limit of normal, during pregnancy, while breast-feeding, and in women of child-bearing potential not using appropriate contraceptive measures.

*Special warnings and special precautions for use:*

*Liver effects:* Liver function tests should be performed before the initiation of treatment and periodically thereafter. Patients who develop any signs or symptoms suggestive of liver injury should have liver function tests performed. Patients who develop increased transaminase levels should be monitored until the abnormality(ies) resolve. Should an increase in ALT or AST of greater than 3 times the upper limit of normal persist, reduction of dose or withdrawal of Lipitor is recommended.

Lipitor should be used with caution in patients who consume substantial quantities of alcohol and/or have a history of liver disease.

*Skeletal muscle efects:* Uncomplicated myalgia has been reported in Lipitor-treated patients. Lipitor therapy should be discontinued if markedly elevated CPK levels occur or myopathy is diagnosed or suspected. Patients who develop any signs or symptoms suggestive of myopathy should have CPK levels measured. Should significant increases in CPK persist, reduction of dose or withdrawal of Lipitor is recommended.

These CPK elevations should be considered when evaluating the possibility of myocardial infarction in the differential diagnosis of chest pain.

Rhabdomyolysis with renal dysfunction secondary to myoglobinuria has been reported with other drugs in this class.

*Interactions with other medicaments and other forms of interaction:* The risk of myopathy during treatment with other drugs in this class is increased with concurrent administration of cyclosporin, fibric acid derivatives, erythromycin, azole antifungals, or niacin. This increase in risk may also occur when combining these drugs with Lipitor.

Phenazone (antipyrine) is a non-specific model for evaluation of drug metabolism by the hepatic microsomal enzyme system. Administration of multiple doses of Lipitor with phenazone showed little or no detectable effect on the pharmacokinetics of phenazone in healthy subjects (no change in the clearance of phenazone but the formation clearance of 4-hydroxyphenazone increased by 20% and that of norphenazone by 8%).

More specific *in vitro* studies using human hepatic microsomes and cells expressing human cytochrome P450 isozymes show that atorvastatin, like other HMG-CoA reductase inhibitors, is metabolised by cytochrome P450 3A4 indicating the possibility of an interaction with drugs also metabolised by this isozyme. When combining Lipitor with other drugs which are the substrate of this isozyme (eg, immunomodulators, many antiarrhythmic agents, some calcium channel antagonists and some benzodiazepines) the possibility of a change in the plasma drug levels of either drug should be considered. In clinical studies in which Lipitor was administered with antihypertensives (including ACE inhibitors, beta-blockers, calcium channel antagonists, and diuretics) or hypoglycaemic agents no clinically significant interactions were seen.

Based on experience with other HMG-CoA reductase inhibitors caution should also be exercised when Lipitor is administered with inhibitors of cytochrome P450 3A4 (eg, macrolide antibiotics and azole antifungals). The effect of inducers of cytochrome P450 3A4 (eg, rifampicin or phenytoin) on Lipitor is unknown.

*Digoxin:* Administration of multiple doses of Lipitor with digoxin increased steady-state plasma digoxin concentrations by approximately 20%. Patients taking digoxin should be monitored appropriately.

*Erythromycin:* In healthy individuals, administration of Lipitor with erythromycin (500 mg QID), a known inhibitor of cytochrome P450 3A4, was associated with higher plasma concentrations of atorvastatin.

*Oral contraceptives:* Administration of Lipitor with an oral contraceptive containing norethisterone and ethinyl oestradiol produced increases in plasma concentrations of norethisterone and ethinyl oestradiol. These increased concentrations should be considered when selecting oral contraceptive doses.

*Colestipol:* Plasma concentrations of atorvastatin were lower (approximately 25%) when colestipol was administered with Lipitor. However, lipid effects were greater when Lipitor and colestipol were administered together than when either drug was given alone.

*Antacid:* Administration of Lipitor with an oral antacid suspension containing magnesium and aluminium hydroxides decreased atorvastatin plasma concentrations approximately 35%; however, LDL-C reduction was not altered.

*Warfarin:* Administration of Lipitor with warfarin caused a minimal decrease in prothrombin time (mean ± SE of 1.7±0.4 seconds) during the first 4 days of dosing with 80 mg Lipitor. Dosing continued for 15 days and prothrombin time returned to normal by the end of Lipitor treatment. Nevertheless, patients receiving warfarin should be closely monitored when Lipitor is added to their therapy.

*Cimetidine:* An interaction study with cimetidine and Lipitor was conducted, and no interaction was seen.

*Pregnancy and lactation:* Lipitor is contraindicated in pregnancy and while breast feeding. Women of child-bearing potential should use appropriate contraceptive measures.

An interval of 1 month should be allowed from stopping Lipitor treatment to conception in the event of planning a pregnancy.

In animal studies atorvastatin had no effect on fertility and was not teratogenic, however, at maternally toxic doses foetal toxicity was observed in rats and rabbits. The development of the rat offspring was delayed and post-natal survival reduced during exposure of the dams to atorvastatin equivalent to 6 and 21 times that expected in man, respectively.

In rats, plasma concentrations of atorvastatin are similar to those in milk. It is not known whether this drug or its metabolites is excreted in human milk.

*Effects on ability to drive or use machines:* There is no pattern of reported adverse events suggesting that patients taking Lipitor will have any impairment of ability to drive and use hazardous machinery.

*Adverse effects:* Lipitor is generally well-tolerated.

Adverse reactions have usually been mild and transient. Less than 2% of patients were discontinued from clinical trials due to side effects attributed to Lipitor.

The most frequent (1% or more) adverse effects associated with Lipitor therapy, in patients participating in controlled clinical studies are constipation, flatulence, dyspepsia, abdominal pain, headache, nausea, myalgia, asthenia, diarrhoea, and insomnia.

Elevated serum ALT levels have been reported in 1.3% of patients receiving Lipitor. Clinically important (>3 times upper normal limit) elevations in serum ALT levels occurred in 19 of the 2483 (0.8%) patients on Lipitor. It was dose related and was reversible in all 19 patients. In 10 cases, the increase was first observed within 12 weeks of starting the treatment. Only 1 case occurred after 36 weeks and only 1 patient had symptoms suggestive of hepatitis. Treatment was discontinued in only 9 of these 19 cases.

Elevated serum CPK levels (>3 times upper normal limit) occurred in 62 of the 2452 (2.5%) patients on Lipitor compared with 3.1% with other HMG-CoA reductase inhibitors in clinical trials. Levels above 10 times the normal upper range occurred in only 11 (0.4%) Lipitor-treated patients. Only 3 (0.1%) of these 11 patients had concurrent muscle pain, tenderness, or weakness.

The following additional adverse effects have been reported in clinical trials. Not all effects listed have necessarily been associated with Lipitor therapy: muscle cramps, myositis, myopathy, paraesthesia, peripheral neuropathy, pancreatitis, hepatitis, cholestatic jaundice, anorexia, vomiting, alopecia, pruritus, rash, impotence, hyperglycaemia, and hypoglycaemia. Chest pain, dizziness, angina, and allergic reactions have also been reported in isolated cases.

*Overdose:* Specific treatment is not available for Lipitor overdosage. Should an overdose occur, the patient should be treated symptomatically and supportive measures instituted, as required. Liver function tests and serum CPK levels should be monitored. Due to extensive drug binding to plasma proteins, haemodialysis is not expected to significantly enhance atorvastatin clearance.

### Pharmacological properties

*Pharmacodynamic properties:* Atorvastatin is a selective, competitive inhibitor of HMG-CoA reductase, the rate-limiting enzyme responsible for the conversion of 3-hydroxy-3-methyl-glutaryl-coenzyme A to mevalonate, a precursor of sterols, including cholesterol. Triglycerides and cholesterol in the liver are incorporated into VLDL and released into the plasma for delivery to peripheral tissues. Low-density lipoprotein (LDL) is formed from VLDL and is catabolised primarily through the high affinity LDL receptor.

Atorvastatin lowers plasma cholesterol and lipoprotein levels by inhibiting HMG-CoA reductase and cholesterol synthesis in the liver and increases the number of hepatic LDL receptors on the cell surface for enhanced uptake and catabolism of LDL.

Atorvastatin reduces LDL production and the number of LDL particles. Atorvastatin produces a profound and sustained increase in LDL receptor activity coupled with a beneficial change in the quality of circulating LDL particles.

Approximately 70% of circulating inhibitory activity for HMG-CoA reductase is attributed to active metabolites (see *Pharmacokinetic properties*).

Atorvastatin has been shown to reduce total-C, LDL-C, apolipoprotein B, and triglycerides while producing variable increases in HDL-C in a dose-response study as shown in Table 2 below.

TABLE 2. Dose Response in Patients With Primary Hypercholesterolaemia

| Lipitor Dose (mg) | N | Total-C | LDL-C | Apo B | TG | HDL-C |
|---|---|---|---|---|---|---|
| Placebo | 12 | 5 | 8 | 6 | -1 | -2 |
| 10 | 11 | -30 | -41 | -34 | -14 | 4 |
| 20 | 10 | -35 | -44 | -36 | -33 | 12 |
| 40 | 11 | -38 | -50 | -41 | -25 | -3 |
| 80 | 11 | -46 | -61 | -50 | -27 | 3 |

Adjusted mean % change from baseline

These results are consistent in patients with heterozygous familial hypercholesterolaemia, nonfamilial forms of hypercholesterolaemia, and mixed hyperlipidaemia, including patients with noninsulin-dependent diabetes mellitus.

Atorvastatin produced a variable but small increase in apolipoprotein AI. However, there was no clear dose response effect.

Lipitor is effective in reducing LDL-C in patients with homozygous familial hypercholesterolaemia, a population that has not usually responded to lipid-lowering medication. In a compassionate use study, 41 patients aged 6 to 51 years with homozygous familial hypercholesterolaemia or with severe hypercholesterolaemia, who had ≤15% reduction in LDL-C

in response to previous maximum dose combination drug therapy, received daily doses of 40 to 80 mg of Lipitor. Twenty four patients with homozygous familial hypercholesterolaemia received 80 mg Lipitor. Nineteen of these 24 patients responded with a greater than 15% reduction of LDL-C (mean 26%, range 18% to 42%).

*Pharmacokinetic properties: Absorption:* Atorvastatin is rapidly absorbed after oral administration; maximum plasma concentrations occur within 1 to 2 hours. Extent of absorption increases in proportion to atorvastatin dose. Lipitor tablets are bioequivalent to atorvastatin solutions. The absolute bioavailability of atorvastatin is approximately 12% and the systemic availability of HMG-CoA reductase inhibitory activity is approximately 30%. The low systemic availability is attributed to presystemic clearance in gastrointestinal mucosa and/or hepatic first-pass metabolism.
*Distribution:* Mean volume of distribution of atorvastatin is approximately 565 L. Atorvastatin is ≥98% bound to plasma proteins.

*Metabolism:* Atorvastatin is metabolised by cytochrome P450 3A4 to ortho- and parahydroxylated derivatives and various beta-oxidation products. In vitro inhibition of HMG-CoA reductase by ortho- and parahydroxylated metabolites is equivalent to that of atorvastatin. Approximately 70% of circulating inhibitory activity for HMG-CoA reductase is attributed to active metabolites.

*Excretion:* Atorvastatin is eliminated primarily in bile following hepatic and/or extrahepatic metabolism. However, the drug does not appear to undergo significant enterohepatic recirculation. Mean plasma elimination half-life of atorvastatin in humans is approximately 14 hours. The half-life of inhibitory activity for HMG-CoA reductase is approximately 20 to 30 hours due to the contribution of active metabolites.

*Special populations:*
*Geriatric:* Plasma concentrations of atorvastatin are higher in healthy elderly subjects than in young adults while the lipid effects were comparable to those seen in younger patient populations.
*Paediatric:* Pharmacokinetic data in the paediatric population are not available.
*Gender:* Concentrations of atorvastatin in women differ (approximately 20% higher for Cmax and 10% lower for AUC) from those in men. These differences were of no clinical significance, resulting in no clinically significant differences in lipid effects among men and women.
*Renal insufficiency:* Renal disease has no influence on the plasma concentrations or lipid effects of atorvastatin.
*Hepatic insufficiency:* Plasma concentrations of atorvastatin are markedly increased (approximately 16-fold in Cmax and 11-fold in AUC) in patients with chronic alcoholic liver disease (Childs-Pugh B).

*Pre-clinical safety data:* Atorvastatin was not carcinogenic in rats. The maximum dose used was 63-fold higher than the highest human dose (80 mg/day) on a mg/kg body-weight basis and 8 to 16-fold higher based on AUC(0-24) values as determined by total inhibitory activity. In a 2-year study in mice, incidences of hepatocellular adenoma in males and hepatocellular carcinomas in females were increased at the maximum dose used, and the maximum dose used was 250-fold higher than the highest human dose on a mg/kg body-weight basis. Systemic exposure was 6 to 11-fold higher based on AUC(0-24). Atorvastatin did not demonstrate mutagenic or clastogenic potential in 4 in vitro tests with and without metabolic activation and in 1 in vivo assay.

### Pharmaceutical particulars

*List of excipients:* The 10, 20, and 40 mg dosage forms each contain the following excipients: Calcium Carbonate, Microcrystalline Cellulose, Lactose (Hydrous), Croscarmellose Sodium, Polysorbate 80, Hydroxypropyl Cellulose, Magnesium Stearate, Opadry White YS-1-7040 (Hydroxypropyl methylcellulose, Polyethylene glycol, Titanium dioxide, Talc), Simethicone Emulsion (Simethicone, Stearate emulsifiers, Sorbic acid, Water), Candelilla Wax

*Incompatibilities:* None.

*Shelf-life:* Two years.

*Special precautions for storage:* None.

*Nature and contents of container:* Foil/foil blisters consisting of a polyamide/aluminium foil/polyvinyl chloride unit-dose blister and a paper/polyester/aluminium foil/vinyl heat-seal coated backing or an aluminium foil/vinyl heat-seal coated backing.
Lipitor is supplied in packs of 28 tablets.

*Instructions for use/handling:* No special requirements needed.

*Marketing authorisation holder:* Parke, Davis & Company, Usk Road, Pontypool, NP4 0YH

### Marketing authorisation numbers
Lipitor Tablets 10 mg 0018/0240
Lipitor Tablets 20 mg 0018/0241
Lipitor Tablets 40 mg 0018/0242

**Date of approval/revision of SPC** 7 November 1996

**Legal category** POM

## LOESTRIN*

**Qualitative and quantitative composition** Each Loestrin 20 tablet contains: Norethisterone Acetate BP 1 mg and Ethinyloestradiol PhEur 20 micrograms.

Each Loestrin 30 tablet contains: Norethisterone Acetate BP 1.5 mg and Ethinyloestradiol PhEur 30 micrograms.

**Pharmaceutical form** Loestrin 20: Pale blue grey film coated tablets. Loestrin 30: Green film coated tablets

**Clinical particulars** *Therapeutic indications:* For the prevention of pregnancy in women who elect to use oral contraceptives. The efficacy of any contraceptive method, except sterilisation, depends on the reliability with which it is used. Correct and consistent use of methods can result in lower failure rates.

*Posology and method of administration:* For Oral administration.

One Loestrin tablet should be taken daily at approximately the same time of day for three weeks, starting on the first day of menstrual bleeding, and then an interval of one week allowed before commencing the second course of tablets. If starting on the fourth day of the cycle or later, additional contraceptive precautions should be used for the first seven days. Second and subsequent courses should be taken for three weeks with one week without tablets between courses. Thus each new course of tablets is always started on the same day of the week. It is important that the tablets are taken as directed and should be taken without regard to menstrual bleeding except in the initial cycle.

*Missed pills:* If a tablet is not taken at the usual time, it must be taken as soon as possible and the next tablet taken at the normal time. If the delay exceeds twelve hours, additional contraception (barriers and spermicides) should be used for the next 7 days whilst continuing to take Loestrin. Additionally, therefore, if pills have been missed during the last 7 days of a pack, there should be no break before the next pack is started.

*Gastrointestinal upset:* Vomiting or diarrhoea may reduce efficacy by preventing full absorption. Barriers and spermicides should therefore be used during and for 7 days after recovery and if these 7 days overrun the end of a pack, the next pack should be started without a break. In this case, a withdrawal bleed should not be expected until the end of the second pack. If the patient does not have a withdrawal bleed at the end of the second pack, she must return to the doctor to exclude the possibility of pregnancy.

*Changing from another 21 day combined oral contraceptive to Loestrin:* The first Loestrin tablet should be taken on the first day immediately after the end of the previous oral contraceptive course. Additional contraception is not required. A withdrawal bleed should not be expected until the end of the first Loestrin pack.

*Changing from an every day (ED) 28 day combined oral contraceptive to Loestrin:* The first tablet of Loestrin should be taken on the day immediately after the day on which the last active pill in the ED pack has been taken. The remaining (inactive) tablets in the ED pack should be discarded. Additional contraception is not required. A withdrawal bleed should not be expected until the end of the first pack of Loestrin.

*Changing from a progestogen-only-pill (POP) to Loestrin:* The first tablet of Loestrin should be taken on the first day of menstruation, even if the POP for that day has already been taken. The remaining tablets in the POP pack should be discarded. Additional contraception is not required.

*Post-partum and post-abortum use:* After pregnancy combined oral contraception can be started in non-lactating women 21 days after a vaginal delivery, provided that the patient is fully ambulant and there are no puerperal complications.

If the pill is started later than 21 days after delivery, then barriers and spermicides should be used until oral contraception is started and for the first 7 days of pill-taking. If unprotected intercourse has taken place after 21 days post partum, then oral contraception should not be started until the first menstrual bleed after childbirth.

After a miscarriage or abortion, oral contraceptives may be started immediately.

*Contra-indications:* (1) Known or suspected pregnancy and lactation

(2) Thrombo-embolic disorders, or a past history of these conditions, ischaemic heart disease, severe hypertension or coagulation abnormalities.

(3) Liver disease including disorders of hepatic

excretion eg. Dublin Johnson or Rotor syndromes, infective hepatitis (until liver function returns to normal), known or suspected disorders of lipid metabolism, porphyria, liver adenoma or carcinoma, gall stones or jaundice with prior pill use.

(4) Sickle cell anaemia

(5) Known or suspected carcinoma of the breast or oestrogen dependent neoplasms

(6) Undiagnosed abnormal vaginal bleeding

(7) History during pregnancy of idiopathic jaundice, severe pruritus, chorea, herpes or deterioration of otosclerosis.

(8) Focal, severe or crescendo migraine or transient cerebral ischaemic attacks without headaches

*Special warnings and special precautions for use:* The following information is principally based on studies in patients who used oral contraceptives with higher concentrations of oestrogens and progestogens than those in common use today. The effect of long-term use of the oral contraceptive with lower concentrations of both oestrogens and progestogens remains to be determined. The efficacy of any contraceptive method, except sterilisation, depends upon the reliability with which it is used. Correct and consistent use of methods can result in lower failure rates.

*Thrombo-embolism:* The use of oral contraceptives has been shown to be associated with an increased risk of thrombo-embolic disorders. The physician should be alert to the earliest manifestations of these disorders (thrombophlebitis, cerebrovascular disorders, pulmonary embolism, and retinal thrombosis). Should any of these occur or be suspected, Loestrin should be discontinued immediately.

Certain factors may predispose to the development of thrombosis eg. smoking, obesity, age, the presence of varicose veins, cardiovascular disease, diabetes and migraine. The suitability of combined oral contraceptives for patients with any of these conditions should be discussed with the patient before a final decision is taken.

Cigarette smoking increases the risk of serious cardiovascular side effects from oral contraceptive use. This risk increases with age and with heavy smoking (15 or more cigarettes a day) and is quite marked in women over 35 years of age. Women who use oral contraceptives should be strongly advised not to smoke.

*Hepatic tumours:* Benign hepatic tumours have been associated with oral contraceptive usage. Malignant hepatic tumours have also been reported on rare occasions in long term users of oral contraceptives. A hepatic tumour should be considered in the differential diagnosis when upper abdominal pain, enlarged liver or signs of intra-abdominal haemorrhage occur.

*Ovarian, endometrial, cervical and breast cancer:* Numerous epidemiological studies have been reported on the risks of ovarian, endometrial, cervical and breast cancer in women using combined oral contraceptives. The evidence is clear that combined oral contraceptives offer substantial protection against both ovarian and endometrial cancer.

An increased risk of cervical cancer in long term users of combined oral contraceptives has been reported in some studies, but there continues to be controversy about the extent to which this is attributable to the confounding effects of sexual behaviour and other factors.

The evidence linking combined oral contraceptive use and breast cancer remains inconclusive. The results of some studies suggest an increased risk of breast cancer presenting below the age of about 35, the risk rising with duration of use. Any possible increased risk of breast cancer with combined oral contraceptives is however likely to be small, and may be expected to be less with low dosage pills. This possible risk should be weighed against the many benefits of combined oral contraceptives, including their protective effects against ovarian and endometrial cancers.

*Reasons for stopping Loestrin immediately:* (1) Occurrence of migraine in patients who have never previously suffered from it. Any unusually frequent or severe headaches.

(2) Any kind of visual disturbance eg. proptosis or diplopia and migraine.

(3) Suspicion of thrombosis or infarction.

(4) Combined oral contraceptives should be stopped at least six weeks before elective surgery and during and following prolonged immobilisation eg. after accidents etc.

(5) Loestrin should be discontinued if the patient becomes jaundiced or has a significant rise in blood pressure.

(6) Patients with a history of depression should be carefully observed and the drug discontinued if the depression recurs to a serious degree.

(7) Since the safety of Loestrin in pregnancy has not been demonstrated, it is recommended that for any patient who has missed a period, the absence of pregnancy should be established before continuing the contraceptive regimen.

(8) Clear exacerbation of conditions known to be capable of deteriorating during oral contraception or pregnancy.

A complete medical history and physical examination should be undertaken prior to the initiation or re-institution of oral contraceptives and periodically thereafter. The physical examination may be deferred until after initiation of the oral contraceptive if requested by the patient and judged appropriate by the clinician.

The pre-treatment and periodic physical examination should include special reference to blood pressure, breast, abdomen and pelvic organs, including relevant laboratory tests and Papanicolaou smear since oestrogens have been known to produce tumours, some of them malignant in five species of subprimate animals.

In case of undiagnosed, persistent or recurrent abnormal vaginal bleeding, appropriate diagnostic measures should be conducted to rule out malignancy. Women with a strong family history of breast cancer or who have breast nodules should be monitored with particular care.

Oestrogen-progestogen preparations should be used with caution in patients with a history of hypertension and some women experience an increase in blood pressure following the administration of contraceptive steroids. Pregnancy should be excluded before starting treatment. Because these agents may cause some degree of fluid retention, patients with conditions which might be influenced by this such as epilepsy, migraine, asthma and cardiac or renal dysfunction should be carefully monitored.

A decrease in glucose tolerance has been observed in a significant percentage of patients on oral contraceptives. The mechanism of this decrease is obscure. For this reason, prediabetic and diabetic patients should be carefully observed whilst receiving Loestrin.

Under the influence of oestrogen-progestogen preparations, pre-existing uterine fibroleiomyomata may increase in size. Loestrin may mask the onset of the climacteric.

*The following conditions also require careful consideration:* multiple sclerosis, porphyria, tetany, disturbed liver function, gall stones, cardiovascular disease, renal disease, chloasma, the wearing of contact lenses or any disease that is prone to worsen during pregnancy. The deterioration or first appearance of any of these conditions may indicate that the oral contraceptive should be stopped. Contact lens wearers who develop visual changes or changes to lens tolerance should be assessed by an optometrist.

*Interference with laboratory tests:* The following laboratory results may be altered by the use of oral contraceptives: hepatic function (increased sulphobromophthalein retention and other tests); thyroid function (increased thyroid binding globulin (TBG) leading to increased circulating total thyroid hormone as measured by protein-bound iodine (PBI), T4 by column, or by radioimmunoassay. Free T3 resin uptake is decreased, reflecting the elevated TBG. Free T4 concentration is unaltered.); haematological tests (increased prothrombin and factors VII, VIII, IX and X, decreased antithrombin 3 and increased adrenaline induced platelet aggregation); measurement of pregnanediol excretion (reduced). Other binding proteins may be elevated in the serum, sex-binding globulins are increased, triglycerides may be increased and serum folate levels may be depressed. Therefore, if such tests are abnormal in a patient taking Loestrin, it is recommended that they be repeated after Loestrin has been withdrawn for two months. The pathologist should be advised of the administration of Loestrin when relevant specimens are submitted. Any influence of prolonged administration of Loestrin on pituitary, ovarian, adrenal, hepatic and uterine functions is unknown at present.

*Interactions with other medicaments and other forms of interaction:* The effectiveness of combined oral contraceptives may be considerably reduced by interaction with drugs that induce hepatic enzyme activity eg. carbamazepine, griseofulvin, phenytoin, phenobarbitone, primidone and rifampicin. Other drugs suspected of having the capacity to reduce the efficacy of oral contraceptives include ampicillin and other broad-spectrum antibiotics.

Additional contraceptive precautions should be taken whilst taking enzyme inducing drugs and some antibiotics and for at least seven days after stopping them. If these seven days run beyond the end of the packet the new packet should be started immediately without a break. Rifampicin is such a potent inducer that even if a course lasts for less than 7 days, the additional contraceptive precautions should be continued for at least 4 weeks after stopping it.

*Pregnancy and lactation:* Loestrin is not recommended for use during pregnancy, suspected pregnancy and in lactating mothers. Studies do not suggest a teratogenic effect, paticularly in so far as cardiac anomalies and limb reduction defects are concerned, when oral contraceptives are taken inadvertently during early pregnancy. The administration of oral contraceptives to induce withdrawal bleeding should not be used as a test for pregnancy. Oral contraceptives should not be used during pregnancy to treat threatened or habitual abortion.

*Effects on ability to drive or use machines:* None expected.

*Undesirable efects:* The following adverse effects which have been reported in patients receiving oral contraceptives are believed to be drug-related.

Nausea, vomiting, gastro-intestinal symptoms (such as abdominal cramps and bloating), breakthrough bleeding, spotting, change in menstrual flow, amenorrhoea during and after treatment, oedema, chloasma, or melasma, breast changes (tenderness, enlargement and secretion), change in weight, cervical erosion and changes in cervical secretion, suppression of lactation when given immediately post-partum, cholestastic jaundice, migraine, rash (allergic), rise in blood pressure, depression, and thrombo-embolic disorders, temporary infertility after discontinuation of treatment, reduced tolerance to carbohydrates, vaginal candidiasis, change in corneal curvature (steepening) and intolerance to contact lenses.

Although the following adverse effects have been reported in women taking oral contraceptives, an association has been neither confirmed nor refuted: prolonged amenorrhoea after discontinuing oral contraceptives, pre-menstrual like syndrome, headache, nervousness, dizziness, fatigue, cataract, backache, hirsutism, loss of scalp hair, erythema multiforme, erythema nodusum, haemorrhagic eruption, itching, changes in appetite, cystitis-like syndrome, vaginitis, porphyria, impaired renal function, haemolytic uraemic syndrome, Budd-Chiari syndrome, acne, changes in libido and colitis.

*Menstrual changes:* Breakthrough bleeding happens more often in the first two or three cycles after starting the tablets. The patient should continue taking the tablets according to the schedule if breakthrough bleeding occurs. Probably it will amount to no more than spotting and will not last more than a day or two. If breakthrough bleeding is experienced after the third cycle, the patient should consult her physician.

*Overdose:* The usual effects in children are nausea and drowsiness. Slight vaginal bleeding occasionally occurs in girls. In view of the low toxicity following overdosage with oral contraceptives, it is suggested that treatment should be conservative.

**Pharmacological properties.**

*Pharmacodynamic properties:* Loestrin achieves contraceptive effect primarily by inhibition of ovulation through gonadotrophin suppression. It is thought that other sites of action such as changes in cervical mucus and in the endometrium may contribute to the efficacy of combined oral contraceptives.

*Pharmacokinetic properties: Ethinyloestradiol* is rapidly and almost completely absorbed and peak serum levels are usually attained within an hour of oral administration. At this time, the majority of drug is already conjugated, largely as the sulphate. These conjugates have a primary serum half-life of approximately 7 hours and a terminal half-life of 48 hours, and are excreted in urine and faeces.

*Norethisterone aceate* undergoes rapid absorption with peak serum concentrations ocurring at one hour after oral administration. Less than 5% is cleared as unchanged norethisterone; glucuronide and sulphate conjugates are excreted in urine and faeces. the terminal half-life for norethisterone conjugates has been estimated at 70 hours (range: 42–84 hours).

*Pre-clinical safety data:* Pre-clinical safety data does not add anything of significance to the prescriber.

**Pharmaceutical particulars**

*List of excipients:* Each Loestrin 20 tablet contains the following excipients: Lactose, sucrose, maize starch, talc, powdered acacia, magnesium stearate, industrial methylated spirit*, purified water*, dichloromethane (technical grade)*, propylene glycol*, hypromellose 15, carnauba wax (powdered) and Opaspray Blue [K-IF-4375] (contains E104, E127, E132, E171, industrial methylated spirit* and hydroxypropylcellulose)

Each Loestrin 30 tablet contains the following excipients: Lactose, sucrose, maize starch, talc, powdered acacia, magnesium stearate, E104, E131, industrial methylated spirit*, purified water*, dichloromethane (technical grade)*, propylene glycol*, hypromellose 15, carnauba wax (powdered) and Opaspray Green [K-IF-5920] (contains E104, E110, E131, E171, industrial methylated spirit* and hydroxypropylcellulose).

* not present in final product

*Incompatibilities:* Not known.

*Shelf-life:* 36 months.

*Special precautions for storage:* Store at a temperature not exceeding 30°C.

*Nature and contents of container:* Printed aluminium foil blister-pack containing 21 tablets in a cardboard carton, together with a product leaflet or a cardboard carton containing three printed aluminium foil blister-packs, each containing 21 tablets, and one product leaflet.

*Instructions for use/handling:* Not applicable.

*Marketing authorisation holder:* Parke, Davis & Company, Usk Road, Pontypool, NP4 0YH.

**Marketing authorisation numbers**
Loestrin 20 0018/0086
Loestrin 30 0018/0087

**Date of approval/revision of SPC** July 1995

**Legal category** POM

## LOPID*

**Presentation** 300 mg capsule: A white powder in a No 0 hard gelatin capsule with a white body and maroon cap, overprinted 'LOPID 300'.

600 mg tablet: A white, elliptical, film-coated tablet debossed with 'LOPID' on one side.

*Composition:* Each capsule contains: gemfibrozil 300 mg. Each tablet contains: gemfibrozil 600 mg

### Uses
*Action:* LOPID is a lipid-regulating agent which decreases total serum cholesterol and serum triglycerides. These decreases occur in the low density lipoprotein (LDL) fraction and in the very low density lipoprotein (VLDL) fraction. In addition, Lopid increases high density lipoprotein (HDL) cholesterol.

*Indications:* Lopid is indicated for the primary prevention of coronary heart disease in men between 40-55 years of age and with hyperlipidaemias who have not responded to diet and other appropriate measures.

Lopid is also indicated for the treatment of patients with hyperlipidaemias of Fredrickson Type IIa (hypercholesterolaemia), Fredrickson Type IIb (mixed hyperlipidaemia), Fredrickson Type III (familial dysbetalipoproteinaemia), Fredrickson Type IV (hypertriglyceridaemia) and Type V (hypertriglyceridaemia). Lopid should be prescribed only for patients with lipid or lipoprotein abnormalities demonstrated by laboratory tests and where diet alone is insufficient to correct the condition.

### Dosage and administration
*Adult:* 1200 mg daily in divided doses usually twice daily. 900 mg as a total daily dose may be given in cases of intolerance at normal dosage. When maximum triglyceride reduction is desired as in Type V patients, up to 1500 mg daily may be needed.

*Elderly:* As for adults. Patients 60 years or older with lipid levels consistent with increased risk of coronary heart disease should be treated with diet for at least three months. If diet therapy is not effective, treatment with gemfibrozil in this age group should be considered. The incidence of side effects associated with treatment with Lopid has not been shown to be different in elderly subjects compared with younger ones.

*Children:* Not recommended.

### Contra-indications, warnings, etc
*Contra-indications:* Hypersensitivity to gemfibrozil, alcoholism, hepatic dysfunction, pre-existing gall stones.

*Use in pregnancy and lactation:* Safe use in human pregnancy has not been established. It is not known whether gemfibrozil is secreted in human milk. Like most drugs, gemfibrozil should normally be avoided during pregnancy and lactation.

*Warnings and precautions:* Before instituting treatment with Lopid, attempts should be made to control serum lipids with appropriate diet, exercise, cessation of smoking, limitation of alcohol intake, weight loss in obese patients, and treatment of the causes of secondary hyperlipidaemias such as hypothyroidism and diabetes mellitus.

Since long-term administration of Lopid is recommended, all baseline values including lipid profile, blood count and liver function tests, should be measured before treatment and periodic determinations of serum lipids should be obtained. The drug should be withdrawn or additional therapy instituted if the lipid response is inadequate after 3 months. In addition, Lopid should be withdrawn if after 3 months the response is paradoxical. Paradoxical response has been occasionally observed, usually in patients with alcoholic hepatic disease. The blood level of LDL cholesterol occasionally rises on treatment with Lopid. A further estimation of LDL cholesterol should there-

fore be made during treatment to confirm that the desired therapeutic effect has been achieved.

Adverse effects have not been reported in patients with renal disease, but such patients should start treatment at 900 mg daily, which may be increased after careful assessment of response and renal function.

Long-term toxicity studies in rats and mice were carried out at one and ten times the human dose on a weight for weight basis. In male rats receiving ten times the human dose, there was a significant increase in incidence of benign liver nodules and liver carcinomas. Male rats receiving a dose equivalent to the human dose had no statistically significant increase in the incidence of liver carcinomas. In high dose female rats there was a significant increase in the combined incidence of benign and malignant liver neoplasms. In mice (both male and female), there were no statistically significant differences from controls in the incidence of liver tumours. Electron microscopy demonstrated a marked hepatic peroxisome proliferation following Lopid administration to the male rat. Similar changes have been sought but not found in the human liver at up to 27 months' continuous gemfibrozil therapy. Male rats had a dose-related increase of benign Leydig cell tumours. Subcapsular bilateral cataracts occurred in 10%, and unilateral cataracts in 6.3% of the high dose males.

Lopid may increase cholesterol excretion into the bile raising the potential for gallstone formation. If cholelithiasis is suspected, gallbladder studies are indicated. Lopid therapy should be discontinued if gallstones are found.

Elevated liver function tests (AST and ALT) increased alkaline phosphatase, LDH, creatine kinase (CK) and bilirubin have occasionally been reported with Lopid administration. These are usually reversible when Lopid is discontinued. Therefore liver function tests are recommended during the first year of therapy and treatment with Lopid should be terminated if abnormalities persist.

Significant mild haemoglobin, haematocrit and white cell decreases have been observed, unrelated to dosage and not progressive beyond six months' treatment. Eosinophilia has been occasionally reported. Rarely, severe anaemia, leucopenia, thrombocytopenia and bone marrow hypoplasia have been reported. Therefore periodic blood counts are recommended during the first 12 months of treatment.

There have been reports of myositis, myopathy and marked elevations of creatine phosphokinase associated with Lopid. Rhabdomyolysis has also been reported rarely. Patients who develop signs of muscle toxicity should be monitored closely and CPK levels checked. Treatment with Lopid should be stopped if myopathy is suspected or if CPK rises to > 10 times the upper limit of normal. The risk of serious muscle toxicity is increased if Lopid is used concomitantly with HMG-CoA reductase inhibitors or other fibrates. Combination therapy should be used with caution and patients monitored closely for signs of muscle toxicity.

*Drug interactions:* Concomitant anticoagulant dosage may need to be reduced and frequent determinations of prothrombin carried out to confirm that the desired prothrombin level has been re-established.

Reduced bioavailability of gemfibrozil may result when given simultaneously with resin-granule drugs such as colestipol. Administration of the drugs two hours or more apart is recommended.

*Adverse effects:* Significant side effects in decreasing order of frequency were abdominal pain, diarrhoea, nausea, epigastric pain, vomiting and flatulence. Occasionally and possibly attributable to Lopid are rash, dermatitis, pruritus, urticaria, impotence, headache, dizziness, blurred vision, cholestatic jaundice, angioedema, laryngeal oedema, atrial fibrillation, pancreatitis, myaesthenia, myopathy, rhabdomyolysis, painful extremities and myalgia accompanied by increases in creatine kinase.

Other reactions where a causal relationship is difficult to establish to which the physician should be alert : dry mouth, constipation, anorexia, dyspepsia, back pain, arthralgia, muscle cramps, swollen joints, vertigo, insomnia, paraesthesia, tinnitus, leucopenia, hypokalaemia, fatigue, malaise, syncope, peripheral neuritis, and acute appendicitis. Viral and bacterial infections (common cold, cough and urinary tract infections) were more common in Lopid than in placebo-treated patients.

*Overdose:* Overdosage has been reported with gemfibrozil. In one case of accidental overdosage, where a child ingested nine grams of gemfibrozil, non specific symptoms of nausea and vomiting were reported. The patient fully recovered.

Symptomatic supportive measures should be taken should overdose occur.

**Pharmaceutical precautions** Store in a dry place at a temperature not exceeding 30°C.

**Legal category** POM

**Package quantities** Lopid 300 mg–Blister packs containing 100 & 112 capsules.
Lopid 600 mg–Blister packs containing 56 tablets.

**Further information** Nil

**Product licence numbers**
Lopid 300 mg 0018/0153
Lopid 600 mg 0018/0157

## NARDIL*

**Presentation** Orange film-coated tablets, each containing 15 mg phenelzine (as the sulphate BP).

### Uses
*Indications:* Phenelzine is a monoamine oxidase inhibitor (MAOI). It has been found to be effective in depressed patients clinically characterised as 'atypical', 'nonendogenous', 'neurotic' or where treatment with other antidepressants has failed. These patients often have mixed anxiety and depression and phobic or hypochondriacal features. There is less conclusive evidence of its usefulness with severely depressed patients with endogenous features.

**Dosage and administration** Oral administration.

*Adults:* One 15 mg tablet three times a day. A response is usually seen within the first week. If no response is evident after two weeks, the dosage may be increased to a maximum of one 15 mg tablet four times a day. Doses of up to two 15 mg tablets three times a day may be used in hospitals. The effectiveness of the drug may not become apparent in less than 4 weeks' therapy. After a satisfactory response has been achieved, the dosage may be reduced very gradually to a suitable maintenance level. This may be as low as one 15 mg tablet every other day.

*Elderly (over 65 years):* As for adults. Postural hypotension may be an unwanted effect of MAOIs in the elderly. Elderly patients as a group tend to receive multiple drug therapies and the possibility of increased risk of drug interactions should be borne in mind. Nardil should only be used with great caution in elderly patients. Despite these problems, MAOIs (including Nardil) have been found to be useful in the treatment of depression in the elderly.

*Children:* Nardil is not indicated for children under 16 years of age.

### Contra-indications, warnings, etc
*Contra-indications:* Nardil should not be used in patients who are hypersensitive to phenelzine or with phaeochromocytoma, cerebrovascular disease, congestive heart failure, a history of liver disease or with abnormal liver function tests.

Phenelzine sulphate should not be administered at the same time as, or within 14 days of treatment with other MAOIs, buspirone, or dibenzazaepine derivative drugs (including tricyclic antidepressant agents, perphenazine or carbamazepine). It is recognised that there is some division of consultant opinion with respect to concomitant use of MAOIs and tricyclic antidepressants. There have been reports of serious reactions (including hyperthermia, rigidity, myoclonic movements and death) when serotonin reuptake inhibitors or serotonin/noradrenaline inhibitors (e.g. venlafaxine) have been combined with MAOIs. Therefore, Nardil should not be used in combination with these drugs and before initiating Nardil, a sufficent amount of time must be allowed for clearance of the drugs and its metabolites. For example, five weeks in the case of fluoxetine and two weeks with paroxetine. Conversely, these drugs should not be started within 14 days of discontinuing phenelzine.

Phenelzine sulphate should not be used in combination with guanethidine, dextromethorphan, or with CNS depressants such as alcohol and narcotic analgesics. Death has been reported in patients receiving a single dose of pethidine.

*Use in pregnancy and lactation:* Do not use during pregnancy, especially during the first and last trimesters, unless there are compelling reasons. There is no evidence as to drug safety in human pregnancy nor is there evidence from animal work that it is free from hazard.

It is not known if phenelzine is excreted in breast milk. Because of the potential for serious adverse effects to the infant, a decision should be made whether to discontinue the drug or not to breast-feed.

*Precautions:* Nardil should be withdrawn two weeks before elective surgery/dentistry. Nardil should not be given with cocaine or local anaesthesia containing sympathomimetic vasoconstrictors and the possible combined hypotensive effects of Nardil and spinal anaesthesia should be kept in mind.

Potentially suicidal patients should be carefully observed until control of depresssion is attained.

Patients should be warned against self medication, particularly cold cures, and about potential food interactions.

Patients under treatment with Nardil should avoid

high protein food that has undergone breakdown by ageing, fermentation, pickling, smoking or bacterial contamination. Patients should avoid cooked or plain cheese, oxo, bovril, marmite, brewer's yeast etc. during treatment and up to 14 days after ceasing treatment. Flavoured textured vegetable protein, hung game, pickled herrings, dry sausage (salami, pepperoni etc), liver, yoghurt and broad bean pods may also present a hazard Patients should not consume alcoholic drinks or non-alcoholic beers, lagers or wines and excessive amounts of tea and coffee should be avoided.

Where a reaction between Nardil and certain foodstuffs occurs the intensity of the reaction is usually related to the tyramine content of the food. The reaction is now well recognised and serious hypertensive episodes are extremely rare. Should such a reaction occur, the hypertension should be controlled promptly by slow administration of phentolamine 5-10 mg i.v. repeated if necessary. Care should be taken to administer this drug slowly to avoid an excessive hypotensive effect.

Nardil should only be used with great caution in agitated patients or those who have cardiovascular disease, epilepsy, blood dyscrasias, porphyria, or diabetes; and in patients taking diuretics.

Blood pressure should be observed frequently to detect any pressor response and therapy discontinued if palpitations or frequent headaches occur.

Patients should also be closely followed for symptoms of postural hypotension. Hypotensive side effects have occured in hypertensive as well as normotensive and hypotensive patients.

Nardil may also potentiate the effects of alcohol.

*Drug interactions:* See *Contra-indications*. Nardil may potentiate the action of pethidine, morphine, adrenaline, amphetamines and other sympathomimetic amines such as fenfluramine, ephedrine, phenylpropanolamine, dopamine and levodopa.

Nardil may also potentiate the effects of antihypertensives, hypoglycaemic agents, sympathomimetics, anti-Parkinson drugs, local anaesthetics and CNS depressants, including barbiturates.

The combination of MAOIs and tryptophan has been reported to cause behavioural and neurological symptoms.

*Side-effects:* Side-effects tend to be mild or moderate in severity, often subside as treatment continues, and can be minimised by adjusting dosage; rarely is it necessary to discontinue Nardil.

The most important reaction associated with Nardil is the occurrence of hypertensive crises, which have been associated with intracranial bleeding and have sometimes been fatal.

Common side-effects include: dizziness, drowsiness, weakness and fatigue, oedema and gastrointestinal disturbances (nausea, vomiting, dryness of the mouth, constipation), insomnia, blurred vision, adverse effects on driving ability, postural hypotension, twitching, myoclonic movement, hyperreflexia, elevated serum transaminases and anorgasmia.

Less common side-effects are headache, nervousness, euphoria, paraesthesia, sweating, increased appetite and weight, rash, pruritus, difficulty in micturition, muscle tremor, peripheral neuritis, behavioural changes, arrhythmias, convulsions, impotence and delayed ejaculation, purpura, blood dyscrasias, jitteriness, palilalia, nystagmus, hypernatraemia and glaucoma.

Although reported less frequently, sometimes only once, additional severe side effects include: Ataxia, shock-like coma, toxic delirium, manic reaction, acute anxiety reaction, precipitation of schizophrenia, transient respiratory and cardiovascular depression following ECT, fatal progressive necrotising hepatocellular damage, reversible jaundice, hypermetabolic syndrome, oedema of the glottis and fever associated with increased muscle tone.

Withdrawal may be associated with nausea, vomiting and malaise.

An uncommon withdrawal syndrome following abrupt withdrawal of Nardil has been infrequently reported. Signs and symptoms of this syndrome generally commence 24 to 72 hours after drug discontinuation and may vary from vivid nightmares with agitition to frank psychosis and convulsions. This syndrome generally responds to reinstitution of low-dose Nardil therapy followed by cautious downward titration and discontinuation.

*Overdosage:* Signs and symptoms may be absent or minimal during the initial 12 hour period following ingestion and may develop slowly thereafter, reaching a maximum in 24-48 hours. Death has been reported following overdosage. Therefore immediate hospitalisation with continuous patient observation and monitoring throughout this period is essential.

Large doses may produce hypomania, euphoria, followed by coma with hypotension, or acute hypertension sometimes with sub-arachnoid haemorrhage. In a few cases extra-pyramidal symptoms have been recorded.

Other symptoms may be: drowsiness, dizziness, faintness, irritability, hyperactivity, agitation, severe headache, hallucinations, trismus, opisthotonos, rigidity, convulsions, rapid and irregular pulse, precordial pain, respiratory depression and failure, hyperpyrexia, diaphoresis and cool, clammy skin.

*Treatment:* Gastric lavage with instillation of charcoal slurry may be helpful in early poisoning (tablets dissolve slowly in stomach).

Absolute bed rest, raise feet in hypotension. Vasopressors are best avoided. Hypertension should be urgently controlled with phentolamine IV. Avoid hypnotics, such as morphine, pethidine, barbiturates. Body temperature should be monitored, and fever managed by cooling.

Use intravenous therapy to maintain fluid and electrolyte balance and use a slow IV injection of diazepam for any CNS stimulation. In deep coma and severe hypotension, hydrocortisone by injection may be tried.

There is no specific antidote for Nardil.

Haemodialysis, peritoneal dialysis and charcoal haemoperfusion may be of value in massive overdosage, but sufficent data is not available to recommend their routine use in these cases.

**Pharmaceutical precautions** Store in a dry place at a temperature not exceeding 25°C.

**Legal category** POM.

**Package quantities** Bottles of 100 tablets.

**Further information** Nil

**Product licence numbers** 0018/0177

# NEURONTIN* ▼

**Qualitative and quantitative composition** Neurontin Capsules 100 mg contain 100 mg gabapentin per capsule. Neurontin Capsules 300 mg contain 300 mg gabapentin per capsule. Neurontin Capsules 400 mg contain 400 mg gabapentin per capsule.

**Pharmaceutical form** Neurontin is supplied in capsules containing 100 mg, 300 mg, and 400 mg of gabopentin for oral administration.

**Clinical particulars** *Therapeutic indications:* Neurontin is an antiepileptic drug indicated as add-on therapy for partial seizures and partial seizures with secondary generalisation in patients who have not achieved satisfactory control with or who are intolerant to standard anticonvulsants used alone or in combination.

*Posology and method of administration:* For oral administration only.

*Adults:* The anti-epileptic effect of Neurontin generally occurs at 900-1200 mg/day. It is not necessary to monitor Neurontin plasma concentrations to optimise Neurontin therapy.

Titration to an effective dose can progress rapidly and can be accomplished over a few days by administering 300 mg once a day on day 1, 300 mg twice a day on day 2, and 300 mg three times a day on day 3.

Thereafter, the dose can be increased to 1200 mg per day given in three equally divided doses, and if necessary, further titration can occur using increments of 300 mg per day given in three equally divided doses up to a maximum of 2400 mg per day.

The maximum time between doses in a three times daily schedule should not exceed 12 hours.

If Neurontin is discontinued and/or an alternate anticonvulsant medication is added to the therapy, this should be done gradually over a minimum of one week.

*Elderly:* Elderly patients may require dosage adjustment because of declining renal function with age (see table 1 below).

*Dosage in patients with compromised renal function or those undergoing haemodialysis:* Dosage adjustment is recommended in patients with compromised renal function or those undergoing haemodialysis (see table 1 below).

*Table 1. Maintenance dosage of Neurontin in adults with reduced renal function*

| Renal Function Creatinine Clearance (ml/min) | Total Daily Dose (mg/day) | Dose Regimen (mg) |
|---|---|---|
| 60-90 | 1200 mg | 400 mg three times a day |
| 30-60 | 600 mg | 300 mg twice daily |
| 15-30 | 300 mg | 300 mg once daily |
| < 15 | 150 mg | 300 mg once daily every other day |
| Haemodialysis[a] | - | 200-300[b] |

[a] Loading dose of 300 to 400 mg
[b] Maintenance dose of 200 to 300 mg gabapentin following each 4 hours of haemodialysis

*Children under 12 years of age:* Not recommended.

*Contra-indications:* Neurontin is contraindicated in patients who are hypersensitive to Neurontin or to the product's components.

*Special warnings and special precautions for use:* Although there is no evidence of rebound seizures with Neurontin, abrupt withdrawal of anticonvulsant agents in epileptic patients may precipitate status epilepticus. When in the judgement of the clinician there is a need for dose reduction, discontinuation, or substitution of alternative anticonvulsant medication, this should be done gradually over a minimum of one week.

Neurontin is not generally considered effective in the treatment of absence seizures.

Patients with epilepsy can be the subject of mood and behavioural disturbances. Such reports have been noted in patients on Neurontin although a causal link has not been established.

*Interactions with other medicaments and other forms of interaction:* Neurontin may be used in combination with other anti-epileptic drugs without concern for alteration of the plasma concentrations of Neurontin or serum concentrations of other anti-epileptic drugs.

There is no interaction between Neurontin and phenytoin, valproic acid, carbamazepine, or phenobarbital. Neurontin steady-state pharmacokinetics are similar for healthy subjects and patients with epilepsy receiving antiepileptic agents.

Coadministration of Neurontin with oral contraceptives including norethisterone and/or ethinyl estradiol does not influence the steady-state pharmacokinetics of either component.

In a clinical study where Neurontin and an aluminium and magnesium containing antacid were given at the same time, Neurontin's bio-availability was reduced by up to 24%. It is recommended that Neurontin is taken about two hours following any such antacid administration.

Renal excretion of Neurontin is unaltered by probenecid. The slight decrease in renal excretion of Neurontin observed when coadministered with cimetidine is not expected to be of clinical importance.

Food has no effect on Neurontin pharmacokinetics.

Because false positive readings were reported with the Ames N-Multistix SG® dipstick test when Neurontin or placebo was added to other anticonvulsant drugs, the more specific sulphosalicylic acid precipitation procedure is recommended to determine urine protein.

*Pregnancy and lactation:* Safe use in human pregnancy has not been established.

Reproduction studies in mice at doses up to 80 times the human dose and in rats and rabbits at doses up to 40 times the human dose revealed no evidence of impaired fertility or harm to the foetus due to Neurontin administration. However, because animal reproduction studies are not always predictive of human response, this drug should be used during pregnancy only if clearly needed.

It is not known if Neurontin is excreted in human milk. Because many drugs are excreted in human milk, and because of the potential for serious adverse reactions in nursing infants from Neurontin, a decision should be made whether to discontinue nursing or to discontinue the drug, taking into account the importance of the drug to the mother.

*Effects on ability to drive or use machines:* As with all anticonvulsants, Neurontin acts on the central nervous system and may produce drowsiness, dizziness or other related symptoms. These otherwise mild or moderate adverse events could be potentially dangerous in patients driving or operating machinery, particularly until such time as the individual patient's experience with the drug is established.

*Undesirable effects:* Neurontin has been evaluated for safety in more than 2000 subjects and patients and was well tolerated.

Since Neurontin was most often administered in combination with other antiepileptic agents, it is not possible to determine which agents, if any, are associated with adverse events. However, based on placebo-controlled, double blind studies, possible side effects are: somnolence, dizziness, ataxia, fatigue, nystagmus, headache, tremor, diplopia, nausea and/or vomiting, rhinitis and amblyopia. Less common side effects are: pharyngitis, dysarthria, weight increase, dyspepsia, amnesia, nervousness and myalgia.

*Post-marketing surveillance:* As with the other AEDs there have been rare reports of pancreatitis, elevated liver function tests, erythema multiforme, Stevens Johnson Syndrome and sudden unexplained deaths where a causal relationship to treatment has not been established.

*Overdose:* In limited experience with overdoses, dizziness, double vision and slurred speech have been noted. Overdoses of Neurontin, up to 30 g ingested at one time, have been reported. Symptoms were drowsiness and mild diarrhoea with a full recovery. Therefore, acute, life-threatening toxicity has not been observed with Neurontin overdoses of up to 30 g per day. Reduced absorption of Neurontin at higher doses may limit drug absorption at the time of overdosing and, hence, toxicity from overdoses.

Although Neurontin can be removed by haemodialysis, it is not usually required. However, in patients with renal impairment, haemodialysis may be indicated.

### Pharmacological properties

*Pharmacodynamic properties:* Neurontin is an anticonvulsant structurally related to the neurotransmitter gamma-aminobutyric acid (GABA) but its mechanism of action is different from that of several drugs that interact with GABA synapses. The identification and function of the gabapentin binding site remains to be elucidated and the relevance of its various actions to the anticonvulsant effect remains to be established.

*Pharmacokinetic properties:* Mean plasma gabapentin concentrations ($C_{max}$) occurred approximately 3 hours ($T_{max}$) following single oral doses of Neurontin regardless of dose size or formulation. Mean $T_{max}$ values following multiple dose administration were approximately 1 hour shorter than the values following single-dose administration.

Mean $C_{max}$ and AUC values increased with increasing dose; however, the increase was less than dose proportional. Deviation from linearity was very slight up to 600 mg for both parameters and thus should be minimal at doses of 300 mg to 400 mg three times daily where the antiepileptic effect generally occurs.

Following repeated Neurontin administration, steady-state was achieved within 1 to 2 days after the start of the multiple dosing and was maintained throughout the dosing regime.

Plasma gabapentin concentration-time profiles were similar between gabapentin solution and capsule formulations following single doses of 300 and 400 mg. Absolute bioavailability of a 300 mg oral dose of Neurontin was approximately 60%. At doses of 300 mg and 400 mg, Neurontin bioavailability was unchanged following multiple-dose administration.

The presence of food did not influence the bioavailabilty of Neurontin.

Gabapentin is not metabolised in humans and does not induce hepatic mixed function oxidase enzymes.

Gabapentin elimination from plasma following IV administration was best described by linear pharmacokinetics. Elimination half-life ($T\frac{1}{2}$) of gabapentin ranged from 5 to 7 hours. Gabapentin elimination parameters, apparent plasma $T\frac{1}{2}$ and renal clearance ($CL_R$) were independent of dose and remained unchanged following repeated administration. Renal clearance was the sole elimination pathway for gabapentin. Since gabapentin is not metabolised in humans, the amount of drug recovered in urine is indicative of gabapentin bioavailability. Following a single 200 mg oral dose of [$C_{14}$] gabapentin recovery of radioactivity was essentially complete with approximately 80% and 20% of the dose recovered in urine and faeces, respectively.

As renal function (as determined by creatinine clearance) decreases with increasing age, gabapentin oral clearance, renal clearance and elimination-rate constant decrease proportionally.

*Pre-clinical safety data:* Gabapentin was given in the diet to mice at 200, 600, and 2000 mg/kg/day and to rats at 250, 1000, and 2000 mg/kg/day for two years. A statistically significant increase in the incidence of pancreatic acinar cell tumors was found only in male rats at the highest dose. Peak plasma drug concentrations and areas under the concentration time curve in rats at 2000 mg/kg is 20 times higher than the therapeutic concentrations in humans given the recommended maximum therapeutic dose and is 14 times higher than the therapeutic concentrations in humans given the recommended maximum tolerated dose (2400 mg/day).

The pancreatic acinar cell tumors in male rats are low grade malignancies, did not affect survival, did not metastasise or invade surrounding tissue, and were similar to those seen in concurrent controls. The relevance of these pancreatic acinar cell tumours in male rats to carcinogenic risk in humans is therefore of uncertain significance.

Gabapentin has no genotoxic potential. It was not mutagenic in the Ames bacterial plate incorporation assay or at the HGPRT locus in mammalian cells in the presence or absence of metabolic activation. Gabapentin did not induce structural chromosome aberrations in mammalian cells in vitro or in vivo, and did not induce micronucleus formation in the bone marrow of hamsters.

### Pharmaceutical particulars

*List of excipients:* The 100 mg, 300 mg and 400 mg capsules contain the following excipients: lactose (hydrous), corn starch, and talc. The capsule shells for

Neurontin 100 mg, 300 mg and 400 mg consist of Gelatin. The capsule shell for Neurontin 100 mg also contain E171 (Titanium Dioxide). The capsule shell for Neurontin 300 mg also contains E171 (Titanium Dioxide) and E172 (Yellow Iron Oxide). The capsule shell for Neurontin 400 mg also contains (E171) (Titanium Dioxide), E172 (Yellow Iron oxide) and E172 (Red Iron Oxide).

*Incompatibilities:* None.

*Shelf-life:* 3 years

*Special precautions for storage:* Store in a dry place at a temperature between 15–30°C.

*Nature and contents of container:* Neurontin Capsules 100 mg, 300 mg and 400 mg are packed in PVC/PVDC blister packs with vinyl heat seal/aluminium coating backing containing 100 capsules

*Instructions for use/handling:* None.

**Marketing authorisation holder:** Parke, Davis & Company, Usk Road, Pontypool, NR4 0YH.

**Marketing authorisation numbers**
Neurontin Capsules 100 mg 0018/0202
Neurontin Capsules 300 mg 0018/0203
Neurontin Capsules 400 mg 0018/0204

**Date of approval/revision of SPC**   March 1997

**Legal category**   POM

## OPILON*

**Presentation**   Pale yellow film-coated tablets. Each tablet contains: Thymoxamine Hydrochloride BP (Moxisylyte Hydrochloride INN) equivalent to Thymoxamine base 40 mg

**Uses**   Thymoxamine is an alpha-adrenergic blocking agent. Opilon is indicated in the short term control of the symptoms of primary Raynaud's Phenomenon.

**Dosage and administration**   Oral administration.

*Adults:* Initially one tablet to be taken four times a day. This may be increased to two tablets four times a day if initial response is poor. For patients exposed to the cold during the daytime, one tablet should be administered every three hours during the period when symptoms are most likely to occur. In the event that a response is not evident within 2 weeks, the drug should be discontinued.

*Elderly (over 65 years):* As for adults. No clinical or pharmacokinetic data specific to this age group is available. Whilst at normal dosage no problems have been reported, caution nevertheless is advised when Opilon is prescribed in the elderly.

*Children:* Opilon tablets are not indicated for use in children.

**Contra-indications, warnings, etc**
*Contra-indications:* Hypersensitivity to any of the ingredients. Active liver disease.

*Warnings:* The alpha-adrenergic blocking action of Opilon will produce a vasodilating effect which may theoretically potentiate the effect of a number of drugs used in the management of hypertension. In practice, with the recommended dosage of Opilon, this has not been reported.

*Precautions:* Opilon should be used with caution in diabetes as, theoretically, insulin requirements may be reduced. Tricyclic antidepressants may increase any hypotensive effect produced by alpha blockade.

*Pregnancy and lactation:* The safety of Opilon for use during pregnancy and lactation has not been established. It should not therefore be used by women who are pregnant or breast feeding.

*Side effects:* Occasionally, mild nausea, diarrhoea, vertigo, headache, facial flushing and rash may be encountered. These are, however, rare and transient. There have also been rare reports of hepatotoxicity, including cases of hepatitis and cholestatic jaundice, which are reversible on stopping treatment. Opilon should be withdrawn promptly if hepatic dysfunction develops.

*Overdosage:* In excessive overdosage, a fall in blood pressure is the main symptom. The patient should be nursed in the supine position until the blood pressure has been restored to normal.

**Pharmaceutical precautions**   Store in a cool dry place at a temperature not exceeding 30°C.

**Legal category**   POM.

**Package quantities**   Blister strips of 30 tablets, four strips in a carton (120 tablets).

**Further information**   Nil

**Product licence number**   0018/0179

## PITRESSIN*

**Presentation**   A clear, sterile, colourless solution for injection.

*Composition:* Each 1 ml contains: Argipressin 20 international units.

**Uses**
*Action:* Pitressin has a direct antidiuretic action on the kidney. It also constricts peripheral vessels and causes contraction of the smooth muscle of the intestine, gall bladder and urinary bladder.

*Indications:* For use in diabetes insipidus, when this is not of nephrogenic origin and control of bleeding from oesophageal varices.

**Dosage and administration**   Oral

*Adults: Diabetes insipidus:* 0.25 ml to 1 ml (5 to 20 units) by subcutaneous or intramuscular injection every four hours.

*Oesophageal varices:* For the initial control of variceal bleeding Pitressin should be given intravenously. Pitressin, 20 units diluted in 100 ml Dextrose 5%w/v may be infused over a 15 minute period. (Shields R, Brit J Hosp Med p. 126, February 1977).

*Elderly (over 65 years):* As for adults. No clinical or pharmacokinetic data specific to this age group are available. However, the drug has been used successfully at normal dosage in the elderly.

*Children:* Not recommended.

**Contra-indications, warnings, etc**
*Contra-indications:* Anaphylaxis or hypersensitivity to the drug or its components.

*Warnings:* This drug should not be used in patients with systemic hypertension or vascular disease, especially disease of the coronary arteries, except with extreme caution. In such patients, even small doses may precipitate anginal pain, and with larger doses, the possibility of myocardial infarction should be considered. **If this drug must be used in patients with peripheral vascular disease then the skin should be observed carefully for signs of ischaemia.**

Pitressin may produce water intoxication. The early signs of drowsiness, listlessness, and headaches should be recognized to prevent terminal coma and convulsions.

*Precautions:* Pitressin should be used cautiously in the presence of epilepsy, migraine, asthma, heart failure, or any state in which a rapid addition to extracellular water may produce hazard for an already overburdened system.

Chronic nephritis with nitrogen retention contraindicates the use of Pitressin until reasonable nitrogen blood levels have been attained.

*Adverse Effects:* Local or systemic allergic reactions may occur in hypersensitive individuals. The following side effects have been reported following the administration of Pitressin: tremor, sweating, vertigo, circumoral pallor, 'pounding' in head, abdominal cramps, passage of gas, nausea, vomiting, urticaria, bronchial constriction. Anaphylaxis (cardiac arrest and/or shock) has been observed shortly after injection of Pitressin. Peripheral ischaemia and rarely gangrene have been reported following use of Pitressin.

*Use during pregnancy and lactation:* No animal reproduction studies on Pitressin are available.

Pitressin has been used successfully during pregnancy for the treatment of diabetes insipidus with no adverse effects upon the foetus being reported. Nevertheless, as with all medicines, use during pregnancy should be avoided if possible and the potential benefit to the patient weighed against any possible risk to the foetus.

Pitressin has been administered to breast feeding women without apparent adverse effect on the infant.

*Treatment of overdose:* If water intoxication occurs, no fluids should be given. In severe cases, small amounts of hypertonic saline may be administered. Urea and mannitol infusions may be helpful in cases of cerebral oedema. If a patient should experience anginal pain after administration of Pitressin, amyl nitrate by inhalation, or glyceryl trinitrate sublingually, may be given.

**Pharmaceutical precautions**   Store between 2°C and 8°C. Do not freeze.

**Legal category**   POM.

**Package quantities**   Available in packs of 10 x 1 ml. ampoules.

**Further information**   Nil

**Product licence number**   018/5056R

## ZARONTIN*

**Presentation**   Elixir: A clear, red, raspberry flavoured, syrup.

Capsules: Amber, oblong gelatin capsules containing a clear liquid and imprinted 'P-D' in ivory ink.

*Composition:* Each 5 ml Zarontin Syrup contains: Ethosuximide BP 250 mg in a pleasantly flavoured syrup.

Each soft gelatin capsule contains: Ethosuximide BP 250 mg.

## Uses

*Action:* Ethosuximide suppresses the paroxysmal spike and wave pattern common to absence (petit mal) seizures. The frequency of epileptiform attacks is reduced, apparently by depression of the motor cortex and elevation of the threshold of the central nervous system to convulsive stimuli. Compared with other succinimide anticonvulsants, ethosuximide is more specific for pure absence seizures.

*Indications:* Primarily useful in absence seizures. When generalised tonic clonic seizures (grand mal) and other forms of epilepsy co-exist with absence seizures, Zarontin may be administered in combination with other antiepileptic drugs.

## Dosage and administration   Oral

*Adults and children over six years:* Initially two capsules or two 5 ml spoonfuls daily and adjusted thereafter to the patient's needs; daily dosage should be increased by small increments, for example, by one capsule or 5 ml every 4 to 7 days until control is achieved with minimal side effects. Although four to six capsules or 20-30 ml daily in divided doses often produces control of seizures, higher doses up to 8 capsules or 40 ml daily may occasionally be required.

*Children and infants under 6 years:* The initial dose is 5 ml daily which is adjusted by small increments until control is achieved with minimal side effects. The optimal dose for most children is 20 mg/kg/day. This dose has given average plasma levels within the accepted therapeutic range of 40 to 100 mg/l.

## Contra-indications, warnings, etc

*Contra-indications:* Hypersensitivity to succinimides.

*Use in pregnancy and lactation:* There is some evidence that the succinimides may produce congenital abnormality in the offspring of a small number of epileptic patients and therefore they should only be used in pregnancy if in the judgement of the physician the potential benefits outweigh the risk.

Ethosuximide may be excreted in breast milk therefore breast feeding is best avoided.

*Precautions and warnings:* Ethosuximide is capable of producing morphological and funtional changes in the animal liver. In humans, abnormal liver and renal function studies have been reported. Zarontin should be used with caution in patients with impaired hepatic or renal function. Periodic urinalysis and liver function studies are advised for all patients receiving the drug.

Psychotic states thought to be induced or exacerbated by anticonvulsant therapy have been reported.

Ethosuximide may impair the mental and/or physical abilities required for the performance of potentially hazardous tasks such as driving or other such activities requiring alertness; therefore the patient should be cautioned accordingly.

Blood dyscrasias including some with fatal outcome have been reported to be associated with the use of ethosuximide. Should symptoms or signs of infection (eg., sore throat, fever) develop, blood count determinations should be performed.

In most cases of leucopenia, the blood picture has been restored to normal on reduction of the dosage or discontinuation of the drug. Where leucopenia has occurred with other drugs, the polymorph count has in some cases increased steadily after starting treatment with ethosuximide and discontinuing the previous medication.

Ethosuximide when used alone in mixed types of epilepsy, may increase the frequency of generalised tonic-clonic (grand mal) seizures in some patients.

If the patient has been receiving other antiepileptic medications the sudden withdrawal of these drugs may precipitate a series of attacks before Zarontin has been given in sufficient amounts to exercise control. This may be avoided by gradually replacing the antiepileptic medication previously used with Zarontin.

Sudden withdrawal of Zarontin should be avoided.

*Drug interactions:* Since ethosuximide may interact with concurrently administered antiepileptic drugs, periodic serum level determinations of these drugs may be necessary (e.g., ethosuximide may elevate phenytoin serum levels and valproic acid has been reported to both increase and decrease ethosuximide levels).

*Adverse reactions:* Mild side effects, which are usually transient, may occur initially. These include apathy, drowsiness, depression, mild euphoria, extrapyramidal side effects, headache, ataxia, dizziness, anorexia, gastric upset, nausea and vomiting.

Skin rashes have been seen in a few patients. Systemic lupus erythematosus has occasionally been associated with the use of ethosuximide. Additionally, lupus-like reactions have been reported in children given ethosuximide. They vary in severity from systemic immunological disorders, which include the nephrotic syndrome, to the asymptomatic presence of antinuclear antibodies. The nephrotic syndrome is rare and a complete recovery has usually been reported on drug withdrawal. Stevens-Johnson syndrome has also occurred during administration.

Cases of leucopenia, agranulocytosis, pancytopenia and aplastic anaemia have been reported. Monocytosis, leucocytosis and transitory mild eosinophilia have also been noted.

Other adverse reactions reported include: weight loss, diarrhoea, abdominal pain, gum hypertrophy, swelling of the tongue, hiccoughs, irritability, hyperactivity, lethargy, fatigue, sleep disturbances, night terrors, inability to concentrate, aggressiveness, paranoid psychosis, increased libido, myopia, and vaginal bleeding.

*Overdosage:* Acute overdoses may produce nausea, vomiting and CNS depression including coma with respiratory depression. A relationship between ethosuximide toxicity and its plasma levels has not been established.

If less than 2 g have been taken, fluids should be given by mouth. If a larger dose has been taken the stomach should be emptied, respiration maintained and any other symptoms treated accordingly. Activated charcoal and purgatives are known to be used in the treatment of overdosage. Haemodialysis may be useful. Forced diuresis and exchange transfusions are ineffective.

**Pharmaceutical precautions**   Capsules: Store at a temperature not exceeding 30°C.

Syrup: Store at a temperature not exceeding 25°C.

Recommended diluent–Syrup B.P. When diluted use within 14 days of preparation.

**Legal category**   POM.

**Package quantities**   Capsules 250 mg: 50. Syrup: 300 ml.

**Further information**   Nil

**Product licence numbers**

| | |
|---|---|
| Zarontin Capsules | 0018/0078R |
| Zarontin Syrup | 0018/5040R |

*\*Trade Mark*

# Pasteur Merieux MSD Ltd
Clivemont House
Clivemont Road
Maidenhead
Berkshire
SL6 7BU

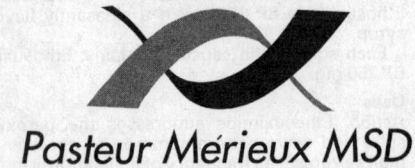

## ACT-HIB*
### Haemophilus type b conjugate vaccine
Pasteur Merieux

**Presentation**  Act-HIB is a sterile solution of inactivated conjugate polysaccharide vaccine against *Haemophilus influenzae* type b invasive disease.

Each 0.5 ml dose contains not less than 10 mcg of lyophilised Haemophilus type b polysaccharide conjugated to tetanus protein, with TRIS and sucrose added as stabilisers. Sodium chloride (0.4%) diluent is supplied with each dose. The product does not contain thiomersal or aluminium hydroxide.

**Uses**  Active immunisation against invasive diseases caused by *Haemophilus influenzae* type b.

**Dosage and administration**  By deep subcutaneous or intramuscular injection.

*Primary immunisation:* The vaccine is indicated for children from 2 months of age. The immunisation schedule is three injections each of 0.5 ml with an interval of 4 weeks between the first and second doses and not less than 4 weeks between the second and third doses.

In cases where both adsorbed diphtheria, tetanus and pertussis vaccine and haemophilus type b conjugate vaccine are indicated, Adsorbed Diphtheria, Tetanus and Pertussis Vaccine BP, Pasteur Mérieux may be used to reconstitute ACT-HIB. The combined vaccine can then be administered as a single injection. No other adsorbed diphtheria, tetanus and pertussis vaccine should be used.

*Haemophilus influenzae* type b conjugate vaccine from the same manufacturer should be used for the whole primary immunisation course.

Children over 13 months should receive a single dose of 0.5 ml of Act-HIB, which may be administered simultaneously with measles, mumps and rubella vaccine, at a different site.

Children of any age may receive Act-HIB but the vaccine would not normally be required in those over 4 years of age.

The vaccine should be reconstituted using the diluent provided.

Record the dose, batch number and date of administration.

*Instructions for mixing adsorbed Diphtheria, Tetanus and Pertussis Vaccine BP, Pasteur Mérieux (DTP Pasteur Mérieux) with ACT-HIB:* Inject the entire contents of an ampoule or pre-filled syringe of DTP Pasteur Mérieux into a vial of ACT-HIB. Shake gently for 30 seconds. Allow the vial to stand, shaking it occasionally. Examine the base of the vial for any remaining undissolved particles of ACT-HIB. Administer the combined vaccine immediately after reconstitution.

### Contra-indications, warnings, etc
*Contra-indications:* Acute infectious illness. Hypersensitivity to the vaccine or any component. Severe reaction to a previous dose of Act-HIB.

*Warnings:* Act-HIB confers protection specific to *Haemophilus influenzae* type b. Immunisation does not protect against other serogroups of *Haemophilus influenzae* or against meningitis caused by meningococci or other organisms.

*Side-effects:* These are normally mild and short lasting with no serious sequelae. Local reactions including erythema, swelling, tenderness or pain may occur at the injection site. Less commonly systemic reactions may occur; reactions reported include fever, headache, malaise, irritability, inconsolable and high pitched crying.

Rarely seizures have been reported. One case of transient cyanosis of the lower limbs, and one case of erythema multiforme have been reported.

*Precautions:* Although anaphylaxis is extremely rare, facilities for its management should always be available during vaccination.

*Use in pregnancy:* No reproductive studies have been conducted in animals. There is no data on the use of this vaccine in pregnancy or lactation. The vaccine

should not normally be used in pregnancy or during lactation.

**Pharmaceutical precautions**  Store at +2°C to +8°C, do not freeze the diluent.

After reconstitution, use within one hour. Any vaccine remaining after this time should be discarded.
Shake before use.

**Legal category**  POM.

**Package quantities**  Box of 1 single vial of lyophilised vaccine + 1 syringe of diluent (0.5 ml).

Box of 10 vials of lyophilised vaccine + 10 syringes of diluent (0.5 ml).

Box of 10 vials of lyophilised vaccine + 10 ampoules of diluent (0.5 ml).

**Further information**  The tetanus protein in the vaccine does not replace the need for routine tetanus immunisation.

**Product licence numbers**

| | |
|---|---|
| Vaccine | 6745/0041 |
| Diluent syringe | 6745/0042 |
| Diluent ampoule | 6745/0054 |

## ACT-HIB* DTP d.c. ▼
### Haemophilus type b conjugate vaccine in a dual chamber syringe with Adsorbed Diphtheria, Tetanus and Pertussis Vaccine BP
(DTP Pasteur Merieux)

### Qualitative and quantitative composition
Purified diphtheria toxoid ≥ 30 IU (≤ 30 Lf)
Purified tetanus toxoid ≥ 60 IU (≤ 12 Lf)
Bordetella pertussis ≥ 4 IU (≤ 16 opacity units)
Haemophilus type b polysaccharide conjugated to tetanus protein equivalent to 10 mcg of polysaccharide
Aluminium (as aluminium hydroxide) ≤ 1.25 mg

The DTP Pasteur Mérieux is a sterile aqueous suspension containing a mixture of the diphtheria, tetanus and pertussis antigens adsorbed onto aluminium hydroxide with thiomersal added as preservative. The ACT-HIB is in lyophilised form to optimise its stability.

**Pharmaceutical form**  The DTP Pasteur Mérieux vaccine is in the form of a sterile liquid suspension; the ACT-HIB is lyophilised. When reconstituted, ACT-HIB DTP d.c. comprises a 0.5 ml dose suspension for intramuscular or deep subcutaneous injection only.

### Clinical particulars
*Therapeutic indications:* Active immunisation against diphtheria, tetanus, pertussis and against invasive diseases caused by Haemophilus influenzae type b (e.g. meningitis, septicaemia, cellulitis, arthritis, epiglottitis).

*Posology and method of administration:* Administer by intramuscular or deep subcutaneous injection only.

*Primary immunisation:* Three injections each of 0.5 ml with an interval of at least 4 weeks between the first and second doses and at least 4 weeks between the second and the third doses. The vaccine may be administered to infants from 2 months of age.

If a primary course is interrupted it should be resumed allowing appropriate intervals between the remaining doses of ACT-HIB DTP d.c.

*Reinforcing doses:* In some children it may have been decided initially not to immunise against pertussis and they may have received one or more doses of adsorbed diphtheria and tetanus vaccine and Haemophilus type b conjugate vaccine. If in such cases, subsequently it is decided to immunise against pertussis, ACT-HIB DTP d.c. may be administered to complete the 3 dose immunisation course of adsorbed diphtheria and tetanus vaccine and Haemophilus type b conjugate vaccine. Monovalent pertussis vaccine may be given thereafter at monthly intervals to complete the 3 dose course of pertussis immunisation.

ACT-HIB DTP d.c. is not recommended for children presenting for their pre-school diphtheria and tetanus

booster. Such children will not normally need Haemophilus type b conjugate vaccine.

*Children aged 4 years and over adults and elderly:* ACT-HIB DTP d.c. vaccine is not recommended for persons aged 4 years or over.

*Other information:* Oral poliomyelitis vaccine BP may be given simultaneously.

Record the dose, batch number and date of administration.

*Contra-indications:* The following recommendations are in line with those of the Department of Health as issued in its 1992 guidelines 'Immunisation against Infectious Diseases' (HMSO).

Hypersensitivity to any vaccine component is a contra-indication to ACT-HIB DTP d.c.

*Specialist advice:* No child should either be immunised or denied immunisation without serious thought as to the consequences, both for the individual and the community. Where there is any doubt, advice should be sought from a Consultant Paediatrician, Consultant in Public Health Medicine or District (Health Board) Immunisation Co-ordinator.

*Alternative vaccination:* If pertussis vaccine is contra-indicated or refused by parents, then DT/Vac/Ads (Child) should be offered.

*Acute illness:* If the child is suffering from any acute illness, immunisation should be postponed until the child has recovered. Minor infections without fever or systemic upset are not reasons to postpone immunisation.

*General reactions:* The following are regarded as severe general reactions: fever equal to or more than 39.5°C within 48 hours of vaccine; anaphylaxis; bronchospasm; laryngeal oedema; generalised collapse. Prolonged unresponsiveness; prolonged inconsolable or high-pitched screaming for more than 4 hours; convulsions or encephalopathy occurring within 72 hours. General reactions to ACT-HIB DTP d.c. are considered most likely to be due to the pertussis component. Children who have a history of severe general reaction to a preceding dose of a pertussis-containing vaccine (including ACT-HIB DTP d.c.) should not receive the whole cell pertussis again. They should receive DT vaccine in one limb and Haemophilus influenzae type b conjugate vaccine in another limb. If another severe general reaction occurs, primary immunisation should be discontinued and expert advice should be sought.

*Local reactions:* The following are regarded as severe local reactions: an extensive area of redness and swelling which becomes indurated and involves most of the antero-lateral surface of the thigh or a major part of the circumference of the upper arm. Since local reactions to ACT-HIB DTP d.c. may be due to one or more of its components, it is recommended that children who have a history of a severe local reaction to a preceding dose of ACT-HIB DTP d.c. be given DTP in one limb and Haemophilus influenzae type b conjugate vaccine in another limb. Despite the previous severe local reaction with ACT-HIB DTP d.c., the need to adequately immunise the child outweighs the risk of a further severe local reaction. If another severe local reaction occurs to one or both of these vaccines, the vaccine(s) concerned should not be re-administered.

*Personal history of epilepsy:* Specialist advice (see above) should be sought prior to performing immunisation on children with a personal history of epilepsy.

*Family history of epilepsy:* In a recent British study, children with a family history of epilepsy were immunised with pertussis vaccine without any significant adverse events. These children's developmental progress has been normal. In children with a close family history (first degree relative) of idiopathic epilepsy, there may be a risk of developing a similar condition, irrespective of vaccine. Immunisation is recommended for these children.

*Febrile convulsions:* When there is a personal or family history of febrile convulsions, there is an increased risk of these occurring after pertussis immunisation. In such children, immunisation is recommended but advice on the prevention of fever should be given at the time of immunisation.

*Evolving neurological disease:* Where there is an on-going evolving neurological problem, immunisation should be deferred until the condition is stable.

*Stable neurological disease:* Stable neurological conditions such as occur in certain patients with cerebral palsy or spina bifida are not a contra-indication to immunisation.

*Cerebral damage in the neonatal period:* When there has been a documented history of cerebral damage in the neonatal period, immunisation should be carried out unless there is evidence of an evolving neurological abnormality. If pertussis immunisation is to be deferred, then this should be stated on the neonatal discharge summary and DT and Haemophilus type b conjugate vaccines given at the appropriate chronological age.

*Allergy:* A personal or family history of allergy is not a contra-indication to immunisation.

*Special warnings and precautions for use:* HIV positive individuals may receive ACT-HIB DTP d.c. but efficacy may be reduced.

Not for intradermal injection.

Although anaphylaxis is rare, facilities for its management should always be available during vaccination.

ACT-HIB DTP d.c. is not recommended for use in individuals aged 4 years or over. Use in individuals aged 10 years or over may be associated with severe hypersensitivity reactions (due to the adsorbed diphtheria, tetanus and pertussis vaccine component).

ACT-HIB DTP d.c. confers protection specific to Haemophilus influenzae type b. It does not protect against other serotypes of Haemophilus influenzae or against meningitis caused by meningococci or other organisms.

*Interactions with other medicaments and other forms of interaction:* ACT-HIB DTP d.c. should not be mixed with other vaccines or drugs prior to administration.

*Pregnancy or lactation:* No reproductive studies have been conducted in animals. There is no data on the use of this vaccine in pregnancy or lactation. The vaccine is not recommended for use in pregnancy or during lactation.

*Effects on ability to drive and use machines:* Not applicable.

*Undesirable effects:* Pain tenderness, swelling or redness may occur at the injection site. Generalised reactions may include headache, fever, malaise, irritability, pallor, crying. Attacks of inconsolable and high pitched screaming, limpness and convulsions may occur.

Rarely seizures, erythema multiforme and transient cyanosis of the lower limbs have been reported.

More severe neurological conditions including encephalopathy and prolonged convulsions have been reported after pertussis vaccine.

Acute allergic reactions may occur, including anaphylaxis, dyspnoea and bronchospasm, urticaria and laryngeal oedema. Peripheral neuropathy has been reported.

A persistent nodule may occur at the site of injection particularly if the vaccine is administered into superficial layers of the subcutaneous tissue.

*Overdose:* Not applicable.

**Pharmacological properties**

*Pharmacodynamic properties:* The Adsorbed Diphtheria, Tetanus and Pertussis vaccine component is a pharmacopoieal product used for active immunisation.

The ACT-HIB component contains the purified capsular polysaccharide (polyribosylribitol phosphate, PRP) of Haemophilus influenzae type b conjugated covalently to tetanus toxin protein.

When administered alone PRP induces a serological response but it is weakly immunogenic in infants. The covalent binding of PRP to tetanus protein renders it a T-cell dependent immunogen which induce a specific IgG anti-PRP response in infants and which can instil an immunological memory.

Immunogenicity studies in infants vaccinated with ACT-HIB DTP d.c. at 2, 3, 4 months of age have shown that a PRP antibody titre of ≥ 0.15 mcg/ml was reached in 97.9–100% of subjects after 3 doses. An anti-PRP titre of ≥ 1.00 mcg/ml was achieved in 82.5–92% after 3 doses. A marked anamnestic response was seen to a single test dose of plain PRP vaccine given at 14 months of age after a primary course using a vial of ACT-HIB reconstituted with a syringe of DTP vaccine at 3, 4, 5 months of age. The geometric mean titre of serum PRP antibody rose 20 fold after the single test dose of plain PRP vaccine given at 14 months.

*Pharmacokinetic properties:* Not applicable.

*Preclinical safety data:* Not applicable.

**Pharmaceutical particulars**

*List of excipients:* Thiomersal, TRIS (hydroxymethyl-aminomethane), sucrose, water for injections, sodium chloride, disodium phosphate, monopotassium phosphate.

*Incompatibilities:* None known.

*Shelf life:* 24 months at +2°C to +8°C.

*Special precautions for storage:* Store at +2°C to +8°C. Do not freeze.

*Nature and contents of container:* ACT-HIB DTP d.c. is supplied in a dual chamber syringe with lyophilised ACT-HIB in the first chamber and DTP Pasteur Mérieux suspension in the second chamber.

The containers are a type I glass dual chamber syringe with a disposable stainless steel needle and a plastic plunger rod. Closures are Elastomer tip-cap and plunger stoppers.

*Instruction for use/handling:* The dual chamber syringe should be shaken well prior to use to achieve a homogenous DTP Pasteur Mérieux suspension. Remove the rubber tip-cap and mount the needle. Whilst holding the syringe upright, depress the plunger carefully and expel the DTP Pasteur Mérieux suspension from the second chamber into the first chamber where it reconstitutes the lyophilised ACT-HIB.

Shake the syringe until a homogeneous suspension is achieved (the suspension is whitish/cloudy) and examine the syringe for any remaining undissolved particles of ACT-HIB. Continue shaking if necessary. Administer ACT-HIB DTP d.c. immediately after reconstitution.

**Marketing authorisation number** 6745/0079.

**Date of approval/revision of SPC** February 1997.

**Legal category** POM.

## ADSORBED DIPHTHERIA AND TETANUS VACCINE BP

**Presentation** Adsorbed diphtheria and tetanus vaccine is a sterile aqueous suspension containing a mixture of purified tetanus and diphtheria toxoids. The toxoids are adsorbed onto aluminium hydroxide with thiomersal added as preservative. Each 0.5 ml dose contains not less than 40 IU of tetanus toxoid and not less than 30 IU of diphtheria toxoid.

**Uses** For active immunisation against diphtheria and tetanus. Reinforcement of immunity to diphtheria and tetanus.

**Dosage and administration** By deep subcutaneous or intramuscular injection. Shake before use.

*(a) Primary immunisation:* 3 injections each of 0.5 ml with an interval of 4 weeks between the first and second doses and 4 weeks between the second and third doses.

*(b) Reinforcing doses:* A single reinforcing dose of adsorbed diphtheria and tetanus vaccine may be administered preferably after at least 3 years from the last dose of the primary immunisation course.

*Children aged 10 years and over, adults, elderly:* Adsorbed diphtheria and tetanus vaccine is *not* normally administered to persons aged 10 years or over. In this age group, if immunisation against diphtheria is indicated, an adult (low dose) diphtheria preparation should be used without the need for prior Schick testing.

**Contra-indications, warnings, etc**

*Contra-indications:* Aged 10 years or over. Acute infectious illness. Severe reaction to a previous dose. Hypersensitivity to any component of the vaccine.

*Warnings:* Not for intradermal injection.

*Side-effects:* Local reactions such as transient erythema, swelling, tenderness or pain at the injection site or rarely systemic effects such as fever, headache, malaise and pallor may occur. Acute allergic reactions have been reported after administration of adsorbed diphtheria and tetanus vaccines, including dyspnoea, urticaria, angioneurotic oedema, peripheral neuropathy and rarely, anaphylaxis. A persistent nodule at the site of vaccination may occur with all adsorbed vaccines, particularly if administered into the superficial layers of the subcutaneous tissue.

*Precautions:* Although anaphylaxis is extremely rare, facilities for its management should always be available during vaccination.

*Use in pregnancy:* Not recommended as there is insufficient data on the use of this type of vaccine in pregnancy.

*Overdosage:* Not applicable.

**Pharmaceutical precautions** Store in a refrigerator between +2°C and +8°C. Do not freeze. Shake well immediately before use.

**Legal category** POM.

**Package quantities** 0.5 ml single dose prefilled syringe (unit pack). 0.5 ml single dose ampoule (pack of 5).

**Further information** Use of Adsorbed Diphtheria and Tetanus Vaccine BP in individuals aged 10 years or over may be associated with severe hypersensitivity reactions.

**Product licence number** 6745/0046.

## ADSORBED DIPHTHERIA TETANUS AND PERTUSSIS VACCINE, BP PASTEUR MERIEUX

**Presentation** Adsorbed diphtheria, tetanus and pertussis vaccine is a sterile aqueous suspension containing a mixture of purified diphtheria and tetanus toxoids and killed *Bordetella pertussis* organisms adsorbed onto aluminium hydroxide with thiomersal added as preservative. Each 0.5 ml dose has a potency of not less than 30 IU of diphtheria toxoid, not less than 60 IU of tetanus toxoid and not less than 4 IU of *Bordetella pertussis* cells.

**Uses** For active immunisation against diphtheria, tetanus and pertussis.

**Dosage and administration** Administer by intramuscular or deep subcutaneous injection.

*Primary immunisation:* Three injections each of 0.5 ml with an interval of at least 4 weeks between the first and second doses and at least 4 weeks between the second and the third doses. The vaccine may be administered to infants from 2 months of age.

In cases where both adsorbed diphtheria, tetanus and pertussis vaccine and haemophilus type b conjugate vaccine are indicated, Adsorbed Diphtheria, Tetanus and Pertussis Vaccine BP, Pasteur Mérieux may be used to reconstitute ACT-HIB. The combined vaccine can then be administered as a single injection. No other adsorbed diphtheria, tetanus and pertussis vaccine should be used.

If a primary course is interrupted it should be resumed allowing appropriate intervals between the remaining doses.

*Reinforcing doses:* Once primary immunisation is completed, a single reinforcing dose of adsorbed diphtheria and tetanus vaccine may be administered preferably at least 3 years after the last dose of the primary course.

Where adsorbed diphtheria and tetanus vaccine (DT/Vac/Ads (child)) has been administered at the start of a primary course, adsorbed diphtheria, tetanus and pertussis vaccine may be administered for subsequent doses. Once three doses of adsorbed diphtheria and tetanus have been administered, monovalent pertussis vaccine may be given at monthly intervals to complete the course.

Children presenting for their pre-school diphtheria and tetanus booster who have not previously been immunised against pertussis may be given a single dose of adsorbed diphtheria, tetanus and pertussis vaccine with 2 subsequent doses of monovalent pertussis vaccine given at monthly intervals.

*Children aged 10 years and over, adults and elderly:* Adsorbed diphtheria, tetanus and pertussis vaccine is not recommended for persons aged 10 years or over.

*Instructions for mixing adsorbed Diphtheria, Tetanus and Pertussis Vaccine BP, Pasteur Mérieux (DTP Pasteur Mérieux) with ACT-HIB:* Inject the entire contents of an ampoule or pre-filled syringe of DTP Pasteur Mérieux into a vial of ACT-HIB. Shake gently for 30 seconds. Allows the vial to stand, shaking it occasionally. Examine the base of the vial for any remaining undissolved particles of ACT-HIB. Administer the combined vaccine immediately after reconstitution.

**Contra-indications, warnings, etc**

*Department of Health recommendations:* These recommendations are from the 1992 guidelines "immunisation against Infectious Diseases" (HMSO).

*Specialist advice:* No child should be either immunised or denied immunisation without serious thought as to the consequences, both for the individual child and the community. Where there is any doubt, advice should be sought from a Consultant Paediatrician, Consultant in Public Health Medicine or District (Health Board) Immunisation Co-ordinator.

*Alternative vaccination:* If pertussis vaccine is contra-indicated or refused by parents, then DT/Vac/Ads should be offered.

*Acute illness:* If the child is suffering from any acute illness, immunisation should be postponed until the child has recovered. Minor infections without fever or systemic upset are not reasons to postpone immunisation.

*Local or general reactions:* Immunisation should not be carried out in children who have a history of severe local or general reaction to a preceding dose. Immunisation should be completed with DT vaccine. The following reactions should be regarded as severe:

*Local:* An extensive area of redness and swelling which becomes indurated and involves most of the antero-lateral surface of the thigh or a major part of the circumference of the upper arm.

*General:* Fever equal to or more than 39.5°C within 48 hours of vaccine; anaphylaxis; bronchospasm; laryngeal oedema; generalised collapse. Prolonged unresponsiveness; prolonged inconsolable or high-pitched screaming for more than 4 hours; convulsions or encephalopathy occurring within 72 hours.

*Personal history of epilepsy:* Specialist advice should be sought prior to performing immunisation on children with a personal history of epilepsy (see above).

*Family history of epilepsy:* In a recent British study, children with a family history of epilepsy were immunised with pertussis vaccine without any significant adverse events. These children's developmental progress has been normal. In children with a close family history (first degree relative) of idiopathic epilepsy, there may be a risk of developing a similar condition, irrespective of vaccine. Immunisation is recommended for these children.

*Febrile conclusions:* When there is a personal or family history of febrile convulsions, there is an increased risk of these occurring after pertussis immunisation. In such children, immunisation is recommended but advice on the prevention of fever should be given at the time of immunisation.

*Evolving neurological disease:* Where there is an ongoing evolving neurological problem, immunisation should be deferred until the condition is stable.

*Stable neurological disease:* Stable neurological conditions such as occur in certain patients with cerebral palsy or spina bifida are not a contraindication to immunisation.

*Cerebral damage in the neonatal period:* When there has been a documented history of cerebral damage in the neonatal period, immunisation should be carried out unless there is evidence of an evolving neurological abnormality. If immunisation is to be deferred, then this should be stated on the neonatal discharge summary.

*Allergy:* A personal or family history or allergy is not a contraindication to immunisation.

*HIV:* HIV positive individuals may receive DTP vaccine but pertussis efficacy may be reduced.

*Warnings:* Not for intradermal injection.

*Side-effects:* Pain, tenderness, swelling or redness may occur at the injection site. Generalised reactions may include headache, malaise, pallor, crying, screaming and fever. Attacks of high pitched screaming, limpness and convulsions may occur.

More severe neurological conditions including encephalopathy and prolonged convulsions have been reported after pertussis vaccine.

Acute allergic reactions may occur, including anaphylaxis, dyspnoea and bronchospasm, urticaria and laryngeal oedema. Peripheral neuropathy has been reported.

A persistent nodule may occur at the site of injection particularly if the vaccine is administered into superficial layers of the subcutaneous tissue.

*Precautions:* Although anaphylaxis is rare, facilities for its management should always be available during vaccination.

*Use in pregnancy and lactation:* No reproductive studies have been conducted in animals. There are no data on the use of this vaccine in pregnancy or lactation. The vaccine should not normally be used in pregnancy or during lactation.

*Treatment of overdose:* Not applicable.

**Pharmaceutical precautions** Store at +2°C to +8°C. Do not freeze. Shake before use.

**Legal category** POM.

**Package quantities** 0.5 ml single dose pre-filled syringe (unit pack). 0.5 ml single dose ampoule (pack of 5).

**Further information** Use of adsorbed diphtheria, tetanus and pertussis vaccine in individuals aged 10 years or over may be associated with severe hypersensitivity reactions.

Oral poliomyelitis vaccine may be given simultaneously.

**Product licence number** 6745/0043.

## Adsorbed Tetanus Vaccine BP Pasteur Merieux (Tet/Vac/Ads)

**Presentation** A sterile aqueous suspension of purified tetanus toxoid. The toxoid is adsorbed onto aluminium hydroxide with thiomersal added as preservative.

Each 0.5 ml dose contains not less than 40 International Units (IU) of tetanus toxoid.

**Uses** Active immunisation against tetanus. Reinforcement of immunity to tetanus.

**Dosage and administration** By deep subcutaneous or intramuscular injection. Shake before use.

*Primary immunisation:* 3 injections each of 0.5 ml with an interval of 4 weeks between the first and second doses and 4 weeks between the second and third doses.

*Reinforcing doses:* Following primary immunisation, a reinforcing dose of 0.5 ml is recommended after 10 years and a further 0.5 ml dose 10 years later.

*Management of tetanus prone wounds:* Following a tetanus prone injury, a single dose of the vaccine should be administered to persons who have not received a booster dose nor completed a primary course during the preceding 10 years. Persons who have never received a primary course or in whom the immunisation history is not known, should commence or complete a primary course in addition to tetanus immunoglobulin, as appropriate.

Adsorbed tetanus vaccine may be administered simultaneously with tetanus immunoglobulin but must be given at a separate site.

**Contra-indications, warnings, etc**

*Contra-indications:* Acute infectious illness except when used in the management of tetanus prone injuries. The vaccine should not be given to persons who have had a severe reaction to a previous dose.

*Warnings:* Not for intradermal injection.

In immunised adults, booster doses at less than 10 year intervals are unnecessary and may cause excess reactions.

*Side effects:* General reactions are uncommon but may include transient pyrexia, headache, malaise, local swelling, redness and tenderness (especially in adults), acute allergic reactions, pallor, dyspnoea, urticaria, angioneurotic oedema, acute anaphylactic reactions and rarely, peripheral neuropathy. A small painless nodule may form at the injection site especially if administered into the superficial layers of subcutaneous tissue.

*Precautions:* Although anaphylaxis is extremely rare, facilities for its management should always be available during vaccination.

**Pharmaceutical precautions** Store in a refrigerator between +2° and +8°C. Do not freeze. Shake well immediately before use.

Multidose containers which are partly used should be discarded at the end of the vaccination session.

**Legal category** POM.

**Package quantities** Single dose pre-filled syringe (unit pack and pack of 10); single dose ampoule (pack of 5).

**Further information** Active immunisation against tetanus is recommended for everybody. Adsorbed tetanus vaccine may be administered to persons of any age.

**Product licence number** 6745/0045

## AVAXIM* ▼
### Inactivated Hepatitis A vaccine

**Qualitative and quantitative composition** Each 0.5 ml dose contains:

*Active ingredient:*
Inactivated hepatitis A virus†     160 antigen units**

*Other components:*
Aluminium hydroxide (expressed as aluminium)
                                         0.3 mg
2-phenoxyethanol                      2.5 µl
Formaldehyde                         12.5 mcg
Medium 199***, water for injections up to    0.5 ml

This vaccine contains polysorbate 80 and undetectable traces of neomycin.

†     GBM strain cultured on $MRC_5$ human diploid cells.

**   in the absence of an international standardised reference, the antigen content is expressed using an in-house reference.

*** Medium 199 is a mixture of aminoacids, mineral salts, vitamins and other components.

**Pharmaceutical form** Suspension for injection.

**Clinical particulars**

*Therapeutic indications:* Avaxim is indicated for active immunisation against infection caused by hepatitis A virus in adults and adolescents (of 16 years and over).

Individuals having grown up in areas of high endemicity and/or with a history of jaundice may be immune to hepatitis A, in which case the vaccine is unnecessary. Testing for antibodies to hepatitis A prior to a decision on immunisation should be considered in such situations. If not, seropositivity against hepatitis A is not a contra-indication. Avaxim is as well tolerated in seropositive as in seronegative subjects (see *Undesirable Effects* section).

*Posology and method of administration:* recommended dosage is 0.5 ml for each injection.

Primary immunisation is achieved with one single dose of vaccine. In order to provide long term protection, a booster should be given six months later. The long term duration of serum antibodies to hepatitis A virus is unknown. Long term antibody persistence data following vaccination with Avaxim are not currently available. It is predicted that HAV antibodies persist for many years (at least 10 years). In cases of doubt the serum hepatitis antibody titre should be determined.

As Avaxim is adsorbed, the vaccine must be injected by the intramuscular route (i.m.) in order to minimise local reactions.

Avaxim should be administered by intramuscular injection in the deltoid region. Avaxim must not be administered intradermally or intravenously. Before using Avaxim, shake the syringe well.

In exceptional circumstances (e.g. in patients with thrombocytopenia or in patients at risk of haemorrhage), the vaccine may be injected by the subcutaneous route.

In the event of a case contact, Avaxim may be given simultaneously with human immunoglobulin at different sites, after consideration of whether or not the subject is likely to be at long term risk of exposure.

*Contra-indications:* Usual contra-indications to any immunisation: vaccination should be delayed in subjects with current severe febrile infections.

True hypersensitivity to any Avaxim component.

*Special warnings and special precautions for use:* Injection of Avaxim should only be performed by a physician or health care worker trained in the administration of vaccines.

As Avaxim has not been extensively studied in subjects less than or equal to 15 years of age, it is not indicated in this age group.

Do not administer Avaxim by intradermal or intravenous injection. Ensure that the needle does not penetrate a blood vessel.

As with all vaccines, appropriate facilities and medication should be readily availble for immediate use in case of anaphylaxis or hypersensitivity following injection.

Individuals who develop symptoms suggestive of hypersensitivity after an injection of Avaxim should not receive further injections of the vaccine (see *Contra-indications*).

The vaccine should not be administered into the buttocks, due to the varying amount of fatty tissue in this region, contributing to variability in effectiveness of the vaccine.

Following vaccination with Avaxim, protection develops against infection caused by hepatitis A virus. This protection does not occur immediately but over 90% of individuals will have protective levels of antibodies after 2 weeks. As with any vaccine, vaccination may not result in a protective response in all susceptible vaccinees.

Avaxim does not provide protection against infection caused by hepatitis B virus, hepatitis C virus, hepatitis E virus or by other liver pathogens.

In the event that the booster vaccination has been delayed, there may be a decreased anti-hepatitis A antibody response. If long term protection is required the serum anti-hepatitis A antibody titre may be determined after Avaxim administration.

Avaxim has not been studied in patients with impaired immunity. Immunogenicity of Avaxim could be impaired by immunosuppressive treatment or in immunodeficiency. In such cases, it is recommended to measure the antibody response to be sure of protection and, if necessary, to wait for the end of any suppressive treatment before vaccination. Neverthe-less, vaccination of subjects with chronic immunodeficiency such as HIV infection is recommended if the underlying pathology allows the induction of an antibody response, even if limited.

Because of the incubation period of hepatitis A infection may be present but not clinically apparent at the time of vaccination. The effect of Avaxim on individuals late in the incubation period of hepatitis A has not been documented.

As no studies have been performed with Avaxim in subjects with liver disease, the use of this vaccine in such subjects should be considered with care.

*Interaction with other medicaments and other forms of interaction:* Concomitant administration of immunoglobulin and Avaxim at two separate sites may be performed. Seroconversion rates are not modified but antibody titres could be lower than after vaccination with Avaxim alone.

As Avaxim is inactivated, association with other

inactivated vaccine(s) given at another injection site is unlikely to interfere with immune responses. When concurrent administration is considered necessary, Avaxim must not be mixed with other vaccines in the same syringe, and other vaccines should be administered at different sites with different syringes and needles. Studies on the current administration of Avaxim with concurrent recombinant hepatitis B virus vaccine have not been performed.

No interaction with other medicinal products is currently known.

*Pregnancy and lactation:* The effect of Avaxim on embryofoetal development has not been assessed. Avaxim is not recommended in pregnancy unless there is a clear risk of hepatitis A infection. The vaccine should be given to a pregnant woman only if clearly needed.

There is no data on the effect of administration of Avaxim during lactation. Avaxim is therefore not recommended during lactation.

*Effects on ability to drive and use machines:* None known.

*Undesirable effects:* In clinical trials, adverse reactions were usually mild and confined to the first few days after vaccination with spontaneous recovery. As with all pharmaceuticals, however it is possible that expanded commercial use of the vaccine could reveal rare adverse effects.

The most common reactions with an incidence of 1% to 10% were mild local pain (10% of injections), asthenia (10%), myalgia/arthralgia (7.9%), headache (7.2%), gastrointestinal tract disorders (nausea, vomiting, decreased appetite, diarrhoea, abdominal pain) (4.3%) and mild fever (3.7%).

Those with an incidence less than 1% included redness at the injection site (0.5%). On rare occasions a nodule was observed at the injection site (less than 0.1%).

Mild reversible elevation of serum transaminases has been observed on rare occasions.

Reactions were less frequently reported after the booster dose than after the first dose. In subjects seropositive against hepatitis A virus, Avaxim was as well tolerated as in seronegative subjects.

Although there have been no observations of allergic reactions or neurological manifestations following administration of Avaxim, such events have occurred with related vaccines.

*Overdosage effects:* None known.

**Pharmacological properties**

*Pharmacodynamic properties:* Avaxim is prepared from hepatitis A virus cultured, purified and then inactivated by formaldehyde. Avaxim confers immunity against hepatitis A virus by inducing antibody titres greater than those obtained after passive immunisation with immunoglobulin. Immunity appears shortly after the first injection and 14 days after vaccination more than 90% of immunocompetent subjects are protected (titre above 20 mIU/ml).

One month after first injection 100% of subjects are protected. Immunity persists for at least six months and is reinforced after a first booster dose.

Long term protection of serum antibodies to hepatitis A virus after booster dose of Avaxim is under evaluation. Nevertheless, antibody titres obtained two years after the first booster are consistent with a projected 10 year protection.

*Pharmacokinetic properties:* Not relevant.

*Preclinical safety data:* Preclinical safety data reveal no special hazard to humans based on conventional studies of acute toxicity, repeated dose toxicity, local tolerance and hypersensitivity.

**Pharmaceutical particulars**

*List of excipients:* Aluminium hydroxide, 2-phenoxyethanol, formaldehyde, Medium 199.

*Incompatibilities:* None known.

*Shelf life:* 2 years.

*Special precautions for storage:* Store between +2°C and +8°C (in a refrigerator).

The vaccine must not be frozen. If frozen, the vaccine should be discarded.

*Nature and contents of container:* Glass type I container: One dose (0.5 ml) prefilled syringe. Closure: Elastomer plunger-stopper.

*Instructions for use/handling:* Shake before injection to obtain a homogeneous suspension.

**Marketing authorisation number** 6745/0070.

**Date of approval/revision of SPC** February 1997.

**Legal category** POM.

## DIFTAVAX*
## Adsorbed Diphtheria and Tetanus Vaccine for Adults and Adolescents BP

**Presentation** Sterile aqueous suspension containing purified tetanus and low dose diphtheria toxoids. Each 0.5 ml dose contains not less than 40 IU of tetanus toxoid and not less than 4 IU of diphtheria toxoid. The toxoids are adsorbed onto aluminium hydroxide; thiomersal is added as preservative.

**Uses** Active immunisation against tetanus and diphtheria for persons over ten years.

**Dosage and administration** By deep subcutaneous or intramuscular injection.

*Primary immunisation:* Three injections each of 0.5 ml, with an interval of at least 4 weeks between the first and the second doses, and at least 4 weeks between the second and third doses. If a course is interrupted it may be resumed; there is no need to recommence a primary course.

*Reinforcing doses:* A reinforcing dose of 0.5 ml is recommended after 10 years.

*Use in children:* Adsorbed Diphtheria and Tetanus Vaccine for Adults and Adolescents BP would not normally be administered to children under 10 years. Children under this age may receive Adsorbed Diphtheria and Tetanus Vaccine BP (DT/Vac/Ads (child)) which contains a higher amount of diphtheria toxoid.

*Use in elderly:* No special comment.

**Contra-indications, warnings, etc**

*Contra-indications:* Acute infectious illness. Severe reaction to a previous dose, or known hypersensitivity to any component of the vaccine. Immunisation with either diphtheria or tetanus toxoid within the preceding month.

*Precautions:* Adults and adolescents over 10 years requiring combined diphtheria and tetanus immunisation must always receive vaccine containing low dose diphtheria (not less than 4 IU).

Although anaphylaxis is extremely rare, facilities for its management should always be available during vaccination.

*Warnings:* Not for intradermal injection.

Schick testing is not necessary prior to immunisation.

Primary immunisation should only be considered for adults and adolescents who have not received a primary DTP or DT immunisation series in childhood.

Routine reinforcing doses at intervals of less than 10 years are not normally indicated and may be associated with an increased incidence and severity of reactions.

When diphtheria immunisation is indicated for subjects immunised against tetanus within the previous 10 years, the benefits of immunisation should be assessed against the possible risk of reactions.

Adsorbed Diphtheria and Tetanus Vaccine for Adults and Adolescents BP may normally be given to subjects requiring tetanus toxoid for wound management, to help ensure continuing diphtheria immunity, unless they have received a diphtheria toxoid containing vaccine in the last 10 years.

*Adverse reactions:* Local reactions such as transient erythema, swelling, tenderness or pain at the injection site or rarely systemic effects such as fever, headache, malaise and pallor may occur. Acute allergic reactions have been reported after administration of adsorbed diphtheria and tetanus vaccines, including dyspnoea, urticaria, angioneurotic oedema, peripheral neuropathy and rarely, anaphylaxis. A persistent nodule at the site of vaccination may occur with all adsorbed vaccines, particularly if administered into the superficial layers of the subcutaneous tissue.

*Use in pregnancy and lactation:* No reproductive studies have been conducted in animals. There are no data on the use of this vaccine in pregnancy or lactation. The vaccine should not normally be used in pregnancy or during lactation unless the benefit outweighs the risk.

**Pharmaceutical precautions** Store in a refrigerator between +2°C and +8°C. Do not freeze. Shake well immediately before use.

**Legal category** POM.

**Package quantities** 0.5 ml single dose pre-filled syringe unit pack.

**Further information** Nil.

**Product licence number** 6745/0055

## FLUZONE*
## Inactivated Influenza Vaccine (Split Virion) BP

**Qualitative and quantitative composition** *Each 0.5 ml dose contains:*

*Active ingredients:* 15 mcg haemagglutinin antigen of each of the following strains as recommended by the World Health Organisation (WHO) for the 1996/97 season:

| | |
|---|---|
| A/Texas/36/91 ($H_1N_1$) | [AA/Singapore/6/86-like strain] |
| A/Nanchang/933/95 ($H_3N_2$) | [A/Wuhan/359/95-like strain] |
| B/Harbin/7/94 | [B/Beijing/184/93-like strain] |

*Other components*

| | | |
|---|---|---|
| Thiomersal | | 0.01% |
| Gelatin | | 0.05% |
| Phosphate Buffered Saline | | |
| containing sodium chloride | | 4.35 mg |
| | monobasic sodium phosphate | 0.10 mg |
| | dibasic sodium phosphate | 0.33 mg |
| | water for injections | qs 0.5 ml |
| Formaldehyde | Not more than 200 mcg/ml | |
| Sucrose | Not more than 2.0% | |
| Triton* X-100 | Not more than 0.02% | |

**Pharmaceutical form** The vaccine is available as a sterile suspension that is to be injected intramuscularly or subcutaneously in the anterolateral aspect of the mid-thigh (vastus lateralis muscle) or the deltoid. The recommended dosage is 0.5 ml.

The vaccine is packaged in 1 × 0.5 ml syringe or 10 × 0.5 ml syringes.

**Clinical particulars**

*Therapeutic indications:* Fluzone is indicated as an active immunising agent for use in adults and children (six months and older) for the prevention of influenza.

*Posology and method of administration:* The recommended dose of Fluzone is one 0.5 ml dose. Adults and children over the age of 13 years, should receive one 0.5 ml dose. Children between the ages of four and twelve years should receive two 0.5 ml doses at least four weeks apart, unless the individual received any influenza vaccine in the previous year, when one dose would be sufficient. Infants six to forty-seven months of age should receive two 0.25 ml doses at least four weeks apart, unless the individual received any influenza vaccine in the previous year, when one dose would be sufficient.

Administration should be in accordance with the local recommended vaccination schedule.

*Contra-indications:* Do not administer to persons with known hypersensitivity (allergy) to eggs or egg products or to thiomersal. Do not administer to patients with acute respiratory or other active infections or illnesses.

*Special warnings and precautions for use:* Adrenaline injection (1:1000) should be immediately available for control of anaphylactic reactions that may occur. The vaccine may not result in sero-conversion of all patients, and protection is only against the strains of virus contained in the vaccine or closely related strains.

*Interactions with other medicaments and other forms of interaction:* None.

*Pregnancy and lactation:* Animal reproduction studies have not been conducted. It is not known if influenza virus vaccine can cause foetal harm or affect reproduction capacity. The vaccine should be given to a pregnant woman only if needed. Lactation is not a contra-indication.

*Effects on ability to drive and use machines:* The ability of individuals to drive and use machines should not be affected by the receipt of immunisation with Fluzone.

*Undesirable effects:* Local side effects such as transient erythema, swelling, tenderness or pain at the injection site lasting 1–2 days have been reported. Rarely systemic effects such as headache, mild fever, malaise and myalgia/arthralgia lasting 1–2 days.

*Overdose:* Not applicable.

**Pharmacological properties**

*Pharmacodynamic properties:* Since Fluzone is a vaccine, ordinary measures of pharmacodynamics and pharmacokinetics do not apply.

Most of the information on pharmacological effects and mode of action has been gained through human clinical studies.

*Pharmacokinetic properties:* See *Pharmacodynamic Properties.*

*Preclinical safety data:* Preclinical studies have not been conducted on Fluzone as these are not applicable for a product of this nature.

**Pharmaceutical particulars**

*List of excipients:* Thiomersal, gelatin, phosphate buffered saline, sucrose.

*Incompatibilities:* Do not inject intravenously.

*Shelf life:* 12 months between +2°C and +8°C.

*Special precautions for storage:* Store between +2°C and +8°C.

Do not freeze the vaccine. Potency is destroyed by freezing. Do not use vaccine if it has been frozen.

*Nature and contents of container:* Fluzone is supplied,

ready for use, in pre-filled single dose (0.5 ml) glass (Type 1) syringes.

*Instructions for use/handling:* Shake the syringe well to uniformly distribute the suspension before administering the dose.

**Marketing authorisation number** 6745/0080.

**Date of approval/revision of SPC** September 1996.

**Legal category** POM.

## HB-VAX* II
## Recombinant Hepatitis B Vaccine 10 mcg/ml, suspension for injection (IM), adults and adolescents

**Qualitative and quantitative composition**

Ag HBs†

| | |
|---|---|
| Hepatitis B surface antigen, recombinant | 10 mcg |
| Thiomersal (Sodium Mercurothiolate) | 50 mcg |
| Aluminium hydroxide (expressed as Al) | $0.50 \times 10^3$ mcg |
| Sodium chloride | $9.00 \times 10^3$ mcg |
| Formaldehyde | < 20 mcg |
| Potassium thiocyanate | < 0.50 mcg |
| Water for Injections | qs 1 ml |

For a vial and prefilled syringe.

† Surface antigen of hepatitis B virus produced from recombinant strain of the yeast *Saccharomyces cerevisiae.*

**Pharmaceutical form** Suspension for intramuscular administration

**Clinical particulars**

*Therapeutic indications:* This vaccine is indicated for active immunisation against hepatitis B virus infection caused by all known subtypes in subjects of all ages considered at risk of exposure to HBV.

*Groups identified at increased risk of infection:*

*Health care personnel.* Oral surgeons, dentists, physicians and surgeons, nurses, dental hygienists, paramedical personnel in close contact with patients, staff in haemodialysis, haematology and oncology units, laboratory personnel handling blood and other clinical specimens, emergency and first aid workers, ambulance staff, blood bank and plasma fractionation workers, cleaning staff in hospitals handling waste, chiropodists, morticians and embalmers.

*Patients frequently receiving blood products.* Patients in haemodialysis and oncology units, patients suffering from thalassaemia, sickle cell anaemia, liver cirrhosis, haemophilia, and patients receiving frequent blood transfusion or clotting factor concentrates, patients receiving organ transplants.

*Personnel collecting, sorting out, handling the specific waste and household rubbish.*

*Personnel and residents of institutions.* Persons with frequent and/or close contacts with high risk groups, prisoners and prison staff, residents and staff of institutions for mentally handicapped.

*Personnel at increased risk due to their sexual behaviour.* Persons with multiple sexual partners, patients with a Sexually Transmitted Disease (STD), persons seeking treatment for an STD, prostitutes and male homosexuals.

*Illicit users of addictive injectable drugs.*

*Travellers to areas with a high endemicity of HBV.*

*Persons originating from areas with a high endemicity of HBV.* Adoptees, immigrants and refugees.

*Others:* police personnel, fire brigade personnel, armed forces personnel and anybody who through their work or personal lifestyle may be exposed to HBV.

*Household contacts of any of the above groups and contacts with acute or chronic HBV infection.*

Nevertheless, the recommendations should be adjusted in line with national vaccination policies since in some countries generalisation of vaccination is highly recommended.

*Posology and method of administration:*

*Posology:* Adolescents and adults (16 years of age and older): The volume and dose of vaccine recommended for each injection is 10 mcg in 1 ml.

A course of vaccination should include at least three doses as follows:

1st injection: at elected date

2nd injection: ≥ 1 month after the first immunisation

3rd injection: ≥ 1 month after the second immunisation

This schedule allows the incorporation of several schemes in national vaccination recommendations.

*The most commonly used schedules in Europe are:*

*0, 1, 6 months:* two injections with an interval of one month; a third injection 6 months after the first administration

*0, 1, 2, 12 months:* three injections with an interval of one month; a fourth dose should be administered at 12 months

The accelerated schedule (0, 1, 2, 12 months) may induce protective antibody levels earlier in a slightly larger proportion of vaccinees.

The timing of successive injections in a vaccination series may need to be adjusted to local programmes, especially where hepatitis B vaccine is integrated with the administration of other paediatric vaccines.

*Booster:* Immunocompetent vaccinees: The duration of the protective effect of HB-VAX II in healthy vaccinees is unknown at present and the need for booster doses is not yet defined. However, some national vaccination schedules currently include recommendations for periodic booster doses.

Immunoincompetent vaccinees (e.g. dialysis patients).

A booster dose may be considered in these vaccinees if the anti-HBs level is less than 10 IU/L.

*Special dosage recommendations: Recommendations for known or presumed exposure to HBV (e.g. needlestick with contaminated needle);* Hepatitis B immunoglobulin (HBIG) should be given as soon as possible after exposure (with 24 hours).

The first dose of the vaccine should be given within 7 days of exposure and can be given simultaneously with hepatitis B immunoglobulin, however it must be administered at a separate injection site.

Subsequent doses of vaccine, if necessary (i.e. according to the serologic status of the patient), should be given as the recommended schedule for this vaccine.

*Method of administration:* This vaccine is for intramuscular injection. The deltoid muscle is the preferred site for injection.

Exceptionally, the vaccine may be administered subcutaneously in patients with thrombocytopenia or to persons at risk of haemorrhage.

*Contra-indications:* Severe febrile illness. Known hypersensitivity to any component of the vaccine or allergic reaction after previous vaccine administration.

*Special warnings and precautions for use:* Because of the long incubation period of hepatitis B, it is possible for unrecognised hepatitis B infection to be present at the time of immunisation. The vaccine may not prevent hepatitis B infection in such cases.

The vaccine will not prevent infection caused by other agents such as hepatitis A; hepatitis C and hepatitis E and other pathogens known to infect the liver.

In dialysis patients and persons with an impaired immune system, administration of additional doses of vaccine may be needed to obtain a protective anti-HBs titre.

As with all injectable vaccines, appropriate medical treatment should always be readily available in case of rare anaphylactic reactions following the administration of the vaccine.

Exceptionally, the vaccine may be administered subcutaneously in patients with thrombocytopenia or to persons at risk of haemorrhage.

This vaccine contains thiomersal (sodium mercurothiolate) as a preservative.

*Interaction with other medicaments and other forms of interaction:* This vaccine can be administed with hepatitis B immunoglobulin, at a separate injection site.

This vaccine can be used to complete a primary immunisation course or as a booster dose in subjects who have previously received another HBV vaccine.

*Pregnancy and lactation:* The effect of the HBsAg on foetal development has not been assessed. However, as with all inactivated viral vaccines, one does not expect harm for the foetus. Utilisation during pregnancy requires that the potential benefit justifies the potential risk to the foetus.

The effect on breast fed infants of the administration of this vaccine has not been assessed; nevertheless, this situation is not a contra-indication.

*Effects on ability to drive and use machines:* There are no specific data. Some of the rare effects mentioned under *Undesirable effects,* such as dizziness, headache, may effect the ability to drive or operate machinery.

*Undesirable effects:* The following undesirable effects have been reported following the widespread use of the vaccine. As with other hepatitis B vaccines, in many instances, the causal relationship to the vaccine has not been established.

*Common reactions:* Local reactions at injection site: transient soreness, erythema, induration.

*Rare:*

- elevation of liver enzymes, fatigue, fever, malaise, influenza-like symptoms, bronchospasm-like symptoms, serum sickness, thrombocytopenia.
- dizziness, headache, paraesthesia.
- nausea, vomiting, diarrhoea, abdominal pain
- athralgia, myalgia
- rash, pruritus, urticaria, anaphylaxis
- hypotension, syncope
- paralysis (Bell's palsy), neuropathy, neuritis (including Guillain-Barré Syndrome), myelitis (including transverse myelitis), encephalitis, optic neuritis
- angioedema, erythema multiforme
- lymphadenopathy

*Overdose:* There are no data with regard to overdosage.

**Pharmacological properties** Anti-infectious. Vaccines/hepatitis B.

*Pharmacodynamic properties:* The vaccine induces specific humeral antibodies against HBsAg (anti-HBs). Development of an anti-HBs titre above 10 IU/L measured 1–2 months after the last injection correlates with protection to HBV infection.

*Pharmacokinetic properties:* Not applicable.

*Preclinical safety data:* Each lot of vaccine must pass the Abnormal Toxicity Test of the European Pharmacopoeia in mice and guinea pigs; a single dose acute toxicity test has been conducted in mice. Animal reproduction studies have not been conducted.

*Relevant information for vaccines:* In clinical trials, 96% of 1497 healthy infants, children, adolescents and adults given a 3 dose course of HB-VAX II developed a protective level of anti-HBs (≥ 10 IU/L).

The protective efficacy of a dose of HBIG at birth followed by 3 doses of HB-VAX II has been demonstrated for neonates born to mothers positive for both HBsAg and HBeAg. Among 130 vaccinated infants, the estimated efficacy in prevention of chronic hepatitis B infection was 95% as compared to the infection rate in untreated historical controls.

Although the duration of the protective effect of HB-VAX II in healthy vaccinees is unknown, follow-up over 5–9 years of approximately 3000 high-risk subjects given a similar plasma-derived vaccine has revealed no cases of clinically apparent hepatitis B infection.

In addition, persistence of vaccine-induced immunologic memory for HBsAg has been demonstrated through an anamnestic antibody response to a booster dose of HB-VAX II in healthy adults given plasma-derived vaccine 5 to 7 years earlier.

**Pharmaceutical particulars**

*List of excipients:* See *Qualitative and quantitative composition.*

*Incompatibilities:* The vaccine should not be mixed in the same syringe with other vaccines or parenterally administered drugs.

*Shelf life:* Three years for the vial presentation. One year for the prefilled syringe presentation.

*Special precautions for storage:* The vaccine should be stored between: +2°C to +8°C.

Do not freeze.

*Nature and contents of container:* Vial of 1 ml of suspension Type I USP glass 2 ml vial with West n° 888 butyl rubber stopper and aluminium seal. Flip-off plastic cap.

Prefilled syringe (glass) 1 ml of suspension.

*Instructions for use handling:* Before use, the vaccine should be well shaken to obtain a slightly opaque white suspension.

**Marketing authorisation holder:** Merck Sharp and Dohme Limited, Hertford Road, Hoddesdon, Hertfordshire EN11 9BU.

**Marketing authorisation number** 0025/0294.

**Date of approval/revision of SPC** August 1996.

**Legal category** POM.

## HB-VAX* II PAEDIATRIC
## Recombinant Hepatitis B Vaccine 5 mcg/0.5 ml, suspension for injection (IM), paediatric

**Qualitative and quantitative composition**

Ag HBs†

| | |
|---|---|
| Hepatitis B surface antigen, recombinant | 5 mcg |
| Thiomersal (Sodium Mercurothiolate) | 25 mcg |
| Aluminium hydroxide (expressed as Al) | $0.25 \times 10^3$ mcg |
| Sodium chloride | $4.50 \times 10^3$ mcg |
| Formaldehyde | < 10 mcg |
| Potassium thiocyanate | < 0.25 mcg |
| Water for Injections | qs 0.5 ml |

For a prefilled syringe.

† Surface antigen of hepatitis B virus produced from recombinant strain of the yeast *Saccharomyces cerevisiae.*

**Pharmaceutical form** Suspension for intramuscular administration

**Clinical particulars**

*Therapeutic indications:* This vaccine is indicated for active immunisation against hepatitis B virus infection caused by all known subtypes in subjects of all ages considered at risk of exposure to HBV.

*Groups identified at increased risk of infection:*

*Children frequently receiving blood products.* Children in haemodialysis and oncology units, children suffering from thalassaemia, sickle cell anaemia, haemophilia, and children receiving frequent blood transfusions or clotting factor concentrates, organ transplants.

*Infants born of mothers who are HBV carriers.*

*Children residents of institutions.* Children residents of institutions for mentally handicapped.

*Travellers' children to areas with a high endemicity of HBV.*

*Children originating from areas with a high endemicity of HBV.* Adoptees, immigrants and refugees.

*Others:* Children through their personal lifestyle may be exposed to HBV.

*Household contacts of any of the above groups and contacts with acute or chronic HBV infection.*

Nevertheless, the recommendations should be adjusted in line with national vaccination policies since in some countries generalisation of vaccination is highly recommended.

*Posology and method of administration:*

*Posology:* Neonates and children (birth through 15 years of age).

The volume and dose of vaccine recommended for each injection is 5 mcg in 0.5 ml.

A course of vaccination should include at least three doses as follows:

1st injection: at elected date
2nd injection: ≥ 1 month after the first immunisation
3rd injection: ≥ 1 month after the second immunisation

This schedule allows the incorporation of several schemes in national vaccination recommendations.

*The most commonly used schedules in Europe are:*

*0, 1, 6 months:* two injections with an interval of one month; a third injection 6 months after the first administration

*0, 1, 2, 12 months:* three injections with an interval of one month; a fourth dose should be administered at 12 months

The accelerated schedule (0, 1, 2, 12 months) may induce protective antibody levels earlier in a slightly larger proportion of vaccinees.

The timing of successive injections in a vaccination series may need to be adjusted to local programmes, especially where hepatitis B vaccine is integrated with the administration of other paediatric vaccines.

*Booster:*

*Immunocompetent vaccinees:* The duration of the protective effect of HB-VAX II in healthy vaccinees is unknown at present and the need for booster doses is not yet defined. However, some national vaccination schedules currently include recommendations for periodic booster doses.

*Immunoincompetent vaccinees (e.g. dialysis patients):* A booster dose may be considered in these vaccinees if the anti-HBs level is less than 10 IU/L.

*Special dosage recommendations:*

*Neonates born of mothers who are HBV carriers:* At birth, one dose of hepatitis B immunoglobulin (within 24 hours).

The first dose of the vaccine should be given within 7 days of birth and can be given simultaneously with HB immunoglobulin at birth, but administered at a separate injection site.

Subsequent doses of vaccine should be given at 0–1–6 months (or possible at 0–1–2–12 months).

*Method of administration:* The vaccine is for intramuscular injection. The anterolateral thigh is the preferrred site for injection in neonates, infants and young children.

Exceptionally, the vaccine may be administered subcutaneously in patients with thrombocytopenia or to persons at risk of haemorrhage.

*Contra-indications:* Severe febrile illness.

Known hypersensitivity to any component of the vaccine or allergic reaction after previous vaccine administration.

*Special warnings and precautions for use:* Because of the long incubation period of hepatitis B, it is possible for unrecognised hepatitis B infection to be present at the time of immunisation. The vaccine may not prevent hepatitis B infection in such cases.

The vaccine will not prevent infection caused by other agents such as hepatitis A, hepatitis C and hepatitis E and other pathogens known to infect the liver.

In dialysis patients and persons with an impaired immune system, administration of additional doses of vaccine may be needed to obtain a protective anti-HBs titre.

As with all injectable vaccines, appropriate medical treatment should always be readily available in case of rare anaphylactic reactions following the administration of the vaccine.

Exceptionally, the vaccine may be administered subcutaneously in patients with thrombocytopenia or to persons at risk of haemorrhage.

This vaccine contains thiomersal (sodium mercurothiolate) as a preservative.

*Interaction with other medicaments and other forms of interaction:* This vaccine can be administered with hepatitis B immunoglobulin, at a separate injection site.

This vaccine can be used to complete a primary immunisation course or as a booster dose in subjects who have previously received another HBV vaccine.

*Pregnancy and lactation:* Not relevant.

*Effects on ability to drive and use machines:* Not relevant.

*Undesirable effects:* The following undesirable effects have been reported following the widespread use of the vaccine. As with other hepatitis B vaccines, in many instances, the causal relationship to the vaccine has not been established.

*Common reactions:* Local reactions at injection site: transient soreness, erythema, induration.

*Rare:*
 – elevation of liver enzymes, fatigue, fever, malaise, influenza-like symptoms, bronchospasm-like symptoms, serum sickness, thrombocytopenia
 – dizziness, headache, paraesthesia
 – nausea, vomiting, diarrhoea, abdominal pain
 – arthralgia, myalgia
 – rash, pruritis, urticaria, anaphylaxis
 – hypotension, syncope
 – paralysis (Bell's palsy), neuropathy, neuritis (including Guillain-Barré Syndrome), myelitis (including transverse myelitis), encephalitis, optic neuritis
 – angioedema, erythema multiforme
 – lymphadenopathy

*Overdose:* There are no data with regard to overdosage.

**Pharmacological properties** Anti-infectious. Vaccines/hepatitis B.

*Pharmacodynamic properties:* The vaccine induces specific humoral antibodies against HBsAg (anti-HBs). Development of an anti-HBs titre above 10 IU/L measured 1–2 months after the last injection correlates with protection to HBV infection.

*Pharmacokinetic properties:* Not applicable.

*Preclinical safety data:* Each lot of vaccine must pass the Abnormal Toxicity Test of the European Pharmacopoeia in mice and guinea pigs. A single dose acute toxicity test has been conducted in mice. Animal reproduction studies have not been conducted.

*Relevant information for vaccines:* In clinical trials, 96% of 1497 healthy infants, children, adolescents and adults given a 3 dose course of HB-VAX II developed a protective level of anti-HBs (≥ 10 IU/L).

The protective efficacy of a dose of HBIG at birth followed by 3 doses of HB-VAX II has been demonstrated for neonates born to mothers positive for both HBsAg and HBeAg. Among 130 vaccinated infants, the estimated efficacy in prevention of chronic hepatitis B infection was 95% as compared to the infection rate in untreated historical controls.

Although the duration of the protective effect of HB-VAX II in healthy vaccinees is unknown, follow-up over 5–9 years of approximately 3000 high-risk subjects given a similar plasma-derived vaccine has revealed no cases of clinically apparent hepatitis B infection.

In addition, persistance of vaccine-induced immunologic memory for HBsAg has been demonstrated through an anamnestic antibody response to a booster dose of HB-VAX II in healthy adults given plasma-derived vaccine 5 to 7 years earlier.

**Pharmaceutical particulars**

*List of excipients:* See *Qualitative and quantitative composition* section above.

*Incompatibilities:* The vaccine should not be mixed in the same syringe with other vaccines or parenterally administered drugs.

*Shelf life:* 12 months.

*Special precautions for storage:* The vaccine should be stored between: +2°C to +8°C. Do not freeze.

*Nature and contents of container:* 0.5 ml of suspension in prefilled syringes (glass).

*Instructions for use/handling:* Before use, the vaccine should be well shaken to obtain a slightly opaque white suspension.

**Marketing authorisation holder:** Merck Sharp & Dohme Limited, Hertford Road, Hoddesdon, Hertfordshire EN11 9BU.

**Marketing authorisation number** 0025/0295.

**Date of approval/revision of SPC** August 1996.

**Legal category** POM.

## Inactivated Influenza Vaccine (Split Virion) BP Pasteur Merieux

### Qualitative and quantitative composition

| Active ingredient | Quantity per dose |
|---|---|
| A/Wuhan/359/95 (H₃N₂)-like strain | 15 mcg/Haemagglutinin antigen |
| A/Singapore/6/86 (H₁N₁)-like strain | 15 mcg/Haemagglutinin antigen |
| B/Beijing/184/93-like strain | 15 mcg/Haemagglutinin antigen |

**Please note:**
A/Wuhan/359/95-like strain is a new strain for the 1996/1997 season.
A/Nanchang/933/95 is the A/Wuhan/359/95-like strain, A/Texas/36/91 is the A/Singapore 6/86-like strain and B/Harbin/7/94 is the B/Beijing/184/93-like strain.

*Excipients:*

| | |
|---|---|
| Thiomersal preservative | 0.01% w/v |
| Sterile buffered saline solution† | 0.50 ml |
| †Consisting of Sodium Chloride | 4.00 mg |
| Potassium Chloride | 0.10 mg |
| Sodium phosphate (dibasic) | 0.575 mg |
| Potassium phosphate (monobasic) | 0.10 mg |
| Bulk Water for Injections | qs 0.50 ml |

**Pharmaceutical form** Prefilled unit dose syringe containing a sterile colourless aqueous suspension for deep subcutaneous or intramuscular injection.

### Clinical particulars

*Therapeutic indications:* Prophylaxis against influenza.

*Posology and method of administration:* Administer by intramuscular or deep subcutaneous injection.

*Adults, elderly and children over 13 years of age:* Single dose of 0.5 ml.

*Children:*
 13 years and older: one 0.5 ml dose.
 4–12 years of age: 0.5 ml repeated 4–6 weeks later if receiving influenza vaccine for the first time.
 6–47 months of age: 0.25 ml repeated 4–6 weeks later if receiving influenza vaccine for the first time.

*Contra-indications:* The vaccine is contra-indicated in persons hypersensitive to egg products.

Immunisation should be postponed in patients with febrile illness.

*Special warnings and precautions for use:* Use with caution in patients with a history of allergy. Even though allergic reactions are extremely rare it is important to have facilities for the management of anaphylaxis available as a safeguard.

This vaccine may contain traces of residual neomycin.

*Interactions with other medicaments and other forms of interaction:* None known.

*Pregnancy and lactation:* Animal reproduction studies have not been conducted. It is not known if influenza virus vaccine can cause foetal harm or affect reproduction capacity. The vaccine should be given to a pregnant woman only if needed.

Lactation is not a contra-indication.

*Effects on ability to drive and use machines:* None known.

*Undesirable effects:* Local reactions at the injection site have been rarely known.

*Overdose:* Not applicable.

### Pharmacological properties

*Pharmacodynamic properties:* While most vaccines are antigenically stable, the influenza viruses A and B (especially A) are constantly altering their antigenic structure as indicated by changes in the haemagglutinins and neuraminidases on the surface of the viruses. Suitable strains of influenza vaccine for inclusion in the vaccine are recommended each year by the WHO. The vaccine contains these type A and B strains, in which the integrity of the virus particles has been disrupted.

The strains are grown in the allantoic cavity of fertile incubated chick embryos and inactivated so that they are non-infective but retain their antigenic properties.

*Pharmacokinetic properties:* Not applicable.

*Preclinical safety data:* Not applicable.

### Pharmaceutical particulars

*List of excipients:* See *Qualitative and quantitative composition* section above.

*Incompatibilities:* None known.

*Shelf life:* 12 months at +2°C to +8°C.

*Special precautions for storage:* Store at +2°C to +8°C. Do not freeze. Protect from light.

*Nature and contents of container:* Prefilled unit dose (0.5 ml) Glass (Type 1 PhEur), one millilitre syringe fitted with 25×5/8 stainless steel needle.

Siliconised elastomer piston stopper and protective needle guard.

Supplier: Becton Dickinson or Bunder Glass.

*Instruction for Use/Handling:* See *Special precautions for storage.*

**Marketing authorisation number**   6745/0081.

**Date of approval/revision of SPC**   August 1996.

**Legal category**   POM.

## MENGIVAC (A+C)*
## Meningococcal Polysaccharide Vaccine BP

**Presentation**   An inactivated polysaccharide vaccine against *Neisseria meningitidis* Serogroups A and C.

Each 0.5 ml dose contains not less than 50 µg each of lyophilised, Group A and Group C polysaccharides and 2 mg of lactose as stabiliser. Isotonic buffered diluent is supplied with each dose.

**Uses**   Active immunisation against meningococcal meningitis caused by N. meningitidis Serogroups A and C.

*(a) Travel:* Vaccination should be offered to travellers visiting parts of the world where the risk of meningococcal meningitis is high. These regions include countries within the African Meningitis Belt (countries whose borders are between the Equator and latitude 15° North), parts of the Middle East and parts of the Indian Sub-Continent.

*(b) Contacts of cases:* Family members and close contacts of disease cases of Group A and Group C meningococcal meningitis should be immunised. The vaccine does not protect against Group B disease.

*(c) Local outbreaks:* To help control local outbreaks of meningococcal Group A and Group C disease, vaccination may be recommended by appropriate Public Health Authorities.

Post vaccination immunity lasts at least 3 years.

**Dosage and administration**   0.5 ml reconstituted vaccine by deep subcutaneous or intramuscular injection. The vaccine should be reconstituted using the diluent provided.

Shake before use.

Record the dose, batch number and date of administration.

**Contra-indications, warnings, etc**
*Contra-indication:* Acute infectious illness. Hypersensitivity to the vaccine or any component.

*Precautions:* Mengivac A+C confers protection specific to meningococci of Groups A and C. Immunisation does not protect against meningococci of other serogroups or against meningitis caused by other organisms.

*Warnings:* Facilities for the management of anaphylaxis should always be available during vaccination.

*Adverse reactions:* These are normally mild and short lasting. Local reactions may occur at the injection site and less commonly, systemic reactions may occur. Pyrexial reactions may occur more frequently in young children.

Use in pregnancy and lactation is not routinely recommended.

**Pharmaceutical precautions**   Store at +2°C to +8°C. Do not freeze the diluent. After reconstitution, use within 1 hour. Shake before use.

**Legal category**   POM.

**Package quantities**   Carton of 1 single dose vial of lyophilised vaccine + 1 syringe of diluent (0.5 ml).

**Further information**   Young children and infants respond less well to the vaccine than older children and adults, with little response to the Group C polysaccharide under 18 months of age and a poor response to Group A polysaccharide under 3 months of age.

Additionally, protection in infants under 18 months of age is of shorter duration.

**Product licence numbers**
Diluent   6745/0029
Lyophilised vaccine 6745/0048.

## MMR* II
## Measles, Mumps and Rubella vaccine, Live, Attenuated

**Qualitative and quantitative composition**   Each 0.5 ml dose when reconstituted contains not less than equivalent of:

1,000 TCID$_{50}$† of Measles Vaccine Live (the more attenuated Enders Line of the Edmonston strain).
20,000 TCID$_{50}$ of Mumps Vaccine Live (Jeryl Lynn* Level B strain).

1,000 TCID$_{50}$ of Rubella Vaccine Live (Wistar, RA 27/Strain).
† Tissue Culture Infectious Dose.

**Pharmaceutical form**   A lyophilised powder for subcutaneous or intramuscular injection, after reconstitution with sterile water.

**Clinical particulars**   *Therapeutic indications:* For simultaneous immunisation against measles, mumps and rubella in the following groups:

*Children:* Recommended for both primary and booster immunisation of both boys and girls 12 months of age or older.

*Non-pregnant adolescent and adult females:* Immunisation of susceptible non-pregnant adolescent and adult females of childbearing age is indicated when the potential vaccinee agrees not to become pregnant for the next 3 months after vaccination and is informed of the reason, and is told of the frequent occurrence of generally self-limiting arthralgia and/or arthritis beginning 2–4 weeks after vaccination.

*International travellers:* Individuals planning travel abroad who are known to be susceptible to one or more of these diseases can receive either a single antigen vaccine (measles, mumps or rubella) or a combined antigen vaccine as appropriate. MMR II is preferred for persons likely to be susceptible to mumps and rubella as well as measles.

*Posology and method of administration:* The vaccine is administered by subcutaneous or intramuscular injection preferably into the outer aspect of the arm.

*Adults and children:* After suitably cleansing the injection site, 0.5 ml of reconstituted vaccine should be injected. MMR II must not be given intravenously.

*Do not give immunoglobulin with MMR II.*

*Warning:* A sterile syringe and epinephrine (adrenaline) injection should be available for immediate use should an anaphylactic reaction occur.

*Elderly:* No special comment.

*Revaccination:* A second dose of MMR vaccine is recommended in the national immunisation schedule.

Children receiving their first dose of MMR vaccine younger than 12 months of age should be revaccinated at 15 months of age. They may still receive a further dose at the time indicated in the national immunisation schedule (MMR II is not recommended for infants under 12 months of age).

*Use with other vaccines:* Vaccines containing diphtheria, tetanus and pertussis antigens and/or oral poliomyelitis vaccine can be administered at the same time as MMR II. For concurrent parenteral vaccination, separate syringes and separate sites for injection should be used. MMR II should not be given less than one month before or after immunisation with other vaccines.

*Contra-indications:* Do not give MMR II to pregnant females; the possible effects of the vaccine on foetal development are unknown at this time. Pregnancy must be avoided for three months following vaccination of post-pubertal females.

Anaphylactic or anaphylactoid reactions to a previous dose of vaccine or to neomycin or any other vaccine constituent. (Each dose of reconstituted vaccine contains approximately 25 mcg neomycin.)

History of anaphylactic or anaphylactoid reactions to eggs (see *Hypersensitivity to eggs, chicken, or chicken feathers*).

Any febrile respiratory illness, or other active or suspected infection.

Those with impaired immune responsiveness, whether occurring naturally or as a result of therapy with steroids, radiotherapy, cytotoxic or other agents. This contra-indication does not apply to patients receiving corticosteroids as replacement therapy, e.g. for Addison's disease.

Patients with active untreated tuberculosis, blood dyscrasias such as thrombocytopenia, leukaemia, malignant disease including lymphomas of any type or other malignant neoplasms affecting the bone marrow or lymphatic systems.

Primary and acquired immunodeficiency states, including patients who are immunosuppressed in association with AIDS or other clinical manifestations with human immunodeficiency viruses; cellular immune deficiencies; and hypogammaglobulinaemic and dysgammaglobulinaemic states.

Those patients with a family history of congenital hereditary immunodeficiency until their immune competence has been demonstrated.

*Hypersensitivity to eggs, chickens, or chicken feathers:* Live measles and live mumps vaccine are produced in cell cultures of chick embryo.

Patients with a history of anaphylactic, anaphylactoid or other immediate reactions to eating eggs (e.g. hives, swelling of the mouth and throat, difficult breathing, hypotension and shock) should not be vaccinated. Evidence indicates, however, that patients with egg allergies that are not anaphylactic or anaphy-

lactoid may be vaccinated in the usual way. There is no evidence to suggest that allergy to chicken or feathers increases the risk of reaction.

*Children below 12 months of age:* Children below 12 months of age should not normally be given MMR II unless they are at special risk, since the presence of maternal antibody may interfere with their ability to respond. They may be given human normal immunoglobulin. However, where immunisation below the age of 12 months is deemed necessary, a second dose of vaccine should be given at 15 months of age and a further dose may still be given at the usual time.

*Special warnings and special precautions for use:* Epinephrine (adrenaline) should be available for immediate use should an anaphylactic or anaphylactoid reaction occur.

MMR II should be given with caution to those with an individual or family history of cerebral injury or any other condition in which stress due to fever should be avoided. The physician should be alert to the rise in temperature that may follow vaccination.

Children and young adults who are known to be infected with, or have a history of immunodeficiency viruses, but without overt clinical manifestations of immunosuppression, may be vaccinated; however, the vaccinees should be closely monitored for exposure to vaccine-preventable diseases because immunisation may be less effective than for uninfected persons. In selected cases, confirmation of circulating antibody levels may be indicated to help guide appropriate protective measures, including immunoprophylaxis if immunity has waned to non-protective levels.

Excretion of small amounts of live attenuated rubella virus from the nose and throat has occurred in the majority of susceptible individuals 7–28 days after vaccination. There is no definite evidence to indicate that such a virus is transmitted to susceptible persons who are in contact with vaccinated individuals. Consequently transmission, while accepted as a theoretical possibility, has not been regarded as a significant risk. However, transmission of the vaccine virus via breast milk has been documented.

There are no reports of transmission of live attenuated measles or mumps viruses from vaccinees to susceptible contacts.

Children under treatment for tuberculosis have not experienced exacerbation of the disease when immunised with live measles virus vaccine; no studies have been reported to date of the effect of measles virus vaccines on untreated tuberculous children.

Parents of children with a personal or family history of convulsions or idiopathic epilepsy should be advised that such children have a small increased risk of seizures following vaccination and be informed in advance of procedures for their management.

*Interactions with other medicaments and other forms of interaction:* Vaccination should be deferred for at least three months following blood or plasma transfusions or administration of any human immune serum globulin. If any of these substances has been used near to the time of vaccination with MMR II, a test should subsequently be made to confirm successful seroconversions.

Where anti-Rho (D) globulin (human) and rubella vaccine are required in the immediate post-partum period, rubella vaccine alone and not MMR II should be used.

It has been reported that live attenuated measles, mumps and rubella vaccine may temporarily depress tuberculin skin sensitivity. If a tuberculin test is to be done, it should be administered before or simultaneously with MMR II.

*Pregnancy and lactation:* Pregnant females must NOT be given MMR II. Furthermore, pregnancy should be avoided for three months following vaccination (see *Contra-indications*).

Animal reproduction studies have not been conducted with MMR II. It is also not known whether MMR II can cause foetal harm when given to pregnant women or affect reproductive capacity.

If a woman is inadvertently vaccinated or if she becomes pregnant within three months of vaccination, she should be counselled by her physician. It has been established that: (1) in a ten-year study involving 700 pregnant women who received rubella vaccination within three months of conception, none of their new-born infants had abnormalities compatible with a congenital rubella syndrome; (2) although mumps virus is capable of infecting the placenta and foetus, there is no good evidence that it causes congenital malformations in humans.

Mumps vaccine virus has also been shown to affect the placenta, but the virus has not been isolated from foetal tissues taken from susceptible women who were vaccinated and underwent elective abortions; and (3) reports indicate that contracting natural measles during pregnancy increases the rates of spontaneous abortion, stillbirth, congenital defects and prematurity. Although there are no adequate studies on the attenuated (vaccine) strain in pregnancy, it would be prudent to assume that the strain of the virus in the vaccine is also capable of inducing adverse foetal effects.

*Breast-feeding mothers:* Caution should be exercised when MMR II is given to a breast-feeding mother. Although it is not known whether measles or mumps vaccine virus is secreted in human milk, studies have shown that breast-feeding mothers immunised with live attenuated RA 27/3 strain rubella vaccine transmit the virus via breast milk. In those babies with serological evidence of rubella, none showed clinical disease.

*Effects on ability to drive and use machines:* None reported.

*Undesirable effects:* Adverse reactions: Adverse reactions associated with MMR II are similar to those to be expected from the administration of monovalent vaccines given separately.

The following adverse reactions occur commonly: Burning and/or stinging at the injection site for a short period.

The following adverse reactions occur occasionally: *Body as a whole:* Fever (101°F [38.3°C] or higher).

*Skin:* Rash, usually minimal but may be generalised. Generally, fever, rash or both appear between the 5th and the 12th days.

Mild, local reactions such as erythema; induration and tenderness.

The following adverse reactions occur rarely: *Body as a whole:* Sore throat, malaise.

*Digestive:* Parotitis, nausea, vomiting, diarrhoea.

*Haematologic/lymphatic:* Regional lymphadenopathy, thrombocytopenia, purpura.

*Hypersensitivity:* Allergic reactions such as wheal and flare at injection site, anaphylaxis and anaphylactoid reactions, urticaria.

*Musculoskeletal:* Arthralgia and/or arthritis (usually transient and rarely chronic), myalgia.

*Nervous/psychiatric:* Febrile convulsions in children, afebrile convulsion or seizures, headache, dizziness, paraesthesia, polyneuritis, Guillain-Barré syndrome, ataxia. Encephalitis/encephalopathy have been reported approximately once for every 3 million doses. In no cases has it been shown that reactions were actually caused by vaccine. The risk of such serious neurological disorders following live measles virus vaccine administered remains for less than that for encephalitis and encephalopathy with natural measles (1 per 2000 reported cases).

*Skin:* Erythema multiforme.

*Special senses:* Forms of optic neuritis, including retrobulbar neuritis, papillitis, and retinitis; ocular palsies, otitis media, nerve deafness, conjunctivitis.

*Urogenital:* Orchitis.

There have been reports of subacute sclerosing panencephalitis (SSPE) in children who did not have a history of natural measles but did receive measles vaccine. Some of these cases may have resulted from unrecognised measles in the first year of life or possibly from the measles vaccination. Based on the estimated nationwide measles vaccine distribution in the USA, the association of SSPE cases to measles vaccination is about one case per million vaccine doses distributed. This is far less than the association with natural measles: 6–22 cases of SSPE per million cases of measles.

A study suggests that the overall effect of measles vaccine has been to protect against SSPE by preventing measles with its inherent higher risk of SSPE.

Local reactions characterised by marked swelling, redness and vesiculation at the injection site of attenuated live measles virus vaccines and systemic reactions including atypical measles have occurred in vaccinees who had previously received killed measles vaccine. Rarely, there have been reports of more severe reactions, including prolonged high fevers and extensive local reactions requiring hospitalisation. Panniculitis has also been reported rarely following vaccination with measles vaccine.

Arthralgia or arthritis or both are usually transient and rarely chronic features of natural infection, their frequency and severity vary with age and sex, begin greatest in adult females and least in prepubertal children.

The chronic arthritis associated with natural rubella has been related to virus and/or viral antigen found in body tissues. Only rarely have vaccinees developed chronic joint symptoms and causal relationship is unknown.

Following vaccination in children, reactions in joints are uncommon and generally of brief duration. In women, incidence rates for arthritis are generally higher than those seen in children (children 0–3%; women 12–20%) and the reactions tend to be more marked and of longer duration. Symptoms may persist for a matter of months or, on rare occasions, for years. In adolescent girls, the rections appear to be intermediate in incidence between those seen in children and in adult women. Even in older women (35–45 years) these reactions are generally well tolerated and rarely interfere with normal activities. Such reactions occur much less frequently after revaccination than primary vaccination.

*Overdose:* Poisoning is unlikely. Swallowing MMR II would render the live attenuated vaccine benign, and the content of the neomycin (25 mcg/ml) is not likely to cause toxicity. No case of overdosage has been reported.

### Pharmacological properties

*Pharmacodynamic properties:* MMR II Vaccine is a mixture of live attenuated measles, mumps and rubella viruses to provide active immunisation against these diseases.

Clinical studies in 279 triple seronegative children aged 11 months to 7 years, showed that MMR II is highly immunogenic and generally well-tolerated. In these studies, a single injection of the vaccine induced measles haemogglutination-inhibition (HI) antibodies in 95%, mumps neutralising antibodies in 96% and rubella HI antibodies in 99% of susceptible persons.

Based on available evidence a second dose of MMR vaccine in the national immunisation schedule has the potential to prevent epidemics of measles and overall is as well-tolerated as primary immunisation.

Vaccine induced antibody levels following administration of MMR II have been shown to persist for over 11 years.

*Pharmacokinetic properties:* Not applicable.

*Preclinical safety data:* No further information available.

### Pharmaceutical particulars

*List of excipients:* Before lyophilisation each unit of vaccine comprises the component virus in 0.5 ml of a medium with the following composition:

The quantities shown are of initial amounts of materials. Nutrients used for viral growth will be depleted in the final vehicle of the viruses.

| | |
|---|---|
| Albumin, Human USP | 300.0 mcg |
| Dipotassium Hydrogen Phosphate USP | 30.0 mcg |
| Disodium Hydrogen Phosphate PhEur | 30.0 mcg |
| Gelatine, Hydrolysed HSE | 14.5 mg |
| Medium 199 HSE | 3.4 mg |
| Minimum Essential Medium, Eagle HSE | 140.0 mcg |
| Monosodium L-Glutamate USP | 20.0 mcg |
| Neomycin Sulphate USP | 25.0 mcg |
| Phenol Red HSE | 3.4 mcg |
| Potassium Dihydrogen Phosphate USP | 100.0 mcg |
| Sodium Bicarbonate PhEur | 400.0 mcg |
| Sodium Dihydrogen Phosphate PhEur | 100.0 mg |
| Sorbitol | 14.5 mg |
| Sucrose | 1.9 mg |

*Incompatibilities:* None known.

*Shelf life:* 18 months

*Special precautions for storage:* Store between +2°C to +8°C.

*Nature and contents of container:* 3 ml type 1 glass tubing vials with 13 mm (West Co gray butyl 1816) lyophilisation stoppers and 13 mm 1 piece flip-off aluminium seal with plastic cap.

*Instructions for use/handling:* To reconstitute the vaccine, all the diluent provided should be injected into a vial of lyophilised vaccine, and this agitated to ensure thorough mixing. All the reconstituted vaccine is then drawn into the syringe and injected subcutaneously or intramuscularly.

Only the diluent supplied should be used for reconstitution, since it is free of preservatives and other antiviral substances that may inactivate the vaccine.

A separate sterile disposable needle and syringe should be used for each vaccinee.

It is good practice to record title, dose and batch number of all vaccines and dates of administration.

**Pharmaceutic particulars** During shipment, the vaccine must be maintained at a temperature of 10°C (50°F) or less to ensure no loss of potency.

Before reconstitution, MMR II should be stored between +2°C to +8°C (35.6°F to 46.4°F) and protected from light. Do not freeze.

MMR II retains at least 8 times the minimum immunising dose even after 6 weeks at 22°C or 1 week at 37°C. Storage at tempeatures above +2°C to +8°C cannot be recommended due to the difficulty in monitoring the exact temperature and monitoring repeated exposures to time out of refrigeration.

When reconstituted, the vaccine is yellow. It is acceptable for use only when clear and free from particulate matter.

The vaccine should be used as soon as possible and not later than one hour after reconstitution. Protect from light at all times, since exposure may inactivate the virus.

**Marketing authorisation number** 6745/0076.

**Date of approval/revision of SPC** September 1996.

**Legal category** POM.

## PNEUMOVAX II*
### Pneumococcal Vaccine, Polyvalent

**Presentation** Single-dose vial containing, in 0.5 ml, 25 mcg of each polysaccharide type derived from capsules of the 23 most prevalent pneumococci dissolved in isotonic saline containing 0.25% phenol.

**Uses** A pneumococcal vaccine.

Pneumovax II is a sterile liquid vaccine consisting of a mixture of highly purified capsular polysaccharides from the 23 most prevalent or invasive pneumococcal types accounting for at least 90% of pneumococcal blood isolates and at least 85% of all pneumococcal isolates from usually sterile sites determined by ongoing surveillance (see chart).

**23 pneumococcal capsular types included in Pneumovax II**

| Nomenclature | Pneumococcal types | | | | | | | | | | |
|---|---|---|---|---|---|---|---|---|---|---|---|
| Danish | 1 | 2 | 3 | 4 | 5 | 6B | 7F | 8 | 9N | 9V | |
| U.S. | 1 | 2 | 3 | 4 | 5 | 26 | 51 | 8 | 9 | 68 | |
| Danish | 10A | 11A | 12F | 14 | 15B | 17F | 18C | 19F | 19A | 20 | |
| U.S. | 34 | 43 | 12 | 14 | 54 | 17 | 56 | 19 | 57 | 20 | |
| Danish | 22F | 23F | 33F | | | | | | | | |
| U.S. | 22 | 23 | 70 | | | | | | | | |

Protective capsular type-specific antibody levels usually develop by the third week following vaccination.

Pneumovax II is indicated for immunisation against pneumococcal disease caused by those pneumococcal types included in the vaccine. Pneumovax II will not immunise against capsular types of pneumococcus other than those contained in the vaccine. It should be considered for all persons 2 years of age or older in whom there is an increased risk of morbidity and mortality from pneumococcal pneumonia.

Pneumovax II may not be effective in preventing infection resulting from basilar skull fracture or from external communication with cerebrospinal fluid.

**Dosage and administration** *Do not inject intravenously; avoid intradermal administration.*

Administer a single 0.5 ml dose of Pneumovax II subcutaneously or intramuscularly (preferably in the deltoid muscle or lateral mid-thigh) with appropriate precautions to avoid intravascular administration.

*Revaccination*

*Adults:* Routine vaccination of adults with Pneumovax II is not recommended because of an increased incidence and severity of adverse reactions among healthy adults revaccinated with pneumococcal vaccines at intervals under three years. This was probably due to sustained high antibody levels. Also, persons who received the 14-valent vaccine should not be routinely revaccinated with the 23-valent vaccine, as increased coverage is modest and duration of protection is not well defined.

Although routine revaccination is not recommended, revaccination is recommended for adults with chronic conditions which increase the risk of fatal pneumococcal infection and for those shown to have a rapid decline in pneumococcal antibody levels (e.g. patients with nephrotic syndrome, renal failure, or transplant recipients).

Based on clinical study results, revaccination with Pneumovax II is recommended for adults at highest risk of fatal pneumococcal infection who were initially vaccinated with Pneumovax (Pneumococcal Vaccine, Polyvalent, MSD) four or more years previously without a serious or severe reaction.

In addition, it is recommended that revaccination should be considered for adults at highest risk who received the 23-valent vaccine six or more years previously.

*Children:* It is recommended that revaccination after three to five years should be considered for children at highest risk for pneumococcal infection (e.g. children with asplenia, sickle cell disease, or nephrotic syndrome) who would be 10 years old or younger at revaccination. Such children should not, however, be revaccinated within three years.

Children at highest risk for pneumococcal infection may have lower peak antibody levels and/or more rapid antibody decline than do healthy adults. There is evidence that some of these high-risk children (e.g. asplenic children) benefit from revaccination with vaccine containing antigen 7F, 8, 19F.

**Contra-indications, warnings, etc**

*Contra-indications:* Hypersensitivity to any component of the vaccine. Adrenaline injection BP (1:1,000) must be immediately available should an acute anaphylactoid reaction occur.

Revaccination with Pneumovax II is contra-indicated, except as described under 'Revaccination'.

Do not use Pneumovax II less than ten days prior to or during immuno-suppressive therapy.

Patients with Hodgkin's disease who have received extensive chemotherapy and/or nodal irradiation.

Pneumovax II should not be given to pregnant women, since it is not known whether the vaccine can cause fetal harm, or affect the outcome of pregnancy.

Breast-feeding mothers should not be given Pneumovax II.

*Warnings:* The expected serum antibody response may not be obtained in patients receiving immuno-suppressive therapy.

Intradermal administration may cause severe local reactions.

*Precautions:* Caution and appropriate care should be exercised in administering Pneumovax II to individuals with severely compromised cardiac and/or pulmonary function in whom a systemic reaction would pose a significant risk.

Delay the use of Pneumovax II in any febrile respiratory illness or other active infection, except when this delay may involve even greater risk.

Required prophylactic antibiotic therapy against pneumococcal infection should not be stopped after immunisation with Pneumovax II.

It is recommended that a clear note of vaccination with Pneumovax II be kept in the patient's hospital and general practitioner records.

*Children under 2 years of age:* Pneumovax II is not recommended because antibody response to capsular types that most often cause pneumococcal disease in this age group may be poor. Safety and efficacy in children under 2 years have not been established.

*Adverse reactions:* Adverse reactions occurring commonly are:

Local injection site soreness, erythema, and induration.

Adverse reactions occurring occasionally are: *Body as a whole*—Low-grade fever (<100.9°F/38.3°C).

Adverse reactions occurring rarely are: *Body as a whole*—Headache, fever (>102°F/38.9°C), malaise, asthenia; *Haematologic/Lymphatic*—Adenitis; *Hypersensitivity*—Anaphylactoid reactions, serum sickness; *Musculoskeletal*—Arthralgia, myalgia, arthritis; *Skin*—Rash, urticaria.

On rare occasions, patients with otherwise stabilised idiopathic thrombocytopenic purpura have relapsed with a thrombocytopenia that has recurred 2–14 days after vaccination, and lasted for up to two weeks.

Reactions of greater severity, duration, or extent are unusual. Neurological disorders such as paraesthesiae and acute radiculoneuropathy, including the Guillain-Barré syndrome, have rarely been reported at the time of vaccination, but with no established cause-and-effect relationship.

**Pharmaceutical precautions** Store in a refrigerator between +2°C and +8°C. The vaccine is used directly as supplied. No dilution or reconstitution is necessary. Phenol 0.25% is present as preservative. All vaccine must be discarded after the expiration date.

Pneumovax II should be inspected before injection to see that it is a clear, colourless liquid without suspended particles.

**Legal category** POM.

**Package quantities** A single-dose vial.

**Further information** Invasive pneumococcal disease causes high morbidity and mortality in spite of effective antimicrobial control by antibiotics. These effects of pneumococcal disease appear to be due to irreversible pathological damage caused by bacteria during the first five days following onset of illness, irrespective of antimicrobial therapy.

Although the duration of the protective effect of Pneumovax II is presently unknown, previous studies with other pneumococcal vaccines suggest that induced antibodies may persist for five years. Type-specific antibody levels induced by 14-valent Pneumovax decline over a 42-month period of observation, but remain significantly higher than prevaccination levels in almost all recipients who responded initially.

**Product licence number**  0025/0293.

*Product licence holder:* Merck Sharp & Dohme Limited, Hertford Road, Hoddesdon, Hertfordshire, EN11 9BU.

*Distributed by:* Pasteur Mérieux MSD Ltd, Clivemont House, Clivemont Road, Maidenhead, Berkshire, SL6 7BU.

## RABIES VACCINE BP PASTEUR MERIEUX
### Human Diploid Cell Rabies Vaccine

**Presentation** The vaccine is a lyophilised, stabilised suspension of inactivated Wistar rabies virus strain PM/WI38 1503–3M, cultured on human diploid cells (MRC$_5$) and inactivated by beta-propiolactone. The dry vaccine is coloured off-white but, after reconstitution with the diluent supplied, it turns a pinkish colour due to the presence of phenol red. The potency of the reconstituted vaccine is not less than 2.5 International Units per dose (1 ml).

**Uses**
(a) Prophylactic immunisation against rabies.
(b) Treatment of patients following suspected rabies contact.

**Dosage and administration** The dose of reconstituted vaccine in all cases is 1 ml given by deep subcutaneous or intramuscular injection. The vaccine should be administered into the deltoid region but not the gluteal region. Reconstitution: Inject the diluent from the syringe into the vial, agitate to ensure complete reconstitution and withdraw the contents back into the syringe.

*(a) Prophylaxis:* Three injections each of 1 ml given on days 0, 7 and 28. A single reinforcing dose should be given at two or three year intervals to those at continued risk. If, for whatever reason, it has not been possible to give a full course of three injections, it is probable that, in the majority of subjects, two doses may be adequate to confer protection, provided these were given four weeks apart. Subjects receiving only two injections who remain at continued risk should receive a reinforcing dose 6–12 months later, with further reinforcing doses given at two to three year intervals.

*(b) Treatment:*
    (i) *In persons known to have adequate prophylaxis.* In the event of contact with a suspected rabid animal, two further boosters should be given on day 0 and on day 3 to 7.
    (ii) *In persons with no, or possibly inadequate, prophylaxis.* The first injection of rabies vaccine should be given as soon as possible after the suspected contact (day 0) and followed by five further doses on days 3, 7, 14, 30 and 90. The use of Human Rabies Immunoglobulin on day 0 should be considered but only in persons with no adequate prophylaxis. The treatment schedule may be stopped if the animal concerned is found conclusively to be free of rabies.

**Contra-indications, warnings, etc** There are no absolute contra-indications to HDCV, although if there were evidence of severe hypersensitivity, subsequent doses should not be given except for treatment. Redness, swelling or tenderness at the site of injection may occur during the first 48 hours. A mild fever, malaise and influenza-like symptoms have been reported.

Although anaphylaxis is extremely rare remedial facilities such as adrenaline should always be available during vaccination.

The vaccine contains traces of neomycin.

*Use in pregnancy:* Because of the potential consequences of inadequately treated rabies exposure and because there is no indication that foetal abnormalities have been associated with rabies vaccination, pregnancy is not considered a contra-indication to post-exposure prophylaxis. If there is substantial risk of exposure to rabies, pre-exposure prophylaxis may also be indicated during pregnancy.

**Pharmaceutical precautions** Store at +2°C to +8°C. Do not freeze. Use immediately after reconstituting

the vaccine. Discard any vaccine unused one hour after reconstitution.

**Legal category** POM.

**Package quantities** A vial of lyophilised vaccine containing one dose together with a disposable syringe containing 1 ml of diluent. The diluent is Water for Injections with no added preservatives.

**Further information** The British National Formulary and DoH Immunisation against Infectious Disease (HMSO) both contain reference to rabies.

**Product licence number**  6745/0053

## TYPHIM Vi*
### Vi Capsular Polysaccharide Typhoid Vaccine Pasteur Merieux

**Presentation** Clear, colourless, liquid vaccine. Each 0.5 ml dose contains 25 micrograms of the Vi polysaccharide antigen of *Salmonella typhi*, preserved with phenol.

**Uses** Active immunisation against typhoid fever.

**Dosage and administration** A single dose of 0.5 ml administered by deep subcutaneous or intramuscular injection.

*Use in children:* Children under 18 months of age may show a suboptimal response to polysaccharide antigen vaccines. Typhoid is rare in children aged under 2 years; the decision to use the vaccine in this age group should be based upon the risk of exposure to disease.

*Use in elderly:* No special comment.

**Contra-indications, warnings, etc**
*Contra-indications:* Acute infectious illness. Hypersensitivity to the vaccine or any component.

*Precautions:* The vaccine protects against typhoid fever caused by *Salmonella typhi*. Protection is not conferred against paratyphoid fever or illness caused by non-invasive Salmonellae.

*Warnings:* Facilities for the management of anaphylaxis should always be available during vaccination.

*Adverse reactions:* Local reactions including minor degrees of pain, swelling or erythema may be reported in approximately one-fifth of vaccinees. These reactions are normally only reported during the first 48–72 hours after immunisation.

Systemic reactions are also transient, and may include fever, headache, malaise or nausea, and only occur in approximately 8% of subjects.

*Use in pregnancy and lactation:* No reproductive studies have been conducted in animals. There is no data on the use of this vaccine in pregnancy or lactation. The vaccine should not normally be used in pregnancy or during lactation unless the benefit outweighs the risk.

**Pharmaceutical precautions** Store at +2°C to +8°C. Do not freeze. Shake before use.

**Legal category** POM.

**Package quantities** Single dose pre-filled syringe, unit pack.

**Further information** Antibody seroconversion is observed in >90% of recipients after administration of a single dose of typhoid Vi capsular polysaccharide vaccine. In young children antibody responses may be sub-optimal. In adults and children over 5 years, immunity persists for at least 3 years. Subjects who remain at risk from typhoid fever should be revaccinated using a single dose of vaccine every three years.

The importance of scrupulous personal, food and water hygiene must be emphasised to all persons at risk of typhoid fever.

**Product licence number**  6745/0039

*Trade Mark

# Penn Pharmaceuticals Ltd
## Tafarnaubach Industrial Estate
## Tredegar
## Gwent NP2 3AA

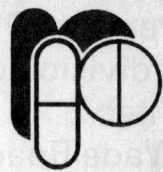

## CARBOMIX*

**Presentation** Black, odourless, tasteless granules for mixing with water before administration.

Carbomix is available in bottles containing activated charcoal 25 g and 50 g.

Carbomix granules also contain citric acid, acacia and glycerol.

**Uses** Emergency treatment of acute oral poisoning or drug overdose. Carbomix absorbs toxic substances and reduces or prevents systemic absorption. The shorter the time interval between ingestion of the toxicant and the administration of Carbomix, the greater is the benefit to the patient. However, as the absorption of massive drug overdoses is often retarded in acute conditions of intoxication, even the delayed administration of Carbomix may be beneficial.

In severe intoxications, repeated administration of Carbomix is recommended to prevent absorbed drug being released (in an unbound state) in the lower intestinal tract or to expedite the elimination and prevent the re-absorption of any drug undergoing entero-hepatic circulation.

### Dosage and administration

*Adults (including the elderly):* 50 g activated charcoal (one standard treatment pack), repeated if necessary.

*Children under 12 years:* 25 g activated charcoal (one small treatment pack or half the contents of the standard pack), repeated if necessary. If a large quantity of toxicant has been ingested, and where there is a risk to life, a dose of 50 g is recommended.

Carbomix should be given as soon as possible after the ingestion of the potential poison.

The contents of the bottle are made up to the red band with water and shaken thoroughly. The suspension is then taken orally or given by intragastric tube using the applicator provided. Carbomix may be administered after emesis or gastric lavage and may be used concurrently with parenteral antidotes such as acetylcysteine.

### Contra-indications, warnings, etc

*Contra-indications:* There are no contra-indications to the use of Carbomix but see under *Precautions* for inappropriate concomitant use.

*Precautions:* The value of Carbomix in the treatment of poisoning by strong acids, alkalis and other corrosive substances is limited. It should also be borne in mind that the presence of charcoal will render difficult any immediate endoscopy that may be required. Carbomix is poor in binding cyanide, iron salts and some solvents including methanol, ethanol and ethylene glycol.

In cases where the toxicant has diuretic properties or has been ingested with alcohol, plenty of fluid should be given after the administration of Carbomix.

Carbomix should not be used concurrently with systemically active oral emetics or oral antidotes such as methionine since such agents would be absorbed by the charcoal.

*Pregnancy and lactation:* There is no evidence to suggest that Carbomix should not be used during pregnancy or lactation. The product is not systemically absorbed.

*Side-effects:* In general, Carbomix is well tolerated. Some patients may however experience constipation or diarrhoea. Faecal impaction has been reported in a patient treated for an overdose of a diuretic with alcohol.

*Interactions:* The purpose of the product is to interact with other medicaments and toxicants taken in overdosage. There are no systemic interactions because the product is not absorbed from the gut.

*Overdose:* Not applicable. In theory, severe constipation would result from excessive use and this could be treated with laxatives.

**Pharmaceutical precautions** Store below 25°C. Dispose of any unused suspension after 24 hours.

**Legal category** P.

**Package quantities** Treatment packs containing 50 g activated charcoal in 61.5 g granules (standard pack) and 25 g activated charcoal in 30.75 g granules.

**Further information** Activated charcoal has well-documented adsorptive properties and is effective in reducing the absorption of a wide variety of toxicants, including drugs taken in overdose, from the gut. In addition, there is evidence that the administration of activated charcoal can enhance the elimination of some compounds by creating an effective concentration gradient from the circulation to the gut. Activated charcoal is not systemically absorbed.

**Product licence number** 4351/0002.

*Date of preparation:* September 1994.

## PARADOTE*

**Qualitative and quantitative composition** Paracetamol 500 mg and DL-Methionine 100 mg (co-methiamol 100/500).

**Pharmaceutical form** White, capsuloid, film-coated tablets, marked 'CM'.

### Clinical particulars

*Therapeutic indications:* Paradote tablets are indicated for use in most painful and febrile conditions such as headache, toothache, colds, influenza, rheumatic pain and dysmenorrhoea. Methionine is added to this preparation as it may prevent liver damage occurring if an overdose is taken.

*Posology and method of administration:* Paradote tablets are for oral administration only.

*Adults (including the elderly):* Two tablets to be taken every four hours as required. No more than eight tablets should be taken in 24 hours.

*Children aged 12 and under:* Not recommended.

*Contra-indications:* Hypersensitivity to paracetamol, methionine or any of the other constituents. The product should not be used by patients taking mono-amine-oxidase inhibitors (MAOIs) or in the presence of hepatic diseases as there is an increased risk of psychosis or encephalopathy.

*Special warnings and special precautions for use:* Care is advised in the administration of paracetamol to patients with severe renal or hepatic impairment. The hazard of overdose is greater in those with non-cirrhotic alcoholic liver disease.

Patients should be advised not to exceed the recommended dose and not to take other paracetamol-containing products concurrently.

*Interactions with other medicaments and other forms of medication:* The speed of absorption of paracetamol may be increased by metoclopramide or domperidone and absorption reduced by cholestyramine. The anticoagulant effect of warfarin and other coumarins may be enhanced by prolonged regular daily use of paracetamol with increased risk of bleeding; occasional doses have no significant effect. Concurrent administration of methionine may inhibit the effect of levodopa.

*Use in pregnancy and lactation:* Epidemiological studies in human pregnancy have shown no ill effects due to paracetamol used in the recommended dosage and methionine is an essential amino acid. Paracetamol is excreted in breast milk but not in a clinically significant amount. Available data do not contraindicate breast feeding. However, the product should be used with caution during pregnancy and lactation.

*Effects on ability to drive and to use machines:* None.

*Undesirable effects:* Adverse effects of paracetamol are rare but hypersensitivity, including skin rash, may occur. There have been a few reports of blood dyscrasias, including thrombocytopenia and agranulocytosis, but these were not necessarily related to paracetamol.

*Overdose:* Symptoms of paracetamol overdosage in the first 24 hours are pallor, nausea, vomiting, anorexia and abdominal pain. Liver damage may become apparent 12 to 48 hours after ingestion. Abnormalities of glucose metabolism and metabolic acidosis may occur. Acute renal failure with acute tubular necrosis may develop even in the absence of severe liver damage. Cardiac arrhythmias and pancreatitis have been reported.

Liver damage is possible in adults who have taken 10 g or more of paracetamol. It is considered that

excess quantities of a toxic metabolite, usually adequately detoxified by glutathione when normal doses of paracetamol are ingested, become irreversibly bound to liver tissue. Death may result from paracetamol overdosage when liver glutathione stores are exhausted so that hepatic necrosis results. Concurrent ingestion of methionine (which enables the liver cells to manufacture more glutathione) in Paradote tablets is designed to help protect the liver against the hepatotoxic effects of excessive amounts of paracetamol.

Immediate treatment is essential in the management of paracetamol overdose and this should still be followed in the case of Paradote tablets. Despite lack of early symptoms, patients should be referred to hospital urgently for immediate medical attention and any patient who has ingested around 7.5 g or more of paracetamol in the preceding 4 hours should undergo gastric lavage or be given activated charcoal. Administration of additional oral methionine or intravenous acetylcysteine, which may have a beneficial effect up to at least 48 hours after the overdose, may be required, taking into account the amount of methionine already ingested. General supportive measures must be available.

### Pharmacological properties

*Pharmacodynamic properties:* Paracetamol possesses analgesic and antipyretic properties but has no useful anti-inflammatory activity. DL-methionine is a racemic mixture of the essential amino acid L-methionine and its D-isomer. Methionine enhances hepatic synthesis of glutathione which is used to inactivate the toxic quinone metabolite of paracetamol by conjugation.

*Pharmacokinetic properties:* Paracetamol is rapidly absorbed from the small intestine, the rate of absorption being dependent on the rate of gastric emptying. Peak plasma levels occur between 30 minutes and 2 hours after ingestion. It has been shown for this preparation that the presence of DL-methionine does not significantly alter the bioavailability of paracetamol. The plasma half-life of paracetamol varies between 1.5 and 2.5 hours; it is extensively metabolised in the liver and excreted in the urine, mainly as the sulphate and glucuronide conjugates. A small proportion (5–10%) is converted to a highly reactive quinone metabolite which is normally inactivated by conjugation with liver glutathione.

Methionine is rapidly and completely absorbed. The plasma half-life of methionine is about 2 hours which is similar to that of paracetamol. Utilisation of L-methionine is 100%. About 50% of the D-methionine is excreted in the urine and, although the remaining 50% is not directly available for synthesis of glutathione, its sulphur moiety is transferred to serine to form L-cysteine which can be used for glutathione synthesis. In the event of overdose, all the L-methionine and about half the D-methionine can provide a source of glutathione.

*Preclinical safety data:* No findings have been reported from pre-clinical safety studies which add to the prescribing information given in other sections.

### Pharmaceutical particulars

*List of excipients:* Sodium Starch Glycollate BP; Colloidal Silicon Dioxide NF (Aerosil 200); Magnesium Stearate PhEur; Povidone PhEur (Kollidon 90); stearic acid; acrylic polymer coating (Eudragit E); Talc BP; Titanium Dioxide BP; Polyethylene Glycol 300 BP.

*Incompatibilities:* None.

*Shelf life:* 24 months, unopened.

*Special precautions for storage:* Store below 25°C in a dry place.

*Nature and contents of container:* The product is blister-packed in strips of 12 and presented in cartons of 12, 24 and 96 tablets.

*Instructions for use/handling:* None.

**Marketing authorisation number** 04351/0017.

**Date of approval/revision of SPC** November 1995.

**Legal category** P.

*\*Trade Mark*

# Perstorp Pharma

a division of Perstorp Ltd
Intec 2
Wade Road
Basingstoke
Hampshire
RG24 8NE

## IODOSORB* Ointment

**Presentation** Tubes of sterile cadexomer iodine (INN) ointment containing Iodine PhEur at a concentration of 0.9% w/w for topical application. The cadexomer iodine, a modified starch gel microbead, is formulated in an inert ointment base. Each tube is for a single application only.

**Uses** For the treatment of chronic leg ulcers. When applied to the wound, Iodosorb Ointment absorbs pus and exudate, cleans the wound surface and reduces bacterial count. In chronic ulcers it stimulates granulation, reduces pain and accelerates healing.

The ointment formulation improves the ease of application on awkward wound sites.

**Dosage and administration** Iodosorb Ointment is applied topically to the wound surface to a depth of approximately 3 mm (1/8"). A single application should not exceed 50 g. The total amount of Iodosorb Ointment used in one week must not exceed 150 g. The preparation should be changed approximately three times per week or when the Iodosorb Ointment has become saturated with wound exudate, indicated by a loss of colour. Each time the dressing is changed and at the end of treatment, the remaining Iodosorb should be gently removed from the ulcer surface either with a stream of sterile water or saline, or with a sterile wet swab. The duration of treatment should not exceed 3 months in any single course of treatment. When venous insufficiency is a contributory factor, support bandages or stockings can be applied in conjunction with the use of Iodosorb Ointment.

**Contra-indications, warnings, etc**
*Contra-indications:* As Iodosorb Ointment contains 0.9% w/w iodine it should not be used in patients with known or suspected iodine sensitivity. Iodosorb Ointment is contra-indicated in Hashimoto's thyroiditis.

In patients with a prior history of Graves' disease it is not recommended to use iodine containing products, which includes Iodosorb Ointment.

The ointment should not be used in the case of non-toxic nodular goitre.

*Warnings:* Patients with a past history of any thyroid disorder are more susceptible to alteration in thyroid metabolism with chronic Iodosorb therapy.

Iodine is absorbed systemically especially when large wounds are treated.

In endemic goitre there have been isolated reports of hyperthyroidism associated with Iodosorb.

There is a potential for interaction of iodine with the following drugs and therefore co-administration is not recommended, lithium, sulphafurazoles and sulphonylureas.

It has been observed occasionally that an adherent crust can form when the dressing is not changed with significant frequency.

*Pregnancy:* Iodine can cross the placental barrier and is secreted into milk. Do not use Iodosorb in pregnant or lactating women.

**Pharmaceutical precautions** Store in a dry place below 25°C.

**Legal category** P

**Package quantities** Four unit dose tubes containing 10 g of ointment per pack. Two unit dose tubes containing 20 g of ointment per pack.

**Further information** On contact with wound exudate, the ointment absorbs fluid, removing exudate, pus and debris from the wound surface. Iodine is physically immobilised within the matrix of the ointment and is slowly released in an active form during uptake of wound fluid. This mechanism of release provides antibacterial activity both at the wound surface and within the formed gel. The gel can be removed with a stream of water without damaging the fragile new epithelium.

**Product licence number** 3863/0004

## IODOSORB* POWDER

**Presentation** Sterile sachets of cadexomer iodine, a dry yellow-brown powder of modified starch gel microbeads containing Iodine PhEur at a concentration of 0.9% w/w for topical application.

**Uses** Treatment of moist wounds including decubitus ulcers and chronic leg ulcers associated with venous disease.

**Dosage and administration** Cadexomer iodine is applied to the wound surface to form a layer approximately 3 mm deep and then covered with a dry dressing of gauze. The dressing should be changed daily, or when all applied cadexomer iodine has become saturated with wound exudate. Each time the dressing is changed and at the end of treatment, the remaining cadexomer iodine gel should be gently washed from the surface either with a gentle stream of sterile water or saline, or with a sterile wet swab.

To avoid the risk of cross-contamination, it is recommended that the use of a single sachet of cadexomer iodine be confined to one patient.

Cadexomer iodine is a dressing for the wound and has no influence on the underlying cause of the chronic wound.

**Contra-indications, warnings, etc** Iodine is absorbed systemically, especially when large wounds are treated. This should be taken into consideration in patients in whom thyroid function is under investigation. Cadexomer iodine contains 0.9% iodine and must not be used in patients with known or suspected iodine sensitivity. Iodine can cross the placental barrier and is secreted into milk. Use of cadexomer iodine should therefore be avoided in pregnant or lactating women.

It has been observed occasionally that an adherent crust can form when the dressing is not changed with sufficient frequency.

**Pharmaceutical precautions** Store in a dry place below 25°C.

**Legal category** P

**Package quantities** Unit dose sachet of 3 g in boxes of 7 sachets.

**Further information** One gram cadexomer iodine can absorb up to 6 ml of fluid. Iodine is physically immobilised within the matrix of the dry cadexomer iodine and is slowly released in an active form during uptake of wound fluid. This mechanism of release provides antibacterial activity at the wound surface and within the formed gel. The gel can be removed with a stream of water without damaging the fragile new epithelium beneath.

**Product licence number** 3863/0001

## IODOFLEX*

**Qualitative and quantitative composition** 1 gram unit-dose paste contains Cadexomer iodine 600 mg equivalent to:

| | |
|---|---|
| Iodine PhEur | 9 mg |
| Cadexomer | 591 mg |

**Pharmaceutical form** Unit-dose paste with gauze backing for topical application.

**Clinical particulars**
*Therapeutic indications:* For the treatment of chronic wounds, eg leg ulcers. When applied to wounds, Iodoflex reduces the bacterial count. In chronic leg ulcers it accelerates healing and reduces pain. For topical application.

*Posology and method of administration:* In adults and the elderly, Iodoflex is applied to the wound surface and then covered with a dry gauze dressing. The frequency of change depends on the exudation from the wound. Changes should be made when the Iodoflex has become saturated with wound exudate, indicated by loss of colour, usually two to three times

a week. If the wound is exudating heavily, daily changes may be needed. Each time the unit-dose paste is changed and at the end of treatment the remaining Iodoflex should be gently removed from the wound surface with a stream of water or saline.

A single application should not exceed 50 g. The total amount of Iodoflex used in one week should not exceed 150 g.

The duration of treatment should not exceed 3 months in any single course of treatment.

There is no experience in children, therefore Iodoflex is not recommended.

*Contra-indications:* As Iodoflex contains 0.9% w/w iodine it should not be used in patients with known or suspected iodine sensitivity. Iodoflex is contra-indicated in Hashimoto's thyroiditis and in cases of non-toxic nodular goitre.

*Special warnings and special precautions for use:* Iodine may be absorbed systemically, especially when large wounds are treated. Patients with a past history of any thyroid disorder are more susceptible to alterations in thyroid metabolism with chronic Iodoflex therapy. In endemic goitre, there have been isolated reports of hyperthyroidism associated with exogenous iodine. It has been observed occasionally that an adherent crust can form when Iodoflex is not changed with sufficient frequency.

*Interaction with other medicaments and other forms of interaction:* There is a potential risk of interaction with lithium.

*Pregnancy and lactation:* Iodine crosses the placental barrier and is secreted into breast milk. Use of Iodoflex should therefore be avoided in pregnant or lactating women.

*Effects on ability to drive and use machines:* It is unlikely to have an effect.

*Undesirable effects:* About 5% of patients treated with Iodoflex experience a transient smarting or pain within the first hour after application. Contact allergy, alteration in thyroid function and local oedema have been reported in rare cases. Minor reddening or swelling around the wound may occur without necessarily being an allergic reaction.

*Overdose:* There have been no reported overdosages. In case of excessive topical use of Iodoflex, the treatment should be stopped, the area washed and symptomatic treatment introduced.

**Pharmacological properties**
*Pharmacodynamic data:* Iodoflex consists of cadexomer iodine in a macrogol base applied to a polyester gauze carrier. In contact with wound exudate Iodoflex absorbs fluid, removes exudate, pus and debris from the wound surface. One gram of cadexomer iodine can absorb up to 6 ml of fluid. Iodine is physically immobilised within the matrix of the dry cadexomer iodine and is slowly released in an active form during uptake of wound fluid. This mechanism of release provides antibacterial activity both at the wound surface and within the formed gel. There is no evidence of the development of bacterial resistance to iodine. The formed gel can easily be removed without damaging the fragile new epithelium underneath.

*Pharmacokinetic properties:* Systemically absorbed iodine from Iodoflex is rapidly and almost exclusively excreted into the urine. Cadexomer is biodegradable by amylases, normally present in wound fluid.

*Preclinical safety data:* In preclinical studies, Iodoflex has been shown not to interfere with normal wound healing. Toxicity studies with daily skin applications of Iodoflex for 6 months in rabbits showed no evidence of local or systemic toxic effect. Iodoflex did not cause sensitisation in animals.

**Pharmaceutical particulars**
*List of excipients:* Lanogen*1500 40% consisting in equal parts of: Macrogol 300 PhEur and Macrogol 1500 PhEur.

*Incompatibilities:* No incompatibilities have been encountered in normal use.

*Shelf life:* 24 months.

*Special precautions for storage:* The product should be stored below 25°C.

*Nature and contents of container:* The Iodoflex unit-dose paste is provided with a polyester gauze backing. Each unit is packed in a heat-sealed sachet of polyethylene or ionomer on the inside, aluminium, polyethylene and paper outside.

The following pack sizes are available:

5 sterile unit-doses of 5 g (6 x 4cm) in an outer carton

3 sterile unit-doses of 10 g (8 x 6cm) in an outer carton

2 sterile unit-doses of 17 g (10 x 8cm) in an outer carton

*Instructions for use:*

1. Clean the wound and let the wound surface stay moist. Dry the surrounding area.

2. Remove the backing gauze and apply Iodoflex directly on the wound surface. Cover with a suitable dressing.

3. Change the dressing when Iodoflex has lost its colour. Irrigate to remove as much remaining Iodoflex as possible.

4. Support bandages or stockings can be applied in conjunction with the use of Iodoflex.

*Marketing authorisation holder* Perstorp Pharma, Perstorp AB, S-223 70 Lund, Sweden.

**Marketing authorisation number** 3863/0005

**Date of approval/revision of SPC** September 1996

**Legal category** P

## SPRILON*

**Presentation** An aerosol containing Zinc Oxide PhEur 12.5% and Dimethicone 350 PhEur 1.04%. Base to 60 g (wool fat, wool alcohols, cetostearyl alcohol, dextran, liquid paraffin, white soft paraffin, purified water). Propellant: butane/propane mix 4518.

**Uses** For prophylaxis and treatment of pressure sores, skin maceration due to faeces or urine, or around fistulae and ileostomies. For the protection and treatment of fissures, leg ulcers, moist eczemas. For the protection of skin beneath plaster casts.

**Dosage and administration** Shake can well. Spray surface at right angles from distance of eight inches. Two to three seconds should be sufficient for an area the size of the buttocks.

*Elderly:* No special instructions.

*Children:* Avoid the eyes in infants

**Contra-indications, warnings, etc**
*Precautions:* Protect the eyes. Keep out of the reach of children. Do not use on cases allergic to wool fat.

*Warning:* Do not puncture, incinerate or heat can over 50°C even when empty. Highly flammable.

**Pharmaceutical precautions** Store away from heat.

**Legal category** GSL.

**Package quantities** 115 g.

**Further information** The spray rapidly forms a white, durable, flexible film which while protecting the skin and assisting healing also allows normal transepidermal water loss.

**Product licence number** 12045/0001

## WARTICON*
## WARTICON FEM*

**Qualitative and quantitative composition** Podophyllotoxin 5 mg/ml (0.5% w/v). The quality of podophyllotoxin fulfils in-house specification.

**Pharmaceutical form** Topical solution.

**Clinical particulars**
*Therapeutic indications:*
*Warticon:* For the treatment of condylomata acuminata affecting the penis.

*Warticon Fem:* For the treatment of condylomata acuminata affecting the external female genitalia.

*Posology and method of administration:* Warticon is applied twice daily for 3 days. If residual warts persist, this 3-day treatment may be repeated weekly, if necessary, for a total of 4 weeks of treatment.

*Contra-indications:* Open wounds following surgical procedures should not be treated with podophyllotoxin. Hypersensitivity to podophyllotoxin is a contra-indication.

*Special warnings and precautions for use:* Avoid contact with the eyes.

*Interaction with other medicaments and other forms of interaction:* None presently known.

*Pregnancy and lactation:* The product is not for use in pregnancy or lactation.

*Effects on ability to drive and use machines:* None presently known.

*Undesirable effects:* Local irritation may occur on the second or third day of application associated with the start of wart necrosis. In most cases the reactions are mild. Tenderness, itching, smarting, erythema, superficial epithelial ulceration and balanoposthitis have been reported. Local irritation decreases after treatment.

*Overdose:* There have been no reported overdosages with Warticon Solution. However, excessive use of podophyllotoxin 0.5% solution has been reported as causing two cases of severe local reactions. In cases of excessive use of Warticon Solution resulting in severe local reaction, the treatment should be stopped, the area washed and symptomatic treatment introduced. No specific antidote is known. In the event of accidental ingestion, give emetic or stomach washout. Treatment should be symptomatic and in severe oral overdose ensure the airway is clear and give fluids. Check and correct electrolyte balance, monitor blood gases and liver function. Blood count should be monitored for at least 5 days.

**Pharmacological properties**
*Pharmacodynamic properties:* Pharmaco-therapeutic group: D06B B Antivirals.

Podophyllotoxin is a metaphase inhibitor in dividing cells binding to at least one binding site on tubulin. Binding prevents tubulin polymerisation required for microtubule assembly. At higher concentrations, podophyllotoxin also inhibits nucleoside transport through the cell membrane.

The chemotherapeutic action of podophyllotoxin is assumed to be due to inhibition of growth and the ability to invade the tissue of the viral infected cells.

*Pharmacokinetic properties:* Topical administration of a 0.5% solution of ethanolic podophyllotoxin in the majority of cases only requires volumes in the range of 0.1 ml to 0.2 ml. Studies monitoring serum drug level reveal that topical application of a twice daily dose of 100MCL to the penile preputial cavity in 10 patients resulted in a maximum serum concentration of 0.25ng/ml.

*Preclinical safety data:* No relevant findings.

**Pharmaceutical particulars**
*List of excipients:* Phosphoric acid PhEur; Ethanol BP; Purified Water PhEur; Patent Blue V (E131).

*Incompatibilities:* None known.

*Shelf life:* 36 months

*Special precautions for storage:* Should be stored below 25°C.

*Nature and contents of container:* An amber glass bottle with plastic child-proof cap. Each bottle contains 3 ml of Warticon Solution. The outer carton also includes a tube containing plastic applicators. Each loop will carry approximately 5μl Warticon Solution.

Warticon Fem also contains a free-standing mirror to facilitate more accurate application.

*Instructions for use/handling:* The solution is applied by the plastic applicators provided.

*Administrative data:*

*Marketing authorisation holder:* Perstorp AB, T/A Perstorp Pharma, S-284 80 Perstorp, Sweden.

**Marketing authorisation number** 3863/0007

**Date of approval/revision of SPC** April 1997

**Legal category** POM

## WARTICON CREAM*

**Qualitative and quantitative composition** Podophyllotoxin 1.5 mg/g (0.15% w/w). The quality of podophyllotoxin fulfils in-house specification.

**Pharmaceutical form** Topical cream

**Clinical particulars**
*Therapeutic indications:* For the topical treatment of condylomata acuminata affecting the penis and the external female genitalia.

**Posology and method of administration:** The affected area should be thoroughly washed with soap and water, and dried prior to application.

Using a fingertip, the cream is applied twice daily for 3 days using only enough cream to just cover each wart.

Residual warts should be treated with further courses of twice daily applications for three days at weekly intervals, if necessary for a total of 4 weeks of treatment.

Where lesions are greater than 4cm², it is recom-

mended that treatment takes place under the direct supervision of medical staff.

*Contra-indications:* Open wounds eg. following surgical procedures. Use in children. Hypersensitivity to podophyllotoxin. Concomitant use with other podophyllotoxin containing preparations. Pregnancy and lactation.

*Special warnings and special precautions for use:* Avoid contact with the eyes. Should the cream accidentally come into the eye, the eye should be thoroughly rinsed with water.

The hands should be thoroughly washed after each application. Prolonged contact with healthy skin must be avoided since the cream contains an active pharmaceutical substance which could be harmful on healthy skin.

*Interactions:* None presently known.

*Pregnancy and lactation:* The product is not for use in pregnancy or lactation.

Reproduction toxicity studies in animals have not given evidence of an increased incidence of fetal damage or other deleterious effects on the reproductive process. However, since podophyllotoxin is a mitosis inhibitor, Warticon Cream should not be used during pregnancy or lactation.

It is not known if the substance is excreted into breast milk.

Observations in man indicate that podophyllin, a crude mixture of lignans, can be harmful to pregnancy. Such observations have not been reported in patients treated with podophyllotoxin.

*Effects on ability to drive and use machines:* None presently known.

*Undesirable effects:* Local irritation may occur on the second or third day of application associated with the start of wart necrosis. In most cases the reactions are mild. Tenderness, itching, smarting, erythema, superficial epithelial ulceration and balanoposthitis have been reported. Local irritation decreases after treatment.

*Overdose:* There have been no reported overdosages with Warticon cream. However, excessive use of podophyllotoxin 0.5% solution has been reported as causing two cases of severe local reactions. In cases of excessive use of Warticon cream resulting in severe local reaction, the treatment should be stopped, the area washed and symptomatic treatment introduced. No specific antidote is known. In the event of accidental ingestion, give emetic or stomach washout. Treatment should be symptomatic and in severe oral overdose ensure the airway is clear and give fluids. Check and correct electrolyte balance, monitor blood gases and liver function. Blood count should be monitored for at least 5 days.

**Pharmacological properties**
*Pharmacodynamic data:* Pharmaco-therapeutic group: D06B B Antivirals.

Podophyllotoxin is a metaphase inhibitor in dividing cells binding to at least one binding site on tubulin. Binding prevents tubulin polymerisation required for microtubule assembly. At higher concentrations, podophyllotoxin also inhibits nucleoside transport through the cell membrane.

The chemotherapeutic action of podophyllotoxin is assumed to be due to inhibition of growth and the ability to invade the tissue of the viral infected cells.

*Pharmacokinetic data:* Systemic absorption of podophyllotoxin after topical application with a higher strength, 0.3% is low. Thus no study was performed on the present strength, 0.15%. The $C_{max}$ (1.0–4.7ng/ml) and $T_{max}$ (0.5–36hrs) are comparable for the 0.3% cream and 0.5% solution in both males and females.

*Preclinical safety data:* No relevant findings.

**Pharmaceutical particulars**
*List of excipients:* Purified water PhEur; Methylparaben PhEur; Propylparaben PhEur; Sorbic Acid PhEur; Phosphoric Acid PhEur; Stearyl alcohol PhEur; Cetyl Alcohol PhEur; Isopropyl Alcohol PhEur; Paraffin, Lquid PhEur; Fractionated Coconut Oil PhEur; Butylated Hydroxyanisole (BHA) PhEur.

Emulgator E 2155, a fixed combination of the following non-ionic emulsifiers: Stearyl Alcohol USP/NF; Steareth-7; Steareth-10 (Stearomacrogol-400).

*Incompatibilities:* None known.

*Shelf life:* 36 months

*Special precautions for storage:* Warticon Cream should be stored at room temperature.

*Nature and contents of container:* A collapsible aluminium tube with imperforate nozzle membrane and internally coated with a protective lacquer. Tube cap of polyethylene with a spike on the upper end aimed to perforate the membrane when opening the tube for the first time. Size 5 g.

*Instructions for use:* The cream is applied with the fingertip.

*Name and address of marketing authorisation holder:*
Perstorp Pharma, Perstorp AB, S-223 70 Lund, Sweden

**Marketing authorisation number** 3863/0010

**Date of approval/revision of SPC** December 1996

**Legal category** POM

## ZIPZOC*

**Qualitative and quantitative composition** Zipzoc is a sterile rayon stocking impregnated with an ointment containing 20% Zinc Oxide PhEur. Each stocking contains a mean value of 41.5 g ointment.

**Pharmaceutical form** Medicated stocking for topical application.

### Clinical particulars
*Therapeutic indications:* Treatment of chronic leg ulcers. Where chronic venous insufficiency exists the medicated stocking can be used as a primary contact layer under compression bandaging or hosiery.

*Posology and method of administration:* For topical application. Zipzoc should be applied to cover the lower leg from the base of the toes to below the knee. All folds should be smoothed out. To protect clothes from Zipzoc a suitable outer bandage should be worn. If chronic venous insufficiency exists, Zipzoc can be used as a primary contact layer under suitable compression bandaging and may be applied for one week. The duration and frequency of application will depend on the clinical circumstances.

*Contra-indications:* There are no known contraindications to Zipzoc.

*Special warnings and special precautions for use:* If arterial insufficiency is an underlying condition then compression bandaging should not be used in conjunction with Zipzoc.

*Interaction with other medicaments and other forms of interaction:* None known.

*Pregnancy and lactation:* There is no evidence to suggest Zipzoc should not be used during pregnancy.

*Effects on ability to drive and use machines:* It is unlikely to have an effect.

*Undesirable effects:* The skin of leg ulcer patients is easily sensitised to some topical medications. Zipzoc contains no preservatives thereby reducing the risk of skin reactions. Reactions reported include, rash, erythema, itching and maceration of the wound edge. If the outer bandage is inappropriate or the medicated stocking is not changed with sufficient frequency it can cause the stocking to dry out. Because Zipzoc is preservative free it must be changed no less frequently than weekly, to avoid the possible risk of infection.

*Overdose:* None stated

### Pharmacological properties
*Pharmacodynamic properties:* The medicated stocking consists of a tubular rayon gauze impregnated with Zinc Oxide PhEur 20% in an ointment base. Zinc oxide has a soothing and protective effect and has been shown to have a role in wound healing. Zipzoc has no effect on the underlying condition but can be

used under appropriate compression bandaging where chronic venous insufficiency is the problem.

*Pharmacokinetic properties:* Not applicable

*Pre-clinical safety data:* Nothing relevant to add to the prescribing information.

### Pharmaceutical particulars
*List of excipients:* Ointment base consists of: Liquid Paraffin PhEur; White Soft Paraffin BP.

*Incompatibilities:* None reported.

*Shelf life:* 2 years.

*Special precautions for storage:* Store at or below 25°C. Keep all medicines out of reach of children.

*Nature and contents of container:* Polyethylene aluminium foil laminated pouches each pouch containing a single medicated stocking. The outer carton will contain either 4 or 10 pouches.

*Instructions for use:* Zipzoc should be applied to cover the lower leg from the base of the toes to below the knee. All folds should be smoothed out. A suitable outer bandage or dressing should be used to prevent soiling of clothes. If chronic venous insufficiency exists, Zipzoc can be used as a primary contact layer under suitable compression and may be applied for one week.

*Marketing authorisation holder* Perstorp AB, Trading as Perstorp Pharma, S-223 70 Lund, Sweden.

**Marketing authorisation number** 03863/0017

**Date of approval/revision of SPC** October 1996

**Legal category** P

*Trade Mark

# Pfizer Limited
## Sandwich
## Kent CT13 9NJ

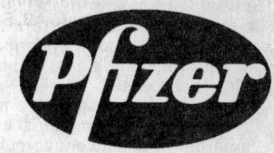

## ATARAX*

**Presentation** Atarax (hydroxyzine hydrochloride) is available as:

10 mg sugar-coated tablets, coloured orange and coded on one side with 'Pfizer'.

25 mg sugar-coated tablets, coloured green and coded on one side with 'Pfizer'.

Inactive excipients: Atarax tablets include lactose, sucrose, butyl parahydroxybenzoate and an azo dye sunset yellow. In addition, Atarax 10 mg tablets contain erythrosine and Atarax 25 mg tablets contain quinoline yellow and patent blue V.

**Uses** *Actions:* Atarax is unrelated chemically to phenothiazine, reserpine, and meprobamate.

Atarax has been shown clinically to be a rapid-acting anxiolytic with a wide margin of safety. It induces a calming effect in anxious, tense adults. It is not a cortical depressant, but its action may be due to a suppression of activity in certain key regions of the subcortical area of the central nervous system.

Antihistamine effects have been demonstrated experimentally and confirmed clinically; it is highly effective in alleviating pruritus.

Atarax is rapidly absorbed from the gastro-intestinal tract and effects are usually noted within 15 to 30 minutes after oral administration.

*Indications:* Atarax is indicated to assist in the management of anxiety in adults.

Atarax is indicated for the management of pruritus associated with acute and chronic urticaria, including cholinergic and physical types, and atopic and contact dermatoses in adults and children.

**Dosage and administration** Anxiety: Adults, 50–100 mg four times daily.

Pruritus: Adults, starting dose of 25 mg at night increasing as necessary to 25 mg three or four times daily; children from 6 months to 6 years 5–15 mg rising to 50 mg daily in divided doses and for children over 6 years, 15–25 mg rising to 50–100 mg daily in divided doses.

As with all medications, the dosage should be adjusted according to the patient's response to therapy.

*Use in elderly patients:* Atarax may be used in elderly patients with no special precautions other than the care always necessary in this age group. The lowest effective maintenance dose and careful observation for side effects are important.

**Contra-indications, warnings, etc**
*Contra-indications:* Atarax is contra-indicated in patients who have shown a previous hypersensitivity to it.

*Use in pregnancy:* Atarax is contra-indicated in early pregnancy. Hydroxyzine, when administered to the pregnant mouse, rat and rabbit, induced foetal abnormalities at doses substantially above the human therapeutic range. Clinical data in humans are inadequate to establish safety in early pregnancy. There is inadequate evidence of safety in the later stages of pregnancy. Use in later pregnancy only when there is no safer alternative or when the disease itself carries risks for the mother or child.

*Warnings: Use in nursing mothers:* It is not known whether Atarax is excreted in human milk. Since many drugs are so excreted, Atarax should not be given to nursing mothers.

*Use in renal insufficiency:* Atarax should be used with caution in patients with impaired renal function. It is uncertain whether the drug may accumulate or have other adverse effects in such patients.

Patients should be warned that Atarax may impair their ability to perform activities requiring mental alertness or physical co-ordination such as operating machinery or driving a vehicle.

Patients should be warned that Atarax may enhance their response to alcohol, barbiturates and other CNS depressants.

*Side-effects:* Therapeutic doses of Atarax seldom produce marked impairment of mental alertness. Drowsiness may occur; if so, it is usually transitory and may disappear after a few days of continued therapy or upon reduction of the dose. Dryness of the mouth may be encountered at higher doses. Dizziness, weakness, headache and confusion have been reported.

Extensive clinical use has substantiated the absence of toxic effects on the liver or bone marrow when administered in recommended doses for over four years of uninterrupted therapy. The absence of side-effects has been further demonstrated in experimental studies in which excessively high doses were administered.

Involuntary motor activity, including rare instances of tremor and convulsions, have been reported, usually with doses considerably higher than those recommended. Continuous therapy with over 1 g/day has been employed in some patients without these effects having been encountered.

*Overdosage:* The most common manifestation of Atarax overdosage is hypersedation. As in the management of overdosage with any drug, it should be borne in mind that multiple agents may have been taken.

If vomiting has not occurred spontaneously in conscious patients, it should be induced. Immediate gastric lavage is also recommended. General supportive care, including frequent monitoring of the vital signs and close observation of the patient is indicated. Hypotension, though unlikely, may be controlled with intravenous fluids and noradrenaline, or metaraminol. Adrenaline should not be used in this situation as Atarax counteracts its pressor action.

There is no specific antidote. It is doubtful whether haemodialysis has any value in the treatment of overdosage with Atarax. However, if other agents such as barbiturates have been ingested concomitantly, haemodialysis may be indicated.

**Pharmaceutical precautions** Store below 25°C.

**Legal category** POM.

**Package quantities**
*Tablets 10 mg:* Original packs of 84 tablets (in blister strips of 6×14 tablets).
*Tablets 25 mg:* Original packs of 28 tablets (in blister strips of 2×14 tablets).

**Further information** Nil.

**Product licence numbers**
Tablets 10 mg     0057/5003R
Tablets 25 mg     0057/5004R

## DELTACORTRIL* ENTERIC

**Qualitative and quantitative composition** Prednisolone 2.5 mg or 5 mg.

**Pharmaceutical form** Tablets 2.5 mg, uniformly brown in colour and coded 'Pfizer'.

Tablets 5 mg, uniformly red in colour and coded 'Pfizer'.

**Clinical particulars**
*Therapeutic indications:*

*Allergy and anaphylaxis:* Bronchial asthma, drug hypersensitivity reactions, serum sickness, angioneurotic oedema, anaphylaxis.

*Arteritis/collagenosis:* Giant cell arteritis/polymyalgia rheumatica, mixed connective tissue disease, polyarteritis nodosa, polymyositis.

*Blood disorders:* Haemolytic anaemia (auto-immune), leukaemia (acute and lymphocytic), lymphoma, multiple myeloma, idiopathic thrombocytopenic purpura.

*Cardiovascular disorders:* Post myocardial infarction syndrome, rheumatic fever with severe carditis.

*Endocrine disorders:* Primary and secondary adrenal insufficiency, congenital adrenal hyperplasia.

*Gastro-intestinal disorders:* Crohn's disease, ulcerative colitis, persistent coeliac syndrome (coeliac disease unresponsive to gluten withdrawal), auto-immune chronic active hepatitis, multisystem disease affecting liver, biliary peritonitis.

*Hypercalcaemia:* Sarcoidosis, vitamin D excess.

*Infections (with appropriate chemotherapy):* Helminthic infestations, Herxheimer reaction, infectious mononucleosis, miliary tuberculosis, mumps orchitis (adult), tuberculous meningitis, rickettsial disease.

*Muscular disorders:* Polymyositis, dermatomyositis.

*Neurological disorders:* Infantile spasms, Shy-Drager syndrome, sub-acute demyelinating polyneuropathy.

*Ocular disease:* Scleritis, posterior uveitis, retinal vasculitis, pseudo tumours of the orbit, giant cell arteritis, malignant ophthalmic Graves disease.

*Renal disorders:* Lupus nephritis, acute interstitial nephritis, minimal change glomerulonephritis.

*Respiratory disease:* Allergic pneumonitis, asthma, occupational asthma, pulmonary aspergillosis, pulmonary fibrosis, pulmonary alveolitis, aspiration of foreign body, aspiration of stomach contents, pulmonary sarcoid, drug induced lung disease, adult respiratory distress syndrome, spasmodic croup.

*Rheumatic disorders:* Rheumatoid arthritis, polymyalgia rheumatica, juvenile chronic arthritis, systemic lupus erythematosus, dermatomyositis, mixed connective tissue disease.

*Skin disorders:* Pemphigus vulgaris, bullous pemphigoid, systemic lupus erythematosus, pyoderma gangrenosum.

*Miscellaneous:* Sarcoidosis, hyperpyrexia, Behçets disease, immunosuppression in organ transplantation.

*Posology and method of administration:* The initial dosage of Deltacortril Enteric may vary from 5 mg to 60 mg daily depending on the disorder being treated. Divided daily dosage is usually used.

The following therapeutic guidelines should be kept in mind for all therapy with corticosteroids:

Corticosteroids are palliative symptomatic treatment by virtue of their anti-inflammatory effects; they are never curative.

The appropriate individual dose must be determined by trial and error and must be re-evaluated regularly according to activity of the disease.

As corticosteroid therapy becomes prolonged and as the dose is increased, the incidence of disabling side-effects increases.

Abrupt cessation of prolonged, high dosage corticosteroid therapy is associated with a significant risk of potentially life-threatening adrenal insufficiency.

In general, initial dosage shall be maintained or adjusted until the anticipated response is observed. The dose should be gradually reduced until the lowest dose which will maintain an adequate clinical response is reached. Use of the lowest effective dose may also minimise side-effects – see *Special warnings and special precautions for use.*

During prolonged therapy, dosage may need to be temporarily increased during periods of stress or during exacerbations of the disease.

When the drug is to be stopped, it must be withdrawn gradually and not abruptly.

If there is lack of a satisfactory clinical response to Deltacortril Enteric, the drug should be gradually discontinued and the patient transferred to alternative therapy.

*Intermittent dosage regimen:* A single dose of Deltacortril Enteric in the morning on alternate days or at longer intervals is acceptable therapy for some patients. When this regimen is practical, the degree of pituitary-adrenal suppression can be minimised.

*Specific dosage guidelines:* The following recommendations for some corticosteroid-responsive disorders are for guidance only. Acute or severe disease may require initial high dose therapy with reduction to the lowest effective maintenance dose as soon as possible. Dosage reductions should not exceed 5–7.5 mg daily during chronic treatment.

*Allergic and skin disorders:* Initial doses of 5–15 mg daily are commonly adequate.

*Collagenosis:* Initial doses of 20–30 mg daily are frequently effective. Those with more severe symptoms may require higher doses.

*Rheumatoid arthritis:* The usual initial dose is 10–15 mg daily. The lowest daily maintenance dose compatible with tolerable symptomatic relief is recommended.

*Blood disorders and lymphoma:* An initial daily dose of 15–60 mg is often necessary with reduction after an adequate clinical or haematological response. Higher doses may be necessary to induce remission in acute leukaemia.

*Use in children:* Although appropriate fractions of the actual dose may be used, dosage will usually be determined by clinical response as in adults (see also *Precautions*). Alternate day dosage is preferable where possible.

*Use in elderly:* Treatment of elderly patients, particularly if long-term, should be planned bearing in mind the more serious consequences of the common side-effects of corticosteroids in old age (see also *Special warnings and special precautions for use*).

*Contra-indications:* Systemic infections unless specific anti-infective therapy is employed. Hypersensitivity to any ingredient. Ocular herpes simplex because of possible perforation.

*Special warnings and special precautions for use:* Caution is necessary when oral corticosteroids, including Deltacortril Enteric, are prescribed in patients with the following conditions, and frequent patient monitoring is necessary.

– Tuberculosis: Those with a previous history of, or X-ray changes characteristic of, tuberculosis. The emergence of active tuberculosis can, however, be prevented by the prophylactic use of antituberculous therapy.
– Hypertension.
– Congestive heart failure.
– Liver failure.
– Renal insufficiency.
– Diabetes mellitus or in those with a family history of diabetes.
– Osteoporosis: This is of special importance in postmenopausal females who are at particular risk.
– Glaucoma or in those with a family history of glaucoma.
– Patients with a history of severe affective disorders and particularly those with a previous history of steroid-induced psychoses.
– Epilepsy.
– Peptic ulceration.
– Previous Steroid Myopathy.

A Patient Information Leaflet is supplied with this product.

Undesirable effects may be minimised by using the lowest effective dose for the minimum period and by administering the daily requirement as a single morning dose on alternate days. Frequent patient review is required to titrate the dose appropriately against disease activity (see *Dosage* section).

*Adrenal suppression:* Adrenal cortical atrophy develops during prolonged therapy and may persist for years after stopping treatment. Withdrawal of corticosteroids after prolonged therapy must therefore always be gradual to avoid acute adrenal insufficiency, being tapered off over weeks or months according to the dose and duration of treatment. During prolonged therapy any intercurrent illness, trauma, or surgical procedure will require a temporary increase in dosage; if corticosteroids have been stopped following prolonged therapy they may need to be temporarily reintroduced.

Patients should carry 'Steroid treatment' cards which give clear guidance on the precautions to be taken to minimise risk and which provide details of prescriber, drug, dosage and the duration of treatment.

*Anti-inflammatory/immunosuppressive effects and infection:* Suppression of the inflammatory response and immune function increases the susceptibility to infections and their severity. The clinical presentation may often be atypical and serious infections such as septicaemia and tuberculosis may be masked and may reach an advanced stage before being recognised.

*Chickenpox:* Chickenpox is of particular concern since this normally minor illness may be fatal in immunosuppressed patients. Patients (or parents of children) without a definite history of chickenpox should be advised to avoid close personal contact with chickenpox or herpes zoster and if exposed they should seek urgent medical attention. Passive immunisation with varicella-zoster immunoglobulin (VZIG) is needed by exposed non-immune patients who are receiving systemic corticosteroids or who have used them within the previous 3 months; this should be given within 10 days of exposure to chickenpox. If a diagnosis of chickenpox is confirmed, the illness warrants specialist care and urgent treatment. Corticosteroids should not be stopped and the dose may need to be increased.

The effect of corticosteroids may be enhanced in patients with hypothyroidism and in those with chronic liver disease with impaired hepatic function.

*Use in children:* Corticosteroids cause growth retardation in infancy, childhood and adolescence, which may be irreversible. Treatment should be limited to the minimum suppression of the hypothalamo-pituitary adrenal axis and growth retardation. Treatment should be administered where possible as a single dose on alternate days.

*Use in the elderly:* Treatment of elderly patients, particularly if long term, should be planned bearing in mind the more serious consequences of the common side-effects of corticosteroids in old age, especially osteoporosis, diabetes, hypertension, hypokalaemia, susceptibility to infection and thinning of the skin. Close clinical supervision is required to avoid life threatening reactions.

*Interactions with other medicaments and other forms of interaction:*
*Hepatic microsomal enzyme inducers:* Drugs which can cause liver enzyme induction such as phenobarbitone, phenytoin, rifampicin, rifabutin, carbamazepine, primidone and aminoglutethimide may reduce the therapeutic efficacy of corticosteroids by increasing the rate of metabolism. Lack of expected response

may be observed and dosage of Deltacortril Enteric may need to be increased.

*Non-steroidal anti-inflammatory drugs:* Concomitant administration of ulcerogenic drugs such as indomethacin during corticosteroid therapy may increase the risk of GI ulceration. Aspirin should be used cautiously in conjunction with glucocorticoids in patients with hypoprothrombinaemia. Although concomitant therapy with salicylate and corticosteroids does not appear to increase the incidence or severity of GI ulceration, the possibility of this effect should be considered.

Serum salicylate concentrations may decrease when corticosteroids are administered concomitantly. The renal clearance of salicylates is increased by corticosteroids and steroid withdrawal may result in salicylate intoxication. Salicylates and corticosteroids should be used concurrently with caution. Patients receiving both drugs should be observed closely for adverse effects of either drug.

*Anticoagulants:* Response to anticoagulants may be reduced or, less often, enhanced by corticosteroids. Close monitoring of the INR or prothrombin time is required to avoid spontaneous bleeding.

*Vaccines:* Live vaccines should not be given to individuals with impaired immune responsiveness. The antibody response to other vaccines may be diminished.

*Oestrogens:* Oestrogens may potentiate the effects of glucocorticoids and dosage adjustment may be required if oestrogens are added to or withdrawn from a stable dosage regimen.

*Other:* The desired effects of hypoglycaemic agents (including insulin), anti-hypertensives and diuretics are antagonised by corticosteroids and the hypokalaemic effect of acetazolamide, loop diuretics, thiazide diuretics and carbenoxolone are enhanced.

*Pregnancy and lactation:*
*Use in pregnancy:* There may be a small risk of cleft palate and intra-uterine growth retardation in the foetus. Hypoadrenalism may occur in the neonate. There is evidence of harmful effects on pregnancy in animals. When corticosteroids are essential however, patients with normal pregnancies may be treated as though they were in the non-gravid state. Patients with pre-eclampsia or fluid retention require close monitoring.

*Use in lactation:* Corticosteroids are excreted in small amounts in breast milk and infants of mothers taking pharmacological doses of steroids should be monitored carefully for signs of adrenal suppression.

*Effects of ability to drive and use machines:* Deltacortril Enteric is unlikely to affect ability to drive and use machines.

*Undesirable effects:* The incidence of predictable undesirable effects, including hypothalmic-pituitary adrenal suppression correlates with the relative potency of the drug, dosage, timing of administration and the duration of treatment. (See *Special warnings and special precautions for use*).

*Gastro-intestinal:* Dyspepsia, peptic ulceration with perforation and haemorrhage, abdominal distension, oesophageal ulceration, oesophageal candidiasis, acute pancreatitis.

*Musculo-skeletal:* Proximal myopathy, osteoporosis, vertebral and long bone fractures, avascular osteonecrosis, tendon rupture.

*Fluid and electrolyte disturbance:* Sodium and water retention, hypertension, hypokalaemic alkalosis.

*Dermatological:* Impaired healing, skin atrophy, bruising, striae, telangiectasia, acne.

*Endocrine/metabolic:* Suppression of the hypothalamo-pituitary adrenal axis, growth suppression in infancy, childhood and adolescence, menstrual irregularity and amenorrhoea. Cushingoid facies, hirsutism, weight gain, impaired carbohydrate tolerance with increased requirement for antidiabetic therapy, negative nitrogen and calcium balance. Increased appetite.

*Neuropsychiatric:* Euphoria, psychological dependence, depression, insomnia. Raised intracranial pressure with papilloedema (pseudotumor cerebri) in children, usually after treatment withdrawal . Aggravation of schizophrenia. Aggravation of epilepsy.

*Ophthalmic:* Increased intra-ocular pressure, glaucoma, papilloedema, posterior subcapsular cataracts, corneal or scleral thinning, exacerbation of ophthalmic viral or fungal disease.

*Anti-inflammatory and immunosuppressive effects:* Increased susceptibility to, and severity of infections with suppression of clinical symptoms and signs, opportunistic infections, recurrence of dormant tuberculosis (see Other special warnings and precautions).

*General:* Leucocytosis, hypersensitivity including anaphylaxis, thromboembolism, nausea, malaise.

*Withdrawal symptoms:* Too rapid a reduction of corticosteroid dosage following prolonged treatment can lead to acute adrenal insufficiency, hypotension and death (see *Special warnings and special precautions for use*). A 'withdrawal syndrome' may also occur including: fever, myalgia, arthralgia, rhinitis,

conjunctivitis, painful itchy skin nodules and loss of weight.

*Overdose:* Reports of acute toxicity and/or death following overdosage of glucocorticoids are rare. No specific antidote is available; treatment is supportive and symptomatic. Serum electrolytes should be monitored.

## Pharmacological properties

*Pharmacodynamic properties:* Naturally occurring glucocorticoids (hydrocortisone and cortisone), which also have salt-retaining properties, are used as replacement therapy in adrenocortical deficiency states. Their synthetic analogs are primarily used for their potent anti-inflammatory effect in disorders of many organ systems.

Glucocorticoids cause profound and varied metabolic effects. In addition, they modify the body's immune responses to diverse stimuli.

*Pharmacokinetic properties:* Prednisolone is rapidly and apparently almost completely absorbed after oral administration; it reaches peak plasma concentrations after 1–3 hours. There is however wide inter-subject variation suggesting impaired absorption in some individuals. Plasma half-life is about 3 hours in adults and somewhat less in children.

Although peak plasma prednisolone levels are somewhat lower after administration of Deltacortril Enteric and absorption is delayed, total absorption and bioavailability are the same as after plain prednisolone.

Prednisolone shows dose dependent pharmacokinetics, with an increase in dose leading to an increase in volume of distribution and plasma clearance. The degree of plasma protein binding determines the distribution and clearance of free, pharmacologically active drug. Reduced doses are necessary in patients with hypoalbuminaemia. Liver disease prolongs the half-life of prednisolone and, if the patients has hypoalbuminaemia, also increases the proportion of unbound drug and may thereby increase adverse effects.

## Pharmaceutical particulars

*List of excipients:* 5 mg tablets: acacia, azo-dye (E124), beeswax, calcium carbonate, carnauba wax, cellulose acetate phthalate, citroflex A-2, kaolin, lactose, magnesium stearate, maize starch, shellac, sucrose and talc.

2.5 mg tablets: acacia, red/brown iron oxide (E172), beeswax, calcium carbonate, carnauba wax, cellulose acetate phthalate, citroflex A-2, kaolin, lactose, magnesium stearate, maize starch, shellac, sucrose and talc.

*Incompatibilities:* None.

*Shelf life:* 24 months.

*Special precautions for storage:* Store below 25°C.

*Nature and contents of container:* Polypropylene tablet container with HDPE Child-Resistant screw cap.

30 or 100 tablets per container in a carton box containing a Patient Information Leaflet.

*Instructions for use/handling:* None.

**Marketing authorisation numbers**
2.5 mg   0057/5012R
5 mg     0057/0128

**Date of approval/revision of the SPC**   19 November 1996.

**Legal category**   POM.

## DIFLUCAN*

**Presentation**   *Diflucan 50 mg capsules* are light turquoise blue and white, coded 'FLU 50' and 'PFIZER', containing 50 mg fluconazole.

*Diflucan 150 mg capsules* are light turquoise blue, coded 'FLU 150' and 'PFIZER', containing 150 mg fluconazole.

*Diflucan 200 mg capsules* are purple and white, coded 'FLU 200' and 'PFIZER', containing 200 mg fluconazole.

*Diflucan Intravenous Infusion* contains fluconazole 2 mg/ml in a 0.9% aqueous sodium chloride solution.

*Diflucan Powder for Oral Suspension* is a dry white to off-white powder which yields, on reconstitution with water, an orange flavoured suspension containing the equivalent of 50 mg or 200 mg fluconazole per 5 ml.

*Inactive excipients:* Capsules (all strengths): Colloidal silicon dioxide, magnesium stearate, maize starch, lactose and sodium lauryl sulphate. In addition, capsule shells contain:

50 mg and 150 mg – gelatin, patent blue V and titanium dioxide.

200 mg – erythrosine, gelatin, indigotine and titanium dioxide.

Powder for Oral Suspension – citric acid, colloidal silicon dioxide, natural orange flavour, sodium benzoate, sodium citrate dihydrate, sucrose, titanium dioxide, xanthan gum.

Intravenous infusion – sodium chloride, water for injection.

**Uses** Fluconazole, a member of the triazole class of antifungal agents, is a potent and selective inhibitor of fungal enzymes necessary for the synthesis of ergosterol.

Diflucan is indicated for:

1. Vaginal candidiasis, acute or recurrent. Candidal balanitis. The treatment of partners who present with symptomatic genital candidiasis should be considered.

2. Mucosal candidiasis. These include oropharyngeal, oesophageal, non-invasive bronchopulmonary infections, candiduria, mucocutaneous and chronic oral atrophic candidiasis (denture sore mouth). Normal hosts and patients with compromised immune function may be treated.

3. Tinea pedis, tinea corporis, tinea cruris, tinea versicolor and dermal Candida infections. Diflucan is not indicated for nail infections.

4. Systemic candidiasis including candidaemia, disseminated candidiasis and other forms of invasive candidal infection. These include infections of the peritoneum, endocardium and pulmonary and urinary tracts. Candidal infections in patients with malignancy, in intensive care units or those receiving cytotoxic or immunosuppressive therapy, may be treated.

5. Cryptococcosis, including cryptococcal meningitis and infections of other sites (e.g. pulmonary, cutaneous). Normal hosts and patients with acquired immune deficiency syndrome (AIDS), organ transplants or other causes of immunosuppression may be treated. Diflucan can be used as maintenance therapy to prevent relapse of cryptococcal disease in patients with AIDS.

6. For the prevention of fungal infections in immunocompromised patients considered at risk as a consequence of neutropenia following cytotoxic chemotherapy or radiotherapy, including bone marrow transplant patients.

**Dosage and administration** Diflucan may be administered either orally or by intravenous infusion at a rate of approximately 5–10 ml/min, the route being dependent on the clinical state of the patient. On transferring from the intravenous to the oral route or vice versa, there is no need to change the daily dose. Diflucan intravenous infusion is formulated in 0.9% sodium chloride solution, each 200 mg (100 ml bottle) containing 15 mmol each of Na+ and Cl-.

The daily dose of fluconazole should be based on the nature and severity of the fungal infection. Most cases of vaginal candidiasis respond to single dose therapy. Therapy for those types of infections requiring multiple dose treatment should be continued until clinical parameters or laboratory tests indicate that active fungal infection has subsided. An inadequate period of treatment may lead to recurrence of active infection. Patients with AIDS and cryptococcal meningitis usually require maintenance therapy to prevent relapse.

*Adults*

1. Candidal balanitis or vaginitis: 150 mg single oral dose.

2. Mucosal candidiasis.

Oropharyngeal candidiasis: The recommended dose is 50 mg once daily for 7–14 days. Treatment should not normally exceed 14 days except in severely immunocompromised patients.

Atrophic oral candidiasis associated with dentures: The recommended dose is 50 mg once daily for 14 days administered concurrently with local antiseptic measures to the denture.

For other candidal infections of mucosa (except vaginal candidiasis see above), e.g. oesophagitis, non-invasive bronchopulmonary infections, candiduria, mucocutaneous candidiasis etc.: The recommended dose is 50 mg daily, given for 14 to 30 days.

In unusually difficult cases of mucosal candidal infections the dose may be increased to 100 mg daily.

3. For tinea pedis, corporis, cruris, versicolor and dermal Candida infections the recommended dosage is 50 mg once daily. Duration of treatment is normally 2 to 4 weeks but tinea pedis may require treatment for up to 6 weeks. Duration of treatment should not exceed 6 weeks.

4. For candidaemia, disseminated candidiasis and other invasive candidal infections: The recommended dose is 400 mg on the first day followed by 200 mg once daily. Depending on the clinical response the dose may be increased to 400 mg once daily. Duration of treatment is based upon the clinical response.

5a. For cryptococcal meningitis and cryptococcal infections at other sites: The recommended dose is 400 mg on the first day followed by 200 mg–400 mg once daily. Duration of treatment for Cryptococcal infections will depend on the clinical and mycological response, but is usually at least 6 to 8 weeks for cryptococcal meningitis.

5b. For the prevention of relapse of cryptococcal meningitis in patients with AIDS, after the patient receives a full course of primary therapy, Diflucan may be administered indefinitely at a daily dose of 100–200 mg.

6. For the prevention of fungal infections in immunocompromised patients considered at risk as a consequence of neutropenia following cytotoxic chemotherapy or radiotherapy, the dose should be 50–400 mg daily based on the patient's risk for developing fungal infection. For patients at high risk of systemic infection, e.g. patients who are anticipated to have profound or prolonged neutropenia such as during bone marrow transplantation, the recommended dose is 400 mg daily. Start dosage several days before anticipated onset of neutropenia and continue for seven days after the neutrophil count rises above 1000 cells per mm³.

*Use in children:* As with similar infections in adults, the duration of treatment is based on the clinical and mycological response.

*Children over four weeks of age:*
Mucosal candidiasis: The recommended dose of fluconazole is 3 mg/kg daily. A loading dose of 6 mg/kg may be used on the first day to achieve steady state levels more rapidly.

Systemic candidiasis and cryptococcal infection: The recommended dosage of fluconazole is 6–12 mg/kg daily, depending on the severity of the disease.

For the prevention of fungal infections in immunocompromised patients considered at risk as a consequence of neutropenia following cytotoxic chemotherapy or radiotherapy, the dose should be 3–12 mg/kg daily depending on the extent and duration of the induced neutropenia.

*Children below four weeks of age:* Neonates excrete fluconazole slowly. In the first two weeks of life the same mg/kg dosing as in older childen should be used but administered every 72 hours. During weeks 2–4 of life the same dose should be given every 48 hours.

For children with impaired renal function the daily dose should be reduced in accordance with the guidelines given for adults, dependent on the degree of renal impairment.

To facilitate accurate measurement of doses less than 10 mg, fluconazole should only be administered to children in hospital using the 50 mg/5 ml suspension orally or the intravenous infusion, depending on the clinical condition of the child. A suitable measuring device should be used for administration of the suspension. Once reconstituted, the suspension should not be further diluted.

*Use in elderly:* The normal dose should be used if there is no evidence of renal impairment. In patients with renal impairment (creatinine clearance less than 40 ml/min) the dosage schedule should be adjusted as described below.

*Use in renal impairment:* Fluconazole is excreted predominantly in the urine as unchanged drug. No adjustments in single dose therapy are required. In multiple dose therapy of patients with renal impairment, normal doses should be given on days 1 and 2 of treatment and thereafter the dosage intervals or daily dose should be modified in accordance with creatinine clearance as follows:

| Creatinine clearance (ml/min) | Dosage interval/daily dose |
|---|---|
| >40 | 24 hours (normal dosage regimen) |
| 21–40 | 48 hours *or* half normal daily dose |
| 10–20 | 72 hours *or* one-third normal daily dose |
| Patients receiving regular haemodialysis | One dose after every dialysis session |

*Compatibility of intravenous infusion:* Although further dilution is unnecessary Diflucan intravenous infusion is compatible with the following administration fluids:

(a) Dextrose 20%
(b) Ringer's solution
(c) Hartmann's solution
(d) Potassium chloride in dextrose
(e) Sodium bicarbonate 4.2%
(f) Normal saline (0.9%)

Diflucan may be infused through an existing line with one of the above listed fluids. No specific incompatibilities have been noted, although mixing with any other drug prior to infusion is not recommended.

**Contra-indications, warnings, etc**
*Contra-indications:* Diflucan should not be used in patients with known hypersensitivity to fluconazole or to related azole compounds.

Co-administration of terfenadine and cisapride is contra-indicated in patients receiving Diflucan (see *Drug interactions*).

*Use in pregnancy:* Adverse foetal effects have been seen in animals only at dose levels associated with maternal toxicity. These levels are many times in excess of those recommended for therapeutic use. There has been little use during human pregnancy. Accordingly, Diflucan should not be used in pregnancy, or in women of child-bearing potential unless adequate contraception is employed.

*Warnings:* In some patients, particularly those with serious underlying diseases such as AIDS and cancer, abnormalities of hepatic, renal, haematological and other biochemical function tests have been observed during treatment with Diflucan but the clinical significance and relationship to treatment is uncertain.

Very rarely, patients who died with severe underlying disease and who have received multiple dose Diflucan, had post-mortem findings which included hepatic necrosis. These patients were receiving multiple concomitant medications, some known to be potentially hepatotoxic, and/or had underlying diseases which could have caused the hepatic necrosis. Consequently, because a causal relationship with Diflucan cannot be excluded, the risk-benefit ratio of continued Diflucan treatment should be assessed in those patients in whom a significant rise of liver enzymes occurs.

Patients have rarely developed exfoliative cutaneous reactions, such as Stevens-Johnson Syndrome and toxic epidermal necrolysis, during treatment with fluconazole. AIDS patients are more prone to the development of severe cutaneous reactions to many drugs.

If a rash develops in a patient treated for a superficial fungal infection which is considered attributable to Diflucan, further therapy with this agent should be discontinued. In patients with invasive/systemic fungal infections who develop rashes, they should be monitored closely and Diflucan discontinued if bullous lesions or erythema multiforme develop.

*Use during lactation:* Fluconazole is found in human breast milk at concentrations similar to plasma, hence its use in nursing mothers is not recommended.

*Driving/use of machinery:* Experience with Diflucan indicates that therapy is unlikely to impair a patient's ability to drive or use machinery.

*Drug interactions:* The following drug interactions relate to the use of multiple-dose Diflucan, and the relevance to single-dose Diflucan 150 mg has not yet been established.

*Anticoagulants:* In an interaction study, Diflucan increased the prothrombin time after warfarin administration in healthy males. Though the magnitude of change was small (12%), careful monitoring of prothrombin time in patients receiving coumarin-type anticoagulants is recommended.

*Sulphonylureas:* Diflucan has been shown to prolong the serum half-life of concomitantly administered oral sulphonylureas (chlorpropamide, glibenclamide, glipizide and tolbutamide) in healthy volunteers. Diflucan and oral sulphonylureas may be co-administered to diabetic patients, but the possibility of a hypoglycaemic episode should be borne in mind.

*Hydrochlorothiazide:* In a kinetic interaction study, co-administration of multiple-dose hydrochlorothiazide to healthy volunteers receiving Diflucan increased plasma concentrations of fluconazole by 40%. An effect of this magnitude should not necessitate a change in the Diflucan dose regimen in subjects receiving concomitant diuretics, although the prescriber should bear it in mind.

*Phenytoin:* Concomitant administration of Diflucan and phenytoin may increase the levels of phenytoin to a clinically significant degree. If it is necessary to administer both drugs concomitantly, phenytoin levels should be monitored and the phenytoin dose adjusted to maintain therapeutic levels.

*Rifampicin:* Concomitant administration of Diflucan and rifampicin has resulted in a 25% decrease in the AUC and 20% shorter half-life of fluconazole. In patients receiving concomitant rifampicin, an increase in the Diflucan dose should be considered.

*Oral contraceptives:* Two kinetic studies with combined oral contraceptives have been performed using multiple doses of Diflucan. There were no relevant effects on either hormone level in the 50 mg Diflucan study, while at 200 mg daily the AUCs of ethinyl estradiol and levonorgestrel were increased 40% and 24% respectively. Thus multiple dose use of Diflucan at these doses is unlikely to have an effect on the efficacy of the combined oral contraceptive.

*Endogenous steroid:* Diflucan 50 mg daily does not affect endogenous steroid levels in females: 200–400 mg daily has no clinically significant effect on endogenous steroid levels or on ACTH stimulated response in healthy male volunteers.

*Cyclosporin:* A kinetic study in renal transplant patients found Diflucan 200 mg daily to slowly increase cyclosporin concentrations. However, in another multiple dose study with 100 mg daily, Diflucan did not affect cyclosporin levels in patients with bone marrow transplants. Cyclosporin plasma concentration monitoring in patients receiving Diflucan is recommended.

*Theophylline:* In a placebo-controlled interaction study, the administration of Diflucan 200 mg for 14 days resulted in an 18% decrease in the mean plasma clearance of theophylline. Patients who are receiving high doses of theophylline or who are otherwise at increased risk for theophylline toxicity should be observed for signs of theophylline toxicity while receiving Diflucan, and the therapy modified appropriately if signs of toxicity develop.

*Terfenadine:* Because of the occurrence of serious dysrhythmias secondary to prolongation of the QTc interval in patients receiving other azole antifungals in conjunction with terfenadine, interactions studies have been performed. One study at a 200 mg daily dose of Diflucan failed to demonstrate a prolongation in QTc interval. Another study at a 400 mg and 800 mg daily dose of Diflucan demonstrated that Diflucan taken in multiple doses of 400 mg per day or greater significantly increased plasma levels of terfenadine when taken concomitantly. There have been spontaneously reported cases of palpitations, tachycardia, dizziness and chest pain in patients taking concomitant Diflucan and terfenadine where the relationship of the reported adverse events to drug therapy or underlying medical conditions was not clear. Because of the potential seriousness of such an interaction, it is recommended that terfenadine not be taken in combination with Diflucan (see *Contra-indications*).

*Cisapride:* There have been reports of cardiac events including torsades de pointes in patients to whom Diflucan and cisapride were co-administered. In most of these cases, the patients appear to have been predisposed to arrhythmias or had serious underlying illnesses, and the relationship of the reported events to a possible Diflucan-cisapride drug interaction is unclear. There have been no formal drug interaction studies with Diflucan and cisapride. Because of the potential seriousness of such an interaction, it is recommended that cisapride not be taken in combination with Diflucan (see *Contra-indications*).

*Astemizole:* The use of Diflucan in patients concurrently taking astemizole or other drugs metabolised by the cytochrome P-450 system may be associated with elevations in serum levels of these drugs. In the absence of definitive information, caution should be used when co-administering Diflucan.

*Zidovudine:* Two kinetic studies resulted in increased levels of zidovudine most likely caused by the decreased conversion of zidovudine to its major metabolite. One study determined zidovudine levels in AIDS or ARC patients before and following Diflucan 200 mg daily for 15 days. There was a significant increase in zidovudine AUC (20%). A second randomised, two-period, two-treatment cross-over study examined zidovudine levels in HIV infected patients. On two occasions, 21 days apart, patients received zidovudine 200 mg every eight hours either with or without Diflucan 400 mg daily for seven days. The AUC of zidovudine significantly increased (74%) during co-administration with Diflucan. Patients receiving this combination should be monitored for the development of zidovudine-related adverse reactions.

Interaction studies have shown that when oral Diflucan is co-administered with food, cimetidine, antacids or following total body irradiation for bone marrow transplantation, no clinically significant impairment of fluconazole absorption occurs.

Physicians should be aware that drug-drug interaction studies with other medications have not been conducted, but that such interactions may occur.

*Side-effects:* Diflucan is generally well tolerated. The commonest side-effects associated with Diflucan are symptoms associated with the gastro-intestinal tract; these include nausea, abdominal discomfort, diarrhoea and flatulence. Other adverse events such as rash are rarely encountered (incidences less than 1%). In rare cases, as with other azoles, anaphylaxis has been reported.

See 'Warnings' for information on hepatic necrosis and cutaneous reactions in AIDS patients.

*Overdosage:* In the event of overdosage, supportive measures and symptomatic treatment, with gastric lavage if necessary, may be adequate.

As fluconazole is excreted largely in the urine, forced volume diuresis would probably increase the elimination rate. A three hour session of haemodialysis decreases plasma levels by approximately 50%.

### Pharmaceutical precautions

*Capsules:* Store below 30°C.

*Intravenous Infusion:* Do not freeze. The infusion does not contain any preservatives. It is for single use only. Discard any remaining solution.

*Powder for Oral Suspension:* Store below 30°C. Reconstituted suspension should be stored at 5°C–30°C. Do not freeze. Any remaining suspension should be discarded after 14 days. Where doses of less than 5 ml are required, a suitable measuring device should be used. Dilution is not appropriate.

**Legal category** POM

**Package quantities**

Single dose therapy: Blister pack containing 1 × 150 mg Diflucan capsule.

Multiple dose therapy: Calendar blister packs containing 7 × 50 mg or 7 × 200 mg Diflucan capsules.

Diflucan Intravenous Infusion 2 mg/ml: Bottle of 25 ml (50 mg). Bottle of 100 ml (200 mg).

Diflucan Powder for Oral Suspension 50 mg/5 ml or 200 mg/5 ml: 35 ml pack after reconstitution with 24 ml of water.

**Further information** Nil.

**Product licence number**

| | |
|---|---|
| Diflucan Capsules 50 mg | 0057/0289 |
| Diflucan Capsules 150 mg | 0057/0290 |
| Diflucan Capsules 200 mg | 0057/0317 |
| Diflucan Intravenous Infusion 2 mg/ml | 0057/0315 |
| Diflucan Powder for Oral Suspension: | |
| 50 mg/5 ml: | 0057/0343 |
| 200 mg/5 ml: | 0057/0344 |

## FASIGYN*

**Presentation** Fasigyn (tinidazole) is available as 500 mg film coated white tablets.

Inactive excipients: alginic acid, hydroxypropylmethyl cellulose, magnesium stearate, maize starch, microcrystalline cellulose, propylene glycol, sodium lauryl sulphate and titanium dioxide.

### Uses

*Actions:* Fasigyn is rapidly and completely absorbed following oral administration. In studies with healthy volunteers receiving 2 g tinidazole orally, peak serum levels of 40–51 micrograms/ml were achieved within two hours and decreased to between 11–19 micrograms/ml at 24 hours. Plasma levels decline slowly and tinidazole can be detected in plasma at concentrations of up to 1 microgram/ml at 72 hours after oral administration. The plasma elimination half-life for tinidazole is between 12–14 hours.

Tinidazole is widely distributed in all body tissues and also crosses the blood brain barrier, obtaining clinically effective concentrations in all tissues. The apparent volume of distribution is about 50 litres. About 12% of plasma tinidazole is bound to plasma protein.

Tinidazole is excreted by the liver and kidneys. Studies in healthy patients have shown that over 5 days, 60–65% of an administered dose is excreted by the kidneys with 20–25% of the administered dose excreted as unchanged tinidazole. Approximately 12% of the administered dose is excreted in the faeces.

Studies in patients with renal failure (creatinine clearance <22 ml/min) indicate that there is no statistically significant change in tinidazole pharmacokinetic parameters in these patients. Thus no adjustments in dosing are required in these patients.

Fasigyn is active against both protozoa and obligate anaerobic bacteria. The activity against protozoa involves *Trichomonas vaginalis, Entamoeba histolytica* and *Giardia lamblia.*

Fasigyn is active against *Gardnerella vaginalis* and most anaerobic bacteria including *Bacteroides fragilis, Bacteroides melaninogenicus,* Bacteroides spp., Clostridium spp., Eubacterium spp., Fusobacterium spp., Peptococcus spp., Peptostreptococcus spp., and Veillonella spp.

The mode of action of Fasigyn against anaerobic bacteria and protozoa involves penetration of the drug into the cell of the micro-organism and subsequent damage of DNA strands or inhibition of their synthesis.

*Indications:*

1. Prophylaxis: The prevention of post-operative infections caused by anaerobic bacteria, especially those associated with colonic, gastro-intestinal and gynaecological surgery.

2. Treatment of anaerobic infections such as:

Intraperitoneal infections: peritonitis, abscess.

Gynaecological infections: endometritis, endomyometritis, tubo-ovarian abscess.

Bacterial septicaemia.

Post-operative wound infections.

Skin and soft tissue infections.

Upper and lower respiratory tract infections: pneumonia, empyema, lung abscess.

3. Non-specific vaginitis.

4. Acute ulcerative gingivitis.

5. Urogenital trichomoniasis in both male and female patients.

6. Giardiasis.

7. Intestinal amoebiasis.

8. Amoebic involvement of the liver.

### Dosage and administration

1. *Prevention of post-operative infections: Adults:* A single oral dose of 2 g approximately 12 hours before surgery.

*Children less than 12 years:* Data are not available to allow dosage recommendations for children below

the age of 12 years in the prophylaxis of post-operative infections.

2. *Treatment of anaerobic infections: Adults:* An initial dose of 2 g the first day followed by 1 g daily given as a single dose or as 500 mg twice daily.

Treatment for 5 to 6 days will generally be adequate but clinical judgement must determine the duration of therapy, particularly when eradication of infection from certain sites may be difficult.

Regular clinical and laboratory observation is advised if it is considered necessary to continue therapy for more than 7 days.

*Children less than 12 years:* Data are not available to allow dosage recommendations for children below the age of 12 years in the treatment of anaerobic infections.

3. *Non-specific vaginitis: Adults:* Non-specific vaginitis is treated with a single oral dose of 2 g. Higher cure rates have been achieved with 2 g single daily doses for two consecutive days (total dosage 4 g).

4. *Acute ulcerative gingivitis: Adults:* A single oral dose of 2 g.

5. *Urogenital trichomoniasis:* When infection with *Trichomonas vaginalis* is confirmed, simultaneous treatment of the consort is recommended.

*Adult preferred regimen:* A single dose of 2 g.

*Children:* A single dose of 50 to 75 mg/kg of body weight. It may be necessary to repeat this dose once in some cases.

6. *Giardiasis: Adults:* A single dose of 2 g.

*Children:* A single dose of 50 to 75 mg/kg of body weight. It may be necessary to repeat this dose once in some cases.

7. *Intestinal amoebiasis: Adults:* A single daily dose of 2 g for two or three days.

*Children:* A single dose of 50 to 60 mg/kg of body weight per day for three successive days.

8. *Amoebic involvement of the liver: Adults:* Total dosage varies from 4.5 to 12g, depending on the virulence of the *Entamoeba histolytica.*

For amoebic involvement of the liver, the evacuation of pus may be required in addition to therapy with Fasigyn.

Initiate treatment with 1.5 to 2 g as a single oral daily dose for 3 days. Occasionally when a three-day course is ineffective, treatment may be continued for up to six days.

*Children:* A single daily dose of 50 to 60 mg/kg of body weight per day for five successive days.

It is recommended that Fasigyn be taken during or after a meal.

*Use in the elderly:* There are no special recommendations for this age group.

### Contra-indications, warnings, etc

*Contra-indications:* Use of Fasigyn is contra-indicated during the first trimester of pregnancy, in nursing mothers, in patients with organic neurologic disorders and in patients with known hypersensitivity to any of the components of Fasigyn. As with other drugs of similar structure, Fasigyn is also contra-indicated in patients having a history of or with blood dyscrasias, although no persistent haematologic abnormalities have been noted in clinical or animal studies with tinidazole.

*Use in pregnancy:* Fertility studies in rats receiving 100 mg or 300 mg tinidazole/kg had no effect on fertility, adult and pup weights, gestation, viability or lactation. There was a slight, not significant, increase in resorption rate at the 300 mg/kg dose.

Tinidazole crosses the placental barrier. Since the effects of compounds of this class on foetal development are unknown, the use of tinidazole during the first trimester is contra-indicated. There is no evidence that Fasigyn is harmful during the latter stages of pregnancy, but its use during the second and third trimesters requires that the potential benefits be weighed against possible hazards to mother or foetus.

*Use in nursing mothers:* Tinidazole is excreted in breast milk. Tinidazole may continue to appear in breast milk for more than 72 hours after administration. Women should not nurse until at least 3 days after having discontinued taking Fasigyn.

*Precautions:* As with related compounds, alcoholic beverages should be avoided during Fasigyn therapy because of the possibility of a disulfiram-like reaction (flushing, abdominal cramps, vomiting, tachycardia). Alcohol should be avoided until 72 hours after discontinuing Fasigyn.

Drugs of similar chemical structure have also produced various neurological disturbances such as dizziness, vertigo, inco-ordination and ataxia. If, during therapy with Fasigyn, abnormal neurological signs develop, therapy should be discontinued.

*Side-effects:* Reported side-effects have generally been infrequent, mild and self-limiting. Gastro-intestinal side-effects include nausea, vomiting, anorexia, diarrhoea, metallic taste and abdominal pain.

Hypersensitivity reactions, occasionally severe,

may occur in rare cases in the form of skin rash, pruritus, urticaria and angioneurotic oedema.

Neurological disturbances associated with Fasigyn include dizziness, vertigo, ataxia, peripheral neuropathy (paraesthesia, sensory disturbances, hypaesthesia) and rarely convulsions.

As with related compounds, Fasigyn may produce transient leucopenia. Other rarely reported side-effects are headache, tiredness, furry tongue and dark urine.

*Overdosage:* In acute animal studies with mice and rats, the $LD_{50}$ for mice was >3600 mg/kg and >2300 mg/kg for oral and intraperitoneal administration, respectively. For rats, the $LD_{50}$ was >2000 mg/kg for both oral and intraperitoneal administration.

There are no reported overdoses in humans with Fasigyn.

There is no specific antidote for treatment of overdosage with tinidazole. Treatment is symptomatic and supportive. Gastric lavage may be useful. Tinidazole is easily dialysable.

**Pharmaceutical precautions**  Store below 25°C in a dry place, away from light.

**Legal category**  POM.

**Package quantities**  20×500 mg tablets.

**Further information**  Nil.

**Product licence number**  0057/0150.

# FELDENE* CAPSULES
# FELDENE* 20 CAPSULES
# FELDENE* DISPERSIBLE TABLETS
# FELDENE* SUPPOSITORIES
# FELDENE* I.M. INTRAMUSCULAR INJECTION
# FELDENE MELT*

**Presentation**  Feldene capsules are available in two strengths: 10 mg-maroon and blue capsules, coded 'Pfizer' and 'FEL 10' containing 10 mg piroxicam. Feldene 20 capsules are maroon capsules coded 'Pfizer' and 'FEL 20' containing 20 mg piroxicam.

Feldene dispersible tablets are available in two strengths: 10 mg – white to off-white flat round tablets coded 'FEL' and '10' on one side, with an incised line between and 'Pfizer' on the other. 20 mg – white to off-white capsular tablets coded 'FEL 20' on one side and lettered 'PFIZER' on the other.

Feldene Melt tablets: Off-white, round, freeze-dried, fast dissolving tablets containing 20 mg piroxicam.

Feldene suppositories (white to off-white) containing 20 mg piroxicam.

Feldene I.M.: Sterile, pyrogen-free, clear solution in ampoule containing 1 ml of piroxicam solution (20 mg/ml) for intramuscular injection.

*Inactive excipients:* Feldene capsules (both strengths): lactose, maize starch, magnesium stearate, sodium lauryl sulphate. In addition, capsule shells contain erythrosine, gelatin, indigotine and titanium dioxide.

Feldene dispersible tablets (both strengths); lactose, microcrystalline cellulose, hydroxypropyl cellulose, sodium stearyl fumarate.

Feldene Melt tablets: aspartame, citric acid anhydrous, gelatin, mannitol.

Feldene suppositories: Lunacera M, propyl gallate, suppocire AM.

Feldene IM: benzyl alcohol, ethanol, nicotinamide, propylene glycol and other ingredients.

**Uses**  Feldene is a non-steroidal anti-inflammatory drug indicated for a variety of conditions requiring anti-inflammatory and/or analgesic activity.

Capsules; dispersible tablets; suppositories; melt tablets: Rheumatoid arthritis, osteoarthritis (arthrosis, degenerative joint disease), ankylosing spondylitis, acute musculoskeletal disorders and acute gout.

Dispersible tablets: Children with definitely diagnosed juvenile chronic arthritis (Still's disease).

Intramuscular injection: Initial treatment of acute conditions (acute gout, acute musculoskeletal disorders) and acute exacerbations of chronic conditions (rheumatoid arthritis, osteoarthritis, ankylosing spondylitis).

## Dosage and administration

*Adults:*

*Rheumatoid arthritis, osteoarthritis, ankylosing spondylitis:* The recommended starting dose is 20 mg given as a single daily dose. The majority of patients will be maintained on 20 mg daily. A relatively small group of patients may be maintained on 10 mg daily. Some patients may require up to 30 mg daily given in single or divided doses. Administration of doses exceeding 20 mg daily (of more than several days duration) carries an increased risk of gastro-intestinal side-effects.

*Acute gout:* Therapy should be initiated by a single dose of 40 mg, followed on the next four to six days with 40 mg daily, given in single or divided doses. Feldene is not indicated for the long-term management of gout.

*Acute musculoskeletal disorders:* Therapy should be initiated with 40 mg daily for the first two days, given in single or divided doses. For the remainder of the seven to fourteen day treatment period, the dose should be reduced to 20 mg daily.

*Children:*

*Juvenile chronic arthritis (Still's disease):* As little data are available in very young children, it is recommended that only children aged 6 years and older are treated with Feldene dispersible tablets according to the following dosage schedule:

| Body weight (kg) | Once-daily dose |
| --- | --- |
| less than 15 | 5 mg |
| 16–25 | 10 mg |
| 26–45 | 15 mg |
| 46 and above | 20 mg |

Dosage recommendations and indications for use in children other than in juvenile chronic arthritis have not been established.

*Feldene dispersible tablets:* These can be swallowed whole with a fluid, or may be dispersed in a minimum of 50 ml of water and then swallowed.

*Feldene Melt tablets:* These should be placed on the tongue to disperse and then swallowed with the saliva. Feldene Melt dissolves almost instantly in the mouth in the presence of saliva.

*Feldene Suppositories:* For each indication (excluding juvenile chronic arthritis), the dosage of Feldene suppositories when used alone, is identical with the dosage of Feldene capsules or dispersible tablets.

*Feldene I.M. intramuscular injection:* The dosage of Feldene I.M. intramuscular injection is identical to the dosage of oral Feldene. For continuation of treatment oral or suppository dose forms should be used. Feldene I.M. intramuscular injection should be administered by deep intramuscular injection into the upper, outer quadrant of the buttock. Feldene I.M. intramuscular injection should not be administered intravenously.

*Combined administration:* The total daily dosage of Feldene administered as capsules, dispersible tablets, melt tablets, suppositories and intramuscular injection should not exceed the maximum recommended daily dosage as indicated above.

*Use in the elderly:* Elderly, frail or debilitated patients may tolerate side-effects less well and such patients should be carefully supervised.

As with other non-steroidal anti-inflammatory drugs, caution should be used in the treatment of elderly patients who are more likely to be suffering from impaired renal, hepatic or cardiac function.

## Contra-indications, warnings, etc
*Contra-indications:*

1. Active peptic ulceration or a history of recurrent ulceration.

2. Feldene should not be used in those patients who have previously shown a hypersensitivity to the drug. The potential exists for cross sensitivity to aspirin and other non-steroidal anti-inflammatory drugs. Feldene should not be given to patients in whom aspirin and other non-steroidal anti-inflammatory drugs induce the symptoms of asthma, nasal polyps, angioneurotic oedema or urticaria.

3. Feldene suppositories should not be used in patients with any inflammatory lesions of the rectum or anus, or in patients with a recent history of rectal or anal bleeding.

*Warnings:*

*Use in pregnancy:* Although no teratogenic effects were seen in animal testing, the use of Feldene during pregnancy is not recommended. Feldene inhibits prostaglandin synthesis and release through a reversible inhibition of the cyclo-oxygenase enzyme. This effect, as with other non-steroidal anti-inflammatory drugs has been associated with an increased incidence of dystocia and delayed parturition in pregnant animals when drug administration was continued into late pregnancy. Non-steroidal anti-inflammatory drugs are also known to induce closure of the ductus arteriosus in infants.

*Nursing mothers:* A study indicates that piroxicam appears in breast milk at about 1% to 3% of the maternal plasma concentrations. No accumulation of piroxicam occurred in milk relative to that in plasma during treatment for up to 52 days. Feldene is not recommended for use in nursing mothers as clinical safety in neonates has not been established.

*Precautions:* Drug administration should be closely supervised in patients with a history of upper gastrointestinal disease. Feldene should be withdrawn if peptic ulceration or gastro-intestinal bleeding occurs.

In rare cases, non-steroidal anti-inflammatory drugs may cause interstitial nephritis, glomerulonephritis, papillary necrosis and the nephrotic syndrome. Such agents inhibit the synthesis of renal prostaglandin which plays a supportive role in the maintenance of renal perfusion in patients whose renal blood flow and blood volume are decreased. In these patients, administration of a non-steroidal anti-inflammatory drug may precipitate overt renal decompensation which is typically followed by recovery to pretreatment state upon discontinuation of non-steroidal anti-inflammatory therapy. Patients at greatest risk of such a reaction are those with congestive heart failure, liver cirrhosis, nephrotic syndrome and overt renal disease. Such patients should be carefully monitored whilst receiving therapy with a non-steroidal anti-inflammatory drug.

Patients with phenylketonuria: Due to aspartame content of Feldene Melt each tablet contains 0.14 mg phenylalanine.

Because of reports of adverse eye findings with non-steroidal anti-inflammatory drugs, it is recommended that patients who develop visual complaints during treatment with Feldene have ophthalmic evaluation.

*Drug interactions:* Non-steroidal anti-inflammatory drugs may cause sodium, potassium and fluid retention and may interfere with the natriuretic action of diuretic agents. These properties should be kept in mind when treating patients with compromised cardiac function or hypertension since they may be responsible for a worsening of those conditions.

As with other non-steroidal anti-inflammatory drugs, bleeding has been reported rarely when Feldene has been administered to patients on coumarin-type anticoagulants. Patients should be monitored closely if Feldene and oral anticoagulants are administered together.

Feldene, like other non-steroidal anti-inflammatory drugs, decreases platelet aggregation and prolongs bleeding time. This effect should be kept in mind when bleeding times are determined.

As with other non-steroidal anti-inflammatory drugs, the use of Feldene in conjunction with aspirin or the concomitant use of two non-steroidal anti-inflammatory drugs is not recommended because data are inadequate to demonstrate that the combination produces greater improvement than that achieved with the drug alone and the potential for adverse reactions is increased.

Studies in man have shown that the concomitant administration of Feldene and aspirin resulted in a reduction of plasma levels of piroxicam to about 80% of the normal values. Concomitant administration of antacids had no effect on piroxicam plasma levels. Neither did concurrent therapy with Feldene and digoxin, or Feldene and digitoxin, affect the plasma levels of either drug.

Feldene is highly protein-bound and therefore might be expected to displace other protein-bound drugs. The physician should closely monitor patients for change in dosage requirements when administering Feldene to patients on highly protein-bound drugs.

Non-steroidal anti-inflammatory drugs, including Feldene, have been reported to increase steady state plasma lithium levels. It is recommended that these levels are monitored when initiating, adjusting and discontinuing Feldene.

Results of two separate studies indicate a slight but significant increase in absorption of piroxicam following cimetidine administration but no significant changes in elimination rate constants or half-life. The small increase in absorption is unlikely to be clinically significant.

*Side-effects: Gastro-intestinal:* These are the most commonly encountered side-effects but in most instances do not interfere with the course of therapy. They include stomatitis, anorexia, epigastric distress, nausea, constipation, abdominal discomfort, flatulence, diarrhoea, abdominal pain and indigestion, rare cases of pancreatitis have been reported. Objective evaluations of gastric mucosal appearances and intestinal blood loss show that 20 mg/day of Feldene administered either in single or divided daily doses is significantly less irritating to the gastro-intestinal tract than aspirin. Peptic ulceration, perforation and gastro-intestinal bleeding, in rare cases fatal, have been reported with Feldene.

Some epidemiological studies have suggested that piroxicam is associated with a higher risk of gastro-intestinal adverse reactions compared with some other NSAIDS, but this has not been confirmed in all studies. Administration of doses exceeding 20 mg daily (of more than several days duration) carries an increased risk of gastro-intestinal side-effects, but they may also occur with lower doses. See Dosage and Administration.

Ano-rectal reactions to suppositories have presented as local pain, burning, pruritus and tenesmus. Rare instances of rectal bleeding have occurred.

*Oedema:* As with other non-steroidal anti-inflammatory drugs, oedema, mainly of the ankle, has been reported in a small percentage of patients and the possibility of precipitating congestive cardiac failure in elderly patients or those with compromised cardiac function should therefore be borne in mind.

*CNS:* Dizziness, headache, somnolence, insomnia, depression, nervousness, hallucinations, mood alterations, dream abnormalities, mental confusion, paraesthesias and vertigo have been reported rarely.

*Dermal hypersensitivity:* Rash and pruritus. Onycholysis and alopecia have rarely been reported. Photosensitivity reactions occur infrequently. As with other non-steroidal anti-inflammatory drugs, toxic epidermal necrolysis (Lyell's disease) and Stevens-Johnson syndrome may develop in rare cases. Vesiculo-bullous reactions have been reported rarely.

*Hypersensitivity reactions:* Hypersensitivity reactions such as anaphylaxis, bronchospasm, urticaria/angioneurotic oedema, vasculitis and serum sickness have been reported rarely.

*Renal function:* Interstitial nephritis, nephrotic syndrome, renal failure and renal papillary necrosis have been reported rarely. (See Precautions).

*Haematological:* Decreases in haemoglobin and haematocrit, unassociated with obvious gastro-intestinal bleeding, have occurred. Anaemia, thrombocytopenia, non-thrombocytopenic purpura (Henoch-Schoenlein), leucopenia and eosinophilia have been reported. Cases of aplastic anaemia, haemolytic anaemia and epistaxis have rarely been reported.

*Liver function:* Changes in various liver function parameters have been observed. As with most other non-steroidal anti-inflammatory drugs, some patients may develop increased serum transaminase levels during treatment with Feldene. Severe hepatic reactions, including jaundice and cases of fatal hepatitis have been reported. Although such reactions are rare, if abnormal liver function tests persist or worsen, if clinical signs and symptoms consistent with liver disease develop, or if systemic manifestations occur (e.g. eosinophilia, rash), Feldene should be discontinued.

*Other:* The following have been reported rarely: palpitations and dyspnoea, anecdotal cases of positive ANA, anecdotal cases of hearing impairment, metabolic abnormalities such as hypoglycaemia, hyperglycaemia, weight increase or decrease.

Swollen eyes, blurred vision and eye irritations have been reported. Routine ophthalmoscopy and slit-lamp examination have revealed no evidence of ocular changes. Malaise and tinnitus may occur.

*Intramuscular:* Transient pain upon injection has occasionally been reported. Local adverse reactions (burning sensations) or tissue damage (sterile abscess formation, fatty tissue necrosis) may occasionally occur at the site of injection.

*Overdosage:* In the event of overdosage with Feldene, supportive and symptomatic therapy is indicated. Studies indicate that administration of activated charcoal may result in reduced absorption and re-absorption of piroxicam thus reducing the total amount of active drug available.

**Pharmaceutical precautions**
Capsules: Store below 30°C.
Dispersible Tablets: Store below 30°C.
Suppositories: Store below 25°C. Do not refrigerate.
Intramuscular injection: Store below 25°C.
Melt Tablets: Store below 25°C.

**Legal category** POM.

**Package quantities**
Feldene Capsules 10 mg: Containers of 56 (Original pack).
Feldene 20 Capsules 20 mg: Containers of 28 (Original pack).
Feldene Dispersible Tablets 10 mg: Containers of 56 (Original pack).
Feldene Dispersible Tablets 20 mg: Containers of 28 (Original pack).
Feldene Suppositories 20 mg: Foil strip of 10 (Original pack).
Feldene I.M. Intramuscular injection 20 mg/ml: Pack of 1×1 ml ampoule.
Feldene Melt Tablets 20 mg: Containers of 28 (Original pack).

**Further information** Feldene pharmacokinetics are similar following oral or rectal administration. Following oral administration with food there is a slight delay in the rate but not the extent of absorption. The plasma half-life is approximately 50 hours in man and stable plasma concentrations are maintained throughout the day on once-daily dosage. Continuous treatment with 20 mg/day for periods of one year produces similar blood levels to those seen once steady state is first achieved.

Feldene Melt and Feldene capsules are bioequivalent. A multiple dose study of the pharmacokinetics and the bioavailability of Feldene Melt compared to oral capsules for 14 days has shown that after once daily administration the piroxicam concentration time profiles were nearly superimposable. Single dose studies demonstrated bioequivalent with capsules when Feldene Melt is taken with or without water.

Feldene I.M. intramuscular injection and Feldene capsules are bioequivalent. However, Feldene intramuscular injection provides significantly higher plasma levels of piroxicam during the first 45 minutes on the first day and 30 minutes on the second day.

Feldene is extensively metabolised and less than 5% of the daily dose is excreted unchanged in urine and faeces. One important metabolic pathway is hydroxylation of the pyridyl ring of the piroxicam side chain, followed by conjugation with glucuronic acid and urinary elimination.

**Product licence numbers**

| | |
|---|---|
| Feldene Capsules 10 mg | 0057/0145 |
| Feldene 20 Capsules 20 mg | 0057/0146 |
| Feldene Dispersible Tablets 10 mg | 0057/0240 |
| Feldene Dispersible Tablets 20 mg | 0057/0242 |
| Feldene Suppositories 20 mg | 0057/0219 |
| Feldene I.M. Intramuscular injection 20 mg/ml | 0057/0320 |
| Feldene Melt Tablets 20 mg | 0057/0352 |

# FELDENE* GEL
# FELDENE* GEL STARTER PACK

**Presentation** Topical Feldene is available as a clear pale yellow gel containing 5 mg piroxicam in each gram. Topical Feldene is available in three tube sizes: 7.5 g Feldene Gel Starter Pack, 60 g Feldene Gel and 112 g Feldene Gel.

Inactive excipients: These are benzyl alcohol, carbopol 940, di-isopropanolamine, ethyl alcohol, hydroxyethyl cellulose, propylene glycol and water.

**Uses** Feldene Gel and Feldene Gel Starter Pack contain piroxicam, a non-steroidal anti-inflammatory agent indicated for a variety of conditions characterised by pain and inflammation, or stiffness.

Feldene Gel is effective in the treatment of osteoarthritis of superficial joints such as the knee, acute musculoskeletal injuries, periarthritis, epicondylitis, tendinitis and tenosynovitis. Feldene Gel is available as a 7.5 g Starter Pack to provide 2–3 days initial treatment of the above conditions.

Feldene Gel and Feldene Gel Starter Pack are for topical use only.

**Dosage and administration** Feldene Gel and Feldene Gel Starter Pack are for external use only. No occlusive dressings should be employed. Apply 1 g of the Gel, corresponding to 3 cms, (approximately 1¼ inches) and rub into the affected site three to four times daily leaving no residual material on the skin. Therapy should be reviewed after four weeks.

*Use in children:* Dosage recommendations and indications for the use of Feldene Gel and Feldene Gel Starter Pack in children have not been established.

*Use in the elderly:* No special precautions are required.

**Contra-indications, warnings, etc**
*Contra-indications:* Feldene Gel and Feldene Gel Starter Pack should not be used in those patients who have previously shown a hypersensitivity to the Gel or piroxicam in any of its forms. The potential exists for cross sensitivity to aspirin and other non-steroidal anti-inflammatory agents.

Feldene Gel and Feldene Gel Starter Pack should not be given to patients in whom aspirin and other non-steroidal anti-inflammatory agents induce the symptoms of asthma, nasal polyps, angioneurotic oedema or urticaria.

*Precautions:* If local irritation develops, the use of the Gel should be discontinued and appropriate therapy instituted as necessary.

Keep away from the eyes and mucosal surfaces. Do not apply to any sites affected by open skin lesions, dermatoses or infection.

*Use in Pregnancy:* Although no teratogenic effects were seen when Feldene was orally administered in animal testing, the use of Feldene Gel during pregnancy or during lactation is not recommended.

*Nursing mothers:* Feldene Gel and Feldene Gel Starter Pack are not recommended for use in nursing mothers as clinical safety has not been established.

*Side-effects:* Feldene Gel is well tolerated. Mild to moderate local irritation, erythema, pruritus and dermatitis may occur at the application site. The systemic absorption of Feldene Gel is very low. In common with other topical NSAIDs, systemic reactions occur infrequently and have included minor gastro-intestinal side-effects such as nausea and dyspepsia. Cases of abdominal pain and gastritis have been reported rarely. There have been isolated reports of bronchospasm and dyspnoea (see also Contra-indications).

*Overdosage:* Overdosage is unlikely to occur with this topical preparation.

**Pharmaceutical precautions** None.

**Legal category** POM.

**Package quantities**
Feldene Gel: 112 g tube.
Feldene Gel: 60 g tube.
Feldene Gel Starter Pack: 7.5 g tube.

**Further information** On the basis of various pharmacokinetic and tissue distribution studies in animals, with the Gel, the highest concentrations of piroxicam were achieved in the tissues below the site of application with low concentrations being reached in the plasma. The Gel was continuously and gradually released from the skin to underlying tissues, equilibrium between skin and muscle or synovial fluid appeared to be reached rapidly, within a few hours of application.

From a pharmacokinetic study in man, 2 g of the Gel was applied to the shoulders of normal volunteers twice daily (corresponding to 20 mg piroxicam/day) for 14 days, plasma levels of piroxicam rose slowly, reaching steady state after about 11 days. The plasma levels at this time were between 300–400 ng/ml, or one-twentieth of those observed in subjects receiving 20 mg orally.

The Gel was well tolerated in volunteers with a history of contact allergy.

**Product licence number**
Feldene Gel (60 g and 112 g) and
Feldene Gel Starter Pack:              0057/0284

# GASTROMAX*

**Qualitative and quantitative composition** Active ingredient: Metoclopramide Hydrochloride PhEur 30 mg.

**Pharmaceutical form** Opaque orange/yellow capsules for oral administration. Controlled release formulation.

**Clinical particulars**
*Therapeutic indications:* For the relief of upper gastro-intestinal symptoms in patients aged over 20 years, including heartburn, dyspepsia and flatulence associated with such conditions as peptic ulcer, reflux oesophagitis, gastric reflux, gastritis, duodenitis and hiatus hernia.

For the relief of nausea and vomiting due to gastrointestinal disorders. Also for use as an anti-emetic for nausea and vomiting associated with cytotoxic drugs.

*Posology and method of administration:*
*Adults over 20 years of age:* Gastromax should be swallowed whole with liquid, preferably before a meal. Dosage is one capsule, once daily, either morning or evening dependent upon timing of symptoms.

For example, in cases of nocturnal reflux and heartburn, the capsule should be taken in the evening. If symptoms are mainly associated with daytime activity e.g. after meals, bending, stooping, etc., the capsule should be taken in the morning.

One capsule (30 mg) is the maximum recommended dose and should not be exceeded.

*Children and young adults under 20 years of age:* Not recommended.

*Elderly:* The usual adult dose is recommended. Since tardive dyskinesia is more likely to occur in the elderly, especially during long term therapy, treatment should be regularly reviewed.

*Use in hepatic or renal impairment:* In patients with clinically significant hepatic or renal impairment, the clearance of Gastromax may be impaired. Such patients should be observed carefully, and treatment discontinued if side-effects occur.

*Contra-indications:* Gastromax is contra-indicated in patients under 20 years of age, in nursing mothers and during the first trimester of pregnancy (see *Pregnancy and lactation*).

Gastromax is contra-indicated in patients with phaeochromocytoma.

Gastromax is also contra-indicated in patients who have shown hypersensitivity to metoclopramide or any component of the product.

*Special warnings and special precautions for use:* If vomiting persists, the patient should be assessed to exclude the possibility of underlying disease.

Patients with hepatic or renal insufficiency should be observed carefully. Treatment should be discontinued if side-effects occur.

Cases of neuroleptic malignant syndrome, an idiosyncratic response characterised by hyperthermia, muscle rigidity, altered consciousness including coma and elevated CPK have been reported with metoclopramide. Tardive dyskinesia may occur principally in the elderly, after prolonged treatment. The dose in the elderly should be strictly adhered to and treatment should be regularly reviewed.

Gastromax should not be administered to patients undergoing gastrointestinal surgery, e.g. gut anastomosis, until a sufficient period for healing has elapsed.

Metoclopramide has been classified as porphyrinogenic and is potentially unsafe in patients with acute porphyria.

*Interaction with other medicaments and other forms of interaction:* The absorption of any orally co-administered medication may be affected by the effects of Gastromax on gastro-intestinal motility. Drugs known to be affected in this way include: asprin, paracetamol, digoxin and alcohol.

The effects of Gatromax on the gastro-intestinal tract are antagonised by anti-muscarinics and by opioid analgesics.

Since extrapyramidal symptoms may occur with both Gatromax and other centrally acting medication (e.g. lithium, phenothiazines, anticonvulsants), particularly care should be exercised in the event of co-administration of these drugs.

Gastromax should be used with care in association with other drugs acting at central dopamine receptors, such as levodopa and bromocriptine.

Gastromax should be used with care in association with drugs that enhance sympathomimetic activity such as MAOIs.

*Pregnancy and lactation:* Gastromax is contra-indicated during the first trimester of pregnancy. In later stages of pregnancy, Gastromax should only be used where there are compelling reasons to do so.

Since metoclopramide is found in breast milk, Gastromax is contra-indicated in nursing mothers.

*Effects of ability to drive and use machines:* Rarely, Gastromax may cause drowsiness and affect reaction times. Patients should be warned of the possibility and cautioned against driving a car or operating machinery if so affected.

*Undesirable effects:* Gastromax is well tolerated. Fatigue, dizziness, drowsiness, restlessness and diarrhoea have been reported.

Raised prolactin levels manifesting as mammary engorgement or galactorrhoea may occur. These symptoms are usually associated with long-term therapy and disappear on discontinuation of therapy. Depression has been reported very rarely.

Various extrapyramidal reactions usually of the dystonic type have been reported. Symptoms which can occur include: spasm of facial, extra-ocular or cervical muscles which may be constant or rhythmic. There may also be a generalised increase in muscle tone. Should treatment of a dystonic reaction be required, an anticholinergic anti-Parkinsonian drug may be used.

Tardive dyskinesia may occur principally in the elderly after prolonged treatment (see other *Special warnings and special precautions for use*).

*Overdose:* Gastric lavage and intensive supportive therapy should be initiated. Dystonic symptoms should be treated with atropine, benztropine or other anticholinergic agents.

**Pharmacological properties**
*Pharmacodynamic properties:* Metoclopramide increases lower oesophageal sphincter pressure, accelerates gastric emptying and increases the amplitude of gastric contractions. As well as a central effect on the 'vomit centre' metoclopramide exerts an increase in gastric motor activity and encourages normal peristaltic action. This anti-emetic effect is useful in post-operative nausea and vomiting, drug-induced vomiting, radiation sickness and non-specific vomiting.

*Pharmacokinetic properties:* Following administration, the Gastromax capsule disintegrates to release pellets into the gastrointestinal tract. Metoclopramide is released from these pellets by a controlled delivery system.

One 30 mg Gastromax capsule, once daily, can replace 10 mg metoclopramide three times daily, minimising peaks and troughs in plasma metoclopramide concentration.

**Pharmaceutical particulars**
*List of excipients:* The capsules contain the following inert ingredients: Colloidal silicon dioxide, sucrose PhEur, maize starch PhEur, talc PhEur, shellac, ethyl cellulose, titanium dioxide (E171), iron (II) oxide yellow (E172), erythrosine (E127), gelatin BP.

*Incompatibilities:* None known.

*Shelf life:* 36 months.

*Special precautions for storage:* None.

*Nature and contents of container:* Packs of 28 capsules. Aluminium/PVC blister strips, 14 capsules/strip, 2 strips in a carton box.

*Instructions for use/handling:* None.

**Marketing authorisation number** 0057/0395.

**Date of approval/revision of SPC** March 1996.

**Legal category** POM.

## GLIBENESE*

**Presentation** Glibenese (glipizide) is available as white oblong tablets marked GBS/5 on the scored side and 'Pfizer' on the other. Each tablet contains 5 mg glipizide.

**Uses** *Actions:* Glibenese is an orally active sulphonylurea which effectively reduces blood glucose to the normal range in properly selected patients with non-insulin-dependent diabetes mellitus (NIDDM). It eliminates or diminishes glycosuria and ameliorates symptoms such as polyuria, polydipsia and pruritus.

The primary mode of action of Glibenese in experimental animals is the stimulation of insulin secretion from the beta-cells of pancreatic islet tissue. In man, stimulation of insulin secretion by Glibenese in response to a meal is undoubtedly of major importance. Fasting insulin levels are not elevated even on long-term Glibenese administration, but the postprandial insulin response continues to be enhanced after at least 6 months of treatment. The insulinotropic response to a meal occurs within 30 minutes after an oral dose of Glibenese in diabetic patients, but elevated insulin levels do not persist beyond the time of the meal challenge. There is also increasing evidence that extrapancreatic effects involving potentiation of insulin action form a significant component of the activity of Glibenese.

Blood sugar control persists for up to 24 hours after a single dose of Glibenese even though plasma levels have declined to a small fraction of peak levels by that time. Once-daily administration of doses up to 15 mg has been shown to be safe and effective maintenance therapy in selected patients.

Some patients fail to respond initially, or gradually lose their responsiveness to sulphonylurea drugs, including Glibenese. Alternatively, Glibenese, may be effective in some patients who have not responded or have ceased to respond to other sulphonylureas.

Gastrointestinal absorption of Glibenese in man is uniform, rapid and essentially complete. Peak plasma concentrations occur 1–3 hours after a single oral dose. The half-life of elimination ranges from 2–4 hours in normal subjects, whether given intravenously or orally. The metabolic and excretory patterns are similar with the two routes of administration, indicating that first-pass metabolism is not significant. Glibenese does not accumulate in plasma on repeated oral administration. Total absorption and disposition of an oral dose was unaffected by food in normal volunteers, but absorption was delayed by about 40 minutes. Thus, Glibenese was more effective when administered about 30 minutes before, rather than with a test meal in diabetic patients. Protein binding was studied in serum from volunteers who received either oral or intravenous Glibenese and found to be 98–99% one hour after either route of administration. The apparent volume of distribution of Glibenese after intravenous administration was 11 litres, indicative of localisation within the extracellular fluid compartment.

The metabolism of Glibenese is extensive and occurs mainly in the liver. The primary metabolites are inactive hydroxylation products and polar conjugates and are excreted mainly in the urine. Less than 10% unchanged Glibenese is found in the urine.

In a placebo-controlled, crossover study in normal volunteers, Glibenese showed no antidiuretic activity, and, in fact, led to a slight increase in free water clearance.

*Indications:* Glibenese is indicated as an adjunct to diet to lower the blood glucose in patients with non-insulin-dependent diabetes mellitus (type II, NIDDM), formerly known as maturity onset diabetes, whose hyperglycaemia cannot be controlled by diet alone.

In initiating treatment for non-insulin dependent diabetes, diet should be emphasised as the primary form of treatment. Caloric restriction and weight loss are essential in the obese diabetic patient. Proper dietary management alone may be effective in controlling the blood glucose and symptoms of hyperglycaemia. The importance of regular physical activity should also be stressed, cardiovascular risk factors should be identified and corrective measures taken where possible.

Use of Glibenese must be viewed by both the physician and patient as a treatment in addition to diet, and not as a substitute for diet or as a convenient mechanism for avoiding dietary restraint. Furthermore, loss of blood glucose control on diet alone also may be transient, thus requiring only short-term administration of Glibenese.

During maintenance programmes, Glibenese should be discontinued if satisfactory lowering of blood glucose is no longer achieved. Judgments should be based on regular clinical and laboratory evaluation.

In considering the use of Glibenese in asymptomatic patients, it should be recognised that controlling the blood glucose in non-insulin-dependent diabetes, has not been definitely established to be effective in preventing the long-term cardiovascular or neurological complications of diabetes.

*Patient selection:* The most likely patient for therapy is one in whom diabetes is of the NIDDM type, stable, and not controlled by dietary regulation alone. A past history of diabetic coma does not necessarily preclude successful therapeutic control with Glibenese. A trial period may be indicated in certain patients who might be expected to respond to this type of medication, but who failed in initial trials with, or after having been on other oral sulphonylurea agents, or in patients whose diabetic control on such agents has not been satisfactory. Glibenese may prove effective and provide improved control of the diabetes. The final evaluation of response in patients who qualify as candidates for Glibenese is a therapeutic trial for a period of at least seven days. During the trial period, the absence of ketonuria together with a satisfactory control, indicates that the patient is responsive and amenable to control with the drug. However, the development of ketonuria within 24 hours after withdrawal of insulin usually will be indicative of a poor response. The patient is considered unresponsive if he fails to achieve satisfactory lowering of blood sugar levels or fails to obtain objective or subjective clinical improvement and if he develops ketonuria or glycosuria. Insulin is indicated for the therapy of such patients.

**Dosage and administration** There is no fixed dosage regimen for the management of diabetes mellitus with Glibenese or any other hypoglycaemic agent. In addition to the usual monitoring of urinary glucose, the patient's blood glucose must also be monitored periodically to determine the minimum effective dose for the patient, to detect primary failure: i.e. inadequate lowering of blood glucose at the maximum recommended dose of medication, and to detect secondary failure; i.e. loss of adequate blood-glucose-lowering response after an initial period of effectiveness. Glycosylated haemoglobin levels may also be of value in monitoring the patient's response to therapy.

Short term administration of Glibenese may be sufficient during periods of transient loss of control in patients usually controlled well on diet.

In general, Glibenese should be given approximately 30 minutes before a meal to achieve the greatest reduction in post-prandial hyperglycaemia.

*Initial dose:* The recommended starting dose is 5 mg, given before breakfast or the midday meal. Mild diabetics, elderly patients or those with liver disease may be started on 2.5 mg.

*Titration:* Dosage adjustments should ordinarily be in increments of 2.5 to 5 mg, as determined by blood glucose response. At least several days should elapse between titration steps. The maximum recommended single dose is 15 mg. Doses above 15 mg should ordinarily be divided.

*Maintenance:* Some patients may be effectively controlled on a once-a-day regimen. Total daily dosage above 15 mg should ordinarily be divided. Total daily dosage above 30 mg has been given safely on a twice daily basis to long term patients. Patients can usually be stabilised on a dosage ranging from 2.5 to 30 mg daily. The maximum recommended daily dosage is 40 mg.

*Use in the elderly:* Elderly diabetics are more sensitive to the hypoglycaemic effect of sulphonylurea drugs and should therefore be prescribed a low starting dose of 2.5 mg daily. The elderly are also particularly susceptible to the effects of hypoglycaemia. Hypoglycaemia may be difficult to recognise in the elderly.

In elderly, debilitated or malnourished patients, and patients with an impaired renal or hepatic function, the initial and maintenance dosing should be conservative to avoid hypoglycaemic reactions (see Precautions section).

*Use in children:* Safety and effectiveness in children have not been established.

*Patients receiving insulin:* As with other sulphonylurea class hypoglycaemics, many stable non-insulin-dependent diabetic patients receiving insulin may be safely placed on Glibenese. When transferring patients from insulin to Glibenese, the following general guidelines should be considered.

For patients whose daily insulin requirement is 20 units or less, insulin may be discontinued and Glibenese therapy begun at usual dosages. Several days should elapse between Glibenese titration steps.

For patients whose daily insulin requirement is greater than 20 units, the insulin dose should be reduced by 50% and Glibenese therapy initiated at usual dosages. Subsequent reductions in insulin dosage should depend on individual patient response. Several days should elapse between Glibenese steps.

During the insulin withdrawal period, the patient should test urine samples for sugar and ketone bodies at least three times daily. Patients should be instructed to contact the prescriber immediately if these tests are abnormal. In some cases, especially when the patient has been receiving greater than 40 units of insulin daily, it may be advisable to consider hospitalisation during the transition period.

*Patients receiving other oral hypoglycaemic agents:* As with other sulphonylurea class hypoglycaemics, no transition period is necessary when transferring patients to Glibenese. Patients should be observed carefully (1–2 weeks) for hypoglycaemia when being transferred from longer half-life sulphonylureas (e.g. chlorpropamide) to Glibenese due to potential overlapping of drug effect.

*Concurrent biguanide therapy:* As with other sulphonylureas, a proportion of patients who do not achieve optimal control with Glibenese alone, or who experience secondary failure, may be expected to have their control improved or restored by the addition of a biguanide.

For such patients, it is suggested that the dosage of Glibenese should be maintained and the biguanide chosen should be added using low doses initially and increasing the dosage of the biguanide progressively until adequate control is achieved or restored. Should gastrointestinal side-effects appear, an attempt should be made to reduce the dosage of the biguanide.

### Contra-indications, warnings, etc
*Contra-indications:* Glibenese is contra-indicated in the following conditions:
1. Known hypersensitivity to Glibenese.
2. Diabetic ketoacidosis, with or without coma. This condition should be treated with insulin.
3. Insulin dependent (juvenile-onset) diabetes.
4. Severe renal, hepatic or thyroid impairment; coexistent renal and hepatic disease.

*Warnings:* The metabolism and excretion of Glibenese may be slowed in patients with impaired renal and/or hepatic function. If hypoglycaemia should occur in such patients, it may be prolonged.

*Precautions*
*General:* Hypoglycaemia: All sulphonylurea drugs are capable of producing severe hypoglycaemia. Proper patient selection, dosage, and instructions are important to avoid hypoglycaemic episodes. Renal or hepatic insufficiency may cause elevated blood levels of Glibenese and the latter may also diminish gluconeogenic capacity, both of which increase the risk of serious hypoglycaemic reactions. Elderly, debilitated or malnourished patients, and those with adrenal or pituitary insufficiency are particularly susceptible to the hypoglycaemic action of glucose-lowering drugs. Hypoglycaemia may be difficult to recognise in the elderly, and in people who are taking beta-adrenergic blocking drugs. Hypoglycaemia is more likely to occur when caloric intake is deficient, after severe or prolonged exercise, when alcohol is ingested, or when more than one glucose-lowering drug is used.

*Loss of control of blood glucose:* When a patient stabilised on any diabetic regimen is exposed to stress such as fever, trauma, infection, or surgery, a loss of control may occur. At such times, it may be necessary to discontinue Glibenese and administer insulin.

The effectiveness of any oral hypoglycaemic drug, including Glibenese, in lowering blood glucose to a desired level decreases in many patients over a period of time, which may be due to progression of the severity of the diabetes or to diminished responsiveness to the drug. This phenomenon is known as secondary failure, to distinguish it from primary failure in which the drug is ineffective in an individual patient when first given.

*Information for patients:* Patients should be informed of the potential risks and advantages of Glibenese and of alternative modes of therapy. They should also be informed about the importance of adherence to dietary instructions, of a regular exercise programme, and of regular testing of urine and/or blood glucose.

The risk of hypoglycaemia, its symptoms and treatment, and conditions that predispose to its development should be explained to patients and responsible family members. Primary and secondary failure should also be explained.

*Laboratory tests:* Blood and urine glucose should be monitored periodically. Measurement of glycosylated haemoglobin may be useful.

*Driving/use of machinery:* Clinical experience with Glibenese indicates that it is unlikely to impair a patient's ability to drive or use machinery.

*Use in pregnancy:* Glibenese is contra-indicated during pregnancy. Diabetes in pregnancy should be treated with insulin and not sulphonylureas. Recent evidence suggests that hyperglycaemia in pregnancy is associated with a higher incidence of congenital abnormalities.

*Nursing mothers:* Although it is not known whether Glibenese is excreted in human milk, some sulphonylurea drugs are known to be excreted in human milk. Caution is therefore necessary if a sulphonylurea drug is prescribed because of the possibility of hypoglycaemia in the infant.

*Use in renal insufficiency:* Glibenese is not recommended in patients with renal insufficiency.

*Drug interactions:* The hypoglycaemic action of sulpho-nylureas may be potentiated by certain drugs including nonsteroidal anti-inflammatory agents and other drugs that are highly protein bound, salicylates, sulphonamides, chloramphenicol, probenecid, coumarins, monoamine oxidase inhibitors and beta-adrenergic blocking agents. When such drugs are administered to a patient receiving Glibenese, the patient should be observed closely for hypoglycaemia. When such drugs are withdrawn from a patient receiving Glibenese, the patient should be observed closely for loss of control.

Certain drugs tend to produce hyperglycaemia and may lead to loss of control. These drugs include the thiazides and other diuretics, corticosteroids, phenothiazines, thyroid products, oestrogens, oral contraceptives, phenytoin, nicotinic acid, sympathomimetics, calcium antagonists and isoniazid. When such drugs are administered to or withdrawn from a patient receiving Glibenese, the patient should be closely observed for loss of control.

In the mouse, Glibenese pre-treatment did not cause an accumulation of acetaldehyde after ethanol administration. Clinical experience has confirmed the virtual absence of an alcohol interaction in man.

*Side-effects:* The majority of side-effects have been dose related, transient, and have responded to dose reduction or withdrawal of the medication. However, clinical experience thus far has shown that, as with other sulphonylureas some side-effects associated with hypersensitivity may be severe and deaths have been reported in some instances.

*Hypoglycaemia:* See 'Precautions' and 'Overdosage' sections.

*Gastrointestinal:* Gastrointestinal complaints include nausea, diarrhoea, constipation and gastralgia. They appear to be dose related and usually disappear on division or reduction of dosage.

*Dermatological:* Allergic skin reactions including erythema, morbilliform or maculopapular reactions, urticaria, pruritus and eczema have been reported. They frequently disappear with continued therapy. However, if they persist, the drug should be discontinued.

*Miscellaneous:* Dizziness, drowsiness and headache have each been reported in patients treated with Glibenese. They are usually transient and seldom require discontinuance of therapy.

*Laboratory tests:* The pattern of laboratory test abnormalities observed with Glibenese is similar to that for other sulphonylureas. Occasional mild to moderate elevations of AST (SGOT), LDH, alkaline phosphatase, BUN and creatinine were noted. One case of jaundice was reported. The relationship of these abnormalities to Glibenese is uncertain, and they have rarely been associated with clinical symptoms.

*Overdosage:* There is no well documented experience with Glibenese overdosage. The acute oral toxicity was extremely low in all species tested ($LD_{50}$ greater than 4g/kg).

Overdosage of sulphonylureas including Glibenese can produce hypoglycaemia. Mild hypoglycaemic symptoms without loss of consciousness or neurological findings should be treated aggressively with oral glucose and adjustments in drug dosage and/or meal patterns. Close monitoring should continue until the physician is assured that the patient is out of danger. Severe hypoglycaemic reactions with coma, seizure, or other neurological impairment occur infrequently, but constitute medical emergencies requiring immediate hospitalisation. If hypoglycaemic coma is diagnosed or suspected, the patient should be given a rapid intravenous injection of concentrated (50%) glucose solution. This should be followed by continuous infusion of a more dilute (10%) glucose solution at a rate that will maintain the blood glucose at a level above 5.6 mmol/l (100 mg/dl). Patients should be closely monitored for a minimum of 24 to 48 hours since hypoglycaemia may recur after apparent clinical recovery. Clearance of Glibenese from plasma would be prolonged in persons with liver disease. Because of the extensive protein binding of Glibenese, dialysis is unlikely to be of benefit.

**Pharmaceutical precautions**  Store below 25°C.

**Legal category**  POM.

**Package quantities**  Glibenese tablets 5 mg: Original packs of 56 tablets (in blister strips of 4 × 14 tablets).

**Further information**  Nil.

**Product licence number**  0057/0113R.

## ISTIN*

**Qualitative and quantitative composition**  Active ingredient: amlodipine. The tablets contain amlodipine besylate (equivalent to 5 and 10 ml amlodipine).

**Pharmaceutical form**  Tablet for oral administration.
5 mg tablets coded 'ITN5' on one side and 'PFIZER' on the other.
10 mg tablets coded 'ITN10' on one side and 'PFIZER' on the other.

**Clinical particulars**
*Therapeutic indications:* Hypertension.
Prophylaxis of chronic stable angina pectoris.
Prinzmetal's (variant) angina when diagnosed by a cardiologist.

In hypertensive patients, Istin has been used in combination with a thiazide diuretic, alpha blocker, beta-adrenoceptor blocking agent, or an angiotensin converting enzyme inhibitor. For angina, Istin may be used as monotherapy or in combination with other antianginal drugs in patients with angina that is refractory to nitrates and/or adequate doses of beta blockers.

Istin is well tolerated in patients with heart failure and a history of hypertension of ischaemic heart disease.

*Posology and method of administration:*
*In adults:* For both hypertension and angina the usual initial dose is 5 mg Istin once daily which may be increased to a maximum dose of 10 mg depending on the individual patient's response.

No dose adjustment of Istin is required upon concomitant administration of thiazide diuretics, beta blockers, and angiotensin-converting enzyme inhibitors.

*Use in children:* Not recommended.

*Use in the elderly:* The time to reach peak plasma concentrations of amlodipine is similar in elderly and younger subjects. Amlodipine clearance tends to be decreased with resulting increases in AUC and elimination half-life in elderly patients. Increases in AUC and elimination half-life in patients with congestive heart failure were as expected for the patient age group studied. Istin, used at similar doses in elderly or younger patients, is equally well tolerated. Therefore normal dosage regimens are recommended.

*Patients with hepatic impairment:* As with all calcium antagonists, amlodipine's half-life is prolonged in patients with impaired liver function and dosage recommendations have not been established. The drug should therefore be administered with caution in these patients.

*Patients with renal impairment:* Amlodipine is extensively metabolised to inactive metabolites with 10% excreted as unchanged drug in the urine. Changes in amlodipine plasma concentrations are not correlated with degree of renal impairment, therefore the normal dosage is recommended. Amlodipine is not dialysable.

*Contra-indications:* Istin is contra-indicated in patients with a known sensitivity to dihydropyridines.
Istin should not be used in cardiogenic shock, clinically significant aortic stenosis, unstable angina (excluding Prinzmetal's angina).
Pregnancy and lactation.

*Special warnings and precautions for use:* There are no data to support the use of Istin alone, during or within one month of a myocardial infarction.
The safety and efficacy of Istin in hypertensive crisis has not been established.

*Interactions with other medicaments and other forms of interaction:* Istin has been safely administered with thiazide diuretics, alpha blockers, beta blockers, angiotensin-converting enzyme inhibitors, long-acting nitrates, sublingual glyceryl trinitrate, non-steroidal anti-inflammatory drugs, antibiotics, and oral hypoglycaemic drugs.

Pharmacokinetic studies with cyclosporin have demonstrated that amlodipine does not significantly alter the pharmacokinetics of cyclosporin.

Special studies have indicated that the co-administration of Istin with digoxin did not change serum digoxin levels or digoxin renal clearance in normal volunteers, and that co-administration of cimetidine did not alter the pharmacokinetics of amlodipine.

In healthy male volunteers, the co-administration of Istin does not significantly alter the effect of warfarin on prothrombin response time.

*In vitro* data from studies with human plasma, indicate that amlodipine has no effect on protein binding of digoxin, phenytoin, warfarin or indomethacin.

Grapefruit juice may interact with Istin to increase the plasma concentration. However this increase is too small to significantly alter blood pressure or heart rate.

*Pregnancy and lactation:* Although some dihydropyridine compounds have been found to be teratogenic in animals, data in the rat and rabbit for amlodipine provide no evidence for a teratogenic effect. There is, however, no clinical experience with the preparation in pregnancy or lactation. Accordingly, Istin should not be administered during pregnancy, or lactation, or to women of childbearing potential unless effective contraception is used.

*Effects on ability to drive and use machines:* Clinical experience with Istin indicates that therapy is unlikely to impair a patient's ability to drive or use machinery.

*Undesirable effects:* The most commonly reported side-effects of Istin are headache, oedema, rash, fatigue, nausea, flushing and dizziness. Gingival hyperplasia has been reported after Istin. The following adverse reactions have been reported rarely: pruritus, palpitations, dyspnoea, abdominal pain, dyspepsia, muscle cramps, asthenia, somnolence, altered bowel habit, myalgia, arthralgia, mood changes, increased urinary frequency, impotence and visual disturbances. The following adverse reactions have been reported very rarely: abnormal liver function tests, jaundice, erythema multiforme and gynaecomastia.

As with other calcium channel blockers the following adverse events have been rarely reported and cannot be distinguished from the natural history of the underlying disease: myocardial infarction, arrhythmia (including ventricular tachycardia and atrial fibrillation) and chest pain.

*Overdose:* In humans, experience with intentional overdose is limited. Gastric lavage may be worthwhile in some cases. Available data suggest that gross overdosage could result in excessive peripheral vasodilatation with subsequent marked and probably prolonged systemic hypotension. Clinically significant hypotension due to Istin overdosage calls for active cardiovascular support including frequent monitoring of cardiac and respiratory function, elevation of extremities, and attention to circulating fluid volume and urine output. A vasoconstrictor may be helpful in restoring vascular tone and blood pressure, provided that there is no contra-indication to its use. Intravenous calcium gluconate may be beneficial in reversing the effects of calcium channel blockade. Since Istin is highly protein-bound, dialysis is not likely to be of benefit.

### Pharmacological properties

*Pharmacodynamic properties:* Istin is a calcium ion influx inhibitor of the dihydropyridine group (slow channel blocker or calcium ion antagonist) and inhibits the transmembrane influx of calcium ions into cardiac and vascular smooth muscle.

The mechanism of the antihypertensive action of Istin is due to a direct relaxant effect on vascular smooth muscle. The precise mechanism by which Istin relieves angina has not been fully determined but Istin reduces total ischaemic burden by the following two actions:

(1) Istin dilates peripheral arterioles and thus, reduces the total peripheral resistance (afterload) against which the heart works. Since the heart rate remains stable, this unloading of the heart reduces myocardial energy consumption and oxygen requirements.

(2) The mechanism of action of Istin probably involves dilatation of the main coronary arteries and coronary arterioles, both in normal and ischaemic regions. This dilatation increases myocardial oxygen delivery in patients with coronary artery spasm (Prinzmetal's or variant angina).

In patients with hypertension, once daily dosing provides clinically significant reductions of blood pressure in both the supine and standing positions throughout the 24 hour interval. Due to the slow onset of action, acute hypotension is not a feature of Istin administration.

In patients with angina, once daily administration of Istin increases total exercise time, time to angina onset, and time to 1 mm ST segment depression, and decreases both angina attack frequency and glyceryl trinitrate tablet consumption.

Istin has not been associated with any adverse metabolic effects or changes in plasma lipids and is suitable for use in patients with asthma, diabetes and gout.

Haemodynamic studies and a controlled clinical trial in Class II–IV heart failure patients have shown that Istin did not lead to clinical deterioration as measured by exercise tolerance, left ventricular ejection fraction and clinical symptomatology.

A placebo controlled study (PRAISE) designed to evaluate patients in NYHA Class III-IV heart failure receiving digoxin, diuretics and ACE inhibitors has shown that Istin did not lead to an increase in risk of mortality or combined mortality and morbidity with heart failure.

*Pharmacokinetic properties*

*Absorption, distribution, plasma protein binding:* After oral administration of therapeutic doses, amlodipine is well absorbed with peak blood levels between 6–12 hours post dose. Absolute bioavailability has been estimated to be between 64 and 80%. The volume of distribution is approximately 21 l/kg. *In vitro* studies have shown that approximately 97.5% of circulating amlodipine is bound to plasma proteins.

*Biotransformation/elimination:* The terminal plasma elimination half life is about 35–50 hours and is consistent with once daily dosing. Amlodipine is extensively metabolised by the liver to inactive metabolites with 10% of the parent compound and 60% of metabolites excreted in the urine.

*Preclinical safety data:* None.

### Pharmaceutical particulars

*List of excipients:* Microcrystalline Cellulose PhEur, dibasic calcium phosphate anhydrous NF, Sodium Starch Glycollate BP and Magnesium Stearate PhEur.

*Incompatibilities:* None stated.

*Shelf life:* 60 months.

*Special precautions for storage:* None specified.

*Nature and contents of container:* Istin is available as: Calendar packs of 28 tablets. Aluminium/PVC blister strips, 14 tablets/strip, 2 strips in a carton box.

*Instructions for use/handling:* No special requirements.

### Marketing authorisation numbers

Istin Tablets 5 mg     0057/0297
Istin Tablets 10 mg    0057/0298

**Date of approval/revision of SPC**   April 1997.

**Legal category**   POM.

## NEPHRIL* TABLETS

**Qualitative and quantitative composition**   Active ingredient: Polythiazide equivalent to 1 mg.

**Pharmaceutical form**   Tablets. White round tablets scored and marked NEP/1 on one side and Pfizer on the reverse.

### Clinical particulars

*Therapeutic indications:* Nephril is indicated as adjunctive therapy in oedema associated with congestive heart failure, hepatic cirrhosis and corticosteroid and oestrogen therapy.

Nephril has also been found useful in oedema due to various forms of renal dysfunction such as nephrotic syndrome, acute glomerulonephritis and chronic renal failure.

Nephril is indicated in the management of hypertension either as the sole therapeutic agent or to enhance the effectiveness of other antihypertensive drugs in the more severe forms of hypertension.

*Posology and method of administration:* Nephril is administered by the oral route.

The usual dosage of Nephril for diuretic therapy is 1 to 4 mg daily.

For antihypertensive therapy the usual maintenance dose is between 2 mg and 4 mg daily although some patients may be optimally controlled on 500 micrograms or 1 mg daily.

*Use in children:* Nephril is not recommended for children.

*Use in the elderly:* Elderly patients are especially liable to the adverse effects of diuretic agents. It is therefore particularly important that the dose should be the lowest possible consistent with adequate effect (see dosage above). The possibility of drug interactions should also be considered in view of the frequency of multiple drug therapy in this age group.

*Use in renal insufficiency:* Thiazides should be used with caution in severe renal disease. In patients with renal disease, thiazides may precipitate azotaemia. Cumulative effects of the drug may develop in patients with impaired renal function. If progressive renal impairment becomes evident, as indicated by a rising non-protein nitrogen or blood urea nitrogen, a careful reappraisal of therapy is necessary with probably cessation of treatment.

*Use in hepatic disease:* Thiazides should be used with caution in patients with impaired hepatic function or progressive liver disease, since minor alterations of fluid and electrolyte balance may precipitate hepatic coma.

*Contra-indications:* Anuria, hypersensitivity to polythiazide and other thiazide diuretics and other sulphonamide derived drugs.

*Special warnings and precautions for use:* All patients receiving thiazide therapy should have periodic determinations of serum electrolytes at appropriate intervals to detect possible electrolyte imbalance. Such patients should also be observed for clinical signs of fluid or electrolyte imbalance; namely hyponatraemia, hypochloraemic alkalosis and hypokalaemia. Serum and urine electrolyte determinations are particularly important when the patient is vomiting or receiving parenteral fluids. Warning signs of possible electrolyte imbalance, irrespective of cause, are: dryness of mouth, thirst, weakness, lethargy, drowsiness, restlessness, muscle pains or cramps, muscular fatigue, hypotension, oliguria, tachycardia and gastro-intestinal disturbances such as nausea and vomiting.

Hypokalaemia may develop with thiazides as with any other potent diuretics, especially with brisk diuresis, when severe cirrhosis is present, or during concomitant use of corticosteroids or ACTH.

Interference with adequate oral electrolyte intake will also contribute to hypokalaemia.

Hypokalaemia may exaggerate metabolic effects of digitalis therapy especially with reference to myocardial activity.

Any chloride deficit is generally mild and usually does not require specific treatment except under extraordinary circumstances (as in liver disease or renal disease). Dilutional hyponatraemia may occur in oedematous patients in hot weather; appropriate therapy is water restriction, rather than administration of salt except in those rare instances, when the hyponatraemia is life threatening. In actual salt depletion, appropriate replacement is the therapy of choice.

Hyperuricaemia may occur or frank gout may be precipitated in certain patients receiving thiazide therapy.

Insulin requirements in diabetic patients may be increased, decreased or unchanged. Latent diabetes mellitus may become manifest during thiazide administration.

Thiazide drugs may increase the responsiveness to tubocurarine.

The antihypertensive effects of thiazides may be enhanced in the post-sympathectomy patient. Thiazides may decrease arterial responsiveness to noradrenaline. This diminution is not sufficient to preclude effectiveness of the pressor agent for therapeutic use.

If progressive renal impairment becomes evident, as indicated by a rising non-protein nitrogen or blood urea nitrogen a careful reappraisal of therapy is necessary with probable discontinuation of therapy with Nephril.

Thiazides may decrease serum protein-bound iodine levels without signs of thyroid disturbance.

*Interactions with other medicaments and other forms of interaction:*

*Corticosteroids or ACTH:* When co-prescribed with polythiazide, corticosteroids or ACTH may enhance total potassium loss. It is recommended that electrolyte balance is carefully monitored.

*Cardiac glycosides/antiarrhythmics:* The possibility that the toxicity of cardiac glycosides, e.g. digitoxin or antiarrhythmics may be enhanced by polythiazide induced hypokalaemia should be borne in mind. Additional care should be taken in prescribing quinidine since plasma levels may be raised due to the urine alkalizing effect of thiazides.

*Antihypertensive drugs:* thiazides may add to or potentiate the action of other antihypertensive drugs. Potentiation occurs with ganglionic or peripheral adrenergic blocking drugs.

*Antidiabetic drugs:* requirement for antidiabetic therapy may be increased, decreased or unchanged. Diabetic patients should be monitored for possible decreased diabetic control.

*Tubocurarine:* thiazide drugs may increase responsiveness to tubocurarine.

*Pregnancy and lactation:*

*Use in pregnancy:* The routine use of diuretics in healthy pregnant women is inappropriate and may expose mother and foetus to unnecessary hazard. Diuretics do not prevent development of toxaemia of pregnancy and there is no satisfactory evidence that they are useful in the treatment of established toxaemia.

Oedema during pregnancy may arise from pathological cause or from physiological and mechanical consequences of pregnancy. Physiological hypervolaemia during pregnancy may be associated with generalised oedema including dependent oedema. This oedema is properly treated by recumbency and support hose. Thiazides may be indicated in pregnancy when oedema is due to pathological causes other than toxaemia. Rarely, short courses of thiazides are indicated where physiological oedema is unrelieved by rest and where the oedema causes extreme discomfort.

Thiazides cross the placental barrier and appear in cord blood. The use of thiazides in pregnant women requires that the anticipated benefit be weighed against possible hazards to the foetus. These hazards include foetal or neonatal jaundice, thrombocytopenia and other side-effects which have occurred in the adult.

*Use in lactation:* Thiazides appear in breast milk. If use of Nephril is deemed essential, breast feeding should be discontinued.

*Effects on ability to drive and use machines:* None stated

*Undesirable effects:*

*Gastrointestinal:* anorexia, gastric irritation, nausea, vomiting, cramping, diarrhoea, constipation, jaundice (intrahepatic cholestatic jaundice), pancreatitis.

*Central nervous system:* dizziness, vertigo, paraesthesia, headache, xanthopsia.

*Haematological:* leucopenia, agranulocytosis, thrombocytopenia, aplastic anaemia.

*Dermatological:* purpura, photosensitivity, rash, urticaria, necrotising angiitis (vasculitis) (cutaneous vasculitis).

*Cardiovascular:* orthostatic hypotension may occur and be aggravated by alcohol, barbiturates or narcotics.

*Other:* hyperglycaemia, glycosuria, hyperuricaemia, muscle spasm, weakness, restlessness.

Whenever adverse reactions are moderate or severe, thiazide dosage should be reduced or therapy withdrawn.

Thiazides may add to or potentiate the action of other hypertensive drugs. Potentiation occurs with ganglionic or peripheral adrenergic blocking drugs.

Sensitivity reactions may occur in patients with a history of allergy or bronchial asthma. The possibility of exacerbation or activation of systemic lupus erythematosus has been reported.

*Overdose:* Gastric lavage and supportive therapy. Treatment of acute renal failure if present. Potassium supplements.

**Pharmacological properties**

*Pharmacodynamic properties:* Nephril (polythiazide) is one of the thiazide diuretics, all of which have an identical mode of action as diuretic agents. The chief mechanism of action is interference with the distal renal tubular mechanism of electrolyte reabsorption and, in particular, at the cortical diluting site. Thiazides are also antihypertensive agents although their mode of action is uncertain. Their use as antihypertensive agents is initially associated with a fall in plasma volume and in the longer term, with a modest reduction in total peripheral resistance.

The therapeutic effects, mode of action and adverse effects of the thiazide diuretics are identical. Such differences as exist between the various compounds are related to milligram potency and duration of action.

*Pharmacokinetic properties:* Nephril has a long duration of action in man (24–48 hours) and an elimination half-life of approximately 26 hours. It is rapidly absorbed from the gastrointestinal tract and usually shows an effect within 1 hour of administraiton.

Increased lipid solubility, compared with other thiazides, is associated with larger apparent volume of distribution, lower renal clearance and binding to tissue elements.

*Preclinical safety data:* None.

**Pharmaceutical particulars**

*List of excipients:* Calcium phosphate dibasic, lactose, maize starch, vanillin, magnesium stearate, sodium lauryl sulphate, purified water for starch paste (not present in final product).

*Incompatibilities:* None stated.

*Shelf life:* 5 years.

*Special precautions for storage:* Store below 25°C.

*Nature and contents of container:* White opaque HDPE bottle with child resistant cap, containing 28 tablets.

*Instructions for use/handling:* None.

**Marketing authorisation number** 0057/5024R.

**Date of approval/revision of SPC** 7 October 1996.

**Legal category** POM.

## SINEQUAN*

**Presentation** Sinequan (doxepin hydrochloride) is available in capsules of four strengths. All capsules bear the name 'Pfizer'.

The four sizes of capsules are distinguished by their colour and coding as follows:

Sinequan 10 mg capsule coded 'SQN 10' (opaque red).

Sinequan 25 mg capsule coded 'SQN 25' (opaque blue cap/opaque red body).

Sinequan 50 mg capsule coded 'SQN 50' (opaque blue).

Sinequan 75 mg capsule coded 'SQN 75' (opaque blue cap/opaque rich yellow body).

*Inactive excipients:*

Sinequan 10 mg capsule: Core: lactose, magnesium stearate, maize starch and sodium lauryl sulphate. Shell: amaranth, erythrosine, gelatin, sunset yellow and titanium dioxide.

Sinequan 25 mg capsule: Core: lactose, magnesium stearate, maize starch, and sodium lauryl sulphate. Shell: amaranth, erythrosine, gelatin, patent blue V, sunset yellow and titanium dioxide.

Sinequan 50 mg capsule: Core: lactose, magnesium stearate, maize starch and sodium lauryl sulphate. Shell: erythrosine, gelatin, patent blue V and titanium dioxide.

Sinequan 75 mg capsule: Core: magnesium stearate, maize starch and sodium lauryl sulphate. Shell: erythrosine, gelatin, patent blue V, quinoline yellow and titanium dioxide.

**Uses** *Actions:* Sinequan is a tricyclic antidepressant. The mechanism of action of Sinequan is not definitely known. It is not a central nervous stimulant nor a monoamine oxidase inhibitor. The current hypothesis is that the clinical effects are due, at least in part, to influences on the adrenergic activity at the synapses so that deactivation of noradrenaline by re-uptake into the nerve terminals is prevented. In animal studies anticholinergic, antiserotonin and antihistamine effects on smooth muscle have been demonstrated. At higher than usual clinical doses, adrenaline response was potentiated in animals. This effect was not demonstrated in humans.

Doxepin is well absorbed from the gastrointestinal tract. Approximately 55–87% of orally administered doxepin undergoes first pass metabolism in the liver, forming the primary active metabolite desmethyldoxepin.

In healthy volunteers, a single oral dose of 75 mg resulted in peak plasma concentrations for doxepin ranging from 8.8–45.8 ng/ml (mean 26.1 ng/ml). Peak levels were reached between 2 and 4 hours (mean 2.9 hours) after administration. Peak levels for the primary metabolite desmethyldoxepin ranged from 4.8–14.5 ng/ml (mean 9.7 ng/ml) and were achieved between 2 and 10 hours after administation. The mean apparent volume of distribution for doxepin is approximately 20 l/kg. The protein binding for doxepin is approximately 76%.

In healthy volunteers, the plasma elimination half-life of doxepin ranged from 8 to 24 hours (mean 17 hours). The half-life of desmethyldoxepin ranged from 33–80 hours (mean 51 hours). Mean plasma clearance for doxepin is approximately 0.84 l/kg.hr. Paths of metabolism of doxepin include demethylation, N-oxidation, hydroxylation and glucuronide formation. Doxepin is excreted primarily in the urine, mainly as its metabolites, either free or in conjugate form.

*Indications:* Symptoms of depressive illness, especially where sedation is required.

Sinequan may be used with benefit where symptoms are of short or long duration prior to treatment and in patients with a wide range of intensity of illness.

As with other psychotherapeutic agents, the degree of response varies with each patient. In patients exhibiting a beneficial response, this may be seen within a few days of commencing therapy, while others may not respond for two weeks or longer.

Due to its excellent toleration, Sinequan is particularly useful in ambulatory patients seen in general practice as well as in the treatment of hospitalised patients.

**Dosage and administration** The optimum oral dose depends on the severity of the condition and the individual patient's response. The dose varies from 30–300 mg daily. Doses up to 100 mg daily may be given on a divided or once daily schedule. Should doses over 100 mg daily be required, they should be administered in three divided doses daily. 100 mg is the maximum dose recommended at any one time. This dose may be given at bedtime.

For the majority of patients with moderate or severe symptoms, it is recommended that treatment commences with an initial dose of 75 mg daily. Many of these patients will respond satisfactorily at this dose level. For patients who do not, the dosage may be adjusted according to individual response. In more severely ill patients, it may be necessary to administer a dose of up to 300 mg, in three divided doses daily, to obtain a clinical response.

In patients where insomnia is a troublesome symptom, it is recommended that the total daily dose be divided so that a higher proportion is given for the evening dose; similarly, if drowsiness is experienced as a side effect of treatment, Sinequan may be administered by this regimen, or the dosage may be reduced.

It is often possible, having once obtained a satisfactory therapeutic response, to reduce the dose for maintenance therapy.

The optimal antidepressant effect may not be evident for two to three weeks.

*Use in children:* The use of Sinequan in children under 12 years is not recommended, because safe conditions for its use have not been established.

*Use in the elderly:* In general, lower dosages are recommended. Where the presenting symptoms are mild in nature, it is advisable to initiate treatment at a dose of 10–50 mg daily. A satisfactory clinical response is obtained in many of these patients at a daily dose of 30–50 mg. The dosage may be adjusted according to the individual response.

*Use in hepatic impairment:* Dosage reduction may be required in patients with hepatic impairment.

**Contra-indications, warnings, etc**

*Contra-indications:* Hypersensitivity, mania, severe liver disease, lactation, glaucoma, tendency to urinary retention.

*Precautions:* The once-a-day dosage regimen of Sinequan in patients with intercurrent illness or patients taking other medications should be carefully adjusted. This is especially important in patients receiving other medications with anticholinergic effects.

The use of Sinequan on a once-a-day dosage regimen in geriatric patients should be adjusted carefully on the basis of the patient's condition. The elderly are particularly liable to experience toxic effects, especially agitation, confusion and postural hypotension. The initial dose should be increased with caution under close supervision. Half the normal maintenance dose may be sufficient to produce a satisfactory clinical response.

Patients should be warned that drowsiness may occur with the use of Sinequan. Patients should also be cautioned that their response to alcohol may be potentiated.

Use with caution in patients with severe cardiovascular disease, including patients with heart block, cardiac arrhythmia and those who have experienced a recent myocardial infarction.

Use with caution in patients with hepatic and/or renal impairment.

Use with caution in patients with a history of epilepsy.

Since suicide is an inherent risk in any depressed patient until significant improvement has occurred, patients should be closely supervised during early therapy.

*Drug interactions:* Combined use with other antidepressants, alcohol or anti-anxiety agents should be undertaken with due recognition of the possibility of potentiation. It is known, for example, that monoamine oxidase inhibitors may potentiate other drug effects, therefore Sinequan should not be given concurrently, or within two weeks of cessation of therapy, with monoamine oxidase inhibitors.

Cimetidine has been reported to produce clinically significant fluctuations in steady-state serum concentrations of various tricylic antidepressants.

Sinequan should not be given with sympathomimetic agents, such as ephedrine, isoprenaline, noradrenaline, phenylephrine and phenylpropanolamine.

General anaesthetics and local anaesthetics (containing sympathomimetics) given during tricyclic or tetracyclic antidepressant therapy may increase the risk of arrhythmias and hypotension or hypertension. If surgery is necessary, the anaesthetist should be informed that a patient is being so treated.

Sinequan may decrease the antihypertensive effect of agents such as debrisoquine, bethanidine, guanethidine and possibly clonidine. It usually requires daily doses of Sinequan in excess of 150 mg before any effect on the action of guanethidine is seen. It would be advisable to review all antihypertensive therapy during treatment with tricyclic antidepressants.

Barbiturates may increase the rate of metabolism of Sinequan.

The dose of thyroid hormone medication may need reducing if Sinequan is being given concurrently.

Tolazamide: A case of severe hypoglycaemia 11 days after the addition of doxepin (75 mg/day) has been reported in a non-insulin dependent diabetic patient maintained on tolazamide (1 g/day).

*Driving/use of machinery:* Since drowsiness may occur with the use of Sinequan, patients should be warned of the possibility and cautioned against driving a car or operating machinery while taking this drug.

*Use in pregnancy and lactation:*

*Pregnancy:* Doxepin crosses the placenta. Reproduction studies have been performed in rats, rabbits and monkeys and there was no evidence of harm to the animal foetus. The relevance to humans is not known. Since there is insufficient experience in pregnant women who have received this drug, its safety in pregnancy has not been established.

*Lactation:* Doxepin and its active metabolite desmethyldoxepin are excreted in breast milk. There has been a report of apnoea and drowsiness occurring in a nursing infant whose mother was taking doxepin. The use of Sinequan is contra-indicated during lactation.

*Side-effects:* Sinequan is well tolerated. Most side-effects are mild and generally disappear with continued treatment, or if necessary a reduction in dose.

*Note:* Some of the side-effects noted below have not been specifically reported with Sinequan. However, due to the close pharmacological similarities amongst the tricyclics, the reactions should be considered when prescribing Sinequan.

The most common side-effects to Sinequan are drowsiness, dry mouth and constipation. For further details see below under *Central nervous system effects* and *Anticholinergic effects.*

*Anticholinergic effects:* Anticholinergic effects are relatively common and may occur immediately following the first dose of a tricyclic antidepressant. Dry mouth and constipation are the most common anticholinergic effects. Blurred vision and sweating occur occasionally. Urinary retention is rare except in predisposed males who have an enlarged prostate gland. Tolerance is often achieved if treatment is continued. If these undesirable effects do not subside with continued therapy, or if they become severe, it may be necessary to reduce the dosage.

*Central nervous system effects:* Drowsiness is the most commonly noticed side effect. This tends to disappear as therapy is continued. Other infrequently reported CNS side effects are confusion, disorientation, agitation, numbness or paraesthesiae, tremor (which is usually mild). But at high doses, in susceptible individuals (particularly the elderly) other extrapyramidal symptoms may occur including tardive dyskinesia. Rarely reported are hallucinations, ataxia (generally where mixtures of CNS drugs have been given), and convulsions. Convulsions are unlikely except in people predisposed to seizure activity by brain damage or alcohol and drug abuse.

Psychotic manifestations, including mania and paranoid delusions may be exacerbated during treatment with tricyclic antidepressants.

*Cardiovascular:* Although Sinequan carries less risk than other tricyclic antidepressants, caution should be observed in the treatment of patients with heart block or cardiac arrhythmias. Cardiovascular effects including postural hypotension and tachycardia have been reported occasionally.

*Allergic:* Allergic reactions to tricylic antidepressants are uncommon. They include skin rash, facial oedema, photosensitisation and pruritus.

*Haematological:* Rare cases of eosinophilia and bone marrow depression manifesting as agranulocytosis, leucopenia, thrombocytopenia and purpura.

*Gastro-intestinal:* Nausea, vomiting, indigestion, taste disturbances, diarrhoea, anorexia and aphthous stomatitis have been reported. (See Anticholinergic effects.)

*Endocrine:* Occasional reports of raised or lowered libido, testicular swelling, raised or lowered blood sugar levels. Rarely the syndrome of inappropriate antidiuretic hormone secretion, gynaecomastia, enlargement of breasts and galactorrhoea in the female.

*Other:* Dizziness, weight gain, chills, fatigue, weakness, flushing, alopecia, headache, exacerbation of asthma and hyperpyrexia (in association with chlorpromazine) have been occasionally observed. Rare reports of jaundice and of tinnitus.

*Withdrawal:* Withdrawal symptoms may occur on abrupt cessation of tricyclic antidepressant therapy and include insomnia, irritability, and excessive perspiration. Withdrawal symptoms in neonates whose mothers received tricyclic antidepressants during the third trimester have also been reported and include respiratory depression, convulsions and 'jitteriness' (hyper-reflexia).

*Overdosage:*

A. *Signs and Symptoms:*
1. Mild: Drowsiness, stupor, blurred vision, excessive dryness of mouth.
2. Severe: Respiratory depression, hypotension, coma, convulsions, cardiac arrhythmias and tachycardias.

Also: urinary retention (bladder atony), decreased gastrointestinal motility (paralytic ileus), hyperthermia (or hypothermia), hypertension, dilated pupils, hyperactive reflexes.

B. *Management and Treatment:*
1. Mild: Observation and supportive therapy is all that is usually necessary.
2. Severe: Medical management of severe Sinequan overdosage consists of aggressive supportive therapy. If the patient is conscious, gastric lavage, with appropriate precautions to prevent pulmonary aspiration, should be performed even though Sinequan is rapidly absorbed. The use of activated charcoal has been recommended, as has been continuous gastric lavage with saline for 24 hours or more. An adequate airway should be established in comatose patients and assisted ventilation used if necessary. ECG monitoring may be required for several days, since relapse after apparent recovery has been reported. Arrhythmias should be treated with the appropriate anti-arrhythmic agent. It has been reported that many of the cardiovascular and CNS symptoms of tricyclic antidepressant poisoning in adults may be reversed by the slow intravenous administration of 1 mg to 3 mg of physostigmine salicylate. Because physostigmine is rapidly metabolised, the dosage should be repeated as required. Convulsions may respond to standard anticonvulsant therapy. However, barbiturates may potentiate any respiratory depression. Dialysis and forced diuresis generally are not of value in the management of overdosage due to high tissue and protein binding of Sinequan.

**Pharmaceutical precautions**   Store below 25°C.

**Legal category**   POM.

**Package quantities**
*Capsules 10 mg:* Original packs of 56 capsules (in blister strips of 4×14 capsules).
*Capsules 25 mg:* Original packs of 28 capsules (in blister strips of 2×14 capsules).
*Capsules 50 mg:* Original packs of 28 capsules (in blister strips of 2×14 capsules).
*Capsules 75 mg:* Original packs of 28 capsules (in blister strips of 2×14 capsules).

**Further information**   Nil.

**Product licence numbers**
10 mg capsules   0057/5032R
25 mg capsules   0057/5033R
50 mg capsules   0057/5034R
75 mg capsules   0057/0133

## TERRAMYCIN*

**Presentation**   Terramycin (oxytetracycline) is available as:

*Tablets 250 mg:* Sugar-coated yellow tablets, containing 250 mg Oxytetracycline Dihydrate PhEur and coded 'Pfizer'.

*Capsules 250 mg:* Hard gelatin capsules, opaque yellow cap and body printed TER250 and 'Pfizer', each containing 250 mg Oxytetracycline as the Hydrochloride PhEur.

*Inactive excipients:* Terramycin capsules: magnesium stearate, maize starch and sodium lauryl sulphate. In addition the capsule shell contains: erythrosine, gelatin, quinoline yellow and titanium dioxide.

Terramycin tablets: alginic acid, magnesium stearate and maize starch. In addition, the tablet coating contains: beeswax white, carnauba wax, gelatin, gum acacia, kaolin, methyl hydroxybenzoate, quinoline yellow, shellac orange, sucrose, sunset yellow, talc and titanium dioxide.

**Uses**   *Actions:* Oxytetracycline is primarily bacteriostatic and is thought to exert its antimicrobial effect by the inhibition of protein synthesis. Terramycin is active against a wide range of Gram-negative and Gram-positive organisms.

The drugs in the tetracycline class have closely similar antimicrobial spectra, and cross resistance among them is common.

Oxytetracycline and its salts are readily absorbed orally and are 10–40% bound to plasma proteins. Between 40 and 70% is excreted unchanged in the urine via glomerular filtration. A serum half-life of 6–10 hours has been reported for Terramycin in patients with normal renal function.

Oxytetracycline diffuses readily through the placenta into the foetal circulation, into the pleural fluid and, under some circumstances, into the cerebrospinal fluid. It appears to be well concentrated in the hepatic system and excreted in the bile, so that it appears in the faeces, as well as in the urine, in a biologically active form.

*Indications:* Respiratory tract infections: Pneumonia and other lower respiratory tract infections due to susceptible strains of *Streptococcus pneumoniae*, *Haemophilus influenzae*, *Klebsiella pneumoniae* and other organisms. *Mycoplasma pneumoniae* pneumonia. Treatment of chronic bronchitis.

Urinary tract infections: caused by susceptible strains of the Klebsiella species. Enterobacter species, *Escherichia coli*, *Streptococcus faecalis* and other organisms.

Sexually transmitted diseases: Infections due to *Chlamydia trachomatis* including uncomplicated urethral, endocervical or rectal infections. Non-gonococcal urethritis caused by *Ureaplasma urealyticum*. Terramycin is also indicated in chancroid, granuloma inguinale and lymphogranuloma venereum. Terramycin is an alternative drug in the treatment of gonorrhoea and syphilis.

Skin infections: Acne vulgaris when antibiotic therapy is considered necessary and severe rosacea.

Ophthalmic infections: Trachoma, although the infectious agent, as judged by immunofluorescence, is not always eliminated. Inclusion conjunctivitis may be treated with oral Terramycin alone or in combination with topical agents.

Rickettsial infections: Rocky Mountain spotted fever, typhus group, Q fever and Coxiella endocarditis and tick fevers.

Other infections: Stagnant loop syndrome. Psittacosis, brucellosis (in combination with streptomycin), cholera, bubonic plague, louse and tick-borne relapsing fever, tularaemia, glanders, melioidosis and acute intestinal amoebiasis (as an adjunct to amoebicides).

Terramycin is an alternative drug in the treatment of leptospirosis, gas-gangrene and tetanus.

**Dosage and administration**   The usual daily dose of Terramycin is 1–2 g, given in four equal doses, depending on the severity of the infection.

Therapy should be continued for at least 24–48 hours after symptoms and fever have subsided.

Food, milk and some dairy products interfere with absorption. Tetracyclines should be given one hour before or two hours after meals.

Administration of adequate amounts of fluid along with capsules and tablet forms of drugs in the tetracycline class is recommended to reduce the risk of oesophageal irritation and ulceration.

Dosage recommendation in specific infections:
Acne vulgaris and severe rosacea: Terramycin 250–500 mg daily in single or divided doses.
Brucellosis: Terramycin 500 mg, four times daily in combination with streptomycin.
Sexually Transmitted Diseases: Terramycin 500 mg four times daily for 7 days is recommended in the following infections: uncomplicated gonococcal infections (except anorectal infections in man); uncomplicated urethral, endocervical or rectal infection caused by *Chlamydia trachomatis*; non-gonococcal urethritis caused by *Ureaplasma urealyticum*.
Acute epididymo-orchitis caused by *Chlamydia trachomatis*, or *Neisseria gonorrhoeae*, Terramycin 500 mg, four times daily for 10 days.
Primary and secondary syphilis: Terramycin 500 mg, four times daily for 15 days. Syphilis of more than 1 year's duration, (latent syphilis of uncertain or more than 1 year's duration, cardiovascular or late benign syphilis) except neurosyphilis, should be treated with Terramycin 500 mg, four times daily for 30 days. Patient compliance with this regimen may be difficult so care should be taken to encourage optimal compliance. Close follow-up, including laboratory tests, is recommended.

*Use in the elderly:* See 'Precautions' section.

*Use in children:* Terramycin is contra-indicated in children under the age of 12 years. See 'Contra-indications' section.

**Contra-indications, warnings, etc**
*Contra-indications:* Terramycin is contra-indicated in persons who have shown hypersensitivity to any of the tetracyclines.

*Pregnancy:* Terramycin is contra-indicated in pregnancy. If this drug is used during pregnancy, or if the patient becomes pregnant while taking this drug, the patient should be apprised of the potential hazard to the foetus.

Results of animal studies with the tetracycline family of antimicrobials indicate that tetracyclines cross the placenta, are found in foetal tissues and can have toxic effects on the developing foetus. Evidence of embryo-toxicity has also been noted in animals treated early in pregnancy.

It appears that the risks associated with the use of tetracyclines during pregnancy are predominantly due to effects on teeth and skeletal development. (See below about use during tooth development.)

*Nursing mothers:* Tetracyclines are excreted into milk and are therefore contra-indicated in nursing mothers.

*Children:* Terramycin is contra-indicated in children under the age of 12 years. As with other tetracyclines, Terramycin forms a stable calcium complex in any bone-forming tissue. A decrease in the fibula growth rate has been observed in premature infants given oral tetracyclines in doses of 25 mg/kg every six hours. This reaction was shown to be reversible when the drug was discontinued.

The use of drugs of the tetracycline class during tooth development (pregnancy, infancy and childhood up to the age of 12 years) may cause permanent discolouration of the teeth (yellow-grey-brown) and enamel hypoplasia. This adverse reaction is more common during long-term use of the drug but has been observed following repeated short-term courses.

*Renal impairment:* Administration of usual doses may lead to excessive systemic accumulation of the drug and liver toxicity.

The anti-anabolic action of the tetracyclines may cause an increase in blood urea; while this is not a problem in those with normal renal function, in patients with significantly impaired renal function, higher levels of tetracycline may lead to azotaemia, hyperphosphataemia and acidosis.

*Precautions:* Terramycin should be administered with caution to patients with hepatic impairment or those receiving potentially hepatotoxic drugs.

The use of antibiotics may occasionally result in the overgrowth of nonsusceptible organisms including Candida. Constant observation of the patient is essential. If a resistant organism appears, the antibiotic should be discontinued and appropriate therapy instituted.

When treating venereal disease, where co-existent syphilis is suspected, proper diagnostic procedures should be utilized. In all such cases monthly serological tests should be made for at least four months.

Terramycin should not be given concurrently with bactericidal drugs such as penicillins.

In long term therapy, periodic laboratory evaluation of organ systems, including haematopoietic, renal and hepatic studies should be performed.

All infections due to Group A beta-haemolytic streptococci should be treated for at least 10 days.

*Use in the elderly:* Terramycin may be given in the usual adult dosage. The possibility of sub-clinical renal insufficiency should be kept in mind, as it may lead to drug accumulation (see 'Contra-indications').

*Drug interactions:* Antacids containing aluminium, calcium, magnesium, zinc or iron salts, may impair absorption of oxytetracycline.

In long term therapy, tetracyclines depress plasma prothrombin activity and reduced doses of concomitant anticoagulants may be necessary.

A few cases of pregnancy or breakthrough bleeding have been attributed to the concurrent use of tetracycline or oxytetracycline with oral contraceptives.

The concurrent use of tetracyclines and methoxyflurane has been reported to result in fatal renal toxicity.

*Side-effects:* Gastro-intestinal: Anorexia, nausea, vomiting, diarrhoea, glossitis, dysphagia, enterocolitis, and inflammatory lesions (with candidial overgrowth) in the anogenital regions. Rare instances of oesophagitis and oesophageal ulceration have been reported in patients receiving capsule and tablet forms of drugs in the tetracycline class. Most of these patients took medication immediately before going to bed.

Skin: Maculopapular and erythematous rashes. Exfoliative dermatitis has been reported but is uncommon. Photosensitivity manifested by an exaggerated sunburn reaction has been observed in some individuals taking tetracyclines. Patients likely to be exposed to direct sunlight or ultraviolet light should be advised that this reaction can occur with tetracyclines and treatment should be discontinued at the first evidence of skin erythema.

Hypersensitivity reactions: Urticaria, angioneurotic oedema, anaphylaxis, anaphylactoid purpura, pericarditis, and exacerbation of systemic lupus erythematosus.

Bulging fontanelles in infants and benign intracranial hypertension in adults have been reported in individuals receiving full therapeutic dosages of tetracyclines. These conditions disappeared rapidly when the drug was discontinued.

Blood: Haemolytic anaemia, thrombocytopenia, neutropenia and eosinophilia have been reported with tetracyclines.

When given over prolonged periods, tetracyclines have been reported to produce brown-black microscopic discolouration of thyroid tissue. No abnormalities of thyroid function are known to occur.

*Overdosage:* Acute overdosage with antibiotics is rare. In the event of overdosage, gastric lavage plus appropriate supportive treatment is indicated.

**Pharmaceutical precautions** Store below 25°C. Protect from light.

**Legal category** POM.

**Package quantities** Tablets 250 mg: Original packs of 28 tablets. Capsules 250 mg: Original packs of 28 capsules.

**Further information** Nil.

**Product licence numbers**
Tablets 250 mg 0057/5080R
Capsules 250 mg 0057/5036R

## TERRA-CORTRIL* TOPICAL OINTMENT

**Presentation** Terra-Cortril Topical Ointment contains 30 mg Oxytetracycline as the Hydrochloride PhEur and 10 mg Hydrocortisone PhEur in each gram of paraffin base, comprising white soft and liquid paraffin.

**Uses**
*Actions:* Terra-Cortril Topical Ointment possesses both the anti-inflammatory activity of hydrocortisone and the broad-spectrum antibacterial activity of oxytetracycline, which is active against a wide variety of Gram-positive and Gram-negative organisms.

Where topical therapy with hydrocortisone is of value the concurrent use of oxytetracycline may help eradicate secondary bacterial infection.

*Indications:* Terra-Cortril Topical Ointment is indicated in the following disorders: exudative and secondarily infected eczema including atopic eczema, primary

---

irritant dermatitis, allergic and seborrhoeic dermatitis. Secondarily infected insect bite reactions.

In exudative flexural intertrigo Terra-Cortril Topical Ointment can be used for up to seven days.

Like other tetracyclines, oxytetracycline is generally ineffective against Pseudomonas and Proteus species. Because these are recognised secondary infecting organisms in exudative dermatoses, preliminary identification of the organism and determination of antibiotic sensitivity is important.

Terra-Cortril Topical Ointment is for topical administration only.

**Dosage and administration**
*Adults:* After thorough cleansing of the affected skin areas, a small amount of the ointment should be applied gently two to four times daily.

*Use in the elderly:* No special precautions.

*Use in children:* Not recommended. See 'Contra-indications'.

**Contra-indications, warnings, etc**
*Contra-indications:*
1. Hypersensitivity to any of the components of the preparation.
2. Primary bacterial infections, e.g. impetigo, pyoderma, furunculosis.
3. Acute herpes simplex, vaccinia and varicella.
4. Tuberculosis of the skin.
5. Fungal diseases of the skin.
6. Pregnancy, and in infants and small children because of the theoretical risk of damage to permanent dentition.

*Precautions:* If irritation develops, the product should be discontinued.

Terra-Cortril Topical Ointment should not be continued for more than seven days in the absence of any clinical improvement, since in this situation occult extension of infection may occur due to the masking effect of the steroid.

Extended or recurrent application may increase the risk of contact sensitization and should be avoided.

The use of oxytetracycline and other antibiotics may result in an overgrowth of resistant organisms – particularly Candida and Staphylococci. Careful observation of the patient for this possibility is essential. If new infections due to nonsusceptible bacteria or fungi appear during therapy, Terra-Cortril Topical Ointment should be discontinued.

If extensive areas are treated or if the occlusive technique is used, there may be increased systemic absorption of the corticosteroid and suitable precautions should be taken.

Terra-Cortril Topical Ointment is not recommended for ophthalmic use.

*Side-effects:* Hydrocortisone and oxytetracycline are well tolerated by the epithelial tissues and may be used topically with minimal untoward effects. Allergic reactions may occur occasionally, but are rare.

The following local side-effects have been reported with topical corticosteroids, especially under occlusive dressings: burning, itching, irritation, dryness, folliculitis, hypertrichosis, acneiform eruptions, hypopigmentation, perioral dermatitis, allergic contact dermatitis, maceration of the skin, secondary infection, skin atrophy, striae, miliaria.

The use of Terra-Cortril Topical Ointment should be discontinued if such reactions occur.

*Overdosage:* No cases of overdosage with Terra-Cortril Topical Ointment have been reported. No special antidotes are required following accidental ingestion.

**Pharmaceutical precautions** Store below 25°C.

**Legal category** POM.

**Package quantities** 15 g tube; 30 g tube.

**Further information** Nil.

**Product licence number** 0057/5076R.

## TERRA-CORTRIL* NYSTATIN CREAM

**Presentation** Terra-Cortril Nystatin Cream contains 30 mg Oxytetracycline as Oxytetracycline Calcium BP., 10 mg Hydrocortisone PhEur and 100,000 units Nystatin BP in each gram of perfumed homogeneous yellow cream.

Inactive excipients: These are sodium metabisulphite, polysorbate 80, soft white paraffin, liquid paraffin, stearyl alcohol, stearic acid, cetomacrogol 1000, di-sodium hydrogen ortho-phosphate, sodium hydroxide, propyl and methyl hydroxybenzoates, propylene glycol, fragrance lavender-citrus and water.

**Uses** *Actions:* Terra-Cortril Nystatin Cream is ideal for use in conditions where topical, non-systemic action is desired. The oxytetracycline present will prevent or overcome superficial infections caused by organisms susceptible to it. Concomitantly, the concentration of hydrocortisone supplied is ample for

---

inflammatory reactions resulting from allergy, infection or trauma. Nystatin is an antifungal antibiotic which is both fungistatic and fungicidal *in vitro* against a wide variety of yeasts and yeast-like fungi. It is effective for the treatment of cutaneous infections caused by *Candida albicans* and other Candida as well as other yeasts.

Thus this product provides the combined broad-spectrum activity of oxytetracycline against the primarily causative or secondarily infecting organisms, and the effectiveness of hydrocortisone, an anti-allergic, anti-inflammatory hormone, which controls excessive tissue reaction to infections, allergens and trauma along with nystatin which prevents or eradicates secondary fungal infections.

*Indications:* The use of Terra-Cortril Nystatin Cream is indicated in the treatment of steroid-responsive dermatoses. The added presence of oxytetracycline and nystatin will serve to prevent or eradicate secondary bacterial and fungal complications. Since varying degrees of bacterial and/or fungal infection frequently complicate those skin conditions for which hydrocortisone topical therapy is indicated, this combined preparation may offer therapeutic advantages over the use of hydrocortisone alone.

*Among these conditions are: Atopic dermatitis:* including allergic eczema, both disseminated and circumscribed neurodermatitis, pruritus with lichenification, eczematoid dermatitis and food eczema.

*Cutaneous infections:* including superficial pyogenic infections, pyoderma, pustular dermatitis, and infections associated with minor burns or wounds.

*Contact dermatitis:* due to plants, drugs, cosmetics, clothing material and miscellaneous substances.

*Non-specific pruritus:* of the anus, vulva or scrotum.

**Dosage and administration**
*Adults:* After thorough cleansing of the affected skin areas, a small amount of the cream should be applied gently. Applications should be made two to four times daily. When actual infection is present, the cream may be applied on sterile gauze and, by this means, kept in contiguous contact with the affected area. Care should be taken not to discontinue therapy too soon after the initial response has been obtained.

Supplementary therapy with oral antibiotics is advisable in the treatment of severe infections or those which may become systemic.

*Use in the elderly:* No special precautions.

*Use in children:* Not recommended. See 'Contra-indications'.

**Contra-indications, warnings, etc**
*Contra-indications:*
1. Acute herpes simplex, vaccinia and varicella.
2. Tuberculosis of the skin.
3. Hypersensitivity to any of the components of the cream.
4. Acute purulent infections.
5. Pregnancy, and in infants and small children because of the theoretical risk of damage to permanent dentition.

*Precautions:* The use of oxytetracycline and other antibiotics may result in an overgrowth of resistant organisms. Observation of the patient for this possibility is required.

If irritation develops, the product should be discontinued and appropriate therapy instituted.

If a favourable response does not occur promptly, the corticosteroid should be discontinued until the infection has been adequately controlled.

If extensive areas are treated or if the occlusive technique is used there will be increased systemic absorption of the corticosteroid and suitable precautions should be taken.

Terra-Cortril Nystatin Cream is not for ophthalmic use.

*Side-effects:* Oxytetracycline, hydrocortisone and nystatin are well tolerated by the epithelial tissues and may be used topically with minimal untoward effects. Allergic reactions may occur occasionally, but are rare.

The following local side-effects have been reported with topical corticosteroids, especially under occlusive dressings: burning, itching, irritation, dryness, folliculitis, hypertrichosis, acneiform eruptions, hypopigmentation, perioral dermatitis, allergic contact dermatitis, maceration of the skin, secondary infection, skin atrophy, striae, miliaria.

The use of Terra-Cortril Nystatin Cream should be discontinued if such reactions occur.

*Overdosage:* No cases of overdosage with Terra-Cortril Nystatin Cream have been reported. No special antidotes are required following accidental ingestion.

**Pharmaceutical precautions** Store below 25°C.

**Legal category** POM.

**Package quantities** 30 g tube.

**Further information** Nil.

**Product licence number** 0057/0099.

# TROSYL* NAIL SOLUTION

**Presentation** Trosyl Nail Solution is a clear, slightly yellow solution containing 28% w/w tioconazole. Each ml of solution contains 280 mg tioconazole.

**Uses** Tioconazole is a broad spectrum imidazole antifungal agent. Trosyl Nail Solution is indicated for the topical treatment of nail infections due to susceptible fungi (dermatophytes and yeasts).

## Dosage and administration

*Adults:* The solution should be applied to the affected nails and immediately surrounding skin every twelve hours using the applicator brush supplied.

The duration of treatment is up to six months but may be extended to twelve months.

*Use in the elderly:* No special precautions are required. Use the adult dose.

*Use in children:* No special precautions are required. Use the adult dose.

## Contra-indications, warnings, etc

*Contra-indications:* Trosyl Nail Solution is contra-indicated in individuals who have been shown to be hypersensitive to imidazole antifungal agents, or to any of the components of the solution.

*Use in pregnancy:* In animal studies tioconazole was not teratogenic. At high doses it increased the incidence of renal abnormalities in rat embryos, but this effect was minor and transient and was not evident in weaned animals. There is insufficient evidence as to the drug's safety in human pregnancy, although absorption after topical administration is negligible. Because of the extensive duration of treatment required for nail infections, the use of Trosyl Nail Solution is contra-indicated throughout pregnancy.

*Precautions:* Trosyl Nail Solution is not for ophthalmic use.

*Side-effects:* Trosyl Nail Solution is well tolerated following local application and no systemic adverse reactions have been observed. Symptoms of local irritation have been reported by some patients, but are usually seen during the first week of treatment and are transient and mild.

However, if a sensitivity reaction develops with the use of Trosyl Nail Solution, treatment should be discontinued and appropriate therapy instituted.

*Overdosage:* No cases of overdosage with Trosyl Nail Solution have been reported. In the event of excessive oral ingestion, gastrointestinal symptoms may occur. Appropriate means of gastric lavage should be considered.

**Pharmaceutical precautions** Store between 4° and 30°. Avoid flame and heat.

**Legal category** POM.

**Package quantities** Amber glass bottles containing 12 ml of solution.

**Further information** Nil.

**Product licence number** 0057/0236.

*\*Trade Mark*

# Pfizer Consumer Healthcare
Wilsom Road
Alton, Hampshire GU34 2TJ

*Pfizer* **Consumer Healthcare**

## ISOGEL*

**Presentation** Isogel is a preparation of Ispaghula Husk BP, which consists of the epidermis and collapsed adjacent layers removed from the dried ripe seeds of Plantago ovata Forssk.

Isogel is supplied as small, reddish-brown granules in containers of 200 g.

**Uses** Isogel is not absorbed from the gastrointestinal tract, but it absorbs water to form a mucilaginous mass. This results in a purely mechanical stimulus to mass peristalsis without any purgative effect. It is for this reason that Isogel is not only an effective remedy for constipation but is also of value in the treatment of diarrhoea, irritable bowel syndrome and the management of patients with a colostomy. Isogel is indicated in habitual constipation, including cases due to spastic colon, dietary insufficiencies and in patients with haemorrhoids or diabetes. It can be used to normalise bowel movement in patients with mucous or ulcerative colitis.

Isogel is of help to patients with a colostomy as the formation of a well-formed, easily passed stool assists in the maintenance of cleanliness and the establishment of control.

**Dosage and administration** The required quantity of Isogel should be stirred briskly into half a glass of water and swallowed at once. Carbonated water is frequently preferred and may make swallowing easier.

*Adults and the elderly:* Two teaspoonfuls once or twice daily, preferably at mealtimes. Elderly or debilitated patients should be supervised whilst taking Isogel.

*Children:* One teaspoonful once or twice daily, preferably at mealtimes.

The above dosage is only a general guide and it should be adjusted to suit the needs of each individual patient.

In diarrhoea the dose, usually one teaspoonful, is taken three times daily until symptoms abate.

**Contra-indications, warnings, etc**
*Contra-indications:* Nil.

*Precautions:* A few cases of inhalation of the mucilaginous mass which forms on allowing an Isogel/water mixture to stand have been reported. In consequence, it is important that Isogel should be swallowed immediately after mixing, and elderly or debilitated patients should be supervised whilst taking it.

*Use in pregnancy:* No known adverse effects in pregnancy. However, as with all medicines, care should be taken during pregnancy, particularly during the first trimester. No adverse effects in lactation.

*Side-effects:* Nil.

*Overdosage:* As Isogel is not absorbed and it has no purgative action the problem of overdosage does not arise.

**Pharmaceutical precautions** Store below 25 deg C in a dry place.

**Legal category** GSL.

**Package quantities** Isogel is supplied in containers of 200 g.

**Further information** Nil.

**Product licence number** 1906/0008.

## MIGRALEVE*

**Presentation** *Migraleve 1:* Blister-packed, pink, capsule-shaped, film-coated tablets, engraved 'MGE' on one face, each containing:

| | |
|---|---|
| Buclizine Hydrochloride BP | 6.25 mg |
| Paracetamol PhEur | 500 mg |
| Codeine Phosphate PhEur | 8 mg |

*Migraleve 2:* Blister-packed, yellow, capsule-shaped, film-coated tablets, engraved 'MGE' on one face, each containing:

| | |
|---|---|
| Paracetamol PhEur | 500 mg |
| Codeine Phosphate PhEur | 8 mg |

**Uses** For the treatment of migraine attacks which can include the symptoms of migraine headache, nausea and vomiting.

**Dosage and administration** *Adult: Treatment:* two pink Migraleve 1 immediately it is known that a migraine attack has started or is imminent. If symptoms persist, two yellow Migraleve 2 every four hours. Maximum eight tablets (two Migraleve 1 and six Migraleve 2) in 24 hours.

*Children 10–14 years:* One pink Migraleve 1 initially. If required, one yellow Migraleve 2 every four hours. Maximum four tablets (one Migraleve 1 and three Migraleve 2) in 24 hours.

*Elderly (over 65 years):* As for adults. No clinical or pharmacokinetic data specific to this age group is available. However at normal dosages no problems have been reported.

**Contra-indications, warnings, etc** Hypersensitivity to any of the ingredients.

*Precautions:* Migrainous patients suffering from high blood pressure should first be treated for this condition independently. Because of the possibility of drowsiness, consideration should be given to patients involved in hazardous occupations. Migraleve should be used with caution in patients with liver or kidney dysfunction.

*Side-effects:* Paracetamol may rarely cause allergic reactions such as skin rashes, hives or itching. Codeine may cause constipation. Buclizine hydrochloride may cause drowsiness.

*Use in pregnancy:* Migraleve has been in wide use for many years without apparent ill consequence. Although experiments in some species gave rise to adverse effects following the administration of buclizine to pregnant animals e.g. foetal abnormalities and maternal deaths, these occurred at doses in excess of 120 times the human daily dose. Whilst there are no specific reasons for contra-indicating Migraleve during pregnancy, as with all drugs it is recommended that Migraleve be used in pregnancy only when the physician has considered the need in respect of the patients' welfare.

Insignificant levels of the active ingredients pass into breast milk, therefore Migraleve is not contra-indicated in breast-feeding mothers.

*Treatment of overdosage:* Symptoms of paracetamol overdosage are often delayed for at least 24 hours but to prevent hepatic damage, treatment should be given as soon as possible and within 10 hours of ingestion. Treatment is by the administration of i.v. acetylcysteine. Oral methionine may be used but is less certain in its effect because of its need for GI absorption. Once hepatic failure has developed, standard measures of management should be employed. Patients on enzyme-inducing agents (such as barbiturates) and chronic non-cirrhotic alcoholics may be more susceptible to the toxicity of paracetamol overdosage.

Symptoms of codeine overdosage include nausea and vomiting and circulatory and respiratory depression. Initial treatment includes gastric lavage. If CNS depression is severe, artificial respiration, oxygen and parenteral naloxone may be required.

**Pharmaceutical precautions** Nil.

**Legal category** P.

**Package quantities** 48 (32 pink Migraleve 1 and 16 yellow Migraleve 2) tablets. Also continuation packs of 48 pink Migraleve 1 and 48 yellow Migraleve 2 tablets.

**Further information** Nil.

**Product licence numbers**

| | |
|---|---|
| Migraleve 1 | 0232/0027 |
| Migraleve 2 | 0232/0028 |
| Migraleve (duo pack) | 0232/5008R. |

## PANCREOLAURYL* TEST

**Qualitative and quantitative composition** Each blue capsule contains: 174.25 mg (=0.25 mmol) fluorescein dilaurate. Each red capsule contains: 94.07 mg (=0.25 mmol) Fluorescein Sodium BP.

**Pharmaceutical form** Capsules.

**Clinical particulars**
*Therapeutic indications:* Pancreolauryl Test is used to detect abnormally low pancreatic exocrine function in patients who have symptoms associated with disturbances of pancreatic function. These symptoms include recurrrent diarrhoea, increased flatulence, fat intolerance and recurrent upper abdominal pain.

In these cases, the Pancreolauryl Test is a simple screening procedure and should be carried out before more complex and/or sophisticated diagnostic tests are performed.

Route of administration – oral.

*Posology and method of administration:*

*Adults and the elderly:* The patient can eat and drink as usual on the evening prior to the test, but no medicines containing vitamins should be taken. It is recommended that Pfizer Consumer Healthcare (see: Interactions) are consulted prior to the concomitant administration of digestive aids and Pancreolauryl Test.

*Test Day No 1:* For 10 hours after the start of the test, i.e. administration of 2 blue capsules with the standard meal, all urine is collected including a final emptying of the bladder at exactly 10 hours after the start of the test. The total quantity of urine collected can be tested by the laboratory immediately. If there is any delay the contained should be stored in a refrigerator; preservatives need not be added.

*Test Day No 2:* Two red control capsules can be taken the following day ensuring that the same procedure is followed.

*Children:* Although satisfactory results have been obtained in children, the test is not currently recommended for children.

*Contra-indications:* Acute necrotizing pancreatitis. Pregnancy.

*Special warnings and special precautions for use:* Although satisfactory results have been obtained in children, the test is not currently recommended for children.

*Interactions with other medicaments and other forms of interaction:* No drug interactions known. However, test results may be affected by concomitant use of vitamins. Sulphasalazine can interfere with photometric measurements. Digestive aids sold in the U.K. as of June 1992 may continue to be taken during the test. However, if in doubt it is advisable to check with Pfizer Consumer Healthcare before recommending continued use of digestive aids to prevent interference with test results.

*Pregnancy and lactation:* Contra-indicated in pregnancy. No information in lactation.

*Effects on ability to drive and use machines:* No known effects.

*Undesirable effects:* No side-effects have been reported.

*Overdosage:* General supportive measures. Administration of activated charcoal.

**Pharmacological particulars**
*Pharmacodynamic properties:* Cholesterol ester hydrolase, secreted by the pancreas, is able to break down fluorescein dilaurate into free, water-soluble fluorescein and lauric acid. Absence of the enzyme, as in cases of pancreatic insufficiency will result in a T/K ratio 20 of or below, when the urinary fluorescein concentration after fluorescein dilaurate capsules is compared to urinary fluorescein concentration after water-soluble fluorescein sodium capsules.

*Pharmacokinetic properties:* The blue capsules contain fluorescein dilaurate which has low water solubility and is not absorbed systemically. When administered with a standard meal, pancreatic exocrine function is stimulated and enzymes secreted. The pancreatic enzymes lyse the fluorescein dilaurate releasing fluorescein which is absorbed and excreted in the urine.

The urine is collected for a period of ten hours following administration of the test capsules and the total quantity of fluorescein dye excreted is determined by direct measurement of fluorescein concentration.

The amount of fluorescein excreted in the urine depends on pancreatic function and on individual variations in gastro-intestinal absorption and renal excretion.

To assess the absorption and excretion characteristics for individual patients; a repeat test using the control capsules is carried out the next day. The control capsules are red and contain unesterified fluorescein (Fluorescein Sodium).

The quantity of fluorescein excreted from the test capsules is expressed as a percentage of the quantity of fluorescein excreted from the control capsules. This value is termed the T/K ratio, and is used as a parameter of pancreatic function.

*Pre-clinical safety data:* No further data presented.

**Pharmaceutical particulars**
*List of excipients:*
*Fluorescein dilaurate capsules:* Povidone BP; Microcrystalline cellulose DAB; Gelatin DAB; Titanium Dioxide (E171); Indigotin (E132).

*Fluorescein sodium capsules:* Povidone BP; Lactose

PhEur; Zinc Stearate DAC '79; Gelatin DAB; Indigotin (E132); Titanium Dioxide (E171); Erythrosine (E127).

*Incompatibilities:* None known.

*Shelf-life:* 36 months.

*Special precautions for storage:* Store in a cool, dry place.

*Nature of contents and container:* 20 um aluminium foil strips, yellow, heat sealable, lacquered.

Packs of 4 capsules (2 Test plus 2 Control); and 10×4 capsules (10×2 Test plus 2 Control); and 6×4 capsules (6×2 Test plus 2 Control).

*Instructions for use/handling:* None.

**Marketing authorisation number** 1906/0020.

**Date of approval/revision of SPC** February 1996.

**Legal category** POM.

*\*Trade Mark*

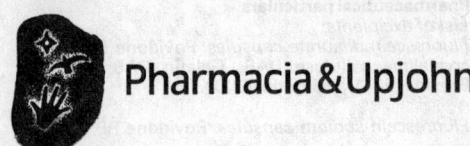
## ADDIPHOS*

**Presentation** Sterile colourless solution containing phosphate, potassium and sodium for addition to infusion fluids. Addiphos corresponds to the following formula:

| | |
|---|---|
| Monobasic potassium phosphate | 170.1 mg |
| Sodium phosphate $2H_2O$ | 133.5 mg |
| Potassium hydroxide | 14.0 mg |
| Sorbitol | 1.0 mg |
| Water for injections to 1 ml | |
| pH: 6.3–6.4 | |

One vial (20 ml Addiphos) provides the following:

| | |
|---|---|
| Phosphate | 40 mmol |
| Potassium | 30 mmol |
| Sodium | 30 mmol |

**Uses** Addiphos may be added to infusion solutions such as Vamin solutions and glucose solutions to provide phosphate during complete intravenous nutrition. This also provides potassium and sodium. For precise details on compatibility with individual infusion solutions see *Pharmaceutical precautions* section.

**Dosage and administration** *Recommended dosage for adults:* A daily requirement for phosphate during complete intravenous nutrition would normally be within the range 10–40 mmol. This can be met by using 5–20 ml of Addiphos. 5–20 ml Addiphos also provides 7.5–30 mmol each of potassium and sodium. The infusion should be given intravenously at a rate corresponding to not more than 10 mmol K+ per hour so as to avoid hyperkalaemia and also within the maximum infusion rate for the Vamin or Intrafusin.

*Recommended dosage for infants:* Dosage should be reduced appropriately according to age and weight.

**Contra-indications, warnings, etc** This preparation must not be administered undiluted. For information on rate of infusion see dosage recommendations above. Addiphos should not be used in patients with hyperkalaemia such as is associated with adrenal insufficiency or severe renal insufficiency, nor should it be given in the presence of dehydration without fluid replacement.

*Use during pregnancy and lactation:* Addiphos is a solution for use as a supplement in TPN regimens, providing phosphate, potassium and sodium. No hazard is expected if used in pregnancy at the recommended dosage.

No animal studies have been performed. However, successful outcomes with administration during pregnancy have been recorded.

*Precautions:* Care should be exercised in patients with cardiac disease, diabetes mellitus, renal dysfunction or hepatic insufficiency. Infusion of potassium may depress cardiac function and counteract the effects of digitalis. Simultaneous infusion of potassium and glucose will lower the serum potassium levels otherwise attainable. Plasma levels and clinical signs suggesting hyperkalaemia require discontinuation of the infusion.

*Overdosage:* Addiphos in overdosage may lead to hyperkalaemia, depressing cardiac function. Insulin may be required to reverse this effect, administered intravenously concomitant with glucose.

**Pharmaceutical precautions**
1. Store at 5° to 25°C.
2. The addition of Addiphos should be performed aseptically immediately before the start of the infusion and should be used within 24 hours.

Compatibility has been demonstrated with the following solutions up to the maximum levels indicated:

| Infusion solution (500 ml volume) | Maximum volume of Addiphos which may be added to 500 ml of infusion solution |
|---|---|
| Vamin 9 | 30 ml |
| Vamin 9 Glucose | 30 ml |
| Vamin 14 | 20 ml |
| Vamin 14 Electrolyte-Free | 30 ml |
| Vamin 18 Electrolyte-Free | 30 ml |
| Glucose 5–60% | 30 ml |

Addiphos must not be added to the foregoing undiluted solutions in the presence of Additrace because of the risk of precipitation.

3. Addiphos must only be added to solutions where compatibility is known.

4. Each vial is for single use only. It should be mixed well immediately after addition to the infusion solution.

5. A cloudy solution or one containing a precipitate must not be used.

**Legal category** POM.

**Package quantities** Boxes of 10×20 ml vials.

**Further information** In regimens including Intralipid, it should be noted that 500 ml Intralipid provides approximately 7.5 mmol organic phosphate. The manufacturer can be consulted for full information on complete and balanced intravenous nutrition regimens.

**Product licence number** 0022/0050.

## ADDITRACE*

**Presentation** A clear, almost colourless solution containing trace elements for addition to Vamin amino acid solutions in the intravenous nutrition of adults. Additrace corresponds to the following formula:

| | |
|---|---|
| Ferric chloride $6H_2O$ | 0.54 mg |
| Zinc chloride | 1.36 mg |
| Manganese chloride $4H_2O$ | 99.0 micrograms |
| Copper chloride $2H_2O$ | 0.34 mg |
| Chromic chloride | 5.33 micrograms |
| Sodium selenite $5H_2O$ | 10.5 micrograms |
| Sodium molybdate $2H_2O$ | 4.85 micrograms |
| Sodium fluoride | 0.21 mg |
| Potassium iodide | 16.6 micrograms |
| Xylitol | 300 mg |
| Water for injections to 1 ml | |
| pH 2.2 | |

One ampoule (10 ml Additrace) contains the following amounts of trace elements;

| | |
|---|---|
| $Fe^{3+}$ | 20 micromol |
| $Zn^{2+}$ | 100 micromol |
| $Mn^{2+}$ | 5 micromol |
| $Cu^{2+}$ | 20 micromol |
| $Cr^{3+}$ | 0.2 micromol |
| $Se^{4+}$ | 0.4 micromol |
| $Mo^{6+}$ | 0.2 micromol |
| $F^-$ | 50 micromol |
| $I^-$ | 1 micromol |

One ampoule of Additrace contains less than 1 mmol of both potassium and sodium.

**Uses** Additrace is used as part of a complete intravenous nutrition regimen providing a source of trace elements for adults and children over 40 kg.

**Dosage and administration**
*Recommended dosage for adults:* 1 ampoule (10 ml) of Additrace is added to either 500 ml or 1000 ml of a solution listed in the table below. Where higher amounts of trace elements are considered necessary, 2 ampoules of Additrace may be added to 1000 ml solution. Additrace should not be added to Vamin 9 amino acid solution directly. Where a regimen includes Vamin 9, Additrace should be added to the glucose infusion first.

Additrace does not contain calcium, magnesium or phosphate. These minerals should be added to the intravenous nutrition regimen if appropriate. (Vamin 9 Glucose, Vamin 9 and Vamin 14 contain calcium and magnesium. See appropriate data sheet). Similarly Additrace does not contain significant amounts of potassium or sodium (see *Presentation* above) since the requirements for these electrolytes vary with different clinical conditions. Potassium and sodium salts should therefore be added as appropriate to the individual patient's regimen. (Vamin 9 Glucose, Vamin 9 and Vamin 14 contain potassium and sodium. See appropriate data sheet).

| Infusion solution | Volume to which 10 ml Additrace may be added (ml) | |
|---|---|---|
| Vamin 9 Glucose | 500–1000 | |
| Vamin 14 | 500–1000 | Infusion should |
| Vamin 14 Electrolyte-Free | 500–1000 | be completed |
| Vamin 18 Electrolyte-Free | 500–1000 | within 24 hours of addition. |
| Glucose 5–50% | 500–1000 | |

Additrace must only be added to solutions where compatibility is known.

The above mixtures containing Vamin should be infused at an appropriate rate for the amino acid solution and the infusion completed not more than 24 hours after preparation. If Additrace is added to a solution other than those listed above, then ensure that the solution is administered over a period of not less than 2 hours, so as to minimise renal losses.

*Recommended dosage for infants and children under 40 kg:* The trace element solution Peditrace should be used.

**Contra-indications, warnings, etc**
*Contra-indications:* Should not be administered undiluted.

*Use in pregnancy and lactation:* Additrace is a solution of trace elements indicated as a supplement in parenteral nutrition (PN) regimens. It contains the following elements: $Fe^{3+}$, $Zn^{2+}$, $Mn^{2+}$, $Cu^{2+}$, $Cr^{3+}$, $Se^{4+}$, $Mo^{6+}$, $F^-$, $I^-$ in amounts per ampoule not exceeding daily recommended requirements where these exist. No hazard is expected if used in pregnancy at the recommended dosage. No animal studies have been performed. There are, however, published reports on safe and successful use of trace elements as part of a PN regimen during pregnancy in the human.

*Other special warnings and precautions:* Care should be taken in the administration of Additrace to patients with impaired liver function (especially cholestasis). Manganese toxicity is more likely to occur in patients with impaired liver function and cholestasis as manganese is almost entirely dependent on the biliary route for excretion. Manganese blood levels and liver function should be monitored regularly (monthly) in such patients. Additrace should be stopped if manganese levels rise into the potentially toxic range (please refer to appropriate reference ranges for the testing laboratory).

Additrace should be used with caution in patients with impaired renal function when the excretion of some trace elements (zinc, selenium, fluoride, chromium and molybdenum) may be significantly decreased.

*Overdosage:* In general overdosage with Additrace is extremely unlikely as the quantity of trace elements per ampoule lies well below known toxic levels of administration.

Chronic overdosage may very rarely occur secondary to an unsuspected idiosyncratic deficiency in metabolism or excretion for a specific trace element. In this case, signs may be observed such as nail dystrophy with insidious onset of symptoms secondary to haematological changes or tissue deposition. Diagnosis would be confirmed by biochemical and haematological tests and treatment should be withdrawal of Additrace.

**Pharmaceutical precautions** No other additions should be made to solutions containing Additrace unless compatibility is known.
1. Store at room temperature (25°C or below).
2. The addition of Additrace should be performed

aseptically immediately before the start of the infusion and should be used within 24 hours.

**Legal category** POM.

**Package quantities** Boxes of 20×10 ml, polypropylene ampoules.

**Further information** The manufacturer can be consulted for full information on complete and balanced intravenous nutrition regimens.

**Product licence number** 0022/0064.

## AMINOGLUTETHIMIDE

**Presentation** Practically white, round, scored tablets, containing 250 mg aminoglutethimide.

**Uses** Aminoglutethimide is indicated for treatment of metastatic carcinoma of the breast in post-menopausal or oophorectomised women.

Aminoglutethimide is also indicated in Cushing's syndrome due to malignant disease, where surgical treatment is inappropriate or as an adjunct to surgery, either pre-operatively in the management of metabolic disturbances or post-operatively for the treatment of relapse.

### Dosage and administration

*Adults:* Metastatic carcinoma of the breast: administration should start at 250 mg twice daily for two weeks. In the absence of severe side-effects the dose may be increased to 250 mg four times daily.

Cushing's syndrome due to malignant disease: treatment should be started at 250 mg daily, increasing gradually up to 1 g daily. In some cases, especially ectopic ACTH syndrome, higher doses may be necessary to achieve adequate suppression.

*Elderly:* The adult dosage schedules may be given without modification.

*Children:* Not recommended.

### Contra-indications, warnings, etc

*Contra-indications:* Use during pregnancy and lactation is contra-indicated as foetal abnormalities have been seen in animal studies and cases of pseudohermaphroditism have been reported in neonates of women treated with aminoglutethimide.

*Warnings:* Aminoglutethimide suppresses production of glucocorticoids and in patients with breast carcinoma supplementary glucocorticoids will be needed.

During initial treatment of Cushing's syndrome due to malignant disease, no corticosteroids should be necessary. Plasma cortisol levels should be monitored regularly and if adrenocortical insufficiency occurs supplementary glucocorticoids may be given.

The suppression of aldosterone synthesis may lead to hyponatraemia, hyperkalaemia, hypotension and dizziness, in which case a mineralocorticoid should be given.

Blood count and plasma electrolytes should be checked regularly. Aminoglutethimide has been found occasionally to diminish thyroid function. If, during treatment of breast carcinoma signs of Cushing's syndrome appear which are due to concomitant glucocorticoid medication, the dosage of the glucocorticoid should be reduced.

Aminoglutethimide may increase the rate of metabolism of some drugs such as coumarin anticoagulants, oral hypoglycaemic agents and dexamethasone and dosage of these may need adjustment.

*Side-effects:* Aminoglutethimide tolerability varies greatly and CNS side-effects such as dizziness, somnolence and lethargy are relatively common and dose dependent; unsteadiness occurs only in the highest dosage range. Gastrointestinal effects are less frequent but usually dose-dependent. A drug rash, sometimes accompanied by fever, may develop after 7–14 days. This usually subsides within 7–10 days even though treatment is continued: if it should not subside, treatment should be stopped temporarily. Alternatively the dose of concomitant glucocorticoid may be increased. Rarely pancytopenia, leucopenia and agranulocytosis have been reported.

*Overdosage:* Following overdosage of aminoglutethimide, no serious outcome has been reported. However, gastric lavage should be performed as soon as possible and full supportive measures should be employed. In severe cases, haemodialysis or charcoal haemoperfusion may be useful. Steroid replacement should be maintained or initiated, as necessary.

**Pharmaceutical precautions** Protect from heat, light and moisture.

**Legal category** POM.

**Package quantities** Cartons of 100 tablets.

**Further information** Aminoglutethimide inhibits steroid biosynthesis in the adrenal cortex causing a chemical adrenalectomy. This inhibition occurs at an early stage in the biosynthesis. Suppression of oestrogen production in peripheral tissue may also occur.

**Product licence number** 3433/0104.

## CABASER* ▼

**Qualitative and quantitative composition** Cabergoline INN 1, 2 and 4 mg

**Pharmaceutical form**
1 mg tablets: oval, 4.58 x 7.12 mm, scored, white tablets
2 mg tablets: convex, capsule-shaped, 5 x 10 mm, scored, white tablets
4 mg tablets: oval, biconvex 7.14 x 12.7 mm, scored white tablets.
Container: Type I amber glass bottles with aluminium tamper resistant screw caps, containing silica gel desiccant.
Each bottle contains 20 tablets of either 1 mg or 2 mg strength, or 16 tablets of 4 mg strength, and is enclosed in an outer cardboard carton.
The tablets are for oral administration.

**Clinical particulars**

*Therapeutic indications:* Treatment of Parkinson's disease.

Cabaser is indicated for the treatment of symptoms of Parkinson's disease, as adjuvant therapy to levodopa plus dopa-decarboxylase inhibitor, in patients affected by ''on-off'' mobility problems with daily fluctuations in motor performance.

Controlled clinical studies have demonstrated that cabergoline administered once daily at an average dose of 4 mg/day following titration (up to 5–6 mg/day in the different studies) is effective in decreasing daily fluctuations in motor performance in Parkinsonian patients receiving levodopa/carbidopa therapy. Improvement of motor deficit has been demonstrated, while substantially decreasing the levodopa/carbidopa dose.

*Posology and method of administration:* Cabaser is for oral administration. Since the tolerability of dopaminergic agents is improved when administered with food, it is recommended that Cabaser be taken with meals.

Cabaser is intended for chronic, long term treatment.

*Adults and elderly patients:* As expected for dopamine agonists, dose response for both efficacy and side effects appears to be linked to individual sensitivity. Optimization of dose should be obtained through slow initial dose titration, from starting doses of 1 mg daily. The dosage of concurrent levodopa may be gradually decreased, while the dosage of Cabaser is increased, until the optimum balance is determined. In view of the long half-life of the compound, increments of the daily dose of 0.5–1 mg should be done at weekly (initial weeks) or bi-weekly intervals, up to optimal doses.

The recommended therapeutic dosage is 2 to 6 mg/day as adjuvant therapy to levodopa/carbidopa. Cabaser should be given as a single daily dose. Maximum doses higher than 6 mg/day and up to 20 mg/day have been administered in a small proportion of patients during clinical studies.

*Use in children:* The safety and efficacy of Cabaser have not been investigated in children as Parkinson's disease does not affect this population.

*Contra-indications:* Hypersensitivity to any ergot alkaloid.

*Special warnings and special precautions for use:* While renal insufficiency has been shown not to modify cabergoline kinetics, hepatic insufficiency of severe degree (> 10 Child-Pugh score, maximum score 12) has been shown to be associated with an increase of AUC, thus indicating that dose regimens in Parkinsonian patients with severe hepatic insufficiency should be modified accordingly.

Pleural effusion/fibrosis has been infrequently reported following long term administration of Cabaser, and usually when given to patients previously treated with ergolinic DA agonists. Therefore Cabaser should be given with caution to patients with a history or clinical symptoms of respiratory disorders linked to fibrotic tissue degeneration. A chest x-ray examination is recommended if clinical symptoms of respiratory disorders are observed. Where x-ray examination indicates pleural effusion/fibrosis, discontinuation of Cabaser is expected to lead to immediate improvement of symptoms.

Erythrocyte sedimentation rate has been found to be abnormally increased in association with pleural effusion/fibrosis. Chest x-ray examination is recommended in cases of unexplained ESR increases to abnormal values.

In addition, by analogy with other ergot derivatives, Cabaser should be given with caution to patients suffering from severe cardiovascular disease, Raynaud's syndrome, peptic ulcer, gastrointestinal bleeding or a history of serious, particularly psychotic mental disease. Symptomatic hypotension can occur following adminstration of Cabaser: particular attention should be paid when administering Cabaser concomitantly with other drugs known to lower blood pressure.

The effects of alcohol on overall tolerability of Cabaser are currently unknown.

*Interaction with other medicaments and other forms of interaction:* No pharmacokinetic interaction with L-Dopa or selegiline was observed in the studies carried out in parkinsonian patients. The concomitant use of other drugs, particularly other antiparkinsonian non-dopamine-agonist agents, was not associated with detectable interactions modifying the efficacy and safety of Cabaser.

No other information is available about possible interaction between Cabaser and other ergot alkaloids: therefore the concomitant use of these medications during long term treatment with Cabaser is not recommended.

Since Cabaser exerts its therapeutic effect by direct stimulation of dopamine receptors, it should not be concurrently administered with drugs which have dopamine antagonist activity (such as phenothiazines, butyrophenones, thioxanthenes, metoclopramide) since these might reduce the therapeutic effect of Cabaser.

By analogy with other ergot derivatives, Cabaser should not be used in association with macrolide antibiotics (e.g erythromycin) since the systemic bioavailability of Cabaser and adverse effects could increase.

*Pregnancy and lactation:* Cabaser has been shown to cross the placenta in rats: it is unknown whether this occurs also in humans.

Animal studies in rats and mice have not demonstrated any teratogenic effect or any effect of the compound on global reproductive performance. In clinical studies there have been over 100 pregnancies in women treated with cabergoline for hyperprolactinemic disorders. The compound was generally taken during the first 8 weeks after conception. Among the pregnancies evaluable so far, there were approximately 85% live births and about 10% spontaneous abortions. Three cases of congenital abnormalities (Down's syndrome, hydrocephalus, malformation of lower limbs) which led to therapeutic abortion and three cases of minor abnormalities in live births were observed.

These incidence rates are comparable with those quoted for normal populations and for women exposed to other ovulation-inducing drugs. Based on the above data, the use of the product does not appear to be associated with an increased risk of abortion, premature delivery, multiple pregnancy or congenital abnormalities.

Because clinical experience is still limited and the drug has a long half-life, as a precautionary measure it is recommended that women seeking pregnancy discontinue Cabaser one month before intended conception, in order to prevent possible foetal exposure to the drug. If conception occurs during therapy, treatment is to be discontinued as soon as pregnancy is confirmed, to limit foetal exposure to the drug.

In rats cabergoline and/or its metabolites are excreted in milk. Lactation is expected to be inhibited/suppressed by Cabaser, in view of its dopamine-agonist properties. Therefore, while no information on the excretion of cabergoline in maternal milk in humans is available, puerperal women should be advised not to breast-feed in case of failed lactation inhibition/suppression by the product.

*Effects on ability to drive and use machines:* During treatment with Cabaser, patients should be cautioned about engaging in activities requiring rapid and precise responses, such as driving or operating machinery.

*Undesirable effects:* About 1070 parkinsonian patients have received Cabaser as adjuvant therapy to L-dopa in clinical studies; of these 74% had at least one adverse event, mainly of mild to moderate severity and transient in nature, and requiring discontinuation in a small proportion of cases.

In the majority of cases (51%), events were related to the nervous system: most frequently reported events were dyskinesia, hyperkinesia, hallucinations or confusion. The gastrointestinal system was involved in 33% of cases: events most frequently reported were nausea, vomiting, dyspepsia and gastritis. The cardiovascular system was involved in 27% of cases, most frequently reported events being dizziness and hypotension. The respiratory system was involved in 13% of cases, symptomatic pleural effusion/fibrosis being reported with a frequency <2%.

Other adverse events expected for the pharmacological class, in view of the vasoconstrictive properties, include angina (reported in about 1% of the patients on cabergoline) and erythromelalgia (observed in 0.4% of the patients). Similarly expected for the pharmacological class, peripheral oedema occurred in 6% of patients.

Gastric upset was more frequent in female than in male patients, while CNS events were more frequent in the elderly.

A blood pressure decrease of clinical relevance was observed mainly on standing in a minority of patients. The effect was mainly evident in the first weeks of therapy. Neither modification of heart rate nor consistent changes of ECG tracing were observed during Cabaser treatment.

Alterations in standard laboratory tests are uncommon during long term therapy with Cabaser.

*Overdose:* The acute toxicity studies carried out in animals indicate very low toxicity, with a wide safety margin with respect to pharmacologically active doses. Clinical signs and cause of death, if any, were related to CNS stimulation.

There is no experience in humans of overdosage with Cabaser in the proposed indication: it is likely to lead to symptoms due to over-stimulation of dopamine receptors. These might include nausea, vomiting, gastric complaints, hypotension, confusion/psychosis or hallucinations. The vomiting stimulating properties of dopamine agonists are expected to favour removal of unabsorbed drug. Supportive measures should be directed to maintain blood pressure, if necessary. In addition, in case of pronounced central nervous system effects (hallucinations) the administration of dopamine antagonist drugs may be advisable.

### Pharmacological properties

*Pharmacodynamic properties:* Cabaser is a dopaminergic ergoline derivative endowed with potent and long-lasting dopamine D2 receptor agonist properties. In rats the compound, acting at D2 dopamine receptors on pituitary lactotrophic cells, decreases PRL secretion at oral doses of 3-25 mcg/kg, and *in vitro* at a concentration of 45 pg/ml. In addition, Cabaser exerts a central dopaminergic effect via D2 receptor stimulation at doses higher than those effective in lowering serum PRL levels. Improvement of motor deficit in animal models of parkinson's disease was present at oral daily doses of 1–2.5 mg/kg in rats and at s.c. doses of 0.5–1 mg/kg in monkeys.

In healthy volunteers the administration of Cabaser at single oral doses of 0.3–2.5 mg was associated with a significant decrease in serum PRL levels. The effect is prompt (within 3 hours of administration) and persistent (up to 7–28 days). The PRL-lowering effect is dose-related both in terms of degree of effect and duration of action.

The pharmacodynamic actions of Cabaser not linked to the therapeutic effect relate only to blood pressure decrease. The maximal hypotensive effect of Cabaser as a single dose usually occurs during the first 6 hours after drug intake and is dose-dependent both in terms of maximal decrease and frequency.

*Pharmacokinetic properties:* The pharmacokinetic and metabolic profiles of Cabaser have been studied in healthy volunteers of both sexes, in female hyperprolactinemic patients and in parkinsonian patients. After oral administration of the labelled compound, radioactivity was rapidly absorbed from the gastrointestinal tract as the peak of radioactivity in plasma was between 0.5 and 4 hours. Ten days after administration about 18/20% and 55/72% of the radioactive dose ($^3$H-cabergoline/$^{14}$C-cabergoline) was recovered in urine and faeces, respectively. Unchanged drug in urine accounted for 2–3% of the dose.

In urine, the main metabolite identified was 6-allyl-8b-carboxy-ergoline, which accounted for 4–6% of the dose. Three additional metabolites were identified in urine, which accounted overall for less than 3% of the dose. The metabolites have been found to be much less potent than Cabaser as $D_2$ dopamine receptor agonists *'in vitro'*.

The low urinary excretion of unchanged Cabaser has been confirmed also in studies with non-radioactive product. The elimination half-life of Cabaser, estimated from urinary excretion rates, is long (63–68 hours in healthy volunteers, 79–115 hours in hyperprolactinemic patients).

The pharmacokinetics of Cabaser seem to be dose-independent both in healthy volunteers (doses of 0.5–1.5 mg) and parkinsonian patients (steady state of daily doses up to 7 mg/day).

On the basis of the elimination half-life, steady state conditions should be achieved after 4 weeks, as confirmed by the mean peak plasma levels of Cabaser obtained after a single dose (37±8 pg/ml) and after a 4 week multiple-regimen (101±43 pg/ml). *In vitro* experiments showed that the drug at concentrations of 0.1–10 ng/ml is 41–42% bound to plasma proteins.

Food does not appear to affect absorption and disposition of Cabaser.

While renal insufficiency has been shown not to modify cabergoline kinetics, hepatic insufficiency of severe degree (> 10 Child-Pugh score, maximum

---

score 12) has been shown to be associated with an increase of AUC.

*Preclinical safety data:* Almost all the findings noted throughout the series of preclinical safety studies are a consequence of the central dopaminergic effects or the long-lasting inhibition of PRL in rodents with a specific hormonal physiology different to man.

Preclinical safety studies of Cabaser indicate a consistent safety margin for this compound in rodents and in monkeys, as well as a lack of teratogenic, genotoxic or carcinogenic potential.

### Pharmaceutical particulars

*List of excipients:* Lactose anhydrous NF USP; Leucine PhEur.

*Incompatibilities:* Not applicable

*Shelf life:* 24 months at room temperature (25°C).

*Special precautions for storage:* There are no special precautions for storage.

*Nature and contents of container:* The tablets are contained in Type I amber glass bottles with tamper resistant screw caps which contain silica gel desiccant.

Each bottle contains 20 tablets of either 1 mg or 2 mg strength or 16 tablets of 4 mg strength and is enclosed in an outer cardboard carton.

*Instructions for use/handling:* Bottles of Cabaser are supplied with desiccant in the caps. This desiccant must not be removed.

### Marketing authorisation numbers

| | |
|---|---|
| 1 mg tablets | 0022/0169 |
| 2 mg tablets | 0022/0170 |
| 4 mg tablets | 0022/0171 |

**Date of approval/revision of SPC** January 1997

**Legal category:** POM

## CAVERJECT* POWDER FOR INJECTION

**Qualitative and quantitative composition** Alprostadil USP 5, 10 or 20 micrograms

**Pharmaceutical form** Powder for injection.

### Clinical particulars

*Therapeutic indications:* Caverject is indicated for the treatment of erectile dysfunction in adult males due to neurogenic, vasculogenic, psychogenic or mixed aetiology.

Caverject may be a useful adjunct to other diagnostic tests in the diagnosis of erectile dysfunction.

*Posology and method of administration:* Caverject is administered by direct intracavernous injection. A 1/2-inch, 27- to 30-gauge needle is generally recommended. The dose of Caverject should be individualised for each patient by careful titration under supervision by a physician.

The intracavernosal injection must be done under sterile conditions. The site of injection is usually along the dorsolateral aspect of the proximal third of the penis. Visible veins should be avoided. Both the side of the penis that is injected and the site of injection must be alternated; prior to the injection, the injection site must be cleansed with an alcohol swab.

To reconstitute Caverject using the prefilled diluent syringe: flip off the plastic cap from the vial, and use one of the swabs to wipe the rubber cap. Fit the 22 gauge needle to the syringe.

Inject the 1 ml of diluent into the vial, and shake to dissolve the powder entirely. Withdraw slightly more than the required dose of Caverject solution, remove the 22 gauge needle, and fit the 30 gauge needle. Adjust volume to the required dose for injection. Following administration, any unused contents of the vial and syringe should be discarded.

*As an aid to aetiologic diagnosis:* Subjects without evidence of neurological dysfunction; 20 micrograms alprostadil to be injected into the corpus cavernosum and massaged through the penis. Should an ensuing erection persist for more than one hour detumescent therapy (please refer to Overdose section) should be employed to prevent a risk of priapism prior to the subject leaving the clinic. Over 80% of subjects may be expected to respond to a single 20 micrograms dose of alprostadil. At the time of discharge from the clinic, the erection should have subsided entirely and the penis must be in a completely flaccid state.

Subjects with evidence of neurological dysfunction; these patients can be expected to respond to lower doses of alprostadil. In subjects with erectile dysfunction caused by neurologic disease/trauma the dose for diagnostic testing must not exceed 10 micrograms and an initial dose of 5 micrograms is likely to be appropriate. Should an ensuing erection persist for more than one hour detumescent therapy (please refer to Overdose section ) should be employed to prevent a risk of priapism prior to the subject leaving the clinic. At the time of discharge from the clinic, the

---

erection should have subsided entirely and the penis must be in a completely flaccid state.

*Treatment:* The initial dose of alprostadil in patients with erectile dysfunction of neurogenic origin secondary to spinal cord injury is 1.25 micrograms, with a second dose of 2.5 micrograms, a third of 5 micrograms, and subsequent incremental increases of 5 micrograms until an optimal dose is achieved. For erectile dysfunction of vasculogenic, psychogenic, or mixed aetiology, the initial dose is 2.5 micrograms. The second dose should be 5 micrograms if there is a partial response, and 7.5 micrograms if there is no response. Subsequent incremental increases of 5 – 10 micrograms should be given until an optimal dose is achieved. If there is no response to the administered dose, then the next higher dose may be given within 1 hour. If there is a response, there should be at least a 1 day interval before the next dose is given. The usual maximum recommended frequency of injection is no more than once daily and no more than three times weekly.

The first injections of alprostadil must be done by medically trained personnel. After proper training and instruction, alprostadil may be injected at home. If self-administration is planned, the physician should make an assessment of the patient's skill and competence with the procedure. It is recommended that patients are regularly monitored (e.g. every 3 months) particularly in the initial stages of self injection therapy when dose adjustments may be needed.

The dose that is selected for self-injection treatment should provide the patient with an erection that is satisfactory for sexual intercourse. It is recommended that the dose administered produces a duration of the erection not exceeding one hour. If the duration is longer, the dose should be reduced. The majority of patients achieve a satisfactory response with doses in the range of 5 to 20 micrograms. Doses of greater than 60 micrograms of alprostadil are not recommended. The lowest effective dose should be used.

*Contra-indications:* Caverject should not be used in patients who have a known hypersensitivity to any of the constituents of the product; in patients who have conditions that might predispose them to priapism, such as sickle cell anaemia or trait, multiple myeloma, or leukaemia; or in patients with anatomical deformation of the penis, such as angulation, cavernosal fibrosis, or Peyronie's disease. Patients with penile implants should not be treated with Caverject.

Caverject should not be used in men for whom sexual activity is inadvisable or contra-indicated.

*Special warnings and precautions for use:* Prolonged erection and/or priapism may occur. Patients should be instructed to report to a physician any erection lasting for a prolonged time period, such as 4 hours or longer. Treatment of priapism should not be delayed more than 6 hours (please refer to Overdose section).

Painful erection is more likely to occur in patients with anatomical deformations of the penis, such as angulation, phimosis, cavernosal fibrosis, Peyronie's disease or plaques. Penile fibrosis, including angulation, fibrotic nodules and Peyronie's disease may occur following the intracavernosal administration of Caverject. The occurrence of fibrosis may increase with increased duration of use. Regular follow-up of patients, with careful examination of the penis, is strongly recommended to detect signs of penile fibrosis or Peyronie's disease. Treatment with Caverject should be discontinued in patients who develop penile angulation, cavernosal fibrosis, or Peyronie's disease.

Patients on anticoagulants such as warfarin or heparin may have increased propensity for bleeding after the intracavernous injection.

Underlying treatable medical causes of erectile dysfunction should be diagnosed and treated prior to initiation of therapy with Caverject.

Use of intracavernosal alprostadil offers no protection from the transmission of sexually transmitted diseases. Individuals who use alprostadil should be counselled about the protective measures that are necessary to guard against the spread of sexually transmitted diseases, including the human immunodeficiency virus (HIV). In some patients, injection of Caverject can induce a small amount of bleeding at the site of injection. In patients infected with blood-born diseases, this could increase the transmission of such diseases to their partner.

Reconstituted solutions of Caverject are intended for single use only, they should be used immediately and not stored.

*Interactions with other medicaments and other forms of interaction:* No known interactions. Caverject is not intended for co-administration with any other agent for the treatment of erectile dysfunction.

*Pregnancy and lactation:* Not applicable. (High doses of alprostadil (0.5 to 2.0 mg/kg subcutaneously) had an adverse effect on the reproductive potential of male rats, although this was not seen with lower doses (0.05 to 0.2 mg/kg). Alprostadil did not affect rat spermatogenesis at doses 200 times greater than the proposed human intrapenile dose.)

*Effects on ability to drive and operate machines*: Not applicable.

*Undesirable effects*: The most frequent adverse reaction after intracavernosal injection of Caverject is penile pain. In studies, 37% of the patients reported penile pain at least once; however, this event was associated with only 11% of the administered injections. In the majority of the cases, penile pain was rated mild or moderate in intensity. 3% of patients discontinued treatment because of penile pain.

Prolonged erection (defined as an erection that lasts for 4 to 6 hours) after intracavernosal administration of Caverject was reported in 4% of patients. The frequency of priapism (defined as an erection that lasts 6 hours or longer) was 0.4%. (Please refer to *Special warnings and precautions for use* section). In the majority of cases, spontaneous detumescence occurred.

Penile fibrosis, including angulation, fibrotic nodules and Peyronie's disease was reported in 3% of clinical trial patients overall, however, in one self-injection study in which the duration of use was up to 18 months, the incidence of penile fibrosis was 7.8% (please refer to Section 4.4).

Haematoma and ecchymosis at the site of injection, which is related to the injection technique rather than to the effects of alprostadil, occurred in 3% and 2% of patients, respectively. Penile oedema or rash was reported by 1% of alprostadil treated patients.

The following local adverse reactions were reported by fewer than 1% of patients in clinical studies following intracavernosal injection of Caverject: balanitis, injection site haemorrhage, injection site inflammation, injection site itching, injection site swelling, injection site oedema, urethral bleeding and penile warmth, numbness, yeast infection, irritation, sensitivity, phimosis, pruritus, erythema, venous leak, painful erection and abnormal ejaculation.

In terms of systemic events, 2 to 4% of alprostadil-treated patients reported headache, hypertension, upper respiratory infection, flu-like syndrome, prostatic disorder, localised pain (buttocks pain, leg pain, genital pain, abdominal pain), trauma, and sinusitis. One percent of patients reported each of the following: dizziness, back pain, nasal congestion and cough. The following were reported for less than 1% of patients in clinical trials and were judged to be possibly related to Caverject use: testicular pain, scrotal disorder (redness, pain, spermatocele), scrotal oedema, haematuria, testicular disorder (warmth, swelling, mass, thickening), impaired urination, urinary frequency, urinary urgency, pelvic pain, hypotension, vasodilatation, peripheral vascular disorder, supraventricular extrasystoles, vasovagal reactions, hypaesthesia, non-generalised weakness, diaphoresis, rash, non-application site pruritus, skin neoplasm, nausea, dry mouth, increased serum creatinine, leg cramps and mydriasis.

Haemodynamic changes, manifested as decreases in blood pressure and increases in pulse rate, were observed during clinical studies, principally at doses above 20 micrograms and above 30 micrograms of Caverject, respectively and appeared to be dose-dependent. However, these changes were usually clinically unimportant; only three patients (0.2%) discontinued the treatment because of symptomatic hypotension.

Caverject had no clinically important effect on serum or urine laboratory tests.

*Overdose*: The pharmacotoxic signs of alprostadil are similar in all animal species and include depression, soft stools or diarrhoea and rapid breathing. In animals, the lowest acute $LD_{50}$ was 12 mg/kg which is 12,000 times greater than the maximum recommended human dose of 60 micrograms.

In man, prolonged erection and/or priapism are known to occur following intracavernous administration of vasoactive substances, including alprostadil. Patients should be instructed to report to a physician any erection lasting for a prolonged time period, such as 4 hours or longer.

The treatment of priapism (prolonged erection) should not be delayed more than 6 hours. Initial therapy should be by penile aspiration. Using aseptic technique, insert a 19–21 gauge butterfly needle into the corpus cavernosum and aspirate 20–50 ml of blood. This may detumesce the penis. If necessary, the procedure may be repeated on the opposite side of the penis until a total of up to 100 ml blood has been aspirated. If still unsuccessful, intracavernous injection of alpha-adrenergic medication is recommended. Although the usual contra-indication to intrapenile administration of a vasoconstrictor does not apply in the treatment of priapism, caution is advised when this option is exercised. Blood pressure and pulse should be continuously monitored during the procedure. Extreme caution is required in patients with coronary heart disease, uncontrolled hypertension, cerebral ischaemia, and in subjects taking monoamine oxidase inhibitors. In the latter case, facilities should be available to manage a hypertensive crisis. A 200 microgram/ml solution of phenylephrine should be prepared, and 0.5 to 1.0 ml of the solution injected every 5 to 10 minutes. Alternatively, a 20 microgram/ml solution of adrenaline should be used. If necessary, this may be followed by further aspiration of blood through the same butterfly needle. The maximum dose of phenylephrine should be 1 mg, or adrenaline 100 micrograms (5 ml of the solution). As an alternative metaraminol may be used, but it should be noted that fatal hypertensive crises have been reported. If this still fails to resolve the priapism, urgent surgical referral for further management, which may include a shunt procedure, is required.

**Pharmacological properties**

*Pharmacodynamic properties*: Alprostadil is present in various mammalian tissues and fluids. It has a diverse pharmacologic profile, among which some of its more important effects are vasodilation, inhibition of platelet aggregation, inhibition of gastric secretion, and stimulation of intestinal and uterine smooth muscle. The pharmacologic effect of alprostadil in the treatment of erectile dysfunction is presumed to be mediated by inhibition of $alpha_1$-adrenergic activity in penile tissue and by its relaxing effect on cavernosal smooth muscle.

*Pharmacokinetic properties*: Following intracavernous injection of 20 micrograms of alprostadil, mean peripheral levels of alprostadil at 30 and 60 minutes after injection are not significantly greater than baseline levels of endogenous $PGE_1$. Peripheral levels of the major circulating metabolite, 15-oxo-13,14-dihydro-$PGE_1$, increase to reach a peak 30 minutes after injection and return to pre-dose levels by 60 minutes after injection. Any alprostadil entering the systemic circulation from the corpus cavernosum will be rapidly metabolized. Following intravenous administration, approximately 80% of the circulating alprostadil is metabolized in one pass through the lungs, primarily by beta- and omega-oxidation.The metabolites are excreted primarily by the kidney and excretion is essentially complete within 24 hours. There is no evidence of tissue retention of alprostadil or its metabolites following intravenous administration.

**Pharmaceutical particulars**

*List of excipients*: lactose, sodium citrate.

*Incompatibilities*: Caverject is not intended to be mixed or coadministered with any other products.

The presence of benzyl alcohol in the reconstitution vehicle decreases the degree of binding to package surfaces. Therefore, a more consistent product delivery is produced when Bacteriostatic Water for Injection containing benzyl alcohol is used.

*Shelf life*: 24 months. Reconstituted solutions should be used immediately and not stored.

*Special precautions for storage*: Store at room temperature (at or below 25°C). Reconstituted solutions are intended for single use only, they should be used immediately and not stored.

*Nature and contents of container*: Single packs containing a vial of Caverject 5, 10 or 20 microgram powder and a syringe of diluent.

Packs also each contain a sterile 22 G and a 30 G needle plus pre-injection swab.

**Marketing authorisation numbers**

| | |
|---|---|
| Caverject Powder for Injection 5 micrograms | 0032/0214 |
| Caverject Powder for Injection 10 micrograms | 0032/0203 |
| Caverject Powder for Injection 20 micrograms | 0032/0188 |
| Bacteriostatic Water for Injections diluent | 0032/0193 |

**Date of approval/revision of SPC** 4 September 1996

**Legal category** POM

## CEDOCARD RETARD*-20

**Presentation** Round yellow sustained-release tablets, embossed CCSR and scored on reverse side, each containing 20 mg isosorbide dinitrate.

**Uses** For the prophylaxis of angina pectoris.

The active principle of Cedocard Retard-20 is isosorbide dinitrate which relaxes vascular smooth muscle and produces coronary vasodilation, reduction in peripheral resistance and venous return, alteration of myocardial metabolism, and reduction of the myocardial oxygen demand.

**Dosage and administration** For oral administration.

*Adult dose:* One tablet in the morning and 1 tablet before retiring to sleep. Onset of action 20–30 minutes and the duration of action is 10–12 hours.

*Dosage for the elderly:* The dosage of nitrates in cardiovascular disease is usually determined by patient response and stabilisation. Clinical experience has not necessitated alternative advice for use in elderly patients. The pharmacokinetics of isosorbide dinitrate in patients with severe renal failure and liver cirrhosis are similar to those in normal subjects.

There is no recommended dose for children.

**Contra-indications, warnings, etc**

*Contra-indication:* A history of sensitivity to the drug.

*Precautions:* Tolerance and cross-tolerance to other nitrates may occur.

*Adverse reactions:* Cutaneous vasodilation with flushing, transient episodes of dizziness and weakness, and other signs of cerebral ischaemia, may occur with postural hypotension.

*Use in pregnancy:* No data have been reported which would indicate the possibility of adverse effects resulting from the use of isosorbide dinitrate in pregnancy. Safety in pregnancy, however, has not been established. Isosorbide dinitrate should only be used in pregnancy if, in the opinion of the physician, the possible benefits of treatment outweigh the possible hazards.

*Treatment of overdosage:* In rare cases of overdosage, gastric lavage is indicated. Passive exercise of the extremities of the recumbent patient will promote venous return.

**Pharmaceutical precautions** *Storage:* Protect from heat and moisture.

**Legal category** P.

**Package quantities** Blister strips of 60 (OP) tablets.

**Further information** Nil.

**Product licence number** 0424/0007.

## CEDOCARD* RETARD-40

**Presentation** Round, orange/red, sustained-release tablets, embossed CCSR and scored on reverse side, each containing 40 mg isosorbide dinitrate.

**Uses** For the prophylaxis of angina pectoris. The active principle of Cedocard Retard-40 is isosorbide dinitrate which relaxes vascular smooth muscle and produces coronary vasodilation, reduction in peripheral resistance and venous return, alteration of myocardial metabolism, and reduction of the myocardial oxygen demand.

**Dosage and administration** For oral administration.

*Adult dose:* 1–2 tablets in the morning and 1–2 tablets before retiring to sleep. Onset of action is 20–30 minutes and the duration of action is 10–12 hours.

There is no dose recommendation for children.

**Contra-indications, warnings, etc**

*Contra-indications:* A history of sensitivity to the drug.

*Precautions:* Tolerance and cross-tolerance to other nitrates may occur.

*Adverse reactions:* Headache; cutaneous vasodilation with flushing; transient episodes of dizziness, weakness and other signs of cerebral ischaemia associated with hypotension may occur.

*Treatment of overdosage:* In rare cases of overdosage, gastric lavage is indicated. Passive exercise of the extremities of the recumbent patient will promote venous return.

**Pharmaceutical precautions** *Storage:* Protect from heat and moisture.

**Legal category** P.

**Package quantities** Blister strips of 60 tablets (OP).

**Further information** Nil.

**Product licence number** 0424/0050.

## CISPLATIN

**Presentation** Cisplatin powder for injection: Yellowish-white freeze-dried cake in vials containing 10 mg or 50 mg cisplatin (cis-diamminedichloroplatinum). The formulation also contains sodium chloride and mannitol.

**Uses** Cisplatin has antitumour activity either as a single agent or in combination chemotherapy particularly in the treatment of testicular and metastatic ovarian tumours, also cervical tumours, lung carcinoma and bladder cancer.

**Dosage and administration** Cisplatin powder should be dissolved in Water for Injections such that the reconstituted solution contains 1 mg/ml of cisplatin. Cisplatin reconstituted powder should be diluted in 2 litres of 0.9% saline or a dextrose/saline solution (to which 37.5 g of mannitol may be added) and administration should be over a 6–8 hour period.

*Single agent therapy:* Adults and children: The usual dose regimen given as a single agent is 50–120 mg/m² by infusion once every 3 to 4 weeks or 15–20 mg/m² by infusion daily for five consecutive days, every 3 to 4 weeks.

*Combination chemotherapy:* Dosage may be adjusted if the drug is used in combination with other anti-tumour chemotherapy.

With multiple drug treatment schedules cisplatin is usually given in doses from 20 mg/m² upward every 3 to 4 weeks. Dosage should be reduced for patients with renal impairment or depressed bone marrow function (see *Contra-indications, warnings etc*).

Pre-treatment hydration with 1 to 2 litres of fluid infused for 8 to 12 hours prior to the cisplatin will initiate diuresis. Adequate subsequent hydration should maintain diuresis during the 24 hours following administration.

### Contra-indications, warnings, etc

*Contra-indications:* Cisplatin is contra-indicated in patients who have had previous allergic reactions to cisplatin or other platinum compounds as anaphylactic-like reactions have been reported. Relative contra-indications are pre-existing renal impairment, hearing disorders and depressed bone marrow function which may increase toxicity (see Warnings).

*Warnings:* This agent should only be administered under the direction of physicians experienced in cancer chemotherapy.

Nephrotoxicity of cisplatin is cumulative and serum creatinine, BUN and creatinine clearance should be measured before starting each course of therapy. Repeat courses of cisplatin should not be given unless levels of serum creatinine are below 1.5 mg/100 ml (100 mcmol/l) or blood urea below 55 mg/100 ml (9 mmol/l) and circulating blood elements are at an acceptable level.

Diuresis should be controlled and serum electrolyte levels monitored regularly. Adequate pre-treatment and 'during treatment' hydration should be ensured and such agents as mannitol given to minimise hazards of renal toxicity. In addition, adequate post-treatment hydration and urinary output should be monitored. Concomitant use of nephrotoxic drugs may seriously impair kidney function.

Ototoxicity is cumulative and occurs with high dose regimens. Hearing function should be evaluated before, and regularly during therapy (see *Adverse reactions*).

Haematologic toxicity is dose-related and may be cumulative; RBC, WBC and platelet counts should be monitored.

The nephrotoxicity, ototoxicity and myelosuppression induced by cisplatin will be additive to existing impairment or to the similar toxicity of agents such as cephaloridine, frusemide, aminoglycosides, etc. administered concurrently.

Anaphylactic-like reactions to cisplatin have been observed. These reactions can be controlled by administration of antihistamines, adrenaline and/or glucocorticoids.

Neurotoxicity secondary to cisplatin administration has been reported and therefore neurological examinations are recommended (see *Adverse reactions*). Cisplatin has been shown to be mutagenic. It may also have an anti-fertility effect. Other antineoplastic substances have been shown to be carcinogenic and this possibility should be borne in mind in long term use of cisplatin.

Cisplatin has been shown to be teratogenic and embryotoxic in animals. The use of the drug should be avoided in pregnant or nursing women if possible.

### Adverse reactions:

*Nephrotoxicity:* Immediate renal toxicity is greatly reduced when extensive saline hydration is used but cumulative toxicity may remain a problem and requires careful monitoring when repeat courses of cisplatin are administered.

Renal function impairment is evidenced by an increase in blood urea nitrogen, creatinine and serum uric acid levels and by a decreased creatinine clearance.

Cisplatin induces pathological lesions in the distal renal tubules and the collecting ducts.

*Gastrointestinal toxicity:* Nausea and vomiting occur in the majority of patients, usually starting within 1 hour of treatment and lasting up to 24 hours. Anorexia, nausea and occasional vomiting may persist for up to a week.

*Myelosuppression:* Cisplatin can cause suppression of all three blood elements.

Leucopenia is dose-related, possibly cumulative, usually reversible. The onset of leucopenia occurs usually between days 6 and 26 and the time of recovery ranges from 21 to 45 days. Thrombocytopenia is also a dose-limiting effect of cisplatin but is usually reversible. The onset of thrombocytopenia is

usually from days 10 to 26 and the time of recovery ranges from about 28 to 45 days.

The incidence of cisplatin-induced anaemia (haemoglobin drop of 2 g/100 ml) ranges from 9% to 40%, although this is a difficult toxic effect to assess because it may have a complex aetiology in cancer patients.

*Ototoxicity:* Unilateral or bilateral tinnitus, which is usually reversible, and/or hearing loss in the high frequency range may occur.

The overall incidence of audiogram abnormalities is 24%, but large variations exist. These abnormalities usually appear within 4 days after drug administration and consist of at least a 15 decibel loss in pure tone threshold. The damage seems to be cumulative and is not reversible. The audiogram abnormalities are most common in the 4000–8000 Hz frequencies.

*Neurotoxicity:* Peripheral neuropathies with paraesthesia in both upper and lower extremities, tremor and loss of taste have been observed in some patients, generally those treated with repeated courses.

*Anaphylactic-like reactions:* Anaphylactic-like reactions such as flushing, facial oedema, wheezing, tachycardia and hypotension may occur within a few minutes after intravenous administration. Antihistamines, adrenaline and/or glucocorticoids control all these reactions.

*Hyperuricaemia:* Hyperuricaemia occurring with cisplatin is more pronounced with doses greater than 50 mg/m². Allopurinol effectively reduces uric acid levels.

*Hypomagnesaemia:* Asymptomatic hypomagnesaemia has been documented in a certain number of patients treated with cisplatin. Symptomatic hypomagnesaemia has been observed in a limited number of cases.

**Pharmaceutical precautions** The unopened vials of the freeze-dried powder should be stored at room temperature protected from light. Solutions of cisplatin must not be cooled or refrigerated as cooling may result in precipitation; they should be stored at room temperature protected from light and used within 20 hours. It is recommended that diluted infusion solutions of cisplatin be protected from light during administration.

Any unused solution should be discarded.

Cisplatin is degraded on contact with aluminium. Aluminium containing equipment should not be used for administration of cisplatin.

It is recommended that personnel handling cisplatin wear protective gloves. Spillage or leakage should be mopped up wearing protective gloves and all cleaning materials should be placed in high-risk, waste-disposal bags and then incinerated. Contaminated surfaces should be washed with copious amounts of water.

**Legal category** POM.

**Package quantities** Cisplatin 10, 50: Individual vials.

**Further information** Nil.

**Product licence numbers**
Cisplatin 10     3433/0061
Cisplatin 50     3433/0063

# COLESTID* GRANULES AND COLESTID ORANGE

### Presentation

*Colestid Granules:* Light yellow, tasteless and odourless granules consisting of colestipol hydrochloride with 0.2% colloidal silicon dioxide. Each sachet contains 5 g colestipol hydrochloride.

*Colestid Orange:* Yellow powder with orange particles and an odour of orange/vanilla, which forms a yellow-orange suspension with a distinct orange aroma when mixed with water. Each sachet contains 5 g colestipol hydrochloride. Also contains mannitol, methylcellulose, citric acid, orange durarome, aspartame, maltol, ethyl vanillin, beta carotene and glycerol.

**Uses** Ion-exchange resin which lowers plasma cholesterol levels through binding with bile acids in the intestinal lumen.

Colestid is indicated as adjunctive therapy to diet in the management of patients with elevated cholesterol levels who have not responded adequately to diet. It may be used alone or in combination with additional lipid lowering agents.

Dietary therapy specific for the type of hypercholesterolaemia should be the initial treatment of choice. Excess body weight may be an important factor and weight reduction should be attempted prior to drug therapy in the overweight. The use of drugs should be considered only when reasonable attempts have been made to obtain satisfactory results with non-drug methods. When drug therapy is begun, the patient should be instructed on the importance of adhering to the correct diet.

Although Colestid is effective in all types of hypercholesterolaemia, it is medically most appropriate in

patients with Fredrickson's type II hyperlipoproteinaemia.

### Dosage and administration

*Preparation:* Colestid Orange is best mixed with plain water. Colestid Granules should always be taken mixed in a liquid such as orange or tomato juice, water, skimmed milk or non-carbonated beverage. The contents of the sachet should be added to 100 ml or more of the preferred aqueous vehicle and mixed thoroughly until dispersed. Colestid may also be taken in soups or with cereals, pulpy fruits with a high water content or yoghurt.

The recommended initial daily adult dosage of colestipol hydrochloride is 5 grams either once or twice daily.

For adults, colestipol hydrochloride is recommended in doses of 5–30 grams taken as one dose or two divided doses. Initiation of therapy is recommended at 5 grams either once or twice daily with 5 gram increments at one month intervals. Appropriate use of lipid profiles including LDL-cholesterol and triglycerides is advised so that optimal but not excessive doses are used to obtain the desired therapeutic effect on LDL-cholesterol level. If the desired therapeutic effect is not obtained at a dose of 5–30 grams/day with good compliance and acceptable side-effects, combined therapy or alternate treatment should be considered. Patients should take other drugs at least one hour before or four hours after Colestid to minimise possible interference with their absorption. However, Colestid and gemfibrozil may be used in the same patient when administered 2 hours apart. (See *Precautions*.)

*Elderly patients:* At present there are no extensive clinical studies with colestipol in patients over the age of 65. Review of available data does not suggest that the elderly are more predisposed to side-effects attributable to colestipol than the general population; however, therapy should be individualised and based on each patient's clinical characteristics and tolerance to the medication.

### Contra-indications, warnings, etc.

*Contra-indications:* Colestipol hydrochloride is contra-indicated in individuals who have previously demonstrated hypersensitivity to its use.

*Warnings:* Before instituting therapy with Colestid, diseases contributing to increased blood cholesterol such as hypothyroidism, diabetes mellitus, nephrotic syndrome, dysproteinaemias and obstructive liver diseases should be looked for and specifically treated.

To avoid accidental inhalation or oesophageal distress, Colestid should not be taken in its dry form.

Colestid Orange contains 32.5 mg aspartame (18.2 mg phenylalanine) per sachet. This should be taken into consideration in patients suffering from phenylketonuria since excessive amounts of aspartame may interfere with the control of this condition.

Safety for use in pregnant women has not been established. The use of Colestid in pregnancy or lactation or by women of childbearing age requires that the potential benefits of treatment be weighed against the possible hazards to the mother and child.

Colestid may elevate serum triglyceride levels when used as sole therapy. This elevation is generally transient but may persist in some individuals. A significant rise in triglyceride level should be considered as an indication for dose reduction, drug discontinuation or combined or alternate therapy.

The use of Colestid in children has been limited; however, it does appear to be effective in lowering serum cholesterol in older children and young adults. Because bile acid sequestrants may interfere with the absorption of fat-soluble vitamins, appropriate monitoring of growth and development is essential. Dosage and long-term safety in children have not been established.

*Precautions:* In man, Colestid may delay or reduce the absorption of certain concomitant oral drugs (digitalis and its glycosides, propranolol, chlorothiazide and hydrochlorothiazide, tetracycline hydrochloride, penicillin G and gemfibrozil). Particular caution should be taken with digitalis preparations since conflicting results have been obtained for the effect of Colestid on the availability of digoxin and digitoxin. Colestid has been shown not to interfere with the absorption of clindamycin, clofibrate, aspirin, tolbutamide, warfarin, methyldopa and phenytoin. The clinical response to concomitant medication should be closely monitored and appropriate adjustments made.

Repeated doses of Colestid given prior to a single dose of propranolol in human trials have been reported to decrease propranolol absorption. However, in a follow-up study in normal subjects, single dose administration of Colestid and propranolol or multiple dose administration of both agents did not affect the extent of propranolol absorption. Effects on the absorption of other beta-blockers have not been determined. Patients on propranolol should be observed when Colestid is either added or deleted from a therapeutic regimen.

Because it sequesters bile acids, Colestid may interfere with normal fat absorption and thus may alter absorption of fat soluble vitamins such as A, D, E and K. A study in humans found only one patient in whom a prolonged prothombin time was noted. Most studies did not show a decrease in vitamin A, D or E levels during the administration of Colestid; however, if Colestid is to be given for a long period, these vitamin levels should be monitored and supplements given if necessary.

Both clinical usage and animal studies with Colestid have provided no evidence of drug related intestinal neoplasms. Colestid is not mutagenic in the Ames test.

*Side-effects:* The most common adverse reactions reported with Colestid have been of a functional gastro-intestinal nature. The most frequent is constipation, which is usually mild, transient and responsive to the usual adjunctive measures. At times, constipation can be severe and may be accompanied by impaction. As such, haemorrhoids can be aggravated and infrequent blood in the stools has been reported. Less frequent gastro-intestinal complaints are abdominal discomfort, belching, flatulence, indigestion, nausea, vomiting and diarrhoea. Rarely, peptic ulceration and bleeding, cholelithiasis and cholecystitis have been reported, although these are not necessarily drug related.

Transient and modest elevation of SGOT and alkaline phosphatase have been observed. No medical significance is attached to these observed changes.

Although not necessarily drug-related, the following non-gastro-intestinal medical events have been reported during clinical trials at a similar incidence to placebo.

*Cardiovascular:* Chest pain, angina and tachycardia have been infrequently reported.

*Hypersensitivity:* Rash has been infrequently reported. Urticaria and dermatitis have been rarely noted.

*Musculoskeletal:* Musculoskeletal pain, aches and pains in the extremities, joint pain and arthritis and backache have been reported.

*Neurological:* Headache, migraine headache and sinus headache have been reported. Other infrequently reported complaints include dizziness, lightheadedness and insomnia.

*Miscellaneous:* Anorexia, fatigue, weakness, shortness of breath and swelling of the hands or feet, have been infrequently reported.

*Overdosage:* No toxic effects due to overdosage have been reported. Should overdosage occur, obstruction of the gastro-intestinal tract would be expected to occur. Treatment would be determined by the location and degree of obstruction.

**Pharmaceutical precautions** None

**Legal category** POM

**Package quantities** Colestid Granules: Box containing 30 x 5 gram foil sachets. Colestid Orange: Box containing 30 x 5 gram foil sachets.

**Further information** Colestid is not absorbed; its action is limited to the lumen of the gastro-intestinal tract and it is passed in the faeces. It binds bile acids in the intestinal lumen and causes them to be excreted in the faeces together with the polymer. When the enterohepatic circulation of bile acids is interrupted, cholesterol conversion to bile acids is enhanced and plasma cholesterol levels are thereby lowered.

**Product licence numbers**

| | |
|---|---|
| Colestid Granules | 0032/0055 |
| Colestid Orange | 0032/0172 |

## COLPERMIN*

**Presentation** A light blue/dark blue enteric-coated hard gelatin capsule size 1, with a blue band between cap and body. Each capsule contains 0.2 ml standardised peppermint oil BP in a sustained-release gel matrix.

**Uses** For the treatment of symptoms of discomfort and of abdominal colic and distension experienced by patients with irritable bowel syndrome. Also for the treatment of intestinal spasm secondary to other gastro-intestinal disorders e.g. diverticular disease.

**Dosage and administration** For oral administration.

*Adult dose:* One capsule three times a day, taken 30–60 minutes before food with a small quantity of water. The capsules should *not* be taken immediately after food.

The dose may be increased to two capsules, three times a day when discomfort is more severe.

The capsules should be taken until symptoms resolve, usually within one or two weeks. At times when symptoms are more persistent, the capsules can be continued for longer periods of between 2 to 3 months.

*Dosage for the elderly:* The mode of action of peppermint oil is local rather than systemic. Clinical experience and known pharmacology do not necessitate alternative advice for elderly patients.

*Children:* There is no experience in the use of these capsules in children under the age of 15 years.

**Contra-indications, warnings, etc**
*Precautions:* Patients should be instructed not to break or chew the capsules because this would release the peppermint oil prematurely, possibly causing local irritation of the mouth and oesophagus.

Patients who already suffer from heartburn, sometimes experience an exacerbation of these symptoms when taking the capsule. Treatment should be discontinued in these patients.

Antacids should not be administered at the same time of day as Colpermin.

There are no data available to establish the safety of Colpermin in pregnancy, therefore, it should be used only if, in the opinion of the physician, the benefits of treatment outweigh the possible hazards.

*Adverse effects:* Occasional heartburn, perianal irritation; allergic reactions to menthol, which are rare, and include erythematous skin rash, headache, bradycardia, muscle tremor and ataxia.

*Treatment of overdosage:* If capsules have been recently ingested, the stomach should be emptied by gastric lavage. Patients should be observed and symptomatic treatment carried out if necessary.

**Pharmaceutical precautions** Store in a cool place. Avoid direct sunlight.

**Legal category** P.

**Package quantities** Containers of 20 or 100 capsules.

**Further information** The enteric-coating of the capsule delays release of the peppermint oil until it reaches the distal small bowel. The oil exerts local effects of colonic relaxation and a fall of intracolonic pressure. The gel matrix ensures the sustained release of the peppermint oil thus exposing the entire bowel to the carminative action of menthol. These local effects have been used for post-operative wind pain and for masking the odour of colostomies.

**Product licence number** 00032/0218.

## CONVULEX*

**Presentation** Enteric-coated soft gelatin capsules containing 150, 300 and 500 mg Valproic Acid USP.

**Uses** For the treatment of epilepsy, both generalised and partial seizures, by oral medication.

**Dosage and administration** Convulex capsules should be swallowed whole.

*Adults:* Starting with a daily dose of 15 mg/kg body weight the dosage should be slowly increased by 5–10 mg/kg body weight up to 30 mg/kg body weight or until the patient no longer suffers from seizures.

*Children:* Starting with a daily dose of 15 mg/kg body weight the dosage should be slowly increased by 5–10 mg/kg body weight up to 30 mg/kg body weight or until the patient no longer suffers from seizures.

*Elderly:* Dosage should be determined by seizure control.

It is recommended that Convulex be given as a divided dose i.e. half the daily dose b.d. In some circumstances the daily dose can be split into 3 or 4 administrations.

Substitution: A one to one dose relationship of Convulex and products containing sodium valproate has been demonstrated in pharmacokinetic trials. In patients previously receiving sodium valproate therapy, Convulex should be initiated at the same total daily dose.

Combination therapy: During therapy with concurrently administered anticonvulsant drugs, Convulex dosages may have to be increased or decreased to maintain seizure control.

**Contra-indications, warnings, etc**
*Contra-indications:* Disturbances of hepatic function, known hypersensitivity to valproic acid and sodium valproate.

*Warnings and precautions:* The following laboratory tests should be determined before the start of therapy, subsequently at two-monthly intervals and before dosage increase; liver function tests, blood coagulation time, thrombocyte aggregation and fibrinogen levels.

Valproic acid should be discontinued or not started if the following abnormalities occur; hypofibrinogenaemia and/or coagulation disturbances, a threefold increase of transaminase values, an increase of alkaline phosphatase and bilirubin in serum in connection with clinical symptoms of toxic hepatitis. If only a slight increase in transaminase values is discovered the dosage should be reduced and liver function and coagulation tests should be monitored. If severe abdominal pain and vomiting occurs serum amylase values should be determined. If the results show pathological values, valproic acid should be discontinued. During treatment with valproic acid urine analysis for ketones may be false-positive. The platelet counts and bleeding time should be measured prior to surgical interventions.

Convulex may enhance the sedating effect of other preparations, especially that of the barbiturates. It may potentiate the CNS depressant action of alcohol, neuroleptics and antidepressants and may interact with concurrently administered anti-epileptic drugs. The effect of drugs affecting coagulation may be enhanced.

*Adverse effects:*
*Hepatic:* Liver function disturbances may occur during Convulex therapy. Rarely non-dose related severe hepatic damage has been reported within the first six months of treatment.

Minor abnormalities of liver function tests may occur during therapy but usually normalise after dosage adaption.

Valproic acid should be discontinued after the occurrence of clinical symptoms of hepatic damage eg recurrent epigastric complaints, anorexia etc. The patient should be instructed to report immediately any such symptoms to the treating physician.

*Pancreatic:* Pancreatic effects (acute pancreatitis) have been observed in rare cases. The treatment should be stopped immediately if symptoms and laboratory tests suggest pancreatitis. Patients should be instructed to report acute abdominal pain to the treating physician.

*Haematological:* Thrombocytopenia and inhibition of platelet aggregation have been observed. Monitoring of platelet function is therefore recommended especially prior to surgical intervention. The treatment should be stopped immediately after the manifestation of any coagulation disturbances.

*Neurological:* Sedation, aggression, hyperactivity, ataxia and tremor may occur rarely. In isolated cases states of confusion, stupor and and coma have been observed some days after reaching therapeutic plasma levels.

*Effects on ability to drive and to use machinery:* Patients should be advised not to drive or use machinery if fatigue occurs.

*Gastro-intestinal:* Gastro-intestinal disturbances are among the most frequent side effects. Minor gastric irritation and nausea occur mostly at the onset of therapy and disappear with dose adjustment and/or taking the capsules during meals. Increased appetite and weight gain have been observed.

*Dermatological:* Allergic skin reactions occur very rarely. Transient loss of hair has been observed in isolated cases.

*Use during pregnancy and lactation:* In pregnancy, the possible benefits should be weighed against possible risks. Up to the 40th day, dosage should be as low as possible (15–20 mg/kg of body weight). Combination with other drugs is to be avoided as much as possible. There is no contra-indication to its use in lactating mothers.

*Treatment of overdosage:* At plasma concentrations of up to 5–6 times the maximum therapeutic levels there are unlikely to be any symptoms other than nausea, vomiting and dizziness.

In massive overdose, ie with plasma concentrations 10–20 times maximum therapeutic levels, there may be serious CNS depression and respiration may be impaired. Full recovery is usual following treatment including induced vomiting, gastric lavage, assisted ventilation and other supportive measures. Naloxone 0.01 mg/kg i.v. has been reported to reverse the CNS depressant effect of Valproic acid.

**Pharmaceutical precautions** Do not store above 25°C. Protect from light.

**Legal category** POM

**Package quantities** Blister packs of 100 capsules.

**Further information** Nil

**Product licence numbers**

| | |
|---|---|
| 150 mg | 8298/0004 |
| 300 mg | 8298/0002 |
| 500 mg | 8298/0003 |

*Product licence holder:* Gerot Pharmaceuticals, Austria.

## CYCLOPHOSPHAMIDE

**Presentation:** Pink, biconvex, sugar coated tablets containing 53.5 mg Cyclophosphamide BP (equivalent to 50 mg anhydrous cyclophosphamide).

Cyclophosphamide for injection is a sterile white powder in clear glass vials, with rubber caps and aluminium seals, containing 107 mg, 214 mg, 535 mg or 1070 mg Cyclophosphamide BP (equivalent to 100 mg, 200 mg, 500 mg or 1000 mg anhydrous cyclophosphamide) with sodium chloride.

**Uses:** Alkylating, antineoplastic agent. Cyclophosphamide has been used successfully to induce and maintain regressions in a wide range of neoplastic conditions, including leukaemias, lymphomas, soft tissue and osteogenic sarcomas, paediatric malignancies and adult solid tumours; in particular, breast and lung carcinomas.

Cyclophosphamide is frequently used in combination chemotherapy regimens involving other cytotoxic drugs.

**Dosage and administration** The dosage regimen should be tailored to the individual requirements of the patient, depending on his general condition, concurrent therapy, the type and state of tumour, and the patient's response. Three samples regimens may serve as guides:

| | |
|---|---|
| Low dose: | 80 to 240 mg/m² (2 to 6 mg/kg) as a single dose weekly i.v., or in divided doses orally. |
| Medium dose: | 400 to 600 mg/m² (10 to 15 mg/kg) as a single dose weekly i.v |
| High dose: | 800 to 1,600 mg/m² (20 to 40 mg/kg) as a single dose i.v. at 10–20 day intervals. |

Higher doses should be used only at the discretion of a physician experienced in cytotoxic chemotherapy.

It is recommended that the calculated dose of cyclophosphamide be reduced when it is given in combination with other anti-neoplastic agents or radiotherapy, and in patients with bone marrow depression.

Cyclophosphamide tablets should be swallowed whole, preferably on an empty stomach, but if gastric irritation is severe, they may be taken with meals.

Cyclophosphamide injection should be reconstituted with Water for Injections, 5 ml for each 100 mg of anhydrous cyclophosphamide. After reconstitution the solution should will remain stable at room temperature for 2–3 hours. It should be given by slow intravenous injection over a period of 2–3 minutes or into the tubing of a freely running intravenous infusion over a period of 2–3 minutes.

A minimum output of 100 ml/hour should be maintained during therapy with conventional doses to avoid cystitis. If the larger doses are used, an output of at least this level should be maintained for 24 hours following administration, if necessary by forced diuresis. Alkalinisation of the urine is not recommended. Cyclophosphamide should be given early in the day and the bladder voided frequently. The patient should be well hydrated and maintained in fluid balance.

Mesna (Uromitexan) can be used concurrently with Cyclophosphamide to reduce urotoxic effects (for dosage see Uromitexan data sheet). If mesna (Uromitexan) is used to reduce uroethelial toxicity, frequent emptying of the bladder should be avoided.

If the leucocyte count is below 4,000/mm³ or the platelet count is below 100,000/mm³, treatment with Cyclophosphamide should be temporarily withheld until the blood count returns to normal levels.

**Contra-indications, warnings, etc** Cyclophosphamide should be used only under the direction of physicians experienced in cytotoxic or immunosuppressant therapy.

*Contra-indications:* Hypersensitivity and haemorrhagic cystitis.

*Warnings:* Cyclophosphamide should be withheld in the presence of severe bone marrow depression and reduced doses should be used in the presence of lesser degrees of bone marrow depression. Single doses will produce a leucopenia which may be severe but usually returns to normal within 21 days. Regular blood counts should be performed in patients who are pregnant or to mothers who are breastfeeding. It should not normally be given to patients with severe infections and should be withdrawn if such infections become life-threatening.

Cyclophosphamide should be used with caution in debilitated patients and those with renal and/or hepatic failure. Cyclophosphamide is not recommended in patients with a plasma creatinine greater than 120 μ mol/l (1.5 mg/100 ml) bilirubin greater than 17 μ mol (1 mg/100 ml); or serum transaminases or alkaline phosphatase more than 2–3 times the upper limit of normal. In all such cases, dosage should be reduced. Oral hypoglycaemic agents may be potentiated by cyclophosphamide.

Amenorrhoea and azoospermia often occur during treatment with cyclophosphamide but in most cases are reversible. Alkylating agents, including cyclophosphamide, have been shown to possess mutagenic, teratogenic and carcinogenic potential. Pregnancy should therefore be avoided during cyclophosphamide therapy and three months thereafter.

Cyclophosphamide is excreted mainly in the urine,

largely in the form of active metabolites. These may give rise to a chemical cystitis which may be haemorrhagic. Because of this, a high fluid intake should be maintained with frequent emptying of the bladder. However, cyclophosphamide may give rise to fluid retention with subsequent water intoxication. Should this arise, a diuretic may be given. Cyclophosphamide may cause myocardial toxicity, especially at high dosage.

Cyclophosphamide may induce permanent sterility in children.

*Adverse reactions:* In addition to those noted above, the following may accompany cyclophosphamide therapy: hair loss, which may be total, although generally reversible; mucosal ulceration, anorexia, nausea and vomiting, pigmentation typically affecting the palms and nails of the hands and the soles of the feet, and interstitial pulmonary fibrosis.

Haematuria may occur during or after therapy with Cyclophosphamide. Acute sterile haemorrhagic cystitis may occur in up to 10% of patients not given mesna (Uromitexan) in conjunction with Cyclophosphamide. Late sequelae of this cystitis are bladder contracture and fibrosis.

Cyclophosphamide therapy may lead to inappropriate secretion of anti-diuretic hormone, fluid retention and hyponatremia, with subsequent water intoxication. Should this occur, diuretic therapy should be instigated.

*Overdosage:* Myelosuppression (particularly granulocytopenia) and haemorrhagic cystitis are the most serious consequences of overdosage. Recovery from myelosuppression will occur by the 21st day after the overdose in the great majority of patients (at doses up to 200 mg/kg i.v.) while granulocytopenia is usually seen by day 6 and lasts for a mean period of 12 days up to 18 days. A broad spectrum antibiotic may be administered until recovery occurs. Transfusion of whole-blood, platelets or white cells and reverse barrier nursing may be necessary.

If the drug has been taken in the form of tablets, early gastric lavage may reduce the amount of drug absorbed. During the first 24 hours and possibly up to 48 hours after overdosage, i.v. mesna may be beneficial in ameliorating damage to the urinary system. Normal supportive measures such as analgesics and maintenance of fluid balance should be instituted. If the cystitis does not resolve, more intensive treatment may be necessary. No further courses should be given until the patient has fully recovered.

**Pharmaceutical precautions** *Tablets:* Store in a cool dry place and protect from light.

*Injection:* Store in a cool place and protect from light. If heated above 32°C, cyclophosphamide may decompose to a damp-looking gel. It is, therefore, recommended that this product is never stored where heat build-up may occur such as near radiators, etc.

**Legal category** POM

**Package quantities** *Tablets:* Containers of 100 tablets of 50 mg

*Injection:* Vials of 100 mg in packs of 10. Vials of 200 mg in packs of 10. Vials of 500 mg in packs of 10. Vials of 1000 mg in packs of 5. Each vial contains dry powder for reconstitution.

**Further information** The dosage regimen for mesna (Uromitexan) varies according to the dose of Cyclophosphamide administered. In general i.v. Uromitexan is given as 60% w/w of the dose of i.v. Cyclophosphamide in three equal doses of 20% at 0, 4 and 8 hours. With the higher doses of Cyclophosphamide, the dose and frequency of administration may need to be increased. Uromitexan Tablets are also available; full prescribing information for both presentations is available on the appropriate data sheet.

**Product licence numbers**

| | |
|---|---|
| Cyclophosphamide tablets 50 mg | 3433/0036 |
| Cyclophosphamide Injection 100 mg | 3433/0037 |
| Cyclophosphamide Injection 200 mg | 3433/0038 |
| Cyclophosphamide Injection 500 mg | 3433/0039 |
| Cyclophosphamide Injection 1000 mg | 3433/0040 |

# CYKLOKAPRON* INJECTION

**Qualitative and quantitative composition** *Active ingredient:* Tranexamic Acid BP/PhEur 500 mg

**Pharmaceutical form** Ampoules containing 5 ml colourless solution.

## Clinical particulars

*Therapeutic indications:*
*Local fibrinolysis:* For short term use in prophylaxis and treatment in patients at high risk of per- and post-operative haemorrhage following: prostatectomy; conisation of the cervix; surgical procedures and dental extractions in haemophiliacs.

*General fibrinolysis:* Haemorrhagic complications in association with thrombolytic therapy. Haemor-

rhage associated with disseminated intravascular coagulation with predominant activation of the fibrinolytic system.

*Posology and method of administration:* Route of administration: by slow intravenous injection.

*Local fibrinolysis:* the recommended standard dose is 5–10 ml (500–1000 mg) by slow intravenous injection (1 ml/min), three times daily. If treatment continues for more than three days, consideration should be given to the use of Cyklokapron tablets or syrup. Alternatively, following an initial intravenous injection, subsequent treatment may proceed by intravenous infusion. Following addition to a suitable diluent (see *Interaction with other medicaments and other forms of interaction* section), Cyklokapron may be administered at a rate of 25–50 mg/kg body wt/day. *Children:* According to body weight (10 mg/kg body wt/ 2–3 times daily)

*Elderly patients:* No reduction in dosage is necessary unless there is evidence of renal failure.

*General fibrinolysis:* In disseminated intravascular coagulation with predominant activation of the fibrinolytic system, usually a single dose of 10 ml (1 g) is sufficient to control bleeding.

Neutralisation of thrombolytic therapy; 10 mg/kg body wt by slow intravenous injection.

*Contra-indications:* Cyklokapron is contra-indicated in patients with a history of thromboembolic disease.

*Special warnings and precautions for use:* In patients with renal insufficiency, because of the risk of accumulation. The dose should be reduced according to the following table:

| Serum Creatinine | Dose iv | Dose Frequency |
|---|---|---|
| 120–250 mcmol/l | 10 mg/kg | Twice daily |
| 250–500 mcmol/l hour | 10 mg/kg | Every 24th |
| > 500 mcmol/l hour | 5 mg/kg | Every 24th |

In massive haematuria from the upper urinary tract (especially in haemophilia) since, in a few cases, ureteric obstruction has been reported. In patients with disseminated intravascular coagulation (DIC) treatment must be restricted to those in whom there is predominant activation of the fibrinolytic system with acute severe bleeding. Characteristically, the haematological profile approximates to the following: reduced euglobulin clot lysis time; prolonged prothrombin time; reduced plasma levels of fibrinogen, factors V and VIII, plasminogen and alpha-2 macroglobulin; normal plasma levels of P and P complex; ie factors II (prothrombin), VIII and X; increased plasma levels of fibrinogen degradation products; a normal platelet count. The foregoing presumes that the underlying disease state does not modify the various elements in this profile. In such acute cases a single dose of 1 g tranexamic acid is frequently sufficient to control bleeding. The fibrinolytic activity in the blood will be reduced for about 4 hours if renal function is normal. Anticoagulation with heparin should be instigated in order to prevent further fibrin deposition. Administration of Cyklokapron in DIC should be considered only when appropriate haematological laboratory facilities and expertise are available. Cyklokapron must not be administered in DIC with predominant activation of the coagulation system.

*Interactions with other medicaments and other forms of interaction:* The solution for injection may be mixed with the following solutions: isotonic sodium chloride; isotonic glucose; 20% fructose; 10% invertose; dextran 40; dextran 70; ringer's solution.

Cyklokapron solution for injection may be mixed with Heparin.

*Pregnancy and lactation:* Although there is no evidence from animal studies of a teratogenic effect, the usual caution with the use of drugs in pregnancy should be observed.

Tranexamic acid passes into breast milk to a concentration of approximately one hundreth of the concentration in the maternal blood. An antifibrinolytic effect in the infant is unlikely.

*Effects on ability to drive and use machines:* None known.

*Undesirable effects:* Gastro-intestinal disorders (nausea, vomiting, diarrhoea) may occur but disappear when the dosage is reduced. Rapid intravenous injection may cause dizziness and/or hypotension.

*Overdose:* No cases of overdosage have been reported. Symptoms may be nausea, vomiting, orthostatic symptoms and/or hypotension. Maintain a high fluid intake to promote renal excretion.

**Pharmacological properties**

*Pharmacodynamic properties:* Tranexamic acid is an antifibrinolytic agent which competitively inhibits the activation of plasminogen to plasmin.

*Pharmacokinetic properties:* Approximately 90% of an intravenously administered tranexamic acid dose is excreted, largely unchanged, in the urine within 24 hours. The plasma half-life is approximately 2 hours.

*Preclinical safety data:* There are no preclinical data of relevance to the prescriber which are additional to that already included in other sections of the Summary of Product Characteristics.

**Pharmaceutical particulars**

*List of excipients:* Water for injections

*Incompatibilities:* Cyklokapron solution for injection should not be added to blood for transfusion, or to injections containing penicillin.

*Shelf life:* 3 years.

*Special precautions for storage:* None.

*Nature and contents of container:* Type I glass 5 ml ampoules packed in outer cardboard carton.

*Instructions for use/handling:* See *Posology and method of administration* section.

**Marketing authorisation number** 0022/0004R

**Date of approval/revision of SPC** *February 1992*

**Legal category** POM

## CYKLOKAPRON* SYRUP

**Qualitative and quantitative composition** *Active ingredient:* Tranexamic Acid PhEur 500 mg/5 ml

**Pharmaceutical form** A colourless or slightly yellow syrup with an orange taste.

**Clinical particulars**

*Therapeutic indications:* Short-term use for haemorrhage or risk of haemorrhage in increased fibrinolysis or fibrinogenolysis. Local fibrinolysis as occurs in the following conditions:

- Prostatectomy and bladder surgery
- Menorrhagia
- Epistaxis
- Conisation of the cervix
- Traumatic hyphaema
- Hereditary angioneurotic oedema
- Management of dental extraction in haemophiliacs

*Posology and method of administration:* Route of administration: Oral.

*Local fibrinolysis:* The recommended standard dosage is 15–25 mg/kg bodyweight (10–15 ml syrup) 2–3 times daily. For the indications listed below the following doses may be used:

*Prostatectomy:* Prophylaxis and treatment of haemorrhage in high risk patients should commence per- or post-operatively with Cyklokapron Injection; thereafter 10 ml syrup 3–4 times daily until macroscopic haematuria is no longer present.

*Menorrhagia:* 10–15 ml syrup 3–4 times daily for 3–4 days. Cyklokapron therapy should be initiated only after heavy bleeding has started.

*Epistaxis:* Where recurrent bleeding is anticipated oral therapy (10 ml syrup 3 times daily) should be administered for 7 days.

*Conisation of the cervix:* 15 ml syrup 3 times daily.

*Traumatic hyphaema:* 10-15 ml syrup 3 times a day. The dose is based on 25 mg/kg 3 times a day.

*Hereditary angioneurotic oedema:* Some patients are aware of the onset of the illness; suitable treatment for these patients is intermittently 10–15 ml syrup 2–3 times daily for some days. Other patients are treated continuously at this dosage.

*Haemophilia:* In the management of dental extractions 10–15 ml syrup every eight hours. The dose is based on 25 mg/kg.

*Children:* Dosage should be calculated according to body weight at 25 mg/kg/dose.

*Elderly patients:* No reduction in dosage is necessary unless there is evidence of renal failure (please refer to section Special Warnings and Precautions for use).

*Contra-indications:* Patients with a history of thromboembolic disease.

*Special warnings and precautions for use:* In patients with renal insufficiency, because of the risk of accumulation. By extrapolation from clearance data relating to the intravenous dosage form, the following reduction in the oral dosage is recommended:

| Serum Creatinine | Oral Dose | Dose Frequency |
|---|---|---|
| 120–250 mmol/l | 25 mg/kg | Twice daily |
| 250–500 mmol/l | 25 mg/kg | Every 24 hours |
| > 500 mmol/l | 12.5 mg/kg | Every 24 hours |

In massive haematuria from the upper urinary tract (especially in haemophilia) since, in a few cases, ureteric obstruction has been reported.

In the long-term treatment of patients with hereditary angioneurotic oedema, regular eye examinations (e.g. visual acuity, slit lamp, intraocular pressure, visual fields) and liver function tests should be performed.

*Interactions with other medicaments and other forms of interaction:* Cyklokapron will counteract the thrombolytic effect of fibrinolytic preparations.

*Pregnancy and lactation*

*Pregnancy:* Although there is no evidence from animal studies of a teratogenic effect, the usual caution with the use of drugs in pregnancy should be observed.

*Lactation:* Tranexamic acid passes into breast milk to a concentration of approximately one hundredth of the concentration in the maternal blood. An antifibrinolytic effect in the infant is unlikely.

*Effects on ability to drive and use machines:* None known.

*Undesirable effects:* Gastrointestinal disorders (nausea, vomiting, diarrhoea) may occur but disappear when the dosage is reduced. Rare instances of colour vision disturbances have been reported. Patients who experience disturbance of colour vision should be withdrawn from treatment.

*Overdose:* No cases of overdosage have been reported. Symptoms may be nausea, vomiting, orthostatic symptoms and/or hypotension. Initiate vomiting, then stomach lavage, and charcoal therapy. Maintain a high fluid intake to promote renal excretion.

**Pharmacological properties**

*Pharmacodynamic properties:* Tranexamic acid is an antifibrinolytic compound which is a potent competitive inhibitor of the activation of plasminogen to plasmin. At much higher concentrations it is a non-competitive inhibitor of plasmin. The inhibitory effect of tranexamic acid in plasminogen activation by urokinase has been reported to be 6–100 times and by streptokinase 6–40 times greater than that of aminocaproic acid. The antifibrinolytic activity of tranexamic acid is approximately ten times greater than that of aminocaproic acid.

*Pharmacokinetic properties:* Following oral administration, 1.13% and 39% of the administered dose were recovered after 3 and 24 hours respectively. Tranexamic acid administered parenterally is distributed in a two compartment model. Tranexamic acid crosses the placenta, and may reach one hundredth of the serum peak concentration in the milk of lactating women. Tranexamic acid crosses the blood brain barrier.

Following intravenous administration, the biological half-life of tranexamic acid has been determined to be 1.9 hours and 2.7 hours.

*Preclinical safety data:* There are no preclinical data of relevance to the prescriber which are additional to that already included in other sections of the Summary of Product Characteristics.

**Pharmaceutical particulars**

*List of excipients:* xylitol; citric acid anhydrous; methyl parahydroxybenzoate; propyl parahydroxybenzoate; orange aroma 3174; purified water.

*Incompatibilities:* None known.

*Shelf life:* Unopened: 24 months. Opened: 3 months.

*Special precautions for storage:* Store below 25°C.

*Nature and contents of container:* 300 ml, brown soda-lime glass bottles (Type III, PhEur) with white polypropylene tamper-proof closure consisting of lip and pour part or 300 ml, amber PET bottles with polypropylene screw caps.

*Instructions for use/handling:* Cyklokapron Syrup may be diluted with Syrup BP and the resulting mixture stored for up to 14 days.

**Marketing authorisation number** 0022/0044

**Date of approval/revision of SPC** March 1996

**Legal category** POM

## CYKLOKAPRON* TABLETS

**Presentation** White, film-coated oblong tablets, 8×18 mm, engraved CY with an arc above and below the lettering. Each tablet contains Tranexamic Acid 500 mg.

**Uses**

*Action:* Tranexamic acid is an antifibrinolytic agent which competitively inhibits the activation of plasminogen to plasmin.

*Indications:* Short-term use for haemorrhage or risk of haemorrhage in increased fibrinolysis or fibrinogenolysis.

1. Local fibrinolysis as occurs in the following conditions:
 (a) Prostatectomy
 (b) Menorrhagia
 (c) Epistaxis
 (d) Conisation of the cervix
 (e) Traumatic hyphaema
2. Management of dental extraction in haemophiliacs.

3. Hereditary angioneurotic oedema.

**Dosage and administration**

*Local fibrinolysis:* The recommended standard dose is 15–25 mg/kg body wt, i.e. 2–3 tablets two to three times daily. For the indications listed below the following doses may be used:

1a. *Prostatectomy:* Prophylaxis and treatment of haemorrhage in high risk patients should commence per- or post-operatively with Cyklokapron Injection; thereafter 2 tablets, three to four times daily until macroscopic haematuria is no longer present.

1b. *Menorrhagia:* 2–3 tablets three to four times daily for three to four days. Cyklokapron therapy is initiated only after heavy bleeding has started.

1c. *Epistaxis:* Where recurrent bleeding is anticipated oral therapy (2 tablets three times daily) should be administered for seven days.

1d. *Conisation of the cervix:* 3 tablets three times daily.

1e. *Traumatic hyphaema:* 2–3 tablets three times daily. The dose is based on 25 mg/kg three times a day.

2. *Haemophilia:* In the management of dental extractions 2–3 tablets every eight hours. The dose is based on 25 mg/kg.

3. *Hereditary angioneurotic oedema:* Some patients are aware of the onset of the illness; suitable treatment for these patients is intermittently 2–3 tablets two to three times daily for some days. Other patients are treated continuously at this dosage.

*Children's dosage:* This should be calculated according to body weight, at 25 mg/kg per dose.

*Elderly patients:* No reduction in dosage is necessary unless there is evidence of renal failure (see guidelines below).

**Contra-indications, warnings, etc** Cyklokapron is contra-indicated in patients with a history of thromboembolic disease.

*Precautions:*

1. In patients with renal insufficiency, because of the risk of accumulation. By extrapolation from clearance data relating to the intravenous dosage form, the following reduction in the oral dosage is recommended.

| Serum creatinine | Oral dose | Dose frequency |
|---|---|---|
| 120–250 micromol/l | 25 mg/kg | twice daily |
| 250–500 micromol/l | 25 mg/kg | every 24th hour |
| >500 micromol/l | 12.5 mg/kg | every 24th hour |

2. In massive haematuria from the upper urinary tract (especially in haemophilia) since, in a few cases, ureteric obstruction has been reported.

3. When disseminated intravascular coagulation is in progress.

4. In the long-term treatment of patients with hereditary angioneurotic oedema regular eye examination (e.g. visual acuity, slit lamp, intra-ocular pressure, visual fields) and liver function tests should be performed.

*Pregnancy:* Although there is no evidence from animal studies of a teratogenic effect, the usual caution with use of drugs in pregnancy should be observed.

*Lactation:* Tranexamic acid passes into breast milk to a concentration of approximately one hundredth of the concentration in the maternal blood. An antifibrinolytic effect in the infant is unlikely.

*Side-effects:* Gastro-intestinal disorders (nausea, vomiting, diarrhoea) may occur but disappear when the dosage is reduced. Rare instances of transient colour vision disturbance have been reported. Patients who experience disturbance of colour vision should be withdrawn from treatment.

*Overdosage:* No cases of overdosage have been reported. Symptoms may be nausea, vomiting, orthostatic symptoms and/or hypotension. Initiate vomiting, then stomach lavage and charcoal therapy. Maintain a high fluid intake to promote renal excretion.

**Legal category** POM.

**Package quantities** Carton containing 5 blister strips of 12 tablets each.

**Further information** Absorption of tranexamic acid from the gastro-intestinal tract is 30–40%. The plasma half-life is approximately 2 hours.

**Product licence number** 0022/0003R.

## CYSTRIN* 3 mg

**Qualitative and quantitative composition** Oxybutynin hydrochloride 3.06 mg equivalent to oxybutynin 3.00 mg.

**Pharmaceutical form** Tablet.

**Clinical particulars**

*Therapeutic indications:* Cystrin is indicated for urinary incontinence, urgency and frequency in unstable bladder conditions due either to idiopathic detrusor instability or neurogenic bladder disorders ( detrusor hyperreflexia) in conditions such as spina bifida and multiple sclerosis.

In addition, for children over 5 years of age, oxybutynin may be used in nocturnal enuresis in conjunction with non-drug therapy where this alone, or in conjunction with other drug treatment, has failed.

*Posology and method of administration:*

*Children under 5 years of age:* Not recommended

*Children over 5 years of age:*
*Neurogenic bladder disorders:* The usual dose is 5 mg twice a day. This may be increased to a maximum of 5 mg three times a day to obtain a clinical response provided that the side effects are tolerated.

*Nocturnal enuresis:* The usual dose is 5 mg two or three times a day. The last dose should be given before bedtime.

In children the maintenance dose may be achieved by upward titration from an initial dose of 3 mg twice daily.

*Adults:* The usual dose is 5 mg two or three times a day. This may be increased to a maximum dosage of 5 mg four times a day (20 mg) to obtain a satisfactory clinical response provided that the side effects are tolerated.

*Elderly:* The elimination half-life may be increased in some elderly patients, therefore, dosage should be individually titrated commencing at 3 mg twice a day. The final dosage will depend on response and tolerance to side-effects. As with other anticholinergic drugs, caution should be observed in frail and elderly patients.

*Contra-indications:* Cystrin is contra-indicated in patients who are hypersensitive to the drug. It is also contraindicated in patients with a significant degree of bladder outflow obstruction where precipitation of urinary retention may occur.

Cystrin is contra-indicated in myasthenia gravis, glaucoma (since it may raise intra-ocular pressure) and in patients with intestinal atony, severe ulcerative colitis, toxic megacolon and other functional or organic gastrointestinal obstructive disorders, including hiatus hernia.

*Special warnings and precautions:* Cystrin should be used with caution in the frail elderly and in patients with autonomic neuropathy, hepatic or renal disease.

The symptoms of hyperthyroidism, coronary artery disease, congestive cardiac failure, cardiac arrhythmias and prostatic hypertrophy may be aggravated following administration of Cystrin.

Special care should be taken in patients with hiatus hernia associated with reflux oesophagitis, as anticholinergic drugs can aggravate this condition.

*Interaction with other medicines and other forms of interaction:* Care should be taken if other anticholinergic agents are administered together with Cystrin, as potentiation of anticholinergic effects can occur.

Occasional cases of interaction between anticholinergics and phenothiazines, amantidine, butyrophenones, L-dopa, digitalis and tricyclic antidepressants have been reported and care should be taken if Cystrin is administered concurrently with such drugs.

Cystrin by reducing gastro-intestinal motility may affect absorption of other drugs.

*Pregnancy and lactation:* There is no experience of the use of oxybutynin during pregnancy in humans, however, in foetal toxicity and fertility studies in animals, effects were seen on reproductive processes at dosages associated with maternal toxicity. Cystrin should, therefore, only be prescribed during pregnancy if considered essential. In the absence of animal data on the levels of oxybutynin in milk, Cystrin should not be administered to women who are breast-feeding.

*Effects on ability to drive and use machinery:* As Cystrin may produce drowsiness or blurred vision, the patient should be cautioned regarding activities requiring mental alertness such as driving, operating machinery or performing hazardous work while taking this drug.

*Other undesirable effects:* The most frequently reported side effects to oxybutynin are: dry mouth, constipation, blurred vision, nausea, abdominal discomfort, facial flushing and difficulty in micturition. The incidence of facial flushing is more marked in children than adults. The occurrence of these effects may be reduced by lowering the dose. Side effects reported less frequently include: headache, urinary retention, dizziness, drowsiness, skin reactions including rash, angioedema and photosensitivity, diarrhoea, cardiac arrhythmias, excitatory effects on CNS including restlessness, disorientation and hallucinations. Children may be more liable to such effects. Convulsions.

*Overdose:* The symptoms of overdosage with Cystrin progress from an intensification of the usual side-

effects of CNS disturbances (from restlessness and excitement to psychotic behaviour), circulatory changes (flushing, fall in blood pressure, circulatory failure etc), respiratory failure, paralysis and coma.

Measures to be taken are: (1) immediate gastric lavage and (2) physostigmine 1.0 to 2.0 mg by slow intravenous injection, repeated as necessary up to a total of 5.0 mg.

Fever should be treated symptomatically with tepid sponging or ice packs.

In pronounced restlessness or excitation, diazepam 10 mg may be given by intravenous injection. Tachycardia may be treated with intravenous propanolol and urinary retention managed by bladder catheterization.

In the event of progression of the curare-like effect to paralysis of the respiratory muscles, mechanical ventilation will be required.

**Pharmacological properties**

*Pharmacodynamic properties:* Oxybutynin hydrochloride is an anticholinergic agent which also exerts a direct antispasmodic effect on smooth muscle. It inhibits bladder contractions and relieves spasm induced by various stimuli; it increases bladder volume, diminishes the frequency of contractions and delays the desire to void in the disturbance of neurogenic bladder. The relaxation of smooth muscle results from the papaverin like effect of the antagonism of the processes distal to the neuromuscular junction in addition to the anticholinergic blocking action of the muscarinic type receptors. In addition oxybutynin hydrochloride has local anaesthetic properties.

*Pharmacokinetic properties:* Pharmacodynamic reports show oxybutynin to be rapidly absorbed from the gastrointestinal tract following oral administration with maximum plasma concentrations reached in less than 1 hour subsequently falling bioexponentially with a half-life of between 2 and 3 hours. Maximum effect can be seen within 3 – 4 hours with some effect still evident after 10 hours.

Repeated oral administration achieved steady state after eight days. Oxybutynin does not appear to accumulate in elderly patients and the pharmacokinetics are similar to those in other adults.

*Preclinical safety data:* No additional data available.

**Pharmaceutical particulars**

*List of excipients:*

| | |
|---|---|
| Lactose | PhEur |
| Maize starch | PhEur |
| Polyvidone 25000 | PhEur |
| Talc | PhEur |
| Magnesium stearate | PhEur |
| Purified water | PhEur |

*Film-coating ingredients:*

| | |
|---|---|
| Methylhydroxypropylcellulose | PhEur |
| Methylhydroxypropylcellulose phthalate | PhEur |
| Ethanol 96% v/v* | FDS |
| Purified water | PhEur |

\* Finnish Drug Standards

*Incompatibilities:* None known.

*Shelf-life:* 3 years

*Special precautions for storage:* To be stored in a dry place below 25°C.

*Nature and contents of container:* Pack size of 56. Containers are of pigmented high density polyethylene each fitted with a tamper-evident tear strip closure of pigmented low density polyethylene; or alternatively, in aluminium/PVC blister strips which are contained within a printed cardboard carton.

*Instructions for use/handling:* No relevance.

**Marketing authorisation number** 3433/0145

**Date of approval/revision of the SPC** 05 November 1996

**Legal category** POM

## CYSTRIN 5 mg

**Qualitative and quantitative composition** Oxybutynin hydrochloride 5.1 mg equivalent to oxybutynin 5.0 mg.

**Pharmaceutical form** Tablet.

**Clinical particulars**

*Therapeutic indications:* Cystrin is indicated for urinary incontinence, urgency and frequency in unstable bladder conditions due either to idiopathic detrusor instability or neurogenic bladder disorders (detrusor hyperreflexia) in conditions such as spina bifida and multiple sclerosis.

In addition, for children over 5 years of age, oxybutynin may be used in nocturnal enuresis in

conjunction with non-drug therapy where this alone, or in conjunction with other drug treatment, has failed.

*Posology and method of administration:*

*Children under 5 years of age:* Not recommended

*Children over 5 years of age:*
*Neurogenic bladder disorders:* The usual dose is 5 mg twice a day. This may be increased to a maximum of 5 mg three times a day to obtain a clinical response provided that the side effects are tolerated.

*Nocturnal enuresis:* The usual dose is 5 mg two or three times a day. The last dose should be given before bedtime.

In children the maintenance dose may be achieved by upward titration from an initial dose of 3 mg twice daily.

*Adults:* The usual dose is 5 mg two or three times a day. This may be increased to a maximum dosage of 5 mg four times a day (20 mg) to obtain a satisfactory clinical response provided that the side effects are tolerated.

*Elderly:* The elimination half-life may be increased in some elderly patients, therefore, dosage should be individually titrated commencing at 3 mg twice a day. The final dosage will depend on response and tolerance to side-effects. As with other anticholinergic drugs, caution should be observed in frail and elderly patients.

*Contra-indications:* Cystrin is contra-indicated in patients who are hypersensitive to the drug. It is also contraindicated in patients with a significant degree of bladder outflow obstruction where precipitation of urinary retention may occur.

Cystrin is contraindicated in myasthenia gravis, glaucoma (since it may raise intra-ocular pressure) and in patients with intestinal atony, severe ulcerative colitis, toxic megacolon and other functional or organic gastrointestinal obstructive disorders, including hiatus hernia.

*Special warnings and precautions:* Cystrin should be used with caution in the frail elderly and in patients with autonomic neuropathy, hepatic or renal disease.

The symptoms of hyperthyroidism, coronary artery disease, congestive cardiac failure, cardiac arrhythmias and prostatic hypertrophy may be aggravated following administration of Cystrin.

Special care should be taken in patients with hiatus hernia associated with reflux oesophagitis, as anticholinergic drugs can aggravate this condition.

*Interaction with other medicines and other forms of interaction:* Care should be taken if other anticholinergic agents are administered together with Cystrin, as potentiation of anticholinergic effects can occur.

Occasional cases of interaction between anticholinergics and phenothiazines, amantidine, butyrophenones, L-dopa, digitalis and tricyclic antidepressants have been reported and care should be taken if Cystrin is administered concurrently with such drugs.

Cystrin by reducing gastro-intestinal motility may affect absorption of other drugs.

*Pregnancy and lactation:* There is no experience of the use of oxybutynin during pregnancy in humans, however, in foetal toxicity and fertility studies in animals, effects were seen on reproductive processes at dosages associated with maternal toxicity. Cystrin should, therefore, only be prescribed during pregnancy if considered essential. In the absence of animal data on the levels of oxybutynin in milk, Cystrin should not be administered to women who are breast-feeding.

*Effects on ability to drive and use machines:* As Cystrin may produce drowsiness or blurred vision, the patient should be cautioned regarding activities requiring mental alertness such as driving, operating machinery or performing hazardous work while taking this drug.

*Other undesirable effects:* The most frequently reported side effects to oxybutynin are: dry mouth, constipation, blurred vision, nausea, abdominal discomfort, facial flushing and difficulty in micturition. The incidence of facial flushing is more marked in children than adults. The occurrence of these effects may be reduced by lowering the dose. Side effects reported less frequently include: headache, urinary retention, dizziness, drowsiness, skin reactions including rash, angioedema and photosensitivity, diarrhoea, cardiac arrhythmias, excitatory effects on CNS including restlessness, disorientation and hallucinations. Children may be more liable to such effects. Convulsions.

*Overdose:* The symptoms of overdosage with Cystrin progress from an intensification of the usual side-effects of CNS disturbances (from restlessness and excitement to psychotic behaviour), circulatory changes (flushing, fall in blood pressure, circulatory failure etc), respiratory failure, paralysis and coma.

Measures to be taken are: (1) immediate gastric lavage and (2) physostigmine 1.0 to 2.0 mg by slow intravenous injection, repeated as necessary up to a total of 5.0 mg.

Fever should be treated symptomatically with tepid sponging or ice packs.

In pronounced restlessness or excitation, diazepam 10 mg may be given by intravenous injection. Tachycardia may be treated with intravenous propanolol and urinary retention managed by bladder catheterization.

In the event of progression of the curare-like effect to paralysis of the respiratory muscles, mechanical ventilation will be required.

## Pharmacological properties

*Pharmacodynamic properties:* Oxybutynin hydrochloride is an anticholinergic agent which also exerts a direct antispasmodic effect on smooth muscle. It inhibits bladder contractions and relieves spasm induced by various stimuli; it increases bladder volume, diminishes the frequency of contractions and delays the desire to void in the disturbance of neurogenic bladder. The relaxation of smooth muscle results from the papaverin like effect of the antagonism of the processes distal to the neuromuscular junction in addition to the anticholinergic blocking action of the muscarinic type receptors. In addition oxybutynin hydrochloride has local anaesthetic properties.

*Pharmacokinetic properties:* Pharmacodynamic reports show oxybutynin to be rapidly absorbed from the gastrointestinal tract following oral administration with maximum plasma concentrations reached in less than 1 hour subsequently falling bioexponentially with a half-life of between 2 and 3 hours. Maximum effect can be seen within 3 – 4 hours with some effect still evident after 10 hours.

Repeated oral administration achieved steady state after eight days. Oxybutynin does not appear to accumulate in elderly patients and the pharmacokinetics are similar to those in other adults.

*Preclinical safety data:* No additional data available.

## Pharmaceutical particulars

*List of excipients:*

| | |
|---|---|
| Lactose | PhEur |
| Maize starch | PhEur |
| Polyvidone 25000 | PhEur |
| Talc | PhEur |
| Magnesium stearate | PhEur |
| Purified water | PhEur |

*Film-coating ingredients*

| | |
|---|---|
| Methylhydroxypropylcellulose | PhEur |
| Methylhydroxypropylcellulose phthalate | PhEur |
| Ethanol 96% v/v* | FDS |
| Purified water | PhEur |

* Finnish Drug Standards

*Incompatibilities:* None known.

*Shelf-life:* 3 years

*Special precautions for storage:* To be stored in a dry place below 25°C.

*Nature and contents of container:* Pack size of 84. Containers are of pigmented high density polyethylene each fitted with a tamper-evident tear strip closure of pigmented low density polyethylene; or alternatively, in aluminium/PVC blister strips which are contained within a printed cardboard carton.

*Instructions for use/handling:* No relevance.

**Marketing authorisation number** 3433/0146

**Date of approval/revision of SPC** 05 November 1996

**Legal category** POM

# CYTOSAR 100 mg and 500 mg

**Qualitative and quantitative composition** Cytarabine PhEur 100 mg or 500 mg.

**Pharmaceutical form** Powder for injection.

**Clinical particulars**

*Therapeutic indications:* Cytotoxic for induction of remission in acute myeloid leukaemia in adults and for other acute leukaemias of adults and children.

*Posology and method of administration:* By intravenous infusion or injection, or subcutaneous injection. Water for Injections, 0.9% saline or 5% dextrose should be used for preparing a solution of cytarabine in the vial. When the accompanying diluent (Water for Injections) is used, such solution contains 20 mg/ml (100 mg vial) or 50 mg/ml (500 mg vial) cytarabine.

The physician is reminded that in practice Cytosar has been administered in combination with a variety of other cytotoxic agents using a number of different dosage schedules, and reference to the current literature before commencing treatment is recommended.

Dosage recommendations may be converted from those in terms of bodyweight to those related to surface area by means of nomograms such as are presented in Documenta Geigy.

*(1) Remission induction:*
  (a) Continuous treatment:
    (i) Rapid injection – 2 mg/kg/day is a judicious starting dose. Administer for 10 days. Obtain daily blood counts. If no antileukaemic effect is noted and there is no apparent toxicity, increase to 4 mg/kg/day and maintain until therapeutic response or toxicity is evident. Almost all patients can be carried to toxicity with these doses.
    (ii) 0.5 – 1.0 mg/kg/day may be given in an infusion of up to 24 hours duration. Results from one-hour infusions have been satisfactory in the majority of patients. After 10 days this initial daily dose may be increased to 2 mg/kg/day subject to toxicity. Continue to toxicity or until remission occurs.
  (b) Intermittent treatment:
    3 – 5 mg/kg/day are administered intravenously on each of five consecutive days. After a two to nine-day rest period, a further course is given. Continue until response or toxicity occurs.

The first evidence of marrow improvement has been reported to occur 7 – 64 days (mean 28 days) after the beginning of therapy.

In general, if a patient shows neither toxicity nor remission after a fair trial, the cautious administration of higher doses is warranted. As a rule, patients have been seen to tolerate higher doses when given by rapid intravenous injection as compared with slow infusion. This difference is due to the rapid metabolism of Cytosar and the consequent short duration of action of the high dose.

*(2) Maintenance therapy:* Remissions which have been induced by cytarabine, or by other drugs, may be maintained by intravenous or subcutaneous injection of 1 mg/kg once or twice weekly.

*Children:* Children appear to tolerate higher doses than adults and, where dose ranges are quoted, the children should receive the higher dose and the adults the lower.

*Elderly patients:* There is no information to suggest that a change in dosage is warranted in the elderly. Nevertheless, the elderly patient does not tolerate drug toxicity as well as the younger patient, and particular attention should thus be given to drug induced leucopenia, thrombocytopenia, and anaemia, with appropriate initiation of supportive therapy when indicated.

*Contra-indications:* Therapy with Cytosar should not be considered in patients with pre-existing drug-induced bone marrow suppression, unless the clinician feels that such management offers the most hopeful alternative for the patient. Cytosar should not be used in the management of non-malignant disease, except for immunosuppression.

*Special warnings and special precautions for use:* Cytosar is a potent bone marrow suppressant. Therapy should be started cautiously in patients with pre-existing drug-induced bone marrow suppression. Patients receiving this drug must be under close medical supervision and, during induction therapy, should have leucocyte and platelet counts performed daily. Bone marrow examinations should be performed frequently after blasts have disappeared from the peripheral blood. Facilities should be available for management of complications, possibly fatal, of bone marrow suppression (infection resulting from granulocytopenia and other impaired body defences, and haemorrhage secondary to thrombocytopenia). One case of anaphylaxis that resulted in acute cardiopulmonary arrest and required resuscitation has been reported. This occurred immediately after the intravenous administration of Cytosar.

Severe and at times fatal CNS, GI and pulmonary toxicity (different from that seen with conventional therapy regimens of Cytosar) has been reported following some experimental Cytosar dose schedules. These reactions include reversible corneal toxicity; cerebral and cerebellar dysfunction, usually reversible; severe gastro-intestinal ulceration, including pneumatosis cystoides intestinalis, leading to peritonitis; sepsis and liver abscess; and pulmonary oedema.

Cytosar has been shown to be carcinogenic in animals. The possibility of a similar effect should be borne in mind when designing the long-term management of the patient.

Patients receiving Cytosar must be monitored closely. Frequent platelet and leucocyte counts are mandatory. Suspend or modify therapy when drug-induced marrow depression has resulted in a platelet count under 50,000 or a polymorphonuclear count under 1,000 per cubic mm. Counts of formed elements in the peripheral blood may continue to fall after the drug is stopped, and reach lowest values after drug-free intervals of five to seven days. If indicated, restart therapy when definite signs of marrow recovery appear (on successive bone marrow studies). Patients whose drug is withheld until 'normal' peripheral blood values are attained may escape from control.

When intravenous doses are given quickly, patients are frequently nauseated and may vomit for several hours afterwards. This problem tends to be less severe when the drug is infused.

The human liver apparently detoxifies a substantial fraction of an administered dose. Use the drug with caution and at reduced dose in patients whose liver function is poor.

Periodical checks of bone marrow, liver and kidney functions should be performed in patients receiving Cytosar.

The safety of this drug for use in infants is not established.

Like other cytotoxic drugs, Cytosar may induce hyperuricaemia secondary to rapid lysis of neoplastic cells. The clinician should monitor the patient's blood uric acid level and be prepared to use such supportive and pharmacological measures as may be necessary to control this problem.

*Interaction with other medicaments and other forms of interaction:* None have been reported.

*Pregnancy and lactation:* Cytosar is known to be teratogenic in some animal species. The use of Cytosar in women who are, or who may become, pregnant should be undertaken only after due consideration of the potential benefits and hazards.

This product should not normally be administered to patients who are pregnant or to mothers who are breast-feeding.

*Effects on ability to drive and use machines:* No adverse effect has been reported.

*Undesirable effects:* Adverse reactions seen with cytarabine treatment have included those seen with cytotoxic agents having an effect on bone marrow, such as: leucopenia, thrombocytopenia, anaemia, bone marrow suppression and megaloblastosis. Other side-effects have included: nausea, vomiting, diarrhoea, oral ulceration, hepatic dysfunction. Occasional adverse experiences have been reported as follows: renal dysfunction, anorexia, sepsis, gastrointestinal haemorrhage, irritation or sepsis at site of injection, neuritis or neurotoxicity, rash, freckling, oesophagitis, skin and mucosal bleeding, chest pain, joint pain and reduction in reticulocytes.

A Cytosar syndrome has been described. It is characterised by fever, myalgia, bone pain, occasionally chest pain, maculopapular rash, conjunctivitis and malaise. It usually occurs 6–12 hours following drug administration. Corticosteroids have been shown to be beneficial in treating or preventing this syndrome. If the symptoms of the syndrome are serious enough to warrant treatment, corticosteroids should be contemplated as well as continuation of therapy with Cytosar.

Cytosar is not recommended for intrathecal use; however, the following side-effects have been reported with such use. Expected systemic reactions: bone marrow depression, nausea, vomiting. Occasionally, severe spinal cord toxicity even leading to quadriplegia and paralysis, necrotising encephalopathy, blindness and other isolated neurotoxicities have been reported.

*Overdose:* Cessation of therapy, followed by management of ensuing bone marrow depression including whole blood or platelet transfusion and antibiotics as required.

**Pharmacological properties**

*Pharmacodynamic properties:* Cytarabine, a pyrimidine nucleoside analogue, is an antineoplastic agent which inhibits the synthesis of deoxyribonucleic acid. It also has antiviral and immunosuppressant properties. Detailed studies on the mechanism of cytotoxicity *in vitro* suggests that the primary action of cytarabine is inhibition of deoxycytidine synthesis, although inhibition of cytidylic kinases and incorporation of the compound into nucleic acids may also play a role in its cytostatic and cytocidal actions.

*Pharmacokinetic properties:* Cytarabine is deaminated to arabinofuranosyl uracil in the liver and kidneys. After intravenous administration to humans, only 5.8% of the administered dose is excreted unaltered in the urine within 12–24 hours, 90% of the dose is excreted as the deaminated product. Cytosar appears to be metabolised rapidly, primarily by the liver and perhaps by the kidney. After single high intravenous doses, blood levels fall to unmeasurable levels within 15 minutes in most patients. Some patients have in demonstrable circulating drug as early as 5 minutes after injection.

**Pharmaceutical particulars**

*List of excipients:* None.

*Incompatibilities:* None.

*Shelf-life:* Shelf-life of the medicinal product as packaged for sale: 60 months.

Solutions reconstituted with Water for Injections, 0.9% saline, or 5% dextrose must be used immediately and not stored. When reconstituted with the accompanying diluent, solutions should be stored at room temperature and used within 48 hours.

Discard any solution in which a slight haze develops.

*Special precautions for storage:* Store at room temperature.

*Nature and contents of container:* Type I flint glass vial with butyl rubber plug and aluminium flip off seal.

Each vial contains 100 mg or 500 mg of cytarabine.

*Instructions for use/handling:* No special requirements.

**Marketing authorisation numbers**
100 mg          0032/5037
500 mg          0032/0109

**Date of approval/revision of SPC**  August 1996

**Legal category** POM

## DALACIN* C CAPSULES 75 MG, 150 MG
## DALACIN* C PAEDIATRIC

**Presentation** Hard-filled, gelatin capsules (lavender/lavender) containing clindamycin hydrochloride equivalent to 75 mg clindamycin. Also contains: lactose, maize starch, talc, magnesium stearate, gelatin, E132 and E127.

Hard-filled, gelatin capsules (maroon/lavender) containing clindamycin hydrochloride equivalent to 150 mg clindamycin. Also contains: lactose, maize starch, talc, magnesium stearate, gelatin, E132, E127 and E171.

Off-white, sucrose-based granules for paediatric suspension, with pineapple flavour. Each 5 ml reconstituted suspension contains clindamycin palmitate hydrochloride equivalent to 75 mg clindamycin. Also contains: sucrose, pluronic F-68, sorbic acid, dimethicone and pineapple flavour.

**Uses**  *Indications:* Antibacterial. Serious infections caused by susceptible Gram-positive organisms, staphylococci (both penicillinase- and non-penicillinase-producing), streptococci (except *Streptococcus faecalis*) and pneumococci. It is also indicated in serious infections caused by susceptible anaerobic pathogens.

Clindamycin does not penetrate the blood/brain barrier in therapeutically effective quantities.

*Mechanism of action:* Lincosamides such as clindamycin bind to the 50S subunit of the bacterial ribosome similarly to macrolides such as erythromycin and inhibit the early stages of protein synthesis. The action of clindamycin is predominantly bacteriostatic although high concentrations may be slowly bactericidal against sensitive strains.

*Pharmacology:* Clindamycin is a lincosamide antibiotic with a primarily bacteriostatic action against Gram-positive aerobes and a wide range of anaerobic bacteria. Most Gram-negative aerobic bacteria, including the Enterobacteriaceae, are resistant to clindamycin. Clindamycin demonstrates cross-resistance with lincomycin. When tested by *in vitro* methods, some staphylococcal strains originally resistant to erythromycin rapidly developed resistance to clindamycin. The mechanisms for resistance are the same as for erythromycin, namely methylation of the ribosomal binding site, chromosomal mutation of the ribosomal protein and in a few staphylococcal isolates, enzymic inactivation by a plasmid-mediated adenyltransferase.

*Pharmacokinetics:* About 90% of a dose of clindamycin hydrochloride is absorbed from the gastro-intestinal tract; concentrations of 2 to 3 micrograms per ml occur within one hour after a 150 mg dose of clindamycin, with average concentrations of about 0.7 micrograms per ml after 6 hours. After doses of 300 and 600 mg, peak plasma concentrations of 4 and 8 micrograms per ml, respectively, have been reported. Absorption is not significantly diminished by food in the stomach, but the rate of absorption may be reduced.

Clindamycin is widely distributed in body fluids and tissues including bone, but it does not reach the cerebrospinal fluid in significant concentrations. It diffuses across the placenta into the fetal circulation and appears in breast milk. High concentrations occur in bile. It accumulates in leucocytes and macrophages. Over 90% of clindamycin in the circulation is bound to plasma proteins. The half-life is 2 to 3 hours, although this may be prolonged in pre-term neonates and patients with severe renal impairment.

Clindamycin undergoes metabolism, presumably in the liver, to the active *N*-demethyl and sulphoxide metabolites and also some inactive metabolites. About 10% of the drug is excreted in the urine as active drug or metabolites and about 4% in the faeces;

the remainder is excreted as inactive metabolites. Excretion is slow and takes place over several days. It is not effectively removed from the blood by dialysis.

**Dosage and administration**

*Oral:* Absorption of Dalacin C is not appreciably modified by the presence of food.

*Capsules: Adults:* moderately severe infection, 150 – 300 mg every six hours; severe infection, 300 – 450 mg every six hours. Dalacin C Capsules should always be taken with a glass of water.

*Paediatric:* to each 100 ml bottle of granules add 74 ml purified water and shake.

*Children:* 3 – 6 mg/kg every six hours depending on the severity of the infection.

In children under one year or weighing 10 kg or less the minimum recommended dose is 2.5 ml (37.5 mg) every eight hours.

The following paediatric dose regime is recommended as a guide:

*Moderately severe infection:* 0–11 months: 3.5 – 9.0 kg: 2.5 ml every eight hours.
1 – 3 years: 10 – 15 kg: 2.5 ml every six hours.
4 – 7 years: 16 – 25 kg: 5 ml every six hours.
8 – 12 years: 26 – 38 kg: 7.5 ml every six hours.
*Severe infection:* 0 – 11 months: 3.5 – 9.0 kg: 2.5 ml every six hours.
1 – 3 years: 10 – 15 kg: 5 ml every six hours.
4 – 7 years: 16 – 25 kg: 7.5 ml every six hours.
8 – 12 years: 26 – 38 kg: 10 ml every six hours.

*Adults:* moderately severe infection: 10 ml every six hours; severe infection: 20 ml every six hours.

Note: In cases of beta-haemolytic streptococcal infection, treatment with Dalacin C should continue for at least 10 days to diminish the likelihood of subsequent rheumatic fever or glomerulonephritis.

*Elderly patients:* The half-life, volume of distribution and clearance and extent of absorption after administration of clindamycin hydrochloride are not altered by increased age. Analysis of data from clinical studies has not revealed any age-related increase in toxicity. Dosage requirements in elderly patients, therefore, should not be influenced by age alone. See *Precautions* for other factors which should be taken into consideration.

**Contra-indications, warnings, etc.**

*Contra-indications:* Dalacin C is contra-indicated in patients previously found to be sensitive to clindamycin or lincomycin.

*Interactions with other medicaments:* Clindamycin has been shown to have neuromuscular blocking properties that may enhance the action of other neuromuscular blocking agents. It should be used with caution, therefore, in patients receiving such agents.

Antagonism has been demonstrated between clindamycin and erythromycin in vitro. Because of possible clinical significance the two drugs should not be administered concurrently.

*Effects on ability to drive and to use machines:* Not applicable

*Other undesirable effects: Gastro-intestinal tract:* Nausea, vomiting, abdominal pain and diarrhoea (see *Warnings*).

*Haematopoietic:* Transient neutropenia (leucopenia), eosinophilia, agranulocytosis and thrombocytopenia have been reported. No direct aetiologic relationship to concurrent clindamycin therapy could be made in any of the foregoing.

*Skin and mucous membranes:* Pruritus, vaginitis and rare instances of exfoliative and vesiculobullous dermatitis have been reported.

*Hypersensitivity reactions:* Maculopapular rash and urticaria have been observed during drug therapy. Generalised mild to moderate morbilliform-like skin rashes are the most frequently reported reactions. Rare instances of erythema multiforme, some resembling Stevens-Johnson syndrome, have been associated with clindamycin. A few cases of anaphylactoid reactions have been reported.

*Liver:* Jaundice and abnormalities in liver function tests have been observed during clindamycin therapy.

*Use in pregnancy and lactation:* Safety for use in pregnancy has not yet been established.

Clindamycin is excreted in human milk. Caution should be exercised when Dalacin C is administered to a nursing mother. It is unlikely that a nursing infant can absorb a significant amount of clindamycin from its gastro-intestinal tract.

*Other special warnings and precautions:*

*Warnings:* Dalacin C should only be used in the treatment of serious infections. In considering the use of the product, the practitioner should bear in mind the type of infection and the potential hazard of the diarrhoea which may develop, since cases of colitis have been reported during, or even two or three weeks following, the administration of clindamycin.

Studies indicate a toxin(s) produced by clostridia (especially *Clostridium difficile*) is the principal direct cause of antibiotic-associated colitis. These studies also indicate that this toxigenic clostridium is usually sensitive in vitro to vancomycin. When 125 mg to 500 mg of vancomycin are administered orally four times a day for 7 – 10 days, there is a rapid observed disappearance of the toxin from faecal samples and a coincident clinical recovery from the diarrhoea. (Where the patient is receiving cholestyramine in addition to vancomycin, consideration should be given to separating the times of administration).

Colitis is a disease which has a clinical spectrum from mild, watery diarrhoea to severe, persistent diarrhoea, leucocytosis, fever, severe abdominal cramps, which may be associated with the passage of blood and mucus. If allowed to progress, it may produce peritonitis, shock and toxic megacolon. This may be fatal.

The appearance of marked diarrhoea should be regarded as an indication that the product should be discontinued immediately. The disease is likely to follow a more severe course in older patients or patients who are debilitated. Diagnosis is usually made by the recognition of the clinical symptoms, but can be substantiated by endoscopic demonstration of pseudomembranous colitis. The presence of the disease may be further confirmed by culture of the stool for *Clostridium difficile* on selective media and assay of the stool specimen for the toxin(s) of *C. difficile.*

*Precautions:* Caution should be used when prescribing Dalacin C to individuals with a history of gastrointestinal disease, especially colitis.

Periodic liver and kidney function tests should be carried out during prolonged therapy. Such monitoring is also recommended in neonates and infants.

The dosage of Dalacin C may require reduction in patients with renal or hepatic impairment due to prolongation of the serum half-life.

Prolonged administration of Dalacin C, as with any anti-infective, may result in super-infection due to organisms resistant to clindamycin.

Care should be observed in the use of Dalacin C in atopic individuals.

*Overdosage:* In cases of overdosage no specific treatment is indicated.

The serum biological half-life of clindamycin is 2.4 hours. Clindamycin cannot readily be removed from the blood by dialysis or peritoneal dialysis.

If an allergic adverse reaction occurs, therapy should be with the usual emergency treatments, including corticosteroids, adrenaline and antihistamines.

*Incompatibilities:* None known.

**Pharmaceutical precautions:** Capsules: Store below 25°C.

Dalacin C Paediatric Granules are stable at room temperature (18–25°C) for at least 24 months.

Following reconstitution the paediatric suspension is stable for up to two weeks at room temperature.

Where further dilution is required use purified water.

**Legal category**  POM

**Package quantities**  75 mg capsules in packs of 24, 150 mg capsules in packs of 24 and 100, Paediatric granules to make 100 ml suspension.

**Product licence numbers**
Dalacin C Capsules 75 mg          0032/5006
Dalacin C Capsules 150 mg         0032/5007
Dalacin C Paediatric              0032/0023

## DALACIN* C PHOSPHATE

**Qualitative and quantitative composition**  Each ml of solution contains Clindamycin Phosphate BP equivalent to 150 mg clindamycin.

**Pharmaceutical form**  Clear, colourless, sterile solution for intramuscular or intravenous use.

**Clinical particulars**

*Therapeutic indications:* Antibacterial. Serious infections caused by susceptible Gram-positive organisms, staphylococci (both penicillinase- and non-penicillinase-producing), streptococci (except *Streptococcus faecalis*) and pneumococci. It is also indicated in serious infections caused by susceptible anaerobic pathogens such as Bacteroides spp, Fusobacterium spp, Propionibacterium spp, Peptostreptococcus spp. and microaerophilic streptococci.

Clindamycin does not penetrate the blood/brain barrier in therapeutically effective quantities.

*Posology and method of administration:* Parenteral (i.m. or iv administration). Dalacin C Phosphate must be diluted prior to iv administration and should be infused over at least 10–60 minutes.

*Adults:* Serious infections: 600 mg – 1.2 g/day in two, three or four equal doses.

More severe infections: l.2–2.7 g/day in two, three or four equal doses.

Single i.m. injections of greater than 600 mg are not recommended nor is administration of more than 1.2 g in a single one-hour infusion.

For more serious infections, these doses may have to be increased. In life-threatening situations, doses as high as 4.8 g daily have been given intravenously to adults.

Alternatively, the drug may be administered in the form of a single rapid infusion of the first dose followed by continuous iv infusion.

*Children (over 1 month of age):* Serious infections: 15–25 mg/kg/day in three or four equal doses.

More severe infections: 25–40 mg/kg/day in three or four equal doses. In severe infections it is recommended that children be given no less than 300 mg/day regardless of body weight.

*Elderly patients:* The half-life, volume of distribution and clearance and extent of absorption after administration of clindamycin phosphate are not altered by increased age. Analysis of data from clinical studies has not revealed any age-related increase in toxicity. Dosage requirements in elderly patients should not be influenced, therefore, by age alone. See *Precautions* for other factors which should be taken into consideration.

Treatment for infections caused by beta-haemolytic streptococci should be continued for at least 10 days to guard against subsequent rheumatic fever or glomerulonephritis.

*Contra-indications:* Dalacin C Phosphate is contra-indicated in patients previously found to be sensitive to clindamycin or lincomycin.

*Special warnings and special precautions for use:*
*Warnings:* This product contains benzyl alcohol. Benzyl alcohol has been reported to be associated with a fatal 'Gasping syndrome' in premature infants.

Dalacin C Phosphate should only be used in the treatment of serious infections. In considering the use of the product, the practitioner should bear in mind the type of infection and the potential hazard of the diarrhoea which may develop, since cases of colitis have been reported during, or even two or three weeks following, the administration of clindamycin.

Studies indicate a toxin(s) produced by clostridia (especially *Clostridium difficile*) is the principal direct cause of antibiotic-associated colitis. These studies also indicate that this toxigenic clostridium is usually sensitive *in vitro* to vancomycin. When 125 mg to 500 mg of vancomycin are administered orally four times a day for 7 – 10 days, there is a rapid observed disappearance of the toxin from faecal samples and a coincident clinical recovery from the diarrhoea. (Where the patient is receiving cholestyramine in addition to vancomycin, consideration should be given to separating the times of administration).

Colitis is a disease which has a clinical spectrum from mild, watery diarrhoea to severe, persistent diarrhoea, leucocytosis, fever, severe abdominal cramps, which may be associated with the passage of blood and mucus. If allowed to progress, it may produce peritonitis, shock and toxic megacolon. This may be fatal. The appearance of marked diarrhoea should be regarded as an indication that the product should be discontinued immediately. The disease is likely to follow a more severe course in older patients or patients who are debilitated. Diagnosis is usually made by the recognition of the clinical symptoms, but can be substantiated by endoscopic demonstration of pseudomembranous colitis. The presence of the disease may be further confirmed by culture of the stool for *C. difficile* on selective media and assay of the stool specimen for the toxin(s) of *C. difficile.*

*Precautions:* Caution should be used when prescribing Dalacin C Phosphate to individuals with a history of gastro-intestinal disease, especially colitis.

Periodic liver and kidney function tests should be carried out during prolonged therapy. Such monitoring is also recommended in neonates and infants. Safety and appropriate dosage in infants less than one month old have not been established.

The dosage of Dalacin C Phosphate may require reduction in patients with renal or hepatic impairment due to prolongation of the serum half-life.

Prolonged administration of Dalacin C Phosphate, as with any anti-infective, may result in super-infection due to organisms resistant to clindamycin.

Care should be observed in the use of Dalacin C Phosphate in atopic individuals.

*Interaction with other medicaments and other forms of interaction:* Clindamycin has been shown to have neuromuscular blocking properties that may enhance the action of other neuromuscular blocking agents. It should be used with caution, therefore, in patients receiving such agents.

Antagonism has been demonstrated between clindamycin and erythromycin *in vitro.* Because of possible clinical significance, the two drugs should not be administered concurrently.

*Pregnancy and lactation:* Safety for use in pregnancy has not been established.

Clindamycin is excreted in human milk. Caution should be exercised when Dalacin C Phosphate is administered to a nursing mother. It is unlikely that a nursing infant can absorb a significant amount of clindamycin from its gastro-intestinal tract.

*Effects on ability to drive and use machines:* None known

*Undesirable effects: Gastro-intestinal tract:* Nausea, vomiting, abdominal pain and diarrhoea (See *Warnings*).

*Haematopoietic:* Transient neutropenia (leucopenia), eosinophilia, agranulocytosis and thrombocytopenia have been reported. No direct aetiologic relationship to concurrent clindamycin therapy could be made in any of the foregoing.

*Skin and mucous membranes:* Pruritus, vaginitis and rare instances of exfoliative and vesiculobullous dermatitis have been reported.

*Hypersensitivity reactions:* Maculopapular rash and urticaria have been observed during drug therapy. Generalised mild to moderate morbilliform-like skin rashes are the most frequently reported reactions. Rare instances of erythema multiforme, some resembling Stevens-Johnson syndrome, have been associated with clindamycin. A few cases of anaphylactoid reactions have been reported.

*Liver:* Jaundice and abnormalities in liver function tests have been observed during clindamycin therapy.

*Cardiovascular:* Rare instances of cardiopulmonary arrest and hypotension have been reported following too rapid intravenous administration (see *Dosage and administration* section).

*Local reactions:* Local irritation, pain, abscess formation have been seen with i.m. injection. Thrombophlebitis has been reported with iv injection. These reactions can be minimized by deep i.m. injection and avoiding the use of an indwelling catheter.

*Overdose:* In cases of overdosage no specific treatment is indicated.

The serum biological half-life of clindamycin is 2.4 hours. Clindamycin cannot readily be removed from the blood by dialysis or peritoneal dialysis.

If an allergic adverse reaction occurs, therapy should be with the usual emergency treatments, including corticosteroids, adrenaline and antihistamines.

**Pharmacological properties**

*Pharmacodynamic properties:* Clindamycin is a lincosamide antibiotic with a primarily bacteriostatic action against Gram-positive aerobes and a wide range of anaerobic bacteria. Lincosamides such as clindamycin bind to the 50S subunit of the bacterial ribosome similarly to macrolides such as erythromycin and inhibit the early stages of protein synthesis. The action of clindamycin is predominantly bacteriostatic although high concentrations may be slowly bactericidal against sensitive strains.

Most Gram-negative aerobic bacteria, including the Enterobacteriaceae, are resistant to clindamycin. Clindamycin demonstrates cross-resistance with lincomycin. When tested by *in vitro* methods, some staphylococcal strains originally resistant to erythromycin rapidly developed resistance to clindamycin. The mechanisms for resistance are the same as for erythromycin, namely methylation of the ribosomal binding site, chromosomal mutation of the ribosomal protein and in a few staphylococcal isolates, enzymic inactivation by a plasmid-mediated adenyltransferase.

*Pharmacokinetic properties: General characteristics of active substance:* Following parenteral administration, the biologically inactive clindamycin phosphate is hydrolysed to clindamycin. When the equivalent of 300 mg of clindamycin is injected intramuscularly, a mean peak plasma concentration of 6 microgram/ml is achieved within three hours; 600 mg gives a peak concentration of 9 microgram/ml. In children, peak concentration may be reached within one hour. When the same doses are infused intravenously, peak concentrations of 7 and 10 micrograms per ml respectively are achieved by the end of infusion.

Clindamycin is widely distributed in body fluids and tissues including bone, but it does not reach the cerebrospinal fluid in significant concentrations. It diffuses across the placenta into the fetal circulation and appears in breast milk. High concentrations occur in bile. It accumulates in leucocytes and macrophages. Over 90% of clindamycin in the circulation is bound to plasma proteins. The half-life is 2 to 3 hours, although this may be prolonged in pre-term neonates and patients with severe renal impairment.

Clindamycin undergoes metabolism, to the active *N*-demethyl and sulphoxide metabolites and also some inactive metabolites. About 10% of the drug is excreted in the urine as active drug or metabolites and about 4% in the faeces; the remainder is excreted as inactive metabolites. Excretion is slow and takes place over several days, It is not effectively removed from the blood by dialysis.

*Characteristics in patients:* No special characteristics. See *Special warnings and special precautions for use* for further information.

**Pharmaceutical particulars**

*List of excipients:* Benzyl alcohol, disodium edetate, sterilised water for injections.

*Incompatibilities:* Solutions of clindamycin salts have a low pH and incompatibilities may reasonably be expected with alkaline preparations or drugs unstable at low pH. Incompatibility has been reported with: ampicillin sodium, aminophylline, barbiturates, calcium gluconate, ceftriaxone sodium, idarubicin hydrochloride, magnesium sulphate, phenytoin sodium and ranitidine hydrochloride.

*Shelf life:* Dalacin C Phosphate has a shelf-life of 24 months when stored below 25°C, avoiding refrigeration.

*Special precautions for storage for product and admixture storage:* Store below 25°C.

*Nature and contents of container:* Type 1 flint glass ampoule containing 2 ml or 4 ml sterile, aqueous solution, packed in cardboard carton, together with a leaflet.

*Instructions for use/handling:* Dalacin C Phosphate has been known to be physically and chemically compatible for at least 24 hours in dextrose 5% water and sodium chloride injection solutions containing the following antibiotics in usually administered concentrations: Amikacin sulphate, aztreonam, cefamandole nafate, cephazolin sodium, cefotaxime sodium, cefoxitin sodium, ceftazidime sodium, ceftizoxime sodium, gentamicin sulphate, netilmicin sulphate, piperacillin and tobramycin.

The compatibility and duration of stability of drug admixtures will vary depending upon concentration and other conditions.

**Marketing authorisation number** 0032/0042R

**Date of approval/revision of SPC** February 1996

**Legal category** POM

## DALACIN* T TOPICAL LOTION AND DALACIN* T TOPICAL SOLUTION

**Presentation** *Dalacin T Topical Solution:* Clear, colourless solution containing clindamycin phosphate (equivalent to clindamycin 10 mg/ml). The solution contains isopropyl alcohol, propylene glycol and water.

*Dalacin T Topical Lotion:* White to off-white emulsion containing clindamycin phosphate (equivalent to clindamycin 10 mg/ml), in an aqueous base containing glycerol, sodium lauroyl sarcosinate, stearic acid, tegin, cetostearyl alcohol, isostearyl alcohol and methylparaben.

**Uses** Treatment of acne vulgaris.

**Dosage and administration** Apply a thin film of Dalacin T Topical Solution or Lotion twice daily to the affected area.

**Contra-indications, warnings, etc**

*Contra-indications:* Dalacin T is contra-indicated in patients previously found to be hypersensitive to this antibiotic. Although cross-sensitisation to lincomycin has not been demonstrated, it is recommended that Dalacin T is not used in patients who have demonstrated lincomycin sensitivity.

*Warnings and precautions:* Oral and parenteral clindamycin, as well as most other antibiotics, have been associated with severe pseudomembranous colitis. However, post-marketing studies have indicated a very low incidence of colitis with Dalacin T Topical Solution. The physician should, nonetheless, be alert to the development of antibiotic-associated diarrhoea or colitis. If diarrhoea occurs, the product should be discontinued immediately.

Studies indicate a toxin(s) produced by *Clostridium difficile* is the major cause of antibiotic-associated colitis. Colitis is usually characterized by persistent, severe diarrhoea and abdominal cramps. Endoscopic examination may reveal pseudomembranous colitis. Stool culture for *C. difficile* and/or assay for *C. difficile* toxin may be helpful to diagnosis.

Vancomycin is effective in the treatment of antibiotic-associated colitis produced by *C. difficile.* The usual dose is 125 – 500 mg orally every 6 hours for 7 – 10 days. Additional supportive medical care may be necessary.

Mild cases of colitis may respond to discontinuance of clindamycin alone. Cholestyramine and colestipol resins have been shown to bind *C. difficile* toxin *in vitro* and cholestyramine has been effective in the treatment of some mild cases of antibiotic-associated colitis. Cholestyramine resins have been shown to bind vancomycin; therefore, when both cholestyramine and vancomycin are used concurrently, their administration should be separated by at least two hours.

Dalacin T Topical Solution contains an alcohol base which can cause burning and irritation of the eye. In the event of accidental contact with sensitive surfaces (eye, abraded skin, mucous membranes) bathe with copious amounts of cool tap water. Both the Solution and Lotion have an unpleasant taste and caution should be exercised when applying medication around the mouth.

Safety for use in pregnancy has not been established.

Reproduction studies have been performed in rats and mice using subcutaneous and oral doses of clindamycin ranging from 100 to 600 mg/kg/day and have revealed no evidence of impaired fertility or harm to the foetus due to clindamycin. There are, however, no adequate and well-controlled studies in pregnant women. Because animal reproduction studies are not always predictive of human response, this drug should be used during pregnancy only if clearly needed.

It is not known whether clindamycin is excreted in human milk following use of Dalacin T. However, orally and parenterally administered clindamycin has been reported to appear in breast milk. As a general rule, breastfeeding should not be undertaken while a patient is on a drug since many drugs are excreted in breast milk.

Products containing benzoyl peroxide should not be used concurrently with Dalacin T Topical Solution.

*Side-effects:* With the solution, skin dryness is the most common side-effect reported. Other side-effects include skin irritation, contact dermatitis, oily skin, stinging of the eye, Gram-negative folliculitis, gastrointestinal disturbances and abdominal pain. For the lotion, adverse reactions reported in clinical trials have been minor and of a similar incidence to placebo.

**Pharmaceutical precautions**  Store at room temperature. Dalacin T Topical Solution is flammable.

**Legal category**  POM

**Package quantities**  30 and 50 ml bottle with integral applicator.

**Further information**  Clindamycin in vitro inhibited all *Propionibacterium acnes* cultures tested (MIC 0.4 microgram/ml). The mean concentration of clindamycin in comedone samples from patients treated for 4 weeks with Dalacin T was 597 microgram/g.

Dalacin T Topical Lotion does not contain alcohol. It is non-drying and particularly useful for those with dry skins or who live in cold climates.

**Product licence numbers**
Dalacin T Topical Solution        0032/0135
Dalacin T Topical Lotion          0032/0156

## DALACIN* CREAM 2%

**Presentation**  Dalacin Cream is a white, semi-solid cream containing Clindamycin Phosphate BP equivalent to clindamycin 20 mg per gram and benzyl alcohol 10 mg per gram as preservative. The base contains sorbitan monostearate, polysorbate 60, propylene glycol, stearic acid, cetostearyl alcohol, cetyl palmitate and liquid paraffin.

**Uses**  Antibiotic for the treatment of bacterial vaginosis.

**Dosage and administration**  One applicator full (approximately 5 grams) intravaginally at bedtime for 3-7 days.

*Children and the elderly:* No clinical studies have been conducted in populations younger than 15 or older than 60. Dalacin Cream is not recommended in children under 12 years of age.

**Contra-indications, warnings, etc**
*Contra-indications:* Dalacin Cream is contra-indicated in patients previously found to be hypersensitive to preparations containing clindamycin or any of the components of the cream base (see *Presentation*). Although cross-sensitisation to lincomycin has not been demonstrated, it is recommended that Dalacin Cream should not be used in patients who have demonstrated lincomycin sensitivity.

*Warnings:* As there are no data available on the use of Dalacin Cream in patients younger than 12 years of age, it should not be used in this population.

The use of clindamycin may result in the overgrowth of non-susceptible organisms, particularly yeasts.

Virtually all antibiotics have been associated with diarrhoea and in some cases pseudomembranous colitis. Therefore, even though only a minimal amount of drug is absorbed, if significant diarrhoea occurs, the drug should be discontinued and appropriate diagnostic procedures and treatment provided as necessary.

*Pregnancy and lactation:* Reproduction studies have been performed in rats and mice using subcutaneous and oral doses of clindamycin ranging from 20 to 600 mg/kg/day and have revealed no evidence of impaired fertility or harm to the foetus due to clindamycin. In one mouse strain, cleft palates were observed in treated foetuses; this response was not produced in other mouse strains or in other species and is, therefore, considered to be a strain specific effect.

There are no adequate and well-controlled studies in pregnant women during their first trimester and because animal reproduction studies are not always predictive of human response, this drug should be used during the first trimester of pregnancy only if clearly needed.

In a clinical trial in pregnant women during the second trimester, Dalacin Cream was effective in treating bacterial vaginosis and no drug-related medical events were reported in the neonates. However, as with any drug used during pregnancy, a careful risk-benefit assessment should take place beforehand.

It is not known if clindamycin is excreted in breast milk following the use of vaginally administered clindamycin phosphate. However, orally and parenterally administered clindamycin has been reported to appear in breast milk. Therefore, a full assessment of benefit-risk should be made when consideration is given to using vaginal clindamycin phosphate in a nursing mother.

*Side-effects:* In clinical trials medical events judged to be related probably related, or possibly related to vaginally administered clindamycin phosphate cream were reported for (24%) of patients as indicated below:

*Genital tract:* cervicitis/vaginitis (14%); vulvo-vaginal irritation (6%).

*Central nervous system:* dizziness, headache, vertigo.

*Gastro-intestinal:* heartburn, nausea, vomiting, diarrhoea, constipation, abdominal pain.

*Dermatological:* rash, exanthema.

*Hypersensitivity:* urticaria.

(Events without percentages were reported by less than 1% of the patients.)

*Overdose:* Intravaginal overdose is not possible. Accidental ingestion of the product could be accompanied by effects related to therapeutic levels of oral clindamycin.

*Interactions:* Cross resistance has been demonstrated between clindamycin and lincomycin and erythromycin and clindamycin. Antagonism has been demonstrated between clindamycin and erythromycin *in vitro.*

*Incompatibilities:* No information is available on concomitant use with other intra-vaginal products, which is not recommended.

*Effect on condoms and diaphragms:* Dalacin Cream contains oil-based components. Some of these have been shown to weaken the rubber of condoms and diaphragms and make them less effective as a barrier method of contraception or as protection from sexually transmitted diseases, including AIDS. Do not rely on condoms or contraceptive diaphragms when using Dalacin Cream.

**Pharmaceutical precautions**  Store at controlled room temperature (15–30°C). Protect from freezing.

**Legal category**  POM

**Package quantities**  Dalacin Cream is supplied in 40 gram tubes with 7 measured–dose disposable applicators.

**Further information**  Clindamycin has been shown to be active *in vitro* against the following organisms which have been associated with bacterial vaginosis: *Gardnerella vaginalis, Mobiluncus spp, Bacteroides spp, Mycoplasma hominis, Peptostreptococcus spp.* Approximately 4% (range 0.8–8%) of the administered dose of clindamycin (100 mg in 5 g of cream) is absorbed after vaginal administration.

**Product licence number** 0032/0176

## DEBRISAN*

**Presentation**  Sterile, straw-coloured spherical beads of dextranomer of 0.1–0.3 mm diameter, packed in plastic castors.

**Uses**  A dressing for moist wounds and indolent ulcers, whether clean or infected and small area burns.

**Dosage and administration**  A 3 mm layer of Debrisan should be sprinkled onto the wound and kept in place by a pad of lint or a perforated plastic sheet. Debrisan is hydrophilic and the tissue exudate is drawn up into the layer. The Debrisan should be renewed before saturation occurs. Depending on the rate of exudation this may be necessary from one to five times a day. Once or twice daily is usually adequate. When Debrisan is changed the old material

is readily rinsed off with water or saline and new material may then be sprinkled onto the wound.

Shallow wounds, or those in awkward positions, may be dressed more easily by using Debrisan Paste, or by mixing four parts of Debrisan with one part of sterile glycerol to form a stiff paste. This should be spread into the wound with a spatula to a depth of 3 mm or more. Dressing continues as above. The paste should be prepared freshly at each application. Once the wound is clean and poorly secreting, change therapy to an antiseptic dressing, e.g. chlorhexidine tulle, or a sterile pad.

Full instructions for use are enclosed with each pack. Treated in this manner the wound will remain soft and pliable during healing.

*Elderly:* No special instructions.

**Contra-indications, warnings, etc**
1. Do not leave Debrisan for more than 24 hours on wounds with a very low exudation rate as it may dry and form a crust which may be difficult to wash off.
2. Occlusive dressings may lead to maceration of skin round the wound under treatment.
3. When deep infected wounds are treated, care must be taken to wash Debrisan from the depths of the wound.
4. No side-effects have been reported.

*Warning:* Debrisan spillage can render surfaces very slippery. Clear spillages promptly.

*Precautions:*
1. Not to be used on dry wounds.
2. When exudate has been markedly removed by Debrisan alternative treatment should be substituted.
3. In order to avoid cross-infection it is recommended that the contents of a castor be confined to the treatment of a single patient for one day.

**Pharmaceutical precautions**  Keep in a dry place in well-closed containers.

**Package quantities**  Castors of 60 g.

**Legal category**  P.

**Further information**  Each gram of Debrisan absorbs 4 grams of exudate. Capillary action carries debris and bacteria away from the wound surface. Local oedema is reduced so that the wound may look larger initially. Debrisan is non sensitising and controls malodour.

**Product licence number** 0022/0144

## DEBRISAN* PASTE

**Presentation**  Foil-plastic laminate pouches containing 10 g of a sterile soft, white, granular paste consisting of: Dextranomer 6.4 g, polyethylene glycol 600 and water to 10 g.

**Uses**  Treatment of exudative and infected wounds such as surgical or post-traumatic wounds, decubital ulcers and leg ulcers. As the paste is adherent it may be preferred to Debrisan beads on shallow wounds, or those where retention of the beads is a problem.

**Dosage and administration**  After cleaning the wound with sterile water or saline the Paste is applied firmly with a spatula to a depth of not less than 3 mm. The wound is covered and the Paste changed at intervals governed by the exudation rate of the wound, the Paste being renewed before it is entirely discoloured and saturated with secretion and debris. Debrisan Paste should be changed from twice daily to every two days according to the rate of exudation. Stop Debrisan Paste once the wound is granulating and free of exudate, changing to sterile or antiseptic dressings.

*Elderly:* No special instructions.

**Contra-indications, warnings, etc**  Use with caution: When applied near the eyes; in deep fistulae etc. with a narrow opening where paste removal might be difficult.

Occasionally pain may be experienced in the wound after application. This can be avoided by wetting the wound before applying the Paste.

**Pharmaceutical precautions**  Stored at room temperature the shelf life is 3 years.

**Legal category**  P.

**Package quantities**  6×10 g.

**Further information**  Nil.

**Product licence number** 0022/0146.

## DEPO-MEDRONE*

**Qualitative and quantitative composition**  Methylprednisolone Acetate BP 40 mg/ml.

**Pharmaceutical form**  Sterile, aqueous suspension.

## Clinical particulars

*Therapeutic indications:* Depo-Medrone may be used locally or systemically, particularly where oral therapy is not feasible.

Depo-Medrone may be used by any of the following routes: intramuscular, intra-articular, periarticular, intrabursal, intralesional or into the tendon sheath. It **must not** be used by the intrathecal or intravenous routes (see Contra-indications and Undesirable effects).

*Intramuscular administration:*
*Rheumatic disorders:* Rheumatoid arthritis
  *Collagen diseases/arteritis:* Systemic lupus erythematosus
  *Dermatological diseases:* Severe erythema multiforme (Stevens-Johnson syndrome)
  *Allergic states:* Bronchial asthma; severe seasonal and perennial allergic rhinitis; drug hypersensitivity reactions; angioneurotic oedema.
  *Gastro-intestinal diseases:* Ulcerative colitis; Crohn's disease.
  *Respiratory diseases:* Fulminating or disseminated tuberculosis (with appropriate antituberculous chemotherapy); aspiration of gastric contents.
  *Miscellaneous:* TB meningitis (with appropriate antituberculous chemotherapy).

*Intra-articular administration:* Rheumatoid arthritis; osteo-arthritis with an inflammatory component.

*Soft tissue administration (intrabursal, periarticular, into tendon sheath):* Synovitis not associated with infection; epicondylitis; tenosynovitis; plantar fasciitis; bursitis.

*Intralesional:* Keloids; localized lichen planus; localized lichen simplex; granuloma annulare; discoid lupus erythematosus; alopecia areata.

*Posology and method of administration:* Depo-Medrone should not be mixed with any other suspending agent or solution. Parenteral drug products should be inspected visually for particulate matter and discoloration prior to administration, whenever suspension and container permit. Depo-Medrone may be used by any of the following routes: intramuscular, intra-articular, periarticular, intrabursal, intralesional and into the tendon sheath. It must not be used by the intrathecal or intravenous routes (see *Contra-indications and Undesirable effects*).

Undesirable effects may be minimised by using the lowest effective dose for the minimum period (see *Special warnings and special precautions for use*).

Depo-Medrone vials are intended for single dose use only.

*Intramuscular*–for sustained systemic effect: Allergic conditions (severe seasonal and perennial allergic rhinitis, asthma, drug reactions), 80 – 120 mg (2 – 3 ml).

Dermatological conditions, 40 – 120 mg (1 – 3 ml).

Rheumatic disorders and collagen diseases (rheumatoid arthritis, SLE), 40 – 120 mg (1 – 3 ml) per week.

Dosage must be individualized and depends on the condition being treated and its severity.

Note: Depo-Medrone is not intended for the prophylaxis of severe seasonal and perennial allergic rhinitis or other seasonal allergies and should be administered only when symptoms are present.

The frequency of intramuscular injections should be determined by the duration of clinical response.

In the case of seasonal allergic rhinitis a single injection is frequently sufficient. If necessary, however, a second injection may be given after two to three weeks.

On average the effect of a single 2 ml (80 mg) injection may be expected to last approximately two weeks.

*Intra-articular:* Rheumatoid arthritis, osteo-arthritis. The dose of Depo-Medrone depends upon the size of the joint and the severity of the condition. Repeated injections, if needed, may be given at intervals of one to five or more weeks depending upon the degree of relief obtained from the initial injection. A suggested dosage guide is: large joint (knee, ankle, shoulder), 20 – 80 mg (0.5 – 2 ml); medium joint (elbow, wrist), 10 – 40 mg (0.25 – 1 ml); small joint (metacarpophalangeal, interphalangeal, sternoclavicular, acromioclavicular), 4 – 10 mg (0.1 – 0.25 ml).

*Intrabursal:* Subdeltoid bursitis, prepatellar bursitis, olecranon bursitis. For administration directly into bursae, 4 – 30 mg (0.1 – 0.75 ml). In most cases, repeat injections are not needed.

*Intralesional:* Keloids, localised lichen planus, localized lichen simplex, granuloma annulare, alopecia areata, and discoid lupus erythematosus. For administration directly into the lesion for local effect in dermatological conditions, 20 – 60 mg (0.5 – 1.5 ml). For large lesions, the dose may be distributed by repeated local injections of 20 – 40 mg (0.5 – 1 ml). One to four injections are usually employed. Care should be taken to avoid injection of sufficient material to cause blanching, since this may be followed by a small slough.

*Peri-articular:* Epicondylitis. Infiltrate 4–30 mg (0.1 – 0.75 ml) into the affected area.

*Into the tendon sheath:* Tenosynovitis, epicondylitis. For administration directly into the tendon sheath, 4 – 30 mg (0.1 – 0.75 ml). In recurrent or chronic conditions, repeat injections may be necessary.

Special precautions should be observed when administering Depo-Medrone. Intramuscular injections should be made deeply into the gluteal muscles. The usual technique of aspirating prior to injection should be employed to avoid intravascular administration. Doses recommended for intramuscular injection must not be administered superficially or subcutaneously.

Intra-articular injections should be made using precise, anatomical localisation into the synovial space of the joint involved. The injection site for each joint is determined by that location where the synovial cavity is most superficial and most free of large vessels and nerves. Suitable sites for intra-articular injection are the knee, ankle, wrist, elbow, shoulder, phalangeal and hip joints. The spinal joints, unstable joints and those devoid of synovial space are not suitable. Treatment failures are most frequently the result of failure to enter the joint space. Intra-articular injections should be made with care as follows: ensure correct positioning of the needle into the synovial space and aspirate a few drops of joint fluid. The aspirating syringe should then be replaced by another containing Depo-Medrone. To ensure position of the needle, synovial fluid should be aspirated and the injection made. After injection the joint is moved slightly to aid mixing of the synovial fluid and the suspension. Subsequent to therapy care should be taken for the patient not to overuse the joint in which benefit has been obtained. Negligence in this matter may permit an increase in joint deterioration that will more than offset the beneficial effects of the steroid.

Intrabursal injections should be made as follows: the area around the injection site is prepared in a sterile way and a wheal at the site made with 1 per cent procaine hydrochloride solution. A 20 to 24 gauge needle attached to a dry syringe is inserted into the bursa and the fluid aspirated. The needle is left in place and the aspirating syringe changed for a small syringe containing the desired dose. After injection, the needle is withdrawn and a small dressing applied. In the treatment of tenosynovitis care should be taken to inject Depo-Medrone into the tendon sheath rather than into the substance of the tendon. Due to the absence of a true tendon sheath, the Achilles tendon should not be injected with Depo-Medrone.

*Children:* Dosage may be reduced for infants and children but should be governed more by the severity of the condition and response of the patient, than by age or size.

*Elderly patients:* When used according to instructions, there is no information to suggest that a change in dosage is warranted in the elderly. However, treatment of elderly patients, particularly if long-term, should be planned bearing in mind the more serious consequences of the common side-effects of corticosteroids in old age and close clinical supervision is required (see *Special warnings and special precautions for use*).

*Contra-indications:* Depo-medrone is contra-indicated where there is known hypersensitivity to components and in systemic infection unless specific anti-infective therapy is employed.

Due to its potential for neurotoxicity, Depo-Medrone **must not** be given by the intrathecal route. In addition, as the product is a suspension it **must not** be given by the intravenous route (see *Undesirable effects*).

*Special warnings and special precautions for use*
*Warnings and precautions:* A Patient Information Leaflet is provided in the pack by the manufacturer.

Undesirable effects may be minimised by using the lowest effective dose for the minimum period. Frequent patient review is required to appropriately titrate the dose against disease activity (see *Posology and method of administration*).

Patients should carry 'Steroid Treatment' cards which give clear guidance on the precautions to be taken to minimise risk and which provide details of prescriber, drug, dosage and the duration of treatment.

Depo-Medrone vials are intended for single dose use only. Any multidose use of the product may lead to contamination.

Depo-Medrone is not recommended for epidural, intranasal, intra-ocular, or any other unapproved route of administration. See *Undesirable effects* section for details of side-effects reported from some non-recommended routes of administration.

Due to the absence of a true tendon sheath, the Achilles tendon should not be injected with Depo-Medrone.

While crystals of adrenal steroids in the dermis suppress inflammatory reactions, their presence may cause disintegration of the cellular elements and physiochemical changes in the ground substance of the connective tissue. The resultant infrequently occurring dermal and/or subdermal changes may form depressions in the skin at the injection site. The degree to which this reaction occurs will vary with the amount of adrenal steroid injected. Regeneration is usually complete within a few months or after all crystals of the adrenal steroid have been absorbed. In order to minimize the incidence of dermal and subdermal atrophy, care must be exercised not to exceed recommended doses in injections. Multiple small injections into the area of the lesion should be made whenever possible. The technique of intra-articular and intramuscular injection should include precautions against injection or leakage into the dermis. Injection into the deltoid muscle should be avoided because of a high incidence of subcutaneous atrophy.

Intralesional doses should not be placed too superficially, particularly in easily visible sites in patients with deeply pigmented skins, since there have been rare reports of subcutaneous atrophy and depigmentation.

Systemic absorption of methylprednisolone occurs following intra-articular injection of Depo-Medrone. Systemic as well as local effects can therefore be expected.

Intra-articular corticosteroids are associated with a substantially increased risk of inflammatory response in the joint, particularly bacterial infection introduced with the injection. Charcot-like arthropathies have been reported particularly after repeated injections. Appropriate examination of any joint fluid present is necessary to exclude any bacterial infection, prior to injection.

Following a single dose of Depo-Medrone, plasma cortisol levels are reduced and there is evidence of hypothalamic-pituitary-adrenal (HPA) axis suppression. This suppression lasts for a variable period of up to 4 weeks. The usual dynamic tests of HPA axis function can be used to diagnose evidence of impaired activity (e.g. Synacthen test).

Adrenal cortical atrophy develops during prolonged therapy and may persist for months after stopping treatment. Withdrawal of corticosteroids after prolonged therapy must therefore always be gradual to avoid acute adrenal insufficiency, being tapered off over weeks or months according to the dose and duration of treatment. During prolonged therapy any intercurrent illness, trauma or surgical procedure will require a temporary increase in dosage; if corticosteroids have been stopped following prolonged therapy they may need to be temporarily re-introduced.

Since mineralocorticoid secretion may be impaired, salt and/or a mineralocorticoid should be administered concurrently.

Because rare instances of anaphylactic reactions have occurred in patients receiving parenteral corticosteroid therapy, appropriate precautionary measures should be taken prior to administration, especially when the patient has a history of drug allergy.

Corticosteroids may mask some signs of infection, and new infections may appear during their use. Suppression of the inflammatory response and immune function increases the susceptibility to fungal, viral and bacterial infections and their severity. The clinical presentation may often be atypical and may reach an advanced stage before being recognised.

Chickenpox is of serious concern since this normally minor illness may be fatal in immunosuppressed patients. Patients (or parents of children) without a definite history of chickenpox should be advised to avoid close personal contact with chickenpox or herpes zoster and if exposed they should seek urgent medical attention. Passive immunization with varicella/zoster immunoglobin (VZIG) is needed by exposed non-immune patients who are receiving systemic corticosteroids or who have used them within the previous 3 months; this should be given within 10 days of exposure to chickenpox. If a diagnosis of chickenpox is confirmed, the illness warrants specialist care and urgent treatment. Corticosteroids should not be stopped and the dose may need to be increased.

Live vaccines should not be given to individuals with impaired immune responsiveness. The antibody response to other vaccines may be diminished.

The use of Depo-Medrone in active tuberculosis should be restricted to those cases of fulminating or disseminated tuberculosis in which the corticosteroid is used for the management of the disease in conjunction with an appropriate antituberculous regimen. If corticosteroids are indicated in patients with latent tuberculosis or tuberculin reactivity, close observation is necessary as reactivation of the disease may occur. During prolonged corticosteroid therapy, these patients should receive chemoprophylaxis.

Care should be taken for patients receiving cardioactive drugs such as digoxin because of steroid induced electrolyte disturbance/potassium loss (see *Undesirable effects*).

*The following precautions apply for parenteral*

*corticosteroids:* Following intra-articular injection, the occurrence of a marked increase in pain accompanied by local swelling, further restriction of joint motion, fever, and malaise are suggestive of septic arthritis. If this complication occurs and the diagnosis of sepsis is confirmed, appropriate antimicrobial therapy should be instituted.

Local injection of a steroid into a previously infected joint is to be avoided.

Corticosteroids should not be injected into unstable joints.

Sterile technique is necessary to prevent infections or contamination.

The slower rate of absorption by intramuscular administration should be recognised.

*Special precautions:* Particular care is required when considering the use of systemic corticosteroids in patients with the following conditions and frequent patient monitoring is necessary.

Osteoporosis (post-menopausal females are particularly at risk).

Hypertension or congestive heart failure.

Existing or previous history of severe affective disorders (especially previous steroid psychosis).

Diabetes mellitus (or a family history of diabetes).

History of tuberculosis.

Glaucoma (or a family history of glaucoma).

Previous corticosteroid-induced myopathy.

Liver failure or cirrhosis.

Renal insufficiency.

Epilepsy.

Peptic ulceration.

Fresh intestinal anastomoses.

Predisposition to thrombophlebitis.

Abscess or other pyogenic infections.

Ulcerative colitis.

Diverticulitis.

Myasthenia gravis.

Ocular herpes simplex, for fear of corneal perforation.

Hypothyroidism.

*Use in children:* Corticosteroids cause growth retardation in infancy, childhood and adolescence which may be irreversible. Treatment should be limited to the minimum dosage for the shortest possible time.

*Use in the elderly:* The common adverse effects of systemic corticosteroids may be associated with more serious consequences in old age, especially osteoporosis, hypertension, hypokalaemia, diabetes, susceptibility to infection and thinning of the skin. Close clinical supervision is required to avoid life-threatening reactions.

*Interaction with other medicaments and other forms of interaction:* Convulsions have been reported with concurrent use of methylprednisolone and cyclosporin. Since concurrent administration of these agents results in a mutual inhibition of metabolism, it is possible that convulsions and other adverse effects associated with the individual use of either drug may be more apt to occur.

Drugs that induce hepatic enzymes, such as rifampicin, rifabutin, carbamazepine, phenobarbitone, phenytoin, primidone, and aminoglutethimide enhance the metabolism of corticosteroids and its therapeutic effects may be reduced.

Drugs such as erythromycin and ketoconazole may inhibit the metabolism of corticosteroids and thus decrease their clearance.

Steroids may reduce the effects of anticholinesterases in myasthenia gravis. The desired effects of hypoglycaemic agents (including insulin), anti-hypertensives and diuretics are antagonised by corticosteroids, and the hypokalaemic effects of acetazolamide, loop diuretics, thiazide diuretics and carbenoxolone are enhanced.

The efficacy of coumarin anticoagulants may be enhanced by concurrent corticosteroid therapy and close monitoring of the INR or prothrombin time is required to avoid spontaneous bleeding.

The renal clearance of salicylates is increased by corticosteroids and steroid withdrawal may result in salicylate intoxication. Salicylates and non-steroidal anti-inflammatory agents should be used cautiously in conjunction with corticosteroids in hypothrombinaemia.

Steroids have been reported to interact with neuromuscular blocking agents such as pancuronium with partial reversal of the neuromuscular block.

*Pregnancy and lactation:* Corticosteroids cross the placenta. There may be a very small risk of cleft palate and intra-uterine growth retardation in the fetus; there is evidence of harmful effects on pregnancy in animals. Neonates of mothers who received such therapy during pregnancy should be observed for signs of hypoadrenalism and appropriate measures instituted if such signs exist. When corticosteroids are essential however, patients with normal pregnancies may be treated as though they were in the non-gravid state. Patients with pre-eclampsia or fluid retention require close monitoring.

Methylprednisolone is excreted in breast milk and infants of mothers taking pharmacological doses of steroids should be monitored carefully for signs of adrenal suppression.

*Effects on ability to drive and use machines:* None stated.

*Undesirable effects:* The incidence of predictable undesirable side-effects associated with the use of corticosteroids, including hypothalamic-pituitary-adrenal suppression correlates with the relative potency of the drug, dosage, timing of administration and duration of treatment (see Special warnings and special precautions for use).

*Paremteral corticosteroid therapy:* Anaphylactic reaction or allergic reactions, hypopigmentation or hyperpigmentation, subcutaneous and cutaneous atrophy, sterile abscess, post injection flare (following intra-articular use), Charcot-like arthropathy, rare instances of blindness associated with intralesional therapy around the face and head.

*Gastro-intestinal:* Dyspepsia, peptic ulceration with perforation and haemorrhage, abdominal distension, oesophageal ulceration, oesophageal candidiasis, acute pancreatitis, perforation of bowel.

Increases in alanine transaminase (ALT, SGPT) aspartate transaminase (AST, SGOT) and alkaline phosphatase have been observed following corticosteroid treatment. These changes are usually small, not associated with any clinical syndrome and are reversible upon discontinuation.

*Anti-inflammatory and immunosuppressive effects:* Increased susceptibility and severity of infections with suppression of clinical symptoms and signs, opportunistic infections, may suppress reactions to skin tests, recurrence of dormant tuberculosis (see *Special warnings and special precautions for use*).

*Musculoskeletal:* Proximal myopathy, osteoporosis, vertebral and long bone fractures, avascular osteonecrosis, tendon rupture, aseptic necrosis, muscle weakness.

*Fluid and electrolyte disturbance:* Sodium and water retention, potassium loss, hypertension, hypokalaemic alkalosis, congestive heart failure in susceptible patients.

*Dermatological:* Impaired healing, petechiae and ecchymosis, thin fragile skin, skin atrophy, bruising, striae, telangiectasia, acne.

*Endocrine/metabolic:* Suppression of the hypothalamo-pituitary-adrenal axis, growth suppression in infancy, childhood and adolescence, menstrual irregularity and amenorrhoea. Cushingoid facies, hirsutism, weight gain, impaired carbohydrate tolerance with increased requirement for antidiabetic therapy, negative nitrogen and calcium balance. Increased appetite.

*Neuropsychiatric:* Euphoria, psychological dependence, mood swings, depression, personality changes, insomnia. Increased intra-cranial pressure with papilloedema in children (pseudotumour cerebri), usually after treatment withdrawal. Psychosis, aggravation of schizophrenia, seizures.

*Ophthalmic:* Increased intra-ocular pressure, glaucoma, papilloedema, cataracts with possible damage to the optic nerve, corneal or scleral thinning, exacerbation of ophthalmic viral or fungal disease, exophthalmos.

*General:* Leucocytosis, hypersensitivity including anaphylaxis, thrombo-embolism, nausea, vertigo.

*Withdrawal symptoms:* Too rapid a reduction of corticosteroid dosage following prolonged treatment can lead to acute adrenal insufficiency, hypotension and death. However, this is more applicable to corticosteroids with an indication where continuous therapy is given (see *Special warnings and special precautions for use*).

A 'withdrawal syndrome' may also occur including, fever, myalgia, arthralgia, rhinitis, conjunctivitis, painful itchy skin nodules and loss of weight.

*Certain side-effects reported with some non-recommended routes of administration:*

*Intrathecal:* Usual systemic corticoid adverse reactions, headache, meningismus, meningitis, paraplegia, spinal fluid abnormalities, nausea, vomiting, sweating, arachnoiditis, convulsions.

*Extradural:* Wound dehiscence, loss of sphincter control.

*Intranasal:* Permanent/temporary blindness, rhinitis.

*Ophthalmic:* (Subconjunctival)–Redness and itching, abscess, slough at injection site, residue at injection site, increased intra-ocular pressure, decreased vision–blindness, infection.

*Miscellaneous injection sites:* Scalp, tonsillar fauces, sphenopalatine ganglion: blindness.

*Overdose:* There is no clinical syndrome of acute overdosage with Depo-Medrone. Following overdosage the possibility of adrenal suppression should be guarded against by gradual diminution of dose levels over a period of time. In such event the patient may require to be supported during any further traumatic episode.

**Pharmacological properties**

*Pharmacodynamic properties:* Methylprednisolone acetate is a synthetic glucocorticoid. An aqueous suspension may be injected directly into joints and soft tissues in the treatment of rheumatoid arthritis, osteoarthritis, bursitis and similar inflammatory conditions. For prolonged systemic effect it may be administered intramuscularly.

*Pharmacokinetic properties:* Methylprednisolone acetate is absorbed from joints in a few days, with peak serum levels being reached 2–12 hours after injection.

It is more slowly absorbed following deep intramuscular injection with plasma levels detected up to 17 days afterwards.

Methylprednisolone acetate is less soluble than methylprednisolone.

**Pharmaceutical particulars**

*List of excipients:* Polyethylene glycol, sodium chloride, myristyl-gamma-picolinium chloride and sterile water for injections.

*Incompatibilities:* None stated.

*Shelf-life:* Shelf-life of the medicinal product as packaged for sale: 60 months.

Depo-Medrone should not be mixed with any other fluid. Discard any remaining suspension after use.

*Special precautions for storage:* Depo-Medrone should be protected from freezing.

*Nature and contents of container:* Type I flint glass vial with a butyl rubber plug and metal seal. Each vial contains 1 ml, 2 ml, or 3 ml of Depo-Medrone 40 mg/ml.

*Instructions for use/handling:* No special requirements.

**Marketing authorisation number** 0032/5038

**Date of approval/revision of SPC** August 1996

**Legal category** POM

## DEPO-MEDRONE* WITH LIDOCAINE

**Qualitative and quantitative composition** Methylprednisolone acetate 40 mg/ml, lidocaine hydrochloride 10 mg/ml.

**Pharmaceutical form** White, sterile aqueous suspension for injection

**Clinical particulars**

*Therapeutic indications:* Corticosteroid (glucocorticoid). Depo-Medrone with Lidocaine is indicated in conditions requiring a glucocorticoid effect: e.g. anti-inflammatory or anti-rheumatic. It is recommended for local use where the added anaesthetic effect would be considered advantageous.

Depo-Medrone with Lidocaine may be used as follows:

*Intra-articular administration:* Rheumatoid arthritis; osteo-arthritis with an inflammatory component.

*Periarticular administration:* Epicondylitis.

*Intrabursal administration:* Subacromial bursitis; prepatellar bursitis; olecranon bursitis.

*Tendon sheath administration:* Tendinitis; tenosynovitis; epicondylitis.

Therapy with Depo-Medrone with Lidocaine does not obviate the need for the conventional measures usually employed. Although this method of treatment will ameliorate symptoms, it is in no sense a cure and the hormone has no effect on the cause of the inflammation.

*Posology and method of administration:* Depo-Medrone with Lidocaine should not be mixed with any other preparation as flocculation of the product may occur. Parenteral drug products should be inspected visually for particulate matter and discoloration prior to administration whenever suspension and container permit. Depo-Medrone with Lidocaine may be used by any of the following routes: intra-articular, periarticular, intrabursal, and into the tendon sheath. It **must not** be used by the intrathecal or intravenous routes (see *Contra-indications* and *Side-effects*)

*Adults:*

*Intra-articular:* Rheumatoid arthritis, osteo-arthritis. The dose of Depo-Medrone with Lidocaine depends on the size of the joint and the severity of the condition. Repeated injections, if needed, may be given at intervals of one to five or more weeks depending upon the degree of relief obtained from the initial injection. A suggested dosage guide is: large joint (knee, ankle, shoulder), 0.5 – 2 ml (20 – 80 mg of steroid); medium joint (elbow, wrist), 0.25 – 1 ml (10 – 40 mg of steroid); small joint (metacarpophalangeal, interphalangeal, sternoclavicular, acromioclavicular), 0.1 – 0.25 ml (4 – 10 mg of steroid).

*Periarticular:* Epicondylitis. Infiltrate 0.1 – 0.75 ml (4 – 30 mg of steroid) into the affected area.

*Intrabursal:* Subdeltoid bursitis, prepatellar bursitis, olecranon bursitis. For administration directly into bursae, 0.1 – 0.75 ml (4 – 30 mg of steroid). In most acute cases, repeat injections are not needed.

*Into the tendon sheath:* Tendinitis, tenosynovitis, epicondylitis. For administration directly into the tendon sheath, 0.1 -- 0.75 ml (4 – 30 mg of steroid). In recurrent or chronic conditions, repeat injections may be necessary.

*Children:* For infants and children, the recommended dosage should be reduced, but dosage should be governed by the severity of the condition rather than by strict adherence to the ratio indicated by age or body weight.

*Elderly:* When used according to instructions, there is no information to suggest that a change in dosage is warranted in the elderly. However, treatment of elderly patients, particularly if long-term, should be planned bearing in mind the more serious consequences of the common side-effects of corticosteroids in old age and close clinical supervision is required (see *Other special warnings and precautions*).

Special precautions should be observed when administering Depo-Medrone with Lidocaine:

Intra-articular injections should be made using precise, anatomical localisation into the synovial space of the joint involved. The injection site for each joint is determined by that location where the synovial cavity is most superficial and most free of large vessels and nerves. Suitable sites for intra-articular injection are the knee, ankle, wrist, elbow, shoulder, phalangeal and hip joints. The spinal joints, unstable joints and those devoid of synovial space are not suitable. Treatment failures are most frequently the result of failure to enter the joint space. Intra-articular injections should be made with care as follows: ensure correct positioning of the needle into the synovial space and aspirate a few drops of joint fluid. The aspirating syringe should then be replaced by another containing Depo-Medrone with Lidocaine. To ensure position of the needle synovial fluid should be aspirated and the injection made.

After injection the joint is moved slightly to aid mixing of the synovial fluid and the suspension. Subsequent to therapy care should be taken for the patient not to overuse the joint in which benefit has been obtained. Negligence in this matter may permit an increase in joint deterioration that will more than offset the beneficial effects of the steroid.

Intrabursal injections should be made as follows: the area around the injection site is prepared in a sterile way and a wheal at the site made with 1 percent procaine hydrochloride solution. A 20 to 24 gauge needle attached to a dry syringe is inserted into the bursa and the fluid aspirated. The needle is left in place and the aspirating syringe changed for a small syringe containing the desired dose. After injection, the needle is withdrawn and a small dressing applied. In the treatment of tenosynovitis and tendinitis, care should be taken to inject Depo-Medrone with Lidocaine into the tendon sheath rather than into the substance of the tendon. Due to the absence of a true tendon sheath, the Achilles tendon should not be injected with Depo-Medrone with Lidocaine.

*Contra-indications:* Depo-Medrone with Lidocaine is contra-indicated where there is known hypersensitivity to components or to any local anaesthetics of the amide type and in systemic infection unless anti-infective therapy is employed.

Due to its potential for neurotoxicity, Depo-Medrone with Lidocaine **must not** be given by the intrathecal route. In addition, as the product is a suspension it **must not** be given by the intravenous route (see *Side-effects*).

*Special warnings and special precautions for use:* Undesirable effects may be minimised by using the lowest effective dose for the minimum period. Frequent patient review is required to appropriately titrate the dose against disease activity (see *Posology and method of administration*).

Patients should carry 'Steroid Treatment' cards which give clear guidance on the precautions to be taken to minimise risk and which provide details of prescriber, drug, dosage and the duration of treatment.

Depo-Medrone with Lidocaine vials are intended for single dose use only. Any multidose use of the product may lead to contamination.

Depo-Medrone with Lidocaine is not recommended for epidural, intranasal, intra-ocular, or any other unapproved route of administration. See *Side-effects* section for details of side-effects reported from some non-recommended routes of administration.

Due to the absence of a true tendon sheath, the Achilles tendon should not be injected with Depo-Medrone with Lidocaine.

While crystals of adrenal steroids in the dermis suppress inflammatory reactions, their presence may cause disintegration of the cellular elements and physiochemical changes in the ground substance of the connective tissue. The resultant infrequently occurring dermal and/or subdermal changes may form depressions in the skin at the injection site and the possibility of depigmentation. The degree to which this reaction occurs will vary with the amount of adrenal steroid injected. Regeneration is usually complete within a few months or after all crystals of the adrenal steroid have been absorbed. In order to minimize the incidence of dermal and subdermal atrophy, care must be exercised not to exceed recommended doses in injections. Multiple small injections into the area of the lesion should be made whenever possible. The technique of intra-articular injection should include precautions against injection or leakage into the dermis.

Systemic absorption of methylprednisolone occurs following intra-articular injection of Depo-Medrone with Lidocaine. Systemic as well as local effects can therefore be expected.

Intra-articular corticosteroids are associated with a substantially increased risk of inflammatory response in the joint, particularly bacterial infection introduced with the injection. Charcot-like arthropathies have been reported particularly after repeated injections. Appropriate examination of any joint fluid present is necessary to exclude any bacterial infection, prior to injection.

Following a single dose of Depo-Medrone with Lidocaine, plasma cortisol levels are reduced and there is evidence of hypothalamic-pituitary-adrenal axis (HPA) suppression. This suppression lasts for a variable period of up to 4 weeks. The usual dynamic tests of HPA axis function can be used to diagnose evidence of impaired activity (e.g. Synacthen test).

Adrenal cortical atrophy develops during prolonged therapy and may persist for months after stopping treatment. Withdrawal of corticosteroids after prolonged therapy must therefore always be gradual to avoid acute adrenal insufficiency, being tapered off over weeks or months according to the dose and duration of treatment. During prolonged therapy any intercurrent illness, trauma or surgical procedure will require a temporary increase in dosage; if corticosteroids have been stopped following prolonged therapy they may need to be temporarily re-introduced.

Since mineralocorticoid secretion may be impaired, salt and/or a mineralocorticoid should be administered concurrently.

Because rare instances of anaphylactic reactions have occurred in patients receiving parenteral corticosteroid therapy, appropriate precautionary measures should be taken prior to administration, especially when the patient has a history of drug allergy.

Corticosteroids may mask some signs of infection, and new infections may appear during their use. Suppression of the inflammatory response and immune function increases the susceptibility to fungal, viral and bacterial infections and their severity. The clinical presentation may often be atypical and may reach an advanced stage before being recognised.

Chickenpox is of serious concern since this normally minor illness may be fatal in immunosuppressed patients. Patients (or parents of children) without a definite history of chickenpox should be advised to avoid close personal contact with chickenpox or herpes zoster and if exposed they should seek urgent medical attention. Passive immunization with varicella/zoster immunoglobin (VZIG) is needed by exposed non-immune patients who are receiving systemic corticosteroids or who have used them within the previous 3 months; this should be given within 10 days of exposure to chickenpox. If a diagnosis of chickenpox is confirmed, the illness warrants specialist care and urgent treatment. Corticosteroids should not be stopped and the dose may need to be increased.

Live vaccines should not be given to individuals with impaired immune responsiveness. The antibody response to other vaccines may be diminished.

If corticosteroids are indicated in patients with latent tuberculosis or tuberculin reactivity, close observation is necessary as reactivation of the disease may occur. During prolonged corticosteroid therapy, these patients should receive chemoprophylaxis.

This product contains benzyl alcohol. Benzyl alcohol has been reported to be associated with a fatal 'Gasping Syndrome' in premature infants.

Care should be taken for patients receiving cardioactive drugs such as digoxin because of steroid induced electrolyte disturbance/potassium loss (see Side-effects).

*The following precautions apply for parenteral corticosteroids:* Following intra-articular injection, a marked increase in pain accompanied by local swelling, further restriction of joint motion, fever, and malaise are suggestive of septic arthritis. If this complication occurs and the diagnosis of sepsis is confirmed, appropriate antimicrobial therapy should be instituted.

No additional benefit derives from the intramuscular administration of Depo-Medrone with Lidocaine. Where parenteral corticosteroid therapy for sustained systemic effect is desired, plain Depo-Medrone should be used.

Local injection of a steroid into a previously infected joint is to be avoided.

Corticosteroids should not be injected into unstable joints.

Sterile technique is necessary to prevent infections or contamination.

*Special precautions:* Particular care is required when considering the use of systemic corticosteroids in patients with the following conditions and frequent patient monitoring is necessary.

Osteoporosis (post-menopausal females are particularly at risk).

Hypertension or congestive heart failure.

Existing or previous history of severe affective disorders (especially previous steroid psychosis).

Diabetes mellitus (or a family history of diabetes).

History of tuberculosis.

Glaucoma (or a family history of glaucoma).

Previous corticosteroid-induced myopathy.

Liver failure or cirrhosis.

Renal insufficiency.

Epilepsy.

Peptic ulceration.

Fresh intestinal anastomoses.

Predisposition to thrombophlebitis.

Abscess or other pyogenic infections.

Ulcerative colitis.

Diverticulitis.

Myasthenia gravis.

Ocular herpes simplex, for fear of corneal perforation.

Hypothyroidism.

*Use in children:* Corticosteroids cause growth retardation in infancy, childhood and adolescence which may be irreversible. Treatment should be limited to the minimum dosage for the shortest possible time.

*Use in the elderly:* The common adverse effects of systemic corticosteroids may be associated with more serious consequences in old age, especially osteoporosis, hypertension, hypokalaemia, diabetes, susceptibility to infection and thinning of the skin. Close clinical supervision is required to avoid life-threatening reactions.

*Interaction with other medicaments and other forms of interaction*

Convulsions have been reported with concurrent use of methylprednisolone and cyclosporin. Since concurrent administration of these agents results in a mutual inhibition of metabolism, it is possible that convulsions and other adverse effects associated with the individual use of either drug may be more apt to occur.

Drugs that induce hepatic enzymes, such as rifampicin, rifabutin, carbamazepine, phenobarbitone, phenytoin, primidone, and aminoglutethimide enhance the metabolism of corticosteroids and its therapeutic effects may be reduced.

Drugs such as erythromycin and ketoconazole may inhibit the metabolism of corticosteroids and thus decrease their clearance.

Steroids may reduce the effects of anticholinesterases in myasthenia gravis. The desired effects of hypoglycaemic agents (including insulin), anti-hypertensives and diuretics are antagonised by corticosteroids, and the hypokalaemic effects of acetazolamide, loop diuretics, thiazide diuretics and carbenoxolone are enhanced.

The efficacy of coumarin anticoagulants may be enhanced by concurrent corticosteroid therapy and close monitoring of the INR or prothrombin time is required to avoid spontaneous bleeding.

The renal clearance of salicylates is increased by corticosteroids and steroid withdrawal may result in salicylate intoxication. Salicylates and non-steroidal anti-inflammatory agents should be used cautiously in conjunction with corticosteroids in hypothrombinaemia.

Steroids have been reported to interact with neuromuscular blocking agents such as pancuronium with partial reversal of the neuromuscular block.

*Pregnancy and lactation:* Corticosteroids cross the placenta. There may be a very small risk of cleft palate and intra-uterine growth retardation in the foetus; there is evidence of harmful effects on pregnancy in animals. Neonates of mothers who received such therapy during pregnancy should be observed for signs of hypoadrenalism and appropriate measures instituted if such signs exist. When corticosteroids are essential however, patients with normal pregnancies may be treated as though they were in the non-gravid state. Patients with pre-eclampsia or fluid retention require close monitoring.

Methylprednisolone is excreted in breast milk and infants of mothers taking pharmacological doses of steroids should be monitored carefully for signs of adrenal suppression.

The use of local anaesthetics such as lidocaine during labour and delivery may be associated with adverse effects on mother and foetus. Lidocaine readily crosses the placenta.

It is not known whether lidocaine is excreted in human breast milk.

*Effects on ability to drive and use machines:* None stated.

*Undesirable effects:* The incidence of predictable undesirable side-effects associated with the use of corticosteroids, including hypothalamic-pituitary-adrenal suppression correlates with the relative potency of the drug, dosage, timing of administration and duration of treatment (see other special warnings and precautions).

Side-effects for the Depo-Medrone component may be observed including:

*Parenteral corticosteroid therapy:* Anaphylactic reaction or allergic reactions, hypopigmentation or hyperpigmentation, subcutaneous and cutaneous atrophy, sterile abscess, post injection flare (following intra-articular use), charcot-like arthropathy.

*Gastro-intestinal:* Dyspepsia, peptic ulceration with perforation and haemorrhage, abdominal distension, oesophageal ulceration, oesophageal candidiasis, acute pancreatitis, perforation of bowel.

Increases in alanine transaminase (ALT, SGPT) aspartate transaminase (AST, SGOT) and alkaline phosphatase have been observed following corticosteroid treatment. These changes are usually small, not associated with any clinical syndrome and are reversible upon discontinuation.

*Anti-inflammatory and immunosuppressive effects:* Increased susceptibility and severity of infections with suppression of clinical symptoms and signs, opportunistic infections, may suppress reactions to skin tests, recurrence of dormant tuberculosis (see *Other special warnings and precautions*).

*Musculoskeletal:* Proximal myopathy, osteoporosis, vertebral and long bone fractures, avascular osteonecrosis, tendon rupture, aseptic necrosis, muscle weakness.

*Fluid and electrolyte disturbance:* Sodium and water retention, potassium loss, hypertension, hypokalaemic alkalosis, congestive heart failure in susceptible patients.

*Dermatological:* Impaired healing, petechiae and ecchymosis, thin fragile skin, skin atrophy, bruising, striae, telangiectasia, acne.

*Endocrine/metabolic:* Suppression of the hypothalamo-pituitary-adrenal axis; growth suppression in infancy, childhood and adolescence; menstrual irregularity and amenorrhoea. Cushingoid facies, hirsutism, weight gain, impaired carbohydrate tolerance with increased requirement for antidiabetic therapy, negative nitrogen and calcium balance. Increased appetite.

*Neuropsychiatric:* Euphoria, psychological dependence, mood swings, depression, personality changes, insomnia. Increased intra-cranial pressure with papilloedema in children (pseudotumour cerebri), usually after treatment withdrawal. Psychosis, aggravation of schizophrenia, seizures.

*Ophthalmic:* Increased intra-ocular pressure, glaucoma, papilloedema, cataracts with possible damage to the optic nerve, corneal or scleral thinning, exacerbation of ophthalmic viral or fungal disease, exophthalmos.

*General:* Leucocytosis, hypersensitivity including anaphylaxis, thrombo-embolism, nausea, vertigo.

*Withdrawal symptoms:* Too rapid a reduction of corticosteroid dosage following prolonged treatment can lead to acute adrenal insufficiency, hypotension and death. However, this is more applicable to corticosteroids with an indication where continuous therapy is given (see *Other special warnings and precautions*).

A 'withdrawal syndrome' may also occur including, fever, myalgia, arthralgia, rhinitis, conjunctivitis, painful itchy skin nodules and loss of weight.

*Side-effects for the Lidocaine component include:*

*Central nervous system:* Lightheadedness, nervousness, apprehension, euphoria, confusion, dizziness, drowsiness, tinnitus, blurred or double vision, vomiting, sensation of heat, cold, numbness, twitching, tremors, convulsions, loss of consciousness, respiratory depression, respiratory arrest.

*Cardiovascular system:* Bradycardia, hypotension, cardiovascular collapse, cardiac arrest.

*Allergic reactions:* Cutaneous lesions, urticaria, oedema, anaphylactic reactions.

*Certain side-effects reported with some non-recommended routes of administration:*

*Intrathecal:* Usual systemic corticoid adverse reactions, headache, meningismus, meningitis, paraplegia, spinal fluid abnormalities, nausea, vomiting, sweating, arachnoiditis, convulsions.

*Extradural:* Wound dehiscence, loss of sphincter control.

*Intranasal:* Permanent/temporary blindness, allergic reactions, rhinitis.

*Ophthalmic (Subconjunctival):* Redness and itching, abscess, slough at injection site, residue at injection site, increased intra-ocular pressure, decreased vision–blindness, infection.

*Miscellaneous:* Scalp, tonsillar fauces, sphenopalatine ganglion, blindness.

*Overdose:* There is no clinical syndrome of acute overdosage with Depo-Medrone with Lidocaine. Following overdosage the possibility of adrenal suppression should be guarded against by gradual diminution of dose levels over a period of time. In such event the patient may require to be supported during any further traumatic episode.

**Pharmacological properties**

*Pharmacodynamic properties:* Methylprednisolone acetate is a synthetic glucocorticoid with the actions and use of natural corticosteroids. However the slower metabolism of the synthetic corticosteroid with their lower protein-binding affinity may account for their increased potency compared with the natural corticosteroids.

Lidocaine has the actions of a local anaesthetic.

*Pharmacokinetic properties:* Administration of methylprednisolone acetate 40 mg intramuscularly produced measurable plasma concentrations of methylprednisolone for 11–17 days. The average peak plasma concentration was 14.8 ng per ml and occurred after 6–8 hours.

Plasma concentrations of lidocaine decline rapidly after an intravenous dose with an initial half life of less than 30 minutes; the elimination half life is 1–2 hours.

*Preclinical safety data:* Due to the age and well established safety nature of this product, preclinical data has not been included.

**Pharmaceutical particulars**

*List of excipients:* Sodium chloride, myristyl-gamma-picolinium chloride, benzyl alcohol, polyethylene glycol, sodium hydroxide, hydrochloric acid and water for injection.

*Incompatibilities:* None

*Shelf life:* 24 months

*Special precautions for storage:* Store below 25°C.

*Nature and contents of container:* Glass vials with rubber cap containing 1 or 2 ml of suspension.

*Instructions for use/handling:* None

**Marketing authorisation number** 0032/0076

**Date of approval/revision of SPC** July 1996.

**Legal categoray** POM

## DEPO-PROVERA 150 mg/ml

**Qualitative and quantitative composition** Each ml of suspension contains 150 mg Medroxyprogesterone Acetate PhEur.

**Pharmaceutical form** Sterile suspension for injection.

**Clinical particulars**

*Therapeutic indications:* Progestogen: for contraception.

Depo-Provera is a long-term contraceptive agent suitable for use in women who have been appropriately counselled concerning the likelihood of menstrual disturbance and the potential for a delay in return to full fertility.

Depo-Provera may also be used for short-term contraception in the following circumstances:

For partners of men undergoing vasectomy, for protection until the vasectomy becomes effective.

In women who are being immunised against rubella, to prevent pregnancy during the period of activity of the virus.

In women awaiting sterilisation.

It is of the greatest importance that adequate explanations of the long-term nature of the product, of its possible side-effects and of the impossibility of immediately reversing the effects of each injection are given to potential users and that every effort is made to ensure that each patient receives such counselling as to enable her to fully understand these explanations. Patient information leaflets are supplied by the manufacturer. It is recommended that the doctor uses these leaflets to aid counselling of the patient.

Consistent with good clinical practice a general medical as well as gynaecological examination should be undertaken before administration of Depo-Provera and at appropriate intervals thereafter.

*Posology and method of administration:* The sterile aqueous suspension of Depo-Provera should be vigorously shaken just before use to ensure that the dose being given represents a uniform suspension of Depo-Provera.

Doses should be given by deep intramuscular injection.

*Adults:*

*First injection:* To provide contraceptive cover in the first cycle of use, an injection of 150 mg i.m. should be given during the first five days of a normal menstrual cycle. If the injection is carried out according to these instructions, no additional contraceptive cover is required.

*Post partum:* To increase assurance that the patient is not pregnant at the time of first administration, this injection should be given within 5 days post partum if not breast feeding.

There is evidence that women prescribed Depo-Provera in the immediate puerperium can experience prolonged and heavy bleeding. Because of this, the drug should be used with caution in the puerperium. Women who are considering use of the product immediately following delivery or termination should be advised that the risk of heavy or prolonged bleeding may be increased. Doctors are reminded that in the non breast feeding post partum patient, ovulation may occur as early as week 4.

If the puerperal woman will be breast-feeding, the initial injection should be delayed until six weeks post partum, when the infant's enzyme system is more fully developed. Further injections should be given at 12 week intervals.

*Further doses:* These should be given at 12 week intervals, however, as long as the injection is given no later than five days after this time, no additional contraceptive measures (e.g. barrier) are required. (N.B. For partners of men undergoing vasectomy a second injection of 150 mg i.m. 12 weeks after the first may be necessary in a small proportion of patients where the partner's sperm count has not fallen to zero.) If the interval from the preceding injection is greater than 89 days (12 weeks and five days) for any reason, then pregnancy should be excluded before the next injection is given and the patient should use additional contraceptive measures (e.g. barrier) for fourteen days after this subsequent injection.

*Elderly:* Not appropriate.

*Children:* Not appropriate.

*Contra-indications:* Depo-Provera is contra-indicated in patients with a known sensitivity to medroxyprogesterone acetate or any ingredient of the vehicle.

Depo-Provera should not be used during pregnancy, either for diagnosis or therapy.

Depo-Provera is contra-indicated as a contraceptive at the above dosage in known or suspected hormone-dependent malignancy of breast or genital organs.

Whether administered alone or in combination with oestrogen, Depo-Provera should not be employed in patients with abnormal uterine bleeding until a definite diagnosis has been established and the possibility of genital tract malignancy eliminated.

*Special warnings and special precautions for use:*

*Warnings:*

*Menstrual irregularity:* The administration of Depo-Provera usually causes disruption of the normal menstrual cycle. Bleeding patterns include amenorrhoea (present in up to 30% of women during the first 3 months and increasing to 55% by month 12 and 68% by month 24); irregular bleeding and spotting; prolonged (>10 days) episodes of bleeding (up to 33% of women in the first 3 months of use decreasing to 12% by month 12). Rarely, heavy prolonged bleeding may occur. Evidence suggests that prolonged or heavy bleeding requiring treatment may occur in 0.5–4 occasions per 100 women years of use. If abnormal bleeding persists or is severe, appropriate investigation should take place to rule out the possibility of organic pathology and appropriate treatment should be instituted when necessary. Excessive or prolonged bleeding can be controlled by the co-administration of oestrogen. This may be delivered either in the form of a low dose (30 micrograms oestrogen) combined oral contraceptive pill or in the form of oestrogen replacement therapy such as conjugated equine oestrogen (0.625–1.25 mg daily). Oestrogen therapy may need to be repeated for 1–2 cycles. Long-term co-administration of oestrogen is not recommended.

*Return to fertility:* There is no evidence that Depo-Provera causes permanent infertility. Pregnancies have occurred as early as 14 weeks after a preceding injection, however, in clinical trials, the mean time to return of ovulation was 5.3 months following the preceding injection. Women should be counselled that there is a potential for delay in return to full fertility following use of the method, regardless of the duration of use, however, 83% of women may be expected to conceive within 12 months of the first 'missed' injection (i.e. 15 months after the last injection administered). The median time to conception was 10 months (range 4–31) after the last injection.

*Cancer risks:* Long-term case-controlled surveillance of Depo-Provera users found no overall increased risk of ovarian, liver, or cervical cancer and a prolonged, protective effect of reducing the risk of endometrial cancer in the population of users. In women under the age of 35, an increased relative risk of breast cancer was noted in women with a history of use in the 4 years preceding diagnosis (2.19, 95%CI 1.23–3.89) and prolonged use, however, there was no evidence that risk of breast cancer differed between short-term and long-term users in this group of women under age 35. The overall relative risk for ever-users of the drug was 1.2 (95%CI 0.96–1.52) which was not statistically significant. As with oral contraceptives, the evidence linking progestogen contraceptive use and breast cancer remains inconclusive. The possible risk should be weighed against the many benefits of progestogen contraceptives.

*Bone mineral density changes:* Data from a small cross-sectional study has given rise to a concern that Depo-Provera may be considered among the risk factors for osteoporosis. There is evidence that bone loss is reversible in premenopausal women and that structure and bone mass is restored after Depo-Provera usage ends. Pending the result of larger well controlled studies, women who reach the menopause and have a history of prolonged usage of Depo-Provera could be considered candidates for hormone replacement therapy.

*Weight gain:* There is a tendency for women to gain weight while on Depo-Provera therapy. Studies indicate that over the first 1–2 years of use, average weight gain was 5–8 lbs. Women completing 4–6 years of therapy gained an average of 14–16.5 lbs. There is evidence that weight is gained as a result of increased fat and is not secondary to an anabolic effect or fluid retention.

*Anaphylaxis:* Very few reports of anaphylactoid reactions have been received.

*Thrombo-embolic disorders:* Should the patient experience pulmonary embolism, cerebrovascular disease or retinal thrombosis while receiving Depo-Provera, the drug should not be readministered.

*Psychiatric disorders:* Patients with a history of endogenous depression should be carefully monitored. Some patients may complain of premenstrual-type depression while on Depo-Provera therapy.

*Precautions:* History or emergence of the following conditions require careful consideration and appropriate investigation: migraine or unusually severe headaches, acute visual disturbances of any kind, pathological changes in liver function and hormone levels. Patients with thromboembolic or coronary vascular disease should be carefully evaluated before using Depo-Provera.

A decrease in glucose tolerance has been observed in some patients treated with progestogens. The mechanism for this decrease is obscure. For this reason, diabetic patients should be carefully monitored while receiving progestogen therapy.

Rare cases of thrombo-embolism have been reported with use of Depo-Provera, but causality has not been established.

The effects of medroxyprogesterone acetate on lipid metabolism have been studied with no clear impact demonstrated. Both increases and decreases in total cholesterol, triglycerides and low-density lipoprotein (LDL) cholesterol have been observed in studies. The use of Depo-Provera appears to be associated with a 15–20% reduction in serum high density lipoprotein (HDL) cholesterol levels which may protect women from cardiovascular disease. The clinical consequences of this observation are unknown. The potential for an increased risk of coronary disease should be considered prior to use.

Doctors should carefully consider the use of Depo-Provera in patients with recent trophoblastic disease before levels of human chorionic gonadotrophin have returned to normal.

Physicians should be aware that pathologists should be informed of the patient's use of Depo-Provera if endometrial or endocervical tissue is submitted for examination.

The results of certain laboratory tests may be affected by the use of Depo-Provera. These include gonadotrophin levels (decreased), plasma progesterone levels (decreased), urinary pregnanediol levels (decreased), plasma oestrogen levels (decreased), plasma cortisol levels (decreased), glucose tolerance test, metyrapone test, liver function tests (may increase), thyroid function tests (protein bound iodine levels may increase and T3 uptake levels may decrease). Coagulation test values for prothrombin (Factor II), and Factors VII, VIII, IX and X may increase.

*Interaction with other medicaments and other forms of interaction:* Aminoglutethimide administered concurrently with Depo-Provera may significantly depress the bioavailability of Depo-Provera.

Interactions with other medicinal treatments (including oral anticoagulants) have rarely been reported, but causality has not been determined. The possibility of interaction should be borne in mind in patients receiving concurrent treatment with other drugs.

The clearance of medroxyprogesterone acetate is approximately equal to the rate of hepatic blood flow. Because of this fact, it is unlikely that drugs which

induce hepatic enzymes will significantly affect the kinetics of medroxyprogesterone acetate. Therefore, no dose adjustment is recommended in patients receiving drugs known to affect hepatic metabolising enzymes.

*Pregnancy and lactation:* Doctors should check that patients are not pregnant before initial injection of Depo-Provera, and also if administration of any subsequent injection is delayed beyond 89 days (12 weeks and five days).

Infants from accidental pregnancies that occur 1–2 months after injection of Depo-Provera may be at an increased risk of low birth weight, which in turn is associated with an increased risk of neonatal death. The attributable risk is low because such pregnancies are uncommon.

Children exposed to medroxyprogesterone acetate *in utero* and followed to adolescence, showed no evidence of any adverse effects on their health including their physical, intellectual, sexual or social development.

Medroxyprogesterone acetate and/or its metabolites are secreted in breast milk but there is no evidence to suggest that this presents any hazard to the child. Infants exposed to medroxyprogesterone via breast milk have been studied for developmental and behavioural effects to puberty. No adverse effects have been noted.

*Effects on ability to drive and use machines:* None

*Undesirable effects:* In a large clinical trial of over 3900 women, who were treated with Depo-Provera for up to 7 years, the following adverse events were reported.

The following adverse events were commonly (by more than 5% of subjects) reported: menstrual irregularities (bleeding and/or amenorrhoea), weight changes, headache, nervousness, abdominal pain or discomfort, dizziness, asthenia (weakness or fatigue).

Adverse events reported by 1% to 5% of subjects using Depo-Provera were: decreased libido or anorgasmia, backache, leg cramps, depression, nausea, insomnia, leucorrhoea, acne, vaginitis, pelvic pain, breast pain, no hair growth or alopecia, bloating, rash, oedema, hot flushes.

Other events were reported infrequently (by fewer than 1% of subjects), and included: galactorrhoea, melasma, chloasma, convulsions, changes in appetite, gastrointestinal disturbances, jaundice, genitourinary infections, vaginal cysts, dyspareunia, paraesthesia, chest pain, pulmonary embolus, allergic reactions, anaemia, syncope, dyspnoea, thirst, hoarseness, pain at injection site, blood dyscrasia, rectal bleeding, changes in breast size, breast lumps or nipple bleeding, axillary swelling, prevention of lactation, sensation of pregnancy, lack of return to fertility, paralysis, facial palsy, scleroderma, osteoporosis, uterine hyperplasia, varicose veins, dysmenorrhoea, thrombophlebitis, deep vein thrombosis.

*Overdose:* No positive action is required other than cessation of therapy.

**Pharmacological properties**

*Pharmacodynamic properties:* Medroxyprogesterone acetate exerts anti-oestrogenic, anti-androgenic and antigonadotrophic effects.

*Pharmacokinetic properties:* Parenteral medroxyprogesterone acetate (MPA) is a long acting progestational steroid. The long duration of action results from its slow absorption from the injection site. Immediately after injection of 150 mg/ml MPA, plasma levels were 1.7 ± 0.3 nmol/l. Two weeks later, levels were 6.8 ± 0.8 nmol/l. Concentrations fell to the initial levels by the end of 12 weeks. At lower doses, plasma levels of MPA appear directly related to the dose administered. Serum accumulation over time was not demonstrated. MPA is eliminated via faecal and urinary excretion. Plasma half-life is about six weeks after a single intramuscular injection. At least 11 metabolites have been reported. All are excreted in the urine, some, but not all, conjugated.

**Pharmaceutical particulars**

*List of excipients:* Excipients are methylparaben, polyethylene glycol, polysorbate 80, propylparaben, sodium chloride, hydrochloric acid, sodium hydroxide and water for injections.

*Incompatibilities:* None known.

*Shelf-life:* 36 months.

*Special precautions for storage:* Store below 25˚C. Protect from freezing.

*Nature and contents of container:* Disposable syringe with plunger stopper and tip cap.

*Instructions for use/handling:* No special instructions are applicable.

**Marketing authorisation number**   0032/0082

**Date of approval/revision of SPC**   January 1997

**Legal category:** POM

# DEPO-PROVERA 150 mg/ml

**Presentation**   White sterile aqueous suspension. Each 1 ml contains 150 mg medroxyprogesterone acetate. Also contains methylparaben, propylparaben, polyethylene glycol, sodium chloride, polysorbate and water.

**Uses**   Progestogen.

A proportion of certain classes of malignant tumours have been shown to respond to hormone administration or ablative hormonal surgery. These classes include carcinoma of endometrium, carcinoma of kidney and carcinoma of breast. Depo-Provera has been shown to be effective as adjunctive therapy in carcinoma of endometrium, carcinoma of kidney and carcinoma of breast in post-menopausal women.

**Dosage and administration**   The sterile aqueous suspension of Depo-Provera should be vigorously shaken just before use to ensure that the dose being given represents a uniform suspension of Depo-Provera.

Doses should be given by deep intramuscular injection.

*Endometrial or renal carcinoma:* The normal initial dose lies in the range 400 – 1000 mg per week, but doses in excess of 1000 mg per day have been used without serious adverse effects. If improvement is noted within a few weeks or months and the disease appears stabilised, it may be possible to maintain the improvement with as little as 400 mg per month. Depo-Provera is not recommended as primary therapy but as adjunctive and palliative treatment in advanced inoperable cases including those with recurrent or metastatic disease.

*Breast carcinoma:* The recommended schedule is 500 mg/day for 28 days. The patient should then be placed on a maintenance schedule of 500 mg twice weekly as long as the patient is responding to treatment.

Progression of disease at any time during therapy indicates treatment with Depo-Provera should be terminated, although response to hormonal therapy may not be evident until after at least 8 – 10 weeks of therapy.

Where large doses are being administered consideration should be given to dividing the dose between two separate sites.

*Elderly patients:* Depo-Provera has been extensively used in both the young (20 – 35) and older age groups (ages 50 – 75). Its use in the young has been primarily for contraception while its use in the older age group has been for the treatment of malignancies. There appears to be no evidence to suggest that the older aged patient is less well prepared to handle the drug metabolically than is the younger aged patient. Therefore, the same dosage, contra-indications, and precautions would apply to either age group.

*Children:* Not appropriate.

**Contra-indications, warnings, etc**

*Contra-indications:* Depo-Provera is contra-indicated in patients with a known sensitivity to medroxyprogesterone acetate or any ingredient of the vehicle. It should not be used during pregnancy, either for diagnosis or therapy.

Depo-Provera is contra-indicated in cancer patients with liver dysfunction or disease.

*Warnings and precautions:* In the treatment of carcinoma of breast occasional cases of hypercalcaemia have been reported.

Any patient who develops an acute impairment of vision, proptosis, diplopia or migraine headache should be carefully evaluated ophthalmologically to exclude the presence of papilloedema or retinal vascular lesions before continuing medication.

Animal studies show that Depo-Provera possesses adrenocorticoid activity. This has also been reported in man, therefore, patients receiving large doses continuously and for long periods should be observed closely.

Because progestogens may cause some degree of fluid retention, conditions which might be influenced by this factor, such as epilepsy, migraine, asthma, cardiac or renal dysfunction, require careful observation.

Gynaecomastia, hirsutism and other evidence of virilisation may develop after prolonged courses of Depo-Provera.

This form of therapy should only be administered under the direction of specialist units having facilities for appropriate surveillance of the patient.

A very low incidence of anaphylactoid reactions has been reported.

A decrease in glucose tolerance has been observed in some patients on progestogens. The mechanism for this decrease is obscure. For this reason, diabetic patients should be carefully observed while receiving progestogen therapy.

For patients with a history of endogenous depression, the physician should bear in mind the prolonged action of the product when considering the use of Depo-Provera.

Rare cases of thromboembolism have been reported with use of Depo-Provera, but causality has not been established.

Physicians should be aware that pathologists should be informed of the patient's use of Depo-Provera if endometrial or endocervical tissue is submitted for examination.

The results of certain laboratory tests may be affected by the use of Depo-Provera. These include gonadotrophin levels (decreased), plasma progesterone levels (decreased), urinary pregnanediol levels (decreased), plasma oestrogen levels (decreased), plasma cortisol levels (decreased), glucose tolerance test, metyrapone test, liver function tests (may increase), thyroid function tests (protein bound iodine levels may increase and T3 uptake levels may decrease). Coagulation test values for prothrombin (factor II) and factors VII, VIII, IX and X may increase.

Discard any remaining contents after use.

*Use in pregnancy and lactation:* Depo-Provera should not be used during pregnancy, either for diagnosis or therapy. Doctors should, therefore, check that patients are not pregnant before initial injection of Depo-Provera and also if administration of any subsequent injection is overdue. Congenital anomalies, including female foetal masculinization and clitoral hypertrophy, have been observed following larger doses of progestogens.

Medroxyprogesterone acetate and/or its metabolites are secreted in breast milk but there is no evidence to suggest that this presents any hazard to the child.

*Interactions:* Aminoglutethimide administered concurrently with Depo-Provera may significantly depress the bioavailability of Depo-Provera.

Interactions with other medicinal treatments (including oral anticoagulants) have rarely been reported, but causality has not been determined. The possibility of interaction should be borne in mind in patients receiving concurrent treatment with other drugs.

The clearance of medroxyprogesterone acetate is approximately equal to the rate of hepatic blood flow. Because of this fact, it is unlikely that drugs which induce hepatic enzymes will significantly affect the kinetics of medroxyprogesterone acetate. Therefore, no dose adjustment is recommended in patients receiving drugs known to affect hepatic metabolising enzymes.

*Side-effects:* Depending on the volume injected, some patients may be expected to show undesirable sequelae at the site of injection such as residual lump, change in colour of skin or sterile abscess. Other adverse reactions noted, particularly with large doses have been:

*Breast:* In a few instances, breast tenderness or galactorrhoea has occurred.

*Psychic:* An occasional patient has experienced nervousness, insomnia, somnolence, fatigue or dizziness.

*Skin and mucous membranes:* sensitivity reactions ranging from pruritus, urticaria, angioneurotic oedema, to generalised rash and anaphylaxis, have occasionally been reported. Acne, alopecia or hirsutism have been reported in a few cases.

*Gastro-intestinal:* Rarely nausea has been reported. Jaundice has been noted in a few instances.

*Miscellaneous:* hyperpyrexia, weight gain and moon facies.

*Overdosage:* No action required other than cessation of therapy.

**Pharmaceutical precautions** Store below 25°C and protect from freezing. Do not mix with other agents. Discard any remaining contents after use.

**Legal category** POM

**Package quantity** 3.3 ml vial.

**Further information** A 1 ml presentation of Depo-Provera 150 mg/ml is available for contraceptive use.

**Product licence number** 0032/0082

## DIPENTUM*

**Presentation** Caramel coloured capsules containing 250 mg olsalazine sodium.

Yellow capsule shaped tablets containing 500 mg olsalazine sodium with 'KPh' on one side and code '110' and score line on the other.

**Uses** Oral treatment of acute mild ulcerative colitis and the maintenance of remission. Olsalazine consists of two molecules of 5-amino-salicylic acid (5-ASA) joined through an azo-bond. The systemic absorption of olsalazine is minimal. 99% of an oral dose will reach the colon. Olsalazine is activated in the colon where it is converted into 5-ASA. The release of 5-ASA is neither pH nor time dependent. 5-ASA acts topically on the colonic mucosa and local colonic concentrations of 5-ASA are more than 1000 time that found in the serum.

**Dosage and administration**

*General:* Olsalazine taken on an empty stomach may sometimes lead to loose stools or diarrhoea. By taking the drug at the end of a meal, this may be avoided.

*Acute mild disease:*

*Adults including the elderly:* Commence on 1 g daily in divided doses taken at the end of meals. Depending on the patient's response, the dose may be titrated upwards over a period of 1 week to a maximum of 3 g daily.

A single dose should not exceed 1 g.

*Remission:*

*Adults including the elderly:* A dose of 0.5 g should be taken twice daily, at the end of meals.

Olsalazine has been used concomitantly with gluco-corticosteroids.

**Contra-indications, warnings, etc**

*Contra-indications:* Hypersensitivity to salicylates.

There is no experience of the use of olsalazine in patients with significant renal impairment. Olsalazine is contra-indicated in patients with significant renal impairment.

*Precautions:* Serious blood dyscrasias have been reported very rarely with olsalazine. Haematological investigations should be performed if the patient develops unexplained bleeding, bruising, purpura, anaemia, fever or sore throat. Treatment should be stopped if there is a suspicion or evidence of a blood dyscrasia.

*Pregnancy and lactation:* Reproduction studies performed in mice, rats and rabbits have revealed no evidence of impaired fertility, harm to the foetus or teratogenic effects due to olsalazine administration. However, the experience of use in pregnant women is limited.

Dipentum should not be used during pregnancy unless the clinician considers that the potential benefit outweighs the possible risk to the foetus.

*Adverse reactions:* As with sulphasalazine and mesalazine gastrointestinal side-effects are the most common. The most frequently reported adverse reactions are diarrhoea, arthralgia and rash.

A watery diarrhoea occurs in some patients. This is usually controlled by taking the drug at the end of a meal, as directed. Dose reduction or titration may also help.

Blood dyscrasias have been reported in a few patients: leucopenia, neutropenia, aplastic anaemia, pancytopenia, thrombocytopenia, anaemia and haemolytic anaemia.

*Treatment of overdosage:* There is no specific antidote to olsalazine. Treatment should be supportive.

**Pharmaceutical precautions** Store in a dry place.

**Legal category** POM

**Package quantities** Containers of 60 tablets. Containers of 112 capsules.

**Further information** Olsalazine has been used concomitantly with gluco-corticosteroids.

**Product licence numbers**

| | |
|---|---|
| Capsules | 0022/0134 |
| Tablets | 0022/0135 |

## DOSTINEX*

**Presentation** Flat, capsule-shaped, 4×8 mm, scored, white tablets, each containing 0.5 mg cabergoline, in type I amber glass bottles with tamper resistant screw caps and containing silica gel dessicant. Each bottle contains 8 tablets and is enclosed in an outer cardboard carton. The tablets are for oral administration.

**Uses**

*Inhibition/suppression of physiological lactation:* Dostinex is indicated for the inhibition of physiological lactation soon after delivery and for suppression of already established lactation:

(1) After parturition, when the mother elects not to breast feed the infant or when breast feeding is contraindicated due to medical reasons related to the mother or the newborn.

(2) After stillbirth or abortion.

*Treatment of hyperprolactinemic disorder:* Dostinex is indicated for the treatment of dysfunctions associated with hyperprolactinemia, including amenorrhea, oligomenorrhea, anovulation and galactorrhea. Dostinex is indicated in patients with prolactin-secreting pituitary adenomas (micro- and macroprolactinomas), idiopathic hyperprolactinemia, or empty sella syndrome with associated hyperprolactinemia, which represent the basic underlying pathologies contributing to the above clinical manifestations.

**Dosage and administration** Dostinex is to be administered by the oral route. Since in clinical studies Dostinex has been mainly administered with food and since the tolerability of this class of compounds is improved with food, it is recommended that Dostinex be preferably taken with meals for all the therapeutic indications.

*Inhibition/suppression of physiological lactation:* For INHIBITION of lactation Dostinex should be administered during the first day post-partum. The recommended therapeutic dosage is 1 mg (two 0.5 mg tablets) given as a single dose.

For SUPPRESSION of established lactation the recommended therapeutic dosage regimen is 0.25 mg (one-half 0.5 mg tablet) every 12 hours for two days (1 mg total dose). This dosage regimen has been demonstrated to be better tolerated than the single dose regimen in women electing to suppress lactation having a lower incidence of adverse events, in particular of hypotensive symptoms.

*Treatment of hyperprolactinemia disorders:* The recommended initial dosage of Dostinex is 0.5 mg per week given in one or two (one-half of one 0.5 mg tablet) doses (e.g. on Monday and Thursday) per week. The weekly dose should be increased gradually, preferably by adding 0.5 mg per week at monthly intervals until an optimal therapeutic response is achieved. The therapeutic dosage is usually 1 mg per week and ranges from 0.25 mg to 2 mg per week. Doses of Dostinex up to 4.5 mg per week have been used in hyperprolactinemic patients. The weekly dose may be given as a single administration or divided into two or more doses per week according to patient tolerability. Division of the weekly dose into multiple administrations is advised when doses higher than 1 mg per week are to be given since the tolerability of doses greater than 1 mg taken as a single weekly dose has been evaluated only in a few patients. Patients should be evaluated during dose escalation to determine the lowest dosage that produces the therapeutic response. Monitoring of serum prolactin levels at monthly intervals is advised since, once the effective therapeutic dosage regimen has been reached, serum prolactin normalisation is usually observed within two to four weeks. After Dostinex withdrawal, recurrence of hyperprolactinemia is usually observed. However, persistent suppression of prolactin levels has been observed for several months in some patients. Of the group of women followed-up 23–29 had ovulatory cycles which continued for greater than 6 months.

*Use in children:* The safety and efficacy of Dostinex has not been established in subjects less than 16 years of age.

*Use in the elderly:* As a consequence of the indications for which Dostinex is presently proposed, the experience in elderly is very limited. Available data do not indicate a special risk.

**Contra-indications, warnings, etc**

*Contra-indications:* Hypersensitivity to any ergot alkaloid. Dostinex is contra-indicated in patients with hepatic insufficiency and with toxaemia of pregnancy. Dostinex should not be co-administered with antipsychotic medications or administered to women with a history of puerperal psychosis.

*Precautions:* The safety and efficacy of Dostinex have not yet been established in patients with renal and hepatic disease. Dostinex should be given with caution to subjects with cardiovascular disease, Raynaud's syndrome, renal insufficiency, peptic ulcer, gastrointestinal bleeding or a history of serious, particularly psychotic, mental disease. Particular care should be taken when patients are taking concomitant psychoactive medication. Symptomatic hypotension can occur with Dostinex administration for any indication. Care should be exercised when administering Dostinex concomitantly with other drugs known to lower blood pressure. The effects of alcohol on overall tolerability of Dostinex are currently unknown. Before Dostinex administration, pregnancy should be excluded and after treatment pregnancy should be prevented for at least one month.

*Inhibition/suppression of physiological lactation:* By analogy with other ergot derivatives, Dostinex should not be used in women with pre-eclampsia and should be used with caution in patients with post-partum hypertension. In post-partum studies with Dostinex, blood pressure decreases were mostly symptomatic and were frequently observed on a single occasion 2 to 4 days after treatment. Since decreases in blood pressure are frequently noted during the puerperium, independently of drug therapy, it is likely that many of the observed decreases in blood pressure after Dostinex administration were not drug-induced. However, periodic monitoring of blood pressure, particularly during the first days after Dostinex administration, is advised. Dostinex should not be administered as a single dose greater than 0.25 mg in nursing women treated for suppression of established lactation since a clinical study exploring the efficacy and tolerability of 0.5 mg of Dostinex given as a single dose for suppression of lactation has shown that the risk of side effects is approximately doubled in this indication if the drug is administered as a single dose of 0.5 mg. In rats Dostinex and/or its metabolites are excreted in milk. Therefore, while no information on the excretion of Dostinex in maternal milk in humans is available, puerperal women should be advised not to breast-feed in case of failed lactation inhibition/suppression by Dostinex.

*Treatment of hyperprolactinemic disorders:* Since hyperprolactinemia with amenorrhea/galactorrhea and infertility may be associated with pituitary tumours, a complete evaluation of the pituitary is indicated before treatment with Dostinex is initiated. Dostinex restores ovulation and fertility in women with hyperprolactinemic hypogonadism: since pregnancy might occur prior to reinitiation of menses, a pregnancy test is recommended at least every four weeks during the amenorrheic period and, once menses are reinitiated, every time a menstrual period is delayed by more than three days. Women not seeking pregnancy should be advised to use mechanical contraception during treatment and after Dostinex withdrawal until recurrence of anovulation. Because of the still limited experience on the safety of fetal exposure to Dostinex, until further data become available it is advisable that women seeking pregnancy conceive at least one month after Dostinex discontinuation given that ovulatory cycles persist in some patients for 6 months after drug withdrawal. Should pregnancy occur during treatment, Dostinex is to be discontinued. As a precautionary measure, women who become pregnant should be monitored to detect signs of pituitary enlargement since expansion of pre-existing pituitary tumours may occur during gestation. Regular gynaecological assessment, including cervical and endometrial cytology, is recommended for patients taking Dostinex for extensive periods.

*Interactions:* The concomitant use of other drugs during early puerperium, particularly of ergot alkaloids, was not associated with detectable interactions modifying the efficacy and safety of Dostinex. Although there is no conclusive evidence of an interaction between Dostinex and other ergot alkaloids the concomitant use of these medications during long term treatment with Dostinex is not recommended. Since Dostinex exerts its therapeutic effect by direct stimulation of dopamine receptors, it should not be concurrently administered with drugs which have dopamine antagonist activity (such as phenothiazines, butyrophenones, thioxanthenes, metoclopramide) since these might reduce the prolactin-lowering effect of Dostinex. By analogy with other ergot derivatives, Dostinex should not be used in association with macrolide antibiotics (e.g. erythromycin) since the systemic bioavailability and also adverse effects could increase.

*Pregnancy and lactation:* Dostinex crosses the placenta in rats: it is unknown whether this occurs also in humans. Studies in animal models have not demonstrated any teratogenic effect. In clinical studies there have been over 100 pregnancies in women treated for hyperprolactinemic disorders. Dostinex was generally taken during the first 8 weeks after conception. Among the pregnancies evaluable so far, there were approximately 85% live births and about 10% spontaneous abortions. Three cases of congenital abnormalities (Down's syndrome, hydrocephalus, malformation of lower limbs) which led to therapeutic abortion and three cases of minor abnormalities in live births were observed. These incidence rates are comparable with those quoted for normal populations and for women exposed to other ovulation-inducing drugs. Based on the above data, the use of Dostinex does not appear to be associated with an increased risk of abortion, premature delivery, multiple pregnancy, or congenital abnormalities. Because clinical experience is still limited and the drug has a long half life, as a precautionary measure it is recommended that once regular ovulatory cycles have been achieved women seeking pregnancy discontinue Dostinex one month before intended conception. This will prevent possible fetal exposure to the drug and will not interfere with the possibility of conception since ovulatory cycles persist in some cases for six months after withdrawal. If conception occurs during therapy, treatment is to be discontinued as soon as pregnancy is confirmed to limit fetal exposure to the drug. Before Dostinex administration, pregnancy should be excluded and after treatment pregnancy should be prevented for at least one month. Dostinex should not be administered to mothers who elect to breast-feed their infants since it prevents lactation and no information is available on excretion of the drug in maternal milk.

*Effects on ability to drive and use machines:* During the first days of Dostinex administration, patients should be cautioned about re-engaging in activities requiring rapid and precise responses such as driving an automobile or operating machinery.

*Undesirable effects: Inhibition suppression of lactation:* Approximately 14% of women treated with a single 1 mg Dostinex for inhibition of physiological lactation complained of at least one side effect. All side effects were mild to moderate in severity and of a transient nature. The most frequently occurring adverse events were dizziness/vertigo, headache, nausea and abdominal pain. In addition, rarely palpitations, epigastric pain, somnolence, epistaxis and transient hemianopsia were reported. Asymptomatic decreases in blood pressure (no greater or lesser than ≥20 mm Hg systolic and no greater or lesser than ≥10 mm Hg diastolic) may occur usually once during the first 3–4 days post-partum. Adverse effects have been observed in approximately 14% of nursing women treated with 0.25 mg of Dostinex every 12 hours for two days for *suppression of lactation.* The most frequent symptoms were dizziness/vertigo, headache, nausea, somnolence, abdominal pain. In addition, rarely, vomiting, syncope, asthenia, and hot flushes were reported. Most side effects were transient and mild to moderate in severity.

*Hyperprolactinemic disorders:* Data obtained in a controlled clinical trial of 6 months therapy with doses ranging between 1 and 2 mg per week given in two weekly administrations, indicate a 68% incidence of adverse events during Dostinex therapy; this was significantly lower than the incidence observed for the reference standard compound. Moreover, the symptoms were generally mild to moderate in degree, mainly appearing during the first two weeks of therapy, and mostly disappearing despite continued therapy. Severe adverse events were reported at least once during therapy by 14% of patients but therapy was discontinued because of adverse events in only approximately 3% of patients. Dostinex withdrawal results in reversal of side effects, usually within a few days after discontinuation. The most common symptoms in decreasing rank of frequency were nausea, headache, dizziness/vertigo, abdominal pain/dyspepsia/gastritis, asthenia/fatigue, constipation, vomiting, breast pain, hot flushes, depression and paraesthesia. Dostinex generally exerts a hypotensive effect in patients treated chronically: however, symptomatic hypotension or fainting have been rarely reported. Being an ergot derivative, Dostinex may also act in some patients as a vasoconstrictor: digital vasospasm and leg cramps have been occasionally reported. Side effects are generally dose-related. In patients known to be intolerant of dopaminergic drugs, side effects may be lessened by starting Dostinex therapy with reduced doses (e.g. 0.25 mg once a week) with subsequent gradual increase until the therapeutic range is reached. In case of persistent or severe adverse events, temporary reduction of dosage followed by a more gradual increase (e.g. in steps of 0.25 mg per week fortnightly) may result in reversal of side effects once they have occurred. Alterations in standard laboratory tests are uncommon during long term therapy with Dostinex: a decrease in haemoglobin values have been observed in amenorrheic women during the first few months after menses resumption.

*Overdose:* There is no experience in humans of overdosage of Dostinex in the proposed indications: it is likely to lead to symptoms due to over-stimulation of dopamine receptors. These might include nausea, vomiting, gastric complaints, hypotension, confusion/psychosis or hallucinations. General supportive measures should be undertaken to remove any unabsorbed drug and maintain blood pressure if necessary. In addition, the administration of dopamine antagonist drugs may be advisable.

**Pharmaceutical precautions** Bottles of Dostinex are supplied with dessicant in caps. This dessicant must not be removed.

**Legal category** POM.

**Package quantities** Bottles of 8 tablets.

**Further information** Nil.

**Product licence number** 3433/0169.

## DOXORUBICIN RAPID DISSOLUTION

**Presentation** Sterile, pyrogen-free, orange-red, freeze-dried powder in vials containing 10 and 50 mg of doxorubicin hydrochloride with lactose and hydroxybenzoate.

**Uses** Antimitotic and cytotoxic. Doxorubicin has been used successfully to produce regression in a wide range of neoplastic conditions including acute leukaemia, lymphomas, soft-tissue and osteogenic sarcomas, paediatric malignancies and adult solid tumours, in particular breast and lung carcinomas.

Doxorubicin is frequently used in combination chemotherapy regimens involving other cytotoxic drugs. Doxorubicin cannot be used as an antibacterial agent.

**Dosage and administration** For reconstitution the contents of the 10 mg vial may be dissolved in 5 ml Water for Injections or Sodium Chloride Injection and those of the 50 mg vial in 25 ml of the same solvents.

After adding the diluent, the vial contents will dissolve with gentle shaking, without inversion, within 30 seconds. The approximate displacement value of the contents of a 50 mg vial, after 25 ml of solvent have been added, is 0.15 ml.

*Adults and children:*

*Intravenous administration:* This is the most frequently used route of administration. The reconstituted solution is given via the tubing of a freely-running intravenous infusion, taking 2–3 minutes over the injection. This technique minimises the risk of thrombosis or perivenous extravasation which can lead to severe cellulitis and vesication. Commonly used acceptable solutions are Sodium Chloride Injection, Dextrose Injection 5% or Sodium Chloride and Dextrose Injection.

Dosage is usually calculated on the basis of body surface area. On this basis, 60–75 mg/m² may be given every three weeks when doxorubicin is used alone. If it is used in combination with other antitumour agents having overlapping toxicity, the dosage of doxorubicin may need to be reduced to 30–40 mg/m² every three weeks. If dosage is to be calculated on the basis of body weight, 1.2–2.4 mg/kg should be given as a single dose every three weeks.

It has been shown that giving doxorubicin as a single dose every three weeks greatly reduces the distressing toxic effect, mucositis; however, there are still some who believe that dividing the dose over three successive days (0.4–0.8 mg/kg or 20–25 mg/m² on each day) gives greater effectiveness even though at the cost of higher toxicity.

Administration of doxorubicin in a weekly regimen has been shown to be as effective as the 3-weekly regimen. The recommended dosage is 20 mg/m² weekly although objective responses have been seen at 6–12 mg/m². Weekly administration leads to a reduction in cardiotoxicity.

Dosage may need to be reduced for patients who have had prior treatment with other cytotoxic agents.

Dosage may also need to be reduced in children and the elderly.

If hepatic function is impaired, doxorubicin dosage should be reduced according to the following table:

| *Serum bilirubin levels* | *BSP retention* | *Recommended dose* |
|---|---|---|
| 1.2–3.0 mg/100 ml | 9–15% | normal dose |
| | 50% | |
| >3.0 mg/100 ml | >15% | 25% normal dose |

*Intra-arterial administration:* Intra-arterial injection has been used in attempts to produce intense local activity while keeping the total dose low and therefore reducing general toxicity. It should be emphasised that this technique is potentially extremely hazardous and can lead to widespread necrosis of the perfused tissue unless due precautions are taken.

Intra-arterial injection should only be attempted by those fully conversant with this technique.

*Intravesical administration:* Doxorubicin is being increasingly used by intravesical administration for the treatment of transitional cell carcinoma, papillary bladder tumours and carcinoma-in-situ. It should not be employed in this way for the treatment of invasive tumours which have penetrated the bladder wall. It has also been found useful to instil doxorubicin into the bladder at intervals after transurethral resection of a tumour in order to reduce the probability of recurrence. While at present many regimens are in use, making interpretation difficult, the following may be helpful guides: The concentration of doxorubicin in the bladder should be 50 mg per 50 ml. To avoid undue dilution with urine, the patient should be instructed not to drink any fluid in the 12 hours prior to instillation. This should limit urine production to approximately 50 ml per hour. The patient should be rotated a quarter turn every 15 minutes while the drug is in situ. Exposure to the drug solution for one hour is generally adequate and the patient should be instructed to void at the end of this time.

**Contra-indications, warnings, etc** Doxorubicin Rapid Dissolution is intended for use under the direction of those experienced in cytotoxic therapy.

Hypersensitivity to hydroxybenzoates is a contra-indication.

Dosage should not be repeated in the presence of bone-marrow depression or buccal ulcerations. The latter may be preceded by premonitory buccal burning sensations and repetition in the presence of this symptom is not advised.

Haematological monitoring should be undertaken regularly in both haematological and non-haematological conditions, because of the possibility of bone-marrow depression which may become evident around ten days from the time of administration.

Cardiotoxicity may be manifested in tachycardia, including supra-ventricular tachycardia and ECG changes. Routine ECG monitoring is recommended and caution should be exercised in patients with impaired cardiac function.

A cumulative dose of 450–550 mg/m² should only be exceeded with extreme caution. Above this level, the risk of irreversible congestive cardiac failure increases greatly. The total dose of doxorubicin administered to the individual patient should also take account of any previous or concomitant therapy with other potentially cardiotoxic agents such as high-dose i.v. cyclophosphamide, mediastinal irradiation or related anthracycline compounds such as daunorubicin. Administration of doxorubicin weekly has been shown to be associated with reduced cardiotoxicity compared with a 3-weekly schedule allowing patients to be treated to a higher cumulative dose. It should be noted that cardiac failure may also occur several weeks after administration and may not respond to treatment.

Baseline and follow-up ECGs during and immediately after drug administration are advisable. Transient ECG changes, such as T-wave flattening, S-T segment depression and arrhythmias, are not considered indications for the suspension of doxorubicin therapy. A reduction of the QRS wave is considered more indicative of cardiac toxicity. If this change occurs, the benefit of continued therapy must be carefully evaluated against the risk of producing irreversible cardiac damage.

Severe cardiac failure may occur suddenly, without premonitory ECG changes.

Doxorubicin Rapid Dissolution may impart a red colour to the urine, particularly to the first specimen passed after the injection and patients should be advised that this is no cause for alarm.

Alopecia occurs frequently, including the interruption of beard-growth, but all hair growth normally resumes after treatment is stopped.

Nausea, vomiting and diarrhoea may also occur.

The risk of thrombophlebitis at the injection site may be minimised by following the procedure for administration recommended above. A stinging or burning sensation at the site of administration signifies a small degree of extravasation and the infusion should be stopped and re-started in another vein.

*Pregnancy and lactation:* There is no conclusive information as to whether doxorubicin may adversely affect human fertility, or cause teratogenesis. Experimental data, however, suggest that doxorubicin may harm the foetus and should, therefore, not be administered to pregnant women or to mothers who are breast-feeding.

*Overdosage:* Single doses of 250 mg and 500 mg of doxorubicin have proved fatal. Such doses may cause acute myocardial degeneration within 24 hours and severe myelosuppression, the effects of which are greatest between 10 and 15 days after administration. Treatment should aim to support the patient during this period and should utilise such measures as blood transfusions and reverse barrier nursing. Delayed cardiac failure may occur up to six months after the overdose. Patients should be observed carefully and should signs of cardiac failure arise, be treated along conventional lines.

**Pharmaceutical precautions** The vial contents are under a negative pressure to minimise aerosol formation during reconstitution; particular care should be taken when the needle is inserted. Inhalation of any aerosol produced during reconstitution must be avoided.

The following protective recommendations are given due to the toxic nature of this substance:
— Personnel should be trained in good technique for reconstitution and handling.
— Pregnant staff should be excluded from working with this drug.
— Personnel handling Doxorubicin Rapid Dissolution should wear protective clothing: goggles, gowns and disposable gloves and masks.
— A designated area should be defined for reconstitution (preferably under a laminar flow system). The work surface should be protected by disposable, plastic-backed, absorbent paper.
— All items used for reconstitution, administration or cleaning, including gloves, should be placed in high-risk, waste-disposal bags for high-temperature incineration.

The reconstituted solution is stable when stored for up to 48 hours at room temperature in normal artificial light, however, in line with good pharmaceutical practice it is recommended that it should normally be stored at 2°–8°C, protected from light and used within 24 hours. The reconstituted solution is chemically stable for at least 24 hours at room temperature in strong sunlight.

The reconstituted solution contains 0.02% hydroxybenzoate. This is not a preservative solution. Discard any unused solution.

Prolonged contact with any solution of an alkaline pH should be avoided as it will result in hydrolysis of the drug. Doxorubicin Rapid Dissolution should not be mixed with heparin as a precipitate may form and it is not recommended that Doxorubicin Rapid Dissolution be mixed with other drugs.

Accidental contact with the skin or eyes should be treated immediately by copious lavage with water, or soap and water, or sodium bicarbonate solution: medical attention should be sought.

Spillage or leakage should be treated with dilute sodium hypochlorite (1% available chlorine) solution, preferably by soaking, and then water. All cleaning materials should be disposed of as indicated previously.

**Legal category** POM.

**Package quantities** 10 mg and 50 mg vials for injection.

**Further information** Nil.

**Product licence number** 3433/0110

# DOXORUBICIN SOLUTION FOR INJECTION

**Presentation** Sterile, red, mobile solution in vials containing 10 mg and 50 mg of doxorubicin hydrochloride as a 2 mg/ml solution in 0.9% Sodium Chloride Injection.

**Uses** Antimitotic and cytotoxic. Doxorubicin has been used successfully to produce regression in a wide range of neoplastic conditions, including acute leukaemia, lymphomas, soft-tissue and osteogenic sarcomas, paediatric malignancies and adult solid tumours; in particular, breast and lung carcinomas.

Doxorubicin is frequently used in combination chemotherapy regimens with other cytotoxic drugs. Doxorubicin cannot be used as an antibacterial agent.

**Dosage and administration** Adults and children.
*Intravenous administration:* The solution is given via the tubing of a freely-running intravenous infusion, taking 2–3 minutes over the injection. This technique minimises the risk of thrombosis or perivenous extravasation which can lead to severe cellulitis and vesication.

Dosage is usually calculated on the basis of body surface area. On this basis, 60–75 mg/m² may be given every three weeks when doxorubicin is used alone. If it is used in combination with other antitumour agents having overlapping toxicity, the dosage of doxorubicin may need to be reduced to 30–40 mg/m² every three weeks. If dosage is calculated on the basis of body weight, 1.2–2.4 mg/kg should be given as a single dose every three weeks.

It has been shown that giving doxorubicin as a single dose every three weeks greatly reduces the distressing toxic effect, mucositis; however there are still some who believe that dividing the dose over three successive days (0.4–0.8 mg/kg or 20–25 mg/m² on each day) gives greater effectiveness though at the cost of higher toxicity.

Administration of doxorubicin in a weekly regimen has been shown to be as effective as the 3-weekly regimen. The recommended dosage is 20 mg/m² weekly although objective responses have been seen at 6–12 mg/m². Weekly administration leads to a reduction in cardiotoxicity.

Dosage may need to be reduced for patients who have had prior treatment with other cytotoxic agents.

Dosage may also need to be reduced in children and the elderly.

If hepatic function is impaired, doxorubicin dosage should be reduced according to the following table:

| Serum bilirubin levels | BSP retention | Recommended dose |
|---|---|---|
| 1.2–3.0 mg/100 ml | 9–15% | 50% normal dose |
| >3.0 mg/100 ml | >15% | 25% normal dose |

**Contra-indications, warnings, etc** Doxorubicin Solution for Injection is intended for use under the direction of those experienced in cytotoxic therapy.

Dosage should not be repeated in the presence of bone-marrow depression or buccal ulcerations. The latter may be preceded by premonitory buccal burning sensations and repetition in the presence of this symptom is not advised.

Haematological monitoring should be undertaken regularly in both haematological and non-haematological conditions, because of the possibility of bone-marrow depression which may become evident around ten days from the time of administration.

Cardiotoxicity may be manifested in tachycardia, including supraventricular tachycardia, and ECG changes. Routine ECG monitoring is recommended and caution should be exercised in patients with impaired cardiac function.

A cumulative dose of 450–550 mg/m² should only be exceeded with extreme caution. Above this level, the risk of irreversible congestive cardiac failure increases greatly. The total dose of doxorubicin administered to the individual patient should also take account of any previous or concomitant therapy with other potentially cardiotoxic agents such as high-dose i.v. cyclophosphamide, mediastinal irradiation or related anthracycline compounds such as daunorubicin.

Administration of doxorubicin weekly has been shown to be associated with reduced cardiotoxicity compared with a 3-weekly schedule allowing patients to be treated to a higher cumulative dose.

It should be noted that cardiac failure may also occur several weeks after administration and may not respond to treatment.

Baseline and follow-up ECGs during and immediately after drug administration are advisable. Transient ECG changes, such as T-wave flattening, S-T segment depression and arrhythmias, are not considered indications for the suspension of doxorubicin therapy. A reduction of the QRS wave is considered more indicative of cardiac toxicity. If this change occurs, the benefit of continued therapy must be carefully evaluated against the risk of producing irreversible cardiac damage.

Severe cardiac failure may occur suddenly, without premonitory ECG changes.

Doxorubicin Solution for Injection may impart a red colour to the urine, particularly to the first specimen passed after the injection and patients should be advised that this is no cause for alarm.

Alopecia occurs frequently, including the interruption of beard growth, but all hair growth normally resumes after treatment is stopped.

Nausea, vomiting and diarrhoea may also occur.

The risk of thrombophlebitis at the injection site may be minimised by following the procedure for administration recommended above. A stinging or burning sensation at the site of administration signifies a small degree of extravasation and the infusion should be stopped and re-started in another vein.

The occurrence of secondary acute myeloid leukaemia with or without a pre-leukaemic phase has been reported rarely in patients concurrently treated with doxorubicin in association with DNA-damaging antineoplastic agents. Such cases could have a short (1–3 year) latency period.

*Pregnancy and lactation:* There is no conclusive information as to whether doxorubicin may adversely affect human fertility, or cause teratogenesis. Experimental data, however, suggest that doxorubicin may harm the foetus and should, therefore, not be administered to pregnant women or to mothers who are breast-feeding.

*Overdosage:* Single doses of 250 mg and 500 mg of doxorubicin have proved fatal. Such doses may cause acute myocardial degeneration within 24 hours and severe myelosuppression, the effects of which are greatest between 10 and 15 days after administration. Treatment should aim to support the patient during this period and should utilise such measures as blood transfusions and reverse barrier nursing. Delayed cardiac failure may occur up to six months after the overdose. Patients should be carefully observed and should signs of cardiac failure arise, be treated along conventional lines.

**Pharmaceutical precautions** The following protective recommendations are given due to the toxic nature of this substance:
— Personnel should be trained in good technique for handling.
— Pregnant staff should be excluded from working with this drug.
— Personnel handling Doxorubicin Solution for Injection should wear protective clothing: goggles, gowns and disposable gloves and masks.
— All items used for administration or cleaning, including gloves, should be placed in high-risk, waste-disposal bags for high-temperature incineration.

Doxorubicin Solution for Injection should be stored at 2°C–8°C.

Discard any unused solution.

Prolonged contact with any solution of an alkaline pH should be avoided as it will result in hydrolysis of the drug. Doxorubicin Solution for Injection should not be mixed with heparin as a precipitate may form and it is not recommended that Doxorubicin Solution for Injection be mixed with other drugs.

Accidental contact with the skin or eyes should be treated immediately by copious lavage with water, or soap and water, or sodium bicarbonate solution: medical attention should be sought.

Spillage or leakage should be treated with dilute sodium hypochlorite (1% available chlorine) solution, preferably by soaking, and then water. All cleaning materials should be disposed of as indicated previously.

**Legal category** POM.

**Package quantities** 10 mg and 50 mg vials for injection.

**Further information** Doxorubicin Solution for Injection is adjusted to pH 3 with 0.5 N hydrochloric acid.

**Product licence number** 3433/0127.

## EDRONAX* ▼

**Qualitative and quantitative composition** Reboxetine 4.0 mg (equivalent to 5.224 mg reboxetine methanesulphonate).

**Pharmaceutical forms** 4.0 mg strength: white, round, convex, 8 mm diameter tablet with a breakline on one side. A "P" will be marked on the left side of the breakline. A "U" will be marked on the right side of the breakline. The side opposite the breakline will be marked "7671".

The tablets are contained in aluminium-PVDC/PVC-PVDC opaque blisters.

Each pack contains 60 tablets in blisters.

The tablets are for oral administration.

**Clinical particulars**

*Therapeutic indications:* Reboxetine is indicated for the treatment of depressive illness.

Controlled clinical studies carried out in adult and elderly (>65 years) patients suffering mainly from Major Depressive Disorders, have demonstrated that reboxetine is effective in the therapy of acute episodes of depression as well as in the prevention of re-emergence of symptoms of depressive illness when administered on long-term therapy.

The results of the studies indicate that the primary effect of reboxetine is on the nuclear symptom (depressed mood) of depressive illness. However, the positive effect is also seen on accessory symptoms related to arousal (insomnia, decreased activity level) and on anxiety and somatic symptoms.

The remission of the acute phase of the depressive illness is associated with an improvement in the patient's quality of life in terms of social adaptation.

*Posology and method of administration:*

*Use in adults:* The recommended therapeutic dose is 4 mg b.i.d. (8 mg/day) administered orally. The full therapeutic dose can be given upon starting treatment. After 3–4 weeks, this dose can be increased to 10 mg/day in case of incomplete clinical response.

*Use in the elderly:* As with other antidepressants, in elderly subjects and in elderly depressed patients, particularly in the presence of concomitant systemic illnesses and medications, systemic exposure appeared higher than that usually observed in young healthy volunteers. The recommended therapeutic dose is 2 mg b.i.d. (4 mg/day) administered orally.

This dose can be increased to 6 mg/day in case of incomplete clinical response after 3 weeks from starting reboxetine. This dose regimen has been shown to allow adequate clinical response in the majority of the patients studied.

*Use in children:* The use of reboxetine in children is not recommended since safety and efficacy have not been evaluated in this population.

*Contra-indications:* Hypersensitivity to the compound.

*Special warnings and special precautions for use:* As expected on the basis of preferential elimination route, plasma levels and half-lives appear to increase in subjects with renal impairment and especially in severe renal impairment ($CL_{CR}$ < 20 ml/min) where a dose adjustment is required. Similar findings, though less relevant and not consistently observed, were apparent in elderly subjects and patients with hepatic insufficiency.

As reboxetine has not been tested in patients with convulsive disorders in clinical studies and since rare cases of seizures have been reported in clinical studies, it should be given under close supervision to subjects with a history of convulsive disorders and it must be discontinued if the patient develops seizures.

Combined usage of MAO inhibitors and reboxetine has not been studied in the clinical trials to date. Therefore, as for other antidepressants, concomitant use should be avoided until further data are available.

As with all antidepressants, switches to mania/hypomania have occurred during the clinical studies. Close supervision of bipolar patients is, therefore, recommended.

The risk of a suicidal attempt is inherent in depression and may persist until significant remission occurs: close patient supervision during initial drug therapy is, therefore, recommended.

Clinical experience with reboxetine in patients affected by serious concomitant systemic illnesses is limited. Close supervision should be applied in patients with current evidence of urinary retention and glaucoma.

At doses higher than the maximum recommended, orthostatic hypotension has been observed with greater frequency. Particular attention should be paid when administering reboxetine with other drugs known to lower blood pressure.

Clinical experience with Reboxetine in the long-term treatment of elderly patients is, at present, limited. In this population, lowering of mean potassium levels was found starting from week 14; the magnitude of this reduction did not exceed 0.8 mmol/litre and potassium levels never dropped below normal limits.

*Interactions with other medicaments and other forms of interaction:* Reboxetine is extensively bound to plasma proteins; the available data indicate that the drug is almost exclusively bound to $\alpha_1$ acid glycoprotein. Therefore, the concurrent administration of drugs with a high affinity for this fraction of plasma proteins (such as dipyridamole, propranolol, alprenolol, methadone, lidocaine and other local anaesthetics, but also imipramine and chlorpromazine) may cause a shift in plasma concentration of either drug, potentially resulting in an adverse reaction.

Plasma pharmacokinetics of reboxetine are not significantly modified when Cytochrome P450 2D6 activity is blocked. Therefore, no modification of reboxetine metabolism is expected in poor metabolisers with deficiency of this isoenzyme.

Repeated doses of reboxetine do not affect Cytochrome P450 3A activity as documented by the unmodified urinary excretion of 6-β-hydroxycortisol. As a consequence, no modification is expected in the metabolism of oral contraceptives or other steroids, triazolam, alprazolam, terfenadine, nifedipine, erythromycin, lidocaine, cyclosporine A, when they are co-administered with reboxetine.

No significant reciprocal pharmacokinetic interaction has been found between reboxetine and lorazepam. During their co-administration in healthy volunteers, mild to moderate drowsiness and short lasting orthostatic acceleration of heart rate have been observed.

Reboxetine does not appear to potentiate the effect of alcohol on cognitive functions in healthy volunteers.

Concomitant use of reboxetine with other antidepressants (tricyclics, MAO Inhibitors, SSRIs and Lithium) has not been evaluated during clinical studies.

The extent of absorption of reboxetine is not significantly influenced by concomitant food intake.

Although data are not available from clinical studies, the possibility of hypokalaemia with concomitant use of potassium losing diuretics should be considered.

*Pregnancy and lactation:* Studies in animals have not demonstrated any teratogenic effect or any effect of the compound on global reproductive performance. In humans experience is very limited. Therefore, administration during pregnancy should be avoided. If conception occurs during therapy, treatment is to be discontinued as soon as pregnancy is confirmed to limit foetal exposure to the drug.

In rats reboxetine is excreted in milk. Therefore, while no information on the excretion of reboxetine in maternal milk in humans is available, reboxetine administration is not recommended in breast feeding women.

*Effects on ability to drive and use machines:* Reboxetine is not sedative per se. No cognitive or psychomotor impairment has been observed with reboxetine in clinical studies, also when the compound was co-administered with alcohol. However, as with all psychoactive drugs, patients should be cautioned about operating machinery and driving.

*Undesirable effects* : About 1500 patients received reboxetine in clinical studies, 200 of which received reboxetine for up to 1 year.

Taking into account the placebo-controlled studies, in acute depression 373 adult patients received reboxetine and 373 received placebo. In these studies adverse events were reported in 69% of reboxetine-treated patients and in 57% of placebo-treated patients. Adverse events were the main reason for discontinuation in 8% of the reboxetine treated patients and 7.5% of the placebo treated patients. Adverse events associated with discontinuation of reboxetine with a frequency at least twice that on placebo were: insomnia (1.3% *vs* 0.5% of the exposed patients), increased sweating (1.1% *vs* 0.3%), dizziness or hypotension (0.8% *vs* 0%), paraesthesia (0.8% *vs* 0.3%), impotence, urinary tract infection or dysuria (0.5% *vs* 0%).

Adverse events with statistically significantly higher risk of development on reboxetine than on placebo included: dry mouth (reported in 27% *vs* 16% of the patients on reboxetine and placebo, respectively), constipation (17% *vs* 8%), insomnia (14% *vs* 5%), increased sweating (14% *vs* 7%), tachycardia (5% *vs* 2%), vertigo (2% *vs* 0%), urinary hesitancy/retention (5% *vs* 2%; of which, retention is 2% *vs* 1%), impotence (5% *vs* 0%), the latter mainly observed in patients treated with doses higher than 8 mg/day.

As for long-term tolerability, 143 reboxetine-treated and 140 placebo-treated adult patients participated in a long term placebo-controlled study. Adverse events newly emerged on long-term treatment in 28% of the reboxetine-treated patients and 23% of the placebo-treated patients and caused discontinuation in 4% and 1% of the cases, respectively. There was a similar risk of the development of individual events with reboxetine and placebo. Among events seen more than occasionally, no individual events not seen on short term treatment were apparent.

The most relevant between gender difference in adverse event rate was related to the frequency of urinary hesitancy/retention complained of mainly by male patients (10% *vs* 2% in females on short term treatment; 14% *vs* 1% in females on long term treatment).

In the elderly population, frequency of total adverse events, as well as of individual events, was never higher than that reported above.

No indication of withdrawal syndrome upon reboxetine discontinuation emerged from the results of the clinical trials: signs and symptoms newly reported on abrupt discontinuation were infrequent and less frequent in patients treated with reboxetine (4%) than in those treated with placebo (6%).

Vital signs, including blood pressure and heart rate, body weight and body temperature, were evaluated in the majority of reboxetine treated patients and the only modification observed was related to heart rate, particularly on standing, significantly increased *vs* baseline (>20%, to values ≥ 100 beats/min) mainly in adult patients (20% of the patients on short-term treatment compared with 6% on placebo and 23% of the patients on long-term treatment compared with 17% on placebo).

Apart from tachycardia in a minority of cases, no consistent changes of ECG tracings were observed during reboxetine treatment in adult patients. Similarly, no consistent changes were observed at the ophthalmological examination, carried out upon long-term treatment. In the elderly population, newly observed rhythm disorders (mainly tachycardia) and conduction disorders were apparent at ECG in a minority of cases.

Abnormal laboratory test values have been uncommon during reboxetine therapy.

*Overdose:* The acute toxicity studies carried out in animals indicate a very low toxicity, with a wide safety margin with respect to the pharmacologically active doses. Clinical signs and cause of death were related to CNS stimulation (mainly convulsive symptoms).

In a few cases doses higher than those recommended were administered to patients (12 mg to 20 mg/day) for a period ranging from a few days to some weeks during clinical studies: newly reported complaints include postural hypotension, anxiety and hypertension.

Two cases of self-overdosing with reboxetine were reported by the patients during the clinical studies. No major adverse events were observed.

In case of overdose, monitoring of cardiac function and vital signs is recommended. General symptomatic supportive and/or emetic measures might be required.

**Pharmacological properties**

*Pharmacodynamic properties:* Reboxetine is a highly selective and potent inhibitor of norepinephrine reuptake.

Norepinephrine reuptake inhibition and the consequent increase of norepinephrine availability in the synaptic cleft and modification of noradrenergic transmission, reportedly is among the most relevant mechanisms of action of known antidepressant drugs.

*In vitro*, studies have shown that reboxetine has no significant affinity for adrenergic ($\alpha_1$, $\alpha_2$, β) and muscarinic receptors; antagonism of such receptors has been described to be associated with cardiovascular, anticholinergic and sedative side effects of other antidepressant drugs.

In healthy volunteers the administration of reboxetine single doses of 1 and 3 mg was followed by dose-dependent CNS effects with EEG modifications (decreased power of theta and fast beta-waves in the fronto central derivative) and performance improvement (peg-board test).

*Pharmacokinetic properties:* The pharmacokinetics of reboxetine after single or multiple oral doses have been studied in healthy young or elderly volunteers, in depressed patients and in subjects with renal or liver insufficiency. After oral administration of a single 4 mg reboxetine dose to healthy volunteers, peak levels of about 130 ng/ml are achieved within 2 h post-dosing. Data indicate that absolute bioavailability is at least 60%. Reboxetine plasma levels decay monoexponentially with a half-life of about 13 h. Steady-state conditions are observed within 5 days. Linearity of the pharmacokinetics was shown in the range of single oral doses in the clinically recommended dose-ranges.

The drug appears to be distributed into total body water. Reboxetine is 97 % bound to human plasma proteins (with affinity markedly higher for $\alpha_1$ acid glycoprotein than albumin), with no significant dependence of the concentration of drug.

The amount of radioactivity excreted in urine accounts for 78 % of the dose. Even though unchanged drug is predominant in the systemic circulation (70% of total radioactivity, in terms of AUC), only 10% of the dose is excreted as unchanged drug in urine. These findings suggest that biotransformation rules the overall elimination of reboxetine and that metabolites excretion is limited by their formation. The main metabolic pathways identified are 2-O-dealkylation, hydroxylation of the ethoxyphenoxy ring and oxidation of the morpholine ring, followed by partial or complete glucuro- or sulphoconjugation.

The drug is available as a racemic compound (with both enantiomers being active in the experimental models): no chiral inversion, nor reciprocal pharmacokinetic interferences between enantiomers have been observed. Plasma levels of the more potent SS enantiomer are about two times lower and urinary excretion two times higher than those of the enantiomeric counterpart. No significant differences were observed in the terminal half-lives of the two enantiomers.

Some increase in systemic exposure and half-life up to two fold are observed in patients with renal insufficiency; similar findings, though less relevant and not consistently observed, were apparent in elderly subjects and patients with hepatic insufficiency.

*Preclinical safety data:* Preclinical safety studies of reboxetine indicate a satisfactory safety margin for this compound in humans, as well as a lack of teratogenic, genotoxic or carcinogenic potential.

**Pharmaceutical particulars**

*List of excipients:* Cellulose microcrystalline; Dibasic calcium phosphate dihydrate; Crospovidone; Silicon dioxide; Magnesium stearate

*Incompatibilities:* None known.

*Shelf life:* 36 months at room temperature

*Special precautions for storage:* Storage below 25° C.

*Nature and contents of container:* The tablets are contained either in aluminium-PVDC / PVC-PVDC opaque blisters.

Each pack contains 60 tablets in blisters.

*Instructions for use/handling:* There are no special instructions for handling.

**Marketing authorisation number** 0032/0216

**Date of approval/revision of SPC** December 1996

**Legal category** POM

## ESTRACYT* CAPSULES

**Presentation** Off-white gelatin capsules marked with KPh 750 on one side and Estracyt on the other. Each contains 140 mg estramustine phosphate as the disodium salt.

*Active ingredient:* 140 mg estramustine phosphate – oestra -1,3,5 (10)-triene-3,17β-diol-3-bis-(2-chloroethyl) carbamate-17-disodium phosphate.

**Uses** *Pharmacology:* Estracyt is a chemical compound of oestradiol and normustine and has both oestrogenic and cytotoxic activity. Its oestrogenic effect is weaker than that of oestradiol and this is reflected by the lower incidence of gynaecomastia and other feminising side-effects in patients treated with Estracyt for prostatic carcinoma. Estracyt also has antioestrogenic activity in that it antagonises the uterotrophic effect of oestrone in juvenile mice, antigonadotrophic activity in that it causes atrophy of the testes and accessory sex organs in rats, and antiandrogenic activity in that it inhibits testosterone-induced growth of the ventral prostate of castrated animals.

The cytotoxic activity of Estracyt is weaker than that of conventional alkylating agents. It is concentrated ten times more efficiently than oestradiol in prostatic tissue and has a greater affinity for prostatic than for other tissue. Though active against experimental animal tumours (rat DMBA-induced mammary tumour and hepatoma AH130), Estracyt has weak general cytostatic effects and causes little or no marrow depression at conventional therapeutic dosage. It has no immunosuppressant effect.

Estracyt appears to lose its phosphate moiety in the gut, liver and in phosphatase-rich human tissue, and following breakage of the carbamate linkage the steroid and alkylating moieties are excreted independently. Absorption of Estracyt from the gut is about 75% complete.

**Indications** Carcinoma of the prostate, especially in cases unresponsive to, or relapsing after, treatment by conventional oestrogens (stilboestrol, polyoestradiol phosphate (Estradurin), etc) or by orchidectomy. The response rate to Estracyt in such oestrogen-resistant cases is about 30% to 50%.

**Dosage and administration** *Adults including the elderly:* Dosage range may be from 1 to 10 capsules a day by mouth. The capsules should be taken not less than 1 hour before or 2 hours after meals. The capsules should not be taken with milk or milk products. Standard starting dosage is 4 a day in divided doses with later adjustment according to response and gastrointestinal tolerance.

*Children:* Adenocarcinoma of the prostate is almost unknown in young boys and no relevant clinical studies of Estracyt have been carried out. Estracyt should not be administered to children.

**Contra-indications, warnings, etc**
*Contra-indications:*

Known hypersensitivity to either oestradiol or to nitrogen mustard.

Peptic ulceration.

Severe hepatic or cardio-vascular disease.

*Interactions:* Milk, milk products or drugs containing calcium may impair the absorption of Estracyt and should not be taken simultaneously with Estracyt.

*Effects on ability to drive or operate machinery:* No adverse effects on a patient's ability to drive or operate machinery have been reported.

*Other undesirable effects:* Gastro-intestinal disturbances (most commonly transient nausea, but occasionally vomiting and rarely diarrhoea) sometimes occur at the beginning of therapy. In a few cases thrombocytopenia, leukopenia and elevated transaminases/bilirubin have been noted. Cardiovascular effects including oedema, worsening angina, congestive cardiac failure. Myocardial infarction has rarely been reported. Thromboembolic disorders, gynaecomastia, reduced libido and potency may occur as with other oestrogenic drugs. Occasionally allergy (manifest as rash and/or fever) is encountered.

*Other special warnings and precautions:* Use with caution in patients with moderate to severe bone marrow depression, thrombophlebitis, thrombosis, thromboembolic disorders, cerebrovascular disease, coronary artery disease and congestive cardiac failure.

Caution should also be exercised in patients with diabetes, hypertension, epilepsy, hepatic and renal impairment and diseases associated with hypercalcaemia. Blood counts, liver function tests and serum calcium in hypercalcaemia should be performed at regular intervals.

*Overdosage:* There is no specific antidote. Treatment is symptomatic and supportive and in the event of dangerously low levels of red cell, white cell or platelet count, whole blood should be given as necessary. Liver function should be monitored.

*Incompatibilities* (major): None reported.

**Pharmaceutical precautions** Store at room temperature. The preparation has a shelf life of three years from the date of manufacture.

**Legal category** POM.

For use in hospitals and hospital clinics, and supplied to retail pharmacies for dispensing prescriptions for patients whose treatment has been initiated in hospital practice. Estracyt capsules are available on prescription only.

**Package quantities** Bottles of 100 capsules each containing 140 mg estramustine phosphate as the disodium salt.

**Further information** Nil.

**Product licence number** 0022/0106.

## ESTRADURIN* INJECTION

**Presentation** Estradurin Injection contains 80 mg polyoestradiol phosphate per vial, for reconstitution with water for injection.

*Estradurin 80 mg vial:*

| | |
|---|---|
| Polyoestradiol phosphate | 80 mg |
| Mepivacaine | 5 mg |
| Nicotinamide | 40 mg |

**Uses** *Pharmacology:* Estradurin is a water-soluble polymer in which molecules of oestradiol-17β alternate with phosphate groups. After intramuscular injection it acts primarily as a long-acting form of oestradiol, but it also has an inhibitory action on acid and alkaline phosphatases.

The prolonged action of Estradurin is attributed to the slow progressive breakdown of the polymer by phosphatases *in vivo.* Since Estradurin has an inhibiting effect on phosphatases this breakdown is very slow, providing sustained oestrogen activity for up to four weeks after a single injection.

*Indications:* The treatment of oestrogen-responsive carcinoma of the prostate, particularly in men suspected of unreliability in the taking of conventional oral oestrogen.

**Dosage and administration** *Adults:* The recommended starting dose is 80–160 mg every four weeks for two to three months. Thereafter the dose may be reduced, in accordance with the patient's clinical and biochemical progress, to 40–80 mg every four weeks.

NB. Estradurin must be administered by *deep* intramuscular injection.

*Children:* Estradurin should not be administered to children.

**Contra-indications, warnings, etc**
*Contra-indications:* Estradurin should not be used in patients with any of the following conditions:

Known hypersensitivity to oestradiol
Seriously impaired liver function
Active thrombophlebitis or thromboembolic disorders
Dubin-Johnson syndrome
Rotor syndrome
Sickle cell anaemia
Jaundice
Oestrogen-dependent neoplasms (known or suspected).

*Interactions:* Thyroid hormone binding globulin may be increased leading to increased circulating total thyroid hormone, therefore care must be taken in interpreting thyroid function tests.

Risk of deep vein thrombosis is temporarily increased when undergoing major surgery of prolonged immobilisation, therefore treatment should be stopped before surgery.

*Effects on ability to drive and to use machines:* None known.

*Other undesirable effects:*
*Gastro-intestinal tract:* Nausea, vomiting, cholelithiasis, cholestatic jaundice.

*Cardiovascular system:* Hypertension, thrombosis, thrombophlebitis, thromboembolism.

*CNS:* Headache, migraine, mood changes (elation or depression).

*Metabolic:* Sodium and water retention, reduced glucose tolerance, change in body weight.

*Hormonal:* Gynaecomastia, feminisation, testicular atrophy.

*Behavioural:* Change in libido or potency.

*Skin:* Erythema.

*Other special warnings and precautions*
*Warnings:* Estradurin may cause fluid retention; patients with conditions which may be influenced by this factor, such as epilepsy, migraine or cardiac or renal dysfunction need careful observation.

Patients with severe varicose veins, sickle cell haemoglobinopathy, untreated polycythaemia or pulmonary hypertension. The benefits of Estradurin treatment must be weighed against the possible risk of exacerbating these conditions.

*Precautions:* Estradurin may be poorly metabolised in patients with impaired liver function and should be administered with caution in such patients. Liver function tests should be performed at regular intervals.

Because glucose tolerance may be decreased, diabetic patients should be carefully observed while receiving Estradurin.

Hypertension may occur hence blood pressure should be monitored.

Caution is recommended in patients with a history of hyperlipoproteinaemia, thrombophlebitis, thrombosis, thromboembolic disorders, otosclerosis, porphyria or cerebral vascular or coronary artery disease.

*Overdose:* Reversible feminisation most likely sign. There is no specific antidote, treatment should be symptomatic.

*Incompatibilities:* None known.

**Pharmaceutical precautions** Store at room temperature.

The product has a shelf life of five years from the date of manufacture. Estradurin solution is prepared by adding 2 ml water for injection to the vial and shaking until solution is complete.

It is recommended that solutions of Estradurin be prepared immediately before use.

**Legal category** POM.

**Package quantities** 10×80 mg vials: (with 10×2 ml ampoules water for injection).

**Further information** Mepivacaine, a local anaesthetic, is included to minimise discomfort at the site of injection.

Nicotinamide is included to enhance solubility of the polymer.

**Product licence number** 0458/5001

*Product licence holder:* Lundbeck Ltd, Sunningdale House, Caldecotte Lake Business Park, Caldecotte, Milton Keynes, MK7 8BR

## ESTRING*

**Presentation** Estradiol vaginal ring is a slightly opaque ring, made of a silicone elastomer, with a whitish core, containing a drug reservoir of 2 mg Estradiol Hemihydrate PhEur. The product has the following dimensions: outer diameter – 55 mm; cross sectional diameter – 9 mm; core diameter – 2 mm.

**Uses**
*Action:* Estring is a vaginal ring which delivers approximately 7.5 micrograms/24 hours of 17β-oestradiol for 3 months.

The oestradiol from the ring acts locally to eliminate or reduce symptoms and signs of postmenopausal urogenital oestrogen deficiency.

*Indications:* Treatment of postmenopausal atrophic vaginitis. Estring is only suitable for the treatment of urogenital complaints due to oestrogen deficiency. Its pharmacokinetic profile shows that there is no significant systemic effect and therefore it is not suitable for postmenopausal complaints which require a systemically active dose of oestrogen (e.g. vasomotor symptoms), neither is it suitable for osteoporosis prophylaxis.

**Dosage and administration**
*Adults including the elderly:* One ring to be inserted into the upper third of the vagina, to be worn continuously for 3 months, then replaced by a new ring as appropriate. The maximum recommended duration of continuous therapy is two years.

Instructions for use are available in a Patient Information Leaflet enclosed in each pack.

Estring is only intended for treatment of postmenopausal women.

*Children:* Estring is not recommended for use in children.

**Contra-indications, warnings, etc**
*Contra-indications:* Known or suspected oestrogen-dependent malignancy, e.g. endometrial carcinoma or other oestrogen-dependent tumours.

Undiagnosed abnormal genital bleeding.

Known or suspected pregnancy.

*Precautions:* Some women may be unsuitable for treatment with Estring, in particular those with short narrow vaginas due to previous surgery or the effect of atrophy, or those with a degree of uterovaginal prolapse severe enough to prevent retention of the ring. During long-term treatment with oestrogens, periodic medical examinations are advisable.

In addition, any woman with symptoms/signs of abnormal vaginal discharge, vaginal discomfort, or any vaginal bleeding should be examined fully to exclude ulceration, infection, or unresponsive atrophic vaginitis.

Minor signs of irritation are often transient. Any woman experiencing persistent or severe discomfort due to the presence of the ring or excessive movement of the ring should be withdrawn from treatment.

Patients with signs of ulceration or severe inflammation due to unresponsive atrophic vaginitis should also be withdrawn from treatment.

Patients with vaginal infection should be treated appropriately. In the case of systemic therapy, Estring treatment may continue without interruption. However, removal of Estring should be considered while using vaginal preparations.

Treatment with Estring will result in very low plasma levels of oestradiol, similar to those seen in untreated postmenopausal women. It has been estimated that approximately 4 μg of 17-β oestradiol are absorbed systemically per 24 hours. It is unlikely that this level of oestradiol would be associated with any of the known risks of systemic oestrogen treatment.

However, it is advisable that patients with endometrial hyperplasia; thromboembolic disease; acute or chronic liver disease (including Dubin Johnson Syndrome and Rotor Syndrome) or acute intermittent porphyria should be treated with caution. Accordingly, these patients should be carefully assessed prior to treatment and monitored during therapy including measurement of appropriate parameters.

Patients on long-term corticosteroid treatment or those with conditions causing poor skin integrity, e.g. Cushing's Disease, may be unsuitable for treatment as they may have vaginal atrophy unresponsive to oestrogen therapy.

There have been incidences of both the ring falling out and movement of the ring, generally at defaecation. Therefore, if the woman is constipated she should remove the ring before defaecation. There may also be other instances when some women wish to remove the ring, e.g. prior to sexual intercourse. Comprehensive advice for removal and reinsertion of the ring are provided in the Patient Information Leaflet which is included in every pack.

*Pregnancy and lactation:* Estring is indicated for postmenopausal treatment. Women of child bearing potential and lactating women should, therefore, not be prescribed Estring.

*Side-effects:* Adverse reactions with Estring are rare. Adverse reactions reported with a frequency of 1% or more in clinical trials, in order of decreasing frequency, were vaginal irritation, abdominal pain/lower abdominal pain/abdominal discomfort, vulvovaginal infection, urogenital pruritus, pressure symptoms in vagina/on bladder/on rectum, generalised pruritus, urinary tract infection and increased sweating. However, some of these symptoms occur more frequently in untreated postmenopausal women, e.g. vaginal irritation, urinary tract infection, urogenital pruritus, vulvovaginal infection and increased sweating.

A few cases of vaginal ulceration were reported in clinical trials. While these were minor and transient it is recommended that any patient who develops an ulcer should be withdrawn from treatment.

In the Patient Information Leaflet, patients are advised that if they experience any undesirable effects they should consult their doctor. Furthermore, if these effects are severe the leaflet gives instructions on how to remove the ring themselves, if they wish, before seeing their doctor.

*Overdosage:* This is not relevant due to the mode of administration.

*Interactions:* As the oestrogen is administered vaginally and due to the low levels released, it is unlikely that any clinically relevant drug interactions will occur with Estring.

Removal of Estring should be considered when using other vaginal preparations.

**Pharmaceutical precautions** Store at room temperature (below 30°C).

**Legal category** POM.

**Package quantities** Carton containing one vaginal ring in a foil pouch and a Patient Information Leaflet.

**Further information**
*Pharmacokinetics:* After a brief initial peak, the release of oestradiol from Estring is constant (7.5 micrograms/24 hours) for at least 90 days. Following ring insertion, plasma oestradiol levels reach 200 pmol/l within 3 hours. However, after this initial peak, concentrations decline rapidly and constant levels are achieved after 2–3 days. These levels are maintained at, or near, the quantification limit (20–30 pmol/l) throughout the rest of the treatment period.

*Pharmacodynamics:* Estring therapy restores vaginal pH to premenopausal values and returns the histology and physiology of the vaginal and urethral epithelia to premenopausal states. The very low, constant release of oestradiol from Estring does not exert adverse systemic effects, i.e. induces no increase in SHBG (Sex Hormone Binding Globulin) or alpha$_2$-PAG (Pregnancy Zone Protein). Therefore, theoretically, it should not cause endometrial proliferation. Estring can, therefore, be used continuously without the addition of progestogens and consequently, no uterine bleeding will result from treatment.

**Product licence number** 0022/0115.

## FARLUTAL*

**Presentation** *Injection:* White, sterile suspension for i.m. injection, which settles on standing and readily disperses on shaking, containing 500 mg of medroxyprogesterone acetate in 2.5 ml, or 1000 mg in 5.0 ml.

*Tablets:* White, uncoated, round, biconvex, scored tablets, diameter 9 mm (100 mg) or 11 mm (250 mg), stamped '100' or '250' diametrically and containing 100 mg or 250 mg of medroxyprogesterone acetate, respectively.

White, uncoated, capsule-shaped tablets, measuring about 22 mm×7 mm, scored on both faces and stamped 'FCE' and '500' on one face, containing 500 mg of medroxyprogesterone acetate.

**Uses** Palliative treatment of hormone-sensitive malignancies. Farlutal has been successfully used to produce regressions in breast, endometrial, prostatic and renal cell carcinoma. High dose Farlutal therapy has proved especially useful in breast carcinoma and in achieving subjective improvements in terminally ill patients, notably pain relief and improved performance status.

**Dosage and administration** Suggested dosage schemes are as follows:

Breast carcinoma

| | |
|---|---|
| Initial dose | 500—1000 mg/day i.m. for 4 weeks. |
| Maintenance | 500 mg i.m. twice a week. |

*Alternatively,* 1000–1500 mg daily, orally, is recommended, although doses of up to 2000 mg daily have been used. Daily oral administration, to be effective, must be at least 2–3 times the recommended i.m. dosage.

*Endometrial carcinoma*

| | |
|---|---|
| Initial dose | 500 mg i.m. twice weekly for 3 months. |
| Maintenance | 500 mg i.m. weekly. |
| Alternatively | 100–500 mg/day orally. |

*Renal adenocarcinoma*

| | |
|---|---|
| Initial dose | 500 mg i.m. on alternate days for 30 days. |
| Maintenance | 500 mg i.m. twice weekly until 60th day, then 250 mg i.m. weekly. |
| Alternatively | 100–500 mg/day orally. |

Prostatic adenocarcinoma

| | |
|---|---|
| Initial dose | 500 mg i.m. twice weekly. |
| Maintenance | 500 mg i.m. weekly. |
| Alternatively | 100–500 mg/day orally. |

Intramuscular administration should be by deep injection into alternate gluteal muscles using a long wide-bore needle such as 21 G×1½ (8/10 40 mm). Narrow-bore or short needles must not be used.

Large tablets, and in this case particularly Farlutal 500, should be taken while sitting or standing and with copious amounts of liquid. The tablets may be broken in half before administration, if necessary.

**Contra-indications, warnings, etc**
*Contra-indications:* Thrombophlebitis, thrombo-embolic disorders, severe hepatic insufficiency and hypercalcaemia as may occur in patients with osseous metastases; also, suspected or early breast carcinoma, missed abortion, metrorrhagia, pregnancy and known hypersensitivity to medroxyprogesterone acetate or, for the injectable formulation, hydroxybenzoates (excipients).

*Warnings:* Farlutal should be used under the direction of those experienced in cancer chemotherapy.

Since medroxyprogesterone acetate appears to enhance blood clotting potential, treatment should be discontinued upon the appearance of thrombo-embolic episodes, migraine or associated ocular problems such as sudden or partial or total loss of vision, diplopia or vascular lesions of the retina.

In the event of vaginal bleeding occurring, an accurate diagnosis should be made. If a histological examination is indicated, the laboratory should be informed that the patient has been receiving a progestogen.

*Precautions:* Animal studies have shown that medroxyprogesterone acetate possesses adrenocorticoid activity and this effect has also been observed in humans. Patients treated with high doses continuously over long periods should be carefully observed for signs normally associated with adrenocorticoid therapy, such as hypertension, sodium retention, oedema, etc. Care is needed in treating patients with cardiovascular, renal or hepatic impairment, diabetes mellitus, asthma, epilepsy, migraine or other conditions which may be aggrevated by fluid retention, porphyria and patients with a history of mental depression.

It should be noted that long term administration of medroxyprogesterone acetate to beagle dogs has resulted in the development of mammary nodules which were occasionally found to be malignant. The relevance of these findings to humans has, however, not been established.

Farlutal may raise plasma calcium levels; some cases of hypercalcaemia have been reported in the treatment of breast carcinoma.

*Pregnancy and lactation:* Administration of progesterone during the first months of pregnancy may possibly be associated with the occurrence of congenital cardiac malformations in the neonate. In addition, instances of masculinisation of female foetuses have been reported following high dose therapy during pregnancy. For these reasons, Farlutal is contra-indicated during pregnancy.

It is known from literature that medroxyprogesterone acetate is secreted in breast milk and although no adverse effect on the newborn child has been reported, it is advisable to avoid breast feeding during the treatment with Farlutal.

*Interactions:* Progestogens may inhibit the metabolism of cyclosporin, leading to increased plasma cyclosporin concentrations. Rifampicin may accelerate the metabolism of progestogens, leading to decreased efficacy.

*Adverse reactions:* As is generally found after intramuscular administration of large volumes of suspension, the i.m. preparation may cause local lesions at the injection site, such as sterile abscesses or inflammatory infiltrates. The suspension should, therefore, be well shaken before use and injected deeply into healthy gluteal muscle.

In common with other progestogens, Farlutal may cause mastodynia, galactorrhoea, vaginal bleeding, changes in menstrual flow, amenorrhoea, cervical erosions and modifications of cervical secretions. Farlutal also exerts a corticoid-like effect which may lead to facies lunaris, Cushingoid syndrome and weight changes; and an adrenergic-like action which may result in fine hand tremors, sweating and cramps in the calves at night. Other effects may include gastro-intestinal disturbances, changes in appetite, fluid retention, acne, melasma or chloasma, allergic skin rashes, urticaria, mental depression, changes in libido hair loss or hirsutism, fatigue, drowsiness or insomnia, fever and headache. Anaphylaxis ornaphylactoid reactions may occur rarely. Alterations in liver function tests have been reported and cholestatic jaundice occasionally been reported.

**Pharmaceutical precautions** The vials for injection should be well shaken before use and the contents should not be mixed with other agents. The vials are for single dose administration only, should be stored between 15°–30°C and should not be frozen.

The tablets should be stored in a dry place.

### Package quantities

Farlutal 100: Cartons containing blister packs of 100 tablets.

Farlutal 250:Cartons containing blister packs of 50 tablets.

Farlutal 500:Cartons containing calendar blister packs of 56 tablets.

Farlutal 500 for Injection Vials in individual cartons.

Farlutal 1000 for Injection Vials in individual cartons.

### Legal category POM.

**Further information** Analysis of the various i.m. dosage schedules so far employed indicates that higher response rates may be obtained by attainment and maintenance of high plasma levels. The intramuscular injection of Farlutal as a 20% suspension of medroxyprogesterone acetate, enables these levels to be achieved while minimising the local side effects associated with high dose therapy using formulations of lower concentrations.

After oral administration of medoxyprogesterone acetate, absorption is rapid. The plasma half life is of the order of 2 days and with repeated dosing once daily a steady state concentration is reached in about 10 days. Plasma concentrations are usually proportional to the administered dose, but considerable individual variation occurs. In general, to obtain concentrations comparable to those achieved after 4 weeks i.m. administration, at least twice the daily i.m. dose should be given.

### Product licence numbers

| | |
|---|---|
| Farlutal 100 | 3433/0056 |
| Farlutal 250 | 3433/0058 |
| Farlutal 500 | 3433/0080 |
| Farlutal 500 for Injection and | |
| Farlutal 1000 for Injection | 3433/0045 |

## FRAGMIN* AMPOULES

### Qualitative and quantitative composition

*Active ingredient.* Dalteparin sodium (INN).

Quality according to PhEur and in-house specification. Potency is described in International anti-Factor Xa units (IU) of the 1st International Standard for Low Molecular Weight Heparin.

*Content of active ingredient:* Fragmin 10,000 IU/4 ml: Ampoules containing dalteparin sodium corresponding to 2,500 IU (anti-Factor Xa)/ml.

Fragmin 10,000 IU/1 ml: Ampoules containing dalteparin sodium, 10,000 IU (anti-Factor Xa) in 1 ml.

**Pharmaceutical form** Solution for injection for intravenous or subcutaneous administration.

### Clinical particulars

*Therapeutic indications:* Prevention of clotting in the extracorporeal circulation during haemodialysis or haemofiltration, in patients with chronic renal insufficiency or acute renal failure.

Treatment of acute deep venous thrombosis.

Unstable coronary artery disease, defined as newly developed or increased angina or ongoing chest pain, with the electrocardiogram changes of non Q-wave myocardial infarction.

*Posology and method of administration:*

*Recommended dosage for adults*

*Prevention of clotting during haemodialysis and haemofiltration:* In chronic renal insufficiency for patients with no known additional bleeding risk, the dosage is:

Long-term haemodialysis or haemofiltration–duration of haemodialysis/haemofiltration more than 4 hours;

An i.v bolus injection of Fragmin 30–40 IU (anti-Factor Xa)/kg bodyweight, followed by an infusion of 10–15 IU (anti-Factor Xa)/kg bodyweight/hour.

Short-term haemodialysis or haemofiltration–duration of haemodialysis/haemofiltration less than 4 hours;

Either as above, or, a single i.v bolus injection of Fragmin 5000 IU (anti-Factor Xa).

Both for long and short-term haemodialysis and haemofiltration, the plasma anti-Factor Xa levels should be within the range 0.5–1.0 IU (anti-Factor Xa)/ ml.

In acute renal failure, or chronic renal failure in patients with a high risk of bleeding, the dosage is:

An i.v bolus injection of Fragmin 5–10 IU (anti-Factor Xa)/kg bodyweight, followed by an infusion of 4–5 IU (anti-Factor Xa)/kg bodyweight/hour.

The plasma anti-Factor Xa levels should be within the range 0.2–0.4 IU (anti-Factor Xa)/ml.

When considered necessary, it is recommended that the antithrombotic effect of Fragmin be monitored by analysing anti-Factor Xa activity using a suitable chromogenic substrate assay. This is because Fragmin has only a moderate prolonging effect on clotting time assays such as APTT or thrombin time.

*Treatment of deep venous thrombosis (10,000 IU/1 ml presentation):* Fragmin can be administered subcutaneously either as a single daily injection or as twice daily injections.

*Once daily administration:* 200 IU/kg body weight is administered s.c once daily. Monitoring of the anticoagulant effect is not necessary. The single daily dose should not exceed 18,000 IU.

*Twice daily administration:* A dose of 100 IU/kg body weight administered s.c twice daily can be used for patients with increased risk of bleeding. Monitoring of the treatment is generally not necessary but can be performed with a functional anti-Factor Xa assay. Maximum plasma levels are obtained 3–4 hours after s.c injection, when samples should be taken. Recommended plasma levels are between 0.5–1.0 IU (anti-Factor Xa)/ml.

Simultaneous anticoagulation with oral vitamin K antagonists can be started immediately. Treatment with Fragmin is continued until the prothrombin complex levels (factor II, VII, IX and X) have decreased to a therapeutic level. At least five days of combined treatment is normally required.

*Unstable coronary artery disease (10,000 IU/1 ml presentation):* 120 IU/kg body weight subcutaneously twelve hourly. The maximum dose is 10,000 IU/12 hours.

The recommended treatment period is 5–8 days. Concomitant therapy with low dose aspirin is recommended.

*Children:* Not recommended for children.

*Elderly:* Fragmin has been used safely in elderly patients without the need for dosage adjustment.

*Contra-indications.* Known hypersensitivity to Fragmin; acute gastroduodenal ulcer; cerebral haemorrhage; known haemorrhagic diathesis; subacute endocarditis; injuries to and operations on the central nervous system, eyes and ears; thrombocytopenia in patients with a positive result in the *in-vitro* aggregation test in the presence of dalteparin sodium. In patients being treated with Fragmin for acute deep venous thrombosis, regional anaesthesia is contraindicated due to an increased risk of bleeding.

*Special warnings and special precautions for use:* Do not administer by the intramuscular route.

Caution should be exercised in patients in whom there is an increased risk of bleeding complications, e.g. following surgery or trauma, haemorrhagic stroke, severe liver failure, thrombocytopenia or defective platelet function, uncontrolled hypertension, hypertensive or diabetic retinopathy, patients receiving concurrent anticoagulant/antiplatelet agents (see interactions section), and also patients with known hypersensitivity to heparin and/or to other low molecular weight heparin.

Fragmin induces only a moderate prolongation of the APTT and thrombin time. Accordingly, dosage increments based upon prolongation of the APTT may cause overdosage and bleeding. Therefore, prolongation of the APTT should only be used as a test of overdosage.

Anti-Factor Xa levels should be regularly monitored in new patients on chronic haemodialysis during the first weeks, later less frequent monitoring is generally required. Patients undergoing acute haemodialysis have a narrower therapeutic dose range and should be monitored frequently in accordance with the individual course of the disease.

Patients with severely disturbed hepatic function may need a reduction in dosage and should be monitored accordingly.

If a transmural myocardial infarction occurs in patients with unstable coronary artery disease, thrombolytic treatment might be appropriate. This does not necessitate discontinuation of treatment with Fragmin, but might increase the risk of bleeding.

As individual low molecular weight (mass) heparins have differing characteristics, switching to an alternative low molecular weight heparin should be avoided. The directions for use relating to each specific product must be observed as different dosages may be required.

*Interaction with other medicaments and other forms of interaction:* The possibility of the following interactions with Fragmin should be considered:

An enhancement of the anticoagulant effect by anticoagulant/antiplatelet agents e.g. aspirin/ dipyridamole, vitamin K antagonists, NSAIDs e.g. indomethacin, cytostatics, dextran, sulphinpyrazone, probenecid, and ethacrynic acid. However, unless specifically contraindicated, patients with unstable coronary artery disease should receive oral low dose aspirin.

A reduction of the anticoagulant effect may occur with concomitant administration of antihistamines, cardiac glycosides, tetracycline and ascorbic acid.

*Pregnancy and lactation.* This medicinal product has been assessed in pregnant women and no harmful effects are known with respect to the course of pregnancy and the health of the unborn and neonate.

No information is available as to whether Fragmin passes into breast milk.

*Effects on ability to drive and use machines.* Fragmin does not affect the ability to drive or operate machinery.

*Undesirable effects.* Bleeding may be provoked, especially at high dosages corresponding with anti-Factor Xa levels greater than 1.5 IU/ml. However, at recommended dosages bleeding rarely occurs.

Transient, slight to moderate, elevation of liver transaminases (ASAT, ALAT) has been observed, but no clinical significance has been demonstrated.

Commonly reported side-effects include subcutaneous haematomas at the injection site. Thrombocytopenia and allergic reactions (urticaria, pruritus, hair loss and skin necrosis) occur rarely. Few cases of anaphylactoid reactions have been observed.

Osteoporosis has been associated with long-term heparin treatment and therefore cannot be excluded with Fragmin.

*Overdose.* The anticoagulant effect (i.e. prolongation of the APTT) induced by Fragmin is inhibited by protamine. Since protamine itself has an inhibiting effect on primary haemostasis it should be used only in an emergency.

The prolongation of the clotting time induced by Fragmin may be fully neutralised by protamine, but the anti-Factor Xa activity is only neutralised to about 25–50%. 1 mg of protamine inhibits the effect of 100 IU (anti-Factor Xa) of Fragmin.

### Pharmacological properties

*Pharmacodynamic properties:* Dalteparin sodium is a low molecular weight heparin fraction (average molecular weight 4000-6000 Daltons) produced from porcine-derived sodium heparin.

Dalteparin sodium is an antithrombotic agent, which acts mainly through its ability to potentiate the inhibition of Factor Xa and thrombin by antithrombin. It has a relatively higher ability to potentiate Factor Xa inhibition than to prolong plasma clotting time (APTT).

Compared with standard, unfractionated heparin, dalteparin sodium has a reduced adverse effect on platelet function and platelet adhesion, and thus has only a minimal effect on primary haemostasis. Some of the antithrombotic properties of dalteparin sodium are thought to be mediated through the effects on vessel walls or the fibrinolytic system.

*Pharmacokinetic properties:* The half life following i.v and s.c administration is 2 hours and 3.5–4 hours respectively, twice that of unfractionated heparin.

The bioavailability following s.c injection is approximately 87 per cent and the pharmacokinetics are not dose dependent. The half life is prolonged in uraemic patients as dalteparin sodium is eliminated primarily through the kidneys.

*Preclinical safety data:* The acute toxicity of dalteparin sodium is considerably lower than that of heparin. The only significant finding, which occurred consistently throughout the toxicity studies after subcutaneous administration of the higher dose levels was local haemorrhage at the injection sites, dose-related in incidence and severity. There was no cumulative effect on injection site haemorrhages.

The haemorrhagic reaction was reflected in dose related changes in the anticoagulant effects as measured by APTT and anti-Factor Xa activities.

It was concluded that dalteparin sodium did not have a greater osteopenic effect than heparin since at equivalent doses the osteopenic effect was comparable.

The results revealed no organ toxicity irrespective of the route of administration, doses or the duration of treatment. No mutagenic effect was found. No embryotoxic or teratogenic effects and no effect on fertility reproductive capacity or peri- and postnatal development was shown.

### Pharmaceutical particulars

*List of excipients:* Sodium chloride (PhEur), Water for injections (PhEur)

*Incompatibilities:* The compatibility of Fragmin with products other than those mentioned under Instructions for use/handling has not been investigated.

*Shelf life:* 36 months.

*Special precautions for storage:* Store at room temperature (below 30°C).

*Nature and contents of container:* Clear glass ampoules (PhEur Type 1) containing dalteparin sodium, 10,000 IU (anti-factor Xa) in 1 ml or 10,000 IU (anti-factor Xa) in 4 ml.

*Instructions for use/handling:* Fragmin solution for injection is compatible with isotonic sodium chloride (9 mg/ml) or isotonic glucose (50 mg/ml) infusion solutions in glass bottles and plastic containers for up to 24 hours. Compatibility between Fragmin and other products has not been studied.

**Marketing authorisation numbers**
Fragmin 10,000 IU/4 ml    0022/0074
Fragmin 10,000 IU/1 ml    0022/0075

**Date of approval/revision of SPC**  December 1996

**Legal category** POM

## FRAGMIN* MULTIDOSE VIAL

### Qualitative and quantitative composition

*Active ingredient:* Dalteparin sodium (INN).

Quality according to PhEur. Potency is described in International anti-Factor Xa units (IU) of the 1st International Standard for Low Molecular Weight Heparin.

*Content of active ingredient:* Fragmin 100,000 IU/4 ml: Multidose vial containing dalteparin sodium corresponding to 25,000 IU (anti-Factor Xa)/ml.

**Pharmaceutical form**  Solution for injection for subcutaneous administration.

### Clinical particulars

T*herapeutic indications:*  Treatment of acute deep venous thrombosis.

*Posology and method of administration:*
*Recommended dosage for adults*
Treatment of deep venous thrombosis: Fragmin can be administered subcutaneously either as a single daily injection or as twice daily injections.

*Once daily administration:* 200 IU/kg body weight is administered s.c once daily. Monitoring of the anticoagulant effect is not necessary. The single daily dose should not exceed 18,000 IU.

*Twice daily administration:* A dose of 100 IU/kg body weight administered s.c twice daily can be used for patients with increased risk of bleeding. Monitoring of the treatment is generally not necessary but can be performed with a functional anti-Factor Xa assay. Maximum plasma levels are obtained 3–4 hours after s.c injection, when samples should be taken. Recommended plasma levels are between 0.5–1.0 IU (anti-Factor Xa)/ml.

Simultaneous anticoagulation with oral vitamin K antagonists can be started immediately. Treatment with Fragmin is continued until the prothrombin complex levels (factor II, VII, IX and X) have decreased to a therapeutic level. At least five days of combined treatment is normally required.

*Children:* Not recommended for children.

*Elderly:* Fragmin has been used safely in elderly patients without the need for dosage adjustment.

*Contra-indications:* Known hypersensitivity to Fragmin or benzyl alcohol; acute gastroduodenal ulcer; cerebral haemorrhage; known haemorrhagic diathesis; subacute endocarditis; injuries to and operations on the central nervous system, eyes and ears; thrombocytopenia in patients with a positive result in the in-vitro aggregation test in the presence of dalteparin sodium. In patients treated with Fragmin for acute deep venous thrombosis, regional anaesthesia is contraindicated due to an increased risk of bleeding.

*Special warnings and special precautions for use:* Do not administer by the intramuscular route.

Caution should be exercised in patients in whom there is an increased risk of bleeding complications, e.g. following surgery or trauma, haemorrhagic stroke, severe liver failure, thrombocytopenia or defective platelet function, uncontrolled hypertension, hypertensive or diabetic retinopathy, patients receiving concurrent anticoagulant/antiplatelet agents (see interactions section), and also patients with known hypersensitivity to heparin and/or to other low molecular weight heparin.

Fragmin induces only a moderate prolongation of the APTT and thrombin time. Accordingly, dosage increments based upon prolongation of the APTT may cause overdosage and bleeding. Therefore, prolongation of the APTT should only be used as a test of overdosage.

Patients with severely disturbed hepatic function may need a reduction in dosage and should be monitored accordingly.

As individual low molecular weight (mass) heparins have differing characteristics, switching to an alternative low molecular weight heparin should be avoided. The directions for use relating to each specific

product must be observed as different dosages may be required.

*Interaction with other medicaments and other forms of interaction:* The possibility of the following interactions with Fragmin should be considered:

An enhancement of the anticoagulant effect by anticoagulant/antiplatelet agents e.g. aspirin/ dipyridamole, vitamin K antagonists, NSAIDs e.g. indomethacin, cytostatics, dextran, sulphinpyrazone, probenecid, and ethacrynic acid.

A reduction of the anticoagulant effect may occur with concomitant administration of antihistamines, cardiac glycosides, tetracycline and ascorbic acid.

*Pregnancy and lactation:* Fragmin multidose vial contains benzyl alcohol as a preservative and is not recommended for use during pregnancy. Benzyl alcohol may cross the placenta. One should bear in mind the potential toxicity for premature infants.

No information is available as to whether Fragmin passes into breast milk.

*Effects on ability to drive and use machines:* Fragmin does not affect the ability to drive or operate machinery.

*Undesirable effects:* Bleeding may be provoked, especially at high dosages corresponding with anti-Factor Xa levels greater than 1.5 IU/ml. However, at recommended dosages bleeding rarely occurs.

Transient, slight to moderate, elevation of liver transaminases (ASAT, ALAT) has been observed, but no clinical significance has been demonstrated.

Commonly reported side-effects include subcutaneous haematomas at the injection site. Thrombocytopenia and allergic reactions (urticaria, pruritus, hair loss and skin necrosis) occur rarely. Few cases of anaphylactoid reactions have been observed.

Osteoporosis has been associated with long-term heparin treatment and therefore cannot be excluded with Fragmin.

*Overdose:* The anticoagulant effect (i.e. prolongation of the APTT) induced by Fragmin is inhibited by protamine. Since protamine itself has an inhibiting effect on primary haemostasis it should be used only in an emergency. The prolongation of the clotting time induced by Fragmin may be fully neutralised by protamine, but the anti-Factor Xa activity is only neutralised to about 25–50%. 1 mg of protamine inhibits the effect of 100 IU (anti-Factor Xa) of Fragmin.

### Pharmacological properties

*Pharmacodynamic properties:* Dalteparin sodium is a low molecular weight heparin fraction (average molecular weight 4000-6000 Daltons) produced from porcine-derived sodium heparin.

Dalteparin sodium is an antithrombotic agent, which acts mainly through its ability to potentiate the inhibition of Factor Xa and thrombin by antithrombin. It has a relatively higher ability to potentiate Factor Xa inhibition than to prolong plasma clotting time (APTT).

Compared with standard, unfractionated heparin, dalteparin sodium has a reduced adverse effect on platelet function and platelet adhesion, and thus has only a minimal effect on primary haemostasis.

Still some of the antithrombotic properties of dalteparin sodium are thought to be mediated through the effects on vessel walls or the fibrinolytic system.

*Pharmacokinetic properties:* The half life following i.v and s.c administration is 2 hours and 3.5–4 hours respectively, twice that of unfractionated heparin.

The bioavailability following s.c injection is approximately 87 per cent and the pharmacokinetics are not dose dependent. The half life is prolonged in uraemic patients as dalteparin sodium is eliminated primarily through the kidneys.

*Preclinical safety data:* The acute toxicity of dalteparin sodium is considerably lower than that of heparin. The only significant finding, which occurred consistently throughout the toxicity studies after subcutaneous administration of the higher dose levels was local haemorrhage at the injection sites, dose-related in incidence and severity. There was no cumulative effect on injection site haemorrhages.

The haemorrhagic reaction was reflected in dose related changes in the anticoagulant effects as measured by APTT and anti-Factor Xa activities.

It was concluded that dalteparin sodium did not have a greater osteopenic effect than heparin since at equivalent doses the osteopenic effect was comparable.

The results revealed no organ toxicity irrespective of the route of administration, doses or the duration of treatment. No mutagenic effect was found. No embryotoxic or teratogenic effects and no effect on fertility reproductive capacity or peri- and postnatal development was shown.

### Pharmaceutical particulars

*List of excipients:* Benzyl Alcohol PhEur, Water for injections PhEur.

*Incompatibilities:* Not applicable.

*Shelf life:* 24 months. Once opened, the solution should be used within 14 days.

*Special precautions for storage:* Store at room temperature (below 30°C).

*Nature and contents of container:* Multidose vial (PhEur Type 1) with bromobutyl rubber stopper, secured with aluminium overseal with flip off cap, containing dalteparin sodium 100,000 IU (anti-Factor Xa) in 4 ml.

*Instructions for use/handling:* As with other multidose preparations, care should be taken to avoid any risk of cross-contamination during use.

**Marketing authorisation number**  0022/0177

**Date of approval/revision of SPC** 31 July 1996.

**Legal category**  POM

## FRAGMIN* 2500 IU AND 5000 IU SYRINGES

### Qualitative and quantitative composition
*Active ingredient:* Dalteparin sodium (INN). Quality according to Ph.Eur. and in-house specification.

Potency is described in International anti-Factor Xa units (IU) of the 1st International Standard for Low Molecular Weight Heparin.

*Content of active ingredient:* Fragmin 2500 IU: single dose syringe containing dalteparin sodium 2,500 IU (anti-Factor Xa) in 0.2 ml solution.

Fragmin 5000 IU: single dose syringe containing dalteparin sodium 5000 IU (anti-Factor Xa) in 0.2 ml solution.

Fragmin syringes do not contain preservatives.

**Pharmaceutical form**  Solution for injection for subcutaneous administration.

### Clinical particulars
*Therapeutic indications:* Peri- and post-operative surgical thromboprophylaxis.

*Posology and method of administration*
*Adults*
Surgical thromboprophylaxis in patients at moderate risk of thrombosis: 2,500 IU is administered subcutaneously 1–2 hours before the surgical procedure and thereafter 2,500 IU subcutaneously each morning until the patient is mobilised, in general 5–7 days or longer.

*Surgical thromboprophylaxis in patients at high risk of thrombosis:* 2,500 IU is administered subcutaneously 1–2 hours before the surgical procedure and 2,500 IU subcutaneously 8–12 hours later. On the following days, 5,000 IU subcutaneously each morning.

As an alternative, 5,000 IU is administered subcutaneously the evening before the surgical procedure and 5,000 IU subcutaneously the following evenings.

Treatment is continued until the patient is mobilised, in general 5–7 days or longer.

*Prolonged thromboprophylaxis in hip replacement surgery:* 5,000 IU is given subcutaneously the evening before the operation and 5,000 IU subcutaneously the following evenings. Treatment is continued for five post-operative weeks.

*Children:* Not recommended for children.

*Elderly:* Fragmin has been used safely in elderly patients without the need for dosage adjustment.

*Method of Administration:* By subcutaneous injection, preferably into the abdominal subcutaneous tissue anterolaterally or posterolaterally, or into the lateral part of the thigh. Patients should be supine and the total length of the needle should be introduced vertically, not at an angle, into the thick part of a skin fold, produced by squeezing the skin between the thumb and forefinger; the skin fold should be held throughout the injection.

*Contra-indications:* Known hypersensitivity to Fragmin; acute gastroduodenal ulcer; cerebral haemorrhage; known haemorrhagic diathesis; subacute endocarditis; injuries to and operations on the central nervous system, eyes and ears; thrombocytopenia in patients with a positive result in the in-vitro aggregation test in the presence of dalteparin sodium.

*Special warnings and special precautions for use:* Caution should be exercised in patients in whom there is an increased risk of bleeding complications, e.g. following trauma, haemorrhagic stroke, severe liver or renal failure, thrombocytopenia or defective platelet function, uncontrolled hypertension, hypertensive or diabetic retinopathy, patients receiving concurrent anticoagulant/anitplatelet agents (see Interactions section), and also patients with known hypersensitivity to heparin and/or to other low molecular weight heparin.

Fragmin when administered in a dose of 2,500–5,000 IU (anti-Factor Xa)/day does not generally accumulate, and therefore monitoring of the effect is not usually required. However, if considered necessary, chromogenic substrate assays can be used to measure anti-Factor Xa activity (Fragmin has only a moderate prolonging effect on clotting time assays such as APTT or thrombin time).

As individual low molecular weight (mass) heparins have differing characteristics, switching to an alternative low molecular weight heparin should be avoided. The directions for use relating to each specific product must be observed as different dosages may be required.

Do not administer by the intramuscular route.

*Interaction with other medicaments and other forms of interaction:* The possibility of the following interactions with Fragmin should be considered:

An enhancement of the anticoagulant effect by anticoagulant/antiplatelet agents e.g. aspirin/dipyridamole, Vitamin K antagonists, NSAIDS e.g. indomethacin, cytostatics, dextran, sulphinpyrazone, probenecid, and ethacrynic acid.

A reduction of the anticoagulant effect may occur with concomitant administration of antihistamines, cardiac glycosides, tetracycline and ascorbic acid.

*Pregnancy and lactation:* This medicinal product has been assessed in pregnant women and no harmful effects are known with respect to the course of pregnancy and the health of the unborn and neonate.

No information is available as to whether Fragmin passes into breast milk.

*Effects on ability to drive and use machines:* Fragmin does not affect the ability to drive or operate machinery.

*Undesirable effects:* Bleeding may be provoked, especially at high dosages corresponding with anti-Factor Xa levels greater than 1.5 IU/ml. However, at recommended dosages bleeding rarely occurs.

Transient, slight to moderate, elevation of liver transaminases (ASAT, ALAT) has been observed, but no clinical significance has been demonstrated.

Commonly reported side-effects include subcutaneous haematomas at the injection site. Thrombocytopenia and allergic reactions (urticaria, pruritus, hair loss and skin necrosis) occur rarely. Few cases of anaphylactoid reactions have been observed.

Osteoporosis has been associated with long-term heparin treatment and therefore cannot be excluded with Fragmin.

*Overdose:* The anticoagulant effect (i.e. prolongation of the APTT) induced by Fragmin is inhibited by protamine. Since protamine itself has an inhibiting effect on primary haemostasis it should be used only in an emergency. The prolongation of the clotting time induced by Fragmin may be fully neutralised by protamine, but the anti-Factor Xa activity is only neutralised to about 25-50%. 1 mg of protamine inhibits the effect of 100 IU (anti-Factor Xa) of Fragmin.

**Pharmacological properties**

*Pharmacodynamic properties:* Dalteparin sodium is a low molecular weight heparin fraction (average molecular weight 4000-6000 daltons) produced from porcine-derived sodium heparin.

Dalteparin sodium is an antithrombotic agent, which acts mainly through its ability to potentiate the inhibition of Factor Xa and thrombin by antithrombin. It has a relatively higher ability to potentiate Factor Xa inhibition than to prolong plasma clotting time (APTT).

Compared with standard, unfractionated heparin, dalteparin sodium has a reduced adverse effect on platelet function and platelet adhesion, and thus has only a minimal effect on primary haemostasis. Still some of the antithrombotic properties of dalteparin sodium are thought to be mediated through the effects on vessel walls or the fibrinolytic system.

*Pharmacokinetics:* The half-life following i.v. and s.c. administration is 2 hours and 3.5-4 hours respectively, twice that of unfractionated heparin.

The bioavailability following s.c. injection is approximately 87 per cent and the pharmacokinetics are not dose dependent. The half life is prolonged in uraemic patients as dalteparin sodium is eliminated primarily through the kidneys.

*Preclinical safety data:* The acute toxicity of dalteparin sodium is considerably lower than that of heparin. The only significant finding, which occurred consistently throughout the toxicity studies after subcutaneous administration of the higher dose levels was local haemorrhage at the injection sites, dose-related in incidence and severity. There was no cumulative effect on injection site haemorrhages.

The haemorrhagic reaction was reflected in dose related changes in the anticoagulant effects as measured by APTT and anti-Factor Xa activities.

It was concluded that dalteparin sodium did not have a greater osteopenic effect than heparin since at equivalent doses the osteopenic effect was comparable.

The results revealed no organ toxicity irrespective of the route of administration, doses or duration of treatment. No mutagenic effect was found. No embryotoxic or teratogenic effects and no effect on fertility, reproductive capacity or peri- and post natal development was shown.

**Pharmaceutical particulars**

*List of excipients:* Sodium chloride PhEur (2,500 IU presentation only). Water for Injections PhEur (2,500 IU and 5,000 IU presentations)

*Incompatibilities:* Not applicable.

*Shelf life:* 36 months

*Special precautions for storage:* Store at room temperature (below 30°C)

*Nature and contents of container:* Single dose syringe (glass Ph. Eur. Type I) with chlorobutyl rubber stopper containing dalteparin sodium 2500 IU (anti-Factor Xa) in 0.2 ml or 5000 IU (anti-Factor Xa) in 0.2 ml.

*Instructions for use/handling:* Not applicable

**Marketing authorisation numbers**

Fragmin 2,500 IU 0022/0076
Fragmin 5,000 IU 0022/0077

**Date of approval/revision of SPC** January 1997

**Legal category** POM

## GENOTROPIN* 2IU, 3IU, 4IU KABIQUICK, GENOTROPIN* 4IU, GENOTROPIN* 4IU KABIVIAL MULTIDOSE, GENOTROPIN* 16IU, GENOTROPIN* 36IU

**Qualitative and quantitative composition**

*Active constituent:* Somatropin (rbe) 2, 3, 4, 16 or 36 IU.

**Pharmaceutical form** Powder for injection prepared with the supplied diluent (with or without preservative) for subcutaneous administration.

***Clinical particulars***

*Therapeutic indications:* Treatment of growth disturbance due to insufficient secretion of growth hormone or associated with gonadal dysgenesis (Turner syndrome).

Treatment of growth disturbance in prepubertal children with chronic renal insufficiency.

Genotropin is indicated for replacement therapy in adults with pronounced growth hormone deficiency as diagnosed in two different dynamic tests for growth hormone deficiency. Patients must also fulfil the following criteria:

*Childhood onset:* Patients, who were diagnosed as growth hormone deficient during childhood, must be retested and their growth hormone deficiency confirmed before replacement therapy with Genotropin is started.

*Adult onset:* Patients must have growth hormone deficiency as a result of hypothalamic or pituitary disease and at least one other hormone deficiency diagnosed (except for prolactin) and adequate replacement therapy instituted, before replacement therapy using growth hormone may begin.

*Posology and method of administration:* The dosage and administration schedule should be personalised for each individual.

The weekly dose should be divided into 7 subcutaneous injections. The injection site should be varied to prevent lipoatrophy.

*Insufficient secretion of growth hormone in children:* Generally a dose of 0.5–0.7IU/kg body weight/week or 14–20IU/m² body surface area/week is recommended. Higher doses have been used.

*Gonadal dysgenesis (Turner syndrome):* A dose of 1.0IU/kg body weight/week or 28IU/m² body surface area/week is recommended.

*Chronic renal insufficiency:* A dose of 30IU/m² body surface area/week (approximately 1.0IU/kg body weight/week) is recommended. Higher doses may be needed if growth velocity is too low. Dose correction may be required after six months of treatment.

*Growth hormone deficient adult patients:* The recommended dosage at the start of therapy is 0.125 IU/kg per week given as a daily subcutaneous injection. The dose should be gradually increased according to individual patient requirements to a maximum of 0.25 IU/kg per week. Side effects of the patient as well as determination of insulin-like growth factor-I (IGF-1) in serum should be used as guidance for dose titration. The minimum effective dose should be used and dose requirements may decline with increasing age.

*Contra-indications:* Genotropin should not be used when evidence of tumour activity exists; intracranial lesions must be inactive and antitumour therapy completed before treatment begins.

Genotropin should not be used for growth promotion in children with closed epiphyses.

*Special warnings and special precautions for use:* Diagnosis and therapy with Genotropin should be initiated and monitored by physicians who are appropriately qualified and experienced in the diagnosis and management of patients with growth hormone deficiency.

Patients suffering from diabetes mellitus may require adjustment of their insulin dose when Genotropin therapy is instituted.

A state of hypothyroidism may develop during somatropin treatment. Since untreated hypothyroidism may interfere with the response to somatropin, patients should have periodic thyroid function tests and should be treated with thyroid hormone when indicated.

In cases where growth hormone deficiency is secondary to treatment of malignant disease, it is recommended to pay attention to signs of malignancy relapse.

In patients with endocrine disorders, including growth hormone deficiency, slipped epiphyses of the hip may occur more frequently. Any child limping during treatment with growth hormone should be clinically examined.

In patients with (pan) hypopituitarism, standard replacement therapy has to be monitored closely.

In cases of severe or recurrent headache, visual problems, nausea and/or vomiting, a funduscopy for papilloedema is recommended. If papilloedema is confirmed, a diagnosis of benign intracranial hypertension should be considered and, if appropriate, growth hormone treatment should be discontinued.

At present there is insufficient evidence to guide clinical judgement in patients with resolved intracranial hypertension. If growth hormone treatment is restarted, patients must be carefully monitored for the symptoms of intracranial hypertension.

No information is available regarding the final height of treated patients with Turner syndrome.

In chronic renal insufficiency, renal function should have decreased to below 50 per cent of normal before therapy is instituted. To verify the growth disturbance, growth should have been followed for a year preceding institution of therapy. Conservative treatment for renal insufficiency should have been established and should be maintained during treatment. Treatment should be discontinued after renal transplantation.

Experience in patients above 60 years is lacking.

Experience with prolonged treatment in adults is limited.

*Interaction with other medicaments and other forms of interaction:* Patients with diabetes mellitus may require adjustment of their antidiabetic therapy.

*Pregnancy and lactation:*

*Pregnancy:* No clinical experience of the use in pregnant women is available. Animal experimental data are incomplete. Treatment with Genotropin should be interrupted if pregnancy occurs.

*Lactation:* No information is available as to whether peptide hormones pass into breast milk, but absorption of intact protein from the gastrointestinal tract of the infant is extremely unlikely.

*Effects on ability to drive and use machines:* The ability to react is not influenced by Genotropin.

*Undesirable effects:* Side-effects have been noted in approximately 10% of the patients participating in clinical trials in children with short stature.

In clinical trials in adults, side effects have been noted in approximately 30–40% of the patients primarily related to symptoms of fluid retention. These events have an early onset after initiation of therapy with a reduction in incidence and prevalence over time and rarely influencing daily activities.

Common (> 1/100) side-effects are: Transient local skin reactions at the injection site. The symptoms of fluid retention (peripheral oedema, arthralgia/myalgia).

Genotropin has given rise to the formation of antibodies in a few patients. The binding capacity of these antibodies has been low.

It has been reported that patients may develop hypothyroidism during treatment with Genotropin and this should be considered.

*In vitro* chromosome aberrations have been reported during growth hormone therapy; the clinical significance is unknown.

Some cases of leukaemia have been reported in growth hormone deficient children, untreated as well as treated with growth hormone, and might possibly represent a slightly increased incidence compared with non growth hormone deficient children. A causal relationship to growth hormone therapy has not been established.

Some rare cases of benign intracranial hypertension have been reported.

*Overdose:* No cases of overdose or intoxication are known.

Acute overdosage could lead initially to hypoglycaemia and subsequently to hyperglycaemia. Long-term overdosage could result in signs and symptoms consistent with the known effects of human growth hormone excess.

### Pharmacological properties

*Pharmacodynamic properties:* Genotropin stimulates linear growth and increases growth rate in children who lack adequate endogenous growth hormone. In adults with growth hormone deficiency, Genotropin reduces fat mass, increases muscle mass and improves energy, vitality and subjective well-being.

Treatment of growth hormone deficient patients with Genotropin normalises serum IGF-I (Insulin-like Growth Factor-I/Somatomedin C) concentrations.

The primary and secondary pharmacological effects of Genotropin have been studied and are equal to those of pituitary growth hormone.

In addition, the following actions have been demonstrated for Genotropin and/or somatropin.

*Tissue growth:* Stimulation of skeletal muscle growth in patients with growth hormone deficiency (GHD). It also increases the number and size of muscle cells.

*Protein metabolism:* Nitrogen retention demonstrated by decreased urinary nitrogen excretion and decreased serum urea nitrogen.

*Carbohydrate metabolism:* Children with hypopituitarism sometimes experience fasting hypoglycaemia that is improved by treatment with Genotropin. Large doses of human growth hormone may impair glucose tolerance.

*Lipid metabolism:* In GHD patients, administration of somatropin has resulted in lipid mobilisation, reduction in body fat stores and increased plasma fatty acids.

*Mineral metabolism:* Retention of sodium, potassium and phosphorus is induced by somatropin. Serum concentrations of inorganic phosphate are increased in patients with GHD after therapy with Genotropin or somatropin. Serum calcium is not significantly altered by either Genotropin or somatropin.

*Pharmacokinetic properties:* Approximately 80% of Genotropin is absorbed following s.c. injection and maximum serum concentrations are achieved after 3–4 hours.

*Preclinical safety data:* The general toxicity, local tolerance and genotoxicity of Genotropin has been studied using pituitary growth hormone as the reference. Genotropin has a toxicological profile equivalent to pituitary growth hormone. Based on the experimental studies, the treatment of growth failure has a large safety margin. Preclinical studies on point mutations and induction of chromosome aberrations have been negative.

### Pharmaceutical particulars

*List of excipients:* (Each complying to the requirements of the European Pharmacopoeia, excluding M-cresol)

*Genotropin 2IU, 3IU, 4IU KabiQuick respectively:* Glycine 12.0 mg, 18.0 mg, 24.0 mg, Sodium dihydrogen phosphate anhydrous (as monohydrate) 0.13 mg, 0.20 mg, 0.26 mg, Disodium phosphate anhydrous (added as dodecahydrate) 0.13 mg, 0.19 mg, 0.26 mg, Water for injections to 0.5 ml, 0.75 ml, 1.0 ml

*Genotropin 4IU:* Glycine 2.0 mg, Sodium dihydrogen phosphate anhydrous (as monohydrate) 0.26 mg, Disodium phosphate anhydrous (added as dodecahydrate) 0.26 mg

*Genotropin 4IU KabiVial Multidose:* Glycine 24.0 mg, Sodium dihydrogen phosphate anhydrous (as monohydrate) 0.26 mg, Disodium phosphate anhydrous (added as dodecahydrate) 0.26 mg, M-cresol 3.0 mg, Water for injections to 1.0 ml

*Genotropin 16IU:* Glycine 2.0 mg, Mannitol 41.0 mg, Sodium dihydrogen phosphate anhydrous (as monohydrate) 0.29 mg, Disodium phosphate anhydrous (added as dodecahydrate) 0.28 mg, M-cresol 3.0 mg, Water for injections to 1.0 ml

*Genotropin 36IU:* Glycine 2.0 mg, Mannitol 40.0 mg, Sodium dihydrogen phosphate anhydrous (as monohydrate) 0.41 mg, Disodium phosphate anhydrous (added as dodecahydrate) 0.40 mg, M-cresol 3.0 mg, Water for injections to 1.0 ml

*Incompatibilities:* Should only be reconstituted with the diluent supplied.

*Shelf life:* The powder for injection is assigned a shelf life of 24 months (Genotropin 36IU–18 months) when stored cold at 2–8°C. Storage for one month can take place at room temperature.

*Genotropin 2IU, 3IU, 4IU KabiQuick and Genotropin 4IU:* The reconstituted product has been assigned a shelf life of 24 hours when stored at 2–8°C and protected from light.

*Genotropin 4IU KabiVial Multidose:* The reconstituted product has been assigned a shelf life of two weeks when stored at 2–8°C and protected from light.

*Genotropin 16IU and Genotropin 36IU:* The reconstituted product may be stored cold at 2–8°C for three weeks protected from light.

*Special precautions for storage:* Genotropin cartridges and vials should be stored at 2–8°C and protected from light. The reconstituted product should be stored in the same way.

*Nature and contents of container:*

*Genotropin 2IU, 3IU, 4IU KabiQuick:* Dual chamber cartridge containing lyophilised powder and liquid for reconstitution and injection supplied in a KabiQuick.

*Genotropin 4IU:* Glass vial containing lyophilised powder together with glass ampoule containing 1 ml water for injection for reconstitution.

*Genotropin 4IU KabiVial Multidose:* Dual chamber cartridge containing lyophilised powder and liquid for reconstitution and injection supplied in a KabiVial.

*Genotropin 16IU:* Dual chamber cartridge containing lyophilised powder and liquid for reconstitution and injection using either a Genotropin Pen 16 or KabiMixer injection device, or intact in a KabiVial device.

*Genotropin 36IU:* Dual chamber cartridge containing lyophilised powder and liquid for reconstitution and injection using either a Genotropin Pen 36 or KabiMixer injection device.

*Instructions for use/handling:*

*Genotropin 4IU:* Genotropin solution is prepared by adding the diluent to the vial containing lyophilised powder. Gently dissolve the powder using a slow, swirling motion. Do not shake vigorously as this might denature the active ingredient.

*Genotropin 2IU, 3IU, 4IU KabiQuick, Genotropin 4IU KabiVial Multidose, Genotropin 16IU, Genotropin 36IU:* Genotropin solution is prepared by screwing the device together so that the diluent is mixed with the powder in the dual chamber cartridge. Gently dissolve the powder using a slow, swirling motion. Do not shake vigorously as this might denature the active ingredient.

### Marketing authorisation numbers

| | |
|---|---|
| Genotropin 2IU, 3IU, 4IU KabiQuick | 0022/0089-91 |
| Genotropin 4IU | 0022/0071 |
| Genotropin 4IU KabiVial Multidose | 0022/0088 |
| Genotropin 16IU | 0022/0085 |
| Genotropin 36IU | 0022/0098 |

**Date of approval/revision of SPC** February 1997

**Legal category CD   (Sch 4), POM**

## GLAMIN*

**Qualitative and quantitative composition:** 1000 ml of the infusion solution contains:

| Active ingredients | Quantity | Reference to standards |
|---|---|---|
| Alanine | 16.00 g | PhEur |
| Aspartic acid | 3.40 g | PhEur |
| Glutamic acid | 5.60 g | PhEur |
| Glycyl-Glutamine H₂O (corresponding to Glycine 10.27 g corresponding to Glutamine 20.0 g) | 30.27 g | in-house specification |
| Glycyl-Tyrosine 2H₂O (corresponding to Glycine 0.94 g corresponding to Tyrosine 2.28 g) | 3.45 g | in-house specification |
| Histidine | 6.80 g | PhEur |
| Isoleucine | 5.60 g | PhEur |
| Leucine | 7.90 g | PhEur |
| Lysine-Acetate (corresponding to Lysine 9.0 g) | 12.70 g | USP |
| Methionine | 5.60 g | DAB |
| Phenylalanine | 5.85 g | PhEur |
| Proline | 6.80 g | PhEur |
| Serine | 4.50 g | PhEur |
| Threonine | 5.60 g | DAB |
| Tryptophan | 1.90 g | DAB |
| Valine | 7.30 g | PhEur |

| Other Ingredients | | |
|---|---|---|
| Citric acid | to pH 5.8 | PhEur |
| Water for injections | to 1000 ml | PhEur |
| Amino acids/dipeptides | 134 g/l | |
| Total nitrogen | 22.4 g/l | |
| Energy content | 2300 kJ (540 kcal)/l | |
| Theoretical osmolarity | 1040 mosm/l | |
| Theoretical osmolality | 1140 mosm/kg | |
| Titration acidity to pH 7.4 | approx. 60 mmol/l | |
| pH | approx 5.8 | |
| Density | 1.0414 g/cm³ | |

**Pharmaceutical form** Solution for infusion.

Electrolyte-free, clear, colourless to slightly yellow solution of free amino acids and dipeptides for intravenous nutrition.

### Clinical particulars

*Therapeutic indications:* Glamin provides amino acids as part of parenteral nutrition therapy, when oral or enteral nutrition is impossible, insufficient or contraindicated, especially in patients with a moderate to severe catabolic status.

In parenteral nutrition regimens amino acid solutions should always be administered in combination with appropriate energy-supplying infusion solutions.

*Posology and method of administration:* The dosage depends on the amino acid requirements.

Generally, 1-2 g amino acids/ dipeptides (corresponding to 0.17-0.34 g N) per kg body weight per day are recommended. This corresponds to 7-14 ml Glamin/kg body weight/day or to 500-1000 ml Glamin/day for a patient weighing 70 kg.

Recommended infusion rate: 0.6-0.7 ml (corresponding to 0.08-0.09 g amino acids/dipeptides)/kg body weight/hour. This corresponds to 500 ml in 10-12 hours or 1000 ml in 20-24 hours for a patient weighing 70 kg.

Dosage to be adjusted individually for patients with renal or liver disease.

*Method and duration of administration:* Intravenous infusion. Glamin should be administered by the central venous route due to its osmolarity above 800 mosm/l.

Infusion may be continued for as long as required by the patient's clinical condition. No experience is available so far for administration over more than 2 weeks.

*Contra-indications:* Patients with inborn errors of amino acid metabolism (e.g phenylketonuria), severe liver failure and severe renal failure.

General contra-indications of parenteral nutrition are: unstable life-threatening circulatory conditions (shock), metabolic acidosis, insufficient cellular oxygen supply, hyperhydration, hyponatraemia, hypokalaemia, hyperlactataemia, increased serum osmolarity, pulmonary oedema, decompensated cardiac insufficiency and known hypersensitivity to any of the ingredients.

*Special warnings and special precautions for use:* See also *Incompatibilities* and *Instructions for use/handling.*

*Monitoring advice:* Serum electrolytes, serum osmolarity, water balance, acid-base status as well as liver function tests (alkaline phosphatase, GPT, GOT) should be monitored.

*Use in paediatric patients:* Glamin is not indicated for use in children below the age of 2 years since its composition is not adapted to the requirements of these patients. For older children experience is lacking, the use of Glamin can therefore not be recommended.

*Interaction with other medicaments and other forms of interaction:* Not investigated, however no interactions are known to date.

*Pregnancy and lactation:* No human data are available on the use of Glamin during pregnancy and lactation. The use of Glamin during pregnancy and lactation should be subject to a benefit-risk evaluation.

However, an evaluation of experimental animal studies (embryotoxicity study in rabbit) does not indicate direct or indirect harmful effects with respect to reproduction.

*Effects on ability to drive and use machines:* Not applicable.

*Undesirable effects:* Not to be expected, if used as directed.

See also *Posology and method of administration, Method and duration of administration* and *Special warnings and special precautions for use.*

*Overdose:* When infusion rates exceed the recommended maximum rate, signs of intolerance may occur: nausea, vomiting, flushing, sweating in combination with renal excretion of amino acids and dipeptides.

Therapy if symptoms of overdose occur: Reduce infusion rate or, if necessary, interrupt infusion.

### Pharmacological properties

Glamin is an infusion solution for parenteral nutrition containing 18 essential and non-essential amino acids, three of which are in the form of the dipeptides glycyl-glutamine and glycyl-tyrosine.

The solution is suitable to support protein synthesis and to improve nitrogen balance during intravenous nutrition. In order to ensure optimal utilisation of the infused amino acids and dipeptides, the patient's requirements of energy (carbohydrates, fat), electrolytes, trace elements and vitamins should be covered.

*Pharmacodynamic properties:* Pharmacological effects, except nutritive ones, are not expected from amino acid solutions as long as they are infused according to the recommended dosage for parenteral nutrition. Both dipeptides, glycyl-glutamine and glycyl-tyrosine, are included to improve availability of glutamine and tyrosine and to stimulate protein synthesis. The dipeptides are not expected to exert other specific pharmacodynamic effects than those of the corresponding free amino acids. Only in rats it has been shown that glutamine decreases clearance of methotrexate.

*Pharmacokinetic properties:* The two dipeptides glycyl-glutamine and glycyl-tyrosine are rapidly and quantitatively hydrolysed to their constituent amino acids when infused intravenously in animals and humans. Several tissues participate in the hydrolysis of the dipeptides, but the kidneys play the quantitatively most important role. The liver, skeletal muscle and intestine also participate in the clearance of the dipeptides. Finally, hydrolysis of the dipeptides also takes place in plasma.

*Preclinical safety data: Local tolerance:* Due to the osmolarity of 1040 mosm/l, Glamin should be administered by the central venous route. However, peripheral-venous infusion of Glamin in the dog for 28 days (6 hours daily) induced no macroscopic or microscopic changes at the infusion site. In clinical phase I studies no regional vascular complications were observed during peripheral venous infusion.

*Single dose toxicity:* No evidence of toxicity was apparent in rats or mice after a bolus injection of Glamin at a dosage corresponding to 2-3 times the daily recommended dose for patients to be infused over 10-20 hours.

Nor were any signs of toxicity observed in rats when the individual dipeptide glycyl-glutamine or glycyl-tyrosine was infused for 8 hours at a dosage of 5.1 and 5.9 g/kg, respectively.

*Repeated dose toxicity:* Subchronic toxicity studies with Glamin in rats and dogs for 28 days revealed no drug-related changes in the clinical observations, laboratory investigations or post-mortem examinations.

*Mutagenic potential:* No mutagenic potential was demonstrated for the individual dipeptides.

*Oncogenic/carcinogenic potential:* For the intended indication conventional carcinogenicity studies are not considered mandatory. The lack of mutagenic activity of the dipeptides would not imply any carcinogenic potential. Moreover, the dipeptides are rapidly hydrolysed to their constituent amino acids and there are many years of experience for amino acids as physiological substrates.

*Reproduction toxicity:* No embryotoxic or teratogenic effects were observed in rabbits infused with the maximum tolerable volume of 24 ml of Glamin/kg (4 hours daily).

Additional studies are not considered necessary in view of the clinical use, the pharmacokinetic properties and the lack of adverse reproductive effects in the rabbit as well as of changes in reproductive organs in the subchronic toxicity studies.

**Pharmaceutical particulars**

*List of excipients:* Citric acid (pH adjustment), water for injections

*Incompatibilities:* Amino acid solutions should not be used as carrier solutions for drugs.

Glamin may only be mixed with other solutions where compatibility is documented.

*Shelf life:* The shelf life is 2 years

*Special precautions for storage:* Store below +25°C (room temperature).

*Nature and contents of container:* Glass bottles of hydrolytic class II according to PhEur sealed with butyl rubber stoppers.

Bottle sizes: 250 ml and 500 ml.

*Instructions for use/handling:* Use only clear solutions in intact containers.

To achieve a complete parenteral nutrition regimen, Glamin should be administered in combination with carbohydrates and/or fat as well as electrolytes, trace elements and vitamins.

*Compatibility:* Compatibility is documented for the following mixture: 1000 ml Glamin with 20% fat emulsion (up to 1000 ml Intralipid 20%*), up to 1000 ml glucose 40%, 80 mmol NaCl, 5 mmol $CaCl_2$, 60 mmol KCl, 3.5 mmol Mg-L-hydrogen-glutamate, phosphate supplement (15 ml Addiphos*), trace elements (10 ml Additrace*), fat soluble vitamins (10 ml Vitlipid N Adult*) and water soluble vitamins (1 vial Solivito N*).

* used for compatibility testing

Additions should be performed aseptically immediately before the start of the infusion. Discard any residual contents.

The manufacturer can be contacted for full information on complete and balanced intravenous nutrition regimens.

**Marketing authorisation number** 0022/0179

**Date of approval/revision of SPC** 5 April 1996

**Legal category** POM

## HARMOGEN* 1.5 MG TABLETS

**Presentation** Peach-coloured, flat, elongated, scored tablets marked U and 3773 on either side of the score. Each tablet contains 1.5 mg Estropipate USP (piperazine oestrone sulphate), equivalent to 0.93 mg oestrone.

Also contains lactose, dibasic potassium phosphate, tromethamine, hydroxypropyl cellulose, sodium starch glycollate, microcrystalline cellulose, colloidal silicon dioxide, magnesium stearate, hydrogenated vegetable oil wax and E110.

**Uses** Menopausal and post-menopausal oestrogen replacement therapy for vasomotor symptoms, senile atrophic vaginitis, vulvitis. Harmogen is also indicated in the prophylaxis of postmenopausal osteoporosis in women identified to be at risk of this condition. These women include those suffering from an early menopause, receiving recent prolonged corticosteroid therapy, having a family history of osteoporosis, of small frame, who are thin, smokers and those with an excess alcohol intake.

In women with an intact uterus the addition of a progestogen is essential.

**Dosage and administration** Oral

*Adults: Postmenopausal osteoporosis:* 1.5 mg daily.

*Other indications:* 1.5 mg – 3.0 mg daily taken as a single or divided dose.

Harmogen should be given continuously and, in women with an intact uterus, a progestogen should be added for 10–13 days at the end of each 28-day cycle. If the patient has undergone hysterectomy, the addition of a progestogen is not necessary.

*Elderly:* As for adults

*Children:* Not recommended

**Contra-indications, warnings, etc**

*Contra-indications:* Known or suspected pregnancy; cardiovascular or cerebrovascular disorders, e.g. thrombophlebitis, thrombosis or thromboembolic disorders, moderate to severe hypertension, hyperlipoproteinaemia or a history of these conditions; known or suspected oestrogen dependent tumours; endometrial hyperplasia, uterine fibromyomata, undiagnosed vaginal bleeding; severe liver disease including Rotor syndrome and Dubin-Johnson syndrome; porphyria.

*Side-effects:* The incidence of side-effects with Harmogen is low. The following adverse reactions have been reported with oestrogen therapy:

*Genito-urinary tract:* Endometrial neoplasia, intermenstrual bleeding, increase in the size of uterine fibromyomata, endometrial proliferation or aggravation of endometriosis, changes in cervical eversion and excessive production of cervical mucus.

*Breast:* Tenderness, pain, enlargement or secretion.

*Gastro-intestinal tract:* Nausea, vomiting, cholelithiasis, cholestatic jaundice, abdominal cramp, bloating.

*Cardiovascular system:* Hypertension, thrombosis, thrombophlebitis, thrombo-embolism.

*Skin:* Chloasma which may persist when the drug is discontinued, erythema multiforme, erythema nodosum, rash, loss of scalp hair, hirsutism.

*Eyes:* Steepening of corneal curvature, intolerance to contact lenses.

*CNS:* Headache, migraine, dizziness, mood changes (elation or depression), chorea.

*Miscellaneous:* Sodium and water retention, reduced glucose tolerance, change in body weight, aggravation of porphyria, changes in libido.

*Use in pregnancy and lactation:* The indications for Harmogen are such that it is not likely to be used in pregnant or lactating women. Harmogen is contraindicated in known or suspected pregnancy. In the unlikely event of the use of Harmogen in breastfeeding women, it should be remembered that oestrogens are excreted in breast milk and inhibit milk flow.

*Warnings:* Prolonged exposure to unopposed oestrogens increases the risk of endometrial neoplasia, however, the addition of a progestogen to the oestrogen regimen reduces the incidence of endometrial hyperplasia and cancer.

Severe varicose veins: the benefits of oestrogen-containing preparations must be weighed against the possible risks.

Cardiac failure, latent or overt.

Epilepsy or migraine, or a history of these conditions.

Sickle cell haemoglobinopathy, since under certain circumstances, e.g. infections or anoxia, oestrogen-containing preparations may induce thromboembolic processes in patients with this condition.

Untreated polycythaemia or pulmonary hypertension.

*Precautions:* Before initiation of therapy, a complete medical and family history should be taken. The pretreatment and periodic physical examination should include special emphasis on blood pressure, breasts, abdomen and pelvic organs including cervical cytology and endometrial assessment where possible. Regular follow-up examinations are recommended every 6–12 months. The benefit of continued treatment should be reviewed periodically.

Caution should be exercised when administering Harmogen to women with a family history of breast cancer or who have breast nodules, fibrocystic disease or abnormal mammograms. There is suggestive evidence of a small increased risk of breast cancer with oestrogen replacement therapy used for long-term (greater than 5 years). Some studies have reported an increased risk of breast cancer in long-term users. Others, however, have not shown this relationship. It is not known whether concurrent progestogen use influences the risk of breast cancer in post-menopausal women taking hormone replacement therapy. Women on long-term therapy should have regular breast examinations.

Mild hypertension or a history of it. If hypertension develops in patients receiving Harmogen, treatment should be stopped.

Studies to date do not indicate that there is an increased risk of thrombembolic disease including stroke, myocardial infarction and thrombophlebitis with oestrogen replacement therapy at the current recommended low dosages in apparently normal women. If an acute vascular thromboembolism occurs coincidentally during therapy, current opinion suggests that treatment should be discontinued. There is no evidence that a past history of deep vein thrombosis, pulmonary embolism, stroke or myocardial infarction should be contra-indications to hormone replacement therapy. However, in the absence of sufficient data, Harmogen should be used with caution in these patients. Consideration should be given to discontinuing treatment at least 4 weeks prior to surgery or during periods of prolonged immobilisation.

Pre-existing uterine fibromyomata may increase in size during oestrogen therapy. The pathologist should be advised of the patient's use of Harmogen when submitting relevant samples.

Glucose tolerance may be lowered and may, therefore, increase the need for insulin or other antidiabetic drugs in diabetics.

Thyroid hormone binding globulin may be increased leading to increased circulating total thyroid hormone, therefore, care must be taken in interpreting thyroid function tests.

History of gall stones, cholestatic jaundice in pregnancy or jaundice due to oral contraceptives. If jaundice develops or liver function tests become abnormal in any patient receiving Harmogen, the medication should be stopped while the cause is investigated.

Renal dysfunction.

Major depression

Contact lens wearers.

*Overdosage:* Overdosage is unlikely to cause serious problems, though the following symptoms may be present i.e. nausea and withdrawal bleeding in women. However, gastric lavage or emesis may be used when considered appropriate.

**Pharmaceutical precautions** None

**Legal category** POM

**Package quantities** Packs of 28 tablets.

**Further information** Metabolisable carbohydrate content: approx. 0.2 g per tablet.

The amount of piperazine in Harmogen is not sufficient to exert a pharmacological action, but its addition ensures stability, solubility and uniform potency.

**Product licence number** 0037/5064R

*Product licence holder:* Abbott Laboratories Limited, Queenborough, Kent, ME11 5EL.

## HEALONID*

**Presentation** Disposable single use cartridge/syringe assemblies containing a sterile isotonic buffered solution of sodium hyaluronate:

| | |
|---|---|
| Sodium hyaluronate (5000) | 10 mg |
| Sodium chloride | 8.5 mg |
| Disodium hydrogen phosphate dihydrate | 0.28 mg |
| Sodium dihydrogen phosphate hydrate | 0.04 mg |
| Water for injection | to 1 ml |

**Uses**

*Properties:* Sodium hyaluronate is a polysaccharide normally found in the aqueous humour. Presented as Healonid, the solution has viscoelastic properties, being a clear viscous solution at rest yet under pressure able to pass easily through a fine needle or cannula. The average molecular weight of sodium hyaluronate in Healonid is approximately 4 million.

*Indications:* Introduction into the eye during anterior segment surgery helps maintain the shape of the anterior chamber and the space in which to work. The solution can be used as a soft tool to move tissues and objects. During surgery Healonid protects tissues from trauma and dehydration and reduces endothelial cell loss. Healonid may also be used in posterior segment surgery.

At close of surgery Healonid should be removed by aspiration or irrigation. Excess residues left in the eye may cause a rise in intraocular pressure a few hours after closure.

**Dosage and administration** The volume of Healonid will vary according to the procedure and technique employed.

The volume will be increased if the viscoelastic is used to coat the intraocular lens or tips of instruments, or where bleeding necessitates replacement on one or more occasions. At close of surgery Healonid should be aspirated or irrigated out. Excessive residues in the eye may lead to raised intraocular pressure postoperatively.

As a guide to volumes used, the anterior chamber has a volume of 0.2–0.3 ml.

No special directions are given for use in the elderly or children.

Prior to use, Healonid should be allowed to warm to room temperature over 30–60 minutes.

**Contra-indications, warnings, etc**
*Warnings:*

(i) Rarely inflammatory reactions have been reported; their connection with Healonid has not been established.

(ii) With traces of avian protein being present in Healonid there is the remote possibility of an idiosyncratic reaction.

*Precautions:* Healonid is viscous and thus residues left in the eye may impair drainage of aqueous humour through the trabecular meshwork. Consequently at close of surgery Healonid should be irrigated or aspirated out and intraocular pressure monitored over the first 24 hours, rises being most likely after 4–8 hours. In keratoplasty and trabeculectomy it is permissible to leave some Healonid *in situ* to prevent 'shallowing' of the anterior chamber due to leakage or excessive drainage. Again, intraocular pressure should be monitored. Excessive rises in pressure may be treated with appropriate therapy such as beta blockers or carbonic anhydrase inhibitors.

*Pregnancy and lactation:* There is no adverse animal evidence and Healonid has been widely used for many years without apparent ill consequence. Considering also the small amounts entering the body from what may be an isolated procedure, safety in pregnancy and lactation is likely.

*Interactions and incompatibilities:* Do not use with hyaluronidase. Healonid may become turbid due to precipitation in the presence of cationic agents such as benzalkonium chloride or detergents residual in some recycled cannulae. Avoid recycled cannulae.

*Pharmaceutical precautions:* Healonid has a shelf life of three years when stored at 2–8°C, protected from light and freezing. These conditions should be adhered to routinely. Healonid should be allowed to warm to room temperature over 30–60 minutes before use.

**Legal category** POM.

**Package quantities** Disposable cartridge/syringe assemblies containing 0.50 or 0.85 ml. A sterile cannula (27 G) is supplied.

**Further information** Healonid may be used in anterior segment surgery in situations such as trauma; intra- and extra-capsular lens extraction; corneal graft; glaucoma surgery; intraocular lens insertion; to facilitate manipulation within the eye; to protect the corneal endothelium and other sensitive tissues; to manoeuvre and separate tissues and bodies within the eye; to control vitreous bulge; to maintain a deep anterior chamber; to provide a support for corneal graft at suturing. Posterior segment surgery may include procedures for vitreal replacement and retinal detachment repair.

Evidence from animals suggests that Healonid is no longer present in the anterior chamber six days after introduction.

**Product licence number** 0022/0131.

## HEALONID* GV

**Presentation** Disposable single use cartridge/syringe assembly containing a sterile isotonic buffered solution of high viscosity:

| | |
|---|---|
| Sodium hyaluronate (7000) | 14 mg |
| Sodium chloride | 8.5 mg |
| Disodium hydrogen phosphate dihydrate | 0.28 mg |
| Sodium dihydrogen phosphate hydrate | 0.04 mg |
| Water for injection | to 1 ml |

**Uses**
*Properties:* Sodium hyaluronate is a polysaccaharide normally found in the aqueous humour. By virtue of a greater concentration of a higher molecular weight sodium hyaluronate, the resting viscosity is considerably greater than that of Healonid. Although extremely viscous at rest, its viscoelasticity allows it, under pressure, to pass readily through a fine needle or cannula. The average molecular weight of the sodium hyaluronate in Healonid GV is approximately 5 million.

*Indications:* Healonid GV (GV=Greater Viscosity) is used intraocularly in anterior segment surgery such as cataract extraction, intraocular lens insertion and corneal transplant surgery where the surgeon requires greater visco-elastic properties to achieve his purpose than Healonid offers.

Residues in the eye may lead to raised intraocular pressure post operatively (Healonid GV may be more prone to this effect than Healonid), so particular care should be taken in its removal.

**Dosage and administration** The volume of Healonid GV will vary according to the procedure and technique employed. The volume will be increased if the viscoelastic is used to coat the intraocular lens or tips of instruments, or where bleeding necessitates replacement on one or more occasions. At close of surgery Healonid GV should be aspirated or irrigated out, the texture facilitating the procedure.

Residues in the eye may lead to raised intraocular pressure postoperatively and particular care in removal should be taken because this effect maybe more pronounced than with Healonid or Healonid Yellow.

As a guide to volumes used, the anterior chamber has a volume of 0.2–0.3 ml.

No special directions are given for use in the elderly or children.

Prior to use Healonid GV should be allowed to warm to room temperature over 30–60 minutes.

**Contra-indications, warnings, etc**
*Warnings:*

(i) Rarely inflammatory reactions have been reported; their connection with Healonid GV has not been established.

(ii) With traces of avian protein being present in Healonid GV, there is the remote possibility of an idiosyncratic reaction.

*Precautions:* Healonid GV is very viscous and thus residues left in the eye may impair drainage of aqueous humour through the trabecular meshwork. Consequently at close of surgery Healonid GV should be irrigated or aspirated out of the eye (the texture of the product is helpful here) and the intraocular pressure monitored over the first 24 hours, rises being most likely after 4–8 hours. Healonid GV may be more prone to cause such rises than Healonid or Healonid Yellow. Excessive rises in intraocular pressure may be treated with appropriate therapy such as beta blockers or carbonic anhydrase inhibitors.

*Pregnancy and lactation:* There has been limited use of Healonid GV in humans, but there is no adverse animal evidence and Healonid has been in wide use for many years without apparent ill consequence. Considering also the small amounts entering the body from what may be an isolated procedure, safety in pregnancy and lactation is likely.

*Interactions and incompatibilities:* Do not use with hyaluronidase. Healonid GV may beome turbid due to precipitation in the presence of cationic agents such as benzalkonium chloride or detergents residual in some recycled cannulae. Avoid recycled cannulae.

**Pharmaceutical precautions** Healonid GV has a shelf life of two years when stored at 2–8°C, protected from light and freezing. These conditions should be adhered to routinely. Healonid GV should be allowed to warm to room temperature over 30–60 minutes before use.

**Legal category** POM.

**Package quantities** Disposable cartridge/syringe assemblies containing 0.55 ml. A sterile cannula (27 G) is supplied.

**Further information** Evidence from animals suggests that sodium hyaluronate is no longer in the anterior chamber six days after introduction.

**Product licence number** 0022/0132.

## HEMABATE* STERILE SOLUTION

**Presentation** Colourless, sterile, aqueous solution containing carboprost tromethamine equivalent to carboprost 250 micrograms/ml.

The product also contains benzyl alcohol, sodium chloride, tromethamine and water.

**Uses** Treatment of post-partum haemorrhage due to uterine atony and refractory to conventional methods of treatment with oxytocic agents and ergometrine used either alone or in combination.

Conventional therapy should usually consist of 0.5 – 1 mg ergometrine with up to 50 units of oxytocin infused intravenously over periods of time from 20 minutes to 12 hours. The dosage and duration of administration should reflect the seriousness of the clinical situation.

**Dosage and administration** Parenteral drug products should be inspected visually for particulate matter and discolouration prior to administration whenever solution and container permit.

An initial dose of 250 micrograms (1.0 ml) of Hemabate should be administered as a deep intramuscular injection.

If necessary, further doses of 250 micrograms may be administered at intervals of approximately 1.5 hours. In severe cases the interval between doses may be reduced at the discretion of the attending physician, but it should not be less than 15 minutes. The total dose of Hemabate should not exceed 2 mg (8 doses).

*Elderly:* Not applicable

*Children:* Not applicable

**Contra-indications, warnings, etc.**
*Contra-indications:* There are no absolute contra-indications to the use of Hemabate, however, its use is not recommended in the following circumstances:

(1) Hypersensitivity to any of the components of the preparation.

(2) Acute pelvic inflammatory disease.

(3) Patients with known cardiac, pulmonary, renal or hepatic disease.

*Interactions with other medicaments and other forms of interaction:* Since prostaglandins may potentiate the effect of oxytocin, it is recommended that the use of these drugs simultaneously or in sequence should be carefully monitored.

*Effects on ability to drive and to use machines:* None

*Other undesirable effects:* The adverse effects of Hemabate are generally transient and reversible when therapy ends.

The most frequent side-effects observed with the use of Hemabate are related to its contractile effect on smooth muscle. Thus nausea, vomiting and diarrhoea have been reported as commonly encountered. The incidence of vomiting and diarrhoea may be decreased by pre-treatment and concomitant use during treatment of anti-emetic and antidiarrhoeal agents.

Hyperthermia and flushing have been observed after intramuscular Hemabate, but if not complicated by endometritis, the temperature will usually return to normal within several hours of the last injection.

Asthma and wheezing have been noted with Hemabate treatment.

Less frequent, but potentially more serious adverse effects are elevated blood pressure, dyspnoea and pulmonary oedema. Other less serious adverse effects noted include chills, headache, diaphoresis, dizziness and injection site erythema and pain.

*Use in pregnancy and lactation:* Not applicable

*Other special warnings and precautions*

*Warnings:* This preparation should not be used for induction of labour.

Hemabate, as with other potent oxytocic agents, should be used only with strict adherence to recommended dosages. Hemabate should be used by medically trained personnel and is available only to hospitals and clinics with specialised obstetric units where 24 hour resident medical cover is provided.

Hemabate must not be given intravenously.

Very rare cases of cardiovascular collapse have been reported following the use of prostaglandins. This should always be considered when using Hemabate.

*Precautions:* Hemabate should be used with caution in patients with a history of glaucoma or raised intraocular pressure, asthma, hypertension or hypotension, cardiovascular disease, renal disease, hepatic disease, anaemia, jaundice, diabetes or epilepsy.

As with other oxytocic agents, Hemabate should be used with care in patients with compromised (scarred) uteri. The possibility of uterine rupture should be borne in mind where high tone myometrial contractions are sustained.

Animal studies lasting several weeks at high doses have shown that prostaglandins of the E and F series can induce proliferation of bone. Such effects have also been noted in newborn infants who have received prostaglandin E1 during prolonged treatment. There is no evidence that short-term administration of Hemabate can cause similar bone effects.

Decreases in maternal arterial oxygen content have been observed in patients treated with carboprost tromethamine. A causal relationship to carboprost tromethamine has not been established, however, it is recommended that patients with pre-existing cardio-pulmonary problems receiving Hemabate are monitored during treatment and given additional oxygen if necessary.

*Overdosage:* Treatment of overdosage must be, at this time, symptomatic, as clinical studies with prostaglandin antagonists have not progressed to the point where recommendations may be made.

If evidence of excessive uterine activity or side-effects appear, the rate of infusion or frequency of administration should be decreased or discontinued.

In cases of massive overdosage resulting in extreme uterine hypertonus, appropriate obstetric procedures are indicated.

*Incompatibilities:* None.

**Pharmaceutical precautions** Hemabate must be stored in a refrigerator between 2 and 8°C. At 4°C it has a shelf-life of 48 months.

**Legal category** POM

**Package quantities** Pack containing 10 x 1 ml ampoules of Hemabate Sterile Solution 250 micrograms/ml.

**Further information** Carboprost tromethamine stimulates the myometrium of the gravid uterus to contract in a manner that is similar to that observed in the term uterus during labour. Whether or not this action results from a direct effect of carboprost tromethamine on the myometrium has not been determined with certainty at this time.

When Hemabate is given post-partum, the resulting myometrial contractions provide haemostasis at the site of placentation and hence prevent further blood loss.

**Product licence number** 0032/0152

## IMPROVERA*

**Qualitative and quantitative composition** Each estropipate tablet 1.5 mg contains Estropipate USP (piperazine oestrone sulphate) equivalent to 0.93 mg oestrone. Each medroxyprogesterone acetate tablet 10 mg contains 10 mg Medroxyprogesterone Acetate PhEur.

**Pharmaceutical form** Tablets for oral administration

**Clinical particulars**

*Therapeutic indications:* For oral use.

The treatment in this combination pack is recommended for women with intact uteruses only.

Hormone replacement therapy (HRT) for the treatment of the climacteric syndrome.

Prevention of postmenopausal osteoporosis in women identified to be at risk of this condition, e.g. early menopause, family history of osteoporosis, thin/small body frame, cigarette smoker, recent long-term use of systemic corticosteroids.

For maximum prophylactic benefit in the prevention of osteoporosis, treatment should begin as soon as possible after the menopause.

*Posology and method of administration:* The peach tablets contain 1.5 mg estropipate. The white tablets contain 10 mg medroxyprogesterone acetate.

*Adults:* Patients should start on day 1 of the calendar pack, taking one peach-coloured tablet daily until day 16, thereafter, one peach-coloured and one white-coloured tablet until day 28. Treatment should be continuous so that the next pack is started immediately after the previous pack without a break

Patients who are still menstruating: treatment should begin on the fifth day of menstruation.

Patients who are menstruating very infrequently or who are post-menopausal: treatment may be started at any time, provided pregnancy has been excluded.

During treatment , bleeding usually occurs within the last few days of one pack and the first week of the next.

The addition of a progestogen for the last 12 days of each cycle is to prevent the development of endometrial hyperplasia in those women who have an intact uterus.

*Elderly:* As for adults

*Children:* Not applicable

*Contra-indications:* Use in patients who are sensitive to medroxyprogesterone acetate, estropipate or any of the tablets' constituents; known or suspected pregnancy and lactation; known or suspected hormone dependent neoplasia, such as breast cancer; untreated endometrial hyperplasia (with nuclear atypia); undiagnosed abnormal vaginal bleeding; active thrombo-embolic disease; porphyria; acute or chronic liver disease; severe cardiac and renal diseases.

*Special warnings and special precautions for use:* A complete family and medical history and a careful examination including an examination of the breasts and pelvis should be performed before prescribing hormone replacement therapy. Women on long-term therapy for the prophylaxis of osteoporosis should be kept under regular review directed at the early diagnosis and treatment of breast and/or endometrial disease. As with all long-term treatment, the continuing need for such therapy should be intermittently reviewed.

HRT is not contraceptive and, if appropriate, the use of adequate, non-hormonal, methods of contraception should be advised.

*Endometrial hyperplasia and carcinoma:* Prolonged exposure to unopposed oestrogens increases the risk of endometrial neoplasia. For this reason this pack contains a progestogen for 12 days in each cycle. Bleeding, similar to that experienced during menstruation, can be expected to occur following the addition of the progestogen. In the first 3–6 cycles of use, bleeding may not follow a cyclical pattern. Erratic or irregular bleeding persisting after the first 6 cycles of use, should give rise to a suspicion of endometrial disease. In this event, appropriate diagnostic tests should be employed to assess the state of the endometrium. Endometrial hyperplasia, with atypia, should be adequately treated prior to continuation of oestrogen therapy. Similarly, irregular or break-through bleeding occurring *de novo* during therapy, should be investigated and the presence of endometrial disease ruled out. Patients with a past history of endometrial hyperplasia should be carefully monitored in order to detect any recurrence of the condition during therapy.

*Breast disease:* There is conflicting evidence on the relationship between oestrogen-containing HRT and breast cancer. At the present time, there is some evidence to suggest a slight increase in the risk of breast cancer in post-menopausal women who receive long-term (ie more than 5 –10 years) therapy. HRT can be used in patients with non-oestrogen dependent fibrocystic disease of the breast for up to 10 years before any increase in risk is likely to occur.

*Cardiovascular disease and hypertension:* There is no evidence that oestrogen replacement therapy will exacerbate pre-existing cardiovascular disease or hypertension. It has been estimated that the lifetime risk of death from cardiovascular disease (myocardial infarction and stroke) could be reduced by HRT. Fluid retention, which can occur in the early cycles of use, could exacerbate cardiovascular disease and pre-existing hypertension. Therefore, patients with such conditions should be carefully monitored during therapy.

*Thromboembolic disease:* There is no evidence that HRT is associated with an increase in risk of thromboembolism. HRT should not be started until any active thromboembolism has resolved. In patients with a past history of thromboembolism occurring *de novo,* a careful risk/benefit analysis should be considered prior to the commencement of therapy. Consideration should be given to discontinuing treatment at least 4 weeks before surgery or during prolonged periods of immobilisation.

*Diabetes:* There is no evidence that HRT exacerbates glucose intolerance. Blood sugar should be carefully monitored in diabetic patients beginning therapy, as transient alterations in control may occur.

*Liver disease:* Patients with congenital liver disorders exacerbated by oestrogens may become jaundiced during therapy. Such jaundice will fade on withdrawal from therapy. In the event that jaundice appears, treatment should be discontinued.

*Chronic diseases:* Some chronic disease conditions may be adversely affected by HRT such as otosclerosis, multiple sclerosis, melanoma, epilepsy and asthma. Patients with pre-existing migraine should be carefully monitored during therapy. Patients with systemic lupus erythematosus can be considered candidates for HRT unless they have severe unstable disease with renal impairment.

*Gallbladder disease:* It has been reported that there is an increase in the risk of surgically confirmed gallbladder disease in oestrogen-treated post-menopausal women.

*Laboratory tests:* Altered oestrogen concentrations may affect certain endocrine and liver function tests.

Endometriosis may recur during HRT. Patients experiencing recurrence of symptoms of the condition should be discontinued from oestrogen therapy.

Oestrogen administration has been associated with the growth of uterine fibromyomata.

*Interaction with other medicaments and other forms of interaction:* Patients on anticonvulsants may require a dose adjustment of their HRT, depending on the type of anticonvulsant taken. The active ingredients of this combination pack do not affect the pharmacokinetics of anticonvulsants.

Interactions with other medicinal treatments (including oral anti-coagulants) have rarely been reported, but causality has not been determined. The possibility of interaction should be borne in mind in patients receiving concurrent treatment with other drugs.

*Pregnancy and lactation:* This combination product is contra-indicated during pregnancy and lactation.

*Effects on ability to drive and use machines:* None

*Undesirable effects:* Side-effects associated with the use of oestrogens and/or progestogens may be observed. The incidence of side-effects reported with either medroxyprogesterone acetate or estropipate is low. The most commonly reported side-effect is nausea. Less frequently reported effects include breast tenderness, dysmenorrhoea, irregular vaginal bleeding/spotting, headaches, migraine, galactorrhoea, fluid retention, anorexia and vomiting, acneiform rashes and changes in liver function. Rare reactions include allergies, jaundice, changes in glucose metabolism and alterations of libido.

It is possible that fluid retention during adjustment to HRT may cause changes in corneal curvature leading to intolerance of contact lenses.

*Overdose:* Overdosage is unlikely to cause serious problems, although minor problems such as nausea and withdrawal bleeding may occur.

**Pharmacological properties**

*Pharmacodynamic properties:* Medroxyprogesterone acetate has actions and uses similar to those of progesterone. It has minimal androgenic activity compared with progesterone and virtually no oestrogenic activity.

Estropipate is a semi-synthetic oestrogen conjugate. Its action is due to oestrone, to which it is hydrolysed in the body. Oestrogens are important in the development and maintenance of the female reproductive system and secondary sex characteristics. They promote growth and development of the vagina, uterus and fallopian tubes and enlargement of the breasts. Indirectly, they contribute to the shaping of the skeleton, maintenance of tone and allow for the pubertal growth spurt and its termination, growth of axillary and pubic hair and pigmentation of the nipples and genitals. Along with other hormones such as progesterone, oestrogens are intricately involved in the process of menstruation. Oestrogens also affect the release of pituitary gonadotrophins. A depletion of endogenous oestrogens occurs postmenopausally as a result of a decline in ovarian function and may cause symptomatic vulvovaginal epithelial atrophy and other symptoms associated with its deficiency.

*Pharmacokinetic properties*

*General characteristics of active substance:* Medroxyprogesterone acetate (MPA) is rapidly absorbed from the gastro-intestinal tract. With a single oral dose of 10–250 mg, the time taken to reach the peak serum concentration ($T_{MAX}$) was 2–6 hours and the average peak serum concentration ($C_{MAX}$) was from 13–46.89 mg/ml. Unmetabolised MPA is highly plasma protein bound. MPA is metabolised in the liver and is primarily eliminated by faecal excretion as a glucuronide conjugated metabolite. Metabolised MPA is excreted more rapidly and in a greater percentage following oral doses than after aqueous intramuscular injection.

Oestradiol is rapidly hydrolysed in the body to oestrone which in turn may be hydrated to the less active oestriol. These transformations occur readily, mainly in the liver where there is also free interconversion between oestrone and oestradiol. Gastro-intestinal absorption of orally administered (tablets) oestrogens is usually prompt and complete. Inactivation of oestrogens in the body occurs mainly in the liver. During cyclic passage through, oestrogens in the body are degraded to less active oestrogenic compounds and conjugated with sulphuric and glucuronic acids. Oestrone is 50–80% bound as it circulates in the blood, primarily as a conjugate with sulphate.

*Characteristics in patients:* As both medroxyprogesterone acetate and estropipate are metabolised in the liver, any form of liver impairment results in reduced metabolism. See *Special warnings and special precautions for use* for further information.

*Preclinical safety data:* No special information. See *Special warnings and special precautions for use* for further information.

**Pharmaceutical particulars**

*List of excipients: Estropipate tablets:* lactose, dibasic potassium phosphate, tromethamine, hydroxypropyl cellulose, sodium starch glycollate, microcrystalline cellulose, colloidal silicon dioxide, magnesium stearate, hydrogenated vegetable oil wax, dye E110

*Medroxyprogesterone acetate tablets:* lactose, sucrose, maize starch, liquid paraffin, talc, calcium stearate, purified water

*Incompatibilities:* None known

*Shelf life:* Two years at 25°C

*Special precautions for product and admixture storage:* Store below 25°C.

*Nature and contents of container:* One or three PVC/aluminium foil strips packed in a carton, together with a Patient Information Leaflet. Each strip holds 28 peach-coloured estropipate tablets and 12 white medroxyprogesterone acetate tablets.

*Instructions for use/handling:* No special instructions

**Marketing authorisation number** 0032/0206

**Date of approval/revision of SPC** November 1995

**Legal category** POM

# INDOMOD*

## Presentation
*Indomod 25 mg:* Hard gelatin orange capsules with the imprint AB27 in light type, containing 25 mg indomethacin, in modified release form (Repro-Dose).

*Indomod 75 mg:* Hard gelatin brown capsules with imprint AB26 in light type, containing 75 mg indomethacin, in modified release form (Repro-Dose).

**Uses** Inflammatory rheumatic diseases such as rheumatoid arthritis, ankylosing spondylitis and gout. Inflammatory phases in osteoarthrosis. Inflammatory conditions such as bursitis, tendinitis, and tenosynovitis.

## Dosage and administration
*Dosage:* Use as directed by physician. The dose should be adjusted individually. In chronic rheumatoid disease the initial daily dose is normally 50–75 mg, which is increased by 25 mg or 50 mg at weekly intervals until a satisfactory effect is achieved. The daily dose should never exceed 200 mg.

In acute conditions, e.g. gouty arthritis, a dose of 100 mg is given initially, followed by 75 mg b.i.d. for controlling the pain. Then the dose is rapidly reduced and medication is discontinued. (See 'Further information').

Paediatric usage not established.

## Contra-indications, warnings, etc
*Contra-indications:* Active peptic ulcer or a history of recurrent gastrointestinal lesions; ulcerative colitis.

Haemophilia and other bleeding disorders. Allergy to non-steroidal anti-inflammatory drugs (salicylates, etc.).

*Warnings and precautions:* To be used with caution in patients with psychiatric disturbances, parkinsonism, or epilepsy. NSAIDs have been reported to cause nephrotoxicity in various forms and their use can lead to interstitial nephritis, nephrotic syndrome and renal failure. The symptoms of infection may be masked by indomethacin. The use of indomethacin is not recommended during pregnancy or lactation. Serum levels of indomethacin are raised by the concurrent administration of probenicid. Indomethacin reduces the natriuretic effect of frusemide.

*Side-effects:* Headache, dizziness, light-headedness, confusion and other reactions from the central nervous system are correlated to plasma concentrations and less likely to occur when high peak levels are avoided, as in the case with Indomod. Dyspepsia is another frequent side-effect of indomethacin likely to be modified by Indomod, due to the bypass of the stomach. Gastrointestinal bleeding and ulceration, fluid retention, disturbed renal or hepatic function, fatigue, tinnitus, drowsiness or insomnia may occur.

In patients with renal, cardiac or hepatic impairment caution is required since the use of NSAIDs may result in deterioration of renal function. The dose should be kept as low as possible and renal function should be monitored.

Anaphylactic reactions in hypersensitive patients.

**Pharmaceutical precautions** No special requirements or precautions.

**Legal category** POM.

## Package quantities
*Indomod 25 mg:* Blister packs of 120 modified release capsules.

*Indomod 75 mg:* Blister packs of 30 modified release capsules.

**Further information** Due to the special indomethacin plasma profile obtained with Indomod, doses may be taken at intervals of 8–12 hours, and a capsule of 75 mg taken at bedtime can be expected to relieve the next day's morning stiffness.

## Product licence numbers
Indomod 25 mg    4338/0006
Indomod 75 mg    4338/0007

**Product licence holder:** Benzon Pharma A/S, 29 Halmtorvet, DK-1700 Copenhagen, Denmark.

# INTRAFUSIN* 22

**Presentation** A clear, sterile solution of amino acids which provide a high level of nitrogen in a low fluid volume, for intravenous nutrition.

*Active ingredients*

| Amino acids | g/litre |
| --- | --- |
| Isoleucine | 4.20 |
| Leucine | 5.70 |
| Lysine-L-glutamate.2H$_2$O | 15.15 |
| Methionine | 5.40 |
| Phenylalanine | 4.10 |
| Threonine | 5.40 |
| Tryptophan | 2.10 |
| Valine | 4.70 |
| Arginine | 14.00 |
| Histidine | 3.50 |
| N-Acetyl-L-cysteine | 0.70 |
| Glycine | 15.60 |
| Alanine | 26.00 |
| Glutamic acid | 15.30 |
| Proline | 14.10 |
| Serine | 14.10 |
| N-Acetyl-L-tyrosine | 2.25 |
| TOTAL | 152.30 |

| | |
| --- | --- |
| Total Nitrogen g/litre | 22.8 |
| kcal/litre approximately | 600.0 |
| pH | 5.2 |
| Osmolality (mosmol/kg water) | 1,400.0 |
| Acetate | Nil |

**Uses** To be used for use as part of an intravenous parenteral nutrition regimen which is indicated whenever oral feeding is impossible or inadequate.

**Dosage and administration** The amount of Intrafusin 22 to be administered daily is calculated according to individual patients' requirements of nitrogen, fluid, etc.

*Recommended dosage for adults (including the elderly):* Adults should receive 1.0–2.0 g amino acids/kg body weight/day which equates to approximately 6.5–13 ml/kg body weight/day of Intrafusin 22. In a 70 kg patient this would result in an infusion volume of 450–900 ml/day.

Pregnant women and post-operative patients should receive 1.6–2.0 g amino acids/kg body weight daily.

An infusion rate of 0.9–1.3 ml/kg body weight/hour is recommended, which in a 70 kg patient corresponds to 63-91 ml/hour. The infusion rate should not exceed 1.3 ml/kg body weight/hour.

*Recommended dosage for children:* The product is not recommended for use in children.

## Contra-indications, warnings, etc
*Contra-indications:* Intrafusin 22 is contra-indicated in patients suffering from severe shock, hyperkalaemia, severe disturbances of liver or kidney function and disturbance of amino acid metabolism.

*Precautions:* The effects of Intrafusin 22 should be carefully controlled when administered to patients with a tendency to elevated serum potassium or urea levels. Too rapid an infusion may result in renal losses and nausea in sensitive patients.

A pre-existing deficiency of vitamins and in particular, folic acid and Vitamin B$_{12}$ may become clinically evident during intravenous nutrition with amino acids. Regular checks of the patients' Vitamin B$_{12}$ status and folate demand are therefore recommended. Prophylactic administration of adequate vitamins should be given if required.

*Overdosage:* In the event of fluid or solute overload during parenteral therapy, re-evaluate the patient's condition and institute appropriate corrective treatment.

**Pharmaceutical precautions** Store between 15°C and 25°C. Protect from light.

Do not use if the bottle is leaking or if the solution is cloudy or contains a precipitate.

Discard any unused contents.

Additions of drugs to the bottle of amino acid solution or giving set should be avoided.

**Legal category** POM.

**Package quantities** 500 ml and 1000 ml glass bottles.

**Further information** Intrafusin 22 is an electrolyte-free solution in which the L-lysine content is freely soluble and stable. This is achieved by utilisation of L-lysine-L-glutamate.2H$_2$O which is water soluble and dissociates in aqueous solution to free the lysine base.

Similarly N-acetyl L-tyrosine is used rather than L-tyrosine as the N-acetylated form is more easily soluble.

**Product licence number** 0022/0128.

# INTRALIPID* 10%
# INTRALIPID* 20%

**Presentation** A white, oil in water emulsion containing:

| | Intralipid 10% | Intralipid 20% |
| --- | --- | --- |
| Purified soybean oil | 50 g | 100 g |
| Fractionated egg phospho-lipids | 6 g | 6 g |
| Glycerol | 11 g | 11 g |
| Water for injections to | 500 ml | |
| pH 7 | | |

The emulsion is sterile and pyrogen-free.

## Uses
1. Intralipid is a concentrated source of energy for complete intravenous nutrition. Provision of a sufficient amount of energy in the form of carbohydrate is often restricted by such considerations as hypertonicity, hypervolaemia, tendency to thrombophlebitis and the limit beyond which further carbohydrate cannot be utilised. By the use of Intralipid it is possible to provide a high energy intake in a relatively small volume. One litre of Intralipid 20% provides 2,000 kcal (8.4 MJ) and one litre of Intralipid 10% 1,100 kcal (4.6 MJ).

2. Intralipid is a rich source of the essential fatty acids; linoleic and linolenic acids.

3. Intralipid has a protein-sparing effect when given in conjunction with amino acid and carbohydrate solutions.

4. Intralipid 20% has an osmolality of ~350 mosmol per kg water.

Intralipid 10% has an osmolality of ~300 mosmol per kg water. (Plasma ~290).

Therefore both these preparations are suitable for infusion into peripheral veins.

*Indications:* Intralipid should be used as part of a balanced intravenous feeding regimen in patients who are unable to receive sufficient amounts of nutrients enterally. Intralipid is especially valuable in providing a high energy intake to compensate for increased energy expenditure following trauma, infections, severe burns, etc.

**Dosage and administration** The dosage and infusion rate should be within the ranges recommended below and should be governed by the patient's ability to utilise fat.

*Recommended dosage for adults:* Intralipid 20%: 500–1000 ml per 24 hours in conjunction with intravenous administration of amino acid and carbohydrate solutions. For lesser energy requirements Intralipid 10% 500–1500 ml per 24 hours in conjunction with amino acid and carbohydrate solutions.

*Essential fatty acid deficiency:* When Intralipid is administered to prevent or correct essential fatty acid deficiency, 4–8% of non protein calories should be supplied as Intralipid to provide sufficient amounts of linoleic and linolenic acids.

When EFAD is associated with stress, the amount of Intralipid needed to correct the deficiency may be substantially increased.

*Recommended dosage for infants:* Dosage is governed by the maturity and birth-weight of the infant. In mature infants dosage scheme 1 should be used. In small gestational age and low birth-weight infants where the ability to handle fat may be impaired, dosage scheme 2 should be utilised.

In all cases, the infant's ability to eliminate infused fat from the circulation should be checked daily. Measuring serum triglycerides is the only reliable method. If lipaemia is present re-testing should be carried out after an interval of four hours.

When administered to infants Intralipid should, if possible, be infused continuously over 24 hours and to maintain a constant rate of infusion it is essential that an appropriate pump is used.

(1) Infants: 0.5–4 g fat per kg body weight in 24 hours. In practice 0.02–0.17 g/kg body weight should be administered each hour. The equivalent volumes of Intralipid are 10% 0.21–1.70 ml/kg/hour; 20% 0.10–0.85 ml/kg/hour. The dosage should be gradually increased during the first week of administration.

(2) To premature and low birth weight infants, Intralipid should be administered continuously during 24 hours/day. The initial infusion rate should be 0.5–1.0 g/kg/24 hours (2.5–5.0 ml Intralipid 20%/kg/24 hours). The dose is then increased by the same amount (0.5–1.0 g/kg) every 24 hour period up to 2.0 g/kg/24 hours (10 ml Intralipid 20%/kg/24 hours). The dose can only be increased above that level and up to a maximum of 4.0 g/kg/24 hours (20 ml Intralipid 20%/kg/24 hours) by concomitant careful monitoring by following the triglyceride levels, liver function tests and oxygen saturation.

The rates given are maximum rates and no attempt

should be made to exceed these in order to compensate for missed doses.

*Recommended dosage for the elderly:* Age per se requires no adjustment of the adult dosage. However, caution should be exercised in the 'frail' elderly and indeed in all patients with poor renal, cardiac or liver function, where smaller volumes should be used depending on the individual's requirements and condition.

**Administration:** Intralipid 10% and 20% are administered by slow intravenous infusion. During the first 10 minutes the drip should be adjusted to 20 drops per minute and then gradually increased to a final rate after half an hour of 25–40 drops per minute for Intralipid 20% and 40–60 drops per minute for Intralipid 10%. 500 ml of Intralipid 20% should be given over a period of not less than five hours. 500 ml of Intralipid 10% should be given over a period of not less than three hours. On the first day of infusion it is advisable to administer 5 ml Intralipid 20% per kg body weight or 10 ml Intralipid 10% per kg bodyweight. Subsequently the dose is usually doubled and when a larger intake is indicated the dosage may be increased to a maximum of 3 g fat per kg body weight per 24 hours.

Intralipid may be given as a separate infusion or as an admixture. When separate infusion is preferred the fat emulsion may be infused into the same central or peripheral vein as carbohydrates/amino acid solutions by means of a y-connector near the infusion site.

Intralipid can also be given as part of an all in one admixture containing carbohydrates, amino acids, electrolytes, vitamins and trace elements. The admixture must be approved for physical stability.

As with all infusions, care should be taken to avoid complications or catheterisation including air embolism and central venous thrombosis. The risk of serious thoracic complications can be avoided by the use of a peripheral catheter. The provision of intravenous nutrition via a peripheral catheter is facilitated by the near isotonicity of Intralipid. Strict asepsis should be maintained, especially in the immunosuppressed patient.

**Monitoring:** Electrolyte, fluid, acid-base imbalance and shock should be corrected prior to commencement of intravenous nutrition. In the metabolic and nutritional management of the seriously ill patient, specific preliminary investigations and continuous monitoring are essential, particularly of electrolyte levels. Monitoring of vitamin and trace element levels should be included, especially in patients receiving long-term intravenous nutrition.

**Contra-indications, warnings, etc** Intralipid is contra-indicated in severe disorders of fat metabolism such as in severe liver damage and acute shock.

*Other special warnings and precautions:* Intralipid should be given with caution in conditions of impaired lipid metabolism such as renal insufficiency, uncompensated diabetes mellitus, pancreatitis, certain forms of liver insufficiency, hypothyroidism (if hypertriglyceridemic), metabolic disorders and sepsis. Fat embolism has been reported in a few cases when the recommended infusion rate has been exceeded in these patients.

If intravenous administration of fat is considered in patients with the above mentioned disorders, the elimination of fat should be checked daily.

Patients known to be allergic to soy protein, should be given Intralipid with caution and only after hypersensitivity tests.

In newborns with neonatal hyperbilirubinaemia Intralipid should be used with caution, especially in low birth-weight infants, because of the risk of free fatty acids displacing bilirubin from albumin. Intralipid should be administered with caution to infants with known or suspected pulmonary hypertension. In neonates, particularly prematures on long term parental nutrition, platelet count, liver test and serum triglyceride concentration should be monitored.

Intralipid may interfere with certain laboratory measurements (bilirubin, lactate dehydrogenase, oxygen saturation, Hb etc) if blood is sampled before fat is adequately cleared from the blood stream. Fat is cleared after a fat-free interval of 4 to 6 hours in most patients.

*Interaction with other medicaments and other forms of interaction:* Some drugs, like insulin, may interfere with the body's lipase system. However, this kind of interaction seems to be of only limited clinical importance.

Heparin in clinical doses, causes a transient increase in lipolysis in plasma, resulting in a transient decrease in triglyceride due to depletion of lipoprotein lipase.

Soybean oil has a natural content of vitamin $K_1$. This is considered important only for patients treated with coumarin derivatives which interfere with vitamin $K_1$.

*Fat elimination:* The ability to eliminate fat should be closely monitored in patients with conditions mentioned under special warnings (this section), but also in patients given Intralipid for more than one week.

This is done by collecting a blood sample after a fat-free clearance period of 4–6 hours. Blood cells are then separated from plasma by centrifugation (1200–1500 rotations per minute, rpm). If the plasma is opalescent, the infusion should be postponed. The sensitivity of the method is such that hypertriglyceridaemia can pass undetected. Therefore, it is recommended that serum triglyceride concentrations are measured in patients who are likely to have an impaired fat tolerance.

*Other undesirable effects (frequency and seriousness):* In rare instances, initial administration of Intralipid has produced a rise in temperature and less frequently, shivering, chills and nausea/vomiting (incidence <1%). Infusion of Intralipid should be discontinued in such cases.

Other adverse event reports are extremely rare, occurring in less than one in one million infusions.

The following have been reported occurring immediately or soon after commencing infusion: hypersensitivity reactions (anaphylaxis, skin rash, urticaria), respiratory symptoms (e.g. tachypnoea), circulatory effects (e.g. hyper/hypotension), haemolysis, reticulocytosis, abdominal pain, headache, tiredness and priapism.

Increased levels of transaminases, alkaline phosphatases and bilirubin have been observed in patients receiving intravenous nutrition, with or without Intralipid. If the dosage is reduced values usually return to normal. Cholestasis has also been reported.

Thrombocytopenia has been reported in association with prolonged treatment with Intralipid in infants.

*Use in pregnancy and lactation:* Animal reproduction studies have not been carried out with Intralipid. There are, however, published reports of its successful and safe administration during pregnancy in the human.

*Overdosage (symptoms, emergency procedures, antidotes):* Overdosage leading to fat overload syndrome may occur, acutely as a result of too rapid an infusion rate, or chronically at recommended rates of infusion in association with a change in the patient's clinical condition, e.g. renal function impairment or infection. Fat overload syndrome is characterised by hyperlipidaemia, fever, fat infiltration, organ dysfunction and coma. All symptoms are usually reversible if the infusion is discontinued.

**Pharmaceutical precautions**

1. Store below 25°C. Do not freeze. After long periods of storage the bottle of Intralipid should be gently inverted two or three times before use.

2. Do not use if the bottle is leaking.

3. Discard any unused contents.

4. Additives may only be added to Intralipid where compatibility is known. The following additions can be recommended:

(i) Vitlipid N Adult or Vitlipid N Infant.
(ii) Solivito N (see Solivito N data sheet for details on reconstitution).
(iii) Diazemuls.
(iv) Heparin.

**Legal category** POM.

**Package quantities**
Intralipid 10%: 100 or 500 ml
Intralipid 20%: 100, 250 or 500 ml

**Further information** Intralipid, Vamin or Intrafusin solutions can be infused simultaneously, centrally or peripherally when the mixture reaches the vein through the same cannula. Intralipid can be mixed with other solutions in a single container (e.g. 3-litre bag). Such mixing must follow defined formulae and mixing techniques, details of which are available on request. The manufacturer can be consulted for full information on complete and balanced intravenous nutrition regimens.

Intralipid 10% and 20% contain 15 mmol organic phosphate per litre. This phosphate is considered to be bioavailable.

**Product licence numbers**
Intralipid 10%    0022/0027R
Intralipid 20%    0022/0028R

## INTRALIPID* 30%

**Qualitative and quantitative composition** 1000 ml of the emulsion contains:
*Active ingredient:* Purified Soybean Oil PhEur. *Quantity:* 300 g.

**Pharmaceutical form** Intralipid 30% is a sterile non-pyrogenic fat emulsion for intravenous infusion.

**Clinical particulars**

*Therapeutic indications:* Intralipid should be used as part of a balanced intravenous feeding regimen in patients who are unable to receive sufficient amounts of nutrients enterally. Intralipid is especially valuable in providing a high energy intake to compensate for increased energy expenditure following trauma, infections, severe burns.

*Posology and method of administration:* The ability to utilise and eliminate fat should govern the dosage elimination and infusion rate. See fat elimination.

*Adults (including the elderly):*
*For supply of energy and essential fatty acids:* The daily supplementation of 333 ml Intralipid 30% (100 g fat) is recommended for a patient weighing 70 kg with basal energy requirements and on total parenteral nutrition. On the first day of infusion it is advisable to administer 3 ml Intralipid 30% per kg/bw. The recommended maximum dosage is 3 g triglycerides/kg body weight/day.

*In essential fatty acid deficiency:* When Intralipid 30% is administered to prevent or correct essential fatty acid deficiency, 4 to 8% of non protein calories should be supplied as Intralipid 30% to provide sufficient amounts of linoleic and linolenic acids.

When EFAD is associated with stress, the amount of Intralipid 30% needed to correct the deficiency may be substantially increased.

*Infants and children:* There are no clinical data to support the use of Intralipid 30% in infants and children. Theoretically, tolerance of Intralipid 30% is expected to be similar to Intralipid 10% and 20%, (PL 0022/0027-0028R) but until data are available Intralipid 30% should be used with caution in infants and children.

*Administration:* Intralipid 30% should be administered by slow intravenous infusion, where the rate for the first half-hour is half the final administration rate. The infusion rate should not exceed 333 ml Intralipid 30% in 5 hours.

Intralipid 30% may be given as a separate infusion or as an admixture. When separate infusion is preferred the fat emulsion may be infused into the same central or peripheral vein as carbohydrates/amino acid solutions by means of a Y-connector near the infusion site.

Intralipid 30% can also be given as part of an All in One admixture containing carbohydrates, amino acids, electrolytes, vitamins and trace elements. The admixture must be approved for physical stability.

As with all infusions, care should be taken to avoid complications of catheterisation including air embolism and central venous thrombosis. The risk of serious thoracic complications can be avoided by the use of a peripheral catheter. The provision of intravenous nutrition via a peripheral catheter is facilitated by the near isotonicity of Intralipid. Strict asepsis should be maintained, especially in the immunosuppressed patient.

*Monitoring:* Electrolyte, fluid, acid-base imbalance and shock should be corrected prior to commencement of intravenous nutrition. In the metabolic and nutritional management of the seriously ill patient, specific preliminary investigations and continuous monitoring are essential, particularly of electrolyte levels. Monitoring of vitamin and trace element levels should be included, especially in patients receiving long-term intravenous nutrition

*Contra-indications:* Intralipid should be contra-indicated in severe disorders of fat metabolism such as in severe liver damage and acute shock.

*Special warnings and special precautions for use:* Intralipid 30% should be given with caution in conditions of impaired lipid metabolism as in renal insufficiency, uncompensated diabetes mellitus, pancreatitis, impaired liver function, hypo-thyroidism (if hypertriglyceridemic) and sepsis. Fat embolism has been reported in a few cases when the recommended infusion rate has been exceeded in these patients.

If Intralipid 30% is given to patients with these conditions, close monitoring of the serum triglyceride concentration and liver function is required.

Patients known to be allergic to soy protein, should be given Intralipid 30% with caution and only after hypersensitivity tests.

Intralipid 30% may interfere with certain laboratory measurements (bilirubin, lactate dehydrogenase, oxygen saturation, Hb etc) if blood is sampled before fat has been adequately cleared from the bloodstream. Fat is normally cleared after a period of 4 to 6 hours in most patients.

*Fat elimination:* The ability to eliminate fat should be closely monitored in patients with conditions mentioned under *Special warnings* but also in patients given Intralipid 30% for more than one week. This is done by collecting a blood sample after a fat clearance period of 4-6 hours. Blood cells are then separated from plasma by centrifugation (1200-1500 rotations per minute, rpm). If the plasma is opalescent the infusion should be postponed. The sensitivity of this method is such that hypertriglyceridaemia can pass undetected. Therefore, it is recommended that serum triglyceride concentrations are measured in patients who are likely to have an impaired fat tolerance.

*Interaction with other medicaments and other forms of interaction:* Some drugs, like insulin, may interfere with the body's lipase system. However, this kind of interaction seems to be of only limited clinical importance.

Heparin in clinical doses, causes a transient increase in lipolysis in plasma, resulting in a transient decrease in triglyceride clearance due to depletion of lipoprotein lipase.

Soybean oil has a natural content of vitamin $K_1$. This is considered important only for patients treated with coumarin derivatives which interfere with vitamin $K_1$.

*Pregnancy and lactation:* Animal reproduction studies have not been performed with Intralipid 30%. However, Intralipid 30% is expected to be tolerated similarly to Intralipid 10% and 20%, (PL 0022/0027-0028R) on which there are published reports on safe and successful administration during pregnancy in the human.

*Effects on ability to drive and use machines:* Not applicable.

*Undesirable effects:* In rare instances initial administration of Intralipid has produced a rise in temperature, and less frequently, shivering, chills and nausea/vomiting (incidence < 1%).

Other adverse event reports are extremely rare, occurring in less than one in one million infusions.

The following have been described occurring immediately or soon after commencing infusion: Hypersensitivity reactions (anaphylaxis, skin rash, urticaria), respiratory symptoms (e.g. tachypnoea), circulatory effects (e.g. hyper/hypotension), haemolysis, reticulocytosis, abdominal pain, headache, tiredness and priapism.

Increased levels of transaminases, alkaline phosphatase and bilirubin have been observed in patients receiving intravenous nutrition, with or without Intralipid. Cholestasis has also been reported. These changes are reversible and usually return to normal when intravenous nutrition is interrupted.

Thrombocytopenia has been reported in association with prolonged treatment with Intralipid in infants.

*Overdose:* Overdose leading to fat overload syndrome may occur, acutely as a result of too rapid an infusion rate, or chronically at recommended rates of infusion in association with a change in the patients clinical condition, eg. renal function impairment or infection. Fat overload syndrome is characterised by hyperlipaemia, fever, fat infiltration, organ dysfunction and coma. All symptoms are usually reversible if the infusion is discontinued.

**Pharmacological properties**

*Pharmacodynamic properties:* The pharmacodynamic effects of Intralipid 30% are limited due to the nature of the product. No significant effects were observed in cardiovascular parameters in the anaesthetised cat over 3.5 hours. In comparison, the recommended dose in man is up to 3 g fat/kg bw/24 hours. At considerably higher doses, (e.g 9.75 g fat/kg/2 hours) blood flow was decreased to approximately 76 ± 6% of the preinfusion flow but there was no significant effect on blood pressure. The pharmacodynamic profile is comparable with Intralipid 10% and 20%, (PL 0022/0027-0028R).

*Pharmacokinetic properties:* The elimination of Intralipid 30% is comparable with Intralipid 10% and 20%, (PL 0022/0027-0028R). Intralipid, which is administered intravenously is distributed within the blood vessels. It is eliminated from the blood stream by the enzyme lipoprotein lipase (LPL) and after association with apolipoproteins is metabolised in a similar way to chylomicrons. The half-life is approximately 9.00 ± 0.64 minutes and the clearance mechanism is concentration dependent, with saturation above 1.1 mm in blood, which corresponds to a dose of approximately 0.1 g fat/kg bw. Below this concentration elimination follows first order kinetics.

Intralipid as such is not excreted. The metabolites, carbon dioxide, water and phosphate are excreted via lungs, lungs and urine and urine respectively.

*Preclinical safety data:* During the preclinical animal studies there were no findings which were of relevance to the prescriber, in relation to the safety profile of Intralipid 30%. The pharmaco-toxicological properties of Intralipid 30% are comparable to Intralipid 10% and 20%, (PL 0022/ 0027-0028R).

**Pharmaceutical particulars**

*List of excipients:* Purified egg phospholipids, glycerol, sodium hydroxide, water for injections.

*Incompatibilities:* There are no known incompatibilities with Intralipid 30%. However, additives may only be added to Intralipid 30% where compatibility is known. Such mixing must follow defined formulae and mixing techniques, details of which are available on request from the manufacturer. The following additions can be recommended: Vitlipid N Adult or Vitlipid N Infant, Solivito N (see Solivito N data sheet for details of reconstitution).

*Shelf life:* The shelf life is 24 months.

*Special precautions for storage:* Store below 25°C. Do not freeze.

*Nature and contents of container:* Colourless glass bottles of hydrolytic class II according to PhEur.

Glass bottle sizes: 250 ml, 350 ml, 500 ml and 1000 ml.

The bottles are sealed with butyl rubber stoppers. The bottles are filled with Intralipid 30% to volumes of 250, 333, 500 and 1000 ml respectively.

*Instructions for use/handling:* There are no special instructions on handling of the product.

**Marketing authorisation number** 0022/0110

**Date of approval/revision of SPC** November 1996

**Legal category** POM

## KABIGLOBULIN*

**Presentation** Ampoules containing Human Normal Immunoglobulin solution 16%, a clear pale straw colour. The active constituent is gamma globulin.

**Uses** *Main pharmacological action:* The immunoglobulins present in Kabiglobulin may be used prophylactically and therapeutically to provide passive immunity against infectious diseases.

*Indications:* Prophylaxis against infectious hepatitis (Hepatitis A). Prophylaxis against Rubella following exposure during pregnancy. Prevention, or modification of symptoms, following measles exposure in susceptible individuals. Antibody deficiency syndromes; to reduce the incidence and severity of infections in agammaglobulinaemia, hypogammaglobulinaemia and dysgammaglobulinaemia. Following burns injury.

**Dosage and administration** *Route of administration:* By intramuscular injection only.

*Recommended dosage: Infectious hepatitis (Hepatitis A):* for prophylaxis against infectious hepatitis for up to 3 months, in adults and children, 0.02–0.04 ml per kg body weight is recommended by WHO. In massive exposure, e.g. to people visiting highly endemic areas, 0.06–0.12 ml per kg body weight is recommended. The effect of the larger injection lasts for a period of at least four months.

*Rubella in pregnancy:* 20 ml is administered as soon as possible following exposure. The effect of an injection lasts about 3 weeks and therefore the dosage should be repeated after this time in the case of renewed exposure to the disease.

*Measles prevention:* 0.2 ml per kg body weight is injected within five days of exposure. The preventive effect of an injection normally lasts three weeks. The dosage should therefore be repeated after that period of time in the case of renewed exposure to the disease.

*Measles modification:* 0.04 ml per kg body weight is injected within five days of exposure.

*Antibody deficiency syndromes:* agammaglobulinaemia, hypogammaglobulinaemia, dysgammaglobulinaemia. As an initial dosage, 1.3 ml per kg body weight (maximum 60 ml) injected in divided doses over 48 hours. Half this dosage, 0.65 ml per kg (maximum 30 ml), is then given every three to four weeks.

*Burns injury:* during the first week following the trauma a total of about 50 g gamma globulin in the form of Kabiglobulin should be given in addition to plasma and blood. From the third up to the tenth day, 15–30 ml (2.5–5.0 g gamma globulin) per day is administered.

**Contra-indications, warnings, etc** Kabiglobulin should not be given at the same time as live vaccines, such as measles, mumps, rubella and oral polio vaccines (Sabin). If Kabiglobulin (2 ml) has been administered these vaccines should not be given for 3 months. This period should be increased to 4 months for the 5 ml injection. Following administration of live vaccines a period of 2–3 weeks should elapse before giving Kabiglobulin. Kabiglobulin may be given at the same time as tetanus, typhoid, diphtheria, cholera, polio [the inactivated form (Salk)] and yellow fever; although a live vaccine, Kabiglobulin donors are unlikely to possess the antibody to yellow fever.

*Pregnancy and lactation:* There is no evidence of safety nor of toxicity of Kabiglobulin in human pregnancy or lactation, but it has been commonly used for many years without apparent ill consequence. If such therapy is needed in pregnancy or lactation, Kabiglobulin can be used if there is no alternative course of action.

*Side-effects:* In exceptional cases, intramuscular injections of gamma globulin may give rise to adverse reactions of the following types:

*Local reactions:* at the site of injection such as erythema, swelling, tenderness and induration, which generally subside within a few days after the injection.

*General reactions:* such as fever (38–40°C), chills and general malaise. These symptoms have appeared 6–8 hours after the injection and have generally subsided by the following day.

*Hypersensitivity reactions:* such as exanthema and pruritus. Flush, tachycardia and shock are rare. The reactions are more frequent in patients with hypogammaglobulinaemia or dysgammaglobulinaemia and may be delayed for some hours following administration.

*Overdosage:* There have been no reports of overdosage with Kabiglobulin. There is no specific antidote and in the unlikely event of any reactions occurring following overdosage, they should be treated symptomatically.

**Pharmaceutical precautions** Store between 2°C and 8°C.

**Legal category** POM.

**Package quantities** Ampoules of 2.0 and 5.0 ml.

**Further information** The IgA content of Kabiglobulin does not exceed 0.01% of the total protein content. Kabiglobulin contains no preservative agents. Based on results from model experiments and from clinical follow-up, several organisations such as the Food and Drug Administration, Centers for Disease Control and World Health Organisation have drawn the conclusion that immunoglobulin preparations, manufactured according to standard methods are safe with respect to transmission of HIV infectivity.

**Product licence number** 0022/5009.

## KABIKINASE*

**Presentation** Vial containing a straw coloured lyophilised powder, containing 250,000 iu of streptokinase. Human albumin and buffering agents are present as stabilisers.

**Uses** *Action:* By activating the fibrinolytic system streptokinase induces dissolution of intravascular thrombi and emboli.

*Indications:* Thrombolytic therapy by intravenous Kabikinase infusion is indicated in the treatment of deep vein thrombosis, acute major pulmonary embolism, acute arterial thromboembolism.

Additionally, thrombolytic therapy by local streptokinase administration is indicated in the treatment of myocardial infarction (see b, below) and in the clearance of clotted haemodialysis shunts (see c, below).

**Dosage and administration** *Routes of administration:* By intravascular infusion; intracoronary infusion.

*Recommended dosage for adults:*

*(a) Standard intravenous infusion regimen:* The standard intravenous dosage scheme includes a loading dose sufficient to neutralise circulating streptococcal antibody, followed by a maintenance dose to maintain an appropriate degree of fibrinolysis.

*Loading dose:* Streptokinase 600,000 iu is infused via a peripheral vein over a period of 30–60 minutes.

*Maintenance dose:* Streptokinase 100,000 iu/hour is infused for 72 hr. If further treatment is considered necessary it should be continued for not more than a further 3 days.

*(b) Intracoronary administration in myocardial infarction:* Intracoronary thrombolysis is performed using standard techniques for selective coronary angiography by either the brachial or femoral approach. Early intervention is recommended, ideally within 6 hours following onset of chest pain.

Using a standard 7 or 8 French catheter, angiography is used to identify the presence and location of the thrombus. Nitroglycerin (100–400 micrograms) is administered into the involved vessel, to relieve coronary artery spasm. Initially a bolus dose of streptokinase 10,000–25,000 iu is administered followed by a continuous infusion of 4,000 iu/minute, which is continued until vessel patency is restored, or for 60–75 minutes (total dose 240,000–300,000 iu). If reperfusion is achieved prior to this time then the infusion rate may be reduced when patency is restored, and infusion should continue for an additional 30–60 minutes (80,000–100,000 iu streptokinase) in order to lyse any remaining residual thrombus.

Subsequent anticoagulant treatment with heparin is necessary in order to prevent rethrombosis in the infarct-related coronary artery. However, in the majority of patients intracoronary streptokinase administration produces significant fibrinogen (and plasminogen) depletion. Additionally, circulating fibrin/fibrinogen degradation products exert an anticoagulant effect. Accordingly heparin should be administered incrementally and judiciously during the first 24 hr following treatment. The partial thromboplastin time should be monitored at regular intervals, and the heparin dosage adjusted to maintain the former within the range 2–2.5 times normal.

*(c) Local application in occluded haemodialysis shunts:* Kabikinase 100,000 iu is dissolved in normal saline 100 ml. 10,000–25,000 iu (10–25 ml) is deposited in the clotted portion of the shunt, which is then sealed on the venous side with forceps. A sterile single-dose syringe is attached on the arterial side to form an air cushion against which the artery can pulsate. If required, the treatment may be repeated after 30–45 minutes.

*Recommended dosage for infants:* Although the standard dosage scheme may be reduced proportionally to circulating volume, it may be preferable to titrate the initial dose followed by a maintenance dose of 1300–1400 iu/kg body weight/hr for 3 days. Response normally occurs within this period but if further therapy is considered it should not be for more than an additional 3 days.

*Preparation of solution:* The contents of a vial of Kabikinase are dissolved at room temperature in 5 ml water for injections carefully avoiding the formation of a foam. The concentrated solution thus obtained is transferred aseptically into an infusion bottle of glucose or saline of suitable volume, according to the needs of the patient. The rate of infusion is then adjusted to give the required dosage rate.
*Standard intravenous infusion regimen:* For the loading dose; 600,000 iu Kabikinase is made up in 100 ml 5% glucose or physiological saline and is administered over 30 minutes.

For the maintenance dose; 600,000 iu is made up in 500 ml 5% glucose or physiological saline, and is administered at a rate of 80 ml per hr (100,000 iu hourly). If desired, smaller volumes can be employed, to enable the use of a syringe pump.

*Intracoronary administration:* The contents of a reconstituted vial are added to a volume of 5% glucose or physiological saline in order to achieve a final streptokinase concentration of not less than 1,000 iu/ml.

*Control of therapy (standard intravenous infusion regimen):* Therapy is controlled by the thrombin clotting time performed at intervals and should be within the limits of two to four times the normal value.

**Contra-indications, warnings, etc**
*Contra-indications:* Kabikinase should not be administered intramuscularly. Since thrombolytic therapy increases the risk of bleeding, Kabikinase is contra-indicated in the following:
1. Surgery within the last 10 days.
2. Invasive procedures during the last 10 days.
3. Gastrointestinal bleeding within the last six months.
4. Thrombocytopenia or other evidence of defective haemostasis.
5. Liver or kidney disease.
6. Cerebrovascular accident.
7. Severe hypertension treated and untreated.
8. Parturition (within the last 10 days).
9. Ulcerative colitis.
10. Visceral carcinoma.
11. Menstrual bleeding.
12. During the first 18 weeks of pregnancy (see note below).
13. Sub-acute bacterial endocarditis.

*Precautions and warnings:* Following 7–10 days' treatment with streptokinase, the patient's anti-streptokinase antibody titre increases considerably, and returns to normal only after up to 6 months. Normally, a second treatment with streptokinase should not be considered within 6 months of the first. If a second treatment is considered necessary within 6 months then the initial loading dose should be individually determined. The titrated initial dose may be calculated following determination of the smallest quantity of Kabikinase required to lyse a clot, formed from 1.0 ml of the patient's blood within 10 minutes.

If heparin or oral anticoagulants have been given before commencing Kabikinase thrombolytic therapy, further administration should cease (it is not advisable to give Kabikinase and heparin simultaneously). The Kabikinase infusion can then be started after 4 hours. If immediate Kabikinase therapy is required the heparin in the blood should be neutralised with protamine sulphate.

On termination of Kabikinase treatment, the patient should be given anticoagulants in an attempt to prevent rethrombosis. Preferably heparin should be used, starting four hours after the end of thrombolysis, and then oral anticoagulants may be introduced in the usual manner. Drugs which affect blood platelet function, such as salicylic acid preparations, pyrazolone, or indole derivatives, should not be administered concurrently with Kabikinase since the risk of bleeding will be increased.

Streptokinase should be used with caution in patients with haemorrhagic retinopathy.

*Pregnancy:* Thrombolytic therapy with Kabikinase during the first 18 weeks of pregnancy should be avoided, since there may be a risk of placental separation.

Negligible amounts of streptokinase cross the placenta. The foetal blood concentration reaches about one thousandth of the maternal blood concentration. Fibrinolytic effects in the foetus are unlikely.

*Elderly patients:* The incidence of cerebral haemorrhage resulting from thrombolytic therapy is increased in elderly patients. Therapy should be restricted to those patients in whom the benefit of treatment outweighs this additional hazard.

*Side-effects:* Kabikinase therapy may be accompanied by a slight to moderate elevation in body temperature. Mild allergic reactions such as urticaria occur uncommonly. Anaphylaxis occurs extremely rarely. These reactions may be controlled by the prior administration of corticosteroids (25 mg prednisolone or a corresponding amount of another glucocorticoid).

Streptokinase administration has been associated with low back pain. This may indicate an allergic response and it may be appropriate to discontinue the infusion. In some cases, without other features of allergy, infusion has been continued with analgesic cover, without adverse consequence.

A few allergic reactions such as polyneuropathy and uveitis have been temporally related to the administration of streptokinase. Guillain-Barre Syndrome has been reported after streptokinase treatment.

Haemorrhage can occur in any tissue and organ in the body and can present with symptoms affecting any body system, including the abdomen, cardiovascular system, joints and CNS. Haemorrhage should be considered as a potential cause of unusual symptoms occurring after administration.

Minor oozing or bleeding occurring at injection sites may be controlled by applying local pressure.

Exceptionally there may be severe haemorrhage, in which case administration of Kabikinase must be discontinued. If necessary, the antifibrinolytic agent Cyklokapron (tranexamic acid-10 mg/kg body weight) should be given immediately by slow intravenous injection. Cryoprecipitate may be used to correct haemostatic deficiency.

*Antidote:* Tranexamic acid 10 mg/kg body weight by slow intravenous injection.

**Pharmaceutical precautions** Vials of Kabikinase should be stored below 25˚C before reconstitution. Reconstituted vials may be stored for up to 24 hr when kept in a refrigerator. Kabikinase solutions diluted for infusion should be used within 12 hours of preparation.

**Legal category** POM.

**Package quantities** Vial of 250,000 iu.

**Further information** Kabikinase is a highly purified streptokinase preparation. It is prepared from beta-haemolytic streptococci culture filtrates. Subsequent purification ensures that Kabikinase is virtually free from streptodornase, streptolysin, hyaluronidase and other enzymes. Kabikinase is soluble in water, is non-toxic and is non-pyrogenic, but is weakly antigenic. Kabikinase is stabilised with sterile human albumin and this imparts a faint straw colour to the preparation.

**Product licence number** 0022/5012R.

## KABIKINASE* 750,000 IU

**Presentation** Vial of straw coloured lyophilised powder containing 750,000 iu of streptokinase. Human albumin and buffering agents are present as stabilisers.

**Uses**
*Action:* By activating the fibrinolytic system, streptokinase induces dissolution of intravascular thrombi and emboli.

*Indication:* Acute myocardial infarction.

**Dosage and administration**
*Recommended dosage for adults:* Streptokinase 1.5 million iu in physiological saline or dextrose 5% is administered as an intravenous infusion, at a constant rate, over 60 minutes.

*Preparation of solution:* Dissolve the contents of 2 vials of Kabikinase 750,000 iu by adding 5 ml Water for Injections, to each vial.

The solution should be prepared at room temperature. Care should be taken to avoid the formation of foam. The concentrated solution thus obtained is transferred aseptically into an infusion bottle or PVC bag, containing 100 ml of physiological saline, or dextrose 5%.

**Contra-indications, warnings, etc**
*Contra-indications:* Kabikinase should not be administered intramuscularly. Since thrombolytic therapy

increases the risk of bleeding, Kabikinase is contra-indicated in the following:

1. *Invasive or traumatic procedures within the previous 10 days* including the following: surgery; central venous cannulation, or puncture of a non-compressible vessel; external cardiac compression; endotracheal intubation; biopsy.
2. *Defective haemostasis* including: thrombocytopenia or any other platelet disorder; coagulation disorder (including those caused by hepatic or renal impairment); acute systemic infection, bacteraemia or septicaemia; oral or intravenous anticoagulant therapy (see under Precautions, paragraph 2).
3. *Potential for gastrointestinal haemorrhage* including: oesophageal varices; history of peptic ulceration; visceral carcinoma; ulcerative colitis; diverticulitis.
4. *Increased risk of cerebral haemorrhage/infarction* as evidenced by any of the following: stroke; cerebral tumour; hypertension (treated or untreated); hypertensive or diabetic retinopathy; transient ischaemic attacks.
5. *Obstetric or gynaecological conditions likely to predispose to haemorrhage,* including: menstruation; pregnancy – see also Pregnancy section; parturition within the previous 18 weeks.
6. *Potential for cardiac thromboemboli,* including: active or recent infective endocarditis; atrial valve disease with atrial fibrillation.
7. *Increased risk of pulmonary haemorrhage,* including: active tuberculosis; pneumothorax.
8. *Previous streptokinase therapy,* more than 5 days and up to 6 months previously, or recent streptococcal infection, since an elevated titre of anti-streptokinase antibody may render the treatment ineffective.
9. *Coma.*

*Precautions: Patients should not receive streptokinase unless they will be managed within a hospital setting, under expert medical supervision. It is recommended that patients should be treated in a coronary care (or intensive care) unit.*

1. The *diagnosis* of acute myocardial infarction should initially be based upon both clinical signs and ECG evidence. Specific ECG changes diagnostic of recent myocardial infarction should be present. The following diagnoses, which can be associated with ECG changes, and in which administration of thrombolytic therapy might result in life-threatening haemorrhage MUST be excluded: aortic dissection; acute pericarditis, oesophageal rupture; acute abdominal emergencies, including pancreatitis and perforation of the duodenum; intracranial haemorrhage; (see also 2., below).

A chest X-ray should be performed in order to assist in eliminating ruptured oesophagus (pneumomediastinum) or duodenum (air under the diaphragm) and aortic dissection (wide mediastinum). Aortic dissection should be suspected particularly when pain radiates into the back, aortic regurgitation is evident on auscultation or there are absent pulses. Pericarditis should be suspected when ST-segment elevation occurs in all ECG leads. Raised blood amylase is an indication of pancreatitis.

2. Thrombolytic therapy should be considered only in the case of patients for whom a well documented *medical history* is available. It is essential that thrombolytic therapy is not instituted in patients with co-existing medical conditions likely to exacerbate the risk of haemorrhage (e.g. peptic ulceration, history of cerebro-vascular accident, cerebral tumour, visceral carcinoma, see also *Contra-indications*). Additionally, caution should be exercised in patients who are receiving other drug therapies which are likely to predispose to increased risk of haemorrhagic complications.

3. In most patients, infarction probably is complete within 4–6 hrs and, accordingly, only patients in whom therapy can be initiated within this time interval should be considered for treatment. (But see statement on Q waves below.) *Myocardial salvage* is possible only when recanalisation of the infarct-related artery is effected within a critical time interval following coronary occlusion. The rate of progression of myocardial necrosis is inversely related to the extent of residual perfusion of the ischaemic myocardium. When infarction is due to sub-total coronary occlusion (ca 10–25% of patients) and there is some residual antegrade perfusion, the rate of necrosis is less than when infarction results from complete coronary occlusion. Similarly, in some patients (ca 5–10%) a well developed collateral circulation may retard the progress and reduce the severity of ischaemia. The maximum time delay commensurate with myocardial salvage and reduction in mortality is not known. In patients treated within one hour following symptomatic onset, the risk of death is halved. Generally, the presence of marked pathological Q waves in the ECG should be considered as evidence that transmural infarction is complete and that appreciable myocardial salvage is not possible.

Conversely, benefit may be derived up to 18 hours following symptom onset, in patients in whom pathological Q waves are absent, or symptoms are intermittent.

4. *Hypokalaemia* predisposes to ventricular arrhythmias and, if present should be corrected.

5. If *venous access* is considered necessary (e.g. for cardiac pacing) the risk of haemorrhage from central venous cannulation must be considered, and preference should be given to the antecubital route.

6. Thrombolytic therapy with Kabikinase induces a *systemic fibrinolytic state.* The presence of circulating free plasmin results in consumption of fibrinogen and of coagulation factors (predominantly Factors V, VIII and XII). Additionally, circulating degradation products of fibrinogen and fibrin exert an anticoagulant effect. Accordingly thrombolytic therapy increases the risk of haemorrhage both throughout the period of streptokinase infusion, and for approximately 12–24 hours thereafter, i.e. until the serum fibrinogen exceeds 100 mg%.

7. Care should be exercised when moving the patient to avoid trauma-induced haematomas. Unnecessary venepunctures should be avoided.

8. Streptokinase should be used with caution in patients with haemorrhagic retinopathy.

9. *Reperfusion* is usually accompanied by relief of chest pain. Occasionally, reperfusion is preceded by a period of fluctuation in the severity of chest pain. Reperfusion is followed by resolution of the ischaemic ST segment changes. An ECG lead with distinct ST segment elevation should be selected for continuous monitoring, and the initial positions of the ST segment and the peak of the T waves marked. The time of reperfusion may then be recorded. In patients who have sustained minimal necrosis there may be no development of Q waves. However, development of Q waves may not imply complete necrosis, since myocardium subjected to prolonged ischaemia ('stunned myocardium') may take several days to recover.

10. In some patients with inferior wall infarction reperfusion is associated with *vagal reactions* of nausea, vomiting, sinus bradycardia and hypotension. It has been proposed that these result from the triggering of the Bezold-Jarisch reflex by the restoration of perfusion to the inferior and posterior wall of the left ventricle. These vagal reactions usually respond to intravenous atropine.

11. Accelerated idioventricular rhythm occurs at the time of reperfusion or shortly thereafter in approximately 50–60% of patients. Reperfusion is also associated with ventricular ectopic beats occurring late in diastole. These may be single or may give rise to ventricular bigeminy or trigeminy, or may form fusion beats. These ventricular arrhythmias (frequently referred to as 'reperfusion arrhythmias') are probably related to increased automaticity. Sustained ventricular tachycardia and ventricular fibrillation are rare, occurring no more commonly than in patients receiving standard management, and should be managed in the normal way.

12. The titre of circulating antistreptokinase antibody rises abruptly at 5–7 days following Kabikinase administration, and may reach levels sufficient to neutralise subsequent Kabikinase dosages administered within the following 3–6 months.

Accordingly, (a) Information relating to the administration of Kabikinase therapy should be recorded clearly in the patient's notes.

(b) Kabikinase therapy should not be repeated within the period of 5 days to 6 months following the initial treatment.

(c) Patients with on-going, or recent, streptococcal infections may be resistant to Kabikinase therapy.

13. Subsequent *anticoagulant treatment* with heparin is generally considered necessary in order to prevent rethrombosis in the infarct-related coronary artery, since following thrombolysis, the thrombogenic segment is again exposed to circulating blood, and may again induce thrombosis in the affected artery. Reocclusion occurs in approximately 10–20% of successfully reperfused patients. If anticoagulant treatment is considered appropriate, then heparin should be administered incrementally and judiciously during the first 24 hr following treatment. The partial thromboplastin time should be monitored at regular intervals, and the heparin dosage adjusted to maintain the former within the range 2–2.5 times normal. The optimal duration of anticoagulant therapy is not known. The use of thrombolytic therapy should not necessarily lead to any change in the normal patient management of acute myocardial infarction.

14. Successful thrombolytic therapy will not obviate the requirement for further expert cardiological assessment and patient management.

*Side-effects:* Kabikinase therapy may be accompanied by a slight to moderate pyrexia. Mild allergic reactions such as urticaria are uncommon, particularly when the total duration of infusion is less than 2 hours. Anaphylaxis occurs extremely rarely (ca 0.1%). These reactions may be controlled by the prior intravenous administration of corticosteroids (e.g. hydrocortisone

100 mg, or prednisolone 25 mg). If streptokinase infusion is to be administered for more than 2 hours, or is to be repeated within 6 months, the prior administration of intravenous corticosteroid and/or an antihistamine should be considered, in order to reduce the incidence of allergic reactions.

Streptokinase administration has been associated with low back pain. This may indicate an allergic response and it may be appropriate to discontinue the infusion. In some cases, without other features of allergy, infusion has been continued with analgesic cover, without adverse consequences.

A few allergic reactions such as polyneuropathy and uveitis have been temporally related to the administration of streptokinase. Guillain-Barre Syndrome has been reported after streptokinase treatment.

Haemorrhagic complications largely result from inappropriate anticoagulant therapy, rather than from fibrinolysis *per se.*

Haemorrhage can occur in any tissue and organ in the body and can present with symptoms affecting any body system, including the abdomen, cardiovascular system, joints and CNS. Haemorrhage should be considered as a potential cause of unusual symptoms occurring after administration. Minor bleeding, predominantly at puncture sites, occurs with an incidence of approximately 3–4%. Major haemorrhagic episodes requiring transfusion of 2 or more units of blood (gastrointestinal and retroperitoneal haemorrhage) occur with an incidence of approximately 0.3%. Cerebral haemorrhage and stroke occurs with a frequency of approximately 0.1%. Though there is a theoretical risk of haemorrhagic infarction and haemorrhage into the pericardium, these are extremely rarely encountered. In cases of severe haemorrhage administration of Kabikinase must be discontinued. If necessary, the antifibrinolytic agent Cyklokapron (tranexamic acid – 10 mg/kg body weight), should be given immediately by slow intravenous injection. Fresh frozen plasma, or preferably cryoprecipitate, should be administered, to correct haemostatic deficiencies.

*Antidote:* Tranexamic acid 10 mg/kg body weight by slow intravenous injection.

*Pregnancy:* Thrombolytic therapy with Kabikinase is contraindicated during pregnancy, since there may be increased risk of placental separation.

*Elderly patients:* The incidence of cerebral haemorrhage may be increased in elderly compared with young patients.

*Children:* Not recommended.

**Pharmaceutical precautions** Vials of Kabikinase should be stored below 25°C before reconstitution. The overall reconstituted shelf life is 12 hours. The concentrate should be stored at 2–8°C. Diluted material should be used as soon as possible and not longer than 12 hours after initial reconstitution.

**Legal category** POM.

**Package quantities** Vials containing 750,000 iu streptokinase.

**Further information** Kabikinase is a highly purified streptokinase preparation. It is prepared from beta-haemolytic streptococci culture filtrates. Subsequent purification ensures that Kabikinase is virtually free from streptodornase, streptolysin, hyaluronidase and other enzymes. Kabikinase is soluble in water, is non-toxic and is non-pyrogenic but is weakly antigenic.

Kabikinase is stabilised with sterile human albumin and this imparts a faint straw colour to the preparation.

**Product licence number** 0022/0069.

## KABIKINASE* 1.5 Million IU

**Presentation** Vial of straw coloured lyophilised powder containing 1.5 million iu of streptokinase. Human albumin and buffering agents are present as stabilisers.

### Uses
*Action:* By activating the fibrinolytic system, streptokinase induces dissolution of intravascular thrombi and emboli.

*Indication:* Acute myocardial infarction.

### Dosage and administration
*Recommended dosage for adults:* Streptokinase 1.5 million iu in physiological saline or dextrose 5% is administered as an intravenous infusion, at a constant rate, over 60 minutes.

*Preparation of solution:* Dissolve the contents of the vial by adding 10 ml Water for Injections.

The solution should be prepared at room temperature. Care should be taken to avoid the formation of foam. The concentrated solution thus obtained is transferred aseptically into an infusion bottle or PVC

bag, containing 100 ml of physiological saline, or dextrose 5%.

**Contra-indications, warnings, etc**
*Contra-indications:* Kabikinase should not be administered intramuscularly. Since thrombolytic therapy increases the risk of bleeding, Kabikinase is contraindicated in the following:

*Invasive or traumatic procedures within the previous 10 days* including the following: Surgery; central venous cannulation, or puncture of a non-compressible vessel; external cardiac compression; endotracheal intubation biopsy.

*Defective haemostasis* including: Thrombocytopenia or any other platelet disorder; coagulation disorders (including those caused by hepatic or renal impairment); acute systemic infection, bacteraemia or septicaemia; oral or intravenous anticoagulant therapy (see under *Precautions,* paragraph 2).

*Potential for gastro-intestinal haemorrhage* including: Oesophageal varices; history of peptic ulceration; visceral carcinoma; ulcerative colitis; diverticulitis.

*Increased risk of cerebral haemorrhage/infarction* as evidenced by any of the following: Stroke; cerebral tumour; hypertension (treated or untreated); hypertensive or diabetic retinopathy; transient ischaemic attacks.

*Obstetric or gynaecological conditions likely to predispose to haemorrhage,* including: Menstruation; pregnancy – see also *Pregnancy* section; parturition within the previous 18 weeks.

*Potential for cardiac thromboemboli,* including: Active or recent infective endocarditis; atrial valve disease with atrial fibrillation.

*Increased risk of pulmonary haemorrhage,* including: Active tuberculosis; pneumothorax.

*Previous streptokinase therapy,* more than 5 days and up to 6 months previously, or recent streptococcal infection, since an elevated titre of anti-streptokinase antibody may render the treatment ineffective.

*Coma.*

*Precautions: Patients should not receive streptokinase unless they will be managed within a hospital setting, under expert medical supervision. It is recommended that patients should be treated in a coronary care (or intensive care) unit.*

1. The *diagnosis* of acute myocardial infarction should initially be based upon both clinical signs and ECG evidence. Specific ECG changes diagnostic of recent myocardial infarction should be present. The following diagnoses, which can be associated with ECG changes, and in which administration of thrombolytic therapy might result in life-threatening haemorrhage **MUST** be excluded:

aortic dissection; acute pericarditis; oesophageal rupture; acute abdominal emergencies, including pancreatitis and perforation of the duodenum; intracranial haemorrhage; (see also (2) below).

A chest X-ray should be performed in order to assist in eliminating ruptured oesophagus (pneumomediastinum) or duodenum (air under the diaphragm) and aortic dissection (wide mediastinum). Aortic dissection should be suspected particularly when pain radiates into the back, aortic regurgitation is evident on auscultation or there are absent pulses. Pericarditis should be suspected when ST-segment elevation occurs in all ECG leads. Raised blood amylase is an indication of pancreatitis.

2. Thrombolytic therapy should be considered only in the case of patients for whom a well documented *medical history* is available. It is essential that thrombolytic therapy is not instituted in patients with co-existing medical conditions likely to exacerbate the risk of haemorrhage (e.g. peptic ulceration, history of cerebro-vascular accident, cerebral tumour, visceral carcinoma, see also 'Contra-indications'). Additionally, caution should be exercised in patients who are receiving other drug therapies which are likely to predispose to increased risk of haemorrhagic complications.

3. In most patients, infarction probably is complete within 4–6 hrs and, accordingly, only patients in whom therapy can be iniated within this time interval should be considered for treatment. (But see statement on Q waves below.) *Myocardial salvage* is possible only when recanalisation of the infarct-related artery is effected within a critical time interval following coronary occlusion. The rate of progression of myocardial necrosis is inversely related to the extent of residual perfusion of the ischaemic myocardium. When infarction is due to sub-total coronary occlusion (ca 10–25% of patients) and there is some residual antegrade perfusion, the rate of necrosis is less than when infarction results from complete coronary occlusion. Similarly, in some patients (ca 5–10%) a well developed collateral circulation may retard the progress and reduce the severity of ischaemia. The maximum time delay commensurate with myocardial salvage and reduction in mortality is not known. In patients treated within one hour following symptomatic onset, the risk of death is halved. Generally, the presence of

marked pathological Q waves in the ECG should be considered as evidence that transmural infarction is complete and that appreciable myocardial salvage is not possible.

Conversely, benefit may be derived up to 18 hours following symptoms onset, in patients in whom pathological Q waves are absent, or symptoms are intermittent.

4. *Hypokalaemia* predisposes to ventricular arrhythmias and, if present should be corrected.

5. If *venous access* is considered necessary (e.g. for cardiac pacing) the risk of haemorrhage from central venous cannulation must be considered, and preference should be given to the antecubital route.

6. Thrombolytic therapy with Kabikinase induces a *systemic fibrinolytic state*. The presence of circulating free plasmin results in consumption of fibrinogen and of coagulation factors (predominantly Factors V, VIII and XII). Additionally, circulating degradation products of fibrinogen and fibrin exert an anticoagulant effect. Accordingly thrombolytic therapy increases the risk of haemorrhage both throughout the period of streptokinase infusion, and for approximately 12–24 hours thereafter, i.e. until the serum fibrinogen exceeds 100 mg%.

7. Care should be exercised when moving the patient to avoid trauma-induced haematomas. Unnecessary venepunctures should be avoided.

8. Streptokinase should be used with caution in patients with haemorrhagic retinopathy.

9. *Reperfusion* is usually accompanied by relief of chest pain. Occasionally, reperfusion is preceded by a period of fluctuation in the severity of chest pain. Reperfusion is followed by resolution of the ischaemic ST segment changes. An ECG lead with distinct ST segment elevation should be selected for continuous monitoring, and the initial positions of the ST segment and the peak of the T waves marked. The time of reperfusion may then be recorded. In patients who have sustained minimal necrosis there may be no development of Q waves. However, development of Q waves may not imply complete necrosis, since myocardium subjected to prolonged ischaemia ('stunned myocardium') may take several days to recover.

10. In some patients with inferior wall infarction reperfusion is associated with *vagal reactions*, of nausea, vomiting, sinus bradycardia and hypotension. It has been proposed that these result from the triggering of the Bezold-Jarisch reflex by the restoration of perfusion to the inferior and posterior wall of the left ventricle. These vagal reactions usually respond to intravenous atropine.

11. Accelerated idioventricular rhythm occurs at the time of reperfusion or shortly thereafter in approximately 50–60% of patients. Reperfusion is also associated with ventricular ectopic beats occurring late in diastole. These may be single or may give rise to ventricular bigeminy or trigeminy, or may form fusion beats. These ventricular arrhythmias (frequently referred to as '*reperfusion arrhythmias*') are probably related to increased automaticity. Sustained ventricular tachycardia and ventricular fibrillation are rare, occurring no more commonly than in patients receiving standard management, and should be managed in the normal way.

12. The titre of circulating antistreptokinase antibody rises abruptly at 5–7 days following Kabikinase administration, and may reach levels sufficient to neutralise subsequent Kabikinase dosages administered within the following 6 months.

Accordingly,

a. Information relating to the administration of Kabikinase therapy should be recorded clearly in the patient's notes.

b. Kabikinase therapy should not be repeated within the period of 5 days to 6 months following the initial treatment.

c. Patients with on-going, or recent, streptococcal infections may be resistant to Kabikinase therapy.

13. Subsequent *anticoagulant treatment* with heparin is generally considered necessary in order to prevent rethrombosis in the infarct-related coronary artery, since following thrombolysis, the thrombogenic segment is again exposed to circulating blood, and may again induce thrombosis in the affected artery. Reocclusion occurs in approximately 10–20% of successfully reperfused patients. If anticoagulant treatment is considered appropriate, then heparin should be administered incrementally and judiciously during the first 24 hr following treatment. The partial thromboplastin time should be monitored at regular intervals, and the heparin dosage adjusted to maintain the former within the range 2–2.5 times normal. The optimal duration of anticoagulant therapy is not known. The use of thrombolytic therapy should not necessarily lead to any change in the normal patient management of acute myocardial infarction.

14. Successful thrombolytic therapy will not obviate the requirement for further expert cardiological assessment and patient management.

*Side-effects:* Kabikinase therapy may be accompanied by a slight to moderate pyrexia. Mild allergic reactions such as urticaria are uncommon, particularly when the total duration of infusion is less than 2 hours. Anaphylaxis occurs extremely rarely (ca 0.1%). These reactions may be controlled by the prior intravenous administration of corticosteroids (e.g. hydrocortisone 100 mg, or prednisolone 25 mg). If streptokinase infusion is to be administered for more than 2 hours, or is to be repeated within 6 months, the prior administration of intravenous corticosteroid and/or an antihistamine should be considered, in order to reduce the incidence of allergic reactions.

Streptokinase administration has been associated with low back pain. This may indicate an allergic response and it may be appropriate to discontinue the infusion. In some cases, without other features of allergy, infusion has been continued with analgesic cover, without adverse consequences.

A few allergic reactions such as polyneuropathy and uveitis have been temporally related to the administration of streptokinase. Guillain-Barre Syndrome has been reported after streptokinase treatment.

Haemorrhagic complications largely result from inappropriate anticoagulant therapy, rather than from fibrinolysis *per se*. Haemorrhage can occur in any tissue and organ in the body and can present with symptoms affecting any body system, including the abdomen, cardiovascular system, joints and CNS. Haemorrhage should be considered as a potential cause of unusual symptoms occurring after administration. Minor bleeding, predominantly at puncture sites, occurs with an incidence of approximately 3–4%. Major haemorrhagic episodes requiring transfusion of 2 or more units of blood (gastro-intestinal and retroperitoneal haemorrhage) occur with an incidence of approximately 0.3%. Cerebral haemorrhage and stroke occurs with a frequency of approximately 0.1%. Though there is a theoretical risk of haemorrhagic infarction and haemorrhage into the pericardium, these are extremely rarely encountered. In cases of severe haemorrhage administration of Kabikinase must be discontinued. If necessary, the antifibrinolytic agent Cyklokapron, (tranexamic acid – 10 mg/kg body weight) should be given immediately by slow intravenous injection. Fresh frozen plasma, or preferably cryoprecipitate, should be administered, to correct haemostatic deficiencies.

*Antidote:* Tranexamic acid 10 mg/kg body weight by slow intravenous injection.

*Pregnancy:* Thrombolytic therapy with Kabikinase is contra-indicated during pregnancy, since there may be an increased risk of placental separation.

*Elderly patients:* The incidence of cerebral haemorrhage may be increased in elderly compared with young patients.

*Children:* Not recommended.

**Pharmaceutical precautions** Vials of Kabikinase should be stored below 25°C before reconstitution. The overall reconstituted shelf life is 12 hours. The concentrate should be stored at 2–8°C. Diluted material should be used as soon as possible and not longer than 12 hours after initial reconstitution.

**Legal category:** POM.

**Package quantities** Vials containing 1.5 million iu streptokinase.

**Further information** Kabikinase is a highly purified streptokinase preparation. It is prepared from beta-haemolytic streptococci culture filtrates. Subsequent purification ensures that Kabikinase is virtually free from streptodornase, streptolysin, hyaluronidase and other enzymes. Kabikinase is soluble in water, is non-toxic and is non-pyrogenic, but is weakly antigenic.

Kabikinase is stabilised with sterile human albumin and this imparts a faint straw colour to the preparation.

**Product licence number** 0022/0070.

## KABIMIX* 9

**Qualitative and quantitative composition** 2580 ml of KabiMix 9 contains:

| *Active Ingredients* | *Quantity* |
|---|---|
| Intralipid 20% | 500.00 ml |
| Glucose monohydrate | 165.00 g |
| corresponding to | |
| Glucose (anhydrous) | 150.00 g |
| L-Alanine | 8.00 g |
| L-Arginine | 5.60 g |
| L-Aspartic Acid | 1.70 g |
| L-Cysteine(+ Cystine) | 0.28 g |
| L-Glutamic Acid | 2.80 g |
| Glycine (Aminoacetic Acid) | 4.00 g |
| L-Histidine | 3.40 g |
| L-Isoleucine | 2.80 g |
| L-Leucine | 4.00 g |
| L-Lysine Acetate | |
| corresponding to | 6.30 g |
| L-Lysine | 4.50 g |
| L-Methionine | 2.80 g |
| L-Phenylalanine | 4.00 g |
| L-Proline | 3.40 g |
| L-Serine | 2.20 g |
| L-Threonine | 2.80 g |
| L-Tryptophan | 0.95 g |
| L-Tyrosine | 0.12 g |
| L-Valine | 3.70 g |
| Sodium Glycerophosphate (anhydrous) | 3.24 g |
| Magnesium Chloride $6H_2O$ | 1.02 g |
| corresponding to Magnesium Chloride | 0.48 g |
| Sodium Hydroxide (100%) | 2.00 g |
| Potassium Hydroxide (86.5%) | 3.89 g |
| corresponding to Potassium Hydroxide (100%) | 3.36 g |

*Content per bag (2580 ml)*

| | | |
|---|---|---|
| Triglycerides | | 100.00 g |
| Phospholipids | | 6.00 g |
| Glycerol | | 11.00 g |
| Amino Acids | | 57.00 g |
| Nitrogen | | 9.00 g |
| Glucose | | 150.00 g |
| Energy, non-protein | | 1600 kcal |
| Energy, total | | 1830 kcal |
| Osmolality | | 770 mosm/ kg $H_2O$ |
| pH | | approx 5.6 |
| Electrolytes: | Na | 80 mmol |
| | K | 60 mmol |
| | Ca | 5 mmol |
| | Mg | 5 mmol |
| | P | 28 mmol |
| | Cl | 80 mmol |

**Pharmaceutical form** KabiMix is a sterile mixture for intravenous nutrition containing amino acids, fat emulsion, glucose and electrolytes in a 3 litre EVA (Ethylenevinylacetate) plastic bag.

**Clinical particulars**

*Therapeutic indications:* KabiMix should be used to supply energy, essential fatty acids, essential and non-essential amino acids and electrolytes to patients needing intravenous nutrition. KabiMix 9 is particularly suitable for patients with basal nutritional requirements.

*Posology and method of administration:* The ability to utilise and eliminate fat should govern the dosage and infusion rate. See fat elimination.

*Adults (including the elderly):* The content of one bag KabiMix 9 is infused slowly during 8-24 hours in a peripheral or central vein to patients with basal needs of energy and protein. The infusion time should be at least 8 hours.

*Recommended dosage for children:* For children the product KabiMix 14 (PL 0022/0123) is recommended as the composition is more suited to their nutritional requirements.

*Administration:* KabiMix 9 can be supplemented with trace elements, vitamins and extra electrolytes in certain ranges according to individual patient requirements and following recommendations on compatibility from the manufacturer (see section 6.6). These additions should be made aseptically to the bag before infusion and the admixture should be infused within 24 hours. However, if the additions are made in the hospital pharmacy under laminar air flow, the admixture may be stored for 6 days at 2-8°C before being used. (These 6 days at 2-8°C + 1 day at room temperature must be within the shelf-life (180 days) given for the finished product KabiMix 9. Any admixture remaining after infusion must be discarded.

*Monitoring:* Electrolyte, fluid acid base imbalance and shock should be corrected prior to commencement of intravenous nutrition.

In the metabolic and nutritional management of the seriously ill patient, specific preliminary investigations and continuous monitoring are essential, particularly of electrolyte levels. Monitoring of vitamin and trace element levels should be included, especially in patients receiving long term intravenous nutrition.

*Contra-indications:* KabiMix may be contraindicated in acute shock and severe disturbances in lipid metabolism such as pathological hyperlipemia. Inborn errors of amino acid metabolism. Irreversible liver damage. Severe uremia when dialysis facilities are not available.

*Special warnings and precautions for use:* KabiMix should be given with caution in conditions of impaired lipid metabolism as in renal insufficiency, uncompensated diabetes mellitus, pancreatitis, impaired liver function, hypothyroidism (if hypertriglyceridaemic, and sepsis. If KabiMix is given to patients with these conditions, close monitoring of the serum triglyceride concentration and liver function is required.

Patients known to be allergic to soy protein, should

be given KabiMix with great caution and only after hypersensitivity tests.

KabiMix may interfere with certain laboratory measurements (bilirubin, lactate dehydrogenase, oxygen saturation, haemoglobin etc.) If blood is sampled before fat has been adequately cleared from the bloodstream. Fat is normally cleared after a period of 4-6 hours in most patients.

Intravenous infusion of amino acids is accompanied by increased urinary excretion of the trace elements copper and, in particular zinc. This should be considered particularly during long term intravenous nutrition.

Care should be taken in the administration of amino acids to patients with disturbances in protein metabolism.

As with all infusions, care should be taken to avoid complications of catheterisation including air embolism and central venous thrombosis. Strict asepsis should be maintained especially in the immunosuppressed patient.

Care should be exercised in the administration of large volume infusion fluids to patients with cardiac insufficiency. Potassium replacement therapy should be controlled as plasma potassium levels may not be directly related to tissue levels.

In patients with renal insufficiency, phosphate intake should be carefully controlled to prevent accumulation of phosphate in the circulation.

*Fat elimination*: The ability to eliminate fat should be closely monitored in patients with conditions mentioned under *Special Warnings* but also in patients given Intralipid for more than one week. This is done by collecting a blood sample after a fat clearance period of 4-6 hours. Blood cells are then separated from plasma by centrifugation (1200-1500 rotations per minute, rpm). If the plasma is opalescent the infusion should be postponed. The sensitivity of this method is such that hypertriglyceridaemia can pass undetected. Therefore, it is recommended that serum triglyceride concentrations are measured in patients who are likely to have an impaired fat tolerance.

*Interaction with other medicaments and other forms of interaction*: Amino acid solutions may precipitate acute folate deficiency, and folic acid should be given daily.

*Use during pregnancy and lactation*: Animal reproduction studies have not been performed with KabiMix. There are, however, published reports of the successful and safe administration of its components (Intralipid, glucose, amino acids, and electrolytes) during pregnancy in the human.

*Effects on ability to drive and use machines*: Not applicable.

*Undesirable effects*: Undesirable effects with the components of KabiMix are rare. Those that do occur are usually reversible and regress when therapy is discontinued. The following have been observed. Initial administration of Intralipid has produced a rise in temperature (incidence < 3%), and less frequently shivering, chills and nausea/vomiting (incidence < 1%).

Similar effects have been observed with infusion of amino acids, particularly when the recommended rate of infusion is exceeded.

Increased levels of transaminases, alkaline phosphatase and bilirubin have been observed in patients receiving intravenous nutrition. Cholestasis has also been reported. These changes are reversible and usually return to normal when intravenous nutrition is interrupted.

Hypersensitivity reactions, haemolysis, reticulocytosis, abdominal pain, headache, tiredness and priapism have been reported.

Overdosage: In general, significant overdose with KabiMix is unlikely to occur.

Overdose would arise from fluid overload, with symptoms such as nausea, vomiting, flushing and sweating being observed.

There are no specific antidotes for overdosage. In case of suspicion of overdosage the infusion should be stopped. Emergency procedures should be general supportive measures, respiratory and cardiovascular. Close biochemical monitoring would be essential and specific abnormalities treated appropriately.

**Pharmacological properties**
*Pharmacodynamic properties*: The pharmacodynamic effects of KabiMix are limited due to the nature of the product. No significant effects were observed in cardiovascular parameters in the anaesthetised cat.

*Pharmacokinetic properties*: The pharmacokinetic profile of the components of KabiMix are well known. Intralipid is eliminated from the blood stream by the enzyme lipoprotein lipase (lpl), and after association with apolipoproteins is metabolised in a similar way to chylomicrons. The half-life is approximately 9.00 ± 0.64 minutes, and the clearance mechanism is concentration dependent, with saturation above 1.1 mmol in

blood, which corresponds to a dose of approximately 0.1 g fat/kg/bw. Below this concentration elimination follows first order kinetics. Intralipid as such is not excreted. The metabolites, carbon dioxide, water and phosphate are excreted via lungs, lungs and urine, and urine respectively.

The distribution and metabolism of intravenously infused amino acids are well known. In the body the infused amino acids are subject to metabolic reactions such as protein synthesis and oxidation. Nitrogen may be utilised for synthesis of non-essential amino acids, or eliminated as urea.

Sodium glycerophosphate is hydrolysed completely in plasma. Hydrolysis rate is concentration dependent, with enzyme saturation at increasing glycerophosphate concentration reaching a maximum at plasma concentrations from 0.7 mmol/l. The mean in vitro hydrolysis rate is approximately 0.09 mmol/l/hr.

*Preclinical safety data*: During the preclinical animal studies there were no findings which were of relevance to the prescriber, in relation to the safety profile of KabiMix.

**Pharmaceutical particulars**
*List of excipients*:

| | |
|---|---|
| Hydrochloric Acid | QS |
| Acetic Acid | QS |
| Water for injections to | 2580 ml |
| Helium | QS |

*Incompatibilities*: There are no known incompatibilities with the components of KabiMix. However, additions to KabiMix should be avoided unless compatibility is known.

*Shelf-life*:
*Shelf-life of the product as packaged for sale*: KabiMix is assigned a shelf-life of 180 days when stored at a temperature between 2-8°C. KabiMix is stable for 24 hours after removal from the refrigerator.

**NB**: This day at room temperature must be within the shelf-life of 180 days.

*Shelf-life after dilution or reconstitution according to directions*: Not applicable.

*Shelf-life after first opening the container*: KabiMix should be used immediately after opening. Any remaining solution should be discarded.

*Special precautions for storage*: KabiMix should be stored between 2-8°C. KabiMix is stable at room temperature for 24 hours following removal from the refrigerator.

*Nature and contents of container*: KabiMix is contained in a 3 litre I.V bag made from Ethylenevinylacetate co-polymer (EVA). The bag is overwrapped with aluminium to reduce oxidation of the contents.

In addition helium gas is inserted between the bag and aluminium overwrap.

*Instructions for use/handling*: Admixture Guidelines are available on request from Pharmacia & Upjohn Ltd.

The following additions can be made to KabiMix:

*Limits for additions to KabiMix 9 (per bag)*:

| | Highest possible amount: | |
|---|---|---|
| Addition | Added | Total |
| Vitlipid N Adult* | 10 ml | 10 ml |
| Solivito N* | 1 vial | 1 vial |
| Additrace* | 10 ml | 10 ml |
| Na | 120 mmol | 200 mmol |
| K | 90 mmol | 150 mmol |
| Mg | 4 mmol | 9 mmol |
| Ca | 8 mmol | 13 mmol |
| Phosphate (as Addiphos* or Acidic Phosphate) | 10 mmol (5.0 ml Addiphos) | 38 mmol |

To ensure a homogenous admixture, the bags should be inverted a couple of times immediately before the infusion.

* These products are licensed to Pharmacia Laboratories Limited.

| | |
|---|---|
| Vitlipid N Adult | 0022/0062 |
| Solivito N | 0022/0061 |
| Additrace | 0022/0064 |
| Addiphos | 0022/0050 |

**Marketing authorisation number** 0022/0122

**Date of approval/revision of SPC** November 1992.

**Legal category** POM

## KABIMIX* 14

**Qualitative and quantitative composition** 2580 ml of KabiMix 14 contains:

| Active Ingredients | Quantity |
|---|---|
| Intralipid 20% | 500.00 ml |
| Glucose Monohydrate corresponding to | 330.00 g |
| Glucose (anhydrous) | 300.00 g |
| L-Alanine | 12.00 g |

| | |
|---|---|
| L-Arginine | 8.40 g |
| L-Aspartic Acid | 2.50 g |
| L-Cysteine(+ Cystine) | 0.42 g |
| L-Glutamic Acid | 4.20 g |
| Glycine (Aminoacetic Acid) | 5.90 g |
| L-Histidine | 5.10 g |
| L-Isoleucine | 4.20 g |
| L-Leucine | 5.90 g |
| L-Lysine Acetate corresponding to | 9.50 g |
| L-Lysine | 6.80 g |
| L-Methionine | 4.20 g |
| L-Phenylalanine | 5.90 g |
| L-Proline | 5.10 g |
| L-Serine | 3.40 g |
| L-Threonine | 4.20 g |
| L-Tryptophan | 1.40 g |
| L-Tyrosine | 0.17 g |
| L-Valine | 5.50 g |
| Calcium Glycerophosphate (anhydrous) | 1.05 g |
| Sodium Glycerophosphate (anhydrous) | 3.24 g |
| Magnesium Chloride 6H$_2$0 | 1.02 g |
| corresponding to | |
| Magnesium Chloride | 0.48 g |
| Sodium Hydroxide (100%) | 2.00 g |
| Potassium Hydroxide (86.5%) | 3.89 g |
| corresponding to | |
| Potassium Hydroxide (100%) | 3.36 g |

| Content per bag (2580 ml) | |
|---|---|
| Triglycerides | 100.00 g |
| Phospholipids | 6.00 g |
| Glycerol | 11.00 g |
| Amino Acids | 85.30 g |
| Nitrogen | 13.50 g |
| Glucose | 300.00 g |
| Energy, non-protein | 2200 kcal |
| Energy, total | 2550 kcal |
| Osmolality | 1330 mosm/kg water |
| pH | approx 5.6 |
| Electrolytes: | Na |

| | | |
|---|---|---|
| | Na | 80 mmol |
| | K | 60 mmol |
| | Ca | 5 mmol |
| | Mg | 5 mmol |
| | P | 28 mmol |
| | Cl | 80 mmol |

**Pharmaceutical form** KabiMix is a sterile mixture for intravenous nutrition containing amino acids, fat emulsion, glucose and electrolytes in a 3 litre EVA (Ethylenevinylacetate) plastic bag.

**Clinical particulars**
*Therapeutic indications*: KabiMix should be used to supply energy, essential fatty acids, essential and non-essential amino acids and electrolytes to patients needing intravenous nutrition. KabiMix 14 is particularly suitable for patients with moderately increased nutritional requirements.

*Posology and method of administration*: The ability to utilise and eliminate fat should govern the dosage and infusion rate. See fat elimination.

*Adults (including the elderly)*: The content of one bag KabiMix 14 is infused slowly during 8-24 hours in a **central vein** to patients with moderately increased needs of energy and protein. The infusion time should be at least 8 hours.

*Recommended dosage for children*:

| Age (years) | Dose (ml/kg) |
|---|---|
| 1-6 | 50-70 |
| 6-12 | 50-60 |
| 12-18 | 30-40 |

*Administration*: KabiMix 14 can be supplemented with trace elements, vitamins and extra electrolytes in certain ranges according to individual patient requirements and following recommendations on compatibility from the manufacturer (see section 6.6). These additions should be made aseptically to the bag before infusion and the admixture should be infused within 24 hours. However, if the additions are made in the hospital pharmacy under laminar air flow, the admixture may be stored for 6 days at 2-8°C before being used. (These 6 days at 2-8°C + 1 day at room temperature must be within the shelf-life (180 days) given for the finished product KabiMix 14. Any admixture remaining after infusion must be discarded.

*Monitoring*: Electrolyte, fluid acid base imbalance and shock should be corrected prior to commencement of intravenous nutrition.

In the metabolic and nutritional management of the seriously ill patient, specific preliminary investigations and continuous monitoring are essential, particularly of electrolyte levels. Monitoring of vitamin and trace element levels should be included, especially in patients receiving long term intravenous nutrition.

*Contraindications*: KabiMix may be contraindicated in acute shock and severe disturbances in lipid metabolism such as pathological hyperlipemia. Inborn errors of amino acid metabolism. Irreversible liver damage. Severe uremia when dialysis facilities are not available.

*Special warnings and precautions for use:* KabiMix should be given with caution in conditions of impaired lipid metabolism as in renal insufficiency, uncompensated diabetes mellitus, pancreatitis, impaired liver function, hypothyroidism (if hypertriglyceridaemic) and sepsis. If KabiMix is given to patients with these conditions, close monitoring of the serum triglyceride concentration and liver function is required

Patients known to be allergic to soy protein, should be given KabiMix with great caution and only after hypersensitivity tests.

KabiMix may interfere with certain laboratory measurements (bilirubin, lactate dehydrogenase, oxygen saturation, haemoglobin etc.) If blood is sampled before fat has been adequately cleared from the bloodstream. Fat is normally cleared after a period of 4-6 hours in most patients.

Intravenous infusion of amino acids is accompanied by increased urinary excretion of the trace elements copper and, in particular zinc. This should be considered particularly during long term intravenous nutrition.

Care should be taken in the administration of amino acids to patients with disturbances in protein metabolism.

As with all infusions, care should be taken to avoid complications of catheterisation including air embolism and central venous thrombosis. Strict asepsis should be maintained especially in the immunosuppressed patient.

Care should be exercised in the administration of large volume infusion fluids to patients with cardiac insufficiency.

Potassium replacement therapy should be controlled as plasma potassium levels may not be directly related to tissue levels.

In patients with renal insufficiency, phosphate intake should be carefully controlled to prevent accumulation of phosphate in the circulation.

*Fat elimination:* The ability to eliminate fat should be closely monitored in patients with conditions mentioned under special warnings but also in patients given Intralipid for more than one week. This is done by collecting a blood sample after a fat clearance period of 4-6 hours. Blood cells are then separated from plasma by centrifugation (1200-1500 rotations per minute, rpm). If the plasma is opalescent the infusion should be postponed. The sensitivity of this method is such that hypertriglyceridaemia can pass undetected. Therefore, it is recommended that serum triglyceride concentrations are measured in patients who are likely to have an impaired fat tolerance.

*Interaction with other medicaments and other forms of interaction:* Amino acid solutions may precipitate acute folate deficiency, and folic acid should be given daily.

*Use during pregnancy and lactation:* Animal reproduction studies have not been performed with KabiMix. There are, however, published reports of the successful and safe administration of its components (Intralipid, glucose, amino acids, and electrolytes) during pregnancy in the human.

*Effects on ability to drive and use machines:* Not applicable.

*Undesirable effects:* Undesirable effects with the components of KabiMix are rare. Those that do occur are usually reversible and regress when therapy is discontinued. The following have been observed. Initial administration of Intralipid has produced a rise in temperature (incidence < 3%), and less frequently shivering, chills and nausea/vomiting (incidence < 1%).

Similar effects have been observed with infusion of amino acids, particularly when the recommended rate of infusion is exceeded.

Increased levels of transaminases, alkaline phosphatase and bilirubin have been observed in patients receiving intravenous nutrition. Cholestasis has also been reported. These changes are reversible and usually return to normal when intravenous nutrition is interrupted.

Hypersensitivity reactions, haemolysis, reticulocytosis, abdominal pain, headache, tiredness and priapism have been reported.

*Overdosage:* In general, significant overdose with KabiMix is unlikely to occur.

Overdose would arise from fluid overload, with symptoms such as nausea, vomiting, flushing and sweating being observed.

There are no specific antidotes for overdosage. In case of suspicion of overdosage the infusion should be stopped. Emergency procedures should be general supportive measures, respiratory and cardiovascular. Close biochemical monitoring would be essential and specific abnormalities treated appropriately.

**Pharmacological properties**

*Pharmacodynamic properties:* The pharmacodynamic effects of KabiMix are limited due to the nature of the product. No significant effects were observed in cardiovascular parameters in the anaesthetised cat.

*Pharmacokinetic properties:* The pharmacokinetic profile of the components of KabiMix are well known. Intralipid is eliminated from the blood stream by the enzyme lipoprotein lipase (lpl), and after association with apolipoproteins is metabolised in a similar way to chylomicrons. The half-life is approximately 9.00 ± 0.64 minutes, and the clearance mechanism is concentration dependent, with saturation above 1.1 mmol in blood, which corresponds to a dose of approximately 0.1 g fat/kg/bw. Below this concentration elimination follows first order kinetics. Intralipid as such is not excreted. The metabolites, carbon dioxide, water and phosphate are excreted via lungs, lungs and urine, and urine respectively.

The distribution and metabolism of intravenously infused amino acids are well known. In the body the infused amino acids are subject to metabolic reactions such as protein synthesis and oxidation.

Nitrogen may be utilised for synthesis of non-essential amino acids, or eliminated as urea.

Sodium glycerophosphate is hydrolysed completely in plasma. Hydrolysis rate is concentration dependent, with enzyme saturation at increasing glycerophosphate concentration reaching a maximum at plasma concentrations from 0.7 mmol/l. The mean in vitro hydrolysis rate is approximately 0.09 mmol/l/hr.

*Preclinical safety data:* During the preclinical animal studies there were no findings which were of relevance to the prescriber, in relation to the safety profile of KabiMix.

**Pharmaceutical particulars**

*List of excipients:*

| | |
|---|---|
| Hydrochloric Acid | QS |
| Acetic Acid | QS |
| Water for injections to | 2580 ml |
| Helium | QS |

*Incompatibilities:* There are no known incompatibilities with the components of KabiMix. However, additions to KabiMix should be avoided unless compatibility is known.

*Shelf-life:*

*Shelf-life of the product as packaged for sale:* KabiMix is assigned a shelf-life of 180 days when stored at a temperature between 2-8°C. KabiMix is stable for 24 hours after removal from the refrigerator.

NB: This day at room temperature must be within the shelf-life of 180 days.

*Shelf-life after dilution or reconstitution according to directions:* Not applicable.

*Shelf-life after first opening the container:* KabiMix should be used immediately after opening. Any remaining solution should be discarded.

*Special precautions for storage:* KabiMix should be stored between 2-8°C. KabiMix is stable at room temperature for 24 hours following removal from the refrigerator.

*Nature and contents of container:* KabiMix is contained in a 3 litre I.V bag made from Ethylenevinylacetate co-polymer (EVA). The bag is overwrapped with aluminium to reduce oxidation of the contents.

In addition helium gas is inserted between the bag and aluminium overwrap.

*Instructions for use/handling:* Admixture Guidelines are available on request from Pharmacia & Upjohn Ltd.

The following additions can be made to KabiMix:

*Limits for additions to KabiMix 14 (per bag):*

| *Addition* | Highest possible amount *Added* | *Total* |
|---|---|---|
| Vitlipid N Adult* | 10 ml | 10 ml |
| Solivito N* | 1 vial | 1 vial |
| Additrace* | 10 ml | 10 ml |
| Na | 120 mmol | 200 mmol |
| K | 90 mmol | 150 mmol |
| Mg | 4 mmol | 9 mmol |
| Ca | 8 mmol | 13 mmol |
| Phosphate (as Addiphos* or acidic phosphate) | 10 mmol (5.0 ml addiphos) | 38 mmol |

To ensure a homogenous admixture, the bags should be inverted a couple of times immediately before the infusion.

* These products are licensed to Pharmacia Laboratories Limited.

| | |
|---|---|
| Vitlipid N Adult | 0022/0062 |
| Solivito N | 0022/0061 |
| Additrace | 0022/0064 |
| Addiphos | 0022/0050 |

**Marketing authorisation number** 0022/0123

**Date of approval/revision of SPC** November 1992

**Legal category** POM

## KAOPECTATE* SUSPENSION

**Qualitative and quantitative composition** Each 5 ml contains 1.03 g light kaolin BP.

**Pharmaceutical form** Suspension for oral administration.

**Clinical particulars**

*Therapeutic indications:* Anti-diarrhoeal. Diarrhoea of non-specific origin.

*Posology and method of administration*

*Adults:* 10 –30 ml every 4 hours.

*Elderly:* There is no information to suggest that change in dosage is warranted in the elderly. Side-effects do not appear to be more common or severe in elderly patients.

*Children:* Children up to 1 year of age : 5 ml every 4 hours

*Children 1–5 years of age*: 10 ml every 4 hours

*Contra-indications:* Intestinal obstruction

*Special warnings and special precautions for use:*

*Special warnings:* The label on the Kaopectate 180 ml (OTC) pack will state: 'If no improvement within 48 hours consult your doctor'.

*Special precautions for use:* None.

*Interaction with other medicaments and other forms of interaction:* The absorption of other drugs from the gastro-intestinal tract may be reduced if given concomitantly. Other medicines should be taken either one to two hours before or after Kaopectate.

*Pregnancy and lactation:* No restrictions.

*Effects on ability to drive and use machines:* None stated

*Undesirable effects:* None stated.

*Overdose:* The possibility of intestinal obstruction should be investigated.

**Pharmacological properties**

*Pharmacodynamic properties:* Kaolin is a natural hydrated aluminium silicate which absorbs toxic and other substances from the alimentary tract, increases the bulk of faeces and reduces water loss.

*Pharmacokinetic properties:* Kaolin is not absorbed from the gastro-intestinal tract.

**Pharmaceutical particulars**

*List of excipients:* Sorbic acid; methylparaben; saccharin sodium granular; citric acid; pectin pure citrus; product no. 167 contains: vanilla extract, ethyl alcohol, oleoresin vanilla, glycerin, peppermint oil, bentonite powder, purified water, sodium citrate, citric acid.

*Incompatibilities:* None stated

*Shelf life:* 60 months

*Special precautions for storage:* Use within three months of opening the bottle

*Nature and contents of container:* Polyethylene bottle with tamper-evident polyethylene screw cap 180 ml–OTC pack.

*Instructions for use/handling:* No special instructions.

**Marketing authorisation number** 0032/5040R

**Date of approval/revision of SPC** February 1997

**Legal category** GSL

## KELFIZINE W*

**Presentation** White, uncoated tablets each containing sulfametopyrazine 2 g stamped 'Kelfizine W' obverse, and 'Weekly Dose' reverse.

**Uses** The treatment of infections due to sulphonamide-sensitive organisms. Kelfizine W is recommended in the management of chronic bronchitis (including prophylaxis), it is also indicated for use in urinary tract infections.

**Dosage and administration**

*Adults:* 2 g once weekly by mouth.

*Children:* Not recommended.

*Elderly:* As hepatic conjugation and renal clearance occur at a reduced rate in the elderly, caution is advised when prescribing the drug for long periods of time, to avoid accumulation.

The tablet should be stirred into half a tumblerful o water or orange squash.

**Contra-indications, warnings, etc**

*Contra-indications:* Not to be taken by persons sensi tive to sulphonamides.

*Warnings:* Occasionally severe reactions such as erythema multiforme and the Stevens–Johnson syn drome, epidermal necrolysis, eosinophilia, agranulo cytosis, granulocytopenia, purpura and leucopenia have been reported in patients treated with sulphonamides.

Sulphonamides, and thus sulfametopyrazine, may potentiate the effects of coumarin derivatives, some oral antidiabetic agents (sulphonylureas) and some diaminopyrimidine derivatives (trimethoprim, pyrimethamine). Paraminobenzoic acid can antagonize the antibacterial activity of sulfametopyrazine.

*Adverse reactions:* Other side-effects reported with the use of sulphonamides include nausea, vomiting and rashes: these are usually mild and transient with Kelfizine W.

*Precautions:* Sulfametopyrazine should be used with caution in patients with renal or hepatic dysfunction, dehydration, or blood dyscrasias.

*Use in pregnancy and lactation:* There is no evidence of the drug's safety in human pregnancy nor is there evidence from animal work that it is free from hazard. Kelfizine W is contra-indicated during the third trimester of pregnancy and during breast-feeding.

*Overdosage:* Doses up to 8 g have been taken over 36 hours without evidence of ill effects. To increase excretion a high fluid intake should be maintained for seven days and the urine rendered alkaline with Potassium Citrate mixture BP or sodium bicarbonate. The sulphonamide will then be retained in the urine in higher concentrations in the form of the alkali metal salt.

**Legal category** POM.

**Package quantities** Pack of 5 tablets individually foil wrapped.

**Further information** Sulfametopyrazine has a long half-life. This is due not to a high degree of serum protein binding (which is only 60%) but to a high degree of renal tubular re-absorption coupled with a low rate of hepatic metabolism of the drug.

**Product licence number** 3433/5916R.

## KEMICETINE* SUCCINATE

**Presentation** Individual glass vials of chloramphenicol sodium succinate for injection containing the equivalent of 1 g of chloramphenicol.

**Uses** Kemicetine (chloramphenicol) is a broad-spectrum antibiotic and is active against many gram-positive and gram-negative organisms, spirillae and rickettsia. Kemicetine should not be used for trivial infections due to the possibility of severe blood dyscrasias, which may prove fatal.

Kemicetine succinate is indicated for typhoid, meningitis caused by *H. influenzae* infections and other serious infections. It is also indicated wherever chloramphenicol is deemed the antibiotic of choice and oral administration is not possible, or higher than usual blood concentrations are required.

**Dosage and administration**

In order to ensure rapid attainment of high blood levels, Kemicetine succinate is best administered by i.v. injection. Where this is not possible, however, intramuscular administration may be used, although it should be borne in mind that absorption may be slow and unpredictable.

The injection should be reconstituted with Water for Injections, Sodium Chloride Injection, or Dextrose Injection 5%. The following dilution table may be useful for the administration of a proportion of the contents of a vial:

| Concentration | Solution strength | Volume of diluent to be added | Total volume after dilution |
|---|---|---|---|
| 40% | 400 mg/ml | 1.7 ml | 2.5 ml |
| 25% | 250 mg/ml | 3.2 ml | 4.0 ml |
| 20% | 200 mg/ml | 4.2 ml | 5.0 ml |
| 10% | 100 mg/ml | 9.2 ml | 10.0 ml |

The dose administered and the concentration used is dependent on the severity of the infection. The recommended standard dosage is as follows:

*Adults:* The equivalent of 1 g chloramphenicol every 6–8 hours.

*Children:* The equivalent of 50 mg/kg chloramphenicol, according to body weight, daily in divided doses every 6 hours (this dose should not be exceeded). The patient should be carefully observed for signs of toxicity.

*Elderly:* The usual adult dosage should be given subject to normal hepatic and renal function.

*Neonates and premature infants:* 25 mg/kg in divided doses.

Certain infections, such as meningitis or septicaemia, may require substantially higher doses.

The 10% solution should be given by intravenous injection over a period of about a minute, or in a larger volume of fluid, by slow intravenous infusion.

The concurrent administration of i.v. Kemicetine succinate with topical treatment has been found to be very effective in the treatment of osteomyelitic foci, abscesses, empyema and skin and urinary infections.

**Contra-indications, warnings, etc** Kemicetine succinate is contra-indicated in patients with a previous history of sensitivity and/or toxic reaction to chloramphenicol. It is also contra-indicated in pregnancy and whilst breast feeding. Kemicetine is to be administered only under the direction of a medical practitioner. Chloramphenicol may cause severe bone marrow depression which may lead to agranulocytosis, thrombocytopenic purpura or aplastic anaemia. These effects on the haemopoietic system are usually associated with a high dose, prolonged administration, or repeated courses, but they may occur at relatively low doses. Chloramphenicol should not be used in the treatment of any infection for which a less toxic antibiotic is available. It is also advisable to perform blood tests in the case of prolonged or repeated administration. Evidence of any detrimental effect on blood elements is an indication to discontinue therapy immediately.

Other adverse reactions which may become apparent after chloramphenicol treatment are: dryness of the mouth, nausea and vomiting, diarrhoea, urticaria, optic neuritis with blurring or temporary loss of vision, peripheral neuritis, headache and depression. Superinfection by fungi, e.g. *C. albicans* in the gastrointestinal tract, or vagina, may also occur due to the disturbance of normal bacterial flora.

Chloramphenicol has been shown to interact with, and enhance the effects of, coumarin anticoagulants, some hypoglycaemic agents (e.g. tolbutamide) and phenytoin. When given concurrently, a dose reduction of these agents may, therefore, be necessary. Plasma concentrations of chloramphenicol may be reduced with concomitant usage of phenobarbitone and rifampicin. Chloramphenicol may also impede the development of immunity and should therefore not be given during active immunisation.

The drug should be used with great caution in patients with impairment of hepatic or renal function. The dosage should be reduced in these patients. 'The Grey Syndrome' may occur after administration, in patients with immature hepatic metabolic capacity, i.e. infants and neonates, usually in those treated with doses substantially in excess of those recommended.

Because of its toxic nature, it is important to monitor serum levels of this antibiotic particularly in newborn and premature infants, in the elderly, in patients with renal or hepatic disease and in those receiving other drugs with which chloramphenicol may interact.

*Overdosage:* General supportive therapy should be given.

**Pharmaceutical precautions** Any Kemicetine succinate solution remaining in the vial after use should be discarded, as chloramphenicol sodium succinate is not bactericidal or bacteriostatic.

**Legal category** POM.

**Package quantities** Cartons containing 25 individual vials.

**Further information** Nil.

**Product licence number** 3433/5903R.

## LONITEN* TABLETS 2.5 mg, 5 mg, and 10 mg

**Qualitative and quantitiative composition** Each Loniten Tablet contains 2.5 mg, 5 mg or 10 mg Minoxidil USP.

**Pharmaceutical form:** Tablet

**Clinical particulars**

*Therapeutic indications:* Loniten is indicated for the treatment of severe hypertension.

It should not be used as the sole agent to initiate therapy. It is a peripheral vasodilator and should be given in conjunction with a diuretic, to control salt and water retention and a beta-adrenergic blocking agent or appropriate substitute, to control reflex tachycardia.

*Posology and method of administration:* Oral administration

*Adults and patients over 12 years of age:* An initial daily dose of 5 mg, which may be given as a single or divided dosage, is recommended. This dose may first be increased to 10 mg daily and subsequent increases should be by increments of 10 mg in the daily dose. Dosage adjustments should be made at intervals of not less than three days, until optimum control of blood pressure is achieved. It is seldom necessary to exceed 50 mg per day although, in exceptional circumstances, doses up to 100 mg per day have been used.

Twice-daily dosage is satisfactory. Where diastolic pressure reduction of less than 30 mm Hg is required, once daily dosing has been reported as effective.

Dosage requirements may be lower in dialysis patients. Minoxidil is removed from the blood by dialysis, but its pharmacological action, once established is not reversed. Therefore, haemodialysis patients should take Loniten either after or at least two hours before dialysis.

*Children:* For patients of 12 years of age or under, the initial dose should be 200 micrograms per kilogram (0.2 mg/kg) given as a single or divided daily dosage. Incremental increases of 100 – 200 micrograms per kilogram (0.1–0.2 mg/kg) in the daily dose are recommended at intervals of not less than three days until optimum blood pressure control has been achieved, or the maximum daily dose of 1.0 mg/kg has been reached.

*Rapid reduction of blood pressure:* Under hospital monitoring conditions, rapid reduction of blood pressure can be achieved using continuous blood pressure monitoring and incremental doses of 5 mg every six hours.

*Concomitant antihypertensive therapy:* It is recommended that, where possible, antihypertensive therapy, other than a beta-adrenergic blocking agent and a diuretic be discontinued before Loniten treatment is started. It is recognised that some antihypertensive agents should not be abruptly discontinued. These drugs should be gradually discontinued during the first week of Loniten treatment.

Loniten causes sodium retention and, if used alone, can result in several hundred milli-equivalents of salt being retained together with a corresponding volume of water.

Therefore, in all patients who are not on dialysis, Loniten must be given in conjunction with a diuretic in sufficient dosage to maintain salt and water balance. Examples of the daily dosages of diuretics commonly used when starting therapy with Loniten include: hydrochlorothiazide (100 mg) or other thiazides at equi-effective dosage; chlorthalidone (100 mg); frusemide (80 mg).

If excessive water retention results in a weight gain of more than 3 pounds when a thiazide or chlorthalidone is being used, diuretic therapy should be changed to frusemide, the dose of which may be increased in accordance with the patient's requirements. Diuretic dosage in children should be proportionally less in relation to weight.

Patients will require a sympathetic nervous system suppressant to limit a Loniten-induced rise in heart rate. The preferred agent is a beta-blocker equivalent to an adult propranolol dosage of 80–160 mg/day. Higher doses may be required when pre-treated patients have an increase in heart rate exceeding 20 beats per minute or when simultaneous introduction causes an increase exceeding 10 beats per minute. When beta-blockers are contra-indicated, alternatives such as methyldopa may be used instead and should be started 24 hours prior to Loniten.

*Elderly patients:* At present there are no extensive clinical studies with minoxidil in patients over age 65. There is data indicating that elevated systolic and diastolic pressures are important risk factors for cardiovascular disease in individuals over age 65. However, elderly patients may be sensitive to the blood pressure lowering effect of minoxidil and thus caution is urged in initiating therapy as orthostatic hypotension may occur. It is suggested that 2.5 mg per day be used as the initial starting dose in patients over 65 years of age.

*Contra-indications:* Loniten is contra-indicated in patients with a phaeochromocytoma.

*Special warnings and special precautions for use:* If used alone, Loniten can cause a significant retention of salt and water leading to positive physical signs such as oedema and to clinical deterioration of some patients with heart failure. Diuretic treatment alone or in combination with restricted salt intake is, therefore, necessary for all patients taking Loniten.

Patients who have had myocardial infarction should only be treated with Loniten after a stable post-infarction state has been established.

The physician should bear in mind that if not controlled by sympathetic suppressants, the rise in cardiac rate and output that follows the use of potent vasodilators may induce anginal symptoms in patients with undiagnosed coronary artery disease or may aggravate pre-existing angina pectoris.

The effect of Loniten may be additive to concurrent antihypertensive agents. The interaction of Loniten with sympathetic-blocking agents such as guanethidine or bethanidine may produce excessive blood pressure reduction and/or orthostasis.

Hypertrichosis occurs in most patients treated with Loniten and all patients should be warned of this possibility before starting therapy. Spontaneous reversal to the pre-treatment state can be expected one to three months after cessation of therapy.

Soon after starting Loniten therapy approximately 60% of patients exhibit ECG alterations in the direction and magnitude of their T waves. Large changes may encroach on the ST segment, unaccompanied by evidence of ischaemia. These asymptomatic changes usually disappear with continuing Loniten treatment. The ECG reverts to the pre-treatment state if Loniten is discontinued.

Pericardial effusion has been detected in patients treated with a Loniten-containing regime. A cause and effect relationship has not been established. Most effusions have either been present before Loniten was given or occurred among uraemic patients. However, it is suggested that Loniten-treated patients should be periodically monitored for signs or symptoms of pericardial effusion and appropriate therapy instituted if necessary.

Salt and water retention in excess of 2 to 3 pounds may diminish the effectiveness of Loniten. Patients should, therefore, be carefully instructed about compliance with diuretic therapy and a detailed record of body weight should be maintained.

*Interaction with other medicaments and other forms of interaction:* The effect of Loniten may be additive to concurrent antihypertensive agents. The interaction of Loniten with sympathetic-blocking agents such as guanethidine or bethanidine may produce excessive blood pressure reduction and/or orthostasis.

*Pregnancy and lactation:* The safety of Loniten in pregnancy remains to be established. Minoxidil has been shown to reduce the conception rate in rats and to show evidence of increased fetal absorption in rabbits. There was no evidence of teratogenic effects in rats and rabbits. Minoxidil has been reported to be secreted in breast milk. Therefore, breast-feeding should not be undertaken while a patient is on Loniten Tablets.

*Effects on ability to drive and use machines:* No adverse effects reported.

*Undesirable effects:* Most patients receiving Loniten experience a diminution of pre-existing side-effects attributable to their disease or previous therapy. New events or side-effects likely to increase include peripheral oedema, associated with or independent of weight gain; increases in heart rate; hypertrichosis; and a temporary rise in creatinine and blood urea nitrogen. Gastro-intestinal intolerance, rash and breast tenderness are infrequently reported side-effects of Loniten therapy.

*Overdose:* If exaggerated hypotension is encountered, it is most likely to occur in association with residual sympathetic nervous system blockade (guanethidine-like effects or alpha-adrenergic blockade). Recommended treatment is intravenous administration of normal saline. Sympathomimetic drugs, such as noradrenaline or adrenaline, should be avoided because of their excessive cardiac-stimulating action. Phenylephrine, angiotensin II and vasopressin, which reverse the effect of Loniten, should be used only if inadequate perfusion of a vital organ is evident.

**Pharmacological properties**

*Pharmacodynamic properties:* Minoxidil is an antihypertensive agent which acts predominantly by causing direct peripheral vasodilation of the arterioles.

*Pharmacokinetic properties:* About 90% of an oral dose of minoxidil has been reported to be absorbed from the GI tract.

Following oral administration the maximum hypotensive effect usually occurs after 2–3 hours. The action may persist for up to 75 hours. The plasma half life is about 4.2 hours.

Minoxidil is not bound to plasma proteins. It is extensively metabolised in the liver primarily by conjugation with glucuronic acid and is excreted in the urine mainly in the form of metabolites.

**Pharmaceutical particulars**

*List of excipients:* Lactose hydrous, microcrystalline cellulose, starch, colloidal silicon dioxide and magnesium stearate.

*Incompatibilities:* None

*Shelf-life:* Shelf-life of the medicinal product as packaged for sale: 36 months.

*Special precautions for storage:* Store below 25°C.

*Nature and contents of container:* High density polyethylene (HDPE) bottles with LDPE caps. Each bottle contains 100 tablets.

20–25 micron aluminium foil/250 micron opaque pvc blister. Pack contains 60 tablets.

*Instructions for use/handling:* No special requirements.

**Marketing authorisation numbers**

| | |
|---|---|
| 2.5 mg | 0032/0064 |
| 5 mg | 0032/0065 |
| 10 mg | 0032/0066 |

**Date of approval/revision of SPC** March 1995

**Legal category** POM

## MAXTREX*

**Presentation** *Maxtrex tablets:* Round, uncoated, convex tablets diameter 6 mm, containing 2.5 mg (pale yellow tablets marked 'M2.5') and 10 mg (deep yellow tablets marked 'M10' on one side and scored on the other) methotrexate.

**Uses** Methotrexate is a folic acid antagonist and is classified as an antimetabolite cytotoxic agent.

Methotrexate has been used to produce regression in a wide range of neoplastic conditions including acute leukaemias, non-Hodgkin's lymphoma, soft-tissue and osteogenic sarcomas, and solid tumours particularly breast, lung, head and neck, bladder, cervical, ovarian, and testicular carcinoma.

Methotrexate has also been used in the treatment of severe, uncontrolled psoriasis which is not responsive to other therapy.

**Dosage and administration** Single doses, not exceeding 30 mg/m², on not more than 5 successive days. A rest period of at least two weeks is recommended between treatments, in order to allow the bone marrow to return to normal.

Methotrexate has been used both alone and in combination chemotherapy with radiotherapy and surgery. Dosage regimens may therefore vary considerably. Leucovorin rescue regimens are discussed briefly under 'Further information'.

If methotrexate is administered in combination chemotherapy regimens, the dosage should be reduced, taking into consideration any overlapping toxicity of the other drug components.

*Dosage for psoriasis:* For the treatment of severe psoriasis 10–25 mg orally, once weekly, is recommended. Dosage should be adjusted according to the patient's response and the haematological toxicity.

**Contra-indications, warnings, etc** Maxtrex is usually intended for use under the direction of those experienced in cytotoxic therapy.

*Contra-indications:* Methotrexate is contra-indicated in the presence of severe renal or hepatic impairment and serious anaemia, leucopenia or thrombocytopenia.

*Warnings:* Methotrexate should be used with extreme caution in patients with haematological depression, renal impairment, diarrhoea, ulcerative disorders of the G.I. tract and psychiatric disorders and in the elderly and very young. Hepatic toxicity has been observed. Renal lesions may develop if the urinary flow is impeded and urinary pH is low, especially if large doses have been administered.

The administration of low doses of methotrexate for prolonged periods may give rise, in particular, to hepatic toxicity. Liver function tests should be periodically carried out and abnormalities are an indication for discontinuing treatment for at least a period of 2 weeks.

Particular care and possible cessation of treatment are indicated if stomatitis or G.I. toxicity occurs as haemorrhagic enteritis and intestinal perforation may result.

After intrathecal administration, leucoencephalopathies have been observed, especially with concomitant cerebral radiotherapy.

Reversible eosinophilic pulmonary reactions and treatment-resistant, interstitial fibrosis may occur, particularly after long-term treatment.

Methotrexate is teratogenic and should not ordinarily be administered to patients who are pregnant or to mothers who are breast-feeding. The drug affects spermatogenesis and oogenesis and may therefore decrease fertility. The effect appears to be reversible after discontinuation of therapy. Conception should be prevented for at least 6 months after administration has ceased.

There are isolated reports in the literature of tumours occurring in patients following treatment with methotrexate, and in some studies in animals. However controlled animal studies and human epidemiological surveys have not demonstrated carcinogenicity. Nevertheless, the possibility of such an effect should be borne in mind when designing long-term management.

Methotrexate is immunosuppressive and may therefore reduce immunological response to concurrent vaccination. Severe antigenic reactions may occur if a live vaccine is given concurrently.

*Precautions:* Before, during and after treatment with methotrexate a complete haematological analysis should be performed, together with renal and hepatic function tests. Haemopoietic depression may occur suddenly even with low doses. A severe reduction of any blood element requires immediate cessation of treatment and suitable supportive measures such as blood transfusion and reverse barrier nursing. During therapy urine should be kept alkaline, if necessary, by giving oral or i.v. sodium bicarbonate, to prevent crystal deposition.

The disappearance of methotrexate from plasma should be monitored, if possible. This is recommended in particular when high, or very high doses are administered, in order to permit calculation of an adequate dose of leucovorin rescue (see under *Further information*).

Radiotherapy to the CNS should not be given concomitantly with intrathecally administered methotrexate.

After intrathecal administration the drug is transported into the general circulation and may therefore still give rise to systemic toxicity, particularly myelosuppression.

*Drug interactions:* Methotrexate is extensively protein bound and may displace, or be displaced by, other acidic drugs. The concurrent administration of agents such as aminobenzoic acid, chloramphenicol, phenytoin, propionic acid anti-inflammatory agents, salicylates, sulphonamides, tetracyclines, thiazide diuretics, probenecid or sulphinpyrazone will decrease the methotrexate transport function of renal tubules, thereby reducing excretion and almost certainly increasing methotrexate toxicity.

*Side-effects:* Common side-effects are leucopenia and thrombocytopenia (which are usually reversible), nausea and vomiting, diarrhoea and stomatitis. Other side-effects include G.I. ulceration, alopecia, erythematous skin reactions and suppression of ovarian and testicular function.

Megaloblastic anaemia has been reported. Renal and hepatic damage may occur, particularly after high doses or prolonged administration, respectively. Reversible, eosinophilic pulmonary reactions and treatment-resistant interstitial fibrosis have been recorded.

CNS side-effects that may follow intrathecal or intraventricular use are headache, drowsiness, blurred vision, ataxia and, rarely, dementia and convulsions.

*Overdosage:* Leucovorin is a specific antidote for methotrexate and, following accidental overdosage, should be administered within one hour at a dosage equal to, or greater than, the methotrexate dose. It may be administered by i.v. bolus or infusion. Further doses may be required. The patient should be observed carefully and blood transfusions, renal dialysis and reverse barrier nursing may be necessary.

**Pharmaceutical precautions** Maxtrex should be stored at room temperature protected from light.

**Legal category** POM.

**Package quantities**

| | |
|---|---|
| Maxtrex 2.5 tablets: | Bottles of 100 tablets. |
| Maxtrex 10 tablets: | Bottles of 100 tablets. |

**Further information** Methotrexate is a folic acid antagonist and its major site of action is the enzyme dihydrofolate reductase. Its main effect is inhibition of DNA synthesis, but it also acts directly both on RNA and protein synthesis. Methotrexate is a phase specific substance, the main effect being directed during the S-phase of cell division.

The inhibition of dihydrofolate reductase can be circumvented by the use of leucovorin (folinic acid; citrovorum factor) and protection of normal tissues can be carried out by properly timed administration of leucovorin calcium. Dosage regimens for leucovorin rescue vary, depending on the dose of methotrexate administered. Up to 120 mg are generally given (as the calcium salt), usually in divided doses over 12–24 hours, by i.m., or i.v. bolus, or intravenous infusion in normal saline. This is followed by 12–15 mg i.m. or 15 mg orally every 6 hours for 48 hours.

**Product licence numbers**

| | |
|---|---|
| Maxtrex 2.5 | 3433/0071 |
| Maxtrex 10 | 3433/0072 |

## MEDRONE* TABLETS 2 mg and 4 mg

**Qualitative and quantitative composition** Each Medrone Tablet contains 2 mg or 4 mg methylprednisolone PhEur.

**Pharmaceutical form** Tablet

**Clinical particulars**

*Therapeutic indications:* Medrone is indicated for conditions requiring glucocorticoid activity such as:
*Endocrine disorders:* Primary and secondary adrenal insufficiency; congenital adrenal hyperplasia.

*Rheumatic disorders:* Rheumatoid arthritis; juvenile chronic arthritis; ankylosing spondylitis

*Collagen diseases/arteritis:* Systemic lupus erythematosus; systemic dermatomyositis (polymyositis); rheumatic fever with severe carditis; giant cell arteritis/ polymyalgia rheumatica.

*Dermatological diseases:* Pemphigus vulgaris.

*Allergic states:* Severe seasonal and perennial allergic rhinitis; drug hypersensitivity reactions; serum sickness; allergic contact dermatitis; bronchial asthma.

*Ophthalmic diseases:* Anterior uveitis (iritis, iridocyclitis); posterior uveitis; optic neuritis.

*Respiratory diseases:* Pulmonary sarcoid; fulminating or disseminated tuberculosis (with appropriate anti-tuberculous chemotherapy); aspiration of gastric contents.

*Haematological disorders:* Idiopathic thrombocytopenic purpura; haemolytic anaemia (autoimmune).

*Neoplastic diseases:* Leukaemia (acute and lymphatic); malignant lymphoma.

*Gastro-intestinal diseases:* Ulcerative colitis; Crohn's disease.

*Miscellaneous:* Tuberculous meningitis (with appropriate antituberculous chemotherapy); transplantation

*Posology and method of administration:* The dosage recommendations shown in the table below are suggested initial daily doses and are intended as guides. The average total daily dose recommended may be given either as a single dose or in divided doses (excepting in alternate day therapy when the minimum effective daily dose is doubled and given every other day at 8.00 am).

Undesirable effects may be minimised by using the lowest effective dose for the minimum period (see *Special warnings and special precautions for use*).

The initial suppressive dose level may vary depending on the condition being treated. This is continued until a satisfactory clinical response is obtained, a period usually of three to seven days in the case of rheumatic diseases (except for acute rheumatic carditis), allergic conditions affecting the skin or respiratory tract and ophthalmic diseases. If a satisfactory response is not obtained in seven days, re-evaluation of the case to confirm the original diagnosis should be made. As soon as a satisfactory clinical response is obtained, the daily dose should be reduced gradually, either to termination of treatment in the case of acute conditions (e.g. seasonal asthma, exfoliative dermatitis, acute ocular inflammations) or to the minimal effective maintenance dose level in the case of chronic conditions (e.g. rheumatoid arthritis, systemic lupus erythematosus, bronchial asthma, atopic dermatitis). In chronic conditions, and in rheumatoid arthritis especially, it is important that the reduction in dosage from initial to maintenance dose levels be accomplished as clinically appropriate. Decrements of not more than 2 mg at intervals of 7 – 10 days are suggested. In rheumatoid arthritis, maintenance steroid therapy should be at the lowest possible level.

In alternate-day therapy, the minimum daily corticoid requirement is doubled and administered as a single dose every other day at 8.00 am. Dosage requirements depend on the condition being treated and response of the patient.

*Elderly patients:* Treatment of elderly patients, particularly if long-term, should be planned bearing in mind the more serious consequences of the common side-effects of corticosteroids in old age and close clinical supervision is required (see *Special warnings and special precautions for use*).

*Children:* In general, dosage for children should be based upon clinical response and is at the discretion of the clinician. Treatment should be limited to the minimum dosage for the shortest period of time. If possible, treatment should be administered as a single dose on alternate days (see *Special warnings and special precautions for use*).

*Dosage recommendations:*

| Indications | Recommended initial daily dosage |
| --- | --- |
| Rheumatoid arthritis: | |
| severe | 12 – 16 mg |
| moderately severe | 8 -- 12 mg |
| moderate | 4 -- 8 mg |
| children | 4 -- 8 mg |
| Systemic dermatomyositis | 48 mg |
| Systemic lupus erythematosus | 20 -- 100 mg |
| Acute rheumatic fever | 48 mg until ESR normal for one week |
| Allergic diseases | 12 -- 40 mg |
| Bronchial asthma | up to 64 mg single dose/alternate day up to 100 mg maximum |
| Ophthalmic diseases | 12 -- 40 mg |
| Haematological disorders and leukaemias | 16 -- 100 mg |
| Malignant lymphoma | 16 -- 100 mg |
| Ulcerative colitis | 16 -- 60 mg |
| Crohn's disease | up to 48 mg per day in acute episodes |
| Organ transplantation | up to 3.6 mg/kg/day |
| Pulmonary sarcoid | 32 -- 48 mg on alternate days |

| Indications | Recommended initial daily dosage |
| --- | --- |
| Giant cell arteritis/ polymyalgia rheumatica | 64 mg |
| Pemphigus vulgaris | 80 -- 360 mg |

*Contra-indications:* Medrone is contra-indicated where there is known hypersensitivity to components and in systemic infection unless specific anti-infective therapy is employed.

*Special warnings and special precautions for use:*
*Warnings and precautions:* A Patient Information Leaflet is provided in the pack by the manufacturer.

Undesirable effects may be minimised by using the lowest effective dose for the minimum period, and by administering the daily requirement as a single morning dose or whenever possible as a single morning dose on alternative days. Frequent patient review is required to appropriately titrate the dose against disease activity (see *Posology and method of administration*).

Adrenal cortical atrophy develops during prolonged therapy and may persist for months after stopping treatment. Withdrawal of corticosteroids after prolonged therapy must therefore always be gradual to avoid acute adrenal insufficiency, being tapered off over weeks or months according to the dose and duration of treatment. During prolonged therapy any intercurrent illness, trauma or surgical procedure will require a temporary increase in dosage; if corticosteroids have been stopped following prolonged therapy they may need to be temporarily re-introduced.

Since mineralocorticoid secretion may be impaired, salt and/or a mineralocorticoid should be administered concurrently.

Patients should carry 'Steroid Treatment' cards which give clear guidance on the precautions to be taken to minimise risk and which provide details of prescriber, drug, dosage and the duration of treatment.

Corticosteroids may mask some signs of infection, and new infections may appear during their use. Suppression of the inflammatory response and immune function increases the susceptibility to fungal, viral and bacterial infections and their severity. The clinical presentation may often be atypical and may reach an advanced stage before being recognised.

Chickenpox is of serious concern since this normally minor illness may be fatal in immunosuppressed patients. Patients (or parents of children) without a definite history of chickenpox should be advised to avoid close personal contact with chickenpox or herpes zoster and if exposed they should seek urgent medical attention. Passive immunization with varicella/zoster immunoglobulin (VZIG) is needed by exposed non-immune patients who are receiving systemic corticosteroids or who have used them within the previous 3 months; this should be given within 10 days of exposure to chickenpox. If a diagnosis of chickenpox is confirmed, the illness warrants specialist care and urgent treatment. Corticosteroids should not be stopped and the dose may need to be increased.

Live vaccines should not be given to individuals with impaired immune responsiveness. The antibody response to other vaccines may be diminished.

The use of Medrone in active tuberculosis should be restricted to those cases of fulminating or disseminated tuberculosis in which the corticosteroid is used for the management of the disease in conjunction with an appropriate antituberculous regimen. If corticosteroids are indicated in patients with latent tuberculosis or tuberculin reactivity, close observation is necessary as reactivation of the disease may occur. During prolonged corticosteroid therapy, these patients should receive chemoprophylaxis.

Care should be taken for patients receiving cardioactive drugs such as digoxin because of steroid induced electrolyte disturbance/potassium loss (see *Undesirable effects*).

*Special precautions:* Particular care is required when considering the use of systemic corticosteroids in patients with the following conditions and frequent patient monitoring is necessary:

Osteoporosis (post-menopausal females are particularly at risk).
Hypertension or congestive heart failure.
Existing or previous history of severe affective disorders (especially previous steroid psychosis).
Diabetes mellitus (or a family history of diabetes).
History of tuberculosis.
Glaucoma (or a family history of glaucoma).
Previous corticosteroid-induced myopathy.
Liver failure or cirrhosis.
Renal insufficiency.
Epilepsy.
Peptic ulceration.
Fresh intestinal anastomoses.
Predisposition to thrombophlebitis.
Abscess or other pyogenic infections.
Ulcerative colitis.

Diverticulitis.
Myasthenia gravis.
Ocular herpes simplex, for fear of corneal perforation.
Hypothyroidism.

*Use in children:* Corticosteroids cause growth retardation in infancy, childhood and adolescence, which may be irreversible. Treatment should be limited to the minimum dosage for the shortest possible time. In order to minimise suppression of the hypothalamo-pituitary-adrenal axis and growth retardation, treatment should be administered where possible as a single dose on alternate days.

*Use in the elderly:* The common adverse effects of systemic corticosteroids may be associated with more serious consequences in old age, especially osteoporosis, hypertension, hypokalaemia, diabetes, susceptibility to infection and thinning of the skin. Close clinical supervision is required to avoid life-threatening reactions.

*Interaction with other medicaments and other forms of interaction:* Convulsions have been reported with concurrent use of methylprednisolone and cyclosporin. Since concurrent administration of these agents results in a mutual inhibition of metabolism, it is possible that convulsions and other adverse effects associated with the individual use of either drug may be more apt to occur.

Drugs that induce hepatic enzymes, such as rifampicin, rifabutin, carbamazepine, phenobarbitone, phenytoin, primidone, and aminoglutethimide enhance the metabolism of corticosteroids and its therapeutic effects may be reduced.

Drugs such as erythromycin and ketoconazole may inhibit the metabolism of corticosteroids and thus decrease their clearance.

Steroids may reduce the effects of anticholinesterases in myasthenia gravis. The desired effects of hypoglycaemic agents (including insulin), anti-hypertensives and diuretics are antagonised by corticosteroids, and the hypokalaemic effects of acetazolamide, loop diuretics, thiazide diuretics and carbenoxolone are enhanced.

The efficacy of coumarin anticoagulants may be enhanced by concurrent corticosteroid therapy and close monitoring of the INR or prothrombin time is required to avoid spontaneous bleeding.

The renal clearance of salicylates is increased by corticosteroids and steroid withdrawal may result in salicylate intoxication. Salicylates and non-steroidal anti-inflammatory agents should be used cautiously in conjunction with corticosteroids in hypothrombinaemia.

Steroids have been reported to interact with neuromuscular blocking agents such as pancuronium with partial reversal of the neuromuscular block.

*Pregnancy and lactation:* Corticosteroids cross the placenta. There may be a very small risk of cleft palate and intra-uterine growth retardation in the fetus; there is evidence of harmful effects on pregnancy in animals. Neonates of mothers who received such therapy during pregnancy should be observed for signs of hypoadrenalism and appropriate measures instituted if such signs exist. When corticosteroids are essential however, patients with normal pregnancies may be treated as though they were in the non-gravid state. Patients with pre-eclampsia or fluid retention require close monitoring.

Methylprednisolone is excreted in breast milk and infants of mothers taking pharmacological doses of steroids should be monitored carefully for signs of adrenal suppression.

*Effects on ability to drive and use machines:* None stated.

*Undesirable effects:* The incidence of predictable undesirable side-effects associated with the use of corticosteroids, including hypothalamic-pituitary-adrenal suppression correlates with the relative potency of the drug, dosage, timing of administration and duration of treatment (see *Special warnings and special precautions for use*).

*Gastro-intestinal:* Dyspepsia, peptic ulceration with perforation and haemorrhage, abdominal distension, oesophageal ulceration, oesophageal candidiasis, acute pancreatitis, perforation of bowel.

Increases in alanine transaminase (ALT, SGPT) aspartate transaminase (AST, SGOT) and alkaline phosphatase have been observed following corticosteroid treatment. These changes are usually small, not associated with any clinical syndrome and are reversible upon discontinuation.

*Anti-inflammatory and immunosuppressive effects:* Increased susceptibility and severity of infections with suppression of clinical symptoms and signs, opportunistic infections, may suppress reactions to skin tests, recurrence of dormant tuberculosis (see Special warnings and special precautions for use).

*Musculoskeletal:* Proximal myopathy, osteoporosis, vertebral and long bone fractures, avascular osteonecrosis, tendon rupture, muscle weakness.

*Fluid and electrolyte disturbance:* Sodium and water

retention, hypertension, hypokalaemic alkalosis, potassium loss, congestive heart failure in susceptible patients.

*Dermatological:* Impaired healing, skin atrophy, bruising, striae, telangiectasia, acne, petechiae and ecchymosis.

*Endocrine/metabolic:* Suppression of the hypothalamo-pituitary-adrenal axis, growth suppression in infancy, childhood and adolescence; menstrual irregularity and amenorrhoea. Cushingoid facies, hirsutism, weight gain, impaired carbohydrate tolerance with increased requirement for antidiabetic therapy, negative nitrogen and calcium balance. Increased appetite.

*Neuropsychiatric:* Euphoria, psychological dependence, mood swings, depression, personality changes, insomnia. Increased intra-cranial pressure with papilloedema in children (pseudotumour cerebri), usually after treatment withdrawal. Psychosis, aggravation of schizophrenia, seizures.

*Ophthalmic:* Increased intra-ocular pressure, glaucoma, papilloedema, cataracts with possible damage to the optic nerve, corneal or scleral thinning, exacerbation of ophthalmic viral or fungal disease, exophthalmos.

*General:* Leucocytosis, hypersensitivity reactions including anaphylaxis, thrombo-embolism, nausea, malaise.

*Withdrawal symptoms:* Too rapid a reduction of corticosteroid dosage following prolonged treatment can lead to acute adrenal insufficiency, hypotension and death (see *Special warnings and special precautions for use*).

A 'withdrawal syndrome' may also occur including, fever, myalgia, arthralgia, rhinitis, conjunctivitis, painful itchy skin nodules and loss of weight.

*Overdose:* Administration of Medrone should not be discontinued abruptly but tailed off over a period of time. Appropriate action should be taken to alleviate the symptoms produced by any side-effect that may become apparent. It may be necessary to support the patient with corticosteroids during any further period of trauma occurring within two years of overdosage.

There is no clinical syndrome of acute overdose with Medrone. Methylprednisolone is dialysable.

## Pharmacological properties

*Pharmacodynamic properties:* Medrone is a potent corticosteroid with an anti-inflammatory activity at least five times that of hydrocortisone. An enhanced separation of glucocorticoid and mineralocorticoid effect results in a reduced incidence of sodium and water retention.

*Pharmacokinetic properties:* Corticosteroids are absorbed from the gastro-intestinal tract. In the circulation they are extensively bound to plasma proteins and are metabolised mainly in the liver but also in the kidney and are excreted in the urine.

The half-life of methylprednisolone has been reported to be slightly longer than that of prednisolone.

## Pharmaceutical particulars

*List of excipients:* Lactose, sucrose, maize starch and calcium stearate. Medrone Tablets 2 mg also contain E123 and E127.

*Incompatibilities:* None stated.

*Shelf-life:* Blister packs–36 months.

*Special precautions for storage:* Store below 25°C.

*Nature and contents of container:* 20–25 micron hard tempered aluminium foil/lacquer, 250 micron opaque polyvinyl chloride film blister. Pack contains 30 tablets.

*Instructions for use/handling:* No special requirements.

**Marketing authorisation numbers**
2 mg     0032/5017
4 mg     0032/5018

**Date of approval/revision of SPC** July 1996

**Legal category** POM

## MEDRONE* TABLETS 16 mg

**Presentation** Oval single-scored white tablet marked 'UPJOHN 73' containing 16 mg methylprednisolone. Medrone Tablets 16 mg also contain lactose, sucrose, maize starch, mineral oil and calcium stearate.

**Uses** Medrone is a potent corticosteroid with an anti-inflammatory activity at least five times that of hydrocortisone. An enhanced separation of glucocorticoid and mineralocorticoid effect results in a reduced incidence of sodium and water retention.

These products are indicated for conditions requiring glucocorticoid activity such as:

*Collagen diseases/arteritis:* Systemic lupus erythematosus; systemic dermatomyositis (polymyositis); rheumatic fever with severe carditis; giant cell arteritis/polymyalgia rheumatica.

*Dermatological diseases:* Pemphigus vulgaris.

*Allergic states:* Bronchial asthma.
*Respiratory diseases:* Pulmonary sarcoid.
*Haematological disorders:* Idiopathic thrombocytopenic purpura; haemolytic anaemia (autoimmune).
*Neoplastic diseases:* Leukaemia (acute and lymphatic); malignant lymphoma.
*Gastro-intestinal diseases:* Crohn's disease.
*Miscellaneous:* Tuberculous meningitis (with appropriate antituberculous chemotherapy); transplantation.

**Dosage and administration** The dosage recommendations shown in the table below are suggested initial daily doses and are intended as guides. The average total daily dose recommended may be given either as a single dose or in divided doses (excepting in alternate day therapy when the minimum effective daily dose is doubled and given every other day at 8.00 a.m.).

Undesirable effects may be minimised by using the lowest effective dose for the minimum period (see *Other special warnings and precautions*).

The initial suppressive dose level may vary depending on the condition being treated. As soon as a satisfactory clinical response is obtained, the daily dose should be reduced gradually, either to termination of treatment in the case of acute conditions or to the minimal effective maintenance dose level in the case of chronic conditions. In chronic conditions it is important that the reduction in dosage from initial to maintenance dose levels be accomplished as clinically appropriate.

In alternate-day therapy, the minimum daily corticoid requirement is doubled and administered as a single dose every other day at 8.00 a.m. Dosage requirements depend on the condition being treated and response of the patient.

*Elderly patients:* Treatment of elderly patients, particularly if long-term, should be planned bearing in mind the more serious consequences of the common side-effects of corticosteroids in old age and close clinical supervision is required (see *Other special warnings and precautions*).

*Children:* In general, dosage for children should be based upon clinical response and is at the discretion of the clinician. Treatment should be limited to the minimum dosage for the shortest period of time. If possible, treatment should be administered as a single dose on alternate days (see *Other special warnings and precautions*).

*Dosage recommendations:*

| Indications | Recommended initial daily dosage |
|---|---|
| Systemic lupus erythematosus | 20--100 mg |
| Systemic dermatomyositis | 48 mg |
| Acute rheumatic fever | 48 mg until ESR normal for one week. |
| Giant cell arteritis/polymyalgia rheumatica | 64 mg |
| Pemphigus vulgaris | 80--360 mg |
| Bronchial asthma | up to 64 mg single dose/alternate day up to 100 mg maximum. |
| Pulmonary sarcoid | 32--48 mg on alternate days. |
| Haematological disorders and leukaemias | 16--100 mg |
| Malignant lymphoma | 16--100 mg |
| Crohn's disease | up to 48 mg per day in acute episodes. |
| Organ transplantation | up to 3.6 mg/kg/day |

**Contra-indications, warnings, etc.**

*Contra-indications:* Medrone is contra-indicated where there is known hypersensitivity to components and in systemic fungal infection unless specific anti-infective therapy is employed.

*Interactions:* Convulsions have been reported with concurrent use of methylprednisolone and cyclosporin. Since concurrent administration of these agents results in a mutual inhibition of metabolism, it is possible that convulsions and other adverse effects associated with the individual use of either drug may be more apt to occur.

Drugs that induce hepatic enzymes, such as rifampicin, rifabutin, carbamazepine, phenobarbitone, phenytoin, primidone, and aminoglutethimide enhance the metabolism of corticosteroids and its therapeutic effects may be reduced.

Drugs such as erythromycin and ketoconazole may inhibit the metabolism of corticosteroids and thus decrease their clearance.

Steroids may reduce the effects of anticholinesterases in myasthenia gravis. The desired effects of hypoglycaemic agents (including insulin), anti-hypertensives and diuretics are antagonised by corticosteroids, and the hypokalaemic effects of acetazolamide, loop diuretics, thiazide diuretics and carbenoxolone are enhanced.

The efficacy of coumarin anticoagulants may be enhanced by concurrent corticosteroid therapy and close monitoring of the INR or prothrombin time is required to avoid spontaneous bleeding.

The renal clearance of salicylates is increased by corticosteroids and steroid withdrawal may result in salicylate intoxication. Salicylates and non-steroidal anti-inflammatory agents should be used cautiously in conjunction with corticosteroids in hypothrombinaemia.

Steroids have been reported to interact with neuromuscular blocking agents such as pancuronium with partial reversal of the neuromuscular block.

*Effects on ability to drive and to use machines:* None stated.

*Other undesirable effects (frequency and seriousness):*
*Side-effects:* The incidence of predictable undesirable side-effects associated with the use of corticosteroids, including hypothalamic-pituitary-adrenal suppression correlates with the relative potency of the drug, dosage, timing of administration and duration of treatment (see Other special warnings and precautions).

*Gastro-intestinal:* Dyspepsia, peptic ulceration with perforation and haemorrhage, abdominal distension, oesophageal ulceration, oesophageal candidiasis, acute pancreatitis, perforation of bowel.

Increases in alanine transaminase (ALT, SGPT) aspartate transaminase (AST, SGOT) and alkaline phosphatase have been observed following corticosteroid treatment. These changes are usually small, not associated with any clinical syndrome and are reversible upon discontinuation.

*Anti-inflammatory and immunosuppressive effects:* Increased susceptibility and severity of infections with suppression of clinical symptoms and signs, opportunistic infections, may suppress reactions to skin tests, recurrence of dormant tuberculosis (see *Other special warnings and precautions*).

*Musculoskeletal:* Proximal myopathy, osteoporosis, vertebral and long bone fractures, avascular osteonecrosis, tendon rupture, muscle weakness.

*Fluid and electrolyte disturbance:* Sodium and water retention, hypertension, hypokalaemic alkalosis, potassium loss, congestive heart failure in susceptible patients.

*Dermatological:* Impaired healing, skin atrophy, bruising, striae, telangiectasia, acne, petechiae and ecchymosis.

*Endocrine/metabolic:* Suppression of the hypothalamo-pituitary-adrenal axis; growth suppression in infancy, childhood and adolescence; menstrual irregularity and amenorrhoea. Cushingoid facies, hirsutism, weight gain, impaired carbohydrate tolerance with increased requirement for antidiabetic therapy, negative nitrogen and calcium balance. Increased appetite.

*Neuropsychiatric:* Euphoria, psychological dependence, mood swings, depression, personality changes, insomnia. Increased intra-cranial pressure with papilloedema in children (pseudotumour cerebri), usually after treatment withdrawal. Psychosis, aggravation of schizophrenia, seizures.

*Ophthalmic:* Increased intra-ocular pressure, glaucoma, papilloedema, cataracts with possible damage to the optic nerve, corneal or scleral thinning, exacerbation of ophthalmic viral or fungal disease, exophthalmos.

*General:* Leucocytosis, hypersensitivity reactions including anaphylaxis, thrombo-embolism, nausea, malaise.

*Withdrawal symptoms:* Too rapid a reduction of corticosteroid dosage following prolonged treatment can lead to acute adrenal insufficiency, hypotension and death (see Other special warnings and precautions).

A 'withdrawal syndrome' may also occur including, fever, myalgia, arthralgia, rhinitis, conjunctivitis, painful itchy skin nodules and loss of weight.

*Other special warnings and precautions:*
Warnings and precautions: A Patient Information Leaflet is provided in the pack by the manufacturer.

Undesirable effects may be minimised by using the lowest effective dose for the minimum period, and by administering the daily requirement as a single morning dose or whenever possible as a single morning dose on alternative days. Frequent patient review is required to appropriately titrate the dose against disease activity (see Dosage and administration).

Adrenal cortical atrophy develops during prolonged therapy and may persist for months after stopping treatment. Withdrawal of corticosteroids after prolonged therapy must therefore always be gradual to avoid acute adrenal insufficiency, being tapered off over weeks or months according to the dose and duration of treatment. During prolonged therapy any intercurrent illness, trauma or surgical procedure will require a temporary increase in dosage; if corticosteroids have been stopped following prolonged therapy they may need to be temporarily re-introduced.

Since mineralocorticoid secretion may be impaired, salt and/or a mineralocorticoid should be administered concurrently.

Patients should carry 'Steroid Treatment' cards which give clear guidance on the precautions to be taken to minimise risk and which provide details of prescriber, drug, dosage and the duration of treatment.

Corticosteroids may mask some signs of infection, and new infections may appear during their use. Suppression of the inflammatory response and immune function increases the susceptibility to infections and their severity.

Chickenpox is of serious concern since this normally minor illness may be fatal in immunosuppressed patients. Patients (or parents of children) without a definite history of chickenpox should be advised to avoid close personal contact with chickenpox or herpes zoster and if exposed they should seek urgent medical attention. Passive immunization with varicella/zoster immunoglobin (VZIG) is needed by exposed non-immune patients who are receiving systemic corticosteroids or who have used them within the previous 3 months; this should be given within 10 days of exposure to chickenpox. If a diagnosis of chickenpox is confirmed, the illness warrants specialist care and urgent treatment. Corticosteroids should not be stopped and the dose may need to be increased.

Live vaccines should not be given to individuals with impaired immune responsiveness. The antibody response to other vaccines may be diminished.

The use of Medrone in active tuberculosis should be restricted to those cases of fulminating or disseminated tuberculosis in which the corticosteroid is used for the management of the disease in conjunction with an appropriate antituberculous regimen. If corticosteroids are indicated in patients with latent tuberculosis or tuberculin reactivity, close observation is necessary as reactivation of the disease may occur. During prolonged corticosteroid therapy, these patients should receive chemoprophylaxis.

Care should be taken for patients receiving cardioactive drugs such as digoxin because of steroid induced electrolyte disturbance/potassium loss (see Side-effects).

*Special precautions:* Particular care is required when considering the use of systemic corticosteroids in patients with the following conditions and frequent patient monitoring is necessary.

Osteoporosis (post-menopausal females are particularly at risk).

Hypertension or congestive heart failure.

Existing or previous history of severe affective disorders (especially previous steroid psychosis).

Diabetes mellitus (or a family history of diabetes).

History of tuberculosis.

Glaucoma (or a family history of glaucoma).

Previous corticosteroid-induced myopathy.

Liver failure or cirrhosis.

Renal insufficiency.

Epilepsy.

Peptic ulceration.

Fresh intestinal anastomoses.

Predisposition to thrombophlebitis.

Abscess or other pyogenic infections.

Ulcerative colitis.

Diverticulitis.

Myasthenia gravis.

Ocular herpes simplex, for fear of corneal perforation.

Hypothyroidism.

*Use in pregnancy and lactation:* Corticosteroids cross the placenta. There may be a very small risk of cleft palate and intra-uterine growth retardation in the fetus; there is evidence of harmful effects on pregnancy in animals. Neonates of mothers who received such therapy during pregnancy should be observed for signs of hypoadrenalism and appropriate measures instituted if such signs exist. When corticosteroids are essential however, patients with normal pregnancies may be treated as though they were in the non-gravid state. Patients with pre-eclampsia or fluid retention require close monitoring.

Methylprednisolone is excreted in breast milk and infants of mothers taking pharmacological doses of steroids should be monitored carefully for signs of adrenal suppression.

*Use in children:* Corticosteroids cause growth retardation in infancy, childhood and adolescence. Treatment should be limited to the minimum dosage for the shortest possible time. In order to minimise suppression of the hypothalamo-pituitary-adrenal axis and growth retardation, treatment should be administered where possible as a single dose on alternate days.

*Use in the elderly:* The common adverse effects of systemic corticosteroids may be associated with more serious consequences in old age, especially osteoporosis, hypertension, hypokalaemia, diabetes, susceptibility to infection and thinning of the skin. Close clinical supervision is required to avoid life-threatening reactions.

*Overdosage:* Administration of Medrone should not be discontinued abruptly but tailed off over a period of time. Appropriate action should be taken to alleviate the symptoms produced by any side-effect that may become apparent. It may be necessary to support the patient with corticosteroids during any further period of trauma occurring within two years of overdosage.

There is no clinical syndrome of acute overdose with Medrone. Methylprednisolone is dialysable.

*Incompatibilities (major):* None stated.

**Pharmaceutical precautions** Medrone Tablets 16 mg–store below 25°C.

**Legal category** POM

**Package quantities** Packs of 30 tablets

**Further information** Medrone has achieved a clinically acceptable split between glucocorticoid effect and undesired mineralocorticoid effect. Weight for weight, methylprednisolone has five times the anti-inflammatory activity of hydrocortisone but has little tendency to cause salt and water retention. The 16 mg tablet gives opportunity for use of alternate day therapy in long term use in chronic conditions.

A separate data sheet is available for Medrone Tablets 2 mg and 4 mg and includes additional indications in which low dose therapy is appropriate.

**Product licence number** 0032/0024

## MEDRONE* TABLETS 100 mg

**Qualitative and quantitative composition** Each Medrone Tablet contains 100 mg Methylprednisolone PhEur.

**Pharmaceutical form** Tablet

**Clinical particulars**

*Therapeutic indications:* Medrone is a potent corticosteroid with an anti-inflammatory activity at least five times that of hydrocortisone. An enhanced separation of glucocorticoid and mineralocorticoid effect results in a reduced incidence of sodium and water retention.

Medrone is indicated for conditions requiring glucocorticoid activity such as:

*Collagen diseases/arteritis:* Systemic lupus erythematosus; systemic dermatomyositis (polymyositis); rheumatic fever with severe carditis; giant cell arteritis/polymyalgia rheumatica.

*Dermatological diseases*: Pemphigus vulgaris.

*Allergic states:* Bronchial asthma.

*Respiratory diseases:* Pulmonary sarcoid.

*Haematological disorders:* Idiopathic thrombocytopenic purpura; haemolytic anaemia (autoimmune).

*Neoplastic diseases:* Leukaemia (acute and lymphatic); Malignant lymphoma

*Gastro-intestinal diseasess*: Crohn's disease.

*Miscellaneous:* Tuberculous meningitis (with appropriate antituberculous chemotherapy); transplantation.

*Posology and method of administration:* The dosage recommendations shown in the table below are suggested initial daily doses and are intended as guides. The average total daily dose recommended may be given either as a single dose or in divided doses (excepting in alternate day therapy when the minimum effective daily dose is doubled and given every other day at 8.00 a.m.). It is envisaged that the 100 mg tablet will be used for high initial daily or alternate day doses in acute situations, with tapering of dosage achieved by using the 16 mg tablet.

Undesirable effects may be minimised by using the lowest effective dose for the minimum period (see *Special warnings and special precautions for use*).

The initial suppressive dose level may vary depending on the condition being treated. As soon as a satisfactory clinical response is obtained, the daily dose should be reduced gradually, either to termination of treatment in the case of acute conditions or to the minimal effective maintenance dose level in the case of chronic conditions. In chronic conditions it is important that the reduction in dosage from initial to maintenance dose levels be accomplished as clinically appropriate.

In alternate-day therapy, the minimum daily corticoid requirement is doubled and administered as a single dose every other day at 8.00 a.m. Dosage requirements depend on the condition being treated and response of the patient.

*Elderly patients:* Treatment of elderly patients, particularly if long-term, should be planned bearing in mind the more serious consequences of the common side-effects of corticosteroids in old age and close clinical supervision is required (see *Special warnings and special precautions for use*).

*Children:* In general, dosage for children should be based upon clinical response and is at the discretion of the clinician. Treatment should be limited to the minimum dosage for the shortest period of time. If possible, treatment should be administered as a single dose on alternate days (see *Special warnings and special precautions for use*).

*Dosage recommendations:*

| *Indications* | *Recommended initial daily dosage* |
|---|---|
| Systemic lupus erythematosus | 20--100 mg |
| Systemic dermatomyositis | 48 mg |
| Acute rheumatic fever | 48 mg until ESR normal for one week. |
| Giant cell arteritis/polymyalgia rheumatica | 64 mg |
| Pemphigus vulgaris | 80--360 mg |
| Bronchial asthma | up to 64 mg single dose/alternate day up to 100 mg maximum. |
| Pulmonary sarcoid | 32--48 mg on alternate days. |
| Haematological disorders and leukaemias | 16--100 mg |
| Malignant lymphoma | 16--100 mg |
| Crohn's disease | up to 48 mg per day in acute episodes |
| Organ transplantation | up to 3.6 mg/kg/day |

*Contra-indications:* Medrone is contra-indicated where there is known hypersensitivity to components and in systemic fungal infection unless specific anti-infective therapy is employed.

*Special warnings and special precautions for use:* *Warnings and* precautions: A Patient Information Leaflet is provided in the pack by the manufacturer.

Undesirable effects may be minimised by using the lowest effective dose for the minimum period, and by administering the daily requirement as a single morning dose or whenever possible as a single morning dose on alternative days. Frequent patient review is required to appropriately titrate the dose against disease activity (see *Posology and method of administration*).

Adrenal cortical atrophy develops during prolonged therapy and may persist for months after stopping treatment. Withdrawal of corticosteroids after prolonged therapy must therefore always be gradual to avoid acute adrenal insufficiency, being tapered off over weeks or months according to the dose and duration of treatment. During prolonged therapy any intercurrent illness, trauma or surgical procedure will require a temporary increase in dosage; if corticosteroids have been stopped following prolonged therapy they may need to be temporarily re-introduced.

Since mineralocorticoid secretion may be impaired, salt and/or a mineralocorticoid should be administered concurrently.

Patients should carry 'Steroid Treatment' cards which give clear guidance on the precautions to be taken to minimise risk and which provide details of prescriber, drug, dosage and the duration of treatment.

Corticosteroids may mask some signs of infection, and new infections may appear during their use. Suppression of the inflammatory response and immune function increases the susceptibility to infections and their severity.

Chickenpox is of serious concern since this normally minor illness may be fatal in immunosuppressed patients. Patients (or parents of children) without a definite history of chickenpox should be advised to avoid close personal contact with chickenpox or herpes zoster and if exposed they should seek urgent medical attention. Passive immunization with varicella/zoster immunoglobin (VZIG) is needed by exposed non-immune patients who are receiving systemic corticosteroids or who have used them within the previous 3 months; this should be given within 10 days of exposure to chickenpox. If a diagnosis of chickenpox is confirmed, the illness warrants specialist care and urgent treatment. Corticosteroids should not be stopped and the dose may need to be increased.

Live vaccines should not be given to individuals with impaired immune responsiveness. The antibody response to other vaccines may be diminished.

The use of Medrone in active tuberculosis should be restricted to those cases of fulminating or disseminated tuberculosis in which the corticosteroid is used for the management of the disease in conjunction with an appropriate antituberculous regimen. If corticosteroids are indicated in patients with latent tuberculosis or tuberculin reactivity, close observation is necessary as reactivation of the disease may occur. During prolonged corticosteroid therapy, these patients should receive chemoprophylaxis.

Care should be taken for patients receiving cardioactive drugs such as digoxin because of steroid induced electrolyte disturbance/potassium loss (see Undesirable effects).

*Special precautions*: Particular care is required when considering the use of systemic corticosteroids in patients with the following conditions and frequent patient monitoring is necessary.

Osteoporosis (post-menopausal females are particularly at risk).

Hypertension or congestive heart failure.

Existing or previous history of severe affective disorders (especially previous steroid psychosis).

Diabetes mellitus (or a family history of diabetes).

History of tuberculosis.

Glaucoma (or a family history of glaucoma).

Previous corticosteroid-induced myopathy.

Liver failure or cirrhosis.

Renal insufficiency.

Epilepsy.

Peptic ulceration.

Fresh intestinal anastomoses.

Predisposition to thrombophlebitis.

Abscess or other pyogenic infections.

Ulcerative colitis.

Diverticulitis.

Myasthenia gravis.

Ocular herpes simplex, for fear of corneal perforation.

Hypothyroidism.

*Use in children:* Corticosteroids cause growth retardation in infancy, childhood and adolescence. Treatment should be limited to the minimum dosage for the shortest possible time. In order to minimise suppression of the hypothalamo-pituitary-adrenal axis and growth retardation, treatment should be administered where possible as a single dose on alternate days.

*Use in the elderly:* The common adverse effects of systemic corticosteroids may be associated with more serious consequences in old age, especially osteoporosis, hypertension, hypokalaemia, diabetes, susceptibility to infection and thinning of the skin. Close clinical supervision is required to avoid life-threatening reactions.

*Interaction with other medicaments and other forms of interaction:* Convulsions have been reported with concurrent use of methylprednisolone and cyclosporin. Since concurrent administration of these agents results in a mutual inhibition of metabolism, it is possible that convulsions and other adverse effects associated with the individual use of either drug may be more apt to occur.

Drugs that induce hepatic enzymes, such as rifampicin, rifabutin, carbamazepine, phenobarbitone, phenytoin, primidone, and aminoglutethimide enhance the metabolism of corticosteroids and its therapeutic effects may be reduced.

Drugs such as erythromycin and ketoconazole may inhibit the metabolism of corticosteroids and thus decrease their clearance.

Steroids may reduce the effects of anticholinesterases in myasthenia gravis. The desired effects of hypoglycaemic agents (including insulin), anti-hypertensives and diuretics are antagonised by corticosteroids, and the hypokalaemic effects of acetazolamide, loop diuretics, thiazide diuretics and carbenoxolone are enhanced.

The efficacy of coumarin anticoagulants may be enhanced by concurrent corticosteroid therapy and close monitoring of the INR or prothrombin time is required to avoid spontaneous bleeding.

The renal clearance of salicylates is increased by corticosteroids and steroid withdrawal may result in salicylate intoxication. Salicylates and non-steroidal anti-inflammatory agents should be used cautiously in conjunction with corticosteroids in hypothrombinaemia.

Steroids have been reported to interact with neuromuscular blocking agents such as pancuronium with partial reversal of the neuromuscular block.

*Pregnancy and lactation:* Corticosteroids cross the placenta. There may be a very small risk of cleft palate and intra-uterine growth retardation in the fetus; there is evidence of harmful effects on pregnancy in animals. Neonates of mothers who received such therapy during pregnancy should be observed for signs of hypoadrenalism and appropriate measures instituted if such signs exist. When corticosteroids are essential however, patients with normal pregnancies may be treated as though they were in the non-gravid state. Patients with pre-eclampsia or fluid retention require close monitoring.

Methylprednisolone is excreted in breast milk and infants of mothers taking pharmacological doses of steroids should be monitored carefully for signs of adrenal suppression.

*Effects on ability to drive and use machines:* None stated.

*Undesirable effects:* The incidence of predictable undesirable side-effects associated with the use of corticosteroids, including hypothalamic-pituitary-adrenal suppression correlates with the relative potency of the drug, dosage, timing of administration and duration of treatment (see *Special warnings and special precautions for use*).

*Gastro-intestinal:* Dyspepsia, peptic ulceration with perforation and haemorrhage, abdominal distension, oesophageal ulceration, oesophageal candidiasis, acute pancreatitis, perforation of bowel.

Increases in alanine transaminase (ALT, SGPT) aspartate transaminase (AST, SGOT) and alkaline phosphatase have been observed following corticosteroid treatment. These changes are usually small, not associated with any clinical syndrome and are reversible upon discontinuation.

*Anti-inflammatory and immunosuppressive effects:* Increased susceptibility and severity of infections with suppression of clinical symptoms and signs, opportunistic infections, may suppress reactions to skin tests, recurrence of dormant tuberculosis (see Special warnings and special precautions for use).

*Musculoskeletal:* Proximal myopathy, osteoporosis, vertebral and long bone fractures, avascular osteonecrosis, tendon rupture, muscle weakness.

*Fluid and electrolyte disturbance:* Sodium and water retention, hypertension, hypokalaemic alkalosis, potassium loss, congestive heart failure in susceptible patients.

*Dermatological:* Impaired healing, skin atrophy, bruising, striae, telangiectasia, acne, petechiae and ecchymosis.

*Endocrine/metabolic:* Suppression of the hypothalamo-pituitary-adrenal axis, growth suppression in infancy, childhood and adolescence, menstrual irregularity and amenorrhoea. Cushingoid facies, hirsutism, weight gain, impaired carbohydrate tolerance with increased requirement for antidiabetic therapy, negative nitrogen and calcium balance. Increased appetite.

*Neuropsychiatric:* Euphoria, psychological dependence, mood swings, depression, personality changes, insomnia. Increased intra-cranial pressure with papilloedema in children (pseudotumour cerebri), usually after treatment withdrawal. Psychosis, aggravation of schizophrenia, seizures.

*Ophthalmic:* Increased intra-ocular pressure, glaucoma, papilloedema, cataracts with possible damage to the optic nerve, corneal or scleral thinning, exacerbation of ophthalmic viral or fungal disease, exophthalmos.

*General:* Leucocytosis, hypersensitivity reactions including anaphylaxis, thrombo-embolism, nausea, malaise.

*Withdrawal symptoms:* Too rapid a reduction of corticosteroid dosage following prolonged treatment can lead to acute adrenal insufficiency, hypotension and death (see *Special warnings and special precautions for use*).

A 'withdrawal syndrome' may also occur including, fever, myalgia, arthralgia, rhinitis, conjunctivitis, painful itchy skin nodules and loss of weight.

*Overdose:* Administration of Medrone should not be discontinued abruptly but tailed off over a period of time. Appropriate action should be taken to alleviate the symptoms produced by any side-effect that may become apparent. It may be necessary to support the patient with corticosteroids during any further period of trauma occurring within two years of overdosage.

There is no clinical syndrome of acute overdose with Medrone. Methylprednisolone is dialysable.

**Pharmacological properties**

*Pharmacodynamic properties:* Methylprednisolone is a potent anti-inflammatory steroid. It has greater anti-inflammatory potency than prednisolone and less tendency than prednisolone to induce sodium and water retention. The relative potency of methylprednisolone to hydrocortisone is at least four to one.

*Pharmacokinetic properties:* The mean elimination half-life ranges from 2.4 to 3.5 hours in normal, healthy adults and appears to be independent of the route of administration.

Methylprednisolone is metabolised in the liver to inactive metabolites, the major ones being 20 β-hydroxymethylprednisolone and 20 β-hydroxy-α-methylprednisolone.

Methylprednisolone clearance is altered by concurrent administration of troleandomycin, erythromycin, rifampicin, anticonvulsants and theophylline. No dosing adjustments are necessary in renal failure. Methylprednisolone is haemodialyzable.

**Pharmaceutical particulars**

*List of excipients:* Methylcellulose, sodium starch glycolate, microcrystalline cellulose, magnesium stearate and E132.

*Incompatibilities:* None stated.

*Shelf-life:* 48 months.

*Special precautions for storage:* Store below 25°C.

*Nature and contents of container:* Amber glass bottle with LDPE cap and bulb each bottle contains 20, tablets.

*Instructions for use/handling:* No special requirements.

**Marketing authorisation number** 0032/0145

**Date of approval/revision of SPC** September 1996

**Legal category** POM

## MINODIAB*

**Presentation** Minodiab is available as white, biconvex, 8 mm tablets containing 2.5 or 5 mg of glipizide. The 5 mg tablets are scored.

**Uses** Minodiab is an orally active hypoglycaemic sulphonylurea and has been shown to be effective in the treatment of diabetes mellitus Type II. In certain patients receiving insulin, the concurrent use of Minodiab allows a reduction in the daily dose of insulin.

**Dosage and administration** The usual dose range of Minodiab is 2.5–30 mg daily but if control is not achieved within this range then it may be increased to a total daily dose of 40 mg, although the additional proportion of patients responding to this higher dosage may not be large.

*Patients previously untreated:* The initial dose is 2.5–5 mg daily. Doses of 2.5 mg daily should be taken as a single dose before breakfast. Doses of 5 mg daily may be taken as a single dose before breakfast or as two doses; one in the morning and one in the evening before meals.

*Patients changing from other oral antidiabetics:* The recommended starting dose is 5 mg daily taken as a single dose or in two divided doses.

Dosage adjustments in all patients, either upwards or downwards, should be in 2.5–5 mg steps at weekly intervals until good control is achieved. The maximum recommended single dose is 15 mg. Doses above 15 mg should ordinarily be taken in 2 divided doses before meals. Multiple divided doses (2 or 3 daily) are recommended for patients who experience particularly high post-prandial blood glucose peaks.

Concomitant food intake may delay absorption and administration should therefore be 15–20 minutes before a main meal: therapeutic effects are usually seen within 30 minutes and peak at about 60 minutes. Glipizide is rapidly metabolised and excreted mainly in the urine and therefore it is unlikely that delayed hypoglycaemic episodes will occur.

When administered in divided daily doses glipizide can be considered as having a physiological action as its peak effect coincides with post-prandial peak blood-sugar levels.

A biguanide may be added to the treatment if control is not achieved with Minodiab.

**Contra-indications, warnings, etc**

*Contra-indications:* Minodiab is contra-indicated in pregnancy, juvenile diabetes, diabetic ketoacidosis, diabetic coma, severe renal or hepatic insufficiency, infections and febrile conditions, gangrene and in severe trauma and major surgical procedures.

*Warnings:* Concurrent use of MAOIs, phenylbutazone, β-blockers, sulphonamides, coumarin derivatives or salicylates may enhance the hypoglycaemic effect. Conversely the effect may be diminished in the presence of adrenaline, corticosteroids, oral contraceptives and thiazide diuretics.

Patients should be instructed to take their meals regularly and not to exercise excessively without additional calorie intake. Failure to do so may result in a hypoglycaemic episode. The hypoglycaemia is controlled by giving carbohydrates.

*Adverse reactions:* Side-effects are not common with Minodiab. Those that do occur are associated with the gastro-intestinal tract, and include nausea, vomiting, anorexia, gastric pain, etc. Skin reactions have been reported, e.g. rash, urticaria, pruritus, etc. Other reactions include headache, dizziness and vertigo.

*Overdosage:* Gastric lavage should be performed as soon as possible. Hypoglycaemia should be treated as it occurs with appropriate measures including oral or i.v. glucose.

**Pharmaceutical precautions** None.

**Legal category** POM.

**Package quantities** Cartons containing 60 tablets.

**Further information** Glipizide is almost completely absorbed from the GI tract and appears to act by stimulating insulin secretion from pancreatic β cells, but may also act by potentiating peripheral insulin action. Peak concentrations in blood are achieved within 60 minutes and the half-life is approximately 3½ hours.

**Product licence numbers**
Minodiab 2.5  3433/0022.
Minodiab 5  3433/0023.

## MONO-CEDOCARD*-10

**Presentation**  Round orange tablets, embossed 'C MONO C', reverse side scored, containing 10 mg isosorbide-5-mononitrate.

**Uses**  For the prophylaxis of angina pectoris.

Isosorbide Mononitrate, the active constituent of Mono-Cedocard-10, is the major active metabolite of isosorbide dinitrate. It has significant vasodilator activity, the strongest effect being exerted on the venous system and a lesser effect on the arterial circulation. As a consequence, the heart has less work to perform against diminished resistance and therefore oxygen requirement is reduced.

**Dosage and administration**  For oral administration.

*Adult dose:* One tablet two to three times a day. The tablet should be swallowed (without chewing) with a little water. The daily dosage may be increased to 120 mg if necessary, taken in divided doses. Mono-Cedocard-10 is suitable when lower dosage is used at the start of treatment.

*Dosage for the elderly:* The dosage of nitrates in cardiovascular disease is usually determined by patient response and stabilisation. Clinical experience has not necessitated alternative advice for use in elderly patients.
*There is no dose recommendation for children.*

**Contra-indications, warnings, etc**
*Contra-indications:* Acute myocardial infarction with low filling pressures. Acute circulatory failure (shock, vascular collapse). When blood pressure is very low. During the first three months of pregnancy.

*Warnings/precautions:* Some of the effects of alcohol and the action of hypotensive agents may be potentiated by isosorbide dinitrate.

*Adverse effects:* Generally, no serious adverse effects are to be expected. Headache, dizziness, fatigue, palpitations, orthostatic hypotension and flushing may occur, especially at the beginning of treatment. These reactions can usually be controlled by a temporary dosage reduction.

Patients who experience throbbing headache and dizziness, should be advised not to drive or operate machinery, if so affected.

*Use in pregnancy:* Mono-Cedocard-10 should not be used in the first trimester of pregnancy. Although no data have been reported which would indicate the possibility of adverse effects resulting from the use of isosorbide mononitrate during pregnancy, safety has not been established. Use of the drug in the second and third trimesters of pregnancy, should only occur if considered essential by the physician.

*Treatment of overdosage:* Gastric lavage: passive exercise of the extremities of the recumbent patient will promote venous return.

**Pharmaceutical precautions**
*Storage:* Protect from heat and moisture.

**Legal category**  P.

**Package quantities**  Packs of 60 tablets (OP).

**Further information**  The plasma half-life of isosorbide mononitrate is 4.2 hours. After oral administration, isosorbide mononitrate is well absorbed, a haemodynamic effect being measurable within 15–20 minutes. In contrast to isosorbide dinitrate, the mononitrate is not subject to first-pass metabolism.

**Product licence number** 0424/0072.

## MONO-CEDOCARD*-20

**Presentation**  Round white tablets, embossed 'MONO CC', reverse side scored, containing 20 mg isosorbide 5-mononitrate.

**Uses**  For the prophylaxis of angina pectoris.

Isosorbide mononitrate, the active constituent of Mono-Cedocard-20, is the major active metabolite of isosorbide dinitrate. It has significant vasodilator activity, the strongest effect being exerted on the venous system and a lesser effect on the arterial circulation. As a consequence, the heart has less work to perform against diminished resistance and therefore oxygen requirement is reduced.

**Dosage and administration**  For oral administration.

*Adult dose:* One tablet two or three times a day taken after meals. The tablet should be swallowed (without chewing) with a little water. The dosage may be increased to two tablets three times a day.

*Dosage for the elderly:* The dosage of nitrates in cardiovascular disease is usually determined by pa-

tient response and stabilisation. Clinical experience has not necessitated alternative advice for use in elderly patients.

There is no dose recommendation for children.

**Contra-indications, warnings, etc**
*Contra-indications:* In acute myocardial infarction with low filling pressures. Acute circulatory failure (shock, vascular collapse). When blood pressure is very low. During the first three months of pregnancy.

*Warnings/precautions:* Consumption of alcohol should be avoided during treatment, as reaction capacity may be reduced, and the vasodilator activity of isosorbide mononitrate may be enhanced. Symptoms of circulatory collapse can arise in patients already taking ACE inhibitors.

*Adverse effects:* Generally, no serious adverse effects are to be expected. Headache, dizziness, fatigue, palpitations, orthostatic hypotension and flushing may occur, especially at the beginning of treatment. These reactions can usually be controlled by a temporary dosage reduction.

*Treatment of overdosage:* Gastric lavage; passive exercise of the extremities of the recumbent patient will promote venous return.

**Pharmaceutical precautions**  *Storage:* Protect from heat and moisture.

**Legal category**  P.

**Package quantities**  Packs of 100 tablets (OP).

**Further information**  The plasma half-life of isosorbide mononitrate is 4.2 hours.

After oral administration, isosorbide mononitrate is well absorbed, a haemodynamic effect being measurable within 15–20 minutes. In contrast to isosorbide dinitrate, the mononitrate is not subject to first-pass metabolism.

**Product licence number**  0424/0040.

## MONO-CEDOCARD*-40

**Qualitative and quantitative composition**  Isosorbide-5-mononitrate-lactose 40 mg

**Pharmaceutical form**  Round, flat, bevel edged, white tablet, scored on one side and imprinted 40 MONO 40 on the other side.

**Clinical particulars**
*Therapeutic indications:* For the prophylaxis and maintenance of angina pectoris.

*Posology and method of administration:* By oral administration:
*Children:* There is no recommended dose for children.
*Adults:* One tablet to be taken twice daily after meals.
*Elderly adults:* As for adult dose.

*Contra-indications:* Acute myocardial infarction with low filling pressures; acute circulatory failure (shock and vascular collapse). Severe hypotension. During the first trimester of pregnancy.

*Special warnings:* Consumption of alcohol should be avoided during treatment, as reaction capacity may be reduced and the vasodilator activity of isosorbide mononitrate may be enhanced.

*Interaction with other medicaments and other forms of interaction:* Nitrates may potentiate the effects of anti-hypertensive agents. The vasodilator activity of isosorbide mononitrate may be enhanced by alcohol.

*Use during pregnancy and lactation:* No data have been reported which would indicate the possibility of adverse effects resulting from the use of nitrates in pregnancy. However, safety in pregnancy has not been established. Isosorbide mononitrate should only be used in pregnancy if, in the opinion of the practitioner, the possible benefits of treatment outweigh the possible hazards.

*Effects on ability to drive and use machines:* Side effects include throbbing headache and dizziness. Patients are advised not to drive or operate machinery if so affected.

*Undesirable effects:* Most commonly transient headaches which can usually be controlled by temporary dosage reduction. Less frequently, cutaneous vasodilation with flushing, transient episodes of dizziness and weakness and other signs of cerebral ischaemia can occur with postural hypotension.

*Overdosage:* Symptoms and signs of overdosage include vomiting, hypotension, restlessness, syncope, cyanosis, headache, flushing, dizziness, collapse, convulsions and methaemoglobinaemia. Treatment should include emesis or gastric lavage, if appropriate. Symptomatic and supportive measures should be provided. Syncope should be treated by keeping the patient in recumbent position. Fluid replacement with or without vasopressors may be indicated. Methae-

moglobinaemia should be treated with intravenous injection of 1 mg to 4 mg/kg of methylene blue.

**Pharmacological properties**
*Pharmacodynamic properties:* Isosorbide-5-mononitrate is a vasodilator.

*Pharmacokinetic properties:* Isosorbide-5-mononitrate is readily absorbed from the gastrointestinal tract following oral administration; it does not undergo first-pass hepatic metabolism and it is eliminated more slowly than is isosorbide dinitrate.

*Preclinical safety data:* Isosorbide mononitrate is a well established drug for which there are adequate published safety data.

**Pharmaceutical particulars**
*Excipients:*

| | |
|---|---|
| Lactose | PhEur |
| Talc | PhEur |
| Colloidal Silicon Dioxide (Aerosil 200) | DAB |
| Microcrystalline Cellulose | DAB |
| Potato starch | PhEur |
| Aluminium stearate | HSE |

*Incompatibilities:* None stated.

*Shelf life:* 5 years when stored at room temperature

*Special precautions for storage:* To be protected from heat and moisture.

*Nature and contents of container:* The tablets are presented in aluminium/PVC blisters, strips of which are contained within a printed cardboard carton.

*Instructions for use and handling:* No specific statement

**Marketing authorisation number**  0424/0054

**Date of approval/revision of SPC**  8 July 1996

**Legal category**  POM

## MCR-50* (MONO CEDOCARD RETARD-50)

**Presentation**  Hard gelatin slow release capsules (size 3) containing 50 mg isosorbide mononitrate. Each capsule contains white micro pellets which are specially formulated to release 30% of the dose initially and the remaining 70% as a maintenance dose.

**Uses**  For the prophylaxis of angina pectoris.

**Dosage and administration**  The capsules are for oral administration and should be swallowed whole.

*Adults:* One capsule to be taken in the morning.

*Elderly patients:* The dosage of nitrates in cardiovascular disease is usually determined by patient response and stabilisation. Clinical experience has not necessitated alternative advice for use in elderly patients.

*Children:* The safety and efficacy of MCR-50 in children has yet to be established.

For patients with higher nitrate requirements the dose may be increased to two capsules daily.

**Contra-indications, warnings, etc**
*Contra-indications:* MCR-50 should not be used in cases of acute myocardial infarction with low filling pressures, acute circulatory failure (shock, vascular collapse) or very low blood pressure.

This product should not be given to patients with a known sensitivity to nitrates.

MCR-50 should not be used in patients with marked anaemia, head trauma, cerebral haemorrhage, severe hypotension or hypovolaemia.

*Precautions and warnings:* This preparation may give rise to postural hypotension and syncope at higher doses. This may be avoided if treatment is started with the lowest dose possible.

Some of the effects of alcohol and the action of hypotensive agents may be potentiated by this product. MCR-50 should be used with caution in patients who are pre-disposed to closed angle glaucoma.

A headache may occur at the start of the treatment but this usually disappears after a few days.

This product should not be used during pregnancy or lactation unless considered essential by the physician. MCR-50 should be used with caution in patients suffering from hypothyroidism, hypothermia, malnutrition, severe liver or renal disease.

Symptoms of circulatory collapse may arise after the first dose, particularly in patients with labile circulation.

**Pharmaceutical precautions**  None.

**Legal category**  P.

**Package quantities**  MCR-50 is calendar packed in cartons of 28 capsules (OP).

**Further information**  MCR-50 is a long-acting nitrate which is effective for twenty four hours. The total amount of drug is divided into micro pellets which distribute themselves throughout the gastro-intestinal tract, thus giving a controlled and predictable release of isosorbide 5-mononitrate.

Each micro pellet releases 30% of the dose initially and the remaining 70% as a maintenance dose.

Isosorbide mononitrate is the British Approved Name for isosorbide 5-mononitrate.

MCR-50 lacks any significant first pass metabolism providing consistently uniform plasma levels of isosorbide mononitrate thereby laying the foundation for improved clinical response.

**Product licence number** 0424/0081.

## MOTRIN*

**Presentation** Film-coated tablets containing Ibuprofen BP:

200 mg – round, biconvex, yellow tablet marked U on one side;

400 mg – round, biconvex, orange tablet marked U on one side;

600 mg – elliptical, peach tablet marked U on one side;

800 mg – elliptical, capsule shaped, white tablet marked MOTRIN 800 on one side.

Motrin Tablets 200 mg, 400 mg, 600 mg also contain maize starch, colloidal silicon dioxide, pregelatinised starch, stearic acid and carnauba wax. In addition, Motrin Tablets 200 mg contain E110, E104; Motrin Tablets 400 mg and 600 mg contain hydroxypropyl methylcellulose, propylene glycol and E110.

Motrin Tablets 800 mg contain silicon dioxide, croscarmellose sodium, magnesium stearate, microcrystalline cellulose, talc, E464, E171, propylene glycol and carnauba wax.

**Uses** Non-steroidal, anti-inflammatory agent with analgesic and antipyretic properties. Motrin is indicated for the relief of the signs and symptoms of rheumatoid arthritis (including Still's Disease), osteoarthritis, ankylosing spondylitis and seronegative (non-rheumatoid) arthropathies. It may also be used in non-articular rheumatic conditions and soft tissue injuries; these include low back pain, capsulitis, bursitis, tenosynovitis, sprains and strains.

### Dosage and administration

*Adults:* 1200 – 1800 mg daily in three divided doses; up to 2400 mg daily may be given in severe conditions.

*Children:* 20 mg/kg daily in divided doses. In juvenile rheumatoid arthritis, up to 40 mg/kg daily in divided doses may be taken. In those children weighing less than 30 kg, the total dose in 24 hours should not exceed 500 mg.

If gastro-intestinal complaints occur, administer Motrin with food or milk.

*Elderly patients:* It appears that advanced age has a minimal influence on the pharmacokinetics of ibuprofen. However, the following should be considered:

Ibuprofen may increase levels of digoxin concentration, presumably from reduced renal excretion of digoxin.

Ibuprofen has been reported to have an antagonistic effect on frusemide-induced diuresis in cardiac failure.

Ibuprofen has been reported to be associated with cognitive dysfunction in the elderly.

Ibuprofen should be used with caution in association with anti-coagulants (warfarin).

### Contra-indications, warnings etc

*Contra-indications:* Active peptic ulceration. Motrin Tablets should not be given to patients who have previously shown hypersensitivity to the drug, or to those patients in whom aspirin, Motrin or other non-steroidal anti-inflammatory drugs induce the syndrome of nasal polyps, bronchospastic reactivity or angioedema. Fatal asthmatic and anaphylactoid reactions have occurred in such patients.

*Warnings:* Use with extreme caution in those patients with asthma. Fatal asthmatic and anaphylactic reactions have been reported.

Serious gastro-intestinal toxicity such as bleeding, ulceration and perforation of the stomach, small intestine or large intestine, have been reported in patients receiving ibuprofen. Motrin should be given under close supervision to patients with a history of upper gastro-intestinal tract disease.

Treatment should be discontinued in patients reporting blurred or diminished vision, scotomata and/or changes in colour vision.

*Precautions:* Administration of Motrin is not recommended during pregnancy. Reproductive studies conducted in rats and rabbits at doses somewhat less than the clinical maximum dose did not demonstrate any evidence of developmental abnormalities. As there are no adequate and well-controlled studies in pregnant women, this drug should be used during pregnancy only if clearly needed. Because of the known effects of non-steroidal anti-inflammatory drugs on the foetal cardiovascular system (closure of ductus arteriosus), use during late pregnancy should

be avoided. As with other drugs known to inhibit prostaglandin synthesis, an increased incidence of dystocia and delayed parturition occurred in rats.

In limited studies, an assay capable of detecting 1 microgram/ml did not demonstrate ibuprofen in the milk of lactating women. However, due to the limited nature of the studies and the possible adverse effects of prostaglandin-inhibiting drugs on neonates, Motrin is not recommended for use in nursing mothers.

Pre-existing asthma: About 10% of patients with asthma may have aspirin-sensitive asthma. The use of aspirin in patients with aspirin-sensitive asthma has been associated with severe bronchospasm which can be fatal. Since cross-reactivity, including bronchospasm, between aspirin and other non-steroidal anti-inflammatory drugs has been reported in such aspirin-sensitive patients, Motrin Tablets should not be administered to patients with this form of aspirin-sensitivity and should be used with caution in all patients with pre-existing asthma.

Fluid retention and oedema have been reported in association with Motrin; therefore, the drug should be used with caution in patients with a history of cardiac decompensation or hypertension.

As with other non-steroidal anti-inflammatory drugs, long-term administration of ibuprofen to animals has resulted in renal papillary necrosis and other abnormal renal pathology. In humans, there have been reports of acute interstitial nephritis with haematuria, proteinuria and occasionally nephrotic syndrome.

A second form of renal toxicity has been seen in patients with prerenal conditions leading to a reduction in renal blood flow or blood volume, where the renal prostaglandins have a supportive role in the maintenance of renal perfusion. In these patients, administration of a non-steroidal anti-inflammatory drug may cause a dose dependent reduction in prostaglandin formation and may precipitate overt renal decompensation. Patients at greatest risk of this reaction are those with impaired renal function, heart failure, liver dysfunction, those taking diuretics and the elderly. Discontinuation of non-steroidal anti-inflammatory drug therapy is typically followed by recovery to the pre-treatment state.

Since ibuprofen is eliminated primarily by the kidneys, patients with significantly impaired renal function should be closely monitored and a reduction in dosage should be anticipated to avoid drug accumulation.

Those patients at high risk of developing renal dysfunction during long-term treatment should have renal function monitored periodically.

Ibuprofen, like other non-steroidal anti-inflammatory drugs, can inhibit platelet aggregation, but the effect is quantitatively less and of shorter duration than that seen with aspirin. Motrin has been shown to prolong bleeding time (but within the normal range) in normal subjects. Because this prolonged bleeding effect may be exaggerated in patients with underlying haemostatic defects, Motrin should be used with caution in persons with intrinsic coagulation defects and those on anticoagulant therapy.

Patients on Motrin should report to their physicians signs or symptoms of gastro-intestinal ulceration or bleeding, blurred vision or other eye symptoms, skin rash, weight gain or oedema.

The antipyretic and anti-inflammatory activity of ibuprofen may reduce fever and inflammation, thus diminishing their utility as diagnostic signs in detecting complications of presumed non-infectious, non-inflammatory painful conditions.

*Drug interactions:*

*Coumarin-type anticoagulants:* Several short-term controlled studies failed to show that Motrin significantly affected prothrombin times, or a variety of other clotting factors, when administered to individuals on coumarin-type anticoagulants.

*Aspirin:* Animal studies show that aspirin given with non-steroidal anti-inflammatory drugs, including Motrin, causes a net decrease in anti-inflammatory activity with lowered blood levels of the non-aspirin drug.

*Methotrexate:* Motrin and other non-steroidal anti-inflammatory drugs have been reported to reduce renal tubular secretion of methotrexate *in vitro*. This may lead to enhanced toxicity of methotrexate. Caution should be used if Motrin is administered concomitantly with methotrexate.

*Diuretics:* Motrin has been shown to reduce the natriuretic effect of frusemide, thiazide or other diuretics in some patients, probably due to inhibition of renal prostaglandin synthesis by Motrin and other non-steroidal anti-inflammatory drugs. Patients being treated concomitantly with Motrin and frusemide, thiazide or other diuretics should therefore be observed closely.

*Anti-hypertensive agents:* Antagonism of the anti-hypertensive effect of beta-adrenergic blocking agents by non-steroidal anti-inflammatory drugs including Motrin has been reported. During the co-administra-

tion of these drugs, as well as other anti-hypertensive medications, care should be taken to monitor blood pressure.

*Lithium:* Motrin has been shown to produce a clinically relevant elevation of plasma lithium levels and a reduction in renal lithium clearance in a volunteer study. This effect has been attributed to inhibition of renal prostaglandin synthesis. Thus, when Motrin and lithium are administered concurrently, subjects should be carefully observed for signs of lithium toxicity.

*Cardiac glycosides:* Increased plasma levels of cardiac glycosides may occur during concomitant administration with ibuprofen.

*Quinolones:* The CNS excitatory effects of 4-quinolones may be increase by concomitant administration of non-steroidal anti-inflammatory drugs.

*Adverse reactions:* A decrease in haemoglobin content of 1 gram or more has been observed in 20% of patients.

Gastro-intestinal effects are a frequent adverse reaction to Motrin Tablets.

The following adverse reactions may occur in 3–9% of patients taking Motrin Tablets: nausea, epigastric pain, dizziness, non-specific rash, elevated serum creatinine levels and anaemia.

The following rarely occurring adverse reactions have been reported in patients taking Motrin Tablets: renal failure, lupus erythematosus syndrome with aseptic meningitis, jaundice, abnormal liver function tests, blood dyscrasias including thrombocytopenia, colitis, exacerbation of inflammatory bowel disease, perforation of the colon, inflammation of the small intestine with loss of blood and protein, collagenous colitis, small bowel perforation, ulcer or stricture, complications of colonic diverticula (perforation, fistula). Aseptic meningitis is probably more common in patients with systemic lupus erythematosus and related connective tissue diseases.

*Treatment of overdosage:* Gastric lavage. No specific antidote. It is theoretically advantageous to administer alkali and induce diuresis as the drug is acidic and excreted in the urine.

**Pharmaceutical precautions** Motrin Tablets 200 mg, 400 mg and 600 mg should be stored below 25°C in a well-closed container. Motrin Tablets 800 mg should be stored below 25°C.

**Legal category** POM

**Package quantities** 200 mg, 400 mg, 600 mg and 800 mg strengths–packs of 90 tablets.

**Further information** The absorption profile shows Motrin to be of particular value in relieving morning stiffness.

**Product licence numbers**

| | |
|---|---|
| 200 mg | 0032/0104 |
| 400 mg | 0032/0105 |
| 600 mg | 0032/0106 |
| 800 mg | 0032/0134 |

## MYCIFRADIN* SULPHATE TABLETS 0.5 g

**Qualitative and quantitiative composition** Each tablet contains 500 mg neomycin sulphate.

**Pharmaceutical form:** An off-white, biconvex oval tablet for oral use.

**Clinical particulars**

*Therapeutic indications:* Antibacterial.

For pre-operative suppression of bacterial bowel flora. Also for reduction of ammonia-forming bacteria in the intestine in hepatic coma.

*Posology and method of administration:* Oral.

*Adults:* Bowel surgery: One gram every 4 hours. Dosage should not continue longer than 72 hours.

Hepatic coma: 4 – 12 grams per day in divided doses for up to 6 days.

*Elderly patients:* It should be borne in mind that elderly patients may have some degree of renal impairment and thus not excrete neomycin normally. See *Special warnings and special precautions for use* section for other factors which should be taken into consideration.

*Children:* Safety and efficacy in patients under 18 years of age have not been established.

*Contra-indications:* The product is contra-indicated in patients who are receiving or have received, other ototoxic medications such as aminoglycosides or potent diuretics, in patients with ulcerative colitis, malabsorption syndrome or intestinal obstruction, in patients with renal insufficiency and in patients hypersensitive to neomycin.

*Special warnings and special precautions for use:*
*Warnings:* Systemic absorption of neomycin occurs following oral administration and toxic reactions may occur.

Neurotoxicity (including ototoxicity) and nephrotoxicity have been reported following oral administration of neomycin even when used in recommended doses. Higher doses of neomycin or administration for longer periods than recommended may give rise to ototoxicity and nephrotoxicity even in patients with normal renal function. The risk of hearing loss continues after drug withdrawal. The risk of ototoxicity and nephrotoxicity is greater in patients with impaired renal function. Use in such patients should be considered only when alternative therapy is clearly contra-indicated.

Neuromuscular blockade and respiratory paralysis have been reported following the oral use of neomycin. Concurrent administration of neomycin with a neuromuscular blocking agent may enhance neuromuscular blockade and lead to respiratory paralysis. Thus, the use of neomycin in patients receiving such agents or in patients with myasthenia gravis, should be avoided.

Concurrent and/or sequential systemic, oral or topical use of other aminoglycoside antibiotics and other potentially nephrotoxic or neurotoxic drugs should be avoided because the toxicity may be additive.

The concurrent use of neomycin with potent diuretics such as ethacrynic acid or frusemide should be avoided since certain diuretics by themselves may cause ototoxicity. In addition, when administered intravenously, diuretics may enhance neomycin toxicity by altering the antibiotic concentration in serum and tissue.

*Precautions:* As with other antibiotics, use of neomycin may result in the overgrowth of nonsusceptible organisms, particularly fungi.

Cross allergenicity among aminoglycosides has been demonstrated.

*Laboratory tests:* Patients with renal insufficiency may develop toxic neomycin blood levels unless doses are properly regulated. If renal insufficiency develops during treatment, the dosage should be reduced or the antibiotic discontinued. To avoid nephrotoxicity and eighth nerve damage associated with high doses and prolonged treatment, the following should be performed prior to and periodically during therapy: urinalysis for increased excretion of protein, decreased specific gravity, casts and cells; renal function tests such as serum creatinine, BUN or creatinine clearance; tests of the vestibulocochlearis nerve (eighth cranial nerve) function. During prolonged treatment, neomycin serum concentrations should be monitored to detect the presence of systemic absorption. Ototoxicity has been reported in cases with neomycin blood levels as low as 0.4 – 1.2 microgram/ml.

Serial vestibular and audiometric tests should be performed (especially in high risk patients). Since elderly patients may have reduced renal function which may not be evident in the results of routine screening tests such as BUN or serum creatinine, a creatinine clearance determination may be more useful.

*Interaction with other medicaments and other forms of interaction:* Oral neomycin at high doses may produce a malabsorption syndrome for a variety of substances including fat, nitrogen, cholesterol, carotene, glucose, xylose, lactose, sodium, calcium, cyanocobalamin and iron.

Although the clinical significance has not been established clearly, neomycin has been reported to decrease the gastro-intestinal absorption of penicillin, methotrexate and 5-fluorouracil and digoxin. Oral neomycin may enhance the effect of coumarin in anticoagulation by decreasing vitamin K availability.

*Pregnancy and lactation:* Some aminoglycosides cross the placenta and although serious side-effects to the foetus or newborn have not been reported in the treatment of the pregnant woman with neomycin, the potential for harm exists. Because of this risk, use in pregnancy is not recommended unless clearly indicated based on an assessment of benefit-risk.

Aminoglycosides are excreted in human milk. Administration to nursing mothers is not recommended unless it is clearly indicated based on an assessment of benefit-risk.

*Effects on ability to drive and use machines:* None

*Undesirable effects:* The most common adverse reactions to oral neomycin are nausea, vomiting and diarrhoea.

*Overdose:* In the event of signs or symptoms of ototoxicity or nephrotoxicity occurring, discontinue treatment immediately.

**Pharmacological properties**

*Pharmacodynamic properties:* Neomycin is a broad spectrum bactericidal aminoglycoside antibiotic, with activity against both Gram-positive and Gram-negative organisms.

*Pharmacokinetic properties:* About 97% of an oral

dose is excreted unchanged with faeces and a daily intake of 10 g for 3 days yields a blood level below that associated with systemic toxicity. Approximately 0.7% of the total oral dose is excreted in the urine within 24 hours. Gastro-intestinal ulceration does not seem to affect absorption, although gastroenteritis in children may augment it.

**Pharmaceutical particulars**

*List of excipients:* Povidone, calcium stearate.

*Incompatibilities:* None

*Shelf-life:* 60 months

*Special precautions for storage:* Keep container tightly closed. Store below 25°C.

*Nature and contents of container:* Amber glass tablet bottle with screw cap containing 100 tablets. High density polyethylene bottle with white LDPE tamper evident cap containing 100 or 500 tablets.

*Instructions for use/handling:* None

**Marketing authorisation number:** 0032/5012R

**Date of approval/revision of SPC** October 1995.

**Legal category** POM

# MYCOBUTIN*

**Qualitative and quantitative composition** Rifabutin INN 150.0 mg.

**Pharmaceutical form** Opaque, red-brown, hard gelatin capsules Size No.0 containing 150 mg rifabutin in transparent PVC/Al blisters or in amber glass bottles.
The capsules are for oral administration.

**Clinical particulars**

*Therapeutic indications:* Mycobutin is indicated for:
- the prophylaxis of M. avium intracellulare complex (MAC) infections in patients with HIV disease with CD4 counts lower than 75 cells/mcl.
- the treatment of non-tuberculous mycobacterial disease (such as that caused by MAC and M. xenopi).
- pulmonary tuberculosis.

*Posology and method of administration:* Mycobutin can be administered as a single, daily, oral dose at any time independently of meals.

*Adults:*
Prophylaxis of M. avium intracellulare complex (MAC) infections in patients with HIV disease with CD4 counts lower than 75 cells/mcl: 300 mg (2 capsules) as a single agent.
Treatment of non-tuberculous mycobacterial disease: 450 – 600 mg (3 – 4 capsules) in combination regimens for up to 6 months after negative cultures are obtained.
When Mycobutin is given in association with clarithromycin (or other macrolides) and/or fluconazole (or related compounds) the Mycobutin dosage may need to be reduced to 300 mg (see Interactions with other medicaments and other forms of interaction section).
Treatment of pulmonary tuberculosis: 150 – 450 mg (1 – 3 capsules) in combination regimens for at least 6 months.
In accordance with the commonly accepted criteria for the treatment of mycobacterial infections, Mycobutin should always be given in combination with other anti-mycobacterial drugs not belonging to the family of rifamycins.

*Children:* There are inadequate data to support the use of Mycobutin in children at the present time.

*Elderly:* No specific recommendations for dosage alterations in the elderly are suggested.

*Contra-indications:* Mycobutin is contra-indicated in patients with a history of hypersensitivity to rifabutin or other rifamycins (e.g. rifampicin).
Due to insufficient clinical experience in pregnant and breast-feeding women and in children, Mycobutin should not be used in these patients.

*Special warnings and special precautions for use:* Before starting Mycobutin prophylaxis, patients should be assessed to ensure that they do not have active disease caused by pulmonary tuberculosis or other mycobacteria.
Prophylaxis against MAC infection may need to be continued throughout the patient's lifetime.
Mycobutin may impart a red-orange colour to the urine and possibly to skin and body secretions. Contact lenses, especially soft, may be permanently stained.
Mild hepatic impairment does not require a dose modification. Mycobutin should be used with caution in cases of severe liver insufficiency. Mild to moderate renal impairment does not require any dosage adjustment.
Severe renal impairment (creatinine clearance below 30 ml/min) requires a dosage reduction of 50%.
It is recommended that white blood cell and platelet

counts and liver enzymes be monitored periodically during treatment.

Because of the possibility of occurrence of uveitis, patients should be carefully monitored when rifabutin is given in combination with clarithromycin (or other macrolides) and/or fluconazole (and related compounds). If such an event occurs, the patient should be referred to an ophthalmologist and, if considered necessary, Mycobutin treatment should be suspended.

Uveitis associated with Mycobutin must be distinguished from other ocular complications of HIV.

*Interactions with other medicaments and other forms of interaction:* Rifabutin has been shown to induce the enzymes of the cytochrome P450 3A subfamily and therefore may affect the pharmacokinetic behaviour of drugs metabolised by the enzymes belonging to this subfamily. Upward adjustment of the dosage of such drugs may be required when administered with Mycobutin. For this reason, during Mycobutin therapy oral contraception may not be adequate and patients should be advised to use other forms of contraception.

Similarly, Mycobutin might reduce the activity of analgesics, anticoagulants, corticosteroids, cyclosporin, digitalis (although not digoxin), dapsone, oral hypoglycaemics, narcotics, phenytoin and quinidine.

Although pharmacokinetic data have shown that Mycobutin when given in combination with zidovudine reduces the plasma levels of the latter, a large controlled clinical study has shown that these changes are of no clinical relevance. Clinical studies have shown that Mycobutin does not affect the pharmacokinetics of didanosine (DDI), isoniazid (for the latter refer also to *Undesirable effects*). On the basis of the above metabolic considerations no significant reaction may be expected with ethambutol, theophylline, sulphonamides, pyrazinamide and zalcitabine (DDC).

An interaction, leading to an increase in rifabutin plasma levels, occurs when Mycobutin is administered together with clarithromycin and/or fluconazole. This may apply to drugs of the same classes (refer to *Undesirable effects* and *Special precautions*). However, Mycobutin does not affect the pharmacokinetics of fluconazole.

As p-aminosalicylic acid has been shown to impede GI absorption of rifamycins it is recommended that when it and Mycobutin are both to be administered they be given with an interval of 8 – 12 hours.

*Pregnancy and lactation:* Due to lack of data in pregnant women, as a precautionary measure, Mycobutin should not be administered to pregnant women or those breast-feeding children even though in experimental animal studies the drug was not teratogenic.

Mycobutin may interact with oral contraceptives (see *Interactions with other medicaments and other forms of interaction* section).

*Effects on ability to drive and use machines:* There have been no reports of adverse effects on ability to drive and use machines.

*Undesirable effects:* The tolerability of Mycobutin in multiple drug regimens, was assessed in both immunocompetent and immunocompromised patients, suffering from tuberculosis and non-tuberculous mycobacteriosis in long term studies with daily dosages up to 600 mg.

Bearing in mind that Mycobutin was often given in these studies as part of a multidrug regimen it is not possible to define with certainty a drug-event relationship. Treatment discontinuation was necessary only in a very few cases. The most commonly reported adverse events, were primarily related to:
– the gastro-intestinal system, such as nausea, vomiting, increase of liver enzymes, jaundice;
– the blood and lymphatic system, such as leucopenia, neutropenia, thrombocytopenia and anemia, where the frequency and severity of haematologic reactions could be increased by combined administration of isoniazid;
– the musculo-skeletal system: arthralgia and myalgia.

Also, fever, rash and rarely other hypersensitivity reactions such as eosinophilia, bronchospasm and shock might occur as has been seen with other antibiotics.

In addition, mild to severe, reversible uveitis has been reported. The risk appears to be low, when Mycobutin is used at 300 mg as monotherapy in MAC prophylaxis, but increases when Mycobutin is administered at higher doses in combination with clarithromycin (or other macrolides) for MAC treatment (see *Special warnings and special precautions for use* section). The possible role of fluconazole (and related compounds) has not been established yet. Asymptomatic corneal opacities have been reported after long term therapy. Pseudojaundice (yellow skin discolouration with normal plasma bilirubin) has been reported with high doses of rifabutin. Flu-like syndrome, chest pressure or pain with dyspnoea and rarely hepatitis and haemolysis. *Clostridium difficile* diarrhoea has been reported rarely.

*Overdose:* Gastric lavage and diuretic treatment should be carried out. Supportive care and symptomatic treatment should be administered.

**Pharmacological properties**
*Pharmacodynamic properties: In vitro* activity of rifabutin against laboratory strains and clinical isolates of *M. tuberculosis* has been shown to be very high. *In vitro* studies carried out so far have shown that from one-third to half of *M.tuberculosis* strains resistant to rifampicin are susceptible to rifabutin, indicating that cross-resistance between the two antibiotics is incomplete.

The *in vivo* activity of rifabutin on experimental infections caused by *M. tuberculosis* was about 10 times greater than that of rifampicin in agreement with the *in vitro* findings.

Rifabutin was seen to be active against non-tuberculous (atypical) mycobacteria including *M. avium-intracellulare* (MAC), *in vitro* as well as in experimental infections caused by these pathogens in mice with induced immuno-deficiency.

*Pharmacokinetic properties:* In man, rifabutin is rapidly absorbed and maximum plasma concentrations are reached around 2 – 4 hours after oral administration. The pharmacokinetics of rifabutin is linear after single administration of 300, 450, and 600 mg to healthy volunteers. With these doses, C max is in the range of 0.4 – 0.7 microgram/ml. Plasma concentrations are maintained above the MIC values for *M. tuberculosis* up to about 30 hours from administration.

Rifabutin is widely distributed in various animal organs with the exception of the brain. In particular, in human lung tissue the concentrations measured up to 24 hours after dosing were about 5 – 10 times higher than the plasma levels.

The intracellular penetration of rifabutin is very high as demonstrated by intracellular/extracellular concentration ratios which ranged from 9 in neutrophils to 15 in monocytes, both obtained from human sources.

The high intracellular concentration is likely to play a crucial role in sustaining the efficacy of rifabutin against intracellular pathogens such as mycobacteria.

Rifabutin and its metabolites are eliminated mainly by the urinary route. The $t_{\frac{1}{2}}\beta$ of rifabutin in man is approximately 35 – 40 hours.

*Preclinical safety data: Preclinical safety studies of rifabutin indicate a good safety margin in rodents and in monkeys.*

In repeated dose studies, target organs were identified at doses producing blood levels higher than those achieved with recommended doses for human therapy. The main target organs are liver and, to a lesser degree, erythrocytes.

Rifabutin did not show any teratogenic, mutagenic or carcinogenic potential.

**Pharmaceutical particulars**
*List of excipients:* Microcrystalline cellulose; sodium lauryl sulphate; magnesium stearate; silica gel

*Incompatibilities:* None known.

*Shelf life:* 24 months at room temperature.

*Special precautions for storage:* None.

*Nature and contents of container:* Transparent PVC/Al blisters in cardboard cartons containing 30 capsules or amber glass bottles containing 30 or 100 capsules.

*Instructions for use/handling:* There are no special instructions for handling.

**Marketing authorisation number** 3433/0168

**Date of approval/revision of SPC** 30 July 1997

**Legal category** POM

## NICORETTE*

**Presentation** Square pieces of chewing gum containing 2 mg nicotine in a chewing gum base.

**Uses**
*Pharmacology:* When Nicorette is chewed, nicotine is slowly released into the mouth and is absorbed through the buccal mucosa, the desired action is relief of unpleasant symptoms associated with smoking cessation. A proportion, by the swallowing of nicotine-containing saliva, reaches the stomach and intestine where it is inactivated.

*Indications:* Nicorette is intended to help smokers who want to give up smoking, but experience great difficulty in doing so because of their nicotine dependence.

**Dosage and administration**
*Adults (including the elderly):* The rate of gum use should depend upon the previous smoking habits of the individual.

Nicorette should be chewed slowly when there is an urge to smoke, up to a maximum of 15 pieces per day; however the patient's individual need may be considerably less than this. If more than 15 pieces of Nicorette per day are required, treatment with 4 mg nicotine gum (Nicorette Plus) may be considered. Most patients require about 10 pieces of gum per day initially. All available nicotine is released from a piece of gum after about 30 minutes chewing. Since effective absorption is through the buccal mucosa, the rate of chewing should be adjusted to minimise the swallowing and inactivation of nicotine contained in saliva.

After 3 months ad libitum dosage, Nicorette should be gradually withdrawn.

*Children:* Not to be administered to children.

**Contra-indications, warnings, etc**
*Contra-indications:* Nicotine in any form is contra-indicated in pregnancy.

*Precautions:* Swallowed nicotine may exacerbate symptoms in patients suffering from gastritis or peptic ulcers.

Nicotine's cardiovascular effects may be deleterious to patients with angina or a history of coronary artery disease. Nicorette presents a lesser hazard, however, than smoking, which introduces carbon monoxide as an additional toxic factor.

*Warnings and adverse effects:* Nicorette in the recommended dose has not been found to cause any serious adverse effects. Nicotine from the gum may sometimes cause a slight irritation of the throat at the start of treatment, and may also cause increased salivation. Allergic reactions such as angiodema and urticaria, and ulcerative stomatitis have been reported.

Excessive swallowing of dissolved nicotine may, at first, cause hiccuping. Those with a tendency of indigestion may suffer initially from minor degrees of indigestion or heartburn, slower chewing will usually overcome this problem.

Dependence is a rare side-effect and is both less harmful and easier to break than smoking dependence.

Excessive consumption of Nicorette by patients who have not been in the habit of inhaling tobacco smoke could possibly lead to nausea, faintness or headaches (as may be experienced by such a patient if tobacco smoke is inhaled).

Smokers who wear dentures may experience difficulty in chewing Nicorette.

*Overdosage:* Overdosage of Nicorette can occur only if many pieces are chewed simultaneously. The fatal acute dose of nicotine in man is probably about 60 mg. Risk of overdosage with Nicorette is, however, small since nausea or vomiting usually occurs at an early stage.

Risk of poisoning by swallowing the gum is also small, since the release of nicotine from the gum is slow. Therefore very little nicotine is absorbed from the stomach and intestine and any that is will be inactivated in the liver. Nicotine is excreted in acid urine four times as rapidly as in alkaline urine.

*Treatment of overdosage:* In the event of overdosage vomiting should be induced with syrup of ipecacuanha or gastric lavage carried out (wide bore tube). A suspension of activated charcoal should then be passed through the tube and left in the stomach. Artificial respiration with oxygen should be instituted if needed and continued for as long as necessary. Other therapy, including treatment of shock, is purely symptomatic.

**Pharmaceutical precautions** No special storage conditions are necessary. The preparation has a shelf-life at room temperature of 30 months from the date of manufacture.

**Legal category** P.

**Package quantities** Packages of 30 or 105 pieces, in the form of blister-packed strips each containing 15 pieces.

**Further information** Nicorette should be chewed slowly. Sufficient nicotine may be released from the gum by chewing intermittently and leaving the gum under the lip or in the corner of the mouth between chews. Nicorette is sugar-free.

**Product licence number** 0022/0101

## NICORETTE PLUS*

**Presentation** Square pieces of chewing gum containing 4 mg nicotine in a chewing gum base.

**Uses**
*Pharmacology:* When Nicorette Plus is chewed, nicotine is slowly released into the mouth and is absorbed through the buccal mucosa, the desired action is relief of unpleasant symptoms associated with smoking cessation. A proportion, by the swallowing of nicotine-containing saliva, reaches the stomach and intestine where it is inactivated.

*Indications:* Nicorette Plus is intended to help smokers who want to give up smoking, but experience great difficulty in doing so because of their nicotine dependence, particularly those patients who are heavy smokers or who require more than 15 pieces of 2 mg nicotine gum (Nicorette) per day.

**Dosage and administration**
*Adults (including the elderly):* The rate of gum use should depend upon the previous smoking habits of the individual.

Nicorette Plus should be chewed slowly when there is an urge to smoke, up to a maximum of 15×4 mg pieces per day; however the patient's individual need may be considerably less than this. All available nicotine is released from a piece of gum after about 30 minutes chewing. Since effective absorption is through the buccal mucosa, the rate of chewing should be adjusted to minimise the swallowing and inactivation of nicotine contained in saliva.

After 3 months ad libitum dosage, Nicorette Plus should be gradually withdrawn.

*Children:* Not to be administered to children.

**Contra-indications, warnings, etc**
*Contra-indications:* Nicotine in any form is contra-indicated in pregnancy.

*Precautions:*
1. Swallowed nicotine may exacerbate symptoms in patients suffering from gastritis or peptic ulcers.
2. Nicotine's cardiovascular effects may be deleterious to patients with angina or a history of coronary artery disease. Nicorette Plus presents a lesser hazard, however, than smoking, which introduces carbon monoxide as an additional toxic factor.

*Warnings and adverse effects:* Nicorette Plus in the recommended dose has not been found to cause any serious adverse effects. Nicotine from the gum may sometimes cause a slight irritation of the throat at the start of treatment, and may also cause increased salivation. Allergic reactions such as angiodema and urticaria, and ulcerative stomatitis have been reported.

Excessive swallowing of dissolved nicotine may, at first, cause hiccuping. Those with a tendency of indigestion may suffer initially from minor degrees of indigestion or heartburn if Nicorette Plus is used; slower chewing and the use of 2 mg nicotine gum (Nicorette) (if necessary more frequently) will usually overcome this problem.

Dependence is a rare side-effect and is both less harmful and easier to break than smoking dependence.

Excessive consumption of Nicorette Plus by patients who have not been in the habit of inhaling tobacco smoke could possibly lead to nausea, faintness or headaches (as may be experienced by such a patient if tobacco smoke is inhaled).

Smokers who wear dentures may experience difficulty in chewing Nicorette Plus.

*Overdosage:* Overdosage of Nicorette Plus can occur only if many pieces are chewed simultaneously. The fatal acute dose of nicotine in man is probably about 60 mg. Risk of overdosage with Nicorette Plus is, however, small since nausea or vomiting usually occurs at an early stage.

Risk of poisoning by swallowing the gum is also small, since the release of nicotine from the gum is slow. Therefore very little nicotine is absorbed from the stomach and intestine and any that is will be inactivated in the liver. Nicotine is excreted in acid urine four times as rapidly as in alkaline urine.

*Treatment of overdosage:* In the event of overdosage vomiting should be induced with syrup of ipecacuanha or gastric lavage carried out (wide bore tube). A suspension of activated charcoal should then be passed through the tube and left in the stomach. Artificial respiration with oxygen should be instituted if needed and continued for as long as necessary. Other therapy, including treatment of shock, is purely symptomatic.

**Pharmaceutical precautions** No special storage conditions are necessary. The preparation has a shelf-life at room temperature of 30 months from the date of manufacture.

**Legal category** P.

**Package quantities** Blister packed strips each containing 15 pieces supplied in packs of 105 pieces.

**Further information** Nicorette Plus should be chewed slowly. Sufficient nicotine may be released from the gum by chewing intermittently and leaving the gum under the lip or in the corner of the mouth between chews. Nicorette Plus is sugar-free.

**Product licence number** 0022/0102

## NICORETTE* MINT

**Presentation** Square pieces of chewing gum containing 2 mg nicotine in a mint flavoured chewing gum base.

## Uses

*Pharmacology:* When Nicorette Mint is chewed, nicotine is slowly released into the mouth and is absorbed through the buccal mucosa, the desired action is relief of unpleasant symptoms associated with smoking cessation. A proportion, by the swallowing of nicotine-containing saliva, reaches the stomach and intestine where it is inactivated.

*Indications:* Nicorette Mint is intended to help smokers who want to give up smoking, but experience great difficulty in doing so because of their nicotine dependence.

## Dosage and administration

*Adults (including the elderly):* The rate of gum use should depend upon the previous smoking habits of the individual.

Nicorette Mint should be chewed slowly when there is an urge to smoke, up to a maximum of 15 pieces per day; however the patient's individual need may be considerably less than this. If more than 15 pieces of Nicorette Mint per day are required, treatment with 4 mg nicotine gum (Nicorette Mint Plus) may be considered. Most patients require about 10 pieces of gum per day initially. All available nicotine is released from a piece of gum after about 30 minutes chewing. Since effective absorption is through the buccal mucosa, the rate of chewing should be adjusted to minimise the swallowing and inactivation of nicotine contained in saliva.

After 3 months ad libitum dosage, Nicorette Mint should be gradually withdrawn.

*Children:* Not to be administered to children.

## Contra-indications, warnings, etc

*Contra-indications:* Nicotine in any form is contra-indicated in pregnancy.

*Precautions:* Swallowed nicotine may exacerbate symptoms in patients suffering from gastritis or peptic ulcers.

Nicotine's cardiovascular effects may be deleterious to patients with angina or a history of coronary artery disease. Nicorette Mint presents a lesser hazard, however, than smoking, which introduces carbon monoxide as an additional toxic factor.

*Warnings and adverse effects:* Nicorette Mint in the recommended dose has not been found to cause any serious adverse effects. Nicotine from the gum may sometimes cause a slight irritation of the throat at the start of treatment, and may also cause increased salivation. Allergic reactions such as angiodema and urticaria, and ulcerative stomatitis have been reported.

Excessive swallowing of dissolved nicotine may, at first, cause hiccuping. Those with a tendency of indigestion may suffer initially from minor degrees of indigestion or heartburn, slower chewing will usually overcome this problem.

Dependence is a rare side-effect and is both less harmful and easier to break than smoking dependence.

Excessive consumption of Nicorette Mint by patients who have not been in the habit of inhaling tobacco smoke could possibly lead to nausea, faintness or headaches (as may be experienced by such a patient if tobacco smoke is inhaled).

Smokers who wear dentures may experience difficulty in chewing Nicorette Mint.

*Overdosage:* Overdosage of Nicorette Mint can occur only if many pieces are chewed simultaneously. The fatal acute dose of nicotine in man is probably about 60 mg. Risk of overdosage with Nicorette Mint is, however, small since nausea or vomiting usually occurs at an early stage.

Risk of poisoning by swallowing the gum is also small, since the release of nicotine from the gum is slow. Therefore very little nicotine is absorbed from the stomach and intestine and any that is will be inactivated in the liver. Nicotine is excreted in acid urine four times as rapidly as in alkaline urine.

*Treatment of overdosage:* In the event of overdosage vomiting should be induced with syrup of ipecacuanha or gastric lavage carried out (wide bore tube). A suspension of activated charcoal should then be passed through the tube and left in the stomach. Artificial respiration with oxygen should be instituted if needed and continued for as long as necessary. Other therapy, including treatment of shock, is purely symptomatic.

**Pharmaceutical precautions** No special storage conditions are necessary. The preparation has a shelf-life at room temperature of 30 months from the date of manufacture.

**Legal category** P.

**Package quantities** Packages of 15, 30 or 105 pieces, in the form of blister-packed strips each containing 15 pieces.

**Further information** Nicorette Mint should be chewed slowly. Sufficient nicotine may be released from the gum by chewing intermittently and leaving the gum under the lip or in the corner of the mouth between chews. Nicorette Mint is sugar-free.

**Product licence number** 0022/0112

## NICORETTE MINT PLUS*

**Presentation** Square pieces of chewing gum containing 4 mg nicotine in a mint flavoured chewing gum base.

## Uses

*Pharmacology:* When Nicorette Mint Plus is chewed, nicotine is slowly released into the mouth and is absorbed through the buccal mucosa, the desired action is relief of unpleasant symptoms associated with smoking cessation. A proportion, by the swallowing of nicotine-containing saliva, reaches the stomach and intestine where it is inactivated.

*Indications:* Nicorette Mint Plus is intended to help smokers who want to give up smoking, but experience great difficulty in doing so because of their nicotine dependence, particularly those patients who are heavy smokers or who require more than 15 pieces of 2 mg nicotine gum (Nicorette Mint) per day.

## Dosage and administration

*Adults (including the elderly):* The rate of gum use should depend upon the previous smoking habits of the individual.

Nicorette Mint Plus should be chewed slowly when there is an urge to smoke, up to a maximum of 15×4 mg pieces per day; however the patient's individual need may be considerably less than this. All available nicotine is released from a piece of gum after about 30 minutes chewing. Since effective absorption is through the buccal mucosa, the rate of chewing should be adjusted to minimise the swallowing and inactivation of nicotine contained in saliva.

After 3 months ad libitum dosage, Nicorette Mint Plus should be gradually withdrawn.

*Children:* Not to be administered to children.

## Contra-indications, warnings, etc

*Contra-indications:* Nicotine in any form is contra-indicated in pregnancy.

*Precautions:*

1. Swallowed nicotine may exacerbate symptoms in patients suffering from gastritis or peptic ulcers.

2. Nicotine's cardiovascular effects may be deleterious to patients with angina or a history of coronary artery disease. Nicorette Mint Plus presents a lesser hazard, however, than smoking, which introduces carbon monoxide as an additional toxic factor.

*Warnings and adverse effects:* Nicorette Mint Plus in the recommended dose has not been found to cause any serious adverse effects. Nicotine from the gum may sometimes cause a slight irritation of the throat at the start of treatment, and may also cause increased salivation. Allergic reactions such as angiodema and urticaria, and ulcerative stomatitis have been reported.

Excessive swallowing of dissolved nicotine may, at first, cause hiccuping. Those with a tendency of indigestion may suffer initially from minor degrees of indigestion or heartburn if Nicorette Mint Plus is used; slower chewing and the use of 2 mg nicotine gum (Nicorette Mint) (if necessary more frequently) will usually overcome this problem.

Dependence is a rare side-effect and is both less harmful and easier to break than smoking dependence.

Excessive consumption of Nicorette Mint Plus by patients who have not been in the habit of inhaling tobacco smoke could possibly lead to nausea, faintness or headaches (as may be experienced by such a patient if tobacco smoke is inhaled).

Smokers who wear dentures may experience difficulty in chewing Nicorette Mint Plus.

*Overdosage:* Overdosage of Nicorette Mint Plus can occur only if many pieces are chewed simultaneously. The fatal acute dose of nicotine in man is probably about 60 mg. Risk of overdosage with Nicorette Mint Plus is, however, small since nausea or vomiting usually occurs at an early stage.

Risk of poisoning by swallowing the gum is also small, since the release of nicotine from the gum is slow. Therefore very little nicotine is absorbed from the stomach and intestine and any that is will be inactivated in the liver. Nicotine is excreted in acid urine four times as rapidly as in alkaline urine.

*Treatment of overdosage:* In the event of overdosage vomiting should be induced with syrup of ipecacuanha or gastric lavage carried out (wide bore tube). A suspension of activated charcoal should then be passed through the tube and left in the stomach. Artificial respiration with oxygen should be instituted if needed and continued for as long as necessary. Other therapy, including treatment of shock, is purely symptomatic.

**Pharmaceutical precautions** No special storage conditions are necessary. The preparation has a shelf-life at room temperature of 30 months from the date of manufacture.

**Legal category** P.

**Package quantities** Packages of 15, 30 or 105 pieces, in the form of blister-packed strips each containing 15 pieces.

**Further information** Nicorette Mint Plus should be chewed slowly. Sufficient nicotine may be released from the gum by chewing intermittently and leaving the gum under the lip or in the corner of the mouth between chews. Nicorette Mint Plus is sugar-free.

**Product licence number** 0022/0113

## NICORETTE* NASAL SPRAY

**Presentation** A metered spray bottle containing 10 ml of a 10 mg/ml solution of nicotine for intranasal use. Each 50 microlitre spray contains 0.5 mg nicotine.

## Uses

*Pharmacology:* Nicotine solution applied to the nasal passages is rapidly absorbed into the circulation, reaching a maximum in 10–15 minutes. About 50% is absorbed.

*Indications:* Nicorette Nasal Spray is for the rapid relief of nicotine withdrawal symptoms in the treatment of nicotine dependent persons as a part of a supervised smoking cessation programme. It may be of particular use in the most heavily dependent smokers.

## Dosage and administration

*Children and young adults:* The product is not for use by any person under the age of 16 years.

*Adults and elderly:* Use of Nicorette Nasal Spray should be restricted to 3 months. The spray is to be used as part of a supervised smoking cessation programme for nicotine dependency. Counselling should be part of this procedure.

The method of use of the spray is illustrated in the package insert.

A 50 µl dose of solution is sprayed into the nostril when the unit is activated. This is described as a 'spray' and dosage is described using this term. Each spray delivers 0.5 mg of nicotine, about half of which is absorbed.

On commencing treatment the patient uses the spray to treat craving as required, subject to a limit of one spray to each nostril twice an hour. The daily limit of use is 32 mg of nicotine (64 sprays) which is the equivalent of two sprays to each nostril every hour for 16 hours.

*The 3 month course should take the following pattern:*

a. For 8 weeks the patient uses the spray as required, subject to the maxima described above, to relieve craving.

b. After this period the patient reduces usage until after 4 more weeks treatment has ended. It is suggested that after 2 weeks into this period usage will have been reduced by a half and usage be zero by the last day.

c. In order to avoid substituted dependence, treatment should be limited to 3 months within the rehabilitation programme. No other nicotine containing drugs, or tobacco products should be used during the treatment. The patient should understand the aim of decreasing the use of the spray to make a final break with nicotine at the end of the course.

## Contra-indications, warnings, etc

*Contra-indications:*

(i) The product should not be administered to non tobacco users or to patients known to be allergic to components of the spray.

(ii) Nicotine in any form should be avoided during pregnancy and lactation.

(iii) Nicorette Nasal Spray is contra-indicated in persons up to 16 years of age.

(iv) Other nicotine-containing preparations or tobacco products must not be used during the Nicorette Nasal Spray course.

*Interactions with other medicaments and other forms of interactions:*

| May require a decrease in dose at cessation of smoking | Possible mechanism of action |
|---|---|
| Paracetamol, caffeine, imipramine, oxazepam, pentazocine, propranolol, theophylline. | Deinduction of hepatic enzymes on smoking cessation. |
| Insulin. | Increase of subcutaneous insulin absorption with smoking cessation. |

| May require a decrease in dose at cessation of smoking | Possible mechanism of action |
|---|---|
| Adrenergic antagonists (e.g. prazosin, labetalol). | Decrease in circulating catecholamines with smoking cessation. |

| May require an increase in dose at cessation of smoking | Possible mechanism of action |
|---|---|
| Adrenergic agonists (e.g. isoprenaline, phenylephrine). | Decrease in circulating catecholamines with smoking cessation. |

*Effects on ability to drive and use machinery:* The nasal spray should not be used whilst the user is driving or operating machinery as sneezing and watering eyes can contribute to accidents which may result in serious injury.

*Other undesirable effects:* Nicorette Nasal Spray may cause adverse reactions similar to those produced by nicotine given by other means, including smoking.

*Principal adverse effects:* These occur commonly at start of therapy but usually decline within the first couple of weeks or treatment.

*Local:* Nasal irritation (sneezing, running nose), watering eyes and throat irritation.

*Systemic:* Headache and dizziness.

*Other:* Additionally an incidence greater than 1% compared with placebo was noted in clinical studies for the following: Sore nose, ear sensations, increased urination, tingling or burning sensation in the head, nose bleed, dyspepsia.

*Pregnancy and lactation:* Nicotine in any form is contra-indicated in pregnancy. As nicotine passes freely into breast milk, it should also be avoided by nursing mothers.

*Other special warnings and special precautions for use:* The patient should be urged to stop smoking completely when initiating therapy with the product. Patients who continue smoking when using the spray may experience adverse effects due to peak nicotine levels higher than those experienced from smoking alone. Similarly adverse effects may occur if nicotine products are used at the same time as nasal spray.

The cardiovascular effects of nicotine may be deleterious to patients with a history of angina pectoris. Nicorette Nasal Spray should be used with caution in patients with a history of peptic ulcer and chronic nasal disorders (polyposis, vasomotor rhinitis, perennial rhinitis), recent myocardial infarction, serious cardiac arrhythmias, systemic hypertension or peripheral vascular disease.

Nicotine can stimulate production of adrenaline; Nicorette Nasal Spray should be used with caution in patients with diabetes mellitus, hyperthyroidism or phaeochromocytoma.

*Substituted dependence:* The practitioner should be aware of the possibility of substituted dependence and accordingly limit treatment to 3 months.

*Concomitant disease:* Only severe renal impairment would be expected to affect the clearance of nicotine or its metabolites from the circulation. In patients smoking and undergoing haemodialysis elevated nicotine levels have been seen.

*Overdosage:* Overdosage with nicotine can only occur, if the patient has very low nicotine dependence or uses other forms of nicotine concomitantly. Should Nicorette Nasal Spray be used orally, the risk of poisoning is small due to high first pass metabolism. Due to the nature of the container it will not be possible to take the product without using the spraying device.

Symptoms of overdosage are those of acute nicotine poisoning and include nausea, salivation, abdominal pain, diarrhoea, sweating, headache, dizziness, disturbed hearing and marked weakness. In extreme cases, these symptoms may be followed by hypotension, rapid, weak, irregular pulse, breathing difficulties, prostration, circulatory collapse and terminal convulsions.

The acute minimum lethal oral dose of nicotine in man is believed to be 40–60 mg.

*Management of overdosage:* All nicotine intake should cease immediately and the patient should be treated symptomatically. Artificial respiration with oxygen should be instituted if necessary.

**Pharmaceutical precautions** Protect from light. Shelf life is 2 years at room temperature.

**Legal category** POM.

**Package quantities** Metered spray bottle, 10 ml in packs of one.

**Further information** Contains methyl and propyl parabens as preservatives.

**Product licence number** 0022/0141

## NICORETTE* PATCH

**Presentation** Nicorette Patch is a transdermal delivery system for topical application, available in sizes of 30, 20 and 10 cm² each containing 0.83 mg/cm² of nicotine, releasing 15 mg, 10 mg and 5 mg respectively over 16 hours. Each patch is rectangular in shape and comprises 3 distinct layers; an outer beige matt finish backing layer, a patterned silvery middle layer and an inner clear release liner, which is removed prior to use. Each patch is packaged in a heat sealed multilaminate sachet.

**Uses**

*Pharmacology:* When the patch is applied, nicotine is slowly released and absorbed through the skin. Blood levels of nicotine are lower than the peaks associated with smoking but sufficient to relieve smoking withdrawal symptoms. The patch is designed to be applied during waking hours only (16 hours).

*Pharmacokinetics:* Taking into account the residual concentration of nicotine in the transdermal system, the nicotine released from the system is efficiently absorbed: a bioavailability of between 80–108% has been reported. There is no clinically significant difference in bioavailability when the patch is applied to the hip, upper arm or chest.

Steady state concentrations of plasma nicotine in volunteers were examined during a study period of six days. Although nicotine was detectable 24 hours after the first dose, the data did not indicate any accumulation.

Tmax of nicotine after application of a 30 cm² nicotine transdermal system has been shown to vary between 6±2 and 9±3 hours; Cmax has been shown to vary between 13±3 and 16±5 ng/ml. No differences in these pharmacokinetic parameters have been observed between males and females.

All Nicorette Patches are labelled by the average amount of nicotine absorbed by the patient over 16 hours.

*Indications:* The treatment of nicotine dependence, and the relief of withdrawal symptoms associated with smoking cessation.

**Dosage and administration**

*Adults (including elderly):* The recommended treatment programme for Nicorette Patch should occupy 3 months. Nicorette Patch should not be used concurrently with any other nicotine products and patients must stop smoking completely when starting treatment.

The daily dose is one patch delivering 15 mg, 10 mg or 5 mg nicotine as appropriate, with application limited to 16 hours in a 24 hour period in each case.

Daily treatment commences with one 15 mg (30 cm²) patch, applied on waking (usually in the morning) and removed 16 hours later (usually at bedtime). Treatment should continue at this dose for an initial period of 8 weeks. Patients who have successfully abstained from smoking during this 8 week period should be supported through a further 4 week weaning period, using the lower strength patches. Downward titration of dose is achieved by applying one 10 mg (20 cm²) patch daily for 2 weeks followed by one 5 mg (10 cm²) patch daily for a further 2 weeks. Patients should be reviewed at 3 months. Following this review, if abstinence has not been achieved, further courses of treatment may be recommended if it is considered that the patient would benefit.

Nicorette Patch should be applied to clean, dry intact areas of hairless skin, for example on the hip, upper arm, or chest. These areas should be varied each day and the same site should not be used on consecutive days.

There is no clinically significant difference in bioavailability of nicotine when the patch is applied to the hip, upper arm or chest.

After removal, used patches should be disposed of carefully (see below).

Experience with treatment of nicotine dependence shows that success rates are improved if patients also receive supportive therapy and counselling.

*Children:* Nicorette Patches should not be administered to individuals under 18 years of age.

**Contra-indications, warnings, etc**

*Contra-indications:* Not to be administered to non-tobacco users. Nicorette Patch should not be administered to patients with known hypersensitivity to nicotine or any component of the patch.

*Pregnancy and lactation:* Nicotine in any form, is contra-indicated during pregnancy or whilst breast feeding. Nicotine has been shown in animal studies to cause harm to the foetus including non-specific retardation of growth and skeletal abnormalities. It is therefore presumed nicotine could cause harm to the human foetus if administered to pregnant women. The effect of nicotine delivered by Nicorette Patch has not been examined in pregnancy, although the harmful effects of smoking on maternal and foetal health are clearly established.

*Precautions:* Due to the cardiovascular effects of nicotine, Nicorette Patch should be used with caution in patients with a history of angina, recent myocardial infarction or cerebrovascular accident, serious cardiac arrythmias, systemic hypertension or peripheral vascular disease. Nicorette Patch should be used with caution in patients with a history of peptic ulcer.

Nicotine can stimulate production of adrenaline; Nicorette Patch should be used with caution in patients with diabetes mellitus, hyperthyroidism or phaeochromocytoma.

Patients with chronic generalised dermatological disorders such as psoriasis, chronic dermatitis or urticaria should not use Nicorette Patch.

After removal, the patch should be folded in half, adhesive side innermost, and placed inside the opened sachet, or in a piece of aluminium foil. The used patch should then be disposed of carefully, away from the reach of children or animals.

*Warnings:* Erythema may occur. If it is severe or persistent, treatment should be discontinued.

*Drug interactions:* Smoking cessation, with or without nicotine replacement, may alter the pharmacokinetics of certain concomitant medications.

| May require a decrease in dose at cessation of smoking | Possible mechanism |
|---|---|
| Paracetamol, caffeine, imipramine, oxazepam, pentazocine, propranolol, theophylline, warfarin, oestrogens, lignocaine, phenacetin. | Deinduction of hepatic enzymes on smoking cessation. |
| Insulin. | Increase of subcutaneous insulin absorption with smoking cessation. |
| Adrenergic antagonists (e.g. prazosin, labetalol). | Decrease in circulating catecholamines with smoking cessation. |

| *May require an increase in dose at cessation of smoking* | *Possible mechanism* |
|---|---|
| Adrenergic agonists (e.g. isoprenaline, phenylephrine). | Decrease in circulating catecholamines with smoking cessation. |

Other effects, associated with smoking, include reduced analgesic efficacy with propoxyphene, reduced diuretic response to frusemide and reduced rates of ulcer healing with $H_2$ antagonists.

*Side-effects:* Nicorette patch may cause adverse reactions similar to those associated with nicotine administered by other means.

During controlled clinical studies, the following adverse events were reported at an incidence of greater than 1% and more frequently with active than with placebo treatment: application site reactions (e.g. erythema and itching), headache, dizziness, nausea, palpitations, dyspepsia and myalgia.

Other subjective sensations associated with smoking cessation may occur, such as impaired concentration, fatigue, anxiety, irritability and increased appetite.

Concurrent smoking may be associated with symptoms of nicotine overdose.

*Overdosage:* Overdosage with nicotine can occur if many patches are used simultaneously, or if the patient has very low nicotine dependence or uses other forms of nicotine concomitantly. Should Nicorette Patch be swallowed, the risk of poisoning is small due to slow release of nicotine and high first pass metabolism.

Symptoms of overdosage are those of acute nicotine poisoning and include, nausea, salivation, abdominal pain, diarrhoea, sweating, headache, dizziness, disturbed hearing and marked weakness. In extreme cases, these symptoms may be followed by hypotension, rapid weak irregular pulse, breathing difficulties, prostration, circulatory collapse and terminal convulsions.

The acute minimum lethal oral dose of nicotine in man is believed to be 40–60 mg.

*Treatment of overdosage:* All nicotine patches should be removed and the patient should be treated symptomatically. Artificial respiration with oxygen should be instituted if necessary.

**Pharmaceutical precautions** No special storage conditions are necessary. The storage sachet should remain unopened until Nicorette Patch is administered.

**Legal category** P.

**Package quantities** Cartons containing Nicorette Patches in single sachets in the following quantities:
Nicorette Patch 15 mg boxes of 7
Nicorette Patch 10 mg boxes of 7
Nicorette Patch 5 mg boxes of 7

**Further information** Nil.

**Product licence numbers**
Nicorette Patch 15 mg   0022/0105
Nicorette Patch 10 mg   0022/0104
Nicorette Patch 5 mg    0022/0103

# NOVAGARD*

**Presentation** Novagard is an intrauterine device consisting of pure copper wire with a silver core, surface area approximately 200 mm², wound on to the vertical arm of a T-shaped plastic carrier. The plastic carrier is composed of polyethylene impregnated with barium sulphate to render it radio-opaque, with a polyethylene thread attached to the base of the vertical arm. The device is presented partially loaded in its inserter tube and instructions for use are included with each sterile pack.

Novagard dimensions – Transverse arms 32 mm, Vertical arm 32 mm.

**Uses** Intrauterine contraception.

**Dosage and administration** Novagard is recommended for women with a uterine size measurement from external os to fundus greater than 5.5 cm. Novagard should be replaced at least every five years. The procedure for insertion is fully detailed in the instructions for use leaflet included with each sterile pack.

Although IUCDs may be inserted at any time during the menstrual cycle, insertion during or shortly after the menstrual period reduces the possibility of an existing undiagnosed pregnancy. Postpartum insertion is usually delayed until involution of the uterus is complete. The benefits of immediate post abortion insertion should be weighed against the risks due to the relatively soft structure of the uterus.

**Contra-indications, warnings, etc**
*Contra-indications:* Contra-indications are pregnancy; history of ectopic pregnancy; postpartum endometritis or septic abortion within the past three months; abnormalities of the uterine cavity including developmental abnormalities; large or multiple fibroids; acute pelvic inflammatory disease; a history of repeated, recent or severe pelvic inflammatory disease; acute cervicitis; cervical dysplasia; endometrial disease such as hyperplasia or uterine polyps; suspected or proven malignancy of the genital organs, including unresolved abnormal Papanicolaou smear; severe dysmenorrhoea; menorrhagia and/or intermenstrual bleeding; significant anaemia; heart disease; leukaemia; use of chronic corticosteroid therapy because of the increased susceptibility to infection with certain micro-organisms which may possibly be introduced at the time of an IUCD insertion; Wilson's disease or a hypersensitivity to copper.

Medical diathermy to the abdominal and sacral regions is contra-indicated because of the possibility of heat injury to the surrounding tissues.

*Warnings:* An increased incidence of pelvic inflammatory disease and menorrhagia associated with the use of IUCDs has been reported. Pelvic infection may result in future infertility. Women with certain known or suspected heart disease are more susceptible to development of subacute bacterial endocarditis. Use of an IUCD in these women may represent a potential source of septic emboli. Appropriate precautions including administration of antibiotics should be observed when inserting an IUCD in such cases.

Syncope or bradycardia may occur in some women during insertion or removal of an IUCD. In the event of early signs of a vasovagal attack, insertion may need to be abandoned or the device removed. The woman should be kept supine, the head lowered and the legs elevated to the vertical position if necessary in order to restore cerebral blood flow. A clear airway must be maintained; an airway should always be at hand. Persistent bradycardia may be controlled with intravenous atropine in a dose of 0.6 mg. If oxygen is available it may be administered by using an Ambu bag. In the very rare emergency situation where the woman fails to regain consciousness she should be transferred to hospital intensive care.

Post-insertion cramps are usually of only a few minutes duration, but some women may experience cramps for several hours or days. Spotting, intermenstrual bleeding or increased menstrual flow may occur. If heavy or persistent bleeding or persistent abdominal cramps occur, removal of the device may be indicated.

Novagard should be removed in the event of partial expulsion and a new device inserted. If perforation of the uterus or cervix is suspected, the device should be removed as soon as medically feasible. Adhesions, foreign body reactions and intestinal obstruction may result if an IUCD is left within the peritoneal cavity. Removal is also indicated in cases of pelvic infection resistant to treatment, menorrhagia producing significant anaemia, or intractable pain.

*Precautions:* A complete gynaecological examination, including measurement of the uterus, should precede insertion of the device. Ideally the woman should be re-examined within the first three months after insertion and annually thereafter. After insertion the woman should be taught to examine herself to ascertain the continued presence of the retrieval thread. Advise her to consult her doctor if pregnancy is suspected.

Intrauterine devices should be used with caution in women with anaemia, menorrhagia, hypermenorrhoea, a history of a previous uterine incision or perforation of the uterus and those receiving anticoagulants, steroid therapy or having a coagulopathy.

The possibility of a seizure being precipitated in an epileptic, at or shortly after the insertion of an IUCD should also be borne in mind.

It has been reported that IUCDs may be less effective in insulin-dependent diabetics.

*Lost threads:* If the retrieval thread is not visible at the cervix on follow-up examination, it may have been drawn up into the uterus or cervical canal and may reappear during the next menstrual period. The thread may usually be located by gently probing with a suitable instrument. If it cannot be found, it may have broken off, or the device may have been expelled. Ultrasound or X-ray may be used to locate the device.

*Pregnancy:* The risk of ectopic pregnancy is reported to be greater in women who conceive with an IUCD in situ than in those without an IUCD. Therefore, if a woman becomes pregnant with an IUCD in situ, she should be carefully evaluated for possible ectopic pregnancy. There have been reports of an increased incidence of septic abortion, associated in some instances with septicaemia, septic shock and death, in women who become pregnant with an IUCD in situ. Women who are pregnant with an IUCD in situ should be closely observed and told to report immediately all abnormal symptoms such as 'flu-like symptoms, fever, cramp-like pain, bleeding or excessive discharge, as the onset of septicaemia associated with septic abortion may be insidious with general symptoms rather than initial signs of spontaneous abortion. Also, the incidence of spontaneous abortion appears to be increased over that in unprotected women when conception occurs with an IUCD in situ. If pregnancy occurs with an IUCD in situ and the thread is visible then the device should be removed. If the thread is not visible or device removal would be difficult, the IUCD may be left in situ until the pregnancy goes to term or until a decision is made to terminate the pregnancy. If the woman elects to continue the pregnancy, careful observation is required. The long term effects of intrauterine copper on the foetus are unknown.

*Adverse effects:* Uterine or cervical perforation, vaginal discharge, embedment and allergic reactions have been reported.

**Pharmaceutical precautions** Novagard is supplied in a sterile pack which should not be opened until required for insertion. Each device should be handled with aseptic precautions and it is advisable that the folded device in the inserter tube should not be left for more than two minutes, as this may prevent the transverse arms from reassuming the correct position.

Care should be taken not to damage the sterile package which should be stored below 30°C (86°F).

**Legal category** POM.

**Package quantities**
Pack containing one sterile device.
Pack containing ten sterile devices.

**Further information** The average amount of copper eluted from copper IUCDs is well below the daily dietary intake of copper. Small increases of endometrial copper levels have been noted in the presence of copper IUCDs, but these are not cumulative. No changes in blood levels of copper have been detected.

**Product licence number 0022/0046.**

# OLBETAM*

**Presentation** Red-brown/dark-pink, hard gelatin capsules stamped 'Farmitalia Carlo Erba' containing acipimox 250 mg (capsule size No. 1) as a white to cream powder.

**Uses** Olbetam is indicated for the treatment of lipid disorders characterised, according to Fredrickson, by elevated plasma levels of triglycerides (Type IV hyperlipoproteinaemia), or cholesterol (Type IIa hyperlipoproteinaemia), and of both triglycerides and cholesterol (Type IIb hyperlipoproteinaemia).

Olbetam inhibits the release of fatty acids from adipose tissue and reduces the blood concentration of very low density lipoproteins (VLDL or pre-beta) and low density lipoproteins (LDL or beta) with a subsequent overall reduction in triglyceride and cholesterol levels.

The drug also has a favourable effect on high density lipoproteins (HDL or alpha) which increase during treatment.

**Dosage and administration**
The daily dosage should be adjusted individually depending on plasma triglyceride and cholesterol levels.

The recommended dosage is one 250 mg capsule 2 or 3 times daily to be taken with or after meals. The lower dose is advised in Type IV and the higher dose in Type IIa and IIb hyperlipoproteinaemias. The daily dose should be divided and taken with main meals.

Daily dosages of up to 1200 mg have been safely administered for long periods. Improvement in the plasma lipids' picture is usually seen within the first month of therapy.

In patients with renal impairment it is advisable to reduce the dosage on the basis of creatinine clearance values. For guidance the following is suggested:

Clearance between 60 and 30 ml/min – 150 mg twice daily

Clearance between 30 and 10 ml/min – 150 mg once daily

Clearance below 10 ml/min – 150 mg every other day

(Capsules containing 150 mg are available on request).

**Contra-indications, warnings, etc**
*Contra-indications:* Olbetam is contra-indicated in patients who are hypersensitive to the drug and those with peptic ulceration.

*Warnings and precautions:* Modification of hyperlipidaemia is recommended only for patients with hyperlipidaemia of a degree and type considered appropriate for treatment. Low-cholesterol and low-fat diets, together with cessation of alcohol consumption, are preferable therapeutic approaches to be tried before starting treatment with Olbetam.

The absorption of Olbetam is not affected by the concomitant administration of cholestyramine.

Evidence of clinical efficacy in the prevention of heart disease has not been established.

The possible beneficial, and adverse, long-term consequences of some drugs used in the hyperlipidaemias are still the subject of scientific discussion.

*Pregnancy and lactation:* There is no evidence from the animal studies that acipimox is teratogenic. However, a higher incidence of immature and underweight foetuses was seen in pregnant animals given high doses of acipimox. This effect may be due to maternal toxicity.

There is only limited experience to date of administration of acipimox to humans therefore epidemiological data are not available.

Taking into account the present experience of administration to humans of acipimox and that the safety of acipimox in human pregnancy has not yet been ascertained it is recommended, therefore, that acipimox not be administered to women who are, or may be, pregnant.

In the absence of animal data on the levels of acipimox excreted in milk, Olbetam should not be administered to women who are breast-feeding

*Adverse reactions:* The drug may induce skin vasodilation giving rise to a sensation of heat, flushing or itching, especially at the beginning of therapy and also rash and erythema. These reactions usually disappear rapidly during the first days of treatment. Moderate gastric disturbances (heartburn, epigastric pain, nausea and diarrhoea) have been reported occasionally, as well as headache, malaise, eye symptoms (dry or gritty eye) and urticaria. On rare occasions patients have developed angioedema and bronchospasm; and anaphylactoid reactions have also been reported.

*Overdosage:* If toxic effects are observed, supportive care and symptomatic treatment should be administered.

**Pharmaceutical precautions** Store below 30°C in a dry place.

**Legal category** POM

**Package quantities** Blister packs of 100 capsules.

**Further information** Acipimox is rapidly absorbed orally, reaching peak plasma levels within two hours. The half-life is about two hours. It does not bind to plasma proteins, it is not significantly metabolised and is eliminated almost completely intact by the urinary route.

**Product licence number 3433/0097**

# PEDITRACE*

**Qualitative and quantitative composition** 1 ml of Peditrace contains:

| Active Ingredients | Quantity | Reference to Standard |
| --- | --- | --- |
| Zinc chloride | 521 micrograms | PhEur |

| Active Ingredients | Quantity | Reference to Standard |
|---|---|---|
| Copper chloride 2H₂0 | 53.7 micrograms | USP |
| Manganese chloride 4H₂0 | 3.60 micrograms | USP |
| Sodium selenite 5H₂0 | 6.66 micrograms | |
| Sodium fluoride | 126 micrograms | BP |
| Potassium iodide | 1.31 micrograms | PhEur |

The active ingredients in 1 ml correspond to:

| | | |
|---|---|---|
| Zn | 250 micrograms | 3.82 µmol |
| Cu | 20 micrograms | 0.315 µmol |
| Mn | 1 micrograms | 18.2 nmol |
| Se | 2 micrograms | 25.3 nmol |
| F | 57 micrograms | 3.00 µmol |
| I | 1 micrograms | 7.88 nmol |

| Other ingredients | Quantity | Reference to Standard |
|---|---|---|
| Hydrochloric Acid | to pH 2.0 | PhEur |
| Water for Injections | to 1 ml | PhEur |

**Pharmaceutical form** A 10 ml polypropylene vial of a sterile clear colourless solution containing trace elements for addition to certain infusion fluids in the intravenous nutrition of paediatric patients.

**Clinical particulars**

*Therapeutic Indications:* Peditrace is an integral part of the complete intravenous nutrition of infants and children. It is intended to meet basal requirements for trace elements and should be used in conjunction with Vaminolact*, Vamin*14 Electrolyte-Free (at physician's discretion: see data sheet) or a glucose solution.

As the requirements of trace elements may vary in different clinical conditions, these substances may have to be added as appropriate in the individual patient.

Peditrace administration should not be started until kidney function is established usually during the second day of life.

It is not to be given undiluted.

*Posology and method of administration:*

*Adults and elderly:* Peditrace is designed for paediatric use.

Additrace should be used in adults and elderly.

*Infants and children (weighing 15 kg or less):* Basal requirements of the included trace elements are covered by 1 ml Peditrace per kg body weight per day to a maximum dose of 15 ml.

*Children (weighing 15 kg or more):* A daily dose of 15 ml Peditrace should meet basic trace element requirements. However, for patients weighing more than 40 kg the adult preparation Additrace should be used.

Patients who are likely to lose higher than average amounts of trace elements, or those requiring prolonged intravenous nutrition should be monitored biochemically to confirm that requirements are being appropriately met. Peditrace can be added to either an amino acid solution or glucose solution and in these cases, up to 6 ml Peditrace can be added to 100 ml Vaminolact®, Vamin® 14 Glucose-Free (at physician's discretion: see data sheet) or glucose solution (50-500 mg/ml). It may also be administered as a paediatric admixture but only admixtures in which compatibility has been documented are to be used.

The infusion should be given at a very slow rate (minimum infusion period -8 hours) and is best done with an appropriate pump or an automatic drop rate counter.

The requirements of potassium and sodium vary with different patient conditions. Peditrace is not intended to meet these requirements.

*Contra-indications:* Peditrace must not be given undiluted.

*Special warnings and precautions for use:* Administration should be carried out only under specialist surveillance especially in patients with pre-existing imbalances, in renal failure or in hepatic disease.

Peditrace should be used with caution in conditions where excretion in the bile is reduced, particularly when cholestatic liver disease is present and/or when urinary excretion is markedly reduced. Patients with such conditions require careful biochemical monitoring as the excretion of trace elements may also be significantly decreased. (Copper and manganese being normally excreted in bile; selenium and zinc, especially in patients receiving parenteral nutrition, being excreted mainly in the urine).

Patients requiring long term total parenteral nutrition (TPN) (defined as longer than one month) should have a baseline whole blood or serum manganese level within or below the normal range and normal liver function before receiving Peditrace.

Manganese levels and liver function should be monitored regularly (monthly) while the patient is maintained on Peditrace.

Peditrace should be stopped if manganese levels rise into the potentially toxic range (please refer to appropriate reference ranges for the testing laboratory), or if cholestasis develops.

Addition of other drugs to be avoided due to the risk of precipitation.

A cloudy solution or one containing a precipitate must not be used.

The addition of Peditrace must be done aseptically within one hour before the start of infusion. To minimise the risk of infection the infusate should be used within 24 hours.

*Interactions with other medicaments and other forms of interaction:* No interactions with other drugs have been observed.

*Pregnancy and lactation:* Not appropriate to the use of this product.

*Effects on ability to drive and use machines:* Not appropriate to the use of this product.

*Undesirable effects:* Impaired renal or hepatic excretion may lead to chronic overdose of one or more trace elements.

*Overdose:* In recommended doses Peditrace supplies trace elements at the level of normal daily requirements.

*Acute:* Acute overdose of these trace elements is unlikely to be hazardous.

*Chronic:* Chronic overdose of manganese has been recorded as causing Parkinsonism and psychosis.

Chronic overdosage may very rarely occur secondary to an unsuspected idiosyncratic deficiency in metabolism or excretion for a specific trace element. In this case, signs may be observed such as nail dystrophy with insidious onset of symptoms secondary to haematological changes or tissue deposition. Diagnosis would be confirmed by biochemical and haematological tests and treatment should be withdrawal of Peditrace.

**Pharmacological properties**

*Pharmacodynamic properties:* Peditrace is a concentrated trace element solution formulated to cover the requirements of neonates and infants receiving total parenteral nutrition. Potassium, magnesium and calcium are not included in the formulation as individual requirements vary from patient to patient.

*Pharmacokinetic properties:* The trace elements in Peditrace, when infused in physiological amounts, should be utilised in the same way as elements absorbed from an oral diet. No pharmacokinetic studies with Peditrace have been performed.

*Preclinical safety data:* No toxic effects were observed during the pre-clinical studies.

**Pharmaceutical particulars**

*List of excipients:*

| | |
|---|---|
| Hydrochloric acid | PhEur |
| Water for injections | PhEur |

*Incompatibilities:* Do not add drugs with Peditrace to infusion solutions unless the compatibility profile is satisfactory.

Do not add Peditrace to infusion solutions other than those recommended unless the compatibility profile is satisfactory.

*Shelf life:* The shelf life is 36 months when stored in room temperature (below 25°C).

*Special precautions for storage:* Do not freeze. Protect vials from light. Store below 25°C.

*Nature and contents of container:* Peditrace is supplied in 10 ml polypropylene plastic vials for injection, which fulfil the tests according to PhEur. The vials are sealed with a chlorobutyl rubber stopper coated with a steel blue fluoropolymer and flip-off caps.

*Instruction for use/handling:* Must not be given undiluted. Peditrace can be added to either an amino acid solution or glucose solution (see below) and given during a minimum infusion period of 8 hours. The infusion should be given at a very slow rate and is best done with an appropriate pump or an automatic drop rate counter. Only admixtures in which compatability has been documented are to be used.

The addition of Peditrace must be done aseptically within one hour before the start of infusion. To minimise the risk of infection the infusate should be used within 24 hours.

*Compatibility:* Up to 6 ml of Peditrace can be added to 100 ml Vaminolact, Vamin 14 Electrolyte-Free or glucose solution (50-500 mg/ml).

**Marketing authorisation number**   0022/0160

**Date of approval/revision of SPC**   March 1997

**Legal category**   POM

## PHARMORUBICIN* RAPID DISSOLUTION

**Presentation** Sterile, pyrogen-free, red, freeze-dried powder in vials containing 10 mg, 20 mg and 50 mg of epirubicin hydrochloride with lactose and hydroxybenzoate.

**Uses** Pharmorubicin has produced responses in a wide range of neoplastic conditions, including breast, ovarian, gastric, lung and colorectal carcinomas, malignant lymphomas, leukaemias and multiple myeloma.

Intravesical administration of Pharmorubicin has been found to be beneficial in the treatment of papillary transitional cell carcinoma of the bladder, carcinoma-in-situ and in the prophylaxis of recurrences after transurethral resection.

**Dosage and administration** For reconstitution the contents of the 10 mg vial should be dissolved in 5 ml of Water for Injections or Sodium Chloride Injection, the 20 mg vial in 10 ml of Water for Injections or Sodium Chloride Injection and the 50 mg vial in 25 ml of Water for Injections or Sodium Chloride Injection.

After adding the diluent the vial contents will dissolve with gentle shaking, without inversion, within 30 seconds. The approximate displacement value of the contents of a 50 mg vial after 25 ml of solvent have been added is 0.15 ml.

*Intravenous administration:* Pharmorubicin is not active when given orally and should not be injected intramuscularly or intrathecally.

It is advisable to give the drug via the tubing of a freely-running i.v. saline infusion after checking that the needle is well placed in the vein. This method minimises the risk of drug extravasation and makes sure that the vein is flushed with saline after the administration of the drug. Extravasation of Pharmorubicin from the vein during injection may give rise to severe tissue lesions, even necrosis. Venous sclerosis may result from injection into small vessels or repeated injections into the same vein.

*Conventional doses:* When Pharmorubicin is used as a single agent, the recommended dosage in adults is 60–90 mg/m² body area; the drug should be injected i.v. over 3–5 minutes and, depending on the patient's haematomedullary status, the dose should be repeated at 21 day intervals.

*High doses:* Pharmorubicin as a single agent for the treatment of lung cancer at high doses should be administered according to the following regimens:

Small cell lung cancer (previously untreated): 120 mg/m² day 1, every 3 weeks.

Non-small cell lung cancer (squamous, large cell, and adenocarcinoma previously untreated): 135 mg/m² day 1 or 45 mg/m² day 1, 2, 3, every 3 weeks.

The drug should be given as an i.v. bolus over 3–5 minutes or as an infusion up to 30 minutes. Lower doses (60–75 mg/m² for conventional treatment and 105–120 mg/m² for high dose schedules) are recommended for patients whose bone marrow function has already been impaired by previous chemotherapy or radiotherapy, by age, or neoplastic bone-marrow infiltration. The total dose per cycle may be divided over 2–3 successive days. When the drug is used in combination with other antitumour agents, the doses need to be adequately reduced. Since the major route of elimination of Pharmorubicin is the hepatobiliary system, the dosage should be reduced in patients with impaired liver function, in order to avoid an increase of overall toxicity.

Moderate liver impairment (bilirubin: 1.4–3 mg/100 ml) requires a 50% reduction of dose, while severe impairment (bilirubin>3 mg/100 ml) necessitates a dose reduction of 75%.

Moderate renal impairment does not appear to require a dose reduction in view of the limited amount of Pharmorubicin excreted by this route.

*Intravesical administration:* For the treatment of papillary transitional cell carcinoma of the bladder, a therapy of 8 weekly instillations of 50 mg is recommended.

In the case of local toxicity (chemical cystitis) a dose reduction to 30 mg is advised. For carcinoma-in-situ, depending on the individual tolerability of the patient, the dose may be increased up to 80 mg.

It should not be used in this way for the treatment of invasive tumours which have penetrated the bladder wall where systemic therapy or surgery is more appropriate.

For prophylaxis of recurrences after transurethral resection of superficial tumours, 4 weekly administrations of 50 mg followed by 11 monthly instillations at the same dosage are recommended.

Pharmorubicin, to be instilled using a catheter, should be retained intravesically for 1 hour. The patient should be instructed to void at the end of this time. To avoid undue dilution with urine, the patient should be instructed not to drink any fluid in the 12 hours prior to instillation. During instillation, the pelvis of the patient should be rotated to ensure extensive contact of the solution with the vesical mucosa.

**Contra-indications, warnings, etc**

*Contra-indications:* Pharmorubicin Rapid Dissolution is contra-indicated in patients with marked myelosuppression induced by previous treatment with other antitumour agents or by radiotherapy and in patients already treated with maximal cumulative doses of other anthracyclines such as doxorubicin or daunorubicin. The drug is contra-indicated in patients with a current or previous history of cardiac impairment.

*Warnings:* Pharmorubicin Rapid Dissolution should be administered only under the supervision of a qualified physician experienced in antiblastic and cytotoxic therapy.

Treatment with high dose Pharmorubicin in particular requires the availability of facilities for the care of patients with possible clinical complications due to myelosuppression.

Initial treatment calls for careful baseline monitoring of various laboratory parameters and cardiac function.

*Precautions:* During each cycle of treatment with Pharmorubicin Rapid Dissolution, patients must be carefully and frequently monitored. Red and white blood cells, neutrophils and platelet counts should be carefully assessed both before and during each cycle of therapy. Leukopenia and neutropenia are usually transient both with conventional and high doses, reaching a nadir between the 10th and 14th day and returning to normal values by the 21st day: they are more severe with high dose schedules. Very few patients, even receiving high doses, experience thrombocytopenia (<100,000 platelets/mm$^3$).

Before starting therapy and if possible during treatment, liver function should be evaluated (SGOT, SGPT, alkaline phosphatase, bilirubin). A cumulative dose of 900–1000 mg/m$^2$ should only be exceeded with extreme caution with both conventional and high doses. Above this level the risk of irreversible congestive cardiac failure increases greatly. There is objective evidence that cardiac toxicity may rarely occur below this range. However, cardiac function must be carefully monitored during treatment to minimize the risk of heart failure of the type described for other anthracyclines.

Heart failure can appear even several weeks after discontinuing treatment and may prove unresponsive to specific medical treatment. The potential risk of cardiotoxicity may increase in patients who have received concomitant, or prior, radiotherapy to the mediastinal pericardial area.

In establishing the maximal cumulative doses of Pharmorubicin, any concomitant therapy with potentially cardiotoxic drugs should be taken into account.

It is recommended that an ECG before and after treatment cycle should be carried out. Alterations in the ECG tracing, such as flattening or inversion of the T wave, depression of the S-T segment, or the onset of arrhythmias, generally transient and reversible, need not necessarily be taken as indications to discontinue treatment.

Cardiomyopathy induced by anthracyclines is associated with a persistent reduction of the QRS voltage, prolongation beyond normal limits of the systolic interval (PEP/LVET) and a reduction of the ejection fraction. Cardiac monitoring of patients receiving Pharmorubicin treatment is highly important and it is advisable to assess cardiac function by non-invasive techniques such as ECG, echocardiography and, if necessary, measurement of ejection fraction by radionuclide angiography.

Like other cytotoxic agents, Pharmorubicin may induce hyperuricemia as a result of rapid lysis of neoplastic cells. Blood uric acid levels should therefore be carefully checked so that this phenomenon may be controlled pharmacologically.

Pharmorubicin Rapid Dissolution may impart a red colour to the urine for 1–2 days after administration.

*Adverse reactions:* Apart from myelosuppression and cardiotoxicity (described under Precautions) the following adverse reactions have been described:

- alopecia, normally reversible, appears in 60–90% of treated cases; it is accompanied by lack of beard growth in males.
- mucositis may appear 5–10 days after the start of treatment and usually involves stomatitis with areas of painful erosions, mainly along the side of the tongue and on the sublingual mucosa.
- gastro-intestinal disturbances, such as nausea, vomiting and diarrhoea.
- hyperpyrexia.

Fever, chills and urticaria have been rarely reported; anaphylaxis may occur.

High doses of Pharmorubicin have been safely administered in a large number of untreated patients having various solid tumours and has caused adverse events which are no different from those seen at conventional doses with the exception of reversible severe neutropenia (<500 neutrophils/mm$^3$ for <7 days) which occurred in the majority of patients. Only a few patients have required hospitalization and supportive therapy for severe infectious complications at high doses.

During intravesical administration, as drug absorption is minimal, systemic side effects are rare; more frequently chemical cystitis, sometimes haemorrhagic, has been observed.

The occurrence of secondary acute myeloid leukaemia with or without a pre-leukaemic phase has been reported rarely in patients concurrently treated with epirubicin in association with DNA-damaging antineoplastic agents. Such cases should have a short (1–3 year) latency period.

*Use during pregnancy and lactation:* There is no conclusive information as to whether epirubicin may adversely affect human fertility or cause teratogenesis. Experimental data, however, suggest that epirubicin may harm the foetus. This product should not normally be administered to patients who are pregnant or to mothers who are breast-feeding. Like most other anticancer agents, epirubicin has shown mutagenic and carcinogenic properties in animals.

*Overdosage:* Very high single doses of Pharmorubicin may be expected to cause acute myocardial degeneration within 24 hours and severe myelosuppression within 10–14 days. Treatment should aim to support the patient during this period and should utilise such measures as blood transfusions and reverse barrier nursing. Delayed cardiac failure has been seen with the anthracyclines up to 6 months after the overdose. Patients should be observed carefully and should, if signs of cardiac failure arise, be treated along conventional lines.

**Pharmaceutical precautions** The following protective recommendations are given due to the toxic nature of this substance:

— personnel should be trained in good technique for reconstitution and handling.
— pregnant staff should be excluded from working with this drug.
— personnel handling Pharmorubicin Rapid Dissolution should wear protective clothing: goggles, gowns and disposable gloves and masks.
— a designated area should be defined for reconstitution (preferably under a laminar flow system). The work surface should be protected by disposable, plastic-backed, absorbent paper.
— all items used for reconstitution, administration or cleaning, including gloves, should be placed in high-risk, waste-disposal bags for high temperature incineration.

The reconstituted solution is chemically stable when stored for up to 48 hours at 2°C to 8°C or 24 hours at room temperature; however, it is recommended that, in line with good pharmaceutical practice, the solution should not normally be stored for longer than 24 hours at 2°C to 8°C. Avoid exposure of the product to sunlight or direct light. Discard any unused solution.

Prolonged contact with any solution of an alkaline pH should be avoided as it will result in hydrolysis of the drug. Pharmorubicin should not be mixed with heparin due to chemical incompatibility which may lead to precipitation when the drugs are in certain proportions.

Pharmorubicin can be used in combination with other antitumour agents, but it is not recommended that it be mixed with these drugs in the same syringe.

Accidental contact with the skin or eyes should be treated immediately by copious lavage with water, or soap and water, or sodium bicarbonate solution; medical attention should be sought.

Spillage or leakage should be treated with dilute sodium hypochlorite (1% available chlorine) solution, preferably by soaking, and then water.

All cleaning materials should be disposed of as indicated previously.

**Legal category** POM.

**Package quantities** 10 mg, 20 mg, 50 mg and 200 mg vials for injection.

**Further information** In patients with normal hepatic and renal function, plasma levels, after i.v. injection of 60–150 mg/m$^2$ of the drug, follow a tri-exponential decrease with a very fast first phase and a slow terminal phase corresponding to a half-life of about 40 hours. These doses are within the limits of pharmacokinetic linearity both in terms of plasma clearance values and metabolic pathway. Plasma levels of the main metabolite, the 13-OH derivative, are constantly lower and virtually parallel those of the unchanged drug. Pharmorubicin is eliminated mainly through the liver; high plasma clearance values (0.9 l/min) indicate that the slow elimination is due to extensive tissue distribution. The drug does not cross the blood–brain barrier.

When Pharmorubicin is administered intravesically, the systemic absorption is minimal.

**Product licence number** 3433/0082

## PHARMORUBICIN* SOLUTION FOR INJECTION

**Qualitative and quantitative composition** Epirubicin hydrochloride HSE 0.2% w/v.

**Pharmaceutical form** Sterile red mobile solution in vials containing 10 mg , 50 mg and 200 mg of epirubicin hydrochloride as a 2 mg/ml solution in 0.9% sodium chloride.

**Clinical particulars**

*Therapeutic indications:* Pharmorubicin has produced responses in a wide range of neoplastic conditions, including breast, ovarian, gastric, lung, and colorectal carcinomas, malignant lymphomas, leukaemias and multiple myeloma.

Intravesical administration of epirubicin has been found to be beneficial in the treatment of papillary transitional cell carcinoma of the bladder, carcinoma-in-situ and in the prophylaxis of recurrences after transurethral resection.

*Posology and method of administration:* Pharmorubicin is not active when given orally and should not be injected intramuscularly or intrathecally.

It is advisable to give the drug via the tubing of a freely-running i.v. saline infusion after checking that the needle is well placed in the vein. This method minimises the risk of drug extravasation and makes sure that the vein is flushed with saline after the administration of the drug. Extravasation of Pharmorubicin from the vein during injection may give rise to severe tissue lesions, even necrosis. Venous sclerosis may result from injection into small vessels or repeated injections into the same vein.

*Conventional doses:* When Pharmorubicin is used as a single agent, the recommended dosage in adults is 60–90 mg/m$^2$ body area; the drug should be injected i.v. over 3–5 minutes and depending on the patient's haematomedullary status, the dose should be repeated at 21-day intervals.

*High doses:* Pharmorubicin as a single agent for the treatment of lung cancer at high doses should be administered according to the following regimens:

Small cell lung cancer (previously untreated): 120 mg/m$^2$ day 1, every 3 weeks.

Non small cell lung cancer (squamous, large cell, and adenocarcinoma previously untreated): 135 mg/m$^2$ day 1, 2, 3, every 3 weeks.

The drug should be given as an i.v. bolus over 3–5 minutes or as an infusion up to 30 minutes. Lower doses (60–75 mg/m$^2$ for conventional treatment and 105–120 mg/m$^2$ for high dose schedules) are recommended for patients whose bone marrow function has already been impaired by previous chemotherapy or radiotherapy, by age, or neoplastic bone-marrow infiltration. The total dose per cycle may be divided over 2–3 succesive days.

When the drug is used in combination with other anti-tumour agents, the doses need to be adequately reduced. Since the major route of elimination of Pharmorubicin is the hepatobiliary system, the dosage should be reduced in patients with impaired liver function, in order to avoid an increase of overall toxicity. Moderate liver impairment (bilirubin: 1.4–3 mg/100 ml) requires a 50% reduction of dose, while sever impairment (>3 mg/100 ml) necessitates a dose reduction of 75%.

Moderate renal impairment does not appear to require a dose reduction in view of the limited amount of Pharmorubicin excreted by this route.

*Intravesical administration:* Pharmorubicin can be given by intravesical administration for the treatment of papillary carcinoma of the bladder and carcinoma-in-situ. It should not be used in this way for the treatment of invasive tumours which have penetrated the bladder wall where systemic therapy or surgery is more appropriate. Epirubicin has also been successfully used intravesicularly as a prophylactic agent after transurethral resection of superficial tumours in order to prevent recurrences.

While many regimens have been used, the following may be helpful as a guide: for therapy, 8 x weekly instillations of 50 mg/50 ml (diluted with saline or distilled sterile water). In the case of local toxicity (chemical cystitis), a dose reduction to 30 mg/50 ml is advised. For carcinoma-in-situ, depending on the individual tolerability of the patient, the dose may be increased up to 80 mg/50 ml. For prophylaxis, 4 x weekly administrations of 50 mg/ 50 ml followed by 11 x monthly instillations at the same dosage, is the schedule most commonly used.

The solution should be retained intravesically for 1 hour. To avoid undue dilution with urine, the patient should be instructed not to drink any fluid in the 12 hours prior to instillation. During the instillation, the patient should be rotated occasionally and should be instructed to void at the end of the instillation time.

*Contra-indications:* Pharmorubicin Solution for Injection is contraindicated in patients with marked myelosuppression induced by previous treatments with other anti-tumour agents or by radiotherapy and in patients already treated with maximal cumulative doses of other anthracyclines such as doxorubicin or daunorubicin. The drug is contraindicated in patients with a current or previous history of cardiac impairment.

*Special warnings and special precautions for use:* Pharmorubicin Solution for Injection should be administered only under the supervision of qualified physicians experienced in antiblastic and cytotoxic therapy. Treatment with high dose Pharmorubicin in particular requires the availability of facilities for the care of possible clinical complications due to myelosuppression.

Initial treatment calls for a careful baseline monitoring of various laboratory parameters and cardiac function.

During each cycle of treatment with Pharmorubicin Solution for Injection, patients must be carefully and frequently monitored. Red and white blood cells, neutrophils and platelet counts should be carefuilly assessed both before and during each cycle of therapy. Leukopenia and neutropenia are usually transient with conventional and high-dose schedules, reaching a nadir between the 10th and 14th day and returning to normal values by the 21st day; they are more severe with high dose schedules. Very few patients, even receiving high doses, experience thrombocytopenia (< 100,000 platelets/mm³).

Before starting therapy and if possible during treatment, liver function should be evaluated (SGOT, SGPT, alkaline phosphatase, bilirubin). A cumulative dose of 900–1000 mg/m² should only be exceeded with extreme caution with both conventional and high doses.

Above this level the risk of irreversible congestive cardiac failure increases greatly. There is objective evidence that the cardiac toxicity may occur rarely below this range. However, cardiac function must be carefully monitored during treatment to minimise the risk of heart failure of the type described for other anthracyclines.

Heart failure can appear even several weeks after discontinuing treatment, and may prove unresponsive to specific medical treatment. The potential risk of cardiotoxicity may increase in patients who have received concomitant, or prior, radiotherapy to the mediastinal pericardial area.

In establishing the maximal cumulative doses of Pharmorubicin, any concomitant therapy with potentially cardiotoxic drugs should be taken into account. It is recommended that an ECG before and after each treatment cycle should be carried out. Alterations in the ECG tracing, such as flattening or inversion of the T-wave, depression of the S-T segment, or the onset of arrhythmias, generally transient and reversible, need not necessarily be taken as indications to discontinue treatment.

Cardiomyopathy induced by anthracyclines, is associated with a persitent reduction of the QRS voltage, prolongation beyond normal limits of the systolic interval (PEP/LVET) and a reduction of the ejection fraction. Cardiac monitoring of patients receiving Pharmorubicin treatment is highly important and it is advisable to assess cardiac function by non-invasive techniques such as ECG, echocardiography and, if necessary, measurement of ejection fraction by radionuclide angiography.

Like other cytotoxic agents, Pharmorubicin may induce hyperuricaemia as a result of rapid lysis of neoplastic cells. Blood uric acid levels should therefore be carefully checked so that this phenomenon may be controlled pharmacologically.

Pharmorubicin Solution for Injection may impart a red colour to the urine for 1–2 days after administration.

*Interaction with other medicaments and other forms of interaction*: It is not recommended that Pharmorubicin Solution for Injection be mixed with other drugs. But Pharmorubicin can be used in combination with other anticancer drugs.

*Pregnancy and lactation:* There is no conclusive information as to whether epirubicin may adversely affect human fertility or cause teratogenesis. Experimental data, however, suggest that epirubicin may harm the foetus. This product should not normally be administered to patients who are pregnant or to mothers who are breast-feeding. Like most other anticancer agents, epirubicin has shown mutagenic and carcinogenic properties in animals.

*Effects on ability to drive and use machines*: There have been no reports of particular adverse events relating to effects on ability to drive and to use machines.

*Undesirable effects*: Apart from myelosuppression and cardiotoxicity, the following adverse reactions have been described:

Alopecia, normally reversible, appears in 60–90% of treated cases; it is accompanied by lack of beard growth in males.

Mucositis may appear 5–10 days after the start of treatment, and usually involves stomatitis with areas of painful erosions, mainly along the side of the tongue and on the sublingual mucosa.

Gastro-intestinal disturbances, such as nausea, vomiting and diarrhoea.

Hyperpyrexia.

Fever, chills and urticaria have been rarely reported; anaphylaxis may occur.

High doses of Pharmorubicin have been safely administered in a large number of untreated patients having various solid tumours and has caused adverse events which are no different from those seen at conventional doses with the exception of reversible severe neutropenia (<500 neutrophils/mm³ for <7 days) which occurred in the majority of patients. Only a few patients have required hospitalisation and supportive therapy for severe infectious complications at high doses.

During intravesical administration, as drug absorption is minimal, systemic side effects are rare; more frequently chemical cystitis, sometimes haemorrhagic, has been observed.

*Haematologic:* The occurrence of secondary acute myeloid leukaemia with or without a pre-leukaemic phase has been reported rarely in patients concurrently treated with epirubicin in association with DNA-damaging antineoplastic agents, such cases could have a short (1–3 year) latency period.

*Overdose:* Very high single doses of epirubicn may be expected to cause acute myocardial degeneration within 24 hours and severe myelosuppression within 10–14 days. Treatment should aim to support the patient during this period and should utilise such measures as blood transfusion and reverse barrier nursing. Delayed cardiac failure has been seen with the anthracyclines up to 6 months after the overdose. Patients should be obserbved carefully and should, if signs of cardiac failure arise, be treated along conventional lines.

**Pharmacological properties**

*Pharmacodynamic properties*: The mechanism of action of Pharmorubicin is related to its ability to bind to DNA. Cell culture studies have shown rapid cell penetration, localisation in the nucleus and inhibition of nucleic acid symthesis and mitosis. Pharmorubicin has proved to be active on a wide spectrum of experimental tumours including L1210 and P388 leukaemias, sarcomas SA180 (solid and ascitic forms), B16 melanoma, mammary carcinoma, Lewis lung carcinoma and colon carcinoma 38. It has also shown activity against human tumours transplanted into athymic nude mice (melanoma, mammary, lung, prostatic and ovarian carcinomas).

*Pharmacokinetic:* In patients with normal hepatic and renal function, plasma levels after i.v. injection of 60–150 mg/m² of the drug follow a tri-exponential decreasing pattern with a very fast first phase and a slow terminal phase with a mean half-life of about 40 hours. These doses are within the limits of pharmacokinetic linearity both in terms of plasma clearance values and metabolic pathway. The major metabolites that have been identified are epirubicinol (13-OH epirubicin) and glucuronides of epirubicin and epirubicinol.

The 4'-O-glucuronidation distinguishes epirubicin from doxorubicin and may account for the faster elimination of epirubicin and its reduced toxicity. Plasma levels of the main metabolite, the 13-OH derivative (epirubicinol) are consistently lower and virtually parallel those of the unchanged drug.

Pharmorubicin is eliminated mainly through the liver; high plasma clearance values (0.9 l/min) indicate that this slow elimination is due to extensive tissue distribution. Urinary excretion accounts for approximately 9–10% of the administered dose in 48 hours.

Biliary excretion represents the major route of elimination, about 40% of the administered dose being recovered in the bile in 72 hours. The drug does not cross the blood brain-barrier.

*Preclinical safety data*: No further information is given.

**Pharmaceutical particulars**

*List of excipients*

| | |
|---|---|
| Hydrochloric acid | PhEur |
| Sodium hydrochloride | PhEur |
| Water for Injections | PhEur |

Incompatibilities: Prolonged contact with any solution of an alkaline pH should be avoided as it will result in hydrolysis of the drug.

Pharmorubicin should not be mixed with heparin due to chemical incompatibility which may lead to precipitation when the drugs are in certain proportions.

Pharmorubicin can be used in combination with other antitumour agents, but it is not recommended that it be mixed with other drugs.

*Shelf life*: The shelf-life shall not exceed 36 months from the time of manufacture.

*Special precautions for storage*: Store at 2°C–8°C.

*Nature and contents of container*: Colourless glass vial (type I), with teflon-faced chlorobutyl rubber bung and aluminium cap with inset grey polypropylene disk.

*Instructions for use/handling:* The following protective recommendations are given due to the toxic nature of this substance:

Personnel should be trained in good technique for handling.

Pregnant staff should be excluded from working with this drug.

Personnel handling Pharmorubicin Solution for Injection should wear protective clothing: goggles, gowns and disposable gloves and masks.

All items used for administration or cleaning, including gloves, should be placed in high-risk, waste disposal bags for high temperature incineration.

Spillage or leakage should be treated with dilute sodium hypochlorite (1% available chlorine) solution, preferably by soaking, and then water. All cleaning materials should be disposed of as indicated previously. Accidental contact with the skin or eyes should be treated immediately by copious lavage with water, or soap and water, or sodium bicarbonate solution; medical attention should be sought.

The drug should be used within 24 hours of first penetration of the rubber stopper. Pharmorubicin Solution for Injection should be stored at 2–8°C. Discard any unused solution.

**Marketing authorisation number** 3433/0135

**Date of approval/revision of SPC** 18 March 1996

**Legal category** POM

## PREPIDIL* GEL 500 micrograms

**Presentation** Translucent, thixotropic, sterile gel containing 500 micrograms dinoprostone per 3 g (2.5 ml). Also contains silicon dioxide and triacetin.

**Uses** Pre-induction cervical softening and dilation in pregnant women with at term or near term, gestation and unfavourable induction features, when there are no fetal or maternal contra-indications.

**Dosage and administration** The entire contents of the syringe are administered into the cervical canal just below the level of the internal cervical os using the accompanying catheter. The patient should be instructed to remain recumbent for 10–15 minutes.

**Contra-indications, warnings, etc.**

*Contra-indications:* Prepidil Gel 0.5 mg should not be used where the patient is sensitive to prostaglandins or other constituents of the gel.

Prepidil Gel 0.5 mg is not recommended in the following circumstances: For patients in whom oxytocic drugs are generally contra-indicated or where prolonged contractions of the uterus are considered inappropriate such as: cases with a history of Caesarean section or major uterine surgery; cases where there is cephalopelvic disproportion; cases in which fetal malpresentation is present; cases where there is clinical suspicion or definite evidence of pre-existing fetal distress; cases in which there is a history of difficult labour and/or traumatic delivery; grand multiparae with over five previous term pregnancies.

Patients with ruptured membranes.

In patients with a past history of, or existing, pelvic inflammatory disease, unless adequate prior treatment has been instituted.

In patients where there is clinical suspicion or definite evidence of placenta praevia or unexplained vaginal bleeding during this pregnancy.

Patients with active cardiac, pulmonary, renal or hepatic disease.

*Special warnings and special precautions for use:*

This product is only available to hospitals and clinics with specialised obstetric units and should only be used where 24-hour resident medical cover is provided.

Use the total contents of the syringe for one patient only. Discard after use. Use caution in handling this product to prevent contact with skin. Wash hands thoroughly with soap and water after administration.

Care should be taken not to administer Prepidil Gel 0.5 mg above the level of the internal os, as placement of the gel into the extra-amniotic space has been associated with uterine hyperstimulation.

Caution should be exercised in the administration of Prepidil Gel 0.5 mg in patients with: asthma or a history of asthma; epilepsy or a history of epilepsy; glaucoma or raised intra-ocular pressure; compromised cardiovascular, hepatic or renal function; hypertension.

As with any oxytocic agent, Prepidil Gel 0.5 mg

should be used with caution in patients with compromised (scarred) uteri.

Cephalopelvic relationships should be carefully evaluated before use of Prepidil Gel 0.5 mg. During use, uterine activity, fetal status and the cervical dilation and effacement should be carefully monitored to detect possible evidence of undesired responses, e.g. hypertonus, sustained uterine contractions or fetal distress.

In cases where there is a known history of hypertonic uterine contractility or tetanic uterine contractions, it is recommended that uterine activity and the state of the fetus (where applicable) should be continuously monitored throughout labour. The possibility of uterine rupture should be borne in mind where high-tone uterine contractions are sustained.

Animal studies lasting several weeks at high doses have shown that prostaglandins of the E and F series can induce proliferation of bone. Such effects have also been noted in newborn infants who received prostaglandin $E_1$ during prolonged treatment. There is no evidence that short-term administration of prostaglandin $E_2$ can cause similar bone effects.

*Interaction with other medicaments and other forms of interaction:* Since it has been found that prostaglandins potentiate the effect of oxytocin, it is recommended that if these drugs are used in sequence, the patient's uterine activity should be carefully monitored.

*Pregnancy and lactation:* Prepidil Gel 0.5 mg is only used during pregnancy, for pre-induction of labour.

Prostaglandins are excreted in breast milk. This is not expected to be a hazard given the circumstances in which the product is used.

*Effects on ability to drive and use machines:* Not applicable

*Undesirable effects:* The most commonly reported events are vomiting, nausea and diarrhoea. Certain rare events that should be especially noted are: hypersensitivity to the drug; uterine rupture and cardiac arrest. Other adverse events, in decreasing order of severity, reported with use of dinoprostone are: pulmonary/amniotic fluid embolism; abruptio placenta; stillbirth, neonatal death; uterine hypercontractility or hypertonus; fetal distress; hypertension – systemic (maternal); bronchospasm/asthma; rapid cervical dilation; fever; backache; rash; vaginal symptoms – warmth, irritation, pain.

In addition, other adverse reactions that have been seen with the use of prostaglandin $E_2$ for term labour induction have included: uterine hypercontractility with fetal bradycardia; uterine hypercontractility without fetal bradycardia and low Apgar scores in the newborn.

*Overdose:* Uterine hypertonus or unduly severe uterine contractions have rarely been encountered, but might be anticipated to result from overdosage. Where there is evidence of fetal distress or uterine hypertonus, then prompt delivery is indicated. Treatment of overdosage must be, at this time, symptomatic, since clinical studies with prostaglandin antagonists have not progressed to the point where recommendations may be made.

*Incompatibilities:* None known

**Pharmaceutical precautions** Store in a refrigerator at 2˚C – 8˚C. Use the total contents of the syringe for one patient only. Discard after use.

**Legal category** POM

**Package quantities** Prepidil Gel is supplied as a 2.5 ml pre-filled disposable syringe containing 500 micrograms dinoprostone.

**Further information** Prepidil Gel exhibits the capacity of other prostaglandins to influence uterine activity at any stage of gestation. Other forms of dinoprostone (Prostin E2) are available for induction of labour (oral, vaginal and i.v. routes), fetal death in utero (i.v. route), therapeutic termination of pregnancy (i.v. and extra-amniotic routes), missed abortion and hydatidiform mole (i.v. route).

**Product licence number** 0032/0138

## PROSTIN* E2 ORAL TABLETS 0.5 MG

**Qualitative and quantitative composition** Each tablet contains 500 micrograms (0.5 mg) dinoprostone (plus 5% overage).

**Pharmaceutical form** White, roughly rectangular tablets embossed on one side to resemble the letter 'U' and marked '76' on the other side.

### Clinical particulars

*Therapeutic indications:* Oxytocic. Prostin E2 Oral Tablets 0.5 mg are indicated for the induction of labour when there are no fetal or maternal contra-indications.

*Posology and method of administration: Adults:* The

dosage of Prostin E2 Oral Tablets 0.5 mg must be adapted to the patient's response and should always be maintained at the lowest level which will produce satisfactory uterine response. All doses should be taken with a small glass of water.

An initial dose of 500 micrograms (1 tablet) should be given. Thereafter, doses should be given hourly. The usual dose will be 500 micrograms (1 tablet), but if uterine activity is inadequate, 1 mg (2 tablets) may be given hourly until such time as adequate uterine activity is established. Thereafter, it may be possible to reduce the dosage to 500 micrograms (1 tablet) hourly. It is recommended that a total single dose of 1.5 mg (3 tablets) is not exceeded.

*Elderly:* Not applicable

*Children:* Not applicable

*Contra-indications:* Prostin E2 Oral Tablets 0.5 mg should not be used where the patient is sensitive to prostaglandins or any other constituents of the tablet.

Prostin E2 Oral Tablets 0.5 mg are not recommended in the following circumstances:

For patients in whom oxytocic drugs are generally contra-indicated or where prolonged contractions of the uterus are considered inappropriate such as: cases with a history of Caesarean section or major uterine surgery; cases where there is cephalopelvic disproportion; cases in which fetal malpresentation is present; cases where there is clinical suspicion or definite evidence of pre-existing fetal distress; cases in which there is a history of difficult labour and/or traumatic delivery; grand multiparae with over five previous term pregnancies.

In patients with a past history of, or existing, pelvic inflammatory disease, unless adequate prior treatment has been instituted.

In patients where there is clinical suspicion or definite evidence of placenta praevia or unexplained vaginal bleeding during this pregnancy.

Patients with active cardiac, pulmonary, renal or hepatic disease.

*Special warnings and special precautions for use:* This product is only available to hospitals and clinics with specialised obstetric units and should only be used where 24-hour resident medical cover is provided.

Use caution in handling this product to prevent contact with skin. Wash hands thoroughly with soap and water after administration.

Caution should be exercised in the administration of Prostin E2 Oral Tablets 0.5 mg for the induction of labour in patients with: asthma or a history of asthma; epilepsy or a history of epilepsy; glaucoma or raised intra-ocular pressure; compromised cardiovascular, hepatic, or renal function; hypertension

As with any oxytocic agent, Prostin E2 Oral Tablets 0.5 mg should be used with caution in patients with compromised (scarred) uteri.

In labour induction, cephalopelvic relationships should be carefully evaluated before use of Prostin E2 Oral Tablets 0.5 mg. During use, uterine activity, fetal status and the progression of cervical dilation should be carefully monitored to detect possible evidence of undesired responses, e.g. hypertonus, sustained uterine contractions or fetal distress. In cases where there is a known history of hypertonic uterine contractility or tetanic uterine contractions, it is recommended that uterine activity and the state of the fetus (where applicable) should be continuously monitored throughout labour. The possibility of uterine rupture should be borne in mind where high-tone uterine contractions are sustained.

Animal studies lasting several weeks at high doses have shown that prostaglandins of the E and F series can induce proliferation of bone. Such effects have also been noted in newborn infants who received prostaglandin $E_1$ during prolonged treatment. There is no evidence that short-term administration of prostaglandin $E_2$ can cause similar bone effects.

*Interaction with other medicaments and other forms of interaction:* Since it has been found that prostaglandins potentiate the effect of oxytocin, it is not recommended that these drugs are used together. If used in sequence, the patient's uterine activity should be carefully monitored.

*Pregnancy and lactation:* Prostin E2 Oral Tablets 0.5 mg are only used during pregnancy, to induce labour.

Prostaglandins are excreted in breast milk. This is not expected to be a hazard given the circumstances in which the product is used.

*Effects on ability to drive and use machines:* Not applicable

*Undesirable effects:* The most commonly reported events are vomiting, nausea and diarrhoea. Certain rare events that should be especially noted are: hypersensitivity to the drug; uterine rupture and cardiac arrest. Other adverse events, in decreasing order of severity, reported with use of dinoprostone are: pulmonary/amniotic fluid embolism; abruptio placenta; stillbirth, neonatal death; uterine hypercon-

tractility or hypertonus; fetal distress; hypertension – systemic (maternal); bronchospasm/asthma; rapid cervical dilation; fever; backache; rash.

In addition, other adverse reactions that have been seen with the use of prostaglandin $E_2$ for term labour induction have included: altered fetal heart rate patterns; uterine hypercontractility with fetal bradycardia; uterine hypercontractility without fetal bradycardia and low Apgar scores in the newborn.

*Overdose:* Uterine hypertonus or unduly severe uterine contractions have rarely been encountered, but might be anticipated to result from overdosage. Where there is evidence of fetal distress or uterine hypertonus, then prompt delivery is indicated. Treatment of overdosage must be, at this time, symptomatic, since clinical studies with prostaglandin antagonists have not progressed to the point where recommendations may be made. It is currently believed that vomiting produced by overdosage may act as a self-limiting factor in protecting the patient.

**Pharmacological properties**

*Pharmacodynamic properties:* Dinoprostone is a prostaglandin of the E series with actions on smooth muscle; the endogenous substance is termed prostaglandin E2 (PGE₂). It induces contraction of uterine muscle at any stage of pregnancy and is reported to act predominantly as a vasodilator on blood vessels and as a bronchodilator on bronchial muscle.

*Pharmacokinetic properties: General characteristics of active substance*

Following ingestion of the tablet, PGE₂ absorption (as measured by the presence of PGE₂ metabolites) was detectable at 15 minutes, with a peak level occurring at about 45 minutes after the first oral dose. There was little evidence of accumulative effects when a second dose was administered after one hour.

There is a possibility that oral prostaglandin $E_2$ is converted in the stomach into prostaglandin $A_2$ and subsequently into its metabolites, which may contribute to uterine action.

There has been found to be considerable inter-patient variability in the time courses and in the absolute levels of PGE₂ metabolites in plasma following the administration of oral PGE₂ tablets. This seems likely to reflect differences in the rates of absorption of PGE₂ and in its metabolic transformations, but it may also incorporate varying contributions from endogenous prostaglandin production–although this is unlikely to be significant.

*Characteristics in patients:* No special characteristics. See 'Special warnings and special precautions for use' for further information.

*Preclinical safety data:* In mice and rats, the oral $LD_{50}$ values were >500 mg/kg and 141–513 mg/kg respectively.

Three month oral administration to rats resulted in significantly heavier stomach weights for treated compared with untreated rats, which effect was reversible on treatment cessation. Treated rats had a dose related acanthotic squamous glandular junction and thickened glandular gastric mucosal epithelium. No significant alterations were recognized in routine evaluation of the sternebrae and the femur.

A fourteen day oral toxicity study in dogs showed a maximum tolerated dose of 6–20 mg/kg/day. All treated dogs had microscopic evidence of increased fundic and pyloric mucus. The fundic and pyloric mucosa were thickened, having a cobblestone appearance and had an increased gastric mucus in both 20 mg/kg/day treated dogs and the 60 mg/kg/day male dog. These were the only gross and microscopic drug related changes observed.

Satisfactory results were obtained in intravenous and intramuscular tolerability tests performed in dog and monkey.

Teratogenic effects were observed in rats injected subcutaneously with 0.5 mg/animal. No teratogenic effects were seen in the rabbit at dosage levels of up to 1.5 mg/kg day.

No evidence of mutagenicity was obtained using the Ames Assay, the DNA Damage/Alkaline Elution Assay and the micronucleus test.

**Pharmaceutical particulars**

*List of excipients:* Lactose, microcrystalline cellulose, maize starch, magnesium stearate and colloidal silicon dioxide.

*Incompatibilities:* None known

*Shelf life:* Prostin E2 Oral Tablets 0.5 mg have a shelf-life of 24 months when stored at 4˚C.

*Special precautions for product and admixture storage:* Store in a refrigerator. The tablets should be used within three months of opening the bottle.

*Nature and contents of container:* Amber glass bottle with screw cap and tac seal. Each bottle contains a desiccant capsule.

*Instructions for use/handling:* Use caution in handling

this product to prevent contact with skin. Wash hands thoroughly with soap and water after administration.

**Marketing authorisation number** 0032/0040R

**Date of approval/revision of SPC** September 1995

**Legal category** POM

## PROSTIN* E2 STERILE SOLUTION 1 mg/ml

**Presentation** Colourless, sterile solution containing 1 mg/ml dinoprostone (prostaglandin E2). Also contains ethanol.

**Uses** *Indications:* Oxytocic agent. Prostin E2 Sterile Solution 1 mg/ml is indicated for the induction of labour.

*Mechanism of action:* Dinoprostone induces contraction of uterine muscle.

*Pharmacology:* Dinoprostone is a prostaglandin of the E series with actions on smooth muscle. It induces contraction of uterine muscle at any stage of labour.

*Pharmacokinetics:* Dinoprostone is rapidly metabolised in the body. Intravenous administration results in very rapid distribution and metabolism, with only 3% of unchanged drug remaining in the blood after 15 minutes. At least nine prostaglandin E2 metabolites have been identified in human blood and urine.

**Dosage and administration** Prostin E2 Sterile Solution 1 mg/ml is administered by the intravenous route.

The ampoule contents must be diluted before use and full instructions on method of dilution and dosage are given on the package insert which should be consulted prior to initiation of therapy. The dose of Prostin E2 used, normally depends not only upon the indication, but also on patient response.

The following is a guide to dosage:

Dilute with normal saline or 5% dextrose according to the package insert to produce a 1.5 micrograms/ml solution. The 1.5 micrograms/ml solution is infused at 0.25 micrograms/minute for 30 minutes and then maintained or increased. Cases of fetal death *in utero* may require higher doses. An initial rate of 0.5 micrograms/minute may be used with stepwise increases, at intervals of not less than one hour.

The appearance of fetal distress or uterine hypertonus requires cessation of therapy until the state returns to normal. The situation should be re-assessed and, if necessary, the infusion can be recommenced but at lower dosage rates, 50% of the last dose level used.

If no response is seen within the first 12–24 hours of treatment, the medication should be discontinued.

*Children and elderly patients:* Not applicable

**Contra-indications, warnings etc.**

*Contra-indications:* Prostin E2 Sterile Solution 1 mg/ml should not be used where the patient is sensitive to prostaglandins.

Prostin E2 Sterile Solution 1 mg/ml is not recommended in the following circumstances:

For patients in whom oxytocic drugs are generally contra-indicated or where prolonged contractions of the uterus are considered inappropriate, such as: cases with a history of Caesarean section or major uterine surgery; cases in which there is cephalopelvic disproportion; cases in which fetal malpresentation is present; cases in which there is clinical suspicion or definite evidence of pre-existing fetal distress; cases in which there is a history of difficult labour and/or traumatic delivery; grand multiparae with six or more previous term pregnancies.

In patients with a past history of, or existing, pelvic inflammatory disease, unless adequate prior treatment has been instituted.

In patients where there is clinical suspicion or definite evidence of placenta praevia or unexplained vaginal bleeding during this pregnancy.

Patients with active cardiac, pulmonary, renal or hepatic disease.

*Interactions with other medicaments:* Since it has been found that prostaglandins potentiate the effect of oxytocin, it is not recommended that these drugs are used together. If used in sequence, the patient's uterine activity should be carefully monitored.

*Effects on ability to drive and to use machines:* Not applicable.

*Other undesirable effects:* The most commonly reported events are vomiting, nausea and diarrhoea. Certain rare events that should be especially noted are: hypersensitivity to the drug; uterine rupture and cardiac arrest. Other adverse events,in decreasing order of severity, reported with use of dinoprostone are: Pulmonary/amniotic fluid embolism; abruptio placenta; stillbirth, neonatal death; uterine hypercontractility or hypertonus; fetal distress; hypertension – systemic (maternal); bronchospasm/asthma; rapid cervical dilation; fever; back ache; rash.

Transient vasovagal symptoms , including flushing, shivering, headache and dizziness, have been recorded with intravenous use of Prostin E2. Local tissue irritation and erythema have occurred. No evidence of thrombophlebitis has been recorded and local tissue erythema at the infusion site has disappeared within two to five hours after infusion. A temporary pyrexia and elevated WBC are not unusual, but both have reverted after termination of infusion.

In addition, other adverse reactions that have been seen with the use of prostaglandin $E_2$ for term labour induction have included: altered fetal heart rate patterns; uterine hypercontractility with fetal bradycardia; uterine hypercontractility without fetal bradycardia and low Apgar scores in the newborn.

*Use in pregnancy and lactation:* Prostin E2 Sterile Solution 1 mg/ml is only used during pregnancy, to induce labour.

Prostaglandins are excreted in breast milk. This is not expected to be a hazard given the circumstances in which the product is used.

*Other special warnings and precautions:*

*Warnings:* This product is available only to hospitals and clinics with specialised obstetric units and should only be used where 24-hour resident medical cover is provided.

It is advised that Prostin E2 Sterile Solution 1 mg/ml should not be administered by the intramyometrial route since there have been reports of a possible association between this route of administration and cardiac arrest in severely ill patients.

*Precautions:* Use caution in handling this product to prevent contact with skin. Wash hands thoroughly with soap and water after administration. Caution should be exercised in the administration of Prostin E2 Sterile Solution 1 mg/ml for the induction of labour in patients with: asthma or a history of asthma; epilepsy or a history of epilepsy; glaucoma or raised intra-ocular pressure; compromised cardiovascular, hepatic or renal function; hypertension.

As with any oxytocic agent, Prostin E2 Sterile Solution should be used with caution in patients with compromised (scarred) uteri.

In labour induction, cephalopelvic relationships should be carefully evaluated before use of Prostin E2 Sterile Solution 1 mg/ml. During use, uterine activity, fetal status and the progression of cervical dilation should be carefully monitored to detect possible evidence of undesired responses, e.g. hypertonus, sustained uterine contractions or fetal distress.

In cases where there is a known history of hypertonic uterine contractility or tetanic uterine contractions, it is recommended that uterine activity and the state of the fetus (where applicable) should be continuously monitored throughout labour. The possibility of uterine rupture should be borne in mind where high-tone uterine contractions are sustained.

Animal studies lasting several weeks at high doses have shown that prostaglandins of the E and F series can induce proliferation of bone. Such effects have also been noted in newborn infants who received prostaglandin $E_1$ during prolonged treatment. There is no evidence that short-term administration of prostaglandin $E_2$ can cause similar bone effects.

*Overdose:* Uterine hypertonus or unduly severe uterine contractions have rarely been encountered, but might be anticipated to result from overdosage. In the rare instance where temporary discontinuation of therapy is not effective in reversing fetal distress or uterine hypertonus, then prompt delivery is indicated. Treatment of overdosage must be, at this time, symptomatic, since clinical studies with prostaglandin antagonists have not progressed to the point where recommendations may be made.

*Incompatibilities:* None known

**Pharmaceutical precautions** Prostin E2 Sterile Solution 1 mg/ml must be refrigerated at 4°C. It should be diluted before use only with the diluents stated. Diluted solutions should be used within 24 hours (48 hours for extra-amniotic).

**Legal category** POM

**Package quantities** Pack containing 1 × 0.75 ml ampoule of Prostin E2 Sterile Solution 1 mg/ml

**Further information** Oral Prostin E2 Tablets, Prostin E2 Vaginal Tablets and Prostin E2 Vaginal Gel are also available for the induction of labour.

**Product licence number** 0032/0020R

## PROSTIN* E2 STERILE SOLUTION 10 MG/ML

**Presentation** Colourless sterile solution containing 10 mg/ml dinoprostone (prostaglandin E2). Also contains ethanol.

**Uses** *Indications:* Oxytocic agent. Prostin E2 Sterile Solution 10 mg/ml is indicated for the therapeutic termination of pregnancy, missed abortion and hydatidiform mole.

*Mechanism of action:* Dinoprostone induces contraction of uterine muscle

*Pharmacology:* Dinoprostone is a prostaglandin of the E series with actions on smooth muscle. It induces contraction of uterine muscle at any stage of labour.

*Pharmacokinetics:* Dinoprostone is rapidly metabolised in the body. Intravenous administration results in very rapid distribution and metabolism, with only 3% of unchanged drug remaining in the blood after 15 minutes. At least nine prostaglandin E2 metabolites have been identified in human blood and urine.

**Dosage and administration** Prostin E2 Sterile Solution 10 mg/ml is administered by the intravenous route.

The ampoule contents must be diluted before use and full instructions on method of dilution and dosage are given in the package insert which should be consulted prior to initiation of therapy. The dose of Prostin E2 Sterile Solution 10 mg/ml used, normally depends not only upon the indication, but also on patient response. Increase in dosage above that recommended is possible, but may produce excessive uterine activity and be governed by the unacceptable appearance of dose-related side-effects, such as nausea and vomiting.

The following is a guide to dosage:

Dilute with normal saline or 5% dextrose according to package insert to produce a 5 micrograms/ml solution. The 5 micrograms/ml solution is infused at 2.5 micrograms/minute for 30 minutes and then maintained or increased to 5 micrograms/minute. The rate should be maintained for at least four hours before increasing further.

Continuous administration of the drug for more than 2 days is not recommended.

*Children and elderly patients:* Not applicable

**Contra-indications, warnings etc.**

*Contra-indications:* Prostin E2 Sterile Solution 10 mg/ml should not be used where the patient is sensitive to prostaglandins.

Prostin E2 Sterile Solution 10 mg/ml is not recommended in the following circumstances:

For patients in whom oxytocic drugs are generally contra-indicated or where prolonged contractions of the uterus are considered inappropriate such as: cases with a history of Caesarean section or major uterine surgery; cases where there is evidence of a potential for obstructed labour;

In therapeutic termination of pregnancy where known pelvic infection exists, unless adequate prior treatment has been instituted.

Patients with active cardiac, pulmonary, renal or hepatic disease.

*Interactions with other medicaments and other forms of interaction:* Since it has been found that prostaglandins potentiate the effect of oxytocin, it is not recommended that these drugs are used together. If used in sequence, the patient's uterine activity should be carefully monitored.

*Effects on ability to drive and to use machines:* Not applicable.

*Other undesirable effects:* The most commonly reported events are vomiting, nausea and diarrhoea. Certain rare events that should be especially noted are: hypersensitivity to the drug; uterine rupture; and cardiac arrest. Other adverse events, in decreasing order of severity, reported with use of dinoprostone are: pulmonary/amniotic fluid embolism; uterine hypercontractility or hypertonus; hypertension – systemic (maternal); bronchospasm/asthma; rapid cervical dilation; fever; back ache; rash.

In addition, with intravenous use, transient vasovagal symptoms, including flushing, shivering, headache and dizziness, have been recorded. Local tissue irritation and erythema have occurred. No evidence of thrombophlebitis has been recorded and local tissue erythema at the infusion site has disappeared within two to five hours after infusion. A temporary pyrexia and elevated WBC are not unusual, but both have reverted after termination of infusion.

*Use in pregnancy and lactation:* Prostin E2 Sterile Solution 10 mg/ml is only used during pregnancy for therapeutic termination of pregnancy, missed abortion and hydatidiform mole. There has been some evidence in animals of a low order of teratogenic activity, Therefore, if abortion does not occur or is suspected to be incomplete as a result of prostaglandin therapy, (as in spontaneous abortion, where the process is sometimes incomplete), the appropriate treatment for complete evacuation of the pregnant uterus should be instituted in all instances.

Prostaglandins are excreted in breast milk. This is

not expected to be a hazard given the circumstances in which the product is used.

*Other special warnings and precautions:*

*Warnings:* This product is only available to hospitals and clinics with specialised obstetric units and should only be used where 24-hour resident medical cover is provided.

It is advised that Prostin E2 Sterile Solution should not be administered by the intramyometrial route since there have been reports of a possible association between this route of administration and cardiac arrest in severely ill patients.

*Precautions:* Use caution in handling this product to prevent contact with skin. Wash hands thoroughly with soap and water after administration.

Caution should be exercised in the administration of Prostin E2 Sterile Solution 10 mg/ml to patients with asthma or a history of asthma; epilepsy or a history of epilepsy; glaucoma or raised intra-ocular pressure; compromised cardiovascular, hepatic or renal function; hypertension.

As with any oxytocic agent, Prostin E2 should be used with caution in patients with compromised (scarred) uteri.

Animal studies lasting several weeks at high doses have shown that prostaglandins of the E and F series can induce proliferation of bone. Such effects have also been noted in newborn infants who received prostaglandin $E_1$ during prolonged treatment. There is no evidence that short-term administration of prostaglandin $E_2$ can cause similar bone effects.

*Overdosage:* Uterine hypertonus or unduly severe uterine contractions have rarely been encountered, but might be anticipated to result from overdosage. Treatment of overdosage must be, at this time, symptomatic, as clinical studies with prostaglandin antagonists have not progressed to the point where recommendations may be made. If evidence of excessive uterine activity or side-effects appears, the rate of infusion should be decreased or discontinued. In cases of massive overdosage resulting in extreme uterine hypertonus, appropriate obstetric procedures are indicated.

**Pharmaceutical precautions**  Prostin E2 Sterile Solution 10 mg/ml must be refrigerated at 4°C. It should be diluted before use only with the diluents stated. Diluted solutions should be used within 24 hours.

**Legal category**  POM

**Package quantities**  Pack containing 1 x 0.5 ml ampoule of Prostin E2 Sterile Solution 10 mg/ml.

**Product licence number** 0032/0021R

## PROSTIN* E2 STERILE SOLUTION 10 mg/ml (EXTRA-AMNIOTIC PACK)

**Qualitative and quantitative composition**  Each ml contains 10 mg dinoprostone.

**Pharmaceutical form**  colourless, sterile solution, which after appropriate dilution is intended for extra-amniotic administration to human beings

**Clinical particulars**

*Therapeutic indications:* Oxytocic agent. The therapeutic termination of pregnancy by the extra-amniotic route.

*Posology and method of administration:*

*Adults:* Ampoule contents must be diluted before use and full instructions on method of dilution and dosage are given on the package insert which should be consulted prior to initiation of therapy. The following is a guide to dosage:

Dilute with the 50 ml of diluent provided according to the package insert to produce a 100 micrograms/ml solution. The 100 micrograms/ml solution is instilled via a 12-14 french gauge foley catheter. Initial instillation is 1 ml, then dependent on uterine response, 1 or 2 ml usually at two hour intervals.

*Elderly:* Not applicable

*Children:* Not applicable

*Contra-indications:* Prostin E2 Sterile Solution should not be used where the patient is sensitive to prostaglandins.

Prostin E2 Sterile Solution 10 mg/ml is not recommended in the following circumstances:

For patients in whom oxytocic drugs are generally contra-indicated or where prolonged contractions of the uterus are considered inappropriate such as:

Cases with a history of Caesarean section or major uterine surgery;

Cases where there is evidence of a potential for obstructed labour;

In patients with a past history of, or existing, pelvic inflammatory disease, unless adequate prior treatment has been instituted.

In patients with cervicitis or vaginal infections.

Patients with active cardiac, pulmonary, renal or hepatic disease.

*Special warnings and special precautions for use:*

**This product is only available to hospitals and clinics with specialised obstetric units and should only be used where 24-hour resident medical cover is provided**

Use caution in handling this product to prevent contact with skin. Wash hands thoroughly with soap and water after administration.

It is advised that Prostin E2 Sterile Solution should not be administered by the intramyometrial route since there have been reports of a possible association between this route of administration and cardiac arrest in severely ill patients

Caution should be exercised in the administration of Prostin E2 Sterile Solution to patients with:

asthma or a history of asthma;

epilepsy or a history of epilepsy;

glaucoma or raised intra-ocular pressure;

compromised cardiovascular, hepatic, or renal function;

hypertension.

As with any oxytocic agent, Prostin E2 Sterile Solution should be used with caution in patients with compromised (scarred) uteri.

Animal studies lasting several weeks at high doses have shown that prostaglandins of E and F series can induce proliferation of bone. Such effects have also been noted in newborn infants who received prostaglandin $E_1$ during prolonged treatment. There is no evidence that short-term administration of prostaglandin $E_2$ can cause similar bone effects.

*Interaction with other medicaments and other forms of interaction:* Since it has been found that prostaglandins potentiate the effect of oxytocin, it is not recommended that these drugs are used together. If used in sequence, the patient's uterine activity should be carefully monitored.

*Pregnancy and lactation:* Prostin E2 Sterile Solution 10 mg/ml is only used during pregnancy for therapeutic termination of pregnancy. There has been some evidence in animals of a low order of teratogenic activity, therefore, if abortion does not occur or is suspected to be incomplete as a result of prostaglandin therapy, (as in spontaneous abortion, where the process is sometimes incomplete), the appropriate treatment for complete evacuation of the pregnant uterus should be instituted in all instances.

Prostaglandins are excreted in breast milk. This is not expected to be a hazard given the circumstances in which the product is used.

*Effects on ability to drive and use machines:* Not applicable

*Undesirable effects:* The most commonly reported events are vomiting, nausea and diarrhoea. Certain rare events that should be especially noted are: hypersensitivity to the drug; uterine rupture; and cardiac arrest. Other adverse events, in decreasing order of severity, reported with use of dinoprostone are:

Pulmonary/amniotic fluid embolism;

Uterine hypercontractility or hypertonus;

Hypertension—systemic (maternal);

Bronchospasm/asthma;

Rapid cervical dilation;

Fever;

Back ache;

Rash.

A temporary pyrexia and elevated WBC are not unusual, but both have reverted after termination of therapy. In extra-amniotic therapy, the possibility of local infection must be considered and appropriate therapy initiated if necessary.

*Overdose:* Uterine hypertonus or unduly severe uterine contractions have rarely been encountered, but might be anticipated to result from overdosage. Treatment of overdosage must be, at this time, symptomatic, as clinical studies with prostaglandin antagonists have not progressed to the point where recommendations may be made. If evidence of excessive uterine activity or side-effects appears, the rate of infusion should be decreased or discontinued. In cases of massive overdosage resulting in extreme uterine hypertonus, appropriate obstetric procedures are indicated.

**Pharmacological properties**

*Pharmacodynamic properties:* Dinoprostone is a prostaglandin of the E series with actions on smooth muscle. It induces contraction of uterine muscle at any stage of pregnancy.

*Pharmacokinetic properties:*

*General characteristics of active substance:* Dinoprostone is rapidly metabolised in the body. Intravenous administration results in very rapid distribution and metabolism, with only 3% of unchanged drug remaining in the blood after 15 minutes. At least nine

prostaglandin $E_2$ metabolites have been identified in human blood and urine.

*Characteristics in patients:* No special characteristics. See *Special warnings and special precautions for use* for further information.

*Preclinical safety data:* In mice and rats, the oral $LD_{50}$ values were >500 mg/kg and 141-513 mg/kg respectively.

Three month oral administration to rats resulted in significantly heavier stomach weights for treated compared with untreated rats, which effect was reversible on treatment cessation. Treated rats had a dose related acanthotic squamous glandular junction and thickened glandular gastric mucosal epithelium. No significant alterations were recognized in routine evaluation of the sternebrae and the femur

A fourteen day oral toxicity study in dogs showed a maximum tolerated dose of 6-20 mg/kg/day. All treated dogs had microscopic evidence of increased fundic and pyloric mucus. The fundic and pyloric mucosa were thickened, having a cobblestone appearance and had an increased gastric mucus in both 20 mg/kg/day treated dogs and the 60 mg/kg/day male dog. These were the only gross and microscopic drug related changes observed.

Satisfactory results were obtained in intravenous and intramuscular tolerability tests performed in dog and monkey.

Teratogenic effects were observed in rats injected subcutaneously with 0.5 mg/animal. No teratogenic effects were seen in the rabbit at dosage levels of up to 1.5 mg/kg day.

No evidence of mutagenicity was obtained using the Ames Assay, the DNA Damage/Alkaline Elution Assay and the micronucleus test.

**Pharmaceutical particulars**

*List of excipients:* Dehydrated Alcohol BP.

*Incompatibilities:* None known.

*Shelf life:* 24 months.

*Special precautions for product and admixture storage:* Store in a refrigerator at 4°C. Once diluted, the diluted solution should be stored in a refrigerator and used within 48 hours.

*Nature and contents of container:* PhEur. Type I glass ampoule, containing 0.5 ml sterile solution, packed in a carton, together with a vial containing diluent.

*Instructions for use/handling:* Use caution in handling this product to prevent contact with skin. Wash hands thoroughly with soap and water after administration.

**Marketing authorisation number**  0032/0026R

**Date of approval/revision of SPC**  March 1997

**Legal category**  POM

Animal studies lasting several weeks at high doses have shown that prostaglandins of the E and F series can induce proliferation of bone. Such effects have also been noted in newborn infants who received prostaglandin $E_1$ during prolonged treatment. There is no evidence that short-term administration of prostaglandin $E_2$ can cause similar bone effects

## PROSTIN* E2 VAGINAL GEL 1 mg and 2 mg

**Presentation**  Translucent thixotropic gel containing 1 or 2 mg dinoprostone per 3 g (2.5 ml). Also contains silicon dioxide and triacetin.

**Uses**  Oxytocic. Prostin E2 Vaginal Gel is indicated for the induction of labour, when there are no fetal or maternal contra-indications.

**Dosage and administration**  In primigravida patients with unfavourable induction features (Bishop score of 4 or less), an initial dose of 2 mg should be administered vaginally. In other patients an initial dose of 1 mg should be administered vaginally.

In both groups of patients, a second dose of 1 mg or 2 mg may be administered after 6 hours as follows:

1 mg should be used where uterine activity is insufficient for satisfactory progress of labour.

2 mg may be used where response to the initial dose has been minimal.

Maximum dose 4 mg in unfavourable primigravida patients or 3 mg in other patients (see *Precautions*).

The gel should be inserted high into the posterior fornix avoiding administration into the cervical canal. The patient should be instructed to remain recumbent for at least 30 minutes.

**Contra-indications, warnings, etc.**

*Contra-indications:* Prostin E2 Vaginal Gel should not be used where the patient is sensitive to prostaglandins or other constituents of the gel.

Prostin E2 Vaginal Gel is not recommended in the following circumstances: For patients in whom oxytocic drugs are generally contra-indicated or where prolonged contractions of the uterus are considered inappropriate such as: cases with a history of caesarean section or major uterine surgery; cases where there is cephalopelvic disproportion; cases in which fetal malpresentation is present; cases where there is clinical suspicion or definite evidence of pre-existing fetal distress; cases in which there is a history of difficult labour and/or traumatic delivery; grand multiparae with over five previous term pregnancies.

Patients with ruptured membranes.

In patients with a past history of, or existing, pelvic inflammatory disease, unless adequate prior treatment has been instituted.

In patients where there is clinical suspicion or definite evidence of placenta praevia or unexplained vaginal bleeding during this pregnancy.

Patients with active cardiac, pulmonary, renal or hepatic disease.

*Interactions with other medicaments:* Since it has been found that prostaglandins potentiate the effect of oxytocin, it is not recommended that these drugs are used together. If used in sequence, the patient's uterine activity should be carefully monitored.

*Effects on ability to drive and use machines:* Not applicable

*Other undesirable effects (frequency and seriousness):* The most commonly reported events are vomiting, nausea and diarrhoea. Certain rare events that should be especially noted are: hypersensitivity to the drug; uterine rupture and cardiac arrest. Other adverse events, in decreasing order of severity, reported with use of dinoprostone, are: pulmonary/amniotic fluid embolism; abruptio placenta; stillbirth, neonatal death; uterine hypercontractility or hypertonus; fetal distress; hypertension – systemic (maternal); bronchospasm/asthma; rapid cervical dilation; fever; back ache; rash; vaginal symptoms – warmth, irritation, pain.

In addition, other adverse reactions that have been seen with the use of prostaglandin E$_2$ for term labour induction have included: altered fetal heart rate patterns; uterine hypercontractility with fetal bradycardia; uterine hypercontractility without fetal bradycardia and low Apgar scores in the newborn.

*Use in pregnancy and lactation:* Prostin E2 Vaginal Gel is only used during pregnancy, to induce labour.

Prostaglandins are excreted in breast milk. This is not expected to be a hazard given the circumstances in which the product is used.

*Other special warnings and precautions:* This product is only available to hospitals and clinics with specialised obstetric units and should only be used where 24- hour resident medical cover is provided.

Use the total contents of the syringe for one patient only. Discard after use. Use caution in handling this product to prevent contact with skin. Wash hands thoroughly with soap and water after administration.

Prostin E2 Vaginal Gel and Prostin E2 Vaginal Tablets are not bioequivalent.

Caution should be exercised in the administration of Prostin E2 Vaginal Gel for the induction of labour in patients with: asthma or a history of asthma; epilepsy or a history of epilepsy; glaucoma or raised intra-ocular pressure; compromised cardiovascular, hepatic, or renal function; hypertension.

As with any oxytocic agent, Prostin E2 Vaginal Gel should be used with caution in patients with compromised (scarred) uteri.

In labour induction, cephalopelvic relationships should be carefully evaluated before use of Prostin E2 Vaginal Gel. During use, uterine activity, fetal status and the progression of cervical dilation should be carefully monitored to detect possible evidence of undesired responses, e.g. hypertonus, sustained uterine contractions or fetal distress.

In cases where there is a known history of hypertonic uterine contractility or tetanic uterine contractions, it is recommended that uterine activity and the state of the fetus (where applicable) should be continuously monitored throughout labour. The possibility of uterine rupture should be borne in mind where high-tone uterine contractions are sustained.

Animal studies lasting several weeks at high doses have shown that prostaglandins of the E and F series can induce proliferation of bone. Such effects have also been noted in newborn infants who received prostaglandin E$_1$ during prolonged treatment. There is no evidence that short-term administration of prostaglandin E$_2$ can cause similar bone effects.

*Overdose:* Uterine hypertonus or unduly severe uterine contractions have rarely been encountered, but might be anticipated to result from overdosage. Where there is evidence of fetal distress or uterine hypertonus, then prompt delivery is indicated. Treatment of overdosage must be, at this time, symptomatic, since clinical studies with prostaglandin antagonists have not progressed to the point where recommendations may be made.

*Incompatibilities:* None known

**Pharmaceutical precautions** Store in a refrigerator

at 2–8°C. The contents of one syringe to be used for one patient. Discard after use.

**Legal category** POM

**Package quantities** Prostin E2 Vaginal Gel is available in single packs of 1 mg or 2 mg.

**Further information** Unlike other oxytocics, Prostin E2 exhibits the capacity of the prostaglandins to influence uterine activity at any stage of gestation. Other Prostin E2 dosage forms are available for induction of labour (oral, vaginal and i.v. routes), foetal death in utero (i.v. route), therapeutic termination of pregnancy (i.v. and extra-amniotic routes), missed abortion and hydatidiform mole (i.v. route).

**Product licence numbers**
| | |
|---|---|
| Prostin E2 Vaginal Gel 1 mg | 0032/0123 |
| Prostin E2 Vaginal Gel 2 mg | 0032/0124 |

## PROSTIN* E2 VAGINAL TABLETS

**Presentation** Prostin E2 Vaginal Tablets are presented as white, biconvex, oblong tablets with radiused corners marked 'UPJOHN' and '715' on one side. Each tablet contains 3 mg dinoprostone. Also contains: lactose, microcrystalline cellulose, silicon dioxide, maize starch and magnesium stearate.

**Uses** Oxytocic. Prostin E2 Vaginal Tablets are indicated for the induction of labour, especially in patients with favourable induction features, when there are no fetal or maternal contra-indications.

**Dosage and administration** One tablet (3 mg) to be inserted high into the posterior fornix. A second tablet may be inserted after six to eight hours if labour is not established. Maximum dose 6 mg.

**Contra-indications, warnings, etc**
*Contra-indications:* Prostin E2 Vaginal Tablets should not be used where the patient is sensitive to prostaglandins or other constituents of the tablet.

Prostin E2 Vaginal Tablets are not recommended in the following circumstances: For patients in whom oxytocic drugs are generally contra-indicated or where prolonged contractions of the uterus are considered inappropriate such as: cases with a history of caesarean section or major uterine surgery; cases where there is cephalopelvic disproportion; cases in which fetal malpresentation is present; cases where there is clinical suspicion or definite evidence of pre-existing fetal distress; cases in which there is a history of difficult labour and/or traumatic delivery; grand multiparae with over five previous term pregnancies.

Patients with ruptured membranes.

In patients with a past history of, or existing, pelvic inflammatory disease, unless adequate prior treatment has been instituted.

In patients where there is clinical suspicion or definite evidence of placenta praevia or unexplained vaginal bleeding during this pregnancy.

Patients with active cardiac, pulmonary, renal or hepatic disease.

*Interactions with other medicaments:* Since it has been found that prostaglandins potentiate the effect of oxytocin, it is not recommended that these drugs are used together. If used in sequence, the patient's uterine activity should be carefully monitored.

*Effects on ability to drive and use machines:* Not applicable

*Other undesirable effects (frequency and seriousness):* The most commonly reported events are vomiting, nausea and diarrhoea. Certain rare events that should be especially noted are: hypersensitivity to the drug; uterine rupture and cardiac arrest. Other adverse events, in decreasing order of severity, reported with use of dinoprostone, are: pulmonary/amniotic fluid embolism; abruptio placenta; stillbirth, neonatal death; uterine hypercontractility or hypertonus; fetal distress; hypertension– systemic (maternal); bronchospasm/asthma; rapid cervical dilation; fever; back ache; rash; vaginal symptoms – warmth, irritation, pain.

In addition, other adverse reactions that have been seen with the use of prostaglandin E$_2$ for term labour induction have included: altered fetal heart rate patterns; uterine hypercontractility with fetal bradycardia; uterine hypercontractility without fetal bradycardia and low Apgar scores in the newborn.

*Use in pregnancy and lactation:* Prostin E2 Vaginal Tablets are only used during pregnancy, to induce labour.

Prostaglandins are excreted in breast milk. This is not expected to be a hazard given the circumstances in which the product is used.

*Other special warnings and precautions:* This product is only available to hospitals and clinics with specialised obstetric units and should only be used where 24- hour resident medical cover is provided.

Use caution in handling the product to prevent

contact with skin. Wash hands thoroughly with soap and water after administration.

Caution should be exercised in the administration of Prostin E2 Vaginal Tablets for the induction of labour in patients with: asthma or a history of asthma; epilepsy or a history of epilepsy; glaucoma or raised intra-ocular pressure; compromised cardiovascular, hepatic or renal function; hypertension

As with any oxytocic agent, Prostin E2 Vaginal Tablets should be used with caution in patients with compromised (scarred) uteri.

In labour induction, cephalopelvic relationships should be carefully evaluated before use of Prostin E2 Vaginal Tablets. During use, uterine activity, fetal status and the progression of cervical dilation should be carefully monitored to detect possible evidence of undesired responses, e.g. hypertonus, sustained uterine contractions or fetal distress.

In cases where there is a known history of hypertonic uterine contractility or tetanic uterine contractions, it is recommended that uterine activity and the state of the fetus (where applicable) should be continuously monitored throughout labour. The possibility of uterine rupture should be borne in mind where high-tone uterine contractions are sustained.

Animal studies lasting several weeks at high doses have shown that prostaglandins of the E and F series can induce proliferation of bone. Such effects have also been noted in newborn infants who received prostaglandin E$_1$ during prolonged treatment. There is no evidence that short-term administration of prostaglandin E$_2$ can cause similar bone effects.

*Overdose:* Uterine hypertonus or unduly severe uterine contractions have rarely been encountered, but might be anticipated to result from overdosage. Where there is evidence of fetal distress or uterine hypertonus, then prompt delivery is indicated. Treatment of overdosage must be, at this time, symptomatic, since clinical studies with prostaglandin antagonists have not progressed to the point where recommendations may be made.

*Incompatibilities:* None known

**Pharmaceutical precautions** Prostin E2 Vaginal Tablets have a shelf-life of 24 months when stored at 4°C. Store in a refrigerator.

**Legal category** POM

**Package quantities** Prostin E2 Vaginal Tablets are supplied in packs of 8 tablets.

**Further information** Tablet disintegration and release of prostaglandin is moisture dependent. In a small proportion of women, tablet remains may be seen in the vagina a few hours after insertion and may contain some prostaglandin. However, this is rarely of clinical significance.

Unlike other oxytocics, Prostin E2 exhibits the capacity of the prostaglandins to influence uterine activity at any stage of gestation. Other Prostin E2 dosage forms are available for a number of indications, including induction of labour.

**Product licence number** 0032/0074

## PROSTIN* VR STERILE SOLUTION

**Qualitative and quantitative composition** Each 1 ml contains 500 micrograms (0.5 mg) alprostadil.

**Pharmaceutical form** Sterile solution for injection.

**Clinical particulars**

*Therapeutic indications:* Prostin VR is indicated to temporarily maintain the patency of the ductus arteriosus until corrective or palliative surgery can be performed in infants who have congenital defects and who depend upon the patent ductus for survival. Such congenital heart defects include pulmonary atresia, pulmonary stenosis, tricuspid atresia, tetralogy of Fallot, interruption of the aortic arch, co-arctation of the aorta, aortic stenosis, aortic atresia, mitral atresia, or transposition of the great vessels with or without other defects.

*Posology and method of administration:* For administration by intravenous drip or constant rate infusion pump.

In infants with lesions restricting pulmonary blood flow (blood is flowing through the ductus arteriosus from the aorta to the pulmonary artery), Prostin VR may be administered by continuous infusion through an umbilical artery catheter placed at or just above the junction of the descending aorta and the ductus arteriosus, or intravenously. Adverse effects have occurred with both routes of administration, but the types of reactions are different. A higher incidence of flushing has been associated with intra-arterial than with intravenous administration.

The infusion is generally initiated at a rate of 0.05 to 0.1 micrograms alprostadil per kilogram of body weight per minute. The most experience has been with 0.1 micrograms/kg/min. After a therapeutic response (an increase in $pO_2$ in neonates with restricted pulmonary blood flow or an increase in systemic blood pressure and blood pH in neonates with restricted systemic blood flow) has been obtained, the infusion rate should be reduced to the lowest possible dosage that will maintain the desired response.

*Dilution instructions:* To prepare infusion solutions, dilute 1 ml of Prostin VR Sterile Solution with sterile 0.9% Sodium Chloride Intravenous Infusion or sterile 5% Dextrose Intravenous Infusion. If undiluted Prostin VR Sterile Solution comes in direct contact with a plastic container, plasticisers are leached from the sidewalls. The solution may turn hazy and the appearance of the container may change. Should this occur, the solution should be discarded and the plastic container should be replaced. This appears to be a concentration-dependent phenomenon. To minimize the possibility of haze formation, Prostin VR Sterile Solution should be added directly to the intravenous infusion solution, avoiding contact with the walls of plastic containers. Dilute to volumes appropriate for the delivery system available. Prepare fresh infusion solutions every 24 hours. Discard any solution more than 24 hours old.

PARTICULAR CARE SHOULD BE TAKEN IN CALCULATING AND PREPARING DILUTIONS OF PROSTIN VR

*Contra-indications:* None.

*Special warnings and special precautions for use:* *Warnings:* Only the recommended Prostin VR dosages should be administered and only by medically trained personnel in hospitals or other facilities with immediately available intensive care.

Approximately 10–12% of neonates with congenital heart defects treated with Prostin VR Sterile Solution experienced apnoea. Apnoea is most often seen in neonates weighing less than 2 kg at birth and usually appears during the first hour of drug infusion. Therefore, Prostin VR Sterile Solution should be used where ventilatory assistance is immediately available.

*Precautions:* Prostin VR Sterile Solution (alprostadil) should be infused for the shortest time and at the lowest dose which will produce the desired effects. The risk of long-term infusion of Prostin VR should be weighed against the possible benefits that critically ill infants may derive from its administration.

Cortical proliferation of the long bones has followed long-term infusions of alprostadil in infants and dogs. The proliferation in infants regressed after withdrawal of the drug.

Use Prostin VR Sterile Solution cautiously in neonates with histories of bleeding tendencies.

Care should be taken to avoid the use of Prostin VR Sterile Solution in neonates with respiratory distress syndrome (hyaline membrane disease), which sometimes can be confused with cyanotic heart disease. If full diagnostic facilities are not immediately available, cyanosis (pO2 less than 40 mm Hg) and restricted pulmonary blood flow apparent on an X-ray are good indicators of congenital heart defects.

In all infants, commencing when infusion starts, intermittently monitor arterial pressure by umbilical artery catheter, auscultation, or with a Doppler transducer. Should arterial pressure fall significantly, decrease the rate of infusion immediately.

A weakening of the wall of the ductus arteriosus and pulmonary artery has been reported, particularly during prolonged administration.

The administration of alprostadil to neonates may result in gastric outlet obstruction secondary to antral hyperplasia. This effect appears to be related to duration of therapy and cumulative dose of the drug. Neonates receiving alprostadil at recommended doses for more than 120 hours should be closely monitored for evidence of antral hyperplasia and gastric outlet obstruction.

Long-term carcinogenicity and fertility studies have not been done. The Ames and Alkaline Elution assays reveal no potential for mutagenesis.

*Interaction with other medicaments and other forms of interaction:* No drug interactions have been reported to occur between Prostin VR and the standard therapy employed in neonates with congenital heart defects. Standard therapy includes antibiotics, such as penicillin or gentamicin; vasopressors, such as dopamine or isoproterenol; cardiac glycosides; and diuretics, such as frusemide.

*Pregnancy and lactation:* This product is for use in children only.

*Effects on ability to drive and use machines:* Not applicable

*Undesirable effects:* The most frequent adverse reactions observed with Prostin VR infusion in neonates with ductal-dependent congenital heart defects are related to the drug's known pharmacological effects. These include, in decreasing frequency, transient pyrexia, apnoea, bradycardia, seizures, hypotension, tachycardia, and diarrhoea. The relationship of the following adverse events, in decreasing frequency, to the drug is unknown: sepsis, cardiac arrest, disseminated intravascular coagulation, hypokalaemia, and oedema. Cutaneous vasodilation (flushing) is the only event related to the route of administration, occurring more frequently during intra-arterial administration.

*Overdose:* Apnoea, bradycardia, pyrexia, hypotension and flushing may be signs of drug overdose. If apnoea or bradycardia occur, the infusion should be discontinued and the appropriate medical treatment initiated. Caution should be used if the infusion is restarted. If pyrexia or hypotension occur, the infusion rate should be reduced until these symptoms subside. Flushing is usually attributed to incorrect intra-arterial catheter placement and is usually alleviated by repositioning the tip of the catheter.

**Pharmacological properties**

*Pharmacodynamic properties:* Prostaglandins are potent vasoactive derivatives of arachadonic acid that exert vasomotor, metabolic and cellular effects on the pulmonary and coronary circulation. The E series of prostaglandins produces vasodilation of the systemic and coronary circulation in most species: these prostaglandins have been used for maintaining the patency of the ductus arteriosus in children.

*Pharmacokinetic properties:* Based on studies in several animal species, intravenous or arterially administered prostaglandin $E_1$ is very rapidly metabolised and distributed throughout the entire body, with the exception of the CNS, where distribution, though detectable, is markedly reduced. The primary organisms for metabolism and inactivation of prostaglandin $E_1$ are probably the lung, liver and kidney which remove and metabolise 40–95% of the prostaglandin $E_1$ in a single pass through the organ. A number of other tissues possess lesser, but significant, capacity to metabolise prostaglandin $E_1$. The predominant metabolites found in plasma, 15-oxo-prostaglandin $E_1$ and 13,14-dihydro-15 oxo-prostaglandin $E_1$ are extensively metabolised by $\beta$ and $\omega$-oxidation prior to excretion, primarily by the kidney. Few urinary metabolites of prostaglandin $E_1$ have been characterised, but are widely believed to be analogous to those reported in detail for prostaglandin $E_2$ and prostaglandin $F_{2\alpha\zeta s10}$. Excretion is essentially complete within 24 hours after dosing, with no intact prostaglandin $E_1$ being found in urine and no evidence of tissue retention of prostaglandin $E_1$ or metabolites. In three species, rat, rabbit and lamb, the prostaglandin metabolising activity of lung from near-term fetal animals has been shown to be at least as effective as that of adults.

*Preclinical safety data:* See section *Undesirable effects.*

**Pharmaceutical particulars**

*List of excipients:* Dehydrated ethanol

*Incompatibilities:* Diluted solutions of Prostin VR should be infused from glass or hard plastic containers, or PVC infusion bags. If undiluted Prostin VR Sterile Solution comes in direct contact with a plastic container, plasticisers are leached from the sidewalls. This appears to be a concentration-dependent phenomenon.

*Shelf life:* Three years (36 months).

*Special precautions for product storage:* Store in a refrigerator.

*Nature and contents of container:* Glass ampoule, containing 1 ml solution.

*Instructions for use/handling:* Diluted solutions should be used within 24 hours.

**Marketing authorisation number** 0032/0083

**Date of approval/revision of SPC** 1 April 1997

**Legal category** POM

## PROVERA TABLETS 2.5 mg and 5 mg

**Presentation** 2.5 mg: Orange, compressed tablets scored on one face and marked U64 on the other face, containing 2.5 mg medroxyprogesterone acetate.

Also contains: lactose, sucrose, maize starch, liquid paraffin, talc, calcium stearate and E110.

5 mg: Blue, compressed tablets scored on one face, marked 286 on either side of the score and marked 'U' on the other face, containing 5 mg medroxyprogesterone acetate.

Also contains: lactose, sucrose, maize starch, liquid paraffin, talc, calcium stearate and E132.

**Uses** Progestogen.

Indicated for dysfunctional (anovulatory) uterine bleeding, secondary amenorrhoea and for mild to moderate endometriosis.

**Dosage and administration** Oral.

*Dysfunctional (anovulatory) uterine bleeding:* 2.5 – 10 mg daily for 5 – 10 days commencing on the assumed or calculated 16th – 21st day of the cycle. Treatment should be given for two consecutive cycles. When bleeding occurs from a poorly developed proliferative endometrium, conventional oestrogen therapy may be employed in conjunction with medroxyprogesterone acetate in doses of 5 – 10 mg for 10 days.

*Secondary amenorrhoea:* 2.5 – 10 mg daily for 5 – 10 days beginning on the assumed or calculated 16th to 21st day of the cycle. Repeat the treatment for three consecutive cycles. In amenorrhoea associated with a poorly developed proliferative endometrium, conventional oestrogen therapy may be employed in conjunction with medroxyprogesterone acetate in doses of 5 – 10 mg for 10 days.

*Mild to moderate endometriosis:* Beginning on the first day of the menstrual cycle, 10 mg three times a day for 90 consecutive days. Breakthrough bleeding, which is self-limiting, may occur. No additional hormonal therapy is recommended for the management of this bleeding.

**Contra-indications, warnings, etc**

*Contra-indications:* Use in patients with a known sensitivity to medroxyprogesterone acetate.

Use in patients with impaired liver function or with active liver disease.

Before using Provera, the general medical condition of the patient should be carefully evaluated. This evaluation should exclude the presence of genital or breast neoplasia before considering the use of Provera.

*Warnings:* Doses of up to 30 mg a day may not suppress ovulation and patients should be advised to take adequate contraceptive measures, where appropriate.

*Precautions:* A negative pregnancy test should be demonstrated before starting therapy with Provera.

Whether administered alone or in conjunction with oestrogens, Provera should not be employed in patients with abnormal uterine bleeding until a definite diagnosis has been established and the possibility of genital malignancy eliminated.

Provera, especially in high doses, may cause weight gain and fluid retention. With this in mind, caution should be exercised in treating any patient with a pre-existing medical condition, such as epilepsy, migraine, asthma, cardiac or renal dysfunction, that may be adversely affected by weight gain or fluid retention.

Some patients receiving Provera may exhibit a decreased glucose tolerance. The mechanism for this is not known. This fact should be borne in mind when treating all patients, especially known diabetics.

Rare cases of thrombo-embolism have been reported with use of Provera, especially at higher doses. Causality has not been established.

Patients with a history of treatment for mental depression should be carefully monitored while receiving Provera therapy. Some patients may complain of premenstrual-like depression while on Provera therapy.

Medroxyprogesterone acetate and its metabolites are secreted in breast milk, however, there is no evidence to suggest that this presents any hazard to the child.

*Interactions:* Aminoglutethimide administered concurrently with Provera may significantly depress the bioavailability of Provera.

Interactions with other medicinal treatments (including oral anti-coagulants) have rarely been reported, but causality has not been determined. The possibility of interaction should be borne in mind in patients receiving concurrent treatment with other drugs.

*Side-effects:* The following medical events, listed in order of seriousness rather than frequency of occurrence, have been associated occasionally to rarely with the use of progestogens:

Rare anaphylactoid-like reactions.

Psychic: nervousness, insomnia, somnolence, fatigue, depression, dizziness and headache.

Skin and mucous membranes: urticaria, pruritus, rash, acne, hirsutism and alopecia.

Gastro-intestinal: nausea.

Breast tenderness and galactorrhoea.

Miscellaneous: change in weight.

*Overdosage:* In animals, Provera has been shown to be capable of exerting an adreno-corticoid effect: this has not been reported in the human, following usual dosages. The oral administration of Provera at a rate of 100 mg per day has been shown to have no effect on adrenal function.

**Pharmaceutical precautions** None.

**Legal category** POM

**Package quantities** 2.5 mg: Packs of 30. 5 mg: Packs of 10 and 100.

**Further information** Pathologists should be informed of the patient's ingestion of Provera if endometrial or endocervical tissue is submitted for examination.

The results of certain laboratory tests may be affected by the use of Provera; these include gonadotrophin levels, plasma progesterone levels, urinary pregnanediol levels, plasma testosterone levels (in the male), plasma oestrogen levels (in the female), plasma cortisol levels, glucose tolerance test and metyrapone tests.

**Product licence numbers**
2.5 mg   0032/0168
5 mg   0032/5035R

## PROVERA TABLETS 10 mg

**Qualitative and quantitative composition** Each tablet contains 10 mg Medroxyprogesterone Acetate PhEur.

**Pharmaceutical form** Tablets for oral use

**Clinical particulars**

*Therapeutic indications:* Progestogen. Indicated for dysfunctional (anovulatory) uterine bleeding, secondary amenorrhoea and for mild to moderate endometriosis.

*Posology and method of administration:* Oral.
*Adults: Dysfunctional (anovulatory) uterine bleeding:* 2.5 – 10 mg daily for 5 – 10 days commencing on the assumed or calculated 16th – 21st day of the cycle. Treatment should be given for two consecutive cycles. When bleeding occurs from a poorly developed proliferative endometrium, conventional oestrogen therapy may be employed in conjunction with medroxyprogesterone acetate in doses of 5 – 10 mg for 10 days.

*Secondary amenorrhoea:* 2.5 -- 10 mg daily for 5 – 10 days beginning on the assumed or calculated 16th to 21st day of the cycle. Repeat the treatment for three consecutive cycles. In amenorrhoea associated with a poorly developed proliferative endometrium, conventional oestrogen therapy may be employed in conjunction with medroxyprogesterone acetate in doses of 5 – 10 mg for 10 days.

*Mild to moderate endometriosis:* Beginning on the first day of the menstrual cycle, 10 mg three times a day for 90 consecutive days. Breakthrough bleeding, which is self-limiting, may occur. No additional hormonal therapy is recommended for the management of this bleeding.

*Elderly:* Not applicable

*Children:* Not applicable

*Contra-indications:* Use in patients with a known sensitivity to medroxyprogesterone acetate.

Use in patients with impaired liver function or with active liver disease.

Before using Provera, the general medical condition of the patient should be carefully evaluated. This evaluation should exclude the presence of genital or breast neoplasia before considering the use of Provera.

*Special warnings and special precautions for use:* Whether administered alone or in conjunction with oestrogens, Provera should not be employed in patients with abnormal uterine bleeding until a definite diagnosis has been established and the possibility of genital malignancy eliminated.

Rare cases of thrombo-embolism have been reported with use of Provera, especially at higher doses. Causality has not been established.

Doses of up to 30 mg a day may not suppress ovulation and patients should be advised to take adequate contraceptive measures, where appropriate.

Provera, especially in high doses, may cause weight gain and fluid retention. With this in mind, caution should be exercised in treating any patient with a pre-existing medical condition, such as epilepsy, migraine, asthma, cardiac or renal dysfunction, that might be adversely affected by weight gain or fluid retention.

Some patients receiving Provera may exhibit a decreased glucose tolerance. The mechanism for this is not known. This fact should be borne in mind when treating all patients and especially known diabetics.

Patients with a history of treatment for mental depression should be carefully monitored while receiving Provera therapy. Some patients may complain of premenstrual like depression while on Provera therapy.

*Interaction with other medicaments and other forms of interaction:* Aminoglutethimide administered concurrently with Provera may significantly depress the bioavailability of Provera.

Interactions with other medicinal treatments (including oral anti-coagulants) have rarely been reported, but causality has not been determined. The possibility of interaction should be borne in mind in patients receiving concurrent treatment with other drugs.

*Pregnancy and lactation:* A negative pregnancy test should be demonstrated before starting therapy. Medroxyprogesterone acetate and its metabolites are secreted in breast milk, but there is no evidence to suggest that this presents any hazard to the child.

*Effects on ability to drive and use machines:* No adverse effect has been reported.

*Undesirable effects:* The following medical events, listed in order of seriousness rather than frequency of occurrence, have been occasionally to rarely associated with the use of progestogens:
Rare anaphylactoid-like reactions:
*Psychic:* nervousness, insomnia, somnolence, fatigue, depression, dizziness and headache.
*Skin and mucous membranes:* urticaria, pruritus, rash, acne, hirsutism and alopecia.
*Gastro-intestinal:* nausea.
*Breast:* tenderness and galactorrhoea.
*Miscellaneous:* change in weight.

*Overdose:* In animals Provera has been shown to be capable of exerting an adreno-corticoid effect, but this has not been reported in the human, following usual dosages. The oral administration of Provera at a rate of 100 mg per day has been shown to have no effect on adrenal function.

**Pharmacological properties**

*Pharmacodynamic properties:* Medroxyprogesterone acetate has actions and uses similar to those of progesterone.

MPA has minimal androgenic activity compared to progesterone and virtually no oestrogenic activity.

Progestogens are used in the treatment of dysfunctional uterine bleeding, secondary amenorrhoea and endometriosis.

*Pharmacokinetic properties:* MPA is rapidly absorbed from the GI tract with a single oral dose of 10 –250 mg. The time taken to reach the peak serum concentration ($T_{max}$) was 2 – 6 hours and the average peak serum concentration ($C_{max}$) was 13 – 46.89 mg/ml.

Unmetabolised MPA is highly plasma protein bound. MPA is metabolised in the liver.

**Pharmaceutical particulars**

*List of excipients:* Lactose, Sucrose, Maize starch, Liquid paraffin, Talc, Calcium stearate.

*Incompatibilities:* None known.

*Shelf life:* Five years.

*Special precautions for storage:* None.

*Nature and contents of container:* HDPE tamper-evident bottles with LDPE push-fit tamper evident caps, containing 50 tablets.
Aluminium foil/PVC blisters, containing 10, 90 and 100 tablets.

*Instructions for use/handling:* None.

**Marketing authorisation number** 0032/0151

**Date of approval/revision of SPC** 8 January 1996

**Legal category** POM

## PROVERA* TABLETS 100 mg, 200 mg and 400 mg

**Presentation** 100 mg: White, circular, flat bevelled tablets marked 'U 467' on one side and scored on the reverse, containing 100 mg medroxyprogesterone acetate.

200 mg: White, circular, biconvex tablets marked 'U 320' on one side and scored on the reverse, containing 200 mg medroxyprogesterone acetate.

400 mg: White, capsule shaped, compressed tablets marked 'Upjohn 421' on one side only, containing 400 mg medroxyprogesterone acetate.

Provera Tablets (all strengths) also contain microcrystalline cellulose, maize starch, byco C, polyethylene glycol, sodium starch glycollate, docusate sodium, sodium benzoate and magnesium stearate.

**Uses** Progestogen.
Indicated for the treatment of certain hormone dependent neoplasms, such as endometrial carcinoma, renal cell carcinoma and carcinoma of breast in post-menopausal women.

**Dosage and administration** Oral.

*For endometrial and renal cell carcinoma:* 200 – 400 mg daily.

*For breast carcinoma:* 400 – 800 mg per day. Doses of 1000 mg daily have been given although the incidence of minor side-effects, such as indigestion and weight gain, increase with the increase in dose. Response to hormonal therapy may not be evident until after at least 8 – 10 weeks of therapy.

*Elderly patients:* These products have been used primarily in the older age group for the treatment of malignancies. There is no evidence to suggest that the older aged group is any less prepared to handle the drug metabolically than is the younger aged patient. Therefore, the same dosage, contra-indications and precautions would apply to either age group.

**Contra-indications, warnings, etc**
*Contra-indications:* Use in patients with a known sensitivity to medroxyprogesterone acetate.

Use in patients with impaired liver function or active liver disease.

*Warnings:* In the treatment of carcinoma of breast, occasional cases of hypercalcaemia have been reported.

Any patient who develops an acute impairment of vision, proptosis, diplopia or migraine headache should be carefully evaluated ophthalmologically to exclude the presence of papilloedema or retinal vascular lesions before continuing medication.

Medroxyprogesterone acetate and/or its metabolites are secreted in breast milk but there is no evidence to suggest that this presents any hazard to the child.

*Precautions:* Animal studies show that Provera possesses adrenocorticoid activity. This has also been reported in man, therefore, patients receiving large doses continuously and for long periods should be observed closely.

The administration of large doses to pregnant women has resulted in the observation of some instances of female foetal masculinization. Doctors should, therefore, check that patients are not pregnant before commencing treatment.

Because progestogens may cause some degree of fluid retention, conditions which might be influenced by this factor, such as epilepsy, migraine, asthma, cardiac or renal dysfunction, require careful observation.

Rare cases of thrombo-embolism have been reported with use of Provera, but causality has not been established.

Patients who have a history of mental depression should be carefully observed and the drug discontinued if the depression recurs to a serious degree.

A decrease in glucose tolerance has been observed in some patients on progestogens. The mechanism of this decrease is obscure. For this reason, diabetic patients should be carefully observed while receiving progestogen therapy.

Before using Provera, the general medical condition of the patient should be carefully evaluated.

This product should be used under the supervision of a specialist and the patients kept under regular surveillance.

*Interactions:* Aminoglutethimide administered concomitantly with Provera may significantly depress the bioavailability of Provera.

Interactions with other medicinal treatments (including oral anti-coagulants) have rarely been reported, but causality has not been determined. The possibility of interaction should be borne in mind in patients receiving concurrent treatment with other drugs.

*Side-effects:* Reactions occasionally associated with the use of progestogens, particularly in high doses, are:
*Breast:* tenderness or galactorrhoea.
*Psychic:* nervousness, insomnia, somnolence, fatigue, dizziness, depression and headache.
*Skin and mucous membranes:* sensitivity reactions ranging from pruritus, urticaria, angioneurotic oedema to generalised rash and anaphylaxis have occasionally been reported. Acne, alopecia or hirsutism have been reported in a few cases.
*Gastro-intestinal:* nausea and indigestion have been noted particularly with the higher doses.
*Miscellaneous:* hyperpyrexia, weight gain, moon facies, increased blood pressure.

*Overdosage:* No action required other than cessation of therapy.

**Pharmaceutical precautions** Keep containers tightly closed.

Provera Tablets should be stored at controlled room temperature (15 – 30°C).

**Legal category** POM

**Package quantities**
Provera Tablets 100 mg in packs of 60 and 100 tablets.
Provera Tablets 200 mg in packs of 30 (OP) and 100 tablets.
Provera Tablets 400 mg in packs of 30 tablets (OP).

**Further information** The results of certain laboratory tests may be affected by the use of Provera; these include gonadotrophin levels, plasma progesterone levels, urinary pregnanediol levels, plasma testosterone levels (in the male), plasma oestrogen levels (in the female), plasma cortisol levels, glucose tolerance and metyrapone tests.

Pathologists should be informed of the patient's ingestion of Provera if endometrial or endocervical tissue is submitted for examination.

**Product licence numbers**
100 mg Tablet     0032/0111
200 mg Tablet     0032/0112
400 mg Tablet     0032/0131

## REFOLINON*

**Presentation**   Clear, pale yellow liquid for injection containing leucovorin 3 mg/ml (as the calcium salt) in ampoules of 10 ml.

Pale yellow, round, convex, uncoated tablet marked with an 'F' on one side and 'CF' on the other; diameter 9 mm containing 15 mg leucovorin (as the calcium salt).

**Uses**   Leucovorin (folinic acid) is the formyl derivative of tetrahydrofolic acid and is an intermediate product of the metabolism of folic acid. Leucovorin is used in cytotoxic therapy as an antidote to folic acid antagonists such as methotrexate. Leucovorin is effective in the treatment of megaloblastic anaemia due to folate deficiency.

**Dosage and administration**   (Adults and children)

*Leucovorin rescue:* Depending upon the dose of methotrexate administered, dosage regimens of leucovorin calcium vary. Up to 120 mg leucovorin calcium are generally given, usually in divided doses over 12–24 hours by intramuscular injection, bolus intravenous injection or intravenous infusion in normal saline. This is followed by 12–15 mg intramuscularly or 15 mg orally every 6 hours for 48 hours. Rescue therapy is usually started 24 hours after the commencement of methotrexate administration.

If overdosage of methotrexate is suspected, the dose of leucovorin calcium should be equal to or greater than the dose of methotrexate and should be administered within one hour of the methotrexate administration.

*Megaloblastic anaemia (folate deficiency):* 15 mg (one tablet) leucovorin per day.

**Contra-indications, warnings, etc**   Calcium folinate should not be used for the treatment of pernicious anaemia or other megaloblastic anaemia where vitamin B12 is deficient.

Leucovorin should not be given simultaneously with a folic acid antagonist, for the purpose of reducing or preventing clinical toxicity, as the therapeutic effect of the antagonist may be nullified.

High-dose methotrexate therapy together with leucovorin rescue should only be carried out under the direction of physicians experienced in antitumour chemotherapy.

Adverse reactions to leucovorin calcium are rare, but following parenteral administration occasional pyrexial reactions have been reported.

**Pharmaceutical precautions**   Protect from light.

Refolinon for injection has been shown to be compatible with 0.9% sodium chloride solution. Under normal light conditions and at room temperature solutions of calcium folinate in 0.9% sodium chloride have been shown to be stable for 24 hours.

**Legal category**   POM.

**Package quantities**
Refolinon for Injection: 5×10 ml ampoules.
Refolinon Tablets: Containers of 30 tablets.

**Further information**   Nil.

**Product licence numbers**
Refolinon for Injection     3433/0079
Refolinon Tablets     3433/0078

## REGAINE* TOPICAL SOLUTION 2%

**Presentation**   Clear, colourless to light yellow liquid containing minoxidil 20 mg per ml in a solution of ethanol, propylene glycol and water.

**Uses**   Regaine Topical Solution is indicated for the treatment of alopecia androgenetica. There is also evidence that Regaine slows hair loss in patients with diagnosed male pattern baldness.

After only four months of treatment, little regrowth of terminal hair should be expected (the average length of the scalp hair cycle is three years). Physicians observed 8% of subjects to have moderate or dense terminal hair regrowth after four months, increasing to 39% of the subjects after treatment for 12 months. Twenty-six percent of patients assessed themselves as having moderate to dense hair regrowth after four months, increasing to 48% of subjects treated for 12 months. At 12 months, 36% of patients had minimal regrowth as assessed by both the patients themselves as well as the treating physicians. In these, patients

loss of hair from affected areas was considered to be reduced. Onset and degree of hair regrowth may be variable among patients and it may take at least four months of continuous twice daily use before evidence of hair regrowth can be expected. Although trends in the data suggest that those patients who are younger, who have been balding for a shorter period of time or who have a smaller area of baldness on the vertex are more likely to respond to Regaine, individual response cannot be predicted. If hair regrowth occurs, twice daily applications of Regaine are necessary for continued hair growth. Anecdotal reports indicate that regrown hair may disappear three to four months after stopping Regaine application and the balding process will continue. Patients should discontinue treatment if there is no improvement after one year.

**Dosage and administration**   Hair and scalp should be thoroughly dry prior to topical application of Regaine. A dose of 1 ml Regaine Topical Solution should be applied to the total affected areas of the scalp twice daily. The total dosage should not exceed 2 ml. If fingertips are used to facilitate drug application, hands should be washed afterwards.

The method of application varies according to the disposable applicator used:

*Pump spray applicator:* This is useful for large areas. Aim the pump at the centre of the bald area, press once and spread with fingertips over the entire bald area. Repeat for a total of 6 times to apply a dose of 1 ml. Avoid breathing spray mist.

*Extended spray tip applicator:* This is useful for small areas or under hair. The pump spray applicator must be in place in order to use this additional applicator. Use in the same way as the pump spray.

*Rub-on applicator:* Squeeze the upright bottle once to fill the 1 ml chamber to the black line. Invert bottle, dab on scalp and spread Regaine over the entire bald area until chamber is empty.

**Contra-indications, warnings, etc**

*Contra-indications:* Regaine is contra-indicated in patients with a history of sensitivity to minoxidil, ethanol or propylene glycol.

*Warnings:* Use of Regaine Topical Solution results in slight absorption (an average of 1.4% of the applied topical dose) of minoxidil from the skin surface. Although not causally related to the use of Regaine in clinical trials, the following potential systemic effects should be considered: sodium and water retention, tachycardia, aggravation of pre-existing angina pectoris or the induction of anginal symptoms in patients with undiagnosed coronary artery disease. Patients should be instructed to discontinue use of Regaine and contact their physician if any of the above systemic effects occur.

*Precautions:* Patients with hypertension, including those under treatment with antihypertensive agents, should be monitored closely when treated with Regaine Topical Solution.

Regaine contains an alcohol base which will cause burning and irritation of the eye. In the event of accidental contact with sensitive surfaces (eye, abraded skin and mucous membranes), the area should be bathed with large amounts of cool tap water.

Inhalation of the spray mist should be avoided. Regaine should not be used in conjunction with other topical agents including corticosteroids, retinoids and petrolatum or agents that are known to enhance cutaneous drug absorption.

As is the case with other topically applied drugs, decreased integrity of the epidermal barrier caused by inflammation or disease processes in the skin (e.g. excoriations of the scalp, scalp psoriasis or severe sunburn) may increase percutaneous absorption of minoxidil.

Regaine is for external use only. Do not apply to areas of the body other than the scalp.

The safety and effectiveness of Regaine in patients under 18 or over 65 years of age has not been established.

There is no evidence as to drug safety in human pregnancy nor is there evidence from animal work that it is free from hazard. Regaine should not be used during pregnancy or lactation.

*Side-effects:* When incidences of medical events in placebo-controlled trials of topical minoxidil were compared, they revealed that only reports involving the dermatological system were present at a significantly greater level in the minoxidil group than in the placebo group. In both groups in all body systems, the overall incidence of medical events reported by females was approximately five times that of males.

Details of percentage occurrences after 4–8 months treatment with minoxidil (n=3857) or placebo (n=2717) were as follows:-

| Body system | Minoxidil % occurrence | Placebo % occurrence |
|---|---|---|
| Respiratory (bronchitis, URTI, sinusitis) | 7.16 | 8.58 |
| Dermatological (irritant dermatitis, allergic contact dermatitis) | 7.36 | 5.41 |
| Gastro-intestinal (diarrhoea, nausea, vomiting) | 4.33 | 6.55 |
| Neurology (headache, dizziness, faintness, lightheadedness) | 3.42 | 3.46 |
| Musculoskeletal (fractures, back pain, tendinitis, aches and pains) | 2.59 | 2.21 |
| Cardiovascular (oedema, chest pain, blood pressure increases/decreases, palpitations, pulse rate increases/decreases) | 1.53 | 1.55 |

In other systems monitored (allergy, special senses, metabolic-nutritional, urinary tract, genital tract, psychiatric, haematology, endocrine) occurrences were all below 1.5% (range 0.31– 1.29).

*Interactions:* There are currently no known drug interactions associated with the use of Regaine Topical Solution. Although it has not been clinically demonstrated, there exists the theoretical possibility of absorbed minoxidil potentiating orthostatic hypotension caused by guanethidine.

*Overdosage:* Increased systemic absorption of minoxidil may potentially occur if higher-than-recommended doses of Regaine are applied to larger surface areas of the body or areas other than the scalp. There are no known cases of minoxidil overdosage resulting from topical administration of Regaine.

Because of the concentration of minoxidil in Regaine, accidental ingestion has the potential of producing systemic effects related to the pharmacological action of the drug (5 ml of Regaine contains 100 mg minoxidil, the maximum recommended adult dose for oral minoxidil administration in the treatment of hypertension). Signs and symptoms of minoxidil overdosage would most likely be cardiovascular effects associated with sodium and water retention and tachycardia. Fluid retention can be managed with appropriate diuretic therapy. Clinically significant tachycardia can be controlled by administration of a beta adrenergic blocking agent.

If encountered, hypotension should be treated by intravenous administration of normal saline. Sympathomimetic drugs, such as noradrenaline and adrenaline, should be avoided because of their excessive cardiac stimulating activity.

**Pharmaceutical precautions**   Regaine Topical Solution should be stored at room temperature. The solution is flammable.

**Legal category**   P

**Package quantities**   Regaine Topical Solution is supplied in bottles of 60 ml with one or more of the following disposable applicators: pump spray, extended tip or rub-on assemblies.

**Further information**   The mechanism of action of minoxidil in the treatment of male pattern baldness is currently not known.

Following application of Regaine, minoxidil is poorly absorbed from normal intact skin with an average of 1.4% (range 0.3 – 4.5%) of the total applied dose reaching the systemic circulation. Therefore, a 1 ml dose of Regaine Topical Solution, delivering 20 mg of minoxidil solution to the skin, would result in absorption of approximately 0.28 mg minoxidil. This compares with greater than 95% absorption from the gastro-intestinal tract of orally administered minoxidil as tablets. Serum levels resulting from administration of Regaine are governed by the drug's percutaneous absorption rate. Following cessation of topical dosing of Regaine, approximately 95% of systemically absorbed minoxidil is eliminated within four days.

**Product licence number**   0032/0136

## REGAINE* TOPICAL SOLUTION 5%

**Qualitative and quantitative composition**   Minoxidil 50 mg/ml.

**Pharmaceutical form**   Topical Solution

**Clinical particulars**

*Therapeutic indications*: Regaine Topical Solution 5% is indicated for the treatment of alopecia androgenetica. There is also evidence that Regaine slows hair loss in patients with diagnosed male pattern baldness.

Onset and degree of hair regrowth may be variable among patients and it may take at least four months of continuous twice daily use before evidence of hair regrowth can be expected. Although trends in the data suggest that those patients who are younger, who have been balding for a shorter period of time or who have a smaller area of baldness on the vertex are more likely to respond to Regaine, individual response cannot be predicted. If hair regrowth occurs, twice daily applications of Regaine are necessary for continued hair growth. Anecdotal reports indicate that regrown hair may disappear three to four months after stopping Regaine application and the balding process will continue. Patients should discontinue treatment if there is no improvement after one year.

*Posology and method of administration*: Hair and scalp should be thoroughly dry prior to topical application of Regaine. A dose of 1 ml Regaine topical solution should be applied to the total affected areas of the scalp twice daily. The total dosage should not exceed 2 ml. If fingertips are used to facilitate drug application, hands should be washed afterwards.

The method of application varies according to the disposable applicator used:

*Pump spray applicator*: this is useful for large areas. Aim the pump at the centre of the bald area, press once and spread with fingertips over the entire bald area. Repeat for a total of 6 times to apply a dose of 1 ml. Avoid breathing spray mist.

*Extended spray tip applicator*: this is useful for small areas, or under hair. The pump spray applicator must be in place in order to use this additional applicator. Use in the same way as the pump spray.

*Rub-on applicator*: squeeze the upright bottle once to fill the 1 ml chamber to the black line. Invert bottle, dab on scalp, and spread Regaine over the entire bald area until chamber is empty.

*Children and the elderly*: Not recommended. The safety and effectiveness of Regaine in patients under 18 or over 65 years of age has not been established.

*Contra-indications:* Regaine is contra-indicated in patients with a history of sensitivity to minoxidil, ethanol, and propylene glycol.

*Special warnings and special precautions for use*: Patients with hypertension, including those under treatment with anti-hypertensive agents, should be monitored closely when treated with Regaine Topical Solution.

Regaine Topical Solution contains alcohol, which will cause burning and irritation of the eye. In the event of accidental contact with sensitive surfaces (eye, abraded skin and mucous membranes) the area should be bathed with large amounts of cool tap water.

Regaine Topical Solution should not be used in conjunction with other topical agents including corticosteroids, retinoids and petrolatum or agents that are known to enhance cutaneous drug absorption.

As is the case with other topically applied drugs, decreased integrity of the epidermal barrier caused by inflammation or disease processes in the skin (eg. excoriations of the scalp, scalp psoriasis, or severe sunburn) may increase percutaneous absorption of minoxidil.

Regaine is for external use only. Do not apply to areas of the body other than the scalp.

Hands should be washed thoroughly after applying the solution.

*Interaction with other medicaments and other forms of interaction*: There are currently no known drug interactions associated with the use of Regaine Topical Solution. Although it has not been clinically demonstrated, there exists the theoretical possibility of absorbed minoxidil potentiating orthostatic hypotension caused by peripheral vasodilators.

*Pregnancy and lactation*: There is no evidence as to drug safety in human pregnancy nor is there evidence from animal work that it is free from hazard. Regaine should not be used during pregnancy or lactation.

*Effects on ability to drive and use machines*: Based on the pharmacodynamic and overall safety profile of minoxidil, it is not expected that Regaine would interfere with the ability to drive or operate machinery.

*Undesirable effects*: Use of Regaine Topical Solution 5% results in slight absorption (an average of 1.7% of the applied topical dose) of minoxidil from the skin surface. Although not causally related to the use of Regaine in clinical trials, the following potential systemic effects should be considered: sodium and water retention, tachycardia, aggravation of pre-existing angina pectoris or the induction of anginal symptoms in patients with undiagnosed coronary artery disease. Patients should be instructed to discontinue use of Regaine and contact their physician if any of the above systemic effects occur.

When incidences of medical events in placebo-controlled trials of topical minoxidil were compared, they revealed that only reports involving the dermatological system were present at a significantly greater level in the minoxidil group than in the placebo group. In both groups in all body systems, the overall incidence of medical events reported by females was approximately five times that of males.

Details of percentage occurrences after 4–8 months treatment with minoxidil (n=3857) or placebo (n=2717) were as follows:-

| *Body System* | *Minoxidil % occurrence* | *Placebo % occurrence* |
|---|---|---|
| Respiratory (bronchitis, URTI, sinusitis) | 7.16 | 8.58 |
| Dermatological (irritant dermatitis, allergic contact dermatitis) | 7.36 | 5.41 |
| Gastro-intestinal (diarrhoea, nausea, vomiting) | 4.33 | 6.55 |
| Neurology (headache, dizziness, faintness, lightheadedness) | 3.42 | 3.46 |
| Musculoskeletal (fractures, back pain, tendinitis, aches and pains) | 2.59 | 2.21 |
| Cardiovascular (oedema, chest pain, blood pressure increases/decreases, palpitations, pulse rate increases/decreases) | 1.53 | 1.55 |

In other systems monitored (allergy, special senses, metabolic-nutritional, urinary tract, genital tract, psychiatric, haematology, endocrine) occurrences were all below 1.5% (range 0.31 – 1.29).

In a comparative trial between Regaine Topical Solution 5%, Regaine Topical Solution 2% and placebo, dermatological events were more frequent in the 5% group. The events were of similar type and severity in the 5% and 2% groups, but the incidence was greater in the 5% group.

*Overdose:* Increased systemic absorption of minoxidil may potentially occur if higher-than-recommended doses of Regaine are applied to larger surface areas of the body or areas other than the scalp. There are no known cases of minoxidil overdosage resulting from topical administration of Regaine.

Because of the concentration of minoxidil in Regaine, accidental ingestion has the potential of producing systemic effects related to the pharmacological action of the drug (2 ml of Regaine contains 100 mg minoxidil, the maximum recommended adult dose for oral minoxidil administration in the treatment of hypertension). Signs and symptoms of minoxidil overdosage would most likely be cardiovascular effects associated with sodium and water retention and tachycardia. Fluid retention can be managed with appropriate diuretic therapy. Clinically significant tachycardia can be controlled by administration of a beta adrenergic blocking agent.

**Pharmacological properties**

*Pharmacodynamic properties:* Minoxidil is a powerful vasodilator. It was noticed that in patients with severe hypertension, about 80% developed hypertrichosis as a side-effect. The mode of action of minoxidil in causing hair growth has not been elucidated. It does not appear to be due to vasodilatation or a hormonal action. Early studies indicate that it appears to induce growth in previously dormant hair follicle cells.

*Pharmacokinetic properties*: Following application of Regaine Topical Solution 5%, minoxidil is poorly absorbed from normal intact skin, with an average of 1.7% (range 0.3–4.5%) Of the total applied dose ultimately reaching the systemic circulation. Maximum serum concentrations average 2.9 ng/ml (range 0.3–20.0). In contrast, minoxidil is almost completely absorbed from the gastrointestinal tract following oral administration of minoxidil tablets. Following cessation of topical dosing of Regaine, approximately 95% of systemically absorbed minoxidil is eliminated within 4 days. The effects of concomitant dermal diseases on absorption are unknown.

The metabolic biotransformation of minoxidil absorbed following topical application has not been fully determined. Orally administered minoxidil is metabolised predominately by conjugation with glucuronic acid at the n-oxide position in the pyrimidine ring but also by conversion to more polar products. Known metabolites exert much less pharmacologic effect than minoxidil itself. Minoxidil does not bind to plasma proteins and its renal clearance corresponds to the glomerular filtration rate. Minoxidil does not cross the blood brain barrier. Minoxidil and its metabolites are haemodialysable, and are excreted principally in the urine.

**Pharmaceutical particulars**

*List of excipients*: Propylene glycol, ethanol, water.

*Incompatibilities:* None known.

*Shelf-life:* 24 months

*Special precautions for storage*: Regaine Topical Solution 5% is flammable.

*Nature and contents of container*: Polyethylene bottle containing 60 ml of solution. A pump spray, extended spray nozzle, and dab-on applicators are supplied.

*Instructions for use/handling:* As Regaine Topical Solution 5% is flammable, avoid smoking whilst applying.

**Marketing authorisation number** 0032/0183

**Dates of approval/revision of SPC** 18 October 1995

**Legal category** POM

## SALAZOPYRIN* TABLETS, ENEMAS, SUPPOSITORIES AND SUSPENSION

**Presentation**

Tablets: Yellow, 13.5 mm diameter tablets, tasteless, scored deeply on one side, with KPh on one side and 101 on the other, containing Sulphasalazine PhEur 0.5 g. Excipients: Maize starch, PVP, magnesium stearate, colloidal silicon dioxide.

*Enema:* Round, soft, polyethylene 135 ml enema bottle with screw-on cap/spout (elastomer valve in spout) containing sulphasalazine 3 g, vehicle to 100 mls. Excipients: Normal saline, methyl and propyl parabens.

*Suppositories:* Yellow, odourless, torpedo-shaped containing sulphasalazine 0.5 g. Excipients: PVP, hard fat.

*Suspension:* Yellow suspension, orange-lemon flavour 250 mg/5 ml in polythene bottle with tamper evident cap. Excipients: Xanthan gum, microcrystalline cellulose, sucrose, orange/lemon flavouring, polysorbate 80, sodium benzoate, water.

**Uses** Treatment of ulcerative colitis and Crohn's disease.

**Dosage and administration**

*Adults and elderly:* The dose is adjusted according to the severity of the disease and the patient's tolerance to the drug, as detailed below.

1. Tablets: Induction and maintenance of remission of ulcerative colitis; treatment of active Crohn's disease.

*Severe attack:* Salazopyrin 2–4 tablets four times a day may be given in conjunction with steroids as part of an intensive management regime. Rapid passage of the tablets may reduce effect of the drug. Night-time interval between doses should not exceed eight hours.

*Mild-moderate attack:* 2–4 tablets four times a day may be given in conjunction with steroids.

*Maintenance therapy:* With induction of remission reduce the dose gradually to 4 tablets per day. This dosage should be continued indefinitely, since discontinuance even several years after an acute attack is associated with a four fold increase in risk of relapse.

2. Enemas: Treatment of ulcerative colitis and Crohn's colitis.

One enema should be given daily, preferably at bedtime.

3. Suppositories: Treatment of ulcerative colitis and Crohn's colitis affecting the rectum.

Two suppositories to be inserted in the morning and two at bedtime after defaecation. After three weeks it may be possible to gradually reduce the dosage as the patient improves.

Adjunct to oral therapy: In severe generalised disease affecting the rectum or rectosigmoid, and in cases slow to respond to oral therapy, one or two suppositories may be given morning and evening in addition.

4. Suspension: Dosage as for tablets, 10 ml being taken instead of each 0.5 g tablet.

*Children*

1. Tablets: The dose is reduced in proportion to body weight.

| | |
|---|---|
| Severe attack: | 40–60 mg/kg per day |
| Mild–moderate attack: | 40–60 mg/kg per day |
| Maintenance: | 20–30 mg/kg per day |

2. Enema: The enema presentation contains an adult dose and is not recommended for children.
3. Suppositories: Reduce the adult dosage on the basis of body weight.

4. Suspension: 5 ml contains 250 mg sulphasalazine.
   Reduce adult dosage on the basis of body weight.

   | | |
   |---|---|
   | Severe attack: | 0.8–1.2 ml/kg per day |
   | Mild–moderate attack: | 0.8–1.2 ml/kg per day |
   | Maintenance therapy: | 0.4–0.6 ml/kg per day |

**Contra-indications, warnings, etc**
*Contra-indications:*

a. History of sensitivity to sulphonamides or salicylates.
b. Infants under 2 years of age.
c. In the case of the Enema, subjects sensitive to methyl or propyl parabens.
d. In the case of Suspension, subjects sensitive to sodium benzoate.

*Precautions:* Haematological and hepatic side effects may occur. Differential white cell, red cell and platelet counts should be performed initially and at least monthly for a minimum of the first three months of treatment. The patient should also be counselled to report immediately with any sore throat, fever, malaise or unexpected non specific illness. The treatment should be stopped immediately if there is suspicion or laboratory evidence of a potentially serious blood dyscrasia.

A patient information leaflet should be supplied specifically advising patients on blood dyscrasias.

Liver function tests should be carried out at monthly intervals for the first three months of treatment. Kidney function should be checked initially and at regular intervals during treatment.

Patients with allergy, or renal or hepatic disease should be treated with caution. Patients with glucose-6-phosphate dehydrogenase deficiency should be closely observed for signs of haemolytic anaemia (Heinz body anaemia).

The uptake of digoxin and folate may be reduced. An acute attack may be precipitated in patients with porphyria.

*Adverse effects:* Overall, about 75% of ADRs occur within 3 months of starting therapy, and over 90% by 6 months. Some undesirable effects are dose dependent and symptoms can often be alleviated by reduction of the dose.

Since sulphasalazine is metabolised to sulphapyridine and 5-amino salicylic acid, side-effects of sulphonamides or salicylates may occur. Patients with slow acetylator status are more likely to experience adverse effects due to sulphapyridine. The most commonly encountered reactions are nausea, headache, rash, loss of appetite and raised temperature.

The following adverse reactions have been reported:

*Haematological:* Potentially fatal leucopenia, neutropenia, agranulocytosis, aplastic anaemia and thrombocytopenia. Leucopenia, which is normally mild and transient, may occur in up to 1.5% of patients and agranulocytosis in up to 1 in 700 patients during the second month of therapy.

Heinz body anaemia, methaemoglobinaemia, hypoprothrombinaemia, haemolytic anaemia, megaloblastic anaemia.

*Hypersensitivity reactions:* Generalised skin eruptions, Stevens–Johnson syndrome, exfoliative dermatitis, epidermal necrolysis, pruritus, urticaria, photosensitisation, anaphylaxis, serum sickness, drug fever, periorbital oedema, conjunctival and scleral injection, arthralgia, allergic myocarditis, polyarteritis nodosa, LE-phenomenon and lung complications with dyspnoea, fever, cough, eosinophilia, fibrosing alveolitis.

*Gastro-intestinal reactions:* Stomatitis, parotitis, pancreatitis, hepatitis.

*CNS reactions:* Vertigo, tinnitus, peripheral neuropathy, ataxia, convulsions, insomnia, mental depression, aseptic meningitis and hallucinations.

*Fertility:* Oligospermia, reversible on discontinuance of drug.

*Renal reactions:* Crystalluria, haematuria, proteinuria and nephrotic syndrome. An acute attack may be precipitated in patients with porphyria.

*Overdosage:* There is no specific antidote to Salazopyrin.

*Pregnancy and lactation:* Long term clinical usage and experimental studies have failed to reveal any teratogenic or icteric hazards. The amounts of drug present in the milk should not present a risk to a healthy infant.

**Pharmaceutical precautions** Store suppositories in a cool place.

**Legal category** POM.

**Package quantities**

| | |
|---|---|
| Tablets: | Bottles of 112 |
| Suppositories: | Boxes of 10 |
| Enemas: | Boxes of 7×100 mls. |
| Suspension: | Bottles of 500 ml. |

**Further information** The drug may colour the urine orange-yellow.

Extended-wear soft contact lenses (Bausch and Lomb 70) have been reported as being permanently stained during sulphasalazine treatment. Daily-wear soft contact and gas-permeable types should respond to standard cleansing.

When gastro-intestinal intolerance to Salazopyrin tablets occurs, Salazopyrin EN-tabs may be used instead. These film-coated enteric tablets are subject to a separate Data Sheet.

The suspension contains 33 g/100 ml sucrose.

**Product licence numbers**

| | |
|---|---|
| Tablets: | 0022/0158 |
| Suppositories: | 0022/0156 |
| Enemas: | 0022/0154 |
| Suspension: | 0022/0157 |

## SALAZOPYRIN* EN-TABS

**Presentation** Yellow elliptical convex film coated enteric tablets, containing 0.5 g of sulphasalazine. One side of the tablet has KPh with 102 on the reverse. Excipients: maize starch, P.V.P., magnesium stearate, enteric coating, colloidal silicon dioxide.

**Uses**

1. The treatment of Rheumatoid Arthritis which has failed to respond to non-steroidal anti-inflammatory drugs (NSAIDs).
2. Induction and maintenance of remission of Ulcerative Colitis.
3. The treatment of active Crohn's disease.

**Dosage and administration**
*Rheumatoid arthritis*
*Adults including the elderly:* Commence treatment with 0.5 g daily (one tablet) for one week, thereafter increasing the dose by one tablet each week, to a maximum of 3 g/day (six tablets) as in the following table.

| | 1st Week | 2nd Week | 3rd Week | 4th Week |
|---|---|---|---|---|
| Morning — | | 1 tablet | 1 tablet | 2 tablets |
| Evening | 1 tablet | 1 tablet | 2 tablets | 2 tablets† |

†etc to 3 g/day maximum.

Should a patient experience nausea, the dose should be reduced to a previously tolerated dose for one week and then increased. EN-tabs should not be broken or crushed. Alternatively, the total daily dose may be divided and taken three times or four times daily.

In rheumatoid arthritis Salazopyrin EN-tabs have a 'disease-modifying' action: clinical and haematological response is often seen after one month but may be delayed for up to 12 weeks following the commencement of treatment.

Salazopyrin EN-tabs do not possess analgesic activity, therefore NSAIDs or analgesic treatment should not be reduced or stopped abruptly until clinical response has been achieved.

Patients have been maintained on Salazopyrin EN-tabs for several years.

No recommendations are made for the treatment of children with rheumatoid arthritis.

*Ulcerative colitis*
*Adults:*
*Severe:* 2–4 tablets four times a day may be given in conjunction with steroids as part of an intensive management regime. The night-time interval between doses should not exceed eight hours. In severe disease rapid passage of the tablets may reduce the effect of the drug.

*Mild–moderate:* 2–4 tablets four times a day may be given in conjunction with steroids.

*Maintenance:* With induction of remission reduce the dose gradually to four tablets per day in divided doses. This dosage should be continued indefinitely, since discontinuance even several years after an acute attack has been shown to be associated with a four fold increase in the risk of relapse.

Salazopyrin EN-tabs should not be broken or crushed.

*Children:* The dose is reduced in proportion to body weight.

| | |
|---|---|
| Severe: | 40–60 mg/kg per day |
| Mild–Moderate: | 40–60 mg/kg per day |
| Maintenance: | 20–30 mg/kg per day |

*Crohn's Disease:* In active Crohn's disease, Salazopyrin EN-tabs should be administered as for severe ulcerative colitis.

**Contra-indications, warnings, etc**
*Contra-indications:*

a. History of sensitivity to sulphonamides or salicylates.
b. Infants under 2 years of age.

*Precautions:* Haematological and hepatic side effects may occur. Differential white cell, red cell and platelet counts should be performed initially and at least monthly for a minimum of the first three months of treatment. The patient should also be counselled to report immediately with any sore throat, fever, malaise or unexpected non specific illness. Treatment should be stopped immediately if there is suspicion or laboratory evidence of a potentially serious blood dyscrasia.

A patient information leaflet should be supplied specifically advising patients on blood dyscrasias.

Liver function tests should be carried out at monthly intervals for the first three months of treatment. Kidney function should be checked initially and at intervals during treatment.

Patients with allergy, or renal or hepatic disease should be treated with caution. Patients with glucose-6-phosphate dehydrogenase deficiency should be closely observed for signs of haemolytic anaemia (Heinz body anaemia).

The uptake of digoxin and folate may be reduced. An acute attack may be precipitated in patients with porphyria.

*Adverse effects:* Overall, about 75% of ADRs occur within 3 months of starting therapy, and over 90% by 6 months. Some undesirable effects are dose dependent and symptoms can often be alleviated by reduction of the dose.

Since sulphasalazine is metabolised to sulphapyridine and 5-amino salicylic acid, effects of sulphonamides or salicylates may occur. Patients with slow acetylator status are more likely to experience adverse effects due to sulphapyridine. The most commonly encountered reactions are nausea, headache, rash, loss of appetite and raised temperature.

The following adverse reactions have been reported:

*Haematological:* Potentially fatal leucopenia, neutropenia, agranulocytosis, aplastic anaemia and thrombocytopenia. Leucopenia, which is normally mild and transient, may occur in up to 1.5% of patients and agranulocytosis in up to 1 in 700 patients during the second month of therapy.

The risk of sulphasalazine associated blood disorders is substantially higher in patients treated for rheumatoid arthritis than it is for patients treated for inflammatory bowel disease.

Heinz body anaemia, methaemoglobinaemia, hypoprothrombinaemia, haemolytic anaemia, megaloblastic anaemia.

*Hypersensitivity reactions:* Generalised skin eruptions, Stevens–Johnson syndrome, exfoliative dermatitis, epidermal necrolysis, pruritus, urticaria, photosensitisation, anaphylaxis, serum sickness, drug fever, periorbital oedema, conjunctival and scleral injection, arthralgia, allergic myocarditis, polyarteritis nodosa, LE-phenomenon and lung complications with dyspnoea, fever, cough, eosinophilia, fibrosing alveolitis.

*Gastro-intestinal reactions:* Stomatitis, parotitis, pancreatitis, hepatitis.

*CNS reactions:* Vertigo, tinnitus, peripheral neuropathy, ataxia, convulsions, insomnia, mental depression, aseptic meningitis and hallucinations.

*Fertility:* Oligospermia, reversible on discontinuance of drug.

*Renal reactions:* Crystalluria, haematuria, proteinuria and nephrotic syndrome.

*Overdosage:* There is no specific antidote to Salazopyrin EN-tabs.

*Pregnancy and lactation:* Long term clinical usage and experimental studies have failed to reveal any teratogenic or icteric hazards. The amounts of drug present in the milk should not present a risk to a healthy infant.

**Legal category** POM.

**Package quantities** EN-tabs: Containers of 112 (special easily-opened pack for the disabled).

**Further information** The drug may colour the urine orange-yellow.

Extended-wear soft contact lenses (Bausch and Lomb 70) have been reported as being permanently stained during sulphasalazine treatment. Daily-wear soft contact and gas-permeable types should respond to standard cleansing.

**Product licence number** 0022/0155

## SOLIVITO* N

**Presentation** A yellow lyophilised mixture of water-soluble vitamins to be added, after reconstitution, to glucose solution or Intralipid for intravenous infusion. One vial of Solivito N corresponds to the following formula:

| Thiamine mononitrate | 3.1 mg |
|---|---|
| Sodium riboflavine phosphate | 4.9 mg |
| Nicotinamide | 40 mg |
| Pyridoxine hydrochloride | 4.9 mg |
| Sodium pantothenate | 16.5 mg |
| Biotin | 60 micrograms |
| Folic acid | 0.4 mg |
| Cyanocobalamin | 5.0 micrograms |
| Sodium ascorbate | 113 mg |
| Glycine | 300 mg |
| Sodium edetate | 0.5 mg |
| Methyl hydroxybenzoate | 0.5 mg |

One vial of Solivito N contains the following quantities of water-soluble vitamins:

| Vitamin B$_1$ | 2.5 mg |
|---|---|
| Vitamin B$_2$ | 3.6 mg |
| Nicotinamide | 40 mg |
| Vitamin B$_6$ | 4.0 mg |
| Pantothenic acid | 15.0 mg |
| Biotin | 60 micrograms |
| Folic acid | 0.4 mg |
| Vitamin B$_{12}$ | 5.0 micrograms |
| Vitamin C | 100 mg |

**Uses** Solivito N is intended as a supplement in intravenous nutrition in order to cover the daily requirements of the water-soluble vitamins in both adults and infants.

**Dosage and administration** The daily requirements of the majority of adult patients and children weighing 10 kg or more are met by the contents of one vial.

Children weighing less than 10 kg should receive 1/10 of the contents of one vial per kg bodyweight.

*Recommended dosage for adults and children weighing 10 kg or more:* The contents of one vial of Solivito N are dissolved by the aseptic addition of 10 ml of one of the following:

(i)   Vitlipid N Adult or, for children under 11 years of age, Vitlipid N Infant
(ii)  Intralipid 10%, 20% or 30%
(iii) Glucose intravenous infusion (5–60%)
(iv)  Water for Injections

The reconstituted mixtures (i) or (ii) should be aseptically transferred to Intralipid 10%, 20% or 30% for infusion. The reconstituted mixtures (iii) and (iv) should be added to either glucose solution (5–60%) or Intralipid 10%, 20% or 30%. In this way the basal requirements of the water-soluble vitamins are provided.

*Recommended dosage for infants and children weighing under 10 kg:* The contents of one vial are dissolved by the aseptic addition of 10 ml of one of the following:

(i)   Vitlipid N Infant
(ii)  Intralipid 10%, 20% or 30%
(iii) Glucose intravenous infusion (5–60%)
(iv)  Water for injections

The basal requirements for water-soluble vitamins in children are provided by 1.0 ml of this reconstituted mixture per kg bodyweight.

The reconstituted mixtures (i) and (ii) should be aseptically transferred to Intralipid 10%, 20% or 30% for infusion. The reconstituted mixtures (iii) and (iv) should be added to either glucose solution (5–60%) or to Intralipid 10%, 20% or 30%.

1 vial of Solivito N should be infused over a minimum period of 2–3 hours in patients with normal renal function so as to minimise renal losses.

**Contra-indications, warnings, etc** Known hypersensitivity to any of the components, e.g. thiamine (vitamin B$_1$) or methyl hydroxybenzoate.

*Precautions:* Pyridoxine (vitamin B$_6$) can reduce the effect of levodopa. Some of the optic neuropathies appear to respond to massive doses of hydroxocobalamin and have been claimed to be adversely affected by administration of cyanocobalamin. Folic acid may lower the serum concentration of phenytoin and obscure pernicious anaemia.

*Pregnancy and lactation:* Solution is a supplement in TPN regimens, providing water soluble vitamins. No hazard is expected if used in pregnancy at the recommended dosage, covering the daily requirements of vitamins B$_1$, B$_2$, B$_6$, B$_{12}$ and C.

No animal studies have been performed. There are, however, published reports on the safe and successful use of vitamins as part of a TPN regimen during pregnancy in the human.

**Pharmaceutical precautions** Store the lyophilised powder before reconstitution at 2–8˚C, protected from light. The addition of Solivito N should be performed aseptically immediately before the start of the infusion and the solution should be used within 24 hours of preparation.

**Legal category** POM.

**Package quantities** Boxes of 10 vials.

**Further information** The manufacturer can be consulted for full information on complete and balanced intravenous nutrition regimens.

**Product licence number** 0022/0061.

## SOLU-CORTEF*

**Qualitative and quantitative composition** Hydrocortisone sodium succinate 133.7 mg equivalent to hydrocortisone 100.0 mg.

**Pharmaceutical form:** White, freeze dried powder for parenteral use.

**Clinical particulars**

*Therapeutic indications:* Anti-inflammatory agent.

Solu-Cortef is indicated for any condition in which rapid and intense corticosteroid effect is required such as:

*Endocrine disorders:* primary or secondary adrenocortical insufficiency
*Collagen diseases:* systemic lupus erythematosus
*Dermatological diseases:* severe erythema multiforme (Stevens-Johnson syndrome)
*Allergic states:* bronchial asthma, anaphylactic reactions
*Gastro-intestinal diseases:* ulcerative colitis, Crohn's disease
*Respiratory diseases:* apiration of gastric contents
*Medical emergencies:* Solu-Cortef is indicated in the treatment of shock secondary to adrenocortical insufficiency or shock unresponsive to conventional therapy when adrenocortical insufficiency may be present.

*Posology and method of administration:* Solu-Cortef may be administered by intravenous injection, by intravenous infusion or by intramuscular injection, the preferred method for initial emergency use being intravenous injection. Following the initial emergency period, consideration should be given to employing a longer-acting injectable preparation or an oral preparation.

Dosage usually ranges from 100 mg to 500 mg depending on the severity of the condition, administered by intravenous injection over a period of one to ten minutes. This dose may be repeated at intervals of 2, 4 or 6 hours as indicated by the patient's response and clinical condition.

In general, high-dose corticosteroid therapy should be continued only until the patient's condition has stabilised – usually not beyond 48 to 72 hours. If hydrocortisone therapy must be continued beyond 48 to 72 hours hypernatraemia may occur. Therefore, it may be preferable to replace Solu-Cortef with a corticosteroid such as methylprednisolone sodium succinate as little or no sodium retention occurs. Although adverse effects associated with high dose, short-term corticoid therapy are uncommon, peptic ulceration may occur. Prophylactic antacid therapy may be indicated.

Patients subjected to severe stress following corticoid therapy should be observed closely for signs and symptoms of adrenocortical insufficiency.

Corticosteroid therapy is an adjunct to and not a replacement for, conventional therapy.

*Elderly patients:* Solu-Cortef is primarily used in acute short-term conditions. There is no information to suggest that a change in dosage is warranted in the elderly. However, treatment of elderly patients should be planned bearing in mind the more serious consequences of the common side-effects of corticosteroids in old age and close clinical supervision is required (see Special warnings and special precautions for use).

*Children:* While the dose may be reduced for infants and children, it is governed more by the severity of the condition and response of the patient than by age or body weight but should not be less than 25 mg daily (see *Special warnings and special precautions for use*).

*Preparation of solutions:* For intravenous or intramuscular injection prepare the solution aseptically by adding not more than 2 ml of Sterile Water for Injections to the contents of one vial of Solu-Cortef 100 mg, shake and withdraw for use.

For intravenous infusion, first prepare the solution by adding not more than 2 ml of Sterile Water for Injections to the vial; this solution may then be added to 100 ml – 1000 ml (but not less than 100 ml) of 5% dextrose in water (or isotonic saline solution or 5% dextrose in isotonic saline solution if patient is not on sodium restriction).

When reconstituted as directed, the pH of the solution will range from 7.0 to 8.0.

**Contra-indications:** Solu-Cortef is contra-indicated where there is known hypersensitivity to components and in systemic fungal infection unless specific anti-infective therapy is employed.

*Special warnings and special precautions for use:*

*Warnings and precautions:* A Patient Information Leaflet is provided in the pack by the manufacturer.

Undesirable effects may be minimised by using the lowest effective dose for the minimum period. Frequent patient review is required to appropriately titrate the dose against disease activity (see Posology and method of administration).

Adrenal cortical atrophy develops during prolonged therapy and may persist for months after stopping treatment. Withdrawal of corticosteroids after prolonged therapy must, therefore, always be gradual to avoid acute adrenal insufficiency, being tapered off over weeks or months according to the dose and duration of treatment. During prolonged therapy any intercurrent illness, trauma or surgical procedure will require a temporary increase in dosage; if corticosteroids have been stopped following prolonged therapy, they may need to be temporarily re-introduced.

Patients should carry 'Steroid Treatment' cards which give clear guidance on the precautions to be taken to minimise risk and which provide details of prescriber, drug, dosage and the duration of treatment.

Corticosteroids may mask some signs of infection and new infections may appear during their use. Suppression of the inflammatory response and immune function increases the susceptibility to fungal, viral and bacterial infections and their severity. The clinical presentation may often be atypical and may reach an advanced stage before being recognised.

Chickenpox is of serious concern since this normally minor illness may be fatal in immunosuppressed patients. Patients (or parents of children) without a definite history of chickenpox should be advised to avoid close personal contact with chickenpox or herpes zoster and, if exposed, they should seek urgent medical attention. Passive immunization with varicella/zoster immunoglobin (VZIG) is needed by exposed non-immune patients who are receiving systemic corticosteroids or who have used them within the previous 3 months; this should be given within 10 days of exposure to chickenpox. If a diagnosis of chickenpox is confirmed, the illness warrants specialist care and urgent treatment. Corticosteroids should not be stopped and the dose may need to be increased.

Live vaccines should not be given to individuals with impaired immune responsiveness. The antibody response to other vaccines may be diminished.

The use of Solu-Cortef in active tuberculosis should be restricted to those cases of fulminating or disseminated tuberculosis in which the corticosteroid is used for the management of the disease in conjunction with an appropriate antituberculosis regimen. If corticosteroids are indicated in patients with latent tuberculosis or tuberculin reactivity, close observation is necessary as reactivation of the disease may occur. During prolonged corticosteroid therapy, these patients should receive chemoprophylaxis.

Rarely, anaphylactoid reactions have been reported following parenteral Solu-Cortef therapy. Physicians using the drug should be prepared to deal with such a possibility. Appropriate precautionary measures should be taken prior to administration, especially when the patient has a history of drug allergy.

Care should be taken with patients receiving cardioactive drugs such as digoxin because of steroid induced electrolyte disturbance/potassium loss (see Undesirable effects).

*Special precautions:* Particular care is required when considering the use of systemic corticosteroids in patients with the following conditions and frequent patient monitoring is necessary: osteoporosis (postmenopausal females are particularly at risk); hypertension or congestive heart failure; existing or previous history of severe affective disorders (especially previous steroid psychosis); diabetes mellitus (or a family history of diabetes).

History of tuberculosis; glaucoma (or a family history of glaucoma); previous corticosteroid-induced myopathy; liver failure or cirrhosis; renal insufficiency; epilepsy; peptic ulceration; fresh intestinal anastomoses; predisposition to thrombophlebitis; abscess or other pyogenic infections; ulcerative colitis; diverticulitis; myasthenia gravis; ocular herpes simplex for fear of corneal perforation; hypothyroidism.

*Use in children:* Corticosteroids cause growth retardation in infancy, childhood and adolescence, which may be irreversible. Treatment should be limited to the minimum dosage for the shortest possible time. The use of steroids should be restricted to the most serious indications.

*Use in the elderly:* The common adverse effects of systemic corticosteroids may be associated with more serious consequences in old age, especially osteoporosis, hypertension, hypokalaemia, diabetes, susceptibility to infection and thinning of the skin. Close clinical supervision is required to avoid life-threatening reactions.

*Interaction with other medicaments and other forms*

*of interaction:* Convulsions have been reported with concurrent use of corticosteroids and cyclosporin. Since concurrent administration of these agents results in a mutual inhibition of metabolism, it is possible that convulsions and other adverse effects associated with the individual use of either drug may be more apt to occur.

Drugs that induce hepatic enzymes, such as rifampicin, rifabutin, carbamazepine, phenobarbitone, phenytoin, primidone and aminoglutethimide enhance the metabolism of corticosteroids and its therapeutic effects may be reduced.

Drugs such as erythromycin and ketoconazole may inhibit the metabolism of corticosteroids and thus decrease their clearance.

Steroids may reduce the effects of anticholinesterases in myasthenia gravis. The desired effects of hypoglycaemic agents (including insulin), anti-hypertensives and diuretics are antagonised by corticosteroids and the hypokalaemic effects of acetazolamide, loop diuretics, thiazide diuretics and carbenoxolone are enhanced.

The efficacy of coumarin anticoagulants may be enhanced by concurrent corticosteroid therapy and close monitoring of the INR or prothrombin time is required to avoid spontaneous bleeding.

The renal clearance of salicylates is increased by corticosteroids and steroid withdrawal may result in salicylate intoxication. Salicylates and non-steroidal anti-inflammatory agents should be used cautiously in conjunction with corticosteroids in hypothrombinaemia.

Steroids have been reported to interact with neuromuscular blocking agents such as pancuronium with partial reversal of the neuromuscular block.

*Pregnancy and lactation:* Corticosteroids cross the placenta. There may be a very small risk of cleft palate and intra-uterine growth retardation in the fetus; there is evidence of harmful effects on pregnancy in animals. Neonates of mothers who received such therapy during pregnancy should be observed for signs of hypoadrenalism and appropriate measures instituted if such signs exist. When corticosteroids are essential, however, patients with normal pregnancies may be treated as though they were in the non-gravid state. Patients with pre-eclampsia or fluid retention require close monitoring.

Because prednisolone is excreted in breast milk, it is reasonable to assume that all corticosteroids are. Infants of mothers taking pharmacological doses of steroids should be monitored carefully for signs of adrenal suppression.

*Effects on ability to drive and use machines:* None stated.

*Undesirable effects:* Since Solu-Cortef is normally employed on a short-term basis it is unlikely that side-effects will occur; however, the possibility of side-effects attributable to corticosteroid therapy should be recognised (see Special warnings and special precautions for use). Such side-effects include:

*Parenteral corticosteroid therapy* – Anaphylactoid reaction e.g. bronchospasm, hypopigmentation or hyperpigmentation, subcutaneous and cutaneous atrophy, sterile abscess, laryngeal oedema and urticaria.

*Gastro-intestinal*– Dyspepsia, peptic ulceration with perforation and haemorrhage, abdominal distension, oesophageal ulceration, oesophageal candidiasis, acute pancreatitis, perforation of bowel.

Increases in alanine transaminase (ALT, SGPT) aspartate transaminase (AST, SGOT) and alkaline phosphatase have been observed following corticosteroid treatment. These changes are usually small, not associated with any clinical syndrome and are reversible upon discontinuation.

*Anti-inflammatory and immunosuppressive effects* – Increased susceptibility and severity of infections with suppression of clinical symptoms and signs, opportunistic infections, may suppress reactions to skin tests, recurrence of dormant tuberculosis (see Special warnings and special precautions for use).

*Musculoskeletal* – Proximal myopathy, osteoporosis, vertebral and long bone fractures, avascular osteonecrosis, tendon rupture, aseptic necrosis, muscle weakness.

*Fluid and electrolyte disturbance* – Sodium and water retention, potassium loss, hypertension, hypokalaemic alkalosis, congestive heart failure in susceptible patients.

*Dermatological – Impaired healing, petechiae and ecchymosis, skin atrophy, bruising, striae, increased sweating, telangiectasia, acne.*

*Endocrine/metabolic* – Suppression of the hypothalamo-pituitary-adrenal axis; growth suppression in infancy, childhood and adolescence; menstrual irregularity and amenorrhoea, Cushingoid facies, hirsutism, weight gain, impaired carbohydrate tolerance with increased requirement for antidiabetic therapy, negative nitrogen and calcium balance, increased appetite.

*Neuropsychiatric* – Euphoria, psychological dependence, mood swings, depression, personality changes, insomnia, convulsions, increased intra-cranial pressure with papilloedema in children (pseudotumour cerebri), usually after treatment withdrawal. Psychosis, aggravation of schizophrenia, seizures.

*Ophthalmic* – Increased intra-ocular pressure, glaucoma, papilloedema, cataracts with possible damage to the optic nerve, corneal or scleral thinning, exacerbation of ophthalmic viral or fungal disease, exophthalmos.

*General* – Leucocytosis, hypersensitivity reactions including anaphylaxis, thrombo-embolism, nausea, malaise.

*Withdrawal symptoms* – Too rapid a reduction of corticosteroid dosage following prolonged treatment can lead to acute adrenal insufficiency, hypotension and death. However, this is more applicable to corticosteroids with an indication where continuous therapy is given (see *Special warnings and special precautions for use*).

A 'withdrawal syndrome' may also occur including, fever, myalgia, arthralgia, rhinitis, conjunctivitis, painful itchy skin nodules and loss of weight.

*Overdose:* There is no clinical syndrome of acute overdosage with Solu-Cortef. Hydrocortisone is dialysable.

**Pharmacological properties**

*Pharmacodynamic properties:* Hydrocortisone sodium succinate has the same metabolic and anti-inflammatory actions as hydrocortisone. It is a glucocorticosteroid. Used in pharmacological doses, its actions supress the clinical manifestations of disease in a wide range of disorders.

*Pharmacokinetic properties:* Twelve normal subjects received 100, 200 or 400 mg Solu-Cortef intravenously. Radio-immunoassay results were as follows:-

| *DOSE (mg)* | *CMAX (µg 100 ml)* | *TMAX (hr)* | *12-HR AUC (mG/ 100 ml x hr)* |
|---|---|---|---|
| 100 | 132.3 | 0.35 | 418.0 |
| 200 | 231.8 | 0.25 | 680.0 |
| 400 | 629.8 | 0.37 | 1024.0 |

In another study, a 1 mg/kg i.m. dose of Solu-Cortef peaked in 30-60 minutes, with a plasma $C_{max}$ of 80 mg/ 100 ml.

In analysing hydrocortisone metabolism, a 25 mg IV dose resulted in higher plasma concentrations in females than in males.

**Pharmaceutical particulars**

*List of excipients:* Sodium biphosphate, sodium phosphate.

*Incompatibilities:* None stated.

*Shelf-life:* Shelf-life of the medicinal product as packaged for sale: 60 months.

After reconstitution with Sterile Water for Injections, use immediately, discard any remainder.

*Special precautions for storage:* Store below 25°C.

Refer to Section 'Dosage and Administration'. No diluents other than those referred to are recommended. Parenteral drug products should be inspected visually for particulate matter and discoloration prior to administration.

*Nature and contents of container:* Type I flint glass vials with a butyl rubber plug and metal seal. Each vial of Solu-Cortef 100 mg contains the equivalent of 100 mg hydrocortisone as the sodium succinate for reconstitution with 2 ml of Sterile Water for Injections.

*Instructions for use/handling:* No special requirements.

**Marketing authorisation number** 0032/5019

**Date of approval/revision of SPC** June 1995

**Legal category** POM

## SOLU-MEDRONE*

**Qualitative and quantitative composition**

Solu-Medrone 40 mg : Methylprednisolone sodium succinate 53.0 mg equivalent to 40 mg of methylprednisolone.

Solu-Medrone 125 mg : Methylprednisolone sodium succinate 165.8 mg equivalent to 125 mg of methylprednisolone.

Solu-Medrone 500 mg : Methylprednisolone sodium succinate 663.0 mg equivalent to 500 mg of methylprednisolone.

Solu-Medrone 1 gram : Methylprednisolone sodium succinate 1.326 gm equivalent to 1.0 g of methylprednisolone.

**Pharmaceutical form** Powder for injection.

**Clinical particulars**

*Therapeutic indications:* Solu-Medrone is indicated to treat any condition in which rapid and intense corticosteroid effect is required such as:

*Dermatological disease:* Severe erythema multiforme (Stevens-Johnson syndrome)

*Allergic states:* Bronchial asthma; Severe seasonal and perennial allergic rhinitis; Angioneurotic oedema; Anaphylaxis

*Gastro-intestinal diseases:* Ulcerative colitis; Crohn's disease

*Respiratory diseases:* Aspiration of gastric contents; Fulminating or disseminated tuberculosis (with appropriate antituberculous chemotherapy)

*Neurological disorders:* Cerebral oedema secondary to cerebral tumour; Acute exacerbations of multiple sclerosis superimposed on a relapsing-remitting background.

*Miscellaneous:* T.B. meningitis (with appropriate antituberculous chemotherapy); Transplantation

*Posology and method of administration:* Solu-Medrone may be administered intravenously or intramuscularly, the preferred method for emergency use being intravenous injection given over a suitable time interval. When administering Solu-Medrone in high doses intravenously it should be given over a period of at least 30 minutes. Doses up to 250 mg should be given intravenously over a period of at least five minutes.

For intravenous infusion the initially prepared solution may be diluted with 5% dextrose in water, isotonic saline solution, or 5% dextrose in isotonic saline solution. To avoid compatibility problems with other drugs Solu-Medrone should be administered separately, only in the solutions mentioned.

Undesirable effects may be minimised by using the lowest effective dose for the minimum period (see *Other special warnings and precautions*).

Parenteral drug products should wherever possible be visually inspected for particulate matter and discoloration prior to administration.

*Adults:* Dosage should be varied according to the severity of the condition, initial dosage will vary from 10 to 500 mg. In the treatment of graft rejection reactions following transplantation, a dose of up to 1 g/day may be required. Although doses and protocols have varied in studies using methylprednisolone sodium succinate in the treatment of graft rejection reactions, the published literature supports the use of doses of this level, with 500 mg to 1 g most commonly used for acute rejection. Treatment at these doses should be limited to a 48–72 hour period until the patient's condition has stabilised, as prolonged high dose corticosteroid therapy can cause serious corticosteroid induced side-effects (see *Undesirable effects* and *Special warnings and special precautions for use*).

*Children:* In the treatment of high dose indications, such as haematological, rheumatic, renal and dermatological conditions, a dosage of 30 mg/kg/day to a maximum of 1 g/day is recommended. This dosage may be repeated for three pulses either daily or on alternate days. In the treatment of graft rejection reactions following transplantation, a dosage of 10 to 20 mg/kg/day for up to 3 days, to a maximum of 1 g/ day, is recommended. In the treatment of status asthmaticus, a dosage of 1 to 4 mg/kg/day for 1–3 days is recommended.

*Elderly patients:* Solu-Medrone is primarily used in acute short-term conditions. There is no information to suggest that a change in dosage is warranted in the elderly. However, treatment of elderly patients should be planned bearing in mind the more serious consequences of the common side-effects of corticosteroids in old age and close clinical supervision is required (see *Special warnings and special precautions for use*).

*Detailed recommendations for adult dosage are as follows:*

*In anaphylactic reactions* adrenaline or noradrenaline should be administered first for an immediate haemodynamic effect, followed by intravenous injection of Solu-Medrone (methylprednisolone sodium succinate) with other accepted procedures. There is evidence that corticosteroids through their prolonged haemodynamic effect are of value in preventing recurrent attacks of acute anaphylactic reactions.

*In sensitivity reactions* Solu-Medrone is capable of providing relief within one half to two hours. In patients with status asthmaticus Solu-Medrone may be given at a dose of 40 mg intravenously, repeated as dictated by patient response. In some asthmatic patients it may be advantageous to administer by slow intravenous drip over a period of hours.

*In graft rejection reactions following transplantation* doses of up to 1 g per day have been used to suppress rejection crises, with doses of 500 mg to 1 g most commonly used for acute rejection. Treatment should be continued only until the patient's condition has stabilised; usually not beyond 48–72 hours.

*In cerebral oedema* corticosteroids are used to

reduce or prevent the cerebral oedema associated with brain tumours (primary or metastatic).

In patients with oedema due to tumour, tapering the dose of corticosteroid appears to be important in order to avoid a rebound increase in intracranial pressure. If brain swelling does occur as the dose is reduced (intracranial bleeding having been ruled out), restart larger and more frequent doses parenterally. Patients with certain malignancies may need to remain on oral corticosteroid therapy for months or even life. Similar or higher doses may be helpful to control oedema during radiation therapy.

The following are suggested dosage schedules for oedemas due to brain tumour:

| Schedule A (1) | Dose (mg) | Route | Interval in hours | Duration |
|---|---|---|---|---|
| Pre-operative | 20 | IM | 3--6 | |
| During surgery | 20--40 | IV | hourly | |
| Post-operative | 20 | IM | 3 | 24 hours |
| | 16 | IM | 3 | 24 hours |
| | 12 | IM | 3 | 24 hours |
| | 8 | IM | 3 | 24 hours |
| | 4 | IM | 3 | 24 hours |
| | 4 | IM | 6 | 24 hours |
| | 4 | IM | 12 | 24 hours |

| Schedule B (2) | Dose (mg) | Route | Interval in hours | Days Duration |
|---|---|---|---|---|
| Pre-operative | 40 | IM | 6 | 2–3 |
| Post-operative | 40 | IM | 6 | 3–5 |
| | 20 | oral | 6 | 1 |
| | 12 | oral | 6 | 1 |
| | 8 | oral | 8 | 1 |
| | 4 | oral | 12 | 1 |
| | 4 | oral | | 1 |

Aim to discontinue therapy after a total of 10 days.

*References:* Fox JL, MD. 'Use of Methylprednisolone in Intracranial Surgery' Medical Annals of the District of Columbia, 34:261–265,1965.

Cantu RC, MD Harvard Neurological Service, Boston, Massachusetts. Letter on file, The Upjohn Company (February 1970).

In the treatment of *acute exacerbations of multiple sclerosis* in adults, the recommended dose is 1 g daily for 3 days. Solu-Medrone should be given as an intravenous infusion over at least 30 minutes.

*In other indications*, initial dosage will vary from 10 to 500 mg depending on the clinical problem being treated. Larger doses may be required for short-term management of severe, acute conditions. The initial dose, up to 250 mg, should be given intravenously over a period of at least 5 minutes, doses exceeding 250 mg should be given intravenously over a period of at least 30 minutes. Subsequent doses may be given intravenously or intramuscularly at intervals dictated by the patient's response and clinical condition. Corticosteroid therapy is an adjunct to, and not replacement for, conventional therapy.

*Contra-indications:* Solu-Medrone is contra-indicated where there is known hypersensitivity to components, in systemic infection unless specific anti-infective therapy is employed and in cerebral oedema in malaria.

*Special warnings and special precautions for use:* Warnings and precautions: A Patient Information Leaflet is provided in the pack by the manufacturer.

Undesirable effects may be minimised by using the lowest effective dose for the minimum period. Frequent patient review is required to appropriately titrate the dose against disease activity (see *Posology and method of administration*).

Adrenal cortical atrophy develops during prolonged therapy and may persist for months after stopping treatment. Withdrawal of corticosteroids after prolonged therapy must therefore always be gradual to avoid acute adrenal insufficiency, being tapered off over weeks or months according to the dose and duration of treatment. During prolonged therapy any intercurrent illness, trauma or surgical procedure will require a temporary increase in dosage; if corticosteroids have been stopped following prolonged therapy they may need to be temporarily re-introduced.

Patients should carry 'Steroid Treatment' cards which give clear guidance on the precautions to be taken to minimise risk and which provide details of prescriber, drug, dosage and the duration of treatment.

Although Solu-Medrone is not approved in the UK for use in any shock indication, the following warning statement should be adhered to. Data from a clinical study conducted to establish the efficacy of Solu-Medrone in septic shock, suggest that a higher mortality occurred in subsets of patients who entered the study with elevated serum creatinine levels or who developed a secondary infection after therapy

began. Therefore this product should not be used in the treatment of septic syndrome or septic shock.

There have been a few reports of cardiac arrhythmias and/or circulatory collapse and/or cardiac arrest associated with the rapid intravenous administration of large doses of Solu-Medrone (greater than 500 mg administered over a period of less than 10 minutes). Bradycardia has been reported during or after the administration of large doses of methylprednisolone sodium succinate, and may be unrelated to the speed and duration of infusion.

Corticosteroids may mask some signs of infection, and new infections may appear during their use. Suppression of the inflammatory response and immune function increases the susceptibility to fungal, viral and bacterial infections and their severity. The clinical presentation may often be atypical and may reach an advanced stage before being recognised. Chickenpox is of serious concern since this normally minor illness may be fatal in immunosuppressed patients. Patients (or parents of children) without a definite history of chickenpox should be advised to avoid close personal contact with chickenpox or herpes zoster and if exposed they should seek urgent medical attention. Passive immunization with varicella/zoster immunoglobin (VZIG) is needed by exposed non-immune patients who are receiving systemic corticosteroids or who have used them within the previous 3 months; this should be given within 10 days of exposure to chickenpox. If a diagnosis of chickenpox is confirmed, the illness warrants specialist care and urgent treatment. Corticosteroids should not be stopped and the dose may need to be increased.

Live vaccines should not be given to individuals with impaired immune responsiveness. The antibody response to other vaccines may be diminished.

The use of Solu-Medrone in active tuberculosis should be restricted to those cases of fulminating or disseminated tuberculosis in which the corticosteroid is used for the management of the disease in conjunction with an appropriate anti-tuberculous regimen. If corticosteroids are indicated in patients with latent tuberculosis or tuberculin reactivity, close observation is necessary as reactivation of the disease may occur. During prolonged corticosteroid therapy, these patients should receive chemoprophylaxis.

Rarely anaphylactoid reactions have been reported following parenteral Solu-Medrone therapy. Physicians using the drug should be prepared to deal with such a possibility. Appropriate precautionary measures should be taken prior to administration, especially when the patient has a history of drug allergy.

Care should be taken for patients receiving cardioactive drugs such as digoxin because of steroid induced electrolyte disturbance/potassium loss (see *Undesirable effects*).

*Special precautions:* Particular care is required when considering the use of systemic corticosteroids in patients with the following conditions and frequent patient monitoring is necessary:

Osteoporosis (post-menopausal females are particularly at risk).

Hypertension or congestive heart failure.

Existing or previous history of severe affective disorders (especially previous steroid psychosis).

Diabetes mellitus (or a family history of diabetes).

History of tuberculosis.

Glaucoma (or a family history of glaucoma).

Previous corticosteroid-induced myopathy.

Liver failure or cirrhosis.

Renal insufficiency.

Epilepsy.

Peptic ulceration.

Fresh intestinal anastomoses.

Predisposition to thrombophlebitis.

Abscess or other pyogenic infections.

Ulcerative colitis.

Diverticulitis.

Myasthenia gravis.

Ocular herpes simplex, for fear of corneal perforation.

Hypothyroidism.

*Use in children:* Corticosteroids cause growth retardation in infancy, childhood and adolescence, which may be irreversible. Treatment should be limited to the minimum dosage for the shortest possible time. In order to minimise suppression of the hypothalamo-pituitary-adrenal axis and growth retardation, treatment should be administered where possible as a single dose on alternate days.

*Use in the elderly:* The common adverse effects of systemic corticosteroids may be associated with more serious consequences in old age, especially osteoporosis, hypertension, hypokalaemia, diabetes, susceptibility to infection and thinning of the skin. Close clinical supervision is required to avoid life-threatening reactions.

*Interaction with other medicaments and other forms of interaction:* Convulsions have been reported with

concurrent use of methylprednisolone and cyclosporin. Since concurrent administration of these agents results in a mutual inhibition of metabolism, it is possible that convulsions and other adverse events associated with the individual use of either drug may be more apt to occur.

Drugs that induce hepatic enzymes, such as rifampicin, rifabutin, carbamazepine, phenobarbitone, phenytoin, primidone, and aminoglutethimide enhance the metabolism of corticosteroids and its therapeutic effects may be reduced.

Drugs such as erythromycin and ketoconazole may inhibit the metabolism of corticosteroids and thus decrease their clearance.

Steroids may reduce the effects of anticholinesterases in myasthenia gravis. The desired effects of hypoglycaemic agents (including insulin), anti-hypertensives and diuretics are antagonised by corticosteroids, and the hypokalaemic effects of acetazolamide, loop diuretics, thiazide diuretics and carbenoxolone are enhanced.

The efficacy of coumarin anticoagulants may be enhanced by concurrent corticosteroid therapy and close monitoring of the INR or prothrombin time is required to avoid spontaneous bleeding.

The renal clearance of salicylates is increased by corticosteroids and steroid withdrawal may result in salicylate intoxication. Salicylates and non-steroidal anti-inflammatory agents should be used cautiously in conjunction with corticosteroids in hypothrombinaemia.

Steroids have been reported to interact with neuromuscular blocking agents such as pancuronium with partial reversal of the neuromuscular block.

*Pregnancy and Lactation:* Corticosteroids cross the placenta. There may be a very small risk of cleft palate and intra-uterine growth retardation in the fetus; there is evidence of harmful effects on pregnancy in animals. Neonates of mothers who received such therapy during pregnancy should be observed for signs of hypoadrenalism and appropriate measures instituted if such signs exist. When corticosteroids are essential however, patients with normal pregnancies may be treated as though they were in the non-gravid state. Patients with pre-eclampsia or fluid retention require close monitoring.

Methylprednisolone is excreted in breast milk and infants of mothers taking pharmacological doses of steroids should be monitored carefully for signs of adrenal suppression.

*Effects on ability to drive and use machines:* None stated.

*Undesirable effects:* Under normal circumstances Solu-Medrone therapy would be considered as short-term. However, the possibility of side-effects attributable to corticosteroid therapy should be recognised, particularly when high-dose therapy is being used (see *Special warnings and special precautions for use*). Such side-effects include:

*Parenteral corticosteroid therapy* - Anaphylactic reaction with or without circulatory collapse, cardiac arrest, bronchospasm, cardiac arrhythmias, hypotension or hypertension.

*Gastro-intestinal* - Dyspepsia, peptic ulceration with perforation and haemorrhage, abdominal distension, oesophageal ulceration, oesophageal candidiasis, acute pancreatitis. Nausea, vomiting and bad taste in mouth may occur especially with rapid administration.

Increases in alanine transaminase (ALT, SGPT) aspartate transaminase (AST, SGOT) and alkaline phosphatase have been observed following corticosteroid treatment. These changes are usually small, not associated with any clinical syndrome and are reversible upon discontinuation.

*Anti-inflammatory and immunosuppressive effects*–Increased susceptibility and severity of infections with suppression of clinical symptoms and signs, opportunistic infections, may suppress reactions to skin tests, recurrence of dormant tuberculosis (see *Special warnings and special precautions for use*).

*Musculoskeletal* - Proximal myopathy, osteoporosis, vertebral and long bone fractures, avascular osteonecrosis, tendon rupture.

*Fluid and electrolyte disturbance* - Sodium and water retention, potassium loss, hypertension, hypokalaemic alkalosis, congestive heart failure in susceptible patients.

*Dermatological* - Impaired healing, petechiae and ecchymosis, skin atrophy, bruising, striae, telangiectasia, acne.

*Endocrine/metabolic* - Suppression of the hypothalamo-pituitary-adrenal axis, growth suppression in infancy, childhood and adolescence, menstrual irregularity and amenorrhoea. Cushingoid facies, hirsutism, weight gain, impaired carbohydrate tolerance with increased requirement for antidiabetic therapy, negative nitrogen and calcium balance. Increased appetite.

*Neuropsychiatric*- Euphoria, psychological dependence, mood swings, depression, personality changes, insomnia. Increased intra-cranial pressure with papilloedema in children (pseudotumour cerebri), usually after treatment withdrawal. Psychosis, aggravation of schizophrenia, seizures.

*Ophthalmic* - Increased intra-ocular pressure, glaucoma, papilloedema, cataracts with possible damage to the optic nerve, corneal or scleral thinning, exacerbation of ophthalmic viral or fungal disease.

*General* - Leucocytosis, hypersensitivity including anaphylaxis, thrombo-embolism, malaise.

*Withdrawal symptoms* - Too rapid a reduction of corticosteroid dosage following prolonged treatment can lead to acute adrenal insufficiency, hypotension and death. However, this is more applicable to corticosteroids with an indication where continuous therapy is given (see Special warnings and special precautions for use).

A 'withdrawal syndrome' may also occur including, fever, myalgia, arthralgia, rhinitis, conjunctivitis, painful itchy skin nodules and loss of weight.

*Overdose:* There is no clinical syndrome of acute overdosage with Solu-Medrone. Methylprednisolone is dialysable. Following chronic overdosage the possibility of adrenal suppression should be guarded against by gradual diminution of dose levels over a period of time. In such event the patient may require to be supported during any further stressful episode.

### Pharmacological properties

*Pharmacodynamic properties:* Medrone is a corticosteroid with an anti-inflammatory activity at least five times that of hydrocortisone. An enhanced separation of glucocorticoid and mineralocorticoid effect results in a reduced incidence of sodium and water retention.

*Pharmacokinetic properties:* Methylprednisolone is extensively bound to plasma proteins, mainly to globulin and less so to albumin. Only unbound corticosteroid has pharmacological effects or is metabolised. Metabolism occurs in the liver and to a lesser extent in the kidney. Metabolites are excreted in the urine.

Mean elimination half-life ranges from 2.4 to 3.5 hours in normal healthy adults and appears to be independent of the route of administration.

Total body clearance following intravenous or intramuscular injection of methylprednisolone to healthy adult volunteers is approximately 15–16 l/hour. Peak methylprednisolone plasma levels of 33.67 mcg/100 ml were achieved in 2 hours after a single 40 mg i.m. injection to 22 adult male volunteers.

### Pharmaceutical particulars

*List of excipients:* Sodium biphosphate and sodium phosphate.

The 40 mg vial also contains lactose.

*Incompatibilities:* None stated.

*Shelf life:* Shelf life of the medicinal product as packaged for sale: 60 months.

After reconstitution with Sterile Water for injections, use immediately, discard any remainder.

*Special precautions for storage:* Store below 25°C.

Refer to *Posology and method of administration* Section. No diluents other than those referred to are recommended. Parenteral drug products should be inspected visually for particulate matter and discoloration prior to administration.

*Nature and contents of container:* Type I clear glass vial with butyl rubber plug and flip top seal.

Each vial of Solu-Medrone 40 mg contains the equivalent of 40 mg of methylprednisolone as the sodium succinate for reconstitution with 1 ml of Sterile Water for Injections.

Each vial of Solu-Medrone 125 mg contains the equivalent of 125 mg of methylprednisolone as the sodium succinate for reconstitution with 2 ml of Sterile Water for Injections.

Each vial of Solu-Medrone 500 mg contains the equivalent of 500 mg of methylprednisolone as the sodium succinate for reconstitution with 7.8 ml of Sterile Water for Injections.

Each vial of Solu-Medrone 1 g contains the equivalent of 1 g of methylprednisolone as the sodium succinate for reconstitution with 15.6 ml of Sterile Water for Injections.

*Instructions for use/handling:* No special requirements.

### Marketing authorisation numbers

Solu-Medrone 40 mg    0032/0033
Solu-Medrone 125 mg    0032/0034
Solu-Medrone 500 mg    0032/0035
Solu-Medrone 1 g    0032/0039

**Date of approval/revision of SPC** August 1996

**Legal category** POM

## SOLU-MEDRONE* 2 gram

**Qualitative and quantitative composition** Methylprednisolone sodium succinate 2.652 grams equivalent to 2 grams of methylprednisolone.

**Pharmaceutical form** Powder for injection.

### Clinical particulars

*Therapeutic indications:* Solu-Medrone is indicated to treat any condition in which rapid and intense corticosteroid effect is required such as:

*Dermatological disease:* severe erythema multiforme (Stevens-Johnson syndrome)

*Allergic states:* bronchial asthma, severe seasonal and perennial allergic rhinitis, angioneurotic oedema, anaphylaxis

*Gastro-intestinal diseases:* ulcerative colitis, Crohn's disease

*Respiratory diseases:* aspiration of gastric contents, fulminating or disseminated tuberculosis (with appropriate antituberculous chemotherapy)

*Neurological disorders* : cerebral oedema secondary to cerebral tumour

*Miscellaneous:* T.B. meningitis (with appropriate antituberculous chemotherapy), transplantation; acute spinal cord injury. The treatment should begin within eight hours of injury.

*Posology and method of administration:* Solu-Medrone may be administered intravenously or intramuscularly, the preferred method for emergency use being intravenous injection given over a suitable time interval. When administering Solu-Medrone in high doses intravenously, it should be given over a period of at least 30 minutes. Doses up to 250 mg should be given intravenously over a period of at least five minutes.

For intravenous infusion the initially prepared solution may be diluted with 5% dextrose in water, isotonic saline solution or 5% dextrose in isotonic saline solution. To avoid compatibility problems with other drugs, Solu-Medrone should be administered separately, only in the solutions mentioned.

Undesirable effects may be minimised by using the lowest effective dose for the minimum period (see *Special warnings and special precautions for use*).

Parenteral drug products should wherever possible be visually inspected for particulate matter and discoloration prior to administration.

*Adults:* Dosage should be varied according to the severity of the condition, initial dosage will vary from 10 to 500 mg. In the treatment of graft rejection reactions following transplantation, a dose of up to 1 g/day may be required. Although doses and protocols have varied in studies using methylprednisolone sodium succinate in the treatment of graft rejection reactions, the published literature supports the use of doses of this level, with 500 mg to 1 g most commonly used for acute rejection. Treatment at these doses should be limited to a 48–72 hour period until the patient's condition has stabilised, as prolonged high dose corticosteroid therapy can cause serious corticosteroid induced side-effects (see *Undesirable effects* and *Special warnings and special precautions for use*).

*Children:* In the treatment of high dose indications, such as haematological, rheumatic, renal and dermatological conditions, a dosage of 30 mg/kg/day to a maximum of 1 g/day is recommended. This dosage may be repeated for three pulses either daily or on alternate days. In the treatment of graft rejection reactions following transplantation, a dosage of 10 to 20 mg/kg/day for up to 3 days, to a maximum of 1 g/day, is recommended. In the treatment of status asthmaticus, a dosage of 1 to 4 mg/kg/day for 1–3 days is recommended.

Solu-Medrone is not recommended for use in spinal cord injury in children.

*Elderly patients:* Solu-Medrone is primarily used in acute short-term conditions. There is no information to suggest that a change in dosage is warranted in the elderly. However, treatment of elderly patients should be planned bearing in mind the more serious consequences of the common side-effects of corticosteroids in old age and close clinical supervision is required (see *Special warnings and special precautions for use*).

*Detailed recommendations for adult dosage are as follows:*

*In anaphylactic reactions:* adrenaline or noradrenaline should be administered first for an immediate haemodynamic effect, followed by intravenous injection of Solu-Medrone with other accepted procedures. There is evidence that corticosteroids through their prolonged haemodynamic effect are of value in preventing recurrent attacks of acute anaphylactic reactions.

*In sensitivity reactions:* Solu-Medrone is capable of providing relief within one half to two hours. In patients with status asthmaticus Solu-Medrone may

be given at a dose of 40 mg intravenously, repeated as dictated by patient response. In some asthmatic patients it may be advantageous to administer by slow intravenous drip over a period of hours.

*In graft rejection reactions following transplantation:* doses of up to 1 g per day have been used to suppress rejection crises, with doses of 500 mg to 1 g most commonly used for acute rejection. Treatment should be continued only until the patient's condition has stabilised; usually not beyond 48–72 hours.

*In cerebral oedema:* corticosteroids are used to reduce or prevent the cerebral oedema associated with brain tumours (primary or metastatic).

In patients with oedema due to tumour, tapering the dose of corticosteroid appears to be important in order to avoid a rebound increase in intracranial pressure. If brain swelling does occur as the dose is reduced (intracranial bleeding having been ruled out), restart larger and more frequent doses parenterally. Patients with certain malignancies may need to remain on oral corticosteroid therapy for months or even life. Similar or higher doses may be helpful to control oedema during radiation therapy.

The following are suggested dosage schedules for oedemas due to brain tumour.

| Schedule A (1) | Dose (mg) | Route | Interval in hours | Duration |
|---|---|---|---|---|
| Pre-operative | 20 | IM | 3--6 | |
| During surgery | 20 to 40 | IV | hourly | |
| Post-operative | 20 | IM | 3 | 24 hours |
| | 16 | IM | 3 | 24 hours |
| | 12 | IM | 3 | 24 hours |
| | 8 | IM | 3 | 24 hours |
| | 4 | IM | 3 | 24 hours |
| | 4 | IM | 6 | 24 hours |
| | 4 | IM | 12 | 24 hours |

| Schedule B (2) | Dose (mg) | Route | Interval in hours | Days Duration |
|---|---|---|---|---|
| Pre-operative | 40 | IM | 6 | 2--3 |
| Post-operative | 40 | IM | 6 | 3--5 |
| | 20 | Oral | 6 | 1 |
| | 12 | Oral | 6 | 1 |
| | 8 | Oral | 8 | 1 |
| | 4 | Oral | 12 | 1 |
| | 4 | Oral | | 1 |

Aim to discontinue therapy after a total of 10 days.

*References:* Fox JL, MD. 'Use of Methylprednisolone in Intracranial Surgery' Medical Annals of the District of Columbia, 34:261--265,1965.

Cantu RC, MD Harvard Neurological Service, Boston, Massachusetts. Letter on file, The Upjohn Company (February 1970).

*For treatment of acute spinal cord injury:* administer intravenously 30 mg methylprednisolone per kilogram of body weight in a bolus dose over a 15 minute period, followed by a 45 minute pause, and then a continuous infusion of 5.4 mg/kg per hour for 23 hours. There should be a separate intravenous site for the infusion pump. The treatment should begin within eight hours of injury.

*In other indications:* initial dosage will vary from 10 to 500 mg depending on the clinical problem being treated. Larger doses may be required for short-term management of severe, acute conditions. The initial dose, up to 250 mg, should be given intravenously over a period of at least 5 minutes, doses exceeding 250 mg should be given intravenously over a period of at least 30 minutes. Subsequent doses may be given intravenously or intramuscularly at intervals dictated by the patient's response and clinical condition. Corticosteroid therapy is an adjunct to and not replacement for, conventional therapy.

*Contra-indications:* Solu-Medrone is contra-indicated where there is known hypersensitivity to components, in systemic fungal infections unless specific anti-infective therapy is employed and in cerebral oedema in malaria.

*Special warnings and special precautions for use: Warnings and precautions:* A Patient Information Leaflet is provided in the pack by the manufacturer.

Undesirable effects may be minimised by using the lowest effective dose for the minimum period. Frequent patient review is required to appropriately titrate the dose against disease activity (see *Posology and method of administration*).

Adrenal cortical atrophy develops during prolonged therapy and may persist for months after stopping treatment. Withdrawal of corticosteroids after prolonged therapy must, therefore, always be gradual to avoid acute adrenal insufficiency, being tapered off over weeks or months according to the dose and duration of treatment. During prolonged therapy any intercurrent illness, trauma or surgical procedure will require a temporary increase in dosage; if corticosteroids have been stopped following prolonged therapy they may need to be temporarily re-introduced.

Patients should carry 'Steroid Treatment' cards which give clear guidance on the precautions to be taken to minimise risk and which provide details of prescriber, drug, dosage and the duration of treatment.

Although Solu-Medrone is not approved in the UK for use in any shock indication, the following warning statement should be adhered to. Data from a clinical study conducted to establish the efficacy of Solu-Medrone in septic shock, suggest that a higher mortality occurred in subsets of patients who entered the study with elevated serum creatinine levels or who developed a secondary infection after therapy began. Therefore, this product should not be used in the treatment of septic syndrome or septic shock.

There have been a few reports of cardiac arrhythmias and/or circulatory collapse and/or cardiac arrest associated with the rapid intravenous administration of large doses of Solu-Medrone (greater than 500 mg administered over a period of less than 10 minutes). Bradycardia has been reported during or after the administration of large doses of methylprednisolone sodium succinate and may be unrelated to the speed and duration of infusion.

Corticosteroids may mask some signs of infection, and new infections may appear during their use. Suppression of the inflammatory response and immune function increases the susceptibility to fungal, viral and bacterial infections and their severity. The clinical presentation may often be atypical and may reach an advanced stage before being recognised.

Chickenpox is of serious concern since this normally minor illness may be fatal in immunosuppressed patients. Patients (or parents of children) without a definite history of chickenpox should be advised to avoid close personal contact with chickenpox or herpes zoster and, if exposed, they should seek urgent medical attention. Passive immunization with varicella/zoster immunoglobin (VZIG) is needed by exposed non-immune patients who are receiving systemic corticosteroids or who have used them within the previous 3 months; this should be given within 10 days of exposure to chickenpox. If a diagnosis of chickenpox is confirmed, the illness warrants specialist care and urgent treatment. Corticosteroids should not be stopped and the dose may need to be increased.

Live vaccines should not be given to individuals with impaired immune responsiveness. The antibody response to other vaccines may be diminished.

The use of Solu-Medrone in active tuberculosis should be restricted to those cases of fulminating or disseminated tuberculosis in which the corticosteroid is used for the management of the disease in conjunction with an appropriate anti-tuberculous regimen. If corticosteroids are indicated in patients with latent tuberculosis or tuberculin reactivity, close observation is necessary as reactivation of the disease may occur. During prolonged corticosteroid therapy, these patients should receive chemoprophylaxis.

Rarely anaphylactoid reactions have been reported following parenteral Solu-Medrone therapy. Physicians using the drug should be prepared to deal with such a possibility. Appropriate precautionary measures should be taken prior to administration, especially when the patient has a history of drug allergy.

Care should be taken for patients receiving cardioactive drugs such as digoxin because of steroid induced electrolyte disturbance/potassium loss (see Undesirable effects).

*Special precautions*: Particular care is required when considering the use of systemic corticosteroids in patients with the following conditions and frequent patient monitoring is necessary: osteoporosis (postmenopausal females are particularly at risk); hypertension or congestive heart failure; existing or previous history of severe affective disorders (especially previous steroid psychosis); diabetes mellitus (or a family history of diabetes); history of tuberculosis; glaucoma (or a family history of glaucoma); previous corticosteroid-induced myopathy; liver failure or cirrhosis; renal insufficiency; epilepsy; peptic ulceration; fresh intestinal anastomoses; predisposition to thrombophlebitis; abscess or other pyogenic infections; ulcerative colitis; diverticulitis; myasthenia gravis; ocular herpes simplex for fear of corneal perforation; hypothyroidism.

*Use in children*: Corticosteroids cause growth retardation in infancy, childhood and adolescence, which may be irreversible. Treatment should be limited to the minimum dosage for the shortest possible time. In order to minimise suppression of the hypothalamo-pituitary-adrenal axis and growth retardation, treatment should be administered where possible as a single dose on alternate days.

*Use in the elderly*: The common adverse effects of systemic corticosteroids may be associated with more serious consequences in old age, especially osteopo-

rosis, hypertension, hypokalaemia, diabetes, susceptibility to infection and thinning of the skin. Close clinical supervision is required to avoid life-threatening reactions.

*Interaction with other medicaments and other forms of interaction*: Convulsions have been reported with concurrent use of methylprednisolone and cyclosporin. Since concurrent administration of these agents results in a mutual inhibition of metabolism, it is possible that convulsions and other adverse events associated with the individual use of either drug may be more apt to occur.

Drugs that induce hepatic enzymes, such as rifampicin, rifabutin, carbamazepine, phenobarbitone, phenytoin, primidone and aminoglutethimide enhance the metabolism of corticosteroids and its therapeutic effects may be reduced.

Drugs such as erythromycin and ketoconazole may inhibit the metabolism of corticosteroids and thus decrease their clearance.

Steroids may reduce the effects of anticholinesterases in myasthenia gravis. The desired effects of hypoglycaemic agents (including insulin), anti-hypertensives and diuretics are antagonised by corticosteroids and the hypokalaemic effects of acetazolamide, loop diuretics, thiazide diuretics and carbenoxolone are enhanced.

The efficacy of coumarin anticoagulants may be enhanced by concurrent corticosteroid therapy and close monitoring of the INR or prothrombin time is required to avoid spontaneous bleeding.

The renal clearance of salicylates is increased by corticosteroids and steroid withdrawal may result in salicylate intoxication. Salicylates and non-steroidal anti-inflammatory agents should be used cautiously in conjunction with corticosteroids in hypothrombinaemia.

Steroids have been reported to interact with neuromuscular blocking agents such as pancuronium with partial reversal of the neuromuscular block.

*Pregnancy and lactation*: Corticosteroids cross the placenta. There may be a very small risk of cleft palate and intra-uterine growth retardation in the fetus; there is evidence of harmful effects on pregnancy in animals. Neonates of mothers who received such therapy during pregnancy should be observed for signs of hypo-adrenalism and appropriate measures instituted if such signs exist. When corticosteroids are essential, however, patients with normal pregnancies may be treated as though they were in the non-gravid state. Patients with pre-eclampsia or fluid retention require close monitoring.

Methylprednisolone is excreted in breast milk and infants of mothers taking pharmacological doses of steroids should be monitored carefully for signs of adrenal suppression.

*Effects on ability to drive and use machines*: None stated.

*Undesirable effects:* Under normal circumstances, Solu-Medrone therapy would be considered as short-term. However, the possibility of side-effects attributable to corticosteroid therapy should be recognised, particularly when high-dose therapy is being used (see Special warnings and special precautions for use). Such side-effects include:

*Parenteral corticosteroid therapy* – Anaphylactic reaction with or without circulatory collapse, cardiac arrest, bronchospasm, cardiac arrhythmias, hypotension or hypertension.

*Gastro-intestinal* – Dyspepsia, peptic ulceration with perforation and haemorrhage, abdominal distension, oesophageal ulceration, oesophageal candidiasis, acute pancreatitis. Nausea, vomiting and bad taste in mouth may occur especially with rapid administration.

Increases in alanine transaminase (ALT, SGPT) aspartate transaminase (AST, SGOT) and alkaline phosphatase have been observed following corticosteroid treatment. These changes are usually small, not associated with any clinical syndrome and are reversible upon discontinuation.

*Anti-inflammatory and immunosuppressive effects* – Increased susceptibility and severity of infections with suppression of clinical symptoms and signs, opportunistic infections, may suppress reactions to skin tests, recurrence of dormant tuberculosis (see *Special warnings and special precautions for use*).

*Musculoskeletal* – Proximal myopathy, osteoporosis, vertebral and long bone fractures, avascular osteonecrosis, tendon rupture.

*Fluid and electrolyte disturbance* – Sodium and water retention, potassium loss, hypertension, hypokalaemic alkalosis, congestive heart failure in susceptible patients.

*Dermatological* -- Impaired healing, petechiae and ecchymosis, skin atrophy, bruising, striae, telangiectasia, acne.

*Endocrine/metabolic* – Suppression of the hypothalamo-pituitary-adrenal axis; growth suppression in infancy, childhood and adolescence; menstrual irregularity and amenorrhoea. Cushingoid facies, hirsut-

ism, weight gain, impaired carbohydrate tolerance with increased requirement for antidiabetic therapy, negative nitrogen and calcium balance, increased appetite.

*Neuropsychiatric* – Euphoria, psychological dependence, mood swings, depression, personality changes, insomnia. Increased intra-cranial pressure with papilloedema in children (pseudotumour cerebri), usually after treatment withdrawal. Psychosis, aggravation of schizophrenia, seizures.

*Ophthalmic* – Increased intra-ocular pressure, glaucoma, papilloedema, cataracts with possible damage to the optic nerve, corneal or scleral thinning, exacerbation of ophthalmic viral or fungal disease.

*General* – Leucocytosis, hypersensitivity including anaphylaxis, thrombo-embolism, malaise.

*Wtihdrawal symptoms* – Too rapid a reduction of corticosteroid dosage following prolonged treatment can lead to acute adrenal insufficiency, hypotension and death. However, this is more applicable to corticosteroids with an indication where continuous therapy is given (see *Special warnings and special precautions for use*).

A 'withdrawal syndrome' may also occur including, fever, myalgia, arthralgia, rhinitis, conjunctivitis, painful itchy skin nodules and loss of weight.

*Overdose:* There is no clinical syndrome of acute overdosage with Solu-Medrone. Methylprednisolone is dialysable. Following chronic overdosage the possibility of adrenal suppression should be guarded against by gradual diminution of dose levels over a period of time. In such event the patient may require to be supported during any further stressful episode.

**Pharmacological properties**

*Pharmacodynamic properties:* Methylprednisolone is a corticosteroid with an anti-inflammatory activity at least five times that of hydrocortisone. An enhanced separation of glucocorticoid and mineralocorticoid effect results in a reduced incidence of sodium and water retention.

*Pharmacokinetic properties:* Methylprednisolone is extensively bound to plasma proteins, mainly to globulin and less so to albumin. Only unbound corticosteroid has pharmacological effects or is metabolised. Metabolism occurs in the liver and to a lesser extent in the kidney. Metabolites are excreted in the urine.

Mean elimination half-life ranges from 2.4 to 3.5 hours in normal healthy adults and appears to be independent of the route of administration.

Total body clearance following intravenous or intramuscular injection of methylprednisolone to healthy adult volunteers is approximately 15–16l/hour. Peak methylprednisolone plasma levels of 33.67 microgram/100 ml were achieved in 2 hours after a single 40 mg i.m. injection to 22 adult male volunteers.

**Pharmaceutical particulars**

*List of excipients:* Sodium biphosphate and sodium phosphate.

*Incompatibilities:* None stated.

*Shelf-life:* Shelf-life of the medicinal product as packaged for sale: 60 months.

After reconstitution with Sterile Water for Injections, use immediately, discard any remainder.

*Special precautions for storage:* Store below 25°C.

Refer to section *Posology and method of administration*. No diluents other than those referred to are recommended. Parenteral drug products should be inspected visually for particulate matter and discoloration prior to administration.

*Nature and contents of container:* Type I clear glass vial with butyl rubber plug and flip top seal. Each vial contains 2 grams of methylprednisolone as the sodium succinate for reconstitution with 31.2 ml of Sterile Water for Injections.

*Instructions for use/handling:* No special requirements.

**Marketing authorisation number**    0032/0073

**Date of approval/revision of SPC**    June 1995

**Legal category**    POM

## SULPITIL*

**Qualitative and quantitiative composition:** Each tablet contains 200 mg sulpiride.

**Pharmaceutical form:** Round, white tablet with bevelled edge, marked 'L113' on one side and scored on the reverse.

**Clinical particulars**

*Therapeutic indications:* For the treatment of acute and chronic schizophrenia.

*Posology and method of administration:* For oral administration.

*Adult dose:* In mild cases, 400 mg to 800 mg daily given as one or two tablets twice daily. In severe cases, a maximum dosage of 1200 mg to 1800 mg per day may be given. A maintenance dose of 400 mg to 800 mg is recommended.

*Children:* 3 – 5 mg/kg body weight daily is recommended. Clinical experience in children under the age of 14 years is insufficient to permit specific recommendations.

*Dosage in the elderly:* Elderly patients are usually more sensitive to all centrally-acting drugs, therefore an initial dose of 50 mg to 100 mg is recommended, increasing gradually to the normal adult dose. Reduced dosage should be used in patients with renal impairment.

*Contra-indications:* Phaeochromocytoma. Severe hepatic, renal or blood disease. Alcoholic intoxication and other disorders which depress CNS function.

*Special warnings and special precautions for use:* Sulpiride should be given with caution to patients suffering from extrapyramidal disturbances, hypertension, and to patients with tumours.

As with all drugs, of which the kidney is a major elimination pathway, the usual precautions should be taken in cases of renal failure.

Patients should be warned against taking alcohol with sulpiride as reaction capacity may be impaired.

Increased motor agitation has been reported at high doses in a small number of patients, i.e. in excessively agitated or excited phases of the disease process, this drug may aggravate symptoms. Care should be exercised when hypomania is present. If warranted, reduction in dosage or anti-parkinsonian medication is sufficient.

*Interaction with other medicaments and other forms of interaction:* Although no drug interactions are known, unnecessary polypharmacy should be avoided. Patients should be warned against taking alcohol with sulpiride, as reaction capacity may be impaired. Sulpiride has no anticholinergic or significant cardiovascular activity.

*Pregnancy and lactation:* Despite the negative results of teratogenicity studies in animals sensitive to the effects of thalidomide and the lack of teratogenic effect during widespread clinical use in other countries, this drug should not be considered an exception to the general principle of avoiding drug treatment during pregnancy, particularly during the first sixteen weeks, with potential benefits being weighed against probable hazards.

*Effects on ability to drive and use machines:* Patients should be advised not to drive or operate machinery if they experience symptoms of slowing of reaction time or loss of concentration.

*Undesirable effects:* Extrapyramidal symptoms can occur: tremor, tardive dyskinesia (rare), and akathisia. Insomnia and other sleep disturbances have been reported.

As is usual with neuroleptic and psychotropic drugs, sulpiride increases serum prolactin levels, sometimes causing gynaecomastia and galactorrhoea.

Sulpiride has a low toxicity and, unlike other neuroleptics, does not produce serious adverse effects on the autonomic nervous system.

Cases of convulsions, sometimes in patients with no previous history, have been reported.

Hepatic reactions have been reported.

*Overdose:* Overdosage may be treated with alkaline osmotic diuresis and anti-parkinsonian drugs to treat any extrapyramidal symptoms. An overdose of more than 7 g may cause coma which has been observed to last for up to four days and which should receive suitable treatment.

## Pharmacological properties

*Pharmacodynamic properties:* Sulpiride belongs to a new class of neuroleptics, the benzamides, and has both antidepressant and neuroleptic properties. In high doses it controls florrid positive symptoms but in lower doses it has an alerting effect on apathetic withdrawn schizophrenics; further reductions in dosage increase this alerting effect.

*Pharmacokinetic:* The plasma half-life of sulpiride is 8 – 9 hours.

*Preclinical safety data:* In long-term animal studies with neuroleptic drugs, including sulpiride, an increased incidence of various endocrine tumours, some of which have been malignant, has been found in some, but not all, strains of rats and mice studied. The significance of these findings to man is not known. There is no current evidence of an association between neuroleptic use and tumour risk in man.

## Pharmaceutical particulars

*List of excipients:* Microcrystalline Cellulose USP; Maize Starch PhEur; Lactose PhEur; Gelatin BP; Talc PhEur; Sodium Stearyl Fumarate (PRUV) HSE.

*Incompatibilities:* None stated.

*Shelf life:* 60 months.

*Special precautions for storage:* Store in a dry place below 25°C.

*Nature and contents of container:* Polyethylene containers each fitted with a tamper-evident strip closure and enclosed within a printed cardboard carton, containing either 28 or 112 tablets.

*Instructions for use/handling:* None stated.

**Marketing authorisation number:** 0424/0066

**Date of approval/revision of SPC** 2 January 1996

**Legal category** POM

# SUPRANE* ▼

**Qualitative and quantitative composition** Desflurane, supplied as pure drug substance.

**Pharmaceutical form** Volatile liquid for administration by inhalation.

**Clinical particulars**

*Therapeutic indications:* Desflurane is indicated as an inhalation agent for induction and/or maintenance of anaesthesia for inpatient and outpatient surgery in adults and maintenance of anaesthesia for inpatient and outpatient paediatric surgery.

*Posology and method of administration:*
*Method of administration:* Desflurane is administered by inhalation. The concentration of desflurane should be delivered from a vaporizer specifically designed and designated for use with desflurane.

*Premedication:* Premedication should be selected according to the needs of the individual patient taking into account that salivary secretions are stimulated. The use of anticholinergic drugs is a matter of choice for the anaesthetist.

*Dosage:* The minimum alveolar concentration (MAC) of desflurane is age-specific and has been determined as listed below:

| Age | MAC 100% Oxygen | 60% Nitrous Oxide |
|---|---|---|
| 0 – 1 year | 8.95 – 10.65% | 5.75 – 7.75%* |
| 1 – 12 years | 7.20 – 9.40% | 5.75 – 7.00%** |
| 18 – 30 years | 7.25 – 7.25% | 3.75 – 4.25% |
| 30 – 65 years | 5.75 – 6.25% | 1.75 – 3.25% |
| over 65 years | NA*** | NA*** |

\* 3–12 months  ** 1–5 years  *** NA = data not available

*Induction:* Inspired concentrations of 4–11% of desflurane usually produce surgical anaesthesia in 2–4 minutes. However, concentrations of up to 15% have been used in clinical trials. Suprane is not recommended for paediatric induction.

*Maintenance:* Surgical levels of anaesthesia may be sustained with 2–6% concentration of desflurane when nitrous oxide is used concomitantly. Desflurane at 2.5–8.5% may be required when administered using oxygen or oxygen enriched air. Although concentrations of up to 18% desflurane have been administered for short periods of time, if high concentrations are used with nitrous oxide it is important to ensure that the inspired mixture contains a minimum of 25% oxygen. Desflurane concentrations of greater than 17% are therefore not recommended.

If added relaxation is required, supplemental doses of muscle relaxants may be used.

*Dosage in renal and hepatic impairment:* Concentrations of 1–4% desflurane in nitrous oxide/ oxygen have been used successfully in patients with chronic renal or hepatic impairment and during renal transplantation surgery.

*Contra-indications:* Desflurane should not be used for patients in whom general anaesthesia is contraindicated. Desflurane is also contraindicated in patients with known sensitivity to halogenated agents and in patients with known or genetic susceptibility to malignant hyperthermia.

*Special warnings and special precautions for use:* Desflurane should only be administered by persons trained in the administration of general anaesthesia using a vaporizer specifically designed and designated for use with desflurane. Facilities for maintenance of

a patent airway, artificial ventilation, oxygen enrichment and circulatory resuscitation must be immediately available. Hypotension and respiratory depression increase as anaesthesia is deepened.

Desflurane is not recommended for use as an inhalation induction agent in paediatric patients because of the frequent occurrence of cough, breath holding, apnoea, laryngospasm and increased secretions in children under 12 years.

Due to limited experience in neurosurgical patients, desflurane cannot be recommended in this group.

Desflurane, as with other volatile anaesthetics, may increase CSF or intracranial pressure in patients with space occupying lesions.

Use of desflurane in hypovolaemic, hypotensive and debilitated patients has not been extensively investigated. As with other potent inhaled anaesthetics, a lower concentration is recommended for use in these patients.

Desflurane has been reported to interact with dry carbon dioxide absorbents to form carbon monoxide. In order to minimise the risk of formation of carbon monoxide in rebreathing circuits and the possibility of elevated carboxyhaemoglobin levels, carbon dioxide absorbents should not be allowed to dry out.

As with other halogenated anaesthetic agents, desflurane may cause sensitivity hepatitis in patients who have been sensitized by previous exposure to halogenated anaesthetics.

*Interaction with other medicaments and other forms of interaction:* Commonly used muscle relaxants are potentiated by desflurane. Lower doses of desflurane are required in patients receiving opioids, benzodiazepines or other sedatives. These interactions are illustrated below. In addition, concomitant nitrous oxide reduces desflurane MAC, as illustrated under dosage, above.

*Non-depolarizing and depolarizing muscle relaxants:* The doses of pancuronium, atracurium and suxamethonium needed to produce 95% (ED$_{95}$) depression in neuromuscular transmission at different concentrations of desflurane are given in Table 1. (These doses are similar to isoflurane.)

*Opioids and benzodiazepines:* Patients anaesthetized with different concentrations of desflurane who received increasing doses of fentanyl showed a marked reduction in the anaesthetic requirements or MAC. The administration of increasing doses of intravenous midazolam showed a small reduction in MAC. Results are reported in Table 2. These MAC reductions are similar to those observed with isoflurane. It is anticipated that there will be a similar influence on MAC with other opioid and sedative drugs.

*Table 2–Desflurane 0.6–0.8 MAC/O$_2$*

| | *MAC (%) | % MAC reduction |
|---|---|---|
| No Fentanyl | 6.33 – 6.35 | — |
| Fentanyl (3 mg/kg) | 3.12 – 3.46 | 46 – 51 |
| Fentanyl (6 mg/kg) | 2.25 – 2.97 | 53 – 64 |
| No Midazolam | 5.85 –6.86 | — |
| Midazolam (25 mg/kg) | 4.93 | 15.7 |
| Midazolam (50 mg/kg) | 4.88 | 16.6 |

\* Includes values for ages 18 – 65 years

*Pregnancy and lactation:* Developmental toxicity studies with desflurane, administered at 1 MAC to rats and rabbits have shown a possible anaesthetic-related fetotoxic effect at approximately 40 cumulative MAC-hours of exposure. No adverse effects were observed following 10 cumulative MAC-hours of exposure.

Increased post-implantation loss and reduced offspring weight gain during lactation were observed in rats following maternal desflurane exposure of 4 MAC-hours per day throughout gestation and lactation (approximately 37 days). No adverse effects on these parameters were observed following maternal exposure of 1 MAC-hour per day over this time course. All fetal or offspring effects observed were restricted to groups where maternal toxicity (mortalities and reduced weight gain) was noted, and therefore offspring effects may reflect the pharmacological effect of desflurane on the dams.

There are no adequate and well-controlled studies in pregnant women, therefore desflurane is not indicated for use during pregnancy.

Desflurane is not indicated for use in nursing

*Table 1–Dosage (mg/kg) of muscle relaxant causing 95% depression in neuromuscular transmission*

| Desflurane concentration | Pancuronium | Atracurium | Suxamethonium |
|---|---|---|---|
| 0.65 MAC/60%N$_2$O/O$_2$ | 0.026 | 0.133 | *NA |
| 1.25 MAC/60%N$_2$O/O$_2$ | 0.018 | 0.119 | *NA |
| 1.25 MAC/O$_2$ | 0.022 | 0.120 | 0.360 |

*NA = not available

mothers because it is not known whether it is excreted in human milk.

*Effects on ability to drive and use machines*: There is no information on the effects of desflurane on the ability to drive or operate machinery. However, patients should be advised that the ability to perform tasks such as driving or operation of machinery may be impaired after general anaesthesia, and it is advisable to avoid such tasks for a period of 24 hours.

*Undesirable Effects*: As with all potent inhaled anaesthetics desflurane may cause dose-dependent cardio-respiratory depression. Most other adverse events are mild and transient. Nausea and vomiting have been observed in the postoperative period, common sequelae of surgery and general anaesthesia, which may be due to inhalational anaesthetic, other agents administered intraoperatively or post-operatively and to the patient's response to the surgical procedure.

Hepatitis may occur in patients sensitized by prior exposure to halogenated anaesthetics.

In adults, adverse reactions associated with desflurane during its use for inhaled induction of anaesthesia include cough, breath holding, salivation, apnoea and laryngospasm.

Desflurane is not recommended for use as an inhalation induction agent in paediatric patients because of the frequent occurrence of cough, breath holding, apnoea, laryngospasm and increased secretions in children under 12 years.

As with all other general anaesthetics, transient elevations in white blood count have been observed even in the absence of surgical stress.

As with other agents of this type, in a susceptible animal model, desflurane anaesthesia has been shown to trigger a skeletal muscle hypermetabolic state leading to high oxygen demand and the clinical syndrome known as malignant hyperthermia (MH).

The syndrome includes non-specific features such as hypercapnia, muscle rigidity, tachycardia, tachypnoea, cyanosis, arrhythmias and unstable blood pressure and an increase in overall metabolism may be reflected in an elevated temperature. Treatment includes discontinuation of triggering agents, administration of intravenous dantrolene sodium and application of supportive therapy. This effect has not been observed in man with desflurane anaesthesia, but desflurane should not be used in subjects known to be susceptible to MH.

*Overdose:*
*Acute experience in animals*: Preclinical toxicology data for desflurane suggest that it produces concentration related respiratory and cardiovascular depression which is predictable and controllable. It does not produce target organ toxicity or pathology.

*Human experience*: There is no experience of overdosage in humans.
*Symptoms and treatment of overdosage*: The symptoms of overdosage of desflurane are anticipated to be similar to those of other volatile agents with a deepening of anaesthesia, cardiac and/or respiratory depression in spontaneous breathing patients, and hypotension in ventilated patients in whom hypercarbia and hypoxia may occur only at a late stage.

In the event of overdosage or what may appear to be overdosage, the following actions should be taken: stop desflurane, establish a clear airway and initiate assisted or controlled ventilation with pure oxygen. Support and maintain adequate haemodynamics.

**Pharmacological properties**

*Pharmacodynamic properties*: Desflurane is one of a family of halogenated methylethylethers which are administered by inhalation producing a dose-related, reversible loss of consciousness and of pain sensations, suppression of voluntary motor activity, reduction of autonomic reflexes and sedation of respiration and the cardiovascular system. Other members of the series include enflurane and its structural isomer isoflurane which are halogenated with chlorine as well as fluorine. Desflurane is halogenated exclusively with fluorine. As suggested by its structure, the low blood/gas partition coefficient of desflurane (0.42) is lower than that of other potent inhaled anaesthetics such as isoflurane (1.4) and even lower than that of nitrous oxide (0.46). These data indicate that desflurane would meet the need for an agent characterized by rapid recovery and that it is particularly suited for use in outpatient anaesthesia where this is an important property. Animal studies showed a more rapid induction and recovery from anaesthesia than for isoflurane, with a similar cardiorespiratory profile.

There were no signs of epileptogenic or other untoward effects on EEG, and adjuvant drugs produced no unanticipated or toxic EEG responses during anaesthesia with desflurane.

Studies in pigs bred to be susceptible to malignant hyperthermia (MH) indicated that desflurane is a potential trigger for MH.

*Pharmacokinetic properties:*

*General characteristics:* As predicted from its physicochemical profile, pharmacokinetic studies in animals as in man indicate that desflurane washes into the body more rapidly than other volatile anaesthetic agents, suggesting a more rapid induction of anaesthesia. It also washes out of the body more rapidly, allowing quick recovery and flexibility in adjustment of the depth of anaesthesia. Desflurane is eliminated via the lungs, undergoing only minimal metabolism (0.02%).

*Characteristics in patients:* The pharmacological effect is proportional to the inspired concentration of desflurane. The main adverse effects are extensions of the pharmacological action.

MAC decreases with increasing age. A reduction of dosage is recommended in hypovolaemic, hypotensive and debilitated patients, as discussed under Warnings above.

*Preclinical safety data:* In swine, desflurane does not sensitize the myocardium to exogenously administered adrenaline. Desflurane appears to produce coronary vasodilation at arteriolar level in selected animal models, in a similar fashion to that of isoflurane. In an animal model simulating coronary artery disease with conscious, chronically instrumented dogs, desflurane does not appear to divert blood from collateral dependent myocardium to normally perfused areas ('coronary steal'). Clinical studies to date evaluating myocardial ischaemia, infarction and death as outcome parameters have not established that the coronary arteriolar property of Suprane is associated with coronary steal or myocardial ischaemia in patients with coronary artery disease.

**Pharmaceutical particulars**

*List of excipients:* Not applicable.

*Incompatibilities:* None.

*Shelf life:* Two years.

*Special precautions for storage:* The product should be stored in an upright position at room temperature (25°C).

*Nature and contents of container:* Suprane is presented in amber glass bottles, containing 240 ml of desflurane. The closure is constructed of black, moulded phenol resin, fitted with a conical insert of polypropylene. Alternatively the glass bottle may be closed with a crimped-on valve directly compatible with the filling port of the desflurane vaporizer.

*Instructions for use/handling:* Desflurane should only be administered by persons trained in the administration of anaesthesia, using a vaporizer specifically designed and designated for use with desflurane.

**Marketing authorisation number** 0022/0120

**Date of approval/revision of SPC** June 1996

**Legal category** POM

# TAMOFEN-10*

**Presentation** Round, convex, off-white tablets, scored on one side and marked T10 on the reverse. Each tablet contains 15.2 mg Tamoxifen Citrate BP equivalent to 10 mg tamoxifen.

**Uses** For the treatment of: (i) Breast cancer; (ii) Anovulatory infertility.

Tamoxifen is an anti-oestrogenic drug which binds to oestrogen receptors preventing the stimulating effects of oestrogen on nucleic acid synthesis. The metabolites of tamoxifen are also anti-oestrogens.

**Dosage and administration** For oral administration.

*Adults:*

*(1) Breast cancer:* The recommended daily dose for tamoxifen is 20 mg. No additional benefit, in terms of delayed reccurrence or improved survival in patients, has been demonstrated with higher doses. Substantive evidence supporting the use of treatment with 30–40 mg per day is not available, although these doses have been used in some patients with advanced disease.

*(2) Anovulatory infertility:* The possibility of pregnancy must be excluded before the commencement of treatment. In women with regular menstruation but with anovular cycles treatment should commence with 20 mg daily in either one or two doses administered on the second, third, fourth and fifth days of the menstrual cycle. If treatment is unsuccessful further courses may be given during subsequent menstrual periods, increasing the dosage to 20 mg twice daily and then 40 mg twice daily.

In women with irregular menstruation, the commencement of treatment may take place on any day. If this initial course is not successful then a further course may be initiated after an interval of 45 days with the higher dosage level (30 mg to 40 mg twice daily). If a patient responds with menstruation then

the next course of treatment should be initiated on the second day of the cycle.

*Elderly:* The adult dosage range has been used in elderly patients with breast cancer.

*Children:* Not applicable.

**Contra-indications, warnings, etc**
*Contra-indications:* Pregnancy.

*Precautions:* Tamoxifen may be given to pre-menopausal women only after thorough examination has excluded the possibility of pregnancy.

Tamoxifen increases the dopaminergic effect of bromocriptine. Significant increases in anti-coagulant effect may occur if tamoxifen is used in combination with coumarin type anti-coagulant (e.g. warfarin). Careful monitoring of patients is recommended if co-administration is initiated.

*Adverse effects:* Side-effects are generally mild. The following effects have been reported – hot flushes, mild nausea, mild thrombocytopenia and leucopenia.

Occasionally occurring side-effects are pruritus vulvae, skin rash, fluid retention, gastrointestinal pain, pain from metastases and tumour pain.

A number of cases of visual disturbance including corneal changes, cataracts and retinopathy have been described in patients receiving tamoxifen therapy.

In breast cancer patients, temporary reductions in platelet count (usually to 80,000–90,000 but sometimes lower) have been observed during treatment with tamoxifen. The platelet counts have recovered during treatment and no haemorrhagic tendency has been reported.

Hypercalcaemia has been reported in patients with bone metastases.

The adverse reactions can sometimes be controlled by a reduction of dosage.

In a proportion of pre-menopausal women treated for breast cancer, there is a suppression of menstruation; reversible cystic ovarian swelling has occasionally been observed in this group of patients receiving 40 mg of tamoxifen twice a day for short periods. A small number of endometrial hyperplasia and endometrial polyps have been reported in association with tamoxifen treatment. A definitive relationship to tamoxifen therapy has not been established. An increased incidence of endometrial cancer has been reported in association with tamoxifen treatment. Abnormal vaginal bleeding including menstrual irregularities, vaginal discharge and symptoms such as pelvic pain or pressure in patients who are receiving tamoxifen should be promptly investigated. Tamoxifen has been associated with changes in liver enzyme levels and rarely with more severe liver abnormalities including fatty liver, cholestasis and hepatitis.

*Treatment of overdosage:* Overdosage causes antioestrogenic effects. In animals, extremely high doses (over 100 times the recommended daily dose) have caused oestrogenic effects. There is no specific antidote to overdosage and treatment should therefore be symptomatic.

**Pharmaceutical precautions** *Storage:* Protect from moisture and heat (store below 25°C).

**Legal category** POM.

**Package quantities** Containers of 30 (OP).

**Further information** Maximum plasma levels of tamoxifen occur at 4–7 hours after administration. The elimination half-life is about 7 days. Considerable enterohepatic circulation is a probable reason for the slow elimination.

**Product licence number** 0424/0031.

# TAMOFEN-20*

**Presentation** Round, convex, off-white tablets marked T20 on one side. Each tablet contains 30.4 mg Tamoxifen Citrate BP equivalent to 20 mg tamoxifen.

**Uses** For the treatment of: (i) Breast cancer; (ii) anovulatory infertility.

Tamoxifen is an anti-oestrogenic drug which binds to oestrogen receptors preventing the stimulating effects of oestrogen on nucleic acid synthesis. The metabolites of tamoxifen are also anti-oestrogens.

**Dosage and administration** For oral administration.

*Adults:*

*(1) Breast cancer:* The recommended daily dose for tamoxifen is 20 mg. No additional benefit, in terms of delayed recurrence or improved survival in patients, has been demonstrated with higher doses. Substantive evidence supporting the use of treatment with 30–40 mg per day is not available, although these doses have been used in some patients with advanced disease.

*(2) Anovulatory infertility:* The possibility of pregnancy must be excluded before the commencement of treatment. In women with regular menstruation but

with anovular cycles treatment should commence with 20 mg daily in either one or two doses administered on the second, third, fourth and fifth days of the menstrual cycle. If treatment is unsuccessful further courses may be given during subsequent menstrual periods, increasing the dosage to 20 mg twice daily and then 40 mg twice daily.

In women with irregular menstruation, the commencement of treatment may take place on any day. If this initial course is not successful then a further course may be initiated after an interval of 45 days with the higher dosage level (30 mg to 40 mg twice daily). If a patient responds with menstruation then the next course of treatment should be initiated on the second day of the cycle.

*Elderly:* The adult dosage range has been used in elderly patients with breast cancer.

*Children:* Not applicable.

**Contra-indications, warnings, etc**
*Contra-indications:* Pregnancy.

*Precautions:* Tamoxifen may be given to pre-menopausal women only after thorough examination has excluded the possibility of pregnancy.

Tamoxifen increases the dopaminergic effect of bromocriptine. Significant increases in anti-coagulant effect may occur if tamoxifen is used in combination with coumarin type anti-coagulants (e.g. warfarin). Careful monitoring of patients is recommended if co-administration is initiated.

*Adverse effects:* Side-effects are generally mild. The following effects have been reported – hot flushes, mild nausea, mild thrombocytopenia and leucopenia.

Occasionally occurring side-effects are pruritus vulvae, skin rash, fluid retention, gastro-intestinal pain, pain from metastases and tumour pain.

A number of cases of visual disturbance including corneal changes, cataracts and retinopathy have been described in patients receiving tamoxifen therapy.

In breast cancer patients, temporary reductions in platelet count (usually to 80,000–90,000 but sometimes lower) have been observed during treatment with tamoxifen. The platelet counts have recovered during treatment and no haemorrhagic tendency has been reported.

Hypercalcaemia has been reported in patients with bone metastases.

The adverse reactions can sometimes be controlled by a reduction of dosage.

In a proportion of pre-menopausal women treated for breast cancer, there is a suppression of menstruation; reversible cystic ovarian swelling has occasionally been observed in this group of patients receiving 40 mg of tamoxifen twice a day for short periods.

A small number of endometrial hyperplasia and endometrial polyps have been reported in association with tamoxifen treatment. A definitive relationship to tamoxifen therapy has not been established. An increased incidence of endometrial cancer has been reported in association with tamoxifen treatment. Abnormal vaginal bleeding including menstrual irregularities, vaginal discharge and symptoms such as pelvic pain or pressure in patients who are receiving tamoxifen should be promptly investigated. Tamoxifen has been associated with changes in liver enzyme levels and rarely with more severe liver abnormalities including fatty liver, cholestasis and hepatitis.

*Treatment of overdosage:* Overdosage causes anti-oestrogenic effects. In animals, extremely high doses (over 100 times the recommended daily dose) have caused oestrogenic effects. There is no specific antidote to overdosage and treatment should therefore be symptomatic.

**Pharmaceutical precautions** *Storage:* protect from moisture and heat.

**Legal category** POM.

**Package quantities** Containers of 30 (OP).

**Further information** Maximum plasma levels of tamoxifen occur at 4–7 hours after administration. The elimination half-life is about 7 days. Considerable enterohepatic circulation is a probable reason for the slow elimination.

**Product licence number** 0424/0043.


## TAMOFEN-40*

**Presentation** Round, convex, off white tablets marked T40 on one side. Each tablet contains 60.8 mg Tamoxifen Citrate BP equivalent to 40 mg tamoxifen.

**Uses** For the treatment of: (i) Breast cancer; (ii) anovulatory infertility.

Tamoxifen is an anti-oestrogenic drug which binds to oestrogen receptors preventing the stimulating effects of oestrogen on nucleic acid synthesis. The metabolities of tamoxifen are also anti-oestrogens.

**Dosage and administration** For oral administration

*Adults:*

*(1) Breast cancer:* The recommended daily dose for tamoxifen is 20 mg. No additional benefit, in terms of delayed recurrence or improved survival in patients, has been demonstrated with higher doses. Substantive evidence supporting the use of treatment with 30–40 mg per day is not available, although these doses have been used in some patients with advanced disease.

*(2) Anovulatory infertility:* The possibility of pregnancy must be excluded before the commencement of treatment. In women with regular menstruation but with anovular cycles treatment should commence with 20 mg daily in either one or two doses administered on the second, third, fourth and fifth days of the menstrual cycle. If treatment is unsuccessful, further courses may be given during subsequent menstrual periods, increasing the dosage to 20 mg twice daily and then 40 mg twice daily.

In women with irregular menstruation, the commencement of treatment may take place on any day. If this initial course is not successful then a further course may be initiated after an interval of 45 days with the higher dosage level (30 mg to 40 mg twice daily). If a patient responds with menstruation then the next course of treatment should be initiated on the second day of the cycle.

*Elderly:* The adult dosage range has been used in elderly patients with breast cancer.

*Children:* Not applicable.

**Contra-indications, warnings, etc**
*Contra-indications:* Pregnancy.

*Precautions:* Tamoxifen may be given to pre-menopausal women only after thorough examination has excluded the possibility of pregnancy.

*Adverse effects:* Side effects are generally mild. The following effects have been reported – hot flushes, mild nausea, mild thrombocytopenia and leucopenia.

Occasionally occurring side effects are vaginal bleeding, pruritus vulvae, skin rash, fluid retention, gastro-intestinal pain, pain from metastases and tumour pain.

A number of cases of visual disturbance including corneal changes, cataracts and retinopathy have been described in patients receiving tamoxifen therapy.

In breast cancer patients, temporary reductions in platelet count (usually to 80,000–90,000 but sometimes lower) have been observed during treatment with tamoxifen. The platelet counts have recovered during treatment and no haemorrhagic tendency has been reported.

Hypercalcaemia has been reported in patients with bone metastases.

The adverse reactions can sometimes be controlled by a reduction of dosage.

In a proportion of pre-menopausal women treated for breast cancer, there is a suppression of menstruation; reversible cystic ovarian swelling has occasionally been observed in this group of patients receiving 40 mg of tamoxifen twice a day for short periods.

A small number of endometrial hyperplasia, endometrial polyps and endometrial carcinomas have been reported in association with tamoxifen treatment. A definitive relationship to tamoxifen therapy has not been established. An increased incidence of endometrial cancer has been reported in association with tamoxifen treatment. Abnormal vaginal bleeding including menstrual irregularities, vaginal discharge and symptoms such as pelvic pain or pressure in patients who are receiving tamoxifen should be promptly investigated. Tamoxifen has been associated with changes in liver enzyme levels and rarely with more severe liver abnormalities including fatty liver, cholestasis and hepatitis.

*Treatment of overdosage:* Overdosage causes anti-oestrogenic effects. In animals, extremely high doses (over 100 times the recommended daily dose) have caused oestrogenic effects. There is no specific antidote to overdosage and treatment should therefore be symptomatic.

**Pharmaceutical precautions** Protect from moisture and heat. Store below 25°C.

**Legal category** POM.

**Package quantities** Containers of 30 tablets (OP).

**Further information** Maximum plasma levels of tamoxifen occur at 4–7 hours after administration. The elimination half-life is about 7 days. Considerable enterohepatic circulation is a probable reason for the slow elimination.

**Product licence number** 0424/0055.


## TEMAZEPAM* GELTHIX CAPSULES

**Presentation**

Temazepam Gelthix Capsules 10 mg: Green gel filled, soft gelatin capsules marked '10' in white on one side and 'Gelthix' on the other, containing temazepam 10 mg.

Temazepam Gelthix Capsules 15 mg: Green gel filled, soft gelatin capsules marked '15' in white on one side and 'Gelthix' on the other, containing temazepam 15 mg.

Temazepam Gelthix Capsules 20 mg: Green gel filled, soft gelatin capsules marked '20' in white on one side and 'Gelthix' on the other, containing temazepam 20 mg.

Temazepam Gelthix Capsules 30 mg: Green gel filled, soft gelatin capsules marked '30' in white on one side and 'Gelthix' on the other, containing temazepam 30 mg.

**Uses** Temazepam Gelthix Capsules 10, 15, 20 and 30 mg are indicated for the short-term treatment of sleep disturbances considered severe or disabling or where insomnia is subjecting the individual to extreme distress. This product is especially useful in those patients for whom the persistence of hypnotic effect after rising would be undesirable.

**Dosage and administration**

*Insomnia:* Treatment should be as short as possible. Generally the duration of treatment should vary from a few days to two weeks with a maximum, including the tapering off process, of four weeks. In certain cases extension beyond the maximum treatment period may be necessary; if so, it should not take place without re-evaluation of the patient's status. The product should be taken on retiring or up to 30 minutes before going to bed.

*Adults:* 10–20 mg. In exceptional circumstances the dose may be increased to 30–40 mg.

Elderly: 10 mg. In exceptional circumstances the dose may be increased to 20 mg.

Treatment should be started with the lowest recommended dose. The maximum dose should not be exceeded. Patients with impaired liver function should have a reduced dose.

**Contra-indications, warnings, etc**

*Contra-indications:* Hypersensitivity to benzodiazepines, severe respiratory insufficiency, myasthenia gravis, sleep apnoea syndrome, children, severe hepatic insufficiency.

*Warnings:* Temazepam Gelthix Capsules should not be taken in concomitant intake of alcohol. The sedative effect may be enhanced when the product is used in combination with alcohol. This affects the ability to drive or use machines.

Take into account combination with CNS depressants. Enhancement of the central depressive effect may occur during concomitant use with antipsychotics (neuroleptics), hypnotics, anxiolytics/sedatives, antidepressant agents, narcotic analgesics, antiepileptic drugs, anaesthetics and sedative antihistamines. In the case of narcotic analgesics enhancement of the euphoria may also occur leading to an increase in psychic dependence.

Sedation, amnesia, impaired concentration and impaired muscular function may adversely affect the ability to drive or to use machines. If insufficient sleep duration occurs, the likelihood of impaired alertness may be increased.

*Use in pregnancy:* Insufficient data are available on temazepam to assess its safety during pregnancy and lactation. If the product is prescribed to a woman of child-bearing age, she should be warned to contact her physician about stopping the product if she intends to become, or suspects that she is, pregnant. If for compelling medical reasons, temazepam is administered during the late phase of pregnancy, or during labour, effects on the neonate, such as hypothermia, hypotonia and moderate respiratory depression, can be expected due to the pharmacological action of the product. Moreover, infants born to mothers who took benzodiazepines chronically during the later stages of pregnancy may have developed physical dependence and may be at some risk of developing withdrawal symptoms in the postnatal period.

Since benzodiazepines are found in breast milk, temazepam should not be administered to breast-feeding mothers.

*Adverse effects:* Drowsiness during the day, numbed emotions, reduced alertness, confusion, fatigue, headaches, muscle weakness, ataxia, or double vision. These phenomena occur predominantly at the start of therapy and usually disappear thereafter. Other side effects like gastrointestinal disturbances, changes in libido or skin reactions have been reported occasionally. Anterograde amnesia may occur using therapeutic dosages, the risk increasing at higher dosages. Amnesia may be associated with inappropriate behaviour (see also 'Precautions'). Pre-existing depression may be unmasked during benzodiazepine use. Reactions like restlessness, agitation, irritability, aggressiveness, delusion, rages, nightmares, hallucinations, psychoses, inappropriate behaviour and other adverse behavioral effects are known to occur when using benzodiazepines. Should this occur, use of the product should be discontinued. These reactions are more likely to occur in children and the elderly.

Use (even at therapeutic doses) may lead to the development of physical dependence: discontinuation of therapy may result in withdrawal or rebound phenomena (see also precautions). Psychic dependence may occur. Abuse has been reported in polydrug users.

*Precautions: Tolerance:* Some loss of efficacy to the hypnotic effects of short acting benzodiazepines may develop after repeated use for a few weeks.

*Dependence:* Use of benzodiazepines may lead to the development of physical and psychic dependence upon the products. The risk of dependence increases with dose and duration of treatment; it is also greater in patients with a history of alcohol and drug abuse. Once physical dependence has developed, abrupt termination of treatment will be accompanied by withdrawal symptoms. These may consist of headaches, muscle pain, extreme anxiety, tension, restlessness, confusion and irritability. In severe cases the following symptoms may occur: derealisation, depersonalisation, hyperacusis and tingling of the extremities, hypersensitivity to light, noise and physical contact, hallucinations or epileptic seizures.

*Rebound insomnia:* A transient syndrome whereby the symptoms that led to treatment with a benzodiazepine recur in an enhanced form, may occur on withdrawal of hypnotic treatment. It may be accompanied by other reactions including mood changes, anxiety and restlessness. Since the risk of withdrawal phenomena/rebound phenomena is greater after abrupt discontinuation of treatment it is recommended that the dosage is decreased gradually.

*Duration of treatment:* The duration of treatment should be as short as possible (see dosage), but should not exceed 4 weeks, including the tapering off process. Extension beyond this period should not take place without re-evaluation of the situation. It may be useful to inform the patient at the start of treatment that it will be of limited duration and to explain precisely how the dosage will be progressively decreased. Moreover, it is important that the patient should be made aware of the possibility of rebound phenomena to minimise anxiety over such symptoms should they occur while the medicinal product is being discontinued. There is some evidence to suggest that for benzodiazepines with a short duration of action, withdrawal phenomena can occur within the dosage interval, especially when the dosage is high.

*Amnesia:* Benzodiazepines may induce anterograde amnesia. The condition occurs most often several hours after ingesting the product and therefore to reduce the risk, patients should ensure that they will be able to have an uninterrupted sleep of 7–8 hours (see also adverse effects).

*Psychiatric and 'paradoxical reactions':* Reactions like restlessness, agitation, irritability, aggressiveness, delusion, rages, nightmares, hallucinations, psychoses, inappropriate behaviour and other adverse behavioral effects are known to occur when using benzodiazepines. Should this occur, use of the product should be discontinued. These reactions are more likely to occur in children and in the elderly.

*Specific patient groups:* For the elderly see the dosage recommendation. A lower dose is also recommended for patients with a chronic respiratory insufficiency due to risk of respiratory depression. Benzodiazepines are contra-indicated in patients with severe hepatic insufficiency as their use may precipitate encephalopathy. Benzodiazepines are not recommended for the primary treatment of psychotic illness. Benzodiazepines should not be used alone to treat depression or anxiety associated with depression (suicide may be precipitated in such patients). Benzodiazepines should be used with extreme caution in patients with a history of alcohol or drug abuse.

*Overdosage:* As with other benzodiazepines, overdose should not present a threat to life unless combined with other CNS depressants (including alcohol). In the management of overdose with any medicinal product, it should be borne in mind that multiple agents may have been taken.

Following overdose with oral benzodiazepines, vomiting should be induced (within one hour) if the patient is conscious or gastric lavage undertaken with the airway protected if the patient is unconscious. If there is no advantage in emptying the stomach, activated charcoal should be given to reduce absorption. The value of dialysis has not been determined for temazepam. 3-OH benzodiazepines are, as a rule not dialysable and their metabolites (glucuronides) only dialysable with difficulty. Special attention should be paid to respiratory and cardiovascular function in intensive care.

Overdose of benzodiazepines is usually manifested by degrees of central nervous system depression ranging from drowsiness to coma. In mild cases, symptoms include drowsiness, mental confusion and lethargy; in more serious cases, symptoms may include ataxia, hypotonia, hypotension, respiratory depression, rarely coma and very rarely death. Flumazenil may be used as an antidote.

**Pharmaceutical precautions** Dispense in glass or plastic containers.

**Legal category** CD(Sch.3) POM

**Package quantities**

Temazepam Gelthix Capsules 10 mg: Containers of 500 and 1000 capsules

Temazepam Gelthix Capsules 15 mg: Containers of 60 capsules

Temazepam Gelthix Capsules 20 mg: Containers of 250 and 500 capsules

Temazepam Gelthix Capsules 30 mg: Containers of 60 capsules.

**Further information** The formulation of temazepam as a gel in soft gel capsules ensures rapid and complete absorption which, with its short half-life and lack of active metabolites, results in prompt induction of sleep and a low incidence of hangover effects.

Temazepam is a short-acting benzodiazepine. As accumulation tends not to occur, patients are less likely to experience excessive drowsiness or impairment in the performance of skilled tasks. The short half-life of this drug may offer advantages in the treatment of the elderly, in patients with impaired renal or liver function, and in situations where daytime alertness is desirable.

**Product licence numbers**

| | |
|---|---|
| Temazepam Gelthix Capsules 10 mg | 3433/0094 |
| Temazepam Gelthix Capsules 15 mg | 3433/0105 |
| Temazepam Gelthix Capsules 20 mg | 3433/0095 |
| Temazepam Gelthix Capsules 30 mg | 3433/0106 |

## TEMAZEPAM ELIXIR

**Presentation** A clear, green, lemon-mint flavoured elixir containing 10 mg temazepam per 5 ml in a sugar free base.

**Uses** Temazepam Elixir is indicated for the short-term treatment of sleep disturbances considered severe or disabling or where insomnia is subjecting the individual to extreme distress. This product is especially useful in those patients for whom the persistence of hypnotic effect after rising would be undesirable.

**Dosage and administration**

*Insomnia:* Treatment should be as short as possible. Generally the duration of treatment should vary from a few days to two weeks with a maximum, including the tapering off process, of four weeks. In certain cases extension beyond the maximum treatment period may be necessary; if so, it should not take place without re-evaluation of the patient's status. The product should be taken on retiring or up to 30 minutes before going to bed.

*Adults:* 10–20 mg. In exceptional circumstances the dose may be increased to 30–40 mg.

*Elderley:* 10 mg. In exceptional circumstances the dose may be increased to 20 mg.

Treatment should be started with the lowest recommended dose. The maximum dose should not be exceeded. Patients with impaired liver function should have a reduced dose.

**Contra-indications, warnings, etc**

*Contra-indications:* Hypersensitivity to benzodiazepines, severe respiratory insufficiency, myasthenia gravis, sleep apnoea syndrome, children, severe hepatic insufficiency.

*Warnings:* Temazepam Elixir should not be taken in concomitant intake of alcohol. The sedative effect may be enhanced when the product is used in combination with alcohol. This affects the ability to drive or use machines.

Take into account combination with CNS depressants. Enhancement of the central depressive effect may occur during concomitant use with antipsychotics (neuroleptics), hypnotics, anxiolytics/sedatives, antidepressant agents, narcotic analgesics, antiepileptic drugs, anaesthetics and sedative antihistamines. In the case of narcotic analgesics enhancement of the euphoria may also occur leading to an increase in psychic dependence.

Sedation, amnesia, impaired concentration and impaired muscular function may adversely affect the ability to drive or to use machines. If insufficient sleep duration occurs, the likelihood of impaired alertness may be increased.

*Use in pregnancy:* Insufficient data are available on temazepam to assess its safety during pregnancy and lactation. If the product is prescribed to a woman of child-bearing age, she should be warned to contact her physician about stopping the product if she intends to become, or suspects that she is, pregnant. If for compelling medical reasons, temazepam is administered during the late phase of pregnancy, or during labour, effects on the neonate, such as hypothermia, hypotonia and moderate respiratory depression, can be expected due to the pharmacological action of the product. Moreover, infants born to mothers who took benzodiazepines chronically during the later stages of pregnancy may have developed physical dependence and may be at some risk of developing withdrawal symptoms in the postnatal period.

Since benzodiazepines are found in breast milk, temazepam should not be administered to breast-feeding mothers.

*Adverse effects:* Drowsiness during the day, numbed emotions, reduced alertness, confusion, fatigue, headaches, muscle weakness, ataxia, or double vision. These phenomena occur predominantly at the start of therapy and usually disappear thereafter. Other side effects like gastrointestinal disturbances, changes in libido or skin reactions have been reported occasionally. Anterograde amnesia may occur using therapeutic dosages, the risk increasing at higher dosages. Amnesia may be associated with inappropriate behaviour (see also *Precautions*). Pre-existing depression may be unmasked during benzodiazepine use. Reactions like restlessness, agitation, irritability, aggressiveness, delusion, rages, nightmares, hallucinations, psychoses, inappropriate behaviour and other adverse behavioral effects are known to occur when using benzodiazepines. Should this occur, use of the product should be discontinued. These reactions are more likely to occur in children and the elderly.

Use (even at therapeutic doses) may lead to the development of physical dependence: discontinuation of therapy may result in withdrawal or rebound phenomena (see also precautions). Psychic dependence may occur. Abuse has been reported in polydrug users.

*Precautions:* Tolerance – some loss of efficacy to the hypnotic effects of short acting benzodiazepines may develop after repeated use for a few weeks.

Dependence – use of benzodiazepines may lead to the development of physical and psychic dependence upon the products. The risk of dependence increases with dose and duration of treatment; it is also greater in patients with a history of alcohol and drug abuse. Once physical dependence has developed, abrupt termination of treatment will be accompanied by withdrawal symptoms. These may consist of headaches, muscle pain, extreme anxiety, tension, restlessness, confusion and irritability. In severe cases the following symptoms may occur: derealisation, depersonalisation, hyperacusis and tingling of the extremities, hypersensitivity to light, noise and physical contact, hallucinations or epileptic seizures.

Rebound insomnia – a transient syndrome whereby the symptoms that led to treatment with a benzodiazepine recur in an enhanced form, may occur on withdrawal of hypnotic treatment. It may be accompanied by other reactions including mood changes, anxiety and restlessness. Since the risk of withdrawal phenomena/rebound phenomena is greater after abrupt discontinuation of treatment it is recommended that the dosage is decreased gradually.

Duration of treatment – the duration of treatment should be as short as possible (see dosage), but should not exceed 4 weeks, including the tapering off process. Extension beyond this period should not take place without re-evaluation of the situation. It may be useful to inform the patient at the start of treatment that it will be of limited duration and to explain precisely how the dosage will be progressively decreased. Moreover, it is important that the patient should be made aware of the possibility of rebound phenomena to minimise anxiety over such symptoms should they occur while the medicinal product is being discontinued. There is some evidence to suggest that for benzodiazepines with a short duration of action, withdrawal phenomena can occur within the dosage interval, especially when the dosage is high.

Amnesia – benzodiazepines may induce anterograde amnesia. The condition occurs most often several hours after ingesting the product and therefore to reduce the risk, patients should ensure that they will be able to have an uninterrupted sleep of 7 – 8 hours (see also adverse effects).

Psychiatric and 'paradoxical reactions' – reactions like restlessness, agitation, irritability, aggressiveness, delusion, rages, nightmares, hallucinations, psychoses, inappropriate behaviour and other adverse behavioral effects are known to occur when using benzodiazepines. Should this occur, use of the product should be discontinued. These reactions are more likely to occur in children and in the elderly.

Specific patient groups – for the elderly see the dosage recommendation. A lower dose is also recommended for patients with a chronic respiratory insufficiency due to risk of respiratory depression.

Benzodiazepines are contraindicated in patients with severe hepatic insufficiency as their use may precipitate encephalopathy. Benzodiazepines are not recommended for the primary treatment of psychotic illness. Benzodiazepines should not be used alone to treat depression or anxiety associated with depression (suicide may be precipitated in such patients). Benzodiazepines should be used with extreme caution in patients with a history of alcohol or drug abuse.

*Overdosage:* As with other benzodiazepines, overdose should not present a threat to life unless combined with other CNS depressants (including alcohol). In the management of overdose with any medicinal product, it should be borne in mind that multiple agents may have been taken.

Following overdose with oral benzodiazepines, vomiting should be induced (within one hour) if the patient is conscious or gastric lavage undertaken with the airway protected if the patient is unconscious. If there is no advantage in emptying the stomach, activated charcoal should be given to reduce absorption. The value of dialysis has not been determined for temazepam. 3-OH benzodiazepines are, as a rule not dialysable and their metabolites (glucuronides) only dialysable with difficulty. Special attention should be paid to respiratory and cardiovascular function in intensive care.

Overdose of benzodiazepines is usually manifested by degrees of central nervous system depression ranging from drowsiness to coma. In mild cases, symptoms include drowsiness, mental confusion and lethargy; in more serious cases, symptoms may include ataxia, hypotonia, hypotension, respiratory depression, rarely coma and very rarely death. Flumazenil may be used as an antidote.

**Pharmaceutical precautions** Store below 25°C and protect from light. Temazepam Elixir is sugar-free being based on a glycerol vehicle. If dilution of the elixir is required, glycerol BP is a suitable diluent.

**Legal category** CD(Sch.4), POM

**Package quantities**

Single dose containers of 5 ml (10 mg) and 10 ml (20 mg).

Bottles of 300 ml.

**Further information** The formulation of temazepam as an elixir ensures rapid and complete absorption which, with its short half-life and lack of active metabolites, results in prompt induction of sleep and a low incidence of hangover effects.

Temazepam is a short-acting benzodiazepine. As accumulation tends not to occur, patients are less likely to experience excessive drowsiness or impairment in the performance of skilled tasks. The short half-life of this drug may offer advantages in the treatment of the elderly, in patients with impaired renal or liver function, and in situations where daytime alertness is desirable.

**Product licence number** 3433/0054

## TOLANASE* TABLETS 100 mg

**Qualitative and quantitative composision** Each tablet contains 100 mg tolazamide

**Pharmaceutical form** Tablet for oral use

**Clinical particulars**

*Therapeutic indications:* Sulphonylurea. Indicated in maturity-onset diabetes of mild to moderate severity.

*Posology and method of administration:* Oral.

*Adults:* 100--250 mg daily, or up to 1 g daily in divided doses if necessary. It is doubtful whether doses greater than 1 g daily will result in improved control. (For dose conversion from other oral hypoglycaemic agents see literature).

Depending on the results of urinary glucose tests and blood sugar determinations, the daily dose should be either raised or lowered by amounts of one tablet (100 mg or 250 mg) at weekly intervals.

*Elderly patients:* These agents have had their primary use in the older aged group. The contra-indications and precautions that appear below in this Summary of Product Characteristics should be carefully observed for all aged patients and any patient with significantly compromised liver or renal function should be very carefully followed if it is the election of the physician to use oral agents.

*Contra-indications:* Tolanase is not indicated in juvenile or labile (brittle) diabetes, or in patients with infections or those undergoing surgery or trauma. It is contra-indicated in patients with ketosis, acidosis or in coma, or who have a history of such.

Since Tolanase has not been studied extensively in diabetes complicated by pregnancy nor in diabetics with liver, kidney or endocrine disease, it is not recommended in these instances.

*Special warnings and special precautions for use:* The appearance of significant acetonuria in a patient transferred from insulin to tolazamide makes return to insulin therapy mandatory.

*Interaction with other medicaments and other forms of interaction:* The hypoglycaemic action of sulphonylureas may be potentiated by certain drugs including phenylbutazone, oxyphenbutazone, salicylates, sulphonamides, chloramphenicol, probenecid, coumarins, monoamine oxidase inhibitors and beta adrenergic blocking agents. When such drugs are administered to a patient receiving Tolanase, the patient should be closely observed for hypoglycaemia. When such drugs are withdrawn from a patient receiving Tolanase, the patient should be observed closely for loss of control.

Certain drugs tend to produce hyperglycaemia and may lead to loss of control. These drugs include the thiazides and other diuretics, corticosteroids, phenothiazines, thyroid products, oestrogens, oral contraceptives, phenytoin, nicotinic acid, sympathomimetics and isoniazid. When such drugs are administered to a patient receiving Tolanase, the patient should be observed for loss of control. When such drugs are withdrawn from a patient receiving Tolanase, the patients should be observed closely for hypoglycaemia.

*Pregnancy and lactation:* See *Contra-indications* section, above.

*Effects on ability to drive and use machines:* No information

*Undesirable effects:* The most commonly encountered symptoms are gastro-intestinal (1.8%), including nausea, anorexia, diarrhoea. Other minor occurrences, such as dizziness, weakness, insomnia, lethargy, have been reported. A disulfiram-like action after taking alcohol has been reported.

*Overdose:* Action should be taken to counteract the ensuing hypoglycaemic period. No known antidote.

**Pharmacological properties**

*Pharmacodynamic properties:* Tolazamide is a sulphonylurea which stimulates the islet tissue to secrete insulin. It is approximately 7 times as potent as tolbutamide in normal subjects, and 5 times in diabetics, on a milligram, single dose, basis. Hypoglycaemic effects begin 20 minutes after administration and peak at 2–4 hours. Hypoglycaemia is still apparent after 20 hours in fasted non-diabetics. With fasting diabetics, the peak effect occurs at 4–6 hours, with a duration of maximal effect of about 10 hours. Blood glucose levels begin to rise at 14–16 hours.

*Pharmacokinetic properties:* Peak serum concentrations occur 3–4 hours after a single oral dose. The average half-life is 7 hours. Accumulation stops after the first 4–6 doses, and peak and nadir values do not change after this time.

Tolazamide is metabolised to 5 major metabolites, with hypoglycaemic activity from 0–70%. They are excreted principally in the urine.

**Pharmaceutical particulars**

*List of excipients:* Calcium sulphate; docusate sodium; methyl cellulose; sodium alginate; magnesium stearate.

*Incompatibilities:* None known.

*Shelf-life:* 60 months (36 months in blisters).

*Special precautions for storage:* Store at room temperature (at or below 25°C).

*Nature and contents of container:* Amber glass bottle or HDPE bottle with tamper-evident LDPE cap containing 100 or 500 tablets.

PVC blister/aluminium foil strip of 15 tablets with two or six strips in a carton.

*Instructions for use/handling:* None.

**Marketing authorisation number** 0032/5043R

**Date of approval/revision of SPC** October 1996

**Legal category** POM

## TOLANASE* TABLETS 250 mg

**Qualitative and quantitative composision** Each tablet contains 250 mg tolazamide.

**Pharmaceutical form** Tablet for oral use.

**Clinical particulars**

*Therapeutic indications:* Sulphonylurea. Indicated in maturity-onset diabetes of mild to moderate severity.

*Posology and method of administration:* Oral.

*Adults:* 100--250 mg daily, or up to 1 g daily in divided doses if necessary. It is doubtful whether doses greater than 1 g daily will result in improved control. (For dose conversion from other oral hypoglycaemic agents see literature).

Depending on the results of urinary glucose tests and blood sugar determinations, the daily dose should be either raised or lowered by amounts of one tablet (100 mg or 250 mg) at weekly intervals.

*Elderly patients:* These agents have had their primary use in the older aged group. The contra-indications and precautions that appear below in this Summary of Product Characteristics should be carefully observed for all aged patients and any patient with significantly compromised liver or renal function should be very carefully followed if it is the election of the physician to use oral agents.

*Contra-indications:* Tolanase is not indicated in juvenile or labile (brittle) diabetes, or in patients with infections or those undergoing surgery or trauma. It is contra-indicated in patients with ketosis, acidosis or in coma, or who have a history of such.

Since Tolanase has not been studied extensively in diabetes complicated by pregnancy nor in diabetics with liver, kidney or endocrine disease, it is not recommended in these instances.

*Special warnings and special precautions for use:* The appearance of significant acetonuria in a patient transferred from insulin to tolazamide makes return to insulin therapy mandatory.

*Interaction with other medicaments and otherfForms of interaction:* The hypoglycaemic action of sulphonylureas may be potentiated by certain drugs including phenylbutazone, oxyphenbutazone, salicylates, sulphonamides, chloramphenicol, probenecid, coumarins, monoamine oxidase inhibitors and beta adrenergic blocking agents. When such drugs are administered to a patient receiving Tolanase, the patient should be closely observed for hypoglycaemia. When such drugs are withdrawn from a patient receiving Tolanase, the patient should be observed closely for loss of control.

Certain drugs tend to produce hyperglycaemia and may lead to loss of control. These drugs include the thiazides and other diuretics, corticosteroids, phenothiazines, thyroid products, oestrogens, oral contraceptives, phenytoin, nicotinic acid, sympathomimetics and isoniazid. When such drugs are administered to a patient receiving Tolanase, the patient should be observed for loss of control. When such drugs are withdrawn from a patient receiving Tolanase, the patients should be observed closely for hypoglycaemia.

*Pregnancy andlLactation:* See *Contra-indications* section, above.

*Effects on ability to drive and use machines:* No information

*Undesirable effects:* The most commonly encountered symptoms are gastro-intestinal (1.8%), including nausea, anorexia, diarrhoea. Other minor occurrences, such as dizziness, weakness, insomnia, lethargy, have been reported. A disulfiram-like action after taking alcohol has been reported.

*Overdose:* Action should be taken to counteract the ensuing hypoglycaemic period. No known antidote.

**Pharmacological properties**

*Pharmacodynamic properties:* Tolazamide is a sulphonylurea which stimulates the islet tissue to secrete insulin. It is approximately 7 times as potent as tolbutamide in normal subjects, and 5 times in diabetics, on a milligram, single dose, basis. Hypoglycaemic effects begin 20 minutes after administration and peak at 2–4 hours. Hypoglycaemia is still apparent after 20 hours in fasted non-diabetics. With fasting diabetics, the peak effect occurs at 4–6 hours, with a duration of maximal effect of about 10 hours. Blood glucose levels begin to rise at 14–16 hours.

*Pharmacokinetic properties:* Peak serum concentrations occur 3–4 hours after a single oral dose. The average half-life is 7 hours. Accumulation stops after the first 4–6 doses, and peak and nadir values do not change after this time.

Tolazamide is metabolised to 5 major metabolites, with hypoglycaemic activity from 0–70%. They are excreted principally in the urine.

**Pharmaceutical particulars**

*List of excipients:* Calcium sulphate; docusate sodium; methyl cellulose; sodium alginate; magnesium stearate.

*Incompatibilities:* None known.

*Shelf-life:* 60 months (36 months in blisters)

*Special precautions for storage:* Store at room temperature (at or below 25ºC).

*Nature and contents of container:* Amber glass bottle or HDPE bottle with tamper-evident LDPE cap containing 100 or 500 tablets.

PVC blister/aluminium foil strip of 10 tablets with three or nine strips in a carton.

*Instructions for use/handling:* None.

**Marketing authorisation number** 0032/5044R

Date of approval/revision of SPC   March 1997

Legal category   POM

# TROBICIN*

**Presentation**   Vial containing Spectinomycin Hydrochloride BP, equivalent to spectinomycin 2 g, as a sterile powder. Also ampoule containing Water for Injections PhEur, for use as diluent.

**Uses**   Antibiotic for intramuscular injection in the treatment of ano-genital gonorrhoea.

**Dosage and administration**   Add 3.2 ml water for injections to the vial containing Trobicin as the sterile powder. Shake the vial vigorously immediately after adding diluent and before withdrawing dose. When reconstituted according to direction, each vial yields 5 ml of a suspension containing 400 mg spectinomycin per millilitre.

*Adults:* A single dose of 2 grams (5 ml) by deep intramuscular injection. Up to 4 grams (10 ml) have been administered in difficult-to-treat cases and in areas where antibiotic resistance is known to occur. Intramuscular injections should be made deep into the upper outer quadrant of the gluteal muscle. The dose may be divided between two injection sites.

*Elderly:* There is no evidence to suggest that Trobicin is less well tolerated by patients of advanced age. The normal adult dose should be given.

*Children:* There are insufficient data to recommend the use of Trobicin in children. Doses of 40 mg/kg are reported to be effective in children of over 2 years of age and may be used where no alternative therapy exists. There are no data to support the use of Trobicin in infants.

**Contra-indications, warnings, etc**

*Contra-indications:* Trobicin is contra-indicated for patients previously found to be hypersensitive to it. Trobicin is not indicated for the treatment of syphilis.

*Interactions with other medicaments:* Spectinomycin increases lithium effect and toxicity due to decreased lithium clearance. This interaction is clinically significant.

*Effects on ability to drive and to use machines:* None

*Other undesirable effects:* The following reactions have been observed during single dose clinical trials: soreness at the injection site; urticaria; dizziness; nausea; chills; fever and a reduction in urine output (without renal function changes indicative of renal toxicity).

The following reactions have been observed during multiple-dose tolerance studies in healthy volunteers: a decrease in haemoglobin, haematocrit and creatinine clearance and an elevation of alkaline phosphatase, blood urea nitrogen and serum glutamic pyruvic transaminase.

Anaphylaxis and anaphylactoid reactions have been reported on rare occasions.

*Use in pregnancy and lactation:* There are no adequate or well-controlled studies in pregnant women. Trobicin has been used successfully, at the standard adult dose level, to treat gonorrhoea in pregnant women either where the strain of *Neisseria gonorrhoeae* was resistant to penicillin or in whom penicillin had produced an allergic reaction. Reproductive studies conducted in rats, mice and rabbits, at doses above the clinical dose level, did not demonstrate any evidence of developmental abnormalities. Nevertheless, Trobicin should only be used during pregnancy if clearly needed.

Animal studies have demonstrated that only minute quantities of Trobicin are excreted in breast milk. There are, however, insufficient data to support the use of Trobicin in nursing mothers.

*Other special warnings and precautions:* Spectinomycin is excreted renally and where renal impairment exists, there has been shown to be a significant prolonging of the excretion time. As Trobicin is given as single-dose therapy, the increased excretion time is not considered to be a contra-indication to its use in renally impaired patients, nevertheless, Trobicin should be used only where alternative therapies are inappropriate. The standard adult dosage should be used.

The safety of use in patients with hepatic dysfunction has not been established.

Antibiotics used in high doses for short periods of time to treat gonorrhoea may mask or delay the symptoms of incubating syphilis. Since the treatment of acute syphilis demands prolonged therapy with an effective antibiotic, patients being treated for gonorrhoea should be closely observed clinically for a period of four to six weeks. Appropriate serological follow-up for at least four months should be instituted if a diagnosis of syphilis is suspected.

Development of resistance to antibiotics has been observed with *N. gonorrhoeae*. This appears, so far, to occur only rarely with Trobicin, however, the clinical effectiveness of Trobicin should be monitored to detect evidence of resistance development.

*Overdosage:* Overdosage is unlikely to be a problem in practice.

*Incompatibilities:* None known

**Pharmaceutical precautions**   Shake vial vigorously immediately after adding diluent and before withdrawing dose. Dilution of the reconstituted suspension should not be necessary. Prepare suspension immediately before use. Discard any unused suspension.

**Legal category**   POM

**Package quantities**   1 x 2 g vial plus diluent.

**Further information**   Trobicin bears no structural or antigenic relationship to the penicillins. It is an inhibitor of protein synthesis in the bacterial cell, the site of action being the 30 S ribosomal subunit. Trobicin is rapidly absorbed after intramuscular injection, a single 2 g dose producing peak serum concentrations averaging 103 microgram/ml at one hour. Serum concentrations inhibitory to most gonococcal strains persist for up to eight hours. Up to 100% of the administered dose is excreted in the urine within 48 hours in a biologically active form.

**Product licence number** 0032/0032

# VAMIN* 9

**Presentation**   A clear, colourless to straw-coloured solution of amino acids in the physiological L-form together with electrolytes for intravenous nutrition:

| | | |
|---|---|---|
| Alanine | 3.0 g | |
| Arginine | 3.3 g | |
| Aspartic acid | 4.1 g | |
| Cysteine/cystine | 1.4 g | |
| Glutamic acid | 9.0 g | |
| Glycine | 2.1 g | |
| Histidine | 2.4 g | |
| Isoleucine | 3.9 g | |
| Leucine | 5.3 g | |
| Lysine | 3.9 g | 70.2 g |
| Methionine | 1.9 g | |
| Phenylalanine | 5.5 g | |
| Proline | 8.1 g | |
| Serine | 7.5 g | |
| Threonine | 3.0 g | |
| Tryptophan | 1.0 g | |
| Tyrosine | 0.5 g | |
| Valine | 4.3 g | |
| Sodium | 50 mmol | |
| Potassium | 20 mmol | |
| Calcium | 2.5 mmol | |
| Magnesium | 1.5 mmol | |
| Chloride | 50 mmol | |

in each 1,000 ml. pH 5.2. Free from antioxidant additives.

*Osmolality:* 700 mosmol per kg water.

*Nitrogen per litre:* 9.4 g corresponding to about 60 g of first-class protein.

*Acetate content per litre:* Nil.

*Energy content per litre:* 250 kcal (1.0 MJ).

**Uses**   Vamin 9 provides a balanced mixture of all essential and non-essential amino acids. Electrolytes are present, but may need supplementing according to patient needs. Vamin 9 is indicated in conditions of protein depletion where sufficient enteral nutrition is impossible or impracticable.

**Dosage and administration**   Electrolyte, fluid, acid-base imbalance and shock should be corrected prior to commencement of intravenous nutrition. In the metabolic and nutritional management of the seriously ill patient, specific preliminary investigations and continuous monitoring are essential, particularly of electrolyte levels. Monitoring of vitamin and trace element levels should be included, especially in patients receiving long-term intravenous nutrition.

To achieve an optimal utilisation of administered amino acids, adequate energy sources, e.g. glucose solutions and fat emulsion (Intralipid) should be provided, together with electrolytes, trace elements (Additrace) and vitamins (Solivito N and Vitlipid N).

Hypertonic preparations such as amino acid solutions and concentrated glucose solutions are commonly infused into a central vein. As with all infusions, care should be taken to avoid complications of catheterisation including air embolism and central venous thrombosis. The risk of serious thoracic complications can be avoided by the use of a peripheral catheter if Vamin 9 is given simultaneously with Intralipid through the same cannula, since the reduced osmolality of the overall mixture may reduce the risk of thrombophlebitis.

Strict asepsis should be maintained especially in the immunosuppressed patient. For safe administration of intravenous fluids from non-collapsible containers, a giving set with an integral airway is recommended.

*Recommended dosage for adults:* Depending upon patient requirements 0.5–2.0 litres intravenously per 24 hours.

Vamin 9 is administered by slow intravenous infusion at approx. 40–55 drops per minute (2.1–2.8 ml/min) corresponding to an infusion time of six to eight hours per litre. For long-term feeding (i.e. a period of longer than one week) or in short-term feeding if a deficiency of trace elements exists, a trace element solution should be given i.e. Additrace.

*Recommended dosage for infants:* 30 ml per kg body weight in 24 hours to be achieved gradually during first week of administration. (If a supply of trace elements and electrolytes is required, the recommended regimen is Peditrace with Vaminolact or Vamin 9 Glucose)

*Recommended dosage for the elderly:* Age per se requires no adjustment of the adult dosage.

However, caution should be exercised in the 'frail' elderly, and indeed in all patients with poor renal, cardiac or liver function, where smaller volumes should be used depending on the individual patients' requirements and condition.

**Contra-indications, warnings, etc**   Vamin 9 is contra-indicated in patients with irreversible liver damage and in severe uraemia when dialysis facilities are not available.

*Precautions:* It should not be given to patients with hyperkalaemia – Vamin 14 Electrolyte-Free and Vamin 18 Electrolyte-Free may be suitable alternatives.

Care must be exercised in the administration of large volume infusion fluids to patients with cardiac insufficiency. Amino acid infusions must also be administered with caution to patients with disturbances in protein metabolism.

Hyperkalaemia, hypernatraemia, and acidosis should be corrected prior to commencement of intravenous nutrition. Serum electrolytes, blood glucose levels and acid-base balance should be regularly monitored. Fluid balance should also be monitored since hypertonic dehydration may occur. Amino acid solutions may precipitate acute folate deficiency and folic acid should be given daily.

Vamin 9 should be given with caution to patients with electrolyte retention e.g. impaired renal function and to those with cardiac disease requiring electrolyte restriction or drug therapy e.g. Digitalis. Vamin 14 Electrolyte-Free or Vamin 18 Electrolyte-Free may be suitable in such patients. In particular, potassium replacement therapy should be carefully controlled as plasma potassium levels may not be directly related to tissue levels.

Animal reproduction studies have not been carried out with Vamin 9. There are, however, published reports on the successful and safe infusion of amino acid solutions during pregnancy in the human.

*Interactions with other medicaments and other forms of interaction:* Amino acid solutions may precipitate acute folate deficiency and folic acid should be given daily.

*Side-effects:* Vamin 9 is well tolerated. In exceptional cases, nausea may occur. As with all hypertonic infusion solutions, thrombophlebitis may occur when peripheral veins are used. The incidence could be reduced by the simultaneous infusion of Intralipid as described above.

Vomiting, flushing and sweating may occur if the recommended rate of infusion is exceeded. Abnormal liver function tests have been observed during intravenous nutrition but all values return to normal on cessation of artificial feeding. Cholestasis has been reported in some patients receiving intravenous nutrition.

*Overdosage:* (In general significant overdosage with Vamin 9 does not occur). Excessive infusion rates may result in nausea, vomiting, flushing and sweating.

The effects of overdosage are likely to be due to the volume infused and the hypertonicity of the solution, i.e. circulating overload. The amount required to produce this effect will vary depending on the patient's condition, cardiac and renal status.

There are no specific antidotes for overdosage.

In case of suspicion of overdosage the infusion should immediately be stopped.

Emergency procedures should be general supportive measures: respiratory and cardiovascular. Close biochemical monitoring would be essential and specific abnormalities treated appropriately, perhaps by the careful infusion of hypotonic solutions and concomitant diuretic therapy, and administration of Na bicarbonate for metabolic acidosis.

**Pharmaceutical precautions**
1. Store at 5° to 25°C.
2. Do not use if the bottle is leaking or if the solution is cloudy or contains a precipitate.

3. Discard any unused contents.

4. For long-term feeding (i.e. a period of longer than one week) or in short-term feeding if a deficiency of trace elements exists, a trace element solution should be added.

Additives may only be added to Vamin 9 where compatibility is known.

**Legal category** POM.

**Package quantities** Bottles of 500 ml and 1000 ml.

**Further information** The manufacturer can be consulted for full information on complete and balanced intravenous nutrition regimens.

**Product licence number** 0022/0031R.

## VAMIN* 9 GLUCOSE

**Presentation** A clear, pale yellow to yellow solution of amino acids in the physiological L-form together with glucose and electrolytes for intravenous nutrition:

| | | |
|---|---|---|
| Alanine | 3.0 g | 70.2 g |
| Arginine | 3.3 g | |
| Aspartic acid | 4.1 g | |
| Cysteine/cystine | 1.4 g | |
| Glutamic acid | 9.0 g | |
| Glycine | 2.1 g | |
| Histidine | 2.4 g | |
| Isoleucine | 3.9 g | |
| Leucine | 5.3 g | |
| Lysine | 3.9 g | |
| Methionine | 1.9 g | |
| Phenylalanine | 5.5 g | |
| Proline | 8.1 g | |
| Serine | 7.5 g | |
| Threonine | 3.0 g | |
| Tryptophan | 1.0 g | |
| Tyrosine | 0.5 g | |
| Valine | 4.3 g | |
| Glucose anhydrous | 100 g | |
| Sodium | 50 mmol | |
| Potassium | 20 mmol | |
| Calcium | 2.5 mmol | |
| Magnesium | 1.5 mmol | |
| Chloride | 50 mmol | |

in each 1,000 ml. pH 5.2. Free from antioxidant additives.

*Osmolality:* 1350 mosmol per kg water.

*Nitrogen per litre:* 9.4 g corresponding to about 60 g of first-class protein.

*Acetate content per litre:* Nil.

*Energy content per litre:* 650 kcal (2.7 MJ), of which 400 kcal (1.7 MJ) are provided by the glucose.

**Uses** Vamin 9 Glucose provides a balanced mixture of all essential and non-essential amino acids. Glucose is included to meet part of the carbohydrate requirements. Electrolytes are present, but may need supplementing according to patient needs. Vamin 9 Glucose is indicated in conditions of protein depletion where sufficient enteral nutrition is impossible or impracticable.

**Dosage and administration** Electrolyte, fluid, acid-base imbalance and shock should be corrected prior to commencement of intravenous nutrition. In the metabolic and nutritional management of the seriously ill patient, specific preliminary investigations and continuous monitoring are essential, particularly of electrolyte levels. Monitoring of vitamin and trace element levels should be included, especially in patients receiving long-term intravenous nutrition.

To achieve an optimal utilisation of administered amino acids, adequate energy sources, e.g. glucose solutions and fat emulsion (Intralipid) should be provided, together with electrolytes, trace elements (Additrace) and vitamins (Solivito N and Vitlipid N).

Hypertonic preparations such as amino acid solutions and concentrated glucose solutions are commonly infused into a central vein. As with all infusions, care should be taken to avoid complications of catheterisation including air embolism and central venous thrombosis. The risk of serious thoracic complications can be avoided by the use of a peripheral catheter if Vamin 9 Glucose is given simultaneously with Intralipid through the same cannula, since the reduced osmolality of the overall mixture may reduce the risk of thrombophlebitis.

Strict asepsis should be maintained especially in the immunosuppressed patient. For safe administration of intravenous fluids from non-collapsible containers, a giving set with an integral airway is recommended.

*Recommended dosage for adults:* Depending upon patient requirements 0.5–2.0 litres intravenously per 24 hours.

Vamin 9 Glucose is administered by slow intravenous infusion at approx. 40–55 drops per minute (2.1–2.8 ml/min) corresponding to an infusion time of six to eight hours per litre.

*Recommended dosage for the elderly:* Age per se requires no adjustment of the adult dosage.

However, caution should be exercised in the 'frail' elderly, and indeed in all patients with poor renal, cardiac or liver function, where smaller volumes should be used depending on the individual patients' requirements and condition.

*Recommended dosage for infants:* 30 ml per kg body weight in 24 hours to be achieved gradually during first week of administration.

**Contra-indications, warnings, etc** Vamin 9 Glucose is contra-indicated in patients with irreversible liver damage and in severe uraemia when dialysis facilities are not available. It should not be given to patients with hyperkalaemia – Vamin 14 Electrolyte-Free and Vamin 18 Electrolyte-Free may be suitable alternatives.

Care must be exercised in the administration of large volume infusion fluids to patients with cardiac insufficiency. Amino acid infusions must also be administered with caution to patients with disturbances in protein metabolism.

*Precautions:* Hyperkalaemia, hypernatraemia, and acidosis should be corrected prior to commencement of intravenous nutrition. Serum electrolytes, blood glucose levels and acid-base balance should be regularly monitored. Fluid balance should also be monitored since hypertonic dehydration may occur. Amino acid solutions may precipitate acute folate deficiency and folic acid should be given daily.

Vamin 9 Glucose should be given with caution to patients with electrolyte retention e.g. impaired renal function and to those with cardiac disease requiring electrolyte restriction or drug therapy e.g. Digitalis. Vamin 14 Electrolyte-Free or Vamin 18 Electrolyte-Free may be suitable in such patients. In particular, potassium replacement therapy should be carefully controlled as plasma potassium levels may not be directly related to tissue levels.

Animal reproduction studies have not been carried out with Vamin 9 Glucose. There are, however, published reports on the successful and safe infusion of amino acid solutions during pregnancy in the human.

*Interactions with other medicaments and other forms of interaction:* Amino acid solutions may precipitate acute folate deficiency and folic acid should be given daily.

*Side-effects:* Vamin 9 Glucose is well tolerated. In exceptional cases, nausea may occur. As with all hypertonic infusion solutions, thrombophlebitis may occur when peripheral veins are used. The incidence could be reduced by the simultaneous infusion of Intralipid as described above.

Vomiting, flushing and sweating may occur if the recommended rate of infusion is exceeded. Abnormal liver function tests have been observed during intravenous nutrition but all values return to normal on cessation of artificial feeding. Cholestasis has been reported in some patients receiving intravenous nutrition.

*Overdosage:* (In general significant overdosage with Vamin 9 Glucose does not occur). Excessive infusion rates may result in nausea, vomiting, flushing and sweating.

The effects of overdosage are likely to be due to the volume infused and the hypertonicity of the solution, i.e. circulating overload. The amount required to produce this effect will vary depending on the patient's condition, cardiac and renal status.

There are no specific antidotes for overdosage.

In case of suspicion of overdosage the infusion should immediately be stopped.

Emergency procedures should be general supportive measures: respiratory and cardiovascular. Close biochemical monitoring would be essential and specific abnormalities treated appropriately, perhaps by the careful infusion of hypotonic solutions and concomitant diuretic therapy, and administration of Na bicarbonate for metabolic acidosis.

**Pharmaceutical precautions**

1. Store at 5° to 25°C.

2. Do not use if the bottle is leaking or if the solution is cloudy or contains a precipitate.

3. Discard any unused contents.

4. Additives may only be added to Vamin 9 Glucose where compatibility is known.

**Legal category** POM.

**Package quantities** Bottles of 100 ml, 500 ml and 1,000 ml.

**Further information** The manufacturer can be consulted for full information on complete and balanced intravenous nutrition regimens.

**Product licence number** 0022/0030.

## VAMIN* 14

**Presentation** A clear, colourless to slightly yellow solution of amino acids in the physiological L-form with electrolytes, for intravenous nutrition:

| | | |
|---|---|---|
| Alanine | 12.0 g | 85 g |
| Arginine | 8.4 g | |
| Aspartic acid | 2.5 g | |
| Cysteine/cystine | 420 mg | |
| Glutamic acid | 4.2 g | |
| Glycine | 5.9 g | |
| Histidine | 5.1 g | |
| Isoleucine | 4.2 g | |
| Leucine | 5.9 g | |
| Lysine | 6.8 g | |
| Methionine | 4.2 g | |
| Phenylalanine | 5.9 g | |
| Proline | 5.1 g | |
| Serine | 3.4 mg | |
| Threonine | 4.2 g | |
| Tryptophan | 1.4 g | |
| Tyrosine | 170 mg | |
| Valine | 5.5 g | |
| Sodium | 100 mmol | |
| Potassium | 50 mmol | |
| Calcium | 5 mmol | |
| Magnesium | 8 mmol | |
| Chloride | 100 mmol | |
| Sulphate | 8 mmol | |
| Acetate | 135 mmol | |

in each 1,000 ml. pH 5.6. Free from antioxidant additives.

*Osmolality:* 1145 mosmol per kg water.

*Nitrogen per litre:* 13.5 g corresponding to about 84 g of protein.

*Energy content per litre:* 350 kcal (1.4 MJ).

**Uses** Vamin 14 provides a concentrated and balanced mixture of all essential and non-essential amino acids. Electrolytes are present, but may need supplementing according to patient needs. See under Dosage and administration for information on compatibility. Vamin 14 is indicated for the prophylaxis or therapeutic treatment of protein depletion, where sufficient enteral nutrition is impossible or impracticable. It is particularly suited to meet moderately increased requirements for nitrogen in patients in whom fluid intake is a limiting factor.

**Dosage and administration** Electrolyte, fluid, acid-base imbalance and shock should be corrected prior to commencement of intravenous nutrition. In the metabolic and nutritional management of the seriously ill patient specific preliminary investigations and continuous monitoring are essential, particularly of electrolyte levels. Monitoring of vitamin and trace element levels should be included, especially in patients receiving long-term intravenous nutrition.

To achieve an optimal utilisation of administered amino acids, adequate energy sources, e.g. glucose solutions and fat emulsion (Intralipid) should be provided, together with electrolytes, trace elements (Additrace) and vitamins (Solivito N and Vitlipid N Adult).

Hypertonic preparations such as amino acid solutions and concentrated glucose solutions are commonly infused into a central vein. As with all infusions, care should be taken to avoid complications of catheterisation including air embolism and central venous thrombosis. The risk of serious thoracic complications can be avoided by the use of a peripheral catheter if Vamin 14 is given simultaneously with Intralipid through the same cannula, since the reduced osmolality of the overall mixture may reduce the risk of thrombophlebitis.

Strict asepsis should be maintained especially in the immuno-suppressed patient. For safe administration of intravenous fluids from non-collapsible containers, a giving set with an integral airway is recommended.

*Recommended dosage for adults:* Depending upon patient requirements, up to 1 litre intravenously per 24 hours. In severe catabolism, Vamin 18 Electrolyte-Free or Intrafusin may be used. Vamin 14 is administered by slow intravenous infusion at a rate not exceeding 2 ml per minute corresponding to approximately 40 drops per minute or to an infusion time of at least 8 hours per litre.

*Infant dosage:* Can be administered at the physician's discretion. An amino acid solution containing larger amounts of cysteine/cystine and tyrosine may be considered more appropriate in infants e.g. Vaminolact.

*Recommended dosage for the elderly:* Age per se requires no adjustment of the adult dosage.

However, caution should be exercised in the 'frail' elderly, and indeed in all patients with poor renal, cardiac or liver function, where smaller volumes should be used depending on the individual patients' requirements and condition.

**Contra-indications, warnings, etc** Vamin 14 is contra-indicated in patients with irreversible liver damage and in severe uraemia when dialysis facilities are not available. It should not be given to patients with hyperkalaemia – Vamin 14 Electrolyte-Free is a suitable alternative.

Care must be exercised in the administration of large volume infusion fluids to patients with cardiac insufficiency. Amino acid infusions must also be administered with caution to patients with disturbances in protein metabolism.

*Precautions:* Hyperkalaemia, hypernatraemia, and acidosis should be corrected prior to commencement of intravenous nutrition. Serum electrolytes, blood glucose levels and acid-base balance should be regularly monitored. Fluid balance should also be monitored since hypertonic dehydration may occur. Amino acid solutions may precipitate acute folate deficiency and folic acid should be given daily.

Vamin 14 should be given with caution to patients with electrolyte retention, e.g. impaired renal function and to those with cardiac disease requiring electrolyte restriction or drug therapy, e.g. Digitalis. Vamin 14 Electrolyte-Free is recommended in such patients. In particular, potassium replacement therapy should be carefully controlled as plasma potassium levels may not be directly related to tissue levels.

Animal reproduction studies have not been carried out with Vamin 14. There are, however, published reports on the successful and safe infusion of amino acid solutions during pregnancy in the human.

*Interactions with other medicaments and other forms of interaction:* Amino acid solutions may precipitate acute folate deficiency and folic acid should be given daily.

*Side-effects:* Vamin 14 is well tolerated. Rarely, nausea may occur. As with all hypertonic infusion solutions, thrombophlebitis may occur when peripheral veins are used. The incidence could be reduced by the simultaneous infusion of Intralipid as described above. Vomiting, flushing and sweating may occur if the recommended rate of infusion is exceeded. Abnormal liver function tests have been observed during intravenous nutrition but all values return to normal on cessation of artificial feeding. Cholestasis has been reported in some patients receiving intravenous nutrition.

*Overdosage:* (In general significant overdosage with Vamin 14 does not occur). Excessive infusion rates may result in nausea, vomiting, flushing and sweating.

The effects of overdosage are likely to be due to the volume infused and the hypertonicity of the solution, i.e. circulating overload. The amount required to produce this effect will vary depending on the patient's condition, cardiac and renal status.

There are no specific antidotes for overdosage.

In case of suspicion of overdosage the infusion should immediately be stopped.

Emergency procedures should be general supportive measures: respiratory and cardiovascular. Close biochemical monitoring would be essential and specific abnormalities treated appropriately, perhaps by the careful infusion of hypotonic solutions and concomitant diuretic therapy, and administration of Na bicarbonate for metabolic acidosis.

**Pharmaceutical precautions**

1. Store at 5–25°C.
2. Do not use if the bottle is leaking or if the solution is cloudy or contains a precipitate.
3. Discard any unused contents.
4. Vamin 14 contains electrolytes, but additional electrolytes and trace elements may be required according to patient needs. Up to 20 ml Additrace can be added to one litre Vamin 14 without risk of precipitation. Phosphate may be added to one litre Vamin 14 as up to 40 ml Addiphos (containing 80 mmol phosphate, 60 mmol $Na^+$ and 60 mmol $K^+$) provided Additrace is not present. All additions should be performed aseptically immediately before the start of the infusion and should be used within 24 hours unless the mixture is refrigerated when it may be used within 48 hours of preparation.

Additives may only be added to Vamin 14 where compatibility is known.

**Legal category** POM.

**Package quantities** Bottles of 500 ml and 1000 ml.

**Further information** The manufacturer can be consulted for full information on complete and balanced intravenous nutrition regimens.

**Product licence number** 0022/0053.

## VAMIN* 14 ELECTROLYTE-FREE

**Presentation** A clear, colourless to slightly yellow solution of amino acids in the physiological L-form for intravenous nutrition:

| | | |
|---|---|---|
| Alanine | 12.0 g | 85 g |
| Arginine | 8.4 g | |
| Aspartic acid | 2.5 g | |
| Cysteine/cystine | 420 mg | |
| Glutamic acid | 4.2 g | |
| Glycine | 5.9 g | |
| Histidine | 5.1 g | |
| Isoleucine | 4.2 g | |
| Leucine | 5.9 g | |
| Lysine | 6.8 g | |
| Methionine | 4.2 g | |
| Phenylalanine | 5.9 g | |
| Proline | 5.1 g | |
| Serine | 3.4 g | |
| Threonine | 4.2 g | |
| Tryptophan | 1.4 g | |
| Tyrosine | 170 mg | |
| Valine | 5.5 g | |

in each 1,000 ml. pH 5.6. Free from antioxidant additives.

*Osmolality:* 810 mosmol per kg water.

*Nitrogen per litre:* 13.5 g corresponding to about 84 g of protein.

*Acetate content per litre:* 90 mmol.

*Energy content per litre:* 350 kcal (1.4 MJ).

**Uses** Vamin 14 Electrolyte-Free provides a concentrated and balanced mixture of all essential and non-essential amino acids. It is free from chlorides and other inorganic electrolytes, and electrolyte requirements can therefore be met by the addition of individually adjusted doses. See under *Pharmaceutical precautions* for information on compatibility. Vamin 14 Electrolyte-Free is indicated for the prophylaxis or therapeutic treatment of protein depletion, where sufficient enteral nutrition is impossible or impracticable. It is particularly suited to meet moderately increased requirements for nitrogen in patients in whom fluid intake is a limiting factor.

**Dosage and administration** Electrolyte, fluid, acid-base imbalance and shock should be corrected prior to commencement of intravenous nutrition. In the metabolic and nutritional management of the seriously ill patient, specific preliminary investigations and continuous monitoring are essential, particularly of electrolyte levels. Monitoring of vitamin and trace element levels should be included, especially in patients receiving long-term intravenous nutrition.

To achieve an optimal utilisation of administered amino acids, adequate energy sources, e.g. glucose solutions and fat emulsions (Intralipid) should be provided, together with electrolytes, trace elements (Additrace) and vitamins (Solivito N and Vitlipid N Adult).

Hypertonic preparations such as amino acid solutions and concentrated glucose solutions are commonly infused into a central vein. As with all infusions, care should be taken to avoid complications of catheterisation including air embolism and central venous thrombosis. The risk of serious thoracic complications can be avoided by the use of a peripheral catheter if Vamin 14 Electrolyte-Free is given simultaneously with Intralipid through the same cannula, since the reduced osmolality of the overall mixture may reduce the risk of thrombophlebitis.

Strict asepsis should be maintained especially in the immunosuppressed patient. For safe administration of intravenous fluids from non-collapsible containers, a giving set with an integral airway is recommended.

*Recommended dosage for adults:* Depending upon patient requirements, up to 1 litre intravenously per 24 hours. In severe catabolism, Vamin 18 Electrolyte-Free or Intrafusin may be used. Vamin 14 Electrolyte-Free is administered by slow intravenous infusion at a rate not exceeding 2 ml per minute corresponding to approximately 40 drops per minute or an infusion time of at least 8 hours per litre.

*Recommended dosage for infants:* Can be administered at the physician's discretion. An amino acid solution containing larger amounts of cysteine/cystine and tyrosine may be considered more appropriate in infants.

*Recommended dosage for the elderly:* Age per se requires no adjustment of the adult dosage.

However, caution should be exercised in the 'frail' elderly, and indeed in all patients with poor renal, cardiac or liver function, where smaller volumes should be used depending on the individual patients' requirements and condition.

**Contra-indications, warnings, etc** Vamin 14 Electrolyte-Free is contra-indicated in patients with irreversible liver damage and in severe uraemia when dialysis facilities are not available.

Care must be exercised in the administration of large volume infusion fluids to patients with cardiac insufficiency. Amino acid infusions must also be administered with caution to patients with disturbances in protein metabolism.

*Precautions:* Hyperkalaemia, hypernatraemia and acidosis should be corrected prior to commencement of intravenous nutrition. Serum electrolytes, blood glucose levels and acid-base balance should be regularly monitored. Fluid balance should also be monitored since hypertonic dehydration may occur. Amino acid solutions may precipitate acute folate deficiency and folic acid should be given daily.

Animal reproduction studies have not been carried out with Vamin 14 Electrolyte-Free. There are, however, published reports on the successful and safe infusion of amino acid solutions during pregnancy in the human.

*Interactions with other medicaments and other forms of interaction:* Amino acid solutions may precipitate acute folate deficiency and folic acid should be given daily.

*Side-effects:* Vamin 14 Electrolyte-Free is well tolerated. Rarely, nausea may occur. As with all hypertonic infusion solutions, thrombophlebitis may occur when peripheral veins are used. The incidence could be reduced by the simultaneous infusion of Intralipid as described above. Vomiting, flushing and sweating may occur if the recommended rate of infusion is exceeded. Abnormal liver function tests have been observed during intravenous nutrition but all values return to normal on cessation of artificial feeding. Cholestasis has been reported in some patients receiving intravenous nutrition.

*Overdosage:* (In general significant overdosage with Vamin 14 Electrolyte-Free does not occur). Excessive infusion rates may result in nausea, vomiting, flushing and sweating.

The effects of overdosage are likely to be due to the volume infused and the hypertonicity of the solution, i.e. circulating overload. The amount required to produce this effect will vary depending on the patient's condition, cardiac and renal status.

There are no specific antidotes for overdosage.

In case of suspicion of overdosage the infusion should immediately be stopped.

Emergency procedures should be general supportive measures: respiratory and cardiovascular. Close biochemical monitoring would be essential and specific abnormalities treated appropriately, perhaps by the careful infusion of hypotonic solutions and concomitant diuretic therapy, and administration of Na bicarbonate for metabolic acidosis.

**Pharmaceutical precautions**

1. Store at 5–25°C.
2. Do not use if the bottle is leaking or if the solution is cloudy or contains a precipitate.
3. Discard any unused contents.
4. Vamin 14 Electrolyte-Free contains no electrolytes. Electrolyte and trace element requirements can be met by the addition of individually adjusted doses. Laboratory studies have shown that the maximum levels of electrolytes which are compatible with 1 litre of Vamin 14 Electrolyte-Free are as follows: 20 ml Additrace, 480 mmol $Na^+$(as NaCl), 480 mmol $K^+$ (as KCl), 24 mmol $Ca^{2+}$(as calcium glubionate or gluconate) and 48 mmol $Mg^{2+}$ (as $MgSO_4$) which can be added either singly or in any combination. Phosphate may be added to 1 litre Vamin 14 Electrolyte-Free as up to 60 ml Addiphos (containing 120 mmol phosphate, 90 mmol $Na^+$ and 90 mmol $K^+$) with or without addition of up to 480 mmol $Na^+$ and 480 mmol K as chlorides and 48 mmol $Mg^{2+}$ as sulphate, provided Additrace is not present. All additions should be performed aseptically immediately before the start of the infusion and should be used within 24 hours unless the mixture is refrigerated when it may be used within 48 hours of preparation.

Additives may only be added to Vamin 14 Electrolyte-Free where compatibility is known.

**Legal category** POM.

**Package quantities** Bottles of 500 ml and 1000 ml.

**Further information** The manufacturer can be consulted for full information on complete and balanced intravenous nutrition regimens.

**Product licence number** 0022/0052.

## VAMIN* 18 ELECTROLYTE-FREE

**Presentation** A clear, colourless to slightly yellow solution of amino acids in the physiological L-form for intravenous nutrition:

| | | |
|---|---|---|
| Alanine | 16.0 g | |
| Arginine | 11.3 g | |
| Aspartic acid | 3.4 g | |
| Cysteine/cystine | 560 mg | |
| Glutamic acid | 5.6 g | |
| Glycine | 7.9 g | |
| Histidine | 6.8 g | |
| Isoleucine | 5.6 g | |
| Leucine | 7.9 g | |
| Lysine | 9.0 g | 114 g |
| Methionine | 5.6 g | |
| Phenylalanine | 7.9 g | |
| Proline | 6.8 g | |
| Serine | 4.5 mg | |
| Threonine | 5.6 g | |
| Tryptophan | 1.9 g | |
| Tyrosine | 230 mg | |
| Valine | 7.3 g | |

in each 1,000 ml. pH 5.6. Free from antioxidant additives.

***Osmolality:*** 1130 mosmol per kg water.

*Nitrogen per litre:* 18.0 g corresponding to 112 g of protein.

*Acetate content per litre:* 110 mmol.

*Energy content per litre:* 460 kcal (1.9 MJ).

**Uses** Vamin 18 Electrolyte-Free provides a concentrated and balanced mixture of all essential and non-essential amino acids. It is free from chlorides and other inorganic electrolytes, and electrolyte requirements can therefore be met by the addition of individually adjusted doses. See under *Pharmaceutical precautions* for information on compatibility.

Vamin 18 Electrolyte-Free is indicated for the prophylaxis or therapeutic treatment of protein depletion, where sufficient enteral nutrition is impossible or impracticable. It is particularly suited to meet increased requirements for nitrogen in patients in whom fluid intake is a limiting factor.

**Dosage and administration** Electrolyte, fluid, acid-base imbalance and shock should be corrected prior to commencement of intravenous nutrition. In the metabolic and nutritional management of the seriously ill patient, specific preliminary investigations and continuous monitoring are essential, particularly of electrolyte levels. Monitoring of vitamin and trace element levels should be included, especially in patients receiving long-term intravenous nutrition.

To achieve an optimal utilisation of administered amino acids, adequate energy sources, e.g. glucose solutions and fat emulsions (Intralipid) should be provided, together with electrolytes, trace elements (Additrace) and vitamins (Solivito N and Vitlipid N Adult).

Hypertonic preparations such as amino acid solutions and concentrated glucose solutions are commonly infused into a central vein. As with all infusions, care should be taken to avoid complications of catheterisation including air embolism and central venous thrombosis. The risk of serious thoracic complications can be avoided by the use of a peripheral catheter if Vamin 18 Electrolyte-Free is given simultaneously with Intralipid through the same cannula, since the reduced osmolality of the overall mixture may reduce the risk of thrombophlebitis.

Strict asepsis should be maintained especially in the immunosuppressed patient. For safe administration of intravenous fluids from non-collapsible containers, a giving set with an integral airway is recommended.

*Recommended dosage for adults:* Depending upon patient requirements, up to 1 litre intravenously per 24 hours. Vamin 18 Electrolyte-Free is administered by slow intravenous infusion at a rate not exceeding 2 ml per minute corresponding to approximately 40 drops per minute or an infusion time of at least 8 hours per litre.

*Recommended dosage for infants:* Can be administered at the physician's discretion. An amino acid solution containing larger amounts of cysteine/cystine and tyrosine may be considered more appropriate in infants.

*Recommended dosage for the elderly:* Age per se requires no adjustment of the adult dosage.

However, caution should be exercised in the 'frail' elderly, and indeed in all patients with poor renal, cardiac or liver function, where smaller volumes should be used depending on the individual patients' requirements and condition.

**Contra-indications, warnings, etc** Vamin 18 Electrolyte-Free is contra-indicated in patients with irreversible liver damage and in severe uraemia when dialysis facilities are not available.

Care must be exercised in the administration of large volume infusion fluids to patients with cardiac insufficiency. Amino acid infusions must also be administered with caution to patients with disturbances in protein metabolism.

*Precautions:* Hyperkalaemia, hypernatraemia and acidosis should be corrected prior to commencement of intravenous nutrition. Serum electrolytes, blood glucose levels and acid-base balance should be regularly monitored. Fluid balance should also be monitored since hypertonic dehydration may occur. Amino acid solutions may precipitate acute folate deficiency and folic acid should be given daily.

Animal reproduction studies have not been carried out with Vamin 18 Electrolyte-Free. There are, however, published reports on the successful and safe infusion of amino acid solutions during pregnancy in the human.

*Side-effects:* Vamin 18 Electrolyte-Free is well tolerated. Rarely, nausea may occur. As with all hypertonic infusion solutions, thrombophlebitis may occur when peripheral veins are used. The incidence could be reduced by the simultaneous infusion of Intralipid as described above. Vomiting, flushing and sweating may occur if the recommended rate of infusion is exceeded. Abnormal liver function tests have been observed during intravenous nutrition but all values return to normal on cessation of artificial feeding. Cholestasis has been reported in some patients receiving intravenous nutrition.

*Interactions with other medicaments and other forms of interaction:* Amino acid solutions may precipitate acute folate deficiency and folic acid should be given daily.

*Overdosage:* (In general significant overdosage with Vamin 18 Electrolyte-Free does not occur). Excessive infusion rates may result in nausea, vomiting, flushing and sweating.

The effects of overdosage are likely to be due to the volume infused and the hypertonicity of the solution, i.e. circulating overload. The amount required to produce this effect will vary depending on the patient's condition, cardiac and renal status.

There are no specific antidotes for overdosage.

In case of suspicion of overdosage the infusion should immediately be stopped.

Emergency procedures should be general supportive measures: respiratory and cardiovascular. Close biochemical monitoring would be essential and specific abnormalities treated appropriately, perhaps by the careful infusion of hypotonic solutions and concomitant diuretic therapy, and administration of Na bicarbonate for metabolic acidosis.

**Pharmaceutical precautions**

1. Store at 5–25°C.
2. Do not use if the bottle is leaking or if the solution is cloudy or contains a precipitate.
3. Discard any unused contents.
4. Vamin 18 Electrolyte-Free contains no electrolytes. Electrolyte requirements can be met by the addition of individually adjusted doses. Laboratory studies have shown that the maximum levels of electrolytes which are compatible with 1 litre of Vamin 18 Electrolyte-Free are as follows: 20 ml Additrace, 480 mmol $Na^+$ (as NaCl), 480 mmol $K^+$ (as KCl), 24 mmol $Ca^{2+}$ (as calcium glubionate or gluconate) and 48 mmol $Mg^{2+}$ (as $MgSO_4$) which can be added either singly or in any combination. Phosphate may be added to 1 litre Vamin 18 Electrolyte-Free as up to 60 ml Addiphos (containing 120 mmol phosphate, 90 mmol $Na^+$ and 90 mmol $K^+$) with or without addition of up to 480 mmol $Na^+$, and 480 mmol $K^+$ as chlorides and 48 mmol $Mg^{2+}$ as sulphate providing Additrace is not present. All additions should be performed aseptically immediately before the start of the infusion and should be used within 24 hours unless the mixture is refrigerated when it may be used within 48 hours of preparation.

Additives may only be added to Vamin 18 Electrolyte-Free where compatibility is known.

**Legal category** POM.

**Package quantities** Bottles of 500 ml and 1000 ml.

**Further information** The manufacturer can be consulted for full information on complete and balanced intravenous nutrition regimens.

**Product licence number** 0022/0054.

## VAMINOLACT*

**Presentation** A clear, colourless to slightly yellow solution of amino acids in the physiological L-form for intravenous nutrition, specifically formulated for paediatric use.

| | | |
|---|---|---|
| Alanine | 6.3 g | |
| Arginine | 4.1 g | |
| Aspartic acid | 4.1 g | |
| Cysteine/cystine | 1.0 g | |
| Glutamic acid | 7.1 g | |
| Glycine | 2.1 g | |
| Histidine | 2.1 g | |
| Isoleucine | 3.1 g | |
| Leucine | 7.0 g | |
| Lysine | 5.6 g | 65.3 g |
| Methionine | 1.3 g | |
| Phenylalanine | 2.7 g | |
| Proline | 5.6 g | |
| Serine | 3.8 g | |
| Taurine | 0.3 g | |
| Threonine | 3.6 g | |
| Tryptophan | 1.4 g | |
| Tyrosine | 0.5 g | |
| Valine | 3.6 g | |

in each 1000 ml. pH 5.2. Free from antioxidant additives.

*Osmolality:* 510 mosmol per kg water.

*Nitrogen per litre:* 9.3 g corresponding to 58 g of protein.

*Energy content per litre:* 240 kcal (1.0 MJ).

**Uses** Vaminolact provides a balanced mixture of all essential and non-essential amino acids, with a profile similar to that of breast milk protein. This profile includes cysteine and tyrosine which seem to be essential for premature neonates. In addition it contains taurine, an amino sulphonic acid. The ratio between taurine and total amino acid nitrogen in Vaminolact corresponds to that in human breast milk.

*Indications:* Vaminolact is indicated for the prophylaxis and therapeutic treatment of protein depletion in neonates and infants, where sufficient enteral nutrition is impossible or impracticable. It is free from chlorides and other inorganic electrolytes so as to allow administration in a dosage adjusted to the individual needs of the patient (see under 'Pharmaceutical precautions' for information on compatibility).

**Dosage and administration** Electrolyte, fluid, acid-base imbalance and shock should be corrected prior to commencement of intravenous nutrition. In the metabolic and nutritional management of the seriously ill patient specific preliminary investigations and continuous monitoring are essential, particularly of electrolyte levels. Monitoring of vitamin and trace element levels should be included, especially in patients receiving long-term intravenous nutrition.

To achieve an optimal utilisation of administered amino acids, adequate energy sources, e.g. glucose solutions and fat emulsions should be provided, together with electrolytes, trace elements and vitamins.

Hypertonic preparations such as amino acid solutions and concentrated glucose solutions are commonly infused into a central vein. Vaminolact may also be infused into a peripheral vein when given simultaneously with Intralipid through the same cannula, since the reduced osmolality of the overall mixture may reduce the risk of thrombophlebitis.

As with all infusions, care should be taken to avoid complications of catheterisation including air embolism and central venous thrombosis. Strict asepsis should be maintained especially in the immunosuppressed patient. For safe administration of intravenous fluids from non-collapsible containers, a giving set with an integral airway is recommended.

*Recommended dosage for infants:* The full dosage should be increased gradually during the first week of administration to a final daily dose of up to 35 ml Vaminolact per kg body weight. It should be given as a continuous infusion using a suitable pump, ideally over 24 hours and in any case, not less than 8 hours.

*Recommended dosage for children:* The full dosage should be increased gradually during the first week of administration to the final dose ranges indicated below and should be infused over 24 hours:

| | *Body weight kg* | *Dosage ml/kg bw/24 hours* |
|---|---|---|
| Neonates (including LBW) and Infants | up to 10 | 8–35 (to be increased gradually during the first week of life). |
| Children | 10 | 24 |
| | 20 | 18.5 |
| | 30 | 16 |
| | 40 | 14.5 |
| | >40 | ** |

** (0.5–2.0 litres per 24 hours or 0.8–1.6 g amino acids/kg bw/day. Infusion should be at a rate of 2.0–2.8 ml per minute (40–55 drops per minute). This corresponds to an infusion time of approximately 6–8 hours per litre).

*Caution:* The recommended infusion rate should not be exceeded.

**Contra-indications, warnings, etc** Vaminolact is contra-indicated in patients with irreversible liver damage and in severe uraemia when dialysis facilities are not available.

*Precautions:* Hyperkalaemia, hypernatraemia and acidosis should be corrected prior to commencement of intravenous nutrition. Serum electrolytes, blood glucose levels and acid-base balance should be regularly monitored. Fluid balance should also be monitored since hypertonic dehydration may occur. Amino acid solutions may precipitate acute folate deficiency and folic acid should be given daily.

In extremely sick, premature and small babies requiring neonatal intensive care, liver function is likely to be immature and/or disturbed. Amino acids which, to a large extent, are metabolized by the liver may therefore accumulate in plasma. In this clinical condition, monitoring of amino acid concentration during therapy is advisable.

Care must be exercised in the administration of large volume infusion fluids to patients with cardiac insufficiency. Amino acid infusions must also be administered with caution to patients with disturbances in protein metabolism.

*Side-effects:* Vaminolact is well tolerated. Rarely, nausea may occur. As with all hypertonic solutions, thrombophlebitis may occur when peripheral veins are used. The incidence could be reduced by the simultaneous infusion of Intralipid as described earlier. Abnormal liver function tests have been observed during intravenous nutrition but all values return to normal on cessation of artificial feeding. Cholestasis has been reported in some patients receiving intravenous nutrition.

*Overdosage:* Infusion rates and volumes should be carefully monitored in infants. Excessive infusion rates may result in nausea, vomiting, flushing and sweating. The effects of overdosage are likely to be due to the volume infused and the hypertonicity of the solution, i.e. circulatory overload. The amount required to produce this effect will vary depending on the patients age, weight and general condition. There are no specific antidotes for overdosage.

In cases of suspicion of overdosage the infusion should be stopped. Emergency procedures should be general supportive measures, i.e. respiratory and cardiovascular. Close biochemical monitoring would be essential and specific abnormalities treated appropriately, perhaps by the careful infusion of hypotonic solutions and concomitant diuretic therapy and administration of sodium bicarbonate for metabolic acidosis.

As endogenous formation of taurine is either absent or limited, due to lack of necessary enzymes, taurine is considered an essential amino acid.

**Pharmaceutical precautions** Store at 5 to 25°C.

Do not use if the bottle is leaking or if the solution is cloudy or contains a precipitate.

Discard any unused contents.

Vaminolact contains no electrolytes.

Additions to Vaminolact should only be made where compatibility is known.

Electrolyte requirements should be individually assessed. Laboratory studies have shown the following electrolytes may be mixed with 500 ml Vaminolact either singly or in any combination: up to 200 mmol $Na^+$ (as NaCl) up to 160 mmol $K^+$ (as KCl), up to 35 mmol $Ca^{2+}$ (as $CaCl_2$ or calcium gluconate) and up to 15 mmol $Mg^{2+}$ (as $MgCl_2$ or $MgSO_4$).

All additions should be performed aseptically immediately prior to infusion and the regimen used within 24 hours.

**Legal category** POM.

**Package quantities** Bottles of 100 ml and 500 ml.

**Further information** The manufacturer can be consulted for full information on complete and balanced intravenous nutrition regimens.

**Product licence number** 0022/0092.

## VISTIDE* ▼

**Qualitative and quantitative composition** Each vial contains cidofovir equivalent to 375 mg/5 ml (75 mg/ml) cidofovir anhydrous. The formulation is adjusted to pH 7.4.

**Pharmaceutical form** Concentrate for solution for infusion.

**Clinical particulars**

*Therapeutic indications:* Cidofovir is indicated for the treatment of CMV retinitis in patients with acquired immunodeficiency syndrome (AIDS) and without renal dysfunction. Until further experience is gained, cidofovir should be used only when other agents are considered unsuitable.

*Posology and method of administration:* Before each administration of cidofovir, serum creatinine and urine protein levels should be investigated.

The recommended dosage, frequency, or infusion rate must not be exceeded. Cidofovir must be diluted in 100 millilitres 0.9% (normal) saline prior to administration. To minimise potential nephrotoxicity, oral probenecid and intravenous saline prehydration must be administered with each cidofovir infusion.

*Dosage in adults:*

*Induction Treatment:* The recommended dose of cidofovir is 5 mg/kg body weight (given as an intravenous infusion at a constant rate over 1 hour) administered once weekly for two consecutive weeks.

*Maintenance treatment:* Beginning two weeks after the completion of induction treatment, the recommended maintenance dose of cidofovir is 5 mg/kg body weight (given as an intravenous infusion at a constant rate over 1 hour) administered once every two weeks.

Cidofovir therapy should be discontinued and intravenous hydration is advised if serum creatinine increases by ≥ 44 μmol/l (≥ 0.5 mg/dl), or if persistent proteinuria ≥ 2+ develops.

*Probenecid:* A course of probenecid, administered orally with each cidofovir dose may reduce the potential for nephrotoxicity. All clinical trials relevant to clinical efficacy evaluation were performed using probenecid concomitantly with cidofovir. Therefore to minimise the potential for nephrotoxicity, a course of probenecid should be administered orally with each cidofovir dose. Two grams should be administered 3 hours prior to the cidofovir dose and one gram administered at 2 hours and again at 8 hours after the completion of the 1 hour cidofovir infusion (for a total of 4 grams). In order to reduce the potential for nausea and/or vomiting associated with the administration of probenecid, patients should be encouraged to eat food prior to each dose of probenecid. The use of an anti-emetic may be necessary. In patients who develop allergic or hypersensitivity symptoms to probenecid (e.g., rash, fever, chills and anaphylaxis), prophylactic or therapeutic use of an appropriate antihistamine and/or paracetamol should be considered (see *Contra-indications*).

*Hydration:* To minimise the potential for nephrotoxicity, patients should receive a total of one litre of 0.9% (normal) saline solution intravenously immediately prior to each infusion of cidofovir. Patients who can tolerate the additional fluid load may receive up to a total of 2 litres of 0.9% saline intravenously with each dose of cidofovir. The first litre of saline solution should be infused over a 1 hour period immediately before the cidofovir infusion, and the second litre, if given, infused over a 1-3 hour period beginning simultaneously with the cidofovir infusion or starting immediately after the infusion of cidofovir.

*Dosage in elderly:* The safety and efficacy of cidofovir have not been established for the treatment of CMV disease in patients over 60 years of age. Since elderly individuals frequently have reduced glomerular function, particular attention should be paid to assessing renal function before and during administration of cidofovir.

*Dosage in children and neonates:* The safety and efficacy of cidofovir have not been established for the treatment of CMV disease in patients under 18 years of age. Therefore, cidofovir is not recommended for use in children and neonates.

*Dosage in renal insufficiency:* Renal insufficiency is a contraindication for the use of cidofovir (see *Contra-indications.*) Treatment with cidofovir should not be initiated in patients with serum creatinine > 133 μmol/l (> 1.5 mg/dl), creatinine clearance ≤ 0.92 ml/s (≤ 55 ml/min), or ≥ 2+ proteinuria (≥ 100 mg/dl), as the optimum induction and maintenance doses for patients with moderate to severe renal impairment are not known.

*Dosage in Hepatic Insufficiency:* The safety and efficacy of cidofovir have not been established in patients with hepatic disease.

*Monitoring Advice:* Proteinuria appears to be an early and sensitive indicator of cidofovir-induced nephrotoxicity. Patients receiving cidofovir must have their serum creatinine and urine protein levels determined on specimens obtained within 24 hours prior to the administration of each dose of cidofovir. In patients exhibiting ≥ 2+ proteinuria, intravenous hydration should be performed and the test repeated. If following hydration, a ≥ 2+ proteinuria is still observed, cidofovir therapy should be discontinued. Continued administration of cidofovir to patients with persistent ≥ 2+ proteinuria following intravenous hydration may result in further evidence of proximal tubular injury, including glycosuria, decreases in serum phosphate, uric acid and bicarbonate, and elevations in serum creatinine.

During treatment, these parameters should be investigated prior to the administration of each infusion, and the treatment should be stopped in case of abnormality. In case of complete recovery, the reintroduction of cidofovir has not yet been evaluated.

White blood cell counts, including the differential neutrophil count, should also be performed prior to each dose of cidofovir.

Patients receiving cidofovir should be advised to have regular follow-up ophthalmologic examinations.

*Contra-indications:* Cidofovir is contra-indicated in patients with renal impairment [serum creatinine > 133 μmol/l (> 1.5 mg/dl) or creatinine clearance ≤ 0.92 ml/s (≤ 55 ml/min) or proteinuria ≥ 100 mg/dl (≥ 2+ proteinuria)]. The safety of cidofovir has not been evaluated in patients receiving other known potentially nephrotoxic agents such as aminoglycosides, amphotericin B, foscarnet, intravenous pentamidine and vancomycin. Concomitant administration of cidofovir and these agents is contra-indicated. Cidofovir is also contra-indicated in patients with hypersensitivity to the drug.

Direct intraocular injection of cidofovir is contraindicated; direct injection may be associated with significant decreases in intraocular pressure and impairment of vision.

*Special warnings and special precautions for use:* Cidofovir is formulated for intravenous infusion only and should not be administered by intraocular injection. Cidofovir should be infused only into veins with adequate blood flow to permit rapid dilution and distribution. Therapy should be accompanied by administration of oral probenecid and adequate intravenous saline prehydration. In patients unable to receive probenecid because of a clinically significant hypersensitivity to the drug or to other sulpha-containing medications, cidofovir administration should only be considered if the potential benefits of therapy outweigh the potential risks. Such use of cidofovir without concomitant probenecid has not been clinically investigated. A probenecid desensitization program is not recommended for use.

Renal function (serum creatinine and urine protein) must be monitored prior to each dose of cidofovir. Interruption, and possibly discontinuation, is required for changes in renal function (see *Posology* section).

*Renal impairment:* Dose-dependent nephrotoxicity is the major dose-limiting toxicity related to administration of cidofovir. Proteinuria, as measured by urinalysis in a clinical laboratory, may be an early indicator of nephrotoxicity. Patients receiving weekly intravenous cidofovir at a dose of 0.5 mg/kg or 1.0 mg/kg, without concomitant probenecid, with or without intravenous saline prehydration, did not show evidence of significant drug-related nephrotoxicity (as defined by serum creatinine ≥ 177 μmol/l (≥ 2.0 mg/dl), while patients treated at 3.0 mg/kg, 5.0 mg/kg or 10.0 mg/kg without concomitant probenecid developed evidence of proximal tubular cell injury, including glycosuria, and decreases in serum phosphate, uric acid and bicarbonate, and elevations in serum creatinine. The signs of nephrotoxicity were partially reversible in some patients.

*Haematology:* Reversible neutropenia has been observed in patients receiving cidofovir. This has not been associated with clinical sequelae and does not appear to be dose-dependent. Resolution has occurred in some cases while on continued cidofovir therapy and in others following discontinuation of the drug.

*Laboratory tests:* Renal function tests (routine urinalysis and serum creatinine) must be measured, and the results reviewed, prior to administration of each cidofovir dose. Neutrophil counts also should be monitored regularly.

*Other:* Cidofovir should be considered a potential carcinogen in humans. (see *Preclinical Safety* section)

Caution should be applied when considering cidofovir treatment of patients with diabetes mellitus due to the potential increased risk of developing ocular hypotony.

Male patients should be advised that cidofovir caused reduced testes weight and hypospermia in animals. Although not observed in clinical studies of cidofovir, such changes may occur in humans and cause infertility. Men should be advised to practice barrier contraceptive methods during and for 3 months after treatment with cidofovir.

*Interaction with other medicaments and other forms of interaction:* Probenecid is known to interact with the metabolism or renal tubular secretion of many drugs (e.g., paracetamol, acyclovir, angiotensin-converting enzyme inhibitors, aminosalicylic acid, barbiturates, benzodiazepines, bumetanide, clofibrate, methotrexate, famotidine, frusemide, nonsteroidal anti-inflammatory agents, theophylline, and zidovudine).

Patients who are being treated with zidovudine should temporarily discontinue zidovudine administration or decrease their zidovudine dose by 50% on days when cidofovir is administered, because probenecid reduces the clearance of zidovudine.

Interactions of cidofovir, probenecid, and anti-HIV drugs, including anti-HIV protease inhibitors, have not been investigated in clinical trials.

*Use during pregnancy and lactation:* Cidofovir is embryotoxic in rats and rabbits at subtherapeutic dose levels. A significantly increased foetal incidence of external, soft tissue and skeletal anomalies occurred in rabbits at 1.0 mg/kg/day, which was also maternally toxic.

There are no studies of cidofovir in pregnant women. The drug should not be used during pregnancy.

Women of childbearing potential should be advised to use effective contraception during and after treatment with cidofovir.

It is not known whether cidofovir is excreted in human milk. Because many drugs are excreted in human milk, nursing mothers should be instructed to discontinue cidofovir or discontinue nursing if they continue to receive cidofovir. Passage of the placenta barrier of drug-related compound was observed in pregnant rats. Excretion of drug-related material into milk of lactating animals was not examined.

Refer to *Special warnings and special precautions for use* section for further information.

*Effects on ability to drive and use machines:* Adverse effects such as asthenia may occur during cidofovir therapy. The physician is advised to discuss this issue with the patient, and based upon the condition of the disease and the tolerance of medication, give his recommendation in the individual case.

*Undesirable effects:* In controlled clinical trials with cidofovir in patients with AIDS and CMV retinitis, the most frequently reported adverse events were: proteinuria 51%, fever 43%, asthenia 32%, nausea with vomiting 26%, and rash 19%. These incidence figures were calculated independent of relationship to study drugs (cidofovir or probenecid) or severity. The adverse events reported as serious and which occurred in at least 5% of patients were: proteinuria 13%, neutropenia 10%, fever 9%, death 8%, infection 8%, creatinine increase 8%, dyspnea 7%, pneumonia 7%, asthenia 6%, and nausea with vomiting 5%. All deaths occurring during study were attributed to complications of AIDS and not to cidofovir.

The adverse events which occurred in at least 10% of the patients and were possibly or probably related to cidofovir were: proteinuria 41%, neutropenia 18%, asthenia 15%, creatinine increase 14%, fever 13%, alopecia 12%, and nausea without vomiting 10%.

The serious adverse events which occurred in at least 5% of patients and were possibly or probably related to cidofovir were: proteinuria 11%, neutropenia 9%, and creatinine increase 7%.

The adverse events which occurred in at least 10% of the patients and were possibly or probably related to probenecid were: fever 18%, rash 13%, nausea with vomiting 12%, and nausea without vomiting 10%.

The incidence of decreased intraocular pressure (≥ 50% decrease from pretreatment baseline) was 9%.

*Overdose:* Two cases of cidofovir overdose have been reported. In both cases, the overdose occurred during the first induction dose and no additional cidofovir therapy was administered. One patient received a single dose of 16.4 mg/kg and the other patient received a single dose of 17.3 mg/kg. Both patients were hospitalised and received prophylactic oral probenecid and vigorous hydration for 3 to 7 days. One of these patients experienced a minor transient change in renal function, while the other patient had no change in renal function.

### Pharmacologocal properties

*Pharmacodynamic properties:* Antiviral for Systemic Use (ATC Code J05)

*General:* Cidofovir is a cytidine analogue with in vitro and in vivo activity against human cytomegalovirus (HCMV). HCMV strains resistant to ganciclovir may still be susceptible to cidofovir.

*Mechanism of action:* Cidofovir suppresses CMV replication by selective inhibition of viral DNA synthesis. Biochemical data support selective inhibition of HSV-1, HSV-2 and CMV DNA polymerases by cidofovir diphosphate, the active intracellular metabolite of cidofovir.

Cidofovir diphosphate inhibits these viral polymerases at concentrations that are 8- to 600-fold lower than those needed to inhibit human cellular DNA polymerases alpha, beta, and gamma. Incorporation of cidofovir into viral DNA results in reductions in the rate of viral DNA synthesis.

Cidofovir enters cells by fluid-phase endocytosis and is phosphorylated to cidofovir monophosphate and subsequently to cidofovir diphosphate. In addition, a cidofovir phosphate-choline adduct is formed. In contrast to ganciclovir, the metabolism of cidofovir is neither dependent on, nor facilitated by, viral infections. Prolonged antiviral effects of cidofovir are related to the half-lives of metabolites; cidofovir diphosphate persists inside cells with a half-life of 17-65 hours. Additionally, the phosphate-choline species has a half-life of 87 hours.

*Antiviral activity:* Cidofovir is active in vitro against CMV, a member of the herpesviridae family. Antiviral activity is seen at concentrations significantly below those which cause death in cell monolayers. The in

vitro sensitivity to cidofovir is shown in the following table:

Cidofovir Inhibition of Virus Multiplication in Cell Culture

| Virus | IC$_{50}$ (µM) |
| --- | --- |
| Wild-type CMV isolates | 0.7 (±0.6) |
| Ganciclovir-resistant CMV isolates | 7.5 (±4.3) |
| Foscarnet-resistant CMV isolates | 0.59 (±0.07) |

In vivo activity against human CMV was confirmed with controlled clinical studies of cidofovir for the treatment of CMV retinitis in patients with AIDS, which demonstrated statistically significant delays in time to CMV retinitis progression for patients on cidofovir when compared to control patients. The median times to retinitis progression in the two studies relevant for efficacy assessment (studies GS-93-106 and GS-93-105, both conducted in patients previously untreated for CMV retinitis) were 120 days and not reached for the treatment arms vs. 22 days and 21 days for the untreated (deferred treatment) arms, respectively.

In study GS-93-107 conducted in patients who had relapsed after treatment with other agents, the median time to retinitis progression was 115 days.

*Viral resistance:* Following in vitro selection of ganciclovir-resistant human CMV isolates, cross-resistance between ganciclovir and cidofovir was seen with ganciclovir-selected mutations in the CMV DNA polymerase gene but not with mutations in the UL97 gene. No cross-resistance between foscarnet and cidofovir was seen with foscarnet-selected mutants. Cidofovir-selected mutants had a mutation in the DNA polymerase gene and were cross-resistant to ganciclovir, but susceptible to foscarnet.

*Pharmacokinetic properties:* The major route of elimination of cidofovir was by renal excretion of unchanged drug by a combination of glomerular filtration and tubular secretion. In patients with normal renal function, 80 to 100% of the intravenous dose was recovered in the urine over 24 hours as unchanged cidofovir. No metabolites of cidofovir have been detected in serum or urine of patients.

At the end of a one-hour infusion of cidofovir 5 mg/kg administered with concomitant oral probenecid, the mean (± SD) serum concentration of cidofovir was 19.6 (± 7.18) mg/ml. The mean values of total serum clearance, volume of distribution at steady-state and terminal elimination half-life were 138 (± 36) ml/hr/kg, 388 (± 125) ml/kg and 2.2 (± 0.5) hour, respectively.

Dose-independent kinetics were demonstrated with single doses of cidofovir given over the dose range 3 to 7.5 mg/kg.

*In vitro protein binding:* In vitro protein binding of cidofovir to plasma or serum protein was 10% or less over the cidofovir concentration range 0.25 to 25 mg/ml.

*Preclinical safety data:* Preclinical animal studies demonstrated that nephrotoxicity was the major dose-limiting toxicity of cidofovir. Evidence for a nephroprotective effect for probenecid was shown in a 52-week study conducted in cynomolgus monkeys administered cidofovir 2.5 mg/kg once weekly intravenously with 1 gram of probenecid given orally.

*Carcinogenesis:* In a 26-week intravenous toxicity study, a significant increase in incidence of mammary adenocarcinomas was seen in female rats and of Zymbal's gland carcinomas in male and female rats at subtherapeutic plasma levels of cidofovir. In a separate study, once weekly subcutaneous injections of cidofovir for 19 consecutive weeks resulted in mammary adenocarcinomas in female rats at doses as low as 0.6 mg/kg/week. In both studies, tumors were observed within 3 months of dosing. No tumours were observed in cynomolgus monkeys administered cidofovir intravenously once weekly for 52 weeks at doses up to 2.5 mg/kg/week.

*Mutagenicity and reproductive toxicology:* Studies have shown that cidofovir is clastogenic in vitro at 100 µg/ml and is embryotoxic in rats and rabbits.

No mutagenic response was elicited by cidofovir at dose levels up to 5 mg/plate, in the presence and absence of metabolic activation by rat liver S-9 fraction, in microbial assays involving Salmonella typhimurium for base pair substitutions or frameshift mutations (Ames) and Escherichia coli for reverse mutations.

An increase in formation of micronucleated polychromatic erythrocytes was observed in vivo in mice receiving a high, toxic intraperitoneal dose of cidofovir (≥ 2000 mg/kg).

Cidofovir induced chromosomal aberrations in human peripheral blood lymphocytes in vitro without metabolic activation (S-9 fraction). At the 4 cidofovir levels (12.5 to 100 µg/ml) tested, the percentage of damaged metaphases and number of aberrations per cell increased in a concentration-dependent manner.

No adverse effects on fertility or general reproduction were seen following once weekly intravenous injections of cidofovir in male rats for 13 consecutive

weeks at doses up to 15 mg/kg/week. Female rats dosed intravenously once weekly at 1.2 mg/kg/week or higher for up to 6 weeks prior to mating and for 2 weeks post mating had decreased litter sizes and live births per litter and increased early resorptions per litter. Peri- and post-natal development studies in which female rats received subcutaneous injections of cidofovir once daily at doses up to 1.0 mg/kg/day from day 7 of gestation through day 21 postpartum (approximately 5 weeks) resulted in no adverse effects on viability, growth, behavior, sexual maturation or reproductive capacity in the offspring. Daily intravenous administration of cidofovir during the period of organogenesis led to reduced fetal body weights when administered to pregnant rats at 1.5 mg/kg/day and to pregnant rabbits at 1.0 mg/kg/day. The no-observable-effect dosages for embryotoxicity was 0.5 mg/kg/day in rats and 0.25 mg/kg/day in rabbits.

### Pharmaceutical particulars

*List of excipients:* Sodium Hydroxide; Hydrochloric Acid; Water for Injection

*Incompatibilities:* The chemical and physical stability of Vistide admixed with saline has been demonstrated in glass bottles, in infusion bags composed of either polyvinyl chloride (PVC) or ethylene/propylene copolymer, and in PVC based vented I.V. administration sets. Other types of I.V. set tubing and infusion bags have not been studied.

No data are available to support the addition of other drugs or supplements to the recommended admixture for intravenous infusion. Compatibility with Ringer's Solution, Lactated Ringer's Solution or bacteriostatic infusion fluids has not been evaluated.

*Shelf life:* Vistide vials are stable for 2 years when stored between 15°C and 30°C.

*Special precautions for storage:* Store at a temperature between 15°C and 30°C.

If not intended for use immediately after preparation, Vistide infusion admixtures may be stored temporarily for up to 24 hours in a refrigerator (2-8°C) when reconstitution is performed under aseptic conditions. Storage beyond 24 hours or freezing is not recommended. Refrigerated solutions should be allowed to warm to room temperature prior to use.

Vistide is supplied in single-use vials. Partially used vials should be discarded.

*Nature and contents of container:* Sterile cidofovir solution is supplied in single use 5 ml clear glass vials with a 5 ml nominal fill volume. The container/closure components include: Type I clear borosilicate glass vials, Teflon™ faced grey butyl plug stoppers, and aluminum crimp seals with a flip off plastic tab. Each pack contains one 5 ml vial together with the package leaflet.

*Instructions for use and handling:*

*Method of preparation and administration:* As with all parenteral products, Vistide vials should be visually inspected for particulate matter and discolouration prior to administration.

With a syringe, transfer under aseptic conditions the appropriate dose of Vistide from the vial to an infusion bag containing 100 ml 0.9% (normal) saline solution, and mix thoroughly. The entire volume should be infused intravenously into the patient at a constant rate over a period of 1 hour by use of a standard infusion pump. Vistide should be administered by health care professionals adequately experienced in the care of AIDS patients.

*Handling and disposal:* Adequate precautions including the use of appropriate safety equipment are recommended for the preparation, administration and disposal of Vistide. The preparation of Vistide should be done in a laminar flow biological safety cabinet. Personnel preparing the drug should wear surgical gloves, safety glasses and a closed front surgical-type gown with knit cuffs. If Vistide contacts the skin, wash membranes and flush thoroughly with water. Excess Vistide and all other materials used in the admixture preparation and administration should be placed in a leak-proof, puncture-proof container for disposal.

*Marketing authorisation holder:* Gilead Sciences Limited, UK, Springfield House, Hyde Street, Leeds.

**Marketing authorisation number** EU/1/97/037/001

**Date of approval/revision of SPC** April 1997

**Legal category** POM

## VITLIPID* N ADULT

**Presentation** A white, oil in water emulsion containing the fat soluble vitamins A, D$_2$, E and K$_1$, in the oil phase of the emulsion with a composition corresponding to that of Intralipid 10%. Vitlipid N Adult is intended for addition to Intralipid 10%, 20% or 30% and for use in adults and children over 11 years of age receiving intravenous nutrition. One ampoule of Vitlipid N Adult contains:

| | |
|---|---|
| Retinol palmitate | 990 micrograms |
| corresponding to retinol | (3,300 i.u.) |
| Ergocalciferol | 5 micrograms |
| | (200 i.u.) |
| dl-alpha-tocopherol | 9.1 mg (10 i.u.) |
| Phytomenadione | 150 micrograms |
| Fractionated soybean oil | 1 g |
| Fractionated egg | |
| phospholipids | 120 mg |
| Glycerol | 225 mg |
| Water for injections to 10 ml | |

**Uses** Vitlipid N Adult is indicated as a supplement to Intralipid 10%, 20% or 30% in intravenous nutrition of adults and older children in order to cover the daily requirements of the fat soluble vitamins A, $D_2$, E and $K_1$.

**Dosage and administration** *Recommended dosage for adults and children over 11 years of age:* One ampoule (10 ml) of Vitlipid N Adult is added to 500 ml of Intralipid 10%, 20% or 30%. After gentle shaking, the emulsion is infused as described for Intralipid. The daily maintenance dosages of the vitamins A, $D_2$, E and $K_1$ are thereby supplied.

*Recommended dosage for infants and younger children:* For patients under 11 years of age the preparation Vitlipid N Infant should be used.

**Contra-indications, warnings, etc** Should not be given undiluted. Vitlipid N Adult contains vitamin $K_1$, which may interact with anticoagulants of the coumarin type.

*Use in pregnancy and lactation:* Vilipid N adult is an emulsion indicated as a supplement in TPN regimens, providing the fat soluble vitamins $A_1$, $D_2$, E and $K_1$. No hazard is expected if used in pregnancy at the recommended dosage, covering the daily requirement of $A_1$, $D_2$, E and $K_1$. No animal studies have been performed. There are, however, published reports on safe and successful use of vitamins as part of a TPN regimen during pregnancy in the human.

*Overdosage:* In general overdosage with Vitlipid N adult is unlikely. If chronic overdosage occurred symptoms such as headache, nausea, vomiting and drowsiness may be observed. Treatment should be symptomatic along with withdrawal of Vitlipid N adult. Spontaneous reversal of any symptoms should occur without requiring a specific antidote.

**Pharmaceutical precautions** Store at 2 to 8°C protected from light. The addition of Vitlipid N Adult should be performed aseptically immediately before the start of infusion and should be used within 24 hours.

**Legal category** POM.

**Package quantities** Boxes of 10×10 ml ampoules.

**Further information** Vitlipid N Adult is specially formulated for addition to Intralipid 10%, 20% or 30%. It may be used for the reconstitution of Solivito N before addition to Intralipid (see Solivito N data sheet for details).

The manufacturer can be consulted for full information on complete and balanced intravenous nutrition regimens.

**Product licence number** 0022/0062.

## VITLIPID* N INFANT

**Presentation** A white, oil in water emulsion containing the fat soluble vitamins A, $D_2$, E and $K_1$, in the oil phase of the emulsion with a composition corresponding to that of Intralipid 10%. Vitlipid N Infant is intended for addition to Intralipid 10% or 20% and for use in infants and children receiving intravenous nutrition. One ml contains:

| | |
|---|---|
| Retinol palmitate | 135 micrograms |
| corresponding to retinol | 69 micrograms |
| | (230 i.u.) |
| Ergocalciferol | 1.0 micrograms |
| | (40 i.u.) |
| dl-alpha-tocopherol | 0.64 mg (0.7 i.u.) |
| Phytomenadione | 20 micrograms |
| Fractionated soybean oil | 100 mg |
| Fractionated egg | |
| phospholipids | 12 mg |
| Glycerol | 22.5 mg |
| Water for injections to 1 ml | |

**Uses** Vitlipid N Infant is indicated as a supplement to Intralipid 10% or 20% in intravenous nutrition of infants and children under 11 years of age in order to cover the daily requirements of the fat soluble vitamins A, $D_2$, E and $K_1$.

**Dosage and administration** *Recommended dosage for infants and children under 11 years of age:* Vitlipid N Infant in a dosage of 1 ml per kg bodyweight per day is added to Intralipid 10% or 20%. The daily

dosage must not exceed 10 ml. After gentle shaking the emulsion is infused as stated for Intralipid.

*Recommended dosage for adults and older children:* The preparation Vitlipid N Adult is recommended for use in patients 11 years of age and older.

**Contra-indications, warnings, etc**
*Contra-indications:* Should not be given undiluted.

*Precautions:* Vitlipid N Infant contains vitamin $K_1$, which may interact with anticoagulants of the coumarin type.

*Overdosage:* In general overdosage with Vitlipid N Infant is unlikely. If chronic overdosage occurs symptoms such as headache, nausea, vomiting and drowsiness may be observed. Treatment should be symptomatic along with withdrawal of Vitlipid N Infant. Spontaneous reversal of any symptoms should occur without requiring a specific antidote.

**Pharmaceutical precautions** Store at 2 to 8°C protected from light. The addition of Vitlipid N Infant should be performed aseptically immediately before the start of the infusion and should be used within 24 hours.

**Legal category** POM.

**Package quantities** Boxes of 10×10 ml ampoules.

**Further information** Vitlipid N Infant is specially formulated for addition to either Intralipid 10% or 20%. It may be used for the reconstitution of Solivito N before addition to Intralipid (see Solivito N data sheet for details).

The manufacturer can be consulted for full information on complete and balanced intravenous nutrition regimens.

**Product licence number** 0022/0063.

## VITRIMIX KV*

**Presentation** A combination pack containing a 250 ml bottle of Intralipid* 20% and a 1000 ml bottle partially filled with 750 ml of Vamin 9 Glucose which, when aseptically mixed via the transfer set provided, produces an intravenous nutrition mixture suitable for infusion via a peripheral or central vein.

*The mixture contains:*

| | |
|---|---|
| Alanine | 2.2 g |
| Arginine | 2.5 g |
| Aspartic acid | 3.1 g |
| Cysteine/cystine | 1.0 g |
| Glutamic acid | 6.8 g |
| Glycine | 1.6 g |
| Histidine | 1.8 g |
| Isoleucine | 2.9 g |
| Leucine | 4.0 g |
| Lysine | 2.9 g |
| Methionine | 1.4 g |
| Phenylalanine | 4.1 g |
| Proline | 6.1 g |
| Serine | 5.6 g |
| Threonine | 2.2 g |
| Tryptophan | 0.75 g |
| Tyrosine | 0.38 g |
| Valine | 3.2 g |
| Glucose anhydrous | 75 g |
| Fractionated soybean oil | 50 g |
| Fractionated egg phospholipids | 3.0 g |
| Glycerol | 5.5 g |
| Sodium | 38 mmol |
| Potassium | 15 mmol |
| Calcium | 1.9 mmol |
| Magnesium | 1.1 mmol |
| Chloride | 38 mmol |

in each 1000 ml pH 5.2. Free from antioxidant additives.

*Osmolality:* 1130 mosmol per kg. water.

*Nitrogen per litre:* 7.0 g corresponding to about 45 g of protein.

*Energy content per litre:* approximately 1000 kcal (4.18 MJ) of which 800 kcal (3.34 MJ) is provided as nonprotein energy. Glucose provides 300 kcal (1.25 MJ) and Intralipid provides 500 kcal (2.09 MJ).

**Uses** The use of Vitrimix KV is indicated in conditions where sufficient enteral nutrition is impossible or impracticable and is likely to remain so for a short period of time. Vitrimix KV provides a balanced mixture of essential and non-essential amino acids together with energy in the form of Intralipid (62% of non-protein energy) and glucose (38% of non-protein energy). Electrolytes are present but may need supplementing according to patient needs, as will fluid. Electrolytes should not be added directly to the Vitrimix KV bottle but may be added to any additional fluid that is given.

*Note:* For conditions requiring intravenous nutrition as the sole source of nutrition for a longer period,

complete intravenous nutrition including trace elements and vitamins will be more appropriate.

**Dosage and administration** Electrolyte, fluid, acid-base imbalance and shock should be corrected prior to commencement of intravenous nutrition. Vitrimix KV can be infused via a peripheral vein with reduced risk of thrombophlebitis. As with all infusions, strict asepsis should be maintained and care should be taken to avoid complications of catheterisation including air embolism and central venous thrombosis. For safe administration of intravenous fluids from noncollapsible containers, use of a giving set with an integral airway is recommended.

*Recommended dosage for adults:* 1–2 litres Vitrimix KV per 24 hours administered by slow intravenous infusion via either a peripheral or central vein at a rate of approximately 60 drops per minute (2.8 ml/min), corresponding to an infusion time of at least six hours per litre. Fluid intake may be supplemented by separate infusions; additional electrolytes and intravenous drugs may be given in these solutions if required.

*Recommended dosage for infants:* Not recommended.

*Recommended dosage for the elderly:* Age per se requires no adjustment of the adult dosage.

However, caution should be exercised in the 'frail' elderly, and indeed in all patients with poor renal, cardiac or liver function, where smaller volumes should be used depending on the individual patients' requirements and condition.

**Contra-indications, warnings, etc** Vitrimix KV is a mixture of Vamin 9 Glucose and Intralipid 20%. The precautions which should be observed in its use are therefore similar to those required when these two preparations are simultaneously infused from individual containers, with the exception of considerations relevant to long term total parenteral nutrition (such as folate deficiency) which are not likely to be complicating factors in the short term use of Vitrimix.

*Contra-indications:* Vitrimix KV is contra-indicated in patients with severe or irreversible liver damage, acute shock or other severe disorders of fat metabolism, or severe uraemia, when dialysis facilities are not available.

*Precautions:* Hyperkalaemia, hypernatraemia and acidosis should be corrected prior to commencement of intravenous nutrition. Serum electrolytes, blood glucose levels and acid-base balance should be regularly monitored, as should fluid balance. In patients with electrolyte retention, e.g. impaired renal function, and to those with cardiac disease requiring electrolyte restriction or drug therapy, e.g. digitalis, alternative regimens incorporating electrolyte-free amino acid solutions may be more suitable.

Fat metabolism may be disturbed in conditions such as renal insufficiency, uncompensated diabetes, certain forms of hepatic insufficiency, metabolic disorders and sepsis. If intravenous administration of fat is considered in patients with these disorders, the elimination of fat should be checked daily. Care must be exercised in the administration of large volume infusion fluids to patients with cardiac insufficiency. Amino acid-containing infusions must also be administered with caution to patients with disturbances in protein metabolism.

Animal reproduction studies have not been carried out with Vitrimix KV or its components. There are, however, published reports on the successful and safe infusion of amino acid solutions and fat emulsions during pregnancy in the human.

*Caution:* Interference with certain laboratory measurements may occur if blood samples are taken before fat has been adequately cleared from the bloodstream.

*Side-effects:* The components of Vitrimix KV are well tolerated. In exceptional cases nausea may occur due to the Vamin 9 Glucose component and, rarely, initial administration of Intralipid has produced a rise in temperature with shivering. Infusion of Vitrimix KV should be discontinued in such cases.

Vomiting, flushing and sweating may occur if the recommended rate of infusion is exceeded. Abnormal liver function tests have been observed during intravenous nutrition but all values return to normal on cessation of artificial feeding. Cholestasis has been reported in some patients receiving intravenous nutrition. The infusion of Intralipid has been associated with an altered lipoprotein profile. The significance of these changes is not known.

**Pharmaceutical precautions** Store kit at 5–25°C. Do not freeze.

Do not use if either bottle is leaking or if the Vamin 9 Glucose solution is cloudy or contains a precipitate.

After long periods of storage the bottle of Intralipid 20% should be gently inverted two or three times before use.

Vitrimix KV should be prepared immediately prior to use and infusion should be completed within 24 hours.

No additions should be made to the individual

Vamin 9 Glucose and Intralipid 20% bottles prior to mixing, nor should any additions be made to the final mixture.

Discard any unused contents.

**Legal category** POM.

**Package quantities** Combined pack consisting of one 250 ml bottle of Intralipid 20% and one 1000 ml bottle containing 750 ml of Vamin 9 Glucose, together with a sterile transfer set and directions for use, and a self-adhesive label for application to the bottle containing the final mixture.

**Further information** Vitrimix KV is intended to provide nutritional support for a limited period of time, where sufficient enteral nutrition is impossible or impracticable. The manufacturer can be consulted for full information on complete intravenous nutrition regimens suitable for patients requiring longer term intravenous nutritional support.

**Product licence number** 0022/0067.

# XALATAN* ▼

## Qualitative and quantitative composition

|  | 1 ml | One Bottle with 2.5 ml |
|---|---|---|
| Latanoprost | 50 micrograms | 125 micrograms |
| Benzalkonium chloride | 0.20 mg | 0.50 mg |

Sodium chloride, sodium dihydrogen phosphate monohydrate, disodium phosphate anhydrous, water for injections.

One drop contains approximately 1.5 micrograms latanoprost.

**Pharmaceutical form** Eye drops.

## Clinical particulars

*Therapeutic indications:* Reduction of elevated intraocular pressure in patients with open angle glaucoma and ocular hypertension who are intolerant or insufficiently responsive to another intraocular pressure lowering medication.

To date, the majority of clinical trials have investigated use of Xalatan as monotherapy, although short term studies suggest that the effect of Xalatan is additive when used in combination with other agents (see *Posology and method of administration* section).

*Posology and method of administration:* Recommended dosage for adults (including the elderly):

Recommended therapy is one eye drop in the affected eye(s) once daily. Optimal effect is obtained if Xalatan is administered in the evening.

If one dose is missed treatment should continue with the next dose as normal.

*Administration:* Pivotal studies have demonstrated that Xalatan is effective as a single drug therapy. Although definitive clinical trials of combination use have not been done, a three month study shows that latanoprost is effective in combination with beta-adrenergic antagonists (timolol).

Short term (1 or 2 weeks) studies suggest that the effect of latanoprost is additive in combination with adrenergic agonists (dipivalyl epinephrine), carbonic anhydrase inhibitors (acetazolamide) and at least partly additive with cholinergic agonists (pilocarpine).

In case of combined therapy the eye drops should be administered with an interval of at least five minutes.

The dosage of Xalatan should not exceed once daily since it has been shown that more frequent administration decreases the intraocular pressure lowering effect.

Reduction of the intraocular pressure in man starts about three to four hours after administration and maximum effect is reached after eight to twelve hours. Pressure reduction is maintained for at least 24 hours.

*Children:* Safety and effectiveness in children has not been established.

*Contra-indications:* Known hypersensitivity to any component in Xalatan. Use of all contact lenses.

*Special warnings and special precautions for use:* Xalatan may gradually change the eye colour by increasing the amount of brown pigment in the iris. This effect has predominantly been seen in patients with mixed coloured irides, i.e. blue-brown, grey-brown, green-brown or yellow-brown, and is due to increased melanin content in the stromal melanocytes of the iris. Typically the brown pigmentation around the pupil spreads concentrically towards the periphery in affected eyes, but the entire iris or parts of it may become more brownish. This effect has been seen in 16% of patients during 12 months of treatment in clinical trials (based on evidence from consecutive photographs). In patients with homogenously blue, grey, green or brown eyes, the change has only rarely been seen during two years of treatment in clinical trials.

The change in iris colour occurs slowly and may not be noticeable for several months to years. It has not been associated with any symptom or pathological changes in clinical trials to date.

No further increase in brown iris pigment has been observed after discontinuation of treatment, but the resultant colour change may be permanent. Neither naevi nor freckles of the iris have been affected by treatment.

Accumulation of pigment in the trabecular meshwork or elsewhere in the anterior chamber has not been observed in clinical trials, but until further long term experience regarding increased iris pigmentation is available, patients should be examined regularly and, depending on the clinical situation, treatment may be stopped if increased iris pigmentation ensues. The effects of continuous treatment with Xalatan after the appearance of iris pigmentation are currently not known.

Before treatment is instituted patients should be informed of the possibility of a change in eye colour. Unilateral treatment can result in permanent heterochromia.

There is no experience of Xalatan in inflammatory, neovascular, angle closure or congenital glaucoma and only limited experience in open angle glaucoma of pseudophakic patients and in pigmentary glaucoma. Xalatan has no or little effect on the pupil but there is no experience in acute attacks of closed angle glaucoma. Therefore it is recommended that Xalatan should be used with caution in these conditions until more experience is obtained.

Latanoprost has not been found to affect the pulmonary function of patients suffering from moderate asthma but there is no experience from patients with severe or brittle asthma. Such patients should therefore be treated with caution until there is sufficient experience.

*Interaction with other medicaments and other forms of interaction:* The intraocular pressure reducing effect of Latanoprost has been shown to be additive to that of beta-adrenergic antagonists (timolol), adrenergic agonists (dipivalyl epinephrine), carbonic anhydrase inhibitors (acetazolamide) and at least partly additive with cholinergic agonists (pilocarpine) in short term clinical trials. Interactions with other medications have not been investigated.

*Pregnancy and lactation:* This medicinal product does not increase the spontaneous incidence of birth defects, but it has potential hazardous pharmacological effects with respect to the course of pregnancy, to the unborn or the neonate.

Latanoprost has been shown to cause embryofoetal toxicity in rabbits characterised by increased incidences of late resorption and abortion and reduced foetal weight when given in intravenous doses approximately 100 times the human dose.

Xalatan should be used during pregnancy only if the potential benefit justifies the potential risk to the foetus.

*Lactation:* The active substance in Xalatan and its metabolites may pass into breast milk and Xalatan should therefore be used with caution in nursing women.

*Effects on ability to drive and use of machines:* In common with other eye preparations, instillation of eye drops may cause transient blurring of vision.

*Undesirable effects:* A slight foreign body sensation during the first two to three days of treatment has been noted in about 13% of patients.. Mild conjunctival hyperaemia has been noted in about 10% and moderate hyperaemia in about 1% of patients undergoing chronic treatment. Transient punctate epithelial erosions, mostly without symptoms, have been noted in about 8% of patients. Skin rash of unknown etiology has been reported rarely during Xalatan treatment.

Xalatan has caused an increase in brown pigmentation of the iris, predominantly in patients with mixed coloured irides, (i.e blue-brown, grey-brown, green-brown, yellow-brown) and is due to increased melanin content in the stromal melanocytes of the iris. This effect has been seen in 16% of patients during 12 months of treatment in clinical trials (based on evidence from consecutive photographs). The change in iris colour occurs slowly and may not be noticeable for several months to years. It has not been associated with any symptom or pathological changes in clinical trials. No further increase in brown iris pigment has been seen after discontinuation of treatment, but the resultant colour change may be permanent. The change has been seen only rarely in patients with homogenously blue, grey, green or brown eyes during two years of clinical trials, see also Special Warnings and Special Precautions for use section.

*Overdose:* Apart from ocular irritation and conjunctival hyperaemia no other ocular side effects are known if Xalatan is overdosed.

If Xalatan is accidentally ingested the following information may be useful: One bottle contains 125 micrograms latanoprost. More than 90% is metabolised during the first pass through the liver. Intravenous infusion of 3 micrograms/kg in healthy volunteers induced no symptoms but a dose of 5.5–10 micrograms/kg caused nausea, abdominal pain, dizziness, fatigue, hot flushes and sweating. In monkeys latanoprost has been infused intravenously in doses of up to 500 micrograms/kg without major effects on the cardiovascular system.

Intravenous administration of latanoprost in monkeys has been associated with transient bronchoconstriction. However, in patients with moderate bronchial asthma, bronchoconstriction was not induced by latanoprost when applied topically on the eyes in a dose of seven times the clinical dose of Xalatan.

If overdosage with Xalatan occurs, treatment should be symptomatic.

**Pharmacological properties**

*Pharmacodynamic properties:* The active substance latanoprost, a prostaglandin F$_{2a}$ analogue, is a selective prostanoid FP receptor agonist which reduces the intraocular pressure by increasing the outflow of aqueous humour. Studies in animals and man indicate that the main mechanism of action is increased uveoscleral outflow, although some increase in outflow facility (decrease in outflow resistance) has been reported in man.

Clinical trials have shown that latanoprost has no significant effect on the production of aqueous humour. Latanoprost has not been found to have any effect on the blood-aqueous barrier.

Latanoprost has no or negligible effects on the intraocular blood circulation when used at the clinical dose and studied in monkeys. However, mild to moderate conjunctival or episcleral hyperaemia may occur during topical treatment.

Chronic treatment with latanoprost in monkey eyes which had undergone extracapsular lens extraction did not affect the retinal blood vessels as determined by fluorescein angiography.

Latanoprost has not induced fluorescein leakage in the posterior segment of pseudophakic human eyes during short term treatment.

Latanoprost in clinical doses has not been found to have any significant pharmacological effects on the cardiovascular or respiratory system.

*Pharmacokinetic properties:* Latanoprost (mw 432.58) is an isopropyl ester prodrug which per se is inactive, but after hydrolysis to the acid of latanoprost becomes biologically active.

The prodrug is well absorbed through the cornea and all drug that enters the aqueous humour is hydrolysed during the passage through the cornea.

Studies in man indicate that the peak concentration in the aqueous humour is reached about two hours after topical administration. After topical application in monkeys latanoprost is distributed primarily in the anterior segment, the conjunctivae and the eye lids. Only minute quantities of the drug reach the posterior segment.

Reduction of the intraocular pressure in man starts about three to four hours after administration and maximum effect is reached after eight to twelve hours. Pressure reduction is maintained for at least 24 hours.

There is practically no metabolism of the acid of latanoprost in the eye. The main metabolism occurs in the liver. The half life in plasma is 17 minutes in man. The main metabolites, the 1, 2-dinor and 1, 2, 3, 4 tetranor metabolites, exert no or only weak biological activity in animal studies and are excreted primarily in the urine.

*Preclinical safety data:* The ocular as well as systemic toxicity of latanoprost has been investigated in several animal species. Generally latanoprost is well tolerated with a safety margin between clinical ocular dose and systemic toxicity of at least 1000 times. High doses of latanoprost, approximately 100 times the clinical dose/kg body weight, administered intravenously to unanaesthetised monkeys have been shown to increase the respiration rate probably reflecting bronchoconstriction of short duration. In animal studies latanoprost has not been found to have sensitising properties.

In the eye no toxic effects have been detected with doses of up to 100 micrograms/ eye/day in rabbits or monkeys (clinical dose is approximately 1.5 micrograms/eye/day). In monkeys, however, latanoprost has been shown to induce increased pigmentation of the iris.

The mechanism of increased pigmentation seems to be stimulation of melanin production in melanocytes of the iris with no proliferative changes observed. The change in iris colour may be permanent or slowly reversible.

In chronic ocular toxicity studies administration of latanoprost 6 micrograms/eye/day has also been shown to induce increased palpebral fissure. This effect is reversible and occurs at doses above the clinical dose level. The effect has not been seen in humans.

Latanoprost was found negative in reverse mutation tests in bacteria, gene mutation in mouse lymphoma and mouse micronucleus test. Chromosome aberrations were observed *in vitro* with human lymphocytes. Similar effects were observed with prostaglandin $F_{2\alpha}$, a naturally occurring prostaglandin, and indicates that this is a class effect.

Additional mutagenicity studies on *in vitro/in vivo* unscheduled DNA synthesis in rats were negative and indicate that latanoprost does not have mutagenic potency. Carcinogenicity studies in mice and rats were negative.

Latanoprost has not been found to have any effect on male or female fertility in animal studies. In the embryotoxicity study in rats no embryotoxicity was observed at intravenous doses (5, 50 and 250 micrograms/kg/day) of latanoprost. However, latanoprost induced embryolethal effects in rabbits in doses of 5 micrograms/kg/day and above.

The dose of 5 micrograms/kg/day (approximately 100 times the clinical dose) caused significant embryofoetal toxicity characterised by increased incidence of late resorption and abortion and by reduced foetal weight.

No teratogenic potential has been detected.

**Pharmaceutical particulars**

*List of excipients:* Sodium chloride; benzalkonium chloride; sodium dihydrogen phosphate monohydrate; disodium phosphate anhydrous; water for injections.

*Incompatibilities: In vitro* studies have shown that precipitation occurs when eye drops containing thiomersal are mixed with Xalatan.

If such drugs are used the eye drops should be administered with an interval of at least five minutes.

*Shelf life:* Shelf life: 2 years

Shelf life after opening of container: 4 weeks

*Special precautions for storage:* Store in a cold place (+2°C to 8°C).

Protect from light.

Once opened the container should be used within four weeks and may be stored at room temperature up to 25°C.

*Nature and contents of container:* Bottle (5 ml), dropper applicator (dropper tip), screw cap, tamper evident overcap of polyethylene

Each bottle contains 2.5 ml eye drop solution corresponding to approximately 80 drops of solution.

*Instructions for use/handling:* The tamper evident overcap should be removed before use.

**Marketing authorisation number** 0032/0220

**Date of approval/revision of SPC** November 1996

**Legal category** POM

## XANAX* TABLETS

**Presentation** White, oval, biconvex tablets with bevelled edges containing 250 micrograms (0.25 mg) alprazolam, scored on one side and marked 'Upjohn 29' on the other. Also contains lactose, microcrystalline cellulose, maize starch, magnesium stearate, docusate sodium, colloidal silicon dioxide and sodium benzoate.

Pink, oval, biconvex tablets with bevelled edges containing 500 micrograms (0.5 mg) alprazolam, scored on one side and marked 'Upjohn 55' on the other. Also contains lactose, microcrystalline cellulose, maize starch, magnesium stearate, docusate sodium, colloidal silicon dioxide, sodium benzoate and E127.

**Uses** Xanax is indicated for the short-term treatment of moderate or severe anxiety states and anxiety associated with depression. Xanax should not be used to treat short-term mild anxiety, such as anxiety or tension associated with the stress of everyday life. As the efficacy of Xanax in depression and in phobic or obsessional states has yet to be established, specific treatment may have to be considered.

Xanax tablets are recommended for short-term use. It is recommended that the patient be reassessed at the end of no longer than 4 weeks' treatment and the need for continued treatment be established. As with all benzodiazepines, physicians should be aware that long-term use may lead to dependence in certain patients.

**Dosage and administration**

*Adults:* The optimum dosage of Xanax should be based upon the severity of the symptoms and individual patient response. The lowest dose which can control symptoms should be used. Dosage should be reassessed at intervals of no more than 4 weeks. Xanax should not be used for long-term chronic treatment. The usual dosage is stated below; in the few patients who require higher doses, the dosage should be increased cautiously to avoid adverse effects. When higher dosage is required, the evening dose should be increased before the daytime doses. In general, patients who have not previously received psychotropic medications will require lower doses than those so treated or those with a history of chronic alcoholism. Treatment should always be tapered off gradually. Patients who have taken benzodiazepines for a long time may require a longer period during which doses are reduced.

There is a reduced clearance of the drug and, as with other benzodiazepines, an increased sensitivity to the drug in elderly patients.

Anxiety: 250 micrograms (0.25 mg) to 500 micrograms (0.5 mg) three times daily increasing, if required, to a total of 3 mg daily.

Geriatric patients or in the presence of debilitating disease:

250 micrograms (0.25 mg) two to three times daily to be gradually increased if needed and tolerated.

If side-effects occur, the dose should be lowered. It is advisable to review treatment regularly and to discontinue use as soon as possible. Should longer term treatment be necessary, then intermittent treatment may be considered to minimize the risk of dependence.

*Children:* Not recommended

**Contra-indications, warnings etc**

*Contra-indications:* Xanax should not be used in patients with a known sensitivity to benzodiazepines or in patients with acute pulmonary insufficiency.

*Interactions with other medicaments and other forms of interaction:* Potentiation of the sedative effect may be seen when the product is used in combination with alcohol. The concurrent use of other CNS depressant drugs should be avoided.

*Effects on ability to drive and to use machines:* Performance at skilled tasks and alertness may be impaired. Patients should be warned of this hazard and advised not to drive or operate machinery during treatment. These effects are potentiated by alcohol.

*Other undesirable effects (frequency and seriousness):* Products should be used with caution in chronic pulmonary insufficiency and chronic renal or hepatic disease.

The safety and efficacy of Xanax in patients less than 18 years of age has not been established.

Administration to severely depressed or suicidal patients should be done with appropriate precautions and appropriate size of prescriptions.

In cases of loss or bereavement, psychological adjustment may be inhibited by benzodiazepines.

Common adverse effects include drowsiness, sedation, blurring of vision, unsteadiness and ataxia. These effects occur following single as well as repeated dosage and may persist well into the following day. Performance at skilled tasks and alertness may be impaired. The elderly are particularly liable to experience these symptoms together with confusion, especially if organic brain symptoms are present. Amnesia may occur.

As with other benzodiazepines, reactions such as concentration difficulties, confusion, hallucinations, stimulation and adverse behavioural effects such as irritability, agitation, rage and aggressive or hostile behaviour have been reported rarely. In many of the spontaneous case reports of adverse behavioural effects, patients were receiving other CNS drugs concomitantly and/or were described as having underlying psychiatric conditions. Isolated published reports involving small numbers of patients have suggested that patients who have borderline personality disorder, a prior history of violent or aggressive behaviour or alcohol or substance abuse may be at risk for such events.

As with other benzodiazepines, disinhibiting effects and aggressive behaviour towards self and others may be manifested in various ways. Extreme caution should be used, therefore, in prescribing benzodiazepines in patients with personality disorders.

Other rare adverse effects including hypotension, gastro-intestinal and visual disturbances, skin rashes, urinary retention, headache, vertigo, changes in libido, blood dyscrasias and jaundice have been reported also.

*Use in pregnancy and lactation:* There is no evidence as to drug safety in human pregnancy nor is there evidence from animal work that it is free from hazard. Do not use during pregnancy, especially during the first and last trimesters, unless there are compelling reasons.

In labour, high single doses or repeated low doses have been reported to produce hypotonia, poor sucking and hypothermia in the neonate and irregularities in the fetal heart.

Avoid if possible in lactation.

*Other special warnings and precautions:* Xanax is not recommended as the primary treatment for psychotic patients and should not be used in lieu of appropriate treatment for psychosis.

In general the dependence potential of benzodiazepines is low, but this increases when high dosage is attained, especially when given over long periods. This is particularly so in patients with a history of alcoholism, drug abuse or in patients with marked personality disorders. Regular monitoring of treatment in such patients is essential and routine repeat prescriptions should be avoided.

Treatment in all patients should be withdrawn gradually as symptoms such as depression, nervousness, rebound insomnia, irritability, sweating and diarrhoea have been reported following abrupt cessation of treatment, even in patients receiving normal therapeutic doses for short periods of time.

Abrupt withdrawal following excessive dosage may produce confusion, toxic psychosis, convulsions or a condition resembling delirium tremens.

*Overdose:* Manifestations of Xanax overdosage include extensions of its pharmacological activity, namely ataxia and somnolence. Induced vomiting and/or gastric lavage are indicated. As in all cases of drug overdosage, respiration, pulse and blood pressure should be monitored and supported by general measures when necessary. Intravenous fluids may be administered and an adequate airway maintained.

Animal experiments have suggested that forced diuresis or haemodialysis are probably of little value in treating overdosage.

As with the management of any overdosage, the physician should bear in mind that multiple agents may have been ingested.

*Incompatibilities:* None known.

**Pharmaceutical precautions** Bottle packs should be kept tightly closed and protected from light.

**Legal category** CD (Sch 4), POM

**Package of quantities** Packs of 60 tablets

**Further information** Alprazolam is readily absorbed. Following oral administration, peak concentrations in the plasma occur after 1--2 hours. The mean half-life is 12-15 hours. Repeated dosage may lead to accumulation and this should be borne in mind in elderly patients and those with impaired renal or hepatic function. Alprazolam and its metabolites are excreted primarily in the urine. Xanax did not affect the prothrombin times or plasma warfarin levels in male volunteers administered sodium warfarin orally.

**Product licence numbers**

| | |
|---|---|
| 250 micrograms (0.25 mg) tablet | 0032/0092 |
| 500 micrograms (0.5 mg) tablet | 0032/0093 |

## ZAVEDOS*

**Presentation** Sterile, pyrogen-free, orange-red, freeze-dried powder in vials containing 5 and 10 mg of idarubicin hydrochloride with 50 mg and 100 mg of lactose, respectively.

**Uses** Antimitotic and cytotoxic agent. Acute non-lymphocytic leukaemia (ANLL) in adults for remission induction in untreated patients or for remission induction in relapsed or refractory patients.

Acute lymphocytic leukaemia (ALL) as second line treatment in adults and children.

Zavedos may be used in combination chemotherapy regimens involving other cytotoxic agents.

**Dosage and administration** For reconstitution, the contents of the 5 mg vial should be dissolved in 5 ml of Water for Injections (PhEur) and the 10 mg vial in 10 ml of Water for Injections. Zavedos must be administered only by the intravenous route and the reconstituted solution should be given via the tubing of a freely running intravenous infusion of 0.9% Sodium Chloride Injection taking 5 to 10 minutes over the injection. This technique minimises the risk of thrombosis or perivenous extravasation which can lead to severe cellulitis and necrosis. Venous sclerosis may result from injection into small veins or repeated injections into the same vein.

Dosage is usually calculated on the basis of body surface area.

*Acute non-lymphocytic leukaemia (ANLL):* In adult ANLL the dose schedule suggested is 12 mg/m² i.v. daily for 3 days in combination with cytarabine.

Another dose-schedule which has been used in ANLL as a single agent and in combination is 8 mg/m² i.v. daily for 5 days.

*Acute lymphocytic leukaemia (ALL):* As single agent in ALL the suggested dose in adults is 12 mg/m² i.v. daily for 3 days and in children is 10 mg/m² i.v. daily for 3 days.

All of these dosage schedules should, however, take into account the haematological status of the patient and the dosages of other cytotoxic drugs when used in combination.

**Contra-indications, warnings, etc**

*Contra-indications:* Zavedos therapy should not be started in patients with severe renal and liver impairment or patients with uncontrolled infections. See also *Use during pregnancy and lactation.*

*Warnings:* Zavedos is intended for use under the direction of those experienced in leukaemia chemotherapy. The drug should not be given to patients with pre-existing bone marrow suppression induced by previous drug therapy or radiotherapy unless the benefit warrants the risk. Pre-existing heart disease and previous therapy with anthracyclines at high cumulative doses or other potentially cardiotoxic agents are co-factors for increased risk of idarubicin-induced cardiac toxicity and the benefit to risk ratio of Zavedos therapy in such patients should be weighed before starting treatment with Zavedos.

Like most other cytotoxic agents, idarubicin has mutagenic properties and it is carcinogenic in rats.

*Bone marrow:* Zavedos is a potent bone marrow suppressant. Myelosuppression, primarily of leukocytes, will therefore occur in all patients given a therapeutic dose of this agent and careful haematologic monitoring including granulocytes, red cells and platelets is required. Facilities with laboratory and supportive resources adequate to monitor drug tolerability and protect and maintain a patient compromised by drug toxicity should be available. It must be possible to treat rapidly and effectively a severe haemorrhagic condition and/or a severe infection.

*Cardiac effects:* Myocardial toxicity as manifested by potentially fatal congestive heart failure, acute life-threatening arrhythmias or other cardiomyopathies may occur during therapy or several weeks after termination of therapy. Treatment with digitalis, diuretics, sodium restriction and bed-rest is indicated.

Cardiac function should be carefully monitored during treatment in order to minimise the risk of cardiac toxicity of the type described for other anthracycline compounds. The risk of such myocardial toxicity may be higher following concomitant or previous radiation to the mediastinal-pericardial area or treatment with other potentially cardiotoxic agents or in patients with a particular clinical situation due to their disease (anaemia, bone marrow depression, infections, leukaemic pericarditis and/or myocarditis).

On the basis of the recommended dosage schedules the total cumulative dose administered over two courses can be expected to reach 60–80 mg/m². Although a cumulative dose limit cannot yet be defined, a specific cardiological evaluation in cancer patients showed no significant modifications of cardiac function in patients treated with Zavedos at a mean cumulative dose of 93 mg/m².

While there is no reliable method for predicting acute congestive heart failure, cardiomyopathy induced by anthracyclines is usually associated with persistent QRS voltage reduction, increase beyond normal limits of the systolic time interval (PEP/LVET) and decrease of the left ventricular ejection fraction (LVET) from pre-treatment baseline values. An electrocardiogram or echocardiogram and a determination of left ventricular ejection fraction should be performed prior to starting therapy and during treatment with Zavedos. Early clinical diagnosis of drug-induced myocardial damage appears to be important for pharmacological treatment to be useful.

*Evaluation of hepatic and renal function:* Since hepatic and/or renal function impairment can affect the disposition of idarubicin, liver and kidney function should be evaluated with conventional clinical laboratory tests (using serum bilirubin and serum creatinine as indicators) prior to, and during, treatment. In a number of Phase III clinical trials, treatment was not given if bilirubin and/or creatinine serum levels exceeded 2 mg%. With other anthracyclines, a 50% dose reduction is generally employed if bilirubin and creatinine levels are in the range 1.2–2.0 mg%.

*Precautions:* Therapy with Zavedos requires close observation of the patient and laboratory monitoring. Patients aged over 55 years should be given vigorous supportive treatment during the aplastic period.

Hyperuricemia secondary to rapid lysis of leukaemic cells may be induced: blood uric acid levels should be monitored and appropriate therapy initiated if hyperuricemia develops. Appropriate measures must be taken to control any systemic infection before beginning therapy.

Extravasation of Zavedos at the site of i.v. injection can cause severe local tissue necrosis. The risk of thrombophlebitis at the injection site may be minimised by following the recommended procedure for administration. A stinging or burning sensation at the site of administration signifies a small degree of extravasation and the infusion should be stopped and re-started in another vein.

*Adverse reactions:* Severe myelosuppression and cardiac toxicity are the two major adverse effects. Other adverse reactions include: reversible alopecia in most patients; acute nausea and vomiting; mucositis, usually involving the oral mucosa and appearing 3–10 days after starting treatment; oesophagitis and diarrhoea; fever, chills, skin rash; elevation of liver enzymes and bilirubin in about 20–30% of cases. Severe and sometimes fatal infections have been associated with Zavedos alone or in combination with cytarabine.

Zavedos may impart a red colour to the urine for 1–2 days after administration and patients should be advised that this is no cause for alarm.

*Use in pregnancy and lactation:* There is no information as to whether idarubicin may adversely affect human fertility, or cause teratogenesis. However, in rats (but not rabbits) it is teratogenic and embryotoxic. Women of child bearing potential should be advised to avoid pregnancy.

If Zavedos is to be used during pregnancy, or if the patient becomes pregnant during therapy, the patient should be informed of the potential hazard to the foetus. Mothers should be advised not to breast-feed while undergoing chemotherapy with this drug.

*Interactions:* Zavedos is a potent myelosuppressant and combination chemotherapy regimens which contain other agents having a similar action may be expected to lead to additive myelosuppressive effects.

*Overdose:* Very high doses of Zavedos may be expected to cause acute myocardial toxicity within 24 hours and severe myelosuppression within one or two weeks. Treatment should aim to support the patient during this period and should utilise such measures as blood transfusions and reverse-barrier nursing. Delayed cardiac failure has been seen with the anthracyclines up to several months after the overdose. Patients should be observed carefully and if signs of cardiac failure arise, should be treated along conventional lines.

**Pharmaceutical precautions** The vial contents are under a negative pressure to minimise aerosol formation during reconstitution: particular care should be taken when the needle is inserted. Inhalation of any aerosol produced during reconstitution must be avoided.

The following protective recommendations which are valid for all cytotoxic agents are given:

— Personnel should be trained in good technique for reconstitution and handling.
— Pregnant staff should be excluded from working with this drug.
— Personnel handling the drug should wear protective clothing: goggles, gowns and disposable gloves and masks.
— A designated area should be defined for reconstitution (preferably under a vertical laminar flow system). The work surface should be protected by disposable, plastic-backed, absorbent paper.
— All items used for reconstitution, administration or cleaning, including gloves, should be placed in high-risk, waste disposal bags for high temperature incineration.

Accidental contact with the skin or eyes should be treated immediately by copious lavage with water: medical attention should be sought.

Spillage or leakage should be treated with dilute sodium hypochlorite (1% available chlorine) solution, preferably by soaking, and then water. All cleaning materials should subsequently be disposed of as indicated previously.

The reconstituted solution is chemically stable when stored for at least 48 hours at 2°C–8°C and 24 hours at room temperature; however, it is recommended that, in line with good pharmaceutical practice, the solution should not normally be stored for longer than 24 hours at 2°C–8°C.

Discard any unused solution.

Prolonged contact with any solution of an alkaline pH should be avoided as it will result in degradation of the drug. Zavedos should not be mixed with heparin as a precipitate may form and it is not recommended that it be mixed with other drugs.

**Legal category** POM.

**Package quantities** 5 mg and 10 mg vials for injection.

**Further information** Nil.

**Product licence numbers**
Zavedos 5 mg 3433/0133
Zavedos 10 mg 3433/0134

## ZAVEDOS* CAPSULES

**Presentation** *5 mg dosage:* opaque, red cap and red body, self-locking, hard gelatin capsule, marked with the trademark Zavedos, size No 4, containing idarubicin hydrochloride as an orange powder.

*10 mg dosage:* opaque, red cap and white body, self-locking, hard gelatin capsule, marked with the trademark Zavedos, size No 4, containing idarubicin hydrochloride as an orange powder.

*25 mg dosage:* opaque, white cap and white body, self-locking, hard gelatin capsule, marked with the trademark Zavedos, size No 2, containing idarubicin hydrochloride as an orange powder.

**Uses** Whenever intravenous idarubicin cannot be employed e.g. for medical, psychological or social reasons, oral idarubicin can be used for remission induction in patients with previously untreated, relapsed or refractory acute non-lymphocytic leukaemia (ANLL).

Zavedos capsules may be used in combination chemotherapy regimens involving other cytotoxic agents.

Zavedos can also be used as a single agent to treat advanced breast cancer after failure of frontline chemotherapy not including anthracyclines.

**Dosage and administration** Dosage is usually calculated on the basis of body surface area.

In adult ANLL the recommended dose schedule is 30 mg/m² orally given daily for 3 days as a single agent, or between 15 and 30 mg/m² orally daily for 3 days in combination with other anti-leukaemic agents.

In advanced breast cancer the recommended dose schedule as single agent is 45 mg/m² orally given either on a single day or divided over 3 consecutive days, to be repeated every 3 or 4 weeks based on the haematological recovery.

A maximum cumulative dose of 400 mg/m² is recommended.

These dosage schedules should, however, take into account the haematological status of the patient and the dosages of other cytotoxic drugs when used in combination.

In patients with hepatic impairment a dose reduction of Zavedos should be considered (see Special Warnings).

The capsules should be swallowed whole with some water and should not be sucked, bitten or chewed.

Zavedos Capsules may also be taken with a light meal.

**Contra-indications, warnings, etc**
*Contra-indications:* Zavedos should not be administered to individuals with hypersensitivity to idarubicin and/or other anthracyclines.

Zavedos therapy should not be started in patients with severe renal and liver impairment or patients with uncontrolled infections. See also Use during Pregnancy and Lactation.

*Warnings:* Zavedos is intended for use under the direction of those experienced in leukaemia chemotherapy. The drug should not be given to patients with pre-existing bone marrow suppression induced by previous drug therapy or radiotherapy unless the benefit warrants the risk. Pre-existing heart disease and previous therapy with anthracyclines at high cumulative doses or other potentially cardiotoxic agents are co-factors for increased risk of idarubicin-induced cardiac toxicity and the benefit to risk ratio of Zavedos therapy in such patients should be weighed before starting treatment with Zavedos. In absence of sufficient data, the use of oral idarubicin is not recommended in patients with prior total body irradiation or bone marrow transplantation.

Like most other cytotoxic agents, idarubicin has mutagenic properties and it is carcinogenic in rats.

*Bone marrow:* Zavedos is a potent bone marrow suppressant. Myelosuppression, primarily of leukocytes, will therefore occur in all patients given a therapeutic dose of this agent and careful haematologic monitoring including granulocytes, red cells and platelets is required. Facilities with laboratory and supportive resources adequate to monitor drug tolerability and protect and maintain a patient compromised by drug toxicity should be available. It must be possible to treat rapidly and effectively a severe haemorrhagic condition and/or a severe infection.

*Cardiac effects:* Myocardial toxicity as manifested by potentially fatal congestive heart failure (CHF), acute life-threatening arrhythmias or other cardiomyopathies may occur during therapy or several weeks after termination of therapy. Although a cumulative dose limit cannot yet be defined, available data on patients treated with Zavedos capsules indicate that total cumulative doses up to at least 400 mg/m² have a low probability of cardiotoxicity.

Should CHF occur, treatment with digitalis, diuretics, sodium restriction and bed-rest is indicated.

Cardiac function should be carefully monitored during treatment in order to minimise the risk of cardiac toxicity of the type described for other anthracycline compounds. The risk of such myocardial toxicity may be higher following concomitant or previous radiation to the mediastinal-pericardial area or treatment with other potentially cardiotoxic agents or in patients with a particular clinical situation due to their disease (anemia, bone marrow depression, infections, leukaemic pericarditis and/or myocarditis).

While there is no reliable method of predicting acute congestive heart failure, cardiomyopathy induced by anthracyclines is usually associated with persistent QRS voltage reduction, increase beyond normal limits of the systolic time interval (PEP/LVET) and a significant decrease of the left ventricular ejection fraction (LVET) from pretreatment baseline values.

An electrocardiogram or echocardiogram and a determination of left ventricular ejection fraction should be performed prior to starting therapy and during treatment with Zavedos. Early clinical dignosis of drug-induced myocardial damage appears to be important for pharmacological treatment to be useful.

*Evaluation of hepatic function:* Since hepatic function impairment can affect the disposition of idarubicin, liver function should be evaluated with conventional clinical laboratory tests (using serum bilirubin as indicator) prior to, and during, treatment.

In a number of clinical trials, treatment was not given if bilirubin serum levels exceeded 2 mg/100 ml. With other anthracyclines a 50% dose reduction has been employed if bilirubin levels are in the range 1.2–2.0 mg/100 ml in acute leukaemias. In some studies in breast cancer the oral idarubicin dose was reduced by 50% if bilirubin rose to 2–3 mg/100 ml during treatment or withdrawn with a bilirubin level >3 mg/100 ml.

Occasionally episodes of serious gastro-intestinal events (such as perforation or bleeding) have been observed in patients receiving oral idarubicin who had either acute leukaemia or a history of other pathologies/medications that might have led to GI complications. Therefore in the case of patients with active GI disease with increased risk of bleeding and/or perforation the physician must balance the benefit of Zavedos therapy against the risk.

*Precautions:* Therapy with Zavedos requires close observation of the patient and laboratory monitoring. Patients over 55 years of age should be given vigorous supportive treatment during the aplastic period. Hyperuricemia secondary to rapid lysis of leukaemic cells may be induced: blood uric acid levels should be monitored and appropriate therapy initiated if hyperuricemia develops. Appropriate measures must be taken to control any systemic infections before beginning therapy.

*Adverse reactions:* Severe myelosuppression and cardiac toxicity are the two major adverse effects. Other adverse reactions include: reversible alopecia in most patients treated at the dosage recommended in leukaemia and in about half of the patients treated at the doses recommended for breast cancer; acute nausea and vomiting; mucositis, usually involving the oral mucosa and appearing 3–10 days after starting treatment; oesophagitis; diarrhoea; fever and chills; skin rash; elevation of liver enzymes and bilirubin in about 10–20% of cases. Severe and sometimes fatal infections have been associated with idarubicin alone or in combination. Severe enterocolitis with perforation has been reported very rarely.

Idarubicin may impart a red colour to the urine for 1–2 days after administration and patients should be advised that this is no cause for alarm.

*Use in pregnancy and lactation:* There is no information as to whether idarubicin may adversely affect human fertility, or cause teratogenesis. However, in rats (but not in rabbits) it is teratogenic and embryotoxic. Women of child bearing potential should be advised to avoid pregnancy. If Zavedos is to be used during pregnancy, or if the patient becomes pregnant during therapy, the patient should be informed of the potential hazard to the foetus.

Mothers should be advised not to breast-feed while undergoing chemotherapy with this drug.

*Interactions:* Zavedos is a potent myelosuppressant and combination chemotherapy regimens which contain other agents having a similar action may be expected to lead to additive myelosuppressive effects.

An additive myelosuppressant effect is to be expected also with radiotherapy to metastases given concomitantly or within 2–3 weeks prior to treatment with Zavedos.

Food does not appear to reduce idarubicin absorp-tion and Zavedos may therefore be given with a light meal.

*Overdosage:* Although the single-dose packaging is designed to minimise the risk of overdosage and no data on overdosage exists, should this occur gastric lavage should be carried out as soon as possible. The patient should be observed for possible gastrointestinal hemorrhage and severe mucosal damage.

Very high doses of idarubicin may be expected to cause acute myocardial toxicity within 24 hours and severe myelosuppression within one or two weeks. Treatment should further aim to support the patient during this period and should utilise such measures as blood transfusions and reverse-barrier nursing. Delayed cardiac failure has been seen with the anthracyclines up to several months after an overdose. Patients should be observed carefully and if signs of cardiac failure arise, should be treated along conventional lines.

**Pharmaceutical precautions** Before administration it should be ensured that the capsules are intact. They should be swallowed whole with some water and should not be sucked, bitten or chewed.

In case of accidental contact of the powder from the capsule with eye, skin or mucosa, the area should be immediately and thoroughly rinsed with water: medical attention should be sought.

Store in a dry place.

**Legal category** POM.

**Package quantities** 5 mg, 10 mg and 25 mg Capsules placed singly in bottles.

**Further information** Nil.

**Product licence numbers**
Zavedos 5 mg    3433/0158
Zavedos 10 mg   3433/0159
Zavedos 25 mg   3433/0160

*\*Trade Mark*

# Pharmax Limited
Bourne Road
Bexley
Kent DA5 1NX

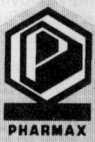

## COLOMYCIN* INJECTION

**Qualitative and quantitative composition** Each vial contains either 1.0 or 0.5 mega units (MU) of Colistin Sulphomethate Sodium BP. 1 mg of colistin sulphomethate sodium is approximately 12,500 units.

**Pharmaceutical form** Sterile creamy-white crystalline powder for reconstitution.

### Clinical particulars
*Therapeutic indications:* Colomycin Injection should only be used to treat severe systemic or localised infections caused by sensitive Gram-negative organisms, e.g. respiratory infection and septicaemia.

By aerosol inhalation, as adjunct therapy in patients already receiving standard antibiotic therapy. Parenterally or via other routes where routine antibiotic therapy has been unsuccessful.

*Posology and method of administration:* Colomycin Injection is administered by aerosol, intramuscularly or intravenously following reconstitution with sterile water or saline, but when indicated can be introduced via other routes such as subconjunctivally (used with 0.5% lidocaine) and by local instillation. Normal recommendations for systemic treatment are:

*Children (up to 60 kg):* 50,000 units/kg/body weight in 24 hours, divided into three eight-hourly doses. Serum levels should be measured if used in the newborn.

*Adults (including elderly) (over 60 kg):* 6,000,000 units in 24 hours (i.e. 2 x 1MU vials every eight hours)

*Infusion therapy:* Daily dosage as above. Infusion should preferably be completed within six hours.

*Aerosol therapy:* Daily dosage as above, concomitant with parenteral administration. For the aerosol, colistin is dissolved in water or saline for use in a suitable nebuliser attached to an air/oxygen supply.

*Bladder irrigation:* 1,000,000 units are dissolved in 50 ml water or saline and instilled during catheterisation. In the presence of infection administration is carried out twice daily.

The above are expressed as average doses. Should clinical or bacteriological response be slow, dosage may be increased as indicated by the patient's condition. Minimum of five days treatment is recommended.

Where there is moderate or severe renal impairment excretion of the antibiotic is delayed. Therefore, size of dose and dosage interval should be adjusted in relation to renal function. The table below is a guide to dosage modifications in order to prevent accumulation of Colomycin. It is stressed that adjustments may still have to be made on evaluation of the individual patient.

Blood level estimations are recommended : 10–15 micrograms/ml should be adequate.

*Contra-indications:* Colomycin Injection is contra-indicated in patients with known sensitivity to colistin.

*Special warnings and precautions for use:* None stated

*Interaction with other medicaments and other forms of interaction:* Curariform muscle relaxants should be used with extreme caution in patients receiving Colomycin Injection.

*Pregnancy and lactation:* Safety in human pregnancy has not been established. Animal studies do not indicate teratogenic properties; however, single dose studies in human pregnancy show that Colomycin crosses the placental barrier and there is a risk of foetal toxicity if repeated doses are given to pregnant patients.
Colomycin is secreted in breast milk and patients to whom the drug is administered should not breast-feed an infant.

*Effects on ability to drive and use machines:* None stated.

*Undesirable effects:* Adverse effects on renal function have been reported, usually following use of higher than recommended doses in patients with normal renal function, or failure to reduce the dosage in patients with renal impairment or during concomitant use of other nephrotoxic antibiotics. The effects are usually reversible on discontinuation of therapy. Other reversible adverse effects may include transient sensory disturbances such as facial paraesthesia and vertigo, and rarely, vasomotor instability, slurred speech, visual disturbances, confusion or psychosis. Neurotoxicity has been reported in association with overdosage, failure to reduce dosage in patients with renal insufficiency and concomitant use of either curariform agents or antibiotics with similar neurotoxic effects. Therapy need not be discontinued and reduction of dosage may alleviate symptoms.

Bronchospasm may occur on antibiotic inhalation; this may be treated with beta₂-agonists.

Permanent nerve damage such as deafness or vestibular damage has not been reported. Local irritation at the site of injection is minimal.

*Overdose:* Overdosage can result in renal insufficiency, muscle weakness and apnoea. There is no specific antidote. Management is by supportive treatment and measures to increase the rate of elimination of colistin e.g. mannitol diuresis, prolonged haemodialysis or peritoneal dialysis.

### Pharmacological properties
*Pharmacodynamic properties:* Colistin is a polypeptide antibiotic derived from *Bacillus polymyxa var. colistinus*. It possesses a rapid bactericidal activity against a number of Gram-negative organisms including *Pseudomonas aeruginosa* and is largely free from the development or transference of resistance.

*Pharmacokinetic properties:* Colomycin Injection is a sterile powder for reconstitution using sterile water or saline prior to administration primarily via intravenous or intramuscular injection, or aerosol inhalation. Peak serum levels are usually attained within 2–3 hours following intramuscular injection and demonstrable amounts of Colomycin persist for at least 8 hours. Transpulmonary absorption has been reported following administration of Colomycin via aerosol inhalation and appears to be influenced by aerosol particle size. Clinical studies have, however, demonstrated the effectiveness of Colomycin in the lungs even in the absence of detectable serum levels of the antibiotic. Distribution of injected Colomycin occurs throughout the body fluids with excretion taking place via the kidneys thus producing high urine levels of Colomycin. Peak urine levels are obtained after 2–3 hours and up to 80% of the administered dose is recovered within approximately 8 hours.

*Preclinical safety data:* There are no preclinical data of relevance to the prescriber which are additional to those already included in other sections of the SPC.

### Pharmaceutical particulars
*List of excipients:* None

*Incompatibilities:* None stated.

*Shelf life:* 36 months.

*Special precautions for storage:* Store below 25°C protected from light.

*Nature and contents of container:* Neutral glass vials in packs of 10.

*Instructions for use/handling:* Solutions of Colomycin Injection for parenteral administration should preferably be freshly prepared. Compatible infusion solutions are: normal saline, 5% dextrose, 5% fructose, Ringer's solution. Infusions should be completed within 6 hours. Mixed infusions or injections involving Colomycin should be avoided.

**Marketing authorisation numbers**
0.5 MU        0108/5005

1.0 MU        0108/5006

**Date of approval/revision of SPC** January 1996
**Legal category** POM

## COLOMYCIN* STERILE POWDER

**Qualitative and quantitative composition** Vial containing 1 g Colistin Sulphate BP. 1 mg of colistin sulphate is approximately 19,500 units.

**Pharmaceutical form** A white to cream coloured powder.

### Clinical particulars
*Therapeutic indications:* For the treatment of topical infections caused by sensitive Gram-negative organisms.

*Posology and method of administration:* For adults, children and the elderly: Colomycin Sterile Powder is applied topically as a 1% solution, dispersed powder or ointment according to the site of infection, as follows:

1% solution in water or saline for use as eye and ear drops, in wound irrigation, and for application to dressings.

1% dispersed powder in lactose or biosorb for application for infected leg ulcers and in other skin infections. Undiluted powder should not be applied topically.

1% ointment in Simple Cream BP, simple cream plus hydrous lanolin (90:10), Hydrous Ointment BP, Macrogel Ointment BPC, for use in skin infections.

**Colomycin Sterile Powder must not be used for the preparation of injectable solutions.**

*Contra-indications:* The preparation is contra-indicated in patients with known sensitivity to colistin. Colomycin Sterile Powder should not be used for the treatment of otitis externa if the tympanic membrane is perforated.

*Special warnings and special precautions for use:* Colistin absorption has not been detected following limited topical application. Absorption may, however, increase with prolonged use and absorption may be enhanced if colistin is applied to large areas of broken skin. Caution should be employed in the use of the preparation in patients with renal failure and in patients receiving curariform muscle relaxants.

*Interaction with other medicaments and other forms of interaction:* Neurotoxicity has been reported with concomitant use of either curariform agents or antibiotics with similar neurotoxic effects and systemic administration of colistin. Therapy need not be discontinued and reduction of dosage may alleviate symptoms.

*Pregnancy and lactation:* Safety in human pregnancy has not been established. Animal studies do not indicate teratogenic properties; however, parenteral single dose studies in human pregnancy show that colomycin crosses the placental barrier and there is a risk of foetal toxicity if repeated doses are given to pregnant patients. Colomycin is secreted in breast milk and patients to whom the drug is administered should not breast-feed an infant.

*Effects on ability to drive and use machines:* None stated.

*Undesirable effects:* Topical therapy is well tolerated. Transient irritation at the site of application has been reported infrequently. Allergic sensitisation has not been reported.

Systemic side effects have not been reported following topical administration. Following systemic therapy with colistin, adverse effects on renal function have been reported, usually following use of higher than recommended dose in patients with normal renal function, or failure to reduce the dosage in patients with renal impairment or during concomitant use of nephrotoxic antibiotics. The effects are usually reversible on discontinuation of therapy. Other adverse effects following systemic administration may include transient sensory disturbances such as perioral paraesthesia and vertigo. Neurotoxicity has been reported in association with overdosage, failure to reduce dosage in patients with renal insufficiency and a concomitant use of either curariform agents or antibiotics with similar neurotoxic effects. Therapy

| Creatinine clearance (ml/min) | B.U.N. (mg/100 ml) | (mmol/l) | Adult Dosage | Childrens' Dosage |
|---|---|---|---|---|
| 20–72 | > 6 | >10 | 1–2 million units every 8 hr | 12,500–16,000 units/kg every 8 hr |
| 10–20 | > 100 | > 16.5 | 1 million units every 12–18 hr | 12,500 units/kg every 12–18 hr |
| < 10 | > 200 | > 33 | 1 million units every 18–24 hr | 8,000 units/kg every 18–24 hr |

need not be discontinued and reduction of dosage may alleviate symptoms. Permanent nerve damage such as deafness or vestibular damage has not been reported.

*Overdose:* No symptoms of overdosage have been reported following topical use of colistin. However, use of the undiluted powder causes stinging and is not recommended. Following systemic administration overdosage can result in renal insufficiency, muscle weakness and apnoea. There is no specific antidote. Manage by supportive treatment and measures to increase the rate of elimination of colistin, e.g. mannitol diuresis, prolonged haemodialysis or peritoneal dialysis.

### Pharmacological properties
*Pharmacodynamic properties:* Colistin is a polmyxin antibiotic derived from *Bacillus polymyxa var. colistinus.* It has a bactericidal action on most Gram-negative bacilli, including *Pseudomonas aeruginosa,* and use is largely free from the development or transference of resistance. It is not recommended for Proteus spp.

*Pharmacokinetic properties:* There is almost complete lack of absorption when colistin is applied to intact or denuded skin; it is poorly absorbed from mucus membranes and the surface of large burns.

*Preclinical safety data:* There are no preclinical data of relevance to the prescriber that might add to the safety data provided in other sections of this SPC.

### Pharmaceutical particulars
*List of excipients:* None

*Incompatibilities:* None stated.

*Shelf-life:* Unopened product as packaged for sale: 60 months. Colomycin Sterile Powder solutions should be used within 24 hours of preparation and stored at 2°-8°C. Ointments or dispersed powders may be stored for up to 1 month at room temp. (25°C), as may preserved solutions.

*Special precautions for storage:* Unopened product should be stored below 25°C, protected from light.

*Nature and contents of container:* Neutral glass vial closed with an aluminium crimp ring. Each vial is individually packed in a cardboard carton.

*Instructions for use/handling:* Colomycin Sterile Powder should be formulated as a 1% solution, 1% dispersed powder or 1% ointment, according to the site of infection. Suitable formulations include:1% solution prepared by dissolving 1 g of powder in 100 ml water or saline; 1% dispersed powder in lactose or Biosorb; a 1% ointment prepared by the addition of 1 g of powder to 100 ml of either Simple Cream BP, simple cream plus hydrous lanolin (90:10), Hydrous Ointment BP or Macrogel Ointment BPC. Colomycin Sterile Powder may be given orally as an alternative to Colomycin Tablets or Syrup by dissolving in a suitable vehicle.

**Marketing authorisation number** 0108/0101

**Date of approval/revision of SPC** November 1995

**Legal category** POM

## COLOMYCIN* SYRUP
## COLOMYCIN* TABLETS

### Qualitative and quantitative composition
*Colomycin Syrup:* Each bottle contains 4 MU of Colistin Sulphate BP, equivalent to 250,000 units/5 ml when dispensed.

*Colomycin Tablets:* Each tablet contains 1.5 MU Colistin Sulphate BP.

**Pharmaceutical form** White powder for reconstitution into syrup and a white bevelled edge tablet with 'P' in a hexagon on one face and two crossed score marks on the reverse.

### Clinical particulars
*Therapeutic indications:* For the treatment of gastro-intestinal infections caused by sensitive Gram-negative organisms. Also for bowel preparation.

Colistin sulphate is not absorbed from the gastro-intestinal tract, except in infants under the age of 6 months, and must not be given orally for the treatment of systemic infection in any age group.

*Posology and method of administration:*
*Adults over 30 kg (including the elderly):* 1,500,000 to 3,000,000 units taken every 8 hours.

*Children (15-30 kg):* 750,000 to 1,500,000 units every 8 hours.

*Children (up to 15 kg):* 250,000 to 500,000 units every 8 hours.

A minimum of 5 days treatment is recommended. Dosage may be increased when clinical or bacteriological response is slow. For bowel preparation, a 24 hour course at the normal dosage above is given. Treatment should preferably finish 12 hours before surgery.

*Contra-indications:* Patients with known sensitivity to colistin.

*Special warnings and special precautions for use:* Colistin is subject to limited and unpredictable absorption from the G.I. tract in infants under 6 months. Studies in older children and adults have demonstrated no systemic absorption of colistin following oral administration. Nevertheless, caution should be employed in the use of these preparations in patients with renal failure and in patients receiving curariform muscle relaxants

*Interaction with other medicaments and other forms of interaction:* Neurotoxicity has been reported in association with the concomitant use of either curariform agents or antibiotics with similar neurotoxic effects. Therapy need not be discontinued and reduction of dosage may alleviate symptoms.

*Pregnancy and lactation:* Safety in human pregnancy has not been established. Animal studies do not indicate teratogenic properties however, parenteral single dose studies in human pregnancy show that Colomycin crosses the placental barrier and there is a risk of foetal toxicity if repeated doses are given to pregnant patients.

Colomycin is secreted in breast milk and patients to whom the drug is administered should not breast-feed an infant.

*Effects on ability to drive and use machines:* None stated.

*Undesirable effects:* No significant systemic absorption has been found to occur in older children and adults following oral administration nor have any systemic side effects been reported.

However, since the use of colistin may be associated with unpredictable, albeit limited, absorption in infants under 6 months, the potential adverse effects of systemic administration should be noted for this patient population. These adverse effects may include transient sensory disturbances such as perioral parasthesia and vertigo.

Neurotoxicity and adverse effects on renal function have been reported in association with systemic overdosage, failure to reduce dosage in patients with renal insufficiency and the concomitant use of either curariform agents or antibiotics with similar neurotoxic effects.

Therapy need not be discontinued and reduction of dosage may alleviate symptoms. Permanent nerve damage such as deafness or vestibular damage has not been reported.

*Overdose:* No symptoms of overdosage have been reported following oral use of colistin. However, following systemic administration overdosage can result in renal insufficiency, muscle weakness and apnoea and this should be borne in mind in the oral therapy of infants under 6 months old.

There is no specific antidote. Manage by supportive treatment and measures to increase the rate of elimination of colistin, e.g. mannitol diuresis, prolonged haemodialysis or peritoneal dialysis.

### Pharmacological properties
*Pharmacodynamic properties:* Colistin is a polymyxin antibiotic derived from *Bacillus polymyxa var. colistinus.* It has a bactericidal action on most Gram-negative bacilli, including *Pseudomonas aeruginosa,* and use is largely free from the development or transference of resistance. It is not recommended for Proteus spp.

*Pharmacokinetic properties:* In adults and older children, colistin sulphate taken orally is not absorbed from the G.I. tract. However, in small infants less than 6 months old, some very limited and unpredictable absorption may occur.

*Preclinical safety data:* There are no preclinical data of relevance to the prescriber that might add to the safety data provided in other sections of this SPC.

### Pharmaceutical particulars
*List of excipients: Syrup:* Sucrose PhEur, Sodium Citrate PhEur, Cherry flavour, Benzoic Acid BP, Sodium Methyl Hydroxybenzoate BP.

*Tablets:* Microcrystalline Cellulose BPC, Maize Starch PhEur, Colloidal Silicon Dioxide NF, Cutina HR.

*Incompatibilities:* None stated.

*Shelf life:* Syrup: 36 months. Tablets: 60 months

*Special precautions for storage:* Store below 25°C in a dry place, protected from light.

*Nature and contents of container: Syrup:* Amber glass bottle for preparation of 80 ml of syrup. *Tablets:* Plastic containers of 50 tablets.

*Instructions for use/handling:* Colomycin Syrup Powder is reconstituted by adding 58 ml of water, and shaking the bottle until the powder is dissolved.

**Marketing authorisation numbers**
Colomycin Syrup       0108/5009
Colomycin Tablets     0108/5008

**Date of approval/revision of SPC**
Colomycin Syrup: November 1995
Colomycin Tablets: July 1996

**Legal category** POM

## FLETCHERS' ARACHIS OIL RETENTION ENEMA*

**Presentation** Ready-to-use, self-contained, single-dose, disposable enema containing Arachis Oil BP 130 ml.

**Uses** To soften impacted faeces.

**Dosage and administration** For rectal administration only.
*Adults and elderly patients:* 1 enema as required.

*Children:* Reduce adult dose in proportion to body-weight.

*Children under 3 years:* Not recommended.

The enema should be warmed before use by placing in warm water.

### Contra-indications, warnings, etc
*Contra-indications:* Hypersensitivity to arachis oil or peanuts. Inflammatory bowel disease except under the instruction of a medical practitioner.

*Precautions and warnings:* Not for use in children unless under medical supervision. Use with caution in patients with intestinal obstruction.

Care should be taken not to use undue force in administration of the enema especially in elderly or debilitated patients or those with neurological disorders.

*Use in pregnancy and lactation:* The use of enemas is not recommended during pregnancy except under medical advice.

*Side-effects:* Like other rectally applied substances arachis oil may produce local irritation.

**Pharmaceutical precautions** Store at room temperature.

**Legal category** P

**Package quantities** Box of 10 enemas.

**Further information** Contains peanut oil.

**Product licence number** 0108/5016

## FLETCHERS' ENEMETTE*

**Presentation** Ready-to-use, self-contained single-dose, disposable microenema of 5 ml liquid containing: Docusate Sodium BP 90 mg, Glycerol PhEur 3780 mg.

This product also contains sorbic acid and polyethylene glycol.

**Uses** Routine treatment of constipation. Pre- and post-operative cleansing of the bowel, in obstetrics and prior to proctoscopy, sigmoidoscopy or X-ray examination.

**Dosage and administration** For rectal administration only.
*Adults, elderly and children over 3 years:* 1 enema as required.

*Children under 3 years:* Not recommended.

### Contra-indications, warnings, etc
*Contra-indications:* Nil

*Precautions:* Use with caution in patients with intestinal obstruction.

Care should be taken not to use undue force in administration of the enema especially in elderly or debilitated patients or those with neurological disorders.

**Pharmaceutical precautions** Store below 25°C. Protect from heat.

**Legal category** P

**Package quantities** Box of 12 microenemas.

**Further information** The formulation of docusate sodium, a faecal softening agent, in glycerol (which when administered rectally promotes peristalsis and evacuation of the lower bowel) and polyethylene glycol, provides an easy-to-use, efficacious, low-volume enema.

**Product licence number** 0108/0078

## FLETCHERS' PHOSPHATE ENEMA*

**Qualitative and quantitative composition** Each 128 ml enema contains: Sodium Acid Phosphate BP 10.0% w/v and Sodium Phosphate PhEur 8.0% w/v. The formulation is equivalent to Phosphates Enema BP Formula B.

**Pharmaceutical form** Single dose enema

**Clinical particulars**

*Therapeutic indications:* Routine treatment of constipation. Pre- and post-operative cleansing of the bowel, in obstetrics and prior to proctoscopy, sigmoidoscopy or X-ray examination.

*Posology and method of administration:*
*Adults including the elderly:* One enema as required.

*Children over 3 years of age:* Reduce adult dosage in proportion to body weight.

*Children under 3 years of age:* Not recommended.
For rectal administration only. The enema may be administered at room temperature or warmed in water before use.

*Contra-indications:* Use in patients with inflammatory or ulcerative conditions of the bowel, in those with increased colonic absorptive capacity e.g. Hirschsprung's disease and in those with acute gastrointestinal conditions.

*Special warnings and precautions for use:* Prolonged use may lead to irritation of the anal canal. Use with caution in patients requiring a reduced sodium intake and electrolyte balance should be maintained during extended use. Use with caution in patients with intestinal obstruction. Care should be taken not to use undue force in administration of the enema, especially in elderly or debilitated patients or those with neurological disorders.

*Interaction with other medicaments and other forms of interaction:* None known.

*Pregnancy and lactation:* No special warnings.

*Effects on ability to drive and use machines:* Not applicable.

*Undesirable effects:* There have been occasional reports of apparent vasovagal attacks occurring in elderly patients following administration of phosphate enemata.

*Overdose:* There have been no reports of overdose. In the event of overdosage electrolyte levels should be monitored and balance restored where appropriate.

**Pharmacological properties**

*Pharmacodynamic properties:* Fletchers' Phosphate Enema is a solution of sodium acid phosphate and sodium phosphate. The formulation is equivalent to Phosphates Enema BP Formula B. Following rectal administration the active ingredients exert their laxative effect via their osmotic properties. The resulting fluid retention in the bowel encourages evacuation.

*Pharmacokinetic properties:* Saline laxatives are poorly and slowly absorbed following rectal administration. Under normal usage only minimal absorption is likely to occur.

**Pharmaceutical particulars**

*List of excipients:* Benzalkonium Chloride BP, Disodium Edetate BP, Purified Water PhEur.

*Shelf life:* Bag presentation: 12 months. Bottle presentation: 36 months

*Special precautions for storage:* Store below 25°C.

*Nature and contents of container:*
(a) Translucent LDPE bottle with rubber non-return valve, plastic nozzle and nozzle plug containing 128 ml solution packed singly in a cardboard carton.
(b) Translucent PVC bag containing 128 ml solution with a plastic extension tube with nozzle and plug (long-tube enema) in packs of 50.

**Marketing authorisation number** 0108/5015R

**Date of approval/revision of SPC** May 1995

**Legal category** P

# INFACOL*

**Qualitative and quantitative composition** Simethicone USP 40 mg/ml.

**Pharmaceutical form** An orange-flavoured, colourless, translucent suspension for oral administration.

**Clinical particulars**

*Therapeutic indications:* An antiflatulent for the relief of griping pain, colic or wind due to swallowed air.

*Posology and method of administration:* Infants: 20 mg (0.5 ml) administered before each feed. If necessary this may be increased to 40 mg (1 ml). Treatment with Infacol may provide a progressive improvement in symptoms over several days.
*Adults and the elderly:* Not applicable.

*Contra-indications:* None stated.

*Special warnings and precautions for use:* If symptoms persist, seek medical advice.

*Interactions with other medicaments and other forms of interaction:* None stated.

*Pregnancy and lactation:* Not applicable.

*Effects on ability to drive and use machines:* Not applicable.

*Undesirable effects:* None stated.

*Overdose:* In the event of deliberate or accidental overdosage, treat symptoms on appearance.

**Pharmacological properties**

*Pharmacodynamic properties:* Physiologically the active ingredient is a chemically inert, non-systemic, gastric defoaming agent that works by altering the elasticity of interfaces of mucus-embedded bubbles in the gastro-intestinal tract.

The gas bubbles are thus broken down or coalesced and in this form gas is more easily eliminated through eructation or passing flatus.

*Pharmacokinetic properties:* Simethicone is not absorbed from the gastro-intestinal tract.

*Preclinical safety data:* There are no pre clinical data of relevance to the prescriber which are additional to that already included in other sections of the SPC.

**Pharmaceutical particulars**

*List of excipients:* Saccharin Sodium BP, Hydroxypropyl Methylcellulose USP, Orange flavour, Methyl Paraben PhEur, Propyl Paraben PhEur, Purified Water PhEur.

*Incompatibilities:* None stated.

*Shelf life:* 24 months.

*Special precautions for storage:* Store at room temperature (below 25°C).

*Nature and contents of container:* High density polyethylene bottle containing 50 ml of liquid fitted with a low density polyethylene dropper and evoprene teat.

*Instruction for use/handling:* None.

**Marketing authorisation number** 0108/0100

**Date of approval/revision of SPC** July 1996

**Legal category** GSL

# LASMA*

**Qualitative and quantitative composition** Each tablet contains 300 mg Theophylline PhEur.

**Pharmaceutical form** Sustained release tablets for oral administration.

**Clinical particulars**

*Therapeutic indications:* Treatment and prophylaxis of bronchospasm associated with asthma, (including nocturnal asthma) and bronchitis.

*Posology and method of administration:* Tablets should be swallowed and not sucked or chewed.

*Adults (including the elderly):* Therapy should commence with 2 tablets (600 mg). In patients of 70 kg body weight or over the dosage should be increased after 1 week to 3 tablets (900 mg) daily.

The daily dosage is administered as 1 or 1½ tablets every 12 hours, preferably after food. The dosage may be increased, as necessary, by half-tablet increments.

*Children:* Not recommended.

*Nocturnal asthma:* In patients where nocturnal symptoms predominate therapeutic benefit of up to 12 hours duration may be achieved by administration of Lasma Tablets as a single dose in the late evening. This will prevent the characteristic 'early-morning dip' in peak expiratory flow rate, thus allowing patients an uninterrupted night's sleep. Any day-time symptoms may then be controlled by inhaled bronchodilators.

*Contra-indications:* There are no absolute contraindications to theophylline, however caution should be exercised in the treatment of patients with cardiac arrhythmias, peptic ulcers or severe hypertension. Cardiac failure or hepatic dysfunction decreases theophylline clearance and patients with such conditions should be carefully monitored.

*Special warnings and precautions for use:* It is recommended, as with all xanthine preparations, that patients are individually titrated to their correct daily dosage by blood level estimations. Once a patient is stabilised on an effective dosage regime of Lasma Tablets this should not be changed, nor should an alternative product be substituted without re-titration of the dosage by clinical assessment and blood-level estimations.

Theophylline is not recommended for patients with a history of seizure activity as seizures have been reported in children whose theophylline levels are within the therapeutic range.

*Interaction with other medicaments and other forms of interaction:* Lasma should not be used concurrently with other preparations containing xanthine derivatives. Theophylline has been reported to interact with a number of drugs.

The following increase clearance and it may therefore be necessary to increase dosage to ensure a therapeutic effect: phenytoin, carbamazepine, rifampicin, sulphinpyrazone and barbiturates. Smoking and alcohol consumption can also increase clearance of theophylline. The following reduce clearance and a reduced dosage may therefore be necessary to avoid side-effects: the calcium-channel blockers verapamil and diltiazem, allopurinol, cimetidine, erythromycin, thiabendazole, ciprofloxacin, isoprenaline and oral contraceptives. Factors such as viral infections, liver disease and heart failure also reduce theophylline clearance. There are conflicting reports concerning the potentiation of theophylline by influenza vaccine and physicians should be aware that interaction may occur. A reduction of dosage may also be necessary in the elderly patient.

The concomitant use of theophylline and fluvoxamine should usually be avoided. Where this is not possible, patients should have their theophylline dose halved and plasma theophylline should be monitored closely.

The following should also be used with caution in patients taking theophylline preparations: halothane, lomustine and lithium.

Xanthine can potentiate hypokalaemia resulting from beta$_2$ agonist therapy, steroids, diuretics and hypoxia. Particular caution is advised in severe asthma. It is recommended that serum potassium levels are monitored in such situations.

*Pregnancy and lactation:* Safety in human pregnancy has not been established. Theophylline crosses the placental barrier and is secreted in breast milk. Theophylline should be used with caution in pregnancy and lactation.

*Effects on ability to drive and use machines:* None known.

*Undesirable effects:* Reported side-effects include gastro-intestinal disturbances, headache, CNS stimulation and tremor. Side-effects (particularly tremor) are rare at plasma concentrations of less than 20 mg/litre.

*Overdose:* Symptoms may include nausea, vomiting, gastro-intestinal irritation, cramps, convulsions, tachycardia and hypotension.

The stomach contents should be emptied and supportive measures employed to maintain circulation, respiration and fluid and electrolyte balance. Electrocardiographic monitoring should be carried out and in severe poisoning charcoal haemoperfusion should be used.

**Pharmacological properties**

*Pharmacodynamic properties:* Theophylline is a xanthine bronchodilator effecting dilatation of bronchial smooth muscle through as yet unknown mechanisms. Efficacy has been established at blood levels of 3–5 mg/litre with a log-blood level response relationship. The benefit of efficacy at higher levels is curtailed by side-effects which occur above 15 mg/litre and become increasingly serious as blood levels are increased especially above 20 mg/litre.

*Pharmacokinetic properties:* The reported elimination half-life for theophylline is 3½ hrs in children and 6–9 hrs in adults. The apparent volume of distribution is 400–500 ml/kg and plasma protein binding is approx. 50%. Lasma is a sustained release tablet and in a multiple dose kinetic study one tablet given 12 hourly produced a Cmin of 4.54 mg/litre and a Cmax of 8.41 mg/litre, the Tmax was 4.06 hrs. The relative bioavailability of the tablet is 88% of an oral liquid. When given as a 900 mg single daily dose the peak to trough difference was 9 mg/litre and the Cmax 14.9 mg/litre.

*Preclinical safety data:* Theophylline has been in use for many years and there are no preclinical safety data that are of additional value to the prescriber.

**Pharmaceutical particulars**

*List of excipients:* Hydroxypropyl Methylcellulose USP, Stearic Acid NF, Magnesium Stearate NF, Colloidal Silicon Dioxide NF.

*Incompatibilities:* None known.

*Shelf life:* 36 months.

*Special precautions for storage:* None.

*Nature and contents of container:* Amber glass bottle containing 60 tablets.

*Instructions for use/handling:* Not applicable.

**Marketing authorisation number** 0108/0075

**Date of approval/revision of SPC** February 1997

**Legal category** P

# MUCOGEL* SUSPENSION

**Presentation** A white mint flavoured suspension. Each 5 ml contains: Aluminium Hydroxide equivalent to Dried Gel BP 220 mg and Magnesium Hydroxide BP 195 mg. This product also contains methyl and propyl parabens.

**Uses** Antacid therapy in gastric and duodenal ulcer, gastritis, heartburn, gastric hyperacidity. Treatment of indigestion.

Relief of symptoms of heartburn and dyspepsia associated with gastric reflux in hiatus hernia, reflux oesophagitis and similar conditions.

## Dosage and administration
*Adults, elderly and children over 12 years old:* 10–20 ml three times daily 20 minutes to one hour after meals and at bedtime, or as required.

*Children under 12 years:* Not recommended.

## Contra-indications, warnings, etc
*Contra-indications:* Mucogel should not be used in patients who are severely debilitated or suffering from kidney failure. Antacids inhibit the absorption of tetracyclines and vitamins and should not be taken concomitantly.

*Adverse effects:* Gastrointestinal side-effects are uncommon. This formulation minimises the problems of diarrhoea and constipation.

*Use in pregnancy and lactation:* Unnecessary drug therapy should be avoided in the first trimester of pregnancy.

*Overdosage:* Serious symptoms are unlikely to follow overdosage.

**Pharmaceutical precautions** Store below 25°C. Do not freeze. Use within 28 days of opening.

**Legal category** GSL

**Package quantities** Bottles of 500 ml

**Further information** Mucogel is a pleasant-tasting, well tolerated antacid containing balanced quantities of aluminium and magnesium.

**Product licence number** 0108/0074

# PREDENEMA*

**Qualitative and quantitative composition** Each 100 ml enema contains 35 mg prednisolone metasulphobenzoate sodium equivalent to prednisolone 20 mg.

**Pharmaceutical form** Single dose enema.

## Clinical particulars
*Therapeutic indications:* Local treatment of ulcerative colitis.

*Posology and method of administration:*
*Adults (including the elderly):* One enema nightly for 2-4 weeks, the course may be extended when a good response is obtained.
*Children:* Not recommended.
Predenema is to be used for rectal administration only.

*Contra-indications:* In local conditions where the use of Predenema might mask infection or impair healing, such as peritonitis, sinus infection, fistulae, intestinal obstruction, perforation of the bowel.

*Special warnings and special precautions for use:* Symptoms of adrenal insufficiency have not been reported, but prolonged therapy should be carefully monitored. Use with caution in patients with intestinal obstruction.

*Interaction with other medicaments and other forms of interaction:* None stated.

*Pregnancy and lactation:* Topical administration of corticosteroids to pregnant animals can cause abnormalities of foetal development. The relevance of this finding to human beings has not been established. However, physicians should be aware of the possibility of teratogenic effects, and also of potential suppression of the HPA axis, and should weigh up the risk/benefit ratio before using Predenema in pregnancy.

If treatment is instituted with Predenema, the minimum dosage and frequency of administration required for clinical control should be employed and prolonged usage should be avoided.

*Effects on ability to drive and use machines:* None stated.

*Undesirable effects:* Administration of prednisolone via this route, for this indication is seldom associated with adverse effects.

*Overdosage:* Overdose is not likely with this route of administration.

## Pharmacological properties
*Pharmacodynamic properties:* Prednisolone 21-so-dium metasulphobenzoate has the general properties of prednisolone as a potent anti-inflammatory agent with immuno-suppressant glucocorticoid properties. Esterification of prednisolone at the 21 position increases the topical activity of the drug.

*Pharmacokinetic properties:* Following rectal administration of prednisolone 21-sodium metasulphobenzoate in the form of an enema, the action of the drug is predominantly local. The peak plasma levels obtained following this treatment are significantly lower than those obtained following treatment with prednisolone 21-phosphate.

Following absorption, the drug is hydrolysed to *m*-sulphobenzoic acid (and salts) and free prednisolone.

At the low plasma levels obtained, following rectal administration of prednisolone 21-sodium metasulphobenzoate the precautions generally applied to the use of prednisolone are considered to be unnecessary.

*Preclinical safety data:* There are no pre-clinical data of relevance to the prescriber which are additional to those already included in other sections of the SPC.

## Pharmaceutical particulars
*List of excipients:* Disodium Edetate PhEur, Nipastat and Purified Water PhEur.

*Incompatibilities:* None stated.

*Shelf life:* 12 months

*Special precautions for storage:* Store below 25°C, protected from light.

*Nature and contents of container:* Predenema is presented as a ready to use, single dose, disposable plastic enema bag containing 100 ml of solution. It is available with a standard tube in packs of 10 or with an extension tube (long tube) in packs of 7.

*Instructions for use/handling:* Predenema may be administered at room temperature or warmed in warm water before use. Hold the bag with tube upwards and squeeze base of tube where it joins the bag. Remove cap and lubricate tube before inserting into rectum. The patient should lie in bed with knees drawn up. Squeeze bag gently until fluid is expelled and discard container hygienically. The patient should lie face down for a few minutes to retain the fluid before going to sleep in the usual position. The long tube presentation facilitates self-administration.

**Marketing authorisation number** 0108/5018R

**Date of approval/revision of SPC** September 1995.

**Legal category** POM

# PREDFOAM*

**Presentation** A white, mucoadherent aerosol foam containing prednisolone metasulphobenzoate sodium equivalent to 20 mg prednisolone per metered dose.

This product also contains disodium edetate, phenoxyethanol and sorbic acid.

**Uses** Treatment of proctitis and distal ulcerative colitis.

## Dosage and administration
*Adults and elderly patients:* One metered dose inserted rectally once or twice daily for two weeks, extending treatment for a further two weeks when a good response is obtained. Use should be discontinued at the discretion of the physician once the disease is stable and under control.

*Children:* Not recommended.

## Contra-indications, warnings, etc
*Contra-indications:* Local conditions where infection might be masked or healing impaired e.g. peritonitis, fistulae, intestinal obstruction, perforation of the bowel.

*Precautions:* This product should be used with extreme caution in the presence of severe ulcerative colitis. The possible occurrence of masking of local or systemic infection should be borne in mind when using this product. For rectal use only.

*Side-effects:* The consequences of systemic absorption should be considered with extensive use over prolonged periods. As with all rectal corticosteroids, prolonged continuous use is undesirable.

*Use in pregnancy and lactation:* There is inadequate evidence of safety in human pregnancy. Topical administration of corticosteroids to pregnant animals can cause abnormalities of foetal development including cleft palate and intra-uterine growth retardation. There may therefore be a very small risk of such effects in the human foetus.

*Overdosage:* Overdosage by this route is unlikely.

**Pharmaceutical precautions** Pressurised container containing a flammable propellant. Store below 25°C. Protect from sunlight and do not expose to temperatures above 50°C. Do not pierce or burn even after use. Do not spray on naked flame or any incandescent material. Shake before use.

**Legal category** POM

**Package quantities** Carton containing an aerosol canister containing sufficient for 14 applications plus 14 disposable applicators.

**Further information** Nil

**Product licence number** 0108/0101

# SAVENTRINE i.v.*

**Qualitative and quantitative composition** Ampoule containing 2 ml of a 1 mg/ml solution of Isoprenaline Hydrochloride BP.

**Pharmaceutical form** Glass ampoules containing a sterile stabilised solution of Isoprenaline Hydrochloride BP for injection.

## Clinical particulars
*Therapeutic indications:*
1. Cardiogenic or endotoxic shock.
2. Acute Stokes-Adams attacks and other cardiac emergencies.
3. Severe bradycardia precipitated by beta-adrenergic antagonists and disopyramide.
4. Evaluation of congenital heart defects.

*Posology and method of administration:* The usual route is by intravenous infusion in 5% dextrose solution or Water for Injections. Widely varying doses have been used with success.

*Adults and elderly patients:*
1. Shock states: 0.5–10 micrograms/min or alternatively injection of 0.1 mg in 10 ml water.
2. Acute Stokes-Adams attack: 4–8 micrograms/min or alternatively intracardiac injection of 0.1 mg in 10 ml water.
3. Severe bradycardia: 1–4 micrograms/min.
4. Evaluation of congenital cardiac defects: 1.5–4 micrograms/min.

*Children:* Adjust above dosage in proportion to body weight.

*Contra-indications:* Saventrine i.v. is contraindicated in acute coronary disease and in patients prone to episodes of ventricular fibrillation or tachycardia secondary to their slow rate.

Isoprenaline may precipitate ventricular extrasystoles and arrhythmias especially in patients who may be hypersensitive to the drug. In such cases the infusion rate should be reduced or possibly discontinued.

*Special warnings and precautions for use:* Use with caution in patients with hyperthyroidism, diabetes, left ventricular failure, ischaemic heart disease, angina, cardiac arrhythmia or hypertension. This product is not suitable for oral administration.

*Interaction with other medicaments and other forms of interaction:* Do not use in patients who are receiving monoamine oxidase inhibitors or within 14 days of stopping such treatment.

Isoprenaline may induce arrhythmias when administered with halothane, cyclopropane and trichlorethylene. Use with caution if isoprenaline is given concomitantly with digoxin, digitoxin, guanethidine, methyldopa or tricyclic antidepressants.

*Pregnancy and lactation:* Safety during pregnancy and lactation has not been established. The risk to benefit ratio should be assessed in individual circumstances.

*Effects on ability to drive and use machines:* None stated.

*Undesirable effects:* These may include palpitations, tremor, precordial pain, sweats, facial flushing and headache.

*Overdose:* Symptoms of overdosage are listed in the 'Undesirable effects' section above. Fatality may also occur in cases of serious overdosage. A beta-adrenergic blocking drug may diminish toxic effects and should be accompanied by monitoring of heart rhythm.

## Pharmacological properties
*Pharmacodynamic properties:* Isoprenaline hydrochloride is a beta-adrenergic agonist, which has a powerful stimulant action on the heart, increasing cardiac output and cardiac rate.

It also produces peripheral vasodilation, a reduction in diastolic blood pressure and maintains or slightly increases systolic blood pressure.

*Pharmacokinetic properties:* Saventrine i.v. administered by intravenous injection allows isoprenaline to become immediately available within the bloodstream, and has a plasma half-life of one to several minutes dependent on injection rate.

Isoprenaline is excreted mainly in the urine as unchanged isoprenaline and metabolites.

*Preclinical safety data:* There are no preclinical data of relevance to the prescriber which are additional to those already included in other sections of the SPC.

**Pharmaceutical particulars**

*List of excipients:* Ascorbic Acid PhEur, Disodium Edetate BP, Hydrochloric Acid, Water for Injections PhEur.

*Incompatibilities:* None stated.

*Shelf life:* 2 years from the date of manufacture.

*Special precautions for storage:* Store below 25°C, protected from light.

*Nature and contents of container:* 2 ml glass ampoules, packed into cartons of 10.

*Instructions for use/handling:* None stated.

**Marketing authorisation number** 0108/5030R

**Date of approval/revision of SPC** June 1996

**Legal category** POM

## SUSCARD* BUCCAL TABLETS

**Presentation** White biconvex tablets, marked with the dosage strength on one face. Suscard is a controlled release presentation of glyceryl trinitrate in four strengths, 1 mg, 2 mg, 3 mg and 5 mg, for buccal administration (see below).

**Uses** The management and treatment of angina pectoris. This product may also be of benefit in the in-patient management of unstable angina. Acute and congestive cardiac failure.

**Dosage and administration**

*Administration:* Buccal. The Suscard tablet is placed high up between the upper lip and the gum to either side of the front teeth. The diagrams below show the correct placement of the tablet. The onset of action of Suscard tablets is extremely rapid and the tablets may be substituted for sublingual glyceryl trinitrate tablets in the treatment of acute angina pectoris. The duration of action of the Suscard tablet, once in place, correlates with the dissolution time of the tablet. This is normally 3–5 hours. However, the first few doses may dissolve more rapidly until the patient is used to the presence of the tablet. During the dissolution period the tablet will soften and adhere to the gum; in practice the presence of the tablet is not noticeable to the patient after a short time.

Patients should be instructed as to the correct placement of the tablet and should note the following points:

a. The tablet should not be moved about the mouth with the tongue as this will cause it to dissolve more rapidly.

b. A slight stinging sensation (as with sublingual glyceryl trinitrate) may be felt for a few minutes after placement of the tablet.

c. If a tablet is **accidentally** swallowed it may be replaced by a further tablet.

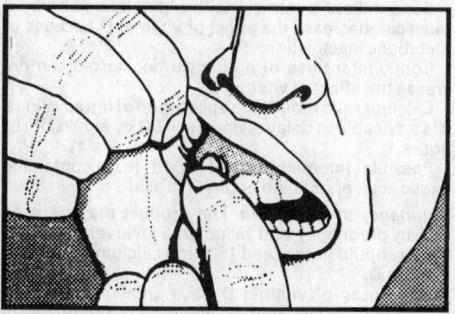

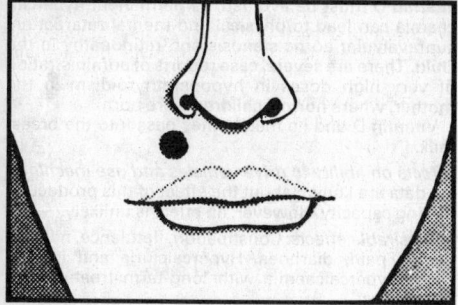

d. In patients who wear dentures the tablet may be placed in any comfortable position between the lip and the gum.

e. The patient may alternate the placement of successive tablets on the right and left sides of the front teeth.

Suscard tablets do not interfere with the ingestion of food or liquids. THE TABLETS SHOULD NOT BE PLACED UNDER THE TONGUE, CHEWED OR INTENTIONALLY SWALLOWED.

*Dosage: Adults and elderly patients:*

*Angina:* Administration of Suscard tablets should start with the 2 mg strength. If angina occurs while the tablet is in place the dosage strength used should be increased to 3 mg where necessary. The 5 mg tablet should be reserved for patients with severe angina pectoris refractory to treatment with the lower dosage strengths. A 1 mg tablet is also available and may be considered for the small number of patients who initially show intolerance to the 2 mg strength as a starting dose.

Suggested dosage frequency in angina:

(a) For patients suffering only occasional angina pectoris the tablets may be administered on a p.r.n. basis, to relieve the acute attack.

(b) For patients suffering angina pectoris in response to known stimuli the tablet may be administered a few minutes prior to encountering the angina-precipitating stimulus.

(c) For patients in whom chronic therapy is indicated the tablet should be administered on a thrice daily basis or as dictated by the dissolution rate of the tablet in an individual patient. If angina occurs during the period between the disappearance of one tablet and the time the next tablet is due to be put in place, dosage frequency should be increased.

Note that if an acute attack of angina pectoris is suffered while a tablet is in place, an additional tablet may be positioned on the opposite side of the mouth.

*Acute heart failure:* Administer 5 mg repeated as indicated by patient response until symptoms abate.

*Unstable angina:* Dosage should be rapidly titrated upwards in order to relieve and prevent symptoms. Suscard Tablets may be used in addition to pre-existing anti-anginal therapy, where considered appropriate. The 5 mg dosage strength may be required to achieve a satisfactory therapeutic response in patients exhibiting severe symptoms. Unstable angina is a serious condition managed under hospitalised conditions and involving continuous monitoring of ECG changes with frequent monitoring of appropriate haemodynamic variables. In common with other nitrate therapy a fall in systolic blood pressure of 10–15 mm Hg may occur.

*Congestive cardiac failure:* Dosage should commence with the 5 mg strength, administered three times daily. In moderately severe or severe cases, particularly where patients have not responded to standard therapy (digitalis/diuretics), the dosage may need to be increased to 10 mg (2 x 5 mg tablets) t.i.d. over a period of three to four days. In such instances one tablet should be placed between the upper lip and the gum, on each side of the front teeth.

**Contra-indications, warnings, etc**

*Contra-indications:* Are as for glyceryl trinitrate. Suscard tablets should not be used in patients with marked anaemia, head trauma, cerebral haemorrhage or closed angle glaucoma or in patients with known hypersensitivity to nitrates.

*Precautions:* Rarely, prolonged use in susceptible individuals with poor dental hygiene and associated plaque may lead to an increased risk of dental caries. Patients should therefore be instructed to alternate the site of application and careful attention should be paid to dental hygiene, particularly in those areas where the tablet is applied. In conditions where xerostomia (dry mouth) may occur e.g. during concomitant medication with drugs having anticholinergic effects, patients should be instructed to moisten the buccal mucosa with the tongue or with a little water, prior to insertion of Suscard.

*Use in pregnancy and lactation:* There is no information on the safety of nitrates in pregnancy and lactation; nitrates should not be administered to pregnant women and nursing mothers unless considered essential by the physician.

*Side-effects:* Side-effects are predominantly headache, dizziness, facial flushing and postural hypotension. In the unlikely event of severe side-effects, the tablet may simply be removed from the mouth.

*Overdosage:* Toxic effects of glyceryl trinitrate include vomiting, restlessness, cyanosis, methaemoglobinaemia and syncope. Overdosage (i.e. if large numbers of tablets have been swallowed) should be treated with gastric aspiration and lavage, plus attention to respiratory and circulatory symptoms.

**Pharmaceutical precautions** Store at room temperature.

**Legal category** P

**Package quantities** Blister strips of 10 tablets in packs of 100 tablets (OP).

**Further information** Nil.

**Product licence numbers**

| | |
|---|---|
| 1 mg | 0108/0067 |
| 2 mg | 0108/0069 |
| 3 mg | 0108/0073 |
| 5 mg | 0108/0071 |

## SUSTAC*

**Presentation** Pink tablets with surface speckling and 'P' in hexagon embossed on one face. Sustac is a prolonged release presentation of glyceryl trinitrate in three strengths; 2.6 mg, 6.4 mg and 10.0 mg. Other ingredients include lactose and sucrose.

**Uses** Prophylactic treatment of angina pectoris.

**Dosage and administration**

*Adults and elderly patients:* Sustac tablets must be swallowed whole and not chewed. They are not for sublingual administration. Dosage should be tailored to the requirements of the individual patient, but it is usually 1 or 2 tablets of the 2.6 mg or 6.4 mg strength taken three times daily, or 1 tablet of the 10 mg strength two or three times daily. Tablets should be taken between meals.

**Contra-indications, warnings, etc**

*Contra-indications:* As for glyceryl trinitrate. Sustac tablets should not be used in patients with marked anaemia, head trauma, cerebral haemorrhage or incipient glaucoma.

*Use in pregnancy and lactation:* There is no evidence relating to the safety of nitrates in pregnancy and lactation; nitrates should not be administered to pregnant women and nursing mothers unless considered essential by the physician.

*Side-effects:* Include facial flushing, headache, hypotension and coldness of the skin.

*Withdrawal from therapy:* As with other drugs for the treatment of angina pectoris, abrupt discontinuation of therapy may lead to an exacerbation of symptoms. When discontinuing long-term treatment, the dosage should be reduced gradually over several days and the patient carefully monitored.

*Overdosage:* In the event of accidental or deliberate overdosage toxic effects of glyceryl trinitrate include vomiting, restlessness, cyanosis, methaemoglobinaemia, tachycardia and syncope. Patients should receive gastric aspiration and lavage and be given respiratory and circulatory support. The physician should be aware that tablets in the intestine will release their content over several hours.

**Pharmaceutical precautions** Can be stored at room temperature.

**Legal category** P

**Package quantities** 2.6 mg and 6.4 mg: Containers of 90 tablets. 10 mg: Containers of 60 tablets.

**Further information** Sustac can be used in combination with reduced beta-blockade dosage to give a patient full anti-anginal support and at the same time reduce the likelihood of beta-blockade side-effects.

**Product licence numbers**

| | |
|---|---|
| 2.6 mg | 0108/5031 |
| 6.4 mg | 0108/5032 |
| 10 mg | 0108/0064 |

*Trade Mark

**Procter & Gamble Pharmaceuticals UK Ltd**
Lovett House
Lovett Road
Staines
Middlesex TW18 3AZ

*Procter&Gamble*

## ALPHADERM* CREAM

**Qualitative and quantitative composition** Alphaderm cream contains the active ingredients Hydrocortisone PhEur 1% w/w and Urea BP 10% w/w.

**Pharmaceutical form** Alphaderm is a translucent white cream containing Hydrocortisone and Urea in a specially formulated base which assists the percutaneous transportation of the active ingredients to the site of action. Due to this formulation Alphaderm acts as a moderately potent topical corticosteroid. The base is self-occlusive and fulfils the functions of both an ointment and a cream.

### Clinical particulars
*Therapeutic indications:* For the treatment of all dry ichthyotic, eczematous conditions of the skin, including atopic, infantile, chronic allergic and irritant eczema, asteatotic, hyperkeratotic and lichenified eczema, neurodermitis and prurigo.

*Posology and method of administration:* Adults and the elderly. A small amount should be applied topically to the preferably dry affected areas twice daily. In resistant lesions occlusive dressings may be used but this is usually unnecessary because of the self occlusive nature of the special base.

*Contra-indications:* Primary bacterial, viral and fungal diseases of the skin and secondarily infected eczemas or intertrigo and, in general, should not be used on weeping surfaces.

Known hypersensitivity to the cream or any of its excipients.

*Special warnings and special precautions for use:* Caution should be exercised when using in children. In infants and children, long term continuous therapy should be avoided, as adrenal suppression can occur even without occlusion. Excessive absorption may occur when applied under napkins.

Application to moist or fissured skin may cause temporary irritation.

As with corticosteroids in general, prolonged application to the face and eyelids is undesirable.

*Interactions with other medicaments and other forms of interaction:* Urea may enhance the absorption of the corticosteroid and this should be borne in mind, especially when long term treatment is contemplated.

*Pregnancy and lactation:* There is inadequate evidence for safety in human pregnancy. Topical administration of corticosteroids to pregnant animals can cause abnormalities of foetal development including cleft palate and intra-uterine growth retardation. There may, therefore, be a very small risk of such effects in the human foetus.

*Effects on ability to drive and use machines:* Alphaderm does not interfere with the ability to drive or use machines.

*Undesirable effects:* If used correctly Alphaderm is unlikely to cause side effects.

*Overdose:* Chronically, grossly excessive over-use on large areas of skin in, for example, children, could result in adrenal suppression of the hypothalamic-pituitary axis (HPA) as well as topical and systemic signs and symptoms of high corticosteroid dosage. In such cases, treatment should not stop abruptly. Adrenal insufficiency may require treatment with systemic hydrocortisone. Ingestion of a large amount of Alphaderm would be expected to result in gastro-intestinal irritation, nausea, and possibly vomiting. Symptomatic and supportive care should be given. Liberal oral administration of milk or water may be helpful.

### Pharmacological properties
*Pharmacodynamic properties:* Hydrocortisone is a naturally occurring glucocorticoid with proven anti-inflammatory and vasoconstrictive properties. Urea has been demonstrated to have hydrating, keratolytic and anti-pruritic properties. As such, urea has additional therapeutic effect in dry hyperkeratotic skin conditions.

*Pharmacokinetic properties:* Therapeutic activity of hydrocortisone depends upon the adequate penetration through the horny layer of skin. The urea in the formulation solubilises part of the hydrocortisone and has a keratolytic effect. Both these factors increase penetration of the hydrocortisone.

### Pharmaceutical particulars
*List of excipients:* White soft paraffin, maize starch, isopropyl myrisate, sycrowax HR-C, palmitic acid, sorbitan monolaurate and Arlatone G.

*Incompatibilities:* See *Interactions with other medicaments.*

*Shelf life:* Two years.

*Special precautions for storage:* Store below 25°C.

*Nature and contents of container:* Supplied in tubes of 30 g and 100 g.

*Instructions for use/handling:* A patient leaflet is provided with details of use and handling of the product.

**Marketing authorisation number** 0364/0019R.

**Date of approval/revision of SPC** June 1996.

**Legal category** POM.

## AQUADRATE* CREAM

**Presentation** Aquadrate is a white to off-white, translucent, unperfumed cream containing Urea BP 10% w/w in a specially formulated base. Because of its keratolytic action it hydrates and penetrates the epidermis. The base is self-occlusive and fulfils the functions of both an ointment and a cream.

**Uses** For the management of ichthyosis, xeroderma, hyperkeratosis and other chronic dry skin conditions.

**Dosage and administration** Aquadrate is applied topically. Wash affected areas well, rinse off all traces of soap, dry, and apply sparingly twice daily. Occlusive dressings may be used but are usually unnecessary because of the self-occlusive nature of the cream.

**Contra-indications, warnings, etc** In some instances, Aquadrate may cause local irritation and oedema when applied to sensitive skin. If the condition is aggravated or there is no improvement the doctor should be consulted.

**Pharmaceutical precautions** Store below 30°C.

**Legal category** P.

**Package quantities** Aquadrate is available in tubes of 30 g and 100 g.

**Further information** Optimum rehydration of dry skin is achieved without the use of occlusive dressings. Aquadrate does not contain lanolin and is preservative free.

**Product licence number** 0364/0018R.

## CACIT* D3

**Qualitative and quantitative composition** Cacit D3 500 mg/440 IU contains 1250 mg of calcium carbonate (equivalent to 500 mg of elemental calcium) and 440 IU of cholecalciferol (vitamin D3) per sachet of 4 g.

**Pharmaceutical form** Effervescent granules for oral solution.

### Clinical particulars
*Therapeutic indications:* For correction of vitamin D and calcium combined deficiency in elderly people. Cacit D3 may be used as an adjunct to specific therapy for osteoporosis, in patients with either established vitamin D and calcium combined deficiencies or in those patients at high risk of needing such therapeutic supplements.

*Posology and method of administration:*

*Dosage:* One or two sachets of Cacit D3 effervescent granules, 500 mg/440 IU per day.

*Method of administration:* Oral, after reconstitution.

Pour the contents of the sachet into a glass, add a large quantity of water, stir, then drink immediately the solution is obtained.

*Contra-indications:*
– hypercalcaemia, hypercalciuria.

– long-term immobilisation accompanied by hyper-calciuria and/or hypercalcaemia.
– calci-lithiasis.
– hypersensitivity to one of the ingredients.

*Special warnings and special precautions for use:* With long-term treatment it is advisable to monitor serum and urinary calcium levels and kidney function, and reduce or interrupt treatment temporarily if urinary calcium exceeds 7.5 mmol/24 hours (300 mg/24 hours).

The product should be used with caution in patients with renal insufficiency and the effects on calcium and phosphate homeostasis should be monitored.

In the case of combined treatment with digitalis, bisphosphonate, sodium fluoride, thiazide diuretics, tetracyclines, see *Interactions with other medicines.*

Allowances should be made for vitamin D/calcium supplements from other sources. Additional administration of vitamin D or calcium should be carried out under strict medical supervision, with weekly monitoring of serum and urinary calcium.

The product should be prescribed with caution in patients with sarcoidosis because of possible increased metabolism of vitamin D to its active form. These patients should be monitored for serum and urinary calcium.

*Interactions with other medicaments and other forms of interaction:* The effects of digitalis and other cardiac glycosides may be accentuated with the oral administration of calcium combined with vitamin D (increases the toxicity of digitalis and therefore the risk of dysrythmia). Strict medical supervision, and if necessary, monitoring ECG and calcaemia are necessary.

In case of concomitant treatment with a bisphosphonate or with sodium fluoride, it is advisable to allow a minimum period of two hours before taking the calcium (risk of reduction of the gastrointestinal absorption of bisphosphonate and sodium fluoride).

Thiazide diuretics increase the renal absorption of calcium, so the risk of hypercalcaemia should be considered. Strict medical supervision of calcaemia is recommended.

Concomitant treatment with phenytoin or barbiturates can decrease the effect of vitamin D because of metabolic inactivation.

Concomitant use of a glucocorticosteroid can decrease the effect of vitamin D.

Calcium salts reduce the absorption of tetracyclines. It is advisable to delay taking Cacit D3 by at least three hours.

Possible interactions with food (e.g. containing oxalic acid, phosphate or phytinic acid).

*Pregnancy and lactation:* The product may be used during pregnancy and lactation. However, the daily intake should not exceed 1500 mg calcium and 600 IU vitamin D.

Overdoses of vitamin D have shown teratogenic effects in pregnant animals. In humans, overdoses of vitamin D must be avoided, as permanent hypercalcaemia can lead to physical and mental retardation, supravalvular aortic stenosis and retinopathy in the child. There are several case reports of administration of very high doses in hypoparathyroidism in the mother, where normal children were born.

Vitamin D and its metabolites pass into the breast milk.

*Effects on ability to drive vehicles and use machines:* No data are known about the effect of this product on driving capacity. However, an effect is unlikely.

*Undesirable effects:* Constipation, flatulence, nausea, gastric pain, diarrhoea. Hypercalciuria and in rare cases hypercalcaemia with long-term treatment at high doses.

*Overdose:* The most serious consequence of acute or chronic overdose would be hypercalciuria and hypercalcaemia due to vitamin D toxicity. Symptoms include nausea, vomiting, thirst, polydipsia, polyuria and constipation. Chronic overdoses can lead to vascular and organ calcifications as a result of hypercalcaemia. Treatment would consist of stopping all intake of calcium and vitamin D and rehydration.

### Pharmacological properties
*Pharmacodynamic properties:* Vitamin D corrects an

insufficient intake of vitamin D and increases intestinal absorption of calcium. The optimal amount of vitamin D in the elderly is 500–1000 IU/day. Calcium corrects an insufficient intake of calcium in the diet. The commonly accepted requirement of calcium in the elderly is 1500 mg/day.

Vitamin D and calcium correct secondary senile hyperparathyroidism.

*Pharmacokinetic properties:* During dissolution the calcium salt contained in Cacit D3 is transformed into calcium citrate. Calcium citrate is well absorbed (approximately 30% to 40% of the ingested dose). Calcium is eliminated in the urine and faeces and secreted in the sweat. Vitamin D is absorbed in the intestine and transported by protein binding in the blood to the liver (first hydroxylation) then to the kidney (second hydroxylation). The non-hydroxylated vitamin D is stored in reserve compartments such as adipose and muscle tissue. Its plasma half-life is several days; it is eliminated in the faeces and the urine.

*Preclinical safety data:* No remarkable findings.

**Pharmaceutical particulars**

*List of excipients:* Citric acid, malic acid, gluconolactone, maltodextrin, sodium cyclamate, saccharin sodium, lemon flavouring (containing: sorbitol, mannitol, D-gluconolactone, dextrin, gum arabic, lemon oil), rice starch, corn starch, potassium carbonate, α-tocopherol, vegetable oils, gelatin, and sucrose.

One sachet of Cacit D3 500 mg/440 IU contains a total of 0.22 mmol of sodium (5 mg).

*Incompatibilities:* None known.

*Shelf life:* 3 years.

*Special precautions for storage:* Store below 25°C.

*Nature and contents of container:* Paper/aluminium/polyethlene sachets packed in boxes of 30.

*Instructions for use:* Pour the contents of the sachet into a glass, add a large quantity of water, stir, then drink immediately the solution obtained.

**Marketing authorisation number**  0364/0060.

**Date of approval/revision of SPC**  January 1997.

**Legal category**  P.

## CACIT* TABLETS

**Presentation**  Cacit tablets are round, flat, white tablets with pink speckles and a distinctive orange odour and flavour. Each tablet contains 1.25 g Calcium Carbonate PhEur which, when dispersed in water, provides 500 mg calcium as calcium citrate.

**Uses**

1. Treatment of calcium deficiency states including osteomalacia, rickets and malabsorption syndromes affecting the upper gastrointestinal tract.

2. An adjunct to conventional therapy in the arrest or slowing down of bone demineralisation in osteoporosis.

3. In the arrest or slowing down of bone demineralisation in osteoporosis, where other effective treatment is contra-indicated.

4. As a therapeutic supplement during times when intake may be inadequate, particularly those associated with the increased demand of childhood, old age, pregnancy and lactation.

**Dosage and administration**  The tablets must be dissolved in a glass of water and the solution should then be drunk immediately after complete dissolution of the tablets.

*Adults and the elderly:* For the simple calcium deficiency states and malabsorption the dosage should be tailored to the individual patient's needs. In osteomalacia 1–3 g per day is recommended.

For the treatment of osteoporosis a dose of up to 1.5 g per day is normally required. In women with adequate dietary calcium intake (at least 1 g/day), 500 mg daily may be sufficient.

Up to 1.5 g of calcium per day is the recommended dosage for therapeutic supplementation.

*Children:* For calcium deficiency states, malabsorption and rickets, the recommendation given under adult dosage should be followed.

For therapeutic supplementation a dose of up to 1 g per day is recommended.

**Contra-indications, warnings, etc**

*Contra-indications:* Hypercalcaemia (e.g. due to hyperparathyroidism, hypervitaminosis D, decalcifying tumours, severe renal failure, bone metastases), severe hypercalciuria and renal calculi.

*Precautions and warnings:* In mild hypercalciuria (exceeding 7.5 mmol/24 hours in adults or 0.12–0.15 mmol/kg/24 hours in children) or renal failure, or where there is evidence of stone formation in the urinary tract; adequate checks must be kept on urinary calcium excretion. If necessary the dosage should be reduced or calcium therapy discontinued.

*Interactions with other drugs:* Concomitant administration with vitamin D causes an increase in calcium absorption and plasma levels may continue to rise after stopping vitamin D therapy.

The effects of digoxin and other cardiac glycosides may be accentuated by calcium and toxicity may be produced, especially in combination with vitamin D.

Calcium salts reduce the absorption of some drugs, in particular tetracyclines. It is therefore recommended that administration of Cacit tablets be separated from these products by at least 3 hours.

Thiazide diuretics increase renal absorption of calcium, so the risk of hypercalcaemia should be considered.

*Side effects:* Mild gastrointestinal disturbances have occurred rarely (e.g. nausea, abdominal pain, constipation, flatulence and eructation).

*Use in pregnancy and lactation:* Calcium supplements have been in wide use for many years without apparent ill consequence.

*Overdosage:* The amount of calcium absorbed will depend on the individuals calcium status. Deliberate overdosage is unlikely with effervescent preparations and acute overdosage has not been reported. It might cause gastro-intestinal disturbance but would not be expected to cause hypercalcaemia, except in patients treated with excessive doses of vitamin D. Treatment should be aimed at lowering serum calcium levels, e.g. administration of oral phosphates.

**Pharmaceutical precautions**  Cacit tablets are hygroscopic and should be dispensed in the original container. Store in a dry place.

**Legal category**  P.

**Package quantities**  Cacit tablets 500 mg are supplied in boxes of 76 (4 tubes each containing 19 tablets).

**Further information**  Cacit tablets contain no sugar and have a low sodium content.

**Product licence number**  0364/0045.

## DANTRIUM* CAPSULES

**Presentation**  Dantrium capsules are available in two strengths, containing either 25 mg or 100 mg dantrolene sodium per capsule.

Dantrium is presented in orange/light brown capsules. The 25 mg capsule carries the monogram Dantrium 25 mg on the cap and 0149, 0030 and a single coding bar on the body. The 100 mg capsule carries the monogram Dantrium 100 mg on the cap and 0149, 0033 and triple coding bars on the body.

**Uses**

*Pharmacological properties:* Dantrium produces relaxation of contracted skeletal muscle by affecting the contractile response at a site beyond the myoneural junction. Dantrium produces a dissociation of excitation contraction coupling, probably by interfering with the release of calcium from the sarcoplasmic reticulum. The effect is seen in both fast and slow fibres but is more pronounced in the former.

*Indication:* For the treatment of chronic, severe spasticity of skeletal muscle in adults.

**Dosage and administration**  The dosage should be titrated against clinical improvement and increased until the maximum benefit compatible with the patient's neurological deficit is achieved. The lowest dose compatible with optimal response is recommended.

A recommended dosage increment scale is shown below:

*Adults and the elderly:*

| Week | Recommended dosage |
| --- | --- |
| First | One 25 mg capsule daily |
| Second | One 25 mg capsule twice daily |
| Third | Two 25 mg capsules twice daily |
| Fourth | Two 25 mg capsules three times daily |
| Fifth | Three 25 mg capsules three times daily |
| Sixth | Three 25 mg capsules four times daily |
| Seventh | One 100 mg capsule four times daily |

Each dosage level should be maintained for seven days, in order to determine the patient's response. The maximum daily dose should not exceed 400 mg.

In view of the potential for hepatotoxicity in long term use, if no observable benefit is derived from the administration of Dantrium after a total of 45 days, therapy should be discontinued.

Many patients experience side-effects such as weakness and fatigue during the first four weeks of therapy whilst they adjust to the changes in muscle tone induced by the drug. They are usually transient and mild in nature. Should it be necessary, the dosage may be reduced and then gradually increased according to the patient's tolerance.

*Children:* Contra-indicated.

**Contra-indications, warnings, etc**

*Contra-indications:* Where spasticity is utilised to sustain upright posture and balance in locomotion, or whenever spasticity is utilised to obtain or maintain increased function.

For the treatment of acute skeletal muscle spasm.

In patients with evidence of hepatic dysfunction.

Dantrium should not be administered to children.

*Precautions and warnings:* There are isolated cases of possibly significant effects of Dantrium on cardiovascular and respiratory systems and therefore Dantrium should be used with caution in patients with cardiovascular or respiratory disease.

Fatal and non fatal liver disorders of an idiosyncratic or hypersensitivity type may occur with Dantrium therapy. The reactions occur at all doses but are more frequent in patients taking over 400 mg/day. The risk of hepatic injury appears to be greater in women over 30 years old. Hence, before beginning therapy, liver function tests should be performed in all patients to establish a base-line, and exclude pre-existing liver disease. These tests should be repeated upon hospital discharge or at six weeks after starting therapy. Further tests may be carried out at the physician's discretion. Generally, if these studies reveal abnormal values, therapy should not be commenced or should be discontinued. In patients with symptoms compatible with hepatitis or where jaundice appears, Dantrium should be discontinued.

*Interactions with other drugs:* The use of Dantrium with other potentially hepatoxic drugs should be avoided. There is also some evidence that hepatic injury is more likely in patients using concomitant oestrogen.

Although the primary pharmacological effect of Dantrium is exerted directly on skeletal muscle, caution should be exercised in the concomitant administration of tranquilising agents and alcohol.

Diazepam and phenobarbitone do not affect the metabolism of Dantrium.

*Side-effects:* Those most frequently reported have been drowsiness, dizziness, weakness, general malaise, fatigue and diarrhoea. These are generally transient and mild. Other side-effects include CNS disturbance, anorexia and skin rash.

Rare reports include tachycardia, labile blood pressure, pericarditis, dyspnoea, pleural effusion, haematuria and crystalluria (unconfirmed), urinary retention and incontinence.

*Use in pregnancy and lactation:* Although teratological studies in animals have proved satisfactory, the use of Dantrium is not advised in pregnant or nursing mothers.

*Overdosage:* For acute overdosage, general supportive measures should be employed along with immediate gastric lavage. Fluids should be administered in large quantities to avert the theoretical possibility of crystalluria.

**Pharmaceutical precautions**  Store at a temperature not exceeding 30°C.

**Legal category**  POM.

**Package quantities**  Dantrium capsules 25 mg and Dantrium capsules 100 mg are supplied in containers of 100 capsules.

**Further information**  The duration and intensity of skeletal muscle relaxation in patients on Dantrium is related to the dosage and blood levels. The mean biological half-life of Dantrium is about nine hours after a 100 mg dose.

**Product licence numbers**
Dantrium capsules 25 mg    0364/0015R
Dantrium capsules 100 mg    0364/0016R

## DANTRIUM* IV

**Presentation**  Dantrium IV is available as a sterile, lyophilized orange powder which is a mixture of 20 mg dantrolene sodium, 3 g mannitol and sufficient sodium hydroxide to yield a pH of approximately 9.5 when reconstituted with 60 ml of Water for Injection PhEur.

**Uses**

*Pharmacological properties:* In isolated muscle preparations, dantrolene sodium uncouples the excitation and contraction of skeletal muscle, probably by interfering with the release of calcium from the sarcoplasmic reticulum.

In the malignant hyperthermia syndrome, evidence points to an intrinsic abnormality of muscle tissue. It has been postulated that 'triggering agents' (i.e. skeletal muscle relaxants and inhalation anaesthetics) induce a sudden rise in myoplasmic calcium, either by preventing the sarcoplasmic reticulum from accumulating calcium adequately, or by accelerating its release. This rise in myoplasmic calcium activates the acute catabolic processes involved in the malignant hyperthermia crisis.

Dantrolene sodium may prevent the increases in myoplasmic calcium and the acute catabolism within the muscle cell by interfering with the release of calcium from the sarcoplasmic reticulum to the myoplasm. Thus the physiological, metabolic and biochemical changes associated with the crisis may be reversed or attenuated.

*Indication:* For the treatment of malignant hyperthermia. It is for intravenous use only.

**Dosage and administration**  As soon as the malignant hyperthermia syndrome is recognised all anaesthetic agents should be discontinued. An initial Dantrium IV dose of 1 mg/kg should be given rapidly into the vein. It must not be mixed with other intravenous infusions. If the physiological metabolic abnormalities persist or reappear, this dose may be repeated up to a cumulative dose of 10 mg/kg. Clinical experience to date has shown that the average dose of Dantrium IV required to reverse the manifestations of malignant hyperthermia has been 2.5 mg/kg. If a relapse or recurrence occurs, Dantrium IV should be readministered at the last effective dose.

**Contra-indications, warnings, etc**
*Contra-indication:* In patients with a known hypersensitivity to dantrolene sodium.
*Precautions and warnings:* In some subjects as much as 10 mg/kg of Dantrium IV has been needed to reverse the crisis. In a 70 kg man this dose would require approximately 36 vials. Such a volume has been administered in approximately one and a half hours.

Because of the high pH of the intravenous formulation of Dantrium, care must be taken to prevent extravasation of the intravenous solution into the surrounding tissues.

In the management of malignant hyperthermia it will be necessary to discontinue the suspect triggering agents, attend to increased oxygen requirements and manage the metabolic acidosis. When necessary institute cooling, attend to urinary output and monitor for electrolyte imbalance.

*Interactions with other drugs:* The combination of therapeutic doses of intravenous dantrolene sodium and verapamil in halothane/alpha-chloralose anaesthetized swine has resulted in ventricular fibrillation and cardiovascular collapse in association with marked hyperkalaemia. Hence, the use of Dantrium IV and calcium channel blockers in combination is not recommended.

*Side-effects:* No side-effects have been attributed to Dantrium IV in patients treated with short term therapy for malignant hyperthermia.

*Use in pregnancy and lactation:* The safety of Dantrium IV in pregnant women has not been established. It should be given only when the potential benefits have been weighed against the possible risk to mother and child.

**Pharmaceutical precautions**  Each vial of Dantrium IV should be reconstituted by adding 60 ml of Water for Injection PhEur, and shaking until the solution is clear. The contents of the vial must be protected from direct light and used within six hours of reconstitution. Protect the reconstituted solutions from temperatures above 30°C and below 15°C.

**Legal category**  POM.

**Package quantities**  Dantrium IV is available in packs of twelve vials each containing 20 mg dantrolene sodium.

**Further information**  Because of the nature of the freeze-drying process used in the manufacture of Dantrium IV, the freeze-dried cake of Dantrium IV may have a mottled orange/white appearance or be in the form of loose aggregates. This is an entirely normal artefact and in no way compromises the stability of the product.

**Product licence number**  0364/0030.

# DIDRONEL* PMO

**Qualitative and quantitative composition**  A two component therapy consisting of 14 Didronel 400 mg tablets and 76 Cacit* 500 mg effervescent tablets (equivalent to 500 mg elemental calcium). Each Didronel tablet contains 400 mg of Etidronate Disodium USP. Each Cacit 500 mg effervescent tablet contains 1250 mg of Calcium Carbonate, PhEur, which when dispersed in water provides 500 mg of elemental calcium as calcium citrate.

**Pharmaceutical form**  Each Didronel 400 mg tablet is white, capsule-shaped and marked with 'NE' on one face and '406' on the other. The Cacit 500 mg effervescent tablet is round, flat, white with pink speckles and has a distinctive orange flavour.

**Clinical particulars**
*Therapeutic indications:* Treatment of osteoporosis, and prevention of bone loss in postmenopausal women considered at risk of developing osteoporosis. Didronel PMO is particularly indicated in patients who are unable or unwilling to take oestrogen replacement therapy. Didronel PMO is also indicated for the prevention and treatment of corticosteroid-induced osteoporosis.

*Posology and method of administration:* Didronel PMO therapy is a long-term cyclical regimen administered in 90-day cycles. Each cycle consists of Didronel 400 mg tablets for the first 14 days, followed by Cacit 500 mg tablets for the remaining 76 days.

The majority of patients have been treated for 3 years, with a small number of patients treated for up to 7 years, with no clinical safety concerns. The optimum duration of treatment has not been established.

*Didronel 400 mg component:* One tablet should be taken each day for 14 consecutive days on an empty stomach. It is recommended that patients take the tablet with water at the midpoint of a four hour fast (i.e. two hours before and two hours after food).

*Cacit 500 mg component:* Following 14 days treatment with Didronel 400 mg tablets, one Cacit tablet should be taken on a daily basis. The Cacit tablet should be dissolved in water and drunk immediately after complete dissolution.

*Adults and elderly:* The patient should adhere to the prescribed regimen above. Modification of the dosage for the elderly is not required.

*Children:* No data exists in the use of this therapy in juvenile osteoporosis.

*Contra-indications:* Known hypersensitivity to etidronate disodium. Treatment of patients with severe renal impairment. Patients with hypercalcaemia or hypercalciuria. Not recommended in patients with clinically overt osteomalacia. Use in pregnancy and lactation.

*Special warnings and special precautions for use:* Clinicians should advise patients to adhere to the recommended treatment regimen, and compliance pack.

In long-term trials no clinical osteomalacia was observed in patients receiving cyclical etidronate. Following long-term therapy in excess of 4 years, analysis of bone biopsies showed an increased prevalence of peritrabecular fibrosis and histologically defined atypical and focal osteomalacia (not to be confused with the syndrome associated with 'cinical osteomalacia' due to vitamin D deficiency). In addition, these laboratory findings were not associated with any clinical consequences. Osteoid, which may accumulate at high doses of continuous etidronate therapy (10–20 mg/kg/day) mineralises normally after discontinuation of therapy.

Therapy should be withheld from patients with enterocolitis because of increased frequency of bowel movements.

Caution should be taken in patients with impaired renal function, or a history of renal stone formation.

Etidronate disodium does not adversely effect serum levels of parathyroid hormone or calcium.

Hyperphosphataemia has been observed in patients receiving etidronate disodium, usually in association with doses of 10–20 mg/kg/day. No adverse effects have been traced to this, and it does not constitute grounds for discontinuing therapy. It is apparently due to a drug-related increase in renal tubular reabsorption of phosphate. Serum phosphate levels generally return to normal 2–4 weeks post therapy.

*Interactions with other medicaments and other forms of interaction:* Food in the stomach or upper gastrointestinal tract, particularly materials with a high calcium content such as milk, may reduce absorption of etidronate disodium. Vitamins with mineral supplements such as iron, calcium supplements, laxatives containing magnesium, or antacids containing calcium or aluminium should not be taken within two hours of dosing etidronate disodium.

A small number of patients in clinical trials (involving more than 600 patients) received either thiazide diuretics or intravaginal oestrogen while on this treatment. The concomitant use of either of these agents did not interfere with the positive effects of the therapy on vertebral bone mass or fracture rates.

Calcium salts may reduce the absorption of some drugs, e.g. tetracyclines. It is therefore suggested that administration of Cacit tablets be separated from these products by at least three hours.

Vitamin D causes an increase in calcium absorption and plasma calcium levels may continue to rise after stopping vitamin D therapy. Concomitant administration of Cacit tablets and vitamin D should therefore be carred out with caution.

The effects of digoxin and other cardiac glycosides may be accentuated by calcium and toxicity may be produced, especially in combination with vitamin D therapy.

*Pregnancy and lactation:* Contra-indicated.

*Effects on ability to drive and use machines:* Etidronate disodium does not interfere with the ability to drive or use machines.

*Undesirable effects:*
*Gastro-intestinal:* In clinical studies of 2–3 years duration, the incidence of these events were comparable to placebo. The most common effects reported in order of incidence were diarrhoea, nausea, flatulence, dyspepsia, abdominal pain, constipation and vomiting.

*Dermatological/hypersensitivity:* Hypersensitivity reactions including angio-oedema, urticaria, rash and/or pruritus have been reported rarely.

*Nervous system:* Headache, paresthesia, peripheral neuropathy.

*Haematological:* There have been rare reports of leucopenia, agranulocytosis and pancytopenia; however a causal relationship has not been established.

*Other:* Occasional mild leg cramps have been reported in less than 5% of patients on the Didronel PMO regimen. These cramps were transient, often nocturnal and generally associated with other underlying conditions.

*Overdose:* Clinical experience of acute overdosage with etidronate is limited and unlikely with this compliance kit. Theoretically it would be manifested as the signs and symptoms of hypocalcaemia and possibly paresthesia of the fingers. Treatment would consist of gastric lavage to remove unabsorbed drug along with correction of hypocalcaemia with administration of $Ca^{2+}$ intravenously.

Prolonged continuous treatment (chronic overdose) has been reported to cause nephrotic syndrome and fractures.

**Pharmacological properties**
*Pharmacodynamic properties:* Etidronate in an intermittent cyclical regimen, works indirectly to increase bone mass. By timing delivery and withdrawal, the etidronate disodium component acts to modulate osteoclasts and reduce the mean resorption depth of the affected basic multicellular units (BMU). Calcium is an essential element which has been shown to help prevent bone loss.

Epidemiological studies have suggested that there are a number of risk factors associated with postmenopausal osteoporosis, such as early menopause, a family history of osteoporosis, prolonged exposure to corticosteroid therapy, small and thin skeletal frame and excessive cigarette smoking.

*Pharmacokinetic properties:* Within 24 hours, about one half of the absorbed dose of etidronate is excreted in the urine. The remainder is chemically absorbed on bone and is slowly eliminated. Unabsorbed drug is excreted in the faeces. Etidronate disodium is not metabolised. After oral doses of up to 1600 mg of the disodium salt, the amount of drug absorbed is approximately 3–4%. In normal subjects, plasma half life ($t\frac{1}{2}$) of etidronate, based on non-compartmental pharmacokinetics is 1–6 hours.

Calcium carbonate is converted into soluble calcium salts in the stomach under the influence of hydrochloric acid. 30–80% of orally ingested calcium is absorbed both by active transport (primarily in the upper small intestine) and by passive diffusion. The distribution of calcium in the body is subject to the mechanism of physiological regulation controlled by parathyroid hormone, calcitonin, calciferol and other hormones.

When calcium effervescent tablets are added to water, insoluble calcium carbonate is converted into calcium citrate.

*Preclinical safety data:* In long-term studies in mice and rats, there was no evidence of carcinogenicity with etidronate disodium. All *in vitro* and *in vivo* assays conducted to assess the mutagenic potential of etidronate disodium have been negative.

**Pharmaceutical particulars**
*List of excipients:* Etidronate disodium tablets contain microcrystalline cellulose, pregelatinised starch and magnesium stearate. Cacit tablets contain citric acid, sodium saccharin, sodium cyclamate, sunset yellow (E110) and orange flavouring.

*Incompatibilities:* None.

*Shelf life:* The expiry date for the compliance pack should not exceed 3 years from the date of its manufacture.

*Special precautions for storage:* Store in a dry place below 30°C. Since Cacit 500 mg tablets are hygroscopic, the stopper should be carefully replaced after use.

*Nature and contents of container:* 14 Didronel 400 mg tablets in a blister plus four polypropylene tubes, each containing 19 Cacit 500 mg tablets, all packaged in a compliance kit.

*Instructions for use/handling:* None.

**Marketing authorisation number**  0364/0051.

**Date of approval/revision of SPC** May 1997.

**Legal category** POM.

## DIDRONEL* TABLETS

**Presentation** Didronel tablets are white, rectangular tablets, marked with 'P&G' on one face and '402' on the other. Each tablet contains Etidronate Disodium USP 200 mg.

**Uses** Paget's disease of bone: Effectiveness has been demonstrated primarily in patients with polyostotic Paget's disease with symptoms of pain and with clinically significant elevations of urinary hydroxyproline and serum alkaline phosphatase. In other circumstances in which there is extensive involvement of the skull or the spine with the prospect of irreversible neurological damage, or when a weight-bearing bone may be involved, the use of Didronel may be considered.

**Dosage and administration** 5 mg/kg/day to 20 mg/kg/day as detailed below.

Didronel should be given on an empty stomach. It is recommended that patients take the therapy with water, at the midpoint of a four hour fast (i.e. two hours before and two hours after food).

*Daily dosage guide*

| Body weight | | Required daily regimen of 200 mg tablets | | |
|---|---|---|---|---|
| Kilograms | Stones | 5 mg/kg* | 10 mg/kg* | 20 mg/kg† |
| 50 | 8 | 1 | 3 | 5 |
| 60 | 9.5 | 2 | 3 | 6 |
| 70 | 11 | 2 | 4 | 7 |
| 80 | 12.5 | 2 | 4 | 8 |
| 90 | 14 | 2 | 5 | 9 |

\* Course of therapy – 6 months
† Course of therapy – 3 months

Paget's disease:

*Adults and elderly:* The recommended initial dose of Didronel for most patients is 5 mg/kg body weight/day, for a period not exceeding six months. Doses above 10 mg/kg should be reserved for use when there is an overriding requirement for suppression of increased bone turnover associated with Paget's disease or when the patient requires more prompt reduction of elevated cardiac output. Treatment with doses above 10 mg/kg/day should be approached cautiously and should not exceed three months duration. Doses in excess of 20 mg/kg/day are not recommended.

Retreatment should be undertaken only after a drug-free period of at least three months and after it is evident that reactivation of the disease has occurred and biochemical indices of the disease have become substantially re-elevated or approach pre-treatment values (approximately twice the upper limit of normal or 75% of pre-treatment value). In no case should duration of retreatment exceed the maximum duration of the initial treatment. Premature retreatment should be avoided. In clinical trials the biochemical improvements obtained during drug therapy have generally persisted for a period of three months to two years after drug withdrawal.

*Children:* Disorders of bone in children, referred to as juvenile Paget's disease, have been reported rarely. The relationship to adult Paget's disease has not been established. Didronel has not been studied in children for Paget's disease.

The recommended oral dose of Didronel for patients who have had hypercalcaemia is 20 mg/kg/day for 30 days. If serum calcium levels remain normal or at clinically acceptable levels, treatment may be extended. Treatment for more than 90 days has not been adequately studied and is not recommended.

*Children:* Safety and efficacy have not been established in children.

**Contra-indications, warnings, etc**
*Contra-indications:* None.

*Precautions and warnings:* In Pagetic patients the physician should adhere to the recommended dose regimen in order to avoid overtreatment with Didronel. The response to therapy may be of slow onset and may continue even for months after treatment when the drug has been discontinued. Dosage should not be increased prematurely nor should treatment be resumed before there is clear evidence of reactivation of the disease process. Retreatment should not be initiated until the patient has had at least a three-month drug-free interval.

It is recommended that serum phosphate, serum alkaline phosphatase and if possible urinary hydroxyproline be measured before commencing medication and at three month intervals during treatment. If after three months of medication the pretreatment levels have not been reduced by at least 25%, the patient may be relatively resistant to therapy. If the serum phosphate level is unchanged in the "resistant"

patient, consideration should be given to increasing the dose since the absorption of pharmacologically active amounts of Didronel is typically accompanied by a rise in serum phosphate. This rise usually correlates with reductions in the biochemical indices of disease activity. If after three or more months of medication elevations of serum phosphate above the upper limit of normal are not accompanied by clinical or biochemical evidence of reduced activity, resistance of the disease to the action of Didronel is probable and termination of Didronel medication should be considered. Patients in whom serum phosphate elevations are high and reductions of disease activity are low may be particularly prone to retarded mineralisation of new osteoid. In those cases where 200 mg per day (a single tablet) may be excessive, doses may be administered less frequently.

Patients with Paget's disease of bone should maintain an adequate intake of calcium and vitamin D. Patients with restricted vitamin D and calcium intake may be particularly sensitive to drugs that affect calcium homeostasis and should be closely monitored during Didronel therapy.

Etidronate disodium does not adversely effect serum levels of parathyroid hormone or calcium.

Hyperphosphataemia has been observed in patients receiving etidronate disodium, usually in association with doses of 10–20 mg/kg/day. No adverse effects have been traced to this, and it does not constitute grounds for discontinuing therapy. It is apparently due to a drug-related increase in renal tubular reabsorption of phosphate. Serum phosphate levels generally return to normal 2–4 weeks post therapy.

Didronel therapy has been withheld from patients with enterocolitis because of increased frequency of bowel movements.

Increased or recurrent bone pain at existing Pagetic sites and/or the appearance of pain at sites previously asymptomatic have been reported at a dose of 5 mg/kg/day.

Fractures are recognised as a common feature in patients with Paget's disease. There has been no evidence of increased risk at the recommended dose of 5 mg/kg/day for six months. At doses of 20 mg/kg/day in excess of three months duration, mineralisation of newly formed osteoid may be impaired and the risk of fracture may be increased. The risk of fracture may also be greater in patients with extensive and severe disease, a history of multiple fractures, and/or rapidly advancing osteolytic lesions. It is therefore recommended that the drug is discontinued when fractures occur and therapy not reinstated until the fracture healing is complete.

The incidence of osteogenic sarcoma is known to be increased in Paget's disease. Pagetic lesions, with or without therapy, may appear by X-ray to progress markedly, possibly with some loss of definition of periosteal margins. Such lesions should be evaluated carefully to differentiate these from osteogenic sarcoma.

*Interactions with other drugs:* Food in the stomach or upper portions of the small intestine, particularly materials with a high calcium content such as milk, may reduce absorption of etidronate disodium. Vitamins with mineral supplements such as iron, calcium supplements, laxatives containing magnesium, or antacids containing calcium or aluminium should not be taken within two hours of dosing etidronate disodium.

*Side-effects:*

Gastro-intestinal—The most common effects reported are diarrhoea and nausea.

Dermatological/hypersensitivity—Hypersensitivity reactions, including angio-oedema/urticaria, rash and/or pruritis, have been reported rarely.

Haematological—In patients receiving etidronate disodium, there have been rare reports of leucopenia, agranulocytosis and pancytopenia; however a causal relationship has not been established.

*Use in pregnancy and lactation:* The safety of this medicinal product for use in human pregnancy has not been established. Reproductive studies have shown skeletal abnormalities in rats. It is therefore recommended that Didronel should not be used in women of childbearing potential unless adequate contraceptive measures are taken.

It is not known whether this drug is excreted in human milk, and therefore caution should be exercised when Didronel is administered to a nursing woman.

*Overdosage:* Overdose would manifest as the signs and symptoms of hypocalcaemia. Treatment should involve cessation of therapy and correction of hypocalcaemia with administration of $Ca^{2+}$ intravenously.

**Pharmaceutical precautions** Store below a temperature of 30°C.

**Legal category** POM.

**Package quantities** 60×200 mg tablets.

**Further information** Didronel is also known as EHDP (the disodium salt of ethane-1-hydroxy-1, 1-diphosphonate).

**Product licence number** 0364/0039.

## FURADANTIN* TABLETS

**Qualitative and quantitative composition** Furadantin Tablets contain 50 mg or 100 mg Nitrofurantoin PhEur.

**Pharmaceutical form** Furadantin Tablets are yellow and pentagonal. Each tablet has a break line on one face and the tablet strength on the opposite face.

**Clinical particulars**
*Therapeutic indications:* For the treatment of and prophylaxis against acute or recurrent, uncomplicated lower urinary tract infections or pyelitis either spontaneous or following surgical procedures.

Nitrofurantoin is specifically indicated for the treatment of infections due to susceptible strains of *Escherichia coli*, enterococci, staphylococci, *Citrobacter*, *Klebsiella* and *Enterobacter*.

Most strains of *Proteus* and *Serratia* are resistant. All *Pseudomonas* strains are resistant.

Furadantin is not indicated for the treatment of associated renal cortical or perinephric abscesses.

*Posology and method of administration*
*Adults and childen over ten years of age:* The dose should be taken with food or milk (e.g. at meal times).

*Acute uncomplicated urinary tract infections:* 50 mg four times daily for seven days.

*Severe chronic recurrent infections:* 100 mg four times daily for seven days. In the event of severe nausea the dose may be reduced, but not below the adult equivalent of 200 mg/day. Should nausea persist the drug should be withdrawn.

*Long term suppressive therapy:* 50–100 mg once a day at bedtime is suggested.

*Surgical prophylaxis:* 50 mg four times daily on the day of the procedure and for the three days after.

*Elderly:* Provided there is no significant renal impairment, the dosage should be that for any normal adult.

*Children over the age of three months: Acute urinary infection:* 3 mg/kg/day in four divided doses for seven days.

*Suppressive therapy:* 1 mg/kg/day once a day.

*Contra-indications:* Patients suffering from renal dysfunction with a creatinine clearance of less than 60 ml/minute or elevated serum creatinine.

In infants under three months of age as well as pregnant patients at term (during labour and delivery) because of the theoretical possibility of haemolytic anaemia in the foetus or in the newborn infant due to immature erythrocyte enzyme systems.

Patients with known hypersensitivity to nitrofurantoin or other nitrofurans.

*Special warnings and special precautions for use:* Gastrointestinal reactions may be minimised by taking the drug with food or milk or by adjustment of dosage.

Nitrofurantoin is not effective for the treatment of parenchymal infections of unilaterally non-functioning kidney.

Nitrofurantoin should be used with caution in patients with pulmonary disease, hepatic dysfunction, neurological disorders, allergic diathesis, anaemia, diabetes mellitus, electrolyte imbalance, and vitamin B (particularly folate) deficiency.

Nitrofurantoin may cause haemolysis in patients with glucose-6-phosphate dehydrogenase deficiency (ten percent of black patients and a variable percentage of ethnic groups of Mediterranean, Near Eastern and Asian origin). Haemolysis ceases when the drug is discontinued.

Discontinue treatment with nitrofurantoin if otherwise unexplained pulmonary, hepatotoxic, haematological or neurologic syndromes occur. For long term treatment monitor patient closely for appearance of hepatic, pulmonary or neurological symptoms and other evidence of toxicity.

*Interactions with other medicaments and other forms of interaction:* Concomitant administration of magnesium trisilicate with nitrofurantoin reduces absorption.

Uricosuric drugs such as probenecid and sulphinpyrazone may inhibit renal tubular secretion of nitrofurantoin. The resulting increase in serum levels may increase toxicity. Decreased urinary levels could reduce efficacy as a urinary tract antibacterial.

Concurrent use with quinolones is not recommended.

There may be decreased antibacterial activity for nitrofurantoin in the presence of carbonic anhydrase inhibitors and urine alkalinising agents.

*Pregnancy and lactation:* Animal studies with nitrofurantoin have shown no teratogenic effects. Nitrofurantoin has been in extensive clinical use since 1952 and its suitability in human pregnancy has been well documented.

Nitrofurantoin is however contraindicated in infants under three months of age and in pregnant women during *labour and delivery*, because of the possible risk of haemolysis of the infants immature red cells.

*Effects on ability to drive and use machines:* Furadantin does not interfere with the ability to drive or use machines.

*Undesirable effects*

*Respiratory:* If the following reactions occur the drug should be discontinued.

Acute pulmonary reactions usually occur within the first week of treatment and are reversible with cessation of therapy.

Subacute reactions may take several months to resolve once the drug has been stopped.

Chronic pulmonary reactions occur rarely in patients who have received continuous therapy for six months or longer and are more common in elderly patients. Changes in ECG have occurred, associated with pulmonary reactions. Minor symptoms such as fever, chills, cough and dyspnoea may be significant. Collapse and cyanosis have seldom been reported. The severity of chronic pulmonary reactions and their degree of resolution appear to be related to the duration of therapy after the first clinical signs appear. It is important to recognise symptoms as early as possible. Pulmonary function may be impaired permanently, even after cessation of therapy.

*Hepatic:* Hepatic reactions including cholestatic jaundice and chronic active hepatitis occur rarely. Fatalities have been reported. Cholestatic jaundice is generally associated with short-term therapy (usually up to two weeks). Chronic active hepatitis, occasionally leading to hepatic necrosis is generally associated with long-term therapy (usually after six months). The onset may be insidious. Treatment should be stopped at the first sign of hepatotoxicity.

*Neurological:* Peripheral neuropathy (including optical neuritis) with symptoms of sensory as well as motor involvement, which may become severe or irreversible, has been reported infrequently. Less frequent reactions of unknown causal relationship are depression, euphoria, confusion, psychotic reactions, nystagmus, vertigo, dizziness, asthenia, headache and drowsiness. Treatment should be stopped at the first sign of neurological involvement.

*Gastrointestinal:* Nausea and anorexia have been reported. Emesis, abdominal pain and diarrhoea are less common gastrointestinal reactions.

*Hypersensitivity:* Exfoliative dermatitis and erythema multiforme (including Stevens-Johnson syndrome) have been reported rarely.

Allergic skin reactions manifesting as angioneurotic oedema, maculopapular, erythematous or eczematous eruptions, urticaria, rash, and pruritis have occurred. Lupus-like syndrome associated with pulmonary reaction to nitrofurantoin has been reported.

Other hypersensitivity reactions include anaphylaxis, sialadenitis, pancreatitis, drug fever, and arthralgia.

*Haematological:* Agranulocytosis, leucopenia, granulocytopenia, haemolytic anaemia, thrombocytopenia, glucose-6-phosphate dehydrogenase deficiency anaemia, megaloblastic anaemia and eosinophilia have occurred. Cessation of therapy has generally returned the blood picture to normal. Aplastic anaemia has been reported rarely.

*Other:* Transient alopecia and benign intercranial hypertension.

Superinfections by fungi or resistant organisms such as *Pseudomonas* may occur. However, these are limited to the genito-urinary tract.

*Overdose:* Symptoms and signs of overdosage include gastric irritation, nausea and vomiting. There is no known specific antidote. Nitrofurantoin can be haemodialysed. Standard treatment is by induction of emesis or by gastric lavage in cases of recent ingestion. Monitoring of full blood count, liver function tests and pulmonary function, are recommended. A high fluid intake should be maintained to promote urinary excretion of the drug.

**Pharmacological properties**

*Pharmacodynamic properties:* Nitrofurantoin is a broad spectrum antibacterial agent, active against the majority of urinary tract pathogens. The mechanism of action of nitrofurantoin is based on reduction to reactive intermediates. These inhibit enzymes involved in energy metablism, such as in the Krebs cycle, interfering with the energy supply for normal growth and maintenance of bacteria. They also bind to bacterial ribosomal proteins at different sites, resulting in disruption of bacterial protein synthesis. Transferable resistance to nitrofurantoin is a rare phenomenon. There is no cross resistance to antibiotics and sulphonamides.

*Pharmacokinetic properties:* Nitrofurantoin is reaidly absorbed in the upper gastrointestinal tract. Intake with food or milk increases absorption. Nitrofurantoin is highly soluble in urine but plasma concentrations are low with peak levels usually less than 1 mcg/ml.

Nitrofurantoin is loosely bound to plasma albumin (60–70%). The molecule is readily distributed into intra and extracellular compartments. However, substantial tissue concentrations are not expected since the drug is rapidly excreted and readily degraded by tissue enzymes. The drug crosses the placenta in small amounts.

The elimination half life in blood or plasma after IV injection is about 20 minutes; and after oral administration of macrocrystals, less than 60 minutes. Following a single dose of nitrofurantoin about 25% is found unchanged in the urine over 24 hours.

**Pharmaceutical particulars**

*List of excipients:* Furadantin Tablets contain lactose, maize starch, talc, alginic acid and magnesium stearate.

*Incompatibilities:* None known.

*Shelf life:* The expiry date for the tablets should not exceed 3 years from the date of manufacture.

*Special precautions for storage:* The tablets should be dispensed in light-proof and preferably moisture-resistant containers. Storage temperatures must not exeed 30°C.

*Nature and contents of container:* Furadantin tablets are supplied in packs of 100 and in polypropylene containers with polythene pilfer-proof caps.

*Instructions for use/handling:* Used as directed by physician.

**Marketing authorisation numbers**

| | |
|---|---|
| 50 mg tablets | 0364/0008R |
| 100 mg tablets | 0364/0009R |

**Date of approval/revision of SPC** September 1995.

**Legal category** POM.

## MACROBID* CAPSULES

**Presentation** Macrobid is a modified release, hard gelatin capsule containing the equivalent of 100 mg of Nitrofurantoin PhEur in the form of nitrofurantoin macrocrystals and nitrofurantoin monohydrate. The 100 mg capsule has an opaque blue cap and opaque yellow body and bears the monogram 'Eaton BID'.

**Uses** For the treatment of acute or recurrent, uncomplicated lower urinary tract infections and pyelitis; and genito-urinary surgical prophylaxis.

Nitrofurantoin is specifically indicated for the treatment of infections when due to susceptible strains of *Escherichia coli*, enterococci, staphylococci, Citrobacter, Klebsiella and Enterobacter.

Most strains of Proteus and Serratia are resistant. All Pseudomonas strains are resistant.

Macrobid is not indicated for the treatment of associated renal cortical or perinephric abscesses.

**Dosage and administration**

*Adults and children over 12 years old:* The dose should be taken with food or milk (e.g. at meal times).

Acute or recurrent uncomplicated urinary tract infections and pyelitis – 100 mg twice daily for 7 days.

Surgical prophylaxis – 100 mg twice daily on the day of the procedure and three days thereafter.

*Elderly patients:* Provided there is no significant renal impairment, the dosage should be that for any normal adult.

*Children under 12 years old:* Macrobid is a fixed dosage and because of this is unsuitable for children under 12 years old. For children under 12 years old, consideration should be given to the use of Furadantin Suspension.

**Contra-indications, warnings, etc**

*Contra-indications:* Patients suffering from renal dysfunction with a creatinine clearance of less than 60 ml/ minute or elevated serum creatinine. In infants under three months of age as well as pregnant patients at term (during labour and delivery) because of the theoretical possibility of haemolytic anaemia in the foetus or in the newborn infant due to immature erythrocyte enzyme systems.

Patients with known hypersensitivity to nitrofurantoin or other nitrofurans.

*Precautions and warnings:* Gastrointestinal reactions may be minimised by taking the drug with food or milk or by adjustment of dosage.

Nitrofurantoin is not effective for the treatment of parenchymal infections of unilaterally non-functioning kidney. Nitrofurantoin should be used with caution in patients with pulmonary disease, hepatic dysfunction, neurological disorders, allergic diathesis, anaemia, diabetes mellitus, electrolyte imbalance, and vitamin B (particularly folate) deficiency. Nitrofurantoin may cause haemolysis in patients with glucose-6-phosphate dehydrogenase deficiency (ten percent of black patients and a variable percentage of ethnic groups of Mediterranean, Near Eastern and Asian origin). Haemolysis ceases when the drug is discontinued.

Discontinue treatment with nitrofurantoin if otherwise unexplained pulmonary, hepatotoxic, haematological or neurologic syndromes occur. For long term treatment monitor patient closely for appearance of hepatic, pulmonary or neurological symptoms and other evidence of toxicity.

*Interactions with other drugs:* Concomitant administration of magnesium trisilicate with nitrofurantoin reduces absorption.

Uricosuric drugs such as probenecid and sulphinpyrazone may inhibit renal tubular secretion of nitrofurantoin. The resulting increase in serum levels may increase toxicity. Decreased urinary levels could lessen its efficacy as a urinary tract antibacterial.

Concurrent use with quinolones is not recommended.

There may be decreased antibacterial activity for nitrofurantoin in the presence of carbonic anhydrase inhibitors and urine alkalinising agents.

*Side-effects:* Respiratory – If the following reactions occur the drug should be discontinued. Acute pulmonary reactions usually occur within the first week of treatment and are reversible with cessation of therapy. Subacute reactions may take several months to resolve once the drug has been stopped.

Chronic pulmonary reactions occur rarely in patients who have received continuous therapy for six months or longer and are more common in elderly patients. Changes in ECG have occurred, associated with pulmonary reactions. Minor symptoms such as fever, chills, cough and dyspnoea may be significant. Collapse and cyanosis have seldom been reported. The severity of chronic pulmonary reactions and their degree of resolution appear to be related to the duration of therapy after the first clinical signs appear. It is important to recognise symptoms as early as possible. Pulmonary function may be impaired permanently, even after cessation of therapy.

Hepatic—Hepatic reactions including cholestatic jaundice and chronic active hepatitis occur rarely. Fatalities have been reported. Cholestatic jaundice is generally associated with short-term therapy (usually up to two weeks). Chronic active hepatitis, occasionally leading to hepatic necrosis is generally associated with long-term therapy (usually after six months). The onset may be insidious. Treatment should be stopped at the first sign of hepatotoxicity.

Neurological—Peripheral neuropathy (including optical neuritis) with symptoms of sensory as well as motor involvement, which may become severe or irreversible, has been reported infrequently. Less frequent reactions of unknown causal relationship are depression, euphoria, confusion, psychotic reactions, nystagmus, vertigo, dizziness, asthenia, headache and drowsiness. Treatment should be stopped at the first sign of neurological involvement.

Gastrointestinal—Nausea and anorexia have been reported. Emesis, abdominal pain and diarrhoea are less common gastrointestinal reactions.

Hypersensitivity—Exfoliative dermatitis and erythema multiforme (including Stevens-Johnson syndrome) have been reported rarely.

Allergic skin rections manifesting as angioneurotic oedema, maculopapular, erythematous or eczematous eruptions, urticaria, rash, and pruritus have occurred. Lupus-like syndrome associated with pulmonary reaction to nitrofurantoin has been reported.

Other hypersensitivity reactions include anaphylaxis, sialadenitis, pancreatitis, drug fever, and arthralgia.

Haematological—Agranulocytosis, leucopenia, granulocytopenia, haemolytic anaemia, thrombocytopenia, glucose-6-phosphate dehydrogenase deficiency anaemia, megaloblastic anaemia and eosinophilia have occurred. Cessation of therapy has generally returned the blood picture to normal. Aplastic anaemia has been reported rarely.

Other—Transient alopecia and benign intercranial hypertension.

Superinfections by fungi or resistant organisms such as Pseudomonas may occur. However, these are limited to the genito-urinary tract.

*Use in pregnancy and lactation:* Animal studies with nitrofurantoin have shown no teratogenic effects. Nitrofurantoin has been in extensive clinical use since 1952 and its suitability in human pregnancy has been well documented. Nitrofurantoin is however contraindicated in infants under three months of age and in pregnant women during labour and delivery, because of the possible risk of haemolysis of the infants immature red cells.

*Overdosage:* Symptoms and signs of overdosage include gastric irritation, nausea and vomiting. There is no known specific antidote. Nitrofurantoin can be haemodialysed. Standard treatment is by induction of emesis or by gastric lavage in cases of recent ingestion. Monitoring of full blood count, liver function tests and pulmonary function, are recommended. A high fluid intake should be maintained to promote urinary excretion of the drug.

**Pharmaceutical precautions** Storage temperature should not exceed 30°C.

**Legal category** POM.

**Package quantities** Blister packs containing 14 capsules.

**Further information** The urine of patients receiving Macrobid may be coloured a dark yellow or brown. This results from the presence of drug and/or metabolite(s) and is quite harmless. Macrobid can interfere with certain laboratory tests. False positive or spuriously high readings may be produced with urine glucose tests utilising the copper sulphate reduction method, e.g. Benedict's reagent, Clinitest (Ames). However, there is no interference with the Clinistix test.

**Product licence number** 0364/0055.

## MACRODANTIN* CAPSULES

**Presentation** Macrodantin is presented in hard gelatin capsules containing 50 mg or 100 mg Nitrofurantoin PhEur in macrocrystalline form.

The 50 mg capsule has an opaque yellow cap and opaque white body marked 'Eaton 008'.

The 100 mg capsule has an opaque yellow cap and body marked 'Eaton 009'.

**Uses** For the treatment of and prophylaxis against acute or recurrent, uncomplicated lower urinary tract infections or pyelitis either spontaneous or following surgical procedures.

Nitrofurantoin is specifically indicated for the treatment of infections when due to susceptible strains of *Escherichia coli*, enterococci, staphylococci, *Citrobacter*, *Klebsiella* and *Enterobacter*.

Most strains of *Proteus* and *Serratia* are resistant. All *Pseudomonas* strains are resistant.

Macrodantin is not indicated for the treatment of associated renal cortical or perinephric abscesses.

**Dosage and administration**

*Adults and children over ten years of age:* The dose should be taken with food or milk (e.g. at meal times).

*Acute uncomplicated urinary tract infections:* 50 mg four times daily for 7 days.

*Severe chronic recurrent infections:* 100 mg four times daily for 7 days. In the event of severe nausea the dose may be reduced, but not below the adult equivalent of 200 mg/day. Should nausea persist the drug should be withdrawn.

*Long-term suppressive therapy:* 50–100 mg once a day at bedtime is suggested.

*Surgical prophylaxis:* 50 mg four times daily on the day of the procedure and for 3 days after.

*Elderly:* Provided there is no significant renal impairment, the dosage should be that for any normal adult.

*Children over the age of three months:*

*Acute urinary tract infections:* 3 mg/kg/day in four divided doses for seven days.

*Suppressive therapy:* 1 mg/kg/day once a day.

**Contra-indications, warnings, etc**

*Contra-indications:* Patients suffering from renal dysfunction with a creatinine clearance of less than 60 ml/minute or elevated serum creatinine.

In infants under three months of age as well as pregnant patients at term (during labour and delivery) because of the theoretical possibility of haemolytic anaemia in the foetus or in the newborn infant due to immature erythrocyte enzyme systems.

Patients with known hypersensitivity to nitrofurantoin or other nitrofurans.

*Precautions and warnings:* Gastrointestinal reactions may be minimised by taking the drug with food or milk or by adjustment of dosage.

Nitrofurantoin is not effective for the treatment of parenchymal infections of unilaterally non-functioning kidney.

Nitrofurantoin should be used with caution in patients with pulmonary disease, hepatic dysfunction, neurological disorders, allergic diathesis, anaemia, diabetes mellitus, electrolyte imbalance, and vitamin B (particularly folate) deficiency.

Nitrofurantoin may cause haemolysis in patients with glucose-6-phosphate dehydrogenase deficiency (ten percent of black patients and a variable percentage of ethnic groups of Mediterranean, Near Eastern and Asian origin). Haemolysis ceases when the drug is discontinued.

Discontinue treatment with nitrofurantoin if otherwise unexplained pulmonary, hepatotoxic, haematological or neurologic syndromes occur. For long term treatment monitor patient closely for appearance of hepatic, pulmonary or neurological symptoms and other evidence of toxicity.

*Interactions with other drugs:* Concomitant administration of magnesium trisilicate with nitrofurantoin reduces absorption.

Uricosuric drugs such as probenecid and sulphinpyrazone may inhibit renal tubular secretion of nitrofurantoin. The resulting increase in serum levels may increase toxicity. Decreased urinary levels could reduce efficacy as a urinary tract antibacterial.

Concurrent use with quinolones is not recommended.

There may be decreased antibacterial activity for nitrofurantoin in the presence of carbonic anhydrase inhibitors and urine alkalinising agents.

*Side-effects:*

Respiratory—If the following reactions occur the drug should be discontinued.

Acute pulmonary reactions usually occur within the first week of treatment and are reversible with cessation of therapy.

Subacute reactions may take several months to resolve once the drug has been stopped.

Chronic pulmonary reactions occur rarely in patients who have received continuous therapy for six months or longer and are more common in elderly patients. Changes in ECG have occurred associated with pulmonary reactions. Minor symptoms such as fever, chills, cough and dyspnoea may be significant. Collapse and cyanosis have seldom been reported. The severity of chronic pulmonary reactions and their degree of resolution appear to be related to the duration of therapy after the first clinical signs appear. It is important to recognise symptoms as early as possible. Pulmonary function may be impaired permanently, even after cessation of therapy.

Hepatic—Hepatic reactions including cholestatic jaundice and chronic active hepatitis occur rarely. Fatalities have been reported. Cholestatic jaundice is generally associated with short-term therapy (usually up to two weeks). Chronic active hepatitis, occasionally leading to hepatic necrosis, is generally associated with long-term therapy (usually after six months). The onset may be insidious. Treatment should be stopped at the first sign of hepatoxicity.

Neurological—Peripheral neuropathy (including optical neuritis) with symptoms of sensory as well as motor involvement, which may become severe or irreversible, has been reported infrequently. Less frequent reactions of unknown causal relationship are depression, euphoria, confusion, psychotic reactions, nystagmus, vertigo, dizziness, asthenia, headache and drowsiness. Treatment should be stopped at the first sign of neurological involvement.

Gastrointestinal—Nausea and anorexia have been reported. Emesis, abdominal pain and diarrhoea are less common gastrointestinal reactions.

Hypersensitivity—Exfoliative dermatitis and erythema multiforme (including Stevens-Johnson syndrome) have been reported rarely.

Allergic skin reactions manifesting as angioneurotic oedema, maculopapular, erythematous or eczematous eruptions, urticaria, rash, and pruritis have occurred. Lupus-like syndrome associated with pulmonary reaction to nitrofurantoin has been reported.

Other hypersensitivity reactions include anaphylaxis, sialadenitis, pancreatitis, drug fever, and arthralgia.

Haematological—Agranulocytosis, leucopenia, granulocytopenia, haemolytic anaemia, thrombocytopenia, glucose-6-phosphate dehydrogenase deficiency anaemia, megaloblastic anaemia and eosinophilia have occurred. Cessation of therapy has generally returned the blood picture to normal. Aplastic anaemia has been reported rarely.

Other—Transient alopecia and benign intercranial hypertension.

Superinfections by fungi or resistant organisms such as Pseudomonas may occur. However, these are limited to the genito-urinary tract.

*Use in pregnancy and lactation:* Animal studies with nitrofurantoin have shown no teratogenic effects. Nitrofurantoin has been in extensive clinical use since 1952 and its suitability in human pregnancy has been well documented. Nitrofurantoin is however contraindicated in infants under three months of age and in pregnant women during labour and delivery, because of the possible risk of haemolysis of the infants immature red cells.

*Overdosage:* Symptoms and signs of overdosage include gastric irritation, nausea and vomiting. There is no known specific antidote. Nitrofurantoin can be haemodialysed. Standard treatment is by induction of emesis or by gastric lavage in cases of recent ingestion. Monitoring of full blood count, liver function tests and pulmonary function, are recommended. A high fluid intake should be maintained to promote urinary excretion of the drug.

**Pharmaceutical precautions** Macrodantin capsules 100 mg should be dispensed in light-proof and preferably moisture-resistant containers. Storage temperatures for both 50 mg and 100 mg capsules must not exceed 30°C.

**Legal category** POM.

**Package quantities** Macrodantin capsules 100 mg are supplied in a blister pack of 100. Macrodantin capsules 50 mg are supplied in a blister pack of 30.

**Further information** The nitrofurantoin macrocrystals of Macrodantin are specially formulated. The crystal size controls the rate of absorption and thus reduces the incidence of nausea. Clinical and animal studies indicate that Macrodantin therapy decreases the likelihood of nausea in patients who might experience these symptoms on nitrofurantoin therapy.

The urine of patients receiving Macrodantin may be coloured a dark yellow or brown. This results from the presence of drug and/or metabolite(s) and is quite harmless. Macrodantin can interfere with certain laboratory tests. False positive or spuriously high readings may be produced with urine glucose tests utilising the copper sulphate reduction method, e.g. Benedict's reagent, Clinitest (Ames). However, there is no interference with the Clinistix test.

**Product licence numbers**

| | |
|---|---|
| Macrodantin Capsules 50 mg | 0364/0005R |
| Macrodantin Capsules 100 mg | 0364/0006R |

## REGULAN* (LEMON/LIME FLAVOUR)
## REGULAN* (ORANGE FLAVOUR)

**Presentation** Premeasured, single-dose sachets containing a lemon/lime or orange flavoured beige fine ground powder. Active ingredient – 3.4 g Ispaghula Husk BP.

**Uses**

*Pharmacological properties:* Regulan acts as a bulking agent which both retains water and promotes microbial growth in the colon, so increasing faecal mass and hence reducing transit time.

*Indication:* For the treatment of constipation and for patients requiring a high fibre regimen (such as IBS and diverticular disease).

**Dosage and administration** The measured dosage should be poured into a glass and 150 ml ($\frac{1}{4}$ pint) of cool water, milk, fruit juice or other liquid added, stirred, and taken immediately. Additional liquid may be taken if required. Adequate fluid intake should be maintained.

*Adults and children over 12 years:* Usual dosage is the entire contents of one sachet taken one to three times daily.

*Elderly:* No alteration in dosage necessary. See *Precautions.*

*Children 6–12 years:* A reduced dosage based upon age and size of the child should be given. $\frac{1}{2}$–1 level 5 ml spoonful one to three times daily.

**Contra-indications, warnings, etc**

*Contra-indications:* Not to be given to patients with intestinal obstruction, faecal impaction, colonic atony, or hypersensitivity to ispaghula.

*Precautions and warnings:* Regulan should always be taken as a liquid suspension and should be drunk immediately after mixing. The last dose should not be taken immediately before going to bed since impaired or reduced gastric motility may impair the intestinal passage and then cause partial obstruction.

May cause allergic reactions in people sensitive to inhaled or ingested ispaghula powder.

It may be advisable to supervise treatment in the elderly or debilitated and patients with intestinal narrowing or decreased motility, as rare instances of gastrointestinal obstruction have been reported with mucilloid preparations when taken with insufficient liquid, contrary to the administration instructions.

Contains 3 mg of phenylalanine and this should be considered by phenylketonuric patients.

*Side-effects:* Allergy, gastrointestinal obstruction or impaction have been reported with hydrophilic mucilloid preparations.

*Use in pregnancy and lactation:* Controlled studies in pregnant and lactating women are not available, but the product has been in wide use for many years without apparent ill consequence and animal studies have shown no hazard. Ispaghula is not thought to be absorbed nor is it thought to enter breast milk. Nevertheless the benefits of therapy should be weighed against the possible risk if used during pregnancy and lactation.

*Overdosage:* No instances of true overdosage have been reported. If overdosage should occur there is no specific treatment and symptomatic measures should be employed.

**Pharmaceutical precautions**  Store in a dry place below 30°C.

**Legal category**  GSL.

**Package quantities**  Boxes of 30 sachets.

**Further information**  Regulan is gluten free and sugar free. Each sachet contains 0.23 mmol of sodium.

**Product licence numbers**
Lemon/Lime Flavour Regulan    0129/0113
Orange Flavour Regulan    0129/0114
*Trade Mark

# Quinoderm Limited
## Manchester Road
## Oldham OL8 4PB

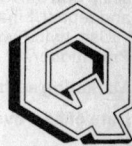

## CEANEL* CONCENTRATE

**Presentation**
*Active constituents:*

| | |
|---|---|
| Phenylethyl Alcohol USP | 7.5% |
| Cetrimide BP | 10% |
| Undecenoic Acid BP | 1% |

*Other constituents:* Lauric diethanolamide, diethanolamine, poly oxy propylene stearyl ether.

*Appearance:* Ceanel Concentrate is a clear, viscous, golden yellow coloured liquid.

**Uses** *Main pharmacological action:* Cetrimide is particularly active against Gram-positive organisms. This feature combined with the bactericidal action of phenylethyl alcohol and the fungicidal properties of undecenoic acid makes Ceanel Concentrate particularly effective in the treatment of dermatological conditions. Ceanel Concentrate is effective in removing debris and scale in seborrhoea capitis, and psoriasis of the scalp.

*Indications:* As an adjunct in the management of psoriasis of the scalp, seborrhoeic dermatitis, dandruff, psoriasis of the trunk and limbs.

**Dosage and administration**
*Adults, children and the elderly: Scalp conditions:* Wet the scalp and hair with warm water. Protect the eyes with a towel to avoid discomfort. Apply ½–1 teaspoonful of Ceanel to the wetted scalp. Then apply a small amount of water and work up into a lather. Rinse and repeat. Finally rinse the hair and scalp *thoroughly.* Use three times in the first week and twice weekly thereafter.

*Other areas of the body:* Wet the area to be treated with warm water; apply sufficient Ceanel Concentrate by gentle massage to cover the wetted area. Allow to remain in contact for two minutes. Remove the Ceanel by thorough rinsing with warm water. Use as required.

**Contra-indications, warnings, etc** *Precaution:* The eyes should be protected during treatment. A simple way to do this is with a towel.

*Overdosage:* Ceanel Concentrate is for external use only. Following accidental ingestion, nausea and vomiting may occur as well as respiratory problems and hypotension. Treatment is supportive and symptomatic avoiding gastric lavage.

*Warning:* There is inadequate evidence of safety in human pregnancy, but it has been in wide use for many years without apparent ill consequence. As with other medicaments it may be used during pregnancy if the anticipated benefits outweigh the risks. No problems are anticipated during lactation.

**Pharmaceutical precautions** *Storage:* No special precaution required.

*Diluents:* Ceanel Concentrate is easily removed by warm water.

**Legal category** P.

**Package quantities** Available in packs of 50 ml, 150 ml and 500 ml.

**Further information** Nil.

**Product licence number** 0291/5002R.


## GELCOSAL*

**Qualitative and quantitative composition**

| | |
|---|---|
| Strong Coal Tar Solution BPC | 2.0% |
| Tar BP (Pine Tar) | 5.0% |
| Salicylic Acid BP | 2.0% |

**Pharmaceutical form** Gelcosal is a light-brown thixotropic gel which spreads easily and cleanly on the skin. It is non-sticky, non-greasy and being water-miscible is easily removed and does not permanently stain the skin.

**Clincial particulars**
*Therapeutic indications:* Gelcosal is indicated in the treatment of psoriasis in the chronic scaling phase and the treatment of dermatitis in the chronic scaling phase.

*Posology and method of administration:*
Route of administration: For topical use only.
*Adults, children and the elderly:* By gentle massage

over all the affected area twice daily. Unless hands are being treated, rinse hands following application.

*Contra-indications:* Patients with known sensitivity or intolerance to any of the ingredients should not use Gelcosal. If sensitivity occurs or infection appears discontinue use and institute appropriate therapy.

*Special warnings and special precautions for use:*
*Precautions:* For topical use only. Contact with eyes and other mucosal surfaces should be avoided.

*Warning:* Prolonged use over large areas of topical preparations containing salicylic acid may result in symptoms of salicylism e.g. tinnitus. In view of this, extra caution should be exercised when treating children.

*Interaction with other medicaments and other forms of interaction:* None known.

*Pregnancy and lactation:* Gelcosal is not contra-indicated in pregnancy or lactation.

*Effects on ability to drive and use machines:* Not applicable.

*Undesirable effects:* None known.

*Overdose:* Not applicable. Gelcosal is for topical use only.

**Pharmacological properties** The combination of two different tars in Gelcosal provides a preparation with antipruritic, keratolytic and antiseptic properites. The combination also provides the usual therapeutic activity of tars.

Salicylic acid provides a keratolytic action.

The salicylic acid constituent of Gelcosal allows removal of scale and thus access of the tar components to the underlying diseased areas.

The base has been developed with the objective of providing a cosmetically acceptable thixotropic formulation at the same time as retaining the therapeutic efficacy of crude tar.

**Pharmaceutical particulars**
*List of excipients:* Poly oxy propylene stearyl ether, Hypromellose BP, Purified Water BP.

*Incompatibilities:* Not applicable.

*Shelf life:* Three years.

*Special precautions for storage:* Gelcosal should be stored in a cool, dry place avoiding extremes of temperature i.e. not less than 5°C and not more than 30°C.

*Nature and contents of container:* Gelcosal is packed in low density polyethylene tubes with flush fitting ribbed cap containing 50 g of product. Each tube is cartoned and contains a patient information leaflet.

*Instructions for use/handling:* By gentle massage over all the affected area twice daily. Unless hands are being treated, rinse hands thoroughly following application.

**Marketing authorisation number** 0291/0019.

**Date of approval/revision of SPC** October 1995.

**Legal category** P.


## GELCOTAR*

**Presentation**
*Active constituents:*

| | |
|---|---|
| Strong Coal Tar Solution BPC | 5% |
| Tar BP (Pine tar) | 5% |

*Other constituents:* Poly oxy propylene stearyl ether, Hypromellose BP.

*Appearance:* Gelcotar is a light-brown thixotropic gel which spreads easily and cleanly on the skin. It is non-sticky, non-greasy and being water-miscible is easily removed and does not permanently stain the skin.

**Uses** *Main pharmacological action:* The combination of two different tars in Gelcotar provides a preparation with antipruritic, keratolytic and antiseptic properties. The combination also provides the usual therapeutic activity of tars.

The base has been developed with the objective of providing a cosmetically acceptable thixotropic formulation at the same time as retaining the efficacy of crude tar.

*Indications:* Treatment of psoriasis.
Treatment of dermatitis in the chronic phase.

**Dosage and administration** *Adults and children:* By gentle massage over all the affected area twice daily.

**Contra-indications, warnings, etc**
*Contra-indications:* Known sensitivity or intolerance to any of the ingredients.

*Precautions:* For external use only. Keep away from the eyes and other mucosal surfaces.

*Overdosage:* Not applicable.

*Main side-effects/adverse reactions:* None reported.

**Pharmaceutical precautions** *Storage:* Store in a cool place.

**Legal category** P.

**Package quantities** 50 g and 500 g.

**Further information** If sensitivity occurs or infection appears discontinue use and institute appropriate therapy.

Gelcotar is water-miscible and does not permanently stain the skin.

**Product licence number** 0291/0011.


## GELCOTAR* LIQUID

**Qualitative and quantitative composition**

| | |
|---|---|
| Strong Coal Tar Solution BP | 1.25% |
| Cade Oil BPC | 0.5% |

**Pharmaceutical form** Gelcotar Liquid is a completely clear deep red/brown viscous liquid.

**Clinical particulars**
*Therapeutic indications:* Psoriasis of the scalp, seborrhoeic dermatitis and dandruff.

*Posology and method of administration:*
Route of administration: For topical use only.
Adults, children and elderly: Wet the scalp and hair with warm water. Sufficient Gelcotar Liquid should be applied to produce a generous lather. Massage the scalp and surrounding area with the fingertips. Rinse and repeat. Finally rinse the hair and scalp thoroughly.
Use twice weekly or as directed by the medical practitioner.

*Contra-indications:* Patients with known sensitivity or intolerance to strong coal tar solution or cade oil should not use Gelcotar liquid.

*Special warnings and special precautions in use:* Contact with eyes and other mucosal surfaces should be avoided. All medicines should be kept out of the reach of children. Gelcotar Liquid can be easily removed by warm water.

*Interaction with other medicaments and other forms of interaction:* None known.

*Pregnancy and lactation:* Gelcotar Liquid is not contra-indicated in pregnancy or lactation.

*Effects on ability to drive and use machines:* Not applicable.

*Undesirable effects:* None known.

*Overdose:* Not applicable. Gelcotar Liquid is for topical use only.

**Pharmacological properties** The combination of strong coal tar solution and cade oil provides a preparation with antiseptic and keratolytic properties to be used as a medicated scalp cleanser.

**Pharmaceutical particulars**
*List of excipients:* Coconut diethanolamide, Chlorocresol BP, poly ethylene mono tallowate, disodium fatty acid monoethanolamide sulpho succinate, ricinoleic propyl amido trimethyl ammonium metho sulphate, triethanolamine lauryl sulphate, lecithin, Purified Water BP.

*Incompatibilities:* Not applicable. Gelcotar Liquid is for topical use only.

*Shelf life:* 2 years.

*Special precautions for storage:* Gelcotar Liquid should be stored in a dry place avoiding extremes of temperature i.e. not less than 5°C and not more than 30°C.

*Nature and contents of container:* Gelcotar Liquid is packed in printed polyethylene bottles of 150 ml and 350 ml.

*Instructions for use/handling:* Wet the scalp and hair with warm water. Sufficient Gelcotar Liquid should be applied to produce a generous lather. Massage the scalp and surrounding area with the fingertips. Rinse and repeat. Finally rinse the hair and scalp thoroughly.

Use twice weekly or as directed by the Medical Practitioner.

**Marketing authorisation number** 0291/0018

**Date of approval/revision of SPC** October 1995.

**Legal category** GSL.

## HIOXYL* CREAM

**Qualitative and quantitative composition** Hydrogen Peroxide 1.50%

**Pharmaceutical form** Hioxyl Cream is a smooth, white, non-greasy cream with virtually no odour.

### Clinical particulars
*Therapeutic indications:* Hioxyl Cream is indicated in the treatment of leg ulcers, pressure sores, minor wounds and infections of the skin.

*Posology and method of administration:*
    *Route of administration:* For topical use only.
    *Adults, children and the elderly:* Hioxyl Cream is applied freely using a piece of lint or gauze. If necessary it may be covered with a dressing. The application is repeated as required.

*Contra-indications:* There are no known contra-indications except true hypersensitivity to the active ingredient.

*Special warnings and special precautions for use:* Care should be taken to avoid usage with other medicaments due to possible interaction negating the active ingredient. Care should be taken to avoid contact with dyed fabrics as this product may adversely affect dye fastness.

*Interaction with other medicaments and other forms of interaction:* Hydrogen peroxide is an oxidising agent and should not be used in conjunction with other topical agents which would react with an oxidising agent.

*Pregnancy and lactation:* Hioxyl Cream is not contra-indicated in pregnancy or lactation.

*Effects on ability to drive and use machines:* Not applicable. Hioxyl Cream is for topical use only.

*Undesirable effects:* Not applicable.

*Overdose:* Not applicable. Hioxyl Cream is for topical use only.

**Pharmacological properties** The antiseptic effect of hydrogen peroxide is a result of its ready release of oxygen when applied to tissues. The effect only lasts as long as oxygen is being released, and for solutions of hydrogen peroxide, this is of only short duration.

Hioxyl Cream is a unique formulation in which hydrogen peroxide has been stabilised in a soothing, easy to apply cream to give prolonged antiseptic action.

**Pharmaceutical particulars**
*List of excipients:* Lactic Acid BP, White Soft Paraffin BP, Sodium Acid Phosphate BP, Maize Starch BP, cetyl stearyl alcohol, sodium cetyl stearyl sulphate, PEG 40 castor oil, Purified Water BP.

*Incompatibilities:* Hioxyl Cream should not be used at the same time as other topical medicaments. It is an oxidising agent and other topical agents may negate the effect of the active ingredient.

*Shelf life:* 18 months.

*Special precautions for storage:* Hioxyl Cream should be stored in a cool, dry place avoiding extremes of temperature i.e. not less than 5˚C and not more than 30˚C.

*Nature and contents of container:* Hioxyl Cream is packed in low density polythene tubes of 25 g and 100 g with flush fitting cap.

*Instructions for use/handling:* For topical use only. *Adults, children and the elderly:* Hioxyl Cream is applied freely using a piece of lint or gauze. If necessary it may be covered with a dressing. The application is repeated as required.

**Marketing authorisation number** 0291/0008.

**Date of approval/revision of SPC** January 1997.

**Legal Category** P.

## HYDROMOL* CREAM

**Presentation**
*Active constituents:*

| | |
|---|---|
| Arachis (Peanut) Oil BP | 10.0% |
| Isopropyl Myristate BP | 5.0% |
| Liquid Paraffin BP | 10.0% |
| Sodium Pyrrolidone Carboxylate | 2.5% |
| Sodium Lactate | 1.0% |

*Other constituents:* Cetomacrogol Emulsifying Wax BP, myristyl myristate, Cetomacrogol 1000 BP, hydroxybenzoates (parabens), phenoxyethanol.

*Appearance:* Hydromol Cream is a soft, white, oil in water cream which can be massaged easily into the skin.

**Uses**
*Main pharmacological action:* The combination of oils in Hydromol Cream helps to lubricate and hydrate the skin. Moisture loss from the stratum corneum is reduced by the formation of an occlusive film by arachis oil and liquid paraffin on the surface of the skin. Isopropyl myristate, a fatty acid ester, is easily absorbed into the skin and helps to improve skin softness.

The combination of sodium pyrrolidone carboxylate and sodium lactate positively aids the hydration of the skin.

*Indications:* Any condition in which 'dry skin' is a feature, including all forms of dermatitis/eczema – all degrees of ichthyosis and senile pruritus.

**Dosage and administration**
*Adults and children:* Apply liberally to the affected area and massage well into the skin. Hydromol Cream may be used as often as required.

Hydromol Cream is especially beneficial when used immediately after washing or bathing, when the resultant warmth of the skin enhances absorption.

**Contra-indications, warnings, etc**
*Contra-indications:* There are no contra-indications except true hypersensitivity to any of the ingredients.

**Pharmaceutical precautions** The formulation is not designed for use as a diluent.

**Legal category** GSL.

**Package quantities** 50 g, 100 g tubes and 500 g pump dispenser.

**Further information** Hydromol Cream provides soothing, antipruritic symptomatic relief in addition to the longer term therapeutic activity outlined above.

Hydromol Cream does not contain lanolin or fragrance and may thus be used on patients sensitive to these substances.

**Product licence number** 0291/0023.

## HYDROMOL* EMOLLIENT

**Presentation**
*Active constituents:*

| | |
|---|---|
| Light Liquid Paraffin BP | 37.8% |
| Isopropyl Myristate BP | 13.0% |

*Other constituents:* C12-C14 alcohol with 3 molecules of ethylene oxide, polyol fatty acid ester, iso-octyl stearate.

*Appearance:* Hydromol Emollient is a clear colourless water-dispersible bath additive resulting in an emulsion of dispersed oils together with an homogenised film on the surface.

*Main pharmacological action:* The combination of oils used in Hydromol Emollient are deposited on the skin surface during bathing and thus reduce moisture loss, provide antipruritic action, lubricate and soften the skin.

Hydromol Emollient is particularly suitable for infant bathing. The preparations can also be used as a cleanser where soaps etc. are best avoided.

*Indications:* For the treatment of dry skin conditions such as eczema, ichthyosis and senile pruritus.

**Dosage and administration** Hydromol Emollient should always be either added to water or applied to wet skin.

*1. For use in the bath*
(a) *Adults, children and the elderly:* Add 1–3 capfuls to an 8 inch bath of water. Soak for 10–15 minutes.
(b) *Infants:* Add ½–2 capfuls to a small bath of water.

*2. For application to the skin as a sponge bath or in the shower*
    *Adults, children and the elderly:* Pour a small quantity on to a wet sponge or flannel and rub onto wet skin. Rinse and pat dry.

**Contra-indications, warnings, etc** Keep away from eyes. Take care to avoid slipping in the bath/shower.

**Pharmaceutical precautions** Nil.

**Legal category** GSL.

**Package quantities** Polyethylene bottles of 150 ml, 350 ml and 1 litre.

**Further information** In order to ensure a complete coverage of the emulsion in patients with large areas of body involvement, Hydromol Emollient should be used as a bath additive. The bath can be easily cleaned after use.

Hydromol Emollient does not contain lanolin, fragrance or preservative and may thus be used on patients sensitive to these substances.

A pump dispenser for the 1 litre bottle is available on request.

**Product licence number** 0291/0022.

## QUINOCORT* CREAM

**Qualitative and quantitative composition**

| | |
|---|---|
| Potassium Hydroxyquinoline Sulphate BP | 0.5% |
| Hydrocortisone BP | 1.0% |

**Pharmaceutical form** Quinocort Cream is a faintly yellow vanishing cream. It is intended for topical use only.

### Clinical particulars
*Therapeutic indications:* The treatment of infected eczema, intertrigo and other steroid-responsive dermatoses where anti-infective cover is appropriate.

*Posology and method of administration:*
    *Route of administration:* For topical use only.
    *Adults, children and the elderly:* By gentle massage over all the affected area two to three times daily.

*Contra-indications:* Patients with known sensitivity or intolerance to any of the ingredients.

*Special warnings and special precautions for use:* Contact with eyes and other mucosal surfaces should be avoided. Caution should be exercised when using this preparation in infants. Long term continuous topical therapy should be avoided in infants – adrenal suppression can occur even without occlusion.

*Interaction with other medicaments and other forms of interaction:* Not applicable.

*Pregnancy and lactation:* In pregnant animals administration of corticosteroids can cause abnormalities of foetal development. The relevance of this finding in human beings has not been established. However, topical steroids should not be used extensively in pregnancy i.e. in large amounts for long periods.

*Effects on ability to drive and use machines:* Not applicable.

*Undesirable effects:* Not applicable.

*Overdose:* Not applicable.

**Pharmacological properties** Hydrocortisone provides anti-inflammatory action yet is the least potent topical corticosteroid available. Potassium hydroxyquinoline sulphate provides broad spectrum antibacterial and anticandidal activity. The combination facilitates treatment of steroid-responsive dermatoses where complication by infection with bacteria or yeasts is evident suspected, or a possibility.

**Pharmaceutical particulars**
*List of excipients:* Lactic Acid BP, White Soft Paraffin BP, EDTA, Sodium Acid Phosphate BP, Maize Starch BP, cetyl stearyl alcohol, sodium cetyl stearyl sulphate, PEG 40 Castor Oil, Chlorocresol BP, Purified Water BP.

*Incompatibilities:* Not applicable.

*Shelf life:* Two years.

*Special precautions for storage:* Quinocort Cream should be stored in a cool, dry place avoiding extremes of temperature i.e. not less than 5˚C and not more than 30˚C.

*Nature and contents of container:* Quinocort Cream is available in heat sealed low density polyethylene tubes with flush fitting cap containing 30 g of product. Each tube is cartoned and contains a patient information leaflet.

*Instructions for use/handling:* For topical use only.

**Marketing authorisation number** 0291/0014.

**Date of approval/revision of SPC** May 1995.

**Legal category** POM.

## QUINODERM* CREAM

**Qualitative and quantitative composition**

| | |
|---|---|
| Benzoyl Peroxide BP | 10.0% |
| Potassium Hydroxyquinoline Sulphate BP | 0.5% |

**Pharmaceutical form** Quinoderm Cream is a creamy white astringent vanishing cream. It is intended for topical use only.

### Clinical particlars
*Therapeutic indications:* Acne vulgaris, acneform eruptions, folliculitis.

*Posology and method of administration:*
    *Route of administration:* For topical use only.
    *Adults, children and the elderly:* By gentle massage over all the affected area two or three times daily.

*Contra-indications:* Acne rosacea. Patients with known sensitivity to either of the active ingredients should not use Quinoderm Cream.

*Special warnings and special precautions for use* Contact with mouth and eyes should be avoided. Care should be taken to avoid contact with dyed fabrics as this product may adversely affect dye fastness.

In a few isolated cases, overreaction to Quinoderm Cream may occur. To minimise this possibility, select a small area of skin behind the ear, apply the cream and leave for twelve hours. If severe irritation or pronounced redness occurs, do not proceed with treatment.

*Interaction with other medicaments and other forms of interaction:* Benzoyl peroxide is an oxidising agent. Hence, Quinoderm Cream should not be used at the same time as other topical agents which would react with an oxidising agent.

*Pregnancy and lactation:* Quinoderm Cream is not contra-indicated in pregnancy or lactation.

*Effects on ability to drive and use machines:* Not applicable.

*Undesirable effects:* Not applicable.

*Overdose:* Not applicable.

**Pharmacological properties**  The combination of the mild keratolytic properties of benzoyl peroxide and the antibacterial and antifungal properties of potassium hydroxyquinoline sulphate in a specially formulated bland water-miscible base make this preparation valuable in the treatment of acne vulgaris, acneform eruptions and folliculitis.

**Pharmaceutical particulars**
*List of excipients:* Lactic Acid BP, White Soft Paraffin BP, EDTA, Sodium Acid Phosphate BP, Maize Starch BP, cetyl stearyl alcohol, sodium cetyl stearyl sulphate, PEG 40 Castor Oil, Purified Water BP.

*Incompatibilities:* Not applicable.

*Shelf life:* Three years.

*Special precautions for storage:* Quinoderm Cream should be stored in a cool, dry place avoiding extremes of temperature i.e. not less than 5°C and not more than 30°C.

*Nature and contents of container:* Quinoderm Cream is available in heat sealed low density polythene tubes with flush fitting cap containing 25 g and 50 g of product. Each tube is cartoned and contains a patient information leaflet.

*Instructions for use/handling:* For topical use only.

**Marketing authorisation number**  0291/5000R.

**Date of approval/revision of SPC**  May 1995.

**Legal category**  P.

## QUINODERM* CREAM 5

**Presentation**
*Active constituents:*
Benzoyl Peroxide BP ..... 5.0%
Potassium Hydroxyquinoline Sulphate BP ..... 0.5%
*Other constituents:* Lactic Acid BP, White Soft Paraffin BP, EDTA, Sodium Acid Phosphate BP, Maize Starch BP, cetyl stearyl alcohol, sodium cetyl stearyl sulphate, PEG 40 castor oil.

*Appearance:* Quinoderm Cream 5 is a creamy white astringent vanishing cream.

**Uses**  *Main pharmacological action:* The combination of the mild keratolytic properties of benzoyl peroxide and the antibacterial and antifungal properties of potassium hydroxyquinoline sulphate in a specially formulated bland water-miscible base make this preparation valuable in the treatment of pustular affections of the skin particularly when associated with staphylococcal infection.

*Indications:* Acne vulgaris, acneform eruptions, folliculitis.

**Dosage and administration**  *Adults, children and the elderly:* By gentle massage over all the affected area, two or three times daily.

**Contra-indications, warnings, etc**
*Contra-indications:* Quinoderm Cream 5 is contra-indicated in acne rosacea. Patients with known sensitivity to either of the active ingredients should not use Quinoderm Cream 5. Quinoderm Cream 5 is used topically.

*Precaution:* In a few isolated cases overreaction to Quinoderm Cream 5 may occur. To minimise this possibility, select a small area of skin behind the ear, apply the cream and leave for 12 hours. If severe irritation or pronounced redness occurs do not proceed.

All medicines should be kept out of the reach of children.

**Pharmaceutical precautions**  *Storage:* Quinoderm Cream 5 should be stored in a cool place, avoiding extremes of temperature.

*Diluents, etc:* Quinoderm Cream 5 can be easily removed by warm water and soap.

**Legal category**  P.

**Package quantities**  Quinoderm Cream 5 is supplied in tubes of 50 g.

**Further information**  Contact with mouth and eyes should be avoided. Care should be taken to avoid contact with dyed fabrics as this preparation may adversely affect dye fastness.

**Product licence number**  0291/0012.

## QUINODERM* LOTIO-GEL 5%

**Qualitative and quantitative composition**
Benzoyl Peroxide BP ..... 5.0%
Potassium Hydroxyquinoline Sulphate BP ..... 0.5%

**Pharmaceutical form**  Quinoderm Lotio-gel 5% is a homogeneous astringent gel formulated to give the colour and consistency of a creamy white lotion. It is intended for topical use only.

**Clinical particulars**
*Therapeutic indications:* Acne.

*Posology and method of administration:*
  *Route of administration:* For topical use only.
  *Adults, children and the elderly:* By gentle massage over all the affected area one to three times daily.

*Contra-indications:* Patients with known sensitivity to either of the active constituents should not use Quinoderm Lotio-gel 5%.

*Special warnings and special precautions for use:* Contact with mouth and eyes should be avoided. Care should be taken to avoid contact with dyed fabrics as this product may adversely affect dye fastness.

In a few isolated cases, overreaction to Quinoderm Lotio-gel 5% may occur. To minimise this possibility, select a small area of skin behind the ear, apply the cream and leave for twelve hours. If severe irritation or pronounced redness occurs, do not proceed with treatment.

*Interaction with other medicaments and other forms of interaction:* Benzoyl peroxide is an oxidising agent. Hence, Quinoderm Lotio-gel 5% should not be used at the same time as other topical agents which would react with an oxidising agent.

*Pregnancy and lactation:* Quinoderm Lotio-gel 5% is not contra-indicated in pregnancy or lactation.

*Effects on ability to drive and use machines:* Not applicable.

*Undesirable effects:* If symptoms persist or if the condition worsens or if irritation, itch or rash occurs, treatment should be discontinued and the Physician or Pharmacist consulted for advice.

*Overdose:* If accidentally ingested symptomatic and supportive management is advised.

**Pharmacological properties**  The main pharmacological action of benzoyl peroxide is considered to be keratolytic and comedolytic. Potassium hydroxyqui-

noline sulphate has broad spectrum antibacterial activity. This combination is formulated in a specifically researched and developed base and is designed to aid the resolution of the polymorphic lesions of acne.

The base has been developed with the objective of providing a stable pharmaceutical form which maximises the advantages of a gel and lotion in a system which does not employ organic solvents and therefore has a correspondingly lower irritancy, toxicity and abuse potential.

**Pharmaceutical particulars**
*List of excipients:* Light Liquid Paraffin BP, EDTA, Sodium Acid Phosphate BP, Maize Starch BP, Lactic Acid BP, Cetomacrogol 1000 BP, cetyl stearyl alcohol, sodium cetyl stearyl sulphate, PEG 40 castor oil, Purified Water BP.

*Incompatibilities:* Any topical agent that would react with an oxidising agent.

*Shelf life:* 3 years.

*Special precautions for storage:* Quinoderm Lotio-gel 5% should be stored in a cool, dry place avoiding extremes of temperature, i.e. not less than 5°C and not more than 30°C.

*Nature and contents of container:* Quinoderm Lotio-gel 5% is available in polyethylene bottles with a flip-top cap containing 30 ml of product. Each bottles is cartoned and contains a package insert.

*Instructions for use/handling:* By gentle massage over all the affected area one to three times daily.

**Marketing authorisation number**  0291/0009

**Date of approval/revision of SPC**  September 1995.

**Legal category**  P.

## QUINOPED* CREAM

**Presentation**
*Active constituents:*
Benzoyl Peroxide BP ..... 5%
Potassium Hydroxyquinoline Sulphate BP ..... 0.5%
*Other constituents:* Lactic Acid BP, White Soft Paraffin BP, EDTA, Sodium Acid Phosphate BP, Maize Starch BP, cetyl stearyl alcohol, sodium cetyl stearyl sulphate, PEG 40 castor oil.

*Appearance:* Quinoped Cream is a cream-coloured astringent cream.

**Uses**  *Main pharmacological action:* Benzoyl peroxide functions as a keratolytic and facilitates the removal of macerated tissue and associated debris. Potassium hydroxyquinoline sulphate has antifungal and deodorant properties.

*Indications:* Athlete's foot (tinea pedis) and related fungal infections.

**Dosage and administration**  *Adults and children:* Spread thinly over all the affected area and gently massage until no trace of the cream can be seen on the skin surface. Apply morning and night.

**Contra-indications, warnings, etc**  Not applicable.

**Pharmaceutical precautions**  *Storage:* Quinoped Cream should be stored in a cool place, avoiding extremes of temperature.

*Diluents:* The cream is easily removed with warm water and soap.

**Legal category**  P.

**Package quantities**  Quinoped Cream is available in tubes of 25 g.

**Further information**  Quinoped Cream is a balanced formulation to counteract the effect of *T. rubrum, T. interdigitale* and *E. floccosum.*

**Product licence number**  0291/0002.

*\*Trade Mark*

# Reckitt & Colman Products
Dansom Lane
Hull HU8 7DS

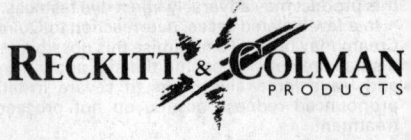

## BONJELA* ORAL PAIN RELIEVING GEL

**Presentation** Bonjela is a clear, almost colourless gel containing choline salicylate 8.7% w/w and cetalkonium chloride 0.01% w/w, in a sugar free base containing ethanol, menthol, glycerol, hypromellose, aniseed oil and sodium cyclamate.

**Uses** For the relief of pain and discomfort of common mouth ulcers, cold sores, denture sore spots and infant teething.

**Dosage and administration** By topical application to the oral mucosa.

*Adults:* Using a clean finger, massage approximately half an inch of the gel onto the sore area, not more than once every three hours.

*Children:* (from 4 months): using a clean finger, massage approximately one quarter inch of gel onto the sore area, not more than once every three hours and not more than six doses in any twenty-four hour period.

*Elderly:* There is no evidence that dosage need be modified for the elderly.

*Denture sore spots:* Apply Bonjela to the gums and leave at least 30 minutes before reinsertion of the dentures. Do not apply this product directly to the dentures.

**Contra-indications, warnings, etc** Preparations containing aspirin should not be given to children under 12 during Bonjela treatment. Unwanted effects are those of salicylates. Bonjela should not be given to patients suffering from active peptic ulceration or known to be allergic to salicylates. Not to be used in infants under four months.

Salicylates may precipitate bronchospasm, and induce attacks of asthma in susceptible subjects.

*Use in pregnancy:* There is clinical evidence of the safety of salicylates in pregnancy but they may prolong bleeding and contribute to maternal and neonatal bleeding and are best avoided at term.

*Use in lactation:* Salicylates are excreted in low concentrations in breast milk but are unlikely to adversely affect the breast fed infant.

*Drug interactions:* Salicylates may enhance the effect of anticoagulants and inhibit the action of uricosurics.

*Interferences with laboratory tests:* Salicylates may produce falsely increased results for blood creatinine, urate (low dose aspirin) and urea. Falsely decreased results may be obtained for blood thyroxine and urate (>4 g/day aspirin) and for urinary 5-HIAA (with nitrosonaphthol method). Urinary VMA (HMMA) levels may be falsely increased or decreased depending on the method of analysis.

*Treatment of overdosage:* The usual procedure for salicylate overdosage should be followed, including general supportive measures and gastric lavage if necessary.

**Pharmaceutical precautions** None.

**Legal category** GSL.

**Package quantities** Tubes of 15 g.

**Product licence number** 0107/5002.

## BUCCASTEM*

**Presentation** Buccastem tablets are circular, biconvex, pale yellow and uncoated with J1 engraved on the face; the reverse is plain. They contain 3 mg prochlorperazine maleate. This product contains sucrose.

**Uses** Buccastem is a potent phenothiazine neuroleptic. It is indicated in the symptomatic treatment of vertigo due to Meniere's disease, labyrinthitis and other causes; for nausea and vomiting from whatever cause and in the treatment of migraine.

### Dosage and administration
*Dosage: Adults and children aged 12 years and over:* One or two 3 mg Buccastem tablets twice a day.

*Elderly patients:* For the indications shown above, there is no evidence that the dosage needs to be modified but the lower dosage is recommended for initial use.

*Administration:* The tablet should be placed high up between the upper lip and the gums to either side of the front teeth, where it will soften and adhere to the gum.

Patients should be instructed as to the correct placement of the tablet and should note the following points:

(a) The tablet should be left undisturbed.
(b) Slight numbness of the gum and tongue may be observed but this is transient.
(c) If a tablet is accidentally swallowed during insertion, it may be replaced by a further tablet.
(d) In patients who wear dentures, the tablet may be placed in any comfortable position between the lip and the gum.

**Contra-indications, warnings, etc**
*Contra-indications:* Buccastem is contra-indicated in patients with impaired renal or liver function, existing blood dyscrasias, known hypersensitivity to the active ingredient, epilepsy, Parkinson's disease, prostatic hypertrophy, and narrow angle glaucoma.

*Use in pregnancy and lactation:* There is inadequate evidence of safety in human pregnancy, although prochlorperazine has been used widely for many years without apparent ill effects. However, as with other drugs, use of Buccastem in the first trimester of pregnancy should be avoided unless absolutely necessary. Since data from animal studies show that prochlorperazine may be found in breast milk, Buccastem should not be used during lactation.

*Warnings:* Hypotension, usually postural, may occur, particularly in elderly or volume depleted subjects.

Parkinsonism or tardive dyskinesia may occur occasionally, although are normally associated with higher doses than are recommended for Buccastem.

Alcohol and other CNS depressants should be used with caution, as should α-adrenoreceptor blocking antihypertensives.

Patients who drive or operate machinery should be warned of the possibility of drowsiness.

*Adverse reactions:* Drowsiness, dizziness, dry mouth, insomnia, agitation and mild skin reactions may occur. Extrapyramidal reactions are very unlikely at the recommended dosage.

Other adverse effects which have occurred rarely with prochlorperazine and other phenothiazine neuroleptics include jaundice, blood dyscrasias and, very rarely, hyperprolactinaemic effects. Neuroleptic malignant syndrome (hyperthermia, rigidity, autonomic dysfunction and altered consciousness) may occur with any neuroleptic.

*Overdosage:* The signs and symptoms will be predominantly extrapyramidal and may be accompanied by either restlessness and agitation or central nervous depression. Hypotension may also occur. Treatment is essentially symptomatic and supportive. There is no specific antidote. Gastric lavage is helpful, particularly when carried out within 6 hours of ingestion. Do not induce vomiting. Particular attention must be directed to maintaining a clear airway, since this may be threatened by the extrapyramidal muscle dystonias. Severe dystonic reactions usually respond to procyclidine (5–10 mg) or orphenadrine (20–40 mg) given i.m. or i.v. If convulsions occur they should be treated using i.v. diazepam. If hypotension is present strict attention to ventilation and posturing of the patient will often secure the desired effect but failing this, consideration should be given to volume expansion by i.v. fluids. If this is insufficient, positive inotropic agents such as dopamine may be tried, but peripheral vasoconstrictor agents are not generally recommended. Adrenaline should *not* be used.

**Pharmaceutical precautions** Protect from light.

**Legal category** POM.

**Package quantities** Packs of 60 tablets, in blister foils of 15 tablets each.

**Further information** Pharmacokinetic studies have shown that prochlorperazine is absorbed via the buccal mucosa. One Buccastem tablet administered twice daily produces steady state plasma levels equivalent to those achieved after oral administration of 5 mg three times daily.

**Product licence number** 0063/0011

## DISPRIN CV*

**Presentation** Modified release tablets in a 28 day calendar pack.
1. White capsule-shaped tablets containing 100 mg Aspirin PhEur impressed on one side with a heart shape and the other a scoreline.
2. White capsule-shaped tablets containing 300 mg Aspirin PhEur impressed on one side with a heart shape and the other with 3C.

**Uses** Disprin CV 100. For the prevention of graft occlusion following aortocoronary by-pass surgery.

Disprin CV 300. To reduce the risk of myocardial infarction in patients who have had a previous attack or in patients with unstable angina and to reduce the risk of occlusive stroke and recurrent transient cerebral ischaemic attacks in patients with a history of such thrombotic events.

**Dosage and administration** Disprin CV is a modified release tablet which should be swallowed whole with water.

*Adults and children over 12:* 1 tablet to be taken every day, preferably at the same time each day.

Not to be given to children under 12 years, unless the expected benefits outweigh the possible risks.

*Elderly:* Risk/benefit ratios in the elderly have not yet been fully evaluated.

**Contra-indications, warnings, etc** The patient should start treatment only after consulting a doctor and is advised to consult a doctor if symptoms which were there before starting treatment persist. Disprin CV should not be given to patients suffering from active peptic ulceration or haemophilia, or patients known to be allergic to aspirin.

Aspirin may induce gastric irritation and gastrointestinal haemorrhage, occasionally major. Disprin CV should not be given to patients with asthma.

*Use in pregnancy and lactation:* There is clinical and epidemiological evidence of the safety of aspirin in pregnancy but it may prolong labour and contribute to maternal and neonatal bleeding and is best avoided in the last trimester of pregnancy unless recommended by a doctor.

Aspirin is excreted in low concentrations in breast milk but it is unlikely to adversely affect the breast-fed infant.

*Drug interactions:* Aspirin may enhance the effects of anticoagulants, oral hypoglycaemics and methotrexate and decrease the action of uricosurics.

*Interference with laboratory tests:* Salicylates may produce falsely increased results for blood creatinine, urate (low dose aspirin) and urea. Falsely decreased results may be obtained for blood thyroxine and urate (>4 g/day aspirin) and for urinary 5-HIAAA (with nitrosonaphthol method). Urinary VMA (HMMA) levels may be falsely increased or decreased depending on the method of analysis.

*Treatment of overdosage:* The major toxic signs of aspirin overdose arise from stimulation and terminal depression of the central nervous system. Symptoms include tinnitus, difficulty in hearing, dizziness, sweating, mental confusion and hyperventilation.

Treat symptomatically. Gastric lavage may be required. Blood tests should be undertaken to determine treatment.

**Pharmaceutical precautions** Store below 25°C.

**Legal category** P.

**Package quantities** Calendar packs of 28 tablets in individual blisters.

**Further information** Nil.

**Product licence numbers**
Disprin CV100 4338/0019
Disprin CV300 4338/0020

## DISPROL* PAEDIATRIC

**Presentation** Disprol Paediatric is a pale yellow suspension contained in an amber glass bottle fitted with an expanded polythene wad and an aluminium roll-on pilfer-proof cap. Each 5 ml dose contains paracetamol PhEur 120 mg in a base containing hydrogenated glucose syrup, glycerol, carbomer, sodium hydroxide, methyl hydroxybenzoate, citric acid, sodium saccharin, banana flavour and riboflavin

**Uses** For the treatment of mild to moderate pain, including headache, migraine, neuralgia, toothache, pain in teething, sore throat, aches and pains. Symptomatic relief of rheumatic aches and pains. Symptomatic relief of influenza, feverishness and feverish colds. Symptomatic relief of reactions due to vaccination or immunisation.

**Dosage and administration**
*Children 3–12 months:* Half to one 5 ml spoonful every four hours.

*1 year to under 6 years:* One to two 5 ml spoonfuls every four hours.

*6 to 12 years:* Two to four 5 ml spoonfuls every four hours.

Dosage for children under 3 months is at a physician's discretion.

Disprol Paediatric may be diluted with an equal volume of boiled then cooled water to produce a 12 mg/ml solution (60 mg/5 ml spoonful) with a 14 day shelf life.

For babies who develop fever following vaccination at 2 months, a 2.5 ml dose is suitable. When prescribed for a baby weighing less than 4.4 kg dose at 0.5 ml/kg (12 mg/kg) using an oral measuring syringe. In all other cases, not to be given to children under 3 months without doctor's advice.

Not more than 4 doses should be administered in any 24-hour period.

Dosage should not be continued for more than 3 days without consulting a doctor.

**Contra-indications, warnings, etc** Disprol Paediatric should not be given to patients with a history of hypersensitivity to paracetamol. It should be used with caution in patients with hepatic or renal dysfunction.

Each 5 ml dose of suspension contains approximately 3.25 g of hydrogenated glucose syrup (up to 12 Kcal). This should be borne in mind when treating diabetic children.

Side-effects from paracetamol administered in normal doses are rare. There have been isolated reports of agranulocytosis, methaemoglobinaemia and thrombocytopenic purpura, and after overdosage or prolonged administration, isolated cases of chronic hepatic necrosis, acute pancreatitis and nephrotoxicity.

*Drug interactions:* Drugs which induce hepatic microsomal enzymes, such as alcohol, barbiturates and tricyclic antidepressants, may increase the hepatotoxicity of paracetamol particularly after overdosage.

*Interferences with laboratory tests:* In paracetamol overdosage, the following tests for blood glucose may be distorted:

Reduction methods and YSI analyser – falsely increased results.

Glucose oxidase method – falsely decreased results.

There is no interference with the hexokinase method.

There may be analytical interference with catechoamine estimations.

*Treatment of overdosage:* Overdosage should be treated promptly by gastric lavage followed by an infusion of N-acetylcysteine or oral methionine since liver damage following overdosage does not become apparent for 1–6 days after ingestion. Initial mild symptoms consist of nausea, vomiting and pallor. Measurement of the blood paracetamol level and the time elapsed since ingestion is important in order to determine whether further therapy with N-acetylcysteine is necessary.

**Pharmaceutical precautions** Store below 25°C and protect from light, avoid freezing.

**Legal category** P.

**Package quantities** 500 ml bottles.

**Product licence number** 0063/0021.

## FYBOGEL*, FYBOGEL* ORANGE and FYBOGEL* LEMON

**Presentation** Fybogel, Fybogel Orange and Fybogel Lemon (hereafter referred to as Fybogel) are buff coloured granules, presented in sachets and enclosed in an outer cardboard carton. The granules form a suspension in water. Each sachet contains Ispaghula Husk BP 3500 mg in a base containing citric acid, potassium bicarbonate, sodium bicarbonate, povidone, aspartame.

The variants are coloured and flavoured as follows:

Fybogel – betacarotene, no flavouring
Fybogel Orange – betacarotene, orange flavouring
Fybogel Lemon – curcumin, lemon flavouring

Fybogel is gluten free and contains no mono or disaccharides. Fybogel is low in sodium and potassium, containing approximately 0.4 mmol sodium and 0.7 mmol potassium per sachet.

**Uses** Fybogel is recommended for the treatment of patients requiring a high-fibre regimen: for example, for the relief of constipation including constipation in pregnancy and the maintenance of regularity; for the management of bowel function in patients with colostomy, ileostomy, haemorrhoids, anal fissure, chronic diarrhoea associated with diverticular disease, irritable bowel syndrome and ulcerative colitis.

**Dosage and administration** Fybogel effervescent granules disperse readily to form a palatable drink in water. The contents of one sachet should be stirred into approximately $\frac{1}{4}$ pint (150 ml) water and taken as quickly as possible, preferably after meals.

*Adults and children over 12 years:* One sachet morning and evening.

*Children 6–12 years:* Half to one level 5 ml spoonful depending on age and size, morning and evening. If there has been no bowel movement after 3 days of treatment a doctor should be consulted.

*Children under 6 years:* To be taken only on medical advice: Dose half to one level 5 ml spoonful, depending on age and size, morning and evening.

*Elderly:* There is no indication that dosage needs to be modified for the elderly.

The unflavoured variant may be added to foods with a high liquid content, as an alternative method of administration.

**Contra-indications, warnings, etc** Fybogel is contraindicated in cases of intestinal obstruction, faecal impaction and colonic atony such as senile megacolon.

Due to its aspartame content, Fybogel should not be given to patients with phenylketonuria.

Fybogel should not be taken in the dry form. Gastrointestinal obstruction or impaction have been reported with hydrophilic mucinoid preparations when taken with insufficient liquid, contrary to administration instructions.

*Use in pregnancy and lactation:* May be used during pregnancy and lactation since the ispaghula is not absorbed from the gastrointestinal tract.

*Drug interactions:* There have been no interactions reported when Fybogel granules have been used with other drugs.

*Interference with laboratory tests:* Fybogel has no known effects on diagnostic laboratory tests.

*Treatment of overdosage:* In the event of overdosage, conservative measures should be taken. The patient may notice abdominal discomfort and flatulence. Attention should be paid to maintaining an adequate fluid intake, particularly if the granules have been taken without water, contrary to the administration instructions.

*Side-effects:* Flatulence and bloating may be experienced during the first few days of treatment but diminish during continued treatment.

**Further information** Ispaghula husk is capable of absorbing up to forty times its own weight of water in vitro, and part of its activity can be attributed to its action as a simple bulking agent. In addition, colonic bacteria are believed to use the hydrated material as a metabolic substrate. This results in an increase in the bacterial cell mass which softens the faeces to allow easy evacuation and avoiding episodes of straining.

**Pharmaceutical precautions** Store below 30°C in a dry place.

**Legal category** GSL

**Package quantities** 30 sachets (prescription pack – all variants). 10 sachets (OTC pack – orange or lemon variants).

**Product licence numbers**

| | |
|---|---|
| Fybogel | 0063/0023 |
| Fybogel Orange | 0063/0026 |
| Fybogel Lemon | 0063/0024 |

## FYBOGEL* MEBEVERINE

**Presentation** Buff coloured granules containing orange spheroids, presented in sachets and enclosed in an outer cardboard carton. The product forms an orange suspension in water. Each individual sachet contains Ispaghula Husk BP 3500 mg and Mebeverine Hydrochloride BP 135 mg, in a base containing microcrystalline cellulose, eudragit, sterilised talc, polyethylene glycol, apocarotenal, citric acid, potassium bicarbonate, povidone, orange flavour, sodium saccharin and beta-carotene. The potassium content is 7 mmol per sachet.

**Uses** Fybogel Mebeverine is indicated for the treatment of the symptoms of abdominal pain and bowel dysfunction associated with irritable bowel syndrome or other gastrointestinal diseases.

**Dosage and administration**
*Adults and children over 12 years:* One sachet morning and evening before meals. An additional sachet may be taken before the midday meal if necessary.

*Children under 12 years:* Not recommended.

*Elderly:* There is no indication that the dosage need be modified for the elderly.

The contents of one sachet should be stirred into a glass of cold water (approx. $\frac{1}{4}$ pint) and taken immediately.

**Contra-indications, warnings, etc** Fybogel Mebeverine is contraindicated in cases of intestinal obstruction, faecal impaction and colonic atony such as senile megacolon.

*Use in pregnancy and lactation:* In common with most drugs, care should be taken in prescribing during pregnancy and lactation.

*Drug interactions:* None known.

*Treatment of overdosage:* In the event of overdosage, conservative measures should be taken. The patient may notice abdominal discomfort and flatulence, and attention should be paid to maintaining an adequate fluid intake, particularly if the product has been taken without water contrary to the administration instructions.

*Interference with laboratory tests:* None known.

**Pharmaceutical precautions** Store below 30°C in a dry place.

**Legal category** POM.

**Package quantities** 10 sachet packs.

**Further information** Studies by Ritchie and Truelove (1979, 1980) have demonstrated that a combination of ispaghula and mebeverine gave better overall relief of the symptoms of irritable bowel syndrome when compared to bran or another antispasmodic agent. Fybogel Mebeverine is presented as effervescent granules which disperse readily in water. References: Ritchie, J. A. & Truelove, S. C. (1979) Br. Med. J. 1, 376, Ritchie. J. A. & Truelove, S. C. (1980) Br. Med J. 281, 1317.

**Product licence number** 0063/0025.

## FYBOZEST* ORANGE

**Qualitative and quantitative composition** A standard does of Fybozest Orange contins 3.5 g Ispaghula Husk BP.

**Pharmaceutical form** Granules for the preparation of an oral suspension.

**Clinical particulars**
*Therapeutic indications:* Primary hypercholesterolaemia. Fybozest Orange is indicated for reduction of mild to moderately elevated total serum cholesterol levels (6.5–7.8 mmol/l) and for the maintenance of lowered levels thereafter.

To be used in conjunction with dietary modification.

*Posology and method of administration:* For oral administration. Fybozest Orange should be stirred into at least 150 ml water and taken as quickly as possible.

*Adults:* The standard dose is 3.5 g ispaghula husk morning and evening (one measure of Fybozest Orange).

*Elderly:* Dosage need not be modified for use in elderly patients.

*Children:* Not recommended.

*For packs to be used to fill prescriptions only:* A higher dose of 5.25 g ispaghula husk morning and evening (one and a half measures of Fybozest Orange) may be taken for the initial two to three months of treatment by patients for whom an earlier onset of maximum serum cholesterol reduction is desirable for either clinical or motivational reasons.

*Contra-indications:* In cases of intestinal obstruction, faecal impaction and colonic atony such as senile megacolon.

Hypersensitivity to any of the ingredients.

Owing to its aspartame content, Fybozest Orange should not be taken by patients with phenylketonuria.

*Special warnings and special precautions for use:* Ispaghula husk should not be taken in the dry form. Gastrointestinal obstruction or impaction have been reported with hydrophilic mucilloid preparations when taken with insufficient liquid contrary to administration instructions.

Patients with diabetes mellitus should only take Fybozest Orange under medical supervision. A reduction in insulin dose may be necessary.

*Interactions with other medicaments and other forms of interaction:*

*Drug interactions:* None known.

*Interference with laboratory tests:* None known.

*Pregnancy and lactation:* Ispaghula husk has no

systemic activity and consequently can be taken during pregnancy and lactation.

*Effects on ability to drive and use machines:* None.

*Undesirable effects:* Flatulence and abdominal bloating may be experienced during the first few days of treatment, but should diminish during continued treatment. If abdominal discomfort is noticed on commencing treatment, the dosage may be reduced to one level measure per day until the effects subside.

*Overdose:* In the event of overdose, symptomatic treatment should be given. The patient may notice abdominal discomfort and flatulence. Attention should be paid to maintaining an adequate fluid intake, especially if the product was taken without fluid, contrary to administration instructions.

**Pharmacological properties**
*Pharmacodynamic particulars:* Ispaghula husk consists of both soluble and insoluble dietary fibre. It exerts a bulking effect in the gut as a result of its ability to absorb and hold water, up to 40 times its own weight of water *in vitro*. The hydrated material is used by bacteria as a metabolic substrate resulting in an increase in bacterial cell mass and enhancement of the bulking effect. Several hypotheses have been proposed to explain the reduction in serum cholesterol levels caused by soluble dietary fibre. These include a reduction in the absorption of cholesterol and fatty acids from the gut due to the viscous nature of the hydrated fibre or as a result of binding between bile acids/lipids and fibre, increased faecal excretion of bile acids and, to a small extent, inhibitiion of cholesterol synthesis by short chain fatty acids produced during fermentation of dietary fibre by colonic bacteria.

*Pharmacokinetic particulars:* Although the majority of isphagula husk passes through the digestive system unchanged, gut fermentation by colonic bacteria may lead to the formation of short chain fatty acids, primarily acetate with some propionate and butyrate. These SCFAs are further metabolised in the colon (mainly butyrate) or passed to the portal vein and cleared by the liver. Acetate and butyrate are converted to acetyl-coenzyme A, whilst propionate is converted to succinyl-coenzyme A. Further metabolism occurs in the same way as that of endogenous acetyl-coenzyme A and succinyl-coenzyme A via the citric acid cycle.

*Preclinical safety data:* No preclinical findings relevant to the prescriber have been reported.

**Pharmaceutical particulars**
*List of excipients:* Povidone K90, citric acid, potassium bicarbonate, sodium bicarbonate, aspartame, betacarotene (E160a), orange flavour.

*Incompatibilities:* None known.

*Shelf life:* Tubs – three years.

*Special precautions for storage:* Store below 30°C.

*Nature and contents of container:* Polyethylene container with a polypropylene flip top lid and containing 265 g Fybozest Orange.

A propylene dose measure sits inside the flip top lid.

*Instructions for use/handling:* No special instructions.

**Marketing authorisation number** 0063/0043

**Date of approval/revision of SPC** October 1996.

**Legal category** P.

## GAVISCON* ADVANCE

**Qualitative and quantitative composition** Each 10 ml dose contains:

| | |
|---|---|
| Sodium Alginate BP | 1000.0 mg |
| Potassium Bicarbonate USP | 200.0 mg |

**Pharmaceutical form** Oral suspension.

**Clinical particulars**
*Therapeutic indications:* Gastric reflux, reflux oesophagitis, heartburn, hiatus hernia, flatulence associated with gastric reflux, heartburn of pregnancy. All cases of epigastric and retrosternal distress where the underlying cause is gastric reflux.

*Posology and method of administration:*
*Adults and children 12 years and over:* 5–10 ml after meals and at bedtime.

*Children under 12 years:* Should be given only on medical advice.

*Elderly:* No dose modification is required for this age group.

*Contra-indications:* Hypersensitivity to any of the ingredients.

*Special warnings and special precautions for use:* Each 10 ml dose has a sodium content of 106 mg (4.6 mmol) and a potassium content of 78 mg (2.0 mmol). This should be taken into account when a highly restricted salt diet is recommended as in some renal and cardiovascular conditions.

If symptoms do not improve after seven days, the doctor should be consulted.

*Interactions with other medicaments and other forms of interaction:* None known.

*Use in pregnancy and lactation:* Alginic acid has no systemic activity and consequently can be taken during pregnancy and lactation.

*Effect on ability to drive and to use machines:* None.

*Undesirable effects:* Very rarely patients sensitive to the ingredients may develop allergic manifestations such as urticaria or bronchospasm.

*Overdose:* In the event of overdosage symptomatic treatment should be given. The patient may notice abdominal distension.

**Pharmacological properties**
*Pharmacodynamic properties:* On ingestion the suspension reacts with gastric acid to form a raft of alginic acid gel having a near-neutral pH and which floats on the stomach contents effectively impeding gastro-oesophageal reflux. In severe cases the raft itself may be refluxed into the oesophagus in preference to the stomach contents and exert a demulcent effect.

*Pharmacokinetic properties:* The mode of action of Gaviscon Advance is physical and does not depend on absorption into the systemic circulation.

*Preclinical safety data:* No preclinical findings of relevance to the prescriber have been reported.

**Pharmaceutical particulars** *List of excipients:* Calcium carbonate, carbomer, ethyl hydroxybenzoate, sodium butyl hydroxybenzoate, saccachrin sodium, fennel flavour, sodium hydroxide, purified water.

*Incompatibilities:* None known.

*Shelf life:* Two years.

*Special precautions for storage:* Store below 30°C. Do not refrigerate.

*Nature and contents of container:* Amber glass bottles with moulded polypropylene cap with polyethylene tamper-evident strip, lined with an expanded polyethylene wad and containing 140 ml or 500 ml of suspension.

*Instructions for use/handling:* To be taken orally. Shake well before use. Check that the cap seal is unbroken before first taking the product.

**Marketing authorisation number** 0063/0097

**Date of approval/revision of SPC** November 1996.

**Legal category** GSL.

## LIQUID GAVISCON*
## LIQUID GAVISCON* PEPPERMINT FLAVOUR

**Presentation** Liquid Gaviscon is a pink suspension with a flavour of fennel (similar to aniseed) and Liquid Gaviscon Peppermint Flavour is a white suspension with a flavour of peppermint. Each 10 ml of liquid contains Sodium Alginate BP 500 mg, Sodium Bicarbonate PhEur 267 mg, Calcium Carbonate PhEur 160 mg in a base containing carbomer, methyl hydroxybenzoate, propyl hydroxybenzoate, sodium saccharin, sodium hydroxide and water. The fennel – flavoured liquid also contains erythrosine and fennel flavour, and the peppermint – flavoured liquid contains peppermint oil.

Liquid Gaviscon is gluten free and sugar free.

**Uses** Liquid Gaviscon and Liquid Gaviscon Peppermint Flavour (hereafter referred to as Gaviscon) alleviate the painful conditions resulting from the reflux of gastric acid and bile into the oesophagus by suppressing the reflux itself.

On ingestion, Gaviscon reacts with gastric acid to produce in the stomach a floating viscous gel of near neutral pH which effectively impedes reflux. In severe cases the gel itself may be refluxed into the oesophagus, where it protects the inflamed mucosa, thus allowing healing to take place and preventing further inflammation. Gaviscon is indicated in heartburn including heartburn of pregnancy, dyspepsia associated with gastric reflux, hiatus hernia, reflux oesophagitis, regurgitation and all cases of epigastric and retrosternal distress where the underlying cause is gastric reflux.

**Dosage and administration**
*Adults, children over 12 years:* 10–20 ml after meals and at bedtime.

*Children 6 years to under 12 years:* 5–10 ml after meals and at bedtime.

*Children 2–6 years:* Should only be given on medical advice.

*Infants:* Not recommended, Infant Gaviscon is available for Infants.

*Elderly:* There is no indication that dosage need be modified for the elderly.

If desired, the standard dose of Liquid Gaviscon may be taken diluted with not more than an equal quantity of water, well stirred.

**Contra-indications, warnings, etc** There are no specific contra-indications.

The sodium content of a dose of 10 ml is 141 mg (6.2 mmol). This may be of importance when a highly restricted salt diet is required as in some renal and cardiovascular conditions.

Very rarely, patients sensitive to the ingredients may develop allergic manifestations such as urticaria or bronchospasm.

*Use in pregnancy:* Liquid Gaviscon is indicated for heartburn in pregnancy.

*Use in lactation:* May be used in lactation since alginate is not absorbed from the gastrointestinal tract.

*Drug interactions:* There have been no interactions reported when Liquid Gaviscon has been used with other drugs.

*Treatment of overdosage:* As Gaviscon's mode of action is physical, overdosage in terms of alginate presents virtually no hazard. The only likely consequence is abdominal distention which is best treated conservatively.

**Pharmaceutical precautions** Store below 30°C; do not refrigerate.

**Legal category** GSL.

**Package quantities** 500 ml bottles.

**Product licence numbers**
Liquid Gaviscon 0063/0031
Liquid Gaviscon Peppermint Flavour 0063/0032

## GAVISCON TABLETS*
## GAVISCON TABLETS* LEMON FLAVOUR

**Presentation** Matt, white, flat and circular tablets with bevelled edges. "GAVISCON", and the sword and circle symbol are impressed on both surfaces. The tablets are presented in polypropylene tubes with snap on caps, inside a cardboard carton. Each tablet contains Alginic Acid BP 500 mg, Sodium Bicarbonate EP 170 mg, Aluminium Hydroxide Gel BP 100 mg and Magnesium Trisilicate EP 25 mg in a base containing mannitol, xylitol, povidone, magnesium stearate, calcium carbonate and sodium saccharin.

Gaviscon Tablets, which are peppermint flavoured also contain vanillin and peppermint oil. Gaviscon Tablets Lemon Flavour also contain lemon flavouring. The tablets are free from gluten, lactose and sugar.

**Uses** Gaviscon Tablets and Gaviscon Tablets Lemon Flavour (hereafter referred to as Gaviscon) alleviate the painful conditions resulting from the reflux of gastric acid and bile into the oesophagus by suppressing the reflux itself.

On ingestion, Gaviscon reacts with gastric acid to produce in the stomach a floating viscous gel of near neutral pH which effectively impedes reflux. In severe cases the gel itself may be refluxed into the oesophagus, where it protects the inflamed mucosa, thus allowing healing to take place and preventing further inflammation. Gaviscon is indicated for heartburn including heartburn of pregnancy, dyspepsia associated with gastric reflux, hiatus hernia, reflux oesophagitis, regurgitation and all cases of epigastric and restrosternal distress where the underlying cause is gastric reflux.

**Dosage and administration**
*Adults and children over 12 years:* One or two tablets after meals and at bedtime.

*Children 6–12 years:* One tablet after meals and at bedtime.

*Children 2–6 years:* Should be given only on medical advice. Dose: One tablet after meals and at bedtime.

*Infants:* Not recommended. Infant Gaviscon is available for infants.

*Elderly:* There is no indication that dosage need be modified for the elderly. Tablets should be thoroughly chewed. It is recommended they be broken in half and chewed a little at a time. This may be followed by a drink of water.

**Contra-indications, warnings, etc** There are no specific contra-indications.

Aluminium hydroxide containing products should be used with caution in patients with renal dysfunction or hypophosphataemia. The sodium content of a tablet is 47 mg (2.04 mmol). This may be of importance when a highly restricted salt diet is required as in some renal and cardiovascular conditions.

*Use in pregnancy:* Gaviscon is indicated for heartburn including heartburn of pregnancy.

*Use in lactation:* May be used during lactation sinc

the alginate is not absorbed from the gastrointestinal tract.

*Drug interactions:* There have been no interactions reported when Gaviscon has been used with other drugs. Although large doses of antacids interfere with the absorption of some drugs, the amount of antacid in the recommended dose of Gaviscon is unlikely to interact with other drugs.

*Interference with laboratory tests:* Gaviscon has no known effects on diagnostic laboratory tests.

*Treatment of overdosage:* As Gaviscon's mode of action is physical, overdosage in terms of the alginate presents virtually no hazard. The only likely consequence is abdominal distension which is best treated conservatively.

**Pharmaceutical precautions** Store below 30°C in a dry place.

**Legal category** GSL.

**Package quantities** Carton containing 60 Tablets (3 tubes of 20 tablets).

**Product licence numbers**
Gaviscon Tablets 0063/0033
Gaviscon Tablets Lemon Flavour 0063/0029

## INFANT GAVISCON*

**Presentation** Infant Gaviscon is a fine, white powder packed in dual sachets (1 dose per sachet) and sterilised. Each dose contains sodium alginate 225 mg, magnesium alginate 87.5 mg and dried Aluminium Hydroxide BP 112.5 mg in a base containing colloidal silica (Aerosil) and Mannitol BP. Infant Gavison is sugar free.

**Uses** Infant Gaviscon reacts with gastric acid to form a viscous gel which when mixed with stomach contents thickens them and helps prevent reflux into the oesophagus.

It is indicated for gastric regurgitation, including that seen when the competence of the cardiac sphincter has not been fully established, gastro-oesophageal reflux and reflux associated with hiatus hernia in infants and young children.

**Dosage and administration** Not to be used except on a doctor's recommendation, or in infants under 1 year except under medical supervision. Mix immediately before use as directed below.

*Breast-fed infants:* Under 10 lb (4.5 kg), one dose. Over 10 lb (4.5 kg), two doses. Add 1 teaspoon (5 ml) of boiled, cooled water to the powder in a glass, mix to a smooth paste, add two more teaspoons of the water and mix. Give after each feed using a spoon or feeding bottle.

*Bottle-fed infants:* Under 10 lb (4.5 kg), one dose to be mixed into not less than 4 fluid oz (115 ml) of each feed in the bottle and shaken well. Over 10 lb (4.5 kg), two doses to be mixed into not less than 8 fluid oz (225 ml) of each feed in the bottle and shaken well.

*Young children:* Two doses, prepared as for breast-fed infants, to be drunk after each meal.

**Contra-indications, warnings etc** Contra-indicated in cases of intestinal obstruction and in cases of established diarrhoea.

Attention should be paid to the dosage instructions to avoid an excessive amount of product per feed and the possible risk of hypernatraemia.

Infant Gaviscon's mode of action is physical resulting in a thickening of the gastric contents. An excessive concentration of Infant Gaviscon may lead to gastric distension.

Not to be used in premature infants or in situations where excessive water loss is likely, e.g. fever, diarrhoea, vomiting or high room temperature. Not to be used in gastroenteritis, where the appropriate treatment is rehydration with fluid replacement.

Not to be used when treating infants with known or suspected impairment of renal function as the sodium content (approximately 21 mg or 0.92 mmol per dose) may add to the risk of hypernatraemia. A medical review of the patient's condition should be undertaken seven days after initiating treatment or before if symptoms worsen.

*Drug interactions:* There have been no interactions reported when Infant Gaviscon was used with other drugs.

*Interference with laboratory tests:* Infant Gaviscon has no known effects on diagnostic laboratory tests.

*Treatment of overdosage:* Rare instances have occurred in which an intragastric mass has developed, comprising Infant Gaviscon and milk proteins. Overdosage may have contributed to the development of such masses. The majority resolved spontaneously when the child was admitted, Infant Gaviscon was discontinued and a regime of adequate fluid intake and monitoring of fluid and electrolyte balance was installed. If spontaneous resolution of the mass does

not occur, removal by surgical or endoscopic means may be required.

If hypernatraemia occurs it should be treated with oral fluids and monitoring of the infant's electrolytes. Severe cases should be treated by the cautious use of hypo-osmotic solutions.

**Pharmaceutical precautions** Nil.

**Legal category** P.

**Package quantities** Carton of 15 dual sachets (30 doses).

**Product licence number** 0063/0030.

## SENOKOT*

**Presentation** *Tablets:* Small brown tablets engraved on one side only with the word Senokot and a sword symbol. One tablet contains standardised senna equivalent to 7.5 mg total sennosides calculated as sennoside B. Senokot tablets contain lactose and parabens.

*Granules:* Brown chocolate-flavoured granules. One 5 ml level spoonful (2.73 g) contains standardised senna equivalent to 15 mg total sennosides calculated as sennoside B. Senokot granules contain sucrose.

*Syrup:* Brown, fruit-flavoured syrup. One 5 ml spoonful contains standardised senna extract equivalent to 7.5 mg total sennosides calculated as sennoside B. Senokot syrup contains sucrose and ethanol.

**Uses** In the management of constipation, including:
Simple constipation, whether self-induced or environmental, e.g. neglect of the call to stool or poor sanitary conditions.
Constipation in old age, especially where maintenance treatment is required.
Constipation in pregnancy and the puerperium.
Idiopathic slow-transit constipation.
Constipation in the irritable bowel syndrome.
Conservative treatment of haemorrhoids.
Avoidance of straining after surgery and in cerebral and cardiovascular disease.

The physiological action of the anthrone glycoside in Senokot is virtually colon specific. The anthroquinones are protected by a natural sugar moiety which safeguards their transport to the large bowel, where bacterial action breaks the sugar-anthrone bond and releases the active fraction. Peristalsis is then stimulated via the submucosal and myenteric plexuses.

Being colon specific, Senokot does not affect the vital nutritional functions of the upper gastro-intestinal tract.

**Dosage and administration** The correct dose of Senokot is the smallest required to produce a comfortable soft-formed motion. It varies between individuals, but is generally found within the following ranges:

*Adults:* 2 tablets (up to 4 on medical advice) or one 5 ml spoonful of granules (up to 10 ml on medical advice) or 10 ml of syrup (up to 20 ml on medical advice) at bedtime.

*Children over 6 years:* Half the adult dosages, taken in the morning.

*Children 2–6 years:* Use Senokot syrup ½ to one 5 ml spoonful. Tablets and Granules are not recommended for children 6 and under.

There is no indication that dosage need be modified for the elderly.

New users should start with the lowest dose of the preferred formulation. These are available from a range of general sales packs advising only the lowest dose and available for self medication as described above. Alternatively the product may be dispensed to allow, if necessary, an increase by half the initial dose each day until a comfortable formed motion is produced. If no bowel action has occurred after three days' progressively increased dosage a medical examination should be considered.

Senokot is best taken as a single dose, at bedtime by adults and in the morning by children. The tablets can be taken with a drink, the granules can be stirred into hot milk, sprinkled on food, or eaten as they are.

Once regularity has been achieved, dosage should be reduced and can usually be stopped.

**Contra-indications, warnings, etc** Senokot like all laxatives, should not be given when any undiagnosed acute or persistent abdominal symptoms are present. Temporary mild griping may occur during adjustment of dosage.

Diabetic patients should use the tablets as these have a negligible sugar content.

*Use in lactation:* Clinical studies have shown that breast fed infants of mothers taking Senokot did not show any side effects of the drug.

*Interference with laboratory tests:* Senokot has no known effects on diagnostic laboratory tests.

*Treatment of overdosage:* In cases of accidental

overdosage, where diarrhoea is severe, conservative measures are usually sufficient: generous amounts of fluid especially fruit drinks should be given.

**Pharmaceutical precautions** The tablets and granules should be kept in closed airtight containers, and the syrup in amber bottles as supplied. Store in a cool place.

**Legal category** GSL, sales restricted to pharmacies.

**Package quantities**
Tablets: 20, 60 and 100 in blisters; 500 in Securitainers.
Granules: 100 g in Securitainers.
Syrup: Bottles of 100 ml and 500 ml.

**Further information** Nil.

**Product licence numbers**
Tablets    0063/5000R
Granules   0063/5002
Syrup      0063/5003

## TEMGESIC* INJECTION

**Presentation** Temgesic Injection is a colourless liquid containing 300 micrograms/ml buprenorphine, as the hydrochloride, in a 5% dextrose solution, adjusted to pH range 3.5–5.5 with hydrochloric acid. Clear glass snap ampoules of 1 ml (300 micrograms).

Temgesic Injection contains 50 mg dextrose per ml, but no sodium, potassium or preservative.

**Uses** As a strong analgesic for the relief of moderate to severe pain.

**Dosage and administration** *Adults and children over 12 years old:* The recommended dosage is 1 to 2 ml (300–600 micrograms buprenorphine), by IM or slow IV injection, every six to eight hours or as required. Temgesic Injection may be employed in balanced anaesthetic techniques as a premedication at a dose of 300 micrograms intramuscularly or as an analgesic supplement at doses of 300–450 micrograms intravenously.

*Children under 12 years:* Temgesic is suitable for children under 12 at a dose of 3–6 micrograms/kg body weight every 6–8 hours. In refractory cases up to 9 micrograms/kg may be administered. There is no clinical experience in infants below the age of six months.

*Elderly:* There is no evidence that dosage need be modified for the elderly though they may be more susceptible to hallucinations and other psychotomimetic effects.

**Contra-indications, warnings, etc** Not to be given to patients who are known to be allergic to Temgesic or other opiates. Controlled human and animal studies indicate that buprenorphine has a substantially lower dependence liability than pure agonist analgesics. In patients abusing opioids in moderate doses substitution with buprenorphine may prevent withdrawal symptoms. In man limited euphorigenic effects have been observed. This has resulted in some abuse of the product and caution should be exercised when prescribing it to patients known to have, or suspected of having, problems with drug abuse.

There is evidence to indicate that therapeutic doses of buprenorphine do not reduce the analgesic efficacy of standard doses of an opioid agonist, and that when buprenorphine is employed within the normal range, standard doses of opioid agonist may be administered before the effects of the former have ended without compromising analgesia. However, in individuals on high doses of opioids, buprenorphine may precipitate abstinence effects due to its properties as a partial agonist.

Temgesic may cause some drowsiness which may be potentiated by other centrally-acting agents, including alcohol, tranquillisers, sedatives and hypnotics. Ambulant patients should be warned not to drive or operate machinery until they are certain they can tolerate Temgesic.

Temgesic occasionally causes significant respiratory depression and, as with other strong centrally acting analgesics, care should be taken when treating patients with impaired respiratory function or patients who are receiving drugs which can cause respiratory depression. Although volunteer studies have indicated that opioid antagonists may not fully reverse the effects of Temgesic, clinical experience has shown that naloxone may be of benefit in reversing a reduced respiratory rate. Respiratory stimulants such as doxapram are also effective.

Since buprenorphine is metabolised in the liver, the intensity and duration of its action may be affected in patients with impaired liver function.

Temgesic should be used with caution in patients receiving monoamine oxidase inhibitors, although animal studies have given no indication of interactions.

*Use in pregnancy and lactation:* Temgesic is not recommended for use during pregnancy. Animal studies indicate that the amounts of buprenorphine excreted in milk are very low and in human use are unlikely to be of clinical significance to the baby. There is indirect evidence in animal studies to suggest that Temgesic may cause a reduction in milk flow during lactation. Although this occurred only at doses well in excess of the human dose, it should be borne in mind when treating lactating women.

*Interference with laboratory tests:* Temgesic has no known effects on diagnostic laboratory tests.

*Overdosage:* Temgesic has a wide safety margin, and in clinical practice doses well in excess of those recommended have been used without untoward effect. Supportive measures should be instituted and, if appropriate, naloxone or respiratory stimulants can be used.

The expected symptoms of overdosage would be drowsiness, nausea and vomiting; marked miosis may occur.

*Side-effects:* Drowsiness, or sleep from which the patient can be easily aroused, may occur particularly in the post-operative period. In common with other strong analgesics, nausea, vomiting, dizziness, sweating and drowsiness have been reported which may be more frequent in ambulant patients. Should nausea and vomiting occur, concurrent administration of an anti-emetic is advised. Hallucinations and other psychotomimetic effects have occurred although more rarely than with other agonist-antagonists. Hypotension leading to syncope may occur. Rashes, headache, urinary retention and blurring of vision have occasionally been reported. Rarely, a serious allergic reaction may occur following a single dose.

**Pharmaceutical precautions** Temgesic Injection, though stable, should be kept cool and protected from light. It may be diluted with 5% Injection Dextrose BP or Injection Sodium Chloride BP.

**Legal category** CD(Sch 3), POM.

**Package quantities** Packs of 5 ampoules (1 ml).

**Product licence number** 0063/0007.

## TEMGESIC* SUBLINGUAL

**Presentation** Temgesic Sublingual is presented as white, biconvex tablets containing 200 micrograms (0.2 mg) or 400 micrograms (0.4 mg) of buprenorphine as the hydrochloride, engraved on one side with a 'L' or 'H' respectively and on the other with a sword symbol. This product contains lactose, mannitol, maize starch, povidone, citrate buffer, and magnesium stearate.

**Uses** As a strong analgesic for the relief of moderate to severe pain.

**Dosage and administration**
*Adults and children over 12:* 200–400 micrograms (0.2–0.4 mg) buprenorphine to be dissolved under the tongue every 6–8 hours or as required. The recommended starting dose for moderate to severe pain of the type typically presenting in general practice is 200–400 micrograms (0.2–0.4 mg) every eight hours. The tablet should not be chewed or swallowed as this will reduce efficacy.

Temgesic Sublingual may be employed in balanced anaesthetic techniques as a premedication at a dose of 400 micrograms.

*Children under 12 years:* Temgesic Sublingual 0.2 mg is suitable for use in children as follows:

16–25 kg (35–55 lb), 100 micrograms (half a 0.2 mg tablet).
25–37.5 kg (55–82.5 lb), 100–200 micrograms (half to one 0.2 mg tablet).
37.5–50 kg (82.5–110 lb), 200–300 micrograms (one to one and a half 0.2 mg tablets).

There is no clinical experience in infants below the age of six months.

*Elderly:* There is no evidence that dosage need be modified for the elderly though they may be more susceptible to hallucinations and other psychotomimetic effects.

**Contra-indications, warnings, etc** Not to be given to patients who are known to be allergic to Temgesic or other opiates. Controlled human and animal studies indicate that buprenorphine has a substantially lower dependence liability than pure agonist analgesics. In patients abusing opioids in moderate doses substitution with buprenorphine may prevent withdrawal symptoms. In man limited euphorigenic effects have been observed. This has resulted in some abuse of the product and caution should be exercised when prescribing it to patients known to have, or suspected of having, problems with drug abuse.

There is evidence to indicate that therapeutic doses of buprenorphine do not reduce the analgesic efficacy of standard doses of an opioid agonist, and clinical studies have shown that when buprenorphine is employed within the normal therapeutic range, standard doses of narcotic agonist may be administered before the effects of the former have ended without compromising analgesia. However, in individuals on high doses of narcotics, buprenorphine may precipitate withdrawal effects due to its properties as a partial agonist.

Temgesic may cause some drowsiness which may be potentiated by other centrally-acting agents, including alcohol, tranquillisers, sedatives and hypnotics. Ambulant patients should be warned not to drive or operate machinery until they are certain they can tolerate Temgesic.

Temgesic occasionally causes significant respiratory depression and, as with other strong centrally acting analgesics, care should be taken when treating patients with impaired respiratory function or patients who are receiving drugs which can cause respiratory depression. Although volunteer studies have indicated that opioid antagonists may not fully reverse the effects of Temgesic, clinical experience has shown that naloxone may be of benefit in reversing a reduced respiratory rate. Respiratory stimulants such as doxapram are also effective.

Since buprenorphine is metabolised in the liver, the intensity and duration of its action may be affected in patients with impaired liver function.

Temgesic should be used with caution in patients who are receiving monoamine oxidase inhibitors, although animal studies have given no indication of interactions.

*Use in pregnancy:* Temgesic is not recommended for use during pregnancy. Animal studies indicate that the amounts of buprenorphine excreted in milk are very low and in human use are unlikely to be of clinical significance to the baby.

*Use in lactation:* There is indirect evidence in animal studies to suggest that Temgesic may cause a reduction in milk flow during lactation. Although this occurred only at doses well in excess of the human dose, it should be borne in mind when treating lactating women.

*Interference with laboratory tests:* Temgesic has no known effects on diagnostic laboratory tests.

*Overdosage:* Temgesic Sublingual has a wide safety margin and in clinical practice doses of buprenorphine well in excess of those recommended have been used without untoward effect. Supportive measures should be instituted and, if appropriate, naloxone or respiratory stimulants can be used. The expected symptoms of overdosage would be drowsiness, nausea and vomiting; marked miosis may occur.

*Side-effects:* Drowsiness, or sleep from which the patient can easily be aroused, may occur particularly in the postoperative period. In common with other strong analgesics, nausea, vomiting, dizziness, sweating and drowsiness have been reported and may be more frequent in ambulant patients. Should nausea and vomiting occur, concurrent administration of an anti-emetic is advised. Hallucinations and other psychotomimetic effects have occurred although more rarely than with other agonist-antagonists. Elderly patients would be expected to be more susceptable to the effects Hypotension leading to syncope may occur. Rashes, headache urinary retention and blurring of vision have occasionally been reported. Rarely, a serious allergic reaction may occur following a single dose.

**Pharmaceutical precautions** Store in a cool place.

**Legal category** CD(Sch 3), POM.

**Package quantities** Cartons of 50 tablets as blisterpacks of 10 each.

**Further information** Nil.

**Product licence numbers**
Temgesic sublingual 0.2 mg    0063/0008
Temgesic sublingual 0.4 mg    0063/0009

## TIMODINE*

**Presentation** A pale yellow cream presented in an internally laquered aluminium tube, in an outer cardboard carton. Each 30 g tube contains w/w Nystatin BP 100,000 i.u./g. Hydrocortisone Ph Eur 0.5 %, Benzalkonium Chloride solution BP 0.2% and Dimethicone 350 BP 10.0%, in a base containing: butylated hydroxyanisole, cetostearyl alcohol, cellulose nitrate, dibutyl phthalate, glyceryl monostearate, methyl and propyl hydroxybenzoate, sorbic acid, stearic acid and sodium metabisulphate.

**Uses** For the treatment of dermatoses, including intertrigo, eczema, seborrhoeic dermatitis, "housewive's eczema" and pruritus ani and vulvae, in which infection with Candida albicans is a factor. For the treatment of severe napkin rash in which Candida albicans is a factor.

Timodine is particularly indicated in the treatment of dermatoses occurring in sites, such as the skin folds, in which the special environmental conditions present predispose to maceration and chafing, leading to secondary infection with Candida albicans and bacteria, and causing additional inflammation and persistent pruritis.

**Dosage and administration** *Dermatoses:* A thin layer of Timodine should be applied to cover the lesion. It should then be massaged into the skin until the cream disappears. The treatment should be repeated three times a day until the lesion has healed.

There is no indication that dosage need be modified for the elderly.

*Napkin rash:* After removal of the soiled napkin, the affected areas should be cleaned and dried and a thin layer of Timodine applied. The treatment should be repeated after every napkin change. In infants the long term continuous topical steroid therapy should be avoided and a course of treatment should not normally exceed seven days.

**Contra-indications, warnings, etc** Use only on the skin. Timodine should not be used by anyone who is allergic to the product or any of its ingredients.

*Precautions:* Keep away from eyes.

*Use in pregancy:* Topical administration of corticosteroids to pregnant animals can cause abnormalities of foetal development. The relevance of this finding to human beings has not been established; however, topical steroids should not be used extensively in pregnancy, ie: in large amounts or for prolonged periods.

*Use in lactation:* There is no information about effects on lactation.

*Side-effects:* None have been reported.

*Interference with laboratory tests:* Timodine has no known effects on diagnostic laboratory tests.

**Pharmaceutical precautions** Store below 15°C.

**Legal category** POM.

**Package quantities** 30 g tubes.

**Further information** Nil.

**Product licence number** 1839/0001

*Product licence holder:* Lloyd-Hamol Limited.

*\*Trade Mark*

# Rhône-Poulenc Rorer Limited
## West Malling
## Kent ME19 4AH

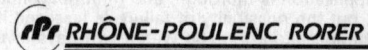

# AEROCROM* INHALER AND SYNCRONER

## Qualitative and quantitative composition

| Ingredients | mg per actuation |
|---|---|
| Sodium cromoglycate, micronised | 1.00 |
| Salbutamol sulphate, micronised | 0.1205 |

(equivalent to 0.10 mg salbutamol base).

**Pharmaceutical form** Aerocrom Inhaler is presented as a metered dose pressurised aerosol containing sodium cromoglycate and salbutamol sulphate as a suspension in chlorofluorocarbon propellants, for inhalation.

## Clinical particulars

*Therapeutic indications:* Aerocrom is indicated for patients who have been shown to require regular doses of sodium cromoglycate and salbutamol for the treatment of asthma. Aerocrom is not intended for first line maintenance treatment but is only for use once the need for regular combination therapy has been established.

*Posology and method of administration: Adults (including the elderly):* Two inhalations (2 mg Sodium cromoglycate and 200 micrograms salbutamol) four times daily. This is the maximum recommended dose for regular treatment with salbutamol.

In patients who experience exercise-induced asthma, one of the scheduled doses may be administered a few minutes prior to exercise. In the event of isolated episodes of breakthrough wheezing an additional dose of two inhalations may be administered. If the patient experiences breakthrough symptoms regularly or notices the effectiveness of the inhaler in relieving bronchospasm is diminishing they should be advised to seek medical advice.

*Children:* Aerocrom is not recommended for use in children.

*Contra-indications:* Aerocrom is contra-indicated in patients with a history of hypersensitivity to any of the ingredients. Not for use in children.

*Special warnings and special precautions for use:* Patients who experience breakthrough wheezing regularly should be advised to obtain medical advice. Aerocrom Inhaler is not for use in acute attacks but for regular maintenance treatment. If the patient notices that the effectiveness of the inhaler in relieving bronchospasm or symptoms is diminishing they should be advised to seek further medical advice.

Aerocrom should be administered with caution to patients suffering from thyrotoxicosis. Potentially serious hypokalaemia may result from beta$_2$-agonist therapy.

If it is necessary to withdraw this treatment, it should normally be done progressively over a period of one week. Symptoms of asthma may recur.

*Interactions with other medicaments and other forms of interaction:* Potentially serious hypokalaemia may result from beta$_2$-agonist therapy. Particular caution is advised in severe asthma as this effect may be potentiated by concomitant treatment with xanthine derivatives, steroids, diuretics and by hypoxia. It is recommended that serum potassium levels be monitored in such situations. Non-selective beta-blockers such as propranolol should not usually be prescribed with Aerocrom.

*Use during pregnancy and lactation:* As with all medicines, administration during pregnancy should only be considered if the expected benefit to the mother is greater than any possible risk to the foetus. Particular caution must be exercised during the first trimester of pregnancy.

Both sodium cromoglycate and salbutamol have been in widespread use for many years without apparent effects on foetal development. However, there is little published evidence concerning safety in early human pregnancy. Animal studies with salbutamol are reported as showing evidence of some harmful effects on the foetus at high dose levels.

It is not known whether sodium cromoglycate is excreted in breast milk. On the basis of animal studies this is unlikely. There is no information to suggest that the use of sodium cromoglycate by nursing mothers has any undesirable effects on the nursing infant. However, as salbutamol is reported as probably being excreted in breast milk the use of Aerocrom in nursing mothers needs to be carefully considered.

The effect of salbutamol on neonates is not known. The use of Aerocrom should be limited to cases where the expected benefit to the mother outweighs any potential risk to the neonate.

*Effects on ability to drive and use machines:* Aerocrom has no known effects on ability to drive or operate machinery.

*Undesirable effects:* Some patients may experience mild tremor, throat irritation, coughing, headache, transient muscle cramps, bronchospasm or rash particularly when treatment is first started.

Very rarely following administration of sodium cromoglycate or salbutamol by inhalation, severe bronchospasm associated with a marked fall in pulmonary function has been reported. Hypersensitivity reactions such as angioedema, urticaria, hypotension and collapse have been reported very rarely in association with the use of salbutamol. In such cases Aerocrom should be stopped immediately and not be reintroduced. Medical advice should be sought. Consideration should be given to the introduction of other anti-inflammatory asthma therapy.

*Overdose:* Overdosage with Aerocrom leading to signs of excessive beta-stimulation may be managed by the administration of a cardioselective beta-blocking agent, but such drugs should be used with caution in patients with a history of bronchospasm. No action other than medical observation should be necessary for overdosage with sodium cromoglycate.

## Pharmacological properties

*Pharmacodynamic properties:* Sodium cromoglycate is believed to act by inhibiting the release of chemical mediators from sensitised mast cells, thereby preventing the allergic reaction in the lung. This inhibition prevents the asthmatic response. Salbutamol is a direct-acting sympathomimetic agent with predominantly beta-adrenergic activity and a selective action on beta$_2$-receptors. When applied topically to the lungs this action is seen as a sustained bronchodilation.

*Pharmacokinetic properties:* Sodium cromoglycate: Following inhalation as a fine powder, about 8% of the dose is reported to be deposited in the lungs, from where it is rapidly absorbed and excreted unchanged in the urine and bile. The majority of an inhaled dose is swallowed and excreted unchanged via the alimentary canal.

Salbutamol: As with sodium cromoglycate much of the inhaled dose is swallowed. Oral salbutamol is well absorbed from the gut giving peak plasma concentrations about 3 hours after administration. Salbutamol is subject to extensive first pass metabolism; 50% is excreted in the urine as an inactive sulphate conjugate. The remainder is excreted unchanged. Absorption from the lung is slower giving peak plasma concentrations about 3–5 hours after administration. The half life is similarly prolonged.

*Preclinical safety data:* Animal studies have shown that sodium cromoglycate has a very low order of local or systemic toxicity. The safety of salbutamol has been established during more than 20 years of worldwide clinical use.

## Pharmaceutical particulars

*List of excipients:* Sorbitan trioleate; propellant mixture 12:114 (dichlorodifluoromethane and dichlorotetrafluoroethane, 60:40% w/w).

*Incompatibilities:* None known.

*Shelf life:* 36 months.

*Special precautions for storage:* Store below 25°C. The aerosol canister is pressurised and should be protected from direct sunlight, heat and frost and must not be punctured or burnt even when empty. As with most other inhaled medications in aerosol canisters, the therapeutic effect of Aerocrom may decrease when the canister is cold.

*Nature and contents of container:*
Aerocrom Inhaler: A pressurised aerosol containing sodium cromoglycate and salbutamol sulphate as a suspension in compressed, liquefied propellant gas mixture. The aluminium can is fitted with a metering valve (delivering 200 actuations) and a plastic valve cover.

Aerocrom Syncroner: The cartoned pack contains an aerosol canister, a moulded polyethylene mouthpiece with a spacer device fitted with a dustcap and instructions for use.

**Marketing authorisation number** PL 0113/0165.

**Date of approval/revision of SPC** January 1995.

Legal category POM.

# ALGICON* TABLETS AND SUSPENSION

## Presentation

*Tablets:* White tablet marked with the product name on one side and 'RORER' on reverse.

Each tablet contains magnesium alginate 500 mg, aluminium hydroxide/magnesium carbonate co-gel 360 mg, Magnesium Carbonate Heavy BP 320 mg, Potassium Bicarbonate USP 100 mg. Other ingredients include sucrose.

*Suspension:* Algicon Suspension–A yellow suspension with odour and taste of lemon and mint.

Each 5 ml contains: magnesium alginate 250 mg, aluminium hydroxide/magnesium carbonate co-gel 140 mg, Magnesium Carbonate BP 175 mg, Potassium Bicarbonate USP 50 mg. Other ingredients include parabens.

**Uses** Heartburn, indigestion, excess stomach acid.

**Dosage and administration** For oral administration. *Tablets: Adult dose:* Chew 1 or 2 tablets four times a day or as directed by a physician. Tablets should be taken after meals and at bedtime, or as needed.

*Suspension:* 10 to 20 ml four times a day or as directed by a physician. The suspension should be taken after meals and at bedtime, or as needed. The bottle should be shaken well before use.

*Children:* Not recommended for children under 12 years.

*Elderly:* No special precautions required.

**Contra-indications, warnings, etc** Algicon should not be administered to patients who are severely debilitated or suffering from kidney disease or to patients who are currently taking an antibiotic drug containing tetracycline. Due to the high sugar content of the tablets, care should be exercised in the treatment of diabetic patients with this dosage presentation.

*Use in pregnancy:* There is no information on the use of Algicon in pregnancy.

*Overdosage:* In overdose, abdominal distension is the most likely occurrence and appropriate conservative measures should be taken.

**Pharmaceutical precautions** *Tablets:* Store below 25°C in a dry place.
*Suspension:* Mix well before use. Do not freeze.

**Legal category** GSL.

**Package quantities** *Tablets:* Cartons containing 60 blister-packed tablets.
*Suspension:* Bottles containing 500 ml of suspension.

**Further information** The product contains an alginate combined with an antacid which, on reaction with the gastric contents of the stomach, forms an insoluble gel-like layer above the stomach contents, which impedes reflux and provides a demulcent action.

The product has a low sodium content of less than 10 mg per tablet, and less than 10 mg per 10 ml of suspension.

**Product licence numbers**
Tablets           5272/0010
Suspension     5272/0009

# ASCABIOL* EMULSION 25% W/V

**Qualitative and quantitative composition** Benzyl benzoate BP 25% w/v.

**Pharmaceutical form** White emulsion.

**Clinical particulars**

*Therapeutic indications:* Ascabiol is an efficient acaricide and is indicated for the treatment of scabies and pediculosis.

*Posology and method of administration:* Topical.

*Adults: Scabies*–after a hot bath and drying, Ascabiol is applied to the whole body except the head and face. If the application is thorough, one treatment should suffice, but the possibility of failure is lessened if a second application is made within five days of the first.

Alternatively Ascabiol can be applied to the whole body, except the head and face, on three occasions at 12-hourly intervals. The patient has a hot bath 12 hours after the last application and changes to clean clothes and sheets.

*Pediculosis*–the affected region is coated with Ascabiol followed by a wash 24 hours later with soap and water. In severe cases this procedure may need to be repeated two or three times. An examination should always be made a week after the last treatment to confirm disinfestation.

*Elderly patients:* No specific recommendations.

*Children:* Ascabiol can be diluted with an equal quantity of water for older children and with three parts of water for babies.

*Contra-indications:* None.

*Special warnings and special precautions for use:* The emulsion may damage plastic or acrylic bathroom furniture, Care should be taken not to splash the emulsion on such surfaces.

*Interaction with other medicaments and other forms of interaction:* Not applicable.

*Pregnancy and lactation:* There is inadequate evidence of the safety of Ascabiol in human pregnancy, but it has been in widespread use for many years without apparent ill consequence. Nevertheless Ascabiol should not be used during pregnancy unless considered essential.

Breast feeding should be suspended during treatment with Ascabiol. Feeding may be restarted after the emulsion has been washed off the body.

*Effects on ability to drive and use machines:* Not applicable.

*Undesirable effects:* Ascabiol causes little skin irritation, but may cause a transient burning sensation. This is usually mild but can occasionally be severe in sensitive individuals. In the event of a severe skin reaction the preparation should be washed off using soap and warm water. Ascabiol is also irritating to the eyes therefore these should be protected if it is applied to the scalp.

*Overdose:* If Ascabiol is accidentally taken by mouth, treatment should consist of gastric lavage or the administration of an emetic. An anticonvulsant should be given if necessary, otherwise treatment is symptomatic.

Urinary retention in adults and convulsions in infants, have been reported following excessive use of topical benzyl benzoate. The body should be washed to remove excess benzyl benzoate. Otherwise treatment is symptomatic.

## Pharmacological properties

*Pharmacodynamic properties:* Benzyl benzoate is lethal to *Sarcoptes scabei* and to the larval and adult forms of head lice.

*Pharmacokinetic properties:* No data available by the topical route.

*Preclinical safety data:* There are no pre-clinical data of relevance to the prescriber which are additional to that already included in other sections of the SPC.

## Pharmaceutical particulars

*List of excipients:* Stearic acid powder, Triethanolamine, Terpineol, Oil Cinnamon Leaf Ceylon, Silicone MS Antifoam A, Demineralised Water,

*Incompatibilities:* Not applicable.

*Shelf life:* 36 months.

*Special precautions for storage:* Store below 25˚C.

*Nature and contents of container:* Amber glass bottles with a screw cap containing 100 ml.

*Instructions for use / handling:* The emulsion may damage plastic or acrylic bathroom furniture. Care should be taken not to splash the emulsion on such surfaces.

**Marketing authorisation number** 0012/5104R.

**Date of approval/revision of SPC** February 1997.

**Legal category** P.

## CALCITARE*

**Presentation** *For intramuscular or subcutaneous use only.* Each vial contains 160 international units Calcitonin (Pork) BP.

**Uses** For short term treatment in
(i) Paget's disease of bone
(ii) *Hypercalcaemia:* The calcium lowering effect of

calcitonin is usually rapid. Treatment should be regarded as an adjunct to more specific long-term measures. The fall in serum calcium is more pronounced in hypercalcaemic patients with a raised bone turnover, e.g. Paget's disease and thyrotoxicosis. Treatment may also be beneficial in patients with hypercalcaemia due to immobilisation in Paget's disease, malignancy, vitamin D intoxication and hyperparathyroidism. Calcitonin is of particular value when such patients have concurrent renal or cardiac failure.

**Dosage and administration** Calcitare can be given subcutaneously or intramuscularly.

1. *Paget's disease of bone:* Clinical and biochemical improvement has been observed with dosage regimens ranging from 80 international units three times a week to 160 international units daily in single or divided doses.

Daily injections of 80 international units or 160 international units are recommended for three to six months in patients with bone pain or nerve compression syndromes.

Clinical improvement is usually seen within three months but may occasionally be delayed for as long as a year. When clinical improvement occurs, an attempt to reduce the dose and/or frequency of injection may be made, consistent with maintaining a remission. Alternatively, treatment can be stopped and restarted at a later date when necessary. Duration of dosage should be a maximum of two six month courses.

Biochemical improvement is shown by a reduction in serum alkaline phosphatase and urinary hydroxyproline excretion, the fall in urinary hydroxyproline often occurring in a matter of days. The fall in serum alkaline phosphatase occurs in a matter of weeks. Serum alkaline phosphatase and urinary hydroxyproline levels return slowly towards pre-treatment values (at different rates) on withdrawal of calcitonin therapy.

When changing from synthetic salmon calcitonin (Calsynar) to porcine calcitonin (Calcitare), 80 international units of Calcitare may be conveniently substituted for 50 international units of Calsynar and 160 international units for 100 international units respectively.

2. *Hypercalcaemia:* The optimum dosage pattern must essentially be gauged by the magnitude of the hypocalcaemic response obtained in a particular patient. In general the greatest response will be observed in cases of rapid bone turnover. Four international units per kg per day of Calcitare may produce a fall in serum calcium. However, larger doses of calcitonin may be necessary, but are inconvenient to administer as Calcitare, in which case treatment with Calsynar is advised.

*Elderly:* No special precautions.

*Children:* Calcitare should not be given to children for more than a few weeks unless the physician considers that longer treatment is indicated on compelling medical grounds; careful surveillance of bone growth is recommended.

**Contra-indications, warnings, etc** A species and strain-specific dose-related increase of pituitary adenomas has been observed in long term toxicity studies in the rat. As the significance of these findings to man is uncertain, long term use is not recommended.

Calcitonin may cause nausea, vomiting, facial flushing and tingling of the hands. An unpleasant taste and inflammatory reactions at the injection site have been reported. The nausea and flushing are usually transient and rarely necessitate withdrawal of treatment. If necessary, the injections can be administered at night with an antiemetic. Administration of Calcitare has been reported in a few cases to cause serious allergic type reactions which should be differentiated from generalised flushing and hypotension.

In any patient with a history of allergy, a scratch (or intradermal) test should be conducted prior to administration of Calcitare using a 1:100 dilution in Sodium Chloride Injection BP. To detect gelatin sensitivity a similar test should be carried out using gelatin diluent in the same dilution.

Some patients will develop porcine calcitonin binding antibodies after several months of treatment. The antibodies are generally of low titre and are more likely to occur in patients on the higher doses. The development of these antibodies is not usually related to loss of clinical efficacy. It is possible that this may be analogous to treated diabetic patients in whom insulin binding antibodies frequently develop, but who rarely manifest clinical resistance to insulin. The presence of these antibodies appears to bear no relationship to allergic reactions which are very rare. Secondary hyperparathyroidism is not thought to occur following calcitonin therapy.

There are several reports of the value of calcitonin in the acute treatment of severe hypercalcaemia in patients with concurrent renal or cardiac failure; however, care should be exercised when treating such patients.

Trace amounts of $T_3/T_4$ are present in Calcitare.

Experience over a number of years has not revealed any significant metabolic effects due to $T_3$ and $T_4$ when Calcitare has been given at the maximum recommended dose for Paget's disease of 160 international units daily. At higher doses (e.g. 4 international units/kg) used in the treatment of hypercalcaemia, the amounts of $T_3/T_4$ normally detected in the product are most unlikely to have any adverse effect, except in highly susceptible patients such as those with significant ischaemic heart disease.

*Use in pregnancy and lactation:* Studies have not been carried out in pregnant patients. Animal studies have suggested a possible relationship between calcitonin and retardation of foetal growth and inhibition of lactation. Unless considered essential, calcitonin should not be used in women of child bearing potential or nursing mothers.

*Treatment of overdosage:* No specific antidote. Following overdosage, e.g., 600 international units as a single injection one might experience flushing of the face and/or extremities or gastrointestinal disturbance. Acute hypocalcaemia is unlikely to occur.

**Pharmaceutical precautions** Calcitare is presented as a sterile, lyophilised powder providing 160 international units porcine calcitonin per vial. Calcitare should normally be used immediately after aseptic reconstitution. The reconstituted product will, however, maintain its potency for up to 24 hours at room temperature or 7 days in a refrigerator (2˚–8˚C) Typically, however, the reconstituted product should be stored at 2˚–8˚C and used within 48 hours.

The lyophilised powder when stored at less than 25˚C will retain its potency for three years.

**Legal category** POM.

**Package quantities** *For intramuscular or subcutaneous use:* Boxes of 5 vials Calcitare 160 international units per vial sterile, lyophilised, with 5 ampoules gelatin diluent, sterile (2 ml).

Boxes of 10 vials Calcitare 160 international units per vial sterile, lyophilised, with 10 ampoules gelatin diluent, sterile (2 ml).

**Further information** The calcium lowering ability of the calcitonins is measured in international units. The international unit is based on a rat bioassay in which one fortieth of the weight of salmon calcitonin, as compared with weights of porcine and human calcitonin, produces the same fall in serum calcium. The weights of pure calcitonin equivalent to 100 international units in this assay are: human calcitonin, 1 mg porcine calcitonin, 1 mg, and salmon calcitonin 0.025 mg.

**Product licence number** 00012/0296

## CALSYNAR*

### Presentation

*Multidose vials:* An aqueous solution containing 400 international units of synthetic Salmon Calcitonin in 2 mls of solution. The injection also contains Sodium Chloride, Sodium Acetate, Acetic Acid and Phenol.

*Ampoule:* An aqueous solution containing 100 international units of Synthetic Salmon Calcitonin in 1 ml of solution. The injection also contains Sodium Chloride, Sodium Acetate and Acetic Acid.

**Uses** For the short term treatment of:
a. Paget's disease of bone.
b. Advancing osteolytic hypercalcaemia of malignancy.
c. Pain associated with advanced metastatic bone cancer: The use of Calsynar has been reported to be beneficial in the relief of pain in some patients with advanced metastatic bone cancer.
d. Postmenopausal osteoporosis: Studies based on total body calcium determinations have indicated that Calsynar may be effective in the prevention of progressive loss of bone mass in the treatment of postmenopausal osteoporosis.

**Dosage and administration** For subcutaneous or intramuscular use only.

*(a) Paget's disease of bone:* Clinical and biochemical improvement has been observed with dosage regimens ranging from 50 international units three times a week to 100 international units daily in single or divided doses.

When clinical improvement occurs, a dosage reduction may maintain a remission in some patients. Alternatively, treatment can be stopped and restarted at a later date when necessary.

Biochemical improvement is shown by a reduction in serum alkaline phosphatase and urinary hydroxyproline excretion, the fall in urinary hydroxyproline often occurring in a matter of days, the fall in serum alkaline phosphatase and urinary hydroxyproline levels return slowly towards pretreatment values (at different rates) on withdrawal of calcitonin therapy.

When changing from porcine calcitonin (Calcitare)

to synthetic salmon calcitonin (Calsynar) 50 international units of Calsynar may be conveniently substituted for 80 international units of Calcitare and 100 international units for 160 international units of Calcitare.

*(b) Advancing osteolytic hypercalcaemia of malignancy:* Treatment should be adjusted to the patient's clinical and biochemical response.

Severe hypercalcaemia may require high doses of Calsynar and initially 400 international units may be given every 6 or 8 hours. Lower doses may be satisfactory in some patients and dosage may be adjusted according to the patient's clinical and biochemical response. There is no additional benefit to be gained from doses in excess of 8 international units per kg given every 6 hours.

*(c) Pain associated with metastatic bone cancer:* The usual dose is 200 international units, 6-hourly or 400 international units 12-hourly for 48 hours. Concomitant analgesic medication may be reduced as appropriate. The treatment course may be repeated at the discretion of the physician.

Many patients with advanced malignant disease already suffer from anorexia and nausea. In these cases, prior administration of anti-emetic therapy may reduce the incidence of nausea and vomiting sometimes associated with calcitonin therapy.

*(d) Post menopausal osteoporosis:* The recommended dose of Calsynar is 100 international units per day. Patients should also receive supplementary calcium (equivalent to 600 mg elemental calcium daily) and vitamin D (400 units daily). An adequate diet is also essential. (See also 'Further Information').

*Elderly:* No special precautions.

*Children:* Calsynar should not be given to children for periods of more than a few weeks unless the physician considers that longer treatment is indicated on compelling medical grounds. Careful surveillance of bone growth is recommended.

### Contra-indications, warnings, etc
*Precautions:* Rat carcinogenicity studies have shown a dose related excess of pituitary tumours. As the significance of this finding is uncertain, long term use is not recommended.

There are several reports of the value of Calcitonin in the acute treatment of severe hypercalcaemia in patients with concurrent renal or cardiac failure, however, care should be exercised when treating such patients.

Following injections of calcitonin serum calcium levels may be transiently lowered to below normal values. This effect is noted most frequently on initiation of therapy where bone turnover is abnormally high, but diminishes as osteoclastic activity is reduced with Calsynar. Whilst this phenomenon does not usually give rise to complications, care should be exercised in patients who are receiving concurrent cardiac glycosides as dosage adjustments of these drugs may be necessary in view of the fact that their effect may be modified by changes in cellular electrolyte concentrations.

Prior to treatment with Calsynar any patients with a history of allergy should undergo a scratch (or intradermal) test using a 1:100 dilution of Calsynar in Sodium Chloride injection BP.

*Side-effects:* Calcitonin may cause nausea, vomiting, facial flushing, tingling of the hands and an unpleasant taste. Inflammatory reactions at the injection site have been reported. The nausea and flushing are usually transient and rarely necessitate withdrawal of treatment. If necessary, the injections can be administered at night with an antiemetic.

Some patients will develop salmon calcitonin binding antibodies after several months of treatment. The antibodies are generally of low titre and are more likely to occur in patients on the higher doses. The development of these antibodies is not usually related to loss of clinical efficacy. It is possible that this may be analogous to treated diabetic patients in whom insulin binding antibodies frequently develop, but who rarely manifest clinical resistance to insulin. The presence of antibodies appears to bear no relationship to allergic reactions which are very rare. Secondary hyperparathyroidism is not thought to occur following calcitonin therapy.

Administration of salmon calcitonin has been reported in a few cases to cause serious allergic type reactions (e.g. bronchospasm, swelling of the tongue or throat and anaphylactic shock). Allergic reactions should be differentiated from generalised flushing and hypotension.

*Use in pregnancy and lactation:* Studies have not been carried out in pregnant women. Animal studies have suggested a possible relationship between Calcitonin and retardation of foetal growth and inhibition of lactation. Hence unless considered essential, Calcitonin should not be used in women of child bearing potential or nursing mothers.

*Treatment of overdosage:* Symptoms following overdosage, e.g. 400 international units administered as a single injection, may include flushing of the face and or extremities, and gastrointestinal disturbance. Acute hypocalcaemia is unlikely to occur. There is no specific antidote.

### Pharmaceutical precautions
*Calsynar multidose vials:* Store between 2–8°C. Do not freeze.

*Calsynar ampoules:* Store between 2–8°C. Do not freeze.

### Legal category   POM.

### Package quantities   Multidose vial: Box of 1 and cartons of 4 vials. Ampoules: Cartons of 5.

### Further information
*Postmenopausal osteoporosis:* There is evidence from published literature on postmenopausal osteoporosis that cyclical therapy may be useful in some patients.

*Units and potency:* The calcium lowering ability of the calcitonins is measured in international units. The international unit is based on a rat bioassay in which one fortieth of the weight of salmon calcitonin, as compared with weights of porcine and human calcitonin, produces the same fall in serum calcium. The weights of pure calcitonin equivalent to 100 international units in this assay are approximately: human calcitonin 1 mg; porcine calcitonin 1 mg and salmon calcitonin 0.025 mg.

### Product licence numbers
Multidose vials:      00012/0297
Ampoules:             00012/0298

## CAMPTO*   ▼

**Qualitative and quantitative composition** Vials of Campto contain 40 mg or 100 mg of irinotecan hydrochloride, trihydrate.

**Pharmaceutical form** Concentrate for infusion.

**Clinical particulars**

*Therapeutic indications:* Campto is indicated for the second-line treatment of adult patients with metastatic colorectal cancer who have failed an established 5-fluorouracil (5FU) containing treatment regimen.

*Posology and method of administration:* Recommended dosage: The recommended dosage of Campto is 350 mg/m² administered as an intravenous infusion over a 30 to 90 minute period every three weeks (see *Instructions For Use/Handling* section).

*Dosage adjustments:* In patients who experienced asymptomatic severe neutropenia (neutrophil count <500 cells/mm³), fever or infections associated with neutropenia (temperature ≤ 38°C and neutrophil count ≥1,000 cells/mm³) or severe diarrhoea (requiring an intravenous rehydration), dosage should be reduced from 350 mg/m² to 300 mg/m² in subsequent cycles. If at 300 mg/m², the patient again experiences severe neutropenia, fever or infections associated with neutropenia as defined above or severe diarrhoea, the dosage should be decreased from 300 mg/m² to 250 mg/m² at the next cycle.

*Delayed dosing:* Campto should not be administered until the neutrophil count returns to above 1,500 cells/mm³. In patients who experienced severe neutropenia or severe gastrointestinal adverse events such as diarrhoea, nausea and vomiting, (see *Special Warnings and Special Precautions for Use* section), dosing of Campto® should be delayed until there has been a full recovery of these symptoms, especially diarrhoea.

*Treatment duration:* Treatment with Campto should be continued until there is an objective progression of the disease or an unacceptable toxicity.

*Special populations: Patients with Impaired Hepatic Function:* In patients with a bilirubin ≤ 1.5 times the upper limit of the normal range (ULN), a dose of 350 mg/m² Campto remains recommended. In patients with a bilirubin > 1.5 times the ULN, patients should not be treated with Campto (see *Contraindications* and *Special warnings and special precautions for use* sections).
*Patients with impaired renal function:* Campto is not recommended for use in patients with impaired renal function, as studies in this population have not been conducted. (see *Special warnings and special precautions for use* and *Pharmacokinetic properties*).
*Elderly:* No specific pharmacokinetic studies have been performed in the elderly. However, the dose should be chosen carefully in this population due to their greater frequency of decreased biological functions, in particular hepatic function (see *Special warnings and special precautions for use*).

*Contra-indications:* Campto is contra-indicated in patients who have chronic inflammatory bowel disease and/or bowel obstruction (see *Special warnings and special precautions for use*). Campto is contra-indicated in patients who have a history of severe

hypersensitivity reactions to irinotecan hydrochloride trihydrate or to one of the excipients of Campto. Campto is contra-indicated during pregnancy and lactation (see *Pregnancy and lactation* and *Special warnings and special precautions for use* sections). Campto is contra-indicated in patients with a bilirubin >1.5 times the upper limit of the normal range (see *Special warnings and special precautions for use* section). Campto is contra-indicated in patients with severe bone marrow failure. Campto is contra-indicated in patients with WHO performance status >2.

*Special warnings and special precautions for use:* The use of Campto should be confined to units specialised in the administration of cytotoxic chemotherapy and it should only be administered under the supervision of a qualified oncologist. It is strongly recommended that Campto be administered only in Healthcare institutions with adequately equipped facilities, including an intensive care unit.

Given the nature and incidence of adverse events, Campto will only be prescribed in the following cases after the expected benefits have been weighed against the possible therapeutic risks: in patients presenting a risk factor, particularly those with a WHO performance status = 2. in the few rare instances where patients are deemed unlikely to observe recommendations regarding management of side effects (need for immediate and prolonged antidiarrheal treatment combined with high fluid intake at onset of delayed diarrhoea). Strict hospital supervision is recommended for such patients.

Campto should not be administered as an intravenous bolus or an intravenous infusion shorter than 30 minutes. and longer than 90 minutes (see *Posology and method of administration* section)

*Delayed diarrhoea:* Patients should be made aware of the risk of delayed diarrhoea occurring more than 24 hours after the administration of Campto and at any time before the next cycle. They should quickly inform their physician of its occurrence and start appropriate therapy immediately. Patients with an increased risk of diarrhoea are those who had a previous abdominal/pelvic radiotherapy, those with baseline hyperleucocytosis and those with performance status ≥ 2. If not properly treated, diarrhoea can be life-threatening, especially if the patient is concomitantly neutropenic. As soon as the first liquid stool occurs, the patient should start drinking large volumes of beverages containing electrolytes and an appropriate antidiarrhoeal therapy must be initiated immediately. This antidiarrhoeal treatment will be prescribed by the department where Campto has been administered. After discharge from the hospital, the patients should obtain the prescribed drugs so that they can treat the diarrhoea as soon as it occurs. In addition, they must inform their physician or the department administering Campto when/if diarrhoea is occurring. The currently recommended antidiarrhoeal treatment consists in high doses of loperamide (2 mg every 2 hours). This therapy should continue for 12 hours after the last liquid stool and should not be modified. In no instance should loperamide be administered for more than 48 consecutive hours at these doses, because of the risk of paralytic ileus. If the diarrhoea is severe (requiring an intravenous rehydration) or accompanied by vomiting or fever, the patient must be hospitalised for treatment (including a broad-spectrum antibiotic) in an intensive care unit. If mild to moderate diarrhoea (≤ 6 stools per day with moderate cramping) does not resolve within the first 48 hours, prophylaxis with oral broad-spectrum antibiotics should be initiated immediately, since there is a high risk of concomitant severe neutropenia in patients with diarrhoea. If at any time, severe neutropenia concomitant with diarrhoea is identified, an oral prophylactic antibiotic should be initiated. Loperamide should not be given prophylactically, even in patients who experienced delayed diarrhoea at previous cycles. In patients who experienced severe diarrhoea, a reduction in dose is recommended (see *Posology and method of administration* section).

*Haematology:* Weekly monitoring of complete blood cell counts is recommended during Campto treatment. Patients should be aware of the risk of neutropenia and the significance of fever. Febrile neutropenia (temperature ≥ 38°C and neutrophil count ≤1,000 cells/mm³) should be urgently treated in the hospital with broad-spectrum intravenous antibiotics. Campto administration should be delayed until the neutrophil count is ≥ 1,500 cells/mm³. In patients who experienced severe asymptomatic neutropenia (< 500 cells/mm³), fever or infections associated with neutropenia (temperature ≥ 38°C and neutrophil count >1,000 cells/mm³), the dose of Campto should be reduced (see *Posology and method of administration* section). There is an increased risk of infections and haematological toxicity in patients with severe diarrhoea. In patients with severe diarrhoea, complete blood cell counts should be performed.

*Liver impairment:* Liver function tests should be

performed at baseline and before each cycle. Patients with impaired liver function (bilirubin 1-1.5 times the ULN and transaminases >5 times the ULN) are at greater risk of developing febrile neutropenia or severe neutropenia. Campto should not be used in patients with a bilirubin 1-1.5 times the ULN (see *Contraindications* section) and the patients with bilirubin 1-1.5 times the ULN should be closely monitored.

*Nausea and vomiting:* A prophylactic treatment with an antiemetic is recommended before each treatment with Campto. Nausea and vomiting have been frequently reported. Patients with vomiting associated with delayed diarrhoea should be hospitalised as soon as possible for treatment.

*Acute cholinergic syndrome:* If acute cholinergic syndrome appears (defined as early diarrhoea plus symptoms such as sweating, abdominal cramping, lachrymation, myosis and salivation), atropine sulphate (0.25 mg subcutaneously) should be administered unless clinically contraindicated (see *Undesirable effects* section). Caution should be exercised in patients with asthma. In patients who experienced an acute and severe cholinergic syndrome, the use of prophylactic atropine sulphate is recommended with subsequent doses of Campto.

*Elderly:* Due to the greater frequency of decreased biological functions, in particular hepatic function, in elderly patients, dose selection with Campto should be cautious in this population (see *Posology and method of administration* section).

*Patients with bowel obstruction:* Patients must not be treated with Campto until resolution of the bowel obstruction (see *Contra-indications*).

*Patients with impaired renal function:* Studies in this population have not been conducted. (see *Posology and method of administration* and *Pharmacokinetic properties*).

*Others:* Contraceptive measures must be taken during and for at least three months after cessation of therapy.

*Interaction with other medicaments and other forms of interaction:* There have been no clinical studies to evaluate the drug interactions of irinotecan with other drugs.

Interaction between irinotecan and neuromuscular blocking agents cannot be ruled out. Drugs with anticholinesterase activity may prolong the neuromuscular blocking effects of suxamethonium and the neuromuscular blockade of non-depolarising drugs may be antagonised.

Loperamide should not be given prophylactically.

*Pregnancy and lactation*
*Pregnancy:* There is no information on the use of Campto in pregnant women. Campto has been shown to be embryotoxic, foetotoxic and teratogenic in rabbits and rats. Therefore, Campto must not be used during pregnancy. Women of childbearing age receiving Campto should be advised to avoid becoming pregnant, and to inform the treating physician immediately should this occur (see *Contra-indications* and *Special warnings and special precautions for use*).

*Lactation:* In lactating rats, $^{14}$C-irinotecan was detected in milk. It is not known whether irinotecan is excreted in human milk. Consequently, because of the potential for adverse reactions in nursing infants, breast-feeding must be discontinued for the duration of Campto therapy (see *Contra-indications*).

*Effects on ability to drive and use machines:* Patients should be warned about the potential for dizziness or visual disturbances which may occur within 24 hours following the administration of Campto, and advised not to drive or operate machinery if these symptoms occur.

*Undesirable effects:* The adverse reactions considered to be possibly or probably related to the administration of Campto at the recommended dose of 350 mg/m², have been obtained from 455 patients (2381 treatment cycles).

*Delayed diarrhoea:* Diarrhoea (occurring more than 24 hours after administration) is a dose-limiting toxicity of Campto. It occurred in 87% of patients (severe in 38.5%) during 61% of the cycles (severe in 14%). In one study including 107 patients who complied strictly with the recommendations for management of delayed diarrhoea, severe diarrhoea occurred in 26% of the patients. The median time of onset of the first liquid stool was on day 5 after the infusion of Campto. Uncommon cases of pseudomembranous colitis have been reported, one of which has been documented bacteriologically (*Clostridium difficile*).

*Haematology* Neutropenia is a dose-limiting toxic effect. Neutropenia was observed in 78.7 % of patients and was severe (neutrophil count < 1,000 cells/mm³) in 39.6% of patients. Of the evaluable cycles, 18% had a neutrophil count below 1,000 cells/mm³ including 7.6% with a neutrophil count <500 cells/mm³. Neutro-

penia was reversible and not cumulative; the median day to nadir was 8 days and total recovery was usually reached by day 22. Fever with severe neutropenia was reported in 6.2% of patients (1.7% of cycles). Infectious episodes occurred in about 10.3% of patients (2.5 % of cycles) and were associated with severe neutropenia in about 5.3 % of patients (1.1 % of cycles) and resulted in death in 2 cases. Anaemia was reported in about 58.7% of patients (8% with haemoglobin < 8 g/dl and 0.9% with haemoglobin < 6.5 g/dl). Thrombocytopenia (≤ 100,000 cells/mm³) was observed in 7.4% of patients and 1.8% of cycles (platelets count ≤ 50,000 cells/mm³ occurred in 0.9% of patients and 0.2% of cycles). Nearly all the patients showed a recovery by day 22. One case of peripheral thrombocytopenia with antiplatelet antibodies has been reported in the post-marketing experience.

*Nausea and vomiting* during the first day of infusion or more than 24 hours after the administration occurred in approximately 84.4% of patients (severe in about 19%) during 56.3% of cycles (severe in 6.9%).

*Acute cholinergic syndrome* Transient acute cholinergic syndrome was observed in about 83% of patients (49.1% of cycles) and was rarely severe. The main symptoms were defined as early diarrhoea plus symptoms such as abdominal pain, conjunctivitis, rhinitis, hypotension, vasodilation, sweating, chills, malaise, dizziness, visual disturbances, myosis, lachrymation and increased salivation occurring during or within the first 24 hours after the infusion of Campto.

*Laboratory tests* Transient and mild to moderate increases in serum levels of either transaminases, alkaline phosphatase or bilirubin were observed in 9.2%, 8.1% and 1.8% of the patients, respectively, in the absence of progressive liver metastasis. Transient and mild to moderate increases of serum levels of creatinine have been observed in 7.3% of the patients.

*Other effects* Early effects such as dyspnoea, muscular contraction or cramps and paresthesia have been reported. Asthenia was experienced by approximately 73.4% of patients and was severe in 17.6% of patients. The causal relationship to Campto has not been clearly established. Alopecia was observed in about 86% of the patients. Constipation relative to Campto and/or loperamide has been observed in about 3.3% of patients (1.1% of cycles). Fever in the absence of infection or severe neutropenia occurred in 12% of the patients. Episodes of dehydration commonly associated with diarrhoea and/or vomiting have been reported. Other mild effects include anorexia, cutaneous reactions, abdominal pain and mucositis. Allergy and infusion site reactions have been reported, although uncommonly.

*Overdose:* There have been no reports of overdosage. Doses as high as 750 mg/m² have been used in a phase I study under careful monitoring. The most significant adverse reactions reported were severe neutropenia and diarrhoea. Consequently, in case of overdosage, the patients should be kept in a specialised unit. There is no known antidote for Campto.

### Pharmacological properties

*Pharmacodynamic properties:* Cytostatic topoisomerase I inhibitor.
*Experimental data:* Irinotecan is a semi-synthetic derivative of camptothecin. It is an antineoplastic agent which acts as a specific inhibitor of DNA topoisomerase I. It is metabolised by carboxylesterase in most tissues to SN-38, which was found to be more active than irinotecan in inhibiting purified topoisomerase I and more cytotoxic than irinotecan against several murine and human tumour cell lines. The inhibition of DNA topoisomerase I by irinotecan or SN-38 induces single-strand DNA lesions which blocks the DNA replication fork and are responsible for the cytotoxicity. This cytotoxic activity was found to be time-dependent and was specific to the S phase. *In vitro*, irinotecan and SN-38 were not found to be significantly recognised by the P-glycoprotein$^{MDR}$, and displays cytotoxic activities against doxorubicin and vinblastine resistant cell lines. Furthermore, irinotecan has a broad antitumour activity *in vivo* against murine tumour models (P03 pancreatic ductal adenocarcinoma, MA16/C mammary adenocarcinoma, C38 and C51 colon adenocarcinomas) and against human xenografts (Co-4 colon adenocarcinoma, Mx-1 mammary adenocarcinoma, C38 and C51 colon adenocarcinomas) and against human xenografts (Co-4 colon adenocarcinomas, Mx-1 mammary adenocarcinomas, ST-15 and SC-16 gastric adenocarcinomas). Irinotecan is also active against tumours expressing the P-glycoprotein$^{MDR}$ (vincristine- and doxorubicin-resistant P388 leukaemia's). Beside the antitumour activity of Campto, the most relevant pharmacological effect of irinotecan is the inhibition of acetylcholinesterase.

*Clinical data:* Clinical data from 4 phase II studies involving a total of 455 patients in 63 centers support the use of Campto in patients with metastatic colorectal cancer who have failed a previous 5-FU regimen. These studies were designed to evaluate the activity on tumour growth in patients with documented

progression on 5-FU at study entry. At 6 months, the progression-free survival was 30%. This illustrates the lack of clinical cross-resistance of Campto to 5-fluorouracil. Due to the lack of data from comparative studies, the definite clinical benefit, in terms of survival and quality of life, has not yet been established.

*Pharmacokinetic/Pharmacodynamic data:* The intensity of the major toxicities encountered with Campto (e.g., leuconeutropenia and diarrhoea) are related to the exposure (AUC) to parent drug and metabolite SN-38. Significant correlations were observed between haematological toxicity (decrease in white blood cells and neutrophils at nadir) or diarrhoea intensity and both irinotecan and metabolite SN-38 AUC values.

*Pharmacokinetic properties:* The pharmacokinetic properties of both irinotecan and SN-38 (its active metabolite) were evaluated in 60 patients during phase I studies using the recommended dosage regimen, i.e. 30-minute intravenous infusion of 100 to 750 mg/m². The kinetic profile of irinotecan is dose independent. The different irinotecan administration schedules investigated were pharmacokinetically similar in patients enrolled in the clinical trials.

The plasma decay was either biphasic or triphasic. The mean plasma half-life of the first phase of the triphasic model was 12 minutes, the second phase was 2.5 hours, and the terminal phase half-life was 14.2 hours. The mean irinotecan and SN-38 peak plasma concentrations, achieved at the end of the infusion at the recommended dose of 350 mg/m², were 7.7μg/ml and 56ng/ml, respectively, with corresponding area under the curve (AUC) values of 34μg.h/ml and 451ng.h/ml. The volume of distribution at steady state (Vdss) was large and remained relatively stable as a function of dose with a mean value of 157 l/m². The total body clearance had a mean value of 15 l/h/m², and did not vary between cycles in the same patient. A wide interindividual variability of pharmacokinetic parameters is observed mainly for SN-38. The mean 24 hour-urinary excretion of irinotecan and SN-38 was 19.9% and 0.25% of the administered dose, respectively. A pharmacokinetic phase II analysis has been performed with irinotecan in 72 cancer patients. Pharmacokinetic parameters estimated by a limited sampling model were very close to those estimated from phase I studies. *In vitro*, the plasma protein binding for irinotecan and SN-38 were approximately 65% and 95% respectively.

*Preclinical safety data::* Irinotecan and SN-38 have been shown to be mutagenic *in vitro* in the chromosomal aberration test on CHO-cells as well as in the *in vivo* micronucleus test in mice. However, they have been shown to be devoid of any mutagenic potential in the Ames test. In rats treated once a week during 13 weeks at the maximum dose of 150 mg/m² (which is less than half the human recommended dose), no treatment related tumours were reported 91 weeks after the end of treatment. Single- and repeated-dose toxicity studies with Campto have been carried out in mice, rats and dogs. The main toxic effects were seen in the haematopoietic and lymphatic systems. In dogs, delayed diarrhoea associated with atrophy and focal necrosis of the intestinal mucosa was reported. Alopecia was also observed in the dog. The severity of these effects was dose-related and reversible.

### Pharmaceutical particulars

*List of excipients:* Sorbitol, lactic acid and water for injections. The pH of the solution is adjusted to 3.5 with sodium hydroxide.

*Incompatibilities:* None known. Do not admix with other medications.

*Shelf life:* The shelf-life of unopened vials is 24 months. The Campto solution should be used immediately after reconstitution as it contains no antibacterial preservative. If reconstitution and dilution are performed under strict aseptic conditions (e.g. on laminar air flow bench) Campto solution should be used (infusion completed) within 12 hours at room temperature or 24 hours if stored 2°-8°C after the first breakage.

*Special precautions for storage* Vials of Campto concentrate for infusion should be protected from light.

*Nature and contents of container:*
Campto 40 mg 2-ml brown glass vial, with a halobutyl rubber closure coated with teflon on the inner side.

Campto 100 mg 5-ml brown glass vial, with a halobutyl rubber closure coated with teflon on the inner side.

*Instructions for use/handling:* As with other antineoplastic agents, Campto must be prepared and handled with caution. The use of glasses, mask and gloves is required. If Campto solution or infusion solution should come into contact with the skin, wash immediately and thoroughly with soap and water. If Campto solution or infusion solution should come into contact with the mucous membranes, wash immediately with water.

*Preparation for the intravenous infusion administration* As with any other injectable drugs, Campto solution must be prepared aseptically (see *Shelf life*). Aseptically withdraw the required amount of Campto solution from the vial with a calibrated syringe and inject into a 250 ml infusion bag or bottle containing either 0.9% sodium chloride solution or 5% dextrose solution. The infusion should then be thoroughly mixed by manual rotation.

Campto infusion solution should be infused into a peripheral or central vein.

Campto should not be delivered as an intravenous bolus or an intravenous infusion shorter than 30 minutes or longer than 90 minutes.

*Disposal:* All materials used for dilution and administration should be disposed of according to hospital standard procedures applicable to cytotoxic agents.

**Marketing authorisation numbers**
Campto 40 mg/2 ml 0012/0302
Campto 100 mg/5 ml 0012/0303

**Date of approval/revision of SPC** 17 October 1996

**Legal category** POM

## CELECTOL* AND CELECTOL* 400

**Qualitative and quantitative composition** Celectol tablets contain 200 mg Celiprolol hydrochloride. Celectol 400 contain 400 mg celiprolol hydrochloride.

**Pharmaceutical form** Celectol tablets are yellow film coated biconvex heart shaped tablets engraved with 200 and a breakline on one face and the Celectol logo on the other face. Celectol 400 are white film coated heart shaped tablets engraved with the Celectol logo on one side and a break line on the other.

**Clinical particulars**
*Therapeutic indications:* The management of mild to moderate hypertension.

*Posology and method of administration:* Oral.
*Adults:* The initial dose is 200 mg orally taken once daily with a glass of water. Celectol should be taken on rising, half an hour before food. If response is inadequate, the dose may be increased to 400 mg once daily. *Elderly:* Dosage as for adults. *Children:* Not recommended.

*Contra-indications:* Second or third degree heart block, severe bradycardia, overt heart failure, cardiogenic shock, severe renal impairment with creatinine clearance less than 15 ml per minute and acute episodes of asthma. Although cardio selective beta blockers may have less effect on lung function than non selective beta blockers, as with all beta blockers these should be avoided in patients with reversible obstructive airways disease unless there are compelling clinical reasons for use. Celectol tablets should not be prescribed for patients being treated with theophylline.

*Special warnings and special precautions for use*: The pharmacokinetics are not significantly different in the elderly, however these patients should be regularly monitored and due regard made for decreased renal and liver function in this age group. Celectol may be used in patients with mild to moderate degrees of reduced renal function as celiprolol is cleared by both renal and non-renal excretory pathways. A reduction in dosage by half may be appropriate in patients with creatinine clearances in the range of 15 to 40 ml per minute. However, careful surveillance of such patients is recommended until steady state blood levels are achieved which typically would be within one week. Celectol is not recommended for patients with creatinine clearance less than 15 ml per minute. Patients with hepatic impairment should also be carefully monitored after commencing therapy.

Sudden withdrawal of beta-adrenoceptor blocking agents in patients with ischaemic heart disease may result in the appearance of anginal attacks of increased frequency or severity or deterioration in cardiac state. Although no adverse effects due to abrupt cessation of Celectol have been seen in clinical trials, gradual discontinuation of therapy is recommended.

Celectol should only be used with caution in patients with controlled congestive cardiac failure. Evidence of decompensation should be regarded as a signal to discontinue therapy.

Celectol therapy must be reported to the anaesthetist prior to general anaesthesia. If it is decided to withdraw the drug before surgery, 48 hours should be allowed to elapse between the last dose and anaesthesia. In the event of continuation of Celectol treatment special care should be exercised when using anaesthetic agents such as ether, cyclopropane or trichloroethylene.

*Interaction with other medicaments and other forms of interaction*: Care should be taken in prescribing a beta- adrenoceptor blocking agent with class I antiarrhythmic agents such as disopyramide.

It has been shown that the bioavailability of celiprolol is impaired when it is given with food. Co-administration of chlorthalidone and hydrochlorothiazide also reduces the bioavailability of celiprolol.

Verapamil and beta blockers both slow A-V conduction and depress myocardial contractility through different mechanisms. When changing from verapamil to celiprolol and vice versa, a period between stopping one and starting the other is recommended. Concomitant administration of both drugs is not recommended and should only be initiated with ECG monitoring. Patients with pre existing conduction abnormalities should not be given the two drugs together.

*Pregnancy and lactation:* The safety of this medicinal product for use in human pregnancy have not been established. An evaluation of experimental animal studies does not indicate direct or indirect harmful effects with respect to reproduction, development of the embryo or foetus, the course of gestation and peri- and post-natal development.

The use of Celectol is not recommended in breast-feeding mothers.

*Effects on ability to drive and use machines:* It has been shown that driving ability is unlikely to be impaired in patients taking Celectol.

*Undesirable effects:* Occasional side effects, which are usually mild and transient have occurred. These include headache, dizziness, fatigue, nausea and somnolence. Additional side effects associated with beta-two agonist activity, tremor and palpitations, have been reported. These effects usually do not require withdrawal of therapy. Depression and hypersensitiviypneumonitis have been reported rarely.

Bronchospasm, skin rashes and/or ocular changes have been reported in association with the use of beta blockers. Celectol should be discontinued if these effects occur.

*Overdose:* No data are available regarding overdose in humans. In the event of excessive bradycardia, intravenous atropine sulphate should be administered without delay to a total dose of 2 mg. Inadequate response requires administration of a bolus dose of glucagon 10 mg intravenously. If required this may be repeated or followed by an intravenous infusion of glucagon 1–10 mg/hr, depending on response. If no response, or glucagon is unavailable, a slow intravenous infusion of isoprenaline with close cardiac monitoring is suggested. Cardiac pacing should be considered in refractory bradycardia and heart block. Hypotension should be treated with intravenous catecholamines including dopamine and dobutamine.

**Pharmacological properties**
*Pharmacodynamic properties:* Celiprolol is a vasoactive beta-1 selective adrenoceptor antagonist with partial beta-2 agonist activity indicated in mild to moderate hypertension. The beta-2 agonist activity is thought to account for its mild vasodilating properties. It lowers blood pressure in hypertensive patients at rest and on exercise. The effects on heart rate and cardiac output are dependant on the pre-existing background level of sympathetic tone.

Under conditions of stress such as exercise celiprolol attenuates chronotropic and inotropic responses to sympathetic stimulation. However, at rest minimal impairment of cardiac function is seen.

Celectol therapy has not been shown to adversely effect plasma lipid profiles.

*Pharmacokinetic properties:* Celiprolol is a hydrophilic compound that is incompletely absorbed from the gastrointestinal tract. Plasma half-life is approximately 5-6 hours and pharmacodynamic effects are present for at least 24 hours. After once daily administration celiprolol is only slightly metabolised before excretion in the bile and urine in almost equal quantities.

It has been shown that the bioavailability of celiprolol is impaired when it is given with food. Co-administration of chlorthalidone, hydrochlorothiazide and theophylline also reduces the bioavailability of celiprolol.

**Pharmaceutical particulars**
*List of excipients: Celectol 400:* Mannitol BP, Microcrystalline Cellulose BP, Croscarmellose Sodium NF, Magnesium Stearate BP, Demineralised Water *Film coating:* Opadry Y-1-7000 (White) contains E464, E171 and polyethylene glycol Opadry YS-1-7006 (Clear) contains E464, and polyethylene glycol.

*Celectol Tablets:* Magnesium stearate, Croscarmellose sodium, microcrystalline cellulose, mannitol. *Film coating* Opadry YS-1-7006, Opadry OY-F-6097

*Incompatibilities:* None stated.

*Shelf life:* 36 months

*Special precautions for storage:* Store below 25°C.

*Nature and contents of container:* Blister packs of 28 tablets.

*Instructions for use/handling:* No special Instructions.

**Marketing authorisation numbers**
Celectol tablets 0012/0231
Celectol 400 0012/0247

**Date of approval/revision of SPC** February 1997

**Legal category** POM

## CERUBIDIN*

**Qualitative and quantitative composition** The active ingredient in Cerubidin is daunorubicin hydrochloride PhEur Each vial contains 21.4 mg daunorubicin hydrochloride (equivalent to 20 mg as base).

**Pharmaceutical form** Vial containing a red lyophilised powder for intravenous administration following reconstitution in Water for Injections and dilution with saline.

**Clinical particulars**
*Therapeutic indications:* Cerubidin is indicated for the following: Inducing remissions of acute myelogenous and lymphocytic leukaemias.

*Posology and method of administration*: For intravenous administration. *Adults*: 40-60 mg/m² on alternate days for a course of up to three injections for the induction of remissions.
*Acute myelogenous leukaemia*: The recommended dose is 45 mg/m²/day

*Acute lymphoctyic leukemia:* The recommended dose is 45 mg/m²/day.

*Children: Over 2 years* - Same as for adults. *Under 2 years or if less than 0.5 m² surface area*: 1 mg/m²/day.

*Elderly*: Cerubidin should be used with care in patients with inadequate bone marrow reserves due to old age. A reduction of 50% in dosage is recommended.

The number of injections required varies widely from patient to patient and must be determined in each case according to response and tolerance.

The dosage should be reduced in patients with impaired hepatic or renal function. A 25% reduction is recommended in patients with serum bilirubin concentrations of 20-50µmol/l or creatinine of 105-265 µmol/l. A 50% reduction is recommended in cases with serum bilirubin concentrations of above 50µmol/l or creatinine of above 265µmol/l.

Cerubidin is extremely irritating to tissues and may only be administered intravenously after dilution. Cerubidin should be administered through a large vein and the infusion should be kept free flowing. When second or subsequent injections are given, the doses and time intervals depend on the effect of the previous doses and must be the subject of careful deliberation, examination of the peripheral blood and, under some circumstances, of the bone marrow.

The effect of Cerubidin on the disease process and on normal blood precursors cannot be exactly predicted for any particular case. The difference between incomplete treatment, a satisfactory remission and overdosage with possible irreversible aplasia of the bone marrow depends on the correct choice of dosage, time intervals and total number of doses.

*Contra-indications:* Cerubidin should not be used in patients recently exposed to, or with existing chicken pox or herpes zoster.

Do not administer by the intramuscular or subcutaneous route.

*Special warnings and special precautions for use:* Cerubidin should be used under the direction of a clinician conversant with the management of acute leukaemia and cytotoxic chemotherapy. The haematological status of patients should be monitored regularly.

Cerubidin should be used with care in patients at risk of hyperuricaemia (eg in the presence of gout, urate and renal calculi), tumour cell infiltration of the bone marrow and in patients with inadequate bone marrow reserves due to previous cytotoxic drug or radiation therapy. The cumulative dose of Cerubidin should be limited to 400 mg/m² when radiation therapy to the mediastinum has been previously administered. The dose of Cerubidin should not be repeated in the presence of bone marrow depression or buccal ulceration.

Care should be taken to avoid extravasation during intravenous administration. All steps should be taken to avoid tissuing and bandages should be avoided. Facial flushing or erythematous streaking along veins indicates too rapid injection. If tissue necrosis is suspected, the infusion should be stopped immediately and resumed in another vein. Where extravasation has occurred, an attempt should be made to aspirate the fluid back through the needle., The affected area may be injected with hydrocortisone. Sodium bicarbonate (5 ml of 8.4% w/v solution) may also be injected in the hope that through pH change the drug will hydrolyse. The opinion of a plastic surgeon should be sought as skin grafting may be required.

Application of ice packs may help decrease discomfort and also prevent extension. Liberal application of corticosteriod cream and dressing the area with sterile gauze should then be carried out.

Each patient should be given a clinical and bacteriological examination to determine whether infection is present; any infections should be adequately eliminated before treatment with Cerubidin which might depress the bone marrow to the point where anti-infective agents would no longer be effective. If facilities are available, patients should be treated in a germ-free environment or, where this is not possible, reverse barrier nursing and aseptic precautions should be employed.

Anti-infective therapy should be employed in the presence of suspected or confirmed infection and during a phase of aplasia. It should be continued for some time after the marrow has regenerated. Care should also be used in patients at risk of infection.

*Interactions with other medicaments and other forms of interaction:* None.

*Pregnancy and lactation:* Daunorubicin crosses the placenta and experiments in animals have shown it to be mutagenic, carcinogenic and teratogenic.

There is also the possibility that treatment during pregnancy may produce delayed effects in the offspring. If appropriate, the mother should be offered the opportunity of a therapeutic abortion.

Owing to potential toxic risk to the infant, breast-feeding should be discontinued during treatment.

*Effects on ability to drive and use machines:* Not applicable.

*Undesirable effects:* Bone marrow depression: In every patient bone marrow function will be depressed by treatment with Cerubidin and in a variable proportion of cases, severe aplasia will develop.

Leucopenia is usually more significant than thrombocytopenia. The nadir for leucopenia usually occurs between 10-14 days and recovery occurs gradually over the next 1-2 weeks. Bone marrow depression must be anticipated in every case by eliminating infection before treatment, by isolating the patient from infection during treatment and by means of supportive therapy. This includes the continuous administration of anti-infective agents, the administration of platelet-rich plasma or fresh whole blood transfusion and, under some circumstances, the transfusion of white cell concentrates.

Other less serious reactions have been reported (in order of frequency) are: stomatitis, alopecia, phlebitis, fever, anaemia, nausea, vomiting, mucositis, diarrhoea and rash. The urine may be temporarily coloured red after treatment.

Rapid destruction of a large number of leukaemia cells may cause a rise in blood uric acid or urea and so it is a wise precaution to check these concentrations three or four times a week during the first week of treatment. Fluids should be administered and allopurinol used in severe cases to prevent the development of hyperuricaemia.

Patients with heart disease should not be treated with this potentially cardiotoxic drug. Cardiotoxicity if it occurs is likely to be heralded by either a persistent tachycardia, shortness of breath, swelling of feet and lower limbs or by minor changes in the electrocardiogram and for this reason an electrocardiographic examination should be made at regular intervals during the treatment. Cardiotoxicity usually appears within 1 to 6 months after initiation of therapy. It may develop suddenly and not be detected by routine ECG. It may be irreversible and fatal but responds to treatment if detected early.

The risk of congestive heart failure increases significantly when the total cumulative dosage exceeds 600 mg/m² in adults, 300 mg/m² in children over 2 years or 10 mg/kg in children under 2 years. Cardiotoxicity may be more frequent in children and the elderly. The dosage should be modified if previous or concomitant cardiotoxic drug therapy is used.

*Overdose:* Although no cases of overdosage have been reported to our knowledge, overdosage may result in drastic myelosuppression and severe cardiotoxicity with or without transient reversible ECG changes leading to congestive heart failure. Treatment should be supportive and symptomatic.

**Pharmacological properties**

*Pharmacodynamic properties:* Cerubidin is an anthracycline glycoside antibiotic and is a potent antileukaemic agent. It also has immunosuppressant effects.

The exact mechanism of antineoplastic action is uncertain but may involve binding to DNA by intercalation between base pairs and inhibition of DNA and RNA synthesis by template disordering and steric obstruction. Daunorubicin is most active in the S-phase of cell division but is not cycle phase-specific. Tumour cell cross-resistance has been observed between daunorubicin and doxorubicin.

*Pharmacokinetic properties:* Daunorubicin is rapidly taken up by the tissues, especially by the kidneys, spleen, liver and heart. It does not cross the blood-brain barrier, subsequent release of drug and its metabolites from the tissues is slow (T½=55 hours). Daunorubicin is rapidly metabolised in the liver. The major metabolite daunorubicinol is also active. Daunorubicin is excreted slowly in the urine, mainly as metabolites with 25% excreted in the first 5 days. Biliary excretion also makes a significant (40%) contribution to elimination.

*Preclinical safety data:* No further information available.

**Pharmaceutical particulars**

*List of excipients:* Mannitol.

*Incompatibilities:* The reconstituted solution is incompatible with heparin sodium injection and dexamethasone sodium phosphate injection.

*Shelf life:* The shelf-life of Cerubidin is 3 years. After reconstitution Cerubidin should be used within 24 hours.

*Special precautions for storage:* Cerubidin vials should be stored below 25°C, protected from light. After reconstitution Cerubidin should be stored at 2-8°C, protected from light.

*Nature and contents of container:* Glass vial with rubber cap containing 21.4 mg of daunorubicin hydrochloride (equivalent to 20 mg as base).

*Instructions for use/handling:* The contents of a vial should be reconstituted with 4 ml of Water for Injection giving a concentration of 5 mg per ml. The calculated dose of Cerubidin should be further diluted with normal saline to give a final concentration of 1 mg per ml. The solution should be injected over a 20 minute period into the tubing or side arm, of a well placed, rapidly flowing i.v. infusion of normal saline (to minimise extravasation and possible tissue necrosis).

Alternatively, the Cerubidin may be added to a minibag of sodium chloride injection 0.9% and this solution infused into the side arm of a rapidly flowing infusion of normal saline.

**Marketing authorisation number**    0012/0220

**Date of approval/revision of SPC**    February 1997

**Legal category**    POM

# CLEXANE* INJECTION

**Qualitative and quantitative composition**

*20 mg Injection* Enoxaparin 20 mg (equivalent to 2000IU anti-Xa activity) in 0.2 ml Water for Injections

*40 mg Injection* Enoxaparin 40 mg (equivalent to 4000IU anti-Xa activity) in 0.4 ml Water for Injections

*60 mg Injection* Enoxaparin 60 mg (equivalent to 6000IU anti-Xa activity) in 0.6 ml Water for Injections

*80 mg Injection* Enoxaparin 80 mg (equivalent to 8000IU anti-Xa activity) in 0.8 ml Water for Injections

*100 mg Injection* Enoxaparin 100 mg (equivalent to 10,000IU anti-Xa activity) in 1.0 ml Water for Injections

**Pharmaceutical form** Sterile pyrogen-free solution for injection contained in ready-to-use prefilled syringes.

**Clinical particulars**

*Therapeutic indications:* The prophylaxis of thromboembolic disorders of venous origin, in particular those which may be associated with orthopaedic or general surgery. The treatment of deep vein thrombosis. The prevention of thrombus formation in the extracorporeal circulation during haemodialysis.

*Posology and method of administration: Adults: Prophylaxis of venous thromboembolism:* In patients with a low to moderate risk of venous thromboembolism the recommended dosage is 20 mg (2000 IU) once daily for 7 to 10 days, or until the risk of thromboembolism has diminished. In patients undergoing surgery, the initial dose should be given approximately 2 hours pre-operatively. In patients with a higher risk, such as in orthopaedic surgery, the dosage should be 40 mg (4,000 IU) daily with the initial dose administered approximately 12 hours before surgery. *Treatment of deep vein thrombosis:* A dose of 1 mg/kg (100 IU/kg) should be given subcutaneously every 12 hours. Clexane treatment is usually prescribed for at least 5 days and until adequate oral anticoagulation is established. *Prevention of extracorporeal thrombus formation during haemodialysis:* A dose equivalent to 1 mg/kg (100 IU/kg) introduced into the arterial line at the beginning of a dialysis session is usually sufficient for a 4 hour session. If fibrin rings are found, such as after a longer than normal session, a further dose of 0.5 to 1 mg/kg (50 to 100 IU/kg) may be given. For patients at a high risk of haemorrhage the dose should be reduced to 0.5 mg/kg (50 IU/kg) for double vascular access or 0.75 mg/kg (75 IU/kg) for single vascular access.

*Elderly:* No dose adjustment necessary.

*Children:* Not recommended, as dosage not established.

*Renal impairment:* no adjustment of the prophylaxis dose is required. Patients with severe renal impairment should be closely monitored when receiving treatment doses.

*Hepatic impairment:* In the absence of clinical studies, caution should be exercised.

Clexane is administered by subcutaneous injection for the prevention of venous thromboembolic disease or treatment of deep vein thrombosis and through the arterial line of a dialysis circuit for the prevention of thrombus formation in the extra-corporeal circulation during haemodialysis. It must not be administered by the intramuscular route.

*Subcutaneous injection technique:* The prefilled disposable syringe is ready for immediate use. Clexane should be administered when the patient is lying down by deep subcutaneous injection. The administration should be alternated between the left and right anterolateral or posterolateral abdominal wall. The whole length of the needle should be introduced vertically into a skin fold held between the thumb and index finger. The skin fold should not be released until the injection is complete. Do not rub the injection site after administration.

*Contra-indications:* Contra-indicated in patients with acute bacterial endocarditis; major bleeding disorders; thrombocytopenia in patients with a positive in-vitro aggregation test in the presence of enoxaparin; active gastric or duodenal ulceration; hypersensitivity to enoxaparin; stroke (unless due to systemic emboli); other patients with an increased risk of haemorrhage.

*Special warnings and special precautions for use:* As different low molecular weight heparins may not be equivalent, alternative products should not be substituted during a course of treatment. Enoxaparin is to be used with extreme caution in patients with a history of heparin-induced thrombocytopenia with or without thrombosis. As there is a risk of antibody-mediated heparin-induced thrombocytopenia also occurring with low molecular weight heparins, regular platelet count monitoring should be considered prior to and during therapy with these agents. Thrombocytopenia, should it occur, usually appears between the 5th and the 21st day following the beginning of therapy. If platelet count is significantly reduced (30 to 50 % of the initial value), therapy must be discontinued immediately and an alternative therapy initiated. Enoxaparin injection, as with any other anticoagulant therapy, should be used with caution in conditions with increased potential for bleeding, such as: impaired haemostasis, history of peptic ulcer, recent ischaemic stroke, uncontrolled severe arterial hypertension, diabetic retinopathy, recent neuro- or ophthalmologic surgery. As with other anti-coagulants, there have been rare cases of intra-spinal haematomas reported with the concurrent use of enoxaparin and spinal/epidural anaesthesia resulting in long term or permanent paralysis. The risk of these rare events may be higher with the use of post-operative indwelling catheters.

*Interaction with other medicaments and other forms of interaction:* It is recommended that agents which affect haemostasis should be discontinued prior to enoxaparin therapy unless their use is essential, such as: systemic salicylates, acetylsalicylic acid, NSAIDs including ketorolac, dextran and ticlopidine, systemic glucocorticoids, thrombolytics and anticoagulants. If the combination cannot be avoided, enoxaparin should be used with careful clinical and laboratory monitoring.

*Pregnancy and lactation: Pregnancy:* Animal studies have not shown any evidence of foetotoxicity or teratogenicity. In the pregnant rat, the transfer of ³⁵S-enoxaparin across the maternal placenta to the foetus is minimal. In humans, there is no evidence that enoxaparin crosses the placental barrier during the second trimester of pregnancy. There is no information available concerning the first and the third trimesters. As there are no adequate and well-controlled studies in pregnant women and because animal studies are not always predictive of human response, this drug should not be used in pregnant patients unless no safer alternative is available.
*Lactation:* In lactating rats, the concentration of ³⁵S-enoxaparin or its labelled metabolites in milk is very low. It is not known whether unchanged enoxaparin is excreted in human breast milk. The oral absorption of enoxaparin is unlikely. However, as a precaution, lactating mothers receiving enoxaparin should be advised to avoid breast-feeding.

*Effects on ability of drive and use machines:* Enoxaparin has no effect on the ability to drive and operate machines

*Undesirable effects:* Bleeding may occur during enoxaparin therapy in the presence of associated risk factors such as: organic lesions liable to bleed or the use of medications affecting haemostasis (see *Interactions* section). Mild, transient, asymptomatic thrombocytopenia has been reported during the first days of therapy. Immuno-allergic thrombocytopenia, with or without thrombosis, has rarely been reported. Pain, haematoma and mild local irritation may follow the subcutaneous injection of enoxaparin. Rarely, hard inflammatory nodules which are not cystic enclosures of enoxaparin, have been observed at the injection site. They resolve after a few days and should not cause therapy discontinuation. Exceptional cases of skin necrosis at the injection site have been reported with heparins and low molecular weight heparins. These phenomena are usually preceded by purpura or erythematous plaques, infiltrated and painful. Enoxaparin must be discontinued. Although rare, cutaneous or systemic allergic reactions may occur. In some cases discontinuation of therapy may be necessary. Asymptomatic and reversible increases in platelet counts and liver enzyme levels have been reported. Long term therapy with heparin has been associated with a risk of osteoporosis. Although this has not been observed with enoxaparin the risk of osteoporosis cannot be excluded. There have been rare reports of intra-spinal haematomas with the concurrent use of enoxaparin and spinal/epidural anaesthesia and post-operative indwelling catheters. These events have resulted in varying degrees of neurological injuries including long term or permanent paralysis.

*Overdose:* Orally administered enoxaparin is poorly absorbed and even large oral doses should not lead to any serious consequences. This may be checked by plasma assays of anti-Xa and anti-IIa activities. Accidental overdose following parenteral administration may produce haemorrhagic complications. These may be largely neutralised by slow intravenous injection of protamine sulphate or hydrochloride. The dose of protamine should be equal to the dose of enoxaparin injected, that is, 100 anti-heparin units of protamine should neutralise the anti-IIa activity generated by 1 mg (100 IU) of enoxaparin. However, even with high doses of protamine, the anti-Xa activity of enoxaparin is never completely neutralised (maximum about 60%).

**Pharmacological properties**

*Pharmacodynamic properties:* Enoxaparin is a low molecular weight heparin which has antithrombotic activity. It is characterised by a higher ratio of antithrombotic activity to anticoagulant activity than unfractionated heparin. At recommended does, it does not significantly influence platelet aggregation, binding of fibrinogen to platelets or global clotting tests such as APTT and prothrombin time.

*Pharmacokinetic properties:* Enoxaparin is rapidly and completely absorbed following subcutaneous injection. The maximum plasma anti-Xa activity occurs 1 to 4 hours after injection with peak activities in the order of 0.16 iu/ml and 0.38 iu/ml after doses of 20 mg or 40 mg respectively. The anti-Xa activity generated is localised within the vascular compartments and elimination is characterised by a half life of 4 to 5 hours. Following a 40 mg dose, anti-Xa activity may persist in the plasma for 24 hours. The enoxaparin elimination rate remains unchanged in renal insufficiency. Hepatic metabolism by desulphation and depolymerisation also contributes to elimination. The elimination half life may be prolonged in elderly patients although no dosage adjustment is necessary. Enoxaparin, as detected by anti-Xa activity, does not cross the placental barrier during the second trimester of pregnancy.

*Preclinical safety data:* There are no pre-clinical data of relevance to the prescriber which are additional to that already included in other sections of the SPC

**Pharmaceutical particulars**

*List of excipients:* Water for Injections BP

*Incompatibilities:* Clexane should not be mixed with any other injections or infusions

*Shelf life:* 2 years

*Special precautions for storage:* Store at room temperature (22°C ± 4°C).

*Nature and contents of container:* Hypak SCF prefilled syringes (Becton Dickinson) in packs of 10

*Instructions for use/handling:* See *Posology and method of administration*.

**Marketing authorisation number**  0012/0196

**Date of approval/revision of SPC** February 1997

**Legal category** POM

# DIORALYTE* EFFERVESCENT TABLETS BLACKCURRANT AND CITRUS

**Qualitative and quantitative composition::**

| | |
|---|---|
| Glucose BP | 1.62 g |
| Sodium Bicarbonate BP | 0.336 g |
| Potassium Chloride BP | 0.186 g |
| Citric Acid Anhydrous BP | 0.384 g |
| Sodium Chloride BP | 0.117 g |

**Pharmaceutical form:**  Effervescent tablets

**Clinical particulars** Oral treatment of fluid and electrolyte loss and the management of conditions associated with mild to moderate dehydration in all age groups particularly acute diarrhoea of varying aetiologies.

*Posology and method of administration:* Two tablets should be dissolved in 200 ml (approximately 7 fluid ounces) of drinking water. Use fresh drinking water for adults and children. For infants and where drinking water is unavailable, the water should be freshly boiled and cooled. The solution should be made up immediately before use. If refrigerated, the solution may be stored for up to 24 hours, otherwise any solution remaining an hour after reconstitution should be discarded. The solution must not be boiled.

The actual volume of reconstituted Dioralyte effervescent tablets to be taken should be decided by the clinician, taking into consideration the weight of the patient and the stage and severity of the condition.

A basic principle of treatment of diarrhoea is to replace lost fluid and the electrolytes and then to maintain sufficient fluid intake to replace fluid loss from stools.

Severe dehydration may need to be corrected by parenteral fluids initially followed by oral maintenance with Dioralyte if indicated.

Dioralyte should not be administered to infants under 1 year of age except on medical advice

Daily intake may be based on a volume of 150 ml/kg body weight for infants and 20–40 ml/kg body weight for adults and children. A reasonable approximation is:

*Infants:* One to one and a half times the usual 24 hour feed volume.

*Children:* Two tablets after every loose motion.

*Adults (including elderly):* Two or four tablets after every loose motion.

More may be required initially to ensure early and full volume repletion.

In the initial stages of treatment of diarrhoea all foods, including cow's or artificial milk should be stopped. However, breast milk need not be withheld. In breast fed infants it is suggested that the infant is given the same volume of Dioralyte as the bottle fed baby and then put to the breast until satisfied. Expression of residual milk from the breasts may be necessary during this period. After 24-48 hours, when symptoms are subsiding, the normal diet should be resumed but this should be gradual to avoid exacerbation of the condition.

When vomiting is present with the diarrhoea it is advisable that small amounts of Dioralyte effervescent be taken frequently. However, it is important that the whole of the required volume of Dioralyte is taken. Where the kidneys are functioning normally, it is difficult to overhydrate by mouth and where there is doubt about the dosage more rather than less should be taken.

If no improvement is seen within 36 hours it is recommended that the patient be reassessed.

*Contra-indications* There are no known absolute contra-indications to Dioralyte effervescent. However, there may be a number of conditions where treatment with Dioralyte Effervescent will be inappropriate, e.g., acute abdominal obstructive conditions. Treatment is also inappropriate in renal failure with oliguria or anuria, intractable vomiting and severe dehydration or severe infantile diarrhoea when parenteral therapy is required.

*Special warnings and precautions:* Two tablets should always be dissolved in 200 ml of water. A weaker solution than recommended will not contain the optimal glucose and electrolyte concentration and a stronger solution than recommended may give rise to electrolyte imbalance.

Dioralyte should not be administered to infants under 1 year of age except on medical advice.

In administration to infants the effervescence should be allowed to subside before use.

If diarrhoea persists unremittingly for longer than 36 hours the patient should be reassessed by the physician.

No specific precautions are necessary in the elderly. However, care should be taken when administering glucose electrolyte solutions in cases of severe renal or hepatic impairment or other conditions where the normal electrolyte balance may be disturbed.

*Interactions:* None stated

*Use in pregnancy and lactation:* No special precautions in normal pregnancy and lactation.

*Effects on ability to drive and use machines:* Dioralyte effervescent could not be expected to affect the ability to drive or use machines.

*Undesirable effects:* None stated

*Overdose:* In the event of significant overdose serum electrolytes should be evaluated as soon as possible, appropriate steps taken to correct any abnormalities and levels monitored until return to normal levels is established. This is particularly important in the very young and in cases of severe hepatic or renal failure.

**Pharmacological properties**

*Pharmacodynamic properties:* Dioralyte effervescent tablet is an oral rehydration therapy. The combination of electrolytes stimulates water and electrolyte absorption from the GI tract and therefore prevents or reverses dehydration in diarrhoea.

*Pharmacokinetics properties:* Sodium and glucose are actively transported via the membrane into enterocytes. Sodium is then extruded into the intercellular spaces and the resulting osmotic gradient causes water and electrolyte to be drawn from the gut and then into the circulation.

*Preclinical safety data:* Not applicable

**Pharmaceutical particulars**

*List of excipients:* Saccharin sodium and Blackcurrant flavour (PL5272/0025), saccharin sodium and Lemon/Lime flavour (PL5272/0042).

*Incompatibilities:* None

*Shelf life:* 24 months

*Special precautions for storage:* Store in original container in a cool (below 25°C) and dry place. Immediately after removal of a tablet replace the cap.

*Nature and contents of container:* Plastic tube with a push on/off cap containing a desiccant as a moisture proof seal. Each pack contains 10 tablets, available in packs containing one or four tubes.

*Instructions for use/handling:* Two tablets should be dissolved in 200 ml of drinking water. The tablets should not be reconstituted in other diluents other than water.

**Marketing authorisation numbers**
Dioralyte Blackcurrant Effervescent Tablets 5272/0025
Dioralyte Citrus Effervescent Tablets        5272/0042

**Date of approval/revision of SPC**  February 1997

**Legal category**  P

# DIORALYTE* SACHETS PLAIN, BLACKCURRANT AND CITRUS

**Qualitative and quantitative composition**

| | |
|---|---|
| Sodium Chloride BP | 0.47 g |
| Potassium Chloride BP | 0.30 g |
| Glucose BP | 3.56 g |
| Disodium Hydrogen Citrate BP | 0.53 g |

**Pharmaceutical form** Powder for reconstitution with 200 ml water.

**Clinical particulars**

*Therapeutic indications:* Oral correction of fluid and electrolyte loss in infants, children and adults. Treatment of watery diarrhoea of various aetiologies including gastro-enteritis in all age groups.

*Posology and method of administration:*

*Reconstitution:* The contents of each sachet should be dissolved in 200 ml (approximately 7 fluid ounces) of drinking water. Use fresh drinking water for adults and children. For infants, and where drinking water is unavailable, the water should be freshly boiled and cooled. The solution should be made up immediately before use. If refrigerated, the solution may be stored for up to 24 hours, otherwise any solution remaining an hour after reconstitution should be discarded. The solution must not be boiled.

The actual volume of reconstituted Dioralyte to be taken should be decided by the clinician, taking into consideration the weight of the patient and the stage and severity of the condition. A basic principle of treatment of diarrhoea is to replace lost fluid and electrolytes and then to maintain sufficient fluid intake to replace fluid loss from stools. Severe dehydration may need to be corrected by parenteral fluids initially followed by oral maintenance if indicated.

Dioralyte should not be administered to infants under 1 year of age except on medical advice.

Daily intake may be based on a volume of 150 ml/kg body weight for infants and 20–40 ml/kg body weight for adults and children. A reasonable approximation is:

*Infants:* One to one and a half times the usual 24 hour feed volume.

*Children:* One sachet after every loose motion.

*Adults (including elderly):* One or two sachets after every loose motion.

More may be required initially to ensure early and full volume repletion.

In the initial stage of treatment of diarrhoea all foods, including cow's or artificial milk should be stopped. However, breast milk need not be withheld. In breast fed infants it is suggested that the infant is given the same volume of Dioralyte as the bottle fed baby and then put to the breast until satisfied. Expression of residual milk from the breasts may be necessary during this period. After 24-48 hours, when symptoms are subsiding, the normal diet should be resumed but this should be gradual to avoid exacerbation of the condition.

When vomiting is present with the diarrhoea, it is advisable that small amounts of Dioralyte be taken frequently. However, it is important that the whole of the required volume of Dioralyte be taken. Where the kidneys are functioning normally, it is difficult to overhydrate by mouth and where there is doubt about the dosage, more rather than less should be taken. If no improvement is seen within 36 hours, it is recommended that the patient should be reassessed.

*Contra-indications:* There are no known contra-indications to Dioralyte. However, there may be a number of conditions where treatment with Dioralyte will be inappropriate, e.g. intestinal obstruction requiring surgical intervention.

*Special warnings and precautions for use:* For oral administration only. Dioralyte should not be reconstituted in diluents other than water. Each sachet should always be dissolved in 200 ml water. A weaker solution than recommended will not contain the optimal glucose and electrolyte concentration and a stronger solution than recommended may give rise to electrolyte imbalance.

Dioralyte should not be administered to infants under 1 year of age except on medical advice.

If diarrhoea persists unremittingly for longer than 36 hours the patient should be reassessed by the physician.

No specific precautions are necessary in the elderly. However, care should be taken when administering glucose electrolyte solutions in cases of severe renal or hepatic impairment or other conditions where the normal electrolyte balance may be disturbed.

*Interactions with other medicaments and other forms of interaction:* None stated

*Pregnancy and lactation:* Dioralyte is not contra-indicated in pregnancy or during lactation.

*Effects on ability to drive and use machines:* Dioralyte could not be expected to affect the ability to drive or use machines

*Undesirable effects:* None stated

*Overdose:* In the event of significant overdose, serum electrolytes should be evaluated as soon as possible, appropriate steps taken to correct any abnormalities and levels monitored until return to normal levels is established. This is particularly important in the very young and in cases of severe hepatic or renal failure.

**Pharmacological properties**

*Pharmacodynamic properties:* Dioralyte is an oral rehydration therapy. The combination of electrolytes stimulates water and electrolyte absorption from the gastro-intestinal tract and therefore prevents or reverses dehydration in diarrhoea.

*Pharmacokinetic properties:* Sodium and glucose are actively transported via the membrane into enterocytes. Sodium is then extruded into the intercellular spaces and the resulting osmotic gradient causes water and electrolytes to be drawn from the gut and then into the circulation.

*Preclinical safety data:* Not applicable

**Pharmaceutical particulars**

*List of excipients:* Silicon dioxide PhEur and Saccharin Sodium BP (PL5272/0016).

Silicon dioxide PhEur, Saccharin Sodium BP and Lemon/Lime flavour. (PL5272/0023)

Silicon dioxide PhEur, Saccharin Sodium BP and Blackcurrant flavour(PL5272/0022)

*Incompatibilities:* None

*Shelf life:* 24 months

*Special precautions for storage:* Store in a cool dry place.

*Nature of and contents of container:* Foil/Laminate sachets containing powder for reconstitution with 200 ml water.

**Marketing authorisation numbers**
Dioralyte Plain                    5272/0016
Dioralyte Blackcurrant      5272/0022

Dioralyte Citrus                   5272/0023

**Date of approval/revision of SPC**   February 1997

**Legal category**   P

## FLAGYL* COMPAK

**Qualitative and quantitative composition** The active component of the tablets is metronidazole 400 mg, the active component of the vaginal inserts is nystatin BP 42 mg.

**Pharmaceutical form** *Flagyl tablets 400 mg:* White to off-white, biconvex, circular, film coated tablets impressed 'FLAGYL 400' on one face, plain reverse.
*Nystatin vaginal inserts 100,00 units:* Yellowish-cream, almond shaped, marked M&B on one face, other plain. Both surfaces are slightly convex.

**Clinical particulars**

*Therapeutic indications:* Flagyl is a potent trichomonacide. It is also active against other protozoa and anaerobic bacteria. Nystatin is a fungistatic and fungicidal antibiotic which is actively topically against *Candida albicans.*

Flagyl Compak is indicated in the treatment of vaginitis where a mixed trichomonal/candidal infection is diagnosed or suspected. Presenting symptoms may include vaginal discharge, pruritus vulvae and dyspareunia.

*Posology and method of administration:* Flagyl tablets–for oral administration. Nyastatin inserts–for vaginal administration.
*Adults including the elderly:* One Flagyl 400 tablet to be swallowed whole, with half a glass of water during or after meals, twice daily for seven days. Concurrently, one nystatin vaginal insert to be moistened and introduced high into the vagina, night and morning for seven days. Some physicians may prefer to instruct patients to use one insert nightly, before retiring for fourteen nights. Full patient instructions for use of the applicator are included in each Compak.

This product is not recommended for girls under 10 years of age.

Where cross infection with trichomonas vaginalis is confirmed or suspected the male consort should be treated concurrently with one Flagyl 400 tablet by mouth twice daily for seven days.

*Contra-indications:* Known hypersensitivity to metronidazole.

*Special warnings and special precautions for use:* Regular clinical and laboratory monitoring are advised if administration of Flagyl for more than 10 days is considered to be necessary. There is a possibility that after Trichomonas vaginalis has been eliminated a gonococcal infection might persist. The elimination half-life of metronidazole remains unchanged in the presence of renal failure.. The dosage of metronidazole therefore needs no reduction. Such patients however retain the metabolites of metronidazole. The clinical significance of this is not known at present. Metronidazole is mainly metabolised by hepatic oxidation. Substantial impairment of metronidazole clearance may occur in the presence of advanced hepatic insufficiency. Significant cumulation may occur in patients with hepatic encephalopathy and the resulting high plasma concentrations of metronidazole may contribute to the symptoms of the encephalopathy. Flagyl should therefore, be administered with caution to patients with hepatic encephalopathy. The daily dosage should be reduced to one third and may be administered once daily.

*Interaction with other medicaments and other forms of interaction:* Patients should be advised not to take alcohol during metronidazole therapy and for at least 48 hours afterwards because of the possibility of a disulfiram-like (antabuse effect) reaction. Some potentiation of anticoagulant therapy has been reported when metronidazole has been used with the warfarin type oral anticoagulants. Dosage of the latter may require reducing. Prothrombin times should be monitored. There is no interaction with heparin. Lithium retention accompanied by evidence of possible renal damage has been reported in patients treated simultaneously with lithium and metronidazole. Lithium treatment should be tapered or withdrawn before administering metronidazole. Plasma concentrations of lithium, creatinine and electrolytes should be monitored in patients under treatment with lithium while they receive metronidazole. Patients receiving phenobarbitone metabolise metronidazole at a much greater rate than normally, reducing the half-life to approximately 3 hours.

*Pregnancy and lactation:* There is inadequate evidence of the safety of metronidazole in pregnancy. Flagyl should not, therefore, be given during pregnancy or during lactation unless the physician considers it essential; in these circumstances the short, high-dosage regimens are not recommended.

*Effects on ability to drive and use machines:* None stated.

*Undesirable effects:* During intensive and/or prolonged metronidazole therapy, a few instances of peripheral neuropathy or transient epileptiform seizures have been reported. In most cases neuropathy disappeared after treatment was stopped or when dosage was reduced. A moderate leucopenia has been reported in some patients but the white cell count has always returned to normal before or after treatment has been completed. Serious adverse reactions occur rarely with standard recommended regimens. Unpleasant taste in the mouth, furred tongue, nausea, vomiting, gastro-intestinal disturbances, urticaria and angioedema occur occasionally. Anaphylaxis may occur rarely. Drowsiness, dizziness, headaches, ataxia, skin rashes, pruritus, inco-ordination of movement, darkening of urine (due to metronidazole metabolite), myalgia and arthralgia have been reported but very rarely.

*Overdose:* There is no specific treatment for gross overdosage of Flagyl.

**Pharmacological properties**

*Pharmacodynamic Properties:* Flagyl is a potent trichomonacide. It is also active against other protozoa and anaerobic bacteria. Nystatin is a fungistatic and fungicidal antibiotic which is active topically against *Candida albicans.*

*Pharmacokinetic properties:* Metronidazole is rapidly and almost completely absorbed from the tablets leading to peak plasma concentrations after 20 minutes to 3 hours. Metronidazole is excreted in milk but the intake of a suckling infant of a mother receiving normal dosage would be considerably less than the therapeutic dosage for infants. Nystatin is not absorbed through the skin or mucous membranes when applied topically.

*Preclinical safety data:* There are no pre-clinical data of relevance to the prescriber which are additional to that already included in other sections of the SPC.

**Pharmaceutical particulars**

*List of excipients:*
*Flagyl tablets:* calcium hydrogen phosphate (E341), starch maize, povidone K30 (E1201), magnesium stearate (E572), hydroxypropylmethylcellulose(E464), polyethylene glycol 400, and french chalk powdered (E553(b)).
*Nystatin vaginal inserts:* lactose anhydrous, sodium starch glycollate and magnesium stearate.

*Incompatibilities:* None known.

*Shelf life:* 36 months.

*Special precaution for storage:* Store below 20°C protected from light.

*Nature and contents of container:* blister containing 14 Flagyl 400 tablets and 14 nystatin vaginal inserts.

*Instructions for use/handling:* None stated.

**Marketing authorisation number**   0012/5091

**Date of approval/revision of SPC**   February 1997

**Legal category**   POM

## FLAGYL* INJECTION

**Qualitative and quantitative composition** Metronidazole BP 0.5% w/v.

**Pharmaceutical form:** A clean, bright, pale yellow sterile isotonic solution for intravenous infusion.

**Clinical particulars**

*Therapeutic indications:* Flagyl is indicated in the prophylaxis and treatment of infections in which anaerobic bacteria have been identified or are suspected to be the cause. Flagyl is active against a wide range of pathogenic micro-organisms notably species of *Bacteroides, Fusobacteria, Clostridia, Eubacteria,* anaerobic cocci and *Gardnerella vaginalis.* It is also active against *Trichomonas, Entamoeba histolytica, Giardia lamblia* and *Balantidium coli.*

Used by the intravenous route Flagyl is indicated in the 1. prevention of postoperative infections due to anaerobic bacteria, particularly species of bacteroides and anaerobic streptococci. 2. treatment of established anaerobic infections (septicaemia, bacteraemia, peritonitis, brain abscess, necrotising pneumonia, osteomyelitis, puerperal sepsis, pelvic abscess, pelvic cellulitis, and post-operative wound infections from which pathogenic anaerobes have been isolated).

*Posology and method of administration:* For intravenous use. Flagyl injection should be infused intravenously at a rate of approximately 5 ml/min (see dosage table). Oral medication should be substituted as soon as possible.

Use Flagyl injection in the elderly with caution,

particularly at high doses since there is limited information available on dose modification.

*Contra-indications:* Known hypersensitivity to metronidazole.

*Special warnings and special precautions for use:* Metronidazole has no direct activity against anaerobic or facultative anaerobic bacteria. Regular clinical and laboratory monitoring are advised if administration of Flagyl for more than 10 days is considered to be necessary. There is a possibility that after Trichomonas vaginalis has been eliminated a gonococcal infection might persist. The elimination half-life of metronidazole remains unchanged in the presence of renal failure. The dosage of metronidazole therefore needs no reduction. Such patients however retain the metabolites of metronidazole. The clinical significance of this is not known at present. In patients undergoing haemodialysis metronidazole and metabolites are efficiently removed during an eight hour period of dialysis. Metronidazole should therefore be re-administered immediately after haemodialysis. No routine adjustment in the dosage of Flagyl need be made in patients with renal failure undergoing intermittent peritoneal dialysis (IDP) or continuous ambulatory peritoneal dialysis (CAPD). Metronidazole is mainly metabolised by hepatic oxidation. Substantial impairment of metronidazole clearance may occur in the presence of advanced hepatic insufficiency. Significant cumulation may occur in patients with hepatic encephalopathy and the resulting high plasma concentrations of metronidazole may contribute to the symptoms of the encephalopathy. Flagyl should therefore, be administered with caution to patients with hepatic encephalopathy. The daily dosage should be reduced to one third and may be administered once daily. Aspartate amino transferase assays may give spuriously low values in patients being treated with Metronidazole depending on the method used. Flagyl should be used with caution in patients with active disease of the CNS.

*Interaction with other medicaments and other forms of interaction:* Patients should be advised not to take alcohol during metronidazole therapy and for at least 48 hours afterwards because of the possibility of a disulfiram-like (antabuse effect) reaction. Some potentiation of anticoagulant therapy has been reported when metronidazole has been used with the warfarin type oral anticoagulants. Dosage of the latter may require reducing. Prothrombin times should be monitored. There is no interaction with heparin. Lithium retention accompanied by evidence of possible renal damage has been reported in patients treated simultaneously with lithium and metronidazole. Lithium treatment should be tapered or withdrawn before administering metronidazole. Plasma concentrations of lithium, creatinine and electrolytes should be monitored in patients under treatment with lithium while they receive metronidazole. Patients receiving phenobarbitone metabolise metronidazole at a much greater rate than normally, reducing the half-life to approximately 3 hours.

*Pregnancy and lactation:* There is inadequate evidence of the safety of metronidazole in pregnancy but it has been in wide use for many years without apparent ill consequence. Nevertheless Flagyl, like other medicines, should not be given during pregnancy or during lactation unless the physician considers it essential; in these circumstances the short, high-dosage regimens are not recommended.

*Effects on ability to drive and use machines:* Therapy with Flagyl does not affect a patient's ability to drive or operate machines.

*Undesirable effects* During intensive and/or prolonged metronidazole therapy, a few instances of peripheral neuropathy or transient epileptiform seizures have been reported. In most cases neuropathy disappeared after treatment was stopped or when dosage was reduced. A moderate leucopenia has been reported in some patients but the white cell count has always returned to normal before or after treatment has been completed. Clinicians who contemplate continuous therapy for the relief of chronic conditions for periods longer than those recommended are advised to consider the possible therapeutic benefit against the risk of peripheral neuropathy. Serious adverse reactions occur rarely with standard recommended regimens. Unpleasant taste in the mouth, furred tongue, nausea, vomiting, gastro-intestinal disturbances, urticaria and angioedema occur occasionally. Anaphylaxis may occur rarely. Erythema multiforme may occur, which may be reversed on drug withdrawal. Abnormal liver function tests, cholestatic hepatitis and jaundice, reversible on drug withdrawal, have been reported very rarely. Agranulocytosis, neutropenia, thrombocytopenia and pancytopenia, often reversible on drug withdrawal, have very rarely been reported, although fatalities have occurred. Drowsiness, dizziness, headaches, ataxia, skin rashes, pruritus, inco-ordination of movement, darkening of urine (due to metronidazole metabolite) myalgia and arthralgia have been reported but very rarely.

*Overdose:* There is no specific treatment for gross overdosage of Flagyl

**Pharmacological properties**

*Pharmacodynamic properties:* Metronidazole has antiprotozoal and antibacterial actions and is effective against Trichomonas vaginalis and other protozoa including Entamoeba histolytica and Gardia lambila and against anaerobic bacteria.

*Pharmacokinetic properties:* Metronidazole is widely distributed in body tissues. The plasma half life is of the order of 8.5 hours with at least half the dose being excreted in the urine as Metronidazole and its metabolites. Metronidazole can be used in chronic renal failure; it is rapidly removed from the plasma by dialysis. Metronidazole diffuses across the placenta and is excreted in breast milk with levels equivalent to those seen in serum.

*Preclinical safety data:* There are no pre-clinical data of relevance to the prescriber which are additional to that already included in other sections of the SPC.

**Pharmaceutical particulars**

*List of excipients:* Sodium phosphate, citric acid anhydrous, sodium chloride and water for injections.

*Incompatibilities:* Flagyl injection should not be mixed with cefamandole nafate, cefoxitin sodium, dextrose 10% w/v, compound sodium lactate injection, penicillin G potassium.

*Shelf life:* 24 months.

*Special precautions for storage:* store below 25°C, protect from light.

*Nature and contents of container:* Cartons containing 20 x 100 ml Viaflex minibags.

*Instructions for use/handling:* Cerufoxaime sodium is physically and chemically compatible with Flagyl. The following drugs have been shown to be physically compatible in terms of pH and appearance with Flagyl injection over the normal period of administration, although there is no evidence of chemical stability: amikacin sulphate, ampicillin sodium, carbenicillin sodium, cephazolin sodium, ceftoxamine sodium, cephalothin sodium, chloramphenicol sodium succinate, clindamycin phosphate, gentamicin sulphate, hydrocortisone sodium succinate, latamoxef disodium, netilmicin sulphate and tobramycin sulphate. In patients maintained on intravenous fluids, Flagyl injection may be diluted with appropriate volumes of normal saline, dextrose-saline, dextrose 5% w/v or potassium chloride infusions (20 and 40 mmol/litre). Apart from the above, Flagyl should on no account be mixed with any other substance.

**Marketing authorisation number** 0012/0107

**Date of approval/revision of SPC** February 1997

**Legal category** POM

**Flagyl Injection dosages**

*1. Prevention of post-operative infections due to anaerobic bacteria:*

| | |
|---|---|
| *Adults and children over 10 years* | 500 mg pre-operatively, repeated 8 hourly until substitution of oral medication. |
| *Children* | 7.5 mg/kg (1.5 ml/kg) 8 hourly |

*2. Treatment of established anaerobic infection:*

| | |
|---|---|
| *Adults and children over 10 years* | 500 mg 8 hourly |
| *Children* | 7.5 mg/kg 8 hourly |

## FLAGYL* SUPPOSITORIES

**Qualitative and quantitative composition**
*Flagyl Suppository 500 mg* contain Metronidazole BP 500 mg.

*Flagyl Suppositories 1 g* contain Metronidazole BP 1 g

**Pharmaceutical form:** A cream coloured, smooth, torpedo-shaped suppositories.

**Clinical particulars**

*Therapeutic indications:* Flagyl is indicated in the prophylaxis and treatment of infections in which anaerobic bacteria have been identified or are suspected to be the cause. Flagyl is active against a wide range of pathogenic micro-organisms notably species of *Bacteroides, Fusobacteria, Clostridia, Eubacteria,* anaerobic cocci and *Gardnerella vaginalis.* It is also active against *Trichomonas, Entamoeba histolytica, Giardia lamblia* and *Balantidium coli.*

Used by the rectal route Flagyl is indicated in the : 1. prevention of postoperative infections due to anaerobic bacteria, particularly species of bacteroides and anaerobic streptococci. 2. treatment of established anaerobic infections (septicaemia, bacteraemia, peritonitis, brain abscess, necrotising pneumonia, osteomyelitis, puerperal sepsis, pelvic abscess, pelvic cellulitis, and post-operative wound infections from which pathogenic anaerobes have been isolated).

*Posology and method of administration:* For rectal administration. All dosages are given in terms of metronidazole (see dosage table).

*Contra-indications:* Known hypersensitivity to metronidazole.

*Special warnings and special precautions for use:* Metronidazole has no direct activity against anaerobic or facultative anaerobic bacteria. Regular clinical and laboratory monitoring are advised if administration of Flagyl for more than 10 days is considered to be necessary. There is a possibility that after Trichomonas vaginalis has been eliminated a gonococcal infection might persist. The elimination half-life of metronidazole remains unchanged in the presence of renal failure. The dosage of metronidazole therefore needs no reduction. Such patients however retain the metabolites of metronidazole. The clinical significance of this is not known at present. In patients undergoing haemodialysis metronidazole and metabolites are efficiently removed during an eight hour period of dialysis. Metronidazole should therefore be re-administered immediately after haemodialysis. No routine adjustment in the dosage of Flagyl need be made in patients with renal failure undergoing intermittent peritoneal dialysis (IDP) or continuous ambulatory peritoneal dialysis (CAPD). Metronidazole is mainly metabolised by hepatic oxidation. Substantial impairment of metronidazole clearance may occur in the presence of advanced hepatic insufficiency. Significant cumulation may occur in patients with hepatic encephalopathy and the resulting high plasma concentrations of metronidazole may contribute to the symptoms of the encephalopathy. Flagyl should therefore, be administered with caution to patients with hepatic encephalopathy. The daily dosage should be reduced to one third and may be administered once daily. Aspartate amino transferase assays may give spuriously low values in patients being treated with Metronidazole depending on the method used. Flagyl should be used with caution in patients with active disease of the CNS.

*Interaction with other medicaments and other forms of interaction:* Patients should be advised not to take alcohol during metronidazole therapy and for at least 48 hours afterwards because of the possibility of a disulfiram-like (antabuse effect) reaction. Some potentiation of anticoagulant therapy has been reported when metronidazole has been used with the warfarin type oral anticoagulants. Dosage of the latter may require reducing. Prothrombin times should be monitored. There is no interaction with heparin. Lithium retention accompanied by evidence of possible renal damage has been reported in patients treated simultaneously with lithium and metronidazole. Lithium treatment should be tapered or withdrawn before administering metronidazole. Plasma concentrations of lithium, creatinine and electrolytes should be monitored in patients under treatment with lithium while they receive metronidazole. Patients receiving phenobarbitone metabolise metronidazole at a much greater rate than normally, reducing the half-life to approximately 3 hours.

*Pregnancy and lactation:* There is inadequate evidence of the safety of metronidazole in pregnancy but it has been in wide use for many years without apparent ill consequence. Nevertheless Flagyl, like other medicines, should not be given during pregnancy or during lactation unless the physician considers it essential; in these circumstances the short, high-dosage regimens are not recommended.

*Effects on ability to drive and use machines:* Therapy with Flagyl does not affect a patient's ability to drive or operate machines.

*Undesirable effects:* During intensive and/or prolonged metronidazole therapy, a few instances of peripheral neuropathy or transient epileptiform seizures have been reported. In most cases neuropathy disappeared after treatment was stopped or when dosage was reduced. A moderate leucopenia has been reported in some patients but the white cell count has always returned to normal before or after

## Flagyl Suppositories dosages

### 1. Prevention of post-operative infections due to anaerobic bacteria:

| | |
|---|---|
| Adults and children over 10 years | 1 gram suppository inserted 2 hours before surgery repeated 8 hourly until patient is able to take oral form. |
| Children (5-10 years) | 500 mg 8 hourly until oral medication becomes possible |

### 2. Treatment of established anaerobic infection:

| | |
|---|---|
| Adults and children over 10 years | 1 gram 8 hourly for 3 days. Oral medication should be substituted as soon as possible. If rectal administration continued for more than 3 days dose should be reduced to 1 gram 12 hourly. |
| Children (5-10 years) | 500 mg suppository according to adult schedule. Oral medication should be substituted as soon as feasible |
| Children 1-5 years | 250 mg (one half 500 mg suppository) according to adult schedule. Oral medication should be substituted as soon as feasible. |
| Infants under 1 years | 125 mg (one quarter of 500 mg suppository) according to adult schedule. Oral medication should be substituted as soon as feasible. |

treatment has been completed. Clinicians who contemplate continuous therapy for the relief of chronic conditions for periods longer than those recommended are advised to consider the possible therapeutic benefit against the risk of peripheral neuropathy. Serious adverse reactions occur rarely with standard recommended regimens. Unpleasant taste in the mouth, furred tongue, nausea, vomiting, gastro-intestinal disturbances, urticaria and angioedema occur occasionally. Anaphylaxis may occur rarely. Erythema multiforme may occur, which may be reversed on drug withdrawal. Abnormal liver function tests, cholestatic hepatitis and jaundice, reversible on drug withdrawal, have been reported very rarely. Agranulocytosis, neutropenia, thrombocytopenia and pancytopenia, often reversible on drug withdrawal, have very rarely been reported, although fatalities have occurred. Drowsiness, dizziness, headaches, ataxia, skin rashes, pruritus, inco-ordination of movement, darkening of urine (due to metronidazole metabolite) myalgia and arthralgia have been reported but very rarely.

*Overdose:* There is no specific treatment for gross overdosage of Flagyl

### Pharmacological properties

*Pharmacodynamic properties:* Metronidazole has antiprotozoal and antibacterial actions and is effective against Trichomonas vaginalis and other protozoa including Entamoeba histolytica and Gardia lambila and against anaerobic bacteria.

*Pharmacokinetic properties:* Metronidazole is rapidly absorbed after oral and rectal administration of Flagyl with peak plasma concentrations occurring between 20 min and 3 hours post dose. Metronidazole is widely distributed in body tissues. The plasma half life is of the order of 8.5 hours with at least half the dose being excreted in the urine as Metronidazole and its metabolites. Metronidazole can be used in chronic renal failure; it is rapidly removed from the plasma by dialysis. Metronidazole diffuses across the placenta and is excreted in breast milk with levels equivalent to those seen in serum.

*Preclinical safety data:* There are no pre-clinical data of relevance to the prescriber which are additional to that already included in other sections of the SPC.

### Pharmaceutical particulars

*List of excipients:* Suppository base E75 and suppository base W35

*Incompatibilities:* None known.

*Shelf life:* 36 months.

*Special Precautions for storage:* Store below 20°C, protect from light.

*Nature and contents of container:* Flagyl suppositories are available PVC/polyethylene bandoliers containing 10 suppositories.

*Instructions for use/handling:* None stated.

**Marketing authorisation number** 0012/0113

**Date of approval/revision of SPC** February 1997

**Legal category** POM

# FLAGYL* TABLETS AND FLAGYL* S SUSPENSION

## Qualitative and quantitative composition

*Flagyl Tablets 200 mg* contain metronidazole BP 200 mg.

*Flagyl Tablets 400 mg* contain metronidazole BP 400 mg.

*Flagyl S Suspension* contains 320 mg/5 ml metronidazole benzoate equivalent to 200 mg/5 ml metronidazole

## Pharmaceutical form

*Flagyl tablets:* White to off-white, circular biconvex, film coated tablets. The 200 mg tablets are impressed

'FLAGYL 200' on one face, plain reverse, and the 400 mg tablets are impressed 'FLAGYL 400' on one face, plain reverse.

*Flagyl S Suspension:* White to cream suspension with a slight yellow tinge and an odour of orange and lemon

## Clinical particulars

*Therapeutic indications:* Flagyl is indicated in the prophylaxis and treatment of infections in which anaerobic bacteria have been identified or are suspected to be the cause. Flagyl is active against a wide range of pathogenic micro-organisms notably species of *Bacteroides, Fusobacteria, Clostridia, Eubacteria,* anaerobic cocci and *Gardnerella vaginalis*. It is also active against *Trichomonas, Entamoeba histolytica, Giardia lamblia* and *Balantidium coli*.

Used by the oral route Flagyl is indicated in the 1. prevention of postoperative infections due to anaerobic bacteria, particularly species of bacteroides and anaerobic streptococci. 2. treatment of established anaerobic infections (septicaemia, bacteraemia, peritonitis, brain abscess, necrotising pneumonia, osteomyelitis, puerperal sepsis, pelvic abscess, pelvic cellulitis, and post-operative wound infections from which pathogenic anaerobes have been isolated). 3. treatment of urogenital trichomoniasis in the female (trichomonal vaginitis) and in the male. 4. treatment of bacterial vaginosis (also known as non-specific vaginitis, anaerobic vaginosis or Gardnerella vaginitis). 5. treatment of all forms of amoebiasis (intestinal and extra-intestinal disease and that of symptomless cyst passers). 6. treatment of giardiasis. 7. treatment of acute ulcerative gingivitis. 8. treatment of anaerobically-infected leg ulcers and pressure sores. 9. treatment of acute dental infections (e.g. acute pericoronitis and acute apical infections).

*Posology and method of administration:* For oral administration. All dosages are given in terms of metronidazole or metronidazole equivalent (see dosage table). Flagyl tablets should be swallowed with water (not chewed). It is recommended that the tablets be taken during or after a meal and that Flagyl S suspension be taken at least one hour before a meal.

*Infants and children weighing less than 10 kg* should receive proportionally smaller dosages.

*Elderly:* Flagyl is well tolerated by the elderly but a pharmacokinetic study suggests cautious use of high dosage regimens in this age group.

*Contra-indications:* Known hypersensitivity to metronidazole.

*Special warnings and special precautions for use:* Metronidazole has no direct activity against anaerobic or facultative anaerobic bacteria. Regular clinical and laboratory monitoring are advised if administration of Flagyl for more than 10 days is considered to be necessary. There is a possibility that after Trichomonas vaginalis has been eliminated a gonococcal infection might persist. The elimination half-life of metronidazole remains unchanged in the presence of renal failure. The dosage of metronidazole therefore needs no reduction. Such patients however retain the metabolites of metronidazole. The clinical significance of this is not known at present. In patients undergoing haemodialysis metronidazole and metabolites are efficiently removed during an eight hour period of dialysis. Metronidazole should therefore be re-administered immediately after haemodialysis. No routine adjustment in the dosage of Flagyl need be made in patients with renal failure undergoing intermittent peritoneal dialysis (IDP) or continuous ambulatory peritoneal dialysis (CAPD). Metronidazole is mainly metabolised by hepatic oxidation. Substantial impairment of metronidazole clearance may occur in the presence of advanced hepatic insufficiency. Significant cumulation may occur in patients with hepatic encephalopathy and the resulting high plasma concentrations of metronidazole may contribute to the symptoms of the encephalopathy. Flagyl should therefore, be administered with caution to patients

with hepatic encephalopathy. The daily dosage should be reduced to one third and may be administered once daily. Aspartate amino transferase assays may give spuriously low values in patients being treated with Metronidazole depending on the method used. Flagyl should be used with caution in patients with active disease of the CNS.

*Interaction with other medicaments and other forms of interaction:* Patients should be advised not to take alcohol during metronidazole therapy and for at least 48 hours afterwards because of the possibility of a disulfiram-like (antabuse effect) reaction. Some potentiation of anticoagulant therapy has been reported when metronidazole has been used with the warfarin type oral anticoagulants. Dosage of the latter may require reducing. Prothrombin times should be monitored. There is no interaction with heparin. Lithium retention accompanied by evidence of possible renal damage has been reported in patients treated simultaneously with lithium and metronidazole. Lithium treatment should be tapered or withdrawn before administering metronidazole. Plasma concentrations of lithium, creatinine and electrolytes should be monitored in patients under treatment with lithium while they receive metronidazole. Patients receiving phenobarbitone metabolise metronidazole at a much greater rate than normally, reducing the half-life to approximately 3 hours.

*Pregnancy and lactation:* There is inadequate evidence of the safety of metronidazole in pregnancy but it has been in wide use for many years without apparent ill consequence. Nevertheless Flagyl, like other medicines, should not be given during pregnancy or during lactation unless the physician considers it essential; in these circumstances the short, high-dosage regimens are not recommended.

*Effects on ability to drive and use machines:* Therapy with Flagyl does not affect a patient's ability to drive or operate machines.

*Undesirable effects:* During intensive and/or prolonged metronidazole therapy, a few instances of peripheral neuropathy or transient epileptiform seizures have been reported. In most cases neuropathy disappeared after treatment was stopped or when dosage was reduced. A moderate leucopenia has been reported in some patients but the white cell count has always returned to normal before or after treatment has been completed. Clinicians who contemplate continuous therapy for the relief of chronic conditions for periods longer than those recommended are advised to consider the possible therapeutic benefit against the risk of peripheral neuropathy. Serious adverse reactions occur rarely with standard recommended regimens. Unpleasant taste in the mouth, furred tongue, nausea, vomiting, gastro-intestinal disturbances, urticaria and angioedema occur occasionally. Anaphylaxis may occur rarely. Erythema multiforme may occur, which may be reversed on drug withdrawal. Abnormal liver function tests, cholestatic hepatitis and jaundice, reversible on drug withdrawal, have been reported very rarely. Agranulocytosis, neutropenia, thrombocytopenia and pancytopenia, often reversible on drug withdrawal, have very rarely been reported, although fatalities have occurred. Drowsiness, dizziness, headaches, ataxia, skin rashes, pruritus, inco-ordination of movement, darkening of urine (due to metronidazole metabolite) myalgia and arthralgia have been reported but very rarely.

*Overdose:* There is no specific treatment for gross overdosage of Flagyl

### Pharmacological properties

*Pharmacodynamic properties:* Metronidazole has antiprotozoal and antibacterial actions and is effective against Trichomonas vaginalis and other protozoa including Entamoeba histolytica and Gardia lambila and against anaerobic bacteria.

*Pharmacokinetic properties:* Metronidazole is rapidly absorbed after oral and rectal administration of Flagyl with peak plasma concentrations occurring between 20 min and 3 hours post dose. Metronidazole is widely distributed in body tissues. The plasma half life is of the order of 8.5 hours with at least half the dose being excreted in the urine as Metronidazole and its metabolites. Metronidazole can be used in chronic renal failure; it is rapidly removed from the plasma by dialysis. Metronidazole diffuses across the placenta and is excreted in breast milk with levels equivalent to those seen in serum.

*Preclinical safety data:* There are no pre-clinical data of relevance to the prescriber which are additional to that already included in other sections of the SPC.

### Pharmaceutical particulars

*List of excipients: Flagyl tablets (200 mg and 400 mg):* Calcium hydrogen phosphate (E341), starch maize, Povidone K30 (E1201), magnesium stearate (E572),

## Flagyl Tablets and Flagyl S Suspension dosages

### 1. Prevention of post-operative infections due to anaerobic bacteria†:

| | |
|---|---|
| Adults | 400 mg 8 hourly during 24 hours immediately preceding operation then intravenous or rectal administration until patient is able to take oral form. |
| Children and infants | 7.5 mg/kg 8 hourly |

### 2. Treatment of established anaerobic infection†:

| | |
|---|---|
| Adults | 800 mg followed by 400 mg 8 hourly |
| Children and infants | 7.5 mg/kg 8 hourly |

†For the prevention and treatment of anaerobic infections the duration of dosing is about 7 days but, depending on the seriousness of the patient's condition assessed clinically and bacteriologically, this may be prolonged.

### 3. Treatment of urogenital trichomoniasis (where reinfection of adults is likely the partner should be treated concurrently)

| | |
|---|---|
| Adults | Either: 300 mg three times daily for 7 days |
| | Or: 400 mg twice daily for 7 days |
| | Or: 800 mg morning and 1200 mg evening for 2 days |
| | Or: 2 g as a single dose |
| Children 7-10 years | 100 mg three times daily |
| Children 3-7 years | 100 mg twice daily |
| Children 1-3 years | 50 mg three times daily |

### 4. Treatment of bacterial vaginosis

| | |
|---|---|
| Adults | Either: 400 mg twice daily for 7 days |
| | Or: 2.0 g as a single dose |

### 5. Treatment of amoebiasis
Invasive intestinal disease in susceptible patients

| | |
|---|---|
| Adults | 800 mg three times daily for 5 days |
| Children 7-10 years | 400 mg three times daily for 5 days |
| Children 3-7 years | 200 mg four times daily for 5 days |
| Children 1-3 years | 200 mg three times daily for 5 days |

Intestinal disease in less susceptible patients and chronic amoebic hepatitis

| | |
|---|---|
| Adults | 400 mg three times daily for 5-10 days |
| Children 7-10 years | 200 mg three times daily for 5-10 days |
| Children 3-7 years | 100 mg four times daily for 5-10 days |
| Children 1-3 years | 100 mg three times daily for 5-10 days |

Extra-intestinal amoebiasis

| | |
|---|---|
| Adults | 400 mg three times daily for 5 days |
| Children 7-10 years | 200 mg three times daily for 5 days |
| Children 3-7 years | 100 mg four times daily for 5 days |
| Children 1-3 years | 100 mg three times daily for 5 days |

Symptomless cyst passers

| | |
|---|---|
| Adults | 400-800 mg three times daily for 5-10 days |
| Children 7-10 years | 200-400 mg three times daily for 5-10 days |
| Children 3-7 years | 100-200 mg four times daily for 5-10 days |
| Children 1-3 years | 100-200 mg three times daily for 5-10 days |

### 6. Treatment of gardiasis

| | |
|---|---|
| Adults | 2.0 g once daily for 3 days |
| Children 7-10 years | 1.0 g once daily for 3 days |
| Children 3-7 years | 600-800 mg once daily for 3 days |
| Children 1-3 years | 500 mg once daily for 3 days |

### 7. Treatment of acute ulcerative gingivitis

| | |
|---|---|
| Adults | 200 mg three times daily for 3 days |
| Children 7-10 years | 100 mg three times daily for 3 days |
| Children 3-7 years | 100 mg twice daily for 3 days |
| Children 1-3 years | 50 mg three times daily for 3 days |

### 8. Treatment of anaerobically infected leg ulcers and pressure sores

| | |
|---|---|
| Adults | 400 mg three times daily for 7 days |

### 9. Treatment of acute dental infections

| | |
|---|---|
| Adults | 200 mg three times daily for 3 to 7 days |

hydroxypropylmethylcellulose (E464), polyethylene glycol 400, and demineralised water.
Flagyl S Suspension: Liquid sugar granular. liquors, sodium dihydrogen phosphate or sodium acid phosphate crystalline., Veegum HV, methyl hydroxybenzoate (E218), propyl hydroxybenzoate (E216), ethanol, lemon flavour, oil orange terpenless, demineralised water.

Incompatibilities: None known.

Shelf life:
Flagyl tablets (200 mg and 400 mg): 60 months.
Flagyl S Suspension: 36 months. After dilution with Syrup BP the diluted suspension may be stored for 14 days.

Special precautions for storage:
Flagyl tablets (200 mg and 400 mg): Protect from light.

Flagyl S Suspension: Store below 25°C, protect from light

Nature and contents of container:
Flagyl tablets 200 mg are available in blisters packs of 21 tablets
Flagyl tablets 400 mg are available in blisters packs of 14 tablets
Flagyl S Suspension is available in glass bottles containing 100 ml

Instructions for use/handling: None stated.

**Marketing authorisation numbers**
| | |
|---|---|
| Flagyl tablets 200 mg | 0012/5256 |
| Flagyl tablets 400 mg | 0012/0084 |
| Flagyl S Suspension | 0012/0131 |

**Date of approval/revision of SPC** February 1997

**Legal category** POM

## FRUMIL*

**Qualitative and quantitative composition** *Frumil:* The active ingredient is Frusemide BP (Furosemide INN) 40.0 mg and Amiloride Hydrochloride equivalent to 5.0 mg anhydrous Amiloride Hydrochloride BP. *Frumil LS:* The active ingredient is Frusemide BP (Furosemide INN) 20.0 mg and Amiloride Hydrochloride equivalent to 2.5 mg anhydrous Amiloride Hydrochloride BP. Frumil Forte: The active ingredient is Frusemide BP (Furosemide INN) 80.0 mg and Amiloride Hydrochloride equivalent to 10.0 mg anhydrous Amiloride Hydrochloride BP.

**Pharmaceutical form** Tablets for oral administration.

**Clinical particulars**

*Therapeutic indications:* Frumil is a potassium sparing diuretic which is indicated where a prompt diuresis is required. It is of particular value in conditions where potassium conservation is important: congestive cardiac failure, nephrosis, corticosteriod therapy, oestrogen therapy and for ascites associated with cirrhosis.

*Posology and method of administration: Adults:* Frumil: One or two tablets to be taken in the morning. Frumil LS: One or two tablets to be taken in the morning. Frumil Forte: One tablet to be taken in the morning. *Children:* Not recommended. *Elderly:* The dosage should be adjusted according to the diuretic response; serum electrolytes and urea should be carefully monitored.

*Contra-indications:* Hyperkalaemia (serum potassium >5.3 mmol/litre), Addison's disease, renal failure, anuria, severe progressive renal disease, electrolyte imbalance, precomatose states associated with cirrhosis, concomitant potassium supplements or potassium sparing diuretics, known sensitivity to frusemide or amiloride. Frumil is contraindicated in children as safety in this age group has not been established.

*Special warnings and special precautions for use:* Frumil should be discontinued before a glucose tolerance test. Patients who are being treated with this preparation require supervision, with monitoring of fluid electrolyte states to avoid excessive loss of fluid. Frumil should be used with particular caution in elderly patients or those with potential obstruction of the urinary tract or disorders rendering electrolyte balance precarious.

*Interaction with other medicaments and other forms of Interaction:* Cephaloridine nephrotoxicity may be increased by concomitant administration of potent diuretics such as Frumil. The dosage of concurrently administered cardiac glycosides, lithium, non-depolarising muscle relaxants or antihypertensive agents may require adjustment.

*Pregnancy and lactation:* The safety of Frumil during pregnancy and lactation has not been established. women; therefore, the therapeutic benefit to the mother should outweigh any potential risk to the baby

*Effects on ability to drive and use machines:* None stated.

*Undesirable effects:* Serum uric acid levels may rise during treatment with Frumil and acute attacks of gout may be precipitated. Malaise, gastric upset, nausea, vomiting, diarrhoea and constipation may occur. If skin rashes or pruritis occur treatment should be withdrawn. Rare complications may include minor psychiatric disturbances, disturbances in liver function tests and ototoxicity. Bone marrow depression occasionally complicates treatment, necessitating withdrawal of the product. The haematopoetic state should be regularly monitored during treatment. Hyponatraemia, hypochloraemia and raised blood urea nitrogen may occur during vigorous diuresis, especially in seriously ill patients. Careful monitoring of serum electrolytes and urea should therefore be undertaken in these patients. Hyperkalaemia has been observed in patients receiving amiloride hydrochloride. As ACE inhibitors may elevate serum potassium levels, especially in the presence of renal impairment, combination with Frumil is best avoided in elderly patients or in any others in whom renal function may be compromised. If use of the combination is deemed essential clinical condition and serum electrolytes must be continuously monitored. Frusemide may cause latent diabetes to become manifest. It may be necessary to increase the dose of hypoglycaemic agents in diabetic patients. Patients with prostatic hypertrophy or impairment of microturition have an increased risk of developing acute urinary retention during diuretic therapy.

*Overdose:* Treatment of overdosage should be aimed at reversing dehydration and correcting electrolyte imbalance, particularly hyperkalaemia. Emesis should be induced or gastric lavage performed. Treatment should be symptomatic and supportive. If hyperkalaemia is seen, appropriate measures to reduce serum potassium must be instituted.

## Pharmacological properties

*Pharmacodynamic properties:* Frusemide: Frusemide is a loop diuretic which acts primarily to inhibit electrolyte reabsorption in the thick ascending Loop of Henle. Excretion of sodium, potassium and chloride ions is increased and water excretion enhanced. Amiloride: Amiloride is a mild diuretic which moderately increases the excretion of sodium and chloride and reduces potassium excretion, and appears to act mainly on the distal renal tubules. It does not appear to act by inhibition of aldosterone and does not inhibit carbonic anhydrase. Amiloride adds to the natiuretic but diminishes the kaliuretic effect of other diuretics. A combination of Frusemide and Amiloride is a diuretic which reduces the potassium loss of frusemide alone while avoiding the possible gastro-intestinal disturbances of potassium supplements.

*Pharmacokinetic properties:* Frusemide: Approximately 65% of the dose is absorbed after oral administration. The plasma half-life is biphasic with a terminal elimination phase of about $1\frac{1}{2}$ Hours. Frusemide is up to 99% bound to plasma proteins and is mainly excreted in the urine, largely unchanged, but also excreted in the bile, non-renal elimination being considerably increased in renal failure. Frusemide crosses the placental barrier and is excreted in the milk. Amiloride: Approximately 50% of the dose is absorbed after oral administration and peak serum concentrations are achieved by about 3-4 hours. The serum half-life is estimated to be about 6 hours. Amiloride is not bound to plasma proteins. Amiloride is not metabolised and is excreted unchanged in the urine. Pharmacokinetic studies have been completed on Frumil.

Frusemide:
Cp MAX = 1.14 µg/ml SD = 0.76
Tmax = 3.0 hours
AUC= 3.17 µg/ml hr SD = ± 1.25

Amiloride
Cp MAX = 13.42 ng/ml SD = 5.74
Tmax = 4.0 hours
AUC = 154 ng/ml hr SD = ± 65.2

*Preclinical safety data:* No further information available.

## Pharmaceutical particulars

*List of excipients:* Frumil, Frumil LS and Frumil Forte tablets contain the following excipients: lactose BP, starch maize BP microcrystalline cellulose BP, sodium starch glycollate BP, Sunset yellow dye (E110), French chalk powdered BP, colloidal anhydrous silica BP, magnesium stearate BP.

*Incompatibilities:* None stated.

*Shelf-life:* The shelf-life of Frumil, Frumil LS and Frumil Forte is 36 months.

*Special precautions for storage:* Store below 25°C in a dry place. Protect from light.

*Nature and contents of container:* Frumil–blister packs of 28 and 56 tablets, Frumil LS–blister packs of 28 and 56 tablets, Frumil Forte–blister packs of 28 and 56 tablets.

Instructions for use/handling: None

**Marketing authorisation numbers**
Frumil 5272/0017
Frumil LS 5272/0024
Frumil Forte 5272/0026

**Date of approval/revision of SPC** February 1997

**Legal category** POM

# IKOREL* TABLETS ▼

**Presentation** Ikorel is presented as off-white, bevelled edge, circular tablets which are scored on one face. Ikorel 10 mg tablets contain nicorandil 10 mg and bear the identification code IK10. Ikorel 20 mg tablets contain nicorandil 20 mg and are coded IK20. The tablets are provided in blister packs with an integral silica gel desiccant.

**Uses** *Pharmacology.* Nicorandil provides a dual mode of action leading to relaxation of vascular smooth muscle. A potassium channel opening action provides arterial vasodilation, thus reducing afterload, while the nitrate component promotes venous relaxation and a reduction in preload. Nicorandil has a direct effect on coronary arteries without leading to a steal phenomenon. The overall action improves blood flow to post-stenotic regions and the oxygen balance in the myocardium
*Kinetics:* Nicorandil is well absorbed with no significant first-pass metabolism. Maximum plasma concentrations are achieved in 30 to 60 minutes and are dose related. Metabolism is mainly by denitration of the molecule into the nicotinamide pathway with approximately 20% of an administered dose being excreted in the urine mainly as metabolites. The main phase of

elimination has a half-life of about 1 hour. Nicorandil is only slightly bound to plasma proteins. No clinically relevant modifications in the pharmacokinetic profile have been seen in the elderly or in patients with liver disease or chronic renal failure.

*Indications:* Ikorel tablets are indicated for the prevention and long-term treatment of chronic stable angina pectoris

**Dosage and administration:** *Adults*: The recommended starting dose is 10 mg nicorandil twice daily although 5 mg twice daily may be employed in patients particularly susceptible to headache. Subsequently the dosage should be titrated upward depending on the clinical response. The usual therapeutic dosage is in the range 10 to 20 mg nicorandil twice daily, although up to 30 mg twice daily may be employed if necessary. *Elderly:* There is no special requirement for dosage adjustment in elderly patients. As with all medicines the lowest effective dosage should be used. *Children:* A paediatric dosage has not been established and use of nicorandil is not recommended.

**Contra-indications, warnings, etc**
*Contra-indications:* Ikorel is contraindicated in patients with cardiogenic shock, left ventricular failure with low filling pressures and in hypotension. It is also contraindicated in patients who have demonstrated an idiosyncratic response or hypersensitivity to nicorandil.

*Warnings:* The use of nicorandil should be avoided in patients with depleted blood volume, low systolic blood pressure, acute pulmonary oedema or acute myocardial infarction with acute left ventricular failure and low filling pressures. Therapeutic doses of nicorandil may lower the blood pressure of hypertensive patients and therefore nicorandil, as with other antianginal agents, should be used with care when prescribed with antihypertensive drugs

*Pregnancy:* Animal studies have not revealed any harmful effect of nicorandil on the foetus although there is no experience in humans. It should not be used in pregnant patients unless there is no safer alternative.

*Lactation:* As it is not known whether nicorandil is excreted in human milk, breast feeding should be avoided by lactating patients who require therapy.

*Precautions:* Patients should be warned not to drive or operate machinery until it is established that their performance is unimpaired by nicorandil.

*Interactions:* No pharmacological or pharmacokinetic interactions have been observed in humans or animals with beta-blockers, digoxin, rifampicin, cimetidine, nicoumalone, a calcium antagonist or a combination of digoxin and frusemide. Nevertheless, there is the possibility that nicorandil may potentiate the blood pressure lowering effect of other vasodilators, tricyclic antidepressants or alcohol.

*Adverse effects:* The most frequent effect to be anticipated is headache, usually of a transitory nature, especially when treatment is initiated. Cutaneous vasodilation with flushing is less frequent. Nausea, vomiting, dizziness and a feeling of weakness have been reported occasionally. Myalgia and different types of rash have been reported rarely. Hypotension may occur at high therapeutic doses. An increase in heart rate may occur at high doses.

*Overdosage:* Acute overdosage is likely to be associated with peripheral vasodilation, decreased blood pressure and reflex tachycardia. Cardiac function should be monitored and general supportive measures employed. If necessary, circulating plasma volume should be increased by infusion of suitable fluid. In life-threatening situations administration of vasopressors should be considered. There is no experience of massive overdosage in humans although the $LD_{50}$ in dogs is in the range 62.5 to 125 mg/kg and in rodents it is in the order of 1200 mg/kg.'

**Pharmaceutical precautions** Ikorel tablets should be stored at a temperature not exceeding 25 °C and in a dry place.

**Legal category** POM

**Package quantities** Blister packs of 60 tablets.

**Further information** Nil

**Product licence numbers**
10 mg tablet 0012/0229
20 mg tablet 0012/0230

# INTAL* SPINCAPS

**Presentation** Intal is a presentation for inhalation of Sodium Cromoglycate BP 20 mg in micronised powder form. It is presented in a yellow/colourless, transparent, hard gelatin cartridge, bearing the overprint 'FISONS INTAL P'.

**Uses** Intal is indicated for the preventive treatment of bronchial asthma which may be due to allergy, exercise, cold air or chemical and occupational irritants. Sodium cromoglycate inhibits the release from sensitised mast cells of mediators of the allergic reaction. In the lung this inhibition of mediator release prevents both the immediate and late asthmatic response to immunological stimuli. Sodium cromoglycate also prevents the bronchoconstriction caused by exercise, cold air and chemical irritants.

**Dosage and administration** Intal is presented in a single dose cartridge, the Spincap*, for use in the Spinhaler*. Inhalation of the drug is controlled by the patient's inspiratory effort. Intal is not effective if the Spincap is swallowed because the prevention of the asthmatic attack depends upon local application to the lung.

*Dosage:* Since Intal therapy is essentially preventative, it is important that the patient is instructed to maintain regular dosage, as distinct from inhaling the drug intermittently to relieve symptoms.

*Adults (including the elderly) and children:* The normal dose is one Spincap four times daily, i.e. one night and morning and at intervals of 3-6 hours in between. It may be necessary to increase this to 6–8 times daily in more severe cases or during periods of severe antigen challenge. Additional doses may be taken before exertion to prevent exercise induced asthma or before exposure to other trigger factors.

When the asthmatic condition is stabilised, it may be possible to reduce the dosage provided that adequate control of the asthma is maintained.

*Concomitant steroid therapy:* In patients currently treated with steroids, the addition of Intal to the regime may make it possible to reduce the maintenance dose or to discontinue steroids completely. The patient must be carefully supervised while the steroid dose is reduced: a rate of reduction of 10% weekly is suggested. An increase in steroid dosage may be necessary if symptoms increase and at times of infection, severe antigen challenge or stress. If reduction of steroid dosage has been possible Intal should not be withdrawn until steroid cover has been reinstituted.

*Concomitant bronchodilator therapy:* If bronchodilators are used concomitantly, patients may find that the frequency of bronchodilator usage can be reduced as their asthma is stabilised with Intal.

**Contra-indications, warnings, etc**
*Contra-indications:* Intal Spincaps are contra-indicated in patients with known sensitivity to sodium cromoglycate.

*Side-effects:* Mild throat irritation, coughing and transient bronchospasm may occur. Very rarely severe bronchospasm associated with a marked fall in pulmonary function has been reported. In such cases treatment should be stopped and should not be reintroduced.

*Overdosage:* No action other than medical observation should be necessary.

*Withdrawal of Intal therapy:* Since the therapy acts prophylactically, it is important to continue treatment in those patients who benefit. If it is necessary to withdraw Intal, this should be done progressively over a period of one week. Symptoms of asthma may recur.

*Use in pregnancy and lactation:* As with all medication, caution should be exercised especially during the first trimester of pregnancy. Cumulative experience with sodium cromoglycate suggests that it has no adverse effects on foetal development. It should only be used in pregnancy where there is a clear need.

It is not known whether sodium cromoglycate is excreted in the breast milk but on the basis of its physicochemical properties this is considered unlikely. There is no information to suggest that use of sodium cromoglycate has any undesirable effects on the baby.

**Pharmaceutical precautions** Store in a moisture proof container in a cool, dry place protected from light.

Intal Spincaps can be adversely affected by moisture ingress. To prevent possible deterioration of the product, it is essential that the Spincaps are kept in their original container.

It is acceptable for up to four of the Spincaps to be stored in the Spinhaler Carrying Case for up to 24 hours.

**Legal category** POM.

**Package quantities** Original packs containing 112 Spincaps. Spinhaler Insufflators are supplied in individual containers. Instructions for use are supplied with each pack.

**Further information** Nil.

**Product licence number** 0113/5022R.

## INTAL* INHALER

**Qualitative and quantitative composition** Sodium Cromoglycate BP 5.0 mg

**Pharmaceutical form:** Intal is presented as a metered dose pressurised aerosol containing sodium cromoglycate as a suspension in chlorofluorocarbon propellants, for inhalation.

### Clinical particulars

*Therapeutic indication:* Intal is indicated for the preventative treatment of bronchial asthma, in adults and children.

*Posology and method of administration: Adults and Children:* The initial dose is two inhalations of the aerosol four times daily. Once adequate control of symptoms has been achieved it may be possible to reduce to a maintenance dose of one inhalation four times daily. However, the dose may be increased to two inhalations six or eight times daily in more severe cases or during periods of severe antigen challenge. An additional dose before exercise may also be taken.

*Elderly:* No current evidence for alteration of the recommended adult dose.

*Concomitant Bronchodilator Therapy:* Where a concomitant aerosol bronchodilator is prescribed it is recommended that this be administered prior to Intal.

*Concomitant Steroid Therapy:* In patients currently treated with steroids, the addition of Intal to the regimen may make it possible to reduce the maintenance dose, or discontinue therapy completely. The patient must be carefully supervised while the steroid dose is reduced; a rate of 10% weekly is suggested. If reduction of a steroid dosage has been possible, Intal should not be withdrawn until steroid cover has been reinstituted.

*Contra-indications:* Intal is contra-indicated in patients with known hypersensitivity to sodium cromoglycate, sorbitan trioleate or aerosol propellants.

*Special warnings and special precautions for use:* Intal must not be used for relief of an acute attack of bronchospasm.

*Withdrawal of Intal therapy:* Since the therapy is prophylactic, it is important to continue therapy in those patients who benefit. If it is necessary to withdraw this treatment, it should be done progressively over a period of one week. Symptoms of asthma may recur.

*Interactions with other medicaments and other forms of interaction:* None

*Pregnancy and lactation:* As with all medication, caution should be exercised especially during the first trimester of pregnancy. Cumulative experience with sodium cromoglycate suggests that it has no adverse effects on foetal development. It should only be used in pregnancy where there is a clear need. It is not known whether sodium cromoglycate is excreted in the breast milk but on the basis of its physico-chemical properties this is considered unlikely. There is no evidence to suggest that the use of sodium cromoglycate has any undesirable effects on the baby.

*Effects on ability to drive and use machines:* None.

*Undesirable effects:* Mild throat irritation, coughing and transient bronchospasm may occur. Very rarely severe bronchospasm associated with a marked fall in pulmonary function has been reported. In such cases treatment should be stopped and should not be reintroduced.

*Overdose:* No action other than medical supervision should be necessary.

### Pharmacological properties

*Pharmacodynamic properties:* Sodium cromoglycate has multiple actions in the lung. It inhibits the release from sensitised mast cells of mediators of the allergic reaction. In the lung, this inhibition of mediator release prevents both the immediate and late asthmatic response to immunological stimuli. It is also known that sodium cromoglycate offers protection against many types of immunologic and non-immunologic challenge systems, some of which are thought to produce bronchoconstriction by mechanisms independent of mast cells. It has also been shown that sodium cromoglycate inhibits reflex bronchoconstriction, probably by acting on sensory nerve endings in the lung.

*Pharmacokinetic properties:* Sodium cromoglycate is poorly absorbed from the gastro-intestinal tract. Following inhalation as a fine powder, about 8% of a dose is reported to be deposited in the lungs, from where it is rapidly absorbed and excreted unchanged in the urine and bile..

*Preclinical safety data:* Animal studies have shown that sodium cromoglycate has a very low order of local or systemic toxicity.

### Pharmaceutical particulars

*List of excipients:* Sorbitan trioleate, propellant mixture of dichlorotetrafluoroethane (propellant 114) and dichlorodifluoromethane (propellant 12).

*Incompatibilities:* None known.

*Shelf life:* 36 months.

*Special precautions for storage:* Store below 30°C, not in a refrigerator. The aerosol canister is pressurised and should be protected from direct sunlight, heat and frost and must not be punctured or burnt, even when empty.

*Nature and contents of container:* The aluminium can is fitted with a metering valve which delivers 112 actuations each containing 5 mg of sodium cromoglycate.

*Intal Inhaler:* The cartoned pack consists of an aerosol canister and a plastic adapter with a dustcap.

*Intal Fisonair:* The cartoned pack consists of an aerosol canister and a plastic adapter with a dustcap and a holding chamber.

*Intal Syncroner:* The cartoned pack consists of two aerosol canisters, each with a spacer device and dustcap.

*Instructions for use/handling:* Instructions for use are supplied with each pack.

**Marketing authorisation number**   0113/0109

**Date of approval/revision of SPC** March 1997

**Legal category**   POM

## INTAL* NEBULISER SOLUTION

**Presentation**   Intal Nebuliser Solution is presented in plastic ampoules containing Sodium Cromoglycate BP 20 mg in 2 ml of a clear colourless sterile aqueous solution.

**Uses**   Intal Nebuliser Solution is indicated for the preventive treatment of bronchial asthma which may be due to allergy, exercise, cold air or chemical and occupational irritants. Sodium cromoglycate inhibits the release from sensitised mast cells of the mediators of the allergic reaction. In the lung this inhibition of mediator release prevents both the immediate and late asthmatic response to immunological stimuli. Sodium cromoglycate also prevents the bronchoconstriction caused by exercise, cold air and chemical irritants.

**Dosage and administration**   Intal Nebuliser Solution should be administered from a power-operated (air-driven or ultrasonic) or foot pump operated machine nebuliser, via a face mask or mouthpiece.

*Dosage:* Since Intal Nebuliser Solution therapy is essentially preventative, it is important that regular dosage is maintained, as distinct from intermittent use to relieve symptoms.

*Adults (including the elderly) and children:* The contents of one ampoule are administered by nebulisation four times a day, i.e. night and morning and at intervals of 3–6 hours. In severe cases frequency of administration may be increased to 5 or 6 times daily.

*Concomitant steroid therapy:* In patients currently treated with steroids the addition of Intal Nebuliser Solution to the regime may make it possible to reduce the maintenance dose or discontinue steroids completely. The patient must be carefully supervised whilst the steroid dose is reduced; a rate of reduction of 10% weekly is suggested. An increase in steroid dosage may be necessary if symptoms increase and at times of infection, severe antigen challenge or stress. If reduction of steroid dosage has been possible, Intal Nebuliser Solution should not be withdrawn until steroid cover has been re-instituted.

*Concomitant bronchodilator therapy:* If bronchodilators are used concomitantly, patients may find that the frequency of bronchodilator usage can be reduced as their asthma is stabilised with Intal Nebuliser Solution.

**Contra-indications, warnings, etc**

*Contra-indications:* Known sensitivity to sodium cromoglycate. Intal Nebuliser Solution must not be given by injection.

*Side-effects:* Mild throat irritation, coughing and transient bronchospasm may occur. Very rarely severe bronchospasm associated with a marked fall in pulmonary function has been reported. In such cases treatment should be stopped and should not be reintroduced.

*Overdosage:* No action other than medical observation should be necessary.

*Withdrawal of Intal Nebuliser Solution:* Since the therapy is essentially prophylactic, it is important to continue treatment in those patients who benefit. If it is necessary to withdraw Intal Nebuliser Solution this should be done progressively over a period of one week. Symptoms of asthma may recur.

Intal Nebuliser Solution must not be used for an acute attack of bronchospasm.

*Use in pregnancy and lactation:* As with all medication, caution should be exercised especially during the first trimester of pregnancy. Cumulative experience with sodium cromoglycate suggests that it has no adverse effects on foetal development. It should only be used in pregnancy where there is a clear need.

It is not known whether sodium cromoglycate is excreted in the breast milk but on the basis of its physico-chemical properties this is considered unlikely. There is no evidence to suggest that the use of sodium cromoglycate has any undesirable effects on the baby.

**Pharmaceutical precautions**   Store in a dry place, below 30°C, away from sunlight. Should the physician decide to mix Intal Nebuliser Solution with other agents, the mixture should be prepared just prior to use and discarded if any turbidity develops. Any unused solution should be discarded immediately and the chamber of the nebuliser thoroughly cleaned.

**Legal category**   POM

**Package quantities**   Box containing 60×2 ml ampoules.

**Further information**   Nil.

**Product licence number** 0113/0068R

## INTRAVAL* SODIUM

**Presentation**   Vials or bottles of thiopentone sodium. It is supplied in vials of 0.5 g and bottles of 2.5 g for extemporaneous preparation of 2.5% solutions. A sterile transfer device, with instructions for use, is supplied with each 2.5 g bottle.

**Uses**   Administered intravenously Intraval Sodium produces general anaesthesia of short duration.

Intraval Sodium is indicated for the induction of general anaesthesia; for general anaesthesia of short duration with or without the addition of a muscle relaxant; for the control of convulsive states. It is administered rectally for the induction of basal anaesthesia.

*Other information:* Although bound to plasma proteins it rapidly crosses the blood-brain barrier and reaches maximum concentration in the brain within 30 seconds of injection. It is slowly metabolised by the liver. Only a small proportion of the active drug is excreted in the urine.

**Dosage and administration**   Intraval Sodium is administered usually as a 2.5% solution, but a 5% solution is sometimes used. A 2.5% solution is advised for all elderly and bad-risk patients. The injection may be given through any superficial vein.

Definite dosage cannot be stated for every case. The response of each patient must be observed and the dose regulated according to the onset of unconsciousness. Fractional administration is advised rather than the single-dose method, as this gives close control and greater flexibility of the anaesthetic and helps to prevent overdosage.

Most patients will require not more than 0.5 g otherwise recovery will be prolonged and possibly complicated. The patient should in all cases be premedicated with atropine and if necessary with an analgesic or tranquilliser, although the latter will increase the recovery time. If chlorpromazine or promethazine are used for pre-medication the amount of Intraval Sodium required for induction should be reduced.

Solutions are prepared by adding Water for Injections (BP). They must be used within 24 hours or discarded.

For induction: Inject 2–3 ml of the 5% solution or twice this volume of the 2.5% solution in 10–15 seconds, then pause for 30 seconds to 1 minute to observe the effect of the drug, depending on the state of the patient's circulation. Usually there is loss of consciousness and some relaxation. A further quantity of the solution may then be given if indicated, otherwise anaesthesia should be maintained by an appropriate inhalation agent.

For minor operations: Induction is as described above with additional quantities of the anaesthetic solution being given as required to maintain anaesthesia at a level adequate to obtund pain reflexes. The level of anaesthesia is best judged by the depth of respiration; surgical anaesthesia is usually present when respiration is depressed. It cannot be too strongly emphasised that the airway must be kept open with the patient breathing an adequate concentration of oxygen. In these circumstances the depressed respiration is not dangerous and the patient should remain a good colour with the skin warm and dry.

Intravenous anaesthesia is not recommended for the maintenance of unconsciousness in lengthy procedures, so that for these, after induction, it should always be supplemented by the chosen inhalation agent.

*Children:* Intraval Sodium is suitable for use in children

as well as adults. The dosage is 2–7 mg/kg intravenously.

**Contra-indications, warnings, etc**

*Use in pregnancy:* There is epidemiological and clinical evidence of the safety of barbiturates in pregnancy including thiopentone. This drug readily crosses the placenta and appears in human milk. Dosage in the pregnant female should not exceed 250 mg.

*Contra-indications:* A history of acute intermittent porphyria is an absolute contra-indication to any barbiturate. Special care is required in patients with the following conditions: hypovolaemia; severe haemorrhage; burns; dehydration; severe anaemia; cardiovascular disease; status asthmaticus; severe liver disease; myasthenia gravis and muscular dystrophies; adrenocortical insufficiency even when controlled by cortisone; cachexia and severe toxaemia; raised intracranial pressure; raised blood urea; raised plasma potassium; metabolic disorders, e.g. thyrotoxicosis, myxoedema, diabetes.

*Precautions:* Reduced doses are required in the elderly and in patients heavily pre-medicated with narcotics and other central depressants. On the other hand, those addicted to drugs are difficult subjects to anaesthetise with normal thiopentone dosage and it is advised that supplementary analgesic agents and relaxants be given as necessary.

The jaw drops rapidly after starting the injection and must be supported, since it is imperative to keep the airway open. The patient should always be in a recumbent position to avoid cerebral ischaemia.

If Intraval Sodium is used in dental work a mouth prop is inserted before injection is commenced. The throat must be properly packed to prevent access of blood, etc. to the larynx and the dose employed should not exceed 0.25 g otherwise recovery will be delayed. Facilities for intubation and administration of oxygen under positive pressure must always be available.

To prevent accidental intra-arterial injection the site of administration must be palpated carefully and after insertion of the needle a little blood should be drawn into the syringe to observe its colour. Intra-arterial injection produces severe arterial spasm with intense burning pain in the hand and fingers. The patient can sometimes warn the anaesthetist of this before losing consciousness. In the event of such accident, inject procaine hydrochloride directly into the artery and perform a stellate ganglion block. Early anticoagulant therapy is advisable.

*Side-effects: Adverse effects:* Coughing, sneezing or laryngeal spasm may occur during induction. Extravasation causes pain and possible tissue necrosis. Thrombophlebitis may result from the use of 5% solution. Skin rashes, fever, arthralgia and weakness are rare side-effects. Allergic reactions and hypersensitivity have been documented.

*Toxicity and treatment of overdosage:* Respiratory depression during thiopentone anaesthesia must be treated by artificial ventilation with oxygen, as should cardiac arrhythmia associated with anoxia or hypercarbia. A fall in blood pressure is often noted initially, while overdose may lead to circulatory failure.

Apnoea or serious respiratory depression must be treated by controlled respiration with oxygen. Cardiovascular collapse requires immediate lowering of the head of the table; if the blood pressure fails to rise a pressor agent such as mephentermine or a plasma expander should be given. If the heart stops immediate cardiac massage should be given.

**Pharmaceutical precautions** Aqueous solutions of thiopentone sodium are strongly alkaline; a 2.5% solution has a pH about 10.5. The solution is incompatible with acids, acidic salts and oxidising agents. Solutions decompose on standing giving cloudiness, precipitation or crystallisation; any such solution must not be used.

Solutions should be freshly prepared, stored at 2-8°C, and used within 24 hours or discarded.

**Legal category** POM.

**Package quantities** For the preparation of 2.5% solution:

Boxes of 10×2.5 g.
Boxes of 10×2.5 g+10×100 ml Water for Injection.
Boxes of 25×0.5 g.
Boxes of 25×0.5 g+25×20 ml Water for Injection.

**Further information** Nil.

**Product licence number** 0012/5043.

## LARGACTIL* TABLETS, SYRUP AND FORTE SUSPENSION

**Qualitative and quantitative composition**

*Largactil tablets 10 mg* contain 10 mg chlorpromazine hydrochloride. *Largactil tablets 25 mg* contain 25 mg chlorpromazine hydrochloride. Largactil tablets 50 mg contain 50 mg chlorpromazine hydrochloride. *Largactil tablets 100 mg* contain 100 mg chlorpromazine hydrochloride. Largactil syrup contains 0.5% w/v chlorpromazine hydrochloride BP (25 mg chlorpromazine hydrochloride in 5 ml).

*Largactil Forte Suspension* contains 2.9% w/v chlorpromazine embonate, equivalent to 100 mg/5 ml of chlorpromazine hydrochloride.

**Pharmaceutical form:** Largactil tablets are white to off-white circular, biconvex, film coated tablets: one face impressed LG and the strength , and the reverse face plain. Largactil syrup is a clear, bright golden-brown syrup, Largactil Forte suspension is an orange coloured suspension.

**Clinical particulars**

*Therapeutic indications:* Largactil is a phenothiazine neuroleptic. It is indicated in the following conditions:

Schizophrenia and other psychoses (especially paranoid) mania and hypomania.

Anxiety, psychomotor agitation, excitement, violent or dangerously impulsive behaviour. Largactil is used as an adjunct in the short-term treatment of these conditions

Intractable hiccup.

Nausea and vomiting of terminal illness (where other drugs have failed or are not available).

Childhood schizophrenia and autism.

*Posology and method of administration:* Oral administration should be used whenever possible. Route of administration: oral. Patients unwilling to swallow tablets may be treated with suspension or syrup. Dosages should be low to begin with and gradually increased under close supervision until the optimum dosage within the recommended range, for the individual is reached (see dosage table). Individuals vary considerably and the optimum dose may be affected by the formulation used.

*Contra-indications:* None stated.

*Special warnings and special precautions for use:* Largactil should be avoided in patients with liver or renal dysfunction, epilepsy, Parkinson's disease, hypothyroidism, cardiac failure, phaechromcytoma, myasthenia gravis and prostate hypertrophy. It should be avoided in patients known to be hypersensitive to phenothiazines or with a history of narrow angle glaucoma. It should be used with caution in the elderly, particularly during very hot or cold weather (risk of hyper-, hypothermia). The elderly are particularly susceptible to postural hypotension.

*Interaction with other medicaments and other forms of interaction:* The CNS depressant actions of Largactil and other neuroleptic agents may be intensified (additively) by alcohol, barbiturates and other sedatives. Respiratory depression may occur. The hypotensive effect of most antihypertensive drugs especially alpha adrenceptor blocking agents may be exaggerated by Largactil. The mild anticholinergic effect of Largactil may be enhanced by other anticholinergic drugs possibly leading to constipation, heat stroke, etc. The action of some drugs may be opposed by Largactil; these include amphetamine, levodopa, clonidine, guanethidine, adrenaline. Anticholinergic agents may reduce the antipsychotic effect of Largactil. Some drugs interfere with absorption of neuroleptic agents: antacids, anti-Parkinson, lithium. Increases or decreases in the plasma concentrations of a number of drugs, e.g. propranalol, phenobarbitone have been observed but were not of clinical significance. High doses of Largactil reduce the response to hypoglycaemic agents the dosage of which might have to be raised. Documented adverse clinically significant interactions occur with alcohol. Guanethidine and hypoglycaemic agents. Adrenaline must not be used in patients overdosed with Largactil. Other interactions are of a theoretical nature and not serious. Simultaneous administration of desferroxamine and prochlorperazine has been observed to induce a transient metabolic encephalopathy characterised by loss of consciousness for 48-72 hours. It is possible this may occur with Largactil since it shares many of the pharmacological properties of prochlorperazine.

*Pregnancy and lactation:* There is inadequate evidence of the safety of Largactil in human pregnancy but it has been widely used for many years without apparent ill consequence. There is evidence of harmful effects in animals. Like other drugs it should be avoided in pregnancy unless the physician considers it essential. It may occasionally prolong labour and at such time should be withheld until the cervix is dilated 3-4 cm. Possible adverse effect on the foetus include lethargy or paradoxical hyperexcitability, tremor and low Apgar score. Largactil being excreted in milk, breast-feeding should be suspended during treatment.

*Effects on ability to drive and use machines:* Patients should be warned about drowsiness during the early days of treatment and advised not to drive or operate machinery.

*Undesirable effects:* Minor side effects are nasal stuffiness, dry mouth, insomnia, agitation. *Liver effects:* Jaundice, usually transient, occurs in a very small percentage of patients taking chlorpromazine. A premonitory sign may be a sudden onset of fever after one to three weeks of treatment followed by the development of jaundice. Chlorpromazine jaundice has the biochemical and other characteristics of obstructive jaundice and is associated with obstructions of the canaliculi by bile thrombi; the frequent presence of an accompanying eosinophilia indicates the allergic nature of this phenomenon. Treatment should be withheld on the development of jaundice. *Skin and eyes:* Contact skin sensitisation is a serious but rare complication in those frequently handling preparations of chlorpromazine: the greatest care must be taken to avoid contact of the drug with the skin. Skin rashes of various kinds may also be seen in patients treated with the drug. Patients on high dosage may develop photosensitivity in sunny weather and should avoid exposure to direct sunlight. Ocular changes and the development of a metallic greyish-mauve coloration of exposed skin have been noted in some individuals, mainly females, who have received chlorpromazine continuously for long periods (four to eight years). *Cardiorespiratory:* Hypotension, usually postural, commonly occurs. Elderly or volume depleted subjects are particularly susceptible: it is more likely to occur after intramuscular administration.. Cardiac arrhythmia's including atrial arrhythmia, A-V block, ventricular tachycardia and fibrillation have been reported during neuroleptic therapy, possibly related to dosage. Pre-existing cardiac disease, old age, hypokalaemia and concurrent tricyclic antidepressant may predispose. ECG changes, usually benign, including widened QT interval, ST depression, U-waves and T-wave changes. Respiratory depression is possible in susceptible patients. *Blood picture:* A mild leucopenia occurs in up to 30% of patients on prolonged high dosage. Agranulocytosis may occur rarely; it is not dose related. The occurrence of unexplained infections or fever requires immediate haematological investigation. *Extrapyramidal:* Acute dystonias or dyskenias, usually transitory are more common in children and young adults and usually occur within the first 4 days of treatment or after dosage increases. Akathisia characteristically occurs after large initial doses. Parkinsonism is more common in adults and the elderly. It usually develops after weeks or months of treatment. One or more of the following may be seen: tremor, rigidity, akinesia or other features of Parkinsonism. Commonly just tremor. *Tardive Dyskinesia:* If this occurs it is usually, but not necessarily, after prolonged high dosage. It can even occur after treatment has been stopped. Dosage should therefore be kept low whenever possible. Endocrine: Hyperprolactinaemia which may result in galactorrhoea, gynaecomastia, amenorrhoea and impotence. *Neuroleptic malignant syndrome* (hyperthermia, rigidity, autonomic dysfunction and altered consciousness) may occur with any neuroleptic.

*Overdose:* Symptoms of chlorpromazine overdosage include drowsiness or loss of consciousness, hypotension, tachycardia, ECG changes, ventricular arrhythmia's and hypothermia. Severe extra-pyramidal dyskinesias may occur. If the patient is seen sufficiently soon (up to 6 hours) after ingestion of a toxic dose, gastric lavage may be attempted. Pharmacological induction of emesis is unlikely to be of any use. Activated charcoal should be given. There is no specific antidote. Treatment is supportive. Generalised vasodilation may result in circulatory collapse; raising the patient's legs may suffice. In severe cases, volume expansion by intravenous fluids may be needed; infusion fluids should be warmed before administration in order not to aggravate hypothermia. Positive inotropic agents such as dopamine may be tried if fluid replacement is insufficient to correct the circulatory collapse. Peripheral vasoconstriction agents are not generally recommended; avoid the use of adrenaline. Ventricular or supraventricular tachyarrhythmias usually respond to restoration of normal body temperature and correction of circulatory or metabolic disturbances. If persistent or life threatening, appropriate anti-arrhythmic therapy may be considered. Avoid lignocaine and, as far as possible, long acting anti-arrhythmic drugs. Pronounced central nervous system depression requires airway maintenance or, in extreme circumstances, assisted respiration. Severe dystonic reactions usually respond to procyclidine (5-10 mg) or orphenadrine (20-40 mg) administered intramuscularly or intravenously. Convulsions should be treated with intravenous diazepam. Neuroleptic malignant syndrome should be treated with cooling. Dantrolene sodium may be tried.

**Pharmacological properties**

*Pharmacodynamic properties:* Largactil is a phenothiazine neuroleptic.

*Pharmacokinetic properties:* Chlorpromazine is rap-

## Largactil Tablets, Syrup and Forte Suspension dosages

*Schizophrenia, other psychoses, anxiety, childhood schizophrenia and autism.*

| Adult | Children under 1 year | Children 1–5 years | Children 6 -12 years | Elderly or debilitated patients |
|---|---|---|---|---|
| Initially 25 mg t.d.s. or 75 mg at bedtime increasing by daily amounts of 25 mg to an effective maintenance dose. This is usually in the range 75 to 300 mg daily, but some patients may require up to 1 g daily. | Do not use unless need is life saving. | 0.5 mg/kg bodyweight every 4-6 hours to a maximum recommended dose of 40 mg daily. | 1/3 to 1/2 the adult dose to a maximum recommended dose of 75 mg daily. | Start with 1/3 to 1/2 the usual adult dose with a more gradual increase in dosage. |

*Hiccup:*

| Adult | Children under 1 year | Children 1-5 years | Children 6-12 years | Elderly or debilitated patients |
|---|---|---|---|---|
| 25-50 mg t.d.s or q.d.s | No information available | | | |

*Nausea and vomiting of terminal illness*

| Adults | Children under 1 year | Children 1-5 years | Children 6-12 years | Elderly or debilitated patients |
|---|---|---|---|---|
| 10-25 mg every 4-6 hours | Do not use unless need is life saving | 0.5 mg/kg 4-6 hours. Maximum daily dosage should not exceed 40 mg | 0.5 mg/Kg 4-6 hours. maximum daily dosage should not exceed 75 mg. | Initially 1/3 to 1/2 the adult dose. The physician should then use his clinical judgement to obtain control. |

idly absorbed and widely distributed in the body. It is metabolised in the liver and excreted in the urine and bile. Whilst plasma concentration of chlorpromazine itself rapidly declines excretion of chlorpromazine metabolites is very slow. The drug is highly bound to plasma protein. It readily diffuses across the placenta. Small quantities have been detected in milk from treated women. Children require smaller dosages per kg than adults.

### Pharmaceutical particulars

*List of excipients:*
*Largactil Tablets*: lactose, maize starch, Aerosil 200 (E464), magnesium sterate; Tablet coating: Hydroxypropylmethylcellulose, polyethylene glycol 200, Opaspray M-1-7111B (contains E171 and E646)

*Largactil Syrup:* Liquid sugar gran. liquors, Oil peppermint Chinese, Fruit flavouring, Sodium citrate gran. (E331), Sodium sulphite anhydrous (E221), Caramel flavour, Demineralised water, Tween 20, Oil spearmint, Citric acid anhydrous (E330), Ascorbic acid (E300), Sodium metabisulphite powder (E223), Sodium benzoate (E211),

*Largactil Forte Suspension:* sorbitol solution or sorbitol powder (E420), Sodium benzoate (E211), Sodium citrate gran, Standacol sunset yellow dye (E110), Propylene glycol, Povidone K30 (E1201), Veegum RG, Citric acid anhydrous (E330), Saccharin sodium, Oil Orange terpenless, Sodium alginate (E401), Demineralised water,

*Incompatibilities:* None stated.

*Shelf life:* 36 months.

*Special precautions for storage:* Protect from light. Store below 30°C.

*Nature and contents of container:*
*Largactil Tablets 10 mg 25 mg 50 mg and 100 mg are* available in blisters of 56 tablets.
*Largactil Syrup* is available in glass bottles containing 100, ml.
*Largactil Forte Suspension* is available in glass bottles containing 100 ml.

*Instructions for use/handling:* None

**Marketing authorisation numbers**
| | |
|---|---|
| Largactil tablets 10 mg | 0012/5108R |
| Largactil tablets 25 mg | 0012/5019R |
| Largactil tablets 50 mg | 0012/5110R |
| Largactil Tablets 100 mg | 0012/5111R |
| Largactil Syrup | 0012/5083R |
| Largactil Forte Suspension | 0012/5001R |

**Date of approval/revision of SPC** February 1997

**Legal category** POM

## LARGACTIL* INJECTION

**Qualitative and quantitative composition** Largactil injection contains 2.5% w/v chlorpromazine hydrochloride BP

**Pharmaceutical form** Largactil injection is a sterile solution for injection

### Clinical particulars

*Therapeutic indications:* Largactil is a phenothiazine neuroleptic. It is indicated in the following conditions:
Schizophrenia and other psychoses (especially paranoid) mania and hypomania.
Anxiety, psychomotor agitation, excitement, violent or dangerously impulsive behaviour. Largactil is used as an adjunct in the short-term treatment of these conditions
Intractable hiccup.
Nausea and vomiting of terminal illness (where other drugs have failed or are not available).
Induction of hypothermia is facilitated by largactil which prevents shivering and causes vasodilation.
Childhood schizophrenia and autism.

*Posology and method of administration:* Deep intramuscular injection.
Oral route administration should be used wherever possible.
Parenteral formulations may be used in emergencies. They may only be administered by *deep* intramuscular injection. Largactil is too irritant to give subcutaneously. Repeated injections should be avoided if possible.
*Adults:* A single deep intramuscular injection of 25-50 mg followed by oral therapy will suffice in many cases, but the intramuscular dose may be repeated if required at 6 to 8 hour intervals. As soon as possible oral administration should be substituted.
*Elderly:* Should be started on half or even quarter of the adult dosage.

*Contra-indications:* None

*Special warnings and special precautions for use:* Largactil should be avoided in patients with liver or renal dysfunction, epilepsy, Parkinson's disease, hypothyroidism, cardiac failure, phaechromcytoma, myasthenia gravis and prostate hypertrophy. It should be avoided in patients known to be hypersensitive to phenothiazines or with a history of narrow angle glaucoma. It should be used with caution in the elderly, particularly during very hot or cold weather (risk of hyper-, hypothermia). Postural hypotension with tachycardia as well as local pain or nodule formation may occur after intramuscular administration. The patient should be kept supine and blood pressure monitored when receiving parenteral chlorpromazine. The elderly are particularly susceptible to postural hypotension.

*Interaction with other medicaments and other forms of interaction:* The CNS depressant actions of Largactil and other neuroleptic agents may be intensified (additively) by alcohol, barbiturates and other sedatives. Respiratory depression may occur. The hypotensive effect of most antihypertensive drugs especially alpha adrenceptor blocking agents may be exaggerated by Largactil. The mild anticholinergic effect of Largactil may be enhanced by other anticholinergic drugs possibly leading to constipation, heat stroke, etc. Anticholinergic agents may reduce the antipsychotic effects of Largactil. The action of some drugs may be opposed by Largactil; these include amphetamine, levodopa, clonidine, guanethidine, adrenaline. Some drugs interfere with absorption of neuroleptic agents: antacids, anti-Parkinson, lithium. Increases or decreases in the plasma concentrations of a number of drugs, e.g. propranalol, phenobarbitone have been observed but were not of clinical significance. High doses of Largactil reduce the response to hypoglycaemic agents the dosage of which might have to be raised. Documented adverse clinically significant interactions occur with alcohol, guanethidine and hypoglycaemic agents. Adrenaline must not be used in patients overdosed with Largactil. Other interactions are of a theoretical nature and not serious. Simultaneous administration of desferroxamine and prochlorperazine has been observed to induce a transient metabolic encephalopathy characterised by loss of consciousness for 48-72 hours. It is possible this may occur with Largactil since it shares many of the pharmacological properties of prochlorperazine.

*Pregnancy and lactation:* There is inadequate evidence of the safety of Largactil in human pregnancy but it has been widely used for many years without apparent ill consequence. There is evidence of harmful effects in animals. Like other drugs it should be avoided in pregnancy unless the physician considers it essential. It may occasionally prolong labour and at such a time should be withheld until the cervix is dilated 3-4 cm. Possible adverse effects on the foetus include lethargy or paradoxical hyperexcitability, tremor and low Apgar score. Largactil being excreted in milk, breastfeeding should be suspended during treatment.

*Effects on ability to drive and use machines:* Patients should be warned about drowsiness during the early days of treatment and advised not to drive or operate machinery.

*Undesirable effects:* Minor side effects are nasal stuffiness, dry mouth, insomnia, agitation. *Liver effects:* Jaundice, usually transient, occurs in a very small percentage of patients taking chlorpromazine. A premonitory sign may be a sudden onset of fever after one to three weeks of treatment followed by the development of jaundice. Chlorpromazine jaundice has the biochemical and other characteristics of obstructive jaundice and is associated with obstructions of the canaliculi by bile thrombi; the frequent presence of an accompanying eosinophilia indicates the allergic nature of this phenomenon. Treatment should be withheld on the development of jaundice. *Skin and eyes*: Contact skin sensitisation is a serious but rare complication in those frequently handling preparations of chlorpromazine: the greatest care must be taken to avoid contact of the drug with the skin. Skin rashes of various kinds may also be seen in patients treated with the drug. Patients on high dosage may develop photosensitivity in sunny weather and should avoid exposure to direct sunlight. Ocular changes and the development of a metallic greyish-mauve coloration of exposed skin have been noted in some individuals, mainly females, who have received chlorpromazine continuously for long periods (four to eight years). *Cardiorespiratory*: Hypotension, usually postural, commonly occurs. Elderly or volume depleted subjects are particularly susceptible: it is more likely to occur after intramuscular administration. Cardiac arrhythmia's including atrial fibrillation, A-V block, ventricular tachycardia and fibrillation have been reported during neuroleptic therapy, possibly related to dosage. Pre-existing cardiac disease, old age, hypokalaemia and concurrent tricyclic antidepressant may predispose. ECG changes, usually benign, including widened QT interval, ST depression, U-waves and T-wave changes. Respiratory depression is possible in susceptible patients. *Blood picture*: A mild leucopenia occurs in up to 30% of patients on prolonged high dosage. Agranulocytosis may occur rarely; it is not dose related. The occurrence of unexplained infections or fever requires immediate haematological investigation. *Extrapyramidal*: Acute dystonias or dyskinesias, usually transitory are more common in children and young adults and usually occur within the first 4 days of treatment or after dosage increases. Akathisia characteristically occurs

## Largactil Injection dosages

*Dosage of chlopromazine in schizophrenia, other psychoses, anxiety and agitation, childhood schizophrenias and autism.*
Route: Intramuscular.

| Adult | Children under 1 year | Children 1–5 years | Children 6 -12 years | Elderly or debilitated patients |
|---|---|---|---|---|
| For acute relief of symptoms 25-50 mg every 6-8 hours | Do not use unless need is life saving. | 0.5 mg/kg bodyweight every 6-8 hours. Dosage is not advised to exceed 40 mg daily . | 0.5 mg/kg bodyweight every 6-8 hours. Dosage is not advised to exceed 75 mg daily. | Doses in the lower range for adults should be sufficient to control symptoms. i.e. 25 mg 8 hourly |

*Hiccup. Induction of hypothermia to prevent shivering*

| Indication | Adult dose | Children under 1 year | Children 1-5 years | Children 6-12 years | Elderly or debilitated patients |
|---|---|---|---|---|---|
| Hiccups | 25–50 mg and if this fails 25-50 mg in 500-1000 ml sodium chloride injection by slow intravenous infusion. | No information available | | | |
| Induction of hypothermia to prevent shivering | 25-50 mg every 6-8 hours. | Do not use. | Initial dose 0.5 to 1 mg/kg. Maintenance 0.5 mg/kg every 4-6 hours. | Initial dose 0.5 to 1 mg/kg. Maintenance 0.5 mg/kg every 4-6 hours. | No data available. |

*Nausea and vomiting of terminal illness*

| Adults | Children under 1 year | Children 1-5 years | Children 6-12 years | Elderly or debilitated patients. |
|---|---|---|---|---|
| 25 mg initially then 25-50 mg every 3-4 hours until vomiting stops then drug to be taken orally | Do not use unless need is life saving. | 0.5 mg/kg 6-8 hourly. It is advised that maximum daily dosage should not exceed 40 mg. | 0.5 mg/kg every 6-8 hours. It is advised that maximum daily dosage should not exceed 75 mg. | Not recommended |

after large initial doses. Parkinsonism is more common in adults and the elderly. It usually develops after weeks or months of treatment. One or more of the following may be seen: tremor, rigidity, akinesia or other features of Parkinsonism. Commonly just tremor. *Tardive Dyskinesia*: If this occurs it is usually, but not necessarily, after prolonged high dosage. It can even occur after treatment has been stopped. Dosage should therefore be kept low whenever possible. *Endocrine*: Hyperprolactinaemia which may result in galactorrhoea, gynaecomastia, amenorrhoea and impotence. *Neuroleptic malignant syndrome* (hyperthermia, rigidity, autonomic dysfunction and altered consciousness) may occur with any neuroleptic. Allergic phenomena such as angiodema, bronchospasm, and urticaria have occurred with phenothiazines but anaphylactic reactions have been exceedingly rare.

*Overdose:* Toxicity and treatment of overdosage: Symptoms of chlorpromazine overdosage include drowsiness or loss of consciousness, hypotension, tachycardia, ECG changes, ventricular arrhythmias and hypothermia. Severe extra-pyramidal dyskinesias may occur. If the patient is seen sufficiently soon (up to 6 hours) after ingestion of a toxic dose, gastric lavage may be attempted. Pharmacological induction of emesis is unlikely to be of any use. Activated charcoal should be given. There is no specific antidote. Treatment is supportive. Generalised vasodilation may result in circulatory collapse; raising the patient's legs may suffice. In severe cases, volume expansion by intravenous fluids may be needed; infusion fluids should be warmed before administration in order not to aggravate hypothermia. Positive inotropic agents such as dopamine may be tried if fluid replacement is insufficient to correct the circulatory collapse. Peripheral vasoconstriction agents are not generally recommended; avoid the use of adrenaline. Ventricular or supraventricular tachy-arrhythmias usually respond to restoration of normal body temperature and correction of circulatory or metabolic disturbances. If persistent or life threatening, appropriate anti-arrhythmic therapy may be considered. Avoid lignocaine and, as far as possible, long acting anti-arrhythmic drugs. Pronounced central nervous system depression requires airway maintenance or, in extreme circumstances, assisted respiration. Severe dystonic reactions usually respond to procyclidine (5-10 mg) or orphenadrine (20-40 mg) administered intramuscularly or intravenously. Convulsions should be treated with intravenous diazepam. Neuroleptic malignant syndrome should be treated with cooling. Dantrolene sodium may be tried.

### Pharmacological properties

*Pharmacodynamic properties:* Largactil is a phenothiazine neuroleptic.

*Pharmacokinetic properties:* Chlorpromazine is rapidly absorbed and widely distributed in the body. It is metabolised in the liver and excreted in the urine and bile. Whilst plasma concentration of chlorpromazine itself rapidly declines excretion of chlorpromazine

metabolites is very slow. The drug is highly bound to plasma protein. It readily diffuses across the placenta. Small quantities have been detected in milk from treated women. Children require smaller dosages per kg than adults.

### Pharmaceutical particulars

*List of excipients:* Sodium sulphite anhydrous (E221), Sodium citrate, Sodium metabisulphite powder (E223), , Water for Injections, Sodium chloride .

*Incompatibilities:* Largactil injection solutions have a pH of 5.0-6.5; they are incompatible with benzylpenicillin potassium, phenobarbitone sodium and phenobarbitone sodium.

*Shelf life:* The shelf-life of the Largactil Injection is 60 months.

*Special precaution for storage:* Largactil Injection should be stored protected from light. Discoloured solution should not be used.

*Nature and content of Container:* Largactil Injection 2.5% w/v is supplied in boxes containing 10 x 1 ml or 10 x 2 ml in glass ampoules.

*Instructions for use/handling:* None

**Marketing authorisation number** 0012/5308R

**Date of approval/revision of SPC** February 1997

**Legal category** POM

## MAALOX* SUSPENSION

**Qualitative and quantitative composition:** Dried Aluminium Hydroxide Gel BP 220 mg, and Magnesium Hydroxide BP 195 mg per 5 ml.

**Pharmaceutical form** Suspension.

### Clinical particulars

*Therapeutic indications:* Antacid therapy in gastric and duodenal ulcer, gastritis, heartburn and gastric hyperacidity.

*Posology and method of administration:* Oral.
   *Adult and elderly:* 10–20 ml taken 20 minutes to one hour after meals and at bedtime, or as required. Maalox can be taken with water or milk if required.
   *Children:* Not recommended for children under 14 years.

*Contra-indications:* Maalox should not be used in patients who are severely debilitated or suffering from renal insufficiency or if there is severe abdominal pain and/or the possibility of bowel obstruction.

*Special warnings and special precautions for use:* none stated.

*Interactions with other medicaments and other forms of interaction:* Antacids are known to interfere with the absorption of certain drugs including tetracyclines, vitamins, ciprofloxacin, ketoconazole, hydroxychlororquine, chloroquine, chlorpromazine and rifampicin.

*Pregnancy and lactation:* it is wise to avoid taking

preparations containing antacids in the first trimester of pregnancy and during lactation.

*Effects on ability to drive and use machines:* None stated.

*Undesirable effects:* Gastro-intestinal side effects are uncommon. However, occasional diarrhoea and constipation may occur if use is excessive.

*Overdose:* serious symptoms are unlikely following overdose. Discontinue medication and correct fluid deficiency if necessary.

### Pharmacological properties

*Pharmacodynamic properties:* Maalox is a balanced mixture of two antacids; aluminium hydroxide is a slow acting antacid and magnesium hydroxide is a quick-acting one. The two are frequently combined in antacid mixtures. Aluminium hydroxide on its own is astringent and may cause constipation. This effect is balanced by the effect of magnesium hydroxide, which, in common with other magnesium salts, may cause diarrhoea. Gastro-intestinal side-effects are thus rare with Maalox and makes it especially suitable when long-term therapy is necessary.

*Pharmacokinetic properties:* The absorption of aluminium and magnesium from antacids is small. Aluminium hydroxide is slowly converted to aluminium chloride in the stomach. Some absorption of soluble aluminium salts occurs in the gastro-intestinal tract with urinary excretion. Any absorbed magnesium is likewise excreted in the urine. Aluminium containing antacids should not be administered to patients with renal impairment where increased plasma concentration may occur.

*Preclinical safety data:* No relevant data.

### Pharmaceutical particulars

*List of excipients:* Methylparaben NF, propylparaben NF, citric acid (anhydrous) USP, sodium saccharin (granular) USP, sorbitol solution 70% USP, mannitol powder USP, hydrogen peroxide solution 35%, hydrochloric acid BP, peppermint oil NF and purified water.

*Incompatibilities:* none stated.

*Shelf life:* Unopened: 24 months. After opening: 28 days.

*Special precautions for storage:* Protect from freezing. Store away from direct sunlight.

*Nature and contents of container:* White plastic bottles with polypropylene cap containing 500 ml.

*Instructions for use/handling:* Maalox can be taken with milk of water if required.

**Marketing authorisation number** 0050/5002.

**Date of approval/revision of SPC** February 1997

**Legal category** GSL.

## MAALOX* TC SUSPENSION AND TABLETS

**Presentation**
*Suspension:* White, peppermint flavoured suspension. Each 5 ml contains:

| | |
|---|---|
| Dried Aluminium Hydroxide BP | 600 mg |
| Magnesium Hydroxide BP | 300 mg |

Other ingredients include parabens.

*Tablets:* White, peppermint flavoured tablets marked 'Maalox TC' on one face and 'Rorer' on the other face. Each tablet contains:

| | |
|---|---|
| Dried Aluminium Hydroxide BP | 600 mg |
| Magnesium Hydroxide BP | 300 mg |

Other ingredients include sucrose.

**Uses**
*Indications:* The management of the symptoms of heartburn, gastric hyperacidity and gastritis.
The treatment of duodenal ulcer.
The management of the symptoms of peptic ulceration.
The prevention of duodenal ulcer recurrence.

**Dosage and administration** Maalox TC is administered orally and can be taken with milk or water if required.

*Adult doses* (including elderly):
*Management of heartburn, gastric hyperacidity, gastritis and peptic ulceration:*
*Suspension:* 5–10 ml four times daily taken 20 minutes to 1 hour after meals and at bedtime.
*Tablets:* 1–2 tablets four times daily taken 20 minutes to 1 hour after meals and at bedtime.
*Treatment of duodenal ulcer:*
*Suspension:* 15 ml four times daily taken 1 hour after meals and at bedtime.
*Tablets:* 3 tablets four times daily taken 1 hour after meals and at bedtime.
*Prevention of duodenal ulcer recurrence:*
*Suspension:* 15 ml in the morning, after food, and 15 ml at bedtime.
*Tablets:* 3 tablets in the morning, after food, and 3 tablets at bedtime.

**Contra-indications, warnings, etc** Contra-indicated in hypersensitivity to any of the active or inactive ingredients, alkalosis, hypermagnesaemia or hypophosphataemia, where abdominal distension may be due to partial or complete intestinal obstruction. Not recommended for severely debilitated patients or those with impaired renal function.

*Precautions:* Magnesium salts, in the presence of renal insufficiency may cause CNS depression. Aluminium hydroxide, in the presence of low phosphorus diets, may cause phosphorus deficiency.

Maalox TC is a balanced formulation of antacids which will minimise bowel reaction, however, mild diarrhoea may be experienced at high doses.

Do not administer concomitantly with tetracycline antibiotics or iron preparations as antacids may interfere with the absorption of these drugs.

*Use in pregnancy:* The safety of Maalox TC in pregnancy has not been established.

*Treatment of overdosage:* Serious symptoms are unlikely following overdosage and specific therapy is rarely required.

**Pharmaceutical precautions** The suspension must be kept from freezing and the bottle tightly closed.

**Legal category** GSL.

**Package quantities**
Suspension: Plastic bottle containing 500 ml.
Tablets: Carton containing 100 strip-packed tablets.

**Further information** Nil.

**Product licence numbers**
Suspension 5272/0021
Tablets 5272/0019.

## MENOREST*

**Qualitative and quantitative composition** The active component of the Menorest patch is 17β-oestradiol (17β-estradiol-INN). The remaining components of the patch are pharmacologically inactive.

Three Menorest patches are available (see table).

The composition of the patch per unit area is identical.

| | Nominal delivery (μg/day) | 17β-oestradiol content (mg) | Surface area ($cm^2$) | Shape |
|---|---|---|---|---|
| Menorest 37.5 | 37.5 | 3.29 | 11 | Round |
| Menorest 50 | 50 | 4.33 | 14.5 | Round |
| Menorest 75 | 75 | 6.57 | 22.0 | Oval |

**Pharmaceutical form** Transdermal patch.

**Clinical particulars**

*Therapeutic indications:* The Menorest patch is indicated for the following:

Symptoms of oestrogen deficiency due to natural or surgically induced menopause.

Prevention of postmenopausal osteoporosis in women at risk of developing fractures. Epidemiological studies suggest a number of individual risk factors which contribute to the development of postmenopausal osteoporosis. These include: early menopause; family history of osteoporosis; thin, small frame; cigarette use; prolonged corticosteroid use. If several of these risk factors are present in a patient consideration should be given to oestrogen replacement therapy.

*Posology and method of administration:* Adults and elderly: Menopausal symptoms: Therapy should be initiated with one Menorest 50 patch applied every 3 to 4 days (see *Instructions for use/handling*). The dose should be adjusted monthly depending on efficacy and signs of intolerance (e.g. breast tenderness). Dosage adjustment can be made using Menorest 37.5 and 75 patches. For maintenance therapy the lowest effective dose should be used.

Prevention of postmenopausal osteoporosis: Therapy should be initiated with one Menorest 50 patch applied every 3 to 4 days. The dosage may be adjusted monthly depending on signs of intolerance (e.g. breast tenderness) and yearly based upon bone mineral density assessment. Dosage adjustment can be made using Menorest 75 patch. Doses of less than 50 micrograms/day have not been shown to be effective in the prevention of osteoporosis.

Treatment with Menorest should commence as soon as possible after the onset of menopause and certainly within 2-3 years. Treatment should continue for at least 5 years and probably 10 years. Protection appears to be effective as long as the treatment is continued, however data beyond 10 years is limited. A careful reappraisal of the risk/benefit ratio should be undertaken before treating for longer than 5-10 years. For long term use see also *Special Warnings and Special Precautions for Use.*

Women undergoing a premature menopause, e.g. surgically induced menopause, may need to take Menorest for longer periods.

*Therapeutic regimen:* Menorest should be used as a continuous treatment. In patients with an intact uterus, progestogen therapy should be administered for at least 12 days per month normally during the second half of the month. Bleeding may occur after the progestogen treatment is completed.

*Children:* Menorest is not to be used by children.

*Contra-indications:* Oestrogens should not be used by women with any of the following conditions:
Known or suspected pregnancy.
Lactation.
History of, known or suspected cancer of the breast.
Known or suspected oestrogen-dependant neoplasia.
Undiagnosed abnormal vaginal bleeding.
Acute or chronic liver disease or history of liver disease where the liver function tests are still abnormal. Rotor syndrome or Dubin-Johnson syndrome.
Severe renal or cardiac disease.
Active deep venous thrombosis, thromboembolic disorders, or a past history of these conditions (see also *Special warnings and special precautions for use*).
Hypersensitivity to oestrogen or to components of this product.

*Special warnings and special precautions for use:* A complete medical and family history should be taken prior to the initiation of any oestrogen therapy. The pre-treatment and periodic physical examination should include special reference to blood pressure, breasts, abdomen, and pelvic organs and should include a Papanicolaou smear if not performed recently. Regular examination of the breasts is desirable in patients with a family history of breast cancer. As a general rule, oestrogen should not be prescribed for longer than 1 year without another physical examination being performed.

Some studies have suggested a possible increased incidence of breast cancer in postmenopausal women receiving long term (greater than 5 years) hormone replacement therapy. An assessment of the risk/benefit ratio should be undertaken before treating patients for longer than 5 years. Women on long-term therapy should have regular breast examinations and be instructed on self-breast examination. Regular mammographic investigation should be conducted where considered appropriate.

The long term administration (greater than 1 year) of unopposed oestrogen to women with an intact uterus increases the risk of endometrial hyperplasia and carcinoma. Women with an intact uterus should always receive a progestogen for at least 12 days of the menstrual cycle.

Patients with asthma, epilepsy, migraine, benign breast disease, otosclerosis, melanoma, multiple sclerosis, systemic lupus erythematosis, porphyria or hypophyseal tumours require careful observation as these conditions may be made worse by hormone replacement therapy.

Oestrogens may cause fluid retention and therefore patients with cardiac or renal dysfunction should be carefully observed.

Most studies indicate that oestrogen replacement therapy has little effect on blood pressure and some indicate that oestrogen use may be associated with a small decrease. In addition, most studies of combined therapy indicate that the addition of a progestogen also has little effect on blood pressure. Rarely, idiosyncratic hypertension may occur. When oestrogens are administered to hypertensive women, supervision is necessary and blood pressure should be monitored at regular intervals.

Epidemiological evidence suggests that use of hormone replacement therapy (HRT) is associated with an increased relative risk of developing deep vein thrombosis (DVT) or pulmonary embolism (PE). Although this increase in relative risk is about 2-3, for healthy women the excess absolute risk of either of these conditions is about 1 in 5000 per year while taking HRT. The increased risk of venous thromboembolism (VTE) means that caution should be exercised in using HRT in women who are likely to be at risk of DVT or PE. Women with severe varicose veins, severe obesity (Body Mass Index >30 kg/m²), immobilisation for 3 weeks or more, trauma or surgery requiring bed rest, are at risk of VTE so that the benefits of treatment with HRT will need to be weighed against risk carefully. Where elective surgery is planned requiring subsequent bed rest HRT should be stopped four weeks prior to surgery. If venous thromboembolism develops after initiating therapy the drug should be discontinued. Although Menorest is a transdermal patch, there is no evidence that it is different to the oral forms in respect of the risk of VTE.

Oral oestrogen therapy may be associated with elevations of plasma triglycerides, leading to pancreatitis and other complications in patients with familial defects of lipoprotein metabolism.

Certain patients may develop undesirable manifestations of oestrogenic stimulation, such as irregular uterine bleeding, enlargement of fibroids, and mastodynia.

Changed oestrogen levels may affect certain endocrine and liver function tests.

Menorest is not a contraceptive neither will it restore fertility. If Menorest is administered to women of child bearing potential they should be advised to adhere to non-hormonal contraceptive methods.

*Interactions with other medicaments and other forms of interaction:* Preparations inducing microsomal liver enzymes, e.g. barbiturates, hydantoins, anticonvulsants (including carbamazepine), meprobamate, phenylbutazone, antibiotics (including rifampicin) and activated charcoal, may impair the activity of oestrogens (irregular bleeding and recurrence of symptoms may occur). The extent of interference with transdermally administered oestradiol is not known; these problems may be reduced by the transdermal route of administration which avoids any first pass hepatic metabolism.

*Pregnancy and lactation:* Oestrogens should not be used during pregnancy or while breast feeding.

*Effects on ability to drive and use machines:* On the basis of pharmacodynamic profile of Menorest, it is presumed to be safe or unlikely to produce an effect on driving performance or the operation of machines.

*Undesirable effects:* See *Special warnings and special precautions for use.*

Headache was the most commonly reported adverse reaction during clinical trials. Mild itching and rash were also reported around the application site and transient skin redness was observed after removing the patch.

The following adverse reactions have been reported with oral oestrogen therapy:

*Urogenital system:* Changes in vaginal bleeding pattern and abnormal withdrawal bleeding or flow; breakthrough bleeding; spotting; increase in size of uterine leoimyomata; vaginal candidiasis; change in amount of cervical secretion.

*Breasts.* Tenderness, enlargement.

*Gastrointestinal.* Nausea, vomiting; abdominal cramps, bloating; cholestatic jaundice.

*Skin.* Erythema and pruritus.

*Eyes.* Steepening of corneal curvature; intolerance to contact lenses.

*Central nervous system.* Headache, migraine, dizziness; mental depression, chorea.

*Miscellaneous.* Increase or decrease in weight; reduced carbohydrate tolerance, aggravation of porphyria, oedema; changes in libido.

As in the case with all oestrogens when administered without progestogen treatment, Menorest may induce hyperplasia of the endometrium.

*Overdose:* If signs of overdosage should appear the patch should be removed. The effects of overdosage with oral oestrogens are breast tenderness, nausea, vomiting and/or metrorrhagia.

**Pharmacological properties**

*Pharmacodynamic properties:* The Menorest patch is an efficient and systemic therapy for oestrogen replacement therapy which alleviates the symptoms of oestradiol deficiency in menopausal women as oestradiol is largely responsible for the development and maintenance of the female urogenital system and of secondary sexual characteristics.

Loss of ovarian secretion after menopause can result in instability of thermoregulation causing hot flushes and sweating associated with sleep disturbances.

Oestrogen therapy promotes growth and development of the urogenital epithelium providing an efficient therapy to avoid vaginal discomfort, dyspareunia, urinary urgency and frequency; in particular, vaginal cytology is converted to a pattern similar to that found in the premenopausal women, by increasing the proportion of superficial cells and concomitantly decreasing the number of basal and prebasal cells.

Oral oestrogen therapy changes the plasma lipid metabolism by a decrease in plasma levels of total and low density (LDL) cholesterol and by an increase in plasma high density lipoprotein (HDL) cholesterol. Although such alterations in the lipid profile are consistent with a reduction in the risk of coronary heart disease, plasma concentrations of triglycerides (a risk factor for coronary heart disease) may be elevated.

Oestrogen mainly exerts an anti-resorbitive and thus anti-activating effect on bone, leading to a reduction in bone turnover. Oestrogen therapy significantly reduces urinary calcium, hydroxyproline cross-links and serum alkaline phosphatase which are markers of bone turnover.

Oestrogen exerts a proliferative effect on endometrium which is prevented by concomitant progestogen administration.

*Pharmacokinetic properties:* The transdermal route achieves similar oestradiol plasma levels in the range of those observed in the pre-menopausal women at the early to mid-follicular phase. Following oral administration, oestradiol undergoes extensive first-pass metabolism to less active metabolites. The transdermal absorption of oestradiol avoids this first pass metabolism and thereby produces therapeutic plasma levels with a smaller total daily dose.

In pharmacokinetic studies it has been shown that following the application of Menorest patches delivering 25, 50 and 100µg/day, the average plasma oestradiol concentrations and oestrone to oestradiol ratios were comparable with the physiological range reported for premenopausal women. Following the application of Menorest 50 patch twice-a-week for 3 weeks, the average oestradiol plasma concentration at steady-state was 57pg/ml. At the end of the application period, the average plasma concentration of oestradiol was 29pg/ml. Plasma oestradiol and oestrone concentrations with different dosages of Menorest increases linearly. Plasma concentrations of oestradiol and oestrone declined to baseline levels within 22 hours after removal of the patch.

*Pre-clinical safety data:* There are no pre-clinical data of relevance to the prescriber which are additional to that already included in other sections of the SPC.

**Pharmaceutical particulars**

*List of excipients:* Duro-Tak* adhesive; Morstik* adhesive; polyisobutylene (Vistanex LM-MS-LC*); 1,3 butylene glycol; oleic acid; mineral oil; bentonite; dipropylene glycol; vinyl acetate resin (Elvax 40W*); Alcolec 622/PG*.

*Incompatibilities:* Not applicable

*Shelf life:* The shelf life of the Menorest patch is 2 years when stored below 25°C.

*Special precautions for storage:* The Menorest patch should be stored below 25°C. Do not refrigerate.

*Nature and contents of container:* The Menorest patch is individually heat-sealed in foil laminate pouches of a paper/polyethylene/aluminium foil/polyethylene composite. They are available in packs of 8 patches.

*Instructions for use/handling:* The adhesive side of Menorest patch should be placed on a clean, dry area of the skin of the buttocks, abdomen, back or upper portion of the thighs. The Menorest patch should not be applied on or near to the breasts. The Menorest patch should be replaced every 3 to 4 days. The sites of application must be rotated, with an interval of at least 1 week allowed between applications to a particular site. The area selected should not be oily, abraded, or irritated. The waistline should be avoided, since tight clothing may rub the patch off. The patch should be applied immediately after opening the pouch and removing the protective liner. The patch should be pressed firmly in place with the palm of the hand for about 10 seconds, making sure there is good contact, especially around the edges. In the unlikely event that a patch should fall off, the same patch may be reapplied. If necessary, a new patch may be applied. In either case, the original treatment schedule should be continued. The patch may be worn during exercise or bathing. The patch should not be exposed to direct sunlight.

Menorest either new or used should always be kept out of the reach of children.

The Menorest patch should not be applied to any skin surface that is greasy, as this will affect the adhesive properties of the patch. Creams and lotions should not be used in the area of the patch for similar reasons.

The Menorest patch is used only once; after use the patch should be folded and disposed of with normal household waste.

**Marketing authorisation numbers**
Menorest 0012/0283
37.5
Menorest 50 0012/0268
Menorest 75 0012/0269

**Date of approval/revision of SPC** April 1997

**Legal category** POM.

## MUCODYNE*

**Presentation**
*Mucodyne Capsules:* Opaque yellow capsules marked 'MUCODYNE 375', each containing carbocisteine 375 mg. Other ingredients include lactose. Capsule shell colouring contains tartrazine.

*Mucodyne Syrup:* Clear amber syrup containing carbocisteine 250 mg in each 5 ml. Other ingredients include parabens and sucrose.

*Mucodyne Paediatric Syrup:* Clear red syrup containing carbocisteine 125 mg in each 5 ml. Other ingredients include parabens, sucrose, Ponceau 4R (E124).

**Uses** Mucolytic agent for the adjunctive therapy of respiratory tract disorders, characterised by excessive or viscous mucus, including Glue Ear in children and chronic obstructive airways disease.

**Dosage and administration** *Adults (including elderly):* (Syrup and Capsules.) Dosage is based upon an initial daily dosage of 2250 mg carbocisteine in divided doses reducing to 1500 mg daily in divided doses when a satisfactory response has been obtained, e.g. for normal syrup 15 ml tds reducing to 10 ml tds.

*Children:* The normal daily dose is 20 mg/kg body weight in divided doses. The following dosage is recommended for the Mucodyne Paediatric syrup: 2 to 5 years: 2.5–5 ml four times a day; 5 to 12 years: 10 ml three times a day. Dosage in younger children and infants has not been established.

**Contra-indications, warnings, etc** There have been rare reports of skin rashes or gastro-intestinal bleeding occurring during treatment with Mucodyne. Contra-indicated in active peptic ulceration.

*Use in pregnancy:* Although tests in mammalian species have revealed no teratogenic effects, Mucodyne is not recommended during the first trimester of pregnancy.

*Use in lactation:* Effects not known.

*Treatment of overdosage:* Gastric lavage may be beneficial, followed by observation. Gastro-intestinal disturbance is the most likely symptom of Mucodyne overdosage.

**Pharmaceutical precautions** The syrups should be stored in a cool place below 25°C. Mixture with linctus of pholcodine causes precipitation of carbocisteine from solution. Dilution of Mucodyne Syrup may be effected with unpreserved Syrup BP but diluted preparations should not be kept for more than 14 days.

**Legal category** POM.

**Package quantities** *Mucodyne Capsules:* Containers of 30.

*Mucodyne Syrup:* Bottles of 300 ml with dosage cap.

*Mucodyne Paediatric Syrup:* Bottles of 300 ml with dosage cap.

**Further information** Nil.

**Product licence numbers**

| | |
|---|---|
| *Capsules* | 0012/0238 |
| *Syrup* | 0012/0241 |
| *Paediatric Syrup* | 0012/0240 |

## NALCROM*

**Presentation** Nalcrom is a presentation of sodium cromoglycate for oral use. It is presented in clear/clear hard gelatin capsules printed Fisons 101 in black. Each capsule contains 100 mg Sodium Cromoglycate BP as a white powder.

**Uses** Food allergy (where adequate investigations have been performed to determine sensitivity to one or more ingested allergens) in conjunction with restriction of main causative allergens.

Sodium cromoglycate inhibits the release from mast cells of mediators of the allergic reaction. In gastro-intestinal disease the release of mediators causes a local inflammation which can either result in gastrointestinal symptoms or may allow absorption of antigenic material leading to systemic allergic reactions.

**Dosage and administration**
*Initial dose: Adults (including the elderly):* 2 capsules four times daily before meals.

*Children:* From 2–14 years: 1 capsule four times daily before meals.

For adults and children if satisfactory control is not achieved within two to three weeks the dosage may be doubled but should not exceed 40 mg/kg/day.

*Maintenance dose:* Once a therapeutic response has been achieved the dose may be reduced to the minimum required to maintain the patient free of symptoms.

Patients who are unable to avoid allergenic foods under certain circumstances (e.g. school meals, restaurants) may be able to protect themselves against the effect of these foods by taking a single dose of Nalcrom 15 minutes before the meal. The optimum dosage will need to be determined for each patient and a suitable starting dose would be 200 mg in adults and 100 mg in children.

*Administration:* The capsules may be swallowed whole or the powder contents may be dissolved in a small quantity of very hot water and diluted with cold water to drink. Administration as a solution in water is probably the method of choice.

**Contra-indications, warnings, etc**
*Contra-indications:* Known sensitivity to sodium cromoglycate.

*Warnings:* The safety of Nalcrom for the treatment of children under two years has not yet been established.

*Side-effects:* Nausea, skin rashes and joint pains have been reported in a few cases.

*Use in pregnancy and lactation:* As with all medication caution should be exercised especially during the first trimester of pregnancy. Cumulative experience with sodium cromoglycate suggests that it has no adverse effects on foetal development. It should only be used in pregnancy where there is a clear need.

It is not known whether sodium cromoglycate is excreted in the breast milk but on the basis of its physico-chemical properties this is considered unlikely. There is no information to suggest that the use of sodium cromoglycate has any undesirable effects on the baby.

*Overdosage:* As Nalcrom is absorbed only to a very limited extent, no action other than medical observation should be necessary.

**Pharmaceutical precautions** Store in a dry place. Reclose the container tightly after use.

**Legal category** POM.

**Package quantities** Containers of 100 capsules.

**Further information** If oral steroid therapy is to be reduced or withdrawn this should be done cautiously and not more rapidly than 10% per week.

**Product licence number** 0113/0073.

## NASACORT* ▼

**Qualitative and quantitative composition:** The active component of Nasacort is triamcinolone acetonide. Each bottle of Nasacort contains 9.075 mg triamcinolone acetonide and provides at least 120 actuations each containing 55 micrograms of active compound after initial priming (see Instructions for Use/Handling).

**Pharmaceutical form:** Aqueous Nasal spray. For nasal use only.

**Clinical particulars**

*Therapeutic indications:* Nasacort is indicated for the treatment and prophylaxis of the symptoms of seasonal and perennial allergic rhinitis.

*Posology and method of administration:* Patients aged 12 years and over: The recommended dose is 220 micrograms as 2 sprays in each nostril once daily. Once symptoms are controlled patients can be maintained on 110 micrograms (1 spray in each nostril once daily). The minimum effective dose should be used to ensure continued control of symptoms. Paediatric patients aged 6 to 12 years: The recommended dose is 110 micrograms as 1 spray in each nostril once daily.

*Contra-indications:* Hypersensitivity to any of the ingredients of this preparation contra-indicate its use.

*Special warnings and special precautions for use:* If there is any reason to suppose that adrenal function is impaired, care must be taken while transferring patients from systemic steroid treatment to Nasacort.

In clinical studies with Nasacort administered intranasally, the development of localised infections of the nose and pharynx with *Candida albicans* has rarely occurred. When such an infection develops it may require treatment with appropriate local therapy and discontinuance of treatment with Nasacort.

Because of the inhibitory effect of corticosteriods on wound healing in patients who have experienced recent nasal septal ulcers, nasal surgery or trauma, Nasacort should be used with caution until healing has occurred.

*Interaction with other medicaments and other forms of interaction:* None known.

*Pregnancy and lactation: Pregnancy:* There are no adequate and well-controlled studies in pregnant women with Nasacort. Because animal studies indicate a teratogenic effect, typical of corticosteriods, Nasacort should not be administered during pregnancy unless the benefit to the patient is considered to outweigh the risk to the embryo or foetus (see *Preclinical safety data* section). *Lactation:* It is not known whether triamcinolone acetonide is excreted in human milk. Because other corticosteriods are excreted in human milk, caution should be exercised when Nasacort is administered to nursing women; therefore, the therapeutic benefit to the mother should outweigh any potential risk to the baby.

*Effects on ability to drive and use machines:* Nasacort has no known effect on the ability to drive and operate machines.

*Undesirable effects:* The most commonly reported adverse reactions in clinical trials with Nasacort included those involving mucous membranes of the nose and throat. The three most prevalent adverse reactions considered to be at least possibly drug-related were rhinitis, headache and pharyngitis. The nasopharyngeal-related adverse reactions considered drug-related were; epistaxis, nasal irritation, dry mucous membrane, naso-sinus congestion and sneezing.

These adverse reactions with the exception of epistaxis, were reported at approximately the same or lower incidence as placebo treated patients.

As with other nasally inhaled corticosteriods, nasal septal perforations have been reported in rare instances.

*Overdose:* Like any other nasally administered corticosteroid, acute overdosing with Nasacort is unlikely in view of the total amount of active ingredient present. In the event that the entire contents of the bottle were administered all at once, via either oral or nasal application, clinically significant adverse events would most likely not result. The patient may experience some gastrointestinal upset if taken orally.

**Pharmacological properties**

*Pharmacodynamic properties:* Triamcinolone acetonide is a more potent derivative of triamcinolone and is approximately 8 times more potent than prednisone. Although the precise mechanism of corticosteroid antiallergic action is unknown, corticosteriods are very effective in the treatment of allergic diseases in man. However, when allergic symptoms are very severe, local treatment with recommended doses (microgram) of any available topical corticosteriod are not as effective as treatment with larger doses (milligram) of oral or parenteral formulations.

Nasacort does not have an immediate effect on allergic signs and symptoms. An improvement in some patients symptoms may be seen within the first day of treatment with Nasacort and relief may be expected in 3 to 4 days. When Nasacort is prematurely discontinued symptoms may not recur for several days.

In clinical studies performed in adults and children at doses up to 440 micrograms/day intranasally, no suppression of the Hypothalamic-Pituitary-Adrenal (HPA) axis has been observed.

*Pharmacokinetic properties:* Single dose intranasal administration of 220 micrograms of Nasacort in normal adult subjects and in adult patients with allergic rhinitis demonstrated minimal absorption of triamcinolone acetonide. The mean peak plasma concentration was approximately 0.5ng/mL (range 0.1 to 1 ng/mL) and occurred at 1.5 hours post dose. The mean plasma drug concentrations was less than 0.06 ng/mL at 12 hours and below the assay detection limit at 24 hours. The average terminal half life was 3.1 hours. Dose proportionality was demonstrated in normal subjects and in patients following a single intranasal dose of 110 micrograms or 220 micrograms Nasacort. Following multiple doses in paediatric patients, plasma drug concentrations, AUC, $C_{max}$ and $T_{max}$ were similar to those values observed in adult patients.

*Preclinical safety data:* No genotoxicity studies have been conducted with triamcinolone acetonide. However, other members of this chemical class were not genotoxins. In addition, there are long-term assays which show no evidence for triamcinolone acetonide being a genotoxic carcinogen.

Carcinogenicity assays in rodents show no increase in the incidence of individual tumour types.

Like other corticosteriods, triamcinolone acetonide has been shown to be teratogenic in rats and rabbits. Teratogenic effects which occurred in the rat and in the rabbit included cleft palate and/or internal hydrocephaly and axial skeletal defects. Teratogenic effects, including CNS and cranial malformations, have also been observed in non-human primates.

Administration of triamcinolone acetonide by inhalation (aerosol) to pregnant rats and rabbits produced embryotoxic and foetotoxic effects which were comparable to those produced by administration by other routes.

**Pharmaceutical particulars**

*List of excipients:* Microcrystalline cellulose, carboxymethylcellulose sodium, polysorbate 80, purified water, dextrose, benzalkonium chloride and edetate disodium. Hydrochloric acid or sodium hydroxide may be added to adjust the pH to between 4.5 and 6.0.

*Incompatibilities:* None known.

*Shelf-life:* The shelf-life of Nasacort is 24 months.

*Special precautions for storage:* Store below 25°C.

*Nature and contents of container:* Nasacort is supplied as an unscented, thixotropic, water-based metered-dose pump spray formulation unit containing a microcystalline suspension of triamcinolone acetonide in an aqueous medium. Each bottle of Nasacort provides at least 120 actuations after initial priming and is supplied with a nasal adapter. Each actuation provides 55 micrograms triamcinolone acetonide from the nasal actuator to the patient.

*Instructions for use/handling:* It is important to shake the bottle gently before each use. Each actuation delivers 55 micrograms triamcinolone acetonide from the nasal actuator to the patient (estimated from *in vitro* testing) after an initial priming of 5 sprays. Nasacort will remain adequately primed for 2 weeks. If the product is unused for more than 2 weeks, then it can be adequately reprimed with one spray. Also, the bottle should be discarded after 120 actuations and/or within 2 months of starting treatment. Do not transfer any remaining suspension to another bottle.

**Marketing authorisation number** 0012/0311.

**Date of approval/revision of SPC** February 1997.

**Legal category** POM

## NIVAQUINE* TABLETS AND INJECTION

**Presentation**

*Tablets:* Yellowish buff film-coated tablets containing 200 mg chloroquine sulphate (equivalent to 150 mg chloroquine base) impressed 'Nivaquine 200' on one face, reverse plain. The tablets also contain glucose.

*Injection:* A colourless injection solution of chloroquine sulphate 5.45% w/v equivalent to 40 mg chloroquine base per ml in ampoules of 5 ml.

**Uses** Chloroquine is a 4-aminoquinoline derivative, which has a high degree of activity against the asexual erythrocytic forms of all species of malaria parasites. It is indicated for the suppression and clinical cure of all forms of malaria and, in addition, produces radical cure of falciparum malaria.

Nivaquine exerts a beneficial effect in certain collagen diseases and protects against the effects of solar radiation. It is also indicated in the treatment of rheumatoid arthritis, juvenile rheumatoid arthritis, discoid and systemic lupus erythematosus and skin conditions aggravated by sunlight.

Nivaquine is also active against Entamoeba histolytica and Giardia lamblia and when metronidazole is not available it may be used in hepatic amoebiasis and giardiasis.

**Dosage and administration**

*Suppression of malaria:* It is advisable to start taking Nivaquine 1 week before entering an endemic area and to continue for 4 weeks after leaving.

| *Age group* | *Dose to be taken once a week on the same day each week* |
|---|---|
| Adults | Two Nivaquine tablets (300 mg chloroquine base) |
| Infants and children up to twelve years | 5 mg chloroquine base per kg bodyweight |

These dosages are those recommended by the World Health Organisation.

*Treatment of malaria*
*(1) Non-immune subjects*
*(a) Oral route*

*Adults:*

| *Day of treatment* | Dosage |
|---|---|
| Day 1 | Four Nivaquine tablets (600 mg chloroquine base) in one dose followed by a further two tablets (300 mg chloroquine base) six hours later. |
| Day 2 | Two Nivaquine tablets (300 mg chloroquine base). |
| Day 3 | Two Nivaquine tablets (300 mg chloroquine base). |

The above dosage is intended as a guide in the treatment of Plasmodium falciparum malaria. However, due to variation in the strain sensitivity, it may sometimes be necessary to increase the duration of treatment by administering two Nivaquine tablets (300 mg chloroquine base) daily on days 4 to 7.

*Infants and children:* Nivaquine syrup can be conveniently used in this age group to permit flexibility of dosage.

*(b) Injection*
*Adults and children:* Slow intravenous infusion: 10 mg/kg bodyweight chloroquine base to be administered in sodium chloride 0.9% injection by slow intravenous infusion over eight hours followed by three further 8 hour infusions containing 5 mg base/kg (total dose 25 mg base/kg over 32 hours). The dose should not be modified in renal or hepatic disease.

Exceptionally, where intravenous administration is not possible, Nivaquine may be given by intramuscular or subcutaneous injection in small divided doses of 3.5 mg chloroquine base/kg bodyweight every 6 hours or 2.5 mg base/kg every 4 hours.

*(2) Partially immune subjects*
*Adults:* A single dose of four Nivaquine tablets (600 mg chloroquine base) will provide an effective course of treatment.

*Infants and children:* Repeated infection with many species and strains of malaria parasite prevalent in highly endemic malarial areas eventually produces a high degree of immune response frequently resulting in modification of the symptoms of clinical attack. This is particularly obvious in adults but less so in adolescents and children. Immunity is uncommon in very young age groups with the exception of infants up to the age of about 6 months who are partly protected by trans-placentally derived maternal antibodies. It is therefore advisable to treat previously exposed children in the same way as non-immune children.

*Other indications:*

| *Indication* | *Age group* | *Dose* |
|---|---|---|
| Rheumatoid arthritis | Adults | One Nivaquine tablet (150 mg chloroquine base) daily. |
| | Children | 3 mg/kg bodyweight as base per day |

| Indication | Age group | Dose |
|---|---|---|
| Systemic lupus erythematosus | Adults | One Nivaquine tablet (150 mg chloroquine base) daily until maximum improvement is obtained followed by a smaller maintenance dosage. |
| | Children | 3 mg/kg bodyweight as base per day. |
| Light-sensitive skin eruptions | Adults | One or two Nivaquine tablets (150 mg to 300 mg chloroquine base) daily during the period of maximum light exposure. |
| | Children | 3 mg/kg bodyweight as base per day during the period of maximum light exposure. |

Treatment should be discontinued if no improvement has occurred after 6 months.

Dosage in the elderly: No specific dosage recommendations.

**Contra-indications, warnings, etc**

*Precautions:* Caution is advised in cases of porphyria, severe gastrointestinal, neurological and blood disorders. Nivaquine should be used with care in patients with a history of epilepsy as it has been reported to provoke seizures. Caution should be exercised in patients with hepatic or renal disease. Retinopathy: Irreversible retinal damage may occur with prolonged treatment. Ophthalmological examination should always be carried out before and regularly (3–6 monthly intervals) during treatment. Retinal damage is particularly likely to occur if treatment has been given for longer than one year or if the total dosage has exceeded 1.6 g/kg bodyweight. These precautions also apply to patients receiving chloroquine continuously at weekly intervals as a prophylactic against malarial attack for more than three years.

Nivaquine has a temporary effect on visual accommodation and patients should be warned regarding driving or operating machinery.

*Use in pregnancy:* Nivaquine is generally contraindicated in pregnancy. However, clinicians may decide to administer Nivaquine to pregnant women for the prevention or treatment of malaria. Ocular or inner ear damage may occur in infants born of mothers who receive high doses of chloroquine throughout pregnancy.

*Side-effects:* The more common side-effects include gastro-intestinal disturbances, headache and skin eruptions. Psoriasis may be exacerbated. Retinal damage and depigmentation or loss of hair may also occur. These effects usually disappear on cessation of treatment. Convulsions have been reported rarely (these may result from cerebral malaria, such patients should receive an injection of phenobarbitone to prevent seizures in a dose of 3.5 mg/kg in addition to intravenous administration of Nivaquine). Bone marrow depression, including aplastic anaemia, occurs rarely. Full blood counts should therefore be carried out regularly during extended treatment. Allergic and anaphylactic reactions have occurred rarely.

*Treatment of overdosage:* Chloroquine is highly toxic in overdose; children are particularly susceptible to toxic doses of chloroquine. The chief symptoms of overdosage include circulatory collapse due to a potent cardiotoxic effect, respiratory arrest and coma. Symptoms may progress rapidly after initial nausea and vomiting.

Death may result from circulatory or respiratory failure or cardiac dysrhythmia.

Gastric lavage should be carried out urgently, first protecting the airway and instituting artificial ventilation where necessary. There is a risk of cardiac arrest following aspiration of gastric contents in more serious cases. Activated charcoal left in the stomach may reduce the absorption of any remaining chloroquine from the gut. Circulatory status (with central venous pressure measurement), respiration, plasma electrolytes and blood gases should be monitored, with correction of hypokalaemia and acidosis if indicated. Cardiac arrhythmias should not be treated unless life threatening; drugs with quinidine-like effect should be avoided.

Early administration of the following has been shown to improve survival in cases of serious poisoning:

1. Adrenaline infusion 0.25 micrograms/kg/min initially with increments of 0.25 micrograms/kg/min until adequate systolic blood pressure (more than 100 mm Hg) is restored; adrenaline reduces the effects of chloroquine on the heart through its inotropic and vasoconstrictor effects.

2. Diazepam infusion (2 mg/kg over 30 minutes as a loading dose, followed by 1–2 mg/kg/day for up to 2–4 days). Diazepam may minimise cardiotoxicity.

Acidification of the urine, haemodialysis, peritoneal dialysis or exchange transfusion have not been shown to be of value in treating chloroquine poisoning. Chloroquine is excreted very slowly, therefore symptomatic cases merit observation for several days.

**Pharmaceutical precautions**    Tablets: Protect from light. Injection: Protect from light.

**Legal category**    Nivaquine Tablets POM, but when supplied for prevention of malaria in a container specifically labelled for that purpose, P.
Nivaquine Injection POM.

**Package quantities**    30×200 mg Tablets. Injection: 10 ampoules of 5 ml per carton.

**Further information**    Nil.

**Product licence numbers**
Injection    0012/5048
Tablets    0012/5260

# NIVAQUINE* SYRUP

**Qualitative and quantitative composition** Nivaquine Syrup contains Chloroquine Sulphate BP 68 mg/5 ml.

**Pharmaceutical form** Syrup

**Clinical particulars**

*Therapeutic indications:* Nivaquine is a 4-aminoquinoline compound which has a high degree of activity against the asexual erythrocytic forms of all species of malaria parasites. It is indicated for the suppression and clinical cure of all forms of malaria and, in addition, produces radical cure of flaciparum malaria.

Nivaquine also exerts a beneficial effect in certain collagen diseases and protects against the effects of solar radiation. It is employed in the treatment of rheumatoid arthritis, juvenile arthritis, discoid and systemic lupus erythematosus and skin conditions aggravated by sunlight.

Nivaquine is also active against entamoeba histolica and giardia lamblia and when flagyl (metronidazole) is not available it may be used in hepatic amoebiasis and giardiasis.

Packs for supply directly to the public: For the prevention of malaria.

*Posology and method of administration:* Route of administration oral.

*Rheumatoid arthritis: Adults:* 4 x 5 ml Nivaquine Syrup (150 mg chloroquine base) daily. *Children:* 3 mg/kg bodyweight daily. Treatment should be discontinued if no improvement has occurred after 6 months.

*Systemic lupus erythematosus: Adults:* 4 x 5 ml Nivaquine Syrup (150 mg chloroquine base) daily until maximum improvement is obtained followed by smaller maintenance dosage. *Children:* 3 mg x kg bodyweight daily. Treatment should be discontinued if no improvement has occurred after 6 months.

*Light sensitive skin eruptions: Adults:* 4 to 8 x 5 ml Nivaquine Syrup (150 mg to 300 mg chloroquine base) daily during the period of maximum light exposure. *Children:* 3 mg/kg body weight daily. Treatment should be discontinued if no improvement has occurred after 6 months.

*Suppression of malaria: Adults:* 8 x 5 ml Nivaquine Syrup (300 mg chloroquine base) to be taken once a week on the same day each week. *Infants and children up to 12 years:* 5 mg Chloroquine base per kg bodyweight to be taken once a week on the same day each week. It is advisable to start taking Nivaquine 1 week before entering an endemic area and to continue for 4 weeks after leaving.

*Treatment of malaria:* 1. *Partially immune adults:* A single dose of 16 x 5 ml Nivaquine Syrup (600 mg chloroquine base) will provide a safe and effective course of treatment. 2. *Non-immune adults:* Day 1 16 x 5 ml Nivaquine syrup (600 mg chloroquine base) in one dose followed by a further 8 x 5 ml syrup (300 mg chloroquine base) six hours later. Day 2 8 x 5 ml Nivaquine syrup (300 mg chloroquine base). Day 3 8 x 5 ml Nivaquine Syrup (300 mg chloroquine base). The above dosage is intended as a guide in the treatment of plasmodium falciparum malaria. However, due to a variation in the strain sensitivity, it may sometimes be necessary to increase the duration of treatment by administering 8 x 5 ml Nivaquine Syrup (300 mg chloroquine base) daily on days 4 to 7. 3. *Non-immune or partially immune infants and children:* Nivaquine Syrup can be conveniently used in patients in this age group to permit flexibility of dosage. Day 1 10 mg chloroquine base/kg bodyweight (maximum 600 mg base) followed by 5 mg chloroquine base/kg bodyweight (maximum 300 mg base) six hours later. Day 2 5 mg chloroquine base/kg bodyweight (maximum 300 mg base). Day 3 5 mg chloroquine base/kg bodyweight (maximum 300 mg base).

*Contra-indications:* Nivaquine is generally contraindicated in pregnancy. However, clinicians may decide to administer Nivaquine to pregnant women for the prevention or treatment of malaria. Ocular or inner ear damage may occur in infants born of mothers who receive high doses of chloroquine throughout pregnancy.

*Special warnings and precautions for use:* Nivaquine should be used with care in patients with a history of epilepsy as it has been reported to provoke seizures. Caution is advised in cases of porphyria, hepatic or renal disease, severe gastrointestinal, neurological and blood disorders and in patients receiving anticoagulant therapy.

*Interactions with other medicaments and other forms of interaction:* Caution is advised in patients receiving anticoagulant therapy.

*Pregnancy and lactation:* Nivaquine is generally contraindicated in pregnancy. However, clinicians may decide to administer Nivaquine to pregnant women for the prevention or treatment of malaria. Ocular or inner ear damage may occur in infants born of mothers who receive high doses of chloroquine throughout pregnancy.

*Effects on ability to drive and use machines:* Nivaquine has a temporary effect on visual accommodation and patients should be warned that they should not drive or operate machinery if they are affected.

*Undesirable effects:* The more common side effects include gastrointestinal disturbances, headache, skin eruptions, and disturbance of visual accommodation. Psoriasis may be exacerbated. Depigmentation or loss of hair may also occur. Bone marrow depression, including aplastic anaemia occurs rarely. Full blood counts should therefore be carried out regularly during extended treatment.

Irreversible retinal damage may occur with prolonged treatment. Ophthalmological examination should always be carried out before and regularly (3-6 monthly intervals) during treatment. Retinal damage is particularly likely to occur if treatment has been given for longer than one year, or if the total dosage has exceeded 1.6 g/kg bodyweight. These precautions also apply to patients receiving chloroquine continuously at weekly intervals as a prophylactic against malarial attack for more than three years. Convulsions have been reported rarely (these may result from cerebral malaria. Such patients should receive an injection of phenobarbitone to prevent seizures, in a dose of 3.5 mg/kg in addition to intravenous administration of Nivaquine). Allergic and anaphylactic reactions have occurred rarely.

Changes in liver function, including hepatitis and abnormal liver function tests, have been reported rarely.

*Overdosage:* Chloroquine is highly toxic in overdosage; children are particularly susceptible to toxic doses of chloroquine. The chief symptoms of overdose include circulatory collapse due to a potent cardiotoxic effect, respiratory arrest and coma. Symptoms may progress rapidly after initial nausea and vomiting. Death may result from circulatory or respiratory failure or cardiac dysrhythmia. Gastric lavage should be carried out urgently, first protecting the airways and instituting artificial ventilation where necessary. There is a risk of cardiac arrest following aspiration of gastric contents in more serious cases. Activated charcoal left in the stomach may reduce absorption of any remaining chloroquine from the gut. Circulatory status (with central venous pressure measurement) respiration, plasma electrolytes and blood gases should be monitored, with correction of hypokalaemia and acidosis if indicated. Cardiac arrhythmias should not be treated unless life threatening; drugs with quinidine-like effects should be avoided. Early administration of the following has been shown to improve survival in cases of serious poisoning:

(1) Adrenaline infusion (0.25 micrograms/kg/min initially, with increments of 0.25 micrograms/kg/min until adequate systolic blood pressure (more than 100 mm mercury) is restored; adrenaline reduces the effects of chloroquine on the heart through its inotropic and vasoconstrictor effects.

(2) Diazepam infusion (2 mg/kg over 30 minutes as a loading dose, followed by 1-2 mg/kg/day for up to 2-4 days). Diazepam may minimise cardiotoxicity.

Acidification of the urine, haemodialysis, peritoneal dialysis or exchange transfusions have not been shown to be of value in treating chloroquine poisoning. Chloroquine is excreted very slowly, therefore symptomatic cases merit observation for several days.

### Pharmacological properties

*Pharmacodynamic properties:* Chloroquine is used for the suppression and treatment of malaria. It has rapid schizonticidal effect and appears to affect cell growth by interfering with DNA; its activity also seems to depend on preferential accumulation in the infected erythrocyte. Chloroquine kills the erythrocytic forms of malaria parasites at all stages of development. In addition to its antimalarial properties, it possesses other pharmacological properties. Its anit-inflammatory properties enable Nivaquine to be used in certain collagen diseases and it protects against the effects of solar radiation. Nivaquine is also active against entamoeba histolytica and giardia lamblia. It may be used in hepatic amoebiasis and giardiasis.

*Pharmacokinetic properties:* Chloroquine is readily absorbed from the gastro-intestinal tract and about 55% in the circulation is bound to plasma proteins. It accumulates in high concentrations in some tissues, such as kidneys, liver, lungs and spleen and is strongly bound in melanin containing cells such as those in the eyes and the skin; it is also bound to double stranded DNA, present in red blood cells containing schizonts. Chloroquine in eliminated very slowly from the body and it may persist in tissues for a long period. Up to 70% of a dose may be excreted unchanged in urine and up to 25% may be excreted also in the urine as the desethyl metabolite. The rate of urinary excretion of chloroquine is increased at low pH values.

### Pharmaceutical particulars

*List of excipients:* Liquid sugar gran. liquors, Sodium L glutamate, Saccharin Sodium BP, Propylene Glycol, Methyl Hydroxybenzoate BP, Propyl Hydroxybenzoate BP, Oil peppermint (Chinese), Witham pineapple flavour (F), Caramel HT, Demineralised Water BP.

*Incompatibilities:* None known

*Shelf life:* 36 months

*Special precautions for storage:* Nivaquine should be stored below 25°C, protected from light.

*Nature and contents of container:* Amber glass bottle containing 100 ml.

*Instructions for use/handling:* None stated

**Marketing authorisation number** 0012/5020

**Date of approval/revision of SPC** February 1997

**Legal category** POM. When used solely for the prevention of malaria: P.

## OPTICROM* AQUEOUS EYE DROPS

**Presentation** A clear colourless aqueous solution of Sodium Cromoglycate BP 2% w/v, with benzalkonium chloride 0.01% w/v.

*Inactive ingredients:* Benzalkonium Chloride USNF, Disodium Edetate BP.

**Uses** For the prophylaxis and symptomatic treatment of acute allergic conjunctivitis such as hay fever, chronic allergic conjunctivitis and vernal kerato conjunctivitis. Sodium cromoglycate inhibits the release from sensitised mast cells of mediators of the allergic reaction.

**Dosage and administration** *Adults (including the elderly) and children:* One or two drops into each eye four times daily.

**Contra-indications, warnings, etc**
*Contra-indications:* Opticrom is contra-indicated in patients with known sensitivity to any ingredient.

*Warnings:* As with other ophthalmic solutions containing benzalkonium chloride, soft contact lenses should not be worn during the treatment period.

*Effects on ability to drive and use machinery:* As with all eye drops, instillation of Opticrom may cause a transient blurring of vision.

*Side-effects:* Transient stinging and burning may occur after instillation. Other symptoms of local irritation have been recorded rarely.

*Use in pregnancy and lactation:* As with all medication caution should be exercised especially during the first trimester of pregnancy. Cumulative experience with sodium cromoglycate suggests it has no adverse effects on foetal development. It should only be used in pregnancy where there is a clear need.

It is not known whether sodium cromoglycate is excreted in the breast milk but on the basis of its

physico-chemical properties this is considered unlikely. There is no information to suggest that the use of sodium cromoglycate has any undesirable effects on the baby.

*Overdosage:* No action other than medical observation should be necessary.

**Pharmaceutical precautions** Store below 30°C. Protect from direct sunlight.

**Legal category** POM.

**Package quantities** 13.5 ml.

**Further information** Discard any remaining contents four weeks after opening the bottle.

**Product licence number** 0113/0039R.

## OPTICROM* EYE OINTMENT

**Presentation** Opticrom Eye Ointment is a cream coloured opaque sterile ointment containing 4% w/w Sodium Cromoglycate BP.

*Inactive ingredients:* Liquid Paraffin BP, Yellow Soft Paraffin BP, Modulan (acetylated lanolin)

**Uses** For the prophylactic relief and treatment of allergic conjunctivitis such as hay fever, chronic allergic conjunctivitis and vernal kerato conjunctivitis. Sodium cromoglycate inhibits the release from sensitised mast cells of mediators of the allergic reaction.

**Dosage and administration** *Adults (including the elderly) and children:* To be applied to the eye two to three times daily. Opticrom Ointment should be used regularly to ensure optimal control of symptoms. It is recommended that treatment is continued during the period of exposure to allergen even when free of symptoms.

Care should be taken to avoid direct contact between the eye and the tube nozzle.

**Contra-indications, warnings, etc**
*Contra-indications:* Known sensitivity to any ingredient.

*Warnings:* As with other ophthalmic ointments, transient blurring of vision may occur. The ointment should not be used if contact lenses are being worn.

*Side-effects:* Transient blurring of vision, stinging and burning may occur after application. Other symptoms of local irritation have been reported rarely.

*Use in pregnancy and lactation:* As with all medication caution should be exercised especially during the first trimester of pregnancy. Cumulative experience with sodium cromoglycate suggests that it has no adverse effects on foetal development. It should only be used in pregnancy where there is a clear need.

It is not known whether sodium cromoglycate is excreted in the breast milk but on the basis of its physico-chemical properties this is considered unlikely. There is no information to suggest that the use of sodium cromoglycate has any undesirable effects on the baby.

**Pharmaceutical precautions** Store below 25°C. Protect from direct sunlight. The contents should be discarded four weeks after opening.

**Legal category** POM.

**Package quantities** 5 g.

**Further information** Patients may prefer to use Opticrom Aqueous Eye Drops during the day and Opticrom Eye Ointment at night.

**Product licence number** 0113/0103.

## ORUDIS*

**Presentation** Capsules each containing 50 mg ketoprofen, bicoloured (opaque green/opaque purple) with each half printed 'Orudis 50' in white. Capsules each containing 100 mg ketoprofen (flesh opaque) printed 'Orudis 100' in black. The capsules also contain lactose.

Cream coloured suppositories each containing 100 mg ketoprofen.

**Uses** Orudis is recommended in the management of rheumatoid arthritis, osteoarthritis, ankylosing spondylitis, acute articular and periarticular disorders (bursitis, capsulitis, synovitis, tendonitis), fibrositis, cervical spondylitis, low back pain (strain, lumbago, sciatica, fibrositis), painful musculo-skeletal conditions, dysmenorrhoea, acute gout and control of pain and inflammation following orthopaedic surgery. Orudis suppositories are *not* recommended for treatment of dysmenorrhoea.

Orudis is a potent non-steroidal anti-inflammatory analgesic agent and a strong inhibitor of prostaglandin synthetase.

Orudis reduces joint pain and inflammation, and facilitates increase in mobility and functional independence. As with other non-steroidal anti-inflammatory agents, it does not cure the underlying disease.

*Kinetics:* Ketoprofen is completely absorbed from Orudis capsules and maximum plasma concentration occurs after $\frac{1}{2}$–1 hour. It declines thereafter with an elimination half-life of about 2–3 hours. There is no accumulation on continued daily dosing. Ketoprofen is rapidly absorbed from the suppository dosage form with maximum plasma concentrations at 1–2 hours with an elimination half-life of 2–3 hours. Plasma levels obtained are comparable to those obtained from equal oral doses. Ketoprofen is very highly bound to plasma protein.

**Dosage and administration** Orudis is administered orally and/or rectally; to limit occurrence of gastrointestinal disturbance, capsules should always be taken with food (milk, meals).

Oral dosage is 50–100 mg twice daily, depending on patient weight and on severity of symptoms; medication should be taken early in the morning and late at night.

Rectal dosage is one suppository (100 mg) late at night supplemented as required with Orudis capsules during the daytime.

Orudis suppositories are especially appropriate for controlling overnight symptoms (severity of night and morning pain; duration and severity of morning stiffness). Suppositories administered late at night provide more consistent effective control of overnight symptoms than oral medication.

Best results are obtained by titrating dosage to suit each patient; start with a low dosage in mild chronic disease and a high dosage in acute or severe disease. Some patients derive greater benefit by treatment with capsules only; some with a combined capsule/suppository regimen; and others with a higher dosage at night-time than at early morning. Where patients require a maximum oral dosage initially, an attempt should be made to reduce this dosage for maintenance, since lower dosage might be better tolerated for purposes of long-term treatment.

*Elderly:* As with other medications, it is generally advisable to begin ketoprofen therapy at the lower end of the dose range and to maintain such patients on the lowest effective dosage.

*Paediatric:* Dosage is not established.

**Contra-indications, warnings, etc** Active peptic ulceration; a history of recurrent peptic ulceration or chronic dyspepsia; severe renal dysfunction; disease in children (safety/dosage during long-term treatment has not been established).

Suppositories should not be used following recent proctitis or in association with haemorrhoids.

Ketoprofen should not be given to patients with a known hypersensitivity to ketoprofen or to aspirin or other non-steroidal anti-inflammatory agents. Severe bronchospasm might be precipitated in these subjects, and in patients suffering from, or with a history of, bronchial asthma or allergic disease.

*Precautions*
*Use in pregnancy:* No embryopathic effects have been demonstrated in animals and there is epidemiological evidence of the safety of ketoprofen in human pregnancy. Nevertheless, it is recommended to avoid ketoprofen unless considered essential in which case it should be discontinued within one week of expected confinement when NSAIDs might cause premature closure of the ductus arteriosus or persistent pulmonary hypertension in the neonate. They also may delay labour. Trace amounts of ketoprofen are also excreted in breast milk; avoid use of ketoprofen unless considered essential.

*Warnings:* Inhibition of renal prostaglandin synthesis by non-steroidal anti-inflammatory agents may interfere with renal function especially in the presence of existing renal disease. Ketoprofen should therefore be used with caution in patients with renal impairment.

Orudis capsules should always be prescribed 'To be taken with food' to minimise gastric intolerance.

*Interactions:* Ketoprofen is highly protein-bound. Concomitant use of other protein-binding drugs, e.g. anticoagulants, sulphonamides, hydantoins, might necessitate modification of dosage in order to avoid increased levels of such drugs resulting from competition for plasma protein-binding sites. Similar acting drugs such as aspirin or other non-steroidal anti-inflammatory agents should not be administered concomitantly with ketoprofen as the potential for adverse reactions is increased.

Serious interactions have been recorded after the use of high dose methotrexate with non-steroidal anti-inflammatory agents including ketoprofen.

*Adverse effects:* Minor adverse effects, frequently transient, consist for the most part of gastrointestinal effects such as indigestion, dyspepsia, nausea, constipation, diarrhoea, heartburn and various types of abdominal discomfort. Other minor effects such as headache, dizziness, mild confusion, vertigo, drowsiness, oedema, mood change and insomnia may occur less commonly.

Major gastrointestinal adverse effects such as peptic ulceration, haemorrhage or perforation may rarely occur.

Major adverse effects involving other organ systems such as haematological reactions including thrombocytopenia, hepatic or renal damage, dermatological and photosensitivity reactions, bronchospasm and anaphylaxis are exceedingly rare.

In all cases of major adverse effects Orudis should be withdrawn at once.

Use of suppositories is sometimes associated with change in stool consistency mostly of mild softening. In a study of 64 patients treated for up to six months with one suppository each night (supplemented during daytime with Orudis capsules), local intolerance to suppositories sufficiently severe to discontinue treatment occurred in only four subjects.

*Overdosage:* Like other propionic acid derivatives, ketoprofen is of low toxicity in overdosage; symptoms after acute ketoprofen intoxication are largely limited to drowsiness, abdominal pain and vomiting, but adverse effects seen after overdosage with propionic acid derivatives such as hypotension, bronchospasm and gastrointestinal haemorrhage should be anticipated. Treatment is otherwise supportive and symptomatic.

**Pharmaceutical precautions** Store in a dry place, below 25°C.

**Legal category** POM.

**Package quantities** Orudis 50: Containers of 112×50 mg (OP).
Orudis 100: Containers of 56×100 mg (OP) capsules.
Blister pack of 10×100 mg (OP) suppositories.

**Further information** Nil.

**Product licence numbers**
50 mg capsules 0012/0122
100 mg capsules 0012/0133
100 mg suppositories 0012/0109

## ORUVAIL* GEL

**Presentation** Colourless, non greasy, non staining, transparent gel, with lavender fragrance for topical application, containing Ketoprofen BP 2.5% w/w. The gel also contains carboxypolymethylene 940, ethanol, triethanolamine, lavender oil and water.

**Uses** Oruvail gel is recommended for the relief of acute, painful musculoskeletal conditions caused by trauma such as sports injuries, sprains, strains and contusions. Ketoprofen is a non-steroidal anti-inflammatory drug. It has anti-inflammatory and analgesic actions.

Oruvail gel is for topical use only.

*Pharmacokinetics:* Applied locally as a gel, ketoprofen is absorbed into the blood very slowly and there is no accumulation in the body. The bioavailability of the gel relative to oral forms of ketoprofen is around 5%. The low systemic bioavailability suggests that systemic effects are unlikely.

**Dosage and administration** To be applied two to four times daily to the skin in the painful or inflamed region for up to seven days. After application, the affected area should be well massaged to ensure local absorption of ketoprofen. The usual recommended dose is 15 g per day.

*Elderly:* There are no specific dosage recommendations for the elderly.

*Children:* Not recommended as safety in children has not been established.

**Contra-indications, warnings, etc** *Contra-indications:* Patients with a known hypersensitivity to ketoprofen, aspirin or other non-steroidal anti-inflammatory agents; patients suffering from or with a history of, bronchial asthma or allergic disease. Oruvail gel should be avoided in patients with exudative dermatoses, eczema, sores and infected lesions or broken skin.

Oruvail gel should not be applied to mucous membranes, anal or genital areas, eyes, or used with occlusive dressings.

*Precautions:* Although systemic effects are minimal, the gel should be used with caution in patients with severe renal impairment. Should a skin rash occur after gel application, treatment must be stopped.

*Use in pregnancy and lactation:* No embryopathic effects have been demonstrated in animals and there is epidemiological evidence of the safety of ketoprofen in human pregnancy. Nevertheless, it is recommended that ketoprofen should be avoided during pregnancy. Non-steroidal anti-inflammatory drugs may also delay labour.

Trace amounts of ketoprofen are excreted in breast milk, following oral administration, therefore Oruvail gel should not be used during breastfeeding.

*Interactions:* Interactions are unlikely as serum concentrations following topical administration are low. Serious interactions have been recorded after the use of high dose methotrexate with non-steroidal anti-inflammatory agents, including ketoprofen, when administered by the systemic route.

*Adverse reactions:* Skin reactions including photosensitivity reactions, pruritus and localised erythema have occurred rarely. These are usually mild and resolve after cessation of treatment.

*Overdosage:* Overdose is unlikely to be caused by topical administration. If accidentally ingested, the gel may cause systemic adverse effects depending on the amount ingested. However, if they occur, treatment should be supportive and symptomatic.

**Pharmaceutical precautions** Store below 25°C. Keep the gel away from naked flames. Do not incinerate. Do not dilute the gel. Replace cap after use.

**Legal category** POM.

**Package quantities** Tubes of 100 g.

**Further information** Nil.

**Product licence number** 0012/0243.

## ORUVAIL*CAPSULES

**Qualitative and quantitative composition**
Ketoprofen BP 100 mg
Ketoprofen BP 150 mg
Ketoprofen BP 200 mg

**Pharmaceutical form** Controlled release capsules

**Clinical particulars**

*Therapeutic indications:* Oruvail is recommended in the management of rheumatoid arthritis, osteoarthritis, ankylosing spondylitis, acute articular and periarticular disorders, (bursitis, capsulitis, synovitis, tendinitis), cervical spondylitis, low back pain (strain, lumbago, sciatica, fibrositis), painful musculoskeletal conditions, acute gout, dysmenorrhoea and control of pain and inflammation following orthopaedic surgery.

Oruvail reduces joint pain and inflammation and facilitates increase in mobility and functional independence. As with other non-steroidal anti-inflammatory agents, it does not cure the underlying disease

*Posology and method of administration: Adults*: 100–200 mg once daily, depending on patient weight and on severity of symptoms. *Elderly*: There is no evidence of an excess of adverse reactions in the elderly. However, as with other medication, it is generally advisable in the elderly to begin ketoprofen therapy at the lower end of the dose range and to maintain such patients on the lowest effective dosage. *Paediatric dosage:* not established.

Oruvail capsules are for oral administration.

Oruvail capsules should always be prescribed, 'to be taken with food' to minimise gastric intolerance.

*Contra-indications*: Active peptic ulceration, a history of recurrent peptic ulceration or chronic dyspepsia, severe renal dysfunction.

Ketoprofen should not be given to patients sensitive to aspirin or other non-steroidal anti-inflammatory agents.

Severe bronchospasm might be precipitated in these subjects and in patients suffering from or with a history of, bronchial asthma or allergic disease

*Special warnings special precautions for use*: Inhibition of renal prostaglandin synthesis by non-steroidal anti-inflammatory agents may interfere with renal function especially in the presence of existing renal disease. Ketoprofen should therefore be used with caution in patients with renal impairment.

*Interactions with other medicaments and other forms of interaction*: Ketoprofen is highly protein bound, concomitant use of other protein-binding drugs e.g. anticoagulants, sulphonamides, hydantoins, might necessitate modification of dosage in order to avoid increased levels of such drugs resulting from competition for plasma protein-binding sites.

Similar acting drugs such as aspirin or other NSAIDS should not be administered concomitantly with ketoprofen as the potential for adverse reactions is increased.

Serious interactions have been recorded after the use of high dose methotrexate with non-steroidal anti-inflammatory agents, including ketoprofen.

*Pregnancy and lactation*: No embryopathic effects have been demonstrated in animals and there is epidemiological evidence of the safety of ketoprofen in human pregnancy. Nevertheless, it is recommended to avoid ketoprofen unless considered essential in which case it should be discontinued within one week of expected confinement when NSAIDS might cause premature closure of the ductus arteriosus or persistent pulmonary hypertension in the neonate. They may also delay labour.

Trace amounts of ketoprofen are excreted in breast milk. Avoid use of ketoprofen unless it is considered essential

*Effects on ability to drive and use machines*: CNS side effects have been observed in some patients (see undesirable effects) If affected patients should not drive or operate machinery.

*Undesirable effects:*
*Adverse effects:* minor adverse effects, frequently transient, consist for the most part of gastrointestinal effects such as indigestion, dyspepsia, nausea, constipation, diarrhoea, heartburn and various types of abdominal discomfort. Other minor effects, such as headache, dizziness, mild confusion, vertigo, drowsiness, oedema, mood change and insomnia may occur less commonly.

Major gastrointestinal adverse effects such as peptic ulceration, haemorrhage, or perforation may rarely occur.

Major adverse effects involving other organ systems such as haematological reactions including thrombocytopenia, hepatic or renal damage, dermatological and photosensitivity reactions, bronchospasm and anaphylaxis are exceedingly rare.

In all cases of major effects Oruvail should be withdrawn at once.

*Overdose*: Like other propionic acid derivatives, ketoprofen is of low toxicity in overdosage; symptoms after acute ketoprofen intoxication are largely limited to drowsiness, abdominal pain and vomiting, but adverse effects seen after overdosage with propionic acid derivatives such as hypotension, bronchospasm and gastro-intestinal haemorrhage should be anticipated. Owing to the slow release characteristics of Oruvail, it should be expected that ketoprofen will continue to be absorbed for up to 16 hours after ingestion.

Gastric lavage, aimed at recovering pellets that may still be in the stomach should be performed if the patient is seen soon after ingestion. It should be possible to identify the pellets in the gastric contents. Treatment is otherwise supportive and symptomatic.

Administration of activated charcoal in an attempt to reduce absorption of slowly-released ketoprofen should be considered.

**Pharmacological properties**

*Pharmacodynamic properties*: Ketoprofen overall has the properties of a potent non-steroidal anti-inflammatory agent. It has the following pharmacological effects:

*Anti-inflammatory:* It inhibits the development of carageenan-induced abscesses in rats at 1 mg/kg and UV-radiation induced erythema in guinea pigs at 6 mg/kg. It is also a potent inhibitor of $PGE_2$ and $PGF_{2\alpha}$ synthesis in guinea pig and human chopped lung preparations.

*Analgesic:* Ketoprofen effectively reduced visceral pain in mice caused by phenyl benzoquinone or by bradykinin following p.o. administration at about 6 mg/kg.

*Antipyretic:* Ketoprofen (2 and 6 mg/kg) inhibited hyperthermia caused by s.c injection of brewer's yeast in rats and, at 1 mg/kg hyperthermia caused by i.v. administration of anticoagulant vaccine to rabbits.

Ketoprofen at 10 mg/kg i.v. did not affect the cardiovascular, respiratory, central nervous system or autonomic nervous systems

*Pharmacokinetic properties*: Ketoprofen is slowly but completely absorbed from Oruvail capsules. Maximum plasma concentration occurs after 6–8 hours. It declines thereafter with a half-life of about 8 hours. There is no accumulation on continued daily dosing. Ketoprofen is very highly bound to plasma protein.

*Preclinical safety data*: No additional data of relevance to the prescriber.

**Pharmaceutical particulars**

*List of excipients:*
*Oruvail 100: Pellets*: Sugar spheres NF, Colloidal Silicon dioxide EP, Shellac NF, Ethyl Cellulose NF, Talc EP-*Capsule shell-body*: Erythrocine (EEC127), Gelatin. *Capsule shell-Cap*: Erythrocine (EEC 127), Patent blue V (EEC 131), Titanium dioxide (EEC 171), Gelatin.

*Oruvail 150: Pellets*: : Sugar spheres NF, Colloidal Silicon dioxide EP, Shellac NF, Ethyl Cellulose NF, Talc EP, Industrial methylated spirit BP or Ethanol 95/96% USP, Talc EP. *Capsule shell- body:* Erythrocine (EEC127), Gelatin. *Capsule shell-Cap:* Erythrocine (EEC 127), Titanium dioxide (EEC 171), Gelatin.

*Oruvail 200*: Pellets: Sugar spheres NF, Colloidal Silicon dioxide EP, Shellac NF, Ethyl Cellulose NF, Talc EP *Capsule shell-body*: Erythrocine (EEC127), Gelatin. *Capsule shell-Cap*: Erythrocine (EEC 127), Gelatin.

*Incompatibilities:* None stated

Shelf-life: 36 months

Special Precautions for storage:: Blister pack- Store below 25°C in a dry place and protect from light.

Nature and contents of container: Oruvail 100: Containers of 56 capsules (OP). Oruvail 150: Calendar blister pack of 28 capsules(OP). Oruvail 200: Calendar blister pack of 28 capsules (OP).

Instructions for Use/handling: None stated

**Marketing authorisations numbers**

Oruvail 100    0012/0143
Oruvail 150    0012/0262
Oruvail 200    0012/0158

**Date of approval/revision of SPC**   February 1997

**Legal category**   POM

## ORUVAIL IM INJECTION

**Qualitative and quantitative composition** Ketoprofen BP 100 mg in 2 ml

**Pharmaceutical form** Solution for IM injection

**Clinical particulars**

Therapeutic indications: Oruvail is recommended for management of acute exacerbations of:

Rheumatoid arthritis, osteoarthritis, ankylosing spondylitis, Periarticular conditions such as fibrositis, bursitis, capsulitis, tendinitis and tenosynovitis, Low back pain of musculoskeletal origin, sciatica. Other musculoskeletal conditions. Acute gout Control of pain and inflammation following orthopaedic surgery.

Dosage and administration: Adults: 50 to 100 mg every four hours, repeated up to a maximum of 200 mg in twenty-four hours. Following a satisfactory response, oral therapy should be instituted with Oruvail capsules. It is recommended that the injection should not normally be continued for longer than three days. Elderly: As with other medications it is generally advisable in the elderly to begin ketoprofen therapy at the lower end of the dose range and to maintain such patients on the lowest effective dosage. Paediatric dosage: Not established Oruvail IM injection is for intramuscular injection. It must not be given intravenously.

Contra-indications: Active peptic ulceration, a history of recurrent peptic ulceration or chronic dyspepsia, severe renal dysfunction, sensitivity to aspirin or other non-steroidal anti-inflammatory agents.

Special warnings and precautions for use: Inhibition of renal prostaglandin synthesis by non-steroidal anti-inflammatory agents may interfere with renal function especially in the presence of existing renal disease. Ketoprofen should therefore be used with caution in patients with renal impairment.

Severe bronchospasm might be precipitated in patients with a history of bronchial asthma or allergic disease.

Oruvail injection must not be given intravenously.

Interactions with other medicaments and other forms of interaction: Ketoprofen is highly protein bound. Concomitant use of other protein-binding drugs e.g. anticoagulants, sulphonamides, hydantoins, might necessitate modification of dosage in order to avoid increased levels of such drugs resulting from competition for plasma protein-binding sites.

Similar acting drugs such as aspirin or other NSAIDs should not be administered concomitantly with ketoprofen as the potential for adverse reactions is increased.

Serious interactions have been recorded after the use of high dose methotrexate with non-steroidal anti-inflammatory agents, including ketoprofen.

Pregnancy and lactation: No embryopathic effects have been demonstrated in animals and there is epidemiological evidence of the safety of ketoprofen in human pregnancy. Nevertheless, it is recommended to avoid ketoprofen unless considered essential in which case it should be discontinued within one week of expected confinement when NSAIDs might cause premature closure of the ductus arteriosus or persistent pulmonary hypertension in the neonate. They may also delay labour.

Trace amounts of ketoprofen are excreted in breast milk. Avoid use of ketoprofen unless considered essential.

Effects on ability to drive and use machines: CNS side effects have been observed in some patients (see undesirable effects). If affected patients should not drive or operate machinery.

Undesirable effects: Adverse effects: minor adverse effects, frequently transient, consist for the most part of gastrointestinal effects such as indigestion, dyspepsia, nausea, constipation, diarrhoea, heartburn and various types of abdominal discomfort. Other minor effects such as headache, dizziness, mild confusion,

vertigo, drowsiness, oedema, mood change and insomnia may occur less commonly.

Major gastrointestinal adverse effects such as peptic ulceration, haemorrhage or perforation may rarely occur.

Major adverse effects involving other organ systems such as haematological reactions including thrombocytopenia, hepatic or renal damage, dermatological and photosensitivity reactions, bronchospasm and anaphylaxis are exceedingly rare.

Local reactions at the injection site can occur and may include pain or a burning sensation. In all cases of major adverse effects Oruvail should be withdrawn at once

Overdosage: Like other propionic acid derivatives, ketoprofen is of low toxicity in overdosage. Symptoms after acute ketoprofen intoxication are largely limited to drowsiness, abdominal pain and vomiting, but adverse effects seen after overdosage with propionic acid derivatives such as hypotension, bronchospasm and gastro-intestinal haemorrhage should be anticipated. Treatment is otherwise supportive and symptomatic

**Pharmacological properties**

Pharmacodynamic properties: Ketoprofen is a pharmacopoeial non-steroidal anti-inflammatory drug (NSAID). It is a strong inhibitor of prostaglandin synthetase and potent analgesic agent. Studies in vitro and in vivo show that ketoprofen possesses powerful anti-inflammatory, antipyretic, antibradykinin and lysosomal membrane stabilising properties.

Pharmacokinetic properties: Peak concentrations of approximately 10 mg/L are reached at about 0.5-0.75 H after a 100 mg dose. The elimination half life is approximately 1.88 H. Apart from earlier Tmax values, there are no significant differences between the pharmacokinetics of Oruvail IM injection and conventional release capsules (Orudis)

Preclinical safety data: No additional data of relevance to the prescriber.

**Pharmaceutical particulars**

List of excipients Arginine BP, Benzyl alcohol BP, Citric acid anhydrous (E330) BP, Water for injections BP.

Incompatibilities: None stated

Shelf-life: 36 months

Special precautions for storage: Store below 30°C. Protect form light.

Nature and contents of container: Boxes of 10x2 ml ampoules

Instructions for use/handling: None stated

**Marketing authorisation number**   0012/0186

**Date of approval/revision of SPC**   February 1997

**Legal category**   POM

## PHENERGAN* TABLETS AND ELIXIR

**Qualitative and quantitative composition**
Phenergan Elixir contains Promethazine Hydrochloride BP 5 mg / 5 ml
Phenergan 10 mg tablets contain Promethazine Hydrochloride BP 10 mg
Phenergan 25 mg tablets contain Promethazine Hydrochloride BP 25 mg

**Pharmaceutical form**
Phenergan Elixir is a clear golden syrupy liquid
Phenergan tablets are pale blue and marked PN 10 (10 mg tablets) and PN 25 (25 mg tablets)

**Clinical particulars**
Therapeutic indications: As symptomatic treatment for allergic conditions of the upper respiratory tract and skin including allergic rhinitis, urticaria and anaphylactic reactions to drugs and foreign proteins. As an adjunct in preoperative sedation in surgery and obstetrics. As an antiemetic.

For short term use : Sedation and treatment of insomnia in adults. As a paediatric sedative.

Posology and method of administration: Route of administration: Oral. See table for dosages.

Not for use in children under the age of 2 years because the safety of such use has not been established

Contra-indications: Phenergan should not be used in patients in coma or suffering from CNS depression of any cause. It must not be given to neonates, premature infants or patients hypersensitive to phenothiazines. Phenergan should be avoided in patients taking monoamine oxidase inhibitors up to 14 days previously. The elixir contains hydrogenated glucose and is not suitable for diabetics.

Special warnings and special precautions for use: Phenergan may thicken or dry lung secretions and impair expectoration. It should therefore be used with caution in patients with asthma, bronchitis or bron-

chiectasis. Use with care in patients with severe coronary artery disease, narrow angle glaucoma, epilepsy or hepatic and renal insufficiency. Caution should be exercised in patients with bladder neck or pyloro-duodenal obstruction. Promethazine may mask the warnings signs of ototoxicity caused by ototoxic drugs e.g. salicylates. It may also delay the early diagnosis of intestinal obstruction or raised intracranial pressure through the suppression of vomiting. Phenergan Elixir should not be used for longer than 7 days without seeking medical advice.

Interaction with other medicaments and other forms of interaction: Phenergan will enhance the action of any anticholinergic agent, tricyclic anti-depressant, sedative or hypnotic. Alcohol should be avoided during treatment. Phenergan may interfere with immunological urine pregnancy tests to produce false-positive or false-negative results. Phenergan should be discontinued at least 72 hours before the start of skin tests as it may inhibit the cutaneous histamine response thus producing false negative results.

Pregnancy and lactation: There is epidemiological evidence for the safety of promethazine in pregnancy and animal studies have shown no hazard. Nevertheless, it should not be used in pregnancy unless the physician considers it essential. The use of Phenergan is not recommended in the 2 weeks prior to delivery in view of the risk of irritability and excitement in the neonate. Available evidence suggests that the amount excreted in milk is insignificant. However, there are risks of neonatal irritability and excitement.

Effects on ability to drive and use machines: Because the duration of action may be up to 12 hours, patients should be advised that if they feel drowsy they should not drive or operate heavy machinery.

Undesirable effects: Side effects may be seen in a few patients: drowsiness, dizziness, restlessness, headaches, nightmares, tiredness, and disorientation. Anticholinergic side effects such as blurred vision, dry mouth and urinary retention occur occasionally. Infants are susceptible to the anticholinergic effects of promethazine, while other children may display paradoxical hyperexcitability. The elderly are particularly susceptible to the anticholinergic effects and confusion due to promethazine. Other side-effects include anorexia, gastric irritation, palpitations, hypotension, arrhythmias, extrapyramidal effects, muscle spasms and tic-like movements of the head and face. Anaphylaxis, jaundice and blood dyscrasias including haemolytic anaemia rarely occur. Photosensitive skin reactions have been reported. Strong sunlight should be avoided during treatment.

The preservatives used in Phenergan Elixir have been reported to cause hypersensitivity reactions, characterised by circulatory collapse with CNS depression in certain susceptible individuals with allergic tendencies.

Overdose: Symptoms of severe overdosage are variable. They are characterised in children by various combinations of excitation, ataxia, incoordination, athetosis and hallucinations, while adults may become drowsy and lapse into coma. Convulsions may occur in both adults and children. Coma or excitement may precede their occurrence. Cardiorespiratory depression is uncommon. If the patient is seen soon enough after ingestion, it should be possible to induce vomiting with ipecacuanha despite the antiemetic effect of promethazine; alternatively, gastric lavage may be used.

Treatment is otherwise supportive with attention to maintenance of adequate respiratory and circulatory status. Convulsions should be treated with diazepam or other suitable anticonvulsant.

**Pharmacological properties**

Pharmacodynamic properties: Potent, long acting, antihistamine with additional anti-emetic central sedative and anticholinergic properties.

Pharmacokinetic properties: Promethazine is distributed widely in the body. It enters the brain and crosses the placenta. Promethazine is slowly excreted via urine and bile. Phenothiazines pass into the milk at low concentrations.

Preclinical safety data: No additional pre-clinical data of relevance to the prescriber.

**Pharmaceutical particulars**

List of excipients:
Phenergan Elixir: Hydrogenated glucose syrup, citric acid anhydrous BP (E330), sodium citrate BP (E331), ascorbic acid BP (E300), sodium sulphite anhydrous BP (E221), sodium metabisulphite BP (E223), sodium benzoate BP (E211), Orange juice flavour, Caramel, acesulphame potassium (E950), demineralised water BP.

Phenergan tablets Lactose BP, maize starch BP, Povidone K30 BP, magnesium stearate BP, polyethylene glycol 200, Opaspray M-1-4210A (contains E132 and E171), Pharmacoat 606.

**Phenergan Tablets and Elixir dosages**

| | Elixir | 10 mg tablets | 25 mg tablets |
|---|---|---|---|
| **As an antihistamine in allergy** | | | |
| Children 2-5 years | Either: 5-15 mg as a single dose Or 5 mg bd Maximum daily dose 15 mg | The use of the Elixir is recommended for this age group | The use of the Elixir is recommended for this age group |
| Children 5-10 years | Either 10-25 mg as a single dose Or: 5-10 mg bd Maximum daily dose 25 mg | Either 10 or 20 mg as a single dose† Or 10 mg bd Maximum daily dose 20 mg | 25 mg as a single dose† Maximum daily dose 25 mg |
| Children over 10 years, adults (inc elderly) | Initially 10 mg bd Increasing to a maximum of 20 mg tds as required | Initially 10 mg bd Increasing to a maximum of 20 mg tds as required | 25 mg as a single dose† Increasing to 25 mg bd as required |
| †Single doses best taken at night | | | |
| **As an antiemetic** | | | |
| Children 2-5 years | 5 mg to be taken the night before the journey To be repeated after 6-8 hours as required | The use of the Elixir is recommended for this age group | The use of the Elixir is recommended for this age group |
| Children 5-10 years | 10 mg to be taken the night before the journey To be repeated after 6-8 hours as required | 10 mg to be taken the night before the journey. To be repeated after 6-8 hours as required | The use of the Elixir or 10 mg tablets is recommended for this age group |
| Children over 10 years and adults (including elderly) | 25 mg to be taken the night before the journey To be repeated after 6-8 hours as required. | 20 mg to be taken the night before the journey. To be repeated after 6-8 hours as required | 25 mg to be taken the night before the journey. To be repeated after 6-8 hours as required |
| **Short term sedation** | | | |
| Children 2-5 years | 15 or 20 mg as a single night time dose | The use of Phenergan Elixir is recommended for this age group | The use of Phenergan Elixir is recommended for this age group |
| Children 5-10 years | 20 or 25 mg as a single night time dose | 20 mg as a single night time dose | 25 mg as a single night time dose |
| Children over 10 years and adults (including elderly) | 25 or 50 mg as a single night time dose. The use of Phenergan tablets to provide these doses is recommended. | 20 to 50 mg as a single night time dose | 25 or 50 mg as a single night time dose |

*Incompatibilities:* None stated

*Shelf life:*
*Phenergan Elixir:* 24 months when unopened. 1 month when opened.
*Phenergan tablets:* 60 months.

*Special precautions for storage:*
*Phenergan Elixir:* Protect from light. Store below 25°C.
*Phenergan tablets:* Protect from light. Store below 30°C.

*Nature and contents of container:*
*Phenergan Elixir:* Amber glass bottles containing 100 ml.
*Phenergan tablets:* Blister packs of 56 tablets.

*Instructions for use/handling:* No special instructions.

**Marketing authorisation numbers**
Phenergan Elixir      0012/5025R
Phenergan 10 mg tablets      0012/5285R
Phenergan 25 mg tablets      0012/5286R

**Date of approval/revision of SPC**    August 1997

**Legal category**    P

## PHENERGAN* INJECTION

**Qualitative and quantitative composition** Phenergan Injection contains Promethazine Hydrochloride BP 2.5%w/v.

**Pharmaceutical form** Solution for injection.

**Clinical particulars**

*Therapeutic indications:* A symptomatic treatment for allergic conditions of the upper respiratory tract and skin including allergic rhinitis, urticaria and anaphylactic reactions to drugs and foreign proteins.
Sedation and treatment of insomnia in adults.
As an adjunct in preoperative sedation in surgery and obstetrics.
As a paediatric sedative.
Not for use in children under 2 years of age because the safety of such use has not been established.

*Posology and method of administration:* For intramuscular or intravenous use. The usual dose is 25–50 mg by deep intramuscular injection, or, in emergency, by slow intravenous injection after dilution of the 2.5% solution to 10 times its volume with water for injections immediately before use.
Maximum parenteral dose 100 mg.
*Elderly:* No specific dosage recommendations.
*Children:* 6.25–12.5 mg for children from 5–10 years by deep intramuscular injection.

*Contra-indications:* Phenergan should not be used in patients in coma or suffering from CNS depression of any cause. It must not be given to neonates, premature infants or patients hypersensitive to phenothiazines. Phenergan should be avoided in patients taking monoamine oxidase inhibitors up to 14 days previously.

*Special warnings and precautions for use:* Phenergan may thicken or dry lung secretions and impair expectoration. It should therefore be used with caution in patients with asthma, bronchitis or bronchiectasis. Use with care in patients with severe coronary artery disease, narrow angle glaucoma, epilepsy or hepatic and renal insufficiency. Caution should be exercised in patients with bladder neck or pyloro-duodenal obstruction. Promethazine may mask the warning signs of ototoxicity caused by ototoxic drugs e.g. Salicylates. It may also delay the early diagnosis of intestinal obstruction or raised intracranial pressure through the suppression of vomiting. Accidental intra-arterial injection may lead to peripheral gangrene and necrosis while subcutaneous injections may lead to local necrosis.

*Interactions with other medicaments and other forms of interaction:* Phenergan will enhance the action of any anticholinergic agent, tricyclic anti-depressant, sedative or hypnotic. Alcohol should be avoided during treatment. Phenergan may interfere with immunological urine pregnancy tests to produce false-positive or false-negative results. Phenergan should be discontinued at least 72 hours before the start of skin tests as it may inhibit the cutaneous histamine response thus producing false-negative results. Phenergan injection may increase glucose tolerance.

*Pregnancy and lactation:* There is epidemiological evidence for the safety of promethazine in pregnancy and animal studies have shown no hazard. Nevertheless it should not be used in pregnancy unless the physician considers it essential. The use of Phenergan is not recommended in the 2 weeks prior to delivery in view of the risk of irritability and excitement in the neonate.
Available evidence suggests that the amount excreted in milk is insignificant. However, there are risks of neonatal irritability and excitement.

*Effects on ability to drive and use machines:* Ambulant patients receiving Phenergan for the first time should not be in control of vehicles or machinery for the first few days until it is established that they are not hypersensitive to the central nervous effects of the drug and do not suffer from disorientation, confusion or dizziness.

*Undesirable effects:* Side effects may be seen in a few patients: drowsiness, dizziness, restlessness, headaches, nightmares, tiredness, and disorientation. Anticholinergic side effects such as blurred vision, dry mouth and urinary retention occur occasionally. Newborn and premature infants are susceptible to the anticholinergic effects of promethazine, while other children may display paradoxical hyperexcitability. The elderly are particularly susceptible to the anticholinergic effects and confusion due to promethazine. Other side-effects include anorexia, gastric irritation, palpitations, hypotension, arrhythmias, extrapyramidal effects, muscle spasms and tic-like movements of the head and face. Anaphylaxis, jaundice and blood dyscrasias including haemolytic anaemia rarely occur.

Photosensitive skin reactions have been reported; strong sunlight should be avoided during treatment.
The preservatives used in Phenergan injection have been reported to cause hypersensitivity reactions, characterised by circulatory collapse with CNS depression in certain susceptible individuals with allergic tendencies.

*Overdosage:* Symptoms of severe overdosage are variable. They are characterised in children by various combinations of excitation, ataxia, incoordination, athetosis and hallucinations, while adults may become drowsy and lapse into coma. Convulsions may occur in both adults and children: coma or excitement may precede their occurrence. Cardiorespiratory depression is uncommon. If the patient is seen soon enough after ingestion, it should be possible to induce vomiting with ipecacuanha despite the antiemetic effect of promethazine; alternatively, gastric lavage may be used.
Treatment is otherwise supportive with attention to maintenance of adequate respiratory and circulatory status. Convulsions should be treated with diazepam or other suitable anticonvulsant.

**Pharmacological properties**

*Pharmacodynamic properties:* Potent, long acting, antihistamine with additional anti-emetic central sedative and anti-cholinergic properties.

*Pharmacokinetic properties:* Promethazine is slowly excreted via urine and bile. It is distributed widely in the body. It enters the brain and crosses the placenta. Phenothiazines pass into the milk at low concentrations.

**Pharmaceutical particulars**

*List of excipients:* Sodium Sulphite anhydrous (E221), Sodium Metabisulphite (E223), Water for Injections

*Incompatibilities:* None stated.

*Shelf life:* 60 months.

*Special precautions for storage:* Protect from light.

*Nature and contents of container:* Cardboard carton containing 10 x 1 ml ampoules.

*Instructions for use/handling:* Discoloured solutions should not be used.

**Marketing authorisation number**    0012/5054R

**Date of approval/revision of SPC** February 1997

**Legal category** POM

## PRIMALAN*

**Qualitative and quantitative composition** Primalan tablets contain 5 mg Mequitazine 5 mg.

**Pharmaceutical form:** Primalan tablets are white or almost white with one side impressed 'Primalan'.

**Clinical particulars**

*Therapeutic indications:* Antihistamine for the treatment of allergic conditions such as hay fever, perennial rhinits, urticaria, pruritis of allergic origin and allergic reactions associated with insect bites and stings.

*Posology and method of administration:* For oral use. *Adults:* one 5 mg tablet to be taken orally twice a day. *Elderly patients:* There is no information on specific dosage recommendation in the elderly. Caution should therefore be exercised in this group of patients. *Children:* Primalan is not recommended for children under the age of 12.

*Contra-indications:* Primalan should not be given to patients sensitive to phenothiazines, or given concurrently with monoamine oxidase inhibitors. As with all antihistamines, it should be used with caution in epilepsy, prostatic hypertrophy, glaucoma and hepatic disease.

*Special warnings and special precautions for use:* None stated

*Interaction with other medicaments and other forms of interaction:* Primalan may potentiate sympathomimetic amines. Potentiation of the sedative effects of alcohol may occur in individual patients

*Pregnancy and lactation:* Primalan should not be administered during pregnancy.

*Effects on ability of drive and use machines:* In objective tests Primalan has been shown to have no significant effect on alertness, performance and reaction time. As drowsiness can occur in some patients it is advisable to check individual responses prior to driving or operating machinery.

*Undesirable effects:* Anticholinergic effects such as dryness of the mouth and disturbance of visual accommodation may occasionally occur particularly in the early days of treatment.

*Overdose:* Gastric lavage and supportive therapy. Avoid sedation with other phenothiazine derivatives.

### Pharmacological properties

*Pharmacodynamic properties:* Mequitazine is a phenothiazine derivative with the actions and uses of the antihistamines. Antihistamines diminish or abolish the main actions of histamine in the body by competitive, reversible blockade of histamine receptor sites on tissues; they do not inactivate histamine or prevent its synthesis or release. Antihistamines are used for palliative treatment of allergic reactions. Mequitazine is reported to cause less sedation than promethazine.

*Pharmacokinetic properties:* In general, antihistamines are readily absorbed from the gastrointestinal tract, metabolised in the liver and excreted, usually mainly as metabolites, in the urine.

### Pharmaceutical particulars

*List of excipients:* Lactose BP, Maize starch BP, Colloidal silicon dioxide E551, Magnesium stearate BP, Microcrystalline cellulose BP E460.

*Incompatibilities:* None stated

*Shelf life:* 36 months

*Special precautions for storage:* Store in a cool, dry place, protect from light

*Nature and contents of container:* Blister pack of 56 tablets.

*Instructions for use/handling:* Not applicable

**Marketing authorisation number** 0012/0161

**Date of approval/revision of SPC** February 1997

**Legal category** POM

## RAPITIL*

**Qualitative and quantitative composition:** Nedocromil sodium 2.0% w/v

**Pharmaceutical form:** Rapitil is presented as a 5 ml sterile, preserved, aqueous solution containing 2% nedocromil sodium in a dropper bottle for administration to the eye.

### Clinical particulars

*Therapeutic indications:* Rapitil is recommended for the prevention, relief and treatment of allergic conjunctivitis, perennial allergic conjunctivitis and vernal kerato-conjunctivitis

*Posology and method of administration:* Adults (including the elderly) and children aged 6 years and over: In seasonal allergic conjunctivitis: one drop into each eye twice daily, increasing when necessary to four times daily. In seasonal allergic conjunctivitis: therapy should be restricted to 12 weeks. In vernal kerato-conjunctivitis: one drop into each eye four times daily. Adults (including the elderly): In perennial allergic conjunctivitis: one drop into each eye twice daily, increasing when necessary to four times daily.

Rapitil should be used regularly to ensure optimum control of symptoms.

There is only limited trial evidence with Rapitil in children aged below 6 years, therefore use in this age range cannot be recommended.

*Contra-indications:* Rapitil is contra-indicated in patients with known hypersensitivity to any constituent of the formulation.

*Special warnings and special precautions for use:* Patients who use soft contact lenses should be advised not to wear them during the treatment period. In patients who continue to use hard or gas-permeable contact lenses during Rapitil treatment, the lenses should be taken out of the eye prior to instillation and not inserted again for at least 10 minutes.

*Interactions with other medicaments and other forms of interaction:* None have been reported.

*Pregnancy and lactation:* Studies in pregnant lactating animals have failed to reveal a hazard with nedocromil sodium. However, as with all medications caution should be exercised during pregnancy (especially during the first trimester) and whilst breast feeding.

On the basis of animal studies and its physiochemical properties it is considered that only negligible amounts of nedocromil sodium may pass into human breast milk. There is no information to suggest that the use of nedocromil sodium by nursing mothers has any undesirable effects on the baby.

*Effects on ability to drive and use machines:* No sedative effects have been reported with Rapitil.

*Undesirable effects:* Transient stinging and burning may occur after instillation. Other symptoms of local irritation have been reported rarely. Some patients have reported a distinctive taste.

*Overdose:* Animal studies have not shown evidence of toxic effects of nedocromil sodium even at high dosage, nor have extended human studies revealed any safety hazard with the drug. Overdosage is unlikely, therefore to cause problems. However, if suspected, treatment should be supportive and directed to the control of the relevant symptoms.

### Pharmacological properties

*Pharmacodynamic properties:* Rapitil, the ophthalmic preparation of nedocromil sodium, displays specific anti-allergic and anti-inflammatory properties. Nedocromil sodium has been shown to prevent the release of inflammatory mediators from a range of inflammatory cell types

*Pharmacokinetic properties:* Following topical ophthalmic administration, less than 4% of the dose is absorbed following multiple dosing. Absorption occurs primarily through the nasal mucosa as approximately 80% of the ophthalmic dose drains into the nose via the naso-lachrymal duct, although 1-2% of the dose may be absorbed orally.

Nedocromil sodium is reversibly bound to plasma proteins and is not metabolised, but is excreted unchanged in bile and urine. The drug is rapidly cleared from the plasma (plasma clearance 102±1.3 ml/min/kg-elimination half-life 5.3±0.9 min) and accumulation does not occur.

*Pre-clinical safety data:* Animal studies have failed to reveal toxic effects with nedocromil sodium even at high doses.

### Pharmaceutical particulars

*List of excipients:* Benzalkonium chloride, sodium chloride, disodium edetate.

*Incompatibilities:* None known.

*Shelf life:* 36 months.

*Special precautions for storage:* Store below 25°C, away from direct sunlight. Discard any remaining contents four weeks after opening the bottle.

*Nature and contents of container:* A plastic dropper bottle containing 5 ml of sterile, aqueous Rapitil solution for administration to the eye.

*Instructions for use/handling:* Please refer to enclosed package insert.

**Marketing authorisation number** 0113/0152

**Date of approval/revision of SPC** February 1997

**Legal category** POM

## RILUTEK* ▼

**Qualitative and quantitative composition** Riluzole 50 mg

**Pharmaceutical form** Capsule-shaped, white, film-coated tablets for oral use. The tablets are engraved with « RPR 202 » on one side of the tablet.

### Clinical particulars

*Therapeutic indications:* Riluzole is indicated to extend life or the time to mechanical ventilation for patients with amyotrophic lateral sclerosis (ALS).

Clinical trials have demonstrated that Rilutek ex-

tends survival for patients with ALS. Survival was defined as patients who were alive, not intubated for mechanical ventilation and tracheotomy-free. There is no evidence that riluzole exerts a therapeutic effect on motor function, lung function, fasciculations, muscle strength and motor symptoms. Riluzole has not been shown to be effective in the late stages of ALS. Safety and efficacy of riluzole has only been studied in ALS. Therefore, riluzole should not be used in any other form of motor neurone disease.

*Further information on clinical trials* In a trial, 155 patients were randomised to riluzole 100 mg/day (50 mg twice daily) or placebo and were followed-up for 12 to 21 months. Survival, as defined in the second paragraph of section 4.1., was significantly extended for patients who received riluzole as compared to patients who received placebo. The median survival time was 17.7 months versus 14.9 months for riluzole and placebo, respectively. In a dose-ranging trial, 959 patients with ALS were randomised to one of four treatment groups: riluzole 50, 100, 200 mg/day, or placebo and were followed-up for 18 months. In patients treated with riluzole 100 mg/day, survival was significantly higher compared to patients who received placebo. The effect of riluzole 50 mg/day was not statistically significant compared to placebo and the effect of 200 mg/day was essentially comparable to that of 100 mg/day. The median survival time approached 16.5 months versus 13.5 months for riluzole 100 mg/day and placebo, respectively. In a parallel group study designed to assess the efficacy and safety of riluzole in patients at a late stage of the disease, survival time and motor function under riluzole did not differ significantly from that of placebo. In this study, the majority of patients had a vital capacity ratio less than 60%.

*Posology and method of administration:* The recommended daily dose in adults or elderly is 100 mg (50 mg every 12 hours). No significant increased benefit can be expected from higher daily doses. Treatment with riluzole should only be initiated by specialist physicians with experience in the management of motor neurone diseases. Special populations: Children: Rilutek is not recommended for use in children, as the safety and effectiveness of riluzole in any neurodegenerative process occurring in children or adolescents have not been established (see *Special Warnings and Special Precautions for Use*). Patients with Impaired Renal Function: Rilutek is not recommended for use in patients with impaired renal function, as studies in this population have not been conducted (see *Special Warnings and Special Precautions for Use*). Patients with Impaired Hepatic Function: (see *Contra-indications* and *Special Warnings and Special Precautions for Use*).

*Contra-indications:* Patients who have a history of severe hypersensitivity reactions to riluzole or any of the tablet components. Patients who have hepatic disease or who have baseline transaminases greater than 3 times the upper limit of normal. Patients who are pregnant or lactating.

*Special warnings and special precautions for use:* Liver impairment Riluzole should be prescribed with care in patients with a history of abnormal liver function, or in patients with slightly elevated serum transaminases (ALT/SGPT; AST/SGOT up to 3 times ULN), bilirubin and/or gamma-glutamyl transferase (GGT) levels. Baseline elevations of several liver function tests (especially elevated bilirubin) should preclude the use of riluzole. (see « Undesirable Effects »). It is recommended that serum transaminases, including ALT, be measured before and during therapy with riluzole. ALT should be measured every month during the first 3 months of treatment, every 3 months during the remainder of the first year, and periodically thereafter. ALT levels should be measured more frequently in patients who develop elevated ALT levels. Riluzole should be discontinued if the ALT levels increase to five times the ULN. There is no experience with dose reduction or rechallenge in patients who have developed an increase of ALT to 5 times ULN. Readministration of riluzole to patients in this situation cannot be recommended. Neutropenia: Patients should be warned to report any febrile illness to their physicians. The report of a febrile illness should prompt physicians to check white blood cell counts and to discontinue riluzole in case of neutropenia (see *Undesirable Effects*). Children The safety and effectiveness of riluzole in any neurodegenerative process occurring in children or adolescents have not been studied (see *Posology and Method of Administration*). Patients with Impaired Renal Function: Studies in this population have not been conducted (see *Posology and Method of Administration*).

*Interaction with other medicines and other forms of interaction:* There have been no clinical studies to evaluate the interactions of riluzole with other drugs. *In vitro* studies using human liver microsomal preparations suggest that CYP 1A2 is the principal isozyme involved in the initial oxidative metabolism of riluzole.

Inhibitors of CYP 1A2 (e.g. caffeine, diclofenac, diazepam, nicergoline, clomipramine, imipramine, fluvoxamine, phenacetin, theophylline, amitriptyline and quinolones) could potentially decrease the rate of riluzole elimination, while inducers of CYP 1A2 (e.g. cigarette smoke, charcoal-broiled food, rifampicin and omeprazole) could increase the rate of riluzole elimination.

*Pregnancy and lactation:*
*Pregnancy:* In the pregnant rat, the transfer of $^{14}C$-riluzole across the placenta to the foetus has been detected. In rats, riluzole decreased the pregnancy rate and the number of implantations at exposure levels at least 2 times higher than the systemic exposure of humans given clinical therapy. No malformations were seen in animal reproductive studies.

Clinical experience with riluzole in pregnant women is lacking. Riluzole must not be used in pregnant women.

*Lactation:* In lactating rats, $^{14}C$-riluzole was detected in milk. It is not known whether riluzole is excreted in human milk. Riluzole must not be used in lactating women.

*Effects on ability to drive and use machines:* Patients should be warned about the potential for dizziness or vertigo, and advised not to drive or operate machinery if these symptoms occur.

*Undesirable effects:* The following adverse reactions have been reported in patients enrolled in Phase III studies conducted in Europe and North America.

The most frequent side-effects related to riluzole were asthenia, nausea and elevations in liver function tests. Elevations of alanine-aminotransferase (ALT) levels to more than 3 times the upper limit of the normal range (ULN) were observed in about 11 % of the patients treated with riluzole compared to 4.2 % in the placebo group; levels increased to more than 5 times the ULN in 3.8% of the patients treated with riluzole compared to 1.7 % of the placebo treated patients. The increases in ALT usually appeared within 3 months after the start of therapy with riluzole; they were usually transient and levels returned to below 2 times the ULN after 2 to 6 months while treatment was continued. These increases were rarely associated with jaundice. In patients with increases in ALT to more than 5 times the ULN, treatment was discontinued and the levels returned to less than 2 times the ULN within 2 to 4 months (see *Special Warnings and Special Precautions for Use*). The listing that follows describes all the adverse events that occurred at a frequency of 1% or more among ALS patients receiving riluzole 100 mg/day and were greater than placebo by 1%, or were serious adverse events with frequency greater than placebo.

*Adverse Events Occurring in Placebo-Controlled Clinical Trials—Percentage of patients reporting events\**

| Adverse Event* | Riluzole 100 mg/day (N=395) | Placebo (N=406) |
|---|---|---|
| Asthenia | 17.5 | 11.3 |
| Nausea | 14.2 | 9.1 |
| Headache | 6.8 | 5.7 |
| Abdominal pain | 5.1 | 3.7 |
| Pain | 4.8 | 2.0 |
| Vomiting | 3.8 | 1.5 |
| Dizziness | 3.3 | 2.2 |
| Tachycardia | 3.0 | 1.5 |
| Somnolence | 2.0 | 1.0 |
| Circumoral paresthesia | 1.3 | 0.0 |

\* Where riluzole incidence is greater than placebo by 1%.

Anaphylactoid reaction and angioedema have been reported exceptionally.

*Neutropenia* Among approximately 5000 patients given riluzole for ALS, there were three cases of marked neutropenia (absolute neutrophil count less than 500/mm$^3$), all seen within the first 2 months of riluzole treatment. In one case, neutrophil counts rose on continued treatment. In a second case, counts rose after therapy was stopped. A third case was associated with marked anaemia (see *Special Warnings and Special Precautions for Use*).

*Overdose:* There have been no reports of overdose with riluzole; no specific treatment information or antidote are available. In case of overdosage, treatment is symptomatic and supportive.

**Pharmacological properties** Although the pathogenesis of ALS is not completely elucidated, it is suggested that glutamate (the primary excitatory neurotransmitter in the central nervous system) plays a role for cell death in the disease. Riluzole is proposed to act by inhibiting glutamate processes. The mode of action is unclear.

*Pharmacodynamic properties:* Pharmacotherapeutic class: other nervous system drugs, ATC code N07X.

*Pharmacokinetic properties:* The pharmacokinetics of riluzole have been evaluated in healthy male volunteers after single oral administration of 25 to 300 mg and after multiple dose oral administration of 25 to 100 mg bid. Plasma levels increase linearly with the dose and the pharmacokinetic profile is dose-independent. With multiple dose administration (10 day-treatment at 50 mg riluzole bid), unchanged riluzole accumulates in Cmax plasma by about 2 fold and steady-state is reached in less than 5 days.
*Absorption:* Riluzole is rapidly absorbed after oral administration with maximal plasma concentrations occurring within 60 to 90 minutes (Cmax = 173 ± 72 (SD) ng/ml). About 90% of the dose is absorbed and the absolute bioavailability is 60 ± 18%. The rate and extent of absorption is reduced when riluzole is administered with high-fat meals (decrease in Cmax of 44%, decrease in AUC of 17%). *Distribution:* Riluzole is extensively distributed throughout the body and has been shown to cross the blood brain barrier. The volume of distribution of riluzole is about 245 ± 69 l (3.4 l/kg). Riluzole is about 97% protein bound and it binds mainly to serum albumin and to lipoproteins. *Metabolism:* Unchanged riluzole is the main component in plasma and is extensively metabolised by cytochrome P450 and subsequent glucuronidation. In vitro studies using human liver preparations demonstrated that cytochrome P450 1A2 is the principal isoenzyme involved in the metabolism of riluzole. The metabolites identified in urine are 3 phenolic derivatives, one ureido-derivative and unchanged riluzole. The identified and non-conjugated metabolites do not contribute to the pharmacodynamic profile of riluzole in animals and therefore have not been investigated in humans. *Elimination:* The elimination half-life ranges from 9 to 15 hours. Riluzole is eliminated mainly in the urine. The overall urinary excretion accounts for about 90% of the dose. Glucuronides accounted for more than 85% of the metabolites in the urine. Only 2% of a riluzole dose was recovered in the urine as unchanged drug.

*Preclinical safety data:* Long-term studies to determine the carcinogenic potential of riluzole have not yet been completed.

Conventional genotoxicity assays in vitro, utilising rat liver S9 fraction to model metabolism, gave no evidence of genotoxic potential for riluzole. In vivo assays in rat and mouse also gave no indication of chromosomal damage. There remains the possibility that these models did not generate all metabolites relevant to humans, particularly since no metabolic characterisation of the S9 fraction was conducted. Reductions in red blood cell parameters and/or alterations in liver parameters were noted inconsistently in subacute and chronic toxicity studies in rats and monkeys. In dogs, haemolytic anaemia was observed. In a single toxicity study, the absence of corpora lutea was noted at a higher incidence in the ovary of treated compared to control female rats. This isolated finding was not noted in any other study or species. All these findings were noted at doses which were 2-10 times higher than the human dose of 100 mg/day. Fertility studies in rats revealed slight impairment of reproductive performance and fertility at doses of 15 mg/kg/day, probably due to sedation and lethargy.

**Pharmaceutical particulars**

*List of excipients:* core: dibasic calcium phosphate, anhydrous; micro crystalline cellulose; colloidal silica, anhydrous; magnesium stearate; cross linked carboxymethylcellulose sodium (croscarmellose sodium); coating: hydroxypropylmethyl cellulose; Macrogol 6000 and titanium dioxide (E171).

*Incompatibilities:* None known.

*Shelf life:* 24 months.

*Special precautions for storage:* Rilutek must be kept out of the reach of children.

*Nature and contents of container:* Rilutek tablets are packaged in opaque PVC/Aluminium blister packs. Each package contains 4 blister cards of 14 tablets each.

*Instructions for use/handling:* Not applicable.

**Marketing authorisation number** EU/96/010/001

**Date of approval/revision of SPC:** 10 June 1996

**Legal category** POM

## RYNACROM* 4% NASAL SPRAY

**Qualitative and quantitative composition** Sodium cromoglycate 4%

**Pharmaceutical form** Rynacrom 4% Nasal Spray is presented as an aqueous solution, containing 4% w/v sodium cromoglycate in a metered dose spray pack, for nasal administration.

**Clinical particulars**

*Therapeutic indications:* Rynacrom Nasal Spray is indicated for the preventative treatment of allergic rhinitis (seasonal and perennial)

*Posology and method of administration:* For nasal administration *Adults (including the elderly) and children:* one spray into each nostril two to four times daily. (each actuation of the pump unit delivers approximately 5.2 mg of sodium cromoglycate).

Since therapy is essentially preventative, regular doses, distinct from using drug intermittently to relieve symptoms, should be observed.

*Contra-indications:* Rynacrom 4% Nasal Spray is contraindicated in patients with known sensitivity to sodium cromoglycate or any of the ingredients.

*Special warnings and precautions for use:* None known

*Interactions with other medicaments and other forms of interaction:* There are no known interactions between sodium cromoglycate and other drugs. A reduction in concomitant anti-histamine therapy will often be possible during treatment with Rynacrom Nasal Spray.

*Pregnancy and lactation:* Cumulative experience with sodium cromoglycate suggests that it has no effect on foetal development. It should only be used in pregnancy if there is a clear need. On the basis of animal studies and its physico-chemical properties, sodium cromoglycate is unlikely to pass into human breast milk. There is no evidence to suggest that the use of sodium cromoglycate by nursing mothers has any undesirable effects on the baby.

*Effects on ability to drive and use machines:* None known

*Undesirable effects:* Occasional irritation of the nasal mucosa may occur during the first days of use. In rare cases wheezing or tightness of the chest have been reported in patients.

*Overdose:* No action, other than medical supervision should be necessary.

**Pharmacological properties**

*Pharmacodynamic properties:* sodium cromoglycate inhibits the release of mediators of the allergic reaction from sensitised mast cells. In the nose, the inhibition of mediator release prevents the symptoms of rhinitis.

*Pharmacokinetic properties:* after instillation of Rynacrom Nasal Spray into the nose, less than 7% of the total dose administered is absorbed via the nasal mucosa. This fraction is excreted unchanged in the bile and urine. The remainder of the dose is expelled from the nose, or swallowed and excreted via the alimentary tract.

*Preclinical safety data:* None given

**Pharmaceutical particulars**

*List of excipients:* disodium edetate, benzalkonium chloride, purified water.

*Incompatibilities:* None known

*Shelf life:* 36 months

*Special precautions for storage:* Store below 25°C. Protect from direct sunlight

*Nature and contents of container:* Rynacrom 4% Nasal Spray is presented as a transparent, colourless to pale yellow liquid, in a 22 ml high density polyethylene bottle, fitted with a metered dose pump unit, protected by a polypropylene cover.

*Instructions for use/handling:* None stated

**Marketing authorisation number** 0113/0139

**Date of approval/revision of SPC** February 1997

**Legal category** P

## RYNACROM* COMPOUND

**Presentation** A metered-dose presentation of a clear aqueous solution of Sodium Cromoglycate BP 2% w/v and Xylometazoline Hydrochloride BP 0.025% w/v. The pack contains a bottle of solution and a pump unit ready assembled.

*Inactive ingredients:* Benzalkonium Chloride, Disodium Edetate. Purified water.

**Uses** Rynacrom Compound is indicated for the prophylaxis and treatment of allergic rhinitis (such as hayfever and perennial rhinitis) where this is accompanied by nasal congestion.

Sodium cromoglycate inhibits the release of mediators of the allergic reaction from sensitised mast cells. In the nose, this inhibition of mediator release prevents the symptoms of rhinitis.

Xylometazoline hydrochloride is a sympathomimetic agent with alpha-adrenergic activity. It produces vasoconstriction thus reducing nasal congestion.

**Dosage and administration** *Adults (including the elderly) and children:* One spray to each nostril four times daily.

One spray delivers approximately 2.6 mg of sodium cromoglycate and 0.0325 mg of xylometazoline hydrochloride from the metered-dose device.

### Contra-indications, warnings, etc

*Contra-indications:* Known sensitivity to any ingredient.

*Precautions:* The prolonged use or abuse of decongestants in general may lead to rebound congestion or drug induced rhinitis. This is reported to be less likely with xylometazoline.

*Side-effects:* No serious side effects have been reported. Occasional irritation of the nasal mucosa may occur during the first days of use. In rare cases with sodium cromoglycate solutions alone wheezing and tightness of the chest have been reported. Because a lower dose of xylometazoline is employed in this presentation than in other formulations, the side-effects usually attributed to this drug are expected to be minimal or absent.

Exposure to higher doses of xylometazoline than are likely with the correct use of Rynacrom Compound are reported to cause mild side-effects such as nasal irritation, dryness of the nose, sneezing, headache, insomnia, drowsiness and palpitations.

*Use in pregnancy and lactation:* As with all medicines, caution should be exercised during pregnancy especially during the first trimester.

*Overdosage:* Adults: Generally no action other than medical supervision should be necessary.

Infants and children: Overdosage of decongestants may cause sedation; uneventful recovery is usual, although medical supervision is recommended. Should accidental overdosage lead to convulsions or respiratory depression, gastric lavage and symptomatic therapy should be instituted.

**Pharmaceutical precautions** Store below 30°C. Protect from direct sunlight.

**Legal category** P

**Package quantities** Bottle of 26 ml and pump unit.

**Further information** Nil.

**Product licence number** 0113/0097

## SECADREX*

**Qualitative and quantitative composition** Each tablet contains the equivalent of 200 mg acebutolol (in the form of the hydrochloride) and 12.5 mg hydrochlorothiazide. The tablets also contain lactose.

**Pharmaceutical form** Secadrex tablets are white, round, slightly biconvex, and film-coated, imprinted 'SECADREX' on one face

### Clinical particulars

*Therapeutic Indications:* Secadrex tablets are indicated for the control of mild and moderate hypertension.

*Posology and method of administration:* One tablet once daily, usually in the morning. If response is inadequate dosage may be increased to two tablets daily. Secadrex is not intended for use in children.

*Contra-indications:* Cardiogenic shock is an absolute contra-indication to beta-blockade and caution is required in patients with blood pressures of the order of 100/60 mmHg or below. Heart block: Administration of any beta-adrenoceptor blocking agent is considered inadvisable (except perhaps in first degree block).

Severe kidney and liver failure. Hypersensitivity to hydrochlorothiazide.

Secadrex tablets should not be used with verapamil or within several days of verapamil therapy (and vice versa). Insulin-dependent diabetes. Use in non-insulin dependent diabetics may be inadvisable since thiazide diuretics may cause further impairment of glucose tolerance. Gout or hyperuricaemia.

Reversible obstructive airways disease. Although cardio-selective beta blockers may have less effect on lung function than non-selective beta blockers as with all beta blockers these should be avoided in patients with reversible obstructive airways disease unless there are compelling clinical reasons for their use.

*Special warnings and special precautions for use:* Caution should be exercised: If Secadrex tablets are administered in the presence of bradycardia (depending on the circumstances). If Secadrex tablets are to be prescribed with a catecholamine-depleting drug, such as reserpine. In the presence of signs of heart failure, since acebutolol has a slight but acceptable cardiodepressant action. In anaesthesia, some anaesthetists prefer to discontinue therapy 48 hours before anaesthesia, others do not consider this essential. Withdrawal should be made gradually. Thiazides may increase responsiveness to tubocurarine. If Secadrex and clonidine are given concurrently clonidine should not be discontinued until several days after withdrawal of the beta blocker. *If used in patients with a history*

*of asthma and wheezing.* All patients receiving hydrochlorothiazide therapy (as in Secadrex tablets) should be monitored periodically for clinical signs of fluid or electrolyte imbalance, hypokalaemia, hyponatraemia and hypochloraemic alkalosis. Hypokalaemia can sensitise or exaggerate the response of the heart to the toxic effects of digitalis (e.g. increased ventricular irritability). With the low dose of hydrochlorothiazide present in Secadrex tablets the possibility of significant imbalance becomes less likely.

*Interaction with other medicaments and other forms of interaction:* Tricyclic antidepressants and MAO inhibitors should not be used with Secadrex tablets. Lithium should generally not be given to patients receiving diuretics since the risk of lithium toxicity is very high in such patients.

*Pregnancy and lactation:* Secadrex should not be administered to female patients during the first trimester of pregnancy unless the physician considers it essential. Animal studies with acebutolol have shown no teratogenic hazard. Thiazides are not generally recommended in the treatment of pregnancy hypertension; it may be preferable to use monotherapy with Sectral™ or another suitable antihypertensive drug in pregnant patients.

*Effects on ability to drive and use machines:* Secadrex has no effect on patients' ability to drive and operate machines.

*Undesirable effects:* No serious side effects have been reported with Secadrex treatment. The most common i.e. those related to beta-blockade–hypotension, bradycardia, gastrointestinal effects and depression–have been met with infrequently, and usually do not require interruption or withdrawal of therapy.

There have been reports of skin rashes and/or dry eyes associated with the use of beta-adrenoceptor antagonists. The reported incidence is small and in most cases the symptoms have cleared when treatment was withdrawn. Discontinuation of the drug should be considered if any such reaction is not explicable. Cessation of treatment with a beta-blocker should be gradual. Bronchospasm has occurred rarely with usage of acebutolol.

Skin rashes and photosensitivity due to hydrochlorothiazide have been reported as have blood dyscrasias including thrombocytopenia, but these are rare.

*Overdose:* In the rare event of excessive bradycardia or hypotension, 1 mg atropine sulphate administered intravenously should be given without delay. If this proves insufficient it should be followed by a slow intravenous injection of isoprenaline (5 mcg per minute) with constant monitoring until a response occurs. In cases of severe poisoning with beta-adrenoceptor antagonists an injection of 10 mg glucagon intravenously has produced rapid improvement. If bradycardia becomes severe electrical pacing may be necessary.

### Pharmacological properties

*Pharmacodynamic properties:* Acebutolol is a cardioselective beta adrenoceptor antagonist. Hydrochlorothiazide is a thiazide diuretic/antihypertensive agent.

*Pharmacokinetic properties:* Acebutolol reaches a peak plasma level 2 to 4 hours after dosing, for hydrochlorothiazide the average time to peak plasma levels is about two hours after dosing.

### Pharmaceutical particulars

*Excipients:* Lactose, Starch maize, Povidone K30, Magnesium sterate,

*Incompatibilities:* Not applicable

*Shelf life:* 36 months.

*Special precautions for storage:* Store in a dry place below 30°C.

*Nature and contents of container:* Secadrex is packed in blister strips of 28 tablets

*Instructions for use/handling:* Secadrex should always be kept out of the reach of children.

**Marketing authorisation numbers** 0012/0137

**Date of approval/revision of SPC** February 1997

**Legal category** POM

## SECTRAL*

**Qualitative and quantitative composition** Sectral Capsules 100 mg contains Acebutolol hydrochloride 111.0 mg (equivalent to 100 mg of base). Sectral Capsules 200 mg contains Acebutolol hydrochloride 222.0 mg (equivalent to 200 mg of base). Sectral Tablets 400 mg contains Acebutolol hydrochloride 443.4 mg (equivalent to 400 mg of base).

**Pharmaceutical form** Sectral 100 capsules are hard gelatin capsules, the bodies being opaque yellowish-buff and the caps opaque white in colour. Length approximately 17 mm, diameter of body approxi-

mately 6 mm. Both body and cap are printed in black "Sectral 100" The capsules contain a white or almost white powder. Sectral 200 capsules are hard gelatin capsules, the bodies being opaque yellowish-buff and the caps opaque pink in colour. Length approximately 17 mm, diameter of body approximately 6 mm. Both body and cap are printed in black "Sectral 200." The capsules contain a white or almost white powder. Sectral 400 tablets are white to off-white, circular, biconvex, film-coated tablets with bevel edges, one face impressed 'Sectral 400'. Plain reverse

### Clinical particulars

*Therapeutic indications:* Sectral is indicated for the management of all grades of hypertension, angina pectoris and the control of tachyarrhythmias

*Posology and method of administration:* Hypertension: Initial dosage of 400 mg orally once daily at breakfast or 200 mg orally twice daily. If response is not adequate within two weeks, dosage may be increased up to 400 mg orally twice daily; if the hypertension is still not adequately controlled consideration should be given to adding a second antihypertensive agent such as the calcium antagonist nifedipine or small doses of a thiazide diuretic.

*Angina pectoris:* Initial dosage of 400 mg orally once daily at breakfast or 200 mg twice daily. In severe forms up to 300 mg three times daily may be required. Up to 1200 mg daily has been used.

*Cardiac arrhythmias:* Maximal anti-arrhythmic effect may not be achieved until up to 3 hours after oral administration.

The daily dose requirement for long term anti-arrhythmic activity should lie between 400 and 1200 mg daily. The dose can be gauged by response. Since the presence of more consistent beta-blockade may be necessary for the control of arrhythmias, better control may be achieved by divided doses rather than single daily doses.

*Elderly:* There are no specific dosage recommendations for the elderly with normal glomerular filtration rate. Dose reduction is necessary if moderate to severe renal impairment is present. *Children:* Paediatric dose has not been established.

*Contra-indications:* Cardiogenic shock is an absolute contraindication and caution is required in patients with blood pressures of the order of 100/60 mmHg or below. Sectral is also contraindicated in patients with atrioventricular block, hypersensitivity to acebutolol or beta blockers, marked bradycardia and uncontrolled heart failure. Although cardio-selective beta blockers may have less effect on lung function than non-selective beta blockers as with all beta blockers these should be avoided in patients with obstructive airways disease unless there are compelling clinical reasons for their use.

*Special warnings and special precautions for use:* Renal impairment is not a contraindication to the use of Sectral which has both renal and non-renal excretory pathways. Some caution should be exercised when administering high doses to patients with severe renal failure as cumulation could possibly occur in these circumstances. The dosage frequency should not exceed once daily in patients with renal impairment. As a guide, the dosage should be reduced by 50% when glomerular filtration rates are between 25-50 ml/min and by 75% when they are below 25 ml/min. Drug-induced bronchospasm is usually at least partially reversible by the use of a suitable agonist. Withdrawal of treatment by beta blockers should be achieved by gradual dosage reduction. Beta blockers may mask signs of thyrotoxicosis and hypoglycaemia. *Caution should be exercised if using in patients with a history of wheezing or asthma*

*Interaction with other medicaments and other forms of interaction:* Sectral should not be used with Verapamil or within several days of Verapamil therapy (and vice versa).

Although nifedipine has been successfully combined with β-blockers, the risk of hypotension is increased. There is also a risk of cardiac failure in patients with a latent or an uncontrolled cardiac insufficiency. Blood pressure should be closely monitored in cases of coadministration with dihydropyridine derivatives especially when initiating therapy.

*Diltiazem should be used with caution in combination with beta blockers.*

In patients with labile and insulin-dependent diabetes, the dosage of the hypoglycaemic agent may need to be reduced. However beta blockers have also been known to blunt the effect of glibenclamide. Cross reactions due to displacement of other drugs from plasma protein binding sites are unlikely due to the low degree of plasma protein binding exhibited by acebutolol and diacetolol. If a beta-adrenoceptor antagonist is used concurrently with clonidine the latter should not be withdrawn until several days after the former is discontinued. Acebutolol is a cardioselective beta blocker and it may antagonize the effect of *sympathomimetic* and xanthine bronchodilators but to a lesser extent than non-cardio selective beta blockers. Concurrent use of digoxin and beta blockers may occasionally induce serious bradycardia. The antihypertensive effects of beta blockers may be attenuated by non-steroidal anti-inflammatory agents. There is a theoretical risk that concurrent administration of monoamine oxidase inhibitors and high doses of beta-blockers, even if they are cardio-selective can produce hypertension. Sectral therapy should be brought to the attention of the anaesthetist prior to general anaesthesia. If treatment is continued, special care should be taken when using anaesthetic agents such as ether, cyclopropane and trichlorethylene.

*Pregnancy and lactation: Pregnancy:* Sectral should not be administered to female patients during the first trimester of pregnancy unless the physician considers it essential. Beta blockers administered in late pregnancy may give rise to bradycardia *and* hypoglycaemia of the foetus/neonate. Animal studies have shown no teratogenic hazard. Lactation: Acebutolol and its active metabolite are excreted in breast milk and the half life of acebutolol in the neonate is double that in adults. *The risks of hypoglycemia and bradycardia occurring in the nursing infant have not been evaluated. Therefore, breast-feeding is not recommended during treatment.*

*Effects on ability to drive and use machines:* None stated.

*Undesirable effects:* Sectral possesses antihypertensive effects but these are unlikely to be noted in normotensive subjects. Those common to beta-blockade: bradycardia, gastrointestinal effects, cold extremities, dizziness, headaches, shortness of breath, nightmares, loss of libido and lethargy have been met with infrequently. The low lipid solubility and lack of cumulation in CNS tissues of acebutolol and its active metabolite reduce the likelihood of sleep disturbances, depression or other central effects and such occurrences are rare. There have been reports of skin rashes and/or dry eyes associated with the use of beta-adrenoceptor blocking drugs. The reported incidence is small and in most cases the symptoms have cleared when treatment was withdrawn. Discontinuation of the drug should be considered if any such reaction is not otherwise explicable. Cessation of therapy with a beta-blocker should be gradual. Although some patients have developed anti-nuclear factor titres, the incidence of associated clinical symptoms is rare and when present, these clear promptly on discontinuation of treatment. Bronchospasm has occurred rarely during treatment with acebutolol.

*Overdose:* In the rare event of excessive bradycardia or hypotension, 1 mg atropine sulphate administered intravenously should be given without delay. If this is insufficient it should be followed by a slow intravenous injection of isoprenaline (5 mcg per minute) with constant monitoring until a response occurs. In severe cases of self-poisoning with circulatory collapse unresponsive to atropine and catecholamines the intravenous injection of glucagon 10-20 mg may produce a dramatic improvement. Cardiac pacing may be employed if bradycardia becomes severe.

Judicious use of vasopressors, diazepam, phenytoin, lidocaine, digoxin and bronchodilators should be considered depending on the presentation of the patient. Acebutolol can be removed from blood by haemodialysis. Other symptoms and signs of overdosage include cardiogenic shock, *AV* block, conduction defects, pulmonary edema, depressed level of consciousness, bronchospasm, hypoglycemia and rarely hyperkalaemia

**Pharmacological properties**

*Pharmacodynamic properties:* Mode of action: Sectral is a beta adrenoceptor antagonist which is cardioselective, i.e. acts preferentially on beta-1 adrenergic receptors in the heart. Its principal effects are to reduce heart rate especially on exercise and to lower blood pressure in hypertensive subjects. SECTRAL™ and its equally active metabolite, diacetolol have anti-arrhythmic activity, the combined plasma half-life of the active drug and metabolite being 7-10 hours. Both have partial agonist activity (PAA) also known as intrinsic sympathomimetic activity (ISA). This property ensures that some degree of stimulation of beta receptors is maintained. Under conditions of rest, this tends to balance the negative chronotropic and negative inotropic effects. Sectral blocks the effects of excessive catecholamine stimulation resulting from stress.

*Pharmacokinetic properties:* After oral administration, acebutolol is rapidly and almost completely absorbed. Absorption appears to be unaffected by the presence of food in the gut. There is rapid formation of a major equiactive metabolite, diacetolol, which possesses a similar pharmacological profile to acebutolol. Peak plasma concentrations of active material (i.e. acebutolol plus diacetolol) are achieved within 2-4 hours and the terminal plasma elimination half-life is around 8-10 hours. Because of biliary excretion and direct

transfer across the gut wall from the systemic circulation to the gut lumen, more than 50% of an oral dose of Sectral is recovered in the faeces with acebutolol and diacetolol in equal proportions; the rest of the dose is recovered in the urine, mainly as diacetolol. Both acebutolol and diacetolol are hydrophilic and exhibit poor penetration of the CNS.

**Pharmaceutical particulars**

*List of excipients:* Sectral 100 and 200 capsules contain Starch potato, Aerosil, Magnesium stearate (E572). Opadry OY-L-28900 containing Titanium dioxide (E171) PhEur, Lactose PhEur, HPMC 2910 15cP and Polyethylene glycol 4000NF. The Capsule shell contains Yellow Iron Oxide (E172), Titanium dioxide (E171), Gelatin, Black ink (Opacode s-24-8109). Sectral 200 also contains red iron oxide (E172).

The tablets contain lactose BP, Starch maize BP, French chalk powdered (E553b), aerosil (silicon dioxide E551), Povidone K30 BP, Magnesium stearate (E572) BP, Opadry OY-L-28900 (contains titanium dioxide (E171) Ph. Eur., Lactose Ph. Eur., HPMC 2190 15cP (E464), Polyethylene glycol 4000 NF)

*Incompatibilities:* Not applicable

*Shelf life:* The shelf-life of Sectral Capsules is 60 months. The shelf life for Sectral tablets is 36 months.

*Special precautions for storage:* Capsules only: Store in a dry place below 25°C. Protect from light

*Nature and contents of container:*
 Sectral capsules 100 mg blister packs of 84 tablets.
 Sectral capsules 200 mg blister packs of 56 tablets
 Sectral tablets 400 mg blister packs of 28 tablets

*Instructions for use/handling:* None

**Marketing authorisation numbers**
Sectral Tablets 400 mg     0012/0124
Sectral Capsules 200 mg    0012/0101R
Sectral Capsules 100 mg    0012/0100R

**Date of approval/revision of SPC** February 1997

**Legal category** POM

# STEMETIL Eff*

**Qualitative and quantitative composition** The active component of Stemetil Eff is prochlorperazine mesylate BP 5 mg equivalent to 3.3 mg prochlorperazine base.

**Pharmaceutical form** White effervescent granular powder which dissolves in water to give a lemon flavoured effervescent solution.

**Clinical particulars**

*Therapeutic indications:* Prevention of nausea and vomiting. Treatment of nausea and vomiting. Treatment of vertigo and Meniere's syndrome. Adjunct in the short-term management of anxiety.

*Posology and method of administration:* For oral administration.

*Adults:*

| Indication | Dosage |
| --- | --- |
| Prevention of nausea and vomiting | 5 to 10 mg b.d. or t.d.s. |
| Treatment of nausea and vomiting | 20 mg stat, followed if necessary by 10 mg two hours later. |
| Vertigo and Meniere's syndrome | 5 mg t.d.s increasing if necessary to a total of 30 mg daily. After several weeks dosage may be reduced gradually to 5-10 mg daily. |
| Adjunct in the short-term management of anxiety | 15-20 mg daily in divided doses initially but this may be increased if necessary to maximum of 40 mg daily in divided doses. |

*Children:* Not recommended. *Elderly:* A lower initial dose is recommended. Please see 'Special warnings and special for precautions for use' section.

*Contra-indications:* None stated.

*Special warnings and special precautions for use:* Stemetil should be avoided in patients with liver or renal dysfunction, epilepsy, Parkinson's disease, hypothyroidism, phaeochromocytoma, myasthenia gravis, prostate hypertrophy. It should be avoided in patients known to be hypersensitive to phenothiazines or with a history of narrow angle glaucoma. It should be used with caution in the elderly, particularly during very hot or very cold weather (risk of hyper-, hypothermia).
The elderly are particularly susceptible to postural hypotension.
Stemetil should be used cautiously in the elderly owing to their susceptibility to drugs acting centrally

on the nervous system and a lower initial dosage is recommended. There is an increased risk of drug-induced Parkinsonism in the elderly, particularly after prolonged use. Care should also be taken not to confuse the adverse effects of Stemetil e.g. orthostatic hypotension, with effects due to the underlying disorder.
Due to its aspartame content, Stemetil Eff should not be given to patients with phenylketonuria.
Children: Stemetil has been associated with dystonic reactions particularly after a cumulative dosage of 0.5 mg/kg. It should therefore be used cautiously in children.

*Interaction with other medicaments and other forms of interaction:* Interactions of phenothiazine neuroleptics: The CNS depressant actions of neuroleptic agents may be intensified (additively) by alcohol, barbiturates and other sedatives. Respiratory depression may occur.
The hypotensive effect of most antihypertensive drugs especially alpha adrenoceptor blocking agents may be exaggerated by neuroleptics.
The mild anticholinergic effect of neuroleptics may be enhanced by other anticholinergic drugs possibly leading to constipation, heat stroke, etc.
The action of some drugs may be opposed by phenothiazine neuroleptics; these include amphetamine, levodopa, clonidine, guanethidine, adrenaline.
Anticholinergic agents may reduce the antipsychotic effect of neuroleptics.
Some drugs interfere with absorption of neuroleptic agents: antacids, anti-Parkinson, lithium. Increases or decreases in the plasma concentrations of a number of drugs, e.g. propranolol, phenobarbitone have been observed but were not of clinical significance.
High doses of neuroleptics reduce the response to hypoglycaemic agents the dosage of which might have to be raised.
Adrenaline must *not* be used in patients overdosed with Stemetil. Most of the above interactions are of a theoretical nature and not dangerous.
Simultaneous administration of desferrioxamine and prochlorperazine has been observed to induce a transient metabolic encephalopathy characterised by loss of consciousness for 48-72 hours.

*Pregnancy and lactation:* Stemetil is contra-indicated in pregnancy. There is inadequate evidence of the safety of Stemetil in human pregnancy but it has been widely used for many years without apparent ill consequence. There is evidence of harmful effects in animals. Like other drugs it should be avoided in pregnancy unless the physician considers it essential. Neuroleptics may occasionally prolong labour and at such a time should be withheld until the cervix is dilated 3-4 cm. Possible adverse effects on the neonate include lethargy or paradoxical hyperexcitability, tremor and low Apgar score. Phenothiazines may be excreted in milk, breastfeeding should be suspended during treatment.

*Effects on ability to drive and use machines:* Patients should be warned about drowsiness during the early days of treatment, and advised not to drive or operate machinery.

*Undesirable effects:* Minor side-effects of neuroleptics are nasal stuffiness, dry mouth, insomnia, agitation. Adverse effects of neuroleptics: *Liver function*: Jaundice, usually transient, occurs in a very small percentage of patients taking neuroleptics. A premonitory sign may be a sudden onset of fever after one to three weeks of treatment followed by the development of jaundice. Neuroleptic jaundice has the biochemical and other characteristics of obstructive jaundice and is associated with obstruction of the canaliculi by bile thrombi; the frequent presence of an accompanying eosinophilia indicates the allergic nature of this phenomenon. Treatment should be withheld on the development of jaundice. *Cardiorespiratory:* Hypotension, usually postural, commonly occurs. Elderly or volume depleted subjects are particularly susceptible, it is more likely after intramuscular injection. Cardiac arrhythmias, including atrial arrhythmia, A-V block, ventricular tachycardia and fibrillation have been reported during neuroleptic therapy, possibly related to dosage. Pre-existing cardiac disease, old age, hypokalaemia and concurrent tricyclic antidepressants may pre-dispose. ECG changes, usually benign, include widened QT interval, ST depression, U-waves and T-wave changes. *Respiratory depression* is possible in susceptible patients. *Blood picture*: A mild leucopenia occurs in up to 30% of patients on prolonged high dosage. Agranulocytosis may occur rarely; it is not dose related. The occurrence of unexplained infections or fever requires immediate haematological investigation. *Extrapyramidal*: Acute dystonias or dyskinesias, usually transitory, are more common in children and young adults, and usually occur within the first 4 days of treatment or after dosage increases. Akathisia characteristically occurs after large initial doses. Parkinsonism is more common in adults and the elderly. It usually develops after weeks or months of treatment. One or more of the following may be seen: tremor, rigidity, akinesia or other features of Parkinsonism, commonly just tremor. Tardive dyskinesia: If this occurs it is usually, but not necessarily, after prolonged or high dosage. It can even occur after treatment has been stopped. Dosage should therefore be kept low whenever possible. *Skin and eyes*: Contact skin sensitisation is a serious but rare complication in those frequently handling preparations of certain phenothiazines; the greatest care must be taken to avoid contact of the drug with the skin. Skin rashes of various kinds may also be seen in patients treated with the drug. Patients on high dosage should be warned that they may develop photosensitivity in sunny weather and should avoid exposure to direct sunlight. Ocular changes and the development of a metallic greyish-mauve coloration of exposed skin have been noted in some individuals mainly females, who have received chlorpromazine continuously for long periods (four to eight years). This could possibly happen with Stemetil. *Endocrine:* Hyperprolactinaemia which may result in galactorrhoea, gynaecomastia, amenorrhoea and impotence. Neuroleptic malignant syndrome (hyperthermia, rigidity, autonomic dysfunction and altered consciousness) may occur with any neuroleptic.

*Overdose:* Symptoms of phenothiazine overdosage include drowsiness or loss of consciousness, hypotension, tachycardia, ECG changes, ventricular arrhythmias and hypothermia. Severe extra-pyramidal dyskinesias may occur.

If the patient is seen sufficiently soon (up to 6 hours) after ingestion of a toxic dose, gastric lavage may be attempted. Pharmacological induction of emesis is unlikely to be of any use. Activated charcoal should be given. There is no specific antidote. Treatment is supportive.

Generalised vasodilatation may result in circulatory collapse; raising the patient's legs may suffice. In severe cases, volume expansion by intravenous fluids may be needed; infusion fluids should be warmed before administration in order not to aggravate hypothermia.

Positive inotropic agents such as dopamine may be tried if fluid replacement is insufficient to correct the circulatory collapse. Peripheral vasoconstrictor agents are not generally recommended; avoid the use of adrenaline.

Ventricular or supraventricular tachy-arrhythmias usually respond to restoration of normal body temperature and correction of circulatory or metabolic disturbances. If persistent or life threatening, appropriate anti-arrhythmic therapy may be considered. Avoid lignocaine and, as far as possible, long acting anti-arrhythmic drugs.

Pronounced central nervous system depression requires airway maintenance or, in extreme circumstances, assisted respiration. Severe dystonic reactions usually respond to procyclidine (5–10 mg) or orphenadrine (20–40 mg) administered intramuscularly or intravenously. Convulsions should be treated with intravenous diazepam.

Neuroleptic malignant syndrome should be treated with cooling. Dantrolene sodium may be tried.

**Pharmacological properties**

*Pharmacodynamic properties:* Prochlorperazine (PCP) is a dopamine and histamine antagonist. The mechanism of the anti-emetic is due predominantly to blockade of the histamine $H_1$ and dopamine $D_2$ neurotransmitter receptors in the chemoreceptor trigger zone and vomiting centre. It also has weak anticholinergic effect and prevents acid reflux by increasing the tone of the lower oesphangeal sphincter.

*Pharmacokinetic properties:* Peak prochlorperazine (PCP) concentrations of approximately 1.1ng/ml were reached at 2.8 hours after oral administration of an aqueous solution of prochlorperazine mesylate (Stemetil syrup) to healthy volunteers.

PCP was rapidly metabolised to the S-oxide due to a first pass effect during absorption, thus producing peak metabolite concentrations of 17ng/ml at 0.5 hour. The AUC values for the S-oxide indicate that PCP is well absorbed orally, compared with i.m. injection. Plasma concentrations of PCP and S-oxide fell with half-lives of 6.2 and 8.5 hours, respectively.

PCP is widely distributed throughout the body and diffuses rapidly across the placenta. It is excreted in the urine and faeces mainly as metabolites.

*Preclinical safety data:* There is no pre-clinical data of relevance to the prescriber which are additional to that already included in other sections of the SPC.

**Pharmaceutical particulars**

*List of excipients:* Tartaric acid BP (E334), Povidone K30 BP, sodium bicarbonate BP (E500), fresh lemon juice (Flav-O-Lok 610406E), citric acid anhydrous BP (E330), ascorbic acid BP (E300), sodium carbonate dried 1968 BPC (E500), aspartame (E951).

*Incompatibilities:* None stated.

*Shelf life:* 36 months.

*Special precautions for storage:* Store below 25°C.

*Nature and content of container:* Stemetil Eff is available in sealed sachets consisting of paper/foil/polyethylene laminate in cartons of 21.

*Instructions for use/handling:* None stated.

**Marketing authorisation number** 0012/0177

**Date of approval/revision of SPC** July 1997.

**Legal category** POM

## STEMETIL *TABLETS AND SYRUP

**Qualitative and quantitative composition** The active component of the Stemetil tablets 5 mg is prochlorperazine maleate BP 5 mg. The active component of the Stemetil tablets 25 mg is prochlorperazine maleate BP 25 mg. The active component of the Stemetil syrup is prochlorperazine mesylate BP 5 mg per 5 ml.

**Pharmaceutical form** Stemetil tablets 5 mg: Off-white to pale cream coloured circular tablets for oral use. The tablets are marked on one face 'STEMETIL' around a centrally impressed '5', reverse face plain. Stemetil tablets 25 mg: Off-white to pale cream coloured tablets for oral use. The tablets are marked 'STEMETIL' around a centrally impressed '25', a breakline on the reverse. Stemetil syrup: A dark straw coloured syrup.

**Clinical particulars**

*Therapeutic indications:* Vertigo due to Meniere's Syndrome, labyrinthis and other causes, and for nausea and vomiting from whatever cause including that associated with migraine. It may also be used for schizophrenia (particularly in the chronic stage), acute mania and as an adjunct to the short-term management of anxiety.

*Posology and method of administration:*

*Adults*

| *Indication* | Dosage |
|---|---|
| Prevention of nausea and vomiting | 5 to 10 mg b.d. or t.d.s. |
| Treatment of nausea and vomiting | 20 mg stat, followed if necessary by 10 mg two hours later. |
| Vertigo and Meniere's syndrome | 5 mg t.d.s. increasing if necessary to a total of 30 mg daily. After several weeks dosage may be reduced gradually to 5-10 mg daily. |
| Adjunct in the short term management of anxiety | 15-20 mg daily in divided doses initially but this may be increased if necessary to a maximum of 40 mg daily in divided doses. |
| Schizophrenia and other psychotic disorders | Usual effective daily oral dosage is in the order of 75-100 mg daily. Patients very widely in response. The following schedule is suggested: Initially 12.5 mg twice daily for 7 days, the daily amount being subsequently increased by 12.5 mg at 4 to 7 days interval until a satisfactory response is obtained. After some weeks at the effective dosage, an attempt should be made reduce this dosage. Total daily amounts as small as 50 mg or even 25 mg have sometimes been found to be effective. |

*Children*

| Indication | Dosage |
|---|---|
| Prevention and treatment of nausea and vomiting | If it is considered unavoidable to use Stemetil for a child, the dosage is 0.25 mg/kg bodyweight two or three a day. Stemetil is not recommended for children weighing less than 10 Kg or below 1 year of age. |

*Elderly:* A lower dose is recommended. Please see *Special warnings and special precautions for use* section.

*Contra-indications:* Pregnancy.

*Special warnings and special precautions for use:* Stemetil should be avoided in patients with liver or renal dysfunction, epilepsy, Parkinson's disease, hypothyroidism, phaeochromocytoma, myasthenia gravis, prostate hypertrophy. It should be avoided in patients known to be hypersensitive to phenothiazines or with a history of narrow angle glaucoma. It should be used with caution in the elderly, particularly during very hot or very cold weather (risk of hyper-, hypothermia).

The elderly are particularly susceptible to postural hypotension.

Stemetil should be used cautiously in the elderly owing to their susceptibility to drugs acting centrally on the nervous system and a lower initial dosage is recommended. There is an increased risk of drug-induced Parkinsonism in the elderly particularly after prolonged use. Care should also be taken not to confuse the adverse effects of Stemetil e.g. orthostatic hypotension with effects due to the underlying disorder.

Children: Stemetil has been associated with dystonic reactions particularly after cumulative dosage of 0.5 mg/kg. It should therefore be used cautiously in children.

*Interaction with other medicaments and other forms of interaction:* Interactions of phenothiazine neuroleptics: The CNS depressant actions of neuroleptic agents may be intensified (additively) by alcohol, barbiturates and other sedatives. Respiratory depression may occur.

The hypotensive effect of most antihypertensive drugs especially alpha adrenoceptor blocking agents may be exaggerated by neuroleptics.

The mild anticholinergic effect of neuroleptics may be enhanced by other anticholinergic drugs possibly leading to constipation, heat stroke, etc.

The action of some drugs may be opposed by phenothiazine neuroleptics; these include amphetamine, levodopa, clonidine, guanethidine, adrenaline.

Anticholinergic agents may reduce the antipsychotic effect of neuroleptics.

Some drugs interfere with absorption of neuroleptic agents: antacids, anti-Parkinson, lithium. Increases or decreases in the plasma concentrations of a number of drugs, e.g. propranolol, phenobarbitone have been observed but were not of clinical significance.

High doses of neuroleptics reduce the response to hypoglycaemic agents the dosage of which might have to be raised.

Adrenaline must *not* be used in patients overdosed with Stemetil. Most of the above interactions are of a theoretical nature and not dangerous.

Simultaneous administration of desferrioxamine and prochlorperazine has been observed to induce a transient metabolic encephalopathy characterised by loss of consciousness for 48–72 hours.

*Pregnancy and lactation:* Stemetil is contra-indicated in pregnancy. There is inadequate evidence of the safety of Stemetil in human pregnancy but it has been widely used for many years without apparent ill consequence. There is evidence of harmful effects in animals. Like other drugs it should be avoided in pregnancy unless the physician considers it essential. Neuroleptics may occasionally prolong labour and at such a time should be withheld until the cervix is dilated 3–4 cm. Possible adverse effects on the neonate include lethargy or paradoxical hyperexcitability, tremor and low Apgar score. Phenothiazines may be excreted in milk, breastfeeding should be suspended during treatment.

*Effects on ability to drive and use machines:* Patients should be warned about drowsiness during the early days of treatment, and advised not to drive or operate machinery.

*Undesirable effects:* Minor side-effects of neuroleptics are nasal stuffiness, dry mouth, insomnia, agitation. Adverse effects of neuroleptics: *Liver function*: Jaundice, usually transient, occurs in a very small percentage of patients taking neuroleptics. A premonitory sign may be a sudden onset of fever after one to three weeks of treatment followed by the development of jaundice. Neuroleptic jaundice has the biochemical and other characteristics of obstructive jaundice and is associated with obstruction of the canaliculi by bile thrombi; the frequent presence of an accompanying eosinophilia indicates the allergic nature of this phenomenon. Treatment should be withheld on the development of jaundice. *Cardiorespiratory*: Hypotension, usually postural, commonly occurs. Elderly or volume depleted subjects are particularly susceptible, it is more likely to occur after intramuscular injection. Cardiac arrhythmias, including atrial arrhythmia, A-V block, ventricular tachycardia and fibrillation have been reported during neuroleptic therapy, possibly related to dosage. Pre-existing cardiac disease, old age, hypokalaemia and concurrent tricyclic antidepressants may predispose. ECG changes, usually benign, include widened QT interval, ST depression, U-waves and T-wave changes. Respiratory depression is possible in susceptible patients. *Blood picture*: A mild leucopenia occurs in up to 30% of patients on prolonged high dosage. Agranulocytosis may occur rarely; it is not dose related. The occurrence of unexplained infections or fever requires immediate haematological investigation. *Extrapyramidal*: Acute dystonias or dyskinesias, usually transitory, are more common in children and young adults, and usually occur within the first 4 days of treatment or after dosage increases. Akathisia characteristically occurs after large initial doses. Parkinsonism is more common in adults and the elderly. It usually develops after weeks or months of treatment. One or more of the following may be seen: tremor, rigidity, akinesia or other features of Parkinsonism. Commonly just tremor. Tardive dyskinesia: If this occurs it is usually, but not necessarily, after prolonged or high dosage. It can even occur after treatment has been stopped. Dosage should therefore be kept low whenever possible. *Skin and eyes*: Contact skin sensitisation is a serious but rare complication in those frequently handling preparations of certain phenothiazines; the greatest care must be taken to avoid contact of the drug with the skin. Skin rashes of various kinds may also be seen in patients treated with the drug. Patients on high dosage should be warned that they may develop photosensitivity in sunny weather and should avoid exposure to direct sunlight. Ocular changes and the development of a metallic greyish-mauve coloration of exposed skin have been noted in some individuals mainly females, who have received chlorpromazine continuously for long periods (four to eight years). This could possibly happen with Stemetil. *Endocrine*: hyperprolactinaemia which may result in galactorrhoea, gynaecomastia, amenorrhoea; impotence. Neuroleptic malignant syndrome (hyperthermia, rigidity, autonomic dysfunction and altered consciousness) may occur with any neuroleptic.

*Overdose:* Symptoms of phenothiazine overdosage include drowsiness or loss of consciousness, hypotension, tachycardia, ECG changes, ventricular arrhythmias and hypothermia. Severe extra-pyramidal dyskinesias may occur.

If the patient is seen sufficiently soon (up to 6 hours) after ingestion of a toxic dose, gastric lavage may be attempted. Pharmacological induction of emesis is unlikely to be of any use. Activated charcoal should be given. There is no specific antidote. Treatment is supportive.

Generalised vasodilatation may result in circulatory collapse; raising the patient's legs may suffice. In severe cases, volume expansion by intravenous fluids may be needed; infusion fluids should be warmed before administration in order not to aggravate hypothermia.

Positive inotropic agents such as dopamine may be tried if fluid replacement is insufficient to correct the circulatory collapse. Peripheral vasoconstrictor agents are not generally recommended; avoid the use of adrenaline.

Ventricular or supraventricular tachy-arrhythmias usually respond to restoration of normal body temperature and correction of circulatory or metabolic disturbances. If persistent or life threatening, appropriate anti-arrhythmic therapy may be considered. Avoid lignocaine and, as far as possible, long acting anti-arrhythmic drugs.

Pronounced central nervous system depression requires airway maintenance or, in extreme circumstances, assisted respiration. Severe dystonic reactions usually respond to procyclidine (5–10 mg) or orphenadrine (20–40 mg) administered intramuscularly or intravenously. Convulsions should be treated with intravenous diazepam.

Neuroleptic malignant syndrome should be treated with cooling. Dantrolene sodium may be tried.

**Pharmacological properties**

*Pharmacodynamic properties:* Stemetil is a potent phenothiazine neuroleptic.

*Pharmacokinetic properties:* There is little information about blood levels, distribution and excretion in humans. The rate of metabolism and excretion of phenothiazines decreases in old age.

*Preclinical safety data:* There is no pre-clinical data of relevance to the prescriber which are additional to that already included in other sections of the SPC.

**Pharmaceutical particulars**

*List of excipients: Stemetil tablets:* lactose BP, starch maize, aerosil (E551) and magnesium stearate BP. *Stemetil syrup:* liquid sugar gran. liquors, Tween 80 Ph Eur. (E433), Zimm banana 504, caramel HT (E150a), citric acid anhydrous BP (E330), sodium citrate gran. BP (E331), sodium benzoate BP (E211), sodium sulphite anhydrous BP (E221), sodium metabisulphite powder BP (E223), ascorbic acid L(+) BP (E300) and demineralised water BP.

*Incompatibilities:* None stated.

*Shelf-life: Tablets:* 60 months. *Syrup*: 36 months

*Special precautions for storage*: Store protected from light.

*Nature and content of container:* Stemetil tablets 5 mg are available in PVDC coated UPVC/aluminium foil blisters containing 84 tablets. Stemetil tablets 25 mg are available in PVDC coated UPVC/aluminium foil blisters containing 56 tablets. Stemetil syrup is available in amber glass bottles containing 100 ml.

*Instructions for use/handling:* None.

**Marketing authorisation numbers**

Tablets 5 mg 0012/5263
Tablets 25 mg 0012/5316
Syrup 0012/5022

**Date of approval/revision of SPC** February 1997

**Legal category** POM.

## STEMETIL* INJECTION

**Qualitative and quantitative composition** Each 1 ml of Stemetil Injection contains 12.5 mg prochlorperazine mesylate BP.

**Pharmaceutical form** Colourless sterile solution.

**Clinical particulars**

*Therapeutic indications:* Stemetil is a potent phenothiazine neuroleptic. Uses: The treatment of nausea and vomiting and in schizophrenia (particularly the chronic stage) and acute mania.

*Posology and method of administration:* For deep intramuscular injection.

*Adults*

| *Indication* | Dosage |
|---|---|
| Treatment of nausea and vomiting | 12.5 mg by deep i.m. injection followed by oral therapy medication 6 hours later if necessary. |
| Schizophrenia and other psychotic disorders | 12.5 mg to 25 mg b.i.d. or t.d.s. by deep intramuscular injection until oral treatment becomes possible |

*Children:* Intramuscular Stemetil should not be given to children. *Elderly:* A lower dose is recommended. Please see *Special warnings and special precautions for use* section.

*Contra-indications:* The use of Stemetil injection is contraindicated in children has it has been associated with dystonic reactions after the cumulative dose of 0.5 mg/kg.

*Special warnings and special precautions for use:* Stemetil should be avoided in patients with liver or renal dysfunction, epilepsy, Parkinson's disease, hypothyroidism, phaeochromocytoma, myasthenia gravis, prostate hypertrophy. It should be avoided in patients known to be hypersensitive to phenothiazines or with a history of narrow angle glaucoma. It should be used with caution in the elderly, particularly during very hot or very cold weather (risk of hyper-, hypothermia).

Postural hypotension with tachycardia as well as local pain or nodule formation may occur after i.m. administration.

The elderly are particularly susceptible to postural hypotension.

Stemetil should be used cautiously in the elderly owing to their susceptibility to drugs acting centrally on the nervous system and a lower initial dosage is recommended. There is an increased risk of drug-induced Parkinsonism in the elderly particularly after prolonged use. Care should also be taken not to confuse the adverse effects of Stemetil e.g. orthostatic hypotension with effects due to the underlying disorder.

*Interaction with other medicaments and other forms of interaction:* Interactions of phenothiazine neuroleptics: The CNS depressant actions of neuroleptic agents may be intensified (additively) by alcohol, barbiturates and other sedatives. Respiratory depression may occur.

The hypotensive effect of most antihypertensive drugs especially alpha adrenoceptor blocking agents may be exaggerated by neuroleptics.

The mild anticholinergic effect of neuroleptics may be enhanced by other anticholinergic drugs possibly leading to constipation, heat stroke, etc.

The action of some drugs may be opposed by phenothiazine neuroleptics; these include amphetamine, levodopa, clonidine, guanethidine, adrenaline.

Anticholinergic agents may reduce the antipsychotic effect of neuroleptics.

Some drugs interfere with absorption of neuroleptic agents: antacids, anti-Parkinson, lithium. Increases or decreases in the plasma concentrations of a number of drugs, e.g. propranolol, phenobarbitone have been observed but were not of clinical significance.

High doses of neuroleptics reduce the response to hypoglycaemic agents the dosage of which might have to be raised.

Adrenaline must *not* be used in patients overdosed with Stemetil. Most of the above interactions are of a theoretical nature and not dangerous.

Simultaneous administration of desferrioxamine and prochlorperazine has been observed to induce a transient metabolic encephalopathy characterised by loss of consciousness for 48–72 hours.

*Pregnancy and lactation:* Stemetil is contra-indicated in pregnancy. There is inadequate evidence of the safety of Stemetil in human pregnancy but it has been widely used for many years without apparent ill consequence. There is evidence of harmful effects in animals. Like other drugs it should be avoided in pregnancy unless the physician considers it essential. Neuroleptics may occasionally prolong labour and at such a time should be withheld until the cervix is dilated 3–4 cm. Possible adverse effects on the neonate include lethargy or paradoxical hyperexcitability, tremor and low Apgar score. Phenothiazines may be excreted in milk, breastfeeding should be suspended during treatment.

*Effects on ability to drive and use machines:* Patients should be warned about drowsiness during the early days of treatment, and advised not to drive or operate machinery.

*Undesirable effects:* Minor side-effects of neuroleptics are nasal stuffiness, dry mouth, insomnia, agitation. Adverse effects of neuroleptics: *Liver function*: Jaundice, usually transient, occurs in a very small percentage of patients taking neuroleptics. A premonitory sign may be a sudden onset of fever after one to three weeks of treatment followed by the development of jaundice. Neuroleptic jaundice has the biochemical and other characteristics of obstructive jaundice and is associated with obstruction of the canaliculi by bile thrombi; the frequent presence of an accompanying eosinophilia indicates the allergic nature of this phenomenon. Treatment should be withheld on the development of jaundice. *Cardiorespiratory*: Hypotension, usually postural, commonly occurs. Elderly or volume depleted subjects are particularly susceptible, it is more likely to occur after intramuscular injection. Cardiac arrhythmias, including atrial arrhythmia, A-V block, ventricular tachycardia and fibrillation have been reported during neuroleptic therapy, possibly related to dosage. Pre-existing cardiac disease, old age, hypokalaemia and concurrent tricyclic antidepressants may predispose. ECG changes, usually benign, include widened QT interval, ST depression, U-waves and T-wave changes. Respiratory depression is possible in susceptible patients. *Blood picture*: A mild leucopenia occurs in up to 30% of patients on prolonged high dosage. Agranulocytosis may occur rarely; it is not dose related. The occurrence of unexplained infections or fever requires immediate haematological investigation. *Extrapyramidal*: Acute dystonias or dyskinesias, usually transitory, are more common in children and young adults, and usually occur within the first 4 days of treatment or after dosage increases. Akathisia characteristically occurs after large initial doses. Parkinsonism is more common in adults and the elderly. It usually develops after weeks or months of treatment. One or more of the following may be seen: tremor, rigidity, akinesia or other features of Parkinsonism. Commonly just tremor. Tardive dyskinesia: If this occurs it is usually, but not necessarily, after prolonged or high dosage. It can even occur after treatment has been stopped. Dosage should therefore be kept low whenever possible. *Skin and eyes*: Contact skin sensitisation is a serious but rare complication in those frequently handling preparations of certain phenothiazines; the greatest care must be taken to avoid contact of the drug with the skin. Skin rashes of various kinds may also be seen in patients treated with the drug. Patients on high dosage should be warned that they may develop photosensitivity in sunny weather and should avoid exposure to direct sunlight. Ocular changes and the development of a metallic greyish-mauve coloration of exposed skin have been noted in some individuals mainly females, who have received chlorpromazine continuously for long periods (four to eight years). This could possibly happen with Stemetil. *Endocrine*: hyperprolactinaemia which may result in galactorrhoea, gynaecomastia, amenorrhoea; impotence. Neuroleptic malignant syndrome (hyperthermia, rigidity, autonomic dysfunction and altered consciousness) may occur with any neuroleptic.

*Overdose:* Symptoms of phenothiazine overdosage include drowsiness or loss of consciousness, hypotension, tachycardia, ECG changes, ventricular arrhythmias and hypothermia. Severe extra-pyramidal dyskinesias may occur.

If the patient is seen sufficiently soon (up to 6 hours) after ingestion of a toxic dose, gastric lavage may be attempted. Pharmacological induction of emesis is unlikely to be of any use. Activated charcoal should be given. There is no specific antidote. Treatment is supportive.

Generalised vasodilatation may result in circulatory collapse; raising the patient's legs may suffice. In severe cases, volume expansion by intravenous fluids may be needed; infusion fluids should be warmed before administration in order not to aggravate hypothermia.

Positive inotropic agents such as dopamine may be tried if fluid replacement is insufficient to correct the circulatory collapse. Peripheral vasoconstrictor agents are not generally recommended; avoid the use of adrenaline.

Ventricular or supraventricular tachy-arrhythmias usually respond to restoration of normal body temperature and correction of circulatory or metabolic disturbances. If persistent or life threatening, appropriate anti-arrhythmic therapy may be considered. Avoid lignocaine and, as far as possible, long acting anti-arrhythmic drugs.

Pronounced central nervous system depression requires airway maintenance or, in extreme circumstances, assisted respiration. Severe dystonic reactions usually respond to procyclidine (5–10 mg) or orphenadrine (20–40 mg) administered intramuscularly or intravenously. Convulsions should be treated with intravenous diazepam.

Neuroleptic malignant syndrome should be treated with cooling. Dantrolene sodium may be tried.

**Pharmacological properties**

*Pharmacodynamic properties:* Stemetil is a potent phenothiazine neuroleptic. It is used in vertigo due to Meniere's syndrome, labryrinthitis and other causes, and for nausea and vomiting from whatever cause including that associated with migraine. It may also be used for schizophrenia (particularly the chronic stage), acute mania and as an adjunct to the short term management of anxiety.

*Pharmacokinetic properties:* There is little information about blood levels, distribution and excretion in humans. The rate of metabolism and excretion of phenothiazines decreases in old age.

*Preclinical safety data:* There is no pre-clinical data of relevance to the prescriber which are additional to that already included in other sections of the SPC.

**Pharmaceutical particulars**

*List of excipients:* sodium sulphite anhydrous BP (E221), sodium metabisulphite powder BP (E223), sodium chloride Ph Eur, ethanolamine BP and water for injections (non-sterilised) BP.

*Incompatibilities:* None stated.

*Shelf-life:* 60 months.

*Special precautions for storage:* Protect from light. Discoloured solutions should not be used.

*Nature and content of container:* Stemetil injection is supplied in colourless glass ampoules in packs of 10 x 1 ml.

*Instructions for use/handling:* None.

**Marketing authorisation number** 0012/5008

**Date of approval/revision of SPC** February 1997

**Legal category** POM

## STEMETIL* SUPPOSITORIES

**Qualitative and quantitative composition** Each Stemetil 5 mg suppository contains 0.32% w/w prochlorperazine base, equivalent to 5 mg prochlorperazine maleate. Each Stemetil 25 mg suppository contains 0.78% w/w prochlorperazine base, equivalent to 25 mg prochlorperazine maleate.

**Pharmaceutical form** Cream, smooth, torpedo-shaped suppositories.

**Clinical particulars**

*Therapeutic indications:* Stemetil is a potent phenothiazine neuroleptic. Uses: The treatment of nausea and vomiting, the prevention of post-operative vomiting. The management of nausea and vomiting and in schizophrenia (particularly the chronic stage) and acute mania.

*Posology and method of administration:* Route of administration: Rectal.

*Adults:*

| *Indication* | *Dosage* |
|---|---|
| Treatment of nausea and vomiting | 25 mg followed by oral medication 6 hours later if necessary. |
| For the management of nausea and vomiting due to migraine | One 5 mg suppository three times a day. In acute cases an intramuscular injection may be administered followed by the use of suppositories. |
| Prevention of post-operative vomiting | Two 5 mg suppositories before operation followed by two every 5 hours for up to 20 hours thereafter. |
| Schizophrenia and other psychotic disorders | 25 mg b.d. or t.d.s. until oral treatment becomes possible. |

*Children:* Stemetil suppositories should not be given to children. *Elderly:* A lower dose is recommended. Please see 'Special warnings and special for precautions for use' section.

*Contra-indications:* Pregnancy.

*Special warnings and special precautions for use:* Stemetil should be avoided in patients with liver or renal dysfunction, epilepsy, Parkinson's disease, hypothyroidism, phaeochromocytoma, myasthenia gravis, prostate hypertrophy. It should be avoided in patients known to be hypersensitive to phenothiazines or with a history of narrow angle glaucoma. It should be used with caution in the elderly, particularly during very hot or very cold weather (risk of hyper-, hypothermia).

The elderly are particularly susceptible to postural hypotension.

Stemetil should be used cautiously in the elderly owing to their susceptibility to drugs acting centrally on the nervous system and a lower initial dosage is recommended. There is an increased risk of drug-induced Parkinsonism in the elderly particularly after prolonged use. Care should also be taken not to confuse the adverse effects of Stemetil e.g. orthostatic hypotension with effects due to the underlying disorder.

*Interaction with other medicaments and other forms of interaction:* Interactions of phenothiazine neuroleptics: The CNS depressant actions of neuroleptic agents may be intensified (additively) by alcohol, barbiturates and other sedatives. Respiratory depression may occur.

The hypotensive effect of most antihypertensive drugs especially alpha adrenoceptor blocking agents may be exaggerated by neuroleptics.

The mild anticholinergic effect of neuroleptics may be enhanced by other anticholinergic drugs possibly leading to constipation, heat stroke, etc.

The action of some drugs may be opposed by phenothiazine neuroleptics; these include amphetamine, levodopa, clonidine, guanethidine, adrenaline.

Anticholinergic agents may reduce the antipsychotic effect of neuroleptics.

Some drugs interfere with absorption of neuroleptic agents: antacids, anti-Parkinson, lithium. Increases or decreases in the plasma concentrations of a number of drugs, e.g. propranolol, phenobarbitone have been observed but were not of clinical significance.

High doses of neuroleptics reduce the response to hypoglycaemic agents the dosage of which might have to be raised.

Adrenaline must *not* be used in patients overdosed with Stemetil. Most of the above interactions are of a theoretical nature and not dangerous.

Simultaneous administration of desferrioxamine and prochlorperazine has been observed to induce a transient metabolic encephalopathy characterised by loss of consciousness for 48–72 hours.

*Pregnancy and lactation:* Stemetil is contra-indicated in pregnancy. There is inadequate evidence of the safety of Stemetil in human pregnancy but it has been widely used for many years without apparent ill consequence. There is evidence of harmful effects in animals. Like other drugs it should be avoided in pregnancy unless the physician considers it essential. Neuroleptics may occasionally prolong labour and at such a time should be withheld until the cervix is dilated 3–4 cm. Possible adverse effects on the neonate include lethargy or paradoxical hyperexcitability, tremor and low Apgar score. Phenothiazines may be excreted in milk, breastfeeding should be suspended during treatment.

*Effects on ability to drive and use machines:* Patients should be warned about drowsiness during the early days of treatment, and advised not to drive or operate machinery.

*Undesirable effects:* Minor side-effects of neuroleptics are nasal stuffiness, dry mouth, insomnia, agitation. Adverse effects of neuroleptics: *Liver function:* Jaundice, usually transient, occurs in a very small percentage of patients taking neuroleptics. A premonitory sign may be a sudden onset of fever after one to three weeks of treatment followed by the development of jaundice. Neuroleptic jaundice has the biochemical and other characteristics of obstructive jaundice and is associated with obstruction of the canaliculi by bile thrombi; the frequent presence of an accompanying eosinophilia indicates the allergic nature of this phenomenon. Treatment should be withheld on the development of jaundice. *Cardiorespiratory:* Hypotension, usually postural, commonly occurs. Elderly or volume depleted subjects are particularly susceptible, it is more likely to occur after intramuscular injection. Cardiac arrhythmias, including atrial arrhythmia, A-V block, ventricular tachycardia and fibrillation have been reported during neuroleptic therapy, possibly related to dosage. Pre-existing cardiac disease, old age, hypokalaemia and concurrent tricyclic antidepressants may predispose. ECG changes, usually benign, include widened QT interval, ST depression, U-waves and T-wave changes. Respiratory depression is possible in susceptible patients. *Blood picture:* A mild leucopenia occurs in up to 30% of patients on prolonged high dosage. Agranulocytosis may occur rarely; it is not dose related. The occurrence of unexplained infections or fever requires immediate haematological investigation. *Extrapyramidal:* Acute dystonias or dyskinesias, usually transitory, are more common in children and young adults, and usually occur within the first 4 days of treatment or after dosage increases. Akathisia characteristically occurs after large initial doses. Parkinsonism is more common in adults and the elderly. It usually develops after weeks or months of treatment. One or more of the following may be seen: tremor, rigidity, akinesia or other features of Parkinsonism. Commonly just tremor. Tardive dyskinesia: If this occurs it is usually, but not necessarily, after prolonged or high dosage. It can even occur after treatment has been stopped. Dosage should therefore be kept low whenever possible. *Skin and eyes:* Contact skin sensitisation is a serious but rare complication in those frequently handling preparations of certain phenothiazines; the greatest care must be taken to avoid contact of the drug with the skin. Skin rashes of various kinds may also be seen in patients treated with the drug. Patients on high dosage should be warned that they may develop photosensitivity in sunny weather and should avoid exposure to direct sunlight. Ocular changes and the development of a metallic greyish-mauve coloration of exposed skin have been noted in some individuals mainly females, who have received chlorpromazine continuously for long periods (four to eight years). This could possibly happen with Stemetil. *Endocrine:* hyperprolactinaemia which may result in galactorrhoea, gynaecomastia, amenorrhoea; impotence. Neuroleptic malignant syndrome (hypothermia, rigidity, autonomic dysfunction and altered consciousness) may occur with any neuroleptic.

*Overdose:* Symptoms of phenothiazine overdosage include drowsiness or loss of consciousness, hypotension, tachycardia, ECG changes, ventricular arrhythmias and hypothermia. Severe extra-pyramidal dyskinesias may occur.

If the patient is seen sufficiently soon (up to 6 hours) after ingestion of a toxic dose, gastric lavage may be attempted. Pharmacological induction of emesis is unlikely to be of any use. Activated charcoal should be given. There is no specific antidote. Treatment is supportive.

Generalised vasodilatation may result in circulatory collapse; raising the patient's legs may suffice. In severe cases, volume expansion by intravenous fluids may be needed; infusion fluids should be warmed before administration in order not to aggravate hypothermia.

Positive inotropic agents such as dopamine may be tried if fluid replacement is insufficient to correct the circulatory collapse. Peripheral vasoconstrictor agents are not generally recommended; avoid the use of adrenaline.

Ventricular or supraventricular tachy-arrhythmias usually respond to restoration of normal body temperature and correction of circulatory or metabolic disturbances. If persistent or life threatening, appropriate anti-arrhythmic therapy may be considered. Avoid lignocaine and, as far as possible, long acting anti-arrhythmic drugs.

Pronounced central nervous system depression requires airway maintenance or, in extreme circumstances, assisted respiration. Severe dystonic reactions usually respond to procyclidine (5–10 mg) or orphenadrine (20–40 mg) administered intramuscularly or intravenously. Convulsions should be treated with intravenous diazepam.

Neuroleptic malignant syndrome should be treated with cooling. Dantrolene sodium may be tried.

**Pharmacological properties**

*Pharmacodynamic properties:* Stemetil is a potent phenothiazine neuroleptic.

*Pharmacokinetic properties:* There is little information about blood levels, distribution and excretion in humans. The rate of metabolism and excretion of phenothiazines decreases in old age.

*Preclinical safety data:* There is no pre-clinical data of relevance to the prescriber which are additional to that already included in other sections of the SPC.

**Pharmaceutical particulars**

*List of excipients:* suppository base E75 and suppository base W35.

*Incompatibilities:* None stated.

*Shelf-life:* 36 months.

*Special precautions for storage:* Store below 25°C. Protect from light.

*Nature and content of container:* Suppositories enclosed automatically during filling in preformed strips of PVC and polyethylene being the inner surface in contact with the product. Sealing of bandolier effected by the action of heat and pressure. Stemetil suppositories are available in packs of 10.

*Instructions for use/handling:* None.

**Marketing authorisation numbers**
Suppositories 5 mg 0012/5117
Suppositories 25 mg 0012/5013

**Date of approval/revision of SPC** February 1997

**Legal category** POM

## SUPRAX*

**Presentation**
*Tablets 200 mg:* Rectangular, white, film-coated tablets with a break-line on each side engraved with "SUPRAX" on one side and "LL200" on the other side. Each tablet contains 200 mg of Cefixime.

*Powder for Paediatric Oral Suspension:* Bottles of powder for the preparation of suspension. When reconstituted each 5 ml volume contains 100 mg of Cefixime. The suspension contains 2.5 g of sucrose in 5 ml.

**Uses** Suprax is an orally active cephalosporin antibiotic which has marked in-vitro bactericidal activity against a wide variety of Gram-positive and Gram-negative organisms.

It is indicated for the treatment of the following acute infections when caused by susceptible micro-organisms:

*Upper Respiratory Tract Infections (URTI):* e.g. otitis media; and other URTI where the causative organism is known or suspected to be resistant to other commonly used antibiotics, or where treatment failure may carry significant risk.

*Lower Respiratory Tract Infections*–e.g. bronchitis.

*Urinary Tract Infections:* e.g. cystitis, cystourethritis, pyelonephritis.

Clinical efficacy has been demonstrated in infections caused by commonly occurring pathogens including *Streptococcus pneumoniae, Streptococcus pyogenes, Escherichia coli, Proteus mirabilis, Klebsiella* species, *Haemophilus influenzae* (beta-lactamase positive and negative), *Moraxella catarrhalis* (beta-lactamase positive and negative) and *Enterobacter* species. Suprax is highly stable in the presence of beta-lactamase enzymes.

Most strains of enterococci (*Streptococcus faecalis,* group D *Streptococci*) and *Staphylococci* (including coagulase positive and negative strains and methicillin-resistant strains) are resistant to Suprax. In addition, most strains of *Pseudomonas, Bacteroides fragilis, Listeria monocytogenes* and *Clostridia* are resistant to Suprax

**Dosage and administration** Absorption of Suprax is not significantly modified by the presence of food. The usual course of treatment is 7 days. This may be continued for up to 14 days if required.

*Adults and children over 10 years:* the recommended adult dosage is 200–400 mg daily according to the severity of the infection, given either as a single dose or in two divided doses.

*Elderly:* Elderly patients may be given the same dose as recommended for adults. Renal function should be assessed and dosage should be adjusted in severe renal impairment (See "Dosage in Renal Impairment").

*Children (Use Paediatric Oral Suspension):* the recommended dosage for children is 8 mg/kg day administered as a single dose or in two divided doses. As a general guide for prescribing in children the following daily doses in terms of volume of Paediatric Oral Suspension are suggested:

6 months up to 1 year: 3.75 ml daily
Children 1-4 years: 5 ml daily
Children 5-10 years: 10 ml daily
(A spoon is supplied with the 37.5 ml bottle to aid correct dosing–see *Package quantities*).

Children weighing more than 50 kg or older than 10 years should be treated with the recommended adult dose (200–400 mg daily depending on the severity of infection). The safety and efficacy of Cefixime has not been established in children aged less than 6 months.

*Dosage in Renal Impairment:* Suprax may be administered in the presence of impaired renal function. Normal dose and schedule may be given in patients with creatinine clearances of 20 ml/min or greater. In patients whose creatinine clearance is less than 20 ml/min, it is recommended that a dose of 200 mg once daily should not be exceeded. The dose and regimen for patients who are maintained on chronic ambulatory peritoneal dialysis or haemodialysis should follow the same recommendation as that for patients with creatinine clearances of less than 20 ml/min.

**Contra-indications, warnings, etc**
*Contra-indications:* Patients with known hypersensitivity to cephalosporin antibiotics.

*Warnings and precautions:* Cefixime should be given with caution to patients who have shown hypersensitivity to other drugs. Cephalosporins should be given with caution to penicillin-sensitive patients, as there is some evidence of partial cross-allergenicity between the penicillins and the cephalosporins. Patients have had severe reactions (including anaphylaxis) to both classes of drugs. If an allergic effect occurs with cefixime, the drug should be discontinued and the patient treated with appropriate agents if necessary. Cefixime should be administered with caution in patients with markedly impaired renal function (See "*Dosage in Renal Impairment*"). Treatment with broad spectrum antibiotics alters the normal flora of the colon and may permit overgrowth of clostridia. Studies indicate that a toxin produced by *Clostridium difficile* is a primary cause of antibiotic-associated diarrhoea. Pseudomembraneous colitis is associated with the use of broad-spectrum antibiotics (including macrolides, semi-synthetic penicillins, lincosamides and cephalosporins); it is therefore important to consider its diagnosis in patients who develop diarrhoea in association with the use of antibiotics. Symptoms of pseudomembraneous colitis may occur during or after antibiotic treatment. Management of pseudomembraneous colitis should include sigmoidoscopy, appropriate bacteriologic studies, fluids, electrolytes and protein supplementation. If the colitis does not improve after the drug has been discontinued, or if the symptoms are severe, oral vancomycin is the drug of choice for antibiotic-associated pseudomembraneous colitis produced by *C.difficile.* Other causes of colitis should be excluded.

*Use in pregnancy and lactation:* Reproduction studies have been performed in mice and rats at doses up to 400 times the human dose and have revealed no evidence of impaired fertility or harm to the foetus due to cefixime. In the rabbit, at doses up to 4 times the human dose, there was no evidence of a teratogenic effect; there was a high incidence of abortion and maternal death which is an expected consequence of the known sensitivity of rabbits to antibiotic-induced changes in the population of the microflora of the intestine. There are no adequate and well-controlled studies in pregnant women. Cefixime should therefore not be used in pregnancy or in nursing mothers unless considered essential by the physician.

*Interactions:* A false positive reaction for glucose in the urine may occur with Benedict's or Fehling's solutions or with copper sulphate test tablets, but not with test based on enzymatic glucose oxidase reactions. A false positive direct Coombs test has been reported during treatment with cephalosporin antibiotics, therefore it should be recognised that a positive Coombs test may be due to the drug. In common with other cephalosporins, increases in prothrombin times have been noted in a few patients. Care should therefore be taken in patients receiving anticoagulant therapy.

*Overdose:* There is no experience with overdoses of cefixime. Adverse reactions seen at dose levels up to 2 g cefixime in normal subjects did not differ from the profile seen in patients treated at the recommended doses. Gastric lavage may be indicated in overdosage. No specific antidote exists. Cefixime is not removed from the circulation in significant quantities by dialysis.

*Side-effects:* Suprax is generally well tolerated. The majority of adverse reactions observed in clinical trials were mild and self limiting in nature. *Gastrointestinal Disturbances:* the most frequent side effects seen with cefixime are diarrhoea and stool changes; diarrhoea has been more commonly associated with higher doses. Some cases of moderate to severe diarrhoea have been reported; this has occasionally warranted cessation of therapy. Cefixime should be discontinued if marked diarrhoea occurs. Other gastrointestinal side effects seen less frequently are nausea, abdominal pain, dyspepsia, vomiting and flatulence. Pseudomembraneous colitis has been reported (see above). *Central Nervous System:* headache and dizziness. *Hypersensitivity reactions:* allergies in the form of rash, pruritis, urticaria, drug fever and arthralgia have been observed. These reactions usually subsided upon discontinuation of therapy. *Haematological and Clinical Chemistry:* thrombocytopenia, leukopenia and eosinophilia have been reported. These reactions were infrequent and reversible. Mild transient changes in liver and renal function tests have been observed. *Miscellaneous:* other possible reactions include genital pruritis and vaginitis.

**Pharmaceutical precautions** *Tablets:* Store at controlled room temperature (15-25°C).
*Powder for Paediatric Oral Suspension:* Store unreconstituted product at controlled room temperature (15-25°C). To reconstitute, add 33 ml of water (37.5 ml bottle) or 50 ml of water (75 ml bottle) in two portions shaking after each addition. After reconstitution, the suspension may be stored at room temperature (below 25°C) for 14 days without significant loss of potency. Do not freeze. Keep bottles tightly closed and shake well before use. Discard any unused portion after 14 days. Dilution of the suspension is not recommended.

**Legal category** POM.

**Package quantities** *Tablets 200 mg:* Blister packs of 7 tablets.
*Powder for Paediatric Oral Suspension (100 mg / 5 ml):* Bottles containing powder for preparation of 37.5 ml and 75 ml of suspension. A double ended (3.75 ml / 5 ml) spoon is supplied with the 37.5 ml bottle to enable correct dosing of the younger child (see Dosage and Administration).

**Further information** Nil.

**Product licence numbers**
Powder for Paediatric Oral Suspension 0095/0211
Tablets 200 mg 0095/0212

*Product licence holder:* Cyanamid of Great Britain Ltd, Cyanamid House, Fareham Road, Gosport, Hampshire, PO13 0AS

## SURMONTIL*

**Qualitative and quantitative composition** *Surmontil Tablets 10 mg* contain Trimipramine Maleate EP 14 mg equivalent to 10 mg trimipramine per tablet. *Surmontil tablets 25 mg* contain Trimipramine Maleate EP 35.0 mg equivalent to 25 mg trimipramine per tablet. *Surmontil capsules 50 mg* contain Trimipramine Maleate EP 69.75 mg per capsule.

**Pharmaceutical form** *Surmontil tablets* are compression coated , white. The face is indented with the name and strength; the reverse is plain. *Surmontil capsules* are white opaque with a green cap, printed "SU50".

**Clinical particulars**
*Therapeutic indications:* Surmontil has a potent antidepressant action similar to that of other tricyclic antidepressants. It also possesses pronounced sedative action. It is, therefore, indicated in the treatment of depressive illness, especially where sleep disturbance, anxiety or agitation are presenting symptoms. Sleep disturbance is controlled within 24 hours and true antidepressant action follows within 7 to 10 days.

*Posology and method of administration: For* oral. use *Adults:* For depression 50-75 mg/day initially increasing to 150-300 mg/day in divided doses or one dose at night. The maintenance dose is 75-150 mg/day. *Elderly* 10-25 mg three times a day initially. The initial dose should be increased with caution under close supervision. Half the normal maintenance dose may be sufficient to produce a satisfactory clinical response. *Children:* Not recommended.

*Contra-indications:* Recent myocardial infarction. Any degree of heart block or other cardiac arrhythmias. Mania. Severe liver disease. During breast feeding.

*Special warnings and precautions for use:* The elderly are particularly liable to experience adverse reactions, especially agitation, confusion and postural hypotension. Avoid if possible in patients with narrow angle glaucoma, symptoms suggestive of prostatic hypertrophy and a history of epilepsy.

Patients posing a high suicidal risk require close initial supervision. Tricyclic antidepressants potentiate the central nervous depressant action of alcohol.

Anaesthetics given during tri/tetracyclic antidepressant therapy may increase the risk of arrhythmias and hypotension. If surgery is necessary, the anaesthetist should be informed that a patient is being so treated.

It may be advisable to monitor liver function in patients on long term treatment with Surmontil.

*Interactions with other medicaments and other forms of interaction:* Trimipramine should not be given concurrently with, or within 2 weeks of cessation of, therapy with monoamine oxidase inhibitors. Trimipramine may decrease the antihypertensive effect of guanethidine, debrisoquine, bethanidine and possibly clonidone. It would be advisable to review all antihypertensive therapy during treatment with tricyclic antidepressants.

Trimipramine should not be given with sympathomimetic agents such as adrenaline, ephedrine, isoprenaline, noradrenaline, phenylephrine and phenylpropanolamine.

Barbiturates may increase the rate of metabolism.

Surmontil should be administered with care in patients receiving therapy for hyperthyrodism.

*Pregnancy and lactation:* Do not use in pregnancy especially during the first and last trimesters unless there are compelling reasons. There is no evidence from animal work that it is free from hazard. Trimipramine is contraindicated during lactation.

*Effects on ability to drive and use machines:* Trimipramine may initially impair alertness. Patients should be warned of the possible hazard when driving or operating machinery.

*Undesirable effects:* Cardiac arrhythmias and severe hypotension are likely to occur with high dosage or in deliberate overdosage. They may also occur in patients with pre-existing heart disease taking normal dosage.

The following adverse effects, although not necessarily all reported with trimipramine, have occurred with other tricyclic antidepressants. Atropine-like side effects including dry mouth, disturbance of accommodation, tachycardia, constipation and hesitancy of micturation are common early in treatment but usually lessen. Other common adverse effects include drowsiness, sweating, postural hypotension, tremor and skin rashes. Interference with sexual function may occur. Serious adverse effects are rare; the following have been reported: depression of bone marrow, including agranularcytosis, cholestatic jaundice, hypomania, convulsions and peripheral neuropathy. Psychotic manifestations including mania and paranoid delusions, may be exacerbated during treatment with tricyclic antidepressants. Withdrawal symptoms may occur on abrupt cessation of therapy and include insomnia, irritability and excessive perspiration. Adverse effects such as withdrawal symptoms, respiratory depression and agitation have been reported in neonates whose mothers had taken trimipramine during the last trimester of pregnancy.

*Overdosage:* Acute overdosage may be accompanied by hypotesive collapse, convulsions and coma. Provided coma is not present, gastric lavage should be carried out without delay even though some time may have passed since the drug was ingested. Patients in coma should have an endotracheal tube passed before gastric lavage is started. Absorption of trimipramine is slow but, as cardiac effects may appear soon after the drug is absorbed, a saline purge should be given. Electrocardiography monitoring is essential.

It is important to treat acidosis as soon as it appears with, for example, 20 ml per kg of M/6 sodium lactate injection by slow intravenous injection. Intubation is necessary and the patient should be ventilated before convulsions develop. Convulsions should be treated with diazepam administered intravenously.

Ventricular tachycardia or fibrillation should be treated by electrical defibrillation. If supraventricular tachycardia develops, pyridostigmine bromide 1 mg (adults) intravenously or propranolol 1 mg (adults) should be administered at intervals as required.

Treatment should be continued for at least three days even if the patient appears to have recovered.

**Pharmacological properties**

*Pharmacodynamic properties:* Trimiparamine is a tricyclic antidepressant. It has marked sedative properties.

*Pharmacokinetic properties:* Trimipramine undergoes high first-pass hepatic clearance, with a mean value for bioavailability of about 41% after oral administration.

The absolute volume of distribution is 31 litres/kg and total metabolic clearance is 16 ml/min/kg.

Plasma protein binding of trimipramine is about 95%. The plasma elimination half-life is around 23 hours. Trimipramine is largely metabolised by demethylation prior to conjugation yielding a glucuronide.

**Pharmaceutical particulars**

*List of excipients:* The tablets contain: Maize starch, Heavy Kaolin, White Technical Dextrin, Williams Aravit Indigo Carmine C1 73015, Calcium Hydrogen Phosphate, Starch Potato, Sodium Lauryl Sulphate, Magnesium Stearate.

The capsules contain Maize Starch, Microcrystalline cellulose (E460), Magnesium Stearate, Colloidal Silicon Dioxide. The shell contains Titanium Dioxide, Indigo carmine, Iron oxide Yellow, Gelatine, Iron Oxide Black ink (E172).

*Incompatibilities:* None known

*Shelf life:*
*Tablets* 60 months
*Capsules* 36 months

*Special precautions for storage:*
*Tablets:* Protect from light
*Capsules:* Store in a dry place below 25°C and protect from light

*Nature and contents of container*
*Surmontil tablets 10 mg:* blister packs of 84 tablets.
*Surmontil tablets 25 mg:* blister packs of 84 tablets.
*Surmontil capsules 50 mg:* blister packs of 84 tablets.

*Instructions for use/handling:* None stated.

**Marketing authorisation numbers**

| | |
|---|---|
| Surmontil Tablets 10 mg | 0012/5296R |
| Surmontil Tablets 25 mg | 0012/5297R |
| Surmontil Capsules 50 mg | 0012/5298R |

**Date of approval/revision of SPC** February 1997

**Legal category** POM

## TAXOTERE* ▼

**Qualitative and quantitative composition** Single-dose vials of Taxotere containing 20 mg of docetaxel (anhydrous) in 0.5 ml polysorbate 80 and 80 mg of docetaxel (anhydrous) in 2.0 ml polysorbate 80

The viscous solution contains 40 mg/ml docetaxel (anhydrous).

**Pharmaceutical form** Concentrate for infusion–parenteral preparation to be diluted.

**Clinical particulars**

*Therapeutic indications:* Taxotere (docetaxel) monotherapy is indicated for the treatment of patients with locally advanced or metastatic breast cancer: a) who are resistant or have recurrent disease after a cytotoxic therapy b) who have relapsed during an adjuvant cytotoxic therapy. The cytotoxic therapy should have included an anthracycline.

The use of docetaxel should be confined to units specialised in the administration of cytotoxic chemotherapy and it should only be administered under the supervision of a qualified oncologist.

*Posology and method of administration: Recommended Dosage:* The recommended dosage of docetaxel monotherapy is 100 mg/m² administered as a one-hour infusion every three weeks (see *Instructions For Use/Handling* section). Patients should be observed closely especially during the first and second infusion of docetaxel because of the risk of hypersensitivity reactions (see *Special Warnings and Precautions for Use* section). A premedication consisting of an oral corticosteroid, such as dexamethasone 16 mg per day (e.g. 8 mg bid) for 5 days starting 1 day prior to docetaxel administration, unless contraindicated, can reduce the incidence and severity of fluid retention as well as the severity of hypersensitivity reactions.

*Dosage adjustments during treatment:* Docetaxel should be administered when the neutrophil count is ≥ 1,500 cells/mm³. Patients who experienced either febrile neutropenia, neutrophil < 500 cells/mm³ for more than one week, severe or cumulative cutaneous reactions or severe peripheral neuropathy during docetaxel therapy should have the dosage of docetaxel reduced from 100 mg/m² to 75 mg/m². If the patient continues to experience these reactions at 75 mg/m², the dosage should either be decreased from 75 mg/m² to 55 mg/m² or the treatment should be discontinued.

*Special populations: Patients with hepatic impairment:* Based on pharmacokinetic data, in patients who have both elevations of transaminase (ALT and/or AST) greater than 1.5 times the upper limit of the normal range (ULN) and alkaline phosphatase greater than 2.5 times the ULN, the recommended dose of docetaxel is 75 mg/m² (see *Special Warnings and Special Precautions for Use* and *Pharmacokinetic properties* sections). For those patients with serum bilirubin > ULN and/or ALT and AST > 3.5 times the ULN associated with alkaline phosphatase > 6 times the ULN, no dose-reduction can be recommended and docetaxel should not be used unless strictly indicated. *Children:* The safety and effectiveness of docetaxel in children have not been established. *Elderly:* Based on a population pharmacokinetic analysis, there are no special instructions for the use in elderly.

*Contra-indications:* Docetaxel is contraindicated in patients who have a history of severe hypersensitivity reactions to the drug or polysorbate 80. Docetaxel should not be used in patients with baseline neutrophil count of < 1,500 cells/mm³. Docetaxel must not be used in pregnant or breast-feeding women. Docetaxel should not be used in patients with severe liver impairment since there is no data available (see *Special Warnings and Special Precautions for use* and *Posology and Method of Administration* sections).

*Special warnings and special precautions for use:* A premedication consisting of an oral corticosteroid such as dexamethasone 16 mg per day (e.g. 8 mg BID) for 5 days starting one day prior to docetaxel administration, unless contraindicated, can reduce the incidence and severity of fluid retention as well as the severity of hypersensitivity reactions (see *Posology and Method of Administration* section). Severe hypersensitivity reactions characterised by hypotension or bronchospasm or generalised rash/erythema have occurred in 5.3% of the patients receiving docetaxel.

*Haematology:* Neutropenia is the most frequent adverse reaction of docetaxel. Neutrophil nadirs occurred at a median of 8 days but this interval may be shorter in heavily pretreated patients. Frequent monitoring of complete blood counts should be conducted on all patients receiving docetaxel. Patients should be retreated with docetaxel when neutrophils recover to a level ≥ 1,500 cells/mm³ (see *Posology and Method of Administration* section). In the case of severe neutropenia (<500 cells/mm³ for seven days or more) during a course of docetaxel therapy, a reduction in dose for subsequent courses of therapy or the use of appropriate symptomatic measures are recommended.

*Hypersensitivity reactions:* Patients should be observed closely for hypersensitivity reactions especially during the first and second infusions. Hypersensitivity reactions may occur within a few minutes following the initiation of the infusion of docetaxel, thus facilities for the treatment of hypotension and bronchospasm should be available. If hypersensitivity reactions occur, minor symptoms such as flushing or localised cutaneous reactions do not require interruption of therapy. However, severe reactions, such as severe hypotension, bronchospasm or generalised rash/erythema require immediate discontinuation of docetaxel and appropriate therapy. Patients who have developed severe hypersensitivity reactions should not be rechallenged with docetaxel.

*Cutaneous reactions:* Localised skin erythema of the extremities (palms of the hands and soles of the feet) with oedema followed by desquamation has been observed. Severe symptoms such as eruptions followed by desquamation which lead to interruption or discontinuation of docetaxel treatment were reported in 5.9% of the patients (see *Posology and Method of Administration* section). Bullous epidermolysis has not been observed.

*Fluid retention:* A premedication consisting of an oral corticosteroid such as dexamethasone 16 mg per day (e.g. 8 mg BID) for 5 days starting one day prior to docetaxel administration, unless contraindicated, can reduce the incidence and severity of fluid retention as well as the severity of hypersensitivity reactions (see *Posology and Method of Administration* section). Patients with severe fluid retention such as pleural effusion, pericardial effusion and ascites should be monitored closely.

*Patients with liver impairment:* In patients treated with docetaxel at 100 mg/m² who have serum transaminase levels (ALT and /or AST) greater than 1.5 times the ULN concurrent with serum alkaline phosphatase levels greater than 2.5 times the ULN, there is a higher risk of developing severe adverse reactions such as toxic deaths including sepsis and gastrointestinal haemorrhage which can be fatal, febrile neutropenia, infections, thrombocytopenia, stomatitis and asthenia. Therefore, the recommended dose of docetaxel in patients with elevated liver function test (LFTs) is 75 mg/m² and LFTs should be measured at baseline and before each cycle (see *Posology and Method of Administration* section). For patients with serum bilirubin levels> ULN and/or ALT and AST > 3.5 times the ULN concurrent with serum alkaline phosphatase levels > 6 times the ULN, no dose-reduction can be recommended and docetaxel should not be used unless strictly indicated.

*Nervous System:* The development of severe peripheral neurotoxicity has been observed in 4.1 % of patients and requires a reduction of dose (see *Posology and Method of Administration* section).

*Others:* Contraceptive measures must be taken during and for at least three months after cessation of therapy.

*Interaction with other medicaments and other forms of interaction:* There have been no formal clinical studies to evaluate the drug interactions of docetaxel. In vitro studies have shown that the metabolism of docetaxel may be modified by the concomitant administration of compounds which induce, inhibit or are metabolised by (and thus may inhibit the enzyme competitively) cytochrome P450-3A such as cyclosporin, terfenadine, ketoconazole, erythromycin and troleandomycin. As a result, caution should be exercised when treating patients with these drugs as concomitant therapy since there is a potential for a significant interaction.

Docetaxel is highly protein bound (>95%). Although the possible in vivo interaction of docetaxel with concomitantly administered medication has not been investigated formally, in vitro interactions with tightly protein-bound drugs such as erythromycin, diphenhydramine, propranolol, propafenone, phenytoin, salicylate, sulfamethoxazole and sodium valproate did not affect protein binding of docetaxel. In addition, dexamethasone did not affect protein binding of docetaxel. Docetaxel did not influence the binding of digoxin.

*Pregnancy and lactation:* There is no information on the use of docetaxel in pregnant women. Docetaxel has been shown to be both embryotoxic and foetotoxic in rabbits and rats, and to reduce fertility in rats. As with other cytotoxic drugs, docetaxel may cause foetal harm when administered to pregnant women. Therefore, docetaxel must not be used during pregnancy. Women of childbearing age receiving docetaxel should be advised to avoid becoming pregnant, and to inform the treating physician immediately should this occur.

Docetaxel is a lipophilic substance but it is not known whether it is excreted in human milk. Consequently, because of the potential for adverse reactions in nursing infants, breast feeding must be discontinued for the duration of docetaxel therapy.

*Effects on ability to drive and use machines:* Docetaxel is unlikely to affect the ability to drive or operate machines.

*Undesirable effects:* The adverse reactions considered to be possibly or probably related to the administration of docetaxel have been obtained from 1312 patients with normal LFTs at baseline who received an initial planned dose of 100 mg/m2 over a one-hour infusion regardless of the premedication received. The patients were enrolled in 36 clinical trials conducted in Europe and North America (514 with breast carcinoma and 798 with various other tumour types).

*Haematology:* The most frequent adverse reaction to docetaxel (in patients who did not receive G-CSF) was neutropenia which was reversible and not cumulative. The median day to nadir was 8 days and the median duration of severe neutropenia (<500 cells/mm3) was 7 days. Severe neutropenia occurred in 56.4% of cycles (76.4% of the patients) and lasted for more than 7 days in 3.5 % of evaluable cycles. Fever was associated with neutropenia (<500 cells/mm3) in 11.8% of the patients (3% of the cycles) and the incidence of severe infections associated with neutrophil counts < 500 cells/mm$^3$ was 4.6% of the patients (1.2% of the cycles). Infectious episodes occurred in 20% of the patients (6% of the cycles) and were severe (including sepsis and pneumonia) in 5.7% of the patients (1.4% of the cycles) and were fatal in 1.7% of the patients. Thrombocytopenia (<100,000 cells/mm$^3$) has been reported in 7.8% of the patients. Bleeding episodes were reported in 2.4% of the patients and were rarely associated with severe thrombocytopenia (<50,000 cells/mm$^3$). Anaemia (<11 g/dl) was observed in 90.4% of the patients and was severe (<8 g/dl) in 8.9 % of the cases.

*Hypersensitivity reactions:* Hypersensitivity reactions (HSRs) have occurred in 25.9% of the patients (9.4% of the cycles) generally within a few minutes following the start of the infusion of docetaxel and were usually mild to moderate. The most frequently reported symptoms were flushing, rash with or without pruritus, chest tightness, back pain, dyspnoea and drug fever or chills. Severe reactions characterised by hypotension and/or bronchospasm or generalised rash/erythema were observed in 5.3% of patients. They resolved after discontinuing the infusion and appropriate therapy.

*Cutaneous:* Reversible cutaneous reactions have been observed in 56.6% of the patients and were generally considered as mild to moderate. 73% of these events were reversible within 21 days. The cutaneous reactions were characterised by a rash including localised eruptions mainly on feet, hands, but also on arms, face or thorax, and frequently associated with pruritus. Eruptions generally occurred within one week after the docetaxel infusion, recovered before the next infusion and were not disabling. Less frequently (5.9% of the patients), severe symptoms such as eruptions followed by desquamation which rarely lead to interruption or discontinuation of docetaxel treatment were reported. Nail disorders occurred in 2 7.9% of the patients and were characterised by hypo- or hyperpigmentation and sometimes pain and onycholysis (2.6% of the patients).

*Fluid retention:* Fluid retention has been reported in 50% (5.3% severe) of patients receiving the recommended premedication compared with 81.6% (22.4% severe) in patients without premedication. Events such as peripheral oedema and less frequently pleural effusion, pericardial effusion, ascites, lacrymation with or without conjunctivitis and weight gain have been reported. The peripheral oedema usually starts at the lower extremities and may become generalised with a weight gain of 3 kgs or more. Fluid retention is cumulative in incidence and severity. The onset of moderate and severe retention is delayed (median cumulative dose: 745.6 mg/m$^2$) in patients with premedication compared with patients without premedication (median cumulative dose: 489.7 mg/m$^2$); however, it has been reported in some patients during the early courses of therapy. Discontinuation occurred in 2 % of the patients treated with the recommended premedication. The median time to fluid retention reversibility was 29 weeks (range 0 to 42+ weeks) in patients receiving the recommended premedication. Fluid retention has not been accompanied by acute episodes of oliguria or hypotension. Dehydration has been reported rarely in association with fluid retention.

*Gastrointestinal:* Gastrointestinal effects such as nausea, vomiting, diarrhoea, and abdominal pain were seen in 40.5%, 24.5%, 40.6% and 7.3% of the patients treated respectively with an incidence of severe reactions of 4%, 3%, 4%, and 1%, respectively. Anorexia was reported in 16.8% of the patients and was infrequently severe. Constipation was reported in 9.3% (0.2% severe) of the patients. Stomatitis and oesophagitis were reported in 41.8% (5.3% severe) and 1% (0.4% severe) of the patients, respectively. Taste perversion has been reported in 10.1% of the patients (0.07% severe). Gastrointestinal bleeding has been seen in 1.4% of the patients (0.3% severe).

*Neurologic:* Mild to moderate neuro-sensory signs characterised by paresthesia, dysesthesia or pain including burning were reported in 45.9% of patients and were considered severe in 4.1% of the cases. Neuro-motor events mainly characterised by weakness were reported in 13.8% of patients and were severe in 4% of the patients. The events were spontaneously reversible within 3 months in 35.3% of patients with neurotoxicity for whom data is available.

*Cardiovascular:* Hypotension occurred in 3.8% of the patients and required therapy in 0.7% of the patients. Dysrhythmia occurred in 4.1% of the patients and was severe in 0.7% of the patients. Other meaningful cardiovascular events included hypertension (2.4%) or heart failure (0.46%); the relationship of these findings to the administration of docetaxel has not been clearly defined.

*Infusion site reactions:* Infusion site reactions were generally mild and occurred in 5.6% of the patients, and consisted of hyperpigmentation, inflammation, redness or dryness of the skin, phlebitis or extravasation and swelling of the vein.

*Hepatic:* Increases in serum levels of AST, ALT, bilirubin and alkaline phosphatase greater than 2.5 times the ULN were observed in less than 5% of the patients.

*Others:* Alopecia was observed in a total of 79% of patients but was considered severe in about 67% of the patients. Alopecia was reversible in 13% of the patients for whom data is available; the median recovery time was 22 weeks following the initial hair loss. Asthenia was observed in 62.6% of patients and was severe in 11.2% of the patients. Arthralgias and myalgias were observed in 8.6% and 20% of the patients, respectively and were generally considered mild to moderate. Dyspnea was reported in 16.1% (2.7% severe) of the patients and was frequently associated with acute hypersensitivity reactions, respiratory infections, and cancerous lung involvement. Generalised or localised pain has been observed in 16.5% of the patients and was severe in 0.8% of patients. Chest pain was seen in 4.5% of patients (0.4% severe) without any cardiac or respiratory involvement.

*Overdose:* There were two reports of overdose. One patient received 150 mg/m$^2$ and the other received 200 mg/m$^2$ of docetaxel as a one hour infusion. They both recovered after experiencing severe neutropenia, mild asthenia, cutaneous reactions and mild paresthesia.

In case of overdose, the patient should be kept in a specialised unit and vital functions closely monitored. There is no known antidote for docetaxel overdose. The primary anticipated complications of overdose would consist of bone marrow suppression, peripheral neurotoxicity and mucositis.

**Pharmacological properties**

*Pharmacodynamic properties:* Pharmaco-therapeutic group: Antineoplastic agents.

*Preclinical data:* Docetaxel is an antineoplastic agent which acts by promoting the assembly of tubulin into stable microtubules and inhibits their disassembly which leads to a marked decrease of free tubulin. The binding of docetaxel to microtubules does not alter the number of protofilaments. Docetaxel has been shown *in vitro* to disrupt the microtubular network in cells which is essential for vital mitotic and interphase cellular functions. Docetaxel was found to be cytotoxic *in vitro* against various murine and human tumour cell lines and against freshly excised human tumour cells in clonogenic assays. Docetaxel achieves high intracellular concentrations with a long cell residence time. In addition, docetaxel was found to be active on some but not all cell lines overexpressing the *p*-glycoprotein which is encoded by the multidrug resistance gene. *In vivo*, docetaxel is schedule independent and has a broad spectrum of experimental antitumour activity against advanced murine and human grafted tumours.

*Clinical data: Breast cancer:* Six phase II studies were conducted in patients with locally advanced or metastatic breast carcinoma. A total of 117 patients had received no prior chemotherapy (previously untreated) and 111 patients had received prior chemotherapy (previously treated) which included 83 patients who had progressive disease during anthracycline therapy (anthracycline resistant). In these clinical trials, docetaxel was administered at a 100 mg/m$^2$ dose given as a one-hour infusion every 3 weeks.

The overall response rate (ORR) was 56% in the anthracycline resistant patients with a 4.4% complete response rate (CR). A 46% ORR was observed in the anthracycline refractory patients with 7.3% CR. The median duration of response was 27 weeks in the anthracycline resistant patients and 28 weeks in the anthracycline refractory patients. The median survival time was 11 months in the anthracycline-resistant patients. There was a high response rate in patients with visceral metastases, 53.1% in the 49 anthracycline resistant patients. In anthracycline resistant patients, a significant response rate of 40% was seen in patients with liver metastases and a 63.2 % response rate was observed in patients with soft tissue disease. However, due to lack of data from comparative randomised clinical trials, the exact benefit/risk ratio has not yet been established.

*Pharmacokinetic properties:* The pharmacokinetics of docetaxel have been evaluated in cancer patients after administration of 20-115 mg/m$^2$ in Phase I studies. The kinetic profile of docetaxel is dose independent and consistent with a three-compartment pharmacokinetic model with half lives for the $\alpha$, $\beta$ and $\gamma$ phases of 4 min, 36 min and 11.1 h, respectively. The late phase is due, in part, to a relatively slow efflux of docetaxel from the peripheral compartment. Following the administration of a 100 mg/m$^2$ dose given as a one-hour infusion a mean peak plasma level of 3.7 μg/ml was obtained with a corresponding AUC of 4.6 h.μg/ml. Mean values for total body clearance and *steady-state* volume of distribution were 21 l/h/m$^2$ and 113 l, respectively. Interindividual variation in total body clearance was approximately 50%. Docetaxel is more than 95% bound to plasma proteins. A study of $^{14}$C-docetaxel has been conducted in three cancer patients. Docetaxel was eliminated in both the urine and faeces following cytochrome P450-mediated oxidative metabolism of the tert-butyl ester group, within seven days, the urinary and faecal excretion accounted for about 6% and 75% of the administered radioactivity, respectively. About 80% of the radioactivity recovered in faeces is excreted during the first 48 hours as one major inactive metabolite and 3 minor inactive metabolites and very low amounts of unchanged drug. A population pharmacokinetic analysis has been performed with docetaxel in 577 patients. Pharmacokinetic parameters estimated by the model were very close to those estimated from Phase I studies. The pharmacokinetics of docetaxel were not altered by the age or sex of the patient. In a small number of patients (n=23) with clinical chemistry data suggestive of mild to moderate liver function impairment (ALT, AST ≥1.5 times the ULN associated with alkaline phosphatase ≥ 2.5 times the ULN), total clearance was lowered by 27% on average (see *Posology and Method of Administration* section). Docetaxel clearance was not modified in patients with mild to moderate fluid retention and there is no data available in patients with severe fluid retention.

*Preclinical safety data:* The carcinogenic potential of docetaxel has not been studied. Docetaxel has been shown to be mutagenic in the in vitro micronucleus and chromosome aberration test in CHO-K1 cells and in the in vivo micronucleus test in the mouse. However, it did not induce mutagenicity in the Ames test or the CHO/HGPRT gene mutation assay. These results are consistent with the pharmacological activity of docetaxel.

Adverse effects on the testis observed in rodent toxicity studies suggest that docetaxel may impair male fertility.

**Pharmaceutical particulars**

*List of excipients:* Each ml of docetaxel solution contains 40 mg docetaxel anhydrous and 1040 mg polysorbate 80 and each ml of solvent contains 13% ethanol in water for injections.

*Incompatibilities:* None known.

*Shelf-life:* Vials of Taxotere concentrate for infusion should be stored under refrigeration and protected from bright light. The shelf-life under these conditions is 12 months for Taxotere 20 mg and 15 months for Taxotere 80 mg. Freezing does not adversely affect the product.

*Special precautions for storage:* Vials should be stored under refrigeration and protected from bright light.

*Nature and contents of container:* The Taxotere 20 mg vial is a 7 ml clear glass vial with a green flip-off cap and for 80 mg a 15 ml clear glass vial with a red flip-off cap. The Taxotere 20 mg and 80 mg vials contain a solution of docetaxel in polysorbate 80 at a concentration of 40 mg/ml. Each Taxotere 20 mg vial contains 0.59 ml equivalent to 23.6 mg docetaxel. Each Taxotere 80 mg vial contains 2.36 ml equivalent to 94.4 mg docetaxel. These volumes have been established during the development of Taxotere to compensate for liquid loss during preparation of the premix due to foaming, adhesion to the walls of the vial and 'dead-volume'. Overfilling ensures that after dilution with the entire contents of the accompanying solvent for Taxotere vial, there is minimum extractable premix volume corresponding to the labelled amount per vial.

*Solvent for Taxotere:* The solvent for Taxotere 20 mg vial is a 7 ml clear glass vial and for Taxotere 80 mg a 15 ml clear glass vial with a transparent colourless flip-off cap containing 1.83 ml and 7.33 ml respectively of a 13% w/w solution of ethanol in water for injections.

*Taxotere 20 mg:* Each blister carton contains one single-dose vial of Taxotere (docetaxel) equivalent to 20 mg docetaxel (anhydrous) in 0.5 ml polysorbate 80 (Fill: 23.6 mg/0.59 ml) and one single-dose solvent for Taxotere vial containing 1.83 ml 13% ethanol in water for injections.

*Taxotere 80 mg:* Each blister carton contains one single-dose vial of Taxotere (docetaxel) equivalent to 80 mg docetaxel (anhydrous) in 2 ml polysorbate 80 (Fill: 94.4 mg/2.36 ml) and one single-dose solvent for Taxotere vial containing 7.33 ml 13% ethanol in water for injections.

*Instructions for use/handling:*
*Recommendations for safe handling:* Taxotere is an antineoplastic agent and, as with other potentially toxic compounds, caution should be exercised when handling it and preparing Taxotere solutions. The use of gloves is recommended. If Taxotere concentrate, premix solution or infusion solution should come into contact with skin, wash immediately and thoroughly with soap and water. If Taxotere concentrate, premix solution or infusion solution should come into contact with mucous membranes, wash immediately and thoroughly with water.

*Preparation for intravenous administration:*
(a) *Preparation of the Taxotere premix solution (10 mg docetaxel/ml):* Remove the required number of Taxotere boxes from the refrigerator and allow to stand at room temperature for 5 minutes. Using a syringe fitted with a needle, aseptically withdraw the entire contents of the solvent for Taxotere vial. Inject the entire contents of the syringe into the corresponding Taxotere vial. Remove the syringe and needle and shake the mixture manually for 15 seconds.

Allow the premix vial to stand for 5 minutes at room temperature and then check that the solution is homogenous and clear (foaming is normal even after 5 minutes due to the presence of polysorbate 80 in the formulation).

(b) *Preparation of the infusion solution:* More than one premix vial may be necessary to obtain the required dose for the patient. Based on the required dose for the patient expressed in mg, aseptically withdraw the corresponding premix volume containing 10 mg/ml docetaxel from the appropriate number of premix vials using graduated syringes fitted with a needle. For example, a dose of 140 mg docetaxel would require 14 ml docetaxel premix solution. Inject the required premix volume into a 250 ml infusion bag or bottle containing either 5% glucose solution or 0.9% sodium chloride solution. If a dose greater than 200 mg of docetaxel is required, use a larger volume of the infusion vehicle so that a concentration of 0.9 mg/ml docetaxel is not exceeded. Mix the infusion bag or bottle manually using a rocking motion.

The Taxotere infusion solution should be administered intravenously within four hours including a one hour infusion time under room temperature and normal lighting conditions. As with all parenteral products, Taxotere premix solution and infusion solution should be visually inspected prior to use, solutions containing a precipitate should be discarded.

*Disposal:* All materials that have been used for dilution and administration should be disposed of according to standard procedures.

**Marketing authorisation numbers**
Taxotere 20 mg      EU/1/95/002/001
Taxotere 80 mg      EU/1/95/002/002

**Date of approval/revision of SPC**  April 1997

**Legal category** POM

## TILADE* INHALER AND SYNCRONER

**Qualitative and quantitative composition**  Nedocromil sodium 2.0 mg per actuation.

**Pharmaceutical form**  Tilade is presented as a metered dose pressurised aerosol containing nedocromil sodium as a suspension in chlorofluorocarbon propellants, for inhalation.

**Clinical particulars**

*Therapeutic indications:* Tilade is recommended for the treatment of bronchial asthma where regular preventative anti-inflammatory therapy is indicated and in particular in patients whose asthma is not adequately controlled by bronchodilators alone. Tilade may be given in addition to all existing therapies and in many cases will provide added therapeutic benefit.

*Posology and method of administration:* Adults (including the elderly) and children over the age of 6 years: Initially two actuations (4 mg of nedocromil sodium) four times daily. Once symptomatic control

has been achieved, the usual maintenance dosage is two actuations twice daily.

Tilade is intended for regular daily usage and should not be used for the relief of symptoms in an acute attack.

*Contra-indications:* Tilade is contra-indicated in patients with known hypersensitivity to any constituent of the formulation.

*Special warnings and special precautions for use:* Tilade should not be used for the relief of an acute attack of bronchospasm.

*Interaction with other medicaments and other forms of interaction:* None known.

*Use during pregnancy and lactation:* Studies in pregnant and lactating animals have failed to reveal a hazard. However, as with all medications caution should be exercised, especially during the first trimester of pregnancy.

On the basis of animal studies and its physicochemical properties it is considered that only negligible amounts of nedocromil sodium may pass into human breast milk. There is no information to suggest that the use of nedocromil sodium by nursing mothers has any undesirable effects on the baby.

*Effect on ability to drive and use machines:* Tilade has no known effect on ability to drive or operate machinery.

*Undesirable effects:* The principal side-effects reported are headache and upper gastro-intestinal tract symptoms (nausea, vomiting, dyspepsia and abdominal pain). These are usually mild and transient. In common with other inhaled medications, Tilade may produce cough or bronchospasm.

*Overdose:* Animal studies have not shown evidence of toxic effects of nedocromil sodium even at high dosage, nor have extended human studies revealed any safety hazard with the drug. Overdosage is unlikely, therefore to cause problems.

However, if overdosage is suspected, treatment should be supportive and directed to the control of the relevant symptoms.

**Pharmacological properties**

*Pharmacodynamic properties:* Tilade contains nedocromil sodium, a non-steroid agent, which has anti-inflammatory properties when administered topically in the lung. In-vivo, ex-vivo and in-vitro studies have shown that nedocromil sodium has beneficial effects on cellular, humoral and neuronal mechanisms thought to be involved in the inflammation of bronchial asthma. In the treatment of bronchial asthma, nedocromil sodium reduces bronchospasm, cough and bronchial hyperreactivity and improves objective measurements of lung function.

*Pharmacokinetic properties:* Nedocromil can be detected in the plasma for several hours after administration of a dose of 4 mg by inhalation. Approximately 5% of the inhaled dose was found to be absorbed with a rate of constant which was lower than the elimination rate constant; this means that absorption from the lungs is rate limiting. After oral administration, the extent of absorption was low (0.7 to 1.7%) and was shown to occur over a period of at least 72 hours. Following multiple dosing by inhalation, there was no accumulation, although the slow oral absorption contributed to the small carry-over that occurred from day to day.

Intravenous administration was used to study the elimination process from the body. The results demonstrated nedocromil to have a high clearance (10 ml $min^{-1}$ $kg^{-1}$) due largely to excretion. The major route was via the urine (70%) the remainder via the alimentary tract.

Plasma protein binding was moderate and readily reversible.

No metabolism of the compound was detected.

*Preclinical safety data:* Animal studies have failed to reveal toxic effects with nedocromil sodium even at high doses.

**Pharmaceutical particulars**

*List of excipients:* Dentomint; saccharin sodium; sorbitan trioleate; Propellant mixture 12:114 (dichlorodifluoromethane and dichlorotetrafluoroethane).

*Incompatibilities (major):* None known.

*Shelf life:* Thirty-six months.

*Special precautions for storage:* Store below 30°C, away from direct sunlight, do not freeze. The canister is pressurised and must not be punctured or burnt even when empty.

*Nature and contents of container:* A metered dose pressurised aerosol containing nedocromil sodium with Dentomint and saccharin as a suspension in chlorofluorocarbon propellants.

*Tilade Inhaler:* The aluminium can is fitted with a metering valve delivering 56 actuations (each containing 2 mg of nedocromil sodium per shot from the

valve or 1.75 mg from the adapter mouthpiece). The pack consists of an aerosol can and a plastic adapter with a dust cap.

*Tilade Syncroner:* The aluminium can is fitted with a metering valve delivering 112 actuations. Each pack contains two canisters, each with a spacer device.

*Instructions for use/handling:* Please refer to enclosed package insert.

**Marketing authorisation number**  0113/0140

**Date of approval/revision of SPC**  July 1995.

**Legal category** POM

## TILARIN*

**Presentation**  Tilarin Nasal spray is presented as a preserved aqueous solution containing 1% w/v nedocromil sodium in a metered dose, spray pack for nasal administration.

*Inactive ingredients:* Benzalkonium chloride, disodium edetate, sodium chloride.

**Uses**
*Indications:* Tilarin is indicated for the prophylactic treatment of seasonal allergic rhinitis and for the treatment of symptoms, including rhinorrhoea and sneezing, once they have developed.

*Pharmacology:* Tilarin, a preparation for nasal administration, contains nedocromil sodium which has been demonstrated to possess anti-inflammatory and anti-allergic properties.

Around 4% of a dose of nedocromil sodium 1% nasal spray is absorbed into the systemic circulation. 80% of the absorbed drug is reversibly bound to plasma proteins. Nedocromil sodium is not metabolised but excreted unchanged in bile and urine. The drug is cleared very rapidly from the circulation and accumulation does not occur.

**Dosage and administration**
*Adults (including the elderly) and children over 12 years:* One spray per nostril four times a day. A total daily dose is 10.4 mg.

Tilarin should be used regularly to ensure optimum control of symptoms. It is recommended that Tilarin is continued throughout the period of exposure to allergen.

The safety and efficacy of Tilarin in children under the age of 12 years has not been established. It is recommended that Tilarin should not be used in this age group.

**Contra-indications, warnings, etc**
*Contra-indications:* Known hypersensitivity to nedocromil sodium, benzalkonium chloride or other constituents of the formulation.

*Warnings and precautions:* None.

*Side-effects:* Few side effects have been reported, principally mild nasal irritation (nasal burning, stinging and soreness). Some patients have reported a distinctive taste.

*Use in pregnancy and lactating women:* Studies in pregnant and lactating animals have failed to reveal a hazard with nedocromil sodium. No recommendation can be made at present for the use of this preparation in pregnant and lactating women. As with all medicines caution should be exercised during pregnancy (especially during the first trimester) and whilst breast feeding.

*Overdosage:* Animal studies have not shown evidence of toxic effects of nedocromil sodium even at high doses. In the event of an overdose, no action other than medical supervision should be necessary. Some sensitive individuals may experience a mild facial warmth which is self-limiting.

*Interactions:* None have been reported.

*Effect on ability to drive or operate machinery:* Tilarin has no known affect on the ability to drive or operate machinery. Additionally, no sedative effects have been reported following the administration of Tilarin.

**Pharmaceutical precautions**  Store below 25°C away from direct sunlight. Discard any remaining contents eight weeks after first opening.

**Legal category** POM.

**Package quantities**  Tilarin is presented in a 15 ml opaque white high density polyethylene bottle fitted with a metered dose pump unit and yellow actuator. Instructions for use are included in each pack.

**Further information**  Nil.

**Product licence number** 0113/0150

## UBRETID*

**Presentation:**  White tablets marked 'UBRETID' with single break line on reverse. Each tablet contains 5 mg distigmine bromide. Other ingredients include lactose.

**Uses:** Anticholinesterase. Post-operative urinary retention. Post operative ileus and intestinal atony. To assist emptying of the neurogenic bladder. As an adjunct in the treatment of myasthenia gravis.

Distigmine bromide is an anticholinesterase with a much longer duration of action than neostigmine or pyridostigmine. In man, maximum inhibition of plasma for approximately 24 hours returning to normal after 48 hours. cholinesterase occurs nine hours after a single intramuscular dose of 0.5 mg Ubretid, and persists for approximately 24 hours returning to normal after 48 hours.

**Dosage and administration**
*Adults:*

*In prevention of urinary retention, ileus or intestinal atony following surgery:* 1 Ubretid Tablet may be given daily half-an-hour before breakfast.

*In neurogenic bladder:* 1 Ubretid Tablet daily or on alternate days, half-an-hour before breakfast, on an empty stomach.

*In myasthenia gravis. Adults:* Dosage to be individualised for each patient, dependent upon the severity of the condition, the degree and duration of response and the side-effects encountered. The tablets should always be taken on an empty stomach half an hour before breakfast. Dosage should commence at 1 tablet daily and may be adjusted at intervals of three to four days to a total not exceeding 4 tablets daily.

*Children:* Up to 2 tablets daily, according to age.

*Elderly:* No dosage adjustment is necessary for elderly patients.

Ubretid tablets are for oral administration.

**Contra-indications, warnings etc** Ubretid is contra-indicated in cases of severe postoperative shock, serious circulatory insufficiency, severe constipation, serious spastic and mechanical ileus, asthma and mechanical urinary obstruction.

*Warnings:* Because of the pharmacological action of Ubretid, caution should be taken in conditions where the potentition of the effects of acetylcholine is undesirable eg. cardiac dysfunction, bronchospasm, peptic ulcer, oesophagitis, epilepsy and Parkinsonism. Use with caution in patients receiving concomitantly drugs acting on the cardiovascular system eg. beta blockers, drugs with local anaesthetic properties and muscle relaxants. In myasthenia gravis, where short-acting cholinergic drugs are taken concurrently, their dosage should be reduced to the minimum required to control symptoms. The patient should be supervised in the early stages of dose titration to guard against the possibility of myasthenic crisis or cholinergic crisis.

*Use in pregnancy and lactation:* Ubretid should be avoided during pregnancy. No information is available on lactation.

*Adverse effects:* The pharmacological effects of Ubretid indicate the following side effects may occur infrequently: bradycardia, AV block, hypotension, bronchospasm, dyspnoea, increased bronchial secretions, sweating, salivation and lacrimation, muscle twitching, abdominal cramps, diarrhoea, urinary frequency and miosis. These effects of Ubretid may be controlled with atropine 2 mg intramuscularly; atropinisation should be maintained for at least 24 hours.

*Overdosage:* Excessive doses of Ubretid may also produce skeletal muscle fatigue, weakness and eventually paralysis. The muscarinic effects of overdosage may be controlled with atropine 2 mg intramuscularly repeated at intervals indicated by the clinical response until signs of mild atropinisation (dry mouth, mydriasis) appear. The patient should be kept fully atropinised for at least 24 hours.

**Pharmaceutical precautions** No special precautions.

**Legal category** POM.

**Package quantities** Tablets: Containers of 30 x 5 mg.

**Further information** Nil.

**Product licence number** 5272/0029.

## UNIVER*

**Presentation** Univer capsules are a sustained release formulation of verapamil having clinical efficacy over a full 24 hours with once daily dosing. The product is available in three strengths: 120 mg sustained release Verapamil Hydrochloride BP as a yellow/dark blue capsule, marked V120; 180 mg sustained release Verapamil Hydrochloride BP as a yellow capsule marked V180; and 240 mg sustained release Verapamil Hydrochloride BP as a yellow/dark blue capsule, marked V240.

**Uses**
*Indications:* Univer is recommended for the long term treatment of mild to moderate hypertension and angina pectoris.

*Mode of action:* Calcium antagonists are a group of agents that selectively inhibit calcium influx into cells. In the myocardium two calcium specific channels exist. Fast channels are involved in the initiation of contraction and slow channels in sustaining contraction. Calcium antagonists interfere with calcium movement through slow channels. As a result verapamil tends to increase the refractory period between the contractions of the heart, and reduce excitability.

In smooth vascular muscle this action on calcium channels results in the reduction of muscle tone leading to dilatation of the blood vessels. This effect is most prominent in blood vessels with high tone or in vessels subject to spasm. Verapamil increases arterial blood flow with minimal changes in venous capacitance. This action of verapamil is responsible for the reduction in blood pressure that is observed.

In the coronary artery vasculature verapamil increases blood flow by reducing coronary vessel tone and abolishing vasospasm, increasing oxygen delivery to all areas of the myocardium. This increased level of oxygen delivery results clinically in an effective treatment for angina pectoris.

**Dosage and administration**
*Adults: Hypertension:* Initial dose in patients new to verapamil therapy should be 120 mg o.d. This can be increased to 240 mg o.d., which is the normal maintenance dosage. The dose may be further increased to a maximum of 480 mg o.d. if required. *Angina:* The usual dose is 360 mg once daily. Dosage may be increased to a maximum of 480 mg daily if required.

*Elderly patients:* Elderly patients show enhanced bioavailability of verapamil and therapeutic control may be achieved with lower doses in this patient population.

*Children:* Univer is not recommended in children as no studies have been undertaken.

**Contra-indications, warnings, etc**
*Contra-indications:* Significant bradycardia (less than 50 bpm): second or third degree heart block; sick sinus syndrome or uncontrolled heart failure. Verapamil should not be used when atrial flutter/fibrillation complicates Wolff-Parkinson-White syndrome. Porphyria.

*Precautions:* Verapamil hydrochloride has an action that alters conduction in the heart and should be used with caution in first degree heart block. Patients with atrial flutter/fibrillation in association with Wolff-Parkinson-White Syndrome may develop increased conduction across the anomalous pathway and ventricular tachycardia may be precipitated. It also has an effect that reduces the contractility of the myocardium and this action may aggravate or occasionally precipitate heart failure in borderline cases. In circumstances where there is pre-existing poor ventricular function it is prudent to treat this condition before initiating therapy with Univer.

Special care should be taken in hypotension especially in acute myocardial infarction as this is a condition where atrioventricular conduction defects may develop and contractility may be impaired.

In view of the action of beta-adrenoceptor blocking agents which may tend to interfere with conduction and decrease contractility, verapamil should be used with caution in combination with beta-blocking agents, and a period between stopping beta-blocker therapy and starting Univer Capsules may be advisable.

Verapamil is extensively metabolised in the liver and special care should be taken in cases where liver damage exists, as plasma levels of verapamil may be increased.

Caution is required when verapamil hydrochloride is given with digoxin therapy as the plasma digoxin level may rise.

*Use in pregnancy and lactation:* The use of all therapeutic agents, including verapamil, requires special care in pregnancy. Although there is no evidence of teratogenicity for verapamil hydrochloride, its use in the first trimester should be avoided if at all possible. Verapamil hydrochloride is excreted in breast milk; it is recommended that the product should not be administered to nursing mothers.

*Side-effects:* Few adverse reactions have been reported in patients taking Univer Capsules. Constipation may occur and flushing has been recorded. Headaches are uncommon. Very infrequently nausea, vomiting and allergic reactions have been observed. On very rare occasions, a reversible impairment of liver function characterised by an increase in transaminases and/or alkaline phosphatase may occur during verapamil treatment and is most probably a hypersensitivity reaction.

*Treatment of overdosage:* Normal resuscitation procedures should be initiated in the event of cardiovascular collapse, i.e., if atrioventricular conduction defects such as second or third degree block develop these should be treated in the usual way using atropine, isoprenaline or temporary insertion of a pacemaker, as required. Hypotension may be observed, requiring repositioning of the patient with head tilted down, and if persistent, and in the absence of any conduction defect, treatment with systemic dopaminergic agents, such as dopamine, dobutamine or noradrenaline, should be started.

**Pharmaceutical precautions** Store in a cool, dry place.

**Legal category** POM.

**Package quantities** For both 120 mg and 240 mg presentations: Blister strips of 14 capsules, two strips per carton of 28 capsules (OP).

For the 180 mg presentation: Blister strips of 14 capsules, four strips per carton of 56 capsules (OP).

**Further information** In hypertension, patients new to verapamil therapy may be started on 120 mg once daily. Univer Capsules have been found to give good control of blood pressure, with more than 70% of mild to moderate hypertensives showing a good response with up to 240 mg once daily. Two week intervals should be allowed before changing to higher doses, to a maximum of 480 mg once daily. In the few patients who fail to respond to the highest dose, a thiazide may be introduced to produce an additional fall in blood pressure.

**Product licence numbers**

| | |
|---|---|
| Univer 120 mg Capsules | 5272/0039 |
| Univer 180 mg Capsules | 5272/0040 |
| Univer 240 mg Capsules | 5272/0041 |

## VALLERGAN* TABLETS

**Qualitative and quantitative composition** Trimeprazine tartrate BP (alimemazine tartrate (rINN)) 10 mg

**Pharmaceutical form** Circular, film coated biconvex tablet with bevelled edge, dark blue in colour, one face impressed V/10. The reverse side is plain

**Clinical particulars**

*Therapeutic indications:* Vallergan is used in the management of urticaria and pruritus and in premedication for anaesthesia in children.

*Posology and method of administration:* The product is administered orally. Not recommended for infants less than 2 years old.

*Urticaria and pruritus:* Adults: 10 mg two or three times daily; up to 100 mg per day have been used in intractable cases. Elderly: Dosage should be reduced to 10 mg once or twice daily. Children over 2 years of age: 2.5–5 mg three or four times daily.

*Pre-anaesthetic medication:* The dosage for children is best achieved by use of Vallergan Syrup or Vallergan Forte Syrup.

*Contra-indications:* Vallergan should be avoided in patients with hepatic or renal dysfunction, epilepsy, Parkinson's disease, hypothyroidism, phaeochromocytoma, myasthenia gravis, prostatic hypertrophy. It should be avoided in patients known to be hypersensitive to phenothiazines or with history of narrow angle glaucoma.

*Special warnings and special precautions for use:* Vallergan should be used with caution in the elderly, particularly in very hot or very cold weather (risk of hyper-hypothermia). The elderly are particularly susceptible to postural hypotension.

*Interaction with other medicaments and other forms of interaction:* The CNS depressant actions of phenothiazines may be intensified (additively) by alcohol, barbiturates and other sedatives. Respiratory depression may occur.

The hypotensive effect of most antihypertensive drugs especially alpha adrenoreceptor blocking agents may be exaggerated by phenothiazines.

The mild anticholinergic effect of phenothiazines may be enhanced by other anticholinergic drugs possibly leading to constipation, heat stroke, etc

The action of some drugs may be opposed by phenothiazines; these include amphetamine, levodopa, clonidine, guanethidine, adrenaline.

Anticholinergic agents may reduce the antipsychotic effect of phenothiazines.

Some drugs interfere with absorption of phenothiazines: antacids, anti-Parkinson, lithium. Increases or decreases in the plasma concentrations of a number of drugs, eg propranolol, phenobarbitone have been observed but were not of clinical significance.

High doses of phenothiazines reduce the response to hypoglycaemic agents, the dosage of which may have to be raised. Adrenaline must not be used in patients overdosed with phenothiazines.

Most of the above interactions are of a theoretical nature and not dangerous

*Pregnancy and lactation:* There is inadequate evidence of the safety of Vallergan in human pregnancy, but it has been widely used for many years without apparent ill consequence. Some phenothiazines have shown evidence of harmful effects in animals. Vallergan, like other drugs, should be avoided in pregnancy unless the physician considers it essential. Neuroleptics may occasionally prolong labour and at such a time should be withheld until the cervix is dilated 3-4cm. Possible adverse effects on the neonate include lethargy or paradoxical hyperexcitability, tremor and low Apgar score. Phenothiazines may be excreted in milk: breast feeding should be suspended during treatment.

*Effects on ability to drive and use machines:* Patients should be warned about drowsiness during the early days of treatment, and advised not to drive or operate machinery.

*Undesirable effects:* Minor side-effects of phenothiazines are nasal stuffiness, dry mouth, insomnia, agitation. *Liver function:* Jaundice, usually transient, occurs in a very small percentage of patients taking phenothiazines. A premonitory sign may be a sudden onset of fever after one to three weeks of treatment followed by the development of jaundice. Neuroleptic jaundice has the biochemical and other characteristics of obstructive jaundice and is associated with obstructions of the canaliculi by bile thrombi; the frequent presence of an accompanying eosinophilia indicates the allergic nature of this phenomenon. Treatment should be withheld on the development of jaundice. *Cardiorespiratory:* hypotension, or pallor may occur in children. Elderly or volume depleted subjects are particularly susceptible to postural hypotension. Cardiac arrhythmias, including atrial arrhythmia, A-V block, ventricular tachycardia and fibrillation have been reported during phenothiazine therapy, possibly related to dosage. Pre-existing cardiac disease, old age, hypokalaemia and concurrent tricyclic antidepressants may predispose. ECG changes, usually benign, include widened QT interval, ST depression, U-waves and T-wave changes. Respiratory depression is possible in susceptible patients. *Blood picture:* A mild leukopenia occurs in up to 30% of patients on prolonged high dosage of phenothiazines. Agranulocytosis may occur rarely; it is not dose related. The occurrence of unexplained infections or fever requires immediate haematological investigation. *Extrapyramidal:* Acute dystonias or dyskinesias, usually transitory are commoner in children and young adults and usually occur within the first 4 days of treatment or after dosage increases. Akathisia characteristically occurs after large doses. Parkinsonism is commoner in adults and the elderly. It usually develops after weeks or months of treatment. One or more of the following may be seen: tremor, rigidity, akinesia or other features of Parkinsonism. Commonly just tremor. Tardive dyskinesia: If this occurs it is usually, but not necessarily, after prolonged or high dosage. It can even occur after treatment has been stopped. Dosage should therefore be kept low whenever possible. *Skin and eyes:* contact skin sensitisation is a serious but rare complication in those frequently handling preparations of phenothiazines: Care must be taken to avoid contact of the drug with the skin. Skin rashes of various kinds may also be seen in patients treated with the drug. Patients on high dosage should be warned that they may develop photosensitivity in sunny weather and should avoid exposure to direct sunlight. Ocular changes and the development of a metallic greyish-mauve coloration of exposed skin have been noted in some individuals, mainly females, who have received chlorpromazine continuously for long periods (four to eight years). *Endocrine:* hyperprolactinaemia which may result in galactorrhoea, gynaecomastia, amenorrhoea: impotence. Neuroleptic malignant syndrome (hyperthermia, rigidity, autonomic dysfunction and altered consciousness) may occur with any phenothiazine

*Overdose:* Symptoms of phenothiazine overdosage include drowsiness or loss of consciousness, hypotension, tachycardia, ECG changes, ventricular arrhythmias and hypothermia. Severe extra-pyramidal dyskinesias may occur. If the patient is seen sufficiently soon (up to 6 hours) after ingestion of a toxic dose, gastric lavage may be attempted. Pharmacological induction of emesis is unlikely to be of any use. Activated charcoal should be given. There is no specific antidote. Treatment is supportive. Generalised vasodilatation may result in circulatory collapse; Raising the patient's legs may suffice, in severe cases, volume expansion by intravenous fluids may be needed; infusion fluids should be warmed before administration in order not to aggravate hypothermia. Positive inotropic agents such as dopamine may be tried if fluid replacement is insufficient to correct the circulatory collapse. Peripheral vasoconstrictor agents are not generally recommended; avoid the use of adrenaline. Ventricular or supraventricular tachyarrhythmias usually respond to restoration of normal body temperature and correction of circulatory or metabolic disturbances. If persistent or life-threatening, appropriate anti-arrhythmic therapy may be

considered. Avoid lignocaine and, as far as possible, long acting anti-arrhythmic drugs.

Pronounced central nervous system depression requires airway maintenance or, in extreme circumstances, assisted respiration. Severe dystonic reactions, usually respond to procyclidine (5-10 mg) or orphenadrine (20-40 mg) administered intramuscularly or intravenously. Convulsions should be treated with intravenous diazepam. Neuroleptic malignant syndrome should be treated with cooling. Dantrolene sodium may be tried.

**Pharmacological properties**

*Pharmacodynamic properties:* Trimeprazine has a central sedative effect, comparable to that of chlorpromazine, but largely devoid of the latter's anti-adrenaline action. It has powerful antihistamine and anti-emetic actions.

*Pharmacokinetic properties:* There is little information about blood levels, distribution and excretion in humans. The rate of metabolism and excretion of phenothiazines decreases in old age.

**Pharmaceutical particulars**

*List of excipients:* Microcrystalline cellulose BP, Lactose spray dried BP, Colloidal Silicone Dioxide, Magnesium stearate BP, Sodium starch glycollate BP, Hydroxypropyl Methylcellulose, Polyethylene glycol 200, Blue opaspray M-1-4229 (purified water PhEur, Indigo Carmine, Titanium Dioxide PhEur, Industrial Methylated Spirits 74 OP BP, Hydroxypropyl methylcellulose USP/PhEur), Demineralised water BP

*Incompatibilities:* None stated

*Shelf life:* 36 months

*Special Precautions for storage:* Protect from light. Store below 30 °C

*Nature and contents of container:* Blister pack containing 28 tablets

*Instructions for use/handling:* Not applicable

**Marketing authorisation number** 0012/5303R

**Date of approval/revision of SPC** February 1997

**Legal category** POM

## VALLERGAN*

**Presentation**
*Syrup:* A clear bright straw-coloured apricot-flavoured syrupy liquid containing 7.5 mg trimeprazine tartrate in each 5 ml. It contains 68% w/v sugars, ethanol, sodium sulphite, sodium metabisulphite and sodium benzoate.

*Forte syrup:* A clear colourless/pale yellow apricot-flavoured syrupy liquid containing 30 mg trimeprazine tartrate in each 5 ml. It contains 68% w/v of sugars, ethanol, sodium sulphite, sodium metabisulphite and sodium benzoate.

**Uses** Trimeprazine has a central sedative effect comparable to that of chlorpromazine, but largely devoid of the latter's anti-adrenaline action. It has powerful antihistamine and anti-emetic actions.

Vallergan is used in: Urticaria and pruritus, premedication for anaesthesia.

*Kinetics:* There is little information about blood levels, distribution and excretion in humans. The rate of metabolism and excretion of phenothiazines decreases in old age.

**Dosage and administration** Not recommended for infants less than 2 years old.
*Urticaria and pruritus: Adults:* 10 mg two or three times daily; up to 100 mg per day have been used in intractable cases. *Elderly:* Dosage should be reduced to 10 mg once or twice daily. *Children:* 2.5–5 mg three or four times daily.
*Pre-anaesthetic medication (children aged 2–7 years):* The maximum dosage of Vallergan or Vallergan Forte syrup recommended for this indication is 2 mg per kg bodyweight.

**Contra-indications, warnings, etc**
*Use in pregnancy and lactation:* There is inadequate evidence of the safety of Vallergan in human pregnancy, but it has been widely used for many years without apparent ill consequence. Some phenothiazines have shown evidence of harmful effects in animals. Vallergan, like other drugs, should be avoided in pregnancy unless the physician considers it essential. Neuroleptics may occasionally prolong labour and at such a time should be withheld until the cervix is dilated 3–4 cm. Possible adverse effects on the neonate include lethargy or paradoxical hyperexcitability, tremor and low Apgar score. Phenothiazines may be excreted in milk; breast feeding should be suspended during treatment.

*Contra-indications:* Vallergan should be avoided in patients with hepatic or renal dysfunction, epilepsy, Parkinson's disease, hypothyroidism, phaeochromo-

cytoma, myasthenia gravis, prostatic hypertrophy. It should be avoided in patients known to be hypersensitive to phenothiazines or with history of narrow angle glaucoma.

*Precautions:* It should be used with caution in the elderly, particularly during very hot or very cold weather (risk of hyper-hypothermia). Patients should be warned about drowsiness during the early days of treatment, and advised not to drive or operate machinery. The elderly are particularly susceptible to postural hypotension.

*Interactions of phenothiazines:* The CNS depressant actions of these agents may be intensified (additively) by alcohol, barbiturates and other sedatives. Respiratory depression may occur.

The hypotensive effect of most antihypertensive drugs especially alpha adrenoreceptor blocking agents may be exaggerated by phenothiazines.

The mild anticholinergic effect of phenothiazines may be enhanced by other anticholinergic drugs possibly leading to constipation, heat stroke, etc.

The action of some drugs may be opposed by phenothiazines; these include amphetamine. levodopa, clonidine, guanethidine, adrenaline.

Anticholinergic agents may reduce the antipsychotic effect of phenothiazines.

Some drugs interfere with absorption of phenothiazines: antacids, anti-Parkinson, lithium. Increases or decreases in the plasma concentrations of a number of drugs, e.g. propranolol, phenobarbitone have been observed but were not of clinical significance.

High doses of phenothiazines reduce the response to hypoglycaemic agents, the dosage of which might have to be raised. Adrenaline must not be used in patients overdosed with phenothiazines. Most of the above interactions are of a theoretical nature and not dangerous.

*Adverse effects:* Minor side-effects of phenothiazines are nasal stuffiness, dry mouth, insomnia, agitation. *Liver function:* Jaundice, usually transient, occurs in a very small percentage of patients taking phenothiazines. A premonitory sign may be a sudden onset of fever after one to three weeks of treatment followed by the development of jaundice. Neuroleptic jaundice has the biochemical and other characteristics of obstructive jaundice and is associated with obstructions of the canaliculi by bile thrombi; the frequent presence of an accompanying eosinophilia indicates the allergic nature of this phenomenon. Treatment should be withheld on the development of jaundice. *Cardiorespiratory:* Hypotension, or pallor may occur in children. Elderly or volume depleted subjects are particularly susceptible to postural hypotension. Cardiac arrhythmias, including atrial arrhythmia, A-V block, ventricular tachycardia and fibrillation have been reported during phenothiazine therapy, possibly related to dosage. Pre-existing cardiac disease, old age, hypokalaemia and concurrent tricyclic antidepressants may predispose. ECG changes, usually benign, include widened QT interval, ST depression, U-waves and T-wave changes. Respiratory depression is possible in susceptible patients. *Blood picture:* A mild leukopenia occurs in up to 30% of patients on prolonged high dosage of phenothiazines. Agranulocytosis may occur rarely; it is not dose related. The occurrence of unexplained infections or fever requires immediate haematological investigation. *Extrapyramidal:* Acute dystonias or dyskinesias, usually transitory are more common in children and young adults, and usually occur within the first 4 days of treatment or after dosage increases. Akathisia characteristically occurs after large doses. Parkinsonism is more common in adults and the elderly. It usually develops after weeks or months of treatment. One or more of the following may be seen: tremor, rigidity, akinesia or other features of Parkinsonism. Commonly just tremor. Tardive dyskinesia: If this occurs it is usually, but not necessarily, after prolonged or high dosage. It can even occur after treatment has been stopped. Dosage should therefore be kept low whenever possible. *Skin and eyes:* Contact skin sensitisation is a serious but rare complication in those frequently handling preparations of certain phenothiazines; care must be taken to avoid contact of the drug with the skin. Skin rashes of various kinds may also be seen in patients treated with the drug. Patients on high dosage should be warned that they may develop photosensitivity in sunny weather and should avoid exposure to direct sunlight. Ocular changes and the development of a metallic greyish-mauve coloration of exposed skin have been noted in some individuals mainly females, who have received chlorpromazine continuously for long periods (four to eight years). *Endocrine:* Hyperprolactinaemia which may result in galactorrhoea, gynaecomastia, amenorrhoea; impotence. Neuroleptic malignant syndrome (hyperthermia, rigidity, autonomic dysfunction and altered consciousness) may occur with any phenothiazine.

*Toxicity and treatment of overdosage:* Symptoms of phenothiazine overdosage include drowsiness or loss of consciousness, hypotension, tachycardia, ECG changes, ventricular arrhythmias and hypothermia. Severe extra-pyramidal dyskinesias may occur.

If the patient is seen sufficiently soon (up to 6 hours) after ingestion of a toxic dose, gastric lavage may be attempted. Pharmacological induction of emesis is unlikely to be of any use. Activated charcoal should be given. There is no specific antidote. Treatment is supportive.

Generalised vasodilation may result in circulatory collapse; raising the patient's legs may suffice, in severe cases, volume expansion by intravenous fluids may be needed; infusion fluids should be warmed before administration in order not to aggravate hypothermia.

Positive inotropic agents such as dopamine may be tried if fluid replacement is insufficient to correct the circulatory collapse. Peripheral vasoconstrictor agents are not generally recommended; avoid the use of adrenaline.

Ventricular or supraventricular tachy-arrhythmias usually respond to restoration of normal body temperature and correction of circulatory or metabolic disturbances. If persistent or life threatening, appropriate anti-arrhythmic therapy may be considered. Avoid lignocaine and, as far as possible, long acting anti-arrhythmic drugs.

Pronounced central nervous system depression requires airway maintenance or, in extreme circumstances, assisted respiration. Severe dystonic reactions usually respond to procyclidine (5–10 mg) or orphenadrine (20–40 mg) administered intramuscularly or intravenously. Convulsions should be treated with intravenous diazepam.

Neuroleptic malignant syndrome should be treated with cooling. Dantrolene sodium may be tried.

**Pharmaceutical precautions**  Protect from light. Store below 25°C. Vallergan Syrup and Vallergan Forte Syrup may be diluted if required, using simple syrup (without preservative).

**Legal category**  POM.

**Package quantities**  Syrup: Bottles of 100 ml (OP). Forte syrup: Bottles of 100 ml (OP).

**Further information**  Nil.

**Product licence numbers**
Syrup　　　0012/5019
Forte syrup　0012/5018.

## ZIMOVANE*

### Presentation
*Zimovane:* White, film-coated tablets impressed 'ZM'. Each tablet contains 7.5 mg zopiclone. The tablets also contain lactose, hydroxypropyl methylcellulose, microcrystalline cellulose and sodium equivalant to a maximum of 0.2 mg per tablet.

*Zimovane LS* (low strength): Blue film coated tablets impressed Z. Each tablet contains 3.75 mg zopiclone. The tablets also contain lactose, hydroxypropyl methylcellulose, microcrystalline cellulose and sodium equivalent to 0.1 mg per tablet.

### Uses
*Pharmacology:* Zopiclone is a non-benzodiazepine hypnotic agent, a member of the cyclopyrrolone group of compounds which is structurally unrelated to other hypnotics and tranquillisers. It rapidly initiates and sustains sleep without reduction of total REM sleep and with preservation of slow wave sleep. Negligible residual effects are seen the following morning. Its pharmacological properties include hypnotic, sedative, anxiolytic, anticonvulsant and muscle-relaxant actions. These are related to its high affinity and specific agonist action at central receptors belonging to the GABA macromolecular receptor complex modulating the opening of the chloride ion channel. However, it has been shown that zopiclone and other cyclopyrrolones act on a different site to those of benzodiazepines inducing different conformational changes in the receptor complex.

Zopiclone has a short elimination half life of approximately 5 hours, with no significant accumulation of drug substance or metabolites on repeated dosage.

*Indications:* Zimovane tablets are indicated for the short term treatment of insomnia, including difficulties in falling asleep, nocturnal awakening and early awakening, transient, situational or chronic insomnia, and insomnia secondary to psychiatric disturbances, in situations where the insomnia is debilitating or is causing severe distress for the patient.

Long term continuous use is not recommended. A course of treatment should employ the lowest effective dose .

*Treatment duration:* Transient insomnia 2-5 days. Short term insomnia 2-3 weeks. A single treatment should not continue for longer than 4 weeks including any tapering off.

**Dosage and administration**  Each tablet should be swallowed whole without sucking, chewing or breaking.

*Adults:* The recommended dose is 7.5 mg zopiclone (one Zimovane tablet) by the oral route shortly before retiring.

*Elderly:* A lower dose of 3.75 mg zopiclone (one Zimovane LS tablet) should be employed to start treatment in the elderly. Depending on effectiveness and acceptability, the dosage subsequently may be increased if clinically necessary.

*Patients with hepatic insufficiency:* As elimination of zopiclone may be reduced in patients with hepatic dysfunction a lower dose of 3.75 mg zopiclone nightly is recommended. The standard dose of 7.5 mg zopiclone may be used with caution in some cases, depending on effectiveness and acceptability.

*Renal insufficiency:* Accumulation of zopiclone or its metabolites has not been seen during treatment of insomnia in patients with renal insufficiency. However it is recommended that patients with impaired renal function should start treatment with 3.75 mg.

**Contra-indications, warnings, etc**  Zimovane is contra-indicated in patients with myasthenia gravis, respiratory failure, severe sleep apnoea syndrome, severe hepatic insufficiency and those people with a hypersensitivity to zopiclone.

As with all hypnotics Zimovane should not be used in children

*Use during pregnancy:* Experience of the use of zopiclone during pregnancy in humans is limited although there have been no adverse findings in animals. Use in pregnancy is therefore not recommended. If the product is prescribed to a woman of child bearing potential, she should be advised to contact her physician about stopping the product if she intends to become pregnant, or suspects that she is pregnant.

Moreover, if zopiclone is used during the last three months of pregnancy or during labour, due to the pharmacological action of the product, effects on the neonate, such as hypothermia, hypnotic and respiratory depression can be expected.

Infants born to mothers who took benzodiazepines or benzodiazepine-like agents chronically during the latter stages of pregnancy may have developed physical dependence and may be at some risk of developing withdrawal symptoms in the postnatal period.

*Use during lactation:* Zopiclone is excreted in breast milk and use in nursing mothers must be avoided.

*Use in hepatic insufficiency:* A reduced dosage is recommended, see above.

*Use in renal insufficiency:* A reduced dosage is recommended, see above.

*Risk of dependence:* Clinical experience to date with Zimovane suggests that the risk of dependence is minimal when the duration of treatment is limited to not more than 4 weeks.

Use of benzodiazepines and benzodiazepine-like agents ( even at therapeutic doses) may lead to the development of physical and psychological dependence upon these products. The risk of dependence increases with dose and duration of treatment; it is also greater in patients with a history of alcohol and/ or drug abuse, or those who have marked personality disorders. The decision to use a hypnotic in such patients should be taken only with this clearly in mind. If physical dependence has developed, abrupt termination of treatment will be accompanied by withdrawal symptoms. These may consist of headaches, muscle pain, extreme anxiety, tension, restlessness, confusion and irritability. In severe cases the following symptoms may occur: derealisation, depersonalisation, hyperacusis, numbness and tingling of the extremities, hypersensitivity to light, noise and physical contact, hallucinations or epileptic seizures. Rare cases of abuse have been reported.

*Withdrawal:* The termination of treatment with Zimovane is unlikely to be associated with withdrawal effects when duration of treatment is limited to 4 weeks. Patients may benefit from tapering of the dose before discontinuation.

*Depression:* As with other hypnotics, zopiclone does not constitute a treatment for depression. Any underlying cause of the insomnia should also be addressed before symptomatic treatment.

*Tolerance:* Some loss of efficacy to the hypnotic effect of benzodiazepines and benzodiazepine-like agents may develop after repeated use for a few weeks. However with Zimovane there is an absence of any marked tolerance during treatment periods of up to 4 weeks.

*Rebound insomnia* is a transient syndrome where the symptoms which led to treatment with a benzodiazepine or benzodiazepine-like agent recur in an enhanced form on discontinuation of therapy. It may be accompanied by other reactions including mood changes, anxiety and restlessness. Since the risk of withdrawal/ rebound phenomena may be increased after prolonged treatment, or abrupt discontinuation of therapy decreasing the dosage in a stepwise fashion may be helpful.

A course of treatment should employ the lowest effective dose for the minimum length of time necessary for effective treatment. See above for guidance on possible treatment regimens. A course of treatment should not continue for longer than 4 weeks including any tapering off.

*Amnesia:* Amnesia is rare, but anterograde amnesia may occur, especially when sleep is interrupted or when retiring to bed is delayed after taking the tablet. To reduce the frequency of this possible event, patients should ensure that:
– they take the tablet strictly when retiring for the night
– they are able to have a full nights sleep.

*Interactions:* The sedative effect of zopiclone may be enhanced when used in combination with alcohol. Concomitant use is therefore not recommended. In particular this could affect the patients ability to drive or use machines the next day.

In combination with CNS depressants an enhancement of the central depressive effect may occur. The therapeutic benefit of co-administration with antipsychotics (neuroleptics), hypnotics, anxiolytics/sedatives, antidepressant agents, narcotic analgesics, anti epileptic drugs, anaesthetics and sedative antihistamines should therefore be carefully weighed. Concomitant use of benzodiazepine or benzodiazepine-like agents with narcotic analgesics may enhance their euphoric effect and could lead to an increase in psychic dependence. Compounds which inhibit certain hepatic enzymes (particularly cytochrome P450) may enhance the activity of benzodiazepines and benzodiazepine-like agents.

*Adverse effects:* A mild bitter or metallic after-taste is the most frequently reported adverse effect. Less commonly, mild gastrointestinal disturbances, including nausea and vomiting, dizziness, headache, drowsiness and dry mouth have occurred.

Psychological and behavioural disturbances, such as irritability, aggressiveness, confusion, depressed mood, anterograde amnesia, hallucinations and nightmares have been reported. Rarely these reactions may be severe and may be more likely to occur in the elderly

Rarely allergic and allied manifestations such as urticaria or rashes have been observed and, more rarely, light headedness and incoordination.

Although residual effects are rare and generally of minor significance, patients should be advised not to drive or operate machinery the day after treatment until it is established that their performance is unimpaired.

Withdrawal and rebound insomnia have occasionally been observed on discontinuation of treatment, mainly in association with prolonged treatment.

*Overdosage:* Overdose is usually manifested by varying degrees of central nervous system depression ranging from drowsiness to coma according to the quantity ingested. Overdose should not be life-threatening unless combined with other CNS depressants (including alcohol). Symptomatic and supportive treatment in an adequate clinical environment is recommended. Attention should be paid to respiratory and cardiovascular functions. Gastric lavage is only useful when performed soon after ingestion. Haemodialysis is of no value due to the large volume of distribution of zopiclone. Flumazenil may be a useful antidote.

**Pharmaceutical precautions**  Protect from light. Store in a dry place below 30°C.

**Legal category**  POM

**Package quantities**  Zimovane tablets are available in containers of 100 tablets and blister packs of 28 tablets (OP).

Zimovane LS tablets are available in blister packs of 28 tablets (OP).

**Further information**  Nil.

**Product licence numbers**
Zimovane　　　0012/0259
Zimovane LS　　0012/0260

*Trade Mark

# Richborough Pharmaceuticals
## A Division of Pfizer Limited
## Sandwich
## Kent, CT13 9NJ

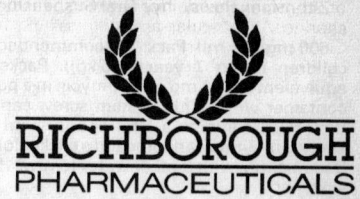

## ZITHROMAX* CAPSULES
## ZITHROMAX* SUSPENSION

**Qualitative and quantitative composition** Active ingredient: azithromycin. Zithromax Capsules contain azithromycin dihydrate equivalent to 250 mg azithromycin.

Zithromax Powder for Oral Suspension is a dry blend of azithromycin dihydrate containing the equivalent of 200 mg azithromycin per 5 ml on reconstitution with water.

**Pharmaceutical form** Zithromax Capsules are white, hard gelatin capsules marked Pfizer and ZTM 250.

Zithromax Powder for Oral Suspension is a dry powder which reconstitutes with water to give a cherry/banana flavoured suspension with a slight vanilla odour.

### Clinical particulars

*Therapeutic indications:* Zithromax is indicated for infections caused by susceptible organisms; in lower respiratory tract infections including bronchitis and pneumonia, skin and soft tissue infections, otitis media and in upper respiratory tract infections including sinusitis and pharyngitis/tonsillitis.

In sexually transmitted diseases in men and women, Zithromax is indicated in the treatment of uncomplicated genital infections due to *Chlamydia trachomatis.*

*Posology and method of administration:* Zithromax should be given as a single daily dose. In common with many other antibiotics Zithromax Capsules should be taken at least 1 hour before or 2 hours after food.

*Adults:* For the treatment of sexually transmitted diseases caused by *Chlamydia trachomatis,* the dose is 1 g given as a single dose.

For all other indications, the dose is 1.5 g which should be given 500 mg daily for 3 days.

*In the elderly:* The same dose range as in younger patients may be used in the elderly.

*In children:* Zithromax Suspension should be used for children under 45 kg. There is no information on children under 6 months of age. The dose in children is 10 mg/kg as a single daily dose for 3 days:

| | |
|---|---|
| Up to 15 kg: (less than 3 years) | Measure the dose as closely as possible using 5 ml oral dosing syringe provided. The syringe is graduated in 0.25 ml divisions, providing 10 mg of azithromycin in every graduation. |

For children weighing more than 15 kg, Zithromax suspension should be administered using the spoon provided according to the following guidance:

| | |
|---|---|
| 15–25 kg: (3–7 years) | 5 ml (200 mg), given as 1×5 ml spoonful, once daily for 3 days. |
| 26–35 kg: (8–11 years) | 7.5 ml (300 mg), given as 2×3.75 ml spoonfuls, once daily for 3 days. |
| 36–45 kg: (12–14 years) | 10 ml (400 mg), given as 2×5 ml spoonfuls, once daily for 3 days. |
| Over 45 kg: | Dose as per adults. |

See *Nature and contents of container* for appropriate pack size to use depending on age/body weight of child.

The specially supplied measure should be used to administer Zithromax suspension to children.

*In patients with renal impairment:* No dosage adjustment is needed in patients with mild renal impairment (creatinine clearance >40 ml/min). For patients with more severe renal impairment see *Special warnings and special precautions for use.*

*In patients with hepatic impairment:* See *Special warnings and special precautions for use.*

Zithromax Capsules and Zithromax Suspension are for oral administration only.

*Contra-indications:* Zithromax is contra-indicated in patients with a known hypersensitivity to azithromycin or any of the macrolide antibiotics.

Because of the theoretical possibility of ergotism, Zithromax and ergot derivatives should not be co-administered.

*Special warnings and special precautions for use:* As with erythromycin and other macrolides, rare serious allergic reactions, including angioneurotic oedema and anaphylaxis, have been reported. Some of these reactions with Zithromax have resulted in recurrent symptoms and required a long period of observation and treatment.

As with any antibiotic preparation, observations for signs of superinfection with non-susceptible organisms, including fungi is recommended.

*Use in renal impairment:* No dose adjustment is needed in patients with mild renal impairment (creatinine clearance >40 ml/min), but there are no data regarding Zithromax in patients with more severe renal impairment, thus caution should be exercised in using Zithromax in these patients.

*Use in hepatic impairment:* As the liver is the principal route of excretion of azithromycin, it should not be used in patients with hepatic disease.

*Interaction with other medicaments and other forms of interaction:*

*Antacids:* In patients receiving Zithromax and antacids, Zithromax should be taken at least 1 hour before or 2 hours after the antacid.

*Carbamazepine:* In a pharmacokinetic interaction study in healthy volunteers, no significant effect was observed on the plasma levels of carbamazepine or its active metabolite.

*Cimetidine:* A single dose of cimetidine administered 2 hours before Zithromax had no effect on the pharmacokinetics of azithromycin.

*Cyclosporin:* Some of the related macrolide antibiotics interfere with the metabolism of cyclosporin. In the absence of conclusive data from pharmacokinetic studies or clinical data investigating potential interactions between Zithromax and cyclosporin, caution should be exercised before coadministration of these two drugs. If coadministration is necessary, cyclosporin levels should be monitored and the dose adjusted accordingly.

*Digoxin:* Some of the macrolide antibiotics have been reported to impair the metabolism of digoxin (in the gut) in some patients. Therefore, in patients receiving concomitant Zithromax and digoxin the possibility of raised digoxin levels should be borne in mind and digoxin levels monitored.

*Ergot derivatives:* Because of the theoretical possibility of ergotism, Zithromax and ergot derivatives should not be co-administered.

*Methylprednisolone:* In a pharmacokinetic interaction study in healthy volunteers, Zithromax had no significant effect on the pharmacokinetics of methylprednisolone.

*Theophylline:* There is no evidence of any pharmacokinetic interaction when Zithromax and theophylline are co-adminstered to healthy volunteers. In general, however, theophylline levels should be monitored.

*Warfarin:* In a pharmacodynamic interaction study, Zithromax did not alter the anticoagulant effect of a single 15 mg dose of warfarin administered to healthy volunteers. Zithromax and warfarin may be co-administered, but monitoring of the prothrombin time should be continued as routinely performed.

*Terfenadine:* Zithromax did not affect the pharmacokinetics of terfenadine administered at the recommended dose of 60 mg every 12 hours. Addition of Zithromax did not result in any significant changes in cardiac repolarisation (QTc interval) measured during the steady state dosing of terfenadine.

*Use during pregnancy and lactation:*

*Use in pregnancy:* Animal reproduction studies have demonstrated that azithromycin crosses the placenta, but have revealed no evidence of harm to the foetus. There are no adequate and well controlled studies in pregnant women. Since animal studies are not always predictive of human response, Zithromax should be used during pregnancy only if adequate alternatives are not available.

*Use in lactation:* No data on secretion of azithromycin in breast milk are available, so Zithromax should only be used in lactating women where adequate alternatives are not available.

*Effects of ability to drive and use machines:* There is no evidence to suggest that Zithromax may have an effect on a patient's ability to drive or operate machinery.

*Undesirable effects:* Zithromax is well tolerated with a low incidence of side effects. Most side effects observed were mild to moderate in severity.

The majority of side effects were gastrointestinal in origin with nausea, abdominal discomfort (pain/cramps), vomiting, flatulence, diarrhoea and loose stools being occasionally observed.

Allergic reactions such as rash or photosensitivity have occurred and there have also been rare reports of serious hypersensitivity reactions – see Special Warnings/Precautions.

Reversible elevations in liver transaminases have been seen with a frequency similar to the comparative macrolides and penicillins used in clinical trials. Rarely, cases of cholestatic jaundice have been observed.

Transient mild reductions in neutrophil counts have occasionally been observed in clinical trials, although a causal relationship to Zithromax has not been established.

Hearing impairment: In investigational studies where higher doses were used for prolonged periods of time, reversible hearing impairment was seen in some patients.

*Overdose:* There are no data on overdosage with Zithromax. Typical symptoms of overdosage with macrolide antibiotics include hearing loss, severe nausea, vomiting and diarrhoea. Gastric lavage and general supportive measures are indicated.

### Pharmacological properties

*Pharmacodynamic properties:* Zithromax is an azalide, derived from the macrolide class of antibiotics. The mode of action of azithromycin is inhibition of protein synthesis in bacteria by binding to the 50s ribosomal subunit and preventing translocation of peptides.

Azithromycin demonstrates activity *in vitro* against a wide variety of Gram-positive and Gram-negative bacteria including: *Staphylococcus aureus, Streptococcus pneumoniae, Streptococcus pyogenes* (Group A) and other Streptococcal species; *Haemophilus influenzae* and *parainfluenzae; Branhamella catarrhalis;* anaerobes including *Bacteroides fragilis; Escherichia coli; Bordetella pertussis; Bordetella parapertussis; Borrelia burgdorferi; Haemophilus ducreyi; Neisseria gonorrhoeae* and *Chlamydia trachomatis.* Azithromycin also demonstrates *in vitro* activity against *Legionella pneumophila, Mycoplasma pneumoniae* and *hominis,* Campylobacter sp., *Toxoplasma gondii* and *Treponema pallidum.*

*Pharmacokinetic properties:* Following oral administration in humans, azithromycin is widely distributed throughout the body; bioavailability is approximately 37%. The time taken to peak plasma levels is 2–3 hours. The plasma terminal elimination half-life closely reflects the tissue depletion half-life of 2 to 4 days.

Kinetic studies have shown markedly higher azithromycin levels in tissue than in plasma (up to 50 times the maximum observed concentration in plasma) indicating that the drug is heavily tissue bound. Concentrations in target tissues such as lung, tonsil, and prostate exceed the MIC90 for likely pathogens after a single dose of 500 mg.

### Pharmaceutical particulars

*List of excipients:* Zithromax Capsules contain: Lactose, magnesium stearate, maize starch, and sodium lauryl sulphate. The capsule shells contain: Gelatin, iron oxide-black (E172), shellac, sulphur dioxide and titanium dioxide.

Zithromax Powder for Oral Suspension contains: Hydroxypropylcellulose, sodium phosphate tribasic anhydrous, sucrose, xanthan gum. Flavours: artificial banana, artificial cherry, artificial creme de vanilla.

*Incompatibilities:* None known.

*Shelf life:* Zithromax Capsules 4 years.

Powder for Oral Suspension 3 years. Once reconstituted with water, Zithromax Suspension has a shelf-life of 5 days.

*Special precautions for storage:* None.

*Nature and contents of container:* Zithromax Capsules are available as:
– Packs of 4 capsules. Aluminium/PVC blister strips, 4 capsules per strip, 1 strip in a carton box.
– Pack of 6 capsules. Aluminium/PVC blister strips, 6 capsules per strip, 1 strip in a carton box.

Zithromax Powder for Oral Suspension is available as:

600 mg (15 ml) Pack: (Recommended for use in children up to 7 years (25 kg)). Packs of powder equivalent to 600 mg azithromycin in a polypropylene container with child resistant screw cap, in a carton box. Pack contains a 5 ml spoon, 5 ml oral dosing syringe, a syringe adaptor and a sticker for the syringe. Reconstitute with 9 ml of water to give 15 ml suspension.

900 mg (22.5 ml) Pack: (Recommended for use in children from 8–11 years (26–35 kg)). Packs of powder equivalent to 900 mg azithromycin in a polypropylene container with child resistant screw cap, in a carton box. Pack contains a 3.75 ml spoon. Reconstitute with 12 ml of water to give 22.5 ml suspension.

1200 mg (30 ml) Pack: (Recommended for use in children aged from 12–14 years (36–45 kg)). Packs of powder equivalent to 1200 mg azithromycin in a polypropylene container with child resistant screw cap, in a carton box. Pack contains a 5 ml spoon. Reconstitute with 15 ml of water to give 30 ml suspension.

*Instructions for use/handling:* When dispensing the 15 ml pack, advice should be given as to whether the dose should be measured using the oral dosing syringe or the spoon provided. If the dose is to be given using the oral dosing syringe, before dispensing the syringe adaptor should be inserted into the bottle neck and the cap replaced. Also, the sticker should be used to mark the syringe at the appropriate level once the correct daily dosage has been calculated.

*Marketing authorisation holder:* Pfizer Limited, Ramsgate Road, Sandwich, Kent CT13 9NJ.

**Marketing authorisation numbers**

| | |
|---|---|
| Zithromax Capsules 250 mg | 0057/0335 |
| Zithromax Powder for Oral Suspension 200 mg/5 ml | 0057/0336 |

**Date of approval/revision of SPC**    April 1996.

**Legal category**    POM.

*Trade Mark

# Roche Products Limited
## PO Box 8
## Welwyn Garden City
## Hertfordshire AL7 3AY

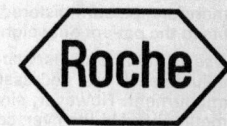

## ALCOBON*

**Presentation** Infusion bottles containing 2.5 g flucytosine PhEur in 250 ml isotonic sodium chloride solution. Other excipients are tromethamine and hydrochloric acid 25%. The solution is colourless to slightly yellow.

**Uses**
*Pharmacological properties:* Alcobon is a fluorinated pyrimidine effective in the treatment of certain systemic fungal infections. In fungi sensitive to the preparation, it acts as a competitive inhibitor of uracil metabolism.

*Pharmacokinetics:* Alcobon is widely distributed in body tissues and fluids (including cerebrospinal fluid). Binding to plasma proteins is minimal. Half-life of elimination is 3–6 hours in patients with normal renal function but this value increases in renal failure. The majority of the dose administered is excreted unchanged in the urine. Flucytosine can be removed by haemodialysis.

*Indications:* Alcobon is indicated for the treatment of systemic yeast and fungal infections due to sensitive organisms: such infections include cryptococcosis, candidiasis, chromomycosis and infections due to *Torulopsis glabrata* and *Hansenula*.

In the treatment of cryptococcal meningitis and severe systemic candidiasis it is recommended that Alcobon should be given in combination with amphotericin-B. Amphotericin-B may also be given in combination with Alcobon in severe or long-standing infections due to other organisms.

**Dosage and administration**
*Adults and children:* Alcobon for Infusion should be administered using a giving set incorporating a 15 micron filter. It may be administered directly into a vein, through a central venous catheter, or by intraperitoneal infusion. The recommended daily dosage in adults and children is 200 mg/kg body-weight divided into four doses over the 24 hours. In patients harbouring extremely sensitive organisms a total daily dose of 100 to 150 mg/kg body-weight may be sufficient. Adequate effects can, however, often be obtained with a lower dose.

It is suggested that the duration of the infusion should be of the order of 20 to 40 minutes provided this is balanced with the fluid requirements of the patient. As a rule, treatment with Alcobon for Infusion should rarely be required for periods of more than one week.

Since Alcobon is excreted primarily by the kidneys, patients with renal impairment should be given smaller doses. The following is suggested as a guide for dosage in patients with severe infection associated with renal impairment:
In patients with:
– creatinine clearance < 40 to > 20 ml/min: 50 mg/kg every 12 hours.
– creatinine clearance < 20 to > 10 ml/min: 50 mg/kg every 24 hours.
– creatinine clearance < 10 ml/min: an initial single dose of 50 mg/kg; subsequent doses should be calculated according to the results of regular monitoring of the serum concentration of the drug, which should not be allowed to exceed 80 micrograms/ml. Blood levels of 25 to 50 micrograms/ml are normally effective.

The duration of treatment should be determined on an individual basis.

The outcome of therapy will be affected by variations in the sensitivity of the infecting organism, its accessibility and its susceptibility to Alcobon, as well as by differences in the response of individual patients. In cases of cryptococcal meningitis, treatment should last for at least four months.

*Use in the elderly:* Although no specific studies have been performed to establish the use of Alcobon in the elderly, documented use indicates that the dosage requirements and side effects profile are similar to those of younger patients. Particular attention should be paid to renal function in this group.

Alcobon for Infusion is for intravenous or intraperitoneal administration.

Alcobon for Infusion may be given concurrently with other infusions of normal saline, glucose or glucose/saline. No other agent should be added to or mixed with Alcobon for Infusion.

**Contra-indications, warnings, etc**
*Contra-indications:* Alcobon is contra-indicated in patients who have shown hypersensitivity to flucytosine or any of the excipients.

*Use in pregnancy and lactation:* Teratogenic effects have been seen in rats, in which species flucytosine is metabolised to fluorouracil. The metabolism may differ in man: nevertheless, the use of Alcobon in pregnancy and in women of childbearing age requires that the potential benefits of therapy be weighed against its possible hazards. The drug should not be given to women breast feeding infants.

*Precautions:* The product should be used with great caution in patients with depression of bone marrow function or blood dyscrasias. Blood counts and tests of renal and hepatic function should be performed before and during treatment. This should occur at least weekly in patients with renal insufficiency or blood dyscrasias.

Alcobon should not be used in patients with impaired renal function in the absence of facilities for monitoring blood levels of the drug.

When measuring drug serum levels, it should be noted that levels of the drug in blood samples, taken during or immediately after administration of Alcobon for Infusion, are not a reliable guide to subsequent levels; it is advisable to remove blood for monitoring of blood levels of Alcobon shortly before starting the next infusion.

In calculating the fluid and electrolyte intake of patients with impaired renal function, cardiac failure or electrolyte imbalance, due allowance should be made for the volume and sodium content (138 millimole/litre) of Alcobon for Infusion.

*Side-effects and adverse reactions:* Nausea, vomiting, diarrhoea and skin rashes may occur but are usually of a transient nature.

Less frequently observed side effects include confusion, hallucinations, convulsions, headache, sedation and vertigo. Alterations in tests of liver function are generally dose related and reversible but hepatitis and hepatic necrosis have been reported. Bone marrow depression with leucopenia, thrombocytopenia, agranulocytosis or aplastic anaemia have been reported. This is more common when serum levels of flucytosine are high in patients with renal impairment and when amphotericin-B has been co-prescribed. Local irritation or phlebitis does not appear to be a problem with Alcobon for Infusion.

*Drug interactions:* There is contradictory evidence concerning a drug interaction between Alcobon and cytarabine. Strict monitoring of blood levels is required if the two medicines are given concurrently.

*Treatment of overdosage:* Haemodialysis produces a rapid fall in the serum concentration of Alcobon.

**Pharmaceutical precautions**
*Storage:* Alcobon for Infusion should be stored between 18°C and 25°C. If stored below 18°C, precipitation of Alcobon substance may occur, which should be redissolved by heating to 80°C for not more than 30 minutes.

Prolonged storage above 25°C could lead to the decomposition of Alcobon resulting in the formation of 5-fluorouracil.

*Additives:* Alcobon for Infusion may be given concurrently with other infusions of Sodium Chloride Intravenous infusion (0.9% w/v) BP, Glucose Intravenous Infusion (5% w/v) BP, or Sodium Chloride (0.18% w/v) and Glucose (4% w/v) Intravenous infusion BP. No other agent should be added to or mixed with Alcobon for Infusion.

**Legal category** POM

**Package quantities** Alcobon for Infusion 2.5 g in 250 ml in packs of 5.

**Further information**
*Availability:* Alcobon for Infusion is available to hospitals only.

*Sensitivity testing:* It is recommended that cultures for sensitivity testing be taken before treatment and repeated at regular intervals during therapy. However, it is not necessary to delay treatment until results of these tests are known.

To determine sensitivities, the methods of Shadomy (Appl. Microbiol., 1969, **17**, 871) and Scholer (Mykosen, 1970, **13**, 179) are recommended.

For sensitivity testing it is essential that culture media are free of antagonists to flucytosine.

**Product licence number** 0031/0094R

## ANEXATE*

**Presentation** Ampoules containing 500 micrograms flumazenil in 5 ml. The ampoule solution is almost colourless.

**Uses** *Properties:* Anexate, an imidazobenzodiazepine, is a specific competitive inhibitor of substances which act via the benzodiazepine receptors, specifically blocking their central effects. The hypnotic-sedative effects of the agonist are rapidly reversed by Anexate and may then reappear gradually within a few hours, depending on the half-life and dose ratio of the agonist and antagonist.

*Pharmacokinetics:* Flumazenil is moderately bound to plasma proteins. The drug's distribution parallels that of the benzodiazepines. It is extensively metabolised in the liver, primarily to the inactive carboxylic acid form, and has an elimination half-life of approximately 50 minutes.

*Indications:* Anexate is indicated for the complete or partial reversal of the central sedative effects of benzodiazepines. It may therefore be used in anaesthesia and intensive care in the following situations:
Termination of general anaesthesia induced and/or maintained with benzodiazepines.
Reversal of benzodiazepine sedation in short diagnostic and therapeutic procedures.
For the specific reversal of the central effects of benzodiazepines, to allow return to spontaneous respiration and consciousness, in patients in intensive care.

**Dosage and administration** Anexate is for slow intravenous injection or infusion. It should only be administered under the supervision of an experienced physician.

Anexate ampoule solution may be diluted with Sodium Chloride Intravenous Infusion BP, Sodium Chloride 0.45% and Dextrose 2.5% Intravenous Infusion BP or Dextrose 5% Intravenous Infusion BP. The resultant infusion solution should be used within 24 hours.

No preparations other than those recommended should be added to the Anexate ampoule or mixed with the Anexate infusion solution.

Anexate may be used concurrently with other resuscitative procedures.

*Adults:* The recommended initial dose is 200 micrograms administered intravenously over 15 seconds. If the desired level of consciousness is not obtained within 60 seconds a further dose of 100 micrograms can be injected and repeated at 60-second intervals where necessary, up to a maximum total dose of 1 mg or in intensive care situations, 2 mg. The usual dose required is 300-600 micrograms.

If drowsiness recurs, an intravenous infusion of 100-400 micrograms per hour may be employed. The rate of infusion should be individually adjusted to achieve the desired level of arousal.

The individually titrated, slow injections or infusions of Anexate should not produce withdrawal symptoms, even in patients exposed to high doses of benzodiazepines for long periods of time. If, however, unexpected signs of overstimulation occur, an individually titrated dose of diazepam (Valium Roche) or midazolam (Hypnovel) should be given by slow intravenous injection.

If a significant improvement in consciousness or respiratory function is not obtained after repeated doses of Anexate, a non-benzodiazepine aetiology must be assumed.

*Elderly:* No specific data are available on the use of Anexate in the elderly, but it should be remembered that this population is more sensitive to the effects of benzodiazepines and should be treated with due caution.

*Children:* There are insufficient data to make dosage recommendations for Anexate in children. It should, therefore, be administered only if the potential benefits to the patient outweigh the possible risks.

*Use in renal and hepatic insufficiency:* No dosage adjustments are necessary in patients with renal impairment. However, since flumazenil is primarily metabolised in the liver, careful titration of dosage is recommended in patients with impaired hepatic function.

### Contra-indications, warnings, etc

*Contra-indications:* Anexate is contra-indicated in patients with known hypersensitivity to benzodiazepines.

The use of Anexate is not recommended in epileptic patients who have been receiving benzodiazepine treatment for a prolonged period. Although Anexate exerts a slight intrinsic anticonvulsant effect, its abrupt suppression of the protective effect of a benzodiazepine agonist can give rise to convulsions in epileptic patients.

In mixed intoxications with benzodiazepines and tricyclic and/or tetracyclic antidepressants, the toxicity of the antidepressants can be masked by protective benzodiazepine effects. In the presence of autonomic (anticholinergic), neurological (motor abnormalities) or cardiovascular symptoms of severe intoxication with tricyclics/ tetracyclics, Anexate should not be used to reverse benzodiazepine effects.

*Use in pregnancy and lactation:* Like other benzodiazepine compounds, Anexate is expected to cross the placenta and to enter into breast milk, although the total quantities involved would be small. There has been little human usage but animal studies have shown no teratogenic potential. The established medical principle of only administering drugs in early pregnancy when considered absolutely necessary should therefore be observed.

Emergency use of Anexate during lactation is not contra-indicated.

*Precautions:* In view of the short duration of action of Anexate and the possible need for repeat doses, the patient should remain under close observation until all possible central benzodiazepine effects have subsided.

Rapid reversal of benzodiazepine sedation may increase the risk of raised intracranial pressure in severely head-injured patients.

Benzodiazepine agonists have a dependence potential when used chronically. Symptoms such as depression, nervousness, rebound insomnia, irritability, sweating and diarrhoea may arise following abrupt cessation of benzodiazepine agonists in patients treated for prolonged periods of time. Rapid injection of Anexate in such patients may trigger these withdrawal symptoms and should therefore be avoided.

Anexate should not be given in anaesthesia reversal until the effects of any neuromuscular blockade have cleared.

In high-risk patients, the advantages of counteracting the central nervous system depression associated with benzodiazepines should be weighed against the drawbacks of rapid awakening.

The dosage of Anexate should be adjusted individually to the needs of patients suffering from pre-operative anxiety or having a history of chronic or episodic anxiety. In anxious patients, particularly those with coronary heart disease, it is preferable to maintain a degree of sedation throughout the early post-operative period rather than bring about complete arousal.

The pain felt by patients in the post-operative period must be taken into account. Following a major intervention, it is preferable to maintain a moderate degree of sedation.

Patients who have received Anexate to reverse the effects of benzodiazepine sedation should be warned not to drive, to operate machinery or to engage in any other physically or mentally demanding activity for at least 24 hours, since the effect of the benzodiazepine may return.

*Side-effects and adverse reactions:* Anexate is generally well tolerated. In post-operative use, nausea and/ or vomiting are occasionally observed, particularly if opiates have also been employed. Flushing has also been noted. If patients are awakened too rapidly, they may become agitated, anxious or fearful. Very rarely, seizures have been reported, particularly in patients known to suffer from epilepsy. Transient increases in blood pressure and heart rate may occur on awakening in intensive care patients.

Any side-effects associated with Anexate usually subside rapidly without the need for special treatment.

Excessive and/or rapidly injected doses of Anexate may induce benzodiazepine withdrawal symptoms such as anxiety attacks, tachycardia, dizziness and sweating in patients on long-term benzodiazepine treatment. Such symptoms may be treated by slow intravenous injection of diazepam or midazolam (see *Dosage and Administration*).

*Drug interactions:* Anexate blocks the central effects of benzodiazepines by competitive interaction at the receptor level; the effects of non-benzodiazepines acting via the benzodiazepine receptor, such as zopiclone, are also blocked by Anexate. However, Anexate is ineffective when unconsciousness is due to other substances.

Interaction with other central nervous system depressants has not been observed. However, particular caution is necessary when using Anexate in cases of intentional overdosage since the toxic effects of other psychotropic drugs (especially tricyclic antidepressants) taken concurrently may increase with the subsidence of the benzodiazepine effect.

The pharmacokinetics of benzodiazepines are unaltered in the presence of Anexate.

*Treatment of overdosage:* Even when given intravenously at doses of 100 mg, no symptoms of overdosage attributable to Anexate have been observed.

### Pharmaceutical precautions   *Storage:* The recommended maximum storage temperature for Anexate ampoules is 30°C.

*Diluents:* Anexate ampoule solution may be diluted with Sodium Chloride Intravenous Infusion BP, Sodium Chloride 0.45% and Dextrose 2.5% Intravenous Infusion BP or Dextrose 5% Intravenous Infusion BP. The resultant infusion solution should be used within 24 hours.

No preparations other than those recommended should be added to the Anexate ampoule or mixed with the Anexate infusion solution.

### Legal category   POM.

### Package quantities   Anexate ampoules 500 micrograms per 5 ml in packs of 5.

### Further information   *Availability:* Anexate ampoules are available through hospitals, clinics or retail pharmacies.

### Product licence number   0031/0228

## CARDENE SR*

### Qualitative and quantitative composition   Nicardipine 45 mg.

### Pharmaceutical form   Sustained release capsules.

### Clinical particulars

*Therapeutic indications:* Treatment of mild to moderate hypertension.

*Posology and method of administration:* Capsules should be swallowed whole and not chewed.

*Adults:*
*Starting dose:* 30 mg every 12 hours titrating upwards as required.
*Usual effective dose:* 45 mg every 12 hours (range 30 to 60 mg every 12 hours).
Individually adjust the dose for each patient. Where appropriate Cardene SR may also be used in combination with beta-blockers and/or diuretics.

*Elderly:*
*Starting dose:* 30 mg every 12 hours. Titrating upwards with care as nicardipine may lower systolic pressure more than diastolic pressure in these patients.

*Children:* Cardene SR is not recommended for use in patients under the age of 18.

*Contra-indications:*
(I) Use in pregnancy and lactation.
(ii) Hypersensitivity to nicardipine hydrochloride, or other dihydropyridines because of the theoretical risk of cross-reactivity.
(iii) As part of the effect of nicardipine is secondary to reduced afterload, the drug should not be given to patients with advanced aortic stenosis. Reduction in diastolic pressure in these patients may worsen rather than improve myocardial oxygen balance.
(iv) Cardene should not be used in cardiogenic shock, clinically significant aortic stenosis, and during or within one month of a myocardial infarction.
(v) Cardene should not be used for secondary prevention of myocardial infarction.

*Special warnings and special precautions for use:* If used in combination with diuretics or beta-blockers, careful titration of Cardene SR is advised to avoid excessive reduction in blood pressure.

If switching from beta-blockers to Cardene SR, gradually reduce the beta-blocker dose (preferably over 8–10 days) since nicardipine gives no protection against the dangers of abrupt beta-blocker withdrawal.

Stop Cardene SR in patients experiencing ischaemic pain within 30 minutes of starting therapy or after increasing the dose.

*Use in patients with congestive heart failure or poor cardiac reserve:* Haemodynamic studies in patients with heart failure have shown that nicardipine reduces

afterload and improves overall haemodynamics. In one study, intravenous nicardipine reduced myocardial contractility in patients with severe heart failure despite increases in cardiac index and ejection fraction noted in the same patients.

Since nicardipine has not been extensively studied in patients with severe left ventricular dysfunction and cardiac failure, one must consider that worsening of cardiac failure may occur.

*Use in patients with impaired hepatic or renal function:* Since Cardene is subject to first pass metabolism, use with caution in patients with impaired liver function or reduced hepatic blood flow. Patients with severe liver disease showed elevated blood levels and the half-life of nicardipine was prolonged. Cardene blood levels may also be elevated in some renally-impaired patients. Therefore, the lowest starting dose and extending the dosing interval should be individually considered in these patients.

*Use in patients following a stroke (infarction or haemorrhage):* Avoid inducing systemic hypotension when administering Cardene SR to these patients.

*Laboratory tests:* Transient elevations of alkaline phosphatase, serum bilirubin, SGPT, SGOT and glucose, have been observed. BUN and creatinine may also become elevated. While out-of-range values were seen in $T_3$, $T_4$, and TSH, the lack of consistent alterations suggest that any changes were not drug-related.

Treatment with short acting nicardipine may induce an exaggerated fall in blood pressure and reflex tachycardia which can cause cardiovascular complications such as myocardial and cerebrovascular ischaemia.

There has been some concern about increased mortality and morbidity in the treatment of ischaemic heart disease using higher than recommended doses of some other short-acting dihydropyridines.

*Interaction with other medicaments and other forms of interaction:*

*Digoxin:* Careful monitoring of serum digoxin levels is advised in patients also receiving Cardene SR as levels may be increased.

*Propanolol, Dipyridamole, Warfarin, Quinidine, Naproxen:* Therapeutic concentrations of these drugs do not change the *in vitro* plasma protein binding of nicardipine.

*Cimetidine:* Cimetidine increases nicardipine plasma levels. Carefully monitor patients receiving both drugs.

*Fentanyl Anaesthesia:* Severe hypotension has been reported during fentanyl anaesthesia with concomitant use of a beta-blocker and calcium blockade. Even though such interactions have not been seen in clinical trials, such hypotensive episodes should be vigorously treated with conventional therapy such as intravenous fluids.

*Cyclosporin:* Monitor cyclosporin plasma levels and reduce dosage accordingly in patients concomitantly receiving nicardipine as elevated cyclosporin levels have been reported.

*Rifampicin:* Rifampicin can interact with other dihydropyridines to substantially reduce their plasma levels and so rifampicin and nicardipine should be used together with caution.

As with other dihydropyridines, nicardipine should not be taken with grapefruit juice because bioavailability may be increased.

Cardene may be used in combination with beta-blocking and other anti-hypertensive drugs but the possibility of an additive effect resulting in postural hypotension should be considered.

*Pregnancy and lactation:* See *Contra-indications.*

*Effects on ability to drive and use machines:* None known.

*Undesirable effects:* Most are expected consequences of the vasodilatory effects of Cardene SR. The most frequent side-effects reported are headache, pedal oedema, heat sensation and/or flushing, palpitations, nausea, and dizziness.

Other side-effects noted in clinical trials include the following:

*Cardiovascular system:* as with the use of other sustained-release, dihydropyridines in patients with ischaemic heart disease, exacerbation of angina pectoris may occur rarely at the start of treatment with Cardene SR. The occurrence of myocardial infarction has been reported although it is not possible to distinguish such an event from the natural course of ischaemic heart disease.

*Central nervous system:* drowsiness, insomnia, tinnitus, paraesthesiae, functional disorders.

*Skin:* itching, rashes.

*Hepato-renal:* impairment, frequency of micturition.

Dyspnoea, gastro-intestinal upset and, rarely, depression, impotence and thrombocytopenia, have also been reported.

*Overdose:* Symptoms may include marked hypotension, bradycardia, palpitations, flushing, drowsiness, confusion and slurred speech. In laboratory animals, overdosage also resulted in reversible hepatic function abnormalities, sporadic focal hepatic necrosis and progressive atrioventricular conduction block.

Use routine measures (e.g. gastric lavage), including monitoring of cardiac and respiratory functions. Position the patient to avoid cerebral anoxia. Frequent blood pressure determinations are essential. Vasopressors are clinically indicated for patients exhibiting the effects of calcium entry blockade.

### Pharmacological properties

*Pharmacodynamic properties:*

*Mode of action:* Cardene is a potent calcium channel blocker. Pharmacological studies suggest it is highly selective for the peripheral vasculature over the myocardium, accounting for its minimal negative inotropic effects and marked peripheral vasodilation when used clinically.

In mild to moderate hypertensive patients, Cardene SR has been shown to reduce blood pressure and maintain control over 24 hours, only if the doses are regularly administered exactly 12 hours apart.

*Electrophysiological effects:* Electrophysiological studies in man show that Cardene does not depress sinus node function or atrial or ventricular conduction in patients with either normal or diseased electrical conduction systems. Refractory periods of the His–Purkinje system were actually shortened slightly by nicardipine and SA conduction time was improved.

*Pharmacokinetic properties:* Cardene capsules are completely absorbed with plasma levels detectable as early as 20 minutes following an oral dose. Maximal plasma levels are generally achieved as a broad peak between one and four hours. The pharmacokinetics of Cardene SR are non-linear due to saturable first-pass metabolism. Following oral administration, increasing doses result in disproportionate increases in plasma levels, increasing the dose two-fold increases maximum plasma levels 4–5 fold. A similar disproportionate increase is observed with AUC. Cardene has somewhat lower bioavailability than the standard capsule formulation of Nicardipine (about 35% following a 30 mg oral standard capsule at steady state) except at the 60 mg dose. Minimum plasma levels produced by equivalent daily doses are similar. Cardene SR thus exhibits significantly reduced fluctuation in plasma levels in comparison to standard nicardipine capsules.

When Cardene SR is taken with a high fat meal, mean $C_{max}$ was 45% lower, AUC was 25% lower and trough levels were 75% higher than when Cardene SR was given in the fasting state. Thus, taking Cardene SR with the meal reduced the fluctuation in plasma levels.

Cardene is extensively metabolised by the liver; none of the metabolites possess significant biological activity.

*Preclinical safety data:* None stated.

### Pharmaceutical particulars

*List of excipients:* Pregelatinised starch BP, Magnesium stearate BP, Microcrystalline cellulose BP, Starch PhEur, Lactose PhEur, Methacrylic acid co-polymer US NF.

*Incompatibilities:* None known.

*Shelf life:* 60 months.

*Special precautions for storage:* Protect from light and excessive humidity. Store below 25°C.

*Nature and contents of container:*
Blister packs of 56.
Blister packs of 14.
Securitainers of 100.

*Instructions for use/handling:* No special instructions required.

**Marketing authorisation number** 0031/0464

**Date of approval/revision of SPC** March 1997

**Legal category** POM

## CARDENE*

**Qualitative and quantitative composition** Nicardipine 20 mg or 30 mg.

**Pharmaceutical form** Capsules.

**Clinical particulars**

*Therapeutic indications:* Cardene is indicated for the prophylaxis of patients with chronic stable angina and for the treatment of hypertension considered to be mild to moderate in severity.

*Posology and method of administration:* Cardene capsules are for oral administration.

Nicardipine should be taken with a little water.

*Prophylaxis of chronic stable angina:* Starting dose: 20 mg every eight hours titrating upwards as required. Usual effective dose: 30 mg every eight hours (range of total dose 60 mg–120 mg per day). Allow at least three days before increasing the dose of Cardene to ensure steady state plasma levels have been achieved.

*Hypertension:* Starting dose: 20 mg every eight hours titrating upwards as required. Usual effective dose: 30 mg every eight hours (range of total dose 60 mg–120 mg per day).

*Elderly:* Starting dose is 20 mg three times a day. Titrate upwards with care as nicardipine may lower systolic pressure more than diastolic pressure in these patients.

*Children:* Cardene is not recommended in patients under the age of 18.

*Contra-indications:*

(i) Pregnancy and lactation.

(ii) Hypersensitivity to nicardipine hydrochloride or other dihydropyridines because of the theoretical risk of cross-reactivity.

(iii) Because part of the effect of nicardipine is secondary to reduced afterload, the drug should not be given to patients with advanced aortic stenosis. Reduction in diastolic pressure in these patients may worsen rather than improve myocardial infarction.

(iv) Cardene should not be used in cardiogenic shock, clinically significant aortic stenosis, unstable angina, and during or within one month of a myocardial infarction.

(v) Cardene should not be used for acute attacks of angina.

(vi) Cardene should not be used for secondary prevention of myocardial infarction.

*Special warnings and special precautions for use:* If used in combination with diuretics or beta-blockers, careful titration of Cardene is advised to avoid excessive reduction in blood pressure.

If switching from beta-blockers to Cardene, gradually reduce the beta-blocker dose (preferably over 8–10 days) since nicardipine gives no protection against the dangers of abrupt beta-blocker withdrawal.

Stop Cardene in patients experiencing ischaemic pain within 30 minutes of starting therapy or after increasing the dose.

*Use in patients with congestive heart failure or poor cardiac reserve:* Haemodynamic studies in patients with heart failure have shown that nicardipine reduces afterload and improves overall haemodynamics. In one study, intravenous nicardipine reduced myocardial contractility in patients with severe heart failure despite increases in cardiac index and ejection fraction noted in the same patients.

Since nicardipine has not been extensively studied in patients with severe left ventricular dysfunction and cardiac failure one must consider that worsening of cardiac failure may occur.

*Use in patients with impaired hepatic or renal function:* Since Cardene is subject to first pass metabolism, use with caution in patients with impaired liver function or reduced hepatic blood flow. Patients with severe liver disease showed elevated blood levels and the half-life of nicardipine was prolonged. Cardene blood levels may also be elevated in some renally impaired patients. Therefore, the lowest starting dose and extending the dosing interval should be individually considered in these patients.

*Use in patients following a stroke (infarction or haemorrhage):* Avoid inducing systemic hypotension when administering Cardene to these patients.

*Laboratory tests:* Transient elevations of alkaline phosphatase, serum bilirubin, SGPT, SGOT and glucose, have been observed. BUN and creatinine may also become elevated. While out-of-range values were seen in T3, T4 and TSH, the lack of consistent alterations suggest that any changes were not drug-related.

Treatment with short-acting nicardipine may induce an exaggerated fall in blood pressure and reflex tachycardia which can cause cardiovascular complications such as myocardial and cerebrovascular ischaemia.

There has been some concern about increased mortality and morbidity in the treatment of ischaemic heart disease using higher than recommended doses of some other short-acting dihydropyridines.

*Interaction with other medicaments and other forms of interaction:*

*Digoxin:* Careful monitoring of serum digoxin levels is advised in patients also receiving Cardene as levels may be increased.

*Propranolol, Dipyridamole, Warfarin, Quinidine, Naproxen:* Therapeutic concentrations of these drugs do not change the *in vitro* plasma protein binding of nicardipine.

*Cimetidine:* Cimetidine increases nicardipine plasma levels. Carefully monitor patients receiving both drugs.

*Fentanyl Anaesthesia:* Severe hypotension has been reported during fentanyl anaesthesia with concomitant use of a beta-blocker and calcium blockade. Even though such interactions have not been seen in clinical trials, such hypotensive episodes should be vigorously treated with conventional therapy such as intravenous fluids.

*Cyclosporin:* Monitor cyclosporin plasma levels and reduce dosage accordingly in patients concomitantly receiving nicardipine as elevated cyclosporin levels have been reported.

*Rifampicin:* Rifampicin can interact with other dihydropyridines to substantially reduce their plasma levels and so rifampicin and nicardipine should be used together with caution.

As with other dihydropyridines, nicardipine should not be taken with grapefruit juice because bioavailability may be increased.

Cardene may be used in combination with beta-blocking and other anti-hypertensive drugs but possibility of an additive effect resulting in postural hypotension should be considered.

*Pregnancy and lactation:* See *Contra-indications*.

*Effects on ability to drive and use machines:* None known.

*Undesirable effects:* The majority are not serious and are expected consequences of the vasodilator effects of Cardene. The most frequent side-effects reported are headache, pedal oedema, heat sensation and/or flushing, palpitations, nausea and dizziness.

Other side-effects noted in clinical trials include the following:

*Cardiovascular system:* As with the use of other short-acting dihydropyridines in patients with ischaemic heart disease, exacerbation of angina pectoris may occur frequently at the start of treatment with nicardipine capsules. The occurrence of myocardial infarction has been reported although it is not possible to distinguish such an event from the natural course of ischaemic heart disease.

*Central nervous system:* Drowsiness, insomnia, tinnitus, paraesthesia, functional disorders.

*Skin:* Itching, rashes.

*Hepatorenal:* Impairment, frequency of micturition.

Dyspnoea, gastro-intestinal upset and, rarely, depression, impotence and thrombocytopenia, have also been reported.

*Overdose:* Symptoms may include marked hypotension, bradycardia, palpitations, flushing, drowsiness, confusion and slurred speech. In laboratory animals, overdosage also resulted in reversible hepatic function abnormalities, sporadic focal hepatic necrosis and progressive atrioventricular conduction block.

Use routine measures (e.g. gastric lavage), including monitoring of cardiac and respiratory functions. Position the patient to avoid cerebral anoxia. Frequent blood pressure determinations are essential. Vasopressors are clinically indicated for patients exhibiting the effects of calcium entry blockade.

### Pharmacological properties

*Pharmacodynamic properties:* Cardene is a potent calcium antagonist. Pharmacological studies demonstrate its preferential high selectivity for the peripheral vasculature over the myocardium which accounts for its minimal negative inotropic effects. Cardene produces smooth muscle relaxation and marked peripheral vasodilatation.

In man Cardene produces a significant decrease in systemic vascular resistance, the degree of vasodilatation being more predominant in hypertensive patients than in normotensive subjects. Haemodynamic studies in patients with coronary artery disease and normal left ventricular function have shown significant increases in cardiac index and coronary blood flow, with little if any increase in left ventricular end-diastolic pressure.

*Electrophysiologic effects:* Electrophysiological studies in man show that Cardene does not depress sinus node function or atrial or ventricular conduction in patients with either normal or decreased electrical conduction systems. Refractory periods of the His-Purkinje system were actually shortened slightly by nicardipine and SA conduction time was improved.

*Pharmacokinetic properties:*

*Pharmacokinetics and metabolism:* Nicardipine is rapidly and completely absorbed with plasma levels detectable 20 minutes following an oral dose. Maximal plasma levels are observed within 30 minutes to two hours (mean Tmax = 1 hour). When given with a high fat meal peak plasma levels are reduced by 30%. Nicardipine is subject to saturable first-pass metabolism and the bioavailability is about 35% following a 30 mg oral dose at steady state.

The pharmacokinetics of Cardene are non-linear due to saturable hepatic first pass metabolism.

Steady-state plasma levels are achieved after about 3 days of dosing at 20 and 30 mg tds and remain relatively constant over 28 days of dosing at 30 mg tds. Considerable intersubject variability in plasma levels is observed. Following dosing to steady state using doses of 30 mg and 40 mg (tds), the terminal plasma half-life of nicardipine averaged 8.6 hours.

Nicardipine is highly protein-bound (> 99%) in human plasma over a wide concentration range.

Nicardipine does not induce its own metabolism and does not induce hepatic microsomal enzymes.

*Preclinical safety data:* None stated.

**Pharmaceutical particulars**

*List of excipients:*
*20 and 30 mg Capsules*: Starch, Pregelatinised; Magnesium Stearate.

*Capsule Shell Body:* Indigotine E132 (30 mg capsules only); Titanium Dioxide E171; Gelatin.

*Capsule Shell Cap:* Indigotine E132; Titanium Dioxide E171; Gelatin.

*Incompatibilities:* None known.

*Shelf life:* 60 months.

36 months: 20 mg capsules x 56; 20 mg capsules x 84; 30 mg capsules x 84.

*Special precautions for storage:* No special precautions.

*Nature and contents of container: 20 and 30 mg Capsules:* Securitainer packs of 50 and 100. PVC/aluminium foil blister strips of 21, 56, 60 (30 mg capsules only), 84, 100 and 200 capsules.

*Instructions for use/handling:* Not applicable.

**Marketing authorisation numbers**
Cardene 20 mg Capsules 0031/0461
Cardene 30 mg Capsules 0031/0462

**Date of approval/revision of SPC** March 1997

**Legal category** POM

## CELLCEPT * ▼

**Qualitative and quantitative composition** Each capsule contains 250 mg mycophenolate mofetil.

**Pharmaceutical form** CellCept capsules: oblong, blue/brown, branded with black 'CellCept 250' on the capsule cap and 'Company logo' on the capsule body.

**Clinical particulars**

*Therapeutic indications:* CellCept is indicated in combination with cyclosporin and corticosteroids for the prophylaxis of acute transplant rejection in patients receiving allogeneic renal transplants.

*Posology and method of administration:* The initial dose of CellCept should be given orally within 72 hours following transplantation. The recommended dose in renal transplant patients is 1.0 g administered twice daily (2 g daily dose). Although daily doses of both 2 g and 3 g were studied in clinical trials, an efficacy advantage for the 3 g dose could not be established. Patients receiving 2 g per day of CellCept had an overall better safety profile than patients receiving 3 g per day.

*Use in children:* Safety and effectiveness in paediatric patients have not been established. Very limited pharmacokinetic data are available for paediatric renal transplant patients.

*Use in elderly:* The recommended dose of 1.0 g administered twice a day is appropriate for elderly patients. Patients in this age group may generally be at increased risk of adverse events compared to younger individuals; this is similarly true for patients receiving CellCept as part of a combination immunosuppressive regimen (see *Undesirable effects*).

*Use in severe renal impairment:* In patients with severe chronic renal impairment (glomerular filtration rate <25 mL/min/1.73 m²), outside of the immediate post-transplant period, doses greater than 1 g administered twice a day should be avoided. These patients should also be carefully observed. No dose adjustments are needed in patients experiencing delayed graft function post-operatively (see *Pharmacokinetic properties*).

*Use in severe hepatic impairment:* No dose adjustments are needed for patients with severe hepatic parenchymal disease.

*Other considerations for use:* If neutropenia develops (absolute neutrophil count <1.3 x 10³/µL), physicians should perform appropriate diagnostic tests, manage the patients appropriately, and consider interrupting dosing with CellCept.

Food has no effect on MPA (mycophenolic acid) AUC (area under the curve), but has been shown to decrease Cmax by 40%. It is recommended that CellCept be administered on an empty stomach.

No dosage reduction or interruption is required in the event of a transplant rejection episode.

Treatment should be initiated by appropriately qualified specialists in renal transplantation and continued treatment should remain under the guidance of similarly qualified specialists.

*Contra-indications:* Allergic reactions to CellCept have been observed. Therefore, CellCept is contraindicated in patients with a hypersensitivity to mycophenolate mofetil or mycophenolic acid. For information on use in pregnancy and contraceptive requirements, see 4.6 Pregnancy and lactation.

*Special warnings and special precautions for use:* As in patients receiving immunosuppressive regimes involving combinations of drugs, patients receiving CellCept as part of an immunosuppressive regime are at increased risk of developing lymphomas and other malignancies, particularly of the skin. The risk appears to be related to the intensity and duration of immunosuppression rather than to the use of any specific agent. Oversuppression of the immune system can also increase susceptibility to infection.

CellCept has been administered in combination with the following agents in clinical trials: antithymocyte globulin, OKT3, cyclosporin, and corticosteroids.

Lymphoproliferative disease or lymphoma developed in patients receiving CellCept in regimens which included some or all of the above mentioned immunosuppressive agents in 1% of the patients receiving 3 g daily and 0.6% in patients receiving 2 g daily in the controlled studies of prevention of rejection.

In the three controlled studies for prevention of rejection, similar rates of fatal infections (<2%) have occurred in patients while receiving CellCept or control therapy in regimens which included some or all of the above mentioned immunosuppressive agents.

Up to 2.0% of patients receiving CellCept 3 g daily for prevention of rejection developed severe neutropenia (absolute neutrophil count <500/µL). A total of 0.5% of patients receiving CellCept 2 g and 0.8% of patients receiving azathioprine developed severe neutropenia. Patients receiving CellCept should be monitored for neutropenia. The development of neutropenia may be related to CellCept itself, concomitant medications, viral infections, or some combination of these causes.

Laboratory monitoring: Patients on CellCept should have complete blood counts, weekly during the first month, twice monthly for the second and third months of treatment, then monthly through the first year. If neutropenia develops (absolute neutrophil count <1.3 x 10³/µL) physicians should perform appropriate diagnostic tests, manage the patients appropriately, and consider interrupting dosing with CellCept.

Gastrointestinal tract haemorrhage has been observed in approximately 3% of patients treated with CellCept 3 g daily and 1.4% in patients treated with CellCept 2 g daily. Gastrointestinal perforations (colonic, gall bladder) have been observed. In the three controlled trials for the prevention of rejection, colonic perforation was reported in 1.0% of patients receiving 3 g daily of CellCept, 0.4% of patients receiving 2 g daily of CellCept, 0.3% in patients receiving azathioprine and in no patients receiving placebo. Because CellCept has been associated with an increased incidence of digestive system adverse events, including infrequent cases of gastrointestinal tract ulceration, and haemorrhage, CellCept should be administered with caution in patients with active serious digestive system disease.

Subjects with severe chronic renal impairment (glomerular filtration rate <25 mL/min/1.73 m²), who have received single doses of CellCept, showed higher plasma mycophenolic acid (MPA) and mycophenolic acid glucuronide (MPAG) AUCs relative to subjects with lesser degrees of renal impairment or normal healthy subjects. Administration of doses greater than 1 g BID to these patients should be avoided and they should be carefully observed (see *Posology and method of administration* and *Pharmacokinetic properties*).

In patients with delayed graft function post-transplant, mean MPA $AUC_{0-12}$ was comparable, but MPAG $AUC_{0-12}$ was 2–3 fold higher, compared to that seen in post-transplant patients without delayed graft function. No dose adjustment is recommended for these patients, however, they should be carefully observed (see *Posology and method of administration* and *Pharmacokinetic properties*).

It is recommended that CellCept not be administered concomitantly with azathioprine because such concomitant administration has not been studied.

In view of the significant reduction in the AUC of MPA by cholestyramine, caution should be used in the concomitant administration of CellCept with drugs that interfere with enterohepatic recirculation because of the potential to reduce the efficacy of CellCept.

*Interaction with other medicaments and other forms of interaction:*
*Acyclovir:* Higher MPAG and acyclovir plasma concentrations were observed when mycophenolate mofetil was administered with acyclovir in comparison to the administration of each drug alone. Because MPAG plasma concentrations are increased in the presence of renal impairment, as are acyclovir concentrations, the potential exists for the two drugs to compete for tubular secretion and thus further increases in concentrations of both drugs may occur.

*Antacids with magnesium and aluminum hydroxides:* Absorption of mycophenolate mofetil was decreased when administered with antacids.

*Cholestyramine:* Following single dose administration of 1.5 g of mycophenolate mofetil to normal healthy subjects pretreated with 4 g TID of cholestyramine for 4 days, there was a 40% reduction in the AUC of MPA.

*Cyclosporin A:* Cyclosporin A pharmacokinetics were unaffected by mycophenolate mofetil.

*Ganciclovir:* No pharmacokinetic interaction was observed between mycophenolate mofetil and IV ganciclovir.

*Oral contraceptives:* No pharmacokinetic interaction was observed between mycophenolate mofetil and 1 mg norethisterone/35µg ethinyloestradiol. This single dose study demonstrates the lack of a gross pharmacokinetic interaction, but cannot exclude the possibility of changes in the pharmacokinetics of the oral contraceptive under long term dosing conditions with CellCept which might adversely affect the efficacy of the oral contraceptive.

*Trimethoprim/sulphamethoxazole:* No effect on the bioavailability of MPA was observed.

*Other interactions:* Co-administration of probenecid with mycophenolate mofetil in monkeys raises plasma AUC of MPAG by 3-fold. Thus, other drugs known to undergo renal tubular secretion may compete with MPAG and thereby raise plasma concentrations of MPAG or the other drug undergoing tubular secretion. Single dose studies of CellCept with ganciclovir and trimethoprim/ sulphamethoxazole did not reveal a pharmacokinetic interaction between either of these agents and CellCept. All these types of compounds operate through inhibition of nucleoside synthesis and therefore one cannot exclude a clinical interaction between them.

*Pregnancy and lactation:* Adverse effects on foetal development (including malformations) occurred when pregnant rats and rabbits were dosed during organogenesis (see *Preclinical safety data*). Because there are no adequate and well controlled studies in pregnant women, CellCept should be used in pregnant women only if the potential benefit outweighs the potential risk to the foetus.

It is recommended that CellCept therapy should not be initiated until a negative pregnancy test has been obtained. Patients should be instructed to consult their physician immediately should pregnancy occur.

Effective contraception must be used before beginning CellCept therapy, during therapy, and for six weeks following discontinuation of therapy. Although the results of a single dose drug interaction study with an oral contraceptive suggest the lack of a gross pharmacokinetic interaction, the results cannot exclude the possibility of changes in the pharmacokinetics of the oral contraceptive under long term dosing conditions with CellCept which might adversely affect the efficacy of the oral contraceptive (see *Interaction with other medicaments and other forms of interaction*).

Studies in rats have shown mycophenolate mofetil to be excreted in milk. It is not known whether this drug is excreted in human milk. Because many drugs are excreted in human milk and because of the potential for serious adverse reactions in nursing infants from mycophenolate mofetil, a decision should be made whether to discontinue nursing or to discontinue the drug, taking into account the importance of the drug to the mother.

*Effects on ability to drive and use machines:* No specific studies have been performed. The pharmacodynamic profile and the reported adverse reactions indicate that an effect is unlikely.

*Undesirable effects:* The adverse event profile associated with the use of immunosuppressive drugs is often difficult to establish owing to the presence of underlying disease and the concurrent use of many other medications. The principal adverse reactions associated with the administration of CellCept include diarrhoea, leucopenia, sepsis and vomiting and there is evidence of a higher frequency of certain types of infections.

Adverse reactions reported in ≥10% of patients treated with CellCept in the three Phase III controlled trials for prevention of rejection are presented below:

*Body as a whole:* sepsis, infection, abdominal pain, fever, chest pain, pain, headache, back pain, asthenia; *Blood and lymphatic:* anaemia, leucopenia, thrombocytopenia, hypochromic anaemia, leukocytosis; *Urogenital:* urinary tract infection, urinary tract disorder, renal tubular necrosis, haematuria; *Cardiovascular:* hypertension; *Metabolic and nutritional:* hyperkalaemia, hyperglycaemia, hypophosphataemia, hypokalemia, hyperchlolesteraemia, peripheral oedema, oedema; *Digestive:* diarrhoea, vomiting, constipation, nausea, nausea and vomiting, dyspepsia, oral moniliasis; *Respiratory:* pneumonia, infection, dyspnoea, bronchitis, pharyngitis, cough increased; *Skin and appendages:* herpes simplex, acne; *Nervous:* dizziness, insomnia, tremor.

In three controlled trials for prevention of rejection, patients receiving 2 g per day of CellCept demonstrated an overall better safety profile than did patients receiving 3 g per day of CellCept. Sepsis, which was generally CMV viraemia, was slightly more common in patients treated with CellCept than in control patients and was slightly more common in patients receiving 3 g per day than those receiving 2 g per day. In the digestive system, diarrhoea was most clearly increased in patients receiving CellCept compared to patients receiving azathioprine or placebo. There was also a slight increase in vomiting. These digestive system events were more common in patients receiving 3 g per day than in patients receiving 2 g per day. Urinary tract infections were common in all treatment groups, but were increased slightly in patients receiving CellCept in comparison to those treated with azathioprine or placebo. Leucopenia was more common in patients treated with CellCept than in control patients, and was most common in patients receiving 3 g per day of CellCept.

Cytomegalovirus (CMV) tissue invasive disease was more common in patients receiving CellCept 3 g per day than in those receiving CellCept 2 g per day or control therapy in three controlled studies for prevention of rejection. Similarly, the incidence of Candidemia and tissue invasive Candida and invasive Aspergillosis was slightly higher in patients receiving CellCept 3 g per day than in those receiving CellCept 2 g per day or control therapy for prevention of rejection. In the three controlled studies for prevention of rejection, similar rates of fatal infections (<2%) have occurred in patients while receiving CellCept or control therapy in combination with other immunosuppressive agents.

The incidence of malignancies among the 1,483 patients enrolled in three controlled trials for the prevention of rejection, who were followed for ≥1 year, was similar to the incidence reported in the literature for renal allograft recipients. There was an increase in the incidence of lymphoproliferative disease in the CellCept treatment groups (0.6% for the 2 g per day and 1.0% for the 3 g per day doses) compared to the placebo (0%) and azathioprine groups (0.3%).

Up to 2.0% of patients receiving CellCept 3 g daily for prevention of rejection developed severe neutropenia (absolute neutrophil count <500/μL). A total of 0.5% of patients receiving CellCept 2 g and 0.8% of patients receiving azathioprine developed severe neutropenia.

There were a relatively small number (7%) of elderly patients among the 1,483 patients enrolled in the three controlled trials for the prevention of rejection. Elderly patients, particularly those who are receiving CellCept as part of a combination immunosuppressive regimen, may be at increased risk of certain infections (including CMV tissue invasive disease) and possibly gastrointestinal haemorrhage and pulmonary oedema, compared to younger individuals. Other events observed at an apparent higher frequency in the elderly included leucopenia, elevated serum creatinine and dyspnoea; however, these events were no more common in the patients receiving CellCept than those who received azathioprine. There was no increase in malignancies or mortality in this age group.

The following adverse events, not mentioned above, were reported with ≥3% and <10% incidence in patients treated with CellCept: *Body as a whole:* cyst (including lymphocele and hydrocele), haemorrhage, hernia, malaise, abdomen enlarged, chills and fever, flu syndrome, pelvic pain, face oedema; *blood and lymphatic:* polycytheaemia, ecchymosis; *urogenital:* albuminuria, hydronephrosis, pyelonephritis, dysuria, pain, impotence, urinary frequency; *cardiovascular:* thrombosis, angina pectoris, atrial fibrillation, hypotension, peripheral vascular disorder, cardiovascular disorder, postural hypotension, tachycardia, palpitation, vasodilatation; *metabolic and nutritional:* creatinine increased, gamma glutamyl transpeptidase increased, hyperlipemia, dehydration, hypoglycaemia, SGPT increased, SGOT increased, hypervolaemia, acidosis, hypocalcaemia, lactic dehydrogenase increased, hypercalcaemia, alkaline phosphatase increased, hypoproteinaemia, hyperuricaemia, weight gain; *digestive:* gastrointestinal haemorrhage, ileus, gastritis, gastroenteritis, oesophagitis, hepatitis, infection, liver function tests abnormal, gastrointestinal moniliasis, rectal disorder, anorexia, flatulence, gum hyperplasia, gingivitis, mouth ulceration; *respiratory:* lung oedema, sinusitis, lung disorder, asthma, pleural effusion, rhinitis; *skin and appendages:* skin carcinoma, skin ulcer, herpes zoster, skin benign neoplasm, skin disorder, skin hypertrophy, sweating, alopecia, rash, hirsutism, fungal dermatitis, pruritis; *nervous:* depression, somnolence, paraesthesia, hypertonia, anxiety; *endocrine:* diabetes mellitus, parathyroid disorder; *musculoskeletal:* arthralgia, myalgia, joint disorder, leg cramps, myasthenia; *special senses:* cataract (not specified), conjunctivitis, amblyopia.

*Overdose:* There has been no reported experience of overdosage of mycophenolate mofetil in humans.

At clinically encountered concentrations, MPA and MPAG are not removed by hemodialysis. However, at high MPAG plasma concentrations (>100μg/mL), small amounts of MPAG are removed. By interfering with enterohepatic circulation of the drug, bile acid sequestrants, such as cholestyramine reduce the MPA AUC.

## Pharmacological properties

*Pharmacodynamic properties:* Mycophenolate mofetil is the 2-morpholinoethyl ester of MPA. MPA is a potent, selective, uncompetitive and reversible inhibitor of inosine monophosphate dehydrogenase, and therefore inhibits the *de novo* pathway of guanosine nucleotide synthesis without incorporation into DNA. Because T- and B-lymphocytes are critically dependent for their proliferation on *de novo* synthesis of purines whereas other cell types can utilise salvage pathways, MPA has more potent cytostatic effects on lymphocytes than on other cells.

*Pharmacokinetic properties:* MPA at clinically relevant concentrations, is 97% bound to plasma albumin.

Following oral administration, mycophenolate mofetil undergoes rapid and extensive absorption and complete presystemic metabolism to the active metabolite, MPA. Mycophenolate mofetil is not measurable systemically in plasma following oral administration.

MPA is metabolized principally by glucuronyl transferase to form the phenolic glucuronide of MPA (MPAG), which is not pharmacologically active.

As a result of enterohepatic recirculation, secondary increases in plasma MPA concentration are usually observed at approximately 6–12 hours post-dose. A reduction in the AUC of MPA of approximately 40% is associated with the co-administration of cholestyramine (4 g TID), indicating that there is a significant amount of enterohepatic recirculation.

Negligible amount of drug is excreted as MPA (<1% of dose) in the urine. Orally administered radiolabeled mycophenolate mofetil resulted in complete recovery of the administered dose; with 93% of the administered dose recovered in the urine and 6% recovered in feces. Most (about 87%) of the administered dose is excreted in the urine as MPAG.

The mean bioavailability of oral mycophenolate mofetil, based on MPA AUC, was 94% relative to IV mycophenolate mofetil.

Food had no effect on the extent of absorption (MPA AUC) of mycophenolate mofetil when administered at doses of 1.5 g b.i.d. to renal transplant patients. However, MPA Cmax was decreased by 40% in the presence of food.

Immediately post-transplant (<40 days), mean MPA AUC and Cmax are approximately 50% lower in renal transplant patients than that observed in healthy volunteers or in stable renal transplant patients.

In a single dose study (6 subjects per group), mean plasma MPA AUC observed in subjects with severe chronic renal impairment (glomerular filtration rate <25 mL/min/1.73 m²) were 28–75% higher relative to the means observed in normal healthy subjects or subjects with lesser degrees of renal impairment. However, the mean single dose MPAG AUC was 3–6 fold higher in subjects with severe renal impairment than in subjects with mild renal impairment or normal healthy subjects, consistent with the known renal elimination of MPAG. Multiple dosing of mycophenolate mofetil in patients with severe chronic renal impairment has not been studied.

In patients with delayed graft function post-transplant, mean MPA AUC$_{0-12}$ was comparable to that seen in post-transplant patients without delayed graft function. Mean plasma MPAG AUC$_{0-12}$ was 2–3 fold higher than in post-transplant patients without delayed graft function.

In volunteers with alcoholic cirrhosis, hepatic MPA glucuronidation processes were relatively unaffected by hepatic parenchymal disease. Effects of hepatic disease on this process probably depend on the particular disease. However, hepatic disease with predominantly biliary damage, such as primary biliary cirrhosis, may show a different effect.

Pharmacokinetic behaviour of CellCept in the elderly has not been formally evaluated.

*Preclinical safety data:* In experimental models, mycophenolate mofetil was not tumorigenic and did not demonstrate mutagenic activity. The highest dose tested in the animal carcinogenicity studies resulted in approximately 2 to 3 times the systemic exposure (AUC or Cmax) observed in renal transplant patients at the recommended clinical dose of 2 g per day.

Mycophenolate mofetil had no effect on fertility of male rats at oral doses up to 20 mg/kg/day. The systemic exposure at this dose represents 2 to 3 times the clinical exposure at the recommended clinical dose of 2 g per day. In a female fertility and reproduction study conducted in rats, oral doses of 4.5 mg/kg/day caused malformations (including anophthalmia,

agnathia, and hydrocephaly) in the first generation offspring in the absence of maternal toxicity. The systemic exposure at this dose was approximately 0.5 times the clinical exposure at the recommended clinical dose of 2 g per day. No effects on fertility or reproductive parameters were evident in the dams or in the subsequent generation.

In teratology studies in rats and rabbits, fetal resorptions and malformations occurred in rats at 6 mg/kg/day (including anophthalmia, agnathia, and hydrocephaly) and in rabbits at 90 mg/kg/day (including cardiovascular and renal anomalies, such as ectopia cordis and ectopic kidneys, and diaphragmatic and umbilical hernia), in the absence of maternal toxicity. The systemic exposure at these levels are approximately equivalent to or less than 0.5 times the clinical exposure at the recommended clinical dose of 2 g per day.

Refer to section *Pregnancy and lactation*.

The haematopoietic and lymphoid systems were the primary organs affected in toxicology studies conducted with mycophenolate mofetil in the rat, mouse, dog and monkey. These effects occurred at systemic exposure levels that are equivalent to or less than the clinical exposure at the recommended dose of 2 g per day. Gastrointestinal effects were observed in the dog at systemic exposure levels equivalent to or less than the clinical exposure at the recommended dose. Gastrointestinal and renal effects consistent with dehydration were also observed in the monkey at the highest dose (systemic exposure levels equivalent to or greater than clinical exposure). The nonclinical toxicity profile of mycophenolate mofetil appears to be consistent with adverse events observed in human clinical trials which now provide safety data of more relevance to the patient population (see *Undesirable effects*).

## Pharmaceutical particulars

*List of excipients:* Excipients of CellCept capsules are pregelatinized maize starch, croscarmellose sodium, polyvidone (K-90) and magnesium stearate. The capsule shells contain gelatin, indigo carmine (FP, E132), yellow iron oxide (FP, E172), red iron oxide (FP, E172), titanium dioxide (PhEur, E171), sodium lauryl sulphate, black iron oxide (FP, E172), potassium hydroxide, shellac and silicon dioxide (PhEur).

*Incompatibilities:* None.

*Shelf life:* CellCept capsules have a shelf-life of two years when stored in opaque polyvinyl chloride blister packs at temperatures not exceeding 30°C.

*Special precautions for storage:* Store at or below 30°C.

*Nature and contents of container:* CellCept 250 mg capsules: 1 carton contains 100 capsules (in blister packs of 10)

Three cartons each of 100 capsules may be shrink wrapped together to form a sales unit containing 300 capsules.

*Instructions for use/handling:* Because mycophenolate mofetil has demonstrated teratogenic effects in rats and rabbits, CellCept capsules should not be opened or crushed. Avoid inhalation or direct contact with skin or mucous membranes of the powder contained in CellCept capsules. If such contact occurs, wash thoroughly with soap and water; rinse eyes with plain water.

**Marketing authorisation number** EU/1/96/005/001

**Date of approval/revision of SPC** Not applicable.

**Legal category** POM

# CYMEVENE* CAPSULES

**Qualitative and quantitative composition** Each capsule contains 250 mg of ganciclovir.

**Pharmaceutical form** Opaque green hard gelatine capsule printed with Syntex logo and "CY 250" on the cap and two partial lines on the body.

**Clinical particulars**

*Therapeutic indications:* Cymevene capsules are indicated for the maintenance treatment of CMV retinitis in AIDS patients, where the retinitis is stable following at least 3 weeks of Cymevene intravenous therapy.

*Posology and method of administration:* Cymevene capsules must be taken with food.

For patients with stable CMV retinitis following at least 3 weeks of treatment with intravenous Cymevene therapy, the recommended maintenance dose of Cymevene capsules is 1000 mg three times a day. Alternatively, the dosing regimen may be 500 mg six times a day.

*Patients with renal impairment:*
A dose reduction of Cymevene capsules is required as follows:

| Creatinine Clearance (ml/min) | Dose |
|---|---|
| ≥ 70 | 1000 mg three times a day |
| 50 to 69 | 1500 mg daily |
| 25 to 49 | 1000 mg daily |
| 10 to 24 | 500 mg daily |
| < 10 | 500 mg three times weekly |

To calculate an estimated creatinine clearance:
For males = (140)–age [years] (body weight [kg])/ (0.81) (Serum creatinine [μmol/L])
For females = 0.85 x male value

*Elderly:* No studies on the safety or efficacy of Cymevene in elderly patients have been conducted. Since elderly individuals often have reduced renal function, Cymevene should be administered to elderly patients with special consideration of their renal status (see above).

*Children:* There has been limited clinical experience in treating patients under the age of 12 years. The use of Cymevene capsules in children warrants careful consideration due to the possibility of long-term carcinogenicity and reproductive toxicity. The benefits of treatment should outweigh the risks. Cymevene IS NOT INDICATED FOR THE TREATMENT OF CONGENITAL OR NEONATAL CMV INFECTIONS.

*Laboratory monitoring and dosage reductions:* Due to the frequency of neutropenia, anaemia and thrombocytopenia in patients receiving orally administered Cymevene, it is recommended that neutrophil counts, haemoglobin levels and platelets counts, are performed every 2 weeks. In patients in whom Cymevene or other nucleoside analogues have previously resulted in leucopenia, or in whom neutrophil counts are less than 1000 cells/mm³ at the beginning of treatment, neutrophil counts should be monitored at least weekly.

Patients with severe neutropenia (< 500 cells/mm³) and/or thrombocytopenia (platelets < 25,000/mm³) require a dose interruption until evidence of marrow recovery is observed (≥ 750 cells/mm³).

As dose reductions are required for patients with renal impairment, serum creatinine or creatinine clearance should be monitored every 2 weeks.

*Contra-indications:*
(i) Pregnancy and lactation.
(ii) Patients with known hypersensitivity to Cymevene or to acyclovir.

*Special warnings and special precautions for use:* The clinical toxicity of Cymevene includes leucopenia, anaemia and thrombocytopenia. In preclinical testing ganciclovir caused mutagenicity, teratogenicity and carcinogenicity. It should therefore be considered a potential teratogen and carcinogen in humans.

Cymevene should not be administered if the absolute neutrophil count is less than 500 cells/mm³ or the platelet count is less than 25,000 cells/mm³. Neutropenia, anaemia and thrombocytopenia have been observed in patients treated with Cymevene.

It is considered likely that Cymevene causes temporary or permanent inhibition of spermatogenesis. Animal data also indicate that suppression of fertility in females may occur.

Women of childbearing potential should be advised to use effective contraception during treatment. Male patients should be advised to practise barrier contraception during and for at least 90 days following treatment with Cymevene.

If renal function is impaired, dosage adjustments based on creatinine clearance are required (see *Posology and method of administration section 4.2*).

*Interaction with other medicaments and other forms of interaction:* Binding of ganciclovir to plasma proteins is only about 1–2% and drug interactions involving binding site displacement are not anticipated.
*Probenecid:* It is possible that probenecid, as well as other drugs which inhibit renal tubular secretion or resorption, may reduce renal clearance (22%) of ganciclovir and could increase the plasma half life (45%) of ganciclovir.
*Additive toxicity:* It is possible that drugs which inhibit replication of rapidly dividing cell populations such as bone marrow, spermatogonia, and germinal layers of skin and gastro-intestinal mucosa might have combined additive toxic effects when used concomitantly with, before or after Cymevene. Because of the possibility of additive toxicity with co-administration of drugs such as dapsone, pentamidine, flucytosine, vincristine, vinblastine, adriamycin, amphotericin B, trimethoprim/sulpha combinations or other nucleoside analogues, combination with Cymevene therapy should be used only if the potential benefits outweigh the risks.
*Zidovudine:* The amount of zidovudine in the blood

may increase (by about 15%) when given concomitantly with ganciclovir.
Since both zidovudine and ganciclovir can cause neutropenia, patients receiving these drugs concomitantly are at an increased risk of developing this condition. Regular monitoring of neutrophil counts should be performed (see *Laboratory monitoring and dosage reductions section 4.2*).
*Didanosine:* As ganciclovir can increase the amount of didanosine in the blood (by about 80%), patients must be closely monitored for didanosine toxicity.
There is a decrease in the amount of ganciclovir in the blood (23%) when given 2 hours prior to didanosine, but there is no effect on ganciclovir when the two drugs are given at the same time.
*Imipenem-cilastatin:* Generalised seizures have been reported in patients taking Cymevene and imipenem-cilastatin concomitantly. Use of these drugs should be avoided.

*Pregnancy and lactation:* There are no adequate and well-controlled studies in pregnant women.
Teratogenicity has been observed in animal studies. Cymevene should not be given to pregnant women as there is a high likelihood of damage to the developing foetus.
It is not known if ganciclovir is excreted in human milk. Since many drugs are, Cymevene should not be given to lactating mothers. The minimum time interval before nursing can safely be resumed after the last dose of Cymevene is unknown.
Intravenous administration of 90 mg/kg of ganciclovir to female mice prior to mating and continued during gestation and lactation caused hypoplasia of the testes and seminal vesicles in the month old offspring, as well as pathologic changes in the non-glandular region of the stomach.

*Effects on ability to drive and use machines:* Not known.

*Undesirable effects:* In three controlled clinical trials, adverse events with orally administered Cymevene (3000 mg daily) occurring at a frequency greater than 1% and thought to be "probably" or "possibly" related to treatment were as follows:
Leucopenia, thrombocytopenia, anaemia, diarrhoea, abdominal pain, dyspepsia, nausea, anorexia, flatulence, vomiting, asthenia, rash, headache, pruritus, fever, abnormal liver function tests, pain and infection.
Adverse events which were thought to be possibly related and occurred in 1% or less of the patients are listed by body systems below.
*Body as a whole:* cellulitis, laboratory test abnormality, abdomen enlarged, chest pain, chills, drug level increased, malaise.
*Digestive system:* eructation, mouth ulceration, constipation, dysphagia, faecal incontinence.
*Haematologic system:* hypochromic anaemia, pancytopenia.
*Respiratory system:* dyspnoea, cough increased.
*Central nervous system:* somnolence, dizziness, paraesthesia, abnormal dreams and thoughts, anxiety, euphoria, insomnia, abnormal gait, ataxia, confusion, dry mouth, hypesthesia, manic reaction.
*Skin and appendages:* alopecia, sweating, acne, maculopapular rash.
*Cardiovascular system:* deep thrombophlebitis, migraine, vasodilation.
*Metabolic and nutritional disorders:* increases in creatinine, alkaline phosphatase, SGPT, creatine phosphokinase and lactic dehydrogenase; hypokalemia.
*Special senses:* abnormal vision, vitreous disorder, eye pain, amblyopia, blindness, conjunctivitis, retinal detachment, retinitis, deafness, taste perversion.
*Urogenital system:* decrease in creatinine clearance, abnormal kidney function, breast pain, urinary frequency, urinary tract infection.
*Musculoskeletal system:* myasthenia, myalgia.
*Overdose:* There have been no reports of overdosage with orally administered Cymevene.
Haemodialysis and hydration may be of benefit in reducing drug plasma levels in patients who receive an overdose of Cymevene.

**Pharmacological properties** Ganciclovir (9-[1,3-dihydroxy-2-propoxymethyl]guanine) is a synthetic analogue of guanine which inhibits replication of herpes viruses *in vitro* and *in vivo*. Sensitive human viruses include cytomegalovirus (CMV), herpes simplex virus-1 and -2 (HSV-1 and HSV-2), Epstein-Barr virus (EBV) and varicella zoster virus (VZV). Clinical studies have been limited to assessment of efficacy in patients with CMV infection.
Intracellular ganciclovir is phosphorylated to ganciclovir monophosphate by a cellular deoxyguanosine kinase. Further phosphorylation to ganciclovir triphosphate occurs by several cellular kinases. In CMV-infected cells there is approximately a 10-fold increased concentration of both cellular kinases and ganciclovir triphosphate. Thus, there is a preferential phosphorylation of ganciclovir in virus-infected cells. In such cells ganciclovir triphosphate is metabolised

slowly, with 60 to 70% remaining 18 hours after removal of ganciclovir from the extracellular fluid. The antiviral activity of ganciclovir is the result of inhibition of viral DNA synthesis by: (1) competitive inhibition of incorporation of deoxyguanosine triphosphate into DNA by DNA polymerase, and (2) incorporation of ganciclovir triphosphate into viral DNA causing termination of, or very limited, viral DNA elongation.
Emergence of viral resistance has been reported based on *in vitro* sensitivity testing of CMV isolates from patients receiving Cymevene treatment.

*Pharmacokinetic properties:* The major route of excretion of ganciclovir is via glomerular filtration of unchanged drug. Administration of Cymevene with food increased its bioavailability by approximately 20%. Multiple dose studies with Cymevene capsules indicated that the absolute bioavailability when taken with food was approximately 6%.
Oral doses of 3 g/day yield maximum and minimum plasma concentrations of 1.0 and 0.2 μg/ml respectively (corresponding plasma concentrations for IV maintenance therapy of 5 mg/kg/day are 8.0 μg/ml and < 0.05 μg/ml).
In patients with severe renal impairment, haemodialysis reduced plasma drug levels by 50%.

*Preclinical safety data:* Refer to *Special warnings and special precautions for use* and *Pregnancy and lactation*.

**Pharmaceutical particulars**

*List of excipients:* The capsules contain the following excipients: croscarmellose sodium, magnesium stearate and povidone.

*Incompatibilities:* None.

*Shelf life:* 3 years in a high density polyethylene bottle. 2 years in foil laminate pouches.

*Special precautions for storage:* Cymevene capsules should be stored below 30°C.

*Nature and contents of container:* 180 or 84 capsules in a high density polyethylene bottle with a polypropylene closure, child resistant overcap and with a tamper evident innerseal.
Foil laminate pouches. Each strip consists of 4 x 3 capsules. Pack size is either 7 or 14 strips (84 or 168 capsules).

*Instructions for use/handling:* As Cymevene has shown carcinogenic and mutagenic activity, caution should be observed in the handling of Cymevene capsules. Avoid inhalation or direct contact of the powder contained in the capsules with the skin or mucous membranes. If such contact occurs, wash thoroughly with soap and water, rinse eyes thoroughly with plain water.

**Cymevene capsules should not be opened or crushed.**

**Marketing authorisation number** 0031/0466

**Date of approval/revision of SPC** April 1997

**Legal category** POM

# CYMEVENE* FOR INTRAVENOUS INFUSION

**Presentation** Each vial of Cymevene contains 546 mg of sterile, freeze-dried ganciclovir sodium equivalent to 500 mg ganciclovir as a white to off-white powder. Reconstitution with 10 ml of sterile Water for Injections BP gives a ganciclovir concentration of 50 mg/ml, pH 11. Further dilution in an appropriate intravenous solution must be performed before infusion (see *Method of administration*).

**Uses**
*Pharmacological properties:* Ganciclovir (9-[1,3-dihydroxy-2-propoxymethyl]guanine) is a synthetic analogue of guanine which inhibits replication of herpes viruses *in vitro* and *in vivo*. Sensitive human viruses include cytomegalovirus (CMV), herpes simplex virus-1 and -2 (HSV-1 and HSV-2), Epstein-Barr virus (EBV) and varicella zoster virus (VZV). Clinical studies have been limited to assessment of efficacy in patients with CMV infection.
Intracellular ganciclovir is phosphorylated to ganciclovir monophosphate by a cellular deoxyguanosine kinase. Further phosphorylation to ganciclovir triphosphate occurs by several cellular kinases. In CMV-infected cells there is approximately a 10-fold increased concentration of both cellular kinases and ganciclovir triphosphate. Thus, there is a preferential phosphorylation of ganciclovir in virus-infected cells. In such cells ganciclovir triphosphate is metabolised slowly, with 60 to 70% remaining 18 hours after removal of ganciclovir from the extracellular fluid. The antiviral activity of ganciclovir is the result of inhibition of viral DNA synthesis by: (1) competitive inhibition of incorporation of deoxyguanosine triphosphate into DNA by DNA polymerase, and (2) incorpo-

ration of ganciclovir triphosphate into viral DNA causing termination of, or very limited, viral DNA elongation.

Emergence of viral resistance has been reported based on *in vitro* sensitivity testing of CMV isolates from patients receiving Cymevene treatment.

*Pharmacokinetics:* The major route of excretion of ganciclovir is via glomerular filtration of unchanged drug. In patients with normal renal function the plasma half-life of ganciclovir following a 1-hour iv infusion of 5 mg/kg averaged 2.9 hours with a mean systemic clearance of 3.64 ml/min/kg.

Twice-daily administration of 5 mg/kg for 14 days did not cause accumulation in plasma.

Renal impairment leads to altered kinetics of ganciclovir as indicated below.

| Serum creatinine (micromol/l) | Ganciclovir | |
|---|---|---|
| | Systemic plasma clearance (ml/min/kg) | Plasma half-life (hours) |
| < 124 (n = 32) | 3.64 | 2.9 |
| 125–225 (n = 9) | 2.01 | 5.3 |
| 226–398 (n = 3) | 1.11 | 9.7 |
| > 398 (n = 5) | 0.33 | 28.5 |

In patients with severe renal impairment, haemodialysis reduced plasma drug levels by 50%.

*Indications:* Cymevene is indicated for the treatment of life-threatening or sight-threatening cytomegalovirus (CMV) infections in immunocompromised individuals. These states include acquired immunodeficiency syndrome (AIDS), iatrogenic immunosuppression associated with organ transplantation, or chemotherapy for neoplasia.

Cymevene may also be used for the prevention of CMV disease, specifically in those patients receiving immunosuppressive therapy secondary to organ transplantation.

## Dosage and administration

*Treatment of CMV infection*
*Initial (Induction) Treatment:* 5 mg/kg infused at a constant rate over 1 hour every 12 hours (10 mg/kg/day) for 14 to 21 days.

*Long-term (Maintenance) Treatment:* For immunocompromised patients at risk of relapse of CMV retinitis a course of maintenance therapy may be given. Intravenous infusion of 6 mg/kg daily 5 days per week, or 5 mg/kg daily 7 days per week is recommended.

*Treatment of Disease Progression:* Indefinite treatment may be required in patients with AIDS, but even with continued maintenance treatment, patients may have progression of retinitis. Any patient in whom the retinitis progresses, either while on maintenance treatment or because treatment with Cymevene has been withdrawn, may be re-treated using the induction treatment regimen.

*Prevention of CMV disease*
*Induction Regimen:* 5 mg/kg infused every 12 hours (10 mg/kg/day) for 7 to 14 days.

*Maintenance Regimen:* Intravenous infusion of 6 mg/kg daily 5 days per week, or 5 mg/kg 7 days per week is recommended.

For patients with renal insufficiency the induction dose should be modified as follows:

| Serum creatinine (micromol/l) | Dose (mg/kg) | Dosing Interval (hours) |
|---|---|---|
| < 124 | 5.0 | 12 |
| 125–225 | 2.5 | 12 |
| 226–398 | 2.5 | 24 |
| > 398 | 1.25 | 24 |

The optimal maintenance dose for patients with renal insufficiency is not known.

Patients undergoing dialysis should be given 1.25 mg/kg/24 hours. On days when dialysis is performed the dose should be given shortly after the dialysis session.

*Use in the elderly:* No studies on the efficacy or safety of Cymevene in elderly patients have been conducted. Since elderly individuals often have reduced renal function, Cymevene should be administered to elderly patients with special consideration of their renal status (see above).

*Children:* There has been limited clinical experience in treating patients under the age of 12 years. Reported adverse events were similar to those seen in adults.

**However, the use of Cymevene in children warrants careful consideration due to the possibility of long-term carcinogenicity and reproductive toxicity. The benefits of treatment should outweigh the risks.**

**Cymevene is not indicated for the treatment of congenital or neonatal CMV infections.**

*Laboratory monitoring and dosage reduction:* Because of individual patient sensitivity to the myelosuppressive effects of Cymevene regular clinical and haematological assessments are recommended. White blood cell and platelet counts should be performed every two days for the first 14 days of treatment. Patients with a history of marrow sensitivity to ganciclovir or other nucleoside analogues, or with white blood cell counts less than 1000 cells/μl at the beginning of treatment should be monitored daily. During maintenance treatment complete blood counts are recommended weekly, or more frequently if counts are low.

Neutropenia typically occurs during the first or second week of treatment. Severe neutropenia (< 500 cells/μl) requires a dose interruption. For less severe neutropenia a reduction in the total daily dose may be adequate. Cell counts usually normalise within 3 to 7 days after discontinuing the drug or decreasing the dose. As evidence of marrow recovery becomes apparent gradual increases in dose, with careful monitoring of white blood cell counts, may be appropriate.

*Method of administration:* **Cymevene must only be given by intravenous infusion, preferably via a plastic cannula, into a vein with adequate blood flow. Infusions are recommended to be given over at least one hour, since rapid intravenous injections may increase the toxicity. Intramuscular or subcutaneous injection may result in severe tissue irritation due to the high pH of the solution.**

*Reconstitution of the vial:* Caution should be exercised in the handling of Cymevene (see Precautions).

1. The contents of the vial should be reconstituted by the addition of 10 ml Water for Injections BP. Do not use bacteriostatic water for injection containing para-hydroxybenzoates, since these are incompatible with ganciclovir and may cause precipitation.

2. The vial should be shaken to dissolve the drug. Typically, reconstitution takes less than one minute, although occasionally for some batches it may take up to 3 minutes.

3. Reconstituted solution should be inspected for particulate matter; if there is any present, the drug should not be administered.

4. Due to the possibility of crystal formation, the contents of the reconstituted vial should be used immediately. It should not be refrigerated.

*Infusion solution preparation and administration:* Based on patient weight and therapeutic indications, the appropriate calculated dose volume should be removed from the vial (ganciclovir concentration 50 mg/ml) and added to 100 ml of a suitable infusion fluid for delivery over the course of one hour. Infusion concentrations greater than 10 mg/ml are not recommended. The following infusion fluids are compatible with ganciclovir: Sodium Chloride Intravenous Infusion BP (0.9% w/v); Glucose Intravenous Infusion BP (5% w/v); Compound Sodium Lactate Intravenous Infusion BP; Ringer's Solution for Injection.

Because non-bacteriostatic infusion fluid must be used with Cymevene, the infusion solution must be used within 24 hours of dilution to reduce the risk of bacterial contamination. The infusion solution should be refrigerated. Freezing is not recommended.

### Contra-indications, warnings, etc

*Contra-indications:*
  (I) Pregnancy and lactation
  (ii) Patients with known hypersensitivity to Cymevene or to aciclovir.

*Use in pregnancy and lactation:* Teratogenicity has been observed in animal studies. Cymevene should not be given to pregnant women as there is a high likelihood of damage to the developing foetus.

Adverse effects were observed in the offspring of lactating animals. It is not known if ganciclovir is excreted in human milk. However, since many drugs are, Cymevene should not be given to lactating mothers. Nursing should not be resumed until 72 hours after the last dose of Cymevene.

*Precautions:* **The clinical toxicity of Cymevene includes leucopenia and thrombocytopenia. In preclinical testing ganciclovir caused aspermatogenesis, mutagenicity, teratogenicity and carcinogenicity. It should therefore be considered a potential carcinogen and teratogen in humans.**

Between approximately 10 and 40% of patients receiving intravenous Cymevene develop neutropenia (neutrophil count less than 1000 cells/μl). Cymevene should, therefore, be used with caution in those patients with a history of cytopenia. In a study of 314 AIDS patients there was no relationship between baseline neutrophil count and the occurrence of neutropenia; therefore, the risk of neutropenia may not be predicted from pre-treatment cell counts. **However, Cymevene should not be administered if**

**the absolute neutrophil count falls below 500 cells/μl.**

Thrombocytopenia (platelet count less than 50,000/microlitre) was observed in 19% of patients treated with Cymevene. Patients being treated with immunosuppressive drugs were more likely to develop lowered platelet counts than patients with AIDS. Patients with platelet counts less than 100,000/microlitre were also at increased risk of thrombocytopenia.

Because of the mutagenic potential of Cymevene, women of childbearing potential should be advised to use effective contraception during treatment. Likewise, men should be advised to practice barrier contraception for 90 days following treatment.

Administration of Cymevene by intravenous infusion should be accompanied by adequate hydration, since Cymevene is excreted by the kidneys and normal clearance depends upon adequate renal function. If renal function is impaired, dosage adjustments are required. Such adjustments should be based on serum creatinine (see *Dosage and Administration*).

*Side-effects and adverse reactions:* Leucopenia and thrombocytopenia are the most frequently observed side-effects (see *Precautions*). Anaemia, fever, rash and abnormal liver function tests have been observed in 2% of patients.

Adverse events which were thought to be possibly related and occurred in 1% or less of the patients are listed by body systems below:
*Body as a whole:* chills, oedema, infections, malaise.
*Cardiovascular System:* arrhythmias, hypertension, hypotension.
*Central Nervous System:* abnormal thoughts or dreams, ataxia, coma, confusion, dizziness, headache, nervousness, paraesthesia, psychosis, somnolence, tremor.
*Digestive System:* nausea, vomiting, anorexia, diarrhoea, haemorrhage, pain.
*Haematologic System:* eosinophilia.
*Laboratory Abnormalities:* decrease in blood glucose.
*Respiratory System:* dyspnoea.
*Skin and Appendages:* alopecia, pruritus, urticaria.
*Special Senses:* retinal detachment in AIDS patients with CMV retinitis.
*Urogenital System:* haematuria, increased serum creatinine, increased blood urea nitrogen (BUN).
*Injection Site:* inflammation, pain, phlebitis.

*Drug interactions:* Binding of ganciclovir to plasma proteins is only about 1–2% and drug interactions involving binding site displacement are not anticipated. It is possible that probenecid, as well as other drugs which inhibit renal tubular secretion or resorption, may reduce renal clearance of ganciclovir and could increase the plasma half-life of ganciclovir. It is also possible that drugs which inhibit replication of rapidly dividing cell populations such as bone marrow, spermatogonia, and germinal layers of skin and gastro-intestinal mucosa might have combined additive toxic effects when used concomitantly with, before, or after Cymevene. Because of the possibility of additive toxicity with co-administration of drugs such as dapsone, pentamidine, flucytosine, vincristine, vinblastine, adriamycin, amphotericin B, trimethoprim/sulpha combinations or other nucleoside analogues, combination with Cymevene therapy should be used only if the potential benefits outweigh the risks.

Patients with AIDS may be receiving, or have received, treatment with zidovudine. **Since both zidovudine and Cymevene can result in neutropenia, it is recommended that these two drugs not be given concomitantly during induction treatment with ganciclovir.** In addition, data from a small number of patients studied to date indicate that maintenance ganciclovir treatment plus zidovudine at the recommended dose resulted in severe neutropenia in most individuals.

Generalised seizures have been reported in patients taking Cymevene and imipenem-cilastatin concomitantly. These drugs should only be used concomitantly with Cymevene after careful consideration of the risks involved.

*Treatment of overdosage:* In the event of overdose, dialysis and hydration may be of benefit in reducing drug plasma levels.

Toxic manifestations seen in animals given very high single intravenous doses of ganciclovir (500 mg/kg) included emesis, hypersalivation, anorexia, bloody diarrhoea, inactivity, cytopenia, abnormal liver function tests and BUN, testicular atrophy and death.

**Pharmaceutical precautions Caution should be observed in the handling of Cymevene. Avoid ingestion, inhalation or direct contact with the skin and mucous membranes. Cymevene should be considered a potential teratogen and carcinogen in humans.**

Cymevene solutions are alkaline (pH approximately 11). If Cymevene contacts the skin or mucous membranes wash thoroughly with soap and water. For eye exposure rinse thoroughly with plain water.

Procedures for the disposal of Cymevene should follow local guidelines or requirements.

*Storage:* Store below 30°C.

**Legal category** POM.

**Package quantities** Pack of 5 vials.

**Further information** Nil.

**Product licence number** 0031/0465

# DALMANE*

**Presentation** Capsules with opaque grey cap and opaque yellow body with ROCHE 15 printed in red on both cap and body, containing 16.4 mg flurazepam monohydrochloride (equivalent to 15 mg flurazepam).

Capsules with black cap and opaque grey body with ROCHE 30 printed in red on both cap and body, containing 32.8 mg flurazepam monohydrochloride (equivalent to 30 mg flurazepam).

**Uses** *Properties:* Dalmane is a benzodiazepine drug with hypnotic properties.

*Indications:* Short-term treatment of insomnia when it is severe, disabling or subjecting the individual to extreme distress. Dalmane is helpful in overcoming difficulties in getting to sleep and also in the problem of frequent nocturnal awakenings. Its properties make it particularly indicated where the total duration of sleep is less than adequate.

**Dosage and administration** *Adults:* The dosage of Dalmane should be determined on an individual basis taking into account the severity of the insomnia and the patient's response to treatment. Dosage is important in determining the duration of effect and the occurrence of residual effects. For most patients the optimum dose is 15 mg - this will ensure a full night's sleep with minimal residual effects on wakening. Patients with severe insomnia may require 30 mg but residual effects on awakening, associated with an anxiolytic effect, are more frequent at this dose.

ELDERLY OR DEBILITATED PATIENTS: THE INITIAL DOSE SHOULD NOT EXCEED 15 mg.

Treatment should, if possible, be on an intermittent basis. The lowest dose which can control symptoms should be used. Treatment should not be continued at full dose beyond four weeks. Long-term chronic use is not recommended. Treatment should always be tapered off gradually. Patients who have taken benzodiazepines for a prolonged time may require a longer period during which doses are reduced. Specialist help may be appropriate.

Dalmane is not for paediatric use.

Dalmane capsules are for oral administration.

**Contra-indications, warnings, etc**

*Contra-indications:* Patients with known sensitivity to benzodiazepines; acute pulmonary insufficiency; respiratory depression; phobic or obsessional states; chronic psychosis.

*Use in pregnancy:* There is no evidence as to drug safety in human pregnancy, nor is there evidence from animal work that it is free from hazard. Do not use during pregnancy, especially during the first and last trimesters, unless there are compelling reasons.

The administration of high doses or prolonged administration of low doses of benzodiazepines in the last trimester of pregnancy has been reported to produce irregularities in the foetal heart rate, and hypotonia, poor sucking and hypothermia in the neonate.

No data regarding the passage of flurazepam into breast milk are available. However, in common with other benzodiazepines, its passage into breast milk might be expected. If possible, the use of Dalmane during lactation should be avoided.

*Precautions:* In patients with chronic pulmonary insufficiency, and in patients with chronic renal or hepatic disease, dosage may need to be reduced.

Dalmane should not be used alone to treat depression or anxiety associated with depression, since suicide may be precipitated in such patients.

In cases of loss or bereavement, psychological adjustment may be inhibited by benzodiazepines.

Patients should be advised that, like all medicaments of this type, Dalmane may modify patients' performance at skilled tasks (driving, operating machinery, etc) to a varying degree depending upon dosage, administration and individual susceptibility. Patients should further be advised that alcohol may intensify any impairment, and should therefore be avoided during treatment. If the patient is awoken during the period of maximum drug activity, recall may be impaired.

The dependence potential of the benzodiazepines is low, particularly when limited to short-term use, but this increases when high doses are used, especially when given over long periods. This is particularly so in patients with a history of alcoholism or drug abuse or in patients with marked personality disorders. Regular monitoring in such patients is essential, routine repeat prescriptions should be avoided and treatment should be withdrawn gradually. Symptoms such as depression, nervousness, rebound insomnia, irritability, sweating, and diarrhoea have been reported following abrupt cessation of treatment in patients receiving even normal therapeutic doses for short periods of time.

In rare instances, withdrawal following excessive dosages may produce confusional states, psychotic manifestations and convulsions.

Abnormal psychological reactions to benzodiazepines have been reported. Rare behavioural effects include paradoxical aggressive outbursts, excitement, confusion and the uncovering of depression with suicidal tendencies. Extreme caution should therefore be used in prescribing benzodiazepines to patients with personality disorders.

If Dalmane is combined with centrally-acting drugs such as neuroleptics, tranquillisers, antidepressants, hypnotics, analgesics and anaesthetics, the sedative effects are likely to be intensified. The elderly require special supervision.

When Dalmane is used in conjunction with anti-epileptic drugs, side-effects and toxicity may be more evident, particularly with hydantoins or barbiturates or combinations including them. This requires extra care in adjusting dosage in the initial stages of treatment.

Known inhibitors of hepatic enzymes, e.g. cimetidine, have been shown to reduce the clearance of benzodiazepines and may potentiate their action and known inducers of hepatic enzymes, e.g. rifampicin, may increase the clearance of benzodiazepines.

*Side-effects and adverse reactions:* Common adverse effects include drowsiness, sedation, unsteadiness and ataxia; these are dose-related and may persist into the following day even after a single dose. The elderly are particularly sensitive to the effects of centrally-depressant drugs and may experience confusion, especially if organic brain changes are present; therefore dosage in these patients should not exceed 15 mg.

Other adverse effects are rare and include headache, vertigo, hypotension, gastro-intestinal upsets, skin rashes, visual disturbances, changes in libido, and urinary retention. Isolated cases of blood dyscrasias and jaundice have also been reported.

Occasionally patients treated with Dalmane experience a bitter after-taste.

*Treatment of overdosage:* When taken alone in overdosage, Dalmane presents few problems in management. Signs may include drowsiness, ataxia and dysarthria, with coma in severe cases. Treatment is symptomatic. Gastric lavage is useful only if performed soon after ingestion. The value of dialysis has not been determined. Anexate is a specific IV antidote for use in emergency situations. Patients requiring such intervention should be monitored closely in hospital (see separate prescribing information). If excitation occurs, barbiturates should not be used.

When taken with centrally-acting drugs, especially alcohol, the effects of overdosage are likely to be more severe and, in the absence of supportive measures, may prove fatal.

**Pharmaceutical precautions** *Storage:* Dalmane capsules in blister packings should be stored in a dry place. The recommended maximum storage temperature is 25°C.

**Legal category** CD (Sch.4), POM.

**Package quantities** Dalmane capsules 15 mg and 30 mg in blister packs of 30.

**Further information** The pharmacokinetic properties of Dalmane make it particularly indicated for patients whose total duration of sleep is less than adequate. The dosage of the drug is important in balancing the duration of effect with the occurrence of residual effects. On repeated dosing there is accumulation of an active metabolite, desalkylflurazepam, with steady state levels being reached within two to three weeks. Psychomotor studies have demonstrated, however, that a dose of 15 mg given for seven consecutive nights did not significantly affect performance on the morning after final administration. However, impairment of performance was recorded on the morning after final administration of 30 mg for seven consecutive nights. This dose is associated with daytime anxiolytic effects.

The elderly, and patients with impaired renal and/or hepatic function, will be particularly susceptible to the adverse effects listed above. It is advisable to review treatment regularly and to discontinue use as soon as possible.

Treatment should be kept to a minimum and given only under close medical supervision. Little is known regarding the efficacy or safety of benzodiazepines in long-term use.

An underlying cause for insomnia should be sought before deciding upon the use of benzodiazepines for symptomatic relief.

**Product licence numbers**
Capsules 15 mg   0031/0065R
Capsules 30 mg   0031/0066R

# EFUDIX*

**Qualitative and quantitative composition** Efudix cream contains 5% w/w fluorouracil.

**Pharmaceutical form** White, opaque cream containing 5% w/w fluorouracil.

**Clinical particulars**

*Therapeutic indications:* Efudix is used for the topical treatment of superficial pre-malignant and malignant skin lesions; keratoses including senile, actinic and arsenical forms; keratoacanthoma; Bowen's disease; superficial basal-cell carcinoma. Deep, penetrating or nodular basal cell and squamous cell carcinomas do not usually respond to Efudix therapy. It should be used only as a palliative therapy in such cases where no other form of treatment is possible.

*Posology and method of administration:* Efudix cream is for topical application.

*Pre-malignant conditions:* The cream should be applied thinly to the affected area once or twice daily; an occlusive dressing is not essential.

*Malignant conditions:* The cream should be applied once or twice daily under an occlusive dressing where this is practicable.

The cream should not harm healthy skin. Treatment should be continued until there is marked inflammatory response from the treated area, preferably with some erosion in the case of pre-malignant conditions. Severe discomfort may be alleviated by the use of topical steroid cream. The usual duration of treatment for an initial course of therapy is three to four weeks, but this may be prolonged. Lesions on the face usually respond more quickly than those on the trunk or lower limbs whilst lesions on the hands and forearms respond more slowly. Healing may not be complete until one or two months after therapy is stopped.

*Elderly:* Many of the conditions for which Efudix is indicated are common in the elderly. No special precautions are necessary.

*Children:* In view of the lack of clinical data available, Efudix is not recommended for use in children.

*Contra-indications:* Efudix is contra-indicated in patients with known hypersensitivity to Efudix or parabens.

*Special warnings and special precautions for use:* Efudix is for topical use only and care should be taken to avoid contact with mucous membranes or the eyes. The hands should be washed carefully after applying the cream.

The total area of skin being treated with Efudix at any one time should not exceed 500cm² (approx. 23 x 23cm). Larger areas should be treated a section at a time.

*Interaction with other medicaments and other forms of interaction:* No significant drug interactions with Efudix have been reported.

*Pregnancy and lactation:* There is evidence from animal work that fluorouracil is teratogenic and there is no evidence as to drug safety in human pregnancy. Therefore the use of Efudix is contra-indicated during pregnancy. It should also be regarded as contra-indicated in mothers who are breast-feeding.

*Effects on ability to drive and use machines:* None known.

*Undesirable effects:* Efudix is well tolerated. Transient erythema may occur in healthy skin surrounding the area being treated. Pre-existing subclinical lesions may become apparent. Exposure to sunlight may increase the intensity of the reaction. Dermatitis, allergic skin reactions and, rarely, erythema multiforme have been reported.

Percutaneous absorption of fluorouracil should not lead to clinically significant systemic toxicity when efudix is administered as directed. However, this possibility should be borne in mind if the product is used excessively, especially on ulcerated or broken skin.

*Overdose:* If Efudix is accidentally ingested, signs of fluorouracil overdosage may include nausea, vomiting and diarrhoea. Stomatitis and blood dyscrasias may occur in severe cases. Appropriate measures should be taken for the prevention of systemic infection and daily white cell counts should be performed.

**Pharmacological properties**

*Pharmacodynamic properties:* Efudix is a topical cytostatic preparation which exerts a beneficial therapeutic effect on neoplastic and pre-neoplastic skin lesions without damaging normal skin. The pattern of response follows this sequence: erythema, vesiculation, erosion, ulceration, necrosis and epithelisation.

*Pharmacokinetic properties:* Animal studies have shown that after topical application of fluorouracil, less than 10% is systemically absorbed. This maybe metabolised by catabolic or anabolic routes which are similar to that of endogenous uracil.

### Pharmaceutical particulars

*List of excipients:* Cetostearyl Alcohol HSE, White Soft Paraffin BP, Polysorbate 60 PhEur, Propylene Glycol PhEur, Methyl Parahydroxybenzoate PhEur, Propyl Parahydroxybenzoate PhEur, Purified Water PhEur.

*Incompatibilities:* None known.

*Shelf life:* The recommended shelf life of Efudix cream is 60 months.

*Special precautions for storage: Storage:* The recommended maximum storage temperature for Efudix cream is 30°C.

*Dilution:* Efudix cream should not be diluted.

*Nature and contents of container:* Efudix cream is supplied in an aluminium tube with a plastic screw cap.

*Instructions for use/handling:* Efudix is for topical use only and care should be taken to avoid contact with mucous membranes or the eyes. The hands should be washed carefully after applying the cream.

**Marketing authorisation number** 0031/0027R

**Date of approval/revision of SPC** September 1995

**Legal category** POM

## FANSIDAR*

**Presentation** Round, white tablets with ROCHE and a hexagon imprinted on one face and two break bars on the other, containing 500 mg sulfadoxine and 25 mg pyrimethamine.

**Uses** Properties: The mode of action of Fansidar is based on the reciprocal potentiation of its two components. Fansidar blocks the action of two enzymes which catalyse consecutive stages in the biosynthesis of folinic acid in malaria parasites. Larger doses of the components of Fansidar are necessary if they are given independently and the effect obtained is inferior to that of the combination.

Fansidar is effective against plasmodial strains which are resistant to chloroquine and/or pyrimethamine and other antifolate preparations.

With Fansidar, the danger of emergence of resistance is reduced. However, in certain malarious areas, particularly South-East Asia and South America, strains of *Plasmodium falciparum* may be encountered which have developed resistance to Fansidar.

Fansidar affects all developmental stages of the parasites. It has a prolonged action, yet effective plasma concentrations are rapidly attained after a single dose. Trophozoites and schizonts quickly disappear from the blood. Pre-erythrocytic stages are also affected and the gametocytes, although increased in number, are rendered much less infective for the vector. A protective effect persists for up to two to four weeks depending on the dose given and the immune state of the subject.

*Indications:* Treatment and prophylaxis of *Plasmodium falciparum* malaria.

*Treatment of malaria:* Fansidar is indicated for the treatment of *Plasmodium falciparum* malaria when the infection is contracted in an area of chloroquine resistance.

*Prophylaxis of malaria:* Malaria prophylaxis with Fansidar is indicated for travellers to areas where chloroquine-resistant *Plasmodium falciparum* malaria is endemic. Whenever malaria prophylaxis is prescribed, the malaria situation and in particular, resistance trends at the traveller's destination and any stop-over point must be considered. At present, there is no antimalarial agent which provides absolute protection against malaria, but conscientiously performed drug prophylaxis can usually prevent serious progression of the disease.

### Dosage and administration

*Curative treatment of malaria:* The appropriate amount of the drug is given in one single dose. This dose should not be repeated for at least seven days.

| Adults (higher dose for persons over 60 kg) | | 2 to 3 tablets |
|---|---|---|
| Children 10–14 years | (31–45 kg) | 2 tablets |
| 7–9 years | (21–30 kg) | 1½ tablets |
| 4–6 years | (11–20 kg) | 1 tablet |
| under 4 years | (5–10 kg) | ½ tablet |

In very severe cases, quinine may be added, preferably parenterally. An adequate supply of fluids and electrolytes should be maintained.

*Prophylactic management:* The following dose of Fansidar should be taken every seven days:

| Adults | | 1 tablet |
|---|---|---|
| Children 9–14 years | (30–45 kg) | ¾ tablet |
| 4-8 years | (11–29 kg) | ½ tablet |
| under 4 years | (5–10 kg) | ¼ tablet |

Regular dosage is important for continuous protection to be maintained. Routine measures to protect against mosquito bites should not be omitted.

Fansidar prophylaxis should be started about one week before entering the endemic area in order to assess tolerance; this will enable an alternative drug to be selected in the infrequent case where Fansidar is poorly tolerated.

IMPORTANT: Fansidar prophylaxis should be continued for four to six weeks after returning to a non-malarious area to ensure elimination of possible falciparum infections (malignant malaria). However, as with other prophylactic drugs, infections of benign malaria (vivax and malariae infections) may give rise to clinical attacks up to several months after return, despite regular prophylaxis.

Travellers should be instructed to report to a doctor any fever that occurs during or after their stay in a malarious area.

*Use in the elderly:* Although no specific studies have been performed to establish the use of Fansidar in the elderly, it has been used extensively and the dosage requirements and side effects appear to be similar to those of younger adults.

Fansidar tablets are for oral administration.

### Contra-indications, warnings, etc

*Contra-indications:* Patients with known sulphonamide hypersensitivity.

Prophylactic (repeated) use of Fansidar is contra-indicated in patients with severe renal insufficiency, marked liver parenchymal damage or blood dyscrasias.

Treatment must be immediately discontinued upon the appearance of any mucocutaneous signs or symptoms such as pruritus, erythema, rash, orogenital lesions or pharyngitis and a medical practitioner consulted. The possibility of an adverse drug reaction should be considered in patients developing a rash, jaundice, fever or severe generalised malaise during treatment with Fansidar.

Like all other preparations containing sulphonamides, Fansidar is contra-indicated in premature babies and during the first two months of life.

*Use in pregnancy:* Foetal damage has been observed in the rat when any drug containing a folate inhibitor, including Fansidar, is administered in early gestation. The damage is caused by the folic acid antagonist, pyrimethamine, a component of Fansidar; the damage can be prevented by the concomitant administration of folinic acid.

However, no such adverse effects attributed to Fansidar have been reported during human clinical use and the preparation is, therefore, not contra-indicated during pregnancy. The usual medical practice of avoiding the use of Fansidar during early pregnancy should be followed unless considered essential by a medical practitioner. Pregnant women should be made aware of the particular risks of contracting malaria during pregnancy, and should be advised not to undertake unnecessary journeys to endemic areas. A folate supplement should be given to pregnant women receiving Fansidar.

Although no cases have been documented to date, there is a possibility that use of Fansidar during pregnancy at term may produce kernicterus in the neonate.

Both pyrimethamine and sulfadoxine are excreted in maternal breast milk. Nursing mothers should not take Fansidar.

*Precautions:* Excessive exposure to the sun should be avoided.

Regular blood counts are recommended during long-term prophylactic use (over three months) of Fansidar.

*Drug interactions:* Concurrent administration of other preparations containing folate antagonists (e.g. co-trimoxazole, methotrexate, anticonvulsants) can result in increased impairment of folic acid metabolism which leads to haematological side effects. Such concomitant therapy should be avoided if possible.

There is evidence which may indicate an increase in incidence and severity of adverse reactions when chloroquine is used with Fansidar, as compared to the use of Fansidar alone.

*Side-effects and adverse reactions:* Fansidar is usually well tolerated at the recommended dosage.

As with other drugs containing sulphonamides and/or pyrimethamine, the following side-effects and hypersensitivity reactions may occur:

*Skin reactions:* Drug rash, pruritus and slight hair loss have been observed. These reactions are usually mild and disappear spontaneously upon withdrawal of the drug. In very rare instances, particularly in hypersensitive patients, cases of erythema multiforme, Stevens-Johnson syndrome and Lyell's syndrome have occurred, some of which have been fatal.

*Gastro-intestinal reactions:* Feeling of fullness, nausea, rarely vomiting, stomatitis. There have been isolated reports of hepatitis occurring conjointly with administration of Fansidar.

*Haematological changes:* In rare cases, leucopenia (usually asymptomatic), thrombocytopenia and megaloblastic anaemia have been observed. In extremely rare cases, they take the form of agranulocytosis or purpura. As a rule, all these changes disappear after withdrawal of the drug.

*Other side-effects:* Fatigue, headache, fever and polyneuritis may occasionally occur.

Pulmonary infiltrates such as eosinophilic or allergic alveolitis have been reported in rare instances. If symptoms such as cough or shortness of breath should occur during Fansidar therapy, the drug should be discontinued.

Adverse reactions occurring after the administration of the sulfadoxine component of Fansidar are not normally more prolonged than those occurring after shorter-acting sulphonamides despite the continued presence of the drug in the body.

*Treatment of overdosage:* Possible symptoms of overdosage include anorexia, nausea, vomiting, signs of excitation, and possibly convulsions and haematological changes (megaloblastic anaemia, leucopenia, thrombocytopenia).

Treatment is symptomatic and may include forced diuresis. Vigorous gastric lavage should be carried out as early as possible after ingestion. Alkalinisation of the urine may aid elimination of the sulfadoxine component of Fansidar. Possible convulsions due to the pyrimethamine component of Fansidar should be watched for and may require anticonvulsant therapy. Hypersensitivity reactions may require treatment with steroids. Calcium folinate may be given to counteract the effects of pyrimethamine on haemopoiesis.

**Pharmaceutical precautions** *Storage:* No special precautions are required.

**Legal category** POM.

**Package quantities** Fansidar tablets are available in foil strips in packs of 12 and 150.

**Further information** *Pharmacokinetics:* Absorption: After administration of 1 tablet, peak plasma levels for pyrimethamine (0.21 mg per litre) and for sulfadoxine (63.2 mg per litre) are reached after about four hours (means obtained from 14 test subjects).

Elimination: A relatively long elimination half-life is characteristic of both components. The mean values are 96 hours for pyrimethamine and 184 hours for sulfadoxine. Both pyrimethamine and sulfadoxine are eliminated mainly via the kidneys.

Accumulation: Patients taking 1 tablet a week (recommended adult dose for malaria prophylaxis) can be expected to have mean steady state plasma concentrations of 0.15 mg per litre for pyrimethamine (after about four weeks) and 98.4 mg per litre for sulfadoxine (after about seven weeks).

Protein binding: The following values were determined for binding to plasma protein: pyrimethamine 84.9% and sulfadoxine 91.4%.

**Product licence number** 0031/5097R

## GENTICIN* EYE/ EAR DROPS

**Qualitative and quantitative composition** Gentamicin Sulphate PhEur ≡ 0.3% w/v gentamicin base.

**Pharmaceutical form** Sterile, isotonic solution in dropper bottles.

### Clinical particulars

*Therapeutic indications:* Genticin eye/ear drops are indicated:

(1) For the treatment of superficial eye and ear infections caused by organisms sensitive to gentamicin.

(2) For prophylaxis against infection in trauma of the eye or ear.

*Posology and method of administration:*
*Adults, including the elderly and children*

*Eyes:* 1 or 2 drops should be instilled in the affected eye up to six times a day, or more frequently if required. (Severe infections may require 1 or 2 drops every fifteen to twenty minutes initially, reducing the frequency of instillation gradually as the infection is controlled.)

*Ears:* The area should be cleaned and 2–3 drops instilled in the affected ear three to four times a day and at night, or more frequently if required.

*Contra-indications:* Hypersensitivity to gentamicin or to any of the ingredients. Cross sensitivity with other aminoglycoside antibiotics may occur. Perforation of the ear drum is a contra-indication to use in otitis externa.

*Special warnings and precautions for use:* Long-term continuous topical therapy should be avoided. Prolonged use may lead to skin sensitisation and the emergence of resistant organisms.

In severe infections, topical use of gentamicin should be supplemented with appropriate systemic antibiotic treatment.

Gentamicin may cause irreversible partial or total deafness when given systemically or when applied topically to open wounds or damaged skin. This effect is dose-related and is enhanced by renal and/or hepatic impairment and is more likely in the elderly.

Topical application of aminoglycoside antibiotics into the middle ear carries a theoretical risk of causing hearing loss due to ototoxicity. The benefits of gentamicin therapy should be considered against the risk of infection itself causing hearing loss.

Contact lenses should be removed during the period of treatment of ocular infections.

*Interaction with other medicaments and other forms of interaction:* None relevant to topical use.

*Pregnancy and lactation:* Safety for use in pregnancy and lactation has not been established. Gentamicin should only be used in pregnancy or lactation when considered essential by the physician, after careful assessment of the potential risks and benefits.

*Effects on ability to drive and use machines:* Patients should be advised that the use of Genticin in the eye may cause transient blurring of vision. If affected, patients should not drive or operate machinery until vision has cleared.

*Undesirable effects:* Irritation, burning, stinging, itching and dermatitis may occur. In the event of irritation, sensitisation or super-infection, treatment should be discontinued and appropriate therapy instituted.

*Overdose:* The oral ingestion of the contents of one bottle is unlikely to cause any significant adverse effect.

**Pharmacological properties**

*Pharmacodynamic properties:* Gentamicin is a bactericidal antibiotic which acts by inhibiting protein synthesis.

*Pharmacokinetic properties:* Topical application of gentamicin can result in some systemic absorption. Treatment of large areas can result in plasma concentrations of up to 1μg/ml.

> 90% Gentamicin is excreted in the urine by glomerular filtration.

< 10% is bound to plasma protein.

$T_{1/2}$ = 2–3 hours in individuals with normal kidney function, but can be increased in cases of renal insufficiency.

*Preclinical safety data:* Not relevant.

**Pharmaceutical particulars**

*List of excipients:* Benzalkonium chloride BP, Borax PhEur, Sodium Chloride PhEur, Water, Purified PhEur.

*Incompatibilities:* None known.

*Shelf life:* 3 years. Discard contents 4 weeks after opening.

*Special precautions for storage:* Store below 25°C. Do not freeze.

*Nature of contents and container:* Genticin eye/ear drops are available in 10 ml dropper bottles.

*Instructions for use/handling:* Not applicable.

**Marketing authorisation number**    0031/0380

**Date of approval/revision of SPC**    May 1996

**Legal category** POM

## GENTICIN* INJECTABLE

**Qualitative and quantitative composition**   Gentamicin Sulphate PhEur ≡ 4.0% w/v (80 mg) gentamicin base.

**Pharmaceutical form**    Solution for injection. Each ampoule contains a sterile, clear, colourless to pale yellow liquid. The solution is preservative free.

**Clinical particulars**

*Therapeutic indications:* Gentamicin Injectable ampoules are indicated for the treatment of systemic infections due to susceptible bacteria, for example, bacteraemia, septicaemia, urinary-tract infections and severe chest infections.

*Posology and method of administration:* Genticin is normally administered intramuscularly but may be given intravenously if required. If intravenous administration is necessary the dose should be given as a bolus injection into the tubing of the giving set or directly into the venous system over a period of 2–3 minutes. Genticin should not be given as a slow infusion or mixed with other drugs before use (see *Incompatibilities*).

With either intramuscular or intravenous administration the following dosage applies for normal renal function:

*Adults:* 3–4 mg/kg body weight daily in divided doses. Typical doses:
   Over 60 kg: 80 mg 8-hourly.
   Less than 60 kg: 60 mg 8-hourly.

In cases of impaired renal function a reduction in dosage frequency is recommended. The following table is a guide to recommended dosage schedules:

| Blood urea (mg/100 ml) | Creatinine clearance (GFR) (ml/min) | Dose and frequency of administration |
| --- | --- | --- |
| < 40 | > 70 | 80 mg† 8-hourly |
| 40–100 | 30–70 | 80 mg† 12-hourly |
| 100–200 | 10–30 | 80 mg† daily |
| > 200 | 5–10 | 80 mg† every 48 hours |
| Twice-weekly intermittent haemodialysis | < 5 | 80 mg† after dialysis |

† 60 mg if body weight < 60 kg.

*Urinary tract infections:* As above. Alternatively, if renal function is not impaired, 160 mg once daily may be used.

In life-threatening infections the frequency of dosage may need to be increased to 6-hourly and the quantity of each dose may also be increased at the discretion of the clinician up to a total dosage of 5 mg/kg in 24 hours. In such cases it is advisable to monitor gentamicin serum levels.

*Elderly:* Adjust dosage according to weight and renal function. Periodic serum monitoring is desirable.

*Children:* In children and in neonates, it can be expected that serum levels will be lower than those found in adults at equivalent dosage per kg body weight.

The recommended paediatric dosage is therefore as follows:

*Up to 12 years:* 6 mg/kg in 24 hours in three equally divided doses (i.e. 2 mg/kg 8-hourly).

In infants up to 2 weeks this dosage should be given in two equally divided doses (i.e. 3 mg/kg 12-hourly).

Serum levels should preferably be monitored daily.

In neonates, infants and children, subsequent dosage will often need to be increased to achieve therapeutic serum levels. Peak levels should be measured about 1 hour after intramuscular or intravenous injection and should reach 4 microgrammes/ml, but not exceed 10 microgrammes/ml.

*Contra-indications:* Hypersensitivity to gentamicin, any other ingredient or to other aminoglycosides. Myasthenia gravis.

*Special warnings and precautions for use:* Where renal function is impaired through disease or old age the frequency, but not the amount, of each dose should be reduced according to the degree of impairment. Gentamicin is excreted by simple glomerular filtration, and dosage frequency may be predicted by assessing creatinine clearance rates or blood urea and reducing the frequency accordingly.

It is also advisable to check serum levels to confirm that peak (1 hour) levels do not exceed 10 microgrammes/ml and that trough levels (before next injection) do not exceed 2 microgrammes/ml.

*Interaction with other medicaments and other forms of interaction:* Concurrent use with other potentially nephrotoxic or ototoxic drug substances should be avoided. The potential nephrotoxicity of cephalosporins may be increased in the presence of gentamicin and kidney monitoring is therefore recommended with this combination.

Frusemide and piretanide may potentiate the ototoxicity of gentamicin, and ethacrynic acid, which is ototoxic in its own right, should be avoided with gentamicin.

Ticarcillin has been shown to reduce the gentamicin activity *in vivo* and, if clinically indicated, should be given at different times from gentamicin.

Neuromuscular blockade and respiratory paralysis have occasionally been reported from administration of aminoglycosides to patients who have received curare-type muscle relaxants during anaesthesia.

Bacteriostatic antibiotics may give an antagonistic interaction, but in some cases (e.g. with clindamycin and lincomycin) the disadvantage of antagonism may be outweighed by the addition of activity against anaerobic organisms. Synergistic action has been demonstrated with penicillin. Cross-sensitivity with aminoglycosides may occur.

*Pregnancy and lactation:* Safety for use in pregnancy and lactation has not been established. Gentamicin crosses the placenta and there is a risk of ototoxicity in the foetus. Gentamicin should only be used where the seriousness of the mother's condition justifies the risk.

*Effects on ability to drive and use machines:* None.

*Undesirable effects:* As with all aminoglycosides, at critical levels gentamicin exhibits toxicity. Nephrotoxicity may occur, resulting in a gradual reduction in creatinine clearance after about 2 weeks of treatment. This is rapidly reversed if the drug is withdrawn. Most cases have pre-existing renal disease or have received other nephrotoxic agents.

Vestibular damage or hearing loss may occur, particularly after exposure to ototoxic drugs or in the presence of renal dysfunction. With gentamicin the vestibular mechanism may be affected when peak serum levels of 10 microgrammes/ml or when a trough level of 2 microgrammes/ml are exceeded. This is usually reversible if observed promptly and the dose adjusted. In the patients with normal renal function it is virtually impossible to achieve these levels at standard dosage.

Gentamicin has rarely been associated with pseudomembranous colitis and usually in these cases other antibiotics are also involved.

*Overdose:* Symptoms include dizziness, vertigo and hearing loss if overdose accidentally given parenterally.

If the reaction is severe consider haemodialysis as treatment.

**Pharmacological properties**

*Pharmacodynamic properties:* Gentamicin is a bactericidal antibiotic which acts by inhibiting protein synthesis.

*Pharmacokinetic properties* Gentamicin is rapidly absorbed following intramuscular injection, giving peak plasma concentrations after 30 minutes–1 hour. Effective concentrations are still present 4 hours after injection. An injection of 1 mg/kg body weight results in a peak plasma concentration of approximately 4 micrograms/ml.

> 90% gentamicin is excreted in the urine by glomerular filtration.

< 10% is bound to plasma protein.

$T_{1/2}$ = 2–3 hours in individuals with normal kidney function, but can be increased in individuals with renal insufficiency.

*Preclinical safety data:* There are no pre-clinical data of relevance to the prescriber which are additional to that already included in other sections of the SPC.

**Pharmaceutical particulars**

*List of excipients:* Water for Injection PhEur, Sulphuric Acid PhEur.

*Incompatibilities:* In general, mixing Genticin Injectable with other drugs prior to administration is not advised. In particular the following are incompatible in mixed solution: penicillins, cephalosporins, erythromycin, lipiphysan, heparins and sodium bicarbonate. In the latter case carbon dioxide may be liberated on addition of the two solutions. Normally this will dissolve in the solution, but under some circumstances small bubbles may form.

Dilution in the body will obviate the danger of physical and chemical incompatibility and enable Genticin Injectable to be given concurrently with the drugs listed above either as a bolus injection into the drip tubing with adequate flushing, or at separate sites. However, in the case of carbenicillin and gentamicin they should only be given at separate sites.

*Shelf life:* 4 years.

*Special precautions for storage:* Maximum recommended storage temperature 25°C.

*Nature of contents and container:* Genticin Injectable is available in colourless, Type I glass ampoules containing 2 ml, in boxes of 10 ampoules.

*Instructions for use/handling:* Not applicable

**Marketing authorisation number**    0031/0381

**Date of approval/revision of SPC**    July 1996

**Legal category**    POM

## GENTISONE* HC EAR DROPS

**Qualitative and quantitative composition** Gentisone HC ear drops is a sterile aqueous suspension in 10 ml dropper bottles containing gentamicin sulphate equivalent to 0.3% w/v gentamicin base and 1.0% w/v hydrocortisone acetate.

**Pharmaceutical form** Sterile aqueous suspension.

## Clinical particulars

*Therapeutic indications:* Gentisone HC ear drops are indicated:

1. For the treatment of eczema and infection of the outer ear (otitis externa).
2. For prophylaxis against otitis externa following trauma.
3. For post-operative local use in surgery to infected mastoid cavities.
4. For chronic suppurative otitis media.

*Posology and method of administration*
*For all ages:* The area should be cleaned and 2–4 drops instilled in the affected ear three to four times a day and at night. Alternatively, wicks medicated with Gentisone HC drops may be placed in the external ear or mastoid cavity.

*Contra-indications:* Hypersensitivity to gentamicin or to any of the ingredients. Cross sensitivity with other aminoglycoside antibiotics may occur. Perforation of the ear drum is a contra-indication to use in otitis externa.

*Special warnings and special precautions for use:* Long-term continuous topical therapy should be avoided. Prolonged use may lead to skin sensitisation and the emergence of resistant organisms.

In severe infections, topical use of Gentisone HC should be supplemented with appropriate systemic antibiotic treatment.

Gentamicin may cause irreversible partial or total deafness when given systemically or when applied topically to open wounds or damaged skin. This effect is dose-related and is enhanced by renal and/or hepatic impairment and is more likely in the elderly.

Topical application of aminoglycoside antibiotics into the middle ear carries a theoretical risk of causing hearing loss due to ototoxicity. The benefits of gentamicin therapy should be considered against the risk of infection itself causing hearing loss.

In infants there is a theoretical risk that sufficient steroid may be absorbed to cause adrenal suppression.

*Interaction with other medicaments and other forms of interaction:* None relevant to topical use.

*Pregnancy and lactation:* Safety for use in pregnancy and lactation has not been established. Topical administration of any corticosteroid to pregnant animals can cause abnormalities of foetal development. Gentisone HC drops should only be used in pregnancy or lactation when considered essential by the physician, after careful assessment of the potential risks and benefits.

*Effects on ability to drive and use machines:* Not applicable.

*Undesirable effects:* In the event of irritation, sensitisation or super-infection, treatment with Gentisone HC should be discontinued and appropriate therapy instituted.

*Overdose:* Not applicable.

## Pharmacological properties

*Pharmacodynamic properties:* Gentamicin is a bactericidal antibiotic which acts by inhibiting protein synthesis.

Corticosteroids, such as hydrocortisone acetate, are used in pharmacological doses for their anti-inflammatory and immuno-suppressant glucocorticoid properties which suppress the clinical manifestation of disease in a wide range of disorders.

*Pharmacokinetic properties:* Topical application of gentamicin can result in some systemic absorption. Treatment of large areas can result in plasma concentrations of up to 1 μg/ml.

> 90% gentamicin is excreted in the urine by glomerular filtration.

< 10% is bound to plasma protein.

$T_{\frac{1}{2}}$ = 2–3 hours in individuals with normal kidney function, but can be increased in cases of renal insufficiency.

Hydrocortisone acetate is not absorbed through the skin as rapidly as hydrocortisone and therefore has a prolonged action. Some is absorbed systemically, where greater than 90% is protein bound.

> 70% hydrocortisone acetate is metabolised by the liver. The metabolites are excreted in the urine.

Plasma $T_{\frac{1}{2}}$ = $1\frac{1}{2}$ hours.

*Preclinical safety data:* See *Pregnancy and lactation.*

## Pharmaceutical particulars

*List of excipients:* Benzalkonium chloride (preservative), povidone, polyethylene glycol 4000, sodium chloride, borax, disodium edetate and purified water.

*Incompatibilities:* None known.

*Shelf life:* 3 years.

*Special precautions for storage:* Store below 25°C. Do not freeze or mix with other liquids.

*Nature and contents of container:* 10 ml dropper bottles.

*Instructions for use/handling:* Not applicable.

**Marketing authorisation number** 0031/0382

**Date of approval/revision of SPC** March 1996

**Legal category** POM

# HIVID* ▼

**Presentation** Hivid contains zalcitabine (approved name), chemically known as 4-amino-1-β-D-2',3'-dideoxyribofuranosyl-2-(1,H)-pyrimidinone (2', 3'-dideoxycytidine, dideoxycytidine, ddC).

Grey to bluish-grey, oval, biconvex, flat-edged, film-coated tablets containing 0.750 mg zalcitabine, printed HIVID 0.750 on one side and ROCHE on the other with black ink.

Beige to bluish-grey, oval, biconvex, flat-edged, film-coated tablets containing 0.375 mg zalcitabine, printed HIVID 0.375 on one side and ROCHE on the other with black ink.

## Uses

*Indications:* Hivid (zalcitabine) is indicated for the management of adult patients with advanced HIV infection who are intolerant to or who have failed on zidovudine (ZDV) therapy.

ZDV Intolerance:

- ZDV haematological intolerance is defined as a haemoglobin level below 7.5 g/dl or symptomatic anaemia or a neutrophil count below 0.75 x 10⁹/l.

- ZDV clinical intolerance can be defined as persistent nausea, headache, vomiting or myopathy which is clearly attributable to ZDV.

ZDV Failure:

- ZDV failure can be defined as progression of disease, as evidenced by deteriorating clinical status and/or rapidly worsening immunological status.

*Pharmacological properties:* Zalcitabine is a synthetic analogue of the naturally occurring nucleoside 2'-deoxycytidine in which the 3'-hydroxyl group is replaced by hydrogen. Within cells, zalcitabine is converted to the active metabolite, dideoxycytidine-5'-triphosphate (ddCTP) by cellular enzymes. Dideoxycytidine-5'-triphosphate serves as an alternative substrate to deoxycytidine triphosphate (dCTP) for HIV-reverse transcriptase and inhibits the *in vitro* replication of HIV by competitive inhibition of viral DNA synthesis due to premature chain termination.

Comparative studies of the antiviral activity of zalcitabine against HIV-1 and HIV-2 *in vitro* revealed no significant difference in sensitivity between the two viruses when activity was determined by measuring viral cytopathic effect. The relationship of the *in vitro* inhibition of HIV by zalcitabine to the inhibition of HIV replication in infected people, or the clinical response to therapy, has not been established.

Hivid has been shown to act additively or synergistically with a number of anti-HIV agents, particularly zidovudine and interferon alpha inhibiting the replication of HIV in cell culture.

*Pharmacokinetics:* The pharmacokinetics of zalcitabine have been evaluated in studies with HIV-infected patients following 0.01 mg/kg, 0.03 mg/kg and 1.5 mg oral doses, and a 1.5 mg intravenous dose administered as a 1-hour infusion.

Following oral administration to HIV-infected patients, the mean absolute bioavailability was >80%. The absorption rate of a 1.5 mg oral dose of zalcitabine was reduced when administered with food. This resulted in a 39% decrease in mean maximum plasma concentrations (Cmax) from 25.2ng/ml to 15.5ng/ml and a twofold increase in time to achieve maximum plasma concentrations from a mean of 0.8 hours under fasting conditions to 1.6 hours when the drug was given with food. The mean extent of absorption (as reflected by AUC) was decreased by 14%. The clinical relevance of this decrease is unknown.

The steady-state volume of distribution following IV administration of a 1.5 mg dose of zalcitabine averaged 0.534 (± 0.127)l/kg.

The drug was <4% bound to plasma proteins, indicating that drug interactions involving binding-site displacement are unlikely.

Cerebrospinal fluid (CSF) obtained 2 to 3.5 hours following 0.06 mg/kg or 0.09 mg/kg IV infusion showed measurable concentrations of zalcitabine. The CSF to plasma concentration ratio ranged from 9% to 37%, demonstrating penetration of the drug through the blood-brain barrier.

Zalcitabine is phosphorylated intracellularly to zalcitabine triphosphate, the active substrate for HIV-reverse transcriptase. Concentrations of zalcitabine triphosphate are too low for quantitation following administration of therapeutic doses to humans.

Zalcitabine metabolism in humans has not been fully evaluated. Zalcitabine does not undergo a significant degree of metabolism by the liver. Renal excretion is the primary route of elimination, and accounted

for approximately 70% of an orally-administered, radiolabelled dose (i.e. total radioactivity) within 24 hours after dosing. The mean elimination half-life is 2 hours and generally ranges from 1 to 3 hours in individual patients. Total mean body clearance following an intravenous dose averages 285 ml/min. Less than 10% of a radiolabeled dose of zalcitabine appears in the faeces.

Results from patients with renal impairment (estimated creatinine clearance rate <55 ml/min) indicate that the half-life was prolonged (up to 8.5 hours) in these patients compared to those with normal renal function. Maximum plasma concentrations were higher in some patients after a single dose. In patients with normal renal function, the pharmacokinetics of zalcitabine was not altered during three times daily multiple dosing. Accumulation of drug in plasma during this regimen was negligible.

## Dosage and administration

*Adults:* The optimal dosage regimen remains unknown. Based on controlled clinical studies a dose of 0.75 mg t.i.d. (2.25 mg total daily dose) is recommended.

Monitoring of patients: Periodic complete blood counts and clinical chemistry tests should be performed. Serum amylase levels should be monitored in those individuals who have a history of elevated amylase, pancreatitis, ethanol abuse, who are on parenteral nutrition or who are otherwise at high risk of pancreatitis. Careful monitoring for signs or symptoms suggestive of peripheral neuropathy is recommended, particularly in individuals with a low $CD_4$ cell count who are at a greater risk of developing peripheral neuropathy while on therapy.

Hivid should only be administered under the supervision of a doctor with experience in treating patients with HIV infection.

*Renal and hepatic impairment:* Recommendations for dose adjustment cannot be given for patients with impaired renal or hepatic function because of limited experience.

In individuals with pre-existing liver disease or with a history of ethanol abuse, the use of Hivid may be associated with exacerbation of hepatic dysfunction.

*Children:* The safety of Hivid in children younger than 13 years of age and in asymptomatic HIV-infected individuals has not been established. Recommendations for the dosage in children younger than 13 years cannot be given since experience in this age group is limited.

*Elderly:* The safety and efficacy of Hivid in the elderly has not been established.

## Contra-indications, warnings, etc

*Contra-indications:* Hivid is contra-indicated in patients with known hypersensitivity to any of the components of the tablets.

Hivid is contra-indicated in patients presenting with peripheral neuropathy, as evidenced by symptoms accompanied by objective findings.

*Use in pregnancy and lactation:* The safety of Hivid for use in human pregnancy has not been established. Although a teratogenic effect has been observed in animals at very high exposure levels of zalcitabine, experimental studies are insufficient to assess the safety with respect to reproduction, development of the embryo or foetus or the course of gestation and peri- and postnatal development.

Hivid should be used during pregnancy only if the potential benefit justifies the potential risk to the foetus.

Fertile women should not receive Hivid unless they are using effective contraception during the therapy period.

It is not known whether zalcitabine is excreted in human milk. Because many drugs are excreted in human milk and because of the potential for serious adverse reactions from zalcitabine in nursing infants, a decision should be made whether to discontinue nursing or to discontinue the drug, taking into account the importance of the drug to the mother.

*Effects on ability to drive and use machines:* There are no data available that demonstrate an effect of Hivid on the ability to drive and use machines.

*Precautions:*
*Peripheral neuropathy:* The major clinical toxicity of Hivid is peripheral neuropathy. Hivid-related peripheral neuropathy is a sensorimotor neuropathy characterised initially by numbness and burning dysesthesia involving the distal extremities. These symptoms may be followed by sharp shooting pains or severe continuous burning pain if the drug is not withdrawn. The neuropathy may progress to severe pain requiring narcotic analgesics and is potentially irreversible, especially if Hivid is not stopped promptly. In some patients, symptoms of neuropathy may initially progress despite discontinuation of Hivid. With prompt discontinuation of Hivid, the neuropathy is usually slowly reversible.

Hivid should be used with extreme caution in patients with a risk of developing peripheral neuropathy. It should also be used with particular caution in patients with low CD$_4$ cell counts (CD$_4$ <50 cells/mm³) for whom the risk of developing peripheral neuropathy while on Hivid therapy is greater. Careful monitoring is strongly recommended for these individuals.

*Pancreatitis:* Fatal pancreatitis has been observed with the administration of Hivid. Pancreatitis is an uncommon complication of therapy, occurring in <1% of patients. The occurrence of asymptomatic elevated serum amylase of any etiology while on Hivid therapy was also <1%. Caution should be exercised when administering Hivid to any patient with a history of pancreatitis or known risk factor for the development of pancreatitis.

Patients with a history of pancreatitis or a history of elevated serum amylase should be followed more closely while on Hivid therapy. Treatment should be interrupted in the setting of a rising serum amylase level associated with dysglycaemia, rising triglyceride level, decreasing serum calcium or other parameters suggestive of impending pancreatitis, until a clinical diagnosis is reached. Treatment should also be interrupted if treatment with another drug known to cause pancreatitis (e.g. intravenous pentamidine) is required. Hivid should be restarted only after pancreatitis has been ruled out. If clinical pancreatitis develops during Hivid administration, it is recommended that Hivid be permanently discontinued.

*Other serious adverse events:* Infrequent cases of oesophageal ulcer and hypersensitivity reactions (anaphylactic reaction, urticaria without other signs of anaphylaxis) have been reported in individuals receiving Hivid therapy. Interruption of Hivid should be considered in patients who develop oesophageal ulcers which do not respond to specific treatment for opportunistic pathogens. Infrequent cases of cardiomyopathy and congestive heart failure have been reported in patients receiving Hivid. Treatment in patients with baseline cardiomyopathy or history of congestive heart failure should be approached with caution.

Rare occurrences of lactic acidosis in the absence of hypoxaemia, and severe hepatomegaly with steatosis have been reported with the use of nucleoside analogues, including zidovudine and Hivid, and are potentially life-threatening. In addition, cases of hepatic failure in association with underlying Hepatitis B and Hivid monotherapy have been reported. Treatment with Hivid in patients with pre-existing liver disease, liver enzyme abnormalities, a history of ethanol abuse or hepatitis, should be approached with caution. Hivid should be interrupted or discontinued in the setting of deterioration of liver function tests, hepatic steatosis, progressive hepatomegaly or unexplained lactic acidosis.

*Information for patients:* Patients should be informed that Hivid is not a cure for HIV infection, that they may continue to develop illnesses associated with advanced HIV infection including opportunistic infections, and that Hivid has not been shown to reduce the incidence or frequency of such illnesses. Since it is frequently difficult to determine whether symptoms are a result of drug effect or underlying disease manifestation, patients should be encouraged to report all changes in their condition to their physician. Patients should be informed that the use of Hivid or other antiretroviral drugs do not preclude the ongoing need to maintain practices designed to prevent transmission of HIV.

Patients should be advised of the early symptoms of peripheral neuropathy and pancreatitis and should be instructed to promptly report them to their physician. Since the development of peripheral neuropathy appears to be dose-related to Hivid, patients should follow their physicians' instructions regarding the prescribed dose. Women of childbearing age should use effective contraception while using Hivid.

*Side-effects and adverse reactions:*
*Frequent adverse events:* In clinical trials, the major adverse event associated with Hivid was peripheral neuropathy (20–23%) (see 'Precautions' section).
*Other frequent adverse events reported were:*
*Gastrointestinal:* Oral ulcers, nausea, dysphagia, anorexia, diarrhoea, abdominal pain, vomiting, constipation.
*Skin and appendages:* Rash, pruritus, sweats.
*Central and peripheral nervous system:* Headache, dizziness.
*Musculoskeletal:* Myalgia, arthralgia.
*Body as a whole:* Weight decrease, fatigue, fever, rigors, chest pain.
*Respiratory:* Pharyngitis.
*Laboratory adverse events:* Anaemia, leukopenia, neutropenia, SGPT elevation, SGOT elevation, eosinophilia, thrombocytopenia, alkaline phosphatase elevation.
*Clinical adverse events that occurred less frequently or rarely were:*
*Body as a whole:* Asthenia, pain, substernal chest pain, malaise, general oedema.
*Cardiovascular:* Heart racing, hypertension, palpi-

tation, syncope, atrial fibrillation, tachycardia, cardiomyopathy.
*Gastrointestinal:* Dry mouth, oesophageal ulcers, dyspepsia, glossitis, oesophageal pain, rectal haemorrhage, haemorrhoids, rectal ulcers, flatulence, tongue ulceration, enlarged abdomen, gum disorder, stomatitis, eructation, gastritis, gastrointestinal haemorrhage, pancreatitis, salivary gland enlargement, jaundice, oesophagitis.
*Hepatic:* Hepatocellular damage, hepatitis, abnormal hepatic function.
*Musculoskeletal:* Shoulder pain, leg cramps, foot pain, arm pain, arthritis, arthropathy, cold extremities, wrist pain, myositis.
*Nervous:* Hypertonia, tremor, hand tremor, twitching, seizures, ataxia, abnormal co-ordination, Bell's palsy, dysphonia, hyperkinesia, hypokinesia, migraine, neuralgia, neuritis, stupor, vertigo.
*Psychiatric:* Confusion, impaired concentration, amnesia, insomnia, somnolence, depression, agitation, depersonalisation, emotional lability, nervousness, anxiety, euphoria, manic reaction, dementia.
*Respiratory:* Coughing, dyspnoea, cyanosis.
*Skin:* Dermatitis, alopecia, urticaria, erythematous papules, skin lesions, acne, bullous eruptions, flushing.
*Special senses and vision:* Taste perversion, xerophthalmia, abnormal vision, eye pain, tinnitus, ear blockage, parosmia, loss of taste, eye abnormalities, deafness.
*Urinary system:* Micturition frequency, abnormal renal function, acute renal failure, renal cyst, gout, toxic nephropathy, polyuria, renal calculus, hyperuricemia.

*Drug interactions:* Possible interactions of Hivid with other concomitant medication have not been formally investigated.

The concomitant use of Hivid with drugs that have the potential to cause peripheral neuropathy should be avoided where possible. Drugs which have been associated with peripheral neuropathy include chloramphenicol, cisplatin, dapsone, disulfiram, ethionamide, glutethimide, gold, hydralazine, iodoquinol, isoniazid, metronidazole, nitrofurantoin, phenytoin, ribavirin and vincristine. Concomitant use of Hivid with didanosine is not recommended.

Drugs such as amphotericin, foscarnet and aminoglycosides may increase the risk of developing peripheral neuropathy or other Hivid-associated adverse events by interfering with the renal clearance of zalcitabine (and thereby raising systemic exposure). Patients who require the use of one of these drugs with Hivid should have frequent clinical and laboratory monitoring with dosage adjustment for any significant change in renal function.

Treatment should be interrupted, when using a drug that may cause pancreatitis. A case of fatal fulminant pancreatitis possibly related to Hivid and intravenous pentamidine has been reported. If intravenous pentamidine is required to treat *Pneumocystis carinii* pneumonia, treatment with Hivid should be interrupted.

*Treatment of overdosage*
*Acute overdosage:* There is little experience with acute Hivid overdosage and the sequelae are unknown. There is no known antidote for overdosage. It is not known whether zalcitabine is dialysable by peritoneal dialysis or haemodialysis.
*Chronic overdosage:* In an initial dose-finding study in which zalcitabine was administered at doses of 25 times (0.25 mg/kg every 8 hours) the currently recommended dose, one patient discontinued Hivid after one and a half weeks of treatment subsequent to the development of a rash and fever. In the early phase I studies, all patients receiving Hivid at approximately six times the current total daily recommended dose experienced peripheral neuropathy by week 10. Eighty percent of the patients who received approximately twice the current total daily recommended dose experienced peripheral neuropathy by week 12.

**Pharmaceutical precautions**
*Storage:* Hivid tablets available in glass bottles should be stored below 30°C.

**Legal category**　POM

**Package quantities**　Hivid tablets are available in glass bottles with a tight screw closure fitted with a desiccant unit, each bottle containing 100 tablets of either 0.375 mg or 0.750 mg strength.

**Further information**　Nil.

**Product licence numbers**
0.375 mg tablets　　0031/0312
0.750 mg tablets　　0031/0313

## HYPNOVEL* AMPOULES 10 mg/2 ml

**Presentation**　Hypnovel contains the substance with the approved name midazolam. It is chemically

described as 8-chloro-6-(2-fluorophenyl)-1-methyl-4H-imidazo [1,5-a][1,4]-benzodiazepine.
Colourless glass ampoules containing 10 mg of midazolam base as the hydrochloride in 2 ml aqueous solution. The solution in the ampoule is colourless.

**Uses**
*Pharmacological properties:* Midazolam is a potent imidazobenzodiazepine, forming water-soluble salts which are stable and well tolerated by injection. Midazolam possesses the typical pharmacological properties of the benzodiazepines, namely hypnotic, anxiolytic, muscle-relaxant and anticonvulsant activity. In clinical use the induction of sleep is the main action.

At sedative and anaesthetic doses, given intravenously, the action is rapid in onset and of short duration; anterograde amnesia frequently accompanies the period of peak sedation.

When given by intramuscular injection, Hypnovel is rapidly absorbed and has a bioavailability of greater than 90%. The onset of action is relatively rapid and may be accompanied by anterograde amnesia. On intramuscular injection, Hypnovel is well tolerated locally.

Midazolam is principally cleared by hepatic enzymes (particularly cytochrome P450 IIIA), with a mean elimination half-life of about 2 hours, but this may be prolonged in critically ill patients.

*Indications:* As intravenous sedative cover before and during minor medical, dental and surgical procedures such as gastroscopy, endoscopy, cystoscopy, bronchoscopy and cardiac catheterisation.

For sedation by intravenous injection (either continuous infusion or intermittent bolus injection) in critically ill patients in intensive care.

As an intramuscular premedication before surgery for patients with the physical status ASA I-IV who are to undergo surgical procedures.

As an alternative intravenous agent for the induction of anaesthesia in high risk and elderly patients, especially where cardiovascular stability is of particular importance. Induction is more reliable when heavy opiate premedication has been administered or when Hypnovel is given with a narcotic analgesic such as fentanyl.

**Dosage and administration**
*Intravenous sedation:* One or more intravenous injections over a single operating session.

In most circumstances, the 10 mg/5 ml formulation is more convenient for titration purposes.

*Adults:* An assessment should be made of the degree of sedation necessary for the planned procedure.

The dose should be titrated against the response of the patient. The desired titration end point will depend upon the procedure. Full sedation will be evident by drowsiness and slurred speech but response to commands will be maintained.

As a guide it is recommended that a bolus dose of 0.4 ml of Hypnovel 10 mg/2 ml solution (equivalent to 2 mg midazolam) be administered intravenously over 30 seconds. If after 2 minutes, sedation is not adequate, incremental doses of 0.1 ml to 0.2 ml of Hypnovel 10 mg/2 ml solution (0.5–1 mg midazolam) should be given.

Usual dosage range 2.5–7.5 mg as a total dose (equivalent to around 0.07 mg/kg body-weight). Dosages greater than 5 mg are not usually necessary.

*Use in the elderly:* The elderly are more sensitive to the effects of benzodiazepines. In these patients, doses greater than 3.5 mg are not usually necessary and low doses as little as 1–2 mg (0.2–0.4 ml) may be adequate. The initial bolus dose should not exceed 1–1.5 mg (0.2–0.3 ml).

*Children:* Hypnovel has not been evaluated for use as an intravenous sedative in children.

*Combination therapy:* Where analgesia is provided by a narcotic analgesic, the latter should be administered first, the dose of Hypnovel should then be carefully titrated and low doses 1–2 mg (0.2–0.4 ml) may be adequate. In the elderly, smaller doses as little as 0.5–1 mg (0.1–0.2 ml) may be adequate.

*Mode of administration:* For the administration of Hypnovel the patient should be placed in a supine position and remain there throughout the procedure. Resuscitation facilities should always be available and a second person, fully trained in the use of such equipment, should always be present. It is recommended that patients should remain under medical supervision until at least 1 hour has elapsed from the time of injection. They should always be accompanied home by a responsible adult.

Patients who have received only Hypnovel for i.v. sedation prior to minor procedures, should be warned not to drive or operate machinery for 12 hours. Where Hypnovel is used concurrently with other central nervous system depressants (e.g. potent analgesics) recovery may be prolonged. Patients should therefore be assessed carefully before being allowed to go home or resume normal activities.

*Sedation in the critically ill patient:* Hypnovel can be given intravenously by two methods for this purpose, either by continuous infusion or by intermittent bolus dose. Both have their own advantages and disadvantages and the appropriate method of giving Hypnovel will need to be determined for each patient.

The dose of Hypnovel needed to sedate critically ill patients varies considerably between patients. The dose of Hypnovel should be titrated to the desired state of sedation. This will depend on clinical need, physical status, age and concomitant medication.

Hypnovel can also be given in combination with an opioid. The opioid may be used for its analgesic effects or as an antitussive agent to help the patient tolerate the tracheal tube and ventilatory support.

Patients receiving Hypnovel for sedation in the intensive care situation should receive ventilatory support.

Safety of the use of Hypnovel for periods of over 14 days in duration has not been established in clinical trials.

After prolonged i.v. administration of Hypnovel, abrupt discontinuation may be accompanied by withdrawal symptoms, therefore a gradual reduction of Hypnovel is recommended.

*Potential drug interactions:* The critically ill patient is exposed to many drugs. Because of this, there is a potential for drug interactions. (See Interactions section under Contra-indications, warnings, etc)

*Preparation of intravenous solutions:* Hypnovel solution is stable both physically and chemically for up to 24 hours at room temperature when mixed with infusion fluids containing 4% Dextrose with 0.18% Sodium Chloride, 5% Dextrose, or 0.9% Sodium Chloride.

*Sedation by intermittent bolus dose in intensive care: Hypnovel only:* The exact dose of Hypnovel needs to be titrated to the individual patient response. Small doses of Hypnovel 1.0–2.0 mg can be given, and repeated, until the required degree of sedation is reached.

*Hypnovel and an opioid:* When Hypnovel and an opioid are used together, the opioid should be given first. Both drugs need to be titrated to the individual patients response and to the level of sedation thought to be necessary. Small doses of Hypnovel 1–2 mg (0.2–0.4 ml) can be given, and repeated, until the required degree of sedation is reached. In the elderly, smaller doses as little as 0.5–1.0 mg (0.1–0.2 ml) may be adequate.

The use of these two groups of drugs can increase the risk of respiratory depression. If the patient is being given ventilatory support, using a mode that depends upon some spontaneous effort by the patient, then the minute volume may decrease.

*Sedation by continuous infusion in intensive care Hypnovel only*

*Adults and children:* Loading dose: For patients already sedated or anaesthetised after an operation, a loading dose of midazolam is unnecessary. In other situations a loading dose of 0.03–0.3 mg/kg is recommended, depending on the level of sedation required. This should be given over a five minute period. The loading dose should be reduced or omitted in hypovolaemic, vasoconstricted or hypothermic patients.

Maintenance dose: A dose between 0.03–0.2 mg/kg/hour is recommended, starting at the lower dose. The dose should be reduced in hypovolaemic, vasoconstricted or hypothermic patients.

*Hypnovel and an opioid:* When opioid analgesics are used, the rate of infusion of Hypnovel should be titrated carefully to the sedative needs of the patient. Low doses of Hypnovel 0.01 to 0.1 mg/kg/hour may be used to start.

The use of these two groups of drugs can increase the risk of respiratory depression. If the patient is being given ventilatory support, using a mode that depends upon some spontaneous effort by the patient, then the minute volume may decrease.

Whenever a continuous infusion of Hypnovel is used (with or without an opioid analgesic), its need should be assessed on a daily basis in order to reduce the risk of accumulation and prolonged recovery. Each day the infusion of Hypnovel should be stopped or its rate reduced and the patient seen to recover from its effect. If recovery is prolonged (> 2hours) a lower dose should be used when it is restarted. A sedation score should be used routinely.

When Hypnovel has been given for a number of days and then gradually withdrawn, patients may be awake but show signs of residual sedation for the next 12 to 24 hours. This can cause difficulties because patients may not cough and expectorate well if they are then weaned from ventilatory support. However, while recovering from the effects of Hypnovel, patients may not be sufficiently sedated to tolerate ventilatory support. In such circumstances sedation may be

provided with a shorter acting agent while there is recovery from the effects of Hypnovel.

The recommended concentration of a solution for infusion in a critically ill adult patient is 1 mg/ml.

*Intravenous induction of anaesthesia:* One or more bolus intravenous injections over a single anaesthetic session.

*Adults:* The dose should be titrated against the individual response of the patient. Hypnovel should be given by slow intravenous injection until there is a loss of eyelid reflex, response to commands and voluntary movements.

In anticipating the required dose of Hypnovel, both the premedication already given and the age of the patient are important. Young, fit unpremedicated patients may need at least 0.3 mg/kg body-weight, whereas patients premedicated with an opiate usually need only 0.2 mg/kg body-weight.

*Use in the elderly:* The elderly are more sensitive to the effects of benzodiazepines. Induction may be adequate with 0.1 mg/kg body-weight in premedicated patients and 0.2 mg/kg body-weight in unpremedicated patients.

*Children over 7 years:* Hypnovel has been shown to be an effective agent for induction of anaesthesia in children over 7 years of age, at a dose of 0.15 mg/kg body-weight.

*Intramuscular premedication*

*Adults:* A single intramuscular injection of 0.07–0.1 mg/kg body-weight, given 30–60 minutes before anaesthesia, has been shown to be adequate in most cases. The usual dose is about 5 mg.

Atropine or hyoscine hydrobromide may be given concomitantly, bearing in mind that hyoscine hydrobromide will enhance and prolong the sedative and amnesic effects of Hypnovel.

Hypnovel can be combined with atropine or hyoscine hydrobromide in the same syringe to be given as a single intramuscular injection.

*Use in the elderly:* The elderly are more sensitive to the effects of benzodiazepines and in these patients a lower dose of 2.5 mg may be adequate.

*Children:* Hypnovel has not been evaluated for use as an intramuscular premedicant in children.

### Contra-indications, warnings, etc

*Contra-indications:* Benzodiazepine sensitivity.

*Use in pregnancy and lactation:* Animal experiments have not indicated any teratogenic risk with Hypnovel but evaluation in human pregnancy has not been undertaken. Therefore, Hypnovel should not be used during pregnancy unless this is considered essential by the physician.

The administration of high single doses of benzodiazepines in the last trimester of pregnancy has been reported to produce irregularities in the foetal heart rate, and hypotonia, poor sucking and hypothermia in the neonate. Hypnovel ampoule solution should not, therefore, be used during the last trimester.

Hypnovel may pass into breast milk and caution should be exercised with its use in lactating mothers.

*Precautions:* After prolonged i.v. administration of Hypnovel, abrupt discontinuation may be accompanied by withdrawal symptoms, therefore a gradual reduction of Hypnovel is recommended.

Hypnovel should be given with caution to patients with pulmonary insufficiency, impairment of renal or hepatic function, to elderly or debilitated patients and to patients with myasthenia gravis. In patients with hepatic impairment there can be a significant prolongation of the elimination half-life of midazolam.

During bolus sedation for operative procedures extreme caution should be exercised in patients with acute pulmonary insufficiency or respiratory depression.

Disinhibiting effects have been noted, even after a single dose. This should therefore be borne in mind if treating patients with a history of personality disorders.

*Side-effects and adverse reactions:* Changes in cardiovascular parameters are slight but can include a decrease in mean arterial pressure, cardiac output, stroke volume and systemic vascular resistance. Such changes may be important in patients with impaired myocardial oxygen delivery capacity and hypovolaemia.

Following intravenous application of Hypnovel, respiratory depression and respiratory arrest have occurred. These life-threatening incidents may occur especially in elderly patients or patients with pre-existing respiratory insufficiency, particularly if excessive or too rapidly injected doses are administered.

Paradoxical reactions, e.g. agitation, restlessness and disorientation have been reported, although these are rare.

Hallucinations, some of a sexual nature, have been reported.

Other side-effects reported include headache, dizziness and hiccoughs. Anterograde amnesia frequently accompanies the period of peak sedation. Local effects

on veins are infrequent. However, pain on injection and thrombophlebitis may occur.

*Drug interactions:* When Hypnovel is given along with central nervous system depressants, such as potent analgesics, the sedative effect may be intensified and the possibility of severe respiratory or cardiovascular depression should be considered.

There is a potentially relevant interaction between midazolam and compounds which inhibit certain hepatic enzymes (particularly cytochrome P450 IIIA). Data clearly indicate that these compounds influence the pharmacokinetics of midazolam and may lead to prolonged sedation. At present this interaction is known to occur with cimetidine, erythromycin, diltiazem, verapamil, ketoconazole and itraconazole. There is also a theoretical possibility that, by competitive inhibition of P450 IIIA, midazolam could potentiate the effects of other drugs which are metabolised by this isoenzyme e.g. cyclosporin, nifedipine. Therefore patients receiving the above compounds or others which inhibit P450 IIIA together with midazolam should be monitored carefully for the first few hours after administration of midazolam. (Studies have shown that ranitidine has no influence on the pharmacokinetics of parenterally given midazolam.)

Patients should be instructed to avoid alcohol before and for at least 8 hours after administration of Hypnovel since the individual response cannot be foreseen.

*Treatment of overdosage:* The symptoms of overdosage are mainly an intensification of the therapeutic effects (sedation, muscle weakness, profound sleep) or paradoxical excitation. Extreme overdosage may lead to coma, areflexia, cardiopulmonary depression and apnoea requiring appropriate counter-measures (ventilation, cardiovascular support). Anexate is a specific i.v. antidote for use in emergency situations. Patients requiring such intervention should be monitored closely in hospital (see separate prescribing information).

### Pharmaceutical precautions

*Additives:* Hypnovel ampoule solution is stable, both physically and chemically, for up to 1 hour at room temperature when mixed in the same syringe with Atropine Sulphate Injection 500 micrograms/ml, or Hyoscine Hydrobromide Injection 0.4 mg/ml.

There is no evidence of the adsorption of midazolam onto the plastic of infusion apparatus or syringes.

**Legal category** CD (Sch.4), POM.

### Package Quantities

Hypnovel ampoules 10 mg/2 ml in packs of 10.

**Further information** The "second peak" effect, which is known to occur following intravenous diazepam, has not been observed with Hypnovel.

The metabolites of Hypnovel do not contribute significantly to the clinical effects of the drug.

Hypnovel ampoule solution is stable, both physically and chemically, for up to 24 hours at room temperature when mixed with 500 ml infusion fluids containing Dextrose 4% with Sodium Chloride 0.18%, Dextrose 5%, or Sodium Chloride 0.9%.

Admixture with Hartmann's solution is not recommended, as the potency of midazolam decreases.

Hypnovel ampoules 10 mg/5 ml are also available, and are recommended especially for intravenous administration of the drug where careful dosage titration is required (see separate prescribing information).

**Product licence numbers** 0031/0126

## HYPNOVEL* AMPOULES 10 mg/5 ml

**Presentation** Hypnovel contains the substance with the approved name midazolam. It is chemically described as 8-chloro-6-(2-fluorophenyl)-1-methyl-4H-imidazo [1,5-a][1,4]-benzodiazepine.

Colourless glass ampoules containing 10 mg of midazolam base as the hydrochloride in 5 ml aqueous solution. The solution in the ampoule is colourless.

### Uses

*Pharmacological properties:* Midazolam is a potent imidazobenzodiazepine, forming water-soluble salts which are stable and well tolerated by injection. Midazolam possesses the typical pharmacological properties of the benzodiazepines, namely hypnotic, anxiolytic, muscle-relaxant and anticonvulsant activity. In clinical use the induction of sleep is the main action.

At sedative and anaesthetic doses, given intravenously, the action is rapid in onset and of short duration; anterograde amnesia frequently accompanies the period of peak sedation.

Midazolam is principally cleared by hepatic enzymes (particularly cytochrome P450 IIIA), with a mean elimination half-life of about 2 hours, but this may be prolonged in critically ill patients.

*Indications:* As intravenous sedative cover before and during minor medical, dental and surgical procedures such as gastroscopy, endoscopy, cystoscopy, bronchoscopy and cardiac catheterisation.

For sedation by intravenous injection (either continuous infusion or intermittent bolus injection) in critically ill patients in intensive care.

As an alternative intravenous agent for the induction of anaesthesia in high risk and elderly patients, especially where cardiovascular stability is of particular importance. Induction is more reliable when heavy opiate premedication has been administered or when Hypnovel is given with a narcotic analgesic such as fentanyl.

### Dosage and administration

*Intravenous sedation:* One or more intravenous injections over a single operating session.

*Adults:* An assessment should be made of the degree of sedation necessary for the planned procedure.

The dose should be titrated against the response of the patient. The desired titration end point will depend upon the procedure. Full sedation will be evident by drowsiness and slurred speech but response to commands will be maintained.

As a guide it is recommended that a bolus dose 1 ml Hypnovel 10 mg/5 ml solution (equivalent to 2 mg midazolam) be administered intravenously over 30 seconds. If after 2 minutes, sedation is not adequate, incremental doses of 0.25 to 0.5 ml of Hypnovel 10 mg/5 ml solution (0.5–1 mg midazolam) should be given.

Usual dosage range 2.5–7.5 mg as a total dose (equivalent to around 0.07 mg/kg body-weight). Dosages greater than 5 mg are not usually necessary.

*Use in the elderly:* The elderly are more sensitive to the effects of benzodiazepines. In these patients, doses greater than 3.5 mg are not usually necessary and low doses as little as 1–2 mg (0.5–1.0 ml) may be adequate. The initial bolus dose should not exceed 1–1.5 mg (0.5–0.75 ml).

*Children:* Hypnovel has not been evaluated for use as an intravenous sedative in children.

*Combination therapy:* Where analgesia is provided by a narcotic analgesic, the latter should be administered first, the dose of Hypnovel should then be carefully titrated and low doses 1–2 mg (0.5–1.0 ml) may be adequate. In the elderly, smaller doses as little as 0.5–1 mg (0.25–0.5 ml) may be adequate.

*Mode of administration:* For the administration of Hypnovel the patient should be placed in a supine position and remain there throughout the procedure. Resuscitation facilities should always be available and a second person, fully trained in the use of such equipment, should always be present. It is recommended that patients should remain under medical supervision until at least 1 hour has elapsed from the time of injection. They should always be accompanied home by a responsible adult.

Patients who have received only Hypnovel for IV sedation prior to minor procedures, should be warned not to drive or operate machinery for 12 hours. Where Hypnovel is used concurrently with other central nervous system depressants (e.g. potent analgesics) recovery may be prolonged. Patients should therefore be assessed carefully before being allowed to go home or resume normal activities.

*Sedation in the critically ill patient:* Hypnovel can be given intravenously by two methods for this purpose, either by continuous infusion or by intermittent bolus dose. Both have their own advantages and disadvantages and the appropriate method of giving Hypnovel will need to be determined for each patient.

The dose of Hypnovel needed to sedate critically ill patients varies considerably between patients. The dose of Hypnovel should be titrated to the desired state of sedation. This will depend on the clinical need, physical status, age and concomitant medication.

Hypnovel can also be given in combination with an opioid. The opioid may be used for its analgesic effects or as an antitussive agent to help the patient tolerate the tracheal tube and ventilatory support.

Patients receiving Hypnovel for sedation in the intensive care situation should receive ventilatory support.

Safety of the use of Hypnovel for periods of over 14 days in duration has not been established in clinical trials.

After prolonged i.v. administration of Hypnovel, abrupt discontinuation may be accompanied by withdrawal symptoms, therefore a gradual reduction of Hypnovel is recommended.

*Potential drug interactions:* The critically ill patient is exposed to many drugs. Because of this, there is a potential for drug interactions. (See *Interactions* section under *Contra-indications, warnings etc*)

*Preparation of intravenous solutions:* Hypnovel solution is stable both physically and chemically for up to 24 hours at room temperature when mixed with infusion fluids containing 4% Dextrose with 0.18% Sodium Chloride, 5% Dextrose, or 0.9% Sodium Chloride.

*Sedation by intermittent bolus dose in intensive care:*
*Hypnovel only:* The exact dose of Hypnovel needs to be titrated to the individual patient response. Small doses of Hypnovel 1.0–2.0 mg (0.5–1.0 ml) can be given, and repeated, until the required degree of sedation is reached.

*Hypnovel and an opioid:* When Hypnovel and an opioid are used together, the opioid should be given first. Both drugs need to be titrated to the individual patients response and to the level of sedation thought to be necessary. Small doses of Hypnovel 1–2 mg can be given, and repeated, until the required degree of sedation is reached. In the elderly, smaller doses as little as 0.5–1.0 mg (0.25–0.5 ml) may be adequate.

The use of these two groups of drugs can increase the risk of respiratory depression. If the patient is being given ventilatory support, using a mode that depends upon some spontaneous effort by the patient, then the minute volume may decrease.

*Sedation by continuous infusion in intensive care*
*Hypnovel only*
  *Adults and children:*
Loading dose: For patients already sedated or anaesthetised after an operation, a loading dose of midazolam is unnecessary. In other situations a loading dose of 0.03–0.3 mg/kg is recommended, depending on the level of sedation required. This should be given over a five minute period. The loading dose should be reduced or omitted in hypovolaemic, vasoconstricted or hypothermic patients.

Maintenance dose: A dose between 0.03–0.2 mg/kg/hour is recommended, starting at the lower dose.
The dose should be reduced in hypovolaemic, vasoconstricted or hypothermic patients.

*Hypnovel and an opioid:* When opioid analgesics are used, the rate of infusion of Hypnovel should be titrated carefully to the sedative needs of the patient. Low doses of Hypnovel, 0.01 to 0.1 mg/kg/hour may be used to start.

The use of these two groups of drugs can increase the risk of respiratory depression. If the patient is being given ventilatory support, using a mode that depends upon some spontaneous effort by the patient, then the minute volume may decrease.

Whenever a continuous infusion of Hypnovel is used (with or without an opioid analgesic), its need should be assessed on a daily basis in order to reduce the risk of accumulation and prolonged recovery. Each day, the infusion of Hypnovel should be stopped or its rate reduced and the patient seen to recover from its effect. If recovery is prolonged (> 2 hours) a lower dose should be used when it is restarted. A sedation score should be used routinely.

When Hypnovel has been given for a number of days and then gradually withdrawn, patients may be awake but show signs of residual sedation for the next 12 to 24 hours. This can cause difficulties because patients may not cough and expectorate well when weaned from ventilatory support. However, while recovering from the effects of Hypnovel, patients may not be sufficiently sedated to tolerate ventilatory support. In such circumstances sedation may be provided with a shorter acting agent while there is recovery from the effects of Hypnovel.

The recommended concentration of a solution for infusion in a critically ill adult patient is 1 mg/ml.

*Intravenous induction of anaesthesia:* One or more bolus intravenous injections over a single anaesthetic session.

*Adults:* The dose should be titrated against the individual response of the patient. Hypnovel should be given by slow intravenous injection until there is a loss of eyelid reflex, response to commands and voluntary movements.

In anticipating the required dose of Hypnovel, both the premedication already given and the age of the patient are important. Young, fit unpremedicated patients may need at least 0.3 mg/kg body-weight, whereas patients premedicated with an opiate usually need only 0.2 mg/kg body-weight.

*Use in the elderly:* The elderly are more sensitive to the effects of benzodiazepines. Induction may be adequate with 0.1 mg/kg body-weight in premedicated patients and 0.2 mg/kg body-weight in unpremedicated patients.

*Children over 7 years:* Hypnovel has been shown to be an effective agent for induction of anaesthesia in children over 7 years of age, at a dose of 0.15 mg/kg body-weight.

### Contra-indications, warnings, etc

*Contra-indications:* Benzodiazepine sensitivity.

*Use in pregnancy and lactation:* Animal experiments have not indicated any teratogenic risk with Hypnovel but evaluation in human pregnancy has not been undertaken. Therefore, Hypnovel should not be used during pregnancy unless this is considered essential by the physician.

The administration of high single doses of benzodiazepines in the last trimester of pregnancy has been reported to produce irregularities in the foetal heart rate, and hypotonia, poor sucking and hypothermia in the neonate. Hypnovel ampoule solution should not, therefore, be used during the last trimester.

Hypnovel may pass into breast milk and caution should be exercised with its use in lactating mothers.

*Precautions:* After prolonged i.v. administration of Hypnovel, abrupt discontinuation may be accompanied by withdrawal symptoms, therefore a gradual reduction of Hypnovel is recommended.

Hypnovel should be given with caution to patients with pulmonary insufficiency, impairment of renal or hepatic function, to elderly or debilitated patients and to patients with myasthenia gravis. In patients with hepatic impairment there can be a significant prolongation of the elimination half-life of midazolam.

During bolus sedation for operative procedures extreme caution should be exercised in patients with acute pulmonary insufficiency or respiratory depression.

Disinhibiting effects have been noted, even after a single dose. This should therefore be borne in mind if treating patients with a history of personality disorders.

*Side-effects and adverse reactions:* Changes in cardiovascular parameters are slight but can include a decrease in mean arterial pressure, cardiac output, stroke volume and systemic vascular resistance. Such changes may be important in patients with impaired myocardial oxygen delivery capacity and hypovolaemia.

Following intravenous application of Hypnovel, respiratory depression and respiratory arrest have occurred. These life-threatening incidents may occur especially in elderly patients or patients with pre-existing respiratory insufficiency, particularly if excessive or too rapidly injected doses are administered.

Paradoxical reactions, e.g. agitation, restlessness and disorientation have been reported, although these are rare.

Hallucinations, some of a sexual nature, have been reported.

Other side-effects reported include headache, dizziness and hiccoughs. Anterograde amnesia frequently accompanies the period of peak sedation. Local effects on veins are infrequent. However, pain on injection and thrombophlebitis may occur.

*Drug interactions:* When Hypnovel is given along with central nervous system depressants, such as potent analgesics, the sedative effect may be intensified and the possibility of severe respiratory or cardiovascular depression should be considered.

There is a potentially relevant interaction between midazolam and compounds which inhibit certain hepatic enzymes (particularly cytochrome P450 IIIA). Data clearly indicate that these compounds influence the pharmacokinetics of midazolam and may lead to prolonged sedation. At present this interaction is known to occur with cimetidine, erythromycin, diltiazem, verapamil, ketoconazole and itraconazole. There is also a theoretical possibility that, by competitive inhibition of P450 IIIA, midazolam could potentiate the effects of other drugs which are metabolised by this isoenzyme e.g. cyclosporin, nifedipine. Therefore patients receiving the above compounds or others which inhibit P450 IIIA together with midazolam should be monitored carefully for the first few hours after administration of midazolam. (Studies have shown that ranitidine has no influence on the pharmacokinetics of parenterally given midazolam.)

Patients should be instructed to avoid alcohol before and for at least 8 hours after administration of Hypnovel since the individual response cannot be foreseen.

*Treatment of overdosage:* The symptoms of overdosage are mainly an intensification of the therapeutic effects (sedation, muscle weakness, profound sleep or paradoxical excitation. Extreme overdosage may lead to coma, areflexia, cardiopulmonary depression and apnoea requiring appropriate counter measures (ventilation, cardiovascular support). Anexate is a specific IV antidote for use in emergency situations. Patients requiring such intervention should be monitored closely in hospital (see separate prescribing information).

### Pharmaceutical precautions

*Additives:* Hypnovel ampoule solution is stable, both physically and chemically, for up to 1 hour at room temperature when mixed in the same syringe with Atropine Sulphate Injection 500 micrograms/ml, or Hyoscine Hydrobromide Injection 0.4 mg/ml.

There is no evidence of the adsorption of midazolam onto the plastic of infusion apparatus or syringes.

**Legal category**    CD (Sch.4), POM.

**Package quantities** Hypnovel ampoules 10 mg/5 ml in packs of 10.

**Further information** The "second peak" effect, which is known to occur following intravenous diazepam, has not been observed with Hypnovel.

The metabolites of Hypnovel do not contribute significantly to the clinical effects of the drug.

Hypnovel ampoule solution is stable, both physically and chemically, for up to 24 hours at room temperature when mixed with 500 ml infusion fluids containing Dextrose 4% with Sodium Chloride 0.18%, Dextrose 5%, or Sodium Chloride 0.9%.

Admixture with Hartmann's solution is not recommended, as the potency of midazolam decreases.

Hypnovel ampoules 10 mg/2 ml are also available, and are recommended especially for use as an intramuscular premedication (see separate prescribing information).

**Product licence number** 0031/0189

## INVIRASE*

**Qualitative and quantitative composition** One capsule of Invirase contains saquinavir mesylate corresponding to 200 mg saquinavir.

**Pharmaceutical form** Capsules

**Clinical particulars**

*Therapeutic indications:* Invirase in combination with antiretroviral nucleoside analogues is indicated for the treatment of HIV-1 infected adult patients with advanced or progressive immunodeficiency.

Clinical benefits of the combination therapy with Invirase and zalcitabine on HIV infection in terms of disease progression and survival have been confirmed in a controlled study recruiting patients with previous prolonged zidovudine therapy. Clinical studies are underway to confirm the clinical benefit of saquinavir in combination with other antiretroviral agents. Refer also to section *Pharmacodynamic properties*.

*Posology and method of administration:*
*Adults and children over the age of 16 years:* The recommended regimen for combination therapy with nucleoside analogues is 600 mg of Invirase three times daily within 2 hours after a meal. For the recommended dose of the nucleoside analogues in combination therapy, please refer to the complete prescribing information for these drugs. For information on special patient groups refer to section *Special warnings and special precautions for use.*

*Dose adjustments:*
*Invirase in combination therapy:* For toxicities that may be associated with Invirase the treatment with Invirase should be interrupted. Invirase at doses less than 600 mg tid is not recommended.

*Hepatic and/or renal impairment:* For information on hepatic and renal impairment refer to section *4.4 Special warnings and special precautions for use.*

*Contra-indications:* Invirase is contra-indicated in patients with hypersensitivity to saquinavir or to any of the other components contained in the capsule.

*Special warnings and special precautions for use:* Patients should be informed that saquinavir is not a cure for HIV infection and that they may continue to acquire illnesses associated with advanced HIV infection, including opportunistic infections. Patients should also be advised that they may experience toxicities associated with co-administered medications such as zalcitabine and zidovudine.
*Hepatic impairment:* In cases of mild to moderate impairment no initial dosage adjustment is necessary at the recommended dose. The use of saquinavir by patients with severe hepatic impairment has not been studied. In the absence of such studies, caution should be exercised, as increases in saquinavir levels may occur.

*Renal impairment:* Renal clearance is only a minor elimination pathway, the principal route of metabolism and excretion for saquinavir being via the liver. Therefore, no initial dose adjustment is necessary for patients with renal impairment. However, patients with severe renal impairment have not been studied and caution should be exercised when prescribing saquinavir in this population.

*Patients with chronic diarrhoea or malabsorption:* No information on safety and efficacy of saquinavir is available for patients suffering from chronic diarrhoea or malabsorption. It is unknown whether patients with such conditions could receive subtherapeutic drug levels.

*Young and elderly patients:* The safety and efficacy of saquinavir in HIV-infected patients (younger than 16 years) have not been established. Only limited experience is available in patients older than 60 years.

*Lactose intolerance:* Each capsule contains lactose (anhydrous) 63.3 mg. This quantity is probably not sufficient to induce specific symptoms of intolerance.

*Use during pregnancy and lactation:* Refer to *Pregnancy and lactation* section.

There have been reports of increased bleeding, including spontaneous skin haematomas and haemarthroses, in haemophiliac patients type A and B treated with protease inhibitors. In some patients additional factor VIII was given. In more than a half of the reported cases, treatment with protease inhibitors was continued or reintroduced if treatment had been discontinued. A causal relationship has been evoked, although the mechanism of action has not been elucidated. Haemophiliac patients should therefore be made aware of the possibility of increased bleeding.

*Interaction with other medicinal products and other forms of interaction:* Concomitant use of saquinavir with zalcitabine and/or zidovudine has been studied in adults. Absorption, distribution and elimination of each of the drugs are unchanged when they are used together.
*Ranitidine:* There was an increase in exposure when saquinavir was dosed in the presence of both ranitidine and food, relative to saquinavir dosed with food alone. This resulted in AUC values which were 67% higher. This increase is not thought to be clinically relevant and no dose adjustment of saquinavir is recommended.

*Grapefruit juice:* Co-administration of saquinavir and grapefruit juice as single administration in healthy volunteers results in a 50% and 100% increase in exposure to saquinavir for normal and double strength grapefruit juice, respectively. This increase is not thought to be clinically relevant and no dose adjustment of saquinavir is recommended.

*Inadvisable associations:* Rifampicin (600 mg once daily) was shown to decrease plasma concentrations of saquinavir by 80%. Since this may result in subtherapeutic concentrations of saquinavir, rifampicin should not be administered concomitantly with saquinavir. Rifabutin also reduces saquinavir plasma concentrations by 40%. Other drugs that induce CYP3A4 (e.g. phenobarbital, phenytoin, dexamethasone, carbamazepine) may also reduce saquinavir plasma concentrations. If therapy with such drugs is warranted, physicians should consider using alternatives when a patient is taking Invirase.

*Associations requiring precautions for use:* Concomitant use of ketoconazole (200 mg once daily) and saquinavir caused a 1.5-fold increase in plasma concentrations of saquinavir, with no increase in the elimination half-life or any change in the absorption rate. Ketoconazole pharmacokinetics are not affected by co-administration with saquinavir at a dose of 600 mg three times daily. No dose adjustment for either drug is required when the two drugs are co-administered at the doses studied.

A similar increase in plasma concentration of saquinavir could occur with other compounds in this class, such as fluconazole, itraconazole and miconazole or with other inhibitors of the CYP3A4 isoenzyme.
*Other potential interactions:* Co-administration of terfenadine, astemizole or cisapride with drugs which are known to be potent inhibitors of the CYP3A pathway (i.e. ketoconazole, itraconazole, etc.) may lead to elevated plasma concentrations of terfenadine, astemizole or cisapride. Pharmacokinetic interaction studies with saquinavir and terfenadine, astemizole or cisapride have not been conducted, and although saquinavir is not a strong inhibitor of CYP3A, physicians should use alternatives to terfenadine, astemizole or cisapride. Other compounds that are substrates of CYP3A4 (e.g. calcium channel blockers, clindamycin, dapsone, quinidine, triazolam, midazolam) may have elevated plasma concentrations when co-administered with saquinavir; therefore, patients should be monitored for toxicities associated with such drugs.

Plasma concentrations of saquinavir are expected to increase if co-administered with ritonavir. At this time, there is insufficient data available on efficacy and safety of this co-administration. As no recommendation on dose and schedule for either of the compounds can be made, these drugs should not be used concomitantly.

It is unknown, whether drugs which reduce the gastrointestinal transit time (e.g. metoclopramide and cisapride) could lead to lower saquinavir plasma concentrations.

*Use during pregnancy and lactation:*
*Pregnancy:* Evaluation of experimental animal studies does not indicate direct or indirect harmful effects with respect to the development of the embryo or fetus, the course of gestation and peri- and postnatal development. Clinical experience in pregnant women is lacking. Until additional data become available, saquinavir should be given to pregnant women only after special consideration.

*Lactation:* There are no laboratory animal or human data available on secretion of saquinavir in breast milk. The potential for adverse reactions to saquinavir in nursing infants cannot be assessed and, therefore, breast-feeding should be discontinued prior to receiving saquinavir. Health experts recommend that HIV-infected women do not breast feed their infants under any circumstances in order to avoid transmission of HIV.

*Effects on ability to drive and use machines:* It is not known whether saquinavir has an effect on the ability to drive and to use machines.

*Undesirable effects:* Saquinavir does not alter or add to the toxicity profile of zalcitabine and/or zidovudine, when given in combination.

For comprehensive dose adjustment recommendations and drug-associated adverse reactions for either zalcitabine or zidovudine or other drugs used in combination, physicians should refer to the complete product information for each of these drugs.

The listing below is based on the pivotal study which included a treatment arm with saquinavir used as single drug. Adverse events (mild, moderate and severe) with an incidence > 2% considered by the investigator at least remotely related to saquinavir are given.
*Skin and appendages:* Rash (4%).
*Central and peripheral nervous system:* Headache (4%), peripheral neuropathy (4%),
*Gastrointestinal system:* Diarrhoea (16%), abdominal discomfort (6%), buccal mucosa ulceration (6%), nausea (4%).
*Body as a whole–general disorders:* Asthenia (4%).
*Combination therapy: Saquinavir and zalcitabine*
Peripheral neuropathy is the major toxicity associated with zalcitabine administration. Saquinavir does not potentiate the development of peripheral neuropathy induced by zalcitabine.
*Combination therapy: Saquinavir with zalcitabine and zidovudine*
There was no increase in the incidence of well-established zidovudine or zalcitabine related toxicities such as myositis, haematological abnormalities, pancreatitis, buccal mucosa ulceration or peripheral neuropathy when saquinavir was given in combination with both zidovudine and zalcitabine.
*Other adverse effects:* Single, rare cases of serious adverse effects considered possibly related to use of study drugs have been reported: Confusion, ataxia and weakness; acute myeloblastic leukaemia; haemolytic anaemia; attempted suicide; Stevens-Johnson syndrome; seizures; severe cutaneous reaction associated with increased liver function tests; thrombophlebitis; thrombocytopenia; exacerbation of chronic liver disease with Grade 4 elevated liver function test, jaundice, ascites; liver injury with icterus and elevated transaminases; drug fever; bullous skin eruption and polyarthritis; nephrolithiasis; pancreatitis leading to death.

*Laboratory abnormalities:*
*Combination therapy: Saquinavir and zalcitabine*
The most common marked laboratory abnormalities were isolated CPK increase, glucose decrease and raised transaminase values. The incidence of laboratory toxicity was similar for zalcitabine monotherapy and for the combination of saquinavir and zalcitabine.
*Combination therapy: Saquinavir and zidovudine*
The most frequent marked laboratory abnormalities were isolated CPK increase, neutropenia and elevated transaminases.
*Combination therapy: Saquinavir with zalcitabine and zidovudine*
The most frequent marked laboratory abnormalities were elevated CPK levels, decreased glucose levels, neutropenia and increased transaminase values. Laboratory abnormalities observed with the triple combination were similar to those of zalcitabine and zidovudine combination.

*Overdose:* One patient exceeded the recommended daily dose of saquinavir (1800 mg daily) by taking 8000 mg at once. The patient was treated with induction of emesis within two hours after ingestion of the overdose. The patient did not experience any sequelae. In an exploratory small study, oral dosing with saquinavir at 3600 mg per day has not shown increased toxicity through the first 16 weeks of treatment.

**Pharmacological properties**
*Pharmacodynamic properties:* Pharmaco-therapeutic group: Antiviral agent, ATC code J05AX06.
*Mechanism of action:* The HIV proteinase carries out specific cleavages of viral precursor proteins in infected cells, as an essential step in the creation of fully formed, infectious virus particles. These viral precursor proteins contain a type of cleavage site which is recognised only by HIV and closely related viral proteinases. Saquinavir has been designed as a peptide-like structural mimetic of such cleavage sites. As a result, saquinavir fits closely into the HIV-1 and HIV-2 proteinase active sites, *in vitro* acting as a reversible and selective inhibitor, with approximately a 50,000-fold lower affinity for human proteinases.

Unlike nucleoside analogues (zidovudine, etc.), saquinavir acts directly on its viral target enzyme. It does not require metabolic activation. This extends its potential effectiveness into resting cells. Saquinavir is active at nanomolar concentrations in lymphoblastoid and monocytic lines and in primary cultures of lymphocytes and monocytes infected with laboratory strains or clinical isolates of HIV-1.

Experiments in cell culture show that saquinavir produces an additive to synergistic antiviral effect against HIV-1 in double and triple combination with various reverse transcriptase inhibitors (including zidovudine, zalcitabine, didanosine) without enhanced cytotoxicity.

*Pharmacodynamic effects:* The effects of saquinavir in combination with zalcitabine and zidovudine on biological markers, $CD_4$ cell counts and plasma RNA, were evaluated in HIV-1 infected patients.

In a study (NV14256) with zidovudine pre-treated patients ($CD_4 \geq 50 \leq 300$ cells/mm³), the combination of saquinavir plus zalcitabine compared to zalcitabine monotherapy prolonged the time to first AIDS-defining illness or death.

The combination therapy reduced the risk of a patient having an AIDS-defining illness or dying by 53%. For death alone the combination therapy reduced the risk by 72%. This corresponds to a reduction in the rate of an AIDS-defining illness or death from 29.4% to 16.0% over 18 months. Similarly for death alone, the rate was reduced from 8.6% to 4.1% over 18 months. In the three treatment groups, median treatment duration was 11 to 13 months and median follow-up has been 17 months.

In this study the median $CD_4$ cell count at baseline over all treatment arms was 156 to 176 cells/mm³. The average change from baseline over 16 weeks (median DAVG16) for saquinavir plus zalcitabine was + 26 cells/mm³ for the $CD_4$ cell count and -0.6 $\log_{10}$ RNA copies/mL of plasma for viral load. The peak mean increase in the $CD_4$ cell count was 47 cells/mm³ at week 16. The peak mean reduction in viral load was 0.7 $\log_{10}$ RNA copies/mL of plasma at week 12.

In a study (V13330) with previously untreated patients ($CD_4 \leq 300$ cells/mm³), the combination with zidovudine reduced viral load and increased $CD_4$ cell counts. The median $CD_4$ cell count at baseline over all treatment arms was 157 to 249 cells/mm³. The average change from baseline over 16 weeks (median DAVG16) for saquinavir plus zidovudine in these anti-retroviral naive subjects was + 52 cells/mm³ for the $CD_4$ cell count and -1.1 $\log_{10}$ RNA copies/mL of plasma for viral load. The peak mean increase in the $CD_4$ cell count was 79 cells/mm³ at week 16. The peak mean reduction in viral load was 1.6 $\log_{10}$ RNA copies/mL of plasma at week 4. A confirmatory phase III study (SV14604) is ongoing in anti-retroviral naive patients (less than 4 months zidovudine-experienced).

Monotherapy is not recommended because anti-viral activity has not been demonstrated.

*Potential for resistance and cross-resistance to saquinavir:*

*Resistance:* HIV isolates with reduced susceptibility to saquinavir have been selected after extensive *in vitro* passage using increasing concentrations of the compound. Analysis of the protease amino acid sequence in these isolates shows substitutions at positions 48 (glycine to valine = G48V) and 90 (leucine to methionine = L90M).

Changes to viral sensitivity to drug in culture (= "phenotypic resistance") or in protease amino acid sequence (= "genotypic resistance") have been investigated in clinical trials. Two particular viral protease mutations (L90M or G48V, the former predominating and the combination rare) are found in those saquinavir treated patients with resistant isolates. The overall incidence of genotypic resistance at about one year in a group of phase I/II patients treated in combination with nucleoside analogues (zalcitabine and/or zidovudine), was 38% (15 out of 39 patients). The clinical significance of phenotypic and genotypic changes associated with saquinavir therapy has not been established.

*Cross-resistance to other antiretrovirals:* Cross-resistance between saquinavir and reverse transcriptase inhibitors is unlikely because of their different enzyme targets. HIV isolates resistant to ZDV are sensitive to saquinavir, and conversely, HIV isolates resistant to saquinavir are sensitive to ZDV.

To date, therapy with saquinavir has demonstrated a distinctive and consistent pattern of mutations. Investigations into cross-resistance are in progress.

*Pharmacokinetic properties:*

*Absorption and bioavailability in adults and effect of food:* In healthy volunteers the extent of absorption (as reflected by AUC) after a 600 mg oral dose of saquinavir was increased from 24ng.h/mL (CV 33%), under fasting conditions, to 161ng.h/mL (CV 35%) when saquinavir was given following a heavy breakfast (48 g protein, 60 g carbohydrate, 57 g fat; 1006kcal).

The presence of food also increased the time taken to achieve maximum concentration from 2.4 hours to 3.8 hours and substantially increased the mean maximum plasma concentrations (Cmax) from 3.0ng/mL to 35.5ng/mL. The effect of food has been shown to persist for up to 2 hours. Therefore, Invirase should be taken within 2 hours after a meal.

Absolute bioavailability averaged 4% (CV 73%, range: 1% to 9%) in 8 healthy volunteers who received a single 600 mg dose (3 x 200 mg) of saquinavir following a heavy breakfast. The low bioavailability is thought to be due to a combination of incomplete absorption and extensive first-pass metabolism. Gastric pH has been shown to be only a minor component in the large increase in bioavailability seen when given with food.

After multiple oral doses (25–600 mg tid) in the presence of food, the increase in exposure (50-fold) was greater than directly proportional to the increase in dose (24-fold). Following multiple dosing (600 mg tid) in HIV-infected patients (n = 29), the steady state area under the plasma concentration versus time curve (AUC) was 2.5 times (95% CI 1.6 to 3.8) higher than that observed after a single dose.

HIV-infected patients administered saquinavir 600 mg tid, with the instructions to take saquinavir after a meal or substantial snack, had AUC and maximum plasma concentration (Cmax) values which were about twice those observed in healthy volunteers receiving the same treatment regimen (see below).

Mean (% CV) AUC and Cmax in patients and healthy volunteers:

| | *AUC8 (dose interval) in ng·h/mL* | *Cmax in ng/mL* |
|---|---|---|
| Healthy volunteers (n = 6) | 359.0 (46) | 90.39 (49) |
| Patients (n = 113) | 757.2 (84) | 253.3 (99) |

*Distribution in adults:* Saquinavir partitions extensively into the tissues. The mean steady-state volume of distribution following intravenous administration of a 12 mg dose of saquinavir was 700L (CV 39%). Saquinavir shows a high degree of protein binding (approximately 98%) which is independent of concentration over the range 15–700ng/mL. In two patients receiving Invirase 600 mg three times daily, cerebrospinal fluid concentrations of saquinavir were negligible when compared to concentrations from matching plasma samples.

*Metabolism and elimination in adults: In vitro* studies using human liver microsomes have shown that the metabolism of saquinavir is cytochrome P450 mediated with the specific isoenzyme, CYP3A4, responsible for more than 90% of the hepatic metabolism. Based on *in vitro* studies, saquinavir is rapidly metabolised to a range of mono- and di-hydroxylated inactive compounds. In a mass balance study using 600 mg 14C-saquinavir (n = 8), 88% and 1% of the orally administered radioactivity, was recovered in faeces and urine, respectively, within 4 days of dosing. In an additional four subjects administered 10.5 mg 14C-saquinavir intravenously, 81% and 3% of the intravenously administered radioactivity was recovered in faeces and urine, respectively, within 4 days of dosing. In mass balance studies, 13% of circulating saquinavir in plasma was present as unchanged drug after oral administration and the remainder present as metabolites. Following intravenous administration, 66% of circulating saquinavir is present as unchanged drug and the remainder as metabolites, suggesting that saquinavir undergoes extensive first pass metabolism.

Systemic clearance of saquinavir was high, 1.14 L/h/kg (CV 12%), slightly above the hepatic plasma flow, and constant after intravenous doses of 6, 36 and 72 mg. The mean residence time of saquinavir was 7 hours (n = 8).

*Preclinical safety data:*

*Acute and chronic toxicity:* Oral acute and chronic toxicity and toxicokinetic studies in the mouse, rat, dog and marmoset have demonstrated good tolerance to saquinavir at high plasma exposure to the drug relative to that seen in man.

*Mutagenesis:* Studies, with and without metabolic activation (as appropriate) have shown that saquinavir has no mutagenic or genotoxic activity.

*Carcinogenesis:* Carcinogenicity studies of saquinavir are ongoing.

*Reproductive toxicity:* Refer to section *4.6 Use during pregnancy and lactation.*

**Pharmaceutical particulars**

*List of excipients:*

*Capsule filling:* Lactose (anhydrous), microcrystalline cellulose, povidone, sodium starch glycollate, talc, magnesium stearate.

*Capsule shell:* Gelatine, iron oxide black, red and yellow (E172), indigocarmine (E132), titanium dioxide (E171).

*Capsule appearance:* Light brown and green, opaque; marking "ROCHE" and the code "0245" on each half of the capsule shell.

*Incompatibilities:* Not applicable.

*Shelf-life:* Two years.

*Special precautions for storage:* Store in the closed original pack.

*Nature and content of container:* Amber glass bottles with plastic screw closure containing 270 capsules of Invirase.

*Instructions for use, handling and disposal (if appropriate):* Not applicable.

**Marketing authorisation number** EU/1/96/026/001

**Date of approval/revision of SPC** September 1996

**Legal category** POM

## KONAKION* AMPOULES

**Qualitative and quantitative composition** Konakion Ampoules contain the substance chemically described as 2-methyl-3-phytyl-1,4-napthoquinone. It has the approved name phytomenadione and is known as vitamin $K_1$.

Each Konakion Ampoule contains 1 mg vitamin $K_1$ (phytomenadione) Ph. Eur.in 0.5 ml.

**Pharmaceutical form** Amber glass ampoules containing 1 mg phytomenadione in 0.5 ml. The ampoule solution is clear to opalescent, greenish-yellow in colour and contains a polyethoxylated castor oil as a non-ionic surfactant.

**Clinical particulars**

*Therapeutic indications:* Konakion is indicated in the treatment of haemorrhage or threatened haemorrhage associated with a low blood level of prothrombin or factor VII. The main indications are:

As an antidote to anticoagulant drugs of the coumarin type.

Prevention and treatment of neonatal haemorrhage.

*Posology and method of administration:*

*Adults: As an antidote to anticoagulant drugs:* For potentially fatal and severe haemorrhages: Konakion MM Ampoules are recommended as treatment in this indication (see separate prescribing information).

Less severe haemorrhage: Konakion is given orally in doses of 10 - 20 mg (1 to 2 tablets). The prothrombin level is estimated 8 to 12 hours later, and if the response has been inadequate, the dose should be repeated. Intramuscular injections of Konakion may also be given in doses of 10 - 20 mg, repeated if necessary.

Lowering of prothrombin to dangerous level but no haemorrhage: A dose of 5 - 10 mg Konakion orally may be given to bring the prothrombin level back to within safe limits. In such instances it is not usually necessary to discontinue the anticoagulant.

*Adults: Other indications:* Doses of 10 - 20 mg as required.

*Use in the elderly:* Elderly patients tend to be more sensitive to reversal of anticoagulation with Konakion, dosage in this group should be at the lower end of the ranges recommended.

*Children:* If, on the recommendation of a physician, a children's dosage is required, then it is suggested that 5 - 10 mg be given.

*Treatment of newborn infants:* Prophylactic: 1 mg by intramuscular injection.

Therapeutic: 1 mg by intramuscular injection, repeated at eight-hourly intervals if necessary.

Konakion ampoules are for intramuscular or intravenous injection.

Konakion ampoule solution should not be diluted.

*Contra-indications:* Use in patients with a known hypersensitivity to any of the constituents.

*Special warnings and special precautions for use* Konakion ampoules contain a polyethoxylated castor oil as a non-ionic surfactant. In animal studies polyethoxylated castor oil can produce severe anaphylactoid reactions associated with histamine release. There is strong circumstantial evidence that similar reactions occurring in patients may have been caused by polyethoxylated castor oil. Polyethoxylated castor oil, when given to patients over a period of several days, can also produce abnormal lipoprotein electrophoretic patterns, alterations in blood viscosity and erythrocyte aggregation.

Large doses of Konakion should be avoided if it is intended to continue with anticoagulant therapy.

Vitamin $K_1$ is not an antidote to heparin.

*Interaction with other medicaments and other forms of interaction:* None known.

*Pregnancy and lactation:* There is no specific evidence regarding the safety of Konakion in pregnancy but, as with most drugs, the administration during pregnancy should only occur if the benefits outweigh the risks.

*Effects on ability to drive and use machines:* None known.

*Undesirable effects:* The too rapid intravenous administration of vitamin K₁ has caused reactions, including flushing of the face, sweating, a sense of chest constriction, cyanosis and peripheral vascular collapse.

Repeated intramuscular injections of vitamin K₁ preparations, usually over prolonged periods in patients with hepatic disease, may give rise to local cutaneous and subcutaneous changes.

*Overdose:* Hypervitaminosis of vitamin K₁ is unknown.

### Pharmacological properties

*Pharmacodynamic properties:* Konakion is a synthetic preparation of vitamin K₁. The presence of vitamin K (i.e. vitamin K₁ itself or substances with vitamin K activity) is essential for the formation within the body of prothrombin, factor VII, factor IX and factor X. Lack of vitamin K leads to increased tendency to haemorrhage. When an antidote to an anticoagulant is necessary it is essential to use vitamin K₁ itself, as vitamin K analogues are much less effective.

*Pharmacokinetic properties:* The fat-soluble vitamin compound phytomenadione (Vitamin K₁) requires the presence of bile for its absorption from the gastro-intestinal tract. Vitamin K accumulates mainly in the liver but is stored in the body only for short periods of time. Vitamin K does not appear to cross the placenta readily and it is poorly distributed into breast milk. Phytomenadione is rapidly metabolised to more polar metabolites and is excreted in bile and urine as glucuronide and sulphate conjugates.

*Preclinical safety data:* LD₅₀ (i.v.) of Konakion MM (10 mg/ml) in mice: 12.1–17.7 ml/kg.

### Pharmaceutical particulars

*List of excipients:* Polyoxyl 35 Castor oil USP; Propylene Glycol PhEur; Phenol PhEur; Water for Injections PhEur.

*Incompatibilities:* None known.

*Shelf-life:* The recommended shelf-life of Konakion Ampoules is 60 months.

*Special precautions for storage:* Konakion ampoule solution should be protected from light; it should not be allowed to freeze. The recommended maximum storage temperature for Konakion ampoules is 30°C.

*Nature and contents of container:* Konakion is supplied in 1 ml amber glass ampoules containing 0.6 ml of solution.

*Instructions for use/handling:* Konakion Ampoules are for intramuscular or intravenous injection. Konakion ampoule solution should not be diluted.

**Marketing authorisation number**  0031/5023R

**Date of approval/revision of SPC**  April 1997

**Legal category**  POM

## KONAKION* MM AMPOULES

**Presentation**  Konakion MM Ampoules contain the substance chemically described as 2-methyl-3-phytyl-1,4-naphthoquinone. It has the approved name phytomenadione and is also known as vitamin K₁.

Amber glass ampoules containing 10 mg phytomenadione in 1 ml. The ampoule solution is clear to slightly opalescent, pale yellow in colour and contains the active constituent in a mixed micelles vehicle of glycocholic acid and lecithin.

### Uses

*Properties:* Phytomenadione (vitamin K₁) is involved in the formation of prothrombin, factor VII, factor IX and factor X in the liver. Lack of vitamin K leads to an increased tendency to haemorrhage. Anticoagulants of the coumarin type interfere with this role of vitamin K in the clotting process. Konakion MM Ampoules reverse the action of oral anticoagulants (but not heparin) and may also be used in other forms of hypoprothrombinaemia.

Konakion MM Ampoules utilise a physiological colloidal system for the solubilization of phytomenadione.

*Pharmacokinetics:* The primary distribution compartment corresponds to the plasma volume. In blood plasma, 90% of vitamin K₁ is bound to lipoproteins (VLDL portion). Vitamin K₁ plasma concentration is normally between 0.4 and 1.2µg per litre.

The elimination half-life in plasma is 1.5–3 hours. After metabolic degradation, vitamin K₁ is bound to glucuronic acid and excreted in the bile and urine.

Less than 10% of the drug is excreted unchanged in the urine. Vitamin K₁ has an active metabolite, vitamin K₁-2,3-epoxide, which is reconverted into vitamin K₁.

*Indications:* Konakion MM is indicated as an antidote to anticoagulant drugs of the coumarin type in the treatment of haemorrhage or threatened haemorrhage associated with a low blood level of prothrombin or factor VII.

### Dosage and administration

*Adults: As an antidote to anticoagulant drugs:* For potentially fatal and severe haemorrhages: Konakion MM therapy should be accompanied by a more immediate effective treatment such as transfusions of whole blood or blood clotting factors. The anticoagulant should be withdrawn and an intravenous injection of Konakion MM given slowly in a dose of 10 - 20 mg. The prothrombin level should be estimated three hours later and, if the response has been inadequate, the dose should be repeated. Not more than 40 mg of Konakion MM should be given intravenously in 24 hours. Coagulation profiles must be monitored on a daily basis until these have returned to acceptable levels; in severe cases more frequent monitoring is necessary and where there is no immediate efficacy, transfusion of whole blood or blood clotting factors should be used.

Less severe haemorrhage: Oral treatment with Konakion tablets may be used.

*Use in the elderly:* Elderly patients tend to be more sensitive to reversal of anticoagulation with Konakion MM; dosage in this group should be at the lower end of the ranges recommended.

*Children:* Konakion MM Ampoules should not be given to infants and children, since no data are yet available on this patient group. Konakion Ampoules 1 mg/0.5 ml may be used in these patients. (See separate prescribing information.)

Konakion MM Ampoules are for intravenous injection and should be diluted with 55 mls of 5% glucose before slowly infusing the product. The solution should be freshly prepared and protected from light. Konakion MM Ampoule solution should not be diluted or mixed with other injectables, but may be injected into the lower part of an infusion apparatus.

### Contra-indications, warnings, etc

*Contra-indications:* Use in patients with a known hypersensitivity to any of the constituents.

*Use in pregnancy and lactation:* There is no specific evidence regarding the safety of Konakion MM in pregnancy but, as with most drugs, the administration during pregnancy should only occur if the benefits outweigh the risks.

*Precautions:* When treating patients with severely impaired liver function, it should be borne in mind that one Konakion MM Ampoule contains 54.6 mg glycocholic acid and this may have a bilirubin displacing effect.

At the time of use, the ampoule contents should be clear. Following incorrect storage, the contents may become turbid or present a phase-separation. In this case the ampoule must not be used.

In potentially fatal and severe haemorrhage due to overdosage of coumarin anticoagulants, intravenous injections of Konakion MM must be administered slowly and not more than 40 mg should be given during a period of 24 hours. Konakion therapy should be accompanied by a more immediate effective treatment such as transfusion of whole blood or blood clotting factors. When patients with prosthetic heart valves are given transfusions for the treatment of severe or potentially fatal haemorrhages, fresh frozen plasma should be used.

Large doses of Konakion MM (more than 40 mg per day) should be avoided if it is intended to continue with anticoagulant therapy because there is no experience with doses above this maximum of 40 mg per day and higher doses may give rise to unexpected adverse events. Clinical studies have shown a sufficient decrease in the prothrombin time with the recommended dosage. If haemorrhage is severe, a transfusion of fresh whole blood may be necessary whilst awaiting the effect of the vitamin K₁.

Vitamin K₁ is not an antidote to heparin.

*Side effects and adverse reactions:* There are only few unconfirmed reports of the occurrence of possible anaphylactoid reactions after intravenous injection of Konakion MM.

*Drug interactions:* No significant interactions are known other than antagonism of coumarin anticoagulants.

*Treatment of overdosage:* Hypervitaminosis of vitamin K₁ is unknown.

### Pharmaceutical precautions

*Storage:* Konakion MM Ampoules should be protected from light. The recommended maximum storage temperature is 25°C and the solution should not be frozen. Do not use if the solution is turbid.

**Legal category**  POM

**Package quantities**  Packs of 10 ampoules.

**Further information**  In the mixed micelles solution, vitamin K₁ is solubilized by means of a physiological colloidal system, also found in the human body, consisting of lecithin and bile acid. Owing to the absence of organic solvents, the Konakion mixed micelles solution is well tolerated on intravenous administration.

**Product licence number**  0031/0254

## KONAKION* MM PAEDIATRIC AMPOULES

**Qualitative and quantitative composition**  Each ampoule contains 2 mg phytomenadione in 0.2 ml.

**Pharmaceutical form**  The ampoule solution is clear to slightly opalescent, pale yellow in colour and contains the active constituent in a mixed micelles vehicle of glycocholic acid and lecithin.

### Clinical particulars

*Therapeutic indications:* Konakion MM is indicated for the prophylaxis and treatment of haemorrhagic disease of the newborn.

*Posology and method of administration: Neonates and Babies:*
*Prophylaxis*

*Healthy neonates of 36 weeks gestation and older:* 2 mg orally at birth or soon after birth. This should be followed by a second dose of 2 mg at 4–7 days.

*Preterm neonates of less than 36 weeks gestation weighing 2.5 kg or greater, and term neonates at special risk:* 1 mg IM or IV at birth or soon after birth, the size and frequency of further doses depending on coagulation status.

*Preterm neonates of less than 36 weeks gestation weighing less than 2.5 kg:* 0.4 mg/kg (equivalent to 0.04 ml/kg) IM or IV at birth or soon after birth. This parenteral dose should not be exceeded (see *Special warnings and special precautions for use*). The frequency of further doses should depend on coagulation status.

*Exclusively breast-fed babies:* In addition to the doses at birth and at 4–7 days, a further 2 mg oral dose should be given 1 month after birth. Further monthly 2 mg oral doses until formula feeding is introduced have been advised, but no safety or efficacy data exist for these additional doses.

*Therapy:* Initially 1 mg IV and further doses as required, depending on clinical picture and coagulation status. Konakion therapy may need to be accompanied by a more immediate effective treatment, such as transfusion of whole blood or blood clotting factors to compensate for severe blood loss and delayed response to vitamin K₁.

*Contra-indications:* Use in patients with a known hypersensitivity to any of the constituents.

*Special warnings and special precautions for use:* At the time of use, the ampoule contents should be clear. Following incorrect storage, the contents may become turbid or present a phase-separation. In this case the ampoule must no longer be used.

*For oral use:* After breaking the ampoule open, 0.2 ml of solution should be withdrawn into the oral dispenser until it reaches the mark on the dispenser (0.2 ml = 2 mg vitamin K). Drop the contents of the dispenser directly into the baby's mouth by pressing the plunger.

*For parenteral use:* Konakion MM paediatric should not be diluted or mixed with other parenteral medications, but may be injected into the lower part of an infusion set.

Parenteral administration to premature babies weighing less than 2.5 kg may increase the risk for the development of kernicterus (bilirubin encephalopathy).

*Interaction with other medicaments and other forms of interaction:* No significant interactions are known other than antagonism of coumarin anticoagulants.

*Pregnancy and lactation:* Not applicable.

*Effects on ability to drive and use machines:* Not applicable.

*Undesirable effects:* There are only few unconfirmed reports on the occurrence of possible anaphylactoid reactions after IV injection of Konakion MM. Local irritation may occur at the injection site but is unlikely due to the small injection volume.

*Overdose:* No overdose effects are known.

### Pharmacological properties

*Pharmacodynamic properties:* Konakion MM is a preparation of synthetic phytomenadione (vitamin K₁). The presence of vitamin K₁ is essential for the formation within the body of prothrombin, factor VII, factor IX and factor X, and of the coagulation inhibitors, protein C and protein S.

Vitamin K₁ does not readily cross the placental barrier from mother to child and is poorly excreted in breast milk.

Lack of vitamin K₁ leads to an increased tendency to haemorrhagic disease in the newborn. Vitamin K₁ administration, which promotes synthesis of the above-mentioned coagulation factors by the liver, can reverse an abnormal coagulation status due to vitamin $K_1$ deficiency.

*Pharmacokinetic properties:* In the mixed micelle solution, vitamin $K_1$ is solubilised by means of a physiological colloidal system consisting of lecithin and a bile acid.

Vitamin $K_1$ is absorbed from the small intestine. Absorption is limited in the absence of bile.

Vitamin $K_1$ accumulates predominantly in the liver, is up to 90% bound to lipoproteins in the plasma and is stored in the body only for short periods of time.

Vitamin $K_1$ is transformed to more polar metabolites, such as phytomenadione-2,3-epoxide.

The half-life of vitamin $K_1$ in plasma is about 1.5 to 3 hours. Vitamin $K_1$ is excreted in bile and urine as the glucuronide and sulphate conjugates.

*Preclinical safety data:* None applicable.

**Pharmaceutical particulars**
*List of excipients:* Glycocholic acid, lecithin, sodium hydroxide, hydrochloric acid and water.

*Incompatibilities:* See *Special warnings and special precautions for use.*

*Shelf life:* 3 years.

*Special precautions for storage:* Konakion MM Paediatric Ampoule solution should be stored below 25°C and be protected from light. The solution should not be frozen. Do not use if the solution is turbid.

*Nature and contents of container:* Amber glass ampoules containing 2 mg phytomenadione in 0.2 ml. Plastic oral dispensers. Packs of 1, 5 or 10.

*Instructions for use/handling:* See *Special warnings and special precautions for use.*

**Marketing authorisation number** 0031/0346

**Date of approval/revision of SPC** June 1996

**Legal category** POM

## KONAKION* TABLETS

**Qualitative and quantitative composition** Each Konakion Tablet contains 10 mg vitamin $K_1$ (phytomenadione) BP.

**Pharmaceutical form** Round off-white sugar-coated tablets.

**Clinical particulars**
*Therapeutic indications:* Konakion is indicated in the treatment of haemorrhage or threatened haemorrhage associated with a low blood level of prothrombin or factor VII. The main indications are:

As an antidote to anticoagulant drugs of the coumarin type.

*Posology and method of administration:* Konakion tablets are for oral administration and should be chewed or allowed to dissolve slowly in the mouth.

*Adults: As an antidote to anticoagulant drugs*
*For potentially fatal and severe haemorrhages:* Konakion intravenous injection (see separate prescribing information).

*Less severe haemorrhage:* Konakion is given orally in doses of 10–20 mg (1 to 2 tablets). The prothrombin level is estimated 8 to 12 hours, and later if the response has been inadequate, the dose should be repeated.

*Lowering of prothrombin to dangerous level but no haemorrhage:* A dose of 5–10 mg Konakion orally may be given to bring the prothrombin level back to within safe limits. In such instances it is not usually necessary to discontinue the anticoagulant.

*Adults: Other indications:* Doses of 10–20 mg as required.

*Elderly:* Elderly patients tend to be more sensitive to reversal of anticoagulation with Konakion; dosage in this group should be at the lower end of the ranges recommended.

*Children:* If, on the recommendation of a physician, a children's dosage is required, then it is suggested that 5–10 mg be given.

*Contra-indications:* Use in patients with a known hypersensitivity to any of the constituents.

*Special warnings and special precautions for use:* Large doses of Konakion should be avoided if it is intended to continue with anticoagulant therapy.

Vitamin $K_1$ is not an antidote to heparin.

*Interaction with other medicaments and other forms of interaction:* None known.

*Pregnancy and lactation:* There is no specific evidence regarding the safety of Konakion in pregnancy but, as with most drugs, the administration during pregnancy should only occur if the benefits outweigh the risks.

*Effects on ability to drive and use machines:* None known.

*Undesirable effects:* None known.

*Overdose:* Hypervitaminosis of vitamin $K_1$ is unknown.

**Pharmacological properties**
*Pharmacodynamic properties:* Konakion is a synthetic preparation of vitamin $K_1$. The presence of vitamin K (i.e. vitamin $K_1$ itself or substances with vitamin K activity) is essential for the formation within the body of prothrombin, factor VII, factor IX and factor X. Lack of vitamin K leads to increased tendency to haemorrhage. When an antidote to an anticoagulant is necessary it is essential to use vitamin $K_1$ itself, as vitamin K analogues are much less effective.

*Pharmacokinetic properties:* The fat-soluble vitamin compound phytomenadione (Vitamin $K_1$) requires the presence of bile for its absorption from the gastrointestinal tract. Vitamin K accumulates mainly in the liver but is stored in the body only for short periods of time. Vitamin K does not appear to cross the placenta readily and it is poorly distributed into breast milk. Phytomenadione is rapidly metabolised to more polar metabolites and is excreted in bile and urine as glucuronide and sulphate conjugates.

*Preclinical safety data:* None stated.

**Pharmaceutical particulars**
*List of excipients:* Silicon Dioxide USP; Sucrose PhEur; Glucose PhEur; Skimmed Milk Powder HSE; Cocoa USP; Cocoa Butter BP; Carob Bean Gum FCC; Glycerol PhEur; Rice Starch PhEur; Titanium Dioxide E171; Ethyl Vanillin USP; Acacia Spray Dried PhEur; Paraffin Light Liquid PhEur; Hard Paraffin BP; Talc PhEur; Sodium Carboxymethylcellulose PhEur.

*Incompatibilities:* None known.

*Shelf life:* The recommended shelf life of Konakion Tablets is 60 months.

*Special precautions for storage:* Konakion tablets should be stored in well-closed containers and protected from light.

*Nature and contents of container:* Konakion Tablets are supplied in white HDPE bottles with tamper evident snap-fit, containing 25 tablets.

*Instructions for use/handling:* None stated.

**Marketing authorisation number** 0031/5022R

**Date of approval/revision of SPC** June 1996

**Legal category** P

## LARIAM*

**Presentation** Tablets containing 274.09 mg mefloquine hydrochloride, equivalent to 250 mg mefloquine base.

**Uses**
*Pharmacological properties:* The effectiveness of Lariam in the therapy and prophylaxis of malaria is due essentially to destruction of the asexual blood forms of the malarial pathogens that affect humans (*Plasmodium falciparum, P. vivax, P. malariae, P. ovale*).

Lariam is also effective against malarial parasites resistant to other antimalarials such as chloroquine and other 4-aminoquinoline derivatives, proguanil, pyrimethamine and pyrimethamine-sulfonamide combinations. However, strains of *P. falciparum* resistant to mefloquine have been reported (e.g. in parts of Indochina). Cross-resistance between mefloquine and halofantrine has been observed.

*In vitro* and *in vivo* studies with mefloquine showed no haemolysis associated with glucose-6-phosphate dehydrogenase deficiency.

*Pharmacokinetics:*
*Absorption:* The maximum plasma concentration is reached within 6 to 24 hours after a single oral dose of Lariam. The level in micrograms per litre is roughly equivalent to the dose in milligrams (for example, approximately 1000μg/l after a single dose of 1000 mg). The presence of food significantly enhances the rate and extent of absorption.

At a dose of 250 mg once weekly, maximum steady state plasma concentrations of 1000–2000μg/l are reached after 7–10 weeks. The RBC concentration is almost twice as high as the plasma level. Plasma protein binding is about 98%. Clinical experience suggests a minimal suppressive plasma concentration of mefloquine in the order of 600μg/l.

*Elimination:* The average half-life of mefloquine in Europeans is 21 days. There is evidence that mefloquine is excreted mainly in the bile and faeces. In volunteers, urinary excretion of unchanged mefloquine and its main metabolite accounted for about 9% and 4% of the dose respectively.

*Special clinical situations:* The pharmacokinetics of mefloquine may be altered in acute malaria. Pharmacokinetic differences have been observed between various ethnic populations. In practice, however, these are of minor importance compared with host immune status and sensitivity of the parasite.

Mefloquine crosses the placenta. Excretion into breast milk appears to be minimal.

*Indications:* Therapy and prophylaxis of malaria.

*Therapy:* Lariam is especially indicated for therapy of *P. falciparum* malaria in which the pathogen has become resistant to other antimalarial agents.

Following treatment of *P. vivax* malaria with Lariam, relapse prophylaxis with an 8-amino-quinoline derivative, for example primaquine, should be considered in order to eliminate parasites in the hepatic phase.

*Prophylaxis:* Malaria prophylaxis with Lariam is particularly recommended for travellers to malarious areas in which multiple resistant *P. falciparum* strains occur.

For current advice on geographical resistance patterns and appropriate chemoprophylaxis, current guidelines or the Malaria Reference Laboratory should be consulted, details of which can be found in the British National Formulary (BNF).

**Dosage and administration**
*Curative treatment:* The recommended total therapeutic dose of mefloquine for non-immune patients is 20–25 mg/kg. A lower total dose of 15 mg/kg may suffice for partially immune individuals.

The recommended total therapeutic dosages of Lariam tablets relative to bodyweight and immune status are presented in the following table*.

| | *Non-immune patients* | *Partially immune patients* |
|---|---|---|
| < 20 kg** | ¼ tablet / 2.5–3 kg<br>1 tablet / 10–12 kg | ¼ tablet / 4 kg<br>1 tablet / 16 kg |
| 20–30 kg | 2–3 tablets | 1¼–2 tablets |
| > 30–45 kg | 3–4 tablets | 2–3 tablets |
| > 45–60 kg | 4–5 tablets | 3–4 tablets |
| > 60 kg*** | 6 tablets | 4–6 tablets |

*Splitting the total curative dosage into 2–3 doses (e.g. 3 + 1, 3 + 2 or 3 + 2 + 1 tablets) taken 6–8 hours apart may reduce the occurrence or severity of adverse effects.
**Experience with Lariam in infants less than 3 months old or weighing less than 5 kg is limited.
***There is no specific experience with total dosages of more than 6 tablets in very heavy patients.

A second full dose should be given to patients who vomit less than 30 minutes after receiving the drug. If vomiting occurs 30–60 minutes after a dose, an additional half-dose should be given.

If a full treatment course with Lariam does not lead to improvement within 48–72 hours, alternative treatments should be considered. When breakthrough malaria occurs during Lariam prophylaxis, physicians should carefully evaluate which antimalarial to use for therapy.

Lariam can be given for severe acute malaria after an initial course of intravenous quinine lasting at least 2–3 days. Interactions leading to adverse events can largely be prevented by allowing an interval of at least 12 hours after the last dose of quinine (see *Drug interactions*).

In areas with multi-resistant malaria, initial treatment with artemisinin or a derivative, if available, followed by Lariam is also an option.

*Malaria prophylaxis:* Prophylaxis of malaria with Lariam should be initiated at least one week and up to 2–3 weeks before arrival in a malarious area. The following dosage schedule is given as a guide:

| | *Dosage* | *Course of prophylaxis* |
|---|---|---|
| *Adults and children of more than 45 kg bodyweight* | 1 tablet | Stated dose to be given once weekly, always on the same day for a minimum of six weeks. |
| *Children and adults weighing less than 45 kg* | | First dose at least one week and up to 2–3 weeks before arrival in malarious area. Further doses at weekly intervals during and for four weeks after visiting the malarious area. |
| 5–19 kg | ¼ tablet | |
| 20–30 kg | ½ tablet | |
| 31–45 kg | ¾ tablet | |

The maximum recommended duration of administration of Lariam is 12 months.

The tablets should be swallowed whole preferably after a meal with plenty of liquid.

*Use in the elderly:* No specific adaptation of the usual adult dosage is required for elderly patients.

**Contra-indications, warnings, etc**
*Contra-indications:* Prophylactic use in patients with severe impairment of liver function should be regarded for the time being as a contra-indication as no experience has been gained in such patients.

Patients with a history of psychiatric disturbances

(including depression) or convulsions should not be prescribed Lariam prophylactically, as it may precipitate these conditions (see *Precautions* and *Drug interactions*).

Lariam should not be administered to patients with a known hypersensitivity to mefloquine or related compounds, e.g. quinine.

Because of the danger of a potentially fatal prolongation of the QTc interval, halofantrine must not be given simultaneously with or subsequent to Lariam. No data are available where Lariam was given after halofantrine.

*Use in pregnancy and lactation:* There is too little clinical experience in humans to assess any possible damaging effects of Lariam during pregnancy. However, mefloquine is teratogenic when administered to rats and mice in early gestation. Therefore, Lariam should be used in pregnancy only if there are compelling medical reasons. In the absence of clinical experience, prophylactic use during pregnancy should be avoided as a matter of principle.

Mefloquine is excreted into breast milk in small amounts, the activity of which is unknown. Nursing mothers should be advised not to breast-feed while taking Lariam.

*Precautions:* Women of childbearing potential travelling to malarious areas in which multiple resistant *P. falciparum* is found and who are receiving Lariam for the treatment and prophylaxis of malaria should take reliable contraceptive precautions for the entire duration of therapy and for three months after the last dose of Lariam (see *Use in pregnancy and lactation*).

Experience with Lariam in infants less than 3 months old or weighing less than 5 kg is limited.

There is no evidence that dose adjustment is necessary for patients with renal insufficiency. However, since clinical evidence in such patients is limited, caution should be exercised when using Lariam in patients with impaired renal function.

In patients with epilepsy, mefloquine may increase the risk of convulsions. Therefore in such cases Lariam should be used only for curative treatment and only if compelling reasons exist (see *Contra-indications* and *Drug interactions*).

Lariam should be taken with caution in patients suffering from cardiac conduction disorders, since transient cardiac conduction alterations have been observed during curative and preventative use.

Patients should not disregard the possibility that re-infection or recrudescence may occur after effective antimalarial therapy.

*Effects on ability to drive and to use machines*
*Treatment:* Mefloquine can cause dizziness or disturbed sense of balance. It is consequently recommended not to drive or to carry out tasks demanding fine co-ordination and spatial discrimination during treatment with mefloquine. Patients should avoid such tasks for at least three weeks following therapeutic use as dizziness, a disturbed sense of balance or neuropsychiatric reactions have been reported up to three weeks after the use of Lariam.

*Prophylactic use:* Caution should be exercised with regard to driving, piloting aircraft and operating machines, as dizziness, a disturbed sense of balance or neuropsychiatric reactions have been reported during and for up to three weeks after use of Lariam.

*Side-effects and adverse reactions:* At the doses given for acute malaria, adverse reactions to Lariam may not be distinguishable from symptoms of the disease itself. In a large study of tourists receiving various prophylactic antimalarials, about 22% of the subjects taking Lariam reported adverse events. Because of the long half-life of mefloquine, adverse reactions to Lariam may occur or persist up to several weeks after the last dose.

Patients should be advised to obtain medical advice before the next weekly dose of Lariam, if any concerning or neuropsychiatric symptoms develop. Discontinuation of Lariam should be considered, particularly if neuropsychiatric reactions occur. The need for alternative antimalarial therapy or prophylaxis can then be evaluated.

*Common adverse reactions:* Nausea, vomiting, dizziness or vertigo, loss of balance, headache, somnolence, sleep disorders (insomnia, abnormal dreams), loose stools or diarrhoea and abdominal pain.

*Uncommon adverse reactions:*

*Psychiatric:* Psychiatric reactions sometimes disabling and prolonged have been reported in association with Lariam. These include depression, anxiety, confusion, hallucinations, panic attacks, restlessness, forgetfulness, psychosis and paranoia, emotional instability, aggression and agitation.

*Neurological:* Convulsions, sensory and motor neuropathies (including paraesthesia), tremor, tinnitus and vestibular disorders, abnormal co-ordination, ataxia and visual disturbances.

*Cardiovascular system:* Circulatory disturbances (hypotension, hypertension, flushing, syncope), tachycardia or palpitations, bradycardia, irregular pulse, extrasystoles and other transient cardiac conduction alterations.

*Skin:* Rash, exanthema, erythema, urticaria, pruritus, hair loss, erythema multiforme, Stevens-Johnson syndrome.

*Musculo-skeletal system:* Muscle weakness, muscle cramps, myalgia, arthralgia.

*General symptoms:* Asthenia, malaise, fatigue, fever, chills, loss of appetite.

*Haematological:* Leucopenia or leucocytosis, thrombocytopenia.

*Laboratory abnormalities:* Transient elevation of transaminases.

*Very rare adverse reactions:*
AV-block and encephalopathy.

Studies *in vitro* and *in vivo* showed no haemolysis associated with G6PD deficiency.

*Drug interactions:* Concomitant administration of Lariam and other related compounds (e.g. quinine, quinidine and chloroquine) may produce electrocardiographic abnormalities and increase the risk of convulsions. There is evidence that the use of halofantrine after mefloquine causes a significant lengthening of the QTc interval. Clinically significant QTc prolongation has not been found with mefloquine alone (see Dosage and Administration).

This appears to be the only clinically relevant interaction of this kind with Lariam, although theoretically co-administration of other drugs known to alter cardiac conduction (e.g. anti-arrhythmic or β-adrenergic blocking agents, calcium channel blockers, antihistamines or $H_1$-blocking agents, tricyclic antidepressants and phenothiazines) might also contribute to a prolongation of the QTc interval.

In patients taking an anticonvulsant (e.g. valproic acid, carbamazepine, phenobarbital or phenytoin), the concomitant use of Lariam may reduce seizure control by lowering the plasma levels of the anticonvulsant. Dosage adjustments of antiseizure medication may be necessary in some cases (see *Contra-indications* and *Precautions*).

When Lariam is taken concurrently with oral live typhoid vaccines, attenuation of immunisation cannot be excluded. Vaccinations with oral attenuated live bacteria should therefore be completed at least 3 days before the first dose of Lariam.

No other drug interactions are known. Nevertheless, the effects of Lariam on travellers receiving comedication, particularly those on anticoagulants or antidiabetics, should be checked before departure.

*Treatment of overdosage:* In cases of overdosage with Lariam, the symptoms mentioned under Side-effects and adverse reactions may be more pronounced. Countermeasures: Induce vomiting or perform gastric lavage as appropriate. Monitor cardiac function (if possible by ECG) and neuropsychiatric status for at least 24 hours. Provide symptomatic and intensive supportive treatment as required, particularly for cardiovascular disorders.

**Pharmaceutical precautions**
*Storage:* Protect from moisture.

**Legal category** POM

**Package quantities** Tablets (cross-scored) in packs of 8.

**Further information** None

**Product licence number** 0031/0236

# LEXOTAN*

**Presentation** Lilac, hexagonal biconvex tablets having L1.5 imprinted on one face and a single break bar on the other, containing 1.5 mg bromazepam. Pink, hexagonal biconvex tablets having L3 imprinted on one face and a single break bar on the other, containing 3 mg bromazepam.

**Uses** *Properties:* Lexotan is a pyridylbenzodiazepine compound with anxiolytic properties.

*Indications:* Lexotan is indicated for the short-term (2-4 weeks) symptomatic treatment of anxiety that is severe, disabling or subjecting the individual to unacceptable distress, occurring alone or in association with insomnia or short-term psychosomatic, organic or psychotic illness.

**Dosage and administration** *Adults:* The optimum dosage and frequency of administration of Lexotan should be based on the individual patient, the severity of symptoms and previous psychotropic drug history.

The usual dosage in general practice is from 3 mg to 18 mg daily in divided doses.

In exceptional circumstances, in hospitalised patients, up to the maximum daily dosage of 60 mg, in divided doses, may be given.

*Use in elderly:* ELDERLY PATIENTS ARE MORE SENSITIVE TO THE ACTIONS OF LEXOTAN; DOSES SHOULD NOT EXCEED HALF THOSE NORMALLY RECOMMENDED.

The lowest dose which can control symptoms should be used. Treatment should not be continued at the full dose beyond four weeks. Long-term chronic use is not recommended. Treatment should always be tapered off gradually. Patients who have taken benzodiazepines for a prolonged time may require a longer period during which doses are reduced. Specialist help may be appropriate.

*Children:* Lexotan is not for paediatric use.
Lexotan tablets are for oral administration.

**Contra-indications, warnings, etc**
*Contra-indications:* Patients with known sensitivity to benzodiazepines; acute pulmonary insufficiency; respiratory depression; phobic or obsessional states; chronic psychosis.

*Use in pregnancy and lactation:* There is no evidence as to drug safety in human pregnancy, nor is there evidence from animal work that it is free from hazard. Do not use during pregnancy, especially during the first and last trimesters, unless there are compelling reasons.

The administration of high doses or prolonged administration of low doses of benzodiazepines in the last trimester of pregnancy has been reported to produce irregularities in the foetal heart rate, and hypotonia, poor sucking and hypothermia in the neonate.

Benzodiazepines have been detected in breast milk. If possible, the use of Lexotan should be avoided during lactation.

*Precautions:* In patients with chronic pulmonary insufficiency, and in patients with chronic renal or hepatic disease, dosage may need to be reduced.

Lexotan should not be used alone to treat depression or anxiety associated with depression, since suicide may be precipitated in such patients.

Amnesia may occur.

In cases of loss or bereavement, psychological adjustment may be inhibited by benzodiazepines.

If Lexotan is combined with centrally-acting drugs such as neuroleptics, tranquillisers, antidepressants, hypnotics, analgesics and anaesthetics, the sedative effects are likely to be intensified. The elderly require special supervision.

Patients should be advised that, like all medicaments of this type, Lexotan may modify patients' performance at skilled tasks (driving, operating machinery, etc.) to a varying degree depending upon dosage, administration and individual susceptibility. Patients should further be advised that alcohol may intensify any impairment and should therefore be avoided during treatment.

The dependence potential of the benzodiazepines is low, particularly when limited to short-term use, but this increases when high doses are used, especially when given over long periods. This is particularly so in patients with a history of alcoholism or drug abuse or in patients with marked personality disorders. Regular monitoring in such patients is essential, routine repeat prescriptions should be avoided and treatment should be withdrawn gradually. Symptoms such as depression, nervousness, rebound insomnia, irritability, sweating, and diarrhoea have been reported following abrupt cessation of treatment in patients receiving even normal therapeutic doses for short periods of time. In rare instances, withdrawal following excessive dosages may produce confusional states, psychotic manifestations and convulsions.

Abnormal psychological reactions to benzodiazepines have been reported. Rare behavioural effects include paradoxical aggressive outbursts, excitement, confusion, and the uncovering of depression with suicidal tendencies. Extreme caution should therefore be used in prescribing benzodiazepines to patients with personality disorders.

When Lexotan is used in conjunction with anti-epileptic drugs, side-effects and toxicity may be more evident, particularly with hydantoins or barbiturates or combinations including them. This requires extra care in adjusting dosage in the initial stages of treatment.

Known inhibitors of hepatic enzymes, e.g. cimetidine, have been shown to reduce the clearance of benzodiazepines and may potentiate their action and known inducers of hepatic enzymes, e.g. rifampicin, may increase the clearance of benzodiazepines.

*Side-effects and adverse reactions:* Common adverse effects include drowsiness, sedation, unsteadiness and ataxia; these are dose-related and may persist into the following day, even after a single dose. Drowsiness may be a particular problem when Lexotan is used in higher dosage in some patients, especially if they are unused to this form of therapy. The elderly are particularly sensitive to the effects of centrally depressant drugs and may experience confusion, especially if organic brain changes are present;

the dosage of Lexotan should not exceed one-half that recommended for other adults.

Other adverse effects are rare and include headache, vertigo, hypotension, gastro-intestinal upsets, skin rashes, visual disturbances, changes in libido, and urinary retention. Isolated cases of blood dyscrasias and jaundice have also been reported.

*Treatment of overdosage:* When taken alone in overdosage Lexotan presents few problems in management. Signs may include drowsiness, ataxia and dysarthria, with coma in severe cases. Treatment is symptomatic. Gastric lavage is useful only if performed soon after ingestion.

The value of dialysis has not been determined. Anexate is a specific IV antidote for use in emergency situations. Patients requiring such intervention should be monitored closely in hospital (see separate prescribing information).

If excitation occurs, barbiturates should not be used.

When taken with centrally-acting drugs, especially alcohol, the effects of overdosage are likely to be more severe and, in the absence of supportive measures, may prove fatal.

**Pharmaceutical precautions** *Storage:* Lexotan tablets should be stored in well-closed containers in a dry place, protected from light.

**Legal category** CD (Sch. 4), POM.

**Package quantities** Lexotan tablets 1.5 mg in packs of 60 (OP).

Lexotan tablets 3 mg in packs of 60 (OP).

**Further information** Lexotan is rapidly absorbed from the gastro-intestinal tract. The mean half-life for elimination of Lexotan in man is about 16 hours. Metabolites of Lexotan do not contribute significantly to the effects of the drug.

The elderly, and patients with impaired renal and/or hepatic function, will be particularly susceptible to the adverse effects listed above. It is advisable to review treatment regularly and to discontinue use as soon as possible.

Treatment should be kept to a minimum and given only under close medical supervision. Little is known regarding the efficacy or safety of benzodiazepines in long-term use.

**Product licence numbers**
Tablets 1.5 mg    0031/0127
Tablets 3 mg      0031/0128

# LIBRIUM

**Qualitative and quantitative composition** Each 10 mg capsule contains 10 mg of the active ingredient chlordiazepoxide hydrochloride BP.

**Pharmaceutical form**    Librium Capsules 10 mg.

**Clinical particulars**

*Therapeutic indications:* Short-term (2–4 weeks) symptomatic treatment of anxiety that is severe, disabling or subjecting the individual to unacceptable distress, occurring alone or in association with insomnia or short-term psychosomatic, organic or psychotic illness.

Muscle spasm of varied aetiology.

Symptomatic relief of acute alcohol withdrawal.

*Posology and method of administration*
Adults

| Anxiety states | Usual dose | Up to 30 mg daily in divided doses. |
|---|---|---|
| | Maximum dose | Up to 100 mg daily in divided doses. Adjusted on an individual basis. |
| Insomnia associated with anxiety | | 10 to 30 mg before retiring. |
| Symptomatic relief of acute alcohol withdrawal | | 25 to 100 mg repeated if necessary in 2 to 4 hours. |
| Muscle spasm of varied aetiology | | 10 to 30 mg daily in divided doses. |

*Elderly or debilitated patients:* doses should not exceed half those normally recommended.

*Children:* Librium is not for paediatric use.

The lowest dose which can control symptoms should be used. Treatment should not be continued at the full dose beyond four weeks.

Long-term chronic use is not recommended.

Treatment should always be tapered off gradually. Patients who have taken benzodiazepines for a prolonged time may require a longer period during which doses are reduced. Specialist help may be appropriate.

Librium capsules are for oral administration.

Treatment should be kept to a minimum and given only under close medical supervision. Little is known

regarding the efficacy or safety of benzodiazepines in long-term use.

*Contra-indications:* Patients with known sensitivity to benzodiazepines; acute pulmonary insufficiency; respiratory depression; phobic or obsessional states; chronic psychosis.

*Special warnings and special precautions for use:* In patients with chronic pulmonary insufficiency, and in patients with chronic renal or hepatic disease, dosage may need to be reduced.

Librium should not be used alone to treat depression or anxiety associated with depression, since suicide may be precipitated in such patients.

Amnesia may occur.

In cases of loss or bereavement, psychological adjustment may be inhibited by benzodiazepines.

The dependence potential of the benzodiazepines is low, particularly when limited to short-term use, but this increases when high doses are used, especially when given over long periods. This is particularly so in patients with a history of alcoholism or drug abuse or in patients with marked personality disorders. Regular monitoring in such patients is essential, routine repeat prescriptions should be avoided and treatment should be withdrawn gradually. Symptoms such as depression, nervousness, rebound insomnia, irritability, sweating, and diarrhoea have been reported following abrupt cessation of treatment in patients receiving even normal therapeutic doses for short periods of time.

In rare instances, withdrawal following excessive dosages may produce confusional states, psychotic manifestations and convulsions.

Abnormal psychological reactions to benzodiazepines have been reported. Rare behavioural effects include paradoxical aggressive outbursts, excitement, confusion, and the uncovering of depression with suicidal tendencies. Extreme caution should therefore be used in prescribing benzodiazepines to patients with personality disorders.

*Interaction with other medicaments and other forms of interaction:* If Librium is combined with centrally-acting drugs such as neuroleptics, tranquillisers, antidepressants, hypnotics, analgesics and anaesthetics, the sedative effects are likely to be intensified. The elderly require special supervision.

When Librium is used in conjunction with anti-epileptic drugs, side-effects and toxicity may be more evident, particularly with hydantoins or barbiturates or combinations including them. This requires extra care in adjusting dosage in the initial stages of treatment.

Known inhibitors of hepatic enzymes, e.g. cimetidine, have been shown to reduce the clearance of benzodiazepines and may potentiate their action and known inducers of hepatic enzymes, e.g. rifampicin, may increase the clearance of benzodiazepines.

*Pregnancy and lactation:* There is no evidence as to drug safety in human pregnancy, nor is there evidence from animal work that it is free from hazard. Do not use during pregnancy, especially during the first and last trimesters, unless there are compelling reasons.

The administration of high doses or prolonged administration of low doses of benzodiazepines in the last trimester of pregnancy has been reported to produce irregularities in the foetal heart rate, and hypotonia, poor sucking and hypothermia in the neonate.

Chlordiazepoxide may appear in breast milk. If possible, the use of Librium should be avoided during lactation.

*Effects on ability to drive and use machines:* Patients should be advised that, like all medicaments of this type, Librium may modify patients' performance at skilled tasks (driving, operating machinery, etc.) to a varying degree depending upon dosage, administration and individual susceptibility. Patients should further be advised that alcohol may intensify any impairment and should therefore be avoided during treatment.

*Undesirable effects:* Common adverse effects include drowsiness, sedation, unsteadiness and ataxia; these are dose-related and may persist into the following day even after a single dose. The elderly are particularly sensitive to the effects of centrally-depressant drugs and may experience confusion, especially if organic brain changes are present; the dosage of Librium should not exceed one-half that recommended for other adults.

Other adverse effects are rare and include headache, vertigo, hypotension, gastro-intestinal upsets, skin rashes, visual disturbances, changes in libido, and urinary retention. Isolated cases of blood dyscrasias and jaundice have also been reported.

*Overdose:* When taken alone in overdosage Librium presents few problems in management. Signs may include drowsiness, ataxia and dysarthria, with coma in severe cases. Treatment is symptomatic. Gastric lavage is useful only if performed soon after ingestion.

The value of dialysis has not been determined. Anexate is a specific IV antidote for use in emergency situations. Patients requiring such intervention should be monitored closely in hospital (see separate prescribing information).

If excitation occurs, barbiturates should not be used.

When taken with centrally-acting drugs, especially alcohol, the effects of overdosage are likely to be more severe and, in the absence of supportive measures, may prove fatal.

**Pharmacological properties**

*Pharmacodynamic properties:* Librium has anxiolytic and central muscle relaxant properties. It has little autonomic activity.

*Pharmacokinetic properties:* Librium is well absorbed, with peak blood levels being achieved one or two hours after administration. The drug has a half-life of 6–30 hours. Steady-state levels are usually reached within three days.

Chlordiazepoxide is metabolised to desmethylchlordiazepoxide. Demoxepam and desmethyldiazepam are also found in the plasma of patients on continuous treatment. The active metabolite desmethylchlordiazepoxide has an accumulation half-life of 10–18 hours; that of demoxepam has been recorded as 21–78 hours.

Steady-state levels of these active metabolites are reached after 10–15 days, with metabolite concentrations which are similar to those of the parent drug.

No clear correlation has been demonstrated between the blood levels of Librium and its clinical effects.

**Pharmaceutical particulars**

*List of excipients:* 10 mg capsules contain the following excipients: gelatin, starch maize white, talc purified, lactose, black iron oxide E172, titanium dioxide E171, yellow iron oxide E172 and indigo carmine E 132.

*Incompatibilities:* None.

*Shelf life:* PVDC blister pack–36 months. HDPE bottle–60 months. Plastic bottle–60 months. Amber glass bottle–60 months.

*Special precautions for storage:* Librium capsules should not be stored above 30°C.

*Nature and contents of container:* PVDC blister pack containing 100 tablets. HDPE bottle with jay-cap (snap-fit) closure containing 100 tablets. Plastic bottle with screw cap containing 100 tablets. Amber glass bottle with screw cap containing 100 tablets.

*Instructions for use/handling:* None.

**Marketing authorisation number**    0031/5026R

**Date of approval/revision of SPC**    January 1997

**Legal category**    POM

# LOCERYL CREAM

**Qualitative and quantitative composition** Loceryl cream contains 0.25% w/w amorolfine in the form of hydrochloride. Amorolfine is chemically described as *cis*-4-[(RS)-3[4-(1,1-Dimethylpropyl)phenyl]-2-methyl-propyl]-2,6-dimethylmorpholine.

**Pharmaceutical form** Cream.

**Clinical particulars**

*Therapeutic indications:* Dermatomycoses caused by dermatophytes: tinea pedis (athlete's foot), tinea cruris, tinea inguinalis, tinea corporis, tinea manuum. Pityriasis versicolor.

*Posology and method of administration:*
Dermatomycoses: Cream: To be applied to affected skin areas once daily following cleansing (in the evening).

The treatment should be continued without interruption until clinical cure, and for 3–5 days thereafter. The required duration of treatment depends on the species of fungi and on the localisation of the infection. In general, treatment should be continued for at least two to three weeks. With foot mycoses, up to six weeks of therapy may be necessary.

*Elderly:* There are no specific dosage recommendations for use in elderly patients.

*Children:* There are no specific dosage recommendations for children owing to the lack of clinical experience available to date.

*Contra-indications:* Loceryl cream must not be reused by patients who have shown hypersensitivity to the treatment.

No experience exists of use during pregnancy and nursing, therefore, the use of Loceryl should be avoided during pregnancy and lactation.

*Special warnings and special precautions for use:* Avoid contact of Loceryl cream with eyes, ears and mucous membranes.

*Interaction with other medicaments and other forms*

*of interaction:* There are no specific studies involving concomitant treatment with other topical medicines. Use of nail varnish or artificial nails should be avoided during treatment.

*Pregnancy and lactation:* Reproductive toxicology studies showed no evidence of teratogenicity in laboratory animals but embryotoxicity was observed at high oral doses. The systemic absorption of amorolfine during and after topical administration is very low and therefore the risk to the human foetus appears to be negligible. However, because there is no relevant experience Loceryl should be avoided during pregnancy and breast feeding.

*Effects on ability to drive and use machines:* None.

*Undesirable effects:* Rarely, skin irritation–presenting as erythema, pruritus or a burning sensation–has occurred during treatment with the cream. In exceptional cases, a slight, transient burning sensation in the area of the nails was observed after the application of nail lacquer.

*Overdose:* Loceryl is for topical use. In the event of accidental oral ingestion, an appropriate method of gastric emptying may be used.

### Pharmacological properties

*Pharmacodynamic properties:* Loceryl is a topical antimycotic. Amorolfine belongs to a new chemical class, and its fungicidal action is based on an alteration of the fungal cell membrane targeted primarily on sterol biosynthesis. The ergosterol content is reduced, and at the same time unusual sterically nonplanar sterols accumulate.

Amorolfine is a broad spectrum antimycotic. It is highly active (MIC < 2 mcg/ml) *in vitro* against:
  yeasts: Candida, Cryptococcus, Malassezia
    dermatophytes: Trichophyton, Microsporum, Epidermophyton
  moulds: Hendersonula, Alternaria, Scopulariopsis
  dematiacea: Cladosporium, Fonsecaea, Wangiella
  dimorphic fungi: Coccidioides, Histoplasma, Sporothrix

With the exception of *Actinomyces*, bacteria are not sensitive to amorolfine. *Propionibacterium acnes* is only slightly sensitive.

*Pharmacokinetic properties:* Amorolfine from cream penetrates into the stratum corneum. Nevertheless, systemic absorption is extremely low during and after therapeutic use.

*Preclinical safety data:* There are no pre-clinical data of relevance to the prescriber which are additional to that already included in other sections of the SPC.

### Pharmaceutical particulars

*List of excipients:* Polyoxyl 40 stearate, stearyl alcohol, paraffin liquid, white soft paraffin, carbomer, sodium hydroxide, disodium edetate, 2 phenoxyethanol.

*Incompatibilities:* None.

*Shelf life:* 3 years.

*Special precautions for storage:* Loceryl cream should be stored below 30°C.

*Nature and contents of container:* 20 g collapsible aluminium tube, sealed with an aluminium membrane and fitted with a plastic screw cap.

*Instructions for use/handling:* No special instructions.

**Marketing authorisation number** 0031/0286

**Date of approval/revision of SPC** January 1997

**Legal category** POM

## LOCERYL NAIL LACQUER*

**Qualitative and quantitative composition** Loceryl nail lacquer contains 5% w/v amorolfine in the form of hydrochloride. Amorolfine is chemically described as *cis*-4-[(RS)-3[4-(1,1-Dimethylpropyl)phenyl]-2-methyl-propyl]-2,6-dimethylmorpholine.

**Pharmaceutical form** Lacquer.

**Clinical particulars**

*Therapeutic indications:* Onychomycoses caused by dermatophytes, yeasts and moulds.

*Posology and method of administration:* The nail lacquer should be applied to the affected finger or toe nails once weekly. Twice weekly application may prove beneficial in some cases.

The patient should apply the nail lacquer as follows:
1. Before the first application of Loceryl, it is essential that the affected areas of nail (particularly the nail surfaces) should be filed down as thoroughly as possible using the nail file supplied. The surface of the nail should then be cleansed and degreased using a cleaning pad (as supplied). Before repeat application of Loceryl, the affected nails should be filed down again as required, following cleansing with a cleaning pad to remove any remaining lacquer.

*Caution:* Nail files used for affected nails must not be used for healthy nails.
2. With one of the reusable applicators supplied, apply the nail lacquer to the entire surface of the affected nails and allow it to dry. After use, clean the applicator with the same cleaning pad used before for nail cleaning. Keep the bottle tightly closed.

For each nail to be treated, dip the applicator into the nail lacquer without wiping off any of the lacquer on the bottle neck.

*Caution:* When working with organic solvents (thinners, white spirit, etc.) wear impermeable gloves in order to protect the Loceryl lacquer on the nails.

Treatment should be continued without interruption until the nail is regenerated and the affected areas are finally cured. The required frequency and duration of treatment depends essentially on intensity and localisation of the infection. In general, it is six months (finger nails) and nine to twelve months (toe nails). A review of the treatment is recommended at intervals of approximately three months.

Co-existent tinea pedis should be treated with an appropriate antimycotic cream.

*Elderly:* There are no specific dosage recommendations for use in elderly patients.

*Children:* There are no specific dosage recommendations for children owing to the lack of clinical experience available to date.

*Contra-indications:* Loceryl nail lacquer must not be reused by patients who have shown hypersensitivity to the treatment.

No experience exists of use during pregnancy and nursing, therefore, the use of Loceryl should be avoided during pregnancy and lactation.

*Special warnings and special precautions for use:* Avoid contact of the lacquer with eyes, ears and mucous membranes.

*Interaction with other medicaments and other forms of interaction:* There are no specific studies involving concomitant treatment with other topical medicines.

Use of nail varnish or artificial nails should be avoided during treatment.

*Pregnancy and lactation:* Reproductive toxicology studies showed no evidence of teratogenicity in laboratory animals but embryotoxicity was observed at high oral doses. The systemic absorption of amorolfine during and after topical administration is very low and therefore the risk to the human foetus appears to be negligible. However, because there is no relevant experience, Loceryl should be avoided during pregnancy and breast feeding.

*Effects on ability to drive and use machines:* None.

*Undesirable effects:* In exceptional cases, a slight, transient burning sensation in the area of the nails was observed after the application of nail lacquer.

*Overdose*
*Accidental oral ingestion:* Loceryl is for topical use. In the event of accidental oral ingestion, an appropriate method of gastric emptying may be used.

**Pharmacological properties**

*Pharmacodynamic properties:* Loceryl is a topical antimycotic. Amorolfine belongs to a new chemical class, and its fungicidal action is based on an alteration of the fungal cell membrane targeted primarily on sterol biosynthesis. The ergosterol content is reduced, and at the same time unusual sterically nonplanar sterols accumulate.

Amorolfine is a broad spectrum antimycotic. It is highly active (MIC < 2 mcg/ml) *in vitro* against
  yeasts: Candida, Cryptococcus, Malassezia
    dermatophytes: Trichophyton, Microsporum, Epidermophyton
  moulds: Hendersonula, Alternaria, Scopulariopsis
  dematiacea: Cladosporium, Fonsecaea, Wangiella
  dimorphic fungi: Coccidioides, Histoplasma, Sporothrix

With the exception of *Actinomyces*, bacteria are not sensitive to amorolfine. *Propionibacterium acnes* is only slightly sensitive.

*Pharmacokinetic properties:* Amorolfine from nail lacquer penetrates into and diffuses through the nail plate and is thus able to eradicate poorly accessible fungi in the nail bed. Systemic absorption of the active ingredient is very low with this type of application.

Following prolonged use of Loceryl Nail Lacquer, there is no indication of drug accumulation in the body.

*Preclinical safety data:* There are no pre-clinical data of relevance to the prescriber which are additional to that already included in other sections of the SPC.

**Pharmaceutical particulars**

*List of excipients:* Methacrylic acid, copolymer, triacetin, butyl acetate, methylene chloride.

*Incompatibilities:* None.

*Shelf life:* 3 years.

*Special precautions for storage:* Loceryl nail lacquer should be stored below 30°C. Protect from heat. Keep bottle tightly closed after use.

*Nature and contents of container:* Amber glass container with screw thread and plastic screw closure.

Each pack contains 1 bottle filled with 2.5 ml or 5 ml of nail lacquer together with cleansing swabs, spatulas and nail files.

*Instructions for use/handling:* No special instructions.

**Marketing authorisation number** 0031/0285

**Date of approval/revision of SPC** January 1997

**Legal category** POM

## MADOPAR CR*

**Qualitative and quantitative composition** Each capsule contains 100.0 mg levodopa and 28.5 mg benserazide hydrochloride (equivalent to 25 mg of the base) in a controlled release formulation.

**Pharmaceutical form** Modified release capsules.

**Clinical particulars**

*Therapeutic indications:* Treatment of all stages of Parkinson's disease. Patients with fluctuations related to levodopa plasma concentrations or timing of dose, e.g. end of dose deterioration or wearing-off effects, are more likely to benefit from switching to Madopar CR.

**Posology and method of administration**

*Adults, including the elderly:* Dosage and administration are very variable and must be titrated to the needs of the individual patient.

Madopar CR capsules must always be swallowed whole, preferably with a little water. They may be taken with or without food but antacid preparations should be avoided.

*Patients not currently treated with levodopa:* In patients with mild to moderate disease, the initial recommended dose is one capsule of Madopar CR three times daily with meals. Higher doses, in general, of Madopar CR will be required than with conventional levodopa-decarboxylase inhibitor combinations as a result of the reduced bioavailability. The initial dosages should not exceed 600 mg per day of levodopa.

Some patients may require a supplementary dose of conventional Madopar, or Madopar Dispersible, together with the first morning dose of Madopar CR to compensate for the more gradual onset of the CR formulation.

In cases of poor response to Madopar CR at total daily doses of Madopar CR plus any supplementary conventional Madopar corresponding to 1,200 mg levodopa, administration of Madopar CR should be discontinued and alternative therapy considered.

*Patients currently treated with levodopa:* Madopar CR should be substituted for the standard levodopa-decarboxylase inhibitor preparation by one capsule Madopar CR 125 per 100 mg levodopa. For example, where a patient previously received daily doses of 200 mg levodopa with a decarboxylase inhibitor, then therapy should be initiated with two capsules Madopar CR 125. Therapy should continue with the same frequency of doses as previously.

With Madopar CR, *on average*, a 50% increase in daily levodopa dosage compared with previous therapy has been found to be appropriate. The dosage should be titrated every 2 to 3 days using dosage increments of Madopar CR 125 capsules and a period of up to 4 weeks should be allowed for optimisation of dosage.

Patients already on levodopa therapy should be informed that their condition may deteriorate initially until the optimal dosage regimen has been found. Close medical supervision of the patient is advisable during the initial period whilst adjusting the dosage.

*Children:* Not to be given to patients under 25 years of age: therefore, no dosage recommendations are made for the administration of Madopar CR to children.

*Contra-indications:* Madopar is contra-indicated in narrow-angle glaucoma (it may be used in wide-angle glaucoma provided that the intra-ocular pressure remains under control); severe psychoneuroses or psychoses; severe endocrine, renal, hepatic or cardiac disorders.

It should not be given in conjunction with monoamine oxidase (MAO) inhibitors except selective MAO-B inhibitors or within 2 weeks of their withdrawal.

It should not be given to patients under 25 years of age.

Suspicion has arisen that levodopa may activate a malignant melanoma. Therefore, Madopar should not be used in persons who have a history of, or who may be suffering from, a malignant melanoma.

*Special warnings and special precautions for use:* When other drugs must be given in conjunction with

Madopar, the patient should be carefully observed for unusual side-effects or potentiating effects.

Drugs which interfere with central amine mechanisms, such as rauwolfia alkaloids (reserpine), tetrabenazine (Nitoman), metoclopramide, phenothiazines, thioxanthenes, butyrophenones, amphetamines and papaverine, should be avoided where possible. If, however, their administration is considered essential, extreme care should be exercised and a close watch kept for any signs of potentiation, antagonism or other interactions and for unusual side-effects.

In the event of general anaesthesia being required, Madopar therapy may be continued as long as the patient is able to take fluids and medication by mouth. If therapy is temporarily interrupted, the usual daily dosage may be administered as soon as the patient is able to take oral medication. Whenever therapy has been interrupted for longer periods, dosage should again be adjusted gradually; however, in many cases the patient can rapidly be returned to his previous therapeutic dosage.

If a patient has to undergo emergency surgery, when Madopar has not been withdrawn, anaesthesia with cyclopropane or halothane should be avoided.

There have been occasional reports of a neuroleptic malignant-like syndrome, involving hyperthermia, on abrupt withdrawal of levodopa preparations. Sudden discontinuation of Madopar, without close supervision, or "drug holidays" should therefore be avoided.

Pyridoxine (vitamin $B_6$) may be given with Madopar since the presence of a decarboxylase inhibitor protects against the peripheral levodopa transformation facilitated by pyridoxine.

Care should be taken when using Madopar in the following circumstances: in endocrine, renal, pulmonary or cardiovascular disease, particularly where there is a history of myocardial infarction or arrhythmia; psychiatric disturbances; hepatic disorder; peptic ulcer; osteomalacia; where sympathomimetic drugs may be required (e.g. bronchial asthma), due to possible potentiation of the cardiovascular effects of levodopa; where antihypertensive drugs are being used, due to possible increased hypotensive action.

Periodic evaluation of hepatic, haemopoietic, renal and cardiovascular functions is advised.

Patients who improve on Madopar therapy should be advised to resume normal activities gradually as rapid mobilisation may increase the risk of injury.

Levodopa may interfere chemically with several diagnostic laboratory tests including those for glucose, ketone bodies, or catecholamines in urine and for glucose or uric acid in blood. Levodopa therapy has been reported to inhibit the response to protirelin in tests of thyroid function.

*Interaction with other medicaments and other forms of interaction:* When Madopar CR is given with antacid preparations the bioavailability of levodopa is reduced, in comparison with conventional Madopar.

*Pregnancy and lactation:* Madopar is contra-indicated in pregnancy, since there is evidence of harmful effects in studies in pregnant rabbits and the benserazide component has been found to be associated with skeletal malformations in the rat. In any woman of childbearing potential the risk of its use, should pregnancy occur, must be weighed against the anticipated benefits of treatment. Patients taking Madopar should not breast-feed their infants.

*Effects on ability to drive and use machines:* Not applicable.

*Undesirable effects:* Tolerance to Madopar varies widely between patients and is often related to the rate of dosage increases. Side-effects such as nausea, vomiting and loss of appetite, which are frequently observed during the initial stages of levodopa therapy, are much less common in patients treated with Madopar. If such side-effects do occur, they can largely be controlled by taking Madopar with, or immediately after, food and by increasing dosage only slowly. Also, cardiovascular disturbances such as arrhythmias and orthostatic hypotension may occur, but are less frequent than in patients treated with levodopa alone.

Psychiatric disturbances are common in Parkinsonian patients, including those being treated with levodopa. They include mild elation, anxiety, agitation, insomnia, depression, aggression, delusions, hallucinations, and "unmasking" of psychoses.

Although there have been rare reports of possible antagonism of levodopa by diazepam, in general diazepam (Valium Roche) and nitrazepam (Mogadon) have been found to be useful in the treatment of anxiety and insomnia, respectively, occurring in Parkinsonism. Depression may be treated with tricyclic antidepressants although isolated cases of hypertensive crisis have been reported with the concomitant use of tricyclic drugs. ECT may be administered if appropriate. MAO inhibitors, except selective MAO-B inhibitors, must not be used.

Involuntary movements, commonly in the form of oral dyskinesias, often accompanied by "paddling" foot movements, or of the choreo-athetoid type, are common, particularly on long-term administration. These are usually dose-dependent and may disappear or become tolerable after dose adjustment.

Other side-effects which have occasionally been reported with levodopa therapy include gastro-intestinal bleeding, flushing, sweating, and drowsiness.

On some occasions the urine passed during Madopar treatment may be altered in colour; usually red-tinged, this will turn dark on standing. These changes are due to metabolites and are no cause for concern.

Transient rises in SGOT, SGPT and alkaline phosphatase values have been noted: serum uric acid and blood urea nitrogen levels are occasionally increased. In rare instances, haemolytic anaemia, mild transient leucopenia and thrombocytopenia have been reported.

*Overdose:* Symptoms of overdosage are qualitatively similar to the side-effects but may be of greater magnitude.

Treatment should include gastric lavage, general supportive measures, intravenous fluids and the maintenance of an adequate airway.

Electrocardiographic monitoring should be instituted and the patient carefully observed for the possible development of arrhythmias. If necessary, anti-arrhythmic therapy should be given and other symptoms treated as they arise.

**Pharmacological properties**

*Pharmacodynamic properties:* Madopar is an anti-Parkinsonian agent. Levodopa is the metabolic precursor of dopamine. The latter is severely depleted in the striatum, pallidum and substantia nigra of Parkinsonian patients and it is considered that administration of levodopa raises the level of available dopamine in these centres. However, conversion of levodopa into dopamine by the enzyme dopa decarboxylase also takes place in extracerebral tissues. As a consequence the full therapeutic effect may not be obtained and side-effects occur.

Administration of a peripheral decarboxylase inhibitor, which blocks the extracerebral decarboxylation of levodopa, in conjunction with levodopa has significant advantages; these include reduced gastro-intestinal side-effects, a more rapid response at the initiation of therapy and a simpler dosage regimen.

*Pharmacokinetic properties:* Madopar consists of levodopa and the peripheral decarboxylase inhibitor benserazide in the ratio 4:1 which in clinical trials has been shown to be the most satisfactory combination. Madopar CR is a controlled-release form which provides more prolonged, but lower, peak plasma concentrations of levodopa than standard Madopar or other conventional formulations of levodopa.

The active ingredients of Madopar CR are released slowly in the stomach and the maximum levodopa plasma concentration is reached approximately 3 hours after ingestion. The plasma concentration-time curve for levodopa shows a longer "half-duration" (= time-span when plasma concentrations are equal to or higher than half the maximum concentration) than that of standard Madopar, which indicates pronounced controlled-release properties. Madopar CR bioavailability is approximately 60% that of standard Madopar.

**Pharmaceutical particulars**

*List of excipients:* Each capsule contains: Hydroxypropyl methylcellulose PhEur; Hydrogenated vegetable oil USP; Calcium phosphate, Dibasic Anhydrous PhEur; Mannitol PhEur; Talc PhEur; Povidone BP; Magnesium stearate PhEur and the colouring agents E132, E171 and E172.

*Incompatibilities:* None known.

*Shelf life:* 3 years.

*Special precautions for storage:* Recommended maximum storage temperature 25°C. Protect from moisture.

*Nature and contents of container:* Amber glass bottles with aluminium screw-cap and desiccant containing 100 capsules.

*Instructions for use/handling:* No special requirements.

**Marketing authorisation number** 0031/0227

**Date of approval/revision of SPC** February 1996

**Legal category** POM

## MADOPAR*

**Presentation** Madopar 62.5 capsules: blue cap and grey body with ROCHE printed in black on both cap and body, containing 50 mg levodopa and 14.25 mg benserazide hydrochloride (equivalent to 12.5 mg of the base).

Madopar 62.5 dispersible tablets: round, white tablets with ROCHE 62·5 imprinted on one face and a single break bar on the other, containing 50 mg levodopa and 14.25 mg benserazide hydrochloride (equivalent to 12.5 mg of the base).

Madopar 125 capsules blue cap and pink body with ROCHE printed in black on both cap and body, containing 100 mg levodopa and 28.5 mg benserazide hydrochloride (equivalent to 25 mg of the base).

Madopar 125 dispersible tablets: round, white tablets with ROCHE 125 imprinted on one face and a single break bar on the other, containing 100 mg levodopa and 28.5 mg benserazide hydrochloride (equivalent to 25 mg of the base).

Madopar 250 capsules: blue cap and caramel body with ROCHE printed in black on both cap and body, containing 200 mg levodopa and 57 mg benserazide hydrochloride (equivalent to 50 mg of the base).

**Uses** *Properties:* Madopar is an anti-Parkinsonian agent. Levodopa is the metabolic precursor of dopamine. The latter is severely depleted in the striatum, pallidum and substantia nigra of Parkinsonian patients and it is considered that administration of levodopa raises the level of available dopamine in these centres. However, conversion of levodopa into dopamine by the enzyme dopa decarboxylase also takes place in extracerebral tissues. As a consequence the full therapeutic effect may not be obtained and side-effects occur.

Administration of a peripheral decarboxylase inhibitor, which blocks the extracerebral decarboxylation of levodopa, in conjunction with levodopa has significant advantages; these include reduced gastro-intestinal side-effects, a more rapid response at the initiation of therapy and a simpler dosage regimen. Madopar is a combination of levodopa and benserazide in the ratio 4:1 which in clinical trials has been shown to be the most satisfactory.

Like every replacement therapy, chronic treatment with Madopar will be necessary.

*Indications:* Parkinsonism - idiopathic, post-encephalitic. Previous neurosurgery is not a contra-indication to Madopar.

**Dosage and administration** Dosage and administration are variable and no more than a guide can be given.

*Patients not previously treated with levodopa:* The recommended initial dose is one capsule or dispersible tablet of Madopar 62.5 three or four times daily. If the disease is at an advanced stage, the starting dose should be one capsule or dispersible tablet of Madopar 125 three times daily.

The daily dosage should then be increased by one capsule or dispersible tablet of Madopar 125, or their equivalent, once or twice weekly until a full therapeutic effect is obtained, or side-effects supervene.

In some elderly patients, it may suffice to initiate treatment with one capsule or dispersible tablet of Madopar 62.5 once or twice daily, increasing by one capsule or dispersible tablet every third or fourth day.

The effective dose usually lies within the range of four to eight capsules or dispersible tablets of Madopar 125 (two to four capsules of Madopar 250) daily in divided doses, most patients requiring no more than six capsules or dispersible tablets of Madopar 125 daily.

Optimal improvement is usually seen in one to three weeks but the full therapeutic effect of Madopar may not be apparent for some time. It is advisable therefore, to allow several weeks to elapse before contemplating dosage increments above the average dose range. If satisfactory improvement is still not achieved, the dose of Madopar may be increased but with caution. It is rarely necessary to give more than ten capsules or dispersible tablets of Madopar 125 (five capsules of Madopar 250) per day.

Treatment should be continued for at least six months before failure is concluded from the absence of a clinical response.

Madopar 62.5 capsules or dispersible tablets may be used to facilitate adjustment of dosage to the needs of the individual patient. Patients who experience fluctuations in response may be helped by dividing the dosage into smaller, more frequent doses with the aid of Madopar 62.5 capsules or dispersible tablets without, however, altering the total daily dose.

Madopar 250 capsules are only for maintenance therapy once the optimal dosage has been determined using Madopar 125 capsules or dispersible tablets.

*Patients previously treated with levodopa:* The following procedure is recommended:

Levodopa alone should be discontinued and Madopar started on the following day. The patient should be initiated on a total of one less Madopar 125 capsule or dispersible tablet daily than the total number of 500 mg levodopa tablets or capsules previously taken (for example, if the patient had previously taken 2 g levodopa daily, then he should start on three capsules or dispersible tablets Madopar 125 daily on the following day). Observe the patient for one week and then, if necessary, increase the dosage in the manner described for new patients.

*Patients previously treated with other levodopa/decarboxylase inhibitor combinations:* Previous therapy should be withdrawn for 12 hours. In order to minimise the potential for any effects of levodopa withdrawal, it may be beneficial to discontinue previous therapy at night and institute Madopar therapy the following morning. The initial Madopar dose should be one capsule or dispersible tablet of Madopar 62.5 three or four times daily. This dose may then be increased in the manner described for patients not previously treated with levodopa.

Other anti-Parkinsonian drugs may be given with Madopar. Existing treatment with other anti-Parkinsonian drugs, e.g. anticholinergics or amantadine, should be continued during initiation of Madopar therapy. However, as treatment with Madopar proceeds and the therapeutic effect becomes apparent, the dosage of the other drugs may need to be reduced or the drugs gradually withdrawn.

*Elderly:* Although there may be an age-related decrease in tolerance to levodopa in the elderly, Madopar appears to be well-tolerated and side-effects are generally not troublesome.

*Children:* Not to be given to patients under 25 years of age: therefore, no dosage recommendations are made for the administration of Madopar to children.

Madopar capsules and dispersible tablets are for oral administration. They should be taken with, or immediately after, meals.

Madopar dispersible tablets may be swallowed whole or dispersed in at least 25 ml water per tablet. They may be taken in dilute orange squash (at least 25 ml per tablet) if preferred. However, orange juice should not be used. Madopar dispersible tablets are particularly suitable for patients who dislike taking capsules or have difficulty in swallowing solid dosage forms.

### Contra-indications, warnings, etc

*Contra-indications:* Madopar is contra-indicated in narrow-angle glaucoma (it may be used in wide-angle glaucoma provided that the intra-ocular pressure remains under control); severe psychoneuroses or psychoses; severe endocrine, renal, hepatic or cardiac disorders.

It should not be given in conjunction with monoamine oxidase (MAO) inhibitors except selective MAO-B inhibitors or within 2 weeks of their withdrawal.

It should not be given to patients under 25 years of age.

Suspicion has arisen that levodopa may activate a malignant melanoma. Therefore, Madopar should not be used in persons who have a history of, or who may be suffering from, a malignant melanoma.

*Use in pregnancy:* Madopar is contra-indicated in pregnancy, since there is evidence of harmful effects in studies in pregnant rabbits and the benserazide component has been found to be associated with skeletal malformations in the rat. In any woman of childbearing potential the risk of its use, should pregnancy occur, must be weighed against the anticipated benefits of treatment. Patients taking Madopar should not breast-feed their infants.

*Precautions:* When other drugs must be given in conjunction with Madopar, the patient should be carefully observed for unusual side-effects or potentiating effects.

Drugs which interfere with central amine mechanisms, such as rauwolfia alkaloids (reserpine), tetrabenazine (Nitoman), metoclopramide, phenothiazines, thioxanthenes, butyrophenones, amphetamines and papaverine, should be avoided where possible. If, however, their administration is considered essential, extreme care should be exercised and a close watch kept for any signs of potentiation, antagonism or other interactions and for unusual side-effects.

In the event of general anaesthesia being required, Madopar therapy may be continued as long as the patient is able to take fluids and medication by mouth. If therapy is temporarily interrupted, the usual daily dosage may be administered as soon as the patient is able to take oral medication. Whenever therapy has been interrupted for longer periods, dosage should again be adjusted gradually; however, in many cases the patient can rapidly be returned to his previous therapeutic dosage.

If a patient has to undergo emergency surgery, when Madopar has not been withdrawn, anaesthesia with cyclopropane or halothane should be avoided. There have been occasional reports of a neuroleptic malignant-like syndrome, involving hyperthermia, on abrupt withdrawal of levodopa preparations. Sudden discontinuation of Madopar, without close supervision, or 'drug holidays' should therefore be avoided.

Pyridoxine (vitamin B₆) may be given with Madopar since the presence of a decarboxylase inhibitor protects against the peripheral levodopa transformation facilitated by pyridoxine.

Care should be taken when using Madopar in the following circumstances: in endocrine, renal, pulmonary or cardiovascular disease, particularly where there is a history of myocardial infarction or arrhythmia; psychiatric disturbances; hepatic disorder; peptic ulcer; osteomalacia; where sympathomimetic drugs may be required (e.g. bronchial asthma), due to possible potentiation of the cardiovascular effects of levodopa; where antihypertensive drugs are being used, due to possible increased hypotensive action.

Periodic evaluation of hepatic, haemopoietic, renal and cardiovascular functions is advised.

Patients who improve on Madopar therapy should be advised to resume normal activities gradually as rapid mobilisation may increase the risk of injury.

*Side-effects and adverse reactions:* Tolerance to Madopar varies widely between patients and is often related to the rate of dosage increases. Side-effects such as nausea, vomiting and loss of appetite, which are frequently observed during the initial stages of levodopa therapy, are much less common in patients treated with Madopar. If such side-effects do occur, they can largely be controlled by taking Madopar with, or immediately after, food and by increasing dosage only slowly. Also, cardiovascular disturbances such as arrhythmias and orthostatic hypotension may occur, but are less frequent than in patients treated with levodopa alone.

Psychiatric disturbances are common in Parkinsonian patients, including those being treated with levodopa. They include mild elation, anxiety, agitation, insomnia, depression, aggression, delusions, hallucinations, and 'unmasking' of psychoses.

Although there have been rare reports of possible antagonism of levodopa by diazepam, in general diazepam (Valium Roche) and nitrazepam (Mogadon) have been found to be useful in the treatment of anxiety and insomnia, respectively, occurring in Parkinsonism. Depression may be treated with tricyclic antidepressants although isolated cases of hypertensive crisis have been reported with the concomitant use of tricyclic drugs. ECT may be administered if appropriate. MAO inhibitors, except selective MAO-B inhibitors must not be used.

Involuntary movements, commonly in the form of oral dyskinesias, often accompanied by 'paddling' foot movements, or of the choreo-athetoid type, are common, particularly on long-term administration. These are usually dose-dependent and may disappear or become tolerable after dose adjustment.

With long-term administration, fluctuations in the therapeutic response may be encountered. They include 'freezing' episodes, end-of-dose deterioration and the so-called 'on-off' effect. Patients may be helped by dosage reduction or by giving smaller and more frequent doses.

Other side-effects which have occasionally been reported with levodopa therapy include gastro-intestinal bleeding, flushing, sweating, and drowsiness.

On some occasions the urine passed during Madopar treatment may be altered in colour; usually redtinged, this will turn dark on standing. These changes are due to metabolites and are no cause for concern.

Transient rises in SGOT, SGPT and alkaline phosphatase values have been noted: serum uric acid and blood urea nitrogen levels are occasionally increased. In rare instances, haemolytic anaemia, mild transient leucopenia and thrombocytopenia have been reported.

Levodopa may interfere chemically with several diagnostic laboratory tests including those for glucose, ketone bodies, or catecholamines in urine and for glucose or uric acid in blood. Levodopa therapy has been reported to inhibit the response to protirelin in tests of thyroid function.

*Treatment of overdosage:* Symptoms of overdosage are qualitatively similar to the side-effects but may be of greater magnitude.

Treatment should include gastric lavage, general supportive measures, intravenous fluids and the maintenance of an adequate airway. Electrocardiographic monitoring should be instituted and the patient carefully observed for the possible development of arrhythmias. If necessary, anti-arrhythmic therapy should be given and other symptoms treated as they arise.

### Pharmaceutical precautions

*Storage:* Madopar capsules and dispersible tablets should be protected from moisture. The recommended maximum storage temperature is 25°C.

### Legal category POM

**Package quantities** Madopar 62.5 capsules containing 50 mg levodopa and 12.5 mg benserazide in bottles of 100.

Madopar 62.5 dispersible tablets containing 50 mg levodopa and 12.5 mg benserazide in bottles of 100.

Madopar 125 capsules containing 100 mg levodopa and 25 mg benserazide in bottles of 100.

Madopar 125 dispersible tablets containing 100 mg levodopa and 25 mg benserazide in bottles of 100.

Madopar 250 capsules containing 200 mg levodopa and 50 mg benserazide in bottles of 100.

**Further information** Low levels of endogenous levodopa are detectable in pre-dose blood samples. After oral administration of Madopar, levodopa and benserazide are rapidly absorbed, mainly in the upper regions of the small intestine. Interaction studies indicate that a higher proportion of levodopa is absorbed intact when administered in combination with benserazide, compared with levodopa administered alone. Maximum plasma concentrations of levodopa are reached approximately one hour after ingestion of Madopar. The elimination half-life of levodopa is about 45 minutes.

**Product licence numbers**

| | |
|---|---|
| Madopar 62.5 capsules | 0031/0125 |
| Madopar 62.5 dispersible tablets | 0031/0220 |
| Madopar 125 capsules | 0031/0073R |
| Madopar 125 dispersible tablets | 0031/0221 |
| Madopar 250 capsules | 0031/0074R |

# MANERIX*

### Qualitative and quantitative composition

1 film-coated 150 mg tablet contains 150 mg moclobemide.

1 film-coated 300 mg tablet contains 300 mg moclobemide.

**Pharmaceutical form** Film-coated tablets containing 150 mg or 300 mg of moclobemide.

### Clinical particulars

*Therapeutic indications:* Major depression.

*Posology and method of administration:* Manerix tablets are for oral administration.

The tablets should be taken at the end of a meal.

*Adults:* The recommended initial dose is 300 mg daily, usually administered in divided doses. The dose may be increased up to 600 mg/day depending on the severity of the depression.

The individual response may allow a reduction of the daily dose to 150 mg.

*Elderly:* Elderly patients do not require a special dose adjustment of Manerix.

*Children:* In view of the lack of clinical data available, Manerix is not recommended for use in children.

*Renal/hepatic impairment:* Patients with reduced renal function do not require a special dose adjustment of Manerix. When hepatic metabolism is severely impaired by hepatic disease or a drug that inhibits microsomal mono-oxygenase activity (e.g. cimetidine), normal plasma levels are achieved by reducing the daily dose of Manerix to half or one third.

*Contra-indications:* Manerix is contra-indicated in patients with known hypersensitivity to the drug, in acute confusional states and in patients with phaeochromocytoma.

Manerix should not be co-administered with pethidine or selegiline.

Manerix should not be co-administered with 5-HT re-uptake inhibitors (including those which are tricyclic antidepressants). After stopping treatment with 5-HT re-uptake inhibitors a time period equal to 4–5 half lives of the drug or any active metabolite should elapse between stopping therapy and starting therapy with Manerix.

Manerix should not be administered to children for the time being as clinical experience in this category is lacking.

*Special warnings and special precautions for use:* Manerix is a reversible inhibitor of monoamine oxidase type A (RIMA). It causes less potentiation of tyramine than traditional irreversible MAOI's, and therefore Manerix does not generally necessitate the special dietary restrictions required for these irreversible MAOI's. However, as a few patients may be especially sensitive to tyramine, all patients should be advised to avoid the consumption of large amounts of tyramine rich food (mature cheese, yeast extracts and fermented soya bean products). Patients should also be advised to avoid ephedrine, pseudoephedrine, phenylpropanolamine and dextromethorphan (contained in many proprietary cough and cold medicines).

Depressive patients with excitation or agitation as the predominant clinical feature should either not be treated with Manerix or only in combination with a sedative (e.g. a benzodiazepine). The sedative should only be used for a maximum of 2 to 3 weeks.

Patients with suicidal tendencies should be closely monitored at the start of treatment.

If a depressive episode is treated in bipolar disorders, manic episodes can be provoked.

Due to the lack of clinical data, patients with

concomitant schizophrenia or schizo-affective organic disorders should not be treated with Manerix.

Theoretical pharmacological considerations indicate that MAO inhibitors may precipitate a hypertensive reaction in patients with thyrotoxicosis. As experience with Manerix in this population group is lacking, caution should be exercised before prescribing Manerix.

*Interaction with other medicaments and other forms of interaction:* In animals, Manerix potentiates the effects of opiates. Morphine and fentanyl should be used with caution. A dosage adjustment may be necessary for these drugs.

Cimetidine prolongs the metabolism of Manerix. The normal dose of Manerix should therefore be reduced to half the dose in patients taking cimetidine.

Treatment with tricyclic antidepressants can be initiated without a wash out period.

There is, to date, no experience with co-administration of moclobemide and buspirone in humans.

*Pregnancy and lactation:* Reproduction studies in animals have not revealed any risk to the foetus, but the safety of Manerix in human pregnancy has not been established. Therefore the benefits of drug therapy during pregnancy should be weighed against possible risk to the foetus.

Since only a small amount of Manerix passes into breast milk (approximately $1/30$ of the maternal dose), the benefits of continuing drug therapy during nursing should be weighed against possible risks to the child.

*Effects on ability to drive and use machines:* Impairment of performance in activities requiring complete mental alertness (e.g. driving a motor vehicle) is generally not to be expected with Manerix. The individual reaction should however be monitored during early treatment.

*Undesirable effects:* The following undesirable effects have been observed: sleep disturbances, agitation, restlessness, irritability, dizziness, headache, paraesthesia, dry mouth, visual disturbances, nausea, diarrhoea, constipation, vomiting, oedema and skin reactions such as rash, pruritus, urticaria and flushing. Confusional states have been observed, but these have disappeared rapidly on discontinuation of therapy.

In clinical trials, there was a low incidence of raised liver enzymes without associated clinical sequelae.

*Overdose:* Experience of overdose in man is so far limited. Signs which have been observed are increasing agitation, aggressiveness and behavioural changes. Treatment of overdose should be aimed primarily at maintenance of the vital functions.

**Pharmacological properties**

*Pharmacodynamic properties:* Manerix is an antidepressant which affects the monoaminergic cerebral neurotransmitter system by means of a reversible inhibition of monoamine oxidase preferentially of type A (RIMA). The metabolism of noradrenaline, dopamine and serotonin (5-HT) is decreased by this effect, and this leads to increased extracellular concentrations of these neuronal transmitters.

*Pharmacokinetic properties*
*Absorption:* After oral administration, moclobemide is completely absorbed from the gastrointestinal tract into the portal blood. A hepatic first-pass effect reduces the systemically available dose fraction (bioavailability F). This reduction is more pronounced after single (F: 60%) than after multiple (F: 80%) doses.

*Distribution:* Due to its lipophilic nature, moclobemide is extensively distributed in the body with an apparent volume of distribution ($V_{ss}$) of about 1.2 l/kg. Binding of the drug to plasma proteins, mainly albumin, is relatively low (50%). Peak plasma concentrations of the drug are reached within one hour of dosage. After multiple dosing, plasma concentrations of moclobemide increase over the first week of therapy and remain stable thereafter. When the daily dose is increased, there is a more than proportional increase in steady-state concentrations.

*Metabolism:* The drug is almost entirely metabolised before its elimination from the body. Metabolism occurs largely via oxidative reactions on the morpholine moiety of the molecule. Degradation products with pharmacological activity in *in vitro* or animal experiments are present in the systemic circulation in man at very low concentrations only. Approximately 2% of the Caucasian population and 15% of the Asian population have been shown to be slow metabolisers with respect to oxidative hepatic metabolism via the cytochrome P4502C9 isozyme. It was found that the maximum plasma concentration (Cmax) and area under the concentration time curve (AUC) was approximately 1.5 times greater in slow metabolisers compared with extensive metabolisers for the same dose of moclobemide.

*Elimination:* Moclobemide is rapidly eliminated from the body. Blood clearance is approximately 20–50 1/hour, the elimination half-life one to four hours.

Less than 1% of a dose is excreted renally in unchanged form. The metabolites formed are eliminated renally.

*Preclinical safety data:* Not applicable.

**Pharmaceutical particulars**

*List of excipients:* Lactose, maize starch, povidone K30, sodium starch glycollate, magnesium stearate, hydroxypropyl methylcellulose, ethylcellulose, polyethylene glycol 6000, talc and titanium dioxide (E171). The 150 mg tablets also contain yellow iron oxide (E172).

*Incompatibilities:* Not applicable.

*Shelf life:* 5 years.

*Special precautions for storage:* Store in a dry place.

*Nature and contents of container:* Blister packing. *Pack sizes:* 28, 30, 84 and 100 tablets (150 mg tablets). 30 and 60 tablets (300 mg tablets).

*Instructions for use/handling:* Not applicable.

**Marketing authorisation numbers**
150 mg tablets     0031/0275
300 mg tablets     0031/0347

**Date of approval/revision of SPC**   January 1997

**Legal category**   POM

## MESTINON*

**Presentation**   Round, white tablets with ROCHE imprinted across one face and with two break bars on the other, containing 60 mg pyridostigmine bromide.

**Uses**   *Properties:* Mestinon is an antagonist to cholinesterase, the enzyme which normally destroys acetylcholine. The action of Mestinon can briefly be described, therefore, as the potentiation of naturally occurring acetylcholine. Mestinon has a more prolonged action than Prostigmin (neostigmine) although it is somewhat slower to take effect (generally taking 30-60 minutes). Because it has a weaker 'muscarinic' action than Prostigmin, it is usually much better tolerated by myasthenic patients in whom the longer action is also an advantage.

*Pharmacokinetics:* Oral pyridostigmine is poorly absorbed. Maximum plasma concentrations occur at 1 to 2 hours and it is eliminated by the kidney largely unchanged with a half-life of 3 to 4 hours.

*Indications:* Myasthenia gravis; paralytic ileus; post-operative urinary retention.

**Dosage and administration**
*Myasthenia gravis: Adults:* Doses of 30 to 120 mg are given at intervals throughout the day when maximum strength is needed (for example, on rising and before mealtimes). The usual duration of action of a dose is 3 to 4 hours in the daytime but a longer effect (6 hours) is often obtained with a dose taken on retiring for bed.

The total daily dose is usually in the range of 5-20 tablets but doses higher than these may be needed by some patients.

*Children:* Children under 6 years old should receive an initial dose of half a tablet (30 mg) of Mestinon; children 6-12 years old should receive one tablet (60 mg). Dosage should be increased gradually, in increments of 15-30 mg daily, until maximum improvement is obtained. Total daily requirements are usually in the range of 30-360 mg.

The requirement for Mestinon is usually markedly decreased after thymectomy or when additional therapy (steroids, immunosuppressant drugs) is given.

When relatively large doses of Mestinon are taken by myasthenic patients it may be necessary to give atropine or other anticholinergic drugs to counteract the muscarinic effects. It should be noted that the slower gastro-intestinal motility caused by these drugs may affect the absorption of Mestinon.

In all patients the possibility of 'cholinergic crisis', due to overdosage of Mestinon, and its differentiation from 'myasthenic crisis' due to increased severity of the disease, must be borne in mind. Both types of crisis are manifested by increased muscle weakness, but whereas myasthenic crisis may require more intensive anticholinesterase treatment, cholinergic crisis calls for immediate discontinuation of this treatment and institution of appropriate supportive measures, including respiratory assistance.

*Other indications: Adults:* The usual dose is 1 to 4 tablets (60-240 mg).

*Children:* 15-60 mg.

The frequency of these doses may be varied according to the needs of the patient.

*Elderly:* There are no specific dosage recommendations for Mestinon in elderly patients.

Mestinon tablets are for oral administration.

**Contra-indications, warnings, etc**
*Contra-indications:* Mestinon should not be given to patients with mechanical gastro-intestinal or urinary obstruction.

Mestinon is contra-indicated in patients with known hypersensitivity to the drug and to bromides.

*Use in pregnancy and lactation:* The safety of Mestinon during pregnancy or lactation has not been established. Although the possible hazards to mother and child must be weighed against the potential benefits in every case, experience with Mestinon in pregnant patients with myasthenia gravis has revealed no untoward effect of the drug on the course of pregnancy.

As the severity of myasthenia gravis often fluctuates considerably, particular care is required to avoid cholinergic crisis, due to overdosage of the drug, but otherwise management is no different from that in non-pregnant patients.

Observations indicate that only negligible amounts of Mestinon are excreted in breast milk; nevertheless due regard should be paid to possible effects on the breast-feeding infant.

*Precautions:* Extreme caution is required when administering Mestinon to patients with bronchial asthma.

Care should also be taken in patients with bradycardia, recent coronary occlusion, hypotension, vagotonia, peptic ulcer, epilepsy or Parkinsonism.

There is no evidence to suggest that Mestinon has any special effects on the elderly. However, elderly patients may be more susceptible to dysrhythmias than the young adult.

Mestinon is mainly excreted unchanged by the kidney, therefore lower doses may be required in patients with renal disease and treatment should be based on titration of drug dosage to effect.

*Side-effects and adverse reactions:* These may include nausea and vomiting, increased salivation, diarrhoea and abdominal cramps.

*Treatment of overdosage:* Signs of overdosage due to muscarinic effects may include abdominal cramps, increased peristalsis, diarrhoea, nausea and vomiting, increased bronchial secretions, salivation, diaphoresis and miosis. Nicotinic effects consist of muscular cramps, fasciculations and general weakness. Bradycardia and hypotension may also occur.

Artificial ventilation should be instituted if respiration is severely depressed. Atropine sulphate 1 to 2 mg intravenously is an antidote to the muscarinic effects.

**Pharmaceutical precautions**
*Storage:* The recommended maximum storage temperature for Mestinon tablets is 25°C.

Mestinon tablets should be protected from light and from moisture.

**Legal category**   POM

**Package quantities**   Mestinon tablets in packs of 200

**Further information**   Nil.

**Product licence number**   0031/5036R

## MOBIFLEX*

**Presentation**   Mobiflex Tablets 20 mg–Red-brown film-coated, pentagonal tablets, imprinted MOBIFLEX on one face, containing 20 mg tenoxicam.

Mobiflex Vials containing 20 mg tenoxicam. Ampoules with 2 ml sterile Water for Injections Ph. Eur.

**Uses**
*Pharmacological properties:* Mobiflex is a non-steroidal anti-inflammatory drug which has marked anti-inflammatory and analgesic activity and some antipyretic activity. As with other non-steroidal anti-inflammatory drugs, the precise mode of action is unknown, though it is probably multifactorial, involving inhibition of prostaglandin biosynthesis and reduction of leucocyte accumulation at the inflammatory site.

*Pharmacokinetics:* Mobiflex is long-acting; a single daily dose is effective.

After oral administration, Mobiflex is rapidly and completely absorbed as unchanged drug. Concomitant food reduces the rate, but not the extent, of absorption of Mobiflex. Tenoxicam penetrates well into synovial fluid to give concentrations approximately half those in plasma. The mean plasma elimination half-life is approximately 72 hours.

Following intravenous administration of 20 mg tenoxicam, plasma levels of the drug decline rapidly during the first two hours mainly due to distribution processes. After this short period, no difference in plasma concentrations between intravenous and oral dosing is seen. Following intramuscular injection, levels at or above 90% of the maximally achieved concentrations are reached as early as 15 minutes after a dose, i.e. earlier than after oral dosing. However, again the difference in blood levels between the two routes of administration is restricted to the first two hours after a dose. The bioavailability after an intramuscular dose is complete and indistinguishable from that determined after oral dosing.

With the recommended dosage regimen of 20 mg once daily, steady-state plasma concentrations are reached within 10–15 days, with no unexpected accumulation.

Mobiflex is strongly bound to plasma proteins.

Mobiflex is cleared from the body almost exclusively by metabolism. Approximately two-thirds of the administered dose is excreted in the urine, mainly as the pharmacologically inactive 5-hydroxypyridyl metabolite, and the remainder in the bile, much of it as glucuronide conjugates of hydroxy-metabolites.

No age-specific changes in the pharmacokinetics of Mobiflex have been found although inter-individual variation tends to be higher in elderly persons.

*Indications:* Mobiflex is indicated for the relief of pain and inflammation in osteoarthritis and rheumatoid arthritis. It is also indicated for the short term management of acute musculoskeletal disorders including strains, sprains and other soft-tissue injuries. IV, IM tenoxicam is also available for these indications in those patients considered unable to take oral tenoxicam.

## Dosage and administration

*Adults (including the elderly):* A single daily dose of 20 mg Mobiflex should be taken orally, at the same time each day. Mobiflex Tablets are for oral administration with water or other fluid. Mobiflex Vials should be given IV or IM. A single daily dose of 20 mg for one to two days initially to be continued with the oral form, with administration at the same time each day. The lyophilisate should be dissolved in 2 ml of the solvent provided (2 ml sterile water for injections). This reconstituted solution should be used immediately. Higher doses should be avoided as they do not usually achieve significantly greater therapeutic effect but may be associated with a higher risk of adverse events.

In acute musculoskeletal disorders treatment should not normally be required for more than 7 days, but in severe cases it may be continued up to a maximum of 14 days.

*Use in the elderly:* As with other non-steroidal anti-inflammatory drugs, Mobiflex should be used with special caution in elderly patients since they may be less able to tolerate side-effects than younger patients. They are also more likely to be receiving concomitant medication or to have impaired hepatic, renal or cardiovascular function.

*Children:* There are insufficient data to make a recommendation for administration of Mobiflex to children.

*Use in renal and hepatic insufficiency*

| Creatinine clearance | Dosage regimen |
| --- | --- |
| Greater than 25 ml/min | Usual dosage but monitor patients carefully (see "Precautions") |
| Less than 25 ml/min | Insufficient data to make dosage recommendations |

Because of the high plasma protein-binding of tenoxicam, caution is required when plasma albumin concentrations are markedly reduced (e.g. in nephrotic syndrome) or when bilirubin concentrations are high.

There is insufficient information to make dosage recommendations for Mobiflex in patients with pre-existing hepatic impairment.

## Contra-indications, warnings, etc

*Contra-indications:*

1. Active peptic ulceration and a past history of peptic ulceration, gastro-intestinal bleeding (melaena, haematemesis) or severe gastritis.

2. Hypersensitivity to Mobiflex. Mobiflex should also be avoided in cases where the patient has suffered hypersensitivity reaction (symptoms of asthma, rhinitis, angioedema or urticaria) to other non-steroidal anti-inflammatory drugs, including aspirin, as the potential exists for cross-sensitivity to Mobiflex.

*Use in pregnancy and lactation:* The safety of Mobiflex during pregnancy and lactation has not been established and the drug should therefore not be given in these conditions.

Although no teratogenic effects were seen in animal studies, Mobiflex, like other non-steroidal anti-inflammatory drugs, is associated with prolonged and delayed parturition and an adverse influence on neonatal viability when administered to animals in late pregnancy. Non-steroidal anti-inflammatory agents are also known to induce closure of the ductus arteriosus in infants.

No information is available on penetration of Mobiflex into milk in humans; animal studies indicate that significant levels may be achieved.

*Precautions:* Any patient being treated with Mobiflex who presents with symptoms of gastro-intestinal disease should be closely monitored. If peptic ulceration or gastro-intestinal bleeding occurs, Mobiflex should be withdrawn immediately.

In rare cases, non-steroidal anti-inflammatory drugs may cause interstitial nephritis, glomerulonephritis, papillary necrosis and the nephrotic syndrome. Such agents inhibit the synthesis of renal prostaglandin which plays a supportive role in the maintenance of renal perfusion in patients whose renal blood flow and blood volume are decreased. In these patients, administration of a non-steroidal anti-inflammatory drug may precipitate overt renal decompensation, which returns to the pre-treatment state upon withdrawal of the drug. Patients at greatest risk of such a reaction are those with pre-existing renal disease (including diabetics with impaired renal function), nephrotic syndrome, volume depletion, hepatic disease, congestive cardiac failure and those patients receiving concomitant therapy with diuretics or potentially nephrotoxic drugs. Such patients should have their renal, hepatic and cardiac functions carefully monitored.

Occasional elevations of serum transaminases or other indicators of liver function have been reported. In most cases these have been small and transient increases above the normal range. If the abnormality is significant or persistent, Mobiflex should be stopped and follow-up tests carried out. Particular care is required in patients with pre-existing hepatic disease.

Mobiflex reduces platelet aggregation and may prolong bleeding time. This should be borne in mind for patients who undergo major surgery (e.g. joint replacement) and when bleeding time needs to be determined.

Particular care should be taken to regularly monitor elderly patients to detect possible interactions with concomitant therapy and to review renal, hepatic and cardiovascular function which may be potentially influenced by non-steroidal anti-inflammatory drugs.

Adverse eye findings have been reported with non-steroidal anti-inflammatory drugs, therefore it is recommended that patients who develop visual disturbances during treatment with Mobiflex have ophthalmic evaluation.

*Side-effects and adverse reactions:* For most patients, any side-effects are transient and resolve without discontinuation of treatment.

The most common side-effects relate to the gastro-intestinal tract. They include dyspepsia, nausea, abdominal pain and discomfort, constipation, diarrhoea, flatulence, indigestion, epigastric distress, stomatitis and anorexia. As with other non-steroidal anti-inflammatory drugs, there is a risk of peptic ulceration and gastro-intestinal bleeding, both of which have been reported with Mobiflex. Should this occur, Mobiflex is to be discontinued immediately and appropriate treatment instituted.

As with other non-steroidal anti-inflammatory drugs, peripheral oedema of mild or moderate degree and without clinical sequelae occurred in a small proportion of patients and the possibility of precipitating congestive cardiac failure in elderly patients or those with compromised cardiac function should therefore be borne in mind.

Central nervous system reactions of headache and dizziness have been reported in a small number of patients. Somnolence, insomnia, depression, nervousness, dream abnormalities, mental confusion, paraesthesias and vertigo have been reported rarely.

Skin reactions of rash and pruritus have been reported. Nail disorders, alopecia, erythema, urticaria and photosensitivity reactions have been reported rarely. As with other non-steroidal anti-inflammatory drugs, Lyell's syndrome and Stevens-Johnson syndrome may develop in rare instances. Vesiculobullous reactions and vasculitis have also been reported rarely. Reversible elevations of blood urea nitrogen and creatinine have been reported (see *Precautions*).

Decreases in haemoglobin, unrelated to gastro-intestinal bleeding, have occurred. Anaemia, thrombocytopenia and non-thrombocytopenic purpura, leucopenia and eosinophilia have been reported. Epistaxis has been reported infrequently. Rare cases of agranulocytosis have been reported.

As with most other non-steroidal anti-inflammatory drugs, changes in various liver function parameters have been observed. Some patients may develop raised serum transaminase levels during treatment. Although such reactions are rare, if abnormal liver function tests persist or worsen, if clinical signs and symptoms consistent with liver disease develop or if systemic manifestations occur (e.g. eosinophilia, rash), Mobiflex should be discontinued.

Palpitations and dyspnoea have also been reported rarely. Metabolic abnormalities, such as weight decrease or increase and hyperglycaemia, have occurred rarely.

Swollen eyes, blurred vision and eye irritation have been reported. Ophthalmoscopy and slit-lamp examination have revealed no evidence of ocular changes. Malaise and tinnitus may occur.

Hepatitis has also been reported in isolated cases.

*Drug interactions:* Antacids may reduce the rate, but not the extent, of absorption of Mobiflex. The differences are not likely to be of clinical significance. No interaction has been found with concomitantly administered cimetidine. In healthy subjects no clinically relevant interaction between Mobiflex and low molecular weight heparin has been observed.

Tenoxicam is highly bound to serum albumin. Although potentiation of warfarin or sulphonylurea compounds such as glibenclamide has not been observed, close monitoring of the effects of anticoagulants or oral hypoglycaemic agents is advised, especially during the initial stages of treatment with Mobiflex. No interaction with digoxin has been observed.

Salicylates can displace tenoxicam from protein-binding sites and so increase the clearance and volume of distribution of Mobiflex. Concurrent treatment with salicylates or other non-steroidal anti-inflammatory drugs should therefore be avoided because of the increased risk of adverse reactions (particularly gastro-intestinal).

Non-steroidal anti-inflammatory drugs have been reported to produce lithium retention. If tenoxicam is prescribed for a patient receiving lithium therapy, the frequency of lithium monitoring should be increased, the patient warned to maintain fluid intake and to be aware of symptoms of lithium intoxication.

Non-steroidal anti-inflammatory drugs may cause sodium, potassium and fluid retention and may interfere with the natriuretic action of diuretic agents. These properties should be kept in mind when treating patients with compromised cardiac function or hypertension since they may be responsible for a worsening of those conditions.

No clinically relevant interaction was found in small numbers of patients receiving treatment with penicillamine or parenteral gold.

*Treatment of overdosage:* There is no reported experience of serious overdosage with Mobiflex. No specific measures are available; administration of $H_2$-antagonist drugs may be of benefit. Gastric lavage should be carried out as soon as possible after drug ingestion and the patient should be closely observed and general supportive measures taken as necessary.

## Pharmaceutical precautions

*Storage:* Mobiflex Tablets–The original pack dispenser should be stored in a dry place, otherwise no special storage precautions are necessary.

Mobiflex Vials–The pack should be stored at a temperature below 25°C. Do not freeze as the water ampoule may burst.

**Legal category** POM

**Package quantities**

Mobiflex Tablets 20 mg in packs of 28 and 500.

Mobiflex Vials 20 mg in packs of 5 vials together with 5 ampoules containing 2 ml of sterile Water for Injections PhEur as diluent.

**Further information** Nil.

**Product licence numbers**

| Tablets 20 mg | 0031/0200 |
| Vials 20 mg | 0031/0330 |
| Ampoules Water for Injections | 0031/0284 |

# MOGADON*

**Presentation** Mogadon contains the substance with the approved name nitrazepam, chemically described as 1,3-dihydro-7-nitro-5-phenyl-2H-1,4-benzodiazepin-2-one.

Round, white tablets with ROCHE and two semicircles imprinted on one face with a single break bar on the other, containing 5 mg nitrazepam and the inactive ingredients lactose, maize starch and magnesium stearate.

## Uses

*Properties:* Mogadon is a benzodiazepine compound with sedative properties. It acts in 30 to 60 minutes to produce sleep lasting six to eight hours.

*Pharmacokinetics:* The drug is well absorbed from the GI tract with peak blood levels being achieved within two hours of administration. The half-life is, on average, 24 hours. Steady-state levels are achieved within five days. Nitrazepam undergoes biotransformation to a number of metabolites, none of which possess significant clinical activity. About 5% is excreted unchanged in the urine together with less than 10% each of the 7-amino-and 7-acetylamino-metabolites in the first 48 hours.

*Indications:* Short-term treatment of insomnia when

it is severe, disabling or subjecting the individual to unacceptable distress, where daytime sedation is acceptable.

**Dosage and administration**

*Adults*: 5 mg before retiring. This dose may, if necessary, be increased to 10 mg.

Dosage should be adjusted on an individual basis. Treatment should, if possible, be on an intermittent basis.

The lowest dose which can control symptoms should be used. Treatment should not be continued at full dose beyond four weeks.

Long-term chronic use is not recommended.

Treatment should always be tapered off gradually. Patients who have taken benzodiazepines for a prolonged time may require a longer period during which doses are reduced. Specialist help may be appropriate.

*Use in the elderly*: ELDERLY OR DEBILITATED PATIENTS: DOSES SHOULD NOT EXCEED HALF THOSE NORMALLY RECOMMENDED.

*Children:* Mogadon is not for paediatric use.

Mogadon tablets are for oral administration.

**Contra-indications, warnings, etc**

*Contra-indications:* Patients with known sensitivity to benzodiazepines; acute pulmonary insufficiency; respiratory depression; phobic or obsessional states; chronic psychosis.

*Use in pregnancy and lactation*: There is no evidence as to drug safety in human pregnancy, nor is there evidence from animal work that it is free from hazard. Do not use during pregnancy, especially during the first and last trimesters, unless there are compelling reasons.

The administration of high doses or prolonged administration of low doses of benzodiazepines in the last trimester of pregnancy has been reported to produce irregularities in the foetal heart rate, and hypotonia, poor sucking and hypothermia in the neonate.

Nitrazepam has been detected in breast milk. If possible, the use of Mogadon should be avoided during lactation.

*Precautions:* In patients with chronic pulmonary insufficiency, and in patients with chronic renal or hepatic disease, dosage may need to be reduced.

Mogadon should not be used alone to treat depression or anxiety associated with depression, since suicide may be precipitated in such patients.

In cases of loss or bereavement, psychological adjustment may be inhibited by benzodiazepines.

Patients should be advised that, like all medicaments of this type, Mogadon may modify patients' performance at skilled tasks (driving, operating machinery, etc.) to a varying degree depending upon dosage, administration and individual susceptibility. Patients should further be advised that alcohol may intensify any impairment, and should, therefore, be avoided during treatment. If the patient is awoken during the period of maximum drug activity, recall may be impaired.

The dependence potential of the benzodiazepines is low, particularly when limited to short-term use, but this increases when high doses are used, especially when given over long periods. This is particularly so in patients with a history of alcoholism or drug abuse or in patients with marked personality disorders. Regular monitoring in such patients is essential; routine repeat prescriptions should be avoided and treatment should be withdrawn gradually. Symptoms such as depression, nervousness, rebound insomnia, irritability, sweating, and diarrhoea have been reported following abrupt cessation of treatment in patients receiving even normal therapeutic doses for short periods of time.

In rare instances, withdrawal following excessive dosages may produce confusional states, psychotic manifestations and convulsions.

Abnormal psychological reactions to benzodiazepines have been reported. Rare behavioural effects include paradoxical aggressive outbursts, excitement, confusion and the uncovering of depression with suicidal tendencies. Extreme caution should therefore be used in prescribing benzodiazepines to patients with personality disorders.

If Mogadon is combined with centrally-acting drugs such as neuroleptics, tranquillisers, antidepressants, hypnotics, analgesics and anaesthetics, the sedative effects are likely to be intensified. The elderly require special supervision.

When Mogadon is used in conjunction with anti-epileptic drugs, side-effects and toxicity may be more evident, particularly with hydantoins or barbiturates or combinations including them. This requires extra care in adjusting dosage in the initial stages of treatment.

Known inhibitors of hepatic enzymes, e.g. cimetidine, have been shown to reduce the clearance of benzodiazepines and may potentiate their action and

known inducers of hepatic enzymes, e.g. rifampicin, may increase the clearance of benzodiazepines.

*Side-effects and adverse reactions:* Common adverse effects include drowsiness, sedation, unsteadiness and ataxia; these are dose-related and may persist into the following day, even after a single dose. The elderly are particularly sensitive to the effects of centrally-depressant drugs and may experience confusion, especially if organic brain changes are present; the dosage of Mogadon should not exceed one-half that normally recommended for other adults. Other adverse effects are rare and include headache, vertigo, hypotension, gastro-intestinal upsets, skin rashes, visual disturbances, changes in libido, and urinary retention. Isolated cases of blood dyscrasias and jaundice have also been reported.

*Treatment of overdosage:* When taken alone in overdosage, Mogadon presents few problems in management. Signs may include drowsiness, ataxia and dysarthria, with coma in severe cases. Treatment is symptomatic. Gastric lavage is useful only if performed soon after ingestion.

The value of dialysis has not been determined. Anexate is a specific IV antidote for use in emergency situations. Patients requiring such intervention should be monitored closely in hospital (see separate prescribing information).

If excitation occurs, barbiturates should not be used.

When taken with centrally-acting drugs, especially alcohol, the effects of overdosage are likely to be more severe and, in the absence of supportive measures, may prove fatal.

**Pharmaceutical precautions**

*Storage:* The recommended maximum storage temperature for Mogadon tablets is 25°C.

Mogadon tablets should be protected from light.

**Legal category**    CD(Sch 4), POM

**Package quantities**    Mogadon tablets 5 mg in packs of 30.

**Further information**   No clear correlation has been demonstrated between the blood levels of Mogadon and its clinical effects.

The elderly and patients with impaired renal and/or hepatic function will be particularly susceptible to the adverse effects listed above. It is advisable to review treatment regularly and to discontinue use as soon as possible.

Treatment should be kept to a minimum and given only under close medical supervision. Little is known regarding the efficacy or safety of benzodiazepines in long-term use.

An underlying cause for insomnia should be sought before deciding upon the use of benzodiazepines for symptomatic relief.

In Ireland further information is available from Roche Pharmaceuticals (Ireland) Limited, 3 Richview, Clonskeagh, Dublin 14.

**Product licence number**    0031/0062R

# NAPROSYN*

**Presentation**   A round, scored, buff, low excipient tablet containing 250 mg of naproxen BP, inscribed NAPROSYN 250 on one side and SYNTEX on the other. It also contains the inactive ingredients povidone, croscarmellose sodium, magnesium stearate, iron oxide (E172) and purified water.

An oblong, scored, buff, low excipient tablet containing 500 mg of naproxen BP inscribed NAPROSYN 500 on one side and SYNTEX on the other. It also contains the inactive ingredients povidone, croscarmellose sodium, magnesium stearate, iron oxide (E172) and purified water.

Suppositories each containing 500 mg naproxen BP. They also contain the inactive ingredient witepsol.

A flavoured orange suspension containing 25 mg/ml naproxen BP. It also contains the inactive ingredients fumaric acid, sodium chloride, methylparahydroxybenzoate, sucrose, sorbitol solution, magnesium aluminium silicate, imitation pineapple flavour, imitation orange flavour and purified water.

**Uses**

*Pharmacological properties:* Naprosyn is a non-steroidal, anti-inflammatory, analgesic compound with antipyretic properties when tested in classical animal test systems. It exhibits its anti-inflammatory effect even in adrenalectomised animals, indicating that its action is not mediated through the pituitary-adrenal axis. It inhibits prostaglandin synthetase, as do other non-steroidal, anti-inflammatory agents. As with other agents, however, the exact mechanism of its anti-inflammatory action is not known.

*Pharmacokinetics*: Naproxen is completely absorbed from the gastro-intestinal tract, and peak plasma levels are reached in 2 to 4 hours. Naproxen is present in the blood mainly as unchanged drug, extensively bound to plasma proteins. The plasma half-life is

between 12 and 15 hours, enabling a steady state to be achieved within 3 days of initiation of therapy on a twice daily dose regimen. The degree of absorption is not significantly affected by either foods or most antacids. Excretion is almost entirely via the urine, mainly as conjugated naproxen, with some unchanged drug. Metabolism in children is similar to that in adults. Chronic alcoholic liver disease reduces the total plasma concentration of naproxen but the concentration of unbound naproxen increases. In the elderly, the unbound plasma concentration of naproxen is increased although total plasma concentration is unchanged.

*Indications*: Naprosyn is indicated for the treatment of rheumatoid arthritis, osteoarthrosis (degenerative arthritis), ankylosing spondylitis, juvenile rheumatoid arthritis, acute gout, acute musculo-skeletal disorders and dysmenorrhoea.

**Dosage and administration**

*Adults: Rheumatoid arthritis, osteoarthritis and ankylosing spondylitis:* The usual dose is 500 mg to 1 g daily taken in two doses at 12-hour intervals or alternatively as a single administration.

In the following cases a loading dose of 750 mg or 1 g per day for the acute phase is recommended:

- In patients reporting severe night-time pain and/or morning stiffness.

- In patients being switched to Naprosyn from a high dose of another anti-rheumatic compound.

- In osteoarthritis where pain is the predominant symptom.

Naprosyn Suppositories are recommended for patients in whom rectal administration may be preferable. One suppository is to be inserted at night. If necessary, another suppository or up to 500 mg oral Naprosyn therapy can be used in the morning.

*Acute gout:* The recommended dosage is 750 mg initially, then 250 mg every eight hours until the attack has passed.

*Acute musculoskeletal disorders and dysmenorrhoea*: The recommended dose is 500 mg initially followed by 250 mg at 6–8 hour intervals as needed, with a maximum daily dose after the first day of 1250 mg.

*Use in the elderly:* Studies indicate that although total plasma concentration of naproxen is unchanged, the unbound plasma fraction of naproxen is increased in the elderly. The implication of this finding for Naprosyn dosing is unknown. As with other drugs used in the elderly it is prudent to use the lowest effective dose. For the effect of reduced elimination in the elderly refer to the section *Use in patients with impaired renal function*.

*Children:* The recommended dose for juvenile rheumatoid arthritis in children over 5 years of age is 10 mg/kg/day taken in two doses at 12-hour intervals. Naprosyn is not recommended for use in any other indication in children under 16 years of age.

**Contra-indications, warnings, etc**

*Contra-indications:* Active peptic ulceration. Hypersensitivity to naproxen or naproxen sodium formulations. Since the potential exists for cross-sensitivity reactions, Naprosyn should not be given to patients in whom aspirin or other non-steroidal anti-inflammatory/analgesic drugs induce asthma, rhinitis or urticaria.

*Use in pregnancy and lactation:* Teratology studies in rats and rabbits at dose levels equivalent on a human multiple basis to those which have produced foetal abnormality with certain other non-steroidal anti-inflammatory agents, e.g. aspirin, have not produced evidence of foetal damage with naproxen. As with other drugs of this type naproxen delays parturition in animals (the relevance of this finding to human patients is unknown) and also affects the human foetal cardiovascular system (closure of the ductus arteriosus). Good medical practice indicates minimal drug usage in pregnancy, and use of this class of therapeutic agent requires cautious balancing of possible benefit against potential risk to the mother and foetus especially in the first and third trimesters.

The use of Naprosyn should be avoided in patients who are breast-feeding.

*Precautions*: Episodes of gastro-intestinal bleeding have been reported in patients with naproxen therapy. Naprosyn should be given under close supervision to patients with a history of gastro-intestinal disease.

Serious gastro-intestinal adverse reactions, can occur at any time in patients on therapy with non-steroidal anti-inflammatory drugs. The risk of occurrence does not seem to change with duration of therapy. Studies to date have not identified any subset of patients not at risk of developing peptic ulcer and bleeding. However, elderly and debilitated patients tolerate gastro-intestinal ulceration or bleeding less well than others. Most of the serious gastro-intestinal events associated with non-steroidal anti-inflammatory drugs occurred in this patient population.

The antipyretic and anti-inflammatory activities of

Naprosyn may reduce fever and inflammation, thereby diminishing their utility as diagnostic signs.

Bronchospasm may be precipitated in patients suffering from, or with a history of, bronchial asthma or allergic disease.

Sporadic abnormalities in laboratory tests (e.g. liver function tests) have occurred in patients on naproxen therapy, but no definite trend was seen in any test indicating toxicity.

Naproxen decreases platelet aggregation and prolongs bleeding time. This effect should be kept in mind when bleeding times are determined.

Mild peripheral oedema has been observed in a few patients receiving naproxen. Although sodium retention has not been reported in metabolic studies, it is possible that patients with questionable or compromised cardiac function may be at a greater risk when taking Naprosyn.

Naprosyn Suspension contains sodium chloride (20 mg/ml). This should be considered in patients whose overall intake of sodium must be restricted.

*Use in patients with impaired renal function*: As naproxen is eliminated to a large extent (95%) by urinary excretion via glomerular filtration, it should be used with great caution in patients with impaired renal function and the monitoring of serum creatinine and/or creatinine clearance is advised in these patients. Naprosyn is not recommended in patients having baseline creatinine clearance less than 20 ml/minute.

Certain patients, specifically those whose renal blood flow is compromised, because of extracellular volume depletion, cirrhosis of the liver, sodium restriction, congestive heart failure, and pre-existing renal disease, should have renal function assessed before and during Naprosyn therapy. Some elderly patients in whom impaired renal function may be expected, as well as patients using diuretics, may also fall within this category. A reduction in daily dosage should be considered to avoid the possibility of excessive accumulation of naproxen metabolites in these patients.

*Use in patients with impaired liver function*: Chronic alcoholic liver disease and probably also other forms of cirrhosis reduce the total plasma concentration of naproxen, but the plasma concentration of unbound naproxen is increased. The implication of this finding for Naprosyn dosing is unknown but it is prudent to use the lowest effective dose.

*Side-effects and adverse reactions:*
*Gastro-intestinal:* The more frequent reactions are nausea, vomiting, abdominal discomfort and epigastric distress. More serious reactions, which may occur occasionally are gastro-intestinal bleeding, peptic ulceration (sometimes with haemorrhage and perforation), non-peptic gastro-intestinal ulceration and colitis.

*Dermatological:* Skin rashes, urticaria, angio-oedema. Alopecia, erythema multiforme, Stevens Johnson syndrome, epidermal necrolysis and photosensitivity reactions (including cases in which the skin resembles porphyria cutanea tarda, 'pseudoporphyria') or epidermolysis bullosa may occur rarely.

*Renal:* Including but not limited to glomerular nephritis, interstitial nephritis, nephrotic syndrome, haematuria, renal papillary necrosis and renal failure.

*CNS:* Convulsions, headache, insomnia, inability to concentrate and cognitive dysfunction have been reported.

*Haematological:* Thrombocytopenia, granulocytopenia including agranulocytosis, aplastic anaemia and haemolytic anaemia may occur rarely.

*Other:* Tinnitus, hearing impairment, vertigo, mild peripheral oedema. Anaphylactic reactions to naproxen and naproxen sodium formulations have been reported in patients with, or without, a history of previous hypersensitivity reactions to NSAIDs. Jaundice, fatal hepatitis, visual disturbances, eosinophilic pneumonitis, vasculitis, aseptic meningitis, hyperkalemia and ulcerative stomatitis have been reported rarely.

*Naprosyn Suppositories:* The following minor side-effects have been reported with the use of Naprosyn Suppositories: rectal discomfort, soreness, burning and itching. Also isolated cases of rectal bleeding, tenesmus and proctitis have been reported. However, the incidence of local side-effects in clinical trials was low.

*Drug interactions* Due to the high plasma protein binding of naproxen, patients simultaneously receiving hydantoins, anticoagulants or a highly protein-bound sulphonamide should be observed for signs of overdosage of these drugs. No interactions have been observed in clinical studies with naproxen and anticoagulants or sulphonylureas, but caution is nevertheless advised since interaction has been seen with other non-steroidal agents of this class.

The natriuretic effect of frusemide has been reported to be inhibited by some drugs of this class.

Inhibition of renal lithium clearance leading to increases in plasma lithium concentrations has also been reported.

Naproxen and other non-steroidal anti-inflammatory drugs can reduce the antihypertensive effect of propranolol and other beta-blockers and may increase the risk of renal impairment associated with the use of ACE-inhibitors.

Probenecid given concurrently increases naproxen plasma levels and extends its half-life considerably.

Caution is advised where methotrexate is administered concurrently because of possible enhancement of its toxicity since naproxen, among other non-steroidal anti-inflammatory drugs, has been reported to reduce the tubular secretion of methotrexate in an animal model.

It is suggested that Naprosyn therapy be temporarily discontinued 48 hours before adrenal function tests are performed, because naproxen may artifactually interfere with some tests for 17-ketogenic steroids. Similarly, naproxen may interfere with some assays of urinary 5-hydroxy-indoleacetic acid.

*Treatment of overdosage:* Significant overdosage of the drug may be characterised by drowsiness, heartburn, indigestion, nausea or vomiting. A few patients have experienced seizures, but it is not clear whether these were naproxen-related or not. It is not known what dose of the drug would be life-threatening.

Should a patient ingest a large amount of Naprosyn accidentally or purposefully, the stomach may be emptied and usual supportive measures employed. Animal studies indicate that the prompt administration of activated charcoal in adequate amounts would tend to reduce markedly the absorption of the drug.

Haemodialysis does not decrease the plasma concentration of naproxen because of the high degree of protein binding. However, haemodialysis may still be appropriate in a patient with renal failure who has taken Naprosyn.

**Pharmaceutical precautions**
*Storage:* Protect from light and store below 30°C. Naprosyn Suppositories should be stored at not more than 15°C in a dry place.

**Legal category** POM.

**Package quantities** Naprosyn Low Excipient Tablets are supplied in packs of 250 tablets.

Naprosyn 500 Low Excipient Tablets are supplied in original packs of 56 tablets, and also packs of 100 tablets.

Naprosyn Suppositories are supplied in packs containing 10 suppositories.

Naprosyn Suspension is supplied in 240 ml bottles.

**Product licence numbers**
Low Excipient Tablets 0031/0471
Low Excipient Tablets (500) 0031/0484
Suppositories 0031/0474
Suspension 0031/0475

# NAPROSYN* EC

**Presentation** A white, circular convex, enteric film-coated, low excipient tablet containing Naproxen PhEur 250 mg printed "NPR EC 250" on one side.

A white, oval, convex, enteric film-coated low excipient tablet containing Naproxen PhEur 375 mg printed "Naprosyn EC" on one side and "SYNTEX 375" on the other.

A white, capsule-shaped, enteric film-coated, low excipient tablet containing Naproxen PhEur 500 mg, printed "NPR EC 500" on one side.

The tablets also contain povidone K-90, croscarmellose sodium (type A), magnesium stearate, purified water, methacrylic acid copolymer (type C), purified talc, sodium hydroxide, triethyl citrate, simethicone emulsion and opacode S-8106.

**Uses**
*Pharmacological properties:* Naproxen has been shown to have anti-inflammatory, analgesic and antipyretic properties when tested in classical animal test systems. It exhibits its anti-inflammatory effect even in adrenalectomised animals, indicating that its action is not mediated through the pituitary-adrenal axis. It inhibits prostaglandin synthetase, as do other non-steroidal anti-inflammatory agents. As with other agents, however, the exact mechanism of its anti-inflammatory action is not known.

*Pharmacokinetics:* Naproxen is completely absorbed from the gastro-intestinal tract, and peak plasma levels are reached in 2 to 4 hours. Naproxen is present in the blood mainly as unchanged drug, extensively bound to plasma proteins. The plasma half-life is between 12 and 15 hours, enabling a steady state to be achieved within 3 days of initiation of therapy on a twice daily dose regimen. The degree of absorption is not significantly affected by either foods or most antacids. Excretion is almost entirely via the urine, mainly as conjugated naproxen, with some unchanged drug. Metabolism in children is similar to that in adults. Chronic alcoholic liver disease reduces

the total plasma concentration of naproxen but the concentration of unbound naproxen increases. In the elderly, the unbound plasma concentration of naproxen is increased although total plasma concentration is unchanged.

When naproxen is administered in the enteric-coated form, the peak plasma levels are delayed compared to those seen with standard tablets. However, the mean areas under the plasma concentration-time curves, and hence bioavailability, are equivalent. The tablets, therefore, perform as would be anticipated for a drug which does not disintegrate until it reaches the small intestine, where dissolution is rapid and complete.

*Indications:* Naprosyn EC is indicated for the treatment of rheumatoid arthritis, osteoarthrosis (degenerative arthritis), ankylosing spondylitis, juvenile rheumatoid arthritis, acute gout, acute musculoskeletal disorders (such as sprains and strains, direct trauma, lumbosacral pain, cervical spondylitis, tenosynovitis and fibrositis) and dysmenorrhoea.

**Dosage and administration**
*Adults:* Naprosyn EC tablets should be swallowed whole and not broken or crushed.

*Rheumatoid arthritis, osteoarthritis and ankylosing spondylitis:* The usual dose is 500 mg to 1 g daily taken in two doses at 12-hour intervals. Where 1 g per day is needed, one 500 mg tablet twice daily or two 500 mg tablets in a single administration (morning or evening) is recommended.

*Acute gout:* The recommended dosage is 750 mg initially, then 250 mg every eight hours until the attack has passed.

*Acute musculoskeletal disorders and dysmenorrhoea:* The recommended dose is 500 mg initially followed by 250 mg at 6–8 hour intervals as needed, with a maximum daily dose after the first day of 1250 mg.

*Use in the elderly:* Studies indicate that although total plasma concentration of naproxen is unchanged, the unbound plasma fraction of naproxen is increased in the elderly. The implication of this finding for Naprosyn EC dosing is unknown. As with other drugs used in the elderly it is prudent to use the lowest effective dose. For the effect of reduced elimination in the elderly refer to the section *Use in patients with impaired renal function.*

*Children:* Naprosyn EC is effective in the treatment of juvenile rheumatoid arthritis in children over 5 years of age at a dose of 10 mg/kg/day taken in two doses at 12-hour intervals. Naprosyn EC is not recommended for use in any other indication in children under 16 years of age.

**Contra-indications, warnings, etc**
*Contra-indications:* Active peptic ulceration or intestinal inflammation. Hypersensitivity to naproxen and naproxen sodium formulations. Since the potential exists for cross-sensitivity reactions, Naprosyn EC should not be given to patients in whom aspirin or other non-steroidal anti-inflammatory/analgesic drugs induce asthma, rhinitis or urticaria.

*Use in pregnancy and lactation:* Teratology studies in rats and rabbits at dose levels equivalent on a human multiple basis to those which have produced foetal abnormality with certain other non-steroidal anti-inflammatory agents, e.g. aspirin, have not produced evidence of foetal damage with naproxen. As with other drugs of this type naproxen delays parturition in animals (the relevance of this finding to human patients is unknown) and also affects the human foetal cardiovascular system (closure of the ductus arteriosus). Good medical practice indicates minimal drug usage in pregnancy, and the use of this class of therapeutic agent requires cautious balancing of possible benefit against potential risk to the mother and foetus, especially in the first and third trimesters.

Naproxen has been found in the milk of lactating mothers. The use of Naprosyn EC should therefore be avoided in patients who are breast-feeding.

*Precautions:* Episodes of gastro-intestinal bleeding have been reported in patients with naproxen therapy. Naprosyn EC should be given under close supervision to patients with a history of gastro-intestinal disease.

Serious gastro-intestinal adverse reactions can occur at any time in patients on therapy with non-steroidal anti-inflammatory drugs. The risk of occurrence does not seem to change with duration of therapy. Studies to date have not identified any subset of patients not at risk of developing peptic ulcer and bleeding. However, elderly and debilitated patients tolerate gastro-intestinal ulceration or bleeding less well than others; most of the serious gastro-intestinal events associated with non-steroidal anti-inflammatory drugs occur in this patient population.

The antipyretic and anti-inflammatory activities of Naprosyn EC may reduce fever and inflammation, thereby diminishing their utility as diagnostic signs.

Bronchospasm may be precipitated in patients

suffering from, or with a history of, bronchial asthma or allergic disease.

Sporadic abnormalities in laboratory tests (e.g. liver function tests) have occurred in patients on naproxen therapy, but no definite trend indicating toxicity was seen in any test.

Naproxen decreases platelet aggregation and prolongs bleeding time. This effect should be kept in mind when bleeding times are determined.

Mild peripheral oedema has been observed in a few patients receiving naproxen. Although sodium retention has not been reported in metabolic studies, it is possible that patients with questionable or compromised cardiac function may be at a greater risk when taking Naprosyn EC.

*Use in patients with impaired renal function:* As naproxen is eliminated to a large extent (95%) by urinary excretion via glomerular filtration, it should be used with great caution in patients with impaired renal function and the monitoring of serum creatinine and/or creatinine clearance is advised in these patients. Naprosyn EC is not recommended in patients having a baseline creatinine clearance of less than 20 ml/minute.

Certain patients, specifically those whose renal blood flow is compromised because of extracellular volume depletion, cirrhosis of the liver, sodium restriction, congestive heart failure or pre-existing renal disease, should have renal function assessed before and during Naprosyn EC therapy. Some elderly patients in whom impaired renal function may be expected, as well as patients using diuretics, may also fall within this category. A reduction in daily dosage should be considered to avoid the possibility of excessive accumulation of naproxen metabolites in these patients.

*Use in patients with impaired liver function:* Chronic alcoholic liver disease and probably also other forms of cirrhosis reduce the total plasma concentration of naproxen, but the plasma concentration of unbound naproxen is increased. The implication of this finding for Naprosyn EC dosing is unknown but it is prudent to use the lowest effective dose.

*Side-effects and adverse reactions:*

*Gastro-intestinal:* The more frequent reactions are nausea, vomiting, abdominal discomfort and epigastric distress. More serious reactions which may occur occasionally are gastro-intestinal bleeding, peptic ulceration (sometimes with haemorrhage and perforation), non-peptic gastro-intestinal ulceration and colitis.

*Dermatological:* Skin rashes, urticaria, angio-oedema. Alopecia, erythema multiforme, Stevens Johnson syndrome, epidermal necrolysis and photosensitivity reactions (including cases in which the skin resembles porphyria cutanea tarda, 'pseudoporphyria') or epidermolysis bullosa may occur rarely.

*Renal:* Including but not limited to glomerular nephritis, interstitial nephritis, nephrotic syndrome, haematuria, renal papillary necrosis and renal failure.

*CNS:* Convulsions, headache, insomnia, inability to concentrate and cognitive dysfunction have been reported.

*Haematological:* Thrombocytopenia, granulocytopenia including agranulocytosis, aplastic anaemia and haemolytic anaemia may occur rarely.

*Other:* Tinnitus, hearing impairment, vertigo, mild peripheral oedema. Anaphylactic reactions to naproxen and naproxen sodium formulations have been reported in patients with, or without, a history of previous hypersensitivity reactions to NSAIDs. Jaundice, fatal hepatitis, visual disturbances, eosinophilic pneumonitis, vasculitis, hyperkalemia, aseptic meningitis and ulcerative stomatitis have been reported rarely.

*Drug interactions:* Due to the high plasma protein binding of naproxen, patients simultaneously receiving hydantoins, anticoagulants or a highly protein-bound sulphonamide should be observed for signs of overdosage of these drugs. No interactions have been observed in clinical studies with naproxen and anticoagulants or sulphonylureas, but caution is nevertheless advised since interaction has been seen with other non-steroidal agents of this class.

The natriuretic effect of frusemide has been reported to be inhibited by some drugs of this class.

Inhibition of renal lithium clearance leading to increases in plasma lithium concentrations has also been reported.

Naproxen and other non-steroidal anti-inflammatory drugs can reduce the antihypertensive effect of propranolol and other beta-blockers and may increase the risk of renal impairment associated with the use of ACE-inhibitors.

Probenecid given concurrently increases naproxen plasma levels and extends its half-life considerably.

Caution is advised where methotrexate is administered concurrently because of possible enhancement of its toxicity, since naproxen, in common with other non-steroidal anti-inflammatory drugs, has been reported to reduce the tubular secretion of methotrexate in an animal model.

It is suggested that Naprosyn EC therapy be temporarily discontinued 48 hours before adrenal function tests are performed, because naproxen may artifactually interfere with some tests for 17-ketogenic steroids. Similarly, naproxen may interfere with some assays of urinary 5-hydroxyindoleacetic acid.

*Treatment of overdosage:* Significant overdosage of the drug may be characterised by drowsiness, heartburn, indigestion, nausea or vomiting. A few patients have experienced seizures, but it is not known whether these were naproxen-related or not. It is not known what dose of the drug would be life-threatening.

Should a patient ingest a large amount of Naprosyn EC accidentally or purposefully, the stomach may be emptied and usual supportive measures employed. Animal studies indicate that the prompt administration of activated charcoal in adequate amounts would tend to reduce markedly the absorption of the drug.

Haemodialysis does not decrease the plasma concentration of naproxen because of the high degree of protein binding. However, haemodialysis may still be appropriate in a patient with renal failure who has taken naproxen.

**Pharmaceutical precautions**
*Storage:* Protect from light and store below 30°C.

**Legal category** POM.

**Package quantities**
Naprosyn EC 250 Tablets in packs of 56 and 250 tablets.
Naprosyn EC 375 Tablets in packs of 56 tablets.
Naprosyn EC 500 Tablets in packs of 56 and 100 tablets.

**Further information** Nil.

**Product licence numbers**

| | |
|---|---|
| 250 mg tablets | 0031/0467 |
| 375 mg tablets | 0031/0468 |
| 500 mg tablets | 0031/0469 |

## NEOTIGASON*

**Presentation** Capsules with brown cap and white body with ROCHE printed in black on both cap and body, containing 10 mg acitretin and the inactive ingredients maltodextrin, sodium ascorbate, gelatin, microcrystalline cellulose, iron oxide black (E172), iron oxide yellow (E172), iron oxide red (E172) and titanium dioxide (E171).

Capsules with brown cap and yellow body with ROCHE printed in black on both cap and body, containing 25 mg acitretin and the inactive ingredients maltodextrin, sodium ascorbate, gelatin, microcrystalline cellulose, iron oxide black (E172), iron oxide yellow (E172), iron oxide red (E172) and titanium dioxide (E171).

**Uses**
*Pharmacological properties:* Retinol (vitamin A) is known to be essential for normal epithelial growth and differentiation, though the mode of this effect is not yet established. Both retinol and retinoic acid are capable of reversing hyperkeratotic and metaplastic skin changes. However, these effects are generally only obtained at dosages associated with considerable local or systemic toxicity. Acitretin, a synthetic aromatic derivative of retinoic acid, has a favourable therapeutic ratio, with a greater and more specific inhibitory effect on psoriasis and disorders of epithelial keratinisation. The usual therapeutic response to acitretin consists of desquamation (with or without erythema) followed by more normal re-epithelialisation.

Acitretin is the main active metabolite of etretinate.

*Pharmacokinetics:* Following oral administration of Neotigason, peak plasma concentrations of acitretin are achieved within 1-6 hours then decline at least 10-fold by 24 hours. Peak levels of the 13-cis acitretin metabolite are lower than those of acitretin, but remain relatively unchanged throughout each dosage interval. During the terminal phase, acitretin and its 13-cis metabolite are interconverted; therefore both compounds are excreted with an elimination half-life of approximately two days. Acitretin is highly bound to plasma protein and is excreted via the bile and urine as polar metabolites. Bioavailability is enhanced by food.

IMPORTANT: Etretinate has been detected in the plasma of some patients treated with Neotigason. The levels seen are generally much lower than those occurring during etretinate (Tigason) therapy. Etretinate has a long elimination half-life (approximately 120 days) due to deposition in adipose tissue. Therefore, the two year post-therapy contraception period for etretinate is required following Neotigason therapy.

In a study with healthy volunteers, concurrent intake of a single dose of acitretin together with ethanol led to formation of etretinate.

*Indications:* Severe extensive psoriasis which is resistant to other forms of therapy. Palmo-plantar pustular psoriasis. Severe congenital ichthyosis. Severe Darier's disease (keratosis follicularis).

**Dosage and administration** Neotigason capsules are for oral administration.

The capsules should be taken once daily with meals or with milk.

There is a wide variation in the absorption and rate of metabolism of Neotigason. This necessitates individual adjustment of dosage. For this reason the following dosage recommendations can serve only as a guide.

*Adults:* Initial daily dose should be 25 mg or 30 mg for two to four weeks. After this initial treatment period the involved areas of the skin should show a marked response and/or side-effects should be apparent. Following assessment of the initial treatment period titration of the dose upwards or downwards may be necessary to achieve the desired therapeutic response with the minimum of side-effects. In general, a daily dosage of 25-50 mg taken for a further six to eight weeks achieves optimal therapeutic results. However it may be necessary in some cases to increase the dose up to a maximum of 75 mg/day.

In patients with Darier's disease a starting dose of 10 mg may be appropriate. The dose should be increased cautiously as isomorphic reactions may occur.

Therapy can be discontinued in patients with psoriasis whose lesions have improved sufficiently. Relapses should be treated as described above.

Patients with severe congenital ichthyosis and severe Darier's disease may require therapy beyond three months. The lowest effective dosage, not exceeding 50 mg/day, should be given.

Continuous use beyond 6 months is contraindicated as only limited clinical data are available on patients treated beyond this length of time.

*Use in the elderly:* Dosage recommendations are the same as for other adults.

*Children:* In view of possible severe side-effects associated with long-term treatment, Neotigason is contra-indicated in children unless, in the opinion of the physician, the benefits significantly outweigh the risks.

The dosage should be established according to bodyweight. The daily dosage is about 0.5 mg/kg. Higher doses (up to 1 mg/kg daily) may be necessary in some cases for limited periods, but only up to a maximum of 35 mg/day. The maintenance dose should be kept as low as possible in view of possible long-term side-effects.

*Combination therapy:* Other dermatological therapy particularly with keratolytics, should normally be stopped before administration of Neotigason. However, the use of topical corticosteroids or bland emollient ointment may be continued if indicated.

When Neotigason is used in combination with other types of therapy, it may be possible, depending on the individual patient's response, to reduce the dosage of Neotigason.

**Contra-indications, warnings, etc**
*Contra-indications:* Neotigason is contra-indicated during pregnancy as it is a known human teratogen.

The use of Neotigason is contra-indicated in women who are breast feeding.

Neotigason is contra-indicated in patients with hepatic or renal impairment.

Rare cases of benign intracranial hypertension have been reported after Neotigason and after tetracyclines. Supplementary treatment with antibiotics such as tetracyclines is therefore contra-indicated.

*Use in pregnancy and lactation:* Neotigason is contra-indicated during pregnancy as it is a known human teratogen.

The use of Neotigason is contra-indicated in women who are breast feeding.

*Precautions:* Neotigason is contra-indicated in women of childbearing potential unless the following criteria are met:

1. Pregnancy has been excluded before instituting therapy with Neotigason (negative pregnancy test within two weeks prior to therapy).

2. She starts Neotigason therapy only on the second or third day of the next menstrual cycle.

3. Having excluded pregnancy, any woman of childbearing potential who is receiving Neotigason must practice effective contraception for at least one month before treatment, during the treatment period and for at least two years following its cessation.

Even female patients who normally do not practice contraception because of a history of infertility should be advised to do so, while taking Neotigason.

4. Contraceptive measures must also be taken in the case of repeated courses of treatment.

5. Any pregnancy occurring during treatment with Neotigason, or in the two years following its cessation

carries a high risk of foetal malformation. This would raise the question of the termination of pregnancy for medical reasons. Therefore, before instituting Neotigason the treating physician must explain clearly and in detail what precautions must be taken. This should include the risks involved and the possible consequences of pregnancy occurring during Neotigason treatment or in the two years following its cessation.

6. She is reliable and capable of understanding the risk and complying with effective contraception, and confirms that she has understood the warnings.

In view of the importance of the above precautions, Neotigason Patient Information Leaflets are available to doctors and it is strongly recommended that these be given to all patients.

Patients should not donate blood either during or for at least one year following discontinuation of therapy with Neotigason. Theoretically there would be a small risk to a woman in the first trimester of pregnancy who received blood donated by a patient on Neotigason therapy.

Acitretin has been shown to affect diaphyseal and spongy bone adversely in animals at high doses in excess of those recommended for use in man. Since skeletal hyperostosis and extraosseous calcification have been reported following long-term treatment with etretinate in man, this effect should be expected with acitretin therapy.

Since there have been occasional reports of bone changes in children, including premature epiphyseal closure, skeletal hyperostosis and extraosseous calcification, after long-term treatment with etretinate, these effects may be expected with acitretin. Neotigason therapy in children is not, therefore, recommended. If, in exceptional circumstances, such therapy is undertaken the child should be carefully monitored for any abnormalities of musculo-skeletal development.

Any patients complaining of atypical musculoskeletal symptoms on treatment with Neotigason should be promptly and fully investigated to exclude possible acitretin-induced bone changes. If clinically significant bone or joint changes are found, Neotigason therapy should be discontinued.

The effects of UV light are enhanced by retinoid therapy, therefore patients should avoid excessive exposure to sunlight and the unsupervised use of sun lamps.

Liver function and blood lipids (fasting value) should be measured at the start of treatment, after the first month of administration and at three-monthly intervals thereafter.

In diabetic patients, retinoids can alter glucose tolerance. Blood sugar levels should therefore be checked frequently at the beginning of the treatment period.

Patients should be warned of the possibility of alopecia occurring (see *Side-effects and adverse reactions*).

*Side-effects and adverse reactions:* Most of the clinical side-effects of Neotigason are dose-related and are usually well-tolerated at the recommended dosages. However, the toxic dose of Neotigason is close to the therapeutic dose and most patients experience some side-effects during the initial period whilst dosage is being adjusted. They are usually reversible with reduction of dosage or discontinuation of therapy.

The skin and mucous membranes are most commonly affected, and it is recommended that patients should be so advised before treatment is commenced. Dryness of the mucous membranes, sometimes with erosion, involving the lips, mouth, conjunctivae and nasal mucosa are seen. Dryness of the skin may be associated with scaling, thinning, erythema (especially of the face) and pruritus. Palmar and plantar exfoliation, epistaxis and epidermal fragility have been reported, as well as paronychia. Granulomatous lesions have occasionally been reported. Dryness of the conjunctivae may lead to mild-to-moderate conjunctivitis and result in intolerance of contact lenses; it may be alleviated by lubrication with artificial tears or topical antibiotics. Hair thinning and frank alopecia may occur, usually noted four to eight weeks after starting therapy, and are reversible following discontinuation of Neotigason. Full recovery usually occurs within six months of stopping treatment in the majority of patients.

Rarely, patients may experience photosensitivity reactions.

Non-specific symptoms such as nausea, headache, malaise, drowsiness and sweating have been reported infrequently. Myalgia and arthralgia may occur and be associated with reduced tolerance to exercise.

Benign intracranial hypertension has been reported.

There have been occasional reports of decreased night vision during Neotigason therapy.

Maintenance treatment may result in hyperostosis and extraskeletal calcification, as observed in long-term systemic treatment with other retinoids.

A rise in serum levels of liver enzymes may occur. When significant, dosage reduction or discontinuation of therapy may be necessary. Jaundice and hepatitis have occurred rarely.

Elevation of serum triglycerides above the normal range has been observed, especially where predisposing factors such as a family history of lipid disorders, obesity, alcohol abuse, diabetes mellitus or smoking are present. The changes are dose-related and may be controlled by dietary means (including restriction of alcohol intake) and/or by reduction of dosage of Neotigason.

*Drug interactions:* Existing data suggest that etretinate is formed from acitretin after ingestion of alcoholic beverages. However, the formation of etretinate without concurrent alcohol intake cannot be excluded. Therefore the post-therapy contraception period in women of childbearing potential must be two years.

Patients should be instructed to avoid taking preparations containing high doses of Vitamin A, i.e. more than the recommended dietary allowance of 4,000 - 5,000 i.u. per day.

An increased risk of hepatitis has been reported following the concomitant use of methotrexate and etretinate. Consequently, the concomitant use of methotrexate and Neotigason should be avoided.

In concurrent treatment with phenytoin, it must be remembered that Neotigason partially reduces the protein binding of phenytoin. The clinical significance of this is as yet unknown.

Interaction studies show acitretin does not interfere with the anti-ovulatory action of the combined oral contraceptives.

Interactions between Neotigason and other substances (e.g. digoxin, cimetidine) have not been observed to date.

*Treatment of overdosage:* Manifestations of acute vitamin A toxicity include severe headache, nausea or vomiting, drowsiness, irritability and pruritus. Signs and symptoms of accidental or deliberate overdosage with Neotigason would probably be similar. They would be expected to subside without need for treatment.

Because of the variable absorption of the drug, gastric lavage may be worthwhile within the first few hours after ingestion.

**Pharmaceutical precautions**
*Storage:* The recommended maximum storage temperature is 25°C. Store in a dry place.

**Legal category** POM.

**Package quantities** Neotigason capsules 10 mg in packs of 56. Neotigason capsules 25 mg in packs of 56.

**Further information**
*Availability:* It is recommended that Neotigason capsules should be given by, or under the supervision of, a consultant dermatologist. They are available through hospital pharmacies for use in hospitals, and hospital clinics or, at the written request of a consultant dermatologist can be supplied to specific retail pharmacies for dispensing prescriptions from the named dermatologist whose bonafide can be identified by the dispensing pharmacist.

**Product licence numbers**
Capsules 10 mg 0031/0262
Capsules 25 mg 0031/0263

## NEUPOGEN* ▼

**Qualitative and quantitative composition** Neupogen is a sterile, clear, colourless liquid. Each single use vial and each single use pre-filled syringe of Neupogen contains 30 million units/ml (300µg/ml) of filgrastim formulated in an aqueous sodium acetate buffer at pH 4.0. The quantitative composition (per ml) of Neupogen is:

Filgrastim (pINN) 30 million units (MU)
Acetate 0.59 mg
Sorbitol 50.0 mg
Polysorbate 80 0.04 mg
Sodium 0.035 mg
Water for Injections to 1.0 ml
(qs ad)

Filgrastim is produced in a laboratory strain of *Escherichia coli* bacteria which has been genetically altered by the addition of a gene for the granulocyte-colony stimulating factor.

**Pharmaceutical form** Neupogen is a sterile, clear, colourless liquid for subcutaneous or intravenous injection presented in vials and pre-filled syringes.

Neupogen 30 contains 30 million units (300µg) of active substance in 1.0ml.

Neupogen 48 contains 48 million units (480µg) of active substance in 1.6ml.

**Clinical particulars**
*Therapeutic indications:* Neupogen is indicated for the reduction in the duration of neutropenia and the incidence of febrile neutropenia in patients treated with established cytotoxic chemotherapy for non-myeloid malignancy and for the reduction in the duration of neutropenia and its clinical sequelae in patients undergoing myeloablative therapy followed by bone marrow transplantation.

Neupogen is indicated for the mobilisation of autologous peripheral blood progenitor cells alone, or following myelosuppressive chemotherapy in order to accelerate haematopoietic recovery by infusion of such cells, after myelosuppressive or myeloablative therapy.

The safety and efficacy of Neupogen are similar in adults and children receiving cytotoxic chemotherapy.

In patients, children or adults, with severe congenital, cyclic, or idiopathic neutropenia with an ANC of ≤ 0.5 x $10^9$/L, and a history of severe or recurrent infections, long-term administration of Neupogen is indicated to increase neutrophil counts and to reduce the incidence and duration of infection-related events.

*Posology and method of administration:*
*Established cytotoxic chemotherapy:* The recommended dose of Neupogen is 0.5 MU (5µg)/kg/day. The first dose of Neupogen should not be administered less than 24 hours following cytotoxic chemotherapy. Neupogen may be given as a daily subcutaneous injection or as a daily intravenous infusion diluted in 5% glucose solution given over 30 minutes (see section 6.6 for instructions on dilutions). The subcutaneous route is preferred in most cases. There is some evidence from a study of single dose administration that intravenous dosing may shorten the duration of effect. The clinical relevance of this finding to multiple dose administration is not clear. The choice of route should depend on the individual clinical circumstance. In randomised clinical trials, a subcutaneous dose of 230µg/m² day (4.0–8.4µg/kg/day) was used.

Daily dosing with Neupogen should continue until the expected neutrophil nadir is passed and the neutrophil count has recovered to the normal range. It is expected that the duration of treatment required to fulfill these criteria will be up to 14 days, depending on the type, dose and schedule of cytotoxic chemotherapy used.

In patients receiving cytotoxic chemotherapy, a transient increase in neutrophil counts is typically seen 1 to 2 days after initiation of Neupogen therapy. However, for a sustained therapeutic response, Neupogen therapy should not be discontinued before the expected nadir has passed and the neutrophil count has recovered to the normal range. Premature discontinuation of Neupogen therapy, prior to the time of the expected neutrophil nadir, is not recommended.

*In patients treated with myeloablative therapy followed by bone marrow transplantation:* The recommended starting dose of Neupogen is 1.0 MU (10µg)/kg/day given as a 30 minutes or 24 hours intravenous infusion or 1.0 MU (10µg)/kg/day given by continuous 24 hours subcutaneous infusion. Neupogen should be diluted in 20ml of 5% glucose solution (see section 6.6 for instructions on dilutions).

The first dose of Neupogen should not be administered less than 24 hours following cytotoxic chemotherapy and within 24 hours of bone marrow infusion.

Once the neutrophil nadir has been passed, the daily dose of Neupogen should be titrated against the neutrophil response as follows:

| *Neutrophil count* | *Neupogen dose adjustment* |
|---|---|
| > 1.0 x $10^9$/L for 3 consecutive days | Reduce to 0.5 MU/kg/day |
| Then, if ANC remains > 1.0 x $10^9$/L for 3 more consecutive days | Discontinue Neupogen |
| If the ANC decreases to < 1.0 x $10^9$/L during the treatment period, the dose of Neupogen should be re-escalated according to the above steps | |

ANC = absolute neutrophil count

**For the mobilisation of PBPCs in patients undergoing myelosuppressive or myeloablative therapy followed by autologous PBPC transplantation with or without bone marrow transplantation**

The recommended dose of Neupogen for PBPC mobilisation when used alone is 1.0 MU (10µg)/kg/day as a 24-hour subcutaneous continuous infusion or a single daily subcutaneous injection for 6 consecutive days. For infusions Neupogen should be diluted in 20 ml of 5% glucose solution (see section 6.6 for instructions on dilutions). Timing of leukapheresis: a total of three consecutive collections is recommended, on days 5, 6 and 7.

The recommended dose of Neupogen for PBPC mobilisation after myelosuppressive chemotherapy is 0.5 MU (5µg)/kg/day given daily by subcutaneous injection from the first day after completion of chemotherapy until the expected neutrophil nadir is passed and the neutrophil count has recovered to the normal range. Leukapheresis should be performed during the period when the ANC rises from < 0.5 x

$10^9$/L to > 5.0 x $10^9$/L. For patients who have not had extensive chemotherapy, one leukapheresis is often sufficient. In other circumstances, additional leukaphereses are recommended.

*In Patients with Severe Chronic Neutropenia:*
*Congenital neutropenia:* The recommended starting dose is 1.2 MU (12µg)/kg/day) subcutaneously as a single dose or in divided doses.

*Idiopathic or cyclic neutropenia:* The recommended starting dose is 0.5 MU (5µg)/kg/day subcutaneously as a single dose or in divided doses.

*Dose adjustment:* Neupogen should be administered daily by subcutaneous injection until the neutrophil count has reached and can be maintained at more than 1.5 x $10^9$/L. When the response has been obtained the minimal effective dose to maintain this level should be established. Long-term daily administration is required to maintain an adequate neutrophil count. After one to two weeks of therapy, the initial dose may be doubled or halved depending upon the patient's response. Subsequently the dose may be individually adjusted every 1–2 weeks to maintain the average neutrophil count between 1.5 x $10^9$/L and 10 x $10^9$/L. A faster schedule of dose escalation may be considered in patients presenting with severe infections. In clinical trials, 97% of patients who responded had a complete response at doses ≤ 24µg/kg/day. The long-term safety of Neupogen administration above 24µg/kg/day in patients with severe chronic neutropenia has not been established.

*Other Particulars:* Neupogen therapy should only be given in collaboration with an oncology centre which has experience in G-CSF treatment and hematology and has the necessary diagnostic facilities. The mobilisation and apheresis procedures should be performed in collaboration with an oncology-haematology centre with acceptable experience in this field and where the monitoring of haematopoietic progenitor cells can be correctly performed.

Clinical trials with Neupogen have included a small number of elderly patients but special studies have not been performed in this group and therefore specific dosage recommendations cannot be made.

*Paediatric Use in the SCN and Cancer settings:* Sixty-five percent of the patients studied in the SCN trial program were under 18 years of age. The efficacy of treatment was clear for this age group, which included most patients with congenital neutropenia. There were no differences in the safety profiles for paediatric patients treated for severe chronic neutropenia.

Data from clinical studies in paediatric patients indicate that the safety and efficacy of Neupogen are similar in both adults and children receiving cytotoxic chemotherapy.

The dosage recommendations in paediatric patients are the same as those in adults receiving myelosuppressive cytotoxic chemotherapy.

*Contra-indications:* Neupogen should not be administered to patients with known hypersensitivity to the product or its constituents. Neupogen should not be used to increase the dose of cytotoxic chemotherapy beyond established dosage regimens.

Neupogen should not be administered to patients with severe congenital neutropenia (Kostman's syndrome) with abnormal cytogenetics (see also *Precautions* section).

*Special warnings and special precautions for use:*
*Malignant Cell Growth:* Granulocyte-colony stimulating factor can promote growth of myeloid cells *in vitro* and similar effects may be seen on some non-myeloid cells *in vitro*.

The safety and efficacy of Neupogen administration in patients with myelodysplasia, acute myelogenous leukaemia, or chronic myelogenous leukaemia have not been established. Therefore because of the possibility of tumor growth, caution should be exercised in using Neupogen in any malignancy with myeloid characteristics.

Clinical trials have not yet established whether Neupogen influences the progression of myelodysplastic syndromes to acute myeloid leukaemia. Caution should be exercised in using Neupogen in any pre-malignant myeloid condition.

*Other special precautions:* Monitoring of bone density may be indicated in patients with underlying osteoporotic bone diseases who undergo continuous therapy with Neupogen for more than 6 months.

Studies have not been performed with Neupogen in patients with severe impairment of renal or hepatic function and therefore its use in this patient group cannot be recommended.

*Special precautions in cancer patients: Leucocytosis* – White blood cell counts of 100 x $10^9$/L or greater have been observed in less than 5% of patients receiving Neupogen at doses above 0.3 MU/kg/day (3µg/kg/day). No adverse events directly attributable to this degree of leucocytosis have been reported. However, in view of the potential risks associated with severe leucocytosis, a white blood cell count should be performed at regular intervals during Neupogen

therapy. If leucocyte counts exceed 50 x $10^9$/L after the expected nadir, Neupogen should be discontinued immediately. However, during the period of administration of Neupogen for PBPC mobilisation, discontinuation of Neupogen is appropriate if the leucocyte counts rise to > 100 x $10^9$/L.

*Risks associated with increased doses of chemotherapy:* Special caution should be used when treating patients with high dose chemotherapy, because improved tumour outcome has not been demonstrated and intensified doses of chemotherapeutic agents may lead to increased toxicities including cardiac, pulmonary, neurologic, and dermatologic effects (please refer to the prescribing information of the specific chemotherapy agents used).

Treatment with Neupogen alone does not preclude thrombocytopenia and anaemia due to myelosuppressive chemotherapy. Because of the potential of receiving higher doses of chemotherapy (e.g., full doses on the prescribed schedule) the patient may be at greater risk of thrombocytopenia and anaemia. Regular monitoring of platelet count and haematocrit is recommended. Special care should be taken when administering single or combination chemotherapeutic agents which are known to cause severe thrombocytopenia.

The use of Neupogen-mobilised PBPCs has been shown to reduce the depth and duration of thrombocytopenia following myelosuppressive or myeloablative chemotherapy.

*Other special precautions:* The effects of Neupogen in patients with substantially reduced myeloid progenitors have not been studied. Neupogen acts primarily on neutrophil precursors to exert its effect in elevating neutrophil counts. Therefore in patients with reduced precursors neutrophil response may be diminished (such as those treated with extensive radiotherapy or chemotherapy).

The effect of Neupogen on graft versus host disease has not been defined.

*Special precautions in patients undergoing peripheral blood progenitor cell mobilisation: Mobilisation:* There are no prospectively randomised comparisons of the two recommended mobilisation methods (filgrastim alone, or in combination with myelosuppressive chemotherapy) within the same patient population. The degree of variation between individual patients and between laboratory assays of CD34+ cells mean that direct comparison between different studies is difficult. It is therefore difficult to recommend an optimum method. The choice of mobilisation method should be considered in relation to the overall objectives of treatment for an individual patient.

*Prior exposure to cytotoxic agents:* Patients who have undergone very extensive prior myelosuppressive therapy may not show sufficient mobilisation of PBPC to achieve the recommended minimum yield (≥ 2.0 x $10^6$ CD34+ cells/kg) or acceleration of platelet recovery, to the same degree.

Some cytotoxic agents exhibit particular toxicities to the haematopoietic progenitor pool, and may adversely affect progenitor mobilisation. Agents such as melphalan, carmustine (BCNU), and carboplatin, when administered over prolonged periods prior to attempts at progenitor mobilisation may reduce progenitor yield. However, the administration of melphalan, carboplatin or BCNU together *with* Neupogen, has been shown to be effective for progenitor mobilisation. When a peripheral blood progenitor cell transplantation is envisaged it is advisable to plan the stem cell mobilisation procedure early in the treatment course of the patient. Particular attention should be paid to the number of progenitors mobilised in such patients *before* the administration of high-dose chemotherapy. If yields are inadequate, as measured by the criteria above, alternative forms of treatment, not requiring progenitor support should be considered.

*Assessment of progenitor cell yields:* In assessing the number of progenitor cells harvested in patients treated with Neupogen, particular attention should be paid to the method of quantitation. The results of flow cytometric analysis of CD34+ cell numbers vary depending on the precise methodology used and recommendations of numbers based on studies in other laboratories need to be interpreted with caution.

Statistical analysis of the relationship between the number of CD34+ cells re-infused and the rate of platelet recovery after high-dose chemotherapy indicates a complex but continuous relationship. Currently the minimum yield of CD34+ cells is not well defined. The recommendation of a minimum yield of ≥ 2.0 x $10^6$ CD34+ cells/kg is based on published experience resulting in adequate haematologic reconstitution. Yields in excess of this appear to correlate with more rapid recovery, those below with slower recovery.

*Special precautions in SCN patients: Blood cell counts:* Platelet counts should be monitored closely, especially during the first few weeks of Neupogen therapy. Consideration should be given to intermittent cessation or decreasing the dose of Neupogen in

patients who develop thrombocytopenia, i.e. platelets consistently < 100,000/cmm.

Other blood cell changes occur, including anaemia and transient increases in myeloid progenitors, which require close monitoring of cell counts.

*Transformation to leukaemia or pre-leukaemia:* Special care should be taken in the diagnosis of severe chronic neutropenias to distinguish from other haematologic disorders such as aplastic anaemia, myelodysplasia, and myeloid leukaemia. Complete blood cell counts with differential and platelet counts, and an evaluation of bone marrow morphology and karyotype should be performed prior to treatment.

There was a low frequency (approximately 3%) of myelodysplastic syndromes (MDS) or leukaemia in patients with severe congenital neutropenia treated with Neupogen. This observation has only been made in patients with congenital neutropenia. MDS and leukaemias are natural complications of the disease and are of uncertain relation to Neupogen therapy. A subset of approximately 12% of patients who had normal cytogenetic evaluations at baseline were subsequently found to have abnormalities, including monosomy 7, on routine repeat evaluation. If patients with severe chronic neutropenia develop abnormal cytogenetics, the risks and benefits of continuing Neupogen should be carefully weighed; Neupogen should be discontinued if MDS or leukaemia occur. It is currently unclear whether long-term treatment of patients with severe congenital neutropenia will predispose patients to cytogenetic abnormalities, MDS or leukaemic transformation. It is recommended to perform morphologic and cytogenetic bone marrow examinations in patients at regular intervals (approximately every 12 months).

Other special precautions: Causes of transient neutropenia, such as viral infections, should be excluded.

Splenic enlargement is a direct effect of treatment with Neupogen. 31% of patients in studies were documented as having palpable splenomegaly. Increases in volume, measured radiographically, occurred early during Neupogen therapy and tended to plateau. Dose reductions were noted to slow or stop the progression of splenic enlargement, and in 3% of patients a splenectomy was required. Spleen size should be evaluated regularly. Abdominal palpation should be sufficient to detect abnormal increases in splenic volume.

Haematuria/proteinuria occurred in a small number of patients. Regular urinalysis should be performed to monitor this event.

The safety and efficacy in neonates and patients with autoimmune neutropenia have not been established.

*Interaction with other medicaments and other forms of interaction:* The safety and efficacy of Neupogen given on the same day as myelosuppressive cytotoxic chemotherapy have not been definitively established. In view of the sensitivity of rapidly dividing myeloid cells to myelosuppressive cytotoxic chemotherapy, the use of Neupogen is not recommended in the period from 24 hours before to 24 hours after chemotherapy. Preliminary evidence from a small number of patients treated concomitantly with Neupogen and 5-Fluorouracil indicate that the severity of neutropenia may be exacerbated. Possible interactions with other haematopoietic growth factors and cytokines have not yet been investigated in clinical trials.

*Pregnancy and lactation:* The safety of Neupogen has not been established in pregnant women. There is no evidence from studies in rats and rabbits that Neupogen is teratogenic. An increased incidence of embryo-loss has been observed in rabbits, but no malformation has been seen. In pregnancy, the possible risk of Neupogen use to the foetus must be weighed against the expected therapeutic benefit.

It is not known whether Neupogen is excreted in human milk. Neupogen is not recommended for use in nursing women.

*Effects on ability to drive and use machines:* No effects have been reported.

*Undesirable effects:*
*In cancer patients:* In clinical trials the most frequent clinical adverse events attributable to Neupogen at the recommended dose were mild or moderate musculoskeletal pain, occurring in 10%, and severe musculoskeletal pain in 3% of patients. Musculoskeletal pain is usually controlled with standard analgesics. Less frequent adverse events include urinary abnormalities predominantly mild or moderate dysuria.

In randomised, placebo-controlled clinical trials, Neupogen did not increase the incidence of clinical adverse events associated with cytotoxic chemotherapy. Adverse events reported with equal frequency in patients treated with Neupogen/chemotherapy and placebo/chemotherapy included nausea and vomiting, alopecia, diarrhoea, fatigue, anorexia, mucositis, headache, cough, skin rash, chest pain, generalised weakness, sore throat, constipation and unspecified pain.

Reversible, dose-dependent and usually mild or moderate elevations of lactate dehydrogenase, alkaline phosphatase, serum uric acid, and gamma-glutamyl transpeptidase occurred with Neupogen in approximately 50%, 35%, 25%, and 10% of patients, respectively at recommended doses.

Transient decreases in blood pressure, not requiring clinical treatment, have been reported occasionally.

Vascular disorders, including veno-occlusive disease and fluid volume disturbances, have been reported occasionally in patients undergoing high dose chemotherapy followed by autologous bone marrow transplantation. The causal association with Neupogen has not been established.

Symptoms suggestive of allergic-type reactions have been reported in rare cases, approximately half of these were associated with the initial dose. Overall, reports were more common after intravenous administration. In some cases, rechallenge resulted in a recurrence of symptoms.

*In severe chronic neutropenia (SCN) patients:* Adverse reactions related to Neupogen therapy in SCN patients have been reported and for some their frequency tend to decrease with time.

The most frequent clinical adverse events attributable to Neupogen were bone pain, and general musculoskeletal pain.

Other events seen include splenic enlargement, which may be progressive in a minority of cases, and thrombocytopenia. Headache, and diarrhoea have been reported shortly after starting Neupogen therapy, typically in less than 10% of patients. Anaemia and epistaxis have also been reported with a similar incidence but only following sustained administration.

Transient increases with no clinical symptoms were observed in serum uric acid, lactic dehydrogenase, and alkaline phosphatase. Transient, moderate decreases in non-fasting blood glucose have also been seen.

Adverse events possibly related to Neupogen therapy and typically occurring in < 2% of SCN patients were injection site reaction headache, hepatomegaly, arthralgia, alopecia, osteoporosis, and rash.

During long-term use cutaneous vasculitis has been reported in 2% of SCN patients. There have been very few instances of proteinuria/haematuria.

*Overdose:* The effects of Neupogen overdosage have not been established. Discontinuation of Neupogen therapy usually results in a 50% decrease in circulating neutrophils within 1 to 2 days, with a return to normal levels in 1 to 7 days.

## Pharmacological properties

*Pharmacodynamic properties:* Human G-CSF is a glycoprotein which regulates the production and release of functional neutrophils from the bone marrow. Neupogen containing r-metHuG-CSF causes marked increases in peripheral blood neutrophil counts within twenty-four hours, with minor increases in monocytes. In some severe chronic neutropenia patients Neupogen can also induce a minor increase in the number of circulating eosinophils and basophils relative to baseline; some of these patients may present with eosinophilia or basophilia already prior to treatment. Elevations of neutrophil counts are dose-dependent at recommended doses. Neutrophils produced in response to Neupogen show normal or enhanced function as demonstrated by tests of chemotactic and phagocytic function. Following termination of Neupogen therapy, circulating neutrophil counts decrease by 50% within 1 to 2 days, and to normal levels within 1 to 7 days.

Use of Neupogen in patients undergoing cytotoxic chemotherapy or myeloablative therapy followed by bone marrow transplantation leads to significant reductions in the incidence, severity and duration of neutropenia and febrile neutropenia.

Use of Neupogen, either alone, or after chemotherapy, mobilises haematopoietic progenitor cells into the peripheral blood. These autologous Peripheral Blood Progenitor Cells (PBPCs) may be harvested and infused after high-dose cytotoxic therapy, either in place of, or in addition to bone marrow transplantation. Infusion of PBPCs accelerates haematopoietic recovery reducing the duration of risk for haemorrhagic complications and the need for platelet transfusions.

Use of Neupogen in patients, children or adults, with severe chronic neutropenia (severe congenital, cyclic, and idiopathic neutropenia) induces a sustained increase in absolute neutrophil counts in peripheral blood and a reduction of infection and related events.

*Pharmacokinetic properties:* Clearance of r-metHuG-CSF has been shown to follow first-order pharmacokinetics after both subcutaneous and intravenous administration. The serum elimination half-life of r-metHuG-CSF is approximately 3.5 hours, with a clearance rate of approximately 0.6ml/min/kg. Continuous infusion with Neupogen over a period of up to 28 days, in patients recovering from autologous bone-marrow transplantation, resulted in no evidence of drug accumulation and comparable elimination half-lives. There is a positive linear correlation between the dose and the serum concentration of r-metHuG-CSF, whether administered intravenously or subcutaneously. Following subcutaneous administration of recommended doses, serum concentrations were maintained above 10ng/ml for 8 to 16 hours. The volume of distribution in blood is approximately 150ml/kg.

*Preclinical safety data:* There are no preclinical data of relevance to the prescriber which are additional to that already included in other sections of the SPC.

## Pharmaceutical particulars

*List of excipients:* Neupogen is a sterile, clear, colourless liquid. Neupogen is formulated in an aqueous sodium acetate buffer containing Sorbitol and Polysorbate 80.

*Incompatibilities:* Neupogen should not be diluted with saline solutions.

*Shelf life:* Under recommended storage conditions, Neupogen is stable for up to 24 months.

*Special precautions for storage:* Neupogen 30 and Neupogen 48 should be stored in a refrigerator at 2–8°C.

Accidental exposure to freezing temperatures does not adversely affect the stability of Neupogen.

Neupogen should not be used after the given expiry date.

Diluted Neupogen solutions should not be prepared more than 24 hours before administration and should be stored refrigerated at 2–8°C.

Neupogen vials and pre-filled syringes are for single dose use only.

*Nature and contents of container:* Neupogen 30 is supplied in colourless glass vials with rubber stoppers and pre-filled syringes containing 30 million units, equivalent to 300μg of filgrastim.

Neupogen 48 is supplied in colourless glass vials with rubber stoppers and pre-filled syringes containing 48 million units, equivalent to 480μg of filgrastim.

*Instructions for use/handling:* If required, Neupogen may be diluted in 5% glucose.

Dilute Neupogen may be absorbed to glass and plastic materials. Dilution to a final concentration less than 0.2 MU (2μg) per ml is not recommended at any time.

For patients treated with Neupogen diluted to concentration below 1.5 MU (15μg) per ml, human serum albumin (HSA) should be added to a final concentration of 2 mg/ml.

*Example:* In a final injection volume of 20 ml, total doses of Neupogen less than 30 MU (300μg) should be given with 0.2 ml of 20% human albumin solution PhEur added.

When diluted in 5% glucose solution, Neupogen is compatible with glass and a variety of plastics included PVC, polyolefin (a co-polymer of polypropylene and polyethylene) and polypropylene.

### Marketing authorisation numbers

| Vials | 0031/0268 |
| Syringes 30 MU | 0031/0450 |
| Syringes 48 MU | 0031/0451 |

**Date of approval/revision of SPC** January 1997

**Legal category** POM

# POSICOR* ▼

**Qualitative and quantitative composition** Posicor is supplied as film-coated tablets, containing the active ingredient mibefradil dihydrochloride (pure enantiomer) equivalent to either 50 or 100 mg of mibefradil.

**Pharmaceutical form** Posicor 50 is supplied as white, hexagonal, biconvex, breakable film-coated tablets.

Posicor 100 is supplied as pink, hexagonal, biconvex, breakable film-coated tablets.

## Clinical particulars
*Therapeutic indications:*

*Hypertension* Posicor is indicated for the treatment of essential hypertension.

*Stable angina pectoris* Posicor is indicated for the treatment of stable angina pectoris.

*Posology and method of administration:*
*Adults:*

*Hypertension:* The recommended initial dose of Posicor is 50 mg once daily. Titration to 100 mg once daily should be based on blood pressure response.

*Stable angina pectoris:* The recommended initial dose of Posicor is 50 mg once daily. Titration to 100 mg once daily should be based on therapeutic response.

Posicor can be administered either before, during or after meals. Film-coated tablets should be swallowed and not chewed.

*Patient groups:* In elderly patients or those with renal impairment, no dose adjustment of Posicor is required.

Since mibefradil is extensively metabolised by the liver, caution should be exercised when administering Posicor to patients with hepatic insufficiency. See *Special warnings and special precautions for use.*

*Children:* Safety and efficacy in children have not been established, therefore, Posicor is not recommended for administration to children.

*Contra-indications:*

1. In patients with sick sinus syndrome or 2nd or 3rd degree AV block, without a pacemaker.

2. In patients with a known sensitivity to mibefradil or to any of the other components of the formulation.

3. Pregnancy, lactation and use in women of child bearing potential unless adequate contraceptive measures are undertaken.

4. Co-administration of terfenadine, astemizole or cisapride with Posicor.

5. Severe hepatic impairment

6. Moderate to severe heart failure (NYHA class III or IV)

7. Acute myocardial infarction within 4 weeks of the event or unstable angina pectoris

*Special warnings and precautions for use:*
*General:* Since the vasodilation induced by mibefradil is gradual in onset of action, hypotension was not seen after first oral administration of Posicor at the recommended doses. However, as with other peripheral vasodilators, caution should be exercised when administering Posicor to patients with severe aortic stenosis.

*Use in patients with congestive heart failure:* Clinical experience in congestive heart failure with the recommended doses of mibefradil is limited. In some patients, deterioration of heart failure may occur at the higher dose. As with many other calcium antagonists, mibefradil should be avoided in patients with symptomatic heart failure, until further data from ongoing long-term studies are available (see *Contra-indications*).

*Patients with hepatic insufficiency:* No clinically relevant change in the pharmacokinetics of mibefradil in patients with mild to moderate liver impairment was observed after single doses of 100 mg Posicor. However, as mibefradil is completely metabolised and eliminated mainly via the biliary route, monitoring of blood pressure and heart rate is advised when administering Posicor to patients with mild to moderate hepatic impairment. As there are no data available, Posicor should not be used in patients with severe hepatic impairment (see *Contra-indications*).

*Cardiac conduction and impulse formation:* Posicor affects sinus and AV node conduction.

The effect on the sinus node results in a dose dependent reduction in heart rate of around 5 bpm with 50 mg and 9 bpm with 100 mg. Patients with a pre-treatment heart rate below 55 beats per minute should be followed regularly. In the absence of sufficient data, mibefradil is not recommended for patients with a pre-treatment heart rate below 50 beats per minute.

The effect on the AV node results in small increases in PR interval of 3 msec (50 mg) and 10 msec (100 mg). Posicor should not be administered to patients with 2nd or 3rd degree AV block, who are without a pacemaker (see *Contra-indications*).

*Use in combination with beta-blockers:* When mibefradil was combined with beta-blockers, additive effects in reducing blood pressure and heart rate, as well as increasing PR-interval, were observed. Care should be taken when combining mibefradil with beta-blockers, and patients should be closely monitored at treatment initiation, particularly when pre-treatment heart rate is below 60 beats per minute and/or if there is first degree AV block. Combination of mibefradil with beta-blockers is not recommended for patients with a pre-treatment heart rate below 55 beats per minute.

*Acute myocardial infarction and unstable angina pectoris:* As there are no data available, Posicor should not be used in acute myocardial infarction within 4 weeks of the event or in unstable angina pectoris (see *Contra-indications*).

*Interaction with other medicaments* and other forms of interaction: Since mibefradil is mainly bound to alpha-1 acid glycoprotein it will not displace drugs which bind to serum albumin e.g. warfarin, phenytoin, digoxin.

In specific interaction studies enalapril, atenolol, metoprolol, theophylline, and cimetidine (low dose of 400 mg bid), had no clinically relevant effect on the plasma pharmacokinetics of mibefradil itself.

In vitro results indicate that some isozymes of the cytochrome P450 (CYP) enzyme system are inhibited in the presence of mibefradil or its metabolites. Co-administration of Posicor with drugs metabolised by these isozymes may result in altered plasma concentrations of these drugs.

*Drugs metabolised by CYP 2D6:* Mibefradil can inhibit the activity of the enzyme CYP 2D6 (debrisoquine hydroxylase) consequently causing previously normal metabolisers of this enzyme to resemble poor CYP 2D6 metabolisers. Depending on the fraction of the drug metabolised by CYP 2D6, the increase in plasma concentration of the drug may be small or quite large. Concomitant use of Posicor with drugs metabolised by CYP 2D6 may require dose adjustment of the other drugs, especially if such drugs have a narrow therapeutic range such as type 1C antiarrhythmics and tricyclic antidepressants (particularly those with high first pass effect e.g. desipramine and imipramine).

*Drugs metabolised by CYP 3A4:* Mibefradil may increase plasma concentrations of co-administered drugs which are primarily metabolised by the cytochrome CYP 3A4 enzyme system and may consequently increase or prolong their therapeutic and adverse effects. Therefore, unless otherwise specified, dosage adjustment of these drugs may be necessary.

*Drugs metabolised by CYP 2D6 and/or CYP 3A4 and which prolong QT:* Since elevation of plasma concentrations of these drugs (eg thioridazine, other neuroleptics and class IA and III antiarrhythmics) could be associated with life threatening arrhythmias co-administration of mibefradil with these drugs should be carefully monitored. No clinically relevant pharmacodynamic interaction was observed for quinidine (see below).

*Specific interaction studies:* In specific studies, no clinically relevant interactions have been observed between the recommended doses of mibefradil and enalapril, atenolol, or cimetidine. Despite in vitro evidence of inhibition of CYP 1A2, no pharmacokinetic interaction was observed with theophylline, a CYP 1A2 substrate. In healthy volunteers, small elevations in digoxin peak plasma levels (20–30%) were found during co-administration with Posicor 50 mg and 100 mg; however, trough plasma levels were unchanged. Additionally, in patients with congestive heart failure, trough plasma concentrations of digoxin remained unchanged. Nevertheless, due to the potential for additive effects on AV conduction, patients receiving chronic digoxin therapy concomitantly with mibefradil should be closely monitored.

The following drug interactions have been identified involving mibefradil and other drugs metabolised by the cytochrome P450 system:

*Terfenadine:* Co-administration of terfenadine with mibefradil in healthy subjects led to elevated plasma concentrations of terfenadine, resulting in a 12% increase in mean QTc interval. Since QTc prolongation due to elevated plasma concentrations of terfenadine can be associated with instances of life threatening cardiac dysrhythmias and death, co-administration of Posicor with terfenadine is contraindicated. By analogy, co-administration of cisapride or astemizole with Posicor is contra-indicated (see *Contra-indications*).

*Cyclosporine A:* Cyclosporine A (Sandimmune\*) levels increased about 2-fold under concomitant treatment with 50 mg Posicor for 8 days. Therefore, cyclosporine A levels should be monitored and its dose adjusted accordingly.

*Quinidine:* In healthy volunteers, elevations in peak quinidine plasma concentrations (15–19%) and AUC (50%) were found during co-administration of single doses of quinidine with Posicor 50 and 100 mg; however, the metabolite which is also active was markedly reduced. No clinically relevant pharmacodynamic interactions were observed.

*Metoprolol:* Co-administration of Posicor with metoprolol in healthy subjects resulted in a 2-fold increase in peak plasma concentrations of metoprolol and about 4–5-fold increase in AUC. Elimination half-life increased from 3 hours to 7 to 8 hours. Although the pharmacodynamic effects in this study appeared to be only additive, dosage adjustment of metoprolol may be required.

In clinical studies, Posicor has been safely administered with commonly used drugs such as diuretics, beta-blockers, ACE-inhibitors, non-steroidal anti-inflammatory drugs, long acting nitrates, sublingual nitroglycerin, oral hypoglycemics, lipid lowering agents, conjugated estrogens, antibiotics, and antithrombotics.

*Pregnancy and lactation:* There are no adequate and well-controlled studies of Posicor in pregnant women.

In the rat and the monkey teratogenic effects were observed. Furthermore a prolongation of gestation and delivery was observed in animals. Mibefradil has also been shown to be excreted in the milk of lactating rats. Therefore Posicor may not be used during pregnancy, lactation nor in women of child bearing potential unless adequate contraceptive measures are undertaken (see also *Contra-indications*).

*Effects on ability to drive and use machines:* There are no specific data available about effects on the ability to drive or operate machinery. In patients in whom dizziness, fatigue or light headed feeling occur, caution should be exercised since reaction time may be adversely affected.

*Undesirable effects:* Posicor is generally well tolerated. In most cases side effects are transient and mild or moderate in degree. In placebo-controlled trials, the rate of discontinuation of Posicor 50 mg and 100 mg due to side effects was similar to that observed in patients treated with placebo. The most common dose related side effects observed with Posicor in these trials were leg edema, fatigue, lightheaded feeling and dizziness. The incidence of each of these side-effects for 50 mg of Posicor was similar to placebo and for 100 mg of Posicor did not exceed 3.5%.

The most common ECG changes arising from treatment with mibefradil were 1st degree AV-block and sinus bradycardia. Placebo subtracted incidences of sinus bradycardia (heart rate < 45 bpm) were 0.7% at 50 mg and 1.4% at 100 mg. Placebo subtracted incidences of 1st degree AV block (PR interval > 200 msec) were 1.1% at 50 mg and 7.4% at 100 mg. Treatment with Posicor has rarely been associated with 2nd degree AV block (0.2% at 50 and 100 mg). Symptomatic bradycardia and sino-atrial node dysfunction were very rarely observed at the recommended doses of Posicor.

Isolated cases of immune thrombocytopenia and angioedema occurred, although a causal relationship could not be established.

*Overdose:* At present there has been no experience with overdosage. Due to the pharmacodynamic properties of mibefradil an overdosage could be expected to cause excessive peripheral vasodilation with marked hypotension, bradycardia and high degree AV block. If an overdosage occurs, active cardiac and respiratory monitoring should be instituted. Frequent blood pressure measurements are essential. Should hypotension occur, cardiovascular support including elevation of the extremities and the judicious administration of fluids should be initiated. If hypotension remains unresponsive to these measures, administration of vasopressors (such as phenylephrine) should be considered with attention to circulating volume and urine output.

Bradycardia and conduction system abnormalities may be treated with atropine followed by isoproterenol. Cardiac pacing may be required if haemodynamically significant bradycardia is unresponsive to these measures.

Intravenous calcium gluconate may help to reverse the effects of calcium antagonists. As mibefradil is highly bound to plasma proteins, it can not be removed by dialysis.

## Pharmacological properties

*Pharmacodynamic properties:* ATC-code: C08CX01.

Pharmacotherapeutic class: Calcium channel blocker.

Mibefradil exerts its pharmacological effect by modulating the transmembrane influx of ionic calcium into vascular smooth muscle and cardiac muscle. Mibefradil belongs to a separate class of calcium antagonists which selectively blocks low voltage dependent T calcium channels in addition to high voltage dependent L calcium channels. The clinical significance of this property has not been fully elucidated, but since T channels are present in vascular smooth muscle cells, sino-atrial node cells and the conduction system of the heart, their blockade might contribute to the vasodilation, the reduction in heart rate and the slowing of AV conduction associated with mibefradil. On the L channel mibefradil binds to a site exerting no interaction with the dihydropyridine binding site.

No negative inotropic effect was observed at therapeutic concentrations in several in vitro and in vivo preclinical studies.

The plasma concentrations of mibefradil are predictive of its pharmacological effects.

Data on the long-term effects of mibefradil on mortality and cardiovascular morbidity are not available.

Hypertension: Mibefradil is a peripheral arterial vasodilator that acts directly on vascular smooth muscle to cause a reduction in peripheral vascular resistance, and thereby a reduction in blood pressure. Mibefradil does not induce reflex tachycardia, but rather causes a slight reduction in heart rate. Additive antihypertensive effects have been observed when mibefradil was combined with diuretics, ACE-inhibitors and beta-blockers.

The antihypertensive efficacy of Posicor was demonstrated in the sitting, standing and supine positions. Blood pressure is smoothly controlled over the 24-hour dosing interval. Onset of action is gradual, with full effect reached within 1–2 weeks. Tolerance does not develop on long-term exposure nor is rebound observed following drug discontinuation.

Posicor was effective in lowering high blood pressure in patients with chronic renal failure complicated by systemic hypertension.

Stable angina pectoris: In patients with chronic stable angina pectoris Posicor reduces heart rate, total peripheral resistance (afterload) and double product (heart rate x systolic blood pressure), resulting in a decrease in cardiac workload and myocardial oxygen demand. Additive anti-anginal and anti-ischemic effects have been observed when mibefradil was combined with nitrates and beta-blockers.

Posicor produces a significant increase in exercise tolerance test parameters: symptom limited exercise duration, time to onset of angina pectoris and time to onset of ischemia (persistent 1 mm ST segment depression). Treatment with Posicor is associated with a dose related decrease in anginal episodes, nitroglycerin consumption and the number and duration of silent ischemic episodes. Tolerance does not develop on long-term exposure nor is rebound observed following drug discontinuation.

Electrocardiology: Mibefradil can cause dose related flattening of the T wave and an increase in the voltage of the U wave. The U wave can sometimes merge with the T wave. At supratherapeutic doses, the resulting pattern has sometimes been misread (especially by automated electrocardiography) as one of QTc prolongation. Similar patterns have been seen in association with high and supratherapeutic doses of some other calcium antagonists. No clinical consequences have been observed.

*Pharmacokinetic properties:*

*Absorption and bioavailability:* Mibefradil is rapidly absorbed after oral administration. Peak plasma levels are reached within 1–2 hours after administration. Bioavailability of a single oral dose (drinking solution) of 80 mg mibefradil was 70%. The presence of food has no effect on rate and extent of absorption.

*Distribution:* Volume of distribution at steady-state ($V_{ss}$) amounts to about 200 L. Mibefradil is highly bound to plasma proteins ($\geq$ 99% at therapeutic concentrations), principally to alpha 1-acid glycoprotein (95%).

*Metabolism:* Metabolism of mibefradil is mediated by two pathways: esterase catalysed hydrolysis of the ester side-chain to yield an alcohol metabolite and cytochrome P450 catalysed oxidation.

Mibefradil inhibits its own metabolism by inhibition of cytochrome P450 3A4 . By that mechanism the plasma level of the alcohol metabolite increases after chronic dosing. In animal models the pharmacological effect of this alcohol metabolite was about 10% of the parent compound.

*Excretion:* The elimination half-life following chronic dosing is 17–35 hours. During once daily dosing, steady-state conditions are reached by around 1 week.

Mibefradil is cleared by metabolic inactivation and excreted into the faeces (75%) and urine (25%). Less than 3% of mibefradil is excreted unchanged into the urine. Mean (% coefficient of variation) oral clearance following chronic doses in the therapeutic range amounts to 9 (30%) L/h. No clinically relevant influence of demographic factors (age, race, gender, bodyweight) on clearance have been found.

*Preclinical safety data:* Gingival overgrowth, characteristic of other calcium antagonists in man and animals, was observed in marmoset and rat toxicity studies.

In a two year study, squamous cell carcinomas have been observed in the gingivae of rats receiving mibefradil mixed in a coarse powdered diet. This diet is known to induce by itself marked periodontitis. Further investigations demonstrated that these tumours probably arose from enhancement of the pre-existing periodontal disease, although a direct effect of mibefradil alone cannot be excluded. These findings are not considered to be relevant to humans where clinical experience shows no evidence of treatment related adverse events in the oral cavity.

There was no evidence of mutagenicity.

In rat and monkey teratogenic effects were observed. (See also *Contra-indications* and *Pregnancy and lactation*).

## Pharmaceutical particulars

*List of excipients:* The excipients in each 50 mg and 100 mg film-coated tablet are: Lactose anhydrous, maize starch, povidone K30, talc, sodium stearyl fumarate, hypromellose, ethylcellulose, triacetine, titanium dioxide (E171), red iron oxide (only for 100 mg) (E 172).

*Incompatibilities:* Not applicable.

*Shelf life:* Film-coated tablets–3 years.

*Special precautions for storage:* 50 mg and 100 mg film-coated tablets. Store below 30°C.

*Nature of contents and container:* PVC/PE/PVDC/A triplex blister strip containing 7 film-coated tablets or 10 film-coated tablets.

*Pack size:* For 50 mg film-coated tablets 7, 10, 14, 20, 28, 50, 98 and 100 film-coated tablets. For 100 mg film-coated tablets 7, 10, 14, 20, 28, 50, 98 and 100 film-coated tablets.

*Instructions for use/handling:* Not applicable.

Marketing authorisation numbers
50 mg tablets      14878/0008
100 mg tablets     14878/0009

Date of approval/revision of SPC   July 1997

Legal category   POM

# PULMOZYME*

**Qualitative and quantitative composition** Pulmozyme (dornase alfa) contains the phosphorylated glycosylated recombinant protein human deoxyribonuclease 1.

The active ingredient in Pulmozyme is dornase alfa, which is similar to human DNase isolated from urine. Pulmozyme is a sterile solution for respiratory use at a concentration of 1000 U/ml (1 mg/ml), where 1 Genentech unit/ml = 1μg/ml. The labelled protein concentration is based solely upon the anhydrous polypeptide content and does not include the mass contribution of the carbohydrate or phosphate.

**Pharmaceutical form** Pulmozyme is a sterile, clear, colourless solution for respiratory use and is administered by means of a compressed air-driven (jet) nebulizer. Each single-unit ampoule of Pulmozyme will deliver to the nebulizer chamber 2,500 U (2.5 mg) of the active ingredient, dornase alfa.

## Clinical particulars

*Therapeutic indications:* Daily administration of Pulmozyme is indicated in the management of cystic fibrosis patients with an FVC of greater than 40% of predicted and over 5 years of age to improve pulmonary function.

*Posology and method of administration:* The recommended dose is 2,500 U (corresponding to 2.5 mg) dornase alfa once daily, i.e. inhale the contents of one ampoule of 2.5 ml solution undiluted.

Most patients gain optimal benefit from continuous daily use of Pulmozyme. Studies in which dornase alfa was given on an intermittent regimen indicate that improvement in pulmonary function rapidly subsides on cessation of therapy. Therefore patients should be instructed to take their medication every day.

For patients on Pulmozyme therapy who experience exacerbation of respiratory tract infection, administration of Pulmozyme can be safely continued.

Pulmozyme should be administered using a jet nebulizer. The patient should continue his/her standard regimen of chest physiotherapy. At present, no recommendation can be made as to the optimal time of day for administration of Pulmozyme.

Patients should continue to receive regular medical care when being treated with Pulmozyme. The safety and efficacy of daily administration has not yet been demonstrated in patients under the age of 5 years, or with FVC less than 40% of predicted. Some patients over the age of 21 years may benefit from twice daily therapy.

*Contra-indications:* Pulmozyme should not be administered to patients with known hypersensitivity to the product or its constituents.

*Special warnings and special precautions for use:* None.

*Interaction with other medicaments and other forms of interaction:* There are no known interactions. Pulmozyme should not be mixed with other drugs or solutions in the nebulizer (see *Incompatibilities*). Mixing of Pulmozyme with other drugs or solutions could lead to adverse structural and/or functional changes in Pulmozyme or the admixed compound.

Pulmozyme can be effectively and safely used in conjunction with standard cystic fibrosis therapies such as antibiotics, bronchodilators, digestive enzymes, vitamins, inhaled and systemic corticosteroids, and analgesics.

*Pregnancy and lactation:* The safety of Pulmozyme has not been established in pregnant women. Studies of dornase alfa in rabbits and rodents show no evidence of impaired fertility, teratogenicity, or effects on development, However, because animal reproduction studies are not always predictive of the human response, Pulmozyme should be used during pregnancy only if clearly needed.

It is not known whether Pulmozyme is excreted in human milk. Because many drugs are excreted in human milk, caution should be exercised when Pulmozyme is administered to a nursing woman. A study performed in lactating cynomolgus monkeys, in which high doses of dornase alfa were given by the intravenous route, low concentrations (< 0.1% of the concentrations seen in the serum of pregnant cynomolgus), were measurable in the maternal milk. When used as directed, there is minimal systemic absorption of dornase alfa; little or no measurable concentrations of dornase alfa would be expected in human milk.

*Effects on ability to drive and use machines:* No effects on the patient's ability to drive and use machines have been reported.

*Undesirable effects:* Few patients experienced adverse events resulting in permanent discontinuation from dornase alfa, and the discontinuation rate was observed similarly between placebo (2%) and dornase alfa (3%).

In controlled clinical trials directly comparing dornase alfa [up to 2,500 U (2.5 mg) BID] to placebo for up to 6 months, most adverse events were the sequelae of the underlying lung disease. There was no significant difference in the incidence or frequency of adverse events when patients continued treatment for an additional 6 months of open-label therapy. Patients who experience adverse events common to cystic fibrosis can, in general, safely continue administration of Pulmozyme as evidenced by the high percentage of patients completing the clinical trials.

Adverse events frequently seen were pharyngitis (inflammation of the throat), chest pain and voice alteration (hoarseness). Occasionally, laryngitis (inflammation of the larynx), conjunctivitis and skin rash, with and without itchiness, were observed. Upon initiation of dornase alfa therapy, as with any aerosol, pulmonary function may decline and expectoration of sputum may increase.

There have been no reports of anaphylaxis attributed to the administration of dornase alfa. Skin rashes and urticaria have been observed, and have been mild and transient in nature. Less than 5% of patients treated with dornase alfa have developed antibodies to dornase alfa, and none of these patients have developed IgE antibodies to dornase alfa. Improvement in pulmonary function tests has still occurred even after the development of antibodies to dornase alfa.

*Overdose:* Pulmozyme overdosage has not been established. Single-dose inhalation studies in rats and monkeys at doses up to 180-fold higher than doses routinely used in clinical studies are well tolerated. Oral administration of dornase alfa in doses up to 200 mg/kg are also well tolerated by rats. In clinical studies, CF patients have received up to 20 mg dornase alfa BID for up to six days and 10 mg BID intermittently (2 weeks on/2 weeks off drug) for 168 days. Both dose regimens were shown to be well tolerated.

## Pharmacological properties

*Pharmacodynamic properties:* Recombinant human DNase is a genetically engineered version of a naturally occurring human enzyme which cleaves extracellular DNA.

Retention of viscous purulent secretions in the airways contributes both to reduced pulmonary function and to exacerbations of infection. Purulent secretions contain very high concentrations of extracellular DNA, a viscous polyanion released by degenerating leukocytes, which accumulate in response to infection. *In vitro*, dornase alfa hydrolyses DNA in sputum and greatly reduces the viscoelasticity of cystic fibrosis sputum.

*Pharmacokinetic properties:* Inhalation studies conducted in rats and non-human primates show a low percentage of dornase alfa systemic absorption, < 15% for rats and < 2% for monkeys. Consistent with the results of these animal studies, dornase alfa administered to patients as an inhaled aerosol shows low systemic exposure.

Studies in rats and monkeys have shown that, following intravenous administration, dornase alfa was cleared rapidly from the serum. The initial volume of distribution was similar to serum volume in these studies.

Studies in rats indicate that, following aerosol administration the disappearance half-life of dornase alfa from the lungs is 11 hours. Absorption of dornase alfa from the gastrointestinal tract following oral administration to rats is negligible.

DNase is normally present in human serum. Inhalation of up to 40 mg of dornase alfa for up to 6 days did not result in a significant elevation of serum DNase concentration above normal endogenous levels. No increase in serum DNase concentration greater than 10ng/ml was observed. Following administration of 2,500 U (2.5 mg) of dornase alfa twice daily for 24 weeks, mean serum DNase concentrations were no different from the mean pre-treatment baseline value of 3.5 ± 0.1ng/ml; suggesting low systemic absorption or accumulation.

Inhalation of 2,500 U (2.5 mg) dornase alfa results in a mean sputum concentration of dornase alfa of approximately 3μg/ml within 15 minutes in CF patients. Concentrations of dornase alfa in sputum rapidly decline following inhalation.

No pharmacokinetic data are available in very young or geriatric animals.

*Preclinical safety data:* Following repeat-daily inhalation exposure for periods of up to 6 months, histopathologic evidence of mild, non-life threatening pulmonary changes were observed in rats and primates at doses to the lungs of 6 to 14 times the clinical dose. The pulmonary changes were reversible following cessation of treatment and were characterized in rodents primarily as an alveolitis and lymphoid hyperplasia. In primates, bronchiolitis and alveolitis were observed in addition to an eosinophilic infiltrate and the presence of hemosiderin-laden macrophages. The treatment-related pulmonary changes are primarily consistent with an expected host response to a foreign protein; evidence of an antibody response to dornase alfa was observed in both species. No evidence of anaphylaxis was observed, despite the presence of significant antibody titers.

High concentrations (up to 10 mg/ml) of dornase alfa in three *in vitro* (Ames, mouse lymphoma, clastogenesis in human PBL) and intravenous doses (up to 10 mg/kg) in one *in vivo* (mouse micronucleus) test systems were shown to be nonmutagenic.

No information regarding carcinogenic potential in animals is currently available. A 2-year inhalation study in rodents is in progress.

## Pharmaceutical particulars

*List of excipients:* The following excipients are contained in a 2.5 ml single-use ampoule of Pulmozyme: Sodium Chloride PhEur; Calcium Chloride Dihydrate PhEur; Water for Injections PhEur. In this formulation, sodium chloride is used as a tonicity modifier, calcium chloride as a stabiliser, and water for injection(s) is the vehicle. Pulmozyme contains no preservatives; the nominal pH is 6.3.

*Incompatibilities:* Pulmozyme is an unbuffered aqueous solution and should not be diluted or mixed with other drugs or solutions in the nebulizer bowl. Mixing of this solution could lead to adverse structural and/or functional changes in Pulmozyme or the admixed compound.

*Shelf life:* Under recommended storage conditions of 2–8°C and protected from strong light, Pulmozyme is stable for up to 24 months.

*Special precautions for storage:* Pulmozyme should be stored in a refrigerator at 2–8°C and protected from strong light. Avoid exposure to excessive heat. A single brief exposure to elevated temperatures (less than or equal to 24 hours at up to 30°C) does not affect product stability.

Pulmozyme should not be used after the given expiry date.

Pulmozyme ampoules are for single administration only.

*Nature and contents of container:* Pulmozyme is supplied in single use, low density polyethylene plastic ampoules. The volume in each ampoule is 2.6 ± 0.1 ml. Each ampoule will deliver 2.5 ml of Pulmozyme to the nebulizer chamber.

*Instructions for use/handling:* The recommended dose for use in patients is one 2,500 U (2.5 mg) single-use ampoule of Pulmozyme inhaled once per day using a recommended nebulizer. Most patients gain optimal benefit from continued daily use of Pulmozyme.

Pulmozyme is provided as a sterile solution for inhalation in single-unit ampoules. At present, only jet nebulizers have been shown to effectively deliver biochemically unaltered dornase alfa. The complete contents of a single ampoule should be placed in the bowl of a jet nebulizer/compressor system, such as the Hudson T Up-draft II/Pulmo-Aide, Airlife Misty/Pulmo-Aide, customised Respirgard/Pulmo-Aide, or AcornII/Pulmo-Aide. Pulmozyme may also be used in conjunction with a reusable jet nebulizer/compressor system, such as the Pari LL/Inhalierboy, Pari LC/Inhalierboy or Master, Aiolos/2 Aiolos.

Current data indicate that ultrasonic nebulizers are unsuitable for delivery of Pulmozyme because they may inactivate Pulmozyme or have unacceptable aerosol characteristics.

The patient should follow the nebulizer and compressor manufacturers' instructions on the use and maintenance of this equipment.

Containment of the aerosol is not necessary.

**Marketing authorisation numbers**   0031/0335

**Date of approval/revision of SPC**   October 1996

**Legal category**   POM

# RIVOTRIL* AMPOULES

**Qualitative and quantitative composition**   Each 1 mg/ml ampoule contains 1 mg of the active ingredient clonazepam.

**Pharmaceutical form**   2 x 1 ml ampoules for injection (active and diluent).

## Clinical particulars

*Therapeutic indications:* Administered intravenously, Rivotril quickly controls status epilepticus in all clinical forms.

*Posology and method of administration:* Rivotril ampoules are for intravenous administration. For the treatment of status epilepticus, the dose and rate of administration are governed by the response of the patient.

*Adults:* 1 mg (one ampoule of active substance mixed with one ampoule of diluent) by slow intravenous injection.

*Elderly:* Care should be taken with the elderly.

*Children:* 0.5 mg (equivalent to half an ampoule of active substance mixed with half an ampoule of diluent) by slow intravenous injection.

*Mode of administration:* Intravenous injection of Rivotril should be into a large vein of the antecubital fossa. The injection should be given slowly–in adults, 1 mg over approximately 30 seconds. This will greatly diminish the rare possibility of hypotension or apnoea occurring. Nevertheless, facilities for resuscitation should always be available.

The contents of the diluent ampoule, which contains 1 ml Water for Injection PhEur, *must* be added to the contents of the other ampoule, which contains 1 mg clonazepam in 1 ml, *immediately* before injection.

Rivotril ampoule solution may be diluted when given in intravenous infusions of saline or dextrose, such as are customary in the treatment of status epilepticus.

Thus, up to 3 mg (3 ampoules) in 250 ml of the following solutions is permissible:

Sodium Chloride Injection BP
Dextrose Injection BP 5% and 10%
Sodium Chloride and Dextrose Injection BP (0.45% sodium chloride and 2.5% dextrose)

This infusion dilution should be made up freshly and used within 12 hours

Maintenance of stability cannot be guaranteed when Rivotril ampoule solution is diluted.

*Contra-indications:* Patients with known sensitivity to benzodiazepines; acute pulmonary insufficiency; respiratory depression.

*Special warnings and special precautions for use:* Rivotril should be used with caution in patients with chronic pulmonary insufficiency, or with impairment of renal or hepatic function, and in the elderly or the debilitated. In these cases dosage may need to be reduced.

As with all other anti-epileptic drugs, treatment with Rivotril even if of short duration, must not be abruptly interrupted, but must be withdrawn by gradually reducing the dose in view of the risk of precipitating status epilepticus. This precaution must also be taken when withdrawing another drug while the patient is still receiving Rivotril therapy.

In cases of loss or bereavement, psychological adjustment may be inhibited by benzodiazepines.

*Interaction with other medicaments and other forms of interaction:* Since alcohol can provoke epileptic seizures, irrespective of therapy, patients should be advised not to drink alcohol while under treatment. In combination with Rivotril, alcohol may modify the effects of the drug, compromise the success of therapy or give rise to unpredictable side-effects.

When Rivotril is used in conjunction with other anti-epileptic drugs, side-effects and toxicity may be more evident, particularly with hydantoins or phenobarbitone and combinations including them. This requires extra care in adjusting dosage in the initial stages of treatment. The combination of Rivotril and sodium valproate has, rarely, been associated with the development of absence status epilepticus. Although some patients tolerate and benefit from this combination of drugs, this potential hazard should be borne in mind when its use is considered.

Known inhibitors of hepatic enzymes, e.g. cimetidine, have been shown to reduce the clearance of benzodiazepines and may potentiate their action and known inducers of hepatic enzymes, e.g. rifampicin, may increase the clearance of benzodiazepines.

*Pregnancy and lactation:* There is little evidence as to the drug safety in human pregnancy nor is there evidence from animal work that it is completely free from hazard. The use of Rivotril during pregnancy or lactation should be avoided unless there are compelling reasons.

The administration of high doses or prolonged administration of low doses of benzodiazepines in the last trimester of pregnancy or during labour has been reported to produce irregularities in the foetal heart rate, and hypotonia, poor sucking and hypothermia in the neonate.

*Effects on ability to drive and use machines:* As a general rule, epileptic patients are not allowed to drive. Even when adequately controlled on Rivotril, it should be remembered that any increase in dosage or alteration in timings of dosage may modify patients' reactions, depending on individual susceptibility. If a patient is allowed to operate machinery, he should also be warned of these possible effects.

*Undesirable effects:* The side-effects observed consist of fatigue, somnolence, occasional muscular hypotonia and co-ordination disturbances. Such effects are usually transitory and disappear spontaneously as treatment continues or with dosage reduction. They tend to occur early in treatment and can be greatly reduced, if not avoided, by commencing with low dosages followed by progressive increases.

Rarely respiratory depression may occur with intravenous Rivotril, particularly if other depressant drugs have been administered.

In infants and small children, and particularly those with a degree of mental impairment, Rivotril may give rise to salivary or bronchial hypersecretion with drooling. Supervision of the airway may be required.

As with other benzodiazepines, isolated cases of blood dyscrasias and abnormal liver function tests have been reported.

Rivotril generally has a beneficial effect on behaviour disturbances in epileptic patients. In certain cases, paradoxical effects such as aggressiveness, irritability, agitation, psychotic disorders and activation of new types of seizures may be precipitated. If these occur, the benefit of continuing the drug should be weighed against the adverse effect. The addition to the regimen of another suitable drug may be necessary or, in some cases, it may be advisable to discontinue Rivotril therapy.

Although Rivotril has been given uneventfully to patients with porphyria, rarely it may induce convulsions in these patients.

*Overdose:* As with other benzodiazepine drugs, overdosage should not present undue problems of management or threat to life. Patients have recovered from overdoses in excess of 60 mg without special treatment. Severe somnolence with muscle hypotonia will be present. Treatment is symptomatic and may include the need to maintain an airway. Gastric lavage may be useful if performed soon after ingestion.

The value of dialysis has not been determined.

Overdosage in non-epileptic patients may be treated with Anexate, a specific IV antidote for use in emergency situations. Patients requiring such intervention should be monitored closely in hospital (see separate prescribing information).

The use of Anexate is not recommended in epileptic patients who have been receiving benzodiazepine treatment for a prolonged period. Although Anexate exerts a slight intrinsic anticonvulsant effect, its abrupt suppression of the protective effect of a benzodiazepine agonist can give rise to convulsions in epileptic patients.

If excitation occurs, barbiturates should not be used.

**Pharmacological properties**

*Pharmacodynamic properties:* Rivotril is a benzodiazepine derivative exhibiting marked anticonvulsant properties. These have been demonstrated in the many tests in animals which are employed to establish the anti-epileptic properties of a drug. Animal experiments and electroencephalographic studies in man have shown that Rivotril prevents generalisation of convulsive activity and raises the seizure threshold. In many cases, abnormal electroencephalograms become normal. Rivotril improves both focal seizures and primarily generalised attacks.

*Pharmacokinetic properties:* Rivotril is widely distributed, then eliminated with a half-life generally between one and two days. Clearance is by metabolism in the liver, by nitro-reduction to the corresponding amine, then acetylation. The metabolites are excreted mainly via the urine. Routine monitoring of plasma concentrations of Rivotril is of unproven value since this does not appear to correlate well with either therapeutic response or side-effects.

*Preclinical safety data:* None stated.

**Pharmaceutical particulars**

*List of excipients: Active substance ampoule:* Ethanol absolute, glacial acetic acid, benzyl alcohol, propylene glycol, nitrogen pure.

*Diluent ampoule:* Water for injections.

*Incompatibilities:* It is recommended that Rivotril is only diluted in accordance with instructions given under posology and method of administration.

*Shelf life:* 60 months.

*Special precautions for storage:* Rivotril ampoules (active and diluent) should be protected from light and stored below 30°C.

*Nature and contents of container:* 2 ml amber glass ampoules. *Twin pack:* 1 active., 1 diluent.

*Instructions for use/handling:* The infusion dilution should be made up freshly and used within 12 hours (see *Mode of administration*).

**Marketing authorisation number** 0031/0078

**Date of approval/revision of SPC** January 1997

**Legal category** POM

## RIVOTRIL*

**Presentation** Round, dull pinkish-buff tablets with RIV 0.5 imprinted on one face and two break bars on the other, containing 0.5 mg clonazepam.

Round, white tablets with RIV 2 imprinted on one face and two break bars on the other, containing 2 mg clonazepam.

Ampoules containing lmg clonazepam in lml solvent, each accompanied by an ampoule containing lml Water for Injection Ph Eur as a diluent. The ampoule solution is colourless.

**Uses** *Properties:* Rivotril is a benzodiazepine derivative exhibiting marked anticonvulsant properties. These have been demonstrated in the many tests in animals which are employed to establish the anti-epileptic properties of a drug. Animal experiments and electroencephalographic studies in man have shown that Rivotril prevents generalisation of convulsive activity and raises the seizure threshold. In many cases, abnormal electroencephalograms become normal. Rivotril improves both focal seizures and primarily generalised attacks. Administered intravenously, Rivotril quickly controls status epilepticus.

Rivotril taken orally is well absorbed to give peak levels within four hours. The drug is widely distributed, then eliminated with a half-life generally between one and two days. Clearance is by metabolism in the liver, by nitro-reduction to the corresponding amine, then acetylation. The metabolites are excreted mainly via the urine. Routine monitoring of plasma concentrations of Rivotril is of unproven value since this does not appear to correlate well with either therapeutic response or side-effects.

*Indications: Tablets:* All clinical forms of epileptic disease and seizures in infants, children and adults, especially absence seizures (petit mal) including atypical absence; primary or secondarily generalised tonic-clonic (grand mal), tonic or clonic seizures; partial (focal) seizures with elementary or complex symptomatology; various forms of myoclonic seizures, myoclonus and associated abnormal movements.

*Indications: Ampoules:* Status epilepticus in all clinical forms.

**Dosage and administration** *Tablets:* Treatment should be started with low doses. If desired the total dose may be given at night for the first four days of treatment. The dose may be increased progressively until the maintenance dose suited to the individual patient has been found.

The dosage of Rivotril must be adjusted to the needs of each individual and depends on the individual response to therapy. The maintenance dosage must be determined according to clinical response and tolerance.

*Adults:* Initial dosage should not exceed 1 mg/day. The maintenance dosage for adults normally falls within the range 4 to 8 mg.

*Infants and children:* Initial dosage should not exceed 0.25 mg/day for infants and small children (1 to 5 years) and 0.5 mg/day for older children. The maintenance dosage normally falls within the ranges:

School children (5 to 12 years): 3 to 6 mg
Small children (1 to 5 years): 1 to 3 mg
Infants (0 to 1 year): 0.5 to 1 mg

In some forms of childhood epilepsy, certain patients may cease to be adequately controlled by Rivotril. Control may be re-established by increasing the dose, or interrupting treatment with Rivotril for two or three weeks. During the interruption in therapy, careful observation and other drugs may be needed.

*Use in the elderly:* The elderly are particularly sensitive to the effects of centrally depressant drugs and may experience confusion. It is recommended that the initial dosage of Rivotril should not exceed 0.5 mg/day.

These are total daily dosages which should be divided into three or four doses taken at intervals throughout the day. If necessary, larger doses may be given at the discretion of the physician. The maintenance dose should be attained after two to four weeks of treatment.

Simultaneous administration of more than one anti-epileptic drug is a common practice in the treatment of epilepsy and may be undertaken with Rivotril. The dosage of each drug may be required to be adjusted to obtain the optimum effect. If status epilepticus occurs in a patient receiving oral Rivotril, intravenous Rivotril may still control the status.

Rivotril tablets are for oral administration.

*Ampoules:* For the treatment of status epilepticus, the dose and rate of administration are governed by the response of the patient. As a guide, we suggest:

*Adults:* 1 mg (one ampoule of active substance mixed

with one ampoule of diluent) by slow intravenous injection. Care should be taken with the elderly.

*Infants and children*: 0.5 mg (equivalent to half an ampoule of active substance mixed with half an ampoule of diluent) by slow intravenous injection.

*Mode of administration:* Intravenous injection of Rivotril should be into a large vein of the antecubital fossa. The injection should be given slowly - in adults, 1 mg over approximately 30 seconds. This will greatly diminish the rare possibility of hypotension or apnoea occurring. Nevertheless, facilities for resuscitation should always be available.

The contents of the diluent ampoule, which contains 1 ml Water for Injection Ph Eur, *must* be added to the contents of the other ampoule, which contains 1 mg clonazepam in 1 ml, *immediately* before injection.

Rivotril ampoule solution may be diluted when given in intravenous infusions of saline or dextrose, such as are customary in the treatment of status epilepticus.

Thus, up to 3 mg (3 ampoules) in 250 ml of the following solutions is permissible:

Sodium Chloride Injection BP.

Dextrose Injection BP 5% and 10%.

Sodium Chloride and Dextrose Injection BP (0.45% sodium chloride and 2.5% dextrose).

This infusion dilution should be made up freshly and used within 12 hours.

Rivotril ampoules are for intravenous administration.

Maintenance of stability cannot be guaranteed when Rivotril ampoule solution is diluted.

**Contra-indications, warnings, etc**

*Contra-indications:* Patients with known sensitivity to benzodiazepines; acute pulmonary insufficiency; respiratory depression.

*Use in pregnancy and lactation:* There is little evidence as to the drug safety in human pregnancy nor is there evidence from animal work that it is completely free from hazard. The use of Rivotril during pregnancy or lactation should be avoided unless there are compelling reasons.

The administration of high doses or prolonged administration of low doses of benzodiazepines in the last trimester of pregnancy or during labour has been reported to produce irregularities in the foetal heart rate, and hypotonia, poor sucking and hypothermia in the neonate.

*Precautions:* Rivotril should be used with caution in patients with chronic pulmonary insufficiency, or with impairment of renal or hepatic function, and in the elderly or the debilitated. In these cases dosage may need to be reduced.

Since alcohol can provoke epileptic seizures, irrespective of therapy, patients should be advised not to drink alcohol while under treatment. In combination with Rivotril, alcohol may modify the effects of the drug, compromise the success of therapy or give rise to unpredictable side-effects.

As a general rule, epileptic patients are not allowed to drive. Even when adequately controlled on Rivotril, it should be remembered that any increase in dosage or alteration in timings of dosage may modify patients' reactions, depending on individual susceptibility. If a patient is allowed to operate machinery, he should also be warned of these possible effects.

When Rivotril is used in conjunction with other anti-epileptic drugs, side-effects and toxicity may be more evident, particularly with hydantoins or phenobarbitone and combinations including them. This requires extra care in adjusting dosage in the initial stages of treatment. The combination of Rivotril and sodium valproate has, rarely, been associated with the development of absence status epilepticus. Although some patients tolerate and benefit from this combination of drugs, this potential hazard should be borne in mind when its use is considered.

Known inhibitors of hepatic enzymes, e.g. cimetidine, have been shown to reduce the clearance of benzodiazepines and may potentiate their action and known inducers of hepatic enzymes, e.g. rifampicin, may increase the clearance of benzodiazepines.

As with all other anti-epileptic drugs, treatment with Rivotril even if of short duration, must not be abruptly interrupted, but must be withdrawn by gradually reducing the dose in view of the risk of precipitating status epilepticus. This precaution must also be taken when withdrawing another drug while the patient is still receiving Rivotril therapy.

In cases of loss or bereavement, psychological adjustment may be inhibited by benzodiazepines.

*Side-effects and adverse reactions:* The side-effects observed consist of fatigue, somnolence, occasional muscular hypotonia and co-ordination disturbances. Such effects are usually transitory and disappear spontaneously as treatment continues or with dosage reduction. They tend to occur early in treatment and can be greatly reduced, if not avoided, by commencing with low dosages followed by progressive increases.

Rarely respiratory depression may occur with intravenous Rivotril, particularly if other depressant drugs have been administered.

In infants and small children, and particularly those with a degree of mental impairment, Rivotril may give rise to salivary or bronchial hypersecretion with drooling. Supervision of the airway may be required.

As with other benzodiazepines, isolated cases of blood dyscrasias and abnormal liver function tests have been reported.

Rivotril generally has a beneficial effect on behaviour disturbances in epileptic patients. In certain cases, paradoxical effects such as aggressiveness, irritability, agitation, psychotic disorders and activation of new types of seizures may be precipitated. If these occur, the benefit of continuing the drug should be weighed against the adverse effect. The addition to the regimen of another suitable drug may be necessary or, in some cases, it may be advisable to discontinue Rivotril therapy.

Although Rivotril has been given uneventfully to patients with porphyria, rarely it may induce convulsions in these patients.

*Treatment of overdosage:* As with other benzodiazepine drugs, overdosage should not present undue problems of management or threat to life. Patients have recovered from overdoses in excess of 60 mg without special treatment. Severe somnolence with muscle hypotonia will be present. Treatment is symptomatic and may include the need to maintain an airway. Gastric lavage may be useful if performed soon after ingestion.

The value of dialysis has not been determined.

Overdosage in non-epileptic patients may be treated with Anexate, a specific IV antidote for use in emergency situations. Patients requiring such intervention should be monitored closely in hospital (see separate prescribing information).

The use of Anexate is not recommended in epileptic patients who have been receiving benzodiazepine treatment for a prolonged period. Although Anexate exerts a slight intrinsic anticonvulsant effect, its abrupt suppression of the protective effect of a benzodiazepine agonist can give rise to convulsions in epileptic patients.

If excitation occurs, barbiturates should not be used.

**Pharmaceutical precautions** *Storage:* Rivotril tablets should be stored in well-closed containers. Rivotril tablets and ampoules should be protected from light. The recommended maximum storage temperature for Rivotril ampoules is 30°C.

**Legal category** CD (Sch. 4), POM.

**Package quantities** Rivotril tablets 0.5 mg and 2 mg in packs of 100 and 500.

Rivotril ampoules lmg in packs of 10, accompanied by 1 ml ampoules Water for Injection Ph Eur as diluent.

**Further information** Nil.

**Product licence numbers**

| | |
|---|---|
| Tablets 0.5 mg | 0031/0076R |
| Tablets 2 mg | 0031/0077R |
| Ampoules 1 mg | 0031/0078R |
| 1 ml ampoules Water for Injections PhEur | 0031/0284 |

## ROACCUTANE*

**Presentation** Oval, soft-gelatin capsules (spherical diameter approximately 5.8 mm), one half pale red violet and the other half white, marked 'R5', containing 5 mg isotretinoin.

Oval, soft-gelatin capsules (spherical diameter approximately 8.2 mm), one-half pale red-violet and the other half white, marked 'R20', containing 20 mg isotretinoin.

**Uses** *Properties*: Isotretinoin is a stereoisomer of tretinoin (all-*trans*-retinoic acid), an established preparation for topical treatment of acne vulgaris. Taken orally, Roaccutane has marked therapeutic efficacy in severe forms of acne, which are difficult to control with other means. The exact mechanism of action of Roaccutane is not known but clinical improvement is associated with a dose-related suppression of the size and activity of sebaceous glands.

*Pharmacokinetics*: Following oral administration of Roaccutane, peak blood levels of isotretinoin are achieved within 1-4 hours, and decline with a mean elimination half-life of approximately 10-20 hours.

Terminal elimination of the major metabolite, 4-oxo-isotretinoin, is formation rate limited so that its apparent half-life is similar to that for isotretinoin. The parent compound is highly bound to plasma protein and is excreted via bile and kidney as polar metabolites.

Bioavailability is enhanced by administration with food.

*Indications:* Roaccutane is indicated for the treatment of cystic and conglobate acne and severe acne which has failed to respond to an adequate course of systemic antimicrobial agent.

**Dosage and administration** The therapeutic response to Roaccutane is dose-related and varies between patients. This necessitates individual adjustment of dosage according to the response of the condition and the patient's tolerance of the drug. In most cases complete or near-complete remission of acne is achieved with a 12- to 16-week course of treatment. It is recommended that repeat courses of treatment should not normally be given.

The daily dosage, to the nearest number of whole capsules, should be taken with food either as a single dose or in two divided doses during the day, whichever is more convenient.

*Adults*: *Initial dose*: All patients initially should receive Roaccutane 0.5 mg/kg body-weight daily for a period of four weeks, when their responsiveness to the drug will usually be apparent. Acute exacerbation of acne is occasionally seen during the initial period but this subsides, usually within 7-10 days, with continued treatment.

*Subsequent dosages*: Patients who show early improvement should continue to receive the initial dosage of 0.5 mg/kg body-weight daily for the remainder of the course.

In patients who show little or no initial improvement, and who are tolerating the drug well, dosage should be increased up to 1 mg/kg body-weight daily for the remainder of the course.

In patients who show intolerance to the initial dosage, treatment should be continued with a reduced dosage of 0.1 to 0.2 mg/kg body-weight daily.

Repeated courses of therapy are not normally indicated. With effective treatment, complete clearing of acne is usually achieved and prolonged remission ensues. However, patients whose acne is not completely cleared at the end of treatment can be expected to show continuing improvement for up to several months thereafter. Only if a definite relapse is seen in the post-treatment period should a repeated course be considered.

*Concomitant therapy*: As a rule, other treatments conventionally used for the treatment of acne, including antibiotics, keratolytics and exfoliants, are not indicated nor is concurrent radiation therapy with ultraviolet light or prolonged exposure to strong sunlight indicated but non-irritant topical preparations may be applied if required.

Patients should be instructed to avoid taking preparations containing high doses of vitamin A, i.e. more than the recommended dietary allowance of 4,000-5,000 i.u. per day.

*Use in the elderly*: Dosage as for other adults. Older subjects may have a greater risk of drug-induced arthralgia.

*Children*: Roaccutane is not indicated for the treatment of prepubertal acne.

Roaccutane capsules are for oral administration.

**Contra-indications, warnings, etc**

*Contra-indications:* Hypersensitivity reactions may occur in susceptible individuals. Use of this drug in patients with a known hypersensitivity to isotretinoin and any of the excipients is contra-indicated.

Roaccutane is contra-indicated in hepatic and renal impairment. It should not be given to breast-feeding mothers. Roaccutane is also contra-indicated in hypervitaminosis A, hyperlipidaemia and hypersensitivity to the drug.

Rare cases of benign intracranial hypertension have been reported after Roaccutane and after tetracyclines. Supplementary treatment with tetracyclines is therefore contra-indicated.

Roaccutane is teratogenic; major foetal abnormalities have been reported in humans. Major foetal abnormalities include: hydrocephalus, microcephalus, abnormalities of the external ear (micropinna, small or absent external auditory canals), microphthalmia, cardiovascular abnormalities, facial dysmorphia, thymus gland abnormalities, parathyroid hormone deficiency and cerebellar malformation. There is also a small risk of spontaneous abortion. Roaccutane is therefore contra-indicated in pregnancy. In any women of childbearing potential the risk of its use must be weighed against the expected therapeutic benefit under all circumstances, taking into account the precautions specified below.

*Precautions:* Roaccutane is contra-indicated in a woman of childbearing potential unless she meets the following criteria:

1. Has severe disfiguring cystic acne resistant to standard therapy.
2. Pregnancy should be excluded before instituting therapy with Roaccutane. A negative pregnancy test within two weeks prior to therapy is obtained.
3. Starts Roaccutane therapy only on the second or third day of the next menstrual cycle.

4. Any woman of childbearing potential who is receiving Roaccutane must practise effective contraception for at least four weeks before treatment, during the treatment period and for at least four weeks following its cessation. Even female patients who normally do not practise contraception because of a history of infertility should be advised to do so, while taking Roaccutane.

5. Contraceptive measures must also be taken in the case of repeated courses of treatment.

6. Any pregnancy occurring during treatment with Roaccutane, or immediately following its completion, carries the risk of foetal malformation. This would raise the question of the termination of pregnancy for medical reasons. Therefore, before instituting Roaccutane therapy in a woman of childbearing potential the treating physician must explain clearly and in detail what precautions must be taken. This should include the risks involved and the possible consequences of a pregnancy occurring during Roaccutane treatment or in the first four weeks following its completion.

7. The woman is reliable and capable of understanding the risks and complying with effective contraception and confirms that she has understood the warnings.

In view of the importance of the foregoing precautions, Roaccutane Patient Information Leaflets are available to doctors and it is strongly recommended that these be given to all patients. Wherever practicable a monthly repetition of the pregnancy test is recommended.

Liver function and blood lipids (fasting value) should be measured in all patients at the start of treatment, after the first month of administration and thereafter at 3-monthly intervals before discontinuation of Roaccutane.

At the completion of a lifespan study in rats there was an increased incidence of phaeochromocytoma in animals given isotretinoin at dosages of 32 and 8 mg/kg/day, but not 2 mg/kg/day. Since rats are particularly prone to develop this tumour type, the significance of this finding for use of Roaccutane in man is uncertain; nevertheless, repeated courses of treatment are not normally recommended.

Patients should not donate blood either during or for at least four weeks following discontinuation of therapy with Roaccutane. Theoretically there would be a small risk to a woman in the first trimester of pregnancy who received blood donated by a patient on Roaccutane therapy.

*Side-effects and adverse reactions:* Most of the clinical side effects of Roaccutane are dose related and are usually well tolerated at the recommended dosages. The side effects may recede during continued treatment and have generally proved reversible with reduction of dosage or discontinuation of therapy.

The skin and mucous membranes are most commonly affected. Dryness of the skin may be associated with scaling, thinning, erythema (especially of the face) and pruritus. An increase in epidermal fragility has been reported, and frictional trauma may lead to epidermal blistering. Dryness of the nasal mucosa may be associated with mild epistaxis and dryness of the pharyngeal mucosa with hoarseness. Granulomatous lesions have occasionally been reported. Dryness of the conjunctivae has been reported and may lead to mild to moderate conjunctivitis which may be alleviated by use of topical antibiotics. Decreased tolerance to contact lenses may occur.

Keratitis in association with Roaccutane treatment is a rare event and possibly related to dry eye syndrome. Therefore patients, particularly those with dry eye syndrome, should be monitored for the development of keratitis.

Acne fulminans has been noted to occur in rare cases.

Facial hyperpigmentation may rarely occur in patients treated with Roaccutane.

There have been occasional reports of visual disturbances, including papilloedema and optic neuritis possibly associated with benign intracranial hypertension; also corneal opacities, cataracts, decreased night vision, photophobia and blurred vision. Patients experiencing visual disturbances should be referred for an expert ophthalmological examination and withdrawal of Roaccutane considered.

Isolated cases of hearing deficiency in certain frequencies have been reported.

Hair thinning may occur but is uncommon at dosages below 1 mg/kg/day and is reversible following discontinuation of Roaccutane. Nevertheless, patients should be warned that this is a possibility during treatment. Hirsutism may rarely occur.

There have been occasional reports of allergic vasculitis associated with the administration of Roaccutane.

Non-specific symptoms such as nausea, headache, malaise, drowsiness and sweating have been reported infrequently. Benign intracranial hypertension has been reported, particularly in association with concomitant antibiotic therapy.

Some patients have experienced mood changes including both reduction and precipitation of depression.

Epileptiform seizures have been reported in patients who are receiving Roaccutane therapy.

Myalgia and arthralgia may occur and may be associated with reduced tolerance to vigorous exercise. Isolated instances of raised serum CPK values have been reported in patients receiving Roaccutane, particularly those undertaking vigorous physical activity. In these cases the clinical significance is unknown.

There have been occasional reports of menstrual irregularities which return to normal after completion of Roaccutane therapy.

A rise in serum levels of liver enzymes may occur. In a few cases significant increases have occurred, necessitating dosage reduction or discontinuation of Roaccutane. Jaundice and hepatitis have occurred rarely.

Elevation of serum triglycerides and cholesterol above the normal range, usually accompanied by decreases in HDL, has been observed, especially where predisposing factors such as a family history of lipid disorders, obesity, alcohol abuse, diabetes mellitus or smoking are present. The changes are dose-related and may be controlled by dietary means (including restriction of alcohol intake) and/or by reduction of dosage of Roaccutane. Isotretinoin-treated patients with high serum triglycerides (>8 g/l) are at risk of developing pancreatitis.

Rarely hyperuricemia and inflammatory bowel disease (e.g. colitis, ileitis) have been reported.

Isolated cases of paronychia and local or systemic infections due to Gram positive micro-organisms have been reported.

Rare instances have been reported of elevated blood glucose levels in diabetic patients receiving Roaccutane, therefore, careful monitoring of glucose levels during treatment is advised.

Isolated cases of thrombocytopenia, thrombocytosis, neutropenia and anaemia have been reported. Lymphadenopathy has been observed in some patients.

Isotretinoin has been shown to affect diaphyseal and spongy bone adversely in animals at high doses in excess of those recommended for use in man. Bone changes, including early epiphyseal closure, have occurred in man after several years administration of Roaccutane in very high doses for disorders of keratinisation. Prospective X-ray examination of some patients treated for severe cystic acne with Roaccutane revealed evidence of skeletal hyperostosis without clinical symptoms.

Haematuria and proteinuria have been associated with Roaccutane treatment and symptoms improve following dose reduction or drug withdrawal.

*Treatment of overdosage:* Isotretinoin is a derivative of vitamin A and overdosage should be expected to induce symptoms of hypervitaminosis A.

Manifestations of acute vitamin A toxicity include severe headache, nausea or vomiting, drowsiness, irritability and pruritus. Signs and symptoms of accidental or deliberate overdosage with Roaccutane would probably be similar. They would be expected to be reversible and to subside without need for treatment. Because of the variable absorption of the drug, gastric lavage may be worthwhile in the first few hours after ingestion.

**Pharmaceutical precautions**
*Storage:* Roaccutane capsules should be stored in a well-closed container and protected from light; the recommended maximum storage temperature is 30°C.

**Legal category** POM.

**Package quantities** Roaccutane capsules 5 mg in packs of 56 (8 x 7 capsule blister strips)(OP).

Roaccutane capsules 20 mg in packs of 56 (8 x 7 capsule blister strips)(OP).

**Further information** *Availability:* It is recommended that Roaccutane capsules should be given by, or under the supervision of, a consultant dermatologist. They are available through hospital pharmacies for use in hospitals, and hospital clinics or, at the written request of a consultant dermatologist can be supplied to specific retail pharmacies for dispensing prescriptions from the named dermatologist whose bona fide can be identified by the dispensing pharmacist.

**Product licence numbers**

| | |
|---|---|
| Capsules 5 mg | 0031/0158 |
| Capsules 20 mg | 0031/0160 |

## ROCALTROL*

**Presentation** Soft gelatine capsules, one length red opaque and the other white opaque, containing 0.25 mcg calcitriol and the inactive ingredients butylated hydroxyanisole, butylated hydroxytoluene, fractionated coconut oil, gelatin, glycerol, hydrogenated products of partially hydrolysed starch, titanium dioxide E 171 and canthaxanthin E 161 g.

Soft gelatine capsules, both lengths red opaque, containing 0.5 mcg calcitriol.

**Uses**
*Pharmacological properties:* Calcitriol has the greatest biological activity of the known vitamin D metabolites and is normally formed in the kidneys from its immediate precursor, 25-hydroxycholecalciferol. In physiological amounts it augments the intestinal absorption of calcium and phosphate and plays a significant part in the regulation of bone mineralisation. The defective production of calcitriol in chronic renal failure contributes to the abnormalities of mineral metabolism found in that disorder.

Rocaltrol is a synthetic preparation of calcitriol. Oral administration of Rocaltrol to patients with chronic renal failure compensates for impaired endogenous production of calcitriol which is decreased when the glomerular filtration rate falls below 30 ml/min. Consequently, intestinal malabsorption of calcium and phosphate and the resulting hypocalcaemia are improved, thereby reversing the signs and symptoms of bone disease.

In patients with established postmenopausal osteoporosis, Rocaltrol increases calcium absorption, elevates circulating levels of calcitriol and reduces vertebral fracture frequency.

The onset and reversal of the effects of Rocaltrol are more rapid than those of other compounds with vitamin D activity and adjustment of the dose can be achieved sooner and more precisely. The effects of inadvertent overdosage can also be reversed more readily.

*Pharmacokinetics:* Rocaltrol is efficiently absorbed following an oral dose, and peak serum levels are reached after 4–6 hours. Calcitriol concentrations return to the basal level with a half-life of 3–6 hours, although the duration of pharmacologic activity is approximately 3–5 days. Following oral administration of 1 mcg radiolabeled calcitriol to normal individuals, approximately 10% of the total radioactivity appears in the urine within 24 hours. Biliary excretion and enterohepatic recirculation also occur.

*Indications:* Rocaltrol is indicated for the correction of the abnormalities of calcium and phosphate metabolism in patients with renal osteodystrophy.

Rocaltrol is also indicated for the treatment of established postmenopausal osteoporosis.

**Dosage and administration** The dose of Rocaltrol should be carefully adjusted for each patient according to the biological response so as to avoid hypercalcaemia.

The effectiveness of treatment depends in part on an adequate daily intake of calcium, which should be augmented by dietary changes or supplements if necessary. The capsules should be swallowed with a little water.

*Adults*
*Renal Osteodystrophy:* The initial daily dose is 0.25 mcg of Rocaltrol. In patients with normal or only slightly reduced calcium levels, doses of 0.25 mcg every other day are sufficient. If no satisfactory response in the biochemical parameters and clinical manifestations of the disease is observed within 2–4 weeks, the dosage may be increased by 0.25 mcg daily at 2–4 week intervals. During this period, serum calcium levels should be determined at least twice weekly. Most patients respond to between 0.5 mcg and 1.0 mcg daily. Higher doses may be necessary if barbiturates or anticonvulsant drugs are administered simultaneously.

*Postmenopausal Osteoporosis:* The recommended dose for Rocaltrol is 0.25 mcg twice daily.

Serum calcium and creatinine levels should be determined at 4 weeks, 3 and 6 months and at 6 monthly intervals thereafter.

*Use in the elderly:* Clinical experience with Rocaltrol in elderly patients indicates that the dosage recommended for use in younger adults may be given without apparent ill-consequence.

*Children:* Dosage in children has not been established. Rocaltrol capsules are for oral administration only.

**Contra-indications, warnings, etc**
*Contra-indications:* Rocaltrol should not be given to patients with hypercalcaemia or evidence of metastatic calcification. The use of Rocaltrol in patients with known hypersensitivity to calcitriol (or drugs of the same class) and any of the constituent excipients is contra-indicated.

*Use in pregnancy and lactation:* The safety of Rocaltrol during pregnancy has not been established. Studies of reproductive toxicology in animals have not yielded unequivocal findings, and no controlled studies on the effect of exogenous calcitriol on pregnancy and foetal development have been performed in human subjects. Consequently, Rocaltrol should be given only when the potential benefit has been weighed against the possible hazard to the foetus. The usual caution in prescribing any drug for women of child-bearing age should be observed.

It should be assumed that exogenous calcitriol passes into breast milk. In view of the possible adverse effects on the infant, mothers should not breast-feed while taking Rocaltrol.

*Precautions:* All other vitamin D compounds and their derivatives, including proprietary compounds or food-stuffs which may be 'fortified' with vitamin D, should be withheld during treatment with Rocaltrol.

Treatment does not obviate the need to control plasma phosphate with phosphate-binding agents. Since Rocaltrol affects phosphate transport in the gut and bone, the dose of phosphate-binding agent may need to be modified.

*Side-effects and adverse reactions:* Hypercalcaemia and hypercalciuria are the major side-effects of Rocaltrol and indicate excessive dosage. Patients with tertiary hyperparathyroidism, renal failure, or on regular haemodialysis are particularly prone to develop hypercalcaemia. The clinical features of hypercalcaemia include anorexia, nausea, vomiting, headache, weakness, apathy and somnolence. More severe manifestations may include thirst, dehydration, polyuria, nocturia, abdominal pain, paralytic ileus and cardiac arrhythmias. Rarely, overt psychosis and metastatic calcification may occur. The relatively short biological half-life of Rocaltrol permits rapid elimination of the compound when treatment is stopped and hypercalcaemia will recede within 2–7 days. This rate of reversal of biological effects is more rapid than when other vitamin D derivatives are used.

Mild, non-progressive and reversible elevations in levels of liver enzymes (SGOT, SGPT) have been noted in a few patients treated with Rocaltrol, but no pathological changes in the liver have been reported.

*Treatment of overdosage:* In acute overdosage gastric lavage should be considered as soon after ingestion as possible provided that the drug was taken within the previous 6–8 hours.

Should hypercalcaemia occur, Rocaltrol should be discontinued until plasma calcium levels have returned to normal. A low-calcium diet will speed this reversal. Rocaltrol can then be restarted at a lower dose or given in the same dose but at less frequent intervals than previously. Severe hypercalcaemia may be treated by ensuring adequate hydration, inducing a diuresis where practicable and by general supportive measures. Calcitonin may increase the rate of fall of serum calcium when bone resorption is increased.

In patients treated by intermittent haemodialysis, a low concentration of calcium in the dialysate may also be used.

**Pharmaceutical precautions**

*Storage:* Rocaltrol capsules should be protected from heat; the recommended maximum storage temperature is 30°C.

**Legal category** POM.

**Package quantities** Rocaltrol capsules 0.25 mcg and 0.5 mcg in packs of 100.

**Further information** Nil.

**Product licence numbers**

Capsules 0.25 mcg) 0031/0122
Capsules 0.5 mcg) 0031/0123

## ROCEPHIN* ▼

**Qualitative and quantitative composition**

Each 250 mg vial contains 250 mg ceftriaxone as 298.3 mg hydrated disodium ceftriaxone.

Each 1 g vial contains 1 g ceftriaxone as 1.19 g hydrated disodium ceftriaxone.

Each 2 g vial contains 2 g ceftriaxone as 2.39 g hydrated disodium ceftriaxone.

**Pharmaceutical form** Vials containing a sterile, crystalline powder for reconstitution for injection.

**Clinical particulars**

*Therapeutic indications:* Pneumonia. Septicaemia. Meningitis.Bone, skin and soft tissue infections. Infections in neutropenic patients. Gonorrhoea. Peri-operative prophylaxis of infections associated with surgery. Treatment may be started before the results of susceptibility tests are known.

*Posology and method of administration:* Rocephin may be administered by deep intramuscular injection, slow intravenous injection, or as a slow intravenous infusion, after reconstitution of the solution according to the directions given below. Dosage and mode of administration should be determined by the severity of the infection, susceptibility of the causative organism and the patient's condition. Under most circumstances a once-daily dose–or, in the specified indications, a single dose–will give satisfactory therapeutic results.

*Adults and children 12 years and over:* Standard therapeutic dosage: 1 g once daily.

Severe infections: 2-4 g daily, normally as a single dose every 24 hours.

The duration of therapy varies according to the course of the disease. As with antibiotic therapy in general, administration of Rocephin should be continued for a minimum of 48 to 72 hours after the patient has become afebrile or evidence of bacterial eradication has been obtained.

Acute, uncomplicated gonorrhoea: a single dose of 250 mg intramuscularly should be administered. Simultaneous administration of probenecid is not indicated.

Peri-operative prophylaxis: usually 1 g as a single intramuscular or slow intravenous dose. In colorectal surgery, 2 g should be given intramuscularly by slow intravenous injection or by slow intravenous infusion, in conjunction with a suitable agent against anaerobic bacteria.

*Use in the elderly:* These dosages do not require modification in elderly patients provided that renal and hepatic function are satisfactory (see below).

*Children under 12 years:* Standard therapeutic dosage: 20-50 mg/kg body-weight once daily.

In severe infections up to 80 mg/kg body-weight daily may be given. Doses of 50 mg/kg or over should be given by slow intravenous infusion over at least 30 minutes.

*Renal and hepatic impairment:* In patients with impaired renal function, there is no need to reduce the dosage of Rocephin provided liver function is intact. Only in cases of pre-terminal renal failure (creatinine clearance < 10 ml per minute) should the daily dosage be limited to 2 g or less.

In patients with liver damage there is no need for the dosage to be reduced provided renal function is intact.

In severe renal impairment accompanied by hepatic insufficiency, the plasma concentration of Rocephin should be determined at regular intervals and dosage adjusted.

In patients undergoing dialysis, no additional supplementary dosing is required following the dialysis. Serum concentrations should be monitored, however, to determine whether dosage adjustments are necessary, since the elimination rate in these patients may be reduced.

Preparation of solutions for injection and infusion

The use of freshly prepared solutions is recommended. These maintain potency for at least 6 hours at room temperature in daylight, or 24 hours at 5°C.

When reconstituted for intramuscular or intravenous injection, the white to yellowish-orange crystalline powder gives a pale yellow to amber solution. The displacement value of 250 mg of Rocephin is 0.194 ml.

Each gram of Rocephin contains approximately 3.6 mmol sodium.

*Intramuscular Injection:* 250 mg Rocephin should be dissolved in 1 ml of 1% Lignocaine Hydrochloride Injection BP, or 1 g in 3.5 ml of 1% Lignocaine Hydrochloride Injection BP. The solution should be administered by deep intramuscular injection. Dosages greater than 1 g should be divided and injected at more than one site.

Solutions in lignocaine should not be administered intravenously.

*Intravenous Injection:* 250 mg Rocephin should be dissolved in 5 ml of Water for Injections BP or 1 g in 10 ml of Water for Injections BP. The injection should be administered over 2-4 minutes, directly into the vein or via the tubing of an intravenous infusion.

*Intravenous Infusion:* 2 g of Rocephin should be dissolved in 40 ml of one of the following calcium-free solutions: Dextrose Injection BP 5% or 10%, Sodium Chloride Injection BP, Sodium Chloride and Dextrose Injection BP (0.45% sodium chloride and 2.5% dextrose), dextran 6% in Dextrose Injection BP 5%, hydroxyethyl starch 6-10% infusions. The infusion should be administered over at least 30 minutes.

Solutions containing Rocephin should not be mixed with or added to solutions containing other agents. In particular, Rocephin is not compatible with calcium-containing solutions such as Hartmann's solution and Ringer's solution.

*Contra-indications:* Rocephin should not be given to patients with a history of hypersensitivity to cephalosporin antibiotics.

Rocephin is contra-indicated in premature infants and in full-term infants during the first 6 weeks of life.

*Special warnings and special precautions for use:* The stated dosage should not be exceeded.

Care is required when administering Rocephin to patients who have previously shown hypersensitivity (especially anaphylactic reaction) to penicillins or other non-cephalosporin beta-lactam antibiotics, as occasional instances of cross-allergenicity between cephalosporins and these antibiotics have been recorded. Anaphylactic shock requires immediate counter measures.

In severe renal impairment accompanied by hepatic insufficiency, dosage reduction is required as outlined under *Posology and method of administration.*

*In vitro* studies have shown that ceftriaxone, like some other cephalosporins, can displace bilirubin from serum albumin. Clinical data obtained in neonates have confirmed this finding. Ceftriaxone should not be given to neonates.

*Interaction with other medicaments and other forms of interaction:* No impairment of renal function has been observed in man after simultaneous administration of Rocephin with diuretics.

No interference with the action or increase in nephrotoxicity of aminoglycosides has been observed during simultaneous administration with Rocephin.

The ceftriaxone molecule does not contain the N-methylthio-tetrazole substituent which has been associated with a disulfiram-like effect when alcohol is taken during therapy with certain cephalosporins.

In an in vitro study, antagonistic effects have been observed with the combination of chloramphenicol and ceftriaxone.

In patients treated with Rocephin, the Coombs-test may rarely become false-positive. Rocephin, like other antibiotics, may result in false-positive tests for galactosaemia. Likewise, non-enzymatic methods for glucose determination in urine may give false-positive results. For this reason, urine-glucose determination during therapy with Rocephin should be done enzymatically.

*Pregnancy and lactation:* Rocephin has not been associated with adverse effects on foetal development in laboratory animals but its safety in human pregnancy has not been established. Therefore it should not be used in pregnancy unless absolutely indicated.

Only minimal amounts of Rocephin are excreted in breast milk. However, caution is advised in nursing mothers.

*Effects on ability to drive and use machines:* None.

*Undesirable effects:* Rocephin has been generally well tolerated, with adverse reactions being relatively infrequent, usually mild and transient.

The most common side-effects are gastro-intestinal, consisting mainly of loose stools and diarrhoea or, occasionally, nausea and vomiting, stomatitis and glossitis. Cutaneous reactions, including maculopapular rash or exanthema, pruritus, urticaria, oedema, erythema multiforme and allergic dermatitis, have occurred.

Haematological reactions have included anaemia (all grades), leucopenia, neutropenia, thrombocytopenia, eosinophilia, agranulocytosis and positive Coombs' test. Regular blood counts should be carried out during treatment. Rocephin has rarely been associated with prolongation of prothrombin time.

Headache and dizziness, drug fever, shivering and transient elevations in liver function tests have been reported in a few cases. Other rarely observed adverse reactions include glycosuria, oliguria, haematuria, increase in serum creatinine, mycosis of the genital tract and anaphylactic type reactions such as bronchospasm.

Very rarely, precipitation of the calcium salt of ceftriaxone in the urine has been observed in patients receiving higher doses than currently recommended.

Shadows which have been mistaken for gallstones have been detected by sonograms of the gallbladder, usually following doses higher than the standard recommended dose. These shadows are, however, precipitates of calcium ceftriaxone which disappear on completion or discontinuation of Rocephin therapy. Rarely, have these findings been associated with symptoms. In symptomatic cases, conservative non-surgical management is recommended. Discontinuation of Rocephin treatment in symptomatic cases should be at the discretion of the clinician.

Superinfections with yeasts, fungi or other resistant organisms may occur. A rare side-effect is pseudomembranous colitis which has resulted from infection with *Clostridium difficile* during treatment with Rocephin. Therefore, it is important to consider this diagnosis in patients who present with diarrhoea subsequent to the administration of antibacterial agents.

Pain or discomfort may be experienced at the site of intramuscular injection immediately after administration but is usually well tolerated and transient. Local phlebitis has occurred rarely following intravenous administration but can be minimised by slow injection over 2-4 minutes.

*Overdose:* In the case of overdosage, drug concentrations would not be reduced by haemodialysis or peritoneal dialysis. There is no specific antidote. Treatment should be symptomatic.

**Pharmacological properties**

*Pharmacodynamic properties:* Rocephin has potent bactericidal activity against a wide range of Gram-positive and, especially, Gram-negative organisms.

The spectrum of activity includes both aerobic and anaerobic species. It has considerable stability against degradation by most bacterial beta-lactamases.

A notable feature of Rocephin is its relatively long plasma elimination half-life of approximately 8 hours, which makes single or once-daily dosage of the drug appropriate for most patients.

*Microbiology:* Ceftriaxone is usually active against the following microorganisms *in vitro* and in clinical infections (see Indications). The list is not exhaustive and focuses on those organisms of particular clinical interest.

*Gram-positive aerobes: Staphylococcus aureus* (including penicillinase-producing strains), *Streptococcus pneumoniae, Streptococcus* group A (*Streptococcus pyogenes*), *Streptococcus* group *B* (*Streptococcus agalactiae*), *Streptococcus viridans, Streptococcus bovis*

Note: Methicillin-resistant *Staphylococcus* spp. are resistant to cephalosporins, including ceftriaxone. Most strains of enterococci (e.g. *Enterococcus faecalis*) are resistant.

*Gram-negative aerobes: Acinetobacter iwoffi* (some strains are resistant), *Aeromonas* spp., *Alcaligenes* spp, *Moraxella catarrhalis* (beta-lactamase negative and positive), *Capnocytophaga* spp., *Citrobacter* spp, *Enterobacter* spp (some strains are resistant), *Escherichia coli, Haemophilus ducreyi,*

*Haemophilus influenzae* (including penicillinase-producing strains), *Haemophilus parainfluenzae, Hafnia alvei, Klebsiella* spp (including *K. pneumoniae*), *Moraxella* spp, *Morganella morganii* (= *Proteus morganii*), *Neisseria gonorrhoeae* (including penicillinase-producing strains), *Neisseria meningitidis, Pasteurella multocida, Plesimonas shigelloides, Proteus mirabilis, Proteus vulgaris, Providencia* spp, *Salmonella* spp (including *S. typhi*), *Serratia* spp (including *S. marcescens*), *Shigella* spp, *Vibrio* spp (including *V. cholerae*), *Yersinia* spp (including *Y. enterocolitica*).

*Anaerobic organisms: Clostridium* spp (except C. difficile), *Fusobacterium* spp (except *F. mortiferum* and *F. varium*), *Peptococcus* spp, *Peptostreptococcus* spp.

*Pharmacokinetic properties:* The pharmacokinetics of Rocephin are largely determined by its concentration-dependent binding to serum albumin. The plasma free (unbound) fraction of the drug in man is approximately 5 per cent over most of the therapeutic concentration range, increasing to 15 per cent at concentrations of 300 mg/l. Owing to the lower albumin content, the proportion of free ceftriaxone in interstitial fluid is correspondingly higher than in plasma.

*Plasma Concentrations:* Mean peak concentrations after bolus intravenous injection are about 120 mg/l following a 500 mg dose and about 200 mg/l following a 1 g dose; mean levels of 250 mg/l are achieved after infusion of 2 g over 30 minutes. Intramuscular injection of 500 mg Rocephin in 1% lignocaine produces mean peak plasma concentrations of 40-70 mg/l within 1 hour. Bioavailability after intramuscular injection is 100 per cent.

*Excretion:* Rocephin is eliminated mainly as unchanged ceftriaxone, approximately 60 per cent of the dose being excreted in the urine (almost exclusively by glomerular filtration) and the remainder via the biliary and intestinal tracts. The total plasma clearance is 10-22 ml/min. The renal clearance is 5-12 ml/min. The elimination half-life in adults is about 8 hours. The half-life is not significantly affected by the dose, the route of administration or by repeated administration.

*Pharmacokinetics in special clinical situations:* In elderly persons aged over 75 years, the average elimination half-life is usually 2 to 3 times longer than in the young adult group. As with all cephalosporins, a decrease in renal function in the elderly may lead to an increase in half-life. Evidence gathered to date with ceftriaxone, however, suggests that no modification of the dosage regimen is needed.

In patients with renal or hepatic dysfunction, the pharmacokinetics of ceftriaxone are only minimally altered and the elimination half-life is only slightly increased. If kidney function alone is impaired, biliary elimination of ceftriaxone is increased; if liver function alone is impaired, renal elimination is increased.

*Cerebrospinal fluid:* Rocephin crosses non-inflamed and inflamed meninges, attaining concentrations 4-17 per cent of the simultaneous plasma concentration.

*Preclinical safety data:* Not applicable.

**Pharmaceutical particulars**

*List of excipients:* None.

*Incompatibilities:* Rocephin should not be mixed in the same syringe with any drug other than 1% Lignocaine Hydrochloride Injection BP (for intramuscular injection only).

Rocephin is not compatible with calcium-containing solutions such as Hartmann's solution and Ringer's solution. Based on literature reports ceftriaxone is not compatible with amsacrine, vancomycin, fluconazole or aminoglycosides.

*Shelf life:* Three years. Reconstituted solutions are stable for 6 hours at room temperature in daylight, or 24 hours at 5°C.

*Special precautions for storage:* The recommended maximum storage temperature for Rocephin vials is 25°C.

*Nature and contents of container:* 250 mg and 1 g Vials: Clear glass 15 ml vial with teflonised rubber stopper and aluminium cap in packs of 5.

2 g Vials: Clear glass 50 ml vial with teflonised rubber stopper and aluminium cap in packs of 1.

*Instructions for use/handling:* A plastic loop is attached to the 2 g vial for suspending the vial for use as an intravenous drip.

**Marketing authorisation numbers**

| | |
|---|---|
| 250 mg vials | 0031/0169 |
| 1 g vials | 0031/0171 |
| 2 g vials | 0031/0172 |

**Date of approval/revision of SPC** February 1995

**Legal category** POM

## ROFERON*-A SOLUTION FOR INJECTION

**Qualitative and quantitative composition** Roferon-A is supplied as a ready-to-use solution for injection. Each vial contains 3, 4.5, 6, 9 or 18 million International Units (IU) interferon alfa-2a*.

Roferon-A solution for injection contains 0.77 mg ammonium acetate, 7.21 mg sodium chloride, 10 mg benzyl alcohol (1%) as a preservative, 0.20 mg polysorbate 80 with buffers of acetic acid (10% w/v) and sodium hydroxide to pH 5.0 and water for injection.

*Contains volume overages of 10% and manufacturing overages.

**Pharmaceutical form** Vials containing 3, 4.5, 6, 9 or 18 million International Units per ml (MIU/ml) or 18 MIU/3 ml interferon alfa-2a in a ready-to-use solution for injection.

Prefilled syringes containing 3, 4.5, 6 or 9 million International Units in 0.5 ml (MIU/0.5 ml) interferon alfa-2a in a ready to use solution for injection.

*Route of administration:*
Vials: Intramuscular (i.m.); subcutaneous (s.c.).
Prefilled syringes: Subcutaneous (s.c.).

**Clinical particulars**

*Therapeutic indications:* Roferon-A is indicated for the treatment of:

(1) Hairy cell leukaemia.

(2) AIDS patients with progressive, asymptomatic Kaposi's sarcoma who have a CD4 count > 250/mm³. AIDS patients with CD4 counts < 250/mm³, or those with a history of opportunistic infections or constitutional symptoms, are unlikely to respond to Roferon-A therapy and therefore should not be treated (see section *Posology and method of administration*).

(3) Chronic phase Philadelphia-chromosome positive chronic myelogenous leukaemia. Roferon-A is not an alternative treatment for CML patients who have an HLA-identical relative and for whom allogeneic bone marrow transplantation is planned or possible in the immediate future. It is still unknown whether Roferon-A can be considered as a treatment with a curative potential in this indication.

(4) Cutaneous T-cell lymphoma. Interferon alfa-2a (Roferon-A) may be active in patients who have progressive disease and who are refractory to, or unsuitable for, conventional therapy.

(5) Adult patients with histologically proven chronic hepatitis B who have markers for viral replication, i.e., those who are positive for HBV-DNA, DNA polymerase or HBeAg.

(6) Adult patients with histologically proven chronic hepatitis C who are positive for HCV antibodies and have elevated serum alanine aminotransferase (ALT) without liver decompensation. There is no evidence of long term benefit on clinical and histological grounds.

(7) Follicular non-Hodgkin's lymphoma.

(8) Advanced renal cell carcinoma.

*Posology and method of administration:*

*1. HAIRY CELL LEUKAEMIA*

*Initial dosage:* Three million IU daily, given by subcutaneous or intramuscular injection for 16–24 weeks. If intolerance develops, either the daily dose should be lowered to 1.5 million IU or the schedule changed to 3 times per week, or both.

*Maintenance dosage:* Three million IU, given 3 times per week by subcutaneous or intramuscular injection. If intolerance develops, the dose should be lowered to 1.5 million IU 3 times per week.

*Duration of treatment:* Patients should be treated for approximately 6 months before the physician decides whether to continue treatment in responding patients or to discontinue treatment in non-responding patients. Patients have been treated for up to 20 consecutive months. The optimal duration of Roferon-A treatment for hairy cell leukaemia has not been determined.

*Note*: Subcutaneous administration is recommended for thrombocytopenic patients (platelet count less than 50 x 10⁹/l) or patients at risk of bleeding.

The minimum effective dose of Roferon-A in hairy cell leukaemia has not been established.

*2. AIDS-RELATED KAPOSI'S SARCOMA*

Roferon-A is indicated for the treatment of AIDS patients with progressive, asymptomatic Kaposi's sarcoma who have a CD4 count > 250/mm³. AIDS patients with CD4 counts < 250/mm³, or those with a history of opportunistic infections or constitutional symptoms, are unlikely to respond to Roferon-A therapy and therefore should not be treated. The optimal posology has not yet been well established.

Roferon-A should not be used in conjunction with protease inhibitors. With the exception of zidovudine, there is a lack of safety data for the combination of Roferon-A with reverse transcriptase inhibitors.

*Initial dosage*: Roferon-A should be given by subcutaneous or intramuscular injection, and escalated to at least 18 million IU daily and if possible to 36 million IU daily for a total of 10 to 12 weeks in patients of 18 years or older. The recommended escalation schedule is as follows:

| | |
|---|---|
| Days 1–3 | 3 million IU daily |
| Days 4–6 | 9 million IU daily |
| Days 7–9 | 18 million IU daily–and, if tolerated, increase to: |
| Days 10–84 | 36 million IU daily |

*Maintenance dosage:* Roferon-A should be given by subcutaneous or intramuscular injection 3 times per week at the maximum dose which is acceptable to the patient, but not exceeding 36 million IU.

Patients with AIDS-related Kaposi's sarcoma treated with 3 million IU of Roferon-A given daily showed a lower response rate than those treated with the recommended dosage.

*Duration of treatment:* The evolution of lesions should be documented to determine response to therapy. Patients should be treated for a minimum of 10 weeks and preferably for at least 12 weeks before the physician decides whether to continue treatment in responding patients or to discontinue treatment in non-responding patients. Patients generally showed evidence of response after approximately 3 months of therapy. Patients have been treated for up to 20 consecutive months. If a response to treatment occurs, treatment should continue at least until there is no further evidence of tumour. The optimal duration of Roferon-A treatment for AIDS-related Kaposi's sarcoma has not been determined.

*Note:* Lesions of Kaposi's sarcoma frequently reappear when Roferon-A treatment is discontinued.

*3. CHRONIC MYELOGENOUS LEUKAEMIA*

Roferon-A is indicated for the treatment of patients with chronic phase Philadelphia-chromosome positive chronic myelogenous leukaemia. Roferon-A is not an alternative treatment for CML patients who have an HLA-identical relative and for whom allogeneic bone marrow transplantation is planned or possible in the immediate future.

Roferon-A produces haematological remissions in 60% of patients with chronic phase CML, independent of prior treatment. Two thirds of these patients have complete haematological responses which occur as late as 18 months after treatment start.

In contrast to cytotoxic chemotherapy, interferon alfa-2a is able to generate sustained, ongoing cytogenetic responses beyond 40 months. It is still unknown whether Roferon-A can be considered as a treatment with a curative potential in this indication.

*Dosage*: It is recommended that Roferon-A should be given by subcutaneous or intramuscular injection for 8 to 12 weeks to patients 18 years or more. The recommended schedule is:

| | |
|---|---|
| Days 1–3 | 3 million IU daily |
| Days 4–6 | 6 million IU daily |
| Days 7–84 | 9 million IU daily |

*Duration of treatment*: Patients should be treated for a minimum of 8 weeks, preferably for at least 12 weeks before the physician decides whether or not to continue treatment in responding patients or to discontinue treatment in patients not showing any changes in haematological parameters. Responding patients should be treated until complete haematological response is achieved or for a maximum of 18 months. All patients with complete haematologic responses should continue treatment with 9 million IU daily (optimum) or 9 million IU 3 times a week (minimum) in order to achieve a cytogenetic response in the shortest possible time. The optimal duration of Roferon-A treatment for chronic myelogenous leukaemia has not been determined, although cytogenetic responses have been observed 2 years after treatment start.

The safety, efficacy and optimal dosage of Roferon-A in children with CML has not yet been established.

*4. CUTANEOUS T-CELL LYMPHOMA (CTCL)*

Interferon alfa-2a (Roferon-A) may be active in patients with progressive cutaneous T-cell lymphoma and who are refractory to, or unsuitable for conventional therapy.

The optimal dosage has not been established.

*Initial dosage*: Roferon-A should be given by subcutaneous or intramuscular injection, and escalated to 18 million IU daily for a total of 12 weeks in patients of 18 years or older. The recommended escalation schedule is as follows:

| | |
|---|---|
| Days 1–3 | 3 million IU daily |
| Days 4–6 | 9 million IU daily |
| Days 7–84 | 18 million IU daily |

*Maintenance dosage*: Roferon-A should be given by subcutaneous or intramuscular injection 3 times per week at the maximum dose which is acceptable to the patient, but not exceeding 18 million IU.

*Duration of treatment*: Patients should be treated for a minimum of 8 weeks and preferably for at least 12 weeks before the physician decides whether to continue treatment in responding patients or to discontinue treatment in non-responding patients. Minimum treatment duration in responding patients should be 12 months in order to maximise the chance to achieve a complete response and improve the chance for a prolonged response. Patients have been treated for up to 40 consecutive months. The optimal duration of Roferon-A treatment for cutaneous T-cell lymphoma has not been determined.

*Warning*: Objective tumour responses have not been observed in approximately 40% of patients with CTCL. Partial responses are usually seen within 3 months and complete responses within 6 months, although it may occasionally take more than one year to reach the best response.

*5. CHRONIC HEPATITIS B*

Roferon-A is indicated for the treatment of adult patients with histologically proven chronic hepatitis B who have markers for viral replication, i.e., those who are positive for HBV-DNA, DNA polymerase or HBeAg.

*Dosage recommendation*: The optimal schedule of treatment has not been established yet. The dose is usually in the range of 2.5 million IU to 5.0 million IU/$m^2$ body surface administered subcutaneously 3 times per week for a period of 4 to 6 months.

The dosage may be adjusted according to the patient's tolerance to the medication. If no improvement has been observed after 3–4 months of treatment, discontinuation of therapy should be considered.

*Children:* Up to 10 million IU/$m^2$ has been safely administered to children with chronic hepatitis B. However efficacy of therapy has not been demonstrated.

*6. CHRONIC HEPATITIS C*

Roferon-A is indicated for the treatment of adult patients with histologically proven chronic hepatitis C who are positive for HCV antibodies and have elevated serum alanine aminotransferase (ALT) without liver decompensation. There is no evidence of long term benefit on clinical and histological grounds.

In responding patients serum ALT will normalize and/or serum HCV-RNA will significantly decrease.

*Initial dosage*: Roferon-A should be administered at a dose of 3 to 6 million IU by subcutaneous or intramuscular injection 3 times a week for 6 months as induction therapy, patient tolerance permitting. In patients who fail to respond after 3 to 4 months of treatment, discontinuation of Roferon-A should be considered.

*Maintenance dosage*: Patients whose serum ALT has normalized require maintenance therapy with 3 million IU Roferon-A 3 times a week for an additional 6 months to consolidate the complete response. The optimal duration of treatment has not yet been determined.

*Note*: The majority of patients who relapse after adequate treatment do so within 4 months of the end of treatment.

*7. FOLLICULAR NON-HODGKIN'S LYMPHOMA*

Roferon-A prolongs disease-free and progression-free survival when used as adjunctive treatment to CHOP-like chemotherapy regimens in patients with advanced (high tumour burden) follicular non-Hodgkin's lymphoma. However, the efficacy of adjunctive interferon treatment on overall long-term survival of these patients has not yet been established.

*Dosage recommendation:* Roferon-A should be administered concomitantly to a conventional chemotherapy regimen (such as the combination of cyclophosphamide, prednisone, vincristine and doxorubicin) according to a schedule such as 6 million IU/$m^2$ given subcutaneously or intramuscularly from day 22 to day 26 of each 28-day cycle.

*8. ADVANCED RENAL CELL CARCINOMA*

Therapy with Roferon-A in combination with vinblastine induces overall response rates of approximately 17–26%, delays disease progression, and prolongs overall survival in patients with advanced renal cell carcinoma.

*Dosage recommendation*: Roferon-A should be given by subcutaneous or intramuscular injection at a dose of 3 million IU 3 times weekly for one week, 9 million IU 3 times weekly for the following week and 18 million IU 3 times weekly thereafter. Concomitantly vinblastine should be given intravenously according to the manufacturer's instructions at a dose of 0.1 mg/kg once every 3 weeks.

If the Roferon-A dosage of 18 million IU 3 times per week is not tolerated the dose may be reduced to 9 million IU 3 times per week.

Treatment should be given for a minimum of 3 months, up to a maximum of 12 months or until the development of progressive disease. Patients who achieve a complete response may stop treatment 3 months after the response is established.

*Contra-indications:* Roferon-A is contra-indicated in patients with:

(1) A history of hypersensitivity to recombinant interferon alfa-2a or any component of the preparation,

(2) Patients with severe pre-existing cardiac disease or with any history of cardiac illness. No direct cardiotoxic effect has been demonstrated, but it is likely that acute, self-limiting toxicities (i.e., fever, chills) frequently associated with administration of Roferon-A may exacerbate pre-existing cardiac conditions,

(3) Severe renal, hepatic or myeloid dysfunction,

(4) Seizure disorders and/or compromised central nervous system function,

(5) Chronic hepatitis with advanced, decompensated hepatic disease or cirrhosis of the liver,

(6) Chronic hepatitis who are being or have recently been treated with immunosuppressive agents,

(7) Benzyl alcohol which is an excipient in Roferon-A solution for injection has on rare occasions been associated with potentially fatal toxicities in neonates. Therefore, Roferon-A solution for injection should not be used in the neonatal period.

*Special warnings and special precautions for use:* Roferon-A should be administered under the supervision of a qualified physician experienced in the management of the respective indication. Appropriate management of the therapy and its complications is possible only when adequate diagnostic and treatment facilities are readily available.

Patients should be informed not only of the benefits of therapy but also that they will probably experience adverse reactions.

When mild to moderate renal, hepatic or myeloid dysfunction is present, close monitoring of these functions is required.

Careful periodic neuropsychiatric monitoring of all patients is recommended. Suicidal behaviour has been observed rarely in patients receiving Roferon-A. Therapy should be discontinued in patients exhibiting suicidal behaviour.

Extreme caution should be exercised when administering Roferon-A to patients with severe myelosuppression as it has a suppressive effect on the bone marrow, leading to a fall in the white blood count, particularly granulocytes, platelet count and, less commonly, haemoglobin concentration. This can lead to an increased risk of infection or of haemorrhage. It is important to monitor closely these events in patients and periodic complete blood counts should be performed during the course of Roferon-A treatment, both prior to therapy and at appropriate periods during therapy.

In transplant patients (e.g., kidney or bone marrow transplant) therapeutic immunosuppression may be weakened because interferons also exert an immunostimulatory action.

Use of alfa interferon has been rarely associated with exacerbation or provocation of psoriasis.

In rare cases, severe hepatic dysfunction and liver failure have been reported after treatment with alfa interferon.

Hyperglycaemia has been observed rarely in patients treated with Roferon-A. All patients who develop symptoms of hyperglycemia should have their blood glucose measured and followed-up accordingly. Patients with diabetes mellitus may require adjustment of their antidiabetic regimen.

The development of different auto-antibodies has been reported during treatment with alfa interferons. Clinical manifestations of autoimmune disease during interferon therapy occur more frequently in subjects predisposed to the development of autoimmune disorders. Autoimmune phenomena such as vasculitis, arthritis, haemolytic anaemia, thyroid dysfunction and lupus erythematosus syndrome have been observed rarely in patients receiving Roferon-A.

The use of Roferon-A in children is not recommended as the safety and effectiveness of Roferon-A in children have not been established.

Efficacy in patients with chronic hepatitis B or C who are on haemodialysis or have haemophilia or are coinfected with human immunodeficiency virus has not been demonstrated.

*Interactions with other medicaments and other forms of interaction:* Since alfa-interferons alter cellular metabolism, the potential to modify the activity of other drugs exists. In a small study, Roferon-A was shown to have an effect on specific microsomal enzyme systems. The clinical relevance of these findings is unknown.

Alfa-interferons may affect the oxidative metabolic process; this should be borne in mind when prescribing concomitant therapy with drugs metabolised by this route. However, as yet no specific information is available.

Roferon-A has been reported to reduce the clearance of theophylline.

As Roferon-A may affect central nervous system functions, interactions could occur following concurrent administration of centrally-acting drugs. The neurotoxic, haematotoxic or cardiotoxic effects of previously or concurrently administered drugs may be increased by interferons.

*Pregnancy and lactation:* Men and women receiving Roferon-A should practise effective contraception. In pregnancy, Roferon-A should be administered only if the benefit to the woman justifies the potential risk to the foetus. Although animal tests do not indicate that Roferon-A is a teratogen, harm to the foetus from use during pregnancy cannot be excluded. When doses greatly in excess of the recommended clinical dose were administered to pregnant rhesus monkeys in the early to mid-foetal period, an abortifacient effect was observed.

It is not known whether this drug is excreted in human milk. A decision must be taken whether to suspend breast feeding or to discontinue the drug, taking into account the importance of the drug to the mother.

*Effects on ability to drive and use machines:* Depending on dose and schedule as well as the sensitivity of the individual patient, Roferon-A may have an effect on the speed of reaction which could impair certain operations, e.g., driving, operation of machinery etc.

*Undesirable effects:* The following data on adverse reactions are based on information derived from the treatment of cancer patients with a wide variety of malignancies and often refractory to previous therapy and suffering from advanced disease, patients with chronic hepatitis B and patients with chronic hepatitis C. Most cancer patients received doses that were significantly higher than the dose now recommended and this probably explains the higher frequency and severity of adverse reactions in this patient group compared with patients with hepatitis B where adverse reactions are usually transient, and patients return to pre-treatment status within 1 to 2 weeks after the end of therapy; increased hair loss may continue for several weeks.

*General symptoms:* The majority of the patients experienced flu-like symptoms such as fatigue, fever, chills, appetite loss, myalgia, headache, arthralgia and diaphoresis. These acute side-effects can usually be reduced or eliminated by concurrent administration of paracetamol and tend to diminish with continued therapy or dose moderation although continuing therapy can lead to lethargy, weakness and fatigue.

*Gastrointestinal tract:* About two thirds of cancer patients experienced anorexia and one half nausea. Emesis, taste alterations, mouth dryness, weight loss, diarrhoea and mild or moderate abdominal pain were less frequently observed. Constipation, flatulence, hypermotility or heartburn occurred rarely, and reactivation of peptic ulcer and non-life-threatening gastrointestinal bleeding have been reported in isolated cases.

*Alterations of hepatic function* shown by an elevation particularly of ALT, but also of alkaline phosphatase, LDH and bilirubin have been observed and generally did not require dose adjustment. In rare cases hepatitis was reported. In hepatitis B patients, changes in transaminases usually signal an improvement in the clinical state of the patient.

*Central nervous system:* Dizziness, vertigo, visual disturbances, decreased mental status, forgetfulness, depression, drowsiness, confusion, behavioural disturbances such as anxiety and nervousness, and sleep disturbances were uncommon. Suicidal behaviour, severe somnolence, convulsions, coma, cerebrovascular adverse events, transient impotence and ischaemic retinopathy were rare complications.

*Peripheral nervous system*: Paresthesia, numbness, neuropathy, itching and tremor occasionally occurred.

*Cardiovascular and pulmonary systems*: Disorders were seen in about one fifth of cancer patients and consisted of transient hypotensive and hypertensive episodes, oedema, cyanosis, arrhythmias, palpitations and chest pain. Coughing and mild dyspnea were rarely observed. Rare cases of pulmonary oedema, pneumonia, congestive heart failure, cardiorespiratory arrest and myocardial infarction have been reported. Cardiovascular problems are very rarely seen in patients with hepatitis B.

*Skin, mucous membranes and adnexa*: Re-exacerbation of herpes labialis, rash, pruritus, dryness of skin and mucous membranes, rhinorrhea and epistaxis were reported rarely. Mild to moderate alopecia occurred in up to one fifth of patients, but this was reversible on discontinuation of treatment.

*Renal and urinary system*: In rare instances, decreased renal function has occurred. Electrolyte disturbances have been seen, generally in association with anorexia or dehydration. Disorders consisted primarily of proteinuria and increased cell count in sediment. Elevation of BUN, serum creatinine and uric acid has been observed in rare cases. Rare cases of acute renal failure have been reported, mainly in cancer patients with renal disease and/or nephrotoxic comedications as concomitant risk factors.

*Haematopoietic system*: Transient leukopenia occurred variably in about one third to over one half of the patients, but rarely required restriction of dosage. In non-myelosuppressed patients, thrombocytopenia was less frequently seen, and decrease of haemoglobin and haematocrit occurred rarely. In myelosuppressed patients, thrombocytopenia and decreased haemoglobin occurred more frequently. Recovery of severe haematological deviations to pre-treatment levels usually occurred within 7 to 10 days after discontinuing Roferon-A treatment.

*Other*: Inconsequential hypocalcemia was reported in about one half of the patients. Hyperglycemia has been observed rarely in patients treated with Roferon-A.

Reactions at injection sites have occurred in patients.

Transient menstrual cycle irregularities including prolonged menstrual periods have been seen in rhesus monkeys administered doses greatly in excess of the recommended clinical dose. The relevance of these findings in man has not been established.

*Anti-interferon antibodies:* Neutralising antibodies to proteins may be formed in some subjects following homologous administration. Antibodies to all interferons, whether natural or recombinant, are therefore likely to be found in a certain proportion of patients. In certain clinical conditions (cancer, systemic lupus erythematosus, herpes zoster) antibodies to human leukocyte interferon may also occur spontaneously in patients who have never received exogenous interferons.

In clinical trials where lyophilised Roferon-A which had been stored at 25°C was used, neutralising antibodies to Roferon-A have been detected in approximately one fifth of patients. In patients with hepatitis C, a trend for responding patients who develop neutralising antibodies to lose response while still on treatment and to lose it earlier than patients who do not develop such antibodies, has been seen. No other clinical sequelae of the presence of antibodies to Roferon-A have been documented. The clinical significance of the development of antibodies has not been fully clarified.

No data on neutralising antibodies yet exist from clinical trials in which lyophilised Roferon-A or Roferon-A solution for injection which is stored at 4°C has been used. In a mouse model, the relative immunogenicity of lyophilised Roferon-A increases with time when the material is stored at 25°C–no such increase in immunogenicity is observed when lyophilised Roferon-A is stored at 4°C, the recommended storage conditions.

*Overdose:* There are no reports of overdosage but repeated large doses of interferon can be associated with profound lethargy, fatigue, prostration and coma. Such patients should be hospitalised for observation and appropriate supportive treatment given.

Patients who experience severe reactions to Roferon-A will usually recover within days after discontinuation of therapy, given appropriate supportive care. Coma has been observed in 0.4% of cancer patients in clinical trials.

**Pharmacological properties**

*Pharmacodynamic properties:* Roferon-A has been shown to possess many of the activities of the so-called natural human alfa-interferon preparations. Roferon-A exerts its antiviral effects by inducing a state of resistance to viral infections in cells and by modulating the effector arm of the immune system to neutralise viruses or eliminate virus infected cells. The essential mechanism for the antitumour action of Roferon-A is not yet known. However, several changes are described in human tumoural cells treated with Roferon-A: HT 29 cells show a significant reduction of DNA, RNA and protein synthesis. Roferon-A has been shown to exert antiproliferative activity against a variety of human tumours *in vitro* and to inhibit the growth of some human tumour xenografts in nude mice. A limited number of human tumour cell lines grown *in vivo* in immunocompromised nude mice has been tested for the susceptibility to Roferon-A. *In vivo* antiproliferative activity of Roferon-A has been studied on tumours including breast mucoid carcinoma, adenocarcinoma of the caecum, colon carcinoma and prostatic carcinoma. The degree of antiproliferative activity is variable.

Unlike other human proteins, many of the effects of interferon alfa-2a are partially or completely suppressed when it is tested in other animal species. However, significant antivaccinia virus activity was induced in rhesus monkeys pre-treated with interferon alfa-2a.

*Pharmacokinetic properties:* The serum concentrations of interferon alfa-2a reflected a large intersubject variation in both healthy volunteers and patients with disseminated cancer. The pharmacokinetics of Roferon-A in animals (monkey, dog and mouse) were similar to those seen in man. The pharmacokinetics of Roferon-A in man were linear over a 3 million to 198 million IU dose range. In healthy man, interferon alfa-2a exhibited an elimination half-life of 3.7–8.5 hours (mean: 5.1 hours), a volume of distribution at steady state of 0.223–0.748 l/kg (mean: 0.4 l/kg) and a total body clearance of 2.14–3.62 ml/min/kg (mean: 2.79 ml/min/kg) after a 36 million IU intravenous infusion. After intramuscular administration of 36 million IU, peak serum concentrations ranged from 1500 to 2580 pg/ml (mean: 2020 pg/ml) at a mean time to peak of 3.8 hours, and after subcutaneous administration of 36 million IU from 1250 to 2320 pg/ml (mean: 1730pg/ml) at a mean time to peak of 7.3 hours.

The apparent fraction of the dose absorbed after intramuscular or subcutaneous injection is greater than 80%.

The pharmacokinetics of interferon alfa-2a after single intramuscular doses to patients with disseminated cancer and chronic hepatitis B were similar to those found in healthy volunteers. Dose-proportional increases in serum concentrations were observed after single doses up to 198 million IU. There were no changes in the distribution or elimination of interferon alfa-2a during twice daily (0.5–36 million IU), once daily (1–54 million IU), or 3 times weekly (1–136 million IU) dosing regimens up to 28 days of dosing. Renal catabolism is the major pathway for Roferon-A elimination. Biliary excretion and liver metabolism are considered to be minor pathways of elimination of Roferon-A.

Intramuscular administration of Roferon-A one or more times daily for up to 28 days to some patients with disseminated cancer resulted in peak plasma concentrations of 2 to 4 times greater than those seen after single doses. However, multiple dosing caused no changes in its distribution or elimination parameters during several dosage regimens studied.

*Preclinical safety data:* Because of species specificity of human interferon, only limited toxicological studies have been carried out with Roferon-A. The acute parenteral toxicity of Roferon-A has been studied in mice rats, rabbits and ferrets at doses up to 30 million IU/kg intravenously, and 500 million IU/kg intramuscularly. No treatment-related mortality was noted in any species studied given Roferon-A by any of the routes of administration. With doses greatly exceeding the recommended clinical dose no significant adverse effects were observed except for an abortifacient effect when administered to pregnant rhesus monkeys in the early to mid-foetal period and transient menstrual cycle irregularities including prolonged menstrual periods in non-pregnant monkeys.

Mutagenic effects of Roferon-A have not been observed experimentally.

**Pharmaceutical particulars**

*List of excipients:* Ammonium acetate; sodium chloride; benzyl alcohol; polysorbate 80; acetic acid; sodium hydroxide; water for injection.

*Incompatibilities:* None observed.

*Shelf life:* 2 years (at 2–8°C).

*Special precautions for storage:* Store vials and prefilled syringes between +2 and +8°C. Protect from light. Do not freeze.

The 18 MIU/3 ml solution for injection is suitable for multiple-dose use. All other strengths (vials and prefilled syringes) are for single dose use.

*Nature and contents of container:*
*Vials:* Vial 2 ml (flint glass), butyl rubber stopper laminated with FPE, aluminium cap (3 MIU/ml, 4.5 MIU/ml, 6 MIU/ml, 9 MIU/ml, 18 MIU/ml)).

Vial 3 ml (flint glass), butyl rubber stopper laminated with FPE, aluminium cap (18 MIU/3 ml).

An injection kit (1 syringe 2 ml, 1 needle for i.m. injection, 1 needle for s.c. injection) may be supplied with the product.

*Prefilled syringes:* Syringe barrel 1 ml (flint glass), butyl rubber stopper laminated with PTFE (fluororesin D-3), tip cap of butyl rubber and laminated with ETFE (fluororesin D), plunger rod, made of polyethylene, injection needle for subcutaneous injection made of stainless steel, needle hub made of polypropylene. Injection swabs may be supplied with the product.

*Instructions for use/handling*
*Vials:* Plastic syringes are recommended for administration of Roferon-A solution for injection.

Only the 18 MIU/3 ml vial is suitable for multidose use and is for single patient use only. The top of the vial should be swabbed with disinfectant using an aseptic technique before withdrawal of a dose and the date of first withdrawal should be written in the space provided on the vial label. A new sterile syringe and needle must be used each time a dose is withdrawn from the multidose vial. Used needles and syringes must not be re-inserted into multidose vials. 18 MIU/3 ml multidose vials should be used within 30 days of the first withdrawal.

**Marketing authorisation numbers**

| | |
|---|---|
| Roferon-A Solution for injection (vials) 3 MIU/ml | 0031/0400 |
| Roferon-A Solution for injection (vials) 4.5 MIU/ml | 0031/0401 |
| Roferon-A Solution for injection (vials) 6 MIU/ml | 0031/0402 |
| Roferon-A Solution for injection (vials) 9 MIU/ml | 0031/0403 |
| Roferon-A Solution for injection (vials) 18 MIU/ml | 0031/0456 |
| Roferon-A Solution for injection (vials) 18 MIU/3 ml | 0031/0404 |
| Roferon-A Prefilled Syringe 3 MIU/0.5 ml | 0031/0485 |
| Roferon-A Prefilled Syringe 4.5 MIU/0.5 ml | 0031/0486 |
| Roferon-A Prefilled Syringe 6 MIU/0.5 ml | 0031/0487 |
| Roferon-A Prefilled Syringe 9 MIU/0.5 ml | 0031/0488 |

**Date of approval/revision of SPC** March 1997

**Legal category** POM

## ROHYPNOL*

**Presentation** Rohypnol contains the substance with the approved name flunitrazepam, chemically described as 5-(*o*-fluorophenyl)-1,3-dihydro-1-methyl-7 nitro- 2*H*-1,4-benzodiazepin-2-one.

A purple, film-coated, bi-convex diamond-shaped tablet with a single break bar on one side and ROHYPNOL on the other side, containing 1 mg flunitrazepam and the inactive ingredients lactose, maize starch, magnesium stearate, hydroxypropylmethylcellulose, de-ionised water, distilled water, industrial methylated spirits, titanium dioxide (E171), the red colour erythrosine (E127) and the purple colour indigocarmine (E132).

**Uses**

*Properties:* Rohypnol is a full benzodiazepine agonist with a high affinity for the benzodiazepine central site. It has anxiolytic, anticonvulsant and sedative properties, and it causes slowing of psychomotor performance, amnesia, muscle relaxation and sleep induction.

*Pharmacokinetics:* Flunitrazepam is rapidly and almost completely absorbed after oral administration. The distribution half-life of flunitrazepam is about 3 hours; the elimination half-life is variable and may be between 16–35 hours. The onset of effect is rapid and the duration of effect is dose-dependent. Flunitrazepam is almost completely metabolised. The main metabolites are the inactive 7-aminoflunitrazepam and N-desmethyl-flunitrazepam which is less active than the parent compound. The steady state level of the active metabolite is below the minimum effective concentration. The volume of distribution is approximately 3.3–5.5 1/kg. Flunitrazepam is approximately 78% bound to plasma proteins.

*Indications:* Short-term treatment of insomnia when it is severe, disabling or subjecting the individual to unacceptable distress, particularly for patients who have difficulty in falling asleep.

May be employed on an intermittent basis for induction of sleep at unusual times on a short-term or irregular basis.

An underlying cause for insomnia should be sought before deciding upon the use of benzodiazepines for symptomatic relief.

Benzodiazepines are not recommended for the primary treatment of psychotic illness.

**Dosage and administration** Treatment should be as short as possible and should be started with the lowest recommended dose. The maximum dose should not be exceeded. Generally the duration of treatment varies from a few days to two weeks with a maximum of four weeks, including the tapering off process. Patients who have taken benzodiazepines for a prolonged time may require a longer period during which doses are reduced. Specialist help may be appropriate. Little is known regarding the efficacy or safety of benzodiazepines in long-term use.

In certain cases, extension beyond the maximum treatment period may be necessary; if so, it should not take place without re-evaluation of the patient's status. Long-term chronic use is not recommended.

The product should be taken just before going to bed. Rohypnol tablets are for oral administration.

*Adults* Usual dose 0.5 - 1 mg; in exceptional circumstances the dose may be increased to 2 mg.

*Elderly or debilitated patients* Usual dose 0.5 mg; in exceptional circumstances the dose may be increased to 1 mg. If organic brain changes are present, the dosage of Rohypnol should not exceed 0.5 mg in these patients.

In patients with chronic pulmonary insufficiency and in patients with chronic renal or hepatic disease, dosage may need to be reduced.

*Children* Rohypnol tablets are contra-indicated for use in children.

### Contra-indications, warnings, etc

*Contra-indications* Acute pulmonary insufficiency; respiratory depression; phobic or obsessional states; chronic psychosis; myasthenia gravis; sleep apnoea syndrome; severe hepatic insufficiency; use in children.

Use of this drug is contra-indicated in patients with a known hypersensitivity to flunitrazepam (or other benzodiazepines) and any of the excipients. Hypersensitivity reactions including rash, angioedema and hypotension have been reported on rare occasions in susceptible patients.

*Use in pregnancy and lactation* There is no evidence as to drug safety in human pregnancy, nor is there evidence from animal work that it is free from hazard. Do not use during pregnancy, especially during the first and last trimesters, unless there are compelling reasons.

Administration of benzodiazepines in the last trimester of pregnancy or during labour has been reported to produce irregularities in the foetal heart rate, and hypotonia, poor sucking, hypothermia and moderate respiratory depression in the neonate.

Infants born to mothers who took benzodiazepines chronically during the latter stages of pregnancy may have developed physical dependence and may be at some risk of developing withdrawal symptoms in the postnatal period.

Flunitrazepam has been detected in breast milk. The use of Rohypnol in mothers who are breast-feeding should be avoided.

*Precautions* Rohypnol should not be used alone to treat depression or anxiety associated with depression, since suicide may be precipitated in such patients.

In cases of loss or bereavement, psychological adjustment may be inhibited by benzodiazepines.

Patients should be advised that, like all medicaments of this type, Rohypnol may modify patients' performance at skilled tasks (driving, operating machinery, etc.) to a varying degree depending upon dosage, administration, sleep pattern and individual susceptibility. Patients should further be advised that alcohol may intensify any impairment and should, therefore, be avoided during treatment.

Use of benzodiazepines may lead to the development of physical and psychological dependence. The dependence potential of the benzodiazepines is low, particularly when limited to short-term use, but this increases when high doses are used, especially when given over long periods. This is particularly so in patients with a history of alcoholism or drug abuse or in patients with marked personality disorders.

Regular monitoring in such patients is essential; routine repeat prescriptions should be avoided and treatment should be withdrawn gradually. Symptoms such as depression, nervousness, extreme anxiety, tension, restlessness, confusion, mood changes, rebound insomnia, irritability, sweating, diarrhoea, headaches and muscle pain have been reported following abrupt cessation of treatment with normal therapeutic doses. In severe cases the following symptoms may occur: derealisation, depersonalisation, hyperacusis, numbness and tingling of the extremities, hypersensitivity to light, noise and physical contact and hallucinations or epileptic seizures. In rare instances, withdrawal following excessive dosages may produce confusional states and psychotic manifestations. Abuse of flunitrazepam has been reported.

Some loss of efficacy to the hypnotic effects of short-acting benzodiazepines may develop after repeated use for a few weeks.

Abnormal psychological reactions to benzodiazepines have been reported. Rare behavioural effects include paradoxical aggressive outbursts, excitement, confusion, restlessness, agitation, irritability, delusion, rages, nightmares, hallucinations, psychoses, inappropriate behaviour and the uncovering of depression with suicidal tendencies. Extreme caution

should therefore be used in prescribing benzodiazepines to patients with personality disorders. If any of these reactions occur, use of the drug should be discontinued. These reactions may be quite severe and are more likely to occur in children and the elderly.

Benzodiazepines may induce anterograde amnesia. The condition usually occurs several hours after ingesting the product and therefore, to reduce the risk, patients should ensure that they will be able to have an uninterrupted sleep of 7 to 8 hours.

*Interactions* Enhancement of the central depressive effect may occur if Rohypnol is combined with centrally-acting drugs such as neuroleptics, tranquillisers, antidepressants, hypnotics, analgesics and anaesthetics, anti-epileptics and sedative anti-histamines. In the case of narcotic analgesics, enhancement of the euphoria may also occur leading to an increase in psychological dependence. The elderly require special supervision.

When Rohypnol is used in conjunction with anti-epileptic drugs, side-effects and toxicity may be more evident, particularly with hydantoins or barbiturates or combinations including them. This requires extra care in adjusting dosage in the initial stages of treatment.

Known inhibitors of hepatic enzymes, e.g. cimetidine, have been shown to reduce the clearance of benzodiazepines and may potentiate their action, and known inducers of hepatic enzymes, e.g. rifampicin, may increase the clearance of benzodiazepines.

*Side-*effects and adverse reactions: Adverse effects include drowsiness during the day, numbed emotions, reduced alertness, confusion, fatigue, headache, dizziness, muscle weakness, ataxia and double vision. These phenomena are dose related and are likely to be uncommon with the recommended dosage; they occur predominantly at the start of therapy and usually disappear with repeated administration. The elderly are particularly sensitive to the effects of centrally-depressant drugs.

Other adverse effects are less common and include vertigo, hypotension, gastro-intestinal upsets, skin rashes, changes in libido, and urinary retention. Isolated cases of blood dyscrasias and jaundice have also been reported.

Anterograde amnesia may occur at therapeutic dosages, the risk increasing at higher dosages. Amnesic effects may be associated with inappropriate behaviour.

Pre-existing depression may be unmasked during benzodiazepine use.

*Treatment of overdosage* When taken alone in overdosage, Rohypnol presents few problems in management and should not present a threat to life unless combined with other CNS depressants (including alcohol).

In the management of overdose with any medicinal product, it should be borne in mind that multiple agents may have been taken.

Following overdose with oral benzodiazepines, vomiting should be induced if the patient is conscious or gastric lavage undertaken with the airway protected if the patient is unconscious. If there is no advantage in emptying the stomach, activated charcoal should be given to reduce absorption. Special attention should be paid to respiratory and cardiovascular functions in intensive care. Overdose of benzodiazepines is usually manifested by degrees of central nervous system depression ranging from drowsiness to coma. In mild cases, symptoms include drowsiness, mental confusion, dysarthria and lethargy; in more serious cases, symptoms may include ataxia, hypotonia, hypotension, respiratory depression, rarely coma and very rarely death.

Anexate is a specific IV antidote to Rohypnol for use in emergency situations. Patients requiring such intervention should be monitored closely in hospital (see separate prescribing information).

The value of dialysis has not been determined.

If excitation occurs, barbiturates should not be used.

### Pharmaceutical precautions

*Storage* Rohypnol tablets should be stored in a dry place and protected from light.

**Legal category** CD (Sch. 4), POM

**Package quantities** Rohypnol tablets 1 mg are blister-packed in packs of 30.

**Product licence number** 0031/0104

## SYNFLEX*

**Presentation** Pale blue, opaque, film coated tablet, containing naproxen sodium 275 mg (equivalent to naproxen 250 mg) and the inactive ingredients povidone K29/32, magnesium stearate, microcrystalline cellulose, purified water and coating opadry YS-1-4215.

### Uses

*Pharmacological properties:* Naproxen sodium is a non-steroidal anti-inflammatory agent. It has analgesic, anti-inflammatory and antipyretic properties.

*Pharmacokinetics:* Naproxen sodium is rapidly and completely absorbed from the gastro-intestinal tract after oral administration. Because of this rapid and complete absorption, significant plasma levels and onset of pain relief are obtained in patients within 20 minutes of administration. Peak plasma levels following each dose of Synflex tablets are attained in 1–2 hours, depending on food intake. Naproxen has a mean biological half-life of approximately 13 hours and at therapeutic levels it is greater than 99% protein bound. Approximately 95% of a naproxen sodium dose is excreted in the urine.

*Indications:* Synflex is an anti-inflammatory analgesic for the treatment of musculoskeletal disorders (including sprains and strains, direct trauma and lumbosacral pain, cervical spondylitis, fibrositis, bursitis and tendinitis); post-operative pain; post-partum pain; uterine pain following IUCD insertion; dysmenorrhoea; rheumatoid arthritis; osteoarthritis; ankylosing spondylitis and acute gout.

Synflex is also indicated for the relief of migraine.

### Dosage and administration

*Adults:* For musculoskeletal disorders, post-operative pain, pain following IUCD insertion rheumatoid arthritis, osteoarthritis and ankylosing spondylitis the recommended dose is 550 mg (2 tablets) twice daily, not more than 1100 mg being taken per day.

For post-partum pain a single dose of 550 mg is recommended.

For dysmenorrhoea and acute gout the recommended dose is 550 mg initially followed by 275 mg at 6–8 hour intervals as needed. This represents a maximum dose on the first day of 1375 mg (5 tablets) and 1100 mg (4 tablets) per day there after.

For the relief of migraine, the recommended dose is 825 mg at the first symptom of an impending attack. 275–550 mg can be taken in addition throughout the day, if necessary, but not before half an hour after the initial dose. A total dose of 1375 mg per day should not be exceeded.

*Use in the elderly:* Studies indicate that although the total plasma concentration of naproxen is unchanged, the unbound plasma fraction of naproxen is increased in the elderly. The implication of this finding for Synflex dosing is unknown. As with other drugs used in the elderly it is prudent to use the lowest effective dose. For the effect of reduced elimination in the elderly refer to the section–*Use in patients with impaired renal function.*

*Children:* Synflex is not recommended for use in children under sixteen years of age.

### Contra-indications, warnings, etc

*Contra-indications:* Active peptic ulceration. Hypersensitivity to naproxen or naproxen sodium formulations. Since the potential exists for cross-sensitivity reactions, Synflex should not be given to patients in whom aspirin or other non-steroidal anti-inflammatory/analgesic drugs induce asthma, rhinitis or urticaria.

*Use in pregnancy and lactation:* Teratology studies in rats and rabbits at dose levels equivalent on a human multiple basis to those which have produced foetal abnormality with certain other non-steroidal anti-inflammatory agents, e.g. aspirin, have not produced evidence of foetal damage with Synflex. As with other drugs of this type Synflex delays parturition in animals (the relevance of this finding to human patients is unknown) and also affects the human foetal cardiovascular system (closure of the ductus arteriosus). Good medical practice indicates minimal drug usage in pregnancy, and use of this class of therapeutic agent requires cautious balancing of possible benefit against potential risk to the mother and foetus, especially in the first and third trimesters.

The use of Synflex should be avoided in patients who are breast-feeding.

*Precautions:* Episodes of gastro-intestinal bleeding have been reported in patients with naproxen or naproxen sodium therapy. Synflex should therefore be given under close supervision to patients with a history of gastro-intestinal disease.

Serious gastro-intestinal adverse reactions can occur at any time in patients on therapy with non-steroidal anti-inflammatory drugs. The risk of occurrence does not seem to change with duration of therapy. Studies to date have not identified any subset of patients not at risk of developing peptic ulcer and bleeding. However, elderly and debilitated patients tolerate gastro-intestinal ulceration or bleeding less well than others. Most of the serious gastro-intestinal events associated with non-steroidal anti-inflammatory drugs occurred in this patient population.

The antipyretic and anti-inflammatory activities of Synflex may reduce fever and inflammation, thereby diminishing their usefulness as diagnostic signs.

Bronchospasm may be precipitated in patients suffering from, or with a history of, bronchial asthma or allergic disease.

Sporadic abnormalities in laboratory tests (e.g. liver function tests) have occurred in patients on naproxen or naproxen sodium therapy, but no definite trend was seen in any test indicating toxicity.

Naproxen decreases platelet aggregation and prolongs bleeding time. This effect should be kept in mind when bleeding times are determined.

Mild peripheral oedema has been observed in a few patients receiving naproxen or naproxen sodium. Although sodium retention has not been reported in metabolic studies, it is possible that patients with questionable or compromised cardiac function may be at a greater risk when taking Synflex.

Each Synflex tablet contains approximately 25 mg (about 1 m Eq) of sodium. This should be considered in patients whose overall intake of sodium must be markedly restricted.

*Use in patients with impaired renal function:* As naproxen is eliminated to a large extent (95%) by urinary excretion via glomerular filtration, it should be used with great caution in patients with impaired renal function and the monitoring of serum creatinine and/or creatinine clearance is advised in these patients. Synflex is not recommended in patients having baseline creatinine clearance of less than 20 ml/minute.

Certain patients, specifically those whose renal blood flow is compromised, such as in extracellular volume depletion, cirrhosis of the liver, sodium restriction, congestive heart failure, and pre-existing renal disease, should have renal function assessed before and during Synflex therapy. Some elderly patients in whom impaired renal function may be expected, as well as patients using diuretics, may also fall within this category. A reduction in daily dosage should be considered to avoid the possibility of excessive accumulation of naproxen metabolites in these patients.

*Use in patients with impaired liver function:* Chronic alcoholic liver disease and probably also other forms of cirrhosis reduce the total plasma concentration of naproxen, but the plasma concentration of unbound naproxen is increased. The implication of this finding for Synflex dosing is unknown but it is prudent to use the lowest effective dose.

*Drug interactions:* Due to the high plasma protein binding of naproxen, patients simultaneously receiving hydantoins, anticoagulants or a highly protein-bound sulphonamide should be observed for signs of overdosage of these drugs. No interactions have been observed in clinical studies with naproxen sodium or naproxen and anticoagulants or sulphonylureas, but caution is nevertheless advised since interaction has been seen with other non-steroidal agents of this class.

The natriuretic effect of frusemide has been reported to be inhibited by some drugs of this class.

Inhibition of renal lithium clearance leading to increases in plasma lithium concentrations has also been reported.

Naproxen and other non-steroidal anti-inflammatory drugs can reduce the antihypertensive effect of propranolol and other beta-blockers and may increase the risk of renal impairment associated with the use of ACE-inhibitors.

Probenecid given concurrently increases naproxen plasma levels and extends its half-life considerably.

Caution is advised when methotrexate is given concurrently because of possible enhancement of its toxicity, since naproxen, among other non-steroidal anti-inflammatory drugs, has been reported to reduce the tubular secretion of methotrexate in an animal model.

It is suggested that Synflex therapy be temporarily discontinued 48 hours before adrenal function tests are performed because naproxen may artifactually interfere with some tests for 17-ketogenic steroids. Similarly, naproxen may interfere with some assays of urinary 5-hydroxyindoleacetic acid.

*Side-effects and adverse reactions:*
*Gastro-intestinal:* The more frequent reactions are nausea, vomiting, abdominal discomfort and epigastric distress. More serious reactions which may occur occasionally are gastro-intestinal bleeding, peptic ulceration (sometimes with haemorrhage and perforation), non-peptic gastro-intestinal ulceration and colitis.

*Dermatological:* Skin rash, urticaria, angio-oedema. Alopecia, erythema multiforme, Stevens Johnson syndrome, epidermal necrolysis and photosensitivity reactions (including cases in which the skin resembles porphyria cutanea tarda, 'pseudoporphyria') or epidermolysis bullosa may occur rarely.

*Renal:* Including but not limited to glomerular nephritis, interstitial nephritis, nephrotic syndrome, haematuria, renal papillary necrosis and renal failure.

*CNS:* Convulsions, headache, insomnia, inability to concentrate and cognitive dysfunction have been reported.

*Haematological:* Thrombocytopenia, granulocytopenia including agranulocytosis, aplastic anaemia and haemolytic anaemia may occur rarely.

*Other:* Tinnitus, hearing impairment, vertigo, mild peripheral oedema. Anaphylactic reactions to naproxen and naproxen sodium formulations have been reported in patients with, or without, a history of previous hypersensitivity reactions to NSAIDs. Jaundice, fatal hepatitis, visual disturbances, eosinophilic pneumonitis, vasculitis, aseptic meningitis, hyperkalemia, and ulcerative stomatitis have been reported rarely.

*Treatment of overdosage:* Significant overdosage of the drug may be characterised by drowsiness, heartburn, indigestion, nausea or vomiting. A few patients have experienced seizures, but it is not clear whether these were naproxen-related or not. It is not known what dose of the drug would be life-threatening.

Should a patient ingest a large amount of Synflex accidentally or purposefully, the stomach may be emptied and usual supportive measures employed. Animal studies indicate that the prompt administration of activated charcoal in adequate amounts would tend to reduce markedly the absorption of the drug.

Haemodialysis does not decrease the plasma concentration of naproxen because of the high degree of its protein binding. However, haemodialysis may still be appropriate in a patient with renal failure who has taken Synflex.

**Pharmaceutical precautions**
*Storage:* Protect from light and moisture.

**Legal category** POM.

**Package quantities** Synflex tablets are supplied in packs of 100 tablets.

**Product licence number** 0031/0478

## SYNTARIS* NASAL SPRAY

**Presentation** Syntaris contains the substance with the approved name flunisolide. It is chemically described as (6α-fluoro-11β, 16α, 17, 21-tetrahydroxypregna-1, 4 diene-3, 20-dione, 16, 17-acetonide).

A buffered, clear, colourless, slightly viscous aqueous solution in a bottle fitted with a metered pump device which delivers 25µg of flunisolide per spray via a nozzle which is inserted into the nostril. Syntaris Nasal Spray also contains: polyethylene glycol 400, propylene glycol, sodium citrate dihydrate, citric acid anhydrous, benzalkonium chloride, butylated hydroxytoluene, disodium edetate, sorbitol, polysorbate and purified water.

**Uses**
*Pharmacological properties:* Flunisolide is a synthetic corticosteroid which has been formulated as a topical nasal spray for the treatment of allergic nasal conditions. In animal studies flunisolide has several hundred times the anti-inflammatory, thymolytic and anti-adrenocorticotrophic hormone activities of hydrocortisone. Because of the small dose applied (topically) and low systemic absorption, there is minimal systemic activity.

In controlled clinical trials flunisolide has been shown to be significantly more effective than placebo in the treatment of perennial and seasonal allergic rhinitis.

*Pharmacokinetics* Flunisolide is rapidly and well absorbed from the gastrointestinal tract. In man peak blood-levels after oral administration occurred within one hour, but the systemic availability was estimated to be only 20%. After intra-nasal administration (approximately 100µg) extremely low plasma levels (less than 1ng/ml) were detected within 10–30 minutes of dosing and these fell to undetectable levels within four hours.

In man flunisolide undergoes rapid and extensive first pass metabolism to a 6β-hydroxylated metabolite, which has less than one hundredth times the potency of flunisolide, and is less than three times as potent as hydrocortisone.

The plasma half-life of flunisolide is 1.5–2 hours and that of the 6β-hydroxylated metabolite is 2–4 hours. Repeated BID administration of flunisolide by oral inhalation did not result in any cumulative effects. Excretion is via the urine and faeces. Only minor amounts of unchanged free or conjugated flunisolide are excreted in the urine. The major excretory product is the free 6β-hydroxylated metabolite. Animal studies indicate that although a large amount is excreted in the bile, neither flunisolide nor its metabolites appear to enter the entero-hepatic circulation.

**Indications** Syntaris Nasal Spray is indicated for the prophylaxis and treatment of perennial and seasonal allergic rhinitis including hay fever.

**Dosage and administration** Syntaris Nasal Spray is for administration by the intranasal route only.

*Adults (including the elderly):* The usual dose is two sprays into each nostril twice daily. If symptoms are severe or if an exacerbation occurs, the physician may recommend two sprays into each nostril three times daily.

*Children:* For children five years of age and over; one spray (approximately 25µg) into each nostril up to three times daily. Continuous treatment of children aged between five and ten years of age should be limited to a period of four weeks.

*Maintenance dose:* After the desired clinical effect is obtained, the maintenance dose should be the smallest amount necessary to control the symptoms. Some patients may be maintained on as little as one spray (approximately 25µg) to each nostril per day.

The maximum daily dose should not exceed six sprays in each nostril for adults, and three sprays in each nostril for children five years of age and over.

Syntaris Nasal Spray is not recommended for use in children under five years of age.

The effect of Syntaris Nasal Spray, unlike that of vasoconstrictor preparations, is not immediate. Full therapeutic benefit requires regular usage. The absence of an immediate effect should be explained to the patient in order to ensure co-operation and continuation of treatment with the regular dosage schedule.

There is no evidence that exceeding the maximum recommended dosage is more effective; higher dosage should therefore be avoided.

For full information on using the device, see patient information leaflet. Patients should be carefully instructed in the correct use of the spray and of its care.

**Contra-indications, warnings, etc**

*Contra-indications:*
  1. Untreated fungal, bacterial or viral infections of the nose or eyes.
  2. Hypersensitivity to the formulation.

*Use in pregnancy and lactation:* Animal studies with systemic corticosteroids, including flunisolide, show teratogenicity. Experience of use in human beings during pregnancy has not as yet revealed such effects.

Not recommended in the first three months of pregnancy. If used in the second or third trimester the expected benefits should be weighed against the potential hazards of the foetus.

Syntaris Nasal Spray should only be used during pregnancy if considered essential by the physician.

*Precautions:* Glucocorticoids may mask some signs of infection and new infections may appear during their use.

Care must be taken when transferring patients from systemic corticosteroid therapy to Syntaris Nasal Spray if there is reason to suspect that their adrenal function is impaired. When used in conjunction with other agents, such as systemic corticosteroids, any readjustment of dosage should be carried out with caution.

Although adrenal suppression or local effects such as atrophy of the nasal mucosa and secondary infection have not been observed in clinical trials, the potential for these effects should be considered with prolonged excessive usage.

Prolonged use may increase the incidence of bacterial and fungal (including candidal) infections of the upper respiratory tract. Patients on long-term therapy should be seen at regular intervals.

Particular caution is required in patients with, or with a history of, tuberculosis.

Because of the inhibitory effect of corticosteroids in wound healing, in patients who have experienced recent nasal septal ulcers, recurrent epistaxis, nasal surgery or trauma, a nasal corticosteroid should be used with caution until healing has occurred.

There have been a few reports in the literature of the development of cataracts in patients who have been using intranasal or inhaled corticosteroids for prolonged periods of time. Although it is not possible to rule out systemic corticosteroids as a known factor, prescribers should be aware of the possible role of intranasal or inhaled corticosteroids in cataract development.

*Side-effects and adverse reactions:* Adverse reactions noted in clinical trials with Syntaris Nasal Spray have been consistent with what would be expected when applying topical medication to an already inflamed membrane. The most frequently observed side-effect was after-taste and a mild transient nasal burning and stinging which was occasionally severe enough to warrant discontinuation of treatment. Other side-effects noted, in order of decreasing prevalence were: nasal irritation, dryness, epistaxis, runny and stuffy nose, sore throat, hoarseness, throat irritation and rarely alteration of smell and/or taste, and nasal septal perforation. Rarely, a permanent loss in the sense of smell and/or taste has been reported. If severe these may require discontinuation of therapy.

*Carcinogenesis* A 22-month study in mice and a 24-month study in rats showed evidence of tumor formation that was not consistent between the two species and was not believed to be biologically meaningful to man.

*Treatment of overdosage* Administration of large amounts of flunisolide over a short period may produce suppression of hypothalamic-pituitary-adrenal function. In such event, Syntaris Nasal Spray should be reduced immediately to the recommended dosage.

**Pharmaceutical precautions**
*Storage* Store at room temperature below 30°C.

**Legal category** POM

**Package quantities** Each pack of Syntaris Nasal Spray contains one 24 ml bottle and the metered pump/nozzle device.

**Further information** Nil

**Product licence number** 0286/0057

## TASMAR* ▼

**Qualitative and quantitative composition**
Tasmar 100 mg is supplied as film-coated tablets containing 100 mg tolcapone.

Tasmar 200 mg is supplied as film-coated tablets containing 200 mg tolcapone

**Pharmaceutical form** Tasmar 100 mg is a pale to light yellow, hexagonal, biconvex, film-coated tablet. "ROCHE" and "100" is engraved on one side.

Tasmar 200 mg is an orange yellow to brown yellow, hexagonal, biconvex, film-coated tablet. "ROCHE" and "200" is engraved on one side.

**Clinical particulars** Since Tasmar should be used only in combination with levodopa/benserazide and levodopa/carbidopa, the prescribing information for these levodopa preparations is also applicable to their concomitant use with Tasmar.

*Therapeutic indications:* Tasmar is indicated in combination with levodopa/benserazide or levodopa/carbidopa for use in patients with Parkinson's disease, who cannot be stabilised on those combinations, especially fluctuating patients with end-of-dose phenomena.

*Posology and method of administration:*
*Method of administration:* Tasmar is administered orally three times daily. The first dose of the day of Tasmar should be taken together with the first dose of the day of a levodopa preparation, and the subsequent doses should be given approximately 6 and 12 hours later.

Tasmar may be taken with or without food (see *Pharmacokinetic properties*).

Tasmar tablets are film-coated and should be swallowed whole because tolcapone has a bitter taste.

Tasmar can be combined with all pharmaceutical formulations of levodopa/benserazide and levodopa/carbidopa (see also *Interaction with other medicinal products and other forms of interaction*).

*Posology:* Therapy with Tasmar should be initiated with 100 mg three times daily. In clinical trials, the majority of patients required a decrease in daily levodopa dose if their daily dose of levodopa was > 600 mg or if patients had moderate or severe dyskinesias. These factors, together with the patient's sensitivity to changes in dose of levodopa preparations, should be considered when deciding whether to decrease the daily levodopa dose on initiation of Tasmar therapy. In clinical trials, the average reduction of daily levodopa dose was about 30% in those patients requiring a levodopa dose adjustment.

During treatment with Tasmar the patient's levodopa dose should be adjusted as appropriate to optimise the clinical benefit of the combination therapy.

After adjustment of levodopa dose, an increase to 200 mg Tasmar three times daily may be attempted, if in the physician's opinion further benefit without limiting dopaminergic adverse reactions may be expected. After increasing Tasmar to 200 mg three times daily, a further readjustment of levodopa may be needed.

The maximum therapeutic dose of 200 mg three times daily should not be exceeded as there is no evidence of additional efficacy at higher doses.

Patients with impaired hepatic or renal function: See also *Pharmacokinetic properties.*

Patients with moderate liver impairment should not be escalated to 200 mg Tasmar three times daily.

No dose adjustment of Tasmar is recommended for patients with mild or moderate renal impairment (creatinine clearance ≥ 30 ml/min).

*Contra-indications:* Tasmar is contra-indicated in patients with known hypersensitivity to tolcapone or any of its other ingredients.

Tasmar should not be given in conjunction with non-selective monoamine oxidase (MAO) inhibitors (e.g. phenelzine and tranylcypromine). The combination of MAO-A and MAO-B inhibitors is equivalent to non-selective MAO-inhibition, therefore they should not both be given concomitantly with Tasmar and levodopa preparations. Selective MAO-B inhibitors should not be used at higher than recommended doses (e.g. selegiline 10 mg/day) when co-administered with Tasmar (see also *Interaction with other medicinal products and other forms of interaction).*

*Special warnings and special precautions for use:*
*Dyskinesia, nausea and other levodopa-associated adverse reactions:* Patients may experience an increase in levodopa-associated adverse reactions. These adverse reactions may often be mitigated by reducing the dose of levodopa (see *Posology*).

*Diarrhoea:* In clinical trials, diarrhoea developed in 16% and 18% of patients receiving Tasmar 100 mg and 200 mg respectively, compared to 8% of patients receiving placebo. Diarrhoea associated with Tasmar usually began 2 to 4 months after initiation of therapy. Diarrhoea led to withdrawal of 5% and 6% of patients receiving Tasmar 100 mg and 200 mg respectively, compared to 1% of patients receiving placebo.

*Elevated liver transaminases:* It is recommended that transaminases be monitored when starting Tasmar treatment and monthly for the first 6 months. If elevations occur, and a decision is made to continue to treat the patient, more frequent monitoring of complete liver function is recommended. Treatment should be discontinued if ALT exceeds 5 x ULN (upper limit of normal) or if clinical jaundice develops.

*Neuroleptic malignant syndrome symptom complex (NMS):* NMS is characterised by rigidity, elevated temperature, mental status changes and elevated serum creatine phosphokinase (CPK). It has been reported following large decreases in anti-Parkinson's Disease medications. If after discontinuing Tasmar, symptoms occur, physicians should consider increasing the patient's levodopa dose. NMS and Serotonergic Syndrome may be related and therefore drugs that increase brain serotonin activity may also be responsible for these symptoms.

*Benserazide interaction:* Due to the interaction between high dose benserazide and tolcapone (resulting in increased levels of benserazide), the prescriber should, until more experience has been gained, be observant of dose-related adverse events (see also *Interaction with other medicinal products and other forms of interaction).*

*MAO-A inhibitors:* There are no data available for the combination of Tasmar and MAO-A inhibitors, therefore this combination should be given with caution.

*Lactose intolerance:* Each tablet contains 7.5 mg lactose; this quantity is probably not sufficient to induce symptoms of lactose intolerance.

*Special populations:* Patients with severe liver impairment and severe renal impairment (creatinine clearance < 30 ml/min) should be treated with caution. No information on the tolerability of tolcapone in these populations is available.

*Hepatic impairment:* See under *Pharmacokinetic properties–Section 5.2.*

*Renal impairment:* See under *Pharmacokinetic properties–Section 5.2.*

*Interaction with other medicaments and other forms of interaction:*
*Protein binding:* Although, tolcapone is highly protein bound, *in vitro* studies have shown that tolcapone did not displace warfarin, tolbutamide, digitoxin and phenytoin from their binding sites at therapeutic concentrations.

*Drugs metabolised by catechol-O-methyltransferase (COMT):* Tolcapone may influence the pharmacokinetics of drugs metabolised by COMT. No effects were seen on the pharmacokinetics of the COMT substrate carbidopa. An interaction was observed with benserazide, which may lead to increased levels of benserazide and its active metabolite. The magnitude of the effect was benserazide dose dependent. The plasma concentrations of benserazide observed after co-administration of tolcapone and benserazide-25 mg/levodopa were still within the range of values observed with levodopa/benserazide alone. On the other hand, after co-administration of tolcapone and benserazide-50 mg/levodopa the benserazide plasma concentrations could be increased above the levels usually observed with levodopa/benserazide alone. The effect of tolcapone on the pharmacokinetics of other drugs metabolised by COMT such as α-methyldopa, dobutamine, apomorphine, adrenaline and isoprenaline have not been evaluated. The prescriber should be observant of adverse effects caused by putative increased plasma levels of these drugs when combined with Tasmar.

*Effect of tolcapone on the metabolism of other drugs:* Due to its affinity for cytochrome CYP2C9 in vitro, tolcapone may interfere with drugs whose clearance is dependent on this metabolic pathway, such as tolbutamide and warfarin. In an interaction study, tolcapone did not change the pharmacokinetics of tolbutamide. Therefore, clinically relevant interactions involving cytochrome CYP2C9 appear unlikely.

Since clinical information is limited regarding the combination of warfarin and tolcapone, coagulation parameters should be monitored when these drugs are co-administered.

Tolcapone did not change the pharmacokinetics of desipramine, even though both drugs share glucuronidation as their main metabolic pathway.

*Drugs that increase catecholamines:* Since tolcapone interferes with the metabolism of catecholamines, interactions with other drugs affecting catecholamine levels are theoretically possible.

Tolcapone did not influence the effect of ephedrine, an indirect sympathomimetic, on haemodynamic parameters or plasma catecholamine levels, either at rest or during exercise. Since tolcapone did not alter the tolerability of ephedrine, these drugs can be co-administered.

When Tasmar was given together with levodopa/carbidopa and desipramine, there was no significant change in blood pressure, pulse rate and plasma concentrations of desipramine. Overall, the frequency of adverse events increased slightly. These adverse events were predictable based on the known adverse reactions to each of the three drugs individually. Therefore, caution should be exercised when potent noradrenaline uptake inhibitors such as desipramine, maprotiline, or venlafaxine are administered to Parkinson's disease patients being treated with Tasmar and levodopa preparations.

In clinical trials, patients receiving Tasmar/levodopa preparations reported a similar adverse event profile independent of whether or not they were also concomitantly administered selegiline (a MAO-B inhibitor).

*Pregnancy and lactation:*
*Pregnancy:* In rats and rabbits, embryofetoxicity was observed after tolcapone administration (see also *Preclinical safety data*).

There is no experience from clinical studies regarding the use of Tasmar in pregnant women. Therefore, Tasmar should be used during pregnancy only if the potential benefit justifies the potential risk to the foetus.

*Lactation:* In animal studies, tolcapone was excreted into maternal milk.

The safety of tolcapone in infants is unknown; therefore, women should not breast-feed during treatment with Tasmar.

*Effects on ability to drive and use machines:* There is no evidence from clinical studies that Tasmar adversely influences a patient's ability to drive and use machines. However, patients should be advised that their ability to drive and operate machines may be compromised due to their Parkinson's disease symptoms.

*Undesirable effects:* The most commonly observed adverse events associated with the use of Tasmar, occurring more frequently than in placebo-treated patients, were dyskinesia, nausea, sleep disorders, anorexia and diarrhoea.

The only adverse event commonly leading to discontinuation of Tasmar in clinical trials was diarrhoea (see also *Special warnings and special precautions for use*).

Isolated cases of patients with symptoms suggestive of Neuroleptic Malignant Syndrome Symptom Complex (see *Special warnings and special precautions for use*) have been reported following reduction or discontinuation of Tasmar and other concomitant dopaminergic medications.

Increases to more than three times the upper limit of normal (ULN) in alanine aminotransferase (ALT) occurred in 1% of patients receiving Tasmar 100 mg three times daily, and 3% of patients at 200 mg three times daily. The increases usually appeared within 6 to 12 weeks of starting treatment, and were not associated with any clinical signs or symptoms. In about half the cases, transaminase levels returned spontaneously to baseline values whilst patients continued Tasmar treatment. For the remainder, when treatment was discontinued, transaminase levels returned to pre-treatment levels.

*Urine discolouration:* Tolcapone and its metabolites are yellow and can cause a harmless intensification in the colour of the patient's urine.

Experience with Tasmar obtained in parallel, placebo-controlled, randomised studies in patients with Parkinson's disease are shown in the following table which lists adverse events, with a potential relationship to Tasmar.

Summary of potentially Tasmar-related adverse events, with crude incidence rates for the phase III placebo-controlled studies:

| Adverse Events | Placebo N = 298 (%) | 100 mg Tolcapone N = 296 (%) | 200 mg Tolcapone N = 298 (%) |
|---|---|---|---|
| † Dyskinesia | 19.8 | 41.9 | 51.3 |
| † Nausea | 17.8 | 30.4 | 34.9 |
| † Sleep disorder | 18.1 | 23.6 | 24.8 |
| † Dystonia | 17.1 | 18.6 | 22.1 |
| † Excessive dreaming | 17.1 | 21.3 | 16.4 |
| † Anorexia | 12.8 | 18.9 | 22.8 |
| † Orthostatic complaints | 13.8 | 16.6 | 16.8 |
| † Somnolence | 13.4 | 17.9 | 14.4 |
| Diarrhoea | 7.7 | 15.5 | 18.1 |
| Dizziness | 9.7 | 13.2 | 6.4 |
| † Confusion | 8.7 | 10.5 | 10.4 |
| Headache | 7.4 | 9.8 | 11.4 |
| † Hallucination | 5.4 | 8.4 | 10.4 |
| † Vomiting | 3.7 | 8.4 | 9.7 |
| Constipation | 5.0 | 6.4 | 8.4 |
| Upper respiratory tract infection | 3.4 | 4.7 | 7.4 |
| Sweating increased | 2.3 | 4.4 | 7.4 |
| Xerostomia | 2.3 | 4.7 | 6.4 |
| Abdominal pain | 2.7 | 4.7 | 5.7 |
| † Syncope | 2.7 | 4.1 | 5.0 |
| Urine discoloration | 0.7 | 2.4 | 7.4 |
| Dyspepsia | 1.7 | 4.1 | 3.0 |
| Influenza | 1.7 | 3.0 | 4.0 |
| Chest pain | 1.3 | 3.4 | 1.0 |
| Hypokinesia | 0.7 | 0.7 | 2.7 |

† Potentially L-DOPA-induced symptoms

*Overdose:* The highest dose of tolcapone administered to humans was 800 mg three times daily, with and without levodopa co-administration, in a one week study in elderly, healthy volunteers. The peak plasma concentrations of tolcapone at this dose were on average 30µg/ml (compared to 3 and 6µg/ml with 100 mg and 200 mg of tolcapone respectively). Nausea, vomiting and dizziness were observed, particularly in combination with levodopa.

The threshold for the lethal plasma concentration for tolcapone based on animal data is > 100µg/ml. Respiratory difficulties were observed in rats at high oral (gavage) and intravenous doses and in dogs with rapidly injected intravenous doses.

*Management of overdose:* Hospitalisation is advised. General supportive care is indicated. Based on the physicochemical properties of the compound, haemodialysis is unlikely to be of benefit.

**Pharmacological properties** Tolcapone is an orally active, selective and reversible catechol-*O*-methyltransferase (COMT) inhibitor. Administered concomitantly with levodopa and an aromatic amino acid decarboxylase inhibitor (AADC-I), it leads to more stable plasma levels of levodopa by reducing metabolism of levodopa to 3-methoxy-4-hydroxy-L-phenylalanine (3-OMD).

High levels of plasma 3-OMD have been associated with poor response to levodopa in Parkinson's disease patients. Tolcapone markedly reduces the formation of 3-OMD.

*Pharmacodynamic properties:*
*Pharmaco-therapeutic group:* Anti-Parkinson drug, ATC code: NO4BX01

*Clinical pharmacology:* Studies in healthy volunteers have shown that tolcapone reversibly inhibits human erythrocyte COMT activity after oral administration. The inhibition is closely related to plasma tolcapone concentration. With 200 mg tolcapone, maximum inhibition of erythrocyte COMT activity is, on average, greater than 80%. During dosing with Tasmar 200 mg three times daily, erythrocyte COMT inhibition at trough is 30% to 45%, with no development of tolerance.

Transient elevation above pretreatment levels of erythrocyte COMT activity was observed after withdrawal of tolcapone. However, a study in Parkinson's patients confirmed that after treatment discontinuation there was no significant change in levodopa pharmacokinetics or in patient response to levodopa compared to pretreatment levels.

When Tasmar is administered together with levodopa, it increases the relative bioavailability (AUC) of levodopa approximately twofold. This is due to a decrease in clearance in L-dopa resulting in a prolongation of the terminal elimination half-life ($t_{\frac{1}{2}}\beta$) of levodopa. In general, the average peak levodopa plasma concentration (Cmax) and the time of its occurrence (tmax) were unaffected. The onset of effect occurs after the first administration. Studies in healthy volunteers and parkinsonian patients have confirmed that the maximum effect occurs with 100–200 mg tolcapone. Plasma levels of 3-OMD were markedly and dose-dependently decreased by tolcapone when given with levodopa/AADC-I (aromatic amino acid decarboxylase–inhibitor) (benserazide or carbidopa).

Tolcapone's effect on levodopa pharmacokinetics is similar with all pharmaceutical formulations of levodopa/benserazide and levodopa/carbidopa: it is independent of levodopa dose, levodopa/AADC-I (benserazide or carbidopa) ratio and the use of sustained-release formulations.

*Clinical studies:* Clinical studies have shown a significant reduction of approximately 20% to 30% in OFF time and a similar increase in ON time, accompanied by reduced severity of symptoms in fluctuating patients receiving Tasmar. Investigator's global assessments of efficacy also showed significant improvement.

In a clinical study in patients without end of dose fluctuations, Tasmar was significantly superior to placebo in improving activities of daily living and motor function.

*Pharmacokinetic properties:* In the therapeutic range, tolcapone pharmacokinetics are linear and independent of levodopa/AADC-I (benserazide or carbidopa) co-administration.

*Absorption:* Tolcapone is rapidly absorbed with a tmax of approximately 2 hours. The absolute bioavailability of an oral administration is around 65%. Tolcapone does not accumulate with three times daily dosing of 100 or 200 mg. At these doses, Cmax is approximately 3 and 6 µg/ml, respectively. Food delays and decreases the absorption of tolcapone, but the relative bioavailability of a dose of tolcapone taken with a meal is still 80% to 90%.

*Distribution:* The volume of distribution (Vss) of tolcapone is small (9 l). Tolcapone does not distribute widely into tissues due to its high plasma protein binding (> 99.9%). In vitro experiments have shown that tolcapone binds mainly to serum albumin.

*Metabolism/elimination:* Tolcapone is almost completely metabolised prior to excretion, with only a very small amount (0.5% of dose) found unchanged in urine. The main metabolic pathway of tolcapone is conjugation to its inactive glucuronide. In addition, the compound is methylated by COMT to 3-O-methyltolcapone and metabolised by cytochromes P450 3A4 and P450 2A6 to a primary alcohol (hydroxylation of the methyl group), which is subsequently oxidised to the carboxylic acid. The reduction to a putative amine, as well as the subsequent N-acetylation, occurs to a minor extent. After oral administration, 60% of drug-related material is excreted into urine, and 40% into faeces.

Tolcapone is a low-extraction-ratio drug (extraction ratio = 0.15), with a moderate systemic clearance of about 7 l/h. The $t_{\frac{1}{2}}\beta$ of tolcapone is approximately 2 hours.

*Hepatic impairment:* A study in patients with hepatic impairment has shown that moderate non-cirrhotic liver disease had no impact on the pharmacokinetics of tolcapone. However, in patients with moderate cirrhotic liver disease, clearance of unbound tolcapone was reduced by almost 50%. This reduction may increase the average concentration of unbound drug twofold (see *Posology*).

*Renal impairment:* The pharmacokinetics of tolcapone have not been investigated in patients with renal impairment. However, the relationship of renal function and tolcapone pharmacokinetics has been investigated using population pharmacokinetics during clinical trials. The data of more than 400 patients have confirmed that over a wide range of creatinine clearance values (30–130 ml/min) the pharmacokinetics of tolcapone are unaffected by renal function. This could be explained by the fact that only a negligible amount of unchanged tolcapone is excreted in the urine, and the main metabolite, tolcapone-glucuronide, is excreted both in urine and in bile (faeces).

*Preclinical safety data:*
*Carcinogenesis, mutagenesis:* 3% and 5% of rats in the mid- and high- dose groups, respectively, of the 24-month carcinogenicity study were shown to have renal epithelial tumours (adenomas or carcinomas). The tumours were considered to be due to single cell necrosis and sustained repair as a consequence of chronic epithelial cell damage in the proximal tubule. First signs of proximal tubule cell toxicity were observed in the 12-month rat toxicity study, at plasma AUC (based on unbound concentrations) about 10 times greater than those in patients. No evidence of renal toxicity was observed in the low-dose group of the rat carcinogenicity study, equivalent to at least two times the therapeutic AUC. There were no similar renal findings in the mouse carcinogenicity study, or in the 12-month toxicity studies in dogs, at the plasma concentrations at least six and seven-fold above therapeutic concentrations, respectively.

An increased incidence of uterine adenocarcinomas was seen in the high-dose group of the rat carcinogenicity study. This is most likely due to a pharmacodynamic action resulting in low prolactin secretion and an oestrogen dominance. The mechanism is specific to rats.

Tolcapone was shown not to be genotoxic in a complete series of mutagenicity studies.

*Toxicity to reproduction:* Tolcapone, when administered alone, was shown to be neither teratogenic nor to have any relevant effects on fertility. Resorptions, a decreased number of pups per litter and reduced performance for female rat pups in a learning test were observed in rats at doses associated with maternal toxicity. In rabbits, an abortifacient effect was revealed.

**Pharmaceutical particulars**

*List of excipients:*
*Tablet core:* Calcium hydrogen phosphate (anhydrous), Microcrystalline cellulose, Polyvidone K30, Sodium starch glycollate, Lactose monohydrate, Talc, Magnesium stearate.

*Film-coat:* Methylhydroxypropylcellulose, Talc, Yellow iron oxide (E 172), Ethylcellulose, Titanium dioxide (E 171), Triacetin, Sodium lauryl sulfate.

*Incompatibilities:* Not applicable.

*Shelf life:* 2 years.

*Special precautions for storage:* Not applicable.

*Nature and contents of container:* Tasmar is available in PVC/PE/PVDC blisters (pack sizes of 30 and 60 film-coated tablets) and in glass bottles (pack sizes of 100 film-coated tablets).

*Instructions for use/handling:* Not applicable.

**Marketing authorisation numbers**

| | |
|---|---|
| Tasmar 100 mg 30 tablet blister | EU/1/97/044/001 |
| Tasmar 100 mg 60 tablet blister | EU/1/97/044/002 |
| Tasmar 100 mg 100 tablet bottles | EU/1/97/044/003 |
| Tasmar 200 mg 30 tablet blister | EU/1/97/044/004 |
| Tasmar 200 mg 60 tablet blister | EU/1/97/044/005 |
| Tasmar 200 mg 100 tablet bottles | EU/1/97/044/006 |

**Date of approval/revision of SPC** August 1997

**Legal category** POM

## TORADOL*

**Qualitative and quantitative composition** Toradol contains ketorolac trometamol 10 mg or 30 mg in ampoules of 1 ml. It also contains ethanol, sodium chloride and water.

**Pharmaceutical form** Toradol is a clear, slightly yellow solution for intramuscular or bolus intravenous injection.

**Clinical particulars**

*Therapeutic indications:* Toradol is indicated for the short-term management of moderate to severe acute postoperative pain.

*Posology and method of administration:* Toradol is for administration by intramuscular or bolus intravenous injection. Bolus intravenous doses should be given over no less than 15 seconds. Toradol should not be used for epidural or spinal administration.

The time to onset of analgesic effect following both IV and IM administration is similar and is approximately 30 minutes, with maximum analgesia occurring within 1 to 2 hours. The median duration of analgesia is generally 4 to 6 hours.

Dosage should be adjusted according to the severity of the pain and the patient response.

The administration of continuous multiple daily doses of ketorolac intramuscularly or intravenously should not exceed 2 days because adverse events may increase with prolonged usage. There has been limited experience with dosing for longer periods since the vast majority of patients have transferred to oral medication, or no longer require analgesic therapy after this time.

*Adults:* The recommended initial dose of Toradol is 10 mg, followed by 10 to 30 mg every 4 to 6 hours as required. In the initial postoperative period, Toradol may be given as often as every 2 hours if needed. The lowest effective dose should be given. A total daily dose of 90 mg for non-elderly and 60 mg for the elderly, renally-impaired patients and patients less than 50 kg should not be exceeded. The maximum duration of treatment should not exceed 2 days.

Reduce dosage in patients under 50 kg.

Opioid analgesics (e.g. morphine, pethidine) may be used concomitantly, and may be required for optimal analgesic effect in the early postoperative period when pain is most severe. Ketorolac does not interfere with opioid binding and does not exacerbate opioid-related respiratory depression or sedation. When used in association with Toradol IM/IV, the daily dose of opioid is usually less than that normally required. However, opioid side-effects should still be considered, especially in day-case surgery.

For patients receiving parenteral Toradol, and who are converted to Toradol oral tablets, the total combined daily dose should not exceed 90 mg (60 mg for the elderly, renally-impaired patients and patients less than 50 kg) and the oral component should not exceed 40 mg on the day the change of formulation is made. Patients should be converted to oral treatment as soon as possible.

*Elderly:* For patients over 65 years, the lower end of the dosage range is recommended; a total daily dose of 60 mg should not be exceeded (see *Special warnings and special precautions for use*).

*Children:* Safety and efficacy in children have not been established. Therefore, Toradol is not recommended for use in children under 16 years of age.

*Renal impairment:* Contra-indicated in moderate to severe renal impairment; reduce dosage in lesser impairment (not exceeding 60 mg/day IV or IM) (see *Contra-indications*).

*Contra-indications:*
- a history of peptic ulcer or gastro-intestinal bleeding.
- suspected or confirmed cerebrovascular bleeding.
- haemorrhagic diatheses, including coagulation disorders.
- hypersensitivity to ketorolac trometamol or other NSAIDs and those patients in whom aspirin or other prostaglandin synthesis inhibitors induce allergic reactions (severe anaphylactic-like reactions have been observed in such patients).
- the complete or partial syndrome of nasal polyps, angio-oedema or bronchospasm.
- concurrent treatment with other NSAIDs, oxpentifylline, probenecid or lithium salts .
- hypovolaemia from any cause or dehydration.
- moderate or severe renal impairment (serum creatinine > 160 micromol/l).
- a history of asthma.
- patients who have had operations with a high risk of haemorrhage or incomplete haemostasis.
- patients on anticoagulants including low dose heparin (2500–5000 units 12-hourly).
- during pregnancy, labour, delivery or lactation.
- children under 16 years of age.

*Special warnings and special precautions for use:* Physicians should be aware that in some patients pain relief may not occur until upwards of 30 minutes after IV or IM administration.

*Use in the elderly:* Patients over the age of 65 years may be at a greater risk of experiencing adverse events than younger patients. This age-related risk is common to all NSAIDs. Compared to young adults, the elderly have an increased plasma half-life and reduced plasma clearance of ketorolac. With Toradol IM/IV, a total daily dose greater than 60 mg is not recommended. With Toradol tablets, a longer dosing interval is advisable (see *Posology and method of administration*).

*Gastro-intestinal effects:* Toradol can cause gastro-intestinal irritation, ulcers or bleeding in patients with or without a history of previous symptoms. Elderly and debilitated patients are more prone to develop these reactions. The incidence increases with dose and duration of treatment.

In a non-randomised, in-hospital post-marketing surveillance study, increased rates of clinically serious GI bleeding were seen in patients < 65 years of age who received an average daily dose of > 90 mg ketorolac IM as compared to those patients receiving parenteral opioids.

*Respiratory effects:* Bronchospasm may be precipitated in patients with a history of asthma.

*Renal effects:* Drugs that inhibit prostaglandin biosynthesis (including non-steroidal anti-inflammatory drugs) have been reported to cause nephrotoxicity, including but not limited to glomerular nephritis, interstitial nephritis, renal papillary necrosis, nephrotic syndrome and acute renal failure. In patients with renal, cardiac or hepatic impairment, caution is required since the use of NSAIDs may result in deterioration of renal function.

As with other drugs that inhibit prostaglandin synthesis, elevations of serum urea, creatinine and potassium have been reported with ketorolac trometamol and may occur after one dose.

*Patients with impaired renal function:* Since ketorolac trometamol and its metabolites are excreted primarily by the kidney, patients with moderate to severe impairment of renal function (serum creatinine greater than 160 micromol/l) should not receive Toradol. Patients with lesser renal impairment should receive a reduced dose of ketorolac (not exceeding 60 mg/day IM or IV) and their renal status should be closely monitored.

Caution should be observed in patients with conditions leading to a reduction in blood volume and/or renal blood flow, where renal prostaglandins have a supportive role in the maintenance of renal perfusion.

In these patients, administration of an NSAID may cause a dose-dependent reduction in renal prostaglandin formation and may precipitate overt renal failure. Patients at greatest risk of this reaction are those who are volume depleted because of blood loss or severe dehydration, patients with impaired renal function, heart failure, liver dysfunction, the elderly and those taking diuretics. Discontinuation of NSAID therapy is typically followed by recovery to the pretreatment state. Inadequate fluid/blood replacement during surgery, leading to hypovolaemia, may lead to renal dysfunction which could be exacerbated when Toradol is administered. Therefore, volume depletion should be corrected and close monitoring of serum urea and creatinine and urine output is recommended until the patient is normovolaemic. In patients on renal dialysis, ketorolac clearance was reduced to approximately half the normal rate and terminal half-life increased approximately three-fold.

*Fluid retention and oedema:* Fluid retention and oedema have been reported with the use of Toradol and it should therefore be used with caution in patients with cardiac decompensation, hypertension or similar conditions.

*Use in patients with impaired liver function:* Patients with impaired hepatic function from cirrhosis do not have any clinically important changes in ketorolac clearance or terminal half-life.

Borderline elevations of one or more liver function tests may occur. These abnormalities may be transient, may remain unchanged, or may progress with continued therapy. Meaningful elevations (greater than 3 times normal) of serum glutamate pyruvate transaminase (SGPT/ALT) or serum glutamate oxaloacetate transaminase (SGOT/AST) occurred in controlled clinical trials in less than 1% of patients. If clinical signs and symptoms consistent with liver disease develop, or if systemic manifestations occur, Toradol should be discontinued.

*Haematological effects:* Patients with coagulation disorders should not receive Toradol. Patients on anticoagulation therapy may be at increased risk of bleeding if given Toradol concurrently. The concomitant use of ketorolac and prophylactic low-dose heparin (2,500–5,000 units 12-hourly) has not been studied extensively and may also be associated with an increased risk of bleeding. Patients already on anticoagulants or who require low-dose heparin should not receive ketorolac. Patients who are receiving other drug therapy that interferes with haemostasis should be carefully observed if Toradol is administered. In controlled clinical studies, the incidence of clinically significant postoperative bleeding was less than 1%.

Ketorolac inhibits platelet aggregation and prolongs bleeding time. In patients with normal bleeding function, bleeding times were raised, but not outside the normal range of 2–11 minutes. Unlike the prolonged effects from aspirin, platelet function returns to normal within 24 to 48 hours after ketorolac is discontinued.

In post-marketing experience, postoperative wound haemorrhage has been reported in association with the immediate peri-operative use of Toradol IM/IV. Therefore, ketorolac should not be used in patients who have had operations with a high risk of haemorrhage or incomplete haemostasis. Caution should be used where strict haemostasis is critical, e.g. in cosmetic or day-case surgery. Haematomata and other signs of wound haemorrhage and epistaxis have been reported with the use of Toradol. Physicians should be aware of the pharmacological similarity of ketorolac to other non-steroidal anti-inflammatory drugs that inhibit cyclo-oxygenase and the risk of bleeding, particularly in the elderly.

Toradol is not an anaesthetic agent and possesses no sedative or anxiolytic properties; therefore it is not recommended as a pre-operative medication for the support of anaesthesia when these effects are required.

*Interaction with other medicaments and other forms of interaction:* Toradol should not be used with other NSAIDs because of the potential for additive side-effects.

Ketorolac is highly bound to human plasma protein (mean 99.2%) and binding is concentration-independent.

Ketorolac did not alter digoxin protein binding. *In vitro* studies indicated that at therapeutic concentrations of salicylate (300 mcg/ml) and above, the binding of ketorolac was reduced from approximately 99.2% to 97.5%. Therapeutic concentrations of digoxin, warfarin, paracetamol, phenytoin and tolbutamide did not alter ketorolac protein binding. Because ketorolac is a highly potent drug and present in low concentrations in plasma, it would not be expected to displace other protein-bound drugs significantly.

There is no evidence in animal or human studies that ketorolac trometamol induces or inhibits the hepatic enzymes capable of metabolising itself or other drugs. Hence Toradol would not be expected to alter the pharmacokinetics of other drugs due to enzyme induction or inhibition mechanisms.

In normovolaemic healthy subjects, ketorolac reduces the diuretic response to frusemide by approximately 20%, so particular care should be taken in patients with cardiac decompensation.

There is an increased risk of renal impairment when ketorolac is administered concurrently with ACE inhibitors, particularly in volume depleted patients.

Caution is advised when methotrexate is administered concurrently, since some prostaglandin synthesis inhibiting drugs have been reported to reduce the clearance of methotrexate, and thus possibly enhance its toxicity.

Probenecid should not be administered concurrently with ketorolac because of increases in ketorolac plasma level and half-life.

Because of an increased tendency to bleeding when oxpentifylline is administered concurrently, this combination should be avoided.

In patients receiving lithium, there is a possible inhibition of renal lithium clearance, increased plasma lithium concentration, and potential lithium toxicity (see *Contra-indications*).

*Pregnancy and lactation:* There was no evidence of teratogenicity in rats or rabbits studied at maternally-toxic doses of ketorolac. Prolongation of the gestation period and/or delayed parturition were seen in the rat. Ketorolac and its metabolites have been shown to pass into the foetus and milk of animals. Ketorolac has been detected in human milk at low levels. Safety in human pregnancy has not been established. Ketorolac is therefore contra-indicated during pregnancy, labour or delivery, or in mothers who are breast-feeding.

*Effects on ability to drive and use machines:* None known.

*Undesirable effects:* The following side-effects have been reported with Toradol.

*Gastro-intestinal:* Nausea, dyspepsia, gastro-intestinal pain, abdominal discomfort, gastritis, diarrhoea, eructation, constipation, flatulence, fullness, melaena, peptic ulcer, rectal bleeding, stomatitis, vomiting, haemorrhage, perforation, pancreatitis.

*Central nervous/musculoskeletal systems:* Drowsiness, dizziness, headache, sweating, dry mouth, nervousness, paraesthesia, functional disorders, abnormal thinking, depression, euphoria, convulsions, excessive thirst, inability to concentrate, insomnia, stimulation, vertigo, abnormal taste and vision, myalgia, abnormal dreams, hallucinations, hyperkinesia, hearing loss, tinnitus, aseptic meningitis.

*Renal:* Increased urinary frequency, oliguria, acute renal failure, hyponatraemia, hyperkalaemia, haemolytic uraemic syndrome, flank pain (with or without haematuria), raised serum urea and creatinine, interstitial nephritis.

*Cardiovascular/haematological:* Flushing, bradycardia, pallor, purpura, thrombocytopenia, hypertension.

*Respiratory:* Dyspnoea, asthma, pulmonary oedema.

*Dermatological:* Pruritus, urticaria, Lyell's syndrome, Stevens-Johnson syndrome, exfoliative dermatitis, maculopapular rash.

*Hypersensitivity reactions:* Anaphylaxis, bronchospasm, laryngeal oedema, hypotension, flushing and rash. Such reactions may occur in patients with or without known sensitivity to Toradol or other non-steroidal anti-inflammatory drugs.

*Bleeding:* Postoperative wound haemorrhage, haematomata, epistaxis.

*Other:* Asthenia, oedema, weight gain, abnormalities of liver function tests. Injection site pain has been reported in some patients.

*Overdose:* Doses of 360 mg given intramuscularly over an 8-hour interval for five consecutive days have

| Type of subjects | Total clearance (l/hr/kg) mean (range) | Terminal half-life (hrs) mean (range) |
| --- | --- | --- |
| Normal subjects (n = 54) | 0.023 (0.010–0.046) | 5.3 (3.5–9.2) |
| Patients with hepatic dysfunction (n = 7) | 0.029 (0.013–0.066) | 5.4 (2.2–6.9) |
| Patients with renal impairment (n = 25) (serum creatinine 160–430 micromol/l) | 0.016 (0.005–0.043) | 10.3 (5.9–19.2) |
| Renal dialysis patients (n = 9) | 0.016 (0.003–0.036) | 13.6 (8.0–39.1) |
| Healthy elderly subjects (n = 13) (mean age 72) | 0.019 (0.013–0.034) | 7.0 (4.7–8.6) |

caused abdominal pain and peptic ulcers which have healed after discontinuation of dosing. Two patients recovered from unsuccessful suicide attempts. One patient experienced nausea after 210 mg ketorolac, and the other hyperventilation after 300 mg ketorolac.

**Pharmacological properties**

*Pharmacodynamic properties:* Toradol is a potent analgesic agent of the non-steroidal, anti-inflammatory class (NSAID). It is not an opioid and has no known effects on opioid receptors. Its mode of action is to inhibit the cyclo-oxygenase enzyme system and hence prostaglandin synthesis, and it demonstrates a minimal anti-inflammatory effect at its analgesic dose.

*Pharmacokinetic properties: IM:* Following intramuscular administration, ketorolac trometamol was rapidly and completely absorbed, a mean peak plasma concentration of 2.2 mcg/ml occurring an average of 50 minutes after a single 30 mg dose. The influences of age, kidney and liver function on terminal plasma half-life and mean total clearance are outlined in the table below (estimated from a single 30 mg IM dose of ketorolac).

*IV:* Intravenous administration of a single 10 mg dose of ketorolac trometamol resulted in a mean peak plasma concentration of 2.4 mcg/ml occurring an average of 5.4 minutes after dosing, with a terminal plasma elimination half-life of 5.1 hours, an average volume of distribution of 0.15 l/kg, and a total plasma clearance of 0.35 ml/min/kg.

The pharmacokinetics of ketorolac in man following single or multiple doses are linear. Steady-state plasma levels are achieved after dosing every 6 hours for one day. No changes in clearance occurred with chronic dosing. The primary route of excretion of ketorolac and its metabolites is renal: 91.4% (mean) of a given dose being found in the urine and 6.1% (mean) in the faeces.

More than 99% of the ketorolac in plasma is protein-bound over a wide concentration range.

*Preclinical safety data:* An 18-month study in mice with oral doses of ketorolac tromethamine at 2 mg/kg/day (0.9 times human systemic exposure at the recommended IM or IV dose of 30 mg qid, based on area-under-the-plasma-concentration curve [AUC]), and a 24-month study in rats at 5 mg/kg/day (0.5 times the human AUC), showed no evidence of tumorigenicity.

Ketorolac tromethamine was not mutagenic in the Ames test, unscheduled DNA synthesis and repair, and in forward mutation assays. Ketorolac tromethamine did not cause chromosome breakage in the *in vivo* mouse micronucleus assay. At 1590 µg/ml and at higher concentrations, ketorolac tromethamine increased the incidence of chromosomal aberrations in Chinese hamster ovarian cells.

Impairment of fertility did not occur in male or female rats at oral doses of 9 mg/kg (0.9 times the human AUC) and 16 mg/kg (1.6 times the human AUC) of ketorolac tromethamine, respectively.

**Pharmaceutical particulars**

*List of excipients:* Ethanol; Sodium Chloride; Water.

*Incompatibilities:* Toradol should not be mixed in a small volume (e.g. in a syringe) with morphine sulphate, pethidine hydrochloride, promethazine hydrochloride or hydroxyzine hydrochloride as precipitation of ketorolac will occur.

It is compatible with normal saline, 5% dextrose, Ringer's, lactated Ringer's or Plasmacyte solutions. Compatibility of Toradol with other drugs is unknown.

*Shelf life:* 24 months.

*Special precautions for storage:* Store at controlled room temperature (15–30°C) and protect from light. Do not use if particulate matter is present.

*Nature and contents of container:* Toradol 10 mg and 30 mg is available in single-dose ampoules containing 1 ml of solution in cartons of 1, 5 or 10.

*Instructions for use/handling:* No special instructions applicable.

**Marketing authorisation numbers**
Ampoules 10 mg/ml 0031/0480
Ampoules 30 mg/ml) 0031/0481

**Date of approval/revision of SPC** December 1996

**Legal category** POM

## VALIUM ROCHE AMPOULES*

**Qualitative and quantitative composition** Valium Roche contains the substance with the approved name diazepam, chemically described as 7-chloro-1,3-dihydro-1-methyl-5-phenyl-*2H*-1,4-benzodiazepin-2-one.

**Pharmaceutical form** Ampoules containing 10 mg diazepam in 2 ml.

**Clinical particulars**

*Therapeutic indications:* Severe acute anxiety or agitation; delirium tremens.

Acute muscle spasm; tetanus.

Acute convulsions including status epilepticus, those due to poisoning, and febrile convulsions.

Pre-operative medication or premedication for a wide variety of procedures, e.g. in dentistry, surgery, radiology, endoscopy, cardiac catheterisation, cardioversion.

*Posology and method of administration:*

*Adults: Severe acute anxiety or agitation:* 10 mg by IV or IM injection which may be repeated after an interval of not less than 4 hours.

*Delirium tremens:* 10 to 20 mg IV or IM. Higher doses may be needed, depending on severity of symptoms.

*Acute muscle spasm:* 10 mg by IV or IM injection which may be repeated after an interval of not less than 4 hours.

*Tetanus:* Initially an IV dose of 0.1 to 0.3 mg/kg body-weight, repeated at intervals of 1 to 4 hours. Continuous IV infusion of 30 to 10 mg/kg body-weight per 24 hours can also be used. Alternatively, the same dose of oral Valium Roche may be administered by nasoduodenal tube. The selected dose should relate to the severity of the case and in extremely severe cases higher doses have been used.

*Status epilepticus, convulsions due to poisoning:* 10 to 20 mg IV or IM, repeated if necessary 30–60 minutes later. If indicated, this may be followed by a slow intravenous infusion (maximum dose: 3 mg/kg body-weight over 24 hours).

*Pre-operative medication or premedication:* 0.2 mg/kg body-weight. The usual adult dose is 10 to 20 mg but higher doses may be necessary according to the clinical response.

*Elderly: Elderly or debilitated patients:* Doses should not exceed half those normally recommended.

*Children: Status epilepticus, convulsions due to poisoning, febrile convulsions:* 0.2 to 0.3 mg/kg body-weight IV (or IM) or 1 mg per year of life.

*Tetanus:* As for adults.

*Pre-operative medication or premedication:* 0.2 mg/kg body-weight.

Treatment should be kept to a minimum and given only under close medical supervision. Little is known regarding the efficacy or safety of benzodiazepines in long-term use.

In order to reduce the likelihood of untoward effects during intravenous sedation the injection should be given slowly (0.5 ml of the solution per half-minute) until the patient becomes drowsy, the eyelids droop and the speech becomes slurred but the patient is still able to respond to requests.

It is strongly recommended that intravenous injections of Valium Roche should be given into a large vein of the antecubital fossa, the patient having been placed in a supine position and kept there throughout the procedure.

If these conditions are adhered to for administration of Valium Roche intravenously the possibility of hypotension or apnoea occurring will be greatly diminished.

Except in emergencies, a second person should always be present during intravenous use and facilities for resuscitation should always be available. It is recommended that patients should remain under medical supervision until at least one hour has elapsed from the time of injection. They should always be accompanied home by a responsible adult, with a warning not to drive or to operate machinery for 24 hours.

Valium Roche ampoule solution should not normally be diluted. An exception to this is when given slowly in large intravenous infusions of normal saline or dextrose, such as are given in the treatment of tetanus and status epilepticus. Not more than 40 mg (8 ml ampoule solution) should be added to 500 ml of infusion solution. The solution should be freshly made up and used within six hours.

Valium Roche ampoule solution should not be mixed with other drugs in the same infusion solution or in the same syringe.

Maintenance of stability cannot be guaranteed if this advice is not followed.

Valium Roche ampoules are for intravenous or intramuscular administration.

*Contra-indications:* Patients with known sensitivity to benzodiazepines; acute pulmonary insufficiency; respiratory depression; phobic or obsessional states; chronic psychosis.

*Special warnings and special precautions for use:* Parenteral Valium Roche should not normally be used in patients with organic brain changes (particularly arteriosclerosis) or with chronic pulmonary insufficiency. However, in emergency or when such patients are treated in hospital, Valium Roche may be given parenterally in reduced dosage. For IV administration, the injection should be given slowly.

In patients with chronic pulmonary insufficiency, and in patients with chronic renal or hepatic disease, dosage may need to be reduced.

Valium Roche should not be used alone to treat depression or anxiety associated with depression, since suicide may be precipitated in such patients.

Amnesia may occur.

In cases of loss or bereavement, psychological adjustment may be inhibited by benzodiazepines.

Abnormal psychological reactions to benzodiazepines have been reported. Rare behavioural effects include paradoxical aggressive outbursts, excitement, confusion, and the uncovering of depression with suicidal tendencies. Extreme caution should therefore be used in prescribing benzodiazepines to patients with personality disorders.

In patients with myasthenia gravis, who are prescribed Valium Roche, care should be taken on account of pre-existing muscle weakness.

After prolonged IV administration, abrupt discontinuation may be accompanied by withdrawal symptoms, therefore a gradual reduction in dosage is recommended.

Extreme care must be used when administering injectable Valium Roche, particularly by the IV route, to the elderly, to very ill patients and to those with limited cardiac or pulmonary reserve because of the possibility that apnoea and/or cardiac arrest may occur. Concomitant use of barbiturates, alcohol or other central nervous system depressants increases cardiac or pulmonary depression with increased risk of apnoea. Resuscitative equipment, including that necessary to support respiration, should be readily available.

*Interaction with other medicaments and other forms of interaction:* If Valium Roche is given concomitantly with centrally-acting drugs such as neuroleptics, tranquillisers, antidepressants, hypnotics, analgesics and anaesthetics, the sedative effects are likely to be intensified. Furthermore, if such centrally-depressant drugs are given parenterally in conjunction with intravenous Valium Roche, severe respiratory and cardiovascular depression may occur. The elderly require special supervision.

When intravenous Valium Roche is to be administered concurrently with a narcotic analgesic agent, e.g. in dentistry, it is recommended that Valium Roche be given after the analgesic and that the dose be carefully titrated to meet the patient's needs.

Pharmacokinetic studies on potential interactions between Valium Roche and anti-epileptic drugs (including valproic acid) have produced conflicting results. Both depression and elevation of drug levels, as well as no change, have been reported. When Valium Roche is used in conjunction with anti-epileptic drugs, side-effects and toxicity may be more evident, particularly with hydantoins or barbiturates or combinations including them. This requires extra care in adjusting dosage in the initial stages of treatment.

Known inhibitors of hepatic enzymes, e.g. cimetidine and omeprazole have been shown to reduce the clearance of benzodiazepines and may potentiate their action and known inducers of hepatic enzymes, e.g. rifampicin, may increase the clearance of benzodiazepines.

*Pregnancy and lactation:* There is no evidence as to drug safety in human pregnancy, nor is there evidence from animal work that it is free from hazard. Do not use during pregnancy, especially during the first and last trimesters, unless there are compelling reasons.

The administration of high doses or prolonged administration of low doses of benzodiazepines in the last trimester of pregnancy or during labour has been reported to produce irregularities in the foetal heart rate, and hypotonia, poor sucking and hypothermia in the neonate.

Diazepam has been detected in breast milk. If possible, the use of Valium Roche should be avoided during lactation.

*Effects on ability to drive and use machines:* Patients should be advised that, like all medicaments of this type, Valium Roche may modify patients' performance at skilled tasks (driving, operating machinery, etc.) to a varying degree depending upon dosage, administration and individual susceptibility. Patients should further be advised that alcohol may intensify any impairment and should, therefore, be avoided during treatment.

*Undesirable effects:* Intravenous injection may be associated with local reactions, and thrombophlebitis and venous thrombosis may occur. In order to minimise the likelihood of these effects, intravenous injections of Valium Roche should be given into a large vein of the antecubital fossa.

Apnoea or hypotension may rarely occur following intravenous injection. The incidence may be minimised by not exceeding the recommended rate of administration. Patients should always be managed in the supine position and kept there throughout the procedure.

Circulatory and respiratory depression may follow rapid intravenous administration of Valium Roche.

Other adverse effects include drowsiness, sedation, unsteadiness and ataxia; these are dose-related and may persist into the following day even after a single dose. The elderly are particularly sensitive to the effects of centrally-depressant drugs and may experience confusion, especially if organic brain changes are present. The dosage of Valium Roche in these patients should not exceed one-half that recommended for other adults.

Rare adverse effects include headache, vertigo, hypotension, gastro-intestinal upsets, skin rashes, visual disturbances, changes in libido, and urinary retention. Isolated cases of blood dyscrasias and jaundice have also been reported.

Hallucinations, some of a sexual nature, have been reported.

The elderly and patients with impaired renal and/or hepatic function, will be particularly susceptible to the adverse effects listed above. It is advisable to review treatment regularly and to discontinue use as soon as possible.

*Overdose:* The symptoms of Valium overdose are mainly an intensification of the therapeutic effects (sedation, muscle weakness, profound sleep) or paradoxical excitation. In most cases only observation of vital functions is required.

Extreme overdosage may lead to coma, areflexia, cardiorespiratory depression and apnoea, requiring appropriate countermeasures (ventilation, cardiovascular support).

The value of dialysis has not been determined. Anexate is a specific IV antidote for use in emergency situations. Patients requiring such intervention should be monitored closely in hospital (see separate prescribing information).

If excitation occurs, barbiturates should not be used.

### Pharmacological properties

*Pharmacodynamics properties:* Valium Roche has anxiolytic, anticonvulsant and central muscle-relaxant properties. It has little autonomic activity.

*Pharmacokinetics properties:* Diazepam is a long-acting benzodiazepine. It is metabolised to the active metabolites, N-desmethyldiazepam and oxazepam. Excretion is via the kidney in the form of conjugated oxazepam and temazepam. The half-life of diazepam varies from 20 to 50 hours whilst that of desmethyldiazepam ranges up to 100 hours, depending on age and liver function.

Repeated doses will lead to accumulation of whole drug and metabolites. The latter may take two weeks to reach steady state and can reach higher concentrations than the parent compound.

Intramuscular injection of Valium Roche can lead to a rise in serum creatine phosphokinase activity, with a maximum level occurring between 12 and 24 hours after the injection. This fact should be taken into account in the differential diagnosis of myocardial infarction.

The absorption from intramuscular injection of Valium Roche may be variable, particularly from the gluteal muscles. This route of administration should only be used when oral or intravenous dosing is not possible or advisable.

*Preclinical safety data:* None stated.

### Pharmaceutical particulars

*List of excipients:* Sodium benzoate, benzoic acid, propylene glycol, 1 m sodium hydroxide, ethanol 94%, benzyl alcohol, water for injection.

*Incompatibilities:* None.

*Shelf life:* Valium Roche ampoules have a shelf-life of 3 years.

*Special precautions for storage:* The recommended maximum storage temperature for Valium Roche ampoules is 30°C. They should be protected from light.

*Nature and contents of container:* Valium Roche ampoules 10 mg in 2 ml, in packs of 10.

*Instructions for use/handling:*

*Dilution, additives and pharmaceutical precautions:* Valium Roche ampoule solutions should not normally be diluted. An exception to this is when given slowly in large intravenous infusions of normal saline or dextrose such as are given in the treatment of tetanus and status epilepticus. Not more than 40 mg (8 ml ampoule solution) should be added to 500 ml of infusion solution. The solution should be freshly made up and used within six hours.

Over 50% of diazepam in solution may be adsorbed onto the walls of plastic containers of infusion solution; these should not therefore be used for diazepam solutions. Adsorption onto plastic drip tubing causes an initial significant reduction of delivered diazepam concentration which then gradually rises over the next few hours. The drip rate should frequently be titrated against the patient's condition.

Bolus injection allows a more accurate and rapid titration of dosage than slow intravenous infusion. It is therefore to be preferred for the management of acute problems.

Valium Roche ampoule solution should not be mixed with other drugs in the same infusion solution or in the same syringe.

Maintenance of stability cannot be guaranteed if this advice is not followed.

**Marketing authorisation number**   0031/0068R

**Date of approval/revision of SPC**   July 1996

**Legal category**   POM

## VALIUM ROCHE TABLETS, SYRUP*

**Presentation**   Round, white tablets with $^{ROCHE}_{2}$ imprinted on one face and a single break bar on the other, containing 2 mg diazepam.

Round, pale yellow tablets with $^{ROCHE}_{5}$ imprinted on one face and a single break bar on the other, containing 5 mg diazepam.

Round, pale blue tablets with $^{ROCHE}_{10}$ imprinted on one face and a single break bar on the other, containing 10 mg diazepam.

Pink, raspberry-flavoured syrup containing 2 mg diazepam in 5 ml.

**Uses**   *Properties:* Valium Roche has anxiolytic, anticonvulsant and central muscle-relaxant properties. It has little autonomic activity.

*Pharmacokinetics:* Valium Roche is well absorbed orally, with peak blood levels being achieved 1 to 2 hours after administration, producing a rapid onset of clinical effects.

Diazepam is a long-acting benzodiazepine. It is metabolised to the active metabolites, N-desmethyldiazepam and oxazepam. Excretion is via the kidney in the form of conjugated oxazepam and temazepam. The half-life of diazepam varies from 20 to 50 hours whilst that of desmethyldiazepam ranges up to 100 hours, depending on age and liver function.

Repeated doses will lead to accumulation of whole drug and metabolites. The latter may take two weeks to reach steady state and can reach higher concentrations than the parent compound.

No clear correlation has been demonstrated between the blood levels of Valium Roche and its clinical effects.

*Indications:* *Adults:* Short-term (2-4 weeks) symptomatic treatment of anxiety that is severe, disabling or subjecting the individual to unacceptable distress, occurring alone or in association with insomnia or short-term psychosomatic, organic or psychotic illness.

Short-term (2-4 weeks) treatment of conditions where anxiety may be a precipitating or aggravating factor, e.g. tension headaches or migraine attacks.

Symptomatic treatment of acute alcohol withdrawal.

Muscle spasm. As an adjunct to the control of muscle spasm in tetanus.

May be useful in the management of cerebral spasticity in selected cases.

As an adjunct to the management of some types of epilepsy, e.g. myoclonus.

Premedication.

*Children:* Night terrors and somnambulism.

May be useful in controlling tension and irritability in cerebral spasticity in selected cases.

As an adjunct to the control of muscle spasm in tetanus.

Premedication.

### Dosage and administration

*Anxiety states: Adults:*

| | |
|---|---|
| Usual dose. | 2 mg three times daily. |
| Maximum dose. | Up to 30 mg daily in divided doses Adjusted on an individual basis. |
| Insomnia associated with anxiety | 5 to 15 mg before retiring. |

The lowest dose which can control symptoms should be used.

Treatment should not be continued at the full dose beyond four weeks.

Long-term chronic use is not recommended.

Treatment should always be tapered off gradually. Patients who have taken benzodiazepines for a prolonged time may require a longer period during which doses are reduced. Specialist help may be appropriate.

| | |
|---|---|
| Symptomatic relief of acute alcohol withdrawal. | 5 to 20 mg, repeated if necessary in 2 to 4 hours |

*Night terrors and somnambulism:*

| | |
|---|---|
| Children | 1 to 5 mg at bedtime |

*Conditions associated with muscle spasm:*
*Adults*

| | |
|---|---|
| Muscle spasm. | 2 to 15 mg daily in divided doses. |
| Management of cerebral spasticity in selected cases. | 2 to 60 mg daily in divided doses. |
| Adjunct to control of muscle spasm in tetanus. | 3 to 10 mg/kg body-weight daily by nasoduodenal tube. The selected dose should relate to the severity of the case and in extremely severe cases higher doses have been used. Intravenous Valium Roche is recommended initially (see separate data sheet). |

*Children*

| | |
|---|---|
| Control of tension and irritability in cerebral spasticity in selected cases. | 2 to 40 mg daily in divided doses. |
| As an adjunct to the control of muscle spasm in tetanus. | As for adults. |

*Adjunct to the management of some types of epilepsy:*

| | |
|---|---|
| Adults. | 2 to 60 mg daily in divided doses. |

*Premedication:*

| | |
|---|---|
| Adults | 5 to 20 mg |
| Children | 2 to 10 mg |

ELDERLY OR DEBILITATED PATIENTS: DOSES SHOULD NOT EXCEED HALF THOSE NORMALLY RECOMMENDED.

Valium Roche tablets and syrup are for oral administration.

Valium Roche syrup may be diluted with Sorbitol Solution BPC or Syrup BP.

Shake well. Following dilution use within three weeks.

### Contra-indications, warnings, etc

*Contra-indications:* Patients with known sensitivity to benzodiazepines; acute pulmonary insufficiency; respiratory depression; phobic or obsessional states; chronic psychosis.

*Use in pregnancy and lactation:* There is no evidence as to drug safety in human pregnancy, nor is there evidence from animal work that it is free from hazard. Do not use during pregnancy, especially during the first and last trimesters, unless there are compelling reasons.

The administration of high doses or prolonged administration of low doses of benzodiazepines in the last trimester of pregnancy or during labour has been reported to produce irregularities in the foetal heart rate, and hypotonia, poor sucking and hypothermia in the neonate.

Diazepam has been detected in breast milk. If possible, the use of Valium Roche should be avoided during lactation.

*Precautions:* In patients with chronic pulmonary insufficiency, and in patients with chronic renal or hepatic disease, dosage may need to be reduced.

Valium Roche should not be used alone to treat depression or anxiety associated with depression, since suicide may be precipitated in such patients.

Amnesia may occur.

In cases of loss or bereavement, psychological adjustment may be inhibited by benzodiazepines.

Patients should be advised that, like all medicaments of this type, Valium Roche may modify patients' performance at skilled tasks (driving, operating machinery, etc.) to a varying degree depending on dosage, administration and individual susceptibility. Patients should further be advised that alcohol may intensify any impairment and should, therefore, be avoided during treatment.

The dependence potential of the benzodiazepines is low, particularly when limited to short-term use, but this increases when high doses are used, especially when given over long periods. This is particularly so in patients with a history of alcoholism or drug abuse or in patients with marked personality disorders. Regular monitoring in such patients is essential, routine repeat prescriptions should be avoided and treatment should be withdrawn gradually. Symptoms such as depression, nervousness, rebound insomnia, irritability, sweating, and diarrhoea have been reported following abrupt cessation of treatment in patients receiving even normal therapeutic doses for short periods of time.

In rare instances, withdrawal following excessive dosages may produce confusional states, psychotic manifestations and convulsions.

Abnormal psychological reactions to benzodiazepines have been reported. Rare behavourial effects include paradoxical aggressive outbursts, excitement, confusion, and the uncovering of depression with suicidal tendencies. Extreme caution should therefore be used in prescribing benzodiazepines to patients with personality disorders.

In patients with myasthenia gravis, who are prescribed Valium Roche, care should be taken on account of pre-existing muscle weakness.

*Drug interactions.* If Valium Roche is given concomitantly with centrally-acting drugs such as neuroleptics, tranquillisers, antidepressants, hypnotics, analgesics and anaesthetics, the sedative effects are likely to be intensified. The elderly require special supervision.

Pharmacokinetic studies on potential interactions between Valium Roche and anti-epileptic drugs have produced conflicting results. Both depression and elevation of drug levels, as well as no change, have been reported. When Valium Roche is used in conjunction with anti-epileptic drugs, side-effects and toxicity may be more evident, particularly with hydantoins or barbiturates or combinations including them. This requires extra care in adjusting dosage in the initial stages of treatment.

Known inhibitors of hepatic enzymes, e.g. cimetidine and omeprazole, have been shown to reduce the clearance of benzodiazepines and may potentiate their action and known inducers of hepatic enzymes, e.g. rifampicin, may increase the clearance of benzodiazepines.

*Side-effects and adverse reactions.* Common adverse effects include drowsiness, sedation, unsteadiness and ataxia, these are dose related and may persist into the following day, even after a single dose. The elderly are particularly sensitive to the effects of centrally-depressant drugs and may experience confusion, especially if organic brain changes are present; the dosage of Valium Roche should not exceed one-half that recommended for other adults.

Other adverse effects are rare and include headache, vertigo, hypotension, gastrointestinal upsets, skin rashes, visual disturbances, changes in libido, and urinary retention. Isolated cases of blood dyscrasias and jaundice have also been reported.

*Treatment of overdosage.* The symptoms of Valium overdose are mainly an intensification of the therapeutic effects (sedation, muscle weakness, profound sleep) or paradoxical excitation. In most cases only observation of vital functions is required.

Extreme overdosage may lead to coma, areflexia, cardiorespiratory depression and apnoea, requiring appropriate countermeasures (ventilation, cardiovascular support).

The value of dialysis has not been determined. Anexate is a specific IV antidote for use in emergency situations. Patients requiring such intervention should be monitored closely in hospital (see separate prescribing information).

If excitation occurs, barbiturates should not be used. When taken with centrally-acting drugs, especially alcohol, the effects of overdosage are likely to be more severe and, in the absence of supportive measures, may prove fatal.

**Pharmaceutical precautions**

*Storage.* The recommended maximum storage temperature for Valium Roche syrup is 30°C.

All Valium Roche presentations should be protected from light.

*Additives and pharmaceutical precautions:* Valium Roche syrup may be diluted with Sorbitol Solution BPC or Syrup BP. Shake well. Following dilution use within 3 weeks.

**Legal category** POM; CD (Sch. 4)

**Package quantities** Valium 2 Roche tablets 2 mg, Valium 5 Roche tablets 5 mg, Valium 10 Roche tablets 10 mg, in packs of 100.

Valium Roche syrup in packs of 100 ml.

**Further information** The elderly, and patients with impaired renal and/or hepatic function, will be particularly susceptible to the adverse effects listed above. It is advisable to review treatment regularly and to discontinue use as soon as possible.

Treatment should be kept to a minimum and given only under close medical supervision. Little is known regarding the efficacy or safety of benzodiazepines in long-term use.

*Availability:* Valium Roche is also available as 10 mg ampoules (see separate prescribing information).

**Product licence numbers**

| Tablets 2 mg | 0031/5121R |
| Tablets 5 mg | 0031/5122R |
| Tablets 10 mg | 0031/5123R |
| Syrup | 0031/5126R |

# VASCACE*

**Qualitative and quantitative composition**

*One film coated tablet 0.5 mg contains:* Cilazapril,

anhydrous 0.5 mg, in the form of the monohydrate (cilazapril 0.522 mg).

*One film coated tablet 1.0 mg contains:* Cilazapril, anhydrous 1.0 mg, in the form of the monohydrate (cilazapril 1.044 mg).

*One film coated tablet 2.5 mg contains:* Cilazapril, anhydrous 2.5 mg, in the form of the monohydrate (cilazapril 2.61 mg).

*One film coated tablet 5.0 mg contains:* Cilazapril, anhydrous 5 mg, in the form of the monohydrate (cilazapril 5.22 mg).

**Pharmaceutical form** Tablets.

**Clinical particulars**

*Therapeutic indications:* Vascace is indicated in treatment of all grades of essential hypertension and renovascular hypertension. Vascace is also indicated in the treatment of chronic heart failure, usually as an adjunctive therapy with digitalis and/or diuretics.

*Posology and method of administration:* Vascace should be administered once-daily. As food intake has no clinically significant influence on absorption, Vascace can be administered before or after a meal. The dose should always be taken at about the same time of day.

*Special Dosage Instructions:*

*Essential hypertension:* The recommended initial dosage is 1–1.25 mg once a day. Dosage should be adjusted individually in accordance with the blood pressure response until control is achieved. Most patients can be maintained on between 2.5 and 5.0 mg/day. If the blood pressure is not adequately controlled with 5 mg Vascace once daily, a low dose of a non-potassium-sparing diuretic may be administered concomitantly to enhance the anti-hypertensive effect.

*Renovascular hypertension:* Treatment with Vascace should be initiated with a dose of 0.5 mg or 0.25 mg once daily since these patients may experience more pronounced decreases in blood pressure in response to ACE inhibitors than patients with essential hypertension. The maintenance dose should be adjusted individually.

*Hypertensive patients receiving diuretics:* The diuretic should be discontinued two to three days before beginning therapy with Vascace to reduce the likelihood of symptomatic hypotension. It may be resumed later if required. The recommended starting dose in these patients is 0.5 mg once daily.

*Chronic heart failure:* Vascace can be used as adjunctive therapy with digitalis and/or diuretics in patients with chronic heart failure. Therapy with Vascace should be initiated with a recommended starting dose of 0.5 mg once daily under close medical supervision. The dose should be increased to the lowest maintenance dose of 1 mg daily according to tolerability and clinical status. Further titration within the usual maintenance dose of 1 mg to 2.5 mg daily should be carried out based on patients response, clinical status and tolerability. The usual maximum dose is 5 mg once daily.

Results from clinical trials showed that clearance of cilazaprilat in patients with chronic heart failure is correlated with creatinine clearance. Thus in patients with chronic heart failure and impaired renal function special dosage recommendation as given under *Impaired Renal Function* should be followed.

*Impaired renal function:* Reduced dosages may be required for patients with renal impairment, depending on their creatinine clearance.

The following dose schedules are recommended:

| Creatinine clearance | Initial dose of Vascace | Maximal dose of Vascace |
| --- | --- | --- |
| > 40 ml/min | 1 mg once daily | 5 mg once daily |
| 10–40 ml/min | 0.5 mg once daily | 2.5 mg once daily |
| < 10 ml/min | 0.25–0.5 mg once or twice a week according to blood pressure response | |

In patients requiring haemodialysis, Vascace should be administered on days when dialysis is not performed and the dosage should be adjusted according to blood pressure response.

*Severe hepatic function disorders (including cirrhosis):* In the unlikely event that patients with severe hepatic function disorders should require treatment with cilazapril, it should be initiated with caution at a dose of 0.5 mg or 0.25 mg once daily, because significant hypotension may occur.

*Elderly:* In the treatment of hypertension, Vascace should be initiated with between 0.50 mg and 1.25 mg once daily. Thereafter, the maintenance dose must be adapted to individual response.

In the treatment of chronic heart failure, Vascace should be initiated with a dose of 0.5 mg daily. The maintenance dose of 1 mg to 2.5 mg must be adapted to individual tolerability, response and clinical status.

In elderly patients with chronic heart failure on high

diuretic dosage the recommended starting dose of Vascace 0.5 mg must be strictly followed.

*Children:* Safety and efficacy in children have not been established therefore there is no recommendation for administration of cilazapril to children.

*Contra-indications:* Vascace is contra-indicated in patients who are hypersensitive to the drug cilazapril or other ACE inhibitors, in patients with ascites and in pregnancy and lactation.

Vascace is also contra-indicated in patients with a history of angioedema after treatment with other ACE inhibitors.

*Special warnings and special precautions for use:* (See also *Special Dosage Instructions* under *Posology and Method of Administration.*)

Vascace should be used with caution in patients with aortic stenosis, hypertrophic cardiomyopathy or outflow obstruction.

In elderly patients with chronic heart failure on high diuretic dosage the recommended starting dose of Vascace 0.5 mg must be strictly followed.

Although the mechanism involved has not been definitely established, there is clinical evidence that haemodialysis with polyacrylonitrile methallyl sulphate high-flux membranes (e.g. AN69), haemofiltration or LDL-apheresis, if performed in patients being treated with ACE inhibitors, including cilazapril, can lead to the provocation of anaphylaxis/anaphylactoid reactions including life-threatening shock. The above-mentioned procedures must therefore be avoided in such patients.

*Symptomatic hypotension:* Occasionally, symptomatic hypotension has been reported with ACE inhibitor therapy, particularly in patients with sodium or volume depletion in connection with conditions such as vomiting, diarrhoea, pre-treatment with diuretics, low sodium diet or after dialysis.

Patients with chronic heart failure, especially those taking high doses of loop diuretics, may experience a pronounced blood pressure decrease in response to ACE inhibitors. This should be treated by having the patient rest in the supine position and may require infusion of normal saline or volume expanders. After volume repletion, Vascace therapy may be continued. However, if symptoms persist, the dosage should be reduced or the drug discontinued.

*Renal impairment:* Reduced dosages may be required for patients with renal impairment, depending on their creatinine clearance (see *Special dosage instructions*). As with other ACE inhibitors, increases in blood urea nitrogen and/or serum creatinine may be observed in hypertensive patients with unilateral or bilateral renal artery stenosis. These alterations are usually reversible upon discontinuation of Vascace and/or diuretic therapy.

For haemodialysis using high-flux polyacrylonitrile ("AN69") membranes please see above statement under the heading of *Special warnings and special precautions for use.*

*Hepatic impairment:* In patients with severe liver function impairment, hypotension may occur.

*Serum potassium:* Concomitant administration of potassium-sparing diuretics, potassium supplements or potassium containing salt substitutes may lead to increases in serum potassium, particularly in patients with renal impairment. Therefore, if concomitant use for such agents is indicated, their dosage should be reduced when Vascace is initiated and serum potassium and renal function should be monitored carefully.

*Surgery anaesthesia:* The use of ACE inhibitors in combination with anaesthetic drugs in surgery that also have blood-pressure-lowering effects, can produce arterial hypotension. If this occurs, volume expansion by means of intravenous infusion or–if resistant to these measures–angiotensin II infusion is indicated.

*Interaction with other medicaments and other forms of interaction:* Vascace has been administered concomitantly with digoxin, nitrates, furosemide, thiazides, oral antidiabetics and H2-receptor blockers. There was no increase in digoxin plasma concentrations and no other clinically significant drug interactions. An additive effect may be observed when Vascace is administered in combination with other blood-pressure-lowering agents.

Potassium-sparing diuretics, potassium supplements or potassium containing salt substitutes administered together with Vascace can lead to increases in serum potassium, particularly in patients with renal impairment (see *Special warnings and special precautions for use*).

As with other ACE inhibitors, use of Vascace concomitantly with a non-steroidal antiinflammatory drug (NSAID) may diminish the anti-hypertensive effect of Vascace.

Anaphylactic reactions can occur in patients undergoing desensitisation therapy with wasp or bee venom while receiving an ACE inhibitor. Cilazapril must therefore be interrupted before the start of desensitisation therapy. Additionally, in this situation, cilazapril must not be replaced by a beta blocker.

Concomitant administration of ACE inhibitors and anti-diabetic medicines (insulin, oral hypoglycaemic agents) may cause an increase blood glucose lowering effect with the risk of hypoglycaemia. This phenomenon may be more likely to occur during the first weeks of combined treatment and in patients with renal impairment.

The concomitant administration of ACE inhibitors with lithium may reduce the excretion of lithium. Serum lithium levels should be monitored frequently.

Concomitant administration of allopurinol, cytostatic or immunosuppressive agents, systemic corticosteroids or procainamide with ACE inhibitors may lead to an increased risk for leucopenia.

*Pregnancy and lactation:* Vascace is contra-indicated in pregnancy since foetotoxicity has been observed for ACE inhibitors in animals. Although there is no experience with Vascace, other ACE inhibitors in human pregnancy have been associated with oligohydramnios and neonatal hypotension and/or anuria. It is not known whether cilazapril passes into human breast milk, but since animal data show the presence of cilazaprilat in rat milk, Vascace should not be administered to nursing mothers.

*Effects on ability to drive and use machines:* As with other ACE inhibitors, impairment of performance in activities requiring complete mental alertness (e.g. driving a motor vehicle) is not to be expected with Vascace.

*Undesirable effects:* Headache, dizziness and coughing are the most frequently reported events in patients taking Vascace. Undesirable effects occurring in < 2% of the patients include fatigue, hypotension, dyspepsia, nausea, and rash. In most cases undesirable effects were transient, mild or moderate in degree, and did not require discontinuation of therapy.

*Idiosyncratic:* ACE-inhibitors have been documented to induce cough in a substantial number of patients. Rarely dyspnoea, sinusitis, rhinitis, glossitis, bronchitis and bronchospasm have been reported.

As with other ACE inhibitors, angioneurotic oedema has been reported, although rarely, in patients receiving Vascace. Angioedema involving the tongue, glottis or larynx may be **fatal**. If involvement of the face, lips, tongue, glottis and/or larynx occurs Vascace should be discontinued without delay and appropriate therapy instituted without delay when involvement of the face, lips, tongue, glottis and/or larynx occurs and replaced by an agent belonging to another class of drugs. Emergency therapy should be given including, but not necessarily limited to, immediate intramuscular adrenalin (epinephrine) solution 1:1000 (0.3 to 0.5 ml) or slow intravenous adrenalin 1 mg/ml (observing dilution instructions) with control of ECG and blood pressure. The patient should be hospitalised and observed for at least 12 to 24 hours and should not be discharged until complete resolution of symptoms has occurred.

Pancreatitis has been reported rarely in patients treated with ACE inhibitors; in some cases this has proved fatal.

*Laboratory test findings:* Clinically relevant changes in laboratory test values possibly or probably related to Vascace treatment have been observed only rarely.

Minor, mostly reversible increases in serum creatinine/urea have been observed in patients treated with Vascace. Such changes are likely to occur in patients with renal artery stenosis or with renal impairment (see *Special warnings and special precautions for use*), but they have also occasionally been observed in patients with normal renal function, particularly in those receiving concomitant diuretics.

In some patients decreases in haemoglobin, haematocrit and/or white blood cell count have been reported, but in no case has a definite causal relationship to Vascace been established.

*Overdose:* While single doses of up to 160 mg Vascace have been administered to normal healthy volunteers without untoward effects on blood pressure, only a few data on overdose are available in patients.

The most likely symptoms of overdosage are severe hypotension, shock, stupor, bradycardia, electrolyte disturbances and renal failure.

After ingestion of an overdose, the patient should be kept under close supervision, preferably in an intensive care unit. Serum electrolytes and creatinine should be monitored frequently. Therapeutic measures depend on the nature and severity of the symptoms. Measurements to prevent absorption such as gastric lavage, administration of adsorbents and sodium sulphate within 30 minutes after intake, and to hasten elimination should be applied if ingestion is recent. If hypotension occurs, the patient should be placed in the shock position and salt and volume supplementation should be given, rapidly. Treatment with angiotensin II should be considered. Bradycardia or extensive vagal reactions should be treated by administering atropine. The use of a pacemaker may be considered. ACE inhibitors may be removed from the circulation by haemodialysis. The use of high-flux polyacrylonitrile membranes should be avoided.

**Pharmacological properties**

*Pharmacodynamic properties:* Vascace (cilazapril) is a specific, long-acting angiotensin-converting enzyme (ACE) inhibitor which suppresses the renin-angiotensin-aldosterone system and thereby the conversion of the inactive angiotensin I to angiotensin II which is a potent vasoconstrictor. At recommended doses, the effect of Vascace in hypertensive patients and in patients with chronic heart failure is maintained for up to 24 hours.

In patients with normal renal function, serum potassium usually remains within the normal range during Vascace treatment. In patients concomitantly taking potassium-sparing diuretics, potassium levels may rise.

*Hypertension:* Vascace induces a reduction of both supine and standing systolic and diastolic blood pressure, usually with no orthostatic component. It is effective in all degrees of essential hypertension as well as in renal hypertension. The anti-hypertensive effect of Vascace is usually apparent within the first hour after administration, with maximum effect observed between three and seven hours after dosing. In general the heart rate remains unchanged. Reflex tachycardia is not induced, although small, clinically insignificant alterations of heart rate may occur. In some patients blood pressure reduction may diminish toward the end of the dosage interval.

The initial dosage seldom achieves the desired therapeutic response. Blood pressure should be assessed and dosage adjusted as required. Should the effect of Vascace at the top of the recommended dose be insufficient it can be combined with non-potassium-sparing diuretics.

The anti-hypertensive effect of Vascace is maintained during long-term therapy. No rapid increase in blood pressure has been observed after abrupt withdrawal of Vascace.

In hypertensive patients with moderate to severe renal impairment, the glomerular filtration rate and renal blood flow remained in general unchanged with Vascace despite a clinically significant blood pressure reduction.

As with other ACE inhibitors, the blood pressure-lowering effect of Vascace in black patients may be less pronounced than in non-blacks. However, racial differences in response are no longer evident when Vascace is administered in combination with hydrochlorothiazide.

*Chronic heart failure:* In patients with chronic heart failure the renin-angiotensin-aldosterone and the sympathetic nervous systems are generally activated leading to enhanced systemic vasoconstriction and to the promotion of sodium and water retention. By suppressing the renin-angiotensin-aldosterone system, Vascace improves loading conditions in the failing heart by reducing systemic vascular resistance (afterload) and pulmonary capillary wedge pressure (preload) in patients on diuretics and/or digitalis. Furthermore, the exercise tolerance of these patients increases significantly showing an improvement in quality of life. The haemodynamic and clinical effects occur promptly and persist.

*Pharmacokinetic properties:* Cilazapril is efficiently absorbed and rapidly converted to the active form, cilazaprilat. Ingestion of food immediately prior to Vascace administration, delays and reduces the absorption to a minor extent which, however, is therapeutically irrelevant. The bioavailability of cilazaprilat from oral cilazapril approximates 60% based on urinary recovery data. Maximum plasma concentrations are reached within two hours after administration and are directly related to dosage.

Cilazaprilat is eliminated unchanged by the kidneys, with an effective half-life of nine hours after once-daily dosing with Vascace. In patients with renal impairment, higher plasma concentrations of cilazaprilat are observed than in patients with normal renal function, since drug clearance is reduced when creatinine clearance is lower. There is no elimination in patients with complete renal failure, but haemodialysis reduces concentrations of both cilazapril and cilazaprilat to a limited extent.

In elderly patients whose renal function is normal for age, plasma concentrations of cilazaprilat may be up to 40% higher, and the clearance 20% lower than in younger patients. Similar changes in the pharmacokinetics occur in patients with moderate to severe liver cirrhosis.

In patients with chronic heart failure the clearance of cilazaprilat is correlated with the creatinine clearance. Thus, dosage adjustments beyond those recommended for patients with impaired renal functions (see *Special Dosage Instructions*) should not be necessary.

**Preclinical safety data:** Please refer to section *Pregnancy and lactation.*

**Pharmaceutical particulars**

*List of excipients:*

In the tablet core for all strengths: Lactose; maize starch; hydroxypropyl methylcellulose 3cp; talc; sodium stearyl fumarate.

*In the film coat for all strengths:* Hydroxypropyl methylcellulose 6cp; talc; titanium dioxide E171; red iron oxide E172 (0.25 mg, 2.5 mg and 5.0 mg only); yellow iron oxide E172 (1.0 mg and 2.5 mg only).

*Incompatibilities:* Not applicable.

*Shelf life:* 3 years.

*Special precautions for storage:* Protect from heat (below 25°C).

*Nature and contents of container:*

*Glass bottles and aluminium blisters in the following quantities:*

0.5 mg: 2, 28, 30 or 100 tablets.
1.0 mg: 2, 28, 30 or 100 tablets.
2.5 mg: 4, 28, 30, 98 or 100 tablets.
5.0 mg: 28, 30, 98 or 100 tablets.

**Marketing authorisation numbers**

| | |
|---|---|
| 0.5 mg Tablets | 0031/0244 |
| 1.0 mg Tablets | 0031/0245 |
| 2.5 mg Tablets | 0031/0246 |
| 5.0 mg Tablets | 0031/0247 |

**Date of approval/revision of SPC** September 1996

**Legal category** POM

## VESANOID* ▼

**Qualitative and quantitative composition** 1 capsule contains 10 mg of tretinoin (all-trans retinoic acid).

**Pharmaceutical form** Capsules.

**Clinical particulars**

*Therapeutic indications:* Vesanoid (tretinoin) is indicated for induction of remission in acute promyelocytic leukaemia (APL; FAB classification AML-M3).

This treatment is intended for previously untreated patients as well as patients who relapse after a standard chemotherapy (anthracycline and cytosine arabinoside or equivalent therapies) or patients who are refractory to chemotherapy.

The association of tretinoin with chemotherapy increases the duration of survival and reduces the risk of relapse compared to chemotherapy alone.

*Posology and method of administration:* A total daily dose of 45 mg/m² body surface divided in 2 equal doses is recommended for oral administration. This is approximately 8 capsules per adult dose.

It is recommended to take the capsules with a meal or shortly thereafter.

There is limited safety and efficacy information on the use of tretinoin in children.

Paediatric patients can be treated with 45 mg/m² unless severe toxicity becomes apparent. Dose reduction should be particularly considered for children with intractable headache.

Treatment should be continued until complete remission has been achieved or up to a maximum of 90 days.

Due to limited information on patients with hepatic and/or renal insufficiency, the dose will be decreased to 25 mg/m² as a precautionary measure.

Full-dose anthracycline-based chemotherapy should be added to the tretinoin regimen as follows (see section 4.4 *Special warnings and special precautions for use*):

When the leukocyte count at start of therapy is greater than 5 x $10^9$/L, chemotherapy should be started together with tretinoin on day one.

When the leukocyte count at start of therapy is less than 5 x $10^9$/L but rapidly increases during tretinoin therapy, chemotherapy should be **immediately** added to the tretinoin regimen if the leukocyte count reaches greater than 6 x $10^9$/L by day 5, or greater than 10 x $10^9$/L by day 10, or greater than 15 x $10^9$/L by day 28.

All other patients should receive chemotherapy immediately after complete remission is attained.

If chemotherapy is added to tretinoin because of hyperleukocytosis, it is not necessary to modify the dose of tretinoin.

After completion of tretinoin therapy and the first chemotherapy course, consolidation anthracycline-based chemotherapy should be given, for example, a further 2 courses at 4 to 6 week intervals.

In some patients the plasma levels of tretinoin may fall significantly in spite of continued administration.

*Contra-indications:* Known allergy to a product in the class of retinoids.

Pregnancy.
Lactation.
Tetracyclines (see *Interactions*).
Low-dose progestogens (see *Interactions*).
Vitamin A (see *Interactions*).

*Special warnings and special precautions for use:*

Tretinoin should be administered to patients with acute promyelocytic leukaemia only under the strict supervision of a physician who is experienced in the treatment of haematological/oncological diseases.

Supportive care appropriate for patients with acute promyelocytic leukaemia, for example prophylaxis for bleeding and prompt therapy for infection, should be maintained during therapy with tretinoin. The patient's haematologic profile, coagulation profile, liver function test results, and triglyceride and cholesterol levels should be monitored frequently.

During clinical trials hyperleukocytosis has been frequently observed (in 75% of the cases), sometimes associated with the "Retinoic Acid Syndrome". Retinoic acid syndrome has been reported in many acute promyelocytic leukaemia patients treated with tretinoin (up to 25% in some centres).

The retinoic acid syndrome is characterized by fever, dyspnoea, acute respiratory distress, pulmonary infiltrates, pleural effusions, hyperleukocytosis, hypotension, edema, weight gain, hepatic, renal and multi-organ failure.

Untreated, this syndrome can be fatal.

The incidence of the retinoic acid syndrome is diminished when full dose chemotherapy is added to the tretinoin regimen based on the white blood cell count. The current therapeutic treatment recommendations and method of administration are detailed in the *Posology and method of administration* section.

Immediate treatment with dexamethasone (10 mg every 12 hours for up to maximum 3 days or until resolution of the symptoms) should be given, if the patient presents any symptom(s) or sign(s) of this syndrome.

There is a risk of thrombosis during the first month of treatment.

*Interaction with other medicaments and other forms of interaction:* The effect of food on the bioavailability of tretinoin has not been characterised. Since the bioavailability of retinoids, as a class, is known to increase in the presence of food, it is recommended that tretinoin be administered with a meal or shortly thereafter.

As tretinoin is metabolised by the hepatic P450 system, there is the potential for alteration of pharmacokinetics parameters in patients administered concomitant medications that are also inducers or inhibitors of this system. Medications that generally induce hepatic P450 enzymes include rifampicin, glucocorticoids, phenobarbital and pentobarbital. Medications that generally inhibit hepatic P450 enzymes include ketoconazole, cimetidine, erythromycin, verapamil, diltiazem and cyclosporine. There are no data to suggest that co-use with these medications increases or decreases either efficacy or toxicity of tretinoin.

There are no data on a possible pharmacokinetic interaction between tretinoin and daunorubicin or AraC.

*Contra-indicated drug associations:*

*Low-dose progestogens:* Tretinoin causes diminution of the contraceptive efficacy of the progestogens.

*Tetracyclines:* Systemic treatment with retinoids may cause elevation of the intracranial pressure. As tetracyclines may also cause elevation of the intracranial pressure, patients must not be treated with tretinoin and tetracyclines at the same time.

*Vitamin A:* As with other retinoids, tretinoin must not be administered in combination with vitamin A because symptoms of hypervitaminosis A could be aggravated.

*Pregnancy and lactation:* All the measures listed below should be considered in relationship to the severity of the disease and the urgency of the treatment.

*Pregnancy:* Tretinoin is teratogenic. Its use is contra-indicated in pregnant women and women who might become pregnant during the treatment with tretinoin and within one month after cessation of treatment, unless the benefit of tretinoin treatment outweighs the risk of foetal abnormalities due to the severity of the patient's condition and the urgency of treatment.

There is a very high risk for any exposed foetus that a deformed infant will result if pregnancy occurs while taking tretinoin, irrespective of the dose or duration of the treatment.

Therapy with tretinoin should only be started in female patients of child-bearing age if each of the following conditions is met:

She is informed by her physician of the hazards of

becoming pregnant during and one month after treatment with tretinoin.

She is willing to comply with the mandatory contraception measures: to use a reliable contraception method without interruption during therapy and for one month after discontinuation of treatment with tretinoin.

Pregnancy tests must be performed at monthly intervals during therapy.

In spite of these precautions, should pregnancy occur during treatment with tretinoin or up to one month after its discontinuation, there is a high risk of severe malformation of the foetus, particularly when tretinoin is given during the first trimester of pregnancy.

*Lactation:* Nursing must be discontinued if therapy with tretinoin is initiated.

*Effects on ability to drive and use machines:* The ability to drive or operate machinery might be impaired in patients treated with tretinoin, particularly if they are experiencing dizziness or severe headache.

*Undesirable effects:* In patients treated with the recommended daily doses of tretinoin the most frequent undesirable effects are consistent with the signs and symptoms of the hypervitaminosis A syndrome (as for other retinoids).

*Skin:* (> 75% of patients) dryness, erythema, rash, pruritus, hair loss, sweating,

*Mucous membranes:* (> 75% of patients) cheilitis, dryness of mouth, nose, conjunctiva and other mucous membranes, with or without inflammatory symptoms.

*Central nervous system:* (> 75% of patients) headache, intra-cranial hypertension, pseudotumor cerebri syndrome (mainly in children), fever, shivering, dizziness, confusion, anxiety, depression, paraesthesias, insomnia, malaise.

*Neuro-sensory system:* (25%–50% of patients) vision and hearing disorders.

*Musculo-skeletal system:* (50%–75% of patients) bone pain, chest pain.

*Gastrointestinal tract:* (> 75% of patients) nausea, vomiting, abdominal pain, diarrhoea, constipation, diminished appetite, pancreatitis.

*Metabolic, hepatic and renal dysfunctions:* (50%–75% of patients) elevation in serum triglycerides, cholesterol, transaminases (ALAT, ASAT), creatinine.

*Respiratory system:* (50%–75% of patients) dyspnoea, respiratory insufficiency, pleural effusion, asthma-like syndrome.

*Cardiovascular system:* (50%–75% of patients) arrhythmias, flushing, oedema. Some cases of thrombosis have also been reported.

These undesirable effects do not seem to represent a permanent or irreversible hazard. The decision to interrupt or continue therapy should be based on an evaluation of the benefit of the treatment versus the severity of the side-effects.

The signs, symptoms and manifestations of the Retinoic Acid Syndrome which could be potentially fatal, as well as its prevention and treatment have been described above (see section 4.4 *Special warnings and special precautions for use*).

*Teratogenicity:* See above.

There is limited safety information on the use of tretinoin in children. There have been some reports of increased toxicity in children treated with tretinoin, particularly increased pseudotumor cerebri.

*Overdose:* No cases of acute overdosage with tretinoin have been reported.

In the event of accidental overdosage of tretinoin, reversible signs of hyper-vitaminosis A (headache, nausea, vomiting) can appear.

The recommended dose in acute promyelocytic leukaemia is one-quarter of the maximum tolerated dose in solid tumour patients and below the maximum tolerated dose in children.

There is no specific treatment in the case of an overdose, however it is important that the patient be treated in a special haematological unit.

**Pharmacological properties**

*Pharmacodynamic properties:* Cytostatic-differentiating agent.

*In vitro* studies with tretinoin have demonstrated induction of differentiation and inhibition of cell proliferation in transformed haemopoietic cell lines, including human myeloid leukaemia cell lines.

The mechanism of action in acute promyelocytic

leukaemia is not known but it may be due to a modification in binding of tretinoin to a nuclear retinoic acid receptor (RAR) given that the α-receptor of retinoic acid is altered by fusion with a protein called PML.

*Pharmacokinetic properties:* Tretinoin is an endogenous metabolite of vitamin A which is normally present in plasma.

After oral administration, tretinoin is absorbed by the digestive tract and maximum plasma concentrations in healthy volunteers are attained after 3 hours.

There is a large inter-patient and intra-patient variation in plasma levels of tretinoin.

Tretinoin is extensively bound to plasma proteins. Following peak levels, plasma concentrations decline with a mean elimination half life of 0.7 hours. Plasma concentrations return to endogenous levels after 7 to 12 hours following a single 40 mg dose. No accumulation is seen after multiple doses and tretinoin is not retained in body tissues.

After an oral dose of radiolabelled tretinoin, about 60% of the radioactivity was excreted in urine and about 30% in faeces. The metabolites found in urine were formed by oxidation and glucuronidation.

During continuous administration a marked decrease in plasma concentration can occur, possibly due to cytochrome P-450 enzyme induction which increases clearance and decreases bioavailability after oral doses.

At present there are no data on a possible interaction between tretinoin and daunorubicin.

The requirement for dosage adjustment in patients with renal or hepatic insufficiency has not been investigated. As a precautionary measure, the dose will be decreased (see section 4.2).

*Preclinical safety data:* Oral administration of tretinoin to animals indicated that the compound had very low acute toxicity in all species investigated.

In animal experimental tests it was shown that in all investigated species the acute toxicity of tretinoin administered orally is low. After a longer period of administration rats exhibit a dose- and time-dependent bone matrix dissolution, a decrease in erythrocyte count and toxic alterations in kidney and testes.

Dogs mainly exhibited disorders concerning spermatogenesis and hyperplasia of the bone marrow.

Subchronic and chronic toxicity studies in rats indicated that the no effect oral dose was at or below 1 mg/kg/day; in dogs, 30 mg/kg/day was associated with toxic effects including weight loss, dermatological and testicular changes.

Reproduction studies in animals have demonstrated the teratogenic activity of tretinoin.

No evidence of mutagenicity has been found.

Tretinoin is a natural metabolite of retinol and belongs to the class of retinoids, comprising natural and synthetic analogs.

**Pharmaceutical particulars**

*List of excipients:*
1 capsule contains the following excipients: Yellow beeswax, hydrogenated soybean oil, partially hydrogenated soybean oil, soybean oil.

1 capsule shell contains the following excipients: Gelatin, glycerol, Karion (sorbitol, mannitol, starch), titanium dioxide (E 171), iron oxide yellow (E 172), iron oxide red (E 172).

A capsule is bi-coloured: Orange yellow/reddish brown.

*Incompatibilities:* None are presently known.

*Shelf life:* 3 years.

*Special precautions for storage:*
Bottles: Keep the bottle tightly closed. Protect from light. Store between 5°C and 30°C.
Blister packs: Protect from light. Store between 5°C and 30°C.

This medicine should not be used after the expiration date (EXP) shown on the outer pack.

*Nature and contents of container:* Amber glass-bottles of 100 capsules.

PVC/PE/PVDC/Aluminium–blister packs of 100 capsules.

*Instructions for use/handling:* Not applicable.

**Marketing authorisation number** 14878/0006

**Date of approval/revision of SPC** October 1996

**Legal category** POM

*\*Trade Mark*

# Rybar Laboratories Limited
East Anton
Andover
Hampshire SP10 5RG

## CAM* MIXTURE

**Presentation** CAM is a clear colourless liquid. Each 5 ml contains: Ephedrine Hydrochloride PhEur 4 mg. Contains parabens in a sugar free base.

**Uses** CAM is indicated in the symptomatic treatment of bronchospasm in children and adults with bronchitis.

**Dosage and administration**
*Children 6 months to 2 years:* 2.5 ml 3 times daily.
2 to 4 years: 5 ml 3 times daily
Over 4 years: 10 mls 3 times daily.
*Adults and elderly:* 20 mls 3 to 4 times daily.

**Contra-indications, warnings, etc**
*Contra-indications:* CAM should be avoided in patients with most types of cardiovascular disorders, hypertension, hyperthyroidism, hyperexcitability, phaeochromocytoma and closed-angle glaucoma. In patients with prostatic enlargement it may increase difficulty with micturition. It should not be given to patients taking monoamine oxidase inhibitors or within 14 days of stopping such treatment.

*Precautions:* Care should be taken in patients with any of the following conditions; diabetes mellitus, ischaemic heart disease and renal impairment.

*Interactions:* When possible CAM should be discontinued prior to giving chloroform, cyclopropane, halothane or other halogenated anaesthetics. The effects of ephedrine are diminished by guanethidine, reserpine and probably methyldopa and may be diminished or enhanced by tricyclic antidepressants. It may also diminish the effects of guanethidine and β blockers and may increase the possibility of arrhythmias in digitalised patients.

*Side-effects:* Although not reported for CAM, the following effects are possible based on experience with other ephedrine containing products: tachycardia, anxiety, restlessness, insomnia, tremor, arrhythmias, dry mouth and cold extremities.

*Use in pregnancy and lactation:* While no evidence of ill-consequences have been reported, as with most drugs, administration should be avoided especially during the first and third trimesters.

*Overdosage:* The effects of overdosage include CNS stimulation, hallucinations and hypertension. Management involves supportive and symptomatic treatment. In severe overdosage the stomach should be emptied by aspiration and lavage, if within 4 hours of ingestion. Diazepam may be given to control CNS stimulation and convulsions. For marked excitement or hallucinations chlorpromazine may be necessary. Severe hypertension may call for administration of an alpha-receptor blocking agent such as phentolamine.

**Pharmaceutical precautions** Store below 25°C. Once opened, use within 4 weeks.

**Legal category** P

**Package quantities** CAM is available in bottles of 200 ml and 1 litre.

**Further information** Does not contain colouring agents or sucrose. Contains parabens.

**Product licence number** 0237/5014R.

## FOLEX* 350 TABLETS

**Presentation** Each pink, sugar-coated Folex-350 tablet is overprinted with the word 'Folex-350' and contains Ferrous Fumarate BP 308 mg (equivalent to 100 mg ferrous iron), Folic Acid BP 350 micrograms. The tablets also contain lactose.

**Uses** The prevention of folic acid and iron deficiency anaemia of pregnancy.

**Dosage and administration** *Adults:* One tablet a day. In pregnancy it is recommended that Folex-350 should be started at the first ante-natal consultation and continued until 3 months after delivery.

*Children:* Not recommended.

**Contra-indications, warnings, etc**
*Contra-indications:* Folex-350 is contra-indicated in megaloblastic anaemia due to vitamin $B_{12}$ deficiency.

*Interactions:* Iron reduces the absorption of tetracyclines, ciprofloxacin, norfloxacin and ofloxacin, penicillamine, trientine, levodopa and zinc. Drugs reducing the absorption of iron include: magnesium trisilicate, tetracyclines, zinc and antacids. Folic acid occasionally reduces plasma phenytoin concentrations.

*Use in pregnancy:* This is a specific indication for Folex-350 therapy.

*Overdosage:* Patients who have taken an overdosage of Folex-350 should have gastric lavage performed, preferably within four hours of the overdosage occurring. In addition, patients should have such symptomatic treatment as appears necessary. In order to eliminate excess free iron, a chelating agent such as desferrioxamine may be administered.

*Side-effects:* Nausea, vomiting, gastro-intestinal symptoms, constipation and diarrhoea have been reported.

**Pharmaceutical precautions** Store in a cool dry place.

**Legal category** P

**Package quantities** In containers of 30, 100 and 1000 tablets.

**Further information** Nil

**Product licence number** 0237/5008R.

## GUAREM* GRANULES

**Presentation** Sachets, each containing guar gum granules 5 g. The fine pale cream granules, which are tasteless, are readily water-miscible, for the preparation of palatable fluid drinks.

**Uses** (i) For use in diabetes to help control postprandial glucose levels, thereby facilitating control, and where appropriate, allowing reduction of insulin or oral hypoglycaemic dosage levels.
(ii) For the relief of the symptoms of the 'dumping syndrome'.

*Action:* Guar gum is a gel-forming type of carbohydrate which resists digestion and absorption by the human alimentary tract; it contains a high percentage (more than 66%) of a high molecular weight hydrocolloid polysaccharide, a galactomannan composed of galactan and mannan units combined through glycoside linkages.
When added to glucose test meals it reduces postprandial glycaemia in healthy volunteers and in diabetic patients. Two mechanisms were suggested to account for these effects–that the gum may delay gastric emptying time and so slow the rate of absorption; alternatively, or in addition, the guar may delay the process of absorption within the small intestine.
A study of paracetamol absorption in humans suggests that the effects of guar could simply be due to alterations in the rate of gastric emptying. However, a study of the influence of guar on glucose transport in vitro, using everted sacs prepared from excised rat jejunum suggest that the action of guar is to inhibit glucose transport, and that this effect is probably due to an increase in the thickness of the unstirred solvent layer at the mucosal surface brought about by the higher viscosity of media containing gel-forming polysaccharide gums.

**Dosage and administration**
*Adults including elderly:* One 5 g sachet to be taken three times daily with each main meal. The contents of a sachet may be simply sprinkled evenly onto or into food ready for eating and must be accompanied by a drink of 200 ml. Alternatively, the contents can be stirred into 200 ml of a suitable fruit flavoured drink and swallowed promptly.
Guarem should not be ingested as dry granules.

*Children (12 and over):* As for adults.

*Children (under 12):* Not recommended.

**Contra-indications, warnings, etc**
*Contra-indications:* To avoid the risk of oesophageal obstruction or rupture this product should not be given to patients with a history of oesophageal disease or of difficulty in swallowing.

*Precautions:* This product should not be ingested as dry granules. It if is taken stirred into food at least a glass of water or other liquid should be drunk. The product can be taken by stirring it into water, juice or milk. During initial therapy, blood glucose levels should be carefully monitored, and concurrent treatment adjusted where necessary, to minimise the danger of hypoglycaemia.
In patients with dumping syndrome, while Guarem may be expected to reduce malabsorption, usual monitoring of nutritional status should be continued.

*Interactions:* When given simultaneously with Guarem, the absorption of other drugs may be slowed; however the total amounts absorbed and excreted do not appear to be significantly affected. A study with digoxin concluded that long term administration of guar gum will not interfere with adequate digitalisation. When it is important to establish maximum serum levels (e.g. penicillin) administration should precede Guarem by one hour.

*Side-effects:* Gastro-intestinal disturbances such as flatulence, abdominal pain and diarrhoea are quite common particularly at the commencement of treatment. These side-effects are rarely severe enough to warrant discontinuation of treatment though that may be necessary in some patients.

*Use in pregnancy and lactation:* There is no experience of the use of this product during pregnancy or lactation.

*Overdose:* There is no experience of overdosage with this product. From the nature of the product, a feeling of bloating and indigestion may be possible.

**Pharmaceutical precautions** Store in a cool dry place.

**Legal category** P

**Package quantities** Cartons of 50 and 100 sachets.

**Further information** Each sachet is individually printed with simple and clear administration instructions. The best way to take the product is to stir it into water, juice or milk. If taken in some other way (for example stirred into food) at least a glass of water or other liquid should be drunk.

**Product licence number** 0237/0023.

*Trade Mark

# Sankyo Pharma UK Limited
Sankyo House
Repton Place
White Lion Road
Little Chalfont
Amersham, Bucks HP7 9LP

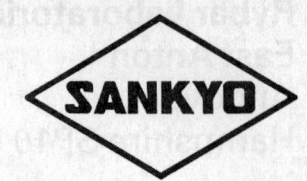

## ANACAL* SUPPOSITORIES
## ANACAL* RECTAL OINTMENT

**Qualitative and quantitative composition**
*Anacal Suppositories:* Each 2 g suppository contains:
Mucopolysaccharide polysulphuric acid
   ester (Heparinoid)                 4.0 mg
Oxypolyethoxydodecane
   (Lauromacrogol-400)           50.0 mg

*Anacal Rectal Ointment:*
Mucopolysaccharide polysulphuric acid
   ester (Heparinoid)           0.2% w/w
Oxypolyethoxydodecane
   (Lauromacrogol-400)      5.0% w/w.

**Pharmaceutical form**   Suppository/rectal ointment.

**Clinical particulars**
*Therapeutic indications:* Anacal Suppositories and Anacal Rectal Ointment are indicated for the treatment of the following conditions: Relief of symptoms associated with haemorrhoids (including perianal haematomas), perianal eczema, pruritus, anal fissure, proctitis, periproctitis, and aftercare of haemorrhoids treated by surgery or injection.

*Posology and method of administration*
*Adults and the elderly: Anacal suppositories:* Insert one suppository once or twice daily. *Anacal Rectal Ointment:* To be applied up to four times daily.
*Children:* Not recommended.

*Contra-indications:* Anacal Suppositories and Anacal Rectal Ointment are contra-indicated in patients with hypersensitivity to one of the ingredients. Not recommended for use in children.

*Special warnings and special precautions for use:* Not to be taken orally. If symptoms persist or worsen, seek medical advice.

*Interactions with other medicaments and other forms of interaction:* None known.

*Pregnancy and lactation:* There is no evidence to suggest that Anacal Suppositories or Anacal Rectal Ointment should not be used during pregnancy and lactation.

*Effects on ability to drive and use machines:* None.

*Undesirable effects:* None known.

*Overdose:* In the absence of any reports of the accidental ingestion of Anacal, no specific advice is available. General supportive measures may be appropriate.

**Pharmacological properties**
*Pharmacodynamic properties:* Mucopolysaccharide polysulphate ester is recognised as having: a weak inhibitory effect on PGE$_2$ synthesis and an indirect effect on LTB$_4$ production (based on *in vitro* studies), anti-coagulant activity (as a heparinoid), Thrombolytic activity (through potentiation of urokinase activity), anti-exudatory activity (through inhibition of hyaluronidase). Oxypolyethoxydodecane has both topical anaesthetic and anti-pruritic properties.

*Pharmacokinetic properties:* Radiochemical studies of absorption following *cutaneous* application of mucopolysaccharide polysulphate have shown that between 0.3 and 4% of the mucopolysaccharide administered is absorbed by various tissues (other than the treated area) within the first 8 hours. Typically between 1.7% and 4.6% will be absorbed within 2 to 4 days. Animal studies have also shown that mucopolysaccharide is bound intracellularly within the subcutis. Peak serum concentrations following *cutaneous* application are below the threshold of physiological relevance for coagulation. Mucopolysaccharide is excreted in the urine partly unchanged and partly as depolymerized, shorter chain length molecules.

**Pharmaceutical particulars**
*List of excipients: Anacal Suppositories:* Miglyol, Hard Fat.
*Anacal Rectal Ointment:* Polyethylene highpolymer 1500, Liquid paraffin, Sorbitan monostearate, Methylhydroxybenzoate (E218).
*Incompatibilities:* None.
*Shelf life:* 3 years.

*Special precautions for storage:* Store below 25°C.

*Nature and contents of container:*
*Anacal Suppositories:* Aluminium foil strips of 10 suppositories.
*Anacal Rectal Ointment:* Aluminium tubes of 30 g.

**Marketing authorisation numbers**
Anacal Suppositories      8265/0005.
Anacal Rectal Ointment    8265/0004.

**Date of approval/revision of SPC**   October 1994.

**Legal category**   P.

## HIRUDOID* CREAM
## HIRUDOID* GEL

**Qualitative and quantitative composition**   Heparinoid 0.3% w/w (Equivalent to 25 000 Units per 100 g cream or gel).

**Pharmaceutical form**   Topical cream or gel.

**Clinical particulars**
*Therapeutic indications:* Hirudoid is indicated for the treatment of superficial thrombophlebitis and the soothing relief of superficial bruising and haematoma.

*Posology and method of administration*
*Adults, the elderly and children over 5 years of age: Hirudoid Cream:* Two to six inches (5–15 cm) to be applied up to four times daily to the affected area and gently massaged into the skin. *Hirudoid Gel:* Two to six inches (5–15 cm) to be applied, as a thin layer, up to four times a day to the affected area. Recommended when its cooling effect and rapid action are required.

*Contra-indications:* Not to be used on large areas of skin, broken skin, sensitive areas of skin or mucous membranes. Not to be used in individuals with a known sensitivity to any active or inactive component of the formulation. Not to be used in childen under 5 years of age.

*Special warnings and special precautions for use:* For external use only. If symptoms persist or worsen, seek medical advice. Do not exceed the stated dose.

*Interactions with other medicaments and other forms of interaction:* None known.

*Pregnancy and lactation:* There is no evidence to suggest that Hirudoid should not be used during pregnancy and lactation.

*Effects on ability to drive and use machines:* None.

*Undesirable effects:* None known.

*Overdose:* In the absence of any reports of the accidental ingestion of Hirudoid, no specific advice is available. General supportive measures may be appropriate.

**Pharmacological properties**
*Pharmacodynamic properties:* Heparinoid is recognised as having: a weak inhibitory effect on PGE$_2$ synthesis and an indirect effect on LTB$_4$ production (based on *in vitro* studies), anti-coagulant activity (as a heparinoid), thrombolytic activity (through potentiation of urokinase activity), anti-exudatory activity (through inhibition of hyaluronidase).

*Pharmacokinetic properties:* Radiochemical studies of absorption following cutaneous application of heparinoid (mucopolysaccharide polysulphate) have shown that between 0.3 and 4% of the mucopolysaccharide administered is absorbed by various tissues (other than the treated area) within the first 8 hours. Typically between 1.7% and 4.6% will be absorbed within 2 to 4 days. Animal studies have also shown that mucopolysaccharide is bound intracellularly within the subcutis. Peak serum concentrations following cutaneous application are below the threshold of physiological relevance for coagulation. Mucopolysaccharide is excreted in the urine partly unchanged and partly as depolymerized, shorter chain length molecules.

**Pharmaceutical particulars**
*List of excipients: Hirudoid Cream:* Anhydrous eucerine, Emulsifying cetostearyl alcohol type A, Glycerol, Isopropyl alcohol, Methyl parahydroxybenzoate (E218), Myristyl alcohol, Potassium hydroxide, Propyl parahydroxybenzoate (E216), Purified water, Stearic acid, Thymol.
*Hirudoid Gel:* Isopropyl alcohol, Perfume oil No 8185, Polyacrylic acid, Propylene glycol, Purified water, Sodium hydroxide.
*Incompatibilities:* None.
*Shelf life:* 5 years.
*Special precautions for storage:* Store below 25°C.
*Nature and contents of container:* Aluminium tubes of 50 g.
*Instructions for use/handling:* Not applicable.

**Marketing authorisation numbers**
Hirudoid Cream    8265/0006
Hirudoid Gel      8265/0007.

**Date of approval/revision of SPC**   March 1995.

**Legal category**   P.

## MOTIFENE* 75 mg

**Presentation**   Size 2, hard gelatin capsules with a light-blue opaque cap and a colourless, transparent body, marked in white print 'D75M', containing white to cream coloured, round lacquered enteric-coated and sustained-release pellets. Each capsule contains 75 mg of diclofenac sodium; 25 mg as enteric-coated pellets and 50 mg as sustained-release pellets.

**Uses**
*Mode of action:* Motifene is a non-steroidal agent with marked analgesic/anti-inflammatory properties. It is an inhibitor of prostaglandin synthetase (cyclo-oxygenase).

*Pharmacokinetics:* Diclofenac sodium is rapidly absorbed from the gut and is subject to first-pass metabolism. Therapeutic plasma concentrations occur about 1/2 hour after administration of Motifene. The active substance is 99.7% protein bound and the plasma half-life for the terminal elimination phase is 1–2 hours. Approximately 60% of the administered dose is excreted via the kidneys in the form of metabolites and less than 1% in unchanged form. The remainder of the dose is excreted via the bile in metabolised form.

Following rapid gastric passage, the enteric-coated pellet component of Motifene ensures quick availability of the active component in the blood stream. The sustained-release pellets cause a delayed release of the active component, which means one single daily dose is usually sufficient.

*Indications: Adults:* Rheumatoid arthritis; osteoarthrosis; low back pain; acute musculo-skeletal disorders and trauma such as periarthritis (especially frozen shoulder), tendinitis, tenosynovitis, bursitis, sprains, strains and dislocations; relief of pain in fractures; ankylosing spondylitis; acute gout; control of pain and inflammation in orthopaedic, dental and other minor surgery.

**Dosage and administration**   For oral administration only. The capsules should be swallowed whole with a liberal quantity of liquid.

*Adults:* One capsule daily. Dose may be increased to two capsules daily if necessary. The first dose should be taken in the morning before breakfast and the second if required 8–12 hours later.

*Children:* Not for use in children.

*Elderly:* The pharmacokinetics of Motifene are not impaired to any clinically relevant extent in elderly patients and the standard adult dose may be used. Non-steroidal anti-inflammatory drugs should be used with particular caution in older patients who are generally more prone to adverse reactions.

**Contra-indications, warnings, etc**
*Contra-indications:* Active or suspected peptic ulcer or gastro-intestinal bleeding. Previous sensitivity to

Motifene. Patients in whom attacks of asthma, urticaria or acute rhinitis are precipitated by aspirin or other non-steroidal anti-inflammatory agents.

*Precautions:* History of gastro-intestinal ulceration, haematemesis or melaena, ulcerative colitis, Crohn's disease, bleeding diathesis or haematological abnormalities.

Patients with severe hepatic, cardiac or renal insufficiency or the elderly should be kept under close surveillance.

The importance of prostaglandins in maintaining renal blood flow should be taken into account in patients with impaired cardiac or renal function, those being treated with diuretics or recovering from major surgery.

Patients who experience dizziness or other central nervous system disturbances while taking NSAIDs should refrain from driving or operating machinery.

All patients who are receiving long-term treatment with non-steroidal anti-inflammatory agents should be monitored as a precautionary measure (e.g. renal, hepatic function and blood counts).

Motifene, in common with other NSAIDs, can reversibly inhibit platelet aggregation.

*Pregnancy and lactation:* Although animal studies have not demonstrated teratogenic effects, Motifene should not be prescribed during pregnancy, unless there are compelling reasons for doing so. If employed, the lowest effective dosage should be used.

Use of prostaglandin synthetase inhibitors may result in premature closure of the ductus arteriosus or uterine inertia. Such drugs are therefore not recommended during the last trimester of pregnancy.

Following oral doses of 50 mg every 8 hours, traces of active substance have been detected in breast milk.

*Interactions:* Motifene may increase plasma concentrations of lithium and digoxin.

Pharmacodynamic studies have shown no potentiation of oral hypoglycaemic and anticoagulant drugs, but caution and adequate monitoring are nevertheless advised (see statement on platelet aggregation in 'Precautions').

Caution should be exercised if NSAIDs and methotrexate are administered within 24 hours of each other, since NSAIDs may increase methotrexate plasma levels, resulting in increased toxicity.

Concomitant therapy with other systemic NSAIDs may increase the frequency of side-effects.

Various NSAIDs are liable to inhibit the activity of diuretics. Concomitant treatment with potassium-sparing diuretics may be associated with increased serum potassium levels, hence serum potassium should be monitored.

Cyclosporin: Cases of nephrotoxicity have been reported in patients receiving concomitant cyclosporin and NSAIDs including diclofenac. This might be mediated through combined renal antiprostaglandin effects of both the NSAID and cyclosporin.

*Side-effects:* If serious side-effects occur, Motifene should be withdrawn.

*Gastro-intestinal tract: Occasional:* epigastric pain, other gastro-intestinal disorders (e.g. nausea, vomiting, diarrhoea). *Rare:* gastro-intestinal bleeding, peptic ulcer. *In isolated cases:* peptic ulcer with perforation, lower gut disorders (e.g. non-specific haemorrhagic colitis and exacerbations of ulcerative colitis).

*Central nervous system: Occasional:* headache, dizziness or vertigo. *Rare:* drowsiness, tiredness. *In isolated cases:* paraesthesia, memory disturbance, disorientation, disturbances of vision (blurred vision, diplopia), impaired hearing, tinnitus, insomnia, irritability, convulsions, depression, anxiety, nightmares, tremor, psychotic reactions.

*Skin: Occasional:* rashes or skin eruption. *Rare:* urticaria. *In isolated cases:* bullous eruptions, eczema, erythema multiforme, Stevens-Johnson syndrome, Lyell's syndrome, loss of hair, photosensitivity reactions.

*Kidney: In isolated cases:* acute renal insufficiency, urinary abnormalities (e.g. haematuria), interstitial nephritis, nephrotic syndrome.

*Liver: Rare:* Liver function disorders including hepatitis (in isolated cases fulminant) with or without jaundice.

*Blood: In isolated cases:* thrombocytopenia, leucopenia, agranulocytosis, haemolytic anaemia, aplastic anaemia.

*Other organ systems: Rare:* oedema, hypersensitivity reactions (e.g. bronchospasm, anaphylactic/anaphylactoid systemic reactions including hypotension).

*Overdosage:* Management of acute poisoning with NSAIDs essentially consists of supportive and symptomatic measures. There is no typical clinical picture resulting from Motifene overdosage. Absorption should be prevented as soon as possible after overdosage by means of gastric lavage and treatment with activated charcoal. Supportive and symptomatic treatment should be given for complications such as hypotension, renal failure, convulsions, gastro-intestinal irritation, and respiratory depression. Specific therapies such as forced diureses, dialysis or haemoperfusion are probably of no help in eliminating NSAIDs due to their high rate of protein binding and extensive metabolism.

**Pharmaceutical precautions**   Store below 25°C.

**Legal category**   POM.

**Package quantities**   56 capsules.

**Further information**   Nil.

**Product licence number**   8265/0003.

**Date of approval/revision of SPC**   July 1994.

# MOVELAT* CREAM
# MOVELAT* GEL

**Qualitative and quantitative composition**
Mucopolysaccharide polysulphate (MPS)   0.2% w/w
Salicylic acid   2.0% w/w

**Pharmaceutical form**   Topical cream or gel.

**Clinical particulars**
*Therapeutic indications:* Movelat is a mild to moderate anti-inflammatory and analgesic topical preparation for the symptomatic relief of muscular pain and stiffness, sprains and strains and pain due to rheumatic and non-serious arthritic conditions.

*Posology and method of administration*
*Adults, the elderly and children over 12 years of age:*
*Movelat Cream:* Two to six inches (5–15 cm) to be massaged into the affected area up to four times a day.

*Movelat Gel:* Two to six inches (5–15 cm) to be applied to the affected area up to four times a day. Children under 12 years of age: Not recommended.

*Contra-indications:* Not to be used on large areas of skin, broken or sensitive skin or on mucous membranes. Not to be used on children under 12 years of age. Not to be used in individuals with a known sensitivity to any active or inactive component of the formulation. Not to be used in susceptible asthmatic patients in whom salicylates can induce allergic bronchial reactions.

*Special warnings and special precautions for use:* For external use only. The stated dose should not be exceeded. If the condition persists or worsens, consult a doctor. Although systemic absorption of topical salicylate is much less than for oral dosage forms, the side-effects of salicylates are theoretically possible.

*Interactions with other medicaments and other forms of interaction:* None known.

*Pregnancy and lactation:* Do not use during the first trimester or during late pregnancy.

*Effects on ability to drive and use machines:* None.

*Undesirable effects:* Allergic skin reactions may occur in individuals sensitive to salicylates.

*Overdose:* Following accidental ingestion of Movelat, individuals may present with the symptoms of salicylate poisoning (hyperventilation, tinnitus, deafness, vasodilation, sweating). The stomach should be emptied and plasma salicylate, plasma pH and electrolytes should be monitored. Forced alkaline diuresis may be required if the plasma salicylate levels are in excess of 500 mg/litre (3.6 mmol/litre) in adults or 300 mg/litre (2.2 mmol/litre) in children.

**Pharmacological properties**
*Pharmacodynamic properties:* Mucopolysaccharide polysulphate ester is recognised as having: a weak inhibitory effect on $PGE_2$ synthesis and an indirect effect on $LTB_4$ production (based on *in vitro* studies), anti-coagulant activity (as a heparinoid), thrombolytic activity (through potentiation of urokinase activity), anti-exudatory activity (through inhibition of hyaluronidase). Salicylic acid is employed in the formulation of Movelat for its keratolytic activity.

*Pharmacokinetic properties:* Radiochemical studies of absorption following cutaneous application of mucopolysaccharide polysulphate have shown that between 0.3 and 4% of the mucopolysaccharide administered is absorbed by various tissues (other than the treated area) within the first 8 hours. Typically between 1.7% and 4.6% will be absorbed within 2 to 4 days. Animal studies have also shown that mucopolysaccharide is bound intracellularly within the subcutis. Peak serum concentrations following cutaneous application are below the threshold of physiological relevance for coagulation.

Mucopolysaccharide is excreted in the urine partly unchanged and partly as depolymerized, shorter chain length molecules. The plasma level of salicylic acid following cutaneous application of Movelat has been shown to remain constant at approximately 0.2 μg/ml even after repeated dosing. The total excretion of salicylate reaches a constant figure of approximately 12 mg/day. Over a seven day period, approximately 6.9% of the administered dose is excreted renally, primarily as salicyluric acid.

**Pharmaceutical particulars**
*List of excipients: Movelat Cream* Glycerol 85%, Stearic acid, Anhydrous eucerine, Myristyl alcohol, Emulsifying cetostearyl alcohol, Ethanolamine, Thymol, Isopropyl alcohol, Purified water.
*Movelat Gel:* Isopropyl alcohol, Mono-ethanolamine, Carbomer, Disodium edetate, Polyethylene glyceryl mono-oleate, Rosemary oil, Purified water.

*Incompatibilities:* None.

*Shelf life:* 5 years.

*Special precautions for storage:* Store below 25°C.

*Nature and contents of container:* Aluminium tubes of 100 g.

*Instructions for use/handling:* Not applicable.

**Marketing authorisation numbers**
Movelat Cream   8265/0008.
Movelat Gel   8265/0009.

**Date of approval/revision of SPC**   May 1997.

**Legal category**   P.

*Trade Mark

**Sanofi Winthrop Limited**
One Onslow Street
Guildford
Surrey GU1 4YS

# sanofi

## AT10*

**Presentation**  A clear, deep straw-coloured, oily solution with a faint nut-like odour containing 250 micrograms/ml Dihydrotachysterol BP.

**Uses**  AT10 is recommended for use in the acute, chronic and latent forms of hypocalcaemic tetany due to hypoparathyroidism where its action is to increase the rate of absorption and utilisation of calcium.

**Dosage and administration**  AT10 is for oral administration only.

*Adults including the elderly:* In acute cases 3–5 ml may be given on each of the first three days of treatment, followed two or three days later by blood and urinary calcium estimations. The maintenance dose of AT10 is usually in the range of 1–7 ml each week, but the precise amount depends on the results of serum and urinary calcium determinations.

In chronic cases an initial dose of 2 ml of AT10 daily, or on alternate days, may be sufficient to maintain normocalcaemia in moderate cases. The dose of AT10 usually has to be increased during menstruation and periods of unusual activity.

*Children:* No specific dosage recommendations.

**Contra-indications, warnings, etc**  As with calciferol, uncontrolled, prolonged administration of AT10 can result in hypercalcaemia which may lead to nephrocalcinosis. Therefore accurate blood calcium determinations must be made at the beginning of treatment and then periodically until the required maintenance dose has been established. The serum calcium level should subsequently be kept between 2.25–2.5 mmol/litre. Serum phosphate, magnesium and alkaline phosphatase should also be measured periodically to monitor progress. If nausea and vomiting are present, serum calcium levels should be checked.

The Sulkowitch test (for urinary calcium) is a convenient supplement to blood calcium determinations, but it should not be regarded as a substitute, because in hypoparathyroid patients treated with AT10, hypercalcuria can occur in the presence of hypocalcaemia.

Certain individuals, particularly those suffering from sarcoidosis, are very sensitive to the effects of vitamin D and it is advisable to consult a physician in cases of doubt.

*Use in pregnancy and lactation:* The safety of AT10 in pregnancy is not established. There is some evidence that its injudicious and unsupervised use during pregnancy could lead to foetal damage and hypercalcaemia in the newborn.

Dihydrotachysterol is excreted in breast milk and may cause hypercalcaemia in the suckling infant.

*Interactions:* Several classes of medicine interact with vitamin D analogues calling for adjustment in the dosage of AT10. Thyroid replacement therapy may increase clearance of dihydrotachysterol; cholestyramine may impair its absorption; thiazide diuretics may enhance the calcaemic response leading to hypercalcaemia; barbiturates, anticonvulsants, rifampicin and isoniazid may reduce the effectiveness of AT10. Hypercalcaemia induced by excessive dosing of AT10 may enhance the toxic effects of cardiac glycosides.

*Side-effects:* Side-effects are most likely to be due to overdosage leading to hypercalcaemia, the first signs of which are loss of appetite, listlessness and nausea. More severe manifestations include vomiting, urgency of micturition, polyuria, dehydration, thirst, vertigo, stupor, headache, abdominal cramps and paralysis. The calcium and phosphorus concentrations of serum and urine are increased. With chronic overdosage, calcium may be deposited in many tissues including arteries and the kidneys, leading to hypertension and renal failure. Plasma cholesterol may also be increased.

*Overdosage:* The symptoms of hypercalcaemia in chronic overdosage will usually respond to withdrawal of medication, bed rest, liberal fluid intake, and the use of laxatives.

In acute overdosage, consideration should be given to recovery of AT10 by emesis or gastric lavage if ingestion is recent. Serum calcium estimations should be helpful in determining management.

In massive overdosage of vitamin D, corticosteroids have been found useful and also neutral phosphate in resistant cases. Several months management may be needed in such cases.

**Pharmaceutical precautions**  Store in well-closed containers protected from heat and light.

**Legal category**  P.

**Package quantities**  AT10 is supplied in bottles containing 15 ml with a 1 ml dropper.

**Further information**  The hypercalcaemic action of AT10 is slower in onset and more prolonged than that of parathyroid hormone, but faster in onset and less persistent in action than calciferol. In patients who have become resistant to large doses of calciferol it may be possible to control blood calcium levels with AT10.

**Product licence number**  11723/0004.

## ADENOCOR*

**Qualitative and quantitative composition**  Adenosine 3 mg/ml.

**Pharmaceutical form**  Injection.

**Clinical particulars**

*Therapeutic indications:* Rapid conversion to a normal sinus rhythm of paroxysmal supraventricular tachycardias, including those associated with accessory by-pass tracts (Wolff-Parkinson-White Syndrome).

*Diagnostic indications:* Aid to diagnosis of broad or narrow complex supraventricular tachycardias. Although Adenocor will not convert atrial flutter, atrial fibrillation or ventricular tachycardia to sinus rhythm, the slowing of AV condition helps diagnosis of atrial activity.

Sensitisation of intra-cavitary electrophysiological investigations.

*Posology and method of administration:* Adenocor is intended for hospital use only. It should be administered by rapid IV bolus injection according to the ascending dosage schedule below. To be certain the solution reaches the systemic circulation administer either directly into a vein or into an IV line. If given into an IV line it should be injected as proximally as possible, and followed by a rapid saline flush.

Adenocor should only be used when facilities exist for cardiac monitoring. Patients who develop high-level AV block at a particular dose should not be given further dosage increments.

*Therapeutic dose*
*Adult:*
  *Initial dose:* 3 mg given as a rapid intravenous bolus (over 2 seconds).
  *Second dose:* If the first dose does not result in elimination of the supraventricular tachycardia within 1 to 2 minutes, 6 mg should be given also as a rapid intravenous bolus.
  *Third dose:* If the second dose does not result in elimination of the supraventricular tachycardia within 1 to 2 minutes, 12 mg should be given also as a rapid intravenous bolus.
  Additional or higher doses are not recommended.

*Children:* No controlled paediatric study has been undertaken. Published uncontrolled studies show similar effects of adenosine in adults and children: effective doses for children were between 0.0375 and 0.25 mg/kg.

*Elderly:* See dosage recommendations for adults.

*Diagnostic dose:* The above ascending dosage schedule should be employed until sufficient diagnostic information has been obtained.

  *Method of administration:* Rapid intravenous injection only.

*Contra-indications:* Adenocor is contra-indicated for patients suffering from:
– Second or third degree AV block (except in patients with a functioning artificial pacemaker).
– Sick sinus syndrome (except in patients with a functional artificial pacemaker).
– Asthma.

*Special warnings and special precautions for use:*
  *Special warnings:* Due to the possibility of transitory electrophysiological phenomena arising during conversion of the supraventricular tachycardia to normal sinus rhythm, administration should be carried out in hospital with electrocardiographic monitoring.

Since neither the kidney nor the liver are involved in the degradation of exogenous adenosine, Adenocor's efficacy should be unaffected by hepatic or renal insufficiency.

*Precautions:* Patients with atrial fibrillation/flutter and an accessory by-pass tract may develop increased conduction down the anomalous pathway. Because of the possible risk of torsade de pointes, Adenocor should be used with caution in patients with a prolonged QT interval, whether this is congenital, drug induced or of metabolic origin.

In patients with chronic obstructive pulmonary disease, adenosine may precipitate or aggravate bronchospasm.

*Interactions with other medicaments and other forms of interaction:* Dipyridamole is a known inhibitor of adenosine uptake and may potentiate the action of Adenocor. Asystole has been reported following concomitant administration. It is suggested that Adenocor should not be administered to patients receiving dipyridamole; if use of Adenocor is essential, dosage should be reduced by a factor of 4 (e.g., initial dosage of 0.5 to 1.0 mg).

Theophylline and other xanthines such as caffeine are known strong inhibitors of adenosine.

Adenocor may interact with drugs tending to impair cardiac conduction.

*Pregnancy and lactation:* Adenosine is a substance which is naturally present in some form in all cells of the body, therefore, no effect on the foetus would be expected. In the absence of evidence that adenosine does not cause foetal harm, Adenocor should only be used during pregnancy where absolutely necessary.

*Effects on ability to drive and use machines:* Not applicable.

*Undesirable effects:* Facial flush, dyspnoea, bronchospasm, a feeling of thoracic constriction, nausea and lightheadedness occur commonly. More rarely observed side-effects have been: feeling of discomfort; sweating; palpitations; hyperventilation, head pressure; apprehension; blurred vision; burning sensation; bradycardia; asystole; chest pains; headache; dizziness; heaviness in arms; arm, back and neck pains; metallic taste. These side-effects were mild, of short duration (usually less than 1 minute) and generally well-tolerated by the patient. Severe bradycardia has been reported and some patients have required temporary pacing. The effects of Adenocor are not blocked by atropine.

One case of worsening of high intracranial pressure has been reported. This was transient (less than 2 minutes) and spontaneously and rapidly reversible. At the time of conversion to normal sinus rhythm, the ECG may show premature ventricular contractions, premature atrial contractions, sinus bradycardia, sinus tachycardia, skipped beats, sinus pause and/or atrioventricular block. The induced bradycardia predisposes to ventricular excitability disorders, including; ventricular fibrillation, and torsade de pointes which justify the recommendations made under *Posology and method of administration.*

*Overdose:* No cases of overdosage have been reported. As the half life of adenosine in blood is very short, the duration of any effects is expected to be limited.

**Pharmacological properties**

*Pharmacodynamic properties:* Antiarrhythmic drug. Adenosine is a purine nucleoside which is present in all cells of the body. Animal pharmacology studies have in several species shown that Adenosine has a negative dromotropic effect on the atrioventricular (AV) node.

In man Adenocor (adenosine) administered by rapid intravenous injection slows conduction through the AV node. This action can interrupt re-entry circuits involving the AV node and restore normal sinus rhythm in patients with paroxysmal supraventricular tachycardias. Once the circuit has been interrupted, the tachycardia stops and normal sinus rhythm is re-established. One acute interruption of the circuit is usually sufficient to arrest the tachycardia.

Since atrial fibrillation and atrial flutter do not involve the AV node as part of a re-entry circuit, adenosine will not terminate these arrhythmias. By transiently slowing AV conduction, atrial activity is easier to evaluate from ECG recordings and therefore the use of adenosine can aid the diagnosis of broad or narrow complex tachycardias.

Adenosine may be useful during electrophysiological studies to determine the site of AV block or to determine in some cases of pre-excitation, whether conduction is occurring by an accessory pathway or via the AV node.

*Pharmacokinetic properties:* Adenosine is impossible to study via classical ADME protocols. It is present in various forms in all cells of the body where it plays an important role in energy production and utilisation systems. An efficient salvage and recycling system exists in the body, primarily in the erythrocytes and blood vessel endothelial cells. The half life *in vitro* is estimated to be < 10 seconds. The *in vivo* half life may be even shorter.

*Pre-clinical safety data:* There are no pre-clinical data of relevance to the prescriber which are additional to that already included in other sections of the SPC.

**Pharmaceutical particulars**

*List of excipients:* Sodium Chloride PhEur and Water for Injections PhEur.

*Incompatibilities:* Compatibility with other medicines is not known.

*Shelf life:* 36 months.

*Special precautions for storage:* Do not refrigerate. Any portion of the vial not used at once should be discarded.

*Nature and contents of container:* Clear, type I glass vials with chlorobutyl rubber closures secured with aluminium caps. Packs of 6 vials in plastic trays in cardboard cartons.

*Instructions for use/handling:* Any portion of the vial not used at once should be discarded.

**Marketing authorisation number** 11723/0005.

**Date of approval/revision of SPC** May 1996.

**Legal category** POM.

## ADENOSCAN*

**Qualitative and quantitative composition** Adenoscan is a sterile solution for intravenous infusion provided in 10 ml clear glass vials containing 30 mg of adenosine.

**Pharmaceutical form** Sterile solution for intravenous infusion.

**Clinical particulars**

*Therapeutic indications:* Intravenous Adenoscan is a coronary vasodilator for use in conjunction with radionuclide myocardial perfusion imaging in patients who cannot exercise adequately or for whom exercise is inappropriate.

*Posology and method of administration:* Adenoscan is intended for use in hospitals. It should be administered following the same procedure as for exercise testing where facilities for cardiac monitoring and cardio-respiratory resuscitation are available. During administration of Adenoscan continuous ECG control is necessary as life-threatening arrhythmia might occur. Heart rate and blood pressure should be monitored every minute.

*Adults*

1. Adenoscan should be administered undiluted as a continuous peripheral intravenous infusion at a dose of 140 micrograms/kg/min for six minutes using an infusion pump. Separate venous sites for Adenoscan and radionuclide administration are recommended to avoid an adenosine bolus effect.

2. After three minutes of Adenoscan infusion, the radionuclide is injected to ensure sufficient time for peak coronary blood flow to occur. The optimal vasodilator protocol is achieved with six minutes of Adenoscan infusion.

3. To avoid an adenosine bolus effect, blood pressure should be measured in the arm opposite to the Adenoscan infusion.

The table below is given as a guide for adjustment of the infusion rate of undiluted Adenoscan, in line with bodyweight (total dose 0.84 mg/kg).

| *Patient weight kg* | *Infusion rate ml/min* |
|---|---|
| 45–49 | 2.1 |
| 50–54 | 2.3 |
| 55–59 | 2.6 |
| 60–64 | 2.8 |
| 65–69 | 3.0 |
| 70–74 | 3.3 |
| 75–79 | 3.5 |
| 80–84 | 3.8 |
| 85–89 | 4.0 |
| 90–94 | 4.2 |
| 95–99 | 4.4 |
| 100–104 | 4.7 |

*Children:* In the absence of data, the use of Adenoscan in children cannot be recommended.

*Elderly:* See dosage recommendations for adults.

*Contra-indications:* Adenoscan is contra-indicated in patients suffering from:
- Known hypersensitivity to adenosine.
- Second or third degree AV block, sick sinus syndrome except in patients with a functioning artificial pacemaker.
- Long QT syndrome.
- Severe hypotension.
- Unstable angina not successfully stabilised with medical therapy.
- Decompensated states of heart failure.
- Chronic obstructive lung disease with evidence of bronchospasm (e.g. asthma bronchiale).
- Concomitant use of dipyridamole.

*Special warnings and special precautions for use:* Because it has the potential to cause significant hypotension, Adenoscan should be used with caution in patients with left main coronary stenosis, uncorrected hypovolemia, stenotic valvular heart disease, left to right shunt, pericarditis or pericardial effusion, autonomic dysfunction or stenotic carotid artery disease with cerebrovascular insufficiency. Adenoscan infusion should be discontinued in any patient who develops persistent or symptomatic hypotension. Adenoscan should be used with caution in patients with recent myocardial infarction or severe heart failure. Adenoscan should be used with caution in patients with minor conduction defects (first degree AV block, bundle branch block) that could be transiently aggravated during infusion.

Adenoscan should be used with caution in patients with atrial fibrillation or flutter and especially in those with an accessory by-pass tract since particularly the latter may develop increased conduction down the anomalous pathway.

Rare cases of severe bradycardia have been reported. Some occurred in early post-transplant patients; in the other cases occult sino-atrial disease was present. The occurrence of severe bradycardia should be taken as a warning of underlying disease and should lead to treatment discontinuation.

Severe bradycardia would favour the occurrence of torsade de pointes, especially in patients with prolonged QT intervals. But to date no case of torsades de pointes has been reported when adenosine is continuously infused.

The occurrence of respiratory failure, asystole, angina or severe hypotension should also lead to treatment discontinuation.

In patients with recent heart transplantation (less than 1 year) an increased sensitivity of the heart to adenosine has been observed.

*Interaction with other medicaments and other forms of interaction:* Dipyridamole inhibits adenosine cellular uptake and metabolism, and potentiates the action of Adenoscan. In one study dipyridamole was shown to produce a 4 fold increase in adenosine actions. It is therefore suggested that Adenoscan should not be administered to patients receiving dipyridamole; if use of Adenoscan is essential, dipyridamole should be stopped 24 hours before hand, or the dose of Adenoscan should be greatly reduced.

Aminophylline, theophylline and other xanthines are competitive adenosine antagonists and should be avoided for 24 hours prior to use of Adenoscan.

Food and drinks containing xanthines (tea, coffee, chocolate and cola) should be avoided for at least 12 hours prior to use of Adenoscan.

Adenosine can safely be co-administered with other cardioactive or vasoactive drugs (see *Pharmacodynamic properties*).

*Pregnancy and lactation:* It is not known whether Adenoscan can cause harm when administered to pregnant or lactating women. Therefore the use during pregnancy is contra-indicated unless the physician considers the benefits outweigh the risk. Adenoscan should not be used during the lactation period.

*Effects on ability to drive and use machines:* None known.

*Undesirable effects:* Effects related to the known pharmacology of adenosine are frequent, but usually self-limiting and of short duration. Flushing, chest pain or pressure and dyspnoea (or the urge to breathe deeply) occur most commonly. Headache, dizziness or feeling lightheaded, abdominal, throat, neck and jaw discomfort have also been reported. Less frequently patients have developed bronchospasm, hypotension, AV block, ST segment depression, arrhythmia (sustained or non-sustained ventricular tachycardia), sweating, nasal congestion, nipple discomfort, nervousness, paraesthesia, tremors, drowsiness, tinnitus, blurred vision, dry mouth, a metallic taste, discomfort in the leg, arm or back, weakness or urinary urgency. Discontinuation of infusion may be necessary if the effect is intolerable.

If sustained second or third degree AV block develops the infusion should be discontinued. If first degree AV block occurs, the patient should be observed carefully as a quarter of patients will progress to a higher degree of block.

Rare cases of severe bradycardia have been reported.

Methylxanthines, such as IV aminophylline have been used to terminate persistent side effects (50–125 mg by slow intravenous injection).

*Overdose:* No cases of overdosage have been reported. Overdosage would cause severe hypotension, bradycardia or asystole. The half life of adenosine in blood is very short, and side-effects of Adenoscan (when they occur) would quickly resolve when the infusion is discontinued. Administration of IV aminophylline or theophylline may be needed.

**Pharmacological properties**

*Pharmacodynamic properties:* Adenosine is a potent vasodilator in most vascular beds, except in renal afferent arterioles and hepatic veins where it produces vasoconstriction. Adenosine exerts its pharmacological effects through activation of purine receptors (cell-surface $A_1$ and $A_2$ adenosine receptors). Although the exact mechanism by which adenosine receptor activation relaxes vascular smooth muscle is not known, there is evidence to support both inhibition of the slow inward calcium current reducing calcium uptake, and activation of adenylate cyclase through $A_2$ receptors in smooth muscle cells. Adenosine may reduce vascular tone by modulating sympathetic neurotransmission. The intracellular uptake of adenosine is mediated by a specific transmembrane nucleoside transport system. Once inside the cell, adenosine is rapidly phosphorylated by adenosine kinase to adenosine monophosphate, or deaminated by adenosine deaminase to inosine. These intracellular metabolites of adenosine are not vasoactive.

Intracoronary Doppler flow catheter studies have demonstrated that intravenous Adenoscan at 140 mcg/kg/min produces maximum coronary hyperaemia (relative to intracoronary papaverine) in approximately 90% of cases within 2–3 minutes of the onset of the infusion. Coronary blood flow velocity returns to basal levels within 1–2 minutes of discontinuing the Adenoscan infusion.

The increase in blood flow caused by Adenoscan in normal coronary arteries is significantly more than that in stenotic arteries. Adenoscan redirects coronary blood flow from the endocardium to the epicardium and may reduce collateral coronary blood flow thereby inducing regional ischaemia.

Continuous infusion of adenosine in man has been shown to produce a mild dose-dependant fall in mean arterial pressure and a dose-related positive chronotropic effect, most likely caused by sympathetic stimulation. The onset of this reflex increase in heart rate occurs later than the negative chronotropic/dromotropic effect. This differential effect is mostly observed after bolus injection thus explaining the potential use of adenosine as a treatment for supraventricular arrhythmias when administered as a bolus or as a coronary vasodilator when administered as an infusion.

Although Adenoscan affects cardiac conduction, it has been safely and effectively administered in the presence of other cardioactive or vasoactive drugs such as beta adrenergic blocking agents, calcium channel antagonists, nitrates, ACE inhibitors, diuretics, digitalis or anti arrhythmics.

*Pharmacokinetic properties:* It is impossible to study adenosine in classical pharmacokinetic studies. It is present in various forms in all the cells of the body where it plays an important role in energy production and utilisation systems. An efficient salvage and recycling system exists in the body, primarily in erythrocytes and blood vessel endothelial cells. The half life *in vitro* is estimated to be less than 10 seconds. The *in vivo* half life may be even shorter.

Since neither the kidney nor the liver are involved in the degradation of exogenous adenosine, the efficacy of Adenoscan should be unaffected by hepatic or renal insufficiency.

*Preclinical safety data:* Because adenosine is naturally present in all living cells, studies in animals to evaluate the carcinogenic potential of Adenoscan (adenosine) have not been performed.

**Pharmaceutical particulars**

*List of excipients:* Sodium chloride, water for injection.

*Incompatibilities:* Compatibility with other medicines is not known.

*Shelf life:* 36 months.

*Special precautions for storage:* Do not refrigerate. Any portion of the vial not used at once should be discarded.

*Nature and contents of container:* Type I glass vials with chlorbutyl rubber stoppers, packs with 6 vials containing 10 ml of solution at 3 mg/ml, i.e. 30 mg of adenosine per vial.

*Instructions for use/handling:* See *Posology and Method of Administration.*

**Marketing authorisation number** 11723/0086.

**Date of approval/revision of SPC** February 1997.

**Legal category** POM.

## BENORAL*

**Presentation** 1. Benoral Suspension is a white suspension, 10 ml of which contains 4 g Benorylate BP. Benoral Suspension contains sorbitol.

2. Benoral Granules: sachets filled with a white, free-flowing powder which disperses readily in water. The contents of each sachet are equivalent to 2 g Benorylate BP. Benoral Granules contain 550 mg sucrose in each sachet.

3. Benoral Tablets are white, capsule-shaped tablets marked 'benoral' on one side only, each containing 750 mg Benorylate BP.

**Uses** Benoral is an anti-inflammatory analgesic and antipyretic. It is recommended for the treatment of rheumatoid arthritis, osteoarthritis and painful musculo-skeletal conditions. It may also be used to treat mild to moderate pain due to many other causes and as an antipyretic in febrile conditions.

**Dosage and administration** Benoral is for oral administration only.

Benoral Suspension may be administered undiluted or taken in hot or cold beverages. Benoral Granules should be stirred into half a glass of water or milk, if preferred and drunk immediately.

*Adults* (except elderly) The maximum daily dosage of benorylate is 8 g.

*Suspension:* To treat active rheumatoid arthritis 10 ml of suspension (4 g benorylate) twice daily is normally required.

For osteoarthritis, quiescent rheumatoid arthritis or soft tissue (non-articular) rheumatism 5 ml (2 g benorylate) twice daily may suffice.

For mild to moderate pain and as an antipyretic the normal dosage is 5 ml suspension (2 g benorylate) twice daily.

*Tablets:* In osteoarthritis, quiescent rheumatoid arthritis and soft tissue rheumatism eight 750 mg tablets (6 g benorylate) per day, in divided doses, are recommended.

*Sachets:* For acute rheumatic conditions up to four sachets (8 g benorylate) daily in divided doses may be required but three sachets (6 g benorylate) daily are often adequate. For milder rheumatic conditions and for the relief of non-rheumatic pain one sachet (2 g benorylate) twice daily is recommended.

*Elderly:* In elderly patients, especially those with impaired renal function, symptoms of salicylism may arise at dosages not normally associated with this effect. In elderly patients it is recommended that the adult dose of Benoral be reduced. For example, dose reduction of Benoral Suspension to a 5 ml (2 g benorylate) morning dose with 10 ml (4 g benorylate) at bedtime may be instituted. Further reduction to 5 ml (2 g benorylate) twice daily may be necessary in some cases.

Dose reduction of Benoral Sachets to three sachets (6 g benorylate) daily in divided doses may be instituted. Further reduction to one sachet (2 g benorylate) twice daily may be necessary in some cases.

*Children:* Benoral is not recommended for children.

**Contra-indications, warnings, etc**
*Contra-indications:* Benoral should not be given to patients with active peptic ulcer, nor to patients known to be sensitive to paracetamol or aspirin including those with asthma, or haemophilia and similar coagulation disorders.

The safety of benorylate has not been established in human pregnancy. Whilst there is clinical and epidemiological evidence that its metabolic products, salicylate and paracetamol, are safe in pregnancy, it is also known that benorylate, in high doses, may have an aspirin-like effect on platelet function. As with aspirin therefore, benorylate should be avoided in the last trimester and at term because of a potential risk of contributing to maternal and neonatal bleeding.

Because salicylate is excreted in breast milk, benorylate should also be avoided by breast feeding mothers.

Because of the possible association between Reye's syndrome and aspirin use, Benoral labelling contains the statement 'Do not give to children under 12 unless your doctor tells you to'.

Patients taking Benoral should be advised against taking analgesics containing aspirin or paracetamol.

*Precautions:* Care is needed in prescribing Benoral for patients with impaired renal or hepatic function and for those with a history of peptic ulcer.

Patients who are taking anticoagulants should have their prothrombin time checked.

Concomitant administration of carbonic anhydrase inhibitors may increase salicylate level and dispose to toxicity, whilst corticosteroids may reduce salicylate level. Salicylate may diminish the diuretic efficiency of frusemide. These possible interactions should be borne in mind in determining respective dosages when initiating or discontinuing concomitant therapy.

*Side-effects:* Overall tolerance is excellent. Minor disturbances including nausea, constipation or diarrhoea, indigestion or heartburn have occurred from time to time and drowsiness and skin rashes have also been reported. The possibility that gastro-intestinal haemorrhage may be induced by Benoral cannot be excluded. The high salicylate levels obtained with Benoral may give rise to dizziness, tinnitus and deafness. If this happens, the dose should be reduced.

There have been a few reports of blood dyscrasias including thrombocytopenia and agranulocytosis but these were not necessarily causally related to paracetamol.

*Overdosage:* Symptoms are likely to resemble those caused by paracetamol overdosage or salicylate overdosage. The hazard of paracetamol overdosage is greater in those with non cirrhotic alcohol liver disease. Treatment should be based on the levels of salicylate and paracetamol in the blood. The possibility that overdosage may cause hepatic necrosis due to accumulation of a highly reactive intermediate metabolite of paracetamol, must be considered. Symptoms of paracetamol overdosage in the first 24 hours are pallor, nausea, anorexia and abdominal pain. Liver damage may become apparent 12 to 48 hours after ingestion. Abnormalities of glucose metabolism and acidosis may occur. In severe poisoning, hepatic failure may progress to encephalopathy, coma and death. Cardiac arrhythmia and pancreatitis have been reported. Liver damage is possible in adults who have taken 10 g or more of paracetamol. It is considered that excess quantities of a toxic metabolite (usually adequately detoxified by glutathione when normal doses of paracetamol are ingested), become irreversibly bound to liver tissue. Immediate treatment is essential in the management of paracetamol and salicylate overdose. Despite a lack of significant early symptoms, patients should be referred to hospital urgently for immediate medical attention and any patient who has ingested around 7.5 g or more of paracetamol in the preceding 4 hours should undergo gastric lavage. Administration of oral methionine or intravenous N-acetylsteine which may have a beneficial effect up to at least 48 hours after the overdose, may be required. General supportive measures must be available. Management may also include forced alkaline diuresis and correction of acid-base balance.

**Pharmaceutical precautions** Nil.

**Legal category** P.

**Package quantities** Benoral Suspension – bottles of 300 ml. Benoral Granules – cartons of 60 sachets (OP). Benoral Tablets – bottles of 100.

**Further information** Benorylate is a prodrug which is metabolised to salicylate and paracetamol by esterases after absorption. It does not give rise to detectable levels of acetylsalicylic acid in the plasma. In chemical terms, 2 g benorylate is equivalent to 1.2 g aspirin and 0.98 g paracetamol.

**Product licence numbers**
Benoral Suspension 11723/0007
Benoral Granules 11723/0006
Benoral Tablets 11723/0008

## BREVIBLOC* 2.5 g and 100 mg

**Presentation** Ampoules (10 ml) containing 2.5 g esmolol hydrochloride (250 mg/ml) in a sterile concentrated aqueous solution to be diluted before intravenous administration.

Vials (10 ml) containing 100 mg esmolol hydrochloride (10 mg/ml) in a sterile aqueous solution for intravenous administration without dilution.

*Action:* Brevibloc is a beta$_1$-selective (cardioselective) adrenergic receptor blocking agent with rapid onset, a very short duration of action and no significant intrinsic sympathomimetic or membrane stabilising activity at therapeutic doses. Its elimination half-life after intravenous infusion is approximately 9 minutes. Brevibloc is metabolised by esterases in the red blood cells.

**Uses** Brevibloc is indicated for the short-term treatment of:

(a) Supraventricular tachyarrhythmias, including atrial fibrillation, atrial flutter and sinus tachycardia.

(b) Tachycardia and hypertension occurring in the perioperative period.

**Dosage and administration** BREVIBLOC IS NOT COMPATIBLE WITH SODIUM BICARBONATE.

BREVIBLOC 2.5 g CONCENTRATE MUST BE DILUTED BEFORE INFUSION.

Dilute the contents of two ampoules to 500 ml with an appropriate intravenous fluid to give a final concentration of 10 mg/ml. See *Pharmaceutical precautions* for appropriate diluents.

Brevibloc 100 mg is a ready-to-use preparation in vials at a concentration of 10 mg/ml. For administration by continuous infusion at the required rate, use a suitable constant infusion control device.

*Supraventricular tachycardia:* The effective dose of Brevibloc for treatment of supraventricular tachycardia is 50 to 200 micrograms/kg/min, although doses as high as 300 micrograms/kg/min have been used. In a few patients a dosage of 25 micrograms/kg/min has been adequate. Brevibloc dosage in supraventricular tachycardia must be individualised by titration in which each step consists of a loading dosage followed by a maintenance dose.

*Flow chart for initiation and maintenance of treatment*
Loading dosage infusion of 500 micrograms/kg/min for 1 minute
THEN maintenance infusion of 50 micrograms/kg/min for 4 minutes*

Response
Maintain infusion at 50 micrograms/kg/min

*Inadequate response within 5 minutes*
Repeat 500 micrograms/kg/min for 1 minute
Increase maintenance infusion to 100 micrograms/kg/min for 4 minutes

Response
Maintain infusion at 100 micrograms/kg/min

*Inadequate response within 5 minutes*
Repeat 500 micrograms/kg/min for 1 minute
Increase maintenance infusion to 150 micrograms/kg/min for 4 minutes

Response
Maintain infusion at 150 micrograms/kg/min

*Inadequate response*
Repeat 500 micrograms/kg/min for 1 minute
Increase maintenance infusion to 200 micrograms/kg/min and maintain

* As the desired heart rate safety end-point (e.g. lowered blood pressure) is approached, OMIT the loading infusion and *reduce* the *incremental* dose in the maintenance infusion from 50 micrograms/kg/min to 25 micrograms/kg/min or lower. If necessary, the interval between titration steps may be increased from 5 to 10 minutes.

*NB.* Maintenance doses above 200 micrograms/kg/min have not been shown to have significantly increased benefits, and the safety of doses above 300 micrograms/kg/min has not been studied.

In the event of an adverse reaction, the dosage of Brevibloc may be reduced or discontinued. Pharmacological adverse reactions should resolve within 30 minutes. If a local infusion site reaction develops, an alternative infusion site should be used and caution should be taken to prevent extravasation.

Abrupt discontinuation of Brevibloc in patients has not been reported to produce the withdrawal effects which may occur with abrupt withdrawal of beta-blockers following chronic use in coronary artery disease (CAD) patients. However, caution should still be used in discontinuing Brevibloc infusions abruptly in CAD patients.

After achieving an adequate control of the heart rate and a stable clinical status in patients with supraventricular tachycardia, transition to alternative antiarrhythmic agents such as verapamil, propranolol or metoprolol, digoxin or quinidine may be accomplished. A recommended guideline for such a transition is given below but the physician should carefully consider the labelling instructions for the alternative agent selected:

| Alternative agent | Dosage |
| --- | --- |
| Propranolol hydrochloride | 10–20 mg 4–6 hourly p.o. |
| Digoxin | 0.125–0.5 mg 6 hourly (p.o. or i.v.) |
| Verapamil | 80 mg 6 hourly p.o. |
| Quinidine | 200 mg 2 hourly p.o. |

The dosage of Brevibloc should be reduced as follows:

(1) Within the first hour after the first dose of the alternative agent, reduce the Brevibloc infusion rate by one-half (50%).

(2) Following the second dose of the alternative agent, monitor the patient's response and if satisfactory control is maintained for the first hour, discontinue the Brevibloc infusion.

The use of Brevibloc infusions for longer than 24 hours has not been thoroughly evaluated. Infusion durations greater than 24 hours should only be used with caution.

*Perioperative tachycardia and hypertension:* When treating tachycardia and/or hypertension in the perioperative setting, the following dose regimens may be used:

(a) For intraoperative treatment – during anaesthesia when immediate control is required, give an 80 mg loading bolus over 15–30 seconds followed by a 150 micrograms/kg/min infusion. Titrate the infusion rate as required up to 300 micrograms/kg/min.

(b) Upon awakening from anaesthesia, administer an infusion of 500 micrograms/kg/min for four minutes followed by a 300 micrograms/kg/min infusion.

(c) For postoperative situations when time for titration is available give the 500 micrograms/kg/min loading dose over one minute before each titration step to produce a rapid onset of action. Use titration steps of 50, 100, 150, 200, 250 and 300 micrograms/kg/min given over four minutes, stopping at the desired therapeutic effect.

Additional dosing information: as the desired therapeutic effect or a safety endpoint (e.g. lowered blood pressure) is approached, omit the loading dose and reduce the incremental infusion to 12.5 from 25 micrograms/kg/min. Also, if desired, increase the interval between titration steps from five to ten minutes. Brevibloc should be discontinued when heart rate or blood pressure rapidly approach or exceed a safety limit, and then restarted without a loading infusion at a lower dose after the heart rate or blood pressure has returned to an acceptable level.

### Contra-indications, warnings, etc

*Contra-indications:* Brevibloc is contra-indicated in patients with severe bradycardia, heart block greater than first degree, cardiogenic shock and overt heart failure.

*Use in pregnancy:* There is no experience with Brevibloc in pregnancy and, although animal tests have shown no teratogenic effect, the use of Brevibloc in women where pregnancy is suspected or confirmed should be avoided.

It is not known whether Brevibloc is excreted in human milk; however, administration of Brevibloc in nursing mothers should be avoided.

*Warnings:* Patients with bronchospastic disease should, in general, not receive beta blockers. Because of its relative beta$_1$ selectivity and titratability, Brevibloc should be used with caution in patients with bronchospastic diseases. However, since beta$_1$ selectivity is not absolute, Brevibloc should be carefully titrated to obtain the lowest possible effective dose. In the event of bronchospasm, the infusion should be terminated immediately and a beta$_2$ agonist should be administered if necessary.

Continued depression of the myocardium with beta-blocking agents over a period of time can, in some cases, lead to cardiac failure. At the first sign or symptom of impending cardiac failure, the dosage should be reduced or Brevibloc should be withdrawn and specific treatment should also be considered.

In clinical trials the most frequently observed side effect was hypotension which was rapidly reversible with dosage reduction or discontinuation. Thus, it is recommended that all patients receiving esmolol should have blood pressure frequently monitored; in the event of a hypotensive episode the infusion rate should be lowered or if necessary the infusion stopped.

Brevibloc should be administered with caution to patients with impaired renal function because the acid metabolite of Brevibloc is primarily excreted unchanged by the kidney.

The use of Brevibloc infusions for longer than 24 hours has not been thoroughly evaluated. Infusion durations greater than 24 hours should only be used with caution.

*Use in children:* The safety and effectiveness of Brevibloc in children have not been established.

*Use in the elderly:* Special studies in the elderly have not been conducted. However, analysis of data from 252 patients over 65 years of age indicated that no variations in pharmacodynamic effects occurred as compared with data from patients under 65.

*Precautions:* Infusion concentrations of 20 mg/ml have been associated with significant venous irritation and thrombophlebitis in animals and man. Extravasation of 20 mg/ml may lead to a serious local reaction and possible skin necrosis. Concentrations greater

than 10 mg/ml or infusion into small veins or through a butterfly catheter should be avoided.

Brevibloc should be used with caution in diabetic patients.

Patients with low pre-treatment systolic pressures should be carefully observed during titration and maintenance infusions with Brevibloc.

*Drug interactions:* Data from an interaction study between Brevibloc and warfarin showed that concomitant administration of Brevibloc and warfarin does not alter warfarin plasma levels. Brevibloc concentrations, however, were equivocally higher when given with warfarin.

When digoxin and Brevibloc were concomitantly administered intravenously to normal volunteers, there was a 10–20% increase in digoxin blood levels at some time points. Digoxin did not affect Brevibloc pharmacokinetics.

When intravenous morphine and Brevibloc interaction was studied in normal subjects, no effect on morphine blood levels was seen. The Brevibloc steady-state blood levels were increased by 46% in the presence of morphine, but no other pharmacokinetic parameters were changed.

The effect of Brevibloc on the duration of succinylcholine-induced neuromuscular blockade has been studied in patients undergoing surgery. The onset of neuromuscular blockade by succinylcholine was unaffected by Brevibloc, but the duration of neuromuscular blockade was prolonged from 5 minutes to 8 minutes.

Although the interactions observed in these studies are not of major clinical importance, Brevibloc should be titrated with caution in patients being treated concurrently with digoxin, morphine, succinylcholine or warfarin.

There exist no data on the interactions of Brevibloc with calcium channel blockers; however, in common with other beta-adrenoceptor antagonists it is recommended that Brevibloc be used with caution in combination with verapamil in patients with impaired ventricular function. The combination should not be given to patients with conduction abnormalities and Brevibloc should not be administered within 48 hours of discontinuing verapamil.

The hypotensive effects of inhalation anaesthetic agents may be increased in the presence of Brevibloc. The dosage of either agent may be modified as needed to maintain the desired haemodynamics.

Catecholamine-depleting drugs, e.g. reserpine, may have an additive effect when given with beta-blocking agents. Patients treated concurrently with Brevibloc and a catecholamine depletor should therefore be closely observed for evidence of hypotension or marked bradycardia, which may result in vertigo, syncope, or postural hypotension.

*Adverse effects:* In the event of an adverse reaction, the dosage of Brevibloc may be reduced or discontinued.

Pharmacological adverse reactions should resolve within thirty minutes of discontinuing the infusion.

The most frequently observed side effect has been hypotension.

Less frequently observed were sweating, nausea, peripheral ischaemia, confusion, somnolence, dizziness, fatigue, agitation, headache, vomiting, inflammation, induration or infiltration at the infusion site, skin discolouration, burning at the infusion site, thrombophlebitis and local skin necrosis from extravasation.

Rarely seen are oedema, wheezing, dyspnoea, anxiety, anorexia, constipation, urinary retention, speech disorder, abnormal vision, rigor and fever.

In the perioperative situation, bradycardia and bronchospasm have also been observed.

*Overdose:* Because of its approximately 9-minute elimination half-life, the first step in the event of toxicity should be to discontinue Brevibloc administration. Then general supportive measures should be instituted as appropriate.

### Pharmaceutical precautions BREVIBLOC 2.5 g CONCENTRATE MUST BE DILUTED BEFORE USE. BREVIBLOC IS NOT COMPATIBLE WITH SODIUM BICARBONATE.

Brevibloc has been shown to be compatible with the following commonly used intravenous fluids, in both glass and PVC containers, at a final concentration of 10 mg esmolol hydrochloride per ml:

Dextrose 5% Injection
Dextrose 5% in Ringer's Injection
Dextrose 5% and Sodium Chloride 0.45% Injection
Dextrose 5% and Sodium Chloride 0.9% Injection
Dextrose 5% in Lactated Ringer's Injection
Lactated Ringer's Injection
Sodium Chloride (0.45%) Injection
Sodium Chloride (0.9%) Injection
Potassium Chloride (40 mEq/l) in Dextrose Injection

Diluted Brevibloc injection is compatible with commonly used PVC giving sets.

There is no information on compatibility of other drugs mixed with Brevibloc infusion.

Store below 25°C.

Exposure to elevated temperatures should be avoided.

After dilution Brevibloc is stable for 24 hours when stored at 2° to 8°C.

**Legal category** POM.

**Package quantities** Brevibloc 250 mg/ml Concentrate, 10 ml ampoule, is supplied individually packed.
Brevibloc 10 mg/ml, 10 ml vial, is supplied in boxes of five.

**Further information** Nil.

**Product licence numbers**
Brevibloc 250 mg/ml Concentrate, 10 ml ampoule
10476/0005
Brevibloc 10 mg/ml, 10 ml vial 10476/0006.

## CALCIPARINE*

**Qualitative and quantitative composition** Heparin Calcium PhEur 25,000 IU/ml.

**Pharmaceutical form** Sterile clear solution of 25,000 International Units of heparin activity per ml as the calcium salt in water for injections.

### Clinical particulars
*Therapeutic indications:* It is indicated for use as an anticoagulant for the prophylaxis and treatment of thromboembolic phenomena, especially myocardial infarction, acute arterial embolism or thrombosis, deep vein thrombosis, thrombophlebitis or pulmonary embolism.

*Posology and method of administration:* For subcutaneous administration using a 26-gauge needle. The best site is the subcutaneous tissue of the lateral abdominal wall. The needle should be inserted perpendicularly into a pinched-up fold of skin and held gently but firmly with the skinfold until injection has been completed. Do not rub the site of injection.

Calciparine is not intended for intramuscular use.

*Adults:*
*Prophylaxis:* A standard prophylactic dose regimen is 5,000 IU by subcutaneous injection 2 hours before operation, followed by 5,000 IU by subcutaneous injection every 8 to 12 hours for seven days. In patients still confined to bed at the end of this period, the same dosage should be continued until they are ambulant.

The standard prophylactic dose following myocardial infarction is 5,000 IU by subcutaneous injection twice daily for 10 days or until the patient is mobile. In other medical conditions in which there is an associated increased risk of thromboembolic phenomena, the same dosage is recommended.

These standard prophylactic regimens do not require routine control in the absence of contra-indications or conditions listed under special warnings and precautions.

If a myocardial infarction is shown to be anterior and therefore has a risk of mural thrombosis of the left ventricle, a higher dose of 12,500 IU twice daily for at least 10 days is recommended. For this dosage regimen, regular monitoring should be considered.

*Treatment:* For the treatment of existing thrombosis the standard dose is 0.1 ml Calciparine (2,500 IU) per 10 kg body weight 12 hourly. To enable dosage to be individually adjusted to maintain a coagulation time in a range of 1.5 to 3 times that of control it is recommended that the thrombin clotting time, whole blood clotting time or the activated partial thromboplastin time be measured on blood withdrawn 5 to 7 hours after the first injection and then at intervals until the patient is stabilised. During long term therapy the test should be repeated at least once each week.

*Children:* Dosage should be individually adjusted according to changes in whole blood clotting time and/or thrombin clotting time and/or APTT. The initial dose should be 0.1 ml Calciparine (2,500 IU) by subcutaneous injection for each 10 kg of body weight. The usual interval between doses is 12 hours, but this also may require individual adjustment.

*Other special groups:* For both prophylaxis and treatment, higher doses are likely to be required in patients of abnormally high body weight and in those suffering from cancer, diabetes mellitus or other diseases associated with marked hypercoagulability. Lower doses are usually indicated in the elderly and in those with low serum albumin or impaired renal or hepatic function. In such patients coagulation times should be checked frequently and dosage adjusted accordingly.

*Use in pregnancy:* There is clinical evidence that heparin does not cause foetal damage and may be the anticoagulant of choice when anticoagulation is indicated during pregnancy. However, the risk of maternal bleeding may be increased. Calciparine should be discontinued if peridural anaesthesia is likely. Individual control is essential and the aim should be to maintain plasma heparin levels between 0.1 and 0.4 units/ml, as assessed by anti-XA assay, and a whole blood clotting time of 15 to 20 minutes.

The standard prophylactic dosage of 5,000 IU by subcutaneous injection every 8 hours is a suitable starting dose in the first 3 or 4 months of pregnancy but higher doses are needed as pregnancy progresses, 10,000 IU two or three times daily being usual in the last trimester. Dosage must be reduced during labour and standard prophylactic dosage is suitable post-partum. Heparin is not excreted into breast milk.

*Contra-indications:* Calciparine is contra-indicated in patients hypersensitive to heparin.

Calciparine is contra-indicated in patients with a condition in which there is an increased danger of haemorrhage. Such conditions include haemorrhagic cerebrovascular accident, haemophilia, thrombocy-topenia and other haemorrhagic diatheses (other than disseminated intra-vascular coagulation not induced by heparin): gastric and duodenal ulcer, sub-acute bacterial endocarditis; threatened abortion and major surgery involving the brain, spinal cord and eye.

Calciparine is contra-indicated in patients with a history of thrombocytopenia associated with any heparin.

Calciparine should not be used in patients with advanced renal or hepatic dysfunction, in severe hypertension or patients in shock.

*Special warnings and special precautions for use:* Special care should be taken in elderly patients, pregnant women and patients with hypertension, history of peptic ulcer or any organic lesion likely to bleed or vascular diseases of the chorio-retina.

Rarely there have been reports of severe thrombo-cytopenia which may be complicated by venous or arterial thrombotic episodes. These complications should be considered in patients with thrombocyto-penia, thrombosis, worsening of initial thrombosis or disseminated intravascular coagulation occurring dur-ing treatment. These reactions may be immuno-allergic in nature and occur mainly between days 5 and 21 of treatment. Platelet count should be meas-ured before treatment and then twice weekly during the first month of treatment; subsequently, monitor-ing can be performed less frequently.

*Interactions with other medicaments and other forms of interaction:* Caution should be observed in patients receiving drugs which interfere with platelet aggre-gation or coagulation, e.g. salicylates, NSAIDs, dex-tran, systemic corticosteroids, oral anticoagulants (during transfer from heparin to oral anticoagulant therapy, clinical monitoring should be particularly vigilant).

*Pregnancy and lactation:* There is clinical evidence that heparin does not cause foetal damage and may be the anticoagulant of choice when anticoagulation is indicated during pregnancy. However, the risk of maternal bleeding may be increased. Calciparine should be discontinued if peridural anaesthesia is likely. Heparin is not excreted into breast milk.

*Effects on ability to drive and to use machines:* None stated.

*Undesirable effects:* Hypersensitivity reactions may occur but are rare. Acute thrombocytopenia, usually reversible, has been reported. Platelet counts should be measured in patients under heparin therapy for longer than 5 days and treatment should be stopped in those who develop significant thrombocytopenia.

Rare cases of skin necrosis occurring generally at the injection site have been reported. This may be preceded by the appearance of purpura and erythem-atous, infiltrated and painful plaques. In this case treatment should be withdrawn immediately.

Overt or concealed haemorrhage from or into any tissue or organ may result from heparin therapy. This can have serious consequences and the presentation may vary.

Raised transaminases, reversible on treatment dis-continuation, have been reported.

Osteoporosis and alopecia have been reported after long term treatment. Subcutaneous heparin may lead to a variety of local effects including pain and bruising. Pain and small haematomas may occur at the injection site as may an inflammatory reaction resulting in firm nodules. The nodules disappear after a few days and are not an indication to withdraw treatment. Rarely, priapism, hypoaldosteronism with hyperkalaemia and/or metabolic acidosis have been noted in patients at risk (e.g. diabetes, renal failure).

*Overdosage:* Haemorrhage is the major clinical sign of overdosage. In case of bleeding, the platelet count and APTT should be determined. Minor bleeding rarely requires specific therapy, and reducing and/or delaying subsequent doses of Calciparine is usually sufficient.

The anticoagulant effect of heparin can be reversed immediately by intravenous administration of a 1% protamine sulphate solution. The dose of protamine

sulphate required for neutralisation should be deter-mined accurately by titrating the patient's plasma.

It is important to avoid overdosage of protamine sulphate because protamine itself has anticoagulant properties. A single dose of protamine sulphate should never exceed 50 mg. Intravenous injection of protamine may cause a sudden fall in blood pressure, bradycardia, dyspnoea and transitory flushing, but these may be avoided or diminished by slow and careful administration.

**Pharmacological properties**

*Pharmacodynamic properties:* Heparin calcium is a preparation containing the calcium salt of sulphated polysaccharide acid present in mammalian tissues. It is an anticoagulant which inhibits the clotting of blood *in vitro* and *in vivo.*

No further data are presented here as the pharma-codynamic properties of heparin calcium are well known and it is the subject of a European Pharmaco-poeial monograph.

*Pharmacokinetic properties:* The slow and regular absorption kinetics of Calciparine (or similar calcium heparins) given subcutaneously makes it especially suitable for low dose prophylactic therapy. Calciparine has been used effectively in the routine prophylaxis of postoperative thromboembolism.

No further data are presented here as the properties of heparin calcium are well known. Heparin calcium is the subject of a European Pharmacopoeial mono-graph.

*Preclinical safety data:* There is no pre-clinical data of relevance to the prescriber which are additional to that already included in other sections of the SPC.

**Pharmaceutical particulars**

*List of excipients:* Calciparine also contains Water for Injection PhEur, Hydrochloric Acid PhEur and Calcium Hydroxide Solution BP.

*Incompatibilities:* Other preparations should not be mixed with Calciparine.

*Shelf life:* 48 months.

*Special precautions for storage:* Store below 25°C but do not freeze.

*Nature and contents of container:* Unit dose disposa-ble syringe 5,000 IU in 0.2 ml, 7,500 IU in 0.3 ml, 12,500 IU in 0.5 ml and syringe graduated 20,000 IU in 0.8 ml. Ampoule with pre-sterilised plastic syringe 12,500 IU in 0.5 ml and 20,000 IU in 0.8 ml.

*Instructions for use/handling:* See *Posology and method of administration.*

**Marketing authorisation number**   11723/0011.

**Date of approval/revision of SPC**   June 1996.

**Legal category**   POM.

# CALCIUM RESONIUM*

**Presentation**   Calcium Resonium contains 99.93% calcium polystyrene sulphonate ground and flavoured to a buff-coloured fine powder with a pleasant vanilla odour and sweet taste.

**Uses**   Calcium Resonium is an ion-exchange resin. It is recommended for the treatment of hyperkalaemia associated with anuria or severe oliguria. It is also used to treat hyperkalaemia in patients requiring dialysis and in patients on regular haemodialysis or on prolonged peritoneal dialysis.

**Dosage and administration**   Calcium Resonium is for oral or rectal administration only. The dosage recom-mendations detailed below are a guide only; the precise requirements should be decided on the basis of regular serum electrolyte determinations.

*Adults, including the elderly:*
1. *Oral:* Usual dose 15 g three or four times a day. The resin is given by mouth in a little water, or it may be made into a paste with some sweetened vehicle.
2. *Rectal:* In cases where vomiting may make oral administration difficult, the resin may be given rectally as a suspension of 30 g resin in 100 ml 2% Methylcel-lulose 450 BP (medium viscosity) and 100 ml water, as a daily retention enema. In the initial stages administration by this route as well as orally may help to achieve a more rapid lowering of the serum potassium level.

The enema should if possible be retained for at least nine hours following which the colon should be irrigated to remove the resin. If both routes are used initially it is probably unnecessary to continue rectal administration once the oral resin has reached the rectum.

*Children:* 1 g/kg body weight daily in divided doses in acute hyperkalaemia. For maintenance therapy dos-age may be reduced to 0.5 g/kg body weight daily in divided doses.

The resin is given orally, preferably with a drink (not a fruit squash because of the high potassium content) or a little jam or honey. When refused by mouth it

should be given rectally using a dose at least as great as that which would have been given orally, diluted in the same ratio as described for adults. Following retention of the enema, the colon should be irrigated to ensure adequate removal of the resin.

*Neonates:* Calcium Resonium should not be given by the oral route. With rectal administration, the mini-mum effective dosage within the range 0.5 g/kg to 1 g/kg should be employed, diluted as for adults and with adequate irrigation to ensure recovery of the resin.

**Contra-indications, warnings, etc**

*Contra-indications:* Calcium Resonium should not be administered orally to neonates and is contraindicated in neonates with reduced gut motility (e.g. post-operatively or drug induced). Calcium Resonium is also contraindicated in patients with hyperparathy-roidism, multiple myeloma, sarcoidosis or metastatic carcinoma who may present with renal failure and hypercalcaemia and in the presence of obstructive bowel disease and in use where plasma potassium levels are below 5 mmol/litre and in patients with a history of hypersensitivity to polystyrene sulphonate resins.

*Drug interactions:* There have been reports of sys-temic alkalosis following concurrent administration of cation-exchange resins and non-absorbable cation-donating antacids and laxatives such as magnesium hydroxide and aluminium carbonate. Intestinal ob-struction due to concretions of aluminium hydroxide has been reported when aluminium hydroxide has been combined with the resins (sodium form). The toxic effects of digitalis on the heart, especially various ventricular arrhythmias and AV nodal dissociation, are likely to be exaggerated if hypokalaemia is allowed to develop. Cation donating agents may reduce the potassium binding effect of Calcium Resonium. Sor-bitol added to enemas may cause colonic necrosis.

*Precautions:* The possibility of severe potassium depletion should be considered and adequate clinical and biochemical control is essential during treatment especially in patients on digitalis.

Administration of the resin should be stopped when the serum potassium falls to 5 mmol/litre. Serum calcium levels should be estimated at weekly intervals to detect the early development of hypercalcaemia, and the dose of resin adjusted to levels at which hypercalcaemia and hypokalaemia are prevented. Like all cation-exchange resins, calcium polystyrene sul-phonate is not totally selective for potassium. Hypo-magnesemia and/or hypercalcaemia may occur. Accordingly, patients should be monitored for all applicable electrolyte disturbances. In the event of clinically significant constipation, treatment should be discontinued until normal bowel movement is resumed. Magnesium-containing laxatives should not be used. The patient should be positioned carefully when ingesting the resin, in order to avoid aspiration, which may lead to bronchopulmonary complications.

The safety and efficacy of sorbitol and Calcium Resonium has not been established and they should not be used together (see *Interactions*).

In children and neonates, particular care is needed with rectal administration as excessive dosage or inadequate dilution could result in impaction of the resin. Cation donating agents may reduce the potas-sium binding effectiveness of Calcium Resonium.

*Pregnancy and lactation:* No data are available regard-ing the use of polystyrene sulphonate resins in pregnancy and lactation. The administration of Cal-cium Resonium in pregnancy and during breast feeding therefore, is not advised unless, in the opinion of the physician, the potential benefits outweigh any potential risks.

*Side-effects:* In accordance with its pharmacological actions, the resin may give rise to sodium retention, hypokalaemia and hypercalcaemia and the related clinical manifestations (see *Warnings and precautions* and *Overdosage*). Gastric irritation, anorexia, nausea, vomiting, constipation and occasionally diarrhoea may occur. Faecal impaction following rectal admin-istration has been reported in children, and gastro-intestinal concretions following oral administration to neonates. Intestinal obstruction has also been re-ported although this has been extremely rare and, possibly, a reflection of co-existing pathology, exces-sive dosage or inadequate dilution of the resin.

Some cases of acute bronchitis and/or broncho-pneumonia associated with inhalation of particles of calcium polystyrene sulphonate have been described.

Hypercalcaemia has been reported in well-dialysed patients receiving calcium resin, and in the occasional patient with chronic renal failure. Many patients in chronic renal failure have low serum calcium and high serum phosphate, but some, who cannot be screened out beforehand, show a sudden rise in serum calcium to high levels after therapy. The risk emphasises the need for adequate biochemical control.

*Overdosage:* Biochemical disturbances from overdos-age may given rise to clinical signs or symptoms of hypokalaemia, including irritability, confusion, delayed thought processes, muscle weakness, hyporeflexia and eventual paralysis. Apnoea may be a serious consequence of this progression. Electrocardiographic changes may be consistent with hypokalaemia; cardiac arrhythmia may occur. Appropriate measures should be taken to correct serum electrolytes and the resin should be removed from the alimentary tract by appropriate use of laxatives or enemas.

**Pharmaceutical precautions** Store in a dry place. Suspensions of the resin should be freshly prepared and not stored beyond 24 hours.

**Legal category** P.

**Package quantities** HDPE containers of 300 g each containing a plastic scoop which, when filled level, contains approximately 15 g.

**Further information** Theoretically, each gram of Calcium Resonium should take up 1.3 to 2 mmol of potassium. However, in vivo, the actual amount of potassium bound will be less than this. The sodium content of Calcium Resonium is less than 1 mg/g. Calcium content is about 8% w/w (1.6–2.4 mmol/g).

**Product licence number** 11723/0010.

# CORDARONE* X 100
# CORDARONE* X 200

## Qualitative and quantitative composition
Cordarone X 100 contain 100 mg of Amiodarone Hydrochloride FP.
Cordarone X 200 contain 200 mg of Amiodarone Hydrochloride FP.

**Pharmaceutical form** Tablet.

**Clinical particulars** Treatment should be initiated and normally monitored only under hospital or specialist supervision. Oral Cordarone X is indicated only for the treatment of severe rhythm disorders not responding to other therapies or when other treatments cannot be used.

*Therapeutic indications:* Tachyarrhythmias associated with Wolff-Parkinson-White Syndrome.

Atrial flutter and fibrillation when other drugs cannot be used.

All types of tachyarrhythmias of paroxysmal nature including: supraventricular, nodal and ventricular tachycardias, ventricular fibrillation; when other drugs cannot be used.

Tablets are used for stabilisation and long term treatment.

*Posology and method of administration:*
*Adults:* It is particularly important that the minimum effective dose be used. In all cases the patient's management must be judged on the individual response and well being. The following dosage regimen is generally effective.

*Initial stabilisation:* Treatment should be started with 200 mg, three times a day and may be continued for 1 week. The dosage should than be reduced to 200 mg, twice daily for a further week.

*Maintenance:* After the initial period the dosage should be reduced to 200 mg daily, or less if appropriate. Rarely, the patient may require a higher maintenance dose. The scored 100 mg tablet should be used to titrate the minimum dosage required to maintain control of the arrhythmia. The maintenance dose should be regularly reviewed, especially where this exceeds 200 mg daily.

*Changeover from intravenous to oral therapy:* As soon as an adequate response has been obtained, oral therapy should be initiated concomitantly at the usual loading dose (200 mg three times a day). Cordarone X Intravenous should than be phased out gradually.

*General considerations*
*Initial dosing:* A high dose is needed in order to achieve adequate tissue levels rapidly.

*Maintenance:* Too high a dose during maintenance therapy can cause side effects which are believed to be related to high tissue levels of amiodarone and its metabolites.

Amiodarone is strongly protein bound and has an average plasma half life of 50 days (reported range 20–100 days). It follows that sufficient time must be allowed for a new distribution equilibrium to be achieved between adjustments of dosage.

It is particularly important that the minimum effective dosage is used and the patient is monitored regularly to detect the clinical features of excess amiodarone dosage. Therapy may then be adjusted accordingly.

*Dosage reduction/withdrawal:* Side effects slowly disappear as tissue levels fall. Following drug withdrawal, residual tissue bound amiodarone may protect the patient for up to a month. However, the likelihood of recurrence of arrhythmia during this

period should be considered. In patients with potentially lethal arrhythmias the long half life is a valuable safeguard as omission of occasional doses does not significantly influence the overall therapeutic effect.

*Elderly:* As with all patients it is important that the minimum effective dose is used. Whilst there is no evidence that dosage requirements are different for this group of patients they may be more susceptible to bradycardia and conduction defects if too high a dose is employed. Particular attention should be paid to monitoring thyroid function. See *Contra-indications and Warnings.*

Cordarone X is for oral administration.

*Contra-indications:* Sinus bradycardia and sino-atrial heart block. In patients with severe conduction disturbances (high grade AV block, bifascicular or trifascicular block) or sinus node disease, Cordarone X should be used only in conjunction with a pacemaker.

Evidence or history of thyroid dysfunction. Thyroid function tests should be performed prior to therapy in all patients.

Known hypersensitivity to iodine or to amiodarone. (One 100 mg tablet contains approximately 37.5 mg iodine, one 200 mg tablet contains approximately 75 mg iodine.)

The combination of Cordarone X with drugs which may induce Torsades de Pointes is contra-indicated (see *Interactions* section).

*Special warnings and special precautions for use:* Too high a dosage may lead to severe bradycardia and to conduction disturbances with the appearance of an idioventricular rhythm, particularly in elderly patients or during digitalis therapy. In these circumstances, Cordarone X treatment should be withdrawn. If necessary beta-adrenostimulants or glucagon may be given.

Oral Cordarone X is not contra-indicated in patients with latent or manifest heart failure but caution should be exercised as, occasionally, existing heart failure may be worsened. In such cases, Cordarone X may be used with other appropriate therapies.

Amiodarone induces ECG changes: QT interval lengthening corresponding to prolonged repolarisation with the possible development of U and deformed T waves; these changes are evidence of its pharmacological action and do not reflect toxicity. Although there have been no literature reports on the potentiation of hepatic adverse effects of alcohol, patients should be advised to moderate their alcohol intake while taking Cordarone X.

*Interactions with other medicaments and other forms of interaction:* Some of the more important drugs that interact with amiodarone include warfarin, digoxin, phenytoin and any drug which prolongs the QT interval.

Amiodarone raises the plasma concentrations of highly protein bound drugs, for example oral anticoagulants and phenytoin. The dose of warfarin should be reduced accordingly. More frequent monitoring of prothrombin time both during and after amiodarone treatment is recommended. Phenytoin dosage should be reduced if signs of overdosage appear, and plasma levels may be measured.

Administration of Cordarone X to a patient already receiving digoxin will bring about an increase in the plasma digoxin concentration and thus precipitate symptoms and signs associated with high digoxin levels. Monitoring is recommeded and digoxin dosage usually has to be reduced. A synergistic effect on heart rate and atrioventricular conduction is also possible.

Combined therapy with the following drugs which prolong the QT interval is contra-indicated (see *Contra-indications* section) due to the increased risk of Torsades de Pointes; for example:
– Class Ia anti-arrhythmic drugs e.g. quinidine, procainamide, disopyramide
– Class III anti-arrhythmic drugs e.g. sotalol, bretylium
– intravenous erythromycin, co-trimoxazole or pentamidine injection
– anti-psychotics e.g. chlorpromazine, thioridazine, pimozide, haloperidol
– lithium and tricyclic anti-depressants e.g. doxepin, maprotiline, amitriptyline
– certain antihistamines e.g. terfenadine, astemizole
– anti-malarials e.g. quinine, mefloquine, chloroquine, halofantrine.
Combined therapy with the following drugs is not recommended: beta blockers and certain calcium channel inhibitors (diltiazem, verapamil); potentiation of negative chronotropic properties and conduction slowing effects may occur.

Caution should be exercised over combined therapy with the following drugs which may cause hypokalaemia: and/or hypomagnesaemia: diuretics, systemic corticosteroids, tetracosactrin, intravenous amphotericin.

In cases of hypokalaemia, corrective action should be taken and QT interval monitored. In case of Torsades de Pointes antiarrhythmic agents should not

be given; pacing may be instituted and IV magnesium may be used.

Caution is advised in patients undergoing general anaesthesia, or receiving high dose oxygen therapy.

Potentially severe complications have been reported in patients taking amiodarone undergoing general anaesthesia: bradycardia unresponsive to atropine, hypotension, disturbances of conduction, decreased cardiac output.

A few cases of adult respiratory distress syndrome, most often in the period immediately after surgery, have been observed. A possible interaction with a high oxygen concentration may be implicated. The anaesthetist should be informed that the patient is taking Cordarone X.

Amiodarone may increase the plasma levels of cyclosporin when used in combination, due to a decrease in the clearance of this drug.

*Pregnancy and lactation:*
*Pregnancy:* Although no teratogenic effects have been observed in animals, there are insufficient data on the use of amiodarone during pregnancy in humans to judge any possible toxicity. However, in view of the pharmacological properties of the drug on the foetus and its effect on the foetal thyroid gland, its administration in pregnancy should be avoided.

*Lactation:* Amiodarone is excreted into the breast milk in significant quantities and breast-feeding is contra-indicated.

*Effects on ability to drive and use machines:* None stated.

*Undesirable effects:* Amiodarone can cause serious adverse reactions affecting the lung, liver, thyroid gland, skin and peripheral nervous system (see below). Because these reactions can be delayed, patients on long-term treatment should be carefully supervised.

*Pulmonary:* Cordarone X can cause pulmonary toxicity (hypersensitivity pneumonitis, alveolar/interstitial pneumonitis or fibrosis, pleuritis, bronchiolitis obliterans organising pneumonia). Sometimes this toxicity can be fatal.

Presenting features can include dyspnoea (which may be severe and unexplained by the current cardiac status), non-productive cough and deterioration in general health (fatigue, weight loss and fever). The onset is usually slow but may be rapidly progressive. Whilst the majority of cases have been reported with long term therapy, a few have occurred soon after starting treatment.

Patients should be carefully evaluated clinically and consideration given to chest X-ray before starting therapy. During treatment, if pulmonary toxicity is suspected, this should be repeated and associated with lung function testing including where possible measurement of transfer factor. Initial radiological changes may be difficult to distinguish from pulmonary venous congestion. Pulmonary toxicity has usually been reversible following early withdrawal of amiodarone therapy, with or without corticosteroid therapy. Clinical symptoms often resolve within a few weeks followed by slower radiological and lung function improvement. Some patients can deteriorate despite discontinuing Cordarone X. A few cases of adult respiratory distress syndrome, most often in the period after surgery, have been observed, resulting sometimes in fatalities (see *Interactions*).

*Cardiac:* Bradycardia which is generally moderate and dose dependent has been reported. In some cases (sinus node disease, elderly patients) marked bradycardia or more exceptionally sinus arrest has occurred. There have been rare instances of conduction disturbances (sino-atrial block, various degrees of AV block). Because of the long half life of amiodarone, if bradycardia is severe and symptomatic the insertion of a pacemaker should be considered. Amiodarone has a low proarrhythmic effect. However arrhythmia (new occurence or aggravation), followed in some cases by cardiac arrest has been reported; with current knowledge, it is not possible to differentiate a drug effect from the underlying cardiac condition or lack of therapeutic efficacy. This has usually occurred in combination with other precipitating factors particularly other antiarrhythmic agents, hypokalaemia and digoxin.

*Hepatic:* Amiodarone may be associated with a variety of hepatic effects, including cirrhosis, hepatitis and jaundice. Some fatalities have been reported, mainly following long-term therapy, although rarely they have occurred soon after starting treatment particularly after Cordarone X intravenous. It is advisable to monitor liver function particularly transaminases before treatment and six monthly thereafter.

At the beginning of therapy, elevation of serum transaminases which can be in isolation (1.5 to 3 times normal) may occur. These may return to normal with dose reduction, or sometimes spontaneously.

Isolated cases of acute liver disorders with elevated serum transaminases and/or jaundice may occur; in such cases treatment should be discontinued.

There have been reports of chronic liver disease.

Alteration of laboratory tests which may be minimal (transaminases elevated 1.5 to 5 times normal) or clinical signs (possible hepatomegaly) during treatment for longer than 6 months should suggest this diagnosis. Routine monitoring of liver function tests is therefore advised. Abnormal clinical and laboratory test results usually regress upon cessation of treatment. Histological findings may resemble pseudo-alcoholic hepatitis, but they can be variable and include cirrhosis.

*Thyroid:* Both hyper and hypothyroidism have occurred during, or soon after, amiodarone treatment. Simple monitoring of the usual biochemical tests is confusing because some tests such as free $T_4$ and free $T_3$ may be altered where the patient is euthyroid. Clinical monitoring is therefore recommended before start of treatment, then six monthly and should be continued for some months after discontinuation of treatment. This is particularly important in the elderly. In patients whose history indicates an increased risk of thyroid dysfunction, regular assessment is recommended.

*Hyperthyroidism:* Clinical features such as weight loss, asthenia, restlessness, increase in heart rate, recurrence of the cardiac dysrhythmia, angina or congestive heart failure, should alert the clinician. The diagnosis may be supported by an elevated serum tri-iodothyronine ($T_3$), a low level of thyroid stimulating hormone (TSH) as measured by high sensitivity methods, and a reduced TSH response to thyrotrophin releasing hormone (TRH). Elevation of reverse $T_3$ ($rT_3$) may also be found.

In the case of hyperthyroidism, therapy should be withdrawn. Clinical recovery usually occurs within a few weeks, although severe cases, sometimes resulting in fatalities, have been reported.

Courses of anti-thyroid drugs have been used for the treatment of severe thyroid hyperactivity; large doses may be required initially. These may not always be effective and concomitant high dose corticosteroid therapy (e.g. 1 mg/kg prednisolone) may be required for several weeks.

*Hypothyroidism:* Clinical features such as weight gain, reduced activity or excessive bradycardia should suggest the diagnosis. This may be supported by an elevated serum TSH level and an exaggerated TSH response to TRH. $T_4$ and $T_3$ levels may be low. Thyroid hypofunction usually resolves within 3 months of cessation of therapy; it may be treated cautiously with L-thyroxine. Concomitant use of Cordarone X should be continued only in life threatening situations, when TSH levels may provide a guide to L-thyroxine dosage.

*Ophthalmological:* Patients on continuous therapy almost always develop microdeposits in the cornea. The deposits are usually only discernible by slit-lamp examinations and may rarely cause subjective symptoms such as visual haloes and blurring of vision. The deposits are considered essentially benign, do not require discontinuation of amiodarone and regress following termination of treatment. Rare cases of impaired visual acuity due to optic neuritis have been reported, although at present, the relationship with amiodarone has not been established. Unless blurred or decreased vision occurs, ophthalmological examination is recommended annually.

*Dermatological:* Patients taking Cordarone X can become unduly sensitive to sunlight and should be warned of this possibility. In most cases, symptoms are limited to tingling, burning and erythema of sun exposed skin but severe phototoxic reactions with blistering may be seen. Photosensitivity may persist for several months after discontinuation of Cordarone X. Photosensitivity can be minimised by limiting exposure to UV light, wearing suitable protective hats and clothing and by using a broad spectrum sun screening preparation. Rarely, a slate grey or bluish discoloration of light exposed skin, particularly on the face, may occur. Resolution of this pigmentation may be very slow once the drug is discontinued. Other types of skin rashes including isolated cases of exfoliative dermatitis have also been reported. Cases of erythema have been reported during radiotherapy.

*Neurological:* Peripheral neuropathy can be caused by Cordarone X. Myopathy has occasionally been reported. Both these conditions may be severe although they are usually reversible on drug withdrawal. Nightmares, vertigo, headaches, sleeplessness and paraesthesia may also occur. Tremor and ataxia have also infrequently been reported usually with complete regression after reduction of dose or withdrawal of the drug. Benign intracranial hypertension (pseudo-tumour cerebri) has been reported.

*Other:* Other unwanted effects occasionally reported include nausea, vomiting, metallic taste (which usually occur with loading dosage and which regress on dose reduction), fatigue, impotence, epididymo-orchitis and alopecia. Isolated cases suggesting a hypersensitivity reaction involving vasculitis, renal involvement with moderate elevation of creatinine levels or thrombocytopenia have been observed. Haemolytic or aplastic anaemia have rarely been reported.

*Overdose:* Animal studies indicate that amiodarone has a high $LD_{50}$, hence it is most unlikely that a patient will ingest an acute toxic dose. In such an event gastric lavage may be employed to reduce absorption in addition to general supportive measures. The patient should be monitored; if bradycardia occurs beta-adrenostimulants or glucagon may be given. Spontaneously resolving attacks of ventricular tachycardia may also occur. Due to the pharmacokinetics of amiodarone, adequate and prolonged surveillance of the patient, particularly cardiac status, is recommended. Neither amiodarone nor its metabolites are dialysable.

## Pharmacological properties

*Pharmacodynamic properties:* Amiodarone hydrochloride is an antiarrhythmic.

*Pharmacokinetic properties:* Amiodarone is strongly protein bound and the plasma half life is usually of the order of 50 days. However there may be considerable inter-patient variation; in individual patients a half life of less than 20 days and a half life of more than 100 days has been reported. High doses of Cordarone X, for example 600 mg/day, should be given initially to achieve effective tissue levels as rapidly as possible. Owing to the long half life of the drug, a maintenance dose of only 200 mg/day, or less is usually necessary. Sufficient time must be allowed for a new distribution equilibrium to be achieved between adjustments of dose.

The long half life is a valuable safeguard for patients with potentially lethal arrhythmias as omission of occasional doses does not significantly influence the protection afforded by Cordarone X.

*Preclinical safety data:* There are no pre-clinical data of relevance to the prescriber which are additional to that already included in other sections of the SPC.

## Pharmaceutical particulars

*List of excipients:* Lactose, maize starch, polyvidone, colloidal silicon dioxide, magnesium stearate.

*Incompatibilities:* None stated.

*Shelf life:* 60 months.

*Special precautions for storage:* The tablets should be protected from light.

*Nature and contents of container:* Cordarone X 100 and 200 tablets are supplied in blister packs of **28** and 30 tablets packed in cardboard cartons. The pack size in **bold** is marketed.

*Instructions for use/handling:* Not applicable.

**Marketing authorisation numbers**
Cordarone X 100   11723/0012.
Cordarone X 200   11723/0013.

**Date of approval/revision of SPC**   June 1996.

**Legal category** POM.

# CORDARONE* X INTRAVENOUS

**Qualitative and quantitative composition** Each ampoule contains 150 mg Amiodarone Hydrochloride FP.

**Pharmaceutical form** Solution for injection.

**Clinical particulars** Treatment should be initiated and normally monitored only under hospital or specialist supervision. Intravenous Cordarone X is indicated only for the treatment of severe rhythm disorders not responding to other therapies or when other treatments cannot be used.

*Therapeutic indications:* Tachyarrhythmias associated with Wolff-Parkinson-White Syndrome.

All types of tachyarrhythmias including: supraventricular, nodal and ventricular tachycardias; atrial flutter and fibrillation; ventricular fibrillation; when other drugs cannot be used. The injection is to be used where a rapid response is required.

*Posology and method of administration:* Cordarone X Intravenous should only be used when facilities exist for cardiac monitoring, defibrillation, and cardiac pacing.

In children, Cordarone X Intravenous normally should be given under the supervision of a paediatric cardiologist.

IV infusion is preferred to bolus due to the haemodynamic effects sometimes associated with rapid injection.

Cordarone X Intravenous may be used prior to DC conversion.

Repeated or continuous infusion via peripheral veins may lead to local discomfort and inflammation. When repeated or continuous infusion is anticipated, administration by a central venous catheter is recommended.

The standard recommended dose is 5 mg/kg bodyweight given by intravenous infusion over a period of 20 minutes to 2 hours. This should be administered as a dilute solution in 250 ml 5% dextrose. This may be followed by repeat infusion up to 1,200 mg (ap-

proximately 15 mg/kg bodyweight) in up to 500 ml 5% dextrose per 24 hours, the rate of infusion being adjusted on the basis of clinical response.

In extreme clinical emergency the drug may, at the discretion of the clinician, be given as a slow injection of 150–300 mg in 10–20 ml 5% dextrose over a minimum of 3 minutes. This should not be repeated for at least 15 minutes.

Patients treated with Cordarone X Intravenous must be closely monitored e.g. in an intensive care unit.

When given by infusion Cordarone X may reduce drop size and, if appropriate, adjustments should be made to the rate of infusion.

*Changeover from intravenous to oral therapy:* As soon as an adequate response has been obtained, oral therapy should be initiated concomitantly at the usual loading dose (200 mg three times a day). Cordarone X Intravenous should then be phased out gradually.

*Elderly:* As with all patients it is important that the minimum effective dose is used. Whilst there is no evidence that dosage requirements are different for this group of patients they may be more susceptible to bradycardia and conduction defects if too high a dose is employed. Particular attention should be paid to monitoring thyroid function. See *Contra-indications* and *Warnings.*

*Contra-indications:* Sinus bradycardia and sino-atrial heart block. In patients with severe conduction disturbances (high grade AV block, bifascicular or trifascicular block) or sinus node disease, Cordarone X should be used only in conjunction with a pacemaker.

Evidence or history of thyroid dysfunction. Thyroid function tests should be performed prior to therapy in all patients.

Severe respiratory failure, circulatory collapse, or severe arterial hypotension; congestive heart failure and cardiomyopathy are also contra-indications when using Cordarone X injection as a bolus injection.

Known hypersensitivity to iodine or to amiodarone. (One ampoule contains approximately 56 mg iodine.)

The combination of Cordarone X with drugs which may induce Torsades de Pointes is contra-indicated (see *Interactions* section).

*Special warnings and special precautions for use:* Too high a dosage may lead to severe bradycardia and to conduction disturbances with the appearance of an idioventricular rhythm, particularly in elderly patients or during digitalis therapy. In these circumstances, Cordarone X treatment should be withdrawn. If necessary beta-adrenostimulants or glucagon may be given.

Caution should be exercised in patients with hypotension and decompensated cardiomyopathy.

Amiodarone induces ECG changes: QT interval lengthening corresponding to prolonged repolarisation with the possible development of U and deformed T waves; these changes are evidence of its pharmacological action and do not reflect toxicity.

Although there have been no literature reports on the potentiation of hepatic adverse effects of alcohol, patients should be advised to moderate their alcohol intake while taking Cordarone X.

*Interaction with other medicaments and other forms of interaction:* Some of the more important drugs that interact with amiodarone include warfarin, digoxin, phenytoin and any drug which prolongs the QT interval.

Amiodarone raises the plasma concentrations of highly protein bound drugs, for example oral anticoagulants and phenytoin. The dose of warfarin should be reduced accordingly. More frequent monitoring of prothrombin time both during and after amiodarone treatment is recommended. Phenytoin dosage should be reduced if signs of overdosage appear, and plasma levels may be measured.

Administration of Cordarone X to a patient already receiving digoxin will bring about an increase in the plasma digoxin concentration and thus precipitate symptoms and signs associated with high digoxin levels. Monitoring is recommended and digoxin dosage usually has to be reduced. A synergistic effect on heart rare and atrioventricular conduction is also possible.

Combined therapy with the following drugs which prolong the QT interval is contra-indicated (see *Contra-indications* section) due to the increased risk of Torsades de Pointes; for example:
- Class Ia anti-arrhythmic drugs e.g. quinidine, procainamide, disopyramide
- Class III anti-arrhythmic drugs e.g. sotalol, bretylium
- intravenous erythromycin, co-trimoxazole or pentamidine injection
- anti-psychotics e.g. chlorpromazine, thioridazine, pimozide, haloperidol
- lithium and tricyclic anti-depressants e.g. doxepin, maprotiline, amitriptyline
- certain antihistamines e.g. terfenadine, astemizole
- anti-malarials e.g. quinine, mefloquine, chloroquine, halofantrine.
Combined therapy with the following drugs is not

recommended: beta blockers and certain calcium channel inhibitors (diltiazem, verapamil); potentiation of negative chronotropic properties and conduction slowing effects may occur.

Caution should be exercised over combined therapy with the following drugs which may cause hypokalaemia: and/or hypomagnesaemia: diuretics, systemic corticosteroids, tetracosactrin, intravenous amphotericin.

In cases of hypokalaemia, corrective action should be taken and QT interval monitored. In case of Torsades de Pointes antiarrhythmic agents should not be given; pacing may be instituted and IV magnesium may be used.

Caution is advised in patients undergoing general anaesthesia, or receiving high dose oxygen therapy.

Potentially severe complications have been reported in patients taking amiodarone undergoing general anaesthesia: bradycardia unresponsive to atropine, hypotension, disturbances of conduction, decreased cardiac output.

A few cases of adult respiratory distress syndrome, most often in the period immediately after surgery, have been observed. A possible interaction with a high oxygen concentration may be implicated. The anaesthetist should be informed that the patient is taking Cordarone X.

Amiodarone may increase the plasma levels of cyclosporin when used in combination, due to a decrease in the clearance of this drug.

*Pregnancy and lactation:*

*Pregnancy:* Although no teratogenic effects have been observed in animals, there are insufficient data on the use of amiodarone during pregnancy in humans to judge any possible toxicity. However, in view of the pharmacological properties of the drug on the foetus and its effect on the foetal thyroid gland, its administration in pregnancy should be avoided.

*Lactation:* Amiodarone is excreted into the breast milk in significant quantities and breast-feeding is contra-indicated.

*Effects on ability to drive and use machines:* None stated.

*Undesirable effects:* Rapid administration of Cordarone X Intravenous has been associated with hot flushes, sweating and nausea. A moderate and transient reduction in blood pressure may occur. Circulatory collapse may be precipitated by too rapid administration or overdosage (atropine has been used successfully in such patients presenting with bradycardia). In cases of respiratory failure, notably in asthmatics, bronchospasm and/or apnoea may also occur. Isolated cases of anaphylactic shock have been reported.

Amiodarone can cause serious adverse reactions affecting the lung, liver, thyroid gland, skin and peripheral nervous system (see below). Because these reactions can be delayed, patients on long-term treatment should be carefully supervised.

*Pulmonary:* Cordarone X can cause pulmonary toxicity (hypersensitivity pneumonitis, alveolar/interstitial pneumonitis or fibrosis, pleuritis, bronchiolitis obliterans organising pneumonia). Sometimes this toxicity can be fatal.

Presenting features can include dyspnoea (which may be severe and unexplained by the current cardiac status), non-productive cough and deterioration in general health (fatigue, weight loss and fever). The onset is usually slow but may be rapidly progressive. Whilst the majority of cases have been reported with long term therapy, a few have occurred soon after starting treatment.

Patients should be carefully evaluated clinically and consideration given to chest X-ray before starting therapy. During treatment, if pulmonary toxicity is suspected, this should be repeated and associated with lung function testing including where possible measurement of transfer factor. Initial radiological changes may be difficult to distinguish from pulmonary venous congestion. Pulmonary toxicity has usually been reversible following early withdrawal of amiodarone therapy, with or without corticosteroid therapy. Clinical symptoms often resolve within a few weeks followed by slower radiological and lung function improvement. Some patients can deteriorate despite discontinuing Cordarone X. A few cases of adult respiratory distress syndome, most often in the period after surgery, have been observed, resulting sometimes in fatalities (see *Interactions*).

*Cardiac:* Bradycardia which is generally moderate and dose dependent has been reported. In some cases (sinus node disease, elderly patients) marked bradycardia or more exceptionally sinus arrest has occurred. There have been rare instances of conduction disturbances (sino-atrial block, various degrees of AV block). Because of the long half life of amiodarone, if bradycardia is severe and symptomatic the insertion of a pacemaker should be considered. Amiodarone has a low proarrhythmic effect. However arrhythmia (new occurrence or aggravation), followed in some cases by cardiac arrest has been reported; with current

knowledge, it is not possible to differentiate a drug effect from the underlying cardiac condition or lack of therapeutic efficacy. This has usually occurred in combination with other precipitating factors particularly other antiarrhythmic agents, hypokalaemia and digoxin.

*Hepatic:* Amiodarone may be associated with a variety of hepatic effects, including cirrhosis, hepatitis and jaundice. Some fatalities have been reported, mainly following long-term therapy, although rarely they have occurred soon after starting treatment particularly after Cordarone X Intravenous. It is advisable to monitor liver function particularly transaminases before treatment and six monthly thereafter.

At the beginning of therapy, elevation of serum transaminases which can be in isolation (1.5 to 3 times normal) may occur. These may return to normal with dose reduction, or sometimes spontaneously.

Isolated cases of acute liver disorders with elevated serum transaminases and/or jaundice may occur; in such cases treatment should be discontinued.

There have been reports of chronic liver disease. Alteration of laboratory tests which may be minimal (transaminases elevated 1.5 to 5 times normal) or clinical signs (possible hepatomegaly) during treatment for longer than 6 months should suggest this diagnosis. Routine monitoring of liver function tests is therefore advised. Abnormal clinical and laboratory test results usually regress upon cessation of treatment. Histological findings may resemble pseudo-alcoholic hepatitis, but they can be variable and include cirrhosis.

*Thyroid:* Both hyper and hypothyroidism have occurred during, or soon after, amiodarone treatment. Simple monitoring of the usual biochemical tests is confusing because some tests such as free $T_4$ and free $T_3$ may be altered where the patient is euthyroid. Clinical monitoring is therefore recommended before start of treatment, then six monthly and should be continued for some months after discontinuation of treatment. This is particularly important in the elderly. In patients whose history indicates an increased risk of thyroid dysfunction, regular assessment is recommended.

*Hyperthyroidism:* Clinical features such as weight loss, asthenia, restlessness, increase in heart rate, recurrence of the cardiac dysrhythmia, angina or congestive heart failure, should alert the clinician. The diagnosis may be supported by an elevated serum $T_3$, a low level of thyroid stimulating hormone (TSH) as measured by high sensitivity methods, and a reduced TSH response to TRH. Elevation of reverse $T_3$ ($rT_3$) may also be found. In the case of hyperthyroidism, therapy should be withdrawn. Clinical recovery usually occurs within a few weeks, although severe cases, sometimes resulting in fatalities, have been reported.

Courses of anti-thyroid drugs have been used for the treatment of severe thyroid hyperactivity; large doses may be required initially. These may not always be effective and concomitant high dose corticosteroid therapy (e.g. 1 mg/kg prednisolone) may be required for several weeks.

*Hypothyroidism:* Clinical features such as weight gain, reduced activity or excessive bradycardia should suggest the diagnosis. This may be supported by an elevated serum TSH level and an exaggerated TSH response to TRH. $T_4$ and $T_3$ levels may be low. Thyroid hypofunction usually resolves within 3 months of cessation of therapy; it may be treated cautiously with L-thyroxine. Concomitant use of Cordarone X should be continued only in life threatening situations, when TSH levels may provide a guide to L-thyroxine dosage.

*Ophthalmological:* Patients on continuous therapy almost always develop microdeposits in the cornea. The deposits are usually only discernible by slit-lamp examinations and may rarely cause subjective symptoms such as visual haloes and blurring of vision. The deposits are considered essentially benign, do not require discontinuation of amiodarone and regress following termination of treatment. Rare cases of impaired visual acuity due to optic neuritis have been reported, although at present, the relationship with amiodarone has not been established. Unless blurred or decreased vision occurs, ophthalmological examination is recommended annually.

*Dermatological:* Patients taking Cordarone X can become unduly sensitive to sunlight and should be warned of this possibility. In most cases, symptoms are limited to tingling, burning and erythema of sun exposed skin but severe phototoxic reactions with blistering may be seen. Photosensitivity may persist for several months after discontinuation of Cordarone X. Photosensitivity can be minimised by limiting exposure to UV light, wearing suitable protective hats and clothing and by using a broad spectrum sun screening preparation. Rarely, a slate grey or bluish discoloration of light exposed skin, particularly on the face, may occur. Resolution of this pigmentation may be very slow once the drug is discontinued. Other types of skin rashes including isolated cases of exfoliative dermatitis have also been reported. Cases of erythema have been reported during radiotherapy.

*Neurological:* Peripheral neuropathy can be caused by Cordarone X. Myopathy has occasionally been reported. Both these conditions may be severe although they are usually reversible on drug withdrawal. Nightmares, vertigo, headaches, sleeplessness and paraesthesia may also occur. Tremor and ataxia have also infrequently been reported usually with complete regression after reduction of dose or withdrawal of the drug. Benign intracranial hypertension (pseudo-tumour cerebri) has been reported.

*Other:* Other unwanted effects occasionally reported include nausea, vomiting, metallic taste (which usually occur with loading dosage and which regress on dose reduction), fatigue, impotence, epididymo-orchitis and alopecia. Isolated cases suggesting a hypersensitivity reaction involving vasculitis, renal involvement with moderate elevation of creatinine levels or thrombocytopenia have been observed. Haemolytic or aplastic anaemia have rarely been reported.

*Overdose:* Animal studies indicate that amiodarone has a high $LD_{50}$, hence it is most unlikely that a patient will ingest an acute toxic dose. In such an event gastric lavage may be employed to reduce absorption in addition to general supportive measures. The patient should be monitored; if bradycardia occurs beta-adrenostimulants or glucagon may be given. Spontaneously resolving attacks of ventricular tachycardia may also occur. Due to the pharmacokinetics of amiodarone, adequate and prolonged surveillance of the patient, particularly cardiac status, is recommended. Neither amiodarone nor its metabolites are dialysable.

**Pharmacological properties**

*Pharmacodynamic properties:* Cordarone X is a product for the treatment of tachyarrhythmias and has complex pharmacological actions. Its effects are anti-adrenergic (partial alpha and beta blockers). It has haemodynamic effects (increased blood flow and systematic/coronary vasodilation). The drug reduces myocardial oxygen consumption and has been shown to have a sparing effect of rat myocardial ATP utilisation, with decreased oxidative processes. Amiodarone inhibits the metabolic and biochemical effects of catecholamines on the heart and inhibits $Na^+$ and $K^+$ activated ATP-ase.

*Pharmacokinetic properties:* Pharmacokinetics of amiodarone are unusual and complex, and have not been completely elucidated. Absorption following oral administration is variable and may be prolonged, with enterohepatic cycling. The major metabolite is desethylamiodarone. Amiodarone is highly protein bound (>95%). Renal excretion is minimal and faecal excretion is the major route. A study in both healthy volunteers and patients after intravenous administration of amiodarone reported that the calculated volumes of distribution and total blood clearance using a two-compartment open model were similar for both groups. Elimination of amiodarone after intravenous injection appeared to be biexponential with a distribution phase lasting about 4 hours. The very high volume of distribution combined with a relatively low apparent volume for the central compartment suggests extensive tissue distribution. A bolus IV injection of 400 mg gave a terminal $T\frac{1}{2}$ of approximately 11 hours.

*Preclinical safety data:* There are no pre-clinical data of relevance to the prescriber which are additional to that already included in other sections of the SPC.

**Pharmaceutical particulars**

*List of excipients:* Benzyl alcohol, polysorbate and water for injections.

*Incompatibilities:* Cordarone X Intravenous is incompatible with saline and should be administered solely in 5% Dextrose solution. Solutions containing less than 2 ampoules Cordarone X Intravenous in 500 ml Dextrose 5% are unstable and should not be used.

*Shelf life:* 24 months.

*Special precautions for storage:* Protect from light.

*Nature and contents of container:* Each carton contains ten glass ampoules.

*Instructions for use/handling:* See *Posology and method of administration* section above.

**Marketing authorisation number**   11723/0014.

**Date of approval/revision of SPC**   October 1993.

**Legal category**   POM.

# CORGARD* TABLETS

**Qualitative and quantitative composition**   The tablets contain Nadolol 40 mg or 80 mg.

**Pharmaceutical form**   Pale blue round biconvex tablets.

## Clinical particulars

*Therapeutic indications:* Corgard is indicated in the management of:

*Angina pectoris:* For the long-term management of patients with angina pectoris by continuous medication.

*Hypertension:* For the long-term management of essential hypertension, either alone or in combination with other antihypertensive agents, especially thiazide-type diuretics.

*Arrhythmias:* For the treatment of cardiac tachyarrhythmias.

*Migraine:* For the prophylactic management of migraine headache. The efficacy of Corgard in the treatment of a migraine attack that has already started has not been established, and Corgard is not indicated for such use.

*Thyrotoxicosis:* For the relief of the symptoms of hyperthyroidism and the pre-operative preparation of patients for surgery. Nadolol may be used in conjunction with conventional antithyroid therapy.

*Posology and method of administration*

*Adults:* Dosage should be titrated gradually with at least a week between increments to assess response; individuals show considerable variation in their response to beta-adrenergic blockade.

Corgard may be given in a once daily dosage without regard to meals. The dosage interval should be increased when creatinine clearance is below 50 ml/min/1.73m².

If Corgard is to be discontinued, reduce dosage over a period of at least two weeks (see Warnings).

*Angina pectoris:* Initially 40 mg once daily. This may be increased at weekly intervals until an adequate response is obtained or excessive bradycardia occurs. Most patients respond to 160 mg or less daily. The value and safety of daily doses exceeding 240 mg have not been established.

*Hypertension:* Initially 80 mg once daily. This may be increased by a weekly increment of 80 mg or less until an optimum response is obtained. Many patients respond to 80 mg daily, and most patients respond to 240 mg or less, daily, but higher doses have been required for a few patients. In some patients it is necessary to administer a diuretic, peripheral vasodilator and/or other antihypertensive agents in conjunction with nadolol in order to achieve satisfactory response.

Treatment of hypertension associated with phaeochromocytoma may require the addition of an alpha-blocking agent.

*Cardiac tachyarrhythmias:* Initially 40 mg once daily. This may be increased if necessary to 160 mg once daily. If bradycardia occurs dosage should be reduced to 40 mg once daily.

*Migraine:* The initial dose of nadolol is 40 mg once daily. Dosage may be gradually increased in 40 mg increments until optimum migraine prophylaxis is achieved. The usual maintenance dose is 80 to 160 mg administered once daily. After 4 to 6 weeks at the maximum dose if a satisfactory response is not obtained, therapy with nadolol should be withdrawn gradually.

*Thyrotoxicosis:* The dosage range is 80–160 mg once daily. It has been found that most patients require a dose of 160 mg once daily. Nadolol may be used together with conventional anti-thyroid treatment. For the preparation of patients for partial thyroidectomy, nadolol should be administered in conjunction with potassium iodide for a period of 10 days prior to operation. Nadolol should be administered on the morning of operation. Post-operatively, nadolol dosage should be slowly reduced and then withdrawn following clinical stability.

*Children:* Safety and effectiveness in children have not been established.

*Elderly:* In elderly patients a low initial dose should be used so that sensitivity to side-effects may be assessed.

*Renal or hepatic impairment:* As with all drugs patients with impaired renal or hepatic function should be monitored.

*Contra-indications:* Like other drugs in this class, nadolol is contra-indicated in bronchial asthma or a history of asthma; sinus bradycardia; 2nd and 3rd degree heart block; cardiogenic shock; right ventricular failure secondary to pulmonary hypertension; congestive heart failure.

*Special warnings and special precautions for use:* Exacerbation of angina and myocardial infarction have occurred after abrupt discontinuation of therapy with beta-adrenergic blocking agents in patients with angina pectoris or other evidence of coronary artery insufficiency. When discontinuing long-term treatment with nadolol, the dosage should be reduced gradually over a period of at least two weeks and the patient carefully monitored.

Beta-adrenergic blockade carries the potential hazard of precipitating cardiac failure. Should this occur and it is not controlled by digitalisation, nadolol should be withdrawn, consideration being given to the foregoing warning.

Beta-blocking impairs the ability of the heart to respond to stress. It has been the usual practice to recommend withdrawal of beta-blockers several days prior to surgery. However, this may render the patient's blood pressure unstable and difficult to control during anaesthesia and the anaesthetist may wish to advise on discontinuation of therapy. In no circumstances should beta-blockers be discontinued prior to surgery in patients with phaeochromocytoma or thyrotoxicosis. In the event of emergency surgery, the effects of nadolol may be reversed by isoprenaline or noradrenaline. However, such patients may be subject to protracted severe hypotension. General anaesthetics which can cause myocardial depression, such as cyclopropane, trichloroethylene, chloroform and ether, should be avoided if nadolol is continued during surgery.

Nadolol should be administered with caution to patients with chronic obstructive airways disease. Discontinue therapy if condition relapses.

Care should be exercised in the administration of nadolol to diabetic patients since early signs of acute hypoglycaemia may be masked. It may also be necessary to adjust the dosage of hypoglycaemic drugs, or insulin doses.

There have been reports of skin rashes (including a psoriasiform type) and/or ocular changes (conjunctivitis and 'dry eye') associated with the use of beta-adrenergic blocking drugs. The reported incidence is small and in most cases the symptoms have cleared when the treatment was withdrawn. Discontinuance of the drug should be considered if any such reaction is not otherwise explicable. Cessation of the therapy with a beta-adrenergic blocker should be gradual.

Beta-blocking may mask certain signs (e.g. tachycardia) of hyperthyroidism. Patients suspected of developing thyrotoxicosis should be managed carefully to avoid abrupt withdrawal of beta-blockade which might precipitate a thyroid storm.

*Precautions:* Occasionally, beta-blockade with drugs such as nadolol may produce hypotension and/or marked bradycardia, resulting in vertigo, syncope or orthostatic hypotension.

Nadolol should be used with caution in patients with impaired renal or hepatic function.

*Administration in renal failure:* In patients with decreased renal function, dosage adjustment is necessary. The recommended dosage intervals are:

| Creatinine clearance (ml/min/1.73 m²) | | Dosage interval (Hours) |
|---|---|---|
| Less than | 10 | 40–60 |
| | 10–30 | 24–48 |
| | 31–50 | 24–36 |
| More than | 50 | 24 |

*Interactions with other medicaments and other forms of interaction*

*General anaesthetics:* Those which cause myocardial depression such as chloroform, cyclopropane, trichloroethylene and ether should be avoided as the patient may be subject to protracted severe hypotension.

*Myocardial depressants:* Myocardial depressants such as lignocaine and procainamide may subject the patient to protracted severe hypotension.

*Adrenoceptor stimulants:* Beta-adrenoceptor stimulants such as isoprenaline and verapamil, or alpha-adrenoceptor stimulants such as noradrenaline and adrenaline, will reverse the hypotensive effects and increase vasoconstrictor activity.

*Catecholamine-depleting drugs:* e.g. Reserpine. Excessive reduction in sympathetic drive to the heart might occur. Close observation is advised.

*Antihypertensives:* e.g. Neurone-blocking drugs, vasodilators, diuretics. Additive hypotensive effect.

*Clonidine:* If Corgard and clonidine are given concurrently, clonidine should not be discontinued until several days after Corgard withdrawal.

*Hypoglycaemics, insulin:* Possible dosage adjustment, see Warnings.

*Monoamine oxidase inhibitors:* Administration of nadolol during and within 2 weeks of administration of adrenergic augmenting psychotropic drugs such as monoamine oxidase inhibitors, should be avoided, although the clinical significance is undetermined.

*Pregnancy and lactation:* The safety of nadolol in pregnancy has not been established and animal studies have shown some foetotoxicity. Use of any drug in pregnancy or by women of childbearing potential requires that the possible risk to mother and/or foetus be weighed against the expected therapeutic benefit.

Nadolol is excreted in human milk; therefore nursing mothers should only receive nadolol if deemed essential.

*Effects on ability to drive and use machines:* None known.

*Undesirable effects:* Most patients tolerate nadolol well. Side-effects resemble those reported with other beta-blocking drugs and rarely require withdrawal of treatment. Those reported infrequently include gastro-intestinal effects, bradycardia, fatigue, light-headedness, cold extremities, insomnia, paraesthesia, dryness of the mouth and alopecia. Cardiac insufficiency, hypotension and AV block have occurred on rare occasions.

*Overdose:* Excessive bradycardia should be treated initially with atropine. If there is no response, isoprenaline may be administered with caution.

Cardiac failure should be managed by digitalisation and diuretics. Glucagon has also been reported to be useful.

Hypotension may be managed with vasopressors such as adrenaline.

Bronchospasm may be counteracted by isoprenaline and aminophylline.

## Pharmacological properties

*Pharmacodynamic properties:* Nadolol is a beta-adrenergic receptor blocking agent with a prolonged activity, permitting once-daily dosage in angina, hypertension, cardiac arrhythmias, the prophylaxis of migraine, and the relief of hyperthyroid symptoms.

Nadolol is not metabolised. It has no membrane stabilising or intrinsic sympathomimetic activity, and its only effect on the autonomic nervous system is one of beta-adrenergic blockade. Nadolol is nonselective.

Receptor blockade by nadolol results in protection from excessive inappropriate sympathetic activity. Nadolol reduces the number and severity of attacks of angina pectoris by blocking response to catecholamine stimulation and thus lowers the oxygen requirement of the heart at any given level of effort.

Nadolol reduces both supine and erect blood pressure. Like other beta-blockers nadolol exerts an antiarrhythmic action. Nadolol has been shown to reduce the rapid ventricular response which accompanies atrial fibrillation/flutter by slowing conduction through the A-V node. Beta-blockade is of particular value in arrhythmias caused by increased levels of, or sensitivity of the heart to, circulating catecholamines, e.g. arrhythmias associated with phaeochromocytoma, thyrotoxicosis, or exercise. Nadolol is effective in reducing ventricular premature beats in selected patients.

Nadolol exerts an effect in the prophylaxis of migraine by a mechanism which may involve prevention of vasoconstriction in the area served by the internal carotid artery and prevention of excessive adrenergic vasodilation in the external carotid artery.

Nadolol alleviates the symptoms of thyrotoxicosis and provides symptomatic control before and during thyroid surgery.

Beta-blocking agents have been shown in large scale studies to reduce mortality by preventing reinfarction and sudden death in patients surviving their first myocardial infarction.

*Pharmacokinetic particulars:* About 30 percent of an oral dose of Corgard is absorbed. Peak serum concentrations usually occur in 3 to 4 hours after drug administration. The presence of food in the gastrointestinal tract does not affect the rate or extent of Corgard absorption. Approximately 30 percent of the Corgard present in serum is reversibly bound to plasma protein. Unlike most available beta-blocking agents, Corgard is not metabolised, and is excreted unchanged principally by the kidneys. The serum half-life of therapeutic doses of Corgard is relatively long, ranging from 20 to 24 hours (permitting once daily dosage). A significant correlation between minimum steady-state serum concentrations of Corgard and total oral daily dose has been demonstrated in hypertensive patients; however, the observed dose-response range is wide and proper dosage requires individual titration.

## Pharmaceutical particulars

*List of excipients:* The tablets also contain citric acid anhydrous, polyvidone, corn starch, microcrystalline cellulose, magnesium stearate, indigo carmine (E132) and indigo carmine aluminium lake.

*Incompatibilities:* Not applicable.

*Shelf life:* 48 months.

*Special precautions for storage:* Store below 25°C.

*Nature and contents of container:* Amber glass bottles containing 100 tablets, foil pouches of 100 tablets and blisters in cartons containing 28 tablets.

**Marketing authorisation numbers**
Corgard tablets 40 mg   11723/0099
Corgard tablets 80 mg   11723/0100

**Date of approval/revision of SPC**   July 1995.

**Legal category**   POM.

# CORGARETIC* TABLETS

**Qualitative and quantitative composition** The 40 mg tablets contain nadolol 40.0 mg and bendrofluazide 5.0 mg. The 80 mg tablets contain nadolol 80.0 mg and bendrofluazide 5.0 mg.

**Pharmaceutical form** Round biconvex tablet.

## Clinical particulars
*Therapeutic indications:* For the treatment of hypertension. The combination of a diuretic and a beta-blocker may be of particular value in patients whose blood pressure has not been adequately controlled with either component given alone.

*Posology and method of administration*
**Adults:** One or two tablets once daily to a maximum of 160 mg nadolol and 10 mg bendrofluazide. For doses of nadolol in excess of 160 mg, the combination product may not be appropriate because an excessive dose of thiazide component may be administered.

Dosage should be titrated gradually with at least a week between increments to assess response; individuals show considerable variation in their response to beta-adrenergic blockade.

Corgaretic may be given in a once daily dosage without regard to meals.

If Corgaretic is to be discontinued, reduce dosage over a period of at least two weeks (see Warnings).

**Children:** Safety and effectiveness in children have not been established.

**Elderly:** In elderly patients a low initial dose should be used so that sensitivity to side-effects may be assessed. As with all drugs, patients with impaired renal or hepatic function should be monitored.

*Administration in renal failure:* Increased blood levels of nadolol occur in the presence of renal failure. Although non-renal elimination does occur, dosage adjustments are necessary in this patient group. The total daily dose of Corgaretic should be reduced or the dose interval increased. Corgaretic, however, would not be appropriate for patients with severe renal impairment since loop diuretics (e.g. frusemide) rather than a thiazide are preferred for such patients.

*Method of administration:* Oral.

*Contra-indications:* In bronchial asthma or a history of asthma; sinus bradycardia and 2nd and 3rd degree heart block; cardiogenic shock; right ventricular failure secondary to pulmonary hypertension; congestive heart failure, anuria, past sensitivity to thiazide diuretics or any sulphonamide-derived drugs.

*Special warnings and special precautions for use*
**Warnings:** Exacerbation of angina and myocardial infarction have occurred after abrupt discontinuation of therapy with beta-adrenergic blocking agents in patients with angina pectoris or other evidence of coronary artery insufficiency. When discontinuing long-term treatment with nadolol, the dosage should be reduced gradually over a period of at least two weeks and the patient carefully monitored.

Beta-adrenergic blockade carries the potential hazard of precipitating cardiac failure. Should this occur and it is not controlled by digitalisation, nadolol should be withdrawn, consideration being given to the foregoing warning. Beta-blockade impairs the ability of the heart to respond to stress. It has been the usual practice to recommend withdrawal of beta-blockers several days prior to surgery. However, this may render the patient's blood pressure unstable and difficult to control during anaesthesia and the anaesthetist may wish to advise on discontinuation of therapy. In no circumstances should beta-blockers be discontinued prior to surgery in patients with phaeochromocytoma or thyrotoxicosis. In the event of emergency surgery, the effects of nadolol may be reversed by isoprenaline or noradrenaline. However, such patients may be subject to protracted severe hypotension. General anaesthetics which can cause myocardial depression such as cyclopropane, trichloroethylene, chloroform and ether, should be avoided if nadolol is continued during surgery.

Nadolol should be administered with caution to patients with chronic obstructive airways disease. Discontinue therapy if condition relapses.

Diabetic patients should be monitored closely as nadolol may mask the early signs of acute hypoglycaemia and thiazide diuretics can lower insulin tolerance. Therefore dosages of hypoglycaemic drugs or insulin doses may need adjustment.

There have been reports of skin rashes (including a psoriasiform type) and/or ocular changes (conjunctivitis and 'dry eye') associated with the use of beta-adrenergic blocking drugs. The reported incidence is small and in most cases the symptoms have cleared when the treatment was withdrawn. Discontinuance of the drug should be considered if any reaction is not otherwise explicable. Cessation of the therapy with a beta-adrenergic blocker should be gradual.

Beta-blockade may mask certain clinical signs (e.g. tachycardia) of hyperthyroidism. Patients suspected of developing thyrotoxicosis should be managed carefully to avoid abrupt withdrawal of beta-blockade which might precipitate a thyroid storm.

*Precautions:* Occasionally, beta-blockade with drugs such as nadolol may produce hypotension and/or marked bradycardia, resulting in vertigo, syncope or orthostatic hypotension.

Nadolol should be used with caution in patients with impaired renal or hepatic function (see Dosage and Administration section for dosage adjustment in renal failure).

Periodic determination of serum electrolytes to detect possible imbalance e.g. hyponatraemia, hypochloric alkalosis and hypokalaemia should be performed at regular intervals.

Potassium depletion is a danger to digitalised patients or those with hepatic cirrhosis with ascites. In patients with renal disease, thiazides may precipitate uraemia and cumulative effects of the drug may develop. In patients with impaired renal function, minor alterations of fluid and electrolyte balance may precipitate hepatic coma.

Thiazide diuretics may raise serum uric acid levels, thus exacerbating gout in susceptible patients.

Pathologic changes in the parathyroid gland with hypercalcaemia and hypophosphataemia have been observed in a few patients during prolonged thiazide therapy.

The possibility that thiazides may exacerbate or activate systemic lupus erythematosus has been reported.

*Interactions with other medicaments and other forms of interaction*
*General anaesthetics:* Those which cause myocardial depression such as chloroform, cyclopropane, trichloroethylene and ether should be avoided as the patient may be subject to protracted severe hypotension.

*Myocardial depressants:* Such as lignocaine and procainamide may potentiate the hypotensive action of Nadolol and lead to severe hypotension.

*Adrenoceptor stimulants:* Beta-adrenoceptor stimulants such as isoprenaline or alpha-adrenoceptor stimulants such as noradrenaline, adrenaline, will reverse the hypotensive effects and increase vasoconstrictor activity. Thiazides may decrease the arterial responsiveness to noradrenaline.

*Catecholamine depleting drugs:* e.g. reserpine. Excessive reduction in sympathetic drive to the heart might occur. Close observation is advised.

*Antihypertensives:* e.g. neurone-blocking drugs, vasodilators, diuretics. Additive hypotensive effect.

*Hypoglycaemic, insulin:* Possible dosage adjustment, see Warnings section.

*Clonidine:* If nadolol and clonidine are given concurrently, clonidine should not be discontinued until several days after nadolol withdrawal.

*Monoamine oxidase inhibitors:* Administration of nadolol during and within two weeks of administration of adrenergic augmenting psychotropic drugs such as monoamine oxidase inhibitors, should be avoided, although the clinical significance is undetermined.

*Tubocurarine:* Thiazides may increase the responsiveness to Tubocurarine.

*Pregnancy and lactation:* The safety of nadolol in pregnancy has not been established and animal studies have shown some foetotoxicity. The use of diuretics in otherwise healthy pregnant women with or without mild oedema is contra-indicated. The hazards of using thiazides include foetal or neonatal jaundice, thrombocytopenia and possibly other adverse reactions which have occurred in the adult. Nadolol and bendrofluazide are excreted in human milk. Corgaretic is therefore not considered suitable for pregnant patients or nursing mothers.

*Effects on ability to drive and use machines:* None.

*Undesirable effects:* Most patients tolerate Corgaretic well.

Nadolol: Side-effects resemble those reported with other beta-blocking drugs and rarely require withdrawal of treatment. Those reported infrequently include gastro-intestinal effects, bradycardia, fatigue, light-headedness, cold extremities, insomnia, paraesthesia, dryness of the mouth and alopecia. Cardiac insufficiency, hypotension and AV block have occurred on rare occasions.

Thiazides: Those reported with the use of thiazides include hypokalaemia, anorexia, gastric irritation, nausea, vomiting, cramping, diarrhoea, intrahepatic cholestatic jaundice, pancreatitis, dizziness, vertigo, headache, xanthopsia, leucopenia, agranulocytosis, thrombocytopenia, aplastic anaemia, purpura, photosensitivity, rash, urticaria, necrotising angiitis, hyperglycaemia, glycosuria, hyperuricaemia, muscle spasm, weakness and restlessness.

*Overdose:* Excessive bradycardia should be treated initially with atropine. If there is no response, isoprenaline may be administered with caution.

Cardiac failure should be managed by digitalisation and diuretics. Glucagon has also been reported to be useful.

Hypotension may be managed with vasopressors such as adrenaline.

Bronchospasm may be counteracted by isoprenaline and aminophylline.

## Pharmacological properties
*Pharmacodynamic properties:* Nadolol is a beta-adrenergic receptor blocking agent. It reduces blood pressure and exerts an antiarrhythmic action. It has no membrane stabilising or intrinsic sympathomimetic activity and its only effect on the autonomic nervous system is one of beta-adrenergic blockade. Nadolol is non-selective. It has a low lipid solubility. It can be efficiently removed from the general circulation by haemodialysis.

Bendrofluazide is a thiazide diuretic which interferes with renal tubular electrolyte reabsorption, thereby increasing sodium and water excretion.

*Pharmacokinetic properties:* About 30 percent of an oral dose of nadolol is absorbed. Peak serum concentrations usually occur in 3 to 4 hours after drug administration. The presence of food in the gastrointestinal tract does not affect the rate or extent of nadolol absorption. Approximately 30 percent of the nadolol present in serum is reversibly bound to plasma protein. Unlike most available beta-blocking agents, nadolol is not metabolised and is excreted unchanged principally by the kidneys. The serum half-life of therapeutic doses of nadolol is relatively long, ranging from 20 to 24 hours (permitting once daily dosage). A significant correlation between minimum steady-state serum concentrations of Nadolol and total oral daily dose has been demonstrated in hypertensive patients, however, the observed dose-response range is wide and proper dosage requires individual titration.

Bendrofluazide is almost completely absorbed from the gastrointestinal tract. It is extensively metabolised, 30 percent being excreted unchanged in the urine. Its plasma half-life is 3 to 4 hours, its biological half-life being much longer.

## Pharmaceutical particulars
*List of excipients:* Microcrystalline Cellulose PhEur, Pregelatinised Maize Starch BP, Povidone K30 BP, Sodium Starch Glycolate BP, Magnesium Stearate PhEur, Blue No 2 Beadlets (E132), lactose anhydrous.

*Incompatibilities:* None known.

*Shelf life:* 36 months.

*Special precautions for storage:* Store below 25°C, avoid excessive heat, protect from moisture and light.

*Nature and contents of container:* Packs of 100 tablets supplied in either amber glass bottles or HDPE bottles.
Packs of 28 tablets supplied in foil strips or PVC blisters.

*Instructions for use/handling:* None.

**Marketing authorisation numbers**
40 mg tablets   11723/0101
80 mg tablets   11723/0102

**Date of approval/revision of SPC** August 1994.

**Legal category** POM.

# DANOL CAPSULES

**Qualitative and quantitative composition**
Danol 100 mg Capsules: Danazol 100 mg.
Danol 200 mg Capsules: Danazol 200 mg.

**Pharmaceutical form** Capsule.

## Clinical particulars
*Therapeutic indications:* Danol capsules are recommended for the treatment of:
(1) Endometriosis, to control pain, pelvic tenderness and other associated symptoms and to resolve or reduce the extent of endometriotic foci. Danol capsules may be used as sole therapy or in preparation for or following surgery.
(2) Dysfunctional uterine bleeding presenting as menorrhagia, to control excessive blood loss and to control associated dysmenorrhoea.
(3) For the treatment of severe cyclical mastalgia with or without nodularity (fibrocystic disease) unresponsive to counselling or simple analgesics, to reduce pain, tenderness and nodularity.
(4) For the control of benign, multiple or recurrent breast cysts in conjunction with aspiration.
(5) Severe symptomatic gynaecomastia, both idiopathic as well as drug induced, to reduce the size of the breast and to control associated pain and tenderness.
(6) Pre-operative thinning of the endometrium prior to hysteroscopic endometrial ablation.

*Posology and method of administration*
**Adults:** The usual range of dosage is 200 mg to 800 mg daily in up to four divided doses.

Danol capsules should be given as a continuous course, dosage being adjusted according to the patient's response. A reduction in dosage once a satisfactory response has been achieved may prove possible. In fertile females, Danol capsules should be started during menstruation, preferably on the first day, to avoid exposing a pregnancy to its possible effects. Where doubt exists, appropriate checks should be made to exclude pregnancy before starting medication. Females of child-bearing age should employ non-hormonal contraception throughout the course of treatment.

In endometriosis, the recommended dosage is initially 400 mg daily in a course of treatment lasting normally six months, although up to nine months may be necessary in some cases. Dosage should be increased if normal cyclical bleeding still persists after two months therapy, a higher dosage may also be needed for severe disease.

For dysfunctional bleeding presenting as menorrhagia, the dosage should be 200 mg daily, normally for 3 months.

In severe cyclical mastalgia, treatment should commence at a dose of 200–300 mg daily, according to the severity of the symptoms, a course of treatment normally lasting 3–6 months.

In benign breast cysts, treatment should commence at a dose of 300 mg daily, a course of treatment normally lasting 3 to 6 months.

In gynaecomastia a six month course of therapy is recommended at a dose of 200 mg daily in adolescents which may be increased to 400 mg daily if no response is obtained after two months. Adults may be given 400 mg daily.

For pre-operative thinning of the endometrium, the usual dose is 400–800 mg daily given as a continuous course normally lasting 3–6 weeks.

*Elderly:* Danol is not recommended.

*Children:* Danol is not recommended.

The capsules are for oral administration.

*Contra-indications:*
1. Pregnancy.
2. Breast feeding: Danol may be excreted in breast milk.
3. Markedly impaired hepatic, renal or cardiac function.
4. Porphyria: Danol can induce ALA synthetase activity and hence porphyrin metabolism.
5. Thromboembolic disease.
6. Androgen dependent tumour.
7. Abnormal vaginal bleeding that has not been fully investigated.

*Special warnings and special precautions for use:* Particular care should be observed when using Danol in patients with hepatic or renal disease, hypertension or other cardiovascular disease and in any state which may be exacerbated by fluid retention as well as in diabetes mellitus, polycythaemia, epilepsy, lipoprotein disorder, in those with a history of thrombosis, and in those who have shown marked or persistent androgenic reaction to previous gonadal steroid therapy. Adjustment in concomitant therapy may be called for particularly in patients with hypertension, diabetes mellitus or epilepsy when introducing or discontinuing Danol as well as during Danol treatment.

Caution is advised in patients with migraine.

Until more is known, caution is advised in the use of Danol in the presence of known or suspected malignant disease (see also *Contra-indications*). The presence of carcinoma should be excluded before continuing Danol therapy if breast nodules persist or enlarge during treatment.

In the event of virilisation, Danol should be withdrawn. Whilst androgenic reactions will generally prove reversible, continued use of Danol in the face of evident virilisation is likely to cause irreversible change.

In addition to clinical monitoring in all patients, appropriate laboratory monitoring should be considered which may include periodic measurement of hepatic function and haematological state.

Experience of long term therapy with Danol is limited. Whilst a course of therapy may need to be repeated, care should be observed. The long-term risk of 17-alkylated steroids (including benign hepatic adenomata and peliosis hepatis), should be considered when danazol, which is chemically related to those compounds, is used for periods longer than those normally recommended.

*Interactions with other medicaments and other forms of interaction:* Anti-convulsant therapy: Danol may affect the plasma level of carbamazepine and possibly the patient's response to this agent and to phenytoin. With phenobarbitone it is likely that similar interaction would occur.

Anti-diabetic therapy: Danol can cause insulin resistance.

Anti-coagulant therapy: Danol can potentiate the action of warfarin.

Anti-hypertensive therapy: Possibly through promotion of fluid retention, Danol can oppose the action of anti-hypertensive agents.

Cyclosporin: Danol can increase the plasma level of cyclosporin.

Concomitant steroids: Although specific instances have not been described, it is likely that interactions will occur between Danol and gonadal steroid therapy.

Migraine therapy: Danol may itself provoke migraine and possibly reduce the effectiveness of medication to prevent that condition.

Ethyl alcohol: Subjective intolerance in the form of nausea and shortness of breath has been reported.

Alpha calcidol: Danol may increase the calcaemic response in primary hypoparathyroidism necessitating a reduction in dosage of this agent.

*Pregnancy and lactation:* There is epidemiological and toxicological evidence of hazard in human pregnancy. Danazol is known to be associated with the risk of virilisation to the female foetus if administered during human pregnancy. Danazol should not be used during pregnancy. Women of childbearing age should be advised to use an effective, non-hormonal, method of contraception. Danazol has the theoretical potential for androgenic effects in breast-fed infants and therefore either danazol therapy or breast-feeding should be discontinued.

*Effects on ability to drive and use machines:* No special warning is felt necessary.

*Undesirable effects:* The possible causal relationship between Danol and many of the following events reportedly associated with its use remains to be defined.

Androgenic effects include weight gain, acne and seborrhoea. Hirsutism, hair loss, voice change, which may take the form of hoarseness, sore throat or instability or deepening of pitch may occur. Hypertrophy of the clitoris is rare.

Other possible endocrine effects include menstrual disturbances in the form of spotting, alteration of the timing of the cycle and amenorrhoea. Although cyclical bleeding and ovulation usually return within 60–90 days after Danol, persistent amenorrhoea has occasionally been reported. Flushing, vaginal dryness and irritation and reduction in breast size may reflect a lowering of oestrogen. In the male a modest reduction in spermatogenesis may be evident during treatment. Insulin resistance may be increased in diabetes mellitus but symptomatic hypoglycaemia in non-diabetic patients has also been reported as has an increase in plasma glucagon level.

Danol may aggravate epilepsy and expose the condition in those so predisposed. Cutaneous reactions include rashes, which may be maculopapular, petechial, or purpuric or may take an urticarial form and may be accompanied by facial oedema. Associated fever has also been reported. Rarely, sun-sensitive rash has been noted. Inflammatory erythematous nodules, changes in skin pigmentation and exfoliative dermatitis have also been reported.

Musculo-skeletal reactions include backache and muscle cramps which can be severe, creatine phosphokinase level may also rise. Muscle tremors, fasciculation, limb pain, joint pain and joint swelling have also been reported.

Cardiovascular reactions may include exacerbation of hypertension, palpitation and tachycardia.

Benign intracranial hypertension, visual disturbances which may take the form of blurring or difficulty in focusing and in wearing contact lenses or need for temporary alteration in refractive correction have been noted.

Haematological responses include an increase in red cell and platelet count. Reversible erythrocytosis or polycythaemia may be provoked. Eosinophilia, leucopenia and thrombocytopenia have also been noted.

Arterial or venous thrombosis is unlikely because danazol activates both the fibrinolytic system and inhibitors in the clotting cascade. Clinical and epidemiological evidence support this conclusion. Rare occurrences of sagittal sinus and cerebrovascular thrombosis have been observed but their association with danazol is unclear.

Hepatic reactions include modest increases in serum transaminase levels and rarely cholestatic jaundice. Benign hepatic adenomata and peliosis hepatis have been observed with long term use.

Fluid retention may explain the occasional reports of carpal tunnel syndrome. Danol capsules may also provoke migraine.

Possible psychical reactions include increased appetite, emotional lability, anxiety, depressed mood, nervousness and changes in libido. Dizziness, vertigo, nausea, headache, fatigue and epigastric and pleuritic pain have also been noted.

A temporary alteration of lipoproteins in the form of an increase in LDL cholesterol, a decrease in HDL, affecting all subfractions, and a decrease in apolipoproteins AI and AII, is likely with Danol in the female. The clinical significance of these changes is not established.

Reduction in thyroid binding globulin, T4, with increased uptake of T3 but without disturbance of thyroid stimulating hormone or free thyroxine index, is also likely during therapy.

Haematuria has rarely been reported with prolonged use in patients with hereditary angioedema.

*Overdose:* In animal tests, doses of 16,000 mg/kg body weight produced no fatalities and it is unlikely that any immediate serious reactions would be seen from a single excessive dose in man.

In the case of acute overdosage, the drug should be removed by emesis or stomach pump (if ingestion is recent) and the patient should be kept under observation in case of any delayed reactions.

**Pharmacological properties**

*Pharmacodynamic properties:* Danazol, 17a-pregna-2,4-dien-20-yno(2,3-d)-isoxazol-17-ol, is a synthetic steroid derived from ethisterone. Its pharmacological properties include:

1. Relatively marked affinity for androgen receptors, less marked affinity for progesterone receptors and least affinity for oestrogen receptors. Danazol is a weak androgen but in addition antiandrogenic, progestogenic, antiprogestogenic, oestrogenic and antioestrogenic actions have been observed.

2. Interference with the synthesis of gonadal steroids, possibly by inhibition of the enzymes of steroidogenesis, including 3B hydroxysteroid dehydrogenase, 17B hydroxysteroid dehydrogenase, 17 hydroxylase, 17,20 lyase, 11B hydroxylase, 21 hydroxylase and cholesterol side chain cleavage enzymes, or alternatively by inhibition of the cyclic AMP accumulation usually induced by gonadotrophic hormones in granulosa and luteal cells.

3. Inhibition of the mid-cycle surge of FSH and LH as well as alterations in the pulsatility of LH. Danazol can also reduce the mean plasma levels of these gonadotrophins after the menopause.

4. A wide range of actions on plasma proteins, including increasing prothrombin, plasminogen, antithrombin III, alpha-2 macroglobulin, C1 esterase inhibitor, and erythropoietin and reducing fibrinogen, thyroid binding and sex hormone binding globulins. Danazol increases the proportion and concentration of testosterone carried unbound in plasma.

*Pharmacokinetic properties:* Danazol is absorbed from the gastrointestinal tract, peak plasma concentrations of 50–80 ng/ml being reached approximately 2–3 hours after dosing. Compared to the fasting state, the bioavailability has been shown to increase 3 fold when the drug is taken with a meal with a high fat content. It is thought that food stimulates bile flow which facilitates the dissolution and absorption of danazol, a highly lipophilic compound.

The apparent plasma elimination half life of danazol in a single dose is approximately 3–6 hours. With multiple doses this may increase to approximately 26 hours.

None of the metabolites of danazol, which have been isolated, exhibits pituitary inhibiting activity comparable to that of danazol.

Few data on excretion routes and rates exist. In the monkey 36% of a radioactive dose was recoverable in the urine and 48% in the faeces within 96 hours.

*Preclinical safety data:* Not applicable.

**Pharmaceutical particulars**

*List of excipients:* Maize starch, lactose, purified talc, magnesium stearate.

*Incompatibilities: None.*

*Shelf life:* 60 months.

*Special precautions for storage:* None.

*Nature and contents of container:* PVC blister pack compound of polyvinyl chloride (thickness 250 μm) sealed to an aluminium foil (thickness 20 μm). The blister are then packed in a cardboard carton.

*Instructions for use/handling:* Not applicable.

**Marketing authorisation numbers**

Danol 100 mg Capsules 11723/0015
Danol 200 mg Capsules 11723/0016

**Date of approval/revision of SPC** April 1996.

**Legal category** POM.

## DERMALEX* SKIN LOTION

**Qualitative and quantitative composition** Dermalex Skin Lotion contains Hexachlorophane USP 0.5 w/v.

**Pharmaceutical form** Skin lotion.

**Clinical particulars**

*Therapeutic indications:* For topical application as an antiseptic emollient for use in areas of unbroken skin where infection is likely; including the sacral area and pressure points in the immobile elderly.

*Posology and method of administration:*

*Adults and children over 2 years:* Apply sparingly as a routine every 4 to 6 hours and after washing.

Dermalex should not be administered except on medical advice to children under 2 years of age.

*Contra-indications:* Dermalex Skin Lotion should not be applied to broken skin, open pressure sores, seriously burnt skin or mucous membranes.

Dermalex Skin Lotion is contra-indicated in pregnancy and in nursing mothers.

Dermalex should not be administered except on medical advice to children under two years of age.

*Special warnings and special precautions for use:* During regular use in the treatment of pressure sores it is inadvisable to apply to areas of the skin in excess of half of the total body surface area.

*Interactions with other medicaments and other forms of interaction:* It is important to ensure that no barrier creams are used on a patient using Dermalex Skin Lotion.

*Pregnancy and lactation:* There is evidence of hazard to neonates. It is therefore advised that the product should not be used during pregnancy or by lactating mothers.

*Effects on ability to drive and to use machines:* None known.

*Undesirable effects:* None known.

*Overdose:* No cases of intoxication with Dermalex Skin Lotion due to deliberate or accidental overdosage have been reported to the company. It is considered that overdosage is unlikely to be a problem.

**Pharmacological properties**
*Pharmacodynamic properties:* Hexachlorophane is a bisphenol anti-bacterial agent which is particularly effective against gram positive organisms.

*Pharmacokinetic properties:* Hexachlorophane is absorbed onto the skin and multiple contact results in sustained degerming activity. It is absorbed through the skin but does not accumulate in the blood with continued use.

The majority of hexachlorophane is probably distributed very rapidly in the lipophilic tissue-compartments. A small amount is slowly excreted unchanged in the urine.

The remainder is metabolised by the liver to glucoronide conjugate which is excreted in the bile and the faeces.

*Preclinical safety data:* There is no pre-clinical data of relevance to the prescriber which are additional to that already included in other sections of the SPC.

**Pharmaceutical particulars**
*List of excipients:* Squalane, allantoin, butylated hydroxyanisole, cetyl alcohol, decyloleate, lanoline anhydrous, octylstearate, propyl paraben, stearic acid, carbomer, triethanolomine, methyl paraben, disodium EDTA, sodium lauryl sulphate, sorbitol powder, perfume, water.

*Incompatibilities:* None known.

*Shelf life:* 36 months.

*Special precautions for storage:* To be stored at a temperature not exceeding 25°C.

*Nature and contents of container:* Blow moulded polyethylene bottle of 60 ml, 100 ml and 250 ml. 60 ml and 100 ml bottles have a polyethylene plug and polyethylene screw cap or a polypropylene screw cap and the 250 ml bottle has a polyethylene or polypropylene dispenser/cap.

*Instructions for use/handling:* Not applicable.

*Marketing authorisation holder:* The Dermalex Company Limited.

**Marketing authorisation number** 1983/5000R

**Date of approval/revision of SPC** October 1996.

**Legal category** P.

# DERMESTRIL*

**Qualitative and quantitative composition** Dermestril is available in three sizes.

*Dermestril 25* has a nominal in vivo release rate of 25 mcg oestradiol per day (active surface area 9 cm²; oestradiol content 2 mg).

*Dermestril 50* has a nominal in vivo release rate of 50 mcg oestradiol per day (active surface area 18 cm²; oestradiol content 4 mg).

*Dermestril 100* has a nominal in vivo release rate of 100 mcg oestradiol per day (active surface are 36 cm²; oestradiol content 8 mg).

The compositions per unit area of the three systems are identical.

**Pharmaceutical form** Dermestril is a transdermal delivery system (transdermal patch) consisting of a transparent backing foil and an oestradiol-containing self-adhesive matrix, covered by a protective liner which is removed prior to use.

**Clinical particulars**
*Therapeutic indications:* For the treatment of symptoms of oestrogen deficiency due to natural or surgically-induced menopause, for example hot flushes, sleep disturbance, urogenital atrophy and emotional instability or mood changes.

*Posology and method of administration:*
*Dosage – Adults and the elderly:* Treatment is usually initiated with one Dermestril 50 patch applied to the skin twice weekly in order to ensure a continuous supply of oestradiol to the body; thus each used system is removed after three or four days and replaced by a new one. The dose should be adjusted individually during treatment, depending on efficacy or symptoms of overdosage (e.g. breast tenderness and/or vaginal bleeding). A maximum dose of 100 mcg per day should not be exceeded. For maintenance therapy, the lowest effective dose should be used. Dermestril is generally used in a continuous pattern. Dermestril should be used in conjunction with a progestogen, in women with an intact uterus i.e., an appropriate dose of progestogen should be administered orally for the last 10–12 days of each month. Vaginal bleeding may occur at the end of treatment with the progestogen.

*Children:* Dermestril is not indicated in children.

*Administration:* The patch should be applied to the skin of the hip, lumbar region or abdomen and pressed firmly over the whole surface and along the edges to ensure good adhesion. The skin of the application site should be clean, dry, non-greasy and free of redness or irritation. Areas of the body which form folds or are subject to friction during movement should be avoided. Patches should not be applied twice consecutively to the same skin site. Dermestril should NOT be applied on or near the breasts.

Dermestril is applied twice weekly on a continuous basis. It is helpful for the patient to establish a routine of changing the patches on the same two days of each week (e.g. Mondays and Thursdays). If the patch is correctly applied, it will adhere to the skin for the required three or four days without problems. In the event that a patch does come off, it should be replaced with a new patch. The patch should then be changed again at the regular time to re-establish the patient's routine schedule. Similarly, if the patch is not changed on the scheduled day, it should be replaced as soon as possible and should be changed again on the next scheduled day to re-establish the patient's normal routine. If the patch is correctly applied, the patient may bathe or shower. However, the patch may become detached after a very hot bath or sauna and should be replaced with a new one, as described above.

*Contra-indications:* Diagnosed or suspected cancer of the breast or genital tract, or other oestrogen-dependent neoplasia; endometriosis; undiagnosed abnormal vaginal bleeding; severe hepatic disease (including Dubin-Johnson or Rotor syndromes); severe renal or cardiac disease; active thrombophlebitis or thromboembolic disorders or history of such events; known or suspected pregnancy.

*Special warnings and special precautions for use:* Before commencing Dermestril therapy, a physical and gynaecological examination of the patient, with particular attention to the pelvic organs and the breasts, is recommended. During prolonged treatment the examination should be repeated at regular intervals, at least once a year.

Presently, there is no definitive evidence that oestradiol replacement therapy increases the risk of breast cancer in postmenopausal women. However, careful monitoring of patients during treatment is advisable and caution is recommended in prescribing oestradiol for women with a family history of breast cancer or with fibrocystic mastopathy.

Since in postmenopausal women with an intact uterus prolonged oestrogen monotherapy may increase the risk of endometrial hyperplasia and carcinoma, it is necessary to adopt sequential therapy with a progestogen in order to protect the endometrium.

Close monitoring and caution are required in patients with cardiac insufficiency, renal or hepatic dysfunction, severe hypertension, epilepsy, oedema, asthma or diabetes, as oestrogens may cause fluid retention and may have anabolic activity.

Close monitoring is also required in patients with multiple sclerosis, porphyria, sickle cell disease or tetany.

The treatment with Dermestril of senile patients or patients with hypogonadism should be undertaken with caution.

If irregular or excessive vaginal bleeding occurs a gynaecological examination is recommended in order to identify possible organic causes.

Since the results of certain endocrine or liver function tests may be altered by oestrogen therapy, such tests should preferably be undertaken after withdrawal of oestrogen administration for at least one cycle.

Therapy should be discontinued immediately if symptoms of thromboembolic disorders (thrombophlebitis, retinal thrombosis, cerebral or pulmonary embolism) occur.

Therapy should be discontinued immediately in case of:
– the onset or aggravation of migraine or frequent or severe headaches;
– any type of visual disturbance;
– trauma (over the whole period of convalescence);
– cholestatic jaundice.
Discontinuation should also be considered prior to surgery.

As chronic treatment with oestrogen may influence the metabolism of calcium and phosphorus, Dermestril should be used with caution in patients with metabolic bone disease associated with hypercalcaemia.

Dermestril is not to be used for contraception.

*Interaction with other medicaments and other forms of interaction:* Drugs causing hepatic enzyme induction, such as barbiturates, phenytoin, carbamazepine, meprobamate, phenylbutazone and rifampicin, may render orally-administered oestrogens less effective. The extent of interaction of these drugs with transdermally-administered oestradiol is not known but such problems are likely to be minimised by use of the transdermal route, which avoids any first-pass metabolism.

Oral oestrogens may reduce the efficacy of anticoagulant and antidiabetic agents; again the effects of transdermal oestradiol are not known.

Transdermally-administered oestradiol does not affect coagulation factors such as fibrinogen and antithrombin III, and has no effects on the serum levels of renin substrate and of sex hormone-, thyroxine- or cortisol-binding globulin.

*Pregnancy and lactation:* Dermestril is not indicated in pregnant or lactating women.

*Effects on ability to drive and use machines:* Dermestril has no known effects on the ability to drive and use machines.

*Undesirable effects:* During treatment with Dermestril, breast tenderness and vaginal bleeding may occur. Other adverse reactions reported with oral oestrogen therapy, such as fluid or sodium retention, oedema, abdominal cramps, meteorism, nausea and headache are infrequent with Dermestril therapy. Increased blood pressure, or alterations of blood coagulation, liver function and glucose tolerance, are unlikely to occur with transdermal oestradiol. There is also no evidence for an increased risk of gallbladder disease (cholelithiasis) with transdermally-administered oestradiol, as may occur with oral oestrogen therapy.

During treatment with Dermestril, as with all oestrogens administered without progestogens, endometrial hyperplasia may develop.

In women with an intact uterus, sequential administration of a progestogen is therefore recommended.

Occasionally, in 5–15% of patients, mild and transient local erythema and pruritus at the application sites have been reported during clinical studies with Dermestril.

*Overdose:* Symptoms of overdosage are breast tenderness and/or vaginal bleeding. If such symptoms occur, a dose reduction should be considered. If necessary, the effects of overdosage can be rapidly reversed by removal of the patch.

**Pharmacological properties**
*Pharmacodynamic properties:* Oestradiol is the physiological oestrogenic hormone produced by the ovarian follicles from menarche to the menopause.

Many organs have cells with specific intracellular receptors for oestradiol, e.g. the uterus, vagina, urethra and mammary glands. There are also receptors for oestradiol in hepatic, hypothalamic and pituitary cells. In these cells oestradiol provokes a series of intracellular reactions and stimulates the synthesis of deoxyribonucleic acid and of proteins.

Oestrogens also have important effects on bone metabolism and they have been shown to inhibit bone resorption reducing postmenopausal bone loss. Oestrogens also have positive effects on lipid metabolism and vessel walls, and consequently in the prevention of coronary artery disease.

At menopause, ovarian function ceases and oestradiol is produced only in small quantities in the liver and in adipose tissue, by conversion from oestrone. The loss of ovarian secretion of oestradiol results in many women in vasomotor and thermoregulation disorders (hot flushes and sweats), sleep disturbance, emotional instability and progressive urogenital atrophy. By means of oestradiol replacement therapy most of these disturbances can be eliminated or alleviated.

The loss of oestradiol secretion leads also to accelerated bone loss and a considerable number of postmenopausal women suffer from osteoporosis, mainly of the spine. Hormone replacement therapy with oestradiol has been shown to prevent or reduce the loss of bone mineral content and hence osteoporosis.

*Pharmacokinetic properties:* The average half-life of

oestradiol in plasma is about one hour. Oestradiol is metabolised mainly in the liver. The most important metabolites are oestriol, oestrone and their conjugates (glucuronides, sulphates), which are much less active than oestradiol. The metabolites of oestradiol are eliminated mainly by the kidney as glucuronides and sulphates.

The majority of orally-administered oestradiol is metabolised to oestrone and its conjugates by the intestine and the liver before reaching the circulation, giving rise to high, unphysiological levels of oestrone in the blood. The consequences of chronic accumulation of oestrone in the body are not yet clear. However, it has been confirmed that prolonged oral administration of oestrogens leads to increased protein synthesis by the liver, in particular of renin substrate, resulting in hypertension.

Following cutaneous application of Dermestril, oestradiol is released from the drug-containing adhesive matrix through the skin and reaches the systemic circulation directly, avoiding first-pass metabolism by the liver, and hence avoiding hepatic protein synthesis stimulation and oestrone accumulation. Consequently, the oestradiol: oestrone ratio in plasma, which falls to values below 1 after the menopause and during oral oestrogen replacement therapy, returns to premenopausal levels (approximately 1) with transdermal oestradiol. The nominal daily in vivo release rates of Dermestril 25, 50 and 100 are 25 mcg, 50 mcg, and 100 mcg of oestradiol, respectively; the system is active for four days. These release rates result in physiological oestradiol serum concentrations, i.e. those of the premenopausal early follicular phase, which are constantly maintained throughout the patch application period.

After a single application of Dermestril with a daily oestradiol release of 100 mcg in postmenopausal women, physiological serum levels of oestradiol were reached approximately four hours after application and mean maximum serum oestradiol levels of 70 pg/mL were obtained. The serum concentration of oestradiol remained within the physiological levels of premenopausal women throughout the 3–4 days of the application period and returned to baseline within 12 hours after removal of Dermestril.

Following repeated applications of Dermestril 50 patches at 84–96 hour intervals, steady-state was reached during application of the second patch and no accumulation was observed thereafter.

*Preclinical safety data:* As oestradiol is a physiological hormone, which has been used for many years in clinical therapy in a variety of pharmaceutical forms and which is very well documented in the scientific literature, only local tolerance to Dermestril has been examined. Local tolerance studies performed in the rabbit after single and repeated applications of Dermestril showed good skin tolerability of the system. A skin sensitisation test performed in the guinea pig did not show any sensitising potential of Dermestril.

Primary skin irritation tests and sensitisation tests performed on the acrylic copolymers that form the adhesive matrix demonstrated the topical safety of these components.

## Pharmaceutical particulars
*List of excipients:* Oestradiol-containing adhesive matrix: acrylic copolymers. Backing foil: polyethylene terephthalate. Each transdermal delivery system is covered by a protective liner (siliconised polyethylene terephthalate) which is removed prior to use.

*Incompatibilities:* No pharmaceutical incompatibilities are known.

*Shelf life:* Two years in the intact sachets, when stored as recommended.

*Special precautions for storage:* Dermestril should be stored below 25°C.

*Nature and contents of container:* Carton of 8 transdermal delivery systems, each sealed individually in protective sachets of heat-sealable material with an internal aluminium layer.

*Instructions for use/handling:* Tear open the sachet at the indentation (do not use scissors to avoid damaging the patch) and remove the patch. Hold the patch between the thumb and index finger at the corner with the pull-off tag. Detach the protective liner with the other hand and discard it.

Do not touch the adhesive side of the patch. Apply the patch to the skin holding between the thumb and index finger the part still covered by the protective liner. Detach the remaining part of the protective liner and press firmly for about 10 seconds on the whole surface of the patch. Pass a finger along the edges to assure good adhesion.

### Marketing authorisation numbers
Dermestril 25　　11723/0218
Dermestril 50　　11723/0219
Dermestril 100　11723/0220

**Date of approval/revision of SPC** April 1997.

**Legal category** POM.

# EPILIM*

## Qualitative and quantitative composition
Epilim 500 Enteric Coated: 500 mg Sodium Valproate PhEur.

Epilim 200 Enteric Coated: 200 mg Sodium Valproate PhEur.

Epilim 100 mg Crushable: 100 mg Sodium Valproate PhEur.

Epilim Syrup and Liquid: 200 mg Sodium Valproate PhEur per 5 ml.

## Pharmaceutical form
Epilim 500 Enteric Coated: Enteric coated tablets.
Epilim 200 Enteric Coated: Enteric coated tablets.
Epilim 100 mg Crushable: Tablets.
Epilim Syrup: Syrup.
Epilim Liquid: Liquid.

## Clinical particulars
*Therapeutic indications:* In the treatment of generalised, partial or other epilepsy. In women of child bearing age, Epilim should be used only in severe cases or in those resistant to other treatment.

*Posology and method of administration:* Epilim tablets, syrup and liquid are for oral administration. Daily dosage requirements vary according to age and body weight.

*Monotherapy:* Usual requirements are as follows:

*Adults:* Dosage should start at 600 mg daily increasing by 200 mg at three day intervals until control is achieved. This is generally within the dosage range 1000 mg to 2000 mg per day, i.e. 20–30 mg/kg body weight. Where adequate control is not achieved within this range the dose may be further increased to 2500 mg per day.

*Children over 20 kg:* Initial dosage should be 400 mg/day (irrespective of weight) with spaced increases until control is achieved; this is usually within the range 20–30 mg/kg body weight per day. Where adequate control is not achieved within this range the dose may be increased to 35 mg/kg body weight per day.

*Children under 20 kg:* 20 mg/kg of body weight per day; in severe cases this may be increased but only in patients in whom plasma valproic acid levels can be monitored. Above 40 mg/kg/day, clinical chemistry and haematological parameters should be monitored.

*Use in the elderly:* Although the pharmacokinetics of valproate are modified in the elderly, they have limited clinical significance and dosage should be determined by seizure control. The volume of distribution is increased in the elderly and because of decreased binding to serum albumin, the proportion of free drug is increased. This will affect the clinical interpretation of plasma valproic acid levels.

In patients where adequate control has been achieved Epilim Chrono formulations are interchangeable with other Epilim conventional or modified release formulations on an equivalent daily dosage basis.

Epilim tablets, syrup and liquid may be given twice daily. Uncoated tablets may be crushed if necessary.

*Combined therapy:* When starting Epilim in patients already on other anticonvulsants, these should be tapered slowly: initiation of Epilim therapy should then be gradual, with target dose being reached after about 2 weeks. In certain cases it may be necessary to raise the dose by 5 to 10 mg/kg/day when used in combination with anticonvulsants which induce liver enzyme activity, e.g. phenytoin, phenobarbitone and carbamazepine. Once known enzyme inducers have been withdrawn it may be possible to maintain seizure control on a reduced dose of Epilim. When barbiturates are being administered concomitantly and particularly if sedation is observed (particularly in children) the dosage of barbiturate should be reduced.

*NB:* In children requiring doses higher than 40 mg/kg/day clinical chemistry and haematological parameters should be monitored.

Optimum dosage is mainly determined by seizure control and routine measurement of plasma levels is unnecessary. However, a method for measurement of plasma levels is available and may be helpful where there is poor control or side effects are suspected.

*Contra-indications:* Hypersensitivity to sodium valproate. Active liver disease, family history of severe hepatic dysfunction, particularly drug related, porphyria.

*Special warnings and special precautions for use:*
*Diabetic patients:* Valproate is eliminated mainly through the kidneys, partly in the form of ketone bodies; this may give false positives in the urine testing of possible diabetics. In addition, care should be taken when treating diabetic patients with Epilim Syrup, as this contains 3.6 g sucrose per 5 ml.

If it is necessary to dilute Epilim Syrup, the recommended diluent is syrup BP, but syrup containing $SO_2$ as a preservative should not be used. The diluted product will have a 14 day shelf life.

*Interactions with other medicaments and other forms of interaction:* Like many other drugs, Epilim may potentiate the effects of neuroleptics, monoamine oxidase inhibitors and other anti-depressants. The enzyme inducing effect of valproate is appreciably less than that of certain other anticonvulsants and loss of efficacy of oral contraceptive agents does not appear to be a problem. Caution is recommended when administering anticoagulants and other products which have anticoagulant properties (e.g. warfarin and salicylates). Aspirin may displace valproate from binding sites resulting in higher free levels of valproate. Valproate decreases protein binding of warfarin but this may not lead to clinically significant effects.

Phenytoin levels may be affected by Epilim and these should be monitored, particularly the free form, which may increase following an initial decrease in total levels.

Valproate may inhibit the metabolism of lamotrigine, dosages should be adjusted (lamotrigine dosage decreased) when appropriate.

Dosage of Epilim may require adjustments when used in combination with other anticonvulsants. See *Dosage, Combined Therapy* section.

There is evidence that cimetidine, (but not ranitidine) and erythromycin may prolong the half life and reduce clearance of valproate, and also that mefloquine may decrease serum levels of valproate.

The absorption of valproate may be decreased in the presence of cholestyramine.

*Pregnancy and lactation:* An increased incidence of congenital abnormalities (including facial dysmorphia, neural tube defects and multiple malformations particularly of the limbs) has been demonstrated in offspring born to mothers with epilepsy both untreated and treated, including those treated with sodium valproate.

The incidence of neural tube defects in women receiving valproate during the first trimester has been estimated to be in the region of 1–2%. Folate supplementation has been demonstrated to reduce the incidence of neural tube defects in the offspring of women at high risk. No direct evidence exists of such effects in women receiving anti-epileptic drugs, however there is no reason to contra-indicate folic acid in these women.

The available evidence suggests that anticonvulsant monotherapy is preferred. Dosage should be reviewed before conception and the lowest effective dose used, in divided doses as abnormal pregnancy outcome tends to be associated with higher total daily dosage. Women of child bearing age should be informed of the risks and benefits of continuing anti-epileptic treatment throughout pregnancy. Pregnancies should be carefully screened by alpha-foetoprotein measurement, ultrasound and other techniques if appropriate.

*Breast feeding:* The concentration of valproic acid found in the breast milk is very low, between 1% and 10% of total maternal plasma levels. There appears to be no contraindication to breast feeding by patients on valproate. The decision to allow the patient to breast feed should be taken with regard to all the known facts.

*Effects on ability to drive and to use machines:* Not applicable. Use of Epilim may provide seizure control such that the patient may again be eligible to hold a driving licence.

*Undesirable effects:*
*Hepatic:* Liver dysfunction, including hepatic failure resulting in fatalities, has occurred in patients whose treatment included valproic acid or sodium valproate. Patients most at risk are children particularly those under the age of three and those with congenital metabolic or degenerative disorders, organic brain disease or severe seizure disorders associated with mental retardation. The incidents mainly occurred during the first 6 months of therapy, the period of maximum risk being 2–12 weeks, and usually involved multiple anticonvulsant therapy. Monotherapy is to be preferred in this group of patients.

Clinical symptoms are more helpful than laboratory investigations in the early stages of hepatic failure. Serious or fatal hepatotoxicity may be preceded by non-specific symptoms, usually of sudden onset, such as loss of seizure control, malaise, weakness, lethargy, oedema, anorexia, vomiting, abdominal pain, drowsiness, jaundice. These are an indication for immediate withdrawal of the drug. Patients should be instructed to report any such signs to the clinician for investigation should they occur. Whilst it is difficult to establish which, if any, investigation is predictive, tests which reflect protein synthesis e.g. prothrombin time may be most relevant.

Routine measurement of liver function should be undertaken before therapy and periodically during the first six months especially in those who seem most at risk, and those with a prior history of liver disease; such patients should have close clinical supervision. Raised liver enzymes are not uncommon during treatment with Epilim and are usually transient or respond to reduction in dosage. Patients with such biochemical abnormalities should be reassessed clinically and tests of liver function including prothrombin time should be monitored until they return to normal. However an abnormally prolonged prothrombin time particularly in association with other relevant abnormalities requires cessation of treatment. Any concomitant use of salicylates should be stopped since they employ the same metabolic pathway.

*Metabolic:* Hyperammonaemia without changes in liver function tests may occur. Isolated and moderate hyperammonaemia may occur frequently, is usually transient and should not cause treatment discontinuation. However, it may present clinically as vomiting, ataxia and increasing clouding of consciousness. Should these symptoms occur Epilim should be discontinued. Oedema has been rarely reported. When an abnormality of the urea cycle is suspected (ornithine transcarbamylase deficiency), pre-treatment ammonia levels should be measured.

*Pancreatic:* There have been reports of pancreatitis including, rarely, fatalities occurring in patients receiving valproic acid or sodium valproate, usually within the first six months of therapy. Patients experiencing acute abdominal pain should have their serum amylase estimated; if these levels are elevated treatment should be discontinued.

*Haematological:* Valproic acid inhibits the second stage of platelet aggregation. Reversible prolongation of bleeding time and frequent occurrence of thrombocytopenia have been reported, but are usually associated with doses above those recommended. Prior to initiation of therapy and also before surgery, clinicians should assure themselves, using the appropriate blood tests, that there is no undue potential for bleeding complications. Spontaneous bruising or bleeding is an indication for withdrawal of medication pending investigations. Red cell hypoplasia, leucopenia and pancytopenia have been reported rarely; the blood picture returned to normal when the drug was discontinued. Isolated reduction of fibrinogen may also occur.

*Neurological:* Ataxia and tremor have been occasionally reported and appear to be dose-related effects.

Sedation has been reported occasionally, usually when in combination with other anticonvulsants. In monotherapy it occurred early in treatment on rare occasions and is usually transient. Rare cases of lethargy and confusion occasionally progressing to stupor, sometimes with associated hallucinations or convulsions have been reported. Coma has very rarely been observed. These cases have often been associated with too high a starting dose or too rapid a dose escalation or concomitant use of other anticonvulsants, notably phenobarbitone. They have usually been reversible on withdrawal of treatment or reduction of dosage.

An increase in alertness may occur; this is generally beneficial but occasionally aggression, hyperactivity and behavioural deterioration have been reported. Hearing loss, either reversible or irreversible has been reported rarely, though a causal relationship has not been established.

*Gastrointestinal:* Increase in appetite may occur and an increase in weight is not uncommon. Minor gastric irritation and, less frequently, nausea may occur frequently in some patients at the start of treatment, but these problems can usually be overcome by administering Enteric Coated Epilim or administering Epilim with or after food.

*Dermatological:* Transient hair loss has often been noted in some patients. This effect does not appear to be dose-related and regrowth normally begins within six months, although the hair may become more curly than previously. Rashes have been rarely reported. Rarely signs of an immune disorder have occurred, therefore caution should be observed when using the drug in patients with features which may suggest systemic lupus erythematosus. The occurrence of vasculitis has occasionally been reported.

*Endocrine:* There have been isolated reports of irregular periods or amenorrhoea. Very rarely gynaecomastia has occurred.

*Overdosage:* Cases of accidental and suicidal overdosage have been reported. At plasma concentrations of up to 5 to 6 times the maximum therapeutic levels, there are unlikely to be any symptoms other than nausea, vomiting and dizziness. In massive overdose, i.e., with plasma concentrations 10 to 20 times maximum therapeutic levels there may be serious CNS depression and respiration may be impaired. The symptoms may however be variable and seizures have been reported in the presence of very high plasma levels. A number of deaths have occurred following large overdoses. Full recovery is usual following treatment including induced vomiting, gastric lavage, assisted ventilation and other supportive measures.

**Pharmacological properties**

*Pharmacodynamic properties:* Sodium valproate is an anticonvulsant. The most likely mode of action for valproate is potentiation of the inhibitory action of gamma amino-butyric acid (GABA) through an action on the further synthesis or further metabolism of GABA.

*Pharmacokinetic properties:* The half life of sodium valproate is usually reported to be within the range 8–20 hours. It is usually shorter in children.

In patients with severe renal insufficiency it may be necessary to alter dosage in accordance with free serum valproic acid levels.

The reported effective therapeutic range for plasma valproic acid levels is 40–100 mg/litre (278–694 micromol/litre). This reported range may depend on time of sampling and presence of co-medication. The percentage of free (unbound) drug is usually between 6% and 15% of the total plasma levels. An increased incidence of adverse effects may occur with plasma levels above the effective therapeutic range. The pharmacological (or therapeutic) effects of Epilim may not be clearly correlated with the total or free (unbound) plasma valproic acid levels.

*Pre-clinical safety data:* There are no pre-clinical data of relevance to the prescriber which are additional to those already included in other sections of the SPC.

**Pharmaceutical particulars**

*List of excipients:*

*Enteric coated tablets:* Polyvidone, talc, calcium silicate, magnesium stearate, hypromellose, citric acid anhydrous, polyethylene glycol, violet lake, methylated spirit†, purified water†, polyvinylacetate phthalate, diethyl phthalate and stearic acid.

*Crushable tablets:* Maize starch, kaolin light (natural), silica hydrated, magnesium stearate and purified water†.

*Epilim Syrup:* Sorbitol powder, sodium methyl hydroxybenzoate, sodium propyl hydroxybenzoate, sodium saccharin, sucrose, flavour IFF cherry 740, Ponceau 4R (E124) and purified water.

*Epilim Liquid:* Hydroxyethyl cellulose, sorbitol powder, sodium methyl hydroxybenzoate, sodium propyl hydroxybenzoate, saccharin sodium, Ponceau 4R (E124), flavour IFF cherry 740, citric acid anhydrous and purified water.

(† not detected in final formulation.)

*Incompatibilities:* None.

*Shelf life:* Epilim Tablets and Syrup: 36 months. Epilim Liquid: 24 months.

*Special precautions for storage:*

Epilim Tablets: Store in a dry place below 30°C.

Epilim Syrup: Store below 30°C.

Epilim Liquid: Store below 30°C and away from direct sunlight. Epilim Liquid should not be diluted.

*Nature and contents of container:* Epilim Enteric Coated tablets are supplied in blister packs further packed into a cardboard carton. Pack sizes of 100 and 112 tablets.

Epilim 100 mg Crushable Tablets are supplied in blister packs further packed into a cardboard carton. Pack sizes of 100 and 112 tablets.

Epilim Syrup and Liquid is supplied in amber glass bottles with polypropylene J-cap and amber polyethylene tetraphthalate bottles with polypropylene tamper evident closure. Bottle size 200 and 300 ml.

*Instructions for use/handling:* None.

**Marketing authorisation numbers**

Epilim 500 Enteric Coated 11723/0020.
Epilim 200 Enteric Coated 11723/0018.
Epilim Crushable 11723/0017.
Epilim Syrup 11723/0025.
Epilim Liquid 11723/0024.

**Date of approval/revision of SPC** April 1996.

**Legal category** POM.

## EPILIM CHRONO*

**Qualitative and quantitative composition**

Epilim Chrono 200 Controlled Release tablets contain 133.2 mg Sodium Valproate PhEur and 58.0 mg Valproic Acid FP equivalent to 200 mg sodium valproate/tablet.

Epilim Chrono 300 Controlled Release tablets contain 199.8 mg Sodium Valproate PhEur and 87.0 mg Valproic Acid FP equivalent to 300 mg sodium valproate/tablet.

Epilim Chrono 500 Controlled Release tablets contain 333 mg Sodium Valproate PhEur and 145 mg Valproic Acid FP equivalent to 500 mg sodium valproate/tablet.

**Pharmaceutical form** Controlled release tablets.

**Clinical particulars**

*Therapeutic indications:* In the treatment of generalised, partial or other epilepsy. In women of childbearing age Epilim should be used only in severe cases or in those resistant to other treatment.

*Posology and method of administration:* Epilim Chrono Controlled Release tablets are for oral administration.

Epilim Chrono is a controlled release formulation of Epilim which reduces peak concentration and ensures more even plasma concentrations throughout the day.

Epilim Chrono may be given once or twice daily. The tablets should be swallowed whole and not crushed.

Daily dosage requirements vary according to age and body weight.

*Monotherapy:* Usual requirements are as follows:

*Adults:* Dosage should start at 600 mg daily increasing by 200 mg at three day intervals until control is achieved. This is generally within the dosage range 1000 mg to 2000 mg per day, i.e. 20–30 mg/kg body weight. Where adequate control is not achieved within this range the dose may be further increased to 2500 mg per day.

*Children over 20 kg:* Initial dosage should be 400 mg/day (irrespective of weight) with spaced increases until control is achieved; this is usually within the range 20–30 mg/kg body weight per day. Where adequate control is not achieved within this range the dose may be increased to 35 mg/kg body weight per day.

*Children under 20 kg:* An alternative formulation of Epilim should be used in this group of patients, due to the need for dose titration.

*Elderly:* Although the pharmacokinetics of valproate are modified in the elderly, they have limited clinical significance and dosage should be determined by seizure control. The volume of distribution is increased in the elderly and because of decreased binding to serum albumin, the proportion of free drug is increased. This will affect the clinical interpretation of plasma valproic acid levels.

In patients where adequate control has been achieved Epilim Chrono formulations are interchangeable with other Epilim conventional or modified release formulations on an equivalent daily dosage basis.

*Combined therapy:* When starting Epilim in patients already on other anticonvulsants, these should be tapered slowly; initiation of Epilim therapy should then be gradual, with target dose being reached after about 2 weeks. In certain cases it may be necessary to raise the dose by 5 to 10 mg/kg/day when used in combination with anticonvulsants which induce liver enzyme activity, e.g. phenytoin, phenobarbitone and carbamazepine. Once known enzyme inducers have been withdrawn it may be possible to maintain seizure control on a reduced dose of Epilim. When barbiturates are being administered concomitantly and particularly if sedation is observed (particularly in children) the dosage of barbiturate should be reduced.

*NB:* In children requiring doses higher than 40 mg/kg/day clinical chemistry and haematological parameters should be monitored. Optimum dosage is mainly determined by seizure control and routine measurement of plasma levels is unnecessary. However, a method for measurement of plasma levels is available and may be helpful where there is poor control or side effects are suspected.

*Contra-indications:* Hypersensitivity to sodium valproate. Active liver disease, family history of severe hepatic dysfunction, particularly drug related, porphyria.

*Special warnings and special precautions for use:*

*Diabetic patients:* Valproate is eliminated mainly through the kidneys, partly in the form of ketone bodies; this may give false positives in the urine testing of possible diabetics.

*Interactions with other medicaments and other forms of interaction:* Like many other drugs, Epilim may potentiate the effect of neuroleptics, monoamine oxidase inhibitors and other antidepressants. The enzyme inducing effect of valproate is appreciably less than that of certain other anticonvulsants and loss of efficacy of oral contraceptive agents does not appear to be a problem.

Caution is recommended when administering anticoagulants and other products which have anticoagulant properties (e.g., warfarin and salicylates). Aspirin may displace valproate from binding sites resulting in higher free levels of valproate. Valproate decreases protein binding of warfarin but this may not lead to clinically significant effects.

Phenytoin levels may be affected by Epilim and these should be monitored, particularly the free form, which may increase following an initial decrease in total levels. Valproate may inhibit the metabolism of lamotrigine, dosages should be adjusted (lamotrigine dosage decreased) when appropriate.

Dosage of Epilim may require adjustment when used in combination with other anticonvulsants. See *Dosage, Combined Therapy* section.

There is evidence that cimetidine, (but not ranitidine) and erythromycin may prolong the half-life and reduce clearance of valproate, and also that mefloquine may decrease serum levels of valproate.

The absorption of valproate may be decreased in the presence of cholestyramine.

*Pregnancy and lactation:* An increased incidence of congenital abnormalities (including facial dysmorphia, neural tube defects and multiple malformations, particularly of the limbs) has been demonstrated in offspring born to mothers with epilepsy both untreated and treated, including those treated with sodium valproate.

The incidence of neural tube defects in women receiving valproate during the first trimester has been estimated to be in the region of 1–2%. Folate supplementation has been demonstrated to reduce the incidence of neural tube defects in the offspring of women at high risk. No direct evidence exists of such effects in women receiving anti-epileptic drugs, however there is no reason to contraindicate folic acid in these women. The available evidence suggests that anticonvulsant monotherapy is preferred. Dosage should be reviewed before conception and the lowest effective dose used, in divided doses, as abnormal pregnancy outcome tends to be associated with higher total daily dosage. Women of child-bearing age should be informed of the risks and benefits of continuing anti-epileptic treatment throughout pregnancy. Pregnancies should be carefully screened by alpha-foetoprotein measurement, ultrasound, and other techniques if appropriate.

*Breast feeding:* The concentration of valproic acid found in the breast milk is very low, between 1% and 10% of total maternal plasma levels. There appears to be no contra-indication to breast feeding by patients on valproate. The decision to allow the patient to breast feed should be taken with regard to all the known facts.

*Effects on ability to drive and to use machines:* Not applicable. Use of Epilim may provide seizure control such that the patient may be eligible to hold a driving licence.

*Undesirable effects: Hepatic:* Liver dysfunction, including hepatic failure resulting in fatalities, has occurred in patients whose treatment included valproic acid or sodium valproate. Patients most at risk are children, particularly those under the age of three and those with congenital metabolic or degenerative disorders, organic brain disease or severe seizure disorders associated with mental retardation. The incidents mainly occurred during the first six months of therapy, the period of maximum risk being 2–12 weeks, and usually involved multiple anticonvulsant therapy. Monotherapy is to be preferred in this group of patients.

Clinical symptoms are more helpful than laboratory investigation in the early stages of hepatic failure. Serious or fatal hepatotoxicity may be preceded by non-specific symptoms, usually of sudden onset, such as loss of seizure control, malaise, weakness, lethargy, oedema, anorexia, vomiting, abdominal pain, drowsiness, jaundice. These are an indication for immediate withdrawal of the drug. Patients should be instructed to report any such signs to the clinician for investigation should they occur. Whilst it is difficult to establish which, if any, investigation is predictive, tests which reflect protein synthesis, e.g. prothrombin time, may be most relevant.

Routine measurement of liver function should be undertaken before therapy and periodically during the first six months, especially in those who seem most at risk, and those with a prior history of liver disease; such patients should have close clinical supervision. Raised liver enzymes are not uncommon during treatment with valproate and are usually transient or respond to reduction in dosage.

Patients with such biochemical abnormalities should be reassessed clinically and tests of liver function including prothrombin time, should be monitored until they return to normal. However an abnormally prolonged prothrombin time, particularly in association with other relevant abnormalities requires cessation of treatment. Any concomitant use of salicylates should be stopped, since they employ the same metabolic pathway.

*Metabolic:* Hyperammonaemia without changes in liver function tests may occur. Isolated and moderate hyperammonaemia may occur frequently, is usually transient and should not cause treatment discontinuation. However, it may present clinically as vomiting, ataxia, and increasing clouding of consciousness. Should these symptoms occur Epilim should be discontinued. Oedema has been rarely reported. When an abnormality of the urea cycle is suspected (Ornithine transcarbamylase deficiency), pre-treatment ammonia levels should be measured.

*Pancreatic:* There have been reports of pancreatitis including, rarely, fatalities occurring in patients receiving valproic acid or sodium valproate, usually within the first six months of therapy. Patients experiencing acute abdominal pain should have their serum amylase estimated; if these levels are elevated treatment should be discontinued.

*Haematological:* Valproic acid inhibits the second

stage of platelet aggregation. Reversible prolongation of bleeding time and frequent occurrence of thrombocytopenia have been reported, but are usually associated with doses above those recommended. Prior to initiation of therapy and also before surgery, clinicians should assure themselves, using the appropriate blood tests, that there is no undue potential for bleeding complications. Spontaneous bruising or bleeding is an indication for withdrawal of medication pending investigations. Red cell hypoplasia, leucopenia and pancytopenia have been reported rarely; the blood picture returned to normal when the drug was discontinued. Isolated reduction of fibrinogen may also occur.

*Neurological:* Ataxia and tremor have been occasionally reported and appear to be dose-related effects.

Sedation has been reported occasionally, usually when in combination with other anticonvulsants. In monotherapy it has occurred early in treatment on rare occasions and is usually transient. Rare cases of lethargy and confusion, occasionally progressing to stupor, sometimes with associated hallucinations or convulsions have been reported. Coma has very rarely been observed. These cases have often been associated with too high a starting dose or too rapid a dose escalation or concomitant use of other anticonvulsants, notably phenobarbitone. They have usually been reversible on withdrawal of treatment or reduction of dosage.

An increase in alertness may occur; this is generally beneficial but occasionally aggression, hyperactivity and behavioural deterioration have been reported. Hearing loss, either reversible or irreversible has been reported rarely, though a causal relationship has not been established.

*Gastrointestinal:* Increase in appetite may occur and an increase in weight is not uncommon. Minor gastric irritation and, less frequently, nausea may occur frequently in some patients at the start of treatment, but these problems can usually be overcome by administering Enteric Coated Epilim or administering Epilim with or after food.

*Dermatological:* Transient hair loss often has been noted in some patients. This effect does not appear to be dose-related and regrowth normally beings within six months, although the hair may become more curly than previously. Rashes have been rarely reported.

Rarely, signs of an immune disorder have occurred, therefore caution should be observed when using the drug in patients with features which may suggest systemic lupus erythematosus. The occurrence of vasculitus has occasionally been reported.

*Endocrine:* There have been isolated reports of irregular periods or amenorrhoea. Very rarely gynaecomastia has occurred.

*Overdosage:* Cases of accidental and suicidal valproate overdosage have been reported. At plasma concentrations of up to 5 to 6 times the maximum therapeutic levels, there are unlikely to be any symptoms other than nausea, vomiting and dizziness.

In massive overdose, i.e. with plasma concentration 10 to 20 times maximum therapeutic levels, there may be serious CNS depression and respiration may be impaired. The symptoms may however be variable and seizures have been reported in the presence of very high plasma levels. A number of deaths have occurred following large overdoses. Full recovery is usual following treatment including induced vomiting, gastric lavage, assisted ventilation, and other supportive measures.

## Pharmacological properties

*Pharmacodynamic properties:* Sodium valproate is an anticonvulsant. The most likely mode of action for valproate is potentiation of the inhibitory action of gamma amino butyric acid (GABA) through an action on the further synthesis or further metabolism of GABA.

*Pharmacokinetic properties:* The half life of sodium valproate is usually reported to be within the range of 8–20 hours. It is usually shorter in children.

In patients with severe renal insufficiency it may be necessary to alter dosage in accordance with free serum valproic acid levels.

The reported effective therapeutic range for plasma valproic acid levels is 40–100 mg/litre (278–694 micromol/litre). This reported range may depend on time of sampling and presence of co-medication. The percentage of free (unbound) drug is usually between 6% and 15% of total plasma levels. An increased incidence of adverse effects may occur with plasma levels above the effective therapeutic range.

The pharmacological (or therapeutic) effects of Epilim Chrono may not be clearly correlated with the total of free (unbound) plasma valproic acid levels.

Epilim Chrono formulations are controlled release formulations which demonstrate in pharmacokinetic studies less fluctuation in plasma concentration compared with other established conventional and modified release Epilim formulations.

In cases where measurement of plasma levels is considered necessary, the pharmacokinetics of Epilim Chrono make the measurement of plasma levels less dependent upon time of sampling.

The Epilim Chrono formulations are bioequivalent to Epilim Liquid and enteric coated (EC) formulations with respect to the mean areas under the plasma concentration time curves. Steady-state pharmacokinetic data indicate that the peak concentration (Cmax) and trough concentration (Cmin) of Epilim Chrono lie within the effective therapeutic range of plasma levels found in pharmacokinetic studies with Epilim EC.

*Pre-clinical safety data:* There are no pre-clinical data of relevance to the prescriber which are additional to that already included in other sections of the SPC.

## Pharmaceutical particulars

*List of excipients:* Hydroxypropylmethyl cellulose, ethylcellulose, hydrated silica.

*Film coat:* Violet coat, containing titanium dioxide (E171), erythrosine BS (E127), indigo carmine (E132), iron oxide black (E172), hydroxypropylmethyl cellulose (E464), polyethylene glycol 400, purified water†. († Not detected in final formulation.)

*Incompatibilities:* None.

*Shelf life:* Epilim Chrono tablets have a shelf-life of 36 months.

*Special precautions for storage:* Store in a dry place below 30°C.

*Nature and contents of container:* Epilim Chrono Controlled Release tablets are supplied in blister packs further packed into a cardboard carton. Pack size 100 tablets.

*Instructions for use/handling:* Not applicable.

**Marketing authorisation numbers**
Epilim Chrono 200 Controlled Release  11723/0078
Epilim Chrono 300 Controlled Release  11723/0021
Epilim Chrono 500 Controlled Release  11723/0079

**Date of approval/revision of SPC**  April 1996.

**Legal category**  POM.

# EPILIM* INTRAVENOUS

**Presentation**  Epilim Intravenous. Off-white sterile, freeze dried Sodium Valproate PhEur 400 mg in a clear glass vial supplied with an ampoule of 4 ml of solvent (Water for Injections PhEur).

**Uses**  Epilim Intravenous may be used for epileptic patients who would normally be maintained on oral sodium valproate, and for whom oral therapy is temporarily not possible.

**Dosage and administration**  Daily dosage requirements vary according to age and body weight.

To reconstitute, inject the solvent provided (4 ml) into the vial, allow to dissolve and extract the appropriate dose. Due to displacement of solvent by sodium valproate the concentration of reconstituted sodium valproate is 95 mg/ml.

Each vial of Epilim Intravenous is for single dose injection only. It should be reconstituted immediately prior to use and infusion solutions containing it used within 24 hours. Any unused portion should be discarded.

Epilim Intravenous may be given by direct slow intravenous injection or by infusion using a separate intravenous line in normal saline, dextrose 5%, or dextrose saline.

Patients already satisfactorily treated with Epilim may be continued at their current dosage using continuous or repeated infusion. Other patients may be given a slow intravenous injection over 3–5 minutes, usually 400–800 mg depending on body weight (up to 10 mg/kg) followed by continuous or repeated infusion up to a maximum of 2500 mg/day.

Epilim Intravenous should be replaced by oral Epilim therapy as soon as practicable.

Daily requirement for children is usually in the range 20–30 mg/kg/day and method of administration is as above. Where adequate control is not achieved within this range the dose may be increased up to 40 mg/kg/day but only in patients in whom plasma valproic acid levels can be monitored. Above 40 mg/kg/day clinical chemistry and haematological parameters should be monitored.

*Use in the elderly:* Although the pharmacokinetics of Epilim are modified in the elderly, they have limited clinical significance and dosage should be determined by seizure control. The volume of distribution is increased in the elderly and because of decreased binding to serum albumin, the proportion of free drug is increased. This will affect the clinical interpretation of plasma valproic acid levels.

*Combined therapy:* When starting Epilim in patients already on other anticonvulsants these should be tapered slowly; initiation of Epilim therapy should then be gradual, with target dose reached after about 2 weeks. In certain cases it may be necessary to raise the dose by 5 to 10 mg/kg/day when used in combination with anticonvulsants which induce liver enzyme activity, e.g. phenytoin, phenobarbitone, and carbamazepine. Once known enzyme inducers have been withdrawn it may be possible to maintain seizure control on a reduced dose of Epilim. When barbiturates are being administered concomitantly and particularly if sedation is observed (particularly in children) the dosage of barbiturate should be reduced.

*NB:* In children requiring doses higher than 40 mg/kg/day clinical chemistry and haematological parameters should be monitored.

*General considerations:* Optimum dosage is mainly determined by seizure control and routine measurement of plasma levels is unnecessary. However, a method for measurement of plasma levels is available and may be helpful where there is poor control or side effects are suspected, see Further Information.

**Contra-indications, warnings, etc**

*Contra-indications:* Hypersensitivity to sodium valproate. Active liver disease, family history of severe hepatic dysfunction, particularly drug-related. Porphyria.

*Side-effects*

*Hepatic:* Liver dysfunction, including hepatic failure resulting in fatalities, has occurred in patients whose treatment included valproic acid or sodium valproate. Patients most at risk are children particularly those under the age of three and those with congenital metabolic or degenerative disorders, organic brain disease or severe seizure disorders associated with mental retardation. The incidents mainly occurred during the first six months of therapy, the period of maximum risk being 2–12 weeks, and usually involved multiple anticonvulsant therapy. Monotherapy is to be preferred in this group of patients.

Clinical symptoms are more helpful than laboratory investigations in the early stages of hepatic failure. Serious or fatal hepatotoxicity may be preceded by non-specific symptoms, usually of sudden onset, such as loss of seizure control, malaise, weakness, lethargy, oedema, anorexia, vomiting, abdominal pain, drowsiness, jaundice. These are an indication for immediate withdrawal of the drug. Patients should be instructed to report any such signs to the clinician for investigation should they occur. Whilst it is difficult to establish which, if any, investigation is predictive, tests which reflect protein synthesis e.g. prothrombin time may be most relevant.

Routine measurement of liver function should be undertaken before therapy and periodically during the first six months especially in those who seem most at risk and those with a prior history of liver disease; such patients should have close clinical supervision. Raised liver enzymes are not uncommon during treatment with Epilim and are usually transient or respond to reduction in dosage of Epilim. Patients with such biochemical abnormalities should be reassessed clinically and tests of liver function including prothrombin time should be monitored until they return to normal. However an abnormally prolonged prothrombin time particularly in association with other relevant abnormalities requires cessation of treatment. Any concomitant use of salicylates should be stopped, since they employ the same metabolic pathway.

*Metabolic:* Hyperammonaemia without changes in liver function tests may occur. Isolated and moderate hyperammonaemia may occur frequently, is usually transient and should not cause treatment discontinuation. However, it may present clinically as vomiting, ataxia and increasing clouding of consciousness. Should these symptoms occur Epilim should be discontinued. Oedema has been reported rarely. When an abnormality of the urea cycle is suspected (ornithine transcarbamylase deficiency), pre-treatment ammonia levels should be measured.

*Pancreatic:* There have been reports of pancreatitis including rarely, fatalities occurring in patients receiving valproic acid or sodium valproate, usually within the first six months of therapy. Patients experiencing acute abdominal pain should have their serum amylase estimated; if these levels are elevated treatment should be discontinued.

*Haematological:* Valproic acid inhibits the second stage of platelet aggregation. Reversible prolongation of bleeding time and thrombocytopenia have been reported, but are usually associated with doses above those recommended. Prior to initiation of therapy and also before surgery, clinicians should assure themselves that there is no undue potential for bleeding complications. Spontaneous bruising or bleeding is an indication for withdrawal of medication pending investigations. Red cell hypoplasia, pancytopenia and leucopenia have been reported rarely; the blood picture returned to normal when the drug was discontinued. Isolated reduction of fibrinogen may also occur.

*Neurological:* Ataxia and tremor have been occasionally reported and appear to be dose-related effects.

Sedation has been reported occasionally, usually when in combination with other anticonvulsants. In Epilim monotherapy it occurred early in treatment on rare occasions and is usually transient. Rare cases of lethargy and confusion occasionally progressing to stupor, sometimes with associated hallucinations or convulsions have been reported.

Coma has very rarely been observed. These cases have often been associated with too high a starting dose or too rapid a dose escalation or concomitant use of other anticonvulsants, notably phenobarbitone. They have usually been reversible on withdrawal of treatment or reduction of dosage.

An increase in alertness may occur; this is generally beneficial but occasionally aggression, hyperactivity and behavioural deterioration have been reported.

Hearing loss, either reversible or irreversible has been reported rarely, though a causal relationship has not been established.

*Gastrointestinal:* Increase in appetite may occur and an increase in weight is not uncommon. Minor gastric irritation and, less frequently, nausea may occur in some patients at the start of treatment.

*Dermatological:* Transient hair loss has often been noted in some patients. This effect does not appear to be dose-related and regrowth normally begins within six months, although the hair may become more curly than previously. Rashes have been rarely reported.

*Endocrine:* There have been isolated reports of irregular periods or amenorrhoea. Very rarely gynaecomastia has occurred.

*Other:* Rarely, signs of an immune disorder have occurred, therefore caution should be observed when using the drug in patients with features which may suggest systemic lupus erythematosus.

*Drug interactions:* Like many other drugs, Epilim may potentiate the effect of neuroleptics, monoamine oxidase inhibitors and other anti-depressants. The enzyme inducing effect of valproate is appreciably less than that of certain other anti-convulsants and loss of efficacy of oral contraceptive agents does not appear to be a problem.

Caution is recommended when administering anticoagulants and other products which have anticoagulant properties (e.g. warfarin and salicylates). Aspirin may displace valproate from binding sites resulting in higher free levels of valproate. Epilim decreases protein binding of warfarin but this may not lead to clinically significant effects. Phenytoin levels may be affected by Epilim and these should be monitored, particularly the free form which may increase following an initial decrease in total levels.

Epilim may inhibit the metabolism of lamotrigine. Dosages should be adjusted (lamotrigine dosage decreased) when appropriate.

Dosage of Epilim may require adjustment when used in combination with other anti-convulsants. See 'Dosage, Combined Therapy Section'.

There is evidence that cimetidine (but not ranitidine) and erythromycin may prolong the half-life and reduce clearance of Epilim and also that mefloquine may decrease serum levels of valproate.

The absorption of Epilim may be decreased in the presence of cholestyramine.

*Diabetic patients:* Epilim is eliminated mainly through the kidneys, partly in the form of ketone bodies; this may give false positives in the urine testing of possible diabetics.

*Pregnancy:* An increased incidence of congenital abnormalities (including facial dysmorphia, neural tube defects and multiple malformations) has been demonstrated in offspring born to mothers with epilepsy both untreated and treated including those treated with sodium valproate.

The incidence of neural tube defects in women receiving valproate during the first trimester has been estimated to be in the region of 1–2%. Folate supplementation has been demonstrated to reduce the incidence of neural tube defects in the offspring of women at high risk. No direct evidence exists of such effects in women receiving anti-epileptic drugs, however there is no reason to contraindicate folic acid in these women.

The available evidence suggests that anticonvulsant monotherapy is preferred. Dosage should be reviewed before conception and the lowest effective dose used, as abnormal pregnancy outcome tends to be associated with higher total daily dosage. Women of childbearing age should be informed of the risks and benefits of continuing anti-epileptic treatment throughout pregnancy. Pregnancies should be carefully screened by alpha-foetoprotein measurement, ultrasound, and other techniques if appropriate.

*Breast feeding:* The concentration of valproic acid found in the breast milk is very low, between 1% and 10% of total maternal plasma levels. Thus there appears to be no contra-indication to breast feeding by patients on Epilim. The decision to allow the patient to breast feed should be taken with regard to all the known facts.

*Overdosage:* Cases of accidental and suicidal overdosage with oral therapy have been reported. At plasma concentrations of up to 5 to 6 times the maximum therapeutic levels, there are unlikely to be any symptoms other than nausea, vomiting and dizziness.

In massive overdose, i.e. with plasma concentrations 10 to 20 times maximum therapeutic levels there may be serious CNS depression and respiration may be impaired. The symptoms may however be variable and seizures have been reported in the presence of very high plasma levels. A number of deaths have occurred following large overdoses. Full recovery is usual following treatment which may include assisted ventilation, and other supportive measures.

**Pharmaceutical precautions** Epilim Intravenous freeze dried powder should be stored below 25°C; infusion solutions at 2–8°C if stored before use, discarding any remaining after 24 hours. Epilim Intravenous should not be administered via the same IV line as other IV additives. The intravenous solution is suitable for infusion in PVC, polythene, or glass containers.

**Legal category** POM.

**Package quantities** Epilim Intravenous is supplied as a pack containing one vial of 400 mg Sodium Valproate PhEur and one ampoule containing 4 ml of solvent.

**Further information** The half life of sodium valproate is usually reported to be within the range 8–20 hours. It is usually shorter in children.

In patients with severe renal insufficiency it may be necessary to alter dosage in accordance with free serum valproic acid levels.

The reported effective therapeutic range for plasma valproic acid levels is 40–100 mg/litre (278–694 micro mol/litre). This reported range may depend on time of sampling and presence of co-medication. The percentage of free (unbound) drug is usually between 6% and 15% of the total plasma levels. An increased incidence of adverse effects may occur with plasma levels above the effective therapeutic range.

The pharmacological (or therapeutic) effects of Epilim may not be clearly correlated with the total or free (unbound) plasma valproic acid levels.

**Product licence numbers**

| | |
|---|---|
| Vial of freeze dried powder | 11723/0022 |
| Ampoule of solvent | 11723/0023 |

## FORTAGESIC*

**Presentation** White tablets with bevelled edges 12.7 mm diameter, marked FORTAGESIC on one side. Each tablet provides Pentazocine BP 15 mg (as the hydrochloride) and Paracetamol PhEur 500 mg. Fortagesic tablets contain sodium metabisulphite.

**Uses** Fortagesic is a compound analgesic for the relief of moderate pain associated with musculoskeletal disorders or injuries, such as bursitis, sprains, strains, fibrositis, sciatica and osteoarthritis, and for rheumatoid arthritis in patients sensitive to aspirin.

**Dosage and administration** Fortagesic is for oral administration only.

*Adults including the elderly:* 2 tablets up to four times daily.

*Children:* 7–12 years: 1 tablet every three to four hours. Not more than 4 doses to be taken in any 24 hour period. Not recommended for children under 7 years of age.

**Contra-indications, warnings, etc**

*Contra-indications:* Fortagesic should not be administered to patients with established respiratory depression, especially in the presence of cyanosis and excessive bronchial secretion and is also contraindicated in the presence of acute alcoholism, head injuries, conditions in which intracranial pressure is raised, acute bronchial asthma, in heart failure, secondary to chronic lung disease and in patients known to be hypersensitive to pentazocine or paracetamol.

*Warnings:*

*Use in pregnancy and lactation:* There is epidemiological evidence for the safety of paracetamol in human pregnancy. No such evidence exists for pentazocine but it has been widely used for many years without apparent ill consequences. In rodents, harmful effects in the foetus have been observed but only at doses high enough to cause maternal toxicity. Pentazocine can enter the foetal circulation and has the potential to cause opioid effects including central depression and abstinence syndrome in the foetus (see below). It does not appear to have significant adverse effects on uterine function at parturition. Nonetheless, careful consideration should be given to the use of Fortagesic during pregnancy, particularly during the first trimester, or at term.

There are insufficient data on the secretion of pentazocine in breast milk so it is recommended that infants of nursing mothers who are receiving high doses of Fortagesic be appropriately monitored.

*Precautions:*
Particular caution should be observed in administering Fortagesic to patients with porphyria, since it may provoke an acute attack in susceptible individuals, as well as in its use in patients who are receiving monoamine oxidase inhibitors or who have received them within the preceding 14 days.

Pentazocine can both depress as well as elevate blood pressure possibly through the release of endogenous catecholamines. Particular caution should be observed therefore in using Fortagesic in the presence of phaeochromocytoma, in the acute phase following myocardial infarction when it may increase pulmonary and systemic blood pressure and vascular resistance and in other clinical situations where alteration of vascular resistance or blood pressure might be particularly undesirable.

Caution should be observed in patients with renal or hepatic impairment and in elderly patients, who may additionally be especially sensitive to the effects of opioids, as both conditions may lead to an increase in bioavailability of pentazocine and call for a reduction in dosage.

Caution should also be observed in patients who are prone to seizures and in the presence of other opioids or opioid-dependence since the weak opioid antagonistic effects of pentazocine may provoke withdrawal symptoms.

Caution should also be observed in patients with hypothyroidism, adrenocortical insufficiency, prostatic hypertrophy and in patients with inflammatory or obstructive bowel disorders.

Pentazocine may produce sedation, so ambulant patients should be warned not to operate machinery or drive if affected.

In chronic usage, care should be exercised to avoid any unnecessary increase in dosage since prolonged use of high doses of pentazocine may produce dependence.

*Interactions:* Monoamine oxidase inhibitors may enhance the opioid effects of pentazocine and the agents may interact through their respective effects on catecholamine breakdown and release. Agents with sedative action including phenothiazines and ethyl alcohol can enhance the central depressant effects of pentazocine which are opposed by respiratory stimulants such as doxapram. Tobacco smoking appears to enhance the metabolic clearance rate of pentazocine reducing the clinical effectiveness of a standard dose of pentazocine.

Pentazocine can antagonise the effects of stronger opioid agonists such as diamorphine, morphine and heroin and is itself antagonised by naloxone.

*Side-effects:* At normal therapeutic doses side-effects are generally of a minor nature. Paracetamol is extremely well tolerated. Any side-effects to Fortagesic are likely to be due to pentazocine which may cause lightheadedness, dizziness, nausea and vomiting, sedation and sweating. Pentazocine may also cause headache, dry mouth, constipation, flushing of the skin, tachycardia, mood changes, nightmares, paraesthesia, pruritus, biliary tract spasm and urinary retention. Respiratory depression, raised intracranial pressure, hypotension, transient hypertension can also occur. Altered uterine contractions, muscle tremor, insomnia, disorientation, hallucinations, disturbances of vision, transient eosinophilia, depression of white blood cells, chills and allergic reactions have also been reported. After large intravenous doses, grand mal convulsions have been noted.

Abrupt discontinuation of pentazocine in patients receiving large parenteral doses over a prolonged period of time may result in withdrawal symptoms, which can also occur in the newborn following prolonged in utero exposure. The abstinence syndrome of pentazocine is not typical of opiate dependence. Symptoms include mild abdominal cramps, nausea, vomiting, nervousness or restlessness, dizziness, fever and chills, but are mild compared with symptoms of opiate withdrawal. Managing the abstinence syndrome of pentazocine has raised few problems. Supportive therapy with tranquillisers may sometimes be required. It should be emphasised that the majority of patients reported to have become dependent on pentazocine had previously been dependent on opiates or had misused other drugs.

*Overdose:* The symptoms and clinical signs of Fortagesic overdose are likely to resemble those of the individual ingredients. Thus with pentazocine, as with morphine and other opioids, there may be somnolence, respiratory depression and hypotension. Circulatory failure and deepening coma may occur in more severe cases, as may convulsions. Adequate measures to maintain ventilation and general circulatory support should be employed. Anti-convulsant therapy may be necessary and the specific antagonist

naloxone should be employed appropriately to reverse any CNS depression.

With paracetamol overdose, patients may appear well for the first three days, then succumb with liver damage. The hepatic changes produced by overdosage of paracetamol result from the accumulation of a highly active intermediate metabolite in the hepatocytes.

N-acetylcysteine intravenously or methionine orally protects the liver if administered within 10–12 hours of ingesting an overdose.

In managing Fortagesic overdose, consideration should be given to gastric lavage and aspiration.

**Pharmaceutical precautions**   Store below 25°C.

**Legal category**   CD (Sch 3) POM.

**Package quantities**   Fortagesic is supplied in bottles of 100 tablets.

**Further information**   Paracetamol is rapidly and completely absorbed from the gastro-intestinal tract, it is relatively uniformly distributed throughout most body fluids and exhibits variable protein binding. Excretion is almost exclusively renal, in the form of conjugated metabolites.

Pentazocine is a strong opioid analgesic with weak opioid antagonist properties. By mouth, pentazocine has a bioavailability of about 47%. In the plasma it is 50–75% bound to protein and has an elimination half-life of about 4.6 hours. Peak plasma concentrations are obtained in 1 to 3 hours. Pentazocine diffuses across the placenta and appears in cerebro-spinal fluid in concentrations reaching 30–50% of those in plasma. It is metabolised by the liver, only a small proportion of a dose being excreted unchanged in the urine.

**Product licence number**   11723/0028.

## FRANOL*

**Presentation**   Franol Tablets are flat, white tablets with bevelled edges, 8.7 mm in diameter, marked Franol on one side. Each tablet contains 120 mg Theophylline PhEur and 11 mg Ephedrine Hydrochloride PhEur.

**Uses**   Franol Tablets are recommended for the management of bronchospasm in reversible airway-obstruction associated with stable asthma or chronic bronchitis.

**Dosage and administration**   Oral administration only.
*Adults:* Dosage varies with individual requirements and should be adjusted accordingly. The usual dosage is 3 tablets daily (morning, midday and evening). For the patient who suffers nocturnal attacks, an extra tablet taken at bedtime is recommended.

*Elderly:* As for adults but see 'Use in special groups'.

*Children:* Not recommended for children under 12 years of age.

If more than four tablets a day are required, it is advisable to monitor plasma theophylline levels during dose titration to ensure that levels are kept below 20 micrograms/ml.

**Contra-indications, warnings, etc**

*Contra-indications:* Franol should not be given to patients who are sensitive to either of its ingredients or to patients with unstable angina, cardiac arrhythmias, severe hypertension, severe coronary artery disease, porphyria or to those receiving other xanthines. Franol should not be used during pregnancy.

*Precautions:* Avoid or use with special caution in patients with cardiovascular disease, hypertension, agitation, phaeochromocytoma, hyperthyroidism, closed-angle glaucoma, prostatic hypertrophy, peptic ulceration, underlying seizure disorders, patients receiving anti-depressant drugs, or patients on MAO inhibitors within the previous 14 days. Special caution is also needed in the elderly, those with hepatic, renal, or cardiac dysfunction and during lactation. Ephedrine has a potential for tachyphylaxis, and abuse with dependence has been reported.

Potentially serious hypokalaemia can result from the use of beta₂ agonists and xanthines in combination particularly when hypoxia is present. The effect may be enhanced by concomitant diuretics or corticosteroids. Care should be observed and serum potassium levels monitored in patients receiving Franol who develop severe asthma, particularly if concomitant diuretic, corticosteroid or beta₂ agonist therapy is being employed.

*Use in special groups:*
Pregnancy: Although caffeine has been implicated as a teratogen, adequate animal teratogenic studies have not been conducted with theophylline nor with ephedrine. The safety of ephedrine and of theophylline, which crosses the placental barrier, have not been established in human pregnancy. Franol should not therefore be prescribed for patients who are pregnant.

Lactation: Theophylline distributes readily into breast milk therefore Franol should be used with caution in nursing women.

Hepatic dysfunction: Theophylline is eliminated primarily by metabolism in the liver. Thus in patients with severe liver disease, theophylline clearance may be decreased. If Franol is used in such patients, dosage may need to be reduced.

Renal dysfunction: Ephedrine is excreted largely unchanged in the urine, therefore Franol should be used with caution in patients with severe renal impairment.

Cardiac dysfunction: Theophylline clearance may be decreased in patients with congestive cardiac failure, acute pulmonary oedema or cor pulmonale, and theophylline may cause arrhythmias or worsen existing arrhythmias, thus caution should be exercised if Franol is used in such patients.

Elderly (over 65 years): Theophylline clearance decreases slightly with age. Elderly patients will tend therefore to have higher serum theophylline levels than younger adults at a given dose. They should be monitored closely for signs of toxicity during dose adjustment.

Others: Theophylline clearance may be increased in heavy smokers, decreased in patients with respiratory infection or those on a high carbohydrate – low protein diet, therefore the dose of Franol may need to be adjusted appropriately in these groups.

*Drug interactions:* Theophylline clearance may be decreased by concurrent administration of cimetidine, macrolide antibiotics, oral contraceptives, interferons, diltiazem, verapamil and viloxazine. Ciprofloxacin also increases plasma theophylline concentrations and if concomitant use is essential, the dose of theophylline should be reduced and plasma concentrations closely monitored to avoid toxicity. The concomitant use of theophylline and fluvoxamine should usually be avoided. When this is not possible, patients should have their theophylline dose halved and plasma theophylline should be monitored closely. Theophylline clearance may be increased by concurrent administration of barbiturates, carbamazepine, phenytoin, rifampicin, sulphinpyrazone, aminoglutethimide, phenobarbitone and primidone.

The effects of ephedrine are diminished by guanethidine, reserpine, and probably methyldopa, and may be diminished or enhanced by tricyclic anti-depressants. Ephedrine may also diminish the effects of guanethidine and may increase the possibility of arrhythmias in digitalised patients.

*Side-effects:* Large doses of Franol may give rise to the following side effects: arrhythmias, tachycardia, palpitation, flushing, giddiness, headache, tremor, anxiety, restlessness, insomnia, muscular weakness, nausea, vomiting, dyspepsia, thirst, sweating, difficulty in micturition.

Some patients may exhibit one or more such symptoms with therapeutic doses.

*Overdosage:* The symptoms and signs of overdosage with Franol are likely to include excessive irritability, sweating, nausea and vomiting, tachycardia, arrhythmias, hypertension, profuse diuresis with fever, flushing and hyperglycaemia, opisthotonus, hallucinations, convulsions and respiratory difficulty. In general the management of overdosage with Franol involves supportive and symptomatic therapy with particular attention being paid to the detection and correction of hypokalaemia, and should include serial assay of plasma potassium and theophylline levels, cardiac monitoring with electro-cardiogram, and maintenance of fluid and electrolyte balance.

Gastric aspiration and lavage may be employed. Convulsions and other CNS stimulation can usually be controlled by intravenous diazepam, or if that fails other anti-convulsants may be used. Marked excitement or hallucinations may be managed with chlorpromazine. Severe hypertension may necessitate the use of an alpha-adrenoreceptor blocking agent and a beta-adrenoreceptor blocking agent may be required to control arrhythmias. Beta 1-receptor agonists such as dopamine should be avoided. Charcoal haemoperfusion may be indicated to remove theophylline, but forced diuresis or peritoneal dialysis are inadequate for this purpose.

**Pharmaceutical precautions**   Store below 25°C.

**Legal category**   P.

**Package quantities**   Franol Tablets are supplied in bottles of 90.

**Further information**   The bronchodilator action of ephedrine is through direct agonism at beta adrenoceptors and, indirectly, through sympathetic amine release. Bronchodilatation with theophylline is attributable to adenosine antagonism or phosphodiesterase inhibition which would be pharmacologically complementary to the action of ephedrine. Theophylline is variably absorbed from the gastrointestinal tract. It is excreted via the urine mainly as 1,3-dimethyluric acid. About 10% is unchanged. Ephedrine is readily absorbed. Its action is evident within one hour. With a plasma elimination half life of about 4 hours, 60–75% is excreted unchanged in the urine.

**Product licence number** 11723/0035.

# FRANOL* PLUS

**Presentation** Franol Plus Tablets are flat, white tablets with bevelled edges, 8.7 mm in diameter, marked F+ on one side. Each tablet contains 120 mg Theophylline PhEur and 15 mg Ephedrine Sulphate USP.

**Uses** Franol Plus Tablets are recommended for the management of bronchospasm in reversible airway-obstruction associated with stable asthma or chronic bronchitis.

**Dosage and administration** Oral administration only.
*Adults:* Dosage varies with individual requirements and should be adjusted accordingly. The usual dosage is 3 tablets daily (morning, midday and evening). For the patient who suffers from nocturnal attacks, an extra tablet at bedtime is recommended.

*Elderly:* As for adults but see 'Use in Special Groups'.

*Children:* Not recommended for children under 12 years of age.

If more than four tablets a day are required, it is advisable to monitor plasma theophylline levels during dose titration to ensure that levels are kept below 20 micrograms/ml.

**Contra-indications, warnings, etc**
*Contra-indications:* Franol Plus should not be given to patients who are sensitive to either of its ingredients or to patients with unstable angina, cardiac arrhythmias, severe hypertension, severe coronary artery disease, porphyria or to those receiving other xanthines. Franol Plus should not be used during pregnancy.

*Precautions:* Avoid or use only with special caution in patients with cardiovascular disease, hypertension, agitation, phaeochromocytoma, hyperthyroidism, closed-angle glaucoma, prostatic hypertrophy, peptic ulceration, underlying seizure disorders, patients receiving anti-depressant drugs, or patients on MAO inhibitors within the previous 14 days. Special caution is also needed in the elderly, those with hepatic, renal, or cardiac dysfunction and during lactation. Ephedrine has a potential for tachyphylaxis, and abuse with dependence has been reported.

Potentially serious hypokalaemia can result from the use of beta₂ agonists and xanthines in combination particularly when hypoxia is present. The effect may be enhanced by concomitant diuretics or corticosteroids. Care should be observed and serum potassium levels monitored in patients receiving Franol Plus who develop severe asthma, particularly if concomitant diuretic, corticosteroid or beta₂ agonist therapy is being employed.

*Use in special groups:*
Pregnancy: Although caffeine has been implicated as a teratogen, adequate animal teratogenic studies have not been conducted with theophylline nor with ephedrine. The safety of ephedrine and of theophylline, which crosses the placental barrier, have not been established in human pregnancy. Franol Plus should not therefore be prescribed for patients who are pregnant.
Lactation: Theophylline distributes readily into breast milk therefore Franol Plus should be used with caution in nursing women.
Hepatic dysfunction: Theophylline is eliminated primarily by metabolism in the liver. Thus in patients with severe liver disease, theophylline clearance may be decreased. If Franol Plus is used in such patients, dosage may need to be reduced.
Renal dysfunction: Ephedrine is excreted largely unchanged in the urine, therefore Franol Plus should be used with caution in patients with severe renal impairment.
Cardiac dysfunction: Theophylline clearance may be decreased in patients with congestive cardiac failure, acute pulmonary oedema or cor pulmonale, and theophylline may cause arrhythmias or worsen existing arrhythmias, thus caution should be exercised if Franol Plus is used in such patients.
Elderly (over 65 years): Theophylline clearance decreases slightly with age. Elderly patients will tend therefore to have higher serum theophylline levels than younger adults at a given dose. They should be monitored closely for signs of toxicity during dose adjustment.
Others: Theophylline clearance may be increased in heavy smokers, decreased in patients with respiratory infection or those on a high carbohydrate – low protein diet, therefore the dose of Franol Plus may need to be adjusted appropriately in these groups.

*Drug interactions:* Theophylline clearance may be decreased by concurrent administration of cimetidine, macrolide antibiotics, oral contraceptives, interferons, diltiazem, verapamil and viloxazine. Ciprofloxacin also increases plasma theophylline concentrations and if concomitant use is essential, the dose of theophylline should be reduced and plasma concentrations closely monitored to avoid toxicity. The concomitant use of theophylline and fluvoxamine should usually be avoided. Where this is not possible, patients should have their theophylline dose halved and plasma theophylline should be monitored closely. Theophylline clearance may be increased by concurrent administration of barbiturates, carbamazepine, phenytoin, rifampicin, sulphinpyrazone, aminoglutethimide, phenobarbitone and primidone. Lithium excretion is accelerated by theophylline.

The effects of ephedrine are diminished by guanethidine, reserpine, and probably methyldopa, and may be diminished or enhanced by tricyclic anti-depressants. Ephedrine may also diminish the effects of guanethidine and may increase the possibility of arrhythmias in digitalised patients.

*Side-effects:* Potentially serious hypokalaemia can result from beta₂ agonists and xanthines in combination particularly when hypoxia is present. Large doses of Franol Plus may give rise to the following side effects: arrhythmias, tachycardia, palpitation, flushing, giddiness, headache, tremor, anxiety, restlessness, insomnia, muscular weakness, nausea, vomiting, dyspepsia, thirst, sweating, difficulty in micturition.

Some patients may exhibit one or more such symptoms with therapeutic doses.

*Overdosage:* The symptoms and signs of overdosage with Franol Plus are likely to include excessive irritability, sweating, nausea and vomiting, tachycardia, arrhythmias, hypertension, profuse diuresis with fever, flushing and hyperglycaemia, opisthotonus, hallucinations, convulsions and respiratory difficulty. In general the management of overdosage with Franol Plus involves supportive and symptomatic therapy with particular attention being paid to the detection and correction of hypokalaemia, and should include serial assay of plasma potassium and theophylline levels, cardiac monitoring with electro-cardiogram, and maintenance of fluid and electrolyte balance.

Gastric aspiration and lavage may be employed. Convulsions and other CNS stimulation can usually be controlled by intravenous diazepam, or if that fails other anti-convulsants may be used. Marked excitement or hallucinations may be managed with chlorpromazine. Severe hypertension may necessitate the use of an alpha-adrenoreceptor blocking agent and a beta-adrenoreceptor blocking agent may be required to control arrhythmias. Beta 1-receptor agonist agents such as dopamine should be avoided. Charcoal haemoperfusion may be indicated to remove theophylline, but forced diuresis or peritoneal dialysis are inadequate for this purpose.

**Pharmaceutical precautions** Nil.

**Legal category** P.

**Package quantities** Franol Plus Tablets are supplied in bottles of 250.

**Further information** The bronchodilator action of ephedrine is through direct agonism at beta adrenoceptors and, indirectly, through sympathetic amine release. Bronchodilatation with theophylline is attributable to adenosine antagonism or phosphodiesterase inhibition which would be pharmacologically complementary to the action of ephedrine. Theophylline is variably absorbed from the gastrointestinal tract. It is excreted via the urine mainly as 1,3-dimethyluric acid and about 10% is unchanged. Ephedrine is readily absorbed. Its action is evident within one hour. With a plasma elimination half life of about 4 hours, 60–75% is excreted unchanged in the urine.

**Product licence number** 11723/0034.

# FRAXIPARINE* ▼

**Qualitative and quantitative composition** Each 1 ml of solution for injection contains Nadroparin Calcium PhEur 9500 AntiXa IU.

**Pharmaceutical form** Sterile, clear, preservative free solution for injection presented in disposable prefilled single use syringes containing:

| Volume (ml) | Type of syringe | Nadroparin Calcium (AntiXa IU PhEur) |
|---|---|---|
| 0.2 | Ungraduated | 1900 |
| 0.3 | Ungraduated | 2850 |
| 0.4 | Ungraduated | 3800 |
| 0.6 | Graduated | 5700 |
| 0.8 | Graduated | 7600 |
| 1.0 | Graduated | 9500 |

**Clinical particulars**
*Therapeutic indications:* Prophylaxis of thromboembolic disorders associated with general or orthopaedic surgery.
Treatment of deep vein thrombosis.
Prevention of clotting during haemodialysis.

*Posology and method of administration:*

*Particular attention should be paid to the specific dosing instructions for each proprietary Low Molecular Weight Heparin as different unit systems (units or mg) are used to express doses and as different strength formulations may exist.*

Graduated syringes are intended for administration of adjusted doses when an adaptation to body weight is necessary.

When given by subcutaneous injection, the usual site for injection is the lateral abdominal wall, but the thigh may be used as an alternative. The needle should be inserted perpendicularly into a pinched-up fold of skin which should be held gently but firmly until injection has been completed. Do not rub the injection site. Fraxiparine is not intended for intramuscular injection.

*Adults:*
*Prophylaxis of thromboembolic disorders in general surgery:* 0.3 ml (2,850 IU AntiXa IU) 2 hours before surgery and 8 hours after the end of surgery, then from the following day as a single daily dose for at least 7 days, and in all cases throughout the risk period until the patient is ambulant.

*Prophylaxis of thromboembolic disorders in orthopaedic surgery:* Initial doses should be administered 12 hours before surgery and 12 hours after the end of surgery, then once daily on subsequent days. Treatment should be for at least 10 days and should continue in all cases throughout the risk period until the patient is ambulant. Doses should be adjusted for body-weight according to the table below, which is based on a target dose of 38 AntiXa IU (0.004 ml)/kg, increased by 50% from the fourth post-operative day.

| Orthopaedic surgery | Volume to be injected subcutaneously | |
|---|---|---|
| Body weight (kg) | 12 hours before surgery, 12 hours after surgery, and once daily on subsequent days to the third post operative day | From the fourth post operative day onwards |
| <60 | 0.2 ml | 0.3 ml |
| 60–74 | 0.3 ml | 0.4 ml |
| 75–90 | 0.3 ml | 0.5 ml |
| >90 | 0.4 ml | 0.6 ml |

*Treatment of deep vein thrombosis:* Fraxiparine should be administered subcutaneously twice daily (every 12 hours) for a usual duration of 10 days. The dose should be adjusted for body-weight according to the table below, which is based on a target dose of 86 AntiXa IU (0.009 ml)/kg.

| Treatment of thromboembolic disorders | |
|---|---|
| Body weight (kg) | Volume to be injected subcutaneously twice daily |
| <55 | 0.5 ml |
| 55–80 | 0.6 ml |
| >80 | 0.7 ml |

Oral anticoagulant therapy should be initiated as soon as possible unless there is a contra-indication. Treatment with Fraxiparine should not be stopped before the International Normalised Ratio (INR) target is reached.

*Prevention of clotting during haemodialysis:* Optimisation of dosage is required for each individual patient and taking into account the technical conditions of the dialysis. Fraxiparine is usually given as a single dose into the arterial line at the start of each session. For patients without increased risk of haemorrhage the following initial doses are suggested according to body-weight and are usually sufficient for a 4-hour session:

| Prevention of clotting during haemodialysis | |
|---|---|
| Body weight (kg) | Volume to be injected into arterial line at start of dialysis |
| <70 | 0.4 ml (3800 AntiXa IU) |
| ≥70 | 0.6 ml (5700 AntiXa IU) |

An additional smaller dose may be given during dialysis for sessions lasting longer than 4 hours. Furthermore, doses should be halved in patients with an increased risk of haemorrhage. The dose in subsequent dialysis sessions should be adjusted as necessary according to the observed effect.

Patients should be carefully monitored throughout each dialysis session for signs of bleeding or clotting in the dialysis circuit.

*Elderly:* No dosage adjustment is necessary in the elderly.

*Children, infants and neonates:* Not recommended as dosage has not been established.

*Special patient groups:* Reduced doses may be considered in patients with moderate to severe renal failure (see *Special precautions*).

*Contra-indications:* Fraxiparine is contra-indicated in patients with known hypersensitivity to heparins, or who have a history of thrombocytopenia with heparin (see *Special warnings*). Fraxiparine is also contra-indicated in patients with active bleeding or an increased risk of haemorrhage including those with bleeding disorders (except for disseminated intravascular coagulation not induced by heparin), organic lesion likely to bleed (such as active peptic ulceration), haemorrhagic cerebrovascular accident or infective endocarditis.

*Special warnings and special precautions for use*
*Special warnings:* Because of the possibility of heparin-induced thrombocytopenia, **regular monitoring of platelet count should be performed throughout the course of treatment with Fraxiparine.**

As with all heparins, acute thrombocytopenia, usually reversible, has been reported. Treatment should be discontinued immediately. Rare cases of severe thrombocytopenia have also been reported and may be associated with arterial or venous thrombosis, exacerbation of the pre-existing thrombosis or disseminated intravascular coagulation; the platelet count should be assessed if these events are suspected. Severe thrombocytopenia is probably immunological in origin and in the case of a first course of heparin treatment usually occur between the 5th and 21st day.

*Special precautions:* Administer with caution in the following cases:
– hepatic failure;
– renal failure (reduced doses may be considered in patients with moderate to severe renal failure);
– uncontrolled arterial hypertension;
– history of peptic ulceration or other organic lesion likely to bleed;
– vascular disorder of the chorio-retina;
– during the post-operative period following surgery of the brain, spinal cord or eye;
– spinal or epidural anaesthesia.

*Interactions with other medicaments and other forms of interaction:* Concomitant use of aspirin (or other salicylates or non steroidal anti-flammatory drugs) is not recommended as they may increase the risk of bleeding. Where such combination cannot be avoided, careful clinical and biological monitoring should be undertaken.

Formal interaction studies with Fraxiparine have not been performed. Nevertheless, as with all heparins, Fraxiparine should be administered with caution in patients receiving other drugs which increase the risk of bleeding such as oral anticoagulants, antiplatelet agents, corticosteroids and dextrans.

As with all heparin preparations, during transfer to oral anticoagulant therapy, clinical monitoring should be particularly vigilant and treatment should be continued until the INR is stabilised at the target value.

*Pregnancy and lactation:*
*Pregnancy:* Studies in animals have not shown any teratogenic or foetotoxic effects. However, there is only limited information and human clinical data concerning transplacental passage. The use of Fraxiparine in pregnancy is not advised.

*Lactation:* Due to limited information on excretion in breast milk and of subsequent absorption in the neonate, use of Fraxiparine during breast feeding is not advised.

*Effects on ability to drive and to use machines:* Not relevant.

*Undesirable effects:* In common with other heparin preparations:

Haemorrhage at various sites, more frequent in patients with other risk factors (see *Contra-indications* and *Interactions with other medicaments and other forms of interaction*).

Acute thrombocytopenia, usually reversible, has been reported. Rare cases of severe thrombocytopenia have also been reported (see *Special warnings*).

Some rare cases of cutaneous necrosis, usually occurring at the injection site, have been reported. They are preceded by purpura or infiltration or painful erythematous blotches, with or without systemic illness. Treatment should be discontinued immediately.

Small haematomas at the injection site are common. The occurrence of pain and bruising upon injection can be minimised by use of a careful injection technique. The potential for haematomas at the surgical site has also been reported.

Rare cutaneous or generalised hypersensitivity reactions, sometimes requiring discontinuation of treatment.

Raised transaminases; usually transient.

Occasional cases of reversible hypoaldosteronism have been reported, either asymptomatic or associated with hyperkalemia and/or hyponatremia.

*Overdosage:* Haemorrhage is the major clinical sign of overdosage. The platelet count and other coagulation parameters should be measured. Minor bleeding rarely requires specific therapy, and reducing or delaying subsequent doses of Fraxiparine is usually sufficient.

The use of protamine sulphate should be considered only in more serious cases. Protamine has a relatively weak neutralising effect on Fraxiparine and some anti-Xa activity will remain. In general, 6 mg of protamine sulphate neutralises about 0.1 ml (950 AntiXa IU) Fraxiparine. The amount of protamine to be injected should take into account the time elapsed from the injection of Fraxiparine; a reduction of the dose may be needed.

**Pharmacological properties**
*Pharmacodynamic properties:* Fraxiparine is a low molecular weight heparin made by depolymerisation of standard heparin. It is a glycosaminoglycan with a mean molecular weight around 4,300 Daltons. It possesses a high ratio of anti-Xa to anti-IIa activity. Fraxiparine has both immediate and prolonged antithrombotic action.

*Pharmacokinetic properties:* These have been determined by measurement of plasma anti-Xa activity. The plasma peak occurs about 3 hours after subcutaneous injection. The elimination half-life is about 3.5 hours. Anti-Xa activity persists for at least 18 hours after injection. Bioavailability is almost complete (around 98 per cent).

*Preclinical safety data:* There are no preclinical data of relevance to the physician which are additional to that already included in the prescribing information.

**Pharmaceutical particulars**
*List of excipients:* Calcium hydroxide solution or dilute hydrochloric acid, water for injections.

*Incompatibilities:* Do not mix with other preparations.

*Shelf life:* 3 years.

*Special precautions for storage:* Store below 25°C, but do not freeze. Do not refrigerate as cold injections may be painful. Discard any unused portion of each syringe.

*Nature and contents of container:* Cartons containing 2 or 10 prefilled glass syringes. Each syringe is individually packed into a PVC blister closed by a plastic-coated paper film.

*Instructions for use/handling:* See *Posology and method of administration.*

**Marketing authorisation number** 11723/0003

**Date of approval/revision of SPC** June 1997.

**Legal category** POM.

# GLURENORM*

**Presentation** Flat, white, bevelled-edged tablets, 9 mm in diameter, scored on one side and with G on the other, each containing 30 mg gliquidone. Glurenorm tablets contain lactose.

**Uses** For the treatment of non-insulin dependent diabetes mellitus which does not respond adequately to dietary measures.

**Dosage and administration** For oral administration only. Glurenorm should be taken up to half an hour before a meal. The dose and frequency of administration should be adjusted, together with the diet, to obtain the best possible control of the diabetes throughout the day.

*Adults including the elderly:* Most patients respond to a total daily dose of 45–60 mg given in two or three divided doses, of which the largest dose is usually taken in the morning with breakfast. The recommended maximum single dose is 60 mg (2 tablets). The maximum daily dose is 180 mg (6 tablets).

During stabilisation, dosage adjustment should be based on frequent blood (random and postprandial) and urinary glucose determinations.

*Stabilisation of previously untreated cases:* Normally, treatment should begin with 15 mg (half a tablet) before breakfast and this should be gradually increased by 15 mg increments prior to mealtimes.

*Change-over in patients previously treated with other oral anti-diabetic agents:* Patients can be changed over from other sulphonylureas to Glurenorm without interruption. It is usual to start with 30 mg Glurenorm before breakfast, increasing as necessary by increments of 15 mg at mealtimes.

In terms of comparative potency of single doses, 30 mg Glurenorm corresponds approximately to 1,000 mg tolbutamide, 5 mg glibenclamide, 250 mg chlorpropamide or 500 mg acetohexamide. However,

in estimating equivalent total daily doses, the half-lives and duration of action of the respective sulphonylureas must be taken into consideration. Thus it will usually be necessary to administer Glurenorm more frequently than a long-acting sulphonylurea.

*Change-over in non-insulin dependent diabetics previously treated with insulin:* In patients treated with up to 30 i.u. of insulin daily, change-over to Glurenorm may be attempted with an initial dose of 30 mg accompanied by a simultaneous gradual reduction of the amount of insulin, provided the pancreas still contains some functioning β cells. Patients who change from insulin to Glurenorm should be strictly supervised and response assessed by frequent and regular blood-glucose determinations.

It may be possible to reduce the insulin requirements of patients who require more than 30 i.u. daily by the concurrent administration of Glurenorm. Blood-glucose should be monitored frequently during the change-over period.

*Combined treatment:* The administration of metformin with Glurenorm to patients who cannot be adequately controlled by Glurenorm alone may achieve satisfactory stabilisation of blood-glucose levels.

*Children:* Not recommended.

**Contra-indications, warnings, etc**
*Contra-indications:* Do not use for diabetes complicated by acidosis or ketosis nor in patients subject to the stress of surgery or acute infections. Glurenorm should not be used in pregnancy or breast feeding nor in patients with severe hepatic or renal failure, or porphyria.

*Precautions:* Patients who miss a meal (particularly the elderly or debilitated) should be warned not to take their dose of Glurenorm, in order to reduce the risk of a hypoglycaemic reaction.

Special care should be observed in the concomitant use of Glurenorm with many other medications because interactions with sulphonylureas are common.

The effect of Glurenorm may be increased by physical exertion.

*Interactions:* The effect of Glurenorm may be increased by alcohol, salicylates, sulphonamides, phenylbutazone, ethionamide, coumarin anticoagulants, chloramphenicol, tetracyclines, cyclophosphamide, MAO inhibitors, tuberculostatics, β-adrenergic blocking agents, azapropazone, co-trimoxazole, miconazole and sulphinpyrazone.

It may be necessary to increase the dose of Glurenorm when any of the following are administered concurrently: oral contraceptives, chlorpromazine, sympathomimetic agents, corticosteroids, thyroid hormones, nicotinic acid preparations, rifampicin, diazoxide and loop or thiazide diuretics.

The effects of barbiturates, vasopressin and oral anticoagulants are potentiated by the administration of Glurenorm.

*Side-effects:* Glurenorm is generally well tolerated, but minor skin allergies, gastric upsets and other nonspecific symptoms have been noted.

Reversible leucopenia has been reported on one occasion and reversible thrombocytopenia twice, but a causal connection with Glurenorm was not established.

Hypoglycaemic reactions are infrequent, but may be accompanied by malaise, impaired concentration and altered consciousness. They may be treated with oral carbohydrate or with intravenous dextrose if the oral route is impractical. Glucagon (1 mg subcutaneously) could also be given.

*Overdosage:* In the conscious patient, hypoglycaemia may be managed by the oral administration of glucose. In the comatose patient, parenteral administration of glucose by intravenous infusion should be instituted. The patient should be kept under observation for further signs of hypoglycaemia. Consideration may be given to the recovery of ingested tablets by gastric lavage.

**Pharmaceutical precautions** Nil.

**Legal category** POM.

**Package quantities** Bottles of 100 tablets.

**Further information** Gliquidone is a sulphonylurea hypoglycaemic agent. Following oral administration it is rapidly absorbed. Its action normally starts within one hour and its optimal effect lasts two to three hours. The plasma elimination half-life is about 1.4 hours. It is almost completely metabolised in the liver by hydroxylation and demethylation, and excreted principally via the bile. Since only approximately 5% of the administered dose appears in the urine, mainly as inactive metabolites, there is little risk of hypoglycaemia due to drug accumulation in patients with impaired renal function.

Sold under licence from Boehringer Ingelheim International GmbH.

Product licence number 11723/0037.

# HEXOPAL* TABLETS AND SUSPENSION HEXOPAL FORTE

**Presentation** 1. Hexopal Tablets are white or almost white, flat tablets with bevelled edges, 12.7 mm in diameter and marked with a stylised Hv on one side and scored on the other. Each tablet contains 500 mg Inositol Nicotinate BP.

2. Hexopal Suspension is a smooth white fluid with a sweet odour and taste which contains 1000 mg Inositol Nicotinate BP in each 5 ml. It also contains a mixture of hydroxybenzoate esters as preservative.

3. Hexopal Forte. White or almost white, oval, biconvex tablets marked HEX750 on one side and scored on the other. Each tablet contains 750 mg Inositol Nicotinate BP.

**Uses** Hexopal is indicated for the symptomatic relief of severe intermittent claudication and Raynaud's phenomenon.

**Dosage and administration** Hexopal is for oral administration only.

*Adults including the elderly:* The usual dose is 3 g daily (5 ml Hexopal Suspension or two Hexopal tablets three times a day or two Hexopal Forte tablets twice daily). The dose may be increased to 4 g daily if necessary.

*Children:* Not recommended.

**Contra-indications, warnings, etc** There are no known contra-indications or precautions associated with the use of Hexopal, and side-effects are uncommon but may include flushing, dizziness, nausea, vomiting and hypotension.

There is no evidence of the safety of Hexopal in human pregnancy, nor is there adequate evidence from animal work that it is free from hazard. The use of Hexopal in pregnancy should therefore be avoided unless there is no safer alternative. Hexopal appears to be virtually non-toxic to animals even in doses up to 100 times the normal therapeutic level.

Despite extensive clinical experience in Britain since 1959, no case of poisoning or overdosage with Hexopal has been reported. In an emergency, it is suggested that the stomach should be emptied by gastric lavage and the patient be treated symptomatically.

**Pharmaceutical precautions** Tablets: Store below 25°C. Suspension: Store at room temperature.

**Legal category** P.

**Package quantities** Hexopal Tablets: Blister packs of 100 and bottles of 500. Hexopal Suspension: Bottles of 300 ml. Hexopal Forte: Bottles of 250 and as Hexopal Forte C-Pak in calendar packs of 112 (OP).

**Further information** Patients with peripheral vascular disease are likely to benefit from stopping or reducing smoking and from control of their weight. It is recommended that patients be so advised.

**Product licence numbers**
Hexopal Tablets      11723/0040
Hexopal Suspension   11723/0039
Hexopal Forte        11723/0038

# HYPAQUE* 25% AND 45%

**Presentation** Hypaque is a sterile, almost colourless aqueous solution in clear glass ampoules or infusion bottles containing either 25% w/v or 45% w/v Sodium Diatrizoate BP. Hypaque 25% and 45% contain sodium calcium edetate.

**Uses** An X-ray radiographic contrast medium suitable for intravenous and retrograde urography, angiography, venography and many other specialised procedures including examination of the gastro-intestinal tract.

**Dosage and administration** The route of administration of Hypaque, which may be parenteral, oral or rectal, and the volume and concentration employed depend on the procedure being undertaken.

*Parenteral administration:* suggested strength and quantity according to procedure.

| Procedure | Strength (%) | Amount of medium used (ml) | |
|---|---|---|---|
| | | Adults and elderly | Children |
| Urography: | | | |
| i.v. | 45 | 0.5–2.0/kg | as adult |
| infusion | 25 | 4.0/kg | as adult |
| retrograde | 25–45 | 5–20 | as adult |
| Cystography | 10–45 | 500–1500 | 100–300 |
| Peripheral arteriography | 45 | 20–40 | 10–20 |
| Haemorrhoidal portal venography | 45 | 30–40 | 15–20 |
| Renal cyst puncture | 25–45 | 5–60 | 5–20 |
| Orbital phlebography | 45 | 2–4 | 1–2 |
| Intraosseous venography | 45 | 20–45 | — |
| Choledochography: | | | |
| percutaneous transhepatic | 25–45 | 15 | 5 |
| operative | 25–45 | 5–20 | 5 |
| post-op. 'T' tube | 25–45 | 5–20 | 5 |
| Hysterosalpingography | 45 | 10 | — |
| Arthrography | 25–45 | 5–20 | 3–10 |
| Sinography | 45 | 20–40 | — |
| Tube screening (gastric including acute abdomen) | 25 | 5–20 | — |
| Abdominal stab wounds | 25 | q.s. | q.s. |
| Dacryocystography | 45 | 1–3 | — |
| Vesiculography | 45 | 1.5–2.0 to a total of 10–12 each side | — |
| Myography | 45 | 3 | — |
| Duct mammography | 25 | 1–2 | — |
| Discography | 45 | 0.5 max. 2.0 | — |

*Oral or rectal administration in examination of the gastro-intestinal tract:* For adults including the elderly, an average dose of 100 ml to 150 ml of a 25–50% solution is suggested when given by mouth or tube. From 500 ml to 1,000 ml of 20–35% solution is suggested as an enema.

For infants or children the dose by mouth or tube may vary from 50 ml to 120 ml of a 10–25% solution, and by enema from 100 ml to 500 ml of a 10–15% solution may be used.

**Contra-indications, warnings, etc**

*Contra-indications:* Hypaque should not be used for myelography. Injection of even a small amount into the subarachnoid space may produce convulsions and result in fatality.

Hypaque should not be used in patients with proven or suspected hypersensitivity to iodine-containing contrast media.

*Precautions:* Particular caution should be exercised in patients with a history of allergy, atopy, asthma, cardiac disease, or a previous adverse reaction with any contrast medium as they may be at higher risk from developing anaphylaxis or cardiovascular collapse. Consideration should be given to the use of low osmolar radiocontrast media in such patients.

Ready availability of emergency resuscitation equipment and familiarity with procedures are prerequisites for the safe use of radiocontrast media.

Recent reports of thyroid storm occurring following the intravascular use of iodinated radio-opaque diagnostic agents in patients with hyperthyroidism or with an autonomously functioning thyroid nodule suggest that this additional risk be evaluated in such patients before use of Hypaque.

In patients with subarachnoid haemorrhage, a rare association between contrast media administration and clinical deterioration, including convulsions and death, has been reported. Therefore, administration of intravascular iodated ionic contrast media to these patients should be undertaken with caution.

Caution should be observed in patients with tuberculosis since it has been suggested that iodine could exacerbate active tuberculosis, although this has not been reported with Hypaque.

Serious, rarely fatal, thromboembolic events causing myocardial infarction and stroke have been reported during angiographic procedures with both ionic and nonionic contrast media. Therefore, meticulous intravascular administration technique is necessary, particularly during angiographic procedures, to minimise thromboembolic events. Numerous factors, including length of procedure, catheter and syringe material, underlying disease state and concomitant medications may contribute to the development of thromboembolic events. For these reasons, meticulous angiographic techniques are recommended including close attention to guidewire and catheter manipulation, use of manifold systems and/or three-way stopcocks, frequent catheter flushing with heparinised saline solutions and minimising the length of the procedure. The use of plastic syringes in

place of glass syringes has been reported to decrease but not eliminate the likelihood of in vitro clotting.

Although Hypaque is not contra-indicated in patients with advanced renal destruction associated with severe uraemia, or in those with severe hepatic disorders, potentially hazardous situations requiring particular care are oliguric renal failure, myeloma and combined renal and hepatic failure. No attempt should be made to dehydrate the uraemic patient, nor should dehydration be carried out in a patient with myeloma. Evidence suggests that, in the latter case, it is dehydration rather than the presence of myeloma protein which has been the cause of adverse effects. Prior purgation should be avoided.

Because of the possibility of inducing a temporary suppression of urine, it is wise to allow an interval of at least 24 hours before repeating excretory or retrograde pyelography in patients with unilateral reduction of normal renal function.

Contrast media may promote sickling in individuals who are homozygous for sickle cell disease when the material is injected intravenously or intra-arterially.

Administration of radio-opaque materials to patients known or suspected of having phaeochromocytoma should be performed with extreme caution. If, in the opinion of the physician, the possible benefits of such procedures outweigh the considered risks, the procedures may be performed; however, the amount of radio-opaque medium injected should be kept to an absolute minimum. The blood pressure should be assessed throughout the procedure and measures for treatment of a hypertensive crisis should be available.

In examinations of the gastro-intestinal tract, Hypaque should be used with caution in infants and debilitated elderly patients because hypovolaemia may develop due to the osmotic activity of the contrast material in the intestines.

*Use in pregnancy and lactation:* X-ray examinations should be avoided during pregnancy. Animal reproduction studies have not been carried out with Hypaque, and it is not known whether it can cause foetal harm when administered to a pregnant woman. Hypaque can be transferred across the placenta to the foetus, and may also appear in breast milk. Hypaque therefore should only be administered to pregnant women when absolutely necessary. Caution should be observed in its administration to nursing mothers.

*Interactions:* Organic iodine contrast media are known to remain in the blood serum of patients for periods varying from two days to several years in concentrations sufficient to interfere with tests of thyroid function such as protein-bound iodine determinations. It has been reported that sodium diatrizoate remains in the serum for four days. It is therefore advisable to perform such thyroid function tests before any examination involving the use of Hypaque.

Other tests which may be affected by sodium diatrizoate, and for which an interval of 2 or 3 days should be allowed between administration and testing include:

*Blood tests:* Diatrizoate salts significantly inhibit all stages of coagulation. The fibrinogen concentration, and factors V, VII and VIII are decreased. Prothrombin time and thromboplastin time are increased.

Platelet aggregation: High levels of plasma diatrizoates inhibit platelet aggregation.

Serum calcium: Diatrizoate salts may decrease serum calcium levels. However, this depletion of serum calcium may also be the result of the addition of chelating agents (edetate disodium) in the preparation of certain contrast media.

Red cell counts: Transitory decreases in red cell counts. Technetium-99m-RBC labelling interference.

Leukocyte counts: Decrease following injection.

Urea nitrogen (BUN): Transitory increase.

Serum creatinine: Transitory increase.

*Urine tests:* Urine osmolarity and specific gravity may be decreased due to induced diuresis. Diatrizoate in urine cultures may inhibit bacterial growth.

Albumin: crystals of diatrizoic acid may separate out on acidification with mineral acid but these crystals are easily distinguished from the amorphous albumin precipitate. Hypaque does not affect the acetic acid or heat coagulation tests.

*Side-effects:* Approximately 95 per cent of adverse reactions accompanying the intravascular use of diatrizoate salts are of mild to moderate severity. However, life-threatening reactions and fatalities, including cardiovascular collapse and anaphylactic shock, have occurred.

Adverse reactions to injectable contrast media fall into two categories: chemotoxic reactions and idiosyncratic reactions.

Chemotoxic reactions result from the physicochemical properties of the contrast media, the dose, and the speed of injection. All haemodynamic disturbances and injuries to organs or vessels perfused by the contrast medium are included in this category.

Idiosyncratic reactions occur more frequently in patients 20 to 40 years old and may or may not be dependent on the amount of dose injected, the speed or the mode of injection, and the radiographic procedure. They are subdivided into minor, intermediate, and severe. The minor reactions are self-limiting and of short duration; the severe reactions are life-threatening and treatment is urgent and mandatory.

Most adverse reactions to injectable contrast media appear within one to three minutes after the start of injection, but delayed reactions may occur.

The reported incidence of adverse reactions to contrast media in patients with a history of allergy is twice that of the general population. Patients with a history of previous reactions to a contrast medium are three times more susceptible than other patients. However, sensitivity to contrast media does not appear to increase with repeated examinations.

Adverse reactions are grouped below by system organ class and are listed in decreasing order of occurrence. Significantly more severe reactions are listed before the other reactions regardless of frequency.

Body as a whole: Reported incidences of death range from 6.6 per 1 million (0.00066 percent) to 1 in 10,000 patients (0.01 percent). Most deaths occur during injection or 5 to 10 minutes later, the main feature being cardiac arrest with cardiovascular disease as the main aggravating factor.

Isolated reports of hypotensive collapse and shock following urography are found in the literature. The incidence of shock is estimated to occur in 1 out of 20,000 (0.005 percent) patients.

*Greater than 1 in 100 patients:* Cardiovascular system: The most frequent adverse reaction to diatrizoate salts is vasodilation (feeling of warmth). The estimated incidence is 49 percent.

Digestive system: Nausea 6 percent, vomiting 3 percent.

Nervous system: Paraesthesia 6 percent, dizziness 5 percent.

Respiratory system: Rhinitis 1 percent, increased cough 2 percent.

Skin and appendages: Urticaria 1 percent. Pain at the injection site is estimated to occur in about 12 percent of the patients undergoing urography. Pain is usually due to extravasation.

Painful hot erythematous swelling above the venipuncture site was estimated to occur in more than one percent of the patients undergoing phlebography.

Special senses: Perversion of taste 11 percent, and numbness.

Urogenital system: Osmotic nephrosis of the proximal tubular cells is estimated to occur in 23 percent of patients following excretory urography.

*Less than 1 in 100 patients*

Other infrequently reported reactions without accompanying incidence rates are listed below, grouped by organ system.

Body as a whole: Malaria relapse, uraemia, high creatinine and BUN, thrombocytopenia, leukopenia and anaemia.

Cardiovascular system: Cerebral haematomas, haemodynamic disturbances, sinus brachycardia, transient electrocardiographic abnormalities, ventricular fibrillation, and petechiae.

Digestive system: Severe unilateral or bilateral swelling of the parotid and submaxillary glands.

Nervous system: Convulsions, paralysis, coma and agitation.

Respiratory system: Asthma, dyspnoea, laryngeal oedema, pulmonary oedema, bronchospasm and respiratory arrest.

Skin and appendages: Extravasation necrosis, urticaria with or without pruritus, mucocutaneous oedema, and angioneurotic oedema.

Special senses: Bilateral ocular irritation, lacrimation, itching, conjunctival chemosis, infection, and conjunctivitis.

Urogenital: Renal failure, pain.

**Pharmaceutical precautions** The sterile aqueous solutions are clear and almost colourless. Hypaque solutions should not be re-autoclaved because of the possibility of free amine production. Solutions should be protected from light.

**Legal category** POM.

**Package quantities** *Hypaque 25%:* 20 ml ampoules in boxes of 5. Infusion bottles of 250 ml or 350 ml. *Hypaque 45%:* 20 ml ampoules in boxes of 20.

**Further information** The radio-opacity of sodium diatrizoate is due to the presence of iodine which absorbs X-rays.

**Product licence numbers**

| | |
|---|---|
| Hypaque 25% | 11723/0041 |
| Hypaque 45% | 11723/0042 |

## HYPAQUE* SODIUM POWDER

**Qualitative and quantitative composition** Active constituents: Sodium Diatrizoate BP 500.0 g.

**Pharmaceutical form** Powder.

**Clinical particulars**

*Therapeutic indications:* Hypaque Sodium Powder is used in the preparation of radiographic contrast media for examination of the gastrointestinal tract and for use in retrograde cystography and micturating urethrography.

*Posology and method of administration:*

*Administration:* Hypaque Sodium Powder is used for the preparation of solutions for oral and rectal administration and for introduction into the bladder via a urinary catheter. Hypaque Sodium Powder is not suitable for the preparation of injectable solutions.

*Recommended dosage:*

*(a) Examination of the gastro-intestinal tract:*

*Adults:* For adults an average dose of from 100 to 150 ml of a 25–50% solution is suggested when given by mouth or by tube. From 500 ml to 1,000 ml of 20–35% solution is suggested as an enema.

*Children:* The oral or tube dose may vary from 50 ml to 120 ml of a 10–25% solution, and as an enema from 100 ml to 500 ml of a 10–15% solution.

*Elderly:* As for adults, but see *Precautions.*

The solvent may be water, saline or Ringer's solution. For oral use, suitable flavouring such as vanilla or chocolate syrup may be helpful in masking the taste of Hypaque.

*(b) Retrograde cystography and micturating urethrography:* There is some variation in the strength and quantity of medium employed. However, for urethrography 5 ml to 20 ml of a 25–45% solution is recommended for both adults and children. For cystography the recommendation for adults is 500 ml to 1500 ml of a 10–45% solution, and the recommendation for children is 100 ml–300 ml of a 10–45% solution. To sterilise, 0.012% w/v sodium calcium edetate should be added to the solution which is then autoclaved at 10 lb per sq in (115–116°C) for 30 minutes.

*Contra-indications:* No specific statement.

*Special warnings and special precautions for use:* A solution of Hypaque Sodium in water greater than 10% is hypertonic. Therefore, care should be taken when such solutions are used to examine the gastrointestinal tracts of infants and debilitated elderly patients, since hypovolaemia may develop due to the osmotic activity of the contrast material in the intestines. It is advisable to correct any electrolyte disturbances before using solutions that are extremely hypertonic.

Patients with a history of allergy, especially to iodine, require careful consideration since Hypaque may be absorbed, though in very small amounts, through the intestinal wall.

Caution is advised in patients with tuberculosis since it has been suggested that iodine could exacerbate active tuberculosis, although this has not been reported with Hypaque.

*Interaction with other medicaments and other forms of interaction:* The presence of sodium diatrizoate in the serum may interfere with tests of thyroid function such as protein bound iodine determinations. It is therefore advisable to perform such thyroid function tests before any examination involving the use of Hypaque.

*Pregnancy and lactation:* X-ray examinations should be avoided during pregnancy. Animal reproduction studies have not been carried out with Hypaque, and it is not known whether Hypaque can cause foetal harm when administered to a pregnant woman. Hypaque can be transferred across the placenta to the foetus, and may also appear in breast milk. Hypaque therefore should only be administered to pregnant women when absolutely necessary. Caution should be observed in its administration to nursing mothers.

*Effects on ability to drive and use machines:* No specific statement.

*Undesirable effects:* Nausea and diarrhoea have been occasionally reported with Hypaque Sodium Powder and dehydration from fluid loss in such cases must be borne in mind. Rarely, the following have been reported: pulmonary oedema following accidental aspiration, colonic overdistension and perforation, mucosal damage due to prolonged contact, and precipitation of the medium as a solid mass in the stomach. Irritation of the urethral and vesicular mucosa has occasionally followed administration into the bladder.

Minor allergic disturbances such as sneezing, rhinorrhoea, lacrimation and pruritus or urticarial rashes may occasionally occur, and should respond to antihistamine treatment.

*Overdosage:* No specific statement.

**Pharmacological properties**

*Pharmacodynamic properties:* Sodium diatrizoate is a radiopaque contrast medium. Its radioopacity is due to the presence of iodine which absorbs X-rays.

*Pharmacokinetic properties:* Hypaque Sodium Powder is diluted to the required concentration and is administered directly into the area to be visualised. Hence its diagnostic value is independent of its pharmacokinetic properties. Following oral administration to adults, Hypaque passes unchanged through the gastrointestinal tract. A very small amount is absorbed through the intestinal wall, since traces of iodine are excreted by the kidney. Absorption from the gastrointestinal tract occurs to a greater extent in infants.

*Preclinical safety data:* There are no pre-clinical data of relevance to the prescriber which are additional to that already included in other sections of the SPC.

**Pharmaceutical particulars**

*List of excipients:* None.

*Incompatibilities:* No specific statement.

*Shelf life:* 60 months.

*Special precautions for storage:* None.

*Nature and contents of container:* Hypaque Sodium Powder is packed in amber round glass bottles with black plastic caps.

*Instructions for use/handling:* No specific statement.

**Marketing authorisation number** 11723/0043

**Date of approval/revision of SPC** July 1996.

**Legal category** P.

## KANNASYN* POWDER

**Qualitative and quantitative composition** Kanamycin Acid Sulphate PhEur, equivalent to 1 g kanamycin base.

**Pharmaceutical form** A white or almost white crystalline sterile powder for reconstitution for injection.

**Clinical particulars**

*Therapeutic indications:* Kannasyn is recommended for the treatment of infections due to Gram-negative organisms resistant to other antibiotics. It may also be used in the treatment of certain staphylococcal infections due to multiple-resistant strains, and in gonorrhoea.

*Posology and method of administration:* For intravenous or intramuscular administration.

*(i) Intramuscular injections:* Kannasyn should be given as a solution containing 250 mg/ml. This can be prepared by dissolving the contents of a 1 g vial in 4 ml of Water for Injections PhEur.

*Adults:* In acute infections: 1 g daily in two or four equally divided doses. Therapy should normally be limited to six days' treatment, and should not exceed a total of 10 g.

In chronic infections: 3 g weekly (1 g on alternate days) or 1 g twice a day, twice weekly (4 g weekly). The total amount administered should not exceed 50 g.

*Children:* In acute infections: 15 mg/kg body weight daily in 2–4 equally divided doses for no more than six days.

In chronic infections: There are no specific dosage recommendations.

*Elderly:* A reduced dosage may be required. See Warnings.

*(ii) Intravenous use:* This route is recommended only for gravely ill patients with overwhelming infections or with impending cardiovascular collapse. Kannasyn may be given as a solution containing 2.5 mg/ml by slow intravenous infusion at the rate of 3–4 ml per minute. This solution may be prepared by dissolving the contents of a 1 g vial in 400 ml Sodium Chloride Intravenous Infusion BP or Glucose Intravenous Infusion BP.

The dosage for both adults and children is 15–30 mg/kg body weight daily in 2 or 3 divided doses.

*Contra-indications:* Kannasyn is contra-indicated in patients with a history of hypersensitivity or toxic reaction to kanamycin or other aminoglycosides.

*Special warnings and special precautions for use:* In cases of impaired renal function, the kidney may be unable to eliminate kanamycin effectively and as a result the serum level will rise quickly. In these conditions reduced doses are necessary to avoid toxic effects. It has been reported that kanamycin is retained in the serum of patients with renal disease for a considerable time. If it is necessary to give the antibiotic to anuric patients, they should not receive increments more frequently than every three to four days and these increments should be one half the loading dose used. The safest procedure, however, is to control the dosage by monitoring the plasma level to prevent it rising above 30 mcg/ml.

Kannasyn should be protected from light. The powder may be stored at room temperature but should be used within three years of assay. Solutions of Kannasyn should be used immediately or stored at 2–8°C for not more than 24 hours.

Kannasyn should always be administered with caution and preferably only in severe or resistant infections caused by organisms known to be sensitive to the compound and blood levels should not be allowed to rise above 30 mcg/ml.

Caution should be observed also in myasthenia gravis because kanamycin has a weak curare-like action.

*Interactions with other medicaments and other forms of interaction:* The use of potent diuretics such as ethacrynic acid or frusemide with kanamycin should be avoided because they are known to potentiate the toxic action of aminoglycoside antibiotics.

As with other aminoglycoside antibiotics, apnoea and respiratory depression have been reported following the intraperitoneal use of kanamycin because of its curare-like effect. In addition, motor and sensory neuropathy has occurred following local application of kanamycin during spinal surgery. It has also produced slight weakening in muscle strength in a patient with myasthenia gravis. Because of these effects, it has been suggested that kanamycin should not be given intraperitoneally during surgery to patients who have received neuro-muscular blocking agents. Calcium gluconate has been suggested to counteract this curare-like action of kanamycin, but neostigmine appears to be more effective.

It has been shown that calcium can inhibit the antibacterial activity of kanamycin against certain organisms and for this reason the routine prophylactic use of calcium solution with intraperitoneal kanamycin should be discouraged.

It should be noted that prior treatment with streptomycin or viomycin may increase the likelihood of a nephrotoxic reaction with kanamycin.

Concurrent aminoglycosides may increase the risk of ototoxicity as may anti-emetics by masking its development. The dose of concurrent oral anticoagulant may require alteration because kanamycin may affect endogenous vitamin K.

*Pregnancy and lactation:* Kanamycin should not be used during pregnancy or lactation.

*Effects on ability to drive and use machines:* There are no specific warnings.

*Undesirable effects:* Local intolerance to intramuscular injection has sometimes been reported, but it is transient and does not require interruption of therapy. Ecchymoses have also been observed at the site of injection in a few patients. It has been suggested that in concentrations above those achieved in the blood at therapeutic dosage, kanamycin has anticoagulant action which may explain haematomas at the site of injection. Sensitivity rashes appear to be uncommon. Intravenous injections are well tolerated and pain is not a problem. Thrombophlebitis has only been reported once in a patient who was receiving 50 million units of penicillin with the kanamycin.

Particular caution should be observed in those with hearing loss. In common with certain other antibiotics, kanamycin can damage the eighth cranial nerve when used in large doses or for long periods. The resultant hearing loss, which may be permanent, is usually but not always preceded by tinnitus. Vestibular damage is less common. Should tinnitus or other sign of auditory toxicity appear, the dose of kanamycin should be reduced or it should be discontinued.

Hyaline and granular casts are sometimes observed in urine samples collected in the first 16 hours after administration in patients who have been given high doses of kanamycin. In these cases no permanent impairment of renal function occurs and the casts disappear within a few days of stopping treatment. Although nephrotoxic effects have been reported in some studies, serious renal toxicicty is not a frequent problem with the doses now used.

*Overdose:* In cases of overdosage or toxic reaction, haemodialysis or peritoneal dialysis will aid the removal of kanamycin from the blood.

### Pharmacological properties

*Pharmacodynamic properties:* Kannasyn is recommended for the treatment of infections due to Gram-negative organisms resistant to other antibiotics. It may also be used in the treatment of certain staphylococcal infections due to multiple-resistant strains, and in gonorrhoea.

*Pharmacokinetic properties:* After intramuscular injection, peak concentrations of kanamycin of about 20 and 30 micrograms per ml are attained in about one hour following doses of 0.5 g and 1 g respectively. A plasma half-life of about 3 hours has been reported.

Kanamycin is rapidly excreted by glomerular filtration and most of a parenteral dose appears in the urine within 24 hours. It has been detected in cord blood and breast milk.

### Pharmaceutical particulars

*List of excipients:* None.

*Incompatibilities:* Infusion solutions containing kanamycin have been reported to be incompatible with the following substances: amphotericin, barbiturates, cephalothin sodium, chlorpromazine, electrolytes ($Ca^{++}$, $Mg^{++}$, citrate or phosphate ions), heparin, hydrocortisone, methicillin sodium, methohexitone, nitrofurantoin, phenytoin, prochlorperazine, sulphafurazole.

*Shelf life:* 36 months.

*Special precautions for storage:* Kannasyn should be protected from light. The powder may be stored at room temperature but should be used within three years of assay. Solutions of Kannasyn should be used immediately or stored at 2–8°C for not more than 24 hours.

*Nature and contents of container:* Amber glass vials containing 1.43 g Kannasyn each, enclosed in cardboard cartons.

*Instructions for use/handling*
*Intramuscular injection:* Prepare by dissolving the contents of a 1 g vial in 4 ml of Water for Injections PhEur.

*Intravenous use:* Prepare by dissolving the contents of a 1 g vial in 400 ml Sodium Chloride Intravenous Infusion BP or Glucose Intravenous Infusion BP.

**Marketing authorisation number** 11723/0044.

**Date of approval/revision of SPC** 12 October 1993.

**Legal category** POM.

## LEVOPHED*

**Presentation** Levophed is a clear, colourless or almost-colourless solution providing 2 mg/ml Noradrenaline Acid Tartrate USP which is equivalent to 1 mg/ml noradrenaline base. Levophed Solution also contains sodium metabisulphite and sodium chloride. This preparation has also been referred to as 1:1,000 noradrenaline base.

**Uses** Levophed is for intravenous use only. It is recommended for use as an emergency measure in the restoration of blood pressure in cases of acute hypotension.

### Dosage and administration
*Route and method of infusion:* Levophed should be administered in a diluted solution via a central venous catheter. The infusion should be at a controlled rate using either a syringe pump or an infusion pump or a drip counter.

*Dilution instructions:* Levophed should be diluted either with dextrose 5%, or with isotonic dextrose saline.

*Adults:* Either add 2 ml of Levophed to 48 ml 5% dextrose for administration by syringe pump, *or* add 20 ml of Levophed to 480 ml 5% dextrose for administration by drip counter.

In both cases the final concentration of the infusion solution is 80 mg/litre noradrenaline acid tartrate, which is equivalent to 40 mg/litre noradrenaline base.

If other dilutions are used check the calculation carefully before starting treatment.

*Initial rate of infusion:* The initial rate of infusion should be between 10 ml/hour and 20 ml/hour (0.16 ml/min to 0.32 ml/min).

This is equivalent to 0.8 mg/hr to 1.6 mg/hr noradrenaline acid tartrate (or 0.4 mg/hr to 0.8 mg/hr noradrenaline base).

*Titration of dose:* Once an infusion of Levophed has been established the dose should be titrated according to the pressor effect observed. There is great individual variation in the dose required to attain and maintain normotension. The aim should be to establish a low normal systolic blood pressure (100–120 mmHg) or to achieve an adequate mean arterial blood pressure (greater than 80 mmHg).

*Duration of treatment/monitoring*
Levophed should be continued for as long as vasoactive drug support is indicated. The patient should be monitored carefully for the duration of Levophed therapy.

*Elderly:* As for adults but see Precautions.

*Children:* Not recommended.

### Contra-indications, warnings, etc
Levophed should be used only in conjunction with appropriate blood volume replacement.

The use of pressor amines during cyclopropane or halothane anaesthesia may cause serious cardiac arrhythmias. Because of the possibility of increasing the risk of ventricular fibrillation, Levophed should be used with caution in patients receiving these or any other cardiac sensitising agent or who exhibit profound hypoxia or hypercarbia.

Levophed should be used with extreme caution in patients receiving monoamine oxidase inhibitors or tricyclic antidepressants because severe, prolonged hypertension may result. The elderly may be especially sensitive to the effects of noradrenaline. Particular caution should be observed in patients with coronary, mesenteric or peripheral vascular thrombosis because noradrenaline may increase the ischaemia and extend the area of infarction. Similar caution should be observed in patients with hypotension following myocardial infarction and in patients with Prinzmetal's variant angina.

When infusing Levophed, the blood pressure and rate of flow should be checked frequently to avoid hypertension.

Extravasation of the solution may cause local tissue necrosis. The infusion site should be checked frequently. If extravasation occurs, the area should be infiltrated with phentolamine without delay. It has been suggested that phentolamine may be added directly to the infusion flask to act as an antidote against sloughing without affecting the vasopressor activity of the Levophed.

*Pregnancy:* Noradrenaline may impair placental perfusion and induce foetal bradycardia. It may also exert a contractile effect on the pregnant uterus and lead to foetal asphyxia in late pregnancy. These possible risks to the foetus should therefore be weighed against the potential benefit to the mother.

*Side-effects:* Hypertension may occur, which may be associated with bradycardia as well as headache and peripheral ischaemia, including gangrene of the extremities. Cardiac arrhythmias may arise when Levophed is used in conjunction with cardiac sensitising agents, and may be more likely in patients with hypoxia or hypercarbia. Prolonged administration may result in plasma volume depletion.

*Overdosage:* Overdosage may result in severe hypertension, reflex bradycardia, marked increase in peripheral resistance and decreased cardiac output. These may be accompanied by violent headache, photophobia, retrosternal pain, pallor, intense sweating and vomiting.

In the event of overdosage, treatment should be withdrawn and appropriate corrective treatment initiated.

**Pharmaceutical precautions** Protect from light. Store below 25°C. The solution should not be used if it is brown in colour. Levophed is best administered in 5% dextrose or dextrose saline solution because the dextrose protects against significant loss of potency due to oxidation. Deterioration occurs more rapidly in normal saline than in dextrose solution.

Infusion solutions containing noradrenaline acid tartrate have been reported to be incompatible with the following substances: alkalis and oxidising agents, barbiturates, chlorpheniramine, chlorothiazide, nitrofurantoin, novobiocin, phenytoin, sodium bicarbonate, sodium iodide, streptomycin.

**Legal category** POM.

**Package quantities** Boxes of six 2 ml or 4 ml ampoules. Boxes of five 20 ml ampoules.

**Further information** Nil.

**Product licence number** 11723/0047

## LEVOPHED* SPECIAL

**Qualitative and quantitative composition** Each ampoule provides 200 micrograms/ml Noradrenaline Acid Tartrate PhEur which is equivalent to 100 micrograms/ml of noradrenaline base. Other ingredients used are sodium metabisulphite and sodium chloride.

**Pharmaceutical form** Clear sterile solution for parenteral use.

### Clinical particulars
*Therapeutic indications:* Levophed Special is for parenteral use only. It is recommended as an emergency measure in the management of cardiac arrest to help restore and maintain blood pressure.

*Posology and method of administration: Adults:* In cases of cardiac standstill the rapid intravenous or intracardiac of 0.50–0.75 ml of Levophed Special may restore a recordable blood pressure for one to four minutes. After intravenous injection the solution should be massaged towards the heart.

A similar dose may be repeated when the blood pressure starts to fall again, or blood pressure can be maintained with a normal Levophed drip. If there is no response to Levophed Special administered intravenously, cardiac massage should be started with the injection of 0.50–0.75 ml Levophed Special into the ascending aorta or into the left atrium. Injection into the ventricle should be avoided because of the possible risk of inducing fibrillation. If the myocardium is fibrillating, a dose of Levophed Special may be injected after normal rhythm has been restored by massage or by electrical defibrillation.

*Elderly:* As for adults but see *Special Precautions.*

*Children:* Not recommended.

*Contra-indications:* The use of pressor amine during cyclopropane or halothane anaesthesia may cause serious cardiac arrhythmias. Because of the possibility of increasing the risk of ventricular fibrillation, Levophed Special should be used with caution in patients receiving these or any other cardiac sensitising agent or who exhibit profound hypoxia or hypercarbia.

*Special warnings and special precautions for use:* Levophed Special should be used in conjunction with appropriate blood volume replacement. There are no special warnings and precautions.

The elderly may be especially sensitive to the effects of noradrenaline. Caution should be observed in patients with coronary, mesenteric or peripheral vascular thrombosis because noradrenaline may increase the ischaemia and extend the area of infarction.

*Interactions with other medicaments and other forms of interaction:* Levophed Special should be used with extreme caution in patients receiving monoamine oxidase inhibitors or tricyclic antidepressants because severe, prolonged hypertension may result.

*Pregnancy and lactation:* Noradrenaline may impair placental perfusion and induce foetal bradycardia. It may also exert a contractile effect on the pregnant uterus and lead to foetal asphyxia in late pregnancy. These possible risks to the foetus should therefore be weighed against the potential benefit to the mother.

*Undesirable effects:* Hypertension may occur, which may be associated with bradycardia as well as headache and peripheral ischaemia, including gangrene of the extremities. Cardiac arrhythmias may arise when Levophed Special is used in conjunction with cardiac sensitising agents and may be more likely in patients with hypoxia or hypercarbia. Extravasation may cause local tissue necrosis.

*Overdosage:* Overdosage may result in severe hypertension, reflex bradycardia, marked increase in peripheral resistance and decreased cardiac output. These may be accompanied by violent headache, photophobia, retrosternal pain, pallor, intense sweating and vomiting.

In the event of overdosage, treatment should be withdrawn and appropriate corrective treatment initiated.

**Pharmacological properties**

*Pharmacodynamic properties:* The vascular effects of noradrenaline in the doses usually used clinically result from the simultaneous stimulation of the alpha and beta adrenergic receptors in the heart and vascular system. Except in the heart, its action is predominantly on the alpha receptors. This results in an increase in the force and (in the absence of vagal inhibition) in the rate of myocardial contraction. Peripheral resistance increases and diastolic and systolic pressures are raised.

*Pharmacokinetic properties:* Up to 16% of an intravenous dose is excreted unchanged in the urine with methylated and deaminated metabolites in free and conjugated forms.

**Pharmaceutical particulars**

*List of excipients:* Levophed Special also contains sodium metabisulphite, sodium chloride and water for injections.

*Incompatibilities:* There are no major incompatibilities.

*Shelf life:* Levophed Special has a shelf life of 24 months.

*Special precautions for storage:* Protect from light. Store below 25°C. The solution should not be used if it is brown in colour.

*Nature and contents of container:* Glass ampoules contained in cardboard cartons.

**Marketing authorisation number** 11723/0048.

**Date of approval/revision of SPC** 31 March 1995.

**Legal category** POM.

## LINGRAINE*

**Presentation** Lingraine Tablets are light green, biconvex tablets, 6.4 mm in diameter, with no markings. Each tablet contains 2.0 mg Ergotamine Tartrate PhEur. Lingraine Tablets also contain lactose.

**Uses** Lingraine Tablets are recommended for the relief of migraine and other vascular headaches.

**Dosage and administration** Lingraine Tablets are for sublingual administration only.

*Adults:* One tablet to be taken at the first sign of an attack of migraine. If necessary another tablet may be taken half an hour to an hour later. No more than three tablets should be taken in 24 hours and not more than six tablets in any one week.

*Elderly:* As for adults but see warnings.

*Children:* Not recommended.

**Contra-indications, warnings, etc** Since (like other ergot alkaloids) ergotamine tartrate causes contraction of uterine muscle it should not be used during pregnancy. Avoid during breast feeding.

Because ergotamine brings about constriction of peripheral blood vessels Lingraine should not be used in the presence of severe arteriosclerosis, coronary artery disease, thrombophlebitis, Raynaud's syndrome or Buerger's disease. Furthermore, Lingraine should not be used where there is liver or kidney dysfunction, nor in the presence of severe hypertension, hyperthyroidism or porphyria. Concomitant use with beta blockers may increase the risk of peripheral vasoconstriction, whilst with erthromycin, the risk of ergotism.

*Side-effects:* These are a relatively minor problem if the dose is carefully regulated. Nausea and vomiting are most frequently reported; other side-effects encountered include abdominal pain, leg cramps, vertigo, diarrhoea and, occasionally, increased headache. If such symptoms are profound or accompanied by cardiovascular or neurological disturbances, they are indicative of chronic overdosage (see below).

Pleural and peritoneal fibrosis may occur with excessive use.

*Overdosage:* Like all the natural amino-acid alkaloids of ergot, ergotamine is a highly toxic substance which may cause chronic or acute poisoning, although the latter is less frequent.

The oral administration of 26 mg over several days has proved fatal, and there have also been deaths from as little as 0.5 mg to 1.5 mg in a single injection.

The principal signs of chronic overdosage are circulatory disturbances, due to vasoconstriction and thrombi-formation, including coldness of the skin, severe muscle pains, and vascular stasis resulting in dry peripheral gangrene. Anginal pain, tachycardia or bradycardia and hypertension or hypotension may occur. Other symptoms include headache, nausea, vomiting, diarrhoea and weakness of the legs. Confusion, drowsiness, hemiplegia and convulsions may also occur.

The main symptoms of acute poisoning consist of nausea, vomiting, diarrhoea, unquenchable thirst, tingling, itching and coldness of the skin, a rapid and weak pulse, confusion and unconsciousness. Treatment: Amyl nitrate inhalations (0.2–0.3 ml) are suggested to counteract arterial spasm.

**Pharmaceutical precautions** Nil.

**Legal category** POM.

**Package quantities** Lingraine Tablets are available in P.P.F.P. laminate strips in boxes of 12 tablets (OP).

**Further information** Ergotamine is an ergot alkaloid, and acts by antagonism of alpha adrenoceptors.

**Product licence number** 11723/0045.

## MICTRAL* SACHETS

**Qualitative and quantitative composition** Nalidixic Acid BP 660 mg, Sodium Citrate PhEur 3750 mg, Citric Acid PhEur 250 mg, Sodium Bicarbonate PhEur 250 mg.

**Pharmaceutical form** Granules which are dissolved in water and suitable for oral administration.

**Clinical particulars**

*Therapeutic indications:* For the treatment of cystitis and lower urinary tract infections caused by pathogens sensitive to nalidixic acid.

*Posology and method of administration:*

*Adults:* The contents of one sachet should be dissolved in a tumblerful of water and taken three times a day. A 3 day course is normally sufficient.

*Elderly:* As for adults.

*Children and Growing Adolescents:* Not recommended.

Mictral sachets are for oral administration.

*Contra-indications:* Nalidixic acid should not be given to patients with a history of convulsive disorders, nor should it be used in patients with renal impairment or porphyria or hypersensitivity to nalidixic acid or related compounds.

*Special warnings and special precautions for use:* Nalidixic acid is mainly metabolised by the liver and should therefore be used with caution in patients with liver disease.

Caution should be observed in patients with severe cerebral arteriosclerosis or glucose-6-phosphate dehydrogenase deficiency. Although care should be exercised in treating patients with renal failure, the full dosage of nalidixic acid may be administered in patients with creatinine clearance of more than 20 ml/min and half the normal dosage in patients with creatinine clearance less than this.

Particular caution is advised in patients with a known allergic disposition. Patients taking nalidixic acid should avoid excessive exposure to sunlight (including sunbathing).

When nalidixic acid is given to patients on anticoagulant therapy, it may be necessary to reduce the anticoagulant dosage.

Caution should be observed and therapy discontinued if patients develop signs or symptoms suggestive of an increase in intracranial pressure, psychosis or other toxic manifestations.

Blood count, renal and liver function should be monitored periodically if treatment is continued for more than two weeks.

Each sachet contains the equivalent of 950 mg (41.3 M Eq) of sodium. This should be taken into account when prescribing for patients for whom sodium restriction is indicated especially the elderly.

*Interactions with other medicaments and other forms of interaction:* If nalidixic acid is given to patients on anticoagulant therapy, it may be necessary to reduce the anticoagulant dosage because nalidixic acid may interact with anticoagulants by competing for protein binding sites. Monitoring of prothrombin time and appropriate adjustment of the anticoagulant dosage following introduction and withdrawal of Mictral is recommended.

Active proliferation of the organisms is a necessary condition for the antibacterial action of nalidixic acid; the action of Mictral may therefore be inhibited by the presence of other antibacterial substances especially bacteriostatic agents such as tetracycline, chloramphenicol and nitrofurantoin which is antagonistic to nalidixic acid in vitro.

There have been reports of serious gastro-intestinal toxicity following the concomitant use of nalidixic acid and melphalan.

Probenecid may reduce the efficacy of Mictral by inhibiting tubular secretion of nalidixic acid.

It is possible that there will be an increased risk of nephrotoxicity with cyclosporins.

When testing for glycosuria in patients receiving Mictral, glucose specific methods based on glucose oxidase should be used since copper reduction methods may give false-positive results.

Nalidixic acid, in therapeutic doses can interfere with the estimation of urinary 17-ketosteroids and may cause high results in the assay of urinary vanilmandelic acid (Pisano method).

It is recognised that convulsions may occur due to an interaction between quinolones and non-steroidal anti-inflammatory drugs. This has not been observed so far with nalidixic acid.

*Pregnancy and lactation:* The safety of nalidixic acid during pregnancy has not been established. Therefore it should be used during pregnancy only if the potential benefits outweigh the potential risks, especially during the first trimester (nalidixic acid crosses the placental barrier and has been shown to be taken up by growing cartilage in several animal species) and during the last month of pregnancy because of the potential risk for the neonate exposure to maternal nalidixic acid in utero may lead to significant blood levels of nalidixic acid in the neonate immediately after birth.

Since nalidixic acid is excreted in breast milk, it is contraindicated during lactation.

*Effects on ability to drive and to use machines:* No specific warnings.

*Undesirable effects:* In keeping with the reduced systemic exposure to nalidixic acid which Mictral therapy entails, it is unlikely that Mictral will give rise to the full spectrum of adverse events reported with conventional oral nalidixic acid therapy, which include:

*Central nervous system:* Drowsiness, weakness headache, dizziness and vertigo; subjective visual disturbances such as over-brightness of lights changed colour perception, difficulty in focusing decreased visual acuity and double vision, which are infrequent and usually disappear promptly on reducing dosage or stopping therapy.

Toxic psychosis or brief convulsions, which are rare, have usually followed excessive dosage in patients predisposed by epilepsy or cerebral arteriosclerosis and, very rarely, 6th cranial nerve palsy has been observed. The mechanism of these reactions being unknown but following withdrawal of treatment rapid resolution without sequelae has usually occurred.

*Gastro-intestinal:* Abdominal pain, nausea, vomiting and diarrhoea.

*Allergic:* Rash, pruritus, urticaria, angio-oedema eosinophilia, arthralgia with joint stiffness and swelling and, rarely, anaphylactoid reactions; photosensitivity reactions which include erythema and bullae on exposed surfaces are likely to resolve within 2–8 weeks of stopping therapy but bullae may continue to appear for up to 12 weeks after therapy, with mild skin trauma or exposure to sunlight (see *Warnings*).

*Other:* Rarely, cholestatis, paraesthesia, metaboli

acidosis, thrombocytopenia, leucopenia or haemolytic anaemia, sometimes associated with glucose-6-phosphate dehydrogenase deficiency.

*Overdosage:* Because of the nature of the product, serious overdose is unlikely. An excessive amount of granules is likely to cause vomiting.

In adults, symptoms of overdose have been noted following single doses of 20 and 25 g. These have included toxic psychosis and convulsions. Occasional reports of metabolic acidosis have occurred in association with overdosage or overdose with concurrent use of probenecid. Vomiting, nausea and lethargy may also occur following overdosage. Reactions are likely to be short-lived because nalidixic acid is normally excreted rapidly.

If systemic absorption has occurred, fluid intake should be promoted; supportive measures such as oxygen and means of artificial respiration should be available. Anti-convulsant therapy may be indicated in a severe case, although it has not been used in the few instances of overdosage that have been reported.

**Pharmacological properties**

*Pharmacodynamic properties:* Nalidixic acid is an antibacterial agent which acts by selectively inhibiting bacterial DNA synthesis. The presence of sodium bicarbonate, citric acid and sodium citrate in the formulation is to maintain the urine at optimal pH for nalidixic acid activity and clearance.

*Pharmacokinetic properties:* Nalidixic acid (0.66 g)+sodium citrate (4 g) was given to healthy male volunteers t.i.d for 3 consecutive days. On day 3 the mean peak plasma concentration of nalidixic acid and hydroxynalidixic acid was 2.8 micrograms/ml and 2.6 micrograms/ml respectively. After undergoing metabolism 80–95% of nalidixic acid and its metabolites were excreted in the urine. The presence of the sodium citrate resulted in the urine of the volunteers becoming more alkaline.

*Pre-clinical safety data:* Not applicable.

**Pharmaceutical particulars**

*List of excipients:* Caster sugar, malic acid, dextrose monohydrate, saccharin sodium, polyvidone, sodium lauryl sulphate, grapefruit flavour 502.107/AP05.51.

*Incompatibilities:* None.

*Shelf life:* The shelf-life of this product is 36 months.

*Special precautions for storage:* Store in a dry place.

*Nature and contents of container:* PPFP sachets containing 7 g of granulate. The sachets are packed into a cardboard carton. Pack sizes of 3 and 9 sachets.

*Instructions for use/handling:* Not applicable.

**Marketing authorisation number** 11723/0049

**Date of approval/revision of SPC** December 1996.

**Legal category** POM.

## MODALIM* TABLETS

**Qualitative and quantitative composition** Each tablet contains 100 mg ciprofibrate.

**Pharmaceutical form** Tablet.

**Clinical particulars**

*Therapeutic indications:* Modalim tablets are recommended for the treatment of primary dyslipoproteinaemias, including types IIa, IIb, III and IV (hypercholesterolaemia, hypertriglyceridaemia and combined forms) – refractory to appropriate dietary treatment. Dietary measures should be continued during therapy.

*Posology and method of administration*

*Adults:* The recommended dosage is one tablet (100 mg ciprofibrate). This dose should not be exceeded (see *Precautions*).

*Elderly patients:* As for adults, but see *Precautions and Warnings.*

*Use in case of impaired renal function:* In moderate renal impairment it is recommended that dosage be reduced to one tablet every other day. Patients should be carefully monitored. Modalim should not be used in severe renal impairment.

*Use in children:* Not recommended since safety and efficacy in children has not been established.

Modalim tablets are for oral administration only.

*Contra-indications:* Modalim is contra-indicated in cases of severe hepatic impairment, cases of renal impairment and in pregnancy and lactation.

*Special warnings and special precautions for use:* Patients should be advised to report unexplained muscle pain, tenderness or weakness immediately.

Doses of 200 mg Modalim per day or greater have been associated with a high risk of rhabdomyolysis. Therefore the daily dose should not exceed 100 mg. Hypoalbuminaemia as seen in nephrotic syndrome, or hypothyroidism may increase the risk of myopathy.

Use with caution in patients with impaired renal or hepatic function. Periodic liver function tests are recommended. Modalim treatment should be halted if liver enzyme abnormalities persist.

Secondary causes of dyslipidaemia, such as hypothyroidism, should be excluded or corrected prior to commencing any lipid lowering drug treatment. If after a period of administration lasting several months, a satisfactory reduction in serum lipid concentrations has not been obtained, additional or different therapeutic measures must be considered.

*Interaction with other medicaments and other forms of interaction:* Ciprofibrate is highly protein bound and is therefore capable of displacing other drugs from plasma protein binding sites. There is evidence that ciprofibrate potentiates the pharmacological response to warfarin in man. Therefore the dose of anticoagulant therapy should be reduced and then gradually re-adjusted by monitoring prothrombin time. Although there are no data to show that ciprofibrate interacts with other classes of drugs, a possible interaction with oral hypoglycaemic agents and oral contraceptive agents should be considered. As with other fibrates, the concomitant use of ciprofibrate with HMG-CoA reductase inhibitors, or other fibrates, may predispose patients to myopathy.

*Pregnancy and lactation:* There is no evidence that ciprofibrate is teratogenic but signs of embryotoxicity were observed at high doses in animals. Ciprofibrate is excreted in the breast milk of lactating rats. There are no data on the use of the drug in human pregnancy of lactation. Therefore the use of ciprofibrate is contraindicated during pregnancy and in nursing mothers.

*Effects on ability to drive and use machines:* Dizziness, drowsiness, or tiredness have only rarely been reported in association with ciprofibrate. It is therefore unlikely to affect the ability to drive or to use machinery.

*Undesirable effects:* There have been occasional reports of headache, vertigo, rashes and gastrointestinal symptoms including nausea, vomiting, diarrhoea and dyspepsia. Generally these side effects were mild to moderate in nature and occurred early on during treatment, becoming less frequent with continuation of dosing. As with other drugs in this class, a low incidence of impotence and hair loss has been reported.

As with other fibrates, elevation of serum creatine phosphokinase (CPK), myalgia and myopathy including rare cases of rhabdomyolysis have been reported. If symptoms of muscle toxicity develop the serum CPK should be measured immediately. Treatment should be discontinued if CPK levels are greater than ten times the upper limit of the normal range, if levels rise progressively or if there is other evidence of myopathy. In the majority of cases muscle toxicity is reversible when treatment is withdrawn. Isolated cases of pneumonitis or pulmonary fibrosis have been reported. As with other fibrates, abnormal liver function tests have been observed occasionally.

*Overdose:* Overdosage with ciprofibrate has been reported rarely. Associated adverse events reflect those seen in routine use. There are no specific antidotes to ciprofibrate. Treatment of overdosage should be symptomatic. Gastric lavage and appropriate supportive care may be instituted if necessary. Ciprofibrate is non-dialysable.

**Pharmacological properties**

*Pharmacodynamic properties:* Ciprofibrate is a new derivative of phenoxyisobutyric acid which has a marked hypolipidaemic action. It reduces both LDL and VLDL and hence the levels of triglyceride and cholesterol associated with these lipoprotein fractions. It also increases levels of HDL cholesterol.

Ciprofibrate is effective in the treatment of hyperlipidaemia associated with high plasma concentrations of LDL and VLDL (types IIa, IIb, III and IV according to the Fredrickson Classification). In clinical studies ciprofibrate has been shown to be effective in complementing the dietary treatment of such conditions.

*Pharmacokinetic properties:* Ciprofibrate is readily absorbed in man, with maximum plasma concentrations occurring mainly between one and four hours following an oral dose. Following a single dose of 100 mg, in volunteers, maximum plasma concentration of ciprofibrate was between 21 and 36 micrograms/ml. In patients on chronic therapy, maximum levels from 53 to 165 micrograms/ml have been measured. Terminal elimination half-life in patients on long term therapy varies from 38 to 86 hours. The elimination half-life in subjects with moderate renal insufficiency was slightly increased compared with normal subjects (116.7 h compared with 81.1 h). In subjects with severe renal impairment, a significant increase was noted (171.9 h).

Approximately 30–75% of a single dose administered to volunteers was excreted in the urine in 72 hours, either as unchanged ciprofibrate (20–25% of the total excreted) or as a conjugate. Subjects with moderate renal impairment excreted on average 7.0% of a single dose as unchanged ciprofibrate over 96 hours, compared with 6.9% in normal subjects. In subjects with severe insufficiency this was reduced to 4.7%.

*Preclinical safety data:* There are no preclinical data of relevance to the prescriber which are additional to that already included in other sections of the SPC.

**Pharmaceutical particulars**

*List of excipients:* Maize Starch PhEur, Lactose PhEur, Microcrystalline Cellulose BP, Hydroxypropyl Methylcellulose USP, hydrogenated vegetable oil, Sodium Lauryl Sulphate PhEur.

*Incompatibilities:* None stated.

*Shelf life:* 48 months.

*Special precautions for storage:* There are no special storage precautions.

*Nature and contents of container:* Clear PVC/Aluminium blister strips in packs of 28 tablets. Amber glass bottles of 100 tablets.

*Instructions for use/handling:* None stated.

**Marketing authorisation number** 11723/0050

**Date of approval/revision of SPC** September 1996.

**Legal category** POM.

## MODECATE*

**Qualitative and quantitative composition** The product contains Fluphenazine Decanoate BP 25 mg/ml.

**Pharmaceutical form** Intramuscular injection for administration to human beings.

**Clinical particulars**

*Therapeutic indications:* For the treatment and maintenance of schizophrenic patients and those with paranoid psychoses.

While Modecate injection has been shown to be effective in acute states, it is particularly useful in the maintenance treatment of chronic patients who are unreliable at taking their oral medication, and also of those who do not absorb their oral phenothiazine adequately.

*Posology and method of administration*

*Adults:* It is recommended that patients be stabilised on the injection in hospital.

*Recommended dosage regimes for all indications:* Patients without previous exposure to a depot fluphenazine formulation: Initially 0.5 ml i.e. 12.5 mg (0.25 ml i.e. 6.25 mg for patients over 60) by deep intramuscular injection into the gluteal region.

The onset of action generally appears between 24 and 72 hours after injection and the effects of the drug on psychotic symptoms become significant within 48 to 96 hours. Subsequent injections and the dosage interval are determined in accordance with the patient's response. When administered as maintenance therapy, a single injection may be effective in controlling schizophrenic symptoms for up to four weeks or longer.

It is desirable to maintain as much flexibility in the dose as possible to achieve the best therapeutic response with the least side-effects; most patients are successfully maintained within the dose range 0.5 ml (12.5 mg) to 4.0 ml (100 mg) given at a dose interval of 2 to 5 weeks.

*Patients previously maintained on oral fluphenazine:* It is not possible to predict the equivalent dose of depot formulation in view of the wide variability of individual response.

*Patients previously maintained on depot fluphenazine:* Patients who have suffered a relapse following cessation of depot fluphenazine therapy may be restarted on the same dose, although the frequency of injections may need to be increased in the early weeks of treatment until satisfactory control is obtained.

*Elderly:* Elderly patients may be particularly susceptible to extrapyramidal reactions. Therefore reduced maintenance dosage may be required and a smaller initial dose (see above).

*Children:* Not recommended for children.

Where a smaller volume of injection is desirable, patients may be transferred directly to the equivalent dose of Modecate Concentrate injection on the basis that 1 ml Modecate Concentrate injection is equivalent to 4 ml Modecate injection.

*Note:* The dosage should not be increased without close supervision and it should be noted that there is a variability in individual response.

The response to antipsychotic drug treatment may be delayed. If drugs are withdrawn, recurrence of symptoms may not become apparent for several weeks or months.

*Route of administration:* Intramuscular.

*Contra-indications:* The product is contra-indicated in the following cases: comatose states; marked cerebral atherosclerosis; phaeochromocytoma; renal failure; liver failure; severe cardiac insufficiency; severely depressed states; existing blood dyscrasias; history of hypersensitivity to any of the ingredients.

*Special warnings and special precautions for use:* Caution should be exercised with the following: liver disease; cardiac arrhythmias, cardiac disease; thyrotoxicosis; severe respiratory disease; epilepsy, conditions predisposing to epilepsy (e.g. alcohol withdrawal or brain damage); Parkinson's disease; patients who have shown hypersensitivity to other phenothiazines; personal or family history of narrow angle glaucoma; in very hot weather; the elderly, particularly if frail or at risk of hypothermia; hypothyroidism; myasthenia gravis; prostatic hypertrophy.

*Interaction with other medicaments and other forms of interaction:* The possibility should be borne in mind that phenothiazines may:

1. Increase the central nervous system depression produced by drugs such as alcohol, general anaesthetics, hypnotics, sedatives or strong analgesics.
2. Antagonise the action of adrenaline and other sympathomimetic agents and reverse the blood-pressure-lowering effects of adrenergic-blocking agents such as guanethidine and clonidine.
3. Impair: the anti-parkinsonian effect of L-dopa; the effect of anticonvulsants; metabolism of tricyclic antidepressants; the control of diabetes.
4. Increase the effect of anticoagulants and antidepressants.
5. Interact with lithium.

Anticholinergic effects may be enhanced by anti-parkinsonian or other anticholinergic drugs.

Phenothiazines may enhance: the cardiac-depressant effects of quinidine, the absorption of corticosteroids, digoxin, and neuromuscular blocking agents.

*Pregnancy and lactation*

*Use in pregnancy:* The safety for the use of this drug during pregnancy has not been established; therefore, the possible hazards should be weighed against the potential benefits when administering this drug to pregnant patients.

*Nursing mothers:* Breast feeding is not recommended during treatment with depot fluphenazines, owing to the possibility that fluphenazine may be excreted in the milk of nursing mothers.

*Effects on ability to drive and use machines:* The use of this drug may impair the mental and physical abilities required for driving a car or operating heavy machinery.

*Undesirable effects*

*Side-effects:* Acute dystonic reactions occur infrequently, as a rule within the first 24–48 hours, although delayed reactions may occur. In susceptible individuals they may occur after only small doses. These may include such dramatic manifestations as oculogyric crises and opisthotonos. They are rapidly relieved by intravenous administration of an anti-parkinsonian agent such as procyclidine.

Parkinsonian-like states may occur particularly between the second and fifth days after each injection, but often decrease with subsequent injection. These reactions may be reduced by using smaller doses more frequently, or by the concomitant use of anti-parkinsonian drugs such as benzhexol, benztropine or procyclidine. Anti-parkinsonian drugs should not be prescribed routinely, because of the possible risks of aggravating anti-cholinergic side-effects or precipitating toxic confusional states, or of impairing therapeutic efficacy.

With careful monitoring of the dose the number of patients requiring anti-parkinsonian drugs can be minimised.

*Tardive dyskinesia:* As with all antipsychotic agents, tardive dyskinesia may appear in some patients on long term therapy or may occur after drug therapy has been discontinued. The risk seems to be greater in elderly patients on high dose therapy, especially females. The symptoms are persistent and in some patients appear to be irreversible.

The syndrome is characterised by rhythmical involuntary movements of the tongue, face, mouth or jaw (e.g. protrusion of tongue, puffing of cheeks, puckering of mouth, chewing movements). Sometimes these may be accompanied by involuntary movements of the extremities. There is no known effective treatment for tardive dyskinesia: anti-parkinsonian agents usually do not alleviate the symptoms of this syndrome. It is suggested that all antipsychotic agents be discontinued if these symptoms appear. Should it be necessary to reinstitute treatment, or increase the dosage of the agent, or switch to a different antipsychotic agent, the syndrome may be masked. It has been reported that fine vermicular movements of the tongue may be an early sign of the syndrome and if the medication is stopped at that time, the syndrome may not develop.

*Other undesirable effects:* As with other phenothiazines, drowsiness, lethargy, blurred vision, dryness of the mouth, constipation, urinary hesitancy or incontinence, mild hypotension, impairment of judgement and mental skills, and epileptiform attacks are occasionally seen.

Blood dyscrasias have rarely been reported with phenothiazine derivatives. Blood counts should be performed if the patient develops signs of persistent infection. Transient leucopenia and thrombocytopenia have been reported. Antinuclear antibodies and SLE have been reported very rarely.

Jaundice has rarely been reported. Transient abnormalities of liver function tests may occur in the absence of jaundice.

A transient rise in serum cholesterol has been reported rarely in patients on oral fluphenazine.

Abnormal skin pigmentation and lens opacities have sometimes been seen following long-term administration of high doses of phenothiazines.

Phenothiazines are known to cause photosensitivity reactions but this has not been reported for fluphenazine. Skin rashes have occasionally been reported.

Elderly or hypothyroid patients may be particularly susceptible to hypothermia. The hazard of hyperpyrexia may be increased by especially hot or humid weather, or by drugs such as anti-parkinsonian agents, which impair sweating.

Rare occurrences of neuroleptic malignant syndrome (NMS) have been reported in patients on neuroleptic therapy. The syndrome is characterised by hyperthermia, together with some or all of the following: muscular rigidity, autonomic instability (labile blood pressure, tachycardia, diaphoresis), akinesia, and altered consciousness, sometimes progressing to stupor or coma. Leucocytosis, elevated CPK, liver function abnormalities, and acute renal failure may also occur. Neuroleptic therapy should be discontinued immediately and vigorous symptomatic treatment implemented since the syndrome is potentially fatal.

Hormonal effects of phenothiazines include hyperprolactinaemia, which may cause galactorrhoea, gynaecomastia and oligomenorrhoea or amenorrhoea. Sexual function may be impaired.

Oedema has been reported with phenothiazine medication.

*Overdose:* Overdosage should be treated symptomatically and supportively, extrapyramidal reactions will respond to oral or parenteral anti-parkinsonian drugs such as procyclidine or benztropine. In cases of severe hypotension, all procedures for the management of circulatory shock should be instituted, e.g. vasconstrictors and/or intravenous fluids. However, only the vasoconstrictors metaraminol or noradrenaline should be used, as adrenaline may further lower the blood pressure through interaction with the phenothiazine.

**Pharmacological properties**

*Pharmacodynamic properties:* Fluphenazine decanoate is an ester of the potent neuroleptic fluphenazine, a phenothiazine derivative of the piperazine type. The ester is slowly absorbed from the intramuscular site of injection and is then hydrolysed in the plasma to the active therapeutic agent, fluphenazine.

Extrapyramidal reactions are not uncommon, but fluphenazine does not have marked sedative or hypotensive properties.

*Pharmacokinetic properties:* Plasma level profiles of fluphenazine following intramuscular injection have shown half-lives of plasma clearance ranging from 2.5–16 weeks, emphasising the importance of adjusting dose and interval to the individual requirements of each patient. The slow decline of plasma levels in most patients means that a reasonably stable plasma level can usually be achieved with injections spaced at 2–4 week intervals.

**Pharmaceutical particulars**

*List of excipients:* Benzyl alcohol and sesame oil.

*Incompatibilities:* None.

*Shelf life:* 24 months. The in use shelf life for the 10 ml vial is 28 days.

*Special precautions for storage:* Store below 25°C. Protect from direct sunlight.

*Nature and contents of container:* Type I Glass ampoules containing 0.5, 1 and 2 ml.

Type I Glass cartridge syringes with Helvoet Pharma rubber plungers and stoppers containing 1 and 2 ml.

Type I Glass vials with pharma-gummi rubber stoppers containing 10 ml.

*Instructions for use/handling:* For intramuscular administration only.

**Marketing authorisation number** 11723/0103.

**Date of approval/revision of SPC** March 1996.

**Legal category** POM.

## MODECATE* CONCENTRATE

**Qualitative and quantitative composition** The product contains Fluphenazine Decanoate BP 100 mg/ml.

**Pharmaceutical form** Intramuscular injection for administration to human beings.

**Clinical particulars**

*Therapeutic indications:* For the treatment and maintenance of schizophrenic patients and those with paranoid psychoses.

While Modecate concentrate injection has been shown to be effective in acute states, it is particularly useful in the maintenance treatment of chronic patients who are unreliable at taking their oral medication, and also of those who do not absorb their oral phenothiazine adequately.

*Posology and method of administration*

*Adults:* It is recommended that patients be stabilised on the injection in hospital.

*Recommended dosage regimes for all indications:*

*Patients without previous exposure to a depot fluphenazine formulation:* Initially 0.125 ml i.e. 12.5 mg (0.0625 ml i.e. 6.25 mg for patients over 60) by deep intramuscular injection into the gluteal region.

The onset of action generally appears between 24 and 72 hours after injection and the effects of the drug on psychotic symptoms become significant within 48 to 96 hours. Subsequent injections and the dosage interval are determined in accordance with the patient's response. When administered as maintenance therapy, a single injection may be effective in controlling schizophrenic symptoms for up to four weeks or longer.

It is desirable to maintain as much flexibility in the dose as possible to achieve the best therapeutic response with the least side-effects; most patients are successfully maintained within the dose range 0.125 ml (12.5 mg) to 1 ml (100 mg) given at a dose interval of 2 to 5 weeks.

*Patients previously maintained on oral fluphenazine:* It is not possible to predict the equivalent dose of depot formulation in view of the wide variability of individual response.

*Patients previously maintained on depot fluphenazine:* Patients who have suffered a relapse following cessation of depot fluphenazine therapy may be restarted on the same dose (as they were receiving formerly), although the frequency of injections may need to be increased in the early weeks of treatment until satisfactory control is obtained.

*Elderly:* Elderly patients may be particularly susceptible to extrapyramidal reactions. Therefore reduced maintenance dosage may be required and a smaller initial dose (see above).

*Children:* Not recommended for children.

Where a very small volume/low concentration of fluphenazine is required patients may be transferred to the equivalent dose of Modecate Injection 25 mg/ml on the basis that 1 ml Modecate Concentrate (100 mg/ml) is equivalent to 4 ml Modecate Injection.

*Note:* The dosage should not be increased without close supervision and it should be noted that there is a variability in individual response.

The response to antipsychotic drug treatment may be delayed. If drugs are withdrawn, recurrence of symptoms may not become apparent for several weeks or months.

*Route of administration:* Intramuscular.

*Contra-indications:* The product is contra-indicated in the following cases: comatose states; marked cerebral atherosclerosis; phaeochromocytoma; renal failure; liver failure; severe cardiac insufficiency; severely depressed states; existing blood dyscrasias; history of hypersensitivity to any of the ingredients.

*Special warnings and special precautions for use:* Caution should be exercised with the following: liver disease; cardiac arrhythmias, cardiac disease; thyrotoxicosis; severe respiratory disease; epilepsy, conditions predisposing to epilepsy (e.g. alcohol withdrawal or brain damage); Parkinson's disease; patients who have shown hypersensitivity to other phenothiazines; personal or family history of narrow angle glaucoma; in very hot weather; the elderly, particularly if frail or at risk of hypothermia; hypothyroidism; myasthenia gravis; prostatic hypertrophy.

*Interaction with other medicaments and other forms of interaction:* The possibility should be borne in mind that phenothiazines may:

1. Increase the central nervous system depression produced by drugs such as alcohol, general anaesthetics, hypnotics, sedatives or strong analgesics.
2. Antagonise the action of adrenaline and other sympathomimetic agents and reverse the blood-pressure-lowering effects of adrenergic-blocking agents such as guanethidine and clonidine.
3. Impair: the anti-parkinsonian effect of L-dopa; the effect of anticonvulsants; metabolism of tricyclic antidepressants; the control of diabetes.
4. Increase the effect of anticoagulants and antidepressants.
5. Interact with lithium.

Anticholinergic effects may be enhanced by anti-parkinsonian or other anticholinergic drugs.

Phenothiazines may enhance: the cardiac-depressant effects of quinidine, the absorption of corticosteroids, digoxin, and neuromuscular blocking agents.

*Pregnancy and lactation*

*Use in pregnancy:* The safety for the use of this drug during pregnancy has not been established; therefore, the possible hazards should be weighed against the potential benefits when administering this drug to pregnant patients.

*Nursing mothers:* Breast feeding is not recommended during treatment with depot fluphenazines, owing to the possibility that fluphenazine is excreted in the milk of nursing mothers.

*Effects on ability to drive and use machines:* The use of this drug may impair the mental and physical abilities required for driving a car or operating heavy machinery.

*Undesirable effects*

*Side-effects:* Acute dystonic reactions occur infrequently, as a rule within the first 24–48 hours, although delayed reactions may occur. In susceptible individuals they may occur after only small doses. These may include such dramatic manifestations as oculogyric crises and opisthotonos. They are rapidly relieved by intravenous administration of an anti-parkinsonian agent such as procyclidine.

Parkinsonian-like states may occur particularly between the second and fifth days after each injection, but often decrease with subsequent injections. These reactions may be reduced by using smaller doses more frequently, or by the concomitant use of anti-parkinsonian drugs such as benzhexol, benztropine or procyclidine. Anti-parkinsonian drugs should not be prescribed routinely, because of the possible risks of aggravating anti-cholinergic side-effects or precipitating toxic confusional states, or of impairing therapeutic efficacy.

With careful monitoring of the dose the number of patients requiring anti-parkinsonian drugs can be minimised.

*Tardive dyskinesia:* As with all antipsychotic agents, tardive dyskinesia may appear in some patients on long term therapy or may occur after drug therapy has been discontinued. The risk seems to be greater in elderly patients on high dose therapy, especially females. The symptoms are persistent and in some patients appear to be irreversible.

The syndrome is characterised by rhythmical involuntary movements of the tongue, face, mouth or jaw (e.g. protrusion of tongue, puffing of cheeks, puckering of mouth, chewing movements). Sometimes these may be accompanied by involuntary movements of the extremities. There is no known effective treatment for tardive dyskinesia: anti-parkinsonian agents usually do not alleviate the symptoms of this syndrome. It is suggested that all antipsychotic agents be discontinued if these symptoms appear. Should it be necessary to reinstitute treatment, or increase the dosage of the agent, or switch to a different antipsychotic agent, the syndrome may be masked. It has been reported that fine vermicular movements of the tongue may be an early sign of the syndrome and if the medication is stopped at that time, the syndrome may not develop.

*Other undesirable effects:* As with other phenothiazines, drowsiness, lethargy, blurred vision, dryness of the mouth, constipation, urinary hesitancy or incontinence, mild hypotension, impairment of judgement and mental skills, and epileptiform attacks are occasionally seen.

Blood dyscrasias have rarely been reported with phenothiazine derivatives. Blood counts should be performed if the patient develops signs of persistent infection. Transient leucopenia and thrombocytopenia have been reported. Antinuclear antibodies and SLE have been reported very rarely.

Jaundice has rarely been reported. Transient abnormalities of liver function tests may occur in the absence of jaundice.

A transient rise in serum cholesterol has been reported rarely in patients on oral fluphenazine.

Abnormal skin pigmentation and lens opacities have sometimes been seen following long-term administration of high doses of phenothiazines.

Phenothiazines are known to cause photosensitivity reactions but this has not been reported for fluphenazine. Skin rashes have occasionally been reported.

Elderly patients may be more susceptible to the sedative and hypotensive effects.

The effects of phenothiazines on the heart are dose-related. ECG changes with prolongation of the QT interval and T-Wave changes have been reported commonly in patients treated with moderate to high dosage; they have been reported to precede serious arrhythmias, including ventricular tachycardia and fibrillation, which have also occurred after overdosage. Sudden, unexpected and unexplained deaths have been reported in hospitalised psychotic patients receiving phenothiazines.

Elderly or hypothyroid patients may be particularly susceptible to hypothermia.

The hazard of hyperpyrexia may be increased by especially hot or humid weather, or by drugs such as anti-parkinsonian agents, which impair sweating.

Rare occurrences of neuroleptic malignant syndrome (NMS) have been reported in patients on neuroleptic therapy. The syndrome is characterised by hyperthermia, together with some or all of the following: muscular rigidity, autonomic instability (labile blood pressure, tachycardia, diaphoresis), akinesia, and altered consciousness, sometimes progressing to stupor or coma. Leucocytosis, elevated CPK, liver function abnormalities, and acute renal failure may also occur. Neuroleptic therapy should be discontinued immediately and vigorous symptomatic treatment implemented since the syndrome is potentially fatal.

Hormonal effects of phenothiazines include hyperprolactinaemia, which may cause galactorrhoea, gynaecomastia and oligomenorrhoea or amenorrhoea. Sexual function may be impaired.

Oedema has been reported with phenothiazine medication.

*Overdose:* Overdosage should be treated symptomatically and supportively, extrapyramidal reactions will respond to oral or parenteral anti-parkinsonian drugs such as procyclidine or benztropine. In cases of severe hypotension, all procedures for the management of circulatory shock should be instituted, e.g. vasconstrictors and/or intravenous fluids. However, only the vasoconstrictors metaraminol or noradrenaline should be used, as adrenaline may further lower the blood pressure through interaction with the phenothiazine.

## Pharmacological properties

*Pharmacodynamic properties:* Fluphenazine decanoate is an ester of the potent neuroleptic fluphenazine, a phenothiazine derivative of the piperazine type. The ester is slowly absorbed from the intramuscular site of injection and is then hydrolysed in the plasma to the active therapeutic agent, fluphenazine.

Extrapyramidal reactions are not uncommon, but fluphenazine does not have marked sedative or hypotensive properties.

*Pharmacokinetic properties:* Plasma level profiles of fluphenazine following intramuscular injection have shown half-lives of plasma clearance ranging from 2.5–16 weeks, emphasising the importance of adjusting dose and interval to the individual requirements of each patient. The slow decline of plasma levels in most patients means that a reasonably stable plasma level can usually be achieved with injections spaced at 2–4 week intervals.

## Pharmaceutical particulars

*List of excipients:* Benzyl alcohol and sesame oil.

*Incompatibilities:* None.

*Shelf life:* 24 months.

*Special precautions for storage:* Store below 25°C. Protect from direct sunlight.

*Nature and contents of container:* Clear type I glass ampoules containing 0.5 ml (packs of 10) and 1 ml (packs of 5).

Prefilled syringe with neoprene or pharma-gummi rubber plunger and stopper containing 0.5 ml (packs of 10 – unmarketed).

*Instructions for use/handling:* For intramuscular administration only.

**Marketing authorisation number** 11723/0104.

**Date of approval/revision of SPC** March 1996.

**Legal category** POM.

# MODITEN* TABLETS

**Qualitative and quantitative composition** Each 5 mg tablet contains Fluphenazine Hydrochloride BP 5.0 mg.

Each 2.5 mg tablet contains Fluphenazine Hydrochloride BP 2.5 mg.

Each 1 mg tablet contains Fluphenazine Hydrochloride BP 1.0 mg.

**Pharmaceutical form** Round biconvex coated tablets.

## Clinical particulars

*Therapeutic indications:* As an adjunct to the short-term management of anxiety, severe psychomotor agitation, excitement, violent or dangerously impulsive behaviour.

In schizophrenia; treatment of symptoms and prevention of relapse.

In other psychoses, especially paranoid.

In mania and hypomania.

*Posology and method of administration*
*Adults:*

*Anxiety and other non-psychotic behavioural disturbances:* Initially 1 mg twice daily rising to 2 mg twice daily, if necessary, according to response.

*Schizophrenia, mania, hypomania and other psychoses:* Initially 2.5–10 mg daily divided into 2 or 3 doses, depending on the severity and duration of symptoms, rising to 20 mg daily, as necessary. Doses exceeding 20 mg daily (10 mg in the elderly) should be used with caution.

*Elderly:* Elderly patients may be extra susceptible to extrapyramidal reactions. Dosage at the lower end of the range is likely to be sufficient for elderly patients.

*Children:* Not recommended for children.

*Note:* The dosage should not be increased without close supervision and it should be noted that there is a variability in individual response.

The response to antipsychotic drug treatment may be delayed. If drugs are withdrawn, recurrence of symptoms may not become apparent for several weeks or months.

*Method of administration:* Oral.

*Contra-indications:* The product is contra-indicated in the following: comatose states; marked cerebral atherosclerosis; phaeochromocytoma; renal failure; liver failure; severe cardiac insufficiency; severely depressed states; existing blood dyscrasias; history of hypersensitivity to any of the ingredients.

*Special warnings and special precautions for use:* Caution should be exercised in patients with the following conditions: liver disease; cardiac arrhythmias, cardiac disease; thyrotoxicosis; severe respiratory disease; epilepsy, conditions predisposing to epilepsy (e.g. alcohol withdrawal or brain damage); Parkinson's disease; patients who have shown hypersensitivity to other phenothiazines; personal or family history of narrow angle glaucoma; in very hot weather; the elderly, particularly if frail or at risk of hypothermia; hypothyroidism; myasthenia gravis; prostatic hypertrophy.

*Interaction with other medicaments and other forms of interaction:* Phenothiazines may:

1. Increase the central nervous system depression produced by drugs such as alcohol, general anaesthetics, hypnotics, sedatives or strong analgesics.

2. Antagonise the action of adrenaline and other sympathomimetic agents and reverse the blood-pressure-lowering effects of adrenergic-blocking agents such as guanethidine and clonidine.

3. Impair: The anti-parkinsonian effect of L-dopa; the effect of anticonvulsants; metabolism of tricyclic antidepressants; the control of diabetes.

4. Increase the effect of anticoagulants and antidepressants.

5. Interact with lithium.

6. Enhance the cardiac-depressant effects of quinidine; the absorption of corticosteroids, digoxin and neuromuscular blocking agents.

Antacids may impair absorption.

Anticholinergic effects may be enhanced by anti-parkinsonian or other anticholinergic drugs.

Tea and coffee produce insoluble precipitates in vitro but the effect on absorption in man is unclear.

*Pregnancy and lactation:* Safety for use during pregnancy has not been established; therefore the possible hazards should be weighed against the potential benefits before administration to pregnant patients. Breast feeding is not recommended during treatment as fluphenazine may be excreted in breast milk.

*Effects on ability to drive and use machines:* May impair the mental and physical abilities required for driving a car or operating heavy machinery.

*Undesirable effects:* Side effects may include: Extrapyramidal reactions, acute dystonias, oculogyric crises, parkinsonian rigidity, tremor, akathisia, tardive dyskinesia, drowsiness, lethargy, blurred vision, dryness of the mouth, constipation, urinary hesitancy, incontinence, mild hypotension, impairment of judgement and mental skills, epileptiform attacks.

Hormonal effects such as hyperprolactinaemia, which may cause galactorrhoea, gynaecomastia and oligo- or amenorrhoea. Impairment of sexual function.

Hypothermia, particularly in elderly or hypothyroid patients.

Hyperpyrexia in hot/humid weather or when given with anti-parkinsonian agents.

Uncommonly: Blood dyscrasias, transient leucopenia, thrombocytopenia, antinuclear antibodies and SLE.

Jaundice, transient abnormalities of liver function, transient rise in serum cholesterol, abnormal skin pigmentation and lens opacities, skin rashes, neuroleptic malignant syndrome (NMS), oedema.

Acute withdrawal symptoms have been described after abrupt cessation of high doses of phenothiazines. Gradual withdrawal is advisable.

*Overdose:* Treat symptomatically and supportively. Extrapyramidal reactions will respond to oral or parenteral anti-parkinsonian drugs such as procyclidine or benztropine. In cases of severe hypotension, all procedures for the management of circulatory shock should be instituted, e.g. vasoconstrictors and/or intravenous fluids. However, only the vasoconstrictors metaraminol or noradrenaline should be used, as adrenaline may further lower the blood pressure through interaction with the phenothiazine.

**Pharmacological properties**

*Pharmacodynamic properties:* Fluphenazine hydrochloride is a salt of the potent neuroleptic fluphenazine, a phenothiazine derivative of the piperazine type. Extrapyramidal reactions are not uncommon but fluphenazine does not have marked sedative or hypotensive properties.

*Pharmacokinetic properties:* The plasma half-life of fluphenazine in patients given the hydrochloride by mouth has been shown to be approximately 14.7 hours.

**Pharmaceutical particulars**

*List of excipients:* The core tablets also contain: corn starch, lactose, talc, sodium benzoate, acacia powder, magnesium stearate.

The 5 mg tablet coating solution is comprised of shellac solution, castor oil, talc, polyvidone, sucrose, chalk, beeswax, carnauba wax, polysorbate and sorbic acid.

The 2.5 mg tablet coating solution is comprised of shellac solution, castor oil, polyvidone, chalk, sucrose, curcumin, titanium dioxide, sodium benzoate, beeswax, carnauba wax, polysorbate and sorbic acid.

The 1 mg tablet coating solution is comprised of shellac solution, castor oil, talc, polyvidone, chalk, sucrose, erythrosine, titanium dioxide, sodium benzoate, beeswax, carnauba wax, polysorbate and sorbic acid.

*Incompatibilities:* None.

*Shelf life:* 60 months.

*Special precautions for storage:* Store below 25°C.

*Nature and contents of container:* Amber glass bottles containing 100 or 500 tablets with one of the following closures:

Wadless polypropylene cap; tin plate cap with pulpboard wad and waxed aluminium facing; black phenolic cap with composition cork wad and tinfoil/melinex lining; roll-on pilfer-proof aluminium cap with polyethylene liner; child-resistant polypropylene cap of the clic-lok type lined with expanded polyethylene with PVDC (saran) facing.

**Marketing authorisation numbers**

| | |
|---|---|
| Moditen 5 mg tablets | 11723/0107 |
| Moditen 2.5 mg tablets | 11723/0106 |
| Moditen 1 mg tablets | 11723/0105 |

**Date of approval/revision of SPC** November 1995.

**Legal category** POM.

## MORCAP SR*

**Qualitative and quantitative composition** Morphine Sulphate BP 20 mg, 50 mg, 100 mg per capsule.

**Pharmaceutical form** Modified release capsule.

**Clinical particulars**

*Therapeutic indications:* Morcap SR is indicated for the prolonged relief of chronic, moderate to severe pain. Morcap SR is intended for use in patients who require repeated dosing with potent opioid analgesics over a period of more than a few days.

*Posology and method of administration* (see: *Pharmacology, Warnings* and *Precautions* sections): Morcap SR capsules are to be administered either twice daily (every 12 hours) or once daily (every 24 hours).

Selection of the initial dose of Morcap SR should take into account the following:

(i) the total daily dose, potency and characteristics of previous opioid analgesics (e.g. pure agonists or mixed agonist/antagonist);

(ii) the reliability of the relative potency estimate used to calculate the dose of morphine required (potency estimates vary with the route of administration);

(iii) the degree of opioid tolerance;

(iv) the patient's general medical condition;

(v) concurrent medication;

(vi) type and severity of pain.

The initial dose of Morcap SR in opioid naive patients should be 20 mg every 12 hours or 40 mg every 24 hours.

The first dose of Morcap SR may be taken with the last dose of any immediate-release opioid medication.

For patients who have difficulty swallowing, Morcap SR pellets may be sprinkled onto a small amount of soft foods (such as yoghurt, apple sauce or jam). This should be taken within 30 minutes of sprinkling. The pellets must not be chewed or crushed and the mouth should be rinsed to ensure that all pellets have been swallowed.

MORCAP SR CAPSULES SHOULD BE SWALLOWED WHOLE. THE CAPSULES AND PELLETS SHOULD NOT BE CHEWED OR CRUSHED.

The use of opioid analgesics for the relief of chronic pain, including cancer pain, should be only part of a complete approach to pain control which should include other types of treatment or drug therapy, non-drug measures and psychosocial support.

If signs of excessive opioid effects are observed early in the dosing interval, the next dose should be reduced. If this adjustment leads to inadequate analgesia, that is, 'breakthrough pain' occurs, a supplemental dose of a short acting analgesic may be given. The dosing interval of Morcap SR should not be reduced below every 12 hours. As experience is gained, adjustments can be made to obtain an appropriate balance between pain relief and opioid side effects.

Because of the sustained release properties of Morcap SR, dosage increases should generally be separated by 24 hours.

The peak morphine plasma levels following administration of Morcap SR once daily (every 24 hours) are significantly higher than the peak morphine plasma levels that follow administration of Morcap SR twice daily (every 12 hours). While clinical studies have not shown any difference in morphine related side effects between the dosage regimens, the possibility of increased side effects with the 24 hourly regimen cannot be discounted. Accordingly, close observation is recommended when converting patients from 12 hourly to 24 hourly administration.

For patients currently receiving opioids, the following dosing recommendations should be considered.

*Conversion from other oral morphine formulations to Morcap SR:* Patients on other oral morphine formulations may be converted to Morcap SR by administering one half of the patient's total daily morphine dose as Morcap SR capsules on an every 12 hours dosing regimen, or by administering the total daily morphine dose as Morcap SR capsules on an every 24 hours dosing regimen. Dose is then adjusted as needed.

*Conversion from parenteral morphine or other parenteral or oral opioids to Morcap SR:* Morcap SR can be administered as the initial oral morphine drug product. However, in this case, particular care must be exercised in the conversion process. Because of uncertainty about and inter-subject variation in relative estimates of opioid potency and cross tolerance, initial dosing regimens should be conservative, that is, an underestimation of the 24 hour oral morphine requirement is preferred to an overestimate. To this end, initial individual doses of Morcap SR should be estimated conservatively.

Estimates of the relative potency of opioids are only approximate and are influenced by route of administration, individual patient differences, and possibly, by an individual's medical condition.

Consequently, it is difficult to recommend any fixed rule for converting a patient to Morcap SR directly. The following general points should be considered:

Parenteral to oral morphine ratio: Estimates of the oral to parenteral potency of morphine vary. Some authorities suggest that a dose of oral morphine only three times the daily parenteral morphine requirement may be sufficient in chronic use settings.

Other parenteral or oral opioids to oral morphine: Because there are no data on these types of analgesic substitutions, specific recommendations are not possible. Physicians are advised to refer to published relative potency data, keeping in mind that such ratios are only approximate (see Table 1). In general, it is safer to underestimate the daily dose of Morcap SR required and rely upon ad hoc supplementation to deal with inadequate analgesia.

*Table 1: Approximate oral opioid potency ratios relative to oral Morphine†*

| | | | |
|---|---|---|---|
| pethidine | 1/8 | methadone | 3–4[2] |
| papaveretum | 2/3 | morphine | 1 |
| oxycodone | 1 | dextromoramide | 2[1] |

[1] Dextromoramide: a single 5 mg dose is equivalent to morphine 15 mg in terms of peak effect but is shorter acting. The overall potency ratio has been adjusted accordingly.

[2] Methadone: a single 5 mg dose is equivalent to morphine 7.5 mg. It has a prolonged plasma half-life, which leads to cumulation when given repeatedly. This means that when given regularly it is several times more potent.

† Adapted from Twycross and Lack, (1989). Oral morphine in advanced cancer. 2nd ed. Beaconsfield.

Conversion from Morcap SR to other Controlled-Release Oral Morphine Formulations.

Morcap SR is not bioequivalent to other controlled-release morphine preparations. Although for a given dose the same amount of morphine is available from Morcap SR as from morphine solution or controlled-release morphine tablets (i.e. AUC is the same), Morcap SR results in reduced maximum and increased minimum plasma morphine concentrations. Conversion from Morcap SR to the same daily dose of other morphine preparations may lead to an initial change in the clinical status of the patient and close observation is recommended.

*Conversion from Morcap SR to parenteral opioids:* When converting a patient from Morcap SR to parenteral opioids, it is best to assume that the parenteral to oral potency is high. NOTE THAT THIS IS THE CONVERSE OF THE STRATEGY USED WHEN THE DIRECTION OF CONVERSION IS FROM THE PARENTERAL TO ORAL FORMULATIONS. IN BOTH CASES, HOWEVER, THE AIM IS TO ESTIMATE THE NEW DOSE CONSERVATIVELY.

For example, to estimate the required 24 hour dose of morphine for i.m. use, one could employ a conversion of 1 mg of morphine i.m. for every 6 mg of morphine as Morcap SR. Of course, the i.m. 24-hour dose would have to be divided by six and administered every 4 hours. This approach is recommended because it is least likely to cause overdose.

Opioid analgesic agents do not effectively relieve dysesthetic pain, post-herpetic neuralgia, stabbing pains, activity-related pain, and some forms of headache. This does not mean that patients with advanced cancer suffering these types of pain should not be given an adequate trial of opioid analgesics. However, such patients may need to be referred early on for other types of pain therapy. Pain without nociception is usually not opioid-responsive.

*Use in children:* The use of Morcap SR in children has not been evaluated.

*Use in the elderly:* Morcap SR should be administered with caution and in reduced dosages in elderly patients.

*Contra-indications:* Morcap SR should not be given to patients with: known hypersensitivity to morphine, morphine salts or any of the capsule components; acute or severe bronchial asthma; respiratory depression; biliary colic; gastrointestinal obstruction, particularly paralytic ileus; concurrent MAO inhibitors or within 14 days of such therapy (see *Interactions*).

*Special warnings and special precautions for use:*
*Warnings: Impaired respiration:* Respiratory depression is the chief hazard of all morphine preparations. Respiratory depression occurs more frequently in elderly and debilitated patients, and in those suffering from conditions accompanied by hypoxia or hypercapnia when even moderate therapeutic doses may significantly decrease pulmonary ventilation.

Morphine should be used with extreme caution in patients with chronic obstructive pulmonary disease or cor pulmonale and in patients having a substantially decreased respiratory reserve, hypoxia, hypercapnia or pre-existing respiratory depression. In such patients, even usual therapeutic doses of morphine may increase airway resistance and decrease respiratory drive to the point of apnoea. Severe pain antagonises the respiratory depressant effects of morphine.

*Head injury and increased intracranial pressure:* The respiratory depressant effects of morphine with carbon dioxide retention and secondary elevation of cerebrospinal fluid pressure may be markedly exaggerated in the presence of head injury, other intracranial lesions, or a pre-existing increase in intracranial pressure. Morphine produces effects which may obscure neurological signs of further increases in pressure in patients with head injuries. Morphine should only be administered under such circumstances when considered essential and then with extreme caution.

*Hypotensive effect:* Morcap SR, like all opioid analgesics may cause severe hypotension in an individual whose ability to maintain blood pressure has already been compromised by a reduced blood volume, or a concurrent administration of drugs such as phenothiazines or general anaesthetics (see *Interactions*).

Morcap SR may produce orthostatic hypotension in ambulatory patients. Morcap SR, like all opioid analgesics should be administered with caution to patients in circulatory shock, as vasodilation produced by the drug may further reduce cardiac output and blood pressure.

*Gastrointestinal motility:* Morcap SR should not be given to patients with gastrointestinal obstruction, particularly paralytic ileus as there is a risk of the product remaining in the stomach for an extended period and the subsequent release of a bolus of morphine when normal gut motility is restored.

As with any other solid dose morphine formulation, diarrhoea may reduce morphine absorption.

*Drug dependence:* Morphine has a potential for physical and psychological dependence. However, this is not a prime concern in the management of terminally ill patients or patients in severe pain. Abrupt cessation or a sudden reduction in dose after prolonged use may result in withdrawal symptoms. If withdrawal is necessary it must be undertaken gradually.

Infants born to mothers who are physically dependent on opioid analgesics may also be physically dependent and may exhibit withdrawal symptoms

These infants may have respiratory depression at birth (see *Precautions*).

*Tolerance:* Tolerance may develop upon repeated administration of morphine. The dose of Morcap SR may need to be increased to maintain adequate pain relief (see *Posology and method of administration*).

*Precautions:*

*General:* Morcap SR is intended for use in patients who require more than several days continuous treatment with a potent opioid analgesic.

As with any potent opioid, it is critical to adjust the dosing regimen of Morcap SR for each patient individually, taking into account the patient's prior analgesic treatment experience. Although it is clearly impossible to enumerate every consideration that is important to the selection of the initial dose of Morcap SR, attention should be given to the points listed under *Posology and method of administration.*

*Cordotomy:* Patients who are scheduled for cordotomy or other interruption of pain transmission pathways should not receive Morcap SR within 24 hours of the procedure.

*Special risk groups:* Morcap SR should be administered with caution, and in reduced dosages in elderly or debilitated patients; patients with severe renal or hepatic insufficiency; patients with Addison's disease; myxoedema; hypothyroidism; prostatic hypertrophy or urethral stricture.

Caution should also be exercised in the administration of Morcap SR to patients with CNS depression; toxic psychosis; acute alcoholism or delerium tremens; severe kyphoscoliosis; convulsive disorders; about to undergo biliary surgery and patients with acute pancreatitis secondary to biliary tract disease.

*Driving and operating dangerous machinery:* Morphine may impair the mental and/or physical abilities needed to perform potentially hazardous activities such as driving a car or operating machinery. Patients must be cautioned accordingly. Patients should also be warned about the potential combined effects of morphine with other CNS depressants, including other opioids, phenothiazines, sedative/hypnotics and alcohol (see *Interactions*).

*Interaction with other medicaments and other forms of interaction: CNS Depressants:* Morphine should be used with great caution and in reduced dosage in patients concurrently receiving other central nervous system depressants including sedatives, hypnotics, general anaesthetics, phenothiazines, other tranquillisers and alcohol because of the risk of respiratory depression, hypotension and profound sedation or coma. When such combined therapy is contemplated, the dose of one or both agents should be reduced.

*Muscle relaxants:* Morphine may enhance the neuromuscular blocking action of skeletal relaxants and produce an increased degree of respiratory depression.

*Mixed Agonist/Antagonist Opioid Analgesics:* From a theoretical perspective, mixed agonist/antagonist opioid analgesics (e.g. pentazocine, and buprenorphine) should NOT be administered to a patient who has received or is receiving a course of therapy with a pure opioid agonist analgesic. In these patients, mixed agonist/antagonist analgesics may reduce the analgesic effect or may precipitate withdrawal symptoms.

*Monoamine oxidase inhibitors (MAOIs):* MAOIs intensify the effects of morphine and other opioid drugs which can cause anxiety, confusion and significant depression of respiration, sometimes leading to coma. Morphine should not be given to patients taking MAOIs or within 14 days of stopping such treatment.

*Cimetidine:* There is a report of confusion and severe respiratory depression when a haemodialysis patient was administered morphine and cimetidine.

*Diuretics:* Morphine reduces the efficacy of diuretics by inducing the release of antidiuretic hormone. Morphine may also lead to acute retention of urine by causing spasm of the sphincter of the bladder, particularly in men with prostatism.

*Food:* The bioavailability of Morcap SR is not significantly affected by food.

*Pregnancy and lactation:*

*Use in pregnancy:* Animal reproduction studies have not been performed using morphine. It is not known whether morphine can cause foetal damage when administered throughout pregnancy or if it can effect reproductive capacity in humans. Pregnant patients should only be given Morcap SR when the benefits clearly outweigh potential risks to the foetus.

*Use in labour/delivery and in nursing mothers:* Morcap SR is not recommended for use in women during and immediately before labour. The effects of opioid analgesics are unpredictable. They may prolong labour by temporarily reducing the strength, duration and frequency of uterine contractions, or conversely they may tend to shorten labour by increasing the rate of cervical dilatation. Infants born to mothers receiving opioid analgesics during labour should be observed closely for signs of respiratory depression. In such infants a specific opioid antagonist, naloxone hydrochloride, should be available for reversal of narcotic-induced respiratory depression. Morphine is excreted in human milk and breast-feeding is not recommended while a patient is receiving Morcap SR. Withdrawal symptoms have been observed in breast-fed infants when maternal administration of morphine sulphate is stopped.

*Effects on ability to drive and use machines:* Morphine may impair mental and/or physical ability required for the performance of potentially hazardous tasks (e.g. driving, operating machinery).

*Undesirable effects:*

*Adverse reactions:* The adverse reactions caused by morphine are essentially the same as those observed with other oral and parenteral opioid analgesics. They include the following major hazards: respiratory depression, apnoea and to a lesser degree circulatory depression, respiratory arrest, shock and cardiac arrest.

*Most common adverse effects:* Constipation, lightheadedness, dizziness, sedation, nausea, vomiting, sweating, dysphoria and euphoria.

*Sedation:* Most patients receiving morphine will experience initial drowsiness. This usually disappears in three to five days and is not a cause for concern unless it is excessive, or accompanied with unsteadiness or confusion. Excessive or persistent sedation should be investigated. Factors to be considered should include: concurrent sedative medications, the presence of hepatic or renal insufficiency, exacerbated respiratory failure, tolerance to the dose used especially in older patients, disease severity and the patient's general condition. If the dose of Morcap SR has been reduced and pain is not adequately controlled, the dose may be carefully increased again after a few days.

Dizziness and unsteadiness may be associated with morphine-induced postural hypotension, particularly in elderly or debilitated patients. The dosage should be adjusted according to individual needs but, because of reduced clearance, dosage may be lower in patients over 50 years of age.

*Nausea and vomiting:* Nausea and vomiting is common after single doses of morphine or as an early undesirable effect of regular opioid therapy. The prescription of a suitable antiemetic should be considered. The frequency of nausea and vomiting usually decreases within a week or so but may persist due to opioid-induced gastric stasis. Metoclopramide is often useful in such patients.

*Constipation:* Virtually all patients suffer from constipation while taking opioids on a chronic basis. Some patients, particularly elderly, debilitated or bedridden patients may become impacted. Patients must be cautioned accordingly and laxatives, softeners and other appropriate treatments should be initiated at the beginning of opioid therapy.

Other adverse reactions include:

*Cardiovascular:* Flushing of the face, chills, tachycardia, bradycardia, palpitations, faintness, syncope, hypotension and hypertension.

*Central nervous system (CNS):* Euphoria, dysphoria, weakness, insomnia, dizziness, confusional symptoms and occasionally hallucinations.

*Gastrointestinal:* Dry mouth, anorexia, constipation, laryngospasm, colic, taste alterations and biliary colic.

*Genitourinary:* Urinary retention or hesitancy, reduced libido or potency.

*Endocrine:* A syndrome of inappropriate antidiuretic hormone secretion characterised by hyponatraemia secondary to decreased free-water excretion may occur (monitoring of electrolytes may be necessary).

*Visual disturbances:* Blurred vision, nystagmus, diplopia and miosis.

*Allergic:* Pruritus, urticaria, other skin rashes and oedema.

*Withdrawal (abstinence) syndrome:* Chronic use of opioid analgesics may be associated with the development of physical dependence. An abstinence syndrome may be precipitated when opioid administration is suddenly discontinued or opioid antagonists administered.

Withdrawal symptoms that may be observed after discontinuation of opioid use include: body aches, diarrhoea, piloerection, anorexia, nervousness or restlessness, rhinorrhoea, sneezing, tremors or shivering, abdominal colic, nausea, sleep disturbance, unusual increase in sweating and yawning, weakness, tachycardia and unexplained fever. With appropriate dose adjustments and gradual withdrawal these symptoms are usually mild.

*Overdose: Symptoms:* Acute overdosage with morphine is manifested by respiratory depression, somnolence progressing to stupor or coma, skeletal muscle flaccidity, cold and clammy skin, constricted pupils, and sometimes bradycardia and hypotension.

*Treatment:* Primary attention should be given to the establishment of a patent airway and institution of assisted or controlled ventilation. The pure opioid antagonist, naloxone hydrochloride, is a specific antidote against respiratory depression which results from opioid overdose. Naloxone (usually 0.4 to 2.0 mg) should be administered intravenously. However, because its duration of action is relatively short, the patient must be carefully monitored until spontaneous respiration is reliably re-established. Morcap SR will continue to release and add to the morphine load for up to 12 hours after administration and the management of morphine overdosage should be modified accordingly. If the response to naloxone is suboptimal or not sustained, additional naloxone may be administered as needed, or given by continuous intravenous infusion to maintain alertness and respiratory function. There is no information available about the cumulative dose of naloxone that may be safely administered.

Naloxone should not be administered in the absence of clinically significant respiratory or circulatory depression secondary to morphine overdosage. Naloxone should be administered cautiously to persons who are known or suspected to be physically dependent on Morcap SR. In such cases, an abrupt or complete reversal of opioid effects may precipitate an acute withdrawal syndrome. The severity of the withdrawal syndrome produced will depend on the degree of physical dependence and the dose of the antagonist administered. If it is necessary to treat serious respiratory depression in the physically dependent patient, the antagonist should be administered with extreme care and by titration with smaller than usually doses of the antagonist.

Supportive measures (including oxygen, vasopressors) should be employed in the management of circulatory shock and pulmonary oedema accompanying overdose as indicated. Cardiac arrest or arrhythmias may require cardiac massage or defibrillation.

Gastric contents may need to be emptied as this can be useful in removing unabsorbed drug, particularly when a sustained-release formulation has been taken. Morphine toxicity may be a result of overdosage but because of the large inter-individual variation in sensitivity to opioids it is difficult to assess the exact dose of any opioid that is toxic or lethal. The toxic effects of morphine tend to be overshadowed by the presence of pain or tolerance. Patients having chronic morphine therapy have been known to take in excess of 3,000 mg/day with no apparent toxic effects being present.

**Pharmacological properties**

*Pharmacodynamic properties:* Morphine is an opioid analgesic which exerts an agonist effect at specific, saturable opioid receptors in the CNS and other tissues. Morphine produces diverse pharmacological effects in man including analgesia, suppression of the cough reflex, respiratory depression due to a reduction in the responsiveness of the respiratory centre to carbon dioxide, nausea and emesis through direct stimulation of the chemoreceptor trigger-zone (CTZ), mood changes including euphoria and dysphoria, sedation, mental clouding, alterations in both the endocrine and autonomic nervous systems, and a decrease in gastrointestinal motility leading to constipation.

*Pharmacokinetic properties:* Morphine is rapidly absorbed from the gastrointestinal tract, nasal mucosa, lung and after subcutaneous (s.c.) and intramuscular (i.m.) injection. When administered orally it is subject to extensive but variable 'first-pass' metabolism and only about 40% of the administered dose reaches the central compartment.

Once absorbed, morphine is distributed to skeletal muscle, kidneys, liver, intestinal tract, lungs, spleen and brain. It crosses the placental membranes and has been found in breast milk. About 30 to 35% of morphine is reversibly protein bound. Although a small fraction of morphine (less than 5%) is demethylated, for all practical purposes, virtually all morphine is converted to glucuronide metabolites including morphine-3-glucuronide and morphine-6-glucuronide. The glucuronide system has very high capacity and is not easily saturated even in disease. Studies in healthy subjects and cancer patients have shown that the glucuronide metabolite to morphine mean molar ratio (based on AUC) are similar following single doses of Morcap SR and morphine sulphate solution, and at steady state for Morcap SR, controlled-release morphine sulphate tablets and morphine sulphate solution. The morphine to morphine-3-glucuronide to morphine-6-glucuronide mean molar ratios (based on AUC) are approximately 1:24:4, similar to those occurring with both morphine sulphate solution and controlled-release morphine tablets following single doses and at steady state.

There has been no evaluation of Morcap SR in patients with impaired hepatic and renal function.

Pharmacokinetic parameters of morphine show considerable inter-subject variation. The average volume of distribution (Vd) is approximately 4 L/kg and the terminal half life is 2 to 4 hours.

Following oral administration the dose normalised extent of absorption (AUC) of morphine from Morcap SR is similar to that obtained from morphine solution or controlled-release tablets. However, the rate of absorption of morphine from Morcap SR is significantly slower.

A single 50 mg oral dose of Morcap SR in 30 healthy male subjects resulted in a mean peak plasma morphine concentration of 8.1 ng/mL (Cmax) at 8.5 hours (Tmax). The extent of absorption was unaffected by food but the Tmax was slightly delayed to 10 hours. However, this is not clinically significant. Morcap SR can be administered with or without food.

When Morcap SR is given on a fixed dosing regimen, steady state is achieved within about two days.

On a 12 hourly dosing schedule Morcap SR at steady state will exhibit a lower mean peak plasma morphine concentration (Cmax) and higher mean trough plasma morphine concentration (Cmin) than the same total daily dose of morphine solution administered on a 4 hourly dosing regimen or controlled-release morphine tablets administered on a 12 hourly dosing regimen. Although there is no clear relationship between analgesic effect or the incidence of adverse reactions and plasma morphine concentrations, the reduced fluctuation in blood morphine concentrations following administration of Morcap SR may reduce adverse reactions and the incidence of breakthrough pain.

Morphine is excreted primarily in the urine as morphine-3-glucuronide and morphine-6-glucuronide. A small amount of the glucuronide metabolites is excreted in the bile and there is some minor enterohepatic cycling. Seven to 10% of administered morphine is excreted in the faeces. Morphine-6-glucuronide has been shown to be pharmacologically active. Because accumulation of this metabolite has been observed in patients with renal disease, caution should be exercised in patients with clinically significant impairment of renal function.

*Preclinical safety data:* Not applicable.

**Pharmaceutical particulars**

*List of excipients:* Sugar spheres (sucrose, maize starch), hypromellose, ethylcellulose, methacrylic acid copolymer, polyethylene glycol, diethyl phthalate, purified talc, gelatin, shellac, black iron oxide (E172), propylene glycol, ammonium hydroxide, potassium hydroxide.

*Incompatibilities:* None known.

*Shelf life:* Blister strips: 30 months from date of manufacture of product cores. HDPE containers: 24 months from date of manufacture of product cores.

*Special precautions for storage:* Store capsules below 25°C. Protect from light and moisture.

*Nature and contents of container:* Blister packs of **30** or **60** capsules. HDPE containers of 60 capsules.

The capsules are transparent, contain creamy-white to light-tan sustained release pellets and are identified as follows:

20 mg capsule – coded K 20 with 2 discontinuous black bands.
50 mg capsule – coded K 50 with 3 discontinuous black bands.
100 mg capsule – coded K 100 with 4 discontinuous black bands.

The pack sizes in bold are marketed.

*Instructions for use/handling:* Take orally with water. No special instructions required.

*Marketing authorisation holder:* Faulding Pharmaceuticals plc, Spartan Close, Tachbrook Park, Warwick CV34 6RS.

**Marketing authorisation numbers**
Morcap SR 20 mg　　4515/0080
Morcap SR 50 mg　　4515/0081
Morcap SR 100 mg　　4515/0082

**Date of approval/revision of SPC**　April 1996.

**Legal category**　CD (Sch2), POM.


## MOTILIUM*

**Presentation**　Motilium tablets are white, film-coated tablets, marked Motilium on one side and containing domperidone maleate, equivalent to 10 mg domperidone base. Motilium tablets contain lactose.

Motilium suppositories are white and each contains domperidone 30 mg.

Motilium suspension is a sweet tasting, sugar free white suspension containing domperidone 1 mg/ml. The suspension also contains methyl and propyl parabens and sorbitol.

**Uses**

*Adults:* 1. The acute treatment of nausea and vomiting of any aetiology, in adults. Motilium is not recommended for chronic use or for the routine prophylaxis of post-operative vomiting.
2. For up to 12 weeks treatment of nausea and vomiting caused by L-dopa and bromocriptine.
3. For the treatment of symptoms of functional dyspepsia.

Motilium is not recommended for chronic administration.

*Children:* Motilium is not recommended for use in children unless indicated for the management of nausea and vomiting following cancer chemotherapy or irradiation.

**Dosage and administration**　Route, dose and frequency of administration should be adjusted according to severity and duration of symptoms.

*For the treatment of nausea and vomiting.*

*Tablets and Suspension:*
Adults (including the elderly): 10–20 mg orally at 4–8 hourly intervals.

*Children:* 0.2–0.4 mg/kg suspension by mouth at 4–8 hourly intervals.

*Suppositories:*
Adults (including the elderly): 1 or 2 suppositories at 4–8 hourly intervals.

*Children aged 2–12 yrs:*

| Weight (kg) | Maximum daily dose suppositories/day (mg/day) |
|---|---|
| 10 –15 | 1 (30 mg) |
| 15.5–25 | 2 (60 mg) |
| 25.5–35 | 3 (90 mg) |
| 35.5–45 | 4 (120 mg) |

*For the treatment of symptoms of functional dyspepsia.*

Adults (including the elderly): Tablets up to 10–20 mg orally 3 times daily before meals and 10–20 mg at night depending on clinical response. A course of treatment should not exceed 12 weeks.

*Children:* Not recommended.

**Contra-indications, warnings, etc**　No specific contra-indications.

*Precautions:* Use in pregnancy: Safe use in pregnant women has not been established, although studies in animals have not demonstrated teratogenic effects. It is therefore not advisable to administer Motilium in pregnancy. Domperidone is excreted into breast milk but at very low levels.

*Interactions:* Whilst adverse interactions have not been reported in general clinical use domperidone has the potential to interact with several classes of agent. Motilium may, therefore, alter the peripheral actions of dopamine agonists such as bromocriptine, including its hypoprolactinaemic action. The actions of Motilium on gastro-intestinal function may be antagonised by antimuscarinics and opioid analgesics. Motilium may enhance the absorption of concomitantly administered drugs particularly in patients with delayed gastric emptying.

*Side-effects:* In common with other dopamine antagonists domperidone produces a rise in serum prolactin which may be associated with galactorrhoea and less frequently with gynaecomastia, breast enlargement or soreness; there have been reports of reduced libido.

Domperidone does not readily cross the normally functioning blood brain barrier and therefore is less likely to interfere with central dopaminergic function. However, acute extrapyramidal dystonic reactions, including rare instances of oculogyric crises, have been reported with Motilium.

Should treatment of dystonic reactions be necessary, domperidone should be withdrawn and an anticholinergic anti-parkinsonian drug, or a benzodiazepine should be used.

Occasional rashes and other allergic phenomena have been reported.

*Overdosage:* No case of overdosage with oral domperidone has been reported. There is no specific antidote to Motilium but in the event of overdosage gastric lavage may be useful.

**Pharmaceutical precautions**　Motilium suppositories should be stored in a cool place. Motilium tablets should be stored below 25°C in a dry place.

**Legal category**　POM.

**Package quantities**　*Motilium tablets:* Cartons of 30 or 100 tablets in blister strips of 10 tablets.
*Motilium Suppositories:* Cartons of 10 suppositories.
*Motilium Suspension:* Bottles of 200 ml (1 mg/ml).

**Further information**　Nil.

**Product licence numbers**
Motilium tablets　　　　11723/0055
Motilium suppositories　11723/0051
Motilium suspension　　11723/0054


## MOTIPRESS* TABLETS
## MOTIVAL* TABLETS

**Qualitative and quantitative composition**
*Active constituents – Motipress*
Fluphenazine Hydrochloride BP　　1.5 mg
Nortriptyline Hydrochloride BP　　34.2 mg
(equivalent to 30 mg Nortriptyline base)

*Active constituents – Motival*
Fluphenazine Hydrochloride BP　　0.5 mg
Nortriptyline Hydrochloride BP　　11.4 mg
(equivalent to 10.0 mg Nortriptyline base)

**Pharmaceutical form**
Motipress: Yellow triangular biconvex tablets
Motival: Coral pink triangular biconvex tablets

**Clinical particulars**
*Therapeutic indications:* The treatment of patients suffering from mild to moderate mixed anxiety depressive states.

*Posology and method of administration*
Adults: One Motipress tablet daily preferably before retiring. One Motival tablet three times daily. The course of treatment should be limited to three months. If the patient does not respond after 4 weeks, an alternative treatment should be given.

*Children:* Not indicated for the treatment of children.

*Elderly:* Elderly patients should be started on one Motival tablet twice daily. If one tablet three times a day is required subsequently, Motipress may be substituted.

Motipress and Motival tablets are for oral administration.

*Contra-indications:* Phenothiazines and tricyclic antidepressants have been shown to lower the threshold for electrically induced convulsions in animals; hence, Motipress and Motival are not recommended for patients with a history of epilepsy or brain damage. They are further contra-indicated in patients with blood dyscrasias, severe cardiac insufficiency, renal or liver damage.

It is inadvisable to give monoamine oxidase inhibitors (MAOIs) with Motipress or Motival, nor should they be given in two weeks after cessation of treatment with MAOIs.

*Special warnings and precautions for use:* Motipress and Motival should be given with caution to patients with glaucoma and to those who have a propensity for urinary retention. Motipress or Motival should be used with caution in patients with cardiac failure especially when there is evidence of rhythm disturbance, and in patients with recent myocardial infarction.

*Interactions with other medicaments and other forms of interaction:* Interactions with barbiturates, alcohol and narcotic drugs may occur, so central nervous depressants should be administered with caution. Motipress and Motival may diminish the anti-hypertensive effect of an adrenergic blocking agent and could potentiate the pressor response to locally injected sympathomimetic agents.

*Pregnancy and lactation:* Do not use during pregnancy, especially in the first and last trimesters unless there are compelling reasons. There is no evidence as to drug safety in human pregnancy, nor are the results of animal studies conclusive. Breast feeding is not recommended for women receiving Motipress and Motival.

*Effects on ability to drive and to use machines:* The use of Motipress or Motival may impair alertness and abilities required for driving a car or operating machinery.

*Undesirable effects:* Tardive dyskinesias have been reported in phenothiazine therapy, usually after prolonged courses given at doses adequate to control psychotic illness. Consequently, Motipress and Motival treatment should be limited to three months.

Dryness of the mouth, drowsiness, faintness and constipation. Occasionally tachycardia, nasal congestion, blurred vision and excitement are seen.

Extrapyramidal reactions are unlikely to occur with this dose of fluphenazine alone, and it is probable that the anticholinergic activity of nortriptyline affords protection against such effects.

As with all neuroleptic drugs the presence of unexplained hyperthermia could indicate neuroleptic malignant syndrome. In this event, Motipress, Motival and associated neuroleptic treatment should be discontinued until the origin of the fever has been determined.

*Overdose:* Overdosage should be treated symptomatically and supportively. If the patient is conscious prompt gastric lavage, dilution of the stomach contents to delay absorption, or stimulation of vomiting should be attempted. An open airway should be maintained. Extrapyramidal symptoms are amenable to anti-parkinsonian drugs.

In severe hypotension, all the standard procedures for the management of circulatory shock should be instituted, e.g. vasoconstrictors and/or intravenous fluids. If vasoconstrictors are required metaraminol, mephentermine or noradrenaline should be administered but not adrenaline, as this will further lower the blood pressure through interaction with the phenothiazine.

## Pharmacological properties
*Pharmacodynamic properties:* Nortriptyline hydrochloride is a tricyclic antidepressant.

Fluphenazine hydrochloride is a tranquilliser of the phenothiazine type with a piperazine side chain.

*Pharmacokinetic properties:* Due to the nature of the two active constituents and the large inter and intra subject variability seen in trials, accurate and consistent pharmacokinetic data are not available. This can be illustrated by the fact that studies of nortriptyline hydrochloride have produced half life values ranging from 16 to 38 hours. In the case of Fluphenazine hydrochloride these values have been 10 to 16 hours.

## Pharmaceutical particulars
*List of excipients:* Tablet core: lactose, dicalcium phosphate, corn starch, magnesium stearate, gelatin.

Coating solutions: Motipress: shellac, castor oil, talc, acacia, gelatin, sugar granular, chalk, magnesium carbonate, titanium dioxide, curcumin, polyvidone, sucrose, sodium benzoate, beeswax, carnauba wax, polysorbate and sorbic acid.

Motival: shellac, castor oil, talc, polyvidone, sugar granular, chalk, erythrosine, curcumin, sucrose, titanium dioxide, sodium benzoate, beeswax, carnauba wax, polysorbate and sorbic acid.

*Incompatibilities:* None known.

*Shelf life:* 24 months.

*Special precautions for storage:* Store below 25°C.

*Nature and contents of container:* Motipress: Packs of 250 tablets supplied in amber glass bottles. Packs of 28 tablets supplied in 250 µm unplasticised PVC/20 µm hard-tempered aluminium (with PVC compatible heat-seal lacquer on the dull side) blister packs further packed into cardboard cartons.

Motival: Packs of 100 and 500 tablets supplied in amber glass bottles with one of the following closures: wadless polypropylene cap; tin plate cap with pulpboard wad and waxed aluminium facing; black phenolic cap with composition cork wad and tin foil/melinex lining; child resistant polypropylene cap of the clik-lock type lined with expanded polyethylene with PVDC (saran) facing. Packs of 30 tablets supplied in 250 µm unplasticised PVC/20 µm hard-tempered aluminium (with PVC compatible heat-seal lacquer on the dull side) blister packs. Further packed into cardboard cartons.

*Instructions for use/handling:* None.

**Marketing authorisation numbers**
Motipress        11723/0109
Motival          11723/0108

**Date of approval/revision of SPC**   November 1995.

**Legal category**  POM.

# MYCARDOL* TABLETS

**Qualitative and quantitative composition**  Mycardol Tablets contain 30 mg of Pentaerythritol Tetranitrate BPC.

**Pharmaceutical form**   Tablets.

**Clinical particulars**
*Therapeutic indications:* Mycardol tablets are indicated for the management of patients with angina pectoris. They are not recommended as a single measure for the treatment of anginal attacks, but rather as an adjunct to glyceryl trinitrate.

*Posology and method of administration:* Mycardol tablets are for oral administration.

*Adults:* The usual dosage is 2 tablets three times a day, though some may need 2 tablets four times daily. If there is nocturnal pain, the last dose should be taken before retiring. The tablets should be taken before meals.

*Elderly:* As for adults.

*Children:* Mycardol Tablets are not recommended for children.

*Contra-indications:* Mycardol should not be used immediately following a coronary thrombosis or in patients with marked anaemia, cerebral haemorrhage or head trauma.

*Special warnings and special precautions for use:* Care should be taken in treating patients liable to hypotension and those with closed-angle glaucoma. Tolerance to nitrates may occur.

*Interactions with other medicaments:* Mycardol may potentiate the effect of anti-hypertensive drugs. Tolerance to glyceryl trinitrate may occur during treatment with Mycardol. Alcohol may enhance some effects of Mycardol.

*Pregnancy and lactation:* There is no evidence of the safety of Mycardol in human pregnancy, nor is there evidence from animal work that it is free from hazard. It should be avoided in pregnancy unless there is no safer alternative.

*Undesirable effects:* Side-effects most commonly reported are headaches (8.3% in one study), nausea (4.6%), rash (3.7%), lethargy and drowsiness. They are usually mild and often resolve on reducing the dose.

*Overdose:* Symptoms of overdose are likely to be similar to those of glyceryl trinitrate: flushing, dizziness, tachycardia, headache, vomiting, restlessness, hypotension, syncope, cyanosis and methaemoglobinaemia, followed by coldness of skin, impairment of respiration and bradycardia. Treatment: gastric lavage, oxygen and assisted ventilation if necessary. Intravenous methylene blue 1–4 mg/kg is given if methaemoglobinaemia is present.

## Pharmacological properties
*Pharmacodynamic properties:* Pentaerythritol tetranitrate has vasodilator activity. It produces coronary vasodilation and increases myocardial perfusion. Its clinical effects may be explained by an improvement in oxygenation of ischaemic areas of the myocardium. Pentaerythritol tetranitrate also produces a decrease in afterload and preload and thereby a reduction in cardiac work. This would reduce the oxygen demand of the myocardium and this could also explain the clinical response.

*Pharmacokinetic properties:* Following oral administration of radio-labelled pentaerythritol tetranitrate, radioactivity was detected in the blood within 15 minutes, peak levels occurring 4 to 8 hours after the dose. Of the 20 mg and 40 mg doses administered, 32% and 41% respectively were eliminated in the faeces, and 60% and 50% in the urine in 48 hours. The main metabolites of the parent compound are pentaerythritol and the mono-, di- and tri-nitrates. The latter is very active and may contribute substantially to the activity of pentaerythritol tetranitrate.

## Pharmaceutical particulars
*List of excipients:* Mycardol tablets also contain lactose, starch (maize), dextrose monohydrate, alginic acid, stearic acid and talc.

*Incompatibilities:* No incompatibilities are known.

*Shelf life:* A shelf life of 60 months is recommended for Mycardol Tablets.

*Special precautions for storage:* Mycardol Tablets should be stored in a cool place and protected from light.

*Nature and contents of container:* Amber glass bottles with wadless polypropylene screw caps.

**Marketing authorisation number**   11723/0057.

**Date of approval/revision of SPC**   18 September 1995.

**Legal category**  P.

# NEGRAM*

**Presentation**  Negram Suspension is a deep pink, viscous suspension with a raspberry odour and taste. It contains 300 mg Nalidixic Acid PhEur per 5 ml dose. Negram Suspension contains methyl, propyl and butyl hydroxybenzoate and amaranth (E123).

Negram Tablets are beige, bi-convex tablets, 12.7 mm in diameter, marked 'NEGRAM' on one side. Each tablet contains 500 mg Nalidixic Acid PhEur.

**Uses**  Negram is recommended for the treatment of acute or chronic infections, especially those of the urinary tract caused by Gram-negative organisms, other than *Pseudomonas* species, sensitive to nalidixic acid. It may also be used for the treatment of selected cases of gastrointestinal Gram-negative infections sensitive to nalidixic acid though relapse rate and treatment failure in gastrointestinal infection may be more common.

**Dosage and administration**  For oral administration only. Nalidixic acid should be taken on an empty stomach, preferably one hour before a meal.

*Adults including the elderly:* For acute infections, 1 g four times daily for at least seven days, reducing to 0.5 g four times a day for chronic infections.

*Children:* For those over the age of three months, the maximum recommended dose is 50 mg/kg body weight per day in divided doses. When prolonged treatment is necessary it may be possible to reduce the dose to 30 mg/kg body weight without loss of therapeutic benefit. Nalidixic acid should not be administered to infants less than three months of age.

**Contra-indications, warnings, etc**
*Contra-indications:* Negram is contra-indicated for patients with a history of convulsive disorders, porphyria or hypersensitivity to nalidixic acid or related compounds.

*Precautions:* Particular caution is advised in patients with a known allergic disposition.

Patients taking Negram should avoid excessive exposure to sunlight (including sunbathing).

Negram is mainly metabolised by the liver and should therefore be used with caution in patients with liver disease. Although care should be exercised in treating patients with renal failure, the full dosage of Negram may be administered in patients with creatinine clearance of more than 20 ml/min and half the normal dosage in patients with creatinine clearance less than this.

Caution should be observed in patients with severe cerebral arteriosclerosis or glucose-6-phosphate dehydrogenase deficiency.

When Negram is given to patients on anticoagulant therapy, it may be necessary to reduce the anticoagulant dosage.

Nalidixic acid has been shown to induce lesions in weight-bearing joints of young animals. The relevance of this to man is unknown. The possible risk of late degenerative joint changes in young patients (children and growing adolescents) receiving nalidixic acid preparations should therefore be considered. If symptoms of arthralgia occur, treatment with Negram should be stopped.

Nalidixic acid should not be administered to infants less than three months of age.

Caution should be observed and therapy discontinued if patients develop signs of symptoms suggestive of an increase in intracranial pressure, psychosis or other toxic manifestations.

Blood count, renal and liver function should be monitored periodically if treatment is continued for more than two weeks.

If the clinical response is unsatisfactory or if relapse occurs, therapy should be reviewed in the light of appropriate culture and sensitivity tests. If bacterial resistance to nalidixic acid develops, it does so usually within 48 hours. Cross-resistance between nalidixic acid and other quinolone derivatives such as oxolinic acid and cinoxacin have been observed.

*Use in pregnancy and lactation:* The safety of nalidixic acid during pregnancy has not been established. Therefore it should be used during pregnancy only if the potential benefits outweigh the potential risks, specially during the first trimester (nalidixic acid crosses the placental barrier and has been shown to be taken up by growing cartilage in several animal species) and during the last month of pregnancy because of the potential risk for the neonate that exposure to maternal nalidixic acid in utero may lead to significant blood levels of nalidixic acid in the neonate immediately after birth.

Since nalidixic acid is excreted in breast milk, it is contraindicated during lactation.

*Interactions:* Negram may interact with anticoagulants due to competition for protein binding sites and it may therefore be necessary to reduce the anticoagulant dosage and monitor the prothrombin time during co-administration, until a satisfactory prothrombin ratio is achieved.

There have been reports of serious gastro-intestinal toxicity following the concomitant use of Negram and melphalan.

Nalidixic acid in therapeutic doses can interfere with the estimation of urinary 17-ketosteroids and may cause high results in the assay of urinary vanilmandelic-acid (Pisano method).

When testing for glycosuria in patients receiving Negram, glucose-specific methods based on glucose oxidase should be used because copper reduction methods may give false-positive results.

Active proliferation of the organisms is a necessary condition for the antibacterial activity of nalidixic acid: the action of Negram may therefore be inhibited by the presence of other antibacterial substances especially bacteriostatic agents such as tetracycline, chloramphenicol, and nitrofurantoin which are antagonistic to nalidixic acid in vitro.

Negram also interacts with probenecid, which inhibits the tubular secretion of nalidixic acid. This may reduce the efficacy of the product in the treatment of urinary tract infections and increase the risk of systemic side-effects.

It is possible that there will be an increased risk of nephrotoxicity with cyclosporin.

It is recognised that convulsions may occur due to an interaction between quinolones and non-steroidal anti-inflammatory drugs. This has not however been observed so far with nalidixic acid.

*Side-effects:* Reactions reported after oral administration of Negram include:

CNS: drowsiness, weakness, headache, and dizziness and vertigo. Reversible subjective visual disturbances without objective findings have occurred infrequently (generally with each dose during the first few days of treatment). These reactions include overbrightness of lights, change in colour perception, difficulty in focusing, decrease in visual acuity, and double vision. They usually disappear promptly when dosage is reduced or therapy is discontinued. Toxic psychosis or brief convulsions have been reported rarely, usually following excessive doses. In general, the convulsions have occurred in patients with predisposing factors such as epilepsy or cerebral arteriosclerosis. In infants and children receiving therapeutic doses of Negram, increased intracranial pressure with bulging anterior fontanelle, papilloedema, and headache has occasionally been observed. A few cases of 6th cranial nerve palsy have been reported. Although the mechanisms of these reactions are unknown, the signs and symptoms usually disappear rapidly with no sequelae when treatment is discontinued.

Gastro-intestinal: abdominal pain, nausea, vomiting and diarrhoea.

Allergic: rash, pruritus, urticaria, angio-oedema, eosinophilia, arthralgia with joint stiffness and swelling, and rarely, anaphylactoid reaction. Photosensitivity reactions consisting of erythema and bullae on exposed skin surfaces usually resolve completely in 2 weeks to 2 months after Negram is discontinued; however, bullae may continue to appear with successive exposures to sunlight or with mild skin trauma for up to 3 months after discontinuation of the drug. (See Warnings).

Other: rarely cholestasis, paraesthesia, metabolic acidosis, thrombocytopenia, leucopenia, or haemolytic anaemia, sometimes associated with glucose-6-phosphate dehydrogenase deficiency.

*Overdosage:* In adults, symptoms of overdosage have been noted following single doses of 20 and 25 g. These have included toxic psychosis and convulsions.

Occasional reports of metabolic acidosis have occurred in association with overdosage, use in infants under the age of three months, or overdose with concurrent use of probenecid.

Vomiting and lethargy may also occur following overdosage. Reactions are likely to be short-lived because nalidixic acid is normally excreted rapidly.

If systemic absorption has occurred, fluid intake should be promoted, supportive measures such as oxygen and means of artificial respiration should be available. Anticonvulsive therapy may be indicated in a severe case, although it has not been used in the few instances of overdosage that have been reported.

**Pharmaceutical precautions** Nil.

**Legal category** POM.

**Package quantities** *Negram Suspension:* Bottles of 150 ml.
*Negram Tablets:* Boxes of 56 tablets (7 strips of 8 tablets) (OP).

**Further information** Nalidixic acid acts by selectively inhibiting bacterial DNA synthesis. It is well absorbed following oral administration, and almost all is excreted by the kidneys, about 80% being recovered in the urine. Effective antibacterial concentrations are readily obtainable in the urine: in human volunteers, single 0.5 and 1 g oral doses produce peak urine levels varying from 25 to 250 microgram/ml.

**Product licence numbers**
Negram Suspenion 11723/0058
Negram Tablets 11723/0059.

## OSSOPAN*

**Presentation** The active ingredient of Ossopan preparations is microcrystalline hydroxyapatite compound (MCHC), which is a source of calcium and phosphorus in a protein base containing trace elements.

*Ossopan 800 tablets:* Pale buff, film-coated tablets. Each tablet contains 830 mg MCHC, providing 178 mg calcium and 82 mg phosphorus.

*Ossopan granules:* Coarse, brown granules, with a taste and odour of malt and cocoa. Each sachet contains 3320 mg MCHC, providing 712 mg calcium and 332 mg phosphorus. Each sachet contains approximately 4 grams, equivalent to 4 Ossopan 800 tablets.

**Uses** Provision of calcium and phosphorus in osteoporosis, rickets and osteomalacia and during lactation.

**Dosage and administration**
*Ossopan 800:* 4–8 tablets to be taken daily in divided doses, before meals.

*Ossopan granules:* One to two sachets daily with or before food.

**Contra-indications, warnings, etc**
*Contra-indications:* Hypercalcaemia, hypercalciuria.

*Precautions:* Care should be exercised in patients with severe immobilisation, e.g. paraplegia, and in patients with a history of renal calcium stone formation.

*Interactions:* None reported but oral calcium administration may reduce the absorption of concomitant oral tetracycline or fluoride preparations. If concomitant administration is required an interval of at least 2 hours should be observed.

*Treatment of overdosage:* No cases of intoxication with Ossopan due to deliberate or accidental overdosage have been reported to the Company. It is considered that overdosage is unlikely to be a problem.

**Pharmaceutical precautions** Tablets: Store in a dry place below 30°C. Granules: Store in a dry place.

**Legal category** P.

**Package quantities**
Ossopan 800: packs of 50 tablets.
Ossopan granules: packs containing 28 sachets (OP).

**Further information** Hydroxyapatite is the complex biological calcium salt which forms the basis of skeletal structure; its overall formula is $Ca_{10}(PO_4)_6(OH)_2$. MCHC contains about 50 per cent hydroxyapatite and X-ray diffraction studies have confirmed the presence and microcrystalline nature of the salt. It also contains many essential trace elements together with natural skeletal protein (collagen), substituent amino acids and glycosaminoglycans. Clinical studies suggest that MCHC may be more readily assimilated than synthetic calcium supplements.

**Product licence numbers**
Ossopan 800 tablets 0376/0001
Ossopan granules 11723/0062

*Product licence holder:* Ossopan tablets – Robapharm AG Basle, Switzerland.

## OXYPERTINE* CAPSULES

**Qualitative and quantitative composition** Oxypertine 10 mg.

**Pharmaceutical form** Capsule.

**Clinical particulars**
*Therapeutic indications:* Oxypertine capsules are recommended for the treatment of acute and chronic anxiety states and psychosomatic conditions whether or not accompanied by depressive overlay, tension, apprehension or sleep disturbance.

In chronic anxiety states, treatment should be restricted to short-term courses.

*Posology and method of administration*
*Adults:* 10 mg three or four times daily, usually after meals. In certain cases up to 60 mg daily in divided doses may be needed.

*Children:* Not recommended.

*Elderly:* Doses lower than those for other adults are recommended.

Oxypertine capsules are for oral administration only.

*Contra-indications:* Bone marrow depression, closed-angle glaucoma and hypersensitivity to phenothiazines. Because oxypertine can bring about the release of small amounts of catecholamines in experimental animals, it would be wise not to give oxypertine with or within three weeks of the use of monoamine oxidase inhibitors.

*Special warnings and special precautions for use:* Should be used cautiously in patients with: cardiovascular disease, respiratory disease, phaeochromocytoma, Parkinsonism, epilepsy, acute infections, renal and hepatic impairment, history of jaundice, hypothyroidism, myasthenia gravis and prostatic hypertrophy. Use with caution in very hot and very cold weather. Elderly patients are more susceptible to side-effects and lower doses are recommended.

*Interactions with other medicaments and other forms of interaction:* Oxypertine can interact with monoamine oxidase inhibitors, leading to CNS excitation and hypertension. Oxypertine may potentiate the central depressant effect of antihypertensives, alcohol and other CNS depressants. There are conflicting reports on the effect of oxypertine on urinary excretion of vanilmandelic acid.

*Pregnancy and lactation:* There is no information on the use of oxypertine in pregnancy and lactation in humans, although tests on pregnant rabbits (Somers' test) have revealed no teratogenic effects. However, the benefits of using oxypertine during the first trimester of pregnancy should be weighed against the possible risks.

Clinical experience with other phenothiazine derivatives has shown that their use in pregnancy is occasionally associated with extra-pyramidal effects in the neonate, and their use during lactation with drowsiness in the suckling infant.

*Effects on ability to drive and to use machines:* Patients should be warned to observe caution in car driving and similar activities. If affected by sedation or drowsiness, patients should not drive or operate machinery.

*Undesirable effects:* Oxypertine would be expected to share the side-effect profiles of phenothiazines. Compared to other phenothiazines, however, oxypertine has fewer sedative, anticholinergic and possibly extra-pyramidal effects. Low doses may produce agitation and hyperactivity, while higher doses are sedative.

Other side-effects reported for either oxypertine or other phenothiazines include gastro-intestinal disturbances, nasal congestion, dry mouth, hypotension, hypothermia, photophobia and photosensitivity, rashes, eosinophilia and other blood dyscrasias, positive LE cell phenomenon, insomnia, dizziness, abnormal liver function tests and jaundice, myalgia and extra-pyramidal signs, disturbances of endocrine function, e.g. hyperglycaemia, hyper-prolactinaemia, menstrual disorders and sexual function. Malignant neuroleptic syndrome, although not reported to date with oxypertine, is a rare but potentially fatal side-effect.

*Overdosage:* Symptoms and signs include CNS depression, respiratory depression, hypotension, arrhythmias, hypothermia, convulsions and severe Parkinsonism. Treatment is gastric lavage but avoid use of emetics. Hypotension is treated by plasma expanders but adrenaline should be avoided. Treatment of other features is symptomatic and supportive. Dialysis is probably not effective at removing the drug.

**Pharmacological properties**
*Pharmacodynamic properties:* It has been reported that oxypertine acts directly on the brain amines and animal studies have shown depletion of brain noradrenaline, serotonin and dopamine.

*Pharmacokinetic properties:* No pharmacokinetic studies in humans have been performed.

**Pharmaceutical particulars**
*List of excipients:* Starch (maize), lactose, magnesium stearate, gelatin, titanium dioxide.

*Incompatibilities:* None.

*Shelf life:* 48 months.

*Special precautions for storage:* Store in a dry place at or below 25°C.

*Nature and contents of container:* Amber glass bottles with wadless polypropylene screw caps containing 100 capsules.

*Instructions for use/handling:* No special warnings.

**Marketing authorisation number** 11723/0185.

**Date of approval/revision of SPC** March 1996.

**Legal category** POM.

## OXYPERTINE* TABLETS

**Qualitative and quantitative composition** Oxypertine 40.0 mg.

**Pharmaceutical form** Tablet.

**Clinical particulars**
*Therapeutic indications:* Oxypertine 40 mg tablets are recommended for the treatment of psychotic patients and are particularly useful in withdrawn schizophrenic patients. Oxypertine 40 mg tablets may also be used in acute incidence of mental disturbances such as acute agitation, behavioural disturbances, delirium and acute or subacute psychoses, including the manic phase of manic depressive psychoses.

*Posology and method of administration*
*Adults:* The usual dose is 2–3 tablets (80–120 mg) daily in divided doses. This may be varied according to the mental state and clinical response of the patient, but the total daily dosage should not exceed 300 mg.

*Children:* There are no dose recommendations for children.

*Elderly:* Doses lower than those for other adults are recommended.

Oxypertine tablets are for oral administration only.

*Contra-indications:* Bone marrow depression, closed-angle glaucoma and hypersensitivity to phenothia zines. Because oxypertine can bring about the release of small amounts of catecholamines in experimental animals, it would be wise not to give oxypertine with or within three weeks of the use of monoamine oxidase inhibitors.

*Special warnings and special precautions for use* Should be used cautiously in patients with: cardiovascular disease, respiratory disease, phaeochromocytoma, Parkinsonism, epilepsy, acute infections renal and hepatic impairment, history of jaundice hypothyroidism, myasthenia gravis and prostatic hypertrophy. Use should be cautious in very hot and very cold weather. Elderly patients are more susceptible to side-effects and lower doses are recommended.

*Interactions with other medicaments and other forms of interaction:* Oxypertine can interact with monoamine oxidase inhibitors, leading to CNS excitation and hypertension. Oxypertine may potentiate the central depressant effect of antihypertensives, alcohol and other CNS depressants. There are conflictin reports on the effect of oxypertine on urinary excretion of vanilmandelic acid.

*Pregnancy and lactation:* There is no information on the use of oxypertine in pregnancy and lactation in humans. Although tests on pregnant rabbits (Somers' test) have revealed no teratogenic effects of oxypertine, the benefits of using oxypertine in the first trimester of pregnancy should be weighed against the possible risks.

Clinical experience with other phenothiazine derivatives has shown that their use in pregnancy is occasionally associated with extra-pyramidal effects in the neonate, and their use during lactation with drowsiness in the suckling infants.

*Effects on ability to drive and to use machines:* Patients should be warned to observe caution in car driving and similar activities. If affected by sedation or drowsiness, patients should not drive or operate machinery.

*Undesirable effects:* Oxypertine would be expected to share the side-effect profiles of phenothiazines. Compared to other phenothiazines, however, oxypertine has fewer sedative, anticholinergic effects and possibly extra-pyramidal effects. Low doses may produce agitation and hyperactivity, while higher doses are sedative.

Other side-effects reported with either oxypertine or with other phenothiazines include gastro-intestinal disturbances, nasal congestion, dry mouth, hypotension, hypothermia, photophobia and photosensitivity, rashes, eosinophilia and other blood dyscrasias, positive LE cell phenomenon, insomnia, dizziness, abnormal liver function tests and jaundice, myalgia and extra-pyramidal signs, disturbances of endocrine function, e.g. hyperglycaemia, hyper-prolactinaemia, menstrual disorders and sexual function. Malignant neuroleptic syndrome, although not reported to date with oxypertine, is a rare but potentially fatal side-effect.

*Overdosage:* Symptoms and signs include CNS depression, respiratory depression, hypotension, arrhythmias, hypothermia, convulsions and severe Parkinsonism. Treatment is gastric lavage but avoid use of emetics. Hypotension is treated by plasma expanders but adrenaline should be avoided. Treatment of other features is symptomatic and supportive. Dialysis is probably not effective at removing the drug.

**Pharmacological properties**

*Pharmacodynamic properties:* It has been reported that oxypertine acts directly on the brain amines and animal studies have shown depletion of brain noradrenaline, serotonin and dopamine.

*Pharmacokinetic properties:* No pharmacokinetic studies in humans have been performed.

**Pharmaceutical particulars**

*List of excipients:* Oxypertine tablets also contain: Magnesium stearate, starch (maize), dibasic calcium phosphate dihydrate, purified talc, pregelatinised starch, lactose, purified water.

*Incompatibilities:* None.

*Shelf life:* 36 months.

*Special precautions for storage:* Store in a dry place at or below 25°C.

*Nature and contents of container:* Amber glass bottles with wadless polypropylene screw caps containing 250 tablets.

*Instructions for use/handling:* No special warnings.

**Marketing authorisation number** 11723/0186.

**Date of approval/revision of SPC** March 1996.

**Legal category** POM.

## pHiso-Med

**Qualitative and quantitative composition** Chlorhexidine Gluconate BP 20% w/v.

**Pharmaceutical form** Solution for topical use.

**Clinical particulars**

*Therapeutic indications:*

1. Pre-operative preparation of surgeons' and nurses' hands and the skin of patients.
2. As an antiseptic skin cleanser for routine hand washing and for spots and acne on the face, shoulders and chest.
3. For use in maternity units by nurses and mothers and for bathing babies, as a measure to prevent cross infection.

*Posology and method of administration:* For topical use only.

*Adults:*

*Pre-operative hand preparation:* Wet the hands and forearms, apply about 5 ml of solution and wash for one minute. Thoroughly clean fingernails with a brush or scaper. Rinse, and repeat the wash for two minutes. Rinse thoroughly and dry.

*Preparation of patients for elective surgery:* Using a sterile swab, the solution is rubbed over the site and surrounding skin for two minutes, adding a little sterile water to work up a lather. Wipe off and dry thoroughly with fresh sterile swabs. Subsequently, at the time of operation, a 0.5% solution of chlorhexidine in alcohol should be applied to the site with sterile gauze swabs. The site and the surrounding skin should be rubbed vigorously for two minutes and until dry.

*As an antiseptic skin cleaner:* Wet the area to be cleaned, apply 5 ml of solution and wash for one minute. Rinse thoroughly and dry.

*Children:*

*For bathing infants in maternity units:* A 1 in 10 dilution of the solution is applied over the body's body with a swab or with the palm of the hand. Rinse thoroughly with warm water and dry in the usual way.

*Elderly:* No special dosage recommendations.

*Contra-indications:* None stated.

*Special warnings and special precautions for use:* Chlorhexidine should not be allowed to come into contact with the brain, meninges or middle ear. During use ensure that the solution is kept away from the eyes and ears. Material which has been in contract with the solution may be stained brown by hypochlorite bleaches.

*Interactions with other medicaments and other forms of interaction:* None stated.

*Pregnancy and lactation:* No special warnings.

*Effects on ability to drive and use machines:* None stated.

*Undesirable effects:* None stated.

*Overdose:* If the solution is swallowed, it should be removed from the stomach by gastric lavage, and symptomatic treatment applied as necessary.

**Pharmacological properties**

*Pharmacodynamic properties:* Chlorhexidine is a disinfectant effective against a wide range of vegetative Gram positive and Gram negative bacteria. It is more effective against Gram positive than Gram negative bacteria, some species of Pseudomonas and Proteus being relatively less susceptible. Chlorhexidine is most active at a neutral or slightly alkaline pH, but its activity is reduced by blood and other organic matter.

*Pharmacokinetic properties:* pHiso-Med is intended for topical use only. Pharmacokinetic details are therefore not relevant.

*Pre-clinical safety data:* There are no pre-clinical data of relevance to the prescriber which are additional to those already in other sections of the SPC.

**Pharmaceutical particulars**

*List of excipients:* Aromox C12W – 30%, Solulan 16, Synchrowax HGLC, polyethylene glycol 6000 distearate, Rewoderm LI 420–70, Varonic LI 67, benzyl alcohol, gluconic acid (50% w/w), and purified water.

*Incompatibilities:* None.

*Shelf life:* 24 months.

*Special precautions for storage:* Protect from heat and light.

*Nature and contents of container:* Polyethylene bottles with polyethylene screw caps, of **150 ml** and 5000 ml capacity.

*Instructions for use/handling:* Not applicable.

**Marketing authorisation number** 11723/0060.

**Date of approval/revision of SPC** November 1996.

**Legal category** GSL.

## PLAQUENIL*

**Presentation** Plaquenil Tablets are smoothly polished, orange-coloured, biconvex, sugar-coated tablets with no markings. Each tablet contains 200 mg Hydroxychloroquine Sulphate BP. They also contain sucrose and dispersed orange (E110).

**Uses** Plaquenil Tablets are recommended for the treatment of rheumatoid arthritis, juvenile chronic arthritis, discoid and systemic lupus erythematosus and dermatological conditions caused or aggravated by sunlight.

**Dosage and administration** Plaquenil tablets are for oral administration only. Each dose should be taken with a meal or glass of milk.

Hydroxychloroquine is cumulative in action and will require several weeks to exert its beneficial effects, whereas minor side-effects may occur relatively early.

For rheumatic diseases treatment should be discontinued if there is no improvement by 6 months. In light-sensitive diseases, treatment should only be given during periods of maximum exposure to light.

*Adults including the elderly:* Initially 400 mg daily in divided doses. The dose can be reduced to 200 mg when no further improvement is evident. The maintenance dose should be increased to 400 mg daily if the response lessens. The minimum effective dose should be employed and should not exceed 6.5 mg/kg/day (calculated from ideal body weight and not actual body weight), or 400 mg whichever is the smaller.

*Children:* The minimum effective doses should be employed and should not exceed 6.5 mg/kg/day based on ideal body weight or 400 mg/day, whichever is smaller. The Plaquenil 200 mg tablet is therefore not suitable for use in children with a body weight of less than 33 kg.

**Contra-indications, warnings, etc**

*Contra-indications:* Plaquenil should not be used in patients with pre-existing maculopathy nor should it be used in those sensitive to 4-aminoquinoline compounds. A chemically related compound, chloroquine phosphate, has been found to cause foetal cochlear damage when taken in high doses during pregnancy; therefore Plaquenil should not be used in pregnancy.

*Precautions:* All patients should have an ophthalmological examination before treatment with Plaquenil is initiated. Thereafter, ophthalmological examinations must be repeated at least every 6 months. The examination should include testing visual acuity, careful ophthalmoscopy and central visual field testing with a red target. Plaquenil should be discontinued immediately in any patient who develops a pigmentary abnormality or visual field defect or any other abnormality not explainable by difficulty in accommodation or presence of corneal opacities. Patients should continue to be observed for possible progression of the changes.

The occurrence of retinopathy is very uncommon if the recommended daily doses are not exceeded. The administration of doses in excess of the recommended maximum is likely to increase the risk of retinopathy and accelerate its onset.

Impaired visual accommodation soon after the start of treatment has been reported and patients should be warned regarding driving or operating machinery. If the condition is not self-limiting it will resolve on reducing the dose or stopping treatment.

Plaquenil should be used with caution in patients taking medicines which may cause adverse ocular or skin reactions. Caution should also be applied when it is used in patients with hepatic or renal disease, in those taking medicines known to affect those organs and in patients with severe gastro-intestinal, neurological or blood disorders. Estimation of plasma hydroxychloroquine levels should be undertaken in patients with severely compromised renal or hepatic function and dosage adjusted accordingly.

Caution is also advised in patients with a sensitivity to quinine, those with glucose-6-phosphate dehydrogenase deficiency, those with porphyria cutanea tarda which can be exacerbated by hydroxychloroquine and in patients with psoriasis since it appears to increase the risk of skin reactions.

Although the risk of bone-marrow depression is low, periodic blood counts are advisable and Plaquenil should be discontinued if abnormalities develop.

Small children are particularly sensitive to the toxic effects of 4-aminoquinolines; therefore, patients should be warned to keep Plaquenil out of the reach of children.

Careful consideration should be given to using hydroxychloroquine during lactation since it has been shown to be excreted in small amounts in human breast milk.

*Interactions:* Plaquenil has been reported to increase plasma digoxin levels; serum digoxin levels should be closely monitored in patients receiving combined therapy.

Plaquenil may also be subject to several of the known interactions of chloroquine even though specific reports have not appeared. These include: potentiation of its direct blocking action at the neuromuscular junction by aminoglycoside antibiotics; inhibition of its metabolism by cimetidine which may increase plasma concentration of the antimalarial; antagonism of effect of neostigmine and pyridostigmine; reduction of the antibody response to primary immunisation with intradermal human diploid-cell rabies vaccine.

As with chloroquine, antacids may reduce absorption of hydroxychloroquine so it is advised that a 4 hour interval be observed between Plaquenil and antacid dosaging.

*Side-effects:* Retinopathy with changes in pigmentation and visual field defects can occur, but appears to be uncommon if the recommended daily dose is not exceeded. In its early form, it appears reversible on discontinuation of Plaquenil. If allowed to develop, there may be a risk of progression even after treatment withdrawal.

Corneal changes including oedema and opacities

have been reported. They are either symptomless or may cause disturbances such as haloes, blurring of vision or photophobia. They may be transient and are reversible on stopping treatment. Blurring of vision due to a disturbance of accommodation which is dose dependant and reversible may also occur.

Skin rashes sometimes occur; pigmentary changes in skin and mucous membranes, bleaching of hair, and hair loss have also been reported. These usually resolve readily on stopping treatment. Isolated cases of exfoliative dermatitis have been reported. Plaquenil may also precipitate or exacerbate porphyria and may precipitate attacks of psoriasis.

Other adverse effects include gastrointestinal disturbances such as nausea, diarrhoea, anorexia, abdominal cramps and, rarely, vomiting. These symptoms usually resolve immediately on reducing the dose or on stopping the treatment. Less frequently, muscle weakness, vertigo, tinnitus, nerve deafness, headache, nervousness and emotional upsets have been reported. Rarely, there have been reports of bone marrow depression, cardiomyopathy, convulsions, neuromyotoxicity, and toxic psychosis.

Isolated cases of abnormal liver function tests have been reported. Rare cases of fulminant hepatic failure have also been reported.

*Overdosage:* Overdosage with the 4-aminoquinolines is particularly dangerous in infants, as little as 1–2 g having proved fatal.

The symptoms of overdosage may include headache, visual disturbance, cardiovascular collapse, and convulsions, followed by sudden and early respiratory and cardiac arrest. Since these effects may appear soon after taking a massive dose, treatment should be prompt and symptomatic. The stomach should be immediately evacuated, either by emesis or by gastric lavage. Finely powdered charcoal in a dose at least five times that of the overdose may inhibit further absorption if introduced into the stomach by tube, following lavage and within 30 minutes of ingestion of the overdose.

Consideration should be given to administration of parenteral diazepam in cases of overdosage; it has been shown to reverse chloroquine cardiotoxicity.

Respiratory support may be needed and need for intubation or tracheostomy considered. Shock should be treated by the administration of fluid (with plasma expanders if necessary) with central venous pressure monitoring. In severe cases, the administration of dopamine should be considered.

A patient who survives the acute phase and is asymptomatic should be closely observed for at least six hours.

**Pharmaceutical precautions** Nil.

**Legal category** POM.

**Package quantities** Plaquenil is supplied in bottles of 56 tablets (OP).

**Further information** Hydroxychloroquine has several pharmacological actions which may be involved in its therapeutic effect. These include interaction with sulphydryl groups, interference with enzyme activity (including phospholipase, NADH – cytochrome C reductase, cholinesterase, proteases and hydrolases), DNA binding, stabilisation of lysosomal membranes, inhibition of prostaglandin formation, polymorphonuclear cell chemotaxis and phagocytosis, possible interference with interleukin 1 production from monocytes and inhibition of neutrophil superoxide release.

Following oral administration, hydroxychloroquine is almost completely absorbed. In one study, mean peak plasma hydroxychloroquine concentrations following a single dose of 400 mg in healthy subjects ranged from 53–208 ng/ml with a mean of 105 ng/ml. The mean time to peak plasma concentration was 1.83 hours.

The mean plasma elimination half-life varied: 5.9 hours (at $C_{max}$–10 hours), 26.1 hours (at 10–48 hours) and 299 hours (at 48–504 hours). The parent compound and metabolites are widely distributed in the body and elimination is mainly via the urine.

**Product licence number** 11723/0063.

# PRIMACOR* INJECTION

**Presentation** Primacor Injection is a sterile, clear, colourless to pale yellow solution, each 10 ml ampoule containing 10 mg milrinone as the lactate. Primacor also contains dextrose and lactic acid.

**Uses** Primacor Injection is indicated for the short-term treatment of severe congestive heart failure unresponsive to conventional maintenance therapy and for the treatment of acute heart failure, including low output states, following cardiac surgery.

Milrinone is a positive inotrope and vasodilator, with little chronotropic activity. It also improves left ventricular diastolic relaxation. It differs in structure and mode of action from the digitalis glycosides, catecholamines or angiotensin-converting enzyme inhibitors.

It is a selective inhibitor of peak III phosphodiesterase isoenzyme in cardiac and vascular muscle. It produces slight enhancement of A–V node conduction, but no other significant electrophysiological effects.

In clinical studies Primacor Injection has been shown to produce improvements in the haemodynamic indices of congestive heart failure, including cardiac output, pulmonary capillary wedge pressure and vascular resistance, without clinically significant effect on heart rate or myocardial oxygen consumption. These improvements are related to both dose and plasma concentration. Haemodynamic improvement during intravenous Primacor therapy is accompanied by clinical symptomatic improvement, as measured by changes in New York Heart Association classification.

**Dosage and administration** For intravenous administration.

*Adults:* Primacor Injection should be given as a loading dose of 50 micrograms/kg administered over a period of 10 minutes followed by continuous maintenance infusion at a dosage titrated between 0.375 micrograms/kg/min and 0.75 micrograms/kg/min according to a haemodynamic and clinical response but should not exceed 1.13 mg/kg/day total dose.

**Note:** In impaired renal function, lower rates of maintenance infusion are advised: See 'Use in impaired renal function.'

The following provides a guide to maintenance infusion delivery rate based upon a solution containing milrinone 200 micrograms/ml.†

| Primacor Injection Dose (micrograms/kg/min) | Maintenance Infusion delivery rate (ml/kg/hr) |
|---|---|
| 0.375 | 0.11 |
| 0.400 | 0.12 |
| 0.500 | 0.15 |
| 0.600 | 0.18 |
| 0.700 | 0.21 |
| 0.750 | 0.22 |

† A 200 micrograms/ml solution is prepared by adding 40 ml diluent per 10 ml ampoule Primacor Injection.

0.45% saline, 0.9% saline or 5% dextrose may be used as diluents.

Solutions of different concentrations may be used according to patient fluid requirements.

The duration of therapy should depend upon the patient's response. In congestive cardiac failure patients have been maintained on treatment for up to 5 days although the usual period is 48 to 72 hours. In acute states following cardiac surgery it is unlikely that treatment need be maintained for more than 12 hours.

*Use in impaired renal function:* Data obtained from patients with severe renal impairment but without congestive heart failure have demonstrated that the presence of renal impairment significantly increases the terminal elimination half-life of milrinone. For patients with clinical evidence of renal impairment, the following maintenance infusion rates are recommended:

| Creatinine Clearance (ml/min/ 1.73m²) | Primacor Injection Dose (micrograms/ kg/min) | Maintenance Infusion delivery rate (for solution of milrinone 200 micrograms/ml) (ml/kg/hr) |
|---|---|---|
| 5 | 0.20 | 0.06 |
| 10 | 0.23 | 0.07 |
| 20 | 0.28 | 0.08 |
| 30 | 0.33 | 0.10 |
| 40 | 0.38 | 0.11 |
| 50 | 0.43 | 0.13 |

Adjustment of the infusion rate should be made according to haemodynamic response.

*Use in elderly patients:* Experience so far suggests that no special dosage recommendations for the elderly patient are necessary.

*Use in children:* Safety and effectiveness in children have not been established.

**Contra-indications, warnings, etc**

*Contra-indications:* Hypersensitivity to Primacor Injection is a contra-indication to its use.

*Precautions:* The use of Primacor Injection is not recommended immediately following acute myocardial infarction until safety and efficacy have been established in this situation.

In patients with severe obstructive aortic or pulmonary valvular disease or hypertrophic subaortic stenosis, Primacor Injection should not be used in place of surgical relief of the obstruction. In these conditions it is possible that a drug with inotropic/vasodilator properties might aggravate outflow obstruction.

Supraventricular and ventricular arrhythmias have been observed in the high risk population treated with Primacor injection. In some patients an increase in non-sustained ventricular tachycardia has been observed which did not affect patient safety or outcome.

As Primacor injection produces a slight enhancement in A–V node conduction, there is a possibility of increased ventricular response rate in patients with uncontrolled atrial flutter/fibrillation. In these patients, prior digitalisation or treatment with other agents to prolong A–V node conduction time should be considered and to discontinuing milrinone therapy if arrythmias occur.

Milrinone may induce hypotension through its vasodilatory actions. Particular caution should therefore be observed when initiating Primacor Injection therapy in patients who are hypotensive and in those in whom prior vigorous diuretic therapy is suspected of causing significant decreases in cardiac filling pressure.

Blood pressure, heart rate, electro-cardiogram, clinical state, fluid balance, electrolytes and renal function should be carefully monitored when initiating and during Primacor Injection therapy. The infusion should be slowed or stopped if arrhythmias develop or an excessive decrease in blood pressure occurs.

Improvement in cardiac output with resultant diuresis may necessitate a reduction in the dose of diuretic. Potassium loss due to excessive diuresis may predispose digitalised patients to arrhythmias. Therefore, hypokalaemia should be corrected by potassium supplementation in advance of, or during, the use of Primacor Injection.

*Use in pregnancy and lactation:* Although animal studies have not revealed evidence of drug-induced foetal damage or other deleterious effects on reproductive function, the safety of milrinone in human pregnancy has not yet been established. It should be used during pregnancy only if the potential benefit justifies the potential risk to the foetus.

Caution should be exercised when Primacor Injection is administered to nursing women, since it is not known whether milrinone is excreted in human milk.

*Side-effects:* Ventricular ectopic activity, supraventricular and ventricular arrhythmias have been reported during treatment with Primacor injection. An increase in ventricular response rate in patients with atrial fibrillation may occur. The incidence of arrhythmias has not been related to dose or plasma levels of milrinone. Other reported side-effects include hypotension, angina/chest pain, headaches, hypokalaemia and tremor. Thrombocytopenia has also been observed but has not been definitely related to the administration of Primacor Injection.

*Drug interactions:* No untoward clinical manifestations of drug interaction have been observed during Primacor Injection therapy.

Whilst there is a theoretical potential interaction with calcium channel blockers, there has been no evidence of a clinically significant interaction to date.

Milrinone has a favourable inotropic effect in fully digitalised patients without causing signs of glycoside toxicity.

*Chemical compatibility:* Precipitation occurs immediately when frusemide or bumetanide is mixed with milrinone solution. Therefore, frusemide or bumetanide should not be administered in intravenous line containing Primacor Injection. Sodium Bicarbonate Intravenous Infusion should not be used for dilution.

Other drugs should not be mixed with Primacor Injection until further compatibility data are available.

*Overdosage:* Overdoses of intravenous Primacor Injection may produce hypotension because of its vasodilatory effect. If this occurs Primacor injection administration should be reduced or temporarily discontinued until the patients condition stabilises. No specific antidote is known, but general measures for circulatory support should be taken.

**Pharmaceutical precautions** Store at room temperature; avoid freezing. Infusion solutions diluted as recommended with 0.45% saline, 0.9% saline or 5% dextrose should be freshly prepared before use.

Parenteral drug products should be examined visually and should not be used if particulate matter or discolouration are present.

**Legal category** POM.

**Package quantities** Boxes of 10 ampoules.

**Further information** In congestive heart failure milrinone, on intravenous administration, has a volume of distribution of about 0.4 l/kg, a terminal elimination half-life of about 2.3 hours and a clearance of about 0.13 l/kg/h. These pharmacokinetic parameters are not dose-dependent. Milrinone is approximately 70% bound to plasma protein and is primarily excreted unchanged via the kidney.

**Product licence number** 11723/0064.

# PROMINAL*

**Presentation** Prominal Tablets 30 mg are white, biconvex tablets, 6.4 mm in diameter, marked P30 on one side and plain on the other. Each tablet contains 30 mg Methylphenobarbitone PhEur.

Prominal Tablets 60 mg are white, biconvex tablets, 7.9 mm in diameter, marked P60 on one side and plain on the other. Each tablet contains 60 mg Methylphenobarbitone PhEur.

Prominal Tablets 200 mg are white, biconvex tablets, 10.3 mm in diameter, marked P200 on one side and plain on the other. Each tablet contains 200 mg Methylphenobarbitone PhEur.

Prominal Tablets 30 mg, 60 mg and 200 mg contain lactose.

## Uses

*Indications:* Prominal Tablets are recommended for the treatment of epilepsy except absence seizures.

*Pharmacology:* Barbiturates reversibly depress the activity of all excitable tissues, the central nervous system being exquisitely sensitive to their effects.

Methylphenobarbitone undergoes N-demethylation by hepatic microsomal enzymes, forming phenobarbitone, to which most of its activity in chronic medication can be attributed.

**Dosage and administration** Prominal is for oral administration only.

*Adults:* The daily dosage must be determined individually. The average range is 200–400 mg. The maximum daily dose is 600 mg.

*Elderly:* As for adults but see 'Precautions'.

*Children:* 5–15 mg/kg/day but see 'Precautions'.

*Dosing:* Dosage should be adjusted carefully with gradual increments at intervals of two to three weeks until fits are controlled or toxicity supervenes. Plateau-state at a given dosage is only achieved after some weeks of medication. Unless serious toxicity dictates otherwise, any reduction in dosage should proceed very gradually to avoid provoking status epilepticus. Monitoring plasma phenobarbitone levels may be helpful when therapy is switched from phenobarbitone to Prominal or vice versa.

## Contra-indications, warnings, etc

*Contra-indications:* Acute intermittent and variegate porphyria; hypersensitivity or idiosyncrasy to barbiturates, states of debilitation, senility, alcohol or other drug abuse or history of abuse; hyperkinetic children; severe renal or hepatic disease.

*Precautions:* Prominal should be avoided or used only with particular caution and appropriate supervision in children and the elderly who are likely to be specially sensitive to its effects and may react paradoxically.

Prominal should also be avoided or used with special care in patients with hepatic or renal disease whose ability to excrete phenobarbitone may be impaired. Similar caution should be observed in patients with respiratory insufficiency who may prove specially sensitive to the depressant effects of barbiturate on respiration.

Patients who drive or operate machinery should be warned that Prominal can reduce alertness and impair performance. If affected, patients should not undertake these tasks.

Alcohol should be avoided when taking Prominal since as with other CNS depressants, its depressant effect is likely to be additive to that of the barbiturate. In view of the extensive range of inter-reactions between barbiturates and other drugs (see below) caution is advised whenever Prominal is to be co-administered with another medication.

Vitamin D supplement may be needed during long-term Prominal therapy, since Vitamin D catabolism may be increased. Vitamin K supplement may be needed for neonates exposed to barbiturate (see below).

*Abuse and dependence:* Prominal, like other barbiturates, may lead to psychical and physical dependence in which tolerance and dose increment may be marked features. Symptoms of chronic intoxication include confusion, poor judgement, irritability, insomnia and somatic complaints. Prominal intake should be reduced with great care and under appropriate supervision. Abrupt cessation may precipitate convulsions and can be fatal. Neonates may also suffer from withdrawal symptoms (see below) even in the face of therapeutic dosaging.

*Use in pregnancy:* Anticonvulsant drugs are as useful to an epileptic during pregnancy as they are at other times and for the individual epileptic mother the chance of an abnormal baby due to drug treatment is small. However, several reports have appeared in the literature suggesting the possible implication of the epileptic state, anticonvulsants and folic acid deficiency as causative agents in certain congenital abnormalities. Scientific knowledge does not yet permit an adequate definition to be made of the respective roles of these three factors. It is recommended therefore, that if anticonvulsant therapy with Prominal is judged necessary during pregnancy, adequate folic acid supplements should be given and the epilepsy controlled as completely as possible with the lowest effective dose.

*Neonates:* Barbiturates may be transferred to the foetus in utero, as well as to the suckling neonate. Therefore the possibility of barbiturate effects in the neonate, including respiratory depression, sedation and withdrawal reaction, and of the need to give Vitamin K to counteract possible hypoprothrombinaemia, should be borne in mind.

*Interactions with other drugs:* Barbiturates can affect the actions of a wide range of other drugs principally through an increase in their disposal by stimulation of hepatic microsomal enzymes with usually a resultant decrease but in some instances, an increase, in their therapeutic effect or toxicity. The interactions may be mutual, the plasma levels and activities of barbiturates being also subject to influence by other drugs. Apart from kinetic and metabolic interactions, there may be an addition of effect, for example, the severe depression that may occur when barbiturates are combined with ethanol or other CNS depressants. For these reasons particular care should be observed when administering Prominal in combination with CNS depressants such as sedatives and antihistamines, coumarin-type anticoagulants, antidepressants, including mono-amine oxidase inhibitors, systemic steroids (including oral contraceptives), anticonvulsants such as phenytoin and valproate, antibiotics such as chloramphenicol, rifampicin, metronidazole, doxycycline and also griseofulvin, antihypertensive agents including beta-blockers such as metoprolol and propranolol, but also frusemide and digoxin, opioids such as pethidine and dextropropoxyphene, and many other agents including theophylline, cimetidine, and some oral hypoglycaemic drugs.

*Side-effects:* Drowsiness and other evidence of sedation is likely to be the most common side effect, but unsteadiness, vertigo and inco-ordination may occur. Paradoxical excitement, restlessness and confusion may occur in the elderly or in the presence of pain; irritability and hyperexcitability may occur in children. Respiratory depression may also occur even at therapeutic dosage and with chronic medication there may be disorientation, mental confusion, ataxia, depression and dependence.

Allergic reactions particularly affecting the skin are not uncommon, including maculopapular rash, fixed drug eruptions and photosensitivity. Occasionally exfoliative dermatitis, erythema multiforme and toxic epidermal necrolysis have been reported. Megaloblastic anaemia associated with folate deficiency has developed during chronic administration and hypoprothrombinaemia may occur in neonates exposed to the barbiturate. Other reported side effects associated with barbiturate include stomatitis, arthritis, acute interstitial nephritis and hepatitis in patients who may be sensitive to this type of drug.

*Overdosage:* The signs and symptoms of acute overdosage include varying degrees of cardiorespiratory depression, hypotension, absent bowel sounds, renal failure, hypothermia, CNS depression including coma and areflexia. In this setting, a flat EEG may not indicate irreversible brain damage. The aims in treating poisoning by Prominal are to maintain respiration, treat any shock and prevent further absorption of the drug. Where patients are seen within four hours of taking an overdose, gastric aspiration or lavage may be beneficial in adults, while children who are conscious may be given an emetic (e.g. Ipecacuanha Emetic Mixture Paediatric BP). Severely poisoned patients who continue to deteriorate despite supportive treatment may require additional active measures including forced alkaline diuresis, peritoneal dialysis, haemodialysis and haemoperfusion.

**Pharmaceutical precautions** Nil.

**Legal category** CD (Sch 3) POM.

**Package quantities** Prominal Tablets (30 mg, 60 mg and 200 mg) are supplied in bottles of 100.

**Further information** Nil.

**Product licence numbers**

| | |
|---|---|
| Prominal Tablets 30 mg | 11723/0066 |
| Prominal Tablets 60 mg | 11723/0067 |
| Prominal Tablets 200 mg | 11723/0065 |

# PYROGASTRONE* LIQUID

**Qualitative and quantitative composition** Active constituents: Carbenoxolone Sodium BP 0.20% w/v, Dried Aluminium Hydroxide PhEur 3.0% w/v and Potassium Bicarbonate BPC 3.0% w/v.

Pyrogastrone Liquid provides 117 mg (3.0 mmol) potassium and 38.8 mg (1.7 mmol) sodium per 10 ml dose.

**Pharmaceutical form** A fine, off white powder with a faint odour of liquorice and aniseed.

**Clinical particulars**

*Therapeutic indications:* For the treatment of oesophageal inflammation, erosions and ulcers due to hiatus hernia or other conditions causing gastro-oesophageal reflux and for the relief of heartburn, flatulence and other symptoms associated with reflux oesophagitis.

*Posology and method of administration:*

*Adults:* 10 ml to be taken three times daily immediately after meals and 20 ml at bedtime. Treatment should be continued for at least six weeks, but up to 12 weeks treatment may be necessary to ensure maximum healing effect.

*Elderly:* Not recommended for patients over 75 years. Otherwise, as for adults but see *Precautions*.

*Children:* Not recommended.

Pyrogastrone liquid is for oral administration only.

*Contra-indications:* Pyrogastrone is contra-indicated in patients over 75 years, in children and in pregnancy. Pyrogastrone should not be administered to patients suffering from cardiac, renal or hepatic failure nor to patients on digitalis glycosides unless serum electrolyte levels are monitored at weekly intervals and measures taken to avoid the development of hypokalaemia. It is contra-indicated in established hypokalaemia.

*Special warnings and special precautions for use:* Special care should be exercised with patients predisposed to sodium and water retention, potassium loss and hypertension (e.g. those with cardiac, renal or hepatic disease) since carbenoxolone can induce similar changes. Potassium supplements should be considered for those at risk from developing hypokalaemia. Regular monitoring of weight, blood pressure and clinical condition is advisable for all patients. Pyrogastrone should be withdrawn if hypokalaemia or oedema develops or a clinically significant rise in blood pressure occurs. Potassium loss should be corrected by the administration of supplements.

*Interactions with other medicaments and other forms of interaction:* Pyrogastrone may provoke digitalis glycoside toxicity by inducing hypokalaemia. There is a theoretical possibility of a pharmacodynamic interaction with anti-hypertensive drugs, carbenoxolone possibly making hypertension more difficult to control.

Most classes of diuretics will induce hypokalaemia which may be exacerbated by concomitant administration of carbenoxolone as may the mineralocorticoid effects of steroids.

Although spironolactone and amiloride will antagonise the hypokalaemia induced by carbenoxolone they also inhibit its healing action and therefore, should not be prescribed with Pyrogastrone.

Antacids can interact with a wide variety of medicaments generally through effects on their absorption or excretion. These include:

Analgesics: the absorption of diflunisal is reduced and urinary excretion of aspirin may be increased.

Antiarrhythmics: the urinary excretion of flecainide, mexiletine and quinidine may be reduced.

Antibacterials: the absorption of ciprofloxacin, ofloxacin, pivampicillin, rifampicin and most tetracyclines may be reduced as may the absorption of itraconazole and ketoconazole.

Other agents: the absorption of chloroquine, hydroxychloroquine, phenothiazines, oral iron, dipyridamole and penicillamine may all be reduced whilst excretion of lithium may be increased.

*Pregnancy and lactation:* Although animal studies have shown no hazard, there is inadequate evidence of the safety of carbenoxolone in human pregnancy. Pyrogastrone should be avoided by patients who are pregnant or are breast-feeding mothers.

*Effects on ability to drive and to use machines:* None.

*Undesirable effects:* Pyrogastrone may induce sodium and water retention and potassium loss provoking hypertension and cardiac failure in those so predisposed. If profound hypokalaemia is permitted to develop it may lead to widespread impairment of neuromuscular function and muscle damage. Prolonged hypokalaemia may cause renal damage.

*Overdosage:* If recently ingested the stomach should be emptied by gastric lavage. Serum electrolytes should be monitored and any dificiency in potassium should be corrected, using the intravenous route if necessary, or slow-release or effervescent tablets of potassium chloride. Should water and sodium retention require correction with a diuretic, careful monitoring of potassium levels is mandatory.

**Pharmacological properties**

*Pharmacodynamic properties:* Carbenoxolone sodium is a derivative of enoxolone with marked anti-inflammatory actions. It appears to act locally on the stomach possibly by stimulant actions upon mucin production and the enzyme process involved in cellular regeneration. Aluminium hydroxide is a slow acting antacid. Potassium bicarbonate is an antacid.

*Pharmacokinetic properties:* Carbenoxolone sodium is absorbed from the gastrointestinal tract, the main site of absorption is the stomach. Absorption is reduced if the gastric pH is above 2. Maximum plasma concentrations are obtained 1 hour after administration in a fasting state but can be delayed for several hours if the dose is taken after food; a second peak appears 2 or 3 hours later probably due to enterohepatic cycling of metabolites. It is bound to proteins in the circulation. Removal of drug from the blood is fairly slow with an elimination half-life of approximately 16 hours. Carbenoxolone is mainly excreted in the faeces via the bile.

Aluminium hydroxide is not generally absorbed from the gastrointestinal tract but patients with renal failure have absorbed aluminium and it has been detected in bone. The hydroxide is converted to chloride in the stomach and reconverted to hydroxide in the intestine. Some insoluble aluminium phosphates are also produced which are excreted in the faeces.

Alginic acid is not absorbed by the body and there is no concentration-effect relationship. It is passed unchanged into the faeces.

**Pharmaceutical particulars**

*List of excipients:* Pyrogastrone liquid also contains sucrose, povidone, dispersible cellulose, sodium methylhydroxybenzoate, sodium propylhydroxybenzoate, sodium alginate, Manugel, liquorice/aniseed flavour and water.

*Incompatibilities:* Not applicable.

*Shelf life:* The shelf-life of the unopened product is 36 months. The shelf-life of the reconstituted product is 3 months.

*Special precautions for storage:* Store below 25°C.

*Nature and contents of container:* The powder is contained in 600 ml glass cylindrical amber glass bottle with a black plastic screw cap. It is reconstituted prior to use with 450 ml of water.

*Instructions for use/handling:* Not applicable.

**Marketing authorisation number**   11723/0069.

**Date of approval/revision of SPC**   September 1993.

**Legal category**   POM.

## PYROGASTRONE* TABLETS

**Presentation**   Pyrogastrone chewable tablets are white, round, strawberry-flavoured chewable tablets, 22.2 mm in diameter, marked PYROGASTRONE on one side. Each tablet contains:

| | |
|---|---|
| Carbenoxolone Sodium BP | 20 mg |
| Dried Aluminium Hydroxide PhEur | 240 mg |
| Magnesium Trisilicate PhEur | 60 mg |

in a base containing 210 mg Sodium Bicarbonate PhEur and 600 mg Alginic Acid PhEur.

Each Pyrogastrone chewable tablet contains approximately 59.2 mg (2.6 mmol) sodium.

**Uses**   For the treatment of oesophageal inflammation, erosions and ulcers due to hiatus hernia or other conditions causing gastro-oesophageal reflux and for the relief of heartburn, flatulence and other symptoms associated with reflux oesophagitis.

**Dosage and administration**   For oral administration only.

*Adults:* 1 tablet to be chewed three times daily immediately after meals and 2 tablets to be chewed at bedtime. The tablets may be followed by a drink of water.

Treatment should be continued for at least six weeks, but up to 12 weeks' treatment may be necessary to ensure maximum healing effect.

*Elderly:* Not recommended for patients over 75 years. Otherwise, as for adults.

*Children:* Not recommended.

**Contra-indications, warnings, etc**

*Contra-indications:* Pyrogastrone is contra-indicated in patients over 75 years, in children and in pregnancy. Pyrogastrone should not be administered to patients suffering from cardiac, renal or hepatic failure nor to patients on digitalis glycosides unless serum electrolyte levels are monitored at weekly intervals and measures taken to avoid the development of hypokalaemia. It is contra-indicated in established hypokalaemia.

*Precautions:* Special care should be exercised with patients pre-disposed to sodium and water retention, potassium loss and hypertension (e.g. the elderly and those with cardiac, renal or hepatic disease) since carbenoxolone can induce similar changes. Potassium supplements should be considered for those at risk from developing hypokalaemia.

Regular monitoring of weight, blood pressure and clinical condition is advisable for all patients. Pyrogastrone should be withdrawn if hypokalaemia or oedema develops or a clinically significant rise in blood pressure occurs. Potassium loss should be corrected by the administration of supplements.

*Pregnancy:* Although animal studies have shown no hazard, there is inadequate evidence of the safety of carbenoxolone in human pregnancy. Pyrogastrone should be avoided in patients who are pregnant.

*Interactions:* Pyrogastrone may provoke digitalis glycoside toxicity by inducing hypokalaemia.

There is a theoretical possibility of a pharmacodynamic interaction with anti-hypertensive drugs, carbenoxolone possibly making hypertension more difficult to control.

Most classes of diuretics will induce hypokalaemia which may be exacerbated by concomitant administration of carbenoxolone as may the mineralocorticoid effects of steroids.

Although spironolactone and amiloride will antagonise the hypokalaemia induced by carbenoxolone they also inhibit its healing action and, therefore, should not be prescribed with Pyrogastrone.

Antacids can interact with a wide variety of medications generally through effects on their absorption or excretion. These include:

Analgesics – the absorption of diflunisal is reduced and urinary excretion of aspirin may be increased.

Antiarrhythmics – the urinary excretion of flecainide, mexiletine and quinidine may be reduced.

Antibacterials – the absorption of ciprofloxacin, ofloxacin, pivampicillin, rifampicin and most tetracyclines may be reduced as may the absorption of itraconazole and ketoconazole.

Other agents – the absorption of chloroquine, hydroxychloroquine, phenothiazines, oral iron, dipyridamole and penicillamine may all be reduced whilst excretion of lithium may be increased.

*Side-effects:* Pyrogastrone may induce sodium and water retention and potassium loss, provoking hypertension and cardiac failure in those so predisposed. If profound hypokalaemia is permitted to develop it may lead to widespread impairment of neuromuscular function and to muscle damage. Prolonged hypokalaemia may cause renal damage.

*Overdosage:* If recently ingested the stomach should be emptied by gastric lavage. Serum electrolytes should be monitored and any deficiency in potassium should be corrected, using the intravenous route if necessary, or slow-release or effervescent tablets of potassium chloride. Should water and sodium retention require correction with a diuretic, careful monitoring of potassium levels is mandatory.

**Pharmaceutical precautions**   Store in a dry place.

**Legal category**   POM.

**Package quantities**   Boxes containing 25 foil strips of 4 tablets.

**Further Information**   The alginate antacid base of Pyrogastrone forms a clinging viscous foam which has buffering capacity. This relieves symptoms, either by coating the oesophageal wall, by impeding gastro-oesophageal reflux, or the foam may reflux instead of the acid gastric contents. The incorporation of carbenoxolone into the formulation has been shown to exert an additional healing effect on oesophageal ulcers possibly by improving mucus synthesis and/or by increasing the life-span of oesophageal epithelium.

Systemic absorption of carbenoxolone is extensive. There is more than 99.95% binding to plasma proteins. There appears to be enterohepatic circulation which delays clearance. Excretion is mainly via the faeces. Plasma elimination half life increases with age. Aluminium hydroxide is not generally absorbed from the gastrointestinal tract, while alginic acid is not digested and passes unchanged into the faeces.

**Product licence number**   11723/0068

## RESONIUM* A

**Presentation**   Resonium A contains 99.93% sodium polystyrene sulphonate ground and flavoured to a buff-coloured powder with a pleasant vanilla odour and sweet taste.

**Uses**   Resonium A is an ion-exchange resin which is recommended for the treatment of hyperkalaemia associated with anuria or severe oliguria. It is also used to treat hyperkalaemia in patients requiring dialysis and in patients on regular haemodialysis or on prolonged peritoneal dialysis.

**Dosage and administration**   Resonium A is for oral or rectal administration only. The dosage recommendations detailed in this section are a guide only, the precise requirements should be decided on the basis of regular serum electrolyte determinations.

*Adults including the elderly:*
1. *Oral:* Usual dose 15 g three or four times a day. The resin is given by mouth in a little water, or it may be made into a paste with some sweetened vehicle.
2. *Rectal:* In cases where vomiting may make oral administration difficult, the resin may be given rectally as a suspension of 30 g resin in 100 ml 2% Methylcellulose 450 BP (medium viscosity) and 100 ml water as a daily retention enema. In the initial stages administration by this route as well as orally may help to achieve a more rapid lowering of the serum potassium level.

The enema should if possible be retained for at least nine hours following which the colon should be irrigated to remove the resin. If both routes are used initially it is probably unnecessary to continue rectal administration once the oral resin has reached the rectum.

*Children:* 1 g/kg body weight daily in divided doses in acute hyperkalaemia. Dosage may be reduced to 0.5 g/kg body weight in divided doses for maintenance therapy. The resin is given orally, preferably with a drink (not a fruit squash because of the high potassium content) or a little jam or honey. When refused by mouth it should be given rectally, using a dose at least as great as that which would have been given orally diluted in the same ratio as described for adults. Following retention of the enema, the colon should be irrigated to ensure adequate removal of the resin.

*Neonates:* Resonium A should not be given by the oral route. With rectal administration, the minimum effective dosage within the range 0.5 g/kg to 1 g/kg should be employed diluted as for adults and with adequate irrigation to ensure recovery of the resin.

**Contra-indications, warnings, etc**

*Contra-indications:* Resonium A should not be administered orally to neonates. It should not be administered to neonates with reduced gut motility (e.g. post operatively or drug induced). Resonium A is also contra-indicated in the presence of obstructive bowel disease, in use where plasma potassium levels are below 5 mmol/litre and in patients with a history of hypersensitivity to polystyrene sulphonate resins.

*Precautions:* The possibility of severe potassium depletion should be considered and adequate clinical and biochemical control is essential during treatment especially in patients on digitalis. Administration of the resin should be stopped when the serum potassium level falls to 5 mmol/litre.

Because the resin may bind calcium and magnesium ions, deficiencies of these electrolytes may occur. Accordingly, patients should be monitored for all applicable electrolyte disturbances.

In the event of clinically significant constipation treatment should be discontinued until normal bowel movement has resumed. Magnesium-containing laxatives should not be used.

The patient should be positioned carefully when ingesting the resin, in order to avoid aspiration, which may lead to bronchopulmonary complications.

Sorbitol added to enemas of sodium polystyrene sulphonate has been implicated in cases of colonic necrosis. The safety and efficacy of sorbitol used with sodium polystyrene sulphonate has not been established and they should not be used together.

In children and neonates particular care is needed with rectal administration as excessive dosage or inadequate dilution could result in impaction of the resin. Care should be taken when administering to patients in whom an increase in sodium load may be detrimental (i.e. congestive heart failure, hypertension, renal damage or oedema). In such cases, Calcium Resonium (calcium polystyrene sulphonate) may be used in place of Resonium A.

*Interactions:* There have been reports of systemic alkalosis following concurrent administration of cation-exchange resins and non-absorbable cation donating antacids such as magnesium hydroxide and aluminium carbonate. Intestinal obstruction due to concretions of aluminium hydroxide has been reported when aluminium hydroxide has been combined with the resin. The toxic effects of digitalis on the heart, especially various ventricular arrhythmias and AV nodal dissociation, are likely to be exaggerated if hypokalaemia is allowed to develop. Cation donating agents may reduce the potassium binding effect of Resonium A. Sorbitol added to enemas may cause colonic necrosis.

*Pregnancy and lactation:* No data are available regarding the use of polystyrene sulphonate resins in pregnancy and lactation. The administration of Resonium A in pregnancy and during breast feeding, therefore, is not advised unless, in the opinion of the physician, the potential benefits outweigh any potential risks.

*Side-effects:* In accordance with its pharmacological actions, the resin may give rise to sodium retention, hypokalaemia and hypercalcaemia and the related clinical manifestations (see *Warnings and precautions* and *Overdosage*). Gastric irritation, anorexia, nausea vomiting, constipation and occasionally diarrhoea may occur. Faecal impaction following rectal administration has been reported in children, and gastro-intestinal concretions following oral administration to neonates, have been reported.

Some cases of acute bronchitis and/or broncho-pneumonia associated with inhalation of particles of calcium polystyrene sulphonate have been described. Colonic necrosis has been reported following administration of sodium polystyrene sulphonate in sorbitol as enemas (see also *Interactions*).

*Overdosage:* Biochemical disturbances from overdosage may give rise to clinical signs or symptoms of hypokalaemia, including irritability, confusion, delayed thought processes, muscle weakness, hyporeflexia and eventual paralysis. Apnoea may be a serious consequence of this progression. Electrocardiographic changes may be consistent with hypokalaemia; cardiac arrhythmia may occur. Hypocalcaemia tetany may occur. Appropriate measures should be taken to correct serum electrolytes and the resin should be removed from the alimentary tract by appropriate use of laxatives or enemas.

**Pharmaceutical precautions** Suspensions of the resin should be freshly prepared and not stored beyond 24 hours.

**Legal category** P.

**Package quantities** Supplied in HDPE containers containing 454 g Resonium A together with a plastic scoop which, when filled level, contains approximately 15 g.

**Further information** Theoretically, each gram of Resonium A should take up 2.8 to 3.4 mmol of potassium. However, in vivo, the actual amount of potassium bound will be less than this. The sodium content of Resonium A is 4.1 to 4.8 mmol/g.

**Product licence number** 11723/0070.

## SKELID* ▼

**Qualitative and quantitative composition** Disodium tiludronate 240.00 mg expressed as tiludronic acid 200.00 mg.

**Pharmaceutical form** Tablet.

**Clinical particulars**

*Therapeutic indications:* Treatment of Paget's disease of bone.

*Posology and method of administration:* Oral route. For use in adults only.

The dosage is 400 mg daily (i.e. 2 tablets) as a single intake for three months (i.e. 12 weeks).

Most patients respond to treatment within the first three months, whether or not they have been previously treated with another bisphosphonate.

Improvements of serum alkaline phosphatase level may last for up to 18 months following discontinuation.

Treatment may be repeated if either biochemical markers (increase in serum alkaline phosphatase with or without an increase in hydroxyprolinuria) or pain suggests relapse. A second course of treatment should be prescribed only after an interval of at least 6 months.

Tablets should be taken in a single dose with a glass of water at least two hours before or after meals.

In the two hours before and after ingestion, patients should refrain from taking food, particularly foods rich in calcium (such as milk and dairy products) and antacid gastric protective agents (cf. interactions).

*Contra-indications:* Patients with a history of allergy to bisphosphonates; Severe renal failure (creatinine clearance less than 30 ml/min); Juvenile Paget's disease; Pregnancy and breast feeding.

*Special warnings and precautions for use:* Tiludronate is not metabolised and is excreted unchanged in the urine. Tiludronate should be administered with caution in cases of mild renal failure (creatinine clearance between 60 and 90 ml/min) and moderate renal failure (creatinine clearance between 30 and 60 ml/min) (regularly monitor renal function).

Patients should ensure that their calcium and Vitamin D intake is adequate; calcium metabolism disorders (hypocalcaemia, vitamin D deficiency) should be corrected before initiating treatment.

*Interactions with other medicaments and other forms of interaction:* Concomitant treatments necessitating additional precautions:

- with calcium salts, gastro-intestinal topical treatments, antacids when administered by the oral route (reduction of gastrointestinal absorption of bisphosphonates).
- with indomethacin (increase of the bioavailability of tiludronic acid).
- tiludronate should not be taken within two hours of these drugs.

The pharmacokinetic parameters of tiludronate are not significantly altered by concomitant treatment with aspirin or diclofenac.

The pharmacokinetic parameters of digoxin are not significantly altered by concomitant treatment with tiludronate.

Concomitant administration of tiludronate and products likely to cause mineralisation disorders is to be avoided.

*Pregnancy and lactation*

*Pregnancy:* The administration of tiludronate is contra-indicated in pregnancy (lack of data).

Whereas tiludronate failed to induce harmful effects in reproduction studies delayed skeletal maturation and ossification of the foetus was reported with other bisphosphonates in experimental animals. Data about transplacental transfer of tiludronate in women are lacking.

*Breast feeding:* The administration of tiludronate is contra-indicated in case of breast feeding (lack of data).

*Effects on ability to drive and use machines:* No special precaution has to be taken in case of driving or using machines.

*Undesirable effects:* The adverse effects are mainly gastro-intestinal: stomach pain, nausea, diarrhoea. These effects are slight to moderate and their incidence is dose-related.

In rare cases there have been reports of asthenia, dizziness, headache and skin reactions.

*Overdose:* In the event of massive overdose, some patients could present with hypocalcaemia and renal failure. Gastric lavage may be useful to remove any unabsorbed tiludronate. Symptomatic treatment of hypocalcaemia (calcium salts by intravenous route, calcium gluconate for example) and/or renal failure should be initiated.

**Pharmacological properties**

*Pharmacodynamic properties:* Medicament for the treatment of bone diseases.
(M05 BA Bisphosphonates)

Tiludronate like other bisphosphonates inhibits the bone resorbing activity of osteoclasts.

Tiludronate slows bone remodelling in Paget's disease, as shown by the reduction in serum alkaline phosphatase. In cases of Paget's disease, preliminary studies of biopsies in a small number of patients have shown that tiludronate reduces excessive remodelling due to this disease.

Data concerning possible long-term mineralisation disorders in clinical use are not available. On the other hand, daily long-term administration (6 months to 1 year) of high doses to rats and baboons did not induce osteomalacia.

*Pharmacokinetic properties:* The absolute bioavailability of tiludronate is low (6% on average) and variable (from 2 to 11%). After repeated administrations of a dose of 400 mg/day, the plasma concentration peaks are very variable (usually between 1 and 5 mg/l and occur 1 to 2 hours after administration). Bioavailability is reduced when administered during or after a meal and greatly reduced in the presence of calcium.

Protein plasma binding is 91% and constant over the therapeutic concentration range. The protein responsible for binding is albumin. Less than 5% is bound to red blood cells. Approximately half of the dose taken undergoes bone fixation.

Tiludronate is excreted in unchanged form by the kidneys. After oral administration of a single dose, the quantities of unchanged tiludronate excreted found after 48 hours are 3.5±1.9%. After treatment withdrawal, the decrease in plasma tiludronate levels is divided into two phases, the second of which is much slower and difficult to determine accurately due to the very low plasma concentrations (half-life greater than 100 hours). The second phase results from bone remodelling and very slow release of tiludronate from the bones.

*Preclinical safety data:* Single-dose toxicity: after oral administration, tiludronate exhibited moderate acute toxicity in rats (LD50 about 550 mg/kg) and low acute toxicity in mice (LD50≥1000 mg/kg). Lesions were observed in the kidney, stomach and lung.

Repeated-dose toxicity: after repeated oral administration of tiludronate mainly to rats and baboons for up to 1 year, gastritis and renal proximal tubulopathy were observed at doses ≥50 mg/kg/d which were substantially higher than pharmacologically effective doses of 5–10 mg/kg/d leading to inhibition of stimulated bone resorption and increase in bone density or metaphyseal trabeculae.

Genotoxicity and carcinogenesis: *in vitro* and *in vivo* investigations with tiludronate to detect gene mutations, chromosomal aberrations or DNA repair processes showed no effect. There was no evidence of carcinogenicity either in mice treated for 80 weeks with up to 50 mg/kg/d tiludronate or in rats treated with up to 25 mg/kg/d tiludronate for 2 years.

Reproduction toxicity: oral tiludronate in doses up to 375 mg/kg/d did not exert teratogenic or direct embryotoxic effects in rats, mice or rabbits. Up to 75 mg/kg/d tiludronate did not affect fertility or peri- and post-natal development of rats. Nevertheless, considering that delayed skeletal maturation and ossification of the foetus was reported with other bisphosphonates in experimental animals and that data about transplacental transfer in women are lacking tiludronate is contra-indicated in pregnancy.

**Pharmaceutical particulars**

*List of excipients:* Sodium lauryl sulphate, methylhydroxypropyl cellulose, crospovidone, magnesium stearate, lactose monohydrate.

*Incompatibilities:* None.

*Shelf life:* Three years.

*Special precautions for storage:* None.

*Nature and contents of container:* 28 tablets in heat-formed blister packs (polyamide – aluminium – PVC/aluminium).

**Marketing authorisation number** 11723/0207.

**Date of approval/revision of SPC** 6 February 1996.

**Legal category** POM.

## SOLPADOL* EFFERVESCENT SOLPADOL CAPLETS*

**Presentation**

1. White bevelled-edged effervescent tablets, plain on the reverse and scored on the obverse, which effervesce vigorously when placed in water. Each tablet is 25.4 mm in diameter and contains Paracetamol PhEur 500 mg and Codeine Phosphate Hemihydrate PhEur 30 mg.

2. White capsule-shaped tablets marked with SOLPADOL on one side and plain on the reverse. Each tablet contains Paracetamol PhEur 500 mg and Codeine Phosphate Hemihydrate PhEur 30 mg.

**Uses** Solpadol is an analgesic, the effect being produced by a combination of the peripheral action of paracetamol and the central action of codeine at opioid binding sites. It is recommended for the relief of severe pain.

**Dosage and administration** Solpadol is for oral administration only.

*Adults:* 1. *Solpadol effervescent tablets:* Two tablets not more frequently than every 4 hours, up to a maximum of 8 tablets in any 24 hour period. Tablets should be dissolved in at least half a tumblerful of water before taking.

2. *Solpadol Caplets:* Two Caplets not more frequently than every 4 hours, up to a maximum of 8 Caplets in any 24 hour period.

*Elderly:* A reduced dose may be required – see warnings.

*Children:* Not recommended for children under 12 years of age.

**Contra-indications, warnings, etc**

*Contra-indications:* Hypersensitivity to paracetamol or codeine, which is rare. Conditions where morphine and opioids are contra-indicated e.g. acute asthma, respiratory depression, acute alcoholism, head injuries, raised intra-cranial pressure and following biliary tract surgery; monoamine oxidase inhibitor therapy, concurrent or within 14 days.

*Warnings:* Patients should be advised not to drive or operate machinery if affected by dizziness or sedation.

Care should be taken in administering the product to any patient whose condition may be exacerbated by opioids, particularly the elderly, who are specially sensitive to their central and gastro-intestinal effects, those on concurrent CNS depressant drugs, those with prostatic hypertrophy and those with inflammatory or obstructive bowel disorders.

Care should also be taken if prolonged therapy is contemplated.

There is inadequate evidence of the safety of codeine in human pregnancy, but there is epidemiological evidence of the safety of paracetamol. Both substances have been used for many years without apparent adverse effect and animal studies have not shown any hazard. Nonetheless, careful consideration should be given before prescribing Solpadol for pregnant patients. Opioid analgesics may depress neonatal respiration and cause withdrawal effects in neonates of dependent mothers.

Each Solpadol effervescent tablet contains 426.8 mg sodium (18.56 mEq). This sodium content should be taken into account when prescribing for patients for whom sodium restriction is indicated. Each Solpadol Caplet contains less than 1 mg of sodium.

*Interactions:* Paracetamol may increase the elimination half-life of chloramphenicol. The absorption of paracetamol may be increased by metoclopramide and decreased by cholestyramine. Oral contraceptives may increase its rate of clearance. The effects of CNS depressants (including alcohol) may be potentiated by codeine.

*Side-effects:* Adverse effects to paracetamol are rare, but hypersensitivity has been reported. Codeine can produce typical opioid effects, including constipation, nausea, vomiting, dizziness, light headedness, confusion, drowsiness and urinary retention. The frequency and severity are determined by dosage, duration of treatment and individual sensitivity.

Tolerance and dependence can occur, especially with prolonged high dosage of codeine.

*Overdosage:* Nausea and vomiting are prominent symptoms of codeine toxicity and there is evidence of circulatory and respiratory depression. Suggested treatment is gastric lavage and catharsis. If CNS depression is severe, assisted ventilation, oxygen and parenteral naloxone may be needed.

Patients who have taken an overdose of paracetamol may appear well for the first three days, then succumb to liver damage. The hepatic changes produced by overdosage of paracetamol result from the accumulation of a highly reactive intermediate metabolite in the hepatocytes. N-acetylcysteine intravenously or methionine orally protects the liver if administered within 12 hours of ingesting an overdose.

Patients in whom oxidative liver enzymes have been induced, including alcoholics and those receiving barbiturates and patients who are chronically malnourished, may be particularly sensitive to the toxic effects of paracetamol in overdosage.

**Pharmaceutical precautions** Solpadol Caplets and effervescent tablets should be stored below 25°C. Solpadol Caplets should be stored in a dry place.

**Legal category** POM.

**Package quantities** Tablets are packed in boxes of 100 tablets (25 laminate strips 4 tablets).

Caplets are packed in foil blisters and supplied in boxes of 100.

**Further information** Nil

**Product licence numbers**

| | |
|---|---|
| Solpadol effervescent tablets | 11723/0072 |
| Solpadol Caplets | 11723/0071 |

## STROMBA*

**Presentation** Stromba Tablets are round, flat, white tablets 9.5 mm in diameter, marked STROMBA on one side and scored in quarters on the other side. Each tablet contains 5 mg Stanozolol BP. Stromba tablets also contain lactose.

**Uses**

1. For the vascular manifestations of Behcet's disease.
2. For the prevention of spontaneous attacks of proven hereditary angio-oedema.

**Dosage and administration** Stromba is for oral administration only.

*1. Behcet's disease*
*Adults:* 10 mg daily.

*2. Hereditary angio-oedema:* The initial dosage should be adjusted to control the occurrence of attacks. Thereafter, the dosage may be reduced for maintenance therapy according to patient response.

*Adults:* Initially 2.5–10 mg daily. Dosage as low as 2.5 mg three times a week has been effective maintenance therapy.

*Children:* Not suitable for children less than one year old. 1–6 years, initially 2.5 mg daily. 6–12 years, initially 2.5–5 mg daily.

**Contra-indications, warnings, etc**

*Contra-indications:* Stromba is not intended for the treatment of loss of appetite, unexplained weight loss or failure to thrive in children. Such cases should be referred to the appropriate centre for investigation.

Because of possible virilising effects on a female foetus, Stromba should not be administered to pregnant women. There are no available data on the excretion of stanozolol in breast milk. Lactating mothers should not breast feed if Stromba treatment is necessary.

Stromba should not be administered to patients with established liver disease. Patients with a history of jaundice should have liver function tests checked prior to commencing treatment.

Stromba should not be used in cases of cancer of the prostate because the condition is androgen-dependent.

Stromba increases ALA synthetase activity and hence porphyrin metabolism. It is therefore not recommended in patients with a history of porphyria as its use may precipitate an acute attack.

Stromba has been used in patients with non-insulin dependent diabetes without adverse consequences. However, it may be advisable to avoid its use in insulin dependent diabetics.

*Precautions:* Prolonged use in children may lead to premature closure of the epiphyses.

In hereditary angio-oedema:

(a) long-term use of Stromba should be restricted to well established cases who have experienced serious attacks.
(b) Stromba should not be used in pre-menopausal women except in life-threatening situations.

Stromba should be used with caution in the presence of impaired renal or cardiac function as it may encourage sodium and water retention that could result in cardiac failure.

Peliosis hepatis and tumours of the liver have been reported occasionally in patients subject to prolonged treatment with androgenic anabolic steroids. The tumours are not typical of primary hepatocellular carcinoma and in some cases discontinuation of steroids has resulted in tumour regression without other therapy. The possibility that Stromba may induce or enhance the development of peliosis hepatis and hepatic tumours cannot be excluded and this should be considered when long-term treatment is carried out.

Caution should also be observed in treating patients with breast cancer since anabolic steroids may induce hypercalcaemia in this condition. Periodic assessment of liver function, haematocrit and haemoglobin is advised during treatment.

*Interactions:* Anabolic steroids increase sensitivity to warfarin type anti-coagulants; therefore, the dose of the latter should be decreased by approximately a half in order to maintain the prothrombin time at the desired therapeutic level.

Dosage of oral hypoglycaemic agents may require adjustment when initiating or discontinuing Stromba therapy.

*Side-effects:* Because of the structural relationship to the male hormones, some androgenic side-effects e.g. acne, hirsutism, amenorrhoea, are to be expected. Because the ratio of anabolic to androgenic properties is high, these effects should be minimal at the recommended dosage and those reported have been generally mild and reversible on stopping treatment. On rare occasions, usually with higher dosage, voice change has been reported; if observed, treatment should be discontinued. Other effects, such as menstrual irregularity, headache, muscle cramp, dyspepsia, skin rash and occasionally hair loss, euphoria and depression have occurred. An increase in haematocrit and haemoglobin level may also occur. There have been occasional reports of cholestatic jaundice, and very rarely, peliosis hepatis and hepatic tumours.

In children, prolonged use may lead to premature closure of the epiphyses.

Stromba may raise levels of aspartate transaminase (AST) and alanine transaminase (ALT) and in some patients these may rise above laboratory normal ranges. These levels return to normal on withdrawing Stromba.

Elevations of creatine phospho-kinase and of alkaline phosphatase have also occasionally been reported.

The use of this preparation may temporarily result in an alteration in the ratio of high and low density lipoproteins. The significance of this is not understood.

Some patients taking Stromba may show increased T3 uptake, decreased T4 levels and a decrease in thyroxine binding globulin although they are clinically euthyroid.

*Overdosage:* There are no reports of chronic or acute overdosage with Stromba. By analogy with other substances of this type, one would expect chronic overdosage to be associated with the signs and symptoms caused by excessive circulating androgens. It is unlikely that any immediate serious reactions would be seen with a single excessive dose (in animals acute toxicity cannot be measured). In such an event, however, the patient should be kept under observation and liver function monitored, in case of delayed reactions.

**Pharmaceutical precautions** Nil.

**Legal category** POM.

**Package quantities** Calendar packs of 56 tablets (OP).

**Further information** Stanozolol is an anabolic agent with fibrinolytic properties which are of therapeutic value in modifying the vascular manifestations of Behcet's disease. In patients with hereditary angio-oedema, stanozolol alters the functional level of plasma C1 esterase inhibitor which is depressed in this condition.

Stanozolol given by mouth is readily absorbed into the bloodstream. Within the serum it is highly protein bound. Metabolism is carried out to a large extent in the liver and the conjugated metabolites are excretec in both the faeces and urine.

**Product licence number** 11723/0073

## TRIDESTRA*

**Qualitative and quantitative composition**

Tridestra tablet (white): Oestradiol valerate 2 mg.
Tridestra tablet (blue): Oestradiol valerate 2 mg anc medroxyprogesterone acetate 20 mg.
Tridestra tablet (yellow): Placebo.

**Pharmaceutical form** Tablets, oral.

**Clinical particulars**

*Therapeutic indications*

(i) The treatment of climacteric symptoms associ ated with the menopause.

(ii) The prevention of postmenopausal osteopo rosis in women considered at risk of developing fractures. Epidemiological studies suggest a numbe of risk factors may contribute to postmenopausa osteoporosis, including: early menopause (either nat ural or surgically induced); family history of osteopo rosis; recent corticosteroid therapy; a small frame thinness; and cigarette smoking.

*Posology and method of administration:* Dosage i according to the calendar pack, one tablet daily continuously, in cycles of 91 days.

Tridestra is an oestrogen-progestogen combinatio product consisting of 91 tablets in a blister pacl bearing calendar markings. The dosage during day 1 to 70 (inclusive) of the cycle is 2 mg oestradio valerate (white tablets). From day 71 to day 8 (inclusive) it is 2 mg of oestradiol valerate and 20 mg of medroxyprogesterone acetate (blue tablets). Fron day 85 to day 91 (inclusive) a placebo preparatio (yellow tablets) is taken.

*Contra-indications:* Tridestra is contra-indicated i pregnancy (known or suspected); severe cardiac o renal disease, severe disturbances of liver function previous or existing liver tumours; jaundice or pruritu during a previous pregnancy; Dubin-Johnson syn drome; Rotor syndrome; existing thromboemboli disorders; sickle cell anaemia; suspected or existin hormone-dependent disorders or tumours of th uterus and breast or other organs; undiagnose abnormal vaginal bleeding; endometriosis; a histor of herpes gestationis; otosclerosis with deterioratio in previous pregnancies; severe diabetes with vascu lar changes.

*Special warnings and special precautions for use* Before starting Tridestra, patients should have thorough general medical and gynaecological exami nataion with special emphasis on body weight, skin legs, blood pressure, heart, breast, pelvic organs wit endometrial assessment if indicated. Regular follow up examinations are recommended during treament at least annually.

Before starting treatment, pregnancy must be ex cluded. If expected withdrawal bleeding fails to occu at about 91 days intervals, treatment should b stopped until pregnancy has been ruled out. In wome of childbearing potential, hormonal contraceptio should be stopped when treatment is started for th first time, and the patient advised to use non-hormona contraception.

If used perimenopausally, breakthrough bleeding may occur due to endogenous sex hormone produc tion. Persistent breakthrough bleeding during treat ment is an indication for endometrial assessmen which may include biopsy. Pre-existing fibroids ma increase in size under the influence of oestrogens. this is observed, treatment should be discontinued.

Thromboembolism has been reported in connec tion with oestrogen replacement therapy, but there i no evidence to date that the overall incidence i increased. However, treatment should be stopped trauma, illness or impending surgery is considered t entail a risk of thrombosis.

In patients with mild chronic liver disease, live function should be checked every 8 to 12 weeks. Som women are predisposed to cholestasis during steroi therapy. Patients with gallstones should be close monitored.

Treatment should be stopped at once and invest gations undertaken if jaundice or pregnancy occurs or if there is a significant rise in blood pressure, th occurrence of thromboembolic disease or epilept seizures.

Diseases that are known to be subject to deteriora tion during pregnancy (e.g. multiple sclerosis, ep lepsy, diabetes, benign breast disease, hypertensio cardiac or renal dysfunction, asthma, porphyria, te any and otosclerosis) and women with a strong famil history of breast cancer should be carefully observe during treatment.

At the present time there is evidence which suggest a slight increase in the relative risk of breast cancer i postmenopausal women receiving long-term ho mone replacement therapy. A careful appraisal of th risk/benefit ratio should be undertaken before treating for longer than 5 to 10 years.

In rare cases, benign and in even rarer cases, malignant liver tumours leading in isolated cases to life-threatening intra-abdominal haemorrhage have been observed after the use of hormonal substances such as those contained in Tridestra. A hepatic tumour should be considered in the differential diagnosis if abdominal pain, enlarged liver, or signs of intra-abdominal haemorrhage occur.

*Interaction with other medicaments and other forms of interaction:* Drugs which induce hepatic microsomal enzymes, for example barbiturates, phenytoin, and rifampicin accelerate the metabolism of oestrogen-progestogen combinations such as Tridestra, and may reduce their efficacy.

*Pregnancy and lactation:* Tridestra is contra-indicated during pregnancy and lactation. Milk/plasma ratio for both E$_2$V and MPA is about 0.5. Use of Tridestra during lactation may induce gynaecomastia and vaginal bleeding in the child, and may also prolong postnatal jaundice.

*Effects on ability to drive and use machines:* None recorded.

*Undesirable effects:* Side-effects are most common in the first months of the treatment. They are usually mild, improving with the continuation of the treatment. Side-effects include: nausea, oedema, breast tenderness or enlargement, headache, migraine, visual disturbances, tiredness, increase in body weight, and changes in mood and libido. Breakthrough bleeding may also occur, particularly during the first year of treatment, but the incidence reduces by the second year of treatment.

The use of oestrogen-progestogen combinations may affect clinical laboratory results. There may be an increase in serum transaminases, alkaline phosphatase, gamma-glutamyltransferase and bilirubin. Thyroid-binding globulin may rise leading to erroneous results in thyroid function tests.

*Overdose:* Overdosage of oestrogen may cause nausea, headache and withdrawal bleeding. Serious ill effects have not been reported following acute ingestion of large doses of oestrogens and progestogens in contraceptive formulations by young children. When needed, therapy is symptomatic.

### Pharmacological properties

*Pharmacodynamic properties:* Oestradiol valerate (E$_2$V) an ester, is absorbed after oral intake and metabolised to free estradiol, a potent natural oestrogen. At a dose of 2 mg/day, E$_2$V is effective in the treatment of postmenopausal symptoms.

Oestradiol valerate exerts its effects through interaction with specific receptors in the cytoplasm or oestrogen sensitive tissues. It is involved in the development and maintenance of the female sex organs, secondary sexual characteristics, control of mammary glands, proliferation of endometrium, development of decidua and cyclic changes in the cervix and vagina.

Medroxyprogesterone acetate (MPA) is a derivative of natural progesterone, a 17-α-hydroxy-6-methylprogesterone acetate. It has a similar effect to progesterone with slight androgenic activity. MPA acts on the endometrium to convert the proliferative phase to secretory phase, and acts by binding to progestogen-specific receptors. MPA is established as a contraceptive, in the treatment of malignant disease (endometrial, ovarian and breast cancer), and in the treatment of dysfunctional uterine bleeding, secondary amenorrhoea and mild to moderate endometriosis.

The progestogen component of Tridestra is added to reduce the risk of endometrial hyperplasia which may occur with unopposed long-term oestrogen therapy. Fixed combinations of oestrogen and progestogens developed to date have been based on a 28-day cycle of use. A major reason for discontinuation of such therapy is the unacceptability of monthly menstruation to some women. Tridestra, which only causes menstruation at the end of a 3-month cycle, is likely to be more acceptable to this group of women, particularly those who are postmenopausal.

In addition of its effect on climacteric symptoms, Tridestra prevents postmenopausal osteoporosis by reducing bone loss.

*Pharmacokinetic properties:* Maximum plasma levels of oestradiol (about 0.2 nmol/l) are reached in about 8 hours. In circulation, natural estrogens are bound to sex hormone binding globulin and albumin. Free estradiol is metabolised in the liver and partly converted to less active oestrogens like oestrone. Maximum plasma levels of estrone (about 2 nmol/l) are reached in 6–7 hours after intake of the tablet. Oestrone is subjected to an enterohepatic cycle and its half-life is 15–20 hours. The majority of oestrogens are excreted via kidneys as conjugates (sulphates or glucuronides).

MPA is well absorbed from the gastrointestinal tract and rapidly distributed from the circulation to extravascular tissues. After the intake of the Tridestra combination tablet, the maximum plasma level of MPA (about 5 µg/l) is reached in 2 hours. The elimination half-life is 40–50 hours. MPA is metabolised in the liver and excreted as glucuronides both in urine and bile. The extent of absorption from the combination tablet is comparable to MPA given alone.

### Pharmaceutical particulars

*List of excipients:* Tridestra tablet (white): Lactose, maize starch, gelatine, purified water, magnesium stearate, talc.

Tridestra tablet (blue): Lactose, maize starch, gelatine, purified water, magnesium stearate, indigo carmine (E132).

Tridestra tablet (yellow): Lactose, maize starch, gelatine, purified water, magnesium stearate, yellow iron oxide (E172).

*Incompatibilities:* None.

*Shelf life:* 3 years.

*Special precautions for storage:* At a temperature not exceeding 25°C in a dry place.

*Nature and contents of container:* A PVC/PVDC/AL thermofoiled blister pack. Quantity: 91.

*Marketing authorisation holder:* Orion Pharma A/S, Bogeskøvvej 9, DK-3490 Kvistgård, Denmark.

**Marketing authorisation number** 13910/0003.

**Date of approval/revision of SPC** 13 February 1995.

**Legal category** POM.

## TRIFYBA*

**Presentation** Trifyba is a light brown particulate powder containing 80% of fibre, derived from the husk of wheat (Testa Triticum Tricum). It is presented as single dose sachets each containing 3.5 g.

**Uses** Colonic and gastro-intestinal disorders where a high-fibre regimen is indicated including simple constipation, uncomplicated diverticular disease, irritable colon, haemorrhoidal disorders and fissures and other conditions where straining at stool should be avoided.

**Dosage and administration**
*Adults:* One sachet two to three times daily.

*Children:* Half to one sachet once or twice daily depending on age and size.

Trifyba should be taken mixed with food. For maximum effect adequate fluids should be taken.

**Contra-indications, warnings, etc** Trifyba is contra-indicated in cases of intestinal obstruction. Some patients may experience transient abdominal distention and flatulence, but this rapidly diminishes and usually disappears within two weeks.

*Overdosage:* Due to the nature of the preparation, overdosage is unlikely. If it does occur, it should be treated conservatively and the patient given copious fluids by mouth.

**Pharmaceutical precautions** Nil.

**Legal category** GSL.

**Package quantities** Cartons containing 56 sachets.

**Further information** Trifyba is 80% fibre, and therefore represents a highly concentrated source of fibre. It is classified as an insoluble bulk forming laxative acting by retaining water in a cellular network with consequent improvement in colonic function. Trifyba contains clinically insignificant levels of phytic acid and does not interfere with mineral absorption from the gastrointestinal tract. Trifyba is free from sugar and other additives, contains no starch and can be used for diabetics and others on a calorie restricted diet. Trifyba contains negligible amounts of sodium, a factor of importance in the treatment of patients with cardiac or renal disease. Trifyba contains a small amount of gluten.

**Product licence number** 5287/0001.

*Product licence holder:* Labaz Ltd.

*Trade Mark

# Schering Health Care Limited
The Brow
Burgess Hill
West Sussex RH15 9NE

**SCHERING**

## ANDROCUR*

**Presentation** Each round, white, 9 mm tablet is impressed on one side with 'BV' in a regular hexagon, and is scored on the other. It contains 50 mg cyproterone acetate.

*Excipients:* lactose, maize starch, povidone 25 000, aerosil, magnesium stearate.

**Uses** Control of libido in severe hypersexuality and/or sexual deviation in the adult male.

**Dosage and administration** The daily dose should be divided and taken after the morning and evening meals. The usual dose is 1 tablet twice daily.

### Contra-indications, warnings, etc
*Contra-indications:* Liver diseases. Malignant tumours (other than prostatic cancer, for which cyproterone acetate is indicated – see data sheet for Cyprostat®) and wasting diseases (because of transient catabolic action). A history of, or existing, thrombosis or embolism. Severe diabetes with vascular changes. Sickle cell anaemia. Severe chronic depression. Androcur should not be given to youths under 18 or those whose bone maturation and testicular maturation are incomplete.

*Warnings/side-effects: Liver:* Direct hepatic toxicity, including jaundice, hepatitis and hepatic failure, which has been fatal in some cases, has been reported in patients treated with 200-300 mg cyproterone acetate. Most reported cases are in men with prostatic cancer. Toxicity is dose-related and develops, usually, several months after treatment has begun. Liver function tests should be performed pre-treatment and whenever any symptoms or signs suggestive of hepatotoxicity occur. If hepatotoxicity is confirmed, cyproterone acetate should normally be withdrawn, unless the hepatotoxicity can be explained by another cause, e.g. metastatic disease, in which case cyproterone acetate should be continued only if the perceived benefit outweighs the risk.

As with other sex steroids, benign and malignant liver changes have been reported in isolated cases. Recognised first-line tests of genotoxicity gave negative results when conducted with cyproterone acetate. However, further tests showed that cyproterone acetate was capable of producing adducts with DNA (and an increase in DNA repair activity) in liver cells from rats and monkeys and also in freshly isolated human hepatocytes. This DNA-adduct formation occurred at exposures that might be expected to occur in the recommended dose regimens for cyproterone acetate. One *in vivo* consequence of cyproterone acetate treatment was the increased incidence of focal, possibly preneoplastic, liver lesions in which cellular enzymes were altered in female rats. The clinical relevance of these findings is presently uncertain. Clinical experience to date would not support an increased incidence of hepatic tumours in man.

In very rare cases, liver tumours may lead to life-threatening intra-abdominal haemorrhage. If severe upper abdominal complaints, liver enlargement or signs of intra-abdominal haemorrhage occur, a liver tumour should be considered in the differential diagnosis.

*Inhibition of spermatogenesis:* The sperm count and the volume of ejaculate are reduced. Infertility is usual, and there may be azoospermia after eight weeks. There is usually slight atrophy of the seminiferous tubules. Follow-up examinations have shown these changes to be reversible, spermatogenesis usually reverting to its previous state about three to five months after stopping Androcur or, in some users, up to 20 months. That spermatogenesis can recover even after very long treatment is not yet known. There is evidence that abnormal sperms which might give rise to malformed embryos are produced during treatment with Androcur.

*Thromboembolism:* In extremely rare cases, the occurrence of thromboembolic events has been reported in temporal association with the use of Androcur. However a causal relationship seems to be questionable.

*Tiredness:* Fatigue and lassitude are common in the first few weeks but become much less from the third month.

*Breathlessness:* A sensation of shortness of breath may occur under high-dosed treatment with Androcur, owing to the known stimulatory effect of progesterone and synthetic progestogens on breathing, which is accompanied by hypocapnia and compensatory alkalosis, and is not considered to require treatment.

*Gynaecomastia:* About one in five patients develops transient or perhaps in some cases permanent enlargement of the mammary glands. In rare cases galactorrhoea and tender benign nodules have been reported. Symptoms mostly subside after discontinuation of treatment or reduction of dosage.

*Osteoporosis:* Rarely cases of osteoporosis have been reported.

*Body weight:* During long-term treatment, changes in body weight have been reported, chiefly weight gains.

Other changes that have been reported include reduction of sebum production and consequently improvement of existing acne vulgaris, transient patchy loss and reduced growth of body hair, increased growth of scalp hair, lightening of hair colour and female type of pubic hair growth.

*Precautions and special information:*
*Adrenocortical function:* During treatment, adrenocortical function should be supervised, since suppression has been observed.

*Diabetes:* Androcur can influence carbohydrate metabolism. Parameters of carbohydrate metabolism should be examined carefully in all diabetics before and regularly during treatment. The requirement for oral antidiabetics or insulin can change.

*Chronic alcoholism:* Alcohol appears to reduce the effect of Androcur, which is of no value in chronic alcoholics.

*Haemoglobin:* Hypochromic anaemia has been found rarely during long-term treatment, and blood counts before and at regular intervals during treatment are advisable.

*Nitrogen balance:* A negative nitrogen balance is usual at the start of treatment, but usually does not persist.

*Spermatogenesis:* A spermatogram should be recorded before starting treatment in patients of procreative age, as a guard against attribution of pre-existing infertility to Androcur at a later stage.

It should be noted that the decline in spermatogenesis is slow, and Androcur should, therefore, not be regarded as a male contraceptive.

*Medico-legal considerations:* Doctors are advised to ensure that the fully informed consent of the patient to Androcur treatment is obtained and can be verified.

*Road safety:* The marked lassitude and asthenia that may be experienced, particularly during the first few weeks of treatment, necessitate especial care whilst driving.

*Overdosage:* There have been no reports of ill-effects from overdosage, which it is, therefore, generally unnecessary to treat. If overdosage is discovered within 2 or 3 hours and is so large that treatment seems desirable, gastric lavage can safely be used. There are no specific antidotes, and treatment should be symptomatic.

**Pharmaceutical precautions** Shelf-life – Five years.

**Legal category** POM

**Package quantities** Original packs containing 56 tablets (4 blister strips of 14 tablets).

**Further information** Cyproterone acetate acts as an antiandrogen by blocking androgen receptors. It also has progestogenic activity which exerts a negative feedback effect on the hypothalamic receptors, so leading to a reduction in gonadotrophin release, and hence to diminished production of testicular androgens.

**Product licence number** 0053/0023

## BETAFERON* ▼

**Qualitative and quantitative composition** Interferon beta-1b 0.25 mg (8.0 million IU) per ml when reconstituted.

The potency is determined using a cytopathic effect (CPE) bioassay using the WHO recombinant interferon beta reference standard.

Betaferon is formulated to contain 0.3 mg (9.6 million IU) of interferon beta-1b per vial at a calculated overfill of 20 %.

Interferon beta-1b is a purified, sterile, lyophilised protein that has 165 amino acids. It is produced by recombinant DNA techniques from a strain of *Escherichia coli* that bears a genetically engineered plasmid containing a modified human interferon beta$_{ser17}$ gene. Interferon beta-1b differs structurally from natural human interferon beta by the presence of serine instead of cysteine in position 17, lack of methionine in position 1 and absence of carbohydrate moieties.

**Pharmaceutical form** Sterile lyophilised white to off white powder for solution for injection.

### Clinical particulars

*Therapeutic indications:* Betaferon is indicated for the reduction of frequency and degree of severity of clinical relapses, in ambulatory patients (i.e. patients who are able to walk unaided) with relapsing, remitting multiple sclerosis, characterised by at least two attacks of neurological dysfunction over the preceding two year period, followed by complete or incomplete recovery.

Patients receiving Betaferon showed a reduction in frequency (30%) and severity of clinical relapses, as well as the number of hospitalisations due to disease. Furthermore, there was a prolongation of the relapse free interval.

There is no evidence of an effect of Betaferon on the duration of exacerbations, on symptoms in between exacerbations, or of the progression of the disease. There are also no data on the effect of Betaferon on performance of daily activities or in the social field.

Betaferon has not yet been investigated in patients with progressive MS.

There is no evidence of an effect on disability.

The clinical studies show that not all patients respond to treatment with Betaferon. Furthermore a deterioration in the bouts was observed in some of the patients despite the treatment. There are no clinical criteria that would allow prediction with regard to non-response or deterioration in the individual patient to be treated.

*Posology and method of administration:* The treatment with Betaferon should be initiated under the supervision of a physician experienced in the treatment of the disease.

The recommended dose of Betaferon is 0.25 mg (8.0 million IU), contained in 1 ml of the reconstituted solution (cf. *Instructions for use/handling*), to be injected subcutaneously every other day.

The optimal dose has not been fully clarified.

At the present time, it is not known for how long the patient should be treated. Efficacy of treatment for longer than two years has not been sufficiently demonstrated.

Full clinical assessment should be made at two years in all patients.

A decision for longer-term treatment should be made on an individual basis by the treating physician.

Exposure data for longer than three years are not available.

Treatment is not recommended in patients with less than 2 exacerbations in the previous 2 years.

If the patient fails to respond, for example: there is steady progression of disability for six months, or treatment with at least 3 courses of ACTH or corticosteroids during a one year period is required despite Betaferon therapy, treatment with Betaferon should be stopped.

Efficacy and safety of Betaferon were not investigated in children and adolescents of less than 18 years of age. Therefore, Betaferon should not be administered to this age group.

*Contra-indications:* Betaferon is contra-indicated in the following conditions:

– Pregnancy (see *Use during pregnancy and lactation*).
– Patients with a history of hypersensitivity to natural or recombinant interferon-β or human albumin.
– Patients with a history of severe depressive disorders and/or suicidal ideation.
– Patients with decompensated liver disease.
– Patients with epilepsy not adequately controlled by treatment.

Serious hypersensitivity reactions (rare but severe

acute reactions such as bronchospasm, anaphylaxis and urticaria) may occur. If reactions are severe, Betaferon should be discontinued and appropriate medical intervention instituted.

*Special warnings and special precautions for use:* Patients to be treated with Betaferon should be informed that depressive disorders and suicidal ideation may be a side effect of the treatment and should report these symptoms immediately to the prescribing physician. In rare cases these symptoms may result in a suicide attempt. Patients exhibiting depressive disorders and suicidal ideation should be monitored closely and cessation of therapy should be considered.

Betaferon should be administered with caution to patients with a history of seizures and of depressive disorders and to those receiving treatment with anti-epileptics (see *Interactions with other medicaments and other forms of interaction*). It should also be used with caution in patients with depressive disorders and to those who suffer from pre-existing cardiac disorders.

Caution should be exercised when administering Betaferon to patients with myelosuppression; patients who develop neutropenia should be monitored closely for the development of fever or infection.

Serious hypersensitivity reactions (rare but severe acute reactions such as bronchospasm, anaphylaxis and urticaria) may occur. If reactions are severe, Betaferon should be discontinued and appropriate medical intervention instituted. Other moderate to severe adverse experiences may require modifications of the Betaferon dosage regimen or even discontinuation of the agent.

Differential WBC, SGOT and SGPT levels should be obtained prior to initiation of Betaferon therapy and regularly during therapy.

There are no data on patients with renal impairment. Renal function should be monitored carefully when such patients receive Betaferon therapy.

In the MS studies, 45 % of the patients developed serum interferon beta-1b neutralising activity on at least one occasion. One third had neutralising activity confirmed by at least two consecutive positive titres. This development of neutralising activity is associated with a reduction in clinical efficacy, becoming evident at 18-24 months.

New adverse events have not been associated with the development of neutralising activity. However, the possibility of cross reactivity with endogenous interferon beta has not been investigated.

There are sparse data in patients who have developed neutralising activity and have completed Betaferon therapy.

Injection site necrosis (ISN) has been reported in patients using Betaferon (see *Undesirable effects*). It can be extensive and may involve muscle fascia as well as fat and therefore can result in scar formation. Occasionally debridement and, less often, skin grafting are required and healing may take up to 6 months.

If the patient has multiple lesions Betaferon should be discontinued until healing has occurred. Patients with single lesions may continue on Betaferon provided the necrosis is not too extensive, as some patients have experienced healing of injection site necrosis whilst on Betaferon.

To minimise the risk of injection site necrosis patients should be advised to:
- use an aseptic injection technique
- rotate the injection sites with each dose.

The procedure for the self-administration by the patient should be reviewed periodically especially if injection site reactions have occurred.

*Interaction with other medicaments and other forms of interaction:* No formal drug interaction studies have been carried out with Betaferon.

The effect of alternate-day administration of 0.25 mg (8.0 million IU) of Betaferon on drug metabolism in MS patients is unknown. Corticosteroid or ACTH treatment of relapses for periods of up to 28 days has been well tolerated in patients receiving Betaferon.

Due to the lack of clinical experience in MS patients use of Betaferon together with immunomodulators other than corticoids or ACTH, is not recommended.

Interferons have been reported to reduce the activity of hepatic cytochrome P450-dependent enzymes in humans and animals. Caution should be exercised when Betaferon is administered in combination with medicinal products that have a narrow therapeutic index and are largely dependent on the hepatic cytochrome P450 system for clearance, e.g. anti-epileptics.

No interaction studies with anti-epileptics have been carried out.

*Influence on laboratory tests/findings:* At the recommended dose, leukopenia (lymphopenia, neutropenia), or elevated SGPT may be seen. Low calcium, high uric acid, or elevated SGOT have appeared to be associated with Betaferon administration.

*Pregnancy and lactation:* It is not known whether Betaferon can cause fetal harm when administered to a pregnant woman or can affect human reproductive capacity. Spontaneous abortions have been reported in subjects with MS in controlled clinical trials. Recombinant human interferon beta-1b in studies with rhesus monkeys has been proven embryotoxic, causing fetal death in the higher dose range. Therefore, Betaferon is contraindicated during pregnancy and women of childbearing potential should take appropriate contraceptive measures. If the patient becomes pregnant or plans to become pregnant while taking Betaferon, she should be informed of the potential hazards and it should be recommended to discontinue therapy (for preclinical results refer to section *Preclinical safety data*).

It is not known whether interferon beta-1b is excreted in human milk. Because of the potential for serious adverse reactions to Betaferon in nursing infants a decision should be made whether nursing or Betaferon should be discontinued.

*Effects on ability to drive and use machines:* This has not been investigated.

Central nervous system-related adverse events associated with the use of Betaferon might influence the ability to drive and use machines in susceptible patients.

*Undesirable effects:* Experience with Betaferon in patients with MS is limited, consequently adverse events with low incidence may not yet have been observed.

Injection site reactions occurred frequently after administration of Betaferon. Redness, swelling, discoloration, inflammation, pain, hypersensitivity, necrosis, and non-specific reactions were significantly associated with 0.25 mg (8.0 million IU) Betaferon treatment. The incidence rate of injection site reactions usually decreased over time.

If the patient experiences any break in the skin, which may be associated with swelling or drainage of fluid from the injection site, the patient should be advised to consult with their physician before continuing injections with Betaferon (see *Special warnings and special precautions for use*).

Flu-like symptom complex (fever, chills, myalgia, malaise, or sweating) has been seen frequently. The incidence rate of the symptoms decreased over time.

Serious hypersensitivity reactions (rare but severe acute reactions such as bronchospasm, anaphylaxis and urticaria) may occur. If reactions are severe, Betaferon should be discontinued and appropriate medical intervention instituted.

Menstrual disorders may occur in premenopausal females.

Central nervous system (CNS) related adverse events including depression, anxiety, emotional lability, depersonalisation, convulsions, suicide attempts, and confusion have been observed.

*Overdose:* Interferon beta-1b has been given without serious adverse events compromising vital functions to adult cancer patients at individual doses as high as 5.5 mg (176 million IU) i.v. three times a week.

**Pharmacological properties**

*Pharmacodynamic properties:* Pharmacotherapeutic group: Cytokines ATC Code L03 AA.

Interferons belong to the family of cytokines, which are naturally occurring proteins. Interferons have molecular weights ranging from 15,000 to 21,000 daltons. Three major classes of interferons have been identified: alpha, beta, and gamma. Interferon alpha, interferon beta, and interferon gamma have overlapping yet distinct biologic activities. The activities of interferon beta-1b are species-restricted and therefore, the most pertinent pharmacologic information on interferon beta-1b is derived from studies of human cells in culture or in human in vivo studies.

Interferon beta-1b has been shown to possess both antiviral and immunoregulatory activities. The mechanisms by which interferon beta-1b exerts its actions in multiple sclerosis (MS) are not clearly understood. However, it is known that the biologic response-modifying properties of interferon beta-1b are mediated through its interactions with specific cell receptors found on the surface of human cells. The binding of interferon beta-1b to these receptors induces the expression of a number of gene products that are believed to be the mediators of the biological actions of interferon beta-1b. A number of these products have been measured in the serum and cellular fractions of blood collected from patients treated with interferon beta-1b. Interferon beta-1b both decreases the binding affinity and enhances the internalisation and degradation of the interferon-$\gamma$ receptor. Interferon beta-1b also enhances the suppressor activity of peripheral blood mononuclear cells.

No separate investigations were performed regarding the influence of Betaferon on the cardiovascular system, respiratory system and the function of endocrine organs.

*Pharmacokinetic properties:* Betaferon serum levels were followed in patients and volunteers by means of a not completely specific bioassay. Maximum serum levels of about 40 IU/ml were found 1–8 hours after subcutaneous injection of 0.5 mg (16.0 million IU) interferon beta-1b. From various studies mean clearance rates and half-lives of disposition phases from serum were estimated to be at most 30 ml·min$^{-1}$·kg$^{-1}$ and 5 hours, respectively. Every other day Betaferon injections do not lead to serum level increases and pharmacokinetics do not seem to change during therapy.

The absolute bioavailability of subcutaneously administered interferon beta-1b was approximately 50 %.

*Preclinical safety data:* No acute toxicity studies have been carried out. As rodents do not react to human interferon beta, repeated dose studies were carried out with rhesus monkeys. Transitory hyperthermia was observed, as well as a significant rise in lymphocytes and a significant decrease in thrombocytes and segmented neutrophils. No long-term studies have been conducted. Reproduction studies with rhesus monkeys revealed maternal and foetal toxicity, resulting in prenatal mortality. No malformations have been observed in the surviving animals. No investigations on fertility have been conducted. No influence on the monkey oestrous cycle has been observed. Experience with other interferons suggests a potential for impairment of male and female fertility.

In one single genotoxicity study (Ames test), no mutagenic effect has been observed. Carcinogenicity studies have not been performed. An in vitro cell transformation test gave no indication of tumorigenic potential. Local tolerance studies after subcutaneous administration were negative. However, in clinical studies local reactions have been observed following use of Betaferon.

**Pharmaceutical particulars**

*List of excipients:* Human albumin PhEur; Dextrose PhEur.

*Incompatibilities:* None known.

*Shelf life:* Of the product as packaged for sale: 18 months at 2-8 °C, starting from the date of sterile filtration of the formulated bulk solution. After reconstitution according to directions: up to 3 hours at 2 - 8 °C.

*Special precautions for storage:* Store at 2 - 8 °C before and after reconstitution.

*Nature and contents of container:* 3 ml clear glass vial with a 13 mm butyl rubber stopper and aluminium overseal.

Each Betaferon vial is provided with a separate solvent vial containing 2 ml sterile sodium chloride solution (0.54% w/v). The solvent is contained in a 3 ml vial with a 13 mm butyl rubber stopper and aluminium overseal.

Each pack of Betaferon contains either 5 or 15 vials of interferon beta-1b and either 5 or 15 vials of 0.54% sodium chloride solution.

*Instructions for use/handling:* To reconstitute lyophilised interferon beta-1b for injection, use a sterile syringe and needle to inject 1.2 ml of the supplied solvent (sodium chloride solution, 0.54 % w/v) into the Betaferon vial. Dissolve the powder completely without shaking. Inspect the reconstituted product visually before use. Discard the product before use if it contains particulate matter or is discoloured. The reconstituted solution contains 0.25 mg (8.0 million IU) of interferon beta-1b per ml.

Store all medicinal products properly and keep them out of reach of children.

*Marketing authorisation holder:* Schering Aktiengesellschaft, D-13342 Berlin

**Marketing authorisation numbers** EU/1/95/003/001, EU/1/95/003/002

**Date of approval/revision of SPC** 20 November 1996

**Legal category** POM

## BILISCOPIN*

**Presentation** Bottles containing sterile solutions of meglumine iotroxate.

*Excipients:* calcium sodium edetate, sodium hydrogen carbonate, sodium chloride, water for injection.

| | *Volume ml* | *Iodine mg/ml* | *Iodine Total, g* | *Osmoles/l at 37°C* |
|---|---|---|---|---|
| *Biliscopin for infusion:* | 100 | 50 | 5.0 | 0.28 |

**Uses** Infusion cholegraphy.

Intravenous cholegraphy should be performed as the first examination only when there is strong evidence of disease involving the biliary tract. In all other cases for diagnosis – especially in obscure upper abdominal complaints – oral cholegraphy is to be preferred.

**Dosage and administration**
*1. Adults:* One 100 ml bottle of Biliscopin for infusion in not less than 15 minutes. The infusion should always be started at a low rate and then increased to the final higher rate after three to five minutes. This technique reduces heterotopic excretion and improves tolerance.

*2. Children:* Because of insufficient experience in the use of Biliscopin in children, optimal paediatric dosages have not been established.

**Contra-indications, warnings, etc**
*Contra-indications:* Severe cardiovascular insufficiency, particularly right ventricular failure or cardiac decompensation. Proven or suspected hypersensitivity to iodine-containing contrast media. Manifest hyperthyroidism. Severe functional disturbance of the liver or kidneys. Monoclonal IgM gammopathy e.g. macroglobulinaemia (Waldenström's disease).

*Warnings/precautions:* For patients with severe impairment of hepatic or renal function, cerebral arteriosclerosis, epileptic conditions, diabetes mellitus requiring drug treatment and/or associated with diabetic complications, pulmonary emphysema, poor general health, latent hyperthyroidism, multiple myeloma or benign nodular goitre the need for examination with X-ray contrast media merits careful consideration. This also applies to patients with a history of allergy, atopy, bronchial asthma, endogenous eczema, cardiac or circulatory insufficiency or a previous adverse reaction with any contrast medium since experience shows that they may be at higher risk from developing anaphylaxis or cardiovascular collapse. Pre-testing does not give a reliable warning of allergic reactions to iodine-containing contrast media. Some radiologists give an antihistamine or a corticoid prophylactically to patients with a history of allergy. Because of the possibility of precipitation, contrast medium and prophylactic agents must not be administered mixed together. X-ray examinations should, if possible, be avoided during pregnancy. It has not yet been proved beyond question that Biliscopin may be used without hesitation in pregnant patients. Therefore an examination with a contrast medium during pregnancy should be carried out only if considered absolutely necessary by the physician. It is not known whether Biliscopin enters the breast milk.

Thyroid hyperfunction can increase for some time after the administration of biliary contrast media.

If iodine isotopes are to be administered for the diagnosis of thyroid disease, it should be borne in mind that the capacity of the thyroid tissue to take up iodine will be reduced for eight to ten weeks or more by iodinated biliary contrast media.

Diabetic nephropathy may predispose to renal impairment following intravascular administration of contrast media. This may precipitate lactic acidosis in patients who are taking biguanides. As a precaution biguanides should be stopped 48 hours prior to the examination and reinstated only after adequate renal function has been regained.

Hypersensitivity reactions can be aggravated in patients on beta-blockers.

The prevalence of delayed reactions (e.g. fever, rash, flu-like symptoms, joint pain and pruritus) to contrast media is higher in patients who have received interleukin.

Some investigators have reported temporary and reversible changes in liver-function tests after Biliscopin. These changes are not thought to reflect liver damage.

The opinion has been expressed that intravenous cholegraphy should not be performed immediately after negative oral cholegraphy. A large number of radiologists do not share this view–provided that the patient is adequately hydrated and renal function is not impaired.

The patient should be recumbent during the administration of Biliscopin. Thereafter, the patient must be kept under close observation for at least 30 minutes, since about 90% of all severe incidents occur within that time. The patient must not be left unsupervised until the end of the examination. If the administration does not take place on the X-ray table, any patient with a labile circulation should be brought to the X-ray machine sitting or lying down. Each bottle of Biliscopin for infusion should be used for one investigation only, and any remaining medium should be discarded.

Delayed reactions following intravascular administration of iodinated contrast media are rare. Nevertheless, driving or operating machinery is not advisable for the first 24 hours.

Particular caution should be exercised in allergic patients who have previously tolerated injectable iodine-containing contrast media without any complication, since they may have become sensitised to these substances. As with any contrast medium, the possibility of hypersensitivity must always be considered. If marked side-effects or suspected allergic reactions occur during infusion or injection and persist or even worsen when the administration is interrupted, it is probable that the patient has such a hypersensitivity. Therefore, the investigation must be abandoned. The needle or cannula should be left in the vein for some time in order to maintain access for intravenous therapy. Even relatively minor symptoms, such as itching of the skin, sneezing, violent yawns, tickling in the throat, hoarseness or attacks of coughing may be early signs of a severe reaction and, therefore, merit careful attention.

*Side-effects:* Side-effects in association with Biliscopin are usually mild to moderate and temporary.

Nausea, vomiting, erythema, a sensation of pain and a general feeling of warmth are the most frequently recorded reactions on intravascular administration. Such reactions are rare if the recommended rate of administration is adhered to. If they do occur, they can usually be ameliorated quite rapidly by reducing the rate of administration still further or by allowing a brief pause in the procedure. Particularly in patients with (manifest of subclinical) cardiovascular insufficiency or poor general health too rapid an administration may even lead to life-threatening reactions. Other symptoms which may occur are: Chills, fever, sweating, headache, dizziness blanching, weakness, gagging and a feeling of suffocation, gasping, a rise or fall of blood pressure, itching, urticaria, other kinds of skin eruption, oedema, tremor, sneezing and lacrimation. These reactions, which can occur irrespective of the amount administered and the mode of administration, may be the first signs of an incipient state of shock. Administration of the contrast medium must be discontinued immediately and – if necessary – specific therapy instituted intravenously. It is therefore advisable to use a flexible indwelling cannula for the administration of the contrast medium.

Very rarely, severe or even life-threatening incidents, such as severe hypotension and collapse, circulatory failure, ventricular fibrillation, cardiac arrest, pulmonary oedema, anaphylactic shock or other allergic manifestations, convulsions or other cerebral symptoms may occur. In some cases these have proved fatal.

To permit immediate countermeasures to be taken in emergencies, appropriate drugs, an endotracheal tube and a ventilator should be ready to hand.

Experience shows that hypersensitivity reactions occur more frequently in patients with an allergic disposition. Temporary renal failure may occur in rare cases especially where risk factors exist e.g. patients with: diabetes mellitus, pre-existing renal insufficiency or multiple myeloma; elderly patients or patients receiving large or repeated doses. In very rare cases also neurological complications such as coma, transient somnolence and convulsions have been described. Delayed reactions can occasionally occur. Paravenous administration of Biliscopin can cause pain, but rarely leads to severe tissue reactions.

**Pharmaceutical precautions**
*Storage:* Protect from light and secondary X-rays.

*Shelf-life:* Five years.

**Legal category** POM

**Package quantities** *Biliscopin for infusion:* Packs of 10 x 100 ml infusion bottles.

**Further information** Nil.

**Product licence number** 0053/0110.

## BILOPTIN*

**Qualitative and quantitative composition** Each capsule contains 500 mg of sodium iopodate.

**Pharmaceutical form** Capsules

**Clinical particulars**

*Therapeutic indications:* Oral contrast medium for cholecystography and cholangiography.

*Posology and method of administration: Preparing the patients:*

(i) On the day before the X-ray examination patients should be put on a diet of light meals, free from fats and from all foods that tend to cause wind. Tea or coffee (without milk), fruit juice or squash, clear fat-free soup, white bread, lean meat or fish grilled or baked without added fat or oil may be eaten. NONE of the following are allowed: fried food, eggs, fruit, oatmeal, pasta, milk or milk products including butter, margarine, cheese, ice-cream and salad dressings, all vegetables, smoked food or wholemeal or freshly baked bread.

(ii) From 6 p.m on the day before the examination, patients should refrain from eating until after the examination the following day. Tea or coffee (without milk), fruit juice or squash is allowed. Smoking shoul also be avoided.

(iii) Biloptin capsules should be swallowed whol with a glassful of cold water or squash.

For oral administration in the following dosages:

*Routine cholecystography:* Biloptin should be take after the last meal on the evening before examinatior Adults and elderly: 6 capsules.

*Other examination techniques in adults only*
Rapid cholecystography: Six capsules or doubl dose of twelve capsules.
Cholangiography: Twelve capsules.
Fractionated oral cholecystography: Six capsule 10-12 hours before the examination and another si capsules 3 hours before the examination.

*Contra-indications:* Manifest hyperthyroidism. Sever impairment of hepatic or renal function.

*Special warnings and special precautions for use* Proven or suspected hypersensitivity to iodine-con taining contrast media, latent hyperthyroidism an benign nodular goitre.

*Interaction with other medicaments and other form of interaction:* If iodine isotopes are to be administere for diagnosing thyroid disease, it should be borne i mind that the capacity of the thyroid tissue to take u iodine will be reduced for 8-10 weeks or more b iodinated biliary X-ray contrast media.

Hypersensitivity reactions can be aggravated i patients on beta-blockers.

The prevalence of delayed reactions (e. g. fever rash, flulike symptoms, joint pain and pruritus) t contrast media is higher in patients who have receive interleukin.

*Pregnancy and lactation:* Apart from the fact that X ray examinations should, if possible, be avoide during pregnancy, it must be pointed out that it ha not yet been proved beyond question that Biloptin may be used without hesitation in pregnant patients Therefore, such an examination with a contras medium during pregnancy should be carried out onl if considered absolutely necessary by the physician.

It is not known whether Biloptin enters the breas milk.

*Effects on ability to drive and use machines:* Non stated.

*Undesirable effects:* Biloptin is well tolerated and side effects even of a trivial nature, are extraordinarily rare Sensitive patients may occasionally complain of mil sensations of pressure in the stomach or nausea Attacks of diarrhoea and vomiting are exceptiona Very few cases of urticaria have been observec Anaphylactoid reactions ranging to shock are possi ble. Thyroid hyperfunction can increase for some tim after the examination with biliary contrast media.

*Overdose:* There have been no reports of ill-effect from overdosage and treatment is generally unnec essary. There are no specific antidotes, and furthe treatment should be symptomatic.

**Pharmacological properties**

*Pharmacodynamic properties:* Sodium iopodate i given by mouth as a cholecystographic contras medium. Following absorption from the gastrointes tinal tract, it appears in the bile where the concentra tion is such that the biliary tract can be examine radiographically.

*Pharmacokinetic properties:* Sodium iopodate is ab sorbed from the gastrointestinal tract and maximur concentrations are found in the gall-bladder about 1 hours after ingestion. It is excreted mainly in the urine

*Preclinical safety data:* None stated.

**Pharmaceutical particulars**

*List of excipients:* Other constituents: Peanut o (arachis oil), butyl hydroxytoluene, soya lecithi disodium edetate. Capsule shell: Karion 83, glyceri 85%, gelatin, methylhydroxybenzoate, propylhydrox ybenzoate, titanium dioxide (E171), iron oxide, yellov (E172) purified water.

*Incompatibilities:* None

*Shelf life:* 3 years.

*Special precautions for storage:* Store below 30°C Protect from light and secondary X-rays.

*Nature and contents of container:* Aluminium bliste packs contained within a cardboard outer. Availabl in packs of 120 capsules.

*Instructions for use/handling:* None

**Marketing authorisation number** 0053/5048R

**Date of approval/revision of SPC** 5 February 1997

**Legal category** P

# CYPROSTAT*

**Presentation** Cyprostat 50 mg: Each round white, 9 mm tablet is impressed on one side with 'BV' in a regular hexagon, and is scored on the other. It contains 50 mg cyproterone acetate.

Cyprostat 100 mg: Each capsule-shaped white tablet of dimensions 15.8 x 5.3 mm is impressed on one side with a regular hexagon and is scored on the other side with "LA" imprinted on both halves of the tablet. It contains 100 mg cyproterone acetate.

Excipients: Maize starch, povidone 25000, magnesium stearate, lactose, aerosil (50 mg only).

**Uses** Management of patients with prostatic cancer (1) to suppress 'flare' with initial LHRH analogue therapy, (2) in long-term palliative treatment where LHRH analogues or surgery are contraindicated, not tolerated, or where oral therapy is preferred, and (3) in the treatment of hot flushes in patients under treatment with LHRH analogues or who have had orchidectomy.

**Dosage and administration** Dosage for suppression of 'flare' with initial LHRH analogue therapy is 300 mg day, which may be reduced to 200 mg if the higher dose is not tolerated. For long-term palliative treatment where LHRH analogues or surgery are contraindicated, not tolerated, or where oral therapy is preferred the dosage is 200-300 mg/day.

For the above two indications the dosage should be divided into 2–3 doses per day and taken after meals.

For the treatment of hot flushes in patients under treatment with LHRH analogues or who have had orchidectomy a 50 mg starting dose, with upward titration if necessary within the range 50-150 mg/day, is recommended. For this indication the dosage should be divided into 1–3 doses per day and taken after meals.

All doses should be taken orally.

**Contra-indications, warnings, etc**
*Contra-indications:* None.

*Warnings, side-effects: Liver:* Direct hepatic toxicity, including jaundice, hepatitis and hepatic failure, which has been fatal in some cases, has been reported in patients treated with 200-300 mg cyproterone acetate. Most reported cases are in men with prostatic cancer. Toxicity is dose-related and develops, usually, several months after treatment has begun. Liver function tests should be performed pre-treatment and whenever any symptoms or signs suggestive of hepatotoxicity occur. If hepatotoxicity is confirmed, cyproterone acetate should normally be withdrawn, unless the hepatotoxicity can be explained by another cause, e.g. metastatic disease, in which case cyproterone acetate should be continued only if the perceived benefit outweighs the risk.

As with other sex steroids, benign and malignant liver changes have been reported in isolated cases. Recognised first-line tests of genotoxicity gave negative results when conducted with cyproterone acetate. However, further tests showed that cyproterone acetate was capable of producing adducts with DNA (and an increase in DNA repair activity) in liver cells from rats and monkeys and also in freshly isolated human hepatocytes. This DNA-adduct formation occurred at exposures that might be expected to occur in the recommended dose regimens for cyproterone acetate. One *in vivo* consequence of cyproterone acetate treatment was the increased incidence of focal, possibly preneoplastic, liver lesions in which cellular enzymes were altered in female rats. The clinical relevance of these findings is presently uncertain. Clinical experience to date would not support an increased incidence of hepatic tumours in man.

In very rare cases, liver tumours may lead to life-threatening intra-abdominal haemorrhage. If severe upper abdominal complaints, liver enlargement or signs of intra-abdominal haemorrhage occur, a liver tumour should be considered in the differential diagnosis.

*Inhibition of spermatogenesis:* The sperm count and the volume of ejaculate are reduced. Infertility is usual, and there may be azoospermia after 8 weeks. There is usually slight atrophy of seminiferous tubules. Follow-up examinations have shown these changes to be reversible, spermatogenesis usually reverting to its previous state about 3-5 months after stopping Cyprostat, or in some users, up to 20 months. That spermatogenesis can recover even after very long treatment is not yet known. There is evidence that abnormal sperms which might give rise to malformed embryos are produced during treatment with Cyprostat.

*Thromboembolism:* Patients with a history of thrombosis may be at risk of recurrence of the disease during Cyprostat therapy.

In patients with a history of thromboembolic processes or suffering from sickle-cell anaemia or severe diabetes with vascular changes, the risk: benefit ratio must be considered carefully in each individual case before Cyprostat is prescribed.

In extremely rare cases, the occurrence of thromboembolic events has been reported in temporal association with the use of Cyprostat. However a causal relationship seems to be questionable.

*Chronic depression:* It has been found that some patients with severe chronic depression deteriorate whilst taking Cyprostat therapy.

*Tiredness:* Fatigue and lassitude are common in the first few weeks of therapy but usually become much less from the third month. The marked lassitude and asthenia necessitate especial care when driving or operating machinery.

*Breathlessness:* Shortness of breath may occur. This may be due to the stimulatory effect of progestogens on breathing, which is accompanied by hypocapnia and compensatory alkalosis, and which is not considered to require treatment.

*Gynaecomastia:* Transient, and perhaps in some cases permanent, enlargement of the mammary glands has been reported. In rare cases, galactorrhoea and tender benign nodules have been reported. Symptoms generally subside after discontinuation of treatment or on reduction of dosage, but this should be weighed against the risk from the tumour of using inadequate doses.

*Body weight:* During long-term treatment, changes in body weight have been reported. Both increases and decreases have been seen.

*Osteoporosis:* Rarely cases of osteoporosis have been reported.

Other changes that have been reported include reduction of sebum production leading to dryness of the skin, transient patchy loss and reduced growth of body hair, increased growth of scalp hair, lightening of hair colour and female type of pubic hair growth.

*Adrenocortical function:* During treatment adrenocortical function should be supervised, since suppression has been observed in children taking cyproterone acetate.

*Diabetes:* Cyprostat can influence carbohydrate metabolism. Parameters of carbohydrate metabolism should be examined carefully in all diabetics before and regularly during treatment. The requirement for oral antidiabetics or insulin can change.

*Haemoglobin:* Hypochromic anaemia has been found rarely during long-term treatment, and blood-counts before and at regular intervals during treatment are advisable.

*Nitrogen balance:* A negative balance is usual at the start of treatment, but does not persist.

*Overdosage:* There have been no reports of ill-effects of overdosage, which it is, therefore, generally unnecessary to treat. There are no specific antidotes, and treatment should be symptomatic.

**Pharmaceutical precautions** Shelf-life: 50 mg tablets, five years. 100 mg tablets, four years.

**Legal category** POM

**Package quantities** 50 mg: Original packs containing 168 tablets (14 blister strips of 12 tablets). 100 mg: Original packs containing 84 tablets (4 blister strips of 21 tablets).

**Further information** Prostatic carcinoma and its metastases are in general androgen-dependent. Cyprostat exerts a direct antiandrogenic action on the tumour and its metastases and in addition it exerts a negative feedback effect on the hypothalamic receptors, so leading to a reduction in gonadotrophin release, and hence to diminished production of testicular androgens.

**Product licence numbers**
50 mg      0053/0133
100 mg    0053/0218

# DIANETTE *

**Qualitative and quantitative composition** Each beige tablet contains 2 milligrams of the anti-androgen, cyproterone acetate and 35 micrograms of the oestrogen, ethinyloestradiol.

**Pharmaceutical form** Sugar-coated tablets.

**Clinical particulars**
*Therapeutic indications:* Dianette is recommended for use in women only for the treatment of (a) severe acne, refractory to prolonged oral antibiotic therapy; (b) moderately severe hirsutism.

Although Dianette also acts as an oral contraceptive, it is not recommended in women solely for contraception, but should be reserved for those women requiring treatment for the androgen-dependent skin conditions described.

Complete remission of acne is to be expected in nearly all cases, often within a few months, but in particularly severe cases treatment for longer may be necessary before the full benefit is seen. It is recommended that treatment be withdrawn when the acne or hirsutism has completely resolved. Repeat courses of Dianette may be given if the condition recurs.

*Posology and method of administration:*
*First treatment course:* One tablet daily for 21 days, starting on the first day of the menstrual cycle (the first day of menstruation counting as Day 1).

*Subsequent courses:* Each subsequent course is started after 7 tablet-free days have followed the preceding course.

When the contraceptive action of Dianette is also to be employed, it is essential that the above instructions be rigidly adhered to. Should bleeding fail to occur during the tablet-free interval, the possibility of pregnancy must be excluded before the next pack is started.

When changing from an oral contraceptive and relying on the contraceptive action of Dianette, follow the instructions given below:
*Changing from 21-day combined oral contraceptives:* The first tablet of Dianette should be taken on the first day immediately after the end of the previous oral contraceptive course. Additional contraceptive precautions are not required.

*Changing from a combined Every Day pill (28 day tablets):* Dianette should be started after taking the last active tablet from the Every Day Pill pack. The first Dianette tablet is taken the next day. Additional contraceptive precautions are not then required.

*Changing from a progestogen-only pill (POP):* The first tablet of Dianette should be taken on the first day of bleeding, even if a POP has already been taken on that day. Additional contraceptive precautions are not then required. The remaining progestogen-only pills should be discarded.

*Post-partum and post-abortum use:* After pregnancy, Dianette can be started 21 days after a vaginal delivery, provided that the patient is fully ambulant and there are no puerperal complications. Additional contraceptive precautions will be required for the first 7 days of pill taking. Since the first post-partum ovulation may precede the first bleeding, another method of contraception should be used in the interval between childbirth and the first course of tablets. Lactation is contra-indicated with Dianette. After a first-trimester abortion, Dianette may be started immediately in which case no additional contraceptive precautions are required.

*Special circumstances requiring additional contraception:*
*Incorrect administration:* A single delayed tablet should be taken as soon as possible, and if this can be done within 12 hours of the correct time, contraceptive protection is maintained. With longer delays, additional contraception is needed. Only the most recently delayed tablet should be taken, earlier missed tablets being omitted, and additional non-hormonal methods of contraception (except the rhythm or temperature methods) should be used for the next 7 days, while the next 7 tablets are being taken. Additionally, therefore, if tablet(s) have been missed during the last 7 days of a pack, there should be no break before the next pack is started. In this situation, a withdrawal bleed should not be expected until the end of the second pack. Some breakthrough bleeding may occur on tablet taking days but this is not clinically significant. If the patient does not have a withdrawal bleed during the tablet-free interval following the end of the second pack, the possibility of pregnancy must be ruled out before starting the next pack.

*Gastro-intestinal upset:* Vomiting or diarrhoea may reduce the efficacy of oral contraceptives by preventing full absorption. Tablet-taking from the current pack should be continued. Additional non-hormonal methods of contraception (except the rhythm or temperature methods) should be used during the gastro-intestinal upset and for 7 days following the upset. If these 7 days overrun the end of a pack, the next pack should be started without a break. In this situation, a withdrawal bleed should not be expected until the end of the second pack. If the patient does not have a withdrawal bleed during the tablet-free interval following the end of the second pack, the possibility of pregnancy must be ruled out before starting the next pack. Other methods of contraception should be considered if the gastro-intestinal disorder is likely to be prolonged.

*Contra-indications:*

1. Pregnancy or lactation
2. Severe disturbances of liver function, jaundice or persistent itching during a previous pregnancy, Dubin-Johnson syndrome, Rotor syndrome, previous or existing liver tumours.
3. Existing or previous arterial or venous thrombotic or embolic processes, conditions which predispose to them e.g. disorders of the clotting processes, valvular heart disease and atrial fibrillation.
4. Sickle-cell anaemia.
5. Mammary or endometrial carcinoma, or a history of these conditions.
6. Severe diabetes mellitus with vascular changes.
7. Disorders of lipid metabolism.

8. History of herpes gestationis.
9. Deterioration of otosclerosis during pregnancy.
10. Undiagnosed abnormal vaginal bleeding.
11. Hypersensitivity to any of the components of Dianette.

*Special warnings and special precautions for use:*
*Warnings:* Like many other steroids, Dianette, when given in very high doses and for the majority of the animal's life-span, has been found to cause an increase in the incidence of tumours, including carcinoma, in the liver of rats. The relevance of this finding to humans is unknown.

In rare cases benign and in even rarer cases malignant liver tumours leading in isolated cases to life-threatening intra-abdominal haemorrhage have been observed after the use of hormonal substances such as those contained in Dianette. If severe upper abdominal complaints, liver enlargement or signs of intra-abdominal haemorrhage occur, a liver tumour should be included in the differential diagnosis.

Animal studies have revealed that feminisation of male foetuses may occur if cyproterone acetate is administered during the phase of embryogenesis at which differentiation of the external genitalia occurs. Although the results of these tests are not necessarily relevant to man, the possibility must be considered that administration of Dianette to women after the 45th day of pregnancy could cause feminisation of male foetuses. It follows from this that pregnancy is an absolute contra-indication for treatment with Dianette, and must be excluded before such treatment is begun.

Although its strong anti-androgenic effect is distinctive, Dianette has many properties in common with combined oral contraceptives, which must not be taken during treatment with Dianette. There is a general opinion, based on statistical evidence, that users of combined oral contraceptives experience, more often than non-users, venous thromboembolism, arterial thrombosis, including cerebral and myocardial infarction, and subarachnoid haemorrhage. Full recovery from such disorders does not always occur, and it should be realised that in a few cases they are fatal. How often these disorders occur in users of the modern low-dose pills is not known, but there are reasons for suggesting that they may occur less often than with older pills.

Certain factors may entail some risk of thrombosis, e.g. smoking, obesity, varicose veins, cardiovascular diseases, diabetes and migraine. The risk of arterial thrombosis associated with combined oral contraceptives increases with age, and this risk is aggravated by cigarette-smoking.

In addition, if there is a history in the family of thromboembolic diseases at a young age (e.g. deep vein thrombosis, heart attack or stroke) disturbances of the coagulation system must be ruled out before Dianette is prescribed. The suitability of Dianette should be judged according to the severity of such conditions in the individual case, and should be discussed with the patient before she decides to take it.

Numerous epidemiological studies have been reported on the risks of ovarian, endometrial, cervical and breast cancer in women using combined oral contraceptives. The evidence is clear that combined oral contraceptives offer substantial protection against both ovarian and endometrial cancer.

An increased risk of cervical cancer in long-term users of combined oral contraceptives has been reported in some studies, but there continues to be controversy about the extent to which this is attributable to the confounding effects of sexual behaviour and other factors.

The evidence linking combined oral contraceptive use and breast cancer remains inconclusive. The results of some studies suggest an increased risk of breast cancer presenting below the age of about 35, the risk rising with duration of use. Any possible increased risk of breast cancer with combined oral contraceptives is, however, likely to be small, and may be expected to be less with low-dosage pills. This possible risk should be weighed against the many benefits of combined oral contraceptives, including their protective effects against ovarian and endometrial cancers. The possibility cannot be ruled out that certain chronic diseases may occasionally deteriorate during the use of Dianette (see *Precautions*).

*Reasons for stopping Dianette immediately:*

1. Occurrence for the first time, or exacerbation, of migrainous headaches or unusually frequent or unusually severe headaches.
2. Sudden disturbances of vision or hearing or other perceptual disorders.
3. First signs of thrombophlebitis or thromboembolic symptoms (e.g. unusual pains in or swelling of the leg(s), stabbing pains on breathing or coughing for no apparent reason). Feeling of pain and tightness in the chest.
4. Six weeks before an elective major operation (e.g.

abdominal, orthopaedic), any surgery to the legs, medical treatment for varicose veins or prolonged immobilisation, e.g. after accidents or surgery. Do not restart until 2 weeks after full ambulation. In case of emergency surgery, thrombotic prophylaxis is usually indicated e.g. subcutaneous heparin.

5. Onset of jaundice, hepatitis, itching of the whole body.
6. Increase in epileptic seizures.
7. Significant rise in blood pressure.
8. Onset of severe depression.
9. Severe upper abdominal pain or liver enlargement.
10. Clear exacerbation of conditions known to be capable of deteriorating during oral contraception or pregnancy.
11. Pregnancy is a reason for stopping immediately because it has been suggested by some investigations that oral contraceptives taken in early pregnancy may slightly increase the risk of foetal malformations. Other investigations have failed to support these findings. The possibility therefore cannot be excluded, but it is certain that if a risk exists at all, it is very small.

*Precautions:* Examination of the pelvic organs, breasts and blood-pressure should precede the prescribing of any combined oral contraceptive and should be repeated regularly. The family medical history should be carefully noted and disturbances of the clotting mechanism ruled out if any member of the family has suffered from thromboembolic disease (e.g. deep vein thrombosis, stroke, myocardial infarction) at a young age. Before starting treatment pregnancy must be excluded.

The following conditions require strict medical supervision during medication with oral contraceptives. Deterioration or first appearance of any of these conditions may indicate that Dianette should be discontinued:

Diabetes mellitus, or a tendency towards diabetes mellitus (e.g. unexplained glycosuria), hypertension, varicose veins, a history of phlebitis, otosclerosis, multiple sclerosis, epilepsy, porphyria, tetany, disturbed liver function, Sydenham's chorea, renal dysfunction, family history of clotting disorders, obesity, family history of breast cancer and patient history of benign breast disease, history of clinical depression, systemic lupus erythematosus, uterine fibroids, an intolerance to contact lenses, migraine, gall-stones, cardiovascular diseases, chloasma, asthma, or any disease that is prone to worsen during pregnancy.

It should be borne in mind that the use of ultraviolet lamps, for the treatment of acne, or prolonged exposure to sunlight, increases the risk of the deterioration of chloasma.

Some women may experience amenorrhoea or oligomenorrhoea after discontinuation of Dianette, especially when these conditions existed prior to use. Women should be informed of this possibility.

*Interaction with other medicaments and other forms of interaction:* Hepatic enzyme inducers such as barbiturates, primidone, phenobarbitone, phenytoin, phenylbutazone, rifampicin, carbamazepine and griseofulvin can impair the contraceptive efficacy of Dianette. For women receiving long-term therapy with hepatic enzyme inducers, another method of contraception should be used. The use of antibiotics may also reduce the contraceptive efficacy of Dianette, possibly by altering the intestinal flora.

Women receiving short courses of enzyme inducers and broad spectrum antibiotics should take additional, non-hormonal (except rhythm or temperature method) contraceptive precautions during the time of concurrent medication and for 7 days afterwards. If these 7 days overrun the end of a pack, the next pack should be started without a break. In this situation, a withdrawal bleed should not be expected until the end of the second pack. If the patient does not have a withdrawal bleed during the tablet-free interval following the end of the second pack, the possibility of pregnancy must be ruled out before resuming with the next pack.

The possibility cannot be ruled out that oral tetracyclines, if used in conjunction with Dianette may reduce its contraceptive efficacy, although it has not been shown. When drugs of these classes are being taken it is, therefore, advisable to use additional non-hormonal methods of contraception (except the rhythm or temperature methods) since an extremely high degree of protection must be provided when Dianette is being taken. With rifampicin, additional contraceptive precautions should be continued for 4 weeks after treatment stops, even if only a short course was administered.

The requirement for oral antidiabetics or insulin can change as a result of the effect on glucose tolerance.

*Pregnancy and lactation:* Contra-indicated.
Animal studies have revealed that feminisation of male foetuses may occur if cyproterone acetate is

administered during the phase of embryogenesis at which differentiation of the external genitalia occurs. Although the results of these tests are not necessarily relevant to man, the possibility must be considered that administration of Dianette to women after the 45th day of pregnancy could cause feminisation of male foetuses. It follows from this that pregnancy is an absolute contra-indication for treatment with Dianette, and must be excluded before such treatment is begun.

*Effects on ability to drive and use machines:* None known.

*Undesirable effects:* In rare cases, headaches, gastric upsets, nausea, vomiting, breast tenderness, changes in body weight, changes in libido, depressive moods can occur.

In predisposed women, use of Dianette can sometimes cause chloasma which is exacerbated by exposure to sunlight. Such women should avoid prolonged exposure to sunlight.

Individual cases of poor tolerance of contact lenses have been reported with use of oral contraceptives. Contact lens wearers who develop changes in lens tolerance should be assessed by an ophthalmologist.
*Menstrual changes:*
*1. Reduction of menstrual flow:* This is not abnormal and it is to be expected in some patients. Indeed, it may be beneficial where heavy periods were previously experienced.
*2. Missed menstruation:* Occasionally, withdrawal bleeding may not occur at all. If the tablets have been taken correctly, pregnancy is unlikely. Should bleeding fail to occur during the tablet-free interval the possibility of pregnancy must be excluded before the next pack is started.
*Intermenstrual bleeding:* 'Spotting' or heavier 'breakthrough bleeding' sometimes occur during tablet taking, especially in the first few cycles, and normally cease spontaneously. Dianette should therefore, be continued even if irregular bleeding occurs. If irregular bleeding is persistent, appropriate diagnostic measures to exclude an organic cause are indicated and may include curettage. This also applies in the case of spotting which occurs at regular intervals in several consecutive cycles or which occurs for the first time after long use of Dianette.
*Effect on blood chemistry:* The use of oral contraceptives may influence the results of certain laboratory tests including biochemical parameters of liver, thyroid, adrenal and renal function, plasma levels of carrier proteins and lipid/lioprotein fractions, parameters of carbohydrate metabolism and parameters of coagulation and fibrinolysis. Laboratory staff should therefore be informed about oral contraceptive use when laboratory tests are requested.
Refer to *Special warnings and special precautions for use* for additional information.

*Overdose:* Overdose may cause nausea, vomiting and, in females, withdrawal bleeding. There are no specific antidotes and further treatment should be symptomatic.

**Pharmacological properties**
*Pharmacodynamic properties:* Dianette blocks androgen-receptors. It also reduces androgen synthesis both by negative feedback effect on the hypothalamo-pituitiary-ovarian systems and by the inhibition of androgen-synthesising enzymes.

Although Dianette also acts as an oral contraceptive it is not recommended in women solely for contraception, but should be reserved for those women requiring treatment for the androgen-dependent skin conditions described.

*Pharmacokinetic properties:*
*Cyproterone acetate:* Following oral administration cyproterone acetate is completely absorbed in a wide dose range. The ingestion of Dianette effects a maximum serum level of 15ng cyproterone acetate, ml at 1.6 hours. Thereafter drug serum levels decrease in two disposition phases characterised by half-lives of 0.8 hours and 2.3 days. The total clearance of cyproterone acetate from serum was determined to be 3.6 ml/min/kg. Cyproterone acetate is metabolised by various pathways including hydroxylations and conjugations. The main metabolite in human plasma is the 15β-hydroxy derivative.

Some dose parts are excreted unchanged with the bile fluid. Most of the dose is excreted in form of metabolites at a urinary to biliary ratio of 3:7. The renal and biliary excretion was determined to proceed with half-life of 1.9 days. Metabolites from plasma were eliminated at a similar rate (half-life of 1.7 days). Cyproterone acetate is almost exclusively bound to plasma albumin. About 3.5–4.0% of total drug levels are present unbound. Because protein binding is non specific changes in sex hormone binding globulin (SHBG) levels do not affect cyproterone acetate pharmacokinetics.

According to the long half-life of the terminal disposition phase from plasma (serum) and the daily intake cyproterone acetate accumulates during one treatment cycle. Mean maximum drug serum levels increased from 15ng/ml (day 1) to 21ng/ml and 24ng/ml at the end of the treatment cycles 1 and 3 respectively. The area under the concentration versus time profile increased 2.2 fold (end of cycle 1) and 2.4 fold (end of cycle 3). Steady state conditions were reached after about 16 days. During long term treatment cyproterone acetate accumulates over treatment cycles by a factor of 2.

The absolute bioavailability of cyproterone acetate is almost complete (88% of dose). The relative bioavailability of cyproterone acetate from Dianette was 109% when compared to an aqueous microcrystalline suspension.

*Ethinyloestradiol:* Orally administered ethinyloestradiol is rapidly and completely absorbed. Following ingestion of Dianette maximum drug serum levels of about 80pg/ml are reached at 1.7 hours. Thereafter ethinyloestradiol plasma levels decrease in two phases characterised by half-lives of 1–2 hours and about 20 hours. For analytical reasons these parameters can only be calculated for higher dosages.

For ethinyloestradiol an apparent volume of distribution of about 5 l/kg and a metabolic clearance rate from plasma of about 5 ml/min/kg were determined.

Ethinyloestradiol is highly but non-specifically bound to serum albumin. 2% of the drug levels are present unbound. During absorption and first liver passage ethinyloestradiol is metabolised resulting in a reduced absolute and variable oral bioavailability. Unchanged drug is not excreted. Ethinyloestradiol metabolites are excreted at a urinary to biliary ratio of 4:6 with a half-life of about 1 day.

According to the half-life of the terminal disposition phase from plasma and the daily ingestion steady state plasma levels are reached after 3–4 days and are higher by 30–40% as compared to a single dose. The relative bioavailability (reference: aqueous microcrystalline suspension) of ethinyloestradiol was almost complete.

The systemic bioavailability of ethinyloestradiol might be influenced in both directions by other drugs. There is, however, no interaction with high doses of vitamin C.

Ethinyloestradiol induces the hepatic synthesis of SHBG and corticosteroid binding globulin (CBG) during continuous use. The extent of SHBG induction, however, is dependent upon the chemical structure and dose of the co-administered progestin. During treatment with Dianette SHBG concentrations in serum increased from about 100nmol/l to 300nmol/l and the serum concentrations of CBG were increased from about 50 micrograms/ml to 95 micrograms/ml.

*Preclinical safety data:* There are no preclinical safety data which could be of relevance to the prescriber and which are not already included in other relevant sections of the SPC.

**Pharmaceutical particulars**

*List of excipients:* Lactose, maize starch, povidone, talc, magnesium stearate (E 572), sucrose, macrogol 6,000, calcium carbonate (E 170), titanium dioxide (E 171), glycerol 85%, montan glycol wax, yellow ferric oxide pigment (E 172).

*Incompatibilities:* None known.

*Shelf life:* 5 years.

*Special precautions for storage:* Not applicable.

*Nature and contents of container:* Outer carton contains aluminium foil and PVC blister memo packs each containing 21 tablets. Each carton contains either 1 or 3 blister memo packs.

*Instructions for use/handling:* Keep out of the reach of children.

**Marketing authorisation number** 0053/0190

**Date of approval/revision of SPC** 16 June 1997

**Legal category** POM

## ECHOVIST* ▼

**Qualitative and quantitative composition** Each vial contains 3 g granules (1 g granules contains 1 g galactose microparticles). 1 ml aqueous solution for production of the suspension contains 200 mg galactose.

**Pharmaceutical form** Microcrystalline suspension for transcervical administration.

**Clinical particulars**

*Therapeutic indications:* Echo-contrast medium for transcervical administration in contrast-enhanced ultrasound investigation of the female genital tract hysterosalpingo-contrast sonography). Echovist can be used to enhance gynaecological ultrasound images and assess tubal patency.

*Posology and method of administration:* To prepare the echo-contrast medium, the galactose solution (13.5 ml) is drawn into a syringe and transferred to

the vial containing 3 g of granules using the 'Mini-Spike' supplied. The vial should then be shaken vigorously for about 5 seconds to suspend the granules in solution, producing a homogenous milky-white suspension. The suspension is then drawn up using the 'Mini-Spike', taking care that recognisable air bubbles are removed. The granules and the galactose solution should be at room temperature at the time the suspension is made up. Warming the suspension (e.g. in the hands) or excessive negative pressure on drawing it up should be avoided as this may result in the decrease of the microbubble concentration or development of larger air bubbles.

For transcervical administration in gynaecological investigations the use of an intrauterine balloon catheter is recommended.

Any suspension not used at one examination session must be discarded.

*Dosage:* For the demonstration of the uterine cavity 2-5 ml of Echovist suspension should be used. In order to demonstrate the Fallopian tubes and to check their patency, additional intermittent administration of doses of 1-2 ml should be given under sonographic control up to a maximum of 30 ml. In general, about 15 ml is normally sufficient.

*Contra-indications:* Galactosaemia. Intact pregnancy. Pelvic inflammatory disease.

*Special warnings and special precautions for use:* Aseptic conditions must be observed to reduce the potential risk of ascending infection.

*Interaction with other medicaments and other forms of interaction:* None so far known.

*Pregnancy and lactation:* The transcervical administration of Echovist is contraindicated in pregnancy. Since galactose is a natural constituent of milk, there is no contraindication to the use of Echovist during lactation, with the exception of women with galactosaemia.

*Effects on ability to drive and use machines:* Not applicable.

*Undesirable effects:* The distension of the uterine cavity and tubes caused by filling with the contrast agent can result in pain which is particularly pronounced in the presence of occluded tubes.

Vasovagal reactions, e.g. outbreaks of sweating, dizziness, nausea and vomiting, may occur in individual cases.

The possibility of ascending genital infection owing to the method itself cannot be ruled out in individual cases.

*Overdose:* Overdose is unlikely with transcervical administration.

**Pharmacological properties**

*Pharmacodynamic properties:* Echovist is an echo-contrast medium for hysterosalpingo-contrast sonography. It consists of a suspension of soluble galactose microparticles in aqueous galactose solution. After transcervical administration this microbubble-microparticle suspension leads to a marked increase of the echo signals from the female genital tract due to the acoustically active inhomogeneities produced.

*Pharmacokinetic properties:* The galactose and small amount of air in the bubbles are completely absorbed after transcervical administration. The galactose first of all becomes dispersed in the extracellular space and is subjected to glucose metabolism independent of insulin. Galactose is stored above all in the liver through the formation of galactose-1-phosphate or is metabolised and broken down to $CO_2$ after isomerisation to glucose-1-phosphate. If the plasma galactose level exceeds about 50 mg/100 ml and, therefore, the elimination rate of the liver, galactose is eliminated via the kidneys. The elimination rate in patients with liver disease is about one third lower than in healthy subjects, in whom the plasma galactose level falls by 10% per minute. Total clearance is about 40% lower in patients with liver disease. In the case of liver damage up to 60% of the amount of galactose administered is eliminated via the kidneys, while about 40% is utilised extrahepatically.

Galactose has a half-life of about 10-11 minutes in adults.

Elimination may be substantially prolonged after consumption of alcohol.

*Preclinical safety data:* Echovist does not pose any risk of acute intoxication even on repeated administration of the diagnostic dose at short intervals of time.

Systemic toxicity studies after repeated daily intravenous administration and after repeated intracardiac (left ventricle) application produced no findings which preclude the usually single transcervical administration in human beings. No unequivocally organ-toxic effects were demonstrable even after very high intravenous dosages.

Studies for embryotoxic and, in particular, teratogenic effects produced no evidence for a teratogenic potential in human beings.

Findings from local tolerance studies on single intravenous, intraarterial, subcutaneous, paravenous intramuscular and, in particular following intrauterine administration, showed that signs of local intolerance are likely only on inadvertent paravenous injection.

No risk of a tumorigenic, mutagenic or sensitising effect to human beings is envisaged on administration of Echovist, since the galactose contained in the medium occurs physiologically and is ingested by human beings with the diet and metabolised, and because no such effects are known for galactose.

**Pharmaceutical particulars**

*List of excipients:* Water for injection.

*Incompatibilities:* None so far known.

*Shelf life:* Echovist solution and Echovist granulate are both stable for five years.

*Special precautions for storage:* Not applicable

*Nature and contents of container:*
Granulate/Galactose solution
Injection vial: Glass type I, siliconized.
Stopper: Chlorinated butyl rubber, grey, fluoropolymer-coated.
Flanged cap: Pure aluminium with polypropylene cover disks.
'Mini-Spike': Plastics.

*Combination pack consisting of*
1 vial of 20 ml with 3 g granulate
1 vial of 15 ml with 13.5 ml galactose solution
1 'Mini-Spike'

*Instructions for use/handling:* The ready-to-use suspension has to be prepared according to instructions. Any suspension not used at one examination session must be discarded. Store all drugs properly and keep them out of reach of children.

**Marketing authorisation number** 0053/0232-3

**Date of approval/revision of SPC** 22 November 1995

**Legal category** POM

## EUGYNON* 30

**Presentation** Each white sugar-coated tablet contains 250 micrograms levonorgestrel and 30 micrograms ethinyloestradiol.
**Excipients:** lactose, maize starch, povidone 25 000, talc, magnesium stearate, sucrose, povidone 700 000, macrogol 6000, calcium carbonate, montan glycol wax.

**Uses** Oral contraception and the recognised gynaecological indications for such oestrogen-progestogen combinations. The mode of action includes the inhibition of ovulation by suppression of the mid-cycle surge of luteinising hormone, the inspissation of cervical mucus so as to constitute a barrier to sperm, and the rendering of the endometrium unreceptive to implantation.

**Dosage and administration**

*First treatment cycle:* 1 tablet daily for 21 days, starting on the first day of the menstrual cycle. Contraceptive protection begins immediately.

*Subsequent cycles:* Tablet taking from the next pack of Eugynon 30 is continued after a 7-day interval, beginning on the same day of the week as the first pack.

*Changing from 21-day combined oral contraceptives:* The first tablet of Eugynon 30 should be taken on the first day immediately after the end of the previous oral contraceptive course. Additional contraceptive precautions are not required.

*Changing from a combined Every Day pill (28 day tablets):* Eugynon 30 should be started after taking the last active tablet from the Every Day Pill pack. The first Eugynon 30 tablet is taken the next day. Additional contraceptive precautions are not then required.

*Changing from a progestogen-only pill (POP):* The first tablet of Eugynon 30 should be taken on the first day of bleeding, even if a POP has already been taken on that day. Additional contraceptive precautions are not then required. The remaining progestogen-only pills should be discarded.

*Post-partum and post-abortum use:* After pregnancy, oral contraception can be started 21 days after a vaginal delivery, provided that the patient is fully ambulant and there are no puerperal complications. Additional contraceptive precautions will be required for the first 7 days of tablet taking to ensure adequate contraceptive cover if early ovulation has occurred. Since the first post-partum ovulation may precede the first bleeding, another method of contraception should be used in the interval between childbirth and the first course of tablets. After a first-trimester abortion, oral contraception may be started immediately, in which case no additional contraceptive precautions are required.

*Pregnancy and lactation:* If pregnancy occurs during medication with oral contraceptives, the preparation should be withdrawn immediately (see *Reasons for stopping oral contraception immediately*).

The use of Eugynon 30 during lactation may lead to a reduction in the volume of milk produced and to a change in its composition. Minute amounts of the active substances are excreted with the milk. Mothers who are breast-feeding may be advised instead to use a progestogen-only pill.

*Special circumstances requiring additional contraception:*
*Incorrect administration:* A single delayed tablet should be taken as soon as possible, and if this can be done within 12 hours of the correct time, contraceptive protection is maintained.

With longer delays, additional contraception is needed. Only the most recently delayed tablet should be taken, earlier missed tablets being omitted, and additional non-hormonal methods of contraception (except the rhythm or temperature methods) should be used for the next 7 days, while the next 7 tablets are being taken. Additionally, therefore, if tablet(s) have been missed during the last 7 days of a pack, there should be no break before the next pack is started. In this situation, a withdrawal bleed should not be expected until the end of the second pack. Some breakthrough bleeding may occur on tablet taking days but this is not clinically significant. If the patient does not have a withdrawal bleed during the tablet-free interval following the end of the second pack, the possibility of pregnancy must be ruled out before starting the next pack.

*Gastro-intestinal upset:* Vomiting or diarrhoea may reduce the efficacy of oral contraceptives by preventing full absorption. Tablet-taking from the current pack should be continued. Additional non-hormonal methods of contraception (except the rhythm or temperature methods) should be used during the gastro-intestinal upset and for 7 days following the upset. If these 7 days overrun the end of a pack, the next pack should be started without a break. In this situation, a withdrawal bleed should not be expected until the end of the second pack. If the patient does not have a withdrawal bleed during the tablet-free interval following the end of the second pack, the possibility of pregnancy must be ruled out before starting the next pack. Other methods of contraception should be considered if the gastro-intestinal disorder is likely to be prolonged.

*Interaction with other drugs:* Hepatic enzyme inducers such as barbiturates, primidone, phenobarbitone, phenytoin, phenylbutazone, rifampicin, carbamazepine and griseofulvin can impair the efficacy of Eugynon 30. For women receiving long-term therapy with hepatic enzyme inducers, another method of contraception should be used. The use of ampicillin and other antibiotics may also reduce the efficacy of Eugynon 30, possibly by altering the intestinal flora. Women receiving short courses of enzyme inducers or broad spectrum antibiotics should take additional, non-hormonal (except rhythm or temperature method) contraceptive precautions during the time of concurrent medication and for 7 days afterwards. If these 7 days overrun the end of a pack, the next pack should be started without a break. In this situation, a withdrawal bleed should not be expected until the end of the second pack. If the patient does not have a withdrawal bleed during the tablet-free interval following the end of the second pack, the possibility of pregnancy must be ruled out before resuming with the next pack. With rifampicin, additional contraceptive precautions should be continued for 4 weeks after treatment stops, even if only a short course was administered.

The requirement for oral antidiabetics or insulin can change as a result of the effect on glucose tolerance.

**Contra-indications, warnings, etc**
*Contra-indications:*

1. Pregnancy
2. Severe disturbances of liver function, jaundice or persistent itching during a previous pregnancy, Dubin-Johnson syndrome, Rotor syndrome, previous or existing liver tumours.
3. Existing or previous arterial or venous thrombotic or embolic processes, conditions which predispose to them e.g. disorders of the clotting processes, valvular heart disease and atrial fibrillation.
4. Sickle-cell anaemia.
5. Mammary or endometrial carcinoma, or a history of these conditions.
6. Severe diabetes mellitus with vascular changes.
7. Disorders of lipid metabolism.
8. History of herpes gestationis.
9. Deterioration of otosclerosis during pregnancy.
10. Undiagnosed abnormal vaginal bleeding.
11. Hypersensitivity to any of the components of Eugynon 30.

*Warnings:* There is a general opinion, based on statistical evidence, that users of combined oral contraceptives experience, more often than non-users, venous thromboembolism, arterial thrombosis, including cerebral and myocardial infarction, and subarachnoid haemorrhage. Full recovery from such disorders does not always occur, and it should be realised that in a few cases they are fatal. How often these disorders occur in users of the modern low-dose pills is not known, but there are reasons for suggesting that they may occur less often than with older pills.

Certain factors may entail some risk of thrombosis, e.g. smoking, obesity, varicose veins, cardiovascular diseases, diabetes, and migraine. The suitability of a combined oral contraceptive should be judged according to the severity of such conditions in the individual case, and should be discussed with the patient before she decides to take it. The risk of arterial thrombosis associated with combined oral contraceptives increases with age, and this risk is aggravated by cigarette-smoking. The use of combined oral contraceptives by women in the older age-group, especially those who are cigarette smokers, should therefore be discouraged and alternative methods used.

In addition if there is a history in the family of thromboembolic diseases at a young age (e.g. deep vein thrombosis, heart attack or stroke) disturbances of the coagulation system must be ruled out before the pill is prescribed.

Numerous epidemiological studies have been reported on the risks of ovarian, endometrial, cervical and breast cancer in women using combined oral contraceptives. The evidence is clear that combined oral contraceptives offer substantial protection against both ovarian and endometrial cancer.

An increased risk of cervical cancer in long-term users of combined oral contraceptives has been reported in some studies, but there continues to be controversy about the extent to which this is attributable to the confounding effects of sexual behaviour and other factors.

The evidence linking the use of combined oral contraceptives and breast cancer remains inconclusive. The results of some studies suggest an increased risk of breast cancer presenting below the age of about 35, the risk rising with duration of use. Any possible increased risk of breast cancer with combined oral contraceptives is however likely to be small, and may be expected to be less with low-dosage pills. This possible risk should be weighed against the many benefits of combined oral contraceptives, including their protective effects against ovarian and endometrial cancers.

The possibility cannot be ruled out that certain chronic diseases may occasionally deteriorate during the use of combined oral contraceptives (see *Precautions*).

In rare cases benign and, in even rarer cases, malignant liver tumours leading in isolated cases to life-threatening intra-abdominal haemorrhage have been observed after the use of hormonal substances such as those contained in Eugynon 30. If severe upper abdominal complaints, liver enlargement or signs of intra-abdominal haemorrhage occur, the possibility of a liver tumour should be included in the differential diagnosis.

*Reasons for stopping oral contraception immediately:*

1. Occurrence for the first time, or exacerbation, of migrainous headaches or unusually frequent or unusually severe headaches.
2. Sudden disturbances of vision or hearing or other perceptual disorders.
3. First signs of thrombophlebitis or thromboembolic symptoms (e.g. unusual pains in or swelling of the leg(s), stabbing pains on breathing or coughing for no apparent reason). Feeling of pain and tightness in the chest.
4. Six weeks before an elective major operation (e.g. abdominal, orthopaedic), any surgery to the legs, medical treatment for varicose veins or prolonged immobilisation, e.g. after accidents or surgery. Do not restart until 2 weeks after full ambulation. In case of emergency surgery, thrombotic prophylaxis is usually indicated e.g. subcutaneous heparin.
5. Onset of jaundice, hepatitis, itching of the whole body.
6. Increase in epileptic seizures.
7. Significant rise in blood pressure.
8. Onset of severe depression.
9. Severe upper abdominal pain or liver enlargement.
10. Clear exacerbation of conditions known to be capable of deteriorating during oral contraception or pregnancy.
11. Pregnancy is a reason for stopping immediately because it has been suggested by some investigations that oral contraceptives taken in early pregnancy may slightly increase the risk of foetal malformations. Other investigations have failed to support these findings. The possibility therefore cannot be excluded, but it is certain that if a risk exists at all, it is very small.

*Precautions:* Examination of the pelvic organs, breasts and blood-pressure should precede the prescribing o any combined oral contraceptive and should b repeated regularly. The family medical history shoul be carefully noted and disturbances of the clotting mechanism ruled out if any member of the family ha suffered from thromboembolic disease (e.g. deep vei thrombosis, stroke, myocardial infarction) at a young age. Before starting treatment pregnancy must b excluded.

The following conditions require strict medica supervision during medication with oral contracep tives. Deterioration or first appearance of any of thes conditions may indicate that use of the oral contracep tive should be discontinued: diabetes mellitus, or a tendency towards diabetes mellitus (e.g. unexplaine glycosuria), hypertension, varicose veins, a history c phlebitis, otosclerosis, multiple sclerosis, epilepsy porphyria, tetany, disturbed liver function, Syden ham's chorea, renal dysfunction, family history o clotting disorders, obesity, family history of breas cancer and patient history of benign breast disease history of clinical depression, systemic lupus erythe matosus, uterine fibroids and migraine, gall-stones cardiovascular diseases, chloasma, asthma, an intol erance of contact lenses, or any disease that is pron to worsen during pregnancy. Some women ma experience amenorrhoea or oligomenorrhoea afte discontinuation of oral contraceptives, especiall when these conditions existed prior to use. Wome should be informed of this possibility.

*Side-effects:* In rare cases, headaches, gastric upsets nausea, vomiting, breast tenderness, changes in bod weight, changes in libido, depressive moods ca occur. In predisposed women, use of Eugynon 30 ca sometimes cause chloasma which is exacerbated b exposure to sunlight. Such women should avoi prolonged exposure to sunlight.

Individual cases of poor tolerance of contact lense have been reported with use of oral contraceptives Contact lens wearers who develop changes in len tolerance should be assessed by an ophthalmologis

*Menstrual changes:*
*1. Reduction of menstrual flow:* This is not abnorma and it is to be expected in some patients. Indeed, may be beneficial where heavy periods were prev ously experienced.

*2. Missed menstruation:* Occasionally, withdrawa bleeding may not occur at all. If the tablets have bee taken correctly, pregnancy is very unlikely. If with drawal bleeding fails to occur at the end of a secon pack, the possibility of pregnancy must be ruled ou before resuming with the next pack.

*Intermenstrual bleeding:* 'Spotting' or heavier 'breal through bleeding' sometimes occur during table taking, especially in the first few cycles, and normall cease spontaneously. Eugynon 30 should therefor be continued even if irregular bleeding occurs. irregular bleeding is persistent, appropriate diagnosti measures to exclude an organic cause are indicate and may include curettage. This also applies in th case of spotting which occurs at irregular intervals i several consecutive cycles or which occurs for th first time after long use of Eugynon 30.

*Effect on blood chemistry:* The use of oral contracep tives may influence the results of certain laborator tests including biochemical parameters of liver, thy roid, adrenal and renal function, plasma levels c carrier proteins and lipid/lipoprotein fractions, para meters of carbohydrate metabolism and paramete of coagulation and fibrinolysis. Laboratory sta should therefore be informed about oral contraceptiv use when laboratory tests are requested.

*Overdosage:* Overdosage may cause nausea, vomi ing and, in females, withdrawal bleeding. There a no specific antidotes and treatment should be symp tomatic.

**Pharmaceutical precautions** *Shelf-life:* Five years.

**Legal category** POM

Package quantities Individual packs containing thre months' supply

**Further information** Nil

**Product licence number** 0053/0049

## FEMODENE*

**Presentation** Each white sugar-coated tablet co tains 75 micrograms gestodene and 30 microgram ethinyloestradiol (ethinylestradiol).

Excipients: lactose, maize starch, povidone 25 00 sodium calcium edetate, magnesium stearate, su crose, povidone 700 000, macrogol 6000, calciu carbonate, talc, montan glycol wax.

**Uses** Oral contraception and the recognised gyna cological indications for such oestrogen-progestoge combinations. The mode of action includes the inh bition of ovulation by suppression of the mid-cyc surge of luteinising hormone, the inspissation of cervical mucus so as to constitute a barrier to sperm, and the rendering of the endometrium unreceptive to implantation.

**Dosage and administration**

*First treatment cycle:* 1 tablet daily for 21 days, starting on the first day of the menstrual cycle. Contraceptive protection begins immediately.

*Subsequent cycles:* Tablet taking from the next pack of Femodene is continued after a 7-day interval, beginning on the same day of the week as the first pack.

*Changing from 21-day combined oral contraceptives:* The first tablet of Femodene should be taken on the first day immediately after the end of the previous oral contraceptive course. Additional contraceptive precautions are not required.

*Changing from a combined Every Day pill (28 day tablets):* Femodene should be started after taking the last active tablet from the Every Day Pill pack. The first Femodene tablet is taken the next day. Additional contraceptive precautions are not then required.

*Changing from a progestogen-only pill (POP):* The first tablet of Femodene should be taken on the first day of bleeding, even if a POP has already been taken on that day. Additional contraceptive precautions are not then required. The remaining progestogen-only pills should be discarded.

*Post-partum and post-abortum use:* After pregnancy, oral contraception can be started 21 days after a vaginal delivery, provided that the patient is fully ambulant and there are no puerperal complications. Additional contraceptive precautions will be required for the first 7 days of tablet taking. Since the first post-partum ovulation may precede the first bleeding, another method of contraception should be used in the interval between childbirth and the first course of tablets. After a first-trimester abortion, oral contraception may be started immediately in which case no additional contraceptive precautions are required.

*Pregnancy and lactation:* If pregnancy occurs during medication with oral contraceptives, the preparation should be withdrawn immediately (see *Reasons for stopping oral contraception immediately*).

The use of Femodene during lactation may lead to a reduction in the volume of milk produced and to a change in its composition. Minute amounts of the active substances are excreted with the milk. Mothers who are breast-feeding may be advised instead to use a progestogen-only pill.

*Special circumstances requiring additional contraception*

*Incorrect administration:* A single delayed tablet should be taken as soon as possible, and if this can be done within 12 hours of the correct time, contraceptive protection is maintained. With longer delays, additional contraception is needed. Only the most recently delayed tablet should be taken, earlier missed tablets being omitted, and additional non-hormonal methods of contraception (except the rhythm or temperature methods) should be used for the next 7 days, while the next 7 tablets are being taken. Additionally, therefore, if tablet(s) have been missed during the last 7 days of a pack, there should be no break before the next pack is started. In this situation, a withdrawal bleed should not be expected until the end of the second pack. Some breakthrough bleeding may occur on tablet taking days but this is not clinically significant. If the patient does not have a withdrawal bleed during the tablet-free interval following the end of the second pack, the possibility of pregnancy must be ruled out before starting the next pack.

*Gastro-intestinal upset:* Vomiting or diarrhoea may reduce the efficacy of oral contraceptives by preventing full absorption. Tablet-taking from the current pack should be continued. Additional non-hormonal methods of contraception (except the rhythm or temperature methods) should be used during the gastro-intestinal upset and for 7 days following the upset. If these 7 days overrun the end of a pack, the next pack should be started without a break. In this situation, a withdrawal bleed should not be expected until the end of the second pack. If the patient does not have a withdrawal bleed during the tablet-free interval following the end of the second pack, the possibility of pregnancy must be ruled out before starting the next pack. Other methods of contraception should be considered if the gastro-intestinal disorder is likely to be prolonged.

*Interaction with other drugs:* Hepatic enzyme inducers such as barbiturates, primidone, phenobarbitone, phenytoin, phenylbutazone, rifampicin, carbamazepine and griseofulvin can impair the efficacy of Femodene. For women receiving long-term therapy with hepatic enzyme inducers, another method of contraception should be used. The use of antibiotics may also reduce the efficacy of Femodene, possibly by altering the intestinal flora.

Women receiving short courses of enzyme inducers or broad spectrum antibiotics should take additional, non-hormonal (except rhythm or temperature method) contraceptive precautions during the time of concurrent medication and for 7 days afterwards. If these 7 days overrun the end of a pack, the next pack should be started without a break. In this situation, a withdrawal bleed should not be expected until the end of the second pack. If the patient does not have a withdrawal bleed during the tablet-free interval following the end of the second pack, the possibility of pregnancy must be ruled out before resuming with the next pack. With rifampicin, additional contraceptive precautions should be continued for 4 weeks after treatment stops, even if only a short course was administered.

The requirement for oral antidiabetics or insulin can change as a result of the effect on glucose tolerance.

**Contra-indications, warnings, etc**

*Contra-indications:*

1. Pregnancy
2. Severe disturbances of liver function, jaundice or persistent itching during a previous pregnancy, Dubin-Johnson syndrome, Rotor syndrome, previous or existing liver tumours.
3. Existing or previous arterial or venous thrombotic or embolic processes, conditions which predispose to them, e.g. disorders of the clotting processes, valvular heart disease and atrial fibrillation.
4. Sickle-cell anaemia.
5. Mammary or endometrial carcinoma, or a history of these conditions.
6. Severe diabetes mellitus with vascular changes.
7. Disorders of lipid metabolism.
8. History of herpes gestationis.
9. Deterioration of otosclerosis during pregnancy.
10. Undiagnosed abnormal vaginal bleeding.
11. Hypersensitivity to any of the components of Femodene.

*Warnings:* There is a general opinion, based on statistical evidence, that users of combined oral contraceptives experience, more often than non-users, venous thromboembolism, arterial thrombosis, including cerebral and myocardial infarction, and subarachnoid haemorrhage. Full recovery from such disorders does not always occur and it should be realised that in a few cases they are fatal. How often these disorders occur in users of the modern low-dose pills is not known, but there are reasons for suggesting that they may occur less often than with older pills.

Certain factors may entail some risk of thrombosis, e.g. smoking, obesity, varicose veins, cardiovascular diseases, diabetes, and migraine. The suitability of a combined oral contraceptive should be judged according to the severity of such conditions in the individual case, and should be discussed with the patient before she decides to take it. The risk of arterial thrombosis associated with oral contraceptives increases with age, and this risk is aggravated by cigarette-smoking. The use of combined oral contraceptives by women in the older age-group, especially those who are cigarette smokers, should therefore be discouraged and alternative methods used.

In addition if there is a history in the family of thromboembolic diseases at a young age (e.g. deep vein thrombosis, heart attack or stroke) disturbances of the coagulation system must be ruled out before the pill is prescribed.

Numerous epidemiological studies have been reported on the risks of ovarian, endometrial, cervical and breast cancer in women using combined oral contraceptives. The evidence is clear that combined oral contraceptives offer substantial protection against both ovarian and endometrial cancer.

An increased risk of cervical cancer in long-term users of combined oral contraceptives has been reported in some studies, but there continues to be controversy about the extent to which this is attributable to the confounding effects of sexual behaviour and other factors.

The evidence linking the use of combined oral contraceptives and breast cancer remains inconclusive. The results of some studies suggest an increased risk of breast cancer presenting below the age of about 35, the risk rising with duration of use. Any possible increased risk of breast cancer with combined oral contraceptives is however likely to be small, and may be expected to be less with low-dosage pills. This possible risk should be weighed against the many benefits of combined oral contraceptives, including their protective effects against ovarian and endometrial cancers.

The possibility cannot be ruled out that certain chronic diseases may occasionally deteriorate during the use of combined oral contraceptives (see *"Precautions"*). The combination of ethinyloestradiol and gestodene, like other contraceptive steroids, is associated with an increased incidence of neoplastic nodules in the rat liver, the relevance of which to man is unknown. Malignant liver tumours have been reported on rare occasions in long-term users of oral contraceptives. In rare cases benign and, in even rarer cases, malignant liver tumours leading in isolated cases to life-threatening intra-abdominal haemorrhage have been observed after the use of hormonal substances such as those contained in Femodene. If severe upper abdominal complaints, liver enlargement or signs of intra-abdominal haemorrhage occur, the possibility of a liver tumour should be included in the differential diagnosis.

*Reasons for stopping oral contraception immediately:*

1. Occurrence for the first time, or exacerbation, of migrainous headaches or unusually frequent or unusually severe headaches.
2. Sudden disturbances of vision or hearing or other perceptual disorders.
3. First signs of thrombophlebitis or thromboembolic symptoms (e.g. unusual pains in or swelling of the leg(s), stabbing pains on breathing or coughing for no apparent reason). Feeling of pain and tightness in the chest.
4. Six weeks before an elective major operation (e.g. abdominal, orthopaedic), any surgery to the legs, medical treatment for varicose veins or prolonged immobilisation, e.g. after accidents or surgery. Do not restart until 2 weeks after full ambulation. In case of emergency surgery, thrombotic prophylaxis is usually indicated e.g. subcutaneous heparin.
5. Onset of jaundice, hepatitis, itching of the whole body.
6. Increase in epileptic seizures.
7. Significant rise in blood pressure.
8. Onset of severe depression.
9. Severe upper abdominal pain or liver enlargement.
10. Clear exacerbation of conditions known to be capable of deteriorating during oral contraception or pregnancy.
11. Pregnancy is a reason for stopping immediately because it has been suggested by some investigations that oral contraceptives taken in early pregnancy may slightly increase the risk of foetal malformations. Other investigations have failed to support these findings. The possibility therefore cannot be excluded, but it is certain that if a risk exists at all, it is very small.

*Precautions:* Examination of the pelvic organs, breasts and blood-pressure should precede the prescribing of any combined oral contraceptive and should be repeated regularly. The family medical history should be carefully noted and disturbances of the clotting mechanism ruled out if any member of the family has suffered from thromboembolic disease (e.g. deep vein thrombosis, stroke, myocardial infarction) at a young age. Before starting treatment pregnancy must be excluded.

The following conditions require strict medical supervision during medication with oral contraceptives. Deterioration or first appearance of any of these conditions may indicate that use of the oral contraceptive should be discontinued:

Diabetes mellitus, or a tendency towards diabetes mellitus (e.g. unexplained glycosuria), hypertension, varicose veins, a history of phlebitis, otosclerosis, multiple sclerosis, epilepsy, porphyria, tetany, disturbed liver function, Sydenham's chorea, renal dysfunction, family history of clotting disorders, obesity, family history of breast cancer and patient history of benign breast disease, history of clinical depression, systemic lupus erythematosus, uterine fibroids, an intolerance of contact lenses, migraine, gall-stones, cardiovascular diseases, chloasma, asthma, or any disease that is prone to worsen during pregnancy.

Some women may experience amenorrhoea or oligomenorrhoea after discontinuation of oral contraceptives, especially when these conditions existed prior to use. Women should be informed of this possibility.

*Side-effects*: In rare cases headaches, gastric upsets, nausea, vomiting, breast tenderness, changes in bodyweight, changes in libido, depressive moods can occur.

In predisposed women, use of Femodene can sometimes cause chloasma which is exacerbated by exposure to sunlight. Individual cases of poor tolerance of contact lenses have been reported with the use of oral contraceptives. Contact lens wearers who develop changes in lens tolerance should be assessed by an ophthalmologist.

*Menstrual changes:*

*1. Reduction of menstrual flow:* This is not abnormal and it is to be expected in some patients. Indeed, it may be beneficial where heavy periods were previously experienced.

*2. Missed menstruation:* Occasionally, withdrawal bleeding may not occur at all. If the tablets have been taken correctly, pregnancy is very unlikely. If withdrawal bleeding fails to occur at the end of a second pack, the possibility of pregnancy must be ruled out before resuming with the next pack.

*Intermenstrual bleeding:* 'Spotting' or heavier 'breakthrough bleeding' sometimes occur during tablet taking, especially in the first few cycles, and normally cease spontaneously. Femodene should therefore be continued even if irregular bleeding occurs. If irregular bleeding is persistent, appropriate diagnostic measures to exclude an organic cause are indicated and may include curettage. This also applies in the case of spotting which occurs at irregular intervals in several consecutive cycles or which occurs for the first time after long use of Femodene.

*Effect on blood chemistry:* The use of oral contraceptives may influence the results of certain laboratory tests including biochemical parameters of liver, thyroid, adrenal and renal function, plasma levels of carrier proteins and lipid/lipoprotein fractions, parameters of carbohydrate metabolism and parameters of coagulation and fibrinolysis. Laboratory staff should therefore be informed about oral contraceptive use when laboratory tests are requested.

*Overdosage:* Overdosage may cause nausea, vomiting and, in females, withdrawal bleeding. There are no specific antidotes and treatment should be symptomatic.

**Pharmaceutical precautions** *Shelf-life* – Five years.

**Legal category** POM

**Package quantities** Individual packs containing three months' supply (OP)

**Further information** Nil

**Product licence number** 0053/0179

## FEMODENE* ED

**Presentation** Each white sugar-coated tablet contains 75 micrograms gestodene and 30 micrograms ethinyloestradiol (ethinylestradiol).

In addition, there are 7 white placebo tablets which are larger.

*Excipients:* lactose, maize starch, povidone 25 000, sodium calcium edetate, magnesium stearate, sucrose, povidone 700 000, macrogol 6000, calcium carbonate, talc, montan glycol wax.

**Uses** Oral contraception and the recognised gynaecological indications for such oestrogen-progestogen combinations. The mode of action includes the inhibition of ovulation by suppression of the mid-cycle surge of luteinising hormone, the inspissation of cervical mucus so as to constitute a barrier to sperm, and the rendering of the endometrium unreceptive to implantation.

**Dosage and administration**

*First treatment cycle:* 1 tablet daily for 28 days, starting in the red sector on the first day of the menstrual cycle. The initial tablet is the one marked with the appropriate day of the week. In the first cycle only, an additional non-hormonal method of contraception (except the rhythm or temperature methods) must be used for the first 14 days of tablet taking.

*Subsequent cycles:* Tablet-taking is continuous, which means that the next pack of Femodene ED follows immediately without a break. A withdrawal bleed usually occurs when the placebo tablets are being taken.

*Changing from another combined oral contraceptive:* The first tablet of Femodene ED should be taken from the red sector immediately after the end of the previous oral contraceptive course. In the first cycle only, an additional non-hormonal method of contraception (except the rhythm or temperature methods) must be used for the first 14 days of tablet taking.

*Changing from a progestogen-only pill (POP):* The first tablet of Femodene ED should be taken from the red sector on the first day of bleeding, even if a POP has already been taken on that day. An additional non-hormonal method of contraception (except the rhythm or temperature methods) must be used for 14 days. The remaining progestogen-only pills should be discarded.

*Post-partum and post-abortum use:* After pregnancy, Femodene ED can be started 21 days after a vaginal delivery, provided that the patient is fully ambulant and there are no puerperal complications. Additional contraceptive precautions will be required for the first 14 days of tablet taking. Since the first post-partum ovulation may precede the first bleeding, another method of contraception should be used in the interval between childbirth and the first course of tablets. After a first-trimester abortion, oral contraception may be started immediately, in which case additional non-hormonal contraceptive precautions are required (except the rhythm or temperature methods) for the first 14 days of tablet taking in the first cycle of Femodene ED.

*Pregnancy and lactation:* If pregnancy occurs during medication with oral contraceptives, the preparation should be withdrawn immediately (see 'Reasons for stopping oral contraception immediately').

The use of Femodene ED during lactation may lead to a reduction in the volume of milk produced and to a change in its composition. Minute amounts of the active substances are excreted with the milk. Mothers who are breast-feeding may be advised instead to use a progestogen-only pill.

*Special circumstances requiring additional contraception:*
*Incorrect administration:* Errors in taking the 7 placebo tablets (i.e. the first 5 tablets in the red section and the 2 immediately before the red section) can be ignored. A single delayed active (small) tablet should be taken as soon as possible, and if this can be done within 12 hours of the correct time, contraceptive protection is maintained.

With longer delays in taking active tablets, additional contraception is needed. Only the most recently delayed tablet should be taken, earlier missed tablets being omitted, and additional non-hormonal methods of contraception (except the rhythm or temperature methods) should be used for *the next 7 days, while the next 7 active (small) tablets are being taken.* Therefore, if the 7 days additional contraception will extend beyond the Friday just before the red section (i.e. the last active tablet) the user should take the tablets up to and including that Friday, and start a new pack next day with the Saturday tablet in the red section i.e. discard the remaining tablets and go to an appropriate active tablet in the next pack. In this situation, a withdrawal bleed should not be expected until the end of the second pack. Some breakthrough bleeding may occur on tablet taking days but this is not clinically significant. If the patient does not have a withdrawal bleed following the end of the second pack, the possibility of pregnancy must be ruled out before starting the next pack.

*Gastro-intestinal upset:* Vomiting or diarrhoea may reduce the efficacy of oral contraceptives by preventing full absorption. Tablet taking from the current pack should be continued. Additional non-hormonal methods of contraception (except the rhythm or temperature methods) should be used during the gastro-intestinal upset and for 7 days following the upset. If these 7 days extend beyond the last active (small) tablet (i.e. the Friday just before the red section), any remaining tablets should be discarded and a new pack of Femodene ED started the next day with the Saturday tablet in the red section (i.e an appropriate active (small) tablet). In this situation, a withdrawal bleed should not be expected until the end of the second pack. If the patient does not have a withdrawal bleed at the end of the second pack, the possibility of pregnancy must be ruled out before starting the next pack. Other methods of contraception should be considered if the gastro-intestinal disorder is likely to be prolonged.

*Interaction with other drugs:* Hepatic enzyme inducers such as barbiturates, primidone, phenobarbitone, phenytoin, phenylbutazone, rifampicin, carbamazepine and griseofulvin can impair the efficacy of Femodene ED. For women receiving long-term therapy with hepatic enzyme inducers, another method of contraception should be used. The use of antibiotics may also reduce the efficacy of Femodene ED, possibly by altering the intestinal flora.

Women receiving short courses of enzyme inducers or broad spectrum antibiotics should take additional, non-hormonal (except rhythm or temperature method) contraceptive precautions during the time of concurrent medication and for 7 days afterwards. If these 7 days extend beyond the last active (small) tablet (i.e. the Friday just before the red section), any remaining tablets should be discarded and a new pack of Femodene ED started the next day with the Saturday tablet in the red section (i.e. an appropriate active (small) tablet). In this situation, a withdrawal bleed should not be expected until the end of the second pack. If the patient does not have a withdrawal bleed at the end of the second pack, the possibility of pregnancy must be ruled out before resuming with the next pack. With rifampicin, additional contraceptive precautions should be continued for 4 weeks after treatment stops, even if only a short course was administered.

The requirement for oral antidiabetics or insulin can change as a result of the effect on glucose tolerance.

**Contra-indications, warnings, etc**
*Contra-indications:*

1. Pregnancy
2. Severe disturbances of liver function, jaundice or persistent itching during a previous pregnancy, Dubin-Johnson syndrome, Rotor syndrome, previous or existing liver tumours.
3. Existing or previous arterial or venous thrombotic or embolic processes, conditions which predispose to them e.g. disorders of the clotting processes, valvula heart disease and atrial fibrillation.
4. Sickle-cell anaemia.
5. Mammary or endometrial carcinoma, or a histor of these conditions.
6. Severe diabetes mellitus with vascular changes.
7. Disorders of lipid metabolism.
8. History of herpes gestationis.
9. Deterioration of otosclerosis during pregnancy.
10. Undiagnosed abnormal vaginal bleeding.
11. Hypersensitivity to any of the components o Femodene ED.

*Warnings:* There is a general opinion, based or statistical evidence, that users of combined ora contraceptives experience, more often than non users, venous thromboembolism, arterial thrombosis including cerebral and myocardial infarction, an subarachnoid haemorrhage. Full recovery from such disorders does not always occur, and it should be realised that in a few cases they are fatal. How ofte these disorders occur in users of the modern low dose pills is not known, but there are reasons fo suggesting that they may occur less often than with older pills.

Certain factors may entail some risk of thrombosis e.g. smoking, obesity, varicose veins, cardiovascula diseases, diabetes, and migraine. The suitability of a combined oral contraceptive should be judged accord ing to the severity of such conditions in the individua case, and should be discussed with the patient befor she decides to take it. The risk of arterial thrombosi associated with combined oral contraceptives in creases with age, and this risk is aggravated by cigarette-smoking. The use of combined oral contra ceptives by women in the older age-group, especiall those who are cigarette smokers, should therefore b discouraged and alternative methods used.

In addition if there is a history in the family o thromboembolic diseases at a young age (e.g. deep vein thrombosis, heart attack or stroke) disturbance of the coagulation system must be ruled out befor the pill is prescribed.

Numerous epidemiological studies have been re ported on the risks of ovarian, endometrial, cervica and breast cancer in women using combined ora contraceptives. The evidence is clear that combine oral contraceptives offer substantial protectio against both ovarian and endometrial cancer.

An increased risk of cervical cancer in long-tern users of combined oral contraceptives has bee reported in some studies, but there continues to b controversy about the extent to which this is attribut able to the confounding effects of sexual behaviou and other factors.

The evidence linking the use of combined ora contraceptives and breast cancer remains inconclu sive. The results of some studies suggest an increase risk of breast cancer presenting below the age o about 35, the risk rising with duration of use. An possible increased risk of breast cancer with combine oral contraceptives is however likely to be small, an may be expected to be less with low-dosage pills. Thi possible risk should be weighed against the man benefits of combined oral contraceptives, includin their protective effects against ovarian and endo metrial cancers.

The possibility cannot be ruled out that certai chronic diseases may occasionally deteriorate during the use of combined oral contraceptives (see '*Precau tions*').

The combination of ethinyloestradiol and gesto dene, like other contraceptive steroids, is associate with an increased incidence of neoplastic nodules i the rat liver, the relevance of which to man is unknown Malignant liver tumours have been reported on rar occasions in long-term users of oral contraceptives.

In rare cases benign and, in even rarer cases malignant liver tumours leading in isolated cases t life-threatening intra-abdominal haemorrhage hav been observed after the use of hormonal substance such as those contained in Femodene ED. If sever upper abdominal complaints, liver enlargement o signs of intra-abdominal haemorrhage occur, th possibility of a liver tumour should be included in th differential diagnosis.

*Reasons for stopping oral contraception immediatel*

1. Occurrence for the first time, or exacerbation, o migrainous headaches or unusually frequent or unu sually severe headaches.
2. Sudden disturbances of vision or hearing or othe perceptual disorders.
3. First signs of thrombophlebitis or thromboem bolic symptoms (e.g. unusual pains in or swelling o the leg(s), stabbing pains on breathing or coughin for no apparent reason). Feeling of pain and tightnes in the chest.
4. Six weeks before an elective major operation (e.g abdominal, orthopaedic), any surgery to the legs medical treatment for varicose veins or prolonge immobilisation, e.g. after accidents or surgery. Do no restart until 2 weeks after full ambulation. In case o

emergency surgery, thrombotic prophylaxis is usually indicated e.g. subcutaneous heparin.

5. Onset of jaundice, hepatitis, itching of the whole body.

6. Increase in epileptic seizures.

7. Significant rise in blood pressure.

8. Onset of severe depression.

9. Severe upper abdominal pain or liver enlargement.

10. Clear exacerbation of conditions known to be capable of deteriorating during oral contraception or pregnancy.

11. Pregnancy is a reason for stopping immediately because it has been suggested by some investigations that oral contraceptives taken in early pregnancy may slightly increase the risk of foetal malformations. Other investigations have failed to support these findings. The possibility therefore cannot be excluded, but it is certain that if a risk exists at all, it is very small.

*Precautions:* Examination of the pelvic organs, breasts and blood-pressure should precede the prescribing of any combined oral contraceptive and should be repeated regularly. The family medical history should be carefully noted and disturbances of the clotting mechanism ruled out if any member of the family has suffered from thromboembolic disease (e.g. deep vein thrombosis, stroke, myocardial infarction) at a young age. Before starting treatment pregnancy must be excluded.

The following conditions require strict medical supervision during medication with oral contraceptives. Deterioration or first appearance of any of these conditions may indicate that use of the oral contraceptive should be discontinued:

Diabetes mellitus, or a tendency towards diabetes mellitus (e.g. unexplained glycosuria), hypertension, varicose veins, a history of phlebitis, otosclerosis, multiple sclerosis, epilepsy, porphyria, tetany, disturbed liver function, Sydenham's chorea, renal dysfunction, family history of clotting disorders, obesity, family history of breast cancer and patient history of benign breast disease, history of clinical depression, systemic lupus erythematosus, uterine fibroids and migraine, gall-stones, cardiovascular diseases, chloasma, asthma, an intolerance of contact lenses, or any disease that is prone to worsen during pregnancy.

Some women may experience amenorrhoea or oligomenorrhoea after discontinuation of oral contraceptives, especially when these conditions existed prior to use. Women should be informed of this possibility.

*Side-effects:* In rare cases, headaches, gastric upsets, nausea, vomiting, breast tenderness, changes in body weight, changes in libido, depressive moods can occur.

In predisposed women, use of Femodene ED can sometimes cause chloasma which is exacerbated by exposure to sunlight. Such women should avoid prolonged exposure to sunlight.

Individual cases of poor tolerance of contact lenses have been reported with use of oral contraceptives. Contact lens wearers who develop changes in lens tolerance should be assessed by an ophthalmologist.

*Menstrual changes:*

*1. Reduction of menstrual flow:* This is not abnormal and it is to be expected in some patients. Indeed, it may be beneficial where heavy periods were previously experienced.

*2. Missed menstruation:* Occasionally, withdrawal bleeding may not occur at all. If the tablets have been taken correctly, pregnancy is very unlikely. If withdrawal bleeding fails to occur at the end of a second pack, the possibility of pregnancy must be ruled out before resuming with the next pack.

*Intermenstrual bleeding:* 'Spotting' or heavier 'breakthrough bleeding' sometimes occur during tablet taking, especially in the first few cycles, and normally cease spontaneously. Femodene ED should therefore, be continued even if irregular bleeding occurs. If irregular bleeding is persistent, appropriate diagnostic measures to exclude an organic cause are indicated and may include curettage. This also applies in the case of spotting which occurs at irregular intervals in several consecutive cycles or which occurs for the first time after long use of Femodene ED.

*Effect on blood chemistry:* The use of oral contraceptives may influence the results of certain laboratory tests including biochemical parameters of liver, thyroid, adrenal and renal function, plasma levels of carrier proteins and lipid/lipoprotein fractions, parameters of carbohydrate metabolism and parameters of coagulation and fibrinolysis. Laboratory staff should therefore be informed about oral contraceptive use when laboratory tests are requested.

*Overdosage:* Overdosage may cause nausea, vomiting and, in females, withdrawal bleeding. There are no specific antidotes and treatment should be symptomatic.

**Pharmaceutical precautions** Shelf-life–Five years.

**Legal category** POM

**Package quantities** Individual packs containing three months' supply (OP)

**Further information** Nil

**Product licence number** 0053/0180

## FLUDARA*

**Qualitative and quantitative composition** Fludarabine phosphate 50 mg per vial (equivalent to 39.05 mg fludarabine per vial). Each vial also contains 50 mg of mannitol and sodium hydroxide which is present to maintain the desired pH.

**Pharmaceutical form** Fludara is supplied as a sterile lyophilised solid cake.

**Clinical particulars**

*Therapeutic indications:* Fludara is indicated for the treatment of patients with B-cell chronic lymphocytic leukaemia (CLL) who have not responded to or whose disease has progressed during or after treatment with at least one standard alkylating-agent containing regimen.

*Posology and method of administration:* Fludara should be administered under the supervision of a qualified physician experienced in the use of antineoplastic therapy.

It is strongly recommended that Fludara should be only administered intravenously. No cases have been reported in which paravenously administered Fludara led to severe local adverse reactions. However, the unintentional paravenous administration must be avoided.

*Adults:* The recommended dose is 25 mg fludarabine phosphate/m² body surface given daily for 5 consecutive days in every 28 days by the intravenous route. Each vial is to be made up in 2 ml water for injection. Each ml of the resulting solution will contain 25 mg fludarabine phosphate.

The required dose (calculated on the basis of the patient's body surface) is drawn up into a syringe. For intravenous bolus injection this dose is further diluted into 10 ml of 0.9 % sodium chloride. Alternatively, the required dose drawn up in a syringe may be diluted into 100 ml 0.9 % sodium chloride and infused over approximately 30 minutes.

The optimal duration of treatment has not been clearly established. It is recommended that Fludara be administered up to the achievement of a maximal response (usually 6 cycles) and then the drug should be discontinued.

*Children:* The safety and effectiveness of Fludara in children has not been established.

*Contra-indications:* Fludara is contra-indicated in those patients who are hypersensitive to this drug or its components and in renally impaired patients with creatinine clearance < 30 ml/min.

Fludara is contra-indicated during pregnancy and lactation.

*Special warnings and special precautions for use:* When used at high doses in dose-ranging studies in patients with acute leukaemia, Fludara was associated with severe neurologic effects, including blindness, coma and death. This severe central nervous system toxicity occurred in 36 % of patients treated with doses approximately four times greater (96 mg/m²/day for 5–7 days) than the dose recommended for treatment of CLL. Similar severe central nervous system toxicity has been rarely (< 0.2 %) reported in patients treated at doses in the range of the dose recommended for CLL. Patients should be closely observed for signs of neurologic side effects.

The effect of chronic administration of Fludara on the central nervous system is unknown. However, patients have received the recommended dose for up to 15 courses of therapy.

Severe bone marrow suppression, notably anaemia, thrombocytopenia and neutropenia, has been reported in patients treated with Fludara. In a Phase I study in solid tumour patients, the median time to nadir counts was 13 days (range, 3–25 days) for granulocytes and 16 days (range, 2–32) for platelets. Most patients had haematologic impairment at baseline either as a result of disease or as a result of prior myelosuppressive therapy. Cumulative myelosuppression may be seen. While chemotherapy-induced myelosuppression is often reversible, administration of fludarabine phosphate requires careful haematologic monitoring.

Fludara is a potent antineoplastic agent with potentially significant toxic side effects. Patients undergoing therapy should be closely observed for signs of haematologic and non-haematologic toxicity. Periodic assessment of peripheral blood counts is recommended to detect the development of anaemia, neutropenia and thrombocytopenia.

Transfusion-associated graft-versus-host disease has been observed rarely (approx. 0.18%) after transfusion of non-irradiated blood in Fludara treated patients. Fatal outcome as a consequence of this disease has been reported with a high frequency. Therefore, patients who require blood transfusion and who are undergoing, or who have received, treatment with Fludara should receive irradiated blood only.

Tumour lysis syndrome associated with Fludara treatment has been reported in CLL patients with large tumour burdens. Since Fludara can induce a response as early as the first week of treatment, precautions should be taken in those patients at risk of developing this complication.

Instances of life-threatening and sometimes fatal autoimmune haemolytic anaemia have been reported to occur during or after treatment with Fludara irrespective of any previous history of autoimmune haemolytic anaemia or Coombs test status. The majority of patients rechallenged with Fludara developed a recurrence in the haemolytic process.

Patients undergoing treatment with Fludara should be closely monitored for signs of autoimmune haemolytic anaemia (decline in haemoglobin linked with haemolysis and positive Coombs test). Discontinuation of therapy with Fludara is recommended in case of haemolysis. Blood transfusion and adrenocorticoid preparations are the most common treatment measures for autoimmune haemolytic anaemia.

The total body clearance of 2-fluoro-ara-A shows a correlation with creatinine clearance, indicating the importance of the renal excretion pathway for the elimination of the compound. So far no clinical data are available in patients with impairment of renal function (creatinine clearance below 70 ml/min). Therefore, if renal impairment is clinically suspected, or in patients over the age of 70 years, creatinine clearance should be measured. If creatinine clearance is between 30 and 70 ml/min, the dose should be reduced by up to 50% and close haematological monitoring should be used to assess toxicity. Fludara treatment is contraindicated, if creatinine clearance is < 30 ml/min.

Since there are limited data for the use of Fludara in elderly persons (> 75 years), caution should be exercised with the administration of Fludara in these patients.

Females of child-bearing potential or males must take contraceptive measures during and at least for 6 months after cessation of therapy.

During and after treatment with Fludara vaccination with live vaccines should be avoided.

*Interaction with other medicaments and other forms of interaction:* In a clinical investigation using Fludara in combination with pentostatin (deoxycoformycin) for the treatment of refractory chronic lymphocytic leukaemia (CLL), there was an unacceptably high incidence of fatal pulmonary toxicity. Therefore, the use of Fludara in combination with pentostatin is not recommended.

The therapeutic efficacy of Fludara may be reduced by dipyridamole and other inhibitors of adenosine uptake.

*Pregnancy and lactation:* There is no experience with the use of Fludara during pregnancy.

Embryotoxicity studies in animals demonstrated an embryotoxic and/or teratogenic potential posing a relevant risk to humans at the envisaged therapeutic dose.

Fludara should not be used during pregnancy.

Women of child-bearing potential should be advised to avoid becoming pregnant and to inform the treating physician immediately should this occur.

*Use during lactation:* It is not known whether this drug is excreted in human milk. Breast-feeding should be discontinued for the duration of Fludara therapy.

*Effects on ability to drive and use machines:* The effect of treatment with Fludara on the patient's ability to drive or operate machinery has not been evaluated.

*Undesirable effects:* The most common adverse events include myelosuppression (neutropenia, thrombocytopenia and anaemia), fever, chills and infection. Other commonly reported events include malaise, fatigue, anorexia, nausea, vomiting and weakness. Serious opportunistic infections have occurred in CLL patients treated with Fludara. Fatalities as a consequence of serious adverse events have been reported.

The most frequently reported adverse events and those reactions which are more clearly related to the drug are arranged below according to body system.

*Haematopoietic system:* Haematologic events (neutropenia, thrombocytopenia, and anaemia) have been reported in the majority of CLL patients treated with Fludara. Myelosuppression may be severe and cumulative.

Clinically significant haemolytic anaemia has been rarely reported in patients receiving Fludara (see *Special warnings and special precautions for use*).

*Metabolic:* Tumour lysis syndrome has been reported in CLL patients treated with Fludara. This complication may include hyperuricaemia, hyperphosphataemia, hypocalcaemia, metabolic acidosis, hyperkalaemia, haematuria, urate crystalluria, and renal failure. The onset of this syndrome may be heralded by flank pain and haematuria.

Changes of hepatic and pancreatic enzymes are possible.

*Nervous system:* In rare cases, weakness, agitation, confusion, visual disturbances occurred in CLL patients. Peripheral neuropathy and coma have been observed.

*Pulmonary system:* Pneumonia has occurred in association with Fludara treatment. Pulmonary hypersensitivity reactions to Fludara characterised by dyspnoea, cough and interstitial pulmonary infiltrate have been observed.

*Gastrointestinal system:* Gastrointestinal disturbances such as nausea and vomiting, anorexia, diarrhoea, stomatitis and gastrointestinal bleeding have been reported in patients treated with Fludara.

*Cardiovascular:* Oedema has been reported frequently.

*Genitourinary system:* Rare cases of haemorrhagic cystitis have been reported in patients treated with Fludara.

*Skin:* Skin rashes have been reported in patients treated with Fludara.

In extremely rare cases a toxic epidermal necrolysis (Lyell's disease) may develop.

*Overdose:* High doses of Fludara have been associated with an irreversible central nervous system toxicity characterised by delayed blindness, coma, and death. High doses are also associated with severe thrombocytopenia and neutropenia due to bone marrow suppression. There is no known specific antidote for Fludara overdosage. Treatment consists of drug discontinuation and supportive therapy.

**Pharmacological properties**

*Pharmacodynamic properties:* Fludara contains fludarabine phosphate, a fluorinated nucleotide analogue of the antiviral agent vidarabine, 9-β-D-arabinofuranosyladenine (ara-A) that is relatively resistant to deamination by adenosine deaminase.

Fludarabine phosphate is rapidly dephosphorylated to 2-fluoro-ara-A which is taken up by cells and then phosphorylated intracellularly by deoxycytidine kinase to the active triphosphate, 2-fluoro-ara-ATP. This metabolite has been shown to inhibit ribonucleotide reductase, DNA polymerase α/δ and ε, DNA primase and DNA ligase thereby inhibiting DNA synthesis. Furthermore, partial inhibition of RNA polymerase II and consequent reduction in protein synthesis occurs.

While some aspects of the mechanism of action of 2-fluoro-ara-ATP are as yet unclear, it is assumed that effects on DNA, RNA and protein synthesis all contribute to inhibition of cell growth with inhibition of DNA synthesis being the dominant factor.

*Pharmacokinetic properties:* Plasma and urinary pharmacokinetics of fludarabine (2F-ara-A):

The pharmacokinetics of fludarabine have been studied after intravenous administration by rapid bolus injection and short-term infusion as well as following continuous infusion of fludarabine phosphate (Fludara, 2F-ara-AMP). 2F-ara-AMP is a water-soluble prodrug of fludarabine, which is rapidly and quantitatively dephosphorylated to the nucleoside 2F-ara-A. After infusion of 25 mg 2F-ara-AMP per m² to CLL patients for 30 minutes 2F-ara-A reached peak concentrations in the plasma of 3.5 +/- 1.2 nmol/ml immediately after the end of the infusion. Postmaximum levels decayed in three disposition phases with an initial half-life of approx. 5 minutes, an intermediate half-life of 1 - 2 hours and a terminal half-life in the range between 10 and approximately 30 hours. Terminal half-lives tended to be longer when a more sensitive analytical method (precolumn derivatization, HPLC and fluorescence detection) was used allowing plasma level determinations up to 72 hours.

The total plasma clearance CL and the distribution volume $V_D$ showed a considerable variance between patients and studies with CL values between 70 and 160 ml/min/m² and distribution volumes between approx. 62 l/m² ($V_{D\gamma}$) and approx. 150 l/m² ($V_{DSS}$). Plasma levels of 2Fara-A and areas under the plasma level time curves increased linearly with the dose, half-lives, plasma clearance and volumes of distribution were independent of the dose indicating a dose linear behaviour.

2F-ara-A elimination is largely by renal excretion. Approximately 60 % of a bolus injection was excreted in the urine within 24 hours. Mass balance studies in laboratory animals with ³H-2F-ara-AMP showed a complete recovery of radio-labelled substances in the urine. Another metabolite, 2F-ara-hypoxanthine, which represents the major metabolite in the dog, was not observed in humans. Individuals with impaired renal function exhibit a reduced total body clearance, indicating the need for a dose reduction.

Cellular pharmacokinetics of fludarabine triphosphate:

2F-ara-A is actively transported into leukaemic cells, whereupon it is rephosphorylated to the monophosphate and subsequently to the di- and triphosphate. The triphosphate 2F-ara-ATP is the major intracellular metabolite of fludarabine and the only metabolite known to have cytotoxic activity. Maximum 2F-ara-ATP levels in leukaemic lymphocytes of CLL patients were observed at a median of 4 hours and exhibited a considerable variation with a median peak concentration of approx. 20 μM. 2F-ara-ATP levels in leukaemic cells were always considerably higher than maximum 2F-ara-A levels in the plasma indicating an accumulation at the target sites. 2F-ara-ATP elimination from CLL target cells likewise showed a considerable scattering with a median half-life of approx. 23 hours.

*Preclinical safety data:* In acute toxicity studies, single intravenous doses of fludarabine phosphate produced severe intoxication symptoms or death at dosages about two orders of magnitude above the therapeutic dose. As expected for a cytotoxic compound, the bone marrow, lymphoid organs, gastrointestinal mucosa, kidneys and male gonads were affected. In patients, severe side effects were observed closer to the recommended therapeutic dose (factor 3 to 4) and included severe neurotoxicity partly with lethal outcome (cf. *Overdose*).

Systemic toxicity studies following repeated administration of fludarabine phosphate showed also the expected effects on rapidly proliferating tissues above a threshold dose. The severity of morphological manifestations increased with dose levels and duration of dosing and the observed changes were generally considered to be reversible. In principle, the available experience from the therapeutic use of Fludara points to a comparable toxicological profile in humans, although additional undesirable effects such as neurotoxicity were observed in patients (cf. *Undesirable effects*).

The results from animal embryotoxicity studies indicated a teratogenic potential of fludarabine phosphate. In view of the small safety margin between the teratogenic doses in animals and the human therapeutic dose as well as in analogy to other antimetabolites which are assumed to interfere with the process of differentiation, the therapeutic use of Fludara is associated with a relevant risk of teratogenic effects in humans (cf. *Pregnancy and lactation*).

Fludarabine phosphate has been shown to induce chromosomal aberrations in an in vitro cytogenetic assay, to cause DNA-damage in a sister chromatid exchange test and to increase the rate of micronuclei in the mouse micronucleus test in vivo, but was negative in gene mutation assays. In view of these results, the known activity of the compound at the DNA-level and in analogy to other antimetabolites, fludarabine phosphate is expected to have a mutagenic potential.

The known activity of fludarabine at the DNA-level and the mutagenicity test results form the basis for the suspicion of a tumorigenic potential. No animal studies which directly address the question of tumorigenicity have been conducted, because the suspicion of an increased risk of second tumours due to Fludara therapy can exclusively be verified by epidemiological data.

According to the results from animal experiments following intravenous administration of fludarabine phosphate, no remarkable local irritation has to be expected at the injection site .Even in case of misplaced injections, no relevant local irritation was observed after paravenous, intraarterial, and intramuscular administration of an aqueous solution containing 7.5 mg fludarabine phosphate/ml.

***Pharmaceutical particulars***

*List of excipients:* Each vial of Fludara contains 50 mg of mannitol. Sodium hydroxide is present to adjust the pH to 7.7.

*Incompatibilities:* None known

*Shelf life:* The shelf life of Fludara stored as a lyophilised solid cake in glass vials is 24 months at up to 30 °C. Reconstituted Fludara should be used within 8 hours of reconstitution. Fludara contains no antimicrobial preservative. Care must be taken to assure the sterility of prepared solutions.

*Special precautions for storage:* Store at room temperature (maximum 30 °C).

*Nature and contents of container:* Fludara is supplied in clear glass single dose vials of 6 ml capacity.

*Instructions for use/handling:* Fludara should be prepared for parenteral use by aseptically adding sterile water for injection. When reconstituted with 2 ml of sterile water for injection, the solid cake should fully dissolve in 15 seconds or less. Each ml of the resulting solution will contain 25 mg of fludarabine phosphate, 25 mg of mannitol, and sodium hydroxide to adjust the pH to 7.7. The pH range for the final product is 7.2–8.2. In clinical studies, the product has been diluted in 100 ml or 125 ml of 5 % dextrose injection or 0.9 % sodium chloride.

*Handling and disposal:* Fludara should not be handled by pregnant staff.

Procedures for proper handling and disposal should be observed. Consideration should be given to handling and disposal according to guidelines used for cytotoxic drugs. Any spillage or waste material may be disposed of by incineration.

Caution should be exercised in the handling and preparation of the Fludara solution. The use of latex gloves and safety glasses is recommended to avoid exposure in case of breakage of the vial or other accidental spillage. If the solution comes into contact with the skin or mucous membranes, the area should be washed thoroughly with soap and water. In the event of contact with the eyes, rinse them thoroughly with copious amounts of water. Exposure by inhalation should be avoided.

**Marketing authorisation number** PL 0053/0239

**Date of approval/revision of SPC** 3 September 1996

**Legal category** POM

## GASTROGRAFIN*

**Presentation** 1 ml Gastrografin contains 100 mg sodium amidotrizoate (sodium diatrizoate) and 660 mg meglumine amidotrizoate (meglumine diatrizoate) in aqueous solution, with added flavouring and wetting agents. The iodine content is 370 mg/ml.

*Excipients:* disodium edetate, saccharin sodium, anise oil, polysorbate 80, water for injection.

**Uses** Gastrografin is designed for investigation of the gastrointestinal tract. It can be used either orally or as an enema. Follow-through examinations with barium can often be improved by combining it with Gastrografin. Gastrografin may be of particular value in the following instances:

1. Suspected partial or complete stenosis.
2. Acute haemorrhage.
3. Threatening perforation (peptic ulcer, diverticulum).
4. Other acute conditions which are likely to require surgery.
5. After resection of the stomach or intestine (danger of perforation or leak).
6 Megacolon.
7. Visualisation of a foreign body or tumour before endoscopy.
8. Visualisation of a gastrointestinal fistula.
9. Before endoscopy.

*Further indications:* Early diagnosis of a radiologically undetectable perforation or anastomotic defect in the oesophagus.

The treatment of uncomplicated meconium ileus Computerised tomography in the abdominal region.

**Dosage and administration** *Oral–Adults and children of 10 years of age or over:* 60 ml Gastrografin are sufficient for the visualisation of the stomach. Up to 100 ml may be needed for a follow-through examination of the gastrointestinal tract.

For computed tomography, 1 to 1.5 litres of a 3% solution of Gastrografin in water (30 ml/litre).

*For elderly or cachetic patients:* Dilution with an equal volume of water is recommended.

*Children up to 10 years of age:* 15-30 ml are usually sufficient. This dose may be diluted with twice its volume of water.

*For infants and young children:* Dilution of 15-30 ml of the contrast medium with three times its volume of water is recommended.

*Rectal–Adults:* The contrast medium should be diluted with three to four times its volume of water. Not more than 500 ml of Gastrografin solution should normally be required.

*Children:* The contrast medium should be diluted with four to five times its volume of water; up to five years of age the weaker dilution should be used.

*Gastrografin and Barium Sulphate:* Oral and rectal administration.

*Adults:* 30 ml Gastrografin plus the usual dose of barium should be adequate.

*Children:* 10 ml Gastrografin may be added to the barium.

*For children up to five years of age:* from 2-5 ml Gastrografin to 100 ml barium may be preferable.

Further dilution which does not affect the contrast may be used if necessary in cases of pylorospasm or pyloric stenosis.

For the early diagnosis of a perforation or investigation of an anastomosis in the oesophagus or gastrointestinal tract, the patient should drink 100 ml Gastrografin. After 30-60 minutes (later, if the defect is suspected of being in the distal gut), a urine specimen should be taken and 5 ml mixed with 5 drops of concentrated hydrochloric acid. The contrast medium which has undergone renal excretion will appear within two hours as a typical crystal formation in the precipitate.

*Technique for the treatment of uncomplicated meconium ileus:* Gastrografin can be given by enema to infants for non-operative treatment of uncomplicated meconium ileus, in the absence of e.g. volvulus, gangrene, perforation, peritonitis or atresia, all of which require immediate operation.

A large syringe and soft rubber catheter, No. 8 French, are recommended. The buttocks can be taped tightly together to minimise leakage but a balloon catheter should not be used. The procedure must be carried out slowly and only under fluoroscopic control. Injection should stop as soon as Gastrografin is seen to enter the ileum. Owing to its high osmolarity, Gastrografin may cause the loss of a large amount of fluid into the intestines. An intravenous drip must therefore be set up before the enema is given and plasma should be infused as required. If the Gastrografin is not expelled during the first hour after removal of the rectal catheter, an X-ray should be taken to ensure that overdistension of the bowel as a result of the high osmolarity of Gastrografin has not occurred.

### Contra-indications, warnings etc
*Contra-indications:*Hypersensitivity to iodine-containing contrast media. Manifest hyperthyroidism.

*Warnings/side-effects:*The need for examination merits particularly careful consideration in the case of latent hyperthyroidism, benign nodular goitre, in dehydrated patients and in babies and young children. Disturbances in water or electrolyte balance must first be corrected.

Because of its high osmolality and minimal absorption, Gastrografin should not be administered to infants in higher doses than those recommended above.

Caution should be observed in patients with thyroid disease. Aspiration of Gastrografin into the lungs may cause pulmonary oedema. Caution is needed with oesophagotracheal fistulae to avoid passage of the medium into the lungs. Systemic effects are rare, since Gastrografin is only minimally absorbed from the alimentary tract.

Nausea and vomiting occur in exceptional cases. Urticarial skin reactions have occasionally been observed, while anaphylactoid reactions and shock are possible.

Owing to its hypertonicity, Gastrografin may occasionally cause diarrhoea, but this ceases as soon as the intestine has been emptied.

Existing enteritis or colitis may be temporarily exacerbated.

Because of the additives (flavourings and a wetting agent), Gastrografin must not be used intravascularly.

If iodine isotopes are to be administered for diagnosing thyroid disease, it should be borne in mind that after the administration of iodised contrast media which are excreted via the kidneys, the capacity of the thyroid tissue to take up iodine will be reduced for 2 weeks and sometimes up to 6 weeks.

Hypersensitivity reactions can be aggravated in patients on beta-blockers.

The prevalence of delayed reactions (e.g. fever, rash, flu-like symptoms, joint pain and pruritus) to contrast media is higher in patients who have received interleukin.

*Use in pregnancy and lactation:* X-ray examinations should, if possible, be avoided during pregnancy. It has not yet been proved beyond question that Gastrografin may be used without hesitation in pregnant patients. Therefore, an examination with a contrast medium during pregnancy should be carried out only if considered absolutely necessary by the physician.

With regard to the use of barium sulphate, attention is drawn to the contra-indications, warnings and possible side-effects relevant to this preparation.

*Overdose:* There are no specific antidotes to Gastrografin. Treatment should be symptomatic.

**Pharmaceutical precautions** *Storage:* Protect from light and X-rays. Store below 25°C. *Shelf-life:* Three years. At temperatures below 7°C Gastrografin tends to crystallize, but this can be reversed by gently warming and shaking the bottle. This phenomenon has no effect on the effectiveness or stability of the preparation.

**Legal category** P

**Package quantities** Bottles 5 x 100 ml

**Further information** Nil

**Product licence number** 0053/5023R

## ISOVIST*

**Presentation** Bottles containing colourless sterile aqueous solutions of various strengths of the non-ionic dimeric contrast medium, iotrolan. Isovist 240 contains 240 mg iodine per ml; Isovist 300 contains 300 mg iodine per ml.

*Excipients:* Isovist 240: calcium disodium edetate, sodium bicarbonate, sodium chloride, water for injection.

Isovist 300: calcium disodium edetate, sodium chloride, sodium bicarbonate, water for injection.

**Uses** Isovist is intended for intrathecal use, i.e. radiculography and myelography of all regions, for ventriculography, evaluation of the circulation of cerebrospinal fluid and cisternography by computed tomography, and for use in other body cavities.

### Dosage and administration
*General information:* The patient should attend for myelographic examination fasting but adequately hydrated. Disorders of water and electrolyte balance must be corrected, particularly in patients prone to this type of disorder.

Nervous patients may be given a suitable sedative (e.g. diazepam) prophylactically. No local anaesthesia is required if thin puncture needles are used. If antiemetics are administered, they should not possess neuroleptic properties.

After myelographic investigations–particularly of higher regions–the patient should be confined to bed with head raised for at least 6 hours, and remain passive for 24 hours.

Patients with a known or suspected low seizure threshold must be kept under careful observation for eight hours.

Isovist should not be drawn up into the syringe until immediately before use. Contrast medium not used in one examination must be discarded.

*Dosage:* The concentration and volume of Isovist chosen depend on the radiological equipment available. If equipment is available that allows films to be taken in all necessary projections without the patient having to move, and with which the injection can be performed under fluoroscopic control, iodine concentrations and volumes of medium at the lower end of the specified range can be used.

Higher concentrations are indicated if it will be necessary to reposition the patient during a myelographic examination, since the medium becomes diluted more quickly as a result of turbulence, and the clarity of detail deteriorates.

*Radiculography* (excluding the medullary cone)–7-10 ml Isovist 240.

*Lumbar myelography* (with thoracic transition)–7-12 ml Isovist 240/300.

*Thoracic myelography*–10–15 ml Isovist 240. 8–12 ml Isovist 300.

*Panmyelography* (injection in the lumbar region)–10–15 ml Isovist 240/300.

*Cervical myelography*–Direct (lateral access between $C_1/C_2$). 8–12 ml Isovist 240. 7–10 ml Isovist 300. *Indirect* (injection in the lumbar region). 15 ml Isovist 240. 8–15 ml Isovist 300.

*Ventriculography*–3–5 ml Isovist 240. 3–5 ml Isovist 300.

*CT-cisternography* (injection in the lumbar region) –4–12 ml Isovist 240, 4-10 ml Isovist 300

Administration of the contrast medium in myelography: After withdrawal of the volume of cerebrospinal fluid (CSF) needed for examination, the appropriate dose of Isovist is injected. N.B. The more the patient moves after the administration of Isovist, the quicker will the medium mix with the CSF and the density of contrast decrease.

*Other body cavities*

Indirect lymphography (e.g. lymphoedema)–5–20 ml Isovist 300.

Arthrography 2–15 ml Isovist 240/300

Hysterosalpingography–10–25 ml Isovist 240/300.

Mammary ducts–1–3 ml Isovist 240/300.

Endoscopic retrograde cholangiopancreatography–10–30 ml Isovist 240/300.

Oesophagus–stomach–bowel–10–100ml Isovist 300.

In the administration of contrast medium for indirect lymphography, multiple simultaneous interstitial (e.g. intracutaneous) injections are to be preferred.

### Contra-indications, warnings etc
*Contra-indications:* Uncontrolled thyrotoxicosis.

Hysterosalpingography must not be carried out during pregnancy or in the presence of acute inflammatory conditions in the pelvic cavity.

*Use in pregnancy:* X-ray examinations should, if possible, be avoided during pregnancy. It has not yet been proved beyond question that Isovist may be used without hesitation in pregnant patients. Therefore, examination with Isovist during pregnancy should be carried out only if considered essential.

*Warnings/side-effects:* Epilepsy is a relative contra-indication for myelography. If, after careful consideration, myelography is considered necessary, equipment and drugs necessary to treat any convulsion that may occur must be readily available. Neuroleptics or antidepressants should be discontinued 48 hours before the examination, because they lower the seizure threshold. Alcoholics and drug addicts may have a lowered seizure threshold. Anticonvulsants (e.g. phenobarbitone 200 mg i.m.) may be given prophylactically.

Hypersensitivity reactions can be aggravated in patients on beta-blockers. The prevalence of delayed reactions to contrast media is higher in patients who have received interleukin.

Hyperthyroidism may be exacerbated. Iodinated contrast media reduce the capacity of the thyroid gland to take up radio-isotopes of iodine for up to 2 weeks, and sometimes longer. Patients with a history of allergy may be particularly susceptible to hypersensitivity reactions. Such reactions are possible in any patient, but are rare in the recommended indications.

The most frequently reported symptoms are headache, nausea and vomiting. However, experience shows that their incidence is no higher than after the loss of pressure in the subarachnoid space that results from a diagnostic tap of CSF from the spinal canal. In view of this, an effort should be made to remove only as much CSF as is being replaced by the Isovist solution. On the other hand, administration of an amount of Isovist greater than the amount of CSF removed does not lead to an increase in CSF pressure.

Severe side-effects are extremely rare when Isovist is administered in the recommended dosages. Minor side-effects include pain or an increase in existing pain in the back, nape or extremities, and, rarely, very brief non-specific EEG changes. Delayed reactions can occasionally occur. Slight muscular tension or paraesthesia has been reported in rare cases 2-6 hours after administration of the medium.

Severe headaches lasting several days occur rarely. If convulsions occur, give 10 mg diazepam immediately by slow i.v. injection, followed, 20-30 minutes after the subsidence of the convulsions, by 200 mg phenobarbitone i.m. to prevent recurrence, unless this has been given prophylactically. Diazepam should be injected i.v. as a precaution at the first signs of hyperactivity or muscular twitching.

As with other myelographic agents, the CSF cell-count increases somewhat after intrathecal injection of Isovist. Very rarely, headaches, nausea, vomiting, stiffness of the neck and an increased cell-count in the CSF may mimic aseptic meningitis. All symptoms have usually disappeared within a week. Arachnoiditis has not been reported.

Isovist is excreted renally. Therefore, for patients with severe impairment of renal function, proven or suspected hypersensitivity to iodine-containing contrast media, latent hyperthyroidism and benign nodular goitre, the need for examination with Isovist merits careful consideration.

Ready availability of all drugs and equipment for emergency treatment and familiarity with the relevant procedures are prerequisites for the effective management of contrast-medium incidents.

*Overdosage:* Acute symptoms of poisoning are unlikely with intrathecal administration. Treatment is symptomatic.

**Pharmaceutical precautions** Protect from light and secondary X-rays. Store below 30°C. Shelf-life–Five years.

Because of possible precipitation, X-ray contrast media and prophylactic agents must not be injected as mixed solutions.

**Legal category** POM

**Package quantities** Isovist 240: Box containing 10 bottles of 10 ml. Box containing 10 bottles of 20 ml. Isovist 300: Box containing 10 bottles of 10 ml.

**Further information** Isovist is a series of non-ionic, dimeric, water-soluble contrast media with osmolalities close to those of normal body fluids. Isovist 240–270 mosm/kg $H_2O$ at 37°C. Isovist 300–320 mosm/kg $H_2O$ at 37°C.

**Product licence numbers**
Isovist 240 0053/0201
Isovist 300 0053/0202

## LEVOVIST*

**Qualitative and quantitative composition** 1 g granules contains 999 mg galactose and 1 mg palmitic acid.

*Physico–chemical properties*
Max. osmolality at 37˚C

| | | |
|---|---|---|
| solution | 200 mg/ml | 1175 mosmol/kg |
| | 300 mg/ml | 1965 mosmol/kg |
| | 400 mg/ml | 2894 mosmol/kg |

"Effective" osmolality
at 25˚C

| | | |
|---|---|---|
| filtrate | 200 mg/ml | 910 mosmol/kg |
| | 300 mg/ml | 980 mosmol/kg |
| | 400 mg/ml | 950 mosmol/kg |

Viscosity at 25˚C

| | | |
|---|---|---|
| filtrate | 200 mg/ml | 1.4 mPa.s |
| | 300 mg/ml | 1.4 mPa.s |
| | 400 mg/ml | 1.4 mPa.s |
| suspension | 200 mg/ml | 1.4 mPa.s |
| | 300 mg/ml | 3.6 mPa.s |
| | 400 mg/ml | 8.0 mPa.s |

**Pharmaceutical form** Sterile granulated powder for injection. For peripheral intravenous administration, after reconstitution with the diluent provided (water for injection) to obtain concentrations of 200, 300 and 400 mg microparticles per ml suspension.

## Clinical particulars

*Therapeutic indications:* One– and two–dimensional Doppler sonographic blood flow imaging in patients, where there is insufficient Doppler signal intensity. B–mode contrast echocardiography.

*Posology and method of administration:* The suspension has to be prepared according to instructions immediately before administration.

The following dosages are recommended:

*Adults:*

ONE– AND TWO–DIMENSIONAL DOPPLER SONOGRAPHY

*Vascular Doppler sonography:* In the case of moderately well detectable but diagnostically unsatisfactory Doppler signals, 10 – 16 ml of the concentration 200 mg/ml.

In the case of weak Doppler signals, e.g. in the presence of small vessels, low blood flow or unfavourable scanning conditions, 5 – 10 ml of the concentration 300 mg/ml.

In the case of very weak or absent Doppler signals, 5 – 8 ml of the concentration 400 mg/ml.

The intravenous injection should be done continuously (approx. 1 – 2 ml/sec.) in order to have homogeneous enhancement effects in the Doppler recording.

A repeat injection of Levovist may be necessary in special cases, e.g. in order to examine several sectional planes. The dose may be increased – particularly by choosing a higher concentration – in order to achieve a stronger effect or longer duration of enhancement. The duration of the increased signal strength is usually 2 – 4 minutes.

Recommended maximum dose: 6 injections of the single dose.

*Doppler echocardiography of the right and left heart chambers:* 10 – 16 ml of the concentration 200 mg/ml

In patients with very weak or non–detectable Doppler signals and for the clarification of mitral insufficiency: 5 – 10 ml of the concentration 300 mg/ml

Examination only of the right heart chambers: 4 – 10 ml of the concentration 200 mg/ml

The intravenous injection should be done continuously (approx. 1 – 2 ml/sec.) in order to have homogeneous enhancement effects in the Doppler recording.

A repeat injection of Levovist may be necessary in special cases, e.g. in order to examine several sectional planes. The dose may be increased – particularly by choosing a higher concentration – in order to achieve a stronger effect or longer duration of enhancement. The duration of the increased signal strength is usually 1 – 2 minutes.

Recommended maximum dose: 6 injections of the single dose.

B–MODE CONTRAST ECHOCARDIOGRAPHY: 10 ml of the concentration 300 mg/ml

In cases of unfavourable sound conduction conditions and for stress echocardiography: 5 – 8 ml of the concentration 400 mg/ml

Examination only of the right heart chambers: 4 – 10 ml of the concentration 300 mg/ml

The intravenous injection should be given as bolus. If desired (e.g. for quantitative evaluations), the reproducibility of the quantitatively measurable contrast effects can be improved by an immediately following injection of 5 to 10 ml of physiological saline to ensure that the total dose of contrast medium is applied. In order to be able to add the injection of saline solution without delay, the use of a 3–way connector is recommended.

Recommended maximum dose: 6 injections of the single dose

*Contra–indications:* Galactosaemia. Use in patients with known or suspected right–to–left shunts.

Use in children is not recommended. There is no experience in patients under 15 years old.

*Special warnings and special precautions for use:* In patients with severe cardiac insufficiency (e.g. NYHA stage IV), the potential risk of the osmotic load caused by the Levovist injections must be considered carefully before administering.

*Interaction with other medicaments and other forms of interaction:* None known.

*Pregnancy and lactation:* No medical objections exist to the peripheral intravenous administration of Levovist as far as the substances contained are concerned. However, no experience is available with the use of Levovist in pregnancy and lactation.

*Effects on ability to drive and use machines:* Not applicable.

*Undesirable effects:* Occasionally, transient pain and a sensation of warmth and cold may occur in the area of the injection site during or shortly after the injection.

Sensations of taste, dyspnoea, changes of blood pressure or pulse, nausea and vomiting as well as headache, dizziness and cutaneous manifestations have been reported in individual cases.

Transient, non–specific irritation of the vascular endothelium may occur due to the hyperosmolality of Levovist.

Pain and tissue irritation may occur following accidental paravascular injection.

*Overdose:* Overdosage is unlikely. Theoretically, the hyperosmolality of the suspension may cause hypervolaemia which would need to be treated by intravenous administration of diuretics (e.g. frusemide) in accordance with symptoms and signs.

Diuresis induced by the osmotic load may affect the serum electrolytes and intravascular volume. These would need to be monitored and controlled as appropriate. Resultant dehydration and possible potassium loss should be treated by oral rehydration or infusion with intravenous fluid and electrolyte replacement.

## Pharmacological properties

*Pharmacodynamic properties:* Levovist is a contrast medium which, after injection into a peripheral vein, leads temporarily to enhanced ultrasound echoes from the heart chambers and blood vessels.

This distinct amplification of the ultrasound echo is caused primarily by micrometre–sized air bubbles, which arise after suspension of the granules in water. Mediated by the palmitic acid additive, they remain stable for several minutes while in transit through the heart and lungs as well as in the subsequent vascular bed before dissolving in the blood stream.

*Pharmacokinetic properties:* The pharmacokinetic investigation of Levovist was performed with the concentration 400 mg/ml and the injection volumes 35 and 70 ml.

After i.v. administration of Levovist, the galactose microparticles quickly dissolve in the blood stream. The galactose becomes distributed in the extracellular space first of all and is subjected to glucose metabolism independently of insulin. Galactose is stored mainly in the liver through the formation of galactose–1–phosphate or is broken down after isomerisation to glucose–1–phosphate and metabolism to $CO_2$. Galactose is excreted via the kidneys if the plasma galactose level exceeds 50 mg/100 ml.

The elimination rate is reduced in patients with liver disease, depending on hepatic function, and a correspondingly prolonged elimination half–life should be expected.

Galactose and palmitic acid are physiological substances with rapid metabolism. The plasma half–lives are in the range of 10 – 11 minutes and 1 – 4 minutes, respectively.

*Preclinical safety data:* The results of animal experiments suggest that an acute adverse reaction to Levovist is unlikely.

Systemic tolerance studies following repeated daily intravenous administration as well as following repeated intercardiac (left ventricle) administration did not result in findings which oppose the intravenous administration to humans. Even after high intravenous doses no organ–toxic findings were observed.

Reproduction toxicological studies produced no indications of either a teratogenic or an embryotoxic potential. Nor were there any indications of an influence on the fertility.

Local tolerance studies following single intravenous, intra–arterial, subcutaneous, intraperitoneal, paravenous and intramuscular administration indicated that slight symptoms of local intolerance may occur in case of inadvertent paravenous administration.

Although no long–term animal studies or mutagenicity testing have been undertaken on Levovist it is

not likely that galactose or palmitic acid possess any mutagenic or carcinogenic potential.

Galactose is a normal constituent of the diet and is readily metabolised. Palmitic acid is contained in human serum (76 – 260 µmol/l).

## Pharmaceutical particulars

*List of excipients:* Water for injection.

*Incompatibilities:* Not applicable.

*Shelf life:* 24 months

*Special precautions for storage:* Protect from light. Store below 30˚C.

*Nature and contents of container:*

| | |
|---|---|
| **Granulate** | |
| Injection vial: | glass type 1 |
| Stopper: | chlorinated butyl rubber, grey, fluoropolymer-covered |
| Flanged cup: | polypropylene covered disk |
| Container for water | 20 ml ampoule made of polyethylene |
| **Equipment** | |
| Mini spike: | plastics |
| Syringe disposable: | 20 ml plastic syringe, double scaled |

*Combination pack consisting of*
1 20 ml injection vial containing 4 g granules
1 mini spike
1 20 ml disposable syringe, scaled for 17, 11 and 8 ml
1 plastic ampoule with 20 ml water for injection

*Combination pack consisting of*
1 20 ml injection vial containing 2.5 g granules
1 mini spike
1 20 ml disposable syringe, scaled for 11, 7 and 5 ml
1 plastic ampoule with 20 ml water for injection

*Instructions for use/handling:* Adhere strictly to the following instructions for the preparation of the suspension. Preparation of the ready–for–use Levovist suspension:

Use only the water for injection included in the package.

1. Bend back the tab on the top of the plastic ampoule containing water for injection.
2. Twist to open.
3. Withdraw the appropriate amount of water for injection using the syringe provided.

*Injection vial with 4 g granules*

| Levovist concentration mg micropart./ml | Volume of water required ml | Resulting* total volume ml |
|---|---|---|
| approx 200 | 17 | 19.5 ml |
| approx 300 | 11 | 13.5 ml |
| approx 400 | 8 | 10.5 ml |

*Injection vial with 2.5 g granules*

| Levovist concentration mg micropart./ml | Volume of water required ml | Resulting* total volume ml |
|---|---|---|
| approx 200 | 11 | 12.5 ml |
| approx 300 | 7 | 8.5 ml |
| approx 400 | 5 | 6.5 ml |

*Withdrawable volume: approx. 1– 2 ml less.

Remove the plastic cap from the vial containing the granules without disturbing the flanged metal cap. Pierce the rubber stopper with the enclosed mini spike.

4. Attach the syringe to the Luer–Lok–connection of the Sterifix mini spike (yellow cap) and transfer the water to the vial. The air–bleed duct with the sterile filter (white cap) permits pressure compensation without removal of the white cap.

5. Prepare the suspension by immediately shaking vigorously for 5 – 10 seconds by hand. Do not use shaking devices or an ultrasound bath. Leave the suspension to stand for two minutes before use.

6. Withdraw the ready–for–use, homogeneous milky Levovist suspension through the mini spike into the syringe and administer within 10 minutes of preparation.

Granules and water for injection should be at room temperature before production of the suspension. Warming the suspension up (e.g. by holding the vial enclosed in the hand for a prolonged period) after it has been prepared for injection and excessive low pressure (e.g. on drawing the suspension up) should be avoided. This is necessary to prevent a decrease of the microbubble concentration and the formation of larger air bubbles due to degassing processes.

It is recommended to perform the injection via a flexible indwelling cannula with a sufficient gauge size (e.g. 19 to 20 G). In addition, the use of a Luer Lok–connection is of practical advantage.

As usual, care must be taken to remove any macroscopically visible air bubbles from the suspension before injection.

Should a slight sedimentation of the microparticles occur during standing time, resuspension of the preparation by gently rotating it immediately before injection is recommended.

Any suspension not used at one examination session must be discarded.

**Marketing authorisation numbers**

Levovist: 0053/0257
Water for injection: 0053/0258

**Date of approval/revision of SPC** 17 July 1996

**Legal category** POM

## LOGYNON*

**Presentation** The memo-pack holds six light brown tablets containing 30 micrograms ethinyloestradiol and 50 micrograms levonorgestrel, five white tablets containing 40 micrograms ethinyloestradiol and 75 micrograms levonorgestrel and ten ochre tablets containing 30 micrograms ethinyloestradiol and 125 micrograms levonorgestrel.

All tablets have a lustrous, sugar coating.

Excipients: lactose, maize starch, povidone 25 000, talc, magnesium stearate, sucrose, povidone 700 000, polyethylene glycol 6000, calcium carbonate, montan glycol wax, titanium dioxide, glycerol, ferric oxide pigment (yellow and red).

**Uses** Oral contraception and the recognised gynaecological indications for such oestrogen-progestogen combinations. The mode of action includes the inhibition of ovulation by suppression of the mid-cycle surge of luteinising hormone, the inspissation of cervical mucus so as to constitute a barrier to sperm, and the rendering of the endometrium unreceptive to implantation.

**Dosage and administration** *First treatment cycle:* 1 tablet daily for 21 days, starting on the first day of the menstrual cycle. Contraceptive protection begins immediately.

*Subsequent cycles:* Tablet taking from the next pack of Logynon is continued after a 7-day interval, beginning on the same day of the week as the first pack.

*Changing from 21-day combined oral contraceptives:* The first tablet of Logynon should be taken on the first day immediately after the end of the previous oral contraceptive course. Additional contraceptive precautions are not required.

*Changing from a combined Every Day pill (28 day tablets):* Logynon should be started after taking the last active tablet from the Every Day Pill pack. The first Logynon tablet is taken the next day. Additional contraceptive precautions are not then required.

*Changing from a progestogen-only pill (POP):* The first tablet of Logynon should be taken on the first day of bleeding, even if a POP has already been taken on that day. Additional contraceptive precautions are not then required. The remaining progestogen-only pills should be discarded.

*Post-partum and post-abortum use:* After pregnancy, oral contraception can be started 21 days after a vaginal delivery, provided that the patient is fully ambulant and there are no puerperal complications. Additional contraceptive precautions will be required for the first 7 days of tablet taking. Since the first post-partum ovulation may precede the first bleeding, another method of contraception should be used in the interval between childbirth and the first course of tablets. After a first-trimester abortion, oral contraception may be started immediately in which case no additional contraceptive precautions are required.

*Pregnancy and lactation:* If pregnancy occurs during medication with oral contraceptives, the preparation should be withdrawn immediately.

The use of Logynon during lactation may lead to a reduction in the volume of milk produced and to a change in its composition. Minute amounts of the active substances are excreted with the milk. Mothers who are breast-feeding may be advised instead to use a progestogen-only pill.

*Special circumstances requiring additional contraception*

*Incorrect administration:* A single delayed tablet should be taken as soon as possible, and if this can be done within 12 hours of the correct time, contraceptive protection is maintained. With longer delays, additional contraception is needed. Only the most recently delayed tablet should be taken, earlier missed tablets being omitted, and additional non-hormonal methods of contraception (except the rhythm or temperature methods) should be used for the next 7 days, while the next 7 tablets are being taken. Additionally, therefore, if tablet(s) have been missed during the last 7 days of a pack, there should be no

break before the next pack is started. In this situation, a withdrawal bleed should not be expected until the end of the second pack. Some breakthrough bleeding may occur on tablet taking days but this is not clinically significant. If the patient does not have a withdrawal bleed during the tablet-free interval following the end of the second pack, the possibility of pregnancy must be ruled out before starting the next pack.

*Gastro-intestinal upset:* Vomiting or diarrhoea may reduce the efficacy of oral contraceptives by preventing full absorption. Tablet-taking from the current pack should be continued. Additional non-hormonal methods of contraception (except the rhythm or temperature methods) should be used during the gastro-intestinal upset and for 7 days following the upset. If these 7 days overrun the end of a pack, the next pack should be started without a break. In this situation, a withdrawal bleed should not be expected until the end of the second pack. If the patient does not have a withdrawal bleed during the tablet-free interval following the end of the second pack, the possibility of pregnancy must be ruled out before starting the next pack. Other methods of contraception should be considered if the gastro-intestinal disorder is likely to be prolonged.

*Interaction with other drugs:* Hepatic enzyme inducers such as barbiturates, primidone, phenobarbitone, phenytoin, phenylbutazone, rifampicin, carbamazepine and griseofulvin can impair the efficacy of Logynon. For women receiving long-term therapy with hepatic enzyme inducers, another method of contraception should be used. The use of antibiotics may also reduce the efficacy of Logynon, possibly by altering the intestinal flora.

Women receiving short courses of enzyme inducers or broad spectrum antibiotics should take additional, non-hormonal (except the rhythm or temperature method) contraceptive precautions during the time of concurrent medication and for 7 days afterwards. If these 7 days overrun the end of a pack, the next pack should be started without a break. In this situation, a withdrawal bleed should not be expected until the end of the second pack. If the patient does not have a withdrawal bleed during the tablet-free interval following the end of the second pack, the possibility of pregnancy must be ruled out before resuming with the next pack. With rifampicin, additional contraceptive precautions should be continued for 4 weeks after treatment stops, even if only a short course was administered.

The requirement for oral antidiabetics or insulin can change as a result of the effect on glucose tolerance.

**Contra-indications, warnings, etc**
*Contra-indications:*

1. Pregnancy

2. Severe disturbances of liver function, jaundice or persistent itching during a previous pregnancy, Dubin-Johnson syndrome, Rotor syndrome, previous or existing liver tumours.

3. Existing or previous arterial or venous thrombotic or embolic processes, conditions which predispose to them e.g. disorders of the clotting processes, valvular heart disease and atrial fibrillation.

4. Sickle-cell anaemia.

5. Mammary or endometrial carcinoma, or a history of these conditions.

6. Severe diabetes mellitus with vascular changes.

7. Disorders of lipid metabolism.

8. History of herpes gestationis.

9. Deterioration of otosclerosis during pregnancy.

10. Undiagnosed abnormal vaginal bleeding.

11. Hypersensitivity to any of the components of Logynon.

*Warnings:* There is a general opinion, based on statistical evidence, that users of combined oral contraceptives experience, more often than non-users, venous thromboembolism, arterial thrombosis, including cerebral and myocardial infarction, and subarachnoid haemorrhage. Full recovery from such disorders does not always occur, and it should be realised that in a few cases they are fatal. How often these disorders occur in users of the modern low-dose pills is not known, but there are reasons for suggesting that they may occur less often than with older pills.

Certain factors may entail some risk of thrombosis, e.g. smoking, obesity, varicose veins, cardiovascular diseases, diabetes, and migraine. The suitability of a combined oral contraceptive should be judged according to the severity of such conditions in the individual case, and should be discussed with the patient before she decides to take it. The risk of arterial thrombosis associated with combined oral contraceptives increases with age, and this risk is aggravated by cigarette-smoking. The use of combined oral contraceptives by women in the older age-group, especially those who are cigarette smokers, should therefore be discouraged and alternative methods used.

In addition if there is a history in the family of

thromboembolic diseases at a young age (e.g. deep vein thrombosis, heart attack or stroke) disturbances of the coagulation system must be ruled out before the pill is prescribed.

Numerous epidemiological studies have been reported on the risks of ovarian, endometrial, cervical and breast cancer in women using combined oral contraceptives. The evidence is clear that combined oral contraceptives offer substantial protection against both ovarian and endometrial cancer.

An increased risk of cervical cancer in long-term users of combined oral contraceptives has been reported in some studies, but there continues to be controversy about the extent to which this is attributable to the confounding effects of sexual behaviour and other factors.

The evidence linking the use of combined oral contraceptives and breast cancer remains inconclusive. The results of some studies suggest an increased risk of breast cancer presenting below the age of about 35, the risk rising with duration of use. Any possible increased risk of breast cancer with combined oral contraceptives is however likely to be small, and may be expected to be less with low-dosage pills. This possible risk should be weighed against the many benefits of combined oral contraceptives, including their protective effects against ovarian and endometrial cancers.

The possibility cannot be ruled out that certain chronic diseases may occasionally deteriorate during the use of combined oral contraceptives (see 'Precautions').

In rare cases benign and, in even rarer cases, malignant liver tumours leading in isolated cases to life-threatening intra-abdominal haemorrhage have been observed after the use of hormonal substances such as those contained in Logynon. If severe upper abdominal complaints, liver enlargement or signs of intra-abdominal haemorrhage occur, the possibility of a liver tumour should be included in the differential diagnosis.

*Reasons for stopping oral contraception immediately:*

1. Occurrence for the first time, or exacerbation, of migrainous headaches or unusually frequent or unusually severe headaches.

2. Sudden disturbances of vision or hearing or other perceptual disorders.

3. First signs of thrombophlebitis or thromboembolic symptoms (e.g. unusual pains in or swelling of the leg(s), stabbing pains on breathing or coughing for no apparent reason). Feeling of pain and tightness in the chest.

4. Six weeks before an elective major operation (e.g. abdominal, orthopaedic), any surgery to the legs, medical treatment for varicose veins or prolonged immobilisation, e.g. after accidents or surgery. Do not restart until 2 weeks after full ambulation. In case of emergency surgery, thrombotic prophylaxis is usually indicated e.g. subcutaneous heparin.

5. Onset of jaundice, hepatitis, itching of the whole body.

6. Increase in epileptic seizures.

7. Significant rise in blood pressure.

8. Onset of severe depression.

9. Severe upper abdominal pain or liver enlargement.

10. Clear exacerbation of conditions known to be capable of deteriorating during oral contraception or pregnancy.

11. Pregnancy is a reason for stopping immediately because it has been suggested by some investigations that oral contraceptives taken in early pregnancy may slightly increase the risk of foetal malformations. Other investigations have failed to support these findings. The possibility therefore cannot be excluded, but it is certain that if a risk exists at all, it is very small.

*Precautions:* Examination of the pelvic organs, breasts and blood-pressure should precede the prescribing of any combined oral contraceptive and should be repeated regularly. The family medical history should be carefully noted and disturbances of the clotting mechanism ruled out if any member of the family has suffered from thromboembolic disease (e.g. deep vein thrombosis, stroke, myocardial infarction) at a young age. Before starting treatment pregnancy must be excluded.

The following conditions require strict medical supervision during medication with oral contraceptives. Deterioration or first appearance of any of these conditions may indicate that use of the oral contraceptive should be discontinued: diabetes mellitus, or a tendency towards diabetes mellitus (e.g. unexplained glycosuria), hypertension, varicose veins, a history of phlebitis, otosclerosis, multiple sclerosis, epilepsy, porphyria, tetany, disturbed liver function, Sydenham's chorea, renal dysfunction, family history of clotting disorders, obesity, family history of breast cancer and patient history of benign breast disease, history of clinical depression, systemic lupus erythematosus, uterine fibroids and migraine, gall-stones, cardiovascular diseases, chloasma, asthma, an intolerance of contact lenses, or any disease that is prone to worsen during pregnancy

Some women may experience amenorrhoea or oligomenorrhoea after discontinuation of oral contraceptives, especially when these conditions existed prior to use. Women should be informed of this possibility.

*Side-effects:* In rare cases, headaches, gastric upsets, nausea, vomiting, breast tenderness, changes in body weight, changes in libido, depressive moods can occur.

In predisposed women, use of Logynon can sometimes cause chloasma which is exacerbated by exposure to sunlight. Such women should avoid prolonged exposure to sunlight.

Individual cases of poor tolerance of contact lenses have been reported with use of oral contraceptives. Contact lens wearers who develop changes in lens tolerance should be assessed by an ophthalmologist.

*Menstrual changes:*
1. *Reduction of menstrual flow:* This is not abnormal and it is to be expected in some patients. Indeed, it may be beneficial where heavy periods were previously experienced.

2. *Missed menstruation:* Occasionally, withdrawal bleeding may not occur at all. If the tablets have been taken correctly, pregnancy is very unlikely. If withdrawal bleeding fails to occur at the end of a second pack, the possibility of pregnancy must be ruled out before resuming with the next pack.

*Intermenstrual bleeding:* 'Spotting' or heavier 'breakthrough bleeding' sometimes occur during tablet taking, especially in the first few cycles, and normally cease spontaneously. Logynon should therefore, be continued even if irregular bleeding occurs. If irregular bleeding is persistent, appropriate diagnostic measures to exclude an organic cause are indicated and may include curettage. This also applies in the case of spotting which occurs at irregular intervals in several consecutive cycles or which occurs for the first time after long use of Logynon.

*Effect on blood chemistry:* The use of oral contraceptives may influence the results of certain laboratory tests including biochemical parameters of liver, thyroid, adrenal and renal function, plasma levels of carrier proteins and lipid/lipoprotein fractions, parameters of carbohydrate metabolism and parameters of coagulation and fibrinolysis. Laboratory staff should therefore be informed about oral contraceptive use when laboratory tests are requested.

*Overdosage:* Overdosage may cause nausea, vomiting and, in females, withdrawal bleeding. There are no specific antidotes and treatment should be symptomatic.

**Pharmaceutical precautions** Shelf-life – Five years

**Legal category** POM

**Package quantities** Individual packs containing three months supply (OP)

**Further information** Nil

**Product licence number** 0053/0085

## LOGYNON* ED

**Qualitative and quantitative composition** Calendar pack containing 6 light brown tablets, 5 white tablets and 10 ochre-coloured tablets containing the following active ingredients.

*Light Brown Tablets*
Levonorgestrel 50 micrograms
Ethinyloestradiol 30 micrograms
*White Tablets*
Levonorgestrel 75 micrograms
Ethinyloestradiol 40 micrograms
*Ochre Tablets*
Levonorgestrel 125 micrograms
Ethinyloestradiol 30 micrograms

Loygnon ED also contains 7 large white placebo tablets.

**Pharmaceutical form** Sugar-coated tablets

**Clinical particulars**

*Therapeutic indications:* Oral contraception and the recognised gynaecological indications for such oestrogen-progestogen combinations.

*Posology and method of administration:*
*First treatment cycle:* 1 tablet daily for 28 days, starting in the red sector on the first day of the menstrual cycle. The initial tablet is the one marked with the appropriate day of the week. In the first cycle only, an additional non-hormonal method of contraception (except the rhythm or temperature methods) must be used for the first 14 days of tablet taking.

*Subsequent cycles:* Tablet taking is continuous, which means that the next pack of Logynon ED follows immediately without a break. A withdrawal bleed usually occurs when the white placebo tablets are being taken.

*Changing from another combined oral contraceptive:* The first tablet of Logynon ED should be taken from the red sector immediately after the end of the previous oral contraceptive course. In the first cycle only, an additional non-hormonal method of contraception (except the rhythm or temperature methods) must be used for the first 14 days of tablet taking.

*Changing from a progestogen-only pill (POP):* The first tablet of Logynon ED should be taken from the red sector on the first day of bleeding, even if a POP has already been taken on that day. An additional non-hormonal method of contraception (except the rhythm or temperature methods) must be used for 14 days. The remaining progestogen-only pills should be discarded.

*Post-partum and post-abortum use:* After pregnancy, Logynon ED can be started 21 days after a vaginal delivery, provided that the patient is fully ambulant and there are no puerperal complications. Additional contraceptive precautions will be required for the first 14 days of tablet taking. Since the first post-partum ovulation may precede the first bleeding, another method of contraception should be used in the interval between childbirth and the first course of tablets. After a first-trimester abortion, oral contraception may be started immediately in which case additional non-hormonal methods of contraception (except the rhythm or temperature methods) should be used for the first 14 days of tablet taking in the first cycle of Logynon ED.

*Special circumstances requiring additional contraception:*

*Incorrect administration:* Errors in taking the 7 inactive white placebo tablets (i.e. the first 5 tablets in the red section and the 2 immediately before the red section) can be ignored. A single delayed active (small) tablet should be taken as soon as possible, and if this can be done within 12 hours of the correct time, contraceptive protection is maintained.

With longer delays in taking active tablets, additional contraception is needed. Only the most recently delayed tablet should be taken, earlier missed tablets being omitted, and additional non-hormonal methods of contraception (except the rhythm or temperature methods) should be used for *the next 7 days, while the next 7 active (small) tablets are being taken.* Therefore, if the 7 days additional contraception will extend beyond the Friday just before the red section (i.e. the last active tablet) the user should take the tablets up to and including that Friday, and start a new pack next day with the Saturday tablet in the red section i.e. discard the remaining tablets and go to an appropriate active tablet in the next pack. In this situation, a withdrawal bleed should not be expected until the end of the second pack. Some breakthrough bleeding may occur on pill taking days but this is not clinically significant. If the patient does not have a withdrawal bleed following the end of the second pack, the possibility of pregnancy must be ruled out before starting the next pack.

*Gastro-intestinal upset:* Vomiting or diarrhoea may reduce the efficacy of oral contraceptives by preventing full absorption. Tablet taking from the current pack should be continued. Additional non-hormonal methods of contraception (except the rhythm or temperature methods) should be used during the gastro-intestinal upset and for 7 days following the upset. If these 7 days extend beyond the last active (small) tablet (i.e. the Friday just before the red section), any remaining tablets should be discarded and a new pack of Logynon ED started the next day with the Saturday tablet in the red section (i.e an appropriate active (small) tablet). In this situation, a withdrawal bleed should not be expected until the end of the second pack. If the patient does not have a withdrawal bleed at the end of the second pack, the possibility of pregnancy must be ruled out before starting the next pack. Other methods of contraception should be considered if the gastro-intestinal disorder is likely to be prolonged.

*Contra-indications:*
1. Pregnancy
2. Severe disturbances of liver function, jaundice or persistent itching during a previous pregnancy, Dubin-Johnson syndrome, Rotor syndrome, previous or existing liver tumours.
3. Existing or previous arterial or venous thrombotic or embolic processes, conditions which predispose to them e.g. disorders of the clotting processes, valvular heart disease and atrial fibrillation.
4. Sickle-cell anaemia.
5. Mammary or endometrial carcinoma, or a history of these conditions.
6. Severe diabetes mellitus with vascular changes.
7. Disorders of lipid metabolism.
8. History of herpes gestationis.
9. Deterioration of otosclerosis during pregnancy.
10. Undiagnosed abnormal vaginal bleeding.
11. Hypersensitivity to any of the components of Logynon ED.

*Special warnings and special precautions for use:*
*Warnings:* There is a general opinion, based on statistical evidence, that users of combined oral contraceptives experience, more often than non-users, venous thromboembolism, arterial thrombosis, including cerebral and myocardial infarction, and subarachnoid haemorrhage. Full recovery from such disorders does not always occur, and it should be realised that in a few cases they are fatal. How often these disorders occur in users of the modern low-dose pills is not known, but there are reasons for suggesting that they may occur less often than with older pills.

Certain factors may entail some risk of thrombosis, e.g. smoking, obesity, varicose veins, cardiovascular diseases, diabetes, and migraine. The suitability of a combined oral contraceptive should be judged according to the severity of such conditions in the individual case, and should be discussed with the patient before she decides to take it. The risk of arterial thrombosis associated with combined oral contraceptives increases with age, and this risk is aggravated by cigarette-smoking. The use of combined oral contraceptives by women in the older age-group, especially those who are cigarette smokers, should therefore be discouraged and alternative methods used.

In addition if there is a history in the family of thromboembolic diseases at a young age (e.g. deep vein thrombosis, heart attack or stroke) disturbances of the coagulation system must be ruled out before the pill is prescribed.

Numerous epidemiological studies have been reported on the risks of ovarian, endometrial, cervical and breast cancer in women using combined oral contraceptives. The evidence is clear that combined oral contraceptives offer substantial protection against both ovarian and endometrial cancer.

An increased risk of cervical cancer in long-term users of combined oral contraceptives has been reported in some studies, but there continues to be controversy about the extent to which this is attributable to the confounding effects of sexual behaviour and other factors.

The evidence linking the use of combined oral contraceptives and breast cancer remains inconclusive. The results of some studies suggest an increased risk of breast cancer presenting below the age of about 35, the risk rising with duration of use. Any possible increased risk of breast cancer with combined oral contraceptives is however likely to be small, and may be expected to be less with low-dosage pills. This possible risk should be weighed against the many benefits of combined oral contraceptives, including their protective effects against ovarian and endometrial cancers.

The possibility cannot be ruled out that certain chronic diseases may occasionally deteriorate during the use of combined oral contraceptives (see 'Precautions').

In rare cases benign and, in even rarer cases, malignant liver tumours leading in isolated cases to life-threatening intra-abdominal haemorrhage have been observed after the use of hormonal substances such as those contained in Logynon ED. If severe upper abdominal complaints, liver enlargement or signs of intra-abdominal haemorrhage occur, the possibility of a liver tumour should be included in the differential diagnosis.

*Reasons for stopping oral contraception immediately:*
1. Occurrence for the first time, or exacerbation, of migrainous headaches or unusually frequent or unusually severe headaches.
2. Sudden disturbances of vision or hearing or other perceptual disorders.
3. First signs of thrombophlebitis or thromboembolic symptoms (e.g. unusual pains in or swelling of the leg(s), stabbing pains on breathing or coughing for no apparent reason). Feeling of pain and tightness in the chest.
4. Six weeks before an elective major operation (e.g. abdominal, orthopaedic), any surgery to the legs, medical treatment for varicose veins or prolonged immobilisation, e.g. after accidents or surgery. Do not restart until 2 weeks after full ambulation. In case of emergency surgery, thrombotic prophylaxis is usually indicated e.g. subcutaneous heparin.
5. Onset of jaundice, hepatitis, itching of the whole body.
6. Increase in epileptic seizures.
7. Significant rise in blood pressure.
8. Onset of severe depression.
9. Severe upper abdominal pain or liver enlargement.
10. Clear exacerbation of conditions known to be capable of deteriorating during oral contraception or pregnancy.
11. Pregnancy is a reason for stopping immediately

because it has been suggested by some investigations that oral contraceptives taken in early pregnancy may slightly increase the risk of foetal malformations. Other investigations have failed to support these findings. The possibility therefore cannot be excluded, but it is certain that if a risk exists at all, it is very small.

*Precautions:* Examination of the pelvic organs, breasts and blood-pressure should precede the prescribing of any combined oral contraceptive and should be repeated regularly. The family medical history should be carefully noted and disturbances of the clotting mechanism ruled out if any members of the family have suffered from thromboembolic disease (e.g. deep vein thrombosis, stroke, myocardial infarction) at a young age. Before starting treatment pregnancy must be excluded.

The following conditions require strict medical supervision during medication with oral contraceptives. Deterioration or first appearance of some of these conditions may indicate that use of the oral contraceptive should be discontinued:

Diabetes mellitus, or a tendency towards diabetes mellitus (e.g. unexplained glycosuria), hypertension, varicose veins, a history of phlebitis, otosclerosis, multiple sclerosis, epilepsy, porphyria, tetany, disturbed liver function, Sydenham's chorea (chorea minor), renal dysfunction, family history of clotting disorders, obesity, family history of breast cancer and patient history of benign breast disease, history of clinical depression, systemic lupus erythematosus, uterine fibroids and migraine, gall-stones, cardiovascular diseases, chloasma, asthma, an intolerance of contact lenses, or any disease that is prone to worsen during pregnancy.

Some women may experience amenorrhoea or oligomenorrhoea after discontinuation of oral contraceptives, especially when these conditions existed prior to use. Women should be informed of this possibility.

*Interaction with other medicaments and other forms of interaction:* Hepatic enzyme inducers such as barbiturates, primidone, phenobarbitone, phenytoin, phenylbutazone, rifampicin, carbamazepine and griseofulvin can impair the efficacy of Logynon ED. For women receiving long-term therapy with hepatic enzyme inducers, another method of contraception should be used. The use of antibiotics may also reduce the efficacy of Logynon ED, possibly by altering the intestinal flora.

Women receiving short courses of enzyme inducers or broad spectrum antibiotics should take additional, non-hormonal (except the rhythm or temperature methods) contraceptive precautions during the time of concurrent medication and for 7 days afterwards. If these 7 days extend beyond the last active (small) tablet (i.e. the Friday just before the red section), any remaining tablets should be discarded and a new pack of Logynon ED started the next day with the Saturday tablet in the red section (i.e. an appropriate active (small) tablet). In this situation, a withdrawal bleed should not be expected until the end of the second pack. If the patient does not have a withdrawal bleed at the end of the second pack, the possibility of pregnancy must be ruled out before resuming with the next pack. With rifampicin, additional contraceptive precautions should be continued for 4 weeks after treatment stops, even if only a short course was administered.

The requirement for oral antidiabetics or insulin can change as a result of the effect on glucose tolerance.

*Pregnancy and lactation:* If pregnancy occurs during medication with oral contraceptives, the preparation should be withdrawn immediately (see 'Reasons for stopping oral contraception immediately').

The use of Logynon ED during lactation may lead to a reduction in the volume of milk produced and to a change in its composition. Minute amounts of the active substances are excreted with the milk. Mothers who are breast-feeding may be advised instead to use a progestogen-only pill.

*Effects on ability to drive and to use machines:* None known.

*Undesirable effects:* In rare cases, headaches, gastric upsets, nausea, vomiting, breast tenderness, changes in body weight, changes in libido, depressive moods can occur.

In predisposed women, use of Logynon ED can sometimes cause chloasma which is exacerbated by exposure to sunlight. Such women should avoid prolonged exposure to sunlight.

Individual cases of poor tolerance of contact lenses have been reported with use of oral contraceptives. Contact lens wearers who develop changes in lens tolerance should be assessed by an ophthalmologist.

*Menstrual changes:*

*1. Reduction of menstrual flow:* This is not abnormal and it is to be expected in some patients. Indeed, it may be beneficial where heavy periods were previously experienced.

*2. Missed menstruation:* Occasionally, withdrawal bleeding may not occur at all. If the tablets have been taken correctly, pregnancy is very unlikely. If withdrawal bleeding fails to occur at the end of a second pack, the possibility of pregnancy must be ruled out before resuming with the next pack.

*Intermenstrual bleeding:* 'Spotting' or heavier 'breakthrough bleeding' sometimes occur during tablet taking, especially in the first few cycles, and normally cease spontaneously. Logynon ED should therefore, be continued even if irregular bleeding occurs. If irregular bleeding is persistent, appropriate diagnostic measures to exclude an organic cause are indicated and may include curettage. This also applies in the case of spotting which occurs at irregular intervals in several consecutive cycles or which occurs for the first time after long use of Logynon ED.

*Effect on blood chemistry:* The use of oral contraceptives may influence the results of certain laboratory tests including biochemical parameters of liver, thyroid, adrenal and renal function, plasma levels of carrier proteins and lipid/lipoprotein fractions, parameters of carbohydrate metabolism and parameters of coagulation and fibrinolysis. Laboratory staff should therefore be informed about oral contraceptive use when laboratory tests are requested.

Refer to 'Special warnings and special precautions for use' section for additional information.

*Overdose:* Overdosage may cause nausea, vomiting and, in females, withdrawal bleeding. There are no specific antidotes and treatment should be symptomatic.

**Pharmacological particulars**

*Pharmacodynamic properties:* Logynon ED is an oestrogen-progestogen combination which acts by inhibiting ovulation by suppression of the mid-cycle surge of luteinizing hormone, the inspissation of cervical mucus so as to constitute a barrier to sperm, and the rendering of the endometrium unreceptive to implantation.

*Pharmacokinetic properties:*

*Levonorgestrel:* Orally administered levonorgestrel is rapidly and completely absorbed. Following ingestion of 0.125 mg levonorgestrel together with 0.03 mg ethinyloestradiol (which represents the combination with the highest levonorgestrel content of the tri-step formulation), maximum drug serum levels of about 4.3ng/ml are reached at 1.0 hour. Thereafter, levonorgestrel serum levels decrease in two phases, characterized by half-lives of 0.4 hours and about 22 hours. For levonorgestrel, a metabolic clearance rate from serum of about 1.5 ml/min/kg was determined. Levonorgestrel is not excreted in unchanged form but as metabolites. Levonorgestrel metabolites are excreted in about equal proportions with urine and faeces. The biotransformation follows the known pathways of steroid metabolism. No pharmacologically active metabolites are known.

Levonorgestrel is bound to serum albumin and to SHBG. Only 1.4% of the total serum drug levels are present as free steroid, but 55% are specifically bound to SHBG. The relative distribution (free, albumin-bound, SHBG-bound) depends on the SHBG concentrations in the serum. Following induction of the binding protein, the SHBG-bound fraction increases while the unbound fractions decrease.

Following daily repeated administration of Logynon ED, levonorgestrel concentrations in the serum increase by a factor of about 4. Steady-state conditions are reached during the second half of a treatment cycle. The pharmacokinetics of levonorgestrel is influenced by SHBG serum levels. Under treatment with Logynon ED, an increase in the serum levels of SHBG by a factor of about 2 occurs during a treatment cycle. Due to the specific binding of levonorgestrel to SHBG, the increase in SHBG levels is accompanied by an almost parallel increase in levonorgestrel serum levels. The absolute bioavailability of levonorgestrel was determined to be almost 100% of the dose administered.

*Ethinyloestradiol:* Orally administered ethinyloestradiol is rapidly and completely absorbed. Following ingestion of 0.03 mg ethinyloestradiol together with 0.125 mg levonorgestrel, maximum drug serum levels of about 116 pg/ml are reached at 1.3 hours. Thereafter, ethinyloestradiol serum levels decrease in two phases characterized by half-lives of 1–2 hours and about 20 hours. For technical reasons, these parameters can only be calculated following the administration of higher doses. For ethinyloestradiol an apparent volume of distribution of about 5 l/kg and a metabolic clearance rate from serum of about 5 ml/min/kg were determined. Ethinyloestradiol is highly but non-specifically bound to serum albumin. About 2% of drug levels are present unbound. During absorption and first liver passage, ethinyloestradiol is metabolized resulting in a reduced absolute and variable oral bioavailability. Unchanged drug is not excreted. Ethinyloestradiol metabolites are excreted at a urinary to biliary ratio of 4:6 with a half-life of about 1 day.

Due to the half-life of the terminal disposition phase from serum and the daily ingestion, steady-state serum levels are reached after 3-4 days and are higher by 30–40% as compared to a single dose. The absolute bioavailability of ethinyloestradiol is subject to a considerable interindividual variation. Following oral administration, the mean bioavailability was found to be about 40–60% of the administered dose.

During established lactation, 0.02% of the daily maternal dose could be transferred to the newborn via milk.

The systemic availability of ethinyloestradiol might be influenced in both directions by other drugs. There is, however, no interaction with high doses of vitamin C. Ethinyloestradiol induces the hepatic synthesis of SHBG and CBG during continuous use. The extent of SHBG induction, however, depends on the chemical structure and the dose of the co-administered progestogen. During treatment with Logynon ED, SHBG concentrations in the serum increased from about 76 nmol/l to 164 nmol/l and the serum concentrations of CBG increased from about 48 μ g/ml to 111 μ g/ml.

*Preclinical safety data:* There are no preclinical safety data which could be of relevance to the prescriber and which are not already included in other relevant sections of the SPC.

**Pharmaceutical particulars**

*List of excipients:* Excipients included in both active and placebo tablets:

| *Active tablets* | *Placebo tablets* |
|---|---|
| lactose | lactose |
| maize starch | maize starch |
| povidone | povidone |
| magnesium stearate (E 572) | magnesium stearate (E 572) |
| sucrose | sucrose |
| polyethylene glycol 6000 | polyethylene glycol 6000 |
| calcium carbonate (E 170) | calcium carbonate (E 170) |
| talc | talc |
| montan glycol wax | montan glycol wax |
| glycerin (E 422) | |
| titanium dioxide (E171) | |
| ferric oxide pigment (red and yellow) (E172) | |

*Incompatibilities:* None known.

*Shelf life: Five years.*

*Special precautions for storage:* Not applicable.

*Nature and contents of container:* Deep drawn strips made of polyvinyl chloride film with counter-sealing foil made of aluminium with heat sealable coating.

Presentation: Cartons containing 3 blister memo-packs. Each memo-pack contains 21 active tablets and 7 placebo tablets (total 28 tablets).

*Instructions for use/handling:* Keep out of the reach of children.

**Marketing authorisation number** 0053/0115

**Date of approval/revison of SPC** 13 December 1995

# MAGNEVIST*

**Qualitative and quantitative composition** Each 1 ml of Magnevist solution contains 469.01 mg of gadopentetic acid, dimeglumine salt. This represents 0.5 moles of Magnevist/l (0.5 mmol/ml).

| | | | |
|---|---|---|---|
| Contrast medium concentration | (mg/ml) 469.01 | | |
| | (mol/l) 0.5 | | |
| Contrast medium content (g) per | | *vial* | *syringe* |
| | 5 ml | 2.3 | - |
| | 10 ml | 4.7 | 4.7 |
| | 15 ml | 7.0 | 7.0 |
| | 20 ml | 9.4 | 9.4 |

| | |
|---|---|
| Properties | |
| Osmolarity at 37°C (mosmol/l solution) | 1440.0 |
| Osmolality at 37°C (mosmol/kg $H_2O$) | 1960.0 |
| Osmotic pressure at 37°C | |
| (atm) | 49.8 |
| (MPa) | 5.06 |
| Density at 20°C (kg/l) | 1.210 |
| at 37°C (kg/l) | 1.195 |
| Viscosity (mPa.s) | |
| at 20°C | 4.9 |
| at 37°C | 2.9 |
| pH | 7.0–7.9 |

**Pharmaceutical form** Solution for injection.

**Clinical particulars**

*Therapeutic indications:* As a paramagnetic contrast medium in cranial, spinal and whole body magnetic resonance imaging (MRI) and for the evaluation of renal function.

*Posology and method of administration:* The patient should fast for 2 hours prior to examination. The usual precautions for MRI (e.g. exclusion of cardiac pacemakers and other ferro-magnetic objects including vascular clips etc) must be observed.

Magnevist should not be drawn up into the syringe until immediately before use. Likewise, the pre-filled syringes must not be taken from the pack and prepared for the injection until immediately before use. Contrast medium not used in one examination must be discarded.

The required dose of Magnevist should be administered as a single intravenous injection. If required, intravenous bolus administration can be used. Ideally the patient should be recumbent during administration, and should be kept under supervision for at least 30 minutes after the injection.

Contrast-enhanced MRI can start immediately after administration of the medium. The timing of optimal opacification after injection of Magnevist varies depending on the tissue and lesion being examined and the MR sequence used. For example, optimal opacification occurs within 5 minutes in the breast, but with cranial and spinal opacification, it is generally observed within 45 minutes. $T_1$- weighted scanning sequences are particularly suitable for contrast-enhanced examinations with Magnevist. In the range of field-strengths, from 0.14 tesla up to 1.5 tesla, (resistive or superconductive magnets) the image contrast was found to be independent of the applied field strength.

The recommended doses are given in ml of Magnevist per kg body weight.

*Cranial and spinal MRI*

*Adults:* In general, the administration of 0.2 ml Magnevist/kg body weight is sufficient to provide diagnostically adequate contrast.

If a strong clinical suspicion of a lesion persists despite a normal scan, a further injection of 0.2 ml or even 0.4 ml Magnevist/kg body weight within 30 minutes may increase the diagnostic yield.

For the exclusion of metastases or recurrent tumours, injection of 0.6 ml Magnevist/kg body weight may increase the diagnostic yield.

*Children (including neonates and infants under the age of 2 years):* 0.2 ml Magnevist/kg body weight is sufficient to provide diagnostically adequate contrast.

If a strong clinical suspicion of a lesion persists despite a normal scan, a further injection of 0.2 ml Magnevist /kg body weight within 30 minutes may increase the diagnostic yield.

*Whole body MRI*

*Adults:* In general, 0.2 ml Magnevist/kg body weight is usually sufficient to provide diagnostically adequate contrast.

In special cases, e.g. in lesions with poor vascularisation and/or a small extracellular space, 0.4 ml Magnevist/kg body weight may be necessary for an adequate contrast especially with relatively less heavily $T_1$-weighted scanning sequences.

For the exclusion of a lesion or tumour recurrences, the injection of 0.6 ml Magnevist/kg body weight may lead to a higher diagnostic confidence.

*Children (over the age of 2 years):* In general, 0.2 ml Magnevist/kg body weight is sufficient to provide diagnostically adequate contrast.

In special cases, e.g. in lesions with poor vascularisation and/or a small extracellular space, 0.4 ml Magnevist/kg body weight may be necessary for an adequate contrast especially with relatively less heavily T1-weighted scanning sequences.

*Neonates and Infants under the age of 2 years:* Experience in children under the age of 2 years is limited. However, this limited experience has shown that 0.2 ml Magnevist/kg body weight may be used in this particular age group.

*Contra-indications:* None stated.

*Special warnings and special precautions for use:* The decision to use Magnevist must be made after particularly careful evaluation of the risk-benefit-ratio in patients with an allergic disposition, since experience shows that these patients suffer more frequently than others from hypersensitivity reactions.

Magnevist is excreted renally and therefore the need for Magnevist-enhanced MRI requires careful consideration in patients with severely impaired renal function in view of the potential retention of Magnevist that may occur in these cases. No further impairment of renal function or reduction in tolerance to the agent has been observed in such patients. However in severe cases consideration should be given to removing Magnevist by haemodialysis.

Slightly elevated levels of iron and bilirubin (within the normal range in the majority of cases) have been observed in the serum in some patients after administration of Magnevist. However, the elevations were seldom sustained for more than 24 hours and there was always a return to the initial values. The clinical

significance of this, if any, is not known, and all patients in whom this effect was observed remained asymptomatic.

The results of serum iron determinations using complexometric methods (e.g. bathophenanthroline) may be reduced for up to 24 hours after the administration of Magnevist because of the free DTPA contained in the contrast-medium solution.

*Interactions with other medicaments and other forms of interaction:* None stated.

*Pregnancy and lactation:* There is as yet no evidence of the safety of Magnevist during human pregnancy. With daily dosage in the rat for 10 days of 12.5 times, and in the rabbit for 13 days of at least 7.5 times, the human dose per unit weight, there was slight retardation of foetal growth and ossification.

It is advisable to avoid using Magnevist during pregnancy, unless an enhanced MR investigation is essential, and no suitable alternative is available.

It is known from animal experiments that minimal amounts of Magnevist (less than 0.2% of the administered dose) enter the breast milk. The clinical relevance of this is not known.

*Effects on ability to drive and use machinery:* None stated.

*Undesirable effects:* Transient sensations of slight warmth at the injection-site, or of pain have been reported very rarely. Transient disturbances of taste may occur after rapid bolus injections.

Inadvertent paravenous injection of Magnevist may cause pain lasting up to 20 minutes. No other tissue reactions have been observed.

Nausea and vomiting and also dermal and mucosal reactions of allergic type have been observed after the administration of Magnevist.

Patients with an allergic disposition suffer more frequently than others from hypersensitivity reactions. In very rare cases anaphylactoid reactions or shock may occur. Familiarity with the practice of emergency measures is essential for prompt efficient action in the event of contrast medium incidents. Appropriate drugs and instruments (e.g. endotracheal tube and ventilator) must be readily available.

In rare cases convulsions have been observed after the administration of Magnevist. However, a causal relationship seems to be questionable.

Transient headaches, vasodilatation, dizziness, chills and syncope following the administration of Magnevist have occasionally been reported. A causal relationship has not been established.

*Overdose:* Acute symptoms of toxicity are unlikely with intravenous administration in adults. Treatment is symptomatic. In infants accidental administration of an entire vial (max 20 ml) may cause the following effects: increase of pulmonary artery pressure; osmotic diuresis; hypervolaemia; dehydration; local vascular pain.

Intoxication due to inadvertent oral ingestion is extremely unlikely due to the low maximum volume (20 ml) and the low gastrointestinal absorption (<1%).

If intoxication occurs due to overdosage or in cases of substantially impaired renal function, Magnevist can be removed by haemodialysis.

**Pharmacological properties**

*Pharmacodynamic properties:* Magnevist is a paramagnetic contrast agent for magnetic resonance imaging. The contrast-enhancing effect is mediated by the di-N-methylglucamine salt of gadopentetate (Gd-DTPA)–the gadolinium complex of pentetic acid (diethylene triamine pentaacetic acid = DTPA). When a suitable scanning sequence (e.g. $T_1$-weighted spin-echo technique) is used in proton magnetic resonance imaging, the gadolinium ion-induced shortening of the spin-lattice relaxation time of excited atomic nuclei leads to an increase in the signal intensity and, hence, to an increase of the image contrast of certain tissues.

Gadopentetate is a highly paramagnetic compound which leads to distinct shortening of the relaxation times even in low concentrations. The paramagnetic efficacy, the relaxivity–determined from the influence on the spin-lattice relaxation time of protons in water– is about 3.8 l/mmol/sec at pH 7 and 39°C and displays only slight dependency on the strength of the magnetic field.

DTPA forms a firm complex with the paramagnetic gadolinium ion with extremely high *in-vivo* and *in-vitro* stability (log K = 22-23). The dimeglumine salt of gadopentetate is a highly water-soluble, extremely hydrophilic compound with a distribution coefficient between n-butanol and buffer at pH 7.6 of about 0.0001. The substance does not display any particular protein binding or inhibitory interaction with enzymes (e.g. myocardial $Na^+$ and $K^+$ ATPase). Magnevist does not activate the complement system and, therefore, probably has a very low potential for inducing anaphylactoid reactions. No impairment of renal function has been observed.

In higher concentrations and on prolonged incubation, gadopentetate has a slight *in-vitro* effect on

erythrocyte morphology. After intravenous administration of Magnevist in man, the reversible process could lead to weak extravascular haemolysis, which might explain the slight increase of serum bilirubin and iron occasionally observed in the first few hours after injection.

The results of the clinical trials do not provide any evidence of an impairment of general well-being or of hepatic, renal or cardiovascular function.

After injection of Magnevist, the resulting opacification of areas with dysfunction of the blood-brain barrier (e.g. glioblastoma) and of intracranial and intraspinal lesions of noncerebral origin provides diagnostic information additional to that obtainable with a plain scan.

*Pharmacokinetic properties:* Gadopentetate behaves in the organism like other highly hydrophilic biologically inert compounds (e.g mannitol or inulin).

After intravenous administration, the compound quickly diffuses in the extracellular space and is eliminated in unchanged form via the kidneys by glomerular filtration. The portion eliminated extrarenally is extremely small. Seven days after intravenous administration of radioactively labelled gadopentetate, distinctly less than 1% of the dose administered was found in the rest of the body of both the rat and the dog. The relatively highest concentrations of the compound were found in the kidneys in the form of the intact gadolinium complex. The compound penetrates and passes neither an intact blood-brain nor the blood-testis barrier. The slight amount which overcomes the placental barrier is quickly eliminated by the foetus.

The pharmacokinetics observed in man were dose-independent. Up to 0.25 mmol Gd-DTPA/kg body weight (= 0.5 ml Magnevist/kg), the plasma level fell after an early distribution phase lasting a few minutes with a half-life of about 90 minutes, identical to the renal elimination rate. At a dose of 0.1 mmol Gd-DTPA/kg (= 0.2 ml Magnevist/kg body weight), 0.6 mmol Gd-DTPA/l plasma were measured 3 minutes after the injection and 0.24 mmol Gd-DTPA/l plasma 60 minutes p.i.; an average of 83% of the dose was eliminated via the kidneys by 6 hours p.i. About 91% of the dose was recovered in the urine within 24 hours of the injection. By the 5th day, the portion of the dose eliminated with the faeces was less than 1%. No cleavage of the paramagnetic ion or metabolic break-down was demonstrable. The renal clearance of gadopentetate referred to 1.73 m² was about 120 ml/min and is therefore comparable to that of inulin or $^{51}$ Cr-EDTA.

Gadopentetate is completely eliminated via the kidneys even in the presence of impaired renal function (creatinine clearance > 20 ml/min); the plasma half-life increases in relation to the degree of renal insufficiency. An increase in the extrarenal elimination was not observed.

Because the serum half-life is prolonged (up to 30 hours) in the presence of greatly impaired renal function (creatinine clearance < 20 ml/min), gadopentetate should be eliminated by means of extracorporeal haemodialysis.

*Preclinical safety data:* Experimental systemic tolerance studies following repeated daily intravenous administration produced no findings which object to a single diagnostic administration of Magnevist to human beings.

Reproduction-toxicological studies with Magnevist gave no indication of a teratogenic or other embryotoxic potential following the administration of Magnevist during pregnancy.

Experimental local tolerance studies with Magnevist following single as well as repeated intravenous administration and single intra-arterial administration gave no indication that adverse local effects are to be expected in blood vessels of human beings.

Experimental local tolerance studies following a single paravenous, subcutaneous as well as intramuscular application indicated that slight local intolerance reactions could occur at the administration site after inadvertent paravenous administration.

Studies into genotoxic effects (gene, chromosomal and genome mutation tests) for gadopentetic acid, dimeglumine *in vivo* and *in vitro* gave no indication of a mutagenic potential.

In a tumorigenicity study with Magnevist in rats, no compound-related tumours were observed.

Due to the absence of genotoxic effects and taking into account the pharmacokinetics and the absence of indications of toxic effects on fast-growing tissues as well as the fact that Magnevist was only administered once, there is no evident risk of a tumorigenic effect on humans.

Studies into contact-sensitizing effect gave no indication of a sensitizing potential for Magnevist.

**Pharmaceutical particulars**

*List of excipients:* Meglumine, pentetic acid (DTPA), water for injection

*Incompatibilities:* Not applicable.

*Shelf-life:* 5 years.

*Special precautions for storage:* Protect from light.

*Nature and contents of container:* Glass vials of 5 ml, 10 ml, 15 ml, 20 ml or glass pre-filled syringes containing 10 ml, 15 ml and 20 ml of Magnevist solution.

*Instructions for use/handling:* Magnevist should not be drawn up into the syringe until immediately before the injection. Likewise, the pre-filled syringes must not be taken from the pack and prepared for the injection until immediately before use. Contrast medium not used in one examination must be discarded.

After preparation, Magnevist remains stable for an examination day. The time indicated does not refer to the physicochemical stability, but to the possibility of microbial contamination.

**Marketing authorisation numbers**
Vials 0053/0206
Pre-filled syringes 0053/0259

**Date of approval/revision of SPC** 4 March 1996

**Legal category** POM

## MAGNEVIST* ENTERAL

**Presentation** Each bottle contains 100 ml of a concentrated colourless aqueous solution of the paramagnetic contrast medium for magnetic resonance imaging, dimeglumine gadopentetate, which is the dimeglumine salt of gadolinium – diethylenetriaminepenta–acetic acid (gadolinium DTPA). A small amount of free DTPA is present to ensure the complete chelation of the gadolinium. 1 ml of Magnevist enteral contains 9.38 mg dimeglumine gadopentetate.

Inactive excipients: sodium citrate dihydrate; diethylenetriaminepenta–acetic acid, sodium salt; mannitol; water.

**Uses** Demonstration and demarcation of the digestive tract from adjacent normal and pathological tissue structures in MRI. Use of Magnevist enteral leads to positive opacification of the gastrointestinal tract after oral or rectal administration. This permits differentiation of the tract from other tissue structures and organs, providing an improved diagnostic yield from MRI.

**Dosage and administration** The patient should fast for 4 hours prior to oral administration. A cleansing enema is recommended before rectal administration. The usual precautions for MRI (eg. exclusion of cardiac pacemakers and other ferro–magnetic objects, including vascular clips etc) must be observed.

Magnevist enteral is not recommended for children below 18 years of age owing to the small amount of clinical experience with this age group as yet.

Ensure that the product is clear before use.

*Dosage:* Magnevist enteral is supplied as a concentrate. The contents of a 100 ml bottle are diluted with 900 ml of tap water immediately before use.

The following guidelines apply to the use of the properly diluted solution in adults:

*Oral:*
100 – 400 ml for oesophagus and stomach
400 – 600 ml for upper abdomen
600 – 1000 ml for lower abdomen and pelvis
Rectal: 100 – 500 ml

For examinations of the oesophagus, stomach and upper abdomen the total dose of diluted solution should be drunk in about 10 minutes and the MRI examination commenced immediately afterwards. For visualisation of bowel segments in the lower abdomen and pelvis the total dose should be drunk over 30–45 minutes and the examination commenced after waiting a further 15–30 minutes.

Complete filling of the bowel segments in the pelvic region is unlikely within 2 hours of oral administration. Rectal administration is advisable if the rectum and distal segments of the colon are to be demonstrated.

T₁–weighted spin–echo sequences, and gradient–echo sequences are the most suitable for low artefact demonstration. In some cases T₂–weighted spin–echo sequences may be necessary to allow demarcation from the abdominal fatty tissue.

Peristalsis increases with increasing doses of the agent and longer examination sequences and may lead to motion artefacts. This can be substantially reduced or even eliminated by the intravenous administration of spasmolytics.

**Contra–indications, warnings, etc.** For oral use: suspected ileus. For rectal use: none known.

*Use in pregnancy and lactation:* There is as yet no evidence of the safety of Magnevist enteral during human pregnancy. Consequently the need for examination merits particularly careful consideration. There have been no studies with Magnevist enteral during lactation. However, since it undergoes minimal enteral absorption it is unlikely that Magnevist enteral enters the breast milk.

*Warnings:* It is known that larger amounts (50–100 g) of mannitol may exacerbate the symptoms of patients with inflammatory gastrointestinal diseases or pre–existing water/electrolyte imbalances. Although such effects have not been observed with Magnevist enteral (maximum mannitol dose 15 g) they should be borne in mind, particularly in elderly patients.

Procedures involving diathermy (polypectomy etc) should not be performed until at least 48 hours after administration of Magnevist enteral as bacterial decomposition of the mannitol can lead to the production of highly inflammable bowel gases.

Ensure that the product is clear before use.

*Side–effects:* Gastrointestinal upsets such as thin stools, increased bowel peristalsis, flatulence and diarrhoea may occur due to the large amount of fluid and mannitol in Magnevist enteral. They are generally mild and short–lived. Nausea and vomiting may occur occasionally.

Cutaneous or mucosal hypersensitivity reactions may occur rarely.

Anaphylactoid reactions or shock have not been observed with Magnevist enteral although they have been reported very rarely with intravenous Magnevist. Familiarity with the practice of emergency measures is essential for prompt efficient action in the event of such incidents.

Appropriate drugs and instruments (eg. endotracheal tube and ventilator) must be readily available.

*Overdosage:* Less than 1% of the usual administered dose of Magnevist enteral is absorbed. Therefore an intoxication due to inadvertent overdosage is unlikely. Treatment is symptomatic.

**Pharmaceutical precautions** Shelf–life–Three years. Magnevist enteral does not contain a preservative. Therefore it is recommended that the solution should be used immediately after opening the 100 ml bottle.

**Legal category** POM

**Package quantities** Bottles of 100 ml

**Further information**
Osmolality at 37°C : 169 mosm/kgH₂0 (dilute solution)
Viscosity at 37°C : 0.75 mPa.s (dilute solution)
Viscosity at 20°C :1.09 mPa.s (dilute solution)
pH 6.5 – 8.0

**Product licence number** 0053/0229

## MICROGYNON* 30

**Presentation** Each beige sugar-coated tablet contains 150 micrograms levonorgestrel and 30 micrograms ethinyloestradiol.
*Excipients:* lactose, maize starch, povidone 25 000, talc, magnesium stearate, sucrose, povidone 700 000, macrogol 6000, calcium carbonate, talc, titanium dioxide, glycerin, montan glycol wax, ferric oxide pigment yellow.

**Uses** Oral contraception and the recognised gynaecological indications for such oestrogen-progestogen combinations. The mode of action includes the inhibition of ovulation by suppression of the mid-cycle surge of luteinising hormone, the inspissation of cervical mucus so as to constitute a barrier to sperm, and the rendering of the endometrium unreceptive to implantation.

**Dosage and administration**
*First treatment cycle:* 1 tablet daily for 21 days, starting on the first day of the menstrual cycle. Contraceptive protection begins immediately.

*Subsequent cycles:* Tablet taking from the next pack of Microgynon 30 is continued after a 7-day interval, beginning on the same day of the week as the first pack.

*Changing from 21-day combined oral contraceptives:* The first tablet of Microgynon 30 should be taken on the first day immediately after the end of the previous oral contraceptive course. Additional contraceptive precautions are not required.

*Changing from a combined Every Day pill (28 day tablets):* Microgynon 30 should be started after taking the last active tablet from the Every Day Pill pack. The first Microgynon 30 tablet is taken the next day. Additional contraceptive precautions are not then required.

*Changing from a progestogen-only pill (POP):* The first tablet of Microgynon 30 should be taken on the first day of bleeding, even if a POP has already been taken on that day. Additional contraceptive precautions are not then required. The remaining progestogen-only pills should be discarded.

*Post-partum and post-abortum use:* After pregnancy, oral contraception can be started 21 days after a vaginal delivery, provided that the patient is fully ambulant and there are no puerperal complications. Additional contraceptive precautions will be required for the first 7 days of tablet taking. Since the first post-

partum ovulation may precede the first bleeding, another method of contraception should be used in the interval between childbirth and the first course of tablets. After a first-trimester abortion, oral contraception may be started immediately, in which case no additional contraceptive precautions are required.

*Pregnancy and lactation:* If pregnancy occurs during medication with oral contraceptives, the preparation should be withdrawn immediately (see *Reasons for stopping oral contraception immediately*).

The use of Microgynon 30 during lactation may lead to a reduction in the volume of milk produced and to a change in its composition. Minute amounts of the active substances are excreted with the milk. Mothers who are breast-feeding may be advised instead to use a progestogen-only pill.

*Special circumstances requiring additional contraception:*
*Incorrect administration:* A single delayed tablet should be taken as soon as possible, and if this can be done within 12 hours of the correct time, contraceptive protection is maintained.

With longer delays, additional contraception is needed. Only the most recently delayed tablet should be taken, earlier missed tablets being omitted, and additional non-hormonal methods of contraception (except the rhythm or temperature methods) should be used for the next 7 days, while the next 7 tablets are being taken. Additionally, therefore, if tablet(s) have been missed during the last 7 days of a pack, there should be no break before the next pack is started. In this situation, a withdrawal bleed should not be expected until the end of the second pack. Some breakthrough bleeding may occur on tablet taking days but this is not clinically significant. If the patient does not have a withdrawal bleed during the tablet-free interval following the end of the second pack, the possibility of pregnancy must be ruled out before starting the next pack.

*Gastro-intestinal upset:* Vomiting or diarrhoea may reduce the efficacy of oral contraceptives by preventing full absorption. Tablet-taking from the current pack should be continued. Additional non-hormonal methods of contraception (except the rhythm or temperature methods) should be used during the gastro-intestinal upset and for 7 days following the upset. If these 7 days overrun the end of a pack, the next pack should be started without a break. In this situation, a withdrawal bleed should not be expected until the end of the second pack. If the patient does not have a withdrawal bleed during the tablet-free interval following the end of the second pack, the possibility of pregnancy must be ruled out before starting the next pack. Other methods of contraception should be considered if the gastro-intestinal disorder is likely to be prolonged.

*Interaction with other drugs:* Hepatic enzyme inducers such as barbiturates, primidone, phenobarbitone, phenytoin, phenylbutazone, rifampicin, carbamazepine and griseofulvin can impair the efficacy of Microgynon 30. For women receiving long-term therapy with hepatic enzyme inducers, another method of contraception should be used. The use of ampicillin and other antibiotics may also reduce the efficacy of Microgynon 30, possibly by altering the intestinal flora. Women receiving short courses of enzyme inducers or broad spectrum antibiotics should take additional, non-hormonal (except rhythm or temperature method) contraceptive precautions during the time of concurrent medication and for 7 days afterwards. If these 7 days overrun the end of a pack, the next pack should be started without a break. In this situation, a withdrawal bleed should not be expected until the end of the second pack. If the patient does not have a withdrawal bleed during the tablet-free interval following the end of the second pack, the possibility of pregnancy must be ruled out before resuming with the next pack. With rifampicin, additional contraceptive precautions should be continued for 4 weeks after treatment stops, even if only a short course was administered.

The requirement for oral antidiabetics or insulin can change as a result of the effect on glucose tolerance.

**Contra-indications, warnings, etc**
*Contra-indications:*
1. Pregnancy
2. Severe disturbances of liver function, jaundice or persistent itching during a previous pregnancy, Dubin-Johnson syndrome, Rotor syndrome, previous or existing liver tumours.
3. Existing or previous arterial or venous thrombotic or embolic processes, conditions which predispose to them e.g. disorders of the clotting processes, valvular heart disease and atrial fibrillation.
4. Sickle-cell anaemia.
5. Mammary or endometrial carcinoma, or a history of these conditions.
6. Severe diabetes mellitus with vascular changes.
7. Disorders of lipid metabolism.
8. History of herpes gestationis.

9. Deterioration of otosclerosis during pregnancy.

10. Undiagnosed abnormal vaginal bleeding.

11. Hypersensitivity to any of the components of Microgynon 30.

*Warnings:* There is a general opinion, based on statistical evidence, that users of combined oral contraceptives experience, more often than non-users, venous thromboembolism, arterial thrombosis, including cerebral and myocardial infarction, and subarachnoid haemorrhage. Full recovery from such disorders does not always occur, and it should be realised that in a few cases they are fatal. How often these disorders occur in users of the modern low-dose pills is not known, but there are reasons for suggesting that they may occur less often than with older pills.

Certain factors may entail some risk of thrombosis, e.g. smoking, obesity, varicose veins, cardiovascular diseases, diabetes, and migraine. The suitability of a combined oral contraceptive should be judged according to the severity of such conditions in the individual case, and should be discussed with the patient before she decides to take it. The risk of arterial thrombosis associated with combined oral contraceptives increases with age, and this risk is aggravated by cigarette-smoking. The use of combined oral contraceptives by women in the older age-group, especially those who are cigarette smokers, should therefore be discouraged and alternative methods used.

In addition if there is a history in the family of thromboembolic diseases at a young age (e.g. deep vein thrombosis, heart attack or stroke) disturbances of the coagulation system must be ruled out before the pill is prescribed.

Numerous epidemiological studies have been reported on the risks of ovarian, endometrial, cervical and breast cancer in women using combined oral contraceptives. The evidence is clear that combined oral contraceptives offer substantial protection against both ovarian and endometrial cancer.

An increased risk of cervical cancer in long-term users of combined oral contraceptives has been reported in some studies, but there continues to be controversy about the extent to which this is attributable to the confounding effects of sexual behaviour and other factors.

The evidence linking the use of combined oral contraceptives and breast cancer remains inconclusive. The results of some studies suggest an increased risk of breast cancer presenting below the age of about 35, the risk rising with duration of use. Any possible increased risk of breast cancer with combined oral contraceptives is however likely to be small, and may be expected to be less with low-dosage pills. This possible risk should be weighed against the many benefits of combined oral contraceptives, including their protective effects against ovarian and endometrial cancers.

The possibility cannot be ruled out that certain chronic diseases may occasionally deteriorate during the use of combined oral contraceptives (see *Precautions*).

In rare cases benign and, in even rarer cases, malignant liver tumours leading in isolated cases to life-threatening intra-abdominal haemorrhage have been observed after the use of hormonal substances such as those contained in Microgynon 30. If severe upper abdominal complaints, liver enlargement or signs of intra-abdominal haemorrhage occur, the possibility of a liver tumour should be included in the differential diagnosis.

*Reasons for stopping oral contraception immediately:*

1. Occurrence for the first time, or exacerbation, of migrainous headaches or unusually frequent or unusually severe headaches.

2. Sudden disturbances of vision or hearing or other perceptual disorders.

3. First signs of thrombophlebitis or thromboembolic symptoms (e.g. unusual pains in or swelling of the leg(s), stabbing pains on breathing or coughing for no apparent reason). Feeling of pain and tightness in the chest.

4. Six weeks before an elective major operation (e.g. abdominal, orthopaedic), any surgery to the legs, medical treatment for varicose veins or prolonged immobilisation, e.g. after accidents or surgery. Do not restart until 2 weeks after full ambulation. In case of emergency surgery, thrombotic prophylaxis is usually indicated e.g. subcutaneous heparin.

5. Onset of jaundice, hepatitis, itching of the whole body.

6. Increase in epileptic seizures.

7. Significant rise in blood pressure.

8. Onset of severe depression.

9. Severe upper abdominal pain or liver enlargement.

10. Clear exacerbation of conditions known to be capable of deteriorating during oral contraception or pregnancy.

11. Pregnancy is a reason for stopping immediately because it has been suggested by some investigations that oral contraceptives taken in early pregnancy may slightly increase the risk of foetal malformations. Other investigations have failed to support these findings. The possibility therefore cannot be excluded, but it is certain that if a risk exists at all, it is very small.

*Precautions:* Examination of the pelvic organs, breasts and blood-pressure should precede the prescribing of any combined oral contraceptive and should be repeated regularly. The family medical history should be carefully noted and disturbances of the clotting mechanism ruled out if any member of the family has suffered from thromboembolic disease (e.g. deep vein thrombosis, stroke, myocardial infarction) at a young age. Before starting treatment pregnancy must be excluded.

The following conditions require strict medical supervision during medication with oral contraceptives. Deterioration or first appearance of any of these conditions may indicate that use of the oral contraceptive should be discontinued: diabetes mellitus, or a tendency towards diabetes mellitus (e.g. unexplained glycosuria), hypertension, varicose veins, a history of phlebitis, otosclerosis, multiple sclerosis, epilepsy, porphyria, tetany, disturbed liver function, Sydenham's chorea, renal dysfunction, family history of clotting disorders, obesity, family history of breast cancer and patient history of benign breast disease, history of clinical depression, systemic lupus erythematosus, uterine fibroids and migraine, gall-stones, cardiovascular diseases, chloasma, asthma, an intolerance of contact lenses, or any disease that is prone to worsen during pregnancy. Some women may experience amenorrhoea or oligomenorrhoea after discontinuation of oral contraceptives, especially when these conditions existed prior to use. Women should be informed of this possibility.

*Side-effects:* In rare cases, headaches, gastric upsets, nausea, vomiting, breast tenderness, changes in body weight, changes in libido, depressive moods can occur. In predisposed women, use of Microgynon 30 can sometimes cause chloasma which is exacerbated by exposure to sunlight. Such women should avoid prolonged exposure to sunlight.

Individual cases of poor tolerance of contact lenses have been reported with use of oral contraceptives. Contact lens wearers who develop changes in lens tolerance should be assessed by an ophthalmologist.

*Menstrual changes:*

1. Reduction of menstrual flow: This is not abnormal and it is to be expected in some patients. Indeed, it may be beneficial where heavy periods were previously experienced.

2. Missed menstruation: Occasionally, withdrawal bleeding may not occur at all. If the tablets have been taken correctly, pregnancy is very unlikely. If withdrawal bleeding fails to occur at the end of a second pack, the possibility of pregnancy must be ruled out before resuming with the next pack.

*Intermenstrual bleeding:* 'Spotting' or heavier 'breakthrough bleeding' sometimes occur during tablet taking, especially in the first few cycles, and normally cease spontaneously. Microgynon 30 should therefore be continued even if irregular bleeding occurs. If irregular bleeding is persistent, appropriate diagnostic measures to exclude an organic cause are indicated and may include curettage. This also applies in the case of spotting which occurs at irregular intervals in several consecutive cycles or which occurs for the first time after long use of Microgynon 30.

*Effect on blood chemistry:* The use of oral contraceptives may influence the results of certain laboratory tests including biochemical parameters of liver, thyroid, adrenal and renal function, plasma levels of carrier proteins and lipid/lipoprotein fractions, parameters of carbohydrate metabolism and parameters of coagulation and fibrinolysis. Laboratory staff should therefore be informed about oral contraceptive use when laboratory tests are requested.

*Overdosage:* Overdosage may cause nausea, vomiting and, in females, withdrawal bleeding. There are no specific antidotes and treatment should be symptomatic.

**Pharmaceutical precautions**    *Shelf-life:* Five years.

**Legal category**   POM

**Package quantities**   Available in packs containing one months' supply

**Product licence number** 0053/0064

## MICROGYNON* 30 ED

**Qualitative and quantitative composition** Each memo-pack contains 21 beige active tablets and 7 white placebo tablets which are larger.

Each active tablet contains 150 micrograms levonorgestrel and 30 micrograms ethinyloestradiol.

**Pharmaceutical form** Sugar-coated tablets

**Clinical particulars**

*Therapeutic indications:* Oral contraception and the recognised gynaecological indications for such oestrogen-progestogen combinations.

*Posology and method of administration:*

*First treatment cycle:* 1 tablet daily for 28 days, starting on the first day of the menstrual cycle. 21 (small) active tablets are taken followed by 7 (larger) placebo tablets. Contraceptive protection begins immediately.

*Subsequent cycles:* Tablet-taking is continuous, which means that the next pack of Microgynon 30 ED follows immediately without a break. A withdrawal bleed usually occurs when the placebo tablets are being taken.

*Changing from 21-day combined oral contraceptives:* The first tablet of Microgynon 30 ED should be taken on the first day immediately after the end of the previous oral contraceptive course. Additional contraceptive precautions are not required.

*Changing from a combined Every Day pill (28 -day pill):* Microgynon 30 ED should be started after taking the last active tablet from the previous Every Day pill pack. The first Microgynon 30 ED tablet is taken the next day. Additional contraceptive precautions are not then required.

*Changing from a progestogen-only pill (POP):* The first tablet of Microgynon 30 ED should be taken on the first day of bleeding, even if a POP has already been taken on that day. Additional contraceptive precautions are not then required. The remaining progestogen only pills should be discarded.

*Post-partum and post-abortum use:* After pregnancy, oral contraception can be started 21 days after a vaginal delivery, provided that the patient is fully ambulant and there are no puerperal complications. Additional contraceptive precautions will be required for the first 7 days of tablet taking to ensure adequate contraceptive cover if early ovulation has occurred. Since the first post-partum ovulation may precede the first bleeding, another method of contraception should be used in the interval between childbirth and the first course of tablets. After a first-trimester abortion, oral contraception may be started immediately in which case no additional contraceptive precautions are required.

*Special circumstances requiring additional contraception*

*Incorrect administration:* Errors in taking the 7 placebo tablets (i.e. the larger white tablets in the last row )can be ignored.

A single delayed active (small) tablet should be taken as soon as possible, and if this can be done within 12 hours of the correct time, contraceptive protection is maintained.

With longer delays in taking active tablets, additional contraception is needed. Only the most recently delayed tablet should be taken, earlier missed tablets being omitted, and additional non-hormonal methods of contraception (except the rhythm or temperature methods) should be used for *the next 7 days, while the next 7 active (small) tablets are being taken.* Therefore, if the 7 days additional contraception extend beyond the last active (small) tablet, the user should finish taking all the active tablets, discard the placebo tablets and start a new pack of Microgynon 30 ED the next day with an appropriate active (small) tablet. Thus, active tablet follows active tablet with no 7 day break. In this situation, a withdrawal bleed should not be expected until the end of the second pack. Some breakthrough bleeding may occur on tablet taking days but this is not clinically significant. If the patient does not have a withdrawal bleed following the end of the second pack, the possibility of pregnancy must be ruled out before starting the next pack.

*Gastro-intestinal upset:* Vomiting or diarrhoea may reduce the efficacy of oral contraceptives by preventing full absorption. Tablet-taking from the current pack should be continued. Additional non-hormonal methods of contraception (except the rhythm or temperature methods) should be used during the gastro-intestinal upset and for 7 days following the upset. If these 7 days extend beyond the last active (small) tablet the user should finish taking all the active tablets, discard the placebo tablets and start a new pack of Microgynon 30 ED the next day with an appropriate active (small) tablet. In this situation, a withdrawal bleed should not be expected until the end of the second pack. If the patient does not have a withdrawal bleed at the end of the second pack, the possibility of pregnancy must be ruled out before starting the next pack. Other methods of contraception should be considered if the gastro-intestinal disorder is likely to be prolonged.

*Children and the elderly:* Microgynon 30 ED is an oral contraceptive and is not applicable in children or the elderly.

*Contra-indications:*

1. Pregnancy
2. Severe disturbances of liver function, jaundice or persistent itching during a previous pregnancy, Dubin-Johnson syndrome, Rotor syndrome, previous or existing liver tumours.
3. Existing or previous arterial or venous thrombotic or embolic processes, conditions which predispose to them e.g. disorders of the clotting processes, valvular heart disease and atrial fibrillation.
4. Sickle-cell anaemia.
5. Mammary or endometrial carcinoma, or a history of these conditions.
6. Severe diabetes mellitus with vascular changes.
7. Disorders of lipid metabolism.
8. History of herpes gestationis.
9. Deterioration of otosclerosis during pregnancy.
10. Undiagnosed abnormal vaginal bleeding.
11. Hypersensitivity to any of the components of Microgynon 30 ED.

*Special warnings and special precautions for use:*

*Warnings:* There is a general opinion, based on statistical evidence, that users of combined oral contraceptives experience, more often than non-users, venous thromboembolism, arterial thrombosis, including cerebral and myocardial infarction, and subarachnoid haemorrhage. Full recovery from such disorders does not always occur, and it should be realised that in a few cases they are fatal. How often these disorders occur in users of the modern low-dose pills is not known, but there are reasons for suggesting that they may occur less often than with older pills.

Certain factors may entail some risk of thrombosis, e.g. smoking, obesity, varicose veins, cardiovascular diseases, diabetes, and migraine. The suitability of a combined oral contraceptive should be judged according to the severity of such conditions in the individual case, and should be discussed with the patient before she decides to take it. The risk of arterial thrombosis associated with combined oral contraceptives increases with age, and this risk is aggravated by cigarette-smoking. The use of combined oral contraceptives by women in the older age-group, especially those who are cigarette smokers, should therefore be discouraged and alternative methods used.

In addition if there is a history in the family of thromboembolic diseases at a young age (e.g. deep vein thrombosis, heart attack or stroke) disturbances of the coagulation system must be ruled out before the pill is prescribed.

Numerous epidemiological studies have been reported on the risks of ovarian, endometrial, cervical and breast cancer in women using combined oral contraceptives. The evidence is clear that combined oral contraceptives offer substantial protection against both ovarian and endometrial cancer.

An increased risk of cervical cancer in long-term users of combined oral contraceptives has been reported in some studies, but there continues to be controversy about the extent to which this is attributable to the confounding effects of sexual behaviour and other factors.

The evidence linking the use of combined oral contraceptives and breast cancer remains inconclusive. The results of some studies suggest an increased risk of breast cancer presenting below the age of about 35, the risk rising with duration of use. Any possible increased risk of breast cancer with combined oral contraceptives is however likely to be small, and may be expected to be less with low-dosage pills. This possible risk should be weighed against the many benefits of combined oral contraceptives, including their protective effects against ovarian and endometrial cancers.

The possibility cannot be ruled out that certain chronic diseases may occasionally deteriorate during the use of combined oral contraceptives (see '*Precautions*').

In rare cases benign and, in even rarer cases, malignant liver tumours leading in isolated cases to life-threatening intra-abdominal haemorrhage have been observed after the use of hormonal substances such as those contained in Microgynon 30 ED. If severe upper abdominal complaints, liver enlargement or signs of intra-abdominal haemorrhage occur, the possibility of a liver tumour should be included in the differential diagnosis.

*Reasons for stopping oral contraception immediately:*

1. Occurrence for the first time, or exacerbation, of migrainous headaches or unusually frequent or unusually severe headaches.
2. Sudden disturbances of vision or hearing or other perceptual disorders.
3. First signs of thrombophlebitis or thromboembolic symptoms (e.g. unusual pains in or swelling of the leg(s), stabbing pains on breathing or coughing for no apparent reason). Feeling of pain and tightness in the chest.
4. Six weeks before an elective major operation (e.g. abdominal, orthopaedic), any surgery to the legs, medical treatment for varicose veins or prolonged immobilisation, e.g. after accidents or surgery. Do not restart until 2 weeks after full ambulation. In case of emergency surgery, thrombotic prophylaxis is usually indicated e.g. subcutaneous heparin.
5. Onset of jaundice, hepatitis, itching of the whole body.
6. Increase in epileptic seizures.
7. Significant rise in blood pressure.
8. Onset of severe depression.
9. Severe upper abdominal pain or liver enlargement.
10. Clear exacerbation of conditions known to be capable of deteriorating during oral contraception or pregnancy.
11. Pregnancy is a reason for stopping immediately because it has been suggested by some investigations that oral contraceptives taken in early pregnancy may slightly increase the risk of foetal malformations. Other investigations have failed to support these findings. The possibility therefore cannot be excluded, but it is certain that if a risk exists at all, it is very small.

*Precautions:* Examination of the pelvic organs, breasts and blood-pressure should precede the prescribing of any combined oral contraceptive and should be repeated regularly. The family medical history should be carefully noted and disturbances of the clotting mechanism ruled out if any member of the family has suffered from thromboembolic disease (e.g. deep vein thrombosis, stroke, myocardial infarction) at a young age. Before starting treatment pregnancy must be excluded.

The following conditions require strict medical supervision during medication with oral contraceptives. Deterioration or first appearance of any of these conditions may indicate that use of the oral contraceptive should be discontinued:

Diabetes mellitus, or a tendency towards diabetes mellitus (e.g. unexplained glycosuria), hypertension, varicose veins, a history of phlebitis, otosclerosis, multiple sclerosis, epilepsy, porphyria, tetany, disturbed liver function, Sydenham's chorea, renal dysfunction, family history of clotting disorders, obesity, family history of breast cancer and patient history of benign breast disease, history of clinical depression, systemic lupus erythematosus, uterine fibroids and migraine, gall-stones, cardiovascular diseases, chloasma, asthma, an intolerance of contact lenses, or any disease that is prone to worsen during pregnancy.

Some women may experience amenorrhoea or oligomenorrhoea after discontinuation of oral contraceptives, especially when these conditions existed prior to use. Women should be informed of this possibility.

*Interaction with other medicaments and other forms of interaction:* Hepatic enzyme inducers such as barbiturates, primidone, phenobarbitone, phenytoin, phenylbutazone, rifampicin, carbamazepine and griseofulvin can impair the efficacy of Microgynon 30 ED. For women receiving long-term therapy with hepatic enzyme inducers, another method of contraception should be used. The use of ampicillin and other antibiotics may also reduce the efficacy of Microgynon 30 ED, possibly by altering the intestinal flora.

Women receiving short courses of enzyme inducers or broad spectrum antibiotics should take additional, non-hormonal (except rhythm or temperature method) contraceptive precautions during the time of concurrent medication and for 7 days afterwards. If these 7 days extend beyond the last active (small) tablet the user should finish taking all the active tablets, discard the placebo (large) tablets and start a new pack of Microgynon 30 ED the next day with an appropriate active (small) tablet. In this situation, a withdrawal bleed should not be expected until the end of the second pack. If the patient does not have a withdrawal bleed at the end of the second pack, the possibility of pregnancy must be ruled out before resuming with the next pack. With rifampicin, additional contraceptive precautions should be continued for 4 weeks after treatment stops, even if only a short course was administered.

The requirement for oral antidiabetics or insulin can change as a result of the effect on glucose tolerance.

*Pregnancy and lactation:* If pregnancy occurs during medication with oral contraceptives, the preparation should be withdrawn immediately (see 'Reasons for stopping oral contraception immediately').

The use of Microgynon 30 ED during lactation may lead to a reduction in the volume of milk produced and to a change in its composition. Minute amounts of the active substances are excreted with the milk. Mothers who are breast-feeding may be advised instead to use a progestogen-only pill.

*Effects on ability to drive and to use machines:* None known.

*Undesirable effects:* In rare cases, headaches, gastric upsets, nausea, vomiting, breast tenderness, changes in body weight, changes in libido, depressive moods can occur.

In predisposed women, use of Microgynon 30 ED can sometimes cause chloasma which is exacerbated by exposure to sunlight. Such women should avoid prolonged exposure to sunlight.

Individual cases of poor tolerance of contact lenses have been reported with use of oral contraceptives. Contact lens wearers who develop changes in lens tolerance should be assessed by an ophthalmologist.

*Menstrual changes:*

*1. Reduction of menstrual flow:* This is not abnormal and it is to be expected in some patients. Indeed, it may be beneficial where heavy periods were previously experienced.

*2. Missed menstruation:* Occasionally, withdrawal bleeding may not occur at all. If the tablets have been taken correctly, pregnancy is very unlikely. If withdrawal bleeding fails to occur at the end of a second pack, the possibility of pregnancy must be ruled out before resuming with the next pack.

*Intermenstrual bleeding:* 'Spotting' or heavier 'breakthrough bleeding' sometimes occur during tablet taking, especially in the first few cycles, and normally cease spontaneously. Microgynon 30 ED should therefore, be continued even if irregular bleeding occurs. If irregular bleeding is persistent, appropriate diagnostic measures to exclude an organic cause are indicated and may include curettage. This also applies in the case of spotting which occurs at irregular intervals in several consecutive cycles or which occurs for the first time after long use of Microgynon 30 ED.

*Effect on blood chemistry:* The use of oral contraceptives may influence the results of certain laboratory tests including biochemical parameters of liver, thyroid, adrenal and renal function, plasma levels of carrier proteins and lipid/lipoprotein fractions, parameters of carbohydrate metabolism and parameters of coagulation and fibrinolysis. Laboratory staff should therefore be informed about oral contraceptive use when laboratory tests are requested.

Refer to 'Special warnings and special precautions for use' section for additional information.

*Overdose:* Overdosage may cause nausea, vomiting and, in females, withdrawal bleeding.

There are no specific antidotes and treatment should be symptomatic.

**Pharmacological particulars**

*Pharmacodynamic properties:* Microgynon 30 ED is an oestrogen-progestogen combination which acts by inhibiting ovulation by suppression of the mid-cycle surge of luteinizing hormone, the inspissation of cervical mucus so as to constitute a barrier to sperm, and the rendering of the endometrium unreceptive to implantation.

*Pharmacokinetic properties*

*Levonorgestrel:* Levonorgestrel is absorbed quickly and completely. Maximum active substance levels of approx. 3 ng/ml were reached in serum just one hour after ingestion of Microgynon 30 ED. The serum concentrations subsequently fell in 2 phases with half-lives of around 0.5 hours and 20 hours. The metabolic clearance rate from plasma is approx. 1.5 ml/min/kg.

Levonorgestrel is eliminated not in unchanged form, but in the form of metabolites with a half-life of around one day and in almost equal proportions via the kidney and bile. Biotransformation takes place via the familiar pathways of steroid metabolism. There are no known pharmacologically active products of metabolism.

Levonorgestrel is bound to serum albumin and SHBG. Only around 1.5% of the respective total concentration is present in unbound form, while approx. 65% is bound to SHBG. The relative proportions (free, albumin-bound, SHBG-bound) depend on the concentration of SHBG. After induction of the binding protein, the portion bound to SHBG increases, while the free portion and that bound to albumin decreases.

After daily repeated ingestion, levonorgestrel accumulates by about the factor 2. A steady state is reached during the second half of the treatment cycle. The pharmacokinetics of levonorgestrel are dependent on the concentration of SHBG in plasma. Under treatment with Microgynon 30 ED, an increase in the serum levels of SHBG effect a concomitant increase in the specific binding capacity and therefore also an increase in levonorgestrel serum levels.

The levonorgestrel serum levels do not change any further after 1–3 cycles of use owing to the fact that SHBG induction is concluded. Compared to a single administration, 3–4 fold higher levonorgestrel serum levels are reached in the steady state.

The absolute bioavailability of levonorgestrel amounts to almost 100%.

Approx. 0.1% of the maternal dose can be passed on to a baby with the breast milk.

*Ethinyloestradiol:* Orally administered ethinyloestradiol is absorbed quickly and completely. Ingestion of Microgynon 30 ED leads to maximum plasma levels of approx. 100 pg/ml after 1–2 hours. The substance concentration then falls in 2 phases for which half-lives of around 1–2 hours and about 20 hours have been determined. For technical reasons, these data can only be calculated at higher dosages.

An imaginary distribution volume of around 5 l/kg and a metabolic clearance rate from plasma of approx. 5 ml/min/kg have been determined for ethinyloestradiol. Ethinyloestradiol is bound non-specifically to serum albumin to the extent of 98%.

Ethinyloestradiol is metabolized even during its absorption phase and during its first liver transit, leading to reduced and individually varying oral bioavailability. Ethinyloestradiol is eliminated not in unchanged form, but in the form of metabolites with a half-life of around one day. The excretion ratio is 40 (urine) : 60 (bile).

Because of the half-life of the terminal elimination phase from plasma, a steady state characterised by a 30–40% higher plasma substance level becomes established after approx. 5–6 daily administrations.

The absolute bioavailability of ethinyloestradiol is subject to considerable interindividual variations. After oral ingestion, it amounts to around 40–60% of the dose.

In women with fully established lactation, around 0.02% of the maternal dose can be passed on to the baby with the breast milk.

Other drugs can have a negative or positive effect on the systemic availability of ethinyloestradiol. No interaction with vitamin C takes place. On continuous use, ethinyloestradiol induces the hepatic synthesis of CBG and SHBG, the extent of SHBG induction being dependent on the type and dose of the simultaneously administered progestogen.

*Preclinical safety data:* There are no preclinical safety data which could be of relevance to the prescriber and which are not already included in other relevant sections of the SPC.

**Pharmaceutical particulars**

*List of excipients:*

*Active tablets:* lactose, maize starch, povidone, magnesium stearate (E 572), sucrose, polyethylene glycol 6000, calcium carbonate (E 170), talc, montan glycol wax, titanium dioxide (E 171), ferric oxide pigment yellow (E 172), glycerin (E 422).

*Placebo tablets:* lactose, maize starch, povidone, magnesium stearate (E 572), sucrose, polyethylene glycol 6000, calcium carbonate (E 170), talc, montan glycol wax.

*Incompatibilities:* None known.

*Shelf life:* 5 years.

*Special precautions for storage:* Not applicable.

*Nature and contents of container:* Deep drawn strips made of polyvinyl chloride film with counter-sealing foil made of aluminium with heat sealable coating.

*Presentation:* Each carton contains 1 or 3 blister memo-packs. Each blister memo-pack contains 21 active tablets and 7 placebo tablets.

*Instructions for use/handling:* Keep out of the reach of children.

**Marketing authorisation number** 0053/0260

**Date of approval/revision of SPC** 12 June 1996

**Legal category** POM.

## MIRENA* ▼

**Qualitative and quantitative composition** Active ingredient: Levonorgestrel 52 mg

**Pharmaceutical form** Levonorgestrel Intrauterine System

**Clinical particulars**

*Therapeutic indications:* Contraception

*Posology and method of administration:* Intrauterine.

The initial release of levonorgestrel is about 20 micrograms/24 hours. Mirena releases levonorgestrel for at least three years.

Mirena is intended for use in women of child-bearing age. Clinical trials were conducted in women of 18 years and over.

Postpartum insertions should be postponed until six weeks after delivery.

*Contra-indications:* Sensitivity to levonorgestrel; known or suspected pregnancy, undiagnosed abnormal genital bleeding; congenital or acquired abnormality of the uterus including fibroids if they distort the uterine cavity; current genital infection; acute or recurrent pelvic inflammatory disease; past attack of bacterial endocarditis or of severe pelvic infection in a woman with an anatomical lesion of the heart or after any prosthetic valve replacement; active or previous severe arterial disease, such as stroke or myocardial infarction; liver tumour; established immunodeficiency; acute malignancies affecting the blood or leukaemias except when in remission; recent trophoblastic disease while hCG levels remain elevated.

*Special warnings and special precautions for use:* Mirena may be used with caution, or removal of the system should be considered, if any of the following conditions exist or arise for the first time:

Confirmed or suspected hormone dependent neoplasia (including breast cancer), malignancies affecting the blood or leukaemias in remission after specialist consultation; hepatic jaundice or other acute or severe liver disease; severe or multiple risk factors for arterial disease; thrombotic arterial or any current embolic disease; use of chronic corticosteroid therapy; past history of symptomatic functional ovarian cysts.

Mirena produces blood levels of levonorgestrel which are lower than in standard progestogen-only pills and is oestrogen-free. Therefore, the following are less likely to occur or to deteriorate:

Past venous thromboembolism; marked increase in blood pressure; and migraine, crescendo migraine, focal migraine with asymmetrical visual loss or other symptoms which are interpretable as being caused by transient cerebral ischaemia.

In general, women using hormonal contraception should be encouraged to give up smoking.

Patients with congenital or acquired cardiac valve defects may be given antibiotic prophylaxis at the time of IUD insertion or removal to prevent endocarditis.

Women with a previous history of ectopic pregnancy carry a higher risk of a further ectopic pregnancy. The possibility of ectopic pregnancy should be considered in the case of lower abdominal pain–especially in connection with missed periods or if an amenorrhoeic woman starts bleeding.

Irregular bleeding may mask symptoms and signs of endometrial cancer.

Functional ovarian cysts have been diagnosed in about 10-12% of patients, and these are also common with progestin-only contraception. In most cases, the enlarged follicles disappear spontaneously during two to three months' observation. Should this not happen, continued ultrasound monitoring and other diagnostic/therapeutic measures are recommended.

Low-dose levonorgestrel may affect glucose tolerance, and the blood glucose concentration should be monitored in diabetic users of Mirena.

Before insertion, the patient must be informed on the efficacy, risks and side-effects of Mirena. A gynaecological examination, including examination of the breasts and exclusion of a pregnancy, should be performed. Cervical infection and sexually transmitted diseases should be excluded. The position of the uterus and the size of the uterine cavity should be determined. The instructions for insertion should be followed carefully. The patient should be re-examined six weeks after insertion and once a year thereafter, or more frequently if clinically indicated.

Syncope or bradycardia may occur in some women during insertion or removal of an IUD. In the event of early signs of a vasovagal attack, insertion may need to be abandoned or the device removed. The woman should be kept supine, the head lowered and the legs elevated to the vertical position if necessary in order to restore cerebral blood flow. A clear airway must be maintained; an airway should always be at hand. Persistent bradycardia may be controlled with intravenous atropine. If oxygen is available it may be administered.

The possibility of pregnancy should be considered if menstruation does not occur within six weeks of the onset of previous menstruation and expulsion should be excluded. A repeated pregnancy test is not necessary in amenorrhoeic subjects unless indicated by other symptoms.

*Pelvic infection:* Known risk factors for pelvic inflammatory disease are multiple sexual partners, frequent intercourse and young age. Mirena should be removed if the woman experiences recurrent endometritis or pelvic infection, or if an acute infection does not respond to treatment within a few days.

*Expulsion:* Symptoms of the partial or complete explusion of any IUD may include bleeding or pain. However, a device can be expelled from the uterine cavity without the woman noticing it. Partial expulsion may decrease the effectiveness of Mirena. As the system decreases menstrual flow, increase of menstrual flow may be indicative of an expulsion.

*Perforation:* Perforation of the uterine corpus or cervix may occur, most commonly during insertion. If perforation is suspected the system should be removed as soon as possible.

*Lost threads:* If the retrieval thread is not visible at the cervix on follow-up examination–first exclude pregnancy. The thread may have been drawn up into the uterus or cervical canal and may reappear during the next menstrual period. If pregnancy has been excluded, the thread may usually be located by gently probing with a suitable instrument. If it cannot be found, it may have broken off, or the system may have been expelled. Ultrasound or X-ray may be used to locate Mirena.

*Post-coital contraception:* Limited experience suggests that Mirena is not suitable for use as a post-coital contraceptive.

*Interaction with other medicaments and other forms of interaction:* The effect of hormonal contraceptives may be impaired by drugs which induce liver enzymes, including barbiturates, phenytoin, carbamazepine and rifampicin. The influence of these drugs on the efficacy of Mirena has not been studied.

*Pregnancy and lactation: Pregnancy:* In case of an accidental pregnancy with Mirena *in situ*, the system must be removed and termination of the pregnancy should be considered. Should these procedures not be possible, the woman should be informed about increased risk of spontaneous abortion or premature labour observed during the use of copper and plastic IUDs. Accordingly, such pregnancies should be closely monitored.

Because of the intrauterine administration and the local exposure to the hormone, teratogenicity (especially virilisation) cannot be completely excluded. It can be expected that the systemic hormone exposure of the foetus through the maternal circulation is lower than with any other hormonal contraceptive method. Because of the rareness of pregnancy with Mirena, there is no clinical experience of the outcome.

*Lactation:* The daily dose and the plasma concentrations of levonorgestrel are lower than with any other hormonal contraceptive method. Concentrations of levonorgestrel have been detected in the breast milk of lactating women. The long-term effects on the nursing infant are unknown.

*Effects on ability to drive and use machines:* There are no known effects on the ability to drive or use machines.

*Undesirable effects:*

*Side-effects:* Subjective side-effects are more common during the first months after the insertion, and subside during prolonged use. Reported conditions elicited by non-specific questioning three months and three years after insertion were as follows:

| *Reported Condition* | *% of Subjects* 3-months | 3-years |
|---|---|---|
| No problems | 46.5 | 71.2 |
| Menstrual problems | 23.9 | 4.0 |
| Lower abdominal pain | 13.2 | 8.4 |
| Headache | 9.8 | 4.9 |
| Acne or other skin problems | 4.7 | 2.7 |
| Back pain | 4.4 | 2.2 |
| Mastalgia | 4.4 | < 1 |
| Nausea | 2.2 | < 1 |
| Other side-effects | 16.7 | 11.1 |

Other subjective side-effects, known to occur with oral contraceptives, may be experienced at a rate of less than 1%.

The average changes in weight and in blood pressure have been similar to those observed for copper IUD patients.

The rate of ectopic pregnancy has been 0.06 per 100 woman-years. This rate is significantly lower than the rate of 1.2-1.6 estimated for patients not using any contraception. The corresponding figure for the copper IUD is 0.12 per 100 woman-years.

*Bleeding patterns:* The most common side-effect of Mirena is a change in menstrual bleeding patterns. The changes may include spotting, shorter or longer menstrual periods, or oligo/amenorrhoea.

During the first month of use, users of Mirena have had on average nine days of spotting. However, spotting decreased gradually and the number of days spotting after six months was less than four, which was comparable to the experience with copper IUDs.

During the first month of use, 20% of users experienced prolonged bleeding (more than eight days). For many women, periods became shorter, and during the third month of use, only 3% of users had prolonged bleeding.

The following cumulative gross discontinuation rates due to menstrual problems have been associated with Mirena during three years of use:

| Event | Cumulative 3-year discontinuation rate per 100 users |
|---|---|
| *Bleeding problems:* | |
| Frequent irregular bleeding | 2.10 |
| Prolonged flow | 1.69 |
| Spotting | 1.78 |
| Heavy flow | 0.35 |
| Other bleeding problems | 0.35 |
| *Oligo/amenorrhoea* | 0.77 |
| *Pain:* | |
| Back pain | 0.40 |
| Dysmenorrhoea | 0.37 |
| Abdominal pain | 4.97 |

Menstrual blood loss is generally reduced during use of Mirena. Scanty blood flow frequently develops into oligo/amenorrhoea. Amenorrhoea is a side-effect that can be positive for some and negative for others. In clinical studies during the first year of use, 17% of women experienced amenorrhoea of at least three months' duration, but the cumulative gross discontinuation rate for amenorrhoea was very low. Amenorrhoea is due to the local effect of levonorgestrel on the endometrium, which-under strong local suppression, does not proliferate in response to oestrogen. Hence, the duration and volume of menstrual bleeding is reduced. The volume of menstrual bleeding was decreased by 88% in menorrhagic women by the end of 3 months use. Reduced bleeding increases the concentration of blood haemoglobin.

Although bleeding patterns may vary from regular scanty menstruation in some women to oligo/amenorrhoea in others, there is no clear difference in follicle development, ovulation or oestradiol and progesterone production in women with different bleeding patterns.

*Overdose:* Not applicable

**Pharmacological properties**

*Pharmacodynamic properties:* Levonorgestrel is a progestin used in gynaecology in various ways: as the progestin component in oral contraceptives, in hormonal replacement therapy or alone for contraception in minipills and subdermal implants. Levonorgestrel can also be administered directly into the uterine cavity as an intrauterine system. This allows a very low daily dosage, as the hormone is released directly into the target organ.

The mechanism of action of Mirena is based on mainly hormonal effects producing the following changes:

- Prevention of proliferation of the endometrium
- Thickening of the cervical mucus thus inhibiting the passage of sperm
- Suppression of ovulation in some women.

The physical presence of the system in the uterus would also be expected to make a minor contribution to its contraceptive effect.

On the basis of more than 12,000 woman-years of use, the pregnancy rate (Pearl Rate) has been 0.14 per 100 woman-years.

Mirena may be particularly useful for contraception in patients with excessive menstrual bleeding, as a marked reduction of menstrual flow is noted after three months use. Some users will become amenorrhoeic.

*Pharmacokinetic properties:* The pharmacokinetics of levonorgestrel itself have been extensively investigated and reported in the literature. One key finding is that the bioavailability of levonorgestrel administered orally is almost 90 per cent. A half life of 20 hours is considered the best estimate although some studies have reported values as short as 9 hours and others as long as 80 hours. Another important finding, although one in agreement with experience with other synthetic steroids, has been marked differences in metabolic clearance rates among individuals, even when administration was by the intravenous route. Levonorgestrel is extensively bound to proteins (mainly sex hormone binding globulin (SHBG)) and extensively metabolised to a large number of inactive metabolites.

The initial release of levonorgestrel from Mirena is 20 micrograms/24 hours, delivered directly into the uterine cavity. Because of the low plasma concentrations, there are only minor effects on the metabolism.

*Preclinical safety data:* Levonorgestrel is a well established progestogen with anti-oestrogenic activity. The safety profile following systemic administration is well documented. A study in monkeys with intrauterine delivery of levonorgestrel for 12 months confirmed local pharmacological activity with good local tolerance and no signs of systemic toxicity. No embryotoxicity was seen in the rabbit following intrauterine administration of levonorgestrel.

**Pharmaceutical particulars**

*List of excipients:* Polydimethylsiloxane elastomer, polydimethylsiloxane tubing, polyethylene, barium sulphate, iron oxide

*Incompatibilities:* None known

*Shelf-life:* Three years

*Special precautions for storage:* Store at a temperature not exceeding +30°C, protected from moisture and direct sunlight.

*Nature and contents of container:* The system with accessories has been packed into a heat sealed TYVEK sterilisation pouch.

*Instructions for use/handling:* Mirena is inserted into the uterine cavity within seven days of the onset of menstruation. It can be replaced by a new system at any time of the cycle.

Mirena can also be inserted immediately after first trimester abortion by curettage. Postpartum insertions should be postponed until six weeks after delivery. Special instructions for insertion are in the package.

Mirena is supplied in a sterile pack which should not be opened until required for insertion. Each device should be handled with aseptic precautions. If the seal of the sterile envelope is broken, the device inside should be discarded.

*Marketing authorisation holder:* Leiras Oy, Pansiontie 47, FIN-20210 Turku, Finland (a subsidiary of Schering AG)

**Marketing authorisation number** 004984/0025

**Date of approval/revision of SPC** 22 February 1995

**Legal category** POM

## NEOGEST*

**Presentation** Each round, dark brown, sugar-coated tablet contains 37.5 micrograms levonorgestrel contained in 75 micrograms norgestrel.

Excipients: lactose, maize starch, povidone 25 000, talc, magnesium stearate, sucrose, povidone 700 000, polyethylene glycol 6000, calcium carbonate, titanium dioxide, ferric oxide pigment (brown), glycerin, montan glycol wax.

**Uses** Oral contraception

*Mode of action:* The contraceptive action of Neogest may be explained as follows.

It changes the cervical mucus so that a barrier is formed against the migration of sperm into the uterine cavity. Nidation is impeded because of changes in the structure of the endometrium. As a rule there is no inhibition of ovulation. Evidence suggests that a reduction in corpus-luteum function may also contribute to the contraceptive action.

**Dosage and administration** *First treatment cycle:* One tablet daily, starting on the first day of the menstrual cycle, at a time of day chosen by the patient. All subsequent tablets must then be taken at this time. The contraceptive effect is likely to be reduced if a tablet is delayed by more than three hours. Additional non-hormonal methods of contraception (except the rhythm or temperature methods) must be used until the first 14 tablets have been taken.

*Subsequent cycles:* The tablets are taken daily and pack follows pack without interruption, and without regard to bleeding.

*Changing from other hormonal contraceptives:* When changing over to Neogest from other hormonal contraceptives, non-hormonal contraceptive measures must be employed additionally until 14 consecutive tablets have been taken regularly.

*Post-partum and post-abortum use:* After pregnancy, Neogest can be started 7 days after a vaginal delivery provided that the patient is fully ambulant and there are no puerperal complications. After a first trimester abortion, Neogest may be started immediately. Additional contraceptive precautions will be required for the first 14 days of pill taking.

*Pregnancy and lactation:* The administration of Neogest during pregnancy is contraindicated.

If pregnancy occurs during medication with Neogest the preparation is to be withdrawn immediately.

There is no evidence that Neogest diminishes the yield of breast milk. However, minute amounts of the active substance are excreted with the milk.

*Special circumstances requiring additional contraception:*

*Incorrect administration:* If a tablet is taken late (i.e. if it is more than 27 hours since the last tablet was taken) or if a tablet is missed, protection against conception may be impaired. Therefore, when such incidents occur, additional, non-hormonal contraceptive methods (except the rhythm or temperature methods) must be employed until 14 consecutive tablets have been taken in the correct manner.

*Gastro-intestinal upset:* Vomiting or diarrhoea may reduce the effectiveness of the tablets by preventing them from being fully absorbed. If the user vomits shortly after taking her daily Neogest tablet, she can maintain protection against contraception by taking a second tablet within 3 hours of the normal time–provided she does not vomit again. For this second intake, the last tablet in the pack should be used.

In the case of repeated vomiting or prolonged diarrhoea, additional, non-hormonal contraceptive methods (except the rhythm or temperature methods) should be continued for a further 14 days after the symptoms have subsided. If the condition reducing the efficacy of the preparation is protracted, other methods of contraception should be considered.

*Interaction with other drugs:* Hepatic enzyme inducers such as barbiturates, primidone, phenobarbitone, phenytoin, phenylbutazone, rifampicin, carbamazepine and griseofulvin can impair the efficacy of Neogest. For women receiving long-term therapy with hepatic enzyme inducers, another method of contraception should be used. The use of antibiotics may also reduce the efficacy of Neogest, possibly by altering the intestinal flora.

Women receiving short courses of enzyme inducers or broad spectrum antibiotics should take additional non-hormonal (except the rhythm or temperature methods) contraceptive precautions during the time of concurrent medication and for 14 days afterwards. With rifampicin, additional contraceptive precautions should be continued for 4 weeks after treatment stops, even if only a short course was administered.

The requirement for oral antidiabetics or insulin can change as a result of an effect on glucose tolerance in diabetes mellitus.

**Contra-indications, warnings etc**
*Contra-indications:*

1. Pregnancy
2. Severe disturbances of liver function
3. Jaundice or persistent itching during a previous pregnancy
4. Dubin-Johnson syndrome
5. Rotor syndrome
6. Previous or existing liver tumours
7. A history of herpes gestationis
8. Mammary carcinoma or a history of this condition
9. Undiagnosed abnormal vaginal bleeding
10. History of or existing thromboembolic processes (e.g. stroke, myocardial infarction)
11. Severe diabetes with vascular changes
12. Sickle-cell anaemia
13. Hypersensitivity to any of the components of Neogest

*Warnings:* Diabetes mellitus or tendency towards diabetes mellitus require careful medical supervision.

There is a general opinion, based on statistical evidence, that users of hormonal contraceptives experience, more often than non-users, venous thromboembolism, arterial thrombosis, including cerebral and myocardial infarction, and subarachnoid haemorrhage. Full recovery from such disorders does not always occur, and it should be realised that in a few cases they are fatal.

If there is a history of ectopic pregnancy or one Fallopian tube is missing, the use of Neogest should be decided on only after carefully weighing the benefits against the risks.

If obscure lower abdominal complaints occur together with an irregular cycle pattern (above all amenorrhoea followed by persistent irregular bleeding), an extrauterine pregnancy must be considered.

According to the present state of knowledge, an association between the use of hormonal contraceptives and an increased risk of venous and arterial thromboembolic diseases cannot be ruled out.

The relative risk of arterial thrombosis (e.g. stroke, myocardial infarction) appears to increase further when heavy smoking, increasing age and the use of hormonal contraceptives coincide.

In rare cases benign, and in even rarer cases, malignant liver tumours leading in isolated cases to life-threatening intra-abdominal haemorrhage have been observed after the use of hormonal substances such as the one contained in Neogest. If severe upper abdominal complaints, liver enlargement or signs of intra-abdominal haemorrhage occur, a liver tumour should be included in the differential diagnosis.

*Reasons for stopping Neogest immediately:*

1. Occurrence for the first time, or exacerbation, of migrainous headaches or unusually frequent or unusually severe headaches
2. Sudden disturbances of vision or hearing or other perceptual disorders
3. First signs of thrombophlebitis or thromboembolic symptoms (for example, unusual pains in or swelling of the legs, stabbing pains on breathing or coughing for no apparent reason), feeling of pain and tightness in the chest
4. Six weeks before an elective major operation (e.g. abdominal, orthopaedic) any surgery to the legs, medical treatment for varicose veins or prolonged

immobilisation e.g. after accidents or surgery. Do not restart until 2 weeks after full ambulation. In case of emergency surgery, thrombotic prophylaxis is usually indicated e.g. subcutaneous heparin

5. Onset of jaundice, hepatitis, itching of the whole body

6. Significant rise in blood pressure

7. Clear exacerbation of conditions known to be capable of deteriorating during oral contraception or pregnancy

8. Pregnancy

Pregnancy is a reason for stopping immediately because it has been suggested by some investigations that oral contraceptives taken in early pregnancy may slightly increase the risk of foetal malformations. Other investigations have failed to support these findings. The possibility therefore cannot be excluded, but it is certain that if a risk exists at all it is very small.

Examination of the pelvic organs, breasts and blood pressure should precede the prescribing of Neogest and should be repeated regularly. Before starting treatment, pregnancy must be excluded.

*Side-effects:* In rare cases, nausea, vomiting, dizziness, headaches, migraine, depressive moods, changes in body weight and libido and allergic reactions can occur. Amenorrhoea and changes in the pattern of the menstrual cycle have also been observed.

*Menstrual changes:* A usual feature of all progestogen-only oral contraceptives is that they can produce an initial irregularity of the bleeding pattern, but such irregularity tends to decrease with time. Some women may experience amenorrhoea.

For these reasons the possibility of such changes in menstrual rhythm should, as a precaution, be pointed out to the patient before the start of tablet taking.

*Missed menstruation:* If no menstrual bleeding has occurred within 6 weeks after the last menstrual bleeding, pregnancy must be excluded before tablet taking is continued. If pregnancy has been excluded and the amenorrhoea lasts longer than 3 months or recurs repeatedly, Neogest should be withheld until normal menstrual bleeding has been restored.

*Procedure in the event of irregular bleeding:* Irregular bleeding is not a medical reason for stopping tablet taking, as long as organic causes for such bleeding and pregnancy can be ruled out and provided it is ensured that the patient is fully compliant.

It is extremely inadvisable to attempt to influence cycle disturbances by the additional administration of an oestrogen. This would only serve to reverse the changes brought about by Neogest in the cervical mucus, thereby seriously reducing the contraceptive effect.

*Effect on blood chemistry:* The use of oral contraceptives may influence the results of certain laboratory tests including biochemical parameters of liver, thyroid, adrenal and renal function, plasma levels of carrier proteins and lipid/lipoprotein fractions, parameters of carbohydrate metabolism and parameters of coagulation and fibrinolysis.

*Overdosage:* Acute toxicity studies did not indicate a risk of acute adverse effects in case of inadvertent intake of a multiple of the daily contraceptive dose. In general it is therefore unnecessary to treat overdosage. There are no specific antidotes and any treatment should be symptomatic.

**Pharmaceutial precautions** *Shelf life:* Five years

**Legal category** POM

**Package quantities** Memo-pack containing 35 tablets (OP).

**Further information** Nil

**Product licence number** 0053/0062

## NERICUR* GEL 5
## NERICUR * GEL 10

**Presentation** Nericur Gel is an aqueous gel containing either 5% or 10% benzoyl peroxide.
*Excipients:* Carbopol 940, polyoxyethylene 23 lauryl ether, propylene glycol, sodium hydroxide, purified water.

**Uses** All stages of acne vulgaris. Benzoyl peroxide has a strong antibacterial action against Propionibacterium acnes. It also has keratolytic and sebostatic actions, which cause some dryness and desquamation.

**Dosage and administration** Treatment should be initiated with Nericur Gel 5%. Once daily, the affected areas should be washed with soap and water and then dried, before Nericur Gel is applied. For stubborn cases treatment may be continued with Nericur Gel 10%, provided that Nericur Gel 5% has been well tolerated. For particularly sensitive skin, Nericur Gel 5% should be applied on alternate days.

For optimal effect, Nericur Gel should be applied in the evening, sufficient time being allowed for it to dry before the patient goes to bed, in order to avoid any bleaching of bed-linen.

**Contra-indications, warnings, etc**
*Contra-indications:* Known hypersensitivity to benzoyl peroxide.

*Precautions:* For external use only. Avoid contact with eyes and mucosae. If the skin is exposed to strong or prolonged sunlight, Nericur Gel should be applied at longer intervals, and a highly protective sun-screening agent should be used. Nericur Gel should only be applied to dry skin, to avoid unnecessary irritation.

*Side-effects:* As with all keratolytic substances, itching, reddening, burning and a feeling of skin tension may occur. This may be relieved by the use of a moisturising cream or by temporary interruption of use.

In rare cases, a contact dermatitis may occur, in which event treatment should be stopped immediately.

**Pharmaceutical precautions** Store below 25°C. *Shelf-life:* two years.

**Legal category** P

**Package quantities** Tubes containing 30 g (OP).

**Further information** Nil.

**Product licence numbers**
Nericur 5   0053/0168
Nericur 10  0053/0169

## NERISONE* CREAM, OILY CREAM AND OINTMENT

**Presentation** *Cream* (oil-in-water emulsion), *oily cream* (water-in-oil emulsion) and *ointment* (anhydrous base): 1 g of each Nerisone presentation contains 1 mg (0.1%) diflucortolone valerate.
*Excipients:* Cream: polyoxyl 40 stearate, stearyl alcohol, liquid paraffin, white soft paraffin, disodium edetate, Carbopol 934 (polyacrylic acid), sodium hydroxide, methylparaben, propylparaben, purified water.

Oily cream: white beeswax, liquid paraffin, white soft paraffin, Dehymuls E, purified water.

Ointment: liquid paraffin, white soft paraffin, Lunacera M (microcrystalline wax), castor oil.

**Uses** Corticoid-responsive dermatoses in the absence of infection.

**Dosage and administration** *Adults and children:* Initially 2-3 applications daily, according to the severity of the condition. For maintenance, one application daily.

*Elderly:* Natural thinning of the skin occurs in the elderly. No special precautions are required, however, when Nerisone Ointment is used in this group of patients.

Nerisone Cream is suitable for weeping skin conditions. Nerisone Cream has a high water and low fat content. In weeping skin diseases it allows secretions to drain away, thus providing for rapid reduction of swelling and drying up of the skin. Nerisone Cream is also suitable for application to moist, exposed and hairy areas of the body.

If the skin dries out too much under protracted use of Nerisone Cream, the patient should be switched to a form which contains more fat (Nerisone Oily Cream or Nerisone Ointment).

Nerisone Oily Cream is suitable for skin conditions which are neither weeping nor very dry. Such conditions require a base with balanced proportions of fat and water. Nerisone Oily Cream makes the skin slightly greasy without retaining heat or fluid.

Nerisone Ointment is suitable in very dry skin conditions which need an anhydrous fatty base. The occlusive effect of the Nerisone Ointment base promotes the healing process.

*Occlusive dressings:* An occlusive dressing may be called for in unusually refractory cases and usually under specialist supervision. If an infection develops under the dressing, occlusive treatment must be terminated.

**Contra-indications, warnings, etc**
*Contra-indications:* Rosacea and peri-oral dermatitis. Acne vulgaris, undiagnosed perianal and genital pruritus, napkin eruptions. Viral infections, primary bacterial or fungal infections of the skin. Secondary infections in the absence of appropriate anti-infective therapy. Nerisone is not suitable for the treatment of ophthalmic conditions.

*Warnings/side-effects:* Long-term continuous therapy with topical corticosteroids should be avoided, irrespective of age. Adrenal suppression can occur, even without occlusion. If used in childhood or on the face, courses should be limited to 5 days and occlusion should not be used.

In common with all other topical corticoids, side-effects may occur when Nerisone is applied to large areas of the body (10% or more) and for long periods of time (more than four weeks), especially if an occlusive dressing is being used. These may be local signs such as atrophy of the skin, telangiectasia, striae, hypertrichosis, peri-oral dermatitis and acneform changes, or systemic corticoid effects caused by absorption. Therefore, caution should be exercised when using occlusive dressings, as there is a possibility that natural steroid production may be depressed.

In rare cases, allergic skin reactions may occur.

Nerisone may be applied under an occlusive dressing. However, each dressing should not be left on for more than 24 hours. Although occlusive dressings may be used repeatedly, it should be noted that systemic corticoid absorption is likely to be increased, with a consequent increased risk of adrenal suppression. If occlusive treatment is expected to be prolonged, it is advisable to change the dressing every 12 hours.

Nerisone should not be allowed to come into contact with the eyes.

Topical corticosteroids may be hazardous in psoriasis for number of reasons including rebound relapses following development of tolerance, risk of generalised pustular psoriasis, and local and systemic toxicity due to impaired barrier function of the skin. Careful patient supervision is important in psoriasis.

Infections or secondarily infected dermatoses require additional therapy with antibiotics or chemotherapeutic agents. This treatment can often be topical, but for heavy infections systemic antibacterial therapy may be necessary. If fungal infections are present, a topically active antimycotic should be applied.

*Pregnancy warning:* There is inadequate evidence of safety in human pregnancy. Topical administration of corticosteroids to pregnant animals can cause abnormalities of foetal development, including cleft palate and intra-uterine growth retardation. There may therefore be a very small risk of such effects on the human foetus and as a general rule, topical preparations containing corticoids should not be applied during the first trimester of pregnancy. In particular, application to large areas of the body or for prolonged periods must be avoided.

Side-effects cannot be excluded in neonates whose mothers have been treated extensively or for a prolonged period of time during pregnancy or while lactating (for example, reduced adrenocortical function, when applied during the last weeks of pregnancy).

*Overdosage:* On the basis of results from acute toxicity studies with both diflucortolone valerate and Nerisone preparations, no acute risk of intoxication is to be expected either after a single dermal application of an overdose (application over a large area under conditions favouring resorption) or even after inadvertent oral intake of a whole tube.

**Pharmaceutical precautions**
Nerisone Cream–Store below 25°C.
Nerisone Oily Cream and Ointment–not applicable Shelf-life–Five years

**Legal category** POM

**Package quantities** 30 g tubes (OP).

**Further information** Nil

**Product licence numbers**
Nerisone Cream 0053/0075
Nerisone Oily Cream 0053/0073
Nerisone Ointment 0053/0074

## NERISONE* FORTE OILY CREAM AND OINTMENT

**Qualitative and quantitative composition** 100 g oily cream contains 0.3 g diflucortolone valerate, 100 g ointment contains 0.3 g diflucortolone valerate

**Pharmaceutical form** Oily cream; fatty ointment.

**Clinical particulars**
*Therapeutic indications:* Initial and intermittent treatment of severe and recalcitrant corticoid-responsive dermatoses in the absence of infection. These include neurodermatitis (endogenous eczema, atopic dermatitis), lichen planus, discoid lupus erythematosus , severe chronic eczema and psoriasis. Nerisone Forte should not be applied to large areas of the body (more than 10%) in psoriasis (see *Special precautions and special warnings for use*).

*Posology and method of administration: Adults and children over the age of four:* Initially, Nerisone Forte should be applied 2-3 times a day. Once the clinical picture has improved, the patient should be changed from Nerisone Forte to Nerisone for maintenance therapy. *Elderly:* Natural thinning of the skin occurs in the elderly. No special precautions are required, however, when Nerisone Forte is used in this group of patients.

Nerisone Forte Oily Cream is suitable for skin conditions which are neither weeping nor very dry. It has a base with balanced proportions of water and fat. It makes the skin slightly greasy without retaining heat or fluid.

Nersione Forte Ointment is suitable for very dry skin conditions. It has an anhydrous fatty base. Its occlusive effect promotes the healing process.

*Contra-indications:* Acne vulgaris, undiagnosed perianal and genital pruritus, napkin eruptions, viral infections, primary bacterial or fungal infections of the skin. Secondary infections in the absence of appropriate anti-infective therapy.

Nerisone Forte is not suitable for the treatment of ophthalmic conditions.

Infants and children up to the age of 4 years must not be treated with Nerisone Forte.

Nerisone Forte should never be applied to the face.

*Special warnings and special precautions for use:* Long-term continuous therapy with topical corticosteroids should be avoided, irrespective of age. Adrenal suppression can occur, even without occlusion.

In view of the high efficacy and potency of Nerisone Forte, no more than 60 g a week should be applied, and it is suggested that treatment for one or two weeks should generally be sufficient to obtain control of even the most refractory lesion, after which a change to Nerisone can usually be made if maintenance therapy is necessary.

Since prolonged therapy with potent topical corticosteroids may cause local atrophic changes such as striae, thinning, hypertrichosis and telangiectasia, particularly in skin folds and where occlusive dressings are used, it is recommended that the progress of patients under treatment for more than one week with Nerisone Forte be reviewed weekly, and that repeat prescriptions be written only when the prescribing physician has seen the patient again.

Topical corticosteroids may be hazardous in psoriasis for a number of reasons including rebound relapses following development of tolerance, risk of generalised pustular psoriasis, and local and systemic toxicity due to impaired barrier function of the skin. Careful patient supervision is important in psoriasis.

Since absorption is increased with the use of occlusive dressings, these should not be left on for more than 24 hours. If secondary infection occurs during treatment, the use of occlusive dressings should be stopped until the infection has been eliminated, and appropriate treatment of the infection should be instituted if it persists.

*Interaction with other medicaments and other forms of interaction:* None known

*Pregnancy and lactation:* There is inadequate evidence of safety in human pregnancy. Topical administration of corticosteroids to pregnant animals can cause abnormalities of foetal development including cleft palate and intra-uterine growth retardation. There may, therefore, be a very small risk of such effects on the human foetus and, as a general rule, topical preparations containing corticoids should not be applied during the first trimester of pregnancy. In particular, application to large areas of the body or for prolonged periods must be avoided.

Side effects cannot be excluded in neonates whose mothers have been treated extensively or for a prolonged period of time during pregnancy or while lactating (for example, reduced adrenocortical function, when applied during the last weeks of pregnancy).

*Effects on ability to drive and use machines:* Not applicable.

*Undesirable effects:* In common with all potent topical corticosteroids, there may be local signs such as atrophy of the skin, striae, thinning, acneform changes, hypertrichosis and systemic effects of the corticoid due to absorption and telangiectasia, particularly in skin folds and where occlusive dressings are used. Side-effects may occur when Nerisone Forte is applied to large areas of the body (10% or more) and for long periods of time (more than 10 days). In rare cases, allergic skin reactions may occur.

*Overdose:* On the basis of results from acute toxicity studies with both diflucortolone valerate and Nerisone Forte preparations, no acute risk of intoxication is to be expected either after a single dermal application of an overdose (application over a large area under conditions favouring resorption) or even after inadvertent oral intake of a whole tube.

**Pharmacological properties**

*Pharmacodynamic properties:* Diflucortolone valerate is a topically acting fluoridated corticosteroid which suppresses inflammation in inflammatory and allergic skin conditions and alleviates the subjective complaints such as itching, burning and pain. Capillary dilatation, intercellular oedema and tissue infiltration regress; capillary proliferation is suppressed. This leads to fading of inflamed skin surfaces.

*Pharmacokinetic properties:* In order to exert its antiproliferative and anti-inflammatory effects, diflucortolone valerate has to diffuse from the preparation into the living epidermis and into the upper dermis. In vitro penetration studies showed that diflucortolone valerate penetrates human skin rapidly. After application to damaged skin–as a model for diseased skin–the local corticosteroid levels were distinctly higher than in the intact skin.

Once in the skin diflucortolone valerate is partly hydrolysed into the similarly effective diflucortolone. Part of the corticosteroid applied to the skin is percutaneously absorbed, distributed into organs and tissues, metabolised and finally excreted. The extent of percutaneous absorption and the resulting systemic load depend on a series of factors: the vehicle, the exposure conditions (skin area dose, treatment area, duration of treatment), condition of treatment (open/occlusive), the status of the penetration barrier and the localisation of the treated area on the body.

After application of the radiolabelled ointment onto an intact and a "stripped" area of skin on the back of 3 volunteers, 0.7% of the dose was percutaneously absorbed during a 7 hour exposure period.

Following percutaneous absorption diflucortolone valerate is hydrolysed very rapidly into diflucortolone and the respective fatty acid. 11-keto-diflucortolone and two further metabolites have been found in the plasma in addition to diflucortolone. Diflucortolone is eliminated from the plasma with a half-life of approximately 4-5 hours, all metabolites together with a half-life of approximately 9 hours (results after i.v. administration). The metabolites are excreted with urine and faeces in a ratio of 75:25.

*Preclinical safety data:* There are no preclinical safety data which could be of relevance to the prescriber and which are not already included in other relevant sections of the SPC.

**Pharmaceutical particulars**

*List of excipients:* Oily Cream: white beeswax, liquid paraffin, white soft paraffin, Dehymuls E, purified water. Ointment: liquid paraffin, white soft paraffin, Lunacera M (microcrystalline wax), hydrogenated castor oil.

*Incompatibilities:* None known.

*Shelf life:* 5 years.

*Special precautions for storage:* None.

*Nature and contents of container:* Aluminium tubes containing 15 g oily cream or ointment

*Instructions for use/handling:* Keep out of the reach of children.

**Marketing authorisation numbers**

| | |
|---|---|
| Oily Cream | 0053/0099 |
| Ointment | 0053/0100 |

**Date of approval/revision of SPC** 1 June 1997

*Legal category* POM

# NORGESTON*

**Presentation** Each round, white, sugar-coated tablet contains 30 micrograms levonorgestrel.

*Excipients:* lactose, maize starch, povidone 25 000, talc, magnesium stearate, sucrose, povidone 700 000, polyethylene glycol 6000, calcium carbonate, montan glycol wax.

**Uses** Oral contraception.

*Mode of action:* The contraceptive action of Norgeston may be explained as follows:

It changes the cervical mucus so that a barrier is formed against the migration of sperm into the uterine cavity. Nidation is impeded because of changes in the structure of the endometrium. As a rule there is no inhibition of ovulation. Evidence suggests that a reduction in corpus-luteum function may also contribute to the contraceptive action.

**Dosage and administration** *First treatment cycle:* One tablet daily, starting on the first day of the menstrual cycle, at a time of day chosen by the patient. All subsequent tablets must then be taken at this time. The contraceptive effect is likely to be reduced if a tablet is delayed by more than three hours. Additional non-hormonal methods of contraception (except the rhythm or temperature methods) must be used until the first 14 tablets have been taken.

*Subsequent cycles:* The tablets are taken daily and pack follows pack without interruption, and without regard to bleeding.

*Changing from other hormonal contraceptives:* When changing over to Norgeston from other hormonal contraceptives, non-hormonal contraceptive measures must be employed additionally until 14 consecutive tablets have been taken regularly.

*Post-partum and post-abortum use:* After pregnancy, Norgeston can be started 7 days after a vaginal delivery provided that the patient is fully ambulant and there are no puerperal complications. After a first trimester abortion, Norgeston may be started immediately. Additional contraceptive precautions will be required for the first 14 days of pill-taking.

*Pregnancy and lactation:* The administration of Norgeston during pregnancy is contraindicated.

If pregnancy occurs during medication with Norgeston the preparation is to be withdrawn immediately.

There is no evidence that Norgeston diminishes the yield of breast milk. However, minute amounts of the active substance are excreted with the milk.

*Special circumstances requiring additional contraception:*

*Incorrect administration:* If a tablet is taken late (i.e. if it is more than 27 hours since the last tablet was taken) or if a tablet is missed, protection against conception may be impaired. Therefore, when such incidents occur, additional, non-hormonal contraceptive methods (except the rhythm or temperature methods) must be employed until 14 consecutive tablets have been taken in the correct manner.

*Gastro-intestinal upset:* Vomiting or diarrhoea may reduce the effectiveness of the tablets by preventing them from being fully absorbed. If the user vomits shortly after taking her daily Norgeston tablet, she can maintain protection against contraception by taking a second tablet within 3 hours of the normal time–provided she does not vomit again. For this second intake, the last tablet in the pack should be used.

In the case of repeated vomiting or prolonged diarrhoea, additional, non-hormonal contraceptive methods (except the rhythm or temperature methods) should be continued for a further 14 days after the symptoms have subsided. If the condition reducing the efficacy of the preparation is protracted, other methods of contraception should be considered.

*Interaction with other drugs:* Hepatic enzyme inducers such as barbiturates, primidone, phenobarbitone, phenytoin, phenylbutazone, rifampicin, carbamazepine and griseofulvin can impair the efficacy of Norgeston. For women receiving long-term therapy with hepatic enzyme inducers, another method of contraception should be used. The use of antibiotics may also reduce the efficacy of Norgeston, possibly by altering the intestinal flora.

Women receiving short courses of enzyme inducers or broad spectrum antibiotics should take additional non-hormonal (except the rhythm or temperature methods) contraceptive precautions during the time of concurrent medication and for 14 days afterwards. With rifampicin, additional contraceptive precautions should be continued for 4 weeks after treatment stops, even if only a short course was administered.

The requirement for oral antidiabetics or insulin can change as a result of an effect on glucose tolerance in diabetes mellitus.

**Contra-indications, warnings etc**

*Contra-indications:*

1. Pregnancy
2. Severe disturbances of liver function
3. Jaundice or persistent itching during a previous pregnancy
4. Dubin-Johnson syndrome
5. Rotor syndrome
6. Previous or existing liver tumours
7. A history of herpes gestationis
8. Mammary carcinoma or a history of this condition
9. Undiagnosed abnormal vaginal bleeding
10. History of or existing thromboembolic processes (e.g. stroke, myocardial infarction)
11. Severe diabetes with vascular changes
12. Sickle-cell anaemia
13. Hypersensitivity to any of the components of Norgeston

*Warnings:* Diabetes mellitus or tendency towards diabetes mellitus require careful medical supervision.

There is a general opinion, based on statistical evidence, that users of hormonal contraceptives experience, more often than non-users, venous thromboembolism, arterial thrombosis, including cerebral and myocardial infarction, and subarachnoid haemorrhage. Full recovery from such disorders does not always occur, and it should be realised that in a few cases they are fatal.

If there is a history of ectopic pregnancy or one Fallopian tube is missing, the use of Norgeston should be decided on only after carefully weighing the benefits against the risks.

If obscure lower abdominal complaints occur together with an irregular cycle pattern (above all amenorrhoea followed by persistent irregular bleeding), an extrauterine pregnancy must be considered.

According to the present state of knowledge, an association between the use of hormonal contraceptives and an increased risk of venous and arterial thromboembolic diseases cannot be ruled out.

The relative risk of arterial thrombosis (e.g. stroke, myocardial infarction) appears to increase further when heavy smoking, increasing age and the use of hormonal contraceptives coincide.

In rare cases benign, and in even rarer cases, malignant liver tumours leading in isolated cases to life-threatening intra-abdominal haemorrhage have been observed after the use of hormonal substances such as the one contained in Norgeston. If severe upper abdominal complaints, liver enlargement or signs of intra-abdominal haemorrhage occur, a liver tumour should be included in the differential diagnosis.

*Reasons for stopping Norgeston immediately:*

1. Occurrence for the first time, or exacerbation, of migrainous headaches or unusually frequent or unusually severe headaches
2. Sudden disturbances of vision or hearing or other perceptual disorders
3. First signs of thrombophlebitis or thromboembolic symptoms (for example, unusual pains in or swelling of the legs, stabbing pains on breathing or coughing for no apparent reason), feeling of pain and tightness in the chest
4. Six weeks before an elective major operation (e.g. abdominal, orthopaedic) any surgery to the legs, medical treatment for varicose veins or prolonged immobilisation e.g. after accidents or surgery. Do not restart until 2 weeks after full ambulation. In case of emergency surgery, thrombotic prophylaxis is usually indicated e.g. subcutaneous heparin
5. Onset of jaundice, hepatitis, itching of the whole body
6. Significant rise in blood pressure
7. Clear exacerbation of conditions known to be capable of deteriorating during oral contraception or pregnancy
8. Pregnancy

Pregnancy is a reason for stopping immediately because it has been suggested by some investigations that oral contraceptives taken in early pregnancy may slightly increase the risk of foetal malformations. Other investigations have failed to support these findings. The possibility therefore cannot be excluded, but it is certain that if a risk exists at all it is very small.

Examination of the pelvic organs, breasts and blood pressure should precede the prescribing of Norgeston and should be repeated regularly. Before starting treatment, pregnancy must be excluded.

*Side-effects:* In rare cases, nausea, vomiting, dizziness, headaches, migraine, depressive moods, changes in body weight and libido and allergic reactions can occur. Amenorrhoea and changes in the pattern of the menstrual cycle have also been observed.

*Menstrual changes:* A usual, feature of all progestogen-only oral contraceptives is that they can produce an initial irregularity of the bleeding pattern, but such irregularity tends to decrease with time. Some women may experience amenorrhoea.

For these reasons the possibility of such changes in menstrual rhythm should, as a precaution, be pointed out to the patient before the start of tablet taking.

*Missed menstruation:* If no menstrual bleeding has occurred within 6 weeks after the last menstrual bleeding, pregnancy must be excluded before tablet taking is continued. If pregnancy has been excluded and the amenorrhoea lasts longer than 3 months or recurs repeatedly, Norgeston should be withheld until normal menstrual bleeding has been restored.

*Procedure in the event of irregular bleeding:* Irregular bleeding is not a medical reason for stopping tablet taking, as long as organic causes for such bleeding and pregnancy can be ruled out and provided it is ensured that the patient is fully compliant.

It is extremely inadvisable to attempt to influence cycle disturbances by the additional administration of an oestrogen. This would only serve to reverse the changes brought about by Norgeston in the cervical mucus, thereby seriously reducing the contraceptive effect.

*Effect on blood chemistry:* The use of oral contraceptives may influence the results of certain laboratory tests including biochemical parameters of liver, thyroid, adrenal and renal function, plasma levels of carrier proteins and lipid/lipoprotein fractions, parameters of carbohydrate metabolism and parameters of coagulation and fibrinolysis.

*Overdosage:* Acute toxicity studies did not indicate a risk of acute adverse effects in case of inadvertent intake of a multiple of the daily contraceptive dose. In general it is therefore unnecessary to treat overdosage. There are no specific antidotes and any treatment should be symptomatic.

**Pharmaceutical precautions** Shelf-life–Five years

**Legal category** POM

**Package quantities** Memo-pack containing 35 tablets (OP).

**Further information** Nil

**Product licence number** 0053/0068

## NORISTERAT*

**Presentation** Norethisterone oenanthate in oily solution for intramuscular administration. Ampoules contain 200 mg in 1 ml.

Excipients: benzyl benzoate, castor oil for injection.

**Uses** Noristerat is a depot contraceptive. It is intended for short-term use when a high level of efficacy independent of possible errors by the patient is required. It has been licensed for short-term use by women whose partners undergo vasectomy, until the vasectomy is effective, and women immunised against rubella, to prevent pregnancy during the period of activity of the virus.

*Use after delivery or abortion:* Noristerat can generally be used immediately after delivery or abortion (but see following *'Use during lactation'*).

*Use during lactation:* Noristerat has not been reported to inhibit milk production, which is an advantage when the mother wishes to breast-feed. However, traces of the hormone appear in the milk, and although considered harmless to a healthy neonate might theoretically, like other steroids, impair the degradation of bilirubin, especially during the first week of life. If the mother has received Noristerat, breast-feeding should therefore be withheld from neonates with severe or persistent jaundice requiring medical treatment.

**Dosage and administration** 200 mg Noristerat intramuscularly provides contraception for eight weeks. The first injection should be given within the first five days of a menstrual cycle (the first day of menstruation counting as day 1), unless it is given so soon after delivery or abortion that no possibility of pregnancy exists. Provided the injection is carried out according to these instructions, no additional contraceptive cover is required. The injection may be repeated once, after eight weeks. Noristerat must always be injected deep into the gluteal muscles, care being taken that no liquid runs back from the injection site, which could result in loss of efficacy. The viscosity of the liquid at low temperatures is high, necessitating considerable pressure of injection. Therefore it is suggested that the ampoule be immersed in warm water before injection. A needle of at least medium bore should be used, and care taken to ensure that the needle is securely attached to the syringe.

**Contra-indications, warnings, etc**

*Contra-indications:*

1. Pregnancy.
2. Acute and severe chronic liver disease.
3. History, during pregnancy, of idiopathic jaundice or general pruritus or of herpes gestationis
4. History of deterioration of otosclerosis during pregnancy.
5. Dubin-Johnson and Rotor syndromes.
6. Sickle-cell anaemia.
7. Severe diabetes with vascular changes.
8. Previous or existing liver tumours.
9. Pathologically increased blood pressure.
10. Twelve weeks before planned operations and during immobilisation (eg: after accidents.)
11. Current thromboembolic disease.
12. Disturbances of lipid metabolism.
13. Existing or treated breast or endometrial cancer.
14. Hypersensitivity to any of the components of Noristerat.

*Warnings:* Noristerat should not be used in patients with abnormal uterine bleeding until a definite diagnosis has been established and the possibility of genital tract malignancy eliminated.

Although there have been so far no observations of thromboembolic disease during the use of Noristerat, as a precaution it is recommended that this preparation should not be used where there is a history of thromboembolic processes.

No further injection should be given if, during treatment, migrainous headaches occur for the first time or recurrent unusually severe headaches develop, if sudden perceptual disorders occur, if first signs of thrombophlebitis or thromboembolic disease are noted, or if a feeling of pain and tightness in the chest, a significant rise in blood pressure, recurrence of earlier depression or pathological changes of liver function and hormone levels are experienced.

There is a general opinion, based on statistical evidence, that users of hormonal contraceptives experience, more often than non-users, venous thromboembolism, arterial thrombosis, including cerebral and myocardial infarction, and subarachnoid haemorrhage. Full recovery from such disorders does not always occur, and it should be realised that in a few cases they are fatal.

The relative risk of arterial thromboses (e.g. stroke and myocardial infarction) appears to increase further when heavy smoking, increasing age and the use of hormonal contraceptives coincide.

A reduction of glucose tolerance has been observed in some women using progestogens. Consequently, diabetics and women with a tendency to diabetes should be carefully supervised during the use of Noristerat. In the case of diabetes, it may be necessary to reassess the required doses of antidiabetics or insulin.

If there is a history of ectopic pregnancy or one Fallopian tube is missing, the use of Noristerat should be decided on only after carefully weighing the benefits against the risks. If obscure lower abdominal complaints occur together with an irregular cycle pattern (above all amenorrhoea followed by persistent irregular bleeding), an extrauterine pregnancy must be considered.

Like all nortestosterone derivatives used for contraception, Noristerat has slight androgenic activity, and a virilising effect on the external genitalia of a female foetus exposed to Noristerat after the first month of pregnancy cannot be totally ruled out on theoretical grounds. However, no such virilisation has been observed after the few pregnancies that have occurred during the use of Noristerat.

Porphyria and existing impairment of liver function might theoretically be exacerbated by Noristerat. In rare cases benign and, in even rarer cases, malignant liver tumours leading in isolated cases to life-threatening intra-abdominal haemorrhage, have been observed after the use of hormonal substances such as the one contained in Noristerat. If severe upper abdominal complaints, liver enlargement or signs of intra-abdominal haemorrhage occur, a liver tumour should be considered in the differential diagnosis.

In rare cases coughing, dyspnoea and circulatory irregularities may occur during or immediately after the injection. Experience has shown that these reactions can be avoided by injecting Noristerat very slowly.

*Precautions:* Examination of the pelvic organs, breasts and blood pressure should precede the prescribing of Noristerat. Before starting treatment, pregnancy must be excluded.

Women with a history of severe depressive states, porphyria, disturbed liver function or any disease that is prone to worsen during pregnancy should be carefully observed during medication.

Amenorrhoea: if, when the second injection is due, bleeding has not occurred in the preceding eight weeks the second injection should not be given until pregnancy has been ruled out.

*Interaction with other drugs:* Some drugs may accelerate the metabolism of Noristerat. Drugs suspected of having this capacity, which may reduce the efficacy of the preparation, include barbiturates, carbamazepine, phenytoin, phenylbutazone, griseofulvin and rifampicin. Reduced substance levels have been observed during the simultaneous use of certain antibiotics (e.g. ampicillin), possibly due to changes in the intestinal flora. The requirement for oral antidiabetics or insulin can change as a result of the effect on glucose tolerance.

*Side-effects:* Subjective symptoms reported consist mainly of bloating, breast discomfort, headaches, dizziness, depressive moods and transient nausea. Marked increases of weight are rare.

The patient should be informed before starting Noristerat that her menstrual pattern is likely to alter. Menstrual changes in the form of spotting, breakthrough bleeding and delayed menstruation are relatively frequent, and generally do not require treatment. With persistent bleeding however, it may be expedient to administer progestogen/oestrogen tablets e.g. combined oral contraceptives, for 10 days to create a withdrawal bleed 1-4 days later.

*Effect on blood chemistry:* No influence of Noristerat on basal plasma cortisol, the ACTH test or the metyrapone test has been observed. In the acute dexamethasone suppression test, however, a higher plasma cortisol value than expected was found in 4 out of 10 women, although there were no clinical indications of disturbed adrenocortical function. A shortening of the recalcification time and of the thromboplastin time (Quick's test) were observed in studies of the blood coagulation system.

*Overdosage:* Acute toxicity studies indicated that even in the case of inadvertent administration of a multiple of the contraceptive dose, no acute toxicity risk is to be expected.

**Pharmaceutical precautions**: Store below 25°C. Protect from light. Shelf-life–Five years

**Legal category** POM

**Package quantities** Single packs of 1 ampoule

**Further information** Nil

**Product licence number** 0053/0095

## NUVELLE*

**Qualitative and quantitative composition** Each white sugar-coated tablet contains: estradiol valerate 2.0 mg.

Each pink sugar-coated tablet contains: estradiol valerate 2.0 mg and levonorgestrel 75 micrograms.

**Pharmaceutical form** Sugar coated tablets for oral use.

**Clinical particulars**

*Therapeutic indications:* Hormone replacement therapy for the treatment of the climacteric syndrome.

Prevention of postmenopausal osteoporosis in women considered at risk of developing fractures. Epidemiological studies suggest a number of risk factors may contribute to postmenopausal osteoporosis including:

- early menopause (either natural or surgically induced);
- family history of osteoporosis;
- recent corticosteroid therapy;
- a small frame;
- thin;
- cigarette consumption.

For maximum prophylactic benefit treatment should commence as soon as possible after the menopause.

Bone mineral density measurements may help to confirm the presence of low bone mass.

Nuvelle is designed to provide hormone replacement therapy during and after the climacteric. The addition of a progestogen in the second half of each course helps to provide good control of the irregular cycles that are characteristic of the premenopausal phase and opposes the production of endometrial hyperplasia. Whilst ovarian hormone production is little affected, Nuvelle abolishes or improves the characteristic symptoms of the climacteric such as hot flushes, sweating attacks and sleep disorders.

Studies of bone mineral content have shown Nuvelle to be effective in the prevention of progressive bone loss following the menopause.

Nuvelle does not consistently inhibit ovulation and is therefore unsuitable for contraception.

*Posology and method of administration:*

*Adults, including the elderly:* If the patient is still menstruating, treatment should begin on the 5th day of menstruation. Patients whose periods are very infrequent or who are postmenopausal may start at any time, provided pregnancy has been excluded. (see Special warnings and special precautions for use).

One white tablet is taken daily for the first 16 days, followed by one pink tablet daily for 12 days. Thus, each pack contains 28 days treatment. Treatment is continuous, which means that the next pack follows immediately without a break. Bleeding usually occurs within the last few days of one pack and the first week of the next.

*Contra-indications:*

- pregnancy (see Special warnings and special precautions for use).
- severe disturbances of liver function
- previous or existing liver tumours
- jaundice or general pruritus during a previous pregnancy
- Dubin-Johnson syndrome
- Rotor syndrome
- existing or previous thromboembolic processes
- sickle-cell anaemia
- suspected or existing hormone-dependent disorders or tumours of the uterus and breast
- undiagnosed irregular vaginal bleeding
- congenital disturbances of lipid metabolism
- a history of herpes gestationis
- otosclerosis with deterioration in previous pregnancies
- endometriosis
- severe diabetes with vascular changes
- mastopathy

*Special warnings and special precautions for use:* Before starting treatment, pregnancy must be excluded. If the expected bleeding fails to occur at about 28-day intervals, treatment should be stopped until pregnancy has been ruled out.

Before starting Nuvelle, patients should have a thorough general medical and gynaecological examination with special emphasis on the body weight, blood pressure, heart, breasts, pelvic organs with an endometrial assessment if indicated, the legs and skin. Follow-up examinations are recommended at least six-monthly during treatment.

Treatment should be stopped at once if migrainous or frequent and unusually severe headaches occur for the first time, or if there are other symptoms that are possible prodromata of vascular occlusion.

Treatment should also be stopped if trauma, illness or impending surgery is considered to entail a risk of thrombosis.

Treatment should be stopped at once if jaundice or pregnancy occurs, or if there is a significant rise in blood pressure, the occurrence of thromboembolic disease or an increase in epileptic seizures.

Pre-existing fibroids may increase in size under the influence of oestrogens. If this is observed treatment should be discontinued.

In patients with mild chronic liver disease, liver function should be checked every 8 – 12 weeks.

Persistent breakthrough bleeding during treatment is an indication for endometrial assessment which may include biopsy.

Prolonged exposure to unopposed oestrogens increases the risk of development of endometrial carcinoma. The general consensus of opinion is that the addition of 12 days progestogen towards the end of the cycle, as in Nuvelle, diminishes the possibility of such a risk, and some investigators consider that it might be protective.

At the present time there is some evidence which suggests a slight increase in the relative risk of breast cancer in postmenopausal women receiving long-term hormone replacement therapy. A careful appraisal of the risk/benefit ratio should be undertaken before treating for longer than 5 to 10 years.

Thromboembolism has been reported in connection with oestrogen replacement therapy but there is no evidence to date that the overall incidence is increased.

Some women are predisposed to cholestasis during steroid therapy. Diseases that are known to be subject to deterioration during pregnancy (e.g. multiple sclerosis, epilepsy, diabetes, benign breast disease, hypertension, cardiac or renal dysfunction, asthma, porphyria, tetany and otosclerosis) and women with a strong family history of breast cancer should be carefully observed during treatment.

In rare cases benign and in even rarer cases malignant liver tumours leading in isolated cases to life-threatening intra-abdominal haemorrhage have been observed after the use of hormonal substances such as those contained in Nuvelle. If severe upper abdominal complaints, enlarged liver, or signs of intra-abdominal haemorrhage occur, a liver tumour should be included in the differential diagnostic considerations.

*Interaction with other medicaments and other forms of interaction:* Hormonal contraception should be stopped when treatment with Nuvelle is started and the patient should be advised to take non-hormonal contraceptive precautions.

Drugs which induce hepatic microsomal enzyme systems e.g. barbiturates, phenytoin, rifampicin, accelerate the metabolism of oestrogen/progestogen combinations such as Nuvelle and may reduce their efficacy.

The requirement for oral antidiabetics or insulin can change.

*Pregnancy and lactation:* Contra-indicated.

*Effects on ability to drive and to use machines:* None known.

*Undesirable effects:* During the first few months of treatment, breakthrough bleeding, spotting and breast tenderness or enlargement can occur. These are usually temporary and normally disappear after continued treatment. Other symptoms known to occur are: anxiety; increased appetite; bloating; palpitations; depressive symptoms; headache; migraine; dizziness; dyspepsia; leg pains; oedema; altered libido; nausea; rashes; vomiting; altered weight; chloasma.

*Overdose:* There have been no reports of ill-effects from overdosage, which it is, therefore, generally unnecessary to treat. There are no specific antidotes, and treatment should be symptomatic.

**Pharmacological particulars**

*Pharmacodynamic properties:* Nuvelle contains estradiol valerate (the valeric acid ester of the endogenous female oestrogen, estradiol) and the synthetic progestogen, levonorgestrel. Estradiol valerate provides hormone replacement during and after the climacteric. The addition of levonorgestrel in the second half of each course of tablets helps to provide good cycle control and opposes the development of endometrial hyperplasia.

Most studies show that oral administration of estradiol valerate to post-menopausal women increases serum high density lipoprotein cholesterol (HDL-C) and decreases low density lipoprotein cholesterol (LDL-C). Although epidemiological data are limited such alterations are recognised as potentially protective against the development of arterial disease. A possible attenuation of these effects may occur with the addition of a progestogen. However, at the doses used in Nuvelle, the 12 days of combined therapy with estradiol valerate and levonorgestrel have not been observed to be associated with any unwanted lipid effects.

*Pharmacokinetic properties:*

*1. Levonorgestrel (LNG):* Orally administered LNG is rapidly and completely absorbed. Following ingestion of one tablet of Nuvelle maximum drug serum levels of 1.9ng/ml were found at 1.3 hours. Thereafter, LNG serum levels decrease in two disposition phases. The first phase is described by a half-life of 0.5–1.5 hours and the terminal phase by a half-life of 20–27 hours. For LNG, a metabolic clearance rate from serum of about 1.5 ml/min/kg was determined. LNG is not excreted in unchanged form but as metabolites. LNG metabolites are excreted at about equal proportions with urine and faeces. The biotransformation follows the known pathways of steroid metabolism. No pharmacologically active metabolites are known.

LNG is bound to serum albumin and to SHBG. Only about 1.5% of the total serum drug levels are present as free steroid, but 65% are specifically bound to SHBG. The relative distribution (free, albumin-bound, SHBG-bound) depends on the SHBG concentrations in the serum. Following induction of the binding protein, the SHBG bound fraction increases while the unbound and the albumin-bound fraction decrease.

Following daily repeated administration, LNG concentrations in the serum increase by a factor of about 2. Steady-state conditions are reached within a few days. The pharmacokinetics of LNG is influenced by SHBG serum levels. Under treatment with Nuvelle SHBG levels will rise by about 40% during the oestrogen phase and remain constant or slightly decrease thereafter. The absolute bioavailability of LNG was determined to be almost 100% of the dose administered. The relative bioavailability was tested against an aqueous microcrystalline suspension and was found to be complete (108%).

About 0.1% of the maternal dose can be transferred via milk to the nursed infant.

*2. Estradiol valerate ($E_2$ val):* $E_2$ val is completely absorbed from the Nuvelle tablet. During absorption and the first passage through the liver the steroid ester is cleaved into estradiol ($E_2$) and valeric acid. At the same time $E_2$ undergoes extensive further metabolism yielding $E_2$ conjugates, estrone ($E_1$) and $E_1$ conjugates. The pharmacologically most active metabolites of $E_2$ Val are $E_2$ and $E_1$. Maximum serum levels of 25 pg $E_2$/ml and 180 pg $E_1$/ml are reached 5–7 hours after the administration of one Nuvelle tablet.

Mean $E_1$ serum levels are 10–12 fold higher than mean $E_2$ serum concentrations. Serum levels of $E_1$ conjugates are about 25 5 fold higher than the $E_1$ serum levels.

$E_2$ is rapidly metabolised and the metabolic clearance rate has been determined to 30 ml/min/kg. After oral intake of $E_2$ the half-life of the terminal disposition phase was about 13 hours for $E_2$. The respective half-life for $E_1$ serum level decline was about 20 hours. The daily use of Nuvelle will lead to an about 50% increase in $E_2$ serum levels and to twofold $E_1$ levels at steady state.

Estradiol is bound to about 97% to serum proteins, about 35% are specifically bound to SHBG. $E_{2=}$ val is not excreted in unchanged form. The metabolites of estradiol are excreted via urine and bile with a half-life of about 1 day at a ratio of 9:1.

The absolute bioavailability of $E_2$ from $E_2$ val is about 3% of oral dose and thus in the same range like oral $E_2$ (5% of dose;).

The relative bioavailability of $E_2$ val (reference: aqueous microcrystalline suspension) from Nuvelle tablets was complete. (111–112%).

Estradiol and its metabolites are excreted into milk only to a minor extent.

*Preclinical safety data:* There are no preclinical data which could be of relevance to the prescriber and which are not already included in other relevant sections of the SPC.

**Pharmaceutical particulars**

*List of excipients:* Nuvelle contains the following excipients: lactose, maize starch, povidone 25 000, povidone 700 000, talcum, magnesium stearate (E572), sucrose, macrogol 6000 (polyethylene glycol 6000), calcium carbonate (E170), glycerol (E422), montan glycol wax, yellow and red ferric iron oxide pigments (E172), titanium dioxide (E171).

*Incompatibilities:* Not applicable.

*Shelf life:* 5 years.

*Special precautions for storage:* None

*Nature and contents of container:* Packs containing aluminium foil and PVC blister strips of 28 tablets.
*Presentation:* Carton containing memo-packs of either 1 x 28 tablets or 3 x 28 tablets.

*Instructions for use/handling:* Not applicable.

**Marketing authorisation number** 0053/0219

**Date of approval/revision of SPC** 17 April 1996
**Legal category** POM

# NUVELLE* TS

**Qualitative and quantitative composition** Estradiol and levonorgestrel transdermal systems:
Nuvelle TS Phase I (4 patches).

Each clear rectangular shaped patch contains 3 mg estradiol (equivalent to 3.1 mg Estradiol Hemihydrate PhEur). The patch is mounted on a shiny polyester protective liner which is removed prior to use. The nominal average absorption rate from the Phase I patch is 80 micrograms of estradiol per 24 hours.

Nuvelle TS Phase II (4 patches)

Each clear rectangular shaped patch contains 2.5 mg estradiol (equivalent to 2.6 mg Estradiol Hemihydrate PhEur) and 1 mg levonorgestrel. The patch is mounted on a paper protective liner which is removed prior to use. The nominal average absorption rate from the Phase II patch is 50 micrograms of estradiol and 20 micrograms of levonorgestrel per 24 hours.

**Pharmaceutical form** Transdermal patches

**Clinical particulars**
*Therapeutic indications:* Hormone replacement therapy for the treatment of the climacteric syndrome.

Nuvelle TS is designed to provide hormone replacement therapy during and after the climacteric. The addition of a progestogen in the second half of each course helps to provide good control of the irregular cycles that are characteristic of the climacteric and opposes the development of endometrial hyperplasia. Whilst endogenous ovarian hormone production is little affected, Nuvelle TS abolishes or improves the characteristic symptoms of the climacteric such as hot flushes, sweating attacks and sleep disorders.

Combined preparations containing an oestrogen and progestogen are only necessary in patients with an intact uterus.

*Posology and method of administration: Adults:* If the patient is still menstruating, treatment should begin any time from the 1st to the 5th day of menstruation. Patients whose periods are very infrequent or who are postmenopausal may start at any time, provided pregnancy has been excluded (see *Special warnings and special precautions for use*).

One cycle of Nuvelle TS therapy consists of four Phase I patches of transdermal estradiol followed by four Phase II patches containing estradiol and levonorgestrel.

One Phase I patch should be applied twice weekly for the first two weeks followed by one Phase II patch twice weekly for the next two weeks. Each used patch is removed after 3 or 4 days and a fresh patch applied to a different site. Thus, two patches are worn consecutively each week and patches are changed on the same days of each week. Recommended application sites are clean, dry and intact areas of skin on the trunk and buttocks. Nuvelle TS should not be applied on or near the breasts. Each pack contains 28 days treatment. Treatment is continuous, which means that the next pack follows immediately without a break. Bleeding usually occurs during the last week of the cycle or within the first few days of the next.

*Children:* Not recommended for children.

*Contra-indications:* pregnancy and lactation (see *Special warnings and special precautions for use*); severe disturbances of liver function (including porphyria), previous or existing liver tumours, jaundice or general pruritus during a previous pregnancy, Dubin-Johnson syndrome, Rotor syndrome; severe cardiac or severe renal disease; existing or previous thromboembolic processes; sickle-cell anaemia; suspected or existing hormone-dependent disorders or tumours; tumours of the uterus or breast; undiagnosed irregular vaginal bleeding; congenital disturbances of lipid metabolism; a history of herpes gestationis; otosclerosis with deterioration in previous pregnancies; endometriosis; severe diabetes with vascular changes; hypersensitivity to any of the ingredients.

*Special warnings and special precautions for use:* Before starting treatment, pregnancy must be excluded. If the expected bleeding fails to occur at about 28-day intervals, treatment should be stopped until pregnancy has been ruled out.

Before starting Nuvelle TS, patients should have a thorough general medical and gynaecological examination with special emphasis on the body weight, blood pressure, heart, pelvic organs with an endometrial assessment if indicated, the legs and skin. Follow-up examinations are recommended at least six-monthly during treatment. Women on therapy should have regular breast examinations and be instructed in self-breast examination. Regular mammographic investigations should be conducted where considered appropriate.

Treatment should be stopped at once if migrainous or frequent and unusually severe headaches occur for the first time, or if there are other symptoms that are possible prodromata of vascular occlusion e.g. sudden visual disturbances. Consideration should be given to discontinuing treatment before operations (6 weeks beforehand) or following immobilisation.

Treatment should be stopped at once if jaundice, cholestasis, hepatitis or pregnancy occurs, or if there is a significant rise in blood pressure, the occurrence of thromboembolic disease or an increase in epileptic seizures.

There is an increased risk of gall bladder disease in women receiving postmenopausal oestrogens.

Pre-existing fibroids may increase in size under the influence of oestrogens. If this is observed, treatment should be discontinued.

In patients with mild chronic liver disease, liver function should be checked every 8-12 weeks. Results of liver function tests may be affected by HRT.

Breakthrough bleeding may occasionally occur and can be the result of poor compliance or concurrent antibiotic use. It may however indicate endometrial pathology and therefore any doubt as to its cause is an indication for endometrial evaluation, including biopsy.

There is an increased risk of endometrial hyperplasia and carcinoma associated with unopposed oestrogen administered long term (for more than one year). However, the appropriate addition of a progestogen to the oestrogen regime statistically lowers the risk.

At the present time there is some evidence which suggests a slight increase in the relative risk of breast cancer in postmenopausal women receiving long-term hormone replacement therapy (more than 5 years). It is not known whether concurrent progestogen use influences this risk. Women on long term therapy should have regular breast examinations and should be instructed in self-examination of the breast. Regular mammographic investigation should be conducted where it is considered appropriate.

Thromboembolism has been reported in connection with oestrogen replacement therapy and it should not be used in women with active or a past history of venous thromboembolism.

Diseases that are known to be subject to deterioration during pregnancy (e.g. multiple sclerosis, epilepsy, diabetes, benign breast disease, hypertension, cardiac or renal dysfunction, asthma, tetany, otosclerosis, systemic lupus erythematosus, and melanoma) and women with a strong family history of breast cancer should be carefully observed during treatment.

Oestrogens may cause fluid retention and therefore patients with cardiac or renal dysfunction should be carefully observed.

Most studies indicate that oestrogen replacement therapy has little effect on blood pressure. Some show that it may decrease blood pressure. In addition studies on combined therapy show that the addition of a progestogen also has little effect on blood pressure. Rarely, idiosyncratic hypertension may occur. When oestrogens are administered to hypertensive women, supervision is necessary and blood pressure should be monitored at regular intervals.

In rare cases benign and in even rarer cases malignant liver tumours leading in isolated cases to life-threatening intra-abdominal haemorrhage have been observed after the use of hormonal substances such as those contained in Nuvelle TS. If severe upper abdominal complaints, enlarged liver, or signs of intra-abdominal haemorrhage occur, a liver tumour should be considered in the differential diagnosis.

Nuvelle TS is not suitable for contraception. Therefore where applicable contraception should be practised with non-hormonal methods with the exception of the rhythm and temperature methods.

*Interaction with other medicaments and other forms of interaction:* Hormonal contraception should be stopped when treatment with Nuvelle TS is started and the patient should be advised to take non-hormonal contraceptive precautions if required.

Drugs which induce hepatic microsomal enzyme systems e.g. barbiturates, carbamazepine, phenytoin, rifampicin, accelerate the metabolism of oestrogen/progestogen combinations such as Nuvelle TS and may reduce their efficacy.

Transdermal therapy avoids the first pass hepatic pathway and therefore the degree of such interactions may be reduced.

The requirement for oral antidiabetics or insulin can change as a result of the effect on glucose tolerance.

There are also some laboratory tests that can be influenced by oestrogens, such as tests for glucose tolerance or thyroid function.

*Pregnancy and lactation:* Contra-indicated.

*Effects on ability to drive and use machines:* None known.

*Undesirable effects:* During the first few months of treatment, breakthrough bleeding, spotting and breast tenderness or enlargement can occur. These are usually temporary and normally disappear after continued treatment. Other symptoms known to occur are: skin irritation at the application site; increased appetite; bloating; palpitations; anxiety/depressive symptoms; headache; migraine; dizziness; dyspepsia; leg pains; oedema; hypertension; altered libido; nausea; rashes; vomiting; altered weight; chloasma.

Some women are predisposed to cholestasis during steroid therapy.

*Overdose:* Overdosage is unlikely with this method of administration. There are no specific antidotes, and treatment should be symptomatic. The patch(es) should be removed.

**Pharmacological properties**

*Pharmacodynamic properties:* Nuvelle TS contains estradiol in the Phase I patch (the endogenous female oestrogen) and a mixture of estradiol and the synthetic progestogen, levonorgestrel in the Phase II patch. Estradiol provides hormone replacement during and after the climacteric. The addition of levonorgestrel in the second half of each cycle helps to provide good cycle control and opposes the development of endometrial hyperplasia. Endometrial protection can be achieved with lower plasma levels of levonorgestrel when administered transdermally than with oral administration.

Most studies show that administration of estradiol to post-menopausal women increases serum high density lipoprotein cholesterol (HDL-C) and decreases low density lipoprotein cholesterol (LDL-C). Although epidemiological data are limited such alterations are recognised as potentially protective against the development of arterial disease. A possible attenuation of these effects may occur with the addition of a progestogen. However, at the doses used in Nuvelle TS, the 14 days of combined therapy with estradiol and levonorgestrel have not been observed to be associated with any unwanted lipid effects.

*Pharmacokinetic properties:* Following transdermal administration to man, estradiol is metabolised in the liver with the formation of sulphuric-acid and glucuronic acid esters (conjugated oestrogens) which are excreted in the urine. Levonorgestrel is similarly absorbed metabolised by the liver and excreted in the urine and faeces as glucuronide and sulphate conjugates.

A pharmacokinetic study showed that the mean serum estradiol concentrations in the steady state following application of the Nuvelle TS phase I patch were in the range of 150 to 260 pmol/L.

In a further pharmacokinetic study the Nuvelle TS Phase II patch was shown to result in mean plasma concentrations of estradiol in the range of 80 to 140 pmol/L, and levonorgestrel concentrations in the range of 50 to 210 pg/ml.

*Preclinical safety data:* Estradiol and levonorgestrel have a long history of safe clinical use in humans and therefore further animal toxicology studies were not considered necessary.

Nuvelle TS contains a number of other constituents including an adhesive copolymer which is unlikely to be absorbed. Therefore neither local nor systemic toxicity would be expected. The patches also contain diethyltoluamide as a residual solvent at a low concentration which is unlikely to result in any local or systemic toxicity.

Dermal irritancy studies in human volunteers have confirmed that Nuvelle TS is well tolerated by human skin and does not possess significant sensitising potential.

**Pharmaceutical particulars**

*List of excipients:* Acrylic adhesive, diethyltoluamide, polyester backing.

*Incompatibilities:* Not applicable.

*Shelf-life:* Two years

*Special precautions for storage:* Keep the patches in their individual blister packs until just before use.
Store below 25°C in a dry place.
Store all drugs properly and keep them out of the reach of children.

*Nature and contents of container:* Each carton contains four Phase I patches and four Phase II patches and a patient information booklet. Each patch is contained in an individual blister pack.

The phase I patch comprises two layers; a clear polyester backing and a matrix of estradiol in an acrylic adhesive. The patch is covered by a protective metallised polyester which must be removed before use.

The phase II patch comprises two layers; a clear polyester backing and a matrix of estradiol and levonorgestrel in an acrylic adhesive. The patch is covered by a protective liner of release coated paper which must be removed before use.

*Instructions for use/handling:* The patch should be used according to the instructions under *Posology and method of administration.*

*Marketing authorisation holder:* Ethical Pharmaceuticals (UK) Ltd., Gemini House, Bartholomew's Walk, Ely, Cambs, CB7 4EA

**Marketing authorisation number** 10013/0036

**Date of approval/revision of SPC** 25 October 1996

**Legal category** POM

## PRIMOLUT N*

**Presentation** Each white, uncoated tablet is impressed with 'AN' in a regular hexagon on one side and contains 5 mg norethisterone BP.

Excipients: lactose, maize starch, magnesium stearate.

**Uses** Metropathia haemorrhagica. Premenstrual syndrome. Postponement of menstruation. Endometriosis. Menorrhagia. Dysmenorrhoea.

A total dose of about 100-150 mg Primolut N (10-15 mg on each of 10 consecutive days) will produce complete secretory transformation of an endometrium that has been subjected to the proliferative effect of oestrogens.

A particular advantage is that menstruation-like withdrawal bleeding occurs consistently two to three days after Primolut N is stopped.

During treatment with Primolut N the basal body temperature rises, as it does under the influence of endogenous progesterone in the second half of the menstrual cycle.

**Dosage and administration** The use of Primolut N is restricted to patients in whom there is no possibility of early pregnancy in the cycle concerned.

*Metropathia haemorrhagica (dysfunctional uterine bleeding):* 1 tablet 3 times daily for 10 days. Bleeding is arrested usually within 1-3 days. A withdrawal bleeding resembling normal menstruation occurs within 2-4 days after discontinuing treatment.

*Prophylaxis against recurrence of dysfunctional bleeding:* If there are no signs of resumption of normal ovarian function (no rise in the second half of the cycle of the morning temperature, which should be measured daily) recurrence must be anticipated. Cyclical bleeding can be established with 1 tablet twice daily from the 19th to the 26th day of the cycle.

*Premenstrual syndrome (including premenstrual mastalgia):* Premenstrual symptoms such as headache, migraine, breast discomfort, water retention, tachycardia and psychological disturbances may be relieved by the administration of 2-3 tablets daily from the 19th to the 26th day of the cycle. Treatment should be repeated for several cycles. When treatment is stopped, the patient may remain symptom-free for a number of months.

*Postponement of menstruation:* In cases of too frequent menstrual bleeding, and in special circumstances (e.g. travel, sports) the postponement of menstruation is possible. 1 tablet Primolut N three times daily, starting 3 days before the expected onset of menstruation. A normal period should occur 2-3 days after the patient has stopped taking tablets.

*Endometriosis* (pseudo-pregnancy therapy): Long-term treatment is commenced on the 5th day of the cycle with 2 tablets Primolut N daily for the first few weeks. In the event of spotting, the dosage is increased to 4, and, if necessary, 5 tablets daily.

After bleeding has ceased, the initial dose is usually sufficient. Duration of treatment: 4-6 months continuously, or longer if necessary.

*Menorrhagia* (hypermenorrhoea): 1 tablet 2-3 times a day from the 19th to the 26th day of the cycle (counting the first day of menstruation as day 1).

*Dysmenorrhoea:* Functional or primary dysmenorrhoea is almost invariably relieved by the suppression of ovulation. 1 tablet three times daily for 20 days, starting on the fifth day of the cycle (the first day of menstruation counting as day 1). Treatment should be maintained for three to four cycles followed by treatment-free cycles. A further course of therapy may be employed if symptoms return.

*Note:* If menstrual bleeding should fail to follow a course of Primolut N, the possibility of pregnancy must be ruled out before a further course is given.

**Contra-indications, warnings, etc**

*Contra-indications:* Pregnancy. Severe disturbances of liver function. Dubin-Johnson and Rotor syndromes. Previous or existing liver tumours. History during pregnancy of idiopathic jaundice, severe pruritus or herpes gestationis. Current thromboembolic processes.

*Reasons for immediate discontinuation of the tablets:* Occurrence for the first time of migrainous headaches or more frequent occurrence of unusually severe headaches, sudden perceptual disorders (e.g. disturbances of vision or hearing), first signs of thrombophlebitis or thromboembolic symptoms, a feeling of pain and tightness in the chest, pending operations

(six weeks beforehand), immobilisation (for instance, following accidents), onset of jaundice, hepatitis, general pruritus, significant rise in blood pressure, pregnancy.

*Warnings:* There is a general opinion, based on statistical evidence that users of combined oral contraceptives experience, more often than non-users, venous thromboembolism, arterial thrombosis, including cerebral and myocardial infarction, and subarachnoid haemorrhage. Full recovery from such disorders does not always occur, and it should be realised that in a few cases they are fatal. Although Primolut N does not contain oestrogen, one should keep the possibility of an increased thromboembolic risk in mind, particularly where there is a history of thromboembolic disease or in the presence of severe diabetes with vascular changes or sickle-cell anaemia.

Primolut N can influence carbohydrate metabolism. Parameters of carbohydrate metabolism should be examined carefully in all diabetics before and regularly during treatment.

In rare cases benign and, in even rarer cases, malignant liver tumours leading in isolated cases to life-threatening intra-abdominal haemorrhage, have been observed after the use of hormonal substances such as the one contained in Primolut N. If severe upper abdominal complaints, liver enlargement or signs of intra-abdominal haemorrhage occur, a liver tumour should be considered in the differential diagnosis.

*Side-effects:* Rarely occur in doses of 15 mg daily. Amongst those recorded are slight nausea, exacerbation of epilepsy and migraine. With extremely high dosage there may be cholestatic liver changes.

*Overdosage:* There have been no reports of ill-effects from overdosage and treatment is generally unnecessary.

There are no special antidotes, and treatment should be symptomatic.

**Pharmaceutical precautions** Shelf-life–Five years.

**Legal category** POM

**Package quantities** Packs containing 3 x 10-tablet blisters.

**Further information** Nil.

**Product licence number** 0053/5033R

## PROGYNOVA* 1MG
## PROGYNOVA* 2MG

**Presentation** Progynova 1 mg: Each beige, sugar-coated tablet contains 1 mg of oestradiol valerate. Progynova 2 mg: Each pale blue, sugar-coated tablet contains 2 mg of oestradiol valerate.

Excipients: lactose, maize starch, povidone 25 000, talc, magnesium stearate, sucrose, povidone 700 000, polyethylene glycol 6000, calcium carbonate, titanium dioxide, glycerol 85%, montan glycol wax, ferric oxide pigment, indigo carmine.

**Uses** In menopausal women who have previously undergone a hysterectomy:

*Progynova 1 mg and 2 mg:* Hormone replacement therapy for the treatment of the climacteric syndrome.

*Progynova 2 mg:* Prophylaxis of osteoporosis in women at risk of developing fractures.

Epidemiological studies suggest a number of risk factors may contribute to postmenopausal osteoporosis including: early menopause (either natural or surgically induced); family history of osteoporosis; recent corticosteroid therapy; a small frame; thin; cigarette consumption.

**Dosage and administration**

*Progynova 1 mg and Progynova 2 mg:*

*Climacteric syndrome:* One tablet of Progynova 1 mg or Progynova 2 mg to be taken daily.

For maintenance the lowest effective dose should be used.

*Progynova 2 mg: Prophylaxis of osteoporosis:* One tablet of Progynova 2 mg to be taken daily. For maximum prophylactic benefit, treatment should commence as soon as possible after onset of the menopause. Bone mineral density measurements may help to confirm the presence of low bone mass.

Treatment is continuous. The next pack follows immediately without a break.

**Contra-indications, warnings, etc**

*Contra-indications:* Severe disturbances of liver function, previous or existing liver tumours, jaundice or general pruritus during a previous pregnancy, Dubin Johnson syndrome, Rotor syndrome, existing or previous thromboembolic processes, sickle-cell anaemia, suspected or existing hormone-dependent disorders or tumours of the breast, congenital disturbances of lipid metabolism, endometriosis, severe diabetes with vascular changes, otosclerosis with

deterioration in previous pregnancies, mastopathy, history of herpes gestationis.

*Warnings/side-effects:* In women with an intact uterus, prolonged exposure to unopposed oestrogens increases the risk of the development of endometrial carcinoma. However, the addition of 12 days progestogen towards the end of the cycle reduces the possibility of such a risk.

During the first few months of treatment, breast tenderness or enlargement can occur. These are usually temporary and normally disappear after continued treatment. Other symptoms known to occur are: anxiety, increased appetite, abdominal pain and bloating, palpitations, depressive symptoms, headache, dizziness, epistaxis, dyspepsia, flatulence, leg pains, oedema, altered libido, nausea, vomiting, hypertension, rashes, thrombophlebitis, mucous vaginal discharge, general pruritus, altered weight.

Some women are predisposed to cholestasis during steroid therapy.

Diseases that are known to be subject to deterioration during pregnancy (e.g. multiple sclerosis, epilepsy, diabetes, benign breast disease, hypertension, cardiac or renal dysfunction, asthma, porphyria, tetany and otosclerosis) and women with a strong family history of breast cancer should be carefully observed during treatment.

*Precautions and special information:* Before starting Progynova, patients should have a thorough general medical and gynaecological examination with special emphasis on the body weight, blood pressure, heart, breasts, pelvic organs, the legs and skin. Follow-up examinations are recommended at least six-monthly during treatment.

Treatment should be stopped at once if migrainous or frequent and unusually severe headaches occur for the first time, or if there are any other symptoms that are possible prodromata of vascular occlusion.

Treatment should also be stopped if trauma, illness or impending surgery is considered to entail a risk of thrombosis.

Treatment should be stopped at once if jaundice occurs, if there is a significant rise in blood-pressure or the occurrence of thromboembolic disease, or an increase in epileptic seizures.

In patients with mild chronic liver disease, liver function should be checked every 8-12 weeks.

At the present time, there is some evidence which suggests a slight increase in the relative risk of breast cancer in postmenopausal women receiving long-term hormone replacement therapy. A careful appraisal of the risk/benefit ratio should be undertaken before treating for longer than 5 to 10 years.

Thromboembolism has been reported in connection with oestrogen replacement therapy but there is no evidence to date that the overall incidence is increased.

In rare cases benign, and in even rarer cases, malignant liver tumours leading in isolated cases to life-threatening intra-abdominal haemorrhage have been observed after the use of hormonal substances such as those contained in Progynova. A hepatic tumour should be considered in the differential diagnosis if upper abdominal pain, enlarged liver or signs of intra-abdominal haemorrhage occur.

*Interaction with other drugs:* Drugs which induce hepatic microsomal enzyme systems e.g barbiturates, phenytoin, rifampicin accelerate the metabolism of oestrogen products such as Progynova and may reduce their efficacy. The requirement for oral antidiabetics or insulin can change.

*Overdosage:* There have been no reports of ill-effects from overdosage, which it is, therefore, generally unnecessary to treat.

There are no specific antidotes, and treatment should be symptomatic.

**Pharmaceutical precautions** None.

Shelf-life: Progynova 1 mg – Five years. Progynova 2 mg – Five years.

**Legal category** POM

**Package quantities** Packs containing 3 x 28 tablet memo-strips

**Further information** Most studies show that oral administration of oestradiol valerate to post-menopausal women increases serum high density lipoprotein cholesterol (HDL-C) and decreases low density lipoprotein cholesterol (LDL-C). Although epidemiological data are limited, such alterations are recognised as potentially protective against the development of arterial disease.

**Product licence numbers**
Progynova 1 mg 0053/0057
Progynova 2 mg 0053/0058

## PROGYNOVA *TS
## PROGYNOVA *TS FORTE

**Qualitative and quantitative composition** Estradiol (oestradiol) transdermal systems:

Progynova TS: 12.5 cm² patch contains 3.9 mg of estradiol. Progynova TS forte: 25.0 cm² patch contains 7.8 mg of estradiol.

Nominal average absorption rates of 50 micrograms/day and 100 micrograms/day were calculated for Progynova TS and Progynova TS Forte respectively.

**Pharmaceutical form** Transdermal delivery system comprising a patch containing estradiol in an acrylate adhesive matrix. The transdermal delivery from a patch is maintained over 7 days.

The active component of the system is estradiol. The remaining components of the system are pharmacologically inactive.

### Clinical particulars

*Therapeutic indications:* Oestrogen replacement therapy for patients with disorders due to natural menopause or surgically induced menopause (only if due to noncarcinomatous diseases) e.g. vasomotor symptoms (hot flushes, sweating), atrophic conditions (such as atrophic vaginitis/vulvitis, and/or atrophic urethritis, trigonitis) caused by deficient endogenous oestrogen production.

*Posology and method of administration: Adults (including the elderly):* Treatment should be initiated with Progynova TS. If considered necessary, Progynova TS forte should be used. Once treatment is established the lowest effective dose necessary for the relief of symptoms should be used.

Treatment can be given either continuously or on a cyclical basis.

Unopposed oestrogen therapy should not be used unless the patient has had a hysterectomy. Where a progestogen is considered necessary the appropriate dose should be administered for 12 days in every month.

The patches should be applied once weekly on a continuous basis, each used system being removed after 7 days and a fresh system applied to a different site. Recommended application sites are clean, dry and intact areas of skin on the trunk and buttocks. Progynova TS and Progynova TS forte should not be applied on or near the breasts.

The patches may also be prescribed on a cyclical basis. Where this is the preferred option, the patches should be applied weekly for 3 consecutive weeks followed by a 7 day interval, without a patch being applied, before the next course.

*Children:* Not recommended for children

*Contra-indications:* Pregnancy; lactation; severe disturbances of liver function (including porphyria); previous or existing liver tumours; Rotor syndrome; Dubin-Johnson syndrome; severe cardiac, severe renal disease; jaundice or general pruritus during a previous pregnancy; existing or previous thromboembolic processes; sickle cell anaemia; severe diabetes with vascular changes; suspected or existing hormone dependent disorders or tumours of the uterus, breast or ovaries; undiagnosed irregular vaginal bleeding; disturbances of lipid metabolism; a history of herpes gestationis; otosclerosis with deterioration in previous pregnancies; endometriosis; hypersensitivity to any of the ingredients.

*Special warnings and special precautions for use:* Before starting treatment pregnancy must be excluded. Prior to treatment, patients should have a thorough general medical and gynaecological examination with special emphasis on the body weight, blood pressure, heart, pelvic organs with an endometrial assessment if indicated, the legs and skin. Follow-up examinations are recommended at least six-monthly during treatment.

Women on therapy should have regular breast examinations and be instructed in self-breast examination. Regular mammographic investigations should be conducted where considered appropriate.

Treatment should be stopped at once if migrainous or frequent and unusually severe headaches occur for the first time, or if there are other symptoms that are possible prodromata of vascular occlusion, e.g. sudden visual disturbances.

Consideration should be given to discontinuing treatment before operations (6 weeks beforehand) or following immobilisation.

There is an increased risk of gall bladder disease in women receiving postmenopausal oestrogens.

Treatment should be stopped at once if jaundice, cholestasis, hepatitis or pregnancy occurs, or if there is a significant rise in blood pressure, the occurrence of thromboembolic disease or an increase in epileptic seizures.

If there is, repeatedly, persistent skin irritation despite application sites being changed according to directions, consideration should be given to discontinuing transdermal treatment.

Pre-existing fibroids may increase in size during oestrogen therapy. If this is observed treatment should be discontinued. In women with an intact uterus, prolonged exposure to unopposed oestrogens increases the risk of the development of endometrial carcinoma. However, the addition of 12 days progestogen towards the end of the month reduces the possibility of such a risk. If irregular bleeding occurs repeatedly during the use of Progynova TS or Progynova TS forte this should be investigated by endometrial biopsy, if necessary.

At the present time there is some evidence which suggests a slight increase in the relative risk of breast cancer in post-menopausal women receiving long-term hormone replacement therapy. A careful appraisal of the risk/benefit ratio should be undertaken before treating for longer than 5 years. Thromboembolism has been reported in connection with oestrogen replacement therapy but there is no evidence to date that the overall incidence is increased.

Diseases that are known to be subject to deterioration during pregnancy (e.g. multiple sclerosis, epilepsy, diabetes, benign breast disease, varicose veins, hypertension, cardiac, hepatic or renal dysfunction, migraine, asthma, chorea minor, tetany and otosclerosis) and women with a strong family history of breast cancer should be carefully observed during treatment.

In rare cases benign, and in even rarer cases, malignant liver tumours leading in isolated cases to life threatening intra-abdominal haemorrhage have been observed after the use of hormonal substances such as those contained in Progynova TS and Progynova TS forte. A hepatic tumour should be considered in the differential diagnosis if upper abdominal pain, enlarged liver, or signs of intra-abdominal haemorrhage occur.

*Interaction with other medicaments and other forms of interaction:* Drugs which induce hepatic microsomal enzyme systems, e.g. barbiturates, carbamazepine, phenytoin, rifampicin, accelerate the metabolism of oestrogens, reducing systemic bioavailability and thus, efficacy. However, it is probable that the transdermally applied oestrogens are less affected by such an interaction than oral oestrogens. The requirement for oral antidiabetics or insulin can change as a result of the effect on glucose tolerance.

There are also some laboratory tests that can be influenced by oestrogens, such as the tests for glucose tolerance or thyroid function.

*Pregnancy and lactation:* Progynova TS and Progynova TS forte are contraindicated during pregnancy and lactation.

*Effects on ability to drive and use machines:* Not applicable.

*Undesirable effects:* Hormonal contraception should be stopped when the use of Progynova TS and Progynova TS forte is started and the patient should be advised to take non-hormonal contraceptive precautions if required. During the first few months of treatment, breakthrough bleeding, spotting and breast tenderness or enlargement can occur. These are usually temporary and normally disappear after continued treatment. Other symptoms known to occur are: skin irritation at the application site; in individual cases an allergic contact dermatitis with post-inflammatory pruritus and generalised exanthema; nausea; abdominal pain; bloating; headache; migraine; anxiety/depressive symptoms; dizziness; alterations in body weight; oedema; hypertension; altered libido; changes in vaginal secretion; growth of pre-existing fibroids; chloasma or melasma which may be persistent. Some women are predisposed to cholestasis during steroid therapy.

*Overdose:* Overdosage is unlikely with this type of application. Nausea, vomiting and withdrawal bleeding may occur in some women. There is no specific antidote and treatment should be symptomatic. The patch(es) should be removed.

### Pharmacological properties

*Pharmacodynamic properties:* The loss of the ovarian function, accompanied by a depletion of oestrogen production, leads to the menopausal syndrome, characterised by vasomotoric-vegetative, and organic symptoms. Hormone replacement therapy aims to eliminate these complaints. Of all physiological oestrogens, estradiol is the most potent one with the highest affinity for the oestrogen receptor. In the oestrogen sensitive target organs, in particular uterus, hypothalamus, pituitary, vagina, urethra, breast, bones (osteoclasts) estradiol exerts its effects, as other steroid hormones, by regulating the transcription of a limited number of genes. After diffusion through the cell membrane, estradiol binds with high affinity to the oestrogen receptor. After activation by the estradiol ligand the hormone receptor complex is translocated into the nucleus where it binds to specific DNA sequences (hormone response elements) that enhance the transcription of adjacent genes. The full number of proteins induced by oestrogen is not known but is estimated to be 50 to 100.

After the menopause the production of estradiol in the female is substantially reduced. The remaining estradiol is mainly synthesised from precursors produced in the adrenal cortex, by aromatisation from androstenedione and to a lesser extent from testosterone by the enzyme aromatase thus forming estrone and estradiol, respectively. Estrone is converted into estradiol via the enzyme 17-hydroxysteriod-dehydrogenase. Both enzymes have been found in the liver and in fat and muscle tissue. The estradiol/estrone ratio in postmenopausal women is approximately 0.2 compared to a ratio of >1 in premenopausal women.

Climacteric disturbances can be treated by oestrogen replacement therapy with mean transdermal doses between 25 and 100 micrograms estradiol per day.

Independent of the route of administration, oestrogen doses, which are necessary for improvement of menopausal complaints, exert a dose dependent stimulating effect on mitosis and proliferation of the endometrium. Oestrogen monotherapy increases the frequency of endometrial hyperplasia and thus the risk of endometrial carcinoma. In order to avoid endometrial hyperplasia the sequential administration of a progestin for 10–12 days is recommended in non-hysterectomised postmenopausal women.

*Pharmacokinetic properties:* The therapy with the once-a-week Progynova TS or Progynova TS forte system is comparable to a continuous low dose intravenous infusion aiming at smooth, stable, plateau-like estradiol serum levels similar to those during the early/mid follicular phase during the reproductive life span. Transdermal administration avoids highly fluctuating estradiol and metabolite levels in the serum seen after oral estradiol substitution and avoids also an inundation of the liver with large amounts of estradiol and its metabolites due to a high presystemic metabolisation of the compound ("first-pass effect") after oral intake. Thus, after transdermal administration of estradiol, no effects on liver protein synthesis have been observed.

During a once-a-week application regimen of Progynova TS or Progynova TS forte, smooth and consistent estradiol and estrone serum level profiles within the desired range are achieved. No accumulation of either substance is observed following multiple 1-week patch applications. The absolute height of the estradiol serum level profile is directly proportional to the area of the patch with mean steady state estradiol serum levels in the range of 35 pg/ml after application of the 12.5 cm² patch and those in the range of approximately 70 pg/ml after application of the 25 cm² patch.

After transdermal administration, the metabolisation of estradiol to estrone and conjugates remains within the physiological range as seen during the early follicular phase in the reproductive life period indicated by an estradiol/estrone serum level ratio of approximately 1. Unphysiologically high estrone levels as a result of the intensive "first pass" metabolisation during oral estradiol hormone replacement therapy, reflected in estradiol/estrone ratios as low as 0.1, are avoided.

The biotransformation and the excretion of the transdermally administered estradiol are the same as that of the endogenous hormone. Estradiol is eliminated from the body with a total serum clearance of approximately 15–30 ml/min/kg by biotransformation mainly in the liver but also extrahepatically, eg. in gut, kidney, skeletal muscles and target organs. These processes involve the formation of estrone, estriol, catecholoestrogens and sulphate and glucuronide conjugates of these compounds, which are all distinctly less oestrogenic or even nonoestrogenic. A certain proportion of estradiol metabolites are excreted in the bile and undergo a so-called enterohepatic circulation. Ultimately estradiol metabolites are mainly excreted as sulphates and glucuronides with the urine.

*Preclinical safety data:* In primary dermal irritation studies, application of Progynova TS or Progynova TS forte resulted in mild irritation related to mechanical trauma at removal. In sensitisation studies, Progynova TS or Progynova TS forte had no dermal sensitising potential.

The components of the adhesive matrix of Progynova TS or Progynova TS forte (monomer and polymer) have been studied extensively and, at many multiples of the projected human exposure, present a low risk. Additional excipients used in the adhesive matrix are either generally regarded as safe for use in food components or considered acceptable as an inactive ingredient for prescription and topical transdermal products.

The adhesive backing and release liner of Progynova TS or Progynova TS forte were tested in biological test methods and were considered to be compatible with biologic systems.

### Pharmaceutical particulars

*List of excipients:* Ethyl oleate, isopropyl myristate, glycerol monolaurate. The adhesive system is an acrylate copolymer.

*Incompatibilities:* None so far known.

*Shelf life:* 2 years.

*Special precautions for storage:* Do not store unpouched. Apply immediately upon removal from the protective pouch.

*Nature and contents of container:* Protective pouch containing a Progynova TS patch with a surface area of 12.5 cm² or a Progynova TS forte patch with a surface area of 25 cm². The patches comprise two layers. From the visible surface to the surface attached to the skin these are: a translucent polyethylene film; a drug reservoir of estradiol in an acrylate adhesive matrix; a protective liner of release-coated polyester film is attached to the adhesive surface and must be removed prior to use. The protective pouch contains a desiccant.

Packs containing 4 patches.

Packs containing 12 patches.

*Instructions for use/handling:* The patch should be used according to the instructions under "Posology and method of administration". Store all drugs properly and keep them out of the reach of children.

**Marketing authorisation numbers**

Progynova TS: 0053 / 0241

Progynova TS forte: 0053/0242

**Date of approval/revision of SPC** June 1996

**Legal category** POM

## PROLUTON*DEPOT

**Presentation** Hydroxyprogesterone hexanoate BP 250 mg and 500 mg in ampoules for intramuscular injection.

Excipients: Benzyl benzoate, castor oil

**Uses** Habitual abortion, when associated with proven progesterone-deficiency.

**Dosage and administration** 250-500 mg Proluton Depot by intramuscular injection at weekly intervals during the first half of pregnancy.

**Contra-indications, warnings etc**

*Contra-indications:* A history of herpes gestationis. Previous or existing liver tumours.

*Warnings:* Many medicinal products, including female sex hormones, have been suspected of being capable of affecting the normal development of a child in the early stages of pregnancy. Many researchers consider that in relation to sex hormones such a suspicion is ill founded but one has to accept that for no medicinal product can teratogenic activity be excluded with absolute certainty. Therefore, the general principle is now widely accepted that inessential use of drugs during pregnancy should be avoided. Following this general principle, Proluton Depot should be used to maintain pregnancy only if it is strictly indicated, i.e. if there is an urgent desire to have a child, and luteal insufficiency is present.

Since Proluton Depot may prevent spontaneous evacuation of a dead foetus (missed abortion) the progress of the pregnancy should be regularly monitored by appropriate means, including immunological tests.

Proluton Depot can influence carbohydrate metabolism. Parameters of carbohydrate metabolism should be examined carefully in all diabetics before and regularly during treatment. The requirement for oral antidiabetics or insulin can change.

In rare cases benign and, in even rarer cases, malignant liver tumours leading in isolated cases to life-threatening intra-abdominal haemorrhage, have been observed after the use of hormonal substances such as the one contained in Proluton Depot. If severe upper abdominal complaints, liver enlargement or signs of intra-abdominal haemorrhage occur, a liver tumour should be considered in the differential diagnosis.

*Side-effects:* Very rarely, local reactions may occur at the site of injection. In rare cases coughing, dyspnoea and circulatory irregularities may occur during or immediately after the injection. Experience has shown that these reactions can be avoided by injecting very slowly.

*Overdosage:* There have been no reports of serious ill-effects from overdosage, which is unlikely to occur with intramuscular administration.

**Pharmaceutical precautions** Protect from light. Shelf-life – Five years.

**Legal category** POM

**Package quantities** 250 mg: Packs of 3 ampoules 1 ml

500 mg: Packs of 3 ampoules 2 ml.

**Further information** Nil

**Product licence numbers**

Proluton Depot 250 mg 0053/5031R

Proluton Depot 500 mg 0053/5032R

## PRO-VIRON*

**Qualitative and quantitative composition** Each tablet contains 25 mg mesterolone.

**Pharmaceutical form** Tablets.

**Clinical particulars**

*Therapeutic indications:* Androgen deficiency or male infertility when associated with primary or secondary male hypogonadism.

*Posology and method of administration:* The following dosages are recommended:

*Adults:* Initially: 3 or 4 tablets daily for several months, followed by maintenance therapy of 2-3 tablets (50-75 mg) daily.

*Children:* Not recommended in children.

*Contra-indications:* Pro-Viron is contra-indicated in the presence of prostatic carcinoma since androgens can stimulate the growth of an existing carcinoma.

Previous or existing liver tumours.

*Special warnings and special precautions for use:* Androgens are not suitable for enhancing muscular development in healthy individuals or for increasing physical ability. Regular examination of the prostate during treatment is advised, in order to exclude prostatic carcinoma. In rare cases benign, and in even rarer cases, malignant liver tumours leading in isolated cases to life-threatening intra-abdominal haemorrhage have been observed after the use of hormonal substances such as the one contained in Pro–Viron. If severe upper abdominal complaints, liver enlargement or signs of intra-abdominal haemorrhage occur, the possibility of a liver tumour should be included in the differential diagnosis.

Frequent or persistent erections of the penis may occur (see *Undesirable effects*).

*Interaction with other medicaments and other forms of interaction:* None known.

*Pregnancy and lactation:* Not applicable.

*Effects on ability to drive and use machines:* None known.

*Undesirable effects:* If, in individual cases, frequent or persistent erections occur, the dose should be discontinued in order to avoid injury to the penis.

*Overdose:* There have been no reports of ill-effects from overdosage and treatment is generally unncessary. If overdosage is discovered within two to three hours and is so large that treatment seems desirable, gastric lavage can safely be used.

**Pharmacological properties**

*Pharmacodynamic properties:* Pro-Viron is an orally active androgen. The presence of a methyl group at C-1 confers special properties on this steroid which, unlike testosterone and all its derivatives that are used for androgen therapy, is not metabolised to oestrogen.

This difference almost certainly accounts for the observation that, in its usual therapeutic dosage in normal men, Pro-Viron does not significantly depress the release of gonadotrophins from the pituitary. Hence (1) spermatogenesis is unimpaired (2) unlike other androgens, which suppress and therefore replace endogenous androgens, Pro-Viron supplements endogenous androgens.

In contrast to other orally active androgens, liver tolerance is excellent (a fact probably related to the absence of 17-alkyl substitution of the steroid nucleus).

*Pharmacokinetic properties:* Following oral ingestion mesterolone is rapidly and almost completely absorbed in a wide dose range of 25–100 mg. The intake of Pro-Viron generates maximum serum drug levels of $3.1 \pm 1.1$ ng/ml after $1.6 \pm 0.6$ hours. Thereafter, drug levels in serum decrease with a terminal half-life of 12–13 hours. Mesterolone is 98% bound to serum proteins, 40% to albumin and 58% to SHBG (sex hormone binding globulin).

Mesterolone is rapidly inactivated by metabolism. The metabolic clearance rate from serum accounts for $4.4 \pm 1.6$ $ml \cdot min^{-1} \cdot kg^{-1}$. There is no renal excretion of unchanged drug. The main metabolite has been identified as 1α-methyl-androsterone, which–in conjugated form–accounts for 55–70 % of renally excreted metabolites. The ratio of the main metabolite glucuronide to sulphate is about 12:1. A further metabolite 1α-methyl-5α-androstane-3α,17β-diol has been recognized, which accounted for about 3 % of renally eliminated metabolites. No metabolic conversion into oestrogens or corticoids has been observed. 77% of the mesterolone metabolites are excreted via the urine and 13% with the faeces. 50% of the dose is excreted in the urine within 24 hours and 90% within 7 days via the faeces and urine.

The absolute bioavailability of mesterolone is about 3 % of the oral dose.

*Preclinical safety data:* There are no preclinical data which could be of relevance to the prescriber and which are not already included in other relevant sections of the SPC.

**Pharmaceutical particulars**

*List of excipients:* Lactose, maize starch, povidone 25 000 (E1201), methyl parahydroxybenzoate (E218), propyl parahydroxybenzoate (E216), magnesium stearate (E572)

*Incompatibilities:* None known.

*Shelf-life:* 5 years.

*Special precautions for storage:* None

*Nature and contents of container:* 3 blister packs of 10 tablets contained in a cardboard outer pack.

*Instructions for use/handling:* Store all drugs properly and keep them out of reach of children.

**Marketing authorisation number** 0053/0030

**Date of approval/revision of SPC** 1 April 1997

**Legal category** CD (Sch.4, Part I),POM

## SCHERING PC4*

**Presentation** Four white sugar-coated tablets, each containing 250 micrograms levonorgestrel (in 500 micrograms dl-norgestrel) and 50 micrograms ethinyloestradiol.

Excipients: lactose, maize starch, povidone 25 000, talc, magnesium stearate, sucrose, povidone 700 000, polyethylene glycol 6000, calcium carbonate, montan glycol wax.

**Uses** Post-coital contraception within 72 hours of unprotected coitus as an occasional emergency measure. Schering PC4 is primarily aimed to prevent implantation of the fertilised ovum in the endometrium.

**Dosage and Administration** The first two tablets should be taken as soon as possible after coitus (up to a maximum of 72 hours afterwards) and the remaining two tablets twelve hours after the first two.

**Contra-indications, warnings, etc**

*Contra-indications:* Pregnancy. Therapy should not be administered in the following circumstances, as pregnancy may already have occurred:

(a) where menstrual bleeding is overdue, and

(b) where the patient has already had unprotected intercourse more than 72 hours previously in the present menstrual cycle.

*Other contra-indications:*

Thrombotic disorders and a history of these conditions;

Sickle-cell anaemia;

Disorders of lipid metabolism and other conditions in which, in individual cases, there is known or suspected to be a much increased risk of thrombosis;

Acute or severe chronic liver diseases;

Dubin-Johnson syndrome;

Rotor syndrome;

Previous or existing liver tumours;

History during pregnancy of idiopathic jaundice or severe pruritus;

History of herpes gestationis;

Mammary or endometrial carcinoma, or a history of these conditions;

Abnormal vaginal bleeding of unknown cause;

Deterioration of otosclerosis during pregnancy;

Severe diabetes with vascular changes;

Hypersensitivity to any of the components of Schering PC4.

*Warnings:* The repeated use of Schering PC4 within a single monthly cycle is to be avoided. Schering PC4 does not appear to be as effective as some regularly-used methods of contraception and is suitable only as an occasional emergency measure. Schering PC4 is not effective if started later than 72 hours after coitus and should not be so used.

There is a general opinion, based on statistical evidence, that users of combined oral contraceptives (oestrogen-progestogen combinations like Schering PC4) experience, more often than non-users, venous thromboembolism, arterial thrombosis, including cerebral and myocardial infarction, and subarachnoid haemorrhage. Full recovery from such disorders does not always occur and it should be realised that in a few cases they are fatal.

Certain factors may entail some risk of thrombosis e.g. smoking, obesity, varicose veins, cardiovascular diseases, diabetes and migraine. The suitability of Schering PC4 should be judged according to the severity of such conditions in the individual case, and should be discussed with the patient before she decides to take it. The risk of arterial thrombosis associated with combined oral contraceptives increases with age, and this risk is aggravated by cigarette smoking. Therefore the use of Schering PC4 by women in the older age-group, especially those who are cigarette smokers, should be discouraged. Caution is also advised before Schering PC4 is prescribed if there is a history in the family of thromboembolic disease at a young age (eg. deep vein thrombosis, heart attack or stroke).

*Pregnancy and lactation:* Patients who become pregnant despite post-coital contraception should be carefully evaluated for possible ectopic pregnancy. Since Schering PC4 appears to affect only endometrial implantation, tubal pregnancy may occur at the expected rate, and it is thus possible that there will be a relative increase in ectopic pregnancy in patients who become pregnant despite the use of Schering PC4.

When Schering PC4 is used during lactation, it must be considered that milk production may be reduced. Furthermore, minute amounts of the active substance are eliminated with the milk.

The effect of Schering PC4 on the conceptus in the event of failure to prevent conception is not definitely known. Some investigators have suggested that sex hormones taken in the first trimester of pregnancy may slightly increase the risk of foetal malformations, but numerous other investigators have failed to support these findings. The consensus of opinion amongst teratologists is that even known teratogens will not produce malformations before organogenesis starts, which is much later than the 72 hours after fertilisation to which the use of Schering PC4 is restricted.

*Malabsorption:* Vomiting, severe diarrhoea or other causes of malabsorption might impair the efficacy of Schering PC4.

*Interaction with other drugs:* The efficacy of Schering PC4 might be impaired by interaction with concurrently-used drugs including barbiturates, primidone, phenytoin, carbamazepine, phenylbutazone, griseofulvin, rifampicin, ampicillin and other antibiotics.

The requirement for oral antidiabetics or insulin can change as a result of an effect on glucose tolerance.

*Precautions:* Examination of the pelvic organs, breasts and blood pressure should normally precede the prescribing of any combined oral contraceptive. The following conditions require careful consideration: a history of severe depressive states, diabetes, hypertension, epilepsy, porphyria, tetany, disturbed liver function, gallstones, cardiovascular diseases, renal diseases, otosclerosis, obesity and migraine.

The importance of follow-up and the possibility of an early or late onset of the next period should be explained to the patient. The practice of abstinence or careful use of a barrier method until the onset of the next period should also be advised. Follow-up should be carried out 3 weeks after administration of therapy to assess the effectiveness of the method, to discuss future management if a period has not occurred, and to counsel the patient about future contraception.

*Side-effects:* Nausea and vomiting are common side-effects, and the latter may reduce the efficacy of therapy if it occurs within about 2 hours after the ingestion of either dose of tablets, in which event consideration should be given to the taking of more pills.

The concomitant administration of an anti-emetic has been favoured by some practitioners.

The pattern of menstrual bleeding is often temporarily disturbed. Breast discomfort and headaches also may occur.

*Overdosage:* There have been no reports of serious ill-effects from overdosage. Treatment is symptomatic.

**Pharmaceutical precautions** Shelf-life—Five years

**Legal category** POM

**Package quantities** Single pack of four tablets (OP)

**Further information** Nil

**Product licence number** 0053/0162

## SCHERIPROCT* OINTMENT AND SUPPOSITORIES

### Presentation

*Scheriproct ointment:* A white ointment containing in 1 g:
Prednisolone hexanoate 1.9 mg
Cinchocaine hydrochloride 5.0 mg
  *Excipients:* polyethylene glycol 400 monoricinoleate, castor oil, 2 octyldodecanol, chypre perfume oil.

*Scheriproct suppositories:* Each white suppository contains:
Prednisolone hexanoate 1.3 mg
Cinchocaine hydrochloride 1.0 mg
  *Excipient:* hard fat

**Uses** For the symptomatic relief of haemorrhoids and pruritus ani in the short term (5-7 days).

**Dosage and administration** *Suppositories:* 1 Scheriproct suppository to be inserted daily. In severe cases 1 suppository two to three times daily at the beginning of treatment. The suppositories should be inserted after defaecation.

*Ointment:* Apply in a thin layer twice daily. In order to obtain a rapid improvement, Scheriproct ointment may be applied three to four times on the first day. The nozzle provided facilitates intra-rectal application.

### Contra-indications, warnings etc

*Contra-indications:* Viral infections, primary bacterial or fungal infections in the treatment area. Secondary infections of the skin in the absence of appropriate anti-infective therapy. Known sensitivity to local anaesthetics.

*Warnings/side-effects:* In infants, long-term continuous therapy with topical corticosteroids should be avoided. Occlusion is not appropriate on the perineum. Adrenal suppression can occur, even without occlusion. As with all topical steroids, there is a risk of developing skin atrophy following extensive therapy. The application of unusually large quantities of topical corticoids may result in the absorption of systemically active amounts of corticoid. Infections or secondarily infected dermatoses definitely require additional therapy with antibiotics or chemotherapeutic agents. This treatment can often be topical, but for heavy infections systemic antibacterial therapy may be necessary. If fungal infections are present, a topically active antimycotic should be applied. Allergic skin reactions may occur.

*Pregnancy warning:* There is inadequate evidence of safety in human pregnancy. Topical administration of corticosteroids to pregnant animals can cause abnormalities of foetal development, including cleft palate and intra-uterine growth retardation. There may therefore be a very small risk of such effects on the human foetus.

**Pharmaceutical precautions** In order to restore the consistency of suppositories which have become soft owing to warm temperature, they should be put into cold water before the covering is removed.
*Suppositories:* Store in cool dry conditions.
*Ointment:* No special storage precautions.
*Ointment and Suppositories:* Shelf-life – Five years.

**Legal category** POM

**Further information** Nil

**Package quantities** *Suppositories:* Packs of 12 (OP).
*Ointment:* Tubes of 30 g (OP).

**Product licence numbers**
Scheriproct Suppositories 0053/5001R
Scheriproct Ointment 0053/5002R

## SKINOREN*

**Presentation** Cream 1 g contains 0.2 g (20%) micronized azelaic acid in an oil-in-water emulsion (approximately 51% water).
Excipients: arlatone 983S, cutina CBS, cetearyl octanoate, propylene glycol, benzoic acid, purified water.

**Uses** Topical treatment of acne vulgaris.

**Dosage and administration** Skinoren should be applied to the affected areas twice daily (mornings and evenings), and rubbed in well. Regular use is important.

The duration of use of Skinoren will vary from person to person and also depends on the severity of the acne. In general, a distinct improvement becomes apparent after about 4 weeks. To obtain the best results, Skinoren should be applied over a period of several months but not for more than 6 months.

Patients with sensitive skin should be advised to use Skinoren only once a day (in the evening) for the first week of treatment and then proceed to twice daily applications.

The amount of Skinoren to be applied will depend on the size of the affected area. As a guide, a daily dose of 2 g (1 g per application) will be sufficient for the treatment of the entire facial area (1 g = 4 cm cream).

If other areas of acne, in addition to the face, require treatment, for example the chest and back, a daily dose of 10 g of cream should not, in general, be exceeded.

Before Skinoren is applied, the skin should be thoroughly washed with water alone, or, if necessary, with a mild cleansing agent.

### Contra-indications, warnings etc

*Contra-indications:* Hypersensitivity to propylene glycol.

*Precautions:* For external use only. Avoid contact with eyes. If Skinoren comes into contact with the eyes, they should immediately be thoroughly irrigated with copious amounts of water.

*Side-effects:* Local skin irritation (e.g. erythema, scaling, itching or burning) occurs in occasional cases, usually at the start of treatment. However, in the majority of cases, the irritation is mild and regresses as treatment continues. If marked skin irritation persists, the amount of cream per application should be reduced, the frequency of application should be reduced, or the treatment temporarily interrupted until the symptoms regress. Photosensitivity reactions have been reported very rarely during the use of Skinoren.

*Use during pregnancy and lactation:* There is no evidence of the safety of azelaic acid during human pregnancy or lactation. It is therefore advisable to avoid using Skinoren during pregnancy or lactation unless essential and no suitable alternative treatment is available. Animal studies have however produced no evidence that would suggest any risk to a foetus from use by a pregnant woman.

**Pharmaceutical precautions** Do not store above 30°C. Shelf-life – Five years.

**Legal category** POM

**Package quantities** Tubes containing 30 g.

**Further information** Azelaic acid inhibits the growth of the propionibacteria involved in the development of acne and their production of acne-promoting fatty acids. Azelaic acid also reduces the multiplication of keratinocytes and their keratinization, and therefore restricts the formation of comedones.

**Product licence number** 0053/0207

## TRAVOGYN*

**Qualitative and quantitative composition** 1 vaginal tablet contains 300 mg isoconazole nitrate

**Pharmaceutical form** Vaginal tablet

### Clinical particulars

*Therapeutic indications:* Fungal infections of the vagina including mixed infections with gram-positive bacteria.

*Posolgy and method of administration:* Two vaginal tablets must be inserted together deep into the vagina. This is best done in a lying position. A suitable time for the application would be in the evening just before going to sleep.
Only one application is required.

*Contra-indications:* None known.

*Special warnings and special precautions for use:* Travogyn should not be the treatment of first choice for pure trichomonal infections.

To prevent reinfection, underclothes (preferably cotton), towels and wash cloths (flannels) that have been in contact with the affected area should be changed frequently.

During treatment and in the following week vaginal douching should be avoided.

To prevent reinfection simultaneous prophylactic treatment of the sexual partner should be considered.

*Interaction with other medicaments and other forms of interaction:* None so far known.

*Pregnancy and lactation:* In order to avoid any possibility of adverse effects on the foetus, the general principle is now widely accepted that the administration of drugs to women during pregnancy should, as far as possible, be avoided. However, nothing that is known about the effect of isoconazole nitrate, either from animal experiments, or from clinical experience, suggests that Travogyn therapy should not be used during pregnancy.

Because of only slight absorption (less than 10% of the dose administered) and the short duration of therapy, adverse effects on the baby from isoconazole nitrate transferred with the breast milk are unlikely.

*Effects on ability to drive and use machines:* Not applicable

*Undesirable effects:* Occasionally, during the first 12 to 24 hours, symptoms of intolerance such as burning or itching of the vagina and vulva may occur.

*Overdose:* According to the results from single dose toxicity studies, the active ingredient isoconazole can be classified as virtually non-toxic. Acute intoxication is unlikely after a single overdose or inadvertent oral intake of a complete pack.

### Pharmacological properties

*Pharmacodynamic properties:* Isconazole nitrate, the active constituent of Travogyn, has a fungicidal action upon yeasts and yeast-like fungi (particularly those belonging to *Candida spp* and *Torulopsis glabrata*) in the vulvo-vaginal region, on dermatophytes and upon hyphomycetes. In addition to this antimycotic activity, isoconazole nitrate is also effective against some gram- positive bacteria, including staphylococci, streptococci and micrococci, which may cause secondary infection of inflammatory fungal lesions of the skin. The broad spectrum of action of isoconazole nitrate has been demonstrated in serial dilution tests and in suspension tests.

In serial dilution tests, Travogyn is also effective against trichomonas vaginalis at concentrations of 25 microgram/ml and against *Staphylococcus aureus* after two hours at a concentration of 100 microgram/ml, and after three hours at 10 microgram/ml.

*Pharmacokinetic properties:* Pharmacokinetic investigations conducted with ³H-labelled isoconazole nitrate in healthy test subjects using a single intravaginal administration of the 100 mg tablet or of two 300 mg tablets demonstrated absorption of 5-10%, on the basis of the elimination with the urine and faeces. This indicates a systemic burden of about 0.2 mg/kg after a single 100 mg tablet and of 1.0 mg/kg after two 300 mg tablets.

The rapid elimination of the ³H activity from the body implies that accumulation of the active substance or its metabolites after repeated administration of the tablets is unlikely.

*Preclinical safety data:* An animal study has shown that there is a risk of conjunctival irritation after inadvertent contamination of the eye.

**Pharmaceutical particulars**

*List of excipients:* Lactose, microcrystalline cellulose (E460), magnesium stearate (E572)

*Incompatibilities:* None known.

*Shelf life:* 5 years

*Special precautions for storage:* None
*Nature and contents of container:* PVC and aluminium foil blister unit packs, each containing two Travogyn tablets 300 mg.
    Presentation: Pack size of 1 x 2 tablets

*Instructions for use/handling:* Store all drugs properly and keep them out of reach of children.

**Marketing authorisation number** 0053/0124

**Date of approval/revision of SPC** 24 February 1997

**Legal category** POM

## TRIADENE*

**Presentation** The memo pack holds six beige tablets containing 30 micrograms ethinyloestradiol and 50 micrograms gestodene, five dark brown tablets containing 40 micrograms ethinyloestradiol and 70 micrograms gestodene, and ten white tablets containing 30 micrograms ethinyloestradiol and 100 micrograms gestodene.

All tablets have a lustrous, sugar-coating.

Excipients: lactose, maize starch, povidone 700 000, calcium disodium edetate, magnesium stearate, sucrose, polyethylene glycol 6000, calcium carbonate, talc, montan glycol wax, glycerin, titanium dioxide, brown and yellow ferric oxide pigment.

**Uses** Oral contraception and the recognised gynaecological indications for such oestrogen-progestogen combinations. The mode of action includes the inhibition of ovulation by suppression of the mid-cycle surge of luteinising hormone, the inspissation of cervical mucus so as to constitute a barrier to sperm, and the rendering of the endometrium unreceptive to implantation.

**Dosage and administration**
*First treatment cycle:* 1 tablet daily for 21 days, starting on the first day of the menstrual cycle. Contraceptive protection begins immediately.

*Subsequent cycles:* Tablet taking from the next pack of Triadene is continued after a 7-day interval, beginning on the same day of the week as the first pack.

*Changing from 21-day combined oral contraceptives:* The first tablet of Triadene should be taken on the first day immediately after the end of the previous oral contraceptive course. Additional contraceptive precautions are not required.

*Changing from a combined Every Day pill (28 day tablets):* Triadene should be started after taking the last active tablet from the Every Day Pill pack. The first Triadene tablet is taken the next day. Additional contraceptive precautions are not then required.

*Changing from a progestogen-only pill (POP):* The first tablet of Triadene should be taken on the first day of bleeding, even if a POP has already been taken on that day. Additional contraceptive precautions are not then required. The remaining progestogen-only pills should be discarded.

*Post-partum and post-abortum use:* After pregnancy, oral contraception can be started 21 days after a vaginal delivery, provided that the patient is fully ambulant and there are no puerperal complications. Additional contraceptive precautions will be required for the first 7 days of tablet taking. Since the first post-partum ovulation may precede the first bleeding, another method of contraception should be used in the interval between childbirth and the first course of tablets. After a first-trimester abortion, oral contraception may be started immediately in which case no additional contraceptive precautions are required.

*Pregnancy and lactation:* If pregnancy occurs during medication with oral contraceptives, the preparation should be withdrawn immediately (see 'Reasons for stopping oral contraception immediately').

The use of Triadene during lactation may lead to a reduction in the volume of milk produced and to a change in its composition. Minute amounts of the active substances are excreted with the milk. Mothers who are breast-feeding may be advised instead to use a progestogen-only pill.

*Special circumstances requiring additional contraception:*
*Incorrect administration:* A single delayed tablet should be taken as soon as possible, and if this can be done within 12 hours of the correct time, contraceptive protection is maintained. With longer delays, additional contraception is needed. Only the most recently delayed tablet should be taken, earlier missed tablets being omitted, and additional non-hormonal methods of contraception (except the rhythm or temperature methods) should be used for the next 7 days, while the next 7 tablets are being taken. Additionally, therefore, if tablet(s) have been missed during the last 7 days of a pack, there should be no break before the next pack is started. In this situation, a withdrawal bleed should not be expected until the end of the second pack. Some breakthrough bleeding may occur on tablet taking days but this is not clinically significant. If the patient does not have a withdrawal bleed during the tablet-free interval following the end of the second pack, the possibility of pregnancy must be ruled out before starting the next pack.

*Gastro-intestinal upset:* Vomiting or diarrhoea may reduce the efficacy of oral contraceptives by preventing full absorption. Tablet taking from the current pack should be continued. Additional non-hormonal methods of contraception (except the rhythm or temperature methods) should be used during the gastro-intestinal upset and for 7 days following the upset. If these 7 days overrun the end of a pack, the next pack should be started without a break. In this situation, a withdrawal bleed should not be expected until the end of the second pack. If the patient does not have a withdrawal bleed during the tablet-free interval following the end of the second pack, the possibility of pregnancy must be ruled out before starting the next pack. Other methods of contraception should be considered if the gastro-intestinal disorder is likely to be prolonged.

*Interaction with other drugs:* Hepatic enzyme inducers such as barbiturates, primidone, phenobarbitone, phenytoin, phenylbutazone, rifampicin, carbamazepine and griseofulvin can impair the efficacy of Triadene. For women receiving long-term therapy with hepatic enzyme inducers, another method of contraception should be used. The use of antibiotics may also reduce the efficacy of Triadene, possibly by altering the intestinal flora.

Women receiving short courses of enzyme inducers or broad spectrum antibiotics should take additional, non-hormonal (except rhythm or temperature method) contraceptive precautions during the time of concurrent medication and for 7 days afterwards. If these 7 days overrun the end of a pack, the next pack should be started without a break. In this situation, a withdrawal bleed should not be expected until the end of the second pack. If the patient does not have a withdrawal bleed during the tablet-free interval following the end of the second pack, the possibility of pregnancy must be ruled out before resuming with the next pack. With rifampicin, additional contraceptive precautions should be continued for 4 weeks after treatment stops, even if only a short course was administered.

The requirement for oral antidiabetics or insulin can change as a result of the effect on glucose tolerance.

**Contra-indications, warnings, etc**
*Contra-indications:*
    1. Pregnancy.
    2. Severe disturbances of liver function, jaundice or persistent itching during a previous pregnancy, Dubin-Johnson syndrome, Rotor syndrome, previous or existing liver tumours.
    3. Existing or previous arterial or venous thrombotic or embolic processes, conditions which predispose to them e.g. disorders of the clotting processes, valvular heart disease and atrial fibrillation.
    4. Sickle-cell anaemia.
    5. Mammary or endometrial carcinoma, or a history of these conditions.
    6. Severe diabetes mellitus with vascular changes.
    7. Disorders of lipid metabolism.
    8. History of herpes gestationis.
    9. Deterioration of otosclerosis during pregnancy.
    10. Undiagnosed abnormal vaginal bleeding.
    11. Hypersensitivity to any of the components of Triadene.

*Warnings:* There is a general opinion, based on statistical evidence, that users of combined oral contraceptives experience, more often than non-users, venous thromboembolism, arterial thrombosis, including cerebral and myocardial infarction, and subarachnoid haemorrhage. Full recovery from such disorders does not always occur, and it should be realised that in a few cases they are fatal. How often these disorders occur in users of the modern low-dose pills is not known, but there are reasons for suggesting that they may occur less often than with older pills.

Certain factors may entail some risk of thrombosis, e.g. smoking, obesity, varicose veins, cardiovascular diseases, diabetes, and migraine. The suitability of a combined oral contraceptive should be judged according to the severity of such conditions in the individual case, and should be discussed with the patient before she decides to take it. The risk of arterial thrombosis associated with combined oral contraceptives increases with age, and this risk is aggravated by cigarette-smoking. The use of combined oral contraceptives by women in the older age-group, especially those who are cigarette smokers, should therefore be discouraged and alternative methods used.

In addition if there is a history in the family of thromboembolic diseases at a young age (e.g. deep vein thrombosis, heart attack or stroke) disturbances of the coagulation system must be ruled out before the pill is prescribed.

Numerous epidemiological studies have been reported on the risks of ovarian, endometrial, cervical and breast cancer in women using combined oral contraceptives. The evidence is clear that combined oral contraceptives offer substantial protection against both ovarian and endometrial cancer.

An increased risk of cervical cancer in long-term users of combined oral contraceptives has been reported in some studies, but there continues to be controversy about the extent to which this is attributable to the confounding effects of sexual behaviour and other factors.

The evidence linking the use of combined oral contraceptives and breast cancer remains inconclusive. The results of some studies suggest an increased risk of breast cancer presenting below the age of about 35, the risk rising with duration of use. Any possible increased risk of breast cancer with combined oral contraceptives is however likely to be small, and may be expected to be less with low-dosage pills. This possible risk should be weighed against the many benefits of combined oral contraceptives, including their protective effects against ovarian and endometrial cancers.

The possibility cannot be ruled out that certain chronic diseases may occasionally deteriorate during the use of combined oral contraceptives (see 'Precautions').

The combination of ethinyloestradiol and gestodene, like other contraceptive steroids, is associated with an increased incidence of neoplastic nodules in the rat liver, the relevance of which to man is unknown. Malignant liver tumours have been reported on rare occasions in long-term users of oral contraceptives.

In rare cases benign and, in even rarer cases, malignant liver tumours leading in isolated cases to life-threatening intra-abdominal haemorrhage have been observed after the use of hormonal substances such as those contained in Triadene. If severe upper abdominal complaints, liver enlargement or signs of intra-abdominal haemorrhage occur, the possibility of a liver tumour should be included in the differential diagnosis.

*Reasons for stopping oral contraception immediately:*
1. Occurrence for the first time, or exacerbation, of migrainous headaches or unusually frequent or unusually severe headaches.
2. Sudden disturbances of vision or hearing or other perceptual disorders.
3. First signs of thrombophlebitis or thromboembolic symptoms (e.g. unusual pains in or swelling of the leg(s), stabbing pains on breathing or coughing for no apparent reason). Feeling of pain and tightness in the chest.
4. Six weeks before an elective major operation (e.g. abdominal, orthopaedic), any surgery to the legs, medical treatment for varicose veins or prolonged immobilisation, e.g. after accidents or surgery. Do not restart until 2 weeks after full ambulation. In case of emergency surgery, thrombotic prophylaxis is usually indicated e.g. subcutaneous heparin.
5. Onset of jaundice, hepatitis, itching of the whole body.

6. Increase in epileptic seizures.
7. Significant rise in blood pressure.
8. Onset of severe depression.
9. Severe upper abdominal pain or liver enlargement.
10. Clear exacerbation of conditions known to be capable of deteriorating during oral ontraception or pregnancy.
11. Pregnancy is a reason for stopping immediately because it has been suggested by some investigations that oral contraceptives taken in early pregnancy may slightly increase the risk of foetal malformations. Other investigations have failed to support these findings. The possibility therefore cannot be excluded, but it is certain that if a risk exists at all, it is very small.

*Precautions:* Examination of the pelvic organs, breasts and blood-pressure should precede the prescribing of any combined oral contraceptive and should be repeated regularly. The family medical history should be carefully noted and disturbances of the clotting mechanism ruled out if any member of the family has suffered from thromboembolic disease (e.g. deep vein thrombosis, stroke, myocardial infarction) at a young age. Before starting treatment pregnancy must be excluded.

The following conditions require strict medical supervision during medication with oral contraceptives. Deterioration or first appearance of any of these conditions may indicate that use of the oral contraceptive should be discontinued:

Diabetes mellitus, or a tendency towards diabetes mellitus (e.g. unexplained glycosuria), hypertension, varicose veins, a history of phlebitis, otosclerosis, multiple sclerosis, epilepsy, porphyria, tetany, disturbed liver function, Sydenham's chorea, renal dysfunction, family history of clotting disorders, obesity, family history of breast cancer and patient history of benign breast disease, history of clinical depression, systemic lupus erythematosus, uterine fibroids and migraine, gall-stones, cardiovascular diseases, chloasma, asthma, an intolerance of contact lenses, or any disease that is prone to worsen during pregnancy.

Some women may experience amenorrhoea or oligomenorrhoea after discontinuation of oral contraceptives, especially when these conditions existed prior to use. Women should be informed of this possibility.

*Side-effects:* In rare cases, headaches, gastric upsets, nausea, vomiting, breast tenderness, changes in body weight, changes in libido, depressive moods can occur.

In predisposed women, use of Triadene can sometimes cause chloasma which is exacerbated by exposure to sunlight. Such women should avoid prolonged exposure to sunlight.

Individual cases of poor tolerance of contact lenses have been reported with use of oral contraceptives. Contact lens wearers who develop changes in lens tolerance should be assessed by an ophthalmologist.

*Menstrual changes:*
1. *Reduction of menstrual flow:* This is not abnormal and it is to be expected in some patients. Indeed, it may be beneficial where heavy periods were previously experienced.

2. *Missed menstruation:* Occasionally, withdrawal bleeding may not occur at all. If the tablets have been taken correctly, pregnancy is very unlikely. If withdrawal bleeding fails to occur at the end of a second pack, the possibility of pregnancy must be ruled out before resuming with the next pack.

*Intermenstrual bleeding:* 'Spotting' or heavier 'breakthrough bleeding' sometimes occur during tablet taking, especially in the first few cycles, and normally cease spontaneously. Triadene should therefore, be continued even if irregular bleeding occurs. If irregular bleeding is persistent, appropriate diagnostic measures to exclude an organic cause are indicated and may include curettage. This also applies in the case of spotting which occurs at irregular intervals in several consecutive cycles or which occurs for the first time after long use of Triadene.

*Effect on blood chemistry:* The use of oral contraceptives may influence the results of certain laboratory tests including biochemical parameters of liver, thyroid, adrenal and renal function, plasma levels of carrier proteins and lipid/lipoprotein fractions, parameters of carbohydrate metabolism and parameters of coagulation and fibrinolysis. Laboratory staff should therefore be informed about oral contraceptive use when laboratory tests are requested.

*Overdosage:* Overdosage may cause nausea, vomiting and, in females, withdrawal bleeding. There are no specific antidotes and treatment should be symptomatic.

**Pharmaceutical precautions** Shelf-life – Five years.

**Legal category** POM

**Package quantities** Individual packs containing three months' supply (OP)

---

**Further information** Nil

**Produce licence number** 0053/0205

## ULTRABASE*

**Qualitative and quantitative composition** There are no active constituents.

**Pharmaceutical form** Cream.

**Clinical particulars**
*Therapeutic indications:* For general use as:
- an emollient
- a diluent for dermatological preparations and
- a vehicle for various dermatological medicaments.

Additionally, it may be alternated with topical corticosteroids when the latter are being gradually withdrawn, and may be continued alone after complete withdrawal of the topical corticosteroid.

*Posology and method of administration:* For topical administration as required.

*Contra-indications:* Hypersensitivity to any of the components of Ultrabase.

*Special warnings and special precautions for use:* None stated.

*Interaction with other medicaments and other forms of interaction:* None known.

*Pregnancy and lactation:* None stated.

*Effects on ability to drive and use machines:* None known.

*Undesirable effects:* None known.

*Overdose:* Not applicable. Ultrabase contains no active ingredients.

**Pharmacological properties**
*Pharmacodynamic properties:* Ultrabase has no specific active ingredient, but the cream formulation has good emollient properties.

*Pharmacokinetic properties:* None stated.

*Preclinical safety data:* There are no preclinical safety data which could be of relevance to the prescriber and which are not already included in other relevant sections of the SPC.

**Pharmaceutical particulars**
*List of excipients:* Polyoxyl 40 stearate [E431], white soft paraffin, liquid paraffin, stearyl alcohol, Carbomer 934, sodium hydroxide, methyl parahydroxybenzoate (methyl paraben) [E218], propyl parahydroxybenzoate (propyl paraben) [E216], disodium edetate [E463], purified water, citrus-rose perfume oil

*Incompatibilities:* None known.

*Shelf life:* 5 years.

*Special precautions for storage:* Not applicable.

*Nature and contents of container:* This product is available in collapsible aluminium tubes (10 g or 50 g). Also available in polypropylene pump dispensers (500 g).

*Instructions for use/handling:* Keep out of the reach of children.

**Marketing authorisation number** 0053/0063

**Date of approval/revision of SPC** 2 June 1997

**Legal category** POM

## ULTRALANUM* OINTMENT PLAIN AND CREAM PLAIN

**Qualitative and quantitative composition** *Ointment:* Each 100 gm of ointment contains 0.25 gm (0.25%) of fluocortolone monohydrate and 0.25 gm (0.25%) of fluocortolone hexanoate.
*Cream:* Each 100 gm of cream contains 0.25 gm (0.25%) of fluocortolone pivalate and 0.25 gm (0.25%) of fluocortolone hexanoate.

**Pharmaceutical form** Ointment and cream

**Clinical particulars**

*Therapeutic indications:* Eczema and dermatitis of all types including atopic eczema, photodermatitis and primary irritant and allergic dermatitis, prurigo nodularis and insect bite reactions. Lichen planus, lichen simplex, discoid lupus erythematosus, necrobiosis lipoidica, pretibial myxoedema, erythroderma, psoriasis of the scalp, chronic plaque psoriasis of hands and feet.

*Posology and method of administration:* Ultralanum is for topical application in children, adults and the elderly as follows:

Initially 2–3 applications daily, according to severity of condition. For maintenance, one application daily.

Skin conditions which are neither weeping nor very dry require a base with balanced proportions of fat

---

and water. Ultralanum Ointment makes the skin slightly greasy without retaining heat or fluid.

Ultralanum Cream has a high water and low fat content. In weeping skin diseases it allows secretions to drain away, thus providing for rapid subsidence and drying up of the skin. Ultralanum Cream is also suitable for application to moist, exposed and hairy areas of the body. If the skin dries out too much under protracted use of Ultralanum Cream, the patient should be switched to Ultralanum Ointment.

*Occlusive dressings.* An occlusive dressing may be called for in unusually refractory cases in adults and usually under specialist supervision.

If an infection develops under the dressing, occlusive treatment must be terminated.

*Contra-indications:*
- Rosacea and peri-oral dermatitis.
- Acne vulgaris, undiagnosed perianal and genital pruritus, napkin eruptions, viral infections, primary bacterial or fungal infections of the skin.
- Secondary infections in the absence of appropriate anti-infective therapy.

Not suitable for the treatment of ophthalmic conditions.

*Special warnings and special precautions for use:* As with all topical steroids, there is a risk of skin atrophy following extensive therapy.

The application of topical steroids may result in the absorption of systemically active amounts of corticoid. If used in childhood or on the face, courses should be limited to 5 days and occlusion should not be used. Long-term continuous therapy should be avoided irrespective of age. Occlusion should be restricted to dermatoses involving limited areas. Adrenal suppression can occur even without occlusion.

Topical corticosteroids may be hazardous in psoriasis for a number of reasons including rebound relapses following development of tolerance, risk of generalised pustular psoriasis, and local and systemic toxicity due to impaired barrier function of the skin. Steroids may have a place in psoriasis of the scalp and chronic plaque psoriasis of the hands and feet. Careful patient supervision is important in psoriasis. Infections or secondarily infected dermatoses definitely require additional therapy with antibiotics or chemotherapeutic agents. This treatment can often be topical, but for heavy infections systemic antibacterial therapy may be necessary. If fungal infections are present, a topically active antimycotic should be applied.

*Interaction with other medicaments and other forms of interactions:* None stated.

*Pregnancy and lactation:* There is inadequate evidence of safety in human pregnancy. Topical administration of corticosteroids to pregnant animals can cause abnormalities of foetal development, including cleft palate and intra-uterine growth retardation. There may therefore be a very small risk of such effects on the human foetus.

Side-effects cannot be excluded in neonates whose mothers have been treated extensively or for a prolonged period of time during pregnancy or while lactating (for example, reduced adrenocortical function, when applied during the last weeks of pregnancy).

*Effects on ability to drive and use machines:* None stated.

*Undesirable effects:* As with all topical steroids, if Ultralanum is applied to large areas of the body and for long periods of time (more than 4 weeks) there is a risk of local effects, such as telangiectasia, striae, acneform changes, hypertrichosis, perioral dermatitis or skin atrophy. The application of unusually large quantities of topical corticoids may result in the absorption of systemically active amounts of corticoid. Allergic skin reactions may occasionally occur.

*Overdose:* None stated.

**Pharmacological properties**

*Pharmacodynamic properties:* Ultralanum suppresses inflammation in inflammatory and allergic skin conditions and alleviates subjective complaints such as itching, burning and pain. Owing to the different speeds with which the two forms of its corticoid component take effect, Ultralanum is both fast-acting and long-lasting in its effectiveness.

Capillary dilatation, intracellular oedema and tissue infiltration regress and capillary proliferation is suppressed. This leads to fading of inflamed skin surfaces.

*Pharmacokinetic properties:* A combination of two corticosteroids (steroid alcohol with ester or two different esters of the same steroid) in a dermatological preparation is pharmacokinetically advantageous since a higher skin concentration of corticosteroids can be achieved and maintained over a longer period of time after application of a combination as compared with a single compound. Due to a different lipophilicity the two compounds distribute in a different way into the horny layer and diffuse at different rates through the skin, leading to a rapid onset of action and a longer duration of activity.

Investigations on the time course of the vasoconstriction in volunteers as well as investigations on the percutaneous absorption indicate that fluocortolone and fluocortolone pivalate penetrate more rapidly into and through human skin than fluocortolone hexanoate, giving evidence that the above mentioned principles hold true with the Ultralanum dermatological preparations.

Measurements of drug recovery on the skin surface at the end of the exposure time in healthy skin volunteers as well as in eczema and psoriasis patients overestimate the extent of the percutaneous absorption and are therefore only of limited value for an assessment of the systemic drug load and for risk assessment. Pharmacodynamic investigations of the effect on the pituitary adrenal axis show only a small risk of systemic effects if large areas of the body are not treated over a long time.

Fluocortolone–21–monoesters are hydrolysed, like other 21–esters of corticosteroids most probably already in the skin, usually immediately after percutaneous absorption, into fluocortolone and the corresponding fatty acid. Fluocortolone itself possesses the shortest plasma half–life of all synthetic corticosteroids (approx. 75–90 minutes determined after i.v. administration) comparable to that of endogenous cortisol. Fluocortolone is inactivated in humans via a series of reduction, oxidation and conjugation reactions with glucuronic and sulphonic acid and is excreted as metabolites mainly in the urine.

*Preclinical safety data:* In systemic tolerance studies following repeated oral and parenteral administration, the effect of fluocortolone, fluocortolone caproate and fluocortolone pivalate was that of a typical glucocorticoid. It can be derived from these results that no systemic side effects further to those which are typical of glucocorticoids are to be expected following therapeutic use of Ultralanum, even under extreme conditions such as application over large areas and/or occlusion.

Specific embryotoxicity studies with the active substances contained in Ultralanum led to results typical of gluocorticoids, i.e. following sufficiently high exposure embryo–lethal and/or teratogenic effects could be induced given the appropriate test systems. A review of the adverse events data has, as yet, given no indications of embryotoxic effects due to systemic glucocorticoid therapy, no embryotoxic effects are to be expected following the therapeutic use of Ultralanum. However, taking animal–experimental results into consideration, particular care should be taken when deciding to use Ultralanum.

Investigation of fluocortolone in a bacterial test system for the detection of point–mutagenic effects gave no indications of a genotoxic potential. Since no relevant indications of genotoxic effects have been found for any of the glucocorticoids, such effects are not to be expected from the active substances in Ultralanum.

Specific tumorigenicity studies have not been carried out with the active substances contained in Ultralanum. On the basis of knowledge concerning the structures, the pharmacological action pattern and the results of systemic tolerance studies with chronic administration, there is no suspicion of tumorigenic potential. Since systemically effective immunosuppressive dosages will not be reached after dermal application of Ultralanum if used as directed, no influence on the occurrence of tumours is to be expected.

Following repeated dermal administration of fluocortolone and the two esters in different combinations and preparations, no substance–related dermal changes were observed.

**Pharmaceutical particulars**

*List of excipients:* Each 100 g of ointment contains:

Bleached wax, lanolin, heavy liquid paraffin, white soft paraffin, Amphocerin K.S., purified water, citrus rose perfume oil (PH No: 65803) and Dehymuls E.

Each 100 g of cream contains: Polyoxyl–40–stearate, stearyl alcohol, heavy liquid paraffin, white soft paraffin, disodium edetate dihydrate, Carbopol 934, sodium hydroxide, methyl parahydroxybenzoate, propyl parahydroxybenzoate, purified water and citrus rose perfume oil (PH No. 65803).

*Incompatibilities:* None so far known.

*Shelf–life:*
Ointment: 18 months.
Cream: 5 years

*Special precautions for storage:*
Ointment: store below 25°C.
Cream: Not applicable

*Nature and contents of container:* Collapsible ointment tubes of pure aluminium lacquered internally. Available in packs of 30 g and 50 g.

*Instructions for use/handling:* Keep out of reach of children.

**Marketing authorisation numbers**
Ointment: 0053/5005R
Cream: 0053/5011R

**Date of approval/revision of SPC** 13 February 1996

**Legal category** POM

## ULTRAPROCT* OINTMENT ULTRAPROCT* SUPPOSITORIES

**Presentation**

*Ultraproct Ointment:* A white ointment containing in 1 g:
Fluocortolone pivalate BP 0.92 mg
Fluocortolone hexanoate BP 0.95 mg
Cinchocaine hydrochloride 5.00 mg

*Excipients:* polyethylene glycol 400 monoricinoleate, castor oil, 2 octyldodecanol, citrus rose perfume oil.

*Ultraproct Suppositories:* Each white suppository contains:
Fluocortolone pivalate BP 0.61 mg
Fluocortolone hexanoate BP 0.63 mg
Cinchocaine hydrochloride 1.00 mg

*Excipient:* solid fat

**Uses** For the symptomatic relief of haemorrhoids and of pruritus ani in the short term (5-7 days).

**Dosage and administration** *Suppositories:* 1 Ultraproct Suppository to be inserted daily. In severe cases 1 suppository two to three times daily at the beginning of treatment. The suppositories should be inserted after defaecation.

*Ointment:* Apply in a thin layer twice daily. In order to obtain a rapid improvement, Ultraproct Ointment may be applied three or four times on the first day. The nozzle provided facilitates intra-rectal application.

**Contra-indications, warnings, etc**
*Contra-indications:* Viral infections, primary bacterial or fungal infections in the treatment area. Secondary infections of the skin in the absence of appropriate anti-infective therapy. Known sensitivity to local anaesthetics.

*Warnings/side-effects:* In infants, long-term continuous therapy with topical corticosteroids should be avoided. Occlusion is not appropriate on the perineum. Adrenal suppression can occur even without occlusion. As with all topical steroids, there is a risk of skin atrophy following extensive therapy. The application of unusually large quantities of topical corticoids may result in the absorption of systemically active amounts of corticoid. Infections or secondarily-infected dermatoses definitely require additional therapy with antibiotics or chemotherapeutics agents. This treatment can often be topical but for heavy infections systemic antibacterial therapy may be necessary. If fungal infections are present, a topically active anti-mycotic should be applied. Allergic skin reactions may occur.

*Pregnancy warning:* There is inadequate evidence of safety in human pregnancy. Topical administration of corticosteroids to pregnant animals can cause abnormalities of foetal development, including cleft palate and intra-uterine growth retardation. There may therefore be a very small risk of such effects on the human foetus.

**Pharmaceutical precautions** In order to restore the consistency of suppositories which have become soft owing to warm temperature, they should be put into cold water before the covering is removed.

Shelf-life: Ointment – Five years (store in a cool dry place). Suppositories – Two years (do not store above 25°C).

**Legal category** POM

**Package quantities** *Suppositories:* Packs of 12 (OP).
*Ointment:* Tubes of 30 g (OP).

**Further information** Nil

**Product licence numbers**
Ultraproct Ointment 0053/5008R
Ultraproct Suppositories 0053/5009R

## ULTRAVIST*

**Presentation** Bottles containing colourless, sterile solutions of various strengths of iopromide. Ultravist 150 contains 150 mg iodine per ml, Ultravist 240 contains 240 mg iodine per ml, Ultravist 300 contains 300 mg iodine per ml, Ultravist 370 contains 370 mg iodine per ml.

*Excipients:* Calcium disodium edetate, tromethamine, hydrochloric acid, water for injection.

**Uses** Non-ionic X-ray contrast media for computed tomography, digital subtraction angiography, intravenous urography, venography, arteriography, visualization of body cavities (e.g. arthrography, hysterosalpingography and fistulography), checking the function of dialysis shunts. Ultravist should not be used for myelography (see *Further information*).

**Dosage and administration:**
*Intravenous urography*

*Adults:* The minimum dose is 0.8 ml/kg body weight Ultravist 370, (1 ml/kg Ultravist 300 or 1.3 ml/kg Ultravist 240). These doses should provide adequate filling of the ureters. It may be necessary to increase the dose in individual cases e.g. obesity or impaired renal function.

*Children:* The poor concentrating ability of the immature nephron of infantile kidneys necessitates the use of relatively high doses of contrast medium, i.e. for Ultravist 300:

| | |
|---|---|
| Neonates: | 4.0 ml/kg body weight |
| Babies: | 3.0 ml/kg body weight |
| Small children: | 1.5 ml/kg body weight |

*Computed tomography*
*Cranial CT:* The following dosages are recommended for cranial CT:

| | |
|---|---|
| Ultravist 240: | 1.5-2.5 ml/kg body weight |
| Ultravist 300: | 1-2 ml/kg body weight |
| Ultravist 370: | 1-1.5 ml/kg body weight |

*Whole-body CT:* For whole-body computed tomography, the doses of the contrast medium and the rates of administration depend on the organs under investigation, the diagnostic problem and, in particular, the different scan and image-reconstruction times of the scanners in use. Infusion is preferable for slow scanners and injection for fast scanners.

*Angiography:* The dosage depends on the age, weight, cardiac output and general condition of the patient, the clinical problem, examination technique and the nature and volume of the vascular region to be investigated.

The following dosages may serve as a guide:

| | |
|---|---|
| *Cerebral angiography:* | |
| Aortic arch angiography | 50-80 ml Ultravist 300/inj. |
| Selective angiography | 6-15 ml Ultravist 300/inj. |
| Retrograde carotid angiography | 30-40 ml Ultravist 300/inj. |
| *Thoracic aortography:* | 50-80 ml Ultravist 300/inj. |
| *Abdominal aortography:* | 40-60 ml Ultravist 300/inj. |
| *Bifemoral arteriography:* | 40-60 ml Ultravist 300/inj. |
| *Peripheral angiography:* | |
| *Upper extremities:* | |
| Arteriography | 8-12 ml Ultravist 300/inj. |
| Venography | 50-60 ml Ultravist 240/inj. |
| | 15-30 ml Ultravist 300/inj. |
| *Lower extremities:* | |
| Arteriography | 20-30 ml Ultravist 300/inj. |
| Venography | 50-80 ml Ultravist 240/inj. |
| | 30-60 ml Ultravist 300/inj. |
| *Angiocardiography:* | |
| Cardiac-ventriculography | 40-60 ml Ultravist 370/inj. |
| Coronary angiography: | 5-8 ml Ultravist 370/inj. |

*Digital subtraction angiography* (DSA): I.V. injection of 30-60 ml Ultravist 300 or 370 as a bolus (flow-rate: 8-12 ml/second into the cubital vein; 10-20 ml/second into the vena cava) is recommended for high-contrast demonstrations of the great vessels, of the pulmonary arteries and of the arteries of the neck, head, kidneys and extremities.

Intra-arterial digital subtraction angiography requires smaller volumes and lower iodine concentrations than the intravenous technique.

The more selective the angiography, the lower the dose of contrast medium can be. This method is therefore recommended for patients with impaired renal function. For high-contrast demonstration of the arteries of the head, neck and limbs, several injections of 10-40 ml Ultravist 150, depending on the size of the vessels, are usually given directly or via a catheter. Larger volumes of contrast medium (about 200 ml) may be necessary in some cases to demonstrate the vessels of the lower limbs, particularly if both legs are to be examined.

*Dialysis shunt:* Ultravist 150 is also suitable for checking the function of a dialysis shunt. About 10 ml of contrast medium is required for this.

**Contra-indications, warnings, etc**
*Contra-indications:* Uncontrolled thyrotoxicosis. Hysterosalpingography must not be carried out during pregnancy or in patients with acute inflammatory conditions in the pelvic cavity.

*Use in pregnancy:* X-ray examinations should, if possible, be avoided during pregnancy. It has not yet been proved beyond question that Ultravist may be used without hesitation in pregnant patients. Therefore, an examination with Ultravist during pregnancy should be carried out only if considered absolutely necessary by the physician.

*Warnings/side-effects:* Use with caution in patients with proven or suspected hypersensitivity to iodine containing contrast media. For patients with severe impairment of hepatic or renal function, cardiac or circulatory insufficiency, cerebral arteriosclerosis, epileptic conditions, diabetes mellitus requiring drug treatment and/or associated with diabetic complications, pulmonary emphysema, poor general health, hyperthyroidism, multiple myeloma and benign nodular goitre, the need for examination with X-ray contrast media merits careful consideration.

This also applies to patients with a history of allergy, e.g. bronchial asthma, since experience shows that they may exhibit hypersensitivity to drugs. Because of possible precipitation, X-ray contrast media and prophylactic agents against hypersensitivity must not be injected as mixed solutions.

Particular caution should be exercised in allergic patients who have previously tolerated an injectable iodine-containing contrast medium without any complications, because they may become sensitised to these substances in the meantime.

Nonionic contrast media have less anticoagulant activity in vitro than ionic media. Meticulous attention should therefore be paid to angiographic technique. Nonionic media should not be allowed to remain in contact with blood in a syringe, and intravascular catheters should be flushed frequently with physiological saline solution (if necessary with heparin added), to minimise the risk of clotting, which rarely has led to serious thromboembolic complications of the procedures.

The patient should be recumbent during the administration of Ultravist, and thereafter, must be kept under close observation for at least 30 minutes, since the majority of severe incidents occur within that time. If the administration does not take place on the X-ray table, any patient with a labile circulation should be brought to the X-ray machine sitting or lying down.

In the case of abdominal angiography, the diagnostic yield is increased if the bowels are emptied of faecal matter and gas. On the two days prior to the examination patients should avoid flatulent food, in particular peas, beans and lentils, salads, fruit, wholemeal and fresh bread and all kinds of uncooked vegetables. On the day before the examination, patients should refrain from eating after 6 p.m. Moreover, it can be appropriate to administer a laxative in the evening.

In babies and young children, however, prolonged fasting and the administration of a laxative before the examination are contraindicated.

Experience shows that pronounced states of excitement, anxiety and pain can be the cause of side-effects or intensify the contrast medium-related reactions. They can be counteracted by calm management of the patient and the use of suitable drugs.

Experience shows that contrast medium is tolerated better if it is warmed to body temperature.

In patients with multiple myeloma, diabetes mellitus, polyuria, oliguria or gout and in babies, small children and patients in a very poor state of health, the fluid supply should not be restricted, and existing disturbances of the balance of water and electrolytes must be corrected before the administration of Ultravist.

Premedication with an alpha-blocker is recommended in patients with phaeochromocytoma, because of blood pressure crises.

Diabetic nephropathy may predispose to renal impairment following intravascular administration of contrast media. This may precipitate lactic acidosis in patients who are taking biguanides. As a precaution biguanides should be stopped 48 hours prior to the examination and reinstated only after control of renal function has been regained.

Hypersensitivity reactions can be aggravated in patients on beta-blockers.

The prevalence of delayed reactions (e.g. fever, rash, flu-like symptoms, joint pain and pruritus) to contrast media is higher in patients who have received interleukin.

If iodine isotopes are to be administered for the diagnosis of thyroid disease, it should be borne in mind that after the administration of iodinated contrast media which are excreted via the kidneys, the capacity of the thyroid tissue to take up iodine will be reduced for two weeks, and sometimes up to six weeks.

Side-effects in association with the intravascular use of iodinated contrast media are usually mild to moderate and temporary, and are less frequent with non-ionic than with ionic preparations. However, severe and life-threatening reactions, even fatal ones, have also been observed.

Nausea, vomiting, erythema, a sensation of pain and a general feeling of warmth are the most frequently recorded reactions on intravascular administration. Subjective complaints such as sensations of warmth or nausea can usually be alleviated quickly by reducing the rate of administration or interrupting the administration briefly.

If marked side-effects or suspected allergic reactions occur during injection and do not disappear, or even get worse, when the injection is briefly interrupted, it is probable that the patient is hypersensitive and the investigation must be abandoned. Even relatively minor symptoms such as itching of the skin, sneezing, violent yawns, tickling in the throat, hoarseness or attacks of coughing may be early signs of a severe reaction and, therefore, merit careful attention. Delayed reactions can occasionally occur. Temporary renal failure may occur in rare cases.

Other symptoms which may occur are: chills, fever, sweating, headache, dizziness, blanching, weakness, gagging and a feeling of suffocation, gasping, a rise or fall of blood pressure, itching, urticaria, other kinds of skin eruption, oedema, cramp, tremor, sneezing and lacrimation. These reactions, which can occur irrespective of the amount administered may be the first signs of an incipient state of shock. Administration of the contrast medium must be discontinued immediately and–if necessary–specific therapy instituted via a venous access. It is therefore advisable to use a flexible indwelling cannula for intravenous contrast medium administration. To permit immediate countermeasures to be taken in emergencies, appropriate drugs, an endotracheal tube and a ventilator should be ready to hand. Experience shows that hypersensitivity reactions occur more frequently in patients with an allergic disposition.

Very rarely, severe or even life-threatening side-effects such as severe hypotension and collapse, circulatory failure, ventricular fibrillation, cardiac arrest, pulmonary oedema, anaphylactic shock or other allergic manifestations, convulsions, or other cerebral symptoms may occur.

Ready availability of all drugs and equipment for emergency treatment and familiarity with the respective procedures are prerequisites for the effective management of contrast-medium incidents. Some guidance in the treatment of such incidents is contained in the leaflet supplied with the pack.

Paravascular administration of the contrast medium rarely leads to severe tissue reactions.

Neurological complications such as coma, temporary states of confusion and somnolence, transient paresis, disturbed vision or facial muscle paresis and epileptic fits may occur after cerebral angiography and other procedures in which the contrast medium reaches the brain with the arterial blood. In very rare cases the induction of fits has been observed after intravenous administration of contrast media in epileptics and patients with focal brain damage.

*Overdosage:* Acute symptoms of poisoning are unlikely with intravascular administration. In special cases, e.g. if renal function is impaired, the contrast medium may be removed by dialysis, and, in cases of intravascular administration of 300 ml or more, the balance of water and electrolytes should be corrected.

**Pharmaceutical precautions:** *Shelf-life:* Ultravist 150: 2 years; Ultravist 240, Ultravist 300 and Ultravist 370: 3 years

Protect from light and secondary X-rays. Store below 30°C. Because of possible precipitation, X-ray contrast media and prophylactic agents must not be injected as mixed solutions.

**Legal category** POM

**Package quantities**

| | |
|---|---|
| Ultravist 150: | Bottles of 50 ml |
| Ultravist 240: | Bottles of 50 ml |
| Ultravist 300: | Bottles of 20 ml, 50 ml, 75 ml, 100 ml and 200 ml |
| Ultravist 370: | Bottles of 30 ml, 50 ml, 75 ml, 100 ml and 200 ml |

**Further information** The Ultravist range consists of non-ionic contrast media with osmotic pressures that are relatively low for contrast media.

Ultravist 150: 0.34 osm/kg $H_2O$ at 37°C
Ultravist 240: 0.48 osm/kg $H_2O$ at 37°C
Ultravist 300: 0.62 osm/kg $H_2O$ at 37°C
Ultravist 370: 0.78 osm/kg $H_2O$ at 37°C

Although it showed excellent neural tolerance in animal studies, the intrathecal administration of iopromide has not been investigated in clinical studies. Ultravist should not therefore be used for myelographic examinations.

**Product licence numbers**

| | |
|---|---|
| Ultravist 150 | 0053/0209 |
| Ultravist 240 | 0053/0173 |
| Ultravist 300 | 0053/0174 |
| Ultravist 370 | 0053/0175 |

## UROGRAFIN*

**Presentation** Ampoules, vials or bottles containing colourless sterile solutions of varying strengths of meglumine/sodium diatrizoate.

*Urografin 150:* An intravenous injection or infusion of meglumine diatrizoate 26.1% w/v and sodium diatrizoate 3.9% w/v, containing 146 mg iodine per ml.

*Urografin 325:* An intravenous injection of meglumine diatrizoate 18% w/v and sodium diatrizoate 40% w/v, containing 325 mg iodine per ml.

*Urografin 370:* An intravascular injection of meglumine diatrizoate 66% w/v and sodium diatrizoate 10% w/v, containing 370 mg iodine per ml.

*Excipients:* calcium disodium edetate, water for injection.

**Uses** X-ray contrast media for the delineation of the vascular and renal systems.

**Dosage and administration**

*1. Adults only:* Table 1 overleaf shows the medium/media Schering suggest for each investigation. Schering media may be used at the discretion of the radiologist for other established permutations of medium and examination which, for the sake of simplicity, have been omitted from the table.

(Other indications include selective visceral angiography, limb venography, jugular venography, vesiculography, sialography, sinusography, amniography, lypmhangiography, intramuscular urography, operative cholangiography, percutaneous cholangiography, fistulography, oesophageal and anal atresia).

Urografin media are not suitable for myelography.

*2. Children and neonates*

*Intravenous urography:* The fact that urograms of infants and young children generally show a lower contrast density than those of adults is explained by the physiologically less effective function of the immature nephron. Relatively high doses of media are therefore indicated. (See Table 2).

*Table 2*

| | Urografin 325/370 |
|---|---|
| Up to 1 year | 7–10 ml |
| 1–2 years | 10–12 ml |
| 2–6 years | 12–15 ml |
| 6–12 years | 15–20 ml |
| over 12 years | adult dose |

*Drip–infusion urography:* Dosage of Urografin 150 should not exceed 4 ml/kg body weight.

*Angiocardiography:* In neonates up to 5 kg body weight, 8 ml of Urografin 370. Infants over 5 kg body weight, 1 ml/kg body weight up to 25 ml per injection

*Right and left heart catheterisation:* 1–1.2 ml/kg body weight of Urografin 370, with a maximum of 15 ml per injection for the right heart and 25 ml per injection for the left heart.

*Pulmonary angiography:* 0.5–0.6 ml/kg body weight up to 8 ml Urografin 370 per injection.

**Contra–indications, warnings, etc**

*Contra–indications:* Proven or suspected hypersensitivity to iodine–containing contrast media, uncontrolled thyrotoxicosis and decompensated cardiac insufficiency.

Hysterosalpingography must not be carried out during pregnancy or in patients with acute inflammatory conditions in the pelvic cavity.

*Warnings/side–effects:* For patients with severe impairment of hepatic or renal function, cerebral arteriosclerosis, epileptic conditions, diabetes mellitus requiring drug treatment and/or associated with diabetic complications, pulmonary emphysema, poor general health, hyperthyroidism, multiple myeloma or benign nodular goitre the need for examination with X–ray contrast media merits careful consideration.

This also applies to patients with a history of allergy, atopy, bronchial asthma, endogenous eczema, cardiac or circulatory insufficiency or a previous adverse reaction with any contrast medium since experience shows that they may be at higher risk from developing anaphylaxis or cardiovascular collapse. Consideration should be given to the use of low osmolar radiocontrast media in such patients.

Because of possible precipitation, X–ray contrast media and prophylactic agents must not be injected as mixed solutions.

Particular caution should be exercised in allergic persons who have previously tolerated an injectable iodine–containing contrast medium without any complication because they may have become sensitized to these substances in the meantime.

The patient should be recumbent during the administration of Urografin. Thereafter, the patient must be kept under close observation for at least 30 minutes since about 90% of all severe incidents occur within that time. If the administration does not take place on the X–ray table, any patient with a labile circulation should be brought to the X–ray machine sitting or lying down.

In patients with multiple myeloma, juvenile–onse

Table 1

| Examination (Adults) | 150 | 325 | 370 |
|---|---|---|---|
| Intravenous urography | | Up to 70 ml | Up to 70 ml |
| High–dose urography | | 100 ml | |
| Drip-infusion urography | 2–4 ml/kg body wt up to 250 ml | | |
| Retrograde urography | 5–10 ml | | |
| Cystography | Up to 500 ml | | |
| Angiocardiography | | | 30–50 ml |
| Right–heart catheterisation | | | 40–80 ml |
| Left–heart catheterisation | | | 40–60 ml |
| Pulmonary angiography | | | 30–40 ml |
| Coronary arteriography | | | 4–8 ml per artery[a] |
| Renal arteriography | | | 5–8 ml |
| Coeliac–axis arteriography | | | 35–80 ml |
| Thoracic aortography | | | 30–60 ml |
| Pelvic aortography | | | 20–25 ml |
| Translumbar abdominal aortography | | | 20–30 ml |
| Placentography | | | 25 ml |
| Pelvic venography | | 25–30 ml | |
| Venacavography | | | |
|   Inferior | | 30–50 ml | |
|   Superior | | 25–35 ml | |
| Splenoportography | | | 40–50 ml |
| Hysterosalpingography | | | 4–7 ml |
| Arthrography | | 1–10 ml | |

[a]100 ml bottles are available for coronary arteriography.

diabetes, long-standing diabetes, polyuria, oliguria or gout, and in infants, young children and marasmic patients the fluid supply should not be restricted. Existing disturbances of the balance of water and electrolytes must be corrected before the administration of a hypertonic contrast–medium solution.

Premedication with an alpha–blocker is recommended in patients with phaeochromocytoma, because of the risk of hypertensive crisis.

Diabetic nephropathy may predispose to renal impairment following intravascular administration of contrast media. This may precipitate lactic acidosis in patients who are taking biguanides. As a precaution biguanides should be stopped 48 hours prior to the examination and reinstated only after adequate renal function has been regained.

Hypersensitivity reactions can be aggravated in patients on beta-blockers. The prevalence of delayed reactions to contrast media is higher in patients who have received interleukin.

X–ray examinations should if possible be avoided during pregnancy. It has not yet been proved beyond question that Urografin may be used without hesitation in pregnant patients. Therefore, an examination with a contrast medium during pregnancy should be carried out only if considered absolutely necessary by the physician.

If iodine isotopes are to be administered for the diagnosis of thyroid disease, it should be borne in mind that after the administration of iodinated contrast media which are excreted via the kidneys, the capacity of the thyroid tissue to take up iodine will be reduced for 2 weeks, and sometimes up to 6 weeks.

Mild subjective symptoms, such as a feeling of heat and nausea, occur very seldom and disappear rapidly when the injection is slowed down or briefly interrupted. Transient pain may occur, in particular during the examination of peripheral vascular regions. Extravasations give rise to serious tissue reactions only in very rare cases.

Other symptoms which may occur are: Chills, fever, sweating, headache, dizziness, blanching, weakness, gagging and a feeling of suffocation, gasping, a rise or fall of blood pressure, itching, urticaria, other kinds of skin eruption, oedema, cramp, tremor, sneezing and lacrimation. These reactions, which can occur irrespective of the amount administered and the mode of administration, may be the first signs of incipient shock. Administration of the contrast medium must be discontinued immediately and – if necessary – specific therapy instituted intravenously. It is therefore advisable to use a flexible indwelling cannula for intravenous contrast medium administration. To permit immediate countermeasures to be taken in emergencies, appropriate drugs, an endotracheal tube and a ventilator should be ready to hand.

If marked side–effects or suspected allergic reactions occur during injection and do not disappear, or even get worse, when the injection is briefly interrupted, it is probable that the patient is hypersensitive and the investigation must be abandoned. Even relatively minor symptoms such as itching of the skin, sneezing, violet yawns, tickling in the throat, hoarseness or attacks of coughing may be early signs of a severe reaction and, therefore, merit careful attention. Delayed reactions can occasionally occur.

Very rarely, severe or even life–threatening side–effects such as severe hypotension and collapse, circulatory failure, ventricular fibrillation, cardiac arrest, pulmonary oedema, anaphylactic shock or other allergic manifestations, convulsions, or other cerebral symptoms may occur. In some cases these have proved fatal.

Paravascular administration of the contrast medium rarely leads to severe tissue reactions.

Neurological complications such as coma, temporary states of confusion and somnolence, transient paresis, disturbed vision or facial muscle paresis and epileptic fits may occur after cerebral angiography and other procedures in which the contrast medium reaches the brain with the arterial blood. In very rare cases the induction of fits has been observed after intravenous administration of Urografin in epileptics and patients with focal brain damage. However, a causal relationship seems to be questionable. Acute renal failure may occur in rare cases.

Ionic iodinated contrast media inhibit blood coagulation in vitro more than non–ionic contrast media. Nevertheless medical personnel performing vascular catheterisation procedures should pay meticulous attention to the angiographic technique and catheter flushing so as to minimise the risk of procedure–related thrombosis and embolisation.

Ready availability of all drugs and equipment for emergency treatment and familiarity with the respective procedures are prerequisites for the effective management of contrast–medium incidents. Some guidance in the treatment of such incidents is contained in the leaflet supplied with the pack.

Overdosage: Acute symptoms of poisoning are unlikely with intravascular administration. On inadvertent overdosage or in greatly impaired renal function, the contrast medium may be removed by dialysis, and the balance of water and electrolytes should be corrected. Acute toxicity studies do not suggest a risk of acute intoxication.

**Pharmaceutical precautions**

Storage: Protect from light and secondary X–rays. Shelf–life 5 years. Because of possible precipitation, X–ray contrast media and prophylactic agents must not be injected as mixed solutions.

**Legal category** POM

**Package quantities** Urografin 150: Packs of 10 x 10 ml ampoules and 10 x 20 ml ampoules.

Urografin 150 for infusion: Packs of 1 x 250 ml bottles and 1 x 500 ml bottles.

Urografin 325: Packs of 10 x 20 ml ampoules and 10 x 50 ml bottles.

Urografin 370: Packs of 10 x 20 ml ampoules and 10 x 50 ml bottles. In addition packs of 1 x 100 ml bottles.

**Further information** Nil

**Product licence numbers**

| | |
|---|---|
| Urografin 150 | 0053/5041R |
| Urografin 150 for infusion | 0053/5007R |
| Urografin 325 | 0053/5006R |
| Urografin 370 | 0053/5044R |

*Trade Mark

# Schering-Plough Ltd
## Schering-Plough House
## Shire Park
## Welwyn Garden City
## Herts AL7 1TW


Schering-Plough

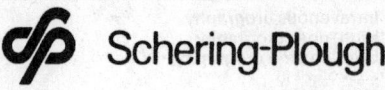

## CAELYX* ▼

**Qualitative and quantitative composition** Each 10 ml vial of Caelyx contains doxorubicin hydrochloride, 2 mg/ml, concentrate for infusion.

Pharmaceutical form Caelyx, a liposome formulation, is doxorubicin hydrochloride encapsulated in liposomes with surface-bound methoxypolyethylene glycol (MPEG). This process is known as pegylation and protects liposomes from detection by the mononuclear phagocyte system (MPS), which increases blood circulation time. Caelyx is a concentrate for infusion presented as a sterile, translucent, red suspension in 10 ml glass vials for single-use intravenous infusion.

Clinical particulars

*Therapeutic indications:* Caelyx is indicated for AIDS-related Kaposi's sarcoma (KS) in patients with low CD4 counts (< 200 CD4 lymphocytes/mm³) and extensive mucocutaneous or visceral disease.

Caelyx may be used as first-line systemic chemotherapy, or as second line chemotherapy in AIDS-KS patients with disease that has progressed with, or in patients intolerant to, prior combination systemic chemotherapy comprising at least two of the following agents: a vinca alkaloid, bleomycin and doxorubicin (or other anthracycline).

*Posology and method of administrtation:*
*Dosage:* Caelyx should be administered intravenously at 20 mg/m² every two-to-three weeks. Intervals shorter than 10 days should be avoided as drug accumulation and increased toxocity cannot be ruled out. Patients should be treated for two-to-three months to achieve a therapeutic response. Treatment should be continued as needed to maintain a therapeutic response.

*Administration:* Caelyx, diluted in 250 ml 5% Glucose Intravenous infusion, is administered by intravenous infusion over 30 minutes. DO NOT administer as a bolus injection or undiluted solution. It is recommended that the Caelyx infusion line be connected through the side port of an intravenous infusion of 5% Glucose Intravenous Infusion to achieve further dilution and minimise the risk of thrombosis and extravasation. Caelyx must not be given by the intramuscular or subcutaneous route.

*Patients with impaired hepatic function:* In a small number of patients with impaired hepatic function (bilirubin values up to 4 mg/dl) administered 20 mg/m² of Caelyx, there appeared to be no change in the clearance and terminal half-life of Caelyx. However, until further experience is gained, the Caelyx dosage should be reduced in patients with impaired hepatic function, based on experience with conventional doxorubicin HCl. Prior to Caelyx administration, hepatic function should be evaluated using conventional clinical laboratory tests such as ALT/AST, alkaline phosphatase, and bilirubin. It is recommended that the Caelyx dosage be reduced if the bilirubin is elevated as follows: at serum bilirubin 1.2–3.0 mg/dl, give $\frac{1}{2}$ the normal dose; at >3 mg/dl, give $\frac{1}{4}$ the normal dose.

*Patients with impaired renal function:* As doxorubicin is metabolised by the liver and excreted in the bile, dose modification should not be required with Caelyx.

*Patients with splenectomy:* As there is no experience with Caelyx in patients with splenectomy, treatment with Caelyx is not recommended.

*Paediatric patients:* The safety and effectiveness in patients less than 18 years of age have not been established.

*Elderly patients:* The safety and effectiveness in patients over 60 years of age have not been established.

*Contra-indications:* Caelyx is contra-indicated in patients who have a history of hypersensitivity reactions to its components or to doxorubicin HCl. Caelyx should not be administered during pregnancy or while breast-feeding.

Caelyx should not be used to treat AIDS-KS that may be effectively treated with local therapy or systemic alfa-interferon.

*Special warnings and special precautions for use:*
*Cardiac risk:* All patients receiving Caelyx should routinely undergo frequent ECG monitoring. Transient ECG changes such as T-wave flattening, S-T segment depression and benign arrhythmias are not considered mandatory indications for the suspension of Caelyx therapy. However, reduction of the QRS complex is considered more indicative of cardiac toxicity. If this change occurs, the most definitive test for anthracycline myocardial injury, i.e., endomyocardial biopsy, should be considered.

More specific methods for the evaluation and monitoring of cardiac functions as compared to ECG are a measurement of left ventricular ejection fraction by echocardiography or preferably by Multiple Gated Arteriography (MUGA). These methods should be applied routinely before the initiation of Caelyx therapy and should be repeated periodically during treatment. The evaluation of left ventricular function is considered to be mandatory before each additional administration of Caelyx which exceeds a cumulative dose of 450 mg/m². Whenever cardiomyopathy is suspected, i.e., the left ventricular ejection fraction has decreased relatively as compared to pre-treatment values and/or (at the same time) left ventricular ejection are lower than a prognostically relevant value (e.g. < 45%), endomyocardial biopsies should be performed and the benefit of continued therapy must be carefully evaluated against the risk of producing irreversible cardiac damage.

Congestive heart failure due to cardiomyopathy may occur suddenly, without prior ECG changes and may also be encountered several weeks after discontinuation of therapy.

The evaluation tests and methods mentioned above concerning the monitoring of cardiac performance during anthracycline therapy should be employed in the following order, ECG monitoring, measurement of left ventricular ejection fraction, endomyocardial biopsy. If a test result indicates possible cardiac injury associated with Caelyx therapy, the benefit of continued therapy must be carefully weighed against the risk of myocardial injury.

Patients with a history of cardiovascular disease should receive Caelyx only when the benefit outweighs the risk to the patient.

Caution should be exercised in patients with impaired cardiac function who receive Caelyx.

Caution should be observed in patients who have received other anthracyclines. The total dose of doxorubicin HCl should also take into account any previous or concomitant) therapy with cardiotoxic compounds such as other anthracyclines/anthraquinones or e.g. 5-FU.

*Myelosuppression:* Many AIDS-KS patients treated with Caelyx have baseline myelosuppression due to such factors as their HIV disease or numerous concomitant medications. In this population, myelosuppression appears to be the dose-limiting adverse event (see 4.8 Undesirable Effects). Because of the potential for bone marrow suppression, periodic blood counts should be performed frequently during the course of Caelyx therapy, and at a minimum, prior to each dose of Caelyx. Persistent severe myelosuppression may result in superinfection or haemorrhage.

*Infusion-associated reactions:* See *Undesirable effects.*

*Diabetic patients:* It should be noted that each vial of Caelyx contains sucrose and is administered in 5% Glucose Intravenous Infusion.

*Interaction with other medicaments and other forms of interaction:* No formal drug interaction studies have been conducted with Caelyx. Caution should be exercised in the concomitant use of drugs known to interact with doxorubicin HCl. Although not formally studied, Caelyx, like other doxorubicin HCl preparations, may potentiate the toxicity of other anti-cancer therapies. Exacerbation of cyclophosphamide-induced haemorrhage cystitis and enhancement of the hepatotoxicity of 6-mercaptopurine have been reported with doxorubicin HCl. Caution should be exercised when giving any other cytotoxic agents, especially myelotoxic agents, at the same time.

*Pregnancy and use during lactation: Pregnancy:* Caelyx is embryotoxic in rats and embryotoxic and abortifacient in rabbits. Teratogenicity cannot be ruled out. There is no experience in pregnant women with Caelyx. Caelyx therefore, should not be administered to pregnant women. Women of child-bearing potential should be advised to avoid pregnancy while they or their male partner are receiving Caelyx and in the six months following discontinuation of Caelyx therapy. (see 5.3 Carcinogenesis, Mutagenesis and Reproductive toxicity.)

*Lactation:* It is not known whether this drug is excretred in human milk and because of the potential for serious adverse reactions in nursing infants from Caelyx, mothers should discontinue nursing prior to taking this drug.

*Effect on the ability to drive and use machines:* Although Caelyx should not effect driving performance, in studies to date, dizziness and somnolence were associated infrequently (< 5%) with the administration of Caelyx. Patients who suffer from these effects should avoid driving and operating machinery.

*Undesirable effects:* Open-label and controlled clinical studies on AIDS-KS patients treated with Caelyx show that myelosuppression was the most frequent side effect considered related to Caelyx occurring in approximately half of the patients.

Leucopenia is the most frequent adverse event experienced with Caelyx in this population; and anaemia and thrombocytopenia can also be expected. These events may occur early on in treatment and are usually transient. In clinical trials patients rarely discontinued treatment due to myelosuppression. Haematological toxicity may require dose reduction or suspension or delay of therapy.

Caelyx treatment should be temporarily suspended in patients when the ANC count is < 1000/mm³ and/or the platelet count is < 50,000/mm³. G-CSF (or GM-CSF) may be given as concomitant therapy to support the blood count when the ANC count is < 1000/mm³. Clinically significant laboratory abnormalities frequently (≥ 5%) occurred in clinical studies with Caelyx. These included increases in alkaline phosphatase; and increases in AST and bilirubin which are believed to be related to the underlying disease and not Caelyx. Reduction in haemoglobin and platelets were less frequently (< 5%) reported. Sepsis related to leucopenia was rarely (< 1%) observed. Some of these abnormalities may have been related to the underlying HIV infection and not Caelyx.

Other frequently (≥ 5%) observed side effects were nausea, asthenia, alopecia, fever, diarrhoea, infusion-associated acute reactions, and stomatitis.

Infusion-associated reactions are characterised by flushing, shortness of breath, facial oedema, headache, chills, back pain, tightness in the chest and throat and/or hypotension. In most cases, the side effect occurs during the first cycle of treatment. Temporarily stopping the infusion or slowing the rate of the infusion resolves these reactions over the course of several hours, regardless of whether any symptomatic treatment is used.

Stomatitis has been repoted in patients receiving continuous infusions of conventional doxorubicin HCl and was frequently reported in patients receiving Caelyx. It did not interfere with patients completing therapy and no dosage adjustments are generally required, unless stomatitis is affecting a patient's ability to eat. In this case, the dose interval may be extended by 1–2 weeks or the dose reduced. Respiratory side effects frequently (≥ 5%) occurred in clinical studies of Caelyx and may be related to opportunistic infections in the AIDS population. Opportunistic infections (OI's) are observed in KS patients after administration with Caelyx, and are frequently observed in patients with HIV-induced immunodeficiency. The most frequently observed OI's in clinical studies were candidiasis, cytomegalovirus, herpes simplex, Pneumocystis carinii pneumonia, and myobacterium avium complex.

Other less frequently (< 5%) observed side effects included palmarplantar erythrodysesthesia, oral monoliasis, nausea and vomiting, vomiting, weight loss, rash, mouth ulceration, dyspnoea, abdominal pain, allergic reaction, vasodilatation, anorexia, glossitis, constipation, paresthesia and retinitis.

Palmar-plantar erythrodysesthesia is characterised

by painful, macular reddening skin eruptions. In patients experiencing this event, it is generally seen after six or more weeks of treatment. In most patients it clears in one or two weeks, with or without treatment with corticosteroids. It appears to be dose and schedule related and can be reduced by extending the dose interval 1–2 weeks or reducing the dose. This reaction can be severe and debilitating in some patients, however, and may require discontinuation of treatment. An increased incidence of congestive heart failure is associated with standard doxorubicin therapy. Although, endomyocardial biopsies on nine of ten AIDS-KS patients receiving cumulative doses of Caelyx greater than 460 mg/m² indicate no evidence of anthracycline-induced cardiomyopathy, until further clinical data are available, the risk of developing cardiomyopathy is assumed to be similar to that of standard doxorubicin. The recommended dose of Caelyx for AIDS-KS patients is 20 mg/m² every two-to-three weeks. The cumulative dose at which cardiotoxicity would become a concern (> 400 mg/m²) would require more than 20 courses of Caelyx therapy over 40 to 60 weeks. Although no local necrosis following extravasation has been observed to date, Caelyx should be considered an irritant. Animal studies indicate that administration of doxorubicin HCl as a liposomal formulation reduces the potential for extravasation injury. If any signs or symptoms of extravasation occur (e.g., stinging, erythema) the infusion should be immediately terminated and restarted in another vein. The application of ice over the site of extravasation for approximately 30 minutes may be helpful in alleviating the local reaction. Caelyx must not be given by the intramuscular or subcutaneous route.

Recall of skin reaction due to prior radiotherapy has rarely occurred with Caelyx administration.

*Overdose:* Acute overdosage with doxorubicin HCl worsens the toxic effects of mucositis, leucopenia and thrombocytopenia. Treatment of acute overdosage of the severely myelosuppressed patient consists of hospitalisation, antibiotics, platelet and granulocyte transfusions and symptomatic treatment of mucositis.

**Pharmacological properties**

*Pharmacodynamic properties:* Pharmaco-therapeutic group: Cytotoxic agents (anthracyclines and related substances), ATC code L01DB.

The active ingredient of Caelyx is doxorubicin HCl, a cytotoxic anthracycline antibiotic obtained from *Stretomyces peucetius* var. *caesius*. The exact mechanism of the antitumour activity of doxorubicin is not known. It is generally believed that inhibition of DNA, RNA and protein synthesis is responsible for the majority of the cytotoxic effects. This is probably the result of intercalation of the anthracycline between adjacent base pairs of the DNA double helix thus preventing their unwinding for replication.

*Pharmacokinetic properties:* Caelyx is a long-circulating pegylated liposomal formulation of doxorubicin HCl that provides greater concentration of doxorubicin in KS tumours than in normal skin. Pegylated liposomes contains surface-grafted segments of the hydrophilic polymer methoxypolyethylene glucol (MPEG). These linear MPEG groups extend from the liposome surface creating a protective coating that reduces interactions between the lipid bilayer membrane and the plasma components. This allows the Caelyx liposomes to circulate for prolonged periods in the blood stream. Pegylated liposomes are small enough (average diameter of approximately 100 nm) to pass intact (extravasate) through defective blood vessels supplying tumours. Evidence of penetration of pegylated liposomes from blood vessels and their entry and accumulation in tumours has been seen in mice with C-26 colon carcinoma tumours and in transgenic mice with KS-like lesions. The pegylated liposomes also have a low permeability lipid matrix and internal aqueous buffer system that combine to keep doxorubicin HCl encapsulated during liposome residence time in circulation.

The plasma pharmacokinetics of Caelyx were evaluated in 23 patients with Kaposi's sarcoma who received single doses of 20 mg/m² administered by a 30-minute infusion. The pharmacokinetic parameters of Caelyx (primarily representing liposome-encapsulated doxorubicin HCl and low levels of unencapsulated doxorubicin HCl) observed after the 20 mg/m² doses are presented in the following table.

The plasma pharmacokinetics of Caelyx in humans differ significantly from those reported in the literature for standard doxorubicin HCl preparations. Caelyx displayed linear pharmacokinetics. Disposition occurred in two phases after Caelyx administration, with a relatively short first phase (~ 5 hours) and a prolonged second phase (~ 55 hours) that accounted for the majority of the area under the curve (AUC). Doxorubicin HCl displays extensive tissue distribution (volume of distribution, 700 to 1100 L/m² and a rapid elimination clearance (24 to 73 L/h/m²). In contrast, the pharmacokinetic profile of Caelyx indicates that

*Pharmacokinetic parameters in Caelyx-treated patients*

| Parameter | Mean ± Standard Error<br>20 mg/m² (n = 23) |
|---|---|
| Maximum Plasma Concentration[a] (µg/ml) | 8.34 ± 0.49 |
| Plasma Clearance (L/h/m²) | 0.041 ± 0.004 |
| Volume of Distribution (L/m²) | 2.72 ± 0.120 |
| AUC (µg/ml h) | 590 ± 58.7 |
| $\lambda_1$ half-live (hours) | 5.2 ± 1.4 |
| $\lambda_2$ half-live (hours) | 55.0 ± 4.8 |

[a] Measured at the end of a 30-minute infusion

Caelyx is confined mostly to the vascular fluid volume and that the clearance of doxorubicin from the blood is dependent upon the liposomal carrier. Doxorubicin becomes available after the liposomes are extravasated and enter the tissue compartment. At equivalent doses, the plasma concentration and AUC values of Caelyx which represent mostly liposome-encapsulated doxorubicin HCl (containing 90% to 95% of the measured doxorubicin) are significantly higher than those achieved with standard doxorubicin HCl preparations. Kaposi's sarcoma lesion and normal skin biopsies were obtained 48 and 96 hours post-infusion. In patients receiving 20 mg/m² Caelyx the concentration of total (liposome encapsulated and unencapsulated) doxorubicin in the KS lesions was a median of 19 (range 3–53) times higher than in normal skin at 48 hours post treatment.

*Preclinical safety data:* In repeat dose studies conducted in animals, the toxicity profile of Caelyx appears very similar to that reported in humans who receive long-term infusions of doxorubicin hydrochloride. With Caelyx, the encapsulation of doxorubicin hydrochloride in pegylated liposomes results in these effects having a differing strength, as follows:

*Cardiotoxicity:* Studies in rabbits have shown that the cardiotoxicity of Caelyx is reduced compared with conventional doxorubicin HCl preparations.

*Dermal toxicity:* In studies performed after the repeated administration of Caelyx to rats and dogs, serious dermal inflammations and ulcer formations were observed at clinically relevant dosages. In the study in dogs, the occurrence and severity of these lesions was reduced by lowering the dose or prolonging the intervals between doses. Similar dermal lesions, which are desribed as palmar-plantar erythrodsesthesia were also observed in patients after long-term intravenous infusion (see *Undesirable effects*).

*Anaphylactoid response:* During repeat dose toxicology studies in dogs, an acute response characterised by hypotension, pale mucous membranes, salivation, emesis and periods of hyperactivity followed by hypoactivity and lethargy was observed following administration of pegylated liposomes (placebo). A similar, but less severe response was also noted in dogs treated with Caelyx and doxorubicin.

The hypotensive response was reduced in magnitude by pretreatment with antihistamines. However, the response was not life-threatening and the dogs recovered quickly upon discontinuation of treatment.

*Local toxicity:* Subcutaneous tolerance studies indicate that Caelyx, as against doxorubicin HCl, causes slighter local irritation or damage to the tissue after a possible extravasation.

*Mutagenicity and carcinogenicity:* Although no studies have been conducted with Caelyx, doxorubicin HCl, the pharmacologically active ingredient of Caelyx, is mutagenic and carcinogenic. Pegylated placebo liposomes are neither mutagenic or genotoxic.

*Reproductive toxicity:* Caelyx resulted in mild moderate ovarian and testicular atrophy in mice after a single dose of 36 mg/kg. Decreased testicular weights and hypospermia were present in rats after repeat doses ≥ 0.25 mg/kg/day and diffuse degeneration of the semniferous tubules and a marked decrease in spermatogenesis were observed in dogs after repeat doses of 1 mg/kg/day (see *Pregnancy and lactation*).

**Pharmaceutical particulars**

*List of excipients:* The following excipients are contained in each vial of product: α-2(2-[1,2-distearoyl-*sn*-glycero(3)phosphooxy]ethylcarbamoyl)-ω-methoxypoly(oxyethylen -40, sodium salt (MPEG-DSPE) fully hydrogenated soy phosphatidylcholine (HSPC); Cholesterol NF; ammonium sulphate ACS; sucrose PhEur; histidine PhEur; water for injections PhEur; hydrochloric acid PhEur; sodium hydroxide PhEur.

*Incompatibilities:* DO NOT MIX WITH OTHER DRUGS.

*Shelf-life:* Unopened vials of material have a shelf-life of 18 months and should be stored at 2°C to 8°C. After dilution with 5% Glucose Intravenous Infusion, the diluted Caelyx solution should be used immediately. Diluted product not for immediate use should be prepared under aseptic conditions and in line with good pharmaceutical practice should be stored at 2°C to 8°C for no longer than 24 hours. Partially used vials should be discarded.

*Special precautions for storage:* Store at 2°C to 8°C. Avoid freezing.

*Nature and contents of container:* The container is a Type 1 glass vial, with a siliconised grey bromobutyl stopper, and an aluminium seal. Caelyx is supplied as a single pack or packs of ten. Each 10 ml vial of Caelyx contains doxorubicin hydrochloride 2 mg/ml; concentrate for infusion.

*Instructions for use/handling:* DO NOT USE MATERIAL THAT SHOWS EVIDENCE OF PRECIPITATION OR ANY OTHER PARTICULTE MATTER.

Determine the dose of Caelyx to be administered (based upon the recommended dose and the patient's surface area). Take the appropriate volume of Caelyx up into a sterile syringe. Aseptic technique must be strictly observed since no preservative or bacteriostatic agent is present in Caelyx. The appropriate dose of Caelyx must be diluted in 250 ml of 5% Glucose Intravenous prior to administration.

The use of any diluent other than 5% Glucose Intravenous Infusion, or the presence of any bacteriostatic agent such as benzyl alcohol may cause precipitation of Caelyx.

It is recommended that the Caelyx infusion line be connected through the side port of an intravenous infusion of 5% Glucose Intravenous Infusion.

Caution should be exercised in handling Caelyx solution. The use of gloves is required. If Caelyx comes into contact with skin or mucosa, wash immediately and thoroughly with soap and water. Caelyx should be handled and disposed of in a manner consistent with that of other anti-cancer drugs.

*Marketing authorisation holder:* SP Europe, Rue de Stalle 73, 1180 Brussels, Belgium.

**Marketing authorisation numbers**
EU/1/96/011/001
EU/1/96/011/002

**Date of approval/revision of SPC** 31 October 1996

Legal category POM.

## CEDAX*

**Qualitative and quantitative composition**

Capsules: 400 mg ceftibuten† per capsule

Powder for Oral Suspension: 90 mg ceftibuten† per 5 ml, when reconstituted
180 mg ceftibuten† per 5 ml, when reconstituted

† charged as ceftibuten dihydrate equivalent to the stated amount of ceftibuten.

**Pharmaceutical form** Oral capsules and powder for oral suspension.

**Clinical particulars**

*Therapeutic indications:* Cedax is indicated in the treatment of the following infections when caused by strains of susceptible microorganisms:

*Respiratory tract infections:* Pharyngitis, tonsillitis in adults and/or children; otitis media in children. Acute episodes of bronchitis and acute exacerbations of chronic bronchitis in adults.

*Urinary tract infections:* In adults and children, both complicated and uncomplicated infections.

*Posology and method of administration:* Duration of treatment generally ranges from five to fourteen days. For treatment of infections due to *Streptococcus pyogenes*, a therapeutic dosage of Cedax should be administered for at least 10 days.

*Adults:* The recommended dose of Cedax is 400 mg daily. For treatment in the following indications this may be administered at a dosage of 400 mg once daily: acute bronchitis, acute exacerbations of chronic bronchitis and complicated or uncomplicated urinary tract infections.

*Adult patients with renal impairment:* Cedax pharmacokinetics are not affected sufficiently to require dosage modification unless creatinine clearance values are lower than 50 ml/min. Guidelines for dose modification in these patients are provided in the following table.

*Modification of Cedax dose in adult patients with renal dysfunction.*

| | | | |
|---|---|---|---|
| Creatinine clearance ml/min | >50 | 30–49 | 5–29 |
| Cedax dose per 24 hours | 400 mg | 200 mg | 100 mg |

If alteration of dosage frequency is preferred, a 400 mg dose of Cedax may be administered every 48 hours (every 2 days) to a patient with a creatinine clearance of 30–49 ml/min, and every 96 hours (every 4 days) if creatinine clearance is 5–29 ml/min.

In patients receiving haemodialysis two or three times weekly, a single dose of Cedax 400 mg may be administered at the end of each haemodialysis session.

*Geriatric patients:* The usual adult dosage recommendations may be followed for patients in this age group.

*Children:* The recommended dose is 9 mg/kg/day of the oral suspension. The dose may be administered as a single daily dose for treatment in the following indications: pharyngitis with or without tonsillitis, acute otitis media with effusion, and complicated or uncomplicated urinary tract infections.

Children weighing more than 45 kg or older than 10 years may receive the recommended adult dosage.

As a general guide the following volume/day may be used:

| | 90 mg/5 ml | 180 mg/5 ml |
|---|---|---|
| 6 months–1 year | 5 ml | — |
| 1–3 years | 8 ml | — |
| 3–6 years | 10 ml | 5 ml |
| 6–10 years | — | 8 ml |
| > 10 yeas | — | 10 ml |

using the graduated syringe provided.

*Contra-indications:* Cedax is contra-indicated in patients with known allergy to cephalosporins.

*Special warnings and precautions for use:* The dosage of Cedax may require adjustment in patients with renal insufficiency (creatinine clearance less than 50 ml per minute), as well as patients undergoing dialysis. Cedax is readily dialyzable. Dialysis patients should be monitored carefully, and Cedax administration should be timed to occur immediately following dialysis.

Cedax should be prescribed with caution in individuals with a history of complicated gastrointestinal disease, particularly chronic colitis.

*Paediatric use:* Safety and efficacy of Cedax in infants less than six months of age have not been established.

Cephalosporin antibiotics should be administered with extreme caution in patients with known or suspected allergy to penicillins. Approximately 5% of patients with documented penicillin allergy experience crossreactivity to the cephalosporin antibiotics. Serious acute hypersensitivity reactions (anaphylaxis) have been reported in individuals receiving both penicillins and cephalosporins, and cross-hyperreactivity with anaphylaxis has been known to occur. If an allergic reaction to Cedax occurs, discontinue use and administer appropriate therapy. Serious anaphylaxis requires appropriate emergency treatment as indicated clinically.

During therapy with broad-spectrum antibiotics like Cedax, alteration of the intestinal flora may result in antibiotic-associated diarrhoea, including pseudomembranous colitis due to *Clostridium difficile* toxin. Patients may experience moderate to severe or life-threatening diarrhoea, with or without dehydration, either during or after treatment with the associated antibiotic. It is important to consider this diagnosis in any patient noted to have persistent diarrhoea while taking any broad-spectrum antibiotic like Cedax.

*Interactions with other medicaments and other forms of interaction:* No known chemical or laboratory test interactions have been noted with Cedax. A false positive direct Coombs test has been reported during the use of other cephalosporins. However, the results of assays using red cells of healthy persons to test the ability of Cedax to cause direct Coombs *in vitro* reactions, showed no positive reactions even at concentrations as high as 40 mg/ml.

*Pregnancy and lactation:* There is inadequate evidence of safety of Cedax in human pregnancy. Studies in rats have not indicated that ceftibuten produces any adverse effects on fertility or reproductive performance at doses equivalent to 25 times those used in man. In addition ceftibuten was not teratogenic in rats or rabbits at doses giving exposure equivalent to 50 and 0.3 times those expected in man, respectively. As animal studies are not always predictive of human response, administration of Cedax during pregnancy should be weighed in terms of potential risk and benefit to both mother and foetus.

Levels of Cedax in the milk of nursing mothers have been below the levels of detection by standard methods.

*Effects on ability to drive and use machines:* None known.

*Undesirable effects:* The most frequently reported adverse events were gastrointestinal, including nausea (≤3%) and diarrhoea (3%), and headache (2%).

Rarely reported adverse events included dyspepsia, gastritis, vomiting, abdominal pain and dizziness. Very rarely, the growth of *Clostridium difficile* in association with moderate to severe diarrhoea was reported in adult patients; hospitalisation was not required. Convulsions were also reported, but were not definitely attributed to therapy.

Most adverse events responded to symptomatic treatment or ceased upon discontinuation of Cedax therapy.

Hypersensitivity reactions in the form of skin rash, or drug allergy may occur and usually subside on discontinuation of treatment.

Clinical laboratory abnormalities including leukopenia, eosinophilia and thrombocytosis have been reported rarely. Transient elevations in AST (SGOT), ALT (SGPT) and LDH have also been reported rarely.

In addition to the adverse events listed above in patients treated with Cedax, the following adverse reactions and altered laboratory tests have been reported for the cephalosporin antibiotic class: Adverse Reactions: Allergic reactions, including anaphylaxis, Stevens-Johnson syndrome; erythema multiforme, toxic epidermal necrolysis, severe diarrhoea and antibiotic-associated colitis, superinfection, renal dysfunction, toxic nephropathy, hepatic dysfunction, aplastic anemia, haemolytic anemia and haemorrhage. Abnormal Laboratory Tests: Elevated bilirubin, positive direct Coombs test, glycosuria, ketonuria, pancytopenia, neutropenia and agranulocytosis.

*Overdose:* No toxic manifestations have been seen following accidental overdosage with Cedax. Gastric lavage may be indicated, otherwise no specific antidote exists. Significant quantities of Cedax can be removed from the circulation by haemodialysis. Effective removal by peritoneal dialysis has not been determined.

In healthy volunteers receiving single doses of up to 2 gm of Cedax, no serious adverse reactions were observed and all clinical and laboratory findings were within normal range.

**Pharmacological properties**

*Pharmacodynamic properties:* Ceftibuten is a semi-synthetic, third generation cephalosporin antibiotic for oral administration.

*Microbiology:* As with most beta-lactam antibiotics, the bactericidal activity of ceftibuten results from the inhibition of bacterial cell wall synthesis. Due to its chemical structure, ceftibuten is highly stable to beta-lactamases. Many beta-lactamase-producing microorganisms, which are resistant to penicillins or other cephalosporins, may be inhibited by ceftibuten.

Ceftibuten is highly stable toward plasmid-mediated penicillinases and cephalosporinases. However, it is not stable to some cephalosporinases that are chromosomally mediated in organisms such as *Citrobacter*, *Enterobacter* and *Bacteroides*. Ceftibuten binds preferentially to PBP-3 of *E.coli*, resulting in formation of filamentous forms at $\frac{1}{4}$ to $\frac{1}{2}$ the minimum inhibitory concentration (MIC) and lysis at two times the MIC. The minimum bactericidal concentration (MBC) for ampicillin-sensitive and -resistant *E.coli* is nearly equal to the MIC.

Ceftibuten has demonstrated activity *in vitro* and in clinical infections against most strains of the following microorganisms: **Gram-positive microorganisms:** *Streptococcus pyogenes*, *Streptococcus pneumoniae*; Gram-negative microorganisms: *Haemophilus influenzae* (both beta-lactamase positive and negative strains); *Haemophilus parainfluenzae* (beta-lactamase positive and negative); *Moraxella (Branhamella) catarrhalis* (most of which are beta-lactamase positive); *Escherichia coli*; *Klebsiella* spp (including *K. pneumoniae*, and *K. oxytoca*); indole-positive *Proteus* (including *P. vulgaris*) as well as other species of *Proteae*, i.e., *Providencia* (including *P. rettgeri* and *P. stuartii*); *P. mirabilis*; *Enterobacter* spp (including *E. cloacae* and *E. aerogenes*); *Salmonella* spp; *Shigella* spp.

Ceftibuten has demonstrated *in vitro* activity against most strains of the following microorganisms, however clinical efficacy has not been firmly established: Gram-positive microorganisms: Group C streptococci. Gram-negative microorganisms: *Morganella morganii*; *Citrobacter freundii*; *Serratia* spp. (including *S. marcescens*); *Hafnia alvei*; *Edwardsiella tarda*; *Yersinia enterocolitica*.

Ceftibuten has no significant activity against Staphylococci, Enterococci, Acinetobacter, Listeria, Flavobacterium and Pseudomonas spp. In addition, it shows little activity against most anaerobes, including most species of Bacteroides. **Penicillin-resistant strains of *Strep. pneumoniae* are also resistant to ceftibuten.**

*Susceptibility testing:* Diffusion technique: Laboratory results of testing a single disc containing 30 mcg ceftibuten should be interpreted according to the following criteria: a zone diameter ≥ 21 mm is Susceptible (S); 18–20 mm, Moderately Susceptible (MS); ≤ 17 mm, Resistant (R). Standard procedures require the use of laboratory control microorganisms. The 30 mcg disc should give a zone diameter of 29–35 mm for *E.coli* ATCC 25922.

The 30 mcg ceftibuten disc should be used for all *in vitro* testing of isolates. The class disc (cephalothin) for cephalosporin susceptibility testing is not appropriate because of spectrum differences with ceftibuten.

*Dilution technique:* Microorganisms may be considered susceptible to ceftibuten if the MIC value for ceftibuten is ≤ 8 mcg/ml and resistant if the MIC is ≥ 32 mcg/ml. Microorganisms having an MIC of 16 mcg/ml are moderately susceptible.

As with standard diffusion methods, dilution procedures require the use of laboratory control microorganisms. Standard ceftibuten powder should give MIC values in range of 0.125–0.5 mcg/ml for *E.coli* ATCC 25922 and ≥ 32 mcg/ml for *S.aureus* ATCC 29213.

*Pharmacokinetic properties:* Ceftibuten given orally, is almost completely absorbed (≥ 90%), based on urinary recovery. In one study, average peak plasma concentration following oral administration of a single 200 mg capsule of ceftibuten was approximately 10 mcg/ml; for a single 400 mg capsule, the average peak concentration was approximately 17 mcg/ml. Peak plasma concentrations occur between 2 and 3 hours following oral administration of a single 200 mg or 400 mg capsule. Ceftibuten is only slightly (62% to 64%) bound to plasma proteins and is not metabolised.

The major circulating ceftibuten-derived compound, ceftibuten-trans, appears to be formed by direct conversion of ceftibuten (cis-form). Generally, in either plasma or urine, the concentration of ceftibuten-trans is approximately 10% or less of ceftibuten concentration. Ceftibuten-bioavailability is dose-independent within the indicated therapeutic dose range (≤ 400 mg).

In young adult volunteers, ceftibuten plasma concentrations are at steady-state by the fifth dose of a b.i.d. dosage regimen. No appreciable drug accumulation occurs with multiple dosing. Ceftibuten plasma elimination half-life **has** a mean of 2.5 hours, regardless of dose or dosage regimen.

Studies demonstrate that ceftibuten penetrates readily into body fluids and tissues. In blister fluid, ceftibuten concentrations were similar to or higher than those in plasma, based on the areas under the concentration-time curve (AUC) data. Ceftibuten penetrated into the middle ear fluid of paediatric patients with acute otitis media achieving concentrations approximately equal to or greater than those in plasma.

Ceftibuten pulmonary concentrations were approximately 40% of plasma concentrations. In nasal secretion, tracheal secretion, bronchial secretion, bronchial alveolar lavage fluid and its cell button, concentrations were approximately 46%, 20%, 24%, 6% and 81% of plasma concentrations, respectively.

Although a study in hospitalised paediatric patients suggested an age-related increase in ceftibuten bioavailability in the age range of 6 months to 17 years, this trend was not confirmed in paediatric volunteers.

In geriatric volunteers, ceftibuten concentrations were at steady-state by the fifth b.i.d. dose. The average AUC in the population was slightly higher than the average AUC in young adults. Only a slight drug accumulation occurs with multiple dosing in the elderly population.

Ceftibuten pharmacokinetics are not altered significantly by the presence of chronic active hepatitis, cirrhosis of the liver, alcoholic liver disease or other hepatic disorders associated with hepatocellular necrosis.

Ceftibuten AUC and plasma half-life increase with increased severity of renal insufficiency. In physiologically anephric patients (creatinine clearance < 5 ml/min) the AUC and half-life were seven to eight times higher than in normal subjects. A single hemodialysis procedure removed approximately 65% of plasma ceftibuten.

Ceftibuten is not detected in the milk of nursing mothers following single oral doses of 200 mg.

High-calorie, high-fat meals lower the bioavailability of ceftibuten by approximately 20%. In clinical trials, however, Cedax was administered without regard to mealtime with no apparent loss of efficacy.

*Preclinical safety data:* Effects of single oral doses of ceftibuten were observed in juvenile and adult mice and rats. The LD 50 was ≥ 5000 mg/kg in both species; in one rat study, the LD 50 was ≥ 10,000 mg/kg (no deaths reported).

Single and repeated dose studies of ceftibuten were conducted in rats and dogs. When administered orally for up to six months, minimal toxicity was observed in rats at doses ≤ 1000 mg/kg/day and in dogs at doses ≤ 600 mg/kg/day.

Ceftibuten did not reveal any mutagenic potential in genetic toxicity studies including the Ames Plate test and Noumi's IMF test in bacteria and *in vitro* and *in vivo* chromosome aberration tests in mammalian cells.

Long-term animal studies have not been conducted to evaluate the carcinogenic potential of ceftibuten.

**Pharmaceutical particulars**

*List of excipients: Capsule:* Microcrystalline cellulose, sodium starch glycolate and magnesium stearate. The capsule shell contains titanium dioxide E171.

sodium lauryl sulphate and gelatin. The band seal contains polysorbate 80 and gelatin.

*Powder:* Xanthan gum, sucrose, simethicone, silicon dioxide, titanium dioxide, polysorbate 80 and sodium benzoate. The powder is cherry flavoured.

**Incompatibilities:** None known.

*Shelf life:*
Cedax Capsules: 24 months.
Cedax Powder for Oral Suspension 18 mg/ml: 18 months.
Cedax Powder for oral Suspension 36 mg/ml: 24 months.
Reconstituted suspension: 2 weeks.

*Special precautions for storage:* Store Cedax capsules and powder for oral suspension below 25°C. Store reconstituted suspension at 2–8°C.

*Nature and contents of container:* Cedax capsules 400 mg are supplied in cartons of 5 or 7 capsules. Within the carton each capsule is individually packed in a unit pouch of paper/polyethylene/aluminium foil/LDPE laminate.

Cedax Powder for Oral Suspension 90 mg and 180 mg per 5 ml is supplied in Type 1 amber glass bottles, with two piece plastic child resistant screw cap, pulp/polyethylene/waxed liner and pressure sensitive inner seal of paper/aluminium foil/vinyl adhesive. Each bottle contains sufficient powder for the preparation of 60 ml suspension.

*Instructions for use/handling*
*Preparation of oral suspension:* To reconstitute the suspension the following volume of water should be added. Shake well before use. Final volume 60 ml. Volume of water to be added 50 ml.

**Marketing authorisation numbers**
Cedax Capsules 400 mg                                     0201/0170
Cedax Powder for Oral Suspension
18 mg/ml                                                   0201/0171
Cedax Powder for Oral Suspension
36 mg/ml                                                   0201/0172

**Date of approval/revision of SPC**   4 November 1996.

**Legal category**  POM.

# CLARITYN*

## Presentation
*Clarityn Tablets:* White, oval tablets plain on one side, and deep score, flask and dish logo with number 10 on the other side. Each tablet contains 10 mg micronised loratadine.

*Clarityn Syrup:* A clear, colourless to light yellow syrup with a peach flavour, containing 5 mg loratadine in 5 ml.

## Uses
*Mode of action:* Clarityn is a long acting tricyclic antihistamine with selective peripheral $H_1$-receptor antagonistic activity and no central sedative or anticholinergic effects.

*Indications:* Clarityn Tablets and Syrup are indicated in adults for the relief of symptoms associated with seasonal and perennial allergic rhinitis, such as sneezing, nasal discharge and itching and ocular itching and burning. Nasal and ocular signs and symptoms are relieved rapidly after oral administration. Clarityn products are also indicated for the relief of symptoms associated with idiopathic chronic urticaria.

In children over two years, Clarityn Syrup is indicated for the symptomatic treatment of seasonal allergic rhinitis and allergic skin conditions such as idiopathic urticaria.

## Dosage and administration
*Adults, including the elderly, and children 12 years of age and over:* One Clarityn 10 mg tablet or two 5 ml spoons of Clarityn Syrup once daily.

*Children aged 6–12 years:* 10 mg (two 5 ml spoonfuls) of syrup once daily.

*Children aged 2–5 years:* 5 mg (one 5 ml spoonful) of syrup once daily.

Safety and efficacy of Clarityn below 2 yrs has not been established.

## Contra-indications, warnings, etc
*Contra-indications:* Clarityn presentations are contra-indicated in patients who have shown hypersensitivity or idiosyncrasy to their components.

*Pregnancy and lactation:* Clarityn should not be administered during pregnancy. There is no experience of the use of Clarityn in human pregnancy. In animal studies loratadine was not teratogenic; at high doses some embryotoxic effects were observed. Since loratadine is excreted in breast milk it should not be administered to lactating women.

*Side effects:* During controlled clinical studies the incidence of adverse events, including sedation and anticholinergic effects, observed with 10 mg Clarityn was comparable to that observed with placebo. Other

events, fatigue, nausea and headache were reported rarely. Tachycardia and syncope have been reported rarely. Causality has not been established. Spontaneous adverse events reported rarely include: alopecia, anaphylaxis, abnormal hepatic function and supraventricular tachyarrythmias.

*Interactions:* When administered concurrently with alcohol, Clarityn has no potentiating effects as measured by psychomotor performance studies. Loratadine is metabolised by hepatic cytochromes P450 3A4 and 2D6. Concomitant therapy with drugs which inhibit or are metabolised by either system may therefore elevate plasma concentrations of either drug and adverse reactions might result. Studies indicate that cimetidine, which inhibits both enzymes, and erythromycin or ketoconazole, which inhibit P450 3A4 each increased loratadine concentrations, although no adverse effects, clinical or electrocardiographic, were observed. Other drugs known to inhibit either P450 3A4 or P450 2D6 are quinidine, fluconazole or fluoxetine.

*Drug/laboratory test interactions:* Antihistamines should be discontinued about four days prior to skin testing procedures, since these drugs may prevent or diminish otherwise positive reactions to dermal reactivity indicators.

*Overdosage:* In the event of overdosage, treatment which should be started immediately is symptomatic and supportive. The patient should be induced to vomit, even if emesis has occurred spontaneously (ipecacuanha is a preferred method), but not in patients with impaired consciousness. Administration of activated charcoal as a slurry with water may be attempted following emesis. If vomiting is unsuccessful or contra-indicated, gastric lavage should be performed. Loratadine is not dialysable to any appreciable extent. After emergency treatment, the patient should continue to be under medical supervision.

*Pharmaceutical precautions*   Tablets: None. Syrup: Store between 2–30°C.

**Legal category**  POM.

**Package quantities**   Clarityn Tablets: Blister strips of 10 in OP cartons of 30 tablets.
Clarityn Syrup: Bottles of 100 ml syrup.

**Further information**  Nil.

**Product licence numbers**
Clarityn Tablets 10 mg          0201/0175
Clarityn Syrup                  0201/0173

# DIPROBASE CREAM*

## Qualitative and quantitative composition
Chlorocresol BO 0.10% w/w
Cetomacrogol BP 2.25% w/w
Cetostearyl alcohol BP 7.20% w/w
Liquid paraffin BP 6.0% w/w
White soft paraffin BP 15.0% w/w
Phosphoric acid BP 0.002 w/w
Sodium dihydrogen phosphate BP 0.30% w.w
Purified water PhEur to 100.00% w.w

**Pharmaceutical form**   Cream

## Clincal particulars
*Therapeutic indications:* Diprobase Cream is an emollient, moisturising and protective cream for the follow-up treatment with topical steroids or in spacing such treatment. It may also be used as diluent for topical steroids. Diprobase Cream is recommended for the symptomatic relief of red, inflamed, damaged, dry or chapped skin, the protection of raw skin areas and as a pre-bathing emollient for dry/eczematous skin to alleviate drying areas.

*Posology and method of administration:* The cream should be applied to the dry skin areas as often as is required and rubbed well into the skin.

*Contra-indications:* There are no absolute contra-indications to the use of the cream other than hypersensitivity to any of the ingredients.

*Special warnings and special precautions for use:* None stated

*Interactions with other medicaments and other forms of interaction:* None stated.

*Pregnancy and lactation:* none stated.

*Effects on ability to drive and use machines:* None stated.

*Undesirable effects:* Rarely, mild skin reactions have been observed.

*Overdose:* None stated.

## Pharmacological properties
*Pharmacodynamic properties:* Diprobase Cream contains no active ingredients and has no pharmacological action. The ingredients provide emollient, moisturising action on dry or chapped skin.

*Pharmacoklinetic properties:* Not applicable due to topical administration and direct action on the skin.

*Preclinical safety data:* Not relevant.

## Pharmaceutical particulars
*List of excipients:* Cholorcresol; cetomacrogol; cetostearyl alcohol; liquid paraffin; white soft paraffin; phosphoric acid; sodium dihydrogen phosphate, purified water.

*Incompatibilities:* None known.

*Shelf life:* 60 months.

*Special precautions for storage:* Store below 25°C.

*Nature and contents of containers:* 50 gm aluminium epoxy lined tubes with plastic caps.

500 gm polypropylene piston pack with polyethylene cap and daplen pump, disc and tube or PVC cap, polypropylene pump, polyolefin disc and HDPE tube.

*Instructions for use/handling:* Not applicable.

**Marketing authorisation number**   0201/0076.

**Date of approval/revision of SPC**   29 April 1996

**Legal category**  GSL.

# DIPROBASE* OINTMENT

## Qualitative and quantitative composition
White soft paraffin BP 5.0% w/w
Liquid paraffin BP 95.0% w/w

**Pharmaceutical form**   Ointment

## Clincal particulars
*Therapeutic indications:* Diprobase Ointment is an emollient, moisturising and protective ointment for the follow-up treatment with topical steroids or in spacing such treatment. It may also be used as diluent for topical steroids. Diprobase Ointment is recommended for the symptomatic relief of red, inflamed, damaged, dry or chapped skin, the protection of raw skin areas and as a pre-bathing emollient for dry/eczematous skin to alleviate drying areas.

*Posology and method of administration:*
*Adults and children:* The ointment should be thinly applied to cover the affected area completely, massaging gently and thoroughly into the skin. Frequency of application should be established by the physician. Generally, Diprobase Ointment can be used as often as required.

*Contra-indications:* Hypersensitivity to any of the components of the ointment is a contraindication to its use.

*Special warnings and special precautions for use:* None stated

*Interactions with other medicaments and other forms of interaction:* None stated.

*Pregnancy and lactation:* none stated.

*Effects on ability to drive and use machines:* None stated.

*Undesirable effects:* None stated.

*Overdose:* None stated.

## Pharmacological properties
*Pharmacodynamic properties:* Diprobase Ointment contains no active ingredients and has no pharmacological action. The ingredients have an emollient action on dry or chapped skin.

*Pharmacoklinetic properties:* Not applicable due to topical administration and direct action on the skin.

*Preclinical safety data:* Not relevant.

## Pharmaceutical particulars
*List of excipients:* White soft paraffin and liquid paraffin.

*Incompatibilities:* None known.

*Shelf life:* 60 months.

*Special precautions for storage:* Store below 25°C.

*Nature and copntents of containers:* 50 gm epoxy lined aluminium tubes with plastic caps or polypropylene tubes.

*Instructions for use/handling:* Not applicable.

**Marketing authorisation number**   0201/0075.

**Date of approval/revision of SPC**   29 April 1996

**Legal category**  GSL.

# DIPROBATH*

## Qualitative and quantitative composition
Light liquid paraffin 46.0 w/w
Isopropyl myristate 39.0 w/w
Laureth-4 15.0% w/w

**Pharmaceutical form**   Liquid bath emollient.

## Clinical particulars
*Therapeutic indications:* Treatment of dry skin condi-

tions and other hyperkeratoses, including those associated with dermatitis and eczema.

To be diluted in bath water for external application.

*Posology and method of administation: Adults including elderly patients:* 25 ml or approximately 2.5 capsful to be diluted in bath of water (100 l approximately). for particularly dry skin the quantity of oil emollient may be doubled.

*Children:* 100 ml or one capful is sufficient for children's baths.

Frequency and duration of bathing will depend on the type and severity of the conditions, but generally 2 to 3 baths should be taken weekly.

*Contra-indications:* Known hypersensitivity to any of the ingredients.

*Special warnings and precautions for use:* As Diprobath deposits a film of oil over the skin, care should be taken to avoid slipping in the bath.

The following warning will appear on the label: 'Take care when entering or leaving the bath which may be more slippery than usual'.

*Interactions with other medicaments and other forms of interaction:* None known.

*Pregnancy and lactation:* No special precautions.

*Effects on ability to drive and use machines:* None known.

*Undesirable effects:* None known.

*Overdose:* Not applicable.

**Pharmacological properties**

*Pharmacodynamic properties:* Both active ingredients have established emollient properties which are of relevance to use as a bathing emollient.

*Pharmacokinetic properties:* Pharmacokinetic principles are not involved due to direct topical application.

*Preclinical safety data:* There are no pre-clinical data of relevance to the prescriber which are additional to that already included in other sections of the SPC.

**Pharmaceutical particulars**

*List of excipients:* Laureth-4.

*Incompatibilities:* None known.

*Shelf life:* 24 months.

*Special precautions for storage:* Store upright at a temperature below 30°C.

*Nature and contents of containers:* 500 ml natural opaque HDPE single neck container with polypropylene or urea/formaldehyde, steran or expanded polyethylene wadded screw cap.

*Instructions for use/handling:* Not applicable.

**Marketing authorisation number** 0201/0174.

**Date of approval/revision of SPC** July 1996.

**Legal category** P.

## DIPROSALIC*

**Presentation** DiproSalic Ointment contains 0.05% betamethasone as the dipropionate ester and 3% salicylic acid. It is a smooth white, preservative-free ointment.

DiproSalic Scalp Application contains 0.05% betamethasone as the dipropionate ester and 2% salicylic acid in a preservative-free isopropyl alcohol base. It is formulated to spread easily without adherence to the hair.

**Uses** Betamethasone dipropionate is a synthetic fluorinated corticosteroid. In combination with salicylic acid it is indicated for the treatment of chronic lichenified eczema, lichen planus, lichen simplex, non bullous ichthyosiform erythroderma. It is also effective in the less responsive conditions such as psoriasis of the scalp and chronic plaque psoriasis of the hands and feet but excluding widespread plaque psoriasis.

Topical salicylic acid softens keratin, loosens cornified epithelium and desquamates the epidermis.

**Dosage and administration** Once to twice daily.

*DiproSalic Ointment:* In most cases a thin film should be applied to cover the affected area once or twice daily.

*DiproSalic Scalp Application:* In most cases a few drops should be applied to the affected areas once or twice daily and massaged gently and thoroughly into the skin.

For some patients adequate maintenance therapy may be achieved with less frequent application.

It is recommended that DiproSalic preparations are prescribed for 2 weeks, and that treatment is reviewed at that time. The maximum weekly dose should not exceed 60 g.

**Contra-indications, warnings, etc**

*Contra-indications:* Rosacea, acne, peri-anal and genital pruritus and peri-oral dermatitis. Hypersensitivity to any of the ingredients of the DiproSalic preparations contra-indicates their use as do tuberculous and most viral lesions of the skin, particularly herpes simplex, vaccinia, varicella. DiproSalic Ointment and Lotion should not be used in napkin eruptions, fungal or bacterial skin infections without suitable concomitant anti-infective therapy.

Occlusion must not be used, since under these circumstances the keratolytic action of salicylic acid may lead to enhanced absorption of the steroid.

*Warnings:* Local and systemic toxicity is common, especially following long continued use on large areas of damaged skin, in flexures or with polythene occlusion. If used in children or on the face, courses should be limited to five days. Long term, continuous therapy should be avoided in all patients irrespective of age.

Topical corticosteroids may be hazardous in psoriasis for a number of reasons, including rebound relapses following development of tolerance, risk of generalised, pustular psoriasis and local systemic toxicity due to impaired barrier function of the skin. Careful patient supervision is important.

It is dangerous if DiproSalic presentations come into contact with the eyes. Avoid contact with eyes and mucous membranes.

There is inadequate evidence of safety in human pregnancy. Topical administration of corticosteroids to pregnant animals can cause abnormalities of foetal development including cleft palate and intra-uterine growth retardation. There may therefore be a very small risk of such effects in the human foetus.

The systemic absorption of betamethasone dipropionate and salicylic acid may be increased if extensive body surface areas or skin folds are treated for prolonged periods or with excessive amounts of steroids. Suitable precautions should be taken in these circumstances, particularly with infants and children.

*Side-effects:* DiproSalic skin preparations are generally well tolerated and side-effects are rare. Continuous application without interruption may result in local atrophy of the skin, striae and superficial vascular dilation, particularly on the face. In addition prolonged use of salicylic acid preparations may cause dermatitis.

*Overdosage:* Excessive prolonged use of topical corticosteroids can suppress pituitary-adrenal functions resulting in secondary adrenal insufficiency which is usually reversible. In such cases appropriate symptomatic treatment is indicated.

With topical preparations containing salicylic acid excessive prolonged use may result in symptoms of salicylism. Treatment is symptomatic.

The steroid and salicylic acid content of each tube is so low as to have little or no toxic effect in the unlikely event of accidental oral ingestion.

**Pharmaceutical precautions** Store in a cool place.

**Legal category** POM.

**Package quantities** DiproSalic Ointment is supplied in 30 g and 100 g tubes. DiproSalic Scalp Application is supplied in 100 ml bottles.

**Further information** DiproSalic Ointment and Scalp Application are formulated to avoid the problems of incompatibility normally experienced between steroids and salicylic acid.

**Product licence numbers**

| | |
|---|---|
| Diprosalic Ointment | 0201/0070 |
| Diprosalic Scalp Application | 0201/0069 |

## DIPROSONE*

**Presentation** The DiproSone skin preparations contain 0.05% betamethasone as the dipropionate ester.

DiproSone Cream is a smooth white cream. It contains chlorocresol as the preservative.

DiproSone Ointment is a smooth white preservative free ointment.

DiproSone Lotion is a slightly gelled solution containing isopropyl alcohol, which has antibacterial activity. It is formulated to spread without adherence to hair.

**Uses** Betamethasone dipropionate is a synthetic fluorinated corticosteroid. It is active topically and produces a rapid and sustained response in eczema and dermatitis of all types, including atopic eczema, photo-dermatitis, primary irritant and allergic dermatitis, lichen planus, lichen simplex, prurigo nodularis, discoid lupus erythematosus, necrobiosis lipoidica, pretibial myxoedema and erythroderma. It is also effective in the less responsive conditions such as psoriasis of the scalp and chronic plaque psoriasis of the hands, but excluding widespread plaque psoriasis.

DiproSone Lotion is indicated for serious steroid responsive dermatoses of the scalp.

**Dosage and administration** Once to twice daily. In most cases a thin film of DiproSone Cream or Ointment should be applied to cover the affected area once or twice daily. For some patients adequate maintenance therapy may be achieved with less frequent application.

DiproSone Cream is especially appropriate for moist or weeping surfaces and the Ointment for dry lichenified or scaly lesions but this is not invariably so.

Control over the dosage regimen may be achieved during intermittent and maintenance therapy by using DiproBase Cream or Ointment (PL 0201/0076 and 0201/0075) the base vehicles of DiproSone Cream and Ointment. Such control may be necessary in mild and improving dry skin conditions requiring low dose steroid treatment.

A few drops of DiproSone Lotion should be applied to the affected areas twice daily and massaged gently and thoroughly into the scalp. For some patients adequate maintenance therapy may be achieved with less frequent application.

**Contra-indications, warnings, etc**

*Contra-indications:* Rosacea, acne, perioral dermatitis perianal and genital pruritus. Hypersensitivity to any of the ingredients of the DiproSone preparations contra-indicates their use, as does tuberculous and most viral lesions of the skin, particularly herpes simplex, vaccinia, varicella. DiproSone should not be used in napkin eruptions, fungal or bacterial skin infections without suitable concomitant anti-infective therapy.

*Warnings:* Local and systemic toxicity is common especially following long continued use on large areas of damaged skin, in flexures or with polythene occlusion. If used in children or on the face courses should be limited to five days. Long term continuous therapy should be avoided in all patients irrespective of age. Occlusion must not be used.

Topical corticosteroids may be hazardous in psoriasis for a number of reasons, including rebound relapses following development of tolerance, risk of generalised pustular psoriasis and local systemic toxicity due to impaired barrier function of the skin. Careful patient supervision is important.

There is inadequate evidence of safety in human pregnancy. Topical administration of corticosteroid to pregnant animals can cause abnormalities of foetal development including cleft palate and intra-uterine growth retardation. There may, therefore, be a very small risk of such effects in the human foetus.

*Side effects:* DiproSone skin preparations are generally well tolerated and side effects are rare. The systemic absorption of betamethasone dipropionate may be increased if extensive body surface areas or skin folds are treated for prolonged periods or with excessive amounts of steroids. Suitable precautions should be taken in these circumstances, particularly with infants and children.

Continuous application without interruption may result in local atrophy of the skin, striae and superficial vascular dilatation, particularly on the face.

*Overdosage:* Excessive prolonged use of topical corticosteroids can result in suppression of pituitary adrenal function resulting in secondary adrenal insufficiency which is usually reversible. In such cases appropriate symptomatic treatment is indicated.

The steroid content of each tube is so low as to have little or no toxic effect in the unlikely event of accidental oral ingestion.

**Pharmaceutical precautions** Store in a cool place.

**Legal category** POM.

**Package quantities** DiproSone Cream and Ointment are supplied in 30 g and 100 g tubes.

DiproSone Lotion is supplied in 30 ml and 100 ml plastic bottles.

**Further information** These preparations do not contain lanolin or parabens.

**Product licence numbers**

| | |
|---|---|
| Cream | 0201/0072 |
| Ointment | 0201/0074 |
| Lotion | 0201/0073 |

## DROGENIL TABLETS*

**Qualitative and quantitative composition** Flutamide (INN) 250 mg.

**Pharmaceutical form** Tablets.

**Clincal particulars**

*Therapeutic indications:* Treatment of advanced prostatic carcinoma in which suppression of testosterone effects is indicated: as initial treatment in combination with an LHRH agonist; as adjunctive therapy in patients already receiving LHRH agonist therapy; in surgically castrated patients; in the treatment of patients who have not responded to other forms of hormonal manipulation or in patients who cannot tolerate such treatment.

In combination with LHRH agonists for the manage

ment of locally confined B2–C2 (T2b–T4) prostate carcinoma as initial therapy; bulky primary tumours confined to the prostate (stage B2 or T2b) or extending beyond the capsule (stage C or T3–T4), with or without pelvic node involvement.

*Posology and method of administration:* One 250 mg tablet three times daily at 8 hour intervals.

*Route of administration:* Oral.

When used as initial treatment with an LHRH agonist, a greater reduction in the incidence and severity of the LHRH agonist flare reaction may be achieved if flutamide is introduced before rather than concomitantly with the agonist. It is, therefore, recommended that flutamide one tablet three times daily should be started at least three days prior to initiation of the LHRH agonist and continued thereafter at the same dose.

In the management of locally confined prostatic carcinoma, the recommended dosage is one 250 mg tablet three times a day. Drogenil should be started at least three days prior to initiation of the LHRH agonist. Administration of Drogenil and the LHRH agonist should begin eight weeks prior to radiation therapy and continue through the course of radiation therapy (usually approx. 8 weeks) i.e. a total of approximately 16 weeks.

Dosage adjustment in renal or liver insufficiency: In patients with impaired liver function, long-term treatment with flutamide should only be administered after careful assessment of the individual benefits and risks.

Monitoring advice: Flutamide is highly protein bound and will not be removed by dialysis.

*Contra-indications:* Patients exhibiting sensitivity reactions to flutamide or any component of this preparation.

*Special warnings and precautions for use:* Hepatic injury: Transaminase abnormalities, cholestatic jaundice, hepatic necrosis, and hepatic encephalopathy have been reported with the use of flutamide. The hepatic conditions were usually reversible after discontinuing therapy or dosage reduction, although there have been occasional reports of a fatal outcome following severe hepatic injury in patients receiving flutamide. Periodic liver function tests should be considered in all patients and performed in patients on long-term treatment. Appropriate laboratory testing should be done at the first symptom/sign of liver dysfunction (e.g., pruritus, dark urine, persistent anorexia, jaundice, right upper quadrant tenderness or unexplained 'flue-like' symptoms). If the patient has laboratory evidence of liver injury or jaundice, in the absence of biopsy-confirmed liver metastases, Drogenil therapy should be discontinued or the dosage reduced.

In addition, in patients who have not received medical or surgical castration, periodic sperm count determinations may be considered during long-term treatment. In such patients flutamide administration tends to elevate plasma testosterone and estradiol levels. Fluid retention may occur, thus the drug should be used with caution in cardiac disease.

*Interactions with other medicaments and other forms of interaction:* Increases in prothrombin time have been reported in patients receiving long-term warfarin therapy after flutamide monotherapy was initiated. Therefore, close monitoring of prothrombin time is recommended. Adjustment of the anticoagulant dose may be necessary when flutamide is administered concomitantly with warfarin.

*Pregnancy and lactation:* Drogenil is indicated only for use in male patients. No studies have been conducted in pregnant or lactating women. Therefore, the possibility that Drogenil may cause foetal harm if administered to a pregnant woman, or may be present in the breast milk of a lactating woman, must be considered.

*Effects on ability to drive and use machines:* Flutamide is presumed to be safe, or unlikely to produce an effect.

*Undesirable effects: Monotherapy:* In clinical studies, the most frequently reported adverse reactions to Drogenil Tablets are gynecomastia and/or breast tenderness, sometimes accompanied by galactorrhea. These reactions disappear upon discontinuation of treatment or reduction in dosage.

Drogenil Tablets demonstrate a low potential for cardiovascular liability, and when compared to diethylstilbestrol this liability has been shown to be significantly lower. Less frequent adverse reactions: diarrhoea, nausea, vomiting, increased appetite, insomnia, tiredness, transient abnormal liver function and hepatitis (see *Additional adverse experiences* and *Special warnings*).

Rare adverse reactions: decreased libido, upset stomach, anorexia, ulcer-like pain, heartburn, constipation, oedema, ecchymoses, herpes zoster, pruritus, lupus-like syndrome, headache, dizziness, weakness, malaise, blurred vision, thirst, chest pain, anxiety, depression, lymphoedema.

Reduced sperm counts have been reported rarely.

*Combination therapy:* In clinical studies, the most frequently reported adverse effects experienced during combination therapy of Drogenil Tablets with LHRH agonist were hot flushes, decreased libido, impotence, diarrhoea, nausea and vomiting. With the exception of diarrhoea, these adverse experiences are known to occur with LHRH agonist alone, and at comparable frequency.

The high incidence of gynecomastia observed with flutamide monotherapy was reduced greatly in combination therapy. In clinical trials, no significant difference in gynecomastia incidence was observed between the placebo- and the flutamide-LHRH agonist treatment groups.

Rarely, patients experienced anaemia, leukopenia, unspecified gastro-intestinal disorders, anorexia, injection site irritation and rash, oedema, neuromuscular symptoms, jaundice, genitourinary tract symptoms, hypertension, central nervous system adverse events (drowsiness, depression, confusion, anxiety, nervousness) and thrombocytopenia.

Very rarely, pulmonary symptoms, hepatitis and photosensitivity have occurred.

Additional adverse experiences: In addition, the following adverse experiences have been reported during worldwide marketing of Drogenil tablets: haemolytic anaemia, macrocytic anaemia, methemoglobinemia, photosensitivity reactions—including erythema, ulcerations, bullous eruptions, and epidermal necrolysis—and change in urine colour to amber or yellow-green appearance, which can be attributed to flutamide and/or its metabolites.

Also observed were cholestatic jaundice, hepatic encephalopathy and hepatic necrosis. The hepatic conditions were usually reversible after discontinuing therapy; however, there have been reports of death following severe hepatic injury associated with use of flutamide.

Two reports of malignant male breast neoplasms in patients dosed with Drogenil have been reported. One involved aggravation of a pre-existing nodule which was first detected three or four months before initiation of Drogenil monotherapy in a patient with benign prostatic hypertrophy. After excision, this was diagnosed as a poorly differentiated ductal carcinoma. The other report involved gynecomastia and a nodule noted two and six months, respectively, after initiation of Drogenil monotherapy for treatment of advanced prostatic carcinoma. Nine months after the initiation of therapy the nodule was excised and diagnosed as a moderately differentiated invasive ductal tumour staged T4NOMO, G3, no metastases had advanced.

Abnormal laboratory test values reported include changes in liver function, elevated blood urea nitrogen (BUN) and rarely, elevated serum creatinine values.

Usually these reactions have not been of sufficient severity to require dosage reduction or discontinuation of therapy.

*Overdose:* In animal studies with flutamide alone, signs of overdose included hypoactivity, piloerection, slow respiration, ataxia and/or lacrimation, anorexia, tranquilization, emesis and methemoglobinemia.

The single dose of flutamide ordinarily associated with symptoms of overdose of considered to be life-threatening has not been established. One patient survived after taking more than 5 g as a single dose—no adverse effects were observed.

Since flutamide is highly protein bound, dialysis may not be of any use as treatment for overdose.

**Pharmacological properties**

*Pharmacodynamic properties:* Flutamide is an anilide, nonsteroidal oral antiandrogen. In animal studies flutamide demonstrates potent antiandrogenic effects. It exerts its antiandrogenic action by inhibiting androgen uptake and/or by inhibiting nuclear binding in target tissues. When flutamide is given in combination with surgical or medical castration, suppression of both testicular and adrenal androgen activity is achieved.

*Pharmacokinetic properties:* Flutamide is well absorbed following oral ingestion. Studies with radiolabelled flutamide show rapid and extensive conversion to its metabolites which are detectable in plasma up to 8 hours post dosing. Approximately 45% of the administered dose is excreted in urine and 2% in faeces during the first two days. Metabolism removes the radiolabel resulting in apparent slowing of excretion due to retention of the label as tritiated water. Thus excretion and metabolism is essentially complete within two days.

*Preclinical safety data:* Animal studies to determine tolerance after repeated administration have been performed in monkeys for up to 6 weeks, in rats for up to 52 weeks and in dogs for up to 78 weeks. The daily administered oral doses were up to 90 mg/kg in monkeys, up to 40 mg/kg in dogs and up to 180 mg/kg in rats, corresponding to 1.5 to 18 fold of the dose used in humans. In addition to weight loss and anorexia which occurred in all animal species, vomiting was observed in dogs and monkeys. All other clinical findings showed no abnormalities. The autopsy finding revealed a reduced size of the prostate, testicles and seminal vesicles with suppressed spermatogenesis which correspond to the antiandrogenic effect of flutamide. In addition, an increase in organ weight of the liver in rats and dogs, and increased transaminase levels in dogs were observed without corresponding morphological changes. In rats only, the occurrence of drug-related (but not dose-dependent) adenomas of testicular interstitial cells was observed. This effect is related to the mechanism of action of flutamide and is species-specific. In a long-term study in rats, dose-related increases in mammary gland adenomas or carcinomas were observed.

*Mutagenicity:* In a range of screening tests flutamide did not show any mutagenic potential.

*Reproduction toxicity:* The influence of flutamide on fertility and the development of the progeny has been studied in rats; additional teratogenicity studies have been performed in rabbits. The effects were related to the antiandrogenic actions of flutamide. These effects are not relevant to the clinical use of flutamide in prostate cancer.

**Pharmaceutical particulars**

*List of excipients:* Lactose, sodium lauryl sulphate, microcrystalline cellulose, starch, silica gel, magnesium stearate.

*Incompatibilities:* None known.

*Shelf life:* 60 months.

*Special precautions for storage:* Store below 25°C. Protect from light.

*Nature and contents of container:* Calendar packs of 84 tablets OP.

*Instructions for use/handling:* None.

**Marketing authorisation number** 0201/0062.

**Date of approval/revision of SPC** 23 September 1996

**Legal category** POM.

## ELOCON* CREAM
## ELOCON* OINTMENT

**Qualitative and quantitative composition** Mometasone furoate 0.1% w/w.

**Pharmaceutical form** Cream or ointment.

**Clincal particulars**

*Therapeutic indications:* Elocon Cream and Ointment are indicated for the treatment of inflammatory and pruritic manifestations of psoriasis (excluding widespread plaque psoriasis) and atopic dermatitis.

*Posology and method of administration:*

*Adults, including elderly patients and children:* a thin film of Elocon Cream or Ointment should be applied to the affected areas of skin once daily.

Use of topical corticosteroids in children or on the face should be limited to the least amount compatible with an effective therapeutic regimen and duration of treatment should be no more than 5 days.

*Contra-indications:* Elocon is contra-indicated in facial rosacea, acne vulgaris, perioral dermatitis, perianal and genital pruritus, napkin eruptions, bacterial (e.g. impetigo), viral (e.g. herpes simplex, herpes zoster and chickenpox) and fungal (e.g. candida or dermatophyte) infections, varicella, tuberculosis, syphilis or post-vaccine reactions. Elocon should not be used in patients who are sensitive to mometasone furoate, or to other corticosteroids.

*Special warnings and precautions for use:* If irritation or sensitisation develop with the use of Elocon treatment should be withdrawn and appropriate therapy instituted.

Should an infection develop, use of an appropriate antifungal or antibacterial agent should be instituted. If a favourable response does not occur promptly, the corticosteroid should be discontinued until the infection is adequately controlled.

Local and systemic toxicity is common especially following long continued use on large areas of damaged skin, in flexures and with polythene occlusion. If used in childhood, or on the face, courses should be limited to 5 days and occlusion should not be used. Long term continuous therapy should be avoided in all patients irrespective of age.

Topical steroids may be hazardous in psoriasis for a number of reasons including rebound relapses following development of tolerance, risk of centralised pustular psoriasis and development of local or systemic toxicity due to impaired barrier function of the skin. If used in psoriasis careful patient supervision is important.

Elocon topical preparations are not for ophthalmic use.

*Interactions with other medicaments and other forms of interaction:* None stated.

*Pregnancy and lactation:* There is inadequate evidence of safety in human pregnancy. Topical administration of corticosteroids to pregnant animals can cause abnormalities of foetal development including cleft palate and intra-uterine growth retardation. There may therefore be a very small risk of such effects in the human foetus.

It is not known whether topical administration of corticosteroids could result in sufficient systemic absorption to produce detectable quantities in breast milk. Elocon should be administered to nursing mothers only after careful consideration of the benefit/risk relationship.

*Effects on ability to drive and use machines:* None stated.

*Undesirable effects:* Local adverse reactions, occasionally reported with Elocon included paresthesia, folliculitis, burning, pruritus, tingling, stinging, allergic contact dermatitis, hypopigmentation, hypertrichosis, secondary infection, striae, acneiform reactions and signs of skin atrophy.

Local adverse reactions reported infrequently with other topical corticosteroids include: irritation, perioral dermatitis, maceration of the skin and miliaria.

Paediatric patients may demonstrate greater susceptibility to topical cosrticosteroid-induced hypothalamic-pituitary-adrenal axis suppression and Cushing's syndrome than mature patients because of a larger skin surface area to body weight ratio. Chronic corticosteroid therapy may interfere with the growth and development of children.

*Overdosage:* None stated.

### Pharmacological properties

*Pharmacodynamic properties:* Mometasone furoate exhibits marked anti-inflammatory activity and marked anti-psoriatic activity in standard animal predictive models.

In the croton oil assay in mice, mometasone was equipotent to betamethasone valerate after single application and about 8 times as potent after five applications.

In guinea pigs, mometasone was approximately twice as potent as betamethasone valerate in reducing m.ovalis-induced epidermal acanthosis (i.e. anti-psoriatic activity) after 14 applications.

*Pharmacokinetic properties:* Pharmacokinetic studies have indicated that systemic absorption following topical application of mometasone furoate cream 0.1% is minimal, approximately 0.4% of the applied dose in man, the majority of which is excreted within 72 hours following application. Characterisation of metabolites was not feasible owing to the small amounts present in plasma and excreta.

*Preclinical safety data:* There are no pre-clinical data of relevance to the prescriber which are additional to that already included in other sections of the SPC.

### Pharmaceutical particulars

*List of excipients: Cream:* Hexylene glycol; phosphoric acid; propylene glycolstearate; stearyl alcohol and ceteareth-20; titanium dioxide; aluminium starch octenylsuccinate; white wax; white petrolatum; purified water.

*Ointment:* Hexylene glycol; phosphoric acid; propylene glycolstearate; white wax; white petrolatum; purified water.

*Incompatibilities:* Not known.

*Shelf life:* 36 months.

*Special precautions for storage:* Store between 2 and 30˚C.

*Nature and contents of container:* 30 and 100 gm aluminium tubes with low density polyethylene cap or laminated tubes with high density polyethylene head and polypropylene cap.

*Instructions for use/handling:* Not applicable.

### Marketing authorisation numbers

Elocon Cream         0201/0117
Elocon Ointment     0201/0118

**Date of approval/revision of SPC**   January 1996

**Lega category**   POM.

## ELOCON* LOTION

**Presentation**   White to off white lotion containing 0.1% w/w mometasone furoate.

**Uses**   Mometasone furoate is an active topical corticosteroid, exhibiting anti-inflammatory, anti-pruritic and vasoconstrictive properties.

Elocon Lotion is indicated for the treatment of inflammatory and pruritic manifestations of psoriasis (excluding widespread plaque psoriasis) and atopic dermatitis. Elocon Lotion is also indicated for treatment of scalp psoriasis and seborrhoeic dermatitis.

### Dosage and administration

*Adults, including elderly patients and children:* A few drops of Elocon Lotion should be applied to the affected skin area including scalp sites, once daily; massage gently and thoroughly until the medication disappears.

Use of topical corticosteroids in children should be limited to the least amount compatible with an effective therapeutic regimen and duration of treatment should be no more than 5 days.

### Contra-indications, warnings, etc

*Contra-indications:* Elocon is contra-indicated in facial rosacea, acne vulgaris, perioral dermatitis, perianal and genital pruritus, napkin eruptions, bacterial (e.g. impetigo), viral (e.g. herpes simplex, herpes zoster and chickenpox) and fungal (e.g. candida or dermatophyte) infections, varicella, tuberculosis, syphilis or post-vaccine reactions. Elocon should not be used in patients who are sensitive to mometasone furoate, or to other corticosteroids.

*Precautions:* If irritation or sensitisation develop with the use of Elocon, treatment should be withdrawn and appropriate therapy instituted.

Should an infection develop, use of an appropriate antifungal or antibacterial agent should be instituted. If a favourable response does not occur promptly, the corticosteroid should be discontinued until the infection is adequately controlled.

Local and systemic toxicity is common especially following long continued use on large areas of damaged skin, in flexures and with polythene occlusion. If used in childhood, or on the face, courses should be limited to 5 days and occlusion should not be used. Long term continuous therapy should be avoided in all patients irrespective of age.

Topical steroids may be hazardous in psoriasis for a number of reasons including rebound relapses following development of tolerance, risk of generalised pustular psoriasis and development of local or systemic toxicity due to impaired barrier function of the skin. If used in psoriasis careful patient supervision is important.

Elocon topical preparations are not for ophthalmic use.

*Use in pregnancy and lactation:* There is inadequate evidence of safety in human pregnancy. Topical administration of corticosteroids to pregnant animals can cause abnormalities of foetal development including cleft palate and intra-uterine growth retardation. There may therefore be a very small risk of such effects in the human foetus.

It is not known whether topical administration of corticosteroids could result in sufficient systemic absorption to produce detectable quantities in breast milk. Elocon should be administered to pregnant women or nursing mothers only after careful consideration of the benefit/risk relationship.

*Side-effects:* Local adverse reactions, occasionally reported with Elocon included paresthesia, folliculitis, burning, pruritus, tingling, stinging, allergic contact dermatitis, hypopigmentation, hypertrichosis, secondary infection, striae, acneiform reactions and signs of skin atrophy. Local adverse reactions reported infrequently with other topical corticosteroids include: irritation, perioral dermatitis, maceration of the skin and miliaria.

Paediatric patients may demonstrate greater susceptibility to topical cosrticosteroid-induced hypothalamic-pituitary-adrenal axis suppression and Cushing's syndrome than mature patients because of a larger skin surface area to body weight ratio. Chronic corticosteroid therapy may interfere with the growth and development of children.

*Overdosage:* Excessive prolonged use of topical corticosteroids can suppress pituitary-adrenal function resulting in secondary adrenal insufficiency which is usually reversible. In such cases appropriate symptomatic treatment is indicated.

The steroid content of each presentation is so low as to have little or no toxic effect in the unlikely event of accidental oral ingestion.

**Pharmaceutical precautions**   Store below 25˚C.

**Legal category**   POM.

**Package quantities**   30 ml bottle.

**Further information**   Nil.

**Product licence number**   0201/0156

## ETHYOL* ▼

**Presentation**   Ethyol is a sterile, lyophilised powder for injection. Each vial contains 500 mg amifostine (active ingredient) and 500 mg of mannitol (bulking agent). Ethyol (amifostine) lyophilised powder for injection is prepared as a sterile lyophilised powder mixture with mannitol requiring reconstitution with 9.5 ml of sterile 0.9% sodium chloride solution before intravenous infusion.

### Uses

*Therapeutic indications:* Ethyol is indicated to reduce the neutropenia related risk of infection (e.g. neutropenic fever) due to the combination regimen cyclophosphamide and cisplatinum in patients with advanced (FIGO stage III or IV) ovarian carcinoma.

Ethyol is indicated to protect patients with advanced solid tumours of non-germ cell origin from cumulative nephrotoxicity of cisplatin and cisplatin containing regimens, where unit doses of cisplatin range from 60–120 mg/m² in conjunction with adequate hydration measures.

**Dosage and administration**   Prior to intravenous administration, Ethyol for injection is reconstituted with 9.5 ml of sterile 0.9% sodium chloride solution. The reconstituted solution (500 mg of amifostine/10 ml) may be kept 6 hours at room temperature (15–25˚C) or 24 hours under refrigeration (2–8˚C).

In patients with advanced ovarian carcinoma receiving the combination regimen of cisplatin and cyclophosphamide, the recommended starting dose of Ethyol is 910 mg/m² administered once daily as a 15 minute i.v. infusion starting within 30 minutes prior to chemotherapy with agents given by short infusion.

If Ethyol is intended to reduce nephrotoxicity associated with cisplatin, then the starting dose of Ethyol should be correlated with the dose and schedule of cisplatin. For cisplatin doses of 100–120 mg/m², the recommended starting dose of Ethyol is 910 mg/m² administered as a 15-minute infusion starting within 30 minutes prior to chemotherapy.

If the dose of cisplatin is less than 100 mg/m², but greater than or equal to 60 mg/m², the recommended starting dose of Ethyol is 740 mg/m² administered as a 15-minute infusion starting with 30 minutes prior to chemotherapy.

The 15-minute infusion for the 740–910 mg/m² dose is reportedly better tolerated than more extended infusion durations. Further reduced infusion times have not been systematically explored.

During the infusion of Ethyol, arterial blood pressure should be monitored.

The infusion of Ethyol should be interrupted if the systolic blood pressure decreases significantly from the baseline value as listed in the following guideline:

*Guideline for interrupting amifostine infusion due to decrease in systolic blood pressure.*

| | Baseline systolic blood pressure (mm Hg) | | | | |
| --- | --- | --- | --- | --- | --- |
| | < 100 | 100–119 | 120–139 | 140–179 | ≥ 180 |
| Decrease in systolic blood pressure during infusion of amifostine (mm Hg) | 20 | 25 | 30 | 40 | 50 |

If the blood pressure returns to normal within 5 minutes and the patient is asymptomatic, the infusion may be restarted so that the full dose of Ethyol may be administered. If the full dose of Ethyol cannot be administered, the dose of Ethyol for subsequent cycles should be reduced by 20%. For example, the 910 mg/m² dose would be reduced to 740 mg/m².

It is recommended that antiemetic medication be administered prior to and in conjunction with amifostine especially when used with strongly emetogenic chemotherepy such as cisplatin.

Ethyol should only be used under the supervision of physicians experienced in cancer chemotherapy.

*Use in the elderly and children:* Due to lack of experience, Ethyol is contra-indicated in these groups.

### Contra-indications, warnings, etc

*Contra-indications:* Known sensitivity to aminothiol compounds or mannitol. Patients who are hypotensive or in a state of dehydration should not receive Ethyol.

As Ethyol is to be administered in conjunction with drugs that are known teratogens and mutagens, therapy should not be administered to pregnant or lactating women.

Due to lack of experience in patients with renal or hepatic impairment, children or patients older than 70 years of age, Ethyol is contra-indicated in these groups.

*Precautions and warnings:* Patients should be adequately hydrated prior to Ethyol infusion and kept in a supine position during the infusion of Ethyol reconstituted solution and blood pressure should be monitored during the infusion. Guidelines for interrupting and re-starting amifostine infusion in case of decrease in systolic blood pressure are given under *Dosage and administration.* If hypotension occurs, patients should be placed in the Trendelenburg position and be given an infusion of normal saline. It is important that the infusion of the recommended dose (740–910 mg/m²) be given over 15 minutes. The administration of amifostine as a longer infusion is associated with a higher incidence of side effects.

It is recommended that antiemetic medication be administered prior to and in conjunction with amifostine especially when used with stongly emetogenic chemotherapy such as cisplatin.

When amifostine is administered with highly emetogenic chemotherapy, the fluid balance of the patient should be monitored carefully.

Anti-hypertensive therapy should be interrupted 24 hours prior to the administration of amifostine and these patients should be monitored carefully during treatment.

Although reports of clinically relevant hypocalcemia are very rare, calcium serum levels should be monitored in patients at risk of hypocalcemia, such as those with nephrotic syndrome. If necessary, calcium supplements may be administered as needed. Caution should be exercised during treatment of patients receiving hypocalcemic agents.

No experience is available for the usage of Ethyol in childen as well as patients older than 70 years. Similarly, use of amifostine in patients with severe hepatic or renal impairment is not documented. Hence Ethyol should not be used in children, the elderly (more than 70 years) or patients with renal or hepatic impairment (see *Contra-indications*).

*Pregnancy and lactation:* It is not known if amifostine or its metabolities is excreted in human breast milk. Therefore, it is recommended that breast feeding be discontinued prior to the initiation of Ethyol therapy.

While Ethyol has been shown to have dose related embryotoxicity in rats at doses greater than 200 mg/kg, it is not teratogenic. There are no studies in pregnant women. As this drug is administered in conjunction with known teratogenic agents, this therapy should not be administered to pregnant women. If the patient becomes pregnant while receiving this therapy, the patient should be apprised of the potential hazard to the foetus.

*Drug interactions:* Limited experience from interaction studies is available. The rapid clearance of amifostine from the plasma minimises the risk of interactions between amifostine and other drugs.

Special consideration should be given with respect to the concurrent administration of Ethyol with anti-hypertensive medication or other drugs that could potentiate hypotension.

*Effects on ability to drive and operate machinery:* There is no intrinsic central nervous system toxicity associated with Ethyol administration, but as it is to be administered with chemotherapy and antiemetic regimens, the total therapy regimen might inhibit patients' ability to competently drive or operate machinery.

*Side-effects and adverse reactions:* Hypotension, as manifested by a transient reduction in systolic blood pressure and less frequently by a decrease in diastolic blood pressure, has been reported. The median time to onset was 13 minutes into the 15 minute period of amifostine infusion, and the median duration was 5 minutes. In some cases, the infusion had to be prematurely terminated due to a more pronounced drop in systolic blood pressure. In these cases, the blood pressure returned to normal within 5–15 minutes. Short term and rapidly reversible loss of consciousness has been very rarely reported.

Clinical symptoms of hypotension are quickly reversed by fluid infusion and postural management of the patient. If the blood pressure returns to normal within 5 minutes and the patient is asymptomatic, the infusion may be restarted, so that the dose of Ethyol can be administered.

Nausea and/or vomiting are frequently reported. Amifostine increased the incidence of mild to moderate nausea/vomiting on day 1 of chemotherapy. However, amifostine does not increase the incidence of delayed nausea and vomiting induced by cisplatin-based chemotherapy. Nausea and vomiting are amenable to treatment with standard antiemetics.

Other effects which have been described during or following Ethyol infusion are flushing/feeling of warmth, chills/feeling of coldness, dizziness, somnolence, hiccups and sneezing.

Decrease in serum calcium concentrations is a known pharmacological effect of Ethyol. At the recommended doses, no clinically relevant manifestation of hypocalcemia has been reported. However, clinical hypocalcemia has occurred very rarely in patients who received multiple doses of Ethyol within 24 hours.

Allergic reactions, ranging from mild skin rashes to rigors, have occurred in some patients. There has been no reported occurrence of anaphylaxis with Ethyol.

*Treatment of overdosage:* In Phase I trials, the maximum single dose of Ethyol administered was 1300 mg/m². No information is available on single doses higher than this in adults. In the setting of a clinical trial, children have received single doses of Ethyol up to 2.7 g/m² with no untoward effects. Multiple doses (up to three times the recommended single dose of 740–910 mg/m²) have been safely administered within a 24-hour period under study conditions. Following the repeated administration of Ethyol at 2 and 4 hours after the initial dose, there has not been any evidence of increase or cumulative side effects, especially nausea and vomiting or hypotension. The most likely symptom of overdosage would be hypotension which should be managed by infusion of normal saline or any other symptomatic treatment. The $LD_{50}$ in mice ranges from 554 mg/kg to 1140 mg/kg.

**Pharmaceutical precautions**

*Storage:* The lyophilised dosage form is labelled: 'Store in a refrigerator (between 2°C and 8°C)'.

When reconstituted with 9.5 ml of sterile 0.9% sodium chloride solution, the reconstituted Ethyol solution may be kept 6 hours at room temperature (15–25°C) or 24 hours under refrigeration (2–8°C).

*Incompatibilities:* No known incompatibilities. However it is recommended that no other drug be mixed or administered with the reconstituted Ethyol solution.

**Legal category** POM.

**Package quantities** Boxes of 3 vials.

**Further information** Nil.

**Product licence number** 11284/0004.

*Product licence holder:* U.S. Bioscience Inc., Suites 10 & 12, The Courtyards, Croxley Business Park, Watford WD1 8YH.

## INTRON A*

**Qualitative and quantitative composition** (per vial)

*Intron A Injection, Powder for Injectable Preparation: Active ingredient:* recombinant interferon alfa-2b, 1 million, 3 million, 5 million, 10 million or 18 million, International Units (IU).

*Inactive ingredients:* glycine, sodium phosphate dibasic, sodium phosphate monobasic and human albumin.

*Diluent:* sterile water for injection.

*Intron A Injection, Injectable Solution: Active ingredient:* recombinant interferon alfa-2b, 10 million or 25 million International Units (IU).

*Inactive ingredients:* glycine, sodium phosphate dibasic, sodium phosphate monobasic, human albumin, methylparaben, propylparaben, water for injection q.s. ad 2 ml (10 million IU) or 5 ml (25 million IU).

**Pharmaceutical form** Powder for Injectable preparation + diluent. Injectable solution.

*Route of administration:* intralesional, subcutaneous or intramuscular injection.

**Clinical particulars**

*Therapeutic indications:*

*Hepatitis B:* Treatment of adult patients with chronic active hepatitis B, who have markers for viral replication e.g., those who are positive for HBV-DNA, DNA polymerase of HBeAg.

*Chronic hepatitis C/non-A, non-B:* Reduction of disease activity in adult patients with chronic hepatitis C/Non-A, Non-B, who have elevated liver enzymes without liver decompensation. Studies in these patients demonstrate that Intron A Injection therapy can produce normalisation of serum ALT, clearance of serum HCV-RNA and improvement in liver histology.

Current clinical experience in patients who remain on Intron A Injection for 12–18 months indicates that a higher proportion of patients demonstrated a sustained response after longer durations of therapy than those who discontinued therapy after six months.

*Hairy cell leukaemia:* Treatment of patients with hairy cell leukaemia.

*Chronic myelogenous leukaemia:* Treatment of adult patients with chronic myelogenous leukaemia.

*Multiple myeloma:* As maintenance therapy in patients who achieved objective remission on induction therapy.

**Non-Hodgkin's lymphoma**: Adjuvant treatment of high tumour burden follicular lymphoma (Stage III or IV) in combination with appropriate chemotherapy, such as a CHOP-like regimens.

*AIDS-related Kaposi's sarcoma:* Treatment of patients who have no history of opportunistic infection.

*Condylomata acuminata:* Intralesional treatment of condylomata acuminata in patients who do not respond satisfactorily to other treatment modalities.

*Posology and method of administration:* Intron A Injection may be administered using either sterilised glass or plastic disposable syringes.

Multidose preparations should be for individual patient use only.

During the course of treatment with Intron A Injection for any indication, if adverse reactions develop, the dosage should be modified or therapy should be discontinued temporarily until the adverse reactions abate. If persistent or recurrent intolerance develops following adequate dosage adjustment, or disease progresses, the treatment with Intron A Injection should be discontinued. For maintenance dosage regimens administered subcutaneously, at the discretion of the physician, the patient may self-administer the dose.

*Chronic active hepatitis B:* The optimal schedule of treatment has not been established yet. The dosage is usually in the range of 2.5 million IU to 5.0 million IU/m² of body surface administered subcutaneously three times per week for a period of four to six months.

If markers for viral replication or HBeAg do not decrease after one month of therapy, the dose can be escalated. The dosage may be adjusted further according to the patient's tolerance to the medication.

If no improvement has been observed after three to four months of treatment, discontinuation of therapy should be considered.

*Chronic hepatitis C/non-A, non-B:* The recommended dose is three million IU administered subcutaneously three times a week. Most patients who respond demonstrate improvement in ALT levels within 12 weeks. In these patients therapy should be continued with 3 million IU three times a week for up to 18 months. In patients who fail to respond after 12–16 weeks of treatment, discontinuation of Intron A Injection therapy should be considered.

*Hairy Cell Leukaemia:* The recommended dose is 2 million IU/m² administered subcutaneously three times a week (every other day). The normalisation of one or more haematological variables begins within one month of therapy. Improvement in all three haematological variables (granulocyte count, platelet count and haemoglobin level) may require six months or more. Non-splenectomised patients responded similarly to splenectomised patients and in addition showed similar demonstrable improvement in transfusion requirements. This regimen should be maintained unless the disease progresses rapidly or severe intolerance is manifested.

*Chronic myelogenous leukaemia:* The recommended dosage of Intron A Injection is 4 to 5 million IU/m² administered subcutaneously daily. When the white blood cell count is controlled, the dosage may be administered three times a week (every other day).

*Multiple myeloma:* Maintenance therapy – In patients who are in the plateau phase following induction chemotherapy, Intron A Injection may be administered as monotherapy, subcutaneously, at a dose of 3 million IU/m² three times a week (every other day).

*Non-Hodgkin's lymphoma:* Adjunctively with chemotherapy, Intron A Injection may be administered subcutaneously, at a dose of 5 million IU three times a week (every other day) for a duration of 18 months. CHOP-like regimens are advised. Experience with the combination of doxorubicin, cyclophosphamide, teniposide and prednisolone is limited.

*AIDS-related Kaposi's sarcoma:* The optimal dosage is not yet known. Efficacy has been demonstrated at a dose of 30 million IU/m² three to five times a week, subcutaneously or intramuscularly. Lower doses (i.e., 10 to 12 million IU/m²/day) also have been used without apparent loss of efficacy.

If severe adverse reactions develop, the dosage should be modified (50% reduction) or therapy discontinued temporarily until the adverse reactions abate.

When disease stabilisation or treatment response occurs, treatment should continue until there is no further evidence of tumour or until discontinuation is required by evidence of a severe opportunistic infection or adverse effect.

*Condylomata acuminata:* The lesion of lesions to be injected should be cleaned first with a sterile alcohol pad. The intralesional injection should be made at the base of the lesion using a fine needle (30 gauge). Inject 0.1 ml of reconstituted solution containing 1.0 million IU Intron A Injection into the lesion three times per week on alternate days, for three weeks. As many as five lesions can be treated at one time. The maximum total dose administered each week should not exceed 15 million IU.

Large lesions may be treated by multiple injections (up to a total of 5.0 million IU of Intron A per day) or by sequentially injecting different areas of the lesions.

*Re-treatment:* Improvement usually occurs four to eight weeks after initiation of the first treatment course. If results at this time are not satisfactory, a second course of treatment at the same dosage schedule may be instituted provided that clinical signs and symptoms or changes in laboratory parameters do not preclude re-treatment.

*Treatment of additional lesions:* Immediately following completion of the first three weeks of treatment, a second course may be instituted at the same dosage regimen to treat up to five additional lesions in patients with six to ten condylomata. Patients with greater than ten condylomata may receive treatment sequentially depending on how large a number of condylomata are present.

*Contra-indications:* A history of hypersensitivity to

recombinant interferon alfa-2b or any other component of Intron A Injection;
severe pre-existing cardiac disease;
severe renal or hepatic dysfunction;
epilepsy and/or compromised central nervous system (CNS) function (see *Special precautions for use*);
chronic hepatitis with decompensated hepatic disease or cirrhosis of the liver;
chronic hepatitis in patients who are being or have been recently treated with immunosuppressive agents excluding short-term corticosteroid withdrawal;
autoimmune hepatitis; or history of autoimmune disease; immunosuppressed transplant recipients;
pre-existing thyroid disease unless controlled by conventional treatment.

*Special warnings and precautions for use:* Efficacy in patients with chronic active hepatitis B co-infected with the human immunodeficiency virus (HIV) has not been demonstrated.

Intron A should be used cautiously in patients with debilitating medical conditions, such as those with a history of pulmonary disease (e.g. chronic obstructive pulmonary disease) or diabetes mellitus prone to ketoacidosis. Caution should be observed also in patients with coagulation disorders (e.g. thrombophlebitis, pulmonary embolism) or severe myelosuppression.

Administration of Intron A Injection in combination with other chemotherapeutic agents may lead to increased risk of toxicity (severity and duration), which may be life-threatening or fatal as a result of the concomitantly administered drug. The most commonly reported potentially life-threatening or fatal adverse events include mucositis, diarrhoea, neutropenia, renal impairment, and electrolyte disturbance. Because of the risk of increased toxicity, careful adjustments of doses are required for Intron A Injection and for the concomitant chemotherapeutic agents.

Acute hypersensitivity reactions (e.g., urticaria, angioedema, bronchoconstriction, anaphylaxis) to Intron A Injection have been observed rarely during Intron A Injection therapy. If such a reaction develops, the drug should be discontinued and appropriate medical therapy instituted immediately. Transient rashes do not necessitate interruption of treatment.

Moderate to severe adverse experiences may require modification of the patient's dosage regimen, or in some cases, termination of Intron A Injection therapy. Any patient developing liver function abnormalities during treatment with Intron A Injection should be monitored closely and treatment discontinued if signs and symptoms progress.

Patients with chronic hepatitis B with evidence of decreasing hepatic synthetic function, such as decreasing albumin levels or prolongation of prothrombin time, who nevertheless meet the criteria for therapy, may be at increased risk of clinical decompensation if a flare of aminotransferases occurs during treatment. In considering these patients for Intron A therapy, the potential risks must be evaluated against the potential benefits of treatment.

Hypotension may occur during Intron A Injection therapy or up to two days post-therapy and may require supportive treatment.

Adequate hydration should be maintained in patients undergoing Intron A Injection therapy since hypotension related to fluid depletion has been seen in some patients. Fluid replacement may be necessary.

Patients with a history of congestive heart failure, myocardial infarction and/or previous or current arrhythmic disorders, who require Intron A Injection therapy, should be closely monitored. Those patients who have pre-existing cardiac abnormalities and/or are in advanced stages of cancer should have electrocardiograms taken prior to and during the course of treatment. Cardiac arrhythmias (primarily supraventricular) usually respond to conventional therapy but may require discontinuation of Intron A Injection therapy.

Pulmonary infiltrates, pneumonitis and pneumonia, including fatality, have been observed rarely in interferon-alpha treated patients, including those treated with Intron A Injection. The etiology has not been defined. These symptoms have been reported more frequently when shosaikoto, a Chinese herbal medicine, is administered concomitantly with interferon-alfa. Any patient developing fever, cough, dyspnea or other respiratory symptoms should have a chest X-ray taken. If the chest X-ray shows pulmonary infiltrates or there is evidence of pulmonary function impairment, the patient should be monitored closely, and, if appropriate, interferon-alfa treatment should be discontinued. While this has been reported more often in patients with chronic hepatitis non-A, non-B/C treated with interferon-alfa, it has also been reported in patients with oncologic diseases treated with interferon-alfa. Prompt discontinuation of interferon-alfa administration and treatment with corticosteroids appear to be associated with resolution of pulmonary adverse events.

Patients with a pre-existing psychiatric condition or a history of severe psychiatric disorder should not be treated with Intron A Injection.

If severe CNS effects, particularly depression, are observed, Intron A Injection therapy should be discontinued. CNS effects manifested by depression, confusion and other alterations of mental status have been observed in some patients during Intron A Injection therapy and suicidal ideation and attempted suicide have been observed rarely. These adverse effects have occurred in patients treated with recommended doses as well as in patients treated with higher Intron A doses. More significant obtundation and coma have been observed in some patients, usually elderly, treated at higher doses. While these effects are generally reversible, in a few patients full resolution took up to three weeks. Very rarely, seizures have occurred with high doses of Intron A Injection.

Infrequently, patients treated for chronic hepatitis non-A, non-B/C with Intron A Injection developed thyroid abnormalities, either hypothyroid or hyperthyroid. In clinical trials <1% (4/426) developed thyroid abnormalities. The abnormalities were controlled by conventional therapy for thyroid dysfunction. The mechanism by which Intron A Injection may alter thyroid status is unknown. Prior to initiation of Intron A Injection therapy for the treatment of chronic hepatitis non-A, non-B/C, serum thyroid-stimulating hormone (TSH) levels should be evaluated. Any thyroid abnormality detected at that time should be treated with conventional therapy. Intron A Injection treatment may be initiated if TSH levels can be maintained in the normal range by medication. If, during the course of Intron A Injection therapy, a patient develops symptoms consistent with possible thyroid dysfunction, TSH levels should be evaluated. In the presence of thyroid dysfunction, Intron A treatment may be continued if TSH levels can be maintained in the normal range by medication. Discontinuation of Intron A therapy has not reversed thyroid dysfunction occurring during treatment.

Because of reports of exacerbating pre-existing psoriatic disease, Intron A Injection should be used in patients with psoriasis only if the potential benefit justifies the potential risk.

While fever may be associated with the flu-like syndrome reported commonly during interferon therapy, other causes of persistent fever should be ruled out.

Ocular adverse events (see *Undesirable effects*) appear to occur after use of the drug for several months, but also have been reported after shorter treatment periods. Any patient complaining of changes in visual acuity or visual fields, or reporting other ophthalmologic symptoms during treatment with Intron A should have an eye examination. Because the retinal events may have to be differentiated from those seen with diabetic or hypertensive retinopathy, a baseline ocular examination is recommended prior to treatment with interferon in patients with diabetes mellitus or hypertension.

*Laboratory tests:* Standard haematologic tests and blood chemistries (complete blood count and differential, platelet count, electrolytes, liver enzymes, serum protein, serum bilirubin and serum creatinine) should be conducted in all patients prior to and periodically during systemic treatment with Intron A Injection. In patients treated for hepatitis the recommended testing schedule is at weeks 1, 2, 4, 8, 12, 16, and every other month, thereafter, throughout treatment. If ALT flares during Intron A therapy to ≥ 2 times baseline, Intron A Injection therapy may be continued unless signs and symptoms of liver failure are observed. During ALT flare, liver function tests: ALT, prothrombin time, alkaline phosphatase, albumin and bilirubin should be monitored at two-week intervals.

In patients considered for treatment of hepatitis, a liver biopsy is recommended to document diagnosis and severity of the disease.

*Paediatric use:* Doses of up to 10 million IU/m² have been administered safely to children with chronic active hepatitis B. However, efficacy of therapy has not been demonstrated. Generally, experience in patients below 18 years of age has been limited, and in such cases the expected benefits should be weighed carefully against potential hazards.

*Effect on fertility:* Interferon may impair fertility. In studies of interferon use in non-human primates, abnormalities of the menstrual cycle have been observed. Decreased serum estradiol and progesterone concentrations have been reported in women treated with human leukocyte interferon. Therefore, fertile women should not receive Intron A Injection unless they are using effective contraception during the treatment period. Intron A Injection should be used with caution in fertile men.

*Interaction with other medicaments and other forms of interaction:*
*Drug/drug interactions:* Paracetamol has been used successfully to alleviate the symptoms of fever and headache which can occur with Intron A Injection therapy. The recommended paracetamol dosage is 500 mg to 1 g given 30 minutes before administration of Intron A Injection. The maximum dosage to be given is 1 g four times daily.

Narcotics, hypnotics or sedatives should be administered with caution concomitantly with Intron A Injection.

Interactions between Intron A Injection and other drugs have not been fully evaluated. Caution should be exercised when administering Intron A in combination with other potentially myelosuppressive agents.

Interferons may affect the oxidative metabolic process. This should be considered during concomitant therapy with drugs metabolised by this route such as the xanthine derivatives theophylline or aminophylline. During concomitant therapy with xanthine agents, serum theophylline levels should be monitored and dosage adjusted if necessary.

*Pregnancy and lactation:* Intron A Injection has been shown to have abortifacient effects in *Macaca mulatta* (rhesus monkeys) at 90 and 180 times the recommended intramuscular or subcutaneous dose of 2 million IU/m². Although abortion was observed in all dose groups (7.5 million, 15 million and 30 million IU/kg), it was only statistically significant versus control at the mid- and high-dose groups (corresponding to 90 and 180 times the recommended intramuscular or subcutaneous dose of 2 million IU/m²). There are no adequate and well controlled studies in pregnant women. Intron A Injection should be used during pregnancy only if the potential benefit justifies the potential risk to the foetus.

It is not known whether the components of this drug are excreted in human milk. Because of the potential for adverse reactions from Intron A Injection in nursing infants, a decision should be made whether to discontinue nursing or to discontinue the drug taking into account the importance of the drug to the mother.

*Effects on ability to drive and use machines:* Not applicable.

*Undesirable effects:*
*Systemic administration:* The most commonly reported adverse effects were fever, fatigue, headache and myalgia. Fever and fatigue were reversible within 72 hours of interruption or cessation of treatment and were dose related. In the hepatitis treatment groups these effects were of mild to moderate severity.

Common adverse effects include rigors, anorexia and nausea.

Less common adverse effects include vomiting, diarrhoea, arthralgia, asthenia, somnolence, dizziness, dry mouth, alopecia, flu-like symptoms (unspecified), back pain, depression, malaise, pain, increased sweating, taste alteration, irritability, insomnia, confusion, impaired concentration and hypotension.

Rarely reported adverse reactions include abdominal pain, rash, nervousness, injection site disorders, paresthesia, herpes simplex, pruritus, eye pain, anxiety, epistaxis, coughing, pharyngitis, pulmonary infiltrates, pneumonitis and pneumonia, impaired consciousness, weight decrease, face edema, dyspnea, dyspepsia, tachycardia, hypertension, increased appetite, decreased libido, hypoesthesia, taste perversion, loose stool, gingival bleeding, neuropathy, and polyneuropathy. Hyperthyroidism or hypothyroidism have also been observed rarely. Hepatotoxicity, including fatality has been observed rarely.

Cardiovascular (CVS) adverse reactions, particularly arrhythmia, appeared to be correlated mostly with pre-existing CVS disease and prior therapy with cardiotoxic agents (see *Special warnings and precautions for use*). Transient reversible cardiomyopathy has been reported rarely in patients without prior evidence of cardiac disease.

Retinal haemorrhages, cotton wool spots, and retinal artery or vein obstruction have been observed rarely in patients treated with interferon alfa, including Intron A (recombinant interferon alfa 2-b) Powder for Injection or Injectable Solution (see *Special warnings and precautions for use*).

Clinically significant laboratory abnormalities, most frequently occurring at doses greater than 10 Million IU daily, include reduction in granulocyte and white blood cell counts; decreases in haemoglobin level and platelet count; increases in alkaline phosphatase, LDH, serum creatinine and serum urea nitrogen levels. Increase in serum ALT/AST (SGPT/SGOT) levels have been noted as an abnormality in some non-hepatitis subjects and also in some patients with chronic hepatitis B coincident with clearance of viral DNAp.

*Intralesional administration:* Most reported adverse reactions were mild to moderate, transient and rapidly reversible. The incidence of reported adverse reac tions in the patients treted for condylomata acuminata to increase in proportion to the number of lesions treated and are consequently dose-related.

The most common adverse reactions are flu-like symptoms, (rigors/chills, fever, headache, myalgia and malaise). Other commonly reported side effects include nausea, fatigue, dizziness, arthralgia, back pain and application site reactions. In patients treated for condylomata acuminata application site reactions appear to be due to manipulation of the lesion rather than to Intron A Injection therapy.

Rarely reported side effects include diarrhoea, somnolence, depression, pain, dyspepsia, increased sweating, unspecified flu-like symptoms, confusion, weakness, vomiting, flushing, leg cramps, asthenia, taste perversion, dermatitis and pruritis.

Low white blood cell counts, elevated serum liver enzyme (AST/SGOT) levels and low platelet counts have been reported in some patients with intralesional administration of Intron A Injection. Most of these laboratory findings were transient, rapidly reversible and mild to moderate in severity.

Reported adverse reactions and abnormal laboratory test values observed in patients who were re-treated for condylomata acuminata with Intron A Injection were qualitatively and quantitatively similar to those reported above.

*Overdose:* Overdosing has not been reported with Intron A Injection, but as for any pharmacologically active compound, symptomatic treatment with frequent monitoring of vital signs and close observation of the patient is indicated.

**Pharmacological properties**
*Pharmacodynamic properties:* Intron A Injection is a sterile, stable, lyphilised formulation of highly purified interferon alfa-2b produced by recombinant DNA techniques. Recombinant interferon alfa-2b is a water soluble protein with a molecular weight of approximately 19,300 daltons. It is obtained from a clone of *E.coli* which has a genetically engineered plasmid hybridised with an interferon alfa-2 gene from human leukocytes.

The activity of Intron A Injection is expressed in terms of IU, with 1 mg of recombinant interferon alfa-2b protein corresponding to $2 \times 10^8$ IU. International Units are determined by comparison of the activity of the recombinant interferon alfa-2b with the activity of the international reference preparation of human leukocyte interferon established by the World Health Organisation.

The interferons are a family of small protein molecules with molecular weights of approximately 15,000 to 21,000 daltons. They are produced and secreted by cells in response to viral infections or various synthetic and biological inducers. Three major classes of interferons have been identified: alpha, beta and gamma. These three main classes are themselves not homogeneous and may contain several different molecular species of interferon. More than 14 genetically distinct human alpha interferons have been identified. Intron A Injection has been classified as recombinant interferon alfa-2b.

*Pharmacodynamic properties:* Interferons exert their cellular activities by binding to specific membrane receptors on the cell surface. Human interferon receptors, as isolated from human lymphoblastoid (Daudi) cells, appear to be highly asymmetric proteins. They exhibit selectivity for human but not murine interferons, suggesting species specificity. Studies with other interferons have demonstrated species specificity.

The results of several studies suggest that, once bound to the cell membrane, interferon initiates a complex sequence of intracellular events that include the induction of certain enzymes. It is thought that this process, at least in part, is responsible for the various cellular responses to interferon, including inhibition of virus replication in virus-infected cells, suppression of cell proliferation and such immunomodulating activities as enhancement of the phagocytic activity of macrophages and augmentation of the specific cytotoxicity of lymphocytes for target cells. Any or all of these activities may contribute to interferon's therapeutic effects.

Recombinant interferon alfa-2b has exhibited antiproliferative effects in studies employing both animal and human cell culture systems as well as human tumour xenografts in animals. It has demonstrated significant immunomodulatory activity *in vitro*.

Recombinant interferon alfa-2b also inhibits viral replication *in vitro* and *in vivo*. Although the exact antiviral mode of action of recombinant interferon alfa-2b is unknown, it appears to alter the host cell metabolism. This action inhibits viral replication or if replication occurs, the progeny virions are unable to leave the cell. The specific mechanism of action in the treatment of condylomata acuminata is unknown.

*Pharmacokinetic properties:* The pharmacokinetics of Intron A Injection were studied in healthy volunteers following single 5 million IU/m² and 10 million IU doses administered subcutaneously, intramuscularly and as a 30-minute intravenous infusion. The mean serum interferon concentrations following subcutaneous and intramuscular injections were comparable. Maximum serum levels occurred three to 12 hours after the lower dose and six to eight hours after the higher dose. The elimination half-lives of interferon injections were approximately two to three hours, and six to seven hours respectively. Serum levels were below the detection limit 16 and 24 hours, respectively, post-injection. Both subcutaneous and intramuscular administration resulted in bioavailabilities greater than 100%.

After intravenous administration, serum interferon levels peaked (135 to 273 IU/ml) by the end of the infusion, then declined at a slightly more rapid rate than after subcutaneous or intramuscular drug administration, becoming undetectable four hours after the infusion. The elimination half-life was approximately two hours.

Urine levels of interferon were below the detection limit following each of the three routes of administration.

Interferon neutralising factor assays were performed on serum samples of patients who received Intron A Injection in Schering-Plough monitored clinical trials. Interferon neutralising factors are antibodies which neutralise the antiviral activity of interferon.

The clinical incidence of neutralising factors developing in cancer patients treated systemically is 2.9% and in hepatitis patients is 6.9%. Serum interferon neutralising factors were detected in 0.8% of patients with condylomata acuminata who received Intron A Injection intralesionally. The detected titres are low in almost all cases and have not been regularly associated with loss of response or any other autoimmune phenomenon.

In patients with hepatitis, no loss of response was observed, apparently due to the low titres. No development of neutralising antibodies has been demonstrated in patients who received Intron A Injection intralesionally in the treatment of basal cell carcinoma.

*Preclinical safety data:* Although interferon is generally recognised to be species specific, toxicology studies in mice, rats, rabbits and monkeys were conducted. Injections of human recombinant interferon alfa-2b for up to three months have shown no evidence of toxicity.

Results of animal reproduction studies indicate that recombinant interferon alfa-2b was not teratogenic in rats or rabbits, nor did it adversely effect pregnancy, foetal development or reproductive capacity in offspring of treated rats. Furthermore, animal studies have shown that interferons do not cross the placental barrier.

Mutagenicity studies with Intron A Injection revealed no adverse effects.

**Pharmaceutical particulars**
*List of excipients:* Glycine, anhydrous sodium phosphate dibasic, sodium phosphate monohydrate monobasic and human albumin; methyl and propyl parabens (injectable solution only).

*Incompatibilities:* Apart from the recommended diluent, no other substance or solution should be mixed with Intron A Injection.

*Shelf life: Intron A Injection Powder for Injectable Preparation:* 36 months when stored at 2° to 8°C. The non-reconstituted product can be kept at room temperature (15° to 25°C) for up to 4 weeks while in possession of the patient.

*Intron A Injection, Injectable Solution:* 24 months when stored at 2° to 8°C. The product can be kept at room temperature (15° to 25°C) for up to 4 weeks during use by the patient.

*Special precautions for storage:* Store between 2° to 8°C.

*Nature and contents of container: Intron A Injection, Powder for Injectable Preparation:* 1, 3, 5, 10, or 18 million IU: 2 ml vial, type I flint glass.

*Intron A Injection, Injectable Solution:* 10 million IU: 2 ml vial, type I flint glass. 25 million IU: 5 ml vial, type I flint glass.

*Instructions for use/handling:*
*Reconstitution of Intron A Injection, Powder for Injectable Preparation, for Parenteral or Intralesional Administration*—Intron A Injection is supplied as a powder at strengths of 1, 3, 5, 10 or 18 million IU for single use.

Single-dose vials must be reconstituted with 1 ml of Sterile Water for Injection. The reconstituted solutions are isotonic for parenteral or intralesional administration.

Using a sterile syringe and needle, inject 1 ml Sterile Water for Injection into the vial of Intron A Injection. Agitate gently to hasten complete dissolution of the powder. The appropriate dose should then be withdrawn with a sterile syringe and injected.

*Stability of reconstituted Intron A Injection*—After reconstitution of Lyophilised Intron A Injection with 1 ml of Sterile Water for Injection, the reconstituted solution is stable for 24 hours at room temperature (15° to 25°C). However, storage at 2° to 8°C is recommended. The reconstituted solution is clear and colourless.

The reconstituted material, as for all parenteral drug products, should be inspected visually for particulate matter and discoloration prior to administration.

**Marketing authorisation numbers**

| | |
|---|---|
| Intron A Powder for Injection 1 MIU | 0201/0063 |
| Intron A Powder for Injection 3 MIU | 0201/0064 |
| Intron A Powder for Injection 5 MIU | 0201/0065 |
| Intron A Powder for Injection 10 MIU | 0201/0066 |
| Intron A Powder for Injection 18 MIU | 0201/0210 |
| Intron A Solution for Injection 10 MIU | 0201/0167 |
| Intron A Powder for Injection 25 MIU | 0201/0168 |

**Date of approval/revision of SPC** June 1996

**Legal category** POM.

## LEUCOMAX* ▼

**Presentation** Leucomax contains molgramostim, a recombinant human granulocyte macrophage-colony stimulating factor (rHuGM-CSF), non-glycosylated with isoleucine at position 100.

Molgramostim is a water-soluble, non-glycosylated protein produced by recombinant techniques. Its activity is expressed in International Units (IU) with 1 million IU corresponding to approximately 90 micrograms of molgramostim protein. Each vial of Leucomax contains the labelled quantity of molgramostim in million IU.

**Uses** Leucomax is indicated for reduction of risk of infection and to allow better adherence to the chemotherapeutic regimen, by decreasing the severity of cytotoxic chemotherapy-induced neutropenia (see *Precautions, Laboratory tests*).

Leucomax is also indicated for the acceleration of myeloid recovery in patients following autologous or syngeneic bone marrow transplantation. Leucomax has not been shown to improve overall survival or increase time to relapse.

Leucomax is also indicated as adjuvant therapy in ganciclovir (DHPG)-induced neutropenia in patients with AIDS-related cytomegalovirus (CMV) retinitis in order to maintain recommended DHPG dosage.

**Dosage and administration** Leucomax must be reconstituted before administration (see *Technical instructions*). Leucomax dosing regimens vary according to the indication for therapy. The maximum daily dose should not exceed $0.11 \times 10^6$IU/kg/day (10 micrograms/kg/day).

The recommended dosage regimens are:
*Cancer chemotherapy:* 0.06–$0.11 \times 10^6$IU/kg/day (5 to 10 micrograms/kg/day) administered subcutaneously. Treatment should be initiated 24 hours after the last dose of chemotherapy and continued for 7 to 10 days. Dosing may be initiated at $0.06 \times 10^6$IU/kg/day (5 micrograms/kg/day).

*Bone marrow transplantation (BMT):* $0.11 \times 10^6$IU/kg/day (10 micrograms/kg/day) administered by intravenous infusion over 4 to 6 hours, beginning the day after BMT. Continue until the absolute neutrophil count (ANC) is $\geq 1 \times 10^9$/l. The maximum duration of treatment is 30 days.

*AIDS-related CMV retinitis as adjuvant therapy to ganciclovir (DHPG):* $0.06 \times 10^6$ IU/kg (5 micrograms/kg) once daily by subcutaneous injection. After the fifth Leucomax dose has been administered the dose may be titrated to maintain the ANC and WBC count at the desired levels, usually $\geq 1 \times 10^9$/l and $< 20 \times 10^9$/l respectively.

*Use in children:* The safety of Leucomax has been demonstrated in a limited number of patients below the age of 18 years.

*Use in the elderly:* There are no apparent differences in the safety of Leucomax in elderly patients.

**Contra-indications, warnings, etc**
*Contra-indications:* Leucomax is contra-indicated in patients with a history of hypersensitivity to molgramostim or any component of the injectable formulation.

Leucomax should not be used in patients with myeloid malignancies.

*Precautions:* Leucomax should be used under the supervision of a physician experienced in the treatment of oncologic and haematopoietic disorders or infectious diseases.

The first dose of Leucomax should be administered under medical supervision.

Acute severe, life threatening hypersensitivity reactions, including anaphylaxis, angioedema or bronchoconstriction have occurred in patients receiving Leucomax. If such reactions occur Leucomax should be withdrawn immediately and not reintroduced.

Leucomax has been associated infrequently with pleurisy, or pleural effusion. Pericarditis occurred in 2% (21/1098) and pericardial effusion in <2% (16/1098). If such reactions occur, Leucomax should be withdrawn. Patients with pre-existing pulmonary disease may be predisposed to decreased pulmonary function and dyspnoea, and should be monitored closely when being treated with Leucomax.

In clinical trials, adverse events reported with initiation of dosing were mostly mild to moderate in severity and included rigors, dyspnoea, fever, nausea, vomiting, non-specific chest pain, asthenia, hypotension or flushing. These symptoms, which infrequently required withdrawal of Leucomax were managed symptomatically.

In a few isolated instances, autoimmune disease developed or was exacerbated during rHuGMCSF therapy. Therefore, when administering Leucomax to patients with a history of, or predisposition to autoimmune disease, this should be considered.

*Laboratory tests:* Standard haematologic tests (full blood count with differential white cell count and platelet count) should be performed and serum albumin levels monitored during therapy with Leucomax.

Because of the potential of receiving higher doses of chemotherapy (i.e. full doses on the prescribed schedule), the patients may be at greater risk of thrombocytopenia and anaemia as consequences of increased chemotherapy doses. Regular monitoring of the platelet count and haematocrit is recommended.

*Drug interactions:* Since dosing with Leucomax has been associated with a decrease in serum albumin, drugs that are highly bound to serum albumin may require dosage adjustment.

*Use in pregnancy and lactation:* Safety of Leucomax for use in human pregnancy has not been established. Animal studies have shown reproductive toxicity. In primate models, administration of molgramostim was associated with foetal death and spontaneous abortion at doses of 0.07 and $0.11\times10^6$ IU/kg/day (6 and 10 mcg/kg/day).

In the absence of clinical data in pregnancy, the therapeutic benefit to the patient must be weighed against potential risks to the progress of pregnancy.

It is not known whether Leucomax is excreted in human milk. However, because of the potential for adverse effects in infants, nursing is not recommended in women receiving Leucomax.

*Side-effects:* Since many of the undesirable events reported during Leucomax clinical trials are often associated with underlying or concurrent disease or their treatment, the causal relationship of many of these events to Leucomax cannot be definitively determined. Most adverse reactions were mild to moderate in severity. Rarely were they severe or life threatening.

The most frequently reported undesirable effects across all indications were fever, nausea, dyspnoea, diarrhoea, rash, rigors, injection site reaction (with sc administration), vomiting, fatigue, anorexia, musculoskeletal pain and asthenia.

Less frequently reported events include; non-specific chest pain, stomatitis, headache, increased sweating, abdominal pain, pruritus, dizziness, peripheral oedema, paraesthesia and myalgia.

Serious reactions, which occurred rarely in clinical trials, include: anaphylaxis, bronchospasm, cardiac failure, capillary leak syndrome, cerebrovascular disorders, confusion, convulsions, hypotension, cardiac rhythm abnormalities, intracranial hypertension, pericardial effusion, pericarditis, pleural effusion, pulmonary oedema and syncope.

Laboratory findings – in all patient groups the most frequently occurring changes in laboratory values were decreased platelet count, decreased haemoglobin level, decreased serum albumin level and an increase in eosinophils (absolute count and percent). The causal relationship of these changes to Leucomax cannot be determined definitively.

The frequency of antibodies that bind to molgramostim, measured by enzyme-linked immunosorbent assay (ELISA) and bioassay, was determined to be 1% post treatment. No loss of activity of Leucomax was evident in these patients.

*Overdosage:* Overdosing has not been reported with Leucomax. As for any pharmacologically active compound, symptomatic treatment with frequent monitoring of vital signs and close observation of the patient is indicated if severe reactions occur.

**Pharmaceutical precautions** Leucomax sterile lyophilised powder should be stored at 2°C to 8°C and protected from light.

Following reconstitution with sterile water for injection Leucomax solution can be used for 24 hours when refrigerated at 2 to 8°C. Unused Leucomax solution should be discarded.

*Technical instructions:* Reconstitution of Leucomax – Add 1.0 ml of diluent (sterile water for injection) to the vial of Leucomax. Agitate the vial gently to dissolve the powder completely. This provides the labelled amount of Leucomax as an isotonic solution, which may be used for s.c. administration. When diluted further in accordance with the instructions below, Leucomax may be administered intravenously.

Dilution for i.v. administration – **dilution instructions must be followed carefully to avoid loss of molgramostim as a result of adsorption to the infusion system.**

Reconstitute each of the required number of vials of lyophilised powder to the appropriate strength of molgramostim with 1 ml of sterile water for injection. The reconstituted molgramostim solution may be further diluted in 25 ml, 50 ml or 100 ml infusion bags or bottles of either normal saline solution or 5% dextrose in water. The number and the strength of lyophilised powder vials required must be such that the above infusion admixture solution contains a final concentration of molgramostim of *not less than $0.08\times10^6$ IU (7 micrograms) per ml.* The resulting infusion solution is stable for 24 hours when stored in a refrigerator.

Leucomax infusion solution is compatible with the following infusion sets: Travenol 2C0001 and C0334, Intrafix air, Infusionsgerat R, 87 Plus, Souplix, Steriflex, Intrafix Air Euroklappe-ISO, Soluset and Linfosol sets. *Significant adsorption of Leucomax has been observed in a Port-A-Cath (Pharmacia) system, and its use is not recommended.*

For i.v. administration, the use of an in-line, low protein binding 0.2 or 0.22 micrometer filter is recommended. The reconstituted solution is colourless to light yellow and should be inspected visually for discolouration and particulate matter prior to administration.

**Further information** The excipients contained in Leucomax are mannitol, citric acid, dibasic sodium phosphate, polyethylene glycol and human albumin. Molgramostim has an elimination half-life of one to two hours following intravenous administration and two to three hours following subcutaneous administration.

**Legal category** POM.

**Package quantities** Leucomax sterile lyophilised powder is supplied in Type I glass vials with butyl or halobutyl rubber closures and aluminium seal in the following strengths: $1.67\times10^6$IU/vial (150 micrograms/vial); $3.33\times10^6$IU/vial (300 micrograms/vial); $4.44\times10^6$IU/vial (400 micrograms/vial).

**Product licence numbers**
$1.67\times10^6$IU/vial (150 mcg/vial) 0201/0150
$3.33\times10^6$IU/vial (300 mcg/vial) 0201/0181
$4.44\times10^6$IU/vial (400 mcg/vial) 0201/0151

## NASONEX* ▼

**Qualitative and quantitative composition** Mometasone furoate monohydrate 0.05% w/w suspension.

**Pharmaceutical form** Nasal spray suspension.

**Clinical particulars**
*Therapeutic indications:* Nasonex Aqueous Nasal Spray is indicated for use in adults and children 12 years of age and older to treat the symptoms of seasonal allergic or perennial rhinitis.

In patients who have a history of moderate to severe symptoms of seasonal allergic rhinitis, prophylactic treatment with Nasonex is recommended two to four weeks prior to the anticipated start of the pollen season.

*Posology and method of administration:* After initial priming of the Nasonex Aqueous Nasal Spray pump (usually 6 or 7 actuations, until a uniform spray is observed), each actuation delivers approximately 100 mg of mometasone furoate suspension, containing mometasone fuorate monohydrate equivalent to 50 micrograms mometasone furoate. If the spray pump has not been used for 14 days or longer, it should be reprimed before next use.

Adults (including geriatric patients) and children 12 years of age and older: The usual recommended dose for prophylaxis and treatment is two sprays (50 micrograms/spray) in each nostril once daily (total dose 200 micrograms). Once symptoms are controlled, dose reduction to one spray in each nostril (total dose 100 micrograms) may be effective for maintenance.

If symptoms are inadequately controlled, the dose may be increased to a maximum daily dose of four sprays in each nostril (total 400 micrograms). Dose reduction is recommended following control of symptoms.

Clinically significant onset of action occurs in some patients as early as 12 hours after the first dose.

Regular usage is recommended to achieve full therapeutic benefit.

There are no clinical results on use in children under the age of 12 years and therefore Nasonex is not recommended in this age group.

*Contra-indications:* Hypersensitivity to any ingredients of Nasonex Aqueous Nasal Spray.

Nasonex Aqueous Nasal Spray should not be used in the presence of untreated localised infection involving the nasal mucosa.

Because of the inhibitory effects of corticosteroids on wound healing, patients who have experienced recent nasal surgery or trauma should not use a nasal corticosteroid until healing has occurred.

*Special warnings and precautions for use:* Nasonex Aqueous Nasal Spray should be used with caution, if at all, by patients with active or quiescent tuberculous infections of the respiratory tract, or in untreated fungl, bacterial, systemic viral infections or ocular herpes simplex.

Following 12 months of treatment with Nasonex Aqueous Nasal Spray, there was no evidence of atrophy of the nasal mucosa; also mometasone furoate tended to reverse the nasal mucosa closer to a normal histologic phenotype. As with any long-term treatment, patients using Nasonex Aqueous Nasal Spray over several months or longer should be examined periodically for possible changes in the nasal mucosa. If localised fungal infection of the nose or pharynx develops, discontinuance of Nasonex Aqueous Nasal Spray therapy or appropriate treatment may be required. Persistence of nasopharyngeal irritation may be an indication for discontinuing Nasonex Aqueous Nasal Spray.

Although Nasonex will control the nasal symptoms in most patients, the concomitant use of antihistamines may provide additional relief of other symptoms, particularly ocular symptoms.

There is no evidence of hypothalamic-pituitary-adrenal (HPA) axis suppression following prolonged treatment with Nasonex Aqueous Nasal Spray. However, patients who are transferred from long-term administation of systemically active corticosteroids to Nasonex Aqueous Nasal Spray require careful attention. Systemic corticosteroid withdrawal in such patients may result in adrenal insufficiency for a number of months until recovery of HPA axis function. If these patients exhibit signs and symptoms of adrenal insufficiency, systemic corticosteroid administration should be resumed and other modes of therapy and appropriate measures instituted.

During transfer from systemic corticosteroids to Nasonex Aqueous Nasal Spray, some patients may experience symptoms of withdrawal from systemically active corticosteroids (e.g. joint and/or muscular pain, lassitude, and depression initially) despite relief from nasal symptoms and will require encouragement to continue with Nasonex Aqueous Nasal Spray therapy. Such transfer may also unmask pre-existing allergic conditions, such as allergic conjunctivitis and eczema, previously suppressed by systemic corticosteroid therapy.

Patients receiving corticosteroids who are potentially immunosuppressed should be warned of the risk of exposure to certain infections (e.g. chickenpox, measles) and of the importance of obtaining medical advice if such exposure occurs.

Following the use of intranasal corticosteroids instances of nasal septum perforation or increased intraocular pressure have been reported very rarely.

Full benefit of treatment may not be achieved in the first 48 hours.

*Interaction with other medicaments and other forms of interaction:* (See *Special warnings and special precautions* for use with systemic corticosteroids).

Nasonex Aqueous Nasal Spray has been administered concomitantly with loratadine with no apparent effect on plasma concentrations of loratadine or its major metabolite. Mometasone furoate plasma concentrations were not detectable. The combination therapy was well tolerated.

*Pregnancy and lactation:* There are no adequate or well controlled studies in pregnant women. Following intranasal administration of the maximal recommended clinical dose, mometasone plasma concentrations are not measurable; thus foetal exposure is expected to be negligible and the potential for reproductive toxicity, very low.

As with other nasal corticosteroid preparations Nasonex Aqueous Nasal Spray should be used in pregnant women, nursing mothers or women of childbearing age only if the potential benefit justifies the potential risk to the mother, foetus or infant. Infants born of mothers who received corticosteroids during pregnancy should be observed carefully for hypoadrenalism.

*Effects on ability to drive and use machines:* None known.

*Undesirable effects:* Treatment-related adverse events reported in clinical studies include headache (8%), epistaxis (i.e. frank bleeding, blood-tinged mucus, and blood flecks) (8%), pharyngitis (4%), nasal burning (2%), and nasal irritation (2%) and nasal ulceration

(1%), which are typically observed with use of a corticosteroid nasal spray. Epistaxis was generally self-limiting and mild in severity, and occurred at a higher incidence compared to placebo (5%), but at a comparable or lower incidence compared to the active control nasal corticosteroids studied (up to 15%). The incidence of all other effects was comparable with that of placebo.

*Overdose:* Because of the negligible (≤ 0.1%) systemic bioavailability of Nasonex, overdose is unlikely to require any therapy other than observation, followed by initiation of the appropriate prescribed dosage. Inhalation or oral administration of excessive doses of corticosteroids may lead to suppression of HPA axis function.

**Pharmacological properties**

*Pharmacodynamic properties:* Mometasone furoate is a topical glucocorticosteroid with local anti-inflammatory properties at doses that are not systemically active.

It is likely that much of the mechanism for the anti-allergic and anti-inflammatory effects of mometasone furoate lies in its ability to inhibit the release of mediators of allergic reactions. Mometasone furoate significantly inhibits the release of leukotrienes from leucocytes of allergic patients.

In cell culture, mometasone furoate demonstrated high potency in inhibition of synthesis and release of IL-1, IL-5, IL-6 and TNFα; it is also a potent inhibitor of leukotriene production. In addition, it is an extremely potent inhibitor of the production of the Th2 cytokines IL-4 and IL-5, from human CD4+ T-cells.

In studies utilising nasal antigen challenge, Nasonex Aqueous Nasal Spray has shown anti-inflammatory activity in both early- and late- phase allergic responses. This has been demonstrated by decreases (vs placebo) in histamine and eosinophil activity and reductions (vs baseline) in eosinophils, neutrophils, and epithelial cell adhesion proteins.

In patients with seasonal allergic rhinitis, Nasonex Aqueous Nasal Spray demonstrated a clinically significany onset of action with 12 hours after the first dose.

*Pharmacokinetic properties:* Mometasone furoate, administered as an aqueous nasal spray, has a negligible (≤ 0.1%) systemic bioavailability and is generally undetectable in plasma, despite the use of a sensitive assay with a lower quantitation limit of 50 pg/ml; thus, there are no relevant pharmacokinetic data for this dosage form. Mometasone furoate suspension is very poorly absorbed from the gastro-intestinal tract, and the small amount that may be swallowed and absorbed undergoes extensive first-pass hepatic metabolism prior to excretion in urine and bile.

*Preclinical safety data:* No toxicological effects unique to mometasone furoate exposure were demonstrated. All observed effects are typical of this class of compounds and are related to exaggerated pharmacologic effects of glucocorticoids.

Preclinical studies demonstrate that mometasone furoate is devoid of androgenic, antiandrogenic, estrogenic or antiestrogenic activity but, like other glucocorticoids, it exhibits some antiuterotrophic activity and delays vaginal opening in animal modes at high oral doses of 56 mg/kg/day and 280 mg/kg/day.

Mometasone furoate was nonmutagenic in tests designed to examine mutagenicity potential.

In studies of reproductive function, subcutaneous mometasone furoate, at 15 micrograms/kg prolonged gestation and prolonged and difficult labour occurred with a reduction in offspring survival and body weight or body weight gain. There was no effect on fertility.

Like other glucocorticoids, mometasone furoate is a teratogen in rodents and rabbits. Effects noted were umbilical hernia in rats, clef palate in mice and gall bladder agenesis, umbilical hernia and flexed front paws in rabbits. There were also reductions in maternal body weight gains, effects on foetal growth (lower foetal body weight and/or delayed ossification) in rats, rabbits and mice and reduced offspring survival in mice.

The carcinogenicity potential of inhaled mometasone furoate (aerosol with CFC propellant and surfactant) at concentrations of 0.25 to 2.0 micrograms/l was investigated in 24-month studies in mice and rats. Typical glucocorticoid-related effects, icluding several non-neoplastic lesions, were observed. No statistically significant dose-response relationship was detected for any of the tumour types.

**Pharmaceutical particulars**

*List of excipients:* Dispersible cellulose BP 65 cps, glycerol, sodium citrate dihydrate, citric acid monohydrate, Polysorbate 80, benzalkonium chloride, phenylethyl alcohol, purified water.

*Incompatibilities:* None known.

*Shelf life:* 24 months from date of manufacture. Use within 2 months of first use.

*Special precautions for storage:* Store between 2° and 25°C.

*Nature and contents of container:* Nasonex Aqueous Nasal Spray 18 g is contained in a white, high density polyethylene bottle, supplied with a metered-dose, manual polypropylene spray pump actuator which delivers 50 micrograms per acuation.

*Instruction for use/handling:* Prior to administration of the first dose, shake container well, and actuate pump 6 or 7 times (until a uniform spray is obtained). If a pump is not used for 14 days or longer, reprime the pump as before. Shake container well before each use. The bottle should be discarded after 120 actuations or within 2 months of first use.

**Marketing authorisation number** 0201/0216.

**Date of approval/revision of SPC** April 1997.

**Legal category** POM.

## NETILLIN* Injection

**Presentation** Netillin Injection for parenteral use is an aqueous solution of netilmicin sulphate. Each millilitre contains netilmicin sulphate equivalent to 100 mg, 50 mg or 10 mg of netilmicin base, and is available in ampoules.

**Uses** Netilmicin sulphate is a semi-synthetic, water-soluble antibiotic of the aminoglycoside group. It is a rapidly acting bactericidal antibiotic which probably acts by inhibiting normal protein synthesis in susceptible organisms. It is active at low concentrations against many strains of a wide variety of pathogenic bacteria including *Escherichia coli, Klebsiella-Enterobacter-Serratia* species, *Citrobacter* species, *Proteus* species (indole-positive and indole-negative), including *Proteus mirabilis, Proteus morganii, Proteus rettgeri, Proteus vulgaris; Pseudomonas aeruginosa,* and *Staphylococcus* species (coagulase-positive and coagulase-negative, including penicillin and methicillin-resistant strains).

Netillin Injection is indicated in: bacteraemia, septicaemia (including neonatal sepsis), serious infections of the respiratory tract, kidney and genitourinary tract infections, skin and soft tissue infections, bone and joint infections, burns, wounds and peri-operative infections, intra-abdominal infections (including peritonitis) and infections of the gastro-intestinal tract.

A single Netillin Injection has been shown to be effective in the treatment of gonorrhoea.

Netillin Injection has also been effective in the treatment of infections caused by organisms resistant to other aminoglycosides, such as kanamycin, gentamicin, tobramycin and amikacin.

Netillin Injection is recommended for prophylactic use.

**Dosage and administration** The recommended dosage for intramuscular and intravenous administration is identical and should be calculated on mg/kg lean body weight. Netillin Injection should usually be administered intramuscularly. For i.v. administration see Table.

The usual duration of treatment is seven to fourteen days. Longer courses have been well tolerated but it is important that patients treated beyond the usual period be carefully monitored for changes in renal, auditory and vestibular function. Dosage should be reduced if clinically indicated.

*Serum levels:* The measurement of peak and trough serum levels is of value to assure adequate levels and to avoid potentially toxic levels. Once daily administration of Netillin may lead to transient peak concentrations of 20–30 mcg/ml. Other dosage regimens will result in peak levels generally not exceeding 12 mcg/ml. Prolonged levels above 16 mcg/ml should be avoided. If trough levels are monitored (just prior to next dose) they will usually be 3 mcg/ml or less with the recommended dosage. Trough concentrations above 4 mcg/ml should be avoided.

The regular monitoring of serum levels is particularly important for patients with impaired renal function or where a longer duration of treatment is necessary.

*I.V. administration:* If i.v. administration is required, the dose may be injected directly into a vein or i.v. tubing over a period of 3 to 5 minutes or administered as an infusion. For infusion in adults, a single dose of Netillin Injection may be diluted in 50 to 200 ml of sterile normal saline or in a sterile solution of dextrose 5% in water; in infants and children the volume of diluent should be dependant on the patients fluid requirements. The solution may be infused over a period of one half to two hours.

Netillin Injection should not be physically pre-mixed with other drugs, but should be administered separately in accordance with the recommended route of administration and dosage schedule. Netillin Injection is physically compatible with the following parenteral solutions: Sterile Water for Injections, Normal Saline, 5% and 10% Dextrose in Water.

*Patients with normal renal function:*

*Adults:* Urinary tract or non-life threatening systemic infections: The recommended dose is 4.0–6 mg/kg/day given once daily. The dose may also be given in equal sub doses 12 hourly or 8 hourly. In general within this dose range, lower dosage will be used for urinary tract infections and higher dosage for systemic infections. Dosage should be adjusted for both uses depending on severity of infection and patient condition.

Patients with urinary tract infections may be treated with a single daily dose of 150 mg administered for five days.

Netillin in a single dose of 300 mg may be used in the treatment of gonorrhoea.

Life threatening infections: Dosages up to 7.5 mg/kg/day may be administered in three equal doses every 8 hours. This dosage should be reduced to 6 mg/kg/day or less as soon as clinically indicated, usually within 48 hours.

*Children:* 6.0–7.5 mg/kg/day (2.0 to 2.5 mg/kg administered every 8 hours).

*Infants and neonates:* over one week of age: 7.5 to 9.0 mg/kg/day (2.5 to 3.0 mg/kg administered every 8 hours).

*Premature or full term neonates:* One Week of Age or Less: 6 mg/kg/day (3.0 mg/kg administered every 12 hours).

*Patients with impaired renal function:* The usual daily dose should be given on the first day as a loading dose (divided into three equal doses every 8 hrs). Dosage must then be adjusted. Whenever possible netilmicin serum concentrations should be monitored and used as the basis for dosage adjustment (see serum levels). If serum levels cannot be measured directly, serum creatinine or creatinine clearance rate may be used as a guide to dosage adjustment, as shown in the Table above.

*Haemodialysis:* For patients on haemodialysis the recommended dose is 2 mg/kg at the end of each

*Dosage Adjustment Guide for Patients with Renal Function Impairment*
(Daily dose to be divided into three equal doses every 8 hours)

*Administer the usual dose on the first day as follows:*

1. Adults, urinary tract and systemic infections 4–6 mg/kg/day.
2. Adults, life-threatening infections 7.5 mg/kg/day.
3. Children, 6–7.5 mg/kg/day.
4. Infants and neonates over 1 week of age, 7.5–9 mg/kg/day.
5. Premature or full term neonates one week of age or less, 6 mg/kg/day.

*On subsequent days, administer a percent of the usual dose, based on serum creatinine or creatinine clearance rate as follows:*

| *Approx. creatinine clearance rate (ml/min/1.73 sq m)* | *Serum creatinine level* | | *Percent of usual dose* |
|---|---|---|---|
| | *mg/100 ml* | *S.I. Units µmol/l* | |
| 100 | ≤1.0 | 80 | 100 |
| 71–100 | 1.1–1.3 | 100–120 | 80 |
| 56–70 | 1.4–1.6 | 130–150 | 65 |
| 46–55 | 1.7–1.9 | 160–175 | 55 |
| 41–45 | 2.0–2.2 | 180–190 | 50 |
| 36–40 | 2.3–2.5 | 210–220 | 40 |
| 31–35 | 2.6–3.0 | 230–260 | 35 |
| 26–30 | 3.1–3.5 | 270–310 | 30 |
| 21–25 | 3.6–4.0 | 320–360 | 25 |
| 16–20 | 4.1–5.1 | 365–450 | 20 |
| 10–15 | 5.2–6.6 | 460–580 | 15 |
| <10 | 6.7–8.0 | 600–700 | 10 |

dialysis period. In children a dose of 2–2.5 mg/kg may be administered depending on the severity of infection.

*Peritoneal dialysis:* Netillin has been used sucessfully in doses of 7.5–10 mg/l at each change of dialysing fluid without elevation of serum levels.

*Concomitant therapy:* Dosages recommended above for patients with normal or impaired renal function should not be reduced when netilmicin is administered concomitantly with other antibiotics (but see Warnings).

### Contra-indications, warnings, etc

*Contra-indications:* Hypersensitivity to netilmicin contra-indicates its use. A history of hypersensitivity or serious toxic reactions to other aminoglycosides may also be a contra-indication.

*Warnings:* Patients treated with aminoglycosides should be under close clinical observation because of the potential toxicity associated with their use. Monitoring of renal and eighth cranial nerve functions is desirable during therapy, particularly for patients with known or suspected reduced renal function.

Evidence of ototoxicity requires dosage adjustment or discontinuance of the drug.

Serum concentration assays of aminoglycosides are of value to assure adequate levels and to avoid potentially toxic levels. Once daily administration of Netillin may lead to transient peak concentrations of 20–30 mcg/ml. Other dosages regimens will result in peak levels not exceeding 12 mcg/ml. Prolonged levels above 16 mcg/ml should be avoided. If trough levels are monitored (just prior to next dose) they will usually be 3 mcg/ml or less with the recommended dosage. Increasing trough concentrations above 4 mcg/ml should be avoided.

In patients with extensive body surface burns, altered pharmocokinetics may result in reduced serum concentrations of aminoglycosides. Measurement of netilmicin serum concentrations is particularly important in these patients as a basis for dosage adjustment.

Concurrent and/or sequential systemic or topical use of other potentially neurotoxic and/or nephrotoxic drugs, such as polymyxin B, colistin, cephaloridine, kanamycin, gentamicin, amikacin, tobramycin, neomycin, streptomycin and vancomycin should be avoided. Advanced age and dehydration may also increase the risk of toxicity.

Increased nephrotoxicity has been reported following concomitant administration of aminoglycoside antibiotics and cephalothin.

Neurotoxic or nephrotoxic antibiotics may be absorbed from body surfaces after local irrigation or application. The potential toxic effect of such antibiotics administered in this fashion should be considered.

The concurrent use of netilmicin with potent diuretics, such as ethacrynic acid or frusemide, should be avoided since these diuretics by themselves may cause ototoxicity. In addition, when administered intravenously, diuretics may enhance aminoglycoside toxicity by altering the antibiotic concentrations in serum and tissue.

Patients should be well hydrated during treatment. Neuromuscular blockade has been reported in animals receiving netilmicin at doses considerably above those clinically recommended. The possibility of this phenomenon occurring in man should be considered, particularly if aminoglycosides are administered to patients receiving anaesthetics, neuromuscular blocking agents (such as succinylcholine or tubocurarine), or massive transfusions of citrate-anticoagulated blood. If blockade occurs, calcium salts may reverse it.

Aminoglycosides should be used with caution in patients with neuromuscular disorders, such as myasthenia gravis or Parkinsonism, since these drugs theoretically may aggravate muscle weakness because of their potential curare-like effects on the neuromuscular junction.

Elderly patients may have reduced renal function which might not be evident by routine screening tests, such as BUN or serum creatinine. A creatinine clearance determination may be more useful. Monitoring of renal function during netilmicin treatment, as with other aminoglycosides, is particularly important in these patients.

Cross-allergenicity among aminoglycosides has been demonstrated.

Although the *in vitro* mixing of netilmicin and carbenicillin results in a rapid and significant inactivation of netilmicin, this interaction has not been demonstrated in patients with normal renal function who received both drugs by different routes of administration. In patients with severe renal impairment receiving carbenicillin concomitantly with an aminoglycoside, a reduction in aminoglycoside serum half-life has been reported.

Treatment with netilmicin may result in overgrowth of non-susceptible organisms. If this occurs, appropriate therapy is indicated.

Safety for use in pregnancy has not been established.

Netilmicin is not intended for intrathecal use.

*Side-effects:* Adverse renal effects, generally mild in nature, have been reported infrequently after netilmicin administration. They occur more frequently in patients with a history of renal impairment, in patients treated with larger than the recommended dosage, and are most often reversible. While eighth cranial nerve toxicity has been reported with netilmicin, the incidence is lower and the severity appears milder than with other aminoglycosides. Some clinical studies indicate that at therapeutic dosage, netilmicin may have less effect than other aminoglycosides on eighth cranial nerve function. Adverse effects on both the vestibular and auditory branches of the eighth cranial nerve occur primarily in patients with renal impairment and in patients on high doses and/or prolonged therapy. Symptoms which are often transient may include dizziness, vertigo, tinnitus, roaring in the ears and hearing loss. The latter is usually manifested by diminution of high-tone acuity. Total deafness has not been reported.

Some patients who have had previous ototoxic reactions to other aminoglycosides have been treated safely with Netillin Injection.

Other rarely reported adverse reactions possibly related to netilmicin include: headache, malaise, visual disturbances, disorientation, tachycardia, paraesthesia, rash, chills, fever, fluid retention, vomiting and diarrhoea.

Laboratory abnormalities possibly related to netilmicin include: increased blood sugar, increased alkaline phosphatase, increased SGOT or SGPT; other abnormal liver function studies; decreased haemoglobin, WBCs, and platelets; eosinophilia and increase in prothrombin time.

While local tolerance of Netillin Injection is generally excellent, there has been an occasional report of pain at the injection site or local reaction.

*Overdosage:* In the event of overdose or toxic reaction, haemodialysis or peritoneal dialysis will aid the removal of netilmicin from the blood.

**Pharmaceutical precautions** Netillin Injection should be stored at 2°C to 30°C (35.6°F to 86°F). Protect from freezing.

Netillin Injections should not be physically premixed with other drugs, but should be administered separately in accordance with the recommended route of administration and dosage schedule.

**Legal category** POM.

**Package quantities** All the presentations of Netillin are colour coded on both cartons and the containers. The 100 mg/ml strength is available in 2 ml (colour coded red), 1.5 ml (brown) and 1 ml (yellow) ampoules. The 50 mg/ml and 10 mg/ml strengths are available in 1 ml (green) and 1.5 ml (blue) ampoules respectively. All ampoules are supplied in packs of ten.

**Further information** Nil.

**Product licence numbers**
Netillin Injection 100 mg/ml    3478/0041
Netillin Injection  50 mg/ml    3478/0040
Netillin Injection  10 mg/ml    3478/0039

## NITRO-DUR* TRANSDERMAL DRUG DELIVERY SYSTEMS

### Qualitative and quantitative composition
Nitro-Dur 0.1 mg/h Transdermal Drug Delivery System

Nitro-Dur 0.2 mg/h Transdermal Drug Delivery System

Nitro-Dur 0.4 mg/h Transdermal Drug Delivery System

Nitro-Dur 0.6 mg/h Transdermal Drug Delivery System

*Active ingredient:* Glyceryl trinitrate 37.4% w/w.

*Inactive ingredients:* Butylacrylate Polymer (Polymer C) 28.4% w/w; Butyrylate Polymer (Polymer D) 28.4% w/w; Sodium Polyacrylate (Polymer A) 1.4% w/w; Melamine Formaldehyde Resin Polymer b) 0.3% w/w; Purified Water 4.0% w/w.

Coated onto tan-coloured Saranex* 2014 extruded thermoplastic film 5 cm² (0.1 mg/h); 10.0 cm² (0.2 mg/h); 20 cm² (0.4 mg/h) or 20 cm² (0.6 mg/h).

Adhesive layer covered by PVC Release Liner 5 cm² (0.1 mg/h); 10.0 cm² (0.2 mg/h); 20 cm² (0.4 mg/h) or 20 cm² (0.6 mg/h).

**Pharmaceutical form** Sustained release transdermal system.

### Clinical particulars
*Therapeutic indications:* For prophylaxis of angina pectoris either alone or in combination with other anti-anginal therapy.

*Poslogy and method of administration:*
*Adults, including elderly patients:* The recommended initial dose is one 0.2 mg/h Nitro-Dur patch daily. In some patients dose titration to higher or lower doses may be necessary to achieve optimum therapeutic effect. Nitro-Dur is suitable for continuous or intermittent use. Patients already receiving continuous 24-hour nitrate therapy without signs of nitrate tolerance may continue on this regimen provided clinical response is maintained. Attenuation of effect has however occurred in some patients being treated with sustained release nitrate preparations. In such patients intermittent therapy may be more appropriate. Under these circumstances Nitro-Dur is applied daily for a period of approximately 12 hours. The patch is then removed to provide a nitrate-free interval of 12 hours which may be varied between 8–12 hours to suit individual patients.

Patients experiencing nocturnal angina may benefit from overnight treatment with a nitrate-free interval during the day. In this patient group additional anti-anginal therapy may be needed during the day.

Patients with severe angina may need additional anti-anginal therapy during nitrate-free intervals.

Nitro-Dur transdermal patches may be applied to any convenient skin area; the recommended site is the chest or outer upper arm. Application sites should be rotated and suitable areas may be shaved if necessary. Nitro-Dur patches should not be applied to the distal part of the extremities.

*Children:* Not recommended.

*Contra-indications:* Contra-indicated in patients hypersensitive to nitrates and in patients with marked anaemia. Use is also contra-indicated in severe hypotension, increased cranial pressure and myocardial insufficiency due to valvular or left ventricular outflow tract obstruction.

*Special warnings and precautions for use:* Nitro-Dur should only be used under careful clinical and/or haemodynamic monitoring in patients with acute myocardial infarction or congestive heart failure. Nitro-Dur is not indicated for the immediate treatment of acute anginal attacks.

Nitro-Dur should be removed before attempting defibrillation or cardioversion, to avoid possibility of electrical arcing, and before diathermy.

The possibility of increased frequency of angina during patch-off periods should be considered. In such cases, the use of concomitant anti-anginal therapy is desirable.

In some patients, severe hypotension may occur particularly with upright posture, even with small doses of glyceryl trinitrate. Thus Nitro-Dur should be used with caution in patients who may have volume depletion from diuretic therapy and in patients who have low systolic blood pressure (e.g. below 90 mm Hg).

Paradoxical bradycardia and increased angina may accompany glyceryl-trinitrate-induced hypotension.

Caution should be exercised in patients with arterial hypoxaemia, due to severe anaemia and patients with hypoxaemia and a ventilation/perfusion imbalance due to lung disease or ischaemic heart failure, as biotransformation of GTN may be reduced.

*Interactions with other medicaments and other forms of interaction:* Concomitant use of Nitro-Dur with other vasodilating agents, alcohol, anti-hypertensive agents, beta adrenergic blocking agents, ace inhibitors, phenothiazines or calcium channel blocking agents may cause additive hypotensive effects.

*Pregnancy and lactation:* It is not known whether glyceryl trinitrate in transdermal form can affect reproductive capacity or cause foetal harm. Thus Nitro-Dur should only be administered to pregnant women if the potential benefits to the mother clearly outweigh the potential hazard to the foetus. It is not known whether glyceryl trinitrate is excreted in human milk. Caution should therefore be exercised when Nitro-Dur is administered to nursing mothers.

*Effects on ability to drive and use machines:* None known.

*Undesirable effects:* Headache is the most common side-effect, especially at higher doses. Transient episodes of dizziness and light-headedness which may be related to blood pressure change may also occur. Hypotension occurs infrequently but may be severe enough to warrant discontinuation of therapy. Syncope and reflex tachycardia have been reported but are uncommon. Application site irritation may occur but is rarely severe. Hypersensitivity reactions may occur.

*Overdose:* High doses of glyceryl trinitrate may produce severe hypotension, syncope and methaemoglobinaemia. Increased intracranial pressure with associated cerebral symptoms may occur. Treatment is by removal of the patch or reduction of dose depending on severity. Thorough scrubbing of underlying skin may reduce absorption more quickly after removal. Any fall in blood pressure or signs of collapse that may occur may be managed by general suppor tive or resuscitative measures. Adrenaline and related products are ineffective in reversing the severe hypotensive events associated with overdose.

### Pharmacological properties

*Pharmacodynamic properties:* Glyceryl trinitrate, (as other organic nitrates), is a potent dilator of vascular smooth muscle. The effect on veins predominates over that on arteries resulting in decreased cardiac preload. Systemic vascular resistance is relatively unaffected, heart rate is unchanged or slightly increased and pulmonary vascular resistance is consistently reduced.

In normal individuals or those with coronary artery disease (in the absence of heart failure) glyceryl trinitrate decreases cardiac output slightly. Doses which do not alter systemic arterial pressure often produce arteriolar dilatation in the face and neck resulting in flushing. Dilatation of the meningeal arterioles may explain the headache which is often reported. Rapid administration of high doses of glyceryl trinitrate decreases blood pressure and cardiac output resulting in pallor, weakness, dizziness and activation of compensatory sympathetic reflexes. A marked hypotensive effect may occasionally occur especially in the upright position.

*Pharmacokinetic properties:* Glyceryl trinitrate is rapidly hydrolysed by liver enzymes which are a major factor in bioavailability. Orally administered glyceryl trinitrate is ineffective as a therapeutic agent due to first-pass metabolism and administration has therefore routinely been via the sub-lingual route thus bypassing the hepatic circulation initially. Peak concentrations of glyceryl trinitrate following sub-lingual administration occur within 4 minutes in man with a half-life of 1 to 3 minutes. Transdermal administration, initially with ointment preparations but more recently with sustained-release delivery systems provide an alternative route to bypass the hepatic circulation with longer term concentrations of approximately 200 pg/ml are achieved within approximately 2 h of application of Nitro-Dur and are maintained for 24 h. Rate of absorption is controlled by the skin.

*Preclinical safety data:* There are no pre-clinical data of relevance to the prescriber which are additional to that already included in other sections of the SPC.

### Pharmaceutical particulars

*List of excipients:* Butylacrylate Polymer (Polymer C); Butylacrylate Polymer (Polymer D); Sodium Polyacrylate (Polymer A); Melamine Formaldehyde Resin (Polymer B); Purified Water.

Coated onto tan-coloured Saranex 2014 extruded thermoplastic film. Adhesive layer covered by PVC Release Liner.

*Incompatibilities:* None known.

*Shelf life:* 24 months.

*Special precautions for storage:* Store below 30°C. Do not refrigerate.

*Nature and contents of container:* Sealed pouches consisting of paper lined with polyethylene/foil laminate enclosing individual transdermal patches.

*Instruction for use/handling:* Nitro-Dur patches are applied after removal from the protective pouch. With the brown lines on the backing cover facing the user, edges are bent away to break open the cover along the brown line. The halves of the cover are peeled off and the patch applied firmly to the skin. Hands should be washed thoroughly after application.

Patients should be advised to dispose of patches carefully to avoid accidental application or use.

**Marketing authorisation numbers**
Nitro-Dur 0.1 mg/h     0201/0157
Nitro-Dur 0.2 mg/h     0201/0158
Nitro-Dur 0.4 mg/h     0201/0159
Nitro-Dur 0.6 mg/h     0201/0160.

**Date of approval/revision of SPC**  19 December 1996.

**Legal category**  P.

## OPTIMINE*

**Presentation**  *Optimine Tablets:* Each white tablet, with score mark on one side and Schering Corporation USA Trademark on the other, contains 1.0 mg Azatadine Maleate USP.

*Optimine Syrup:* Each 5 ml of clear, colourless syrup which has the characteristic odour and flavour of blackcurrant, contains 0.5 mg of Azatadine maleate USP.

**Uses**  Optimine Tablets and Syrup are indicated for the symptomatic relief of allergic conditions such as hayfever, vasomotor rhinitis, urticaria, pruritus of allergic origin and allergic reactions associated with insect bites and stings.

**Dosage and administration**
*Adults, the elderly and children over 12 years of age:* In most conditions, 1 mg of azatadine maleate (1

tablet or 10 ml of syrup) in the morning and evening is recommended in the majority of patients. In refractory or more severe cases, 2 mg twice daily may be used.

*Children 6–12 years of age:* 0.5 to 1.0 mg of azatadine maleate ($\frac{1}{2}$ to 1 tablet or 5 to 10 ml of syrup) twice daily.

*Children 1–6 years of age:* 0.25 mg azatadine maleate (2.5 ml of syrup) twice daily.

Optimine Syrup may be diluted with Syrup BP.

Diluted product should not be used beyond 2 weeks.

**Contra-indications, warnings, etc**  Until the safety of azatadine maleate concerning adverse effects on human foetal development has been established, the drug is not recommended for use in pregnant or lactating women.

Patients taking azatadine maleate should be cautioned against ingestion of alcohol. The drug may potentiate central nervous system depressants. Although drowsiness is infrequent and impairment of psychomotor function is not manifested at the recommended dosage, patients should be cautioned against engaging in mechanical operations requiring mental alertness until individual response to azatadine maleate has been determined.

Due to the anticholinergic effect of azatadine maleate, the drug should be used with caution in patients with prostatic hypertrophy, urinary retention, glaucoma, stenosing peptic ulcer or pyloroduodenal obstructions.

Mono-amine oxidase inhibitors, which are known to intensify or prolong the anticholinergic and sedative action of drugs, should not be used concomitantly with azatadine maleate.

*Side-effects:* Azatadine maleate is well tolerated and side-effects are generally dose-related and transient. Among these are: weakness, nervousness, dry mouth, increased appetite, anorexia, nausea, headache, drowsiness, dysuria and blurring of vision.

*Overdosage:* Symptoms may vary from central nervous system depression to stimulation, the latter is particularly likely in children. Atropine-like symptoms may also occur. If vomiting has not occurred spontaneously the patient should be induced to vomit. If unsuccessful the stomach should be emptied by aspiration and lavage. Stimulants should not be used and vasopressors may be used to treat hypotension.

**Pharmaceutical precautions**  None.

**Legal category**  P.

**Package quantities**  Optimine Tablets are supplied in OP cartons of 56 tablets containing 4 blister strips of 14 tablets. Optimine Syrup is supplied in a 120 ml bottle.

**Further information**  Azatadine maleate possesses potent antihistamine and antiserotonin activity. It has an inherently long action which enables effective and sustained control of symptoms from twice a day administration.

**Product licence numbers**
Optimine Tablets     0201/0128
Optimine Syrup       0201/0129

## PALACOS* LV WITH GENTAMICIN

### Qualitative and quantitative composition
*Powder:* Methyl methacrylate co-polymer 33.12 gm (Plex 6613F); gentamicin sulkphate 1.67 gm.
*Liquid:* Methyl methacrylate 18.424 g.

**Pharmaceutical form**  Radio-opaque bone cement.

### Clinical particulars
*Therapeutic indications:* Palacos LV with Gentamicin is indicated for the fixation of prostheses to bone in partial or total arthroplastic procedures of the hip, knee or other joints.

*Posology and method of administration:* A dose is prepared by mixing the entire contents of one packet of powder with one ampoule of liquid. One or two doses will usually suffice, although this will depend upon the specific surgical procedure and the techniques employed. (At least one extra unit of Palacos LV should be available before starting a surgical procedure.) The amount of material required and the timing of insertion are determined by the clinical judgement of the surgeon in each individual case.

*Application:* Low viscosity cements tend to be too fluid for convenient handling, and generally a higher viscosity form of the cement is recommended for manual insertion into the femoral canal and into the prepared acetabulum.

*Hand mixing: The liquid is poured into a boil and the powder then added to prevent air entrapment.*

The mixture is stirred carefully for 20–30 seconds and left to stand until a dough-like mass is formed which does not adhere to rubber gloves. At this stage,

the mass is kneadable and will remain so for about 2–3 minutes.

The ideal working consistency of the Palacos LV for application to bone is best determined by the surgeon's experience. When the desired consistency is obtained, the preparation may be applied to bone and prosthesis as required. To ensure adequate fixation, the prosthesis should be inserted by 5 minutes and held securely in place without movement until the bone cement has fully hardened, generally eight to ten minutes after the start of mixing.

*Vacuum mixing system:* Either powder or liquid may be added first depending on suitability for the system used, as the vacuum system will remove entrapped air.

*Injection from a cement gun:* Mixing in the barrel of the cement gun may be difficult because Palacos LV with Gentamicin is rather liquid in the early stage of mixing and the bottom of the barrel is often not a tight enough fit to prevent leakage.

Hence, when using a cement gun, the same initial procedure for mixing as described above is adopted. A double dose will generally be required. After 1 minute, the cement can be poured into the syringe. Cement can be injected from the gun from about 1.5 minutes onwards, but has to be controlled carefully by the surgeon, or it may flow out of the bony cavity as it is still runny at this stage.

The use of a bone cement restrictor or a bone plug in the femoral canal is recommended. If the femoral canal is filled from the distal end, an air vent is not necessary. The implant should be in place by approximately 5.5 minutes. The cement heats up at about 7.5 minutes and polymerises generally by 9.5 minutes.

Pressure should be applied to the cement, whether applied by hand or cement gun, until the prosthesis is inserted. Excess cement must be removed while it is still soft.

The longer time intervals when using a cement gun are due to reduced handling of the cement. Handling the cement warms it slightly during the early stages of polymerisation and accelerates the process.

The times given above for doughing, working and setting apply at approximately 23°C (73°F). Higher temperatures will shorten these times and lowering temperatures will prolong the times. If, during the surgical procedure, additional cement is required, another packet of powder and ampoule of liquid may be mixed as described above. The kneadable mass must be applied to the hardened cement without delay to form a continuous mass; delay will increase the risk of laminations forming in the relatively unsupported proximal end of the femur, with the possibility of resultant weakness in the cement core.

Since each pack contains premeasured quantities of components, care should be taken to mix the entire contents of one packet with the entire contents of one ampoule.

Kneading of the cement will produce evaporation of the volatile monomer, thereby reducing the amount to which the patient will be exposed; however, if the kneading process is too long, the polymerisation may proceed to a point where the mass is no longer soft and pliable, making manipulation and application to bone difficult.

*Contra-indications:* Palacos LV with Gentamicin is contra-indicated in patients allergic to any of the components including gentamicin sulphate. If gentamicin or other aminoglycosides are needed prior to surgery, monitoring of through serum concentrations should be performed within 24 hours of operation. If serum concentrations are above 1 mcg/ml gentamicin, Palacos LV with Gentamicin should not be used in surgery.

*Special warnings and precautions for use:* Before using Palacos LV with Gentamicin, surgeons should become thoroughly familiar with its properties, handling characteristics and application to arthroplasty.

It is advisable for the surgeon to go through the entire mixing, handling and setting process before using the material in an actual surgical procedure.

The liquid monomer is highly volatile and flammable and appropriate caution should be taken with its use. It is also a potent lipid solvent, may irritate the respiratory tract and eyes and may possibly be harmful to the liver. Direct contact of the monomer with any part of the body or with rubber, including surgical rubber gloves, should be avoided.

Care should be taken during the mixing to prevent excessive exposure to concentrated monomer vapours; mixing should take place in a well ventilated part of the operating theatre, or a vacuum device or protective mask should be used.

The completion of polymerisation occurs in the patient and is associated with the liberation of heat. The long-term effects of this heat on the tissue surrounding the bone cement are not known.

Long-term durability, wearability and stability of the polymerised bone cement *in situ* are unknown. The long-term effects of this preparation are unknown.

Safety of use in children has not been established. This should be considered in light of the expected longevity of the patients for whom the substance will be used. Thus the physician should decide whether the benefits expected from its use outweigh any possible long-term adverse effects.

*Interactions with other medicaments and other forms of interaction:* None known.

*Pregnancy and lactation:* There is no evidence of the safety of use of bone cement, gentamicin or associated surgical procedures in pregnancy or lactation.

*Effects on ability to drive and use machines:* Not applicable.

*Undesirable effects:* Transient fall in blood pressure immediately after implantation of the bone cement and endoprosthesis is frequently observed. Rare cases have been reported in which the hypotension was associated with cardiac arrest and sudden death.

The following adverse reactions have been associated with joint replacement surgery involving acrylic bone cements. The contribution of the cementing procedure to these is not established: thrombophlebitis; pulmonary embolism; superficial wound infection; haemorrhage and haematoma; loosening or displacement of the prosthesis; heterotopic new bone; short-term irregularities in cardiac conduction; deep wound infection; trochanteric bursitis; trochanteric separation; myocardial infarction; cerebrovascular accident.

*Overdose:* Not applicable.

**Pharmacological properties**
*Pharmacodynamic properties:* The methyl methacrylae and Plex 6613F co-polymer provide the components of an acrylic bone cement when mixed. Gentamicin sulphate has antibiotic activity to counteract local infection at the site of operation during this period immediately following the operation.

*Pharmacokinetic properties:* The rate of release of gentamicin sulphate from Palacos LV with Gentamicin is designed to be similar to that of Palacos R with Gentamicin. However as a result of greater interdigitation of the low viscosity cement the surface area over which release takes place is increased and thus is reflected by peak levels of gentamicin achieved with Palacos LV over the first two days following surgery. Generally serum, wound secretion and urine levels of gentamicin were three times higher with Palacos LV than Palacos R. The highest recovery level of gentamicin in urine, 194 mg within 24 hours corresponded to a single normal systemic daily dose and was encountered in only one patient. Mean peak serum levels for Palacos LV with Gentamicin were 1.49 µg/ml compared with 0.44 µg/ml for Palacos R.

Normal serum levels following a systemic dose of 80 mg gentamicin are 3.8 µg/ml with a rande of 1.9–6.0 µg/ml. Concentrations in wound secretions indicate much higher local gentamicin levels than those achievable following systemic administration.

*Preclinical safety data:* There are no pre-clinical data of relevance to the prescriber which are additional to that already included in other sections of the SPC.

**Pharmaceutical particulars**
*List of excipients:* Powder: benzoyl peroxide hydrous 75%; zirconium dioxide; chlorophyll E141.
Liquid: N, N-Dimethyl-p-toluidine; chlorophyll E141.

*Incompatibilities:* Not known.

*Shelf life:* 36 months.

**Special precautions for storage:** Do not store the liquid component above 30˚C (86˚F) or in direct sunlight to prevent premature polymerisation. Sterility is only guaranteed if the containers are undamaged. Resterilisation of any of the components should not be attempted.

*Nature and contents of container:* Powder component: The powder is supplied in a sterile paper/polyethylene coated packet, contained within a polyethylene coated peel pack, the inner surface of which is sterile. This double package is contained within an outer protective aluminium foil sachet.

Liquid component: The liquid component is supplied within a sterile glass ampoule, enclosed in a blister pack, the inner surface of which is sterile.

Pack sizes: 2 × 41.7 g packets of sterilised powder (polymer); 2 × 20 ml ampoules of sterilised liquid monomer.

*Instructions for use/handling:* See *Posology and method of administration.*

**Marketing authorisation number**   0201/0085.

**Date of approval/revision of SPC**   August 1996.

**Legal category**   POM.

## PALACOS* R
**Presentation**
Powder: Methyl/methacrylate—methyacrylate co-polymer 33.80 gm
Liquid: Methyl methacrylate 18.40 gm (stabilised with hydroquinone) (0.06%).

**Pharmaceutical form**   Radio-opaque bone cement.

**Clinical particulars**
*Therapeutic indications:* Palacos R is indicated for fixation of prostheses to bone in partial or total arthroplastic procedures of the hip, knee or other joints.

*Posology and method of administration:* The prepared bone cement is applied whilst still malleable to the surface of the joint during the surgical procedure.

One dose is prepared by mixing the entire contents of one packet of powder polymer (Component 1) with the entire contents of one ampoule of liquid monomer (Component 2) i.e. 40 g powder plus 20 ml liquid. Each dose must be prepared separately. The number of doses prepared will depend on the surgical procedure and technique to be used.

The following items will be required for preparation of the bone cement: sterile working area; sterile porcelain or stainless steel bowls; sterile porcelain or stainless steel mixing spoons or spatulas.

The following steps should be followed:
(1) The polyethylene peel packaging and the blister pack are opened by a circulating nurse or assistant, placing the sterile paper inner packet and ampoule on to a sterile table.
(2) Paper packet and ampoule are opened under sterile conditions.
(3) *Hand mixing:* The liquid is poured into a bowl and the powder then added to prevent air entrapment.
*Vacuum mixing system:* Either powder or liquid may be added first depending on suitability for the system used, as the vacuum system will remove entrapped air
(4) Stir the mixture carefully, for 30–40 seconds until a dough-like mass is formed. At this stage the mass is kneadable and will only remain so for 4–5 minutes. The ideal working consistency of the bone cement for application is best determined by the surgeon's experience with the preparation.
(5) When the desired consistency is obtained the preparation can be applied to bone and prosthesis as required. It is important to apply adequate pressure.
(6) The prosthesis should be held securely in place without movement until the bone cement has fully hardened (7–8 minutes after mixing the powder and liquid).
(7) Excessive cement is removed whilst it is still soft.

The above doughing, working and setting times apply at approximately 23˚C (73˚F). An increase in temperature will shorten and a decrease will lengthen these times.

Kneading of the material will assist in the evaporation of excess monomer, and hence decrease the amount to which the patient will be exposed. However, excessive kneading will produce a non-pliable mass, which is very difficult to manipulate and to apply to bone successfully.

Heat continues to be released when the material has been applied, as polymerisation proceeds and the cement hardens. The long term effects of this heat on surrounding tissues is not known, but irrigation of the site with cool physiological saline solution will help to dissipate the heat more rapidly.

To prepare additional amounts of cement use another whole packet of powder polymer and a whole ampoule of liquid monomer using the procedure described above. The entire contents of each must be used. The kneadable mass should then be applied immediately to previously hardened bone cement to ensure reliable fixation.

*Contra-indications:* Palacos R is contra-indicated in patients allergic to any of its components.

*Special warnings and precautions for use:* Any significant alteration in blood preessure, pulse and respiration should be corrected immediately with appropriate measures. Monitoring of these vital signs should take place during and immediately after implantation of the bone cement.

Prior to using Palacos R surgeons should become thoroughly familiar with its properties, handling characteristics and application to arthroplasty.

Surgeons are advised to perform the entire mixing, handling and setting procedure prior to using the materials in an actual surgical procedure. The liquid monomer is highly volatile and flammable. Care must be exercised during the mixing of the two components, which should take place in a well ventilated area. This will help to prevent excessive exposure to the concentrated vapours of the monomer, which can irritate the respiratory tract, the eyes and may be harmful to the liver. If possible a proprietary vacuum extractor or appropriate masks should be used.

The monomer is also a potent lipid solvent and should not be allowed to come into direct contact with the body. Skin reactions have been reported after contact with the monomer. Contact of the monomer with rubber (including surgical gloves) should also be avoided.

*Interactions with other medicaments and other forms of interaction:* The long-term effects of this preparation are unknown. Thus the physician should decide whether the benefits of its use outweigh any possible adverse effects. The long term durability, stability and wearability of the bone cement *in situ* have not been examined. This should be considered in light of the expected longevity of the prospective patient.

*Pregnancy and lactation:* There is insufficient evidence to establish any effect Palacos may have during pregnancy or lactation. It is therefore inadvisable to use this product unless regarded as absolutely essential by the surgeon.

*Effects on ability to drive and use machines:* Not applicable.

*Undesirable effects:* Transient fall in blood pressure immediately after implantation of bone cement and endo-prosthesis is frequently observed. Rare cases have been reported in which the hypotension was associated with cardiac arrest and sudden death.

The following adverse reactions have been associated with Joint Replacement Surgery: thrombophlebitis; pulmonary embolism; haemorrhage and haematoma; loosening or displacement of the prosthesis; superficial wound infection; deep wound infection; trochanteric bursitis; trochanteric separation.

Others which have been observed: heterotopic new bone; short term irregularities in cardiac conduction; myocardial infarction; cerebrovascular accident.

*Overdose:* Not applicable.

**Pharmacological properties**
*Pharmacodynamic properties:* In the generally accepted sense this bone cement does not comprise any pharmacologically active constituents.

The various components are not new chemicals but known compounds used in other, well-established similar bone cements. They are all self-curing resins based on methyl-methacrylate used originally in dentistry and latterly for bone replacement and augmentation as a bone cement in surgical procedures.

*Pharmacokinetic properties:* Long-term effects of these implantations are unknown either for their effects in the body or the body's effects on them.

*Preclinical safety data:* There are no pre-clinical data of relevance to the prescriber which are additional to that already included in other sections of the SPC.

**Pharmaceutical particulars**
*List of excipients:* Powder: benzolyperoxide; zirconium dioxide; chlorophyll. Liquid: N, N-Dimethyl-p-toluidine; chlorophyll.

*Incompatibilities:* None known.

*Shelf life:* 60 months.

*Special precautions for storage:* To prevent premature polymerisation, do not store components above 30˚C (86˚F) or in direct sunlight.
Resterilisation of any of the components must not be attempted under any circumstances.

*Nature and contents of container:* Cardboard outer carton containing an aluminium foil packet, two double polyethylene coated packets of powder (inner pack is sterile) plus two blister packed sterile ampoules.

Pack sizes: 2 × 40 g packets of radio-opaque sterile powder polymer and 2 × 20 ml ampoules of sterile liquid monomer.

*Instructions for use/handling:* See *Posology and method of administration.*

**Marketing authorisation number**   0201/0125.

**Date of approval/revision of SPC**   August 1996.

**Legal category**   POM.

## PALACOS* R WITH GENTAMICIN
## PALACOS* R-20 WITH GENTAMICIN

**Qualitative and quantitative composition**
*Palacos R with Gentamicin:*
Powder: Methyl methacrylate—methylacrylate co polymer 33.80 gm; Gentamicin sulphate 0.50 gm (to provide gentamicin base).
Liquid: Methyl methacrylate 18.40 gm (stabilised with hydroquinone) (0.06%).

*Palacos R-20 with Gentamicin:*
Powder: Methyl methacrylate—methylacrylate co polymer 16.90 gm; Gentamicin sulphate 0.25 gm (to provide gentamicin base).
Liquid: Methyl methacrylate 9.20 gm (stabilised with hydroquinone) (0.06%).

**Pharmaceutical form** Radio-opaque bone cement.

## Clinical particulars

*Therapeutic indications:* Palacos R with Gentamicin and Palacos R-20 with Gentamicin are indicated for the fixation of protheses to bone in partial or total arthroplastic procedures of the hip, knee or other joints in which infection by gentamicin-sensitive organisms is confirmed or suspected.

*Posology and method of administration:* The prepared bone cement is applied whilst still malleable to the surface of the joint during the surgical procedure.

One dose is prepared by mixing the entire contents of one packet of powder polymer (Component 1) with the entire contents of one ampoule of liquid monomer (Component 2) i.e. 40 g powder plus 20 ml liquid OR 20 g powder plus 10 ml liquid. Each dose must be prepared separately. The number of doses prepared will depend on the surgical procedure and technique to be used.

The following items will be required for preparation of the bone cement: sterile working area; sterile porcelain or stainless steel bowls; sterile porcelain or stainless steel mixing spoons or spatulas.

The following steps should be followed:

(1) The polyethylene peel package and the blister pack are opened by a circulating nurse or assistant, placing the sterile paper inner packet and ampoule on to a sterile table.

(2) Paper packet and ampoule are opened under sterile conditions.

(3) *Hand Mixing:* The liquid is poured into a bowl and the powder then added to prevent air entrapment.

*Vacuum Mixing System:* Either powder or liquid may be added first depending on suitability for the system used, as the vacuum system will remove entrapped air.

(4) Stir the mixture carefully, for 30–40 seconds until a dough-like mass is formed. At this stage the mass is kneadable and will only remain so for 4–5 minutes. The ideal working consistency of the bone cement for application is best determined by the surgeon's experience with the preparation.

(5) When the desired consistency is obtained the preparation can be applied to bone and prosthesis as required. It is important to apply adequate pressure.

(6) The prosthesis should be held securely in place without movement until the bone cement has fully hardened (7–8 minutes after mixing the powder and liquid).

(7) Excessive cement is removed whilst it is still soft.

The above doughing, working and setting times apply at approximately 23°C (73°F). An increase in temperature will shorten and a decrease will lengthen these times.

Kneading of the material will assist in the evaporation of excess monomer, and hence decrease the amount to which the patient will be exposed. However, excessive kneading will produce a non-pliable mass, which is very difficult to manipulate and to apply to bone successfully.

Heat continues to be released when the material has been applied, as polymerisation proceeds and the cement hardens. The long term effects of this heat on surrounding tissues is not known, but irrigation of the site with cool physiological saline solution will help to dissipate the heat even more rapidly.

To prepare additional amounts of cement use another whole packet of powder polymer and a whole ampoule of liquid monomer using the procedure described above. The entire contents of each must be used. The kneadable mass should then be applied immediately to previously hardened bone cement to ensure reliable fixation.

*Contra-indications:* Palacos R with Gentamicin and Palacos R-20 with Gentamicin are contra-indicated in patients allergic to any of its components.

*Special warnings and precautions for use:* Any significant alteration in blood pressure, pulse and respiration should be corrected immediately with appropriate measures. Monitoring of these vital signs should take place during and immediately after implantation of the bone cement.

Prior to using Palacos R with Gentamicin, or Palacos R-20 with Gentamicin, surgeons should be thoroughly familiar with its properties, handling characteristics and application to arthroplasty.

Surgeons are advised to perform the entire mixing, handling and setting procedure prior to using the materials in an actual surgical procedure. The liquid monomer is highly volatile and flammable. Care must be exercised during the mixing of the two components, which should take place in a well ventilated area. This will help to prevent excessive exposure to the concentrated vapours of the monomer, which can irritate the respiratory tract, the eyes and may be harmful to the liver. If possible a proprietary vacuum extractor or appropriate masks can be used.

The monomer is also a potent lipid solvent and should not be allowed to come into direct contact with the body. Skin reactions have been reported after contact with the monomer. Contact of the liquid monomer with rubber (including surgical gloves) should also be avoided.

*Interactions with other medicaments and other forms of interaction:* The long term effects of this preparation are unknown. Thus the physician should decide whether the benefits of its use outweigh any possible adverse effects. The long term durability, stability and wearability of the bone *in situ* have not been examined. This should be considered in light of the expected longevity of the prospective patient.

*Pregnancy and lactation:* There is insufficient evidence to establish any effect Palacos may have during pregnancy or lactation. It is therefore inadvisable to use this product unless regarded as absolutely essential by the surgeon.

*Effects on ability to drive and use machines:* Not applicable.

*Undesirable effects:* Transient fall in blood pressure immediately after implantation of bone cement and endo-prosthesis is frequently observed. Rare cases have been reported in which the hypotension was associated with cardiac arrest and sudden death.

The following adverse reactions have been associated with Joint Replacement Surgery: thrombophlebitis; pulmonary embolism; haemorrhage and haematoma; loosening or displacement of the prosthesis; superficial wound infection; deep wound infection; trochanteric bursitis; trochanteric separation.

Others which have been observed: heterotopic new bone; short term irregularities in cardiac conduction; myocardial infarction; cerebrovascular accident.

Since the concentration of Gentamicin reaching the VIIIth nerve and the kidney will be quite low, ototoxic and nephrotoxic reactions are very unlikely to result from the use of Palacos R with Gentamicin or Palacos R-20 with Gentamicin. No such events have been reported for these products. Hypersensitivity to Gentamicin has been reported very rarely.

*Overdose:* Not applicable.

### Pharmacological properties

*Pharmacodynamic properties:* In the generally accepted sense this bone cement does not comprise any pharmacologically active constituents other than gentamicin sulphate.

The various components are not new chemicals but known compounds used in other, well-established similar bone cements. They are all self-curing resins based on methyl-methacrylate used originally in dentistry and latterly for bone replacement and augmentation as a bone cement in surgical procedures.

In-vitro studies suggest that gentamicin is effectively released from Palacos R and Palacos R-20. The greatest amounts are released during the first 24 hours after incubation in suitable dilution fluid although continual release has been demonstrated to occur over a considerable period at low levels.

Published in-vivo studies suggest implantation of palacos R with Gentamicin or Palacos R-20 with Gentamicin either subcutaneously in rats or in bone canals in dogs and pigs results in release of gentamicin with therapeutic levels in the areas immediately surrounding the implant.

*Pharmacokinetic properties:* Long-term effects of these implantations are unknown either for their effects in the body or the body's effects on them.

The use of bone cements in which a broad spectrum antibiotic has been incorporated gives prophylactic cover against the possibility of deep-seated infection at the site of implant. It would appear from levels found in the blood and urine that the Gentamicin released from Palacos R products is metabolised in the same way as parenterally administered aminoglycoside antibiotices.

*Preclinical safety data:* There are no pre-clinical data of relevance to the prescriber which are additional to that already included in other sections of the SPC.

### Pharmaceutical particulars

*List of excipients:* Powder: benzolyperoxide; zirconium dioxide; chlorophyll.
Liquid: N, N-Dimethyl-p-toluidine; chlorophyll.

*Incompatibilities:* None known.

*Shelf life:* 48 months.

*Special precautions for storage:* To prevent premature polymerisation, do not store components above 30°C (86°F) or in direct sunlight.

Resterilisation of any of the components must not be attempted under any circumstances.

*Nature and contents of container:* Cardboard outer carton with inner polystyrene tray holding: two blister packed sterile ampoules of liquid and two foil packs of powder. Within each foil overwrap the powder is double packaged; the inner pack is sterile.

*Palacos R with Gentamicin:* Pack sizes: 2 × 40 gm packets of radio-opaque sterile powder polymer containing 0.5 g gentamicin base per packet and 2 × 20 ml ampoules of sterile liquid monomer.

*Palacos R-20 with Gentamicin:* Pack sizes: 2 × 20 gm packets of radio-opaque sterile powder polymer containing 0.25 g gentamicin base per packet and 2 × 10 ml ampoules of sterile liquid monomer.

*Instructions for use/handling:* See *Posology and method of administration.*

### Marketing authorisation numbers

| | |
|---|---|
| Palacos R with Gentamicin | 0201/0126 |
| Palacos R-20 with Gentamicin | 0201/0127 |

**Date of approval/revision of SPC** August 1996

**Legal category** POM.

## TINADERM-M* CREAM

### Qualitative and quantitative composition
Tolnaftate 1.0 w/w
Nystatin 100.0% IU

**Pharmaceutical form** Cream.

### Clinical particulars

*Therapeutic indications:* Tinaderm Cream is recommended in the treatment of cutaneous mycotic infections such as Tinea pedis, Tinea cruris, Tinea corporis, Tinea barbae and Tinea manuum due to *Trichophyton rubrum, T. mentagrophytes, T. tonsurans, Microsporum canis, M. audouinii, Epidermophyton floccosum, Candida albicans* and *Tinea versicolor (Malassezia furfur).*

If Candida albicans is the primary cause of infections, such conditions as 'athlete's foot' (dermatophytosis), perleche, paronychia, intertrigo, 'nappy rash' and other cutaneous lesions can be successfully treated with Tinaderm-M.

Tinaderm-M is particularly recommended for the treatment of fungal infections localised in intertriginous and other moist areas of the skin where Candida infections are present or likely to develop.

*Posology and method of administration:* A sufficient quantity of Tinaderm-M should be applied to completely cover the affected area two or three times daily until healing is complete. Lesions generally begin to clear during the first treatment week and disappear after 2–3 weeks of treatment. If thickening of skin has occurred, treatment for as long as 4–6 weeks may be required. The concomitant use of a mild keratolytic agent may be indicated in areas where the skin has become hyperkeratotic. Use of wet compresses prior to application of Tinaderm-M aids in the healing of exudative lesions and does not interfere with the fungicidal action of the medication.

*Contra-indications:* There are no known contra-indications to tolnaftate, however if hypersensitivity to any of the ingredients occurs, treatment should be stopped.

*Special warnings and precautions for use:* Keep away from eyes and mucous membranes. Mycosis complicated by bacterial infections may require additional antibiotic treatment.

Tinaderm-M is for dermatological use only. If sensitivity occurs, discontinue use.

*Interactions with other medicaments and other forms of interaction:* None known.

*Pregnancy and lactation:* Whilst there is no specific evidence of safety of the drug in human pregnancy, both tolnaftate and nystatin have been in widespread topical use for many years without apparent ill consequence.

*Effects on ability to drive and use machines:* Not applicable.

*Undesirable effects:* A few cases of mild irritation and sensitisation have been reported.

*Overdose:* Not applicable.

### Pharmacological properties

*Pharmacodynamic properties:* Tolnaftate is a highly active non-sensitising fungicidal agent that is very effective in the treatment of superficial fungal infections of the skin.

Nystatin, an antibiotic with antifungal activity provides specific therapy for all localised forms of candidiasis.

*Pharmacokinetic particulars:* Not applicable.

The product is applied topically and systemic absorption is negligible.

*Preclinical safety data:* There are no pre-clinical data of relevance to the prescriber which are additional to that already included in other sections of this SPC.

### Pharmaceutical particulars

*List of excipients:* Butylated hydroxytoluene; methylparaben; propylparaben; potassium sorbate; hydrochloric acid; cetomacrogol 1000; cetostearyl alcohol, fractionated coconut oil, perfume no. 66612, purified water.

*Incompatibilities:* None known.

*Shelf life:* 36 months.

*Special precautions for storage:* There are no special precautions for storage.

*Nature and contents of container:* 10 g or 20 g epoxy resin-lined aluminium tubes with low density polyethylene caps.

*Instructions for use/handling:* Not applicable.

**Marketing authorisation number** 0201/0071.

**Date of approval/revision of SPC** February 1997.

**Legal category** POM.

## VIRAFERON* INJECTABLE SOLUTION

**Qualitative and quantitative composition** Viraferon Injectable Solution:

*Active ingredient:* recombinant interferon alfa-2b, 18 million International Units (IU)/vial (6 million IU/ml).

*Inactive ingredients:* sodium phosphate dibasic, sodium phosphate monobasic, edetate disodium, sodium chloride, m-cresol, polysorbate 80, water for injection q.s. ad 3 ml (18 million IU).

**Pharmaceutical form** Injectable solution.

**Clinical particulars**

*Therapeutic indications:*

*Hepatitis B:* Treatment of adult patients with chronic active hepatitis B, who have markers for viral replication e.g., those who are positive for HBV-DNA, DNA polymerase or HBeAg.

*Chronic hepatitis C/non-A, non-B:* Reduction of disease activity in adult patients with chronic hepatitis C/ non-A, non-B who have elevated liver enzymes without liver decompensation. Studies in these patients demonstrate that Viraferon Injection therapy can produce normalisation of serum ALT, clearance of serum HCV-RNA and improvement in liver histology.

Current clinical experience in patients who remain on Viraferon Injection for 12–18 months indicates that a higher proportion of patients demonstrated a sustained response after longer durations of therapy than those who discontinued therapy after six months.

*Posology and method of administration:* Viraferon Injection may be administered using either sterilized glass or plastic disposable syringes.

Multidose presentations should be for individual patient use only.

During the course of treatment with Viraferon Injection for any indication, if adverse reactions develop, the dosage should be modified or therapy should be discontinued temporarily until the adverse reactions abate. If persistent or recurrent intolerance develops following adequate dosage adjustment, or disease progresses, the treatment with Viraferon Injection should be discontinued.

For maintenance dosage regimens administered subcutaneously, at the discretion of the physician, the patient may self-administer the dose.

*Chronic active hepatitis B:* The optimal schedule of treatment has not been established yet. The dosage is usually in the range of 2.5 million IU to 5.0 million IU/m² of body surface administered subcutaneously three times per week for a period of four to six months.

If markers for viral replication or HbeAg do not decrease after one month of therapy, the dose can be escalated. The dosage may be adjusted further according to the patient's tolerance to the medication.

If no improvement has been observed after three to four months of treatment, discontinuation of therapy should be considered.

*Chronic hepatitis C/non-A, non-B:* The recommended dose is 3 million IU administered subcutaneously three times a week. Most patients who respond demonstrate improvement in ALT levels within 12–16 weeks. In these patients (and in fonction of their tolerance, see the introduction of section 4.2: Posology and method of administration), therapy should be continued with 3 million IU three times a week for up to 18 months. In patients who fail to respond after 12–16 weeks of treatment, discontinuation of Viraferon Injection therapy should be considered.

*Contra-indications:*

- A history of hypersensitivity to recombinant interferon alfa-2b or any other component of Viraferon Injection;
- severe pre-existing cardiac disease;
- severe renal or hepatic dysfunction;
- epilepsy and/or compromised central nervous system (CNS) function (see *Special warnings and special precautions for use*);
- chronic hepatitis with decompensated hepatic disease or cirrhosis of the liver;
- chronic hepatitis in patients who are being or have been treated recently with immunosuppressive agents excluding short-term corticosteroid withdrawal;
- autoimmune hepatitis; or history of autoimmune disease; immunosupressed transplant recipients;
- pre-existing thyroid disease unless it can be controlled with conventional treatment.

*Special warnings and special precautions for use:* Efficacy in patients with chronic active hepatitis B co-infected with the human immunodeficiency virus (HIV) has not been demonstrated.

Viraferon should be used cautiously in patients with debilitating medical conditions, such as those with a history of pulmonary disease (e.g. chronic obstructive pulmonary disease) or diabetes mellitus prone to ketoacidosis. Caution should be observed also in patients with coagulation disorders (e.g. thrombophlebitis, pulmonary embolism) or severe myelosuppression.

Acute hypersensitivity reactions (e.g., urticaria, angioedema, broncho-constriction, anaphylaxis) to Viraferon Injection have been observed rarely during Viraferon Injection therapy. If such a reaction develops, the drug should be discontinued and appropriate medical therapy instituted immediately. Transient rashes do not necessitate interruption of treatment.

Moderate to severe adverse experiences may require modification of the patient's dosage regimen, or in some cases, termination of Viraferon Injection therapy. Any patient developing liver function abnormalities during treatment with Viraferon Injection should be monitored closely and treatment discontinued if signs and symptoms progress.

Patients with chronic hepatitis B with evidence of decreasing hepatic synthetic function, such as decreasing albumin levels or prolongation of prothrombin time, who nevertheless meet the criteria for therapy, may be at increased risk of clinical decompensation if a flare of aminotransferases occurs during treatment. In considering these patients for Viraferon therapy, the potential risks must be evaluated against the potential benefits of treatment.

Hypotension may occur during Viraferon Injection therapy or up to two days post-therapy and may require supportive treatment.

Adequate hydration should be maintained in patients undergoing Viraferon Injection therapy since hypotension related to fluid depletion has been seen in some patients. Fluid replacement may be necessary.

Patients with a history of congestive heart failure, myocardial infarction and/or previous or current arrhythmic disorders, who require Viraferon Injection therapy, should be closely monitored. Those patients who have pre-existing cardiac abnormalities and/or are in advanced stages of cancer should have electrocardiograms taken prior to and during the course of treatment. Cardiac arrhythmias (primarily supraventricular) usually respond to conventional therapy but may require discontinuation of Viraferon Injection therapy.

Pulmonary infiltrates, pneumonitis and pneumonia, including fatality, have been observed rarely in interferon-alpha treated patients, including those treated with Viraferon Injection. The etiology has not been defined. These symptoms have been reported more frequently when shosaikoto, a Chinese herbal medicine, is administered concomitantly with interferon-alpha. Any patient developing fever, cough, dyspnea or other respiratory symptoms should have a chest X-ray taken. If the chest X-ray shows pulmonary infiltrates or there is evidence of pulmonary function impairment, the patient should be monitored closely, and, if appropriate, interferon-alpha treatment should be discontinued. While this has been reported more often in patients with chronic hepatitis C/ non-A, non-B treated with interferon-alpha, it has also been reported in patients with oncologic diseases treated with interferon-alpha. Prompt discontinuation of interferon alpha administration and treatment with corticosteroids appear to be associated with resolution of pulmonary adverse events.

Patients with a pre-existing psychiatric condition or a history of severe psychiatric disorder should not be treated with Viraferon Injection.

If severe CNS effects, particularly depression, are observed, Viraferon Injection therapy should be discontinued. CNS effects manifested by depression, confusion and other alterations of mental status have been observed in some patients during Viraferon Injection therapy and suicidal ideation and attempted suicide have been observed rarely. These adverse effects have occurred in patients treated with recommended doses as well as in patients treated with higher Viraferon doses. More significant obtundation and coma have been observed in some patients, usually elderly, treated at higher doses. While these effects are generally reversible, in a few patients full resolution took up to three weeks. Very rarely, seizures have occurred with high doses of Viraferon Injection.

Infrequently, patients treated for chronic hepatitis non-A, non-B/C with Viraferon Injection developed thyroid abnormalities, either hypothyroid or hyperthyroid. In clinical trials < 1% (4/426) developed thyroid abnormalities. The abnormalities were controlled by conventional therapy for thyroid dysfunction. The mechanism by which Viraferon Injection may alter thyroid status is unknown. Prior to initiation of Viraferon Injection therapy for the treatment of chronic hepatitis non-A, non-B/C, serum thyroid-stimulating hormone (TSH) levels should be evaluated. Any thyroid abnormality detected at that time should be treated with conventional therapy. Viraferon Injection treatment may be initiated if TSH levels can be maintained in the normal range by medication. If, during the course of Viraferon Injection therapy, a patient develops symptoms consistent with possible thyroid dysfunction, TSH levels should be evaluated. In the presence of thyroid dysfunction, Viraferon treatment may be continued if TSH levels can be maintained in the normal range by medication. DIscontinuation of Viraferon therapy has not reversed thyroid dysfunction occurring during treatment.

Because of reports of exacerbating pre-existing psoriatic disease, Viraferon Injection should be used in patients with psoriasis only if the potential benefit justifies the potential risk.

While fever may be associated with the flu-like syndrome reported commonly during interferon therapy, other causes of persistent fever should be ruled out.

Ocular adverse events (see section 4.8 *Undesirable effects*) appear to occur after use of the drug for several months, but also have been reported after shorter treatment periods. Any patient complaining of changes in visual acuity or visual fields, or reporting other ophthalmologic symptoms during treatment with Viraferon, should have an eye examination. Because the retinal events may have to be differentiated from those seen with diabetic or hypertensive retinopathy, a baseline ocular examination is recommended prior to treatment with interferon in patients with diabetes mellitus or hypertension.

Viraferon Injectable Solution contains m-cresol; some individuals may have an allergic reaction to this ingredient.

*Laboratory tests:* Standard haematologic tests and blood chemistries (complete blood count and differential, platelet count, electrolytes, liver enzymes, serum protein, serum bilirubin and serum creatinine) should be conducted in all patients prior to and periodically during systemic treatment with Viraferon Injection. In patients treated for hepatitis the recommended testing schedule is at weeks 1, 2, 4, 8, 12, 16, and every other month, thereafter, throughout treatment.

If ALT flares during Viraferon therapy to ≥ 2 times baseline, Viraferon Injection therapy may be continued unless signs and symptoms of liver failure are observed. During ALT flare, liver function tests: ALT, prothrombin time, alkaline phosphatase, albumin and bilirubin should be monitored at two-week intervals.

In patients considered for treatment of hepatitis, a liver biopsy is recommended to document diagnosis and severity of the disease.

*Paediatric use:* Doses of up to 10 million IU/m² have been administered safely to children with chronic active hepatitis B. However, efficacy of therapy has not been demonstrated. Generally, experience in patients below 18 years of age has been limited, and in such cases the expected benefits should be weighed carefully against potential hazards.

*Effect on fertility:* Interferon may impair fertility. In studies of interferon use in non-human primates abnormalities of the menstrual cycle have been observed. Decreased serum estradiol and progesterone concentrations have been reported in women treated with human leukocyte interferon. Therefore fertile women should not receive Viraferon Injection unless they are using effective contraception during the treatment period. Viraferon Injection should be used with caution in fertile men.

*Interaction with other medicaments and other forms of interaction:*

*Drug/drug interactions:* Paracetamol has been used successfully to alleviate the symptoms of fever and headache which can occur with Viraferon Injection therapy. The recommended paracetamol dosage is 500 mg to 1 g given 30 minutes before administration of Viraferon Injection. The maximum dosage of acetaminophen to be given is 1 g four times daily.

Narcotics, hypnotics or sedatives should be administered with caution concomitantly with Viraferon Injection.

Interactions between Viraferon Injection and other drugs have not been fully evaluated. Caution should be exercised when administering Viraferon in combination with other potentially myelosuppressive agents.

Interferons may affect the oxidative metabolic process. This should be considered during concomitant therapy with drugs metabolised by this route such as the xanthine derivatives theophylline or aminophylline. During concomitant therapy with xanthine agents, serum theophylline levels should be monitored and dosage adjusted if necessary.

*Pregnancy and lactation:* Viraferon Injection has been shown to have abortifacient effects in *Macaca mulatta* (rhesus monkeys) at 90 and 180 times the recommended intramuscular or subcutaneous dose of 2 million IU/m². Although abortion was observed in all dose groups (7.5 million, 15 million and 30 million IU/kg), it was only statistically significant versus control at the mid- and high-dose groups (corresponding to 90 and 180 times the recommended intramuscular or subcutaneous dose of 2 million IU/m²).

There are no adequate and well controlled studies in pregnant women. Viraferon Injection should be used during pregnancy only if the potential benefit justifies the potential risk to the foetus. It is not known whether the components of this drug are excreted in human milk. Because of the potential for adverse reactions from Viraferon Injection in nursing infants, a decision should be made whether to discontinue nursing or to discontinue the drug, taking into account the importance of the drug to the mother.

*Effects on ability to drive and use machines:* Not applicable.

*Undesirable effects: Systemic administration:* The most commonly reported adverse effects were fever, fatigue, headache and myalgia. Fever and fatigue were reversible within 72 hours of interruption or cessation of treatment and were dose related. In the hepatitis treatment groups these effects were of mild to moderate severity.

Common adverse effects include anorexia, nausea and rigors.

Less common adverse effects include vomiting, diarrhoea, arthralgia, asthenia, somnolence, dizziness, dry mouth, alopecia, flu-like symptoms (unspecified), back pain, depression, malaise, pain, increased sweating, taste alteration, irritability, insomnia, confusion, impaired concentration and hypotension.

Rarely reported adverse reactions include abdominal pain, rash, nervousness, injection site disorders, paresthesia, herpes simplex, pruritus, eye pain, anxiety, epistaxis, coughing, pharyngitis, pulmonary infiltrates, pneumonitis and pneumonia, impaired consciousness, weight decrease, face oedema, dyspnea, dyspepsia, tachycardia, hypertension, increased appetite, decreased libido, hypoesthesia, taste perversion, loose stool, gingival bleeding, neuropathy, and polyneuropathy. Hyperthyroidism or hypothyroidism have also been observed rarely. Hepatotoxicity, including fatality has been observed rarely.

Cardiovascular (CVS) adverse reactions, particularly arrhythmia, appeared to be correlated mostly with pre-existing CVS disease and prior therapy with cardiotoxic agents. (see *Special warnings and special precautions for use.*) Transient reversible cardiomyopathy has been reported rarely in patients without prior evidence of cardiac disease.

Retinal haemorrhages, cotton wool spots, and retinal artery or vein obstruction have been observed rarely in patients treated with interferon alfa, including Viraferon (recombinant interferon alfa-2b) (see 4.4 *Special warnings and special precautions for use.*).

Clinically significant laboratory abnormalities, most frequently occurring at doses greater than 10 million IU daily, include reduction in granulocyte and white blood cell counts; decreases in haemoglobin level and platelet count; increases in alkaline phosphatase, LDH, serum creatinine and serum urea nitrogen levels.

Increase in serum ALT/AST levels have been noted as an abnormality in some non-hepatitis subjects and also in some patients with chronic hepatitis B coincident with clearance of viral DNAp.

*Overdose:* Overdosing has not been reported with Viraferon Injection, but as for any pharmacologically active compound, symptomatic treatment with fre-quent monitoring of vital signs and close observation of the patient is indicated.

**Pharmacological properties** Viraferon Injection is a sterile, stable, formulation of highly purified interferon alfa-2b produced by recombinant DNA techniques. Recombinant interferon alfa-2b is a water soluble protein with a molecular weight of approximately 19,300 daltons. It is obtained from a clone of *E.coli*, which has a genetically engineered plasmid hybridized with an interferon alfa-2b gene from human leukocytes.

The activity of Viraferon Injection is expressed in terms of IU, with 1 mg of recombinant interferon alfa-2b protein corresponding to $2 \times 10^8$ IU. International Units are determined by comparison of the activity of the recombinant interferon alfa-2b with the activity of the international reference preparation of human leukocyte interferon established by the World Health Organisation.

The interferons are a family of small protein molecules with molecular weights of approximately 15,000 or 21,000 daltons. They are produced and secreted by cells in response to viral infections or various synthetic and biological inducers. Three major classes of interferons have been identified: alpha, beta and gamma. These three main classes are themselves not homogeneous and may contain several different molecular species of interferon. More than 14 genetically distinct human alpha interferons have been identified. Viraferon Injection has been classified as recombinant interferon alfa-2b.

*Pharmacodynamic properties:* Interferons exert their cellular activities by binding to specific membrane receptors on the cell surface. Human interferon receptors, as isolated from human lymphoblastoid (Daudi) cells, appear to be highly asymmetric proteins. they exhibit selectivity for human but not murine interferons, suggesting species specificity. Studies with other interferons have demonstrated species specificity.

The results of several studies suggest that, once bound to the cell membrane, interferon initiates a complex sequence of intracellular events that include the induction of certain enzymes. It is thought that this process, at least in part, is responsible for the various cellular responses to interferon, including inhibition of virus replication in virus-infected cells, suppression of cell proliferation and such immuno-modulating activities as enhancement of the phago-cytic activity of macrophages and augmentation of the specific cytotoxicity of lymphocytes for target cells. Any or all of these activities may contribute to interferon's therapeutic effects.

Recombinant interferon alfa-2b has exhibited anti-pproliferative effects in studies employing both animal and human cell culture systems as well as human tumour xenografts in animals. It has demonstrated significant immunomodulatory activity *in vitro*.

Recombinant interferon alfa-2b also inhibits viral replication *in vitro* and *in vivo*. Although the exact antiviral mode of action of recombinant interferon alfa-2b is unknown, it appears to alter the host cell metabolism. This action inhibits viral replication or if replication occurs, the progeny virions are to leave the cell. The specific mechanism of action in the treatment of condylomata acuminata is unknown.

*Pharacokinetic properties:* The pharmacokinetics of Viraferon Injection were studied in healthy volunteers following single 5 million IU/mls2 and 10 million IU doses administered subcutaneously, intramuscularly and as a 30-minute intravenous infusion. The mean serum interferon concentrations following subcutaneous and intramuscular injections were comparable. Maximum serum levels occurred three to 12 hours after the lower dose and six to eight hours after the higher dose. The elimination half-lives of interferon injections were approximately two to three hours, and six to seven hours, respectively. Serum levels were below the detection limit 16 and 24 hours, respectively, post-injection. Both intramuscular and subcutaneous administration resulted in bioavailabilities greater than 100%.

After intravenous administration, serum interferon levels peaked (135 to 273 IU/ml) by the end of the infusion, then declined at a slightly more rapid rate than after subcutaneous or intramuscular drug administration, becoming undetectable four hours after the infusion. The elimination half-life was approximately two hours.

Urine levels of interferon were below the detection limit following each of the three routes of administration.

Interferon neutralising factor assays were performed on serum samples of patients who received Viraferon Injection in Schering-Plough monitored clinical trials. Interferon neutralising factors are antibodies which neutralise the antiviral activity of interferon. The clinical incidence of neutralising factors developing in cancer patients treated systemically is 2.9% and in hepatitis patients is 6.9%. Serum interferon neutralising factors were detected in 0.8% of patients with condylomata acuminata who received Viraferon Injection intralesionally. The detected titres are low in almost all cases and have not been regularly associated with loss of response or any other auto-immune phenomenon. In patients with hepatitis, no loss of response was observed, apparently due to the low titres. No development of neutralising antibodies has been demonstrated in patients who received Viraferon Injection intralesionally in the treatment of basal cell carcinoma.

*Preclinical safety data:* Although interferon is generally recognised to be species specific, toxicology studies in mice, rats, rabbits and monkeys were conducted. Injections of human recombinant interferon alfa-2b for up to three months have shown no evidence of toxicity.

Results of animal reproduction studies indicate that recombinant interferon alfa-2b was not teratogenic in rats or rabbits, nor did it adversely affect pregnancy, foetal development or reproductive capacity in offspring of treated rats. Furthermore, animal studies have shown that interferons do not cross the placental barrier.

Mutagenicity studies with Viraferon Injection revealed no adverse effects.

**Pharmaceutical particulars**

*List of excipients:* Sodium phosphate dibasic, sodium phosphate monobasic, edetate disodium, sodium chloride, m-cresol, polysorbate 80, water for injection.

*Incompatabilities:* Not applicable.

*Shelf life:* 18 months when stored at 2–8°C. The unopened product may be kept at room temperatures up to 25°C (room temperature) for up to seven days while in possession of the patient.

*Special precautions for storage:* Store between 2° to 8°C.

*Nature and contents of container:* 6 million IU/ml—18 million IU/vial—3 mil vial, type I flint glass.

*Instructions for use/handling:* Following withdrawal of first dose from the vial, the remaining solution is stable for up to four weeks at 2° to 8°C. Any solution remaining after 4 weeks must be discarded.

**Marketing authorisation number** 0201/0214.

**Date of approval/revision of SPC** January 1997.

**Legal category** POM.

*\*Trade Mark*

# Schwarz Pharma Limited
Schwarz House
East Street
Chesham
Bucks HP5 1DG

**SCHWARZ**
P H A R M A

## DEPONIT*

**Qualitative and quantitative composition** Deponit 5: 1 patch contains glyceryl trinitrate 18.7 mg. The average amount of glyceryl trinitrate absorbed from each patch in 24 hours is 5 mg. Deponit 10: 1 patch contains glyceryl trinitrate 37.4 mg. The average amount of glyceryl trinitrate absorbed from each patch in 24 hours is 10 mg.

**Pharmaceutical form** Transdermal drug delivery system, packaged individually in a sealed sachet.

**Clinical particulars**
*Therapeutic indications:* Prophylaxis of angina pectoris alone or in combination with other anti-anginal therapy.

*Posology and method of administration:*
*Deponit 5 mg: Adults:*Treatment should be initiated with one Deponit 5 daily. If necessary the dosage may be increased to two Deponit 5 Patches.

*Deponit 10 mg: Adults:*Treatment should be initiated with one Deponit 10 daily. If necessary the dosage may be increased to two Deponit 10 Patches.

It is recommended that the patch is applied to the lateral chest wall, the skin should be smooth, unbroken and with few hairs. The replacement patch should be applied to a new area of skin. Allow several days to elapse before applying a fresh patch to the same area of skin. Tolerance may occur during chronic nitrate therapy. Tolerance is likely to be avoided by allowing a patch-free period of 8-12 hours each day, usually at night. Additional anti-anginal therapy with drugs not containing nitro compounds should be considered for the nitrate-free interval.

*Elderly:*No specific information on use in the elderly is available, however there is no evidence to suggest that an alteration in dose is required.

*Children:*The safety and efficacy of Deponit in children has yet to be established.

*Contra-indications:*Hypersensitivity to nitrates, severe hypotension, marked anaemia, increased intracranial pressure, myocardial insufficiency due to obstructions (e.g. in the presence of aortic or mitral stenosis or of constrictive pericarditis).

*Special precautions for use:* In recent myocardial infarction or acute heart failure, Deponit should be employed only under careful surveillance. As with all anti-anginal nitrate preparations, withdrawal of long-term treatment should be gradual by replacement with decreasing doses of long-acting oral nitrates. Caution should be exercised in patients with hypoxaemia and a ventilation/perfusion imbalance due to lung disease or ischaemic heart failure. If tolerance to glyceryl trinitrate patches develops, the effect of sublingual glyceryl trinitrate on exercise tolerance may be partially diminished. Nitrate therapy may aggravate the angina caused by hypertropic cardiomyopathy.

*Interactions:* Concomitant treatment with other vasodilators, calcium antagonists, ACE inhibitors, beta blockers, diuretics, antihypertensives, tricyclic antidepressants and major tranquillisers, as well as the consumption of alcohol, may potentiate the hypotensive effect of the preparation. If administered concurrently, Deponit may increase the blood level of dihydroergotamine and lead to coronary vasoconstriction. The possibility that ingestion of acetylsalicylic acid and non-steroidal anti-inflammatory drugs might diminish the therapeutic response to the patch cannot be excluded.

*Pregnancy and lactation:* Deponit should not be used during pregnancy or lactation unless considered absolutely essential by the physician. It is not known whether the active substance passes into the breast milk. Benefits to the mother must be weighed against risk to the child.

*Effects on the ability to drive and use machines:* Postural hypotension has been reported rarely following initiation of treatment with glyceryl trinitrate and care is advised when driving or operating machinery.

*Undesirable effects:* At the beginning of treatment nitrate headaches may occur, but experience has shown that this usually subsides after a few days of continuous use. Slight reddening at the site of application usually disappears without therapeutic measures, after the patch has been removed. Other reported side-effects are facial flushing, faintness, dizziness and postural hypotension which may be associated with reflex-induced tachycardia. Nausea and vomiting may occur rarely.

*Overdose: Symptoms* - high doses of glyceryl trinitrate are known to cause pronounced systemic side effects, e.g. a marked fall in blood pressure and reflex tachycardia resulting in collapse and syncope. *Treatment* - The effect of Deponit can be rapidly terminated by removing the patch. Any fall in blood pressure or signs of collapse that may occur, may be managed by general resuscitative measures.

**Pharmacological properties**
*Pharmacodynamic properties:* The main pharmacological activity of organic nitrates is the relaxation of smooth vascular muscles. The systemic vasodilation induces an increase of venous capacitance. Venous return is reduced. Ventricular volume, filling pressures and diastolic wall tension are diminished (preload reduction). A diminished ventricular radius and reduced wall tension, lower myocardial energy and oxygen consumption, respectively. The dilation of the large arteries near the heart leads to a decrease in both the systemic (reduction of afterload) and the pulmonary vascular resistance. In addition, this relieves the myocardium and lowers oxygen demands. By dilating the large eipicardial coronary arteries, glyceryl trinitrate enhances blood supply to the myocardium, improving its pump function and increasing the oxygen supply. At molecular level, nitrates form nitric oxide (NO), which corresponds to the physical EDRF (endothelium derived relaxing factor). EDRF mediated production of cyclic guanosine monophosphate (CGMP) leads to relaxation of smooth muscle cells.

*Pharmacokinetic properties:*
*General characteristics of the active substance:* The transdermal absorption of glyceryl trinitrate circumvents the extensive hepatic first pass metabolism so the bioavailability is about 70% of that achieved after i.v. administration. The steady-state concentration in the plasma depends on the patch dosage and the corresponding rate of absorption. At a rate of absorption of 0.4 mg/h, the steady-state concentration is about 0.2 µg/h on average. Plasma protein binding is about 60%. Glyceryl trinitrate is metabolized to 1,2- and 1,3 dinitroglycerols. The dinitrates exert less vasodilatory activity than glyceryl trinitrate. The contribution to the overall effect is not known. The dinitrates are further metabolized to inactive mononitrates, glyceryl and carbon dioxide. The elimination half-life of glyceryl trinitrate is 2-4 min. The metabolism of glyceryl trinitrate, which is effected in the liver, but also in many other cells, e.g. the red blood cells, includes the separation of one or more nitrate groups. In addition to the metabolism of glyceryl trinitrate, there is a renal excretion of the catabolites.

*Characteristics in patients:* There is no evidence that a dosage adjustment is required in the elderly or in diseases such as renal failure or hepatic insufficiency.

*Preclinical safety data:* Glyceryl trinitrate is a well-known active substance, established for more than a hundred years. Thus new preclinical studies have not been carried out with Deponit .

**Pharmaceutical particulars**
*List of excipients:* Acrylate/vinyl acetate copolymer, polypropylene.

*Incompatibilities:* No incompatibilities have so far been demonstrated.

*Shelf life:* Shelf life of the product as packaged for sale: 2 years.

*Nature and contents of container:* Multilaminate film/foil pouch with heat-sealed edges. 28 patches per carton.

*Instructions for use/handling:* The Deponit patch should be removed from the package just before application. After removal of the protective foil, the patch should be applied to unbroken, clean and dry skin that is smooth and with few hairs. The same area of skin should not be used again for some days.

**Marketing authorisation numbers**
Deponit 5         4438/0036
Deponit 10        4438/0037

**Date of approval/revision of SPC**   January 1997

**Legal category**   P

## DIOCTYL* CAPSULES

**Presentation**   Yellow and white soft gelatin capsules containing 100 mg Docusate Sodium USP.

**Uses**   To prevent and treat chronic constipation. As an adjunct in abdominal radiological procedures.

**Dosage and administration**
*Adults and elderly:* Up to 500 mg daily in divided doses. Treatment should be commenced with large doses which should be decreased as the condtion of the patient improves.

*Children:* Not recommended.

The capsules should be swallowed whole with a glass of water.

*For use with barium meals:* 400 mg to be taken with the barium meal.

**Contra-indications, warnings, etc**
*Contra-indications:* Docusate sodium should not be administered when abdominal pain, nausea, vomiting or intestinal obstruction is present. Docusate sodium should not be given to infants under 6 months old.

*Interactions:* Concurrent administration with mineral oil is contra-indicated. Anthraquinone derivatives should be taken in reduced dose when administered with docusate sodium as it increases their absorption.

*Pregnancy and lactation:* There is inadequate evidence of the safety of the drug in human pregnancy, and there is no evidence from animal work that it is free from hazard. However it has been in wide use for many years without apparent ill consequence. Therefore Dioctyl should only be used in pregnancy if the benefits outweigh the potential risk. Docusate sodium is excreted in breast milk and should therefore be used with caution in breast-feeding mothers.

*Overdose:* In rare cases of overdose, excessive loss of water and electrolytes may occur. This should be treated by encouraging the patient to drink plenty of fluid.

**Pharmaceutical precautions**   Dioctyl Capsules should be stored in a dry place below 25°C.

**Legal category**   P

**Package quantities**   Dioctyl Capsules are available in packs of 30 and 100 capsules.

**Further information**   Docusate sodium exerts its clinical effect in the gastro-intestinal tract by means of its physical surfactant properties, by allowing penetration of water and fats into hard, dry faeces. There is some evidence to suggest that docusate sodium is absorbed from the gastro-intestinal tract and that it may enhance absorption of compounds administered concomitantly

**Product licence number**   4438/0032

## ELANTAN*

**Presentation**   White tablets with break-score containing the active ingredient isosorbide mononitrate. The tablets are available in three strengths; Elantan 10 (marked E10), Elantan 20 (marked E20) and Elantan 40 (marked E40) containing isosorbide mononitrate 10 mg, 20 mg and 40 mg respectively.

**Uses**   Elantan 10, 20 and 40 are indicated for the prophylaxis of angina pectoris.

Elantan 20 and 40 are indicated as adjunctive therapy in congestive heart failure not responding to cardiac glycosides or diuretics.

**Dosage and administration**   Tablets should be taken unchewed with a little water after meals.

*Adults:*
*Angina prophylaxis:* Elantan 10, 20 and 40, one tablet to be taken two to three times a day. The dosage may be increased up to 120 mg per day. For patients not already receiving prophylactic nitrate therapy it is recommended that the initial dose be one tablet of Elantan 10 twice a day.

*Congestive heart failure:* Elantan 20 and 40, one tablet to be taken two to three times a day. The dosage may be increased up to 120 mg per day.

*Elderly:* There is no evidence to suggest that an adjustment of the dosage is necessary.

*Children:* The safety and efficacy of Elantan has yet to be established in children.

### Contra-indications, warnings etc.
*Contra-indications:* This product should not be given to patients with a known sensitivity to nitrates. Elantan should not be used in patients with acute myocardial infarction with low filling pressure, acute circulatory failure (shock, vascular collapse) or very low blood pressure. Elantan should not be used in patients with marked anaemia, head trauma, cerebral haemorrhage, severe hypotension or hypovolaemia.

*Interactions:* Some of the effects of alcohol may be potentiated by this agent. The effects of Elantan may be potentiated by other hypotensive agents.

*Pregnancy and lactation:* This product should not be used during pregnancy or in women breast feeding infants unless considered essential by the physician.

*Precautions:* This preparation may give rise to symptoms of postural hypotension and syncope. These symptoms can largely be avoided if the treatment is started with one tablet of Elantan 10 morning and night. Elantan should be used with caution in patients suffering from hypothyroidism, hypothermia, malnutrition, severe liver or renal disease.

*Side-effects:* Headaches may occur as a side-effect. It is also a sign of overdose. Usually the headache subsides after a few days.

*Overdose:* Overdosage may lead to vascular collapse and gastric lavage is indicated in severe cases. Further measures to support the circulation are recommended e.g. elevating the legs and/or treatment with hypertensive agents.

### Pharmaceutical precautions   None

### Legal category
Elantan 10   P
Elantan 20 and 40   POM

### Package quantities   Elantan 10, 20 and 40 are blister packed in the following pack sizes:
Elantan 10: 56 and 84 tablets.
Elantan 20: 56 and 84 tablets.
Elantan 40: 50, 56, 84 and 100 tablets (50 and 100 tablets to be phased out in 1998).

### Further information   Nil

### Product licence numbers
| Elantan 10 | 04438/0018 |
| Elantan 20 | 04438/0005 |
| Elantan 40 | 04438/0008 |

## ELANTAN* LA25

### Qualitative and quantitative composition   Isosorbide mononitrate 25 mg

### Pharmaceutical form   Slow release capsules

### Clinical particulars
*Therapeutic indications:* For the prophylaxis of angina pectoris

*Posology and method of administration:* For oral administration.
*Adults:* one capsule to be taken in the morning. For patients with higher nitrate requirements the dose may be increased to two capsules taken simultaneously.

*Children:* the safety and efficacy of Elantan LA25 has yet to be established in children.

*Contra-indications:* Elantan LA25 should not be used in cases of acute myocardial infarction with low filling pressure, acute circulatory failure, shock, vascular collapse, or very low blood pressure. This product should not be given to patients with a known sensitivity to nitrates, marked anaemia, head trauma, cerebral haemorrhage, severe hypotension or hypovolaemia.

*Special warnings and precautions for use:* Elantan LA25 should be used with caution in patients who are suffering from hypothyroidism, hypothermia, malnutrition, severe liver disease or severe renal disease. Symptoms of circulatory collapse may arise after first dose, particularly in patients with labile circulation.

*Interactions with other medicaments and other forms of interaction:* Some of the effects of alcohol and the action of hypotensive agents may be potentiated by this product.

*Pregnancy and lactation:* There is inadequate evidence of safety of the drug in human pregnancy but nitrates have been used widely in the treatment of angina for many years without apparent ill consequence; animal studies having shown no hazard. Nevertheless it is not advisable to use this drug during pregnancy and lactation.

*Effects on ability to drive and use machines:* None known.

*Undesirable effects:* A headache may occur at the start of treatment, but this usually disappears after a few days.

*Overdose:* Overdosage may lead to vascular collapse and gastric lavage is indicated in severe cases. Further measures to support the circulation are recommended, e.g. elevating the legs and/or treatment with hypertensive agents.

### Pharmacological properties
*Pharmacodynamic properties:* The active ingredient is a coronary vasodilator which reduces venous return.

*Pharmacokinetic properties:* The pharmacokinetic profile of Elantan LA25 closely follows that of Elantan LA50 (PL 4438/0015). Mean plasma concentration for Elantan LA25 8 hours post dose was shown to be 228 (±53) ng/ml. * Kinetics are approximately linear around the proposed dose range. The extraction rate is zero (F = 1). In patients with cirrhotic disease or cardiac failure or renal failure, pharmacokinetic parameters were similar to those obtained in healthy volunteers. *Refers to isosorbide mononitrate.

*Preclinical safety data:* None stated

### Pharmaceutical particulars
*List of excipients:* Lactose, talc, ethyl cellulose, polyethylene glycol, hydroxypropyl cellulose, sucrose, starch, gelatin, titanium dioxide, iron oxide red and iron oxide black.

*Incompatibilities:* None known.

*Shelf life:* 3 years.

*Special precautions for storage:* None.

*Nature and contents of container:* Cartons of blister strips of PVC and aluminium or of PP and aluminium. Aluminium foil thickness 20µ m or 16µ m. Pack size: 28 capsules.

*Instruction for use/handling:* None.

### Marketing authorisation number   04438/0028

### Date of approval/revision of SPC   November 1996

### Legal category   P

## ELANTAN* LA50

### Presentation   Brown and flesh coloured, opaque gelatin capsules containing 50 mg isosorbide mononitrate in a slow release formulation. The capsules also contain gelatin, lactose, ethyl cellulose, talc, hydroxypropyl cellulose, polyethylene glycol, sucrose, corn starch and colours E171 and E172.

### Use   For the prophylaxis of angina pectoris.

### Dosage and administration   The capsules are for oral administration and should be swallowed whole.

*Adults and elderly:* One capsule to be taken in the morning. This may be increased to two capsules if required.

*Children:* The safety and efficacy of LA50 has yet to be established in children.

### Contra-indications, warnings, etc
*Contra-indications:* Elantan LA50 should not be used in cases of acute myocardial infarction with low filling pressure, acute circulatory failure, shock, vascular collapse, or very low blood pressure. It should not be given to patients with a known sensitivity to nitrates, marked anaemia, head trauma, cerebral haemorrhage, severe hypotension or hypovalaemia.

*Interactions:* Some of the effects of alcohol and the action of hypotensive agents may be potentiated by this treatment.

*Warnings:* Elantan LA50 should be used with caution in patients who are suffering from hypothyroidism, hypothermia, malnutrition or severe renal disease. Symptoms of circulatory collapse may arise after the first dose, particularly in patients with labile circulation. A headache may occur at the start of treatment, but this usually disappears after a few days.

*Use in pregnancy and lactation:* There is inadequate evidence of safety of the drug in human pregnancy but nitrates have been used widely in the treatment of angina for many years, without apparent ill consequence, animal studies having shown no hazard.

Nevertheless it is not advisable to use this drug during pregnancy and lactation.

*Overdosage:* Overdosage may lead to vascular collapse and gastric lavage is indicated in severe cases. Further measures to support the circulation are recommended, e.g elevating the legs, and/or treatment with hypertensive agents.

### Pharmaceutical precautions   None

### Legal category   P

### Package quantities   Elantan LA50 is available in calendar packs of 28 capsules.

### Further information   Nil

### Product licence number   04438/0015

## ISOKET* 0.05%

### Presentation   Isoket 0.05% (Isosorbide dinitrate 0.5 mg/ml) in 50 ml bottles. Isoket 0.05% contains isosorbide dinitrate in sterile isotonic saline, no other additives are present.

### Uses   The indications for Isoket 0.05% are: Treatment of unresponsive left ventricular failure, secondary to acute myocardial infarction, unresponsive left ventricular failure of various aetiology, severe or unstable angina pectoris, to facilitate or prolong balloon inflation and to prevent or relieve coronary spasm during percutaneous transluminal coronary angioplasty.

*Pharmacological actions:* Isoket is a vasodilator predominantly of peripheral capacitance veins.

### Dosage and administration
*Intravenous route:* The dose employed must be adjusted according to patient response. In general, a dose of between 2 mg and 12 mg per hour is suitable although doses as high as 20 mg per hour may be necessary.

*Intracoronary route:* The usual dose is 1 mg given as a bolus injection prior to balloon inflation. Further doses may be given not exceeding 5 mg within a 30 minute period.

*Elderly:* The dose of nitrates in cardiovascular disease is usually determined by patient response and stabilisation. Clinical experience has not necessitated alternative advice for use in elderly patients.

*Children:* The safety and efficacy of Isoket 0.05% has not yet been established in children.

*Administration:*
*Intravenous:* Isoket 0.05% can be administered undiluted by slow intravenous infusion using a syringe pump. It is compatible with infusion vechicles such as Sodium Chloride injection BP or Dextrose injection BP and can be administered as an admixture if required.
*Intracoronary:* Isoket 0.05% can be injected directly by this route according to the proposed dosage schedule. Bottles of Isoket are for single use only and should not be regarded as multi-dose containers.

### Contra-indications, warnings etc
*Contra-indications:* These are common to all nitrates: Known hypersensitivity to nitrates, marked anaemia, cerebral haemorrhage, trauma, hypovolaemia and severe hypotension. Use in circulatory collapse or low filling pressure is also contra-indicated. Isoket should not be used in the treatment of cardiogenic shock, unless some means of maintaining an adequate diastolic pressure are undertaken.

*Precautions:* Isoket should be used with caution in patients who are suffering from hypothyroidism, malnutrition, severe liver or renal disease or hypothermia. Some of the effects of alcohol may be potentiated by this agent. The effects of anti-hypertensive drugs may be enhanced. Close attention to pulse and blood pressure is necessary during the administration of Isoket infusions.

*Pregnancy and lactation:* No data have been reported which would indicate the possibility of adverse effects resulting from the use of isosorbide dinitrate in pregnancy. Safety in pregnancy however has not been established. Isosorbide dinitrate should only be used in pregnancy and during lactation if, in the opinion of the physician, the possible benefits of treatment outweigh the possible hazards.

*Adverse effects:* In common with other nitrates, headache, nausea and tachycardia may occur during administration. Whilst sharp falls in systemic arterial pressure can give rise to symptoms of cerebral flow deficiency and decreased coronary perfusion, clinical experience with Isoket has shown that this is not normally a problem. This effect is consistent with the known vasodilatory effects of isosorbide dinitrate which occur predominantly on the venous rather than the arterial side of the circulation.

*Treatment of overdosage:* General supportive therapy.

**Pharmaceutical precautions**: Admixtures are stable for approximately 24 hours at room temperature in the recommended containers. Open ampoules or bottles should be used immediately and any unused drug discarded.

*Compatibility:* Isoket contains isosorbide dinitrate in isotonic saline and is compatible with commonly employed infusion fluids, no incompatibilities have so far been demonstrated. Isoket is compatible with glass infusion bottles and infusion packs made from polyethylene. Isoket may be infused slowly using a syringe pump with a glass or plastic syringe. The use of PVC giving sets and containers should be avoided since significant losses of the active ingredient by absorption can occur.

**Legal category** POM

**Package quantities** 50 ml bottle (Isosorbide dinitrate 25 mg/50 ml)

**Further information** Nil

**Product licence number** 4438/0017

## ISOKET* 0.1%

**Qualitative and quantitative composition** Isosorbide Dinitrate PhEur 0.1% w/v.

**Pharmaceutical form** Sterile colourless solution for intravenous infusion.

**Clinical particulars**
*Therapeutic indications:*
*Intravenous:* Isoket is indicated in the treatment of unresponsive left ventricular failure secondary to acute myocardial infarction, unresponsive left ventricular failure of various aetiology and severe or unstable angina pectoris.

*Intra-coronary:* Isoket is indicated during percutaneous transluminal coronary angioplasty to facilitate prolongation of balloon inflation and to prevent or relieve coronary spasm.

*Posology and method of administration:* Adults, including the elderly.
*Intravenous route:* A dose of between 2 mg and 12 mg per hour is usually satisfactory. However, dosages up to 20 mg per hour administered should be adjusted to the patient response.

*Intra-coronary route:* The usual dose is 1 mg given as a bolus injection prior to balloon inflation. Further doses maybe given not exceeding 5 mg within a 30 minute period.

*Children:* The safety and efficacy of Isoket has not yet been established in children.

*Administration:* Isoket is a concentrated solution and should never be injected directly in the form of a bolus except via the intra-coronary route prior to balloon inflation. A dilution of 50% is advocated for intracoronary administration. Isoket can be administered as an intravenous admixture with a suitable vehicle such as Sodium Chloride Injection BP or Dextrose Injection BP. Prepared Isoket admixtures should be given by intravenous infusion or with the aid of a syringe pump incorporating a glass or rigid plastic syringe. During administration the patients blood pressure and pulse should be closely monitored.

*Contra-indications:* These are common to all nitrates; known hypersensitivity to nitrates, marked anaemia, cerebral haemorrhage, head trauma, hypovolaemia, and severe hypotension. Use in circulatory collapse or low filling pressure is also contraindicated. Isoket should not be used in the treatment of cardiogenic shock, unless some means of maintaining an adequate diastolic pressure is undertaken.

*Special warnings and precautions for use:* Isoket should be used with caution in patients who are suffering from hypothyroidism, malnutrition, severe liver or renal disease or hypothermia. Close attention to pulse and blood pressure is necessary during the administration of Isoket infusions.

*Interaction with other medicaments and other forms of interaction:* Some of the effects of alcohol may be potentiated by this agent. The effects of antihypertensive drugs may be enhanced.

*Pregnancy and lactation:* No data have been reported which would indicate the possibility of adverse effects resulting from the use of isosorbide dinitrate in pregnancy. Safety in pregnancy, however, has not been established. Isosorbide dinitrate should only be used in pregnancy and during lactation if, in the opinion of the physician, the possible benefits of treatment outweigh the possible hazards.

*Effects on ability to drive and use machines:* None known.

*Undesirable effects:* In common with other nitrates, headaches, nausea and tachycardia may occur during administration. Whilst sharp falls in systemic arterial pressure can give rise to symptoms of cerebral flow deficiency and decreased coronary perfusion, clinical experience with Isoket has shown that this is not normally a problem.

*Overdose:* General supportive therapy.

**Pharmacological properties**
*Pharmacodynamic properties:* Isosorbide dinitrate is an organic nitrate which, in common with other cardioactive nitrates, is a vasodilator. It produces decreased left and right ventricular end-diastolic pressures to a greater extent than the decrease in systemic arterial pressure, thereby reducing afterload and especially the preload of the heart. Isosorbide dinitrate influences the oxygen supply to ischaemic myocardium by causing the redistribution of blood flow along collateral channels and from epicardial to endocardial regions by selective dilatation of large epicardial vessels. It reduces the requirement of the myocardium for oxygen by increasing venous capacitance, causing a pooling of blood in peripheral veins, thereby reducing ventricular volume and heart wall distension.

*Pharmacokinetic properties:* Isosorbide dinitrate (ISDN) is eliminated from plasma with a short half-life (about 0.7 H). The metabolic degradation of ISDN occurs via denitration and glucuronidation, like all organic nitrates. The rates of formation of the metabolites has been calculated for isosorbide-5-mononitrate (IS-5-MN) with 0.27 $h^{-1}$, and isosorbide (IS) with 0.16 $h^{-1}$. IS-5-MN and IS-2-MN are the primary metabolites which are also pharmacologically active. IS-5-MN is metabolised to isosorbide 5-mononitrate-2-glucuronide (IS-5-MN-2-GLU). The half life of this metabolite (about 2.5 h) is shorter than that of IS-5-MN (about 5.1. h). The half-life of ISDN is the shortest of all and that of IS-2-MN (about 3.2 h) lies in between.

*Preclinical safety data:* None stated.

**Pharmaceutical particulars**
*List of excipients:* Sodium Chloride PhEur. Water for injection PhEur.

*Incompatibilities:* Isoket contains isosorbide dinitrate in isotonic saline and is compatible with commonly employed infusion fluids, no incompatibilities have so far been demonstrated. Isoket is compatible with glass infusion bottles and infusion packs made from polyethylene. Isoket may be infused slowly using a syringe pump with glass or plastic syringe. The use of PVC giving sets and containers should be avoided since significant losses of the active ingredient by adsorption can occur.

*Shelf life:* 5 years, as packaged for sale. Admixtures are stable for approximately 24 hours at room temperature in the recommended containers. Open ampoules or bottles should be used immediately and any unused drug discarded.

*Special precautions for storage:* There are no special precautions for storage of the product as packaged for sale.

*Nature and contents of container:* Marketed pack sizes, 10 ml glass ampoules, 50 ml glass vials with rubber stoppers.

*Instructions for use/handling:* Example of admixture preparation; To obtain a dose of 6 mg per hour add 50 ml of Isoket 0.1% to 450 ml of a suitable vehicle, under aseptic conditions. The resultant admixture (500 ml), contains 100 μ g/ml (1 mg/10 ml) isosorbide dinitrate. An infusion rate of 60 ml per hour (equivalent to 60 paediatric microdrops per minute or 20 standard drops per minute), will deliver the required dose of 6 mg per hour. Should it be necessary to reduce fluid intake, 100 ml of Isoket 0.1% may be diluted to 500 ml using a suitable vehicle. The resultant solution now contains 200 μ g/ml (2 mg/10 ml) isosorbide dinitrate. An infusion rate of 30 ml per hour (equivalent to 30 paediatric microdrops per minute or 10 standard drops per minute), will deliver the required dose of 6 mg per hour. A dilution of 50% is advocated to produce a solution containing 0.5 mg/ml where fluid intake is strictly limited.

**Marketing authorisation number** 04438/0001

**Date of approval/revision of SPC** January 1997

**Legal category** POM

## ISOKET* RETARD

**Qualitative and quantitative composition** Each tablet contains isosorbide dinitrate 20 mg or 40 mg respectively in a slow release formulation.

**Pharmaceutical form** Slow release tablets.

**Clinical particulars**
*Therapeutic indications:* For the prophylaxis and treatment of angina pectoris.

*Posology and method of administration:* For oral administration.

*Adults:* The usual dose is one tablet every 12 hours. No more than four tablets should be taken daily.

*Elderly:* Clinical experience has not necessitated alternative advice for use in elderly patients.

*Children:* The safety and efficacy of Isoket Retard has yet to be established.

The tablets should be swallowed without chewing.

*Contra-indications:* This product should not be given to patients with a known sensitivity to nitrates, very low blood pressure, acute myocardial infarction with low filling pressure, marked anaemia, head trauma, cerebral haemorrhage, acute circulatory failure, severe hypotension or hypovolaemia.

*Special warnings and special precautions for use:* Isoket Retard should be used with caution in patients who are suffering from hypothyroidism, hypothermia, malnutrition and severe liver or renal disease.

*Interactions:* Alcohol intake may enhance vasodilation.

*Pregnancy and lactation:* This product should not be used during pregnancy or lactation unless considered essential by the physician.

*Effects on ability to drive and use machines:* None known.

*Undesirable effects:* Cutaneous vasodilation, postural hypotension and dry skin rashes may occur occasionally. Headache may occur at the onset of treatment, but may be minimised by commencing with low doses and gradually increasing the dose. Tolerance may occur.

*Overdose:* Higher doses may lead to vascular collapse. In rare cases of overdosage, gastric lavage is indicated. Passive exercise of the extremities of the recumbent patient will promote venous return.

**Pharmacological properties**
*Pharmacodynamic properties:* Isosorbide dinitrate is an organic nitrate which, in common with other cardioactive nitrates, is a vasodilator. It produces decreased left and right ventricular end-diastolic pressures to a greater extent than the decrease in systemic arterial pressure, thereby reducing afterload and especially the preload of the heart. Isosorbide dinitrate influences the oxygen supply to ischaemic myocardium by causing the redistribution of blood flow along collateral channels and from epicardial to endocardial regions by selective dilatation of large epicardial vessels. It reduces the requirements of the myocardium for oxygen by increasing venous capacitance, causing a pooling of blood in peripheral veins, thereby reducing ventricular volume and heart wall distension.

*Pharmacokinetic properties:* After administration of one tablet of Isoket Retard 20 at least two peak concentrations of ISDN occurred in the plasma. The initial peak (mean 1.9 ng/ml, range 1.0 to 3.4 ng/ml) occurred during 0.5 to 2 hours and then the mean plasma concentrations declined to 1.3 ng/ml at 3 hours. The concentration then increased again to reach a major peak level (mean 6.2 ng/ml range 1.6 to 12.3 mg/ml) during 4 to 6 hours after dosing. Plasma concentrations of ISDN have been measured after administration of increasing doses in the range 20 to 100 mg as Isoket Retard 20 tablets. Means of peak concentrations of 4.2 ng/ml , 13-1 ng/ml 20.7 ng/ml, 36.8 ng/ml and 34.9 ng/ml were measured after doses of 20 mg, 40 mg, 60 mg, 80 mg and 100 mg respectively.

**Pharmaceutical particulars**
*List of excipients:* Lactose, talc, polyvinyl acetate, magnesium stearate, potato starch, sodium sulphate, sodium chloride, purified water and colours; E110 and E104 (Isoket Retard 20), E110 and E124 (Isoket Retard 40).

*Incompatibilities:* None known.

*Shelf life:* 5 years.

*Special precautions for storage:* None.

*Nature and contents of container:* Cartons of bliste strips of polypropylene (PP) and aluminium or of PP, PP. †Pack sizes 50, **56**, 60, 84 and 90 tablets.

†Only those pack sizes marked in bold are currently marketed

*Instructions for use/handling:* None.

**Marketing authorisation numbers**

| | |
|---|---|
| Isoket Retard 20 | 04438/0004 |
| Isoket Retard 40 | 04438/0002 |

**Date of approval/revision of SPC** December 1996

**Legal category** P

## NITROCINE*

**Presentation** Nitrocine is presented as ampoules containing 10 mg glyceryl trinitrate in 10 ml, or as glass bottles containing 50 mg glyceryl trinitrate in 50 ml. Nitrocine also contains glucose, propylene glycol and water for injection. Nitrocine is an isotonic sterile solution.

**Uses**

*Surgery:* Nitrocine is indicated for: the rapid control of hypertension during cardiac surgery, reducing blood pressure and maintaining controlled hypotension during surgical procedures, controlling myocardial ischaemia during and after cardiovascular surgery.

*Unresponsive congestive heart failure:* Nitrocine may be used to treat unresponsive congestive heart failure secondary to acute myocardial infarction.

*Unstable angina:* Nitrocine may be used to treat unstable angina which is refractory to treatment with beta blockers and sublingual nitrates.

*Pharmacological actions:* Glyceryl trinitrate reduces the tone of vascular smooth muscle, with a more marked effect on the venous capacitance vessels than on the arterial vessels. This reduces venous return to the heart and lowers elevated filling pressure. The lowering of filling pressure reduces the left ventricular end diastolic volume and preload. The net effect is a lowering of myocardial oxygen consumption. Systemic vascular resistance, pulmonary vascular and arterial pressure are also reduced by glyceryl trinitrate and there is a net reduction in afterload. Glyceryl trinitrate improves the myocardial oxygen supply by redistributing blood flow along collateral channels from epicardial to endocardial regions.

**Dosage and administration**

*Adults and elderly:* The dose of Nitrocine should be adjusted to meet the individual needs of the patient. The recommended dosage range is 10–200 µg/min but up to 400 µg/min may be necessary during some surgical procedures.

*Children:* The safety and efficacy of Nitrocine has not yet been established in children.

*Surgery:* A starting dose of 25 µg/min is recommended for the control of hypertension, or to produce hypotension during surgery. This may be increased by increments of 25 µg/min at 5 minute intervals until the blood pressure is stabilized. Doses between 10–200 µg/min are usually sufficient during surgery, although doses of up to 400 µg/min have been required in some cases. The treatment of perioperative myocardial ischaemia may be started with a dose of 15–20 µg/min, with subsequent increments of 10–15 µg/min until the required effect is obtained.

*Unresponsive congestive heart failure:* The recommended starting dose is 20–25 µg/min. This may be decreased to 10 µg/min, or increased in steps of 20-25 µg/min every 15–30 minutes until the desired effect is obtained.

*Unstable angina:* An initial dose of 10 µg/min is recommended with increments of 10 µg/min being made at approximately 30 minute intervals according to the needs of the patient. Nitrocine can be administered undiluted by slow intravenous infusion using a syringe pump incorporating a glass or rigid plastic syringe. Alternatively, Nitrocine may be administered intravenously as an admixture using a suitable vehicle such as Sodium Chloride Injection B.P. or Dextrose Injection B.P.

*Example of admixture preparation:* To obtain an admixture of GTN at a concentration of 100 µg/ml, add 50 ml Nitrocine solution (containing 50 mg glyceryl trinitrate) to 450 ml of infusion vehicle to give a final volume of 500 ml.

A dosage of 100 µg min. can be obtained by giving 60 ml of the admixture per hour. This is equivalent to a drip rate of 60 paediatric microdrops per minute.

For full details it is advisable to consult the dosage chart on the package insert.

Prepared admixtures should be given by intravenous infusion or with the aid of a syringe pump to ensure a constant rate of infusion. During Nitrocine administration there should be close haemodynamic monitoring of the patient.

Bottles of Nitrocine are for single use only and should not be regarded as multi-dose containers.

**Contra-indications, warnings, etc**

*Contra-indications:* These are common to all nitrates: Known hypersensitivity to nitrates, marked anaemia, severe cerebral haemorrhage, head trauma, uncorrected hypovolaemia or severe hypotension.

*Precautions:* Close attention to pulse and blood pressure is necessary during the administration of Nitrocine infusions. Nitrocine should be used with caution in patients suffering from hypothyroidism, severe liver or renal disease, hypothermia and malnutrition. Nitrocine may potentiate the action of other hypotensive agents.

*Pregnancy and lactation:* There is no, or inadequate, evidence of safety of the drug in human pregnancy or lactation, but it has been in widespread use for many years without apparent ill consequence, animal studies having shown no hazard. If drug therapy is needed in pregnancy, this product can be used if there is no safer alternative

*Adverse effects:* In common with other nitrates, headaches and nausea may occur during administration. Other possible adverse reactions include hypotension, tachycardia, retching, diaphoresis, apprehension, restlessness, muscle twitching, retrosternal discomfort, palpitations, dizziness and abdominal pain. Paradoxical bradycardia has also been observed.

*Overdose:* Mild overdose usually results in hypotension and tachycardia. If arterial systolic blood pressure drops below 90 mmHg and if heart rate increases 10% above its initial value, the infusion should be discontinued to allow a return to pre-treatment levels. If hypotension persists, or in more severe cases, this may be reversed by elevating the legs and/or treatment with hypertensive agents.

**Pharmaceutical precautions** Admixtures are stable for approximately 24 hours at room temperature in the recommended containers. Open ampoules or bottles should be used immediately and any unused drug discarded.

*Compatibility:* Nitrocine is compatible with glass infusion bottles and with rigid infusion packs made of polyethylene. Nitrocine may also be infused slowly using a syringe pump with a glass or plastic syringe.

*Incompatibilities:* Nitrocine is incompatible with polyvinylchloride (PVC) and severe losses of glyceryl trinitrate (over 40%) may occur if this material is used. Contact with polyvinylchloride bags should be avoided. Polyurethane also induces a loss of the active ingredient.

**Legal category** POM

**Package quantities**

*Ampoules:* Each pack contains 10 x 10 ml ampoules of Nitrocine

*Bottles:* Each pack contains 1 x 50 ml bottles of Nitrocine

**Further information** Nil

**Product licence number** 4438/0006

## PERDIX* ▼

**Qualitative and quantitative composition**

Each Perdix 7.5 mg tablet contains moexipril hydrochloride 7.5 mg.

Each Perdix 15 mg tablet contains moexipril hydrochloride 15 mg.

**Pharmaceutical form** Film-coated tablets

**Clinical particulars**

*Therapeutic indications:* For the treatment of hypertension as monotherapy. As second line therapy for the treatment of hypertension in combination with diuretics or calcium antagonists, e.g. hydrochlorothiazide or nifedipine.

*Posology and method of administration:*

*Initial therapy:* In patients with uncomplicated essential hypertension not on diuretic therapy, the recommended initial dose is 7.5 mg once daily. Dosage should be adjusted according to blood pressure response. The maintenance dose is 7.5–15 mg moexipril daily administered in a single dose. Some patients may benefit from a further increase to 30 mg/day. Doses over 30 mg have been used, but do not appear to give a greater effect. If blood pressure is not controlled with Perdix alone, a low dose of a diuretic may be added. Hydrochlorothiazide 12.5 mg has been shown to provide an additive effect. With concomitant diuretic therapy, it may be possible to reduce the dose of Perdix.

*Diuretic treated patients:* In hypertensive patients who are currently being treated with a diuretic, symptomatic hypotension may occur occasionally following the initial dose of Perdix. The diuretic should be discontinued, if possible, for two to three days before beginning therapy with Perdix to reduce the likelihood of hypotension (see *Warnings*). The dosage of Perdix should be adjusted according to blood pressure response. If the patient's blood pressure is not controlled with Perdix alone, diuretic therapy may be resumed as described above. If the diuretic cannot be discontinued or the diuretic has recently been withdrawn, an initial dose of 3.75 mg (half 7.5 mg tablet) should be used under medical supervision for at least two hours and until blood pressure has stabilized for at least an additional hour (see *Warnings* and *Precautions*). Concomitant administration of Perdix with potassium supplements, potassium salt substitutes, or potassium-sparing diuretics may lead to increases of serum potassium (see *Precautions*).

*Nifedipine treated patients:* As add-on therapy, Perdix has been investigated in combination with nifedipine. If Perdix is used as add-on therapy to nifedipine, the starting dose of Perdix should be 3.75 mg (half 7.5 mg tablet).

*Elderly patients:* In elderly patients, an initial dosage of 3.75 mg (half 7.5 mg tablet) once daily is recommended followed by titration to the optimal response.

*Children:* Not recommended. Safety and efficacy in children has not been established.

*Renal failure:* In patients with creatinine clearance ≤ 40 ml/min, an initial dose of 3.75 mg of moexipril (half 7.5 mg tablet) is recommended.

*Hepatic cirrhosis:* In patients with hepatic cirrhosis, an initial dose of 3.75 mg of moexipril (half 7.5 mg tablet) is recommended.

*Afro-Caribbean patients:* Where Perdix is used as a single agent in hypertension, Afro-Caribbean patients may show a reduced therapeutic response.

*Contra-indications:* Perdix is contra-indicated in patients who are hypersensitive to this product and in patients with a history of angioedema related to previous treatment with an angiotensin converting enzyme inhibitor. Perdix is contra-indicated in pregnancy since fetotoxicity has been observed for ACE inhibitors in animals. Although there is no experience with Perdix, other ACE inhibitors in human pregnancy have been associated with oligohydramnios and neonatal hypotension and/or anuria. It is not known whether moexipril passes into human breastmilk, but since animal data indicate that moexipril and its metabolites are present in rat milk Perdix should not be given to nursing mothers.

*Special warnings and precautions for use:*

*Warnings;* Angioedema involving the extremities, face, lips, mucous membranes, tongue, glottis or larynx has been reported in patients treated with ACE inhibitors. If angioedema involves the tongue, glottis or larynx, airway obstruction may occur and be fatal. If laryngeal stridor or angioedema of the face, lips mucous membranes, tongue, glottis or extremities occur, treatment with Perdix should be discontinued and appropriate therapy instituted immediately. Where there is involvement of the tongue, glottis, or larynx, likely to cause airway obstruction, appropriate therapy, e.g. subcutaneous epinephrine solution 1:1000 (0.3 ml to 0.5 ml) should be promptly administered (see *Precautions*).

*Hypotension:* Perdix can cause symptomatic hypotension. Like other ACE inhibitors, Perdix has been only rarely associated with hypotension in hypertensive patients receiving monotherapy. Symptomatic hypotension is most likely to occur in patients who have been volume–and/or salt-depleted as a result of prolonged diurectic therapy, dietary salt restriction, dialysis, diarrhoea, or vomiting. Volume and/or salt depletion should be corrected before initiating therapy with Perdix. If hypotension occurs, the patient should be placed in a supine position and, if necessary, treated with intravenous infusion of physiological saline. Perdix treatment usually can be continued following restoration of blood pressure and volume.

*Neutropenia/agranulocytosis:* ACE inhibitors have been shown to cause agranulocytosis and bone marrow depression, rarely in uncomplicated patients, but more frequently in patients with renal impairment, especially if they also have a collagen-vascular disease such as systemic lupus erythematosus or scleroderma. Available data from clinical trials of Perdix are insufficient to show that Perdix does not cause agranulocytosis at similar rates. Monitoring of white blood cell counts should be considered in patients with collagen-vascular disease, especially if the disease is associated with impaired renal function.

*Precautions:*

*Impaired renal function:* As a consequence of inhibiting the renin-angiotensin-aldosterone system, changes in renal function may be anticipated in susceptible individuals. In hypertensive patients with renal artery stenosis in a solitary kidney or bilateral renal artery stenosis, increases in blood urea nitrogen and serum creatinine may occur. Experience with other angiotensin converting enzyme inhibitors suggests that these increases are usually reversible upon discontinuation of ACE inhibitor and/or diuretic therapy. In such patients, renal function should be monitored during the first few weeks of therapy. Some hypertensive patients with no apparent pre-existing renal vascular disease have developed increases in blood urea nitrogen and serum creatinine, usually minor and transient, especially when Perdix has been given concomitantly with a diuretic. This is more likely to occur in patients with pre-existing renal impairment. Dosage reduction of Perdix and/or discontinuation of the diurectic may be required. Evaluation of the hypertensive patient should always include assessment of renal function. Impaired renal function decreases total clearance of moexiprilat and approximately doubles AUC.

*Hyperkalemia:* In clinical trials, hyperkalemia (serum potassium greater than 10% above the upper limit of normal) has occurred in approximately 2.6% of hypertensive patients receiving Perdix. In most cases, these were isolated values which resolved despite continued therapy. In clinical trials, 0.1% of patients (two patients) were discontinued from therapy due to an elevated serum potassium. Risk factors for the development of hyperkalemia include renal insufficiency, diabetes mellitus and the concomitant use of potassium-sparing diuretics, potassium supplements and/or potassium-containing salt substitutes, which should be used cautiously, if at all, with Perdix (see *Precautions*).

*Hepatic cirrhosis*: Since Perdix is primarily metabolized by hepatic and gut wall esterases to its active moiety, moexiprilat, patients with impaired liver function could develop elevated plasma levels of unchanged Perdix. In a study in patients with alcoholic or biliary cirrhosis, the extent of hydrolysis was unaffected, although the rate was slowed. In these patients, the apparent total body clearance of moexiprilat was decreased and the plasma AUC approximately doubled.

*Surgery/anaesthesia:* In patients undergoing surgery or during anaesthesia with agents that produce hypotension, Perdix will block the angiotensin II formation that could otherwise occur secondary to compensatory renin release. Hypotension that occurs as a result of this mechanism can be corrected by volume expansion.

*Interactions:*
*Diuretics:* Excessive reductions in blood pressure, especially in patients in whom diuretic therapy was recently instituted, have been reported with ACE inhibitors. The possibility of hypotensive effects with Perdix can be minimized by discontinuing diuretic therapy or increasing salt intake for several days before initiation of treatment with Perdix. If this is not possible, the starting dose should be reduced (see also *Posology and method of administration* and *Special warnings and precautions for use*).

*Nifedipine:* The co-administration of nifedipine with Perdix gives rise to an enhanced antihypertensive effect.

*Potassium supplements and potassium-sparing diuretics:* Perdix can attenuate potassium loss caused by thiazide diuretics. Potassium-sparing diuretics (spironolactone, triamterene, amiloride, and others) or potassium supplements have been shown to increase the risk of hyperkalemia when used concomitantly with ACE inhibitors. Therefore, if concomitant use of such agents is indicated, they should be given with caution and the patient's serum potassium should be monitored frequently.

*Oral anticoagulants:* Interaction studies with warfarin failed to identify any clinically important effects on the serum concentrations of the anticoagulants or on their anticoagulant effects.

*Lithium:* Increased serum lithium levels and symptoms of lithium toxicity have been reported in patients receiving ACE inhibitors during therapy with lithium. These drugs should be co-administered with caution, and frequent monitoring of serum lithium levels is recommended. If a diuretic is also used, the risk of lithium toxicity may be increased.

*Other agents:* No clinically important pharmacokinetic interactions occurred when Perdix was administered concomitantly with hydrochlorothiazide, digoxin, cimetidine, or nifedipine in healthy volunteers. However, in hypertensive patients, the antihypertensive effect of Perdix was enhanced when given in combination with diuretics, or calcium antagonists.

*Use during pregnancy and lactation:* There is no experience in man. As it is known from other ACE inhibitors that they can adversely affect the fetus, especially during the second and third trimester, for safety reasons a change to a different antihypertensive drug should be made after pregnancy is confirmed in women who are receiving Perdix (see *Contra-indications*) or in women planning to get pregnant. It is not known whether Perdix is excreted in human milk. As animal data indicate that moexipril and its metabolites are present in rat milk, Perdix should not be administered to a nursing woman.

*Effects on ability to drive and use machines:* The intake of ACE inhibitors may, as any antihypertensive therapy, induce hypotension with subsequent impairment of reactivity. Alcohol intake may enhance this effect.

*Undesirable effects:* The most commonly reported undesirable effects (more than 1% of patients treated with Perdix in controlled trials) were cough (4.0%), headache (3.6%), dizziness (3.3%), fatigue (1.2%), flushing (1.2%), and rash (1.0%). Other adverse experiences possibly or probably related, or of uncertain relationship to therapy, reported in controlled or uncontrolled clinical trials occurring in less than 1% of Perdix patients and less frequent clinically significant events which have been attributed to ACE inhibitors include the following:

*Cardiovascular:* Symptomatic hypotension, postural hypotension, or syncope was seen in <1% of patients; these reactions led to discontinuation of therapy in controlled trials in 2 patients (0.1%) who had received Perdix monotherapy and in 1 patient (0.05%) who had received Perdix with hydrochlorothiazide. Other reports included chest pain, angina/myocardial infarction, palpitations, rhythm disturbances, cerebrovascular accident.

*Renal:* Of hypertensive patients with no apparent pre-existing renal disease, 0.8% of patients receiving Perdix alone and 1.5% of patients receiving Perdix with hydrochlorothiazide have experienced increases in serum creatinine to at least 140% of their baseline values.

*Gastrointestinal:* Abdominal pain, dyspepsia, constipation, nausea, vomiting, diarrhoea, appetite/weight change, dry mouth, pancreatitis, hepatitis.

*Respiratory:* Upper respiratory infection, pharyngitis, sinusitis/rhinitis, bronchospasm, dyspnea.

*Urogenital:* Renal insufficiency.

*Dermatologic:* Apparent hypersensitivity reactions manifested by urticaria, pruritus, photosensitivity.

*Neurological and psychiatric:* Drowsiness, sleep disturbances, nervousness, mood changes, anxiety.

*Other:* Angioedema, taste disturbances, tinnitus, sweating, flu syndrome, malaise, arthralgia, myalgia.

*Clinical laboratory test findings:*
*Creatinine and blood urea nitrogen:* As with other ACE inhibitors, minor increases in blood urea nitrogen or serum creatinine, reversible upon discontinuation of therapy, were observed in approximately 1% of patients with essential hypertension who were treated with PERDIX. Increases are more likely to occur in patients receiving concomitant diuretics or in patients with compromised renal function.

*Potassium:* Since moexipril decreases aldosterone secretion, elevation of serum potassium can occur. Potassium supplements and potassium-sparing diuretics should be given with caution and the patient's serum potassium should be monitored frequently.

*Other:* Clinically important changes in standard laboratory tests were rarely associated with Perdix administration. Elevations of liver enzymes and uric acid have been reported. In trials, less than 1% of moexipril-treated patients discontinued Perdix treatment because of laboratory abnormalities.

*Overdose:* Symptoms and treatment. To date, no case of overdosage has been reported. Signs and symptoms expected in cases of overdosage would be related to hypotension and should be relieved by intravenous infusion of isotonic saline solution.

**Pharmacological properties**
*Pharmacodynamic properties:* In animals as well as in humans, interactions between the renin-angiotensin-aldosterone system and the kallikrein-kinin system provide an important biochemical basis for blood pressure homeostasis. In hypertension the normal feedback mechanism formed by the renin-angiotensin system (RAS) may be dysfunctional, resulting in a self-perpetuating hypertensive condition. Angiotensin converting enzyme (ACE) inhibitors were developed to interrupt this system and thereby to lower blood pressure. Perdix potently inhibits ACE and by this the formation of angiotensin II, the active agent of the RAS, thus blocking its vasoconstrictor and sodium-retaining effects with a consequent reduction in blood pressure. Since ACE is identical is kininase II, an enzyme that degrades the potent vasodilator bradykinin, inhibition of ACE leads to an additional, nonrenin-mediated reduction in systemic blood pressure. The antihypertensive effects of ACE inhibitors are accompanied by a reduction in peripheral vascular resistance.

*Pharmacokinetic properties:* The prodrug moexipril is rapidly absorbed and deesterified to the active metabolite moexiprilat. The pharmacokinetic parameters for moexipril and moexiprilat were similar after both, single and multiple does of meoxipril and appear to be dose-proportional. Moexipril and moexiprilat are moderately bound to plasma proteins, predominately albumin. Therefore, concurrently administered drugs are unlikely to interfere with the binding of moexipril and moexiprilat in any clinically significant way. Metabolites of moexipril present in the diketopiperazine derivatives of moexipril and moexiprilat. Both, moexipril and moexiprilat are eliminated in the urine, and moexiprilat is eliminated in the faeces. The pharmacokinetic profile of moexipril and moexiprilat should allow the same dosage recommendation in patients with mild to moderate renal dysfunction ($Cl_{cr}$>40 ml/min) as in patients with normal renal function. With severe renal dysfunction, dosage reduction is recommended. In patients with liver cirrhosis, the pharmacokinetics of moexipril and moexiprilat were significantly altered as compared with normal subjects. In such patients, therapy with Perdix should be started with 3.75 mg (half 7.5 mg tablet). There were no apparent pharmacokinetic drug interactions with HCTZ, digoxin, cimetidine, warfarin or nifedipine.

*Preclinical safety data:*
*Acute toxicity:* Findings of the acute toxicity studies in animals do not raise questions as to the safety of moexipril HCL as well as the main metabolite moexiprilat under the conditions of proposed clinical usage.

*Subacute/chronic toxicity:* Subacute and chronic toxicity studies in rats and dogs with repeated oral administration of moexipril HCL up to 12 months revealed mainly heart and kidney as target organs. The effects are completely comparable with those of other ACE inhibitors and can be interpreted as results of highly exaggerated pharmacological activity. First unspecific drug-related side-effects after long-term administration were seen at 75 mg/kg, i.e. a dose which corresponds 150 times the maximum recommended total daily dose in humans when compared on the basis of body weight.

*Reproduction studies:* Studies in rats and rabbits including all segments of reproduction revealed no direct effects of moexipril HCL on fertility, reproduction and abnormalities in $F_1$–or $F_2$-pups. Regarding precautions in women of child bearing potential and use during pregnancy and lactation see 4.3 and 4.6.

*Mutagenicity:* As conclusion of different 'in vitro and on 'in vivo' mutagencity studies, the mutagenic potential of moexipril HCL for human beings should be extremely low.

*Carcinogenicity:* Neither the long term toxicity studies in rats and dogs nor special carcinogenicity studies in mice and rats over 78 and 104 weeks respectively, indicated neoplastigenic properties of moexipril HCL. Therefore, it can be concluded that the carcinogenic risk for human beings will be extremely low.

**Pharmaceutical particulars**
*List of excipients:* Lactose, crospovidone, light magnesium oxide, gelatine, magnesium stearate, methy hydroxypropylcellulose, hydroxypropylcellulose, titanium dioxide, polyethyleneglycol 6000, ferric oxide purified water (not present in the finished product).

*Incompatibilities:* No incompatibilities have so fa been demonstrated.

*Shelf life:* 3 years

*Special precautions for storage:* Store in a dry place below 25°C.

*Nature and contents of container:* Calendar packs containing 28 tablets, 14 per Al/Al blister pack.

*Instruction for use/handling:* No special instructio necessary.

**Marketing authorisation numbers** 4438/0033 anc 0034

**Date of approval/revision of SPC** December 1996

**Legal category** POM

## TYLEX*

**Qualatitative and quantitative composition** Each capsule and effervescent tablet contains 500 mg o Paracetamol PhEur and 30 mg of Codeine Phosphate PhEur.

**Pharmaceutical form** Capsules and effervescen tablets.

**Clinical particulars**
*Therapeutic indications*: For the relief of severe pain.

*Posology and method of administration:*
*Adults:* The capsules and effervescent tablets are given orally. The effervescent tablets should be dissolved in at least half a tumbleful of water before taking. The usual dose is one or two capsules effervescent tablets every four hours as required. The total daily dose should not exceed 240 mg of codeine phosphate (i.e. not more than four doses (8 capsules tablets) per 24 hours should be taken).

*Elderly:* A reduced dose may be required.

*Children:* Use in children under 12 years of age i not recommended.

Dosage should be adjusted according to the severit of the pain and the response of the patient. Howeve it should be kept in mind that tolerance to codeine ca develop with continued use and that the incidence c untoward effects is dose related. Doses of codein higher than 60 mg fail to give commensurate relief o pain but merely prolong analgesia and are associate with an appreciably increased incidence of undesira ble side effects.

*Contra-indications*: Tylex should not to be adminis tered to patients who have previously exhibite hypersensitivity to either paracetamol or codeine, o to any of its excipients. Tylex is not recommended fo children under the age of 12 years.

*Special warnings and special precautions for use* Because safety and effectiveness in the administratio of paracetamol with codeine in children under 1 years of age have not been established, such use i not recommended. Tylex Capsules contain sodiur metabisulphite, a sulphite that may cause allergic reactions including anaphylactic symptoms and life threatening or less severe asthmatic episodes in certain susceptible people. The overall prevalence of sulphite sensitivity in the general population is unknown and probably low. Sulphite sensitivity is seen more frequently in asthmatic than non-asthmatic people. Tylex Effervescent contains 312.9 mg sodium/tablet and this should be taken into account when prescribing for patients for whom sodium restriction is indicated. Tylex Effervescent also contains 25 mg aspartame/tablet and therefore care should be taken in phenylketonuria. Tylex should be used with caution in patients with head injuries, increased intracranial pressure, acute abdominal conditions, the elderly and debilitated, and those with severe impairment of hepatic or renal function, hypothyroidism, Addison's disease and prostatic hypertrophy or urethral stricture. The hazard of overdose is greater in those with non-cirrhotic alcoholic liver disease. At high doses codeine has most of the disadvantages of morphine, including respiratory depression. Codeine can produce drug dependence of the morphine type, and therefore has the potential for being abused. Codeine may impair the mental/or physical abilities required for the performance of potentially hazardous tasks. Patients should be advised not to exceed the recommended dose, not to take other paracetamol-containing products concurrently, to consult their doctor if symptoms persist and to keep the product out of the reach of children.

*Interaction with other medicaments and other forms of interaction:* Patients receiving other central nervous system depressants (including other opioid analgesics, tranquillisers, sedative hypnotics and alcohol) concomitantly with Tylex may exhibit an additive depressant effect. When such therapy is contemplated, the dose of one or both agents should be reduced. Concurrent use of MAO inhibitors or tricyclic antidepressants with codeine may increase the effect of either the antidepressant or codeine. Concurrent use of anticholinergics and codeine may produce paralytic ileus. The speed of absorption of paracetamol may be increased by metoclopramide or domperidone and absorption reduced by cholestyramine. The anti-coagulant effect of warfarin and other coumarins may be enhanced by prolonged regular daily use of paracetamol with increased risk of bleeding; occasional doses have no significant effect.

*Pregnancy and lactation:* Tylex is not recommended during pregnancy or lactation since safety in pregnant women or nursing mothers has not been established.

*Effects on the ability to drive and use machines:* Patients should be advised not to drive or operate machinery if affected by dizziness or sedation.

*Undesirable effects:* The most frequently observed reactions include light headedness, dizziness, sedation, shortness of breath, nausea and vomiting. These effects seem more prominent in ambulatory than non-ambulatory patients and some of these adverse reactions may be alleviated if the patient lies down. Other adverse reactions include allergic reactions, (including skin rash), euphoria, dysphoria, constipation, abdominal pain and pruritus. In clinical use of paracetamol-containing products, there have been a few reports of blood dyscrasias including thrombocytopenia and agranulocytosis but these were not necessarily causally related to paracetamol.

*Overdose:* Symptoms of paracetamol overdosage in the first 24 hours are pallor, nausea, vomiting, anorexia and abdominal pain. Liver damage may become apparent 12 to 48 hours after ingestion. Abnormalities of glucose metabolism and metabolic acidosis may occur. In severe poisoning, hepatic failure may progress to encephalopathy, coma and death. Acute renal failure with acute tubular necrosis may develop even in the absence of severe liver damage. Cardiac arrhythmias and pancreatitis have been reported. Liver damage is possible in adults who have taken 10 g or more of paracetamol. It is considered that excess quantities of a toxic metabolite (usually adequately detoxified by glutathione when normal doses of paracetamol are ingested), become irreversibly bound to liver tissue. Immediate treatment is essential in the management of paracetamol overdose. Despite a lack of significant early symptoms, patients should be referred to hospital urgently for immediate medical attention and any patient who has ingested around 7.5 g or more of paracetamol in the preceding 4 hours should undergo gastric lavage. Administration of oral methionine or intravenous N-acetylcysteine which may have a beneficial effect up to at least 48 hours after the overdose, may be required. General supportive measures must be available. Serious overdose with codeine is characterised by respiratory depression, extreme somnolence progressing to stupor or coma, skeletal muscle flaccidity, cold and clammy skin and sometimes bradycardia and hypotension. In severe overdose with codeine, apnoea, circulatory collapse, cardiac arrest and death may occur. Primary attention should be given to the re-establishment of adequate respiratory exchange through the provision of a patent airway and the institution of controlled ventilation. Oxygen, intravenous fluids, vasopressors and other supportive measures should be employed as indicated. Opioid antagonists may be employed. Gastric lavage should be considered.

**Pharmacological properties**

*Pharmacodynamic properties:* Paracetamol has analgesic and antipyretic actions similar to those of aspirin with weak anti-inflammatory effects. Paracetamol is only a weak inhibitor of prostaglandin biosynthesis, although there is some evidence to suggest that it may be more effective against enzymes in the CNS than those in the periphery. This fact may partly account for its well documented ability to reduce fever and to induce analgesia, effects that involve actions on neural tissues. Single or repeated therapeutic doses of paracetamol have no effect on the cardiovascular and respiratory systems. Acid-based changes do not occur and gastric irritation, erosion or bleeding is not produced as may occur after salicylates. There is only a weak effect upon platelets and no effect on bleeding time or the excretion of uric acid.

Codeine is an analgesic with uses similar to those of morphine but has only mild sedative effects. The major effect is on the CNS and the bowel. The effects are remarkably diverse and include analgesia, drowsiness, changes in mood, respiratory depression, decreased gastrointestinal motility, nausea, vomiting and alterations of the endocrine and autonomic nervous systems. The relief of pain is relatively selective, in that other sensory modalities, (touch, vibration, vision, hearing etc.) are not obtunded.

*Pharmacokinetic properties:* Paracetamol is readily absorbed from the gastro-intestinal tract with peak plasma concentration occurring about 30 minutes to 2 hours after ingestion. It is metabolised in the liver and excreted in the urine mainly as the glucuronide and sulphate conjugates. Less than 5% is excreted as unchanged paracetamol. The elimination half-life varies from about 1 to 4 hours. Plasma-protein binding is negligible at usual therapeutic concentrations but increases with increasing concentrations. A minor hydroylated metabolite which is usually produced in very small amounts by mixed-function oxidases in the liver and which is usually detoxified by conjugation with liver glutathione may accumulate following paracetamol overdosage and cause liver damage.

Codeine and its salts are absorbed from the gastro intestinal tract. Ingestion of codeine phosphate produces peak plasma codeine concentrations in about one hour. Codeine is metabolised by O- & N-demethylation in the liver to morphine and norcodeine. Codeine and its metabolites are excreted almost entirely by the kidney, mainly as conjugates with glucuronic acid. The plasma half-life has been reported to be between 3 and 4 hours after administration by mouth or intravascular injection.

*Preclinical safety data:* None stated.

**Pharmaceutical particulars**

*List of excipients:*

*Tylex Capsules:* Pregelatinized starch, calcium stearate, aerosol OT-B (dioctyl sodium sulfosuccinate, sodium benzoate (E211)), sodium metabisulphite, gelatin capsule, E171, E127, E132, printing ink: shellac, soya lecithin, 2-ethyoxyethanol, dimethylpolysiloxane, E172.

*Tylex Effervescent:* Citric acid anhydrous, sodium bicarbonate, sodium carbonate anhydrous, aspartame, blackcurrant flavour no. 78004-31, polyethylene glycol 6000, magnesium stearate, ethanol 96% (not detected in the finished product)

*Incompatibilities:* None pertinent

*Shelf life:*
Tylex Capsules: 60 months.
Tylex Effervescent: 36 months.

*Special precautions for storage:* Store at or below 25°C. Protect from light. Store Tylex Effervescent in a dry place.

*Nature and contents of container:*
Tylex Capsules: PVC/aluminium foil blister strips. Marketed pack sizes: 1 x 8, 3 x 8, 5 x 20 capsules.
Tylex Effervescent: Paper/aluminium laminate blister strips. Marketed pack sizes: 4x2 and 15x6 tablets.

*Instructions for use/handling:* None.

**Marketing authorisation numbers**

| | |
|---|---|
| Tylex Capsules | 04438/0046 |
| Tylex Effervescent | 04438/0045 |

**Date of approval/revision of SPC**
Tylex Capsules: March 1996
Tylex Effervescent: November 1996

**Legal category** POM

## VIRIDAL*

**Qualitative and quantitative composition**

Viridal 5: 1 vial of dry substance (47.7 mg) contains: Alprostadil 5 mcg (used as 1:1 clathrate complex with alfadex)

Viridal 10: 1 vial of dry substance (47.8 mg) contains: Alprostadil 10 mcg (used as 1:1 clathrate complex with alfadex)

Viridal 20: 1 vial of dry substance (48.2 mg) contains: Alprostadil 20 mcg (used as 1:1 clathrate complex with alfadex)

**Pharmaceutical form** Vials containing lyophilised powder for reconstitution with the diluent provided.

*Administration devices:* 0.9 % saline (1 ml) prefilled syringe (PL 4438/0043), Plunger, Injection needle 21 Gx2 (0.8 x 50) for drug preparation (colour code: green) Injection needle 30 Gx½ (0.3 x 13) for injection (colour code: colourless) 2 antiseptic swabs.

*Route of administration:* For injection into the penile cavernous body.

**Clinical particulars**

*Indications:* As an adjunct to the diagnostic evaluation of erectile dysfunction in adult males. Treatment of erectile dysfunction in adult males.

*Posology and method of administration:*

*Application:* The drug solution should be prepared shortly before the injection. Prior to injection, the dry substance should be dissolved in 1 ml of 0.9 % saline. To do this, flip off the lid from the vial. Clean the rubber stopper of the vial using one of the sterile swabs. After fixing needle 21 G x 2 (0.8 x 50) (colour code: green) onto the prefilled syringe the saline is injected into the vial. Shake the vial gently until the powder is completely dissolved. Then the whole of the freshly prepared solution is drawn up into the syringe. After pushing the air out of the syringe and getting the correct amount of drug solution, needle 30 G x ½ (0.3 x 13) (colour code: colourless) is fixed onto the syringe and the air has to be pushed out of it prior to intracavernous injection. Unused solution must be discarded immediately. Cavernous body self-injection is done with the thin needle (30 G x ½ (0.3 x 13), colour code: colourless) into either the right or the left cavernous body of the penile shaft. Once the needle is in the cavernous body, the injection should be done within 5 to 10 seconds and is very easy if the needle is in the correct position. It is recommended that a condom be used during intercourse after completing the injection. Re-evaluation should take place at regular intervals by the physician and he will decide whether correction of the dosage is necessary and also about the duration and frequency of the treatment.

*Dosage for injection in the clinic:* Injections for diagnostic evaluation and dose titration must be performed by the attending physician. He will determine an individual dose suitable to produce an erectile response for diagnostic purposes. The recommended starting dose is 2.5 mcg Viridal in patients with primary psychogenic or neurogenic origin of erectile dysfunction. In all other patients 5 mcg Viridal should be used as a starting dose. Dose adjustments may be performed in increments of about 2.5 mcg to 5 mcg Viridal. Most of the patients require between 10 and 20 mcg per injection. Some patients may need to be titrated to higher doses. Doses exceeding 20 mcg should be prescribed with particular care in patients with cardiovascular risk factors. The dose per injection should never exceed 40 mcg.

*Dosage for self-injection therapy at home:* The patient should only use his optimum individual dosage which has been pre-determined by his physician using the above mentioned procedure. This dose should allow the patient to have an erection at home which should not last longer than one hour. If he experiences prolonged erections beyond 2 hours but less than 4 hours, the patient is recommended to contact his physician to re-establish the dose of the drug. Maximum injection frequency recommended is 2 or 3 times a week with an interval of at least 24 hours between the injections.

*Follow-up:* After the first injections and at regular intervals thereafter, the physician should re-evaluate the patient. Any local adverse reaction, e.g. haematoma, fibrosis or nodules should be noted and controlled. Following discussion with the patient, an adjustment of dosage may be necessary.

*Contra-indications:* Hypersensivity to alprostadil and/or alfadex (ingredients of Viridal). Patients with diseases causing prolonged erections eg. sickle-cell disease, leukaemia and multiple myeloma should not use Viridal.

*Special precautions:* Patients, who experience a prolonged erection lasting longer than four hours should contact their physician immediately. Therefore it is recommended that the patient has an emergency telephone number of his attending physician or of a clinic experienced in therapy of erectile dysfunction. Prolonged erection may damage penile erectile tissue and lead to irreversible erectile dysfunction.

Patients with pre-existing scarring, e.g. fibrosis or nodules of the cavernous body or pre-existing penile deviation or Peyronie's disease should be treated with particular care, e.g. more frequent re-evaluation of the patient's condition.

This is due to the increased risk of painful erections. Patients who have to be treated with alpha-adrenergic drugs due to prolonged erections (see: overdose) may in the case of concomitant therapy with monoamino-oxidase-inhibitors, develop a hypertensive crisis.

Other intracavernous drugs e.g. smooth muscle relaxing agents or alpha-adrenergic blocking agents may lead to prolonged erection and must not be used concomitantly.

Patients with blood clotting disorders or patients on therapy influencing blood clotting parameters should be treated with special care, e.g. monitoring of the clotting parameters and advice to the patient to exercise sufficient manual pressure on the injection site. This is because of the increased risk of bleeding.

Sexual stimulation and intercourse can lead to cardiac and/or pulmonary events in patients with coronary heart disease, congestive heart failure or pulmonary disease. Viridal should be used with care in these patient groups and patients should be examined and cleared for stress resistance by a cardiologist before treatment.

To prevent abuse, self-injection therapy with Viridal should not be used by patients with drug addiction and/or disturbances of psychological or intellectual development. For patients with known venereal disease, HIV-infection, or AIDS, Viridal is not recommended.

In any condition that precludes safe self injection like poor manual dexterity, poor visual acuity or morbid obesity, the partner should be trained in the injection technique and should perform the injection. Up to now, there is no clinical experience in patients under 18 and over 75 years of age. Viridal does not interfere with ejaculation and fertility. It is recommended that a condom be used during intercourse after completing the injection.

*Interactions:* Concomitant use of smooth muscle relaxing drugs like papaverine or other drugs inducing erection like alpha-adrenergic blocking agents may lead to prolonged erection and should not be used in parallel with Viridal. Risks exist when using alpha-adrenergic drugs to terminate prolonged erections in patients with cardiovascular disorders or receiving MAO inhibitors. The effects of blood pressure lowering and vasodilating drugs may be increased.

*Use during pregnancy and lactation:* Not applicable.

Alprostadil did not cause any adverse effects on fertility or general reproductive performance in male and female rats treated with 40-200 mcg/kg/day. The high dose of 200 mcg/kg/day is about 300 times the maximum human recommended dose on a body weight basis (MHRD <1 mcg/kg). Alprostadil was not fetotoxic or teratogenic at doses up to 5000 mcg/kg/day (7500 times the MHRD) in rats, 200 mcg/kg/day (300 times the MHRD) in rabbits and doses up to 20 mcg/kg/day (30 times the MHRD) in guinea pigs or monkeys.

*Effects on ability to drive and use machines:* Viridal may rarely induce hypotension with subsequent impairment of reactivity.

*Undesirable effects:* The most frequent adverse effect of Viridal is a burning pain during and after injection due to the injection technique and the feeling of tension occuring with penile erection. Haematomas are frequently seen at the site of injection. There may also be incorrect injections, e.g. subcutaneous or urethral. Further possible local reactions are haemo-siderin deposits, reddening and swelling or bleeding of the injection site, ecchymosis, swelling of foreskin or glans, cavernositis or penile infection.

Prolonged erections lasting longer than four hours occur occasionally, but more often during diagnostic and titration-periods than during the period of self injection once the optimum dose has been determined. Erections lasting longer than six hours are rare after intracavernous injection of Viridal. Prolonged erection may damage penile erectile structures and lead to irreversible erectile dysfunction.

Adverse effects of long-term treatment are fibrotic nodules, spots or plaques with/without penile angulation associated with the injection site which occur occasionally. Fibrotic tissue alterations of the cavernous body with/without loss of function and with/without penile angulation occur in very rare cases during treatment of up to three years. Penile deviations can occur. Systemic circulation effects e.g. hypotension with/without dizziness, cardiac arrythmias, chest pains, headaches and circulatory collapse after intracavernous injection of Viridal have been reported very rarely.

*Overdose:* Symptoms: Full rigid erections lasting more than four hours. If the patient experiences a prolonged erection, he is advised to contact his attending physician or a urologic clinic nearby immediately. Treatment strategy: Treatment of prolonged erection should be done by a physician experienced in the field of erectile dysfunction: If prolonged erection occurs, the following is recommended: If the erection has lasted less than six hours: observation of the erection because spontaneous flaccidityfrequently occurs. If the erection has lasted longer than six hours cavernous body injection of alpha-adrenergic substances (e.g. phenyl ephrine, etilephrine). Risks exist when using drugs in patients with cardiovascular disorders or receiving MAO inhibitors. All patients should be monitored for cardiovascular effects when these drugs are used to terminate prolonged erections or aspiration of blood from the cavernous body.

*Accidental systemic injection of high doses:* Single dose rising tolerance studies in healthy volunteers indicated that single intravenous doses of alprostadil from 1 to 120 mcg were well tolerated. Starting with a 40 mcg bolus intravenous dose, the frequency of drug-related adverse events increased in a dose-dependent manner, characterised mainly by facial flushing.

## Pharmacological properties

*Pharmacodynamic properties:* Alprostadil [Prosta-glandin E1 ($PGE_1$)], the active ingredient of Viridal, is an endogenous compound derived from the essential fatty acid dihomo-gamma-linolenic acid. Alprostadil is a potent smooth muscle relaxant that produces vasodilation and occurs in high concentrations in the human seminal fluid. Precontracted isolated preparations of the human corpus cavernosum, corpus spongiosum and cavernous artery were relaxed by alprostadil, while other prostanoids were less effective. Alprostadil has been shown to bind to specific receptors in the cavernous tissue of human and non-human primates. The binding of alprostadil to its receptors is accompanied by an increase in intracellular cAMP levels. Human cavernosal smooth muscle cells respond to alprostadil by releasing intracellular calcium. Since relaxation of smooth muscle is associated with a reduction of the cytoplasmic free calcium concentration, this effect may contribute to the relaxing activity of this prostanoid. Intracavernous injection of alprostadil in healthy monkeys resulted in penile elongation and tumescence without rigidity. The cavernous arterial blood flow was increased for a mean duration of 20 min. In contrast, intracavernous application of alprostadil to rabbits and dogs caused no erectile response. Systemic intravascular administration of alprostadil leads to a vasodilation and reduction of systemic peripheral vascular resistance. A decrease in blood pressure can be observed after administration of high doses. Alprostadil has also been shown in animal and in vitro tests to reduce platelet reactivity and neutrophil activation. Additional alprostadil activity has been reported: increase in fibrinolytic activity of fibroblasts, improvement of erythrocyte deformability and inhibition of erythrocyte aggregation; inhibition of the proliferative and mitotic activity of non-striated myocytes; inhibition of cholesterol synthesis and LDL-receptor activity; and an increase in the supply of oxygen and glucose to ischaemic tissue along with improved tissue utilization of these substrates.

*Pharmacokinetic properties:* Pharmacokinetics after intracavernous injection; Viridal contains the active ingredient alprostadil ($PGE_1$) in the form of an inclusion compound (clathrate) with alfadex (α-cyclodextrin). During the preparation of the solution for injection the clathrate complex dissociates into the components of alprostadil and alfadex, therefore the pharmacokinetic behaviour of both compounds is independent of the clathrate structure of the dry substance. Preliminary information of the pharmacokinetics of alprostadil alfadex following intracavernous injection are available. There are no significant differences between the systemic plasma concentration of alprostadil and its metabolites $PGE_0$ and 15-keto-$PGE_0$ after intracavernous injection in patients and after intravenous injection in healthy volunteers. Based on the extremely short half-life of alprostadil and the resulting experimental difficulties the pharmacokinetic parameters of systemic alprostadil were measured under steady-state conditions.

Pharmacokinetics after intravenous infusion; Alprostadil is an endogenous substance with an extremely short half-life. After i.v. infusion of 60 mcg alprostadil over two hours (0.5 μg/min) in healthy volunteers, maximum plasma levels of about 5 pg/ml above basal values were measured (basal value 1-2 pg/ml). After cessation of the infusion, the alprostadil concentration dropped to basal values, with half-lives of about 0.2 min (α-phase, estimate) and about 8 min (β-phase). Due to the short half-life, steady state concentrations were reached shortly after the onset of the i.v. infusion.

Alprostadil undergoes biotransformation predominantly in the lungs. During the first pass through the lungs 80-90 % of alprostadil is metabolized. Enzymatic oxidation of the C15-hydroxy-group followed by reduction of the C13, 14-double-bond produces the main metabolites 15-keto-$PGE_1$, $PGE_0$ and 15-keto-$PGE_0$. The compound 15-keto-$PGE_1$ has up to now only been detected in vitro in homogenated lung preparations, whereas $PGE_0$ and 15-keto-$PGE_0$ were found in plasma. After degradation by β-oxidation and ω-oxidation, the main metabolites are eliminated via urine (88 %) and the faeces (12 %). As a result of biotransformation, $PGE_0$ (13, 14-dihydro-$PGE_1$) and 15-keto-$PGE_0$ were detected in plasma. After i.v. infusion of 60 μg alprostadil over two hours, plasma concentrations of $PGE_0$ reached values of about 12 pg/ml above basal value (1-2 pg/ml) and those of 15-keto-$PGE_0$ were 150 pg/ml above basal value of 4-6 pg/ml. Half-lives were about 2 min (α-phase) and 30 min (β-phase) for $PGE_0$ and 1-2 min and 20 min respectively for 15-keto-$PGE_0$. 93 % of the alprostadil in plasma is bound to macromolecular compartments. The alfadex was found to have a half-life of about seven minutes in rats. It is excreted renally as unchanged alfadex. Studies on the concentration of alprostadil and its metabolites in various organs and tissues of the rat revealed no evidence of accumulation.

*Preclinical safety data:* Studies on local tolerance following single and repeated intracavernous injections of alprostadil or alprostadil alfadex in rabbits and/or monkeys, in monkeys up to 6 months with daily injection, revealed in general good local tolerance. Possible adverse effects like hematomas and inflammations are more likely related to the injection procedure. Within the 6 months study in male monkeys, there were no adverse effects of alprostadil alfadex on male reproductive organs. Different mutagenicity studies with alprostadil alfadex revealed no risk of mutagenicity. Chronic toxicity studies in dogs (6 months, daily intravenous infusion) and monkeys (6 months, daily intracavernous injection) indicates that systemic side effects are unlikely to occur following intracavernous injection of 5 to 40 mcg alprostadil (used as clathrate complex with alfadex).

## Pharmaceutical particulars

*List of excipients:* Lactose, alfadex

*Incompatibilities:* No incompatibilities have so far been demonstrated.

*Shelf life:* Shelf life for the product as packaged for sale; Viridal 5 mcg – 24 months, Viridal 10 mcg – 24 months, Viridal 20 mcg – 24 months

*Shelf life after reconstitution:* for immediate use only.

*Special precautions for storage:* Store below 25°C.

*Nature and contents of container:* Cartons containing one colourless glass vial (glass type I), with a rubber stopper, one prefilled (glass type I) glass syringe, two injection needles, 21 G x 2 (0.8 x 50) for drug preparation and 30 G x ½ (0.3 x 13) for injection, two alcohol swabs.

*Instructions for use/handling:* Fix the needle [21 G x 2 (0.8 x 50) (colour code: green)] onto the prefilled syringe. Clean the rubber stopper of the vial using one of the sterile swabs. Inject the saline out of the prefilled syringe into the vial. Shake the vial to dissolve the dry substance. Draw back into the syringe the whole freshly prepared solution. After pushing the air out of the syringe and getting the correct amount of drug solution, the needle [30 G x ½ (0.3 x 13) (colour code: colourless)] is fixed onto the syringe prior to intracavernous injection. After preparation of the solution, the injection must be performed using aseptic procedures, using the 30-gauge needle (colour code: colourless) into either the left or right cavernous body of the penile shaft. Care should be taken not to inject into penile vessels or nerves on the upper side of the penis and into the urethra on the under side. The injection should be completed within 10 to 15 seconds and manual pressure should be applied to the injection site for 2 to 3 minutes. Unused solution must be discarded immediately.

*Advice:* The vial contains a white dry powder, which forms a compact layer of approximately 3 mm thickness. This layer may show cracks, and sometimes may crumble slightly. If the vial is damaged, then the normally dry content becomes moist and sticky and extensive loss of volume results. If this has happened do not use the product.

## Marketing authorisation numbers

| | |
|---|---|
| Viridal 5 | 4438/0040 |
| Viridal 10 | 4438/0041 |
| Viridal 20 | 4438/0042 |

**Date of approval/revivion of SPC** July 1996

**Legal category** POM

*Trade Mark

**Searle**
PO Box 53
Lane End Road
High Wycombe
Bucks HP12 4HL

**SEARLE**

## ALDACTIDE*

**Presentation**

*Aldactide 50:* Buff, film-coated tablets engraved 'SEARLE 180' on one side containing Spironolactone BP 50 mg and Hydroflumethiazide BP 50 mg.

*Aldactide 25:* Buff, film-coated tablets engraved 'Searle 101' on one side containing Spironolactone BP 25 mg and Hydroflumethiazide BP 25 mg.

**Uses** Congestive cardiac failure.

**Dosage and administration** Administration of Aldactide once daily with a meal is recommended.

*Adults:* Most patients will require an initial dosage of four tablets Aldactide 25 or two tablets Aldactide 50 daily. The dosage should be adjusted as necessary and may range from one tablet Aldactide 25 to eight tablets Aldactide 25 or four tablets Aldactide 50 daily.

*Elderly:* It is recommended that treatment is started with the lowest dose and titrated upwards as required to achieve maximum benefit. Care should be taken in severe hepatic and renal impairment which may alter drug metabolism and excretion.

*Children:* Although clinical trials using Aldactide have not been carried out in children, as a guide, a daily dosage providing 1.5 to 3 mg of spironolactone per kilogram body weight, given in divided doses, may be employed.

**Contra-indications, warnings, etc**

*Contra-indications:* Aldactide is contra-indicated in patients with anuria, acute renal insufficiency, rapidly deteriorating or severe impairment of renal function, hyperkalaemia, significant hypercalcaemia, Addison's disease and in patients who are hypersensitive to spironolactone, thiazide diuretics or to other sulphonamide derived drugs.

Aldactide should not be administered with other potassium-conserving diuretics and potassium supplements should not be given routinely with Aldactide as hyperkalaemia may be induced.

*Warnings: Carcinogenicity:* Spironolactone has been shown to produce tumours in rats when administered at high doses over a long period of time. The significance of these findings with respect to clinical use is not certain. However, the long term use of spironolactone in young patients requires careful consideration of the benefits and the potential hazard involved.

Sulphonamide derivatives, including thiazides, have been reported to exacerbate or activate systemic lupus erythematosus.

*Precautions:*

*Fluid and electrolyte balance:* Fluid and electrolyte status should be regularly monitored, particularly in the elderly, in those with significant renal and hepatic impairment and in patients receiving digoxin and drugs with pro-arrhythmic effects.

Hyperkalaemia may occur in patients with impaired renal function or excessive potassium intake and can cause cardiac irregularities which may be fatal. Should hyperkalaemia develop Aldactide should be discontinued, and if necessary, active measures taken to reduce the serum potassium to normal.

Hypokalaemia may develop as a result of profound diuresis, particularly when Aldactide is used concomitantly with loop diuretics, glucocorticoids or ACTH.

Hyponatraemia may be induced, especially when Aldactide is administered in combination with other diuretics.

*Hepatic impairment:* Caution should be observed in patients with acute or severe liver impairment as vigorous diuretic therapy may precipitate encephalopathy in susceptible patients. Regular estimation of serum electrolytes is essential in such patients.

Reversible hyperchloraemic metabolic acidosis usually in association with hyperkalaemia has been reported to occur in some patients with decompensated hepatic cirrhosis, even in the presence of normal renal function.

*Urea and uric acid:* Reversible increases in blood urea have been reported, particularly accompanying vigorous diuresis or in the presence of impaired renal function.

Thiazides may cause hyperuricaemia and precipitate attacks of gout in some patients.

*Diabetes mellitus:* Thiazides may aggravate existing diabetes and the insulin requirements may alter. Diabetes mellitus which has been latent may become manifest during thiazide administration.

*Hyperlipidaemia:* Caution should be observed as thiazides may raise serum lipids.

*Drug Interactions:* Spironolactone has been reported to increase serum digoxin concentration and to interfere with certain serum digoxin assays. In patients receiving digoxin and spironolactone the digoxin response should be monitored by means other than serum digoxin concentrations, unless the digoxin assay used has been proven not to be affected by spironolactone therapy. If it proves necessary to adjust the dose of digoxin patients should be carefully monitored for evidence of enhanced or reduced digoxin effect.

Potentiation of the effect of other antihypertensive drugs occurs and their dosage may need to be reduced when Aldactide is added to the treatment regimen, and then adjusted as necessary. Since ACE inhibitors decrease aldosterone production they should not routinely be used with Aldactide particularly in patients with marked renal impairment.

As carbenoxolone may cause sodium retention and thus decrease the effectiveness of Aldactide, concurrent use should be avoided.

Nonsteroidal anti-inflammatory drugs may attenuate the natriuretic efficacy of diuretics due to inhibition of intrarenal synthesis of prostaglandins.

Concurrent use of lithium and thiazides may reduce lithium clearance leading to intoxication. Spironolactone and thiazides may reduce vascular responsiveness to noradrenaline. Caution should be exercised in the management of patients subjected to regional or general anaesthesia while they are being treated with Aldactide.

In fluorimetric assays spironolactone may interfere with the estimation of compounds with similar fluorescence characteristics.

The absorption of a number of drugs including thiazides is decreased when co-administered with cholestyramine and colestipol.

Thiazides co-administered with calcium and/or vitamin D may increase the risk of hypercalcaemia.

Thiazides may delay the elimination of quinidine.

*Pregnancy:* Spironolactone or its metabolites may, and hydroflumethazide does, cross the placental barrier. With spironolactone feminisation has been observed in male rat foetuses. Thiazides may decrease placental perfusion, increase uterine inertia and inhibit labour. In the foetus or neonate, thiazides may cause jaundice, thrombocytopenia, hypoglycaemia, electrolyte imbalance and death from maternal complications.

The use of Aldactide in pregnant women requires that the anticipated benefit be weighed against the possible hazards to the mother and foetus.

*Nursing mothers:* Metabolites of spironolactone, and hydroflumethiazide, have been detected in breast milk. If use of Aldactide is considered essential, an alternative method of infant feeding should be instituted.

*Adverse effects:* Gynaecomastia may develop in association with the use of spironolactone. Development appears to be related to both dosage level and duration of therapy and is normally reversible when the drug is discontinued. In rare instances some breast enlargement may persist. Other adverse reactions reported in association with spironolactone include: gastrointestinal intolerance, drowsiness, lethargy, headache, mental confusion, ataxia, drug fever, skin rashes, mestrual irregularities, breast soreness, impotence and mild androgenic effects.

Adverse reactions reported in association with thiazides include: gastrointestinal upset, skin rashes, photosensitivity, blood dyscrasias, raised serum lipids, aplastic anaemia, purpura, muscle cramps, weakness, restlessness, headache, dizziness, vertigo, jaundice, orthostatic hypotension, impotence, paraesthesia, and rarely pancreatitis, necrotising vasculitis and xanthopsia. Rarely hypercalcaemia has been reported in association with thiazides, usually in patients with pre-existing metabolic bone disease or parathyroid dysfunction.

*Overdosage:* Acute overdosage may be manifested by drowsiness, mental confusion, nausea, vomiting, dizziness or diarrhoea. Hyponatraemia, hypokalaemia or hyperkalaemia may be induced, or hepatic coma may be precipitated in patients with severe liver disease, but these effects are unlikely to be associated with acute overdosage. Symptoms of hyperkalaemia may manifest as paraesthesia, weakness flaccid paralysis or muscle spasm and may be difficult to distinguish clinically from hypokalaemia. Electrocardiographic changes are the earliest specific signs of potassium disturbances. No specific antidote has been identified. Improvement may be expected after withdrawal of the drug. General supportive measures including replacement of fluids and electrolytes may be indicated.

**Pharmaceutical precautions** Store in a dry place below 30°C (86°F).

**Legal category** POM.

**Package quantities** *Aldactide 50:* Calendar pack of 28 tablets, Securitainer bottles of 100 tablets. *Aldactide 25:* Blister pack of 100 tablets.

**Further information** Hydroflumethiazide induces diuresis usually within two hours, which lasts for 12-18 hours.

Spironolactone, as a competitive aldosterone antagonist, increases sodium excretion whilst reducing potassium loss at the distal renal tubule. It has a gradual and prolonged action. The renal action of single doses of spironolactone reaches its peak after 7 hours, and activity persists for at least 24 hours.

**Product licence numbers**
Aldactide 50:     08821/0012
Aldactide 25:     08821/0013

## ALDACTONE*

**Presentation**

*Aldactone 100 mg:* Buff, film-coated tablets engraved 'SEARLE 134' on one side. Each tablet contains Spironolactone BP 100 mg.

*Aldactone 50 mg:* Off-white, film-coated tablets engraved 'SEARLE 916'. Each tablet contains Spironolactone BP 50 mg.

*Aldactone 25 mg:* Buff, film-coated tablets engraved 'SEARLE 39' on one side. Each tablet contains Spironolactone BP 25 mg.

**Uses**

Congestive cardiac failure.
Hepatic cirrhosis with ascites and oedema.
Malignant ascites.
Nephrotic syndrome.
Diagnosis and treatment of primary aldosteronism.

**Dosage and administration** Administration of Aldactone once daily with a meal is recommended.

*Adults:*

*Congestive cardiac failure:* Usual dose – 100 mg/day. In difficult or severe cases the dosage may be gradually increased up to 400 mg/day. When oedema is controlled, the usual maintenance level is 75–200 mg/day.

*Hepatic cirrhosis with ascites and oedema:* If urinary Na⁺/K⁺ ratio is greater than 1.0, 100 mg/day. If the ratio is less than 1.0, 200–400 mg/day. Maintenance dosage should be individually determined.

*Malignant ascites:* Initial dose usually 100–200 mg/day. In severe cases the dosage may be gradually increased up to 400 mg/day. When oedema is controlled, maintenance dosage should be individually determined.

*Nephrotic syndrome:* Usual dose – 100–200 mg/day. Spironolactone has not been shown to be anti-inflammatory, nor to affect the basic pathological process. Its use is only advised if glucocorticoids by themselves are insufficiently effective.

*Diagnosis and treatment of primary aldosteronism:* Aldactone may be employed as an initial diagnostic measure to provide presumptive evidence of primary hyperaldosteronism while patients are on normal diets.

Long test: Aldactone is administered at a daily dosage of 400 mg for three to four weeks.

Correction of hypokalaemia and of hypertension provides presumptive evidence for the diagnosis of primary hyperaldosteronism.

Short test: Aldactone is administered at daily dosage of 400 mg for four days. If serum potassium increases during Aldactone administration but drops when Aldactone is discontinued, a presumptive diagnosis of primary hyperaldosteronism should be considered.

After the diagnosis of hyperaldosteronism has been established by more definitive testing procedures, Aldactone may be administered in doses of 100 mg to 400 mg daily in preparation for surgery. For patients who are considered unsuitable for surgery, Aldactone may be employed for long term maintenance therapy at the lowest effective dosage determined for the individual patient.

*Elderly:* It is recommended that treatment is started with the lowest dose and titrated upwards as required to achieve maximum benefit. Care should be taken in severe hepatic and renal impairment which may alter drug metabolism and excretion.

*Children:* Initial daily dosage should provide 3 mg of spironolactone per kilogram body weight, given in divided doses. Dosage should be adjusted on the basis of response and tolerance. If necessary a suspension may be prepared by crushing Aldactone tablets.

**Contra-indications, warnings, etc**

*Contra-indications:* Aldactone is contra-indicated in patients with anuria, acute renal insufficiency, rapidly deteriorating or severe impairment of renal function, hyperkalaemia, Addison's disease and in patients who are hypersensitive to spironolactone.

Aldactone should not be administered concurrently with other potassium-conserving diuretics and potassium supplements should not be given routinely with Aldactone as hyperkalaemia may be induced.

*Warnings:*

*Carcinogenicity:* Spironolactone has been shown to produce tumours in rats when administered at high doses over a long period of time. The significance of these findings with respect to clinical use is not certain. However, the long term use of spironolactone in young patients requires careful consideration of the benefits and the potential hazard involved.

*Precautions:*

*Fluid and electrolyte balance:* Fluid and electrolyte status should be regularly monitored, particularly in the elderly, and in those with significant renal and hepatic impairment.

Hyperkalaemia may occur in patients with impaired renal function or excessive potassium intake and can cause cardiac irregularities which may be fatal. Should hyperkalaemia develop Aldactone should be discontinued, and if necessary, active measures taken to reduce the serum potassium to normal.

Hyponatraemia may be induced, especially when Aldactone is administered in combination with other diuretics.

Reversible hyperchloraemic metabolic acidosis usually in association with hyperkalaemia has been reported to occur in some patients with decompensated hepatic cirrhosis, even in the presence of normal renal function.

*Urea:* Reversible increases in blood urea have been reported, in association with Aldactone therapy, particularly in the presence of impaired renal function.

*Drug interactions:* Spironolactone has been reported to increase serum digoxin concentration and to interfere with certain serum digoxin assays. In patients receiving digoxin and spironolactone and digoxin response should be monitored by means other than serum digoxin concentrations, unless the digoxin assay used has been proven not to be affected by spironolactone therapy. If it proves necessary to adjust the dose of digoxin patients should be carefully monitored for evidence of enhanced or reduced digoxin effect.

Potentiation of the effect of antihypertensive drugs occurs and their dosage may need to be reduced when Aldactone is added to the treatment regimen, and then adjusted as necessary. Since ACE inhibitors decrease aldosterone production they should not routinely be used with Aldactone particularly in patients with marked renal impairment.

As carbenoxolone may cause sodium retention and thus decrease the effectiveness of Aldactone, concurrent use should be avoided.

Nonsteroidal anti-inflammatory drugs may attenuate the natriuretic efficacy of diuretics due to inhibition of intrarenal synthesis of prostaglandins.

Spironolactone reduces vascular responsiveness to noradrenaline. Caution should be exercised in the management of patients subjected to regional or general anaesthesia while they are being treated with Aldactone.

In fluorimetric assays spironolactone may interfere with the estimation of compounds with similar fluorescence characteristics.

*Pregnancy:* Spironolactone or its metabolites may cross the placental barrier. With spironolactone, feminisation has been observed in male rat foetuses. The use of Aldactone in pregnant women requires that the anticipated benefit be weighed against the possible hazards to the mother and foetus.

*Nursing mothers:* Metabolites of spironolactone, have been detected in breast milk. If use of Aldactone is considered essential, an alternative method of infant feeding should be instituted.

*Adverse effects:* Gynaecomastia may develop in association with the use of spironolactone. Development appears to be related to both dosage level and duration of therapy and is normally reversible when spironolactone is discontinued. In rare instances some breast enlargement may persist. Other adverse reactions reported in association with spironolactone include: gastrointestinal intolerance, drowsiness, lethargy, headache, mental confusion, ataxia, drug fever, skin rashes, breast soreness, menstrual irregularities, impotence and mild androgenic effects.

*Overdosage:* Acute overdosage may be manifested by drowsiness, mental confusion, nausea, vomiting, dizziness or diarrhoea. Hyponatraemia or hyperkalaemia may be induced but these effects are unlikely to be associated with acute overdosage. Symptoms of hyperkalaemia may manifest as paraesthesia, weakness, flaccid paralysis or muscle spasm and may be difficult to distinguish clinically from hypokalaemia. Electrocardiographic changes are the earliest specific signs of potassium disturbances. No specific antidote has been identified. Improvement may be expected after withdrawal of the drug. General supportive measures including replacement of fluids and electrolytes may be indicated. For hyperkalaemia, reduce potassium intake, administer potassium-excreting diuretics, intravenous glucose with regular insulin, or oral ion-exchange resins.

**Pharmaceutical precautions**   Store in a dry place below 30°C (86°F).

**Legal category**   POM.

**Package quantities**   *Aldactone 100 mg:*  Calendar pack of 28 tablets, blister pack of 100 tablets.
   *Aldactone 50 mg:* Blister pack of 100 tablets.
   *Aldactone 25 mg:* Blister pack of 100 tablets.

**Further information**   Aldactone, as a competitive aldosterone antagonist, increases sodium excretion whilst reducing potassium loss at the distal renal tubule. It has a gradual and prolonged action, maximum response being usually attained after 2–3 days' treatment. Combination of Aldactone with a conventional, more proximally acting diuretic usually enhances diuresis without excessive potassium loss.

**Product licence numbers**

Aldactone 100 mg:    08821/0009
Aldactone 50 mg:     08821/0010
Aldactone 25 mg:     08821/0011

## ARTHROTEC* 50

**Qualitative and quantitative composition**   Each tablet consists of an enteric-coated core containing 50 mg diclofenac sodium surrounded by an outer mantle containing 200 mcg misoprostol.

**Pharmaceutical form**   White, round, biconvex tablets marked ⟡ on one side and 'SEARLE 1411' on the other side.

**Clinical particulars**

*Therapeutic indications:* Arthrotec 50 is indicated for patients who require a non-steroidal anti-inflammatory drug (NSAID) together with misoprostol.

The diclofenac component of Arthrotec 50 is indicated for the treatment of osteoarthritis and rheumatoid arthritis. The misoprostol component of Arthrotec 50 is indicated for the prophylaxis of NSAID-induced gastric and duodenal ulceration.

*Posology and method of administration:*

*Adults:* One tablet to be taken with food, two or three times daily. Tablets should be swallowed whole, not chewed.

*Elderly/renal impairment/hepatic impairment:* No adjustment of dosage is necessary in the elderly or in patients with hepatic impairment or mild to moderate renal impairment as pharmacokinetics are not altered to any clinically relevant extent. Nevertheless patients with severe renal or hepatic impairment should be closely monitored (see also *Undesirable effects*).

*Children:* The safety and efficacy of Arthrotec 50 have not been established.

*Contra-indications:* Arthrotec 50 is contra-indicated in patients with active GI bleeding (see also *Precautions*).

Arthrotec 50 is contra-indicated is in pregna[n] women and in women planning a pregnancy as it ma[y] increase uterine tone and contractions in pregnanc[y] which could produce miscarriage. Also it may caus[e] premature closure of the ductus arteriosus.

Arthrotec 50 is contra-indicated in patients with known hypersensitivity to diclofenac, aspirin, othe[r] NSAIDs, misoprostol or other prostaglandins.

*Special warnings and special precautions for use:*
*Warnings:*

*Use in pre-menopausal women (see also Contra[-]indications):* Arthrotec 50 should not be used in pre[-]menopausal women unless they use effective contra[-]ception and have been advised of the risks of takin[g] the product if pregnant (see *Contra-indications*).

*Precautions:* Use in patients with known gastric [o]r duodenal ulceration should be avoided. If NSAI[D] therapy is still thought to be essential, then Arthrote[c] 50 may be considered. However, gastric and duodena[l] ulceration has been reported although less frequentl[y] than with diclofenac alone and use of Arthrotec 5[0] should be under close supervision.

Arthrotec 50 in common with other NSAIDs, ma[y] decrease platelet aggregation and prolong bleedin[g] time. This effect should be considered when bleedin[g] times are determined.

Fluid retention and oedema have been observed i[n] patients taking NSAIDs, including Arthrotec 50. There[-]fore, Arthrotec 50 should be used with caution i[n] patients with compromised cardiac function or con[-]ditions predisposing to fluid retention.

In patients with renal, cardiac or hepatic impairmen[t] caution is required since the use of NSAIDs may resu[lt] in deterioration of renal function. The dose should b[e] kept as low as possible and renal function should b[e] monitored.

All patients who are receiving long-term treatmen[t] with NSAIDs should be monitored as a precautiona[ry] measure (e.g. renal, hepatic function and bloo[d] counts).

*Interactions with other medicaments and other form[s] of interaction:* NSAIDs may attenuate the natriureti[c] efficacy of diuretics due to inhibition of intraren[al] synthesis of prostaglandins. Concomitant treatmen[t] with potassium-sparing diuretics may be associate[d] with increased serum potassium levels, hence seru[m] potassium should be monitored.

Steady state plasma lithium and digoxin levels ma[y] be increased.

Pharmacodynamic studies with diclofenac hav[e] shown no potentiation of oral hypoglycaemic an[d] anticoagulant drugs. However, as interactions hav[e] been reported with other NSAIDs, caution and ade[-]quate monitoring are nevertheless advised (see state[-]ment on platelet aggregation in *Precautions*).

Caution is advised when methotrexate is adminis[-]tered concurrently with NSAIDs because of possibl[e] enhancement of its toxicity by the NSAID as a resu[lt] of increase in methotrexate plasma levels.

*Pregnancy and lactation*

*Pregnancy:* Contra-indicated (see *Contra-indica[-]tions*).

*Lactation:* Arthrotec 50 should not be administere[d] during breast feeding.

*Effects on ability to drive and use machines:* Non[e] known.

*Undesirable effects:*

Gastrointestinal: Abdominal pain, diarrhoea, nau[-]sea, dyspepsia, flatulence, vomiting, gastritis, const[i]pation and eructation.

Diarrhoea is usually mild to moderate and transien[t] and can be minimised by taking Arthrotec 50 wit[h] food and by avoiding the use of predominant[ly] magnesium-containing antacids.

Liver: Clinically significant elevations of SGP[T,] SGOT, alkaline phosphatase or bilirubin have bee[n] observed in association with Arthrotec 50 withou[t] symptomatic evidence of hepatic disease.

Kidney: As a class NSAIDs have been associate[d] with renal pathology such as papillary necrosi[s,] interstitial nephritis, nephrotic syndrome and ren[al] failure.

Female reproductive system: Menorrhagia, inte[r]menstrual bleeding and vaginal bleeding have bee[n] reported in pre-menopausal women and vagin[al] bleeding in post-menopausal women.

Other adverse effects: Headache, dizziness and sk[in] rashes. Rarely, with NSAIDs, allergic reactions inclu[d]ing anaphylaxis may occur.

*Overdose:* The toxic dose of Arthrotec 50 has not bee[n] determined and there is no experience of overdosag[e.] Intensification of the pharmacological effects ma[y] occur with overdosage. Management of acute poiso[n]ing with NSAIDs essentially consists of supportiv[e] and symptomatic measures. It is reasonable to tak[e] measures to reduce absorption of any recently con[-]sumed drug by forced emesis, gastric lavage [or] activated charcoal.

**Pharmacological properties**

*Pharmacodynamic properties:* Arthrotec 50 is a non[-] steroidal, anti-inflammatory drug which is effective i[n] reating the signs and symptoms of arthritic conditions.

This activity is due to the presence of diclofenac which has been shown to have anti-inflammatory and analgesic properties.

Arthrotec 50 also contains the gastroduodenal mucosal protective component misoprostol which is a synthetic prostaglandin E₁ analogue that enhances several of the factors that maintain gastroduodenal mucosal integrity.

*Pharmacokinetic properties:* The pharmacokinetic profiles of diclofenac and misoprostol administered as Arthrotec 50 are similar to the profiles when the two drugs are administered as separate tablets. No pharmacokinetic interaction between the two drugs has been observed following multiple doses.

**Pharmaceutical particulars**
*List of excipients:* Arthrotec 50 tablets contain: Lactose, microcrystalline cellulose, maize starch, povidone K-30, cellulose acetate phthalate, diethyl phthalate, methylhydroxypropylcellulose, crospovidone, magnesium stearate, hydrogenated castor oil, colloidal anhydrous silica.

*Incompatibilities:* None known.

*Shelf-life:* Arthrotec 50 has a shelf-life of 3 years when stored in cold-formed blisters.

*Special precautions for storage:* Store in a dry place at or below 25°C.

*Nature and contents of container:* Arthrotec 50 is presented in cold-formed aluminium blisters in pack sizes of 60 and 140 tablets.

*Instructions for use/handling:* None.

*Marketing authorisation holder:* Monsanto p.l.c., PO Box 53, Lane End Road, High Wycombe, Bucks HP12 4HL.

**Marketing authorisation number** 08821/0006

**Date of approval/revision of SPC** March 1996.

**Legal category** POM.

## ARTHROTEC* 75

**Qualitative and quantitative composition** Each tablet consists of an enteric-coated core containing 75 mg diclofenac sodium surrounded by an outer mantle containing 200 mcg misoprostol.

**Pharmaceutical form** White, round, biconvex tablets marked ◇ on one side and 'Searle 1421' on the other side.

**Clinical particulars**
*Therapeutic indications:* Arthrotec 75 is indicated for patients who require a non-steroidal anti-inflammatory drug (NSAID) together with misoprostol.

The diclofenac component of Arthrotec 75 is indicated for the treatment of osteoarthritis and rheumatoid arthritis. The misoprostol component of Arthrotec 75 is indicated for the prophylaxis of NSAID-induced gastric and duodenal ulceration.

*Posology and method of administration:*
Adults: One tablet to be taken with food, twice daily. Tablets should be swallowed whole, not chewed.

*Elderly renal impairment/hepatic impairment:* No adjustment of dosage is necessary in the elderly or in patients with hepatic impairment or mild to moderate renal impairment as pharmacokinetics are not altered to any clinically relevant extent. Nevertheless patients with severe renal or hepatic impairment should be closely monitored (see also *Undesirable effects*).

*Children:* The safety and efficacy of Arthrotec 75 in children has not been established.

*Contra-indications:* Arthrotec 75 is contra-indicated in patients with active GI bleeding (see also *Precautions*).

Arthrotec 75 is contra-indicated in pregnant women and in women planning a pregnancy as it may increase uterine tone and contractions in pregnancy which could produce miscarriage. Also it may cause premature closure of the ductus arteriosus.

Arthrotec 75 is contra-indicated in patients with a known hypersensitivity to diclofenac, aspirin, other NSAIDs, misoprostol, other prostaglandins, or any other ingredient of the product.

*Special warnings and precautions for use:*
*Warnings:*
*Use in pre-menopausal women (see also Contra-indications):* Arthrotec 75 should not be used in pre-menopausal women unless they use effective contraception and have been advised of the risks of taking the product if pregnant (see *Contra-indications*).

*Precautions:* Use in patients with known gastric or duodenal ulceration should be avoided. If NSAID therapy is still thought to be essential, then Arthrotec 75 may be considered. However, gastric and duodenal ulceration have been reported, although less frequently than with diclofenac alone, and use of Arthrotec 75 should be under close supervision.

Arthrotec 75 in common with other NSAIDs, may decrease platelet aggregation and prolong bleeding time. This effect should be considered when bleeding times are determined.

Fluid retention and oedema have been observed in patients taking NSAIDs, including Arthrotec 75. Therefore, Arthrotec 75 should be used with caution in patients with compromised cardiac function or conditions predisposing to fluid retention.

In patients with renal, cardiac or hepatic impairment caution is required since the use of NSAIDs may result in deterioration of renal function. The dose should be kept as low as possible and renal function should be monitored.

All patients who are receiving long-term treatment with NSAIDs should be monitored as a precautionary measure (e.g. renal, hepatic function and blood counts).

*Interactions with other medicaments and other forms of interaction:* NSAIDs may attenuate the natriuretic efficacy of diuretics due to inhibition of intrarenal synthesis of prostaglandins. Concomitant treatment with potassium-sparing diuretics may be associated with increased serum potassium levels, hence serum potassium should be monitored.

Steady state plasma lithium and digoxin levels may be increased.

Pharmacodynamic studies with diclofenac have shown no potentiation of oral hypoglycaemic and anticoagulant drugs. However, as interactions have been reported with other NSAIDs, caution and adequate monitoring are nevertheless advised (see statement on platelet aggregation in *Precautions*).

Caution is advised when methotrexate is administered concurrently with NSAIDs because of possible enhancement of its toxicity by the NSAID as a result of increase in methotrexate plasma levels.

*Pregnancy and lactation:*
*Pregnancy:* Contra-indicated (See *Contra-indications*).
*Lactation:* Arthrotec 75 should not be administered during breast feeding.

*Effects on ability to drive and use machines:* None known.

*Undesirable effects:* Gastrointestinal: Abdominal pain, diarrhoea, nausea, dyspepsia, flatulence, vomiting, gastritis, constipation and eructation.

Diarrhoea is usually mild to moderate and transient and can be minimised by taking Arthrotec 75 with food and by avoiding the use of predominantly magnesium-containing antacids.

Liver: Clinically significant elevations of SGPT, SGOT, alkaline phosphatase or bilirubin have been observed in association with Arthrotec 75 without symptomatic evidence of hepatic disease.

Kidney: As a class NSAIDs have been associated with renal pathology such as papillary necrosis, interstitial nephritis, nephrotic syndrome and renal failure.

Female reproductive system: Menorrhagia, inter-menstrual bleeding and vaginal bleeding have been reported in pre-menopausal women and vaginal bleeding in post-menopausal women.

Other adverse effects: Headache, dizziness and skin rashes. Rarely, with NSAIDs, allergic reactions including anaphylaxis may occur.

*Overdose:* The toxic dose of Arthrotec 75 has been determined and there is no experience of overdosage. Intensification of the pharmacological effects may occur with overdosage. Management of acute poisoning with NSAIDs essentially consists of supportive and symptomatic measures. It is reasonable to take measures to reduce absorption of any recently consumed drug by forced emesis, gastric lavage or activated charcoal.

**Pharmacological properties**
*Pharmacodynamic properties:* Arthrotec 75 is a non-steroidal, anti-inflammatory drug which is effective in treating the signs and symptoms of arthritic conditions.

This activity is due to the presence of diclofenac which has been shown to have anti-inflammatory and analgesic properties.

Arthrotec 75 also contains the gastroduodenal mucosal protective component misoprostol which is a synthetic prostaglandin E₁ analogue that enhances several of the factors that maintain gastroduodenal mucosal integrity.

Arthrotec 75 administered BID provides 200 mcg less misoprostol than Arthrotec TID whilst providing the same daily dose (150 mg) of diclofenac and may offer a better therapeutic ratio for some patients.

*Pharmacokinetic properties:* The pharmacokinetic profiles of diclofenac and misoprostol administered as Arthrotec 75 are similar to the profiles when the two drugs are administered as separate tablets. No pharmacokinetic interaction between the two drugs has been observed following multiple doses.

*Preclinical safety data:* In co-administration studies, the addition of misoprostol did not enhance the toxic effects of diclofenac. The combination was also shown not to be teratogenic or mutagenic. The individual components show no evidence of carcinogenic potential.

Misoprostol in multiples of the recommended therapeutic dose in animals has produced gastric mucosal hyperplasia. This characteristic response to E-series prostaglandins reverts to normal on discontinuation of the compound.

**Pharmaceutical particulars**
*List of excipients:* Arthrotec 75 tablets contain: Lactose, microcrystalline cellulose, maize starch, povidone K-30, methylacrylic acid, sodium hydroxide, talc, triethylcitrate, methylhydroxypropylcellulose, crospovidone, magnesium stearate, hydrogenated castor oil, colloidal silicon dioxide.

*Incompatibilities:* None known.

*Shelf life:* Arthrotec 75 has a shelf-life of 3 years when stored in cold-formed blisters.

*Special precautions for storage:* Store in a dry place, at or below 25°C.

*Nature and contents of container:* Arthrotec 75 is presented in cold formed aluminium blisters in pack sizes of 60 tablets.

*Instructions for use/handling:* None.

*Marketing authorisation holder:* Monsanto p.l.c., PO Box 53, Lane End Road, High Wycombe, Bucks HP12 4HL.

**Marketing authorisation number** 08821/0044.

**Date of approval/revision of SPC** February 1996.

**Legal category** POM.

## BREVINOR* TABLETS

**Qualitative and quantitative composition** Each tablet contains 0.5 milligrams Norethisterone BP and 35 micrograms Ethinyloestradiol BP.

**Pharmaceutical form** White, flat, circular, bevel-edged tablet inscribed 'SYNTEX' on one side and 'B' on the other side.

**Clinical particulars**
*Therapeutic indications:* Brevinor is indicated for oral contraception, with the benefit of a low intake of oestrogen.

*Posology and method of administration:*
*Oral administration:* The dosage of Brevinor for the initial cycle of therapy is 1 tablet taken at the same time each day from the first day of the menstrual cycle. For subsequent cycles, no tablets are taken for 7 days, then a new course is started of 1 tablet daily for the next 21 days. This sequence of 21 days on treatment, seven days off treatment is repeated for as long as contraception is required.

Patients unable to start taking Brevinor tablets on the first day of the menstrual cycle may start treatment on any day up to and including the 5th day of the menstrual cycle.

Patients starting on day 1 of their period will be protected at once. Those patients delaying therapy up to day 5 may not be protected immediately and it is recommended that another method of contraception is used for the first 7 days of tablet-taking. Suitable methods are condoms, caps plus spermicides and intra-uterine devices. The rhythm, temperature and cervical-mucus methods should not be relied upon.

*Tablet omissions:* Tablets must be taken daily in order to maintain adequate hormone levels and contraceptive efficacy.

If a tablet is missed within 12 hours of the correct dosage time then the missed tablet should be taken as soon as possible, even if this means taking 2 tablets on the same day, this will ensure that contraceptive protection is maintained. If one or more tablets are missed for more than 12 hours from the correct dosage time it is recommended that the patient takes the last missed tablet as soon as possible and then continues to take the rest of the tablets in the normal manner. In addition, it is recommended that extra contraceptive protection, such as a condom, is used for the next 7 days.

Patients who have missed one or more of the last 7 tablets in a pack should be advised to start the next pack of tablets as soon as the present one has finished (i.e. without the normal seven day gap between treatments). This reduces the risk of contraceptive failure resulting from tablets being missed close to a 7 day tablet free period.

*Changing from another oral contraceptive:* In order to ensure that contraception is maintained it is advised that the first dose of Brevinor tablets is taken on the day immediately after the patient has finished the previous pack of tablets.

*Use after childbirth, miscarriage or abortion:* Providing the patient is not breast feeding the first dose of

Brevinor tablets should be taken on the 21st day after childbirth. This will ensure the patient is protected immediately. If there is any delay in taking the first dose, contraception may not be established until 7 days after the first tablet has been taken. In these circumstances patients should be advised that extra contraceptive methods will be necessary.

After a miscarriage or abortion patients can take the first dose of Brevinor tablets on the next day; in this way they will be protected immediately.

*Contra-indications:* As with all combined progestogen/oestrogen oral contraceptives, the following conditions should be regarded as contra-indications:

(i) Thrombophlebitis, thrombo-embolic disorders, cerebrovascular disorders, coronary artery disease, myocardial infarction, angina, hyperlipidaemia or a history of these conditions.

(ii) Acute or severe chronic liver disease, including liver tumours, Dubin-Johnson or Rotor syndrome.

(iii) History during pregnancy of idiopathic jaundice, severe pruritus or pemphigoid gestationis.

(iv) Known or suspected breast or genital cancer.

(v) Known or suspected oestrogen-dependent neoplasia.

(vi) Undiagnosed abnormal vaginal bleeding.

(vii) A history of migraines classified as classical focal or crescendo.

(viii) Pregnancy.

*Special warnings and special precautions for use:* Women taking oral contraceptives require careful observation if they have or have had any of the following conditions: breast nodules; fibrocystic disease of the breast or an abnormal mammogram; uterine fibroids; a history of severe depressive states; varicose veins; sickle-cell anaemia; diabetes; hypertension; cardiovascular disease; migraine; epilepsy; asthma; otosclerosis; multiple sclerosis; porphyria; tetany; disturbed liver functions; gallstones; kidney disease; chloasma; any condition that is likely to worsen during pregnancy. The worsening or first appearance of any of these conditions may indicate that the oral contraceptive should be stopped. Discontinue treatment if there is a gradual or sudden, partial or complete loss of vision or any evidence of ocular changes, onset or aggravation of migraine or development of headache of a new kind which is recurrent, persistent or severe.

Gastro-intestinal upsets, such as vomiting and diarrhoea, may interfere with the absorption of the tablets leading to a reduction in contraceptive efficacy. Patients should continue to take Brevinor, but they should also be encouraged to use another contraceptive method during the period of gastro-intestinal upset and for the next 7 days.

Progestogen/oestrogen preparations should be used with caution in patients with a history of hepatic dysfunction or hypertension.

A statistical association between the use of oral contraceptives and the occurrence of thrombosis, embolism or haemorrhage has been reported. Patients receiving oral contraceptives should be kept under regular surveillance, in view of the possibility of development of conditions such as thromboembolism.

The risk of coronary artery disease in women taking oral contraceptives is increased by the presence of other predisposing factors such as cigarette smoking, hypercholesterolaemia, obesity, diabetes, history of pre-eclamptic toxaemia and increasing age. After the age of thirty-five years, the patient and physician should carefully re-assess the risk/benefit ratio of using combined oral contraceptives as opposed to alternative methods of contraception.

Brevinor should be discontinued at least four weeks before, and for two weeks following, elective operations and during immobilisation. Patients undergoing injection treatment for varicose veins should not resume taking Brevinor until 3 months after the last injection.

Benign and malignant liver tumours have been associated with oral contraceptive use. The relationship between occurrence of liver tumours and use of female sex hormones is not known at present. These tumours may rupture causing intra-abdominal bleeding. If the patient presents with a mass or tenderness in the right upper quadrant or an acute abdomen, the possible presence of a tumour should be considered.

An increased risk of congenital abnormalities, including heart defects and limb defects, has been reported following the use of sex hormones, including oral contraceptives, in pregnancy. If the patient does not adhere to the prescribed schedule, the possibility of pregnancy should be considered at the time of the first missed period and further use of oral contraceptives should be withheld until pregnancy has been ruled out. It is recommended that for any patient who has missed two consecutive periods, pregnancy should be ruled out before continuing the contraceptive regimen. If pregnancy is confirmed the patient should be advised of the potential risks to the foetus and the advisability of continuing the pregnancy should be discussed in the light of these risks. It is advisable to discontinue Brevinor three months before a planned pregnancy.

The risk of arterial thrombosis associated with combined oral contraceptives increases with age, and this risk is aggravated by cigarette smoking. The use of combined oral contraceptives by women in the older age group, especially those who are cigarette smokers, should therefore be discouraged and alternative methods advised.

The use of this product in patients suffering from epilepsy, migraine, asthma or cardiac dysfunction may result in exacerbation of these disorders because of fluid retention. Caution should also be observed in patients who wear contact lenses.

Decreased glucose tolerance may occur in diabetic patients on this treatment, and their control must be carefully supervised.

The use of oral contraceptives has also been associated with a possible increased incidence of gall bladder disease.

Women with a history of oligomenorrhoea or secondary amenorrhoea or young women without regular cycles may have a tendency to remain anovulatory or to become amenorrhoeic after discontinuation of oral contraceptives. Women with these pre-existing problems should be advised of this possibility and encouraged to use other contraceptive methods.

Numerous epidemiological studies have been reported on the risks of ovarian, endometrial, cervical and breast cancer in women using combined oral contraceptives. The evidence is clear that combined oral contraceptives offer substantial protection against both ovarian and endometrial cancer.

An increased risk of cervical cancer in long-term users of combined oral contraceptives has been reported in some studies, but there continues to be controversy about the extent to which this is attributable to the confounding effects of sexual behaviour and other factors.

The evidence linking combined oral contraceptive use and breast cancer remains inconclusive. The results of some studies suggest an increased risk of breast cancer presenting below the age of about 35, the risk rising with duration of use. Any possible increased risk of breast cancer with combined oral contraceptives is however likely to be small, and may be expected to be less with low dosage pills. The possible risk should be weighed against the many benefits of combined oral contraceptives, including their protective effects against ovarian and endometrial cancers.

*Interactions with other medicaments and other forms of interaction:* Some drugs may modify the metabolism of Brevinor reducing its effectiveness; these include certain sedatives, antibiotics, anti-epileptic and anti-arthritic drugs. During the time such agents are used concurrently, it is advised that mechanical contraceptives also be used.

The results of a large number of laboratory tests have been shown to be influenced by the use of oestrogen containing oral contraceptives, which may limit their diagnostic value. Among these are: biochemical markers of thyroid and liver function; plasma levels of carrier proteins, triglycerides, coagulation and fibrinolysis factors.

*Pregnancy and lactation:* Contra-indicated in pregnancy.

Patients who are fully breast-feeding should not take Brevinor tablets since, in common with other combined oral contraceptives, the oestrogen component may reduce the amount of milk produced. In addition, active ingredients or their metabolites have been detected in the milk of mothers taking oral contraceptives. The effect of Brevinor on breast-fed infants has not been determined.

*Effects on ability to drive and use machines:* None.

*Undesirable effects:* As with all oral contraceptives, there may be slight nausea at first, weight gain or breast discomfort, which soon disappear.

Other side-effects known or suspected to occur with oral contraceptives include gastro-intestinal symptoms, changes in libido and appetite, headache, exacerbation of existing uterine fibroid disease, depression, and changes in carbohydrate, lipid and vitamin metabolism.

Spotting or bleeding may occur during the first few cycles. Usually menstrual bleeding becomes light and occasionally there may be no bleeding during the tablet-free days.

Hypertension, which is usually reversible on discontinuing treatment, has occurred in a small percentage of women taking oral contraceptives.

*Overdose:* Overdosage may be manifested by nausea, vomiting, breast enlargement and vaginal bleeding. There is no specific antidote and treatment should be symptomatic. Gastric lavage may be employed if the overdose is large and the patient is seen sufficiently early (within four hours).

**Pharmacological properties**

*Pharmacodynamic properties:* The mode of action c Brevinor is similar to that of other progestogen oestrogen oral contraceptives and includes the inhibition of ovulation, the thickening of cervical mucus so as to constitute a barrier to sperm and the rendering of the endometrium unreceptive to implantation. Such activity is exerted through a combined effect on one or more of the following hypothalamus, anterior pituitary, ovary, endometrium and cervical mucus.

*Pharmacokinetic properties:* Norethisterone is rapidly and completely absorbed after oral administration peak plasma concentrations occurring in the majority of subjects between 1 and 3 hours. Due to first-pass metabolism, blood levels after oral administration are 60% of those after i.v. administration. The half life of elimination varies from 5 to 12 hours, with a mean of 7.6 hours. Norethisterone is metabolised mainly in the liver. Approximately 60% of the administered dose is excreted as metabolites in urine and faeces.

Ethinyloestradiol is rapidly and well absorbed from the gastro-intestinal tract but is subject to some first pass metabolism in the gut-wall. Compared to many other oestrogens it is only slowly metabolised in the liver. Excretion is via the kidneys with some appearing also in the faeces.

*Preclinical safety data:* The toxicity of norethisterone is very low. Reports of teratogenic effects in animals are uncommon. No carcinogenic effects have been found even in long-term studies.

Long-term continuous administration of oestrogens in some animals increases the frequency of carcinoma of the breast, cervix, vagina and liver.

**Pharmaceutical particulars**

*List of excipients:* Brevinor tablets contain: Maize starch, povidone, magnesium stearate and lactose.

*Incompatibilities:* None stated.

*Shelf life:* The shelf life of Brevinor tablets is 5 years.

*Special precautions for storage:* Store in a dry place below 25°C, away from direct sunlight.

*Nature and contents of container:* Brevinor tablets are supplied in pvc/foil blister packs of 63 tablets.

*Special instructions for use/handling:* None.

*Marketing authorisation holder:* Monsanto p.l.c., PO Box 53, Lane End Road, High Wycombe, Buck HP12 4HL.

**Marketing authorisation number** 08821/0037.

**Date of approval/revision of SPC** March 1996.

**Legal category** POM.

## CYTOTEC*

**Presentation** White/off-white, hexagonal tablet scored on both sides, engraved 'SEARLE 1461' on one side. Each tablet contains misoprostol 200 micrograms.

**Uses**

*Indications:* Cytotec is indicated for the healing of duodenal ulcer and gastric ulcer including those induced by nonsteroidal anti-inflammatory drugs (NSAID) in arthritic patients at risk, whilst continuing their NSAID therapy. In addition Cytotec can be used for the prophylaxis of NSAID-induced ulcers.

*Actions:* Cytotec is an analogue of naturally occurring prostaglandin $E_1$ which promotes peptic ulcer healing and symptomatic relief.

Cytotec protects the gastroduodenal mucosa by inhibiting basal, stimulated and nocturnal acid secretion and by reducing the volume of gastric secretions, the proteolytic activity of the gastric fluid, and increasing bicarbonate and mucus secretion.

**Dosage and administration**

*Adults:*

*Healing of duodenal ulcer, gastric ulcer and NSAID induced peptic ulcer:* 800 micrograms daily in two or four divided doses taken with breakfast and/or each main meal and at bedtime.

Treatment should be given initially for at least weeks even if symptomatic relief has been achieved sooner. In most patients ulcers will be healed in weeks but treatment may be continued for up to weeks if required. If the ulcer relapses further treatment courses may be given.

*Prophylaxis of NSAID-induced peptic ulcer:* 200 micrograms twice daily, three times daily or four times daily. Treatment can be continued as required. Dosage should be individualised according to the clinical condition of each patient.

*Elderly:* The usual dosage may be used.

*Renal impairment:* Available evidence indicates that no adjustment of dosage is necessary in patients with renal impairment.

*Hepatic impairment:* Cytotec is metabolised by fatty acid oxidising systems present in organs throughou the body. Its metabolism and plasma levels are therefore unlikely to be affected markedly in patients with hepatic impairment.

*Children:* Use of Cytotec in children has not yet been evaluated in the treatment of peptic ulceration or NSAID-induced peptic ulcer disease.

**Contra-indications, warnings, etc**

*Contra-indications:* Cytotec is contra-indicated in pregnant women and in women planning a pregnancy as it increases uterine tone and contractions in pregnancy which may cause partial or complete expulsion of the products of conception. It is also contra-indicated in patients with a known allergy to prostaglandins.

*Warnings*

*Use in pre-menopausal women (see also Contra-indications):* Cytotec should not be used in pre-menopausal women unless the patient requires non-steroidal anti-inflammatory (NSAID) therapy and is at high risk of complications from NSAID-induced ulceration.

In such patients it is advised that Cytotec should only be used if the patient:

—takes effective contraceptive measures

—has been advised of the risks of taking Cytotec if pregnant (see Contra-indications).

*Precautions:* The results of clinical studies indicate that Cytotec does not produce hypotension at dosages effective in promoting the healing of gastric and duodenal ulcers. Nevertheless, Cytotec should be used with caution in the presence of disease states where hypotension might precipitate severe complications, eg, cerebrovascular disease, coronary artery disease or severe peripheral vascular disease including hypertension.

There is no evidence that Cytotec has adverse effects on glucose metabolism in human volunteers or patients with diabetes mellitus.

*Drug interactions:* Cytotec is predominantly metabolised via fatty acid oxidising systems and has shown no adverse effect on the hepatic microsomal mixed function oxidase (P450) enzyme system. In specific studies no clinically significant pharmacokinetic interaction has been demonstrated with antipyrine, diazepam and propranolol. In extensive clinical studies no drug interactions have been attributed to Cytotec. Additional evidence shows no clinically important pharmacokinetic or pharmacodynamic interaction with nonsteroidal anti-inflammatory drugs including aspirin, diclofenac and ibuprofen.

*Pregnancy:* See Contra-indications.

*Lactation:* It is not known if the active metabolite of Cytotec is excreted in breast milk, therefore Cytotec should not be administered during breast feeding.

*Adverse effects:*

*Gastrointestinal system:* Diarrhoea has been reported and is occasionally severe and prolonged and may require withdrawal of the drug. It can be minimised by using single doses not exceeding 200 micrograms with food and by avoiding the use of predominantly magnesium containing antacids when an antacid is required.

Abdominal pain with or without associated dyspepsia or diarrhoea can follow misoprostol therapy.

Other gastrointestinal adverse effects reported include dyspepsia, flatulence, nausea and vomiting.

*Female reproductive system:* Menorrhagia, vaginal bleeding and intermenstrual bleeding have been reported in pre- and post-menopausal women.

*Other adverse events:* Skin rashes have been reported. Dizziness has been infrequently reported.

The pattern of adverse events associated with Cytotec is similar when an NSAID is given concomitantly.

*Overdosage:* Intensification of pharmacological effects may occur with overdose. In the event of overdosage symptomatic and supportive therapy should be given as appropriate. In clinical trials patients have tolerated 1200 micrograms daily for three months without significant adverse effects.

**Pharmaceutical precautions** Store in a dry place below 30°C (86°F).

**Legal category** POM.

**Package quantities** Foil/foil blister pack of 60 (OP).

**Further information** Cytotec in multiples of the recommended therapeutic dose in animals has produced gastric mucosal hyperplasia. This characteristic response to E prostaglandins reverts to normal on discontinuation of the compound. In patients, histological examination of gastric biopsies taken before and after treatment with misoprostol after up to one year's duration have shown no adverse tissue response attributable to misoprostol.

Inhibition of gastric secretion by Cytotec is achieved by a combination of local and systemic effects. Cytotec is rapidly absorbed following oral administration, with peak plasma levels of the active metabolite (misoprostol acid) occurring after about 30 minutes. The plasma elimination half-life of misoprostol acid is 20–40 minutes. No accumulation of misoprostol acid in plasma occurs after repeated dosing of 400 micrograms twice daily.

**Product licence number** 08821/0019.

# DRAMAMINE*

**Qualitative and quantitative composition** Each tablet contains 50 mg Dimenhydrinate BP.

**Pharmaceutical form** Tablet.

**Clinical particulars**

*Therapeutic indications:* For OTC pack only: Motion sickness.

For non-OTC packs: Motion sickness, vertigo, nausea and vomiting associated with Meniere's disease and other labyrinthine disorders.

*Posology and method of administration:* For prevention of motion sickness the first dose should be taken 30 minutes before the journey.

*Adults and children over 12 years:* 1–2 tablets two or three times daily.

*Elderly:* Dosage as for adults. The elderly may be more susceptible to anticholinergic side effects.

*Children:* 1–6 years $\frac{1}{4}$–$\frac{1}{2}$ tablet two or three times daily.
7–12 years $\frac{1}{2}$–1 tablet two or three times daily.

*Contra-indications:* Dramamine is contra-indicated in patients with a hypersensitivity to dimenhydrinate, diphenhydramine and other antihistamines of similar chemical structure.

*Special warnings and precautions for use:*

*Warnings:* For OTC pack only: Warning: May cause drowsiness, if affected do not drive or operate machinery.

*Precautions:* Dimenhydrinate should be used with caution in patients having conditions which might be aggravated by anticholinergic therapy i.e. with raised intraocular pressure, stenosing peptic ulcer, pyloroduodenal obstruction, prostatic hypertrophy, asthma, hypertension, hyperthyroidism or severe coronary artery disease.

Dimenhydrinate should be used with caution in patients with hepatic or renal failure due to the risk of accumulation in such patients.

*Interactions with other medicaments and other forms of interaction:* For OTC pack only: Avoid alcoholic drink.

For non-OTC pack: In common with other antihistamines, Dramamine may potentiate the sedative effects of CNS depressants including alcohol, barbiturates, narcotic analgesics, tranquillisers and may enhance the effects of antoicholinergics such as atropine and tricyclic antidepressants. Dramamine may enhance the effect of ephedrine. Monamine oxidase inhibitors may potentiate the anticholinergic and sedative effects of antihistamines.

Dramamine may mask ototoxic symptoms associated with certain antibiotics. Patients should be advised to avoid alcoholic drinks.

Antihistamines may mask the response of the skin to allergenic skin tests.

*Pregnancy and lactation:*

*Pregnancy:* For OTC pack only: Use during pregnancy should be on the advice of your doctor.

For non-OTC pack: Reproduction studies in rats and rabbits at doses up to 20 and 25 times the human dose respectively (on a mg/kg basis) have shown no evidence of hazard.

There is inadequate evidence of safety of the use of Dramamine in human pregnancy although it has been in wide use for many years without apparent ill consequences. In view of this Dramamine should be used during pregnancy only if clearly needed.

*Lactation:* Diphenhydramine, a metabolite of dimenhydrinate, has been detected in breast milk. If a nursing mother is taking Dramamine the infant may exhibit some effects of the drug. In view of this Dramamine should not be administered during breast feeding unless considered essential.

*Effects on ability to drive and use machines:* In common with other antihistamines Dramamine may cause drowsiness. Patients affected in this way should be advised not to drive or operate machinery.

*Undesirable effects:* For OTC pack only: When used for the prevention and treatment of motion sickness, sedation is the most commonly reported effect. Occasionally allergy or anaphylaxis have been reported.

For non-OTC pack only: Sedation is the most commonly reported effect. Incoordination and confusion (particularly in the elderly) may also occur. Occasionally allergy and anaphylaxis have been reported. Atropine-like effects such as blurred vision, dry mouth, tachycardia, constipation, urinary hesitancy, tightness of the chest and thickening of secretions may be associated with antihistamines. Other adverse effects which may occur include: tremors, paradoxical excitability (especially in children), skin rash and photosensitivity.

*Overdose:* Symptoms of overdosage may comprise drowsiness, dizziness and ataxia together with anticholinergic effects such as dry mouth, flushing of the face, dilated pupils, tachycardia, pyrexia, headache and urinary retention.

In massive overdose and in children the central effects of antihistamines may cause convulsions, hallucinations, excitement and respiratory depression. Such symptoms may be delayed. Treatment should consist of gastric aspiration and lavage, administration of activated charcoal and supportive measures. Diazepam may be required for the treatment of convulsions.

**Pharmacological properties**

*Pharmacodynamic properties:* The active ingredient of Dramamine, dimehydrinate is the chlorotheophylline salt of diphenhydramine and is an $H_1$-receptor blocking agent.

*Pharmacokinetic properties:* An unpublished study of dimenhydrinate 50 mg in 12 volunteers demonstrated mean peak plasma concentrations of 72.1 mg/ml at a mean of 2.29 hours.

*Preclinical safety data:* In acute toxicity studies in rats and mice (oral, i.p.) LD50s of 149–203 mg/kg (mouse) and 1,320 mg/kg (rat) were determined. Subacute studies in cats (50–100 mg/kg) produced no pathological changes in major body organs and chronic studies in rodents at a mean dose of 22 mg/kg/day showed no abnormalities. Reproduction studies in rats and rabbits at 20–25 times the human dose (mg/kg) have showed no evidence of foetotoxicity.

**Pharmaceutical particulars**

*List of excipients:* Dramamine contains lactose, corn starch, pre-gelatinised maize starch and magnesium stearate.

*Incompatibilities:* None known.

*Shelf life:* Dramamine tablets have a shelf life of 5 years when packed in foil/PVC blister packs or amber glass bottles and 3 years when packed in HDPE bottles.

*Special precautions for storage:* Store below 30°C.

*Nature and contents of container:* OTC pack: Foil/PVC blister strips containing 10 tablets in a cardboard carton.

Non-OTC pack: 100 or 500 tablets packed in amber glass bottles with screw caps or HDPE bottles with a tamper-evident closure. Bottles are enclosed within a cardboard carton.

*Instructions for use/handling:* Dramamine may be powdered and dissolved in any acceptable aqueous fluid medium, provided that a concentration of 3 mg/ml is not exceeded. Above this concentration not all of the active constituent may dissolve.

*Marketing authorisation holder:* Monsanto p.l.c., PO Box 53, Lane End Road, High Wycombe, Bucks HP12 4HL.

**Marketing authorisation number** 8821/0035.

**Date of approval/revision of SPC** January 1996.

**Legal category** P.

# EFALITH* OINTMENT

**Presentation** Efalith Ointment is a white to off-white water in oil emulsion containing lithium succinate 8% w/w and zinc sulphate 0.05% w/w.

**Uses** Efalith is indicated for the topical treatment and symptomatic relief of seborrheoic dermatitis.

**Dosage and administration** Efalith may be administered to adults, the elderly and children of 12 years of age and over.

The ointment should be applied thinly and evenly to affected areas and rubbed in gently, twice daily in the morning and evening. This dosage regime should be continued until improvement occurs, usually within four weeks. It may then be possible to maintain this improvement in the long-term by applying the ointment less fequently or on an intermittent basis.

**Contra-indications, warnings, etc**

*Contra-indications:* Administration to children under 12 years of age. Known sensitivity to wool alcohols or paraffins.

*Precautions:* Caution should be used when applying Efalith to or near eyelids and mucous membranes. Psoriasis may be exacerbated by oral lithium therapy. No formal studies have been conducted in patients with psoriasis and, therefore, Efalith should be used with caution in such patients.

*Pregnancy and lactation:* As with all medicines, Efalith should not be used during the first trimester of pregnancy if this can be avoided. Teratogenic effects in animals are known to occur following oral administration of lithium salts. However, animal and clinical studies have shown that Efalith, applied topically, is not systemically absorbed or accumulated.

Efalith may be administered to breast-feeding mothers if care is taken not to apply it to the breasts so as to avoid possible oral ingestion by infants.

*Adverse effects:* Mild and transient irritation to skin and eyelids at sites of application have been reported occasionally.

**Pharmaceutical precautions** Store in a cool place.

**Legal category** POM.

**Package quantities** Each tube contains 20 g.

**Further information** Efalith also contains wool alcohols and hard, soft and liquid paraffins as excipients.

**Product licence number** 4382/0009.

## EFAMAST*

**Qualitative and quantitative composition**

| *Active constituent* | *Quantity/dose unit* |
|---|---|
| Gamolenic acid (provided by Evening Primrose Oil) | 40 mg |
| *Other constituents:* | |
| D-alpha tocopherol acetate | 10 mg |
| *Capsule shell* | |
| Gelatin | 166 mg |
| Glycerol | 77 mg |
| Water | qs |

**Pharmaceutical form** Soft gelatin capsules.

**Clinical particulars**

*Therapeutic indications:* Efamast is indicated for the symptomatic relief of pre-menstrual breast pain (cyclical mastalgia) and non-cyclical mastalgia.

*Posology and method of administration: Adults and elderly:* 3–4 capsules should be taken orally twice daily, providing a total dose of 6–8 capsules.

It is suggested that patients start treatment at the highest recommended dose.

Some patients may not begin to show a clinical response to treatment for 8–12 weeks due to the gradual onset of action of Efamast. Once a clinical response has been achieved, the treatment may be stopped or continued at a lower maintenance dose.

*Contra-indications:* None known.

*Special warnings and precautions for use:* Breast pain may occasionally be a symptom of breast cancer. The doctor should be satisfied that the patient does not have breast cancer.

*Interactions with other medicaments and other forms of interaction:* Efamast may have the potential to make manifest undiagnosed temporal lobe epilepsy, especially in schizophrenic patients and/or those who are receiving known epileptogenic drugs such as the phenothiazines. Physicians are advised to monitor carefully the effects of Efamast in patients on epileptogenic drugs, or in any individuals with a history of epilepsy. No epileptic events have been reported in patients not being treated with phenothiazines.

*Pregnancy and lactation:*

*Pregnancy:* No teratogenic effects have been observed in animal studies. However, as with all medicines, caution is advised concerning administration in the first trimester of pregnancy.

*Lactation:* Efamast may be taken while breast feeding.

*Effects on ability to drive and use machines:* None.

*Undesirable effects:* No major adverse effects have been reported. Nausea, indigestion and headache have occurred occasionally. In rare cases, hypersensitivity reactions, including rash, urticaria, pruritus and abdominal pain have been reported. It should be noted that hypersensitivity reactions may require close medical surveillance and that such reactions may occur particularly in patients who have a history of food or other allergies.

*Overdose:* The only symptom noted in a few cases has been loose stools sometimes accompanied by abdominal pains. No special treatment is required.

There is a high degree of tolerance to evening primrose oil. Up to 25 ml of oil (equivalent to 50 capsules) has been administered daily for one year to children aged 5–12 years, without adverse effects other than occasional loose stools.

**Pharmacological properties**

*Pharmacodynamic properties:* Efamast capsules provide an exogenous source of gamolenic acid (GLA), which may be used to restore some subnormal fatty acid levels towards physiologically normal levels.

Clinical studies demonstrate that it improves the symptoms of mastalgia, however the precise pharmacological mode of action is unclear. No undesirable pharmacological effects are known.

*Pharmacokinetic properties:* The pharmacokinetic profile of evening primrose oil follows that of any normal triglycerides from usual dietary sources. It is approximately 95% absorbed, metabolised in the liver and stored principally in adipose tissue.

There are no unusual pharmacokinetic properties. Gamolenic acid is the unusual fatty acid component of evening primrose oil. It is metablised rapidly to dihomogammalinolenic acid (DGLA) in the body. DGLA levels will fall to pre-treatment levels in approximately two weeks following withdrawal of evening primrose oil.

*Preclinical safety data:* None of relevance to the prescriber.

**Pharmaceutical particulars** *List of excipients:* D-alpha tocopherol acetate, gelatin, glycerol, water.

*Incompatibilities:* None known.

*Shelf life:* 3 years in marketed pack.

*Special precautions for storage:* Store in a dry place protected from heat.

*Nature and contents of container:* (1) Marketed pack: PVC/PVDC blister pack (250/40 μm) with lacquered hard temper aluminium foil (20 μm) plus cardboard outer carton.

(2) Sample pack: Blister pack as above, in a plastic wallet.

*Instructions for use/handling:* For oral administration.

*Marketing authorisation holder:* Scotia Pharmaceuticals Limited, Woodbridge Meadows, Guildford, Surrey GU1 1BA.

**Marketing authorisation number** 4382/0010.

**Date of approval/revision of SPC** May 1996.

**Legal category** POM.

## ELLESTE DUET* 1 mg

**Qualitative and quantitative composition** 16 tablets each containing 1 mg oestradiol, 12 tablets each containing 1 mg oestradiol and 1 mg norethisterone acetate.

**Pharmaceutical form** Tablets for oral administration.

**Clinical particulars**

*Therapeutic indications:* The treatment of menopausal symptoms such as sweating, flushes. Prophylaxis and treatment of the postmenopausal sequelae of oestrogen withdrawal, e.g. atrophic vaginitis, atrophic urethritis.

Elleste Duet 1 mg is designed to provide continuous oestrogen and monthly cyclical progestogen therapy after the climacteric. Oestrogen administration is continued without a break in therapy. The addition of a progestogen in the second half of each course helps to provide good control of the irregular cycles that are characteristic of the premenopausal phase and opposes the production of endometrial hyperplasia.

Patients who have undergone a hysterectomy do not require the addition of a progestogen to the treatment regimen and should use an oestrogen only preparation.

*Posology and method of administration:*

*Adults:* One white tablet to be taken daily for the first 16 days followed by one pale green tablet for the next 12 days. A new cycle should then begin without any break. Therapy may start at any time in patients with established amenorrhoea or who are experiencing long intervals between spontaneous menses.

In patients who are menstruating regularly, it is advised that therapy starts on the second day of bleeding. Patients changing from another cyclical preparation should complete the cycle and may then change to Elleste Duet 1 mg without a break in therapy.

*Elderly:* There are no special dosage requirements for elderly patients.

*Children:* Not to be used in children.

*Contra-indications:* Known or suspected pregnancy, lactation.

Active deep venous thrombosis, thromboembolic disorders, or a past history of these conditions.

Known or suspected cancer of the breast except in appropriately selected patients being treated for metastatic disease.

Known or suspected oestrogen-dependent neoplasia.

Abnormal genital bleeding, endometriosis.

Severe cardiac disease.

Severe renal disease.

Sickle cell anaemia.

Congenital disturbances of lipid metabolism.

Severe diabetes mellitus with vascular changes.

Acute or chronic liver disease or a history of liver disease when the liver function tests have failed to return to normal. Previous or existing liver tumours. Rotor syndrome or Dubin-Johnson syndrome. Jaundice or general pruritus during previous pregnancy.

*Special warnings and precautions for use:* Before starting treatment, pregnancy must be excluded. If the expected bleeding fails to occur at about 28-day intervals, treatment should be stopped until pregnancy has been ruled out.

Before starting Elleste Duet patients should have a thorough general medical and gynaecological examination with special emphasis on the body weight, blood pressure, heart, pelvic organs with an endometrial assessment if indicated, the legs and skin. Follow-up examinations are recommended at least six-monthly during treatment.

Breakthrough bleeding may occasionally occur and can be the result of poor compliance or concurrent antibiotic use. It may however indicate endometrial pathology and therefore any doubt as to its cause is an indication for endometrial evaluation, including biopsy.

Epidemiological evidence suggests that use of hormone replacement therapy (HRT) is associated with an increased relative risk of developing deep vein thrombosis (DVT) or pulmonary embolism (PE). Although this increase in relative risk is about 2–3, for healthy women the excess absolute risk of either of these conditions is about 1 in 5000 per year while taking HRT.

The increased risk of VTE means that caution should be exercised in using HRT in women who are likely to be at high risk of DVT or PE. Women with severe varicose veins, severe obesity (Body Mass Index >30 kg/m²), immobilisation for 3 weeks or more, trauma or surgery requiring bed rest, are at increased risk of VTE so that the benefits of treatment with HRT will need to be weighed against risks carefully.

Where elective surgery is planned requiring subsequent bed rest HRT should be stopped four weeks prior to surgery.

If venous thromboembolism develops after initiating therapy the drug should be discontinued.

Treatment should be stopped at once if migrainous or frequent and unusually severe headaches occur for the first time, or if there are other symptoms that are possible prodromata of vascular occlusion e.g. sudden visual disturbances.

Treatment should be stopped at once if jaundice, cholestasis, hepatitis or pregnancy occurs, or if there is a significant rise in blood pressure, the occurrence of thromboembolic disease or an increase in epileptic seizures.

Pre-existing fibroids may increase in size under the influence of oestrogens, and symptoms associated with endometriosis may be exacerbated. If this is observed, treatment should be discontinued.

There is an increased risk of gall bladder disease in women receiving postmenopausal oestrogens.

In patients with mild chronic liver disease, liver function should be checked every 8–12 weeks.

There is an increased risk of endometrial hyperplasia and carcinoma associated with unopposed oestrogen administered long-term (for more than one year). However, the appropriate addition of a progestogen to the oestrogen regimen statistically lowers the risk.

At the present time there is some evidence which suggests a slight increase in the relative risk of breast cancer in postmenopausal women receiving long-term hormone replacement therapy (more than 5 years). It is not known whether concurrent progestogen use influences this risk. Women on long-term therapy should have regular breast examinations and should be instructed in self-examination of the breasts. Regular mammographic investigation should be conducted where it is considered appropriate.

Women with diseases that are known to be subject to deterioration during pregnancy (e.g. multiple sclerosis, epilepsy, diabetes, benign breast disease, hypertension, cardiac or renal dysfunction, asthma, melanoma, systemic lupus erythematosus, tetany and otosclerosis) and women with a strong family history of breast cancer should be carefully observed during treatment.

In rare cases benign and in even rarer cases malignant liver tumours leading in isolated cases to life-threatening intra-abdominal haemorrhage have been observed after the use of hormonal substances such as those contained in Elleste Duet. If severe upper abdominal complaints, enlarged liver, or signs of intra-abdominal haemorrhage occur, a liver tumour should be considered in the differential diagnosis.

Oestrogens may cause fluid retention and therefore patients with cardiac or renal dysfunction should be carefully observed.

Most studies indicate that oestrogen replacement therapy has little effect on blood pressure. Some show that it may decrease blood pressure. In addition studies on combined therapy show that the addition of a progestogen also has little effect on blood pressure. Rarely, idiosyncratic hypertension may occur. When oestrogens are administered to hypertensive women, supervision is necessary and blood pressure should be monitored at regular intervals.

Elleste Duet is not suitable for contraception. Therefore, where applicable, contraception should be practiced with non-hormonal methods.

Interactions with other medicaments and other forms of interaction: Hormonal contraception should be stopped when treatment with Elleste Duet is started and the patient should be advised to take non-hormonal contraceptive precautions if required.

Drugs which induce hepatic microsomal enzyme systems e.g. barbiturates, carbamazepine, phenytoin, rifampicin, accelerate the metabolism of oestrogen-progestogen combinations such as Elleste Duet and may reduce their efficacy.

The requirements for oral antidiabetics or insulin can change as a result of the effect on glucose tolerance.

Some laboratory tests can be influenced by oestrogens, such as tests for glucose tolerance or thyroid function.

Pregnancy and lactation: Not to be used in pregnant or lactating women.

Effects on ability to drive and use machines: No adverse effects have been recorded.

Undesirable effects: The following have been reported during treatment with hormone replacement therapy: dyspepsia, flatulence, nausea, vomiting, abdominal pain and bloating, weight gain, breast tension and pain, epistaxis, biliary stasis, hypertension, urticaria and other rashes, chloasma, thrombophlebitis, mucous vaginal discharge, general pruritus.

Overdose: There have been no reports of ill-effects from overdosage with hormone replacement therapy. If overdosage is discovered within two or three hours and is so large that treatment seems desirable, gastric lavage can safely be used. There are no specific antidotes for overdosage and further treatment should be symptomatic.

## Pharmacological properties
*Pharmacodynamic properties:*

*Oestradiol:* A naturally occurring oestrogen, active in the development and maintenance of the female sex organs, secondary sex characteristics, control of mammary glands, proliferation of the endometrium, development of the decidua and cyclic changes in the cervix and vagina. Used as a replacement therapy when ovarian function declines.

*Norethisterone acetate:* A progestogen which acts on the endometrium by converting the proliferative phase to a secretory phase and preparing the uterus to receive the fertilised ovum. It also suppresses uterine motility and is responsible for further development of the breasts. It is used in this product to reduce the risk of endometrial hyperplasia which may occur with unopposed long-term oestrogen therapy.

*Pharmacokinetic properties:*

*Oestradiol:* Readily and fully absorbed from the GI tract when given orally, peak levels are generally observed 3–6 hours after ingestion, but by 24 hours concentrations have returned to baseline.

Oestradiol undergoes first-pass effect in the liver. It is excreted via the kidney in the form of water-soluble esters.

*Norethisterone acetate:* Norethisterone acetate is absorbed from the GI tract and its effects last for at least 24 hours. Maximum blood concentrations are generally reached 1–4 hours after administration. Norethisterone acetate undergoes first-pass effects with loss of approximately 36% of the dose. Approximately 80% of the dose is excreted in the urine.

*Preclinical safety data:* No preclinical studies have been conducted for this product, since the safety is well recorded and understood for both oestradiol and norethisterone which are active substances defined in pharmacopoeial monographs, and because the tablet formulation contains only known excipients.

## Pharmaceutical particulars
*List of excipients:* Lactose 200 mesh, maize starch, povidone 25, talc (purified), magnesium stearate, hydroxypropylmethylcellulose (E464), titanium dioxide (E171), polyethylene glycol 400, tartrazine (E102), Lissamine green (E412), purified water.

*Incompatibilities:* No incompatibilities have been noted.

*Shelf life:* SA shelf life of 36 months is recommended.

*Special precautions for storage:* Store tablets below 25°C, in a dry place.

*Nature and contents of container:* Container consists of a UPVC blister and aluminium foil, packed in a cardboard carton. Each blister contains 28 tablets.

*Instructions for use/handling:* There are no special instructions for handling.

*Marketing authorisation holder:* Shire Pharmaceutical Contracts Limited, East Anton, Andover, Hants. SP10 5RG.

**Marketing authorisation number** 08081/0028.

**Date of approval/revision of SPC** February 1997.

**Legal category** POM.

# ELLESTE DUET* 2 mg

**Qualitative and quantitative composition** 16 tablets each containing 2 mg oestradiol, 12 tablets each containing 2 mg oestradiol and 1 mg norethisterone acetate.

**Pharmaceutical form** Tablets for oral administration.

## Clinical particulars
*Therapeutic indications:* The treatment of menopausal symptoms such as sweating, flushes.

Prophylaxis and treatment of the postmenopausal sequelae of oestrogen withdrawal, e.g. osteoporosis, atrophic vaginitis, atrophic urethritis.

Elleste-Duet 2 mg is designed to provide continuous oestrogen and monthly cyclical progestogen therapy after the climacteric. Oestrogen administration is continued without a break in therapy. The addition of a progestogen in the second half of each course helps to provide good control of the irregular cycles that are characteristic of the premenopausal phase and opposes the production of endometrial hyperplasia.

In women with an intact uterus, and in particular women with obesity, diabetes, low parity or a familial history of endometrial carcinoma, for whom hormone replacement therapy is required, Elleste-Duet 2 mg should be considered in preference to unopposed oestrogen therapy as it provides a progestogen to avoid endometrial hyperstimulation.

*Posology and method of administration*
*Adults:* One orange tablet is taken daily for the first 16 days, followed by one grey tablet for the next 12 days. A new cycle should then begin without any break. Therapy may start at any time in patients with established amenorrhoea or who are experiencing long intervals between spontaneous menses. In patients who are menstruating regularly, it is advised that therapy starts on the second day of bleeding. Patients changing from another cyclical preparation should complete the cycle and may then change to Elleste-Duet 2 mg without a break in therapy.

*Elderly:* There are no special dosage requirements for elderly patients.

*Children:* Not to be used in children.

*Contra-indications:* Known or suspected pregnancy; lactation; known or suspected cancer of the breast except in appropriately selected patients being treated for metastatic disease; known or suspected oestrogen-dependent neoplasia; abnormal genital bleeding, endometriosis; active thrombophlebitis or thromboembolic disorders (including coronary thrombosis, cerebrovascular accident etc). Severe cardiac disease. Sickle-cell anaemia. Congenital disturbances of lipid metabolism. Severe diabetes with vascular changes. Acute or chronic liver disease or history of liver disease when the liver function tests have failed to return to normal. Previous or existing liver tumours. Rotor syndrome or Dubin-Johnson Syndrome. Jaundice or general pruritus during previous pregnancy. Severe renal disease.

*Special warnings and special precautions for use:* Treatment should be stopped at once if migrainous or frequent unusually severe headaches occur for the first time, or if there are any other symptoms that are possible prodromata of vascular occlusion.

Treatment should also be stopped if trauma, illness or impending surgery is considered to entail a risk of thrombosis. Treatment should be stopped at once if jaundice occurs, or if there is a significant rise in blood pressure.

In patients with mild chronic liver disease, liver function should be checked regularly.

A thorough gynaecological and physical examination is advised before, and periodically during treatment.

Diseases which are known to be subject to deterioration during pregnancy (e.g. multiple sclerosis, epilepsy, diabetes, hypertension, porphyria, tetany and otosclerosis) should be carefully observed during treatment.

Patients with gallstones should be closely monitored.

Caution is advised in women with a history of thromboembolic disorders. Irregular bleeding during tablet taking is common during the first few months, but if it persists it should be investigated.

As Elleste-Duet 2 mg is not an oral contraceptive, adequate non-hormonal measures should be taken to exclude pregnancy. Before starting treatment, pregnancy must be excluded.

*Interaction with other medicaments and other forms of interaction:* There are no recorded interactions with other medicaments.

*Use during pregnancy and lactation:* Not to be used in pregnant or lactating women.

*Effects on ability to drive and use machines:* No adverse effects have been recorded.

*Undesirable effects:* The following have been reported during treatment with hormone replacement therapy: dyspepsia, flatulence, nausea, vomiting, abdominal pain and bloating, weight gain, breast tension and pain, palpitations, cardiac symptoms, changes in libido, headaches, dizziness, vertigo, epistaxis, biliary stasis, hypertension, urticaria and other rashes, thrombophlebitis, mucous vaginal discharge, general pruritus.

*Overdose:* There have been no reports of ill-effects from overdosage with hormone replacement therapy. If overdosage is discovered within two or three hours and is so large that treatment seems desirable, gastric lavage can safely be used. There are no specific antidotes for overdosage, and further treatment should be symptomatic.

## Pharmacological properties
*Pharmacodynamic properties*

*Oestradiol:* A naturally occurring oestrogen, active in the development and maintenance of the female sex organs, secondary sex characteristics, control of mammary glands, proliferation of the endometrium, development of the decidua and cyclic changes in the cervix and vagina. Used as replacement therapy when ovarian function declines.

*Norethisterone acetate:* A progestogen which acts on the endometrium by converting the proliferative phase to a secretory phase and preparing the uterus to receive the fertilised ovum. It also suppresses uterine motility and is responsible for further development of the breasts. It is used in this product to reduce the risk of endometrial hyperplasia which may occur with unopposed long-term oestrogen therapy.

*Pharmacokinetic properties*

*Oestradiol:* Readily and fully absorbed from the GI tract when given orally, peak levels are generally observed 3–6 hours after ingestion, but by 24 hours concentrations have returned to baseline. Oestradiol undergoes first-pass effect in the liver. It is excreted via the kidney in the form of water-soluble esters.

*Norethisterone acetate:* Norethisterone acetate is absorbed from GI tract and its effects last for at least 24 hours. Maximum blood concentrations are generally reached 1–4 hours after administration. Norethisterone acetate undergoes first pass effect with loss of approximately 36% of the dose. Approximately 80% of the dose is excreted in the urine.

*Preclinical safety data:* Oestradiol and norethisterone acetate are well established pharmaceutical active ingredients and are both the subject of pharmacopoeial monographs. No specific preclinical studies have therefore been performed.

## Pharmaceutical particulars
*List of excipients:* Lactose 200 mesh, maize starch, povidone 25, talc (purified), magnesium stearate, Opadry Grey OY-8238, (oestradiol and norethisterone acetate tablets), Opadry White Y-1-7000, Opadry Orange OY-3533, (oestradiol only tablets), potable water.

*Incompatibilities:* No incompatibilities have been noted.

*Shelf life:* A shelf-life of 36 months is recommended.

*Special precautions for storage:* Store the tablets under 25°C, in a dry place.

*Nature and contents of container:* Container consists of a UPVC blister and aluminium foil, packed in a cardboard carton. Each blister contains 28 tablets.

*Instructions for use/handling:* There are no special instructions for handling.

*Marketing authorisation holder:* Shire Pharmaceutical Contracts Limited, Fosse House, East Anton, Andover, Hampshire, SP10 5RG.

**Marketing authorisation number** 8081/0024.

**Date of approval/revision of SPC** October 1995.

**Legal category** POM.

# ELLESTE SOLO*

**Qualitative and quantitative composition** Oestradiol 1 mg or Oestradiol 2 mg.

**Pharmaceutical form** Tablets for oral administration.

## Clinical particulars
*Therapeutic indications:* The treatment of menopausal symptoms such as sweating, flushes in menopausal and postmenopausal women who require oestrogen replacement therapy (and especially in hysterectomised women).

The prophylaxis and treatment of the postmenopausal sequelae of oestrogen withdrawal, e.g. atrophic vaginitis, atrophic urethritis.

Elleste-Solo 2 mg should be used in patients where symptoms are not adequately relieved or who are seeking long-term protection against osteoporosis.

*Posology and method of administration*
*Adults:* One tablet daily to be taken orally. Elleste-Solo 1 mg and Elleste-Solo 2 mg may be taken continuously and without any limit on duration of

treatment in hysterectomised women. In women with a uterus, a progestogen should be added for 12–14 days each cycle to oppose the production of an oestrogen-stimulated hyperplasia of the endometrium, or an appropriate break in therapy between cycle packs should be advised in order to allow recovery of the endometrium.

*Elderly:* There are no special dosage requirements for elderly patients.

*Children:* Not to be used in children.

*Contra-indications:* Known or suspected pregnancy.

Known or suspected cancer of the breast except in appropriately selected patients being treated for metastatic disease.

Known or suspected oestrogen-dependent neoplasia.

Abnormal genital bleeding, endometriosis.

Active thrombophlebitis or thromboembolic disorders (including coronary thrombosis, cerebrovascular accident etc). Severe cardiac or renal disease. Sickle-cell anaemia. Congenital disturbances of lipid metabolism. Severe diabetes with vascular changes. Acute or chronic liver disease or history of liver disease when the liver function tests have failed to return to normal. Previous or existing liver tumours. Rotor syndrome or Dubin-Johnson Syndrome. Jaundice or general pruritus during previous pregnancy.

*Special warnings and special precautions for use:* Treatment should be stopped at once if migrainous or frequent unusually severe headaches occur for the first time, or if there are any other symptoms that are possible prodromata of vascular occlusion.

Treatment should also be stopped if trauma, illness or impending surgery is considered to entail a risk of thrombosis. Treatment should be stopped at once if jaundice occurs, or if there is a significant rise in blood pressure.

In women of child bearing potential hormonal contraception should be stopped when treatment is started and the patient should be advised to take non-hormonal contraceptive precautions. Before starting treatment, pregnancy must be excluded.

In patients with mild chronic liver disease, liver function should be checked every 8–12 weeks.

A thorough gynaecological and physical examination is advised before and periodically during treatment. Prolonged exposure to unopposed oestrogens may increase the risk of development of endometrial carcinoma.

Diseases which are known to be subject to deterioration during pregnancy (e.g. multiple sclerosis, epilepsy, diabetes, hypertension, porphyria, tetany and otosclerosis) should be carefully observed during treatment.

Efficacy of oestradiol may be reduced with the concomitant administration of liver enzyme-inducing medicines.

Patients with gallstones should be closely monitored.

Caution is advised in women with a history of thromboembolic disorders. Irregular bleeding (spotting) is not uncommon in the first few months of treatment, but if it persists it should be investigated.

*Interaction with other medicaments and other forms of interaction:* There are no recorded interactions with other medicaments.

*Use during pregnancy and lactation:* Not to be used in pregnant or lactating women.

*Effects on ability to drive and use machines:* No adverse effects on the ability to drive or operate machines have been recorded.

*Undesirable effects:* The following have been reported during treatment with hormone replacement therapy: dyspepsia, nausea, vomiting, increased appetite, bloating, altered weight, mastalgia, anxiety, depression, dizziness, cardiac symptoms, leg pains and swelling, altered libido, rashes.

*Overdose:* There have been no reports of ill-effects from overdosage with hormone replacement therapy. If overdosage is discovered within two or three hours and is so large that treatment seems desirable, gastric lavage can safely be used. There are no specific antidotes for overdosage, and further treatment should be symptomatic.

**Pharmacological properties**

*Pharmacodynamic properties:* Oestradiol is a naturally occurring oestrogen, active in the development and maintenance of the female sex organs, secondary sex characteristics, control of mammary glands, proliferation of the endometrium, development of the decidua and cyclic changes in the cervix and vagina. It is used as replacement therapy when ovarian function declines. Oestradiol exerts its effects through interaction with specific receptors in cytoplasm of oestrogen sensitive tissues.

*Pharmacokinetic properties:* Oestradiol is absorbed from the GI tract. When given orally, peak levels are generally observed 3–6 hours after ingestion, but by 24 hours concentrations have returned to baseline. Oestradiol undergoes first-pass effect in the liver. It is excreted via the kidney in the form of water-soluble esters.

*Preclinical safety data:* Oestradiol is a well established pharmaceutical active ingredient and is the subject of a pharmacopoeial monograph. No specific preclinical studies have therefore been performed.

**Pharmaceutical particulars**

*List of excipients:* Lactose 200 mesh, maize starch, povidone 25, talc (purified), magnesium stearate, Opadry White Y-1-7000, potable water. Elleste-Solo 2 mg also contains Opadry Orange OY-3533.

*Incompatibilities:* No incompatibilities have been noted.

*Shelf life:* A shelf-life of 36 months is recommended.

*Special precautions for storage:* Store the tablets under 25°C, in a dry place.

*Nature and contents of container:* Container consists of a UPVC blister and aluminium foil, packed in a cardboard carton. Each blister contains 28 tablets.

*Instructions for use/handling:* There are no special instructions for handling.

*Marketing authorisation holder:* Shire Pharmaceutical Contracts Limited, Fosse House, East Anton, Andover, Hampshire, SP10 5RG.

**Marketing authorisation numbers**

Elleste-Solo 1 mg 8081/0020
Elleste-Solo 2 mg 8081/0017

**Date of approval/revision of SPC** October 1995.

**Legal category** POM.

## EPOGAM*

**Qualitative and quantitative composition**

| *Active constituents* | *Quantity/dose unit* |
|---|---|
| Gamolenic acid (provided by Evening Primrose Oil) | 40 mg |

**Pharmaceutical form** Soft gelatin capsules.

**Clinical particulars**

*Therapeutic indications:* Epogam is indicated for the symptomatic relief of atopic eczema. All features of the disease may improve but Epogam is particularly effective in relieving the generalised itch of atopic eczema.

*Posology and method of administration:* For oral administration. When children cannot swallow the capsules the latter may be snipped open and the oil swallowed directly, or mixed with milk, or put onto bread.

*Children:* Aged 1–12 years; 2–4 capsules twice daily.

*Adults:* 4–6 capsules twice daily.

*Elderly:* The usual adult dose.

No formal studies have been carried out in children under the age of 1 year.

Treatment should be started at the highest recommended dose.

Some patients may not begin to show a clinical response to treatment for 8–12 weeks due to the gradual onset of action of Epogam. Once a clinical response has been achieved the treatment may be stopped or continued at a lower maintenance dose.

*Contra-indications:* None known.

*Special warnings and special precautions for use:* None.

*Interactions:* Epogam may have the potential to make manifest undiagnosed temporal lobe epilepsy, especially schizophrenic patients and/or those who are receiving known epileptogenic drugs such as the phenothiazines. Physicians are advised to monitor carefully the effects of Epogam in patients on epileptogenic drugs, or in any individuals with a history of epilepsy.

*Pregnancy and lactation:*

*Pregnancy:* No teratogenic effects have been observed in animal studies. There is no information available on use during pregnancy in human beings. It should only be used during pregnancy if considered essential by the physician.

*Lactation:* Epogam may be taken while breast feeding.

*Effects on ability to drive and use machines:* None

*Undesirable effects:* No major adverse effects have been reported. Nausea, indigestion and headache have occurred occasionally. In rare cases, hypersensitivity reactions, including rash, urticaria and pruritus and abdominal pain have been reported. It should be noted that hypersensitivity reactions may require close medical surveillance and that such reactions may occur particularly in patients who have a history of food or other allergies.

*Overdose:* The only symptom noted in a few cases have been loose stools sometimes accompanied by abdominal pains. No special treatment is required. There is a high degree of tolerance to evening primrose oil. Up to 25 ml of oil (equivalent to 50 capsules) has been administered daily for one year to children aged 5–12 years, without adverse effects other than occasional loose stools.

**Pharmacological properties**

*Pharmacodynamic properties:* Epogam capsules provide an exogenous source of gamolenic acid (GLA) which may be used to restore some subnormal fatty acid levels towards physiologically normal levels. Clinical studies demonstrate that it improves the symptoms of atopic eczema, however the precise pharmacological mode of action is unclear. No undesirable pharmacological effects are known.

*Pharmacokinetic properties:* The pharmacokinetic profile of evening primrose oil follows that of any normal triglycerides from usual dietary sources. It is approximately 95% absorbed, metabolised in the liver and stored principally in adipose tissue.

There are no unusual pharmacokinetic properties. Gamolenic acid is the unusual fatty acid component of evening primrose oil, it is metabolised rapidly to dihomo-gammalinolenic acid (DGLA) in the body. DGLA levels will fall to pretreatment levels in approximately two weeks following withdrawal of evening primrose oil.

*Preclinical safety data:* None of relevance to the prescriber.

**Pharmaceutical particulars**

*List of excipients:* The following excipients are included in Epogam: D-alpha tocopheryl acetate, gelatin, glycerol, Opacode S-1-7020 White or Mastercote F11983 White.

*Incompatibilities:* None known.

*Shelf-life:* 36 months as packaged for sale.

*Special precautions for storage:* Store below 25°C, in a dry place, protected from heat.

*Nature and contents of containers:* (a) HDPE 'Tamper-tainer' containing 240 Epogam capsules with an LDPE tamper evident closure.

(b) Promotional sample pack containing 12 capsules in PVC/PVDC (250/40) blister pack with lacquered hard temper aluminium foil (20 micron) in a cardboard carton.

*Instructions for use/handling:* 'Swallow the capsule whole or you can snip the capsule with a pair of scissors. Squeeze the liquid into your mouth and swallow. If you prefer you can mix the oil with a cold drink or put it on to your food'.

*Marketing authorisation holder:* Scotia Pharmaceuticals Limited, Woodbridge Meadows, Guildford, Surrey GU1 1BA.

**Marketing authorisation number** 4382/0005.

**Date of approval/revision of SPC** February 1997.

**Legal Category** POM.

## EPOGAM* PAEDIATRIC

**Qualitative and quantitative composition**

| *Active constituents* | *Quantity/dose/unit* |
|---|---|
| Gamolenic acid (provided by Evening Primrose Oil) | 80 mg |

**Pharmaceutical form** Soft gelatin capsules.

**Clinical particulars**

*Therapeutic indications:* Epogam Paediatric is indicated for the symptomatic relief of atopic eczema. All features of the disease may improve but Epogam Paediatric is particularly effective in relieving the generalised itch of atopic eczema

*Posology and method of administration:* These capsules have been specifically designed for children (and also incidentally for older people) who have difficulty swallowing the 40 mg Epogam Capsules. The snip off neck should be cut off and the capsule squeezed to express the contents which may be swallowed directly or mixed with milk or put onto bread or other food.

*Children:* Aged 1–12 years; 1–2 capsules twice daily, providing a total daily dose of 2–4 capsules.

*Adults:* 2–3 capsules twice daily, providing a total daily dose of 4–6 capsules.

*Elderly:* The usual adult dose.

No formal studies have been carried out in children under the age of 1 year.

Treatment should be started at the highest recommended dose.

Some patients may not begin to show a clinical response to treatment for 8–12 weeks due to the gradual onset of action of Epogam Paediatric. Once a clinical response has been achieved the treatment may be stopped or continued at a lower maintenance dose.

*Contra-indications:* None known.

*Special warnings and special precautions for use:* None.

*Interactions:* Epogam Paediatric may have the potential to make manifest undiagnosed temporal lobe epilepsy, especially in schizophrenic patients and/or those who are receiving known epileptogenic drugs such as the phenothiazines. Physicians are advised to monitor carefully the effects of Epogam Paediatric in patients on epileptogenic drugs, or in any individuals with a history of epilepsy.

*Pregnancy and lactation:*

*Pregnancy:* No teratogenic effects have been observed in animal studies. However, as with all medicines, caution is advised concerning administration in the first trimester of pregnancy.

*Lactation:* Epogam Paediatric may be taken while breast feeding.

*Effects on ability to drive and use machines:* None.

*Undesirable effects:* No frequent major adverse effects have been reported. Nausea, indigestion and headache occur occasionally. In rare cases, hypersensitivity reactions, including rash, urticaria and pruritus and abdominal pain have been reported. It should be noted that hypersensitivity reactions may require close medical surveillance and that such reactions may occur particularly in patients who have a history of food or other allergies.

*Overdose:* The only symptom noted in a few cases have been loose stools sometimes accompanied by abdominal pains. No special treatment is required.

There is a high degree of tolerance to evening primrose oil. Up to 25 ml of oil (equivalent to 25 capsules) has been administered daily for one year to children aged 5–12 years, without adverse effects other than occasional loose stools.

**Pharmacological properties**

*Pharmacodynamic properties:* Epogam Paediatric capsules provide an exogenous source of gamolenic acid (GLA) which may be used to restore some subnormal fatty acid levels towards physiologically normal levels. Clinical studies demonstrate that it improves the symptoms of atopic eczema, however the precise pharmacological mode of action is unclear. No undesirable pharmacological effects are known.

*Pharmacokinetic properties:* The pharmacokinetic profile of evening primrose oil follows that of any normal trigl/cerides from usual dietary sources. It is approximately 95% absorbed, metabolised in the liver and stored principally in adipose tissue.

There are no unusual pharmacokinetic properties. Gamolenic acid is the unusual fatty acid component of evening primrose oil, it is metabolised rapidly to dihomo-gammalinolenic acid (DGLA) in the body. DGLA levels will fall to pretreatment levels in approximately two weeks following withdrawal of evening primrose oil.

*Preclinical safety data:* None of relevance to the prescriber.

**Pharmaceutical particulars**

*List of excipients:* The following excipients are included in Epogam: D-alpha tocopheryl acetate, gelatin, glycerol, Opacode S-1-7020 White or Mastercote F11983 White.

*Incompatibilities:* None known.

*Shelf life:* 36 months as packaged for sale.

*Special precautions for storage:* Store in a dry place, protected from heat.

*Nature and contents of container:* (a) HDPE 'Tampertainer' containing 60 or 120 Epogam Paediatric capsules with an LDPE tamper evident closure.

(b) Promotional sample pack containing 4 capsules in PVC/PVDC (250/40) blister pack with lacquered hard tamper aluminium foil (20 micron) in a cardboard carton.

*Instructions for use/handling:* 'Do not swallow the capsule whole. Snip off the neck of the capsule with a pair of scissors. Squeeze the liquid into your mouth and swallow. If you prefer you can mix the oil with a cold drink or put it onto your bread'.

*Marketing authorisation holder:* Scotia Pharmaceuticals Limited, Woodbridge Meadows, Guildford, Surrey GU1 1BA.

**Marketing authorisation number** 04382/0013.

**Date of approval/revision of SPC** February 1997.

**Legal category** POM.

## FEMULEN*

**Presentation** White tablets engraved 'SEARLE' on both sides, containing Ethynodiol Diacetate BP 500 micrograms.

**Uses** Oral contraception.

**Dosage and administration** Starting on the first day of menstruation, one tablet every day without a break in medication for as long as contraception is required. Additional contraceptive precautions (a sheath or a cap, plus spermicide) should be taken for the first 14 days of the first pack. Tablets should be taken at the same time each day.

*Missed tablets:* If the woman misses one tablet or takes it later than the usual time, contraceptive efficacy may be reduced and additional contraceptive precautions (a sheath or a cap, plus spermicide) should be used until the next period occurs. Women who miss a single tablet should be instructed to take the missed tablet as soon as they remember, even though this may mean taking two tablets on one single day. The regular tablet for that day should be taken at the usual time. If two or more consecutive tablets are missed Femulen should be discontinued and alternative contraceptive measures should be taken until menstruation occurs and the possibility of pregnancy is excluded.

*Vomiting or diarrhoea:* Vomiting or diarrhoea may reduce the effectiveness of Femulen, particularly if this should occur at or around the time of ovulation. If an episode of vomiting and/or diarrhoea occurs the woman should be advised to use an additional form of contraception (sheath or a cap, plus spermicide) until the next menstrual period occurs.

**Contra-indications, warnings, etc**

*Contra-indications:* The contra-indications for progestogen-only oral contraceptives are: known, suspected, or a past history of breast, genital or hormone dependent cancer; past or present, benign or malignant liver tumours; impaired liver function; active liver disease; history during pregnancy of idiopathic jaundice or severe pruritus; disorders of lipid metabolism; undiagnosed abnormal vaginal bleeding or amenorrhoea; known or suspected pregnancy.

Combined oestrogen/progestogen preparations have been associated with an increase in the risk of thromboembolic and thrombotic disease. Risk has been reported to be related to both oestrogenic and progestogenic activity. In the absence of long term epidemiological studies with progestogen-only oral contraceptives, it is required that the existence, or history of thrombophlebitis, thromboembolic disorders, cerebral vascular disease, myocardial infarction, coronary artery disease, or a haemoglobinopathy be described as a contraindication to Femulen as it is to oestrogen containing oral contraceptives.

*Warnings:* Femulen should be discontinued if there is a gradual or sudden, partial or complete loss of vision or any evidence of ocular changes, onset or aggravation of migraine or development of headache of a new kind which is recurrent, persistent or severe, suspicion of thrombosis or infarction, significant rise in blood pressure or if jaundice occurs.

Malignant hepatic tumours have been reported on rare occasions in long-term users of contraceptives. Benign hepatic tumours have also been associated with oral contraceptive usage. A hepatic tumour should be considered in the differential diagnosis when upper abdominal pain, enlarged liver or signs of intra-abdominal haemorrhage occur.

Progestogen-only oral contraceptives may offer less protection against ectopic pregnancy, than against intrauterine pregnancy.

*Precautions:* Women receiving treatment with Femulen should be kept under regular medical surveillance.

Femulen should be discontinued at least 6 weeks before elective surgery or during periods of prolonged immobilisation. It would be reasonable to resume Femulen two or three weeks after surgery provided the woman is ambulant. Every woman, however, should be considered individually with regard to the nature of the operation, the extent of immobilisation, the presence of additional risk factors and the chance of unwanted conception.

Caution should be exercised where there is the possibility of an interaction between a pre-existing disorder and a known or suspected side effect. The use of Femulen in women suffering from epilepsy, or with a history of migraine or cardiac or renal dysfunction may result in exacerbation of these disorders because of fluid retention. Caution should also be observed in women who wear contact lenses, women with impaired carbohydrate tolerance, depression, gallstones, varicose veins, hypertension, asthma or any disease that is prone to worsen during pregnancy.

*Pregnancy:* Several reports suggest an association between foetal exposure to female sex hormones, including oral contraceptives, and congenital anomalies. If a woman does not have a menstrual period within 45 days of her last menstrual period, pregnancy should be excluded.

*Drug interactions:* Femulen may be rendered less effective and increased incidence of breakthrough bleeding may occur by virtue of drug interaction. At present, drugs suspected to interact in this way include rifampicin, barbiturates, anticonvulsants, and antibiotics.

*Nursing mothers:* There is no evidence that progestogen-only contraceptives diminish the yield of breast milk. In a study of nursing mothers taking Femulen, the median percentage of norethisterone, the principal metabolite of ethynodiol diacetate given to the mother which was ingested by the infant was 0.02%. No adverse effect of the drug on the infants was noted.

*Adverse effects:* Women taking progestogen-only oral contraceptives for the first time may initially experience menstrual irregularity. This may include amenorrhoea, prolonged bleeding and/or spotting and should decrease with time. Clinical investigations with Femulen indicate that side effects are infrequent and tend to decrease as treatment continues. Known or suspected side effects of progestogen-only oral contraceptives include nausea, vomiting, other gastrointestinal symptoms, skin disorders including chloasma, breast and weight changes, ocular changes, headache, migraine, depression, change in libido and appetite, increase in size of uterine myofibromata, and changes in carbohydrate, lipid or vitamin metabolism. Rarely dizziness, hirsutism, haemorrhagic eruption and colitis have been reported in users of progestogen-only oral contraceptives.

The use of oral contraceptives has also been associated with a possible increased incidence of gallbladder disease.

Tests of endocrine, hepatic and thyroid function, as well as coagulation tests may be affected by this preparation.

*Overdosage:* Serious ill effects have not been reported following acute ingestion of large doses of oral contraceptives by young children. Nausea and vomiting may occur and vaginal withdrawal bleeding may present in pre-pubertal girls. In general, treatment of overdosage is not necessary. However, if thought appropriate, as there is no specific antidote, treatment should be symptomatic.

**Pharmaceutical precautions** Store in a dry place below 30°C (86°F).

**Legal category** POM.

**Package quantities** Carton of 28 tablets with instructions.

**Further information** Femulen does not necessarily inhibit ovulation but it is believed to discourage implantation of the fertilised ovum by altering the endometrium. Cervical mucus viscosity is also changed which may render the passage of sperm less likely.

**Product licence number** 08821/0015.

## LOMOTIL* TABLETS

**Presentation** White tablets, engraved 'SEARLE' on one side. Each tablet contains Diphenoxylate Hydrochloride BP 2.5 milligrams with Atropine Sulphate PhEur 25 micrograms.

**Uses** Adjunctive therapy to appropriate rehydration in diarrhoea.

Control of stool formation after colostomy or ileostomy.

Relief of symptoms in chronic mild ulcerative colitis (see *Warnings*).

**Dosage and administration** Caution: The recommended dosage should not be exceeded. Once satisfactory control is achieved, dosage should be reduced to suit the requirements of the individual patient.

*Adults:* The recommended starting dose is four tablets followed by two tablets every six hours.

*Elderly:* Consideration should be given to the presence of other disease and concomitant drug therapy (see *Precautions*).

*Children:* Recommended dose guide

| | |
|---|---|
| Under 4 years – not recommended. | |
| 4–8 years | 1 tablet three times daily. |
| 9–12 years | 1 tablet four times daily. |
| 13–16 years | 2 tablets three times daily. |

**Contra-indications, warnings, etc** Lomotil is contra-indicated in patients with a known hypersensitivity to diphenoxylate hydrochloride or atropine, in patients with jaundice, intestinal obstruction, acute ulcerative colitis, and in the treatment of diarrhoea associated with pseudomembranous enterocolitis.

Appropriate fluid and electrolyte therapy should be given to protect against dehydration. If severe dehydration or electrolyte imbalance is present, Lomotil should be withheld until appropriate corrective therapy has been initiated. In some patients with ulcerative colitis, agents which inhibit intestinal motility or delay intestinal transit time have been reported to induce toxic megacolon. Patients with ulcerative colitis should be observed carefully and Lomotil therapy should be discontinued promptly if abdominal distension or other untoward symptoms develop.

Lomotil should be used with extreme caution in

patients with advanced hepatorenal disease and in all patients with abnormal liver function since hepatic coma may be precipitated.

**Precautions:** Because a subtherapeutic dose of atropine is added to Lomotil, atropinic effects may occur in susceptible individuals or in overdosage. Individuals with Down's syndrome appear to have an increased susceptibility to the actions of atropine.

*Drug interactions:* Since the chemical structure of diphenoxylate hydrochloride resembles that of meperidine hydrochloride, concurrent use with MAO inhibitors could precipitate hypertensive crisis. Close observation is required when these medications are given concomiitantly with diphenoxylate hydrochloride.

Diphenoxylate hydrochloride may potentiate the action of central nervous system depressants such as barbiturates, tranquillisers and alcohol.

*Pregnancy:* Animal teratology and reproduction studies have demonstrated no adverse effects. The safety of Lomotil in pregnancy has not been established. However, as with all drugs, caution is recommended when used in early pregnancy.

*Nursing mothers:* Diphenoxylate hydrochloride and atropine sulphate may be excreted in human milk. If a nursing mother is taking Lomotil, the infant may exhibit some effects of the drug.

*Adverse effects:* Adverse reactions reported include:

Central nervous system: malaise/lethargy/sedation/somnolence, confusion, dizziness, restlessness, depression, euphoria, hallucinations, headache.

Allegic: anaphylaxis, angioedema, urticaria, pruritus.

Gastrointestinal system: paralytic ileus, toxic megacolon, gastrointestinal intolerance such as nausea and vomiting, anorexia, abdominal discomfort.

Atropine effects, such as flushing, dryness of the skin and mucous membranes, tachycardia, hyperthermia and urinary retention may occur, especially in children.

*Overdosage:* Accidental overdosage may produce narcosis with respiratory depression or atropine poisoning or both, particularly in children. Symptoms of overdosage include dryness of the skin and mucous membranes, flushing, hyperthermia and tachycardia, nystagmus, pinpoint pupils, hypotonic reflexes, lethargy, coma and severe respiratory depression. The onset of symptoms of overdosage may be considerable delayed and respiratory depression may not become evident until as late as 12 to 30 hours after ingestion and may recur in spite of an initial response to narcotic antagonists. Continuous observation should be maintained for at least 48 hours.

If respiratory depression develops, naloxone, a specific antidote, should be administered. The duration of action of naloxone hydrochloride is considerably shorter than that of diphenoxylate hydrochloride and repeated injections of the antidote may be required. Establishment of a patent airway and artificial ventilation may be needed. If the patient is not comatose gastric lavage and administration of a slurry of activated charcoal may be indicated.

**Pharmaceutical precautions**   Store below 30°C (86°F).

**Legal category**  POM.

**Package quantities**  Carton containing blister strips of 100 tablets.

**Further information**  Nil.

**Product licence number**  08821/0028.

# MENOPHASE*

**Qualitative and quantitative composition**  Menophase comprises 6 different formulations:

5 pink tablets containing 12.5 micrograms mestranol;

8 orange tablets containing 25 micrograms mestranol;

2 yellow tablets containing 50 micrograms mestranol;

3 green tablets containing 25 micrograms mestranol and 1 milligram norethisterone;

6 blue tablets containing 30 micrograms mestranol and 1.5 milligrams norethisterone;

4 lavender tablets containing 20 micrograms mestranol and 750 micrograms norethisterone

Tablets are inscribed 'SYNTEX' on one side.

**Pharmaceutical form**  Tablets for oral administration.

## Clinical particulars

*Therapeutic indications:* Menophase is indicated for the treatment of menopausal symptoms and allied disorders. These include hot flushes and sweats, depression, lack of concentration, emotional liability, nervousness, lethargy, insomnia, loss of libido, senile vaginitis, pruritis and dry skin. Menophase is also indicated for the prophylaxis of menopausal osteoporosis in females who are at risk from developing fractures.

*Posology and method of administration:*
*Oral administration:* The patient is advised to take her first tablet on a Sunday and thereafter to take one tablet at the same time each day in sequential order round the pack. She starts a new pack the day after she has taken her last lavender tablet from the previous pack. Though menopausal symptoms are likely to improve during the first months of treatment it will be necessary to maintain therapy for 6–12 months. If symptoms recur after discontinuation further courses can be prescribed.

*Tablet omissions:* Since Menophase is not an oral contraceptive, in the event of a missed tablet the patient should be advised to discard the tablet(s) missed and take only the tablet appropriate to the day of the week.

*Contra-indications:* Pregnancy (see also *Precautions*): benign and malignant liver tumours; severe disturbances of liver function; jaundice or general pruritus during a previous pregnancy; Dubin-Johnson syndrome; Rotor syndrome; cardiovascular or cerebrovascular disorders e.g. thrombophlebitis, thromboembolic processes or a history of these conditions; sickle-cell anaemia; porphyria; existing or previous moderate to severe hypertension; existing or previous breast or uterine cancer or oestrogen-dependent neoplasia; undiagnosed irregular vaginal bleeding; congenital disturbances of lipid metabolism; existing or previous hyperlipoproteinaemia; a history of pemphigoid gestationis or otosclerosis made worse by pregnancy.

*Special warnings and special precautions for use:* Menophase is not an oral contraceptive. Menophase provides sequential graded doses of hormones; the post-menopausal patient with an intact uterus may therefore experience a small, regular monthly bleed but if forewarned of this possibility, it usually causes no distress. Hormonal contraception should be stopped when Menophase is started and the patient should be advised to take non-hormonal contraceptive precautions during the prescribing period.

Treatment should be stopped at once if jaundice or pregnancy occurs. If pregnancy is confirmed the patient should be told of the potential risk to the foetus and the advisability of continuing the pregnancy should be discussed.

The use of this product in patients suffering from epilepsy, or with a history of hypertension, migraine, asthma or cardiac dysfunction may result in exacerbation of these disorders because of fluid retention; these patients should be kept under special surveillance. Regular monitoring of blood pressure should be carried out in hypertensive patients. Treatment should be discontinued if there is a consistent rise in blood pressure. Because of the possibility of corneal oedema caution should also be observed in patients who wear contact lenses.

Discontinue treatment if there is gradual or sudden, partial or complete loss of vision or any evidence of ocular changes, onset or aggravation of migraine or development of headache of a new kind which is recurrent, persistent or severe.

Diseases known to deteriorate during pregnancy (e.g. multiple sclerosis, epilepsy, diabetes, hypertension, porphyria, tetany and otosclerosis) should be carefully observed during treatment.

Caution should be exercised in treating women with a history of oestrogen related thrmboembolic disorders (e.g. during pregnancy) or idiopathic thromboembolic disorders without any obvious risk factors present. In such patients, any inherent abnormality of fibrinolysis or coagulation should be excluded before treatment with Menophase is commenced.

Caution should be observed in patients with severe varicose veins, sickle-cell haemoglobinopathy, untreated polycythaema or pulmonary hypertension.

Pregnancy must be excluded before starting treatment with Menophase.

Measurement of blood pressure, along with examination of breasts and pelvic organs is advised before and periodically during treatment. Examination of the endometrium may also be considered. Treatment should be discontinued if there is a consistent rise in blood pressure.

Treatment should be stopped if trauma, illness or impending surgery is considered to entail a risk of thrombosis. Menophase should be discontinued at least six weeks before operations and during immobilisation.

A statistical association between the use of long-term oestrogen therapy (e.g. oral contraceptives) and the occurrence of thrombosis, embolism or haemorrhage (including myocardial infarct and stroke) has been reported. Patients on such treatments should be kept under regular surveillance in view of the possibility of development of such conditions as thromboembolism. This risk is aggravated by cigarette smoking and therefore use of Menophase in this group of women requires careful consideration.

Benign and malignant liver tumours have also been associated with long-term oestrogen therapy. The relationship between occurrence of liver tumours and the use of female sex hormones is not known at present. These tumours are very rare but they may rupture, causing intra-abdominal bleeding. If the patient presents with a mass or tenderness in the right upper quadrant or an acute abdomen, the presence of a tumour should be considered.

Decreased glucose tolerance may occur in diabetic patients on this treatment and their control must be carefully supervised. Changes in lipid metabolism may also be observed.

Thyroid hormone binding globulin may be increased, leading to increased circulating total thyroid hormone. Hence, care must be taken in interpreting thyroid function tests.

Caution should be observed in patients with a history of gall stones. Some women are predisposed to cholestasis during steroid therapy. Caution should also be observed in patients with renal dysfunction.

*Interactions with other medicaments and other forms of interaction:* Menophase may alter the effectiveness of anticonvulsants, antihypertensive agents, beta-blockers, hypnotics, hypoglycaemic agents, oral anticoagulants, theophylline, tranquillisers, tricyclic antidepressants and vitamins.

*Pregnancy and lactation:* Contra-indicated in pregnancy.

*Effects on ability to drive and use machines:* Not applicable.

*Undesirable effects:* The following symptoms have been reported during treatment: anxiety, increased appetite, bloating, breast symptoms, cardiac symptoms, depression, dizziness, headaches, dyspepsia, leg pains and swelling, altered libido, excessive production of cervical mucus, intermenstrual bleeding, nausea, rashes, vomiting and altered weight.

The following have also been observed: endometrial neoplasia, increase in the size of uterine fibromyomata endometrial proliferation and aggravation of endometriosis.

*Overdose:* Overdosage may be manifested by nausea, vomiting, breast enlargement and vaginal bleeding. There is no specific antidote and treatment should be symptomatic. Gastric lavage may be employed if the overdose is large and the patient is seen sufficiently early (within 4 hours).

**Pharmacological properties**
*Pharmacodynamic properties:* Mestranol is a synthetic oestrogen which achieves its oestrogenic effect through conversion to ethinyloestradiol. It is active in the development and maintenance of the female sex organs, secondary sex characteristics, control of mammary glands, proliferation of the endometrium, development of the decidua and cyclic changes in the cervix and vagina.

Norethisterone is a progestogen which acts on the endometrium by converting the proliferative phase to a secretory phase and preparing the uterus to receive the fertilised ovum. It also suppresses uterine motility and is responsible for further development of the breasts. It is used in this product to reduce the risk of endometrial hyperplasia which may occur with unopposed long-term oestrogen therapy.

*Pharmacokinetic properties:* Norethisterone is rapidly and completely absorbed after oral administration, peak plasma cocentrations occurring in the majority of subjects between 1 and 3 hours. Due to first-pass metabolism, blood levels after oral administration are 60% of those after i.v. administration. The half life of elimination varies from 5 to 12 hours, with a mean of 7.6 hours. Norethisterone is metabolised mainly in the liver. Approximately 60% of the administered dose is excreted as metabolites in urine and faeces.

Mestranol is rapidly absorbed and extensively metabolised to ethinyloestradiol. Ethinyloestradiol is extensively metabolised, largely in the gastro-intestinal mucosa and to a lesser extent in the liver. Very little is excreted unchanged. The metabolites are excreted in both urine and bile.

*Pre-clinical safety data:* The toxicity of norethisterone is very low. Reports of teratogenic effects in animals are uncommon. No carcinogenic effects have been found even in long-term studies.

Long-term continuous administration of oestrogens in some animals increases the frequency of carcinoma of the breast, cervix, vagina and liver.

**Pharmaceutical particulars**
*List of excipients:* All of the tablets in the Menophase pack contain: Maize starch, povidone, magnesium stearate and lactose.

The pink tablets also contain E123. The orange tablets contain E110. The yellow tablets contain E104 and E110. The green tablets contain E104 and E132. The blue tablets contain E132. The lavender tablets contain E123 and E132.

*Incompatibilities:* None stated.

*Shelf life:* The shelf life of Menophase tablets is 5 years.

*Special precautions for storage:* Store in a dry place below 25°C away from direct sunlight.

*Nature and contents of container:* Menophase tablets are supplied in pvc/foil blister packs of 28 tablets.

*Instructions for use/handling:* None.

*Marketing authorisation holder:* Monsanto plc, PO Box 53, Lane End Road, High Wycombe, Bucks HP12 4HL.

**Marketing authorisation number** 08821/0038.

**Date of approval/revision of SPC** April 1996.

**Legal category** POM.

## NAPRATEC*

**Presentation** Napratec is a combination pack containing 56 tablets of naproxen and 56 tablets of Cytotec*.

Naproxen is a yellow, oblong tablet engraved SEARLE N.500 with breakline on one side containing 500 mg of Naproxen BP.

Cytotec is a white/off-white hexagonal tablet, scored on both sides, engraved SEARLE 1461 on one side, containing misoprostol 200 micrograms.

**Uses**
*Indications:* Napratec combination pack is indicated for patients who require naproxen 500 mg twice daily and Cytotec 200 micrograms twice daily.

Naproxen is indicated for the treatment of rheumatoid arthritis, osteoarthritis (degenerative arthritis) and ankylosing spondylitis.

Cytotec is indicated for the prophylaxis of nonsteroidal anti-inflammatory drug (NSAID)-induced gastroduodenal ulceration.

*Actions:* Naproxen is a nonsteroidal anti-inflammatory drug (NSAID). Cytotec is an analogue of naturally occurring prostaglandin $E_1$ which protects the gastroduodenal mucosa against ulcers induced by NSAIDs.

**Dosage and administration**
*Adults:* 1 tablet of naproxen and 1 tablet of Cytotec taken together twice daily with food.

*Elderly:* Studies indicate that although total plasma concentration of naproxen is unchanged, the unbound plasma fraction of naproxen is increased in the elderly.

With Cytotec the usual dosage may be used in the elderly.

Napratec should only be used in those patients for whom 500 mg naproxen twice daily is appropriate and in whom no reduction of naproxen dosage is necessary (see also sections on renal and hepatic impairment).

*Renal impairment:* As the final pathway for the elimination of naproxen metabolites is largely (95%) by urinary excretion via glomerular filtration, it should be used with great caution in patients with impaired renal function and the monitoring of serum creatinine and/or creatinine clearance is advised in these patients. Naproxen is not recommended in patients having a baseline creatinine clearance of less than 20 ml/minute.

Certain patients, specifically those whose renal blood flow is compromised, such as in extracellular volume depletion, cirrhosis of the liver, sodium restriction, congestive heart failure, and pre-existing renal disease, should have renal function assessed before and during naproxen therapy. Some elderly patients in whom impaired renal function may be expected could also fall within this category. Where there is a possibility of accumulation of naproxen metabolites, such patients may not be suitable to receive naproxen 500 mg twice daily.

With Cytotec no dosage alteration is necessary in patients with impaired renal function.

*Hepatic impairment:* Chronic alcoholic liver disease and probably also other forms of cirrhosis reduce the total plasma concentration of naproxen, but the plasma concentration of unbound naproxen is increased.

With Cytotec no dosage alteration is necessary in patients with impaired hepatic function.

*Children:* Napratec is not recommended.

**Contra-indications, warnings, etc**
*Contra-indications*
*Use in pregnancy and lactation:* Napratec is contra-indicated in pregnancy. This is on the basis that Cytotec is contra-indicated in pregnancy or women planning a pregnancy as it increases uterine tone and contractions in pregnancy which may cause partial or complete expulsion of the products of conception.

Teratology studies with naproxen in rats and rabbits at dose levels equivalent on a human multiple basis to those which have produced foetal abnormality with certain other NSAIDs, e.g. aspirin, have not produced evidence of foetal damage with naproxen. As with other drugs of this type, naproxen delays parturition in animals (the relevance of this finding to human patients is unknown) and also affects the human foetal cardiovascular system (closure of the ductus arteriosus).

Napratec should not be administered during breast-feeding.

Napratec is contra-indicated in patients with a known allergy to naproxen, naproxen sodium formulations, or prostaglandins.

As the potential exists with naproxen for cross-sensitivity to aspirin and other nonsteroidal anti-inflammatory drugs, Napratec should not be administered to patients in whom aspirin and other NSAIDs induce asthma, rhinitis, urticaria or angioedema.

As Napratec is a 'prevention pack' it should not be used for treating arthritis in patients with active gastric or duodenal ulceration. Such patients may be treated with a healing dose of Cytotec, 800 micrograms daily in divided doses with meals and the NSAID continued or discontinued at the physician's discretion.

*Warnings*
*Use in pre-menopausal women (see also 'Contra-indications'):* Napratec should not be used in pre-menopausal women unless the patient is at high risk of complications from NSAID-induced ulceration. In such patients it is advised that Napratec should only be used if the patient:
– takes effective contraceptive measures
– has been advised of the risks of taking the product if pregnant (see 'Contra-indications').

*Precautions:* Naproxen in common with other NSAIDs decreases platelet aggregation and prolongs bleeding time. This effect should be considered when bleeding times are determined.

Naproxen may precipitate bronchospasm in patients suffering from, or with a history of, bronchial asthma or allergic disease.

Mild peripheral oedema has been observed in a few patients receiving naproxen. Although sodium retention has not been reported in metabolic studies, it is possible that patients with questionable or compromised cardiac function may be at a greater risk when taking naproxen.

Sporadic abnormalities in laboratory tests (e.g. liver function tests) have occurred in patients on naproxen, but no definite trend was seen in any test indicating toxicity.

Cytotec should be used with caution in disease states where hypotension might precipitate severe complications, e.g. cerebrovascular disease, coronary artery disease or severe peripheral vascular disease including hypertension.

*Drug interactions:* Due to the high plasma protein binding of naproxen, patients simultaneously receiving hydantoins, anti-coagulants or a highly protein-bound sulphonamide should be observed for signs of overdosage of these drugs. No interactions have been observed in clinical studies with naproxen and anti-coagulants or sulphonylureas, but caution is nevertheless advised since interaction has been seen with other non-steroidal agents of this class.

NSAIDs may attenuate the natriuretic efficacy of diuretics due to inhibition of intrarenal synthesis of prostaglandins.

NSAIDs including naproxen have been reported to increase steady state plasma lithium levels. It is recommended that these levels are monitored whenever initiating, adjusting or discontinuing naproxen products.

Concomitant administration of naproxen with beta-blockers may reduce their antihypertensive effect.

Probenecid given concurrently increases naproxen plasma levels and extends its plasma half-life considerably.

Caution is advised when methotrexate is administered concurrently because of possible enhancement of its toxicity since naproxen, among other NSAIDs, has been reported to induce the tubular secretion of methotrexate in an animal model.

Naproxen therapy should be temporarily withdrawn before adrenal function tests are performed as it may artificially interfere with some tests for 17-ketogenic steroids. Similarly naproxen may interfere with some assays of urinary 5-hydroxyindoleacetic acid.

Cytotec is predominantly metabolised via fatty acid oxidising systems and has shown no adverse effect on the hepatic microsomal mixed function oxidase (P450) enzyme system. No drug interactions have been attributed to Cytotec, and in specific studies no clinically significant pharmacokinetic or pharmacodynamic interaction has been demonstrated with antipyrine, diazepam, propranolol or NSAIDs.

*Adverse effects*
*Naproxen*
*Gastrointestinal:* The more frequent reactions are nausea, vomiting, abdominal discomfort and epigastric distress. The more serious reaction, colitis, may occasionally occur.

Naproxen also causes gastrointestinal bleeding and gastric and duodenal ulceration, the consequence of which may be haemorrhage and perforation. The inclusion of Cytotec in the combination pack is to prevent naproxen-induced gastric and duodenal ulceration.

*Dermatological/hypersensitivity:* Skin rashes, urticaria, angio-oedema. Anaphylactic reactions to naproxen and naproxen sodium formulations, eosinophilic pneumonitis, alopecia, erythema multiforme, Stevens Johnson syndrome, epidermal necrolysis, photosensitivity reactions, pseudoporphyria and epidermolysis bullosa may occur rarely.

*Central nervous system:* Headache, insomnia, inability to concentrate and cognitive dysfunction have been reported.

*Haematological:* Thrombocytopenia, granulocytopenia, aplastic anaemia, and haemolytic anaemia may occur rarely.

*Other:* Tinnitus, hearing impairment, vertigo, mild peripheral oedema. Jaundice, fatal hepatitis, nephropathy, haematuria, visual disturbances, vasculitis, aseptic meningitis and ulcerative stomatitis have been reported rarely.

*Cytotec*
*Gastrointestinal:* Diarrhoea has been reported and is occasionally severe and prolonged and may require withdrawal of the drug. It can be minimised by taking Cytotec with food and by avoiding the use of predominantly magnesium-containing antacids when an antacid is required. Abdominal pain with or without associated dyspepsia can follow Cytotec therapy. Other gastrointestinal adverse effects reported include dyspepsia, flatulence, nausea and vomiting.

*Female reproductive system:* Menorrhagia, vaginal bleeding and intermenstrual bleeding have been reported in both pre- and post-menopausal women.

*Other adverse effects:* Skin rashes have been reported. Dizziness has been infrequently reported.

*Overdosage*
*Naproxen:* Significant overdosage of the drug may be characterised by drowsiness, heartburn, indigestion, nausea or vomiting. A few patients have experienced seizures, but it is not clear whether these were naproxen-related or not. It is not known what dose of the drug would be life-threatening.

In the event of overdosage with naproxen, the stomach may be emptied and usual supportive measures employed. Animal studies indicate that the prompt administration of activated charcoal in adequate amounts would tend to reduce markedly the absorption of the drug.

Haemodialysis does not decrease the plasma concentration of naproxen because of the high degree of protein binding. However, haemodialysis may still be appropriate in a patient with renal failure who has taken naproxen.

*Cytotec:* Intensification of pharmacological and adverse effects may occur with overdose. In the event of overdosage with Cytotec, symptomatic and supportive therapy should be given as appropriate.

**Pharmaceutical precautions** Store in a dry place below 30°C (86°F).

**Legal category** POM.

**Package quantities** Combination pack containing 4×7 day treatment wallets containing 56 naproxen 500 mg tablets in pvc/foil blisters and 56 Cytotec 200 microgram tablets in cold-formed aluminium blisters.

**Further information** Cytotec in multiples of the recommended therapeutic dose in animals has produced gastric mucosal hyperplasia. This characteristic response to E prostaglandins reverts to normal on discontinuation of the compound. In patients, histological examination of gastric biopsies taken before and after treatment with misoprostol after up to one year's duration have shown no adverse tissue response attributable to misoprostol. Inhibition of gastric secretion by Cytotec is achieved by a combination of local and systemic effects. Cytotec is rapidly absorbed following oral administration, with peak plasma levels of the active metabolite (misoprostol acid) occurring after about 30 minutes. The plasma elimination half-life of misoprostol acid is 20–40 minutes. Increases in the $C_{max}$ and AUC for misoprostol acid have been observed when co-administered with naproxen in a single dose study. These changes are not thought to be clinically significant since the higher values are still well within the variation seen after 200 micrograms misoprostol in other studies. No accumulation of misoprostol acid in plasma occurs after repeated dosing of 400 micrograms twice daily.

**Product licence number** 08821/0021.

## NORIDAY* TABLETS

**Qualitative and quantitative composition** Each tablet contains 350 micrograms Norethisterone BP.

**Pharmaceutical form** White, flat, circular, bevel-edged tablet inscribed 'SYNTEX' on one side and 'NORIDAY' on the other side.

### Clinical particulars

*Therapeutic indications:* Noriday is a progestogen-only oral contraceptive. It is particularly useful for women for whom oestrogens may not be appropriate.

*Posology and method of administration*

*Oral administration:* The first Noriday tablet is taken on the first day of the menstrual cycle. Thereafter, one tablet is taken continuously at the same time every day even during menstrual bleeding.

Patients unable to start taking Noriday tablets on the first day of the menstrual cycle may start treatment on any day up to and including the 5th day of the menstrual cycle.

Patients starting on day 1 of their period will be protected at once. Those patients delaying therapy up to day 5 may not be protected immediately and it is recommended that another method of contraception is used for the first 7 days of tablet-taking. Suitable methods are condoms, caps plus spermicides and intra-uterine devices. The rhythm, temperature and cervical-mucus methods cannot be used.

*Tablet omissions:* Tablets must be taken daily in order to maintain adequate hormone levels and contraceptive efficacy.

If a tablet is missed within 3 hours of the correct dosage time then the missed tablet should be taken as soon as possible; this will ensure that contraceptive protection is maintained. If one (for longer than 3 hours) or more tablets are missed it is recommended that the patient takes the last missed tablet as soon as possible and then continues to take the rest of the tablets in the normal manner. However, to provide continued contraceptive protection it is recommended that an alternative method of contraception, such as a condom, is used for the next 7 days.

*Changing from another oral contraceptive:* In order to ensure that contraception is maintained it is advised that the first dose of Noriday tablets is taken on the day immediately after the patient has finished the previous pack of tablets.

*Use after childbirth, miscarriage or abortion:* The first dose of Noriday tablets should be taken on the 21st day after childbirth. This will ensure the patient is protected immediately. If there is any delay in taking the first dose, contraception may not be established until 7 days after the first tablet has been taken. In these circumstances patients should be advised that extra contraceptive methods will be necessary.

After a miscarriage or abortion patients can take the first dose of Noriday tablets on the next day; in this way they will be protected immediately.

*Contra-indications:* A history during pregnancy of idiopathic jaundice or severe pruritus. Acute or severe chronic liver diseases including liver tumours, Dubin-Johnson or Rotor syndrome. Undiagnosed abnormal vaginal bleeding. Thrombo-embolic disorders, thrombophlebitis, cerebrovascular disorders, coronary artery disease, myocardial infarction, angina, hyperlipidaemia or a history of these conditions. Pregnancy.

*Special warnings and special precautions for use:* Special caution should be observed in the presence of pre-existing breast or genital-tract cancer.

Gastro-intestinal upsets, such as vomiting and diarrhoea, may interfere with the absorption of the tablets leading to a reduction in contraceptive efficacy. Patients should continue to take Noriday, but they should also be encouraged to use another contraceptive method during the period of gastro-intestinal upset and for the next 7 days.

Noriday should be used with caution in patients with a history of hepatic dysfunction or hypertension.

A statistical association between the use of oral contraceptives and the occurrence of thrombosis, embolism or haemorrhage has been reported.

Patients receiving oral contraceptives should be kept under regular surveillance, in view of the possibility of development of conditions such as thromboembolism.

The risk of coronary artery disease in women taking oral contraceptives is increased by the presence of other predisposing factors such as cigarette smoking, hypercholesterolaemia, obesity, diabetes, history of pre-eclamptic toxaemia and increasing age. After the age of thirty-five years, the patient and physician should carefully re-assess the risk/benefit ratio of using oral contraceptives as opposed to alternative methods of contraception.

Noriday should be discontinued at least four weeks before, and for two weeks following, elective operations and during immobilisation.

Benign and malignant liver tumours have been associated with oral contraceptive use. The relationship between occurrence of liver tumours and use of female sex hormones is not known at present. These tumours may rupture causing intra-abdominal bleeding. If the patient presents with a mass or tenderness in the right upper quadrant or an acute abdomen, the possible presence of a tumour should be considered.

An increased risk of congenital abnormalities, including heart defects and limb defects, has been reported following the use of sex hormones, including oral contraceptives, in pregnancy. If the patient does not adhere to the prescribed schedule, the possibility of pregnancy should be considered at the time of the first missed period and further use of oral contraceptives should be withheld until pregnancy has been ruled out. It is recommended that for any patient who has missed two consecutive periods, pregnancy should be ruled out before continuing the contraceptive regimen. If pregnancy is confirmed the patient should be advised of the potential risks to the foetus and the advisability of continuing the pregnancy should be discussed in the light of these risks. It is advisable to discontinue Noriday three months before a planned pregnancy.

Progestogen-only oral contraceptives such as Noriday may offer less protection against ectopic pregnancy than against intra-uterine pregnancy.

*Interactions with other medicaments and other forms of interaction:* Some drugs may modify the metabolism of Noriday reducing its effectiveness; these include certain sedatives, antibiotics, anti-epileptic and anti-arthritic drugs. During the time such agents are used concurrently, it is advised that mechanical contraceptives also be used.

*Pregnancy and lactation:* Contra-indicated in pregnancy.

There is no evidence that Noriday tablets diminish the yield of breast milk. Small amounts of steroid materials appear in the milk; their effect on the breast-fed child has not been determined.

*Effects on ability to drive and use machines:* None.

*Undesirable effects:* The incidence of side-effects in clinical trials was lower than that experienced with oestrogen-containing oral contraceptives. Side-effects which did occur included some cycle irregularity during the first few months of therapy, spotting or breakthrough bleeding, amenorrhoea, breast discomfort, gastro-intestinal symptoms, headaches, migraine, depression, fatigue, nervousness, disturbance of appetite, changes in weight and libido, rash.

Hypertension, which is usually reversible on discontinuing treatment, has occurred in a small percentage of women taking oral contraceptives.

*Menstrual pattern:* A usual feature of all progestogen-only oral contraceptives is that they produce an initial irregularity of the bleeding pattern, but such irregularity tends to decrease with time. The patient should be informed before starting Noriday tablets that her menstrual pattern is likely to alter.

Irregular bleeding is, from a medical point of view, no reason for discontinuation of therapy, as long as organic causes and pregnancy can be ruled out. The patient should be instructed that if two or more consecutive periods are missed, she should consult her physician in order to rule out pregnancy.

*Overdose:* Overdosage may be manifested by nausea, vomiting, breast enlargement and vaginal bleeding. There is no specific antidote and treatment should be symptomatic. Gastric lavage may be employed if the overdose is large and the patient is seen sufficiently early (within four hours).

### Pharmacological properties

*Pharmacodynamic properties:* Norethisterone administration increases the protein and sialic acid content of cervical mucus which prevents penetration of the mucus by spermatozoa. It causes changes in the structure of the endometrium such that implantation of blastocysts is impaired. It also reduces numbers and height of cilia on cells lining the fallopian tube, which could delay tubal transport of ova.

*Pharmacokinetic properties:* Norethisterone is rapidly and completely absorbed after oral administration, peak plasma concentrations occurring in the majority of subjects between 1 and 3 hours. Due to first-pass metabolism, blood levels after oral administration are 60% of those after i.v. administration. The half life of elimination varies from 5 to 12 hours, with a mean of 7.6 hours. Norethisterone is metabolised mainly in the liver. Approximately 60% of the administered dose is excreted as metabolites in urine and faeces.

*Preclinical safety data:* The toxicity of norethisterone is very low. Reports of teratogenic effects in animals are uncommon. No carcinogenic effects have been found even in long-term studies. In subacute and chronic studies only minimal differences between treated and control animals are observed.

### Pharmaceutical particulars

*List of excipients:* Noriday tablets contain: Maize starch, povidone, magnesium stearate and lactose.

*Incompatibilities:* None stated.

*Shelf life:* The shelf life of Noriday tablets is 5 years.

*Special precautions for storage:* Store in a cool, dry place away from direct sunlight.

*Nature and contents of container:* Noriday tablets are supplied in pvc/foil blister packs of 84 tablets. Blister packaging consists of 250 micron PVC and 20 micron aluminium foil.

*Special instructions for use/handling:* None.

*Marketing authorisation holder:* Monsanto p.l.c., PO Box 53, Lane End Road, High Wycombe, Bucks HP12 4HL.

**Marketing authorisation number** 08821/0036.

**Date of approval/revision of SPC** January 1996.

**Legal category** POM.

## NORIMIN*

**Qualitative and quantitative composition** Each tablet contains 1 milligram Norethisterone BP and 35 micrograms Ethinyloestradiol BP.

**Pharmaceutical form** Yellow flat, circular, bevel-edged tablet inscribed 'SYNTEX' on one side.

### Clinical particulars

*Therapeutic indications:* Norimin is indicated for oral contraception, with the benefit of a low intake of oestrogen.

*Posology and method of administration:* Oral administration: The dosage of Norimin for the initial cycle of therapy is 1 tablet taken at the same time each day from the first day of the menstrual cycle. For subsequent cycles, no tablets are taken for 7 days, then a new course is started of 1 tablet daily for the next 21 days. This sequence of 21 days on treatment, seven days off treatment is repeated for as long as contraception is required.

Patients unable to start taking Norimin tablets on the first day of the menstrual cycle may start treatment on any day up to and including the 5th day of the menstrual cycle.

Patients starting on day 1 of their period will be protected at once. Those patients delaying therapy up to day 5 may not be protected immediately and it is recommended that another method of contraception is used for the first 7 days of tablet taking. Suitable methods are condoms, caps plus spermicides and intra-uterine devices. The rhythm, temperature and cervical-mucus methods should not be relied upon.

*Tablet omissions:* Tablets must be taken daily in order to maintain adequate hormone levels and contraceptive efficacy.

If a tablet is missed within 12 hours of the correct dosage time then the missed tablet should be taken as soon as possible, even if this means taking 2 tablets on the same day, this will ensure that contraceptive protection is maintained. If one or more tablets are missed for more than 12 hours from the correct dosage time it is recommended that the patient takes the last missed tablet as soon as possible and then continues to take the rest of the tablets in the normal manner. In addition, it is recommended that extra contraceptive protection, such as a condom, is used for the next 7 days.

Patients who have missed one or more of the last 7 tablets in a pack should be advised to start the next pack of tablets as soon as the present one has finished (i.e. without the normal seven day gap between treatments). This reduces the risk of contraceptive failure resulting from tablets being missed close to a 7 day tablet free period.

*Changing from another oral contraceptive:* In order to ensure that contraception is maintained it is advised that the first dose of Norimin tablets is taken on the day immediately after the patient has finished the previous pack of tablets.

*Use after childbirth, miscarriage or abortion:* Providing the patient is not breast feeding the first dose of Norimin tablets should be taken on the 21st day after childbirth. This will ensure the patient is protected immediately. If there is any delay in taking the first dose, contraception may not be established until 7 days after the first tablet has been taken. In these circumstances patients should be advised that extra contraceptive methods will be necessary.

After a miscarriage or abortion patients can take the first dose of Norimin tablets on the next day; in this way they will be protected immediately.

*Contra-indications:* As with all combined progestogen/oestrogen oral contraceptives, the following conditions should be regarded as contra-indications:

(i) Thrombophlebitis, thrombo-embolic disorders, cerebrovascular disorders, coronary artery disease, myocardial infarction, angina, hyperlipidaemia or a history of these conditions.

(ii) Acute or severe chronic liver disease, including liver tumours, Dubin-Johnson or Rotor syndrome.
(iii) History during pregnancy of idiopathic jaundice, severe pruritus or pemphigoid gestationis.
(iv) Known or suspected breast or genital cancer.
(v) Known or suspected oestrogen-dependent neoplasia.
(vi) Undiagnosed abnormal vaginal bleeding.
(vii) A history of migraines classified as classical focal or crescendo.
(viii) Pregnancy.

*Special warnings and precautions for use:* Women taking oral contraceptives require careful observation if they have or have had any of the following conditions: breast nodules; fibrocystic disease of the breast or an abnormal mammogram; uterine fibroids; a history of severe depressive states; varicose veins; sickle-cell anaemia; diabetes; hypertension; cardiovascular disease; migraine; epilepsy; asthma; otosclerosis, multiple sclerosis; porphyria; tetany; disturbed liver functions; gallstones; kidney disease; chloasma; any condition that is likely to worsen during pregnancy. The worsening or first appearance of any of these conditions may indicate that the oral contraceptive should be stopped. Discontinue treatment if there is a gradual or sudden, partial or complete loss of vision or any evidence of ocular changes, onset or aggravation of migraine or development of headache of a new kind which is recurrent, persistent or severe.

Gastro-intestinal upsets, such as vomiting and diarrhoea, may interfere with the absorption of the tablets leading to a reduction in contraceptive efficacy. Patients should continue to take Norimin, but they should also be encouraged to use another contraceptive method during the period of gastro-intestinal upset and for the next 7 days.

Progestogen/oestrogen preparations should be used with caution in patients with a history of hepatic dysfunction or hypertension.

A statistical association between the use of oral contraceptives and the occurrence of thrombosis, embolism or haemorrhage has been reported. Patients receiving oral contraceptives should be kept under regular surveillance, in view of the possibility of development of conditions such as thromboembolism.

The risk of coronary artery disease in women taking oral contraceptives is increased by the presence of other predisposing factors such as cigarette smoking, hypercholesterolaemia, obesity, diabetes, history of pre-eclamptic toxaemia and increasing age. After the age of thirty-five years, the patient and physician should carefully re-assess the risk/benefit ratio of using combined oral contraceptives as opposed to alternative methods of contraception.

Norimin should be discontinued at least four weeks before, and for two weeks following, elective operations and during immobilisation. Patients undergoing injection treatment for varicose veins should not resume taking Norimin until 3 months after the last injection.

Benign and malignant liver tumours have been associated with oral contraceptive use. The relationship between occurrence of liver tumours and use of female sex hormones is not known at present. These tumours may rupture causing intra-abdominal bleeding. If the patient presents with a mass or tenderness in the right upper quadrant or an acute abdomen, the possible presence of a tumour should be considered.

An increased risk of congenital abnormalities, including heart defects and limb defects, has been reported following the use of sex hormones, including oral contraceptives, in pregnancy. If the patient does not adhere to the prescribed schedule, the possibility of pregnancy should be considered at the time of the first missed period and further use of oral contraceptives should be withheld until pregnancy has been ruled out. It is recommended that for any patient who has missed two consecutive periods, pregnancy should be ruled out before continuing the contraceptive regimen. If pregnancy is confirmed the patient should be advised of the potential risks to the foetus and the advisability of continuing the pregnancy should be discussed in the light of these risks. It is advisable to discontinue Norimin three months before a planned pregnancy.

The risk of arterial thrombosis associated with combined oral contraceptives increases with age, and this risk is aggravated by cigarette smoking. The use of combined oral contraceptives by women in the older age group, especially those who are cigarette smokers should therefore be discouraged and alternative methods advised.

The use of this product in patients suffering from epilepsy, migraine, asthma or cardiac dysfunction may result in exacerbation of these disorders because of fluid retention. Caution should also be observed in patients who wear contact lenses.

Decreased glucose tolerance may occur in diabetic patients on this treatment, and their control must be carefully supervised.

The use of oral contraceptives has also been associated with a possible increased incidence of gall bladder disease.

Women with a history of oligomenorrhoea or secondary amenorrhoea or young women without regular cycles may have a tendency to remain anovulatory or to become amenorrhoeic after discontinuation of oral contraceptives. Women with these pre-existing problems should be advised of this possibility and encouraged to use other contraceptive methods.

Numerous epidemiological studies have been reported on the risks of ovarian, endometrial, cervical and breast cancer in women using combined oral contraceptives. The evidence is clear that combined oral contraceptives offer substantial protection against both ovarian and endometrial cancer.

An increased risk of cervical cancer in long-term users of combined oral contraceptives has been reported in some studies, but there continues to be controversy about the extent to which this is attributable to the confounding effects of sexual behaviour and other factors.

The evidence linking combined oral contraceptive use and breast cancer remains inconclusive. The results of some studies suggest an increased risk of breast cancer presenting below the age of about 35, the risk rising with duration of use. Any possible increased risk of breast cancer with combined oral contraceptives is however likely to be small, and may be expected to be less with low dosage pills. This possible risk should be weighed against the many benefits of combined oral contraceptives, including their protective effects against ovarian and endometrial cancers.

*Interactions with other medicaments and other forms of interaction:* Some drugs may modify the metabolism of Norimin reducing its effectiveness; these include certain sedatives, antibiotics, anti-epileptic and anti-arthritic drugs. During the times such agents are used concurrently, it is advised that mechanical contraceptives also be used.

The results of a large number of laboratory tests have been shown to be influenced by the use of oestrogen containing oral contraceptives, which may limit their diagnostic value. Among these are: biochemical markers of thyroid and liver function; plasma levels of carrier proteins, triglycerides, coagulation and fibrinolysis factors.

*Pregnancy and lactation:* Contra-indicated in pregnancy.

Patients who are fully breast-feeding should not take Norimin tablets since, in common with other combined oral contraceptives, the oestrogen component may reduce the amount of milk produced. In addition, active ingredients or their metabolites have been detected in the milk of mothers taking oral contraceptives. The effect of Norimin on breast-fed infants has not been determined.

*Effects on ability to drive and use machines:* Not applicable.

*Undesirable effects:* As with all oral contraceptives, there may be slight nausea at first, weight gain or breast discomfort, which soon disappear.

Other side-effects known or suspected to occur with oral contraceptives include gastro-intestinal symptoms, changes in libido and appetite, headache, exacerbation of existing uterine fibroid disease, depression and changes in carbohydrate, lipid and vitamin metabolism.

Spotting or bleeding may occur during the first few cycles. Usually menstrual bleeding becomes light and occasionally there may be no bleeding during the tablet-free days.

Hypertension, which is usually reversible on discontinuing treatment, has occurred in a small percentage of women taking oral contraceptives.

*Overdose:* Overdosage may be manifested by nausea, vomiting, breast enlargement and vaginal bleeding. There is no specific antidote and treatment should be symptomatic. Gastric lavage may be employed if the overdose is large and the patient is seen sufficiently early (within four hours).

**Pharmacological properties**

*Pharmacodynamic properties:* The mode of action of Norimin is similar to that of other progestogen/oestrogen oral contraceptives and includes the inhibition of ovulation, the thickening of cervical mucus so as to constitute a barrier to sperm and the rendering of the endometrium unreceptive to implantation. Such activity is exerted through a combined effect on one or more of the following: hypothalamus, anterior pituitary, ovary, endometrium and cervical mucus.

*Pharmacokinetic properties:* Norithisterone is rapidly and completely absorbed after oral administration, peak plasma concentrations occurring in the majority of subjects between 1 and 3 hours. Due to first-pass metabolism, blood levels after oral administration are 60% of those after i.v. administration. The half life of elimination varies from 5 to 12 hours, with a mean of 7.6 hours. Norethisterone is metabolised mainly in the liver. Approximately 60% of the administered dose is excreted as metabolites in urine and faeces.

Ethinyloestradiol is rapidly and well absorbed from the gastro-intestinal tract but is subject to some first-pass metabolism in the gut-wall. Compared to many other oestrogens it is only slowly metabolised in the liver. Excretion is via the kidneys with some appearing also in the faeces.

*Preclinical safety data:* The toxicity of norithisterone is very low. Reports of teratogenic effects in animals are uncommon. No carcinogenic effects have been found even in long-term studies.

Long-term continuous administration of oestrogens in some animals increases the frequency of carcinoma of the breast, cervix, vagina and liver.

**Pharmaceutical particulars**

*List of excipients:* Norimin tablets contain: Maize starch, povidone, magnesium stearate, lactose and E104.

*Incompatibilities:* None stated.

*Shelf life:* The shelf life of Norimin tablets is 5 years.

*Special precautions for storage:* Store in a dry place, below 25°C, away from direct sunlight.

*Nature and contents of container:* Norimin tablets are supplied in pvc/foil blister packs of 21 and 63 tablets.

*Instruction for use/handling:* None.

*Marketing authorisation holder:* Monsanto p.l.c., PO Box 53, Lane End Road, High Wycombe, Bucks HP12 4HL.

**Marketing authorisation number** 00821/0040.

**Date of approval/revision of SPC** March 1996.

**Legal category** POM.

## NORINYL-1*

**Qualitative and quantitative composition** Each tablet contains 1 milligram Norethisterone BP and 50 micrograms Mestranol BP.

**Pharmaceutical form** White, flat, circular, bevel-edged tablet inscribed 'SYNTEX' on one side and 'Norinyl' on the other side.

**Clinical particulars**

*Therapeutic indications:* Norinyl-1 is indicated for oral contraception, with the benefit of a low intake of oestrogen.

*Posology and method of administration:* Oral administration: The dosage of Norinyl-1 for the initial cycle of therapy is 1 tablet taken at the same time each day from the first day of the menstrual cycle. For subsequent cycles, no tablets are taken for 7 days, then a new course is started of 1 tablet daily for the next 21 days. This sequence of 21 days on treatment, seven days off treatment is repeated for as long as contraception is required.

Patients unable to start taking Norinyl-1 tablets on the first day of the menstrual cycle may start treatment on any day up to and including the 5th day of the menstrual cycle.

Patients starting on day 1 of their period will be protected at once. Those patients delaying therapy up to day 5 may not be protected immediately and it is recommended that another method of contraception is used for the first 7 days of tablet taking. Suitable methods are condoms, caps plus spermicides and intra-uterine devices. The rhythm, temperature and cervical-mucous methods should not be relied upon.

*Tablet omissions:* Tablets must be taken daily in order to maintain adequate hormone levels and contraceptive efficacy.

If a tablet is missed within 12 hours of the correct dosage time then the missed tablet should be taken as soon as possible, even if this means taking 2 tablets on the same day, this will ensure that contraceptive protection is maintained. If one or more tablets are missed for more than 12 hours from the correct dosage time it is recommended that the patient takes the last missed tablet as soon as possible and then continues to take the rest of the tablets in the normal manner. In addition, it is recommended that extra contraceptive protection, such as a condom, is used for the next 7 days.

Patients who have missed one or more of the last 7 tablets in a pack should be advised to start the next pack of tablets as soon as the present one has finished (i.e. without the normal seven day gap between treatments). This reduces the risk of contraceptive failure resulting from tablets being missed close to a 7 day tablet free period.

*Changing from another oral contraceptive:* In order to ensure that contraception is maintained it is advised that the first dose of Norinyl-1 tablets is taken on the day immediately after the patient has finished the previous pack of tablets.

*Use after childbirth, miscarriage or abortion:* Providing the patient is not breast feeding the first dose of Norinyl-1 tablets should be taken on the 21st day after childbirth. This will ensure the patient is protected immediately. If there is any delay in taking the first dose, contraception may not be established until 7 days after the first tablet has been taken. In these circumstances patients should be advised that extra contraceptive methods will be necessary.

After a miscarriage or abortion patients can take the first dose of Norinyl-1 tablets on the next day; in this way they will be protected immediately.

*Contra-indications:* As with all combied progestogen/oestrogen oral contraceptives, the following conditions should be regarded as contra-indications:

   (i)  Thrombophlebitis, thrombo-embolic disorders, cerebrovascular disorders, coronary artery disease, myocardial infarction, angina, hyperlipidaemia or a history of these conditions.

   (ii)  Acute or severe chronic liver disease, including liver tumours, Dubin-Johnson or Rotor syndrome.

   (iii)  History during pregnancy of idiopathic jaundice, severe pruritus or pemphigoid gestationis.

   (iv)  Known or suspected breast or genital cancer.

   (v)  Known or suspected oestrogen-dependent neoplasia.

   (vi)  Undiagnosed abnormal vaginal bleeding.

   (vii)  A history of migraines classified as classical focal or crescendo.

   (viii)  Pregnancy.

*Special warnings and precautions for use:* Women taking oral contraceptives require careful observation if they have or have had any of the following conditions: breast nodules; fibrocystic disease of the breast or an abnormal mammogram; uterine fibroids; a history of severe depressive states; varicose veins; sickle-cell anaemia; diabetes; hypertension; cardiovascular disease; migraine; epilepsy; asthma; otosclerosis, multiple sclerosis; porphyria; tetany; disturbed liver functions; gallstones; kidney disease; chloasma; any condition that is likely to worsen during pregnancy. The worsening or first appearance of any of these conditions may indicate that the oral contraceptive should be stopped. Discontinue treatment if there is a gradual or sudden, partial or complete loss of vision or any evidence of ocular changes, onset or aggravation of migraine or development of headache of a new kind which is recurrent, persistent or severe.

Gastro-intestinal upsets, such as vomiting and diarrhoea, may interfere with the absorption of the tablets leading to a reduction in contraceptive efficacy. Patients should continue to take Norinyl-1, but they should also be encouraged to use another contraceptive method during the period of gastro-intestinal upset and for the next 7 days.

Progestogen/oestrogen preparations should be used with caution in patients with a history of hepatic dysfunction or hypertension.

A statistical association between the use of oral contraceptives and the occurrence of thrombosis, embolism or haemorrhage has been reported. Patients receiving oral contraceptives should be kept under regular surveillance, in view of the possibility of development of conditions such as thromboembolism.

The risk of coronary artery disease in women taking oral contraceptives is increased by the presence of other predisposing factors such as cigarette smoking, hypercholesterolaemia, obesity, diabetes, history of pre-eclamptic toxaemia and increasing age. After the age of thirty-five years, the patient and physician should carefully re-assess the risk/benefit ratio of using combined oral contraceptives as opposed to alternative methods of contraception.

Norinyl-1 should be discontinued at least four weeks before, and for two weeks following, elective operations and during immobilisation. Patients undergoing injection treatment for varicose veins should not resume taking Norinyl-1 until 3 months after the last injection.

Benign and malignant liver tumours have been associated with oral contraceptive use. The relationship between occurrence of liver tumours and use of female sex hormones is not known at present. These tumours may rupture causing intra-abdominal bleeding. If the patient presents with a mass of tenderness in the right upper quadrant or an acute abdomen, the possible presence of a tumour should be considered.

An increased risk of congenital abnormalities, including heart defects and limb defects, has been reported following the use of sex hormones, including oral contraceptives, in pregnancy. If the patient does not adhere to the prescribed schedule, the possibility of pregnancy should be considered at the time of the first missed period and further use of oral contracep-

tives should be withheld until pregnancy has been ruled out. It is recommended that for any patient who has missed two consecutive periods, pregnancy should be ruled out before continuing the contraceptive regimen. If pregnancy is confirmed the patient should be advised of the potential risks to the foetus and the advisability of continuing the pregnancy should be discussed in the light of these risks. It is advisable to discontinue Norinyl-1 three months before a planned pregnancy.

The risk of arterial thrombosis associated with combined oral contraceptives increases with age, and this risk is aggravated by cigarette smoking. The use of combined oral contraceptives by women in the older age group, especially those who are cigarette smokers should therefore be discouraged and alternative methods advised.

The use of this product in patients suffering from epilepsy, migraine, asthma or cardiac dysfunction may result in exacerbation of these disorders because of fluid retention. Caution should also be observed in patients who wear contact lenses.

Decreased glucose tolerance may occur in diabetic patients on this treatment, and their control must be carefully supervised.

The use of oral contraceptives has also been associated with a possible increased incidence of gall bladder disease.

Women with a history of oligomenorrhoea or secondary amenorrhoea or young women without regular cycles may have a tendency to remain anovulatory or to become amenorrhoeic after discontinuation of oral contraceptives. Women with these pre-existing problems should be advised of this possibility and encouraged to use other contraceptive methods.

Numerous epidemiological studies have been reported on the risks of ovarian, endometrial, cervical and breast cancer in women using combined oral contraceptives. The evidence is clear that combined oral contraceptives offer substantial protection against both ovarian and endometrial cancer.

An increased risk of cervical cancer in long-term users of combined oral contraceptives has been reported in some studies, but there continues to be controversy about the extent to which this is attributable to the confounding effects of sexual behaviour and other factors.

The evidence linking combined oral contraceptive use and breast cancer remains inconclusive. The results of some studies suggest an increased risk of breast cancer presenting below the age of about 35, the risk rising with duration of use. Any possible increased risk of breast cancer with combined oral contraceptives is however likely to be small, and may be expected to be less with low dosage pills. This possible risk should be weighed against the many benefits of combined oral contraceptives, including their protective effects against ovarian and endometrial cancers.

*Interactions with other medicaments and other forms of interaction:* Some drugs may modify the metabolism of Norinyl-1 reducing its effectiveness; these include certain sedatives, antibiotics, anti-epileptic and anti-arthritic drugs. During the times such agents are used concurrently, it is advised that mechanical contraceptives also be used.

The results of a large number of laboratory tests have been shown to be influenced by the use of oestrogen containing oral contraceptives, which may limit their diagnostic value. Among these are: biochemical markers of thyroid and liver function; plasma levels of carrier proteins, triglycerides, coagulation and fibrinolysis factors.

*Pregnancy and lactation:* Contra-indicated in pregnancy.

Patients who are fully breast-feeding should not take Norinyl-1 tablets since, in common with other combined oral contraceptives, the oestrogen component may reduce the amount of milk produced. In addition, active ingredients or their metabolites have been detected in the milk of mothers taking oral contraceptives. The effect of Norinyl-1 on breast-fed infants has not been determined.

*Effects on ability to drive and use machines:* Not applicable.

*Undesirable effects:* As with all oral contraceptives, there may be a slight nausea at first, weight gain or breast discomfort, which soon disappear.

Other side-effects known or suspected to occur with oral contraceptives include gastro-intestinal symptoms, changes in libido and appetite, headache, exacerbation of existing uterine fibroid disease, depression and changes in carbohydrate, lipid and vitamin metabolism.

Spotting or bleeding may occur during the first few cycles. Usually menstrual bleeding becomes light and occasionally there may be no bleeding during the tablet-free days.

Hypertension, which is usually reversible on discon-

tinuing treatment, has occurred in a small percentage of women taking oral contraceptives.

*Overdose:* Overdosage may be manifested by nausea, vomiting, breast enlargement and vaginal bleeding. There is no specific antidote and treatment should be symptomatic. Gastric lavage may be employed if the overdose is large and the patient is seen sufficiently early (within four hours).

**Pharmacological properties**

*Pharmacodynamic properties:* The mode of action of Norinyl-1 is similar to that of other progestogen/oestrogen oral contraceptives and includes the inhibition of ovulation, the thickening of cervical mucus so as to constitute a barrier to sperm and the rendering of the endometrium unreceptive to implantation. Such activity is exerted through a combined effect on one or more of the following: hypothalamus, anterior pituitary, ovary, endometrium and cervical mucus.

*Pharmacokinetic properties:* Norithisterone is rapidly and completely absorbed after oral administration, peak plasma concentrations occurring in the majority of subjects between 1 and 3 hours. Due to first-pass metabolism, blood levels after oral administration are 60% of those after i.v. administration. The half life of elimination varies from 5 to 12 hours, with a mean of 7.6 hours. Norethisterone is metabolised mainly in the liver. Approximately 60% of the administered dose is excreted as metabolites in urine and faeces.

Mestranol is rapidly absorbed and extensively metabolised to ethinyloestradiol. Ethinyloestradiol is rapidly and well absorbed from the gastro-intestinal tract but is subject to some first-pass metabolism in the gut-wall. Compared to many other oestrogens it is only slowly metabolised in the liver. Excretion is via the kidneys with some appearing also in the faeces.

*Preclinical safety data:* The toxicity of norithisterone is very low. Reports of teratogenic effects in animals are uncommon. No carcinogenic effects have been found even in long-term studies.

Long-term continuous administration of oestrogens in some animals increases the frequency of carcinoma of the breast, cervix, vagina and liver.

**Pharmaceutical particulars**

*List of excipients:* Norinyl-1 tablets contain: Maize starch, povidone, magnesium stearate, and lactose.

*Incompatibilities:* None stated.

*Shelf life:* The shelf life of Norinyl-1 tablets is 5 years.

*Special precautions for storage:* Store in a dry place, below 25°C, away from direct sunlight.

*Nature and contents of container:* Norinyl-1 tablets are supplied in pvc/foil blister packs of 21 and 63 tablets.

*Instruction for use/handling:* None.

*Marketing authorisation holder:* Monsanto p.l.c., PO Box 53, Lane End Road, High Wycombe, Bucks HP12 4HL.

**Marketing authorisation number** 08821/0039.

**Date of approval/revision of SPC** 24 April 1996.

**Legal category** POM.

# POWERGEL

**Presentation** Colourless, non-greasy, non-staining gel with an aromatic fragrance for topical application, containing ketoprofen BP 2.5% w/w. The gel also contains carboxypolymethylene, ethanol, esters of p-hydroxybenzoic acid, neroli oil, lavender oil, diethanolamine and water.

**Uses**

*Indications:* For local relief of pain and inflammation associated with soft tissue injuries and acute strains and sprains.

*Actions:* Ketoprofen is a non-steroidal anti-inflammatory drug. It has anti-inflammatory and analgesic action. Powergel allows the site specific topical delivery of ketoprofen with very low plasma concentrations of drug. Therapeutic levels in the affected tissues provide relief from pain and inflammation, yet will satisfactorily overcome the problem of significant systemic unwanted effects.

**Dosage and administration** Powergel should be applied topically to the affected area two or three times daily. Maximum duration of use should not exceed 10 days. After application Powergel should be rubbed in well to ensure local absorption of ketoprofen.

*Adults and elderly:* Apply 5 to 10 cm of gel (100-200 mg ketoprofen) with each application.

*Children under 12 years of age:* Not recommended as experience in children is limited.

**Contra-indications, warnings, etc**
*Contra-indications:* Hypersensitivity to ketoprofen or aspirin or other non-steroidal anti-inflammatory drugs. Severe bronchospasm might be precipitated in these patients and in those suffering from, or with a history of bronchial asthma or allergic disease. Hence Powergel should not be administered to patients in whom aspirin or other NSAIDs have caused asthma, rhinitis or urticaria.

*Precautions:* Powergel should not be applied to open wounds or lesions of the skin, or near the eyes. Powergel should be used with caution in patients with renal impairment. Keep out of the reach of children.

*Drug interactions:* No interactions of Powergel with other drugs have been reported. It is however advisable to monitor patients under treatment with coumarinic substances.

*Pregnancy and lactation:* No embryopathic effects have been demonstrated in animals and there is no epidemiological evidence of the safety of ketoprofen in human pregnancy. Therefore, it is recommended to avoid ketoprofen unless considered essential in which case it should be discontinued within one week of expected confinement when NSAIDs might cause premature closure of the ductus arteriosus or persistent pulmonary hypertension in the neonate. They may also delay labour. Trace amounts of ketoprofen are excreted in breast milk after systemic administration.

*Adverse effects:* The prolonged use of products for topical administration may cause hypersensitivity phenomena. In such cases the treatment should be discontinued and a suitable alternative therapy instituted. Skin photosensitivity has been reported in isolated cases. Although not known for topical use of ketoprofen, the following adverse events are reported for systemic use: Minor adverse events, frequently transient, consist of gastrointestinal effects such as indigestion, dyspepsia, nausea, constipation, diarrhoea, heartburn and various types of abdominal discomfort. Other minor effects such as headache, dizziness, mild confusion, vertigo, drowsiness, oedema, mood change and insomnia may occur less frequently. Major gastrointestinal adverse events such as peptic ulceration, haemorrhage or perforation may rarely occur. Haematological reactions including thrombocytopenia, hepatic or renal damage, dermatological reactions, bronchospasm and anaphylaxis are exceedingly rare.

*Overdosage:* Considering the low blood levels of ketoprofen by the percutaneous route, no overdosage phenomena have been described yet.

**Pharmaceutical precautions** Store below 25°C.

**Legal category** POM.

**Package quantities** Packs of 50 g and 100 g tubes. Twin pack of 2×50 g tubes.

**Further information** Powergel is particularly beneficial when combined with physical therapies (ultrasound and iontophoresis).

*Product licence holder:* A Menarini s.r.l., 1–3 Via Sette Santi, Florence, Italy.

**Product licence number** 10649/0001.

## REHIDRAT* MULTIPACK

**Presentation** Foil/laminate sachets containing 14 g of fruit flavoured powder. Each sachet contains:

| | |
|---|---|
| Sodium Chloride PhEur | 0.44 g |
| Potassium Chloride PhEur | 0.38 g |
| Sodium Bicarbonate PhEur | 0.42 g |
| Citric Acid PhEur | 0.44 g |
| Glucose | 4.09–4.13 g |
| Sucrose PhEur | 8.07–8.17 g |
| Fructose | 0.01–0.07 g |
| Plus flavourings | |

**Uses** Oral electrolyte mixture for the prevention and correction of mild and moderate dehydration in the management of diarrhoea in infants, children and adults.

Maintenance and replacement of fluid and electrolytes following corrective parenteral therapy for dehydration. As a supplement to corrective parenteral therapy for dehydration.

**Dosage and administration**
*General advice:* The contents of one 14 g sachet should be dissolved in 250 ml of drinking water. For infants the water should be freshly boiled AND COOLED. The solution should be freshly made immediately prior to use. Any unused solution remaining an hour after reconstitution should be discarded unless stored in a refrigerator where it may be kept and used for up to 24 hours. ADVISE PATIENTS THAT THE SOLUTION SHOULD NOT BE BOILED AFTER RECONSTITUTION, AND THAT IT SHOULD BE USED AT THE RECOMMENDED DILUTION. The degree of dehydration should be assessed. Patients with mild or moderate dehydration may appear almost normal; they may be thirsty and may have normal or slightly diminished skin elasticity or, in children, slightly sunken fontanelle. Urine flow may be reduced. Patients with signs of severe dehydration who are usually too weak to drink will initially require parenteral therapy. Oral therapy should only be instituted when shock is corrected. The volume of reconstituted Rehidrat required will depend on the weight of the patient.

*General guidelines for oral therapy*
*1. Rehydration – Replacement of fluid and electrolyte losses. Mild or moderate dehydration:* 50–120 ml per kilogram body weight orally, usually given in divided doses over 4 to 6 hours. Adults may need up to 1000 ml per hour. A continuous nasogastric infusion may be used if necessary.

*2. Maintenance*
*Mild to moderate diarrhoea:* 100–200 ml per kilogram body weight orally over a period of 24 hours in divided doses.

*Continuing diarrhoea:* 15 ml per kilogram body weight orally every hour. Observe carefully to confirm adequate maintenance of hydration.

Where nausea or vomiting is present Rehidrat should be administered in small frequent doses, in sips. If vomiting persists appropriate intravenous therapy should be instituted. The patient instruction leaflet included in each carton advises patients to consult their doctor if there is no improvement in 24–48 hours.

*Elderly:* Administer Rehidrat in amounts appropriate to correct dehydration. Also see *Precautions.*

*Infants and children:* For bottle fed infants advise mothers to make the feed up for a 24 hour period and to store the reconstituted solution in the refrigerator.

Diarrhoea can have serious consequences in children under 3 years old. For this age group, the patient instruction leaflet included in each carton, advises that management should be on medical advice. Breast feeding should continue and Rehidrat should be given after feeds. In other infants and children administration of Rehidrat should begin with discontinuation of cow's milk and solids for 24 hours. Regrading of feeds is advisable and should be adjusted to meet individual needs. Cow's milk should gradually be introduced over a period of about five days as treatment with Rehidrat continues.

A suggested regimen for regrading of feeds in infants is given below. Regrading may be carried out more quickly for older children.

| *Day* | *Volume of Rehidrat Solution (ml)* | *Volume of Milk (ml)* | *Total volume in 24 hours (ml)* |
|---|---|---|---|
| 1 | 150×wt† | 0 | 150×wt |
| 2 | 120×wt | 30×wt | 150×wt |
| 3 | 90×wt | 60×wt | 150×wt |
| 4 | 60×wt | 90×wt | 150×wt |
| 5 | 30×wt | 120×wt | 150×wt |
| 6 | 0 | 150×wt | 150×wt |

† Weight in kilograms

Solids are usually reintroduced when the infant is receiving full strength milk but introduction may be sooner to suit individual needs.

*Simplified oral dosage guidelines:* For mild diarrhoea a simplified dosage scheme may be suggested. Young children may be given Rehidrat solution in quantities usual for their normal feeds, in conjunction with an appropriate graduated feeding regimen.

Older children and adults may be allowed to drink Rehidrat solution to satisfy their thirst.

**Contra-indications, warnings, etc**
*Contra-indications:* Rehidrat is contra-indicated in patients with renal impairment manifesting as oliguria or anuria, intestinal obstruction, paralytic ileus, intractable vomiting and in patients with severe dehydration which requires parenteral fluid therapy.

*Precautions:* When Rehidrat is used as a supplement to parenteral fluid therapy, care must be taken not to exceed the total water and electrolyte requirements.

The sugar content of Rehidrat should be considered when treating diabetics.

Administration of oral sugar-electrolyte solutions to patients with sugar malabsorption may worsen diarrhoea.

*Drug interactions:* Rehidrat should not be mixed or given with electrolyte-containing solutions. Salt or sugar should not be added to Rehidrat.

*Adverse effects:* Incorrect dilution could result in abnormalities of carbohydrate and electrolyte balance.

*Overdosage:* Toxicity resulting from overdosage of oral electrolyte solutions is rare. In the event of overdosage hypernatraemia or hyperkalaemia could occur.

**Pharmaceutical precautions** Store in a dry place below 30°C (86°F).

**Legal category** P.

**Package quantities** Carton of 16 sachets with instructions for use.

Each carton contains 6 sachets each of Rehidrat Orange and Rehidrat Blackcurrent and 4 sachets of Rehidrat Lemon & Lime.

**Further information** When reconstituted with 250 ml of water the solution has the followig composition:

| | mmol/l |
|---|---|
| Sodium | 50 |
| Potassium | 20 |
| Chloride | 50 |
| Bicarbonate | 20 |
| Citrate | 9 |
| Glucose | 91–2 |
| Sucrose | 94–6 |
| Fructose | <1–2 |
| Total osmolarity | 336–337 |

**Product licence number** 8821/0034.

## SYNAREL NASAL SPRAY*

**Qualitative and quantitative composition** Solution containing 2 mg/ml of nafarelin (as acetate) supplied in bottles fitted with a metered spray pump that delivers 200 micrograms of nafarelin base per spray.

**Pharmaceutical form** Solution for nasal inhalation.

**Clinical particulars**
*Therapeutic indications:* The hormonal management of endometriosis, including pain relief and reduction of endometriotic lesions.

Use in controlled ovarian stimulation programmes prior to in-vitro fertilisation, under the supervision of an infertility specialist.

*Posology and method of administration*
*Adult:* Synarel is for administration by the intranasal route only.

Experience with the treatment of endometriosis has been limited to women 18 years of age and older.

*Endometriosis:* In the use of Synarel in endometriosis, the aim is to induce chronic pituitary desensitisation, which gives a menopause-like state maintained over many months.

The recommended daily dose of Synarel is 200 mcg taken twice daily as one spray (200 mcg of nafarelin) to one nostril in the morning and one spray into the other nostril in the evening (400 mcg/day). Treatment should be started between days 2 and 4 of the menstrual cycle. The recommended duration of therapy is six months; only one 6-month course is advised. In clinical studies the majority of women have only received up to six-months treatment with Synarel.

*Controlled ovarian stimulation prior to in vitro fertilisation:* In the use of Synarel associated with controlled ovarian stimulation prior to *in vitro* fertilisation, the long protocol should be employed, whereby Synarel is continued through a period of transient gonadotrophin stimulation lasting 10–15 days (the 'flare effect') through to pituitary desensitisation (down-regulation). Down-regulation may be defined as serum oestradiol ≤50 pg/ml and serum progesterone ≤1 ng/ml, and the majority of patients down-regulate within 4 weeks.

The recommended daily dose of Synarel is 400 mcg taken twice daily as one spray to each nostril in the morning, and one spray to each nostril in the evening. (800 mcg/day).

Once down-regulation is achieved, controlled ovarian stimulation with gonadotrophins, e.g. hMG, is commenced, and the Synarel dosage maintained until the administration of hCG at follicular maturity (usually a further 8–12 days).

If patients do not down-regulate within 12 weeks of starting Synarel, it is recommended that Synarel therapy be discontinued and the cycle cancelled.

Treatment may begin in either the early follicular phase (day 2) or the mid-luteal phase (usually day 21).

If the use of a nasal decongestant is required at the time of nafarelin administration, it is recommended that the nasal decongestant be used at least 30 minutes after nafarelin dosing.

Sneezing during or immediately after dosing may impair absorption of Synarel. If sneezing occurs upon administration, repeating the dose may be advisable.

Bottles contain either 30 or 60 doses and should not be used for a greater number of doses. The 60 dose-unit bottle is sufficient for 30 days' treatment at 400 mcg (2 sprays) per day, and 15 days' treatment at 800 mcg (4 sprays) per day.

The 30 dose-unit bottle is sufficient for 15 days' treatment at 400 mcg (2 sprays) per day, and 7 days' treatment at 800 mcg (4 sprays) per day. Patients should therefore be advised that continued use after this time may result in delivery of an insufficient amount of nafarelin.

*Contra-indications:* A small loss of trabecular bone mineral content occurs during 6 months treatment with nafarelin. Although this is mostly reversible within 6 months of stopping treatment, there are no data on the effects of repeat courses on bone loss. Retreatment with Synarel or use for longer than 6 months is, therefore, not recommended. (See Side-effects section on 'Changes in bone density').

Synarel should not be administered to patients who:
1. are hypersensitive to GnRH, GnRH agonist analogues or any of the excipients in Synarel;
2. have undiagnosed vaginal bleeding;
3. are pregnant or may become pregnant whilst taking Synarel (see 'Use in pregnancy and lactation');
4. are breast-feeding.

*Special warnings and special precautions for use:* When regularly used at the recommended dose, nafarelin inhibits ovulation. Patients should be advised to use non-hormonal, barrier methods of contraception. In the event of missed doses there may be breakthrough ovulation and a potential for conception. If a patient becomes pregnant during treatment, administration of the drug must be discontinued and the patient must be informed of a potential risk to fetal development. NB Synarel treatment will be stopped at least 3 days before fertilised embryos are placed in the uterine cavity.

As with other drugs in this class ovarian cysts have been reported to occur in the first two months of therapy with Synarel. Many, but not all, of these events occurred in patients with polycystic ovarian disease. These cystic enlargements may resolve spontaneously, generally by about four to six weeks of therapy, but in some cases may require discontinuation of drug and/or surgical intervention.

*Controlled ovarian stimulation prior to in vitro fertilisation:* Transient ovarian cyst formation is a recognised complication of GnRH agonist use. These cysts tend to regress spontaneously over a number of weeks and are more common when GnRH agonists are commenced in the follicular phase of the cycle.

There are no clinical data available on the use of Synarel in ovulation induction regimens involving patients with polycystic ovarian syndrome. Caution is advised in this patient group as they are at greater risk of excessive follicular recruitment when undergoing ovulation induction regimens.

Administration of nafarelin in therapeutic doses results in suppression of the pituitary-gonadal system. Normal function is usually restored within 8 weeks after treatment is discontinued. Diagnostic tests of pituitary-gonadal function conducted during the treatment and up to 8 weeks after discontinuation of nafarelin therapy may therefore be misleading.

*Interactions with other medicaments and other forms of interaction:* Nafarelin would not be expected to participate in pharmacokinetic-based drug-drug interactions because degradation of the compound is primarily by the action of peptidases not cytochrome P-450 enzymes. Additionally, because nafarelin is only about 80% bound to plasma proteins (albumin), drug interactions at the protein-binding level would not be expected to occur.

Rhinitis does not impair nasal absorption of nafarelin. Nasal decongestants used 30 minutes before nafarelin administration decrease absorption.

*Pregnancy and lactation:* When administered intramuscularly to rats on days 6–15 of pregnancy at doses of 0.4, 1.6 and 6.4 mcg/kg/day (0.6, 2.5 and 10.0 times the intranasal human dose of 400 mcg per day), 4/80 fetuses in the highest dose group had major fetal abnormalities that were not seen in a repeat study in rats. Moreover, studies in mice and rabbits failed to demonstrate an increase in fetal abnormalities. In rats, there was a dose-related increase in fetal mortality, and a decrease in fetal weight with the highest dose. These effects on rat fetal mortality are logical consequences of the alterations in hormonal levels brought about by nafarelin in this species.

Use of nafarelin in human pregnancy has not been studied.

Synarel should not therefore be used during pregnancy or suspected pregnancy. Before starting treatment with Synarel pregnancy must be excluded. If a patient becomes pregnant during treatment, administration of the drug must be discontinued and the patient must be informed of a potential risk to fetal development.

*Controlled ovarian stimulation prior to in vitro fertilisation:* Pregnancy should be excluded before starting treatment with Synarel, and the medication should be stopped on the day of administration of hCG. Barrier methods of contraception should be employed whilst Synarel is being taken.

It is not known whether or to what extent nafarelin is excreted into human breast milk. The effects, if any, on the breast-fed child have not been determined and

therefore Synarel should not be used by breast-feeding women.

*Effects on ability to drive and use machines:* None.

*Undesirable effects:* In approximately 0.2% of adult patients, symptoms suggestive of drug sensitivity, such as shortness of breath, chest pain, urticaria, rash and pruritus have occurred.

As would be expected with a drug which lowers serum oestradiol levels to menopausal concentrations the most frequently reported adverse reactions are those related to hypo-oestrogenism.

In controlled studies of nafarelin 400 mcg/day, adverse reactions that were most frequently reported are listed in order of decreasing frequency: hot flushes, changes in libido, vaginal dryness, headaches, emotional lability, acne, myalgia, decreased breast size and irritation of the nasal mucosa.

During post-marketing surveillance, depression, paraesthesia, alopecia, migraine, palpitations, blurred vision have been reported. Emotional lability and depression would be expected with a drug that lowers serum oestradiol to post-menopausal levels.

*Changes in bone density:* After six months of Synarel treatment there was a reduction in vertebral trabecular bone density and total vertebral mass, averaging about 9% and 4%, respectively. There was very little, if any, decrease in the mineral content of compact bone of the distal radius and second metacarpal. Substantial recovery of bone occurred during the post-treatment period. Total vertebral bone mass, measured by dual photon absorptiometry (DPA), decreased by a mean of about 6% at the end of treatment. Mean total vertebral mass, re-examined by DPA six months after completion of treatment, was 1.4% below pretreatment levels. These changes are similar to those which occur during treatment with other GnRH agonists.

*Carcinogenesis/mutagenesis:* As seen with other GnRH agonists, nafarelin given parenterally in high doses to laboratory rodents for prolonged periods induced hyperplasia and neoplasia of endocrine organs, including the anterior pituitary (adenoma/carcinoma) of both mice and rats; tumours of the pancreatic islets, adrenal medulla, testes and ovaries occurred only in long-term studies in rats. No metastases of these tumours were observed. Monkeys treated with high doses of nafarelin for one year did not develop any tumours or proliferative changes. Experience in humans is limited but there is no evidence for tumorigenesis of GnRH analogues in human beings.

In vitro studies conducted in bacterial and mammalian systems provided no indication of a mutagenic potential for nafarelin.

*Impairment of fertility:* Reproduction studies in rats of both sexes have shown full reversibility of fertility suppression when drug treatment was discontinued after continuous administration for up to six months.

*Laboratory values:* Increased levels of SGOT/SGPT and serum alkaline phosphatase may rarely occur which are reversible on discontinuing treatment.

*Overdose:* In animals, subcutaneous administration of up to 60 times the recommended human dose (expressed on a mcg/kg basis) had no adverse effects. Orally-administered nafarelin is subject to enzymatic degradation in the gastro-intestinal tract and is therefore inactive. At present there is no clinical experience with overdosage of nafarelin.

Based on studies in monkeys, nafarelin is not absorbed after oral administration.

## Pharmacological properties
*Pharmacodynamic properties:* Nafarelin is a potent agonistic analogue of gonadotrophin releasing hormone (GnRH). Given as a single dose, nafarelin stimulates release of the pituitary gonadotrophins, LH and FSH, with consequent increase of ovarian and testicular steroidogenesis. During repeated dosing this response to stimulation gradually diminishes. Within three to four weeks, daily administration leads to decreased pituitary gonadotrophin secretion and/or the secretion of gonadotrophin secretion and/or the secretion of gonadotrophins with lowered biological activity. There is a consequent suppression of gonadal steroidogenesis and inhibition of functions in tissues that depend on gonadal steroids for their maintenance.

*Pharmacokinetic properties:* Nafarelin is rapidly absorbed into the circulation after intranasal administration. Maximum plasma concentration is achieved 20 minutes after dosing and the plasma half-life is approximately 4 hours. Bioavailability of the intranasal dose averages 2.8% (range 1.2–5.6%).

*Preclinical safety data:* This is discussed in 'Undesirable effects'.

## Pharmaceutical particulars
*List of excipients:* Synarel contains: Sorbitol, benzalkonium chloride, glacial acetic acid and water. Sodium hydroxide or hydrochloric acid to adjust pH.

*Incompatibilities:* None stated.

*Shelf life:* The shelf life of Synarel is 2 years.

*Special precautions for storage:* Store upright below 25°C. Protect from light and freezing.

*Nature and contents of container:* White, high density polyethylene bottles with a 0.1 ml metered spray pump containing 6.5 ml or 10 ml.

PVC-coated glass bottles with an internal conical reservoir in the base and a valois crimp-on pump, containing 4 ml or 8 ml.

*Special instructions for use/handling:* None.

*Marketing authorisation holder:* Monsanto p.l.c., PO Box 53, Lane End Road, High Wycombe, Bucks HP12 4HL.

**Marketing authorisation number**  08821/0042.

**Date of approval/revision of SPC**  May 1996.

**Legal category**  POM.

## SYNPHASE*

**Qualitative and quantitative composition**  Synphase consists of 7 white tablets containing Norethisterone BP 500 micrograms and Ethinyloestradiol BP 35 micrograms, marked 'B' on one side and 'SYNTEX' on the other; 9 yellow tablets containing Norethisterone BP 1.0 milligram and Ethinyloestradiol BP 35 micrograms inscribed 'SYNTEX' on one face; 5 white tablets containing Norethisterone BP 500 micrograms and Ethinyloestradiol BP 35 micrograms, marked 'B' on one side and 'SYNTEX' on the other.

**Pharmaceutical form**  Tablets for oral administration.

**Clinical particulars**
*Therapeutic indications:* Synphase is indicated for oral contraception, with the benefit of a low intake of oestrogen.

*Posology and method of administration:* Oral administration: The dosage of Synphase for the initial cycle of therapy is 1 tablet taken at the same time each day from the first day of the menstrual cycle. For subsequent cycles, no tablets are taken for 7 days, then a new course is started of 1 tablet for the next 21 days. This sequence of 21 days on treatment, seven days off treatment is repeated for as long as contraception is required.

Patients unable to start taking Synphase tablets on the first day of the menstrual cycle may start treatment on any day up to and including the 5th day of the menstrual cycle.

Patients starting on day 1 of their period will be protected at once. Those patients delaying therapy up to day 5 may not be protected immediately and it is recommended that another method of contraception is used for the first 7 days of tablet taking. Suitable methods are condoms, caps plus spermicides and intra-uterine devices.

The rhythm, temperature and cervical-mucus methods should not be relied upon.

*Tablet omissions:* Tablets must be taken daily in order to maintain adequate hormone levels and contraceptive efficacy.

If a tablet is missed within 12 hours of the correct dosage time then the missed tablet should be taken as soon as possible, even if this means taking 2 tablets on the same day, this will ensure that contraceptive protection is maintained. If one or more tablets are missed for more than 12 hours from the correct dosage time it is recommended that the patient takes the last missed tablet as soon as possible and then continues to take the rest of the tablets in the normal manner. In addition, it is recommended that extra contraceptive protection, such as a condom, is used for the next 7 days.

Patients who have missed one or more of the last 7 tablets in a pack should be advised to start the next pack of tablets as soon as the present has finished (i.e. without the normal seven day gap between treatments). This reduces the risk of contraceptive failure from tablets being missed close to a 7 day free period.

*Changing from another oral contraceptive:* In order to ensure that contraception is maintained it is advised that the first dose of Synphase tablets is taken on the day immediately after the patient has finished the previous pack of tablets.

*Use after childbirth, miscarriage or abortion:* Providing the patient is not breast feeding the first dose of Synphase tablets should be taken on the 21st day after childbirth. This will ensure the patient is protected immediately. If there is any delay in taking the first dose, contraception may not be established until 7 days after the first tablet has been taken. In these circumstances patients should be advised that extra contraceptive methods will be necessary.

After a miscarriage or abortion patients can take the first dose of Synphase tablets on the next day; in this way they will be protected immediately.

*Contra-indications:* As with all combined progestogen/oestrogen oral contraceptives, the following conditions should be regarded as contra-indications:

(i) Thrombophlebitis, thrombo-embolic disorders, cerebrovascular disorders, coronary artery disease, myocardial infarction, angina, hyperlipidaemia or history of these conditions.
(ii) Acute or severe chronic liver disease, including liver tumours, Dubin-Johnson or Rotor syndrome.
(iii) History during pregnancy of idiopathic jaundice, severe pruritis or pemphigoid gestationis.
(iv) Known or suspected breast or genital cancer.
(v) Known or suspected oestrogen-dependent neoplasia.
(vi) Undiagnosed abnormal vaginal bleeding.
(vii) A history of migraines classified as classical, focal or crescendo.
(viii) Pregnancy.

*Special warnings and precautions for use:* Women taking oral contraceptives require careful observation if they have or have had any of the following conditions: breast nodules; fibrocystic disease of the breast or an abnormal mammogram; uterine fibroids; a history of severe depressive states; varicose veins; sickle-cell anaemia; diabetes; hypertension; cardiovascular disease; migraine; epilepsy; asthma; otosclerosis; multiple sclerosis; porphyria; tetany; disturbed liver functions; gallstones; kidney disease; chloasma; any condition that is likely to worsen during pregnancy. The worsening or first appearance of any of these conditions may indicate that the oral contraceptive should be stopped. Discontinue treatment if there is a gradual or sudden, partial or complete loss of vision or any evidence of ocular changes, onset or aggravation of migraine or development of headache of a new kind which is recurrent, persistent or severe.

Gastro-intestinal upsets, such as vomiting and diarrhoea, may interfere with the absorption of the tablets leading to a reduction in contraceptive efficacy. Patients should continue to take Synphase, but they should also be encouraged to use another contraceptive method during the period of gastrointestinal upset and for the next 7 days.

Progestogen/oestrogen preparations should be used with caution in patients with a history of hepatic dysfunction or hypertension.

A statistical association between the use of oral contraceptives and the occurrence of thrombosis, embolism or haemorrhage has been reported. Patients receiving oral contraceptives should be kept under regular surveillance, in view of the possibility of development of conditions such as thromboembolism.

The risk of coronary artery disease in women taking oral contraceptives is increased by the presence of other predisposing factors such as cigarette smoking, hypercholesterolaemia, obesity, diabetes, history of pre-eclamptic toxaemia and increasing age. After the age of thirty five years, the patient and physician should carefully re-assess the risk/benefit ratio of using combined oral contraceptives as opposed to alternative methods of contraception.

Synphase should be discontinued at least four weeks before, and for two weeks following, elective operations and during immobilisation. Patients undergoing injection treatment for varicose veins should not resume taking Synphase until 3 months after the last injection.

Benign and malignant liver tumours have been associated with oral contraceptive use. The relationship between occurrence of liver tumours and use of female sex hormones is not known at present. These tumours may rupture causing intra-abdominal bleeding. If the patient presents with a mass or tenderness in the right upper quadrant or an acute abdomen, the possible presence of a tumour should be considered.

An increased risk of congenital abnormalities, including heart defects and limb defects, has been reported following the use of sex hormones, including oral contraceptives, in pregnancy. If the patient does not adhere to the prescribed schedule, the possibility of pregnancy should be considered at the time of the first missed period and further use of oral contraceptives should be withheld until pregnancy has been ruled out. It is recommended that for any patient who has missed two consecutive periods, pregnancy should be ruled out before continuing the contraceptive regimen. If pregnancy is confirmed the patient should be advised of the potential risks to the foetus and the advisability of continuing the pregnancy should be discussed in the light of these risks. It is advisable to discontinue Synphase three months before a planned pregnancy.

The risk of arterial thrombosis associated with combined oral contraceptives increases with age, and this risk is aggravated by cigarette smoking. The use of combined oral contraceptives by women in the older age group, especially those who are cigarette smokers, should therefore be discouraged and alternative methods advised.

The use of this product in patients suffering from epilepsy, migraine, asthma or cardiac dysfunction may result in exacerbation of these disorders because of fluid retention. Caution should also be observed in patients who wear contact lenses.

Decreased glucose tolerance may occur in diabetic patients on this treatment, and their control must be carefully supervised.

The use of oral contraceptives has also been associated with a possible increased incidence of gall bladder disease.

Women with a history of oligomenorrhoea or secondary amenorrhoea or young women without regular cycles may have a tendency to remain anovulatory or become amenorrhoeic after discontinuation of oral contraceptives. Women with these pre-existing problems should be advised of this possibility and encouraged to use other contraceptive methods.

Numerous epidemiological studies have been reported on the risks of ovarian, endometrial, cervical and breast cancer in women using combined oral contraceptives. The evidence is clear that combined oral contraceptives offer substantial protection against both ovarian and endometrial cancer.

An increased risk of cervical cancer in long-term users of combined oral contraceptives has been reported in some studies, but there continues to be controversy about the extent to which this is attributable to the confounding effects of sexual behaviour and other factors.

The evidence linking combined oral contraceptive use and breast cancer remains inconclusive. The results of some studies suggest an increased risk of breast cancer presenting below the age of about 35, the risk rising with duration of use. Any possible increased risk of breast cancer with combined oral contraceptives is however likely to be small, and may be expected to be less with low dosage pills. This possible risk should be weighed against the many benefits of combined oral contraceptives, including their protective effects against ovarian and endometrial cancers.

*Interactions with other medicaments and other forms of interaction:* Some drugs may modify the metabolosm of Synphase reducing its effectiveness; these include certain sedatives, antibiotics, antiepileptic and anti-arthritic drugs. During the time such agents are used concurrently, it is advised that mechanical contraceptives also be used.

The results of a large number of laboratory tests have been shown to be influenced by the use of oestrogen containing oral contraceptives, which may limit their diagnostic value. Among these are: biochemical markers of thyroid and liver function; plasma levels of carrier proteins, triglycerides, coagulation and fibrinolysis factors.

*Pregnancy and lactation:* Contra-indicated in pregnancy.

Patients who are fully breast-feeding should not take Synphase tablets since, in common with other combined oral contraceptives, the oestrogen component may reduce the amount of milk produced. In addition, active ingredients or their metabolites have been detected in the milk of mothers taking oral contraceptives. The effect of Synphase on breastfed infants has not been determined.

*Effects on ability to drive and use machines:* Not applicable.

*Undesirable effects:* As with all oral contraceptives, there may be slight nausea at first, weight gain or breast discomfort, which soon disappear.

Other side-effects known or suspected to occur with oral contraceptives include gastro-intestinal symptoms, changes in libido and appetite, headache, exacerbation of existing uterine fibroid disease, depression, and changes in carbohydrate, lipid and vitamin metabolism.

Spotting or bleeding may occur during the first few cycles. Usually menstrual bleeding becomes light and occasionally there may be no bleeding during the tablet-free days.

Hypertension, which is usually reversible on discontinuing treatment, has occurred in a small percentage of women taking oral contraceptives.

*Overdose:* Overdosage may be manifested by nausea, vomiting, breast enlargement and vaginal bleeding. There is no specific antidote and treatment should be symptomatic. Gastric lavage may be employed if the overdose is large and the patient is seen sufficiently early (within four hours).

**Pharmacological properties**

*Pharmacodynamic properties:* The mode of action of Synphase is similar to that of other progestogen/oestrogen oral contraceptives and includes the inhibition of ovulation, the thickening of cervical mucus so as to constitute a barrier to sperm and the rendering of the endometrium unreceptive to implantation.

Such activity is exerted through a combined effect on one or more of the following: hypothalamus, anterior pituitary, ovary, endometrium and cervical mucus.

*Pharmacokinetic properties:* Norethisterone is rapidly and completely absorbed after oral administration, peak plasma concentrations occurring in the majority of subjects between 1 and 3 hours. Due to first-pass metabolism, blood levels after oral administration are 60% of those afer i.v. administration. The half life of elimination varies from 5 to 12 hours, with a mean of 7.6 hours. Norethisterone is metabolised mainly in the liver. Approximately 60% of the administered dose is excreted as metabolites in urine and faeces.

Ethinyloestradiol is rapidly and well absorbed from the gastrointestinal tract but is subject to some first-pass metabolism in the gut-wall. Compared to many other oestrogens it is only slowly metabolised in the liver. Excretion is via the kidneys with some appearing also in the faeces.

*Preclinical safety data:* The toxicity of norethisterone is very low. Reports of teratogenic effects in animals are uncommon. No carcinogenic effects have been found even in long-term studies.

Long-term continuous administration of oestrogens in some animals increases the frequency of carcinoma of the breast, cervix, vagina and liver.

**Pharmaceutical particulars**

*List of excipients:* Synphase tablets contain: Maize starch, povidine, magnesium stearate and lactose. The yellow tablets also contain E104.

*Incompatibilities:* None stated.

*Shelf life:* The shelf life of Synphase tablets is 5 years.

*Special precautions for storage:* Store in a dry place below 25°C away from direct sunlight.

*Nature and contents of container:* Synphase tablets are supplied in PVC/foil blister packs of 21 and 63 tablets.

*Instruction for use/handling:* None.

*Marketing authorisation holder:* Monsanto plc, PO Box 53, Lane End Road, High Wycombe, Bucks, HP12 4HL.

**Marketing authorisation number** 08821/0041.

**Date of approval/revision of SPC** 24 April 1996.

**Legal category** POM.

## UTOVLAN*

**Qualitative and quantitative composition** Each tablet contains 5 mg Norethisterone BP.

**Pharmaceutical form** White, flat, circular, bevel-edged tablet inscribed 'SYNTEX' on one side.

**Clinical particulars**

*Therapeutic indications:*

At low dose: Dysfunctional uterine bleeding, endometriosis, polymenorrhoea, menorrhagia, metropathia haemorrhagica, postponement of menstruation and premenstrual syndrome.

At high dose: Disseminated carcinoma of the breast.

*Posology and method of administration:* Oral administration.

*Low dose*

*Dysfunctional uterine bleeding, polymenorrhoea, menorrhagia, dysmenorrhoea and metropathia haemorrhagica:* 1 tablet three times daily for 10 days; bleeding usually stops within 48 hours. Withdrawal bleeding resembling true menstruation occurs a few days after the end of treatment. One tablet twice daily, from days 19 to 26 of the two subsequent cycles, should be given to prevent recurrence of the condition.

*Endometriosis:* 1 tablet three times daily for a minimum treatment period of six months. The dosage should be increased to 4 or 5 tablets a day if spotting occurs. The initial dosage should be resumed when bleeding or spotting stops.

*Postponement of menstruation:* 1 tablet three times daily, starting three days before the expected onset of menstruation. Menstruation usually follows within three days of finishing the treatment.

*Pre-menstrual syndrome:* 1 tablet daily from days 16 to 25 of the menstrual cycle.

*High dose:* For disseminated breast carcinoma the starting dose is 8 tablets (40 mg) per day increasing to 12 tablets (60 mg) if no regression is noted.

*Contra-indications:* Pregnancy; disturbance of liver function; history during pregnancy of idiopathic jaundice, severe pruritus, or pemphigoid gestationis; undiagnosed irregular vaginal bleeding.

*Special warnings and special precautions for use:* If menstrual bleeding should fail to follow a course of Utovlan, the possibility of pregnancy must be excluded before a further course is given.

*Interaction with other medicaments and other forms of interaction:* None.

*Pregnancy and lactation:* Contra-indicated in pregnancy.

*Effects on ability to drive and use machines:* None.

*Undesirable effects:* These rarely occur at the usual dosage level of 15 mg per day. Mild nausea has been reported. High dosage treatment, even over long periods, is well tolerated; transient digestive upsets and jaundice have rarely been reported.

*Overdose:* Overdosage may be manifested by nausea, vomiting, breast enlargement and later vaginal bleeding. There is no specific antidote and treatment should be symptomatic.

Gastric lavage may be employed if the overdosage is large and the patient is seen sufficiently early (within four hours).

**Pharmacological properties**

*Pharmacodynamic properties:* Norethisterone given at intermediate doses (5–10 mg) suppresses ovulation via its effect on the pituitary. The endogenous production of oestrogens and progesterones are also suppressed, and the ectopic endometrium is converted to a decidua resembling that of pregnancy. In carcinoma norethisterone may act by pituitary inhibition or by direct action on tumour deposits.

*Pharmacokinetic properties:* Norethisterone is rapidly and completely absorbed after oral administration, peak plasma concentration occurring in the majority of subjects between 1 and 3 hours. Due to first-pass metabolism, blood levels after oral administration are 60% of those after i.v. administration. The half life of elimination varies from 5 to 12 hours, with a mean of 7.6 hours. Norethisterone is metabolised mainly in the liver. Approximately 60% of the administered dose is excreted as metabolites in urine and faeces.

*Preclinical safety data:* The toxicity of norethisterone is very low. Reports of teratogenic effects in animals are uncommon. No carcinogenic effects have been found even in long-term studies.

**Pharmaceutical particulars**

*List of excipients:* Utovlan tablets contain: Maize starch, povidone, magnesium stearate and lactose.

*Incompatibilities:* None stated.

*Shelf life:* The shelf life of Utovlan tablets is 2 years.

*Special precautions for storage:* Store in a dry place, below 25°C, away from direct sunlight.

*Nature and contents of container:* Utovlan tablets are supplied in pvc/foil blister packs of 30 and 90 tablets.

*Instructions for use/handling:* None.

*Marketing authorisation holder:* Monsanto p.l.c., PO Box 53, Lane End Road, High Wycombe, Bucks HP12 4HL.

**Marketing authorisation number** 08821/0043

**Date of approval/revision of SPC** March 1996.

**Legal category** POM.

## ZYDOL* AMPOULES ▼

**Qualitative and quantitative composition** Each ampoule contains 100 mg tramadol hydrochloride in 2 ml colourless aqueous solution.

**Pharmaceutical form** Clear glass ampoules containing injectable solution.

**Clincal particulars**

*Therapeutic indications:* Management (treatment and prevention) of moderate to severe pain.

*Posology and method of administration:* As with all analgesic drugs, the dose of Zydol should be adjusted according to the severity of the pain and the clinical response of the individual patient.

*Adults and children aged 12 years and over*

*Parenteral administration:* Zydol injection may be administered intramuscularly, by slow intravenous injection, or diluted in solution (see *Pharmaceutical particulars*) for administration by infusion or patient controlled analgesia.

The usual dose is 50 or 100 mg 4–6 hourly by the intravenous or intramuscular route. Dosage should be adjusted according to pain severity and response.

Intravenous injections must be given slowly over 2–3 minutes. For post-operative pain administer a bolus of 100 mg. During the 60 minutes following the initial bolus, further doses of 50 mg may be given every 10–20 minutes, up to a total dose of 250 mg including the initial bolus. Subsequent doses should be 50 mg or 100 mg 4–6 hourly up to a total dose of 600 mg.

*Elderly:* The usual dosages may be used although it should be noted that in volunteers aged over 75 years the elimination half-life of tramadol was increased by 17% following oral administration.

*Renal impairment/renal dialysis:* The elimination of tramadol may be prolonged. The usual initial dosage should be used. For patients with creatinine clearance <30 ml/min, the dosage interval should be increased to 12 hours. Tramadol is not recommended for patients with severe renal impairment (creatinine clearance <10 ml/min). As tramadol is only removed very slowly by haemodialysis or haemofiltration, post-dialysis administration to maintain analgesia is not usually necessary.

*Hepatic impairment:* The elimination of tramadol may be prolonged. The usual initial dosage should be used but in severe hepatic impairment the dosage interval should be increased to 12 hours.

*Children under 12 years:* Not recommended.

*Contra-indications:* Zydol should not be administered to patients who have previously demonstrated hypersensitivity to it or in cases of acute intoxication with alcohol, hypnotics, centrally acting analgesics, opioids or psychotropic drugs. In common with other opioid analgesics it should not be administered to patients who are receiving monamine oxidase inhibitors or within two weeks of their withdrawal.

*Special warnings and special precautions for use:*

*Warnings:* At therapeutic doses, Zydol has the potential to cause withdrawal symptoms. Rarely cases of dependence and abuse have been reported.

At therapeutic doses withdrawal symptoms have been reported at a reporting frequency of 1 in 8,000. Reports of dependence and abuse have been less frequent. Because of this potential the clinical need for continued analgesic treatment should be reviewed regularly.

In patients with a tendency to drug abuse or dependence, treatment should be for short periods and under strict medical supervision.

Zydol is not suitable as a substitute in opioid-dependent patients. Although it is an opioid agonist, Zydol cannot suppress morphine withdrawal symptoms.

*Precautions:* Zydol should be used with caution in patients with head injury, increased intracranial pressure, severe impairment of hepatic and renal function and in patients prone to convulsive disorders or in shock.

Convulsions have been reported at therapeutic doses and the risk may be increased at doses exceeding the usual upper daily dose limit. Patients with a history of epilepsy or those susceptible to seizures should only be treated with tramadol if there are compelling reasons. The risk of convulsions may increase in patients taking tramadol and concomitant medication that can lower the seizure threshold (see *Interactions with other medicaments and other forms of interaction*).

Care should be taken when treating patients with respiratory depression, or if concomitant CNS depressant drugs are being administered, as the possibility of respiratory depression cannot be excluded in these situations. At therapeutic doses respiratory depression has infrequently been reported.

In one study using a nitrous oxide/opioid (Zydol) anaesthetic technique (with only intermittent administration of enflurane 'as required') Zydol was reported to enhance intra-operative recall. Hence its use during potentially very light planes of general anaesthesia should be avoided.

Two recent studies of Zydol administration during anaesthesia comprising continuous administration of isoflurane did not show clinically significant lightening of anaesthetic depth or intra-operative recall. Therefore providing the current practice of administering continuous, potent (volatile or intravenous) anaesthetic agents is followed, Zydol may be used intra-operatively in the same way as other analgesic agents are routinely used.

*Interactions with other medicaments and other forms of interaction:* Concomitant administration of Zydol with other centrally acting drugs including alcohol may potentiate CNS depressant effects.

Simultaneous administration with cimetidine is associated with clinically insignificant changes in serum concentrations of tramadol. Therefore no alteration of the Zydol dosage regimen is recommended for patients receiving chronic cimetidine therapy.

Simultaneous administration of carbamazepine markedly decreases serum concentrations of tramadol to an extent that a decrease in analgesic effectiveness and a shorter duration of action may occur.

Tramadol may increase the potential for both selective serotonin reuptake inhibitors (SSRIs) and tricyclic antidepressants (TCAs) to cause convulsions (see *Special warnings and precautions for use* and *Pharmacokinetic properties*).

There is a theoretical possibility that tramadol could interact with lithium. There have been no reports of this potential interaction.

*Pregnancy and lactation:*

*Pregnancy:* Animal studies (rats and rabbits, exposure to tramadol up to 7 times that expected in man) have not revealed teratogenic effects and minimal embryotoxicity (delayed ossification). Fertility, reproductive performance and development of offspring were unaffected. There is inadequate evidence available on the safety of tramadol in human pregnancy, therefore Zydol should not be used in pregnant women.

*Lactation:* tramadol and its metabolites are found in small amounts in human breast milk. An infant could ingest 0.1% of the dose given to the mother. Zydol should not be administered during breast feeding.

*Effects on ability to drive and use machines:* Zydol may cause drowsiness and this effect may be potentiated by alcohol and other CNS depressants. Ambulant patients should be warned not to drive or operate machinery if affected.

*Undesirable effects:* Rapid intravenous administration may be associated with a higher incidence of adverse effects and therefore should be avoided.

*Gastrointestinal system:* Nausea, vomiting and occasionally dry mouth. Both diarrhoea and constipation have been reported. In controlled clinical trials the incidence of constipation is lower than that of comparator agents.

*Central nervous system and psychiatric:* Tiredness, fatigue, drowsiness, somnolence, dizziness, headache, confusion, hallucinations and infrequently respiratory depression. Dependence, dysphoria and convulsions have been reported rarely (see *Interactions*).

*Physical dependence:* Dependence, abuse and withdrawal reactions have been reported. Typical opiate withdrawal reactions include agitation, anxiety, nervousness, insomnia, hyperkinesia, tremor and gastrointestinal symptoms (see *Special warnings and special precautions in use* and *Posology and method of administration*).

*Allergic/anaphylactoid reaction:* Dyspnoea, wheezing, bronchospasm and worsening of existing asthma.

*Other adverse events:* Diaphoresis, urticaria and pruritus have been reported. Skin rashes, tachycardia, orthostatic hypotension, increase in blood pressure, bradycardia, flushing, syncope and anaphylaxis have been rarely reported. Cases of blood dyscrasias have been rarely observed during treatment with tramadol, but causality has not been established.

*Overdose:* Symptoms of overdosage are typical of other opioid analgesics, and include miosis, vomiting, cardiovascular collapse, sedation and coma, seizures and respiratory depression.

Supportive measures such as maintaining the patency of the airway and maintaining cardiovascular function should be instituted; naloxone should be used to reverse respiratory depression; fits can be controlled with diazepam.

Tramadol is minimally eliminated from the serum by haemodialysis or haemofiltration. Therefore treatment of acute intoxication with Zydol with haemodialysis or haemofiltration alone is not suitable for detoxification.

**Pharmacological properties**

*Pharmacodynamic properties:* Zydol is a centrally acting analgesic. It is a non selective pure agonist at mu, delta and kappa opioid receptors with a higher affinity for the mu receptor. Other mechanisms which may contribute to its analgesic effect are inhibition of neuronal reuptake of noradrenaline and enhancement of serotonin release.

*Pharmacokinetic properties:* The half-life of the terminal elimination phase ($t_{\frac{1}{2}}\beta$) was 6.0±1.5 h in young volunteers. Tramadol pharmacokinetics show little age dependence in volunteers up to the age of 75 years. In volunteers aged 75 years, $t_{\frac{1}{2}}\beta$ was 7.0±1.6 h on oral administration.

Since tramadol is eliminated both metabolically and renally, the terminal half-life $t_{\frac{1}{2}}\beta$ may be prolonged in impaired hepatic or renal function. However, the increase in the $t_{\frac{1}{2}}\beta$ values is relatively low if at least one of these organs is functioning normaly. In patients with liver cirrhosis $t_{\frac{1}{2}}\beta$ tramadol was a mean of 13.3±4.9 h; in patients with renal insufficiency (creatinine clearance ≤5 ml/min) it was 11.0±3.2 h.

*Preclinical safety data:* In single and repeat-dose toxicity studies (rodents and dogs) exposure to tramadol 10 times that expected in man is required before toxicity (hepatotoxicity) is observed. Symptoms of toxicity are typical of opioids and include restlessness, ataxia, vomiting, tremor, dyspnoea and convulsions.

Exposure to tramadol (≤ that expected in man) in lifetime toxicity studies in rodents did not reveal any evidence of carcinogenic hazard, and a battery of in-vitro and in-vivo mutagenicity tests were negative.

**Pharmaceutical particulars**

*List of excipients:* Zydoil ampoules contain: water for injection, sodium acetate.

*Incompatibilities:* Precipitation will occur if Zydol injection is mixed in the same syringe with injections of diazepam, diclofenac sodium, indomethacin, midazolam and piroxicam.

*Shelf life:* Zydol ampoules have a shelf life of 5 years.

*Special precautions for storage:* Store in a dry place below 30°C (86°F).

*Nature and contents of container:* Box of 5 ampoules.

*Special instructions for use/handling:* Zydol injection is physically and chemically compatible for up to 24 hours with 4.2% sodium bicarbonate and Ringer's solution and for up to 5 days with the following infusion solutions:

0.9% sodium chloride
0.18% sodium chloride and 4% glucose
sodium lactate compound
5% glucose
Haemaccel

*Marketing authorisation holder:* Monsanto plc, trading as Searle, PO Box 53, Lane End Road, High Wycombe, Bucks HP12 4HL.

**Marketing authorisation number** 08821/0004.

**Date of approval/revision of SPC** 24 March 1997.

**Legal category** POM.

## ZYDOL* CAPSULES ▼

**Qualitative and quantitative composition** Each capsule contains 50 mg tramadol hydrochloride.

**Pharmaceutical form** Green/pale yellow hard gelatine capsules for oral administration.

**Clinical particulars**

*Therapeutic indications:* Management (treatment and prevention) of moderate to severe pain.

*Posology and method of administration:* As with all analgesic drugs, the dose of Zydol should be adjusted according to the severity of the pain and the clinical response of the individual patient.

*Adults and children aged 12 years and over*
*Oral administration*
*Acute pain:* An initial dose of 100 mg is usually necessary. This can be followed by doses of 50 or 100 mg not more frequently than 4 hourly, and duration of therapy should be matched to clinical need.

*Pain associated with chronic conditions:* Use an initial dose of 50 mg and then titrate dose according to pain severity. The need for continued treatment should be assessed at regular intervals as withdrawal symptoms and dependence have been reported (see section *Special warnings and precautions for use*). A total daily dose of 400 mg should not be exceeded except in special clinical circumstances.

*Elderly:* The usual dosages may be used although it should be noted that in volunteers aged over 75 years the elimination half-life of tramadol was increased by 17% following oral administration.

*Renal impairment/renal dialysis:* The elimination of tramadol may be prolonged. The usual initial dosage should be used. For patients with creatinine clearance < 30 ml/min, the dosage interval should be increased to 12 hours. Tramadol is not recommended for patients with severe renal impairment (creatinine clearance < 10 ml/min).

As tramadol is only removed very slowly by haemodialysis or haemofiltration, post-dialysis administration to maintain analgesia is not usually necessary.

*Hepatic impairment:* The elimination of tramadol may be prolonged. The usual initial dosage should be used but in severe hepatic impairment the dosage interval should be increased to 12 hours.

*Children under 12 years:* Not recommended.

*Contra-indications:* Zydol should not be administered to patients who have previously demonstrated hypersensitivity to it or in cases of acute intoxication with alcohol, hypnotics, centrally acting analgesics, opioids of psychotropic drugs. In common with other opioid analgesics it should not be administered to patients who are receiving monoamine oxidase inhibitors or within two weeks of their withdrawal.

*Special warnings and special precautions for use*
*Warnings:* At therapeutic doses, Zydol has the potential to cause withdrawal symptoms. Rarely cases of dependence and abuse have been reported.

At therapeutic doses withdrawal symptoms have been reported at a reporting frequency of 1 in 8,000. Reports of dependence and abuse have been less frequent. Because of this potential the clinical need for continued analgesic treatment should be reviewed regularly.

In patients with a tendency to drug abuse or dependence, treatment should be for short periods and under strict medical supervision.

Zydol is not suitable as a substitute in opioid-dependent patients. Although it is an opioid agonist, Zydol cannot suppress morphine withdrawal symptoms.

*Precautions:* Zydol should be used with caution in patients with head injury, increased intracranial pressure, severe impairment of hepatic and renal function and in patients prone to convulsive disorders or in shock.

Convulsions have been reported at therapeutic doses and the risk may be increased at doses exceeding the usual upper daily dose limit. Patients with a history of epilepsy or those susceptible to seizures should only be treated with tramadol if there are compelling reasons. The risk of convulsions may increase in patients taking tramadol and concomitant medication that can lower the seizure threshold (see *Interactions with other medicaments and other forms of interaction*).

Care should be taken when treating patients with respiratory depression, or if concomitant CNS depressant drugs are being administered, as the possibility of respiratory depression cannot be excluded in these situations. At therapeutic doses respiratory depression has infrequently been reported.

In one study using a nitrous oxide/opioid (Zydol) anaesthetic technique (with only intermittent administration of enflurane 'as required') Zydol was reported to enhance intra-operative recall. Hence its use during potentially very light planes of general anaesthesia should be avoided.

Two recent studies of Zydol administration during anaesthesia comprising continuous administration of isoflurane did not show clinically significant lightening of anaesthetic depth or intra-operative recall. Therefore providing the current practice of administering continuous, potent (volatile or intravenous) anaesthetic agents is followed, Zydol may be used intra-operatively in the same way as other analgesic agents are routinely used.

*Interactions with other medicaments and other forms of interaction:* Concomitant administration of Zydol with other centrally acting drugs including alcohol may potentiate CNS depressant effects.

Simultaneous administration with cimetidine is associated with clinically insignificant changes in serum concentrations of tramadol. Therefore no alteration of the Zydol dosage regimen is recommended for patients receiving chronic cimetidine therapy.

Simultaneous administration of carbamazepine markedly decreases serum concentrations of tramadol to an extent that a decrease in analgesic effectiveness and a shorter duration of action may occur. Tramadol may increase the potential for both selective serotonin reuptake inhibitors (SSRIs) and tricyclic antidepressants (TCAs) to cause convulsions (see section *Special warnings and special precautions for use* and *Pharmacokinetic properties*). There is a theoretical possibility that tramadol could interact with lithium. There have been no reports of this potential interaction.

*Pregnancy and lactation*
*Pregnancy:* Animal studies (rats and rabbits, exposure to tramadol up to 7 times that expected in man) have not revealed teratogenic effects and minimal embryo-
toxicity (delayed ossification). Fertility, reproductive performance and development of offspring were unaffected. There is inadequate evidence available on the safety of tramadol in human pregnancy therefore Zydol should not be used in pregnant women.

*Lactation:* Tramadol and its metabolites are found in small amounts in human breast milk. An infant could ingest 0.1% of the dose given to the mother. Zydol should not be administered during breast feeding.

*Effects on ability to drive and use machines:* Zydol may cause drowsiness and this effect may be potentiated by alcohol and other CNS depressants. Ambulant patients should be warned not to drive or operate machinery if affected.

*Undesirable effects:*
*Gastrointestinal system:* Nausea, vomiting and occasionally dry mouth. Both diarrhoea and constipation have been reported. In controlled trials the incidence of constipation is lower than that of comparator agents.

*Central nervous system and psychiatric:* Tiredness, fatigue, drowsiness, somnolence, dizziness, headache, confusion, hallucinations and infrequently respiratory depression. Dependence, dysphoria and convulsions have been reported rarely (see *Interactions*).

*Physical dependence:* Dependence, abuse and withdrawal reactions have been reported. Typical opiate withdrawal reactions include agitation, anxiety, nervousness, insomnia, hyperkinesia, tremor and gastrointestinal symptoms (see *Special warnings and special precautions in use* and *Posology and method of administration*).

*Allergic/anaphylactoid reaction:* Dyspnoea, wheezing, bronchospasm and worsening of existing asthma.

*Other adverse events:* Diaphoresis, urticaria and

pruritus have been reported. Skin rashes, tachycardia, orthostatic hypotension, increase in blood pressure, bradycardia, flushing, syncope and anaphylaxis have been rarely reported. Cases of blood dyscrasias have been rarely observed during treatment with tramadol, but causality has not been established.

*Overdose:* Symptoms of overdosage are typical of other opioid analgesics, and include miosis, vomiting, cardiovascular collapse, sedation and coma, seizures and respiratory depression.

Supportive measures such as maintaining the patency of the airway and maintaining cardiovascular function should be instituted; naloxone should be used to reverse respiratory depression; fits can be controlled with diazepam.

Tramadol is minimally eliminated from the serum by haemodialysis or haemofiltration. Therefore treatment of acute intoxication with Zydol with haemodialysis or haemofiltration alone is not suitable for detoxification.

**Pharmacological properties**
*Pharmacodynamic properties:* Zydol is a centrally acting analgesic. It is a non selective pure agonist at mu, delta and kappa opioid receptors with a higher affinity for the mu receptor. Other mechanisms which may contribute to its analgesic effect are inhibition of neuronal reuptake of noradrenaline and enhancement of serotonin release.

*Pharmacokinetic properties:* The half life of the terminal elimination phase ($t_{\frac{1}{2}}\beta$) was 6.0±1.5 h in young volunteers. Tramadol pharmacokinetics show little age dependence in volunteers up to the age of 75 years. In volunteers aged over 75 years, $t_{\frac{1}{2}}\beta$ was 7.0±1.6 h on oral administration.

Since tramadol is eliminated both metabolically and renally, the terminal half-life $t_{\frac{1}{2}}\beta$ may be prolonged in impaired hepatic or renal function. However, the increase in the $t_{\frac{1}{2}}\beta$ values is relatively low if at least one of these organs is functioning normally. In patients with liver cirrhosis $t_{\frac{1}{2}}\beta$ tramadol was a mean of 13.3±4.9 h; in patients with renal insufficiency (creatinine clearance ≤5 ml/min) it was 11.0±3.2 h.

*Preclinical safety data:* In single and repeat-dose toxicity studies (rodents and dogs) exposure to tramadol 10 times that expected in man is required before toxicity (hepatotoxicity) is observed. Symptoms of toxicity are typical of opioids and include restlessness, ataxia, vomiting, tremor, dyspnoea and convulsions.

Exposure to tramadol (≤ that expected in man) in lifetime toxicity studies in rodents did not reveal any evidence of carcinogenic hazard, and a battery of in-vitro and in-vivo mutagenicity tests were negative.

**Pharmaceutical particulars**
*List of excipients:* Zydol capsules contain: microcrystalline cellulose, sodium starch glycolate, magnesium stearate, colloidal anhydrous silica. The capsule shell contains: gelatin, and colours E132, E172 and E171.

*Incompatibilities:* None known.

*Shelf life:* Zydol capsules have a shelf life of 5 years when stored in pvc/foil blisters.

*Special precautions for storage:* Store in a dry place below 30°C (86°F).

*Nature and contents of container:* PVC/foil blister packs of 10, 20 and 100 capsules.

*Special instructions for use/handling:* None.

*Marketing authorisation holder:* Monsanto p.l.c., PO Box 53, Lane End Road, High Wycombe, Bucks HP12 4HL.

**Marketing authorisation number** 08821/0005.

**Date of approval/revision of SPC** January 1996.

**Legal category** POM.

## ZYDOLE* SOLUBLE TABLETS ▼

**Qualitative and quantitative composition** Each soluble tablet contains 50 mg tramadol hydrochloride.

**Pharmaceutical form** White, round, flat tablets, scored on one side and engraved 'T4' with manufacturer's logo on the reverse. For oral administration.

**Clinical particulars**
*Therapeutic indications:* Management (treatment and prevention) of moderate to severe pain.

*Posology and method of administration:* As with all analgesic drugs, the dose of Zydol should be adjusted according to the severity of the pain and the clinical response of the individual patient.

*Adults and children aged 12 years and over:* Oral administration.

*Acute pain:* An initial dose of 100 mg is usually necessary. This can be followed by doses of 50 or 100 mg not more frequently than 4 hourly and duration of therapy should be matched to clinical need.

*Pain associated with chronic conditions:* Use an initial dose of 50 mg and then titrate dose according to pain severity. The need for continued treatment should be assessed at regular intervals as withdrawal symptoms and dependence have been reported (see *Special warnings and precautions for use*). A total daily oral dose of 400 mg should not be exceeded except in special clinical circumstances.

The tablets should be dissolved in at least 50 mls water before administration.

*Elderly:* The usual dosages may be used although it should be noted that in volunteers aged over 75 years the elimination half-life of tramadol was increased by 17% following oral administration.

*Renal impairment/renal dialysis:* The elimination of tramadol may be prolonged. The usual initial dosage should be used. For patients with creatinine clearance <30 ml/min, the dosage interval should be increased to 12 hours. Tramadol is not recommended for patients with severe renal impairment (creatinine clearance <10 ml/min).

*Hepatic impairment:* The elimination of tramadol may be prolonged. The usual initial dosage should be used but in severe hepatic impairment the dosage interval should be increased to 12 hours.

*Children under 12 years:* Not recommended.

*Contra-indications:* Zydol should not be administered to patients who have previously demonstrated hypersensitivity to it or in cases of acute intoxication with alcohol, hypnotics, centrally acting analgesics, opioids or psychotropic drugs.

In common with other opioid analgesics it should not be administered to patients who are receiving monamine oxidase inhibitors or within two weeks of their withdrawal.

*Special warnings and special precautions for use:*
*Warnings:* At therapeutic doses, Zydol has the potential to cause withdrawal symptoms. Rarely cases of dependence and abuse have been reported.

At therapeutic doses withdrawal symptoms have been reported at a reporting frequency of 1 in 8,000. Reports of dependence and abuse have been less frequent. Because of this potential the clinical need for continued analgesic treatment should be reviewed regularly.

In patients with a tendency to drug abuse or dependence, treatment should be for short periods and under strict medical supervision.

Zydol is not suitable as a substitute in opioid-dependent patients. Although it is an opioid agonist, Zydol cannot suppress morphine withdrawal symptoms.

*Precautions:* Zydol should be used with caution in patients with head injury, increased intracranial pressure, severe impairment of hepatic and renal function and in patients prone to convulsive disorders or in shock.

Convulsions have been reported at therapeutic doses and the risk may be increased at doses exceeding the usual upper daily dose limit. Patients with a history of epilepsy or those susceptible to seizures should only be treated with tramadol if there are compelling reasons. The risk of convulsions may increase in patients taking tramadol and concomitant medication that can lower the seizure threshold (see *Interactions with other medicaments and other forms of interactions*).

Care should be taken when treating patients with respiratory depression, or if concomitant CNS depressant drugs are being administered, as the possibility of respiratory depression cannot be excluded in these situations. At therapeutic doses respiratory depression has infrequently been reported.

In one study using a nitrous oxide/opioid (Zydol) anaesthetic technique (with only intermittent administration of enflurane 'as required') Zydol was reported to enhance intra-operative recall. Hence its use during potentially very light planes of general anaesthesia should be avoided.

Two recent studies of Zydol administration during anaesthesia comprising continuous administration of isoflurane did not show clinically significant lightening of anaesthetic depth or intra-operative recall. Therefore providing the current practice of administering continuous, potent (volatile or intravenous) anaesthetic agents is followed, Zydol may be used intra-operatively in the same way as other analgesic agents are routinely used.

*Interactions with other medicaments and other forms of interaction:* Concomitant administration of Zydol with other centrally acting drugs including alcohol may potentiate CNS depressant effects.

Simultaneous administration with cimetidine is associated with clinically insignificant changes in serum concentrations of tramadol. Therefore no alteration of the Zydol dosage regimen is recommended for patients receiving chronic cimetidine therapy.

Simultaneous administration of carbamazepine markedly decreases serum concentrations of tramadol to an extent that a decrease in analgesic effectiveness and a shorter duration of action may occur.

Tramadol may increase the potential for both selective serotonin reuptake inhibitors (SSRIs) and tricyclic antidepressants (TCAs) to cause convulsions (see *Special warnings and special precautions for use* and *Pharmacokinetic properties*). There is a theoretical possibility that tramadol could interact with lithium. There have been no reports of this potential interaction.

*Pregnancy and lactation:*
*Pregnancy:* Animal studies (rat and rabbit, exposure to tramadol up to 7 times that expected in man) have not revealed teratogenic effects and minimal embryotoxicity (delayed ossification). Fertility, reproductive performance and development of offspring were unaffected. There is inadequate evidence available on the safety of tramadol in human pregnancy, therefore Zydol should not be used in pregnant women.

*Lactation:* Tramadol and its metabolites are found in small amounts in human breast milk. An infant could ingest about 0.1% of the dose given to the mother. Zydol should not be administered during breast feeding.

*Effects on ability to drive and use machines:* Zydol may cause drowsiness and this effect may be potentiated by alcohol and other CNS depressants. Ambulant patients should be warned not to drive or operate machinery if affected.

*Undesirable effects:*
*Gastrointestinal system:* Nausea, vomiting and occasionally dry mouth. Both diarrhoea and constipation have been reported. In controlled trials the incidence of constipation is lower than that of comparator agents.

*Central nervous system and psychiatric:* Tiredness, fatigue, drowsiness, somnolence, dizziness, headache, confusion, hallucinations and infrequently, respiratory depression. Dependence, dysphoria and convulsions have been reported rarely (see *Interactions*).

*Physical dependence:* Dependence, abuse and withdrawal reactions have been reported. Typical opiate withdrawal reactions include agitation, anxiety, nervousness, insomnia, hyperkinesia, tremor and gastrointestinal symptoms (see *Special warnings and special precautions in use* and *Posology and method of administration*).

*Allergic/anaphylactoid reaction:* Dyspnoea, wheezing, bronchospasm and worsening of existing asthma.

*Other adverse events:* Diaphoresis, urticaria and pruritus have been reported. Skin rashes, tachycardia, orthostatic hypotension, increase in blood pressure, bradycardia, flushing, syncope and anaphylaxis have been rarely reported. Cases of blood dyscrasias have been rarely observed during treatment with tramadol, but causality has not been established.

*Overdose:* Symptoms of overdosage are typical of other opioid analgesics, and include miosis, vomiting, cardiovascular collapse, sedation and coma, seizures and respiratory depression.

Supportive measures such as maintaining the patency of the airway and maintaining cardiovascular function should be instituted; nalaxone should be used to reverse respiratory depression; fits can be controlled with diazepam.

Tramadol is minimally eliminated from the serum by haemodialysis or haemofiltration. Therefore treatment of acute intoxication with Zydol with haemodialysis or haemofiltration alone is not suitable for detoxification.

**Pharmacological properties**
*Pharmacodynamic properties:* Zydol is a centrally acting analgesic. It is a non selective pure agonist at mu, delta and kappa opioid receptors with a higher affinity for the mu receptor. Other mechanisms which may contribute to its analgesic effect are inhibition of neuronal reuptake of noradrenaline and enhancement of serotonin release.

*Pharmacokinetic properties:* After oral administration, Zydol is almost completely absorbed. The absolute bioavailability is approximately 70% following a single dose and increases to approximately 90% at steady state. The pharmacokinetics of Zydol 50 mg soluble tablets are not significantly different from Zydol 50 mg capsules with respect to extent of bioavailability as measured by AUC. There was a 10% difference in $C_{max}$ between oral capsules and soluble tablets. $T_{max}$ was 1.5 hours for soluble tablets and 2.2 hours for capsules, reflecting the faster absorption of the oral solution. Mean absorption time was 0.63 hours for soluble tablets, 0.94 hours for capsules. These differences in $T_{max}$ and MAT were statistically significant.

Tramadol has a linear pharmacokinetic profile within the therapeutic dosage range. The elimination half life $t_{\frac{1}{2}}\beta$ is 5–7 hours irrespective of the mode of administration. In patients over 75 years, the elimination half life was increased by 17% following oral administration.

The terminal half life may be prolonged in impaired hepatic or renal function. In patients with liver cirrhosis $t_{\frac{1}{2}}\beta$ tramadol was a mean of 1.3±4.9 hours and in patients with renal insufficiency (creatinine clearance ≤5 ml/min) it was 11.0±3.2 hours after administration of Zydol capsules.

*Preclinical safety data:* In single and repeat-dose toxicity studies (rodents and dogs) exposure to tramadol 10 times that expected in man is required before toxicity (hepatotoxicity) is observed. Symptoms of toxicity are typical of opioids and include restlessness, ataxia, vomiting, tremor, dyspnoea and convulsions.

Exposure to tramadol (≤ that expected in man) in lifetime toxicity studies in rodents did not reveal any evidence of carcinogenic hazard, and a battery of in-vitro and in-vivo mutagenicity tests were negative.

**Pharmaceutical particulars**
*List of excipients:* Zydol soluble tablets contain: microcrystalline cellulose, maize starch, saccharin sodium, colloidal anhydrous silica, magnesium stearate, peppermint and aniseed flavouring.

*Incompatabilities:* None known.

*Shelf life:* Zydol soluble tablets have a shelf life of 3 years when stored in polypropylene/foil or pvc/pvdc/foil blisters.

*Special precautions for storage:* Store in a dry place below 25°C.

*Nature and contents of container:* Polypropylene foil or PVC/PVDC foil blister packs of 10, 20 or 100 tablets.

*Special instructions for use/handling:* The tablets are formulated to be dissolved in water prior to administration, producing a slightly peppermint/aniseed flavoured oral solution.

*Market authorisation holder:* Monsanto p.l.c., Trading as Searle, PO Box 53, Lane End Road, High Wycombe, Bucks HP12 4HL.

**Marketing authorisation number** 8821/0046.

**Date of approval/revision of SPC** 24 March 1997.

**Legal category** POM.

## ZYDOL SR* ▼

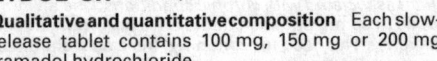

**Qualitative and quantitative composition** Each slow-release tablet contains 100 mg, 150 mg or 200 mg tramadol hydrochloride.

**Pharmaceutical form** White, beige or orange biconvex tablets engraved T1, T2 or T3 (for the 100 mg, 150 mg or 200 mg strengths, respectively) on one side and with manufacturer's logo on the other, for oral administration.

**Clinical particulars**
*Therapeutic indications:* Management (treatment and prevention) of moderate to severe pain.

*Posology and method of administration:* As with all analgesic drugs, the dose of Zydol should be adjusted according to the severity of the pain and the clinical response of the individual patient.

*Adults and children aged 12 years and over*
*Oral administration:* The usual initial dose is one 100 mg tablet twice daily, morning and evening. If pain relief is insufficient, the dosage may be titrated upwards to one 150 mg or one 200 mg tablet twice daily.

Tablets should be swallowed whole.

*Pain associated with chronic conditions:* The need for continued treatment should be assessed at regular intervals as withdrawal symptoms and dependence have been reported (see *Special warnings and precautions for use*).

A total daily oral dose of 400 mg should not be exceeded except in special clinical circumstances.

*Elderly:* The usual dosages may be used although it should be noted that in volunteers aged over 75 years the elimination half-life of tramadol was increased by 17% following oral administration.

*Renal impairment/renal dialysis:* As the elimination of tramadol may be prolonged, use of Zydol capsules may be more appropriate. Tramadol is not recommended for patients with severe renal impairment (creatinine clearance < 10 ml/min). As tramadol is only removed very slowly by haemodialysis or haemofiltration, post-dialysis administration to maintain analgesia is not usually necessary.

*Hepatic impairment:* As the elimination of tramadol may be prolonged use of Zydol capsules may be more appropriate.

*Children under 12 years:* Not recommended.

*Contra-indications:* Zydol should not be administered to patients who have previously demonstrated hypersensitivity to it or in cases of acute intoxication with alcohol, hypnotics, centrally acting analgesics, opioids or psychotropic drugs. In common with other opioid analgesics it should not be administered to patients who are receiving monoamine oxidase inhibitors or within two weeks of their withdrawal.

*Special warnings and special precautions for use*
*Warnings:* At therapeutic doses, Zydol has the potential to cause withdrawal symptoms. Rarely cases of dependence and abuse have been reported.

At therapeutic doses withdrawal symptoms have been reported at a reporting frequency of 1 in 8,000. Reports of dependence and abuse have been less frequent. Because of this potential the clinical need for continued analgesic treatment should be reviewed regularly.

In patients with a tendency to drug abuse or dependence, treatment should be for short periods and under strict medical supervision.

Zydol is not suitable as a substitute in opioid-dependent patients. Although it is an opioid antagonist, Zydol cannot suppress morphine withdrawal symptoms.

*Precautions:* Zydol should be used with caution in patients with head injury, increased intracranial pressure, severe impairment of hepatic and renal function and in patients prone to convulsive disorders or in shock.

Convulsions have been reported at therapeutic doses and the risk may be increased at doses exceeding the usual upper daily dose limit. Patients with a history of epilepsy or those susceptible to seizures should only be treated with Tramadol if there are compelling reasons. The risk of convulsions may increase in patients taking tramadol and concomitant medication that can lower the seizure threshold (see *Interactions with other medicaments and other forms of interaction*).

Care should be taken when treating patients with respiratory depression, or if concomitant CNS depressant drugs are being administered, as the possibility of respiratory depression cannot be excluded in these situations. At therapeutic doses respiratory depression has infrequently been reported.

In one study using a nitrous oxide/opioid (Zydol) anaesthetic technique (with only intermittent administration of enflurane 'as required') Zydol was reported to enhance intra-operative recall. Hence its use during potentially very light planes of general anaesthesia should be avoided.

Two recent studies of Zydol administration during anaesthesia comprising continuous administration of isoflurane did not show clinically significant lightening of anaesthetic depth or intra-operative recall. Therefore providing the current practice of administering continuous, potent (volatile or intravenous) anaesthetic agents is followed, Zydol may be used intra-operatively in the same way as other analgesic agents are routinely used.

*Interactions with other medicaments and other forms of interaction:* Concomitant administration of Zydol with other centrally acting drugs including alcohol may potentiate CNS depressant effects.

Simultaneous administration with cimetidine is associated with clinically insignificant changes in serum concentrations of tramadol. Therefore no alteration of the Zydol dosage regimen is recommended for patients receiving chronic cimetidine therapy.

Simultaneous administration of carbamazepine markedly decreases serum concentrations of tramadol to an extent that a decrease in analgesic effectiveness and a shorter duration of action may occur.

Tramadol may increase the potential for both selective serotonin inhibitors (SSRIs) and tricyclic antidepressants (TCAs) to cause convulsions (see *Special warnings and special precautions for use* and *Pharmacokinetic properties*). There is a theoretical possibility that tramadol could interact with lithium.

There have been no reports of this potential interaction.

*Pregnancy and lactation*
*Pregnancy:* Animal studies (rats and rabbits, exposure to tramadol up to 7 times that expected in man) have not revealed teratogenic effects and minimal embryotoxicity (delayed ossification). Fertility, reproductive performance and development of offspring were unaffected. There is inadequate evidence available on the safety of tramadol in human pregnancy therefore Zydol should not be used in pregnant women.

*Lactation:* Tramadol and its metabolites are found in small amounts in human breast milk. An infant could ingest 0.1% of the dose given to the mother. Zydol should not be administered during breast feeding.

*Effects on ability to drive and use machines:* Zydol may cause drowsiness and this effect may be potentiated by alcohol and other CNS depressants. Ambulant patients should be warned not to drive or operate machinery if affected.

*Undesirable effects:*
*Gastrointestinal system:* Nausea, vomiting and occasionally dry mouth. Both diarrhoea and constipation have been reported. In controlled trials the incidence of constipation is lower than that of comparator agents.

*Central nervous system and psychiatric:* Tiredness, fatigue, drowsiness, somnolence, dizziness, headache, confusion, hallucinations and infrequently respiratory depression. Dependence, dysphoria and convulsions have been reported rarely (see *Interactions*).

*Physical dependence:* Dependence, abuse and withdrawal reactions have been reported. Typical opiate withdrawal reactions include agitation, anxiety, nervousness, insomnia, hyperkinesia, tremor and gastrointestinal symptoms (see *Special warnings and special precautions in use* and *Posology and method of administration*).

*Allergic/anaphylactoid reaction:* Dyspnoea, wheezing, bronchospasm and worsening of existing asthma.

*Other adverse events:* Diaphoresis, urticaria and pruritus have been reported. Skin rashes, tachycardia, orthostatic hypotension, increase in blood pressure, bradycardia, flushing, syncope and anaphylaxis have been rarely reported. Cases of blood dyscrasias have been rarely observed during treatment with tramadol, but causality has not been established.

*Overdose:* Symptoms of overdosage are typical of other opioid analgesics, and include miosis, vomiting, cardiovascular collapse, sedation and coma, seizures and respiratory depression.

Supportive measures such as maintaining the patency of the airway and maintaining cardiovascular function should be instituted; naloxone should be used to reverse respiratory depression; fits can be controlled with diazepam.

Tramadol is minimally eliminated from the serum by haemodialysis or haemofiltration. Therefore treatment of acute intoxication with Zydol with haemodialysis or haemofiltration alone is not suitable for detoxification.

**Pharmacological properties**
*Pharmacodynamic properties:* Zydol is a centrally acting analgesic. It is a non selective pure agonist at mu, delta and kappa opioid receptors with a higher affinity for the mu receptor. Other mechanisms which may contribute to its analgesic effect are inhibition of neuronal reuptake of noradrenaline and enhancement of serotonin release.

*Pharmacokinetic properties:* After oral administration, Zydol SR is almost completely absorbed. The absolute bioavailability is approximately 70% following a single dose and increases to approximately 90% at steady state.

$C_{max}$ (141±40 ng/ml) is reached 4.9 hrs after oral administration of Zydol SR 100 mg and 4.8 hrs ($C_{max}$ 260±62 ng/ml) after oral administration of the 200 mg tablet.

Tramadol has a linear pharmacokinetic profile within the therapeutic dosage range. The elimination half life $t\frac{1}{2}\beta$ is 5–7 hrs irrespective of the mode of administration.

In patients over 75 years the elimination half-life of tramadol was increased by 17% following oral administration. The total clearance is 710 ml/min and may be reduced in elderly patients.

Since tramadol is eliminated both metabolically and renally, the terminal half-life $t\frac{1}{2}\beta$ may be prolonged in impaired hepatic or renal function. However, the increase in the $t\frac{1}{2}\beta$ values is relatively low if at least one of these organs is functioning normally. In patients with liver cirrhosis $t\frac{1}{2}\beta$ tramadol was a mean of 13.3±4.9 hrs; in patients with renal insufficiency (creatinine clearance ≤5 ml/min) it was 11.0±3.2 hrs.

*Preclinical safety data:* In single and repeat-dose toxicity studies (rodents and dogs) exposure to tramadol 10 times that expected in man is required before toxicity (hepatotoxicity) is observed.

Symptoms of toxicity are typical of opioids and include restlessness, ataxia, vomiting, tremor, dyspnoea and convulsions.

Exposure to tramadol (≤ that expected in man) in lifetime toxicity studies in rodents did not reveal any evidence of carcinogenic hazard, and a battery of in-vitro and in-vivo mutagenicity tests were negative.

**Pharmaceutical particulars**
*List of excipients:* Zydol SR 100 mg tablets contain: microcrystalline cellulose, methylhydroxypropylcellulose, magnesium stearate, colloidal anhydrous silica, lactose, polyethylene glycol 6000, Propylene glycol, talc and titanium dioxide (E171).

Zydol SR 150 mg tablets contain: microcrystalline cellulose, methylhydroxypropylcellulose, magnesium stearate, colloidal anhydrous silica, lactose, polyethylene glycol 6000, Propylene glycol, talc, titanium dioxide (E171), quinoline yellow lake (E104), and red iron oxide (E172).

Zydol SR 200 mg tablets contain: microcrystalline cellulose, methylhydroxypropylcellulose, magnesium stearate, colloidal anhydrous silica, lactose, polyethylene glycol 6000, Propylene glycol, talc, titanium dioxide (E171), quinoline yellow (E104), red iron oxide (E172) and brown iron oxide (E172).

*Incompatibilities:* None known.

*Shelf life:* Zydol SR 100 mg has a shelf life of 4 years and Zydol SR 150 mg and 200 mg tablets have a shelf life of 3 years when stored in PVC/PVDC/foil blisters.

*Special precautions for storage:* Store in a dry place below 30°C.

*Nature and contents of container:* PVC/PVDC/foil blister packs of 2, 4 or 10 tablets (sample/starter packs).

PVC/PVDC/foil blister packs of 30 or 60 tablets.

*Special instructions for use/handling:* None.

*Marketing authorisation holder:* Monsanto p.l.c., P.O. Box 53, Lane End Road, High Wycombe, Buckinghamshire, HP12 4HL.

**Marketing authorisation numbers**
Zydol SR 100 mg     08821/0003
Zydol SR 150mg     08821/0002
Zydol SR 200mg     08821/0001

**Date of approval/revision of SPC** March 1997.

**Legal category** POM.

*\*Trade Mark*

# Serono Laboratories (UK) Ltd
99 Bridge Road East
Welwyn Garden City
Hertfordshire AL7 1BG

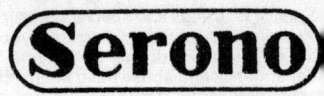

ARES-SERONO GROUP

## CUROSURF*

**Qualitative and quantitative composition** Curosurf is a natural surfactant, prepared from porcine lungs, containing almost exclusively polar lipids, in particular phosphatidylcholine (about 70% of the total phospholipid content) and about 1% of specific low molecular weight hydrophobic proteins SP-B and SP-C.

One 1.5 ml vial contains:
*Active ingredient:* phospholipid fraction from porcine lung 120 mg;
*Excipients:* sodium chloride 13.5 mg, water for injections 1.5 ml.

One 3 ml vial contains:
*Active ingredient:* phospholipid fraction from porcine lung 240 mg;
*Excipients:* sodium chloride 27 mg, water for injections 3 ml.

Composition per ml of suspension: phospholipid fraction from porcine lung 80 mg/ml, equivalent to about 74 mg/ml of total phospholipids and 0.9 mg/ml of low molecular weight hydrophobic proteins.

**Pharmaceutical form** Sterile suspension in single-dose vials for intratracheal administration.

### Clinical particulars
*Therapeutic indications:* Treatment of Respiratory Distress Syndrome (RDS) or hyaline membrane disease in newborn babies with birthweight over 700 g.

Prophylactic use in premature infants between 24 and 31 weeks estimated gestational age at risk from RDS or with evidence of surfactant deficiency.

*Posology and method of administration:* Curosurf should only be administered by those trained and experienced in the care and resuscitation of preterm infants.

Curosurf is available in ready to use vials that should be stored in a refrigerator at +2 to +8°C. The vial should be warmed to 37°C before use e.g., by holding it in an incubator for about one hour or in a thermostated bath for about 3 minutes, and gently turned upside down, without shaking, in order to obtain a uniform suspension.

The suspension should be withdrawn from the vial using a sterile needle and syringe and it should be administered by the intratracheal route in intubated infants.

*Posology*
*Prophylaxis:* a single dose of 100–200 mg/kg should be administered as soon as possible after birth (preferably within 15 minutes). Further doses of 100 mg/kg can be given 6–12 hours after the first dose and then 12 hours later in babies who have persistent signs of RDS and remain ventilator-dependent (maximum total dose: 300–400 mg/kg).

*Rescue treatment:* it is advisable to commence the treatment as soon as possible after diagnosing RDS. Therapy with Curosurf starting more than 48 hours after diagnosing RDS has not been investigated. Initially, a single dose of 100–200 mg/kg (1.25–2.5 ml/kg) is advised.

Further doses of 100 mg/kg, administered at about 12 hourly intervals, may also be indicated in infants who remain intubated and in whom RDS is considered responsible or their persisting or deteriorating respiratory status (maximum total dose of 300–400 mg/kg).

*Method of administration:* Curosurf can be administered either by:
*Disconnecting the baby from the ventilator* – Disconnect the baby momentarily from the ventilator, administer 1.25 to 2.5 ml/kg of suspension, as a single bolus, directly into the lower trachea via the endotracheal tube. Perform approximately one minute of hand-bagging and then reconnect the baby to the ventilator at the same settings as before administration. Further doses (1.25 ml/kg) that may be required can be administered in the same manner.

OR

*Without disconnecting the baby from the ventilator* – Administer 1.25 to 2.5 ml/kg of the suspension, as a single bolus, directly into the lower trachea by passing a catheter through the suction port into the endotracheal tube. Further doses (1.25 ml/kg) that may be required can be administered in the same manner.

After administration of Curosurf, pulmonary compliance (chest expansion) can improve rapidly, thus requiring prompt adjustment of the ventilator settings.

The improvement of alveolar gas exchange can result in a rapid increase of arterial oxygen concentration: therefore a rapid adjustment of the inspired oxygen concentration should be made to avoid hyperoxia. In order to maintain proper blood oxygenation values, in addition to periodic haemo-gasanalysis, continuous monitoring of transcutaneous $P_aO_2$ or oxygen saturation is also advisable.

*Contra-indications:* No specific contra-indications are yet known.

*Special warnings and special precautions of use:* The baby's general conditions should be stabilised. Correction of acidosis, hypotension, anaemia, hypoglycaemia and hypothermia is also recommended.

Babies born following very prolonged rupture of the membranes (greater than 3 weeks) may not show optimal response.

Surfactant administration can be expected to reduce the severity of RDS but cannot be expected to eliminate entirely the mortality and morbidity associated with preterm birth, as preterm babies may be exposed to other complications of their immaturity. After administration of Curosurf a transient depression of cerebro-electrical activity has been recorded lasting 2 to 10 minutes. The impact of this is not clear.

*Interaction with other medicaments and other forms of interaction:* Not known.

*Pregnancy and lactation:* Not applicable.

*Effects on ability to drive and use machines:* Not applicable.

*Undesirable effects:* Pulmonary haemorrhage, the incidence of which increases the more immature the infant is, this is a rare and sometimes fatal complication of preterm delivery. No evidence exists of any increased risk of this event following the administration of Curosurf.

No other undesirable effects have been reported.

*Overdose:* There have been no reports of overdosage following the administration of Curosurf. However, in the unlikely event of accidental overdose, and only if there are clear clinical effects on the infant's respiration, ventilation or oxygenation, as much as the suspension as possible should be aspirated and the baby should be managed with supportive treatment, with particular attention to fluid and electrolyte balance.

### Pharmacological properties
*Pharmacodynamic properties:* Lung surfactant is a mixture of substances, mainly phospholipds and specific proteins, lining the internal surface of alveoli and capable of lowering pulmonary surface tension.

This surface tension lowering activity is essential to stabilise alveoli, and to avoid collapse at end-expiration so that adequate gas exchange is maintained throughout the ventilatory cycle.

Deficiency of lung surfactant, from whatever cause, leads to severe respiratory failure which in preterm babies is known as respiratory distress syndrome (RDS) or hyaline membrane disease (HMD). RDS is a major cause of acute mortality and acute morbidity in the preterm baby and may also be responsible for long term respiratory and neurologic sequelae.

Curosurf was developed to replace this deficiency of endogenous pulmonary surfactant by intratracheal administration of exogenous surfactant.

The surface properties of Curosurf favour its uniform distribution in the lungs and spreading at the air-liquid interfaces in the alveoli. The physiological and therapeutic effects of Curosurf in surfactant deficiency have been documented extensively in various animal models.

In immature rabbit foetuses obtained by hysterectomy and immediately sacrificed the administration of Curosurf caused a marked improvement in lung expansion.

In premature newborn rabbits ventilated with 100% oxygen there was a dramatic improvement of tidal volume and lung-thorax compliance compared to the control animals, after administration of Curosurf via a tracheal cannula.

Also in premature newborn rabbits, treatment with Curosurf (maintaining a standardised tidal volume of about 10 ml/kg) increased the compliance of the lung-thorax system to a level similar to that of mature newborn animals.

*Pharmacokinetic properties:* Curosurf remains mainly in the lungs following intratracheal administration with a half-life of 14C-labelled dipalmitoyl-phosphatidylcholine of 67 hours in newborn rabbits. Only traces of surfactant lipids can be found in serum and organs other than the lungs 48 hours after administration.

*Preclinical safety data:* Acute toxicity studies performed in different animal species by intraperitoneal and intratracheal routes did not elicit signs of lung or systemic toxicity, nor mortality.

The subacute intratracheal toxicity study in the dog, rabbit and rat (14 days) showed no clinical effects or haematological changes, nor macroscopic variations. Moreover, Curosurf did not reveal any evidence of direct toxicity in the rat by intraperitoneal route (4 weeks).

Curosurf by the parenteral route in the guinea pig neither elicits active anaphylactic reactions, nor stimulates the production of antibodies detectable by passive cutaneous anaphylactic reaction. No anaphylactic reaction was observed by intratracheal route. Furthermore there is no evidence of dermal sensitising potential (Magnusson and Kligman test).

Curosurf did not show any evidence of mutagenic or clastogenic activity.

### Pharmaceutical particulars
*List of excipients:* Sodium chloride, water for injections.

*Incompatibilities:* Not known.

*Shelf life:* 12 months. This shelf life refers to the unopened and correctly stored product.

*Special precautions for storage:* The product must be stored in a refrigerator at +2 to +8°C, protected from light, until the moment of use.

Do not use any residual quantity in the vial after the first aspiration.

Warmed vials should not be returned to the refrigerator.

*Nature and contents of container:* Single dose vials in clear colourless glass, provided with a cap in plastic and aluminium and a chlorobutyl rubber stopper.

*Instructions for use/handling:* Not applicable.

**Marketing authorisation number** 3400/0041.

**Date of approval/revision of SPC** May 1997.

**Legal category** POM.

## GEREF* 50

**Presentation** Ampoule containing lyophilised powder of sermorelin acetate corresponding to 50 micrograms of sermorelin INN. Mannitol, sodium phosphate dibasic and sodium phosphate monobasic are added as excipients.

Each ampoule of Geref is accompanied by a solvent ampoule containing 0.9% Sodium Chloride Injection BP.

**Uses** Sermorelin is a synthetic peptide consisting of the 1–29 amino acid sequence of natural GHRF, with a plasma T1/2 of 6–7 minutes after intravenous administration. Response reaches a peak approximately 30 minutes (15–60) post dose and lasts 2–3 hours.

Sermorelin is used for the evaluation of the functional capacity and response of the somatotrophs of the anterior pituitary.

**Dosage and administration**
*Recommended procedure:* A single intravenous injection of 1.0 microgram/kg body weight in the morning following an overnight fast.

Geref should be reconstituted immediately before use with a minimum of 0.5 ml of the accompanying sterile solvent.

Venous blood samples should be drawn 15 minutes before and immediately prior to Geref administration. Venous blood samples are then drawn at 15, 30, 45 and 60 minutes following Geref injection. Samples at 90 and 120 minutes are optional, since, in the majority of patients they do not give additional information.

**Contra-indications, warnings, etc**
*Contra-indications:* Do not use in patients with known

hypersensitivity to sermorelin acetate or any of the excipients of Geref.

Geref should not be used in pregnant or lactating women.

*Warnings:* The Geref test should be conducted in the absence of drugs which affect directly the pituitary secretion of somatotrophin. These would include preparations which contain or induce the release of somatostatin, insulin or glucocorticoids, and cyclo-oxygenase inhibitors such as aspirin and indomethacin.

The somatotrophin levels may be transiently elevated by clonidine, levodopa or insulin-induced hypoglycaemia. The response to Geref may also be blunted by anti-muscarinic agents, such as atropine.

Untreated hypothyroidism or use of anti-thyroid medications such as propylthiouracil or high levels of somatostatin at the time of injection may affect the response to Geref. Obesity, hyperglycaemia and elevated plasma fatty acids are generally associated with a subnormal GH response to Geref.

It is possible that beta adrenoreceptor agonists and blockers may affect response to Geref.

*Precautions:* The test should be carried out and interpreted under specialist supervision.

Patients already on growth hormone therapy should have therapy discontinued one to two weeks pre-test.

The test should be carried out with particular caution in patients with epilepsy or diabetes mellitus.

*Side-effects:* Facial heat, facial flush and injection site pain occasionally occur and usually disappear within a few minutes.

*Overdosage:* No data relating to acute overdosage are available.

**Pharmaceutical precautions** Store at 2–8°C, protect from light. The injection should be reconstituted immediately prior to use with the solvent provided.

Discard any product remaining after use.

**Legal category** POM.

**Package quantities** Boxes containing: 1 ampoule Geref 50 plus 1 ampoule solvent (OP).

**Further information** Nil.

**Product licence numbers**
Geref 50 Injection 3400/0029
Sodium Chloride Injection BP 3400/0024

## GONAL-F* 75 ▼
## GONAL-F* 150 ▼

**Qualitative and quantitative composition** Active ingredient: 75 or 150 IU recombinant human follicle stimulating hormone (follitropin alpha: INN). Follitropin alpha is produced by genetically engineered Chinese Hamster Ovary (CHO) cells and exhibits a specific activity in the range of 7000–14 000 IU–FSH/mg†.

† This range of specific activity is a reflection of the imprecision of the bioassay used to determine potency rather than product variability.

**Pharmaceutical form** Lyophilised sterile powder for injection after reconstitution with accompanying diluent (Water for Injection). After reconstitution with the diluent provided, Gonal-F has a pH in the range of 6.5 to 7.5.

**Clinical particulars**
*Therapeutic indications:* (i) Gonal-F is indicated for anovulation (including polycystic ovarian disease, PCOD) in women who have been unresponsive to treatment with clomiphene citrate.

(ii) Gonal-F is indicated for stimulation of multifollicular development in patients undergoing superovulation for assisted reproductive technologies (ART) such as *in vitro* fertilisation (IVF), gamete intrafallopian transfer (GIFT) and zygote intra-fallopian transfer (ZIFT).

*Posology and method of administration:* Gonal-F is intended for subcutaneous administration. The powder should be reconstituted immediately prior to use with the diluent provided. In order to avoid the injection of large volumes, up to 3 containers of Gonal-F 75 or Gonal-F 150 may be dissolved in 1 ml of diluent.

*Women with anovulation (including PCOD):* The object of Gonal-F therapy is to develop a single mature Graafian follicle from which the ovum will be liberated after the administration of hCG.

Gonal-F may be given as a course of daily injections. In menstruating patients treatment should commence within the first 7 days of the menstrual cycle.

Treatment should be tailored to the individual patient's response as assessed by measuring (i) follicle size by ultrasound and/or (ii) oestrogen secretion. A commonly used regimen commences at 75–150 IU FSH daily and is increased preferably by 37.5 IU, or 75 IU at 7 or preferably 14 day intervals if necessary, to obtain an adequate, but not excessive, response. The maximal daily dose is usually not higher than 225 IU FSH. If a patient fails to respond adequately after 4 weeks of treatment, that cycle should be abandoned and the patient should recommence treatment at a higher starting dose than in the abandoned cycle.

When an optimal response is obtained, a single injection of 5000 IU, up to 10000 IU hCG should be adminsitered 24–48 hours after the last Gonal-F injection. The patient is recommended to have coitus on the day of, and the day following, hCG administration.

If an excessive response is obtained, treatment should be stopped and hCG withheld (see *Warnings*). Treatment should recommence in the next cycle at a dosage lower than that of the previous cycle.

*Women undergoing ovarian stimulation for multiple follicular development prior to in vitro fertilisation or other assisted reproductive technologies:* A commonly used regimen for superovulation involves the administration of 150–225 IU of Gonal-F daily, commencing on days 2 or 3 of the cycle. Treatment is continued until adequate follicular development has been achieved (as assessed by monitoring of serum oestrogen concentrations and/or ultrasound examination), with the dose adjusted according to the patient's response, to usually not higher than 450 IU daily. In general adequate follicular development is achieved on average by the tenth day of treatment (range 5 to 20 days).

A single injection of up to 10 000 IU hCG is administered 24–48 hours after the last Gonal-F injection to induce final follicular maturation.

Down-regulation with a gonadotrophin-releasing hormone (GnRH) agonist is now commonly used in order to suppress the endogenous LH surge and to control tonic levels of LH. In a commonly used protocol, Gonal-F is started approximately 2 weeks after the start of agonist treatment, both being continued until adequate follicular development is achieved. For example, following two weeks of treatment with an agonist, 225 IU Gonal-F are administered for the first 7 days. The dose is then adjusted according to the ovarian response.

Overall experience with IVF indicates that in general the treatment success rate remains stable during the first four attempts and gradually declines thereafter.

The equivalency of the potency of Gonal-F and urinary FSH-containing preparations has not been definitiely proven. However, clinical assessment of Gonal-F indicates that its doses, regimens of administration and treatment monitoring procedures should not be different from those currently used for urinary FSH-containing preparations.

*Contra-indications:* Gonal-F is contra-indicated for safety reasons in:

- pregnancy
- ovarian enlargement or cyst not due to polycystic ovarian disease
- gynaecological haemorrhage of unknown aetiology
- ovarian, uterine or mammary carcinoma
- tumours of the hypothalamus and pituitary gland
- case of prior hypersensitivity reaction to FSH

Gonal-F is contra-indicated when an effective response cannot be obtained, such as:

- primary ovarian failure
- malformations of the sexual organs incompatible with pregnancy
- fibroid tumours of the uterus incompatible with pregnancy.

*Special warnings and precautions for use:* Before starting treatment, the couple's infertility should be assessed as appropriate and putative contra-indications for pregnancy evaluated. In particular, patients should be evaluated for hypothyroidism, adrenocortical deficiency, hyperprolactinemia and pituary or hypothalamic tumours, and appropriate specific treatment given.

Patients undergoing stimulation of follicular growth are at an increased risk of developing hyperstimulation in view of the excessive oestrogen response and multiple follicular development. In ART, aspiration of all follicles, prior to ovulation, may however reduce the incidence of hyperstimulation.

Ovarian hyperstimulation syndrome can become a serious medical event characterised by large ovarian cysts which are prone to rupture. Excessive ovarian response seldom gives rise to significant hyperstimulation unless hCG is administered to induce ovulation. It is therefore prudent to withhold hCG in such cases and advise the patient to refrain from coitus for at least 4 days.

Careful monitoring of ovarian response, based on ultrasound is recommended prior to and during stimulation therapy, especially in patients with Polycystic Ovarian Disease (PCOD).

The risk of multiple pregnancy following assisted reproductive technologies is related to the number of oocytes/embryos replaced. In patients undergoing induction of ovulation, the incidence of multiple pregnancies and births is increased compared with natural conception.

To minimise the risk of OHSS or of multiple pregnancy, ultrasound scans as well as oestradiol measurements are recommended. In anovulation the risk of OHSS is increased by a serum oestradiol >900 pg/ml and more than 3 follicles of 14 mm or more in diameter. In ART there is an increased risk of OHSS with a serum oestradiol >3000 pg/ml and 20 or more follicles of 12 mm or more in diameter. When the oestradiol level is >5500 pg/ml and where there are 40 or more follicles in total, it may be necessary to withhold hCG administration.

Adherence to recommended Gonal-F dosage, regimen of administration and careful monitoring of therapy will minimise the incidence of ovarian hyperstimulation and multiple pregnancy (see the chronic low dose protol in *Posology and method of administration* and *Undesirable effects*).

Pregnancy loss is higher in patients receiving FSH than that in the normal population, but comparable with the rates found in women with other fertility problems.

There have been no reports of hypersensitivity to Gonal-F, however particularly in patients who have a prior history of hypersensitivity to gonadotrophin preparations, there remains the possibility of anaphylactic responses. The first injection of Gonal-F in such patients must be performed under direct medical supervision, with full cardio-pulmonary resuscitation facilities immediately available.

Self-administration of Gonal-F should only be performed by patients who are well-motivated, adequately trained and with access to expert advice.

*Interaction with other medications and other forms of interaction:* Concomitant use of Gonal-F with other agents used to stimulate ovulation may potentiate the follicular response, whereas concurrent use of GnRH agonist-induced pituitary desensitisation may increase the dosage of Gonal-F needed to elicit an adequate ovarian response.

No drug incompatibilities have been reported for Gonal-F.

Gonal-F should not be administered as a mixture with other drugs in the same injection.

*Use during pregnancy and lactation:* Gonal-F should not be administered in case of pregnancy and lactation.

*Effects on ability to drive and use machines:* Gonal-F does not interfere with the patient's ability to drive or use machines.

*Undesirable effects:* Local reactions at the injection site (pain, redness and bruising), have been reported.

During treatment with Gonal-F the possibility of ovarian hyperstimulation must be taken into consideration. This syndrome may occur with a higher incidence in patients with polycystic ovarian disease. First symptoms of ovarian hyperstimulation are pain in the lower abdominal region, possibly in combination with nausea, vomiting and weight gain. In serious, but rare cases, an ovarian hyperstimulation syndrome with clearly enlarged ovaries, can go hand in hand with possible accumulation of fluid in the abdomen or thorax as well as more serious thromboembolic complications. In rare cases the latter can also be found independently of ovarian hyperstimulation syndrome. Should the above mentioned symptoms occur a careful medical and ultrasound examination is indicated.

When the ovarian response is excessive, treatment with Gonal-F should be discontinued and the treatment with hCG for ovulation induction must be abandoned. This will reduce the chances of development of ovarian hyperstimulation syndrome.

The incidence of multiple pregnancies is increased by Gonal-F compared with natural conception. The majority of multiple conceptions have been found to be twins. In IVF, it is related to the number of embryos replaced.

In the initial clinical trial, anovulatory patients were treated with Gonal-F using a 'chronic low dose' protocol i.e. starting dose of 75 IU FSH/day, to be maintained for 14 days unless follicular maturity was reached before that time. If after 14 days of 75 IU FSH/day no response was observed, the daily dose was increased by 37.5 IU FSH.

Each subsequent increase in dose could only be effected after seven days of treatment at any dose, and the increment was not to exceed 37.5 IU FSH on each occasion.

One hundred and ten patients were treated with Gonal-F for a total of 252 cycles. One OHSS was reported (0.4%). Eight percent of clinical pregnancies were multiple and 6% of deliveries were multiple.

In rare instances, arterial thromboembolisms have been associated with menotrophin/human chorionic gonadotrophin therapy. This may also occur with Gonal-F/hCG therapy.

Pregnancy wastage by miscarriage or abortion is

comparable with the rates in women with other fertility problems. Ectopic pregnancy may occur in women with a history of prior tubal disease.

In the course of clinical studies, 24% of patients have reported one or more, moderate or severe local reactions to Gonal-F injections. Pain was the most frequently reported local reaction. It has been observed mainly during the first few days of therapy, did not require specific treatment and did not lead to any interruption of therapy.

*Overdose:* The effects of an overdose of Gonal-F are unknown, nevertheless one could expect ovarian hyperstimulation syndrome to occur, which is further described in Special Warnings and Precautions for Use.

**Pharmacological properties**
*Pharmacodynamic properties:* Gonal-F is a preparation of follicle stimulating hormone produced by genetically engineered Chinese Hamster Ovary (CHO) cells. The most important effect resulting from parenteral administration of FSH is the development of mature Graafian follicles.

*Pharmacokinetic properties:* Following intravenous administration, Gonal-F is distributed to the extracellular fluid space with an initial half-life around 2 hours and eliminated from the body with a terminal half-life of about one day. The steady state volume of distribution and total clearance are 10 L and 0.6 L/h, respectively. One-eighth of the Gonal-F dose is excreted in the urine.

Following subcutaneous administration, the absolute bioavailability is about 70%. Following repeated administration, Gonal-F accumulates 3-fold at steady-state within 3–4 days. In women whose endogenous gonadotrophin secretion is suppressed, Gonal-F has nevertheless been shown to effectively stimulate follicular development and steroidogenesis, despite unmeasurable LH levels.

*Preclinical safety data:* In an extensive range of toxicological, mutagenicity and animal studies (dogs, rats, monkeys), acute and chronic (up to 13 weeks), no significant findings were observed.

Impaired fertility has been reported in rats exposed to pharmacological doses of follitropin ($\geq$40 IU/kg/d) for extended periods, through reduced fecundity.

Given in high doses ($\geq$5 IU/kg/d) follitropin alpha caused a decrease in the number of viable foetuses without being a teratogen, and distocia similar to that observed with urinary hMG.

However, since Gonal-F is contra-indicated in pregnancy, these data are of limited clinical relevance.

**Pharmaceutical particulars**
*List of excipients:* Sucrose, sodium dihydrogen phosphate, disodium phosphate, phosphoric acid, sodium hydroxide.

*Incompatibilities:* There are no known chemical incompatibilities to Gonal-F.

*Shelf-life:* The lyophilised product is stable for 24 months when stored at or below 25°C, protected from light.

*Special precautions for storage:* Store at or below 25°C, protected from light.

*Nature and contents of container:*
*Lyophilised powder:* Nature: Neutral colourless glass ampoules. Content: Follitropin alpha 75 IU or 150 IU, sucrose, sodium dihydrogen phosphate, disodium hydrogen phosphate, phosphoric acid, sodium hydroxide, nitrogen.
*Diluent ampoule:* Nature: Neutral colourless glass ampoules. Content: Water for injection 1 ml.

*Instructions for use/handling:* Gonal-F is for single use only.

To minimise potential losses of FSH due to adsorption onto the syringe, Gonal-F should preferably be administered immediately after reconstitution.

*Marketing authorisation holder:* Ares-Serono (Europe) Ltd, 112 Harley Street, London W1N 1AF.

**Marketing authorisation number** EU/1/95/001.

**Legal category** POM.

# METRODIN HIGH PURITY*

**Qualitative and quantitative composition** Active ingredient: 75 IU or 150 IU human follicle stimulating hormone (urofollitrophin).

**Pharmaceutical form** Lyophilised sterile powder for injection after reconstitution with accompanying NaCl solvent (sodium chloride solution 0.9%).

**Clinical particulars**
*Therapeutic indications:* (i) Metrodin High Purity, followed by chorionic gonadotrophin (hCG), is recommended for the stimulation of follicular development and ovulation in women with hypothalamic-pituitary dysfunction who present with either oligomenorrhoea or amenorrhoea. These women are classified as WHO Group II patients and usually receive clomiphene citrate as primary therapy. They have evidence of endogenous oestrogen production and thus will either spontaneously menstruate or experience withdrawal bleeding after progestagen administration. Polycystic ovarian disease (PCOD) is part of the WHO II classification and is present in the majority of these patients.

(ii) Metrodin High Purity is indicated for stimulation of multifollicular development in patients undergoing superovulation for assisted reproductive technologies (ART) such as *in vitro* fertilisation (IVF), gamete intra-fallopian transfer (GIFT) and zygote intra-fallopian transfer (ZIFT).

(iii) Metrodin High Purity is indicated with concomitant hCG therapy for the stimulation of spermatogenesis in men who have congenital or acquired hypogonadotrophic hypogonadism.

*Posology and method of administration:* Metrodin High Purity is intended for subcutaneous or intramuscular administration. The powder should be reconstituted immediately prior to use with the diluent provided. In order to avoid the injection of large volumes, up to 5 ampoules of Metrodin High Purity may be dissolved in 1 ml of diluent.

*Women with hypothalamic-pituitary dysfunction who present with either oligomenorrhoea or amenorrhoea (WHO Group II):* The object of Metrodin High Purity therapy is to develop a single mature Graafian follicle from which the ovum will be liberated after the administration of hCG.

Metrodin High Purity may be given as a course of daily injections. In menstruating patients treatment should commence within the first 7 days of the menstrual cycle.

Treatment should be tailored to the individual patient's response as assessed by measuring (i) follicle size by ultrasound and/or (ii) oestrogen secretion. A commonly used regimen commences at 75–150 IU FSH daily and is increased or decreased by 37.5 IU (up to 75 IU) at 7 or 14 day intervals if necessary, to obtain an adequate, but not excessive, response. If a patient fails to respond adequately after 4 weeks of treatment, that cycle should be abandoned.

When an optimal response is obtained, single intramuscular injection of up to 1000 IU hCG should be administered 24–48 hours after the last Metrodin High Purity injection. The patient is recommended to have coitus on the day of, and the day following, hCG administration.

If an excessive response is obtained, treatment should be stopped and hCG withheld (see *Warnings*). Treatment should recommence in the next cycle at a dosage lower than that of the previous cycle.

If an excessive response is obtained, treatment should be stopped and hCG withheld (see warnings). Treatment should recommence in the next cycle at a dosage lower than that of the previous cycle.

*Women undergoing superovulation for in-vitro fertilisation and other assisted reproductive technologies:* A regimen for superovulation involves the administration of 150–225 IU of Metrodin High Purity daily, commencing on days 2 or 3 of the cycle. Treatment is continued until adequate follicular development has been achieved (as assessed by monitoring of serum oestrogen concentrations and/or ultrasound examination), with the dose adjusted according to the patient's response, to usually not higher than 450 IU daily.

A single injection of up to 10000 IU hCG is administered 24–48 hours after the last Metrodin High Purity injection to induce final follicular maturation.

Down-regulation with a GnRH agonist is now commonly used in order to suppress the endogenous LH surge and to control tonic levels of LH. In a commonly used protocol, Metrodin High Purity is started approximately 2 weeks after the start of agonist treatment. For example, following two-weeks treatment with an agonist, 225 IU Metrodin High Purity are administered (subcutaneous or intramuscular) for the first 7 days. The dose is then adjusted according to the ovarian repsonse.

*Men with hypogonadotrophic hypogonadism:* Metrodin High Purity should be given, concomitantly, with hCG at the dosage of 150 IU three times a week. This regimen should be continued for a minimum of 4 more months. If after this period, the patient has not responded, the combination treatment (hCG plus Metrodin High Purity 150 IU 3 times a week) may be continued. Current clinical experience indicates that treatment for up to 18 months or more may be necessary to achieve spermatogenesis.

*Contra-indications:* Metrodin High Purity is contra-indicated in women for safety reasons in:

– cases of prior hypersensitivity to menotrophins (or any excipients used in the formulation)
– pregnancy
– ovarian enlargement or cyst not due to polycystic ovarian syndrome

– gynaecological haemorrhages of unknown aetiology
– ovarian, uterine or mammary carcinoma
– tumours of the hypothalamus and pituitary gland

Metrodin High Purity is also contra-indicated in women when an effective response cannot be obtained, such as:

– primary ovarian failure
– malformations of sexual organs incompatible with pregnancy
– fibroid tumors of the uterus incompatible with pregnancy.

Metrodin High Purity is contra-indicated in men for safety reasons in:

– cases of prior hypersensitivity to menotrophins (or any excipients used in the formulation)

Metrodin High Purity is also contra-indicated in men when an effective response cannot be obtained, such as:

– primary testicular insufficiency.

*Special warnings and precautions for use:* Metrodin High Purity may cause local reaction at the injection site. Allergic-type reactions have occasionally been reported, in which lactose intolerance has been suspected, although not proven. It is therefore important to consider the effect of the lactose component of Metrodin High Purity, if administered to lactose-sensitive patients.

*Women:* Before starting treatment, the couple's infertility should be assessed as appropriate and putative contra-indications for pregnancy evaluated. In particular, patients should be evaluated for hypothyroidism, adrenocortical deficiency, hyperprolactinemia and pituitary or hypothalamic tumours, and appropriate specific treatment given.

Although adherence to recommended Metrodin High Purity dosages will minimise the incidence of ovarian hyperstimulation in patients undergoing ovulation induction, the possibility of hyperstimulation and multiple ovulation should be considered and careful monitoring performed during treatment in order to minimise their occurrence. This syndrome can become a serious medical event characterised by large ovarian cysts which are prone to rupture. Excessive oestrogenic response seldom gives rise of significant hyperstimulation unless hCG is administered to induce ovulation. It is therefore prudent to withhold hCG in such case and advise the patient to refrain from coitus for at least 4 days.

Patients undergoing superovulation are at an increased risk of developing hyperstimulation in view of the excessive oestrogen response and multiple follicular development. Aspiration of all follicles, prior to ovulation, may reduce the incidence of hyperstimulation.

The risk of multiple pregnancy following assisted reproductive technologies is related to the number of oocytes/embryos replaced. In other patients the incidence of multiple pregnancies and births is increased by Metrodin High Purity, as with other agents used to stimulate ovulation; however, the majority of multiple conceptions are twins.

Pregnancy loss is higher than that in the normal population, but comparable with the rates found in women with other fertility problems.

In those patients not undergoing super-ovulation the occurrence of smaller, secondary follicles in the presence of more than one dominant follicle, as visualised by ultrasonography, is reported to be associated with an increased incidence of hyperstimulation.

*Men:* Elevated endogenous FSH levels are indicative of primary testicular failure. Such patients are unresponsive to Metrodin High Purity/hCG therapy.

Semen analysis is recommended 4 to 6 months after the beginning of treatment in assessing the response.

*Interaction with other medicaments and other forms of interaction:* No clinically significant adverse drug interactions have been reported during Metrodin High Purity therapy.

Concomitant use of Metrodin High Purity with other agents used to stimulate ovulation may potentiate the follicular response, whereas concurrent use of GnRH agonist-induced pituitary densensitisation may increase the dosage of Metrodin High Purity needed to elicit an adequate ovarian response.

No drug incompatibilities have been reported for Metrodin High Purity. Metrodin High Purity should not be mixed with other drugs in the same syringe.

*Use during pregnancy and lactation:* Metrodin High Purity should not be administered in case of pregnancy and lactation.

*Effects on ability to drive and use machines:* Metrodin High Purity does not interfere with the patient's ability to drive or use machines.

*Undesirable effects:* In clinical trials, headaches have been rarely reported.

Local reactions at the injection site have been reported following urofollitrophin administration.

*Women:* Fever and arthralgias have been reported following urofollitrophin administration.

Under treatment with Metrodin High Purity the possibility of an ovarian hyperstimulation must be taken into consideration. First symptoms of ovarian hyperstimulation are pain in the lower abdominal region, possibly in combination with nausea, vomiting and weight gain. In serious, but rare cases, an ovarian hyperstimulation syndrome with clearly enlarged ovaries, can go hand in hand with a possible accumulation of fluids in the abdomen or thorax as well as more serious thromboembolic complications. In rare cases the latter can also be found independently of an ovarian hyperstimulation syndrome. Should the above mentioned symptoms occur under treatment with Metrodin High Purity, a careful medical examination is indicated. Treatment with Metrodin High Purity should be discontinued in these cases and the treatment with hCG for ovulation induction should be abandoned.

The incidence of multiple pregnancies is increased by Metrodin High Purity, as with other agents used to stimulate ovulation. The majority of multiple conceptions have been found to be twins. In IVF, it is related to the number of embryos replaced.

In rare instances, arterial thromboembolisms have been associated with menotrophin/human chorionic gonadotrophin therapy. This may also occur with Metrodin High Purity/hCG therapy.

Pregnancy wastage by miscarriage or abortion is comparable with the rates in women with other fertility problems. Ectopic pregnancy may occur in women with a history of prior tubal disease.

*Men:* Gynecomastia, acne and weight gain may occur occasionally during Metrodin High Purity/hCG therapy. These are known effects of hCG treatment.

*Overdose:* The effects of an overdose of Metrodin High Purity are unknown, nevertheless one could expect ovarian hyperstimulation syndrome to occur, which is further described in *Special warnings and precautions for use.*

**Pharmacological properties**

*Pharmacodynamic properties: Women:* Metrodin High Purity is a preparation of follicle stimulating hormone (FSH) purified from human menopausal gondaotrophin (hMG). The most important effect resulting from parenteral administration of FSH is the development of mature Graafian follicles.

*Men:* Metrodin High Purity administered concomitantly with hCG for at least 4 months induces spermatogenesis in men deficient in FSH.

*Pharmacokinetic properties:* Following a single s.c. or i.m. administration of Metrodin High Purity (150 IU) to male volunteers:

- Peak serum FSH levels were reached 15±7 (s.c.) and 10±4 (i.m.) hours later with an increase of 4.0±2 IU/1 of FSH over baseline values, for both the s.c. and i.m. routes.
- 72 hours after administration, serum FSH levels were still significantly higher than baseline values. The elimination half-life of FSH was estimated to be between 30–40 hrs.

*Preclinical safety data:* In toxicology and animal studies, no significant findings were observed. Acute toxicology studies were performed in mice and rats at doses exceeding 1500 IU/kg. Subacute toxicology studies in rats and monkeys involved doses up to 100 IU/kg/day for 13 weeks. Metrodin High Purity exhibited no mutagenic activity in a range of mutagenicity studies.

**Pharmaceutical particulars**

*List of excipients:* Lactose.

*Incompatibilities:* There are no known chemical incompatibilities fo Metrodin High Purity.

*Shelf life:* The lyophylised product is stable for two years when stored at or below 25°C, protected from light.

*Special precautions for storage:* Store at or below 25°C, protected from light.

*Nature and contents of containers: Lyophilised powder ampoule:*

| | |
|---|---|
| Nature: | Neutral colourless glass ampoules |
| Content: | Urofollitrophin 75 IU or 150 IU |
| Lactose | 10 mg |

*Diluent ampoule:*

| | |
|---|---|
| Nature: | Neutral colourless glass ampoules |
| Content: | Sodium Chloride (0.9%) in water for injections |

*Instructions for use/handling:* To minimise potential losses of FSH due to adsorption onto the syringe, Metrodin High Purity should preferably be administered immediately after reconstitution. The degree of adsorption which may occur has been shown to have no significant effect on the dose required for clinical efficacy.

**Marketing authorisation numbers**

| | |
|---|---|
| Metrodin High Purity 75 IU | 3400/0038 |
| Metrodin High Purity 150 IU | 3400/0039 |

**Date of approval/revision of SPC** March 1997.

**Legal category** POM.

## PERGONAL*

**Presentation** Pergonal ampoules contain human menopausal gonadotrophin (HMG) in a freeze-dried, sterile powder form (Approved Name: Menotrophin). Each Pergonal ampoule contains:

| | |
|---|---|
| Human follicle-stimulating hormone (FSH) | 75 IU |
| Human luteinising hormone (LH) | 75 IU |
| Lactose | 10 mg |

Each Pergonal ampoule is accompanied by a solvent ampoule containing:

| | |
|---|---|
| Sodium Chloride Injection BP | 1 ml |

**Uses** Pergonal is used for the treatment of infertile patients under the guidance of clinicians familiar with infertility problems.

*(i) Amenorrhoeic/anovulatory women:* Pergonal followed by Chorionic Gonadotrophin (hCG, Profasi*) is indicated for the induction of ovulation in amenorrhoeic patients or anovulatory women with regular or irregular cycles.

*(ii) Women undergoing superovulation for assisted conception techniques such as in vitro fertilisation (IVF):* Pergonal and Profasi are indicated for the induction of multiple follicular development in patients undergoing an assisted conception technique, such as IVF. The induction of multiple follicular growth is also known as 'superovulation'. Tubal occlusion, unexplained infertility and male subfertility are common indications for IVF.

*(iii) Hypogonadotrophic hypogonadism in men:* Pergonal with concomitant Profasi therapy is indicated for the stimulation of spermatogenesis in men who have primary or secondary hypogonadotrophic hypogonadism.

Elevated endogenous FSH levels are indicative of primary testicular failure. Such patients are usually unresponsive to Pergonal/Profasi therapy.

**Dosage and administration** Pergonal is given by intramuscular injection only. In order to avoid the intramuscular injection of large volumes, up to 5 ampoules of Pergonal may be dissolved in 1 ml of solvent.

*(i) Amenorrhoeic/anovulatory women:* The object is to develop a single mature Graafian follicle with individually tailored doses of Pergonal over several days. Stimulated follicles will not always liberate ova spontaneously, therefore follicular rupture has to be achieved by injecting Profasi, which simulates the normal mid-cycle surge of LH.

Pergonal may be given as a course of daily injections or as injections on alternate days. In menstruating patients treatment should commence within the first 7 days of the menstrual cycle.

Two Pergonal dosage schedules are commonly employed:

*Daily therapy:* Treatment with Pergonal should be commenced at 2 ampoules daily (Group I patients) or 1 ampoule daily (Group II patients). This dosage may be increased or decreased at approximately weekly intervals until an adequate, but not excessive, response is obtained (see Monitoring). Up to 10,000 IU Profasi should be given 24–48 hours after the last Pergonal injection. Sexual intercourse is recommended on the day of and that following Profasi injection. If a patient fails to respond adequately after treatment for three weeks that cycle should be abandoned.

The dosage in subsequent cycles should be adjusted if necessary depending upon the patient's response to the previous treatment course.

*Alternate day therapy:* Three equal doses of Pergonal are given on alternate days. This is followed by up to 10,000 IU Profasi one week after the first injection of Pergonal, provided an adequate but not excessive response has been obtained (see 'Monitoring'). Sexual intercourse is recommended on the day of and that following Profasi injection.

The recommended dosage for the initial course of treatment is:

WHO Group I patients (women with little or no evidence of endogenous oestrogen activity)—5 ampoules Pergonal per injection.

WHO Group II patients (women with evidence of some oestrogen activity)—3 ampoules Pergonal per injection.

In both groups of patients, the dosage in subsequent courses should be adjusted if necessary, depending upon the patient's response to the previous course.

*Monitoring of Pergonal therapy:* The dose of Pergonal required to evoke the desired response is critical and varies both from patient to patient and in the same patient from cycle to cycle. Monitoring of Pergonal therapy is, therefore, essential.

Follicular development may be judged by the concentration of oestrogens measured in blood or urine and/or by ultrasonic visualisation of follicle size—ideally both methods should be used concurrently. Local laboratory normal range of values should be taken into consideration.

*Urinary oestrogens:* The amount of oestrogen excreted in a 24 hour collection of urine should be estimated at regular intervals throughout treatment. Urinary oestrogen levels between 180 nmol/24 hr (50 microgram/24 hr) and 514 nmol/24 hr (140 microgram/24 hr) generally indicate an optimum response. Values below this therapeutic range may indicate inadequate follicular development. In cases where the levels are in excess of 514 nmol/24 hr or where a very steep rise in oestrogen levels occur there is an increased risk of hyperstimulation. In cycles in which an excessive oestrogen response has occurred, Profasi should be withheld (see 'Warnings') and the patient should refrain from having sexual intercourse for at least the next 4 days.

*Plasma oestradiol-17β.* The level of plasma oestradiol-17β should be estimated at regular intervals throughout treatment with Pergonal. Levels between 1100 pmol/l (300 pg/ml) and 3000 pmol/l (800 pg/ml) generally indicate an optimum response. Values below this therapeutic range may indicate inadequate follicular development. In cases where the oestradiol-17β level exceeds 3000 pmol/l or where a very steep rise occurs, there is an increased risk of hyperstimulation. Profasi should be withheld (see 'Warnings') and the patient should refrain from having sexual intercourse for at least the next 4 days.

*Ultrasound:* When monitoring Pergonal therapy by serial ultrasonic visualisation of the follicle size, a follicular diameter of 16–25 mm should indicate the presence of a mature follicle and therefore the optimum time for the administration of Profasi. If the follicular diameter of the dominant follicle is less than 16 mm, further Pergonal may be required.

Profasi should not be given if several mature follicles are visualised as there is a risk of multiple ovulation and the occurrence of hyperstimulation syndrome.

*(ii) Women undergoing superovulation for assisted conception techniques such as in vitro fertilisation (IVF):* The objective of superovulation is to stimulate multiple follicular growth, thereby increasing the number of eggs available for fertilisation.

A frequently used regimen for superovulation involves pretreatment with Clomiphene Citrate followed by Pergonal and Profasi. A commonly used combined dosage regimen involves the administration of 100 mg Clomiphene Citrate daily on cycle days 2–6. This is followed by Pergonal at a dosage of 2–3 ampoules daily, commencing on day 5 of the cycle and continuing, at a dose dependent upon the patient's response, until adequate follicular development has been achieved.

An alternative regimen using Pergonal and Profasi involves the administration of Pergonal at a dosage of 2–3 ampoules daily, commencing on day 2 or 3 of the cycle. Treatment is continued, with the dose adjusted according to the patient's response, until adequate follicular development has been achieved.

For both regimens, a single injection of up to 10,000 IU Profasi is administered 24–48 hours after the last Pergonal injection to coincide with the expected onset of the (endogenous) LH surge.

*Monitoring of superovulation:* The administration of Pergonal for superovulation is usually monitored by estimation of plasma oestradiol-17β and ultrasound. One recommendation is that the diameter of at least 3 follicles should be equal to or greater than 15 mm, with the diameter of the leading follicle being 18 mm and the plasma oestradiol-17β level at least 3500 pmol/l (920 pg/ml).

Profasi should not be administered unless there is evidence of adequate follicular development as evidenced by progressively rising oestrogen levels and concomitant follicular growth on ultrasound.

*Egg retrieval:* Egg retrieval is carried out, either by laparoscopy or ultrasound guided aspiration, about 34–36 hours following Profasi injection. Ideally all follicles should be aspirated at egg retrieval (see 'Warnings').

Further details concerning Pergonal dosage and monitoring for both amenorrhoeic/anovulatory women and superovulation are available on request.

*(iii) Hypogonadotrophic hypogonadism in men:* Treatment should commence with Profasi at a dosage of 2,000 IU, twice weekly, to bring about the development of secondary sexual characteristics and a testosterone level within the normal range.

If induction of spermatogenesis is required, but the only response to Profasi has been androgenic, therapy should be continued at a dosage of 2,000 IU, twice weekly and Pergonal 1 ampoule, 3 times a week. This regimen should be continued for a minimum of four months.

If, after four months, the patient has not responded with evidence of increased spermatogenesis, therapy may be continued with Profasi 2,000 IU, twice weekly and Pergonal 1–2 ampoules, three times a week.

Although no specific monitoring is required in the male patient, semen analysis is useful in assessing the response to treatment.

*Children:* Not recommended for use in children.

*Elderly:* Not recommended for use in the elderly.

### Contra-indications, warnings, etc

*Contra-indications:* Pergonal therapy is precluded in women in whom a satisfactory outcome cannot be expected, e.g. women with tubal occlusion (unless they are undergoing superovulation for IVF), ovarian dysgenesis, absent uterus or premature menopause.

Appropriate treatment should first be given for other endocrine disorders, e.g. hypothyroidism, adrenocortical deficiency, hyperprolactinaemia or pituitary tumour and other possible causes of infertility in either partner. An acceptable semen analysis should be available for those couples undergoing ovulation induction or in vitro fertilisation. However, certain types of male infertility can be successfully treated by assisted conception techniques.

Pergonal is contra-indicated in pregnant and lactating women.

*Warnings:* Pergonal may occasionally cause local reactions at the injection site. Fever and joint pains have been reported rarely.

Allergic-type reactions have occasionally been reported, in which lactose intolerance has been suspected, although not proven. It is therefore important to consider the effect of the lactose component of Pergonal if administered to lactose-sensitive patients.

Hyperstimulation: Adherence to recommended Pergonal dosages and monitoring schedules will minimise the possibility of ovarian hyperstimulation in amenorrhoeic and anovulatory women. Excessive oestrogenic responses to Pergonal do not generally give rise to significant side effects unless Profasi is given to induce ovulation. Hormone assays will detect an excessive oestrogen response to Pergonal and ultrasound will reveal any excessive follicular development; Profasi administration should be withheld and sexual intercourse should be avoided (see 'Overdosage').

Patients undergoing superovulation may be at an increased risk of developing hyperstimulation in view of the excessive oestrogen response and multiple follicular development. However aspiration of all follicles, prior to ovulation, may reduce the incidence of hyperstimulation syndrome.

Multiple pregnancy: The incidence of multiple births following Pergonal/Profasi therapy in anovulatory and amenorrhoeic women has been variously reported between 10% and 40%. However, the majority of such multiple conceptions are twins: high order multiple births are extremely rare when accurate monitoring is employed.

The incidence of multiple pregnancies following assisted conception techniques, is related to the number of oocytes/embryos replaced.

There have been reports of ectopic pregnancy in women treated with Pergonal who have undergone assisted conception. Women undergoing such procedures may have tubal disease, which is an important predisposing factor for ectopic pregnancy. A causal relationship between ectopic pregnancy and use of Pergonal has not been established.

Pregnancy loss, in both amenorrhoeic/anovulatory patients and women undergoing assisted conception techniques, is higher than that in the normal population, but comparable with the rates found in women with other fertility problems.

The risks of congenital abnormalities are not increased by Pergonal.

*Precautions:* In amenorrhoeic/anovulatory patients the occurrence of smaller, secondary follicles in the presence of more than one dominant follicle, as visualised by ultrasonography, is reported to be associated with an increased incidence of hyperstimulation syndrome.

*Side-effects:* Local reaction at injection site; allergic-type reaction possibly due to lactose component; fever and joint pains; hyperstimulation; multiple pregnancy.

No adverse reactions have been reported in men.

*Overdosage and treatment:* There are no reports of toxic effects occurring as a result of overdosage. However, hyperstimulation syndrome may result from overdosage with Pergonal. Hyperstimulation is generally categorised as mild, moderate or severe and symptoms usually appear 3–6 days after Profasi administration.

Mild hyperstimulation—Symptoms include some abdominal swelling and pain; ovaries enlarged to about 5 cm diameter. Therapy—rest; careful observa-

tion and symptomatic relief. Ovarian enlargement declines rapidly.

Moderate hyperstimulation—Symptoms include more pronounced abdominal distension and pain; nausea; vomiting; occasional diarrhoea; ovaries enlarged up to 12 cm diameter. Therapy—bed rest; close observation, in the case of conception occurring, to detect any progression to severe hyperstimulation. Pelvic examination of enlarged ovaries should be gentle in order to avoid rupture of the cysts. Symptoms subside spontaneously over 2–3 weeks.

Severe hyperstimulation—This is a rare but serious complication—symptoms include pronounced abdominal distension and pain; ascites; pleural effusion; decreased blood volume; reduced urine output; electrolyte imbalance and sometimes shock; ovaries enlarge to in excess of 12 cm diameter. Therapy—hospitalisation; treatment should be conservative and concentrate on restoring blood volume and preventing shock. Acute symptoms subside over several days and ovaries return to normal over 20–40 days if conception does not occur—symptoms may be prolonged if conception occurs.

**Pharmaceutical precautions**　Pergonal should be stored below 25°C and protected from light. The injection should be reconstituted immediately prior to use with the solvent provided.

**Legal category**　POM.

**Package quantities**　Boxes containing:
(i) 1 ampoule Pergonal plus 1 ampoule solvent (OP).
(ii) 10 ampoules Pergonal plus 10 ampoules solvent (OP).

**Further information**　One IU of human urinary FSH and one IU of human urinary LH are defined as the activities contained in 0.11388 mg and 0.13369 mg of the 1st International Standard, respectively.

**Product licence numbers**
Pergonal 3400/0007
Sodium Chloride Injection BP 3400/0024.

## PROFASI*

**Presentation**　Profasi ampoules contain human chorionic gonadotrophin (hCG) in a sterile, freeze-dried, powder form. The monograph for Chorionic Gonadotrophin Injection BP applies to a hormonal preparation extracted from the urine of pregnant women, which possesses predominantly luteinising properties.

Profasi is available in three strengths (2000, 5000 and 10,000 IU). Ampoules of Profasi contain either:
2,000 IU Chorionic Gonadotrophin+10 mg Lactose
5,000 IU Chorionic Gonadotrophin+10 mg Lactose
10,000 IU Chorionic Gonadotrophin+20 mg Mannitol

Each Profasi ampoule is accompanied by a solvent ampoule containing:

Sodium Chloride Injection BP　　　　　　1 ml

**Uses**　The action of human chorionic gonadotrophin is predominantly luteinising. Profasi is used in the treatment of infertility where its administration forms part of a recognised treatment regimen.

*(i) Anovulatory women:* Follicular development and endometrial proliferation are first stimulated with a suitable agent, e.g. Clomiphene Citrate, Pergonal* (Menotrophin Injection BP, HMG) or Metrodin* High Purity (urofollitrophin, FSH). Profasi is then given to simulate an LH surge and induce ovulation.

*(ii) Women undergoing superovulation for assisted conception techniques such as in vitro fertilisation (IVF):* Profasi is used as part of a superovulation programme in women undergoing an assisted conception technique. Multiple follicular development is stimulated with Pergonal or Metrodin High Purity, either alone or in combination with Clomiphene Citrate. Profasi is then administered to bring about final maturation of the follicles. Follicles are aspirated prior to spontaneous ovulation.

*(iii) Hypogonadotrophic hypogonadism in men:* Profasi stimulates the interstitial (Leydig) cells of the testes and consequently the secretion of androgens and the development of secondary sexual characteristics. With concomitant Pergonal therapy, Profasi stimulates the induction and maintenance of spermatogenesis.

Elevated endogenous FSH levels are indicative of primary testicular failure. Such patients are usually unresponsive to Pergonal/Profasi therapy.

*(iv) Cryptorchidism:* Profasi stimulates the Leydig cells of the testes and effects the secretion of androgens which leads to the descent of cryptorchid testes.

**Dosage and administration**　Profasi is given by subcutaneous or intramuscular injection only.

*(i) Anovulatory women:* Up to 10,000 IU Profasi is given in mid-cycle or as indicated following treatment with Clomiphene Citrate, Pergonal or Metrodin High Purity, according to a recognised scheme, provided

an adequate but not excessive response has been obtained. (See appropriate Data Sheet for details of dosage and monitoring.)

*(ii) Women undergoing superovulation for assisted conception techniques such as in vitro fertilisation (IVF):* Up to 10,000 IU Profasi is given following the induction of multiple follicular development with Pergonal or Metrodin High Purity, either alone or in combination with Clomiphene Citrate, according to a recognised treatment scheme. (See appropriate Data Sheet for details of dosage and monitoring.) Egg retrieval is carried out 34–36 hours following Profasi administration.

*(iii) Hypogonadotrophic hypogonadism in men:* Treatment should commence with Profasi at a dosage of 2,000 IU twice weekly to bring about the development of secondary sexual characteristics and a testosterone level within the normal range.

If induction of spermatogenesis is required, but the only response to Profasi has been androgenic, therapy should be continued at a dosage of 2,000 IU twice weekly, and Pergonal 75 IU three times a week. This regimen should be continued for a minimum of four months.

If, after the four months, the patient has not responded with evidence of increased spermatogenesis, therapy may be continued with Profasi 2,000 IU twice weekly and Pergonal 75 IU–150 IU three times a week.

Although no specific monitoring is required in the male patient, semen analysis is useful in assessing the response to treatment.

*(iv) Cryptorchidism:* 500–1,000 IU Profasi, dependent upon age, on alternate days for several weeks.

*Children:* Not recommended for use in girls.

*Elderly:* Not recommended for use in the elderly.

### Contra-indications, warnings, etc

*Contra-indications:* Profasi is precluded in women in whom stimulation of follicular maturation is not indicated because of the expectations of an unsatisfactory outcome, e.g. women with tubal occlusion unless they are undergoing superovulation for IVF, ovarian dysgenesis, absent uterus or premature menopause.

Appropriate treatment should first be given for other endocrine disorders, e.g. hypothyroidism, adrenocortical deficiency, hyperprolactinaemia or pituitary tumour and other possible causes of infertility in either partner. An acceptable semen analysis should be available, however certain types of male infertility can be successfully treated by assisted conception techniques.

Hyperstimulation: In women undergoing ovulation induction, an excessive response to follicular stimulating agents (e.g. Clomiphene Citrate, Metrodin High Purity or Pergonal) may lead to the development of hyperstimulation syndrome, particularly if Profasi is given to induce ovulation; Profasi should be withheld in such cycles (see 'Overdosage').

*Warnings:* Profasi may occasionally cause local reactions at the injection site.

In men, high doses of Profasi may lead to oedema and in such cases the dosage should be considerably reduced.

Patients undergoing superovulation may be at an increased risk of developing hyperstimulation in view of the excessive oestrogen response and multiple follicular development. However, aspiration of all follicles, may reduce the incidence of hyperstimulation syndrome.

The risk of multiple pregnancy following assisted conception techniques, is related to the number of oocytes/embryos replaced. In other patients the incidence of multiple pregnancies and births is increased by gonadotrophin therapy; however, the majority of such multiple pregnancies are twins.

Profasi may cause sexual precocity. If signs of sexual precocity are observed, treatment should be stopped.

Pregnancy loss, in both anovulatory patients and women undergoing assisted conception techniques is higher than that found in the normal population but comparable with the rates observed in women with other fertility problems.

The risk of congenital abnormalities is not increased by Profasi.

*Precautions:* In those patients not undergoing super ovulation the occurrence of smaller, secondary follicles in the presence of more than one dominant follicle, as visualised by ultrasonography, is reported to be associated with an increased incidence of hyperstimulation.

*Side-effects:* Hyperstimulation (see 'Overdosage') multiple pregnancy; oedema; sexual precocity; local reaction at injection site.

*Overdosage and treatment:* There are no reports of toxic effects occurring as a result of overdosage. However, hyperstimulation syndrome may result from overdosage with follicle stimulating/ovulation inducing agents. Hyperstimulation is generally categorised as mild, moderate or severe and symptoms usually appear 3–6 days after Profasi administration.

Mild hyperstimulation—Symptoms may include some abdominal swelling and pain; ovaries enlarged to about 5 cm diameter. Therapy—rest; careful observation and symptomatic relief. Ovarian enlargement declines rapidly.

Moderate hyperstimulation—Symptoms include more pronounced abdominal distension and pain; nausea; vomiting; occasional diarrhoea; ovaries enlarged up to 12 cm diameter. Therapy—bed rest; close observation, in the case of conception occurring, to detect any progression to severe hyperstimulation. Pelvic examination of enlarged ovaries should be gentle, in order to avoid rupture of the cysts. Symptoms subside spontaneously over 2–3 weeks.

Severe hyperstimulation—This is a rare but serious complication. Symptoms include pronounced abdominal distension and pain; ascites; pleural effusion; decreased blood volume; reduced urine output; electrolyte imbalance and sometimes shock; ovaries enlarge to in excess of 12 cm diameter. Therapy—hospitalisation, treatment should be conservative and concentrate on restoring blood volume and preventing shock. Acute symptoms subside over several days and ovaries return to normal over 20–40 days, if conception has not occurred. Symptoms may be prolonged if conception has occurred.

**Pharmaceutical precautions** Profasi should be stored below 25°C and protected from light. The injection should be reconstituted immediately prior to use with the solvent provided.

**Legal category** POM.

**Package quantities** Boxes containing either:
(i) 3 ampoules of Profasi 2,000 IU plus 3 ampoules solvent.
(ii) 1 ampoule Profasi 5,000 IU plus 1 ampoule solvent.
(iii) 10 ampoules Profasi 5,000 IU plus 10 ampoules solvent.
(iv) 1 ampoule Profasi 10,000 IU plus 1 ampoule solvent.
Available in original packs.

**Further information** One IU of chorionic gonadotrophin is defined as the activity contained in 0.001279 mg of the 2nd International Standard.

**Product licence numbers**
Profasi 2000 3400/0005
Profasi 5000 3400/0006
Profasi 10000 3400/0021
Sodium Chloride Injection BP 3400/0024

# SAIZEN*

**Qualitative and quantitative composition** Saizen vials contain Somatropin (rhGH) in a freeze-dried, sterile powder form.

Each single-use vial of Saizen contains Somatropin PhEur 4 IU (1.33 mg). Each vial is accompanied by an ampoule of solvent containing 1 ml of 0.9% w/v Sodium Chloride Injection BP.

Each multidose vial of Saizen contains Somatropin PhEur 10 IU (3.33 mg). Each vial is accompanied by a sterile solvent vial containing 5 ml saline solvent with benzyl alcohol (0.9% w/v sodium chloride and 0.9% w/v benzyl alcohol).

**Pharmaceutical form** Powder for injection after reconstitution with accompanying solvent.

**Clinical particulars**
*Therapeutic indications:* The treatment of short stature resulting from growth failure caused by decreased or absent secretion of endogenous growth hormone. The diagnosis should be confirmed by appropriate investigations of pituitary function.

Growth failure in patients with gonadal dysgenesis (Turner Syndrome).

It is recommended that Saizen treatment should be initiated/given under the guidance of a physician experienced in the diagnosis and management of GH deficiency.

*Posology and method of administration:* The lyophilised material should be reconstituted with the solvent provided, using a gentle, swirling motion. Vigorous shaking should be avoided. A slightly cloudy solution may be formed, but this is a normal product characteristic.

The 4 IU vial should be reconstituted with 0.5–1 ml of the accompanying solvent. The calculated dose should be withdrawn and the remainder discarded.

The 10 IU vial is intended for multiple dose use. This should be reconstituted with the accompanying bacteriostatic solvent to a concentration of no more than 10 IU/ml.

Administer by subcutaneous or intramuscular injection to patients with growth failure caused by inadequate secretion of endogenous growth hormone, and

by subcutaneous injection to patients with Turner syndrome. The dosage must be individualised for each patient.

*1. Treatment of growth failure due to inadequate secretion of normal endogenous growth hormone:* The recommended dose is as follows:

0.6 IU/kg or 0.20 mg/kg
12 IU/m² or 4.00 mg/m²

If response is poor, the weekly dose may be increased to:

0.8 IU/kg or 0.27 mg/kg
20 IU/m² or 6.67 mg/m²

*(a) Subcutaneous injection:* The weekly dose can be divided as shown below and is expressed per injection:

| 3 single doses | 0.2 IU/kg or 0.07 mg/kg<br>4 IU/m² or 1.33 mg/m² |
|---|---|
| 6 single doses | 0.1 IU/kg or 0.03 mg/kg<br>2 IU/m² or 0.67 mg/m² |
| 7 single doses | 0.085 IU/kg or 0.03 mg/kg<br>1.7 IU/m² or 0.57 mg/m² |

The injection site should be alternated to prevent lipoatrophy.

*(b) Intramuscular injection:* The weekly dose should be divided into 3 single injections:

0.2 IU/kg or 0.07 mg/kg
4 IU/m² or 1.33 mg/m²

*2. Treatment of growth failure due to gonadal dysgenesis (Turner syndrome):* The recommended weekly dose is:

0.6–0.7 IU/kg or 0.20–0.23 mg/kg
18 IU/m² or 6.00 mg/m²

During the second year of treatment, the weekly dose may be increased to:

0.8–1.0 IU/kg or 0.27–0.33 mg/kg
24 IU/m² or 8.00 mg/m²

The weekly dose should be divided in 7 single daily doses corresponding to:

0.09–0.1 IU/kg or 0.03 mg/kg
2.6 IU/m² or 0.87 mg/m²

Some patients with Turner syndrome may require higher growth hormone doses even during the first year of treatment to increase their growth velocity sufficiently.

The concomitant treatment with non-androgenic steroids has shown a further improvement in growth velocity.

Treatment should be continued until the patient has reached a satisfactory adult height or the epiphyses are closed.

*Contra-indications:* Children in whom epiphyseal fusion has occurred should not be treated with Saizen.

Saizen is also contra-indicated in patients who show recurrence or progression of an underlying intracranial lesion.

Saizen is not recommended for use during pregnancy and lactation.

*Special warnings and special precautions for use:* Saizen treatment should be carried out under regular medical supervision.

In patients with diabetes mellitus the treatment should be carried out under strict medical control with laboratory monitoring of their diabetic status; adjustment of anti-diabetic therapy may be required.

The possible appearance of hypothyroidism in the course of the therapy with somatropin should be corrected with thyroid hormone in order to obtain a sufficient growth promoting effect.

Patients with growth hormone deficiency secondary to a treated intracranial lesion should be examined frequently for recurrence of the underlying disease process.

In case of severe or recurrent headache, visual problems, nausea and/or vomiting, a fundoscopy for papilloedema is recommended. If papilloedema is confirmed a diagnosis of benign intracranial hypertension should be considered and if appropriate the somatropin treatment should be discontinued.

At present there is insufficient evidence to guide clinical decision making in patients with resolved intracranial hypertension. If somatropin treatment is restarted, careful monitoring for symptoms of intracranial hypertension is necessary.

When somatropin is administered subcutaneously at the same site over a long period, local tissue atrophy may result. This can be avoided by rotating the injection site daily.

Benzyl alcohol as a preservative in bacteriostatic sodium chloride solution for injection has been associated with toxicity in newborns. Saizen may be reconstituted with Sodium Chloride Injection BP or sterile Water for Injections for immediate use when administering to newborns.

*Interactions with other medicaments and other forms of interaction:* In some individuals concomitant corticosteroid therapy may inhibit the growth promoting

effects of somatropin. Interactions with other medicines are, at present, unknown. Also see *Precautions* re: insulin-dependent diabetes mellitus.

*Pregnancy and lactation:* There are no data from either human or animal studies relating to the use of Saizen during pregnancy. In the event of pregnancy occurring, treatment must be discontinued. There is no knowledge regarding the secretion of somatropin into human breast milk.

*Effects on ability to drive and use machines:* None known.

*Undesirable effects:* Some patients may experience redness and itching at the site of injection, particularly when the subcutaneous route is used.

Antibodies to somatropin can form in some patients; the clinical significance of these antibodies is unknown. In very rare instances, where short stature is due to deletion of the growth hormone gene complex, treatment with growth hormone may induce growth attenuating antibodies.

Intermittent dosage has been associated with the appearance of hypoglycaemia, this has not been reported with the use of uninterrupted, i.e. daily administration.

*Overdose:* Acute overdosage can produce transient hypoglycaemia followed by hyperglycaemia. Long term overdosage may result in the clinical features of acromegaly.

**Pharmacological properties**
*Pharmacodynamic properties:* The administration of Saizen stimulates an increase in growth velocity.

*Pharmacokinetic properties:* Intramuscular (I.M.) administration of 4 IU (1.33 mg)/m² body surface area of Saizen to 12 volunteers produced a peak level after 3 hours (T max). Subcutaneous (S.C.) administration to the same volunteers at the same dosage delayed the mean peak levels to between 4 and 6 hours after administration. The area under the curves for the routes are, however, similar and T max values for Saizen correlate well with those quoted for pituitary growth hormone in the published literature.

*Preclinical safety data:* The documented toxicological profile and the absence of mutagenic activity in a variety of *in vitro* and *in vivo* preclinical tests demonstrates the good safety profile of Saizen.

**Pharmaceutical particulars**
*List of excipients:* Saizen 4 IU – disodium phosphate, sodium dihydrogen phosphate, mannitol, sodium chloride.
Saizen 10 IU – disodium phosphate, sodium dihydrogen phosphate, mannitol.

*Incompatibilities:* No known chemical incompatibilities.

*Shelf life:* 24 months.

*Special precautions for storage:* Store at 2–8°C. Protect from light.
Saizen 4 IU reconstituted with Sodium Chloride Injection BP should be used immediately or within 24 hours when stored at 2–8°C.
Saizen 10 IU reconstituted with saline diluent with benzyl alcohol should be used within 7 days when stored at 2–8°C.

*Nature and contents of container:* Saizen 4 IU – Each box contains: 1 vial of Saizen 4 IU, 1 ml ampoule Sodium Chloride Injection BP.
Saizen 10 IU – Each box contains: 1 vial of Saizen 10 IU, 5 ml vial saline diluent with benzyl alcohol.

*Instructions for use/handling:* The lyophilised material should be reconstituted with the solvent provided. Vigorous shaking should be avoided.

**Marketing authorisation numbers**

| | |
|---|---|
| Saizen 4 IU | 3400/0023 |
| Sodium Chloride Injection BP | 3400/0024 |
| Saizen 10 IU | 3400/0034 |
| Saline diluent with benzyl alcohol | 3400/0035 |

**Date of approval/revision of SPC** 27 May 1997.

**Legal category** CD (Sch 4), POM.

# SEROPHENE*

**Presentation** White, round, flat, bevelled tablet, single score on one side and the letter 'S' imprinted on the other, each containing 50 mg Clomiphene Citrate BP.

**Uses** Serophene is indicated for the induction of ovulation in women with:
(i) hypothalamic-pituitary dysfunction (including polycystic ovarian syndrome (PCOS))
(ii) the induction of multiple follicular development in women undergoing superovulation for assisted conception techniques such as in vitro fertilisation (IVF).

Serophene is prescribable under the supervision of clinicians involved in the treatment of infertility.

**Dosage and administration**

*(i) Hypothalamic pituitary dysfunction (including PCOS):* Serophene is given as a 5 day course of tablets, commencing within the first 5 days of spontaneous or progesterone-induced menstrual bleeding. In patients who have not experienced recent uterine bleeding the commencement date is arbitrary.

A suggested dosage schedule is presented in the following table:

| | *dose mg/day* | *Result after 1 cycle* | | | *Result after 6 cycles—no pregnancy* |
|---|---|---|---|---|---|
| | | *ovulation pregnancy* | *ovulation no pregnancy* | *no ovulation* | |
| Cycle 1 | 50 | cease therapy | continue to 6 cycles (max) | increase dose (cycle 2) | |
| Cycle 2 | 100† | cease therapy | continue to 6 cycles (max) | same dose with hCG may be considered (cycle 3) *or* | reassess patient and consider gonadotrophin therapy |
| Cycle 3 | 100† +hCG | cease therapy | continue to 6 cycles (max) | reassess patient and consider gonadotrophin therapy | |

†This dose of Serophene should not be exceeded.

If ovulation does not occur naturally, a single subcutaneous or intramuscular injection of up to 10,000 IU Profasi* (Chorionic Gonadotrophin, hCG) may be given 7 to 10 days after the last Serophene tablet to simulate an LH surge.

Sexual intercourse is recommended around the expected time of ovulation (approximately 8–12 days after the last dose of Serophene).

*Monitoring of treatment:* Patients should be monitored each cycle at least for the first three cycles, ideally using ultrasound, at the expected time of ovulation, to check for ovulation.

Basal body temperature (BBT) charts have been recommended as a monitoring method in the past. However, it is now felt that this method is inappropriate due to inaccuracy, as the temperature rise occurs after ovulation takes place as well as daily negative reinforcement of the couple's problem.

Home monitoring using ovulation predictor kits based on the LH surge, is more accurate and more acceptable to patients than recording of BBT. Sexual intercourse is recommended at the time of the LH surge as this represents the time of ovulation.

The measurement of mid-luteal plasma progesterone may be used to assess the ovulatory response to treatment. On cycle day 21, serum progesterone levels in excess of 30 nmol/l are suggestive of ovulation.

Local laboratory normal range of values should be taken into consideration.

If a patient shows presumptive evidence of ovulation and menstruation does not follow, pregnancy should be excluded before treatment is recommenced.

*(ii) Superovulation for an assisted conception technique:* The objective of superovulation is to stimulate multiple follicular growth, thereby increasing the number of eggs available for fertilisation.

Serophene is usually administered in combination with gonadotrophins to induce multiple follicular maturation. A commonly used dosage regimen involves the administration of 100 mg (two tablets) Serophene daily on cycle days 2–6, followed by daily gonadotrophins (150–225 IU FSH) commencing on day 5 of the cycle and continuing, at a dose dependent upon the response of the patient, until adequate follicular development has been achieved. (See Pergonal* (Menotrophin Injection BP), Metrodin* High Purity (highly purified urofollitrophin (FSH) injection) and Profasi* Data Sheets for further details).

A single injection of up to 10,000 IU Profasi is administered 24–48 hours after the last gonadotrophin injection to coincide with the expected onset of the (endogenous) LH surge.

*Monitoring of superovulation:* Superovulation is monitored by estimation of plasma oestradiol-17β and by ultrasonography.

One recommendation is that the diameter of at least 3 follicles should be equal to or greater than 15 mm, with the diameter of the leading follicle 18 mm or more and a plasma oestradiol-17β level greater than 3500 pmol/l.

Profasi should not be administered unless there is evidence of adequate follicular development as evidenced by progressively rising oestrogen levels and concomitant follicular growth on ultrasound.

*Egg retrieval:* Egg retrieval is carried out, either by laparoscopy or ultrasound guided aspiration, about 34–36 hours following Profasi injection. Ideally, all follicles should be aspirated at egg retrieval (see Warnings).

Further details concerning Serophene dosage and monitoring, are available on request.

*Children:* Not recommended for use in children.

*Elderly:* Not recommended for use in the elderly.

**Contra-indications, warnings, etc**

*Contra-indications:* Liver disease and liver dysfunction; hereditary defect in bilirubin metabolism; pregnancy; abnormal uterine bleeding; ovarian cysts (except polycystic ovarian syndrome); ovarian endometriosis.

Serophene therapy is precluded in women in whom a satisfactory outcome cannot be expected, e.g., women with tubal occlusion unless thay are undergoing superovulation for IVF, ovarian dysgenesis, absent uterus, premature menopause or hypothalamic pituitary failure.

Serophene is contra-indicated in pregnant and lactating women.

*Warnings*

*Hyperstimulation:*

*(i) Hypothalamic pituitary dysfunction (including PCOS):* Patients receiving Serophene should be instructed to report any abdominal discomfort immediately and undergo appropriate investigations such as ultrasound. Whilst the incidence of clinically significant hyperstimulation is low with the recommended Serophene dosage scheme, the presence of excessive ovarian enlargement may require the dosage scheme to be modified (see Overdosage). Rare occurrences of lutein cyst rupture with intraperitoneal haemorrhage have been reported.

*(ii) Superovulation for an assisted conception technique:* The incidence of hyperstimulation is minimised in patients undergoing superovulation by the aspiration of all follicles.

*Visual symptoms:* Clomiphene citrate should be withdrawn if visual disturbances occur, e.g., blurring, spots or flashes (in rare cases scotomata). Patients should not drive or operate machinery if their vision is adversely affected.

*Multiple pregnancy:* The multiple pregnancy rate in treated patients with hypothalamic pituitary dysfunction or PCOS is approximately 8%, twins representing 90% of this figure.

The multiple pregnancy rate following assisted conception techniques is related to the number of oocytes/embryos replaced.

Although a higher spontaneous abortion rate than that found in the normal population has been reported, this is comparable to the abortion rate in women with other fertility problems. A causal relationship with clomiphene has not been established.

Although Serophene has been shown to be embryotoxic in animals at high doses, there is no evidence to suggest that it increases the incidence of congenital malformations in humans at therapeutic levels. Treatment with Serophene has not been shown to alter the incidence of congenital malformation observed in the offspring of women with fertility problems.

*Precautions;* Appropriate treatment should first be given for other endocrine disorders, e.g., hypothyroidism, adrenocortical deficiency, hyperprolactinaemia or pituitary tumours and other possible causes of infertility in either partner. An acceptable semen analysis should be available for those couples undergoing ovulation induction.

*Side-effects:* Side-effects are usually dose-related and generally reversible on drug withdrawal. The following side-effects have been reported:

Ovarian enlargement and abdominal/pelvic discomfort, vasomotor symptoms (hot flushes).

Nausea, vomiting, breast discomfort and visual symptoms have been reported occasionally.

Nervousness, insomnia, headache, dizziness, increased urination, heavier menses, depression, fatigue, skin reactions (dermatitis and urticaria), weight gain and temporary hair loss have been reported rarely.

Convulsions have been reported: patients with a history of seizures may be predisposed.

There have been rare reports of ovarian cancer with fertility drugs; infertility itself is a primary risk factor. Epidemiological data suggests that prolonged use of Serophene may increase this risk. Therefore the recommended duration of treatment should not be exceeded (see Dosage and administration).

*Overdosage (and treatment):* There is no experience of acute poisoning with Serophene.

Hyperstimulation may occasionally result from an excessive response to clomiphene citrate therapy. Hyperstimulation is categorised as mild, moderate or severe. Generally hyperstimulation will be mild or, very rarely, moderate after clomiphene citrate treatment. Symptoms usually appear 3–6 days after ovulation or Profasi administration.

Mild hyperstimulation—Symptoms may include some abdominal swelling and pain; ovaries enlarged to 5 cm diameter. Therapy—rest; careful observation and symptomatic relief. Ovarian enlargement declines rapidly.

Moderate hyperstimulation—Symptoms include more pronounced abdominal distension and pain; nausea; vomiting; occasional diarrhoea; ovaries enlarged up to 12 cm diameter. Therapy—bed rest; close observation, in the case of conception occurring, to detect any progression to severe hyperstimulation. Pelvic examination should be gentle in order to avoid rupture of the cysts. Symptoms subside spontaneously over 2–3 weeks.

Severe hyperstimulation—A rare but serious complication—symptoms include pronounced abdominal distention and pain; ascites; pleural effusion; decreased blood volume; reduced urine output; electrolyte imbalance and sometimes shock; ovaries enlarged to in excess of 12 cm diameter and may contain cysts. Therapy—hospitalisation, treatment should be conservative concentrating on restoring the blood volume and preventing shock. Acute symptoms subside over several days and ovaries return to normal after 20–40 days if conception does not occur—symptoms may be prolonged if conception has occurred.

**Pharmaceutical precautions** Serophene should be stored below 25°C and protected from light and moisture.

**Legal category** POM.

**Package quantities** Serophene is blister packed in boxes of 10, 30 and 100 tablets (OP).

**Further information** The mode of action of Serophene at the recommended dose appears to be through competition for available oestrogen receptor sites in the hypothalamus. Oestrogen is displaced from these sites and the hypothalamus perceives an apparent lack of circulating oestrogen. This results in gonadotrophin releasing hormone stimulated secretion of FSH and LH, which initiates the normal menstrual cycle.

Patients with very low baseline levels of endogenous gonadotrophins and oestrogens are usually less responsive to Serophene treatment, and consideration should be given to gonadotrophin therapy.

Clomiphene citrate is readily absorbed from the gastrointestinal tract and slowly excreted through the liver into the bile. The biological half-life is reported to be five days. Enterohepatic recirculation takes place.

There is evidence that some women ovulate spontaneously for some cycles after cessation of Serophene treatment.

**Product licence number** 3400/0009

## UKIDAN*

**Qualitative and quantitative composition** Ukidan vials contain urokinase in a sterile, white, freeze-dried powder form. Each vial contains 5,000 IU, 25,000 IU or 100,000 IU of urokinase.

**Pharmaceutical form** Powder for injection after reconstitution with solvent.

**Clinical particulars**

*Therapeutic indications:* Ukidan is indicated for the lysis of clots in the following conditions:

(i) Thromboembolic occlusive vascular disease such as deep vein thrombosis (DVT), pulmonary embolism (PE) and peripheral vascular occlusion.

(ii) Hyphaema (haemorrhage into the anterior chamber of the eye).

(iii) Arterio-venous haemodialysis shunts and intravenous cannulae which are blocked by fibrin clots.

*Posology and method of administration:* Ukidan should be reconstituted with a small amount of sterile Water for Injections or saline and then further diluted with normal saline to the desired volume for administration.

*Adults*

*(i) Thromboembolic Occlusive Vascular Disease:*

*Deep vein thrombosis:* A recommended dosage regimen consists of an initial loading dose of 4,400 IU/kg body weight in 15 ml solution, given over 10 minutes followed by an intravenous infusion of 4,400 IU/kg/hour for 12–24 hours.

*Pulmonary embolism:* A recommended dosage regimen consists of an initial loading dose of 4,400 IU/kg body weight in 15 ml solution, given over 10 minutes followed by an intravenous infusion of 4,400 IU/kg/hour for 12 hours.

Alternatively, a 50 ml bolus injection of Ukidan into the pulmonary artery, repeated for up to 3 doses, at 24 hour intervals, has been employed. The initial dosage of 15,000 IU/kg body weight may be adjusted if necessary for subsequent injections, dependent upon the plasma fibrinogen concentration produced by the previous injection.

*Peripheral vascular occlusion:* A recommended dosage regimen involves the infusion of a 2,500 IU/ml solution of Ukidan (500,000 IU in 200 ml) into the clot, using angiography to monitor the progress of treatment. Ukidan should be infused into the clot at a dose rate of 4,000 IU/minute (96 ml/hr) for 2 hours followed by repeat angiography. The catheter is then advanced into the remaining occluded segment and Ukidan infused at 4,000 IU/min for a further 2 hours; this may be repeated up to 4 times if antegrade flow has not occurred. After lysing a channel through the occlusion the catheter is withdrawn until it is proximal to the remaining clot lining the vessel wall. Ukidan is given at a dose rate of 1,000 IU/min (0.4 ml) until the clot has completely lysed. A dose of 500,000 IU given over approximately 8 hours should be sufficient to achieve this.

If the clot is not reduced in length by more than 25% after the initial infusion of 500,000 IU and by an incremental 10% by subsequent infusions of 500,000 IU, consideration should be given to discontinuation of treatment.

After fibrinolytic therapy has been completed, treatment may be continued with suitable anticoagulant therapy.

*(ii) Hyphaema:* When saline irrigation is unsuccessful in removing the blood clot, Ukidan may be considered for the management of hyphaema, particularly when the clot completely fills the anterior chamber and there is an accompanying rise in intra-ocular pressure. The following general technique is used: an incision of about 3 mm is made inside the temporal limbus of the cornea. 5,000 IU Ukidan is dissolved in Sodium Chloride Injection BP (2 ml) and drawn up into a syringe fitted with a suitable irrigator. The tip of the irrigator is introduced through the incision so as to be over the iris rather than the pupillary space (thus avoiding risk of damage to the lens), with the aperture directed towards the corneal endothelium or parallel to the plane of the iris. The solution is injected and withdrawn repeatedly with minimal pressure. Clot disintegration commonly begins within five minutes, facilitating injection of the solution and aspiration of the clot. The chamber is then washed out with saline. If residual clot remains, a small quantity of the solution (e.g. 0.3 ml) may be left in the anterior chamber to facilitate further dissolution of the clot over the next 24–48 hours.

*(iii) Clotted Arterio-Venous Shunts:* Generally, 5,000–25,000 IU Ukidan in 2–3 ml Sodium Chloride Injection BP is instilled into the affected limb of the shunt which is then clamped off for 2–4 hours. The lysate is then aspirated. This may be repeated if necessary. For the venous side an infusion of 5,000 IU in 200 ml, run in over 30 minutes, has been used but this may be less satisfactory than the use of more concentrated solutions.

*Dosage in the elderly:* Initially no dosage alterations are recommended, however, thereafter, the dosage should be adjusted as necessary, according to response.

*Dosage in children:* Initially no dosage alterations are recommended, however, thereafter, the dosage should be adjusted as necessary, according to response.

*Monitoring of treatment:* The need for haematological monitoring arises only when Ukidan is used systemically to induce a state of whole-body fibrinolysis (e.g.

in the treatment of thromboembolic occlusion). Several tests may be needed to give an overall picture of the coagulation status, because there is no simple way to measure an induced thrombolytic state.

Local use of Ukidan in 'closed situations' does not require haematological monitoring.

*Contra-indications:* Ukidan is contra-indicated in any situation where bleeding has occurred, or is likely to occur.

Recent surgery (including biopsy): administration of Ukidan for thromboembolic occlusive vascular disease is not recommended for 72 hours following surgery because of the risk of bleeding from the operation site.

Severe hypertension (with systolic bp>200 mmHg and/or diastolic bp>120 mmHg): in patients with severe hypertension, administration of Ukidan carries the risk of cerebral haemorrhage.

Ukidan is contra-indicated in pregnancy and the immediate post-partum period.

Severe hepatic or renal insufficiency.

When used in 'local' situations, the above contra-indications may not be relevant.

*Special warnings and special precautions for use:* If bleeding occurs following systemic use, the infusion should be stopped immediately. However, this contra-indication is relative. The benefits of the continued use of Ukidan must be weighed against the risks of stopping therapy, for example, in the situation where vascular occlusion can be life-threatening. For treatment of bleeding see *Overdose* section.

When used in the eye, a normal gonioscopy result should be evident.

Systemic Ukidan should be used with caution in patients with gastrointestinal lesions such as peptic ulceration, which may be prone to haemorrhage, and in patients who have had multiple intracardiac and intravascular punctures as a consequence of cardio-pulmonary resuscitation.

*Interactions with other medicaments and other forms of interaction:* In glucose solution there is a measurable (<10%) reduction in the activity of Ukidan after 8 hours.

Concomitant administration of dextran sulphate may prolong the activity of Ukidan.

*Pregnancy and lactation:* Ukidan is contra-indicated in pregnancy and the immediate post-partum period.

*Effects on ability to drive and use machines:* None known.

*Undesirable effects:* The following side-effects have been associated with Ukidan use in the listed indications.

Hyphaema – none reported;

Arterio-venous shunts – warmth, initial severe pain and dull ache in shunt limb have been reported occasionally;

Thromboembolic occlusive vascular disease – overt bleeding, haemorrhagic complications may occur;

Temporary increase in temperature (when a high yield of lysis degradation products are produced) and haematuria have been reported occasionally.

*Overdose:* If severe haemorrhage occurs, treatment with Ukidan must be stopped. Aprotinin and synthetic inhibitors such as epsilon-aminocaproic acid, tranexamic acid or p-aminomethylbenzoic acid can be used to inhibit the fibrinolytic action of Ukidan. In serious cases, human fibrinogen, Factor XIII, Cohn-Fraction I,

packed red cells or whole blood can be given, as appropriate.

**Pharmacological properties**

*Pharmacodynamic properties:* Ukidan is a preparation of urokinase, which is an enzyme extracted from human adult male urine. As Ukidan is of human origin, it is not antigenic in man.

Ukidan brings about the dissolution of blood clots by promoting the activation of plasminogen; the latter is the inactive precursor of plasmin, the proteolytic enzyme responsible for the breakdown of fibrin into small soluble peptides which are dispersible through the blood stream.

*Pharmacodynamic properties:* Following intravenous administration, urokinase is rapidly cleared from the blood. The *in vivo* half-life of urokinase activity in normal subject is about 10 to 15 minutes.

In cirrhotic patients, the elimination half-life is clearly increased up to about 30 minutes.

In subjects with kidney disease, elimination of endogenous urokinase is markedly decreased, even if the glomerular filtration rate is only moderately impaired.

The liver appears to perform an important function in the metabolism and elimination of urokinase.

The major part of urokinase activity has been found to be excreted in the bile, with peak activity achieved 35 to 60 minutes after injection and falling to unmeasureable levels after 140 to 190 minutes.

*Preclinical safety data:* Being extracted from human urine, urokinase is species-homologous and is free from inherent toxicity in man.

In animal toxicology studies, single i.v. doses up to 1 MIU/kg were not lethal and did not produce symptoms of intoxication or histological changes in any important organs. With repeated administration in increasing doses, no practical relevant toxic changes or lethal effects were observed.

**Pharmaceutical particulars** The activity of Ukidan is expressed in International Units (IU), which are approximately equivalent to one Committee on Thrombolytic Agents (CTA) unit.

*List of excipients:* Mannitol, disodium edetate, disodium hydrogen phosphate.

*Incompatibilities:* None known.

*Shelf life:* 24 months.

*Special precautions for storage:* Ukidan, in the lyophilised form, should be stored below 25°C. When reconstituted, Ukidan is stable for 24 hours when stored below 25°C.

*Nature and contents of container:* 5 ml vials of colourless neutral glass type 1. The product is packed as single vials.

*Instructions for use/handling:* The lyophilised material should be reconstituted with a small amount of saline or Water for Injections, and then further diluted with saline.

**Product licence numbers**
Ukidan 5,000 IU      3400/0001R
Ukidan 25,000 IU     3400/0026R
Ukidan 100,000 IU    3400/0027R

**Date of approval/revision of SPC** 11 July 1996.

**Legal category** POM.

*\*Trade Mark*

# Servier Laboratories Limited
Fulmer Hall
Windmill Road
Fulmer, Slough SL3 6HH

## ADIFAX*

**Qualitative and quantitative composition** Dexfenfluramine hydrochloride 15 mg.

**Pharmaceutical form** Capsule.

**Clinical particulars**

*Therapeutic indications:* Adjunctive therapy to diet, in patients with obesity and a body mass index (BMI) of 30 kg/m² or higher who have not responded to an appropriate weight-reducing regimen alone.

*Note:* a recently conducted, controlled, double-blind study lasting one year, demonstrated a two-fold increase in the number of responders at one year when Dexfenfluramine was combined with a low calorie diet in comparison with a diet alone. A 10% reduction in the initial body weight was observed in 35% and 17% of patients, respectively. Efficacy has only been demonstrated with regard to weight reduction. No significant data on change in morbidity or mortality are yet available.

*Posology and method of administration:* Oral administration.

*Adults:* 2 capsules of 15 mg daily, one capsule in the morning and one capsule in the evening, at meal time.

*Elderly:* Not recommended in absence of clinical studies in elderly.

*Children:* Contra-indicated below 12 years of age.

It is recommended that treatment should be conducted under the care of physicians experienced in the treatment of obesity.

Secondary organic causes of obesity must be excluded by diagnosis before prescribing this agent.

The management of obesity should be undertaken using a global approach, and should include dietary, medical and psychotherapeutic methods.

*Duration of treatment:* Treatment should only be continued beyond 3 months in patients who have responded to treatment as indicated by a weight loss greater than or equal to 10% of the initial weight, within 3 months of the start of treatment.

Unless weight loss is maintained, treatment should not be continued.

No data regarding efficacy of these agents are available beyond one year of treatment.

*Contra-indications:*
– Pulmonary artery hypertension.
– Current or past medical history of cardio-vascular or cerebro-vascular disease, such as myocardial infarction and stroke.
– Current or past medical history of psychiatric disorders including anorexia nervosa, and depression.
– Propensity towards drug abuse, known alcoholism.
– Children below 12 years.
– Dexfenfluramine hydrochloride produces mild mydriasis in some patients and Adifax should not be used in obese patients with glaucoma.
– No specific studies have been carried out in patients with renal or hepatic impairment and in such cases administration of Adifax should be avoided.

*Combination drug therapy with* any other centrally acting anorectic agent is contra-indicated due to the increased risk of potentially fatal pulmonary artery hypertension.

*Special warnings and precautions for use*
*Special warnings:*

Cases of severe, often fatal, pulmonary artery hypertension, have been reported in patients who have received anorectics of the type of this product. An epidemiological study has shown that dexfenfluramine intake is a risk factor involved in the development of pulmonary artery hypertension and that the use of anorectics is strongly associated with an increased risk for this adverse drug reaction. In view of this rare but serious risk, it must be emphasised that:
– careful compliance with the indication and the duration of treatment is required;
– a duration of treatment greater than 3 months and a BMI≥30 kg/m² increase the risk of pulmonary artery hypertension;
– the onset or aggravation of exertional dyspnea suggests the possibility of occurrence of pulmonary artery hypertension. Under these circumstances treatment should be immediately discontinued and the patient referred to a specialist unit for investigation.

*Special precautions for use:* Rarely, cases of cardiac and cerebro-vascular accidents have been reported, often following rapid weight loss. Special care should be taken to ensure gradual and controlled weight loss in obese patients, who are subject to a risk of vascular disease. Adifax should not be prescribed in patients with a current or a past medical history of cardiovascular or cerebro-vascular disease, such as myocardial infarction or stroke.

This anorectic agent must be used carefully in epileptic patients.

Depression has occurred in some patients after abrupt cessation of fenfluramine-containing preparations most commonly about 4 days after cessation of treatment. Therefore steady reduction of dosage of Adifax over one or more weeks is recommended.

Depression has also been reported in patients taking fenfluramine-containing preparations although clinical studies show that incidence of depression was not significantly different in patients taking Adifax compared with placebo.

*Interactions with other medicaments and other forms of interaction:* Dexfenfluramine has a specific serotonergic action and Adifax should not be used concomitantly with monoamine oxidase inhibitors (MAOIs). There should be at least a two week interval after stopping MAOIs before commencing treatment with Adifax.

Adifax should not be used concomitantly with any centrally acting appetite suppressant.

Adifax may potentiate the action of anti-hypertensive, anti-diabetic or sedative drugs and the hypotensive effect of tricyclic anti-depressive drugs.

*Pregnancy and lactation:* Use in pregnancy: animal studies with dexfenfluramine hydrochloride have shown no evidence of teratogenicity; there is, however, no clinical evidence of safety in human pregnancy and Adifax is not therefore recommended in human pregnancy unless the benefits outweigh any possible risk. Also it would not be good clinical practice to treat pregnant women with an anorectic agent.

Use in lactation: dexfenfluramine hydrochloride may be excreted in breast milk and administration of Adifax during lactation is not therefore recommended.

*Effects on ability to drive and use machines:* Adifax may cause drowsiness and dizziness. It may affect the ability to drive or operate machinery.

*Undesirable effects:* Most commonly reported undesirable effects are: dry mouth, nausea, constipation and diarrhoea, disappearing on continuing treatment. The following have been reported but more rarely:
– asthenia, headache, shivering;
– blood pressure variation, tachycardia, faintness, syncope;
– cardiovascular or cerebrovascular accident (mainly arrhythmia and stroke);
– increased transaminases and hepatitis (in exceptional cases);
– drowsiness, dizziness, vertigo, mood disturbance, sleep disorders, nervousness, confusion, agitation;
– depression;
– convulsions;
– diplopia, mydriasis, conjunctivitis;
– skin rash;
– urinary frequency;
– schizophreniform-like reactions have been reported with the racemate fenfluramine (Ponderax*) and there is some evidence that they may also occur with Adifax.

An epidemiological study has shown that dexfenfluramine intake is a risk factor involved in the development of pulmonary artery hypertension and that the use of anorectics is strongly associated with an increased risk for this adverse drug reaction. In addition there have been spontaneous reports of pulmonary artery hypertension in users of these agents. Pulmonary artery hypertension is a severe and often fatal disease. The occurrence or aggravation of exertional dyspnea is usually the first clinical sign and requires treatment discontinuation and investigation in a specialised unit (see *Special warnings*).

Withdrawal reactions including depression, irritability and dizziness have occurred following abrupt discontinuation of Adifax.

*Overdose:* The following symptoms are possible: Drowsiness, agitation, tremor or shivering, abundant sweating, mydriasis, diarrhoea, vomiting, tachycardia, hypertension.

Rarely: Bradycardia, hypotension, nystagmus, muscular cramps, confusion and hallucinations.

Actions to be taken in the event of overdosage:
(i) gastric lavage;
(ii) provoked diuresis with acidification of urine, to accelerate elimination of the drug;
(iii) intensive care, with cardiac monitoring.

(Unlike overdosage with sympathomimetic anorectic drugs, overdosage with Adifax does not necessitate routine administration of a barbiturate.)

**Pharmacological properties**

*Pharmacodynamic properties:* Adifax has been found to be effective adjunctive treatment in severe obesity associated with disorders of eating behaviour (carbohydrate craving).

Experimental studies have shown that the mode of action of dexfenfluramine hydrochloride is specifically serotonergic and that it has no psychostimulating action, no hypertensive effect and no addiction potential (dexfenfluramine hydrochloride, is not subject to control under the Misuse of Drugs Act 1971 nor under the Misuse of Drugs Regulations 1985).

*Pharmacokinetic properties:* After oral administration, the absorption is almost complete. The plasma peak is obtained in approximately 4 hours.

After repeated administration of therapeutic doses (1 capsule in the morning and 1 capsule in the evening) steady state plasma levels of 40 ng/ml are reached within 4 days. Protein binding is low (36%).

The plasma clearance of dexfenfluramine is 45 ml/hour with a half-life of approximately 18 hours. The total radioactivity is mainly eliminated after metabolism into the urine with 90% of the dose recovered in 3 to 4 days. Dexfenfluramine hydrochloride is extensively metabolised with the formation of an active metabolite, d-norfenfluramine.

*Preclinical safety data:* Not applicable.

**Pharmaceutical particulars**

*List of excipients:* Maize starch, microcrystalline cellulose, lactose, pharmaceutical industrial ethanol, purified water, colloidal silica, magnesium stearate, talc.

*Incompatibilities:* None.

*Shelf life:* 36 months.

*Special precautions for storage:* None.

*Nature and contents of container:* Push-through aluminium blister strips containing 30 capsules, enclosed in cardboard carton holding two strips.

*Instruction for use/handling:* Not applicable.

*Marketing authorisation holder:* Les Laboratoires Servier, 22 rue Garnier, 92200 Neuilly-sur-Seine, France.

**Marketing authorisation number** 5815/0003

**Date of approval/revision of SPC** 27 March 1997

**Legal category** POM

## COVERSYL TABLETS

**Qualitative and quantitative composition** Perindopril tert-butylamine salt 2 mg or 4 mg.

**Pharmaceutical form**
Coversyl 2 mg: tablet, white, biconvex.
Coversyl 4 mg: tablet, white, oblong, half-scored on one side.

**Clinical particulars**

*Therapeutic indications:*
*Hypertension:* All grades of essential hypertension and renovascular hypertension.

*Heart failure:* In congestive heart failure Coversyl should be used as an adjunctive therapy with diuretics and, where appropriate, digitalis.

As with other ACE inhibitors, treatment with Coversyl should always be initiated under close medical supervision.

*Severe heart failure:* In severe heart failure treatment with Coversyl should always be initiated in hospital under close supervision.

*Posology and method of administration:*
*Hypertension:* 2 mg once a day is the normal starting dose. Optimum control of blood pressure is achieved by increasing the dose, titrating it against the blood

pressure. The usual maintenance dose is 4 mg given once daily.

The maximum daily dose is 8 mg which may be combined with diuretic therapy. Coversyl should be taken before a meal as ingestion of food decreases conversion to perindoprilat.

*Congestive heart failure:* It is recommended that Coversyl be given with a non-potassium-sparing diuretic and/or digoxin under close medical supervision (in hospital for severe heart failure) with a recommended starting dose of 2 mg taken in the morning. The dose may, in most instances, be increased to 4 mg once daily (once blood pressure acceptability has been demonstrated).

The dose titration of Coversyl may be performed over a two- to four-week period or more rapidly if indicated by the presence of residual signs and symptoms of heart failure. As with other ACE inhibitors, blood pressure and renal function should be monitored closely both before and during treatment with Coversyl. Serum potassium should also be monitored.

In comparative studies versus placebo and other ACE inhibitors, the first administration of 2 mg of Coversyl to patients with mild to moderate heart failure was not associated with any significant reduction of blood pressure as compared to placebo.

However, some patients, other than those with severe heart failure, are considered to be at higher risk when started on an ACE-inhibitor and are recommended for initiation of therapy in hospital. Research data have shown such patients to be: those on multiple or high-dose diuretics (e.g. greater than 80 mg frusemide); patients with hypovolaemia; hyponatraemia (serum sodium less than 130 mmol/l); pre-existing hypotension (systolic blood pressure less than 90 mmHg); patients with unstable cardiac failure; renal impairment (serum creatinine greater than 150 μmol/l); those on high-dose vasodilator therapy; patients aged 70 years and over.

In order to decrease the small possibility of symptomatic hypotension, patients on previous high-dose diuretics should have the diuretic dose reduced before introducing Coversyl. The appearance of hypotension after the initial dose of Coversyl does not preclude subsequent careful dose titration with the drug, following effective treatment of the hypotension.

*Combinations with a diuretic:* Symptomatic hypotension may occur when Coversyl treatment is initiated in patients receiving diuretic treatment, in particular if diuretic treatment was begun only a short time before. It is therefore recommended to discontinue the diuretic 2–3 days before beginning treatment with Coversyl at the starting dose of 2 mg.

Addition of a diuretic potentiates the anti-hypertensive effects of Coversyl.

If co-treatment with a diuretic is thought necessary in patients on Coversyl therapy, the diuretic should be initiated at the lowest dose.

Potassium sparing diuretics should be avoided or used with extreme caution (see *Warnings*).

*Dosage in elderly or in hepatic impairment:* Since elderly patients may have renal impairment and/or other organ dysfunction, Coversyl treatment should be initiated at 2 mg daily under close supervision.

*Dosage in renal impairment and dialysis:* Perindoprilat is excreted by the kidney. Coversyl should therefore be used with caution in patients with renal impairment and the dose adjusted to the degree of renal failure. Normal medical follow-up will include frequent monitoring of potassium and creatinine. The following dosages are recommended:

| *Creatinine clearance* | *Recommended dosage* |
|---|---|
| Between 30 and 60 ml/min | 2 mg per day |
| Between 15 and 30 ml/min | 2 mg every other day |
| Less than 15 ml/min | 2 mg on the day of dialysis On days when the patients are not on dialysis the dose should be tailored to the blood pressure response. |

*Contra-indications:* Patients with a history of hypersensitivity to Coversyl. History of angioneurotic oedema associated with previous other ACE inhibitor therapy.

*Pregnancy:* Coversyl is contra-indicated in pregnancy and should not be used in women of child-bearing potential, unless protected by effective contraception. Maternal and foetal toxicity has been shown at high doses in rodents and rabbits although not in monkeys.

Neither embryotoxicity nor teratogenicity was observed. Oligohydramnios, neonatal hypotension and anuria have been reported following use of ACE inhibitors in the 2nd and 3rd trimester of pregnancy.

*Lactation period:* In animals, very little perindopril crosses into maternal milk. No data are available in humans. Coversyl should not be used in nursing mothers.

*Special warnings and precautions for use:* Renal function should be monitored before and at intervals after treatment.

*Hypotension:* Symptomatic hypotension was seen rarely in uncomplicated hypertensive patients. Symptomatic hypotension with ACE inhibitors is more likely to occur in patients who have been volume depleted by diuretics, salt restriction, dialysis, diarrhoea or vomiting.

Some patients may experience symptomatic hypotension with the first one or two doses. The occurrence of first dose hypotension does not preclude restarting Coversyl cautiously and subsequent dose titration against the blood pressure after correction of hypovolaemia and hypotension.

Exaggerated hypotensive responses may occur after the initial dose of Coversyl in patients receiving diuretic treatment. The possibilities of such occurrences are reduced by discontinuing diuretic therapy 3 days prior to initiating Coversyl.

In most instances, symptoms are relieved simply by the patient lying down, but volume repletion with oral fluids or intravenous infusion with normal saline may be required.

In some patients with congestive heart failure who have normal or low blood pressure, additional lowering of systemic blood pressure may occur with ACE inhibitors.

It has been reported mainly in patients with severe heart failure with or without associated renal insufficiency. This is more likely in patients on high doses of loop diuretics, or those with hyponatraemia or functional renal impairment.

In these patients, treatment should be started under close medical supervision, preferably in the hospital, with low doses and careful dose titration. If possible, diuretic treatment should be discontinued temporarily.

Similar considerations in terms of initiating therapy with a small dose may apply also to patients with ischaemic heart or cerebrovascular disease in whom severe hypotension could result in a myocardial infarct or cerebrovascular accident. If such hypotension becomes symptomatic, a reduction of dose or discontinuation of Coversyl may become necessary.

However, in comparative studies versus placebo and other ACE inhibitors, the first administration of 2 mg of Coversyl to patients with mild to moderate heart failure was not associated with any significant reduction of blood pressure as compared to placebo.

*Patients with renovascular hypertension:* Coversyl can be used when surgery is not indicated or prior to surgery. Renal function of patients with renovascular hypertension should be closely monitored.

*Patients with renal insufficiency:* Renal function of patients with renal failure or insufficiency should be closely monitored. Marked water and sodium depletion (salt-free diet and/or diuretic treatment) or stenosis of the renal arteries stimulate the renin-angiotensin system; blockage of the system by an ACE inhibitor, especially upon initial dosing and during the first 2 weeks of treatment, may lead to an abrupt fall in blood pressure and/or to functional and possibly acute renal failure, although the latter is uncommon and the time interval variable. Discontinuation of Coversyl or discontinuation or reduction of the diuretic may be required.

Patients haemodialysed using high-flux polyacrylonitrile ('AN69') membranes are highly likely to experience anaphylactoid reactions if they are treated with ACE inhibitors. This combination should therefore be avoided, either by use of alternative antihypertensive drugs or alternative membranes for haemodialysis.

*Angioedema:* Angioedema of the face, extremities, lips, mucous membranes, tongue, glottis and/or larynx may occur in patients treated with ACE inhibitors which especially occurs during the first weeks of treatment.

However, in rare cases severe angioedema may develop after long-term treatment with an angiotensin converting enzyme inhibitor. Treatment should promptly be discontinued and replaced by an agent belonging to another class of drugs.

Angioedema involving the tongue, glottis or larynx may be fatal. Emergency therapy should given including, but not necessarily limited to, immediate subcutaneous epinephrine solution 1:1000 (0.3 to 0.5 ml) or slow intravenous epinephrine 1 mg/ml (observe dilution instructions) with control of ECG and blood pressure. The patient should be hospitalised and observed for at least 12 to 24 hours and should not be discharged until complete resolution of symptoms has occurred.

*Cough:* During treatment with an ACE inhibitor a dry and non-productive cough may occur which disappears after discontinuation.

*Patients with liver insufficiency:* Patients with impaired liver function treated with ACE inhibitors primarily metabolised in the liver may develop markedly elevated plasma levels of the drug. Dose adaptation may be necessary, depending on the severity of the liver insufficiency and the way the ACE inhibitor is metabolised.

*Elderly:* Some elderly patients may be more responsive to an ACE inhibitor than younger patients. Administration of low initial doses and evaluation of the renal function at the beginning of the treatment is recommended.

*Children:* Coversyl is not recommended in children as paediatric use has not been studied.

*Hyperkalaemia:* Combination of potassium supplements or potassium-sparing diuretics with Coversyl is not recommended, particularly in patients with renal impairment, since this may lead to a significant increase in plasma potassium. However, if combination with these agents is necessary, caution should be exercised and plasma potassium frequently monitored.

*Surgery/anaesthesia:* In patients undergoing major surgery or during anaesthesia with agents that produce hypotension, Coversyl blocks angiotensin II formation secondary to compensatory renin release. This may lead to hypotension which can be corrected by volume expansion.

*Aortic stenosis/hypertrophic cardiomyopathy:* ACE inhibitors should be used with caution in patients with an obstruction in the outflow tract of the left ventricle.

*Neutropenia/agranulocytosis:* The risk of neutropenia appears to be dose and type-related and is dependent on patient's clinical status. It is rarely seen in uncomplicated patients but may occur in patients with some degree of renal impairment especially when it is associated with collagen vascular disease e.g. systemic lupus erythematosus, scleroderma and therapy with immunosuppressive agents. It is reversible after discontinuation of the ACE inhibitor.

*Proteinuria:* It may occur particularly in patients with existing renal function impairment or on relatively high doses of ACE inhibitors.

*Interactions with other medicaments and other forms of interaction:*

*Not recommended association*

*Potassium sparing diuretics or potassium supplements:* ACE inhibitors attenuate diuretic induced potassium loss. Potassium sparing diuretics e.g. spironolactone, triamterene, or amiloride, potassium supplements, or potassium-containing salt substitutes may lead to significant increases in serum potassium. If concomitant use is indicated because of demonstrated hypokalemia they should be used with caution and with frequent monitoring of serum potassium.

*Precaution for use*

*Diurectics:* Patients on diurectics and especially those who are volume- and/or salt depleted, may experience an excessive reduction of blood pressure after initiation of therapy with an ACE inhibitor. The possibility of hypotensive effects can be reduced by discontinuation of the diuretic, by increasing volume or salt intake prior to intake and by initiation of therapy with lower doses of the ACE inhibitor. Further increases in dosage should be with caution.

*Antidiabetic medicines:* Concomitant administration of ACE inhibitors and antidiabetic medicines (insulin, oral hypoglycaemic agents) may cause an increased blood glucose lowering effect with greater risk of hypoglycaemia. This phenomenon may be more likely to occur during the first weeks of combined treatment and in patients with renal impairment.

*Lithium:* Patients stabilised on lithium therapy who are given an ACE inhibitor concurrently may experience a rise in plasma lithium levels.

*Anaesthetic drugs:* ACE inhibition may enhance the hypotensive effects of certain anaesthetic drugs.

*Narcotic drugs/antipsychotics:* Postural hypotension may occur.

*Antihypertensive agents:* Combination with other antihypertensive agents such as beta-blockers, methyldopa, calcium antagonists or diuretics may increase the antihypertensive efficacy.

*Allopurinol, cytostatic or immunosuppressive agents, systemic corticosteroids or procainamide:* Concomitant administration with ACE inhibitors may lead to an increased risk for leucopenia.

*Take into account*

*Non-steroidal anti-inflammatory drugs:* The administration of a non-steroidal anti-inflammatory agent may reduce the antihypertensive effect of an ACE inhibitor. Furthermore, it has been described that NSAIDs and ACE inhibitors exert an additive effect on the increase in serum potassium, whereas renal function may decrease. These effects are in principle reversible, and occur especially in patients with compromised renal function.

*Antacids:* Induce decreased bioavailability of ACE inhibitors.

*Sympathomimetics:* Sympathomimetics may reduce the antihypertensive effects of ACE inhibitors:

patients should be carefully monitored to confirm that the desired effect is being obtained.

*Pregnancy and lactation:* Appropriate and well-controlled studies have not been done in humans. ACE inhibitors cross the placenta and can cause fetal and neonatal morbidity and mortality when administered to pregnant women.

Fetal exposure to ACE inhibitors during the second and third trimesters has been associated with neonatal hypotension, renal failure, face or skull deformities and/or death. Maternal oligohydramnios has also been reported reflecting decreasing renal function in the fetus. Limb contractures, craniofacial deformities, hyplastic lung development and intrauterine growth retardation have been reported in association with oligohydramnios. Infants exposed in utero to ACE inhibitors should be closely observed for hypotension; oliguria and hyperkalemia. Oliguria should be treated with support of blood pressure and renal perfusion. Intrauterine growth retardation, prematurity, patent ductus arteriorus and fetal death have also been reported but it is not clear whether they are related to the ACE inhibition or the underlying maternal disease.

It is not known whether exposure limited to the first trimester can adversely affect fetal outcome. Women who become pregnant while receiving an ACE inhibitor should be informed of the potential hazard to the fetus.

*Use during lactation:* ACE inhibitors may be excreted in breast milk and their effect on the nursing infant has not been determined. It is recommended that lactating mothers should not breast feed while taking ACE inhibitors.

*Effects on ability to drive and use machines:* There are no studies on the effects of this medicine on the ability to drive. When driving vehicles or operating machines it should be taken into account that occasionally dizziness or weariness may occur.

*Undesirable effects:*

*Cardiovascular system:* Some patients may experience hypotension, usually with the first one or two doses of Coversyl, when the dose is increased, or when a diuretic is also given (see *Posology and method of administration* and *Warnings*).

*Renal system:* Increases of plasma creatinine and urea may occur but are usually reversible. Proteinuria has been observed in some patients.

*Respiratory system:* Cough (described as dry and irritating) may sometimes be observed but is usually mild.

*Gastro-intestinal tract:* Taste impairment, epigastric discomfort, nausea and abdominal pain have been reported. Pancreatitis has been reported rarely in patients treated with ACE inhibitors; in some cases this has proved fatal.

*Skin, vessels:* Localised skin rashes, pruritus or flushing may occur. Angioneurotic oedema has been reported with Coversyl as with other ACE inhibitors.

Where swelling is confined to the face, lips and mouth, the condition will usually resolve on withdrawal of Coversyl without further treatment although antihistamines may be useful in relieving symptoms.

Where there is involvement of the tongue, glottis or larynx, likely to cause airways obstruction, subcutaneous adrenaline (0.5 ml 1:1000) should be administered promptly. The patient should be closely monitored until swelling has resolved.

*Nervous system:* Fatigue, asthenia, malaise, headache, disturbances of mood and/or sleep have been reported. Most of these effects occurred on initiating treatment and were transient.

*Drug/laboratory parameters:* Decreases in haemoglobin and red cells and in platelets have been reported in a few patients with Coversyl as with other inhibitors, but a causal relationship has not been established.

*Overdose:* To date, no case of overdosage has been reported. Signs and symptoms expected in case of overdosage would be related to hypotension and should be relieved by intravenous infusion of isotonic saline solution. Gastric lavage should be considered. Perindopril is dialysable (70 ml/min).

### Pharmacological properties

*Pharmacodynamic properties:* Perindopril is an inhibitor of the enzyme which converts angiotensin I into angiotensin II (ACE inhibitor).

The converting enzyme of Kininase is an exopeptidase which converts angiotensin I into vasoconstrictive angiotensin II and degrades vasodilatory bradykinin into an inactive heptapeptide. Perindopril acts through its active metabolite, perindoprilat, the other metabolites being inactive.

*Systemic hypertension:* Efficacy is sustained throughout the 24 hour cycle. Maximum antihypertensive effect is reached 4 to 6 hours after a single perindopril dose.

The decrease in blood pressure is rapidly achieved; in responding patients, normalisation is achieved within 1 month and is sustained.

Discontinuation of treatment does not lead to a rebound effect.

In man, perindopril has been confirmed to demonstrate vasodilatory properties, to restore elastic properties of the arterial blood vessels and to decrease left ventricular hypertrophy.

*Pharmacokinetic properties:* After oral administration, perindopril is rapidly (peak concentration within 1 hour) and extensively (bioavailability: 65 to 70%) absorbed.

Perindopril is converted into perindoprilat, the active metabolite. The plasma half-life of perindopril is equal to 1 hour. The rate of bioconversion into perindoprilat is approximately 20%. The peak plasma concentration of perindoprilat is achieved within 3 to 4 hours.

Ingestion of food decreases conversion to perindoprilat, hence bioavailability.

The volume of distribution is approximately 0.2 l/kg for unbound perindoprilat. The drug is not extensively bound to protein, the bound fraction is less than 30%, but binding is concentration dependent.

In addition to active perindoprilat, perindopril yields 5 metabolites, all inactive. Perindoprilat is eliminated in the urine, and the half-life of its unbound fraction varies between 3 and 5 hours. Dissociation of the perindoprilat-angiotensin converting enzyme bond yields an 'effective' elimination half-life of 25 hours.

No accumulation of perindopril is observed after repeated administration and the half-life of perindoprilat after repeated administration is equivalent to its active half-life, leading to a state of equilibrium within 4 days.

Elimination of perindopril is slowed in the elderly, and in patients with heart and renal failure. Dosage adjustment is desirable depending on the decrease in creatinine clearance.

Dialysis clearance of perindopril is equal to 70 ml/min.

*Preclinical safety date:* The target organ is the kidney. In rat, administration of perindopril induces arterial anatomical changes which lead to intra-renal haemodynamic changes and to increase in plasma creatinine levels, these effects being reversible when the treatment is stopped.

### Pharmaceutical particulars

*List of excipients:* Microcrystalline cellulose, lactose, hydrophobic colloidal silica, magnesium stearate.

*Incompatibilities:* Not applicable.

*Shelf life:* 2 years.

*Special precautions for storage:* Store below 25°C.

*Nature and contents of container:* PVC aluminium blister strip of 30 tablets packaged in carton box.

*Instruction for use/handling:* Not applicable.

*Marketing authorisation holder:* Les Laboratoires Servier, 22 rue Garnier, 92200 Neuilly-sur-Seine, France.

**Marketing authorisation numbers**
Coversyl 2 mg tablet        5815/0001
Coversyl 4 mg tablet        5815/0002

**Date of approval/revision of SPC**    27 March 1997.

**Legal category**    POM

## DIAMICRON*

**Presentation**    *Diamicron tablets:* White, circular, flat compressed tablets with flat bevelled edges and a cross on one face, each containing 80 mg gliclazide. Gliclazide is 1-(3-azabicyclo (3,3,0) oct-3-yl)-3-(p-tolyl-sulphonyl) urea.

**Uses**
*Indication:* For the treatment of maturity onset diabetes mellitus.

*Mode of action:* Gliclazide is a hypoglycaemic sulphonylurea differing from other related compounds by the addition of an azabicyclo octane ring. The drug is well absorbed and its half-life in man is approximately 10–12 hours. Gliclazide is metabolised in the liver; less than 5% of the dose is excreted unchanged in the urine.

In man, apart from having a similar hypoglycaemic effect to the other sulphonylureas, gliclazide has been shown to reduce platelet adhesiveness and aggregation and increase fibrinolytic activity. These factors are thought to be implicated in the pathogenesis of long term complications of diabetes mellitus.

Gliclazide primarily enhances the first phase of insulin secretion, but also to a lesser degree its second phase. Both phases are diminished in non-insulin dependent diabetes mellitus.

**Dosage and administration**    *Adults:* The total daily dose may vary from 40 to 320 mg taken orally. The dose should be adjusted according to the individual patient's response, commencing with 40–80 mg daily ($\frac{1}{2}$–1 tablet) and increasing until adequate control is achieved. A single dose should not exceed 160 mg (2 tablets). When higher doses are required, Diamicron should be taken twice daily and according to the main meals of the day.

In obese patients or those not showing adequate response to Diamicron alone, additional therapy may be required.

*Elderly:* Plasma clearance of gliclazide is not altered in the elderly and steady state plasma levels can therefore be expected to be similar to those in adults under 65 years. Clinical experience in the elderly to date shows that Diamicron is effective and well tolerated. Care should be exercised, however, when prescribing sulphonylureas in the elderly due to a possible age-related increased risk of hypoglycaemia.

*Children:* Diamicron, as with other sulphonylureas, is not indicated for the treatment of juvenile onset diabetes mellitus.

*Route of administration:* Oral.

**Contra-indications, warnings, etc**
*Contra-Indications:* Diamicron should not be used in:
Juvenile onset diabetes.
Diabetes complicated by ketosis and acidosis.
Pregnancy.
Diabetics undergoing surgery, after severe trauma or during infections.
Patients known to have hypersensitivity to other sulphonylureas and related drugs.
Diabetic pre-coma and coma.
Severe renal or hepatic insufficiency.

*Precautions and warnings:* Care should be exercised in patients with hepatic and/or renal impairment and a small starting dose should be used with careful patient monitoring. As with other sulphonylureas, hypoglycaemia will occur if the patient's dietary intake is reduced or if they are receiving a larger dose of Diamicron than required.

*Interactions with other medicaments:* Care should be taken when giving Diamicron with drugs which are known to alter the diabetic state or potentiate the drug's action. The hypoglycaemic effect of Diamicron may be potentiated by phenylbutazone, salicylates, sulphonamides, coumarin derivatives, MAOIs, beta adrenergic blocking agents, tetracycline compounds, chloramphenicol, clofibrate, disopyramide, miconazole (oral forms) and cimetidine.

It may be diminished by corticosteroids, oral contraceptives, thiazide diuretics, phenothiazine derivatives, thyroid hormones and abuse of laxatives.

*Use in pregnancy and lactation:*
*Pregnancy:* See 'Contra-indications'.
*Nursing mothers:* It has not yet been established whether gliclazide is transferred to human milk. However, other sulphonylureas have been found in milk and there is no evidence to suggest that gliclazide differs from the group in this respect.

*Effects on ability to drive and use machines:* Patients should be informed that their concentration may be affected if their diabetes is not satisfactorily controlled, especially at the beginning of treatment (see other special warnings and precautions).

*Other special warnings and precautions:* Hypoglycaemia: all sulphonylureas drugs are capable of producing moderate or severe hypoglycaemia, particularly in the following conditions:
– in patients controlled by diet alone;
– in cases of accidental overdose;
– when calorie or glucose intake is deficient;
– in patients with hepatic and/or renal impairment, however, in long-term clinical trials, patients with renal insufficiency have been treated satisfactorily, using Diamicron at reduced doses.

In order to reduce the risk of hypoglycaemia it is therefore recommended:
– to initiate treatment for non-insulin dependent diabetics by diet alone, if this is possible;
– to take into account the age of the patient: blood sugar levels not strictly controlled by diet alone might be acceptable in the elderly;
– to adjust the dose of Diamicron according to the blood glucose response and to the 24 hour urinary glucose during the first days of treatment.
Dosage adjustments may be necessary:
– on the occurrence of mild symptoms of hypoglycaemia (sweating, pallor, hunger pangs, tachycardia sensation of malaise. Such findings should be treated with oral glucose and adjustments made in drug dosage and/or meal patterns;
– on the occurrence of severe hypoglycaemic reactions (coma or neurological impairment, see over dose);
– loss of control of blood glucose (hyperglycaemia). When a patient stabilised on any diabetic regimen is exposed to stress such as fever, trauma, infection or surgery, a loss of control may occur. At such times, it may be necessary to progressively increase the dosage of Diamicron and if this is insufficient, to discontinue the treatment with Diamicron and to administer insulin.

*Incompatibilities (major):* None stated.

*Other undesirable effects:* Hypoglycaemia (see other special warnings and precautions).

Abnormalities of hepatic function are not uncommon during gliclazide therapy. There are rare reports of hepatic failure, hepatitis, and jaundice following treatment with gliclazide.

Mild gastro-intestinal disturbances including nausea, dyspepsia, diarrhoea and constipation have been reported, but this type of adverse reaction can be avoided if Diamicron is taken during a meal.

Skin reactions including rash, pruritus, erythema, bullous eruption; blood dyscrasia including anaemia, leucopaenia, thrombocytopaenia and granulocytopaenia have been observed during treatment with Diamicron but are not known to be directly attributable to the drug.

*Overdosage:* The symptom to be expected with an overdose would be hypoglycaemia. The treatment is gastric lavage and correction of the hypoglycaemia by appropriate means with continued monitoring of the patient's blood sugar until the effect of the drug has ceased.

**Pharmaceutical precautions** Nil.

**Legal category** POM.

**Package quantities** Cartons of 60 tablets (containing three push-through blister strips of 20 tablets). OP.

**Further information** Nil.

**Product licence number** 0093/0024.

## LOCABIOTAL*

**Qualitative and quantitative composition** Fusafungine 0.25%. Each metered-dose contains 125 microgrammes fusafungine.

**Pharmaceutical form** Aerosol (metered-dose inhaler).

**Clinical particulars**

*Therapeutic indications:* A topical antibiotic with anti-inflammatory properties for the treatment of infections and inflammatory conditions of the upper respiratory tract.

*Posology and method of administration:* Administration by inhalation (via mouth or nose).

*Duration of treatment:* Depending on severity, one week to ten days, under medical supervision. Should there be no relief of symptoms and signs in one week, alternative treatment should be considered.

| Adults: | Nasal: 3 metered doses in each nostril 5 times a day |
|---|---|
| | Oral: 5 metered doses 5 times a day |

| | No. of metered doses | | |
|---|---|---|---|
| Children: | 3–5 years | 6–12 years | >12 years |
| Nasal (in each nostril 5 times a day) | 1 | 2 | 3 |
| Oral (3 times a day) | 2 | 3 | 4 |

*Contra-indications:* Sensitivity to fusafungine or excipients.

*Special warnings and precautions for use:* Use with caution in patients with allergic tendencies. Prolonged use may encourage superinfection. Avoid directing the spray towards the eyes as the aerosol can cause irritation. If symptoms and signs do not improve in one week, alternative therapy should be considered.

*Interactions with other medicaments and other forms of interactions:* There have been no documented reports of any interactions with fusafungine used topically. In particular no interactions have been reported with systemic antibiotics.

*Pregnancy and lactation:* There are no reports of safety of fusafungine in pregnancy or lactation. In general, fusafungine should be used in these conditions only when benefits clearly exceed potential unknown risks.

*Effects on ability to drive and use machines:* No evidence of any adverse effect on mental alertness.

*Undesirable effects:* Side-effects observed are mainly local reactions including coughing, sneezing, dryness of nose or throat, unpleasant taste in mouth and eye congestion. Very rarely, general reactions have been observed, particularly in patients with allergic tendencies. These include cutaneous allergy, attacks of asthma, urticaria and nausea.

*Overdose:* There are no reports of any overdosage and the management should be symptomatic and supportive.

**Pharmacological properties**

*Pharmacodynamic properties:* Fusafungine is a topical antibiotic produced by Fusanium Luteritium strain 347, with anti-inflammatory properties. It is bacteriostatic.

*Pharmacokinetic properties:* Topical use. No systemic absorption of fusafungine has been shown.

*Preclinical safety data:* No findings in the preclinical testing which could be of relevance for the prescriber.

**Pharmaceutical particulars**

*List of excipients:* Saccharin, eucalyptol, pure alcohol, flavouring substance, dichlorofluoromethane, isopropyl myrustate.

*Incompatibilities:* None known.

*Shelf life:* 3 years.

*Special precautions of storage:* Store at room temperature.

*Nature and contents of container:* Pressurised aerosol into an aluminium canister sealed with a metered-dose plastic valve.

*Instructions for use/handling:*

*(i) Via the nose* – The nose-adaptor will already be attached to the aerosol ready for use.

Clean the nose and place the yellow tip in the nostril.

Hold the container as shown in pack leaflet and press finger and thumb firmly to release one pre-measured dose.

Repeat according to prescription.

*(ii) Via the mouth* – Remove the yellow nose adaptor. Fix on white mouth adaptor as shown.

Place the white adaptor well into the mouth and close lips firmly.

Hold the container as shown in pack leaflet and press finger and thumb firmly to release one pre-measured dose.

Breathe in lightly as dose is released.

Repeat according to prescription.

**Marketing authorisation number** 0093/5003R

**Date of approval/revision of SPC** 7 November 1996

**Legal category** POM

## NATRILIX*

**Presentation** White film coated lenticular tablets each containing 2.5 mg indapamide hemihydrate.

**Uses** For the treatment of essential hypertension. Natrilix may be used as sole therapy or combined with other antihypertensive agents.

*Mode of action:* Natrilix (indapamide) is a non-thiazide sulphonamide with an indole ring, belonging to the diuretic family. At the dose of 2.5 mg per day Natrilix exerts a prolonged antihypertensive activity in hypertensive human subjects.

Dose-effects studies have demonstrated that, at the dose of 2.5 mg per day, the antihypertensive effect is maximal and the diuretic effect is sub-clinical.

At this antihypertensive dose of 2.5 mg per day, Natrilix reduces vascular hyperreactivity to noradrenaline in hypertensive patients and decreases total peripheral resistance and arteriolar resistance.

The implication of an extrarenal mechanism of action in the antihypertensive effect is demonstrated by maintenance of its antihypertensive efficacy in functionally anephric hypertensive patients.

The vascular mechanism of action of Natrilix involves:
– a reduction in the contractility of vascular smooth muscle due to a modification of transmembrane ion exchanges, essentially calcium;
– vasodilatation due to stimulation of the synthesis of prostaglandin PGE 2 and the vasodilator and platelet antiaggregant prostacyclin PGI2;
– potentiation of the vasodilator action of bradykinin.

**Dosage and administration**

*Adults:* The dosage is one tablet, containing 2.5 mg indapamide hemihydrate, daily, to be taken in the morning. The action of Natrilix is progressive and the reduction in blood pressure may continue and not reach a maximum until several months after the start of therapy. A larger dose than 2.5 mg Natrilix is not recommended as there is no appreciable additional antihypertensive effect but a diuretic effect may become apparent. It has been demonstrated that in the short-, medium- and long-term, in hypertensive patients, Natrilix:
– reduces left ventricular hypertrophy;
– does not appear to alter lipid metabolism: triglycerides, LDL-cholesterol and HDL-cholesterol;
– does not appear to alter glucose metabolism, even in diabetic hypertensive patients. Normalisation of blood pressure and a significant reduction in microalbuminuria have been observed after prolonged administration of Natrilix in diabetic hypertensive subjects.

The co-prescription of Natrilix with other antihypertensives (beta-blockers, calcium channel blockers, angiotensin converting enzyme inhibitors) results in an improved control of hypertension with an increased percentage of responders compared to that observed with single-agent therapy.

The co-administration of Natrilix with diuretics which may cause hypokalaemia is not recommended. There is no evidence of rebound hypertension on withdrawal of Natrilix.

*Elderly:* There are no significant changes in the pharmacokinetics of Natrilix in the elderly. Numerous clinical studies have shown that it can be used without problems and indeed has a particular benefit on systolic blood pressure in the elderly.

*Children:* There is no experience of the use of this drug in children.

*Route of administration:* Oral.

**Contra-indications, warnings, etc**

*Contra-indications:* Natrilix is not recommended in patients with recent cerebrovascular accident, severe hepatic failure or a known history of allergy to sulphonamide derivatives.

*Precautions and warnings:* Studies in functionally anephric patients for one month undergoing chronic haemodialysis, have not shown evidence of drug accumulation despite the fact that Natrilix is not dialysable.

Although Natrilix 2.5 mg daily (one tablet) can be safely administered to hypertensive patients with impaired renal function, the treatment should be discontinued if there are signs of increasing renal insufficiency.

*Interactions with other medicaments:* The concomitant administration of the following medicaments with Natrilix is not recommended:
– Diuretics (risk of electrolyte imbalance);
– Antiarrhythmics such as quinidine derivatives, cardiac glycosides, corticoids or laxatives, in case of hypokalaemia;
– Lithium (increase in blood levels due to a diminished urinary excretion of lithium).

*Use in pregnancy and lactation:* Pregnancy: no teratological effects have been seen in animals but because animal reproduction studies are not always predictive of human response, Natrilix should be used during pregnancy only if clearly needed.

Nursing mothers: It is not known if Natrilix is excreted in human milk. Because most drugs are excreted in human milk, if use of Natrilix is deemed essential, the patient should stop nursing.

*Effects on ability to drive and use machines:* No evidence of any adverse effect on mental alertness.

*Other special warnings and precautions:* Blood potassium and urate levels should be closely monitored:
– in patients predisposed or sensitive to hypokalaemia (cardiac patients treated with glycosides, elderly, or patients suffering from hyperaldosteronism);
– in patients suffering from gout.

In case of an aggravation of pre-existing renal insufficiency, it is recommended to interrupt the treatment with Natrilix.

In patients with hyperparathyroidism, the treatment with Natrilix should be interrupted on the occurrence of hypercalcaemia.

*Incompatibilities (major):* None stated.

*Other undesirable effects:* Hypokalaemia, headache, dizziness, fatigue, muscular cramps, nausea, anorexia, diarrhoea, constipation, dyspepsia and cutaneous rash may occur as a result of treatment with Natrilix. There have been some rare reports of orthostatic hypotension, palpitations, increase in liver enzymes, blood dyscrasias including thrombocytopaenia, hyponatraemia, metabolic alkalosis, hyperglycaemia, increase in blood urate levels, paraesthesia, erythema multiforme, epidermal necrolysis, photosensitivity, impotence, renal insufficiency and reversible acute myopia.

*Overdosage:* Symptoms of overdosage would be those associated with a diuretic effect: electrolyte disturbances, hypotension and muscular weakness. Treatment would be symptomatic, directed at correcting the electrolyte abnormalities and gastric lavage or emesis should be considered.

**Pharmaceutical precautions** Nil.

**Legal category** POM.

**Package quantities** Cartons of 30 and 60 tablets (containing respectively 2 and 3 push-through blister strips of 15 and 20 tablets).

**Further information** Nil.

**Product licence number** 0093/0022.

## NATRILIX SR*

**Qualitative and quantitative composition** Indapamide 1.5 mg.

**Pharmaceutical form** Sustained release coated tablet.

**Clinical particulars**

*Therapeutic indications:* Essential hypertension.

*Posology and method of administration:* Oral administration.

One tablet per 24 hours, preferably in the morning. At higher doses the antihypertensive action of indapamide is not enhanced but the saluretic effect is increased.

*Contra-indications:* Hypersensitivity to sulphonamides.

Severe renal failure.

Hepatic encephalopathy or severe impairment of liver function.

Hypokalaemia.

*Special warnings and special precautions for use:* *Warnings:* When liver function is impaired, thiazide-related diuretics may cause hepatic encephalopathy. Administration of the diuretic must be stopped immediately if this occurs.

*Precautions:*

*Water and electrolyte balance: Plasma sodium:* This must be measured before starting treatment, then at regular intervals subsequently. Any diuretic treatment may cause hyponatraemia, sometimes with very serious consequences. The fall in plasma sodium may be asymptomatic initially and regular monitoring is therefore essential, and should be even more frequent in the elderly and cirrhotic patients (see *Adverse reactions* and *Overdose* sections).

*Plasma potassium:* Potassium depletion with hypokalaemia is the major risk of thiazide and related diuretics. The risk of onset of hypokalaemia (<3.4 mmol/l) must be prevented in certain high risk populations, i.e. the elderly, malnourished and/or polymedicated, cirrhotic patients with oedema and ascites, coronary artery disease and cardiac failure patients. In this latter situation, hypokalaemia increases the cardiac toxicity of digitalis preparations and the risks of arrhythmias.

Individuals with a long QT interval are also at risk, whether the origin is congenital or iatrogenic. Hypokalaemia, as well as bradycardia, is then a predisposing factor to the onset of severe arrhythmias, in particular, potentially fatal torsades de pointes.

More frequent monitoring of plasma potassium is required in all the situations indicated above. The first measurement of plasma potassium should be obtained during the first week following the start of treatment. Detection of hypokalaemia requires its correction.

*Plasma calcium:* Thiazide and related diuretics may decrease urinary calcium excretion and cause a slight and transitory rise in plasma calcium. Frank hypercalcaemia may be due to previously unrecognised hyperparathyroidism. Treatment should be withdrawn before the investigation of parathyroid function.

*Blood glucose:* Monitoring of blood glucose is important in diabetics, in particular in the presence of hypokalaemia.

*Uric acid:* Tendency to gout attacks may be increased in hyperuricaemic patients.

*Renal function and diuretics:* Thiazide and related diuretics are fully effective only when renal function is normal or only minimally impaired (plasma creatinine below levels of the order of 25 mg/l, i.e. 220 µmol/l in an adult). In the elderly, this plasma creatinine must be adjusted in relation to age, weight and gender.

Hypovolaemia, secondary to the loss of water and sodium induced by the diuretic at the start of treatment causes a reduction in glomerular filtration. This may lead to an increase in blood urea and plasma creatinine. This transitory functional renal insufficiency is of no consequence in individuals with normal renal function but may worsen preexisting renal insufficiency.

*Athletes:* The attention of athletes is drawn to the fact that this drug contains an active ingredient which may give a positive reaction in doping tests.

*Interactions with other drugs and other types of interactions*

*Inadvisable combinations*

*Lithium:* Increased plasma lithium with signs of overdose, as with a salt-free diet (decreased urinary lithium excretion). However, if the use of diuretics is necessary, careful monitoring of plasma lithium and dose adjustment are required.

*Non-antiarrhythmic drugs prolonging the QT interval or causing torsade de pointes (astemizol, bepridil, IV-erythromycin, halofantrine, pentamidine, sultopride, terfenadine, vincamine):* Torsade de pointes (hypokalaemia is a predisposing factor, the same applying to bradycardia and a preexisting long QT interval). Use substances which do not have the disadvantage of causing torsade de pointes in the presence of hypokalaemia.

*Combinations requiring precautions*

*NSAIDs (systemic), high dose salicylates:* Possible decrease in antihypertensive effect of indapamide. Acute renal failure in dehydrated patients (decreased glomerular filtration). Hydrate the patient; monitor renal function at the start of treatment.

*Other compounds causing hypokalaemia: amphotericin B (IV), gluco- and mineralocorticoids (systemic), tetracosactide, stimulant laxatives:* Increased risk of hypokalaemia (additive effect). Monitoring of plasma potassium and correction if required. Must be particularly borne in mind in case of concomitant digitalis treatment. Use non-stimulant laxatives.

*Baclofen:* Increased antihypertensive effect. Hydrate the patient; monitor renal function at the start of treatment.

*Digitalis preparations:* Hypokalaemia predisposing to the toxic effects of digitalis. Monitoring of plasma potassium, ECG and, if necessary, adjust treatment.

*Combinations which must be taken into consideration*

*Potassium-sparing diuretics (amiloride, spironolactone, triamterene):* Such rational combinations, useful in certain patients, do not eliminate the possibility of hypokalaemia or, in particular in renal failure and diabetic patients, of hyperkalaemia. Monitor plasma potassium, ECG if required and adjust treatment if necessary.

*Angiotensin converting enzyme (ACE) inhibitors:* Risk of sudden hypotension and/or acute renal failure when treatment with a converting enzyme inhibitor is started in the presence of preexisting sodium depletion (in particular in individuals with renal artery stenosis).

*In hypertension,* when prior diuretic treatment may have caused sodium depletion, it is necessary:

- either to stop the diuretic 3 days before starting treatment with the ACE inhibitor, and restart a hypokalaemic diuretic if necessary;
- or give low initial doses of the ACE inhibitor and increase only gradually.

*In congestive cardiac failure,* start with a very low dose of ACE inhibitor, possibly after a reduction in the dose of the combined hypokalaemic diuretic.

*In all cases,* monitor renal function (plasma creatinine) during the first weeks of treatment with an ACE inhibitor.

*Antiarrhythmic agents causing torsade de pointes: Group Ia antiarrhythmic drugs (quinidine, hydroquinidine, disopyramide), amiodarone, bretylium, sotalol:* Torsade de pointes (hypokalaemia is a predisposing factor, the same applying to bradycardia and a preexisting long QT interval). Prevention of hypokalaemia and, if necessary, correction; monitoring of QT interval. In cases of torsade de pointes, do not give antiarrhythmic drugs (management by pacemaker).

*Metformin:* In the presence of functional renal insufficiency related to diuretics and more particularly to loop diuretics, increased risk of metformin induced lactic acidosis.

Do not use metformin when plasma creatinine exceeds 15 mg/litre (135 µmol/litre) in men and 12 mg/litre (110 µmol/litre) in women.

*Iodinated contrast media:* In the presence of dehydration caused by diuretics, increased risk of acute renal failure, in particular when large doses of iodinated contrast media are used.

Rehydration before administration of the iodinated compound.

*Combinations which must be taken into consideration*

*Imipramine-like antidepressants (tricyclics), neuroleptics:* Antihypertensive effect and risk of orthostatic hypotension increased (additive effect).

*Calcium salts:* Risk of hypercalcaemia resulting from decreased urinary calcium elimination.

*Cyclosporin:* Risk of increased plasma creatinine without any change in circulating cyclosporin levels, even in the absence of water/sodium depletion.

*Corticosteroids, tetracosactide (systemic):* Decreased antihypertensive effect (water/sodium retention due to corticosteroids).

*Pregnancy and lactation*

*Pregnancy:* As a general rule, the administration of diuretics should be avoided in pregnant women and should never be used to treat physiological oedema of pregnancy. Diurectics can cause fetoplacental ischaemia, with a risk of impaired fetal growth.

*Breast-feeding:* Breast-feeding is inadvisable (Indapamide is excreted in human milk).

*Effects on ability to drive and use machines:* Natrilix SR does not affect vigilance but different reactions in relation to the decrease in blood pressure may occur in individual cases, especially at the start of the treatment or when another antihypertensive agent is added. As a result the ability to drive vehicles or to operate machinery may be impaired.

*Undesirable effects:* The majority of adverse effects concerning clinical or laboratory parameters are dose-dependent. Thiazide-related diuretics, including indapamide, may cause:

*Regarding laboratory parameters:* Potassium depletion with hypokalaemia, particularly serious in certain high risk populations (see *Precautions*). During clinical trials, hypokalaemia (plasma potassium ≤3.4 mmol/l) was seen in 10% of patients and <3.2 mmol/l in 4% of patients after 4 to 6 weeks' treatment. After 12 weeks' treatment, the mean fall in plasma potassium was 0.23 mmol/l.

Hyponatraemia with hypovolaemia responsible for dehydration and orthostatic hypotension. Concomitant loss of chloride ions may lead to secondary compensatory metabolic alkalosis: the incidence and degree of this effect are slight.

An increase in plasma uric acid and blood glucose during treatment: appropriateness of these diuretics must be very carefully weighed in patients with gout or diabetes.

Haematological events, very rare: thrombocytopenia, leucopenia, agranulocytosis, aplastic anaemia, haemolytic anaemia.

Hypercalcaemia – extremely rare.

*Regarding clinical parameters:* In the presence of hepatic insufficiency, possible onset of hepatic encephalopathy (see *Contra-indications* and *Warnings*).

Hypersensitivity reactions, essentially dermatological, in individuals predisposed to allergic and asthmatic manifestations.

Maculopapular rashes, purpura, possible worsening of preexisting acute disseminated lupus erythematosis.

Nausea, constipation, dry mouth, vertigo, fatigue, paraesthesia, headache, occurring rarely and responding in most instances to a dose reduction.

Very rarely, pancreatitis.

*Overdose:* Indapamide has been found to be free of toxicity at up to 40 mg, i.e. 27 times the therapeutic dose.

Signs of acute poisoning take the form above all of water/electrolyte disturbances (hyponatraemia, hypokalaemia). Clinically, possibility of nausea, vomiting, hypotension, cramps, vertigo, drowsiness, confusion, polyuria or oliguria possibly to the point of anuria (by hypovolaemia). Initial measures involve the rapid elimination of the ingested substance(s) by gastric wash-out and/or administration of activated charcoal, followed by restoration of water/electrolyte balance to normal in a specialised centre.

**Pharmacological properties**

*Pharmacodynamic properties:* Antihypertensive diuretic. Indapamide is a sulphonamide derivative with an indole ring, pharmacologically related to thiazide diuretics, which acts by inhibiting the reabsorption of sodium in the proximal segment of the distal renal tubule. It increases the urinary excretion of sodium and chlorides and, to a lesser extent, the excretion of potassium and magnesium, thereby increasing urine output and having an antihypertensive action.

Phase II and III studies using monotherapy have demonstrated an antihypertensive effect lasting 24 hours. This was present at doses where the diuretic effect was of mild intensity.

The antihypertensive activity of indapamide is related to an improvement in arterial compliance and a reduction in arteriolar and total peripheral resistance. Indapamide reduces left ventricular hypertrophy.

Thiazide and related diuretics have a plateau therapeutic effect beyond a certain dose, while adverse effects continue to increase. The dose should not be increased if treatment is ineffective.

It has also been shown, in the short, mid and long term in hypertensive patients, that indapamide:

- does not interfere with lipid metabolism: tryglycerides, LDL-cholesterol and HDL-cholesterol;
- does not interfere with carbohydrate metabolism, even in diabetic hypertensive patients.

*Pharmacokinetic properties:* Indapamide 1.5 mg is supplied in a sustained release dosage based on a matrix system in which the active ingredient is dispersed in a support which allows sustained release of indapamide.

*Absorption:* The fraction of indapamide released is rapidly and totally absorbed via the gastrointestinal digestive tract.

Eating slightly increases the rapidity of absorption but has no influence on the amount of the drug absorbed.

Peak serum level following a single dose occurs about 12 hours after ingestion, repeated administration reduces the variation in serum levels between 2 doses.

Intra-individual variability exists.

*Distribution:* Binding of indapamide to plasma proteins is 79%. The plasma elimination half-life is 14 to 24 hours (mean 18 hours). Steady state is achieved after 7 days. Repeated administration does not lead to accumulation.

*Metabolism:* Elimination is essentially urinary (70% of the dose) and faecal (22%) in the form of inactive metabolites.

*High risk individuals:* Pharmacokinetic parameters are unchanged in renal failure patients.

*Preclinical safety data:* The highest doses administered orally to different animal species (40 to 8000 times the therapeutic dose) have shown an exacerbation of the saluretic properties of indapamide. The major symptoms of poisoning in acute toxicity studies with indapamide administered intravenously or intraperitoneally were related to the pharmacological action of indapamide, i.e. bradypnoea and peripheral vasodilation.

**Pharmaceutical particulars**

*List of excipients:* Anhydrous colloidal silica, glycerol, hydroxypropylmethylcellulose, lactose, macrogol 6000, magnesium stearate, polyvidone, titanium dioxide.

*Incompatibilities:* Not applicable.

*Shelf life:* 2 years.

*Special precautions for storage:* Store in a dry place at room temperature (15–25°C).

*Nature and contents of container:* Blister sheet (PVC/Aluminium).

*Instructions for use/handling:* Not applicable.

*Marketing authorisation holder:* Les Laboratoires Servier, 905, route de Saran, 45520 Gidy, France.

**Marketing authorisation number** 05815/0010

**Date of approval/revision of SPC** January 1996

**Legal category** POM

## PONDERAX PACAPS*

**Qualitative and quantitative composition** Fenfluramine Hydrochloride BP 60 mg per capsule.

**Pharmaceutical form** Capsule.

Prolonged action formulation in hard gelatine capsule with clear body and opaque blue cap printed in black with Px PA 60 containing small white pellets. Each prolonged action capsule contains 60 mg Fenfluramine Hydrochloride BP.

**Clinical particulars**

*Therapeutic indications:* Adjunctive therapy to diet, in patients with obesity and a body mass index (BMI) of 30 kg/m² or higher who have not responded to an appropriate weight-reducing regimen alone.

*Note:* a recently conducted, controlled, double-blind study lasting one year, demonstrated a two-fold increase in the number of responders at one year when dexfenfluramine (dextro rotatory enantiomer of fenfluramine) was combined with a low calorie diet in comparison with a diet alone. A 10% reduction in the initial body weight was observed in 35% and 17% of patients, respectively. Efficacy has only been demonstrated with regard to weight reduction. No significant data on change in morbidity or mortality are yet available.

*Posology and method of administration:* Oral administration.

*Adults:* One 60 mg capsule daily. Treatment with Ponderax Pacaps should not be stopped suddenly.

Steady reduction of dosage over one or more weeks, e.g. one capsule every other day, is recommended to avoid the possibility of precipitating depression which occasionally has been severe. If possible, capsules should be taken half an hour before food.

*Elderly:* Care should be taken when prescribing for patients over 65 years of age because drowsiness is more likely to occur.

*Children:* Contra-indicated below 12 years of age.

It is recommended that treatment should be conducted under the care of physicians experienced in the treatment of obesity.

Secondary organic causes of obesity must be excluded by diagnosis before prescribing this agent.

The management of obesity should be undertaken using a global approach, and should include dietary, medical and psychotherapeutic methods.

*Duration of treatment:* Treatment should only be continued beyond 3 months in patients who have responded to treatment as indicated by a weight loss greater than or equal to 10% of the initial weight, within 3 months of the start of treatment. Unless weight loss is maintained, treatment should not be continued. No data regarding efficacy of these agents are available beyond one year of treatment.

*Contra-indications:*
– Pulmonary artery hypertension.
– Current or past medical history of cardio-vascular or cerebro-vascular disease, such as myocardial infarction and stroke.
– Current or past medical history of psychiatric disorders including anorexia nervosa, and depression.
– Propensity towards drug abuse, known alcoholism.
– Children below 12 years.

*Combination drug therapy with* any other centrally acting anoretic agent is contra-indicated due to the increased risk of potentially fatal pulmonary artery hypertension.

*Special warnings and precautions for use:*
*Special warnings:*

> Cases of severe, often fatal, pulmonary artery hypertension, have been reported in patients who have received anorectics of the type of this product. An epidemiological study has shown that fenfluramine intake is a risk factor involved in the development of pulmonary artery hypertension and that the use of anorectics is strongly associated with an increased risk for this adverse drug reaction. In view of this rare but serious risk, it must be emphasised that:
> – careful compliance with the indication and the duration of treatment is required;
> – a duration of treatment greater than 3 months and a BMI≥30 kg/m² increase the risk of pulmonary artery hypertension;
> – the onset or aggravation of exertional dyspnea suggests the possibility of occurrence of pulmonary artery hypertension. Under these circumstances treatment should be immediately discontinued and the patient referred to a specialist unit for investigation.

*Special precautions for use:* Rarely, cases of cardiac and cerebro-vascular accidents have been reported, often following rapid weight loss. Special care should be taken to ensure gradual and controlled weight loss in obese patients, who are subject to a risk of vascular disease. Ponderax Pacaps should not be prescribed in patients with a current or past medical history of cardio-vascular or cerebro-vascular disease, such as myocardial infarction or stroke.

This anoretic agent must be used carefully in epileptic patients.

Following sudden withdrawal of Ponderax Pacaps, severe depression has occasionally been reported. This risk may be avoided by a gradual reduction of dosage.

*Interactions with other medicaments and other forms of interaction:* Contra-indicated combinations: Ponderax Pacaps should not be used concomitantly with neuroleptic or antidepressant therapy, especially MAOIs. There should be an interval of three weeks between stopping MAOIs and starting Ponderax.

Ponderax Pacaps should not be used concomitantly with other appetite suppressants. There should be an interval of two weeks between stopping any other appetite suppressant and starting Ponderax to allow for any possible withdrawal symptoms to subside.

Ponderax Pacaps may potentiate the action of anti-hypertensive, anti-diabetic or sedative drugs. The dosage of these drugs should be re-assessed when Ponderax Pacaps is prescribed.

*Pregnancy and lactation:* Medicines should not be used in pregnancy, especially the first trimester unless the benefits outweigh any possible risk. Although no harmful effects on the foetus have been demonstrated, it is not recommended that Ponderax Pacaps be administered during pregnancy. Fenfluramine may be excreted in breast milk and administration during lactation is not recommended.

*Effects on ability to drive and use machines:* Ponderax Pacaps may cause drowsiness. It may affect the ability to drive or operate machinery and increase the effects of alcohol.

*Undesirable effects:* Most commonly reported undesirable effects are: dry mouth, nausea, constipation and diarrhoea, disappearing on continuing treatment. The following have been reported but more rarely:
– asthenia, headache, shivering,
– blood pressure variation, tachycardia, faintness, syncope,
– cardiovascular or cerebrovascular accident (mainly arrhythmia and stroke),
– increased transaminases and hepatitis (in exceptional cases),
– drowsiness, dizziness, vertigo, mood disturbance, sleep disorders, nervousness, confusion, agitation, schizophrenic-like reactions,
– depression,
– convulsions,
– diplopia, mydriasis, conjunctivitis,
– skin rash,
– urinary frequency.

An epidemiological study has shown that fenfluramine intake is a risk factor involved in the development

of pulmonary artery hypertension and that the use of anorectics is strongly associated with an increased risk for this adverse drug reaction. In addition, there have been spontaneous reports of pulmonary artery hypertension in users of these agents. Pulmonary artery hypertension is a severe and often fatal disease. The occurrence or aggravation of exertional dyspnea is usually the first clinical sign and requires treatment discontinuation and investigation in a specialised unit (see *Special warnings*).

Depression may occur after abrupt withdrawal and most commonly about 4 days after cessation of treatment although it also has been reported during therapy. Other withdrawal reactions reported on abrupt discontinuation of the drug include irritability, confusion and dizziness.

*Overdose:* The following symptoms have been reported: dilated pupils, tachycardia, facial flushing, hypertension, agitation, fine tremor; these can progress to vomiting, convulsions, unconsciousness, hyperpyrexia, depression of respiration, cardiac arrhythmia, ventricular fibrillation and death may occur.

Action to be taken in the event of overdosage:
(1) continuously monitor ECG,
(2) use diazepam to control convulsions,
(3) reduce hyperthermia,
(4) use anti-arrhythmic drugs (e.g. beta-blockers) to control cardiac tachyarrhythmias.

**Pharmacological properties**

*Pharmacodynamic properties:* Fenfluramine reduces food intake but at normal therapeutic doses it does not produce the central stimulant action of amphetamine and amphetamine-like appetite suppressants.

Fenfluramine has effects on brain 5-hydroxytryptamine and actions on feeding behaviour centres in the hypothalamus through tryptaminergic mechanisms which probably account for the drug's action. Additionally, the drug increases glucose uptake in muscle which has led to the drug being used in maturity onset diabetes. This action is independent of weight loss and does not produce lactic acidosis.

*Pharmacokinetic properties:*

*Absorption:* Normal half-life absorption of fenfluramine hydrochloride is approximately 1.2 hours and there is an accumulation of fenfluramine in the tissues. This accumulation is reflected in the 3 to 4 days of multiple dosing necessary to achieve steady state plasma levels and also the elapse of 3 to 4 days after dosing cessation for the drug to be eliminated.

*Distribution:* Fenfluramine is widely distributed in all body tissues with substantial storage in brain, fat, muscles and other tissues with limited blood supply. In blood, fenfluramine and its major metabolite norfenfluramine tend to concentrate in red cells rather than in the plasma. If serum protein binding occurs it is minimal.

*Metabolism and excretion:* The dose of Ponderax 60 mg daily achieves a steady state of plasma concentration of 40 to 145 ng/ml fenfluramine and 18 to 80 ng/ml of norfenfluramine after 9 to 14 days. In acute studies the average biological half-life of fenfluramine has been found to be 20.3 hours with a range of 13.8 to 30.1 hours. Urinary elimination of fenfluramine is low when urinary pH is uncontrolled but recovery of fenfluramine increases to 29% with acidic urine. There is extensive metabolism of both fenfluramine and norfenfluramine and more than 85% of an oral dose is excreted in the urine as metabolites.

*Preclinical safety data:* Not applicable.

**Pharmaceutical particulars**

*List of excipients:* Hydroxypropylmethylcellulose, microcrystalline cellulose, sucrose, anhydrous, sodium dihydrogen phosphate, acetyl tributyl citrate, Eudragit retard S, talc, colloidal silicon dioxide, titanium dioxide.

*Solvents:* Purified water, pharmaceutical industrial ethanol, denatured isopropyl alcohol.

*Incompatibilities:* Not applicable.

*Shelf life:* 5 years.

*Special precautions for storage:* Ponderax Pacaps should be stored in a cool, dry place.

*Nature and contents of container:* Push through blister strips of fifteen capsules. Carton of 60 capsules (four strips).

*Instructions for use/handling:* Nil.

**Marketing authorisation number** 0093/0013R

**Date of approval/revision of SPC** 17 April 1997

**Legal category** POM

*Trade Mark

# Seton Healthcare Group plc
Tubiton House
Oldham OL1 3HS

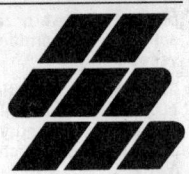

## AQUASEPT* SKIN CLEANSER

**Qualitative and quantitative composition** Triclosan 2.0% w/v .

**Pharmaceutical form** Clear blue solution.

**Clinical particulars**
*Therapeutic indications:* This product has an antibacterial effect and is intended for the following uses:
   Prevention of cross infection
   Prevention of self infection
   Preoperative hand disinfection
   Antiseptic skin cleansing
   Whole body bathing prior to elective surgery
   Whole body bathing to help eliminate the carriage of pathogens

*Posology and method of administration:*
*For preoperative hand disinfection:* (100 ml, 250 ml and 500 ml). Wet area to be cleaned. Apply about 5 ml of Aquasept and wash for one minute, paying particular attention to the area around the fingernails and cuticles and between the fingers. Rinse and repeat for two minutes. Rinse thoroughly and dry hands with a sterile towel.

*For antiseptic skin cleansing :* (100 ml, 250 ml and 500 ml). Wet area to be cleaned and use Aquasept as a liquid soap, washing thoroughly for one minute. Rinse and dry thoroughly.

*For whole body bathing :* (28.5 ml, 100 ml, 250 ml and 500 ml). In shower or bath, use Aquasept as a liquid soap, paying particular attention to the hair, perineum, groin, axillae and nares. Take two baths or showers on the two days prior to surgery. Approximately 28.5 ml of Aquasept will suffice for one shower or bath.

*Contra-indications:* None indicated.

*Special warnings and precautions for use:* For external use only. Avoid contact with eyes. Keep out of the reach of children. Some product excipients may give rise to allergic reactions in some people. In this instance, use and seek medical advice.

*Interactions with other medicaments and other forms of interaction:* None stated.

*Pregnancy and lactation:* None stated.

*Effects on ability to drive and use machines:* None stated.

*Undesirable effects:* None stated.

*Overdose:* Ingestion: Gastric lavage and symptomatic treatment.

**Pharmacological properties**
*Pharmacodynamic properties:* Triclosan is a bactericide.

*Pharmacokinetic properties:* None stated.

*Pre-clinical safety data:* None stated.

**Pharmaceutical particulars**
*List of excipients:* De-ionised water; MEA lauryl sulphate (as 30% w/w active solution); Cocamide DEA; cocamidopropyl betaine (as 30% w/w active solution); isopropyl alcohol; propylene glycol; tetrasodium EDTA and triethanolamide; chlorocresol; perfume ; Cl 42051.

*Incompatibilities:* None stated.

*Shelf life:* 36 months.

*Special precautions for storage:* None stated.

*Nature and contents of container:* HDPE or HDPP container. Polypropylene wadless screw caps or compression moulded screw caps with steran faced pulpboard liners. Sizes: 28.5 ml, 100 ml, 250 ml and 500 ml.

*Instruction for use/handling:* Not applicable.

*Marketing authorisation holder:* Seton Products Limited, Tubiton House, Oldham OL1 3HS.

**Marketing authorisation number** 11314/0096.

**Date of approval/revision of SPC** June 1996.

**Legal category** GSL.

## ASILONE* SUSPENSION

**Qualitative and quantitative composition** Asilone Suspension contains, in each 5 ml, Light Magnesium Oxide BP 70.0 mg, Aluminium Hydroxide BP 420.0 mg and Activated Dimethicone 135.0 mg.

**Pharmaceutical form** Suspension.

**Clinical particulars**
*Therapeutic indications:* Anti-flatulent and antacid; for the relief of dyspeptic symptoms of functional or organic origin, including flatulence and associated abdominal distension, heartburn, including heartburn of pregnancy, hiatus hernia, and oesophagitis, symptomatic management of gastritis and peptic ulceration.

*Posology and method of administration:*
*Adults including the elderly :* One to two 5 ml spoonfuls after meals and at bedtime or when required, up to a maximum of four times daily.
   Use within 28 days of opening.
   *Children:* Not recommended for children under 12 years of age.

*Contra-indications:* Antacid preparations should not be administered in severe debilitation or renal impairment. Do not use during the first trimester of pregnancy.

*Special warnings and precautions for use:* Asilone is not recommended in flatulent abdominal distension possibly related to intestinal obstruction.

*Interactions with other medicaments and other forms of interaction:* Antacids may interfere with the absorption of tetracyclines, rifampicin, warfarin and digoxin if given concomitantly.

*Use in pregnancy and lactation:* Antacid preparations are not recommended during the first trimester of pregnancy.

*Effects on ability to drive and use machines:* None stated.

*Undesirable effects:* Aluminium salts may cause constipation and magnesium salts diarrhoea. However, such bowel disturbances are rare with the formulation of Asilone.

*Overdose:* No cases of overdosage have been reported with Asilone. The components of Asilone are not expected to cause specific local or systemic toxicity even in acute overdosage in healthy individuals. No special treatment, but symptomatic management only if indicated.

**Pharmacological properties**
*Pharmacodynamic properties:* The active ingredients of Asilone Suspension possess antacid and antiflatulent properties which are long established; their actions in a wide variety of gastro-intestinal disorders are well recognised in standard texts. Light magnesium oxide and aluminium hydroxide are potent antacids which increase gastric pH and hence diminish the activity of pepsin in gastric secretion. In addition, aluminium hydroxide has a direct inhibiting effect on pepsin. Silicones are useful anti-foaming agents and the addition of 4-8% of finely divided silicon dioxide increases the anti-foaming activity of dimethicones. Dimethicones activated by silicone dioxide act by changing the surface tension of gas bubbles, thereby causing them to coalesce.

*Pharmacokinetic properties:* No data on pharmacokinetic studies with Asilone are available. Active ingredients aluminium hydroxide and activated dimethicone are not generally absorbed. Some magnesium may be absorbed from magnesium oxide in Asilone Suspension, but is generally rapidly excreted in urine.

*Pre-clinical safety data:* Not stated.

**Pharmaceutical particulars**
*List of excipients:* Potassium Sorbate BP; Sodium Saccharin BP; Sorbitol (or Sorbiton Solution 70 % Non Cryst) BP; Flavex Peppermint/Aniseed Flavour L263; Flavex Flavour Modifier No.12; Hydrogen Peroxide (30% v/v) BP; Methyl Parahydroxybenzoate PhEur; Propyl Parahydroxybenzoate PhEur; Purified Water PhEur.

*Incompatibilities:* None stated.

*Shelf life:* The product has a shelf life of two years but must be used within 28 days of opening.

*Special precautions for storage:* Do not freeze.

*Nature and contents of container:* Bottle of high density polyethylene in blue with a white polypropylene cap or a white polyethylene tamper evident cap with a low density polyethylene inner core liner, containing 500 ml of product.

**Marketing authorisation number** 11314/0034.

**Date of approval/revision of SPC** May 1995.

**Legal category** GSL.

## BETADINE* ALCOHOLIC SOLUTION

**Presentation** A golden brown alcoholic solution containing Povidone Iodine USP 10%w/v.

**Uses** For use as an antiseptic skin cleanser for major and minor surgical procedures where a quick drying effect is desired. For topical administration.

**Dosage and administration**
*Adults:* Apply full strength as an antiseptic skin cleanser.

*Children and the elderly:* As for adults.
   Povidone iodine is not recommended for regular use in neonates and is contra-indicated in very low birth weight infants (below 1500 grams).

**Contra-indications, warnings, etc**
*Contra-indications:* Known or suspected iodine hypersensitivity. Regular use is contra-indicated in patients or users with thyroid disorders (in particular nodular colloid goitre, endemic goitre and Hashimoto's thyroiditis).

*Interactions:* Absorption of iodine from povidone iodine may interfere with thyroid function tests. Contamination with povidone iodine of several types of tests for the detection of occult blood in faeces or blood in urine may produce false-positive results.

*Effect on ability to drive and to use machines:* None known.

*Side effects and adverse reactions:* Povidone iodine may produce local skin reactions although it is considered to be less irritant than iodine. The application of povidone iodine to large wounds or severe burns may produce systemic adverse effects such as metabolic acidosis, hypernatraemia, and impairment of renal function.

*Use in pregnancy and lactation:* Regular use of povidone iodine should be avoided in pregnant or lactating women as absorbed iodine can cross the placental barrier and can be secreted into breast milk. Although no adverse effects have been reported from limited use, caution should be recommended and therapeutic benefit must be balanced against possible effects of the absorption of iodine on foetal thyroid function and development.

*Other special precautions and warnings:* Special caution is needed when regular applications to broken skin are made to patients with pre-existing renal insufficiency. Regular use should be avoided in patients on concurrent lithium therapy. This preparation is flammable and caution is advised during surgical procedures involving hot wire cautery or diathermy.

*Overdose:* Excess iodine can produce goitre and hypothyroidism or hyperthyroidism. Systemic absorption of iodine after repeated application of povidone iodine to large areas of wounds or burns may lead to a number of adverse effects: metallic taste in the mouth, increased salivation, burning or pain in the throat or mouth, irritation and swelling of the eyes, skin reactions, gastrointestinal upset and diarrhoea, and difficulty in breathing due to pulmonary oedema. Metabolic acidosis, hypernatraemia and renal impairment may occur. In the case of accidental ingestion of large quantities of Betadine, symptomatic and supportive treatment should be provided with special attention to electrolyte balance and renal and thyroid function.

**Pharmaceutical precautions**
*Storage:* Store at or below 25˚C. Protect from light.

**Legal category** P

**Package quantities** Container of 500 ml.

**Further information** Betadine Alcoholic Solution has a rapid and prolonged germicidal action and, with repeated use, a cumulative germicidal action. It is active against a wide range of organisms including Gram positive and Gram negative bacteria, fungi, protozoa, viruses, and bacterial spores. In the presence of blood, serum, purulent exudate and necrotic tissue, its activity persists whilst the colour remains.

Product licence number   0223/0010

## BETADINE* ANTISEPTIC PAINT

**Presentation** A golden brown alcoholic solution containing Povidone Iodine USP 10%w/v.

**Uses** Betadine Antiseptic Paint is a broad spectrum, quick drying antiseptic for the treatment and prevention of infection. It is ideal for herpes simplex, herpes zoster, grazes, abrasions, cuts and wounds or any break in the skin which requires protection from infection. Betadine Antiseptic Paint is effective in the treatment of dermal infections caused by bacteria, fungi, yeasts and viruses (e.g. herpes virus types I and II).

**Dosage and administration** Apply Antiseptic Paint undiluted as necessary to affected area and allow to dry. Use twice daily and cover with a dressing if desired. Rinse the brush thoroughly after use.

**Contra-indications, warnings, etc**
*Contra-indications:* Hypersensitivity to iodine. History of abnormal thyroid function or goitre.

*Interactions:* None known.

*Effect on ability to drive and to use machines:* None known.

*Side-effects and adverse reactions:* Povidone iodine may produce local skin reactions although it is less irritant than iodine. The application of povidone iodine to large wounds or severe burns may produce systemic adverse effects such as metabolic acidosis, hypernatraemia, and impairment of renal function.

*Use in pregnancy and lactation:* Use in pregnancy and lactation should be limited to minor lesions only and although no adverse effects are anticipated from such limited use, caution is recommended and the therapeutic benefit must be balanced against the possible effect of the absorption of iodine on foetal thyroid development and function.

*Other special precautions and warnings:* If local irritation or sensitivity develop, then discontinue treatment.

*Overdose:* In the case of deliberate or accidental ingestion of large quantities of Betadine, symptomatic and supportive treatment should be provided with special attention to electrolyte balance and renal and thyroid function.

**Pharmaceutical precautions**
*Storage:* Store at or below 25°C. Protect from light.

**Legal category** P

**Package quantities**   Glass bottle containing 8 ml with an applicator brush.

**Further information**   Betadine Antiseptic Paint has a rapid and prolonged germicidal action against a wide range of organisms including Gram positive and Gram negative bacteria, fungi, protozoa and viruses. It is also active against bacterial spores. In the presence of blood, serum, purulent exudate and necrotic tissue, its activity persists whilst the golden brown colour remains.

Product licence number 0223/0011

## BETADINE* DRY POWDER SPRAY

**Presentation**   A pressurised aerosol can containing a brown powder consisting of Povidone Iodine USP 2.5%w/w.

**Uses** For use as a skin antiseptic for the treatment and prevention of infection in wounds, including ulcers, burns, cuts and other minor injuries.

**Dosage and administration**
*Adults and children:* Shake the can well, spray the required area from a distance of 6-10 inches until coated with powder. If necessary, the treated area may be covered with a dressing.

**Contra-indications, warnings, etc**
*Contra-indications:* Not to be used in serous cavities. Not for use in infants under 2 years. Hypersensitivity to iodine. History of abnormal thyroid function or goitre.

*Warnings:* Avoid inhalation or spraying into the eyes. If local irritation or sensitivity develops, then discontinue treatment. Iodine is absorbed through burns and broken skin and, to a lesser extent, through intact skin. Following prolonged application of Betadine Dry Powder Spray to severe burns or large areas of denuded skin, systemic effects such as metabolic

acidosis, hypernatraemia, renal impairment and thyroid dysfunction may occur.

*Interactions:* None known.

*Effect on ability to drive and to use machines:* None known.

*Use in pregnancy and lactation:* Use in pregnancy and lactation should be limited to minor lesions only and although no adverse effects are anticipated from such limited use, caution is recommended and the therapeutic benefit must be balanced against the possible effect of the absorption of iodine on foetal thyroid development and function.

*Overdose:* In the case of deliberate or accidental ingestion of large quantities of Betadine, symptomatic and supportive treatment should be provided with special attention to electrolyte balance and thyroid and renal function.

**Pharmaceutical precautions**
*Storage:* Store at or below 25°C away from direct heat and sunlight.

**Legal category**   GSL

**Package quantities**   Aerosol can containing 100 ml.

**Further information**   Betadine Dry Powder Spray has a rapid and prolonged germicidal action and, with repeated use, a cumulative germicidal action. It is active against a wide range of organisms including Gram positive and Gram negative bacteria, fungi, protozoa, viruses, and bacterial spores. In the presence of blood, serum, purulent exudate and necrotic tissue, its activity persists whilst the colour remains.

Product licence number 0223/0013

## BETADINE* GARGLE AND MOUTHWASH

**Presentation** A pleasantly flavoured amber coloured solution containing Povidone Iodine USP 1%w/v.

**Uses** For the treatment of acute mucosal infections of the mouth and pharynx. For oral hygiene prior to, during and after dental and oral surgery.

**Dosage and administration**
*Adults and children over 6 years of age:* Use undiluted or diluted with an equal volume of warm water. Gargle or rinse with up to 10 ml for up to 30 seconds without swallowing. Repeat up to four times daily, for up to 14 consecutive days, or as directed.

**Contra-indications, warnings, etc**
*Contra-indications :* Not for use in children under 6 years of age and in patients with a known or suspected iodine hypersensitivity. Regular use is contra-indicated in patients or users with thyroid disorders (in particular nodular colloid goitre, endemic goitre and Hashimoto's thyroiditis) or in pregnant or lactating women.

*Interactions:* Absorption of iodine from povidone iodine may interfere with thyroid function tests. Contamination with povidone iodine of several types of tests for the detection of occult blood in faeces or blood in urine may produce false-positive results.

*Effect on ability to drive and to use machines :* None known.

*Side-effects and adverse reactions:* Idiosyncratic mucosal irritation and hypersensitivity reactions may occur. Excessive absorption of iodine may produce systemic adverse effects such as metabolic acidosis, hypernatraemia and impairment of renal function.

*Use in pregnancy and lactation* Regular use of povidone iodine should be avoided in pregnant or lactating women as absorbed iodine can cross the placental barrier and can be secreted into breast milk. Although no adverse effects have been reported from limited use, caution should be recommended and therapeutic benefit must be balanced against possible effects of the absorption of iodine on foetal thyroid function and development. The use of Betadine Gargle and Mouthwash in pregnant and lactating women should be limited to a single treatment session only.

*Other special precautions and warnings:* Regular use should be avoided as prolonged use may lead to the absorption of a significant amount of iodine. Do not use for more than 14 days. If sores or ulcers in the mouth do not heal within 14 days seek medical or dental advice. Regular use should be avoided in patients on concurrent lithium therapy.

*Overdose:* Excess iodine can produce goitre and hypothyroidism or hyperthyroidism. Acute overdosage may result in symptoms of metallic taste in the mouth, increased salivation, burning or pain in the throat or mouth, irritation and swelling in the eyes, skin reactions, gastrointestinal upset and diarrhoea, and difficulty in breathing due to pulmonary oedema. Metabolic acidosis, hypernatraemia and renal impairment may occur.

In the case of accidental ingestion of large quantities of Betadine, symptomatic and supportive treatment should be provided with special attention to electrolyte balance and renal and thyroid function.

**Pharmaceutical precautions**
*Storage:* Store at or below 25°C. Protect from light.

**Legal category**   P

**Package quantities**   Bottle of 250 ml.

**Further information**   Betadine Gargle and Mouthwash does not stain the skin, mucous membranes or teeth, despite its powerful germicidal action. It is effective against a wide spectrum of organisms including Gram positive and Gram negative bacteria, fungi, protozoa, viruses and bacterial spores. In the presence of blood, serum, purulent exudate and necrotic tissue, its activity persists while the colour remains.

Product licence number 0223/0014

## BETADINE* OINTMENT

**Presentation**   A golden brown water soluble ointment containing Povidone Iodine USP 10%w/w.

**Uses** Betadine Ointment is a broad spectrum antiseptic for the treatment or prevention of infection in minor cuts and abrasions, minor surgical procedures and small areas of burns. Treatment of mycotic and bacterial skin infections and pyodermas. Treatment of infections in decubitus and stasis ulcers.

**Dosage and administration**
*For the treatment of infection :* Apply once or twice daily or at dressing changes for a maximum of 14 days.

*For the prevention of infection:* Apply once or twice a week for as long as necessary. The affected skin should be cleaned and dried. Apply Ointment to the affected area. May be covered with a dressing or bandage.

**Contra-indications, warnings, etc**
*Contra-indications:* Known or suspected iodine hypersensitivity. Regular use is contra-indicated in patients or users with thyroid disorders (in particular nodular colloid goitre, endemic goitre and Hashimoto's thyroiditis). Not for use in infants under 2 years.

*Interactions:* Absorption of iodine from povidone iodine may interfere with thyroid function tests. Contamination with povidone iodine of several types of tests for the detection of occult blood in faeces or blood in urine may produce false-positive results.

*Effect on ability to drive and to use machines:* None known.

*Side-effects and adverse reactions:* Povidone iodine may produce local skin reactions although it is less irritant than iodine. The application of povidone iodine to large wounds or severe burns may produce systemic adverse effects such as metabolic acidosis, hypernatraemia, and impairment of renal function.

*Use in pregnancy and lactation:* Regular use of povidone iodine should be avoided in pregnant or lactating women as absorbed iodine can cross the placental barrier and can be secreted into breast milk. Although no adverse effects have been reported from limited use, caution should be recommended and therapeutic benefit must be balanced against possible effects of the absorption of iodine on foetal thyroid function and development.

*Other special precautions and warnings:* Special caution is needed when regular applications to broken skin are made to patients with pre-existing renal insufficiency. Regular use should be avoided in patients on concurrent lithium therapy. Thyroid function tests should be performed during prolonged use.

*Overdose :* Excess iodine can produce goitre and hypothyroidism or hyperthyroidism. Systemic absorption of iodine after repeated application of povidone iodine to large areas of wounds or burns may lead to a number of adverse effects: metallic taste in the mouth, increased salivation, burning or pain in the throat or mouth, irritation and swelling of the eyes, skin reactions, gastrointestinal upset and diarrhoea, and difficulty in breathing due to pulmonary oedema. Metabolic acidosis, hypernatraemia and renal impairment may occur.

In the case of accidental ingestion of large quantities of Betadine, symptomatic and supportive treatment should be provided with special attention to electrolyte balance and renal and thyroid function.

**Pharmaceutical precautions**
*Storage:* Store at or below 25°C and protect from light.

**Legal category**   GSL.

**Package quantities**   Tube of 20 g and 80 g.

**Further information**   Betadine Ointment has a rapid and prolonged germicidal action and, with repeated use, a cumulative germicidal action. It is active against a wide range of organisms including Gram positive and Gram negative bacteria, fungi, protozoa, viruses, and bacterial spores. In the presence of blood, serum, purulent exudate and necrotic tissue, its activity persists whilst the colour remains.

Product licence number 0223/0015

## BETADINE* SCALP AND SKIN CLEANSER

Presentation A golden brown cleansing and sudsing surfactant solution containing Povidone Iodine USP 7.5%w/v.

Uses Betadine Scalp and Skin Cleanser is a broad spectrum antiseptic for the treatment of seborrhoeic conditions of the scalp and acne vulgaris of the face and neck.

Dosage and administration Adults, the elderly, and children over 2 years:

For the treatment of seborrhoeic conditions of the scalp Use as a shampoo. Allow to remain on the hair for at least 5 minutes. Rinse hair with warm water. Repeat application and rinse again. Repeat twice daily until improvement is noted. Afterwards, use once weekly.

For the treatment of acne vulgaris of the face and neck: Apply directly or with a moistened sponge. Cleanse area thoroughly. Repeat application. Rinse with warm water and dry with a clean or sterile towel or gauze. Repeat daily (morning and evenings) until improvement is noted. Afterwards, use once daily.

Contra-indications, warnings, etc
Contra-indications: Not for use in infants under 2 years. Hypersensitivity to iodine. History of abnormal thyroid function, or goitre.

Interactions: None known.

Use in pregnancy and lactation: Use in pregnancy and lactation should be limited and although no adverse effects are anticipated from such limited use, caution is recommended and the therapeutic benefit must be balanced against possible effects of the absorption of iodine on foetal thyroid function.

Other special precautions and warnings: If local irritation or sensitivity develops, then discontinue treatment. Do not use on broken skin. Iodine is absorbed through burns and broken skin and, to a lesser extent, through intact skin. Restrict use in infants to 2-3 days.

Overdose: In cases of deliberate or accidental ingestion of large quantities of Betadine, symptomatic and supportive treatment should be provided with special attention to electrolyte balance and renal and thyroid function.

Pharmaceutical precautions
Storage: Store at or below 25°C and protect from light.

Legal category GSL.

Package quantities Plastic bottle containing 250 ml.

Further information Betadine Scalp and Skin Cleanser has a highly effective germicidal activity. This activity is maintained in the presence of exfoliative debris and infected scalp lesions, whilst the colour persists. It does not stain the skin.

Product licence number 0223/0016

## BETADINE* SHAMPOO

Presentation A golden brown cleansing and sudsing surfactant solution containing Povidone Iodine USP 4%w/v.

Uses Betadine Shampoo is a broad spectrum antiseptic for the treatment of seborrhoeic conditions of the scalp associated with excessive dandruff, pruritus, scaling, exudation and erythema of the scalp, pityriasis capitis; infected lesions of the scalp–pyodermas (recurrent furunculosis, infective folliculitis and impetigo).

Dosage and administration
Adults, the elderly and children over 12: Having first wetted the hair, apply 2 to 3 capfuls of shampoo, use warm water to lather. Rinse. Apply again 2 to 3 capfuls of shampoo and massage into the scalp with the tips of the fingers. Work up to a golden lather using warm water. Repeat treatment twice weekly until improvement is noted. Afterwards, use shampoo once a week.

Children aged 2 to 12: As for children over 12, substituting 1 or 2 capfuls of shampoo.

Contra-indications, warnings, etc
Contra-indications: Known or suspected iodine hypersensitivity. Regular use is contra-indicated in patients or users with thyroid disorders (in particular nodular

colloid goitre, endemic goitre and Hashimoto's thyroiditis). Not for use in infants under 2 years.

Interactions: Absorption of iodine from povidone iodine may interfere with thyroid function tests. Contamination with povidone iodine of several types of tests for the detection of occult blood in faeces or blood in urine may produce false-positive results.

Effect on ability to drive and to use machines: None known.

Side-effects and adverse reactions: Povidone iodine may produce local skin reactions although it is less irritant than iodine.

Use in pregnancy and lactation: Regular use of povidone iodine should be avoided in pregnant or lactating women as absorbed iodine can cross the placental barrier and can be secreted into breast milk. Although no adverse effects have been reported from limited use, caution should be recommended and therapeutic benefit must be balanced against possible effects of the absorption of iodine on foetal thyroid function and development.

Other special precautions and warnings. : Special caution is needed when regular applications to broken skin are made to patients with pre-existing renal insufficiency. Regular use should be avoided in patients on concurrent lithium therapy.

Overdose: Excess iodine can produce goitre and hypothyroidism or hyperthyroidism. In the case of accidental ingestion of large quantities of Betadine, symptomatic and supportive treatment should be provided with special attention to electrolyte balance and renal and thyroid function.

Pharmaceutical precautions
Storage: Store at or below 25°C and protect from light.

Legal category GSL

Package quantities Plastic bottle containing 250 ml.

Further information Betadine Shampoo has a highly effective germicidal activity. This activity is maintained in the presence of exfoliative debris and infected scalp lesions whilst the colour persists. It does not stain the skin.

Product licence number 0223/0021

## BETADINE* SKIN CLEANSER

Presentation A penetrating golden brown sudsing surfactant solution containing Povidone Iodine USP 4%w/v.

Uses Betadine Skin Cleanser is a broad spectrum antiseptic for the treatment of acne vulgaris of the face and neck. For general disinfection of the skin (as a liquid soap).

Dosage and administration
Adults, the elderly, and children over 2 years: Apply directly with moistened sponge to the affected areas and work up a rich lather. Allow to remain on the skin for 3-5 minutes then rinse off thoroughly with warm water and dry with a clean or sterile towel or gauze. Repeat twice daily.

Contra-indications, warnings, etc
Contra-indications: Not for use in infants under 2 years. Hypersensitivity to iodine. History of abnormal thyroid function, or goitre.

Interactions: None known.

Effect on ability to drive and to use machines: None known.

Use in pregnancy and lactation: Use in pregnancy and lactation should be limited and although no adverse effects are anticipated from such limited use, caution is recommended and the therapeutic benefit must be balanced against possible effects of the absorption of iodine on foetal thyroid function.

Other special precautions and warnings: If local irritation or sensitivity develops, then discontinue treatment. Do not use on broken skin. Iodine is absorbed through burns and broken skin and, to a lesser extent, through intact skin. Restrict use in infants to 2-3 days.

Overdose: In cases of deliberate or accidental ingestion of large quantities of Betadine, symptomatic and supportive treatment should be provided with special attention to electrolyte balance and renal and thyroid function.

Pharmaceutical precautions
Storage: Store at or below 25°C and protect from light.

Legal category GSL.

Package quantities Plastic bottle containing 250 ml.

Further information Betadine Skin Cleanser has a highly effective germicidal activity. This activity is maintained in the presence of exfoliative debris and

infected scalp lesions, whilst the colour persists. It does not stain the skin.

Product licence number 0223/0027

## BETADINE* STANDARDISED ANTISEPTIC SOLUTION

Presentation A golden brown solution containing Povidone Iodine USP 10%w/v.

Uses For use as a pre-operative and post-operative antiseptic skin cleanser for major and minor surgical procedures. For topical application.

Dosage and administration
Adults: Apply full strength as a pre-operative and post-operative antiseptic skin cleanser. Avoid pooling both under the patient and in the skin folds. Wash off excess solution before using occlusive dressings.

Children and the elderly: As for adults.

Povidone iodine is not recommended for regular use in neonates and is contra-indicated in very low birth weight infants (below 1500 grams).

Contra-indications, warnings, etc
Contra-indications: Known or suspected iodine hypersensitivity. Regular use is contra-indicated in patients or users with thyroid disorders (in particular nodular colloid goitre, endemic goitre and Hashimoto's thyroiditis).

Interactions: Absorption of iodine from povidone iodine may interfere with thyroid function tests. Contamination with povidone iodine of several types of tests for the detection of occult blood in faeces or blood in urine may produce false-positive results.

Effect on ability to drive and to use machines: None known.

Side-effects and adverse reactions: Povidone iodine may produce local skin reactions although it is less irritant than iodine. The application of povidone iodine to large wounds or severe burns may produce systemic adverse effects such as metabolic acidosis, hypernatraemia, and impairment of renal function.

Use in pregnancy and lactation: Regular use of povidone iodine should be avoided in pregnant or lactating women as absorbed iodine can cross the placental barrier and can be secreted into breast milk. Although no adverse effects have been reported from limited use, caution should be recommended and therapeutic benefit must be balanced against possible effects of the absorption of iodine on foetal thyroid function and development.

Other special precautions and warnings: Special caution is needed when regular applications to broken skin are made to patients with pre-existing renal insufficiency. Regular use should be avoided in patients on concurrent lithium therapy.

Overdose: Excess iodine can produce goitre and hypothyroidism or hyperthyroidism. Systemic absorption of iodine after repeated application of povidone iodine to large areas of wounds or burns may lead to a number of adverse effects: metallic taste in the mouth, increased salivation, burning or pain in the throat or mouth, irritation and swelling of the eyes, pulmonary oedema, skin reactions, gastrointestinal upset and diarrhoea, metabolic acidosis, hypernatremia and renal impairment.

In the case of accidental ingestion of large quantities of Betadine, symptomatic and supportive treatment should be provided with special attention to electrolyte balance and renal and thyroid function.

Pharmaceutical precautions
Storage: Store at or below 25°C and protect from light.

Legal category P

Package quantities Container of 500 ml.

Further information Betadine Standardised Antiseptic Solution has a rapid and prolonged germicidal action and, with repeated use, a cumulative germicidal action. It is active against a wide range of organisms including Gram positive and Gram negative bacteria, fungi, protozoa, viruses, and bacterial spores. In the presence of blood, serum, purulent exudate and necrotic tissue, its activity persists whilst the colour remains.

Product licence number 0223/0012

## BETADINE* SURGICAL SCRUB

Presentation A golden brown surfactant solution containing Povidone Iodine USP 7.5%w/v with non-ionic surfactants.

Uses For use as an antiseptic skin cleanser for pre-operative scrubbing and washing by surgeons and theatre staff, and pre-operative preparation of patients' skin.

## Dosage and administration
*Adults:* Apply full strength as a pre-operative antiseptic skin cleanser.

*Children and the elderly:* As for adults.

Povidone iodine is not recommended for regular use in neonates and is contra-indicated in very low birth weight infants (below 1500 grams).

## Contra-indications, warnings, etc
*Contra-indications:* Known or suspected iodine hypersensitivity. Regular use is contra-indicated in patients or users with thyroid disorders (in particular nodular colloid goitre, endemic goitre and Hashimoto's thyroiditis).

*Interactions:* Absorption of iodine from povidone iodine may interfere with thyroid function tests. Contamination with povidone iodine of several types of tests for the detection of occult blood in faeces or blood in urine may produce false-positive results.

*Effect on ability to drive and to use machines:* None known.

*Side-effects and adverse reactions:* Povidone iodine may produce local skin reactions although it is less irritant than iodine. The application of povidone iodine to large wounds or severe burns may produce systemic adverse effects such as metabolic acidosis, hypernatraemia, and impairment of renal function.

*Use in pregnancy and lactation:* Regular use of povidone iodine should be avoided in pregnant or lactating women as absorbed iodine can cross the placental barrier and can be secreted into breast milk. Although no adverse effects have been reported from limited use, caution should be recommended and therapeutic benefit must be balanced against possible effects of the absorption of iodine on foetal thyroid function and development.

*Other special precautions and warnings:* Special caution is needed when regular applications to broken skin are made to patients with pre-existing renal insufficiency. Regular use should be avoided in patients on concurrent lithium therapy. Surgical Scrub can permanently discolour white gold jewellery and it is recommended that this type of jewellery should be removed before using Surgical Scrub.

*Overdose:* Excess iodine can produce goitre and hypothyroidism or hyperthyroidism. Systemic absorption of iodine after repeated application of povidone iodine to large areas of wounds or burns may lead to a number of adverse effects: metallic taste in the mouth, increased salivation, burning or pain in the throat or mouth, irritation and swelling of the eyes, pulmonary oedema, skin reactions, gastrointestinal upset and diarrhoea, metabolic acidosis, hypernatremia and renal impairment. In the case of accidental ingestion of large quantities of Betadine, symptomatic and supportive treatment should be provided with special attention to electrolyte balance and renal and thyroid function.

## Pharmaceutical precautions
*Storage:* Store at or below 25°C and protect from light.

## Legal category   P

**Package quantities**   Container of 500 ml.

**Further information**   Betadine Surgical Scrub has a rapid and prolonged germicidal action and, with repeated use, a cumulative germicidal action. It is active against a wide range of organisms including Gram positive and Gram negative bacteria, fungi, protozoa, viruses, and bacterial spores. In the presence of blood, serum, purulent exudate and necrotic tissue, its activity persists whilst the colour remains.

**Product licence number** 0223/0017.

## BETADINE* VAGINAL CLEANSING (VC) KIT

**Presentation** Betadine V.C. Kit consists of V.C. Concentrate, containing 250 ml of Povidone Iodine USP 10% w/v with an applicator squeeze bottle and a plastic vaginal applicator.

**Uses** For vaginitis due to candidal, trichomonal, non-specific or mixed infections, and pre-operative preparation of the vagina.

## Dosage and administration
*Adults and the elderly:* Once a day (preferably in the morning) for a 14 day period, including days of menstruation. The V.C. Concentrate should be diluted 1:10 using the measuring cap, and used according to the patient instruction leaflet provided. The applicators should only be used for the administration of the diluted V.C. Concentrate. May be used in combination with Betadine Vaginal Pessaries or Betadine Vaginal Gel.

*Children:* Contra-indicated for use in pre-puberty children.

## Contra-indications, warnings, etc
*Contra-indications:* Known or suspected iodine hypersensitivity. Regular use is contra-indicated in patients or users with thyroid disorders (in particular nodular colloid goitre, endemic goitre and Hashimoto's thyroiditis).

*Interactions:* Absorption of iodine from povidone iodine may interfere with thyroid function tests. Contamination with povidone iodine of several types of tests for the detection of occult blood in faeces or blood in urine may produce false-positive results.

*Effect on ability to drive and to use machines:* None known.

*Side-effects and adverse reactions:* If local irritation, redness or swelling develops, discontinue treatment. Iodine is absorbed from the vagina and following prolonged use, thyroid dysfunction may develop. The product is spermicidal and should not be used when conception is desired.

*Use in pregnancy and lactation:* Regular use of povidone iodine should be avoided in pregnant or lactating women as absorbed iodine can cross the placental barrier and can be secreted into breast milk. Although no adverse effects have been reported from limited use, caution should be recommended and therapeutic benefit must be balanced against possible effects of the absorption of iodine on foetal thyroid function and development.

*Other special precautions and warnings:* Special caution is needed when regular applications to broken skin are made to patients with pre-existing renal insufficiency. Regular use should be avoided in patients on concurrent lithium therapy.

*Overdose:* Excess iodine can produce goitre and hypothyroidism or hyperthyroidism. In the case of accidental ingestion of large quantities of Betadine, symptomatic and supportive treatment should be provided with special attention to electrolyte balance and renal and thyroid function.

*Incompatibilities (major):* Compatibility with barrier contraceptives has not been established. Therefore this product should not be used with such methods of contraception as their reliability may be affected.

## Pharmaceutical precautions
*Storage:* Store at or below 25°C and protect from light.

## Legal category   P

**Package quantities** Carton containing plastic bottle of 250 ml V.C. Concentrate, an empty applicator squeeze bottle and a plastic vaginal applicator.

**Further information**   Betadine V.C. Kit is fungicidal, trichomonacidal and bactericidal to the pathogenic organisms that cause vaginitis. In the presence of blood, serum and necrotic tissue, its activity persists whilst the colour remains. The preparation is water-soluble and does not stain the skin.

**Product licence number** 0223/0020

## BETADINE* VAGINAL GEL

**Presentation**   A golden brown gel containing Povidone Iodine USP 10% w/w.

**Uses** For vaginitis due to candidal, trichomonal, non-specific or mixed infections, and pre-operative preparation of the vagina.

## Dosage and administration
*Adults and the elderly:* Insert an applicator full of gel (5 g) every night for up to 14 days. The regimen may be varied to combine the use of Betadine Vaginal Gel and Betadine Vaginal Pessaries or in combination with the Betadine V.C. Kit using one in the morning and one at night for up to 14 days. If menstruation occurs during treatment, it is important to continue treatment during the days of the period.

*Children:* Contra-indicated for use in pre-puberty children.

## Contra-indications, warnings, etc
*Contra-indications:* Known or suspected iodine hypersensitivity. Regular use is contra-indicated in patients or users with thyroid disorders (in particular nodular colloid goitre, endemic goitre and Hashimoto's thyroiditis).

*Interactions:* Absorption of iodine from povidone iodine may interfere with thyroid function tests. Contamination with povidone iodine of several types of tests for the detection of occult blood in faeces or blood in urine may produce false-positive results.

*Effect on ability to drive and to use machines:* None known.

*Side-effects and adverse reactions:* If local irritation, redness or swelling develops, discontinue treatment. Iodine is absorbed from the vagina and following prolonged use, thyroid dysfunction may develop. The product is spermicidal and should not be used when conception is desired.

*Use in pregnancy and lactation:* Regular use of povidone iodine should be avoided in pregnant or lactating women as absorbed iodine can cross the placental barrier and can be secreted into breast milk. Although no adverse effects have been reported from limited use, caution should be recommended and therapeutic benefit must be balanced against possible effects of the absorption of iodine on foetal thyroid function and development.

*Other special precautions and warnings:* Special caution is needed when regular applications to broken skin are made to patients with pre-existing renal insufficiency. Regular use should be avoided in patients on concurrent lithium therapy.

*Overdose:* Excess iodine can produce goitre and hypothyroidism or hyperthyroidism. In the case of accidental ingestion of large quantities of Betadine, symptomatic and supportive treatment should be provided with special attention to electrolyte balance and renal and thyroid function.

*Incompatibilities (major):* Compatibility with barrier contraceptives has not been established. Therefore this product should not be used with such methods of contraception as their reliability may be affected.

## Pharmaceutical precautions
*Storage:* Store at or below 25°C.

## Legal category   P

**Package quantities**   80 g with applicator.

**Further information**   Betadine Vaginal Gel is fungicidal, trichomonacidal and bactericidal to the pathogenic organisms that cause vaginitis. In the presence of blood, serum and necrotic tissue, its activity persists whilst the colour remains. The preparation is water-soluble and does not stain the skin.

**Product licence number** 0223/0018

## BETADINE* VAGINAL PESSARIES

**Presentation**   Golden brown in colour, each contain Povidone Iodine USP 200 mg in a water-soluble base.

**Uses** For vaginitis due to candidal, trichomonal, non-specific or mixed infections, and pre-operative preparation of the vagina.

## Dosage and administration
*Adults and the elderly:* Insert one pessary night and morning for up to 14 days. Each pessary should be wetted with water immediately prior to insertion, thus enabling maximum dispersion of the active constituent and avoiding risk of local irritation.. If menstruation occurs during treatment, it is important to continue treatment during the days of the period.

*Children:* Contra-indicated for use in pre-puberty children.

## Contra-indications, warnings, etc
*Contra-indications:* Known or suspected iodine hypersensitivity. Regular use is contra-indicated in patients or users with thyroid disorders (in particular nodular colloid goitre, endemic goitre and Hashimoto's thyroiditis).

*Interactions:* Absorption of iodine from povidone iodine may interfere with thyroid function tests. Contamination with povidone iodine of several types of tests for the detection of occult blood in faeces or blood in urine may produce false-positive results.

*Effect on ability to drive and to use machines:* None known.

*Side-effects and adverse reactions:* If local irritation, redness or swelling develops, discontinue treatment. Iodine is absorbed from the vagina and following prolonged use, thyroid dysfunction may develop. The product is spermicidal and should not be used when conception is desired.

*Use in pregnancy and lactation:* Regular use of povidone iodine should be avoided in pregnant or lactating women as absorbed iodine can cross the placental barrier and can be secreted into breast milk. Although no adverse effects have been reported from limited use, caution should be recommended and therapeutic benefit must be balanced against possible effects of the absorption of iodine on foetal thyroid function and development.

*Other special precautions and warnings:* Special caution is needed when regular applications to broken skin are made to patients with pre-existing renal insufficiency. Regular use should be avoided in patients on concurrent lithium therapy.

*Overdose:* Excess iodine can produce goitre and hypothyroidism or hyperthyroidism. In the case of accidental ingestion of large quantities of Betadine, symptomatic and supportive treatment should be provided with special attention to electrolyte balance and renal and thyroid function.

**Incompatibilities (major):** Compatibility with barrier contraceptives has not been established. Therefore this product should not be used with such methods of contraception as their reliability may be affected.

**Pharmaceutical precautions**

**Storage:** Store at or below 25°C.

**Legal category** P

**Package quantities** 28 with applicator (OP).

**Further information** Betadine Vaginal Pessaries are fungicidal, trichomonacidal and bactericidal to the pathogenic organisms that cause vaginitis. In the presence of blood, serum and necrotic tissue, their activity persists whilst the colour remains. The preparation is water soluble and does not stain the skin.

**Product licence number** 0223/0019

# CARYLDERM* LOTION

**Qualitative and quantitative composition** Carylderm Lotion contains carbaryl 0.5% w/w.

**Pharmaceutical form** Lotion

**Clinical particulars**

*Therapeutic indications:* For the treatment of head lice and pubic lice infestation.

*Posology and method of administration:* For topical external use only.

*Adults, the elderly and children aged six months and above:*

*For head lice* Sprinkle the lotion on the hair and rub gently onto the head until the entire scalp is moistened. Pay special attention to the back of the neck and the area behind the ears. Take care to avoid the eyes. Allow to dry naturally. Use no heat. As all lice and eggs will have been killed, the hair may be shampooed after 2 hours. If a residual effect is desired, however, it is recommended that shampooing be carried out after 12 hours. While still wet, comb the hair with an ordinary comb. A fine toothed metal comb can then be used to remove the dead lice and eggs.

*For pubic lice* Application and dosage etc are as for the head. Apply the lotion to the pubic hair and the hair between the legs and around the anus. Allow to dry naturally, using no heat. Transient, mild stinging may be experienced due to alcohol content.

*Contra-indications:* Known sensitivity to carbaryl.

*Special warnings and precautions for use:* Carylderm Lotion contains isopropyl alcohol which may cause wheezing in asthmatic patients or cause inflammation of the skin in patients with severe eczema.

Contains flammable alcohol. Apply and dry with care. Avoid naked flames or lighted objects. Do not use artificial heat (e.g. electric hairdryers). Dry in a well ventilated room. Do not cover the head before the lotion has dried completely.

Children under the age of six months should only be treated under medical supervision. When Carylderm Lotion is used by a school nurse or other health officers in the mass treatment of large numbers of children, it is advisable that protective plastic or rubber gloves be worn.

The feeding of carbaryl to rats and mice throughout life led to an increased incidence of benign and malignant tumours only at very high doses. However, a range of in vivo and in vitro mutagenicity tests have indicated that carbaryl is not genotoxic.

These findings suggest that use of carbaryl to treat louse infections is unlikely to pose a significant cancer risk in humans.

*Interactions with other medicaments and other forms of interaction:* None known.

*Pregnancy and lactation:* No evidence of safety of this product has been determined in pregnancy and lactation. It is not necessary to contraindicate this product in pregnancy and lactation provided caution is exercised and the directions for use are followed. However, as with all medicines, the advice of a doctor should be sought before the product is used.

*Effects on ability to drive and use machines:* None stated.

*Undesirable effects:* None stated.

*Overdose:* In the event of deliberate or accidental ingestion, empty stomach by gastric lavage and keep patient warm. In the event of massive ingestion, atropine, in doses of 1 or 2 mg intravenously, may be required to counteract cholinesterase inhibition.

**Pharmacological properties**

*Pharmacodynamic properties:* The action of carbamates is to inhibit the acetylcholinesterases present at synaptic junctions within the insect's nervous system.

*Pharmacokinetic properties:* Carylderm Lotion is applied topically to the affected area.

*Preclinical safety data:* None stated.

**Pharmaceutical particulars**

*List of excipients:* Surtic P15413 perfume; isopropyl myristate; isopropanol.

*Incompatibilties:* None stated.

*Shelf life:* Three years.

*Special precautions for storage:* Store at or below 25°C.

*Nature and contents of container:* Cartoned, clear glass bottles with polyethylene caps and polyethylene sprinkler inserts or clear soda glass sprinkler bottles with polypropylene caps containing either 55 or 160 ml of product.

*Instructions for use/handling:* None stated.

**Marketing authorisation number** 11314/0040.

**Date of approval/revision of SPC** June 1997.

**Legal category** POM.

# CARYLDERM* SHAMPOO

**Qualitative and quantitative composition** Carylderm Shampoo contains carbaryl 1.0% w/w.

**Pharmaceutical form** Liquid shampoo.

**Clinical particulars**

*Therapeutic indications :* For the treatment of head lice and pubic lice infestation.

*Posology and method of administration:*

*Adults, the elderly and children aged six months and above :* Treatment should be carried out a total of three times at three day intervals.

*For head lice* Wet the hair thoroughly with warm water and apply sufficient shampoo to work up a rich lather and ensure no part of the scalp is left uncovered. Pay special attention to the back of the neck and the area behind the ears. Take care to avoid the eyes. Leave for at least five minutes. Rinse thoroughly with clean warm water and repeat procedure. While hair is still wet, comb with an ordinary comb. The fine toothed louse comb can then be used to remove the dead lice and eggs.

*For pubic lice* Wet thoroughly and apply the shampoo directly to the pubic hair and the hair between the legs and around the anus. Cover the skin and hair completely with the shampoo. Work up to a lather and leave for at least 5 minutes. Rinse thoroughly. Repeat procedure. The fine toothed louse comb can then be used to remove the dead lice and eggs.

*Contra-indications:* Known sensitivity to carbaryl.

*Special warnings and precautions for use:* As with all shampoos, avoid contact with the eyes. Children under six months of age should only be treated under medical supervision. When Carylderm Shampoo is used by a school nurse or other health officer in the mass treatment of large numbers of children, it is advisable that protective plastic or rubber gloves should be worn. For external use only.

The feeding of carbaryl to rats and mice throughout life led to an increased incidence of benign and malignant tumours only at very high doses. However, a range of in vivo and in vitro mutagenicity test have indicated that carbaryl is not genotoxic.

These findings suggest that use of carbaryl to treat louse infestations is unlikely to pose a significant cancer risk in humans.

*Interactions with other medicaments and other forms of interaction:* None known.

*Pregnancy and lactation:* No evidence of safety of this product has been determined in pregnancy and lactation. It is not necessary to contraindicate this product in pregnancy and lactation provided caution is exercised and the directions for use are followed. However, as with all medicines, the advice of a doctor should be sought before the product is used.

*Effects on ability to drive and use machines:* None stated.

*Undesirable effects:* None stated.

*Overdose:* In the event of deliberate or accidental ingestion, empty stomach contents by gastric lavage and keep patient warm. In the event of massive ingestion, atropine, in doses of 1 or 2 mg intravenously, may be required to counteract cholinesterase inhibition.

**Pharmacological properties**

*Pharmacodynamic properties:* The action of carbamates is to inhibit the acetylcholinesterases present at synaptic junctions within the insect's nervous system.

*Pharmacokinetic properties:* Carylderm Shampoo is applied topically to the affected area.

*Preclinical safety data:* None stated.

**Pharmaceutical particulars**

*List of excipients:* Sodium lauryl ether sulphate (70%); coconut diethanolamide; ethoxylated lanolin (50%); nonoxynol 9; Garland Flora Perfume; alkyl phenol polyglycol ether; polyethylene glycol 400; isopropyl myristate; quinoline yellow; hydrochloric acid (20% w/w); citric acid monohydrate; dibasic sodium phosphate anhydrous; butylated hydroxytoluene; potassium sorbate; phenonip; purified water.

*Incompatibilities:* None stated.

*Shelf life :* Three years.

*Special precautions for storage:* Store at or below 25°C.

*Nature and contents of container:* Cartoned soda glass bottles with plastic containing 100 ml of product.

*Instruction for use/handling :* None stated.

**Marketing authorisation number** 11314/0041.

**Date of approval/revision of SPC** June 1997.

**Legal category** POM

# DERBAC-C* LIQUID

**Qualitative and quantitative composition** Derbac-C Liquid contains Carbaryl 1.0% w/w.

**Pharmaceutical form** Liquid.

**Clinical particulars**

*Therapeutic indications:* For the eradication of head lice and their eggs.

*Posology and method of administration:* Adults, the elderly and children aged six months and above For external use only. As this product does not contain alcohol, it may be more suitable for those with asthma or eczema. Keep the head upright and rub Derbac-C Liquid well into the roots of the hair and scalp, paying particular attention to the partings, back of the neck, fringes and around the ears. Leave the hair to dry naturally and wash in ordinary shampoo the next day or after 12 hours. After shampoo wash, remove the dead eggs with the Derbac Nit Comb while the hair is wet. Family members and close contacts should also be treated simultaneously, if infected. In the event of early re-infestation, Derbac-C Liquid should be applied again, provided seven days have elapsed since the first application. Not to be used on children under the age of 6 months except under medical supervision.

*Contra-indications:* Known sensitivity to carbaryl.

*Special warnings and precautions for use:* Avoid contact with the eyes. Not to be used on infants less than 6 months of age, unless under medical supervision. Nursing staff involved in repeated applications should wear rubber gloves when carrying out treatment. For external use only. Keep out of the reach of children. If Derbac-C is inadvertently swallowed a doctor or casualty department should be contacted at once.

Continued prolonged treatment with Derbac-C Liquid should be avoided. It should not be used more than once a week for three weeks at a time. The feeding of carbaryl to rats and mice throughout life led to an increased incidence of benign and malignant tumours only at very high doses. However, a range of in vivo and in vitro mutagenicity tests have indicated that carbaryl is not genotoxic. These findings suggest that the use of carbaryl to treat louse infestations is unlikely to pose a significant cancer risk in humans.

*Interactions with other medicaments and other forms of interaction:* None known.

*Pregnancy and lactation:* No evidence of the safety of this product has been determined in pregnancy and lactation. It is not necessary to contraindicate this product in pregnancy and lactation provided caution is exercised and the directions for use are followed.

*Effects on ability to drive and use machines:* None stated.

*Overdose:* Accidental ingestion: it is unlikely that a toxic dose of carbaryl will be ingested. Treatment consists of gastric lavage, assisted respiration and, if necessary in the event of massive ingestion, administration of atropine.

**Pharmacological properties**

*Pharmacodynamic properties:* The action of carbamates is to inhibit the acetylcholinesterases present at synaptic junctions within the insect's nervous system.

*Pharmacokinetic properties:* Derbac-C Liquid is applied topically to the affected area.

*Pre-clinical safety data:* None stated

**Pharmaceutical particulars**

*List of excipients*: Potassium Citrate PhEur; Citric Acid PhEur; Lanette Wax SX; Propyl Hydroxybenzoate (E217) PhEur; Methyl Hydroxybenzoate (E219) PhEur; diethylene glycol; Dimethyl Phthalate BP; Colour Blue 1249 (E131); Bronopol BP; water.

*Incompatibilities*: None stated.

*Shelf life*: Three years.

*Special precautions for storage*: Store at or below 25°C and do not refrigerate. Protect from sunlight.

*Nature and contents of container*: Clear or amber glass bottles with polyethylene caps and polypropylene faced wads. The clear glass bottles are contained in cartons. The product is available in bottles containing either 50 or 200 ml of product.

*Instructions for use/handling*: None stated.

**Marketing authorisation number**    11314/0044.

**Date of approval/revision of SPC**    June 1997.

**Legal category**    POM.

## DERBAC-M* LIQUID

**Qualitative and quantitative composition** Malathion 0.5% w/w.

**Pharmaceutical form**    Liquid emulsion.

**Clinical particulars**

*Therapeutic indications*: Eradication of head lice, pubic lice and their eggs. For the treatment of scabies.

*Posology and method of administration*: For topical external use only.

*Adults, the elderly and children aged 6 months and over*: As this product does not contain alcohol, it may be more suitable for those with asthma or eczema. Treatment of head lice Rub the liquid into the scalp until all the hair and scalp is thoroughly moistened. Leave the hair to dry naturally in a warm but well ventilated room. After 12 hours, or the next day, if preferred, shampoo the hair in the normal way. Rinse the hair and comb whilst wet to remove dead lice and eggs (nits) using a fine-toothed louse nit comb.

Treatment of crab lice Apply Derbac-M Liquid to the entire skin surface. Pay particular attention to all hairy areas including beards and moustaches. Avoid any other areas above the neck. Leave on for at least one hour before washing but preferably Derbac-M should be left on overnight. Wash off in the usual manner.

Treatment of scabies Apply Derbac-M Liquid to the entire skin surface. In adults it may not be necessary to apply above the neck but children under the age of two years should have a thin film of Derbac-M Liquid applied to the scalp, face and ears, avoiding the eyes and mouth. Do not wash off or bathe for 24 hours. If hands or any other parts must be washed during this period, the treatment must be reapplied to those areas immediately. No special sterilisation of clothing is necessary, ordinary laundering or dry-cleaning with hot-iron pressing are sufficient.

The infestation is cleared by the treatment. However, the itching and rash may persist for up to 7 days. An anti-irritant cream can be applied if necessary. Family members and close contacts should also be treated simultaneously.

*Children aged 6 months and under*: On medical advice only.

*Contra-indications*: Known sensitivity to malathion. Not to be used on infants less than 6 months except on medical advice.

*Special warnings and precautions for use*: Avoid contact with the eyes. For external use only. Keep out of the reach of children. If inadvertently swallowed, a doctor or casualty department should be contacted at once. When Derbac-M Liquid is used by a school nurse or other health officer in the mass treatment of large numbers of children, it is advisable that protective plastic or rubber gloves be worn. Continued prolonged treatment with this product should be avoided. It should be used not more than once a week and for not more than 3 consecutive weeks. This treatment may affect permed, coloured or bleached hair.

*Interactions with other medicaments and other forms of interaction*: None stated.

*Use in pregnancy and lactation*: No known effects in pregnancy and lactation. However, as with all medicines, use with caution.

*Effects on ability to drive and use machines*: None stated.

*Undesirable effects*: Very rarely, skin irritation has been reported.

*Overdose*: It is most unlikely that a toxic dose of malathion will be ingested. Treatment consists of gastric lavage, assisted respiration and, if necessary

in the event of massive ingestion, administration of atropine together with pralidoxime.

**Pharmacological properties**

*Pharmacodynamic properties*: Derbac-M Liquid contains malathion, a widely used organophosphorous insecticide which is active by cholinesterase inhibition. It is effective against a wide range of insects, but is one of the least toxic organophosphorous insecticides since it is rapidly detoxified by plasma carboxylesterases.

*Pharmacokinetic properties*: None stated. Derbac-M Liquid is applied topically to the affected area.

*Pre-Clinical safety data*: None stated.

**Pharmaceutical particulars**

*List of excipients*: Methyl hydroxybenzoate; propyl hydroxybenzoate; Lanette wax SX; potassium citrate; citric acid; Perfume HT 52; water.

*Incompatibilities*: None stated.

*Shelf life*: Two and a half years.

*Special precautions for storage*: Store at or below 25°C. Protect from sunlight.

*Nature and contents of container*: Cartoned, clear or amber glass bottles with polyethylene caps and polypropylene faced wads containing either 50 or 200 ml of product.

*Instructions for use/handling*: None stated.

**Marketing authorisation number**    11314/0046.

**Date of approval/revision of SPC**    October 1995.

**Legal category**    P.

## FULL MARKS* LOTION

**Qualitative and quantitative composition** Full Marks Lotion contains Phenothrin 0.2% w/v.

**Pharmaceutical form** Lotion.

**Clinical particulars**

*Therapeutic indications*: For the treatment of head lice and pubic lice infestations.

*Posology and method of administration*: For topical external use only. The source of infestation should be sought and treated.

*Adults, the elderly and children aged 6 months and over*:

Treatment of head lice Ensure that the hair is dry before commencing treatment. Sprinkle the lotion on the hair and rub gently onto the head until the entire scalp is moistened. Pay special attention to the back of the neck and the area behind the ears. Take care to avoid the eyes. Allow to dry naturally–use no heat. Ensure that the hair is dry before going to bed. The hair may be washed with a standard shampoo 2 hours after application. While still wet, comb the hair with an ordinary comb. A fine-toothed louse comb can then be used to remove the dead lice and eggs.

Treatment of pubic lice Application and dosage are as for the head. Apply the lotion to the pubic hair and the hair between the legs and around the anus. Allow to dry naturally using no heat. Transient, mild stinging may be experienced due to the alcohol content.

*Contra-indications*: A history of sensitivity to pyrethroid insecticides.

*Special warnings and precautions for use*: Full Marks Lotion contains isopropyl alcohol which may cause wheezing in asthmatic patients or cause inflammation of the skin in patients with severe eczema. If such events are apparent, patients should use a shampoo formulation. Contains flammable alcohol. Apply and dry with care. Avoid naked flames or lighted objects. Do not use artificial heat (e.g. electric hairdryers). Dry in a well ventilated room. Do not cover the head before the lotion has dried completely. The hair should be dry before retiring to bed.

When Full Marks Lotion is used by a school nurse or other health officer in the mass treatment of large numbers of children, it is advisable that protective plastic or rubber gloves be worn. Children under the age of six months should be treated under medical supervision. This treatment may affect permed, coloured or bleached hair.

*Interactions with other medicaments and other forms of interaction*: None stated.

*Use in pregnancy and lactation*: No known effects in pregnancy and lactation. However, as with all medicines, use with caution.

*Effects on ability to drive and use machines*: None stated.

*Undesirable effects*: Some patients may experience stinging or inflammation of the skin due to the alcohol content.

*Overdose*: In the event of deliberate or accidental

ingestion, as for ethyl alcohol, empty the stomach by gastric lavage and treat symptomatically.

**Pharmacological properties**

*Pharmacodynamic properties*: Phenothrin is a synthetic pyrethroid insecticide, highly effective against human lice but with an exceptionally low mammalian toxicity.

*Pharmacokinetic properties*: Full Marks Lotion is applied topically to the affected area. A pharmacokinetic study has shown absorption of the active constituent is negligible.

*Pre-clinical safety data*: None stated.

**Pharmaceutical particulars**

*List of excipients*: Herbal green bouquet P15312; isopropanol; purified water.

*Incompatibilities*: None stated.

*Shelf life*: Three years.

*Special precautions for storage*: Store bottle in carton at or below 30°C protected from light.

*Nature and contents of container*: Cartoned, clear glass or amber bottles with polyethylene caps and polyethylene sprinkler inserts containing either 55 or 160 ml of product.

*Instruction for use/handling*: None stated.

**Marketing authorisation number** 11314/0047.

**Date of approval/revision of SPC**    November 1995.

**Legal category**    P.

## GASTROCOTE* LIQUID

**Qualitative and quantitative composition**
*Active constituents*:
Sodium Alginate BP 220 mg
Dried Aluminium Hydroxide BP 80 mg
Magnesium Trisilicate BP 40 mg
Sodium Bicarbonate BP 70 mg

**Pharmaceutical form**    Oral suspension.

**Clinical particulars**

*Therapeutic indications*: Gastrocote Liquid is indicated in heartburn, including heartburn of pregnancy, reflux oesophagitis, especially where associated with hiatus hernia, and in all cases of epigastric distress associated with gastric reflux or regurgitation. It is also indicated for acid indigestion.

*Posology and method of administration*:
Adults and older children only: One to three 5 ml spoonfuls to be taken four times daily, that is, after main meals and at bedtime.
Infants and young children: Not recommended.

*Contra-indications*: There are no specific contra-indications to the use of Gastrocote Liquid.

*Special warnings and precautions for use*: Each 5 ml contains 42 mg sodium (1.8 mmol) which may be important for patients on a restricted salt intake.

*Interactions with other medicaments and other forms of interaction*: None stated.

*Pregnancy and lactation*: Indicated for use in pregnancy.

*Effects on ability to drive and use machines*: No known effects.

*Undesirable effects*: None stated.

*Overdose*: Acute overdose is virtually free of hazard. Gastric bloating may be anticipated and, if necessary, should be treated symptomatically.

**Pharmacological properties**

*Pharmacodynamic properties*: Alginate antacid products form an alginate raft on top of the gastric contents. The antacid components remain entrained in the alginate raft and exert little or no effect on gastric pH.

The presence of the foam helps to impede gastro-oesophageal reflux. If reflux is forced the alginate antacid foam enters the oesophagus first coating it with a protective demulcent and antacid layer. This coating process is repeated as the reflux subsides. Any refluxed gastric acid is thus rapidly neutralised, the oesophageal mucosa is protected and any pre-existing oesophagitis or ulceration can heal normally.

*Pharmacokinetic properties*: There is very little absorption of aluminium hydroxide from the gastrointestinal tract. Only 5% of magnesium is absorbed. However, there is a theoretical possibility of accumulation of aluminium or magnesium in cases of severe renal failure. There is negligible absorption of alginate.

*Preclinical safety data*: Not applicable.

**Pharmaceutical particulars**

*List of excipients*: Aluminium Magnesium Silicate BP; Sunset Yellow FCF (E110); butterscotch liquid flavour; peppermint liquid; Saccharin Sodium BP; Nipacombin SK; Purified water BP.

*Incompatibilities:* None known.

*Shelf life:* 24 months unopened, one month after opening.

*Special precautions for storage:* Store at or below 25°C.

*Nature and contents of container:* HDPE bottle with tamper evident screw closure or HDPE with screw closure. Bottles of 250 ml and 500 ml.

*Instruction for use/handling:* Not applicable.

**Marketing authorisation number** 11314/0062.

**Date of approval/revision of SPC** July 1996.

**Legal category** GSL.

## GASTROCOTE* TABLETS

**Qualitative and quantitative composition** Alginic Acid BP 200 mg; Dried Aluminium Hydroxide Gel BP 80 mg; Magnesium Trisilicate BP 40 mg; Sodium Bicarbonate BP 70 mg.

**Pharmaceutical form** Tablet uncoated.

### Clinical particulars

*Therapeutic indications:* Gastrocote is indicated in heartburn, including heartburn of pregnancy, reflux oesophagitis, particularly where associated with hiatus hernia, and in all cases of epigastric distress associated with gastric reflux or regurgitation. It is also indicated in acid indigestion.

*Posology and method of administration:*
Adults and older children only: 1 or 2 tablets to be chewed four times a day, that is, after main meals and at bedtime. Not to be given to children under 6 years.
*Important* The tablets must be well chewed before swallowing.

*Contra-indications:* There are no specific contra-indications to the use of Gastrocote.

*Special warnings and precautions for use:* Care should be exercised in treating diabetic patients as the tablets each contain approximately 1 g of sugar. Each tablet also contains 21 mg (0.91 Meq) of sodium which may be important for patients on a low sodium diet. As Gastrocote contains aluminium hydroxide, use with caution in patients with renal dysfunction or on a low phosphate diet.

*Interactions with other medicaments and other forms of interaction:* None stated.

*Pregnancy and lactation:* No special warnings required. Gastrocote is indicated in heartburn, including heartburn of pregnancy.

*Effects on ability to drive and use machines:* None stated.

*Undesirable effects:* None stated.

*Overdose:* Overdose is virtually free of hazard although gastric bloating may occur.

### Pharmacological properties

*Pharmacodynamic properties:* Alginate antacid products form an alginate raft on top of the gastric contents. The antacid components remain entrained in the alginate raft and exert little or no effect on gastric pH.

The presence of the foam helps to impede gastro-oesophageal reflux. If reflux is forced the alginate antacid foam enters the oesophagus first coating it with a protective demulcent and antacid layer. This coating process is repeated as the reflux subsides. Any refluxed gastric acid is thus rapidly neutralised, the oesophageal mucosa is protected and any pre-existing oesophagitis or ulceration can heal normally.

*Pharmacokinetic properties:* There is very little absorption of aluminium hydroxide from the gastrointestinal tract. Only 5% of magnesium is absorbed. However, there is a theoretical possibility of accumulation of aluminium or magnesium in cases of severe renal failure. There is negligible absorption of alginate.

*Pre-clinical safety data:* Not applicable.

### Pharmaceutical particulars

*List of excipients:* Powdered Cellulose NF; Carmellose Sodium BP; Butterscotch Flavour; Magnesium Stearate BP; Directly Compressible Sugar NF.

*Incompatibilities:* None stated.

*Shelf life:* 60 months.

*Special precautions for storage:* Store in a cool dry place below 25°C.

*Nature and contents of container:* Securitainers or high density polyethylene container with tamper evident low density polyethylene lid or blister pack comprised of 20µ aluminium foil and 250µ PVC film. Packs of 20, 40 and 100 tablets.

*Instructions for use/handling:* Not applicable.

**Marketing authorisation number** 11314/0061

**Date of approval/revision of SPC** July 1996.

**Legal category** GSL.

## MANUSEPT*

**Presentation** A clear solution containing 70% v/v Isopropyl Alcohol BP and 0.5% w/v Triclosan.

**Uses** For the disinfection of intact skin. For pre-operative disinfection of physically clean hands. For skin disinfection prior to surgery, injection or venepuncture.

### Dosage and administration

*For the disinfection of physically clean hands:* Dispense approximately 3 ml of Manusept into the palm of one hand. Rub both hands, wrists and forearms together vigorously, paying particular attention to the area around the fingernails. Continue rubbing until dry. Repeat this procedure once more for the pre-operative disinfection.

*For the disinfection of intact skin before surgery, injection or venepuncture:* Apply a quantity of Manusept with a sterile swab. Rub vigorously until dry. Repeat this procedure once more.

**Contra-indications, warnings, etc** *Treatment of overdosage:* If swallowed, gastric aspiration and lavage. Avoid contact with the eyes. For external use only.

**Pharmaceutical precautions** Store at or below normal ambient temperatures. Do not use in the vicinity of naked flames.

**Legal category** GSL.

**Package quantities** 100 ml, 250 ml and 500 ml.

**Further information** Triclosan is compatible with soap which can be used to obtain physically clean hands.

**Product licence number** 11314/0097.

## METROTOP*

**Qualitative and quantitative composition** Metronidazole BP 0.8% w/v .

**Pharmaceutical form** A colourless aqueous gel.

### Clinical particulars

*Therapeutic indications:* For the treatment of malodorous fungating tumours in terminally ill patients.

*Posology and method of administration:* For external use only. Adults: All wounds should be cleaned thoroughly. Flat wounds require a liberal application of the gel over the complete area. Cavities should be loosely packed with paraffin gauze which has been smeared in the gel. All wounds should be covered with a non-adherent dressing and a pad of lint or gauze. Sticking may occur if the appropriate dressing is not used. Use once or twice daily as necessary. Elderly: No specific instructions. Children: Where necessary, instructions apply as for adults.

*Contra-indications:* Known hypersensitivity to metronidazole.

*Special warnings and precautions for use :* The following statements take into the account the possibility that metronidazole may be absorbed after topical application. However, there is no evidence of any significant systemic concentrations of metronidazole following topical applications. Peripheral neuropathy has been reported in association with prolonged use of metronidazole. The elimination half-life of metronidazole remains unchanged in the presence of renal failure. Such patients, however, retain the metabolite of metronidazole. The clinical significance of this is not known at present. However, in patients undergoing dialysis, metronidazole and metabolites are efficiently removed.

*Interactions with other medicaments and other forms of interaction :* Some potentiation of anticoagulant therapy has been reported when metronidazole has been used with the warfarin type oral anticoagulants. Patients receiving phenobarbitone metabolise metronidazole at a much faster rate than normal, reducing the half-life to approximately 3 hours. Patients are advised not to take alcohol during systemic metronidazole therapy because of the possibility of a disulfiram-like reaction.

*Pregnancy and lactation :* There is inadequate evidence of the use of metronidazole in pregnancy. Metronidazole gel cannot therefore be recommended during pregnancy or lactation where significant systemic absorption may occur unless the physician considers it essential.

*Effects on ability to drive and use machines :* None known.

*Undesirable effects:* No adverse effects have been reported. Systemic metronidazole therapy may occasionally cause an unpleasant taste in the mouth, furred tongue, nausea, vomiting, gastrointestinal disturbance, urticaria, angioedema and anaphylaxis. Drowsiness, dizziness, headache, ataxia, skin rash, pruritus, and darkening of the urine has been reported, but rarely.

*Overdose:* There is no specific treatment for gross overdosage of metronidazole. Gastric lavage is recommended in cases of accidental ingestion. Uneventful recovery has followed overdosage of up to 12 g taken orally. Metronidazole is readily removed from the plasma by dialysis.

### Pharmacological properties

*Pharmacodynamic properties:* Metronidazole is a potent agent against the anaerobic bacteria which are believed to produce odorous metabolites as a result of localised tissue colonisation. The aim of the product is to provide a high concentration of metronidazole at and around the site of colonisation in a water-miscible base. This form allows surface spread and penetration within the wound accompanied by ease of aseptic application and up to 24 hours duration of action.

*Pharmacokinetic properties:* There is presently no evidence of any systemic concentrations of metronidazole following topical application.

*Pre-clinical safety data:* No further data given.

### Pharmaceutical particulars

*List of excipients:* Hypromellose (4500) BP; Benzalkonium Chloride Solution BP; Purified Water BP.

*Incompatibilities:* None known.

*Shelf life:* The shelf life shall not exceed 24 months from the date of manufacture.

*Special precautions for storage:* To be stored between 15° and 25°C. Once opened the contents should be used within 24 hours of opening.

*Nature and contents of container:* Polypropylene tubes each fitted with a plastic screw cap and tamper-evident seal and enclosed within a printed cardboard carton. Single tubes may sometimes be supplied without a carton. Pack sizes: 15 mg (packs of 12) and 30 mg (available in single units).

*Instruction for use/handling :* None given.

**Marketing authorisation number** 11314/0090.

**Date of approval/revision of SPC** January 1997.

**Legal category** POM.

## MEDINOL*
## PAEDIATRIC PARACETAMOL ORAL SUSPENSION BP 120 mg/5 ml

**Presentation** A strawberry flavoured sugar and colour free suspension containing 120 mg of Paracetamol BP in each 5 ml dose.

**Uses** For the relief of pain and feverish conditions.

**Dosage and administration** To be taken four times daily. Do not repeat dose more frequently than every 4 hours. Do not take more than four doses in 24 hours.

*Children 1-5 years:* Two 5 ml spoonfuls.

*Infants 3 months to 1 year:* Half to one 5 ml spoonful.

*Infants under 3 months:* A 2.5 ml dose is suitable for babies who develop a fever following vaccination at 2 months. In other cases use only under medical supervision. Not to be given to infants under 2 months except on medical advice. If a baby was born prematurely and is less than 3 months old, the doctor should be consulted before use

**Contra-indications, warnings, etc**
*Contra-indications:* Use with caution in patients with impaired kidney or liver function.

*Drug interactions:* Cholestyramine may reduce absorption of paracetamol. Metoclopramide and domperidone may accelerate the absorption of paracetamol. Alcohol, barbiturates, anticonvulsants and tricyclic antidepressants may increase the hepatotoxicity of paracetamol particularly after an overdose.

*Side-effects and adverse reactions:* If given in therapeutic doses, side effects are rare. Haematological reactions have been reported. Skin reactions and other allergic reactions occur occasionally. Most reports of adverse reactions to paracetamol relate to overdosage with the drug.

*Use in pregnancy and lactation:* There is epidemiological evidence of the safety of paracetamol in human pregnancy. Medinol may be taken during pregnancy and lactation.

*Other special precautions and warnings:* If pain and fever persists for more than 3 days, a doctor should be consulted. Prolonged use without medical supervision may be harmful. In case of accidental overdose medical attention should be sought immediately. The stated dose must not be exceeded.

*Overdose:* An overdose should be treated as soon as possible (within 12 hours) as liver damage from an overdose does not become apparent for 1 to 6 hours after ingestion. Initial symptoms include pallor, nausea, vomiting, anorexia and abdominal pain. Medical attention should be sought. After gastric lavage a suitable antidote such as acetylcysteine or methionine should be given. Acetylcysteine is given by intravenous fluid in an initial dose of 150 mg/kg bodyweight over 15 minutes, followed by 50 mg/kg over 4 hours and then by 100 mg/kg over the next 16 hours. Alternatively, methionine 2.5 g may be given by mouth every 4 hours to a total of four doses. The blood paracetamol levels should be monitored to determine whether further therapy is necessary.

**Pharmaceutical precautions**
*Storage:* Store below 25°C. Extremes of temperature should be avoided.

**Legal category** P.

**Package quantities** Bottles of 100 ml, 150 ml, 200 ml and 1 litre.

**Further information** Medinol is suitable for use by diabetics. Medinol is free of animal fat and alcohol so it is suitable for children with specific dietary requirements.

**Product licence number** 0338/0033
*Name and address of product licence holder:* Cupal Limited (a subsidiary of Seton Healthcare Group plc), King Street, Blackburn BB2 2DX.

## PRIODERM* CREAM SHAMPOO

**Qualitative and quantitative composition** Prioderm Cream Shampoo contains Malathion USP 1.0% w/w.

**Pharmaceutical form** Cream shampoo.

**Clinical particulars**

*Therapeutic indications:* The source of infestation should be sought and treated. For the treatment of head lice and pubic lice infestation.

*Posology and method of administration:* For topical external use only.
*Adults, the elderly and children aged 6 months and over:* As this product does not contain alcohol, it may be more suitable for those with asthma or eczema.

*For head lice:* Wet the hair thoroughly with warm water and apply sufficient shampoo to work up a rich lather and ensure that no part of the scalp is uncovered. Pay special attention to the back of the neck and the area behind the ears. Take care to avoid the eyes. Leave for at least five minutes. Rinse thoroughly with clean warm water and repeat procedure. While hair is still wet, comb with an ordinary comb. The fine-toothed louse comb can then be used to remove the dead lice and eggs. This treatment should be carried out a total of three times at three day intervals, and should not be repeated within a 3 week period.

*For pubic lice:* Application and dosage are as for the head. Apply the lotion to the pubic hair and the hair between the legs and anus.

*Children aged 6 months and under:* On medical advice only.

*Contra-indications:* None stated.

*Special warnings and precautions for use:* As with all shampoos, avoid contact with the eyes. Children under 6 months should only be treated under medical supervision. When Prioderm Cream Shampoo is used by a school nurse or other health officer in the mass treatment of large numbers of children, it is advisable that protective plastic or rubber gloves be worn. Continued prolonged treatment with this product should be avoided. It should not be used for more than three times at three day intervals, and then not repeated within a three week period. Keep out of the reach of children.

*Interactions with other medicaments and other forms of interaction:* None stated.

*Pregnancy and lactation:* Prioderm Cream Shampoo is not known to have any effect on fertility, pregnancy and lactation. Its use in pregnant or lactating women is not recommended unless there is an overdue need.

*Effects on ability to drive and use machines:* None stated.

*Undesirable effects:* None stated.

*Overdose:* In the event of deliberate or accidental ingestion, empty stomach contents by gastric lavage and keep patient warm. In the event of massive ingestion, atropine or pralidoxime may be required to counteract cholinesterase inhibition.

**Pharmacological properties**
*Pharmacodynamic properties:* Prioderm Cream

Shampoo contains malathion, a widely used organophosphorus insecticide which is active by cholinesterase inhibition. It is effective against a wide range of insects, but is one of the least toxic organophosphorus insecticides since it is rapidly detoxified by plasma carboxylesterases.

*Pharmacokinetic properties:* Prioderm Cream Shampoo is applied topically to the affected area.

*Pre-clinical safety data:* None stated.

**Pharmaceutical particulars**
*List of excipients:* sodium lauryl sulphate paste; cetostearyl alcohol; lauric diethanolamide; ethoxylated lanolin (50%); methyl hydroxybenzoate; propyl hydroxybenzoate; hydrochloric acid; citric acid (anhydrous); dibasic sodium phosphate; colour yellow (E110); sodium edetate; perfume M&B 1658; purified water.

*Incompatibilities:* None stated.

*Shelf life:* 18 months.

*Special precautions for storage:* Store at or below 20°C.

*Nature and contents of container:* Cartoned, internally lacquered aluminium tube with polyethylene caps containing 40 g of product.

*Instruction for use/handling:* None stated.

**Marketing authorisation number** 11314/0051.

**Date of approval/revision of SPC** October 1995.

**Legal category** P.

## PRIODERM* LOTION

**Qualitative and quantitative composition** Prioderm Lotion contains Malathion USP 0.5% w/v.

**Pharmaceutical form** Topical solution.

**Clinical particulars**

*Therapeutic indications:* For the treatment of head lice and pubic lice infestation, and scabies.

*Posology and method of administration:*
*Adults, the elderly and children aged 6 months and above:* For topical external use only. The source of infestation should be sought and treated.

*For head lice* Sprinkle the lotion on the hair and rub gently onto the head until the entire scalp is moistened. Pay special attention to the back of the neck and behind the ears. Take care to avoid the eyes. Allow to dry naturally using no heat.
As all lice and eggs will have been killed, the hair may be shampooed after 2 hours. If a residual effect is required, however, it is recommended that shampooing be carried out after 12 hours.
Whilst still wet, comb the hair with an ordinary comb. A fine toothed louse comb can then be used to remove the dead lice and eggs.
*For pubic lice* Application and dosage are as for the head. Apply the lotion to the pubic hair and the hair around the legs and around the anus. Allow to dry naturally using no heat. Transient, mild stinging may be experienced due to the alcohol content.
*For scabies* Use cotton wool to apply the lotion to all parts of the body except the face and scalp. Rub in well and allow to dry naturally. Do not bathe until 12 hours after treatment.
*Infants:* Infants under the age of 6 months should be treated under medical supervision.

*Contra-indications:* None stated.

*Special warnings and precautions for use:* Prioderm Lotion contains isopropyl alcohol which may cause wheezing in asthmatic patients or cause inflammation of the skin in patients with severe eczema.
Contains flammable alcohol. Apply and dry with care. Avoid naked flames or lighted objects. Do not use artificial heat (eg electric hairdryers). Dry in a well ventilated room. Do not cover the head before the lotion has dried completely. The hair should be dry before retiring to bed.
Children under six months should only be treated under medical supervision. When Prioderm Lotion is used by a school nurse or other health officer in the mass treatment of large numbers of children, it is advisable that protective plastic or rubber gloves be worn.
Continued prolonged treatment with this product should be avoided. It should not be used for more than once a week for three weeks at a time.
In the event of contact with the eyes, rinse thoroughly with water. If there is persistent irritation, seek medical advice immediately.

*Interactions with other medicaments and other forms of interaction:* None stated.

*Pregnancy and lactation:* There are no known adverse effects in human pregnancy and lactation. However, as with all drugs, it should be used with caution in pregnant and lactating women.

*Effects on ability to drive and use machines:* None stated.

*Undesirable effects:* Some patients may experience stinging or inflammation of the skin due to the alcohol content.

*Overdose:* In the event of deliberate or accidental ingestion, empty stomach contents by gastric lavage and keep patient warm. In the event of massive ingestion, atropine and pralidoxime may be required to counteract cholinesterase inhibition.

**Pharmacological properties**

*Pharmacodynamic properties:* Prioderm Lotion contains malathion, a widely used organophosphorous insecticide which is active by cholinesterase inhibition. It is effective against a wide range of insects, but is one of the least toxic organophosphorous insecticides since it is rapidly detoxified by plasma carboxylesterases.

*Pharmacokinetic properties:* Prioderm Lotion is applied topically to the affected area.

*Preclinical safety data:* None stated.

**Pharmaceutical particulars**
*List of excipients:* Golden delicious perfume P15498; isopropyl myristate; isopropanol.

*Incompatibilities:* None stated.

*Shelf life:* Two years.

*Special precautions for storage:* Store at or below 20°C.

*Nature and contents of container:* Cartoned, clear glass bottles with polyethylene caps and polyethylene sprinkler inserts or clear soda glass sprinkler bottles with polypropylene caps containing either 55 or 160 ml of product.

*Instructions for use/handling:* None stated.

**Marketing authorisation number** 11314/0052.

**Date of approval/revision of SPC** October 1995.

**Legal category** P.

## PRIPSEN* MEBENDAZOLE TABLETS

**Qualitative and quantitative composition** Pripsen Mebendazole Tablets contain Mebendazole USP 100 mg.

**Pharmaceutical form** Tablets.

**Clinical particulars**

*Therapeutic indications:* For the treatment of threadworm (enterobiasis) infection.

*Posology and method of administration:*
*Adults, the elderly and children over two years of age:* One tablet to be chewed or swallowed whole. The efficacy in threadworm infestations is such that treatment failure will be rare. However, the possibility of re-infection means that some patients may require a second tablet after two weeks, if re-infected. It is strongly recommended that all members of the family are treated at the same time.
*Children under two years of age:* Not recommended.

*Contra-indications:* Pregnancy. Mebendazole has not been studied extensively in children under two years of age—for this reason it is not currently recommended for children under two years of age.

*Special warnings and precautions for use:* Not to be taken during pregnancy or whilst breast feeding. Not recommended for children under two years of age. Keep out of the reach of children. If, after two weeks, you need to take the second tablet, following which your symptoms persist, then consult your doctor.

*Interactions with other medicaments and other forms of interaction:* None stated.

*Pregnancy and lactation:* Mebendazole has shown embryotoxic and teratogenic activity in rats at single oral doses. No such findings have been reported in the rabbit, dog, sheep or horse. Since there is a risk that mebendazole could produce foetal damage if taken during pregnancy, it is contraindicated in pregnant women. No information on secretion into breast milk is available so mothers taking the drug should not breast feed.

*Effects on ability to drive and use machines:* No known effects.

*Undesirable effects:* Side effects reported have been minor. Transient abdominal pain and diarrhoea have been reported only rarely in cases of massive infestation and expulsion of worms. (Slight headache and dizziness have been occasionally reported.)

*Overdose:* No cases of overdose have so far been reported with mebendazole but gastric lavage and/or supportive measures would be recommended. Symptoms of acute overdosage would be expected to include gastrointestinal disturbances, abdominal pain, headache, dizziness, pyrexia and convulsions.

**Pharmacological properties**

*Pharmacodynamic properties:* Mebendazole is an anthelmintic.

*Pharmacokinetic properties:* Mebendazole is poorly absorbed from the gastrointestinal tract (5–10%) and undergoes extensive first pass elimination, being metabolised in the liver, eliminated in the bile as unchanged drug and metabolites and excreted in the faeces. Only about 2% of the drug is excreted unchanged or as metabolites in the urine. Mebendazole is highly protein bound.

*Pre-clinical safety data:* None stated.

**Pharmaceutical particulars**

*List of excipients:* sorbitol; Jaffa Orange 61001E; magnesium stearate; povidone; maize starch; Acdisol; sodium saccharin; water.

*Incompatibilities:* None stated.

*Shelf life:* Three years.

*Special precautions for storage:* Store below 25°C in a dry place.

*Nature and contents of container:* 250 micron white, opaque, rigid, uPVC 20μ aluminium foil blisters in cardboard cartons in packs of two or eight tablets.

*Instruction for use/handling:* Not applicable

*Marketing authorisation holder:* Cupal Limited (A subsidiary of Seton Healthcare Group plc), King Street, Blackburn, Lancashire BB2 2DX.

**Marketing authorisation number** 0338/0084.

**Date of approval/ revision of SPC** February 1997.

**Legal category** P.

## PRIPSEN* PIPERAZINE CITRATE ELIXIR

**Qualitative and quantitative composition** A clear, colourless, orange flavoured liquid containing, in each 5 ml, 750 mg of Piperazine Hydrate (as Citrate).

**Pharmaceutical form** Oral liquid.

**Clinical particulars**

*Therapeutic indications:* To expel enterobiasis (threadworms) and ascariasis (roundworms) from the gastrointestinal tract.

*Posology and method of administration:*

*To expel threadworms:* Dosage to be taken daily for 7 days. It may be necessary to repeat the dosage after 7 days for a further 7 days.
*Adults, the elderly and children over 12 years of age:* Three 5 ml spoonfuls.
  *Children:*
  7-12 years of age: Two 5 ml spoonfuls
  4-6 years of age: One and a half 5 ml spoonfuls
  1-3 years of age: One 5 ml spoonful
  Under 1 year of age: On medical advice only

*To expel roundworms:* Dosage to be taken as a single dose and then repeated after 14 days.
*Adults, the elderly and children over 12 years of age:* Six 5 ml spoonfuls.
  *Children:* 9-12 years of age: Five 5 ml spoonfuls
  6-8 years of age: Four 5 ml spoonfuls
  4-5 years of age: Three 5 ml spoonfuls
  1-3 years of age: Two 5 ml spoonfuls
  Under 1 year of age: On medical advice

*Contra-indications:* Liver disease, epilepsy, and impaired renal function

*Special warnings and precautions for use:* If you are pregnant or think you may be pregnant or if you are currently taking any other medicine, do not take this product without the advice of your doctor. Do not take this product if you have kidney disease or have ever suffered from epilepsy. Keep out of the reach of children.

*Interactions with other medicaments and other forms of interaction:* Piperazine potentiates the extrapyramidal effects of chlorpromazine. Care should therefore be taken when giving piperazine to patients taking phenothiazines.

*Pregnancy and lactation:* The safety of piperazine use in pregnancy has not been established, but foetal toxicity studies in animals and extensive clinical experience have shown rare instances of teratogenicity if used in the first trimester of pregnancy. Therefore, this product should not be taken during pregnancy. Piperazine may be excreted in the breast milk.

*Effects on ability to drive and use machines:* None known.

*Undesirable effects:* These are uncommon but the following reactions have been reported: nausea, vomiting, diarrhoea, abdominal pain, headache, paraesthesia and urticaria. These usually disappear rap-

idly when treatment is stopped. Neurotoxicity has also been reported. Case reports of purpura in a glucose-6-phosphate dehydrogenase deficient individual after piperazine administration appear in the literature.

*Overdose:* Symptoms are similar to the side effects listed under Undesirable effects and can usually be expected to resolve spontaneously. On severe poisoning the stomach may be emptied by aspiration and lavage. Adequate fluids and routine supportive measures should be given. Convulsions can be controlled by intravenous diazepam or a short-acting barbiturate such as thiopentone.

**Pharmacological properties**

*Pharmacodynamic properties* : Pripsen Piperazine Citrate Elixir contains Piperazine Citrate BP equivalent to Piperazine Hydrate BP 750 mg/5 ml. This is an anthelmintic useful for the treatment of enterobiasis and ascariasis infections in children and adults. In ascaris infections, piperazine produces a reversible muscle paralysis and the worms are easily dislodged from the gut by peristaltic motion and expelled in the faeces. Piperazine affects all stages of the parasite in the gut but appears to have little or no effect on larvae in the tissues. Little is known of the effects of piperazine on enterobiasis infections.

*Pharmacokinetic properties:* None stated.

*Pre-clinical safety data:* None stated.

**Pharmaceutical particulars**

*List of excipients:* Sucrose BP; Alcohol (96%) BP; Soluble Jaffa Essence 7300035E; Citric Acid Monohydrate BP; water.

*Incompatibilities:* Alkaloidal salts and salts of copper and iron.

*Shelf life:* Three years.

*Special precautions for storage:* Store below 25°C.

*Nature and contents of container:* Amber glass Sirop bottles with white polypropylene closures with EPE liners in cardboard cartons. Bottles of 140 ml.

*Instruction for use/handling:* Not applicable.

*Marketing authorisation holder:* Cupal Ltd (A subsidiary of Seton Healthcare Group plc), Tubiton House, Oldham OL1 3HS.

**Marketing authorisation number** 0338/5059R.

**Date of approval/revision of SPC** February 1995.

**Legal category** P.

## PRIPSEN* PIPERAZINE PHOSPHATE POWDER

**Qualitative and quantitative composition** Pripsen Powder contains:
  Piperazine Phosphate BP 4.0 mg
  Standardised Senna Pods 15.3 mg (calculated as total sennoside powder).

**Pharmaceutical form** Powder.

**Clinical particulars**

*Therapeutic indications:* For the eradication of enterobiasis (pinworm, threadworm) and ascariasis (roundworm).

*Posology and method of administration:*
*When treating threadworms:* Adults and children over 6: One sachet. Children aged 1-6 years: 1 level 5 ml spoonful of sachet contents. Infants 3 months–1 year: To be taken only when prescribed by a doctor. 1 level 2.5 ml spoonful of sachet contents. There is no indication that dosage be modified for the elderly.

Pripsen should be stirred into a small glass of milk or water and drunk immediately. It should be taken at bed-time by adults and in the morning by children. The dose should be repeated after 14 days. For children under 10 years of age, only one dual dose should be given in any 28 day period without seeking medical advice.

*When treating roundworms:* Adults and children over 6: One sachet. *Children aged 1-6 years:* 1 level 5 ml spoonful of sachet contents. *Infants 3 months–1 year:* To be taken only when prescribed by a doctor. 1 level 2.5 ml spoonful of sachet contents. There is no indication that dosage be modified for the elderly.

Pripsen should be stirred into a small glass of milk or water and drunk immediately. It should be taken at bed-time by adults and in the morning by children. For children under 10 years of age, only one dual dose should be given in any 28 day period without seeking medical advice.

Additional single prophylactic doses at regular monthly intervals up to three months may be necessary to eliminate the risk of re-infection.

*Contra-indications:* Pripsen Piperazine Phosphate Powder is contra-indicated in patients suffering from epilepsy, severe bilateral renal dysfunction, hepatic dysfunction, known sensitivity to piperazine, undi-

agnosed painful abdominal symptoms which may be due to acute appendicitis, and/or other acute surgical conditions, such as intestinal obstruction or acute inflammatory bowel disease, the ileus, and in severe dehydration states with water and electrolyte depletion.

*Other special warnings and precautions::* The product labelling includes the following:

If you believe you may be pregnant, or are taking a prescribed medicine, consult your doctor before using this product. Do not take Pripsen Piperazine Phosphate Powder if you have kidney disease or have ever suffered from epilepsy. Prolonged use of this product should be avoided.

*Interactions with other medicaments and other forms of interaction:* Pyrantel pamoate antagonises the mode of action of piperazine and therefore should not be co-administered. Although caution should be exercised when co-administering phenothiazine or tricyclic anti-depressants due to a possible interaction, this has not been shown to be a problem in clinical practice. Concomitant use of Pripsen Piperazine Phosphate Powder with diuretics, cardiac glycosides or adrenocorticosteroids may enhance electrolyte imbalance.

*Use in pregnancy and lactation:* : Isolated instances of foetal malformation have been reported but no causal relationship to piperazine has ever been established. Use in the first trimester of pregnancy is therefore not advised. Unless symptoms warrant immediate treatment, the administration of Pripsen Piperazine Phosphate Powder should be postponed until after parturition. Piperazine is excreted in breast milk but no unwanted effects in the infant have been reported. To minimise the amount of piperazine ingested by the baby, it is recommended that the infant be fed immediately before taking Pripsen Piperazine Phosphate Powder, then eight hours allowed before breast feeding is resumed. During this eight hour period, milk should be expressed and discarded at the usual feeding interval.

*Effects on ability to drive and use machines:* None known.

*Undesirable effects:* Unwanted effects resulting from Pripsen Piperazine Phosphate Powder therapy are rare. When such reactions do occur, the most frequent are firstly allergic in nature, such as rash, urticaria, itching or rarely bronchospasm, or secondly mild gastrointestinal disturbances such as nausea, vomiting, colic or diarrhoea. A few cases of neurotoxic reactions have been reported, such as drowsiness, confusion, or clonic contractions if administered in the presence of neurological or renal abnormalities. Others such as dizziness, ataxia, tremors, choreoform movement, hyporeflexia, nystagmus, vertigo and blurred vision have been reported in normal subjects. Isolated cases of Stevens Johnson Syndrome and angioneurotic oedema, including arthralgia and fever have also been reported.

*Overdose:* Mild symptoms would be expected from overdose of Pripsen Piperazine Phosphate Powder being either gastrointestinal (diarrhoea, nausea, vomiting) or neurological (muscular hypotonia, ataxia and vertigo). General supportive measures including maintenance of an adequate fluid intake should be adopted and, if necessary, anti-convulsant therapy administered. Particular attention should be paid to correcting electrolyte imbalance.

**Pharmacological properties**

*Pharmacodynamic properties:* The piperazine in Pripsen Powder is believed to paralyse the worms which are then evacuated by the laxative *action of standardised* senna.

*Pharmacokinetic properties:* The therapeutic action of Pripsen occurs within the lumen of the gastrointestinal tract, which is independent of any systemic absorption.

*Preclinical safety data:*
(a) Senna
  *Single dose toxicity:* Senna as crude drug or extracts, as well as sennosides and rhein, showed low acute toxicity in rats and mice after oral treatment.
  *Repeated dose toxicity:* Sennosides showed no specific toxicity when tested at up to 500 mg/kg in dogs for four weeks and up to 100 mg/kg in rats for six months.
  *Reproductive toxicity:* There was no evidence of any embryolethal, teratogenic or fetotoxic actions in rats and rabbits after oral treatment with sennosides. Furthermore, there was no effect on the postnatal development of young rats, on the rearing behaviour of dams or on male and female fertility in rats.
  *Genotoxicity:* Results from in vitro and in vivo genotoxicity studies as well as human and animal pharmacokinetic data indicate no genotoxic risk from senna.
  *Carcinogenicity:* A senna extract given orally for

two years was not carcinogenic in male and female rats.

(b) Piperazine phosphate: Piperazine has very low toxicity in mammals and in the doses used clinically there is no specific organ damage or general toxicity. No adequate teratogenicity studies have been conducted but one dose studies did not produce evidence of foetal malformation in the rat and rabbit. No carcinogenicity tests have been performed.

### Pharmaceutical particulars
List of excipients: vanilla flavour; caramel flavour; raspberry flavour; saccharin; Hexacol natural carmine.

Incompatibilities: None known.

Shelf life: Two years.

Special precautions for storage: Store at or below 25°C in a dry place.

Nature and contents of container: Sachets comprised of polythene/aluminium foil/paper laminate/surlyn, cut into pairs. One pair of sachets in a cardboard outer carton.

Marketing authorisation number    11314/0029.

Date of approval/revision of SPC    October 1994.

Legal category P.

## STERIPOD* CHLORHEXIDINE GLUCONATE 0.05% W/V

Presentation Steripod Chlorhexidine Gluconate is a sterile solution of Chlorhexidine Gluconate 0.05% w/v BP in Purified Water BP. The preparation is a clear pale pink pyrogen-free solution supplied in disposable, sealed, blow-moulded, semi-rigid containers made from polyethylene.

Uses Steripod Chlorhexidine Gluconate is a topical antimicrobial cleansing solution for the swabbing of wounds and burns and in obstetrics.

### Dosage and administration
Adults and children: Apply undiluted.

### Contra-indications, warnings, etc
Contra-indications: Steripod Chlorhexidine Gluconate is not suitable for use as an injection. It is contraindicated in patients who have previously shown a hypersensitivity reaction to chlorhexidine. However, such reactions are rare. Steripod Chlorhexidine Gluconate is for external use only. Do not allow contact with the eyes, brain, meninges or middle ear.

Precautions: Do not use in body cavities, or as an enema. If chlorhexidine solution comes into contact with the eyes, wash out thoroughly and promptly with water.

Drug interactions: Chlorhexidine is incompatible with soaps and other anionic materials. This product will also be incompatible with borates, bicarbonates, carbonates, chlorides, citrates, phosphates and sulphates. Fabrics which have been in contact with chlorhexidine will be stained when bleached with hypochlorite.

Side-effects and adverse reactions: Generalised allergenic reactions to chlorhexidine have been reported but are extremely rare.

Other special precautions and warnings: Do not use unless the product is clear or if there is any evidence of leaking prior to breaking the seal. Check for leaks by squeezing the Steripod before use. Discard any surplus.

Overdose: Chlorhexidine is poorly absorbed following oral ingestion. Do not induce vomiting. Treat with gastric lavage, using milk, egg white, gelatin, or mild soap and employ appropriate supportive measures.

Pharmaceutical precautions Steripod Chlorhexidine Gluconate should be stored between 5 and 25°C.

Legal category P

Package quantities    Cartons of 25 x 20 ml ampoules.

Further information The Steripod is designed to overcome the inherent disadvantages of sachets. Solution application is more controllable and more easily directed to the desired area. The Steripod opening is designed to reduce the risk of touch contamination, and is opened simply by twisting off the top. Once opened, unlike a sachet, a Steripod will stand upright on a flat surface without loss of solution. Simple instructions on the use of the Steripod are reproduced on the carton.

For safe disposal, empty the contents and incinerate at a minimum of 400°C or landfill at an approved site.

Product licence number    11314/0007

## STERIPOD* CHLORHEXIDINE GLUCONATE 0.015% w/v with CETRIMIDE 0.15% w/v

Presentation Steripod Chlorhexidine/Cetrimide is a sterile solution containing Chlorhexidine Gluconate BP 0.015% w/v and Cetrimide PhEur 0.15% w/v in Purified Water BP. The preparation is a clear, yellow, pyrogen-free solution supplied in disposable, sealed, blow-moulded, semi-rigid containers made from polyethylene. Steripod is filled under aseptic conditions.

Uses Steripod Chlorhexidine/Cetrimide is a topical antimicrobial cleansing agent used for the antiseptic treatment of wounds and burns, and for swabbing.

### Dosage and administration
Adults and children: Apply undiluted.

### Contra-indications, warnings, etc
Contra-indications: Steripod Chlorhexidine/Cetrimide is not suitable for use as an injection. It is contraindicated in patients who have previously shown a hypersensitivity to chlorhexidine or cetrimide. However such reactions are extremely rare. For external use only. Do not allow contact with the eyes, brain, meninges or middle ear.

Precautions: If chlorhexidine/cetrimide solutions come into contact with the eyes, wash out thoroughly and promptly with water. Do not use unless the product is clear or if there is any evidence of leaking prior to breaking the seal. Check for leaks by squeezing the Steripod before use. Discard any surplus.

Drug interactions: Chlorhexidine is incompatible with soaps and other anionic agents. This product will also be incompatible with borates, bicarbonates, carbonates, chlorides, citrates, phosphates and sulphates. Fabrics which have been in contact with chlorhexidine will be stained when bleached with hypochlorite.

Side-effects and adverse reactions: Occasional skin sensitivity to chlorhexidine/cetrimide preparations have been reported. Generalised allergenic reactions to chlorhexidine have been reported but are extremely rare. In all cases, stop application of the product.

Overdose: Chlorhexidine is poorly absorbed following oral ingestion. Do not induce vomiting. Treat with gastric lavage, using milk, egg white, gelatin, or mild soap and employ appropriate supportive measures.

Pharmaceutical precautions Steripod Chlorhexidine/Cetrimide should be stored between 5 and 25°C.

Legal category  P

Package quantities Cartons of 25 x 20 ml ampoules.

Further information The Steripod is designed to overcome the inherent disadvantages of sachets. Solution application is more controllable and more easily directed to the desired area. The Steripod opening is designed to reduce the risk of touch contamination, and is opened simply by twisting off the top. Once opened, unlike a sachet, a Steripod will stand upright on a flat surface without loss of solution. Simple instructions on the use of the Steripod are reproduced on the carton. For safe disposal, empty the contents and incinerate at a minimum of 400°C or landfill at an approved site.

Product licence number 11314/0005

## STER-ZAC* BATH CONCENTRATE

Qualitative and quantitative composition Triclosan 2% w/v.

Pharmaceutical form    A clear liquid preparation presented in 28.5 ml and 500 ml.

### Clinical particulars
Therapeutic indications: This product has an antibacterial effect in water and is intended for the prevention of cross infection and secondary infection.

Posology and method of administration: For bathing: Add 28.5 ml of Ster-Zac Bath Concentrate to a bathful of water (approximately 140 litres) immediately prior to the patient entering the water.

For washing: Add 1 ml of Ster-Zac Bath Concentrate to 5 litres of water, prior to use. No dosage recommendations are made for administration to the elderly or children.

Contra-indications: Not to be used for pregnant women.

Special warnings and precautions for use: For external use only. Keep out of the reach of children. Avoid contact with the eyes.

Interactions with other medicaments and other forms of interaction: None stated.

Pregnancy and lactation: Not to be used for pregnant women.

Effects on ability to drive and use machines: None stated.

Undesirable effects: Erythema may arise in some patients with allergy problems.

Overdose: If erythema or other skin rashes occur, rinse thoroughly with water. Seek medical advice if the condition worsens.

### Pharmacological properties
Pharmacodynamic properties: Triclosan is a bactericide.

Pharmacokinetic properties: None stated.

Pre-clinical safety data: None stated.

### Pharmaceutical particulars
List of excipients: Industrial Methylated Spirit BP; Isopropyl Alcohol BP; Dioctyl Sodium Sulphosuccinate 60%; Tetrasodium EDTA and Triethanolamide; Deionised Water.

Incompatibilities: None stated.

Shelf life: Shelf life of the product for sale – 36 months. Shelf life after first opening the container – none stated.

Special precautions for storage: Store in a cool place.

Nature and contents of container: High density polyethylene container with either a polypropylene cap or a compression moulded screw cap with a steran faced liner.

Marketing authorisation number    11314/0098

Date of approval/revision of SPC    May 1997

Legal category    GSL

## STER-ZAC* DC SKIN CLEANSER

Presentation A white cream. Contains 3% Hexachlorophane BP.

Uses Ster-Zac DC has an antibacterial effect and is used for the preoperative preparation of the hands.

Indications For the preoperative disinfection of the hands of surgical personnel.

Dosage and administration For external use only. Apply 3 ml to 5 ml to pre-moistened hands and wash for up to three minutes. Rinse and repeat.

Contra-indications To be administered to children under two years of age on medical advice only. Do not use for whole body bathing. Do not apply to burns and badly damaged skin. For external use only. If swallowed, gastric aspiration and lavage. Not to be used during pregnancy.

Pharmaceutical precautions No special requirements.

Legal category POM

Package quantities 150 ml.

Further information Ster-Zac DC Skin Cleanser is resistant to contamination in use.

Product licence number 0423/0007.
Product licence holder: Houghs Healthcare Ltd, 20-22 Chapel Street, Levenshulme, Manchester M19 3PT.

## STER-ZAC* POWDER

Presentation A white dusting powder containing 0.33% Hexachlorophane BP.

Uses For the prevention of neo-natal staphylococcal cross infection. As an adjunct for the treatment of recurrent furunculosis. For routine whole trunk application for ward use in maternity hospitals and in domicilliary midwifery.

### Dosage and administration
For the prevention of neo-natal staphylococcal cross infection: Immediately after ligature, dust the cord and surrounding area and apply the powder to the perineum, buttocks, flexures and axillae. Repeat at each napkin change until the cord stump has dropped away and the wound has healed.

For the treatment of furunculosis: Dust the affected area and surrounds regularly.

Contra-indications, warnings etc The product should be administered to children under two years of age on medical advice only. The product should not be administered during pregnancy. For external use only. Do not use on badly excoriated skin.

Pharmaceutical precautions No special requirements.

Legal category  P.

Package quantities    Sprinkler tins of 30 g.

Further information May be used on full term and premature infants and low birth weight infants provided that the skin is undamaged.

Product licence number    1314/0100

## SULEO-C* LOTION

**Qualitative and quantitative composition** Suleo-C Lotion contains carbaryl 0.5% w/w.

**Pharmaceutical form** Lotion.

**Clinical particulars**

*Therapeutic indications:* Eradication of head lice infestation.

*Posology and method of administration:*
Adults, the elderly and children aged 6 months and above: For topical external use only.

Rub the lotion gently into the scalp until all the hair and scalp is thoroughly moistened. Allow to dry naturally in a well ventilated room. Do not use a hairdryer or other artificial heat. Live lice will be eradicated after a minimum treatment period of two hours. However the lotion should be left on the head for a period of 10-12 hours to ensure that all eggs are totally eradicated. Shampoo in the normal manner. Rinse and comb the hair while wet to remove the dead lice. In the event of early re-infestation, Suleo-C Lotion may be applied again provided 7 days have elapsed since the first application. Residual protective effect is variable of short duration and should not be relied upon. Not to be used on children under six months of age except on medical advice.

*Contra-indications:* Known sensitivity to carbaryl. Not to be used on infants under six months of age except on medical advice.

*Special warnings and precautions for use:* Avoid contact with the eyes. Do not cover the head until the hair has dried completely. It is advisable that nursing staff involved in repeated applications should wear rubber gloves when carrying out treatment. Suleo-C Lotion is for external use only and should be kept out of reach of children. Keep away from exposed flame or lighted objects (e.g. cigarettes, gas and electric fires) during application and while the hair is wet. Continued prolonged treatment with Suleo-C Lotion should be avoided. It should not be used more than once a week for three weeks at a time. Alcohol based skin products may cause a stinging sensation on patients with sensitive skin.

The feeding of carbaryl to rats and mice throughout life led to an increased incidence of benign and malignant tumours only at very high doses. However, a range of in vivo and in vitro mutagenicity test have indicated that carbaryl is not genotoxic. These findings suggest that use of carbaryl to treat louse infestations is unlikely to pose a significant cancer risk in humans.

*Interactions with other medicaments and other forms of interaction:* None known.

*Pregnancy and lactation:* No evidence of safety of this product has been determined in pregnancy and lactation. It is not necessary to contraindicate this product in pregnancy and lactation provided caution is exercised and the directions for use are followed. However, as with all medicines, the advice of a doctor should be sought before the product is used.

*Effects on ability to drive and use machines :* None stated.

*Undesirable effects :* Very rarely, skin irritation has been reported with carbaryl products.

*Overdose:* Accidental ingestion: gastric lavage, assisted by respiration and, if necessary administration of atropine.

**Pharmacological properties**

*Pharmacodynamic properties:* The action of carbamates is to inhibit the acetylcholinesterases present at synaptic junctions within the insect's nervous system.

*Pharmacokinetic properties:* Suleo-C Lotion is applied topically to the affected area.

*Preclinical safety data:* None stated.

**Pharmaceutical particulars**

*List of excipients:* Isopropyl Alcohol IPSI BP; D-Limonene 17449 ; Terpineol 18689 BP; Shellsol T; Colour Blue 12401; Perfume Loxol P6160; Citric Acid PhEur.

*Incompatibilities:* None stated.

*Shelf life:* Two years.

*Special precautions for storage:* Store at or below 25°C. Protect from sunlight.

*Nature and contents of container:* Clear or amber glass bottles with LDPE caps with HDPE sprinkle plug inserts. The clear glass bottles will be marketed in cartons. Bottles of 50 and 250 ml.

*Instructions for use/handling:* None stated.

**Marketing authorisation number** 11314/0053.

**Date of approval/revision of SPC** June 1997.

**Legal category** POM

## SULEO-M* LOTION

**Qualitative and quantitative composition** Malathion 0.5% w/v.

**Pharmaceutical form** Lotion.

**Clinical particulars**

*Therapeutic indications:* For the eradication of head lice infestation.

*Posology and method of administration:*
Adults, the elderly and children aged 6 months and over : For topical external use only. Rub the lotion gently into the scalp until all the hair and scalp is thoroughly moistened. Allow to dry naturally in a well ventilated room. Do not use a hairdryer or other artificial heat. Live lice will be eradicated after a minimum treatment period of two hours. However the lotion should be left on the head for a further period of 8-10 hours to ensure that all lice eggs are totally eradicated. Shampoo in the normal manner. Rinse and comb the hair while wet to remove the dead lice. In the event of early re-infestation, Suleo-M Lotion may be applied again provided 7 days have elapsed since the first application. Residual protective effect is variable of short duration and should not be relied upon.

*Infants:* Infants under the age of six months should be treated under medical supervision.

*Contra-indications:* Known sensitivity to malathion. Not to be used on infants under six months of age except on medical advice.

*Special warnings and precautions for use:* Suleo-M Lotion contains isopropyl alcohol which may cause wheezing in asthmatic patients or cause inflammation of the skin in patients with severe eczema. Contains flammable alcohol. Apply and dry with care. Avoid naked flames or lighted objects. Do not use artificial heat (e.g. electric hairdryers). Dry in a well ventilated room. Do not cover the head before the lotion has dried completely. The eyes should be well protected during the application and washing of the hair. In the event of contact with the eyes, rinse thoroughly with water. If there is persistent irritation, medical advice should be sought immediately. When Suleo-M Lotion is used by a school nurse or other health officer in the mass treatment of large numbers of children, it is advisable that protective plastic or rubber gloves be worn. Continuous prolonged treatment with this product should be avoided. It should not be used for more than once a week for three weeks at a time. This treatment may affect permed, coloured or bleached hair.

*Interactions with other medicaments and other forms of interaction:* None stated.

*Use in pregnancy and lactation:* No known effects in pregnancy and lactation. However, as with all medicines, use with caution.

*Effects on ability to drive and use machines:* None stated.

*Undesirable effects:* Very rarely skin irritation has been reported with malathion products.

*Overdose:* In the event of deliberate or accidental ingestion, as for ethyl alcohol, empty the stomach by gastric lavage and keep patient warm. In the event of massive ingestion, atropine and pralidoxime may be required to counteract cholinesterase inhibition.

**Pharmacological properties**

*Pharmacodynamic properties:* Suleo-M Lotion contains malathion, a widely used organophosphorous insecticide which is active by cholinesterase inhibition. It is effective against a wide range of insects but is one of the least toxic organophosphorous insecticides since it is rapidly detoxified by plasma carboxylesterases.

*Pharmacokinetic properties:* Suleo-M Lotion is applied topically to the affected area.

*Pre-clinical safety data:* None stated.

**Pharmaceutical particulars**

*List of excipients:* Isopropyl alcohol; D-Limonene 17449; Terpineol 18689; Perfume Loxol P6160; citric acid; Shellsol T.

*Incompatibilities:* None stated.

*Shelf life:* Two years.

*Special precautions for storage:* Store at or below 25°C. Protect from sunlight.

*Nature and contents of container:* Cartoned, clear or amber glass bottles with low density polyethylene caps and high density polyethylene sprinkler inserts containing either 50 or 200 ml of product.

*Instructions for use/handling:* None stated.

**Marketing authorisation number** 11314/0055.

**Date of approval/revision of SPC** November 1995.

**Legal category** P.

## STERETS TISEPT*

**Presentation** Sterets Tisept is a clear, yellow aqueous solution, sterilised by autoclaving and containing Chlorhexidine Gluconate Solution B.P. equivalent to Chlorhexidine Gluconate 0.015% w/v, and Cetrimide PhEur 0.15% w/v.

**Uses** A broad-spectrum antiseptic with detergent properties for swabbing in obstetrics and during dressing changes. For disinfecting and cleansing traumatic and surgical wounds and burns.

**Dosage and administration** Use without further dilution for topical administration only.

**Contra-indications, warnings, etc** For external use only. Not for injection. Tisept should not come into contact with the brain, eyes, meninges or middle ear. When used in antiseptic procedures, the outside of the sachet should be disinfected before opening. Discard any surplus immediately after use. Hypochlorite bleaches may cause brown stains to develop in fabrics that have previously been in contact with Tisept.

*Use in pregnancy and lactation:* Although there are no adverse reports for this product in pregnant or lactating women, care should be exercised when administering the product to pregnant or lactating women.

*Side-effects:* Idiosyncratic skin-reactions can occur but are extremely rare.

**Pharmaceutical precautions** Store at room temperature. Tisept is incompatible with anionic agents.

**Legal category** P

**Package quantities** *25 ml sachets:* 250 sachets in packs of 25. 10 packs per fibreboard outer. *100 ml sachets:* 60 sachets in packs of 10. 6 packs per fibreboard outer.

**Further information** The British Pharmaceutical Codex (1973) recommends that antiseptic solutions applied to broken skin should be sterile. The use of Tisept complies with this recommendation.

**Product licence number** 0303/0017
*Product licence holder:* Seton Prebbles Limited, St John's Road, Bootle L20 8NJ.

## TRANSVASIN* HEAT RUB

**Presentation** Transvasin Heat Rub is a white to pale cream coloured cream with an odour typical of perfume and nicotinates. It contains the following active ingredients: Ethyl Nicotinate 2.0% w/w, Hexyl Nicotinate 2.0% w/w and Tetrahydrofurfuryl Salicylate 14.0% w/w.

**Uses** Transvasin Heat Rub is used for the relief of rheumatic and muscular pain and the symptoms of sprains and strains.

**Dosage and administration**
Adults, the elderly and children: Massage gently into the affected area until the cream is entirely absorbed. Apply at least twice daily until the symptoms abate. For topical application only. Quantities are not critical and the amount used should be consistent with the directions for use and will vary with the size of the treated area.

**Contra-indications, warnings, etc**
*Contra-indications:* Transvasin Heat Rub should not be used by patients with known sensitivity to the product or any of its ingredients.

*Interactions:* None known.

*Effect on ability to drive and to use machines:* None known.

*Side effects and adverse reactions:* Reported effects have taken the form of localised sensitisation reactions and have invariably subsided following withdrawal of medication.

*Use in pregnancy and lactation:* Although there have been no reports of any adverse effects, as with all medicines, care should be taken when administering to pregnant or lactating women.

*Other special precautions and warnings:* Transvasin Heat Rub should not be applied to broken or sensitive skin, for example around the eyes or scrotal skin. Avoid use on mucous membranes. For external use only. Transvasin Heat Rub is a rubefacient, and within a few minutes of application a sensation of warmth is felt, followed by a reddening of the skin. This erythema does not indicate intolerance.

*Overdose:* As this is a topical application with small amounts of actives, adverse systemic effects are unlikely even after oral ingestion. No special measures are necessary.

**Pharmaceutical precautions:** Store at room temperature.

**Legal category** GSL

**Package quantities** Tubes of 40 g and 80 g.

**Further information** None.

**Product licence number** 11314/0001

*Product licence holder:* Seton Products Limited, Tubiton House, Oldham OL1 3HS.

## STERETS UNISEPT*

**Presentation** A clear, pink, aqueous solution, sterilised by autoclaving, which contains Chlorhexidine Gluconate Solution B.P. equivalent to 0.05% w/v Chlorhexidine Gluconate.

**Uses** A potent antibacterial agent for general antiseptic purposes. It is bactericidal to a broad spectrum of organisms and remains bacteriostatic even at high dilutions. Unisept is recommended for use in obstetrics and for swabbing burns and wounds.

**Dosage and administration** Use without further dilution for topical administration only.

**Contra-indications, warnings, etc**

*Contra-indications:* For external use only. Not for injection. Unisept should not come into contact with the brain, eyes, meninges or middle ear.

*Precautions:* When used in antiseptic procedures, the outside of the sachet should be disinfected before opening. Discard any surplus immediately after use.

Hypochlorite bleaches may cause brown stains to develop in fabrics that have previously been in contact with Unisept solutions.

*Use in pregnancy and lactation:* Although there are no adverse reports for this product in pregnant or lactating women, care should be exercised when administering the product to pregnant or lactating women.

*Side-effects:* Idiosyncratic skin reactions can occur but are extremely rare.

*Accidental ingestion:* Gastric lavage should be carried out with milk, egg white, gelatine or mild soap.

**Pharmaceutical precautions** Store at room temperature. Unisept is incompatible with anionic agents.

**Legal category** P

**Package quantities** *25 ml sachets:* 250 sachets in packs of 25. 10 packs per outer fibreboard. *100 ml sachets:* 60 sachets in packs of 10. 6 packs per outer fibreboard.

**Further information** The British Pharmaceutical Codex (1973) recommends that antiseptic solutions applied to broken skin should be sterile. The use of Unisept complies with this recommendation.

**Product licence number** 0303/0016

*Product licence holder:* Seton Prebbles Limited, St John's Road, Bootle L20 8NJ.

*Trade Mark

# Shire Pharmaceuticals Limited
East Anton
Andover
Hampshire SP10 5RG

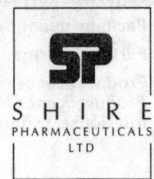

## CALCICHEW*

**Presentation** Round, white slightly speckled, biconvex, chewable tablet with an orange flavour, containing 1250 mg Calcium Carbonate PhEur equivalent to 500 mg calcium.

**Uses** To be chewed, as a supplemental source of calcium in the correction of dietary deficiencies or when normal requirements are high. As an adjunct to conventional therapy in osteoporosis. Phosphate binding agent in the management of renal failure in patients on renal dialysis.

### Dosage and administration
*Adults and elderly:*
Adjunct to osteoporosis therapy: 2 to 3 tablets daily
Dietary deficiency: 2 to 3 tablets daily.
Osteomalacia: 2 to 6 tablets daily
Phosphate binder: Dose as required by the individual patient depending on serum calcium and phosphate levels. Tablets should be taken just before, during or just after each meal.

*Children:*
Dietary deficiency: As for adults.
Phosphate binder: As for adults.

### Contra-indications, warnings etc.
*Contra-indications:* Severe hypercalcaemia and hypercalciuria for example in hyperparathyroidism, vitamin D overdose, decalcifying tumours such as plasmacytoma and skeletal metastases, in severe renal failure untreated by renal dialysis, and in osteoporosis due to immobilisation.

*Precautions:* Patients treated with high doses of vitamin D or who are receiving prolonged calcium treatment, should undergo regulatory measurements of plasma calcium levels which should be interpreted in conjunction with measurements of plasma protein levels.
When used as a phosphate binder in patients on renal dialysis serum phosphate and calcium levels should be monitored regularly.

*Interactions:* May impair absorption of other drugs, for example, tetracyclines and fluoride preparations. Thiazide diuretics reduce urinary calcium excretion so the risk of hypercalcaemia should be considered. Oral calcium supplementation is aimed at restoring normal serum calcium levels. Although it is extremely unlikely that high enough levels will be achieved to adversely affect digitalised patients, this theoretical possibility should be considered. Vitamin D causes an increase in calcium absorption and plasma calcium levels may continue to rise after stopping vitamin D therapy.

*Side effects:* Constipation and wind. Rebound acid production.
Hypercalcaemia–although hypercalcaemia would not be expected in patients unless their renal function were impaired, the following symptoms could indicate the possibility of hypercalcaemia: nausea, vomiting, anorexia, constipation, abdominal pain, bone pain, thirst, polyuria, muscle weakness, drowsiness or confusion. Alkalosis with high doses and in patients on renal dialysis. On long term phosphate binding therapy there are rare reports of tissue calcification.

*Use in pregnancy and lactation:* There is epidemiological and clinical evidence of safety of calcium carbonate in human pregnancy.

*Overdosage:* There are no reports of overdose. Alkalosis is a theoretical risk.

**Pharmaceutical precautions** Store below 25°C.

**Legal category** P

**Package quantities** Containers of 100 tablets.

**Further information** Calcichew contains only the following excipients; sorbitol, polyvinylpyrrolidone, orange oil, magnesium stearate, water, hydrogenated glucose syrup, aspartame, mono, di-fatty acid glycerides.

**Product licence number** 8557/0003

## CALCICHEW* D3

**Qualitative and quantitative composition** Per tablet: Calcium carbonate 1248.75 mg equivalent to 500 mg of elemental calcium; cholecalciferol 200 iu (equivalent to 5 micrograms vitamin $D_3$).

**Pharmaceutical form** Tablets

### Clinical particulars

*Therapeutic indications:* Calcichew $D_3$ should be used only as a therapeutic and not as a food supplement when the diet is deficient or when normal requirements of both components are increased. Calcichew $D_3$ may be used as an adjunct to specific therapy for osteoporosis or as a therapeutic supplement in established osteomalacia, pregnant patients at high risk of needing such a therapeutic supplementation or malnutrition when dietary intake is less than that required.

*Posology and method of administration* Orally.
*Adults and elderly:* Two tablets to be chewed daily
Children: Restrict to over 12 years

*Contra-indications:* Hypercalcaemia, for example, as a result of hyperparathyroidism (primary or secondary), vitamin D overdosage, decalcifying tumours such as myeloma, bone metastases or sarcoidosis. Severe hypercalciuria, renal stones. Osteoporosis due to immobilisation.

*Special warnings and precautions for use:* Hypercalcaemia should particularly be avoided in digitalised patients. Patients with mild to moderate renal failure (commonly found in the elderly) or mild hypercalciuria should be supervised carefully with periodic checks of urinary calcium excretion and plasma calcium levels. Urinary calcium excretion should also be measured in patients with a history of renal stones to exclude hypercalciuria.

*Interaction with other medicaments and other forms of interaction:* Calcium may impair the absorption of tetracyclines, fluoride or iron. At least three hours should intervene between taking Calcichew $D_3$ and these agents.

*Pregnancy and lactation:* Normal requirements for calcium and vitamin D are raised during pregnancy and lactation. If supplementation is necessary, it should be given at a different time from iron supplements. Calcium is excreted in breast milk but not sufficiently to produce an adverse effect in the infant. Allowances should be made for vitamin D/calcium from other sources. During pregnancy and lactation therapy should be under medical supervision.

*Effects on ability to drive and use machinery:* None known

*Undesirable effects:* Mild gastro-intestinal disturbances (e.g. constipation) can occur with calcium supplements, but are infrequent. Rebound secretion of gastric acid is possible, but unlikely to be clinically significant. Milk-alkali syndrome with hypercalcaemia is a rare possibility in chronically treated individuals.

*Overdose:* The most serious consequence of acute or chronic overdosage would be hypercalcaemia due to vitamin D toxicity. This is very unlikely unless extreme sensitivity to vitamin D is present, as in normal people over 200 chewable tablets a day would be required to produce a toxic dose. Features of hypercalcaemia include anorexia, nausea, vomiting, weakness, fatigue and headache. With a plasma calcium of over 2.6 mmol per litre, confusion and coma can develop. Polydipsia and polyuria indicate renal damage. Calcium and vitamin D treatment must be stopped and a high fluid intake and low calcium diet given. Corticosteroid and other specialist treatment may be necessary in severe cases.

### Pharmacological properties

*Pharmacodynamic properties:* Calcium carbonate is a well established medicinal item used as an antacid or calcium supplement in deficient states. Vitamin $D_3$ is a well established medicinal item. Vitamin D compounds are fat-soluble sterols, sometimes considered to be hormones, which are involved in the regulation of calcium and phosphate homeostasis and bone mineralisation.

*Pharmacokinetic properties:* The pharmacokinetics of calcium and its salts are well established. Calcium carbonate is converted into calcium chloride by gastric acid. Some of the calcium is absorbed from the intestines but about 80% is reconverted to insoluble calcium salts such as the carbonate and stearate, and excreted. The pharmacokinetics of vitamin D substances are well established. These are well absorbed from the gastro-intestinal tract; bile must be present for adequate intestinal absorption. Circulation is via specific gamma-globulins, storage can be long term in the adipose and muscle tissue, excretion is mainly in the bile and faeces.

*Preclinical safety data:* Toxic effects would only result from overdosage. Calcium salts by themselves are virtually innocuous in normal subjects. While chronic overdosage with vitamin D is toxic, resulting in hypercalcaemia, the amount present in Calcichew $D_3$ is too small to represent a practical clinical risk.

### Pharmaceutical information

*List of excipients:* Sorbitol, polyvinylpyrrolidone K30, hydrogenated glucose syrup, orange oil, magnesium stearate, aspartame and mono, di-fatty acid glycerides.

*Incompatibilities:* None known

*Shelf life:* 3 years

*Special storage precautions:* Maximum storage temperature of 25°C.

*Nature and contents of container:* Containers of 60 and 100 tablets.

*Instructions for use/handling:* No special conditions.

**Marketing authorisation number** 8557/0021

**Date of approval/revision of SPC** July 1996

**Legal category** P

## CALCICHEW* D3 FORTE

**Qualitative and quantitative composition** Per tablet: Calcium carbonate 1250 mg (equivalent to 500 mg of elemental calcium); cholecalciferol 400 iu (equivalent to 10 micrograms vitamin $D_3$)

**Pharmaceutical form** Tablet

### Clinical particulars

*Therapeutic indications:* Calcichew $D_3$ Forte may be used in: The treatment and prevention of vitamin D/calcium deficiency (characterised by raised serum alkaline phosphatase levels associated with increased bone loss, raised levels of serum PTH and lowered 25-hydroxyvitamin D) particularly in the housebound and institutionalised elderly subjects. The supplementation of vitamin D and calcium as an adjunct to specific therapy for osteoporosis, in pregnancy, in established vitamin D dependent osteomalacia and in other situations requiring therapeutic supplementation of malnutrition.

*Posology and method of administration:* Oral
*Adults and elderly:* 2 chewable tablets per day, preferably one tablet morning and evening.
Children: restrict to over 12 years

*Contra-indications:* Hypercalcaemia, for example as a result of primary hyperparathyroidism, vitamin D overdosage, sarcoidosis or malignant bone diseases such as myeloma, bone metastases. Severe hypercalciuria, renal stones. Osteoporosis due to prolonged immobilisation, for example, paraplegia. Milk alkali syndrome. Severe renal failure.

*Special warnings and precautions for use:* Patients with mild to moderate renal failure or mild hypercalciuria should be supervised carefully with periodic checks of urinary calcium excretion and plasma calcium levels. Urinary calcium excretion should also be measured in patients with a history of renal stones to exclude hypercalciuria.

*Interaction with other medicaments and other forms of interaction:* Calcium may impair the absorption of tetracyclines, fluoride or iron. At least 3 hours should intervene between taking Calcichew $D_3$ Forte and these agents. Thiazide diuretics reduce urinary calcium excretion so the risk of hypercalcaemia should be considered. Hypercalcaemia should particularly be avoided in digitalised patients.

*Pregnancy and lactation:* Normal requirements for calcium and vitamin D are raised during pregnancy and lactation. If supplementation is necessary, it should be given at a different time from iron supplements. Calcium is excreted in breast milk, but not sufficiently to produce an adverse effect in the infant. Allowances should be made for vitamin D/calcium from other sources. During pregnancy and lactation, therapy should be under medical supervision.

*Effects on ability to drive and use machines:* None expected.

*Undesirable effects:* Mild gastrointestinal disturbances, for example, constipation, can occur with calcium supplements, but are infrequent. Rebound secretion of gastric acid is possible, but unlikely to be clinically significant. Milk-alkali syndrome with hypercalcaemia is a rare possibility in chronically treated individuals.

*Overdose:* The most serious consequence of acute or chronic overdosage would be hypercalcaemia due to vitamin D toxicity. This is very unlikely, as in normal people over 100 chewable tablets a day would be required to produce a toxic dose. Features of hypercalcaemia include anorexia, nausea, vomiting, weakness, fatigue and headache. With a plasma calcium of over 2.66 mM., confusion and coma can develop. Polydipsia and polyuria indicate renal damage. Calcium and vitamin D treatment must be stopped and a high fluid intake and low calcium diet given. Corticosteroid and other specialist treatment may be necessary in severe cases.

**Pharmacological properties**

*Pharmacological properties :* Calcium carbonate is a well established medicinal item used as an antacid or calcium supplement in deficiency states. Vitamin $D_3$ is a well established medicinal item. Vitamin D compounds are fat-soluble sterols, sometimes considered to be hormones, which are essential for the proper regulation of calcium and phosphate homeostasis and bone mineralisation.

*Pharmacokinetic properties:* The pharmacokinetics of calcium and its salts are well established. Calcium carbonate is converted to calcium chloride by gastric acid. Some of the calcium is absorbed from the intestines, but about 85% is reconverted to insoluble calcium salts as the carbonate and stearate, and excreted in the faeces. The pharmacokinetics of vitamin D substances are also well established. They are well absorbed from the gastro-intestinal tract; bile must be present for adequate intestinal absorption. Circulation is via specific gamma globulins, storage can be long term in the adipose and muscle tissue, excretion is mainly in the bile and faeces.

*Safety data:* Toxic effects would only result from overdosage. Calcium salts by themselves are virtually innocuous in normal subjects. While chronic overdosage with vitamin D is toxic, resulting in hypercalcaemia, the amount present in Calcichew $D_3$ Forte is too small to represent a practical clinical risk.

**Pharmaceutical particulars**

*List of excipients:* Sorbitol, povidone, hydrogenated glucose, lemon flavouring, fatty acid mono- and diglycerides, aspartame, magnesium stearate, sucrose, gelatin, vegetable fat, tocopherol and maize starch.

*Incompatibility:* Not applicable, oral preparation.

*Shelf life:* 24 months.

*Special storage precautions:* Store at a temperature below 25°C and protect against moisture.

*Nature and contents of container:* White, high density polyethylene bottles. Bottles containing 100 tablets with tamper evident seal.

*Instructions for use/handling* No special conditions.

**Marketing authorisation number** 8557/0029

**Date of approval/revision of SPC** January 1996

**Legal category** P

## CALCICHEW* FORTE

**Presentation** Round, white, slightly speckled, flat, bevel-edged, chewable tablets containing 2.5 g Calcium Carbonate PhEur equivalent to 1 g calcium.

**Uses** To be chewed, as a supplemental source of calcium in the correction of dietary deficiencies or when normal requirements are high. As an adjunct to conventional therapy in osteoporosis. Phosphate binding agent in the management of renal failure in patients on renal dialysis.

**Dosage and administration**

*Adults and elderly:*

Adjunct to osteoporosis therapy: 1 tablet daily
Dietary deficiency: 1 tablet daily
Osteomalacia: 1–3 tablets daily
Phosphate binding: Dose as required by the individual patient depending on serum calcium and phosphate levels. Tablets should be taken just before, during or just after each meal.

*Children:*

Dietary deficiency: As for adults
Phosphate binding: As for adults

**Contra-indications, warnings etc.**

*Contra-indications:* Severe hypercalcaemia and hypercalciuria, for example, in hyperparathyroidism, vitamin D overdose, decalcifying tumours such as multiple myeloma, plasmacytoma and skeletal metastases, in severe renal failure untreated by renal dialysis and in osteoporosis due to immobilisation.

*Precautions:* Patients treated with high doses of vitamin D or who are receiving prolonged calcium treatment, should undergo regulatory measurements of plasma calcium levels which should be interpreted in conjunction with measurements of plasma protein levels. When used as a phosphate binder in patients on renal dialysis serum phosphate and calcium levels should be monitored regularly.

*Interactions:* May impair absorption of other drugs, for example, tetracyclines and fluoride preparations. Thiazide diuretics reduce urinary calcium excretion so the risk of hypercalcaemia should be considered. Oral calcium supplementation is aimed at restoring normal serum calcium levels, although it is extremely unlikely that high enough levels will be achieved to adversely affect digitalised patients, this theoretical possibility should be considered. Vitamin D causes an increase in calcium absorption and plasma calcium levels may continue to rise after stopping vitamin D therapy.

*Side effects:* Constipation and wind. Diarrhoea in a small number of patients. Rebound acid production. Hypercalcaemia–although hypercalcaemia would not be expected in patients unless their renal function was impaired. The following symptoms could indicate the possibility of hypercalcaemia: nausea, vomiting, anorexia, constipation, abdominal pain, bone pain, thirst, polyuria, muscle weakness, drowsiness or confusion. Alkalosis with high doses and in patients on renal dialysis. On long term phosphate binding therapy there are rare reports of tissue calcification.

*Use in pregnancy and lactation:* There is epidemiological and clinical evidence of safety of calcium carbonate in human pregnancy.

*Overdosage:* There are no reports of overdose. Alkalosis is a theoretical risk.

**Pharmaceutical precautions** Store below 25°C.

**Legal category** P

**Package quantities** Containers of 100 tablets.

**Further information** Calcichew Forte contains only the following excipients; sorbitol, polyvinylpyrrolidone K30, hydrogenated glucose syrup, orange oils, magnesium stearate, aspartame, mono, di-fatty acid glycerides.

**Product licence number** 8557/0022

## CALCIDRINK*

**Qualitative and quantitative composition** Calcium carbonate 2.5 g equivalent to 1 g of calcium.

**Pharmaceutical form** Dispersible granules.

**Clinical particulars**

*Therapeutic indications:* Treatment of calcium deficiency. As an adjunct to conventional therapy in osteoporosis.

*Posology and method of administration*
*Adults, elderly and children:* One sachet to be taken dispersed in water daily.

*Contra-indications:* Severe hypercalcaemia and hypercalciuria, for example, in primary hyperparathyroidism, vitamin D overdose, osteoporosis due to immobilisation, decalcifying tumours such as plasmacytoma and skeletal metastases. Severe renal failure.

*Special warnings and precautions for use:* Patients with mild to moderate renal failure or mild calciuria should be supervised carefully with periodic checks of urinary calcium excretion and plasma calcium levels. Urinary calcium excretion should be measured in patients with a history of renal stones to exclude hypercalciuria.

*Interaction with other medicaments and other forms of interaction:* Calcium may impair the absorption of tetracyclines or fluoride. At least 3 hours should intervene between taking Calcidrink and these agents. Calcium salts can reduce the absorption of bisphosphonates and at least 2 hours should intervene between taking these agents. Thiazide diuretics reduce urinary calcium excretion so the risk of hypercalcaemia should be considered. Hypercalcaemia should particularly be avoided in digitalised patients.

*Pregnancy and lactation:* There is epidemiological and clinical evidence of safety of calcium carbonate in human pregnancy. Calcium is secreted in breast milk, but not sufficiently to produce an adverse effect in the infant.

*Effects on ability to drive and use machines:* None expected.

*Undesirable effects* : Mild gastrointestinal disturbances, for example, constipation, can occur with calcium supplements, but are infrequent. Rebound secretion of gastric acid is possible, but unlikely to be clinically significant. Hypercalcaemia would not normally be expected in patients, even at higher doses, unless there is an underlying cause such as impaired renal function/drug interaction.

*Overdose:* No cases of intoxication due to calcium overdose are known.

**Pharmacological properties**

*Pharmacodynamic properties:* Calcium carbonate is a well established medicinal item.

*Pharmacokinetic properties:* The pharmacokinetics of calcium and its salts are well established.

*Preclinical safety data:* Results of preclinical studies are of little relevance for this well established compound.

**Pharmaceutical particulars**

*List of excipients* : Citric acid, sugar, glucose, orange oil, saccharin sodium, lecithin, beta carotene, sodium lauryl sulphate, invert sugar, mono, di-fatty acid glycerides and water.

*Incompatibilities* : Not applicable for an oral preparation.

*Shelf life:* 36 months.

*Special precautions for storage:* No special precautions.

*Nature and contents of container:* Calcidrink is provided in sachets. These are available to pharmacies in boxes of 30.

*Instructions for use/handling:* The contents of a sachet should be added to a glass of water and stirred before drinking.

**Marketing authorisation number:** 8557/0018

**Date of approval/revision of SPC** September 1995

**Legal category:** P

## CALCORT* ▼

**Qualitative and quantitative composition** Active ingredient: Deflazacort HSE 6.0 mg.

**Pharmaceutical form** Deflazacort 6 mg tablets are round, white, uncoated tablets, approximately 8.6 mm diameter, marked with a cross on one face and a '6' on the other face.

**Clinical particulars**

*Therapeutic indications* A wide range of conditions may sometimes need treatment with glucocorticosteroids. The indications include: Anaphylaxis; asthma; severe hypersensitivity reactions. Rheumatoid arthritis; juvenile chronic arthritis; polymyalgia rheumatica. Systemic lupus erythematosus; dermatomyositis; mixed connective tissue disease (other than systemic sclerosis); polyarteritis nodosa; sarcoidosis. Pemphigus; bullous pemphigoid; pyoderma gangrenosum. Minimal change nephrotic syndrome; acute interstitial nephritis. Rheumatic carditis. Ulcerative colitis; Crohn's disease. Uveitis, optic neuritis. Autoimmune haemolytic anaemia, idiopathic thrombocytopenic purpura. Acute and lymphatic leukaemia, malignant lymphoma; multiple myeloma. Immune suppression in transplantation.

*Posology and method of administration* Deflazacort is a glucocorticoid derived from prednisolone and 6 mg of deflazacort has approximately the same anti-inflammatory potency as 5 mg prednisone or prednisolone.

Doses vary widely in different diseases and different patients. In more serious and life-threatening conditions, high doses of deflazacort may need to be given. When deflazacort is used long term in relatively benign chronic diseases, the maintenance dose should be kept as low as possible. Dosage may need to be increased during periods of stress or in exacerbation of illness.

The dosage should be individually titrated according to diagnosis, severity of disease and patient response and tolerance. The lowest dose that will produce an acceptable response should be used (see *Warnings and Precautions*).

*Adults* For acute disorders, up to 120 mg/day deflazacort may need to be given initially. Maintenance doses in most conditions are within the range 3–18 mg/day. The following regimens are for guidance only:

*Rheumatoid arthritis*: The maintenance dose is usually within the range 3–18 mg/day. The smallest effective dose should be used and increased if necessary.

*Bronchial asthma:* In the treatment of an acute attack high doses of 48 to 72 mg/day may be needed, depending on severity, and gradually reduced once the attack has been controlled. For maintenance in chronic asthma, doses should be titrated to the lowest dose that controls symptoms.

*Other conditions:* The dose of deflazacort depends on clinical need titrated to the lowest effective dose for maintenance. Starting dose may be estimated on the basis of ratio of 5 mg prednisone or prednisolone to 6 mg deflazacort.

*Hepatic impairment:* In patients with hepatic impairment, blood levels of deflazacort may be increased. Therefore the dose of deflazacort should be carefully monitored and adjusted to the minimum effective dose.

*Renal impairment:* In renally impaired patients, no special precautions other than those usually adopted in patients receiving glucocorticoid therapy are necessary.

*Elderly* In elderly patients, no special precautions other than those usually adopted in patients receiving glucocorticoid therapy are necessary. The common adverse effects of systemic corticosteroids may be associated with more serious consequences in old age (see Warnings and Precautions).

*Children* There has been limited exposure of children to deflazacort in clinical trials.

In children, the indications for glucocorticoids are the same as for adults, but it is important that the lowest effective dosage is used. Alternate day administration may be appropriate (see *Warnings and Precautions*).

Doses of deflazacort usually lie in the range 0.25–1.5 mg/kg/day. The following ranges provide general guidance:

*Juvenile chronic arthritis*: The usual maintenance dose is between 0.25–1.0 mg/kg/day.

*Nephrotic syndrome*: Initial dose of usually 1.5 mg/kg/day followed by down titration according to clinical need.

*Bronchial asthma*: On the basis of the potency ratio, the initial dose should be between 0.25–1.0 mg/kg deflazacort on alternate days.

*Contra-indications* Systemic infection unless specific anti-infective therapy is employed. Hypersensitivity to deflazacort or any of the ingredients. Patients receiving live virus immunisation.

*Special warnings and special precautions for use*: A patient information leaflet should be supplied with this product. Undesirable effects may be minimised by using the lowest dose for the minimum period, and by administering the daily requirement as a single morning dose, or, whenever possible, as a single morning dose on alternate days. Frequent patient review is required to appropriately titrate dose against disease activity (see *Dosage* section).

*Adrenal suppression:* Adrenal cortical atrophy develops during prolonged therapy and may persist for years after stopping treatment. Withdrawal of corticosteroids after prolonged therapy must therefore always be gradual to avoid acute adrenal insufficiency, being tapered off over weeks or months according to the dose and duration of treatment. During prolonged therapy, any intercurrent illness, trauma or surgical procedure will require a temporary increase in dosage; if corticosteroids have been stopped following prolonged therapy they may need to be temporarily reintroduced.

Patients should carry 'Steroid Treatment' cards which give clear guidance on the precautions to be taken to minimise risk and which provide details of prescriber, drug, dosage and the duration of treatment.

*Anti-inflammatory/immunosuppressive effects and infections:* Suppression of the inflammatory response and immune function increases the susceptibility to infections and their severity. The clinical presentation may often be atypical and serious infections such as septicaemia and tuberculosis may be masked and may reach an advanced stage before being recognised.

Chickenpox is of particular concern since this normally minor illness may be fatal in immunosuppressed patients. Patients (or parents of children) without a definite history of chickenpox should be advised to avoid close personal contact with chickenpox or herpes zoster and, if exposed, they should seek urgent medical attention. Passive immunisation with varicella zoster immunoglobulin (VZIG) is needed by exposed non-immune patients who are receiving systemic corticosteroids or who have used them within the previous 3 months; this should be given within 10 days of exposure to chickenpox. If a diagnosis of chickenpox is confirmed, the illness warrants specialist care and urgent treatment. Corticosteroids should not be stopped and the dose may need to be increased.

Live vaccines should not be given to individuals with impaired responsiveness. The antibody response to other vaccines may be diminished.

Prolonged use of glucocorticoids may produce posterior subcapsular cataracts, glaucoma with possible damage to the optic nerves and may enhance the establishment of secondary ocular infections due to fungi or viruses.

Use in active tuberculosis should be restricted to those cases of fulminating and disseminated tuberculosis in which deflazacort is used for management with appropriate antituberculosis regimen. If glucocorticoids are indicated in patients with latent tuberculosis or tuberculin reactivity, close observation is necessary as reactivation of the disease may occur. During prolonged glucocorticoid therapy, these patients should receive chemoprophylaxis.

*Special precautions:* The following clinical conditions require special caution and frequent patient monitoring is necessary.

– Cardiac disease or congestive heart failure (except in the presence of active rheumatic carditis), hypertension, thromboembolic disorders. Glucocorticoids can cause salt and water retention and increased excretion of potassium. Dietary salt restriction and potassium supplementation may be necessary.

– Gastritis or oesophagitis, diverticulitis, ulcerative colitis if there is probability of impending perforation, abscess or pyogenic infections, fresh intestinal anastomosis, active or latent peptic ulcer.

– Diabetes mellitus or a family history, osteoporosis, myasthenia gravis, renal insufficiency.

– Emotional instability or psychotic tendency, epilepsy.

– Previous corticosteroid-induced myopathy.

– Liver failure;

– Hypothyroidism and cirrhosis, which may increase glucocorticoid effect.

– Ocular herpes simplex because of possible corneal perforation.

*Use in children* Corticosteroids cause dose-related growth retardation in infancy, childhood and adolescence which may be irreversible.

*Use in elderly* The common adverse effects of systemic corticosteroids may be associated with more serious consequences in old age, especially osteoporosis, hypertension, hypokalaemia, diabetes, susceptibility to infection and thinning of the skin. Close clinical supervision is required to avoid life-threatening reactions.

Since complications of glucocorticoid therapy are dependent on dose and duration of therapy, the lowest possible dose must be given and a risk/benefit decision must be made as to whether intermittent therapy should be used.

*Interactions with other medicaments and other forms of interactions* The same precautions should be exercised as for other glucocorticoids. Deflazacort is metabolised in the liver. It is recommended to increase the maintenance dose of deflazacort if drugs which are liver enzyme inducers are co-administered, e.g. rifampicin, rifabutin, carbamazepine, phenobarbitone, phenytoin, primidone and aminoglutethimide. For drugs which inhibit liver enzymes, e.g. ketoconazole, it may be possible to reduce the maintenance dose of deflazacort.

The desired effects of hypoglycaemic agents (including insulin), anti-hypertensives and diuretics are antagonised by corticosteroids and the hypokalaemic effects of acetazolamide, loop diuretics, thiazide diuretics and carbenoxolone are enhanced.

The efficacy of coumarin anticoagulants may be enhanced by concurrent corticosteroid therapy and close monitoring of the INR or prothrombin time is required to avoid spontaneous bleeding.

The renal clearance of salicylates is increased by corticosteroids and steroid withdrawal may result in salicylate intoxication.

As glucocorticoids can suppress the normal responses of the body to attack by micro-organisms, it is important to ensure that any anti-infective therapy is effective and it is recommended to monitor patients closely. Concurrent use of glucocorticoids and oral contraceptives should be closely monitored as plasma levels of glucocorticoids may be increased. This effect may be due to a change in metabolism or binding to serum proteins. Antacids may reduce bioavailability; leave at least 2 hours between administration of deflazacort and antacids.

*Pregnancy and lactation* Human reproduction studies have not been performed with glucocorticoids, but they are known to be teratogenic in animals. Deflazacort was shown to have dose dependent teratogenic effects in rats and rabbits.

Intra-uterine growth retardation in the foetus and a small increased risk of cleft palate have been reported with corticosteroids. Hypoadrenalism may occur in the neonate.

Use during pregnancy or during lactation is not recommended and should only be considered when potential benefit outweighs potential risk. Infants born to mothers receiving glucocorticoids during pregnancy should be carefully observed for signs of hypoadrenalism. Glucocorticoids are excreted in mothers' milk and can cause growth suppression and hypoadrenalism in breast fed infants; therefore mothers taking deflazacort should be advised not to breast feed.

*Effects on ability to drive and use machines* On the basis of the pharmacodynamic profile and reported adverse events, it is unlikely that deflazacort will produce an effect on the ability to drive and use machines.

*Undesirable effects* The incidence of predictable undesirable effects, including hypothalamic-pituitary adrenal suppression correlates with the relative potency of the drug, dosage, timing of administration and the duration of treatment (see *Warnings and Precautions*).

*Endocrine/metabolic* Suppression of the hypothalamic-pituitary-adrenal axis, growth suppression in infancy, childhood and adolescence, menstrual irregularity and amenorrhoea. Cushingoid facies, hirsutism, weight gain, impaired carbohydrate tolerance with increased requirement for anti-diabetic therapy. Negative protein and calcium balance. Increased appetite.

*Anti-inflammatory and immunosuppressive effects* Increased susceptibility and severity of infections with suppression of clinical symptoms and signs, opportunistic infections, recurrence of dormant tuberculosis (see Warnings and Precautions).

*Musculoskeletal* Osteoporosis, vertebral and long bone fractures, avascular osteonecrosis, tendon rupture. Proximal myopathy with wasting and weakness, negative nitrogen balance.

*Fluid and electrolyte disturbance* Sodium and water retention with hypertension, oedema and heart failure, potassium loss, hypokalaemic alkalosis.

*Neuropsychiatric* Headache, vertigo, euphoria, psychological dependence, hypomania or depression, insomnia, restlessness and aggravation of schizophrenia. Increased intra-cranial pressure with papilloedema in children (pseudotumour cerebri), usually after treatment withdrawal. Aggravation of epilepsy.

*Ophthalmic* Increased intra-ocular pressure, glaucoma, papilloedema, posterior subcapsular cataracts especially in children, corneal or scleral thinning, exacerbation of ophthalmic viral or fungal diseases.

*Gastrointestinal* Dyspepsia, peptic ulceration with perforation and haemorrhage, acute pancreatitis (especially in children), candidiasis.

*Dermatological* Impaired healing, skin atrophy, bruising, telangiectasia, striae, acne.

*General* Hypersensitivity including anaphylaxis has been reported. Leucocytosis. Thromboembolism. Rare incidence of benign intracranial hypertension.

*Withdrawal symptoms and signs* Too rapid a reduction of corticosteroid dosage following prolonged treatment can lead to acute adrenal insufficiency, hypotension and death (see Warnings and Precautions).

A "withdrawal syndrome" may also occur including fever, myalgia, arthralgia, rhinitis, conjunctivitis, painful itchy skin nodules and loss of weight. This may occur in patients even without evidence of adrenal insufficiency.

*Overdose* It is unlikely that treatment is needed in cases of acute overdosage. The $LD_{50}$ for the oral dose is greater than 4000 mg/kg in laboratory animals.

**Pharmacological properties**

*Pharmacodynamic properties* Deflazacort is a glucocorticoid. Its anti-inflammatory and immunosuppressive effects are used in treating a variety of diseases and are comparable to other anti-inflammatory steroids. Clinical studies have indicated that the average potency ratio of deflazacort to prednisolone is 0.68–0.89.

*Pharmacokinetic properties* Orally administered deflazacort appears to be well absorbed and is immediately converted to plasma esterases to the pharmacologically active metabolite (D–21–OH) which achieves peak plasma concentrations in 1.5 to 2 hours. It is 40% protein-bound and has no affinity for corticosteroid-binding-globulin (transcortin). It's elimination plasma half-life is 1.1 to 1.9 hours. Elimination takes place primarily through the kidneys; 70% of the administered dose is excreted in the urine. The remaining

30% is eliminated in the faeces. Metabolism of D 21–OH is extensive; only 18% of urinary excretion represents D 21–OH. The metabolite of D 21–OH, deflazacort 6-beta–OH, represents one third of the urinary elimination.

*Preclinical safety data* Safety studies have been carried out in the rat, dog, mouse and monkey. The findings are consistent with other glucocorticoids at comparable doses. Teratogenic effects demonstrated in rodents and rabbits are typical of those caused by other glucocorticoids. Deflazacort was not found to be carcinogenic in the mouse, but studies in the rat produced carcinogenic findings consistent with the findings with other glucocorticoids.

**Pharmaceutical particulars**

*List of excipients* 6 mg tablets–Microcrystalline Cellulose PhEur, Lactose PhEur, Maize Starch PhEur, Magnesium Stearate PhEur, Sucrose PhEur.

*Incompatibilities* None reported.

*Shelf-life* 5 years.

*Special precautions for storage* Store in a dry place below 25°C.

*Nature and contents of container* Deflazacort will be packed in blister packs of polyvinylchloride and aluminium foil presented in cardboard cartons.

60 tablets per pack–6 mg tablets.

*Instructions for use/handling* No special instructions for use or handling are required.

*Marketing authorisation holder:* Marion Merrell Ltd., Broadwater Park, Denham, Uxbridge, Middlesex UB9 5HP.

*Marketing authorisation number* 4426/0125

*Date of approval/revision of SPC* April 1997.

*Legal category* POM

## CARNITOR* INJECTION 1 g

**Presentation** Clear colourless or light straw coloured sterile solution containing levocarnitine inner salt 1 g in 5 ml ampoules.

**Uses** Indicated for the treatment of primary and secondary carnitine deficiency in adults, children, infants and neonates.

*Secondary carnitine deficiency in haemodialysis patients:* Secondary carnitine deficiency should be suspected in long-term haemodialysis patients who have the following conditions:
1. Severe and persistent muscle cramps and/or hypotensive episodes during dialysis.
2. Lack of energy causing a significant negative effect on the quality of life.
3. Skeletal muscle weakness and/or myopathy.
4. Cardiomyopathy.
5. Anaemia of uraemia unresponsive to or requiring large doses of erythropoietin.
6. Muscle mass loss caused by malnutrition.

**Dosage and administration**
*Adults, children, infants and neonates:* For slow intravenous administration over 2–3 minutes.

It is advisable to monitor therapy by measuring free and acyl carnitine levels in both plasma and urine.

*The management of inborn errors of metabolism:* The dosage required depends upon the specific inborn error of metabolism concerned and the severity of presentation at the time of treatment. However, the following can be considered as a general guide.

In acute decompensation, dosages of up to 100 mg/kg/day in 3–4 divided doses are recommended. Higher doses have been used although an increase in adverse events, primarily diarrhoea, may occur.

*Secondary carnitine deficiency in haemodialysis patients:* It is strongly recommended that, before initiating therapy with Carnitor, plasma carnitine is measured. Secondary carnitine deficiency is suggested by a plasma ratio of acyl to free carnitine of greater than 0.4 and/or when free carnitine concentrations are lower than 20 micromol per litre.

A dose of 20 mg per kg should be administered as an intravenous bolus at the end of each dialysis session (assuming three sessions per week). The duration of intravenous treatment should be at least three months which is the time usually required to restore normal muscle levels of free carnitine. The overall response should be assessed by monitoring plasma acyl/free carnitine levels and by evaluating the patient's symptoms. When carnitine supplementation has been stopped there will be a progressive decline in carnitine levels. The need for a repeat course of therapy can be assessed by plasma carnitine assays at regular intervals and by monitoring the patient's symptoms.

*Haemodialysis–maintenance therapy:* If significant clinical benefit has been gained by the first course of

intravenous Carnitor then maintenance therapy can be considered using 1 g of Carnitor orally. On the day of dialysis oral Carnitor has to be administered at the end of the session. (See Data Sheet for Carnitor Paediatric Solution 30% and Single Oral Dose 1 g.)

**Contra-indications, warnings, etc**
*Contra-indications:* Hypersensitivity to any constituent of the product.

*Precautions:* There is limited experience of use in patients with primary and secondary systemic carnitine deficiency suffering from renal failure.

*Pregnancy and lactation:* Reproductive studies were performed in rats and rabbits. There was no evidence of a teratogenic effect in either species. In the rabbit but not in the rat there was a statistically insignificant greater number of post-implantation losses at the highest dose tested (600 mg/kg/ daily) as compared with control animals. The significance of these findings in man is unknown. There is no experience of use in pregnant patients with primary systemic carnitine deficiency.

Taking into account the serious risk if treatment is discontinued, the consequence to a pregnant women who has primary systemic carnitine deficiency requires consideration.

Levocarnitine is a normal component of human milk, use of Carnitor supplementation in nursing mothers has not been studied.

*Side-effects:* Various mild gastrointestinal complaints have been reported during the long term administration of oral levocarnitine, these include transient nausea and vomiting, abdominal cramps and diarrhoea. Decreasing the dosage often diminishes or eliminates drug related patient body odour or gastrointestinal symptoms when present. Tolerance should be monitored very closely during the first week of the administration and after any dosage increase.

*Drug interactions:* There are no known interactions.

*Overdosage:* There have been no reports of toxicity from levocarnitine overdosage. Overdosage should be treated with supportive care.

**Pharmaceutical precautions** Store at a temperature not exceeding 25°C. Protect from light.

**Package quantities** The injections are packed in cardboard cartons of five ampoules.

**Product licence number** 8381/0003

*Product licence holder:* Sigma-Tau Industrie Farmaceutiche Riunite SpA, Viale Shakespeare, 47-00144, Rome, Italy.

## CARNITOR* PAEDIATRIC SOLUTION 30% AND SINGLE ORAL DOSE 1 g

**Presentation**
*Paediatric Solution 30%:* Colourless or slightly yellow solution containing levocarnitine 30%.

*Single Oral Dose 1 g:* A colourless or slightly yellow coloured liquid in a 10 ml amber glass bottle containing levocarnitine inner salt 1 g.

**Uses**
*Paediatric Solution 30%:* Indicated for the treatment of primary and secondary carnitine deficiency in children of under 12 years, infants and newborns.

*Single Oral Dose 1 g:* Indicated for the treatment of primary and secondary carnitine deficiency in adults and children over 12 years of age.

**Dosage and administration** It is advisable to monitor therapy by measuring free and acyl carnitine levels in both plasma and urine.

*The management of inborn errors of metabolism:* The dosage required depends upon the specific inborn error of metabolism concerned and the severity of presentation at the time of treatment. However, the following can be considered as a general guide.

An oral dosage of up to 200 mg/kg/day in divided doses (2 to 4) is recommended for chronic use in some disorders, with lower doses sufficing in other conditions. If clinical and biochemical symptoms do not improve, the dose may be increased on a short term basis. Higher doses of up to 400 mg/kg/day may be necessary in acute metabolic decompensation or the i.v. route may be required.

*Haemodialysis–Maintenance Therapy:* If significant clinical benefit has been gained by a first course of intravenous Carnitor then maintenance therapy can be considered using 1 g per day of Carnitor orally. On the day of the dialysis oral Carnitor has to be administered at the end of the session.

The Paediatric Solution and Single Oral Dose can be drunk directly or diluted further in water or fruit juices.

**Contra-indications, warnings, etc.**
*Contra-indications:* Hypersensitivity to any of the constituents of the product.

*Precautions:* There is limited experience of use in patients with primary and secondary systemic carnitine deficiency suffering from renal failure.

*Pregnancy and lactation:* Reproductive studies were performed in rats and rabbits. There was no evidence of a teratogenic effect in either species. In the rabbit but not in the rat there was a statistically insignificant greater number of post implantation losses at the highest dose tested (600 mg/kg daily) as compared with control animals.

The significance of these findings in man is unknown. There is no experience of use in pregnant patients with primary systemic carnitine deficiency.

Taking into account the serious consequences in a pregnant woman who has primary systemic carnitine deficiency stopping treatment, the risk to the mother of discontinuing treatment seems greater than the theoretical risk to the foetus if treatment is continued.

Levocarnitine is a normal component of human milk. Use of levocarnitine supplementation in nursing mothers has not been studied.

*Side effects:* Various mild gastrointestinal complaints have been reported during the long term administration of oral levocarnitine, these include transient nausea and vomiting, abdominal cramps and diarrhoea.

Decreasing the dosage often diminishes or eliminates drug related patient body odour or gastrointestinal symptoms when present. Tolerance should be monitored very closely during the first week of the administration and after any dosage increase.

*Drug interactions:* There are no known interactions.

*Overdosage:* There have been no reports of toxicity from levocarnitine overdosage. Overdosage should be treated with supportive care.

**Pharmaceutical precautions** Store at a temperature not exceeding 25°C in a dry place. Protect from light.

**Legal category** POM

**Package quantities**
*Paediatric Solution 30%:* 20 ml amber glass bottles
*Single Oral Dose 1 g:* 10 ml amber glass containers in cartons of 10.

**Further information** Nil.

**Product licence numbers**
Carnitor Paediatric Solution 30% 8381/0005
Carnitor Oral Dose 1 g 8381/0004

*Product licence holder:* Sigma Tau Industrie Farmaceutiche Riunite SpA, Viale Shakespeare, 47-00144, Rome, Italy.

## CITRICAL*

**Presentation** Citrical sachets contain granules to prepare a fresh orange flavoured drink containing 1250 mg Calcium Carbonate PhEur equivalent to 500 mg calcium.

**Uses** Orally as a supplemental source of calcium in the correction of dietary deficiencies or when normal requirements are high.

As an adjunct to conventional therapy in osteoporosis.

**Dosage and administration** The contents of each sachet should be dispersed in water.

*Adults and elderly:* Adjunct to osteoporosis therapy: 2–3 sachets daily.
 Dietary deficiency: 2–3 sachets daily.
 Osteomalacia: 2–6 sachets daily.

*Children:* For calcium deficiency states, as adults.

**Contra-indications, warnings, etc**
*Contra-indications:* Severe hypercalcaemia and hypercalciuria, for example in hyperparathyroidism, vitamin D overdose, decalcifying tumours such as plasmacytoma and skeletal metastases, in severe renal failure and in osteoporosis due to immobilisation.

*Precautions:* Oral calcium supplementation is aimed at restoring normal serum calcium levels. Although it is extremely unlikely that high enough levels will be achieved to adversely affect digitalised patients, this theoretical possibility should be considered. Vitamin D causes an increase in calcium absorption and plasma calcium levels may continue to rise after stopping Vitamin D therapy. Patients treated with high doses of vitamin D or who are receiving prolonged calcium treatment should undergo regulatory measurements of plasma calcium levels which should be interpreted in conjunction with measurements of plasma protein levels.

*Interactions:* May impair absorption of other drugs e.g. tetracyclines, fluoride preparations. Thiazide diuretics reduce urinary calcium excretion so the risk of hypercalcaemia should be considered. Gastro-intestinal absorption of aluminium may be enhanced by the presence of citrate. This may be of particular importance in renal patients.

*Side-effects*: Constipation and wind. Rebound acid production. Hypercalcaemia, although hypercalcaemia would not be expected in patients unless their renal function were impaired, the following symptoms could indicate the possibility of hypercalcaemia: nausea, vomiting, anorexia, constipation, abdominal pain, bone pain, thirst, polyuria, muscle weakness, drowsiness or confusion. Alkalosis with high doses.

*Use in pregnancy and lactation*: There is epidemiological and clinical evidence of safety of calcium carbonate in human pregnancy.

*Overdosage*: There are no reports of overdose. Acute hypercalcaemia and alkalosis are a theoretical risk.

**Pharmaceutical precautions** There are no special requirements.

**Legal category** P

**Package quantities** Boxes of 90 sachets.

**Further information** When dispersed in water the calcium carbonate reacts with the citric acid with the formation of calcium citrate in an effervescent drink. Citrical contains no potassium and clinically insignificant amounts of sodium (0.055 mg). The following is a complete list of the excipients in Citrical: citric acid, sugar, glucose, orange oil, saccharin sodium, lecithin, β-carotene 10%, sodium lauryl sulphate, invert sugar, mono, di-fatty acid glycerides, water.

**Product licence number** 8557/0004

## CLINITAR *CREAM 1%

**Qualitative and quantitative composition** Stantar 1% w/w (a coal tar extract)

**Pharmaceutical form** Cream

**Clinical particulars**

*Therapeutic indications:* Subacute and chronic psoriasis and eczema. For use alone or with UVB irradiation.

*Posology and method of administration:* For topical administration. Apply to the affected area(s) once or twice daily. In combined treatment with UVB irradiation, Clinitar should be removed before exposure to light. Suitable for all ages.

*Contra-indications:* Allergy to the ingredients. Contra-indicated in generalised pustular psoriasis and infections of the skin.

*Special warnings and precautions for use:* The patient should be warned against exposing skin areas treated with Clinitar Cream to the sun or any artificial light source unless otherwise prescribed by the doctor.

*Interaction with other medicaments and other forms of interaction:* Sensitises the skin to UV light, which may lead to an unintended sunburn.

*Pregnancy and lactation:* Clinitar has not been tested in classical animal reproduction studies. There are insufficient human data to rule out the possibility of adverse effects in pregnancy and lactation, therefore it is recommended that Clinitar should not be used during pregnancy or lactation.

*Effects on ability to drive and use machinery:* None known.

*Undesirable effects:* Primary irritation and folliculitis. Phototoxic dermatitis has been seen in a few cases.

*Overdose:* Not applicable.

**Pharmacological properties**

*Pharmacodynamic properties*: The toxicology and the pharmacology of coal tar is well-known, coal tar having been used for topical treatment in therapeutic medicine since antiquity. The first clinical reports, however, only date back to the 1920's. Today, preparations containing coal tar are used world-wide in large quantities.

*Pharmacokinetic properties:* Percutaneous absorption of coal tar is assumed to be negligible. There is, however, a risk of absorption of phenols, of which coal tar contains up to 3–4%. Systemic toxicity after human use of coal tar has only been seen very rarely and only in patients who were seriously weakened by immunological and systemic diseases. It is therefore recommended not to apply coal tar to more than 25% of the body surface.

**Pharmaceutical particulars**

*List of excipients:* 1,2 propylene glycol, cetostearyl alcohol, glyceryl stearate, isopropyl palmitate, purified water.

*Incompatibilities:* None known.

*Shelf life:* 3 years.

*Special storage precautions:* No special precautions.

*Nature and contents of container:* 100 g aluminium tubes.

*Instructions for use/handling:* No special conditions.

**Marketing authorisation number** 8557/0024

**Date of approval/revision of SPC** 3 June 1996

**Legal category:** P

## CLINITAR* SHAMPOO 2%

**Qualitative and quantitative composition** Stantar 2% w/w (a coal tar extract).

**Pharmaceutical form** Shampoo

**Clinical particulars**

*Therapeutic indications:* Indicated for the treatment of pityriasis simplex capitis (dandruff). Seborrhoeic dermatitis of the scalp, and psoriasis of the scalp.

**Posology and method of administration:** For topical administration.
Moisten hair and rub a little shampoo into the hair and scalp. Rinse and repeat the treatment, this time producing a heavy lather. Leave in the hair for 5 minutes after the second treatment and then rinse carefully.
Use 1–3 times a week.
Suitable for all ages.

*Contra-indications*: Contains coal tar, therefore should not be used on coal tar sensitive skin, or where there is sensitivity to any of the other ingredients. Do not use in contact dermatitis.

*Special warnings and precautions for use*: If undue irritation occurs, the patient should be advised to discontinue use and see their doctor. Avoid getting shampoo into the eyes.

*Interaction with other medicaments and other forms of interaction*: None stated.

*Pregnancy and lactation*: Clinitar Shampoo has not been tested in classical animal reproduction studies. There are insufficient human data to rule out the possibility of adverse effects in pregnancy and lactation. It is therefore recommended that Clinitar should not be used.

*Effects on ability to drive and use machinery*: None known.

*Undesirable effects*: Coal tar may cause primary irritation and folliculitis.

*Overdose*: None stated.

**Pharmacological properties**

*Pharmacological properties*: Coal tar has been used in medicine for thousands of years. The use of tar preparations in the treatment of eczema, psoriasis and dandruff of the scalp can be considered well established. Tar reduces excess production of skin lipids (seborrhoea) especially from the sebaceous glands. Excessive production of skin surface lipids very often leads to a very troublesome seborrhoea capillitii with greasy hair, dandruff and seborrhoeic dermatitis.

*Pharmacokinetic properties:* Not much is known about the pharmacokinetics of coal tar. Knoth, Herrman and Meyhofer (1959) found that the distribution of tar in the skin showed the highest concentration in the hair follicles and the sebaceous glands, suggesting that these may make up an important route of penetration for the coal tar into the skin.

**Pharmaceutical particulars**

*List of excipients:* Sodium laurylethylsulphate, triethanolamine laurylsulphate, polyoxyethylene glycerolmonostearate, polysorbate 80, cocamidopropyl amine oxide, cocamide DEA, cocamidopropyl betain, perfume mixture and purified water.

*Incompatibilities*: None known

*Shelf life*: 5 years

*Special storage precautions*: No special precautions

*Nature and contents of container:* 100 g polypropylene tubes

*Instructions for use/handling*: No special conditions

**Marketing authorisation number** 8557/0025

**Date of approval/revision of SPC** 3 June, 1996

**Legal category** P

## CYCLOGEST*

**Presentation** White pessaries, suitable for vaginal or rectal insertion. Each 1.85 g pessary contains either 200 mg or 400 mg Progesterone PhEur.

**Uses** Treatment of the symptoms of pre-menstrual syndrome, including pre-menstrual tension and depression.

Treatment of puerperal depression.

**Dosage and administration** 200 mg daily to 400 mg twice a day, by vaginal or rectal insertion. For premenstrual syndrome commence treatment on day 14 of menstrual cycle and continue treatment until onset of menstruation. If symptoms are present at ovulation commence treatment on day 12.

*Children:* Not applicable.

*Elderly:* Not applicable.

**Contra-indications, warning etc** Undiagnosed vaginal bleeding.

*Other undesirable effects:* Menstruation may occur earlier than expected, or, more rarely, menstruation may be delayed. Soreness, diarrhoea and flatulence may occur with rectal administration. As with other vaginal and rectal preparations, some leakage of the pessary base may occur.

*Use in pregnancy and lactation:* Due to the indications of the product, it is anticipated that it will not be administered to pregnant women. As progesterone is a natural hormone, it is not expected to have adverse effects, however, no evidence is available to this effect.

*Other special warnings and precautions:* Use rectally if barrier methods of contraception are used. Use vaginally if patients suffer from colitis or faecal incontinence. Use rectally if patients suffer from vaginal infection (especially moniliasis) or recurrent cystitis. Use rectally in patients who have recently given birth.
Progesterone is metabolised in the liver and should be used with caution in patients with hepatic dysfunction.
Cyclogest contains the hormone progesterone which is present in significant concentrations in women during the second half of the menstrual cycle and during pregnancy. This should be borne in mind when treating patients with conditions that may be hormone-sensitive.

*Overdosage:* There is a wide margin of safety with Cyclogest pessaries, but overdosage may produce euphoria or dysmenorrhoea.

**Pharmaceutical precautions** Store in a cool dry place.

**Legal category** POM

**Package quantities** Packs of 15 pessaries 200 mg (OP). Packs of 15 pessaries 400 mg (OP).

**Further information** It is recommended that the diagnosis and evaluation of the treatment of premenstrual syndrome be monitored using pre-menstrual charts. The vaginal and rectal absorption of progesterone from Cyclogest are equivalent.

**Produce licence numbers**
Cyclogest Pessaries 200 mg    2343/0001
Cyclogest Pessaries 400 mg    2343/0002

*Product licence holder:* L.D. Collins & Co Ltd, Harwood, Mill Hill, London NW7 4HR

## HORMONIN*

**Presentation** Each pink, round, scored tablet contains Oestriol USP 0.27 mg; Oestradiol USP 0.6 mg; Oestrone PhEur 1.4 mg.

**Uses** Hormonin has been designed for replacement therapy in oestrogen-deficiency states, particularly those associated with the menopause such as nocturnal sweating, vasomotor disturbances, atrophic vaginitis and pruritus vulvae.
Prevention of post-menopausal osteoporosis.

**Dosage and administration** Hormonin may be given continuously or cyclically (three weeks out of four).

*Continuous therapy:* 1–2 tablets should be taken daily without a break in therapy. In women with an intact uterus the addition of an adequate dose and duration of progestogen (for 12–13 days) in each 28 day cycle is recommended.

*Cyclical therapy:* Hormonin 1–2 tablets should be taken cyclically (three weeks on followed by one week off). In women with an intact uterus the addition of an adequate dose and duration of progestogen (for 12–13 days) in each 28 day cycle is recommended.
Therapy with Hormonin may be initiated with either dose depending upon severity of symptoms. For maintenance therapy the lowest effective dose is recommended.
If the patient is not menstruating regularly therapy may be started arbitrarily. If the patient is menstruating regularly, therapy is started on day five of bleeding.
Before therapy commences, the patient should have a complete physical and gynaecological examination with special emphasis on blood pressure, breast, abdomen and pelvic organs. In women with an intact uterus, endometrial assessments should be carried

ut whenever possible. Any abnormal bleeding is an ndication for endometrial evaluation.

Regular follow-up examinations to include blood ressure and breast examinations are recommended very 6 months, and a complete physical and gynaeological examination every 12 months.

**ontra-indications, warnings, etc**

*ontra-indications*: Pregnancy and lactation.

Cardiovascular or cerebrovascular disorders, for xample, thrombophlebitis, thrombosis or thromoembolic disorders, moderate to severe hypertenion, hyperlipoproteinaemia, or a history of these onditions.

Cancer of the breast.

Known or suspected oestrogen-dependent tumurs.

Endometrial hyperplasia, uterine fibromyomata, ndiagnosed vaginal bleeding.

Acute or chronic liver disease, where liver function sts had failed to return to normal.

Porphyria.

*recautions:* In patients with mild hypertension or a istory of it, blood pressure should be monitored at egular intervals.

If hypertension develops in patients receiving oesogens, treatment should be stopped.

Risk of deep vein thrombosis is temporarily ineased when undergoing major surgery or prolonged nmobilisation, therefore treatment should be opped before surgery.

If any signs of thrombosis develop in patients eceiving oestrogens, discontinue treatment.

Caution should be exercised in prescribing to omen with a strong familial history of breast arcinoma, breast nodules or abnormal breast mamograms.

Glucose tolerance may be lowered and may, there-re, increase the need for insulin or other antiiabetic drugs in diabetics.

Thyrotoxicosis. Thyroid hormone binding globulin ay be increased leading to increased circulating tal thyroid hormone, therefore care must be taken interpreting thyroid function tests.

History of gall stones, cholestatic jaundice in pregancy or jaundice due to oral contraceptives.

If liver function tests become abnormal during estrogen therapy discontinue treatment.

Endometriosis.

Renal dysfunction. Major depression. Contact lens earers.

*Varnings*: Unopposed oestrogens predispose to ndometrial neoplasia.

Severe varicose veins–the benefits of oestrogenntaining preparations must be weighed against the ossible risks.

Cardiac failure, latent or overt.

Epilepsy, migraine, otosclerosis or a history of these onditions.

Sickle cell haemoglobinopathy, since under certain rcumstances, for example infections or anoxia, estrogen-containing preparations may induce romboembolic processes in patients with this contion.

Untreated polycythaemia or pulmonary hypertenon.

*de-effects*: Genito-urinary tract. Endometrial neoplaa, intermenstrual bleeding, increase in the size of erine fibromyomata, endometrial proliferation or ggravation of endometriosis, excessive production cervical mucus.

Breast: Tenderness, pain, enlargement, secretion.

Gastro-intestinal tract: Nausea, vomiting, cholelithiis, cholestatic jaundice.

Cardiovascular system: Hypertension, thrombosis, rombophlebitis, thromboembolism.

Skin: Erythema nodosum, rash, chloasma, hirsutm, loss of scalp hair.

Eyes: Corneal discomfort if contact lenses are used.

CNS: Headache, migraine, mood changes (elation depression).

Metabolic: Sodium and water retention, reduced ucose tolerance, and change in body weight.

**armaceutical precautions** Store in a closed conner in a dry place, below 25°C.

**gal category** POM

**ckage quantities** Securitainers of 90 tablets.

**rther information** Nil

**oduct licence number** 0271/5000R

*oduct licence holder:* G.W. Carnrick Co. Ltd., 2217 High Street, Orpington, Kent BR6 0NZ

## IDRID*

**esentation** Scarlet capsules, printed with "SP" d "MOI" in black, containing 65 mg Isometheptene ucate BP and 325 mg Paracetamol PhEur.

**Uses** In the treatment of migraine and other vascular headaches. Midrid contains isometheptene mucate, a cerebral vasoconstrictor, which provides prompt relief of migraineous headaches, which stem from dilated cranial vessels. Isometheptene is an indirect adrenergic agent with sympathomimetic properties. The paracetamol in Midrid acts as an analgesic.

**Dosage and administration**

*Adults*: 2 capsules at once, then 1 capsule every hour until relief obtained, up to a maximum of 5 capsules within a 12–hour period.

*Children*: Not recommended.

**Contra-indications, warnings, etc.**

*Contra-indications*: Midrid is contra-indicated in severe renal, hepatic or organic heart disease, severe hypertension, glaucoma, and in those patients who are on monoamine-oxidase inhibitor therapy. Porphyria. Hypersensitivity to paracetamol.

*Precautions*: Cardiovascular disease, diabetes mellitus, hyperthyroidism. Paracetamol should be given with care to patients with impaired liver or kidney function, and to patients taking other drugs that affect the liver. When used in patients with high spinal cord lesions, isometheptene, like other sympathomimetics may cause autonomic dysreflexia.

*Interactions*: On theoretical grounds care should be taken with patients receiving cardiac glycosides, quinidine, antihypertensives and tricyclic antidepressants. Alcohol reduces liver capacity to deal with paracetamol. Chronic use of paracetamol enhances effect of warfarin. Cholestyramine reduces absorption of paracetamol. May interact with chloramphenicol causing increased plasma levels.

*Side-effects*: Transient dizziness may appear in hypersensitive patients. This can usually be eliminated by reducing the dose. Circulatory disturbances may occur. Side effects which may be associated with any paracetamol containing preparation are usually mild, though haematological reactions have been reported. Rashes and other allergic reactions occur occasionally. There are isolated reports of thrombocytopenia purpura, methaemoglobinaemia, and agranulocytosis.

*Use in pregnancy*: There is no evidence of the drug's safety in human pregnancy nor is there evidence from animal work that it is free from hazard. Avoid in pregnancy.

*Overdosage*: Symptoms of paracetamol overdosage in the first 24 hours are pallor, nausea, vomiting, anorexia, and abdominal pain. Liver damage may become apparent 12 to 48 hours after ingestion. Abnormalities of glucose metabolism and metabolic acidosis may occur. In severe poisoning, hepatic failure may progress to encephalopathy, coma and death. Acute renal failure with acute tubular necrosis may develop even in the absence of severe liver damage. Cardiac arrhythmias have been reported. Prompt treatment is essential in the management of paracetamol overdosage. Any patient who has ingested about 7.5 g or more of paracetamol in the preceding 4 hours should undergo gastric lavage. Specific therapy with an antidote such as acetylcysteine or methionine may be necessary. Treatment should be instituted within 15 hours of ingestion. To assess severity of poisoning, paracetamol levels should be measured.

Acetylcysteine may be given either intravenously or by mouth or methionine may be given by mouth. Cysteamine was also formerly used. In adults, hepatic toxicity has rarely been reported with acute overdoses of less than 10 g.

**Pharmaceutical precautions** Store below 25°C.

**Legal category** P

**Package quantities** Securitainers of 100 capsules. Blister packs of 15 capsules.

**Further information** Printed Midrid capsules do not contain azo dyes.

**Product licence number** 0271/5001R.

*Product licence holder:* G.W. Carnrick Co. Ltd., 221-227 High Street, Orpington, Kent BR6 0NZ.

## ROBAXIN* 750

**Presentation** Scored white film-coated capsule-shaped tablet engraved "AHR" containing: Methocarbamol USP 750 mg.

**Uses** As a short-term adjunct to the symptomatic treatment of acute musculoskeletal disorders associated with painful muscle spasms.

**Dosage and administration**

*Oral: Adults:* The usual dosage is 2 tablets four times daily (6.0 g) but therapeutic response has been achieved with doses as low as 1 tablet three times daily.

*Older patients;* Half the maximum adult daily dose, or less, may be sufficient to produce a therapeutic response in the elderly.

*Children*: Not recommended.

**Contra-indications, warnings, etc**

*Contra-indications*: Hypersensitivity to methocarbamol. Coma or pre-coma states. Known brain damage or epilepsy. Myasthenia gravis.

*Use in pregnancy*: There is no evidence of safety in human pregnancy, nor is there evidence from animal work that it is free from hazard. Do not use during pregnancy, especially the first trimester, or lactation, unless there are compelling reasons to do so.

*Precautions and warnings*: Robaxin should be used with caution in patients with renal and hepatic insufficiency.

*Interactions*: This product may potentiate the effects of other central nervous system depressants and stimulants including alcohol, barbiturates, anaesthetics and appetite suppressants. The effects of anticholinergics, e.g. atropine and some psychotropic drugs may be potentiated by methocarbamol. Little is known about the possibility of interaction with other drugs.

*Side-effects*: This product may cause drowsiness and patients receiving it should not drive nor operate machinery unless their physical and mental capacities remain unaffected–especially if other medication capable of causing drowsiness is also being taken.

Robaxin may give rise to manifestations of allergy including skin rash, urticaria and angioneurotic oedema. This product may very rarely give rise to restlessness, anxiety, vertigo, tremor, confusion and convulsions. Light-headedness and dizziness have been reported. Nausea and vomiting have also been reported during use of Robaxin.

*Treatment of overdosage*: Gastric lavage with appropriate supportive therapy for 24 hours as methocarbamol is excreted within that time.

**Pharmaceutical precautions** Nil

**Legal category** POM.

**Package quantities** Bottles of 100 tablets.

**Further information** Nil

**Product licence number** 0100/5026R.

*Product licence holder:* A.H. Robins Company Ltd., Huntercombe Lane South, Taplow, Maidenhead, Berkshire SL6 0PH

## ROBAXISAL* FORTE

**Presentation** A two-layer, pink and white compressed tablet scored and stamped "AHR" containing: Methocarbamol USP 400 mg, Acetylsalicylic Acid PhEur 325 mg

This product also contains erythrosine (E127).

**Uses** In the short term management of pain and skeletal muscle spasm associated with musculoskeletal disorders such as lumbago, fibrositis, sprains, strains, etc.

**Dosage and administration**

*Oral: Adults:* 12 tablets four times daily.

*Older patients:* Half the adult dose may be sufficient to produce a therapeutic response.

*Children*: Not recommended.

**Contra-indications, warnings, etc**

*Contra-indications*: Hypersensitivity to methocarbamol or aspirin. Coma or pre-coma states. Known brain damage or epilepsy. Myasthenia gravis. Active peptic ulceration and haemophilia.

*Use in pregnancy*: There is no evidence of safety in human pregnancy, nor is there evidence from animal work that it is free from hazard. Do not use during pregnancy, especially the first trimester, or lactation, unless there are compelling reasons to do so.

Robaxisal Forte contains aspirin and is therefore best avoided at term because of possible effect on platelet function in the new-born. It may enhance the effects of anticoagulants.

*Precautions and warnings*: Robaxisal Forte should be used with caution in patients with renal and hepatic insufficiency.

Robaxisal Forte contains aspirin and therefore may give rise to gastrointestinal bleeding, and may precipitate bronchospasm especially in asthmatic patients. Patients currently on anti-coagulant therapy should have blood coagulation parameters regularly monitored.

*Interactions*: This product may potentiate the effects of other central nervous system depressants and stimulants including alcohol, barbiturates, anaesthetics and appetite suppressants. The effects of anticholinergics, e.g. atropine and some psychotropic drugs may be potentiated by methocarbamol. Little is known about the possibility of interaction with other drugs.

*Side-effects*: This product may cause drowsiness and patients receiving it should not drive nor operate machinery unless their physical and mental capacities remain unaffected–especially if other medication capable of causing drowsiness is also being taken.

Robaxisal Forte may rarely give rise to manifestations of allergy including skin rash, urticaria and angioneurotic oedema. This product may very rarely give rise to restlessness, anxiety, vertigo, tremor, confusion and convulsions, nausea and vomiting. Light-headedness and dizziness have been reported during use of Robaxisal Forte.

*Treatment of overdosage*: Supportive therapy for 24 hours, as methocarbamol is excreted within that time. If salicylate intoxication occurs, especially in children, the hyperpnoea may be controlled with sodium bicarbonate. Judicious use of 5% $CO_2$ with 95% $O_2$ may be of benefit. Abnormal electrolyte patterns should be corrected with appropriate fluid therapy.

**Pharmaceutical precautions** Store up to 25°C. No other special storage or transport precautions are necessary.

**Legal category** POM.

**Package quantities** Bottles of 100 tablets.

**Further information** Nil

**Product licence number** 0100/5028.

## ROBAXIN* INJECTABLE

**Presentation** 10 ml sterile ampoules each containing: Methocarbamol USP 1 g; vehicle 50% aqueous polyethylene glycol 300. This product also contains Sodium Metabisulphite BP.

**Uses** In the treatment of acute painful muscle spasm, due to musculoskeletal disorders or trauma.

**Dosage and administration** For intravenous use only.

*Adults:* 10–30 ml dependent on the severity of the condition and therapeutic response. Should not exceed 30 ml per day. Not to be administered for more than three consecutive days.

*Older patients:* Half the maximum adult daily dose, or less, may be sufficient for a therapeutic response in the elderly.

*Children*: Not recommended.

*Rate of administration*: Administer by slow intravenous injection or infusion directly into the vein at a maximum rate of 3 ml per minute.

*Diluent*: May be added to an intravenous drip of sterile isotonic saline, or sterile 5% dextrose. 10 ml of Robaxin injectable should not be diluted to more than 250 ml.

**Contra-indications, warnings, etc.**

*Contra-indications*: Hypersensitivity to methocarbamol or sulphite. Coma or pre-coma states. Known brain damage or epilepsy. Myasthenia gravis.

*Use in pregnancy*: There is no evidence of safety in human pregnancy, nor is there any evidence from animal work that it is free from hazard. Do not use during pregnancy, especially the first trimester, or lactation, unless there are compelling reasons to do so.

*Precautions and warnings*: Robaxin Injectable should be used with extreme caution in patients with impaired renal function, as the solvent used may cause raised urea levels and acidosis. Robaxin should be used with caution in patients with hepatic insufficiency.

Since Robaxin Injectable is hypertonic, vascular extravasation must be avoided. A recumbent position will reduce the likelihood of side-effects. Blood aspirated into the syringe does not mix with the hypertonic solution. The blood may be safely injected with the methocarbamol, or the injection may be stopped when the plunger reaches the blood, whichever the physician prefers.

*Interactions*: This product may potentiate the effects of other central nervous system depressants and stimulants including alcohol, barbiturates, anaesthetics and appetite suppressants. The effects of anticholinergics, e.g. atropine and some psychotropic drugs may be potentiated by methocarbamol. Little is known about the possibility of interaction with other drugs.

*Side-effects*: This product may cause drowsiness and patients receiving it should not drive nor operate machinery unless their physical and mental capacities remain unaffected–especially if other medication capable of causing drowsiness is also being taken.

Robaxin may give rise to manifestations of allergy including skin rash, urticaria and angioneurotic oedema. This product may very rarely give rise to restlessness, anxiety, vertigo, tremor, confusion and convulsions. Light-headedness and dizziness have been reported. Nausea and vomiting have also been reported during use of Robaxin.

*Treatment of overdosage*: Appropriate supportive therapy for 24 hours as methocarbamol is excreted within that time.

**Pharmaceutical precautions** Nil

**Legal category** POM.

**Package quantities** Boxes containing 5 ampoules.

**Further information** Nil

**Product licence number** 0100/5027R

*Product licence holder:* A.H. Robins Company Ltd., Huntercombe Lane South, Taplow, Maidenhead, Berkshire SL6 0PH.

## SUPRECUR* INJECTION ▼

**Qualitative and quantitative composition** Suprecur Injection contains 1.00 mg buserelin as buserelin acetate in 1 ml aqueous solution. 1.00 mg buserelin is equivalent to 1.05 mg buserelin acetate.

**Pharmaceutical form** Solution for Injection.

**Clinical particulars**

*Therapeutic indications* Pituitary desensitisation in preparation for ovulation induction regimens using gonadotrophins.

*Posology and method of administration* The total daily dose is usually in the range 200–500 micrograms given as a single injection by the subcutaneous route. Treatment should start in the early follicular phase (day 1) or, provided the existence of an early pregnancy has been excluded, in the mid-luteal phase (day 21). It should continue at least until down-regulation is achieved. e.g. serum oestradiol < 180 pmol/l and serum progesterone < 3 nmol/l. This will usually take about 1–3 weeks. Doses may have to be adjusted for individuals. Occasionally, patients may require up to 500 micrograms twice daily in order to achieve down-regulation. When down-regulation is achieved, stimulation with gonadotrophin is commenced while the dosage of buserelin is maintained. At the appropriate stage of follicular development, gonadotrophin and buserelin are stopped and hCG is given to induce ovulation.

Treatment monitoring, oocyte transfer and fertilisation techniques are performed according to the normal practice of the individual clinic.

Luteal support with hCG or progesterone should be given as appropriate.

*Contra-indications* Hypersensitivity to buserelin, LHRH, or to any of the excipients; pregnancy, lactation, undiagnosed vaginal bleeding; hormone-dependent neoplasms.

*Special warnings and precautions for use* Suprecur Injection is for subcutaneous administration ONLY.

Patients known to suffer from depression should be carefully monitored during treatment with Suprecur.

In patients with hypertension, blood pressure must be monitored regularly.

In diabetic patients, blood glucose levels must be checked regularly.

Whenever the treatment is self-administered, it is strongly recommended that initial doses should be administered under close medical supervision due to the possibility of hypersensitivity reactions. Patients should cease injections and seek medical attention should any adverse event occur which may represent an allergic reaction.

Treatment with Suprecur should be initiated only under the supervision of a specialist with experience of the indication.

Induction of ovulation should be carried out under close medical supervision. Risks specific to IVF/ET and related assisted reproduction procedures such as increase in ectopic and multiple pregnancies are unaltered under adjunctive use of buserelin. However, follicle recruitment may be increased especially in patients with polycystic ovarian disorder (PCOD).

Combined use of buserelin with gonadotrophins may bear a higher risk of ovarian hyperstimulation syndrome (OHSS) than the use of gonadotrophins alone. The stimulation cycle should be monitored carefully to identify patients at risk of developing OHSS, hCG should be withheld if necessary.

Possible clinical signs of ovarian hyperstimulation syndrome (OHSS) include: abdominal pain, feeling of abdominal tension, increased abdominal girth, occurrence of ovarian cysts, nausea, vomiting, as well as massive enlargement of the ovaries, dyspnoea, diarrhoea, oliguria, haemoconcentration, hypercoagulability. Pedicle tension or rupture of the ovary may lead to an acute abdomen. Severe thromboembolic events may also occur. Fatal outcome is possible.

Ovarian cysts have been observed in the initial phase of buserelin treatment. No impact on the stimulation cycle has been reported so far.

*Interactions with other medicaments and other form of interaction* During treatment with Suprecur, th effect of antidiabetic agents may be attenuated.

*Pregnancy and lactation* Pregnancy must be exclude before starting buserelin and the medication shou be stopped on the day of administration of hC Buserelin must not be administered to lactatin mothers; detectable levels of drug are found in milk

*Effects on ability to drive and use machines* Certa adverse events (e.g. dizziness) may impair the abili to concentrate and react, and therefore constitute risk in situations where these abilities are of speci importance (e.g. operating a vehicle or machinery).

*Undesirable effects* After administration of the inje tion, pain or local reaction at the injection site possible. Hypersensitivity reactions may also occu These may become manifest for example, as redde ing of the skin, itching, skin rashes (including urticari and allergic asthma with dyspnoea as well as, isolated cases, anaphylactic/anaphylactoid shock.

Side-effects consequent upon the suppression hormone production occur in most patients. H flushes, increased sweating and loss of libido gene ally occur some weeks after starting treatment ar may be severe in some patients. Dryness of the vagi may also be noticed.

*Changes in bone density*: A decrease in bone minera the magnitude of which relates to the duration therapy, occurs during treatment with buserelin alon The evidence available indicates that six month treatment is associated with a decrease in bo mineral density of the spine of 3.5%. These chang are similar to those seen with other agonists. I creased levels of serum alkaline phosphatase ma occur.

Combined use of buserelin with gonadotrophi may bear a higher risk of ovarian hyperstimulati syndrome (OHSS) than the use of gonadotrophi alone (see Section 4.4).

Other adverse events may include:

*Frequent*: Vaginal discharge, increase or decrea in breast size, breast tenderness, dry skin, acn increase or decrease in scalp hair, headache, palpit tions, nervousness, sleep disturbances, tiredne drowsiness, dizziness, emotional instability, low abdominal pain, stomach ache, nausea, vomitin diarrhoea, constipation, increase or decrease weight, back pain, pains in the limbs, joint discomfo

*Occasional*: Dry eyes (possibly leading to e irritations in women who wear contact lenses), i paired vision (e.g. blurred vision), feeling of pressu behind the eyes, splitting nails, increase or decrea in body hair, lactation, oedema (of face and extren ties), disturbances of memory and concentratio anxiety, depression or worsening of existing depre sion, increased thirst, change in appetite, paraesth sia, increase in serum liver enzyme levels (e transaminases) increase in serum bilirubin.

*Rare*: Increase or decrease in blood lipid leve tinnitus, hearing disorders.

*Very rare*: Deterioration of blood pressure levels patients with hypertension, reduction in gluco tolerance which may lead to worsening of control diabetics, thrombocytopenia, leucopenia.

*Isolated cases*; Severe hypersensitivity reactio with shock.

*Overdose* Overdose may lead to signs and sympto such as asthenia, headache, nervousness, hot flush dizziness, nausea, abdominal pain, oedema of t lower extremities, and mastodynia. Treatment shou be symptomatic

**Pharmacological properties**

*Pharmacodynamic properties:* Buserelin is a synthe peptide. It is a super active analogue of natu gonadotrophin releasing hormone (gonadore LHRH or GNRH). After an initial stimulation of gona otrophin release, it down-regulates the hypothalam pituitary-gonadal (HPO) axis such that a decrease ovarian steroid secretion into the post-menopau range occurs. The time taken to achieve these lev varies between individuals and with the regimen administration, so that close monitoring of circulati levels of oestradiol and progesterone should performed during treatment. This effect provides appropriate setting for the administration of follic stimulating therapy and reduces the incidence premature ovulation by inhibition of surges in LH.

*Pharmacokinetic properties:* The bioavailability buserelin after subcutaneous injection is 100%. Cm occurs at about 1 hour post-injection. The half- after injection is about 80 minutes.

Buserelin accumulates preferentially in the liv kidneys and in the anterior pituitary lobe, the biologi target organ. Buserelin circulates in serum predo nantly in the intact, active form. Protein binding about 15%.

Buserelin is inactivated by peptidases (pyroglu myl peptidase and chymotrypsin-like endopeptidas

the liver and kidneys. In the pituitary gland, receptor-ound buserelin is inactivated by membrane-located nzymes. Buserelin and inactive buserelin metabolites re excreted via the renal and the biliary route.

*reclinical safety data:* No signs of toxicity or histo-athological changes were detected in long term harmacology and toxicology studies with buserelin rats, dogs, and monkeys; the endocrine effects bserved were restricted to the gonads. Pituitary denoma occurred during long-term treatment in rats, is phenomenon has not been found in dogs and onkeys. There are no indications of a mutagenic or arcinogenic potential.

**harmaceutical particulars**

*ist of excipients* Sodium Chloride PhEur, Sodium ihydrogen Phosphate BP, Sodium Hydroxide BP, enzyl Alcohol BP, Water for Injections PhEur.

*compatibilities* Not applicable.

*helf life* Unopened: 36 months (see section 6.6).

*pecial precautions for storage* Store between 2° and 5°C. Do not freeze. Protect from light.

*lature and contents of container* Box of 2 x 5.5 ml ultidose vials each containing 1.05 mg buserelin cetate per 1 ml, corresponding to 1.00 mg buserelin er 1 ml.

*struction for use/handling* Each vial contains enough aterial for 10 doses. After finishing the course of eatment, the vial should be disposed of and a new al started for the next treatment. Do not use if the ontents of the vial are cloudy or discoloured. Patients hould be instructed on the correct handling of the al (aseptic technique) by a doctor or nurse.

*larketing Authorisation Holder:* Hoechst UK Ltd., oechst House, Salisbury Road, Hounslow, Middlesex W4 6JH

**larketing authorisation number** 00086/0195

**ate of approval/revision of SPC** February 1997.

**egal category** POM.

## UPRECUR* NASAL SPRAY

**resentation** Suprecur nasal spray, a colourless to intly yellowish solution, contains 150 micrograms userelin as buserelin acetate in one spray dose. 50 mg buserelin is equivalent to 1.575 mg buserelin etate.

The nasal spray also contains citric acid, sodium trate, sodium chloride and benzalkonium chloride in queous solution.

**ses** The treatment of endometriosis in cases that do ot require surgery as primary therapy.

Pituitary desensitisation in preparation for ovulation duction regimens using gonadotrophins.

**osage and administration**

*ndometriosis:* The total daily dose is 900 micrograms userelin, administered as one spray dose in each ostril in the morning, at mid-day and in the evening. e product may be used before or after meals or at her times, provided that uniform intervals are aintained between doses.

The usual duration of treatment is six months and is should not be exceeded.

Only a single course of treatment is recommended.

*tuitary desensitisation prior to ovulation induction:* e total intranasal dose for this indication is 600 mi-ograms buserelin, given in four divided dosages of 0 micrograms (one application in one nostril) read over the waking hours. Treatment should start the early follicular phase (day 1) or, provided the istence of an early pregnancy has been excluded in e midluteal phase (day 21). It should continue at ast until down-regulation is achieved e.g. serum stradiol <50 ng/l and serum progesterone <1 micro-am/l. This will usually take about 2–3 weeks. In me patients, dosages up to 4 x 300 micrograms ay be required to achieve these levels. When down-gulation is achieved, stimulation with gonadotro-in is commenced while the dosage of buserelin is aintained. At the appropriate stage of follicular velopment, gonadotrophin and buserelin are opped and hCG is given to induce ovulation.

Treatment monitoring, oocyte transfer and fertilis-on techniques are performed according to the rmal practice of the individual clinic.

Luteal support with hCG or progesterone should be ven as appropriate.

If used correctly, reliable absorption of the active gredient takes place via nasal mucous membranes. e drug is absorbed even if the patient has a cold; wever, in such cases the nose should be blown oroughly before administration.

If nasal decongestants are being used concurrently, ey should be administered at least 30 minutes after e buserelin.

*Children:* Suprecur is not suitable for use in children.

*Elderly:* Suprecur is not suitable for use in post-menopausal women.

**Contra-indications, warnings etc**

*Contra-indications:* Pregnancy, lactation, undiagnosed vaginal bleeding, hormone dependent neoplasms, hypersensitivity to buserelin acetate, LHRH or benzalkonium chloride.

*Precautions and warnings:* Patients known to suffer from depression should be carefully monitored during treatment with Suprecur. In patients with hypertension, blood pressure must be checked regularly.

In diabetic patients blood glucose levels must be checked regularly.

*Endometriosis:* Patients should discontinue oral contraceptives before starting treatment. Where appropriate, alternative, non-hormonal methods of contraception should be used. If treatment is interrupted even for only a few days, ovulation may occur and there is a risk of pregnancy.

Suprecur treatment should be started on the first or second day of menstruation in order to exclude pre-existing pregnancy as far as possible. A pregnancy test is advisable if there is any doubt.

A menstruation-like bleed usually occurs during the first few weeks of treatment. Breakthrough bleeding may also occur during continuing courses of treatment in some patients. Recovery of pituitary-gonadal function usually occurs within 8 weeks of discontinuing treatment.

In the initial treatment with buserelin, ovarian cysts may develop.

*Pituitary desensitisation prior to ovulation induction:* Induction of ovulation should be carried out under close medical supervision. Risks specific to IVF/ET and related assisted reproduction procedures such as increase in ectopic and multiple pregnancies are unaltered under adjunctive use of buserelin. In addition, follicle recruitment may be increased especially in patients with PCOD.

Combined use of buserelin with gonadotrophins may bear a higher risk of ovarian hyperstimulation syndrome (OHSS) than the use of gonadotrophins alone. The stimulation cycle should be monitored carefully to identify patients at risk of developing OHSS. hCG should be withheld if necessary. Possible clinical signs of ovarian hyperstimulation syndrome (OHSS) include: abdominal pain, feeling of abdominal tension, increased abdominal girth, occurrence of ovarian cysts, nausea, vomiting, as well as massive enlargement of the ovaries, dyspnoea, diarrhoea, oligurea, haemoconcentration, hypercoagulability. Pedicle tension or rupture of the ovary may lead to an acute abdomen. Severe thromboembolic events may also occur. Fatal outcome is possible.

Ovarian cysts have been observed in the initial phase of buserelin treatment. No impact on the stimulation cycle has been reported so far.

Treatment with Suprecur should be initiated only under the supervision of a specialist with experience of the indication.

*Interactions:* During treatment with buserelin, the effect of antidiabetic agents may be attenuated.

In concomitant treatment with sexual hormones ("add back"), the dosage is to be selected so as to ensure that the overall therapeutic effect is not affected.

*Effects on ability to drive and use machines:* Certain adverse effects (e.g. dizziness) may impair the patients ability to concentrate and react, and therefore, constitute a risk in those situations where these abilities are of special importance (e.g. operating a vehicle or machinery).

*Adverse reactions:* As evidence of the biological response to hormone deprivation, patients may experience menopausal-like symptoms and withdrawal bleeding, which are directly related to the pharmacological action of the drug. Symptoms such as hot flushes, increased sweating, dry vagina, dyspareunia, loss of libido occur some weeks after starting treatment and may be severe in some patients. Withdrawal bleeding may occur during the first few weeks of treatment. Breakthrough bleeding may occur during continuing treatment.

*Changes in bone density:* A decrease in bone mineral, the magnitude of which relates to the duration of therapy, occurs during treatment with buserelin alone. The evidence available indicates that six months' treatment is associated with a decrease in bone mineral density of the spine of 3.5%. These changes are similar to those seen with other agonists. Increased levels of serum alkaline phosphatase may occur. These are reversible on discontinuing treatment.

Other adverse events not directly attributable to the pharmacological effect have been observed. These are changes in breast size (increase/decrease), breast tenderness, splitting nails, acne, dry skin and occasionally vaginal discharge and oedema of the face and extremities (arms and legs).

In addition, vomiting, lactation, stomach ache, lower abdominal pain, paraesthesia may occur, as may dryness of the eyes, leading to eye irritation in wearers of contact lenses.

Buserelin treatment may also lead to:

– changes in scalp and body hair (alopecia, hirsutism),

– deterioration in blood pressure levels in patients with hypertension, hypersensitivity reactions, such as reddening of the skin, itching, skin rashes (including urticaria), and allergic asthma with dyspnoea, as well as in isolated cases leading to anaphylactic/anphylactoid shock,

– reduction in glucose tolerance,

– changes in blood lipids, increase in serum levels of liver enzymes (transaminases) increase in bilirubin; thrombopenia and leucopenia,

– headache (of migranous type in rare instances), palpitations, nervousness, sleep disturbances, fatigue (asthenia), drowsiness, disturbances of memory and concentration, emotional instability, feelings of anxiety. In rare cases depression may develop or existing depression may worsen,

– dizziness, tinnitus, hearing disorders, impaired vision (e.g. blurred vision), feeling of pressure behind the eyes,

– nausea, increased thirst, diarrhoea, constipation, changes in appetite, weight changes (increase or decrease),

– back pain, pain in the limbs and joint discomfort,

The nasal spray may irritate the nasal mucosa. This may lead to nosebleeds and hoarseness as well as to disturbances of smell and taste.

*Pregnancy and lactation:* Suprecur is contra-indicated in pregnancy and lactation, In rats, foetal malformations have been seen after very high doses.

*In endometriosis:* It is unlikely that pregnancy will occur in the later stages of treatment if the recommended doses are taken regularly. However, if treatment is interrupted even for only a few days, ovulation may occur and the patient may become pregnant. In this event, Suprecur must be withdrawn immediately (see also precautions).

*In pituitary desensitisation prior to ovulation induction:* Pregnancy should be excluded before starting Suprecur, and the medication should be stopped on the day of administration of hCG.

Buserelin, in small quantities, is excreted in milk. Suprecur should not be prescribed to lactating mothers, although no effects on the child have been observed so far.

*Overdose:* Overdose may lead to signs and symptoms such as asthenia, headache, nervousness, hot flushes, dizziness, nausea, abdominal pain, oedema of the lower extremities and mastodynia. Treatment should be symptomatic.

**Pharmaceutical precautions** Store between 2 and 25°C. Do not freeze. Once a bottle has been opened, it may be stored at room temperature for five weeks. Any residual material after this time should be discarded.

**Legal category**: POM

**Package quantities**: Cartons containing two bottles and two metered-dose pumps (nebulisers). Each bottle contains 10 g solution.

**Further information**: Buserelin is an analogue of the hypothalamic peptide LHRH. It competes with its parent molecule for binding sites on the anterior pituitary cells secreting LH and FSH. Initial effects are to increase secretion of the gonadotrophins, but provided that sufficient doses are used with sufficient regularity, the activity of the hypothalamic-pituitary-axis is down-regulated. Ovarian activity will be suppressed and oestradiol levels markedly reduced.

**Product licence number**: 0086/0144

*Product licence holder:* Hoechst UK Ltd, Hoechst House, Salisbury Road, Hounslow, Middlesex, TW4 6JH.

## SUPREFACT* INJECTION
## SUPREFACT* NASAL SPRAY

**Presentation** Suprefact injection contains 1.00 mg buserelin as buserelin acetate in 1 ml aqueous solution containing benzyl alcohol as preservative. The solution also contains sodium chloride, sodium dihydrogen phosphate and sodium hydroxide as excipients.

Suprefact nasal spray contains 100 micrograms buserelin as buserelin acetate in one spray dose (100 mg) of aqueous solution containing benzalkonium chloride as preservative. The solution also contains citric acid, sodium chloride and sodium citrate.

1.00 mg buserelin is equivalent to 1.05 mg buserelin acetate.

**Uses** For the treatment of advanced prostatic carcinoma (stage C or stage D according to the classification of Murphy et al, in Cancer, 45, p 1889–95, 1980) in which suppression of testosterone is indicated. Buserelin acts by blockade and subsequent down-regulation of pituitary LHRH receptor synthesis. Gonadotrophin release is consequently inhibited. As a result of this inhibition there is reduced stimulation of testosterone secretion and serum testosterone levels fall to the castration range. Before inhibition occurs there is a brief stimulatory phase during which testosterone levels may rise.

**Dosage and administration**

1. Initiation of therapy: is most conveniently carried out in hospital; 0.5 ml Suprefact injection should be injected subcutaneously at 8 hourly intervals for 7 days.

2. Maintenance therapy: on the 8th day of treatment the patient is changed to intranasal administration of Suprefact. One spray dose is introduced into each nostril 6 times a day according to the following schedule:

1st dose before breakfast
2nd dose after breakfast
3rd and 4th doses before and after midday meal
5th and 6th doses before and after evening meal.

This dosage regimen is to ensure adequate absorption of the material and to distribute the dose throughout the day.

If nasal decongestants are being used concurrently, they should be administered at least 30 minutes after buserelin.

**Contra-indications, warnings, etc**

*Contra-indications*: Suprefact should not be used if the tumour is found to be insensitive to hormone manipulation or after surgical removal of the testes. It is contra-indicated in cases of known hypersensitivity to benzalkonium chloride (nasal spray) or benzyl alcohol (injection) or buserelin.

*Precautions and warnings*: Monitoring of the clinical effect of Suprefact is carried out by the methods generally used in prostatic carcinoma. Initially serum testosterone levels rise and a clinical effect will not be seen until levels start to fall into the therapeutic (castration) range. Disease flare (temporary deterioration of patient's condition) has been reported at the beginning of treatment. The incidence is variable, but of the order of 10%. Symptoms are usually confined to transient increase in pain, but the exact nature depends on the site of the lesions. Neurological sequelae have been reported where secondary deposits impinge upon the spinal cord or CNS.

Disease flare is prevented by the prophylactic use of an anti-androgen, e.g. cyproterone acetate, 300 mg daily. It is recommended that treatment should be started at least 3 days before the first dose of Suprefact and continued for at least 3 weeks after commencement of Suprefact therapy.

Once testosterone levels have started to fall below their baseline concentration, clinical improvement should start to become apparent. If testosterone levels do not reach the therapeutic range within 4 weeks (6 weeks at the latest) the dose schedule should be checked to be sure that it is being followed exactly. It is unlikely that a patient who is taking the full dose will not show a suppression of testosterone to the therapeutic range. If this is the case, alternative therapy should be considered.

After the initial determination, testosterone levels should be monitored at 3-monthly intervals. A proportion of patients will have tumours that are not sensitive to hormone manipulation. Absence of clinical improvement in the face of adequate testosterone suppression is diagnostic of this condition, which will not benefit from further therapy with buserelin.

Patients known to suffer from depression should be carefully monitored during treatment with Suprefact.

If used correctly, reliable absorption of the active ingredient takes place via the nasal mucous membrane. Suprefact Nasal Spray is absorbed even if the patient has a cold.

In patients with hypertension, blood pressure must be monitored regularly.

In diabetic patients blood glucose levels must be checked regularly.

*Interactions:* During treatment with Suprefact, the effect of antidiabetic agents may be attenuated.

*Effects on ability to drive and operate machinery:* Certain adverse effects (e.g. dizziness) may impair the ability to concentrate and react, and therefore constitute a risk in situations where these abilities are of special importance (e.g. operating a vehicle or machinery).

*Side-effects:* At the beginning of treatment, a transient rise in the serum testosterone level usually develops and may lead to temporary activation of the tumour with secondary reactions such as:

– occurrence or exacerbation of bone pain in patients with metastases.
– signs of neurological deficit due to tumour compression with e.g. muscle weakness in the legs.
– impaired micturition, hydronephrosis or lymphostasis.
– thrombosis with pulmonary embolism.

Such reactions can be largely avoided when an anti-androgen is given concomitantly in the initial phase of buserelin treatment (see Precaution and Warnings). However, even with concomitant anti-androgen therapy, a mild but transient increase in tumour pain as well as a deterioration in general well-being may develop in some patients.

Additionally, in most patients, hot flushes and loss of potency or libido (result of hormone deprivation); painless gynaecomastia (occasionally) as well as mild oedema of the ankles and lower legs may occur.

Suprefact treatment may also lead to:
– changes in scalp or body hair (increase or decrease)
– deterioration in blood pressure levels in patients with hypertension.
– hypersensitivity reactions. These may become manifest as, e.g. reddening of the skin, itching, skin rashes (including urticaria) and allergic asthma with dyspnoea as well as, in isolated cases leading to anaphylactic/anaphylactoid shock.
– reduction in glucose tolerance. This may, in diabetic patients, lead to a deterioration of metabolic control.
– changes in blood lipids, increase in serum levels of liver enzymes (e.g. transaminases) increase in bilirubin, thrombopenia and leucopenia.
– headaches, palpitations, nervousness, sleep disturbances, tiredness, drowsiness, disturbance of memory and concentration, emotional instability, feelings of anxiety. In rare cases, depression may develop or existing depression worsen.
– dizziness, tinnitus, hearing disorders, impaired vision (e.g. blurred vision), feeling of pressure behind the eyes.
– nausea, vomiting, increased thirst, diarrhoea, constipation, changes in appetite, weight changes (increase or decrease).
– back pain and pain in the limbs, joint discomfort.

Administration of the nasal spray, may irritate the mucosa in the nasopharynx. This may lead to nosebleeds and hoarseness as well as to disturbances of taste and smell.

After administration of the injection, pain or local reaction at the injection site are possible.

*Overdosage:* Overdose may lead to signs and symptoms such as asthenia, headache, nervousness, hot flushes, dizziness, nausea, abdominal pain, oedema of the lower extremities and mastodynia. Treatment should be symptomatic.

**Pharmaceutical precautions:** Store at room temperature. The spray solution should last for 1 week of treatment. Any residual material after this time should be discarded.

**Legal category:** POM

**Package quantities** *Suprefact for Injection:* Box of 2 x 5.5 ml multidose vials each containing 1.05 mg buserelin acetate per 1 ml, corresponding to 1.00 mg buserelin per 1 ml.

*Suprefact Nasal Spray:* Outer of 4 bottles each containing 10 g solution, and 4 sprays pumps.

**Further information:** The therapeutic effect of Suprefact can only be achieved if the dosage is conscientiously adhered to. It is, therefore, advisable to administer Suprefact nasal spray before and after meals. It can also be used at other times provided uniform intervals are maintained between doses.

**Product licence numbers**

| | |
|---|---|
| Suprefact Nasal Spray | 0086/0101. |
| Suprefact Injection | 0086/0102. |

*Product licence holder:* Hoechst UK Ltd, Hoechst House, Salisbury Road, Hounslow, Middlesex, TW4 6JH.

## URISPAS* 200 Tablets

**Presentation** Each Urispas tablet contains flavoxate hydrochloride 200 mg. The white, sugar-coated tablets are overprinted with the name "URISPAS 200". Urispas tablets also contain lactose, sodium starch glycollate, povidone, talc, magnesium stearate, cellulose microcrystalline, purified water, gelatin, sucrose, maize starch, acacia, light magnesium carbonate, titanium dioxide, opalux AS 7000B, white beeswax, carnauba wax and opacode SI 9005 red.

**Uses**

*Pharmacological properties*: Urispas is an antispasmodic, selective to the urinary tract. In animal and human studies, Urispas has been shown to have a direct antispasmodic action on smooth muscle fibres. In addition, animal studies have shown Urispas t have analgesic and local anaesthetic properties.

*Pharmacokinetics*: Oral studies in man have indicate that flavoxate is readily absorbed from the intestin and converted almost immediately, and to a larg extent, to methyl flavone carboxylic aid, MFCA.

Following an IV dose (equimolar to 100 mg) th following parameters were calculated for flavoxat $T_{\frac{1}{2}}$ 83.3 min.; apparent volume of distribution 2.89 kg. The apparent distribution of MFCA was 0.20 l/k No free flavoxate was found in urine (24 hour however 47% of the dose was excreted as MFCA.

Following single oral dosing to volunteers of 200 m and 400 mg flavoxate, almost no free flavoxate wa detected in the plasma. The peak level of MFCA wa attained at 30–60 min. after the 200 mg dose and round two hours following the 400 mg dose. The AU for the 400 mg dose was approximately twice as larg as the AUC for the 200 mg dose. About 50% of th dose was excreted as MFCA within 12 hours, mo being excreted within the first 6 hours.

After repeated oral dosing (200 mg TDS, 7 days) th cumulative excretion of metabolites stabilised at 60 of the dose on the third day remaining almo unchanged after one week.

*Indications:* Urispas is indicated for the symptomat relief of dysuria, urgency, nocturia, vesical supr pubic pain, frequency and incontinence as may occ in cystitis, prostatis, urethritis, urethro-cystitis ar urethrotrigonitis.

In addition, the preparation is indicated for the reli of vesico-urethral spasms due to catheterisatio cystoscopy or indwelling catheters; prior to cysto copy or catheterisation; sequelae or surgical interve tion of the lower urinary tract.

Where evidence of urinary infection is preser appropriate anti-infective therapy should be institut concomitantly.

**Dosage and administration**

*Adults (including the elderly):* The recommende adult dosage is one tablet three times a day for long as required.

*Children*: Urispas tablets are not recommended f children under 12 years of age.

**Contra-indications, warnings, etc**

*Contra-indications:* The following obstructive con tions: pyloric or duodenal obstruction, obstructi intestinal lesions, or ileus, achalasia, gastro-intestin haemorrhage and obstructive uropathies of the low urinary tract.

*Use in pregnancy and lactation:* Since there is evidence of the drug's safety in human pregnanc nor any evidence from animal work that it is free fro hazard, Urispas should be avoided in pregnan unless there is no safe alternative. It is not know whether flavoxate is excreted in human milk. Becau many drugs are excreted in human milk, cauti should be exercised when Urispas is administer during breast-feeding.

*Precautions*: Urispas should be used with caution patients with suspected glaucoma.

In the event of drowsiness and blurred vision, t patient should not operate a motor vehicle or machi ery.

*Side-effects and adverse reactions:* In clinical tri comparing Urispas with other antispasmodic agen the incidence of side-effects was low. The followi adverse reactions have been observed:

*Gastro-intestinal:* nausea, vomiting, dry mouth, di rhoea.

*CNS:* vertigo, headache, mental confusion, esp cially in the elderly, drowsiness, fatigue and nervo ness.

*Haematologic:* leukopenia (one case which w reversible upon discontinuation of the drug).,

*Cardiovascular:* tachycardia and palpitation.

*Allergic:* urticaria and other dermatoses, eosir philia and hyperpyrexia.

*Ophthalmic:* increased ocular tension, blurred sion, disturbance in eye accommodation.

*Renal:* dysuria.

*Treatment of overdosage:* Patients who have taken overdosage of Urispas should have gastric lava performed within four hours of the overdosa occurring. If overdosage is extreme, or there is a de in removing the drug from the stomach, administ tion of a parasympathomimetic drug should considered.

**Pharmaceutical precautions** *Storage:* No spec precautions are required.

**Legal category** POM

**Package quantities** Urispas tablets are available containers of 90 tablets.

**Further information** Nil.

**Product licence number** 8557/0034

**Trade Mark*

**Smith & Nephew Healthcare Ltd**

Healthcare House
Goulton Street
Hull
HU3 4DJ

**Smith+Nephew**
*Leadership in Worldwide Healthcare*

## AMETOP* GEL

**Qualitative and quantitative composition** Amethocaine base 4.0%w/w

**Pharmaceutical form** Topical, white opalescent gel, each gram containing 40 mg of amethocaine base.

**Clinical particulars**

*Therapeutic indications:* Percutaneous local anaesthetic to produce anaesthesia of the skin prior to venepuncture or venous cannulation.

*Posology and method of administration:*

*Adults (including the elderly) and children over 1 month of age:* Apply the contents of the tube to the centre of the area to be anaesthetised and cover with an occlusive dressing. The contents expellable from 1 tube (approximately 1 gram) are sufficient to cover and anaesthetise an area of up to 30 sq.cm.(6x5cm). Smaller areas of anaesthetised skin may be adequate in infants and small children.

Adequate anaesthesia can usually be achieved following a thirty minute application time for venepuncture, and a forty-five minute application time for venous cannulation, after which the gel should be removed with a gauze swab and the site prepared with an antiseptic wipe in the normal manner.

It is not necessary to apply Ametop gel for longer than 30-45 minutes and anaesthesia remains for 4-6 hours in most patients after a single application.

Not recommended for infants under 1 month of age.

*Contra-indications:* Use in premature babies or in full term infants less than 1 month of age, where the metabolic pathway for amethocaine may not be fully developed.

Known hypersensitivity to local anaesthetics of the ester type.

Do not apply Ametop Gel to broken skin, mucous membranes or to the eyes or ears.

*Special warnings and precautions for use:* Only apply to intact, normal skin. Not to be taken internally. Ametop gel, like other local anaesthetics may be ototoxic and should not be instilled into the middle ear or used for procedures which might involve penetration into the middle ear. Repeated exposure to Ametop gel may increase the risk of sensitisation reactions to amethocaine.

*Interaction with other medicaments and other forms of interaction:* None known

*Pregnancy and lactation:* There is no specific information as to the Safety of amethocaine in pregnancy, although amethocaine has been in wide use for many years without apparent ill-consequence. It is not known whether amethocaine or its metabolites are excreted in breast milk. Therefore the product is not recommended for use on breast feeding mothers.

*Effects on ability to drive and use machines:* No adverse effects on the ability to drive or to use hazardous machinery are expected following use of Ametop Gel.

*Undesirable effects:* Slight erythema is frequently seen at the site of application and is due to the pharmacological action of amethocaine in dilating capillary vessels. This may help delineating the anaesthetised area.

Slight oedema or itching are less frequently seen at the site of application. This may be due to the local release of histamine and 5-HT.

More severe erythema, oedema and/or itching confined to the site of application have rarely been reported.

*Overdose:* Overdosage with Ametop gel is unlikely to result from application to intact skin. If accidentally ingested systemic toxicity may occur, and signs will be similar to those observed after administration of other local anaesthetics.

**Pharmacological properties**

*Pharmacodynamic properties:* Amethocaine is a local anaesthetic and is believed to act by blocking nerve conduction mainly by inhibiting sodium ion flux across the axon membrane. Amethocaine achieves this by acting upon specific receptors that control gating mechanisms responsible for conductance changes in specialised proteinaceous sodium channels.

Blocking sodium ion flux prevents the setting up of an action potential in the nerve axon, thus preventing pain receptors signalling to the central nervous system.

Amethocaine additionally has vasodilatory effects, which commonly results in a localised erythema.

*Pharmacokinetic properties:* The ester type 'caine' anaesthetics are rapidly metabolised in blood mainly by plasma pseudocholinesterase. A 3.33μM (1μg/ml) concentration of amethocaine was fully metabolised in human plasma within 20 seconds.

*In vivo* data has demonstrated that Ametop gel is 15 ± 11% bioavailable when administered to intact normal skin, with a mean absorption and elimination half life of 1.23 ± 0.28 hours.

Peak plasma levels of p-(n-butylamino) benzoic acid (BABA), the major metabolite of amethocaine. are between 3-6 hours post dose.

**Pharmaceutical particulars**

*List of excipients:* In addition to the active ingredient, Ametop Gel contains: Sodium Hydroxide BP, Sodium Methyl-p-hydroxybenzoate BP, Sodium Propyl-p-hydroxybenzoate BP, Monobasic Potassium Phosphate USNF, Xanthan Gum USNF, Sodium Chloride PhEur, Purified Water PhEur

*Incompatibilities:* None known.

*Shelf life:* The shelf-life shall not exceed 24 months from date of manufacture. Within the recommended shelf life of 2 years at 15°C, the product, following dispensing, may be stored for upto 1 month at 25°C at point of use.

*Special precautions for storage:* Store below 15°C. Do not freeze. Do not expose to heat.

*Nature of contents and container:* 1.5 g, internally lacquered, aluminium collapsible tubes, designed to deliver 1.0 g of Ametop gel on squeezing.

*Instructions for use/handling:* As amethocaine can cause contact sensitisation reactions, particularly with repeated contact, healthcare professionals should take care to minimise contact with Ametop gel during application and removal.

**Marketing authorisation number** 14038/0001

**Date of approval/revision of SPC** 10 July 1995

**Legal category** P

## CUPLEX*

**Presentation** A clear, brownish-yellow viscous gel containing Salicylic Acid PhEur 11% w/w, and Lactic Acid PhEur 4% w/w. Other ingredients include copper, collodion, colophony and venice turpentine.

**Uses** Topical treatment of common, juvenile, plantar and mosaic warts; corns and calluses.

**Dosage and administration** Soak the wart nightly for 5 minutes in hot water. Dry with your own towel. Apply just enough Cuplex gel to cover the wart. Let the gel dry. It will form a waterproof elastic film over the wart. Each morning remove the film and apply more gel. Two or three times a week rub the wart surface with emery board or pumice stone before applying Cuplex gel. Suitable for all ages, except infants.

**Contra-indications, warnings, etc** Do not apply to facial or anogenital warts. Not for use in patients sensitive to colophony. Avoid contact with eyes. Only apply to the affected area. Keep away from naked flames.

**Pharmaceutical precautions** Store in a cool place. Highly inflammable.

**Legal category** P

**Package quantities** 5 g tubes. OP.

**Further information** Warts are contagious and any person suffering from warts should always use their own towel.

Most warts will disappear after 6 to 12 weeks of treatment with Cuplex gel providing instructions are carefully and consistently followed. Where, however, the wart continues to increase in size after 6 weeks treatment and the patient has not consulted a doctor, the patient should be advised to do so.

**Product licence number** 13374/0007

*Product licence holder:* Smith & Nephew Pharmaceuticals Ltd, Hessle Road, Hull, HU3 2BN.

## FLAMAZINE* CREAM

**Qualitative and quantitative composition** Silver sulphadiazine 1.0%w/w.

**Pharmaceutical form** Semi-solid oil in water emulsion.

**Clinical particulars**

*Therapeutic indications:* Flamazine cream is indicated for the prophylaxis and treatment of infection in burn wounds. Flamazine cream may also be used as an aid to the short-term treatment of infection in leg ulcers and pressure sores, and as an aid to the prophylaxis of infection in skin graft donor sites and extensive abrasions. Flamazine cream is also indicated for the conservative management of finger-tip injuries where pulp, nail loss and/or partial loss of the distal phalanx has occurred.

*Posology and method of administration:* To be applied topically.

*Burns:* The burn wound should be cleaned and Flamazine cream applied over all the affected areas to a depth of 3-5 mm.

This application is best achieved with a sterile gloved hand and/or sterile spatula. Where necessary, the cream should be re-applied to any area from which it has been removed by patient activity.

In burns, Flamazine cream should be re-applied at least every 24 hours, or more frequently if the volume of exudate is large.

*Hand burns:* Flamazine cream can be applied to the burn and the whole hand enclosed in a clear plastic bag or glove which is then closed at the wrist.

The patient should be encouraged to move the hand and fingers. The dressing should be changed when an excessive amount of exudate has accumulated in the bag.

*Leg ulcers/pressure sores:* The cavity of the ulcer should be filled with Flamazine Cream to a depth of at least 3-5 mm. As Flamazine Cream can cause maceration of normal skin on prolonged contact, care should be taken to prevent spread onto non-ulcerated areas.

Application of Flamazine Cream should be followed by an absorbent pad or gauze dressing, with further application of pressure bandaging as appropriate for the ulcer.

The dressings should normally be changed daily but for wounds which are less exudative, less frequent changes (every 48 hours) may be acceptable. Cleansing and debriding should be performed before application of Flamazine cream.

Flamazine cream is not recommended for use in leg or pressure ulcers that are very exudative.

*Finger-tip injuries:* Haemostasis of the injury should be achieved prior to the application of a 3-5 mm layer of Flamazine cream. A conventional finger dressing may be used. Alternatively the finger of a plastic or unsterile surgical glove can be used and fixed in place with waterproof adhesive tape. Dressings should be changed every 2-3 days.

*Contra-indications:* As sulphonamides are known to cause kernicterus, Flamazine Cream should not be used at, or near term pregnancy, on premature infants or on newborn infants during the first months of life. Flamazine cream is also contraindicated in patients known to be hypersensitive to silver sulphadiazine or to other components of the preparation such as cetyl alcohol or propylene glycol

*Special warnings and precautions for use:* Flamazine cream should be used with caution in the presence of significant hepatic or renal impairment. Caution of use is required in patients known to be sensitive to systemic sulphonamides and in individuals known to have glucose-6-phosphate dehydrogenase deficiency.

Use of Flamazine cream may delay separation of burn eschar and may alter the appearance of the burn wounds.

*Interactions with other medicaments and other forms of interaction:* As silver may inactivate enzymatic debriding agents, their concomitant use may be inappropriate.

In large-area burns where serum sulphadiazine levels may approach therapeutic levels, it should be noted that the effects of systemically administered drugs may be altered. This can especially apply to oral hypoglycaemic agents and to phenytoin. In the case of these drugs, it is recommended that blood levels should be monitored as their effects can be potentiated.

*Pregnancy and lactation:* Safety for use in pregnancy and lactation has not been established. Although animal studies have not shown any hazard, adequate studies in pregnant women have not been performed. Use in pregnancy only if benefit is likely to be greater than the possible risk to the foetus. Since all sulphonamides increase the possibility of kernicterus, caution is required in nursing mothers.

*Effects on ability to drive and to use machines:* None known.

*Undesirable effects:* Local reactions such as burning, itching and skin rash may occur in about 2% of patients.

Leucopenia has been reported in 3–5% of burns patients treated with Flamazine cream. This may be a drug-related effect, and often manifests itself 2–3 days after treatment has commenced. It is usually self-limiting and therapy with Flamazine cream does not usually need to be discontinued, although the blood count must be carefully monitored to ensure that it returns to normal within a few days.

Systemic absorption of silver sulphadiazine may very rarely result in any of the adverse reactions attributable to systemic sulphonamide therapy or clinical argyria.

*Overdose:* Not likely to occur with normal usage

**Pharmacological properties**

*Pharmacodynamic properties:* Silver sulphadiazine has bacteriostatic and bactericidal properties. This combination provides a wide spectrum of antimicrobial activity.

*Pharmacokinetic properties:* There is evidence that in large area wounds and/or after prolonged application, systemic absorption of silver can occur causing clinical argyria. The sulphadiazine readily diffuses across wounds and enters the general circulation. The degree of uptake will significantly depend upon the nature of the wound and the dosing regime. Sulphadiazine is excreted in the urine.

*Preclinical safety data:* None stated.

**Pharmaceutical particulars**

*List of excipients:* In addition to the active ingredient, silver sulphadiazine, Flamazine contains: Polysorbate 60 BP, Polysorbate 80 BP, Glycerol Monostearate BP, Cetyl Alcohol, Liquid Paraffin BP, Propylene Glycol BP, Purified Water PhEur.

*Incompatibilities:* None known.

*Shelf life:* 36 months from date of manufacture.

*Special precautions for storage:* Flamazine should be stored below 25°C. Protect from light. The contents of one container are for the treatment of one person. 250 g and 500 g pots should be discarded 24 hours after opening. Tubes of Flamazine should be discarded 7 days after opening.

*Nature of contents and container:* 15 g, 30 g or 50 g pre-printed cylindrical polyethylene tubes fitted with polyethylene caps.

250 g or 500 g black polypropylene pot fitted with a black polyethylene or polypropylene lid.

All tubes and pots are tamper evident.

*Instructions for use/handling:* None.

*Marketing authorisation holder:* Smith & Nephew Pharmaceuticals Ltd, Hessle Road, Hull, HU3 2BN. Distributed in the UK by Smith & Nephew Healthcare Ltd, Goulton Street, Hull HU3 4DJ

**Marketing authorisation number** 13374/0006

**Date of approval/revision of SPC** 12 March 1997

**Legal category** POM

# WELLDORM* ELIXIR

**Presentation** Welldorm Elixir is a clear red syrup, with a pleasant passion-fruit flavour. Welldorm Elixir contains Chloral Hydrate BP 143 mg/5 ml.

**Uses** Welldorm Elixir is for the short-term treatment of insomnia.

**Dosage and administration**

*Adults:* 15-45 ml taken 15-30 minutes before bedtime with water or milk. Dose should not exceed 2 g chloral hydrate per day.

*Elderly:* Dosage as for adults except in the frail elderly or those with hepatic impairment, where a reduction in dose may be appropriate.

*Children:* 30-50 mg/kg. Dose should not exceed 1 g chloral hydrate per day.

**Contra-indications, warnings, etc** Should not be used in patients with marked hepatic or renal impairment, or in patients with severe cardiac disease. Best avoided in the presence of gastritis and in patients who have previously exhibited an idiosyncracy or hypersensitivy to chloral hydrate. Should not be used in patients susceptible to acute attacks of porphyria.

Interactions may occur in patients taking anticoagulants. When chloral hydrate is added to or withdrawn from the drug regimen, or its dosage changed, careful monitoring of the prothrombin time is required.

Patients should be warned that their ability to drive or use machinery may be impaired by drowsiness.

It is contra-indicated in pregnancy and lactation.

*Side-effects:* Gastric irritation, abdominal distension and flatulence may occur. Excitement, tolerance, allergic skin reactions, headache and ketonuria have occasionally been reported.

Alcohol potentiates the sedative effect. Chloral hydrate followed by intravenous frusemide may result in sweating, hot flushes and variable blood pressure including hypertension due to a hypermetabolic state caused by displacement of thyroid hormone from its bound state. Delerium may occur, especially in the elderly, particularly when used in conjunction with psychotropics or anticholinergics.

*Abuse and chronic intoxication:* There is a danger of abuse or chronic intoxication and the possibility that habituation may develop. In such patients gastritis and parenchymatous renal injury may develop. After long term use sudden withdrawal may result in delirium.

*Overdosage:* The signs and symptoms of overdosage involve the CNS, cardiovascular and respiratory systems. These may include: respiratory depression, arrhythmias, hypothermia, pin-point pupils, hypotension or coma. Gastric irritation may result in vomiting and even gastric necrosis. If the patient survives, icterus due to hepatic damage and albuminuria from renal damage may appear. Serious problems have arisen with doses as little as 4 g and 10 g can be fatal. Overdosage shoud be treated with gastric lavage or inducing vomiting to empty the stomach. Supportive measures must be used. Haemodialysis, and in some cases haemoperfusion, have been reported to be effective in promoting the clearance of trichloroethanol.

**Pharmaceutical precautions** Syrup BP should be used as a diluent. Welldorm elixir should be stored below 25°C in a well-stoppered bottle away from direct sunlight.

**Legal category** POM

**Package quantities** Welldorm elixir is supplied in bottles containing 150 ml. OP.

**Further information** Each 5 ml of Welldorm elixir contains approximately 1.65 g of glucose.

Chloral hydrate and its metabolite trichloroethanol act as a central nervous system depressant.

Chloral hydrate leads to a decrease in sleep latency and in the number of awakenings. A near natural sleep is induced and the REM/NON-REM ratio is not altered.

Chloral hydrate is rapidly absorbed from the stomach and starts to act within 30 minutes. It is widely distributed throughout the body and is metabolised to trichloroethanol, also an active hypnotic, and trichloroacetic acid in the erythrocytes, liver and other tissues. It is excreted partly in the urine as trichloroethanol and its glucuronide, urochloralic acid, and as trichloroacetic acid. Significant amounts are also excreted in bile. Trichloroethanol has a plasma half-life of the order of 8 hours. Trichloroacetic acid has a half-life of several days.

**Product licence number** 13374/0005

*Product licence holder:* Smith & Nephew Pharmaceuticals Ltd, Hessle Road, Hull, HU3 2BN

# WELLDORM* TABLETS

**Presentation** An elongated, oval, film coated tablet. The coated tablet has a uniform smooth, film coat, of bluish-purple. Each tablet contains 707 mg chloral

betaine, equivalent to 414 mg of chloral hydrate. T tablets are packed in opaque blister strips.

**Uses** Welldorm Tablets are used for the short-te treatment of insomnia.

**Dosage and administration**

*Adults:* The hypnotic dose is one to two tablets tak 15-30 minutes before bedtime with water or mi Dose should not exceed 2 g of chloral hydrate p day.

*Elderly:* Dosage as for adults except in the frail elde or those with hepatic impairment, where a reducti in dose may be appropriate.

*Children:* Welldorm tablets are not suitable for use children under the age of 12, for such patie Welldorm Elixir is recommended (please refer separate data sheet for dosage recommendations).

**Contra-indications, warnings, etc** Should not be us in patients with marked hepatic or renal impairme or in patients with severe cardiac disease. Be avoided in the presence of gastritis and in patie who have previously exhibited an idiosyncracy hypersensitivity to chloral hydrate. Should not used in patients susceptible to acute attacks porphyria. Should not be used in pregnancy a lactation.

Interactions may occur in patients taking anticoa ulants. When chloral hydrate is added to or withdrav from the drug regimen, or its dosage changed, care monitoring of the prothrombin time is required.

Patients should be warned that their ability to dri or use machinery may be impaired by drowsiness.

*Side-effects:* Gastric irritation, abdominal distensi and flatulence may occur. Excitement, toleran allergic skin reactions, headache and ketonuria ha occasionally been reported.

Alcohol potentiates the sedative effect. Chlo hydrate followed by intravenous frusemide may res in sweating, hot flushes and variable blood press including hypertension due to a hypermetabolic sta caused by displacement of thyroid hormone from bound state. Delerium may occur, especially in t elderly, particularly when used in conjunction w psychotropics or anticholinergics.

*Abuse and chronic intoxication:* There is a danger abuse or chronic intoxication and the possibility t habituation may develop. In such patients gastr and parenchymatous renal injury may develop. Af long term use sudden withdrawal may result delirium.

*Overdosage:* The signs and symptoms of overdosa involve the CNS, cardiovascular and respiratory s tems. These may include: respiratory depressi arrhythmias, hypothermia, pin-point pupils, hypot sion or coma. Gastric irritation may result in vomiti and even gastric necrosis. If the patient surviv icterus due to hepatic damage and albuminuria fr renal damage may appear. Serious problems ha arisen with doses as little as 4 g and 10 g can be fa Overdosage shoud be treated with gastric lavage inducing vomiting to empty the stomach. Support measures must be used. Haemodialysis, and in so cases haemoperfusion, have been reported to effective in promoting the clearance of trichlor thanol.

**Pharmaceutical precautions** The tablets should stored in a dry place at 15-25°C.

**Legal category** POM

**Package quantities** The tablets are packed in blis strips of 15, two strips (30 tablets) per carton. OP.

**Further information** Chloral hydrate and its metabo trichloroethanol act as central nervous system dep sants.

Welldorm is a chloral hydrate derivative, wh leads to a decrease in sleep latency and in the num of awakenings. A near natural sleep is induced a the REM/NON-REM ratio is not altered.

Chloral hydrate is rapidly absorbed from the sto ach, and starts to act within 30 minutes. It is wid distributed throughout the body, and is metaboli to trichloroethanol, also an active hypnotic, a trichloroacetic acid in the erythrocytes, liver and ot tissues. It is excreted partly in the urine as trichlor thanol and its glucuronide, urochloralic acid, and trichloroacetic acid. Significant amounts are a excreted in bile. Trichloroethanol has a plasma h life of the order of 8 hours. Trichloroacetic acid ha half-life of several days.

**Product licence number** 13374/0004

*Product licence holder:* Smith & Nephew Pharmac ticals Ltd, Hessle Road, Hull, HU3 2BN

*Trade Mark

# mithKline Beecham Pharmaceuticals
Velwyn Garden City
lertfordshire AL7 1EY

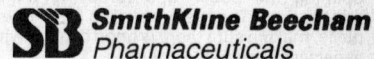

**SmithKline Beecham**
Pharmaceuticals


## C VAX*
### leningococcal vaccine PhEur (groups and C polysaccharides)

**esentation** AC Vax meningococcal meningitis ccine is a lyophilised preparation of purified poly- ccharides from *Neisseria meningitidis* (meningo- ccus) of groups A and C. It is presented as a white llet in a glass vial together with a separate ampoule vial of clear, colourless, sterile diluent. Each 0.5 ml se of reconstituted vaccine contains 50 micrograms group A polysaccharide and 50 micrograms of oup C polysaccharide dissolved in isotonic sodium loride (0.9 per cent).

**ses** Active immunisation against meningococcal eningitis caused by group A and group C meningo- cci.

AC Vax is particularly recommended for subjects at k, for example those living in areas or travelling to untries where the disease is epidemic or highly demic. It is also recommended in epidemic situa- ns and for close contacts of patients with this sease.

**sage and administration**

*dults and children aged two months and over:* 0.5 ml the reconstituted vaccine administered by deep bcutaneous injection only. The vaccine must not be ven intravenously under any circumstances.

The vaccine should be reconstituted with the diluent pplied by adding the entire contents of the diluent al to the vaccine vial.

**ntra-indications, warnings, etc**

*ntra-indications:* Do not use in subjects hypersen- ive to any component of the vaccine or in those th febrile conditions.

*ecautions:* AC Vax gives no protection against eningococcal meningitis caused by meningococci longing to groups other than A and C.

If administered to subjects with impaired immune sponses, the vaccine may not induce an effective sponse.

As with all vaccinations, a solution of 1:1000 renaline should be available for injection should an aphylactic reaction occur.

*se in pregnancy:* No studies in animals have been rformed. Since the effect of the vaccine on the etus is not known, it should not be given during egnancy unless there is a definite risk from groups and C meningococcal disease.

*lverse reactions:* These are mild and short-lasting. cal reactions may consist of erythema, slight duration and tenderness or pain at the site of ection. Febrile reactions and chills have been served rarely in the first 24 hours after vaccination.

**armaceutical precautions** AC Vax should be ored between 2°C and 8°C, its shelf life then being ur years. The reconstituted vaccine should be used mediately, and certainly within one hour.

**gal category** POM.

**ckage quantities** Monodose vials (OP), each with separate ampoule of diluent.

**rther information** One dose of AC Vax will elicit a otective response in over 90 per cent of older ildren and adults within two to three weeks.

n adults and children over five years of age, munity will persist for up to five years. In younger ildren, particularly those below the age of two ars, immunity against group C meningococci is likely to persist for more than one to two years.

Inactive ingredients in the reconstituted vaccine are tose and sodium chloride.

**oduct licence numbers**

| | |
|---|---|
| : Vax vaccine | 10592/0013. |
| line diluent (0.9 per cent) | 0002/0194. |

## LGITEC* SUSPENSION
## LGITEC* CHEWTAB TABLETS

**esentation** A white suspension with an odour of it and mint, each 10 ml of which contains 500 mg dium Alginate BPC and 200 mg cimetidine.

Circular, off-white, flat-faced chewable tablets with odour of butterscotch and with a characteristic ttern and 'Algitec' on both sides. Each tablet contains 500 mg Alginic Acid BPC and 200 mg cimet- idine.

**Uses** Algitec combines sodium alginate or alginic acid, which forms a barrier to the reflux of gastric contents, with cimetidine, an $H_2$-receptor antagonist, which reduces the volume and acidity of gastric juice.

Algitec is indicated in the treatment of gastro- oesophageal reflux disease.

**Dosage and administration**

*Adults only:* Oral: 10 ml suspension or one tablet four times a day, after meals and at bedtime, for four to eight weeks. If the response is inadequate, the dosage may be increased to 20 ml suspension or two tablets four times a day. The tablets should be thoroughly chewed and may be followed by a drink of water.

*Elderly:* The normal adult dosage may be used unless renal function is markedly impaired (see *Precautions* and *Adverse reactions*).

*Children:* Algitec is not recommended for children.

**Contra-indications, warnings, etc**

*Contra-indication:* Hypersensitivity to cimetidine.

*Precautions:* Because of the need to reduce the dose of cimetidine in patients with marked renal impair- ment, Algitec is not recommended for such patients.

Cimetidine can prolong the elimination of drugs metabolised by oxidation in the liver. Although pharmacological interactions with a number of drugs, e.g. diazepam, propranolol, have been demonstrated, only those with oral anticoagulants, phenytoin, the- ophylline and intravenous lignocaine appear, to date, to be of clinical significance. Close monitoring of patients on Algitec receiving oral anticoagulants or phenytoin is recommended and a reduction in the dosage of these drugs may be necessary.

Clinical trials with cimetidine of over six years' continuous treatment and more than 15 years' wide- spread use have not revealed unexpected adverse reactions related to long-term therapy. The safety of prolonged use is not, however, fully established and care should be taken to observe periodically patients given prolonged treatment.

Cimetidine treatment can mask the symptoms and allow transient healing of gastric cancer. The potential delay in diagnosis should particularly be borne in mind in patients of middle age and over with new or recently changed dyspeptic symptoms.

In patients on drug treatment or with illnesses that could cause falls in blood cell count, the possibility that $H_2$-receptor antagonism could potentiate this effect should be borne in mind.

*Use in pregnancy and lactation:* Although tests in animals and clinical evidence have not revealed any hazards from the administration of cimetidine during pregnancy and lactation, both animal and human studies have shown that it does cross the placental barrier and is excreted in milk. As with most drugs, the use of Algitec should be avoided during pregnancy and lactation unless essential.

*Adverse reactions:* Over 56 million patients have been treated with cimetidine worldwide and adverse reac- tions have been infrequent. Diarrhoea, dizziness or rash, usually mild and transient, and tiredness have been reported. Gynaecomastia has been reported and is almost always reversible on discontinuing treat- ment. Biochemical or biopsy evidence of reversible liver damage has been reported occasionally. Revers- ible confusional states have occurred, usually in elderly or already very ill patients, e.g. those with renal failure. Thrombocytopenia and leucopenia, in- cluding agranulocytosis (see *Precautions*), reversible on withdrawal of treatment, have been reported rarely; pancytopenia and aplastic anaemia have been re- ported very rarely. There have been very rare reports of interstitial nephritis, acute pancreatitis, fever, head- ache, myalgia, arthralgia, sinus bradycardia, tachycar- dia and heart block, all reversible on withdrawal of treatment. In common with other $H_2$-receptor antago- nists, there have been very rare reports of anaphylaxis. Alopecia has been reported but no causal relationship has been established. Reversible impotence has also been very rarely reported but no causal relationship has been established at usual therapeutic doses. Isolated increases of plasma creatinine have been of no clinical significance.

*Overdosage:* Acute overdosage of up to 20 grams of cimetidine has been reported several times with no significant ill effects. Overdosage with sodium algin- ate or alginic acid presents virtually no hazard, though abdominal bloating may be present. Induction of vomiting and/or gastric lavage may be employed together with symptomatic and supportive therapy.

**Pharmaceutical precautions** Store the suspension below 25°C but do not refrigerate. Shake the bottle before use. Dilution is not recommended. Store the tablets below 30°C.

**Legal category** POM.

**Package quantities** White plastic bottles containing 600 ml suspension, with Patient Information Leaflet. Cartons (OP) containing 120 Chewtab Tablets in six tubes of 20, with Patient Information Leaflet.

**Further information** Algitec allows the simultaneous use of two distinct and complementary methods, both of proven utility, of treating gastro-oesophageal reflux disease. Alginate and sodium or potassium bicarbon- ate are converted in the stomach to a viscous frothy gel of alginic acid which floats on the gastric contents to prevent reflux. Should reflux still occur, the gel itself may be refluxed to protect the oesophageal mucosa and allow any inflammation to heal. Cimeti- dine inhibits gastric secretion of acid and pepsin, reducing both the damaging gastric acidity and the volume available for reflux.

The absorption of cimetidine is not significantly affected by the sodium alginate or alginic acid in Algitec.

Each 10 ml suspension contains 65.8 mg (2.86 mmol) sodium and 1200 mg sorbitol.

Each tablet contains 47 mg (2.05 mmol) sodium, 330 mg lactose and 680 mg sorbitol.

Inactive ingredients include aspartame in the Chew- tab Tablets and disodium edetate and parabens in the Suspension.

**Product licence numbers**

| | |
|---|---|
| Algitec Suspension | 0002/0176. |
| Algitec Chewtab Tablets | 0002/0149. |

## ANDROPATCH* ▼

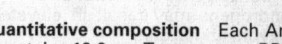

**Qualitative and quantitative composition** Each An- dropatch System contains 12.2 mg Testosterone BP.

**Pharmaceutical form** Andropatch is a transdermal drug delivery system consisting of a self-adhesive patch surrounding a central drug reservoir of testos- terone dissolved in an alcohol-based gel.

Each Andropatch system delivers *in vivo* approxi- mately 2.5 mg of testosterone over 24 hours across skin of average permeability. (Active surface area 7.5 cm²).

Clinical particulars

*Therapeutic indications:* Andropatch is indicated for testosterone replacement therapy in conditions with a deficiency or an absence of endogenous testoster- one associated with primary or secondary hypogon- adism.

*Posology and method of administration:*

*Adults and elderly:* The usual dose is two Andropatch Systems applied nightly (approximately 10pm) and worn for 24 hours, providing approximately 5 mg testosterone per day. The dose can be adjusted up to three systems nightly or down to one system nightly depending on the serum testosterone measured in the morning after application. Measurement of serum testosterone should be repeated taking care to ensure proper system adhesion and correct time of applica- tion before the dose is adjusted. Three systems per day may be required for men with a higher body weight (>130 kg). Treatment in non-virilised patients may be initiated with one system applied nightly. The dose should be adjusted as appropriate.

The duration of treatment and frequency of testos- terone measurements is determined by the physician.

The adhesive side of the Andropatch system should be applied to a clean, dry area of the skin on the back, abdomen, upper arms, or thighs. Bony prominences, such as the shoulder and hip areas, and areas that may be subjected to prolonged pressure during sleeping or sitting should be avoided. Application to these sites has been associated with burn-like blister reactions (see Undesirable effects). Do not apply to the scrotum. The sites of application should be rotated, with an interval of seven days between applications to the same site. The area selected should not be oily, damaged or irritated.

The system should be applied immediately after opening the pouch and removing the protective release liner. The system should be pressed firmly in place, making sure there is good contact with the skin, especially around the edges.

*Children:* Andropatch is not indicated for use in children as there has been no clinical experience of its use below the age of 15.

*Contra-indications:* Androgens are contra-indicated in men with carcinoma of the breast or known or suspected carcinoma of the prostate, nephrotic syndrome, hypercalcaemia and known hypersensitivity to testosterone.

Andropatch is contra-indicated in men with known hypersensitivity to other constituents of the patch.

Andropatch has not been evaluated in women and must not be used in women. Testosterone may be harmful to the foetus.

*Special warnings and special precautions for use:* Elderly men treated with androgens may be at an increased risk for the development of prostatic hyperplasia.

Elderly men and others with an increased risk of developing prostatic cancer, should be assessed before starting testosterone replacement therapy because testosterone may promote the growth of subclinical prostate cancer.

As in men without testosterone deficiency, patients on testosterone replacement therapy should be periodically evaluated for prostate cancer.

Care should be taken in patients with skeletal metastases due to the risk of hypercalcaemia/hypercalcuria developing from androgen therapy.

Testosterone may cause a rise in blood pressure and Andropatch should be used with caution in patients with hypertension.

Oedema, with or without congestive heart failure, may result from androgen treatment in patients with pre-existing cardiac, renal, or hepatic disease. In addition to discontinuation of the drug, diuretic therapy may be required.

Andropatch should be used with caution in patients with ischaemic heart disease, epilepsy and migraine as these conditions may be aggravated.

*Interaction with other medicaments and other forms of interaction:* When given simultaneously with anticoagulants the anticoagulant effect can increase. Patients receiving oral anticoagulants require close monitoring especially when androgens are started or stopped.

Concurrent administration of oxyphenbutazone and androgens may result in elevated serum levels of oxyphenbutazone.

In diabetic patients, the metabolic effects of androgens may decrease blood glucose and, therefore, insulin requirements.

*Pregnancy and lactation:* Andropatch therapy has not been evaluated in and must not be used in women under any circumstances. Testosterone may be harmful to the foetus.

*Effect on ability to drive and use machines:* There is no evidence that Andropatch will affect the ability of a patient to drive or to use machines.

*Undesirable effects:* The following adverse events were observed during clinical trials:

Skin – Transient mild to moderate erythema was observed at the site of application in the majority of patients at some time during treatment. Other application site skin reactions include pruritus; irritation with erythema, induration or burning; and rash. Allergic contact dermatitis and burn-like lesions characterised by blisters, skin necrosis, and ulceration that healed over several weeks with scarring in some cases have also been observed.

The burn-like lesions occurred sporadically, usually only at one site, (most commonly over bony prominences or areas that may have been subjected to prolonged pressure during sleeping or sitting). No patients withdrew from clinical studies due to these reactions. Such lesions should be treated as burns.

As seen with other testosterone treatments, prostate abnormalities, prostate cancer, headache, depression and gastrointestinal bleeding were also observed.

Other known undesirable effects associated with testosterone treatments include hirsuitism, male pattern baldness, seborrhoea, acne, excessive frequency and duration of penile erections, nausea, cholestatic jaundice, increased or decreased libido, anxiety, generalised paraesthesia. Oligospermia may occur at high doses. Prolonged testosterone administration may cause electrolyte disturbances, e.g. retention of sodium, chloride, potassium, calcium, inorganic phosphates and water.

*Overdosage:* This is not likely due to the mode of administration. Serum testosterone has a half-life of 70 minutes and therefore falls rapidly once Andropatch Systems are removed.

**Pharmacological properties**

*Pharmacodynamic properties:* Andropatch delivers physiologic amounts of testosterone producing circulating testosterone concentrations that mimic the normal circadian rhythm of healthy young men.

Testosterone, the primary androgenic hormone is responsible for the normal growth and development of the male sex organs and for maintenance of secondary sex characteristics.

Male hypogonadism results from insufficient secretion of testosterone and is characterised by low serum testosterone concentrations. Symptoms associated with male hypogonadism include the following: impotence and decreased sexual desire; fatigue and loss of energy; mood depression; regression of secondary sexual characteristics.

Androgens promote retention of nitrogen, sodium, potassium and phosphorus, decreases urinary excretion of calcium, increase protein anabolism, decrease protein catabolism, are also responsible for the growth spurt of adolescence and for the eventual termination of linear growth and stimulate the production of red blood cells by enhancing erythropoietin production.

Exogenous administration of androgens inhibits endogenous testosterone release. With large doses of exogenous androgens, spermatogenesis may be suppressed.

*Pharmacokinetic properties:* Following Andropatch application to non-scrotal skin, testosterone is continuously absorbed during the 24-hour dosing period. Daily application of two Andropatch patches at approximately 10 pm results in a serum testosterone concentration profile which mimics the normal circadian variation observed in healthy young men. Maximum concentrations occur in the early morning hours with minimum concentrations in the evening.

In hypogonadal men, application of two Andropatch Systems to the back, abdomen, thighs or upper arms resulted in average testosterone absorption of 4 to 5 mg over 24 hours. Applications to the chest and shins resulted in greater inter-individual variability and average 24-hour absorption of 3 to 4 mg. The serum testosterone concentration profiles during application were similar for all sites.

Normal range morning serum testosterone concentrations are reached during the first day of dosing. There is no accumulation of testosterone during continuous treatment.

Upon removal of the Andropatch Systems, serum testosterone concentrations decrease with an apparent half-life of approximately 70 minutes. Hypogonadal concentrations are reached within 24 hours following system removal.

*Preclinical safety data:* None therapeutically relevant.

**Pharmaceutical particulars**

*List of excipients in drug reservoir:* Alcohol USP, Purified Water PhEur, Glycerin PhEur, glycerol monooleate, methyl laurate, Carbomer 1342 BP, Sodium Hydroxide PhEur.

*Incompatibilities:* No specific incompatabilities.

*Shelf-life:* 24 months.

*Special precautions for storage:* Store below 25°C. Apply to skin immediately upon removal from the protective pouch. Do not store outside the pouch provided.

*Nature and contents of container:* Each Andropatch System contains 12.2 mg testosterone BP for delivery of 2.5 mg testosterone per day. Each Andropatch System is individually pouched and supplied in cartons of 10, 30 and 60 pouches. The pouch is made from paper, low-density polyethylene and aluminium foil.

*Instructions for use/handling:* Andropatch may be discarded with household waste in a manner that avoids accidental contact by others.

Damaged systems should not be used.

The drug reservoir may be burst by excessive heat or pressure.

**Marketing authorisation number** 10592/0069

**Date of approval/revision of SPC** 8 November 1996

**Legal category** POM; CD (Sch.4)

## ASACOL* TABLETS ASACOL* SUPPOSITORIES ASACOL* FOAM ENEMA

**Presentation** Red, oblong tablets containing 400 mg mesalazine (5-aminosalicylic acid) coated with an acrylic based resin (Eudragit S) formulated to release the active ingredient in the terminal ileum and colon.

Opaque, beige suppositories, containing 250 mg or 500 mg mesalazine.

White, aerosol foam enema, containing 1 g mes azine per metered dose.

**Uses**

*Ulcerative colitis:* For the treatment of mild to mod ate acute exacerbations. Tablets, suppositories a foam enema.

The suppositories and foam enema are particula appropriate in patients with distal disease.

For the maintenance of remission. Tablets a suppositories.

*Crohn's ileo-colitis:* For the maintenance of remissic Tablets.

**Dosage and administration**

*Tablets:*

*Adults:* Acute disease: Six tablets a day in divid doses, with concomitant corticosteroid therapy whe clinically indicated.

*Maintenance therapy:* Three to six tablets a day divided doses.

*Children:* There is no dosage recommendation.

*Suppositories:*

*Adults: 250 mg Suppositories:* Three to six suppc tories a day in divided doses, with the last dose bedtime.

*500 mg Suppositories:* A maximum of three suppo tories a day in divided doses, with the last dose bedtime.

*Children:* There is no dosage recommendation.

*Foam enema:*

*Adults:* For disease affecting the rectosigmoid regi one metered dose 1 g a day for four to six weeks; disease involving the descending colon, two mete doses 2 g once a day for four to six weeks.

*Children:* There is no dosage recommendation.

**Contra-indications, warnings, etc**

*Contra-indications:* A history of sensitivity to sali lates or renal sensitivity to sulphasalazine. Sev renal impairment (GFR less than 20 ml/min). Child under two years of age.

*Precautions:* Renal disorder: mesalazine is excre rapidly by the kidney, mainly as its metabolite, acetyl-5-aminosalicylic acid. In rats, large doses mesalazine injected intravenously produce tubu and glomerular toxicity. Asacol is best avoided patients with established renal impairment, bu necessary, it should be used with caution.

Serious blood dyscrasias have been reported v rarely with mesalazine. Haematological investigatic should be performed if the patient develops un plained bleeding, bruising, purpura, anaemia, fe or sore throat. Treatment should be stopped if th is a suspicion or evidence of blood dyscrasia.

Asacol Tablets should not be given with lactul or similar preparations which lower stool pH and m prevent release of mesalazine.

*Use during pregnancy and lactation:* No informat is available with regard to teratogenicity; howe negligible quantities of mesalazine are transfer across the placenta and are excreted in breast m following sulphasalazine therapy. Use of Asacol d ing pregnancy should be with caution, and only if, the opinion of the physician, the potential benefits treatment are greater than the possible hazar Asacol should, unless essential, be avoided by nurs mothers.

*Elderly:* Use in the elderly should be cautious a subject to patients having a normal renal funct (see *Precautions*).

*Adverse reactions:* The side effects are predomina gastrointestinal, including nausea, diarrhoea and dominal pain. Headache has also been reported.

Mesalazine may be associated with an exacerbat of the symptoms of colitis in those patients who h previously had such problems with sulphasalaz There have been rare reports of leucopenia, neut penia, agranulocytosis, aplastic anaemia and thro bocytopenia, pancreatitis, hepatitis, allergic lu reactions, lupus erythematosus-like reactions a rash (including urticaria), interstitial nephritis a nephrotic syndrome with oral mesalazine treatme usually reversible on withdrawal. Renal failure been reported. Mesalazine-induced nephrotoxi should be suspected in patients developing re dysfunction during treatment.

Other side effects observed with sulphasala such as depression of sperm count and function, h not been reported with Asacol.

*Treatment of overdosage:* Following tablet ingesti gastric lavage and intravenous transfusion of elec lytes to promote diuresis. There is no specific antid

**Pharmaceutical precautions** Store tablets in a place not exceeding 25°C and protect from di sunlight. Store suppositories below 25°C and pro from light.

Store the enema below 30°C. This is a pressurised anister, containing a flammable propellant. It should e kept away from any flames or sparks, including garettes. It should be protected from direct sunlight nd must not be pierced or burned even when empty.

**ackage quantities** Tablets in cartons (OP) of 120, ach containing 12 opaque blister packs of 10 tablets r cartons (OP) of 90, each containing six opaque lister packs of 15 tablets.

Suppositories in cartoned plastic moulds (OP), each ontaining 20 suppositories (250 mg) or 10 suppositries (500 mg). Foam enema in cartoned aerosol can, ach carton consisting of one aerosol can containing 4 metered doses, plus 14 disposable applicators and 4 disposable plastic bags.

**egal category:** POM.

**urther information:** Mesalazine is one of the two omponents of sulphasalazine, the other being sulhapyridine. It is the latter which is responsible for e majority of side-effects associated with sulphaalazine therapy whilst mesalazine is known to be the ctive moiety in the treatment of ulcerative colitis. sacol consists only of this active component which released topically in the colon from the tablets or elivered directly by the suppositories and foam nema.

Asacol Tablets contain 400 mg of available mesalane. This is released in the terminal ileum and large owel by the effect of pH. Above pH 7 the Eudragit oat disintegrates and releases the active constituent.

Asacol Tablets contain, in a single tablet, an quivalent quantity of mesalazine to that theoretically vailable from the complete azoreduction of 1 g of ulphasalazine.

Inactive ingredients in the tablets include lactose.

The inactive ingredient in the suppositories is 'itepsol W45 (Hard Fat).

Inactive ingredients in the foam enema include odium metabisulphite, disodium edetate, methyl and ropyl hydroxybenzoate.

**roduct licence numbers**

| | |
|---|---|
| sacol Tablets | 0002/0173. |
| sacol Suppositories 250 mg | 0002/0158. |
| sacol Suppositories 500 mg | 0002/0195. |
| sacol Foam Enema | 0002/0222. |

## UGMENTIN-DUO 400/57

**ualitative and quantitative composition** Augmen-Duo 400/57 contains 400 mg amoxycillin and mg clavulanic acid per 5 ml (co-amoxiclav 400/57). The amoxycillin is present as amoxycillin trihydrate nd the clavulanic acid is present as potassium avulanate.

**harmaceutical form** Dry powder for reconstitution water, at time of dispensing, to form an oral sugar-ee suspension.

**inical particulars**

*herapeutic indications:* Augmentin-Duo 400/57 is an tibiotic agent with a notably broad spectrum of tivity against the commonly occurring bacterial athogens in general practice and hospital. The β-ctamase inhibitory action of clavulanate extends the ectrum of amoxycillin to embrace a wider range of ganisms, including many resistant to other β-lactam tibiotics.

Augmentin-Duo 400/57, for twice-daily (b.i.d.) oral sing, is indicated for short-term treatment of bacrial infections at the following sites when amoxycil-resistant β-lactamase-producing strains are spected as the cause. In other situations, amoxycil-alone should be considered.

*Upper Respiratory Tract Infections (including ENT)* particular sinusitis, otitis media, recurrent tonsillitis. ese infections are often caused by *Streptococcus eumoniae, Haemophilus influenzae*, Moraxella tarrhalis** and *Streptococcus pyogenes.*

*Lower Respiratory Tract Infections* in particular ute exacerbations of chronic bronchitis (especially considered severe), bronchopneumonia. These inctions are often caused by *Streptococcus pneumone, Haemophilus influenzae** and *Moraxella tarrhalis*.*

*Urinary Tract Infections* in particular cystitis (espeally when recurrent or complicated – excluding ostatitis). These infections are often caused by *nterobacteriaceae** (mainly *Escherichia coli**), *aphylococcus saprophyticus, Enterococcus* spe-es.*

*Skin and Soft Tissue Infections* in particular cellulitis, imal bites and severe dental abscess with spreading llulitis. These infections are often caused by *Staphococcus aureus*, Streptococcus pyogenes* and *Bacroides* species*.

A comprehensive list of sensitive organisms is ovided in *Pharmacological properties* section.

* Some members of these species of bacteria produce β-lactamase, rendering them insensitive to amoxycillin alone.

Mixed infections caused by amoxycillin-susceptible organisms in conjunction with Augmentin-Duo 400/57-susceptible β-lactamase-producing organisms may be treated with Augmentin-Duo 400/57. These infections should not require the addition of another antibiotic resistant to β-lactamases.

*Posology and method of administration:* The usual recommended daily dosage is:

25/3.6 mg/kg/day in mild to moderate infections (upper respiratory tract infections e.g. recurrent tonsillitis, lower respiratory infections and skin and soft tissue infections)

45/6.4 mg/kg/day for the treatment of more serious infections (upper respiratory tract infections, e.g. otitis media and sinusitis, lower respiratory tract infections, e.g. bronchopneumonia and urinary tract infections)

The tables below give guidance for children.

*Children over 2 years:*

| | | |
|---|---|---|
| 25/3.6 mg/kg/day | 2–6 years (13–21 kg) | 2.5 ml Augmentin-Duo 400/57 Suspension b.i.d. |
| | 7–12 years (22–40 kg) | 5.0 ml Augmentin-Duo 400/57 Suspension b.i.d. |
| 45/6.4 mg/kg/day | 2–6 years (13–21 kg) | 5.0 ml Augmentin-Duo 400/57 Suspension b.i.d. |
| | 7–12 years (22–40 kg) | 10.0 ml Augmentin-Duo 400/57 Suspension b.i.d. |

*Children aged two months to two years* Children under two years should be dosed according to body weight.

| *Weight (kg)* | *25/3.6 mg/kg/day (ml/b.i.d.*)* | *45/6.4 mg/kg/day (ml/b.i.d.*)* |
|---|---|---|
| 2 | 0.3 | 0.6 |
| 3 | 0.5 | 0.8 |
| 4 | 0.6 | 1.1 |
| 5 | 0.8 | 1.4 |
| 6 | 0.9 | 1.7 |
| 7 | 1.1 | 2.0 |
| 8 | 1.3 | 2.3 |
| 9 | 1.4 | 2.5 |
| 10 | 1.6 | 2.8 |
| 11 | 1.7 | 3.1 |
| 12 | 1.9 | 3.4 |
| 13 | 2.0 | 3.7 |
| 14 | 2.2 | 3.9 |
| 15 | 2.3 | 4.2 |

* The 35 ml presentation is supplied with a syringe dosing device – See *Nature and contents of container* and *Instructions for use/handling* section

There is insufficient experience with Augmentin-Duo to make dosage recommendations for children under two months old.

*Infants with immature kidney function* For children with immature renal function Augmentin-Duo 400/57 is not recommended.

*Renal impairment:* For children with a GFR of >30 ml/min. no adjustment in dosage is required. For children with a GFR of <30 ml/min. Augmentin-Duo 400/57 is not recommended.

*Hepatic impairment:* Dose with caution; monitor hepatic function at regular intervals. There is, as yet, insufficient evidence on which to base a dosage recommendation.

*Method of administration:* To minimise potential gastrointestinal intolerance, administer at the start of a meal. The absorption of co-amoxiclav is optimised when taken at the start of a meal. Duration of therapy should be appropriate to the indication and should not exceed 14 days without review. Therapy can be started parenterally and continued with an oral preparation.

*Contra-indications:* Penicillin hypersensitivity. Attention should be paid to possible cross-sensitivity with other β-lactam antibiotics, e.g. cephalosporins. A previous history of co-amoxiclav- or penicillin-associated jaundice/hepatic dysfunction.

*Special warnings and special precautions for use:* Changes in liver function tests have been observed in some patients receiving co-amoxiclav. The clinical significance of these changes is uncertain but co-amoxiclav should be used with caution in patients with evidence of hepatic dysfunction.

Cholestatic jaundice, which may be severe, but is usually reversible, has been reported rarely. Signs and symptoms may not become apparent for several weeks after treatment has ceased.

In patients with moderate or severe renal impairment Augmentin-Duo 400/57 is not recommended.

Serious and occasionally fatal hypersensitivity (anaphylactoid) reactions have been reported in patients on penicillin therapy. These reactions are more likely to occur in individuals with a history of penicillin hypersensitivity (see *Contra-indications*).

Erythematous rashes have been associated with glandular fever in patients receiving amoxycillin.

Prolonged use may also occasionally result in overgrowth of non-susceptible organisms.

Augmentin-Duo 400/57 contains 12.5 mg aspartame per 5 ml dose and therefore care should be taken in phenylketonuria.

*Interaction with other medicaments and other forms of interaction:* Prolongation of bleeding time and prothrombin time have been reported in some patients receiving co-amoxiclav. Co-amoxiclav should be used with care in patients on anti-coagulation therapy. In common with other broad-spectrum antibiotics, co-amoxiclav may reduce the efficacy of oral contraceptives and patients should be warned accordingly.

Concomitant use of allopurinol during treatment with amoxycillin can increase the likelihood of allergic skin reactions. There are no data on the concomitant use of co-amoxiclav and allopurinol.

*Pregnancy and lactation:*

*Use in pregnancy:* Reproduction studies in animals (mice and rats) with orally and parenterally administered co-amoxiclav have shown no teratogenic effects. There is limited experience of the use of co-amoxiclav in human pregnancy. As with all medicines, use should be avoided in pregnancy, especially during the first trimester, unless considered essential by the physician.

*Use in lactation:* Co-amoxiclav may be administered during the period of lactation. With the exception of the risk of sensitisation, associated with the excretion of trace quantities in breast milk, there are no known detrimental effects for the breast-fed infant.

*Effects on ability to drive and use machines:* Adverse effects on the ability to drive or operate machinery have not been observed.

*Undesirable effects:* Side effects are uncommon and mainly of a mild and transitory nature.

*Gastrointestinal reactions:* Diarrhoea, indigestion, nausea, vomiting, and mucocutaneous candidiasis have been reported. Antibiotic-associated colitis (including pseudomembranous colitis and haemorrhagic colitis) has been reported rarely. Nausea, although uncommon, is more often associated with higher oral dosages. If gastrointestinal side effects occur with oral therapy they may be reduced by taking co-amoxiclav at the start of meals.

Superficial tooth discolouration has been reported rarely, mostly with the suspension. It can usually be removed by brushing.

*Genito-urinary effects:* Vaginal itching, soreness and discharge may occur.

*Hepatic effects:* Moderate and asymptomatic rises in AST and/or ALT and alkaline phosphatases have been reported occasionally. Hepatitis and cholestatic jaundice have been reported rarely. These hepatic reactions have been reported more commonly with co-amoxiclav than with other penicillins.

After co-amoxiclav hepatic reactions have been reported more frequently in males and elderly patients, particularly those over 65 years. The risk increases with duration of treatment longer than 14 days. These reactions have been very rarely reported in children.

Signs and symptoms usually occur during or shortly after treatment but in some cases may not occur until several weeks after treatment has ended. Hepatic reactions are usually reversible but they may be severe and,very rarely, deaths have been reported.

*Hypersensitivity reactions:* Urticarial and erythematous rashes sometimes occur. Rarely erythema multiforme, Stevens-Johnson syndrome, toxic epidermal necrolysis, bullous exfoliative dermatitis, serum sickness-like syndrome and hypersensitivity vasculitis have been reported. Treatment should be discontinued if one of these disorders occurs. In common with other β-lactam antibiotics angioedema and anaphylaxis have been reported. Interstitial nephritis can occur rarely.

*Haematological effects:* As with other β-lactams transient leucopenia, thrombocytopenia and haemolytic anaemia have been reported rarely. Prolongation of bleeding time and prothrombin time has also been reported rarely (see *Interaction with other medicaments and other forms of interaction*).

*CNS effects:* CNS effects have been seen very rarely. These include reversible hyperactivity, dizziness, headache and convulsions. Convulsions may occur with impaired renal function or in those receiving high doses.

*Overdose:* Problems of overdosage with co-amoxiclav are unlikely to occur. If encountered, gastrointestinal symptoms and disturbance of the fluid and electrolyte balances may be evident. They may be treated symptomatically, with attention to the water/electrolyte balance. Co-amoxiclav may be removed from the circulation by haemodialysis.

*Drug abuse and dependence:* Drug dependency, addiction and recreational abuse have not been reported as a problem with this compound.

**Pharmacological properties** Augmentin-Duo 400/57 contains a combination of amoxycillin and clavulanic acid, co-amoxiclav 400/57.

*Pharmacodynamic properties:*
*Microbiology:* Amoxycillin is a semi-synthetic antibiotic with a broad spectrum of antibacterial activity against many Gram-positive and Gram-negative micro-organisms. Amoxycillin is, however, susceptible to degradation by β-lactamases and therefore the spectrum of activity of amoxycillin alone does not include organisms which produce these enzymes.

Clavulanic acid is a β-lactam, structurally related to the penicillins, which possesses the ability to inactivate a wide range of β-lactamase enzymes commonly found in micro-organisms resistant to penicillins and cephalosporins. In particular, it has good activity against the clinically important plasmid mediated β-lactamases frequently responsible for transferred drug resistance. It is generally less effective against chromosomally-mediated type 1 β-lactamases.

The presence of clavulanic acid in Augmentin-Duo 400/57 protects amoxycillin from degradation by β-lactamase enzymes and effectively extends the antibacterial spectrum of amoxycillin to include many bacteria normally resistant to amoxycillin and other penicillins and cephalosporins. Thus Augmentin-Duo 400/57 possesses the distinctive properties of a broad spectrum antibiotic and a β-lactamase inhibitor. Augmentin-Duo 400/57 is bactericidal to a wide range of organisms including:

*Gram-positive:*
Aerobes: *Enterococcus faecalis**, *Enterococcus faecium**, *Streptococcus pneumoniae*, *Streptococcus pyogenes*, *Streptococcus viridans*, *Staphylococcus aureus**, Coagulase negative *staphylococci** (including *Staphylococcus epidermidis**), *Corynebacterium* species, *Bacillus anthracis**, *Listeria monocytogenes*.

Anaerobes: *Clostridium* species, *Peptococcus* species, *Peptostreptococcus*.

*Gram-negative:*
Aerobes: *Haemophilus influenzae**, *Moraxella catarrhalis** (*Branhamella catarrhalis*), *Escherichia coli**, *Proteus mirabilis**, *Proteus vulgaris**, *Klebsiella* species*, *Salmonella* species*, *Shigella* species*, *Bordetella pertussis*, *Brucella* species, *Neisseria gonorrhoeae**, *Neisseria meningitidis**, *Vibrio cholerae*, *Pasteurella multocida*.

Anaerobes: *Bacteroides* species* including *B. fragilis*.

* Some members of these species of bacteria produce β-lactamase, rendering them insensitive to amoxycillin alone.

*Pharmacokinetic properties*
*Absorption:* The two components of Augmentin-Duo 400/57, amoxycillin and clavulanic acid, are each fully dissociated in aqueous solution at physiological pH. Both components are rapidly and well absorbed by the oral route of administration. Absorption of co-amoxiclav is optimised when taken at the start of a meal.

*Pharmacokinetics:* Pharmacokinetic studies have been performed in children, including one study [25000/382] which has compared co-amoxiclav t.i.d. and b.i.d. All of these data indicate that the elimination pharmacokinetics seen in adults also apply to children with mature kidney function.

The mean AUC values for amoxycillin are essentially the same following twice-a-day dosing with the 875/125 mg tablet or three-times-a-day dosing with the 500/125 mg tablet, in adults. No differences between the 875 mg b.i.d. and 500 mg t.i.d. dosing regimens are seen when comparing the amoxycillin $T_{1/2}$, or $C_{max}$ after normalisation for the different doses of amoxycillin administered. Similarly, no differences are seen for the clavulanate $T_{1/2}$, $C_{max}$ or AUC values after appropriate dose normalisation [Study 360].

The time of dosing of co-amoxiclav relative to the start of a meal has no marked effects on the pharmacokinetics of amoxycillin in adults. In a study of the 875/125 mg tablet [Study 362], the time of dosing relative to ingestion of a meal had a marked effect on the pharmacokinetics of clavulanate. For clavulanate AUC and $C_{max}$, the highest mean values and smallest inter-subject variabilities were achieved by administering co-amoxiclav at the start of a meal, compared to the fasting state or 30 or 150 minutes after the start of a meal.

The mean $C_{max}$, $T_{max}$, $T_{1/2}$ and AUC values for amoxycillin and clavulanic acid are given below for an 875 mg/125 mg dose of co-amoxiclav administered at the start of a meal [Study 362].

Amoxycillin serum concentrations achieved with co-amoxiclav are similar to those produced by the oral administration of equivalent doses of amoxycillin alone.

*Distribution:* Following intravenous administration therapeutic concentrations of both amoxycillin and clavulanic acid may be detected in the tissues and interstitial fluid. Therapeutic concentrations of both drugs have been found in gall bladder, abdominal tissue, skin, fat, and muscle tissues; fluids found to

Mean pharmacokinetic parameters

| *Drug administration* | *Dose (mg)* | $C_{max}$ *(mg/l)* | $T_{max}$* *(hours)* | *AUC (mg.h/l)* | $T_{1/2}$ *(hours)* |
|---|---|---|---|---|---|
| Augmentin 1 g | | | | | |
| Amoxycillin | 875 mg | 12.4 | 1.5 | 29.9 | 1.36 |
| Clavulanic acid | 125 mg | 3.3 | 1.3 | 6.88 | 0.92 |

* Median values

have therapeutic levels include synovial and peritoneal fluids, bile and pus.

Neither amoxycillin nor clavulanic acid is highly protein bound, studies show that about 25% for clavulanic acid and 18% for amoxycillin of total plasma drug content is bound to protein. From animal studies there is no evidence to suggest that either component accumulates in any organ.

Amoxycillin, like most penicillins, can be detected in breast milk. There are no data available on the passage of clavulanic acid into breast milk.

Reproduction studies in animals have shown that both amoxycillin and clavulanic acid penetrate the placental barrier. However, no evidence of impaired fertility or harm to the foetus was detected.

*Elimination:* As with other penicillins, the major route of elimination for amoxycillin is via the kidney, whereas for clavulanate elimination is by both non-renal and renal mechanisms. Approximately 60-70% of the amoxycillin and approximately 40-65% of the clavulanic acid are excreted unchanged in urine during the first six hours after administration of a single 375 or 625 mg tablet.

Amoxycillin is also partly excreted in the urine as the inactive penicilloic acid in quantities equivalent to 10-25% of the initial dose. Clavulanic acid is extensively metabolised in man to 2,5-dihydro-4-(2-hydroxyethyl)-5-oxo-1H-pyrrole-3-carboxylic acid and 1-amino-4-hydroxy-butan-2-one and eliminated in urine and faeces and as carbon dioxide in expired air.

*Preclinical safety data*: No further information of relevance.

**Pharmaceutical particulars**

*List of excipients*: Xantham gum, aspartame, succinic acid, colloidal silica, hydroxypropyl methylcellulose, orange dry flavour (61071E), orange dry flavour (9/027108), raspberry dry flavour, golden syrup dry flavour, silicon dioxide.

*Incompatibilities*: None known.

*Shelf life:*
Glass bottles: Dry powder: 18 months when stored at temperatures at or below 25°C.

Reconstituted suspensions: seven days when stored in a refrigerator (2-8°C).

*Sachets*: 18 months when stored at temperatures at or below 25°C.

*Special precautions for storage*: The dry powder should be stored in well-sealed containers in a dry place.

*Nature and contents of container:* Clear, glass bottles with aluminium screw caps, containing an off-white dry powder. The 35 ml presentation is supplied in a carton with a polystyrene syringe dosing device.

Single-dose sachets. Four sachets are supplied in a carton.

When reconstituted, an off-white suspension is formed.

*Instructions for use/handling:*
*Glass bottles:* At time of dispensing, the dry powder should be reconstituted to form an oral suspension, as detailed below:

| *Fill weight* | *Volume of water to be added to reconstitute* | *Nominal bottle size* | *Final volume of reconstituted oral suspension* |
|---|---|---|---|
| 6.3 g | 31 ml | 90 ml | 35 ml |
| 12.6 g | 62 ml | 150 ml | 70 ml |

The 35 ml presentation is provided with a syringe dosing device which should be used in place of the aluminium screw cap following reconstitution. This device is used to dose patients under two years according to the schedule in *Posology and method of administration*.

*Sachets:* Single-dose sachets contain powder for a 2.5 ml dose.

Directions for use: Check that the sachet is intact before use. Cut sachet along dotted line. Empty contents into a glass. Half-fill sachet with water. Pour into the glass, stir well and drink immediately. If two or four sachets have to be taken at once then they can be mixed in the same glass.

**Marketing authorisation number** 10592/0070

**Date of approval/revision of SPC** March 1997

**Legal category** POM

## BACTROBAN* NASAL

**Presentation** Bactroban Nasal Ointment: Calciu mupirocin equivalent to 2% w/w mupirocin in a whi soft paraffin-based ointment containing a glycer ester.

**Uses**
*Action:* Bactroban is a topical antibacterial age active against those organisms responsible for t majority of skin infections, e.g. *Staphylococcus a reus*, including methicillin-resistant strains, oth staphylococci, streptococci. It is also active again Gram-negative organisms such as *Escherichia c.* and *Haemophilus influenzae*.

*Indication:* The elimination of nasal carriage staphylococci, including methicillin-resistant *Staph lococcus aureus* (MRSA).

**Dosage and administration**
*Adults (including the elderly) and children:* Bactrob Nasal Ointment should be applied to the anteri nares two to three times a day, as follows:

A small amount of the ointment (about the size o match-head) should be placed on a cotton bud or the little finger and applied to the anterior part of t inside of each nostril. The nostrils are closed pressing the sides of the nose together; this w spread the ointment throughout the nares. A cotto bud should be used instead of the little finger application in particular to infants or patients who a very ill.

Nasal carriage should normally clear within fiv seven days of treatment.

**Contra-indications, warnings, etc**
*Contra-indications:* Hypersensitivity to any of t constituents of Bactroban Nasal Ointment.

*Use in pregnancy:* Studies on experimental anim have shown mupirocin to be without teratoge effects. However, there is inadequate evidence safety to recommend the use of Bactroban Na Ointment during pregnancy.

*Precautions:* As with all topical preparations ca should be taken to avoid the eyes.

*Side-effects:* During clinical studies some minor a verse effects were noted, such as a transient stingi sensation localised to the area of application in abo 2% of patients.

*Overdosage:* The toxicity of mupirocin is very low. the event of overdose symptomatic treatment shou be given.

**Pharmaceutical precautions** Bactroban Nasal Oi ment may be stored at room temperature (bel 25°C).

Any ointment remaining at the end of treatme should be discarded.

**Legal category** POM.

**Package quantities** *Bactroban Nasal Ointment:* Or inal Pack of 3 g (tube in a sealed carton) with Patie Information Leaflet.

**Further information** Bactroban is a novel antibio both in chemical structure and mode of actio available only for topical application.

Bactroban Nasal Ointment contains a glycerin es to enhance the spreading properties. Such mate has a low potential for sensitisation.

For the treatment of bacterial skin infections Bact ban Ointment should be used. See separate Bactrob SPC for details.

The active ingredient of Bactroban was previou described as pseudomonic acid in the publish literature.

**Product licence number** 0038/0347.

## BACTROBAN* OINTMENT

**Qualitative and quantitative composition** Mupiro 2.0% w/w.

**Pharmaceutical form** Sterile ointment in a wh translucent, water-soluble, polyethylene glycol ba For topical administration.

**Clinical particulars**

*Therapeutic indications:* Bactroban is a topical a bacterial agent, active against those organis responsible for the majority of skin infections, e *Staphylococcus aureus*, including methicillin-res nt strains, other staphylococci, streptococci. It is so active against Gram-negative organisms such as *scherichia coli* and *Haemophilus influenzae*. Bactroban Ointment is used for skin infections, e.g. impetigo, lliculitis, furunculosis.

**osology and method of administration:**

*osage: Adults (including elderly) and children:* Bactroban Ointment should be applied to the affected ea up to three times a day for up to 10 days.

The area may be covered with a dressing or cluded if desired.

*dministration:* Topical.

*ontra-indications:* Hypersensitivity to Bactroban or her ointments containing polyethylene glycols.

This Bactroban Ointment formulation is not suitable r ophthalmic or intranasal use.

*ecial warnings and special precautions for use:* hen Bactroban Ointment is used on the face, care ould be taken to avoid the eyes.

Polyethylene glycol can be absorbed from open ounds and damaged skin and is excreted by the dneys. In common with other polyethylene glycol-sed ointments, Bactroban Ointment should be used th caution if there is evidence of moderate or severe nal impairment.

*teraction with other medicaments and other forms interaction:* None stated.

*egnancy and lactation:* Studies in experimental imals have shown mupirocin to be without teratonic effects. However, there is inadequate evidence safety to recommend the use of Bactroban during egnancy.

*fects on ability to drive and use machines:* None ated.

*ndesirable effects:* During clinical studies some inor adverse effects, localised to the area of application, were seen such as burning, stinging and hing.

*verdose:* The toxicity of mupirocin is very low. In the ent of overdose, symptomatic treatment should be ven.

**armacological properties**

*armacodynamic properties:* Bactroban (mupirocin) tently inhibits bacterial protein and RNA synthesis inhibition of isoleucyl-transfer RNA synthetase.

*armacokinetic properties:* After topical application Bactroban Ointment, mupirocin is only very minially absorbed systemically and that which is abrbed is rapidly metabolised to the antimicrobially active metabolite, monic acid. Penetration of mupicin into the deeper epidermal and dermal layers of e skin is enhanced in traumatised skin and under clusive dressings.

*eclinical safety data:* None stated.

**armaceutical particulars**

*st of excipients:* Polyethylene Glycol 400; Polyethyle Glycol 3350.

*compatibilities:* None stated.

*elf life:* Bactroban Ointment has a shelf-life of two ars.

*ecial precautions for storage:* Store at room temrature (below 25°C).

*ture and contents of container:* Original pack of g (sealed tube in a carton) with Patient Information aflet.

*structions for use/handling:* No special instructions.

**arketing authorisation number** 0038/0319

**ate of approval/revision of SPC** June 1996

**gal category** POM

## ORALESE* TILTAB* TABLETS

**esentation** Pale yellow, biconvex, triangular, film-ated Tiltab tablets, with a small projection on each le. Each tablet contains 20 mg indoramin.

**es** Doralese is an alpha-adrenoceptor antagonist at increases urinary flow rate by acting selectively d competitively on postsynaptic alpha$_1$-receptors.

It is indicated in the management of urinary outflow struction due to benign prostatic hyperplasia, parularly in patients in whom surgery is contralicated or delayed.

**sage and administration**

*ults only:* The recommended dose is 20 mg twice a y.

If necessary the dosage may be increased, in crements of 20 mg at two-weekly intervals, to a aximum of 100 mg a day in divided doses.

*derly:* Since clearance of Doralese may be reduced, mg at night may be adequate.

**Contra-indications, warnings, etc**

*Contra-indications:* Do not use in patients in established cardiac failure or those under treatment with an MAO inhibitor.

*Precautions:* If drowsiness occurs, patients should be warned not to drive or operate machinery and to avoid CNS depressants including alcohol, which can increase both the rate and extent of absorption of indoramin.

Use with caution in patients with hepatic or renal insufficiency, Parkinson's disease (which could be exacerbated), epilepsy, and those with a history of depression. Incipient cardiac failure should be controlled before treatment with Doralese.

At higher dosages indoramin is used in the management of hypertension. Concomitant use of Doralese with thiazide diuretics, β-blockers or other antihypertensive drugs may enhance their hypotensive action. Titration of dosage of the latter may therefore be needed.

*Adverse reactions:* Drowsiness or sedation can occur on starting treatment with Doralese, and also if the dosage is increased too rapidly. This usually responds to a reduction in dosage. Less commonly dry mouth, nasal congestion, weight gain, dizziness, retrograde ejaculation and depression may occur.

*Overdosage:* Experience of overdosage with indoramin is limited but symptoms have included deep sedation, coma, hypotension and convulsions. Animal work suggests that hypothermia may also occur. Suggested treatment includes gastric lavage, assisted ventilation if necessary, circulatory support and control of hypotension, intravenous diazepam for convulsions and slow rewarming if hypothermia occurs.

**Pharmaceutical precautions** Store below 25°C.

**Legal category** POM.

**Package quantities** Opaque blister packs (OP) of 60 (4×15) with Patient Information Leaflet.

**Further information** Postural hypotension has not been shown to be a significant problem. Reflex tachycardia has not been observed in clinical trials with doses of up to 100 mg.

Inactive ingredients include lactose.

**Product licence number** 0002/0168.

## DYAZIDE* TABLETS

**Presentation** Peach-coloured, half-scored, circular tablets bearing the mark SKF E93, each containing 50 mg triamterene and 25 mg hydrochlorothiazide.

**Uses** Dyazide is a potassium-conserving diuretic preparation with antihypertensive activity.

It is recommended for the treatment of mild to moderate hypertension, alone or in combination with other antihypertensive drugs. It is also indicated in the control of oedema in cardiac failure, cirrhosis of the liver or the nephrotic syndrome and in that associated with corticosteroid treatment.

**Dosage and administration**

*Adults only: In hypertension:* Initially one tablet a day after the morning meal, thereafter adjusted to the patient's needs. If Dyazide is added to already established therapy with another antihypertensive drug, the dosage of the latter should be reduced, and later adjusted if necessary. If another antihypertensive drug is added to Dyazide therapy, the dosage of the latter will not normally be reduced.

*In oedema:* The usual starting dosage is one Dyazide tablet twice a day after meals. The optimal dosage may be three tablets a day, two after breakfast and one after lunch. Maintenance dosage: Once a diuresis has been established, dosage should be reduced. Usually one tablet a day, or two tablets on alternate days, will suffice.

A dosage of four tablets a day should not be exceeded; at this level adverse reactions such as raised blood urea are more likely.

*Elderly:* Dosage as above. Dyazide has been widely used and is usually well tolerated in patients over the age of 60 years. The normally occurring reduction in glomerular filtration with age should be borne in mind.

**Contra-indications, warnings, etc**

*Contra-indications:* Do not give Dyazide to patients with hyperkalaemia, progressive renal failure, increasing hepatic dysfunction, hypercalcaemia, diabetic ketoacidosis, Addison's disease or known hypersensitivity to either constituent of the product. Potassium supplements, or other potassium-conserving drugs, including ACE inhibitors, should not be given routinely with Dyazide.

*Precautions:* Use Dyazide with caution in patients with hepatic or renal insufficiency, and in those predisposed to gout since both components can elevate uric acid levels. Folate antagonists combined with triamterene are inadvisable in patients with hepatic cirrhosis because of the increased theoretical risk of folate deficiency. Since thiazide diuretics can provoke hyperglycaemia and glycosuria, diabetic patients should be treated with care, as should patients with diabetic nephropathy due to an increased risk of hyperkalaemia; the dosage of any concomitant sulphonylurea may need increasing. Pancreatitis may be aggravated.

It is advisable to monitor blood urea, serum potassium levels and electrolytes periodically. This is important in the elderly, those with renal impairment and those receiving concomitant treatment with NSAIDs (see *Adverse reactions*).

Triamterene and thiazides reduce excretion of lithium and may thus precipitate intoxication. There may be increased responsiveness to tubocurarine. Cholestyramine may delay or reduce the absorption of many drugs including diuretics.

Caution should be exercised if Dyazide is used in conjunction with hypotensive agents. Also use with caution in conjunction with corticosteroids since an additive effect may result in excess potassium loss: with cardiac glycosides and antiarrhythmic drugs whose toxicity potential is enhanced by hypokalaemia which may result from diuretic treatment; and with carbenoxolone which may antagonise the diuretic action of Dyazide.

*Use in pregnancy and lactation:* Animal studies have not suggested foetal abnormalities. Nevertheless, both triamterene and thiazides have been shown to pass through the placenta in humans and also to pass into breast milk. In rare instances, thrombocytopenia, pancreatitis or hypoglycaemia have been reported in newborn infants of mothers treated with thiazides. Dyazide is best avoided in pregnancy unless used for a pre-existing illness and then only after assessing risk versus benefit. It should also not be used in breast-feeding mothers. Folate antagonists combined with triamterene are inadvisable during pregnancy because of the increased theoretical risk of folate deficiency.

*Adverse reactions:* Nausea, vomiting, diarrhoea, muscle cramps, weakness, dizziness, headache, dry mouth, thirst, undesirable decreases in blood pressure and rash have been reported. Photosensitivity is rare. Anaphylaxis is a remote possibility.

Minor serum electrolyte changes have been observed infrequently, and marked fluctuations in serum potassium levels are uncommon. Long-term use has confirmed that little change occurs in serum potassium and sodium levels in most patients. Metabolic acidosis occasionally occurs. Electrolyte imbalance may also indicate excessive dosage or be secondary to the condition under treatment. Hyperglycaemia, increased uric acid levels which sometimes lead to gout, and hypercalcaemia that does not lead to tertiary hyperparathyroidism may also occur.

In common with most diuretics, Dyazide may reduce glomerular filtration rate and cause a temporary increase in blood urea and creatinine levels; again this may also indicate excessive dosage or be secondary to the condition under treatment. It can also cause increases in plasma lipid levels.

Renal failure, reversible on stopping treatment, has been reported very rarely and has been due to acute interstitial nephritis or an interaction between triamterene and some NSAIDs.

Triamterene has been found in renal stones both alone and in association with other usual calculus components. There is no evidence that stone formation is increased in patients taking triamterene-containing drugs.

Rare cases of thrombocytopenic purpura and megaloblastic anaemia have been reported with triamterene; thiazides alone have caused jaundice, acute pancreatitis and, rarely, blood dyscrasias including agranulocytosis, thrombocytopenia and leucopenia. Very rare cases of SLE have been reported associated with Dyazide.

*Overdosage:* Symptoms of electrolyte imbalance, especially hyperkalaemia, are likely. Symptoms include nausea, vomiting, weakness, lassitude, muscular weakness, hypotension and cardiac arrhythmias. Treatment consists of gastric lavage with careful monitoring of electrolytes and fluid balance. Cardiac rhythm should be monitored and appropriate measures taken to correct hyperkalaemia as necessary. There is no specific antidote. Renal dialysis may be of some benefit in cases of severe overdosage.

**Pharmaceutical precautions** No special storage precautions are required.

**Legal category** POM.

**Package quantities** Calendar packs (OP) of 30 (2×15) with Patient Information Leaflet and containers of 500 tablets.

**Further information** Triamterene may cause a blue fluorescence of the urine under certain light conditions.

Dyazide interferes with some laboratory tests of

thyroid and parathyroid functions and bioassay of folic acid.

Inactive ingredients include aluminium lake of E110.

**Product licence number** 0002/0050R.

## DYSPAMET* CHEWTAB TABLETS
## DYSPAMET* SUSPENSION

**Presentation** White, square, chewable tablets with a surface design consisting of a raised portion towards one side of the tablet and a curved depression over the rest of the surface. Each tablet contains 200 mg cimetidine.

A white vanilla-flavoured suspension. Each 5 ml dose contains 200 mg cimetidine.

**Uses** Cimetidine is a histamine $H_2$-receptor antagonist which rapidly inhibits both basal and stimulated gastric secretion of acid and reduces pepsin output.

Dyspamet is indicated in the treatment of duodenal and benign gastric ulceration, recurrent and stomal ulceration, oesophageal reflux disease and other conditions where reduction of gastric acid by cimetidine has been shown to be beneficial: persistent dyspeptic symptoms with or without ulceration, particularly meal-related upper abdominal pain; the prophylaxis of gastrointestinal haemorrhage from stress ulceration in seriously ill patients; before general anaesthesia in patients thought to be at risk of acid aspiration (Mendelson's) syndrome, particularly obstetric patients during labour; to reduce malabsorption and fluid loss in the short bowel syndrome; and in pancreatic insufficiency to reduce degradation of enzyme supplements. Dyspamet is also recommended in the management of the Zollinger-Ellison syndrome.

**Dosage and administration** Dyspamet Tablets should be chewed thoroughly before swallowing.

The total daily dose should not normally exceed 2.4 g. Dosage should be reduced in patients with impaired renal function (see *Precautions*).

*Adults: Oral:* The usual dosage is 400 mg twice a day with breakfast and at bedtime. For patients with duodenal or benign gastric ulceration, a single daily dose of 800 mg at bedtime is recommended. Other effective regimens are 200 mg three times a day with meals and 400 mg at bedtime (1.0 g/day) and, if inadequate, 400 mg four times a day (1.6 g/day) also with meals and at bedtime.

Symptomatic relief is usually rapid. Treatment should be given initially for at least four weeks (six weeks in benign gastric ulcer). Most ulcers will have healed by that stage, but those which have not will usually do so after a further course of treatment.

Treatment may be continued for longer periods in those patients who may benefit from reduction of gastric secretion and the dosage may be reduced as appropriate to 400 mg at bedtime or 400 mg in the morning and at bedtime.

In patients with benign peptic ulcer disease, relapse may be prevented by continued treatment, usually with 400 mg at bedtime; 400 mg in the morning and at bedtime has also been used.

In oesophageal reflux disease, 400 mg four times a day, with meals and at bedtime, for four to eight weeks is recommended to heal oesophagitis and relieve associated symptoms.

In patients with very high gastric acid secretion (e.g. Zollinger–Ellison syndrome) it may be necessary to increase the dose to 400 mg four times a day, or in occasional cases further.

Antacids can be made available to all patients until symptoms disappear.

In the prophylaxis of haemorrhage from stress ulceration in seriously ill patients, doses of 200–400 mg can be given every four to six hours.

In patients thought to be at risk of acid aspiration syndrome a dose of 400 mg can be given 90–120 minutes before induction of general anaesthesia or, in obstetric practice, at the start of labour. While such a risk persists, a dose of up to 400 mg may be repeated at four-hourly intervals as required up to the usual daily maximum of 2.4 g. The usual precautions to avoid acid aspiration should be taken.

In the short bowel syndrome, e.g. following substantial resection for Crohn's disease, the usual dosage range (see above) can be used according to individual response.

To reduce degradation of pancreatic enzyme supplements, 800–1600 mg a day may be given according to response in four divided doses, one to one and a half hours before meals.

*Elderly:* The normal adult dosage may be used unless renal function is markedly impaired (see *Precautions* and *Adverse reactions*).

*Children:* Experience in children is less than that in adults. In children more than one year old, cimetidine 25–30 mg/kg body weight per day in divided doses may be administered.

The use of cimetidine in infants under one year old is not fully evaluated; 20 mg/kg body weight per day in divided doses has been used.

**Contra-indications, warnings, etc**
*Contra-indication:* Hypersensitivity to cimetidine.

*Precautions:* Dosage should be reduced in patients with impaired renal function according to creatinine clearance. The following dosages are suggested: creatinine clearance of 0–15 ml per minute, 200 mg twice a day; 15–30 ml per minute, 200 mg three times a day; 30–50 ml per minute, 200 mg four times a day; over 50 ml per minute, normal dosage. Cimetidine is removed by haemodialysis, but not to any significant extent by peritoneal dialysis.

Cimetidine can prolong the elimination of drugs metabolised by oxidation in the liver. Although pharmacological interactions with a number of drugs, e.g. diazepam, propranolol, have been demonstrated, only those with oral anticoagulants, phenytoin, theophylline and intravenous lignocaine appear, to date, to be of clinical significance. Close monitoring of patients on Dyspamet receiving oral anticoagulants or phenytoin is recommended and a reduction in the dosage of these drugs may be necessary.

Clinical trials with cimetidine of over six years' continuous treatment and more than 15 years' widespread use have not revealed unexpected adverse reactions related to long-term therapy. The safety of prolonged use is not, however, fully established and care should be taken to observe periodically patients given prolonged treatment.

Cimetidine treatment can mask the symptoms and allow transient healing of gastric cancer. The potential delay in diagnosis should particularly be borne in mind in patients of middle age and over with new or recently changed dyspeptic symptoms.

In patients on drug treatment or with illnesses that could cause falls in blood cell count, the possibility that $H_2$-receptor antagonism could potentiate this effect should be borne in mind.

*Use in pregnancy and lactation:* Although tests in animals and clinical evidence have not revealed any hazards from the administration of cimetidine during pregnancy or lactation, both animal and human studies have shown that it does cross the placental barrier and is excreted in milk. As with most drugs, the use of Dyspamet should be avoided during pregnancy and lactation unless essential.

*Adverse reactions:* Over 56 million patients have been treated with cimetidine worldwide and adverse reactions have been infrequent. Diarrhoea, dizziness or rash, usually mild and transient, and tiredness have been reported. Gynaecomastia has been reported and is almost always reversible on discontinuing treatment. Biochemical or biopsy evidence of reversible liver damage has been reported occasionally. Reversible confusional states have occurred, usually in elderly or already very ill patients, e.g. those with renal failure. Thrombocytopenia and leucopenia, including agranulocytosis (see *Precautions*), reversible on withdrawal of treatment, have been reported rarely; pancytopenia and aplastic anaemia have been reported very rarely. There have been very rare reports of interstitial nephritis, acute pancreatitis, fever, headache, myalgia, arthralgia, sinus bradycardia, tachycardia and heart block, all reversible on withdrawal of treatment. In common with other $H_2$-receptor antagonists, there have been very rare reports of anaphylaxis. Alopecia has been reported but no causal relationship has been established. Reversible impotence has also been very rarely reported but no causal relationship has been established at usual therapeutic doses. Isolated increases of plasma creatinine have been of no clinical significance.

*Overdosage:* Acute overdosage of up to 20 grams cimetidine has been reported several times with no significant ill effects. Induction of vomiting and/or gastric lavage may be employed together with symptomatic and supportive therapy.

**Pharmaceutical precautions** Store tablets in a dry place. Store suspension at a temperature not exceeding 25°C. Dilution of the suspension is not recommended.

**Legal category** POM.

**Package quantities** Chewtab Tablets, 200 mg, in opaque blister packs (OP) of 120 (20×6), with Patient Information Leaflet. Suspension in white plastic bottles (OP) of 600 ml, with Patient Information Leaflet.

**Further information** Inactive ingredients in the tablets include aspartame together with 900 mg lactose and 790 mg sorbitol per tablet, and in the suspension butyl paraben and propyl paraben together with 2.79 g sorbitol per 5 ml.

**Product licence numbers**
Dyspamet Chewtab Tablets 0002/0148.
Dyspamet Suspension 0002/0161.

## ENGERIX* B
## Hepatitis B Vaccine (rby)

**Presentation** Engerix B is a suspension of hepati B surface antigen produced by yeast cells using recombinant DNA technique. It is available as a fi white suspension in the following presentations: ad prefilled syringes (1 ml); adult vials (1 ml); paediat vials (0.5 ml). Each 1 ml contains 20 micrograms protein, comprising at least 95% hepatitis B surfa antigen, adsorbed on aluminium hydroxide adjuva together with thiomersal 1:20,000 as preservative.

**Uses** Active immunisation against infection hepatitis B virus.

Preference should be given to those at increas risk of infection, primarily those likely to be expos to blood, blood products or other body fluids.

Immunisation should be considered for the follo ing risk groups:

Parenteral drug abusers.

Those with multiple sexual partners, particula homosexual and bisexual men and prostitute m and women.

Close family contacts of a case or carrier.

Babies born to mothers who are chronic carriers the hepatitis B virus or who have had acute hepati B during pregnancy.

Haemophiliacs, those receiving regular blood tra fusions or blood products, or relatives responsible the administration of such products.

Patients with chronic renal failure.

Healthcare personnel who have direct contact w blood or blood-stained body fluids or with patie tissues. This includes doctors, surgeons, dentis nurses, midwives, laboratory workers and mortu technicians.

Trainee healthcare workers.

Staff and clients of residential accommodation the mentally handicapped.

Prisoners.

Long-stay travellers and healthcare personnel go to areas of high prevalence.

Police, ambulance, rescue services and staff custodial institutions may have certain individu who are at risk.

In addition, there may be other groups at risk specific circumstances when immunisation should given.

It is not known whether responders will ne booster doses or whether on exposure to virus natu boosting will occur when anti-HBs titres fall below protective level of 10 mIU/ml. Until this is clea known, it would seem wise to recommend a boos dose in those below this 10 mIU/ml level. Howev immunity should persist for at least five years af the last dose of vaccine.

**Dosage and administration** Engerix B is for int muscular use only, and must not be given intra nously or intradermally.

Prior to vaccination, the vaccine should be w shaken and be visually inspected for any col variations or particulate matter. Once shaken, vaccine is slightly opaque.

Engerix B must *not* be mixed in the same syri or injected at the same site as other vaccines.

The immunisation regimen consists of three do of vaccine, the second dose at one month and third at six months after the initial dose. Where m rapid immunisation is required, for example w travellers, the third dose may be given at two mon after the initial dose, with a booster dose at 12 mont Specific humoral antibodies against the surface a gen of hepatitis B appear in almost 100% of th who have received three doses.

*Adults and children over 12 years:* 20 microgra (1 ml) given intramuscularly.

*Neonates and children 12 years and under:* 10 mic grams (0.5 ml) given intramuscularly.

The vaccine should be administered in the delt region though the antero-lateral thigh is the prefer site for infants. Engerix B should not be administe in the buttock since this may result in a lower immu response. In patients with severe bleeding tendenc such as haemophiliacs, subcutaneous injection n be considered.

In neonates born to HBsAg positive mothe hepatitis B immunoglobulin should be given simu neously with the vaccine at different sites within a hours of birth. For other subjects at particular r similar simultaneous administration may be cons ered.

Engerix B may be used as a booster in patie previously immunised with other hepatitis B vaccin

**Contra-indications, warnings, etc**
*Contra-indications:* Hypersensitivity to any com nent of the vaccine. Severe febrile infections.

*Precautions:* In patients having renal dialysis, or th who are immunocompromised, response may impaired and further vaccinations may be necessa

Because of the prolonged incubation period of epatitis B, infection may be present at the time of accination. If so, Engerix B may be ineffective.

As with all vaccinations, a solution of 1:1000 drenaline should be available for injection should an naphylactic reaction occur.

*'se in pregnancy:* No studies in pregnant animals ave been done. Engerix B is not recommended in regnancy unless there is a definite risk of hepatitis B.

*dverse reactions:* These are usually mild. The most ommon reactions, occurring in up to half of vaccinees, are mild transient local soreness, erythema and duration at the injection site.

Local swelling at the injection site and angioedema ave been reported rarely.

Less common systemic complaints, which have een reported, include low-grade fever, malaise, tigue, arthralgia, arthritis, myalgia, headache, dizziess, syncope, nausea, vomiting, diarrhoea, abdomial pain, lymphadenopathy, abnormal liver function sts, and rashes, rarely including urticaria. Thromocytopenic purpura and severe skin disorders such s erythema multiforme have exceptionally occurred. ery rarely, transient arthralgia, pruritus and urticaria ave been reported appearing one week or more after jection.

Neurological manifestations occurring in temporal ssociation have been reported with the vaccine and clude very rarely paraesthesia and extremely rarely aralysis, neuropathy and neuritis (including Guillainarré syndrome, optic neuritis and multiple sclerosis). o causal relationship has been established.

Early onset allergic-type reactions have been reorted rarely.

**harmaceutical precautions** Engerix B should be tored between 2°C and 8°C, its shelf-life then being ree years, and must not be frozen. It should not be luted. Protect from light.

**egal category** POM.

**ackage quantities** Adult prefilled syringes containg 1 ml suspension in packs of one and 10; adult vials ontaining 1 ml suspension in packs of one, three (OP) nd 10; paediatric vials containing 0.5 ml suspension packs of one.

**urther information** Inactive ingredients are dried luminium hydroxide, sodium chloride, sodium moohydrogen phosphate dihydrate, sodium dihydroen phosphate dihydrate, water for injections, and lso thiomersal (see *Presentation*).

**roduct licence number** 10592/0015.

## RVEVAX*
## ubella vaccine, live PhEur
## RA27/3 strain)

**resentation** Ervevax rubella vaccine is a live attenated vaccine prepared in human diploid cells. It is resented as a pink pellet in a glass vial; clear, olourless sterile diluent is provided in a separate ontainer. Each 0.5 ml dose of the reconstituted accine contains not less than 1,000 $TCID_{50}$ of the A27/3 live attenuated strain of rubella virus with not ore than 25 micrograms (17 IU) neomycin sulphate.

**ses** Routine immunisation of pre-pubertal girls gainst rubella. Also indicated in seronegative women f child-bearing age **who are not pregnant** and in hom the possibility of pregnancy can be excluded r at least one month following vaccination, including *ost-partum* mothers, and for immunisation of chilren and adults to prevent transmission of rubella to e at-risk pregnant woman.

**osage and administration**
*dults and children:* A single dose (0.5 ml) of the constituted vaccine administered by deep subcutaeous or intramuscular injection. Do not give intraveously.

The vaccine should be reconstituted using only the erile Water for Injections supplied. The whole of the erile diluent should be transferred into the vial ontaining the vaccine, keeping the latter upright. The accine pellet should be completely dissolved by haking. The vaccine is quickly inactivated by ether, cohol and other detergents and care is needed to void contact with these substances when sterilising kin before vaccination.

**ontra-indications, warnings, etc**
*ontra-indications:* **Never give to pregnant women, r to women of child-bearing age not fully aware of e need to avoid pregnancy for one month after accination,** since theoretically the vaccine virus could ave an effect on the foetus.

Acute febrile illness, whether active or expected llowing exposure to infection (other than rubella).

Ervevax should not be given to subjects with npaired immune responses. These include patients ith primary or secondary immunodeficiencies. However, Ervevax can be given to asymptomatic HIV-infected patients without adverse consequences to their illness and may be considered for those who are symptomatic. Do not give to those with known systemic hypersensitivity to this vaccine or to neomycin. Although anaphylactic reactions are rare, facilities for management should always be available.

*Precautions:* Transmission of vaccine virus to susceptible contacts, whilst accepted as a theoretical possibility, has not been regarded as a significant risk.

Because of the possibility of interference from passive antibodies, the vaccine should not normally be given to subjects who have received blood or human plasma transfusions or human immunoglobulin within the previous three months. If the vaccine is given in these circumstances, serum antibodies should be checked at a later date.

At least three weeks should normally intervene between the administration of any two live vaccines. Ervevax can, however, be given simultaneously with live, oral poliomyelitis vaccine, and with measles and mumps vaccines. In this case the injectable vaccines should be given at different sites.

*Adverse reactions:* Mild rash, temperature elevation and slight enlargement of the posterior cervical glands, transient arthralgia and arthritis with or without joint effusion, and extremely rarely transient polyneuropathy or thrombocytopenic purpura could occur. Such effects are more common and tend to be more marked in adults than in children. Symptoms, when they do occur, usually begin one to three weeks following vaccination and are normally transient.

*Overdosage:* Not a problem.

**Pharmaceutical precautions** Protect from light. The vaccine should be stored between 2°C and 8°C, its shelf-life then being two years (lower temperatures will not harm the vaccine, but may damage the diluent container). At room temperature (20–25°C) the unreconstituted vaccine is stable for up to 10 weeks.

The vaccine should be reconstituted using the sterile Water for Injections provided. For one dose of Ervevax, 0.6 ml of Water for Injections should be withdrawn from the ampoule using a syringe and delivered into the vaccine vial for reconstitution. The reconstituted vaccine should be used immediately, and certainly within one hour.

**Legal category** POM.

**Package quantities** Monodose* vials (OP), each with a separate ampoule of sterile diluent. The diluent is Water for Injections PhEur.

**Further information** Data indicate that satisfactory antibody titres have persisted for up to 20 years so far.

Because of possible interference from persisting maternal antibodies, there is little value in giving the vaccine to infants under one year of age.

Inactive ingredients are human albumin, lactose, sorbitol, dextran 10, aminoacids for injection, and also neomycin sulphate (see *Presentation*).

**Product licence number** 10592/0016.

## ESKAZOLE* TABLETS 400 mg

**Qualitative and quantitative composition** Albendazole 400 mg

**Pharmaceutical form** Tablet

**Clinical particulars**
*Therapeutic indications:* Eskazole is a benzimidazole carbamate anthelmintic for use in the treatment of hydatid cysts caused by:

*Echinococcosis:* Eskazole shows greatest efficacy in the treatment of liver, lung and peritoneal cysts. Experience with bone cysts and those in the heart and central nervous system is limited.

*Cystic echinococcosis* (caused by *Echinococcus granulosus):* Eskazole is used in patients with cystic echinococcosis:

1. Where surgical intervention is not feasible.
2. Prior to surgical intervention.
3. Post-operatively if pre-operative treatment was too short, if spillage has occurred or if viable material was found at surgery.
4. Following percutaneous drainage of cysts for diagnostic or therapeutic reasons.

*Alveolar echinococcosis* (caused by *Echinococcus multilocularis*): Eskazole is used in patients with alveolar echinococcosis:

1. In inoperable disease, particularly in cases of local or distant metastasis.
2. Following palliative surgery.
3. Following radical surgery or liver transplantation.

*Posology and method of administration:*
*Route of administration:* Oral.

*Dosage:* Dosages are dependent on the parasite involved, the weight of the patient, and the severity of the infection:

*Cystic echinococcosis:*
*Patients weighing >60 kg:* Total daily dose: 800 mg given in two divided doses of 400 mg for a total of 28 days.

*Patients weighing <60 kg:* Appropriate dosage adjustment is not possible with the 400 mg tablet presentation.

This 28-day treatment period may be repeated after a 14-day period without treatment for a total of three cycles.

*Alveolar echinococcosis:*
*Patients weighing >60 kg:* Total daily dose: 800 mg given in two equally divided doses for cycles of 28 days with 14 days between cycles.

*Patients weighing <60 kg:* Appropriate dosage adjustment is not possible with the 400 mg tablet presentation.

Treatment may need to be prolonged for months or years. Continuous treatment at the same dose has been used for periods of up to 20 months.

*Method of administration:* Eskazole should be taken with meals.

*Cystic echinococcosis:*

1. Inoperable and multiple cysts: Up to three 28-day cycles of Eskazole may be given for the treatment of liver, lung and peritoneal cysts. More prolonged treatment may be required for sites such as bone and brain.
2. Pre-operative: Two 28-day cycles should be given where possible prior to surgery. Where surgical intervention is necessary before completion of two cycles, albendazole should be given for as long as possible.
3. Post-operative: Where only a short pre-operative course has been given (less than 14 days) and in cases where emergency surgery is required, Eskazole should be given post-operatively for two 28-day cycles separated by 14 drug-free days.

Additionally, where cysts are found to be viable following pre-surgical treatment or where spillage has occurred, a full two-cycle course should be given.

4. After percutaneous cyst drainage: Treatment as for post-surgery above.

*Alveolar echinococcosis:* Treatment is normally given in 28 day cycles as for cystic echinococcosis. It may have to be continued for months or even years. Current follow up suggests that survival times are substantially improved following prolonged treatment. Continuous treatment has been shown in a limited number of patients to lead to apparent cure.

*Children:* There has been limited experience to date with the use of Eskazole in children under six years of age; therefore, usage in children less than six years is not recommended. In older children under 60 kg body weight, although there is clinical experience, appropriate dosage adjustment is not possible with the 400 mg tablet presentation.

*Contra-indications:* Albendazole should not be administered during pregnancy or in women thought to be pregnant. Women of childbearing age should be advised to take effective precautions, with non hormonal contraceptive measures, against conception during and within one month of completion of treatment with Eskazole.

Albendazole is contra-indicated in patients with a known history of hypersensitivity to Eskazole (albendazole or constituents).

*Special warnings and precautions for use:* Eskazole has been associated with mild to moderate elevations of hepatic enzymes in approximately 16% of patients. These have normalised on discontinuation of treatment.

Liver function tests should be obtained before the start of each treatment cycle and at least every two weeks during treatment. If enzymes are significantly increased (greater than twice the upper limit of normal), Eskazole should be discontinued.

Eskazole may be reinstituted when liver enzymes have returned to normal limits, but laboratory tests should be more frequently obtained during repeat therapy.

Eskazole has been shown to cause occasional reversible modest reductions in total white cell counts. Blood counts should be performed at the start and every two weeks during each 28-day cycle. Eskazole may be continued if the decrease appears modest and does not progress.

*Precautions:* In order to avoid administering albendazole during early pregnancy, women of childbearing age should initiate treatment only after a negative pregnancy test. These tests should be repeated at least once before initiating the next cycle.

*Interactions with other medicaments and other forms of interactions:* Albendazole has been shown to induce liver enzymes of the cytochrome P450 system responsible for its own metabolism. There is therefore a theoretical risk of interaction with theophylline, anticonvulsants, anticoagulants, oral contraceptives and oral hypoglycaemics. Care should therefore be exercised during the introduction of Albendazole in patients receiving the above groups of compounds.

Cimetidine and praziquantel have been reported to increase the plasma levels of the albendazole active metabolite.

*Pregnancy and lactation:*
*Pregnancy:* Eskazole should not be administered during pregnancy or in women thought to be pregnant (see *Contra-indications*).

*Lactation:* It is not known whether albendazole or its metabolites are secreted in human breast milk. Thus Eskazole should not be used during lactation unless the potential benefits are considered to outweigh the potential risks associated with treatment.

*Effects on ability to drive and use machines:* Adverse effects on the ability to drive or operate machinery have not been observed.

*Undesirable effects:* As with other benzimidazoles, mild to moderate elevations of hepatic enzymes (around 16% of patients in clinical trials) have occurred during treatment with Eskazole.

Gastrointestinal disturbances (abdominal pain, nausea, vomiting) and leucopenia have been associated commonly (>1%) with Eskazole when treating patients with echinococcosis.

Dizziness and headache have been reported commonly.

As with other benzimidazoles, reversible alopecia (thinning of hair, and moderate hair loss) and fever have been associated commonly (>1%) with Eskazole. Pancytopenia has been reported very rarely (<0.01%).

Hypersensitivity reactions including rash, pruritus and urticaria have been reported very rarely.

*Overdose:* In case of overdosage, symptomatic therapy (gastric lavage) and general supportive measures should be undertaken.

**Pharmacological properties**
*Pharmacodynamic properties:* Albendazole is a benzimidazole carbamate with anthelmintic effects against tissue parasites.

Albendazole exhibits larvicidal, ovicidal and vermicidal activity, and it is thought to exert its anthelmintic effect by inhibiting tubulin polymerisation. This causes the disruption of the helminth metabolism, including energy depletion, which immobilises and then kills the susceptible helminth.

Albendazole is effective in the treatment of tissue parasites including cystic echinococcosis and alveolar echinococcosis caused by infestation of *Echinococcus granulosus* and *Echinococcus multilocularis*, respectively.

In the treatment of cysts due to *E. multilocularis*, a minority of patients were considered to be cured and a majority had an improvement or stabilisation of disease due to albendazole.

*Pharmacokinetic properties:*
*Absorption and metabolism:* In man, albendazole is poorly absorbed (<5%) following oral administration.

Albendazole rapidly undergoes extensive first-pass metabolism in the liver, and is generally not detected in plasma. Albendazole sulfoxide is the primary metabolite, which is thought to be the active moiety in effectiveness against systemic tissue infections. The plasma half-life of albendazole sulfoxide is $8\frac{1}{2}$ hours.

Following oral administration of a single dose of 400 mg albendazole, the pharmacologically active metabolite, albendazole sulfoxide, has been reported to achieve plasma concentrations from 1.6 to 6.0 micromol/litre when taken with breakfast. The systemic pharmacological effect of albendazole is augmented if the dose is administered with a fatty meal, which enhances the absorption by approximately five-fold.

*Excretion:* Albendazole sulfoxide and its metabolites appear to be principally eliminated in bile, with only a small proportion appearing in the urine. Elimination from cysts has been shown to occur over several weeks following high and prolonged dosing.

*Preclinical safety data:* There are no preclinical data of relevance to the prescriber which are additional to that already included in other sections of the SPC.

**Pharmaceutical particulars**
*List of excipients:* Lactose; maize starch; sunset yellow lake; sodium lauryl sulphate; polyvinylpyrrolidone; microcrystalline cellulose; sodium saccharin; sodium starch glycollate; vanilla flavour; orange flavour; passion fruit flavour; magnesium stearate; hydroxypropylmethylcellulose; propylene glycol; purified water.

*Incompatibilities:* None.

*Shelf life:* 36 months.

*Special precautions for storage:* No special storage precautions.

*Nature and contents of container:* Polypropylene 'securitainer' with polyethylene lid, each pack containing 60 tablets

*Instruction for use/handling:* No special instructions.

**Marketing authorisation number** 0002/0202

**Date of approval/revision of SPC** July 1997

**Legal category** POM

## FAMVIR* TILTAB* TABLETS

**Qualitative and quantitative composition** Famciclovir 125, 250, 750 mg.

**Pharmaceutical form** White, round, film-coated 'Tiltab' containing 125 or 250 mg famciclovir for oral administration. White, oval, film-coated 'Tiltab' containing 750 mg famciclovir for oral administration.

**Clinical particulars**
*Therapeutic indications:* Treatment of herpes zoster (shingles) infections, acute genital herpes infections and suppression of recurrent genital herpes infections.

*Posology and method of administration:*
*Dosage: Adults:*
*Herpes zoster infections:* One 750 mg tablet once daily for seven days or alternatively three 250 mg tablets once daily for seven days or alternatively one 250 mg tablet three times daily for seven days. If the tablets are taken once a day they should be taken at approximately the same time each day. Treatment should be initiated as early as possible in the course of the disease, promptly after diagnosis.

*First-episode genital herpes infections:* One 250 mg tablet three times daily for five days. Initiation of treatment is recommended as soon as possible after onset of lesions.

*Recurrent genital herpes infections:*
*Acute treatment:* One 125 mg tablet twice daily for five days. Initiation of treatment is recommended during the prodromal period or as soon as possible after onset of lesions.

*Suppression:* One 250 mg tablet twice daily. Therapy should be interrupted periodically at intervals of six to 12 months in order to observe possible changes in the natural history of the disease.

*Elderly:* Dosage modification is not required unless renal function is impaired.

*Renally impaired:* As reduced clearance of penciclovir is related to reduced renal function, special attention should be given to dosage in patients with impaired renal function (see Overdose section). The following modifications are recommended:

For the treatment of herpes zoster and first-episode genital herpes infections:

| Creatinine clearance (ml/min/1.73 m²) | Dosage |
|---|---|
| 30–59 | 250 mg twice daily |
| 10–29 | 250 mg once daily |

For the treatment of acute recurrent genital herpes infections:

| Creatinine clearance (ml/min/1.73 m²) | Dosage |
|---|---|
| 30–59 | No dose adjustment necessary |
| 10–29 | 125 mg once daily |

For the suppression of recurrent genital herpes infections:

| Creatinine clearance (ml/min/1.73 m²) | Dosage |
|---|---|
| ≥ 30 | 250 mg twice daily |
| 10–29 | 125 mg twice daily |

When only serum creatinine is available, a nomogram or the following formula (Cockcroft and Gault) should be used to estimate creatinine clearance.

Formula to estimate creatinine clearance (ml/min/1.73 m²):

$$\frac{[140\text{–age in years}] \times \text{weight (kg)}}{72 \times \text{serum creatinine } (\mu\text{mol/l})}$$

x **either** 88.5 (for males)
**or** 75.2 (for females)

*Renally impaired patients on haemodialysis:* For a patient on haemodialysis, a dosage interval of 48 hours is recommended for periods between dialysis. Since four hours' haemodialysis results in approximately 75% reduction in plasma concentrations of penciclovir, the full dose of famciclovir should be administered immediately following dialysis.

*Hepatically impaired:* Dosage modification is not required for patients with well compensated chronic liver disease. There is no information on patients with overtly decompensated chronic liver disease; accordingly no precise dose recommendations can be ma[de] for this group of patients.

*Children:* There are currently insufficient data on t[he] safety and efficacy of Famvir in children, therefore, use in children is not recommended.

*Administration:* Oral.

*Contra-indications:* Known hypersensitivity to fam[ci]clovir.

*Special warnings and special precautions for us[e]* Special attention should be paid to patients wi[th] impaired renal function as dosage adjustment may [be] necessary (see *Posology and method of administ[ra]tion* and *Overdose* sections). No special precautio[ns] are required for hepatically impaired or elderly p[a]tients.

Genital herpes is a sexually transmitted disease, t[he] risk of transmission is increased during acute ep[i]sodes. Patients should avoid sexual intercourse wh[en] symptoms are present even if treatment with [an] antiviral has been initiated.

During suppressive treatment with famciclovir, t[he] frequency of viral shedding (both symptomatic a[nd] asymptomatic) may be reduced. However, the risk [of] viral transmission remains even during suppressi[ve] antiviral therapy and with protected intercourse, i.[e.] the use of condoms.

*Interaction with other medicaments and other for[ms] of interaction:* No clinically significant interactio[ns] have been identified. Evidence from preclinical studi[es] has shown no potential for induction of cytochro[me] P450. Probenecid and other drugs that affect re[nal] physiology could affect plasma levels of penciclovi[r].

*Pregnancy and lactation:* Although animal studi[es] have not shown any embryotoxic or teratoge[nic] effects with famciclovir or penciclovir, the safety [of] Famvir in human pregnancy has not been establishe[d.] Famvir should, therefore, not be used during pre[g]nancy or in nursing mothers unless the potent[ial] benefits of treatment outweigh any possible risk.

Studies in rats show that penciclovir is excreted [in] the breast milk of lactating females given oral fam[ci]clovir. There is no information on excretion in huma[n] milk.

*Effects on ability to drive and use machines:* There [is] no evidence that Famvir will affect the ability of [a] patient to drive or to use machines.

*Undesirable effects:* Famciclovir has been well tole[r]ated in human studies. Headache and nausea ha[ve] been reported in clinical trials. These were genera[lly] mild or moderate in nature and occurred at a simi[lar] incidence in patients receiving placebo treatment.

In post-marketing experience, in addition to t[he] above, vomiting, dizziness and skin rash, and con[fu]sion which was predominantly in the elderly, ha[ve] been reported rarely. Hallucinations have been [re]ported very rarely.

*Overdose:* No acute overdosage with Famvir has be[en] reported. Symptomatic and supportive thera[py] should be given as appropriate.

Acute renal failure has been reported rarely [in] patients with underlying renal disease where t[he] Famvir dosage has not been appropriately reduc[ed] for the level of renal function.

Penciclovir is dialysable and plasma concentratio[ns] are reduced by approximately 75% following fo[ur] hours' haemodialysis.

**Pharmacological properties**
*Pharmacodynamic properties:* Famciclovir is the o[ral] form of penciclovir. Famciclovir is rapidly convert[ed] *in vivo* into penciclovir, which has *in vivo* and *in vi[tro]* activity against human herpes viruses including *Va[ri]cella zoster* virus and *Herpes simplex* type 1 and 2.

The antiviral effect of orally administered famcic[lo]vir has been demonstrated in several animal mode[ls;] this effect is due to *in vivo* conversion to penciclo[vir.] In virus-infected cells penciclovir is rapidly and e[ffi]ciently converted into the triphosphate (mediated [by] virus-induced thymidine kinase). Penciclovir tripho[s]phate persists in infected cells for more than 12 hou[rs] where it inhibits replication of viral DNA and has [a] half life of nine, 10 and 20 hours in cells infected w[ith] *Varicella zoster*, *Herpes simplex* virus type 1 a[nd] *Herpes simplex* virus type 2, respectively. In un[in]fected cells treated with penciclovir, concentrations [of] penciclovir-triphosphate are only barely detectab[le.] Accordingly, uninfected cells are unlikely to be [af]fected by therapeutic concentrations of penciclovir.

Penciclovir has been shown to be active agains[t a] recently isolated aciclovir-resistant *Herpes simp[lex]* virus strain which has an altered DNA polymerase.

A placebo-controlled study in patients with imm[u]nodeficiency due to HIV has shown that famciclo[vir] 500 mg b.i.d. significantly decreased the proporti[on] of days of both symptomatic and asymptomatic HS[V] shedding.

*Pharmacokinetic properties:*
*General characteristics:* Following oral administratio[n]

nciclovir is rapidly and extensively absorbed and pidly converted to the active compound, penciclovir. pavailability of penciclovir after oral FAMVIR is 77%. ean peak plasma concentrations of penciclovir, llowing 125 and 250 mg oral doses of famciclovir, ere 0.8 and 1.6 micrograms/ml, respectively, and curred at a median time of 45 minutes post-dose. ean peak plasma concentration of penciclovir, folwing a 750 mg oral dose of famciclovir, was 4.9 mi-ograms/ml and occurred at a median time of minutes post-dose. Plasma concentration-time rves of penciclovir are similar following single and peat (t.i.d.) dosing. The terminal plasma half-life of nciclovir after both single and repeat dosing with nciclovir is approximately 2.0 hours. There is no cumulation of penciclovir on repeated dosing with nciclovir. Penciclovir and its 6-deoxy precursor are orly (<20%) bound to plasma proteins.

Famciclovir is eliminated principally as penciclovir d its 6-deoxy precursor which are excreted in urine changed. Famciclovir has not been detected in ine. Tubular secretion contributes to the renal mination of the compound.

*Characteristics in patients:* Uncomplicated herpes ster infection does not significantly alter the pharacokinetics of penciclovir measured after oral adinistration of Famvir.

*eclinical safety data:* Famciclovir has no significant fects on spermatogenesis or sperm morphology d motility in man. At doses greatly in excess of ose used therapeutically impaired fertility was served in male rats–no such effects being observed female rats.

At a dose level approximately 50 times the normal erapeutic dose there was an increased incidence of ammary adencarcinoma in female rats. No such fect was seen in male rats or mice of either sex.

Additionally, famciclovir was found not to be notoxic in a comprehensive battery of *in vivo* and *vitro* tests designed to detect gene mutation, romosomal damage and repairable damage to NA. Penciclovir, in common with other drugs of this ass, has been shown to cause chromosomal dame, but did not induce gene mutation in bacterial or ammalian cell systems, nor was there evidence of creased DNA repair *in vitro*.

These findings are not considered to have any nical significance.

**armaceutical particulars**

*st of excipients:* Hydroxypropyl Cellulose PhEur; ctose Anhydrous* NF; Sodium Starch Glycollate *; Magnesium Stearate PhEur; Hydroxpropyl Methyl llulose PhEur; Titanium Dioxide PhEur; Polyethyle Glycol NF.

Constituent of Famvir 125 and 250 mg tablets only

*compatibilities:* No specific incompatibilities.

*helf life:* Three years

*pecial precautions for storage:* Famvir 125 and 0 mg tablets–store in a dry place.

Famvir 750 mg tablets–store at or below 30°C in a y place.

*ature and contents of container:*

*erpes zoster treatment:* Famvir is supplied as a ingles patient pack in original blister packs (PVC/ dC with 20 micron aluminium lidding foil) containg 7 x 750 mg tablets or 21 x 250 mg tablets and as a arter pack of 1 x 750 mg tablet. Each pack contains Patient Information Leaflet.

*Genital Herpes treatment:* Famvir is supplied in iginal blister packs (PVC/PVdC with 20 micron aluinium lidding foil) containing 15 x 250 mg tablets r the treatment of first-episode infection, 10 x 125 mg blets for the treatment of acute recurrent infections 56 x 250 mg tablets for suppressive treatment. Each ack contains a Patient Information Leaflet.

*structions for use/handling:* No special instructions

**arketing authorisation numbers**

| | |
|---|---|
| mvir 125 mg Tablets | 10592/0055 |
| mvir 250 mg Tablets | 10592/0035 |
| mvir 750 mg Tablets | 10592/0084 |

**ate of approval/revision of SPC** August 1997

**gal category** POM

## LUARIX* VACCINE

**ualitative and quantitative composition**

*ctive ingredients:* Purified antigen fractions of inacvated Influenza viruses (cultivated in embryonated ens' eggs) corresponding to WHO selected strains 996):

| | |
|---|---|
| Wuhan/359/95 ($H_3N_2$)–like strain | 15 microgram HA |
| Singapore/6/86 ($H_1N_1$)–like strain | 15 microgram HA |
| Beijing/184/93–like strain | 15 microgram HA |

*xcipients:* Thiomersal; Sodium Chloride; Di-sodium ydrogen Phosphate Dodecahydrate; Potassium Dihydrogen Phosphate; Potassium Chloride; Magnesium Chloride; Polysorbate 80; Water for Injections

**Pharmaceutical form** Colourless to slightly opalecent liquid for injection.

**Clinical particulars**

*Therapeutic indications:* Prophylaxis against influenza in adults and children over six months of age.

Fluarix is particularly recommended in those groups regarded as being at special risk, especially the elderly (over 60 years of age) and/or subjects with the following:

Diseases of the cardiovascular system, metabolic disease (diabetes), cystic fibrosis, chronic respiratory diseases and chronic renal insufficiency, congenital or acquired immune deficiency.

Immunisation against influenza is also recommended in school children and the elderly in residential establishments (in which rapid spread is likely to follow the introduction of infection), doctors, nurses and others in contact with influenza sufferers or high-risk individuals.

*Posology and method of administration:*

*Posology:* Fluarix should be administered before the beginning of the influenza season or as required by the epidemiological situation. Vaccination of at-risk individuals should be repeated each year with the appropriate age-related dose.

The vaccine be inspected visually for any foreign particulate matter and/or variation of physical aspects prior to administration. In the event of either being observed, discard the vaccine.

Fluarix can be administered simultaneously with other vaccines. However, different injection sites must be selected.

*For adults and children over six years of age:* One dose of 0.5 ml.

*For children from six months to six years:* Two doses of 0.25 ml with an interval of four to six weeks (if these children have been vaccinated previously, one dose of 0.25 ml suffices).

*Method of administration:* Single dose administered by intramuscular or subcutaneous injection into the deltoid region.

Fluarix should be administered subcutaneously to subjects with thrombocytopenia or a bleeding disorder since bleeding may occur following an intramuscular administration to these subjects.

*Contra-indications:* As with other vaccines, the administration of Fluarix should be postponed in subjects suffering from acute febrile illness. The presence of a minor illness with or without fever should not contra-indicate the use of Fluarix.

Fluarix should not be administered to subjects with known hypersensitivity to egg proteins, or to any other component of the vaccine.

*Special warnings and precautions for use:* Fluarix will only prevent disease caused by influenza viruses. Infection with other agents causing flu-like symptoms are not prevented by the vaccine.

As with all vaccinations, a solution of 1:1000 adrenaline should be available for injection should an anaphylactic reaction occur. Recipients of vaccine should remain under observation until they have been seen to be in good health and not to be experiencing an immediate adverse reaction. It is not possible to specify an exact length of time.

In patients who are receiving immunosuppressive therapy or those who are immunocompromised, response may be impaired.

Fluarix should not under any circumstances be administered intravenously.

*Interactions with other medicaments and other forms of interaction:* None known.

*Pregnancy and lactation:* The effect of Fluarix on foetal development has not been assessed. However, as with all inactivated viral vaccines, the risks to the foetus are considered to be negligible. The vaccine should be used during pregnancy only when clearly needed. There is no known contra-indication to the use of the vaccine during lactation.

*Effects on ability to drive and use machines:* The vaccine is unlikely to produce an effect on the ability to drive and use machines.

*Undesirable effects:* Local adverse effects (pain, redness and swelling) and systemic adverse events such as low grade fever and malaise have been reported in a minority of vaccinees. These symptoms resolved spontaneously.

Allergic reactions in persons with a history of allergy against one of the components of the vaccine have been reported rarely. Serious hypersensitivity reactions (such as anaphylactoid shock) are extremely rare.

*Overdose:* Not applicable.

**Pharmacological properties**

*Pharmacodynamic properties:* Evaluation of pharmacodynamic properties is not required for vaccines.

*Pharmacokinetic properties:* Evaluation of pharmacokinetic properties is not required for vaccines.

*Preclinical safety data:* Not applicable.

**Pharmaceutical particulars**

*List of excipients:* Thiomersal; Sodium Chloride; Disodium Hydrogen Phosphate Dodecahydrate; Potassium Dihydrogen Phosphate; Potassium Chloride; Magnesium Chloride; Polysorbate 80 (trace); Water for Injections.

*Incompatibilities:* None known.

*Shelf-life:* The shelf-life is 12 months when stored under the recommended storage conditions.

*Special precautions for storage:* Store at 2–8°C and protect from light. Do not freeze

*Nature and contents of container:* Colourless, neutral glass ampoules (type 1, PhEur) with break ring system *and/or* Colourless neutral glass vials (type 1, PhEur) with over caps fitted with flip-off tops *and/or* Pre-filled neutral glass syringes (type 1, PhEur), syringe barrel fitted with needle (25 g, 5/8 inch) and rubber shield. Each containing 0.5 ml.

*Instruction for use/handling:* The vaccine should be inspected visually for any foreign particulate matter and/or variation of physical aspects prior to administration. Before use, the vaccine should be shaken well to obtain a colourless to slightly opalescent liquid. Discard if the contents appears otherwise.

**Marketing authorisation number** 10592/0094

**Date of approval/revision of SPC** July 1996

## HALFAN* TABLETS

**Qualitative and quantitative composition** Each tablet contains 250 mg halofantrine hydrochloride (233 mg halofantrine as the base).

**Pharmaceutical form** White to off-white capsule-shaped tablets, with a breakline on one side and enscribed Halfan on the other.

**Clinical particulars**

*Therapeutic indications:* Halfan is an antimalarial indicated in the treatment of acute infection with *Plasmodium falciparum* and *P. vivax*. It is schizonticidal and exerts its action at the erythrocytic stage of the life cycle (trophozoite and schizont). It is not effective against exoerythrocytic (hepatic) schizonts or against the merozoite or gametocyte stages of the life cycle of *Plasmodium* species investigated.

Halfan is especially useful for those likely to be infected with chloroquine or multi-drug-resistant strains.

*Posology and method of administration:* Oral. It is recommended that halofantrine is given on an empty stomach (see *Pharmacokinetic properties*). This is important for all courses of the drug (see *Warnings and precautions*).

All doses are given as halofantrine hydrochloride.

*Adults and children of over 37 kilos:* A total of six tablets (1500 mg) divided into three doses of two tablets given at six-hourly intervals.

*Children of 37 kilos and under:* The usual dosage is 24 mg/kg divided into three doses given at six-hourly intervals according to the following scheme:

*Weight:*

32-37 kg: A total of $4\frac{1}{2}$ tablets (1125 mg) divided into three doses of $1\frac{1}{2}$ tablets given six-hourly.

23-31 kg: A total of three tablets (750 mg) divided into three doses of one tablet given six-hourly.

*Less than 23 kg:* Appropriate dosage adjustment is not possible with the tablet presentation.

*Elderly:* There are no studies on the use of Halfan in the elderly.

Note: In cases where the patient has no previous exposure or minimal exposure to malaria, a second course of therapy is recommended one week after the initial treatment. Higher than recommended doses have been shown to increase the likelihood of prolongation of the QTc interval (see *Warnings and precautions*).

*Contra-indications:* Patients with known hypersensitivity to Halfan. Patients with a known prolonged QTc interval or a family history of congenital QTc prolongation. Pregnancy (see *Pregnancy and lactation*). Do not use for prophylaxis. Unless there are compelling clinical reasons Halfan should not be used in combination with other drugs, e.g. antimalarials (quinine, chloroquine, mefloquine), tricyclic anti-depressants, antipsychotics, some anti-arrhythmic drugs (Vaughan Williams Classes I and III), drugs causing electrolyte disturbance and certain anti-histamines (terfenadine, astemizole), or clinical conditions (e.g. electrolyte abnormalities, particularly hypokalaemia or hypomagnesaemia; thiamine deficiency, ischaemic heart disease, cardiac failure, myocarditis or serious myocardial damage) known to prolong QTc interval, or in patients with known or suspected ventricular dysrhythmias, A–V conduction disorders or unexplained syncopal attacks.

*Special warnings and special precautions for use:* Halfan has been shown to produce a dose-related prolongation of the QTc interval, which usually is reversible within three to four days. This effect has been associated with serious arrhythmias (sometimes with a fatal outcome), even at the recommended therapeutic dose. Therefore, physicians should take a careful history and consider performing an ECG prior to commencing therapy, as halofantrine is not recommended in patients:

- with known QTc prolongation,
- receiving drugs or having clinical conditions known to prolong the QTc interval,
- with ventricular dysrhythmias, A–V conduction disorders, or unexplained syncopal attacks.

Because of the dose-related nature of the effect on the QTc interval, caution should be taken to avoid increased blood levels that may be associated with higher than recommended doses or increased absorption with fatty foods. It is essential to:

- take the recommended dose on an empty stomach;
- avoid fatty food for 24 hours.

This advice is particularly important during a second course of treatment (see dosage section) as the patient is likely to have improved and be eating normally.

There is no experience with the use of halofantrine in the treatment of patients with cerebral malaria and other complicated malarial conditions. Therefore halofantrine should be used with caution in these conditions.

*Interaction with other medicaments and other forms of interaction:* An interaction with mefloquine ($t_{\frac{1}{2}}$ 21 days) has been reported to lead to further prolongation of the QT interval (see *Contra-indications* and *Warnings and Precautions*). No interactions with aspirin or paracetamol have been seen.

*Pregnancy and lactation:* Halfan has been shown to be embryotoxic but not teratogenic in animal tests. Use in women of childbearing age is contra-indicated unless there are compelling clinical grounds.

Animal data suggest that halofantrine may be secreted in breast milk, resulting in reduced rate of weight gain of offspring. Breast feeding should be discontinued whilst the patient is taking Halfan.

*Effects on ability to drive and use machines:* Not applicable.

*Undesirable effects:* Diarrhoea, abdominal pain, nausea and vomiting, pruritus and rash have been observed during or following treatment with Halfan. Transient elevation of serum transaminases has been reported. Serious cardiac adverse effects have been reported (see *Contra-indications* and *Special warnings and special precautions for use*). Haemolytic reactions which have compromised renal function have been reported. There have been isolated case reports of anaphylaxis and angioedema. Extremely rarely convulsions have been reported but no causal relationship has been established.

*Overdose:* There is no experience of acute overdosage with halofantrine. This precludes characterisation of sequelae and assessment of antidotal efficacy at this time. However in case of accidental overdosage, immediate induction of emesis or gastric lavage is recommended in conjunction with appropriate supportive measures which should include ECG monitoring.

**Pharmacological properties**

*Pharmacodynamic properties:* Halofantrine hydrochloride is a blood schizonticidal antimalarial agent.

*Pharmacokinetic properties:* After administration of single doses, Halfan appears in the systemic circulation within one hour. The systemic exposure to halofantrine is increased substantially after a fatty meal. Its elimination half-life from the blood is generally 24 to 48 hours whilst that of its active desbutyl metabolite is approximately twice that time. The major route of elimination is via the faeces.

*Preclinical safety data:* Refer to *Pregnancy and lactation* section.

**Pharmaceutical particulars**

*List of excipients:* Pregelatinised starch; Povidone; Sodium Starch Glycollate; Microcrystalline Cellulose; Purified Talc; Magnesium Stearate; Purified Water.

*Incompatibilities:* None known.

*Shelf-life:* Halfan tablet has a shelf-life of three years.

*Special precautions for storage:* Store in well sealed container at a temperature not exceeding 30°C and protect from light.

*Nature and contents of container:* Blister pack (OP) of 12 tablets (2 x 6).

*Instructions for use/handling:* No special handling instructions.

**Marketing authorisation number** 0002/0203

**Date of approval/revision of SPC** 17 April 1997

**Legal category** POM

## HAVRIX* JUNIOR MONODOSE* VACCINE
### Hepatitis A vaccine (HM 175 strain)

**Qualitative and quantitative composition** Active ingredient: Hepatitis A virus antigen (720* ELISA units/0.5 ml).

* Calculated overage at release: 10%.

*Excipients:* Aluminium hydroxide gel (3% w/w); 2 phenoxyethanol; polysorbate 20; amino acids for injection; disodium phosphate; monopotassium phosphate; sodium chloride; potassium chloride; water for injections.

**Pharmaceutical form** Vaccine for injection.

**Clinical particulars**

*Therapeutic indications:* Havrix Junior Monodose vaccine is indicated for active immunisation against HAV infection. The vaccine is particularly indicated for those at increased risk of infection or transmission.

*Posology and method of administration:* Havrix Junior Monodose vaccine should be injected intramuscularly in the deltoid region. The vaccine should never be administered intravenously.

*Dosage*

Children/adolescents (one to 15 years): Primary immunisation consists of a single dose of Havrix Junior Monodose vaccine (720 ELISA units/0.5 ml) given intramuscularly. This provides anti-HAV antibodies for at least one year.

Havrix Junior Monodose confers protection against hepatitis A within two to four weeks.

In order to obtain more persistent immunity for up to 10 years, a booster dose is recommended between six and 12 months following the initial dose.

Patients who have started a course of Havrix Junior Vaccine at a dose of 360 ELISA unit/0.5 ml are recommended to complete both the primary course and booster at this dosage.

In the event of a subject being exposed to a high risk of contracting hepatitis A within two weeks of the primary immunisation dose, human normal immunoglobulin may be given simultaneously with Havrix Junior Monodose at different injection sites.

*Contra-indications:* Hypersensitivity to any component of the vaccine. Severe febrile illness.

*Special warnings and special precautions for use:* As with all vaccinations, appropriate medication (e.g. adrenaline) should be readily available for immediate use in case of anaphylaxis.

It is possible that subjects may be in the incubation period of a hepatitis A infection at the time of immunisation. It is not known whether Havrix Junior Monodose will prevent hepatitis A in such cases.

In haemodialysis patients and in subjects with an impaired immune system, adequate anti-HAV antibody titres may not be obtained after the primary immunisation and such patients may therefore require administration of additional doses of vaccine.

*Interaction with other medicaments and other forms of interaction:* Simultaneous administration of Havrix with normal immunoglobulin does not influence the seroconversion rate of Havrix, however, it may result in a lower antibody titre. A similar effect could be observed with Havrix Junior Monodose.

Preliminary data on the concomitant administration of Havrix, at a dose of 720 ELISA units/ml, with recombinant hepatitis B virus vaccine suggests that there is no interference in the immune response to either antigen. On this basis and since it is an inactivated vaccine interference with immune response is unlikely to occur when Havrix Junior Monodose is administered with other inactivated or live vaccines. When concomitant administration is considered necessary the vaccines must be given at different injection sites.

Havrix Junior Monodose must not be mixed with other vaccines in the same syringe.

*Pregnancy and lactation:* The effect of Havrix Junior Monodose on foetal development has not been assessed. However, as with all inactivated viral vaccines the risks to the foetus are considered to be negligible. Havrix Junior Monodose should be used during pregnancy only when clearly needed.

The effect on breast-fed infants in the administration of Havrix Junior Monodose to their mothers has not been evaluated in clinical studies. Havrix Junior Monodose should therefore be used with caution in breast-feeding women.

*Effects on ability to drive and use machines:* N applicable.

*Undesirable effects:* These are usually mild a confined to the first few days after vaccination. T most common reactions are mild transient sorene erythema and induration at the injection site. Le common complaints, not necessarily related to vaccination, include headache, fever, malaise, fatig nausea, vomiting and loss of appetite and ra Elevations of serum liver enzymes (usually tr sient) have been reported occasionally. However causal relationship with the vaccine has not be established.

Neurological manifestations occurring in tempo association have been reported extremely rarely w the vaccine and include transverse myelitis, Guilla Barre syndrome and neuralgic amyotrophy. No cau relationship has been established.

*Overdose:* Not applicable.

**Pharmacological properties**

*Pharmacodynamic properties:* Not applicable.

*Pharmacokinetic properties:* Not applicable.

*Preclinical safety data:* Not applicable.

**Pharmaceutical particulars**

*List of excipients:* Aluminium hydroxide gel (3% w/ 2 phenoxyethanol; polysorbate 20; amino acids injection; disodium phosphate; monopotassiu phosphate; sodium chloride; potassium chlori water for injections.

*Incompatibilities:* Not applicable.

*Shelf life:* Havrix Junior Monodose vaccine has shelf-life of three years from the date of manufact when stored at 2–8°C.

*Special precautions for storage:* Store at 2–8°C. Prot from light. Do not freeze.

*Nature and contents of container:* Prefilled neut glass syringes (Type 1, PhEur), syringe barrel fitt with needle and rubber shield.

*Instructions for use handling:* See Technical Packa Leaflet.

**Marketing authorisation number** 10592/0080.

**Date of approval/revision of SPC** February 1997.

**Legal category** POM.

## HAVRIX* MONODOSE* VACCINE
### Hepatitis A vaccine (HM 175 strain)

**Presentation** Havrix Monodose is a formaldehy inactivated vaccine prepared from hepatitis A vir (HAV) HM175 strain grown in human diploid cells is available in prefilled syringes containing a turb white suspension. Each 1 ml contains not less th 1440 ELISA units of hepatitis A viral protein adsorb on aluminium hydroxide adjuvant together with 0. w/v 2-phenoxyethanol as preservative.

**Uses** Active immunisation against infections caus by hepatitis A virus. The vaccine is particula indicated for those at increased risk of infection transmission. For example, immunisation should considered for the following risk groups:

– Travellers visiting areas of medium or high e demicity, i.e. anywhere outside northern and weste Europe, North America, Australia and New Zealand
– Military and diplomatic personnel.
– Haemophiliacs.
– Intravenous drug abusers.
– Homosexual men.
– Laboratory workers working directly with hepati A virus.
– Sanitation workers in contact with untreat sewage.
– Close contacts of hepatitis A cases.

Since virus shedding from infected persons m occur for a prolonged period, active immunisation close contacts may be considered although protective efficacy of the vaccine in such circu stances has not been demonstrated.

Under certain circumstances additional grou could be at increased risk of infection or transmissic Immunisation for such groups should be consider in the light of local circumstances. Such groups mig include:

– Staff and inmates of residential institutions for t mentally handicapped and other institutions whe standards of personal hygiene are poor.
– Staff working in day-care centres and other s tings with children who are not yet toilet-trained.
– Food packagers or handlers.

In addition there may be other groups at risk specific circumstances when immunisation should given.

In the event of a subject being exposed to a hi risk of contracting hepatitis A within two weeks of primary immunisation dose, human normal imm oglobulin may be given simultaneously with Havrix onodose at different injection sites.

**osage and administration** Havrix Monodose is for tramuscular use only and must not be given travenously, subcutaneously or intradermally.

*dults (16 years and over):* Primary immunisation onsists of a single dose of Havrix Monodose vaccine 440 ELISA units/ml) given intramuscularly.

*hildren/adolescents (1-15 years):* Havrix Monodose not recommended. (Havrix Junior should be used).
The immunisation regimen consists of one dose of accine and provides anti-HAV antibodies for at least ne year. Havrix Monodose confers protection against epatitis A within two to four weeks. In order to obtain ore persistent immunity for up to 10 years, a booster ose is recommended between six and 12 months llowing the initial dose.

Patients who have started a course of Havrix Vaccine a dose of 720 ELISA units/ml are recommended to mplete both the primary course and booster at this osage.

Before using Havrix Monodose, the syringe should e well shaken to obtain a slightly opaque white ispension. Discard if the contents of the syringe ppear otherwise. The vaccine should be adminis red into the deltoid region and not in the gluteal gion. In patients with severe bleeding tendencies ich as haemophiliacs, subcutaneous injection may e considered.

**ontra-indications, warnings, etc.**
*ontra-indications:* Hypersensitivity to any compo ent of the vaccine. Severe febrile infections.

*recautions:* As with all vaccinations, appropriate edication (e.g. adrenaline) should be readily availa e for immediate use in case of anaphylaxis following jection.
Because of the incubation period of hepatitis A, fection may be present at the time of vaccination. If , Havrix Monodose may be ineffective.
In haemodialysis patients and in subjects with an paired immune system, adequate antibody titres ay not be obtained after the primary immunisation urse and such patients may therefore require dministration of additional doses of vaccine.

*teractions:* Simultaneous administration of Havrix a dose of 720 ELISA units/ml with human normal munoglobulin does not influence the seroconver on rate to Havrix; however it may result in a lower ntibody titre. A similar effect could be observed with avrix Monodose.
Preliminary data on the concomitant administration Havrix at a dose of 720 ELISA units/ml with combinant hepatitis B virus vaccine suggests that ere is no interference in the immune response to ther antigen. On this basis and since it is an activated vaccine, interference with immune re onse is unlikely to occur when Havrix Monodose is dministered with other inactivated or live vaccines. hen concomitant administration is considered nec ssary, the vaccines must be given at different jection sites.
Havrix Monodose must not be mixed with other accines in the same syringe.

*se in pregnancy and lactation:* The effect of Havrix lonodose on foetal development has not been ssessed. However, as with all inactivated viral vac nes, the risks to the foetus are considered to be egligible. Havrix Monodose is not recommended in regnancy unless there is a definite risk of hepatitis

The effect on breast-fed infants of the administration Havrix Monodose to their mothers has not been valuated in clinical studies. Havrix Monodose should erefore be used with caution in breast-feeding omen.

*dverse reactions:* These are usually mild and con ned to the first few days after vaccination. The most ommon reactions are mild transient soreness, ery ema and induration at the injection site. Less ommon general complaints, not necessarily related vaccination, include fever, malaise, fatigue, head he, nausea, loss of appetite and rash. Elevations of erum liver enzymes (usually transient) have been ported occasionally. However, a causal relationship ith the vaccine has not been established.
Neurological manifestations occurring in temporal ssociation have been reported extremely rarely with e vaccine and include transverse myelitis, Guillain arré syndrome and neuralgic amyotrophy. No causal lationship has been established.

**harmaceutical precautions** Havrix Monodose should stored between 2°C and 8°C and must not be frozen. ne shelf-life is three years. It should not be diluted. rotect from light.

**egal category** POM.

**ackage quantities** Prefilled syringes containing 1 ml ispension in packs of one and 10.

**Further information** In clinical studies involving adults (18–50 years of age) specific humoral antibodies against HAV were detected in more than 88% of vaccinees at day 15 and in 99% at month one.
Inactive ingredients are aluminium hydroxide, 2-phenoxyethanol, polysorbate 20, amino acids for injection, disodium phosphate, monopotassium phosphate, sodium chloride, potassium chloride, water for injections, and also a trace of neomycin B sulphate (maximum 40 ng, 0.028 IU/ml)

**Product licence number** 10592/0037

## HYCAMTIN* ▼

**Qualitative and quantitative composition** Each vial contains topotecan hydrochloride equivalent to 4 mg topotecan.

**Pharmaceutical form** Powder for solution for infusion.

### Clinical particulars

*Therapeutic indications:* Topotecan is indicated for the treatment of patients with metastatic carcinoma of the ovary after failure of first-line or subsequent therapy.

*Posology and method of administration:* The use of topotecan should be confined to units specialised in the administration of cytotoxic chemotherapy and should only be administered under the supervision of a physician experienced in the use of chemotherapy.
*Initial dose:* The recommended dose of topotecan is 1.5 mg/m² body surface area/day administered by intravenous infusion over 30 minutes daily for five consecutive days with a three week interval between the start of each course. A minimum of four courses is recommended since median time to response in clinical trials was 7.6–11.6 weeks.
Prior to administration of the first course of topotecan, patients must have a baseline neutrophil count of ≥ 1.5 x 10⁹/l, and a platelet count of ≥100 x 10⁹/l.
Routine pre-medication for non-haematological adverse events is not required with topotecan.
Topotecan must be reconstituted and further diluted before use *(see section Instructions for use, handling and disposal).*
*Subsequent Doses:* Topotecan should not be re-administered unless the neutrophil count is ≥ 1 x10⁹/l, the platelet count is ≥ 100 x 10⁹/l, and the haemoglobin level is ≥ 9 g/dl (after transfusion if necessary).
Patients who experience severe neutropenia (neutrophil count < 0.5 x 10⁹/l) for seven days or more, or severe neutropenia associated with fever or infection, or who have had treatment delayed due to neutropenia, should be treated as follows:
*either*
be given a reduced dose i.e. 1.25 mg/m²/day (or subsequently down to 1.0 mg/m²/day if necessary)
*or*
be given G-CSF prophylactically in subsequent courses to maintain dose intensity, starting from day six of the course (the day after completion of topotecan administration). If neutropenia is not adequately managed with G-CSF administration, doses should be reduced.
Doses should be similarly reduced if the platelet count falls below 25 x 10⁹/l. In clinical trials, topotecan was discontinued if the dose had been reduced to 1.0 mg/m² and a further dose reduction was required to manage adverse effects.
*Dosage in renally impaired patients:* Insufficient data are available to make a recommendation for patients with a creatinine clearance <20 ml/min. Limited data indicate that the dose should be reduced in patients with moderate renal impairment. The recommended dose in patients with creatinine clearance between 20 and 39 ml/min is 0.75 mg/m² /day.

*Contra-indications:* Topotecan is contra-indicated in patients who
- have a history of severe hypersensitivity reactions to topotecan and/or its excipients
- are pregnant or breast feeding
- already have severe bone marrow depression prior to starting first course, as evidenced by baseline neutrophils < 1.5 x 10⁹/l and/or a platelet count of ≤ 100 x 10⁹/l.

*Special warnings and special precautions for use:* Haematological toxicity is dose-related and full blood count including platelets should be monitored regularly.
As expected, patients with poor performance status have a lower response rate and an increased incidence of complications such as fever and infection.
There is no experience of the use of topotecan in patients with severely impaired renal function (creatinine clearance < 20 ml/min) or severely impaired hepatic function (serum bilirubin ≥ 10 mg/dl) due to cirrhosis. Topotecan is not recommended to be used in these patient groups.

A small number of hepatically impaired patients (serum bilirubin ≥ 1.5 ≤ 10 mg/dl) were able to tolerate 1.5 g/m² for five days every three weeks although a reduction in topotecan clearance was observed. There are insufficient data available to make a dose recommendation for this patient group.

*Interaction with other medicinal products and other forms of interaction:* No *in vivo* human pharmacokinetic interaction studies have been performed.
Topotecan does not inhibit human P450 enzymes (see *Pharmacokinetic properties*). In a population study, the co-administration of granisetron, ondansetron, morphine or corticosteroids did not appear to have a significant effect on the pharmacokinetics of total topotecan (active and inactive form).

*Use during pregnancy and lactation:*
*Pregnancy:* Topotecan is contra-indicated during pregnancy. Topotecan has been shown to be cause embryo-foetal lethality and malformations in preclinical studies.
*Lactation:* Topotecan is contra-indicated during breast-feeding. Although it is not known whether topotecan is excreted in human breast milk, breast-feeding should be discontinued at the start of therapy.

*Effects on ability to drive and use machines:* Caution should be observed when driving or operating machinery if fatigue and asthenia persist.

*Undesirable effects:*
*Haematological:* In dose-finding studies, the dose-limiting toxicity was found to be haematological. Toxicity was predictable, and reversible. No evidence of cumulative toxicity was seen.
*Neutropenia:* Severe, (neutrophil count <0.5 x 10⁹/l) during course 1 was seen in 60% of the patients and with duration ≥ 7 days in 20% and overall in 79% of patients (42% of courses). In association with severe neutropenia, fever or infection occurred in 16% of patients during course 1 and overall in 21% of patients (7% of courses). Median time to onset of severe neutropenia was nine days and the median duration was seven days. Severe neutropenia lasted beyond seven days in 13% of courses overall.
Among all patients treated in clinical studies (including both those with severe neutropenia and those who did not develop severe neutropenia), 13% (5% of courses) developed fever and 27% (10% of courses) developed infection. In addition, 5% of all patients treated (1% of courses) developed sepsis.
*Thrombocytopenia:* Severe, (platelets less than 25 x 10⁹/l) in 23% of patients (9% of courses); moderate (platelets between 25.0 and 49.9 x 10⁹/l) in 20% of patients (13% of courses).
Median time to onset of severe thrombocytopenia was Day 14 and the median duration was five days. Platelet transfusions were given in 4% of courses. Significant sequelae associated with thrombocytopenia were rare.
*Anaemia:* Moderate to severe (Hb ≤ 7.9 g/dl) in 36% of patients (15% of courses). Red cell transfusions were given in 54% of patients (23% of courses).
*Non-haematological:* In clinical trials of 445 ovarian cancer patients, frequently reported non-haematological effects were gastrointestinal such as nausea (68%), vomiting (44%), and diarrhoea (26%), constipation (14%) and stomatitis (20%). Severe (grade 3 or 4) nausea, vomiting, diarrhoea and stomatitis incidence was 6, 4, 3 and 2% respectively.
Mild abdominal pain was also reported amongst 8% of patients.
Fatigue was observed in approximately one-third and asthenia in about one-fifth of patients whilst receiving topotecan. Severe (grade 3 or 4) fatigue and asthenia incidence was 4 and 2% respectively.
Total or pronounced alopecia was observed in 42% of patients and partial alopecia in 17% of patients.
Other severe events occurring in ≥ 1% patients that were recorded as related or possibly related to topotecan treatment were anorexia (1%), malaise (1%) and hyperbilirubinaemia (1%).
Extravasation has been reported rarely. Reactions have been mild and have not generally required specific therapy.
No evidence of significant cardiotoxicity, neurotoxicity or major organ toxicity was observed with topotecan.

**Overdose:** There is no known antidote for topotecan overdosage. The primary complications of overdosage are anticipated to be bone marrow suppression and mucositis.

### Pharmacological properties

*Pharmacodynamic properties:* Pharmaco-therapeutic group: Antineoplastic and immunomodulating agent: ATC-code: L01X X17
The anti-tumour activity of topotecan involves the inhibition of topoisomerase-I, an enzyme intimately involved in DNA replication as it relieves the torsional strain introduced ahead of the moving replication fork. Topotecan inhibits topoisomerase-I by stabilising the covalent complex of enzyme and strand-cleaved

DNA which is an intermediate of the catalytic mechanism. The cellular sequela of inhibition of topoisomerase–I by topotecan is the induction of protein-associated DNA single-strand breaks.

In a comparative study of topotecan and paclitaxel in patients previously treated for ovarian carcinoma with platinum based chemotherapy (n=112 and 114, respectively), the response rate (95% CI) was 20.5% (13, 28) versus 14% (8, 20) and median time to progression 19 weeks versus 15 weeks (hazard ratio 0.7 [0.6, 1.0]), for topotecan and paclitaxel, respectively. Median overall survival was 62 weeks for topotecan versus 53 weeks for paclitaxel (hazard ratio 0.9 [0.6, 1.3]).

The response rate in the whole ovarian carcinoma programme (n=392, all previously treated with cisplatin or cisplatin and paclitaxel) was 16% In patients refractory to, or relapsing within three months after cisplatin therapy (n=186), the response rate was 10%.

These data should be evaluated in the context of the overall safety profile of the drug, in particular to the important haematological toxicity (see *Undesirable effects*).

*Pharmacokinetic properties:* Following intravenous administration of topotecan at doses of 0.5 to 1.5 mg/m$^2$ as a 30-minute infusion daily for five days, topotecan demonstrated a high plasma clearance of 62 l/h (SD 22), corresponding to approximately 2/3 of liver blood flow. Topotecan also had a high volume of distribution, about 132 L, (SD 57) and a relatively short half-life of two to three hours. Comparison of pharmacokinetic parameters did not suggest any change in pharmacokinetics over the five days of dosing. Area under the curve increased approximately in proportion to the increase in dose. The binding of topotecan to plasma proteins was low (35%) and distribution between blood cells and plasma was fairly homogeneous.

In a population study, a number of factors including age, weight and ascites had no significant effect on clearance of total topotecan (active and inactive form).

The elimination of topotecan has only been partly investigated in man. A major route of clearance of topotecan was by hydrolysis of the lactone ring to form the ring-opened hydroxy acid. *In vitro* data using human liver microsomes indicate the formulation of small amounts of N-demethylated topotecan. In man, as in animal species, a significant proportion of the dose (generally 20-60%) was excreted in the urine as topotecan or the open ring form. *In vitro*, topotecan did not inhibit human P450 enzymes CYP1A2, CYP2A6, CYP2C8/9, CYP2C19, CYP2D6, CYP2E, CYP3A, or CYP4A nor did it inhibit the human cytosolic enzymes dihydropyrimidine or xanthine oxidase.

Plasma clearance in patients with hepatic impairment (serum bilirubin ≥ 1.5 ≤ 10 mg/dl) decreased to about 67% when compared with a control group of patients. Topotecan half-life was increased by about 30% but no clear change in volume of distribution was observed. Plasma clearance of total topotecan (active and inactive form) in patients with hepatic impairment only decreased by about 10% compared with the control group of patients.

Plasma clearance in patients with renal impairment (creatinine clearance 41–60 ml/min.) decreased to about 67% compared with control patients. Volume of distribution was slightly decreased and thus half-life only increased by 14%. In patients with moderate renal impairment topotecan plasma clearance was reduced to 34% of the value in control patients. Mean half-life increased from 1.9 hours to 4.9 hours.

*Preclinical safety data:* Resulting from its mechanism of action, topotecan is genotoxic to mammalian cells (mouse lymphoma cells and human lymphocytes) *in vitro* and mouse bone marrow cells *in vivo*. Topotecan was also shown to cause embryo-foetal lethality when given to rats and rabbits.

The carcinogenic potential of topotecan has not been studied

**Pharmaceutical particulars**

*List of excipients:* Tartaric acid, mannitol, hydrochloric acid and sodium hydroxide.

*Incompatibilities:* None known.

*Shelf-life: Vials* 24 months.

*Reconstituted and diluted solutions:* The product should be used immediately after reconstitution as it contains no antibacterial preservative. If reconstitution and dilution is performed under strict aseptic conditions (e.g. an LAF bench) the product should be used (infusion completed) within 12 hours at room temperature or 24 hours if stored at 2–8ºC after the first breakage.

*Special precautions for storage:* Before reconstitution the product must be protected from light during long-term storage by being retained in its carton.

*Nature and content of container:* 5 ml type I flint glass vials, together with 20 mm grey butyl rubber stoppers and 20 mm aluminium seals with plastic flip-off caps.

*Instructions for use/handling and disposal:* Topotecan 4 mg vials must be reconstituted with 4 ml Sterile Water for Injection. Further dilution of the appropriate volume of the reconstituted solution with either 0.9% Sodium Chloride Intravenous Infusion or 5% Dextrose Intravenous Infusion is required to a final concentration of between 25 and 50 microgram/ml.

The normal procedures for proper handling and disposal of anticancer drugs should be adopted, namely:

Personnel should be trained to reconstitute the drug.

Pregnant staff should be excluded from working with this drug.

Personnel handling this drug during reconstitution should wear protective clothing including mask, goggles and gloves.

All items for administration or cleaning, including gloves, should be placed in a high-risk, waste disposal bags for high-temperature incineration. Liquid waste may be flushed with large amounts of water.

Accidental contact with the skin or eyes should be treated immediately with copious amounts of water.

**Marketing authorisation number** EU/1/96/027/001-2

**Date of approval/revision of SPC** November 1996

**Legal category** POM

## KYTRIL* INFUSION
## KYTRIL* TABLETS

**Presentation** Clear glass ampoules, each containing 3 mg granisetron present as the hydrochloride in 3 ml isotonic saline as a clear, colourless or slightly straw-coloured liquid.

White triangular film-coated tablets each containing 1 mg granisetron present as the hydrochloride.

**Uses** Kytril is indicated for the prevention or treatment of nausea and vomiting induced by cytostatic therapy.

Granisetron is a potent and highly selective 5-hydroxytryptamine (5-$HT_3$) receptor antagonist with anti-emetic activity.

**Dosage and administration**

*INFUSION:* Kytril ampoules are for intravenous administration only.

*Adults:* 3 mg Kytril, which should be administered *either* in 15 ml infusion fluid as an intravenous bolus over not less than 30 seconds *or* diluted in 20 to 50 ml infusion fluid and administered over five minutes.

*Prevention:* In clinical trials, the majority of patients have required only a single dose of Kytril to control nausea and vomiting over 24 hours. Up to two additional doses of 3 mg Kytril may be administered within a 24-hour period. There is clinical experience in patients receiving daily administration for up to five consecutive days in one course of therapy. Prophylactic administration of Kytril should be completed prior to the start of cytostatic therapy.

*Treatment:* The same dose of Kytril should be used for treatment as prevention. Additional doses should be administered at least 10 minutes apart.

*Maximum daily dosage:* Up to three doses of 3 mg Kytril may be administered within a 24–hour period. The maximum dose of Kytril to be administered over 24 hours should not exceed 9 mg.

*Concomitant use of dexamethasone:* The efficacy of Kytril may be enhanced by the addition of dexamethasone.

*Elderly:* No special requirements apply to elderly patients.

*Children: Prevention:* A single dose of 40 mcg/kg body weight (up to 3 mg) should be administered as an intravenous infusion, diluted in 10 to 30 ml infusion fluid and administered over five minutes. Administration should be completed prior to the start of cytostatic therapy.

*Treatment:* The same dose of Kytril as above should be used for treatment as prevention.

One additional dose of 40 mcg/kg body weight (up to 3 mg) may be administered within a 24-hour period. This additional dose should be administered at least 10 minutes apart from the initial infusion.

*Patients with renal or hepatic impairment:* No special requirements apply to those patients with renal or hepatic impairment.

*Administration*

*Adults:* To prepare a dose of 3 mg, 3 ml is withdrawn from the ampoule and diluted either to 15 ml with 0.9% w/v Sodium Chloride Injection BP (for bolus administration) or in infusion fluid to a total volume of 20 to 50 ml in any of the following solutions: 0.9% w/v Sodium Chloride Injection BP; 0.18% w/v Sodium Chloride and 4% w/v Glucose Injection BP; 5% w/v Glucose Injection BP; Hartmann's Solution for Injection BP; Sodium Lactate Injection BP; or 10% Mannitol Injection BP (for infusion). No other diluents should be used.

*Children:* To prepare the dose of 40 mcg/kg t appropriate volume (up to 3 ml) is withdrawn fro the ampoule and diluted with infusion fluid (as f adults) to a total volume of 10 to 30 ml.

*TABLETS*

*Adults:* One tablet (1 mg) twice a day during cyt static therapy.

The first dose should be administered within o hour before the start of cytostatic therapy.

Kytril is also available as ampoules for intraveno administration. The maximum dose of Kytril admi istered over 24 hours should not exceed 9 mg.

*Concomitant use of dexamethasone:* The efficacy Kytril may be enhanced by the addition of dexameth sone.

*Elderly:* No special requirements apply to elder patients.

*Children:* There is insufficient evidence on which base appropriate dosage regimens for children und 12 years old. Kytril Tablets are therefore not recor mended in this age group.

*Patients with renal or hepatic impairment:* No speci requirements apply to those patients with renal hepatic impairment.

**Contra-indications, warnings, etc**

*Contra-indication:* Hypersensitivity to granisetron related substances.

*Precautions:* As Kytril may reduce lower bowel mot ity, patients with signs of subacute intestinal obstru tion should be monitored following administration Kytril.

There has been no evidence from human studi that Kytril has any adverse effect on alertness.

Data from two-year carcinogenicity studies ha shown an increase in hepatocellular carcinoma an or adenoma in rats and mice of both sexes giv 50 mg/kg (rat dosage reduced to 25 mg/kg/day at we 59). Increases in hepatocellular neoplasia were al detected at 5 mg/kg in male rats. In both specie drug-induced effects (hepatocellular neoplasia) we not observed in the low-dose group (1 mg/kg).

In several *in vitro* and *in vivo* assays, Kytril w shown to be non-genotoxic in mammalian cells.

*Drug interactions:* In studies in healthy subjects, evidence of any interaction has been indicated b tween Kytril and cimetidine or lorazepam. No eviden of drug interactions has been observed in clinic studies.

*Use in pregnancy and lactation:* Whilst animal studi have shown no teratogenic effects, there is experience of Kytril in human pregnancy. Therefo Kytril should not be administered to women who a pregnant unless there are compelling clinical reasor There are no data on the excretion of Kytril in brea milk. Breast feeding should therefore be discontinu during therapy.

*Adverse reactions:* Kytril has been generally w tolerated in human studies. As reported with oth drugs of this class, headache and constipation ha been the most frequently noted adverse events, b the majority have been mild or moderate in natu Rare cases of hypersensitivity reaction, occasiona severe (e.g. anaphylaxis) have been reported. Oth allergic reactions including minor skin rashes ha also been reported. In clinical trials, transient increas in hepatic transaminases, generally within the norm range, have been seen.

*Overdosage:* There is no specific antidote for Kytril. the case of overdosage, symptomatic treatme should be given. One patient has received 10 tim the recommended intravenous dose of Kytril. T patient reported a slight headache but no oth sequelae were observed.

**Pharmaceutical precautions** Ampoules remov from the pack should be protected from dire sunlight. Do not freeze. Ideally, intravenous infusio of Kytril should be prepared at the time of administ tion. After dilution (see **Dosage and administratio** the shelf life is 24 hours when stored at ambie temperature in normal indoor illumination protect from direct sunlight. It must not be used after hours. If to be stored after preparation, Kytril infusio must be prepared under appropriate aseptic con tions.

As a general precaution, Kytril should not be mix in solution with other drugs.

**Legal category** POM.

**Package quantities** Ampoules in boxes of five a 10. Tablets in boxes of 10.

**Further information** Absorption of Kytril is genera not influenced by food and is rapid and comple though oral bioavailability is reduced to around 60 as a result of first pass metabolism.

Kytril is widely distributed with plasma prote binding of approximately 65%. It is rapidly a extensively metabolised mainly by N-demethylati and aromatic ring oxidation followed by conjugation; excretion is both urinary and faecal.

The inactive ingredients in the infusion are sodium chloride and Water for Injections PhEur. Inactive ingredients in the tablet include lactose.

**Product licence numbers**

| | |
|---|---|
| Kytril Infusion | 10592/0003. |
| Kytril Tablets | 10592/0032. |

## KYTRIL* PAEDIATRIC LIQUID

**Qualitative and quantitative composition** Granisetron hydrochloride equivalent to 200 mcg granisetron (free base equivalent) per 1 ml.

**Pharmaceutical form** An orange coloured and flavoured clear solution equivalent to 200 mcg of granisetron free base per 1 ml.

**Clinical particulars**

*Therapeutic indications:* Kytril Paediatric Liquid is indicated for the prevention of nausea and vomiting induced by cytostatic therapy.

*Posology and method of administration:*
*Children:* A single dose of 20 mcg/kg bodyweight (up to 1 mg) twice a day up to five days during cytostatic therapy. The first dose of Kytril should be administered within one hour before the start of cytostatic therapy.

*Patients with renal or hepatic impairment:* No special requirements apply.

*Contra-indications:* Hypersensitivity to granisetron, or related substances, or any of the other constituents.

*Special warnings and special precautions for use:* As Kytril may reduce lower bowel motility, patients with signs of sub-acute intestinal obstruction should be monitored following administration of Kytril.

*Interaction with other medicaments and other forms of interaction:* In studies in healthy subjects, no evidence of any interaction has been indicated between Kytril and cimetidine or lorazepam. No evidence of drug interactions has been observed in clinical studies.

*Pregnancy and lactation:* Whilst animal studies have shown no teratogenic effects, there is no experience of Kytril in human pregnancy. Therefore Kytril should not be administered to women who are pregnant unless there are compelling clinical reasons. There are no data on the excretion of Kytril in breast milk. Breast feeding should therefore be discontinued during therapy.

*Effects on ability to drive and use machines:* There has been no evidence from human studies that Kytril has any adverse effect on alertness.

*Undesirable effects:* Kytril has been generally well tolerated in human studies. As reported with other drugs of this class, headache and constipation have been the most frequently noted adverse events but the majority have been mild or moderate in nature. Rare cases of hypersensitivity reaction, occasionally severe (e.g. anaphylaxis) have been reported. Other allergic reactions including minor skin rashes have also been reported. In clinical trials transient increases in hepatic transaminases, generally within the normal range, have been seen.

*Overdose:* There is no specific antidote for Kytril. In the case of overdosage, symptomatic treatment should be given. One patient has received 30 mg of Kytril intravenously. The patient reported a slight headache but no other sequelae were observed.

**Pharmacological properties**

*Pharmacodynamic properties:* Kytril is a potent antiemetic and highly selective antagonist of 5-hydroxytryptamine (5-$HT_3$) receptors. Radioligand binding studies have demonstrated that Kytril has negligible affinity for other receptor types including 5-HT and dopamine $D_2$ binding sites.

Kytril is effective orally prophylactically in prevention of the retching and vomiting evoked by cytostatic therapy.

*Pharmacokinetic properties:*
*General characteristics: Absorption:* Absorption of Kytril is rapid and complete, though oral bioavailability is reduced to about 60% as a result of first pass metabolism. Oral bioavailability is generally not influenced by food.

*Distribution:* Kytril is extensively distributed, with a mean volume of distribution of approximately 3 l/kg; plasma protein binding is approximately 65%.

*Biotransformation:* Biotransformation pathways involve N-demethylation and aromatic ring oxidation followed by conjugation.

*Elimination:* Clearance is predominantly by hepatic metabolism. Urinary excretion of unchanged Kytril averages 12% of dose whilst that of metabolites amounts to about 47% of dose. The remainder is excreted in faeces as metabolites. Mean plasma half-life in patients is approximately nine hours, with a wide inter-subject variability.

*Characteristics in patients:* The plasma concentration of Kytril is not clearly correlated with anti-emetic efficacy. Clinical benefit may be conferred even when Kytril is not detectable in plasma.

In elderly subjects after single intravenous doses, pharmacokinetic parameters were within the range found for non-elderly subjects. In patients with severe renal failure, data indicate that pharmacokinetic parameters after a single intravenous dose are generally similar to those in normal subjects. In patients with hepatic impairment due to neoplastic liver involvement, total plasma clearance of an intravenous dose was approximately halved compared to patients without hepatic involvement. Despite these changes, no dosage adjustment is necessary.

In children, after single intravenous doses, pharmacokinetics are similar to those in adults when appropriate parameters (volume of distribution, total plasma clearance) are normalised for body-weight.

*Preclinical safety data:* Data from two-year carcinogenicity studies have shown an increase in hepatocellular carcinoma and/or adenoma in rats and mice of both sexes given 50 mg/kg (rat dosage reduced to 25 mg/kg/day at week 59). Increases in hepatocellular neoplasia were also detected at 5 mg/kg in male rats. In both species, drug-induced effects (hepatocellular neoplasia) were not observed in the low-dose group (1 mg/kg).

In several *in vitro* and *in vivo* assays, Kytril was shown to be non-genotoxic in mammalian cells.

**Pharmaceutical particulars**

*List of excipients:* Sorbitol PhEur; Sodium Benzoate (E211) PhEur; Citric Acid Anhydrous PhEur; Orange Flavour D3798 HSE; Orange Flavour D2362 HSE; F.D. & C Yellow No. 6 (E 110) HSE; Purified Water PhEur.

*Incompatibilities:* Not applicable.

*Shelf-life:* Unopened: two years.
After opening for the first time: one month.

*Special precautions for storage:* Kytril Paediatric Liquid should be stored at or below 30°C and capped after partial use.

*Nature and contents of container:* Kytril Paediatric Liquid is supplied in a 30 ml amber glass bottle with a child-resistant high-density polyethylene cap with a PVdC faced boxboard wad. The bottle contains 30 ml of solution and is enclosed in an outer carton.

*Instructions for use/handling:*
Administering the oral solution: *Children:* To administer the dose of 20 mcg/kg, 0.1 ml of solution per one kilogram of body weight should be withdrawn from the bottle up to a maximum of 5 ml per dose.

An oral dosing syringe should be used. When administering the measured dose, insert the syringe tip into the child's mouth and drip the medicine in slowly.

**Marketing authorisation number** 10592/0077

**Date of approval/revision of SPC** March 1996.

**Legal category** POM

## KYTRIL* TABLETS 2 mg

**Qualitative and quantitative composition** Granisetron hydrochloride equivalent to 2 mg granisetron (free base equivalent).

**Pharmaceutical form** Kytril is presented as white triangular film-coated tablets containing 2 mg granisetron free base equivalent.

**Clinical particulars**

*Therapeutic indications:* Kytril tablets are indicated for the prevention of nausea and vomiting induced by cytostatic therapy.

*Posology and method of administration:*
*Adults:* The dose of Kytril is 1 mg twice a day or 2 mg once a day during cytostatic therapy.

The first dose of Kytril should be administered within one hour before the start of cytostatic therapy.

*Concomitant use of dexamethasone:* The efficacy of Kytril may be enhanced by the addition of dexamethasone.

*Maximum dose and duration of treatment:* Kytril is also available as ampoules for intravenous administration. The maximum dose of Kytril administered orally and/or intravenously over 24 hours should not exceed 9 mg.

*Children:* There is insufficient evidence on which to base appropriate dosage regimens for children under 12 years old. Kytril Tablets are therefore not recommended in this age group.

*Elderly:* As for adults.
*Renally impaired:* As for adults.
*Hepatically impaired:* As for adults.

*Contra-indications:* Kytril is contra-indicated in patients hypersensitive to granisetron or related substances.

*Special warnings and special precautions for use:* As Kytril may reduce lower bowel motility, patients with signs of sub-acute intestinal obstruction should be monitored following administration of Kytril.

*Interaction with other medicaments and other forms of interaction:* In studies in healthy subjects, no evidence of any interaction has been indicated between Kytril and cimetidine or lorazepam. No evidence of drug interactions has been observed in clinical studies.

*Pregnancy and lactation:* Whilst animal studies have shown no teratogenic effects, there is no experience of Kytril in human pregnancy. Therefore Kytril should not be administered to women who are pregnant unless there are compelling clinical reasons. There are no data on the excretion of Kytril in breast milk. Breast feeding should therefore be discontinued during therapy.

*Effects on ability to drive and use machines:* There has been no evidence from human studies that Kytril has any adverse effect on alertness.

*Undesirable effects:* Kytril has been generally well tolerated in human studies. As reported with other drugs of this class, headache and constipation have been the most frequently noted adverse events, but the majority have been mild or moderate in nature. Rare cases of hypersensitivity reaction, occasionally severe (e.g. anaphylaxis), have been reported. Other allergic reactions including minor skin rashes have also been reported. In clinical trials, transient increases in hepatic transaminases, generally within the normal range, have been seen.

*Overdose:* There is no specific antidote for Kytril. In the case of overdosage, symptomatic treatment should be given. One patient has received 30 mg of Kytril intravenously. The patient reported a slight headache but no other sequelae were observed.

**Pharmacological properties**

*Pharmacodynamic properties:* Kytril is a potent antiemetic and highly selective antagonist of 5-hydroxytryptamine (5-$HT_3$) receptors. Radioligand binding studies have demonstrated that Kytril has negligible affinity for other receptor types including 5-HT and dopamine $D_2$ binding sites.

Kytril is effective orally prophylactically in abolishing the retching and vomiting evoked by cytostatic therapy.

*Pharmacokinetic properties:*
*General characteristics – Absorption:* Absorption of Kytril is rapid and complete, though oral bioavailability is reduced to about 60% as a result of first pass metabolism. Oral bioavailability is generally not influenced by food.

*Distribution:* Kytril is extensively distributed, with a mean volume of distribution of approximately 3 l/kg; plasma protein binding is approximately 65%.

*Biotransformation:* Biotransformation pathways involve N-demethylation and aromatic ring oxidation followed by conjugation.

*Elimination:* Clearance is predominantly by hepatic metabolism. Urinary excretion of unchanged Kytril averages 12% of dose whilst that of metabolites amounts to about 47% of dose. The remainder is excreted in faeces as metabolites. Mean plasma half-life in patients is approximately nine hours, with a wide inter-subject variability.

The pharmacokinetics of Kytril demonstrate no marked deviations from linear pharmacokinetics at oral doses up to 2.5-fold of the recommended clinical dose.

*Characteristics in patients:* The plasma concentration of Kytril is not clearly correlated with anti-emetic efficacy. Clinical benefit may be conferred even when Kytril is not detectable in plasma.

In elderly subjects after single intravenous doses, pharmacokinetic parameters were within the range found for non-elderly subjects. In patients with severe renal failure, data indicate that pharmacokinetic parameters after a single intravenous dose are generally similar to those in normal subjects. In patients with hepatic impairment due to neoplastic liver involvement, total plasma clearance of an intravenous dose was approximately halved compared to patients without hepatic involvement. Despite these changes, no dosage adjustment is necessary.

*Preclinical safety:* Data from two-year carcinogenicity studies have shown an increase in hepatocellular carcinoma and/or adenoma in rats and mice of both sexes given 50 mg/kg (rat dosage reduced to 25 mg/kg/day at week 59). Increases in hepatocellular neoplasia were also detected at 5 mg/kg in male rats. In both species, drug-induced effects (hepatocellular neoplasia) were not observed in the low-dose group (1 mg/kg).

In several *in vitro* and *in vivo* assays, Kytril was shown to be non-genotoxic in mammalian cells.

### Pharmaceutical particulars

*List of excipients:* Microcrystalline Cellulose NF; Sodium Starch Glycollate BP; Hydroxypropyl Methylcellulose 2910 USP; Lactose PhEur; Magnesium Stearate PhEur; Film coat: Hydroxypropyl methylcellulose PhEur; Titanium dioxide PhEur. (E171); Polyethylene glycol NF; Polysorbate 80 PhEur.

*Incompatibilities:* None.

*Shelf-life:* Kytril Tablets have a shelf-life of two years.

*Special precautions for storage:* None.

*Nature and contents of container:* Kytril is supplied in opaque blister packs packed in cartons containing five tablets.

*Instructions for use/handling:* None.

**Marketing authorisation number**    10592/0067

**Date of approval/revision of SPC**    January 1996.

**Legal category**    POM

## KYTRIL* VIALS 1 mg/1 ml

**Qualitative and quantitative composition** Vial: Granisetron hydrochloride equivalent to 1.0 mg granisetron (free base equivalent).

**Pharmaceutical form**    A glass vial containing a sterile, clear solution equivalent to 1 mg of granisetron free base per 1 ml of isotonic saline. The content allows withdrawal of 1 ml. A 15% filling overage is included.
    Active constituent INN: Granisetron.

### Clinical particulars

*Therapeutic indications:* Kytril is indicated for the prevention or treatment of nausea and vomiting induced by cytostatic therapy and for the prevention and treatment of post-operative nausea and vomiting.

*Posology and method of administration*
*Cytostatic therapy*
    *Children:* Prevention: A single dose of 40 mcg/kg bodyweight (up to 3 mg) should be administered as an intravenous infusion, diluted in 10 to 30 ml infusion fluid and administered over five minutes. Administration should be completed prior to the start of cytostatic therapy.
    Treatment: The same dose of Kytril as above should be used for treatment as prevention.
    One additional dose of 40 mcg/kg bodyweight (up to 3 mg) may be administered within a 24-hour period if required. This additional dose should be administered at least 10 minutes apart from the initial infusion.
    *Renally impaired:* No special requirements apply.
    *Hepatically impaired:* No special requirements apply.

*Post-operative nausea and vomiting*
    *Adults:* For prevention in adults, a single dose of 1 mg of Kytril should be diluted to 5 ml and administered as a slow intravenous injection (over 30 seconds). Administration should be completed prior to induction of anaesthesia.
    For the treatment of established post-operative nausea and vomiting in adults, a single dose of 1 mg of Kytril should be diluted to 5 ml and administered by slow intravenous injection (over 30 seconds).
    *Maximum dose and duration of treatment:* Two doses (2 mg) in one day.
    *Children:* There is no experience in the use of Kytril in the prevention and treatment of post-operative nausea and vomiting in children. Kytril is not therefore recommended for the treatment of post-operative nausea and vomiting in this age group.
    *Elderly:* As for adults.
    *Renally impaired:* As for adults.
    *Hepatically impaired:* As for adults.

*Contra-indications:* Hypersensitivity to granisetron or related substances.

*Special warnings and special precautions for use:* As Kytril may reduce lower bowel motility, patients with signs of sub-acute intestinal obstruction should be monitored following administration of Kytril.
    No special precautions are required for the elderly or renally or hepatically impaired patient.

*Interaction with other medicaments and other forms of interaction:* In studies in healthy subjects, no evidence of any interaction has been indicated between Kytril and cimetidine or lorazepam. No evidence of drug interactions has been observed in clinial studies conducted.
    No specific interaction studies have been conducted in anaesthetised patients, but Kytril has been safely administered with commonly used anaesthetic and analgesic agents. In addition, *in vitro* human microsomal studies have shown that the cytochrome P$_{450}$ sub-family 3A4 (involved in the metabolism of some of the main narcotic analgesic agents) is not modified by Kytril.

*Pregnancy and lactation:* Whilst animal studies have shown no teratogenic effects, there is no experience of Kytril in human pregnancy. Therefore Kytril should not be administered to women who are pregnant unless there are compelling clinical reasons. There are no data on the excretion of Kytril in breast milk. Breast feeding should therefore be discontinued during therapy.

*Effects on ability to drive and use machines:* There has been no evidence for human studies that Kytril has any adverse effect on alertness.

*Undesirable effects:* Kytril has been generally well tolerated in human studies. As reported with other drugs of this class, headache and constipation have been the most frequently noted adverse events but the majority have been mild or moderate in nature. Rare cases of hypersensitivity reaction, occasionally severe (e.g. anaphylaxis) have been reported. Other allergic reactions including minor skin rashes have also been reported. In clinical trials, transient increases in hepatic transaminases, generally within the normal range, have been seen.

*Overdose:* There is no specific antidote for Kytril. In the case of overdosage, symptomatic treatment should be given. One patient has received 30 mg of Kytril intravenously. The patient reported a slight headache but no other sequelae were observed.

### Pharmacological properties

*Pharmacodynamic properties:* Kytril is a potent anti-emetic and highly selective antagonist of 5-hydroxytryptamine (5-HT$_3$) receptors. Radioligand binding studies have demonstrated that Kytril has negligible affinity for other receptor types including 5-HT and dopamine D$_2$ binding sites.
    Kytril is effective intravenously, either prophylactically or by intervention, in abolishing the retching and vomiting evoked by administration of cytotoxic drugs or by whole body X-irradiation.
    Kytril is effective, intravenously, in the prevention and treatment of post-operative nausea and vomiting.

*Pharmacokinetic properties*
    *General characteristics: Distribution:* Kytril is extensively distributed, with a mean volume of distribution of approximately 3l/kg; plasma protein binding is approximately 65%.
    *Biotransformation:* Biotransformation pathways involve N-demethylation and aromatic ring oxidation followed by conjugation.
    *Elimination:* Clearance is predominantly by hepatic metabolism. Urinary excretion of unchanged Kytril averages 12% of dose whilst that of metabolites amounts to about 47% of dose. The remainder is excreted in faeces as metabolites. Mean plasma half-life in patients is approximately nine hours, with a wide inter-subject variability.

*Characteristics in patients:* The plasma concentration of Kytril is not clearly correlated with antiemetic efficacy. Clinical benefit may be conferred even when Kytril is not detectable in plasma.
    In elderly subjects after single intravenous doses, pharmacokinetic parameters were within the range found for non-elderly subjects. In patients with severe renal failure, data indicate that pharmacokinetic parameters after a single intravenous dose are generally similar to those in normal subjects. In patients with hepatic impairment due to neoplastic liver involvement, total plasma clearance of an intravenous dose was approximately halved compared to patients without hepatic involvement. Despite these changes, no dosage adjustment is necessary.

*Preclinical safety data:* Data from two-year carcinogenicity studies have shown an increase in hepatocellular carcinoma and/or adenoma in rats and mice of both sexes given 50 mg/kg (rat dosage reduced to 25 mg/kg/day at week 59). Increases in hepatocellular neoplasia were also detected at 5 mg/kg in male rats. In both species, drug-induced effects (hepatocellular neoplasia) were not observed in the low-dose group (1 mg/kg).
    In several *in vitro* and *in vivo* assays, Kytril was shown to be non-genotoxic in mammalian cells.

### Pharmaceutical particulars

*List of excipients:* Sodium Chloride PhEur; Water for Injection PhEur. Hydrochloric acid and/or sodium hydroxide may be used to adjust the pH if required.

*Incompatibilities:* As a general precaution, Kytril should not be mixed in solution with other drugs. Prophylactic administration of Kytril should be completed prior to the start of cytostatic therapy or induction of anaesthesia.

*Shelf-life:* Kytril vials have a shelf-life of three years.

*Special precautions for storage:* Kytril vials should be stored protected from light below 30°C. Do not freeze.

*Nature and contents of container:* Kytril is supplied in clear glass vials packaged either individually or in packs of five, with an outer carton.

*Instructions for use/handling*
    *Preparing the infusion: Children:* To prepare the dose of 40 mcg/kg, the appropriate volume is withdrawn and diluted with infusion fluid to a total volume of 10 to 30 ml. Any one of the following solutions may be used: 0.9% w/v Sodium Chloride Injection BP; 0.18% w/v Sodium Chloride and 4% w/v Glucose Injection BP; 5% w/v Glucose Injection BP; Hartmann's Solution for Injection BP; Sodium Lactate Injection BP or 10% Mannitol Injection BP. No other diluents should be used.
    Ideally, intravenous infusions of Kytril should be prepared at the time of administration. After dilution (see above), or when the container is opened for the first time, the shelf life is 24 hours when stored at ambient temperature in normal indoor illumination protected from direct sunlight. It must not be used after 24 hours. If to be stored after preparation, Kytril infusions must be prepared under appropriate aseptic conditions.
    *Adults:* To prepare a dose of 1 mg, 1 ml should be withdrawn from the vial and diluted to 5 ml with 0.9% w/v Sodium Chloride Injection BP. No other diluent should be used.

**Marketing authorisation number**    10592/0063.

**Date of approval/revision of SPC**    September 1995.

**Legal category** POM.

## LISKONUM* TABLETS

**Qualitative and quantitative composition** Liskonum Tablets are available in one strength. Each tablet contains 450 mg lithium carbonate (12.2 mmol Li⁺) in controlled-release form.

**Pharmaceutical form** White, oblong, film-coated tablets, with convex faces and a breakline on both sides.

### Clinical particulars

*Therapeutic indications:* Liskonum is a controlled release tablet, designed to reduce fluctuations in serum lithium levels and the likelihood of adverse reactions.
    It is indicated for the treatment of acute episodes of mania or hypomania and for the prophylaxis of recurrent manic-depressive illness.

*Posology and method of administration:*
*Dosage: Adults only:* Liskonum should be given twice a day.
    *Treatment of acute mania or hypomania:* Patients should be started on one or one-and-a-half tablets twice a day. Dosage should then be adjusted to achieve a serum lithium level of 0.8 to a maximum of 1.5 mmol/l. Serum concentration of lithium should be measured after four to seven days' treatment and then at least once a week until dosage has remained constant for four weeks. When the acute symptoms have been controlled, recommendations for prophylaxis should be followed.
    *Prophylaxis:* The usual starting dosage is one tablet twice a day. Dosage should then be adjusted until a serum level of 0.5 to 1.0 mmol/l is maintained. Serum concentration of lithium should be measured after four to seven days' treatment and then every week until dosage has remained constant for four weeks. Frequency of monitoring may then be gradually decreased to a minimum of once every two months but should be increased following any situation where changes in lithium levels are possible (see *Warnings and precautions*).
    Blood samples for measurement of serum lithium concentration should be taken just before a dose is due and not less than 12 hours after the previous dose.
    Levels of more than 2 mmol/l *must* be avoided.
    *Elderly:* Use with caution. Start with half a tablet twice a day and adjust serum levels to the lower end of the above ranges (see also *Warnings and precautions*).
    The full prophylactic effect of lithium may not be evident for six to 12 months, and treatment should be continued through any recurrence of the illness.
    *Administration:* Oral.

*Contra-indications:* Do not use in patients with impaired renal function, cardiac disease, or untreated hypothyroidism. Lithium should not be given to patients with low body sodium levels, including, for example, dehydrated patients, those on low sodium diets, or those with Addison's disease.

*Special warnings and special precautions for use:* Vomiting, diarrhoea, intercurrent infection, fluid deprivation and drugs likely to upset electrolyte balance such as diuretics, may all reduce lithium excretion and thereby precipitate intoxication; reduction of dosage may be required. In elderly patients, lithium excretion may also be reduced.
    The possibility of hypothyroidism and of renal dysfunction arising during prolonged treatment should be borne in mind and periodic assessment made.
    Patients should be warned of the symptoms of

mpending intoxication (see *Undesirable effects*), of the urgency of immediate action should these symptoms appear, and also of the need to maintain a constant and adequate salt and water intake.

*Interaction with other medicaments and other forms of interaction:* Diuretics should only be used with caution during treatment; thiazides show a paradoxical antidiuretic effect resulting in possible water retention and lithium intoxication. Concomitant use with NSAIDs can increase serum lithium concentrations, possibly resulting in lithium toxicity; serum lithium concentrations should therefore be monitored more frequently if NSAID therapy is initiated or discontinued.

There have been reports of interaction between lithium and some neuroleptics, particularly haloperidol at higher dosages, also between lithium and methyldopa or phenytoin. Fluvoxamine and fluoxetine should be combined with lithium with care.

*Pregnancy and lactation:* Lithium crosses the placental barrier. In animal studies, lithium has been reported to interfere with fertility, gestation and foetal development. There is epidemiological evidence that the drug may be harmful in human pregnancy. Lithium therapy should not be used during pregnancy, especially during the first trimester, unless considered essential. In certain cases where a severe risk to the patient could exist if treatment were to be stopped, lithium has been continued during pregnancy. If given, however, serum levels should be measured frequently because of the changes in renal function associated with pregnancy and parturition.

Since lithium is secreted in breast milk, bottle feeding is advisable.

*Effects on ability to drive and use machines:* None

*Undesirable effects:* At therapeutic serum levels, mild nausea and diarrhoea, fine tremor of the hands, muscle weakness, vertigo, giddiness, weight gain, oedema and a dazed feeling may occur. Hypothyroidism has been reported. Rarely hyperthyroidism may occur and mild hyperparathyroidism has been reported. Mild polyuria and polydipsia are not infrequent and, occasionally, nephrogenic diabetes insipidus may be present. Histological renal changes, with interstitial fibrosis, have been observed in some patients on long-term treatment; whilst there may be an association with impaired reabsorption, a relationship between these changes and a reduction in glomerular filtration rate or development of renal insufficiency has not been established.

Skin reactions including acne or acneiform eruptions, papular skin disorders, rashes, and exacerbation of psoriasis have been reported.

Intoxication: Vomiting, diarrhoea, drowsiness, lack of co-ordination and/or a coarse tremor of the extremities and lower jaw may occur, especially with serum levels above the therapeutic range. Ataxia, giddiness, blurred vision, dysarthria, tinnitus, muscle hyperirritability, choreoathetoid movements and toxic psychosis have also been described.

If any of the above symptoms appear, treatment should be stopped immediately and arrangements made for serum lithium measurement.

*Overdose:* Symptoms are similar to those listed in *Undesirable effects* section under intoxication but more marked, particularly those of central nervous system origin. In severe cases, seizures, coma and death may ensue.

Treatment consists of the induction of vomiting and/or gastric lavage together with supportive and symptomatic measures. Particular attention should be paid to maintenance of fluid and electrolyte balance and of adequate renal function. Where convulsions are present, diazepam may be used. Forced alkaline diuresis, peritoneal dialysis or haemodialysis may help eliminate the lithium ion. The latter method is preferable, particularly where serum lithium exceeds 4 mmol/l.

**Pharmacological properties**

*Pharmacodynamic properties:* Lithium carbonate is used as a source of lithium ions. The mechanism by which it exerts its effect in affective disorders is not known but may be related to inhibition of neurotransmitter receptor mediated processes involving beta-adrenoceptors. It is used in the treatment of acute episodes of mania or hypomania and for prophylaxis of recurrent manic depressive illness.

*Pharmacokinetic properties:* Lithium is readily absorbed from the gastrointestinal tract, and is distributed throughout the body over a period of several hours. Lithium is excreted almost exclusively in the kidneys but can also be detected in sweat and saliva. It is not bound to plasma proteins. It crosses the placenta, and is excreted in breast milk. The half-life of non-sustained lithium varies considerably, but generally is considered to be about 12 to 24 hours following a single dose. It is however increased for example in those with renal impairment and with age,

and may increase significantly during long-term therapy.

*Preclinical safety data:* Not applicable

**Pharmaceutical particulars**

*List of excipients:* Povidone; Maize Starch; Lactose; Gelatin; Calcium Carboxymethylcellulose; Talcum (E553Cb); Calcium Arachinate; Titanium Dioxide (E171); Magnesium Stearate (E572); Polyethylene Glycol 6000; Eudragit (E12.5).

*Incompatibilities:* Not applicable.

*Shelf life:* Liskonum Tablets have a shelf-life of five years.

*Special precautions for storage:* Store in a dry place.

*Nature and contents of container :* Opaque Blister Packs (OP) of 60 (6 x 10) tablets.

*Instructions for use/handling:* Tablets may be halved but should not be chewed or broken up.

**Marketing authorisation number** 0002/0083

**Date of approval/revision of SPC** January 1997

**Legal category** POM

# PARNATE* TABLETS

**Presentation** Geranium-red, sugar-coated tablets, marked SKF, each containing 10 mg tranylcypromine present as the sulphate.

**Uses** Parnate is a non-hydrazine monoamine oxidase inhibitor for the treatment of symptoms of depressive illness especially where phobic symptoms are present or where treatment with other types of antidepressant has failed. It is not recommended for mild depressive states resulting from temporary situational difficulties.

**Dosage and administration** *Adults only:* Initially, one tablet morning and afternoon. If the response is not adequate after the first week, add a further tablet at midday, and continue for at least a week. A dosage of three tablets a day should only be exceeded with caution. When a satisfactory response has been obtained, dosage may be reduced to a maintenance level, often of one tablet a day.

When given with a tranquilliser, the dosage of Parnate is not affected. When given concurrently with electroconvulsive therapy, the usual dosage is one tablet twice a day during the series and one tablet a day afterwards as maintenance therapy.

*Elderly:* Use with great caution (see *Contra-indications* and *Precautions* below).

**Contra-indications, warnings, etc**
*Contra-indications:* Do not give Parnate less than a week after stopping treatment with any other antidepressant drug including other MAO inhibitors, because of persisting effects, then give half the usual dosage for the first week. Similarly, after stopping Parnate, allow at least two weeks to elapse before starting treatment with any drug or ingesting any food that may interact.

Do not give Parnate with indirectly-acting sympathomimetic amines such as amphetamine, fenfluramine or similar anti-obesity agents, ephedrine or phenylpropanolamine (certain 'cold-cures' may contain such agents), or with levodopa or dopamine, as severe hypertensive reactions may result; with pethidine and closely related narcotic analgesics, and nefopam, as potentiation may occur; with dextromethorphan as a similar reaction has been reported; with other MAO inhibitors, as symptoms of overdosage are possible; or with buspirone, since increased blood pressure may occur.

Reports of hyperactivity, hypertonicity, hyperpyrexia, coma and death have been associated with the use of Parnate in combination with tricyclic antidepressants; tetracyclic antidepressants should also be avoided. The use of clomipramine in patients already on Parnate may be particularly hazardous. Use of MAO inhibitors with or after fluvoxamine or fluoxetine has been reported to produce a serotonin syndrome, sometimes fatal.

Do not use Parnate in patients with actual or suspected cerebrovascular disease or severe cardiovascular disease; in those with actual or suspected phaeochromocytoma, or with hyperthyroidism; or in those with known liver damage or blood dyscrasias.

*Dietary precautions:* High levels of tyramine in certain foods have been the cause of severe hypertensive reactions in patients on MAO inhibitor therapy (see *Adverse reactions*). Accordingly, patients must be warned to avoid the following: matured cheeses, hydrolysed protein extracts such as Marmite or Bovril, alcoholic drinks, particularly red wines such as Chianti, non-alcoholic beer and lager, and protein foods that are not fresh or whose preparation involved hydrolysis, fermentation, pickling, or 'hanging'; also broad-

bean pods, which contain levodopa, and banana skins.

*Precautions:* Caution should be exercised when giving Parnate with the following: guanethidine, as its action may be antagonised; reserpine, as hyperactivity may occur; methyldopa, as central excitation may result; other hypotensive agents because of possible additive effects; oral hypoglycaemic agents or insulin, as their action may be potentiated; anticholinergic antiparkinsonism drugs, as potentiation has been reported; narcotic analgesics, except pethidine which is contra-indicated (see above), because of possible potentiation; and carbamazepine, which has similarities with tricyclic antidepressants. Although the effects of barbiturates may be enhanced, and this possibility should be borne in mind, they have frequently been given with Parnate, particularly at night. Metrizamide should be avoided in patients on MAO inhibitors since they may lower the seizure threshold. Although MAO inhibitors have been used therapeutically with L-tryptophan, a neuromotor syndrome has been reported with this combination.

Patients should be specifically asked if they are taking any other medication because of the possibility of drug interactions.

Use Parnate with great caution in elderly patients; in those with cardiovascular disease in whom physical activity should be regulated, as the drug may suppress anginal pain; and in epileptic patients, as tranylcypromine has a variable effect on the convulsive threshold in animals. Parnate may aggravate some co-existing symptoms in depression such as anxiety and agitation. Parnate should preferably be withdrawn at least two weeks before elective surgery because of possible drug interaction.

Caution should be exercised in prescribing Parnate for patients with a previous history of dependence on drugs or alcohol.

In common with other drugs acting on the CNS, Parnate may affect ability to drive or operate machinery.

*Use in pregnancy and lactation:* Do not use in pregnancy, especially during the first and last trimesters, unless there are compelling reasons. There is no evidence as to drug safety in human pregnancy nor is there evidence from animal work that it is free from hazard. Tranylcypromine passes into the milk of lactating dogs.

*Adverse reactions:* Severe hypertensive reactions may occur, notably in association with foods containing tyramine (see *Dietary precautions*). Such reactions may be presaged by palpitations and unusually frequent headaches; patients should be warned to discontinue the drug if such symptoms occur. As well as a rapid rise in blood pressure, severe occipital headache, which may radiate frontally, is virtually always present, and pain and stiffness in the neck are usual; other features include multiple extrasystoles, often with bradycardia though sometimes with tachycardia, other arrhythmias, substernal pain, nausea and vomiting, sweating, pallor, sometimes followed by flushing, mydriasis and photophobia. Rarely, hypotension may dominate the clinical picture. ECG changes may be seen. The symptoms can mimic subarachnoid haemorrhage or may actually be associated with intracranial bleeding. Exceptionally, hemiparesis, hemiplegia or death has resulted.

Severe hypertensive reactions should be treated at once by reducing the blood pressure; slow intravenous injection of 5 mg phentolamine mesylate should be effective. Injectable or oral chlorpromazine is suitable for milder reactions. Acute symptoms generally subside within 24 hours.

Insomnia is the most frequent side-effect; it may usually be overcome by giving the last dose of the day not later than 3 pm, by reducing dosage, or by prescribing a mild hypnotic.

Mild headache, drowsiness, weakness, dizziness, palpitation, transient restlessness, dry mouth, blurred vision, nausea, oedema, weight gain, increased appetite and rash have been reported. Overstimulation, including anxiety and agitation, developing rarely into hypomania, has also been observed; the dosage should be reduced. Hypotension, which may be postural, may occur; it is usually temporary, but if it persists the drug should be stopped. Peripheral neuritis and difficulty in micturition have occurred rarely.

Dependence on Parnate, with tolerance to high doses, has been reported rarely, and can occur in patients without a past history of drug dependence. This should be distinguished from the return of features of the original illness on cessation of treatment.

Liver dysfunction has occurred very rarely, and isolated instances of purpura and blood dyscrasias have been reported.

*Overdosage:* Signs and symptoms are usually of the type already described as adverse reactions, but may be more intense, may include hyperpyrexia, tremor and convulsions, and may follow a latent period. Treatment consists of the induction of vomiting and/or gastric lavage together with supportive and symptomatic measures. External cooling is recommended for hyperpyrexia. Treat hypotension with fluid replacement; if severe or persistent, noradrenaline may be considered. Hypertension, if it occurs, may be relieved by slow intravenous injection of phentolamine mesylate. Pancuronium with mechanical ventilation may help reverse muscle spasm and pyrexia. Beta-adrenergic receptor blockade has been used successfully.

**Pharmaceutical precautions** Store in a dry place at a temperature not exceeding 25°C and protect from light.

**Legal category** POM.

**Package quantities** Containers of 28 tablets.

**Further information** It is generally considered that no particular hazard is attached to the use of local anaesthetics containing small amounts of adrenaline in patients receiving Parnate unless cardiovascular disease is present.

Inactive ingredients include sucrose and aluminium lakes of E122 and E124.

**Product licence number** 0002/5040R.

## PARSTELIN* TABLETS

**Presentation** Leaf-green, sugar-coated tablets, marked SKF, each containing 10 mg tranylcypromine present as the sulphate and 1 mg trifluoperazine present as the hydrochloride.

**Uses** Parstelin is a combination of a non-hydrazine monoamine oxidase inhibitor and a phenothiazine tranquilliser, for the treatment of symptoms of depressive illness complicated by anxiety.

**Dosage and administration** *Adults only:* Initially, one tablet morning and afternoon. If the response is not adequate after the first week, add a further tablet at midday, and continue for at least a week. A dosage of three tablets a day should only be exceeded with caution. When a satisfactory response has been obtained, dosage may be reduced to a maintenance level, often of one tablet a day.

*Elderly:* Use with great caution (see *Contra-indications* and *Precautions* below).

**Contra-indications, warnings, etc**
*Contra-indications:* Do not give Parstelin less than a week after stopping treatment with any other antidepressant drug including other MAO inhibitors, because of persisting effects, then give half the usual dosage for the first week. Similarly, after stopping Parstelin, allow at least two weeks to elapse before starting treatment with any drug or ingesting any food that may interact.

Do not give Parstelin with indirectly-acting sympathomimetic amines such as amphetamine, fenfluramine, or similar anti-obesity agents, ephedrine or phenylpropanolamine (certain 'cold-cures' may contain such agents), or with levodopa or dopamine, as severe hypertensive reactions may result; with pethidine and closely related narcotic analgesics, and nefopam, as potentiation may occur; with dextromethorphan as a similar reaction has been reported; with other MAO inhibitors, as symptoms of overdosage are possible; or with buspirone, since increased blood pressure may occur.

Reports of hyperactivity, hypertonicity, hyperpyrexia, coma and death have been associated with the use of tranylcypromine in combination with tricyclic antidepressants; tetracyclic antidepressants should also be avoided. The use of clomipramine in patients already on Parstelin may be particularly hazardous. Use of MAO inhibitors with or after fluvoxamine or fluoxetine has been reported to produce a serotonin syndrome, sometimes fatal.

Do not use Parstelin in patients with actual or suspected cerebrovascular disease or severe cardiovascular disease; in those with actual or suspected phaeochromocytoma, or with hyperthyroidism; in those with existing blood dyscrasias or known liver damage; or in those hypersensitive to the ingredients.

*Dietary precautions:* High levels of tyramine in certain foods have been the cause of severe hypertensive reactions in patients on MAO inhibitor therapy (see *Adverse reactions*). Accordingly, patients must be warned to avoid the following: matured cheese, hydrolysed protein extracts such as Marmite or Bovril, alcoholic drinks, particularly red wines such as Chianti, non-alcoholic beer and lager, and protein foods that are not fresh or whose preparation involved hydrolysis, fermentation, pickling, or 'hanging'; also broad-bean pods, which contain levodopa, and banana skins.

*Precautions:* Caution should be exercised when giving Parstelin with the following: guanethidine, as its action may be antagonised; reserpine, as hyperactivity may occur; methyldopa, as central excitation may result; other hypotensive agents because of possible additive effects; oral hypoglycaemic agents or insulin, as their action may be potentiated; anticholinergic antiparkinsonism drugs, as potentiation has been reported; narcotic analgesics, except pethidine which is contra-indicated (see above), because of possible potentiation; and carbamazepine, which has similarities with tricyclic antidepressants. Although the effects of barbiturates may be enhanced, and this possibility should be borne in mind, they have frequently been given with Parstelin, particularly at night. Metrizamide should be avoided in patients on MAO inhibitors since they may lower the seizure threshold. Although MAO inhibitors have been used therapeutically with L-tryptophan, a neuromotor syndrome has been reported with this combination. Potentiation may occur if trifluoperazine is used with other CNS depressants.

Patients should be specifically asked if they are taking any other medication because of the possibility of drug interactions.

Use Parstelin with great caution in elderly patients; in those with cardiovascular disease in whom physical activity should be regulated, as tranylcypromine may suppress anginal pain; and in epileptic patients as tranylcypromine has a variable effect on the convulsive threshold in animals. Tranylcypromine may aggravate some co-existing symptoms in depression such as anxiety and agitation. Parstelin should preferably be withdrawn at least two weeks before elective surgery because of possible drug interaction.

Nausea and vomiting as a sign of organic disease may be masked by the anti-emetic action of trifluoperazine.

Caution should be exercised in prescribing Parstelin for patients with a previous history of dependence on drugs or alcohol.

In common with other drugs acting on the CNS, Parstelin may affect ability to drive or operate machinery.

*Use in pregnancy and lactation:* Do not use in pregnancy, especially during the first and last trimesters, unless there are compelling reasons. There is no evidence as to drug safety in human pregnancy nor is there evidence from animal work that it is free from hazard. Both tranylcypromine and trifluoperazine pass into the milk of lactating dogs.

*Adverse reactions:* Severe hypertensive reactions may occur, notably in association with foods containing tyramine (see *Dietary precautions*). Such reactions may be presaged by palpitations and unusually frequent headaches; patients should be warned to discontinue the drug if such symptoms occur. As well as a rapid rise in blood pressure, severe occipital headache, which may radiate frontally, is virtually always present, and pain and stiffness in the neck are usual; other features include multiple extrasystoles, often with bradycardia though sometimes with tachycardia, other arrhythmias, substernal pain, nausea and vomiting, sweating, pallor, sometimes followed by flushing, mydriasis and photophobia. Rarely, hypotension may dominate the clinical picture. ECG changes may be seen. The symptoms can mimic subarachnoid haemorrhage or may actually be associated with intracranial bleeding. Exceptionally, hemiparesis, hemiplegia or death has resulted.

Severe hypertensive reactions should be treated at once by reducing the blood pressure; slow intravenous injection of 5 mg phentolamine mesylate should be effective. Injectable or oral chlorpromazine is suitable for milder reactions. Acute symptoms generally subside within 24 hours.

Insomnia is the most frequent side-effect; it may usually be overcome by giving the last dose of the day not later than 3 pm, by reducing dosage, or by prescribing a mild hypnotic.

Mild headache, drowsiness, weakness, dizziness, palpitation, transient restlessness, dry mouth, blurred vision, nausea, oedema, weight gain, increased appetite and rash have been reported. Overstimulation, including anxiety and agitation, developing rarely into hypomania, has also been observed; the dosage should be reduced. Hypotension, which may be postural, may occur; it is usually temporary, but if it persists the drug should be stopped. Peripheral neuritis and difficulty in micturition have occurred rarely.

Dependence on tranylcypromine, with tolerance to high doses, has been reported rarely, and can occur in patients without a past history of drug dependence. This should be distinguished from the return of features of the original illness on cessation of treatment.

Extrapyramidal symptoms due to the trifluoperazine component are very unlikely at the recommended dosage. Extremely rarely, long-term therapy with trifluoperazine in low dosage has been associated with tardive dyskinesia, which can be long-lasting or even irreversible.

Liver dysfunction has occurred very rarely, and isolated instances of purpura and blood dyscrasia have been reported.

*Overdosage:* Signs and symptoms are usually of th type already described as adverse reactions to trany cypromine, but may be more intense, may includ hyperpyrexia, tremor and convulsions, and ma follow a latent period. In the unlikely event c symptoms from the trifluoperazine component, thes are extrapyramidal in type. Treatment consists c gastric lavage together with supportive and sympto matic measures. Do not induce vomiting. Externa cooling is recommended for hyperpyrexia. Trea hypotension with fluid replacement; if severe c persistent, noradrenaline may be considered; adren aline is contra-indicated. Hypertension, if it occurs may be relieved by slow intravenous injection c phentolamine mesylate. Pancuronium with mechani cal ventilation may help reverse muscle spasm an pyrexia. Beta-adrenergic receptor blockade has bee used successfully.

**Pharmaceutical precautions** Store in a dry place at a temperature not exceeding 25°C and protect fron light.

**Legal category** POM.

**Package quantities** Containers of 28 tablets.

**Further information** It is generally considered tha no particular hazard is attached to the use of loca anaesthetics containing small amounts of adrenalin in patients receiving tranylcypromine unless cardic vascular disease is present.

Inactive ingredients include sucrose and aluminiur lake of E110.

Parstelin should normally only be used on th recommendation of a specialist in psychiatry.

**Product licence number** 0002/5041R.

## POLIOMYELITIS VACCINE, LIVE (ORAL PhEur (TEN DOSE) (Sabin strains)

**Presentation** Poliomyelitis Vaccine, Live (Ora PhEur, as supplied by SmithKline Beecham Pharma ceuticals, is a clear liquid, colourless or light yellow t light red, stabilised with molar magnesium chloride Each dose (3 drops from a 10-dose tube) provides a least $10^{6}$TCID$_{50}$ type 1 (LS-c, 2ab), $10^{5}$TCID$_{50}$ type (P712, Ch, 2ab) and $10^{5.5}$TCID$_{50}$ type 3 (Leon 12a,b) liv attenuated strains of poliomyelitis virus grown i monkey kidney cell cultures, and contains not mor than 7 micrograms (5 IU) neomycin sulphate.

**Uses** Active immunisation against poliomyelitis.

**Dosage and administration**
*Adults and children: For oral use only*: NOT FO INJECTION. Three drops of vaccine from a 10-dos tube constitute one dose which may be given wit syrup or on a lump of sugar to mask the bitter salt taste of the magnesium chloride. Do not administe on foods which contain preservatives.

For a complete schedule, three doses of the vaccin should be given at intervals of at least four weeks (se also *Further information*).

Other unvaccinated members of the same house hold (including adults) should be advised vaccinatio at the same time as the vaccinee.

The vaccine should be inspected for particulat matter or discolouration before administration.

Since the vaccine contains live attenuated polic myelitis virus, care should be taken to avoid transfe or spillage. Care should be taken not to contaminat multidose droppers with vaccinee's saliva.

**Contra-indications, warnings, etc.**
*Contra-indications:* The vaccine should not be used i the presence of acute febrile illness or intercurrer infection, persistent diarrhoea, vomiting or othe gastrointestinal disturbance. (A minor infection is nc a contra-indication). The vaccine should also not b given in the presence of impaired immune respons including leukaemia, lymphoma, generalised malig nancy or treatment with corticosteroids, cytotox drugs or irradiation. HIV infection does not contra indicate immunisation.

*Precautions:* The vaccine may contain trace amount of penicillin and streptomycin and neomycin whic should not contra-indicate its use except in those wit a history of severe anaphylaxis due to either antibioti

Contacts of recent vaccinees should be advised t attend to personal hygiene.

Previous vaccination with inactivated Poliomyeliti Vaccine is not a contra-indication.

Diarrhoea or vomiting (including gastrointestin infections) may interfere with replication ('take' rate)

At least three weeks should normally interven between the administration of any two live vaccine Poliomyelitis vaccine can, however, be given simu taneously with measles, mumps and rubella vaccine and with DTP vaccine. In this case the injectab vaccines should be given at different sites.

No data have been generated on the simultaneous ·dministration of OPV with oral typhoid vaccine herefore the theoretical possibility of an interaction ·etween the two products cannot be ruled out.

Poliomyelitis vaccine has been given at the same ·me as BCG and hepatitis B vaccines.

In some populations and groups of vaccinees lower eroconversion rates have been observed. Due to arious non-specific factors all three vaccine viruses nay not replicate optimally in the gut of susceptible ubjects, even after three doses.

*Jse in pregnancy*: Pregnant women should not be iven oral poliomyelitis vaccine unless they are at efinite risk from poliomyelitis.

*Adverse reactions:* Paralysis temporally associated vith vaccination has been reported very rarely in ecipients or contacts.

*Overdosage*: Occasional reports of overdosage have een received. Overdosage has not resulted in ill ·ffects.

**Pharmaceutical precautions** Protect from light and tore between 2°C and 8°C. Under these conditions here is no significant loss of virus titre for 12 months.

When tubes of vaccine have been opened there is a isk of contamination with bacteria and moulds which nay result in a reduction of vaccine potency. It is ood practice, therefore, to discard vaccine remaining n opened 10-dose tubes at the end of the vaccinating ession. Any unopened vaccine should be returned to torage between 2°C and 8°C as soon as possible.

**Legal category** POM.

**Package quantities** Individual plastic 10-dose dropper tubes.

**Further information** Current policy recommends hat the first dose of oral poliomyelitis vaccine should e given from two months of age. The primary course onsists of three separate doses with intervals of one nonth between each dose, given at the same time as DTP vaccine.

It is currently recommended that a reinforcing dose of poliomyelitis vaccine should be given at school ·ntry and at 15 to 19 years of age. Adults need not be ·ffered a reinforcing dose unless they are at special isk.

Poliomyelitis vaccine has been administered at the ame time as BCG and hepatitis B vaccine.

Inactive ingredients are magnesium chloride, polyorbate 80, purified water, and also neomycin sulphate see *Presentation*).

**Product licence number** 10592/0017.

## POLIOMYELITIS VACCINE, LIVE (ORAL) PhEur (Sabin strains) Monodose* (OPV)

**Presentation** Poliomyelitis Vaccine, Live (Oral) PhEur, as supplied by SmithKline Beecham Pharmaceuticals, is a clear liquid, colourless or light yellow to ight red, stabilised with molar magnesium chloride. Each dose (0.135 ml) provides at least $10^6 TCID_{50}$ type 1 (LS-c, 2ab), $10^5 TCID_{50}$ type 2 (P712, Ch 2ab) and $10^{5.5} TCID_{50}$ type 3 (Leon $12a_1b$) live attenuated strains of poliomyelitis virus grown in monkey kidney cell cultures, and contains not more than 1 microgram 0.7 IU) neomycin sulphate.

**Uses** Active immunisation against poliomyelitis.

**Dosage and administration**

*Adults and children: For oral use only:* NOT FOR INJECTION. Three drops of vaccine from the Monodose tube constitute one dose which may be given with syrup or on a lump of sugar to mask the bitter alty taste of the magnesium chloride. Do not administer on foods which contain preservatives.

For a complete schedule, three doses of the vaccine should be given at intervals of at least four weeks (see also *Further information*).

Other unvaccinated members of the same household (including adults) should be advised vaccination at the same time as the vaccinee.

The vaccine should be inspected for particulate natter or discolouration before administration.

Since the vaccine contains live attenuated poliomyelitis virus, care should be taken to avoid transfer or spillage.

Both parts of the tube and also the spoon (if used) should be carefully disposed of, e.g. by incineration. Alternatively they may be sterilised by immersing for 30 minutes in 0.1% hypochlorite solution yielding 1000 ppm available chlorine (e.g. 1:10 Milton 1%).

Do not administer directly into the vaccinee's mouth as the tube may slip and cause choking.

**Contra-indications, warnings, etc.**

*Contra-indications:* The vaccine should not be used in he presence of acute febrile illness or intercurrent nfection, persistent diarrhoea, vomiting or other gastrointestinal disturbance; (a minor infection is not a contra-indication). The vaccine should also not be given in the presence of impaired immune response including leukaemia, lymphoma, generalised malignancy or treatment with corticosteroids, cytotoxic drugs or irradiation.

*Precautions*: The vaccine may contain trace amounts of penicillin, streptomycin and neomycin which should not contra-indicate its use except in those with a history of severe anaphylaxis due to these antibiotics.

Contacts of recent vaccinees should be advised to attend to strict personal hygiene.

Previous vaccination with inactivated poliomyelitis vaccine is not a contra-indication.

HIV-positive asymptomatic individuals may receive live polio vaccine but excretion of the vaccine virus in the faeces may continue for longer than normal individuals. Household contacts should be warned of this and for the need for strict personal hygiene, including hand-washing after nappy changes for an HIV-positive infant.

For HIV-positive symptomatic individuals, IPV may be used instead of OPV at the discretion of the clinician.

Diarrhoea or vomiting (including gastrointestinal infections) may interfere with replication ('take' rate).

In immunocompetent recipients previous vaccination with inactivated Poliomyelitis Vaccine is not a contra-indication.

At least three weeks should normally intervene between administration of any two live vaccines. Poliomyelitis vaccine can, however, be given simultaneously with measles, mumps and rubella vaccines and with DTP vaccine. In this case the injectable vaccines should be given at different sites.

No data has been generated on the simultaneous administration of OPV with oral typhoid vaccine; therefore the theoretical possibility of an interaction between the two products cannot be ruled out.

Poliomyelitis vaccine has been given at the same time as BCG and Hepatitis B vaccines.

In some populations and groups of vaccinees lower seroconversion rates have been observed. Due to various non-specific factors all three vaccine viruses may not replicate optimally in the gut of susceptible subjects, even after three doses.

*Use in pregnancy:* Pregnant women should not be given oral poliomyelitis vaccine unless they are at definite risk from poliomyelitis.

*Adverse reactions:* Paralysis temporally associated with vaccination has been reported very rarely in recipients or contacts.

*Overdosage:* There have been occasional reports of overdosage but none has resulted in any ill effect.

**Pharmaceutical precautions** Protect from light and store in a refrigerator between 2°C and 8°C.

**Legal category** POM.

**Package quantities** One carton containing 10 individual plastic Monodose tubes.

**Further information** Current policy recommends that the first dose of oral poliomyelitis vaccine should be given from two months of age. The primary course consists of three separate doses with intervals of one month between each dose, given at the same time as DTP vaccine.

It is currently recommended that a reinforcing dose of poliomyelitis vaccine should be given at school entry and at 15 to 19 years of age. Adults need not be offered a reinforcing dose unless they are at special risk.

Inactive ingredients are magnesium chloride, amino acid, polysorbate 80, purified water, and also neomycin sulphate (see *Presentation*).

**Product licence number** 10592/0039.

## RELIFEX* TABLETS
## RELIFEX* SUSPENSION

**Qualitative and quantitative composition**

Tablets: Each tablet contains 500 mg nabumetone.

Suspension: Each 5 ml contains 500 mg nabumetone.

**Pharmaceutical form**

Tablets: Dark red, film-coated tablets marked Relifex on one side and 500 on the other.

Suspension: A white to off-white suspension.

**Clinical particulars**

*Therapeutic indications:* Nabumetone is a non-acidic non-steroidal anti-inflammatory agent which is a relatively weak inhibitor of prostaglandin synthesis. However, following absorption from the gastrointestinal tract it is rapidly metabolised in the liver to the principal active metabolite, 6-methoxy-2-naphthylacetic acid (6-MNA), a potent inhibitor of prostaglandin synthesis.

It is indicated for the treatment of osteoarthritis and rheumatoid arthritis requiring anti-inflammatory and analgesic treatment.

*Posology and method of administration:*

*Adults:* The recommended daily dose is two tablets or 10 ml suspension (1 g) taken as a single dose at bedtime.

For severe or persistent symptoms, or during acute exacerbations, an additional 500 mg-1 g may be given as a morning dose.

*Elderly:* In common with many drugs, blood levels may be higher in elderly patients. The recommended daily dose of 1 g should not be exceeded in this age group and in some cases 500 mg may give satisfactory relief.

*Children:* There are no clinical data to recommend use of Relifex in children.

*Administration:* Oral.

*Contra-indications:* Active peptic ulceration. NSAIDs should not be used in patients with a history of recent or recurrent peptic ulceration. Severe hepatic impairment (e.g. cirrhosis). Patients in whom aspirin or other NSAIDs precipitate asthmatic attacks, urticaria or acute rhinitis. Hypersensitivity to the drug.

*Special warnings and special precautions for use:* It is advisable to avoid the administration of more than one NSAID at a time. Peripheral oedema has been observed in some patients. Relifex should therefore be used with caution in patients with fluid retention, hypertension or heart failure.

Use in patients with impaired renal function: Urine is the major excretion route for the metabolites of Relifex. In patients with impaired renal function (creatinine clearance less than 30 ml/minute), dosage reduction should be considered. It is consistent with good clinical practice that patients with known renal impairment should be monitored regularly during therapy.

Liver function: Fluctuations in some parameters of liver function, particularly alkaline phosphatase, are frequently observed in patients with chronic inflammatory disorders; there is no evidence that Relifex accentuates these changes. However patients with abnormal liver function should be monitored closely.

*Interaction with other medicaments and other forms of interaction:* As the major circulating metabolite of Relifex is highly protein bound, patients receiving concurrent treatment with oral anti-coagulants, hydantoin anticonvulsants or sulphonylurea hypoglycaemics should be monitored for signs of overdosage of these drugs. Dosages should be adjusted if necessary.

Some NSAIDs are known to increase plasma concentrations of cardiac glycosides, lithium and methotrexate and may decrease the therapeutic efficacy of diuretics and antihypertensives. Such drugs may also induce hyperkalaemia when administered with potassium-sparing diuretics. Interaction studies between Relifex and these other drugs have not been performed; caution in co-administration is therefore recommended.

NSAIDs should not be used 8–12 days after mifepristone administration, as they could affect the efficacy of mifepristone treatment.

Aluminium hydroxide gel, paracetamol and aspirin have not affected the bioavailability of Relifex in volunteer subjects.

*Pregnancy and lactation:* Studies in experimental animals have shown no teratogenic potential. As is common with other compounds administered to animals at doses high enough to be maternally toxic, indications of embryotoxicity were noted (studies in the rabbit 300 mg/kg dose). High doses in rats (320 mg/kg) delayed parturition; this effect is considered to be due to inhibition of prostaglandin synthesis. The active metabolite of nabumetone has been found in the milk of lactating animals.

Safety in human pregnancy has not been established. Relifex is not recommended during human pregnancy or in mothers who are breast feeding.

*Effects on ability to drive and use machines:* None known.

*Undesirable effects:* Reported gastrointestinal side effects include dry mouth, faecal occult blood, diarrhoea, dyspepsia, nausea, constipation, abdominal pain, flatulence, gastrointestinal bleeding, ulceration and perforation. Headache, dizziness, fatigue, confusion, sedation, depression, insomnia, tinnitus, abnormal vision, oedema, menorrhagia, anaphylaxis and anaphylactoid reaction have also been reported. Skin reactions including rash, pruritus, urticaria, alopecia and photosensitivity reactions may occur.

As with other NSAIDs, severe skin eruptions, e.g. Stevens Johnson syndrome and toxic epidermal necrolysis have been reported very rarely. Blood dyscrasias including leucopenia and thrombocytopenia have also been reported very rarely.

As with other NSAIDs, there have been rare reports

of renal adverse effects, including nephrotic syndrome and renal failure.

In clinical trials, increases in doses above 1 g did not lead to an increase in the incidence of side effects. However, the lowest effective dose should always be used.

*Overdose:* There is no specific antidote. Treatment is with gastric lavage followed by activated charcoal using up to 60 g orally in divided doses with appropriate supportive therapy.

**Pharmacological properties**

*Pharmacodynamic properties:* Nabumetone is a non-acidic non-steroidal anti-inflammatory agent which is a relatively weak inhibitor of prostaglandin synthesis. A notable feature of the animal pharmacology is the lack of effect on the gastric mucosa. Following absorption from the gastrointestinal tract nabumetone is rapidly metabolised in the liver to the principal active metabolite, 6-methoxy-2-naphthylacetic acid (6-MNA) a potent inhibitor of prostaglandin synthesis.

*Pharmacokinetic properties:* Although nabumetone is absorbed essentially intact through the small intestine, extensive metabolism occurs during the first pass through the liver. As a result, concentrations in plasma of nabumetone are barely detectable after oral dosage. Intravenous studies in rats with nabumetone indicate it to be rapidly distributed throughout the body, in keeping with its highly lipophilic character. The active metabolite, 6-MNA, binds strongly to plasma proteins; it is distributed into inflamed tissue and crosses the placenta into foetal tissue. It is found in the milk of lactating females. 6-MNA is eliminated by metabolism, principally conjugation with glucuronic acid, and O-demethylation followed by conjugation, the main route of excretion being the urine. The plasma elimination half-life is about one day in man.

*Preclinical safety data:* Not applicable.

**Pharmaceutical particulars**

*List of excipients:*
*Tablets*: Sodium starch glycollate; sodium lauryl sulphate; hydroxypropylmethylcellulose; magnesium stearate; microcrystalline cellulose; red carmine; yellow iron oxide; titanium dioxide; talc; polyethylene glycol; saccharin sodium; liquid caramel flavour; purified water

*Suspension:* Methylcellulose; xanthan gum; sorbitol; sodium benzoate; liquid vanilla flavour; liquid buttermint flavour; monoammonium glycyrrhizinate; glycerin; dilute hydrochloric acid; purified water.

*Incompatibilities:* Not applicable.

*Shelf life:* 36 months.

*Special precautions for storage:* Tablets: The tablets should be protected from light. Suspension: None.

*Nature and contents of container:* Tablets: HDPE bottles each containing 56 tablets. Suspension: HDPE bottles each containing 300 ml

*Instructions for use/handling:* None.

**Marketing authorisation numbers**
Tablets 0038/0301
Suspension 0038/0352

**Date of approval/revision of SPC** September 1996.

**Legal category** POM

## REQUIP* TABLETS ▼

**Qualitative and quantitative composition** Ropinirole hydrochloride equivalent to 0.25, 1.0, 2.0 or 5.0 mg ropinirole free base.

**Pharmaceutical form** Film-coated, pentagonal-shaped tablets for oral administration. The tablet strengths are distinguished by colour; 0.25 mg (white), 1.0 mg (green), 2.0 mg (pink) and 5.0 mg (blue).

**Clinical particulars**

*Therapeutic indications:* Treatment of idiopathic Parkinson's disease:

Ropinirole may be used alone (without levodopa) in the treatment of idiopathic Parkinson's disease.

Addition of ropinirole to levodopa may be used to control "on-off" fluctuations and permit a reduction in the total daily dose of levodopa.

*Posology and method of administration:* Individual dose titration against efficacy and tolerability is recommended.

Ropinirole should be taken three times a day, preferably with meals to improve gastrointestinal tolerance.

*Treatment initiation:* The initial dose should be 0.25 mg t.i.d. A guide for the titration regimen for the first four weeks of treatment is given in the table below:

| | Week | | | |
|---|---|---|---|---|
| | 1 | 2 | 3 | 4 |
| Unit dose (mg) | 0.25 | 0.5 | 0.75 | 1.0 |
| Total daily dose (mg) | 0.75 | 1.5 | 2.25 | 3.0 |

*Therapeutic regimen*: After the initial titration, weekly increments of up to 3 mg/day may be given. Ropinirole is usually given in divided doses three times per day.

A therapeutic response may be seen between 3 and 9 mg/day, although adjunct therapy patients may require higher doses. If sufficient symptomatic control is not achieved, or maintained, the dose of ropinirole may be increased until an acceptable therapeutic response is established. Doses above 24 mg/day have not been investigated in clinical trials and this dose should not be exceeded.

When ropinirole is administered as adjunct therapy to L-dopa, the concurrent dose of L-dopa may be reduced gradually by around 20% in total.

When switching treatment from another dopamine agonist to ropinirole, the manufacturer's guidance on discontinuation should be followed before initiating ropinirole.

As with other dopamine agonists, ropinirole should be discontinued gradually by reducing the number of daily doses over the period of one week.

In parkinsonian patients with mild to moderate renal impairment (creatinine clearance 30–50 ml/min) no change in the clearance of ropinirole was observed, indicating that no dosage adjustment is necessary in this population.

The use of ropinirole in patients with severe renal (creatinine clearance <30 ml/min) or hepatic impairment has not been studied. Administration of ropinirole to such patients is not recommended.

*Elderly*: The clearance of ropinirole is decreased in patients over 65 years of age, but the dose of ropinirole for elderly patients can be titrated in the normal manner.

*Children*: Parkinson's disease does not occur in children. The use of ropinirole in this population has therefore not been studied and it should not be given to children.

*Contra-indications:* Hypersensitivity to ropinirole

In light of the results of animal studies and the lack of studies in human pregnancy, ropinirole is contra-indicated in pregnancy, lactation and in women of child-bearing potential unless adequate contraception is used.

*Special warnings and special precautions for use:* Due to the pharmacological action of ropinirole, patients with severe cardiovascular disease should be treated with caution.

Co-administration of ropinirole with anti-hypertensive and anti-arrhythmic agents has not been studied. As with other dopaminergic drugs, caution should be exercised when these compounds are given concomitantly with ropinirole because of the unknown potential for the occurrence of hypotension, bradycardias or other arrhythmias.

Patients with major psychotic disorders should only be treated with dopamine agonists if the potential benefits outweigh the risks (see also *Interactions*).

*Interaction with other medicaments and other forms of interaction:* Neuroleptics and other centrally active dopamine antagonists, such as sulpiride or metoclopramide, may diminish the effectiveness of ropinirole and, therefore, concomitant use of these drugs with ropinirole should be avoided.

No pharmacokinetic interaction has been seen between ropinirole and L-dopa or domperidone which would necessitate dosage adjustment of either drug. No interaction has been seen between ropinirole and other drugs commonly used to treat Parkinson's disease but, as is common practice, care should be taken when adding a new drug to a treatment regimen. Ropinirole should not be given with other dopamine agonists.

In a study in parkinsonian patients receiving concurrent digoxin, no interaction was seen which would require dosage adjustment.

It has been established from *in vitro* experiments that ropinirole is metabolised by the cytochrome P450 enzyme CYP1A2. There is, therefore, the potential for an interaction between ropinirole and substrates (such as theophylline) or inhibitors (such as ciprofloxacin, fluvoxamine and cimetidine) of this enzyme. In patients already receiving ropinirole, the dose of ropinirole may need to be adjusted when these drugs are introduced or withdrawn.

Increased plasma concentrations of ropinirole have been observed in patients treated with high doses of oestrogens. In patients already receiving hormone replacement therapy (HRT), ropinirole treatment may be initiated in the normal manner. However, if HRT is stopped or introduced during treatment with ropinirole, dosage adjustment may be required.

No information is available on the potential for interaction between ropinirole and alcohol. As with other centrally active medications, patients should b cautioned against taking ropinirole with alcohol.

*Pregnancy and lactation:* Ropinirole should not b used during pregnancy. In animal studies, administra tion of ropinirole to pregnant rats at maternally tox doses resulted in decreased foetal body weight a 60 mg/kg (approximately three times the AUC of th maximum dose in man), increased foetal death a 90 mg/kg (~x5) and digit malformations at 150 mg/k (~x9). There was no teratogenic effect in the rat a 120 mg/kg (~x7) and no indication of an effect o development in the rabbit. There have been no studie of ropinirole in human pregnancy.

Ropinirole should not be used in nursing mothe as it may inhibit lactation.

*Effects on ability to drive and use machines:* No dat are available on the effect of ropinirole on the abilit to drive or use machinery. Patients should be cau tioned about their ability to drive or operate machine whilst taking ropinirole because of the possibility c somnolence or dizziness.

*Undesirable effects:* The most common adverse ex periences reported by early therapy patients receivin ropinirole in clinical trials, and not seen at an equiva lent or greater incidence on placebo, were; nause somnolence, leg oedema, abdominal pain, vomitin and syncope.

Similarly, the most common adverse experience reported in adjunct therapy clinical trials were; dysk nesia, nausea, hallucinations and confusion.

The incidence of postural hypotension, an ever commonly associated with dopamine agonists, wa not markedly different from placebo in clinical tria with ropinirole. However, decreases in systolic bloo pressure have been noted; symptomatic hypotensio and bradycardia, occasionally severe, may occur.

*Overdose:* There have been no incidences of inter tional overdose with ropinirole in clinical trials. It anticipated that the symptoms of ropinirole overdos will be related to its dopaminergic activity.

**Pharmacological properties**

*Pharmacodynamic properties:* Ropinirole is a nor ergoline dopamine agonist.

Parkinson's disease is characterised by a marke dopamine deficiency in the nigral striatal syster Ropinirole alleviates this deficiency by stimulatin striatal dopamine receptors.

Ropinirole acts in the hypothalamus and pituitar to inhibit the secretion of prolactin.

*Pharmacokinetic properties:* Oral absorption of rop nirole is rapid and essentially complete. Bioavailabili of ropinirole is approximately 50% and average pea concentrations of the drug are achieved at a media time of 1.5 hours post-dose. Wide inter-individu variability in the pharmacokinetic parameters ha been seen but, overall, there is a proportional increas in the systemic exposure ($C_{max}$ and AUC) to the dru with an increase in dose, over the therapeutic dos range. Consistent with its high lipophilicity, ropinirol exhibits a large volume of distribution (approx. 8 l/kg and is cleared from the systemic circulation with a average elimination half-life of about six hour Plasma protein binding of the drug is low (10-40% Ropinirole is metabolised primarily by oxidative me tabolism and ropinirole and its metabolites are mainl excreted in the urine. The major metabolite is at leas 100 times less potent than ropinirole in animal mode of dopaminergic function.

No change in the oral clearance of ropinirole i observed following single and repeated oral adminis tration. As expected for a drug being administere approximately every half-life, there is, on averag two-fold higher steady-state plasma concentration of ropinirole following the recommended t.i.d. reg men compared to those observed following a singl oral dose.

*Preclinical safety data:*
*General toxicology:* Ropinirole is well tolerated i laboratory animals in the dose range of 15 to 50 mg kg. The toxicology profile is principally determined b the pharmacological activity of the drug (behaviour changes, hypoprolactinaemia, decrease in blood pres sure and heart rate, ptosis and salivation).

*Genotoxicity*: Genotoxicity was not observed in battery of *in vitro* and *in vivo* tests.

*Carcinogenicity*: Two-year studies have been con ducted in the mouse and rat at dosages up to 50 m kg. The mouse study did not reveal any carcinogen effect. In the rat, the only drug-related lesions wer Leydig cell hyperplasia/adenoma in the testis result ing from the hypoprolactinaemic effect of ropinirol These lesions are considered to be a species specif phenomenon and do not constitute a hazard wit regard to the clinical use of ropinirole.

**Pharmaceutical particulars**

*List of excipients:*
*Tablet cores*: hydrous lactose, microcrystalline cellu lose, croscarmellose sodium, magnesium stearate.

The four tablet strengths of ropinirole are distinguished by colour. The composition of the *film coat* therefore varies. All film coats contain hydroxypropyl methylcellulose and polyethylene glycol. The variations are shown in the table below:

| | Tablet strength (mg) and colour | | | |
|---|---|---|---|---|
| | 0.25 | 1.0 | 2.0 | 5.0 |
| Tablet Colour | White | Green | Pink | Blue |
| Titanium Dioxide | ✓ | ✓ | ✓ | ✓ |
| Iron Oxide Yellow | | ✓ | ✓ | |
| Iron Oxide Red | | | ✓ | |
| Indigo Carmine Aluminium | | ✓ | | ✓ |
| Polysorbate 80 | ✓ | | | |
| Talc | | | | ✓ |

*Incompatibilities:* None known.

*Shelf life:* Two years.

*Special precautions for storage:* This product should be stored in a dry place at or below 25°C and protected from light.

*Nature and contents of container:*
Tablets 0.25 mg, in opaque PVC/PVdC blister starting pack of 210.
Tablets 1 mg, in 60 ml HPDE bottle of 84.
Tablets 2 mg, in 60 ml HPDE bottle of 84.
Tablets 5 mg, in 60 ml HPDE bottle of 84.

*Instructions for use/handling:* None.

**Marketing authorisation numbers**
Requip Tablets 0.25 mg 10592/0085
Requip Tablets 1 mg 10592/0087
Requip Tablets 2 mg 10592/0088
Requip Tablets 5 mg 10592/0089

**Date of approval/revision of SPC** 12 July 1996

**Legal category** POM

## SEROXAT* LIQUID

**Qualitative and quantitative composition** Paroxetine hydrochloride equivalent to 20 mg paroxetine free base per 10 ml.

**Pharmaceutical form** Orange-coloured suspension with the smell of oranges and a sweet taste.

**Clinical particulars**

*Therapeutic indications:* Treatment of symptoms of depressive illness of all types including depression accompanied by anxiety.

Treatment of symptoms and prevention of relapse of obsessive compulsive disorder (OCD).

Treatment of symptoms and prevention of relapse of panic disorder with or without agoraphobia.

*Posology and method of administration:* For oral administration.

*Adults:*

*Depression:* The recommended dose is 20 mg daily. In some patients it may be necessary to increase the dose. This should be done gradually by 10 mg increments to a maximum of 50 mg according to the patient's response.

*Obsessive compulsive disorder:* The recommended dose is 40 mg daily. Patients should start on 20 mg and the dose may be increased weekly in 10 mg increments. Some patients will benefit from having their dose increased up to a maximum of 60 mg/day.

*Panic disorder:* The recommended dose is 40 mg daily. Patients should be started on 10 mg per day and the dose increased weekly in 10 mg increments according to the patient's response. Some patients may benefit from having their dose increased up to a maximum of 50 mg per day. As is generally recognised, there is the potential for worsening of panic symptomatology during early treatment of panic disorder; a low initial starting dose is therefore recommended.

It is recommended that Seroxat be administered once daily in the morning with food.

As with all antidepressant drugs, dosage should be reviewed and adjusted if necessary within two to three weeks of initiation of therapy and thereafter as judged clinically appropriate. Patients should be treated for a sufficient period to ensure that they are free from symptoms. This period may be several months for depression and may be even longer for OCD and panic disorder. As with many psychoactive medications, abrupt discontinuation should be avoided (see *Undesirable effects*).

*Elderly:* Increased plasma concentrations of Seroxat occur in elderly subjects.

Dosing should commence at the adult starting dose and may be increased weekly in 10 mg increments to a maximum of 40 mg per day according to patient's response.

*Children:* The use of Seroxat in children is not recommended as safety and efficacy have not been established in this population.

*Renal/hepatic impairment:* Increased plasma concentrations of Seroxat occur in patients with severe renal impairment (creatinine clearance <30 ml/min) or severe hepatic impairment. The recommended dose is 20 mg a day. Incremental dosage, if required, should be restricted to the lower end of the range.

*Contra-indications:* Known hypersensitivity to Seroxat.

*Special warnings and precautions for use:*
*MAO inhibitors:* As with most anti-depressants, Seroxat should not be used in combination with MAO inhibitors or within two weeks of terminating treatment with MAO inhibitors. Thereafter treatment should be initiated cautiously and dosage increased gradually until optimal response is reached. MAO inhibitors should not be introduced within two weeks of cessation of therapy with Seroxat.

*History of mania:* As with all anti-depressants, Seroxat should be used with caution in patients with a history of mania.

*Patients receiving oral anticoagulants:* Seroxat should be administered with great caution to patients receiving oral anticoagulants (see *Interactions*).

*Cardiac conditions:* Seroxat does not produce clinically significant changes in blood pressure, heart rate and ECG. Nevertheless, as with all psychoactive drugs, caution is advised when treating patients with cardiac conditions.

*Epilepsy:* As with other antidepressants, Seroxat should be used with caution in patients with epilepsy.

*Seizures:* Overall, the incidence of seizures is <0.1% in patients treated with Seroxat. Seroxat should be discontinued in any patient who develops seizures.

*ECT:* There is little clinical experience of concurrent administration of Seroxat with ECT.

*Interactions with other medicaments and other forms of interaction:*
*Food/antacids:* The absorption and pharmacokinetics of Seroxat are not affected by food or antacids.

*Tryptophan:* As with other 5-HT reuptake inhibitors, animal studies indicate that an interaction between Seroxat and tryptophan may occur, resulting in a "serotonin syndrome" suggested by a combination of agitation, restlessness and gastrointestinal symptoms including diarrhoea.

*Drug metabolising enzyme inducers/inhibitors:* The metabolism and pharmacokinetics of Seroxat may be affected by drugs which induce or inhibit hepatic drug metabolising enzymes. When Seroxat is to be co-administered with a known drug metabolising inhibitor, consideration should be given to using doses at the lower end of the range. No initial dosage adjustment of Seroxat is considered necessary when it is to be co-administered with known drug metabolising enzyme inducers. Any subsequent dosage adjustment should be guided by clinical effect (tolerability and efficacy).

*Alcohol:* Although Seroxat does not increase the impairment of mental and motor skills caused by alcohol, the concomitant use of Seroxat and alcohol in patients is not advised.

*Haloperidol/amylobarbitone/oxazepam:* Experience in a limited number of healthy subjects has shown that Seroxat did not increase the sedation and drowsiness associated with haloperidol, amylobarbitone or oxazepam when given in combination.

*MAOIs:* As with other 5-HT reuptake inhibitors, animal studies indicate that an interaction between Seroxat and monoamine oxidase (MAO) inhibitors may occur (see *Special warnings and precautions for use*).

*Lithium:* Since there is little clinical experience, and there have been reports of interaction of lithium with other 5-HT reuptake inhibitors, the concurrent administration of Seroxat and lithium should be undertaken with caution. Lithium levels should be monitored.

*Phenytoin/anticonvulsants:* Co-administration with Seroxat and phenytoin is associated with decreased plasma concentrations of Seroxat and increased adverse experiences. Co-administration of Seroxat with other anticonvulsants may also be associated with an increased incidence of adverse experiences.

*Warfarin:* Preliminary data suggest that there may be a pharmacodynamic interaction between Seroxat and warfarin which may result in increased bleeding in the presence of unaltered prothrombin times. Seroxat should therefore be administered with great caution to patients receiving oral anticoagulants.

*Pregnancy and lactation:* Although animal studies have not shown any teratogenic or selective embryotoxic effects, the safety of Seroxat in human pregnancy has not been established and it should not be used during pregnancy or by nursing mothers unless the potential benefit outweighs the possible risk.

*Effects on ability to drive and use machines:* Clinical experience has shown that therapy with Seroxat is not associated with impairment of cognitive or psychomotor function. However, as with all psychoactive drugs, patients should be cautioned about their ability to drive a car and operate machinery.

*Undesirable effects:* In controlled trials the most commonly observed adverse events associated with the use of Seroxat and not seen at an equivalent incidence among placebo-treated patients were: nausea, somnolence, sweating, tremor, asthenia, dry mouth, insomnia, sexual dysfunction (including impotence and ejaculation disorders) dizziness, constipation, diarrhoea and decreased appetite. The majority of these adverse experiences decreased in intensity and frequency with continued treatment and did not generally lead to cessation of therapy.

In addition, there have been spontaneous reports of dizziness, vomiting, diarrhoea, restlessness, hallucinations and hypomania. Rash, including urticaria accompanied by pruritus or angioedema, has been reported. Symptoms suggestive of postural hypotension have been reported, often in patients with other risk factors.

Extrapyramidal reactions have been reported infrequently. Most of these have occurred in patients with underlying movement disorders, or who are using neuroleptic medication. Dystonic movements of the face, tongue and eyes have also been reported.

Abnormalities of liver function tests and hyponatraemia have been described rarely. These usually resolve rapidly on discontinuation of Seroxat.

Seroxat is less likely than tricyclic antidepressants to be associated with dry mouth, constipation and somnolence.

Symptoms including dizziness, sensory disturbance (e.g. paraesthesia), anxiety, sleep disturbances (including intense dreams), agitation, tremor, nausea, sweating and confusion have been reported following abrupt discontinuation of Seroxat. They are usually self-limiting and symptomatic treatment is seldom warranted. No particular patient group appears to be at higher risk of these symptoms; it is therefore recommended that when antidepressive treatment is no longer required, gradual discontinuation by dose-tapering or alternate day dosing be considered.

*Overdose:* A wide margin of safety is evident from available data. Overdose attempts have been reported in patients who took up to 2000 mg alone or in combination with other drugs, including alcohol. Experience of Seroxat in overdose has shown symptoms including nausea, vomiting, tremor, dilated pupils, dry mouth, irritability, sweating and somnolence, but not coma or convulsions.

No specific antidote is known.

Treatment should consist of those general measures employed in the management of overdose with any antidepressant. Early administration of activated charcoal may delay the absorption of Seroxat.

**Pharmacological properties**

*Pharmacodynamic properties:* Seroxat is a potent and selective inhibitor of 5-hydroxytryptamine (5-HT, serotonin) reuptake and its antidepressant action and efficacy in the treatment of OCD and panic disorder is thought to be related to its specific inhibition of 5-HT reuptake in brain neurones.

Seroxat is chemically unrelated to the tricyclic, tetracyclic and other available antidepressants.

The principal metabolites of Seroxat are polar and conjugated products of oxidation and methylation, which are readily cleared. In view of their relative lack of pharmacological activity, it is most unlikely that they contribute to the therapeutic effects of Seroxat.

Seroxat inhibits the hepatic cytochrome P450 isozyme responsible for the metabolism of debrisoquine and sparteine. This may lead to enhanced plasma levels of those co-administered drugs which are metabolised by this isozyme. Such drugs may include certain tricyclic antidepressants, phenothiazine neuroleptics and type Ic anti-arrhythmics.

Long-term treatment with Seroxat has shown that antidepressant efficacy is maintained for periods of at least one year.

In a placebo-controlled trial, the efficacy of paroxetine in the treatment of panic disorder has been maintained for at least one year.

*Pharmacokinetic properties:* Seroxat is well absorbed after oral dosing and undergoes first-pass metabolism.

The elimination half-life is variable but is generally about one day. Steady state systemic levels are attained by seven to 14 days after starting treatment and pharmacokinetics do not appear to change during long-term therapy.

*Preclinical safety data:* Not applicable

**Pharmaceutical particulars**

*List of excipients:* Polacrilin potassium, dispersible cellulose (E460), propylene glycol, glycerol (E422), sorbitol (E420), methyl parahydroxybenzoate (E218), propyl parahydroxybenzoate (E216), sodium citrate (E331), citric acid (E330), sodium saccharin (E954), natural orange flavour, natural lemon flavour, yellow colouring (E110), silicone antifoam, purified water.

*Incompatibilities:* Not applicable.

*Shelf life:* Two years.

*Special precautions for storage:* Store at 25°C or below.

*Nature and contents of container:* Amber glass bottles containing 150 ml, with white HDPE child-resistant cap with tamper evident seal.

*Instruction for use/handling:* None.

**Marketing authorisation number** 10592/0092

**Date of approval/revision of SPC** 22 April 1997

**Legal category** POM

## SEROXAT* TABLETS

**Presentation** *20 mg tablets:* White, film-coated, modified oval, biconvex tablets engraved 'Seroxat 20' on one side and having a breakline on the reverse. Each tablet contains paroxetine hydrochloride equivalent to 20 mg paroxetine free base.

*30 mg tablets:* Blue, film-coated, modified oval, biconvex tablets engraved 'Seroxat 30' on one side and having a breakline on the reverse. Each tablet contains paroxetine hydrochloride equivalent to 30 mg paroxetine free base.

**Uses** Treatment of symptoms of depressive illness of all types including depression accompanied by anxiety. Treatment of symptoms and prevention of relapse of obsessive compulsive disorder (OCD). Treatment of symptoms and prevention of relapse of panic disorder with or without agoraphobia.

**Dosage and administration** For oral administration.

*Adults: Depression:* The recommended dose is 20 mg daily. In some patients it may be necessary to increase the dose. This should be done gradually by 10 mg increments to a maximum of 50 mg according to the patient's response.

*Obsessive compulsive disorder:* The recommended dose is 40 mg daily. Patients should start on 20 mg and the dose may be increased weekly in 10 mg increments. Some patients will benefit from having their dose increased up to a maximum of 60 mg per day.

*Panic disorder:* The recommended dose is 40 mg daily. Patients should be started on 10 mg per day and the dose increased weekly in 10 mg increments according to the patient's response. Some patients may benefit from having their dose increased up to a maximum of 50 mg per day. As is generally recognised, there is the potential for worsening of panic symptomatology during early treatment of panic disorder; a low initial starting dose is therefore recommended.

It is recommended that Seroxat be administered once daily in the morning with food.

The tablet should be swallowed rather than chewed. As with all antidepressant drugs, dosage should be reviewed and adjusted if necessary within two to three weeks of initiation of therapy and thereafter as judged clinically appropriate. Patients should be treated for a sufficient period to ensure that they are free from symptoms. This period may be several months for depression and may be even longer for OCD and panic disorder. As with many psychoactive medications, abrupt discontinuation should be avoided (see *Side-effects*).

*Elderly:* Increased plasma concentrations of Seroxat occur in elderly subjects.

Dosing should commence at the adult starting dose and may be increased in weekly 10 mg increments to a maximum of 40 mg daily according to the patient's response.

*Children:* The use of Seroxat in children is not recommended as safety and efficacy have not been established in this population.

*Renal/hepatic impairment:* Increased plasma concentrations of Seroxat occur in patients with severe renal impairment (creatinine clearance <30 ml/min) or severe hepatic impairment. The recommended dose is 20 mg a day. Incremental dosage, if required, should be restricted to the lower end of the range.

**Contra-indications, warnings, etc**

*Contra-indication:* Known hypersensitivity to paroxetine.

*Use during pregnancy and lactation:* Although animal studies have not shown any teratogenic or selective embryotoxic effects, the safety of Seroxat in human pregnancy has not been established and it should not be used during pregnancy or by nursing mothers unless the potential benefit outweighs the possible risk.

*Warnings:* MAO inhibitors: As with most antidepressants, Seroxat should not be used in combination with MAO inhibitors or within two weeks of terminating treatment with MAO inhibitors. Thereafter treatment should be initiated cautiously and dosage increased gradually until optimal response is reached.

MAO inhibitors should not be introduced within two weeks of cessation of therapy with Seroxat.

History of mania: As with all antidepressants, Seroxat should be used with caution in patients with a history of mania.

Patients receiving oral anticoagulants: Seroxat should be administered with great caution to patients receiving oral anticoagulants (see *Interactions*).

*Precautions:* Cardiac conditions: Seroxat does not produce clinically significant changes in blood pressure, heart rate and ECG. Nevertheless, as with all psychoactive drugs, caution is advised when treating patients with cardiac conditions.

Epilepsy: As with other antidepressants, Seroxat should be used with caution in patients with epilepsy.

Seizures: Overall, the incidence of seizures is <0.1% in patients treated with Seroxat. Seroxat should be discontinued in any patient who develops seizures.

ECT: There is little clinical experience of concurrent administration of Seroxat with ECT.

Ability to drive/use machines: Clinical experience has shown that therapy with Seroxat is not associated with impairment of cognitive or psychomotor function. However, as with all psychoactive drugs, patients should be cautioned about their ability to drive a car and operate machinery.

*Interactions:* Food/antacids: The absorption and pharmacokinetics of Seroxat are not affected by food or antacids.

Tryptophan: As with other 5-HT re-uptake inhibitors, animal studies indicate that an interaction between Seroxat and tryptophan may occur, resulting in a 'serotonin syndrome' suggested by a combination of agitation, restlessness and gastrointestinal symptoms including diarrhoea.

Drug metabolising enzyme inducers/inhibitors: The metabolism and pharmacokinetics of Seroxat may be affected by drugs which induce or inhibit hepatic drug metabolising enzymes.

When Seroxat is to be co-administered with a known drug metabolising inhibitor, consideration should be given to using doses at the lower end of the range. No initial dosage adjustment of Seroxat is considered necessary when it is to be co-administered with known drug metabolising enzyme inducers. Any subsequent dosage adjustment should be guided by clinical effect (tolerability and efficacy).

Alcohol: Although Seroxat does not increase the impairment of mental and motor skill caused by alcohol, the concomitant use of Seroxat and alcohol in depressed patients is not advised.

Haloperidol/amylobarbitone/oxazepam: Experience in a limited number of healthy subjects has shown that Seroxat did not increase the sedation and drowsiness associated with haloperidol, amylobarbitone or oxazepam when given in combination.

MAOIs: As with other 5-HT re-uptake inhibitors, animal studies indicate that an interaction between Seroxat and monoamine oxidase (MAO) inhibitors may occur (see *Warnings*).

Lithium: Since there is little clinical experience, and there have been reports of interaction of lithium with other 5-HT re-uptake inhibitors, the concurrent administration of Seroxat and lithium should be undertaken with caution. Lithium levels should be monitored.

Phenytoin/anticonvulsants: Co-administration of Seroxat and phenytoin is associated with decreased plasma concentrations of Seroxat and increased adverse experiences.

Co-administration of Seroxat with other anticonvulsants may also be associated with an increased incidence of adverse experiences.

Warfarin: Preliminary data suggest that there may be a pharmacodynamic interaction between Seroxat and warfarin which may result in increased bleeding in the presence of unaltered prothrombin times. Seroxat should therefore be administered with great caution to patients receiving oral anticoagulants.

*Side-effects:* In controlled clinical trials the most commonly observed adverse events associated with the use of Seroxat and not seen at an equivalent incidence among placebo-treated patients were: nausea, somnolence, sweating, tremor, asthenia, dry mouth, insomnia, sexual dysfunction (including impotence and ejaculation disorders), dizziness, constipation, diarrhoea and decreased appetite. The majority of these adverse experiences decreased in intensity and frequency with continued treatment and did not generally lead to cessation of therapy.

In addition there have been spontaneous reports of dizziness, vomiting, diarrhoea, restlessness, hallucinations and hypomania. Rash, including urticaria accompanied by pruritus or angioedema, has been reported. Symptoms suggestive of postural hypotension have been reported, often in patients with other risk factors.

Extrapyramidal reactions have been reported infrequently. Most of these have occurred in patients with underlying movement disorders, or who are usin neuroleptic medication. Dystonic movements of th face, tongue and eyes have also been reported.

Abnormalities of liver function tests and hypona traemia have been described rarely. These usuall resolve rapidly on discontinuation of Seroxat.

Seroxat is less likely than tricyclic antidepressant to be associated with dry mouth, constipation an somnolence.

Symptoms including dizziness, sensory disturbanc (e.g. paraesthesia), anxiety, sleep disturbances, (in cluding vivid dreams), agitation, tremor, nause sweating and confusion have been reported followin abrupt discontinuation of Seroxat. They are usuall self-limiting and symptomatic treatment is seldon warranted. No particular patient group appears to b at higher risk of these symptoms; it is therefor recommended that when antidepressant treatment i no longer required, gradual discontinuation by dose tapering or alternate day dosing be considered.

*Overdose:* A wide margin of safety is evident fron available data. Overdose attempts have been reporte in patients who took up to 2000 mg alone or i combination with other drugs, including alcoho Experience of Seroxat in overdose has shown symp toms including nausea, vomiting, tremor, dilate pupils, dry mouth, irritability, sweating and somno lence, but not coma or convulsions.

No specific antidote is known.

Treatment should consist of those general meas ures employed in the management of overdose wit any antidepressant. Early administration of activate charcoal may delay the absorption of Seroxat.

**Pharmaceutical precautions** No special storage pre cautions are required.

**Legal category** POM.

**Package quantities** 20 mg and 30 mg tablets. Avail able in Original Packs of 30 (two calendar strips of 1 tablets).

**Further information** Seroxat is a potent and selectiv inhibitor of 5-hydroxytryptamine reuptake (5-HT, se rotonin) and its antidepressant action and efficacy i the treatment of OCD and panic disorder is thought t be related to its specific inhibition of 5-HT reuptake i brain neurones.

Seroxat is chemically unrelated to the tricycli tetracyclic and other available antidepressants.

The principal metabolites of Seroxat are polar an conjugated products of oxidation and methylatio which are readily cleared. In view of their relative lac of pharmacological activity, it is most unlikely tha they contribute to the therapeutic effects of Seroxat.

Seroxat is well absorbed after oral dosing an undergoes first-pass metabolism.

The elimination half-life is variable but is generall about one day. Steady state systemic levels ar attained by seven to fourteen days after startin treatment and pharmacokinetics do not appear t change during long-term therapy.

Seroxat inhibits the hepatic cytochrome P450 isc zyme responsible for the metabolism of debrisoquin and sparteine. This may lead to enhanced plasm levels of those co-administered drugs which ar metabolised by this isozyme. Such drugs may includ certain tricyclic antidepressants, phenothiazine neu roleptics and type Ic anti-arrhythmics.

Long-term treatment with Seroxat has shown tha antidepressant efficacy is maintained for periods of a least one year.

In a placebo-controlled trial, the efficacy of paroxe tine in the treatment of panic disorders has bee maintained for at least one year.

**Product licence numbers**

| | |
|---|---|
| Seroxat 20 mg Tablets | 10592/0001. |
| Seroxat 30 mg Tablets | 10592/0002. |

## STELAZINE* SPANSULE* CAPSULES
## STELAZINE* SYRUP

**Qualitative and quantitative composition** Stelazin Spansule Capsules are available in three strength Each Spansule capsule contains 2 mg, 10 mg or 15 m trifluoperazine present as the hydrochloride.

Each 5 ml dose of syrup contains 1 mg trifluoper zine present as the hydrochloride.

**Pharmaceutical form** Spansule Capsules: Clear, co ourless capsules, opaque yellow-capped and fille with a mixture of dark and light blue and white pellet

Syrup: A clear, pale yellow, peach-flavoured syrup

**Clinical particulars**

*Therapeutic indications:*

*Low dosage*: Stelazine is indicated as an adjunct i the short-term management of anxiety states, depres sive symptoms secondary to anxiety, and agitatio Orally it is also indicated in the symptomatic treatme of nausea and vomiting.

*High dosage*: Stelazine is indicated for the treatme

of symptoms and prevention of relapse in schizophrenia and in other psychoses, especially of paranoid type, but not in depressive psychoses. It may also be used as an adjunct in the short-term management of severe psychomotor agitation and of dangerously impulsive behaviour in, for example mental subnormality.

**Posology and method of administration:**

*Adults:*

*Low-dosage:* 2–4 mg a day given in divided doses, one or two 2 mg Spansule capsules a day), according to the severity of the patient's condition. If necessary, dosage may be increased to 6 mg a day, but above this level extrapyramidal symptoms are more likely to occur in some patients.

*High-dosage:* The recommended starting dose for physically fit adults is 5 mg twice a day (or one 10 mg Spansule capsule a day); after a week this may be increased to 15 mg a day (which may be given as one 15 mg Spansule capsule a day). If necessary, further increases of 5 mg may be made at three-day intervals, but not more often. When satisfactory control has been achieved, dosage should be reduced gradually, until an effective maintenance level has been established. Stelazine Spansule capsules are particularly useful for such maintenance therapy.

As with all major tranquillisers, clinical improvement may not be evident for several weeks after starting treatment, and there may be delay before recurrence of symptoms after stopping treatment. Gradual withdrawal from high dosage treatment is advisable.

*Children:* Spansule Capsules: *Low dosage:* For children aged 6–12 years, the maximum is 4 mg a day, in divided doses.

*Syrup: Low-dosage:* For children aged 3–5 years, up to 1 mg a day given in divided doses. For children aged 6–12 years, the dosage may be increased to a maximum of 4 mg a day.

*Capsules and Syrup: High-dosage:* For children aged under 12 years, the initial oral dosage should not exceed 5 mg a day, given in divided doses. Any subsequent increase should be made with caution at intervals of not less than three days, and taking into account age, body weight and severity of symptoms.

*Elderly:* The starting dose for elderly or frail patients should be reduced by at least half.

*Administration:* Oral.

*Contra-indications:* Do not use Stelazine in comatose patients, or in those with existing blood dyscrasias or known liver damage, or in those hypersensitive to the active ingredient or related compounds. Patients with uncontrolled cardiac decompensation should not be given Stelazine.

*Special warnings and special precautions for use:* Care should be taken when treating elderly patients, and initial dosage should be reduced. Such patients can be especially sensitive, particularly to extrapyramidal and hypotensive effects. Patients with cardiovascular disease including arrhythmias should also be treated with caution. Because Stelazine may increase activity, care should be taken in patients with angina pectoris.

In patients with Parkinson's disease, symptoms may be worsened, and the effects of levodopa reversed. Since phenothiazines may lower the convulsive threshold, patients with epilepsy should be treated with caution, and metrizamide avoided. Although Stelazine has minimal anticholinergic activity, this should be borne in mind when treating patients with narrow angle glaucoma, myasthenia gravis or prostatic hypertrophy.

Nausea and vomiting as a sign of organic disease may be masked by the anti-emetic action of Stelazine.

*Interaction with other medicaments and other forms of interaction:* Potentiation may occur if antipsychotic drugs are combined with CNS depressants such as alcohol, hypnotics, anaesthetics and strong analgesics, or with antihypertensives or other drugs with hypotensive activity, anticholinergics or antidepressants. Phenothiazines may antagonise the action of guanethidine, avoid drugs that depress leucopoiesis.

Desferrioxamine should not be used in combination with Stelazine, since prolonged unconsciousness has occurred after combination with the related prochlorperazine.

Phenothiazines should be used with care in extremes of temperature since they may affect body temperature control.

Patients on long-term phenothiazine therapy require regular and careful surveillance with particular attention to tardive dyskinesia and possible eye changes, blood dyscrasias, liver dysfunction and myocardial conduction defects, particularly if other concurrently administered drugs have potential effects in these systems.

*Pregnancy and lactation:* Stelazine has been available since 1958. There are some animal studies that indicate a teratogenic effect, but results are conflicting. There is no clinical evidence (including follow-up

surveys in over 800 women who had taken low-dosage Stelazine during pregnancy) to indicate that trifluoperazine has a teratogenic effect in man. Nevertheless, drug treatment should be avoided in pregnancy unless essential, especially during the first trimester. Trifluoperazine crosses the placenta and passes into the milk of lactating dogs; breast feeding should only be allowed at the discretion of the physician.

*Effect on ability to drive and use machines:* Patients who drive or operate machinery should be warned of the possibility of drowsiness.

*Undesirable effects:* Lassitude, drowsiness, dizziness, transient restlessness, insomnia, dry mouth, blurred vision, muscular weakness, anorexia, mild postural hypotension, skin reactions including photosensitivity reactions, weight gain, oedema and confusion may occasionally occur. Tachycardia, constipation, urinary hesitancy and retention, and hyperpyrexia have been reported very rarely. Adverse reactions tend to be dose-related and to disappear. Hyperprolactinaemia may occur at higher dosages with associated effects such as galactorrhoea, amenorrhoea or gynaecomastia; certain hormone-dependent breast neoplasms may be affected. Phenothiazines can produce ECG changes with prolongation of the QT interval and T-wave changes; serious arrhythmias have been reported. Such effects are rare with Stelazine. In some patients, especially non-psychotic patients, Stelazine even at low dosage may cause unpleasant symptoms of being dulled or, paradoxically, of being agitated.

Extrapyramidal symptoms are rare at daily oral dosages of 6 mg or less; they are considerably more common at high-dosage levels. These symptoms include parkinsonism; akathisia, with motor restlessness and difficulty in sitting still; and acute dystonia or dyskinesia, which may occur early in treatment and may present with torticollis, facial grimacing, trismus, tongue protrusion and abnormal eye movements including oculogyric crises. These effects are likely to be particularly severe in children. Such reactions may often be controlled by reducing the dosage or by stopping medication. In more severe dystonic reactions, an anticholinergic antiparkinsonism drug should be given.

Tardive dyskinesia of the facial muscles, sometimes with involuntary movements of the extremities, has occurred in some patients on long-term high dosage and, more rarely, low-dosage phenothiazine therapy, including Stelazine. Symptoms may appear for the first time either during or after a course of treatment; they may become worse when treatment is stopped. The symptoms may persist for many months or even years, and while they gradually disappear in some patients, they appear to be permanent in others. Patients have most commonly been elderly, female or with organic brain damage. Particular caution should be observed in treating such patients. If tardive dyskinesia occurs, the benefit of continued treatment should be balanced against the risk of persisting dyskinesia. Periodic gradual reduction of dosage to reveal persisting dyskinesia has been suggested so that treatment may be stopped if necessary. If re-started, Stelazine could mask symptoms. Anticholinergic antiparkinsonism agents may aggravate the condition. Since the occurrence of tardive dyskinesia may be related to length of treatment and total cumulative dosage, Stelazine should be given for as short a time and at as low a dosage as possible.

The neuroleptic malignant syndrome is a rare but occasionally fatal complication of treatment with various neuroleptic drugs, and is characterised by hyperpyrexia, muscle rigidity, altered consciousness and autonomic instability. Intensive symptomatic treatment should include cooling. Intravenous dantrolene has been suggested for muscle rigidity.

Cholestatic jaundice, and blood dyscrasias such as agranulocytosis, pancytopenia, leucopenia and thrombocytopenia have been reported very rarely. Signs of persistent infection should be investigated.

Very rare cases of skin pigmentation and lenticular opacities have been reported with Stelazine.

*Overdosage:* Signs and symptoms will be predominantly extrapyramidal; hypotension may occur. Treatment consists of gastric lavage together with supportive and symptomatic measures. Do not induce vomiting. Extrapyramidal symptoms may be treated with an anticholinergic antiparkinsonism drug. Treat hypotension with fluid replacement; if severe or persistent, noradrenaline may be considered. Adrenaline is contra-indicated.

**Pharmacological properties**

*Pharmacodynamic properties:* Stelazine is a piperazine phenothiazine tranquilliser with potent antipsychotic, anxiolytic, and anti-emetic activity, and a pharmacological profile of moderate sedative and hypotensive properties, and fairly pronounced tendency to cause extrapyramidal reactions.

*Pharmacokinetic properties:* Trifluoperazine is well

absorbed but undergoes extensive first pass metabolism. Distribution is wide and elimination occurs in the bile and urine.

*Preclinical safety data:* Not applicable.

**Pharmaceutical particulars**

*List of excipients:*
*Spansule Capsules:* Gelatin; Glyceryl Distearate; Microcrystalline Wax; FD&C Blue No. 2 Lake (E132); Dioctyl Sodium Sulphosuccinate; Maize Starch; Talc; Kaolin Heavy; Sugar Granulated; Sugar Caster; Titanium Dioxide (E171); Quinoline Yellow (E104) Black Iron Oxide (E172).

*Syrup:* Sodium Saccharin; Sodium benzoate; Citric acid, anhydrous; Sodium Citrate; Sorbitol solution; Quinoline Yellow (E104); Sunset Yellow (E110); Peach Flavour 85502; Demineralised Water.

*Incompatibilities:* Not applicable.

*Shelf-life:* Stelazine Spansule Capsules have a shelf-life of five years. Stelazine Syrup has a shelf-life of five years.

*Special precautions for storage:* Spansule Capsules: Store in a dry place below 25°C and protect from light. Syrup: Store syrup in carton and protect from light. If it is necessary to dilute the syrup use sorbitol solution BP. The diluted syrup is stable for four weeks. Store diluted syrup in the dark.

*Nature and contents of container:*
Spansule Capsules 2 mg in opaque blister packs (OP) of 60.
Spansule Capsules 10 mg in opaque blister packs (OP) of 30.
Spansule Capsules 15 mg in opaque blister packs (OP) of 30.
Syrup: Amber glass bottle, containing 200 ml of syrup.

*Instructions for use/handling:* None.

**Marketing authorisation numbers**

| | |
|---|---|
| Stelazine Spansule Capsules 2 mg | 0002/5077R |
| Stelazine Spansule Capsules 10 mg | 0002/5078R |
| Stelazine Spansule Capsules 15 mg | 0002/5079R |
| Stelazine Syrup | 0002/5080R |

**Date of approval/revision of SPC** February 1997

**Legal category** POM

## STELAZINE* TABLETS

**Presentation** Blue, aqueous film-coated tablets, marked SKF, containing either 1 mg or 5 mg trifluoperazine present as the hydrochloride.

**Uses** Stelazine is a piperazine phenothiazine tranquilliser with potent antipsychotic, anxiolytic, and anti-emetic activity, and a pharmacological profile of moderate sedative and hypotensive properties, and fairly pronounced tendency to cause extrapyramidal reactions.

*Low dosage:* Stelazine is indicated as an adjunct in the short-term management of anxiety states, depressive symptoms secondary to anxiety, and agitation. Orally it is also indicated in the symptomatic treatment of nausea and vomiting.

*High dosage:* Stelazine is indicated for the treatment of symptoms and prevention of relapse in schizophrenia and in other psychoses, especially of the paranoid type, but not in depressive psychoses. It may also be used as an adjunct in the short-term management of severe psychomotor agitation and of dangerously impulsive behaviour in, for example, mental subnormality.

**Dosage and administration**
*ADULTS*

*Low dosage:* 2–4 mg a day, given in divided doses, according to the severity of the patient's condition. If necessary, dosage may be increased to 6 mg a day, but above this level extrapyramidal symptoms are more likely to occur in some patients.

*High dosage:* The recommended starting dose for physically fit adults is 5 mg twice a day; after a week this may be increased to 15 mg a day. If necessary, further increases of 5 mg may be made at three-day intervals, but not more often. When satisfactory control has been achieved, dosage should be reduced gradually until an effective maintenance level has been established.

As with all major tranquillisers clinical improvement may not be evident for several weeks after starting treatment, and there may also be delay before recurrence of symptoms after stopping treatment. Gradual withdrawal from high-dosage treatment is advisable.

*ELDERLY*
Reduce starting dose in elderly or frail patients by at least half.

*CHILDREN*

*Low dosage:* For children aged 6–12 years, up to a maximum of 4 mg a day given in divided doses.

*High dosage:* For children aged under 12 years, the initial oral dosage should not exceed 5 mg a day, given in divided doses. Any subsequent increase should be made with caution, at intervals of not less than three days, and taking into account age, body weight and severity of symptoms.

**Contra-indications, warnings, etc**

*Contra-indications:* Do not use Stelazine in comatose patients, or in those with existing blood dyscrasias or known liver damage, or in those hypersensitive to the active ingredient or related compounds. Patients with uncontrolled cardiac decompensation should not be given Stelazine.

*Precautions:* Care should be taken when treating elderly patients, and the initial dosage should be reduced. Such patients can be especially sensitive, particularly to extrapyramidal and hypotensive effects. Patients with cardiovascular disease including arrhythmias should also be treated with caution. Because Stelazine may increase activity, care should be taken in patients with angina pectoris.

In patients with Parkinson's disease, symptoms may be worsened, and the effects of levodopa reversed. Since phenothiazines may lower the convulsive threshold, patients with epilepsy should be treated with caution, and metrizamide avoided. Although Stelazine has minimal anticholinergic activity, this should be borne in mind when treating patients with narrow angle glaucoma, myasthenia gravis or prostatic hypertrophy.

Nausea and vomiting as a sign of organic disease may be masked by the anti-emetic action of Stelazine.

Potentiation may occur if antipsychotic drugs are combined with CNS depressants such as alcohol, hypnotics, anaesthetics and strong analgesics or with antihypertensives or other drugs with hypotensive activity, anticholinergics or antidepressants. Phenothiazines may antagonise the action of guanethidine. Avoid drugs that depress leucopoiesis.

Desferrioxamine should not be used in combination with Stelazine, since prolonged unconsciousness has occurred after combination with the related prochlorperazine.

Phenothizines should be used with care in extremes of temperature since they may affect body temperature control.

Patients on long-term phenothiazine therapy require regular and careful surveillance with particular attention to tardive dyskinesia and possible eye changes, blood dyscrasias, liver dysfunction and myocardial conduction defects, particularly if other concurrently administered drugs have potential effects in these systems.

Patients who drive or operate machinery should be warned of the possibility of drowsiness.

*Use in pregnancy and lactation:* Stelazine has been available since 1958. There are some animal studies that indicate a teratogenic effect, but results are conflicting. There is no clinical evidence (including follow-up surveys in over 800 women who had taken low-dosage Stelazine during pregnancy) to indicate that trifluoperazine has a teratogenic effect in man. Nevertheless, drug treatment should be avoided in pregnancy unless essential, especially during the first trimester. Trifluoperazine crosses the placenta and passes into the milk of lactating dogs. Breast feeding should only be allowed at the discretion of the physician.

*Adverse reactions:* Lassitude, drowsiness, dizziness, transient restlessness, insomnia, dry mouth, blurred vision, muscular weakness, anorexia, mild postural hypotension, skin reactions including photosensitivity reactions, weight gain, oedema and confusion may occasionally occur. Tachycardia, constipation, urinary hesitancy and retention, and hyperpyrexia have been reported very rarely. Adverse reactions tend to be dose-related and to disappear. Hyperprolactinaemia may occur at higher dosages with associated effects such as galactorrhoea, amenorrhoea or gynaecomastia; certain hormone-dependent breast neoplasms may be affected. Phenothiazines can produce ECG changes with prolongation of the QT interval and T-wave changes; serious arrhythmias have been reported. Such effects are rare with Stelazine. In some patients, especially non-psychotic patients, Stelazine even at low dosage may cause unpleasant symptoms of being dulled or, paradoxically, of being agitated.

Extrapyramidal symptoms are rare at oral daily dosages of 6 mg or less; they are considerably more common at higher dosage levels. These symptoms include parkinsonism; akathisia, with motor restlessness and difficulty in sitting still; and acute dystonia or dyskinesia, which may occur early in treatment and may present with torticollis, facial grimacing, trismus, tongue protrusion and abnormal eye movements including oculogyric crises. These effects are likely to be particularly severe in children. Such reactions may often be controlled by reducing the dosage or by stopping medication. In more severe dystonic reactions, an anticholinergic antiparkinsonism drug should be given.

Tardive dyskinesia of the facial muscles, sometimes with involuntary movements of the extremities, has occurred in some patients on long-term high dosage and, more rarely, low-dosage phenothiazine therapy, including Stelazine. Symptoms may appear for the first time either during or after a course of treatment; they may become worse when treatment is stopped. The symptoms may persist for many months or even years, and while they gradually disappear in some patients, they appear to be permanent in others. Patients have most commonly been elderly, female or with organic brain damage. Particular caution should be observed in treating such patients. If tardive dyskinesia occurs, the benefit of continued treatment should be balanced against the risk of persisting dyskinesia. Periodic gradual reduction of dosage to reveal persisting dyskinesia has been suggested, so that treatment may be stopped if necessary. If restarted, Stelazine could mask symptoms. Anticholinergic antiparkinsonism agents may aggravate the condition. Since the occurrence of tardive dyskinesia may be related to length of treatment and total cumulative dosage, Stelazine should be given for as short a time and at as low a dosage as possible.

In common with other neuroleptic drugs, the neuroleptic malignant syndrome is a rare but occasionally fatal complication of treatment with Stelazine, and is characterised by hyperpyrexia, muscle rigidity, altered consciousness and autonomic instability. Intensive symptomatic treatment should include cooling. Intravenous dantrolene has been suggested for muscle rigidity.

Cholestatic jaundice, and blood dyscrasias such as agranulocytosis, pancytopenia, leucopenia and thrombocytopenia have been reported very rarely. Signs of persistent infection should be investigated.

Very rare cases of skin pigmentation and lenticular opacities have been reported with Stelazine.

*Overdosage:* Signs and symptoms will be predominantly extrapyramidal; hypotension may occur. Absorption of trifluoperazine from the Spansule capsule is likely to be prolonged, and this should be borne in mind. Treatment consists of gastric lavage together with supportive and symptomatic measures. Do not induce vomiting. Extrapyramidal symptoms may be treated with an anticholinergic antiparkinsonism drug. Treat hypotension with fluid replacement; if severe or persistent, noradrenaline may be considered. Adrenaline is contra-indicated.

**Pharmaceutical precautions** Store tablets in a dry place at or below 25°C and protect from light.

**Legal category** POM.

**Package quantities** Tablets 1 mg, in opaque blister packs of 100 (4 × 25). Tablets 5 mg, in opaque blister packs of 100 (4 × 25).

**Further information** Trifluoperazine is well absorbed but undergoes extensive first pass metabolism. Distribution is wide and elimination occurs in the bile and urine. Inactive ingredients in the tablets include sucrose.

**Product licence numbers**

| | |
|---|---|
| Stelazine tablets, 1 mg | 0002/5081R. |
| Stelazine tablets, 5 mg | 0002/5082R. |

## TAGAMET* TABLETS
## TAGAMET* EFFERVESCENT TABLETS
## TAGAMET* SYRUP
## TAGAMET* INJECTION
## TAGAMET* INFUSION

**Presentation** Pale green, oval, film-coated Tiltab* tablets, engraved SK&F T800 on one side, containing 800 mg cimetidine.

Pale green, oblong, film-coated tablets, engraved TAGAMET on one side and SK&F 400 on reverse, containing 400 mg cimetidine.

Pale green, circular, film-coated Tiltab tablets, engraved TAGAMET on one side and SK&F 200 on reverse, containing 200 mg cimetidine.

White, circular, effervescent tablets with a predominantly orange odour, containing 400 mg cimetidine.

A clear, orange-coloured, peach-flavoured syrup, each 5 ml dose containing 200 mg cimetidine.

Ampoules containing 200 mg cimetidine in 2 ml solution.

Infusion bags (flexible plastic containers) containing 400 mg cimetidine in 100 ml 0.9% w/v sodium chloride.

**Uses** Tagamet is a histamine $H_2$-receptor antagonist which rapidly inhibits both basal and stimulated gastric secretion of acid and reduces pepsin output.

Tagamet is indicated in the treatment of duodenal and benign gastric ulceration, including that associated with non-steroidal anti-inflammatory agent recurrent and stomal ulceration, oesophageal reflu disease and other conditions where reduction gastric acid by Tagamet has been shown to b beneficial: persistent dyspeptic symptoms with without ulceration, particularly meal-related upp abdominal pain, including such symptoms associate with non-steroidal anti-inflammatory agents; the pr phylaxis of gastro-intestinal haemorrhage from stres ulceration in seriously ill patients; before gener anaesthesia in patients thought to be at risk of ac aspiration (Mendelson's) syndrome, particularly o stetric patients during labour; to reduce malabsor tion and fluid loss in the short bowel syndrome; an in pancreatic insufficiency to reduce degradation enzyme supplements. Tagamet is also recommende in the management of the Zollinger-Ellison syndrom

**Dosage and administration** Tagamet is usually give orally, but parenteral or nasogastric dosing may b substituted for all or part of the recommended or dose in cases where oral dosing is impracticable considered inappropriate.

The total daily dose by any route should n normally exceed 2.4 g. Dosage should be reduced patients with impaired renal function (see *Preca tions*).

*ADULTS*

*Oral:* For patients with duodenal or benign gastr ulceration, a single daily dose of 800 mg at bedtime recommended. Otherwise the usual dosage is 400 m twice a day with breakfast and at bedtime. Oth effective regimens are 200 mg three times a day wi meals and 400 mg at bedtime (1.0 g/day) and, inadequate, 400 mg four times a day (1.6 g/day) als with meals and at bedtime.

Symptomatic relief is usually rapid. Treatme should be given initially for at least four weeks (s weeks in benign gastric ulcer, eight weeks in ulc associated with continued non-steroidal anti-inflan matory agents). Most ulcers will have healed by th stage, but those which have not will usually do s after a further course of treatment.

Treatment may be continued for longer periods those patients who may benefit from reduction gastric secretion and the dosage may be reduced appropriate to 400 mg at bedtime or 400 mg in th morning and at bedtime.

In patients with benign peptic ulcer disease, relaps may be prevented by continued treatment, usual with 400 mg at bedtime; 400 mg in the morning an at bedtime has also been used.

In oesophageal reflux disease, 400 mg four times day, with meals and at bedtime, for four to eig weeks is recommended to heal oesophagitis an relieve associated symptoms.

In patients with very high gastric acid secretion (e. Zollinger-Ellison syndrome) it may be necessary increase the dose to 400 mg four times a day, or occasional cases further.

Antacids can be made available to all patients un symptoms disappear.

In the prophylaxis of haemorrhage from stre ulceration in seriously ill patients, doses of 20 400 mg can be given every four to six hours by ora nasogastric or parenteral routes. By direct intraveno injection a dose of 200 mg should not be exceede see below.

In patients thought to be at risk of acid aspiratic syndrome an oral dose of 400 mg can be given 9 120 minutes before induction of general anaesthes or, in obstetric practice, at the start of labour. Wh such a risk persists, a dose of up to 400 mg may b repeated (parenterally if appropriate) at four-hour intervals as required up to the usual daily maximu of 2.4 g. Tagamet syrup should not be used. The usu precautions to avoid acid aspiration should be take

In the short bowel syndrome, e.g. following su stantial resection for Crohn's disease, the usu dosage range (see above) can be used according individual response.

To reduce degradation of pancreatic enzyme su plements, 800–1600 mg a day may be given accordi to response in four divided doses, one to one and half hours before meals.

*Administration of effervescent tablets:* The table should be dissolved in a glass of water.

*Parenteral:* Tagamet may be given intramuscularly intravenously.

The dose by intramuscular injection is norma 200 mg which may be repeated at four- to six-hour intervals.

The usual dosage for intravenous administration 200–400 mg which may be repeated four- to si hourly.

If direct intravenous injection cannot be avoide 200 mg should be given **slowly** over at least tw minutes, and may be repeated four- to six-hourl Rapid intravenous injection has been associated wi cardiac arrhythmias. If there is cardiovascular impai ment, or if a larger dose is needed, the dose shou e diluted and given over at least 10 minutes. In such ases infusion is preferable.

For intermittent intravenous infusion, the contents f one Tagamet Infusion bag (containing cimetidine 00 mg in 100 ml 0.9% w/v sodium chloride) should e infused over 30 minutes to one hour, and may be epeated every four to six hours.

If continuous intravenous infusion is required, agamet may be given at an average rate of 50 to 00 mg/hour over 24 hours.

*LDERLY*

The normal adult dosage may be used unless renal unction is markedly impaired (see *Precautions* and *dverse reactions*).

*HILDREN*

Experience in children is less than that in adults. In hildren more than one year old, Tagamet 25–30 mg/ g body weight per day in divided doses may be dministered by either the oral or parenteral route.

The use of Tagamet in infants under one year old is ot fully evaluated; 20 mg/kg body weight per day in ivided doses has been used.

**ontra-indications, warnings, etc**

*ontra-indication:* Hypersensitivity to cimetidine.

*recautions:* Dosage should be reduced in patients ith impaired renal function according to creatinine earance. The following dosages are suggested: eatinine clearance of 0 to 15 ml per minute, 200 mg vice a day; 15 to 30 ml per minute, 200 mg three mes a day; 30 to 50 ml per minute, 200 mg four times day; over 50 ml per minute, normal dosage. Cimeti- ine is removed by haemodialysis, but not to any gnificant extent by peritoneal dialysis.

Tagamet can prolong the elimination of drugs etabolised by oxidation in the liver. Although harmacological interactions with a number of drugs, g. diazepam, propranolol, have been demonstrated, nly those with oral anticoagulants, phenytoin, the- phylline and intravenous lignocaine appear, to date, be of clinical significance. Close monitoring of atients on Tagamet receiving oral anticoagulants or henytoin is recommended and a reduction in the osage of these drugs may be necessary.

Clinical trials of over six years' continuous treatment nd more than fifteen years' widespread use have not evealed unexpected adverse reactions related to ng-term therapy. The safety of prolonged use is not, owever, fully established and care should be taken observe periodically patients given prolonged eatment.

Tagamet treatment can mask the symptoms and low transient healing of gastric cancer. The potential elay in diagnosis should particularly be borne in ind in patients of middle age and over with new or cently changed dyspeptic symptoms.

Care should be taken that patients with a history of eptic ulcer, particularly the elderly, being treated ith Tagamet and a non-steroidal anti-inflammatory gent are observed regularly.

In patients on drug treatment or with illnesses that ould cause falls in blood cell count, the possibility at $H_2$-receptor antagonism could potentiate this ffect should be borne in mind.

*se in pregnancy and lactation:* Although tests in nimals and clinical evidence have not revealed any azards from the administration of Tagamet during regnancy or lactation, both animal and human udies have shown that it does cross the placental arrier and is excreted in milk. As with most drugs, e use of Tagamet should be avoided during preg- ancy and lactation unless essential.

*dverse reactions:* Over 56 million patients have been eated with Tagamet worldwide and adverse reac- ons have been infrequent. Diarrhoea, dizziness or sh, usually mild and transient, and tiredness have een reported. Gynaecomastia has been reported and almost always reversible on discontinuing treat- ent. Biochemical or biopsy evidence of reversible ver damage has been reported occasionally. Revers- le confusional states have occurred, usually in derly or already very ill patients, e.g. those with nal failure. Thrombocytopenia and leucopenia, in- uding agranulocytosis (see *Precautions*), reversible n withdrawal of treatment, have been reported rarely; ancytopenia and aplastic anaemia have been re- orted very rarely. There have been very rare reports f interstitial nephritis, acute pancreatitis, fever, head- che, myalgia, arthralgia, sinus bradycardia, tachycar- a and heart block, all reversible on withdrawal of eatment. In common with other $H_2$-receptor antago- sts, there have been very rare reports of anaphylaxis. opecia has been reported but no causal relationship as been established. Reversible impotence has also een very rarely reported but no causal relationship as been established at usual therapeutic doses. olated increases of plasma creatinine have been of o clinical significance.

*verdosage:* Acute overdosage of up to 20 grams has een reported several times with no significant ill effects. Induction of vomiting and/or gastric lavage may be employed together with symptomatic and supportive therapy.

**Pharmaceutical precautions** Store effervescent tablets in a dry place, and replace cap after use. Store syrup below 25°C, and ampoules below 30°C, protected from light. Store infusion bags below 25°C, and protect from light except during use.

**Legal category** POM.

**Package quantities** Tiltab Tablets, 800 mg, in opaque calendar packs (OP) of 30 (2 × 15). Tablets, 400 mg, in opaque calendar packs (OP) of 60 (4 × 15) †, ward packs of 1000 (20 × 50). Tiltab Tablets, 200 mg, in opaque blister packs (OP) of 120 (4 × 30) †. Effervescent Tablets, 400 mg, in containers (OP) of 60 (4 tubes each containing 15 tablets) †. Syrup in bottles (OP) containing 600 ml †. Ampoules in boxes of 20 †. Infusion bags in boxes of 20 †.

† with Patient Information Leaflet.

**Further information** Tagamet has been shown to be compatible with electrolyte and dextrose solutions commonly used for intravenous infusion.

Inactive ingredients in the effervescent tablets include aspartame and sodium benzoate. These tablets also contain sodium bicarbonate and the total sodium content per tablet is 415 mg. Inactive ingredients in the syrup include ethanol, methyl paraben, propyl paraben, sucrose and E110. Inactive ingredients in the injection are hydrochloric acid and water for injection and in the infusion are sodium chloride, hydrochloric acid, sodium hydroxide and water for injection.

Tagamet Effervescent Tablets may be particularly suitable for patients with difficulty in swallowing.

**Product licence numbers**

| | |
|---|---|
| Tagamet Tiltab tablets 800 mg | 0002/0128. |
| Tagamet Tablets 400 mg | 0002/0092. |
| Tagamet Tiltab Tablets 200 mg | 0002/0063R. |
| Tagamet Effervescent Tablets 400 mg | 0002/0206. |
| Tagamet Syrup | 0002/0073R. |
| Tagamet Injection | 0002/0059R. |
| Tagamet Infusion | 0002/0112. |

## TRIVAX*-HIB VACCINE ▼ Adsorbed Diphtheria, Tetanus and Pertussis Vaccine BP, DTPer/VAC/Ads (Trivax-AD*) and Haemophilus Type B Conjugate Vaccine (Hib)

**Qualitative and quantitative composition** Trivax-Hib contains Adsorbed Diphtheria, Tetanus and Pertussis Vaccine BP adsorbed on to aluminium hydroxide. It also contains purified polyribosyl-ribitol-phosphate capsular polysaccharide (PRP) of Hib, covalently bound to tetanus toxoid.

The Trivax-AD* components are prepared from chemically detoxified *Corynebacterium diphtheriae* and *Clostridium tetani* exotoxins, and killed whole *Bordetella pertussis* organisms.

The Hib polysaccharide is prepared from Hib, strain 20 752 and after activation with cyanogen bromide and derivatisation with adipic hydrazide spacer is coupled to tetanus toxoid via carbodiimide condensation. After purification the conjugate is lyophilised in the presence of lactose as a stabiliser.

Trivax-Hib meets the World Health Organisation requirements for manufacture of biological substances of Hib conjugate vaccines and of diphtheria, tetanus, pertussis and combined vaccines.

A 0.5 ml dose of the vaccine contains not less than 30 International units (IU) of diphtheria toxoid, not less than 60 IU of tetanus toxoid and not more than 20,000 million *Bordetella pertussis* organisms with a potency of not less than 4 IU adsorbed onto aluminium hydroxide and 10 micrograms of purified capsular polysaccharide of Hib covalently bound to approximately 30 micrograms tetanus toxoid.

**Pharmaceutical form** Hib vaccine (lyophilised) for reconstitution with Trivax-AD vaccine (suspension).

**Clinical particulars**

*Therapeutic indications:* Trivax-Hib is indicated for active immunisation against diphtheria, tetanus, pertussis and *Haemophilus influenzae* type b in infants and children under ten years of age.

*Posology and method of administration*

*Posology:* The primary immunisation course should start at two months of age, and consists of three doses with an interval of at least one month between each dose.

Each dose consists of 0.5 ml of the vaccine by intramuscular injection.

*Method of administration:* Intramuscular injection.

*Contra-indications:* Trivax-Hib should not be administered to subjects with known hypersensitivity to any component of the vaccine, or to subjects that have shown any signs of hypersensitivity after previous administration of diphtheria, tetanus, pertussis or Hib vaccines.

As with other vaccines, the administration of Trivax-Hib should be postponed in subjects suffering from acute severe febrile illness. The presence of a minor non-febrile infection, however, is not a contra-indication to vaccination.

Progressive degenerative neurological disorder.

Severe local reaction to previous dose of the vaccine or one of its components–an area of erythema, swelling and induration involving most of the anterolateral thigh or a major part of the circumference of the upper arm.

Severe general reaction to a previous dose of the vaccine or one of its components–for example:

a. Prolonged inconsolable crying or screaming for over three hours.
b. A convulsion or temperature >40.5°C occurring within 72 hours, for which no other cause was found.
c. Hypotonia–hyporesponsive episode occurring within 72 hours.
d. Severe acute neurological illness occurring within 72 hours.
e. Immediate allergic reaction (severe or anaphylactic) to a previous dose of diphtheria, tetanus or pertussis vaccine.

Any child exhibiting a severe local or significant general reaction to a previous dose of a pertussis-containing vaccine should not be given a further dose of pertussis-containing vaccine. However, protection against diphtheria, tetanus and Hib is advisable and can be accomplished by giving Adsorbed Diphtheria and Tetanus Vaccine (CHILD), and a separate dose of Hib.

The vaccine should not be injected intradermally.

**Trivax-Hib should not be administered to children aged ten years and over, adults and the elderly.**

*Special warnings and precautions for use:* Where there is a family or personal history of febrile convulsions, there is an increased risk of these occurring after pertussis immunisation. In such children, immunisation is recommended but advice on prevention of fever should be given at the time of immunisation.

In a recent British study, children with a personal or family history of epilepsy were immunised with pertussis vaccine without any significant adverse events. These children's developmental progress has been normal. In children with a close family history (first degree relatives) of idiopathic epilepsy there may be a risk of developing this condition irrespective of vaccination. Immunisation is recommended for these children. Children whose epilepsy is well controlled may receive pertussis vaccine.

Advice on the prevention of fever should be given.

When there is still an evolving neurological problem, immunisation should be deferred until the condition is stable. When there has been a documented history of cerebral damage in the neonatal period, immunisation should be carried out unless there is evidence of an evolving neurological abnormality. A personal or family history of allergy is not a contra-indication to immunisation with pertussis nor are stable neurological conditions such as cerebral palsy or spina bifida. Where there is doubt, appropriate advice should be sought from a consultant paediatrician, district (Health Board) Immunisation co-ordinator or a consultant in communicable disease control, rather than withholding the vaccine. HIV-positive individuals may receive pertussis vaccine in the absence of contra-indications.

It is good clinical practice that immunisation should be preceded by a review of the medical history (especially with regard to previous immunisation and possible occurrence of undesirable events) and a clinical examination.

As with all vaccinations, a solution of 1:1000 adrenaline should be available for injection should an anaphylactic reaction occur. Recipients of the vaccine should remain under observation until they have been seen to be in good health and not to be experiencing an immediate adverse reaction. It is not possible to specify an exact length of time.

Antipyretic measures may be indicated in those who experience a febrile convulsion following vaccination.

Use of Trivax-Hib in individuals aged ten years and over may be associated with severe hypersensitivity reactions.

Trivax-Hib should be administered with caution to subjects with thrombocytopenia or a bleeding disorder since bleeding may occur following an intramuscular administration to these subjects. In these subjects Trivax-Hib may be administered by deep subcutaneous injection.

**Trivax-Hib should under no circumstances be administered intravenously or intradermally.**

Excretion of capsular polysaccharide antigen in the urine has been described following receipt of the Hib vaccine and therefore antigen detection may not have a diagnostic value in suspected Hib disease within one to two weeks of vaccination.

*Interactions with other medicaments and other forms of interaction:* Trivax-Hib can be administered simultaneously with oral polio.

As with other vaccines it may be expected that in patients receiving immunosuppressive therapy or patients with immunodeficiency, an adequate response may not be achieved.

*Pregnancy and lactation:* No reproductive studies have been conducted in animals since simultaneous vaccination against diphtheria, tetanus, pertussis and Hib in adults is uncommon. There is no accurate information on the safety of this vaccine in pregnancy therefore this vaccine should not be used in pregnancy or during lactation.

*Effects on ability to drive and use machines:* There is no information available on the effect of Trivax-Hib on driving and use of machines.

*Undesirable effects:* Local reactions, particularly erythema, pain and mild swelling at the site of injection, are commonly seen during the 24 hours following vaccination. They normally subside without treatment. A nodule may be found at the site of the injection, especially if the inoculation is introduced into the superficial layers of subcutaneous tissue.

A transient rise in temperature, restlessness, irritability, crying, loss of appetite, vomiting or diarrhoea may sometimes occur a few hours after vaccination, but does not generally call for treatment. Systemic reactions such as headache, malaise and somnolence have been reported. Allergic manifestations including pallor, dyspnoea and collapse have been observed rarely.

Neurological events have occasionally been observed following the administration of pertussis-containing vaccines. The events reported do not appear to constitute a single, identifiable clinical syndrome but include isolated febrile convulsions, infantile spasms, episodes of persistent screaming and severe encephalopathy resulting in permanent brain damage or death. These events cannot be distinguished from those occurring in unvaccinated children of similar age. In the absence of a common, identifiable pathological mechanism, it is not possible to produce a reliable estimate of the incidence of neurological events attributable to pertussis vaccination *per se*.

An increased incidence of reactions may occur due to failure to shake the container and re-suspend the vaccine before withdrawing a dose, to inadvertent intravenous administration, or to an over-rapid injection.

Since combined diphtheria, tetanus and pertussis vaccines are widely used in populations in which sudden illnesses of undefined origin are not uncommon, intercurrent illness bearing a temporal but not a causal relationship to vaccination may be expected.

Any untoward reactions should be reported to the regulatory authorities and to the manufacturer.

*Overdose:* Not applicable.

**Pharmacological properties**

*Pharmacodynamic properties:* Evaluation of pharmacodynamic properties is not required for vaccines.

*Pharmacokinetic properties:* Evaluation of pharmacokinetic properties is not required for vaccines.

*Preclinical safety data:* Not applicable.

*Relevant Information for vaccines:*

*Trivax-AD Component:* One month after the primary vaccination course 100% of infants vaccinated with Trivax-Hib had antibody titres of ≥ 0.1 IU/ml to tetanus and diphtheria. The vaccine response to the pertussis antigens (PT, FHA, pertactin and agglutinogens II, III) was also 100% i.e. all infants vaccinated at the end of the primary course had a level of antibodies higher than had been present prior to vaccination.

*Haemophilus Influenzae Type b component:* Titres of ≥ 0.15µg/ml have been obtained in 95-100% of infants one month after the completion of a primary vaccination course. Similar titres are seen following primary immunisation with Trivax-Hib.

**Pharmaceutical particulars**

*List of excipients:* Lyophilised Hib vaccine: Lactose.

Trivax-AD vaccine: Aluminium hydroxide, sodium borate, succinic acid, sodium chloride (1.8 mg of elemental sodium per 0.5 ml dose), thiomersal, water for injections.

*Incompatibilities:* Trivax-Hib should not be mixed with other vaccines in the same syringe, unless specified by the manufacturer.

*Shelf life:* The shelf-life of the Trivax-Hib vaccine is two years when stored unopened and unmixed at 2°C to 8°C.

*Special precautions for storage:* Store between 2°C and 8°C. Protect from light. The Trivax-AD vaccine should not be frozen.

*Nature and contents of container:* The lyophilised Hib vaccine is presented as a white pellet in a glass vial.

The Trivax-AD vaccine is a suspension supplied in a prefilled syringe made of neutral glass type 1, which conforms to the European Pharmacopoeia. The prefilled syringe contains an overage to compensate for product loss during reconstitution with lyophilised Hib and should not be used on its own.

*Instructions for use/handling:* The Trivax-AD vaccine and reconstituted Trivax-Hib vaccine should be inspected visually for any foreign particulate matter and/or variation of physical aspect prior to administration. In the event of either being observed, discard the vaccines.

The Hib vaccine must be reconstituted by adding the entire contents of the supplied container of the Trivax-AD vaccine to the vial containing the Hib pellet as follows:

a. Attach the supplied green needle to the prefilled syringe of Trivax-AD.
b. Insert the green needle attached to the prefilled syringe of Trivax-AD through the bung into the Hib vial.
c. Inject the contents of the prefilled syringe of Trivax-AD into the Hib vial.
d. With the needle still inserted, shake the Hib vial vigorously and examine for complete dissolution i.e. a whitish liquid of uniform appearance should be formed.
e. Withdraw the entire mixture back into the syringe.
(f) Replace the green needle with the smaller orange needle supplied and administer the vaccine by intramuscular injection.

After reconstitution, Trivax-Hib should be injected promptly (within one hour).

Disposal should be by incineration at a temperature not less than 1100°C at a registered waste disposal contractor. Trivax-AD vaccine which has been frozen should not be used.

**Marketing authorisation number** 10592/0083

**Date of approval/revision of SPC** 4 July 1997

**Legal category** POM

## TWINRIX* ADULT VACCINE ▼
## Combined inactivated hepatitis A (720 ELISA units) and r DNA hepatitis B (20 mcg) Vaccine

**Qualitative and quantitative composition** Twinrix Adult is a combined vaccine formulated by pooling bulk preparations of the purified, inactivated hepatitis A (HA) virus and purified hepatitis B surface antigen (HBsAg), separately adsorbed on to aluminium hydroxide and aluminium phosphate. The HA virus is propagated in $MRC_5$ human diploid cells. HBsAg is produced by culture, in a selective medium, of genetically engineered yeast cells.

A 1.0 ml dose of vaccine contains not less than 720 ELISA Units of inactivated HA virus and 20 mcg of recombinant HBsAg protein.

**Pharmaceutical form** Suspension for injection.

**Clinical particulars**

*Therapeutic indications:* Twinrix Adult is indicated for use in non-immune adults and adolescents 16 years of age and above who are at risk of both hepatitis A and hepatitis B infection.

*Posology and method of administration:*

*Dosage:* A dose of 1.0 ml is recommended for adults and adolescents 16 years of age and above.

*Primary vaccination schedule:* The standard primary course of vaccination with Twinrix Adult consists of three doses, the first administered at the elected date, the second one month later and the third six months after the first dose. The recommended schedule should be adhered to.

Once initiated, the primary course of vaccination should be completed with the same vaccine.

*Booster dose:* It is not yet fully established whether immunocompetent individuals who have responded to hepatitis A and/or B vaccination(s) will require booster doses as protection in the absence of detectable antibodies may be ensured by immunological memory.

Long-term antibody persistence data following vaccination with Twinrix Adult are not currently available. However, the anti-HBs and anti-HAV antibody titres observed following a primary vaccination course with the combined vaccine are in the range of what is seen following vaccination with the monovalent vaccines. General guidelines for booster vaccination can therefore be drawn from experience with the monovalent vaccines. These guidelines are based on the assumption that a minimal antibody level is required for protection; protective levels (10 mIU/ml) of anti-HBs will persist in the majority of subjects for five years, with anti-HAV predicted to persist for at least 10 years.

Booster vaccination with the combined vaccine ca be recommended five years after initiation of th primary course. If the monovalent vaccines are use as boosters, they can be administered five years aft initiation of the primary course for hepatitis B and 1 years after initiation of the primary course for hepatit A.

Antibody levels of subjects at risk can be assesse at regular intervals and appropriate boosters admi istered when titres fall below minimal levels.

*Method of administration:* Twinrix Adult is f intramuscular injection, preferably in the delto region.

Exceptionally the vaccine may be administere subcutaneously in patients with thrombocytopenia bleeding disorders. However, this route of administr tion may result in suboptimal immune response the vaccine (see *Warnings and precautions*).

*Contra-indications:* Twinrix Adult should not be a ministered to subjects with known hypersensitivity any constituent of the vaccine, or to subjects havir shown signs of hypersensitivity after previous admi istration of Twinrix Adult or the monovalent hepatit A or hepatitis B vaccine.

As with other vaccines, the administration of Twinr Adult should be postponed in subjects suffering fro acute severe febrile illness.

*Special warnings and special precautions for use:* It possible that subjects may be in the incubation peric of a hepatitis A or hepatitis B infection at the time vaccination. It is not known whether Twinrix Adu will prevent hepatitis A and hepatitis B in such case

The vaccine will not prevent infection caused b other agents such as hepatitis C and hepatitis E ar other pathogens known to infect the liver.

Twinrix Adult is not recommended for post-exp sure prophylaxis (e.g. needle-stick injury).

The vaccine has not been tested in patients wi impaired immunity. In haemodialysis patients ar persons with an impaired immune system, adequa anti-HAV and anti-HBs antibody titres may not b obtained after the primary immunisation course a such patients may therefore require administration additional doses of vaccine.

As with all injectable vaccines, appropriate medic treatment and supervision should always be readi available in case of a rare anaphylactic event followi the administration of the vaccine.

Since intradermal injection or intramuscular admi istration into the gluteal muscle could lead to suboptimal response to the vaccine, these rout should be avoided. However, exceptionally Twinr Adult can be administered subcutaneously to subjec with thrombocytopenia or bleeding disorders sin bleeding may occur following an intramuscular a ministration to these subjects (see *Posology a method of administration*).

**Twinrix Adult should under no circumstances b administered intravascularly.**

*Interactions with other medicinal products and oth forms of interaction:* No data on concomitant admi istration of Twinrix Adult with specific hepatitis immunoglobulin or hepatitis B immunoglobulin ha been generated. However, when the monovale hepatitis A and hepatitis B vaccines were administere concomitantly with specific immunoglobulins, influence on seroconversion was observed althou it may result in lower antibody titres.

Although the concomitant administration of Twin Adult and other vaccines has not specifically be studied, it is anticipated that, if different syringes a other injection sites are used, no interaction will observed.

It may be expected that in patients receivi immunosuppressive treatment or patients with i munodeficiency, an adequate response may not achieved.

*Use during pregnancy and lactation:*

*Pregnancy:* The effect of Twinrix Adult on foe development has not been assessed.

However, as with all inactivated vaccines, one do not expect harm to the foetus. Twinrix Adult shou be used during pregnancy only when there is a cle risk of hepatitis A and hepatitis B.

*Lactation:* The effect on breast-fed infants of t administration of Twinrix Adult to their mothers h not been evaluated in clinical studies. Twinrix Ad should therefore be used with caution in brea feeding women.

*Effects on the ability to drive and use machines:* T vaccine is unlikely to produce an effect on the abil to drive and use machines.

*Undesirable effects:* In controlled clinical studi signs and symptoms were actively monitored in subjects for four days following the administration the vaccine. A checklist was used for this purpos The vaccinees were also requested to report a clinical events occurring during the study period. T most common reactions were those at the site injection. They included transient pain, redness and swelling. Systemic adverse events seen were fever, headache, malaise, fatigue, nausea and vomiting. These events were transient, only rarely reported and were considered by the subjects as mild.

In a comparative study it was noted that the frequency of solicited adverse events following the administration of Twinrix Adult is not different from the frequency of solicited adverse events following the administration of the monovalent vaccines.

Following widespread use of the monovalent hepatitis A and/or hepatitis B vaccines, the following undesirable events have been reported in temporal association in the days or weeks after vaccination. In many instances, a causal relationship has not been established.

Flu-like symptoms (such as fever, chills, headache, myalgia, arthralgia), fatigue, dizziness.

Rarely reported: paraesthesia, nausea, vomiting, decreased appetite, diarrhoea, abdominal pain, abnormal liver function tests, rash, pruritus, urticaria.

Very rarely reported: allergic reactions mimicking serum sickness, vasculitis, syncope, hypotension, lymphadenopathy, cases of peripheral and/or central neurological disorders, and may include multiple sclerosis, optic neuritis, myelitis, Bells palsy, polyneuritis such as Guillain-Barré syndrome (with ascending paralysis), meningitis, encephalitis, encephalopathy, thrombocytopenic purpura, erythema exsudativum multiforme.

*Overdose:* No information available.

**Pharmacological properties**

*Pharmacodynamic properties:* Pharmacotherapeutic group: Hepatitis vaccines, ATC code JO7BC.

Twinrix Adult confers immunity against HAV and HBV infection by inducing specific anti-HAV and anti-HBs antibodies.

Protection against hepatitis A and hepatitis B develops within two to four weeks. In the clinical studies, specific humoral antibodies against hepatitis A were observed in approximately 94% of the adults one month after the first dose and in 100% one month after the third dose (i.e. month seven). Specific humoral antibodies against hepatitis B were observed in 70% of the adults after the first dose and approximately 99% after the third dose.

Based on experience with the monovalent vaccines, it is expected that in most vaccinees the antibodies will persist for at least four to five years after the primary vaccination course. To establish long-term protection, booster vaccination with either the monovalent vaccines or the combination vaccine is indicated (see *Posology and method of administration*).

*Pharmacokinetic properties:* Evaluation of pharmacokinetic properties is not required for vaccines.

*Preclinical safety data:* Not applicable.

**Pharmaceutical particulars**

*List of excipients:* Aluminium hydroxide, aluminium phosphate, aminoacids for injection, formaldehyde, neomycin sulphate, 2-phenoxyethanol, polysorbate 20, sodium chloride, residual tris and phosphate buffer and water for injection.

*Incompatibilities:* Twinrix Adult should not be mixed with other vaccines in the same syringe.

*Shelf-life:* The expiry date of the vaccine is indicated on the label and packaging.

Shelf-life is 24 months when stored at +2°C to +8°C.

*Special precautions for storage:* Twinrix Adult should be stored at +2°C to +8°C.

**Do not freeze;** discard if the vaccine has been frozen.

*Nature and contents of container:* Twinrix Adult is presented in a glass prefilled syringe.

The prefilled syringes are made of neutral glass type I, which conforms to European Pharmacopoeia requirements.

The content upon storage may present a fine white deposit with a clear colourless supernatant. Once shaken, the vaccine is slightly opaque.

*Instructions for use/handling:* The vaccine should be inspected visually for any foreign particulate matter and/or variation of physical aspect prior to administration. Before use of Twinrix Adult, the vaccine should be well shaken to obtain a slightly opaque, white suspension. Discard if the content appears otherwise.

**Marketing authorisation numbers**

| | |
|---|---|
| Pack of 1 prefilled syringe | EU/1/96/020/001 |
| Packs 10 prefilled syringes | EU 1/96/020/002 |

**Date of approval/revision of SPC** 20 September 1996

**Legal category** POM.

## TWINRIX* PAEDIATRIC VACCINE ▼
## Combined inactivated hepatitis A (360 ELISA units) and r DNA hepatitis B (10 mcg) Vaccine

**Qualitative and quantitative composition** Twinrix Paediatric is a combined vaccine formulated by pooling bulk preparations of the purified, inactivated hepatitis A (HA) virus and purified hepatitis B surface antigen (HBsAg), separately adsorbed on to aluminium hydroxide and aluminium phosphate.

The HA virus is propagated in $MRC_5$ human diploid cells. HBsAg is produced by culture, in a selective medium, of genetically engineered yeast cells.

A 0.5 ml dose of Twinrix Paediatric contains not less than 360 ELISA Units of inactivated HA virus and 10 mcg of recombinant HBsAg protein.

**Pharmaceutical form** Suspension for injection.

**Clinical particulars**

*Therapeutic indications:* Twinrix Paediatric is indicated for use in non-immune infants, children and adolescents from one year up to and including 15 years who are at risk of both hepatitis A and hepatitis B infection.

Posology and method of administration:

Dosage: The dose of 0.5 ml (360 ELISA Units HA/10 mcg HBsAg) is recommended for infants, children and adolescents from one year up to and including 15 years of age.

*Primary vaccination schedule:* The standard primary course of vaccination with Twinrix Paediatric consists of three doses, the first administered at the elected date, the second one month later and the third six months after the first dose. The recommended schedule should be adhered to. Once initiated, the primary course of vaccination should be completed with the same vaccine.

*Booster dose:* It is not yet fully established whether immunocompetent individuals who have responded to hepatitis A and/or B vaccination(s) will require booster doses as protection in the absence of detectable antibodies may be ensured by immunological memory.

Long-term antibody persistence data following vaccination with Twinrix Paediatric are not currently available. However, the anti-HBs and anti-HAV antibody titres observed following a primary vaccination course with the combined vaccine are in the range of what is seen following vaccination with the monovalent vaccines. General guidelines for booster vaccination can therefore be drawn from experience with the monovalent vaccines. These guidelines are based on the assumption that a minimal antibody level is required for protection; protective levels (10 mIU/ml) of anti-HBs will persist in the majority of subjects for five years, with anti-HAV predicted to persist for at least 10 years.

Booster vaccination with the combined vaccine can be recommended five years after initiation of the primary course. If the monovalent vaccines are used as boosters, they can be administered five years after initiation of the primary course for hepatitis B and 10 years after initiation of the primary course for hepatitis A.

Antibody levels of subjects at risk can be assessed at regular intervals and appropriate boosters administered when titres fall below minimal levels.

*Method of administration:* Twinrix Paediatric is for intramuscular injection, preferably in the deltoid region in adolescents and children or in the anterolateral thigh in infants.

Exceptionally, the vaccine may be administered subcutaneously in patients with thrombocytopenia or bleeding disorders. However, this route of administration may result in suboptimal immune response to the vaccine (see *Warnings and precautions*).

*Contra-indications:* Twinrix Paediatric should not be administered to subjects with known hypersensitivity to any constituent of the vaccine, or to subjects having shown signs of hypersensitivity after previous administration of Twinrix Paediatric or the monovalent hepatitis A or hepatitis B vaccine.

As with other vaccines, the administration of Twinrix Paediatric should be postponed in subjects suffering from acute severe febrile illness.

*Special warnings and special precautions for use:* It is possible that subjects may be in the incubation period of a hepatitis A or hepatitis B infection at the time of vaccination. It is not known whether Twinrix Paediatric will prevent hepatitis A and hepatitis B in such cases.

The vaccine will not prevent infection caused by other agents such as hepatitis C and hepatitis E and other pathogens known to infect the liver.

Twinrix Paediatric is not recommended for post-exposure prophylaxis (e.g. needlestick injury).

The vaccine has not been tested in patients with impaired immunity. In haemodialysis patients, patients receiving immunosuppressive treatment or patients with an impaired immune system, the anticipated immune response may not be achieved after the primary immunisation course. Such patients may require additional doses of vaccine; nevertheless immunocompromised patients may fail to demonstrate an adequate response.

As with all injectable vaccines, appropriate medical treatment and supervision should always be readily available in case of a rare anaphylactic event following the administration of the vaccine.

Since intradermal injection or intramuscular administration into the gluteal muscle could lead to a suboptimal response to the vaccine, these routes should be avoided. However, exceptionally Twinrix Paediatric can be administered subcutaneously to subjects with thrombocytopenia or bleeding disorders since bleeding may occur following an intramuscular administration to these subjects (see *Posology and method of administration*).

**Twinrix paediatric should under no circumstances be administered intravascularly.**

*Interaction with other medicinal products and other forms of interaction:* No data on concomitant administration of Twinrix Paediatric with specific hepatitis A immunoglobulin or hepatitis B immunoglobulin have been generated. However, when the monovalent hepatitis A and hepatitis B vaccines were administered concomitantly with specific immunoglobulins, no influence on seroconversion was observed although it may result in lower antibody titres (see also *Warnings and precautions*).

As the concomitant administration of Twinrix Paediatric and other vaccines has not specifically been studied, it is advised that the vaccine should not be administered at the same time as other vaccines.

*Use during pregnancy and lactation:*

**Pregnancy:** The effect of Twinrix Paediatric on foetal development has not been assessed. However, as with all inactivated vaccines, one does not expect harm to the foetus. Twinrix Paediatric should be used during pregnancy only when there is a clear risk of hepatitis A and hepatitis B.

**Lactation:** The effect on breast-fed infants of the administration of Twinrix Paediatric to their mothers has not been evaluated in clinical studies. Twinrix Paediatric should therefore be used with caution in breast-feeding women.

*Effects on the ability to drive and use machines:* The vaccine is unlikely to produce an effect on the ability to drive and use machines.

*Undesirable effects:* During clinical studies, the most common reactions were those at the site of injection (pain, redness and swelling).

Following widespread use of the monovalent hepatitis A and/or hepatitis B vaccines in adults and in children, the following undesirable events have been reported in temporal association in the days or weeks after vaccination. In many instances, a causal relationship has not been established.

Flu-like symptoms (such as fever, chills, headache, myalgia, arthralgia), fatigue, dizziness.

Rarely reported: paraesthesia, nausea, vomiting, decreased appetite, diarrhoea, abdominal pain, abnormal liver function tests, rash, pruritus, urticaria.

Very rarely reported: allergic reactions mimicking serum sickness, vasculitis, syncope, hypotension, lymphadenopathy, cases of peripheral and/or central neurological disorders, and may include multiple sclerosis, optic neuritis, myelitis, Bell's palsy, polyneuritis such as Guillain-Barré syndrome (with ascending paralysis), meningitis, encephalitis, encephalopathy, thrombocytopenic purpura, erythema exsudativum multiforme.

*Overdose:* No information available.

**Pharmacological properties**

*Pharmacodynamic properties:* Pharmacotherapeutic group: Hepatitis vaccines, ATC code JO7BC.

Twinrix Paediatric confers immunity against HAV and HBV infection by inducing specific anti-HA and anti-HBs antibodies.

Protection against hepatitis A and hepatitis B develops within two to four weeks. In the clinical studies, specific humoral antibodies against hepatitis A were observed in approximately 89% of the subjects one month after the first dose and in 100% one month after the third dose (i.e. month seven). Specific humoral antibodies against hepatitis B were observed in approximately 67% of the subjects after the first dose and 100% after the third dose.

Based on experience with the monovalent vaccines, it is expected that in most vaccinees the antibodies will persist for at least four to five years after the primary vaccination course. To establish long-term protection, booster vaccination with either the monovalent vaccines or the combined vaccine is indicated (see *Posology and method of administration*).

*Pharmacokinetic properties:* Evaluation of pharmacokinetic properties is not required for vaccines.

*Preclinical safety data:* Not applicable.

**Pharmaceutical particulars**

*List of excipients:* Aluminium hydroxide, aluminium phosphate, amino acids for injection, formaldehyde, neomycin sulphate, 2-phenoxyethanol, polysorbate 20, sodium chloride, residual tris and phosphate buffer and water for injection.

*Incompatibilities:* Twinrix Paediatric should not be mixed with other vaccines in the same syringe.

*Shelf life:* The expiry date of the vaccine is indicated on the label and packaging. Shelf-life is 24 months when stored at +2°C to +8°C.

**Special precautions for storage:** Twinrix Paediatric should be stored at +2°C to +8°C.

**Do not freeze;** discard if the vaccine has been frozen.

*Nature and content of container:* Twinrix Paediatric is presented in a glass prefilled syringe.

The prefilled syringes are made of neutral glass type I, which conforms to European Pharmacopoeia requirements.

The content upon storage may present a fine white deposit with a clear colourless supernatant. Once shaken, the vaccine is slightly opaque.

*Instructions for use/handling:* The vaccine should be inspected visually for any foreign particulate matter and/or variation of physical aspect prior to administration. Before use of Twinrix Paediatric, the vaccine should be well shaken to obtain a slightly opaque, white suspension. Discard if the content appears otherwise.

*Marketing authorisation holder:* SmithKline Beecham Biologicals S.A., rue de l'Institut 89, 1330 Rixensart, Belgium.

**Marketing authorisation numbers**
Packs of 1 prefilled syringe        EU 1/97/029/001
Packs of 10 prefilled syringes      EU 1/97/029/002

**Date of approval/revision of SPC**    10 February 1997

**Legal category**   POM

# VECTAVIR* COLD SORE CREAM   ▼

**Qualitative and quantitative composition** Active constituent: Penciclovir 1% - INN penciclovir.

**Pharmaceutical form** White cream for topical application.

**Clinical particulars**

*Therapeutic indications:* Vectavir Cold Sore Cream is indicated for the treatment of cold sores (herpes labialis).

*Posology and method of administration*
*Adults (including ≥ 16 years of age and the elderly):* Vectavir Cold Sore Cream should be applied at approximately two hourly intervals during waking hours. Treatment should be continued for 4 days.

Treatment should be started as early as possible after the first sign of an infection.

*Children (under 16 years):* No work has been carried out in children.

*Contra-indications:* Known hypersensitivity to penciclovir or the other constituents of the formulation, e.g. propylene glycol.

*Special warnings and special precautions for use:* The cream should only be used on cold sores on the lips and around the mouth. It is not recommended for application to mucous membranes. Particular care should be taken to avoid application in or near the eyes.

Severely immunocompromised patients (e.g. AIDS patients or bone marrow transplant recipients) should be encouraged to consult a physician in case oral therapy is indicated.

*Interaction with other medicaments and other forms of interaction:* Clinical trial experience has not identified any interactions resulting from concomitant administration of topical or systemic drugs with Vectavir Cold Sore Cream.

*Pregnancy and lactation:* There is unlikely to be any cause for concern regarding adverse effects when the cream is used in pregnant and/or lactating women as systemic absorption of penciclovir following topical administration of Vectavir Cold Sore Cream has been shown to be minimal (see *Pharmacokinetic properties section*).

Animal studies have not shown any embryotoxic or teratogenic effects with penciclovir given intravenously (at doses greater than 1200 times those recommended for clinical use via topical application), nor were there any effects on male and female fertility and general reproductive performance (at doses greater than 1600 times those recommended for clinical use via topical application). Studies in rats show that penciclovir is excreted in the breast milk of lactating females given oral famciclovir (famciclovir; the oral form of penciclovir, is converted *in vivo* to penciclovir). There is no information on excretion of penciclovir in human milk.

Since the safety of penciclovir in human pregnancy has not been established, Vectavir Cold Sore Cream should only be used during pregnancy or in nursing mothers on the advice of a doctor and if the potential benefits are considered to outweigh the potential risks associated with treatment.

*Effects on ability to drive and use machines:* Adverse effects on the ability to drive or operate machinery have not been observed.

*Undesirable effects:* Vectavir Cold Sore Cream has been well-tolerated in human studies. Clinical trial experience has shown that there was no difference between Vectavir Cold Sore Cream and placebo in the rate or type of adverse reactions reported. In particular, application site reactions (e.g. transient burning, stinging, numbness) occurred in less than 3% of patients in each group in the pivotal clinical trials.

No cases of photosensitivity were reported in the pivotal clinical trials.

*Overdose:* No untoward effects would be expected even if the entire contents of a container of Vectavir Cold Sore Cream were ingested orally; penciclovir is poorly absorbed following oral administration. However, some irritation in the mouth could occur. No

specific treatment is necessary if accidental oral ingestion occurs.

**Pharmacological properties**

*Pharmacodynamic properties:* Penciclovir has demonstrable *in vivo* and *in vitro* activity against herpes simplex viruses (types 1 and 2) and varicella zoster virus. In virus-infected cells penciclovir is rapidly and efficiently converted into a triphosphate (mediated via virus-induced thymidine kinase). Penciclovir triphosphate persists in infected cells for more than 12 hours where it inhibits replication of viral DNA and has a half-life of 9, 10 and 20 hours in cells infected with varicella zoster virus, herpes simplex virus type 1 and herpes simplex virus type 2 respectively. In uninfected cells treated with penciclovir, concentrations of penciclovir triphosphate are only barely detectable. Accordingly, uninfected cells are unlikely to be affected by therapeutic concentrations of penciclovir.

In clinical studies, Vectavir-treated patients healed 30% faster than placebo (up to one day earlier), pain resolution was 25–30% faster (median improvement of up to one day) and infectivity resolved up to 40% faster (one day earlier) than placebo.

*Pharmacokinetic properties:* Following application of Vectavir Cold Sore Cream in a human volunteer study at a daily dose of 180 mg penciclovir (approximately 67 times the proposed daily clinical dose), to occluded and abraded skin for four days, penciclovir was not quantifiable in plasma and urine.

*Pre-clinical safety data*
*General toxicology:* Topical application of 5% Vectavir Cold Sore Cream for four weeks to rats and rabbits was well tolerated. There was no evidence of contact sensitisation in guinea pigs.

A full programme of studies has been conducted using intravenous penciclovir. These studies did not raise any safety concerns regarding topical use of Vectavir Cold Sore Cream. There is a minimal systemic absorption of penciclovir following topical administration.

The results of a wide range of mutagenicity studies *in vitro* and *in vivo* indicate that penciclovir does not pose a genotoxic risk to man.

**Pharmaceutical particulars**

*List of excipients:* White soft paraffin, liquid paraffin, cetostearyl alcohol, propylene glycol, cetomacrogol 1000 and purified water

*Incompatibilities:* No known incompatibilities relevant to topical application of Vectavir Cold Sore Cream.

*Shelf life:* Two years.

*Special precautions for storage:* Store at temperatures not exceeding 30°C. Do not freeze.

*Nature and content of container:* 2 g aluminium tube.

*Instructions for use/handling:* Store at room temperatures not exceeding 30°C. Do not freeze.

**Marketing authorisation number** 10592/0078

**Date of approval/revision of SPC** August 1996.

**Legal category**   POM

*\*Trade Mark*

# Solvay Healthcare Limited
Gaters Hill
West End
Southampton SO18 3JD

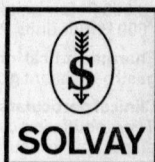

## ALGESAL*

**Presentation** Off white, lavender-scented cream containing diethylamine salicylate 10% w/w. Excipients include glycerol monostearate, ethylene glycol stearate, stearic acid, triethanolamine, liquid and white soft paraffins, microcrystalline wax, Lavandin composition, and purified water.

**Uses** An analgesic cream for the symptomatic relief of rheumatic and minor musculo-skeletal conditions including lumbago, fibrositis, sciatica, bruises and sprains.

**Dosage and administration**
*Adults (including the elderly) and children over 6 years:* Apply three times daily to the affected area, massaging until cream is fully absorbed.

*Children under 6 years:* Not recommended.

**Contra-indications, warnings, etc** Algesal should not be used if the surface of the skin is broken. This product contains a salicylate which is related to aspirin.

*Use in pregnancy:* There is inadequate evidence of safety in human pregnancy, but it has been in wide use for many years without apparent ill consequence. However, it should only be used in pregnancy where there is no safer alternative.

*Treatment of overdosage:* Adverse systemic effects are unlikely even after accidental oral ingestion. No special measures are necessary.

**Pharmaceutical precautions** Store at room temperature.

**Legal category** P.

**Package quantities** Tube containing 50 g.

**Further information** Nil.

**Product licence number** 0512/0066.

## COLOFAC* LIQUID

**Qualitative and quantitative composiiton** Mebeverine pamoate equivalent to 50 mg mebeverine hydrochloride per 5 ml.

**Pharmaceutical form** A yellow, banana flavoured, sugar-free suspension.

**Clinical particulars**
*Therapeutic indications:* For the symptomatic treatment of irritable bowel syndrome and other conditions usually included in this grouping, such as chronic irritable colon, spastic constipation, mucous colitis, spastic colitis. Colofac is effectively used to treat the symptoms of these conditions, such as colicky abdominal pain and cramps, persistent, non-specific diarrhoea (with or without alternating constipation) and flatulence.

For the symptomatic treatment of gastro-intestinal spasm secondary to organic diseases.

*Posology and method of administration:*
*Adults (including the elderly) and children 10 years and over:* 15 ml (150 mg) three times a day preferably 20 minutes before meals.

After a period of several weeks when the desired effect has been obtained, the dosage may be gradually reduced.
*Children under 10 years:* Not applicable.

*Contra-indications:* None known.

*Special warnings and precautions for use:* None.

*Interactions with other medicaments and other forms of interaction:* None known.

*Pregnancy and lactation:* Animal experiments have failed to show any teratogenic effects. However, the usual precautions concerning the administration of any drug during pregnancy should be observed.

*Effects on ability to drive and use machines:* None.

*Undesirable effects:* None known.

*Overdose:* On theoretical grounds it may be predicted that CNS excitability will occur in cases of overdosage. No specific antidote is known; gastric lavage and symptomatic treatment is recommended.

*Pharmacological properties*

*Pharmacodynamic properties:* Mebeverine is a musculotropic antispasmodic with a direct action on the smooth muscle of the gastrointestinal tract, relieving spasm without affecting normal gut motility.

*Pharmacokinetic properties:* Mebeverine is rapidly and completely absorbed after oral administration in the form of tablets or suspension. Mebeverine is not excreted as such, but metabolised completely. The first step in the metabolism is hydrolysis, leading to veratric acid and mebeverine alcohol. Both veratric acid and mebeverine alcohol are excreted into the urine, the latter partly as the corresponding carboxylic acid and partly as the demethylated carboxylic acid.

*Preclinical safety data:* None stated.

**Pharmaceutical particulars**
*List of excipients:* Microcrystalline cellulose, carboxymethylcellulose sodium, citric acid monohydrate, sodium citrate, polysorbate 20, polyoxyl 40 hydrogenated castor oil, disodium pamoate monohydrate, sodium benzoate, saccharin sodium, banana flavour, simethicone emulsion, purified water.
The sodium content is 20.5 mg/5 ml.

*Incompatibilities:* Not applicable.

*Shelf life:* 3 years when stored in the original container.

*Special precautions for storage:* Store at room temperature, protected from light.

*Nature and contents of container:* Amber glass bottle with polyethylene tamper evident cap. Each bottle contains 300 ml.

*Instructions for use/handling:* Shake well before use. Dilution and subsequent storage not recommended. Mebeverine does not produce false positive reactions in standard diagnostic urine tests.

**Marketing authorisation number** 0512/0061

**Date of approval/revision of SPC** February 1997

**Legal category** POM

## COLOFAC* TABLETS

**Presentation** White, round, sugar-coated tablets with no superficial markings each containing 135 mg mebeverine hydrochloride. Excipients include lactose and sucrose.

**Uses** Mebeverine is a musculotropic antispasmodic with a direct action on the smooth muscle of the gastro-intestinal tract, relieving spasm without affecting normal gut motility. Since this action is not mediated by the autonomic nervous system, anticholinergic side-effects are absent. Mebeverine is suitable for patients with prostatic hypertrophy and glaucoma.

*Indications:*

1. For the symptomatic treatment of irritable bowel syndrome and other conditions usually included in this grouping such as: chronic irritable colon, spastic constipation, mucous colitis, spastic colitis. Colofac is effectively used to treat the symptoms of these conditions, such as: colicky abdominal pain and cramps, persistent non-specific diarrhoea (with or without alternating constipation) and flatulence.
2. For the symptomatic treatment of gastro-intestinal spasm secondary to organic diseases.

**Dosage and administration**
*Adults (including the elderly) and children 10 years and over:* One tablet three times a day, preferably 20 minutes before meals.

After a period of several weeks when the desired effect has been obtained, the dosage may be gradually reduced.

*Children under 10 years:* Not applicable.

**Contra-indications, warnings, etc**
*Contra-indications:* None known.

*Warnings:* Animal experiments have failed to show any teratogenic effects. However, the usual precautions concerning the administration of any drug during pregnancy should be observed.

*Treatment of overdosage:* On theoretical grounds it may be predicted that CNS excitability will occur in cases of overdosage. No specific antidote is known;

gastric lavage and symptomatic treatment is recommended.

**Pharmaceutical precautions** Tablets: Store in a dry place, at room temperature, protected from light.

**Legal category** POM.

**Package quantities** Available in packs of 100 (5 strips of 20 blister-packed tablets).

**Further information** Mebeverine does not produce false positive reactions in standard diagnostic urine tests.

**Product licence number** 0512/0044

## CREON*

**Presentation** Brown/yellow hard gelatin capsules containing buff coloured enteric coated granules of pancreatin, equivalent to:
8,000 BP units of lipase
9,000 BP units of amylase
210 BP units of protease

**Uses** Replacement therapy in pancreatic enzyme deficiency states.

*Indications:* Pancreatic exocrine insufficiency.

**Dosage and administration** *Adults (including the elderly) and children:* Initially one to two capsules with meals. Dose increases, if required, should be added slowly, with careful monitoring of response and symptomatology. It is important to ensure adequate hydration of patients at all times whilst dosing Creon.

The capsules can be swallowed whole, or for ease of administration they may be opened and the granules taken with fluid or soft food, but without chewing. If the granules are mixed with food it is important that they are taken immediately, otherwise dissolution of the enteric coating may result.

Colonic damage has been reported in patients with cystic fibrosis taking in excess of 10,000 units of lipase/kg/day (see *Warnings*).

**Contra-indications, warnings, etc**
*Contra-indications:* Substitution with pancreatic enzymes is contra-indicated in the early stages of acute pancreatitis. Patients with known hypersensitivity to porcine proteins.

*Use in pregnancy:* There is inadequate evidence of safety in use during pregnancy.

*Warnings:* The product is of porcine origin.
Rarely cases of hyper-uricosuria and hyper-uricaemia have been reported with very high doses of pancreatin.
Perianal irritation, and rarely, inflammation, could occur when large doses are used.
Stricture of the ileo-caecum and large bowel and colitis has been reported in children with cystic fibrosis taking high doses of pancreatic enzyme supplements. To date, Creon has not been implicated in the development of colonic damage. However, unusual abdominal symptoms or changes in abdominal symptoms should be reviewed to exclude the possibility of colonic damage – especially if the patient is taking in excess of 10,000 units of lipase/kg/day.

*Overdosage:* Most cases respond to supportive measures including stopping enzyme therapy and ensuring adequate rehydration.

**Pharmaceutical precautions** Store below 20°C.

**Legal category** P.

**Package quantities** Available in packs of 100 capsules.

**Further information** This product may be taken by Muslim and Jewish patients.

**Product licence number** 05727/0001

*Product licence holder:* Solvay Pharmaceuticals GmbH, Hans-Böckler-Allee 20, 30173 Hannover, Germany.

## CREON* 10000

**Qualitative and quantitative composition** Each capsule contains:

10,000 PhEur units Lipase
8,000 PhEur units Amylase
600 PhEur units Protease

**Pharmaceutical form** Brown/clear capsules containing gastro-resistant granules.

**Clinical particulars**
*Therapeutic indications*: For the treatment of pancreatic exocrine insufficiency.

*Posology and method of administration:*
*Adults (including the elderly) and children:* Initially one to two capsules with each meal. Dose increases, if required, should be added slowly, with careful monitoring of response and symptomology.

It is important to ensure adequate hydration of patients at all times whilst dosing Creon.

The capsules can be swallowed whole, or for ease of administration they may be opened and the granules taken with fluid or soft food, but without chewing. If the granules are mixed with food it is important that they are taken immediately, otherwise dissolution of the enteric coating may result.

Colonic damage has been reported in patients with cystic fibrosis taking in excess of 10,000 units of lipase/kg/day (see *Undesirable effects*).

*Contra-indications*: Substitution with pancreatic enzymes is contra-indicated in the early stages of acute pancreatitis.

Patients with known hypersensitivity to porcine proteins.

*Special warnings and special precautions for use:* The product is of porcine origin.

*Interaction with other medicaments and other forms of interaction*: None known

*Pregnancy and lactation*: There is inadequate evidence of safety in use during pregnancy and lactation. However, as enzymes are not absorbed, it is unlikely that there would be any effect on the nursing infant.

*Effect on ability to drive and to use machines*: None known

*Undesirable effects*: Rarely cases of hyper-uricosuria and hyper-uricaemia have been reported with very high doses of pancreatin.

Stricture of the ileo-caecum and large bowel and colitis has been reported in children with cystic fibrosis taking high doses of pancreatic enzyme supplements. To date, Creon has not been implicated in the development of colonic damage. However, unusual abdominal symptoms or changes in abdominal symptoms should be reviewed to exclude the possibility of colonic damage–especially if the patient is taking in excess of 10,000 units of lipase/kg/day.

*Overdose*: Most cases respond to supportive measures including stopping enzyme therapy, ensuring adequate rehydration.

**Pharmacological properties**
*Pharmacodynamic properties*: Replacement therapy in pancreatic enzyme deficiency states. The enzymes have hydrolytic activity on fat, carbohydrates and proteins.

*Pharmacokinetic properties*: Pharmacokinetic data are not available as the enzymes act locally in the gastrointestinal tract. After exerting their action, the enzymes are digested themselves in the intestine.

**Pharmaceutical particulars**
*List of excipients*: *Granules*: Polyethylene glycol 4000, liquid paraffin, methylhydroxypropylcellulose phthalate (hp-55), dibutylphthalate, dimethicone 1000.

*Capsule shell*: gelatin, red, yellow and black iron oxides (E172), titanium dioxide (E171).

*Incompatibilities*: Not applicable.

*Shelf life*: 24 months, provided the product is kept in the original undamaged container, at temperatures not exceeding 20°C.

*Special precautions for storage*: Store below 20°C.

*Nature and contents of container*: HDPE container with LDPE cap. Containers hold 100, 250 or 300 capsules.

*Instructions for use/handling*: No special instructions.

*Marketing authorisation holder:* Solvay Pharmaceuticals GmbH, Hans-Böckler-Allee 20, 30173 Hannover, Germany.

**Marketing authorisation number** 05727/0013

**Date of approval/revision of SPC** August 1997

**Legal category** P

## CREON* 25000 ▼

**Presentation** Opaque orange/yellow hard gelatin capsules containing brownish coloured enteric coated pellets of pancreatin, equivalent to:
25,000 PhEur units of lipase
18,000 PhEur units of amylase
1,000 PhEur units of protease

**Uses** Replacement therapy in pancreatic enzyme deficiency states.

*Indications:* For the treatment of pancreatic exocrine insufficiency.

**Dosage and administration** *Adults (including the elderly) and children:* Initially one capsule with meals. Dose increases, if required, should be added slowly, with careful monitoring of response and symptomatology.

It is important to ensure adequate hydration of patients at all times whilst dosing Creon 25000.

The capsules can be swallowed whole, or for ease of administration they may be opened and the granules taken with fluid or soft food, but without chewing. If the granules are mixed with food it is important that they are taken immediately, otherwise dissolution of the enteric coating may result.

Colonic damage has been reported in patients with cystic fibrosis taking in excess of 10,000 units of lipase/kg/day (see *Warnings*).

**Contra-indications, warnings, etc**
*Contra-indications:* Substitution with pancreatic enzymes is contra-indicated in the early stages of acute pancreatitis. Patients with known hypersensitivity to porcine proteins.

*Use in pregnancy:* There is inadequate evidence of safety in use during pregnancy.

*Warnings:* The product is of porcine origin. Rarely cases of hyper-uricosuria and hyper-uricaemia have been reported with very high doses of pancreatin.

Perianal irritation, and rarely, inflammation, could occur when large doses are used.

Stricture of the ileo-caecum and large bowel and colitis has been reported in childen with cystic fibrosis taking high doses of pancreatic enzyme supplements. To date, Creon 25000 has not been implicated in the development of colonic damage. However, unusual abdominal symptoms or changes in abdominal symptoms should be reviewed to exclude the possibility of colonic damage – especially if the patient is taking in excess of 10,000 units of lipase/kg/day.

*Overdosage:* Most cases respond to supportive measures including stopping enzyme therapy and ensuring adequate rehydration.

**Pharmaceutical precautions** Store below 20°C.

**Legal category** POM.

**Package quantities** Available in packs of 50 capsules.

**Further information** This product may be taken by Muslim and Jewish patients.

**Product licence number** 05727/0006

*Product licence holder:* Solvay Pharmaceuticals GmbH, Hans-Böckler-Allee 20, 30173 Hannover, Germany.

## CREON* SACHETS

**Qualitative and quantitative composition** Each sachet contains 750 mg pancreatin equivalent to:
20,000 PhEur units of lipase
22,500 PhEur units of amylase
1,125 PhEur units of protease (total).

**Pharmaceutical form** Sachets containing brownish coloured enteric coated gastro-resistant granules.

**Clinical particulars**

*Therapeutic indications:* For the treatment of pancreatic exocrine insufficiency.

*Posology and method of administration*: Initially the contents of 1 sachet with meals. Dose increases, if required, should be added slowly, with careful monitoring of response and symptomatology. It is important to ensure adequate hydration of patients at all times whilst dosing Creon.

One Creon sachet contains 20,000 PhEur units of lipase, compared to 8,000 BP units per capsule of Creon. Therefore, two sachets of Creon granules are equivalent to five Creon capsules (1BP unit of lipase=1 PhEur unit).

The contents of each sachet can be taken from a spoon or tipped directly onto the tongue, and then washed down with a drink of water or other fluid. The granules can also be sprinkled on soft food, which should then be swallowed without chewing. If the granules are mixed with food, it is important that they are taken immediately, otherwise dissolution of the enteric coating may result. In order to protect the enteric coating, it is important that the granules are not crushed or chewed.

Colonic damage has been reported in patients with cystic fibrosis taking in excess of 10,000 units of lipase/kg/day (see *Undesirable effects*).

*Contra-indications:* Substitution with pancreatic enzymes is contra-indicated in the early stages of acute pancreatitis. Patients with known hypersensitivity to porcine proteins.

*Special warnings and special precautions for use:* The product is of porcine origin.

*Interaction with other medicaments and other forms of interaction:* None known.

*Pregnancy and lactation:* There is inadequate evidence of safety in use during pregnancy. There is inadequate evidence of safety in use during lactation. However, as enzymes are not absorbed, it is unlikely that there would be any effect on the nursing infant.

*Effects on ability to drive and use machines:* None known.

*Undesirable effects:* Rarely cases of hyper-uricosuria and hyper-uricaemia have been reported with very high doses of pancreatin. Perianal irritation, and rarely, inflammation, could occur when large doses are used.

Stricture of the ileo-caecum and large bowel and colitis has been reported in childen with cystic fibrosis taking high doses of pancreatic enzyme supplements. To date, Creon has not been implicated in the development of colonic damage. However, unusual abdominal symptoms or changes in abdominal symptoms should be reviewed to exclude the possibility of colonic damage – especially if the patient is taking in excess of 10,000 units of lipase/kg/day.

*Overdose:* Most cases respond to supportive measures including stopping enzyme therapy and ensuring adequate rehydration.

**Pharmacological properties**

*Pharmacodynamic properties:* Replacement therapy in pancreatic enzyme deficiency states. The enzymes have hydrolytic activity on fat, carbohydrates and proteins.

*Pharmacokinetic properties:* Pharmacokinetic data are not available as the enzymes act locally in the gastrointestinal tract. Afer exerting their action, the enzymes are digested themselves in the intestine.

**Pharmaceutical particulars**

*List of excipients:* Polyethylene glycol 4000, liquid paraffin, methylhydroxypropyl cellulose phthalate (HP-55), dibutyl phthalate, dimethicone 1000.

*Incompatibilities:* None known.

*Shelf life:* 2 years in the original undamaged container.

*Special precautions for storage*: Store at room temperature, protected from heat and moisture.

*Nature and contents of container:* Unit dose sachets consisting of aluminium/paper composite foil, with an internal coating of LDPE. Available in cartons containing 10 or 40 sachets.

*Instructions for use/handling:* This product may be taken by Muslim and Jewish patients.

*Marketing authorisation holder:* Solvay Pharmaceuticals GmbH, Hans-Böckler-Allee 20, 30173 Hannover, Germany.

**Marketing authorisation number** 05727/0007.

**Date of approval/revision of SPC** March 1997

**Legal category** P.

## DUPHALAC* (LACTULOSE SOLUTION BP)

**Presentation** A colourless to brownish yellow, clea[r] or not more than slightly opalescent solution containing lactulose 3.35 g/5 ml. Also contains lactose 0.3 g/5 ml, galactose 0.55 g/5 ml.

**Uses** The action of lactulose in treating constipation depends on the inability of the enzymes in the smal[l] intestine to hydrolyse this synthetic disaccharide into its component molecules of fructose and galactose. Therefore, as lactulose is virtually unabsorbed, i[t] passes into the large bowel chemically unchanged and forms a substrate for commensal saccharolytic bacteria.

The resulting breakdown products, simple organic compounds like lactic and acetic acid, give rise to increased intra-colonic osmotic pressure, with consequent increased faecal bulk, and stimulation of peristalsis. The growth of saccharolytic bacteria is favoured and the normal colonic flora restored.

A soft stool is formed, and normal bowel action encouraged without irritation or direct interference with the gut mucosa.

In patients with hepatic encephalopathy large doses of lactulose are used; a significant reduction in the pH of the colonic contents results, which reduces markedly the formation and absorption of ammonium ions and other nitrogenous toxins into the portal circulation. Rapid decrements in blood ammoni[a] concentration have been reported following lactulose treatment.

*Indications:* 1. Constipation.

2. Hepatic encephalopathy (Portal systemic encephalopathy): hepatic coma.

**Dosage and administration** *Constipation:* Initially lactulose may be given twice daily. In due course the dose should be adjusted to the needs of the individual, but the following serves as a guide.

*Starting dose*

Adults (including the elderly) 15 ml twice daily
Children 5 to 10 years 10 ml twice daily
Children under 5 years 5 ml twice daily
Babies under 1 year 2.5 ml twice daily

Lactulose may, if necessary, be taken with water or fruit juices, etc.

*Hepatic encephalopathy*

*Adults (including the elderly):* Initially 30–50 ml. (6–10×5 ml spoonfuls) three times a day. Subsequently adjust the dose to produce two or three soft stools each day.

*Children:* No dosage recommendations for this indication.

**Contra-indications, warnings, etc**

*Contra-indications:* Galactosaemia. In common with other preparations used for the treatment of constipation, lactulose should not be used when there is evidence of gastro-intestinal obstruction.

*Precaution:* Lactose intolerance.

*Use in pregnancy:* Wide clinical experience, together with data from animal reproduction studies has not revealed any increase in embryotoxic hazard to the fetus, if used in the recommended dosage during pregnancy. If drug therapy is needed in pregnancy the use of this drug is acceptable.

*Side-effects:* During the first few days of treatment meteorism and increased flatulence may occur. These symptoms usually disappear under continued therapy. Diarrhoea may occur especially when using higher dosages, e.g. during treatment of PSE. Dosage should then be adjusted to obtain two or three formed stools per day.

*Treatment of overdosage:* No specific antidote. Symptomatic treatment should be given.

**Pharmaceutical precautions** Store below 20°C. Do not freeze. Dilution and subsequent storage not recommended.

**Legal category** P.

**Package quantities** Available in HDPE containers with tamper evident seals and pack sizes of 200 ml, 300 ml, 500 ml and 1 litre.

**Further information** Because of lactulose's physiological mode of action it may take up to 48 hours before effects are obtained. However, clinical experience has shown that this medicament does exhibit a 'carry-over' effect which may enable the patient to reduce the effective dose gradually over a period of time.

A maintenance dose of 15 ml per day provides only 58 kJ (14 kcals), and is therefore, unlikely to adversely affect diabetics.

**Product licence number** 0512/5001R.

# DUPHALAC* DRY

**Presentation** A white to slightly coloured, crystalline powder containing not less than 95% lactulose. Also contains not more than 5% related substances (lactose, galactose).

**Uses** The active ingredient, lactulose, is metabolised in the colon by the saccharolytic bacteria, producing low molecular weight organic acids, mainly lactic acid, which lower the pH of the colonic contents and promote the retention of water by an osmotic effect, thus increasing peristaltic activity.

In patients with hepatic encephalopathy, larger doses of lactulose are used; a significant reduction in the pH of the colonic content results, which reduces markedly the formation and absorption of ammonium ions and other nitrogenous toxins into the portal circulation. Rapid decrements in blood ammonia concentration have been reported following lactulose treatment.

*Indications:* The relief of constipation.

The treatment and prevention of hepatic encephalopathy (portal systemic encephalopathy): hepatic coma.

**Dosage and administration**

*Constipation:* Initially lactulose may be given twice daily. In due course the dose should be adjusted to the needs of the individual, but the following serves as a guide.

*Starting dose*

Adults (including the elderly) 10 g (1 sachet) twice daily
Children 5 to 10 years 5 g twice daily
Children 5 years and under Lactulose Solution BP is recommended

The dose can be taken from a spoon or tipped directly onto the tongue and then washed down with a drink of water or other fluid. The crystals may also be sprinkled on food, or mixed with water or other fluids before swallowing.

*Hepatic encephalopathy:*

*Adults (including the elderly):* Initially 20–30 g (2–3 sachets) three times daily. Subsequently adjust the dose to produce two or three soft stools each day.

*Children:* No dosage recommendations for this indication.

**Contra-indications, warnings, etc**

*Contra-indications:* Galactosaemia. In common with other preparations used for the treatment of constipation, lactulose should not be used where there is evidence of gastro-intestinal obstruction.

*Precaution:* Lactose intolerance.

*Use in pregnancy:* Wide clinical experience, together with data from animal reproduction studies has not revealed any increase in embryotoxic hazard to the fetus, if used in the recommended dosage during pregnancy. If drug therapy is needed in pregnancy the use of this drug is acceptable.

*Side-effects:* During the first few days of treatment meteorism and increased flatulence may occur. These symptoms usually disappear under continued therapy. Diarrhoea may occur especially when using higher dosages, e.g. during treatment of portal systemic encephalopathy. Dosage should then be adjusted to obtain two or three formed stools per day.

*Treatment of overdosage:* No specific antidote. Symptomatic treatment should be given.

**Pharmaceutical precautions** Store at temperatures up to 25°C.

**Legal category** P.

**Package quantities** 30 unit dose sachets.

**Further information** Because of the physiological mode of action it may take up to 48 hours before effects are obtained.

**Product licence number** 0512/0105.

# DUPHASTON*
# DUPHASTON-HRT*

**Qualitative and quantitative composition** Each tablet contains 10 mg Dydrogesterone BP.

**Pharmaceutical form** Round, white tablet, scored on one side with the imprint '155' on each half of the tablet and imprinted 'S' on the reverse.

**Clinical particulars**

*Therapeutic indications:* To counteract the effects of unopposed oestrogen in Hormone Replacement Therapy; pre-menstrual syndrome, endometriosis, dysmenorrhoea, infertility, irregular cycles, dysfunctional bleeding (with added oestrogen), secondary amenorrhoea (with added oestrogen), threatened and habitual abortion (associated with proven progesterone deficiency).

*Posology and method of administration:*
*Adults:*

*Hormone replacement therapy:* The standard dose is 10 mg Duphaston daily for the last 14 days of each 28-day oestrogen treatment cycle. The dose may be increased to 10 mg twice daily if either early withdrawal bleeding occurs or if endometrial biopsy reveals inadequate progestational response.

*Pre-menstrual syndrome:* 10 mg twice daily from day 12 to 26 of the cycle. The dosage may be increased if necessary.

*Endometriosis:* 10 mg two to three times daily from day 5 to 25 of the cycle, or continuously.

*Dysmenorrhoea:* 10 mg twice daily from day 5 to 25 of the cycle.

*Infertility or irregular cycles:* 10 mg twice daily from day 11 to 25 of the cycle. Treatment should be maintained for at least six consecutive cycles. If the patient conceives, it is advisable to continue treatment for the first few months of pregnancy as described under 'habitual abortion'.

*Dysfunctional bleeding – to arrest bleeding:* 10 mg twice daily together with an oestrogen once daily for five to seven days.

*Dysfunctional bleeding – to prevent bleeding:* 10 mg twice daily together with an oestrogen once daily from day 11 to 25 of the cycle.

*Amenorrhoea:* An oestrogen once daily from day 1 to 25 of the cycle, and Duphaston 10 mg twice daily from day 11 to 25 of the cycle.

*Threatened abortion:* 40 mg at once then 10 mg every eight hours until symptoms remit. If symptoms persist or return during treatment the dose can be increased by one tablet every eight hours. The effective dose must be maintained for a week after symptoms have ceased and can then be gradually decreased unless symptoms return.

*Habitual abortion:* Treatment should be started as early as possible, preferably before conception. 10 mg should be given twice daily from day 11 to 25 of the cycle until conception and then continuously (10 mg twice daily) until the twentieth week of pregnancy, then dosage may be gradually reduced.

*Elderly: Hormone replacement therapy:* Standard adult dosage is recommended.

*Children:* Not applicable.

*Contra-indications:* None known.

*Special warnings and special precautions for use:* None.

*Interaction with other medicaments and other forms of interaction:* None known.

*Pregnancy and lactation:*

*Pregnancy:* There is no known risk in pregnancy. Duphaston is indicated for threatened or habitual abortion, until the twentieth week of pregnancy.

*Lactation:* Small amounts are expected to be excreted, but exact amounts are unknown. There have been no reports of adverse experiences.

*Effects on ability to drive and use machines:* None known.

*Undesirable effects:* Serious side-effects are not expected. Breakthrough bleeding may occur in a few patients. It can, however, be prevented by increasing the dosage. Nausea, breast tenderness, headache, bloated feeling, transient dizziness and skin reactions have occasionally been reported.

*Overdose:*

*Symptoms:* No reports of ill-effects from overdosage have been reported and remedial action is generally unnecessary.

*Treatment:* If a large overdosage is discovered within 2–3 hours and treatment seems desirable, gastric lavage is recommended. There are no special antidotes and treatment should be symptomatic.

**Pharmacological properties**

*Pharmacodynamic properties:* Dydrogesterone is an orally-active progestogen which produces a complete secretory endometrium in an oestrogen-primed uterus thereby providing protection for oestrogen-induced increased risk of endometrial hyperplasia and/or carcinogenesis. It is indicated in all cases of endogenous progesterone deficiency. Duphaston is non-androgenic, non-oestrogenic, non-thermogenic, non-corticoid and non-anabolic.

*Pharmacokinetic properties:* After oral administration of labelled dydrogesterone, on average 63% of the dose is excreted into the urine. Within 72 hours excretion is complete. Dydrogesterone is completely metabolised.

The main metabolite of dydrogesterone is 20α-dihydrodydrogesterone (DHD) and is present in the urine predominantly as the glucuronic acid conjugate. A common feature of all metabolites characterised is the retention of the 4,6 diene-3-one configuration of the parent compound and the absence of 17α-hydroxylation. This explains the lack of oestrogenic and androgenic effects of dydrogesterone.

After oral administration of dydrogesterone, plasma concentrations of DHD are substantially higher as compared to the parent drug. The AUC and $C_{max}$ ratios of DHD to dydrogesterone are in the order of 40 and 25, respectively.

Dydrogesterone is rapidly absorbed. The $T_{max}$ values of dydrogesterone and DHD vary between 0.5 and 2.5 hours.

Mean terminal half lives of dydrogesterone and DHD vary between 5 to 7 and 14 to 17 hours, respectively.

Unlike progesterone, dydrogesterone is not excreted in the urine as pregnanediol. It is therefore possible to analyse production of endogenous progesterone even in the presence of dydrogesterone.

*Preclinical safety data:* Dydrogesterone has been used in several animal models and has been proven to be an entity with low toxicity, not having mutagenic or carcinogenic properties.

No effects were seen in reproduction experiments.

**Pharmaceutical particulars**

*List of excipients:* Lactose, maize starch, methylhydroxypropylcellulose, silica, magnesium stearate, and titanium dioxide (E171).

*Incompatibilities:* None known.

*Shelf life:* Five years.

*Special precautions for storage:* Store in a dry place, at room temperature (25°C) and ambient humidity.

*Nature and contents of container:* Cartons containing 14, 42 or 60 tablets in blister strips.

*Instructions for use/handling:* None.

**Marketing authorisation number** 0512/5004R.

**Date of approval/revision of SPC** June 1997.

**Legal category** POM.

## FAVERIN*

**Presentation** Round, biconvex, scored, white film coated tablets imprinted 'S' on one side, '291' on both sides of the score on the reverse. Each tablet contains 50 mg fluvoxamine maleate.

Oval, biconvex, scored, white film coated tablets imprinted 'S' on one side, '313' on both sides of the score on the reverse. Each tablet contains 100 mg fluvoxamine maleate.

**Uses** The treatment of symptoms of depressive illness. The treatment of symptoms of obsessive-compulsive disorder (OCD).

**Dosage and administration** The tablets should be swallowed without chewing and with water.

*Adults, including the elderly:* The effective dosage usually lies between 100 mg and 200 mg, with some patients requiring up to 300 mg per day. The recommended starting dose is 100 mg per day. The dosage should be increased gradually until the effective dosage is achieved, with a maximum of 300 mg per day. A total daily dosage in excess of 100 mg should be given in divided doses. If no improvement of the OCD symptoms is observed within ten weeks, treatment with Faverin should be reconsidered.

Whilst there are no systematic studies to answer the question of how long to continue Faverin treatment, OCD is a chronic condition and it is reasonable to consider continuation beyond ten weeks in responding patients. Dosage adjustments should be made carefully on an individual patient basis, to maintain the patient at the lowest effective dose. The need for treatment should be reassessed periodically. Some clinicians advocate concomitant behavioural psychotherapy for patients who have done well on pharmacotherapy.

*Children:* There are insufficient data to recommend the use of Faverin in children.

**Contra-indications, warnings, etc**

*Contra-indications:* Faverin should not be given with or within two weeks of terminating treatment with monoamine-oxidase inhibitors. A period of 7 days should elapse before starting an MAOI after discontinuation of Faverin.

*Warnings:* As improvement may sometimes be delayed for two or more weeks, patients should be closely monitored during this initial period. The possibility of a suicide attempt is inherent in patients suffering from depressive illness and may persist until significant improvement occurs.

As with other antidepressants, Faverin should be used with caution in patients with a history of epilepsy. If convulsions occur, Faverin therapy should be discontinued.

There is little clinical experience of concurrent administration of Faverin with ECT.

*Driving:* Faverin has shown no effect on psychomotor skills associated with driving and operating machinery up to and including 150 mg/day. However, as with all psychoactive drugs, patients should be cautioned about their ability to undertake potentially hazardous tasks such as driving or operating machinery.

*Use in pregnancy and lactation:* Although studies in animals have not shown any direct teratogenic effect, the safety of Faverin in human pregnancy has not been established. On basic principles, its use during pregnancy and in nursing mothers should be avoided, unless there are compelling reasons.

*Hepatic/renal impairment:* Patients with hepatic or renal insufficiency should begin treatment with a low dose and be carefully monitored. Rarely treatment with Faverin has been associated with an increase in hepatic enzymes, usually accompanied by symptoms. The drug should be withdrawn in such subjects.

*Drug interactions:* Faverin can prolong the elimination of drugs metabolised by oxidation in the liver. A clinically significant interaction is possible with drugs with a narrow therapeutic index (e.g. warfarin and other coumarin derivative anticoagulants, carbamazepine, clozapine, phenytoin and theophylline). The concomitant use of Faverin and theophylline should usually be avoided. Where this is not possible, patients should have their theophylline dose halved and plasma theophylline levels should be monitored closely.

In interaction studies, increased plasma levels of propranolol, warfarin and oxidatively metabolised benzodiazepines (e.g. bromazepam) were seen during concurrent administration of Faverin. It may therefore be advisable to lower the dose of these drugs when prescribing Faverin. An increase in previously stable plasma levels of tricyclic antidepressants, when used together with Faverin, has been reported. The combination of these drugs is not recommended. No interactions were seen with digoxin or with atenolol.

Faverin has been used in combination with lithium in the treatment of patients with severe drug-resistant depression. However, lithium (and possibly tryptophan) enhances the serotonergic effects of Faverin and the combination should therefore be used with caution.

There are isolated reports of enhanced serotonergic effects, resembling the neuroleptic malignant syndrome, when Faverin has been combined with lithium or neuroleptic medication.

The effects of alcohol may be potentiated by Faverin.

*Side-effects:* Many of the symptoms listed below are often associated with the illness and are not necessarily related to treatment.

*Frequency >10%:* Digestive: nausea.

*Frequency 1–10%:* Body: abdominal pain, headache, malaise.

Cardiovascular: palpitations, tachycardia.

Digestive: anorexia, constipation, diarrhoea, dry mouth, dyspepsia, vomiting.

General: asthenia.

Nervous system: agitation, anxiety, dizziness, insomnia, nervousness, somnolence, tremor.

Skin: sweating.

*Frequency 0.1–1%:* Cardiovascular: (postural) hypotension.

Musculo-skeletal: arthralgia, myalgia.

Nervous system: ataxia, confusion, dystonias, hallucinations.

Urogenital: abnormal (delayed) ejaculation.

Skin: rashes, pruritus.

*Frequency <0.1%:* Digestive: liver function abnormality.

Nervous system: convulsions, mania.

Urogenital: galactorrhoea.

Particularly in the treatment of obsessive compulsive disorder, asthenia, insomnia and abnormal (delayed) ejaculation have been observed.

Faverin may cause a decrease in heart rate. During treatment, limited changes in repolarisation were observed in the ECG, but no causal relationship could be demonstrated.

Anaphylactoid and photosensitivity reactions have been rarely reported in patients taking Faverin.

Hyponatraemia has been reported in association with other antidepressants, though rarely reported with Faverin.

Symptoms, including headache, nausea, dizziness and anxiety, have been rarely reported after abrupt discontinuation of Faverin.

*Treatment of overdosage:* No specific antidote is known. The stomach should be emptied as soon as possible after tablet ingestion and symptomatic treatment should be given. The use of medicinal charcoal is also recommended.

**Pharmaceutical precautions** Store below 25°C, protected from light.

**Legal category** POM.

**Package quantities** 50 mg tablets: available in packs of 60. 100 mg tablets:available in packs of 30.

**Further information** The mechanism of action of Faverin is thought to be related to its selective serotonin re-uptake inhibition in brain neurones, whilst there is minimum interference with noradrenergic or dopaminergic processes. Faverin is chemically unrelated to other currently available antidepressants.

Faverin is indicated for short-term and maintenance treatment.

Faverin is rapidly and completely absorbed after oral administration. The plasma half-life is approximately 15 hours after a single dose and slightly longer (17–22 hours) during repeated dosing, when steady state plasma levels are usually achieved in 10–14 days. It is transformed in the liver into pharmacologically inactive metabolites which are excreted by the kidney. Seventy-seven per cent of fluvoxamine maleate is bound to plasma proteins.

The pharmacokinetic profile in the elderly is similar to that in the general population.

**Product licence numbers**

| | |
|---|---|
| 50 mg | 0512/0070 |
| 100 mg | 0512/0072 |

## FEMAPAK* 40

**Qualitative and quantitative composition** Femapak 40 consists of a pack containing eight Fematrix 40 transdermal patches and a blister strip of 14 Duphaston tablets. Each Fematrix 40 patch contains 1.25 mg estradiol (each patch delivers approximately 40 micrograms of estradiol per 24 hours).

Each Duphaston tablet contains 10 mg Dydrogesterone BP.

**Pharmaceutical form** Fematrix 40 is a self adhesive, flexible transdermal delivery system comprising a layer of clear adhesive sandwiched between a translucent patch and a metallised polyester backing. Fematrix 40 is a rectangular shape with rounded corners and has an active surface area of 14.25 cm².

Duphaston tablets are round and white, marked on one side with an S and on the other scored and marked with 155 on each half of the tablet.

**Clinical particulars**

*Therapeutic indications:* Hormone replacement therapy in female patients who have an intact uterus for the treatment of symptoms of oestrogen deficiency as a result of the natural menopause or oophorectomy. Dydrogesterone is provided to counteract the effects of oestrogen during the second two weeks of each cycle.

*Posology and method of administration:*

*Adults:* Therapy should be initiated with Femapak 40 in women who have menopausal symptoms, who have been oestrogen deficient for a prolonged time or who are likely to be intolerant of high levels of oestradiol. The dosage may be increased if required by using Femapak 80. For maintenance therapy the lowest effective dose should beused.

One Fematrix transdermal patch should be applied twice weekly on a continuous basis. Each patch should be removed after 3 to 4 days and replaced with a new patch applied to a slightly different site. Patches should be applied to clean, dry and intact areas of skin below the waist on the lower back or buttocks. Fematrix should not be applied on or near the breasts.

Women who are having regular periods should commence therapy within five days of the start of bleeding. Women whose periods have stopped or have become very irregular may commence therapy at any time.

During the second two weeks of the cycle, that is from the 15th day after applying the first patch, one Duphaston tablet should be taken each day for the next 14 days. Most patients will commence bleeding towards the end of the Duphaston therapy.

Unopposed oestrogen therapy should not be used unless the patient has undergone a hysterectomy.

*Children:* Femapak is not indicated in children.

*Contra-indications:* Femapak is contra-indicated in women with known or suspected pregnancy, cancer of the breast, genital tract or other oestrogen-dependent neoplasia, undiagnosed vaginal bleeding, endometriosis, severe renal or cardiac disease, acute or chronic liver disease where liver function tests have failed to return to normal, active thrombophlebitis or thromboembolic disorders (see also *Special warnings and precautions*), Dubin-Johnson syndrome or Rotor syndrome or hypersensitivity to lactose or other ingredients of the tablet.

*Special warnings and precautions for use*: It is recommended that the patient should undergo a thorough physical and gynaecological examination before commencing therapy. This should be repeated at regular intervals.

Unopposed oestradiol therapy should not be used in non-hysterectomised women because of the increased risk of endometrial hyperplasia or carcinoma.

At the present time there is suggestive evidence of an overall change in the relative risk of breast cancer in post-menopausal women receiving oestrogen replacement therapy. While some studies have shown that there may be a small increase in risk with treatment for more than 5 years others have shown no such increase. It is not known whether concurrent progestogen use influences the risk of breast cancer in post-menopausal women taking hormone replacement therapy. A careful appraisal of the risk/benefit ratio should be undertaken before treating for longer than 5 to 10 years.

Women with a history of fibrocystic disease, breast nodules, abnormal mammograms or family history of breast cancer should have regular breast examinations.

Certain diseases may be made worse by hormone replacement therapy and patients with these conditions should be closely monitored. These include otosclerosis, multiple sclerosis, systemic lupus erythematosus, cholelithiesis, porphyria, melanoma, epilepsy, migraine, thyrotoxicosis, surgically confirmed gall bladder disease, asthma and diabetes (worsening of glucose tolerance). Pre-existing uterine fibroids may increase in size during oestrogen therapy and symptoms associated with endometriosis may be exacerbated.

There is no indication from published studies of an increased risk of thromboembolic disease or thrombophlebitis in apparently normal women at the current recommended low doses of Hormone Replacement Therapy (HRT).

In the event of an acute thromboembolic event occurring during treatment HRT should be discontinued. However there is no indication to suggest that a history of deep vein thrombosis, pulmonary embolism, stroke or myocardial infarction when associated with recognised risk factors (such as immobilisation or post-trauma or post-operatively) should be a contra-indication to HRT but in the absence of specific data Femapak should be used with caution in these patients.

Consideration should be given to discontinuation of treatment 4 weeks prior to surgery or during periods of prolonged immobilisation. If jaundice or significant hypertension develop, treatment should be discontinued whilst the cause is investigated. As oestrogens may cause fluid retention, patients with cardiac or renal dysfunction should be closely observed. Regular monitoring of blood pressure should be carried out in hypertensive patients.

Women of child bearing potential should be advised to adhere to non-hormonal contraceptive methods.

*Interactions with other Medicaments and other forms of Interaction:* Preparations inducing microsomal liver enzymes, eg barbiturates, hydantoins, anti-convulsants (including carbamazepine), meprobamate, phenylbutazone, antibiotics (including rifampicin), and activated charcoal may impair the activity of oestrogens. Transdermally applied oestrogens are less likely to be affected by such interactions than oral oestrogens since first pass hepatic metabolism is avoided.

Changes in oestrogen serum concentrations may affect the results of certain endocrine or liver function tests.

*Pregnancy and lactation:* Femapak 40 is contra-indicated.

*Effects on ability to drive and use machines:* None.

*Undesirable effects:* Fematrix is generally well tolerated. The most frequent side effects (reported in 10 to 20% of patients, on at least one occasion, in clinical trials with Fematrix 80) which do not normally prevent continued treatment include: breast tenderness, headaches and breakthrough bleeding. Some patients experience mild and transient local erythema at the site of application with or without itching; this usually disappears rapidly on removal of the patch. The overall incidence of general patch irritation in clinical studies is less than 5%. In a clinical study 3% of 102 patients showed well defined erythema (Draize scale) 30 minutes after patch removal. No instances of permanent skin damage have been reported. If unacceptable topical side effects do occur discontinuation of treatment should be considered.

Other side effects associated with oestrogen or oestrogen/progestogen treatment have occasionally been reported (in 1% to 5% of patients in clinical trials with Fematrix 80) include: abdominal cramps, abdominal bloating, oedema, nausea, migraine and weight changes, additional side effects of dydrogesterone include occasional reports of transient dizziness and skin reactions.

More rarely (less than 1% in clinical trials with Fematrix 80) dizziness, dysmenorrhoea, leg cramps and visual disturbances have been reported.

Other side effects which have been rarely reported with oestrogen containing products include: changes in libido or changes in carbohydrate tolerance, vaginal candidiasis, change in vaginal secretions, cystitis like syndrome, cervical erosion, erythema multiforme, erythema nodosa haemorrhagic eruptions, chloasma or melasma which may be persistent, steepening of the corneal curvature, intolerance to contact lenses, mental depression and chorea minor. Cholestasis may be possible in predisposed patients.

*Overdose:* Fematrix 40: This is not likely due to the mode of administration. If it is necessary to stop delivery then the patch can be removed and plasma oestradiol levels will fall rapidly.

*Duphaston: Symptoms:* No reports of ill effects from overdosage have been recorded and remedial action is generally unnecessary.

*Treatment:* If a large overdosage is discovered within 2-3 hours and treatment seems desirable, gastric lavage is recommended. There are no special antidotes and treatment should be symptomatic.

### Pharmacological properties

*Pharmacodynamic properties*
*Oestradiol:* In the female, oestradiol stimulates the accessory reproductive organs and causes development of the secondary sexual characteristics at puberty. It is also responsible for the hypertrophy of the uterus and for the changes in the endometrium during the first half of the menstrual cycle which when acted on by progesterone prepares it for the reception of a fertilised ovum. It furthermore promotes the growth of the ducts of the mammary glands. Large doses inhibit the gonadotropic secretion of the anterior pituitary, thus influencing the normal ovarian cycle.

It is of value in menstrual disorders, ovarian insufficiency, especially at the menopause, and for the treatment of infections of the vagina in children, where it promotes the growth of a cornified and more resistant epithelium; it is also used to terminate lactation, not very successfully, by inhibiting the release of prolactin.

*Dydrogesterone:* Dydrogesterone is an orally-active progestogen which produces a complete secretory endometrium in an oestrogen-primed uterus thereby providing protection for oestrogen-induced increased risk of endometrial hyperplasia and/or carcinogenesis. It is indicated in all cases of endogenous progesterone deficiency. Duphaston is non-androgenic, non-oestrogenic, non-corticoid and non-anabolic.

*Pharmacokinetic properties*

Fematrix 80
*Absorption:* Oestradiol is absorbed from the patch across the stratum corneum and is delivered systemically at a low but constant rate throughout the period of application (3 to 4 days). The estimated delivery of oestradiol is around 40 µg/day.

*Distribution:* Oestrogens circulate in the blood bound to albumin, sex hormone binding globulin (SHBG), cortisol binding globulin and alpha1-glycoprotein. Following diffusion of free oestrogen into the cells of the target tissues in the hypothalamus, pituitary, vagina, urethra, uterus, breast and liver, binding to specific oestrogen receptors occurs. Very little information is currently available on the distribution of oestradiol following transdermal administration.

*Biotransformation:* Inactivation of oestrogens in the body is carried out mainly in the liver. Metabolism of 17β oestradiol is by oxidation to oestrone, which in turn can be hydrated to form oestriol. There is free interconversion between oestrone and oestradiol. Oestrone and oestriol may then undergo conversion to their corresponding sulphate and glucuronide derivatives for excretion in the urine. Oestrone sulphate has a long biologic half-life because of its enterohepatic recirculation and interconversion to oestrone and oestradiol.

*Elimination:* The plasma elimination half-life of oestradiol is approximately 1 hour and is independent of the route of administration. The metabolic plasma clearance rate is between 650 and 900 L/day /m². 

Steady state plasma oestradiol concentrations have been demonstrated in the range of 26 pg/ml to 34 pg/ml for the Fematrix 40 patch and 34 to 62 pg/ml for the Fematrix 80 patch (including baseline levels) and these are maintained throughout the dose interval (for up to four days). Absorption rate may vary between individual patients. After removal of the last patch plasma oestradiol and oestrone concentrations return to baseline values in less than 24 hours.

The median terminal half-life for oestradiol following patch removal has been determined as 5.24h.

*Dydrogesterone:* After oral administration of labelled dydrogesterone on average 63% of the dose is excreted into the urine. Within 72 hours excretion is complete. Dydrogesterone is completely metabolised.

The main metabolite of dydrogesterone is 20 α-dihydrodydrogesterone (DHD) and is present in the urine predominantly as the glucuronic acid conjugate. A common feature of all metabolites characterised is the retention of the 4.6 diene-3-one configuration of the parent compound and the absence of 17 α-hydroxylation. This explains the lack of oestrogenic and androgenic effects of dydrogesterone.

After oral administration of dydrogesterone, plasma concentrations of DHD are substantially higher as compared to the parent drug. The AUC and $C_{max}$ ratios of DHD to dydrogesterone are in the order of 40 and 25, respectively.

Dydrogesterone is rapidly absorbed. The $T_{max}$ values of dydrogesterone and DHD vary between 0.5 and 2.5 hours.

Mean terminal half lives of dydrogesterone and DHD vary between 5 to 7 and 14 to 17 hours, respectively.

Unlike progesterone, dydrogesterone is not excreted in the urine as pregnanediol. It is therefore possible to analyse production of endogenous progesterone even in the presence of dydrogesterone.

*Preclinical safety data*
*Fematrix:* No specific preclinical studies have been conducted on Fematrix. Supraphysiologically high doses (prolonged overdoses) of oestradiol have been associated with the induction of tumours in oestrogen-dependent target organs in rodent species. Pronounced species differences in toxicology, pharmacology and pharmacodynamics exist.

*Dydrogesterone:* Dydrogesterone has been used in several animal models and has been proven to have low toxicity. It does not have mutagenic or carcinogenic properties. No effects were seen in reproduction experiments.

### Pharmaceutical particulars

*List of excipients:*
*Fematrix:* Diethyltoluamide, Acrylic emulsion (Proprietary adhesive and thickener). *Backing:* Polyester film. Release liner: Siliconised/Aluminised/Polyester film (3m Scotchpak 1220).

*Duphaston:* Lactose, maize starch, methylhydroxypropylcellulose, silica, magnesium stearate, and titanium dioxide (E171).

*Incompatibilities:* None known.

*Shelf life:* The shelf-life of the product as packaged for sale is 2 years.

*Special precautions for storage:* Femapak 40 should be stored at room temperature below 25°C in a dry place. Duphaston tablets should also be protected from light.

*Nature and contents of container:*
*Fematrix:* Blister tray with a foil lid containing one transdermal patch.
   *Duphaston:* Blister strip containing 14 tablets.
   Each carton contains eight Fematrix patches and 14 Duphaston HRT tablets sufficient for one 28 day cycle.

*Instruction for use/handling:* Detailed instructions for use are given in the patient leaflet.

*Marketing authorisation holder:* Ethical Pharmaceuticals (UK) Limited, Gemini House, Bartholomew's Walk, Cambridgeshire Business Park, Ely, Cambs CB7 4EA.

**Marketing authorisation number** 10013/0034.

**Date of approval/revision of SPC** June 1997

**Legal category** POM

## FEMAPAK* 80

**Qualitative and quantitative composition** Femapak 80 consists of a pack containing eight Fematrix* 80 transdermal patches and a blister strip of 14 Duphaston* tablets. Each Fematrix 80 patch contains 2.5 mg estradiol (each patch delivers approximately 80 micrograms of estradiol per 24 hours).

Each Duphaston tablet contains 10 mg Dydrogesterone BP.

**Pharmaceutical form** Fematrix 80 is a self adhesive, flexible transdermal delivery system comprising a layer of clear adhesive sandwiched between a translucent patch and a metallised polyester backing. Fematrix 80 is a rectangular shape with rounded corners and has an active surface area of 28.5 cm².

Duphaston tablets are round and white, marked on one side with an S and on the other scored and marked with 155 on each half of the tablet.

**Clinical particulars**
*Therapeutic indications:* Hormone replacement therapy in female patients who have an intact uterus for the treatment of symptoms of oestrogen deficiency as a result of the natural menopause or oophorectomy and for the prevention of osteoporosis in women at risk of developing fractures. Epidemiological studies suggest a number of individual risk factors contribute to post menopausal osteoporosis, including:
   Early menopause (either naturally or surgically)
   Family history of osteoporosis
   Recent prolonged systemic corticosteroid therapy
   A small, thin frame
   Cigarette use
   If several risk factors are present consideration should be given to oestrogen replacement therapy.

For maximum benefit treatment should commence as soon as possible after the menopause.

Dydrogesterone is provided to counteract the effects of estrogen during the second two weeks of each cycle.

*Posology and method of administration:*
*Climateric symptoms:* Therapy should be initiated with Femapak 40 in women who have menopausal symptoms, who have been oestrogen deficient for a prolonged time or who are likely to be intolerant of high levels of oestradiol. The dosage may be increased if required by using Femapak 80 for maintenance therapy the lowest effective dose should be used.

*Prevention of osteoporosis:* Treatment should be with Femapak 80, as the efficacy of Femapak 40 in this indication has yet to be established.

For optimum benefit treatment should continue for 5 to 10 years, protection appears to be effective for as long as treatment continues, however, data beyond 10 years is limited. For long term use see also Precautions and Warnings.

*Dosage schedule (for both indications):* One Fematrix transdermal patch should be applied twice weekly on a continuous basis. Each patch should be removed after 3 to 4 days and replaced with a new patch applied to a slightly different site. Patches should be applied to clean, dry and intact areas of skin below the waist on the lower back or buttocks. Fematrix should not be applied on or near the breasts.

Women who are having regular periods should

commence therapy within five days of the start of bleeding. Women whose periods have stopped or have become very irregular may commence therapy at any time.

During the second two weeks of the cycle, that is from the 15th day after applying the first patch, one Duphaston tablet should be taken each day for the next 14 days. Most patients will commence bleeding towards the end of the Duphaston therapy.

Unopposed oestrogen therapy should not be used unless the patient has undergone a hysterectomy.

*Children:* Femapak 80 is not indicated in children.

*Contra-indications:* Femapak 80 is contra-indicated in women with known or suspected pregnancy, cancer of the breast, genital tract or other oestrogen-dependent neoplasia, undiagnosed vaginal bleeding, endometriosis, severe renal or cardiac disease, acute or chronic liver disease where liver function tests have failed to return to normal, active thrombophlebitis or thromboembolic disorders (see *Special Precautions and Warnings*), Dubin-Johnson syndrome or rotor syndrome or hypersensitivity to lactose or other ingredients of the tablet.

*Special warnings and precautions for use:* It is recommended that the patient should undergo a thorough physical and gynaecological examination before commencing therapy. This should be repeated at regular intervals.

Unopposed estradiol therapy should not be used in non-hysterectomised women because of the increased risk of endometrial hyperplasia or carcinoma.

At the present time there is suggestive evidence of an overall change in the relative risk of breast cancer in post-menopausal women receiving oestrogen replacement therapy. While some studies have shown that there may be a small increase in risk with treatment for more than 5 years others have shown no such increase. It is not known whether concurrent progestogen use influences the risk of breast cancer in post-menopausal women taking hormone replacement therapy. A careful appraisal of the risk/benefit ratio should be undertaken before treating for longer than 5 to 10 years.

Women with a history of fibrocystic disease, breast nodules, abnormal mammograms or family history of breast cancer should have regular breast examinations.

Certain diseases may be made worse by hormone replacement therapy and patients with these conditions should be closely monitored. These include otosclerosis, multiple sclerosis, systemic lupus erythematosus, cholelithiasis, porphyria, melanoma, epilepsy, migrane, thyrotoxicosis, surgically confirmed gall bladder disease, asthma and diabetes (worsening of glucose tolerance). Pre-existing uterine fibroids may increase in size during oestrogen therapy and symptoms associated with endometriosis may be exacerbated.

There is no indication from published studies of an increased risk of thromboembolic disease or thrombophlebitis in apparently normal women at the current recommended low doses of Hormone Replacement Therapy (HRT).

In the event of an acute thromboembolic event occurring during treatment HRT should be discontinued. However there is no indication to suggest that a history of deep vein thrombosis, pulmonary embolism, stroke or myocardial infarction when associated with recognised risk factors (such as immobilisation or post-trauma or post-operatively) should be a contra-indication to HRT but in the absence of specific data Femapak 80 should be used with caution in these patients.

Consideration should be given to discontinuation of treatment 4 weeks prior to surgery or during periods of prolonged immobilisation or in patients who develop hypertension.

If jaundice or significant hypertension develop, treatment should be discontinued whilst the cause is investigated. As oestrogens may cause fluid retention, patients with cardiac or renal dysfunction should be closely observed. Regular monitoring of blood pressure should be carried out in hypertensive patients.

Women who may be at risk of pregnancy should be advised to adhere to non-hormonal contraceptive methods.

*Interactions with other medicaments and other forms of interaction:* Preparations inducing microsomal liver enzymes, e.g. barbiturates, hydantoins, anti-convulsants (including carbamazepine), meprobromate, phenylbutazone, antibiotics (including rifampicin), and activated charcoal may impair the activity of oestrogens. Transdermally applied oestrogens are less likely to be affected by such interactions than oral oestrogens since first pass hepatic metabolism is avoided.

Changes in oestrogen serum concentrations may affect the results of certain endocrine or liver function tests.

*Pregnancy and lactation:* Femapak 80 is contra-indicated.

*Effects on ability to drive and use machines:* None stated.

*Undesirable effects:* The most frequent side effects (reported in 10 to 20% of patients, on at least one occasion in clinical trials with Fematrix 80) which do not normally prevent continued treatment include: breast tenderness, headaches, and breakthrough bleeding. Some patients experience mild and transient local erythema at the site of patch application with or without itching; this usually disappears rapidly on removal of the patch. The overall incidence of general patch irritation in clinical studies in less than 5%. In a clinical study 3% of 102 patients showed well defined erythema (draize scale) 30 minutes after patch removal. No instances of permanent skin damage have been reported. If unacceptable topical side effects do occur discontinuation of treatment should be considered.

Other side effects associated with estrogen or estrogen/progestogen treatment have occasionally been reported (in 1 to 5% of patients in clinical trials with Fematrix 80) include: abdominal cramps, abdominal bloating, oedema, nausea, migraine and weight changes. More rarely (less than 1% in clinical trials with Fematrix 80) dizziness, dysmenorrhoea, leg cramps and visual disturbances have been reported. Additional side effects of dydrogesterone include occasional reports of transient dizziness and skin reactions.

Other side effects which have been rarely reported with oestrogen products include: changes in libido or changes in carbohydrate tolerance, vaginal candidiasis, change in vaginal secretions, cystitis like syndrome, cervical erosion, erythema multiforme, erythema nodosa, haemeorrhagic eruptions, chloasma or melasma which may be persistent when the drug is discontinued, steepening of corneal curvature, intolerance to contact lenses, mental depression and chorea minor. Cholestatis may be possible in predisposed patients.

*Overdose:* Fematrix 80: This is not likely due to the mode of administration. If it is necessary to stop delivery then the patch can be removed and plasma estradiol levels will fall rapidly.

*Duphaston: Symptoms:* No reports of ill effects from overdosage have been recorded and remedial action is generally unnecessary.

*Treatment:* If a large overdosage is discovered within 2–3 hours and treatment seems desirable, gastric lavage is recommended. There are no special antidotes and treatment should be symptomatic.

**Pharmacological properties**

*Pharmacodynamic properties*

*Estradiol:* In the female, estradiol stimulates the accessory reproductive organs and causes development of the secondary sexual characteristics at puberty. It is also responsible for the hypertrophy of the uterus and for the changes in the endometrium during the first half of the menstrual cycle which when acted on by progesterone prepares it for the reception of a fertilised ovum. It furthermore promotes the growth of the ducts of the mammary glands. Large doses inhibit the gonadotropic secretion of the anterior pituitary, thus influencing the normal ovarian cycle.

It is of value in menstrual disorders, ovarian insufficiency, especially at the menopause, and for the treatment of infections of the vagina in childen, where it promotes the growth of a cornified and more resistant epithelium; it is also used to terminate lactation, not very successfully, by inhibiting the release of prolactin.

*Dydrogesterone:* Dydrogesterone is an orally-active progestogen which produces a complete secretory endometrium in an oestrogen-primed uterus thereby providing protection for Oestrogen-induced increased risk of endometrial hyperplasia and/or carcinogenesis. It is indicated in all cases of endogenous progesterone deficiency. Duphaston is non-androgenic, non-oestrogenic, non-corticoid and non-anabolic.

*Pharmacokinetic properties:*

*Fematrix 80:*

*Absorption:* Estradiol is absorbed from the patch across the stratum corneum and is delivered systemically at a low but constant rate throughout the period of application (3 to 4 days). The estimated delivery of estradiol is around 80 µg/day.

*Distribution:* Oestrogens circulate in the blood bound to albumin, sex hormone binding globulin (SHBG), cortisol binding globulin and alpha 1-glycoprotein. Following diffusion of free oestrogen into the cells of the target tissues in the hypothalamus, pituitary, vagina, urethra, uterus, breast and liver, binding to specific oestrogen receptors occurs. Very little information is currently available on the distribution of estradiol following transdermal administration.

*Biotransformation:* Inactivation of oestrogens in the body is carried out mainly in the liver. Metabolism of 17β estradiol is by oxidation to oestrone, which in turn can be hydrated to form oestriol. There is free interconversion between oestrone and estradiol. Oestrone and oestriol may then undergo conversion to their corresponding sulphate and glucuronide derivatives for excretion in the urine. Oestrone sulphate has a long biologic half-life because of its enterohepatic recirculation and interconversion to oestrone and estradiol.

*Elimination:* The plasma elimination half-life of estradiol is approximately 1 hour and is independent of the route of administration. The metabolic plasma clearance rate is between 650 and 900 L/day/m².

Steady state plasma estradiol concentrations have been demonstrated in the range of 34 pg/ml to 62 pg/ml and these are maintained throughout the dose interval (for up to four days). Absorption rate may vary between individual patients. After removal of the last patch plasma estradiol and oestrone concentrations return to baseline values in less than 24 hours. The median terminal half-life for estradiol following patch removal has been determined as 5.24 h.

*Dydrogesterone:* After oral administration of labelled dydrogesterone on average 63% of the dose is excreted into the urine. Within 72 hours excretion is complete. Dydrogesterone is completely metabolised.

The main metabolite of dydrogesterone is 20 α-dihydrodydrogesterone (DHD) and is present in the urine predominantly as the glucuronic acid conjugate. A common feature of all metabolites characterised is the retention of the 4.6 diene-3-one configuration of the parent compound and the absence of 17 α-hydroxylation. This explains the lack of oestrogenic and androgenic effects of dydrogesterone.

After oral administration of dydrogesterone, plasma concentrations of DHD are substantially higher as compared to the parent drug. The AUC and $C_{max}$ ratios of DHD to dydrogesterone are in the order of 40 and 25, respectively.

Dydrogesterone is rapidly absorbed. The $T_{max}$ values of dydrogesterone and DHD vary between 0.5 and 2.5 hours.

Mean terminal half lives of dydrogesterone and DHD vary between 5 to 7 and 14 to 17 hours, respectively.

Unlike progesterone, dydrogesterone is not excreted in the urine as pregnanediol. It is therefore possible to analyze production of endogenous progesterone even in the presence of dydrogesterone.

*Preclinical safety data:*

*Fematrix 80:* No specific preclinical studies have been conducted on Fematrix. Supraphysiologically high doses (prolonged overdoses) of oestradiol have been associated with the induction of tumours in oestrogen dependent target organs in rodent species. Pronounced species differences in toxicology, pharmacology and pharmacodynamics exist.

*Dydrogesterone:* Dydrogesterone has been used in several animal models and has been proven to have low toxicity. It does not have mutagenic or carcinogenic properties. No effects were seen in reproduction experiments.

**Pharmaceutical particulars**

*List of excipients:*

*Fematrix 80:* Diethyltoluamide, Acrylic adhesive). Backing: Polyester film, Release liner: Aluminised/polyester.

*Duphaston:* Lactose, maize starch, methylhydroxypropylcellulose, silica, magnesium stearate, and titanium dioxide (E171).

*Incompatibilities:* None known.

*Shelf life:* The shelf-life of the product as packaged for sale is 2 years.

*Special precautions for storage:* Femapak 80 should be stored at room temperature below 25°C in a dry place. Duphaston tablets should also be protected from light.

*Nature and contents of container:*

*Fematrix 80:* Blister tray with a foil lid containing one transdermal patch.

*Duphaston:* Blister strip containing 14 tablets.

Each carton contains eight Fematrix 80 patches and 14 Duphaston HRT tablets sufficient for one 28 day cycle.

*Instruction for use/handling:* Detailed instructions for use are given in the patient leaflet.

*Marketing authorisation holder:* Ethical Pharmaceuticals (UK) Limited, Gemini House, Bartholomew's Walk, Cambridgeshire Business Park, Ely, Cambs CB7 4EA.

**Marketing authorisation number** 10013/0033.

**Date of approval/revision of SPC** June 1997.

**Legal category** POM.

## FEMATRIX*40

**Qualitative and quantitative composition** Fematrix 40 contains 1.25 mg of oestradiol (Estradiol INN) and each patch delivers approximately 40 micrograms of oestradiol per 24 hours.

**Pharmaceutical form** Fematrix 40 is a self adhesive, flexible transdermal patch comprising a layer of clear adhesive sandwiched between a translucent patch and a metallised polyester backing. Fematrix 40 is a rectangular shape with rounded corners and has an active surface area of 14.25 cm².

**Clinical particulars**
*Therapeutic indications*: Oestrogen replacement therapy in female patients for the treatment of symptoms of oestrogen deficiency as a result of the natural menopause or oophorectomy.

*Posology and method of administration:*
*Adults*: Therapy should be initiated with Fematrix 40 in women who have menopausal symptoms, who have been oestrogen deficient for a prolonged time or who are likely to be intolerant of high levels of oestradiol. The dosage may be increased if required by using Fematrix 80. For maintenance therapy the lowest effective dose should be used.

One Fematrix transdermal patch should be applied twice weekly on a continuous basis. Each patch should be removed after 3 to 4 days and replaced with a new patch applied to a slightly different site. Patches should be applied to clean, dry and intact areas of skin below the waist on the lower back or buttocks. Fematrix should not be applied on or near the breasts.

Women who are having regular periods should commence therapy within five days of the start of bleeding. Women whose periods have stopped or have become very irregular may commence therapy at any time.

In women with a uterus, a progestogen should be added for 12 to 14 days of each cycle. Most patients will commence bleeding towards the end of the progestogen therapy.

Unopposed oestrogen therapy should not be used unless the patient has undergone a hysterectomy.

*Children*: Fematrix is not indicated in children.

*Contra-indications:* Fematrix is contra-indicated in women with known or suspected pregnancy, cancer of the breast, genital tract or other oestrogen-dependent neoplasia, undiagnosed vaginal bleeding, endometriosis, severe renal or cardiac disease, acute or chronic liver disease where liver function tests have failed to return to normal, active thrombophlebitis or thromboembolic disorders, Dubin-Johnson syndrome or rotor syndrome.

*Special warnings and precautions for use:* It is recommended that the patient should undergo a thorough physical and gynaecological examination before commencing therapy. This should be repeated at regular intervals.Unopposed oestradiol therapy should not be used in non-hysterectomised women because of the increased risk of endometrial hyperplasia or carcinoma.

At present time there is suggestive evidence of an overall change in the relative risk of breast cancer in post menopausal women receiving oestrogen replacement therapy. While some studies have shown that there may be a small increase in risk with treatment for more than 5 years others have shown no such increase. It is not known whether concurrent progestogen use influences the risk of breast cancer in postmenopausal women taking hormone replacement therapy. A careful appraisal of the risk/benefit ratio should be undertaken before treating for longer than 5 to 10 years.

Women with a history of fibrocystic disease, breast nodules, abnormal mammograms or family history of breast cancer should have regular breast examinations.

Close monitoring of women with a history of uterine fibroids, cholelithiasis, porphyria, epilepsy, migraine, diabetes is necessary as oestrogen therapy may exacerbate or precipitate these conditions. Regular monitoring of blood pressure should be carried out in hypertensive patients.

Certain diseases may be made worse by hormone replacement therapy and patients with these conditions should be closely monitored. These include otosclerosis, multiple sclerosis, systemic lupus erythematosus, thyrotoxicosis, surgically confirmed gall bladder disease and diabetes (worsening of glucose tolerance). In addition pre-existing uterine fibroids may increase in size during oestrogen therapy and symptoms associated with endometriosis may be exacerbated.

There is no indication from published studies of an increased risk of thromboembolic disease or thrombophlebitis in apparently normal women at the current recommended low doses of Hormone Replacement Therapy (HRT).

In the event of an acute thromboembolic event occurring during treatment HRT should be discontinued. However there is no indication to suggest that a history of deep vein thrombosis, pulmonary embolism, stroke or myocardial infarction when associated with recognized risk factors (such as immobilisation or post-trauma or post-operatively) should be a contraindication to HRT but in the absence of specific data Fematrix should be used with caution in these patients.

Consideration should be given to discontinuation of treatment 4 weeks prior to surgery or during periods of prolonged immobilisation or in patients who develop hypertension.

Women who may be at risk of pregnancy should be advised to adhere to non-hormonal contraceptive methods.

*Interactions with other medicaments and other forms of interaction*: None.

*Pregnancy and lactation*: Fematrix is contra-indicated.

*Effects on ability to drive and use machines*: None.

*Undesirable effects*: Fematrix is generally well tolerated. The most frequent side-effects, (reported in 10 to 20% of patients, on at least one occasion, in clinical trials with Fematrix 80) which do not normally prevent continued treatment include: breast tenderness, headaches and breakthrough bleeding . Some patients experience mild and transient local erythema at the site of application with or without itching; this usually disappears rapidly on removal of the patch. The overall incidence of general patch irritation in clinical studies is less than 5%. In a clinical study 3% of 102 patients showed well defined erythema (Draize scale) 30 minutes after patch removal. No instances of permanent skin damage have been reported. If unacceptable topical side effects do occur discontinuation of treatment should be considered.

Other side effects associated with oestrogen or oestrogen/progestogen treatment have occasionally been reported (in 1% to 5% of patients in clinical trials with Fematrix 80) include: abdominal cramps, abdominal bloating, oedema, nausea, migraine and weight changes.

More rarely (less than 1% in clinical trials with Fematrix 80) dizziness, dysmenorrhoea, leg cramps and visual disturbances and changes in libido or changes in carbohydrate tolerance have been reported with other oestradiol products.

*Overdose*: This is not likely due to the mode of administration. If it is necessary to stop delivery then the patch can be removed and plasma oestradiol levels will fall rapidly.

**Pharmacological properties**
*Pharmacodynamic properties:*
*Pharmacotherapeutic group*: Natural oestrogen.

*Mechanism of action/pharmacodynamic effects*: In the female, oestradiol stimulates the accessory reproductive organs and causes development of the secondary sexual characteristics at puberty. It is also responsible for the hypertrophy of the uterus and for the changes in the endometrium during the first half of the menstrual cycle which when acted on by progesterone prepares it for the reception of a fertilized ovum. It furthermore promotes the growth of the ducts of the mammary glands. Large doses inhibit the gonadotropic secretion of the anterior pituitary, thus influencing the normal ovarian cycle.

It is of value in menstrual disorders, ovarian insufficiency, especially at the menopause, and for the treatment of infections of the vagina in children, where it promotes the growth of a cornified and more resistant epithelium; it is also used to terminate lactation, not very successfully, by inhibiting the release of prolactin.

*Pharmacokinetic properties:*
*General characteristics of the active substance – Absorption*: Oestradiol is absorbed from the patch across the stratum corneum and is delivered systemically at a low but constant rate throughout the period of application (3 to 4 days). The estimated delivery of oestradiol is approximately 40 micrograms per day for Fematrix 40.

*Distribution*: Oestrogens circulate in the blood bound to albumin, sex hormone binding globulin (SHBG), cortisol binding globulin and alpha-1-glycoprotein. Following diffusion of free oestrogen into the cells of the target tissues in the hypothalamus, pituitary, vagina, urethra, uterus, breast and liver, binding to specific oestrogen receptors occurs. Very little information is currently available on the distribution of oestradiol following transdermal administration.

*Biotransformation*: Inactivation of oestrogens in the body is carried out mainly in the liver. Metabolism of 17β-oestradiol is by oxidation to oestrone, which in turn can be hydrated to form oestriol. There is free interconversion between oestrone and oestradiol. Oestrone and oestriol may then undergo conversion to their corresponding sulphate and glucuronide derivatives for excretion in the urine. Oestrone sulphate has a long biologic half-life because of its enterohepatic recirculation and interconversion to oestrone and oestradiol.

*Elimination*: The plasma elimination half-life of oestradiol is approximately 1 hour and is independent of the route of administration. The metabolic plasma clearance rate is between 650 and 900 L/day/m².

Steady state plasma oestradiol concentrations have been demonstrated in the range of 26 pg/ml to 34 pg/ml for the Fematrix 40 patch and 34 to 62 pg/ml for the Fematrix 80 patch (including baseline levels) and these are maintained throughout the dose interval (for up to four days). Absorption rate may vary between individual patients. After removal of the last patch plasma oestradiol and oestrone concentrations return to baseline values in less than 24 hours. The median terminal half-life for oestradiol following patch removal has been determined as 5.24h.

*Preclinical safety data*: No specific preclinical studies have been conducted on Fematrix. Supraphysiologically high doses (prolonged overdoses) of oestradiol have been associated with the induction of tumours in oestrogen-dependent target organs in rodent species. Pronounced species differences in toxicology, pharmacology and pharmacodynamics exist.

**Pharmaceutical particulars**
*List of excipients*: Diethyltoluamide, acrylic emulsion (proprietary adhesive), acrylic emulsion (adhesive thickener). Backing: Polyester. Release liner: Siliconised/aluminised/polyester.

*Incompatibilities:* Not applicable.

*Shelf life*: The shelf-life of the product as packaged for sale is 2 years.

*Special precautions for storage*: Fematrix patches should be stored at room temperature (below 25 °C) in a dry place.

*Nature and contents of container*: PVC/PVDC blister tray with paper/polythene/aluminium foil lid containing one transdermal patch. Each carton contains eight patches, sufficient for one 28 day cycle and a patient leaflet.

*Instruction for use/handling*: Detailed instructions for use are provided in the patient leaflet.

*Marketing authorisation holder*: Ethical Pharmaceuticals (UK) Ltd, Gemini House, Bartholomew's Walk, Cambridgeshire Business Park, Ely, Cambs CB7 4EA

**Marketing authorisation number** 10013/0032

**Date of approval/revision of SPC** 4 January 1996

**Legal category** POM

## FEMATRIX* 80

**Qualitative and quantitative composition** Fematrix 80 contains 2.5 mg of oestradiol (Estradiol INN) and each patch delivers approximately 80 micrograms of oestradiol per 24 hours.

**Pharmaceutical form** Fematrix 80 is a self adhesive, flexible transdermal patch comprising a layer of clear adhesive sandwiched between a translucent patch and a metallised polyester backing. Fematrix 80 is a rectangular shape with rounded corners and has an active surface area of 28.5 cm².

**Clinical particulars**
*Therapeutic indications:* Oestrogen replacement therapy for the relief of postmenopausal symptoms and for the prevention of osteoporosis in women at risk of developing fractures.

Epidemiological studies suggest a number of individual risk factors contribute to postmenopausal osteoporosis, including:

- early menopause (either naturally or surgically)
- family history of osteoporosis
- recent prolonged systemic corticosteroid therapy
- a small, thin frame
- cigarette use

If several risk factors are present consideration should be given to oestrogen replacement therapy.

For maximum benefit treatment should commence as soon as possible after the menopause.

*Posology and method of administration:*
*Climacteric symptoms:* Therapy should be initiated with Fematrix 40 in women who have menopausal symptoms, who have been oestrogen deficient for a prolonged time or who are likely to be intolerant of high levels of oestradiol. The dosage may be increased if required by using Fematrix 80. For maintenance therapy the lowest effective dose should be used.

*Prevention of osteoporosis:* Treatment should be with Fematrix 80, as the efficacy of Fematrix 40 in this indication has yet to be established.

For optimum benefit treatment should continue for 5 to 10 years, protection appears to be effective for as long as treatment continues, however data beyond 10 years is limited. For long term use see also *Precautions and warnings*.

*Dosage schedule:* One Fematrix 80 transdermal patch should be applied twice weekly on a continuous basis. Each patch should be removed after 3 to 4 days and replaced with a new patch applied to a slightly different site. Patches should be applied to clean, dry and intact areas of skin below the waist on the lower back or buttocks. Fematrix should not be applied on or near the breasts.

Women who are having regular periods should commence therapy within five days of the start of bleeding. Women whose periods have stopped or have become very irregular may commence therapy at any time.

In women with a uterus, a progestogen should be added for 12 to 14 days of each cycle. Most patients will commence bleeding towards the end of the progestogen therapy.

Unopposed oestrogen therapy should not be used unless the patient has undergone a hysterectomy.

*Children:* Fematrix is not indicated in children.

*Contra-indications:* Fematrix is contra-indicated in women with known or suspected pregnancy, cancer of the breast, genital tract or other oestrogen-dependent neoplasia, undiagnosed vaginal bleeding, endometriosis, severe renal or cardiac disease, acute or chronic liver disease where liver function tests have failed to return to normal, active thrombophlebitis or thromboembolic disorders (see *Special Precautions and Warnings*), Dubin-Johnson syndrome or rotor syndrome.

*Special warnings and precautions for use:* It is recommended that the patient should undergo a thorough physical and gynaecological examination before commencing therapy. This should be repeated at regular intervals. Unopposed oestradiol therapy should not be used in non-hysterectomised women because of the increased risk of endometrial hyperplasia or carcinoma.

At present time there is suggestive evidence of an overall change in the relative risk of breast cancer in post-menopausal women receiving oestrogen replacement therapy. While some studies have shown that there may be a small increase in risk with treatment for more than 5 years others have shown no such increase. It is not known whether concurrent progestogen use influences the risk of breast cancer in post-menopausal women taking hormone replacement therapy. A careful appraisal of the risk/benefit ratio should be undertaken before treating for longer than 5 to 10 years.

Women with a history of fibrocystic disease, breast nodules, abnormal mammograms or family history of breast cancer should have regular breast examinations.

Certain diseases may be made worse by hormone replacement therapy and patients with these conditions should be closely monitored. These include otosclerosis, multiple sclerosis, systemic lupus erythematosus, cholelithiasis, porphyria, melanoma, epilepsy, migraine, thyrotoxicosis, surgically confirmed gall bladder disease, asthma and diabetes (worsening of glucose tolerance). Pre-existing uterine fibroids may increase in size during oestrogen therapy and symptoms associated with endometriosis may be exacerbated.

There is no indication from published studies of an increased risk of thromboembolic disease or thrombophlebitis in apparently normal women at the current recommended low doses of Hormone Replacement Therapy (HRT).

In the event of an acute thromboembolic event occurring during treatment HRT should be discontinued. However there is no indication to suggest that a history of deep vein thrombosis, pulmonary embolism, stroke or myocardial infarction, when associated with recognised risk factors (such as immobilisation or post-trauma or post-operatively) should be a contra-indication to HRT but in the absence of specific data Fematrix should be used with caution in these patients.

Consideration should be given to discontinuation of treatment 4 weeks prior to surgery or during periods of prolonged immobilisation.

If jaundice or significant hypertension develop, treatment should be discontinued whilst the cause is investigated. As oestrogens may cause fluid retention, patients with cardiac or renal dysfunction should be closely observed. Regular monitoring of blood pressure should be carried out in hypertensive patients.

Women who may be at risk of pregnancy should be advised to adhere to non-hormonal contraceptive methods.

*Interactions with other medicaments and other forms of interaction:* Preparations inducing microsomal liver enzymes, e.g. barbituates, hydantoins, anti-convulsants (including carbamazepine), meprobromate, phenylbutazone, antibiotics (including rifampicin), and activated charcoal may impair the activity of oestrogens. Transdermally applied oestrogens are less likely to be affected by such interactions than oral

oestrogens since first pass hepatic metabolism is avoided.

Changes in oestrogen serum concentrations may affect the results of certain endocrine or liver function tests.

*Pregnancy and lactation:* Fematrix is contra-indicated.

*Effects on ability to drive and use machines:* None.

*Undesirable effects:* Fematrix is generally well tolerated. The most frequent side-effects (reported in 10 to 20% of patients, on at least one occasion, in clinical trials with Fematrix 80), which do not normally prevent continued treatment include: breast tenderness, headaches and breakthrough bleeding. Some patients experience mild and transient local erythema at the site of application with or without itching; this usually disappears rapidly on removal of the patch. The overall incidence of general patch irritation in clinical studies is less than 5%. In a clinical study 3% of 102 patients showed well defined erythema (Draize scale) 30 minutes after patch removal. No instances of permanent skin damage have been reported. If unacceptable topical side-effects do occur discontinuation of treatment should be considered.

Other side-effects associated with oestrogen or oestrogen/progestogen treatment have occasionally been reported (in 1% to 5% of patients in clinical trials with Fematrix 80) include: abdominal cramps, abdominal bloating, oedema, nausea, migraine and weight changes. More rarely (less than 1% in clinical trials with Fematrix 80) dizziness, dysmenorrhoea, leg cramps and visual disturbances have been reported.

Other side effects which have been rarely reported with oestrogen products include: changes in libido or changes in carbohydrate tolerance, vaginal candidiasis, change in vaginal secretions, cystitis like syndrome, cervical erosion, erythema multiforme, erythema nodosa, haemorrhagic eruptions, chloasma or melasma which may be persistent when the drug is discontinued, steepening of corneal curvature, intolerance to contact lenses, mental depression and chorea minor. Cholestasis may be possible in predisposed patients.

*Overdose:* This is not likely due to the mode of administration. If it is necessary to stop delivery then the patch can be removed and plasma oestradiol levels will fall rapidly.

**Pharmacological properties**

*Pharmacodynamic properties:* Pharmacotherapeutic group: Natural oestrogen.

*Mechanism of action/pharmacodynamic effects:* In the female, oestradiol stimulates the accessory reproductive organs and causes development of the secondary sexual characteristics at puberty. It is also responsible for the hypertrophy of the uterus and for the changes in the endometrium during the first half of the menstrual cycle which when acted on by progesterone prepares it for the reception of a fertilised ovum. It furthermore promotes the growth of the ducts of the mammary glands. Large doses inhibit the gonadotropic secretion of the anterior pituitary, thus influencing the normal ovarian cycle.

It is of value in menstrual disorders, ovarian insufficiency, especially at the menopause, and for the treatment of infections of the vagina in childen, where it promotes the growth of a cornified and more resistant epithelium; it is also used to terminate lactation, not very successfully, by inhibiting the release of prolactin.

*Pharmacokinetic properties*
*General characteristics of the active substance –*
*Absorption:* Oestradiol is absorbed from the patch across the stratum corneum and is delivered systemically at a low but constant rate throughout the period of application (3 to 4 days). The estimated delivery of oestradiol is approximately 80 micrograms per day for Fematrix 80.
*Distribution:* Oestrogens circulate in the blood bound to albumin, sex hormone binding globulin (SHBG), cortisol binding globulin and alpha-1-glycoprotein. Following diffusion of free oestrogen into the cells of the target tissues in the hypothalamus, pituitary, vagina, urethra, uterus, breast and liver, binding to specific oestrogen receptors occurs. Very little information is currently available on the distribution of oestradiol following transdermal administration.
*Biotransformation:* Inactivation of oestrogens in the body is carried out mainly in the liver. Metabolism of $17\beta$-oestradiol is by oxidation to oestrone, which in turn can be hydrated to form oestriol. There is free interconversion between oestrone and oestradiol. Oestrone and oestriol may then undergo conversion to their corresponding sulphate and glucuronide derivatives for excretion in the urine. Oestrone sulphate has a long biologic half-life because of its enterohepatic recirculation and interconversion to oestrone and oestradiol.
*Elimination:* The plasma elimination half-life of

oestradiol is approximately 1 hour and is independent of the route of administration. The metabolic plasma clearance rate is between 650 and 900 L/day/m2.

Steady state plasma oestradiol concentrations have been demonstrated in the range of 26 pg/ml to 34 pg/ml for the Fematrix 40 patch and 34 to 62 pg/ml for the Fematrix 80 patch (including baseline levels) and these are maintained throughout the dose interval (for up to four days). Absorption rate may vary between individual patients. After removal of the last patch plasma oestradiol and oestrone concentrations return to baseline values in less than 24 hours. The median terminal half-life for oestradiol following patch removal has been determined as 5.24 h.

*Preclinical safety data:* No specific preclinical studies have been conducted on Fematrix. Supraphysiologically high doses (prolonged overdoses) of oestradiol have been associated with the induction of tumours in oestrogen-dependent target organs in rodent species. Pronounced species differences in toxicology, pharmacology and pharmacodynamics exist.

**Pharmaceutical particulars**

*List of excipients:* Diethyltoluamide, Acrylic adhesive, Backing: Polyester. Release liner: Aluminised/polyester.

*Incompatibilities:* Not applicable.

*Shelf life:* The shelf-life of the product as packaged for sale is 2 years.

*Special precautions for storage:* Fematrix patches should be stored at room temperature (below 25°C) in a dry place.

*Nature and contents of container:* PVC/PVDC blister tray with paper/polythene/aluminium foil lid containing one transdermal patch. Each carton contains eight patches, sufficient for one 28 day cycle and a patient leaflet. An additional pack containing two patches may also be available.

*Instruction for use/handling:* Detailed instructions for use are provided in the patient leaflet.

*Marketing authorisation holder:* Ethical Pharmaceuticals (UK) Ltd, Gemini House, Bartholomew's Walk, Cambridgeshire Business Park, Ely, Cambs CB7 4EA.

**Marketing authorisation numbers** 10013/0021

**Date of approval/revision of SPC** August 1996.

**Legal category** POM.

# FEMOSTON*

**Qualitative and quantitative composition**
*Femoston 1/10 mg:* This product contains estradiol hemihydrate PhEur equivalent to 1 mg estradiol per tablet for the first 14 days of a 28-day cycle (white tablets). For the second 14 days of a 28-day cycle, one tablet contains estradiol hemihydrate PhEur equivalent to 1 mg estradiol and 10 mg dydrogesterone BP (grey tablets).

*Femoston 2/10 mg and Femoston 2/20 mg:* These products contain estradiol hemihydrate PhEur equivalent to 2 mg estradiol per tablet for the first 14 days of a 28-day cycle (orange tablets). For the second 14 days one tablet contains estradiol hemihydrate PhEur equivalent to 2 mg estradiol and 10 mg dydrogesterone BP (yellow tablets) or estradiol hemihydrate PhEur equivalent to 2 mg estradiol and 20 mg dydrogesterone BP (blue tablets).

**Pharmaceutical form** Film-coated tablets for oral use.

**Clinical particulars**

*Therapeutic indications*
*Femoston 1/10:* For the relief of postmenopausal symptoms in women with a uterus.

*Femoston 2/10 and Femoston 2/20:* For the relief of postmenopausal symptoms and prevention of osteoporosis in women with a uterus.

Epidemiological studies suggest a number of risk factors may contribute to postmenopausal osteoporosis, including:

- early menopause (either naturally or surgically induced)
- family history of osteoporosis
- recent prolonged corticosteroid therapy
- a small, thin frame
- excessive cigarette consumption

If several risk factors are present consideration should be given to hormone replacement therapy.

Bone mineral density measurements may help to confirm the presence of low bone mass. For maximum prophylactic benefit, treatment should commence as soon as possible after the menopause.

*Posology and method of administration:* For oral administration.
*Postmenopausal symptoms:* Initial treatment should be with Femoston 1/10 mg. Femoston 2/10 should be

substituted if control of climacteric symptoms is not achieved. The lowest dose compatible with control of symptoms should be used.

One tablet, containing 1 mg or 2 mg estradiol, daily during 14 consecutive days per cycle of 28 days and one tablet, containing 1 mg or 2 mg estradiol and 10 mg dydrogesterone daily during the remaining 14 days has to be taken.

Femoston 2/20 may be prescribed if either early withdrawal bleeding occurs or if endometrial biopsy reveals inadequate progestational response.

Immediately after a 28-day cycle, the next treatment cycle is to be started. Patients should take one tablet a day, according to the sequence indicated on the package. Medication is to be continued without interruption.

If the patient is still menstruating, it is recommended that treatment commences within five days of the start of bleeding.

In patients who had their last period more than approximately 12 months ago, treatment can be started at any time.

*Osteoporosis prevention:* Treatment should be with Femoston 2/10. Femoston 2/20 may be prescribed if either early withdrawal bleeding occurs or if endometrial biopsy reveals inadequate progestational response.

*Contra-indications:* Known or suspected carcinoma of the breast, endometrial carcinoma or other hormone dependent neoplasia.

Acute or chronic liver disease.

History of liver disease where the liver function tests have failed to return to normal.

Deep venous thrombosis, thromboembolic disorders, cerebral vascular accident.

Abnormal genital bleeding of unknown aetiology.

Known or suspected pregnancy.

*Special warnings and precautions for use:* These relate almost exclusively to the oestrogen component of this product: Physical examination and a complete medical and family history should be taken prior to the initiation of any hormone replacement therapy (HRT) with special reference to blood pressure, palpation of the breasts and the abdomen and a gynaecological examination.

Patients who are, or have previously been, treated with unopposed oestrogens should be examined with special care in order to investigate a possible hyperstimulation of the endometrium before commencing therapy.

As a general rule, HRT should not be prescribed for longer than one year without another physical examination, including gynaecological examination. In case of continuing abnormal and/or irregular bleeding, a diagnostic endometrial biopsy should be performed.

This oestrogen-progestogen combination treatment is not contraceptive. Patients in the peri-menopausal phase should be advised to take *non-hormonal* contraceptive precautions.

Consideration should be given to discontinuation of treatment if trauma, illness or impending surgery is considered to entail a risk of thrombosis. Special care should be taken in patients with a past history of deep venous thrombosis, thromboembolic disorders or cerebral vascular accident.

Patients with, or developing epilepsy, migraine, diabetes mellitus, cardiac failure, multiple sclerosis, hypertension, porphyria, haemoglobinopathies or otosclerosis should be carefully observed during treatment, as HRT may worsen these conditions. In patients with a past history of liver disease it is advisable to check liver functions on a regular basis.

Special care should be taken in patients with uterine leiomyomata and patients with a history of endometriosis as oestrogens may influence these conditions.

The indications for immediate withdrawal of therapy are:

- deep venous thrombosis
- thromboembolic disorders
- the appearance of jaundice
- the emergence of migraine-type headache
- sudden visual disturbances
- significant increase in blood pressure
- pregnancy

*Interaction with other medicaments and other forms of interaction:* Oestrogens interact with liver enzyme-inducing drugs with increased metabolism of oestrogens, which may reduce the oestrogen effect. Interactions are documented for the following liver enzyme-inducing drugs: barbiturates, phenytoin, rifampicin, carbamazepine.

No drug interactions are known for dydrogesterone.

*Pregnancy and lactation:* Known, or suspected pregnancy is a contra-indication.

Lactation – this product is not indicated during this period.

*Effects on ability to drive and use machines:* No effects known.

*Undesirable effects:* During the first few months of treatment breast tenderness may occur. Nausea, headache, abdominal pain, dysmenorrhoea, bloating, oedema and dizziness have been reported. Symptoms are normally transient. Skin reactions have been reported.

*Overdose:* There have been no reports of ill-effects from overdosing. If overdosage is discovered within two or three hours and is so large that treatment seems desirable, gastric lavage can safely be used. There is no specific antidote and further treatment should be symptomatic.

**Pharmacological properties**

*Pharmacodynamic properties:* Estradiol is chemically and biologically identical to the endogenous human estradiol and is, therefore, classified as a human oestrogen. Estradiol is the primary oestrogen and the most active of the ovarian hormones. The endogenous oestrogens are involved in certain functions of the uterus and accessory organs, including the proliferation of the endometrium and the cyclic changes in the cervix and vagina.

Oestrogens are known to play an important role for bone and fat metabolism. Furthermore, oestrogens also affect the autonomic nervous system and may have indirect positive psychotropic actions.

Dydrogesterone is an orally-active progestogen having an activity comparable to parenterally administered progesterone.

In the context of HRT, dydrogesterone produces a complete secretory endometrium in an oestrogen-primed uterus thereby providing protection for oestrogen induced increased risk of endometrial hyperplasia and/or carcinoma, without androgenic side-effects.

The beneficial effects of 17β-estradiol on lipoprotein, glucose and insulin metabolism are maintained in the presence of dydrogesterone.

*Pharmacokinetic properties:* Following oral administration, micronised estradiol is readily absorbed, but extensively metabolised. The major unconjugated and conjugated metabolites are oestrone and oestrone sulphate. These metabolites can contribute to the oestrogen activity, either directly or after conversion to estradiol. Oestrone sulphate may undergo enterohepatic circulation. In urine, the major compounds are the glucuronides of oestrone and estradiol.

Oestrogens are secreted in the milk of nursing mothers.

After oral administration of labelled dydrogesterone, on average 63% of the dose is excreted into the urine. Within 72 hours excretion is complete.

In man, dydrogesterone is completely metabolised. The main metabolite of dydrogesterone is 20α-dihydrodydrogesterone (DHD) and is present in the urine predominantly as the glucuronic acid conjugate. A common feature of all metabolites characterised is the retention of the 4,6 diene-3-one configuration of the parent compound and the absence of 17α-hydroxylation. This explains the lack of oestrogenic and androgenic effects of dydrogesterone.

After oral administration of dydrogesterone, plasma concentrations of DHD are substantially higher as compared to the parent drug. The AUC and $C_{max}$ ratios of DHD to dydrogesterone are in the order of 40 and 25, respectively. Dydrogesterone is rapidly absorbed. The $T_{max}$ values of dydrogesterone and DHD vary between 0.5 and 2.5 hours.

Mean terminal half lives of dydrogesterone and DHD vary between 5 to 7 and 14 to 17 hours, respectively.

Dydrogesterone is not excreted in urine as pregnanediol, like progesterone. Analysis of endogenous progesterone production basd on pregnanediol excretion therefore remains possible. No pharmacokinetic interactions occur between estradiol and dydrogesterone.

*Preclinical safety data:* Supraphysiologically high doses (prolonged overdoses) of estradiol have been associated with the induction of tumours in oestrogen-dependent target organs for all rodent species tested. Pronounced species differences in toxicology, pharmacology and pharmacodynamics exist. The changes observed with dydrogesterone in animal toxicity studies are associated with the effects of progesterone-like compounds.

Doses administered to rats and mice sufficient to produce hormone-mediated changes gave no evidence of carcinogenesis.

**Pharmaceutical particulars**

*List of excipients:* Lactose; methylhydroxypropylcellulose; maize starch; colloidal anhydrous silica; magnesium stearate; Opadry Y-1-7000 white (for 1 mg estradiol only tablet) – contains E171; Opadry OY-8243 grey (for combination tablet of 1 mg oestradiol with 10 mg dydrogesterone) – contains E171, E172; Opadry OY-23000 orange (for 2 mg estradiol only tablet) – contains E104, E110, E124, E171; Opadry OY-7915 yellow (for combination tablet of 2 mg oestradiol with 10 mg dydrogesterone) – contains E104, E110, E124, E171; Opadry OY-6535 blue (for combination tablet of 2 mg oestradiol with 20 mg dydrogesterone) – contains E104, E131, E124 and E171.

*Incompatibilities:* Not applicable.

*Shelf life:* Femoston 1/10 mg–2 years at 25°C and ambient humidity in PVC strips. Femoston 2/10 mg and Femoston 2/20 mg–3 years at 25°C and ambient humidity in PVC strips.

*Special precautions for storage:* Store at room temperature (25°C).

*Nature and contents of container:* The tablets are packed in blister strips of 28. The blister strips are made of PVC film with a covering aluminium foil. Each carton contains 28 or 84 tablets.

*Instructions for use/handling:* Instructions for use of the blister package are included in the Patient Information Leaflet.

**Marketing authorisation numbers**

| | |
|---|---|
| Femoston 1/10 mg | 0512/0121 |
| Femoston 2/10 mg | 0512/0113 |
| Femoston 2/20 mg | 0512/0114 |

**Date of approval/revision of SPC** September 1996.

**Legal category** POM.

# INFLUVAC* SUB-UNIT VACCINE

**Qualitative and quantitative composition** Single dose disposable syringes of Inactivated Influenza Vaccine (Surface Antigen) BP.

Each 0.5 ml dose contains the haemagglutinin and neuraminidase antigens prepared from the appropriate quantities of the A and B strains currently recommended by the WHO. The aqueous buffered medium contains traces of sucrose.

**Pharmaceutical form** Sterile colourless opalescent liquid suspension for intramuscular or deep subcutaneous injection.

**Clinical particulars**

*Therapeutic indications:* Prophylaxis of influenza. Particularly recommended in:

- chronic pulmonary disease, e.g. chronic bronchitis and emphysema, asthma, bronchiectasis, pulmonary tuberculosis and fibrosis;
- chronic heart disease, e.g. valvular and hypertensive heart disease;
- chronic renal disease, e.g. chronic nephritis, including patients with renal disease on immuno-suppressive drugs;
- diabetes and possibly other less common endocrine disorders;
- elderly people;
- key personnel;
- chronic furunculosis or other chronic staphylococcal infections;
- persons living in residential establishments in which a rapid spread is likely to follow the introduction of infection.

*Posology and method of administration*
*Adults (including the elderly) and children (over 13 years):* 0.5 ml, single dose.

*Children (4–13 years):* 0.5 ml, two doses†.

*Children (6 months–4 years):* 0.25 ml, two doses†.

† In children under 13 years who have not been previously infected or who have not received trivalent influenza vaccine in the preceding four years, a second dose should be given after an interval of 4–6 weeks.

To be given by intramuscular or deep subcutaneous injection after allowing the vaccine to reach room temperature.

*Contra-indications:* Persons with hypersensitivity to eggs, chicken protein and influenza viral proteins, should not be vaccinated. Immunisation should be postponed in patients with febrile illness.

*Special warnings and special precautions for use:* In the rare event of an unexpected, severe immediate hypersensitivity reaction, Adrenaline Injection BP should be ready for use.

The vaccine may contain minimal amounts of polymyxin, neomycin and gentamicin. Use with caution in patients hypersensitive to these antibiotics.

*Interaction with other medicaments and other forms of interaction:* Influenza vaccine may be given at the same time as other vaccines. Vaccines should however be given at different sites. Influenza vaccine should not be given within 3 days of vaccination with pertussis vaccine.

Adverse events may be aggravated after simultaneous administration of vaccines. Persons known to be sensitive to vaccination should therefore observe a waiting period of 3 weeks, unless the influenza season has already started.

*Pregnancy and lactation:* Although there is no evidence that influenza vaccine has any harmful effect during pregnancy, careful consideration should be given to the use of the vaccine. The vaccine may be given during lactation.

*Effects on ability to drive and use machines:* Not known.

*Undesirable effects:* Because Influvac does not contain infectious particles it cannot cause influenza. Systemic effects, such as pyrexia, fatigue and headache may be experienced. Local effects, such as transient erythema and swelling at the site of injection may also occur, but reactions of both types are usually less frequent than those associated with the administration of whole virus vaccine.

Neurological disorders such as encephalomyelitis and neuritis after influenza vaccination have been rarely reported. An association has not been demonstrated except in the case of Guillain Barré Syndrome (USA Mass-vaccination programme 1976).

*Overdose:* In view of the nature of the product, overdose is unlikely to have any untoward effect. Accidental administration of ten times the normal dose has occurred without adverse effect.

### Pharmacological properties
*Pharmacodynamic properties:* Influvac is a vaccine that offers protection against influenza, normally within ten days after administration. The duration of protection depends on the antibody level post vaccination, which shows a large variation from person to person. Protection is normally effective for one year.

*Pharmacokinetic properties:* Studies have demonstrated that the purified haemagglutinin and neuraminidase antigens in Influvac induce protective titres in a high percentage of vaccines.

*Preclinical safety data:* Non-essential viral components have been removed in order to decrease the reactogenicity. The safety of other components has been established in pre-clinical studies.

### Pharmaceutical particulars
*List of excipients:* The vaccine is preserved with 0.01% thiomersal. Formaldehyde is used to inactivate the viruses. Other ingredients used in the preparation of the vaccine are: potassium dihydrogen phosphate, disodium phosphate, sodium citrate, potassium, sodium, calcium and magnesium chlorides, sucrose, cetyl trimethyl ammonium bromide, sodium deoxycholate and water for injections. The vaccine may also contain traces of the antibiotics polymyxin, neomycin and gentamicin.

*Incompatibilities:* None known.

*Shelf life:* One year from the date of the last determination of the antigen content.

*Special precautions for storage:* Store between +2 and +8°C, protected from light. Do not freeze.

*Nature and contents of container:* 0.5 ml disposable glass syringe. 10×0.5 ml disposable glass syringe.

*Instructions for use/handling:* Expel air by gently pushing the plunger, holding the syringe in upright position.

**Marketing authorisation number** 0512/0146.

**Date of approval/revision of SPC** August 1997.

**Legal category** POM.

## MONOTRIM* INJECTION

**Presentation** Ampoules containing a sterile, clear, colourless, aqueous solution (pH=4.0–4.5), containing trimethoprim lactate equivalent to 20 mg trimethoprim base per ml. Each ampoule contains 5 ml corresponding to 100 mg of trimethoprim base.

**Uses** Trimethoprim is active *in-vitro* against most Gram-positive and Gram-negative aerobic organisms. The antimicrobial activity is due to selective inhibition of bacterial dihydrofolate reductase.

*Indications:* Treatment of susceptible infections caused by trimethoprim-sensitive micro-organisms, particularly infections caused by gram-negative micro-organisms.

### Dosage and administration
*Dosage: Adults (including the elderly) and children over 12 years:* 200 mg every 12 hours.

*Children under 12 years:* The approximate dosage in children is 8 mg trimethoprim per kg body weight per day, divided into two or three equal doses.

In severely ill patients, the initial doses may be higher or given more frequently.

*Dosage advised where there is reduced kidney function:*

| Creatinine clearance (ml/sec) | Plasma creatinine (micromol/l) | | Dosage advised |
|---|---|---|---|
| Over 0.45 | men | <250 | normal |
| | women | <175 | |
| 0.25–0.45 | men | 250–600 | normal for 3 days then half dose |
| | women | 175–400 | |
| Under 0.25 | men | >600 | half the normal dose |
| | women | >400 | |

Trimethoprim is removed by dialysis. However, it should not be administered to dialysis patients unless plasma concentrations can be estimated regularly.

*Administration:* Monotrim Injection may be administered:

1. By direct slow intravenous injection, or
2. Via the tubing (close to the vein) of an established intravenous infusion.

It is compatible with the following commonly used infusion fluids:

Dextran 40 intravenous infusion BP 10% w/v in sodium chloride intravenous infusion 0.9% w/v

Dextran 70 intravenous infusion BP 6% w/v in sodium chloride intravenous infusion 0.9% w/v

Glucose intravenous infusion BP 50 g/l

Fructose intravenous infusion BP 50 g/l

Ringer's Injection USP

Sodium Chloride intravenous infusion BP 0.9% w/v

Sodium Chloride 0.45% w/v and Glucose 2.5% w/v intravenous infusion BP

Sodium Lactate intravenous infusion BP

Compound Sodium Lactate intravenous infusion BP

### Contra-indications, warnings, etc
*Contra-indications:* Pregnancy, hypersensitivity to trimethoprim, blood dyscrasias, severe renal insufficiency where blood levels cannot be monitored.

*Interactions:* Bone marrow depressants: Trimethoprim may increase the potential for bone marrow aplasia. Rifampicin may increase the elimination and shorten the elimination half-life of trimethoprim. Phenytoin and digoxin: The patients should be carefully controlled as trimethoprim may increase the elimination half-life of phenytoin and digoxin.

Cyclosporin may increase the nephrotoxicity of trimethoprim.

*Use in pregnancy and lactation:* Pregnancy is a contra-indication. Although trimethoprim is excreted in breast milk, lactation is not a contra-indication for short-term trimethoprim therapy.

*Precautions:* Caution should be exercised in the administration of trimethoprim to patients with actual or potential folate deficiency (e.g. elderly) and administration of folate supplement should be considered. Although an effect on folic acid metabolism is possible, interference with haematopoiesis rarely occurs at the recommended dose. If any such change is seen, folinic acid should reverse the effect. Elderly people may be more susceptible and a lower dose may be advisable. Regular haematological tests should be undertaken in long term treatment. In neonates, trimethoprim should be used under careful medical supervision.

In patients with impairment of renal function, care should be taken to avoid accumulation.

*Side effects:* Nausea, vomiting and skin rashes have been reported in rare instances: these effects are generally mild and quickly reversible on withdrawal of the drug. Rarely erythema multiforme and toxic epidermal necrolysis have occurred.

Aseptic meningitis has been reported. Trimethoprim may affect haematopoiesis.

*Treatment of overdosage:* Symptomatic treatment and forced diuresis can be used. In cases of oral overdosage, gastric lavage is recommended. Depression of haematopoiesis by trimethoprim can be counteracted by intramuscular administration of calcium folinate.

**Pharmaceutical precautions** Store below 25°C, protected from light.

Monotrim Injection is incompatible with solutions of sulphonamides and should not be mixed with such preparations.

**Legal category** POM.

**Package quantities** Boxes of 5×5 ml ampoules.

**Further information** Trimethoprim is effective *in-vitro* against most Gram-positive and Gram-negative aerobic organisms, including enterobacteria – *E. coli, Proteus, Klebsiella pneumoniae; Streptococcus faecalis; Streptococcus pneumoniae; Haemophilus influenzae;* and *Staphylococcus aureus.*

It is not active against Mycobacterium tuberculosis, Neisseria gonorrhoeae, Pseudomonas aeruginosa, Treponema pallidum, or anaerobic bacteria.

Monotrim Injection may be given in conjunction with, but separately from, other parenterally administered antibacterials, for example, aminoglycosides, metronidazole or sulphonamides whenever such a combination seems suitable.

**Product licence number** 4012/0008.

*Product licence holder:* A/S GEA Farmaceutisk Fabrik, Holger Danskes Vej 89, DK-2000 Frederiksberg, Denmark.

## MONOTRIM* SUSPENSION

**Qualitative and quantitative composition** Trimethoprim 10 mg/ml

**Pharmaceutical form** Suspension

### Clinical particulars
*Therapeutic indications:* Treatment of susceptible infections caused by trimethoprim-sensitive organisms including urinary and respiratory tract infections and for prophylaxis of recurrent urinary tract infections.

### Posology and method of administration
Acute infections:

| | |
|---|---|
| Adults and children over 12 years: | 200 mg (20 ml) twice daily |
| Children 6 years to 12 years: | 100 mg (10 ml) twice daily |
| Children 6 months to 5 years: | 50 mg (5 ml) twice daily |
| Children 6 weeks to 5 months: | 25 mg (2.5 ml) twice daily. |

The approximate dosage in children is 8 mg trimethoprim per kg body weight per day.

Elderly: Depending on kidney function, see special dosage schedule.

Treatment should continue for at least one week but not last longer than two weeks. The first dose can be doubled.

*Long-term treatment and prophylactic therapy:*

| | |
|---|---|
| Adults and children over 12 years: | 100 mg (10 ml) at night |
| Children 6 years to 12 years: | 50 mg (5 ml) at night |
| Children 6 months to 5 years: | 25 mg (2.5 ml) at night |

The approximate dosage in children is 2 mg trimethoprim per kg body weight per day.

Elderly: Depending on kidney function, see special dosage schedule.

Dosage advised where there is reduced kidney function:

| Creatinine clearance (ml/sec) | Plasma creatinine (micromol/l) | | Dosage advised |
|---|---|---|---|
| Over 0.45 | men <250 | | normal |
| | women <175 | | |
| 0.25-0.45 | men 250-600 | | normal for 3 days then half dose |
| | women 175-400 | | |
| Under 0.25 | men >600 | | half the normal dose |
| | women >400 | | |

Trimethoprim is removed by dialysis. However, it should not be administered to dialysis patients unless plasma concentrations can be estimated regularly.

*Contra-indications:* Pregnancy, trimethoprim hypersensitivity, blood dyscrasias, severe renal insufficiency where blood levels cannot be monitored.

*Special warnings and special precautions for use:* Caution should be exercised in the administration of trimethoprim to patients with actual or potential folate deficiency (e.g. elderly) and administration of folate supplement should be considered. Although an effect on folic acid metabolism is possible, interference with haematopoiesis rarely occurs at the recommended dose. If any such change is seen, folinic acid should reverse the effect. Elderly people may be more susceptible and a lower dose may be advisable. Regular haematological tests should be undertaken in long-term treatment.

In neonates, trimethoprim should be used under careful medical supervision.

In patients with impairment of renal function, care should be taken to avoid accumulation.

*Interaction with other medicaments and other forms of interaction:*

*Bone marrow depressants:* Trimethoprim may increase the potential for bone marrow aplasia. Rifampicin may increase the elimination and shorten the elimination half-life of trimethoprim. Phenytoin and digoxin: The patients should be carefully controlled as trimethoprim may increase the elimination half-life of phenytoin and digoxin. Cyclosporin may increase the nephrotoxicity of trimethoprim.

*Pregnancy and lactation:* Pregnancy is a contra-indication. Although trimethoprim is excreted in breast milk, lactation is not a contra-indication for short-term trimethoprim therapy.

*Effects on ability to drive and use machines:* None known.

*Undesirable effects:* Nausea, vomiting, and skin rashes have been reported in rare instances. These effects are generally mild and quickly reversible on withdrawal of the drug. Rarely, erythema multiforme and toxic epidermal necrolysis have occurred. Aseptic meningitis has been reported. Trimethoprim may affect haematopoiesis.

*Overdose:*
*Treatment of overdosage:* Symptomatic treatment, gastric lavage and forced diuresis can be used. Depression of haematopoiesis by trimethoprim can be counteracted by intramuscular administration of calcium folinate.

### Pharmacological properties
*Pharmacodynamic properties:* Trimethoprim is an antimicrobial agent. The antimicrobial activity is due to selective inhibition of bacterial dihydrofolate reductase.

Trimethoprim is effective in-vitro against most Gram-positive and Gram-negative aerobic organisms, including enterobacteria–E. coli, Proteus, Klebsiella pneumoniae, Streptococcus faecalis, Streptococcus pneumoniae, Haemophilus influenzae, and Staphylococcus aureus.

It is not active against Mycobacterium tuberculosis, Neisseria gonorrhoeae, Pseudomonas aeruginosa, Treponema pallidum, or anaerobic bacteria.

*Pharmacokinetic properties:*
*Absorption and half-life:* Trimethoprim is absorbed rapidly and almost completely following oral administration and maximal plasma concentrations are reached after 1-2 hours. Peak plasma concentrations of about 1 μg per ml have been reported after a single dose of 100 mg.

The half-life is about 10 hours in patients with normal renal function but up to 20-50 hours in anuric patients.

*Distribution:* Trimethoprim is rapidly and widely distributed to various tissues and fluids, including kidneys, liver, spleen, bronchial secretions, saliva and prostatic tissue and fluid, and the tissue concentrations are generally higher than the plasma concentration.

*Excretion:* Trimethoprim is predominantly excreted in the urine in unchanged form. Urinary concentrations are generally well above the MIC of common pathogens for more than 24 hours after the last dose.

*Preclinical safety data:* Not relevant (widely used in clinical practice).

### Pharmaceutical particulars
*List of excipients:* Microcrystalline cellulose, carboxymethylcellulose sodium, ammonium glycyrrhizinate, methyl parahydroxybenzoate, sorbitol, anise oil, purified water.

*Incompatibilities:* None known.

*Shelf life:* 3 years.

*Special precautions for storage:* Store below 25˚C.

*Nature and contents of container:* Plastic bottle: 25 ml and 100 ml.

*Instructions for use/handling:* None.

*Marketing authorisation holder:* A/S GEA Farmaceutisk Fabrik, Holger Danskes Vej 89, DK-2000 Frederiksberg, Denmark.

**Marketing authorization number** 4012/0002

**Date of approval/ revision of SPC** 23 January 1996

**Legal category** POM

## MONOTRIM* TABLETS

**Qualitative and quantitative composition** Trimethoprim 100 mg and 200 mg.

**Pharmaceutical form** Tablets.

### Clinical particulars

*Therapeutic indications:* Treatment of susceptible infections caused by trimethoprim-sensitive organisms including urinary and respiratory tract infections and for prophylaxis of recurrent urinary tract infections.

*Posology and method of administration:*

*Acute infections:*
*Adults and children over 12 years:* 200 mg twice daily.
*Children 6 years to 12 years:* 100 mg twice daily.

The approximate dosage in children is 8 mg trimethoprim per kg body weight per day.
*Elderly:* Depending on kidney function, see special dosage schedule.

Treatment should continue for at least one week but not last longer than two weeks. The first dose can be doubled.

*Long-term treatment and prophylactic therapy:*
*Adults and children over 12 years:* 100 mg at night.
The approximate dosage in children is 2 mg trimethoprim per kg body weight per day.
*Elderly:* Depending on kidney function, see special dosage schedule.

*Dosage advised where there is reduced kidney function:*

| Creatinine clearance (ml/sec) | Plasma creatinine (micromol/l) | | Dosage advised |
|---|---|---|---|
| Over 0.45 | men women | <250 <175 | normal |
| 0.25–0.45 | men women | 250–600 175–400 | normal for 3 days then half dose |
| Under 0.25 | men women | >600 >400 | half the normal dose |

*Trimethoprim is removed by dialysis. However, it should not be administered to dialysis patients unless plasma concentrations can be estimated regularly.*

*Contra-indications:* Pregnancy, trimethoprim hypersensitivity, blood dyscrasias, severe renal insufficiency where blood levels cannot be monitored.

*Special warnings and special precautions for use:* Caution should be exercised in the administration of trimethoprim to patients with actual or potential folate deficiency (e.g. elderly) and administration of folate supplement should be considered. Although an effect on folic acid metabolism is possible, interference with haematopoiesis rarely occurs at the recommended dose. If any such change is seen, folinic acid should reverse the effect. Elderly people may be more susceptible and a lower dose may be advisable. Regular haematological tests should be undertaken in long-term treatment.

In neonates, trimethoprim should be used under careful medical supervision.

In patients with impairment of renal function, care should be taken to avoid accumulation.

*Interaction with other medicaments and other forms of interaction:* Bone marrow depressants: Trimethoprim may increase the potential for bone marrow aplasia. Rifampicin may increase the elimination and shorten the elimination half-life of trimethoprim. Phenytoin and digoxin: The patients should be carefully controlled as trimethoprim may increase the elimination half-life of phenytoin and digoxin. Cyclosporin may increase the nephrotoxicity of trimethoprim.

*Pregnancy and lactation:* Pregnancy is a contra-indication. Although trimethoprim is excreted in breast milk, lactation is not a contra-indication for short-term trimethoprim therapy.

*Effects on ability to drive and use machines:* None known.

*Undesirable effects:* Nausea, vomiting, and skin rashes have been reported in rare instances. These effects are generally mild and quickly reversible on withdrawal of the drug. Rarely, erythema multiforme and toxic epidermal necrolysis have occurred. Aseptic meningitis has been reported. Trimethoprim may affect haematopoiesis.

*Overdose:* Treatment of overdosage: Symptomatic treatment, gastric lavage and forced diuresis can be used. Depression of haematopoiesis by trimethoprim can be counteracted by intramuscular administration of calcium folinate.

### Pharmacological properties
*Pharmacodynamic properties:* Trimethoprim is an antimicrobial agent. The antimicrobial activity is due to selective inhibition of bacterial dihydrofolate reductase.

Trimethoprim is effective in-vitro against most Gram-positive and Gram-negative aerobic organisms, including enterobacteria – E. coli, Proteus, Klebsiella pneumoniae, Streptococcus faecalis, Streptococcus pneumoniae, Haemophilus influenzae, and Staphylococcus aureus.

It is not active against Mycobacterium tuberculosis, Neisseria gonorrhoeae, Pseudomonas aeruginosa, Treponema pallidum, or anaerobic bacteria.

*Pharmacokinetic properties:*
*Absorption and half-life:* Trimethoprim is absorbed rapidly and almost completely following oral administration and maximal plasma concentrations are reached after 1–2 hours. Peak plasma concentrations of about 1 μg per ml have been reported after a single dose of 100 mg. The half-life is about 10 hours in

patients with normal renal function but up to 20–50 hours in anuric patients.

*Distribution:* Trimethoprim is rapidly and widely distributed to various tissues and fluids, including kidneys, liver, spleen, bronchial secretions, saliva and prostatic tissue and fluid, and the tissue concentrations are generally higher than the plasma concentration.

*Excretion:* Trimethoprim is predominantly excreted in the urine in unchanged form. Urinary concentrations are generally well above the MIC of common pathogens for more than 24 hours after the last dose.

*Preclinical safety data:* Not relevant (widely used in clinical practice).

### Pharmaceutical particulars
*List of excipients:* Lactose monohydrate, potato starch, gelatin, magnesium stearate, talc.

*Incompatibilities:* None known.

*Shelf life:* 5 years.

*Special precautions for storage:* None.

*Nature and contents of container:* Plastic container. 100 mg: 30, 100, 500 and 5000 tablets. 200 mg: 100, 500 and 2500 tablets.

*Instructions for use/handling:* None.

*Marketing authorisation holder:* A/S GEA Farmaceutisk Fabrik, Holger Danskes Vej 89, DK-2000 Frederiksberg, Denmark.

**Marketing authorisation number** 4012/0001/3.

**Date of approval/revision of SPC** 4 September 1996.

**Legal category** POM.

## PHYSIOTENS* ▼

**Qualitative and quantitative composition** Each tablet contains 200 or 400 micrograms of moxonidine.

**Pharmaceutical form** Round, biconvex, film-coated tablets. The 200 microgram tablet is light pink imprinted '0.2' on one face. The 400 microgram tablet is dull red imprinted '0.4' on one face.

### Clinical particulars
*Therapeutic indications:* Mild to moderate essential or primary hypertension.

*Posology and method of administration*
*Adults (including the elderly):* Treatment should be started with 200 micrograms of Physiotens in the morning. The dose may be titrated after three weeks to 400 micrograms, given as one dose or as divided doses (morning and evening) until a satisfactory response has been achieved. If the response is still unsatisfactory after a further three weeks' treatment, the dosage can be increased up to a maximum of 600 micrograms in divided doses (morning and evening).

A single dose of 400 micrograms of Physiotens and a daily dose of 600 micrograms in divided doses (morning and evening) should not be exceeded.

In patients with moderate renal dysfunction (GFR above 30 ml/min, but below 60 ml/min), the single dose should not exceed 200 micrograms and the daily dose should not exceed 400 micrograms of moxonidine.

The tablets should be taken with a little liquid. As the intake of food has no influence on the pharmacokinetic properties of moxonidine, the tablets may be taken before, during or after the meal.

*Children (under 16 years):* Physiotens should not be given below the age of 16 years as insufficient therapeutic experience exists in this group.

*Contra-indications:* Physiotens should not be used in cases of:

– history of angioneurotic oedema
– hypersensitivity to any of the ingredients
– sick sinus syndrome or sino-atrial block
– 2nd or 3rd degree atrioventricular block
– bradycardia (below 50 beats/minute at rest)
– malignant arrhythmia
– severe heart failure
– severe coronary artery disease or unstable angina
– severe liver disease
– severe renal dysfunction (GFR <30 ml/min, serum creatinine concentration >160 μmol/l)

Physiotens should not be used because of lack of therapeutic experience in cases of

– intermittent claudication
– Raynaud's disease
– Parkinson's disease
– epileptic disorders
– glaucoma
– depression
– pregnancy or lactation
– children below 16 years of age

*Special warnings and special precautions for use:* If Physiotens is used in combination with a beta-blocker and the treatment has to be stopped, the beta-blocker should be stopped first and then Physiotens after a few days have elapsed.

In patients with moderate renal dysfunction (GFR above 30 but below 60 ml/min, serum creatinine above 105 but below 160 μmol), the hypotensive effect of Physiotens should be closely monitored, especially at the start of treatment.

Due to lack of therapeutic experience, the use of Physiotens concomitantly with alcohol or tricyclic antidepressants should be avoided.

In limited studies no rebound effect of the blood pressure after sudden discontinuation of Physiotens treatment has been detected. Nevertheless, it is advised not to interrupt the intake of Physiotens abruptly. Physiotens should be withdrawn gradually over a period of two weeks.

*Interactions with other medicaments and other forms of interaction:* Concurrent administration of other antihypertensive agents enhances the hypotensive effect of Physiotens.

The effect of sedatives and hypnotics may be intensified by Physiotens. The sedative effect of benzodiazepines can be enhanced by concurrent administration of Physiotens.

*Pregnancy and lactation:* As insufficient data are available, Physiotens should not be used during pregnancy. Physiotens should not be used during lactation because it is excreted into breast milk.

*Effects on ability to drive and use machines:* No data are available to suggest that Physiotens adversely affects the ability to drive or operate machines. However, as somnolence and dizziness have been reported, patients should be cautioned about their ability to undertake potentially hazardous tasks such as driving and operating machinery if so affected.

*Undesirable effects:* At the start of treatment dry mouth is frequently observed, while headache, asthenia, dizziness, nausea, sleep disturbances and vasodilatation are observed occasionally. Sedation has been reported in less than 1% of patients. The frequency and intensity of these symptoms often decrease in the course of treatment.

*Overdose:* Oral dosages up to 2.0 mg/day have been tolerated without the occurrence of serious adverse events. Two cases have been reported of accidental overdose with Physiotens by children (2 and 3 years old):

A 2 year old child ingested an unknown quantity of Physiotens. The maximum dosage possibly ingested was 14 mg. The child had the following symptoms: sedation, coma, hypotension, miosis and dyspnoea. Gastric lavage, glucose infusion, mechanically assisted ventilation and rest resulted in the complete disappearance of the symptoms in 11 hours.

A 3 year old child took 3 mg of Physiotens in the morning. The child was hospitalised in the evening for somnolence. There was no hypotension or change in pulse rate. The child was discharged after observation for 24 hours.

Because of the pharmacodynamic properties of Physiotens, the following symptoms can be expected in adults: sedation, hypotension, orthostatic dysregulation, bradycardia, dry mouth. In rare cases emesis and paradoxical hypertension may occur.

No specific antidote is known. Phentolamine (Rogitine) may, depending on the dose, reverse part of the symptoms of moxonidine overdosage. Measures to support blood circulation are recommended.

**Pharmacological properties**

*Pharmacodynamic properties:* In different animal models, Physiotens has been shown to be a potent antihypertensive agent. Available experimental data convincingly suggest that the site of the antihypertensive action of Physiotens is the central nervous system (CNS). Within the brainstem, Physiotens has been shown to selectively interact with $I_1$-imidazoline receptors. These imidazoline-sensitive receptors are concentrated in the rostral ventrolateral medulla, an area critical to the central control of the peripheral sympathetic nervous system. The net effect of this interaction with the $I_1$-imidazoline receptor appears to result in a reduced activity of sympathetic nerves (demonstrated for cardiac, splanchnic and renal sympathetic nerves).

Physiotens differs from other available centrally acting antihypertensives by exhibiting only low affinity for central $\alpha_2$-adrenoceptors as compared with $I_1$-imidazoline receptors; $\alpha_2$-adrenoceptors are considered to be the molecular target via which sedation and dry mouth, the most common undesired effects of the first generation of centrally acting antihypertensives, are mediated.

In humans, Physiotens leads to a reduction of systemic vascular resistance and consequently in arterial pressure.

*Pharmacokinetic properties:* Oral moxonidine treatment of rats and dogs resulted in rapid and almost complete absorption and peak plasma levels within <0.5 hours. Average plasma concentrations were comparable in both species after p.o. and i.v. administration. The elimination half-lives of radioactivity and unchanged compound were estimated to be 1–3 hours. Moxonidine and its two main metabolites (4,5-dehydromoxonidine and a guanidine derivative) were predominantly excreted in the urine. No indication of moxonidine cumulation was observed in either species during chronic toxicity studies after 52 weeks.

In humans, about 90% of an oral dose of moxonidine is absorbed; it is not subject to first-pass metabolism and its bioavailability is 88%. Food intake does not interfere with moxonidine pharmacokinetics. Moxonidine is 10–20% metabolised, mainly to 4,5-dehydromoxonidine and to a guanidine derivative by opening of the imidazoline ring. The hypotensive effect of 4,5-dehydromoxonidine is only 1/10, and that of the guanidine derivative is less than 1/100 of that of moxonidine. The maximum plasma levels of moxonidine are reached 30–180 minutes after the intake of a film-coated tablet.

Only about 7% of moxonidine is bound to plasma protein ($Vd_{ss}$=1.8±0.4 l/kg). Moxonidine and its metabolites are eliminated almost entirely via the kidneys. More than 90% of the dose is eliminated via the kidneys in the first 24 hours after administration, while only about 1% is eliminated via the faeces. The cumulative renal excretion of unchanged moxonidine is about 50–75%.

The mean plasma elimination half-life of moxonidine is 2.2–2.3 hours, and the renal elimination half-life is 2.6–2.8 hours.

*Pharmacokinetics in the elderly:* Small differences between the pharmacokinetic properties of moxonidine in the healthy elderly and younger adults are unlikely to be clinically significant. As there is no accumulation of moxonidine, dosage adjustment is unnecessary provided renal function is normal.

*Pharmacokinetics in children:* No pharmacokinetic studies have been performed in children.

*Pharmacokinetics in renal impairment:* In moderately impaired renal function (GFR 30–60 ml/min), AUC increased by 85% and clearance decreased to 52%. In such patients the hypotensive effect of Physiotens should be closely monitored, especially at the start of treatment, additionally, single doses should not exceed 200 micrograms and the daily dose should not exceed 400 micrograms.

*Preclinical safety data:* Chronic oral treatment for 52 weeks of rats (with dosages of 0.12–4 mg/kg) and dogs (with dosages of 0.04–0.4 mg/kg) revealed significant effects of moxonidine only at the highest doses. Slight disturbances of electrolyte balance (decrease of blood sodium and increase of potassium, urea and creatinine) were found in the high dose rats and emesis and salivation only for the high dose dogs. In addition slight increases of liver weight were obvious for both high dose species.

Reproductive toxicology did not show moxonidine effects (at oral doses up to 6.4 mg/kg) on fertility of rats and development of the embryo and foetus. Neither was evidence seen of embryotoxic and teratogenic properties in the rat at oral doses up to 27 mg/kg and the rabbit up to 4.9 mg/kg, nor on peri- and post-natal development in the rat after oral dosage up to 9 mg/kg.

Five different studies also did not show any indication of mutagenic or genotoxic effects of moxonidine. In addition, carcinogenicity studies in rats and mice at oral dose-ranges of 0.1–7.0 mg/kg did not reveal any evidence of carcinogenic potential.

**Pharmaceutical particulars**

*List of excipients:* Lactose, povidone, crospovidone, magnesium stearate, hydroxypropylmethyl cellulose, ethyl cellulose, polyethyleneglycol 6000, talc, red ferric oxide (E172), titanium dioxide (E171).

*Incompatibilities:* Not applicable.

*Shelf life:* 24 months when stored below 25°C in the original container.

*Special precautions for storage:* None.

*Nature and contents of container:* The tablets are packed in blister strips of 14. The blister strips are made of PVC/PVdC or PVC film with covering aluminium foil. Each carton contains 28 tablets.

*Instructions for use/handling:* No special instructions.

**Marketing authorisation numbers**
200 micrograms 0512/0152
400 micrograms 0512/0154

**Date of approval/revision of SPC** September 1997.

**Legal category** POM.

## SERC* – 8
## SERC* – 16

**Presentation** A round, flat, white to almost white tablet, imprinted '256' on one face and 'S' on the reverse, each tablet containing 8 mg betahistine dihydrochloride.

A round, flat, white to almost white tablet imprinted '267' on one face and 'S' on the reverse, each tablet containing 16 mg betahistine dihydrochloride.

**Uses** Betahistine is an orally effective treatment for Ménière's syndrome, which appears to exert its effect by reducing endolymphatic pressure. It is a histamine analogue which was developed following the successful parenteral use of histamine in patients with Ménière's syndrome. Animal studies have confirmed its specific effect. Clinical experience has demonstrated the efficacy of betahistine on all the principal symptoms of Ménière's syndrome, not only reducing vertiginous episodes and tinnitus but also arresting hearing loss.

*Indications:* Vertigo, tinnitus and hearing loss associated with Ménière's syndrome.

**Dosage and administration** *Adults (including the elderly):* Initially 16 mg three times daily, taken preferably with meals. Maintenance doses are generally in the range 24–48 mg daily.

*Children:* No dosage recommendations are made for children.

**Contra-indications, warnings, etc**
*Contra-indication:* Phaeochromocytoma. Hypersensitivity.

*Interactions:* Although an antagonism beween Serc and antihistamines could be expected on a theoretical basis, no such interactions have been reported.

*Other special warnings and precautions:* Caution is advised in the treatment of patients with a history of peptic ulcer. Clinical intolerance to Serc in bronchial asthma patients has been shown in a relatively few patients and therefore caution should be exercised when administering betahistine to patients with bronchial asthma.

*Use in pregnancy and lactation:* High dosage animal tests have shown no teratogenic properties, but the usual precautions should be observed when administering Serc to patients during pregnancy.

*Other undesirable effects (frequency and seriousness):* Relatively few side effects have been reported. They include gastro-intestinal upset, (including dyspepsia), headache, skin rash and pruritus.

*Treatment of overdosage:* No specific antidote. Gastric lavage and symptomatic treatment is recommended.

**Pharmaceutical precautions** Store at room temperature.

**Legal category** POM.

**Package quantities** 8 mg: Available in packs of 120 tablets.

16 mg: Available in calendar packs of 84 tablets.

**Further information** Betahistine does not produce false positive reactions in standard diagnostic urine tests.

**Product licence numbers**
8 mg: 0512/0076
16 mg: 0512/0088

## YUTOPAR* INJECTION

**Qualitative and quantitative composition** Each ampoule contains 50 mg of ritodrine hydrochloride (10 mg/ml). Aqueous buffered vehicle contains sodium chloride and sodium metabisulphite.

**Pharmaceutical form** Clear, sterile aqueous solution.

**Clinical particulars**

*Therapeutic indications:*
*The management of uncomplicated preterm labour.* Yutopar is a betamimetic drug which stimulates beta receptors, thereby decreasing uterine contractility. The main purpose of giving Yutopar is to delay delivery for at least 48 hours. No statistically significant effect of the drug on peri-natal mortality has as yet been observed in randomised, placebo-controlled trials. Less effect can be expected if the membranes are ruptured or the dilation of the cervix exceeds 4cm.

*IV therapy:* To arrest pre-term labour between 24 and 33 weeks of gestation in patients with no medical or obstetric contra-indication to tocolytic therapy. The most effective use of IV Yutopar is achieved by using the delay in delivery to administer glucocorticosteroids or to implement other measures known to improve peri-natal health.

*IM therapy:* If intravenous administration is considered to be inappropriate, intramuscular administration may be substituted.

*Posology and method of administration: Adults.*

IV: To be administered as early as possible after the diagnosis of pre-term labour, and after evaluation of the patient to rule out contra-indications to the use of ritodrine (see contra-indications). The initial dose is 50 micrograms per minute to be gradually increased according to the response by 50 micrograms/minute every 10 minutes until contractions stop, the maternal heart rate reaches 140 beats per minute or a maximum dose of 350 micrograms/minute is reached. The effective dosage usually lies between 150 micrograms and 350 micrograms/minute; the lowest effective dose should be used. If successful, the infusion should be continued for 12 to 48 hours after uterine contractions have ceased. The infusion should be stopped if labour progresses despite treatment at the maximum dose. Careful control of the level of hydration is essential to avoid the risk of maternal pulmonary oedema (see Special warnings and special precautions for use). The volume of fluid in which the drug is administered should thus be kept to a minimum. A controlled infusion device, preferably a syringe pump should be used.

If a syringe pump is available, the concentration of the drug infused should be 3 mg/ml (i.e. 15 ml of Yutopar solution should be added to 35 ml of infusion fluid to give a total volume of 50 ml). If a syringe pump is not available, the concentration should be 300 micrograms/ml (150 mg in 500 ml fluid). The recommended infusion fluid is 5% dextrose.

Guidance on infusion rates to achieve the required dose is given in the table below:

### I. SYRINGE PUMP

Add 3×5 ml ampoules of Yutopar to 35 ml of 5% w/v dextrose

| Dose | Rate |
| --- | --- |
| 50 micrograms/min | 1 ml/hour |
| 100 micrograms/min | 2 ml/hou |
| 150 micrograms/min | 3 ml/hour |
| 200 micrograms/min | 4 ml/hour |
| 250 micrograms/min | 5 ml/hour |
| 300 micrograms/min | 6 ml/hour |
| 350 micrograms/min | 7 ml/hour |

### II. CONTROLLED INFUSION DEVICE

Add 3×5 ml ampoules of Yutopar to 500 ml of 5% w/v dextrose

| Dose | Rate |
| --- | --- |
| 50 micrograms/min | 10 ml/hour |
| 100 micrograms/min | 20 ml/hour |
| 150 micrograms/min | 30 ml/hour |
| 200 micrograms/min | 40 ml/hour |
| 250 micrograms/min | 50 ml/hour |
| 300 micrograms/min | 60 ml/hour |
| 350 micrograms/min | 70 ml/hour |

The maximum recommended dose is 350 micrograms/minute. The dose should be kept to the minimum required to inhibit uterine contractions.

*IM:* If intravenous administration is considered to be inappropriate, intramuscular administration may be substituted, giving 10 mg intramuscularly every 3 to 8 hours. The intramuscular regime should be continued for 12–48 hours following arrest of labour.

*Elderly:* Not applicable.

*Children:* Not applicable.

*Contra-indications:*

1. Antepartum haemorrhage which demands immediate delivery.
2. Eclampsia and severe pre-eclampsia.
3. Intra-uterine fetal death.
4. Chorioamnionitis.
5. Maternal cardiac disease.
6. Cord compression.

*Special warnings and special precautions for use:* Maternal pulmonary oedema has been reported in patients treated with ritodrine. Therefore, close monitoring of the patient's state of hydration is advised and if pulmonary oedema develops during administration treatment should be discontinued.

It is advisable to screen patients with potential cardiac risk before deciding on ritodrine treatment.

Yutopar should not be administered to patients with mild to moderate pre-eclampsia, hypertension or hyperthyroidism unless the attending physician considers that the benefits clearly outweigh the risks.

In order to minimise the risk of hypotension associated with tocolytic therapy, special care should be taken to avoid vena caval compression by keeping the patient in the left lateral position throughout the infusion.

*Interactions with other medicaments and other forms of interaction:* Careful monitoring is required in patients with suspected heart disease and in those receiving drugs which could interact with ritodrine such as monoamine oxidase inhibitors, tricyclic antidepressants, corticosteroids, sympathomimetic amines, beta-adrenergic blocking drugs, anaesthetics used in surgery:

- corticosteroids used concomitantly may increase the risk of pulmonary oedema.
- other sympathomimetic amines may be potentiated when concurrently administered.
- beta-adrenergic blocking drugs inhibit the action of ritodrine; co-administration of these drugs should therefore be avoided.
- anaesthetics used in surgery may potentiate the hypotensive effect of ritodrine.

Monitoring is also needed in patients receiving potassium-depleting diuretics, as intravenous administration of Yutopar has been shown to decrease plasma potassium levels.

In diabetic patients, glucose levels should be closely monitored and insulin requirements adjusted accordingly during intravenous treatment. On oral treatment no alterations have been reported.

*Pregnancy and lactation:* Animal experiments failed to show a teratogenic effect even in high dosages.

Reproduction studies, in rats and rabbits have revealed no evidence of impaired fertility or harm to the foetus. However, the drug is not recommended during the first 16 weeks of pregnancy.

In a group of children born to ritodrine treated mothers, follow-up of selected variables up to 6 years has not revealed harmful effects on growth, developmental or functional maturation.

*Lactation:* Not applicable.

*Effect on ability to drive and use machines:* Not known.

*Undesirable effects:* Maternal pulmonary oedema has been reported in association with ritodrine usage; in some cases this has proved fatal. Predisposing factors include fluid overload, multiple pregnancy, pre-existing cardiac disease and maternal infection. Close monitoring of the patient's state of hydration is essential. If signs of pulmonary oedema develop (e.g. cough, shortness of breath, haemoptysis), treatment should be discontinued immediately and diuretic therapy instituted.

The maternal pulse rate may progressively increase, usually to a moderate degree. This may lead to palpitations. Any pronounced tachycardia that may arise during intravenous infusion (or oral therapy) with Yutopar disappears after dose reduction or drug withdrawal. Whether the maternal tachycardia is considered acceptable must be determined on a case by case basis, but it is recommended that, in healthy patients, a heart rate of more than 140/min should be avoided. Chest pain or tightness with or without ECG abnormalities, and cardiac arrhythmias have been reported infrequently.

Flushing, sweating, tremor, nausea and vomiting have been reported.

Cases of leucopenia and/or agranulocytosis have been reported with prolonged (i.e. several weeks) intravenous ritodrine treatment. The number of leucocytes returned to normal on drug withdrawal.

Impaired liver function (i.e. increased transaminase levels and hepatitis) has been reported with the use of ritodrine.

Enlargement of the salivary glands and an increased secretion of amylase have been reported infrequently. In most cases, complete recovery occurs within a few days of discontinuation of ritodrine.

*Overdose:*
*Symptoms:* The symptoms of overdosage are those of beta-adrenergic stimulation.

*Treatment:* In cases of overdosage of i.v. Yutopar, discontinue the infusion immediately. A non-selective beta-sympatholytic agent may be given as an antidote.

### Pharmacological properties

*Pharmacodynamic properties:* Ritodrine is beta-sympathomimetic which acts as a uterine relaxant in the management of premature labour. Some chronotropic cardiac effects and peripheral vasodilatation are also seen at therapeutic doses.

*Pharmacokinetic properties:* On average, 90% of a dose of radioactive ritodrine is excreted in the urine, independent of the route of administration.

The distribution volume after intravenous infusion of 9 mg ritodrine hydrochloride (0.15 mg/minute for 60 minutes), was 0.6-0.9 1/kg, while total body clearance was ca.100 1/hour (N=6females).

After intramuscular administration of 10 mg, maximum serum levels are 20-33 ng/ml. The mean area under the serum curve (AUC) was 97 ng/ml/hour, and correlated well with that of the intravenous infusion (95 ng/ml/hour).

*Preclinical safety data:* All toxic effects of ritodrine established by intravenous and oral administration in various animal species, can more or less be ascribed to the beta-adrenergic stimulant properties of the compound. The lowest dose level used (1 mg/kg) was not free from side-effects, such as decreased serum potassium and increased serum glucose, tachycardia, cutaneous vasodilatation. At high dose levels emesis, restlessness and convulsions occurred.

### Pharmaceutical particulars

*List of excipients:* Acetic acid, sodium hydroxide, sodium metabisulphite, sodium chloride, water for injections.

*Incompatibilities:* The injection fluid should not be mixed with other injection fluids, unless the compatibility is proven.

*Shelf life:* 36 months when stored below 30°C in the original, undamaged packaging.

*Special precautions for storage:* None.

*Nature and contents of container:* Boxes of 10×5 ml colourless glass ampoules containing ritodrine hydrochloride 10 mg/ml.

*Instructions for use/handling:* If the solution is discoloured or contains any precipitate or particulate matter, parenteral ritodrine should not be used.

**Marketing authorisation number** 0512/0020R

**Date of approval/revision of SPC** February 1996

**Legal category** POM.

## YUTOPAR* TABLETS

**Presentation** *Tablets:* Round, flat, yellow with bevelled edges, inscribed 'YUTOPAR' on one face and a breakline on the reverse. Each tablet contains 10 mg ritodrine hydrochloride. Excipients include lactose.

### Uses

*The management of uncomplicated preterm labour:* Yutopar is a betamimetic drug which stimulates beta$_2$-receptors, thereby decreasing uterine contractility. The main purpose of giving Yutopar is to delay delivery for at least 48 hours. No statistically significant effect of the drug on perinatal mortality has as yet been observed in randomised, placebo-controlled trials.

For the maintenance of uterine quiescence following successful parenteral therapy. Oral treatment should not be used initially in an attempt to arrest labour.

**Dosage and administration** *Adults:* One tablet (10 mg) may be given approximately 30 minutes before the termination of intravenous therapy. The usual dosage schedule for the first 24 hours of oral maintenance is one tablet (10 mg) every two hours. Thereafter, the usual dose is one or two tablets (10–20 mg) every four to six hours depending on uterine activity and unwanted effects.

The total daily dose of oral ritodrine should not exceed 120 mg. The treatment may be continued as long as the physician considers it desirable to prolong pregnancy.

*Elderly:* Not applicable.

*Children:* Not applicable.

### Contra-indications, warnings, etc
*Contra-indications:*

1. Antepartum haemorrhage which demands immediate delivery.
2. Eclampsia and severe pre-eclampsia.
3. Intra-uterine fetal death.
4. Chorioamnionitis.
5. Maternal cardiac disease.
6. Cord compression.

*Precautions:* Maternal pulmonary oedema has been reported in patients treated with ritodrine. Therefore, close monitoring of the patient's state of hydration is advised and if pulmonary oedema develops during administration treatment should be discontinued.

Careful monitoring is required in patients with suspected heart disease, or those receiving other drugs, in particular those which could interact with ritodrine such as monoamine oxidase inhibitors, tricyclic anti-depressants, corticosteroids, sympathomimetic amines, beta-adrenergic blocking drugs, anaesthetics used in surgery and potassium-depleting diuretics, as intravenous administration of Yutopar has been shown to decrease plasma potassium levels.

Experiments in animals have shown that even in high dosage Yutopar has no teratogenic properties.

In diabetic patients, glucose levels should be closely monitored and insulin requirements adjusted accordingly during intravenous treatment. On oral treatment no alterations have been reported. It is also advisable to screen patients with potential cardiac risk before deciding on ritodrine treatment.

Yutopar should not be administered to patients with mild to moderate pre-eclampsia, hypertension or hyperthyroidism unless the attending physician considers that the benefits clearly outweigh the risks.

In order to minimise the risk of hypotension associated with tocolytic therapy, special care should be taken to avoid vena caval compression by keeping the patient in the left lateral position throughout the infusion.

*Side-effects:* Maternal pulmonary oedema has been reported in association with ritodrine usage; in some cases this has proved fatal. Predisposing factors include fluid overload, multiple pregnancy, pre-existing cardiac disease and maternal infection. Close monitoring of the patient's state of hydration is essential. If signs of pulmonary oedema develop (e.g. cough, shortness of breath, haemoptysis), treatment should be discontinued immediately and diuretic therapy instituted.

The maternal pulse rate may progressively increase, usually to a moderate degree. This may lead to palpitations. Any pronounced tachycardia that may arise during intravenous infusion (or oral therapy) with Yutopar disappears after dose reduction or drug withdrawal. Whether the maternal tachycardia is considered acceptable must be determined on a case by case basis, but it is recommended that, in healthy patients, a heart rate of more than 140/min should be avoided. Chest pain or tightness with or without ECG abnormalities, and cardiac arrhythmias have been reported infrequently.

Flushing, sweating, tremor, nausea and vomiting have been reported.

Cases of leucopenia and/or agranulocytosis have been reported with prolonged (i.e. several weeks) intravenous ritodrine treatment. The number of leucocytes returned to normal on drug withdrawal.

Impaired liver function (i.e. increased transaminase levels and hepatitis) has been reported with the use of ritodrine.

Enlargement of the salivary glands and an increased secretion of amylase have been reported infrequently. In most cases, complete recovery occurs within a few days of discontinuation of ritodrine.

*Treatment of overdosage:* In cases of overdosage of Yutopar, a non-selective beta-sympatholytic agent may be given as an antidote.

**Pharmaceutical precautions**   *Tablets:* Store in a cool dry place, protected from light.

**Legal category**   POM.

**Package quantities**   Tablets: Packs of 90 tablets each containing 10 mg ritodrine hydrochloride.

**Further information**   Less effect can be expected if the membranes are ruptured or the dilatation of the cervix exceeds 4 cm.

Ritodrine does not produce false positive reactions in standard diagnostic urine tests.

**Product licence number**   0512/0018R

## ZUMENON* 1 mg

**Qualitative and quantitative composition**   This product contains 1 mg estradiol hemihydrate PhEur equivalent to 1 mg estradiol per tablet.

**Pharmaceutical form**   White, round, biconvex, film-coated tablets imprinted 'S' on one side and '379' on the other.

**Clinical particulars**

*Therapeutic indications:* For the treatment of symptoms of oestrogen deficiency as a result of natural menopause or oophorectomy, eg hot flushes, nocturnal perspiration and atrophic changes in the genito-urinary tract.

In women with a uterus, a progestogen should be added to Zumenon for 10-14 days each month.

*Posology and method of administration:* One tablet daily without interruption. If clinical response is inadequate, dosage may be increased to two tablets daily, but should be reduced to one tablet daily as soon as practicable.

Treatment of hysterectomized women and post-menopausal women may be started on any convenient day. If the patient is menstruating, treatment is started on day 5 of bleeding.

*Contra-indications:* Known, suspected or past history of carcinoma of the breast, endometrial carcinoma or other hormone dependent neoplasia.

Acute or chronic liver disease or history of liver disease where the liver function tests have failed to return to normal.

Deep venous thrombosis, thromboembolic disorders, cerebral vascular accident.

Abnormal genital bleeding of unknown aetiology.

Known or suspected pregnancy.

*Special warnings and special precautions for use:* Physical examination and a complete medical and family history should be taken prior to the initiation of any oestrogen therapy with special reference to blood pressure, palpation of the breasts and the abdomen and a gynaecological examination.

Patients with an intact uterus who are, or have previously been, treated with unopposed oestrogens should be examined with special care in order to

investigate a possible hyperstimulation of the endometrium before commencing Zumenon therapy.

As a general rule, oestrogens should not be prescribed for longer than 1 year without another physical examination, including gynaecological examination. In case of continuing abnormal and/or irregular bleeding, a diagnostic endometrial biopsy should be performed.

Patients with or developing epilepsy, migraine, diabetes mellitus, cardiac failure, multiple sclerosis, hypertension, porphyria, haemoglobinopathies or otosclerosis should be carefully observed during treatment, as oestrogens may worsen these conditions. In patients with a past history of liver disease it is advisable to check liver functions on a regular basis.

Special care should be taken in patients with uterine leiomyomata and patients with (a history of) endometriosis as oestrogens may influence these conditions.

The indications for immediate withdrawal of therapy are:

– deep venous thrombosis
– thromboembolic disorders
– the appearance of jaundice
– the emergence of migraine–type headache
– sudden visual disturbances
– significant increase in blood pressure
– pregnancy

*Interactions with other medicaments and other forms of interaction:* Oestrogens interact with liver enzyme inducing drugs with increased metabolism of oestrogens, which may reduce the oestrogen effect. Interactions are documented for the following liver enzyme inducing drugs: barbiturates, phenytoin, rifampicin, carbamazepine.

*Pregnancy and lactation:* Known, or suspected pregnancy is a contra-indication to Zumenon therapy.
*Lactation:* This product is not indicated during this period.

*Effects on ability to drive and use machines:* No effects known.

*Undesirable effects:* During the first few months of treatment with Zumenon, breast tenderness may occur. Nausea, headache and oedema occur rarely. Symptoms are normally transient. Furthermore, skin reactions have been reported.

*Overdose:* There have been no reports of ill-effects from overdosing. If overdosage is discovered within two or three hours and is so large that treatment seems desirable, gastric lavage can safely be used. There is no specific antidote and further treatment should be symptomatic.

**Pharmacological properties**

*Pharmacodynamic properties:* Estradiol is chemically and biologically identical to the endogenous human estradiol and is, therefore, classified as a human estrogen. Estradiol is the primary estrogen and the most active of the ovarian hormones. The endogenous estrogens are involved in certain functions of the uterus and accessory organs, including the proliferation of the endometrium and the cyclic changes in the cervix and vagina.

Estrogens are known to play an important role for bone and fat metabolism. Furthermore, estrogens also affect the autonomic nervous system and may have indirect positive psychotropic actions.

*Pharmacokinetic properties:* Following oral administration, micronised estradiol is readily absorbed, but extensively metabolised. The major unconjugated and conjugated metabolites are estrone and estrone sulphate. These metabolites can contribute to the estrogen activity, either directly or after conversion to estradiol. Estrone sulphate may undergo enterohepatic circulation. In urine, the major compounds are the glucuronides of estrone and estradiol.

Estrogens are secreted in the milk of nursing mothers.

*Preclinical safety data:* Supraphysiologically high doses (prolonged overdoses) of estradiol have been associated with the induction of tumors in estrogen-dependent target organs for all rodent species tested. Pronounced species differences in toxicology, pharmacology and pharmacodynamics exist.

**Pharmaceutical particulars**

*List of excipients:* Lactose, methylhydroxypropyl cellulose, maize starch, colloidal anhydrous silica, magnesium stearate, polyethylene glycol 400, E171.

*Incompatibilities:* Not applicable

*Shelf life:* 24 months when stored below 25°C.

*Special precautions for storage:* None.

*Nature and contents of container:* The tablets are packed in blister strips of 28. The blister strips are made of PVC film with covering Aluminium foil. Each carton contains 84 tablets.

*Instruction for use/handling:* Not applicable

**Marketing authorisation number**   0512/0141

**Date of approval/revision of SPC**   May 1996

**Legal category**   POM

## ZUMENON* 2 mg

**Qualitative and quantitative composition**   This product contains 2 mg estradiol hemihydrate PhEur equivalent to 2 mg estradiol per tablet.

**Pharmaceutical form**   Orange, round, biconvex, film-coated tablets imprinted 'S' on one side and '379' on the other.

**Clinical particulars**

*Therapeutic indications:* Hormone replacement therapy for the treatment of symptoms of oestrogen deficiency as a result of natural menopause or oophorectomy, eg hot flushes, nocturnal perspiration and atrophic changes in the genito-urinary tract.

For the prevention of osteoporosis in women at risk of developing fractures.

Epidemiological studies suggest a number of risk factors may contribute to post-menopausal osteoporosis including: early menopause (either naturally or surgically induced); family history of osteoporosis; recent use of corticosteroids; a small frame; a thin frame; cigarette smoking.

If several of these risk factors are present consideration should be given to hormone replacement therapy.

For maximum prophylactic benefit a treatment should commence as soon as possible after the menopause. Bone mineral density measurements may help to confirm the presence of low bone mass.

In women with a uterus, a progestogen should be added to Zumenon for 10-14 days each month.

*Posology and method of administration:* Adults (including the elderly):
*Climacteric symptoms:* Therapy should be initiated with Zumenon 1 mg. The dosage may be increased if required by using Zumenon 2 mg. For maintenance therapy the lowest effective dose should be used.

One tablet daily without interruption. If clinical response is inadequate, dosage may be increased to two tablets daily, but should be reduced to one tablet daily as soon as practicable.

*Prevention of osteoporosis:* One 2 mg tablet daily without interruption. Treatment should start as soon as possible after the onset of menopause and certainly within 2 or 3 years. Protection appears to be effective for as long as treatment continues, however data beyond 10 years are limited. A careful reappraisal of the risk benefit ratio should be undertaken before treating for longer than 5-10 years. For long term use see also Special warnings and special precautions for use.

Treatment of hysterectomised women and post-menopausal women may be started on any convenient day. If the patient is menstruating, treatment is started on day 5 of bleeding.

Before therapy commences it is recommended that the patient is fully informed of all likely benefits and potential risks. She should have a full physical and gynaecological examination with special emphasis on blood pressure, breasts, abdomen and pelvic organs and an endometrial assessment carried out if indicated. Follow-up examinations are recommended every 6-12 months.

Breakthrough bleeding may occasionally occur in the first few weeks after initiating treatment and will usually settle.

*Children:* Zumenon is not indicated in children

*Contra-indications:*

– Known, suspected or past history of carcinoma of the breast, endometrial carcinoma or other hormone dependent neoplasia.
– Acute or chronic liver disease or history of liver disease where the liver function tests
– Active deep venous thrombosis, thromboembolic disorders, or a past history of these conditions (see Special warnings and special precautions for use).
– Cerebral vascular accident.
– Abnormal genital bleeding of unknown aetiology.
– Rotor syndrome or Dubin-Johnson syndrome.
– Severe cardiac or renal disease.
– Known or suspected pregnancy.

*Special warnings and special precautions for use:* Breakthrough bleeding may occasionally occur and can be the result of poor compliance or concurrent antibiotic use. It may however indicate endometrial pathology and therefore any doubt as to the cause of breakthrough bleeding is an indication for endometrial evaluation including endometrial biopsy.

There is an increased risk of endometrial hyperplasia or carcinoma associated with unopposed oestrogen administered long term (for more than 1 year). However, the appropriate addition of a progestogen to an oestrogen regimen lowers this risk.

There is suggestive evidence of a small increased risk of breast cancer with oestrogen replacement therapy used for long term (greater than 5 years). Some studies have reported an increased risk of breast cancer in long term users, others have not shown this relationship. It is not known whether concurrent progestogen use influences the risk of breast cancer in post-menopausal women taking hormone replacement therapy. Women on long-term therapy should have regular breast examinations and should be instructed in self-breast examination. Regular mammographic investigation should be conducted where considered appropriate.

There is need for caution when prescribing oestrogens in women who have a history, or known breast nodules or fibrocystic disease. Breast status should be closely monitored, supported by regular mammography.

Certain diseases may be made worse by hormone replacement therapy and patients with these conditions should be closely monitored. These include otosclerosis, multiple sclerosis, systemic lupus erythematosus, porphyria, melanoma, epilepsy, migraine, asthma, haemoglobinopathies, diabetes mellitus. In patients with a past history of liver disease it is advisable to check liver functions on a regular basis. In addition, pre-existing fibroids may increase in size during oestrogen therapy and symptoms associated with endometriosis may be exacerbated.

Epidemiological evidence suggests that use of hormone replacement therapy (HRT) is associated with an increased relative risk of developing deep vein thrombosis (DVT) or pulmonary embolism (PE). Although this increase in relative risk is about 2-3, for healthy women the excess absolute risk of either of these conditions is about 1 in 5000 per year while taking HRT.

The increased risk of venous thromboembolism (VTE) means that caution should be exercised in using HRT in women who are likely to be at high risk of DVT or PE. Women with severe varicose veins, severe obesity (Body Mass Index >30 kg/m²), immobilisation for 3 weeks or more, trauma or surgery requiring bed rest, are at increased risk of VTE so that the benefits of treatment with HRT will need to be weighed against risks carefully. Where elective surgery is planned requiring subsequent bed rest, HRT should be stopped four weeks prior to surgery.

If venous thromboembolism develops after initiating therapy, the drug should be discontinued.

As oestrogens may cause fluid retention, patients with cardiac or renal dysfunction should be carefully observed.

Zumenon is not an oral contraceptive. Women of child-bearing potential should be advised to use non-hormonal contraceptive methods.

Most studies indicate that oestrogen replacement therapy has little effect on blood pressure and some indicate that oestrogen use may be associated with a small decrease. In addition, most studies on combined therapy indicate that the addition of progestogen also has little effect on blood pressure. Rarely, idiosyncratic hypertension may occur.

When oestrogens are administered to hypertensive women, supervision is necessary and blood pressure should be monitored at regular intervals.

It has been reported that there is an increase in the risk of surgically confirmed gall bladder disease in women receiving post-menopausal oestrogens.

*Interactions with other medicaments and other forms of interaction:* Oestrogens interact with liver enzyme inducing drugs with increased metabolism of oestrogens, which may reduce the oestrogen effect. Interactions are documented for the following liver enzyme inducing drugs: barbiturates, phenytoin, rifampicin, carbamazepine.

Changes in oestrogen serum concentrations may affect the results of certain endocrine or liver function tests.

*Pregnancy and lactation:* Known, or suspected pregnancy is a contra-indication to Zumenon therapy.
*Lactation:* this product is not indicated during this period.

*Effects on ability to drive and use machines:* No effects known

*Undesirable effects:* The following side effects have been reported with oestrogen/progestogen therapy:

– Genito-urinary system–Breakthrough bleeding, spotting, change in menstrual flow, dysmenorrhoea, premenstrual-like syndrome, amenorrhoea, increase in size of uterine fibromyomata, vaginal candidiasis, change in cervical erosion and in degree of cervical secretion, cystitis-like syndrome.
– Breasts–Tenderness, enlargement, secretion.
– Gastrointestinal–Nausea, vomiting, abdominal cramps, bloating, cholestatic jaundice.
– Skin–Chloasma or melasma which may persist when drug is discontinued, erythema multiforme, erythema nodosum, haemorrhagic eruption.
– Eyes–Steepening of corneal curvature, intolerance to contact lenses.
– CNS–Headaches, migraine, dizziness, mental depression, chorea.
– Miscellaneous–Increase or decrease in weight, reduced carbohydrate tolerance, aggravation of porphyria, oedema, changes in libido, leg cramps.

*Overdose:* There have been no reports of ill-effects following overdose. Overdose of oestrogen may cause nausea, and withdrawal bleeding may occur in females.

If overdosage is discovered within two or three hours and is so large that treatment seems desirable, gastric lavage can safely be used. There is no specific antidote and further treatment should be symptomatic.

## Pharmacological properties

*Pharmacodynamic properties:* Estradiol is chemically and biologically identical to the endogenous human estradiol and is, therefore, classified as a human oestrogen. Estradiol is the primary oestrogen and the most active of the ovarian hormones. The endogenous oestrogens are involved in certain functions of the uterus and accessory organs, including the proliferation of the endometrium and the cyclic changes in the cervix and vagina.

Oestrogens are known to play an important role for bone and fat metabolism. Furthermore, oestrogens also affect the autonomic nervous system and may have indirect positive psychotropic actions.

*Pharmacokinetic properties:* Following oral administration, micronised estradiol is readily absorbed, but extensively metabolised. The major unconjugated and conjugated metabolites are estrone and estrone sulphate. These metabolites can contribute to the oestrogen activity, either directly or after conversion to estradiol. Estrone sulphate may undergo enterohepatic circulation. In urine, the major compounds are the glucuronides of estrone and estradiol.

Oestrogens are secreted in the milk of nursing mothers.

*Preclinical safety data:* Supraphysiologically high doses (prolonged overdoses) of estradiol have been associated with the induction of tumours in oestrogen-dependent target organs for all rodent species tested. Pronounced species differences in toxicology, pharmacology and pharmacodynamics exist.

## Pharmaceutical particulars

*List of excipients:* Lactose, methylhydroxypropyl cellulose, maize starch, colloidal anhydrous silica, magnesium stearate, methylcellulose, polyethylene glycol 400, quinoline yellow (E104), sunset yellow (E110), ponceau 4R (E124), titanium dioxide (E171).

*Incompatibilities:* Not applicable

*Shelf life:* 24 months when stored below 25˚C.

*Special precautions for storage:* None.

*Nature and contents of container:* The tablets are packed in blister strips of 28. The blister strips are made of PVC film with covering Aluminium foil. Each carton contains 28 or 84 tablets.

*Instruction for use/handling:* Not applicable

**Marketing authorisation number**   00512/0100

**Date of approval/revision of SPC**   May 1997

**Legal category**   POM

*\*Trade Mark*

# Speywood Pharmaceuticals Ltd
## 1 Bath Road
## Maidenhead
## Berkshire SL6 4UH

# SPEYWOOD

## DE-CAPEPTYL SR* ▼

**Qualitative and quantitative composition** Triptorelin 4.2 mg.

**Pharmaceutical form** A 5 ml slightly tinted transparent Type I glass vial fitted with a crimped elastomer stopper containing a sterile, practically white crumbly cake which when reconstituted as directed with the clear, colourless, sterile liquid in the accompanying 2 ml clear Type I glass ampoule yields a sterile suspension for intramuscular injection.

### Clinical particulars

*Therapeutic indications:* Treatment of advanced prostate cancer. Treatment of endometriosis.

*Posology and method of administration:*
*Advanced prostate cancer:* One intramuscular injection should be administered every 4 weeks (28 days). No dosage adjustment is necessary in the elderly.

*Endometriosis:* One intramuscular injection every 28 days. The treatment must be initiated in the first five days of the cycle. The duration of treatment should be a maximum of 6 months. A second course of treatment by De-capeptyl SR or by other GnRH analogues should not be undertaken due to concerns about bone density losses.

*Contra-indications:* In prostate cancer, De-capeptyl SR should not be prescribed in patients presenting with spinal cord compression or evidence of spinal metastases.

In endometriosis, confirm that the patient is not pregnant before beginning treatment.

*Special warnings and special precautions for use:*
*Advanced prostate cancer:* Initially, De-capeptyl SR causes a transient increase in serum testerone and consequent worsening of symptoms including increase in bone pain (and acid phosphatase levels). Consideration should be given to the use of an anti-androgen for three days prior to De-capeptyl SR treatment, to counteract this initial rise in serum testosterone levels. During the first month of treatment, patients presenting with, or at particular risk of developing, ureteric obstruction should be carefully monitored, as should those at risk of developing spinal cord compression. Continued treatment with De-capeptyl SR leads to suppression of testosterone (and dihydrotestosterone) and consequent improvement in the disease.

*Endometriosis:* Regular administration, every 28 days of one vial of De-capeptyl SR causes a persistent hypogonadotrophic amenorrhoea. During the first month of treatment, a non-hormonal contraception should be given. A supervening metrorrhagia in the course of treatment, other than in the first month, should lead to measurement of plasma oestradiol levels. Should this level be less than 50 pg/ml, possible associated organic lesions should be sought. After withdrawal of treatment, ovarian function resumes and ovulation occurs on average 58 days after the last injection, with first menses occurring on average 70 days after the last injection. Contraception may therefore be required. Due to concerns about bone density losses, De-capeptyl SR should be used with caution in women with known metabolic bone disease.

*Interactions with other medicaments and other forms of interaction:* Drugs which raise prolactin levels should not be prescribed concomitantly as they reduce the level of LHRH receptors in the pituitary.

*Pregnancy and lactation:* Reproductive studies in primates have shown no maternal toxicity or embryotoxicity, and there was no effect on parturition. Inadvertent administration of triptorelin during human pregnancy has not demonstrated a teratogenic or other foetal risk. However, it is recommended that De-capeptyl SR should not be used during pregnancy or lactation.

*Effect on ability to drive and use machines:* There is no evidence that De-capeptyl SR has any effect on the ability to drive or operate machinery.

*Undesirable effects*
*In prostate cancer patients,* the most frequent side-effects of hot flushes, decreased libido, and impotence are a result of the decrease in testosterone levels. Bone pain, as a result of 'disease flare', occurs occasionally. Pain and erythema at injection site, phlebitis and moderate and transient hypertension have been reported. On rare occasions the following have been reported: gynaecomastia, gastralgia, dry mouth, headaches, recurrence of asthma, increased dysuria, fever, pruritus, sweating, paresthesias, dizziness, insomnia, excessive salivation, gastric disturbance, nausea, vertigo, slight hair loss, induration at injection site.

*In endometriosis patients,* adverse effects such as hot flushes, menorrhagia and vaginal dryness, reflect the efficacy of pituitary-ovarian blockade. Cutaneous rash, hair loss, asthenia, headache, weight gain, oedema, arthralgia, myalgia, transient sight disturbances and temporary hypertension may occur. As with any GnRH analogue, a small loss in bone density, specifically trabecular bone density, occurs during six months of De-capeptyl SR treatment. Clinical data suggests that this loss is reversible.

*Overdose:* There is no human experience of overdosage. Animal data do not predict any effects other than those on sex hormone concentration and consequent effect on the reproductive tract. If overdosage occurs, symptomatic management is indicated.

### Pharmacological properties

*Pharmacodynamic properties:* Triptorelin is a decapeptide analogue of LHRH which initially stimulates release of pituitary gonadotrophins.

*Prostate cancer patients:* This results in an increase in peripheral circulating levels of testosterone and dihydrotestosterone. Continued administration (over 7 days) however, leads to suppression of gonadotrophins and a consequent fall in plasma testosterone. In prostate cancer patients, plasma testosterone levels fall to castrate levels after 2–3 weeks of treatment, frequently resulting in an improvement of function and objective symptoms.

*Endometriosis patients:* Continued administration of De-capeptyl SR induces suppression of oestrogen secretion and thus enables resting of ectopic endometrial tissue.

*Pharmacokinetic properties:*
*Subcutaneous form:* In healthy volunteers: Subcutaneously administered triptorelin (100 µg) is rapidly absorbed (Tmax=0.63±0.26 hr for peak plasma concentration=1.85±0.23 ng/ml). Elimination is effected with a biological half-life of 7.6±1.6 hr, after a 3 to 4 hr distribution phase. Total plasma clearance is: 161±28 ml/min. Distribution volume is 104.1±11.7 litres.

In prostate cancer patients: With subcutaneous administration (100 µg), triptorelin blood levels oscillate between maximum values of 1.28±0.24 ng/ml (Cmax) obtained in general one hour after injection (Tmax) and minimum values of 0.28±0.15 ng/ml (Cmin) obtained 24 hrs after injection.

The biological half-life is on average 11.7±3.4 hr but varies according to patients. Plasma clearance (118±32 ml/min) reflects slower elimination in patients, whilst distribution volumes are close to those of healthy volunteers (113.4±21.6 litres).

*Sustained release form: Prostate cancer patients:* Following intramuscular injection of the sustained release form, an initial phase of release of the active principle present on the surface of the microspheres is observed, followed by further fairly regular release (Cmax=0.32±0.12 ng/ml), with a mean rate of release of triptorelin of 46.6±7.1 µg/day. The bioavailability of the microspheres is approximately 53% at one month.

*Endometriosis patients:* After intramuscular injection of De-capeptyl SR in endometriosis patients the maximum blood level of triptorelin is obtained between 2 to 6 hours after injection, the peak value reached is 11 ng/ml. There was no evidence of accumulation of the product following monthly injections over six months. The minimum blood level oscillates between 0.1 and 0.2 ng/ml. The bioavailability of the sustained release product is approximately 50%.

*Preclinical safety data:* Preclinical findings were only those related to the expected pharmacological activity of triptorelin, namely down-regulation of the hypothalamic-pituitary-gonadal axis. These included atrophy of the testes and genital tract, with resultant suppression of spermatogenesis, together with decreased weight of the prostate gland. These findings were largely reversible within the recovery period. In a small number of rats, in a 24 months oncogenity study, a low incidence of benign histological changes were seen in the non-glandular part of the fore stomach. Erosions, ulcers, necrosis and inflammation were seen at varying degrees of severity. The clinical relevance of these findings is unknown. The increased incidence of adenomatous tumours in the rat pituitary observed with De-capeptyl following long-term repeated dosing is thought to be a class specific action of GnRH analogues due to an hormonally-mediated mechanism and has not been found in the mouse nor has it been described in man.

Standard mutagenicity testing revealed no mutagenic activity of triptorelin.

### Pharmaceutical particulars

*List of excipients:*
(a) *Microspheres:* D,L-lactide/glycolide copolymer, mannitol, sodium carboxymethylcellulose, polysorbate 80.
(b) *Suspension vehicle:* mannitol, water for injections.

*Incompatibilities:* None.

*Shelf life:* The shelf-life of the powder for injection shall not exceed 18 months.

The shelf-life of the injection vehicle shall not exceed 3 years.

The product should be used immediately after reconstitution.

*Special precautions for storage:* The product should be stored below 25°C, away from direct heat.

*Nature and contents of container:* A 5 ml slightly tinted, transparent, Type I glass vial with a crimped elastomer stopper containing a sterile, practically white, crumbly cake and a 2 ml, type I glass ampoule containing a clear, colourless, sterile liquid.

*Instructions for use/handling:* The vehicle should be drawn into the syringe provided and transferred to the vial containing the powder for injection. The vial should be gently shaken and the mixture then drawn back into the syringe without inverting the vial. The needle should then be changed and the injection administered immediately.

**Marketing authorisation numbers**
De-capeptyl SR      10829/0002
Mannitol solution      10829/0003

**Date of approval/revision of SPC**    January 1997.

**Legal category**   POM.

## DOPACARD*

**Presentation** A clear glass ampoule containing 5 ml of a 1% aqueous colourless solution of dopexamine hydrochloride (50 mg). The solution is adjusted to pH 2.5. Inactive ingredients: 0.01% Disodium Edetate BP.

### Uses

*Pharmacological action:* The primary actions of Dopacard (dopexamine hydrochloride) are the stimulation of adrenergic β₂-receptors and peripheral dopamine receptors of DA₁ and DA₂ subtypes. In addition, Dopacard is an inhibitor of neuronal reuptake of noradrenaline (Uptake-1). These pharmacological actions result in an increase in cardiac output mediated by afterload reduction (β₂, DA₁) and mild positive inotropism (β₂, Uptake-1 inhibition) together with an increase in blood flow to vascular beds (DA₁) such as the renal and mesenteric beds. Dopacard therefore provides an increase in systemic and regional oxygen delivery. Dopacard is not an α-adrenergic agonist and does not cause vasoconstriction and is not a pressor agent.

*Indications:* Dopacard is indicated for short-term intravenous administration to patients in whom afterload reduction, (through peripheral vasodilation, and or renal and mesenteric vasodilation), combined with a mild positive inotropic effect is required for the treatment of exacerbations of chronic heart failure or heart failure associated with cardiac surgery.

**Dosage and administration** Dopacard must be diluted before use.

*Preparation:* The contents of four ampoules (20 ml

should be injected aseptically into one of the following: 0.9% Sodium Chloride Injection 500 or 250 ml; 5% Dextrose Injection 500 or 250 ml.

These dilutions give a concentration for administration as follows:

4 ampoules of Dopacard diluted to 500 ml = 400 micrograms/ml.

4 ampoules of Dopacard diluted to 250 ml = 800 micrograms/ml.

*Administration:* Dopacard should only be administered intravenously by infusion through a cannula or catheter in a central or large peripheral vein. Contact with metal parts in infusion apparatus should be minimised. A device which provides accurate control of the rate of flow is essential.

*Central administration:* Dopacard can be administered via a cannula or catheter sited in a central vein. The concentration of the infusion solution for administration via this route must not exceed 4 mg/ml.

*Peripheral administration:* Dopacard can be administered via a cannula in a large peripheral vein. The concentration of the infusion solution for administration via this route must not exceed 1 mg/ml. Thrombophlebitis has been reported with peripheral administration using concentrations of Dopacard exceeding 1 mg/ml.

Care should be exercised so as to restrict the sodium and fluid load being administered.

*Recommended dosage for adults including the elderly:* Infusion should begin at a dose of 0.5 microgram/kg/min and may be increased to 1 microgram/kg/min and then in increments (0.5–1 microgram/kg/min) up to 6 micrograms/kg/min at not less than 15 minute intervals according to the patient's haemodynamic and clinical response. Smaller increments (0.5 microgram/kg/min) may be justified in certain patients according to haemodynamic and clinical response.

During the administration of Dopacard, as with any parenteral catecholamine, the rate of administration and duration of therapy should be adjusted according to the patient's response as determined by heart rate and rhythm (ECG), blood pressure, urine flow and, whenever possible, measurement of cardiac output.

It is recommended that the infusion of Dopacard is reduced gradually rather than withdrawn abruptly.

The duration of therapy is dependent upon the patient's overall response to treatment. Extended therapy beyond 48 hours has not been fully evaluated.

*Paediatric use:* The safety and efficacy of Dopacard for use in children have not been established.

**Contra-indications, warnings, etc**
*Contra-indications:* Known hypersensitivity to dopexamine hydrochloride or excipients (disodium edetate). Patients who are receiving monoamine oxidase inhibitors (MAOIs).

Phaeochromocytoma

Thrombocytopenia

Patients with left ventricular outlet obstruction such as hypertrophic obstructive cardiomyopathy or aortic stenosis. In such patients, positive inotropic activity may increase left ventricular outflow obstruction and sudden vasodilatation may cause hypotension.

*Precautions:* If any correction of hypovolaemia is required, this should be achieved before the administration of Dopacard.

*Warnings:* Dopacard should not be administered to patients with severe hypotension or a markedly reduced systemic vascular resistance until specific resuscitative measures have been taken to restore blood pressure to a clinically acceptable level.

In patients with a marked reduction in systemic vascular resistance, Dopacard should not be used as a direct substitute for pressor agents or other inotropes.

As with other catecholamines, Dopacard should be administered with caution to patients with a clinical history of ischaemic heart disease especially following acute myocardial infarction or recent episodes of angina pectoris as a tachycardia may increase myocardial oxygen demand and further exacerbate myocardial ischaemia.

As has been observed with some other $\beta_2$–adrenergic agonists, a small reversible fall in circulating platelet numbers has been observed in some patients. No adverse effects attributable to alterations in platelet count have been seen in clinical studies.

Care must be exercised when administering Dopacard in the presence of hypokalaemia or hyperglycaemia. In common with other $\beta_2$–agonists, Dopacard depresses plasma potassium and raises plasma glucose. These effects are minor and reversible. Monitoring of potassium and glucose is advisable in patients likely to be at risk from such changes e.g. diabetics, patients with myocardial infarction, or patients being treated with diuretics or cardiac glycosides.

Benign arrhythmias such as ventricular premature beats and, more rarely, serious arrhythmias have

been reported in some patients. If excessive tachycardia occurs during Dopacard administration, then a reduction or temporary discontinuation of the infusion should be considered.

As with other parenteral catecholamines, there have been occasional reports of partial tolerance, with some attenuation of the haemodynamic response developing during long term infusions of Dopacard.

The risk of thrombophlebitis and local necrosis may be increased if the concentration of Dopacard administered via a peripheral vein exceeds 1 mg/ml. Thrombophlebitis is rare when the concentration of drug used for peripheral administration is less than 1 mg/ml.

*Use in pregnant and lactating women:* There is no experience of the use of Dopacard in pregnant or lactating women and therefore its safety in these situations has not been established. There is insufficient evidence from animal studies to indicate it is free from hazard. Therefore Dopacard is not currently recommended for use in pregnant and lactating women.

*Side-effects:* The most common undesirable effect reported with Dopacard administration in studies of use in heart failure is tachycardia (11.8% in studies of exacerbations of chronic heart failure; 19.4% in studies of use in cardiac surgery). The increases in heart rate are dose-related and, in most cases, not clinically significant.

Hypertension and transient hypotension have been reported after cardiac surgery (at an incidence of 8.8% and 7.0% respectively). These events, however, are not uncommon as compensatory mechanisms following cardiac surgery. Transient hypotension was reported in studies of exacerbations of chronic heart failure at an incidence of 6.3%.

Other undesirable effects reported in clinical trials in both exacerbations of chronic heart failure and cardiac surgery at an incidence of 1% or more include:

*Cardiovascular:* A number of tachyarrhythmias such as premature ventricular contractions (PVCs) and atrial fibrillation, bradycardia, both sinus and nodal, worsening heart failure leading to asystole and cardiac arrest, angina, myocardial infarction, cardiac enzyme changes and non-specific ECG changes have occurred.

*Non-cardiovascular:* Nausea and vomiting, tremor, headache diaphoresis and dyspnoea. Careful titration of the dose may minimise the incidence of adverse events.

More rarely a number of serious adverse events have been reported in patients undergoing cardiac surgery: renal failure, respiratory failure, acute respiratory distress syndrome (ARDS), pulmonary oedema, pulmonary hypertension, bleeding and septicaemia. However, such events may also be due to the condition of the patients in such populations.

*Interactions:* As Dopacard inhibits the Uptake–1 mechanism, it may potentiate the effects of exogenous catecholamines such as noradrenaline. Caution is recommended when these agents are administered concomitantly with Dopacard or soon after its discontinuation.

In the case of dopamine, there is no evidence of an interaction, other than possible attenuation of the indirect sympathomimetic inotropic effects of higher doses of dopamine due to Uptake–1 blockade by Dopacard.

Concomitant use with $\beta_2$–adrenergic and dopamine receptor antagonists requires caution since attenuation of the pharmacological effects of Dopacard may occur.

*Overdosage:* The half-life of Dopacard in blood is short (approximately 6-7 minutes in healthy volunteers and around 11 minutes in patients with cardiac failure). Consequently, the effects of overdosage are likely to be short-lived provided that administration is discontinued.

Effects of overdosage are likely to be related to the pharmacological actions and include tachycardia, tremulousness and tremor, nausea and vomiting, and anginal pain. Treatment should be supportive and directed to these symptoms.

**Pharmaceutical precautions** Store below 25°C, protect from light.

Ampoules should be discarded if contents are discoloured.

Dopacard should only be diluted with 0.9% Sodium Chloride Injection, 5% Dextrose Injection, Hartmann's Solution (Compound Sodium Lactate Intravenous Infusion) or Dextrose 4% / Saline 0.18% Injection and should not be added to 5% Sodium Bicarbonate or any other strongly alkaline solutions as inactivation will occur.

Prepared intravenous solutions in 0.9% Sodium Chloride Injection or 5% Dextrose Injection are stable for 24 hours at room temperature.

Dopacard, in common with other catecholamines, may turn slightly pink in prepared solutions. There is

no significant loss of potency associated with this change.

Dopacard should not be mixed with any other active agents before administration.

Contact with metal parts, in infusion apparatus for example, should be minimised.

**Legal category** POM.

**Package quantities** Box of 10 clear glass ampoules each containing 5 ml of 1% solution of dopexamine hydrochloride (50 mg per ampoule).

**Further information** The main haemodynamic effects of Dopacard consist of an increase in cardiac output associated with a large reduction in systemic vascular resistance and a smaller decrease of left ventricular filling pressure. Heart rate effects are variable but there is a general tendency for a small increase particularly at high doses. There is little effect on arterial blood pressure.

*Pharmacokinetics:* Dopacard is rapidly eliminated from blood with a half-life of approximately 6-7 minutes in healthy volunteers and around 11 minutes in patients with cardiac failure. Subsequent elimination of the metabolites is by urinary and biliary excretion. The response to Dopacard is rapid in onset and effects subside rapidly on discontinuation of the infusion. Increases in dose may be made at intervals of not less than 15 minutes.

Experience in clinical trials has shown that Dopacard can increase cardiac output by over 100% within the recommended dose range and increases of the order of 50% are frequently achieved at doses of 1–2 micrograms/kg/min without a clinically significant effect on heart rate.

*Use in surgery:* Dopacard has been used in high risk patients undergoing surgery.

**Product licence number** 6958/0008

## DYSPORT*

### Qualitative and quantitative composition

| Active constituent | *per vial* |
|---|---|
| *Clostridium botulinum* type A toxin-haemagglutinin complex | 500U‡ |
| Other constituents | |
| Albumin solution 20% | 125 micrograms |
| Lactose | 2.5 mg |

‡ One unit (U) is defined as the median lethal peritoneal dose in mice.

**Pharmaceutical form** Injection.

### Clinical particulars
*Therapeutic indications:* For the treatment of blepharospasm, hemifacial spasm and spasmodic torticollis.

*Posology and method of administration when treating blepharospasm and hemifacial spasm*
*Adults and elderly:* In the treatment of bilateral blepharospasm the recommended initial dose is 120 units per eye.

Injection of 0.1 ml (20 units) should be made medially and of 0.2 ml (40 units) should be made laterally into the junction between the preseptal and orbital parts of both the upper and lower orbicularis oculi muscles of each eye.

For injections into the upper lid the needle should be directed away from its centre to avoid the levator muscle. A diagram to aid placement of these injections is provided below. The relief of symptoms may be expected to begin within two to four days with maximal effect within two weeks.

Injections should be repeated approximately every eight weeks or as required to prevent recurrence of symptoms. On such subsequent administrations the dose may need to be reduced to 80 units per eye, viz. 0.1 ml (20 units) medially and 0.1 ml (20 units) laterally above and below each eye in the manner previously described. The dose may be further reduced to 60 units per eye by omitting the medial lower lid injection.

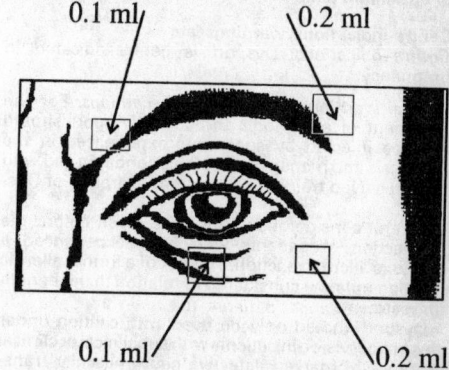

0.1 ml      0.2 ml

0.1 ml      0.2 ml

In cases of unilateral blepharospasm the injections

should be confined to the affected eye. Patients with hemifacial spasm should be treated as for unilateral blepharospasm. The doses recommended are applicable to adults of all ages including the elderly.

*Posology and method of administration when treating spasmodic torticollis:* The doses recommended for torticollis are applicable to adults of all ages providing the adults are of normal weight with no evidence of low neck muscle mass. A reduced dose may be appropriate if the patient is markedly underweight or in the elderly where reduced muscle mass may exist.

The initial recommended dose for the treatment of spasmodic torticollis is 500 units (1 ml) per patient given as a divided dose and administered to the two or three most active neck muscles.

For rotational torticollis distribute the 500 units by administering 350 units into the splenius capitis muscle, ipsilateral to the direction of the chin/head rotation and 150 units into the sternomastoid muscle, contralateral to the rotation.

For laterocollis, distribute the 500 units by administering 350 units into the ipsilateral splenius capitis muscle and 150 units into the ipsilateral sternomastoid muscle. In cases associated with shoulder elevation the ipsilateral trapezoid or levator scapulae muscles may also require treatment, according to visible hypertrophy of the muscle or electromyographic (EMG) findings. Where injections of three muscles are required, distribute the 500 units as follows, 300 units splenius capitis, 100 units sternomastoid and 100 units to the third muscle.

For retrocollis distribute the 500 units by administering 250 units into each of the splenius capitis muscles. This may be followed by bilateral trapezius injections (up to 250 units per muscle) after 6 weeks, if there is insufficient response. Bilateral splenii injections may increase the risk of neck muscle weakness.

All other forms of torticollis are highly dependent on specialist knowledge and EMG to identify and treat the most active muscles. EMG should be used diagnostically for all complex forms of torticollis, for reassessment after unsuccessful injections in non complex cases, and for guiding injections into deep muscles or in overweight patients with poorly palpable neck muscles.

On subsequent administration, the doses may be adjusted according to the clinical response and side effects observed. Doses within the range of 250–1000 units are recommended, although the higher doses may be accompanied by increase in side effects, particularly dysphagia. Doses above 1000 units are not recommended.

The relief of symptoms of torticollis may be expected within a week after the injection. Injections should be repeated approximately every eight to twelve weeks or as required to prevent recurrence of symptoms.

*Children:* The safety and effectiveness of Dysport in children has not been demonstrated.

*Method of administration:* The exposed central portion of the rubber stopper should be cleaned with alcohol immediately prior to piercing the septum. A sterile 23 or 25 gauge needle should be used.

When treating blepharospasm and hemifacial spasm Dysport is reconstituted with 2.5 ml of sodium chloride injection BP (0.9%) to yield a solution containing 200 units per ml of Dysport.

Dysport is administered by subcutaneous injection medially and laterally into the junction between the preseptal and orbital parts of both the upper and lower orbicularis oculi muscles of the eyes.

When treating spasmodic torticollis Dysport is reconstituted with 1 ml of sodium chloride injection BP (0.9%) to yield a solution containing 500 units per ml of Dysport. Dysport is administered by intramuscular injection as above when treating spasmodic torticollis.

**The units of Dysport are specific to the preparation and are not interchangeable with other preparations of botulinum toxin.**

## Contra-indications, warnings, etc

*Contra-indications:* Dysport is contra-indicated in pregnancy.

*Special warnings and special precautions:* For the treatment of spasmodic torticollis, Dysport should only be injected by specialists experienced in the diagnosis and management of this condition and who have received training on the administration of Dysport.

Careful consideration should be given before the re-injection of patients who have experienced a previous allergic reaction. The risk of a further allergic reaction must be considered in relation to the benefit of treatment.

Dysport should only be used with caution under close supervision in patients with subclinical or clinical evidence of marked defective neuromuscular transmission. Such patients may have an increased sensi-

tivity to agents such as Dysport which may result in excessive muscle weakness.

*Training:* Speywood will facilitate training in administration of Dysport injections.

There are no reports of any immune response after the local administration of *Clostridium botulinum* Type A toxin-haemagglutinin complex in accordance with the doses recommended when treating blepharospasm and hemifacial spasm. Antibody formation to botulinum toxin has been noted in a small number of patients receiving therapy with Dysport for torticollis. Clinically, this has been detected by substantial deterioration in response to therapy or a need for consistently increasing high doses.

This product contains a small amount of human albumin. The risk of transmission of viral infection cannot be excluded with absolute certainty following the use of human blood or blood products.

*Interaction with other medicaments and other forms of interaction:* No interactions of clinical significance have been reported.

*Pregnancy and lactation:* Teratological and other reproductive studies have not been performed with Dysport. The safety of its use in pregnant or lactating women has not been demonstrated.

*Effects on ability to drive and use machines:* None known.

*Undesirable effects when treating blepharospasm and hemifacial spasm:* Side-effects may occur from deep or misplaced injections of Dysport, temporarily paralysing other nearby muscle groups. They may also occur from exacerbation of pre-existing eyelid abnormalities or from an initial over-correction. Ptosis is the most common unwanted effect. A few patients may also experience diplopia or symptoms from spread of paralytic effect to mid-facial muscles. These side effects may be expected to resolve within two to four weeks. Keratitis and dry eyes due to reduced blinking have also been reported for which the use of artificial tears could be considered. Minor bruising and lid swelling may occur but are short lived. Reversible external ophthalmoplegia has been reported after excessive dosing.

The injections have been associated with a burning sensation which lasts for 1–2 minutes after injection.

Allergic reactions such as skin rashes and influenza-like symptoms have occasionally been noted.

*Undesirable effects when treating spasmodic torticollis:* Side-effects may occur mainly from deep or misplaced injections temporarily paralysing other nearby muscle groups. The injections have been associated with a burning sensation which lasts for 1–2 minutes after injection.

In patients treated for torticollis dysphagia is the most frequently reported adverse event. In a double-blind placebo controlled trial the incidence of dysphagia was 29% following treatment with 500 units of Dysport and 10% in the placebo group. This appears to be dose related and occurs most frequently following injection into the sternomastoid muscle. A soft diet may be required until symptoms resolve. In those patients severely affected, laryngoscopy has identified pooling of saliva. Aspiration may occur rarely and be of potential concern in those patients with pre-existing respiratory problems. Less frequently reported events include weakness of the neck muscles, dryness of mouth and voice changes. A more generalised weakness and visual disturbances (including diplopia and blurred vision) have occasionally been reported. Respiratory difficulties have been noted on rare occasions in association with high doses.

These side-effects may be expected to resolve within two to four weeks.

Allergic reactions such as skin rashes and influenza-like symptoms have occasionally been noted.

*Overdose:* Excessive doses may produce distant and profound neuromuscular paralysis. Respiratory support may be required where excessive doses cause paralysis of respiratory muscles. There is no specific antidote; antitoxin should not be expected to be beneficial and general supportive care is advised.

## Pharmacological properties

*Pharmacodynamic properties: Clostridium botulinum* type A toxin-haemagglutinin complex blocks peripheral cholinergic transmission at the neuromuscular junction by a presynaptic action at a site proximal to the release of acetylcholine. The toxin acts within the nerve ending to antagonise those events that are triggered by $Ca^{2+}$ which culminate in transmitter release. It does not affect postganglionic cholinergic transmission or postganglionic sympathetic transmission.

The action of toxin involves an initial binding step whereby the toxin attaches rapidly and avidly to the presynaptic nerve membrane. Secondly there is an internalisation step in which toxin crosses the presynaptic membrane, without causing onset of paralysis. Finally the toxin inhibits the release of acetylcholine

by disrupting the $Ca^{2+}$ mediated acetylcholine release mechanism, thereby diminishing the endplate potential and causing paralysis.

Recovery of impulse transmission occurs gradually as new nerve terminals sprout and contact is made with the post synaptic motor endplate, a process which takes 6–8 weeks in the experimental animal.

*Pharmacokinetic properties:* Pharmacokinetic studies with botulinum toxin pose problems in animals because of the high potency, the minute doses involved, the large molecular weight of the compound and the difficulty of labelling toxin to produce sufficiently high specific activity. Studies using $I^{125}$ labelled toxin have shown that the receptor binding is specific and saturable, and the high density of toxin receptors is a contributory factor to the high potency. Dose and time responses in monkeys showed that at low doses there was a delay of 2–3 days with peak effect seen 5–6 days after injection. The duration of action, measured by changes of ocular alignment and muscle paralysis varied between 2 weeks and 8 months. This pattern is also seen in man, and is attributed to the process of binding, internalisation and changes at the neuromuscular junction.

## Pharmaceutical particulars

*List of excipients:* Albumin and lactose.

*Incompatibilities:* None known.

*Shelf life:* The shelf life of the packaged product is 12 months.

The reconstituted product should be used within one hour of reconstitution.

*Special precautions for storage:* Unopened vials must be maintained at temperatures between 2°C and 8°C. Dysport must be stored in a refrigerator at the hospital where the injections are to be carried out and should not be given to the patient to store.

Dysport should not be frozen.

*Nature and contents of container*
*Nature of container/closure:* Type 1 glass vials 3 ml capacity. 13 mm chlorbutyl freeze-drying closures oversealed by 13 mm aluminium overseals with centre hole, crimped over.

*Contents of container:* A white lypophilised powder for reconstitution.

*Instructions for use/handling:* Immediately after treatment of the patient, any residual Dysport which may be present in either vial or syringe should be inactivated with dilute hypochlorite solution (1% available chlorine). Thereafter, all items should be disposed of in accordance with standard hospital practice.

Spillage of Dysport should be wiped up with an absorbent cloth soaked in dilute hypochlorite solution.

**Marketing authorisation number**    6958/0005.

**Date of approval/revision of SPC**    April 1996.

**Legal category**    POM.

# ERWINASE*

**Qualitative and quantitative composition**   Crisantaspase (Asparaginase from *Erwinia chrysanthemi;* Erwinia L-asparaginase), 10,000 Units/vial.

**Pharmaceutical form**   Freeze-dried powder for reconstitution.

## Clinical particulars

*Therapeutic indications:* Erwinase is used in combination with other anti-neoplastic agents to treat acute lymphoblastic leukaemia. It may also be used in other neoplastic conditions where depletion of asparagine might be expected to have a useful effect. Patients receiving treatment with L-asparaginase from *Escherichia coli,* and who develop hypersensitivity to that enzyme may be able to continue treatment with Erwinase as the enzymes are immunologically distinct.

*Dosage and method of administration:* Erwinase solution can be given by intravenous injection or infusion or by intramuscular or subcutaneous injection.

For all patients the usual dose is 6,000 Units/m² body surface area (200 Units/kg of body weight), three times a week for three weeks.

Therapy may be further intensified according to protocol.

Reference to current Medical Research Council protocols on leukaemia therapy should be made for information on dose, route and frequency of treatment.

## Contra-indications, warnings, etc

*Contra-indications:* Previous allergic reaction to Erwinia asparaginase.

*Special warnings and special precautions for use*
*Warnings:* Asparaginase is a bacterial protein and repeated use can, therefore, lead to sensitisation reactions.

*Special precautions for use:* Erwinase should preferably be given without interruption. If, however, an interruption cannot be avoided, treatment should be resumed with a low dose, 10 Units/kg/day, and increased to the full dose over five days if tolerated. Anaphylaxis is rare but facilities should be made available for its management during administration.

*Interaction with other medicaments and other forms of interaction:* Asparaginase must not be mixed with any other drugs prior to administration.

*Pregnancy and lactation:* Asparaginase should not be given to women who are, or likely to become, pregnant.

*Effects on ability to drive and use machinery:* None known.

*Undesirable effects:* Neurotoxicity, life-threatening sepsis and severe hypersensitivity have been described in patients treated with L-asparaginases. Other effects reported with both enzymes include fever; nausea; vomiting; CNS depression; hypersensitivity and various plasma biochemical changes including increased BSP retention and elevation of bilirubin, SGOT, alkaline phosphatase and cholesterol levels; decreases in fibrinogen and some clotting factors. For these reasons, careful monitoring is therefore necessary and urine should be tested for glucose to exclude hyperglycaemia.

Undesirable effects are generally reversible and are less common with Erwinia L-asparaginase than with *E. coli.* asparaginase.

*Overdose:* No specific measures are recommended.

**Pharmacological properties**

*Pharmacodynamic properties:* Neoplastic cells associated with Acute Lymphoblastic Leukaemia (ALL), Acute Myeloid Leukaemia (AML) and Lymphoblastic Lymphosarcoma (LSA) are asparagine-dependent. Reduction of plasma asparagine levels achieved by administration of L-asparaginase produces an antineoplastic effect.

The animal studies carried out with Erwinase provide only an approximate indication of the human dose required when comparisons are made on a mg/kg basis. However, clinical studies have used doses in the range 500 to 60,000 Units/m²/day. The upper dose level is made possible by the intrinsically low toxicity of the Erwinia enzyme.

*Pharmacokinetic properties:* Peak levels of Erwinase are achieved in blood in 1 to 2 hours. The fall in enzyme levels follows first order kinetics with a half-life of 7 to 13 hours.

*Pre-clinical safety data:* No further relevant data.

**Pharamceutical particulars**

*List of excipients:* Sodium chloride BP; dextrose monohydrate BP.

*Incompatibilities:* See '*Interaction with other medicaments and other forms of interaction*'.

*Shelf-life*

*Shelf-life of product as packed for sale:* 3 years.

*Shelf-life following reconstitution according to directions:* 15 minutes in the original container, 8 hours in a glass or polypropylene syringe (See section *Instructions for use/handling*).

*Special precautions for storage:* Store between 2°C and 8°C.

*Nature and contents of container:* Type I clear neutral glass vials of 3 ml nominal capacity, closed with 13 mm halobutyl freeze-drying stoppers and aluminium overseals, containing a white lyophilised solid.

*Instructions for use/handling:* The contents of each vial should be reconstituted in 1 ml to 2 ml of Sodium Chloride for Injection BP and dissolved by gentle mixing.

The solution should be administered within 15 minutes of reconstitution. If a delay of more than 15 minutes between reconstitution and administration is unavoidable, the solution should be withdrawn into a glass or polypropylene syringe for the period of the delay. The solution should be used within 8 hours.

Erwinase is not a cytotoxic drug (such as vincristine or methotrexate) and does not require the special precautions needed for manipulating such agents. It should be handled in the same way as other therapeutic enzymes such as hyaluronidase.

*Name and address of the marketing authorisation holder:* Microbiological Research Authority, Centre for Applied Microbiology and Research, Porton Down, Salisbury, Wiltshire SP4 0JG.

**Marketing authorisation number** 13663/0001

**Date of approval/revision of SPC** January 1996.

**Legal category** POM.

## HEXALEN* CAPSULES ▼

**Qualitative and quantitative composition**

| Active ingredient | Unit and/or percentage formula % w/w | mg/capsule |
|---|---|---|
| Altretamine | 19.6 | 50.0 |

**Pharmaceutical form** Clear transparent capsules containing 50 mg altretamine for oral administration.

**Clinical particulars**

*Therapeutic indications:* Hexalen is indicated for the treatment of advanced ovarian cancer as second line therapy in patients who have failed other treatments.

*Posology and method of administration:* Hexalen is administered orally. Doses are calculated on the basis of body surface area.

Hexalen should be administered only as a single agent for 14 consecutive days in a 28 day cycle at a dose of 260 mg/m²/day. The total daily dose should be rounded to the nearest 50 mg and may be given as 4 divided oral doses, given after meals and at bedtime. Hexalen should be administered for 12 cycles or until disease progression or unacceptable toxicity develops.

For dosage modifications please see *Undesirable effects* section.

*Impaired renal function:* No studies have been conducted in patients with impaired renal function.

*Impaired hepatic function:* There have been no studies of Hexalen metabolism or pharmacokinetics in patients with evidence of liver disease.

*Elderly:* Dose modifications should be based on adult toxicity guidelines described in *Undesirable effects* section, rather than age.

**Contra-indications, warnings, etc**

*Contra-indications:* Hexalen is contra-indicated in patients who have shown hypersensitivity to it. Hexalen should not be used in patients with pre-existing severe bone marrow depression or severe neurological toxicity.

Due to Hexalen's embryotoxic and teratogenic potential it is contra-indicated during pregnancy (see '*Use during pregnancy and lactation*').

*Special warnings and precautions:* Hexalen should only be given under the supervision of a physician experienced in the use of anti-neoplastic agents.

Peripheral blood counts should be monitored at least monthly, prior to the initiation of each course of Hexalen, and as clinically indicated.

Because of the possibility of Hexalen-related neurotoxicity, neurological examination should be performed regularly during Hexalen administration.

Concurrent administration of Hexalen and antidepressants of the monoamine oxidase inhibitor (MAOI) and tricyclic classes may cause severe orthostatic hypotension.

The carcinogenic potential of Hexalen has not been studied in animals, but drugs with similar mechanisms of action have been reported to be carcinogenic. Hexalen was weakly mutagenic when tested in strain TA100 of *Salmonella typhimurium*. With continuous, high dose administration, Hexalen adversely affected fertility in male rats.

*Interactions:* Concurrent administration of Hexalen and antidepressants of the MAO inhibitor or tricyclic classes may cause severe orthostatic hypotension. Cimetidine, an inhibitor of microsomal drug metabolism, increased altretamine's half-life and toxicity in a rat model.

Data from a randomised trial of Hexalen and cisplatin plus or minus pyridoxine in ovarian cancer indicated that pyridoxine significantly reduced neurotoxicity, however, it adversely affected response duration suggesting that pyridoxine should not be administered with Hexalen.

*Use during pregnancy and lactation:* No data are available on the use of Hexalen in human pregnancy. Hexalen has been shown to be embryotoxic and teratogenic in rats and rabbits. Due to Hexalen's embryotoxic and teratogenic potential, it is contraindicated during pregnancy. Women of childbearing potential should be advised to avoid becoming pregnant.

It is not known whether altretamine is excreted in human milk. Because there is a possibility of toxicity in nursing infants secondary to Hexalen treatment of the mother, it is recommended that breast feeding be discontinued if the mother is treated with Hexalen.

*Effects on ability to drive and use machines:* Unless the patient develops neurological toxicity, there is no restriction on driving or operating machinery. Neurological toxicity, manifested principally as peripheral neuropathies may inhibit the patient's ability to competently drive or operate machinery.

*Undesirable effects:* Hexalen should be temporarily discontinued (for 14 days or longer) and subsequently restarted at 200 mg/m²/day for any of the following situations:

1. Gastrointestinal intolerance unresponsive to symptomatic measures.

Nausea and vomiting of gradual onset was shown to occur in 33% of patients. It is recommended that prophylactic anti-emetics be employed.

Approximately 15% of patients may require dose interruptions or reductions and 5–10% of patients may require discontinuation of Hexalen therapy due to nausea and vomiting.

2. Myelosuppression defined as neutrophils $<2\times10^9$/l or platelets $<100\times10^9$/l.

Myelosuppression is dose related to Hexalen. At this dose and schedule Hexalen should not cause significant myelosuppression.

Hexalen should be withheld until neutrophils are $\geq 2\times10^9$/l and platelets $\geq 100\times10^9$/l before restarting at the reduced dose. If at the reduced dose neutrophils are $<1\times10^9$/l or platelets $<50\times10^9$/l Hexalen should be discontinued indefinitely.

Approximately 5% of patients may require dose interruptions or reductions due to neuropenia defined as $<2\times10^9$/l. Less than 1% of patients had neutropenia below $<1\times10^9$/l, following dose reduction. These patients were discontinued from Hexalen therapy.

Approximately 9% of patients may require dose interruptions or dose reductions due to thrombocytopenia defined as platelets $<100\times10^9$/l. Less than 3% of patients had thrombocytopenia below $50\times10^9$/l following dose reduction. These patients were discontinued from Hexalen therapy.

3. Progressive neurotoxicity during therapy.

Approximately 10% of patients may require dose interruptions or reductions. Neurotoxicity is dose and time dependent. If neurological symptoms fail to stabilise on the reduced dose schedule, Hexalen should be discontinued indefinitely.

Peripheral neuropathy and central nervous system symptoms (mood disorders, disorders of consciousness, ataxia, dizziness, vertigo) have been reported. Neurological toxicity may be reversible when therapy is discontinued.

Less than 5% of patients required discontinuation of Hexalen therapy.

4. Renal toxicity, defined as serum creatinine levels ≥1.6 mg/dL.

Dose interruptions or reductions were required in 7% of patients with increased serum creatinine levels (1.6–3.75 mg/dL).

Hexalen should be discontinued indefinitely if renal toxicity (serum creatinine levels ≥1.6 mg/dL) recurs on the reduced dose schedule and known nephrotoxic agents e.g. nephrotoxic anti-biotics have been discontinued.

Following dose interruptions or dose reductions less than 1% of patients required discontinuation of Hexalen therapy due to renal toxicity.

Other toxicities: Rare events included hepatic toxicity, skin rash, pruritus and alopecia; each were reported in <1% of patients treated. Less than 1% of patients had mild to moderate anaemia (haemoglobin 8–10 gm/dl) and less than 1% had severe anaemia (haemoglobin 6.5–7.9 gm/dl).

*Overdose:* No reports of overdosage are available. The most likely reaction would be severe nausea and vomiting and myelosuppression.

In the event of an overdose patients should be observed carefully and should signs of fever and infection arise, be treated along conventional lines.

**Pharmacological properties**

*Pharmacodynamic properties:* The precise mechanism by which Hexalen exerts its cytotoxic effect is unknown, although a number of theoretical possibilities have been studied. Structurally, Hexalen resembles the alkylating agent triethylenemelamine, yet in vitro tests for alkylating activity of Hexalen and its metabolites have been negative. Metabolism of altretamine is a requirement for cytotoxicity. Synthetic monohydroxymethylmelamines and products of altretamine metabolism, in vitro and in vivo, can form covalent adducts with tissue macromolecules including DNA, but the relevance of these reactions to antitumour activity is unknown.

*Pharmacokinetic properties:* Urinary recovery and bioavailability data demonstrate that Hexalen is well absorbed following oral administration in humans, but undergoes rapid and extensive demethylation in the liver, producing variation in Hexalen plasma levels.

After oral administration in doses of 120–300 mg/m², peak plasma levels (as measured by gas-chromatographic assay) varying from 0.2 to 20.8 μg/ml were reached between 0.5 and 3 hours. Half-life of the β-phase of elimination ranged from 4.7 to 10.2 hours. There was no plasma accumulation of $^{14}C$-radiolabelled hexamethylmelamine after daily treatment for 14 to 21 days.

*Preclinical safety data:* After intraperitoneal administration of $^{14}C$-ring-labelled altretamine to mice, tissue distribution was rapid in all organs, reaching a maximum at 30 minutes. The excretory organs (liver and kidney) and the small intestine showed high concentrations of radioactivity, whereas relatively low concentrations were found in other organs, including the brain.

The carcinogenic potential of Hexalen has not been studied in animals, but drugs with similar mechanisms of action have been shown to be carcinogenic. Hexalen was weakly mutagenic when tested in strain TA100 of *Salmonella typhimurium.* Hexalen administered to female rats 14 days prior to breeding through the gestation period had no adverse effect on fertility, but decreased post-natal survival at 120 mg/m²/day and was embryocidal at 240 mg/m²/day. Administration of 120 mg/m²/day Hexalen to male rats for 60 days prior to mating resulted in testicular atrophy, reduced fertility and a possible dominant lethal mutagenic effect. Male rats treated with Hexalen at 450 mg/m²/day for 10 days had decreased spermatogenesis, atrophy of testes, seminal vesicles and ventral prostate.

Treatment of male rats with doses ≥60 mg/m²/day for 60 days produced a marked increase in plasma glucose levels accompanied by morphological changes in pancreatic beta cells (vacuolisation).

**Pharmaceutical particulars**

*List of excipients:* Anhydrous lactose and calcium stearate.

*Incompatibilities:* No major incompatibilities are known.

*Shelf life:* 48 months.

*Special precautions for storage:* Hexalen capsules should be stored at a temperature not exceeding 25°C.

Procedures for the proper handling and disposal of anticancer drugs should be considered.

*Packaging quantities:* Hexalen 50 mg capsules are available in blister packs of 60 capsules. Each pack consists of six blister cards of ten capsules (6 × 10). The blister cards are packaged in a cardboard carton.

*Name and address of holder of the marketing authorisation:* US Bioscience Inc, Suites 9, 10 and 11, Awberry Court, Croxley Business Park, Watford, Hertfordshire WD1 8YJ.

**Marketing authorisation number** 11284/0001.

**Date of approval/revision of SPC** September 1996.

**Legal category** POM.

## HYATE*:C

**Presentation** Hyate:C is a highly purified freeze-dried concentrate of porcine antihaemophilic factor (Porcine Factor VIII:C) for intravenous administration. Hyate:C is in the form of a white lyophilised powder for reconstitution with 20 ml Water for Injections PhEur per vial. Each vial contains between 400 and 700 units of Factor VIII:C. The assayed amount of activity is stated on the label.

**Uses** Hyate:C is intended for the treatment or prevention of bleeding in patients with inhibitory antibodies to human Factor VIII:C. These inhibitors may have developed as a complication of hereditary haemophilia or may have arisen spontaneously in previously non-haemophilic patients (Acquired haemophilia).

Hyate:C has not been known to transmit hepatitis or human immunodeficiency virus (1). It may therefore be justified to consider Hyate:C as a primary treatment option, particularly in patients with spontaneously acquired antibodies to human Factor VIII:C and no previous exposure to human blood products.

**Dosage and administration** The clinical efficiency of Hyate:C has been reported to be as good as that achieved with the administration of human Factor VIII:C in non-antibody patients for similar Factor VIII:C levels and similar bleeding episodes (2, 3). Therefore, the general objectives for treatment with Hyate:C for the prevention or control of bleeding, joint mobilisation, wound healing and surgical cover are essentially the same as those employed with the use of human Factor VIII:C concentrates.

The dosage of Hyate:C varies for individual patients, but is dependent upon the patient's weight, the level of circulating antibody, the type and severity of haemorrhage and the desired plasma Factor VIII:C level.

The required dose is determined by administering an initial dose of Hyate:C and assaying the post-infusion level of Factor VIII:C in the patient's plasma. According to the response, the dosage can then be either increased or decreased for subsequent infusions.

*Initial Dose:* An estimate of the dose of Hyate:C required for the initial infusion can be made in the following ways:

1. It is recommended that the patient's antibody titre against Porcine Factor VIII:C is determined using the Bethesda assay (4).

If the anti-Porcine Factor VIII:C level is less than 20 Bethesda units per ml an initial dose of 25 - 50 units/kg body weight is recommended for a mild to moderate joint or muscle bleed and 50 - 100 units/kg body weight for a severe bleed.

If the anti-Porcine Factor VIII:C inhibitor level is greater than 20 Bethesda units per ml a minimum initial dose of 100 units/kg body weight is suggested for all indications.

2. If the patient's antibody titre against Hyate:C is known, a prediction of the dose of Hyate:C required to neutralise the circulating antibody completely can be made using the formula:

Neutralising dose
= Plasma volume (ml) x antibody titre (Bethesda units/ml)

An incremental dose must then be added to this neutralising dose to increase plasma Factor VIII:C level by the desired amount. This increment can be calculated by assuming that 1 unit of Hyate:C per kg body weight will give rise to a 1.5 units/decilitre increase in plasma Factor VIII:C activity (2).

3. If the patient's antibody titre against Porcine Factor VIII:C is not known but the anti-human Factor VIII:C is less than 50 Bethesda units per ml, an initial dose of 25 - 50 units/kg body weight is recommended for a moderately severe joint or muscle bleed, or 50 - 100 units/kg body weight for a major bleed.

If the patient's antibody titre to human Factor VIII:C is greater than 50 Bethesda units per ml, an initial dose of at least 100 units/kg body weight is suggested (5).

4. If the patient has previously been treated with Hyate:C this may provide a guide to the likely response and therefore assist in estimation of the initial dose.

*Subsequent Dose Administration:* Subsequent doses should be based on the post-infusion levels of Factor VIII:C achieved. It has been reported that recovery of Factor VIII:C can increase during the course of treatment probably as a result of saturation of circulating antibody (2, 5). Monitoring of pre- and post-infusion levels of Factor VIII:C for each dose is therefore recommended.

If measurable post-infusion Factor VIII:C levels are not achieved Hyate:C therapy should still be continued as long as clinical efficacy is judged to be sufficient (6).

*Frequency of Administration:* Based upon the reported half-disappearance time for Hyate:C of 10 - 11 hours (5), it is recommended that the product is administered by intermittent intravenous infusion every 6 - 8 hours.

*Determination of the Activity of Inhibitor Against Hyate:C:* A modification of the Bethesda assay (4) is recommended. Hyate:C should be diluted to 1 unit per ml in Factor VIII depleted plasma and used as a substrate in the Bethesda assay.

*Reconstitution and Administration:* 1. Warm the unopened vials of Hyate:C to between 20°C and 37°C.

2. Clean the exposed central portion of the rubber stopper with antiseptic immediately prior to piercing.

3. Using a sterile needle and syringe slowly inject 20 ml of Water for Injections PhEur into the vial.

4. Withdraw the needle and shake the vial gently, avoiding frothing, until the powder is completely dissolved. This usually takes less than 1 minute.

5. The concentration of Hyate:C in units/ml should be calculated from the units/vial printed on the vial label.

6. Withdraw the solution into a syringe using a filter needle.

7. Replace the filter needle with a sterile injection needle and administer intravenously at a rate of not more than 2 - 5 ml per minute.

**Contra-indications, warnings, etc**

*Contra-indications:* Previous occurrence of an acute infusion reaction.

*Acute Infusion Reactions:* On rare occasions Hyate:C may give rise to acute infusion reactions, such as anaphylactic shock.

Adrenaline, hydrocortisone and facilities for resuscitation should be available in case these reactions occur.

*Mild Infusion Reactions:* Hyate:C may occasionally give rise to reactions such as fever, chills, headache, nausea, vomiting and skin rashes. These reactions are more common after the first infusion of a course of treatment, and tend to lessen in frequency and severity as further infusions are given. Hydrocortisone and/or antihistamine may alleviate these effects and may be prescribed as a precautionary measure.

*Immune Response to Hyate:C:* Infusion of Hyate:C may be followed by a rise in plasma levels of inhibitor to both human and Porcine Factor VIII:C. Inhibitor levels to both human and Porcine Factor VIII:C should be monitored during and after treatment.

*Effect on the platelet count:* A significant fall in the patient's platelet count occurs on rare occasions after infusion of Hyate:C. However, monitoring of platelet count during the treatment period is recommended.

**Pharmaceutical precautions** Hyate:C should be stored between a temperature of minus 15°C to minus 20°C and should be used before the expiry date on the package. Reconstituted Hyate:C must not be stored and should be used within 3 hours.

**Legal category** POM.

**Package quantities** Vials contain between 400 and 700 units of Porcine Factor VIII:C. The number of units in each vial is printed on the vial label.

**Further information** The ease of reconstitution of Hyate:C in 20 ml Water for Injections PhEur makes it suitable for syringe administration facilitating high dose therapy.


References:[1] Lusher J.M Annals N.Y Acad Sci 509:89-102, 1987

[2] Gatti L and Mannucci P.M Thromb and Haemostas 51:379-384, 1984

[3] Ciavarella N et al B.J Haematol 58:641-648, 1984

[4] Kasper C.K et al Thrombos Diathes Haemorrh 34:869-872, 1975

[5] Kernoff P.B.A et al Blood 63:31-41, 1984

[6] Brettler D.B et al Arch Intern Med 149:1381-1385 1989


**Product licence number** 3070/0007

## NEUTREXIN* ▼

**Qualitative and quantitative composition**

| *Active ingredient* | *mg/via* |
|---|---|
| Trimetrexate | 25.0 |

**Pharmaceutical form** Concentrate for infusion.

**Clinical particulars**

*Therapeutic indication:* Neutrexin (trimetrexate glucuronate for injection) with concurrent leucovorin administration (leucovorin protection) is indicated a an alternative therapy for the treatment of moderate to severe *Pneumocystis carinii* pneumonia in patient with Acquired Immunodeficiency Syndrome (AIDS) who are intolerant of or refractory to standard therap or for whom standard therapy is contra-indicated.

In comparative studies as first-line treatment o pneumocystis carinii pneumonia in AIDS patients Neutrexin with concurrent leucovorin was less effective than trimethoprim/sulphamethoxazole. Comparative studies versus IV pentamidine have not yet been performed.

**Caution: Leucovorin must be administered daily during treatment with Neutrexin and for 72 hours past the last dose of Neutrexin in order to avoid potentially serious or life threatening toxicities.**

*Posology and method of administration:* Neutrexin i administered at a dose of 45 mg/m² once daily b intravenous infusion over 60–90 minutes. Leucovori must be administered daily during treatment wit Neutrexin and for 72 hours past the last dose o Neutrexin . Leucovorin may be administered intravenously at a dose of 20 mg/m² over 5 to 10 minute every 6 hours for a total daily dose of 80 mg/m², o orally as 4 doses of 20 mg/m² spaced equally through out the day. The recommended course of therapy i 21 days of Neutrexin and 24 days of leucovorin Leucovorin protection may be administered prior t or following Neutrexin. The daily dosage of leucovori has to be modified according to haematologic toxicities (see '*Dosage modifications*').

Efforts should be made by the physician to continu patients on Neutrexin plus concurrent leucovori therapy for a minimum of 14 days before discontinuation for lack of response to allow sufficient time fo patients to respond. Patients should continue t receive corticosteroid therapy, supplemental oxyge intubation and mechanical ventilation or other sup portive care as necessary throughout Neutrexin therapy. To allow for full therapeutic doses of Neutrexi to be administered, treatment with azidothymidir (AZT) and other myelosuppressive agents should b discontinued during Neutrexin therapy.

Hepatic or renal insufficiency: Patients should b treated with trimetrexate under careful monitorir conditions. Dose modifications should be based o toxicity guidelines described hereafter.

*Dosage modification*

*Haematologic toxicity:* Neutrexin and leucovori doses should be modified for haematologic toxicitie according to the table below. These guidelines we based upon empirical data from clinical trials utilizin initial doses of Neutrexin, 45 mg/m² per day an leucovorin, 20 mg/m², 4 times a day. Therapy shoul then continue with the adjusted dosage for th remainder of the patient's treatment.

*Hepatic toxicity:* Transient elevations of transam nases and alkaline phosphatase have been observe in patients treated with Neutrexin. Interruption treatment is advisable if transaminase levels

**Neutrexin/Leucovorin dose modifications for haematological toxicity**

| Toxicity grade | Neutrophils (Polys and Bands) | Platelets | Recommended dosage of Neutrexin | Recommended dosage of Leucovorin |
|---|---|---|---|---|
| 1 | >1000/mm³ | >75,000/mm³ | 45 mg/m² once daily | 20 mg/m² every 6 hours |
| 2 | 750–1000/mm³ | 50,000–75,000.mm³ | 45 mg/m² once daily | 40 mg/m² every 6 hours |
| 3 | 500–749/mm³ | 25,000–49,999/mm³ | 22 mg/m² once daily | 40 mg/m² every 6 hours |
| 4 | <500/mm³ | <25,000/mm³ | Day 1–9 Discontinue<br>Day 10–21 Interrupt up to 96 hours[a] | 40 mg/m² every 6 hours |

[a] If Grade 4 haematologic toxicity occurs prior to Day 10, Neutrexin should be discontinued. Leucovorin (40 mg/m², q6h) should be administered for an additional 72 hours. If Grade 4 haematologic toxicity occurs at Day 10 or later, Neutrexin may be held up to 96 hours to allow counts to recover. If counts recover to Grade 3 within 96 hours, Neutrexin should be administered at a dose of 22 mg/m² and leucovorin maintained at 40 mg/m², q6h. When counts recover to Grade 2 toxicity, Neutrexin dose may be increased to 45 mg/m², but the leucovorin dose should be maintained at 40 mg/m² for the duration of treatment. If counts do not improve to ≤Grade 3 toxicity within 96 hours, Neutrexin should be discontinued. Leucovorin at a dose of 40 mg/m², q6h should be administered for 72 hours following the last dose of Neutrexin.

alkaline phosphatase levels increase to >5 times the upper limit of normal range.

*Renal toxicity:* Interruption of treatment is advisable if serum creatinine levels increase to >2.5 mg/dL.

*Other toxicities:* Interruption of treatment is advisable in patients who experience severe mucosal toxicity which interferes with oral intake. Treatment should be discontinued for fever (oral temperature ≥105°F/ 40.5°C) that cannot be controlled with antipyretics.

*Elderly:* Dose modifications should be based on toxicity guidelines described above, rather than age.

*Children:* The safety and effectiveness of Neutrexin in children has not been established.

**Contra-indications, warnings, etc**

*Contra-indications:* Neutrexin is contra-indicated in patients with known sensitivity to trimetrexate or to other quinazoline-containing compounds. Neutrexin must not be used without concurrent leucovorin, therefore Neutrexin is contra-indicated in patients with known sensitivity to leucovorin. Due to Neutrexin's fetotoxic and teratogenic potential (see '*Use during pregnancy and lactation*'), it is contra-indicated during pregnancy.

*Special warnings and precautions*

*Warnings:* **Neutrexin must be used with concurrent leucovorin (leucovorin protection) to avoid potentially serious or life threatening complications including bone marrow suppression, oral and gastrointestinal mucosal ulceration, and renal and hepatic dysfunction. Leucovorin therapy must extend for 72 hours past the last dose of Neutrexin.** Patients should be informed that failure to take the recommended dose and duration of leucovorin can lead to fatal toxicity. Patients should be closely monitored for the development of serious haematologic adverse reactions (see '*Precautions*' and '*Posology and method of administration*').

Neutrexin should only be prescribed by clinicians experienced in treating patients with AIDS or with immunocompromised states due to other underlying condition.

Both females of childbearing age and males should take contraceptive measures during and at least 6 months after cessation of therapy.

**Anaphylaxis** In cancer clinical trials, anaphylactoid reactions have been observed very rarely in patients receiving trimetrexate as an intravenous bolus injection. At present, it is not known whether any specific clinical condition or co-indications contributed to the occurrence of these reactions. Therefore, it is recommended that trimetrexate be administered as an intravenous infusion over 60–90 minutes.

*Precautions:* Patients receiving Neutrexin may experience severe haematologic, hepatic, renal and gastrointestinal toxicities; hence these parameters should be closely monitored in all patients. Special caution should be used in treating patients with impaired haematologic, hepatic or renal function. These patients and patients who require concomitant therapy with myelosuppressive, hepatotoxic or nephrotoxic drugs should be treated with Neutrexin under careful monitoring conditions.

*Laboratory tests:* Patients receiving Neutrexin with leucovorin protection should be closely monitored throughout therapy. Blood tests to monitor the following parameters should be performed at least twice a week during therapy: haematology (absolute neutrophil counts [ANC], platelets, haemoglobin), renal function (serum creatinine, BUN), hepatic function (SGOT, SGPT, alkaline phosphatase). In addition, haemoglobin levels should be monitored before, during and after therapy as anaemia may develop in some patients.

*Drug interactions:* The metabolism of trimetrexate both with and without the administration of folinic acid is poorly understood. There is therefore a significant potential for serious drug-drug interactions over a wide range of potential therapeutic agents. This is particularly the case for agents which may utilise, inhibit or induce hepatic cytochrome P450 mechanisms. Such agents may also affect the ratio of trimetrexate to folinic acid in individual tissue subsets. Thus, when ANY comedication is considered mandatory, additional care in monitoring of adverse events, hemopoietic and hepatic toxicities is advised. Agents which may enhance the liver clearance of trimetrexate may also result in diminished efficacy of the trimetrexate-folonic acid combination.

Trimetrexate and its metabolites are partially cleared renally, therefore nephrotoxic agents may also interact with trimetrexate when co-administered. Drugs which may affect protein binding may also affect the pharmacodynamics of trimetrexate and vice versa (see 'Preclinical safety data').

Experience with concomitant corticosteroids and trimetrexate-folinic acid administration has been obtained only in open clinical studies. In these there was no obvious interference with the efficacy of the combination regimen and little or no detectable potentiation of the described toxicities. It is therefore considered that steroids may be co-prescribed in accordance with clinical practice.

*Use during pregnancy and lactation:* The safe use of Neutrexin during pregnancy has not been established. Neutrexin has been shown to be fetotoxic and teratogenic in animals (see 'Preclinical safety data' section); it is therefore contra-indicated during pregnancy.

When Neutrexin is considered to be therapeutically necessary in women of child bearing potential, appropriate procedures should be followed to establish whether pregnancy might have occurred. The patient should be appraised of the risks of becoming pregnant during treatment and take adequate contraceptive measures (see 'Special warnings and precautions' section). Men who are treated with Neutrexin should also take contraceptive measures during treatment and for a period of six months after completing therapy.

It is not known if trimetrexate is secreted in human breast milk. Because there is a possibility of toxicity to nursing infants secondary to Neutrexin treatment of the mother, it is recommended that breast feeding should be terminated and artificial feeding substituted if the mother is treated with Neutrexin.

*Effects on ability to drive and use machines:* Unless the patient develops severe toxicity (see '*Undesirable effects*'), Neutrexin itself, should not impair the patient's ability to drive or operate machinery; this is more likely to be influenced by the patient's overall state of well being.

*Undesirable effects:* As many patients who receive Neutrexin already have complications of advanced HIV disease, it is difficult to distinguish adverse events caused by Neutrexin from those resulting from underlying medical conditions. The toxicities reported hereafter refer to patients with morphologically confirmed PCP who received Neutrexin, 45 mg/m² per day for 21 days and leucovorin, 80 mg/m² per day for 24 days (n=182). These clinical trials included dose modifications to the Neutrexin-Leucovorin combination for toxicity as described under '*Posology and method of administration*'. These toxicities were similar in frequency and severity to the combined analysis of all patients treated in clinical studies.

*Haematological:* The most frequently reported abnormal haematological parameters have been low granulocytes, haemoglobin and platelets. In clinical trials, these effects were classed as severe in approximately 15%, 9% and 3% of patients respectively. However following dose modifications outlined under 'Posology and method of administration', less than 4% of patients had to discontinue Neutrexin therapy due to haematologic toxicity.

*Gastrointestinal:* Emesis and diarrhoea have been reported in 3.8% and 1.6% of patients, occasionally resulting in withdrawal of therapy.

*Cutaneous:* The most common cutaneous reaction reported is rash which occurs in approximately 8% of patients; itching and injection site reaction have been reported rarely.

*Fever:* In clinical trials, this was reported in approximately 11% of patients, but in only 1% of patients was it of sufficient severity to warrant withdrawal of therapy.

*Neurologic:* Confusion was reported in 3% of patients. Seizure has rarely been reported; a causal relationship between seizure and trimetrexate has not been established.

*Hepatic toxicity:* Transiently raised transaminases (SGOT and SGPT) and alkaline phosphatase have been reported; in 14%, 13% and 5% of patients respectively.

*Laboratory abnormalities:* These have rarely been reported, and have included increased and decreased calcium and potassium, magnesium and GGT levels. No clinical signs of hypocalcaemia have been reported.

*Anaphylaxis:* Anaphylactoid reactions have been observed very rarely (see under *Warnings*).

*Overdose:* Neutrexin administered without concurrent leucovorin can cause lethal complications. There has been little experience in humans receiving single intravenous doses of trimetrexate greater than 90 mg/m²/day without concurrent leucovorin. The toxicities seen at this dose were primarily haematologic. In the event of overdose, Neutrexin should be stopped and leucovorin should be administered at a dose of 40 mg/m² every 6 hours for 3 days.

**Pharmacological properties**

*Pharmacodynamic properties:* In vitro studies have shown that trimetrexate is a potent, competitive inhibitor of dihydrofolate reductase (DHFR) from bacterial, protozoan and mammalian sources, including *Pneumocystis carinii.* DHFR catalyzes the reduction of intracellular dihydrofolate to the active cofactor tetrahydrofolate. Inhibition of DHFR results in the depletion of this cofactor, leading directly to interference with thymidylate biosynthesis, as well as interference with folate-dependent formyltransferase, with consequent reduction in purine biosynthesis. The end result is disruption of DNA, RNA and protein synthesis, with consequent cell death.

Leucovorin (folinic acid) is readily transported into mammalian cells by a carrier-mediated active transport process and can be assimilated into cellular folate pools following its metabolism. In vitro studies have shown that leucovorin provides a source of reduced folates necessary for normal cellular biosynthetic processes. Because the *Pneumocystis carinii* organism lacks the reduced folate carrier-mediated transport system, leucovorin is prevented from entering the organism. Therefore, the concurrent administration of leucovorin with trimetrexate protects normal host cells from the cytotoxic effect of trimetrexate without impairing the antifolate's inhibition of *Pneumocystis carinii.* The active transport of leucovorin into mammalian cells but not into the *Pneumocystis carinii* organism allows the concurrent use of leucovorin to protect normal host cells from the cytotoxicity of trimetrexate without inhibiting the antifolate's inhibition of *Pneumocystis carinii.*

*Pharmacokinetic properties*

*Absorption:* No detailed kinetic studies have been performed in patients with AIDS utilising the advised regimen administered by infusion. However, steady-state peak and trough levels were measured in patients administered 30 mg/m²/day by i.v. bolus with leucovorin 80 mg/m²/day (given in 4 equally divided doses). In these subjects the mean 'peak' 1 hour post-dosing level of trimetrexate, using an in-vitro DHFR inhibition assay, was 11.8±6.0 μM. Similarly, the mean 23 hour trough level was 1.9±1.4 μM. In 6 of these patients a terminal half-life in the order of 11 h was observed. More extensive data are available on cancer patients receiving 10–20 hours. Furthermore despite a marked inter-individual variation in pharmacokinetic characteristics a linear relationship between dose and trimetrexate steady state plasma level/AUC was suggested.

*Distribution:* Binding of trimetrexate to plasma proteins is extensive (>97%). The concentration of trimetrexate in the cerebrospinal fluid accounted for less than 2% of the plasma level.

*Metabolism:* The metabolism of trimetrexate in man with or without the coadministration of leucovorin has not yet been completely elucidated. Preclinical data suggest that oxidative O-demethylation, followed by conjugation to either the glucuronide or the sulphate is involved. It appears that N-demethylation and oxidation is a related minor pathway. The exact P450 enzyme catalysing O-demethylation is unknown. Some of the metabolites formed are active in the in vitro cell-free DHFR inhibition assay. Whether these metabolites are also active against *Pneumocystis carinii* infection was not examined. The active metabolites may however contribute to trimetrexate's cytotoxic effects towards host cells.

*Elimination:* Urinary recovery of trimetrexate using an HPLC assay averaged about 10–20% of the dose, over a 24–48 hour period. Part of the trimetrexate metabolites formed, including part of the metabolites that are active in the DHFR-inhibition assay, are renally excreted. Faecal excretion of trimetrexate and its active metabolites appears to be low. To date, the fate of 50% of a trimetrexate dose administered to man remains unknown. Although the low urinary recovery of trimetrexate suggests that clearance is predominantly non-renal, significant retention of trimetrexate may occur in patients with impaired renal function.

No formal studies have evaluated the kinetic behaviour of trimetrexate in patients with renal or hepatic impairment. These patients should be closely monitored.

*Preclinical safety data*

*Drug interactions:* Animal studies suggest that there is a potential for serious drug interactions in man when trimetrexate-folinic acid are prescribed with drugs of the imidazol class (clotrimazole, ketoconazole, micronazole). See *Pharmacodynamic properties* for further details.

*Carcinogenesis and mutagenicity:* Negative results have been observed for trimetrexate in gene mutation systems with bacterial and mammalian cells. Other systems, however, have shown that trimetrexate induces very efficient chromosomal damage, a type of genetic damage which could be expected from the mechanism of action of trimetrexate. Although trimetrexate showed no genotoxic or carcinogenic effects in the limited test procedures utilised in vivo, the compound should be considered as possibly mutagenic and carcinogenic in vivo.

*Impairment of fertility:* No studies have been conducted to evaluate the potential of trimetrexate to impair fertility. However, during standard toxicity studies conducted in mice and rats, degeneration of the testes and spermatocytes including the arrest of spermatogenesis was observed. Therefore, the potential for distribution in male fertility cannot be excluded. As the ova are formed long before ovulation, it is possible that the level of fertility in females will not be affected, but other early stages after fertilisation will be at risk because of the inhibition of DHFR.

*Teratogenic effects:* Maternal and foetal toxicity were observed in both rats and rabbits. Rats administered 1.5 and 2.5 mg/kg/day intravenously on gestational days 6–15 showed substantial post-implantation loss and severe inhibition of maternal weight gain. Trimetrexate administered intravenously to rats at 0.5 and 1.0 mg/kg/day on gestational days 6–15 retarded normal fetal development and was teratogenic. Rabbits administered trimetrexate intravenously at daily doses of 2.5 and 5.0 mg/kg/day on gestational days 6–15 resulted in significant maternal and fetotoxicity. In rabbits, trimetrexate at 0.1 mg/kg/day was teratogenic in the absence of significant maternal toxicity. These effects were observed using doses $\frac{1}{20}$ to $\frac{1}{2}$ the equivalent human therapeutic dose based on a mg/m² basis. Teratogenic effects included skeletal, visceral, ocular and cardiovascular abnormalities.

*Drug interactions:* Based on an in vitro rat liver model, nitrogen substituted imidazole drugs (clotrimazole, ketoconazole, miconazole) were potent, non-competitive inhibitors of trimetrexate metabolism. A number of agents might be co-administered with trimetrexate in AIDS patients for other indications that could elicit this activity including erythromycin, rifampicin, ketoconazole, fluconazole and others.

**Pharmaceutical particulars**

*List of excipients:* D-glucuronic acid 15.35 mg per vial.

*Incompatibilities:* **Caution: Since Neutrexin forms a precipitate instantly upon contact with chloride or Leucovorin, it should not be added to solutions containing sodium chloride or other anions. Neutrexin and Leucovorin solutions must be administered separately. Intravenous lines should be flushed with at least 10 mL of 5% Glucose Injection BP, between Neutrexin and Leucovorin infusions.**

Compatibility with other anions: In a study to determine the potential for precipitation of Neutrexin upon contact with other anions, Neutrexin 2 mg/ml solution in sterile water at ambient temperature for 24 hours precipitated a 1% solution of bicarbonate but did NOT form a precipitate with acetate, lactose or phosphate. However, Neutrexin at a higher concentration of 6.25 mg/ml caused precipitation with all four anions studied.

*Shelf-life:* 24 months for the product as packaged for sale.

After reconstitution, the solution should be used immediately; however, the solution is stable under refrigeration (2–8°C) for 24 hours or at room temperature (15°C–25°C) for up to six hours. [NOTE: This is justified based on acceptable challenge test after incubation with various test organisms.] It must be assumed that like any parenteral product, Neutrexin will be reconstituted aseptically.

*Special precautions for storage:* Neutrexin should be stored at room temperature (15–25°C).

*Nature and contents of container:* Neutrexin is contained in a 5 cc Type I flint glass tubing vial, fitted with a grey rubber stopper and sealed with an aluminium seal, covered with a white polypropylene flip off cap. Each vial of lyophilized powder contains trimetrexate glucuronate equivalent to 25 mg of trimetrexate.

Vials will be supplied in nested white chipboard cartons, shrink wrapped and placed in brown corrugated cartons, in quantities of 10, 25, 50 and 100.

N.B. Only the 25 vial pack presentation will be available in the UK.

*Instructions for use/handling:* Neutrexin should be reconstituted with 2 ml of 5% Glucose Injection BP or Sterile Water for Injection PhEur to yield a concentration of 12.5 mg of trimetrexate per ml (reconstitution time up to two minutes). The reconstituted product must be inspected visually for particulate matter prior to dilution. Do not use if cloudiness or precipitate is observed.

Reconstituted solution should be further diluted with 5% Glucose Injection BP to yield a final concentration of 0.25 to 2 mg of trimetrexate per ml.

Do not freeze reconstituted solution. Discard the unused portion after 24 hours.

If Neutrexin contacts the skin or mucosa, immediately wash thoroughly with soap and water. Procedures for the proper handling and disposal of cytotoxic drugs should be considered.

*Name and address of holder of marketing authorisation:* US Bioscience Inc, Suites 9, 10 and 11, Awberry Court, Croxley Business Park, Watford, Hertfordshire WD1 8YJ.

**Marketing authorisation number** 11284/0006.

**Date of approval/revision of SPC** November 1996.

**Legal category** POM.

*\*Trade Mark*

# E. R. Squibb & Sons Limited
Bristol-Myers Squibb House
Staines Rd
Hounslow TW3 3JA


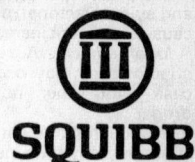

SQUIBB

## ACEPRIL* TABLETS

**Qualitative and quantitative composition** Each tablet contains captopril 12.5 mg, 25 mg or 50 mg.

**Pharmaceutical form** Oral tablet.

**Clinical particulars**

*Therapeutic indications:*
*Hypertension:* Acepril is indicated for the first line treatment of mild to moderate hypertension.

In severe hypertension it should be used where standard therapy is ineffective or inappropriate.

*Congestive heart failure:* Acepril is indicated for the treatment of congestive heart failure. The drug should be used together with diuretics and, where appropriate digitalis.

*Myocardial infarction:* Acepril is indicated following myocardial infarction in clinically stable patients with asymptomatic and symptomatic left ventricular dysfunction to improve survival, delay the onset of symptomatic heart failure, reduce hospitalisations for heart failure, and reduce recurrent myocardial infarction and coronary revascularisation procedures.

Determination of cardiac function by radionuclide ventriculography or echocardiography should be undertaken prior to initiation of preventative treatment with Acepril in post myocardial infarction patients.

*Diabetic nephropathy:* Acepril is indicated for the treatment of diabetic nephropathy (microalbuminuria greater than 30 mg/day) in insulin-dependent diabetics. In these patients, captopril prevents the progression of renal disease and reduces associated clinical events e.g. dialysis, renal transplantation and death.

*Posology and method of administration:*

*Hypertension:* Treatment with Acepril should be at the lowest effective dose which should be titrated according to the needs of the patient.

*Mild to moderate hypertension:* The starting dose is 12.5 mg twice daily. The usual maintenance dose is 25 mg twice daily which can be increased incrementally, at 2–4 week intervals, until a satisfactory response is achieved, to a maximum of 50 mg twice daily.

A thiazide diuretic may be added to Acepril if satisfactory response has not been achieved. The dose of diuretic may be increased at 1-2 week intervals to the level of optimum response or until the maximum dose is reached.

*Severe hypertension:* In severe hypertension where standard therapy is ineffective or inappropriate because of adverse effects, the starting dose is 12.5 mg b.d. The dosage may be increased incrementally to a maximum of 50 mg t.i.d. Acepril should be used together with other anti-hypertensive agents but the dose of these should be individually titrated. A daily dose of 150 mg of Acepril should not normally be exceeded.

*Heart failure:* Acepril therapy must be started under close medical supervision. Acepril should be introduced when diuretic therapy (such as frusemide 40-80 mg or equivalent) is insufficient to control symptoms. A starting dose of 6.25 mg or 12.5 mg may minimise a transient hypotensive effect. The possibility of this occurring can be reduced by discontinuing or reducing diuretic therapy if possible, prior to initiating Acepril.

The usual maintenance dose is 25 mg two or three times a day which can be increased incrementally, with intervals of at least two weeks, until a satisfactory response is achieved. The usual maximum dose is 150 mg daily.

*Myocardial infarction:* Therapy may be initiated as early as three days following a myocardial infarction. After an initial dose of 6.25 mg, captopril therapy should be titrated to a final target dose of 150 mg daily in divided doses over the next several weeks.

Achievement of the target dose of 150 mg should be based on the patient's tolerance to captopril during titration. If symptomatic hypotension occurs, a dosage reduction may be required.

Captopril may be used in patients treated with other post-myocardial infarction therapies, e.g. thrombolytics, aspirin, beta blockers.

*Diabetic nephropathy:* The recommended daily dose of captopril is 75 to 100 mg in divided doses.

If further blood pressure reduction is required, other antihypertensive agents such as diuretics, beta blockers, centrally acting agents or vasodilators may be used in conjunction with captopril.

*Elderly:* The dose should be titrated against the blood pressure response and kept as low as possible to achieve adequate control. Since elderly patients may have reduced renal function and other organ dysfunctions, it is suggested that a low dose of Acepril be used initially.

*Children:* Acepril is not recommended for the treatment of mild to moderate hypertension in children.

Experience in neonates, particularly premature infants, is limited. Because renal function in infants is not equivalent to that of older children and adults, lower doses of Acepril should be used with the patients under close medical supervision.

The starting dose should be 0.3 mg per Kg bodyweight up to a maximum of 6 mg per Kg bodyweight daily in divided doses. The dose should be individualised according to the response and may be given two or three times daily.

*Patients with renal impairment:* Captopril in divided doses of 75 to 100 mg/day was well tolerated in patients with diabetic nephropathy and mild to moderate renal impairment (creatinine clearance at least 30 ml/min/1.73 m²).

Patients with severely impaired renal function will take longer to reach steady-state captopril levels and will reach higher steady-state levels for a given daily dose than patients with normal renal function. These patients may therefore respond to smaller or less frequent doses.

Therefore, patients with severe renal impairment (creatinine clearance less than 30 ml/min/1.73 m²), the initial daily dose should be 12.5 mg b.d. The dose can then be titrated against the response but adequate time should be allowed between dosage adjustments. When concomitant diuretic therapy is required, a loop diuretic rather than a thiazide diuretic should be the diuretic of choice.

Acepril is readily eliminated by haemodialysis.

*Contra-indications:* A history of previous hypersensitivity to the product.

*Pregnancy:* Acepril has been shown to be lethal to rabbit and sheep foetuses. There were no foetotoxic effects to hamster or rat foetuses.

Acepril is contra-indicated in pregnancy and should not be used in women of child bearing potential unless protected by effective contraception.

Exposure of the mother in the second and third trimesters of pregnancy has been associated with oligohydramnios and neonatal hypotension and/or anuria.

*Special warnings and special precautions for use:*

*Precautions:* Evaluation of the patient should include assessment of renal function prior to initiation of therapy and at appropriate intervals thereafter (see *Posology and method of administration* section]

Acepril should not be used in patients with aortic stenosis or outflow tract obstruction.

As limited experience has been obtained in the treatment of acute hypertensive crises, the use of Acepril should be avoided in these patients.

*Warnings:* The incidence of adverse reactions to captopril is principally associated with renal function since the drug is excreted primarily by the kidney. The dose should not exceed that necessary for adequate control and should be reduced in patients with impaired renal function.

*Hypotension:* With the first one or two doses some patients may experience symptomatic hypotension. In most instances, symptoms are relieved simply by the patient lying down.

In patients with severe and renin dependent hypertension (e.g. renovascular hypertension) or severe congestive heart failure who are receiving large doses of diuretic, exaggerated hypotensive responses have occurred usually within one hour of the initial dose of Acepril. In these patients, by discontinuing diuretic therapy or significantly reducing the diuretic dose for four to seven days prior to initiating Acepril the possibility of this occurrence is reduced. By commencing Acepril therapy with small doses (6.25 mg or 12.5 mg) the duration of any hypotensive effect is lessened. Some patients may benefit from an infusion of saline. The occurrence of first dose hypotension does not preclude subsequent dose titration with Acepril. Hypotension has been occasionally reported in patients on Acepril due to causes of acute volume depletion such as vomiting and diarrhoea.

*Serum potassium:* Since Acepril decreases aldosterone production, serum potassium is usually maintained in patients on diuretics. Potassium sparing diuretics or potassium supplements should not therefore be used routinely. In patients with marked renal impairment a significant elevation of serum potassium may occur.

*Renal:* Proteinuria in patients with prior normal renal function is rare.

Where proteinuria has occurred it has usually been in patients with severe hypertension or evidence of prior renal disease. Nephrotic syndrome occurred in some of these patients.

In patients with evidence of prior renal disease, monthly urinary protein estimations (dip stick) are recommended for the first 9 months of therapy.

If repeated determinations show increasing amounts of urinary protein, a 24-hour quantitative determination should be obtained, and if this exceeds 1 g/day, the benefits and risks of continuing Acepril should be evaluated.

In patients with diabetic nephropathy and proteinuria, who received captopril 75 mg/day for a median of 3 years, there was a consistent reduction in proteinuria. It is unknown whether long-term therapy in patients with other types of renal disease would have similar effects.

Although membranous glomerulopathy was found in biopsies taken from some proteinuric patients, a causal relationship to Acepril has not been established.

Some patients with renal disease, particularly those with bilateral renal artery stenosis or unilateral renal artery stenosis in a single functioning kidney, have developed increased concentrations of blood urea and serum creatinine. Acepril dosage reduction and/or discontinuation of diuretic may be required. For some of these patients it may not be possible to normalise blood pressure and maintain adequate renal perfusion.

Recent clinical observations have shown a high incidence of anaphylactoid-like reactions during haemodialysis with high-flux dialysis membranes (e.g. AN69) in patients receiving ACE inhibitors. Therefore, this combination should be avoided.

*Haematological:* Neutropenia/agranulocytosis, thrombocytopenia and anaemia have been reported in patients receiving Acepril.

In patients with normal renal function and no other complicating factors, neutropenia occurs rarely.

Acepril should be used with extreme caution in patients with collagen vascular disease, immunosuppressant therapy, treatment with allopurinol or procainamide, or a combination of these complicating factors especially if there is pre-existing impaired renal function. Some of these patients developed serious infections which in a few instances did not respond to intensive antibiotic therapy.

If Acepril is used in such patients, it is advised that white blood cell count and differential counts should be performed prior to therapy, every 2 weeks during the first 3 months of Acepril therapy, and periodically thereafter.

During treatment all patients should be instructed to report any sign of infection (e.g. sore throat, fever), when a differential white blood cell count should be performed. Acepril and other concomitant medication should be withdrawn if neutropenia (neutrophils less than 1000/mm³) is detected or suspected.

In most patients neutrophil counts rapidly returned to normal upon discontinuing Acepril.

*Surgery/anaesthesia:* In patients undergoing major surgery, or during anaesthesia with agents which produce hypotension, captopril will block angiotensin II formation secondary to compensatory renin release. This may lead to hypotension which can be corrected by volume expansion.

*Clinical chemistry:* Acepril may cause a false-positive urine test for acetone.

*Interactions with other medicaments and other forms of interaction:*
*Diuretics:* Diuretics potentiate the anti-hypertensive effectiveness of Acepril.

Potassium-sparing diuretics (triamterene, amiloride and spironolactone), or potassium supplements may cause significant increase in serum potassium.

*Indomethacin:* A reduction of anti-hypertensive effectiveness may occur. This is probably also the case with other non-steroidal anti-inflammatory drugs.

*Vasodilators:* Acepril has been reported to act synergistically with peripheral vasodilators such as minoxidil. Awareness of this interaction may avert an initial hypotensive response.

*Clonidine:* It has been suggested that the anti-hypertensive effect of Acepril can be delayed when patients treated with clonidine are changed to Acepril.

*Allopurinol and procainamide:* There have been reports of neutropenia and/or Stevens-Johnson syndrome in patients on Acepril plus either allopurinol or procainamide. Although a causal relationship has not been established, these combinations should only be used with caution, especially in patients with impaired renal function.

Immunosuppressants: Azathioprine and cyclophosphamide have been associated with blood dyscrasias in patients with renal failure who were also taking Acepril.

*Probenecid:* The renal clearance of Acepril is reduced in the presence of probenecid.

Lithium: Concomitant use of lithium and ACE-inhibitors may result in an increase of serum lithium concentration.

*Hypoglycaemic agents:* ACE Inhibitors have been shown to enhance insulin sensitivity. There have been rare reports of hypoglycaemic episodes in diabetic patients treated concomitantly with ACE Inhibitors and antidiabetic medicines (insulin or oral hypoglycaemic agents). This phenomenon may be more likely to occur during the first few weeks of treatment. In such cases a reduction in the dose of the antidiabetic medicine may be required.

*Pregnancy and lactation:* Acepril has been shown to be lethal to rabbit and sheep foetuses. There were no foetotoxic effects to hamster or rat foetuses.

Acepril is contra-indicated in pregnancy and should not be used in women of child bearing potential unless protected by effective contraception.

Exposure of the mother in the second and third trimesters of pregnancy has been associated with oligohydramnios and neonatal hypotension and/or anuria.

*Nursing mothers:* Because captopril is excreted in breast milk, Acepril should not be used in nursing mothers.

*Effects on ability to drive and use machines:* See *Warnings* under *Hypotension* section.

*Undesirable effects:*
*Idiosyncratic:* Angioedema involving the extremities, face, lips, mucous membranes, tongue, glottis or larynx has been seen in patients treated with ACE inhibitors, including captopril. In this situation, the ACE inhibitor should be discontinued. Where swelling is confined to the face, lips and mouth the condition will usually resolve without further treatment, although antihistamines may be useful in relieving symptoms. These patients should be followed carefully until the swelling has resolved. However, where there is involvement of the tongue, glottis or larynx, likely to cause airway obstruction, subcutaneous adrenaline (0.5 ml, 1:1,000) should be administered promptly where indicated.

*Haematological:* Neutropenia, anaemia and thrombocytopenia (see Warnings). Rarely a positive ANA has been reported.

*Renal:* Proteinuria, elevated blood urea and creatinine, elevated serum potassium and acidosis (see *Warnings*).

*Cardiovascular:* Hypotension (see *Warnings*), tachycardia.

*Skin:* Rashes, usually pruritic, may occur. They are usually mild, maculopapular, rarely urticarial and disappear within a few days of dosage reduction, short-term treatment with an antihistamine and/or discontinuing therapy. In a few cases the rash has been associated with fever. Pruritus, flushing, vesicular or bullous rash, and photosensitivity have been reported.

*Gastrointestinal:* Reversible and usually self-limiting taste impairment has been reported. Weight loss may be associated with the loss of taste. Stomatitis, resembling aphthous ulcers, has been reported. Elevation of liver enzymes has been noted in a few patients. Rare cases of hepatocellular injury and cholestatic jaundice have been reported. Gastric irritation and abdominal pain may occur. Pancreatitis has been reported rarely in patients treated with ACE Inhibitors; in some cases this has proved fatal.

*Other:* Paraesthesias of the hands, serum sickness, cough, bronchospasm and lymphadenopathy have been reported.

*Overdose:* In the event of overdosage, blood pressure should be monitored and if hypotension develops volume expansion is the treatment of choice. Captopril is removed by dialysis.

**Pharmacological properties**

*Pharmacodynamic properties:* Captopril is a highly specific, competitive inhibitor of angiotensin-I converting enzyme. This enzyme is responsible for the conversion of angiotensin-I to angiotensin-II.

*Pharmacokinetic properties:*

| | | |
|---|---|---|
| Total captopril: | $t_{MAX}$ | 1 hour |
| | $t_{\frac{1}{2}}$ | 8 hours |
| Free captopril: | $t_{MAX}$ | 1 hour |
| | $t_{\frac{1}{2}}$ | 1 hour |

The absolute bioavailability of an oral dose is approximately 65%.

*Preclinical safety data:* No further relevant data

**Pharmaceutical particulars**

*List of excipients:* Lactose, maize starch, microcrystalline cellulose, stearic acid.

*Incompatibilities:* None.

*Shelf life:* 48 Months.

*Special precautions for storage:* Store below 30°C. Protect from moisture.

*Nature and contents of container:* The 12.5 mg tablets are available in blister packs of 56 tablets. The 25 mg and 50 mg tablets are available in blister packs of 56 and 84 tablets.

*Instructions for use/handling:* No special instructions.

**Marketing authorisation numbers**
12.5 mg: 0034/0298
25 mg: 0034/0299
50 mg: 0034/0300

**Date of approval/revision of SPC** 5 November 1996

**Legal category** POM

## ACEZIDE* TABLETS

**Qualitative and quantitative composition** Each tablet contains captopril 50 mg and hydrochlorothiazide 25 mg.

**Pharmaceutical form** Oral tablet.

**Clinical particulars**

*Therapeutic indications:* For the treatment of mild to moderate hypertension in patients who have been stabilised on the individual components given in the same proportions.

*Posology and method of administration:*
*Adults:* The usual dose of Acezide is one tablet daily. A daily dose of two tablets should not be exceeded.

*Elderly:* The dose should be kept as low as possible to achieve adequate blood pressure control. In some patients half a tablet daily may be sufficient.

*Children:* Safety and effectiveness of Acezide has not been established.

*Patients with renal failure:* Acezide is not recommended for use in patients with significant renal impairment.

*Contra-indications:* Acezide is contra-indicated in patients with anuria or hypersensitivity to captopril, thiazides, or any sulphonamide-derived drug.

*Pregnancy:* Captopril has been shown to be lethal to rabbit and sheep foetuses. There were no foetotoxic effects to hamster or rat foetuses.

Acezide is contra-indicated in pregnancy and should not be used in women of child bearing potential unless protected by effective contraception.

Exposure of the mother in the second and third trimester of pregnancy has been associated with oligohydramnios and neonatal hypertension and/or anuria.

*Special warnings and special precautions for use:*
*Precautions:* Acezide should not be used in patients with aortic stenosis or outflow tract obstruction.

Recent clinical observations have shown a high incidence of anaphylactoid-like reactions during haemodialysis with high-flux dialysis membranes (e.g. AN69) in patients receiving ace inhibitors. (see *Contra-indications*).

*Interactions with other medicaments and other forms of interaction:*

Diuretics: Potassium-sparing diuretics (triamterene, amiloride and spironolactone), or potassium supplements may cause significant increase in serum potassium.

Indomethacin: A reduction of anti-hypertensive effectiveness may occur. This is probably also the case with other non-steroidal anti-inflammatory drugs.

Vasodilators: Acezide has been reported to act synergistically with peripheral vasodilators such as minoxidil. This may improve blood pressure control and awareness of this interaction may avert an initial hypotensive response.

Clonidine: It has been suggested that the anti-hypertensive effect of captopril can be delayed when patients treated with clonidine are changed to Acezide.

Allopurinol and procainamide: There have been reports of neutropenia and/or Stevens Johnson syndrome in patients on captopril plus either allopurinol or procainamide. Although a causal relationship has not been established, these combinations should only be used with caution, especially in patients with impaired renal function.

Immunosuppressants: Azathioprine and cyclophosphamide have been associated with blood dyscrasias in patients with renal failure who were also taking captopril.

Probenecid: The renal clearance of captopril is reduced in the presence of probenecid.

*Pregnancy and lactation:* Captopril has been shown to be lethal to rabbit and sheep foetuses. There were no foetotoxic effects to hamster or rat foetuses.

Acezide is contra-indicated in pregnancy and should not be used in women of child bearing potential unless protected by effective contraception.

Exposure of the mother in the second and third trimester of pregnancy has been associated with oligohydramnios and neonatal hypertension and/or anuria.

Acezide should not be used in nursing mothers.

*Effects on ability to drive and use machines:* Not applicable.

*Undesirable effects:*
*Haematological:* Neutropenia/agranulocytosis, thrombocytopenia and anaemia have been reported in patients receiving captopril.

In patients with normal renal function and no other complicating factors, neutropenia occurs rarely.

Captopril should not be used routinely in patients with pre-existing impaired renal function, collagen vascular disease, immunosuppressant therapy, treatment with allopurinol or procainamide, or a combination of these complicating factors. Some of these patients developed serious infections which in a few instances did not respond to intensive antibiotic therapy.

During treatment, all patients should be instructed to report any sign of infection (e.g. persistent sore throat, fever), when a differential white blood cell count should be performed. Acezide and other concomitant medication should be withdrawn if neutropenia (neutrophils less than 1000/mm³) is detected or suspected.

In most patients neutrophil counts rapidly returned to normal upon discontinuing captopril.

*Skin:* With captopril, rashes, usually pruritic, may occur. They are usually mild, transient and maculopapular, rarely urticarial. In a few cases the rash has been associated with fever and some patients have developed angio-neurotic oedema. Pruritus, flushing, vesicular rash, and photosensitivity have been reported.

With thiazides, purpura, photosensitivity, rash, urticaria, necrotising angiitis, Stevens-Johnson syndrome and other hypersensitivity reactions have been observed.

*Gastrointestinal:* Reversible and usually self limiting taste impairment has been reported. Weight loss may be associated with the loss of taste. Stomatitis, resembling aphthous ulcers, has been reported. Elevation of liver enzymes has been noted in a few patients receiving captopril. Rare cases of hepatocellular injury and cholestatic jaundice have been reported. Gastric irritation and abdominal pain may occur. Pancreatitis has been reported rarely in patients treated with ACE Inhibitors; in some cases this has proved fatal.

*Other:* Paraesthesiae of the hands, serum sickness, cough, bronchospasm and lymphadenopathy have been reported.

With thiazides, dizziness, vertigo, headache, xanthopsia, hyperglycaemia, hypokalaemia, glycosuria, hyperuricaemia, hypercalcaemia, muscle spasm, weakness and restlessness have been reported.

*Renal:* Proteinuria is a rare complication of captopril therapy.

Some patients with renal disease, particularly those with bilateral renal artery stenoses or unilateral artery stenoses in a single functioning kidney, have developed increased concentrations of blood urea and serum creatinine. Discontinuation of Acezide may be required.

*Hepatic:* Acezide should be used with caution in patients with impaired hepatic function or progressive liver disease because of the known risks associated with alterations in fluid and electrolyte balance resulting from thiazide treatment in such patients.

*Electrolyte imbalance:* Patients receiving Acezide should be observed for clinical signs of thiazide induced fluid or electrolyte imbalance. In such patients periodic determinations of serum electrolytes should be performed. Because captopril reduces the production of aldosterone, its combination with hydrochlo othiazide may minimise diuretic-induced ıypokalaemia. However, some patients may still equire potassium supplements. Potassium-sparing liuretics should not be used in conjunction with Acezide.

*Surgery/anaesthesia:* In patients undergoing major surgery, or during anaesthesia with agents which produce hypotension, captopril will block Angiotensin I formation secondary to compensatory renin release. This may lead to hypotension which can be corrected by volume expansion.

Thiazides may decrease the arterial response to noradrenaline. In emergency surgery, pre-anaesthetic and anaesthetic agents should be administered in reduced doses. Thiazides may increase the response to tubocurarine.

*Metabolic disorders:* Hyperuricaemia may occur, or frank gout be precipitated by thiazides in certain patients. Insulin requirements in diabetic patients may be altered by thiazides and latent diabetes mellitus may emerge. The captopril component of Acezide has been shown to ameliorate these effects of thiazides.

*Clinical chemistry:* Acezide may cause a false-positive urine test for acetone.

*Side effects:* Haematological: With thiazides, leucopenia, agranuloooocytosis, thrombocytopenia and plastic anaemia have occurred. Cardiovascular: tachcardia.

*Overdose:* In the event of overdosage, blood pressure should be monitored and if hypotension develops volume expansion is the treatment of choice.

Captopril is removed by dialysis.

**Pharmacological properties**

*Pharmacodynamic properties:* Captopril inhibits angiotensin converting enzyme which is responsible for the conversation of Angiotensin I to the pressor substance of Angiotensin II.

Hydrochlorothiazide is a diuretic which increases the excretion of sodium and chloride ions. The resulting fall in blood pressure and blood volume results in an increase in Angiotensin II levels which tend to reduce the hypotensive effect.

*Pharmacokinetic properties:*

Captopril: After oral administration of therapeutic doses of captopril rapid absorption occurs with peak blood levels at about one hour. Average minimal absorption is approximately 75%. In a 24-hour period over 95% of the absorbed dose is eliminated in the urine; 40 to 50% is unchanged drug; most of the remainder is the disulphide dimer of captopril and captopril-cysteine disulphide.

Approximately 25 to 30% of the circulating drug is bound to plasma proteins. The apparent elimination half-life for total radioactivity in blood is probably less than 3 hours. An accurate determination of half-life of unchanged captopril is not, at present, possible but it is probably less than 2 hours. In patients with renal impairment, however, retention of captopril occurs (see dosage and administration).

Hydrochlorothiazide: The mean plasma half-life of hydrochlorothiazide in fasted individuals has been reported to be approximately 2.5 hours. Onset of diuresis occurs in 2 hours and the peak effect at about 4 hours. Its action persists for approximately 6 to 12 hours. Hydrochlorothiazide is eliminated rapidly by the kidney.

*Preclinical safety data:* No further relevant information.

**Pharmaceutical particulars**

*List of excipients:* Lactose, magnesium stearate, maize starch, microcrystalline cellulose, stearic acid.

*Incompatibilities:* None.

*Shelf life:* 36 months.

*Special precautions for storage:* Store below 30°C. Protect from moisture

*Nature and contents of container:* The tablets are packaged in either PVC/PVDC Blister or Foil Strips.

*Instructions for use/handling:* No special instructions.

**Marketing authorisation number** 0034/0301

**Date of approval/revision of SPC** December 1996

**Legal category** POM

## ADCORTYL* CREAM, AND OINTMENT

**Presentation**

*Cream:* White cream containing triamcinolone acetonide 0.1% in an aqueous vanishing cream base.

Other ingredients: Benzyl alcohol, cetyl alcohol, glyceryl monostearate, isopropyl palmitate, polysorbate 60, propylene glycol, water.

*Ointment:* Almost translucent ointment, containing triamcinolone acetonide 0.1% in Plastibase* (liquid paraffin and polyethylene resin).

**Uses**

*Actions:* Triamcinolone acetonide is a potent fluorinated corticosteroid with anti-inflammatory, antipruritic and anti-allergic actions.

*Indications:* Adcortyl Cream and Ointment are recommended in steroid-responsive conditions which include: atopic eczema, contact eczema, follicular eczema, infantile eczema, otitis externa without frank infection, anogenital eczema, nummular eczema, seborrhoeic or flexural eczema, neurodermatitis, psoriasis of the scalp, chronic plaque psoriasis of the palms and soles and in other selected forms of psoriasis (excluding widespread plaque psoriasis) – 'Precautions'.

**Dosage and administration** *Adults and children:*

*Cream:* To be applied to moist, weeping lesions two to four times daily.

*Ointment:* To be applied to dry, scaly lesions two to four times daily.

*Elderly:* Corticosteroids should be used sparingly and for short periods of time, as natural thinning of the skin occurs in the elderly.

**Contra-indications, warnings, etc**

*Contra-indications:* Contra-indicated in patients with a history of hypersensitivity to the product components. In tuberculous and most viral lesions of the skin, particularly herpes simplex and varicella. The products should not be used in fungal or bacterial skin infections without suitable concomitant anti-infective therapy.

Should not be used for facial rosacea, acne vulgaris, perioral dermatitis or napkin eruptions.

*Precautions:* Adrenal suppression can occur, with prolonged use of topical corticosteroids or treatment of extensive areas. These effects are more likely to occur in infants and children and if occlusive dressings are used. If used in childhood, or on the face, courses should be limited to 5 days and occlusion should not be used.

Topical corticosteroids may be hazardous in psoriasis for a number of reasons including rebound relapses following development of tolerance, risk of generalised pustular psoriasis and local and systemic toxicity due to impaired barrier function of the skin. Steroids may have a place in psoriasis of the scalp and chronic plaque psoriasis of the hands and feet. Careful patient supervision is important.

*Children:* In infants, long-term, continuous topical steroid therapy should be avoided. Courses should be limited to 5 days and occlusion should not be used.

*Pregnancy:* There is inadequate evidence of safety in human pregnancy. Topical administration of corticosteroids to pregnant animals can cause abnormalities of foetal development including cleft palate and intra-uterine growth retardation. There may, therefore, be a very small risk of such effects in the human foetus. Caution should be exercised when topical corticosteroids are administered to nursing women.

*Side-effects:* Triamcinolone acetonide is well tolerated. Where adverse reactions occur they are usually reversible on cessation of therapy. However the following side-effects have been reported usually with prolonged usage:

Dermatological: impaired wound healing, thinning of the skin, petechiae and ecchymoses, facial erythema and telangiectasia, increased sweating, purpura, striae, hirsutism, acneiform eruptions, lupus erythematosus-like lesions and suppressed reactions to skin tests.

These effects may be enhanced with occlusive dressings.

The possibility of the systemic effects which are associated with all steroid therapy should be considered.

*Overdosage:* Topically applied corticosteroids can be absorbed in sufficient amounts to produce systemic effects (see Side-effects).

In the event of accidental ingestion, the patient should be observed and treated symptomatically.

**Pharmaceutical precautions**

*Storage:*

*Cream:* At room temperature; avoid freezing.

*Ointment:* At room temperature.

*Dilution:*

*Cream:* Cetomacrogol Cream (formula B) BPC or Aqueous Cream BP. Preservative cover may be reduced depending on the diluent. Diluted creams should be stored below 25°C and should be discarded two weeks after dilution.

*Ointment:* White soft paraffin.

**Legal category** POM.

**Package quantities** *Cream:* Tubes of 30 g (OP). *Ointment:* Tubes of 30 g (OP).

**Further information** Nil.

**Product licence numbers**

Adcortyl Cream 0034/5000R

Adcortyl Ointment 0034/5004R

## ADCORTYL* IN ORABASE*

**Presentation** White to light tan crystalline paste containing triamcinolone acetonide 0.1% in Orabase formulated for adhesion to mucous membrane.

Other ingredients: Gelatin, liquid paraffin, pectin, polyethylene resin, sodium carboxymethylcellulose.

**Uses**

*Actions:* Triamcinolone acetonide is a potent fluorinated corticosteroid with anti-inflammatory, antipruritic and anti-allergic actions.

*Indications:* Adcortyl in Orabase is indicated for aphthous ulcers, ulcerative stomatitis, denture stomatitis, desquamative gingivitis, erosive lichen planus and lesions of the oral mucosa of traumatic origin.

**Dosage and administration** Adults and children. To be applied to the oral lesion two to four times daily. Apply to the affected area; do not rub in.

*Elderly:* Corticosteroids should be used sparingly and for short periods of time.

**Contra-indications, warnings, etc**

*Contra-indications:* Contra-indicated in patients with a history of hypersensitivity to the product components. In tuberculous and most viral lesions, particularly herpes simplex and varicella. The products should not be used in fungal or bacterial infections without suitable concomitant anti-infective therapy.

*Precautions:* Adrenal suppression can occur with prolonged use of topical corticosteroids or with occlusion. These effects are more likely to occur in infants and children and courses of treatment in childhood should be limited to 5 days. Dentures may act in the same way as an occlusive dressing.

*Pregnancy:* There is inadequate evidence of safety in human pregnancy. Topical administration of corticosteroids to pregnant animals can cause abnormalities of foetal development including cleft palate and intra-uterine growth retardation. There may, therefore, be a very small risk of such effects in the human foetus.

*Side-effects:* Triamcinolone acetonide is well tolerated. Where adverse reactions occur they are usually reversible on cessation of therapy.

The possibility of the systemic effects which are associated with all steroid therapy should be considered.

*Overdosage:* Topically applied corticosteroids can be absorbed in sufficient amounts to produce systemic effects (see side-effects).

In the event of accidental ingestion, the patient should be observed and treated symptomatically.

**Pharmaceutical precautions**

*Storage:* At room temperature.

*Dilution:* Should not be diluted.

**Legal category** POM.

**Package quantities** Tubes of 10 g (OP).

**Further information** Nil.

**Product licence number** 0034/5006R.

## ADCORTYL* INTRA-ARTICULAR/ INTRADERMAL INJECTION 10 MG/ML

**Qualitative and quantitative composition** Adcortyl Intra-articular/Intradermal Injection contains triamcinolone acetonide 10 mg per ml of sterile suspension.

**Pharmaceutical form** Sterile aqueous suspension for injection.

**Clinical particulars**

*Therapeutic indications:*

*Intra-articular use:* for alleviating the joint pain, swelling and stiffness associated with rheumatoid arthritis and osteoarthrosis, with an inflammatory component; also for bursitis, epicondylitis, and tenosynovitis.

*Intradermal use:* for lichen simplex chronicus (neuro-dermatitis), granuloma annulare, lichen planus, keloids, alopecia areata and hypertrophic scars.

*Posology and method of administration:* Adcortyl injection is for intra-articular or intra-dermal use only and should not be administered by intravenous, epidural, intrathecal or any other unapproved route of administration. Strict aseptic precautions should be observed. Since the duration of effect is variable, subsequent doses should be given when symptoms recur and not at set intervals.

*Adults:* The dose of Adcortyl injection for intra-articular administration, and injection into tendon sheaths and bursae, is dependent on the size of the joint to be treated and on the severity of the condition. Doses of 2.5-5 mg (0.25-0.5 ml) for smaller joints and 5-15 mg (0.5-1.5 ml) for larger joints usually alleviate the symptoms. Triamcinolone acetonide 40 mg/ml (Kenalog) is available to facilitate administration of larger doses. (See Precautions re Achilles tendon).

Intradermal dosage is usually 2-3 mg (0.2-0.3 ml), depending on the size of the lesion. No more than 5 mg (0.5 ml) should be injected at any one site. If several sites are injected the total dosage administered should not exceed 30 mg (3 ml). The injection may be repeated if necessary, at one or two week intervals.

*Elderly:* Treatment of elderly patients, particularly if long term, should be planned bearing in mind the more serious consequences of the common side effects of corticosteroids in old age, especially osteoporosis, diabetes, hypertension, hypokalaemia, susceptibility to infection and thinning of the skin. Close supervision is required to avoid life-threatening reactions.

*Children:* Adcortyl is not recommended in children under 6 years. Adcortyl intra-articular/intradermal may be used in older children in suitably adjusted dosages. Growth and development of children on prolonged corticosteroid therapy should be carefully observed.

*Contra-indications:* Hypersensitivity to any of the ingredients.

Systemic infections unless specific anti-infective therapy is employed.

*Special warnings and special precautions for use:*
*Warnings (intra-articular Injection):* Patients should be specifically warned to avoid over-use of joints in which symptomatic benefit has been obtained. Severe joint destruction with necrosis of bone may occur if repeated intra-articular injections are given over a long period of time. Care should be taken if injections are given into tendon sheaths to avoid injection into the tendon itself.

Due to the absence of a true tendon sheath, the Achilles tendon should not be injected with depot corticosteroids.

*Precautions:* Administration by non-approved routes (see *Posology and method of administration*).

Intra-articular injection should not be carried out in the presence of active infection in or near joints. The preparation should not be used to alleviate joint pain arising from infectious states such as gonococcal or tubercular arthritis.

Undesirable effects may be minimised using the lowest effective dose for the minimum period, and by administering the daily requirement, whenever possible, as a single morning dose on alternate days. Frequent patient review is required to titrate the dose appropriately against disease activity (see *Dosage* section).

Adrenal cortical atrophy develops during prolonged therapy and may persist for years after stopping treatment. Withdrawal of corticosteroids after prolonged therapy must, therefore, always be gradual to avoid acute adrenal insufficiency and should be tapered off over weeks or months according to the dose and duration of treatment. During prolonged therapy any intercurrent illness, trauma or surgical procedure will require a temporary increase in dosage. If corticosteroids have been stopped following prolonged therapy they may need to be reintroduced temporarily. Patients should carry steroid treatment cards which give clear guidance on the precautions to be taken to minimise risk and which provides details of prescriber, drug, dosage and the duration of treatment.

Suppression of the inflammatory response and immune function increases the susceptibility to infections and their severity. The clinical presentation may often be atypical and serious infections such as septicaemia and tuberculosis may be masked and may reach an advanced stage before being recognised.

Chickenpox is of particular concern since this normally minor illness may be fatal in immunosuppressed patients. Patients (or parents of children receiving Adcortyl tablets) without a definite history of chickenpox should be advised to avoid close personal contact with chickenpox or herpes zoster. If exposed they should seek urgent medical attention. Passive immunisation with varicella zoster immunoglobulin (VZIG) is needed by exposed non- immune patients who are receiving systemic corticosteroids or who have used them within 10 days of exposure to chickenpox. If a diagnosis of chickenpox is confirmed, the illness warrants specialist care and urgent treatment. Corticosteroids should not be stopped and the dose may need to be increased.

During corticosteroid therapy antibody response will be reduced and therefore affect the patient's response to vaccines. Live vaccines should not be administered.

*Special precautions:* Particular care is required when considering use of systemic corticosteroids in patients with the following conditions and frequent patient monitoring is necessary.

Recent intestinal anastomoses, diverticulitis, thrombophlebitis, existing or previous history of severe affective disorders (especially previous steroid psychosis), exanthematous disease, chronic nephritis, or renal insufficiency, metastatic carcinoma, osteoporosis (post-menopausal females are particularly at risk); in patients with an active peptic ulcer (or a history of peptic ulcer). Myasthenia gravis. Latent or healed tuberculosis; in the presence of local or systemic viral infection, systemic fungal infections or in active infections not controlled by antibiotics. In acute psychoses; in acute glomerulonephritis. Hypertension; congestive heart failure; glaucoma (or a family history of glaucoma), previous steroid myopathy or epilepsy. Liver failure.

Corticosteroid effects may be enhanced in patients with hypothyroidism or cirrhosis.

Diabetes may be aggravated, necessitating a higher insulin dosage. Latent diabetes mellitus may be precipitated.

Menstrual irregularities may occur, and this possibility should be mentioned to female patients.

Rare instances of anaphylactoid reactions have occurred in patients receiving corticosteroids, especially when a patient has a history of drug allergies.

All corticosteroids increase calcium excretion

Aspirin should be used cautiously in conjunction with corticosteroids in patients with hypoprothrombinaemia.

*Interactions with other medicaments and other forms of interaction:* Barbiturates, phenytoin, rifampicin, rifabutin, carbamazepine, primidone and aminoglutethimide may enhance the metabolic clearance of corticosteroids, resulting in decreased therapeutic effects.

Corticosteroids antagonise the effects of hypoglycaemic agents (including insulin), anti-hypertensives and diuretics. The hypokalaemic effects of acetazolamide, loop diuretics, thiazide diuretics and carbenoxolone are enhanced.

The efficacy of coumarin anticoagulants may be enhanced by concurrent corticosteroid therapy and close monitoring of the INR or prothrombin time is required to avoid spontaneous bleeding.

The renal clearance of salicylates is increased by corticosteroids and steroid withdrawal may result in salicylate intoxication.

*Pregnancy and lactation:* Corticosteroids are not recommended for pregnant patients, particularly in the first trimester, or for nursing mothers, except when the disease for which they are indicated warrants their use. When corticosteroids are essential however, patients with normal pregnancies may be treated as though they were in the non-gravid state.

There is evidence of harmful effects in pregnancy in animals. There may be a small risk of cleft palate and intra-uterine growth retardation. Hypoadrenalism may occur in the neonate. Patients with pre-eclampsia or fluid retention require close monitoring.

Corticosteroids are found in breast milk.

Infants born of mothers who have received substantial doses of corticosteroids during pregnancy or during breast feeding should be carefully observed for signs of hypoadrenalism. Maternal treatment should be carefully documented in the infant's medical records to assist in follow up.

*Effects on ability to drive and use machines:* None known.

*Undesirable effects:* Where adverse reactions occur they are usually reversible on cessation of therapy. The incidence of predictable side-effects, including hypothalamic-pituitary-adrenal suppression correlate with the relative potency of the drug, dosage, timing of administration and duration of treatment (see *Warnings* and *Precautions*).

Absorption of triamcinolone following Adcortyl injection, especially when given by the intra-articular route, is rare. However, patients should be watched closely for the following adverse reactions which may be associated with any corticosteroid therapy:

Anti-inflammatory and immunosuppressive effects: Increased susceptibility and severity of infections with suppression of clinical symptoms and signs, opportunistic infections, recurrence of dormant tuberculosis (see *Warnings* and *Precautions*).

Fluid and electrolyte disturbances: sodium retention, fluid retention, congestive heart failure in susceptible patients, potassium loss, cardiac arrhythmias or ECG changes due to potassium deficiency, hypokalaemic alkalosis, increased calcium excretion and hypertension.

Musculoskeletal: muscle weakness, fatigue, steroid myopathy, loss of muscle mass, osteoporosis, avascular osteonecrosis, vertebral compression fractures, delayed healing of fractures, aseptic necrosis of femoral and humeral heads, pathological fractures of long bones and spontaneous fractures, tendo rupture.

Gastrointestinal: dyspepsia, peptic ulcer wit possible subsequent perforation and haemorrhage pancreatitis, abdominal distension and ulcerativ oesophagitis, candidiasis.

Dermatological: impaired wound healing, thin frag ile skin, petechiae and ecchymoses, facial erythema increased sweating, purpura, striae, hirsutism, acnei form eruptions, lupus erythematous-like lesions an suppressed reactions to skin tests.

Neurological: euphoria, psychological dependence depression, insomnia, convulsions, increased intra cranial pressure with papilloedema (pseudo-tumou cerebri) usually after treatment, vertigo, headache neuritis or paraesthesias and aggravation of pre existing psychiatric conditions and epilepsy.

Endocrine: menstrual irregularities and amenor rhoea; development of the Cushingoid state; suppres sion of growth in childhood and adolescence secondary adrenocortical and pituitary unresponsive ness, particularly in times of stress (eg. trauma surgery or illness); decreased carbohydrate tolerance manifestations of latent diabetes mellitus and in creased requirements for insulin or oral hypo glycaemic agents in diabetes, weight gain. Negativ protein and calcium balance. Increased appetite.

Ophthalmic: posterior supcapsular cataracts, in creased intraocular pressure, glaucoma, exophtha mos, papilloedema, corneal or scleral thinning exacerbation of ophthalmic viral or fungal diseases.

Others: necrotising angiitis, thrombophlebitis thromboembolism, leucocytosis, insomnia, syncopa episodes and anaphylactoid reactions, particularl where there is a history of drug allergies.

*Withdrawal symptoms and signs:* On withdrawa fever, myalgia, arthralgia, rhinitis, conjunctivitis, pain ful itchy skin nodules and weight loss may occur. To rapid a reduction in dose following prolonged trea ment can lead to acute adrenal insufficiency, hypoter sion and death (see *Warnings* and *Precautions*).

*Intra-articular injection:* Reactions following intra articular administration have been rare. In a fe instances, transient flushing and dizziness have oc curred. Pain and other local symptoms may continu for a short time before effective relief is obtained, bu an increase in joint discomfort has seldom occurre Local fat atrophy may occur if the injection is no given into the joint space, but is temporary an disappears within a few weeks to months.

*Intradermal injection:* Sterile abscesses, hyper- an hypo-pigmentation and subcutaneous and cutaneou atrophy (which usually disappears unless the bas disease process is itself atrophic) have occurred.

*Overdose:* Not applicable.

**Pharmacological properties**

*Pharmacodynamic properties:* Triamcinolone acetor ide is a synthetic glucocorticoid with marked ant inflammatory and anti-allergic actions. Following loc injection, relief of pain and swelling and greate freedom of movement are usually obtained within few hours; such administration avoids the mo severe systemic side-effects which may accompan parenteral or oral corticosteroid administration.

*Pharmacokinetic properties:* Triamcinolone acetonid may be absorbed into the systemic circulation fro synovial spaces. However clinically significant sys temic levels after intra-articular injection are unlike to occur except perhaps following treatment of larg joints with high doses. Systemic effects do n ordinarily occur with intra-articular injections whe the proper techniques of administration and th recommended dosage regimens are observed.

The systemic effects of intradermally administere triamcinolone acetonide have not been extensive studied. The risk of systemic absorption, thoug minimal, should be taken into consideration especial when repeated intralesional administrations may b necessary.

In common with other corticosteroids, triamcin lone is metabolised largely hepatically but also by th kidney and is excreted in urine. The main metabol route is 6-beta-hydroxylation; no significant hydrolyt cleavage of the acetonide occurs. In view of th hepatic metabolism and renal excretion of triamcin lone acetonide, functional impairments of the liver kidney may affect the pharmacokinetics of the dru This may become clinically significant if large frequent doses of intradermal or intra-articular trian cinolone acetonide are given.

*Preclinical safety data:* See *Pregnancy and lactation.*

**Pharmaceutical particulars**

*List of excipients:* Benzyl alcohol. polysorbate 8 sodium carboxymethylcellulose, sodium chlorid water.

*Incompatibilities:* The injection should not be phys cally mixed with other medicinal products.

*Shelf life:* 36 months.

*Special precautions for storage:* In an upright position below 25°C: avoid freezing.

*Nature and contents of container:* Carton containing glass ampoules 5 x 1 ml or individually cartoned multidose vials of 5 ml.

*Instructions for use/handling:* No special handling instructions.

**Marketing authorisation number**  0034/5002R

**Date of approval/revision of SPC**  March 1997

**Legal category**  POM

# ADCORTYL* WITH GRANEODIN* CREAM

**Quantitative and qualitative composition**  Containing in each gram the following: triamcinolone acetonide 0.1%, neomycin (as sulphate) 0.25%, gramicidin 0.025%.

**Pharmaceutical form**  Topical Cream.

**Clinical particulars**

*Therapeutic indications:* The topical treatment of exudative and/or secondarily infected eczema and dermatitis, including: atopic eczema, contact eczema, follicular eczema, otitis externa, nummular eczema, seborrhoeic eczema, intertrigo, neurodermatitis and infected insect bites.

*Posology and method of administration:*
*Adults and children:* Apply to the affected area two to four times daily.

*Elderly:* Corticosteroids should be used sparingly and for short periods of time, as natural thinning of the skin occurs in the elderly.

If, after about 7 days application, little or no improvement has occurred, cultural isolation of the offending organism should be followed by appropriate local or systemic antimicrobial therapy systemic antimicrobial therapy.

*Contra-indications:* In tuberculous and most viral lesions of the skin, particularly herpes simplex and varicella. Also in fungal lesions not susceptible to nystatin.

In patients with hypersensitivity to any of the components.

Should not be used for facial rosacea, acne vulgaris or perioral dermatitis.

Should not be applied to the external auditory canal in patients with perforated eardrums.

The products should not be used for extensive areas because of possible risk of systemic absorption and neomycin-induced ototoxicity.

*Special warnings and special precautions for use:* Adrenal suppression can occur, even without occlusion. The use of occlusive dressings should be avoided because of the increased risk of sensitivity reactions and increased percutaneous absorption. The possibility of sensitivity to neomycin should be taken into consideration.

Steroid-antibiotic combinations should not be continued for more than 7 days in the absence of any clinical improvement, since in this situation occult extension of infection may occur due to the masking effect of the steroid.

Extended or recurrent application may increase the risk of contact sensitisation and should be avoided.

If used on the face, courses should be limited to 5 days and occlusion should not be used.

*Children:* In infants, long-term continuous topical steroid therapy should be avoided. Courses should be limited to 5 days and occlusion should not be used.

*Interactions with other medicaments and other forms of interaction:* Not applicable

*Pregnancy and lactation:* There is inadequate evidence of safety in human pregnancy. Topical administration of corticosteroids to pregnant animals can cause abnormalities of foetal development including cleft palate and intra-uterine growth retardation. There may, therefore, be a very small risk of such effects in the human foetus. There are theoretical risks of neomycin-induced foetal ototoxicity; therefore the product should be used with caution only when the benefit outweighs the potential risk.

*Effects on ability to drive and use machines:* Not applicable.

*Undesirable effects:*
*Triamcinolone acetonide:* The following side effects have been reported. Usually with prolonged usage: dermatologic–impaired wound healing, thinning of the skin, petechiae and ecchymoses, facial erythema and telangiectasia, increased sweating, purpura, striae, hirsutism, acneiform eruptions, lupus erythematosus-like lesions and suppressed reactions to skin tests. These effects may be enhanced with occlusive dressings.

The possibility of the systemic effects which are associated with all steroid therapy should be considered.

*Neomycin:* Sensitivity reactions may occur especially with prolonged use. Ototoxicity and nephrotoxicity have been reported. The product should be used with caution and in small amounts in the treatment of skin infections following extensive burns, open lesions and other conditions where absorption of neomycin is possible particularly children and elderly. The product should also be used with care in patients with established hearing loss and those with renal impairment.

*Gramicidin:* Sensitivity has occasionally been reported.

*Overdose:* Topically applied corticosteroids can be absorbed in sufficient amounts to produce systemic effects (see *Side effects*).

In the event of accidental ingestion, the patient should be observed and treated symptomatically.

**Pharmacological properties**

*Pharmacodynamic properties:* Triamcinolone acetonide is a potent fluorinated corticosteroid with rapid anti-inflammatory, antipruritic and anti-allergic actions.

The combined action of the antibiotics neomycin and gramicidin provides comprehensive antibacterial therapy against a wide range of gram-positive and gram-negative bacteria, including those micro-organisms responsible for most bacterial skin infections.

*Pharmacokinetic properties:* Not applicable.

*Preclinical safety data:* No further relevant data

**Pharmaceutical particulars**

*List of excipients:* Benzyl alcohol, cetyl alcohol, ethanol, glyceryl monostearate, isopropyl palmitate, polysorbate 60, propylene glycol, water.

*Incompatibilities:* None known.

*Shelf life:* 24 months.

*Special precautions for storage:* Store below 25°C. Avoid freezing.

*Nature and contents of container:* Aluminium tubes.

*Instructions for use/handling:* None.

**Marketing authorisation number**  0034/5015R

**Date of approval/revision of SPC**  29th August 1996

**Legal category**  POM

# AZACTAM* FOR INJECTION

**Presentation**  Azactam for Injection is a sterile white to off-white, sodium-free, powder blend of aztreonam and L-arginine (780 mg per g of aztreonam). After reconstitution, Azactam for Injection provides 500 mg, 1.0 g and 2.0 g of aztreonam activity in 15 ml vials.

**Uses**

*Microbiology:* Aztreonam is a monocyclic beta-lactam antibiotic with potent bactericidal activity against a wide spectrum of Gram-negative aerobic pathogens.

Unlike the majority of beta-lactam antibiotics, it is not an inducer *in vitro* of beta-lactamase activity. Aztreonam is usually active *in vitro* against those resistant aerobic organisms whose beta-lactamases hydrolyse other antibiotics.

Aztreonam is active *in vitro* against most strains of the following Gram-negative micro-organisms:

*Escherichia coli, Enterobacter* species, *Klebsiella* species (including *K. pneumoniae* and *K. oxytoca*), *Proteus mirabilis, Proteus vulgaris, Morganella morganii, Providencia* species (including *P. stuartii* and *P. rettgeri*), *Pseudomonas* species (including *Ps. aeruginosa*), *Serratia marcescens, Neisseria gonorrhoeae* (including penicillinase-producing strains), *Haemophilus influenzae* (including ampicillin-resistant and other penicillinase-producing strains), *Neisseria meningitidis, Citrobacter* species.

The majority of these organisms are susceptible to an aztreonam concentration of less than 1 mg/L. Most *Pseudomonas* and *Enterobacter* species are also susceptible but at higher concentrations *in vitro.*

Aztreonam and aminoglycosides are synergistic *in vitro* for many strains of Enterobacteriaceae and for most strains of *Ps. aeruginosa.*

*Indications:* The treatment of the following infections caused by susceptible aerobic Gram-negative micro-organisms:

Urinary tract infections: including pyelonephritis and cystitis (initial and recurrent) and asymptomatic bacteriuria, including those due to pathogens resistant to the aminoglycosides, cephalosporins or penicillins.

Gonorrhoea: acute uncomplicated urogenital or anorectal infections due to beta-lactamase producing or non-producing strains of *N. gonorrhoeae.*

Lower respiratory tract infections: including pneumonia, bronchitis and lung infections in patients with cystic fibrosis.

Bacteraemia/septicaemia.

Meningitis caused by *Haemophilus influenzae* or *Neisseria meningitidis.* Since Azactam provides only Gram-negative cover, it should not be given alone as initial blind therapy, but may be used with an antibiotic active against Gram-positive organisms until the results of sensitivity tests are known.

Bone and joint infections.

Skin and soft tissue infections: including those associated with postoperative wounds, ulcers and burns.

Intra-abdominal infections: peritonitis.

Gynaecological infections: pelvic inflammatory disease, endometritis, and pelvic cellulitis.

Azactam is indicated for adjunctive therapy to surgery in the management of infections caused by susceptible organisms, including abscesses, infections complicating hollow viscus perforations, cutaneous infections and infections of serous surfaces.

Bacteriological studies to determine the causative organism(s) and their sensitivity to aztreonam should be performed. Therapy may be instituted prior to receiving the results of the sensitivity test.

In patients at risk of infections due to non-susceptible pathogens, additional antibiotic therapy should be initiated concurrently with Azactam to provide broad-spectrum coverage before identification and susceptibility testing results of the causative organism(s) are known. Based on these results, appropriate antibiotic therapy should be continued.

Patients with serious Pseudomonas infections may benefit from concurrent use of Azactam and an aminoglycoside because of their synergistic action. If such concurrent therapy is considered in these patients, susceptibility tests should be performed *in vitro* to determine the activity in combination. The usual monitoring of serum levels and renal function during aminoglycoside therapy applies.

**Dosage and administration**  Intramuscular or intravenous injection, or intravenous infusion.

*Adults:* The dose range of Azactam is 1 to 8 g daily in equally divided doses. The usual dose is 3 to 4 g daily. The maximum recommended dose is 8 g daily. The dosage and route of administration should be determined by the susceptibility of the causative organisms, severity of infection, and the condition of the patient.

Dosage Guide: Adults

| Type of infection[1] | Dosage (g) | Frequency (hr) | Route |
|---|---|---|---|
| Urinary tract | 0.5–1 | 8–12 | IM or IV |
| Gonorrhoea/cystitis | 1 | single dose | IM |
| Cystic Fibrosis | 2 | 6–8 | IV |
| Severe or life-threatening infections | 2 | 6–8 | IV |
| Other infections | either 1 | 8 | IM or IV |
| | or 2 | 12 | IV |

[1] Because of the serious nature of infections due to *Pseudomonas aeruginosa*, a dose of 2 g every 6 or 8 hours is recommended, at least for initial therapy in systemic infections caused by this organism.

The intravenous route is recommended for patients requiring single doses greater than 1 g, or those with bacterial septicaemia, localised parenchymal abscess (e.g. intra-abdominal abscess), peritonitis, meningitis or other severe systemic or life-threatening infections.

*Children:* The usual dosage for patients older than one week is 30 mg/kg/dose every 6 or 8 hours. For severe infections in patients 2 years of age or older, 50 mg/kg/dose every 6 or 8 hours is recommended. The total daily dose should not exceed 8 g. Dosage information is not yet available for new-borns less than 1 week old.

*Elderly:* In the elderly, renal status is the major determinant of dosage. Estimated creatinine clearance should be used to determine appropriate dosage, since serum creatinine is not an accurate measurement of renal function in these patients.

Elderly patients normally have a creatinine clearance in excess of 30 ml/min and therefore would receive the normal recommended dose. If renal function is below this level, the dosage schedule should be adjusted (see Renal impairment).

*Renal impairment:* In patients with impaired renal function, the normal recommended initial dose should be given. This should be followed by maintenance doses as shown in the following table.

*Estimated creatinine clearance (ml/min)* — *Maintenance dose*

| | |
|---|---|
| 10–30 | Half the initial dose |
| Less than 10 | One quarter of the initial dose |

The normal dose interval should not be altered.

In patients on haemodialysis a supplementary one eighth of the initial dose should be given after each dialysis.

*Reconstitution:* Azactam for Injection is supplied in 15 ml vials. Upon the addition of the diluent the contents should be shaken immediately and vigorously. Vials of reconstituted Azactam are not intended for multi-dose use, and any unused solution from a single dose must be discarded. Depending on the type and amount of diluent, the pH ranges from 4.5 to 7.5, and the colour may vary from colourless to light straw-yellow, which may develop a slight pink tint on standing; however this does not affect the potency.

*For intramuscular injection:* For each gram of aztreonam add at least 3 ml Water for Injections PhEur or 0.9% Sodium Chloride Injection BP and shake well.

| Single-dose vial size | Volume of diluent to be added |
|---|---|
| 0.5 g | 1.5 ml |
| 1.0 g | 3.0 ml |

Azactam is given by deep injection into a large muscle mass, such as the upper outer quadrant of the gluteus maximus or the lateral part of the thigh.

*For intravenous injection:* To the contents of the vial add 6 to 10 ml Water for Injections PhEur, and shake well. Slowly inject directly into the vein over a period of 3 to 5 minutes.

*For intravenous infusion:* For each gram of aztreonam add at least 3 ml of Water for Injections PhEur and shake well.

Dilute this initial solution with an appropriate infusion solution to a final concentration less than 2% w/v (at least 50 ml solution per gram of aztreonam). The infusion should be administered over 20–60 minutes.

Appropriate infusion solutions include:
0.9% Sodium Chloride Injection BP
5% Glucose Intravenous Infusion BP
5% or 10% Mannitol Intravenous Infusion BP
Sodium Lactate Intravenous Infusion BP
0.9%, 0.45% or 0.2% Sodium Chloride and 5% Glucose Intravenous Infusion BP
Compound Sodium Chloride Injection BPC 1959 (Ringer's Solution for Injection).
Compound Sodium Lactate Intravenous Infusion BP (Hartmanns Solution for Injection).

A volume control administration set may be used to deliver the initial solution of Azactam into a compatible infusion solution being administered. With use of a Y-tube administration set, careful attention should be given to the calculated volume of Azactam solution required so that the entire dose will be infused.

With intermittent infusion of Azactam and another drug via a common delivery tube, the tube should be flushed before and after delivery of Azactam with any appropriate infusion solution compatible with both drug solutions. Except for the antibiotics described below, the drugs should not be delivered simultaneously.

Intravenous infusion solutions of Azactam for Injection prepared with 0.9% Sodium Chloride Injection BP or 5% Glucose Intravenous Infusion BP, in PVC or glass containers, to which clindamycin phosphate, gentamicin sulphate, tobramycin sulphate, or cephazolin sodium have been added at concentrations usually used clinically, are stable for up to 24 hours in a refrigerator (4–7˚C). Ampicillin sodium admixtures with aztreonam in 0.9% Sodium Chloride Injection BP are stable for 24 hours in a refrigerator (4–7˚C); stability in 5% Glucose Intravenous Infusion BP is eight hours under refrigeration.

If aztreonam and metronidazole are to be used together, they should be administered separately as a cherry red colour has been observed after storage of solutions containing combinations of the two products.

### Contra-indications, warnings, etc
*Contra-indications:* Patients with a known hypersensitivity to aztreonam.

Aztreonam is contra-indicated in pregnancy. Aztreonam crosses the placenta and enters the foetal circulation.

*Precautions:* Specific studies have not shown significant cross-reactivity between Azactam and antibodies to penicillins or cephalosporins. The incidence of hypersensitivity to Azactam in clinical trials has been low but caution should be exercised in patients with a history of hypersensitivity to beta-lactam antibiotics until further experience is gained.

Experience in patients with impaired hepatic function is limited. Appropriate liver function monitoring in these patients is recommended.

Concurrent therapy with other antimicrobial agents and Azactam is recommended as initial therapy in patients who are at risk of having an infection due to pathogens that are not susceptible to aztreonam.

Therapy with Azactam may result in overgrowth of

nonsusceptible organisms which may require additional antimicrobial therapy. In comparative studies, the number of patients treated for super-infections was similar to that of the control drugs used.

It is recommended that prothrombin times should be monitored if the patient is on concomitant anticoagulant therapy.

Aztreonam is excreted in breast milk in concentrations that are less than 1% of those in simultaneously obtained maternal serum. Lactating mothers should refrain from breast feeding during the course of therapy.

*Side-effects:* Azactam is generally well tolerated. The following side-effects have been reported from Azactam therapy:

*Dermatological:* Rash; pruritus, urticaria, erythema, petechiae and exfoliative dermatitis.

*Haematological:* Eosinophilia; increases in prothrombin and partial thromboplastin time have occurred. There have been isolated reports of thrombocytopenia, neutropenia, anaemia and bleeding.

*Hepatobiliary:* Jaundice and hepatitis; transient elevations of hepatic transaminases and alkaline phosphatase (without overt signs or symptoms of hepatobiliary dysfunction).

*Gastro-intestinal:* Diarrhoea, nausea and/or vomiting, abdominal cramps, mouth ulcer and altered taste.

*Local reactions:* Phlebitis and discomfort at the i.v. injection site; discomfort at the i.m. injection site.

Rare instances of the following events have been reported: vaginitis, candidosis, anaphylaxis, hypotension, weakness, confusion, dizziness, vertigo, sweating, headache, breast tenderness, halitosis, muscle aches, fever, malaise, sneezing and nasal congestion, transient increases in serum creatinine.

*Treatment of overdosage:* There have been no reported cases of overdosage.

### Pharmaceutical precautions
*Storage before reconstitution:* At room temperature (15–25˚C).

*Stability after reconstitution:* It is good practice to reconstitute immediately before use. If this is not possible, Azactam is stable for 24 hours if stored in a refrigerator (4–7˚C).

Azactam should not be physically mixed with any other drug, antibiotic or diluent except those listed in the 'Dosage and administration' section under reconstitution for intravenous infusion.

### Legal category POM.

### Package quantities
| 500 mg vial: | pack of 5 |
|---|---|
| 1 g vial: | single-dose pack |
| 2 g vial: | single-dose pack |

**Further information** Aztreonam is the first member of a new class of antibiotics, the monobactams. It has been synthesised as a monocylic beta-lactam antibiotic in which the sulphonic acid substituent in the 1-position of the nuclear ring activates the beta-lactam moiety.

Single 30-minute i.v. infusions of 0.5 g, 1.0 g and 2.0 g in healthy volunteers produced peak serum levels of 54, 90 and 204 mg/L, and single 3-minute i.v. injections of the same doses produced peak levels of 58, 125 and 242 mg/L. Peak levels of aztreonam are achieved at about one hour after i.m. administration. After identical single i.m. or i.v. doses, the serum concentrations are comparable at 1 hour (1.5 hours from the start of i.v. infusion), with similar slopes of serum concentrations thereafter.

The serum half-life of aztreonam averaged 1.7 hours in subjects with normal renal function, independent of the dose and route. In healthy subjects 60–70% of a single i.m. or i.v. dose was recovered in the urine by 8 hours, and urinary excretion was essentially complete by 12 hours.

Single-dose pharmacokinetic studies have not shown any significant interaction between aztreonam and gentamicin, cephradine, clindamycin or metronidazole.

As with other antibiotics, in the treatment of acute pulmonary exacerbations in patients with cystic fibrosis, while clinical improvement is usually noted, lasting bacterial eradications may not be achieved.

Unlike broad spectrum antibiotics, aztreonam produces no effects on the normal anaerobic intestinal flora. No disulfiram-like reactions with alcohol ingestion have been reported.

### Product licence numbers
| 500 mg vial | 0034/0250 |
|---|---|
| 1 g vial | 0034/0251 |
| 2 g vial | 0034/0252 |

## CAPOTEN* TABLETS 12.5 mg, 25 mg and 50 mg

**Qualitative and quantitative composition** Capoten tablets 12.5 mg: Slightly mottled, white, flat-faced, bevel-edged, capsule-shaped tablets, each containing captopril 12.5 mg. Engraved with 'Squibb' and '450' on one side with a bisecting bar on the other.

*Capoten tablets 25 mg:* Slightly mottled, white, square, biconvex tablets each containing captopril 25 mg. Engraved with 'Squibb' and '452' on one side and with quadrisect bars on the other.

*Capoten tablets 50 mg:* Slightly mottled, white, oval, biconvex tablets each containing captopril 50 mg. Engraved with 'Squibb' and '482' on one side with a bisecting bar on the other.

**Pharmaceutical form** Oral tablet.

**Clinical particulars**

*Therapeutic indications:*
*Hypertension:* Capoten is indicated for the first line treatment of mild to moderate hypertension.

In severe hypertension it should be used where standard therapy is ineffective or inappropriate.

*Congestive heart failure:* Capoten is indicated for the treatment of congestive heart failure. The drug should be used together with diuretics and, where appropriate digitalis.

*Myocardial infarction:* Capoten is indicated following myocardial infarction in clinically stable patients with asymptomatic and symptomatic left ventricular dysfunction to improve survival, delay the onset of symptomatic heart failure, reduce hospitalisations for heart failure, and reduce recurrent myocardial infarction and coronary revascularisation procedures.

Determination of cardiac function by radionuclide ventriculography or echocardiography should be undertaken prior to initiation of preventative treatment with Capoten in post myocardial infarction patients.

*Diabetic nephropathy:* Capoten is indicated for the treatment of diabetic nephropathy (microalbuminuria greater than 30 mg/day) in insulin-dependent diabetics. In these patients, captopril prevents the progression of renal disease and reduces associated clinical events e.g. dialysis, renal transplantation and death.

*Posology and method of administration:*

*Adults:*
*Hypertension:* Treatment with Capoten should be at the lowest effective dose which should be titrated according to the needs of the patient.

*Mild to moderate hypertension:* The starting dose is 12.5 mg twice daily. The usual maintenance dose is 25 mg twice daily which can be increased incrementally, at 2–4 week intervals, until a satisfactory response is achieved, to a maximum of 50 mg twice daily.

A thiazide diuretic may be added to Capoten if satisfactory response has not been achieved. The dose of diuretic may be increased at 1-2 week intervals to the level of optimum response or until the maximum dose is reached.

*Severe hypertension:* In severe hypertension where standard therapy is ineffective or inappropriate because of adverse effects, the starting dose is 12.5 mg b.d. The dosage may be increased incrementally to a maximum of 50 mg t.i.d. Capoten should be used together with other anti-hypertensive agents but the dose of these should be individually titrated. A daily dose of 150 mg of Capoten should not normally be exceeded.

*Heart failure:* Capoten therapy must be started under close medical supervision. Capoten should be introduced when diuretic therapy (such as frusemide 40-80 mg or equivalent) is insufficient to control symptoms. A starting dose of 6.25 mg or 12.5 mg may minimise a transient hypotensive effect. The possibility of this occurring can be reduced by discontinuing or reducing diuretic therapy if possible, prior to initiating Capoten. The usual maintenance dose is 25 mg two or three times a day which can be increased incrementally, with intervals of at least two weeks until a satisfactory response is achieved. The usual maximum dose is 150 mg daily.

*Myocardial infarction:* Therapy may be initiated as early as three days following a myocardial infarction. After an initial dose of 6.25 mg, captopril therapy should be titrated to a final target dose of 150 mg daily in divided doses over the next several weeks.

Achievement of the target dose of 150 mg should be based on the patient's tolerance to captopril during titration. If symptomatic hypotension occurs, a dosage reduction may be required.

Captopril may be used in patients treated with other post-myocardial infarction therapies, e.g. thrombolytics, aspirin, beta blockers.

*Diabetic nephropathy:* The recommended daily dose of captopril is 75 to 100 mg in divided doses.

If further blood pressure reduction is required, other antihypertensive agents such as diuretics, beta block ers, centrally acting agents or vasodilators may be used in conjunction with captopril.

*Elderly:* The dose should be titrated against the blood pressure response and kept as low as possible to achieve adequate control. Since elderly patients may have reduced renal function and other organ dysfunctions, it is suggested that a low dose of Capoten be used initially.

*Children:* Capoten is not recommended for the treatment of mild to moderate hypertension in children.

Experience in neonates, particularly premature infants, is limited. Because renal function in infants is not equivalent to that of older children and adults, lower doses of Capoten should be used with the patients under close medical supervision.

The starting dose should be 0.3 mg per Kg bodyweight up to a maximum of 6 mg per Kg bodyweight daily in divided doses. The dose should be individualised according to the response and may be given two or three times daily.

*Patients with renal impairment:* Captopril in divided doses of 75 to 100 mg/day was well tolerated in patients with diabetic nephropathy and mild to moderate renal impairment (creatinine clearance at least 30 ml/min/1.73 m²).

Patients with severely impaired renal function will take longer to reach steady-state captopril levels and will reach higher steady-state levels for a given daily dose than patients with normal renal function. These patients may therefore respond to smaller or less frequent doses.

Therefore, patients with severe renal impairment (creatinine clearance less than 30 ml/min/1.73 m²), the initial daily dose should be 12.5 mg b.d. The dose can then be titrated against the response but adequate time should be allowed between dosage adjustments. When concomitant diuretic therapy is required, a loop diuretic rather than a thiazide diuretic should be the diuretic of choice.

Capoten is readily eliminated by haemodialysis.

*Contra-indications:* A history of previous hypersensitivity to the product.

*Pregnancy:* Capoten has been shown to be lethal to rabbit and sheep foetuses. There were no foetotoxic effects to hamster or rat foetuses.

Capoten is contra-indicated in pregnancy and should not be used in women of child bearing potential unless protected by effective contraception.

Exposure of the mother in the second and third trimesters of pregnancy has been associated with oligohydramnios and neonatal hypertension and/or anuria.

*Special warnings and special precautions for use:*

*Precautions:* Evaluation of the patient should include assessment of renal function prior to initiation of therapy and at appropriate intervals thereafter (see Recommended Dosage and Dosage Schedule Section).

Capoten should not be used in patients with aortic stenosis or outflow tract obstruction.

As limited experience has been obtained in the treatment of acute hypertensive crisis, the use of Capoten should be avoided in these patients.

*Warnings:* The incidence of adverse reactions to captopril is principally associated with renal function since the drug is excreted primarily by the kidney. The dose should not exceed that necessary for adequate control and should be reduced in patients with impaired renal function.

*Haematological:* Neutropenia/agranulocytosis, thrombocytopenia and anaemia have been reported in patients receiving Capoten

In patients with normal renal function and no other complicating factors, neutropenia occurs rarely.

Capoten should be used with extreme caution in patients with collagen vascular disease, immunosuppressant therapy, treatment with allopurinol or procainamide, or a combination of these complicating factors especially if there is pre-existing impaired renal function. Some of these patients developed serious infections which in a few instances did not respond to intensive antibiotic therapy.

If Capoten is used in such patients, it is advised that white blood cell count and differential counts should be performed prior to therapy, every 2 weeks during the first 3 months of Capoten therapy, and periodically thereafter.

During treatment all patients should be instructed to report any sign of infection (e.g. sore throat, fever), when a differential white blood cell count should be performed. Capoten and other concomitant medication should be withdrawn if neutropenia (neutrophils less than 1000/mm³) is detected or suspected.

In most patients neutrophil counts rapidly returned to normal upon discontinuing Capoten.

*Renal:* Proteinuria in patients with prior normal renal function is rare.

Where proteinuria has occurred it has usually been in patients with severe hypertension or evidence of prior renal disease. Nephrotic syndrome occurred in some of these patients.

In patients with evidence of prior renal disease, monthly urinary protein estimations (dip stick) are recommended for the first 9 months of therapy. If repeated determinations show increasing amounts of urinary protein, a 24-hour quantitative determination should be obtained, and if this exceeds 1 g/day, the benefits and risks of continuing Capoten should be evaluated.

In patients with diabetic nephropathy and proteinuria, who received captopril 75 mg/day for a median of 3 years, there was a consistent reduction in proteinuria. It is unknown whether long-term therapy in patients with other types of renal disease would have similar effects.

Although membranous glomerulopathy was found in biopsies taken from some proteinuric patients, a causal relationship to Capoten has not been established.

Some patients with renal disease, particularly those with bilateral renal artery stenosis or unilateral renal artery stenosis in a single functioning kidney, have developed increased concentrations of blood urea and serum creatinine. Capoten dosage reduction and/or discontinuation of diuretic may be required. For some of these patients it may not be possible to normalise blood pressure and maintain adequate renal perfusion.

Recent clinical observations have shown a high incidence of anaphylactoid-like reactions during haemodialysis with high-flux dialysis membranes (e.g. AN69) in patients receiving ACE inhibitors. Therefore, this combination should be avoided.

*Hypotension:* With the first one or two doses some patients may experience symptomatic hypotension. In most instances, symptoms are relieved simply by the patient lying down.

In patients with severe and renin dependent hypertension (e.g. renovascular hypertension) or severe congestive heart failure who are receiving large doses of diuretic, exaggerated hypotensive responses have occurred usually within one hour of the initial dose of Capoten. In these patients, by discontinuing diuretic therapy or significantly reducing the diuretic dose for four to seven days prior to initiating Capoten the possibility of this occurrence is reduced. By commencing Capoten therapy with small doses (6.25 mg or 12.5 mg) the duration of any hypotensive effect is lessened. Some patients may benefit from an infusion of saline. The occurrence of first dose hypotension does not preclude subsequent dose titration with Capoten. Hypotension has been occasionally reported in patients on Capoten due to causes of acute volume depletion such as vomiting and diarrhoea.

*Serum potassium:* Since Capoten decreases aldosterone production, serum potassium is usually maintained in patients on diuretics. Potassium sparing diuretics or potassium supplements should not therefore be used routinely. In patients with marked renal impairment a significant elevation of serum potassium may occur.

*Surgery/anaesthesia:* In patients undergoing major surgery, or during anaesthesia with agents which produce hypotension, captopril will block angiotensin II formation secondary to compensatory renin release. This may lead to hypotension which can be corrected by volume expansion.

*Clinical chemistry:* Capoten may cause a false-positive urine test for acetone.

*Interaction with other medicaments and other forms of interaction:*

Diuretics: Diuretics potentiate the anti-hypertensive effectiveness of Capoten. Potassium-sparing diuretics (triamterene, amiloride and spironolactone), or potassium supplements may cause significant increase in serum potassium.

Indomethacin: A reduction of anti-hypertensive effectiveness may occur. This is probably also the case with other non-steroidal anti-inflammatory drugs.

Vasodilators: Capoten has been reported to act synergistically with peripheral vasodilators such as minoxidil. Awareness of this interaction may avert an initial hypotensive response.

Clonidine: It has been suggested that the anti-hypertensive effect of Capoten can be delayed when patients treated with clonidine are changed to Capoten.

Allopurinol and procainamide: There have been reports of neutropenia and/or Stevens-Johnson syndrome in patients on Capoten plus either allopurinol or procainamide. Although a causal relationship has not been established, these combinations should only be used with caution, especially in patients with impaired renal function.

Immunosuppressants: Azathioprine and cyclophosphamide have been associated with blood dyscrasias in patients with renal failure who were also taking Capoten.

Probenecid: The renal clearance of Capoten is reduced in the presence of probenecid.

Lithium: Concomitant use of lithium and ACE-inhibitors may result in an increase of serum lithium concentration.

Hypoglycaemic agents: ACE Inhibitors have been show to enhance insulin sensitivity. There have been rare reports of hypoglycaemic episodes in diabetic patients treated concomitantly with ACE Inhibitors and antidiabetic medicines (insulin or oral hypoglycaemic agents). This phenomenon may be more likely to occur during the first few weeks of treatment. In such cases a reduction in the dose of the antidiabetic medicine may be required.

*Pregnancy and laction:*

*Pregnancy:* See *Contra-indications.*

*Nursing mothers:* Because captopril is excreted in breast milk, Capoten should not be used in nursing mothers.

*Effects on ability to drive and use machines:* See warnings under hypotension section.

*Undesirable effects:*

Idiosyncratic: Angioedema involving the extremities, face, lips, mucous membranes, tongue, glottis or larynx has been seen in patients treated with ACE inhibitors, including captopril. In this situation, the ACE inhibitor should be discontinued. Where swelling is confined to the face, lips and mouth the condition will usually resolve without further treatment, although antihistamines may be useful in relieving symptoms. These patients should be followed carefully until the swelling has resolved. However, where there is involvement of the tongue, glottis or larynx, likely to cause airway obstruction, subcutaneous adrenaline (0.5 ml, 1:1,000) should be administered promptly where indicated.

Haematological: Neutropenia, anaemia and thrombocytopenia (see Warnings). Rarely a positive ANA has been reported.

Renal: Proteinuria, elevated blood urea and creatinine, elevated serum potassium and acidosis (see Warnings).

Cardiovascular: Hypotension (see warnings), tachycardia.

Skin: Rashes, usually pruritic, may occur. They are usually mild, maculopapular, rarely urticarial and disappear within a few days of dosage reduction, short-term treatment with an antihistamine and/or discontinuing therapy. In a few cases the rash has been associated with fever. Pruritus, flushing, vesicular or bullous rash, and photosensitivity have been reported.

Gastrointestinal: Reversible and usually self-limiting taste impairment has been reported. Weight loss may be associated with the loss of taste. Stomatitis, resembling aphthous ulcers, has been reported. Elevation of liver enzymes has been noted in a few patients. Rare cases of hepatocellular injury and cholestatic jaundice have been reported. Gastric irritation and abdominal pain may occur. Pancreatitis has been reported rarely in patients treated with ACE Inhibitors; in some cases this has proved fatal.

Other: Paraesthesias of the hands, serum sickness, cough, bronchospasm and lymphadenopathy have been reported.

*Overdose:* In the event of overdosage, blood pressure should be monitored and if hypotension develops volume expansion is the treatment of choice. Captopril is removed by dialysis.

**Pharmacological properties**

*Pharmacodynamic properties:* Captopril is a highly specific, competitive inhibitor of angiotensin-I converting enzyme. This enzyme is responsible for the conversion of angiotensin-I to angiotensin-II.

*Pharmacokinetic properties:*

| | | |
|---|---|---|
| Total captopril: | $t_{MAX}$ | 1 hour |
| | $t_{\frac{1}{2}}$ | 8 hours |
| Free captopril | $t_{MAX}$ | 1 hour |
| | $t_{\frac{1}{2}}$ | 1 hour |

The absolute bioavailability of an oral dose is approximately 65%.

*Preclinical safety data:* No further relevant data

**Pharmaceutical particulars**

*List of excipients:* Lactose, corn starch, microcrystalline cellulose, stearic acid.

*Incompatibilites:* None.

*Shelf life:* 48 Months.

*Special precautions for storage:* Store below 30°C. Protect from moisture

*Nature and contents of container:* The tablets are packaged in any of the following: amber glass bottles (packs of 100), HDPE bottles (packs of 100), foil strips, PVC/PVDC blisters or PVC/aluminium blisters in packs of 90, 60 or 56's.

*Instructions for use/handling:* No special instructions.

**Marketing authorisation numbers**
12.5 mg: 0034/0221
25 mg: 0034/0193
50 mg: 0034/0194

**Date of approval/revision of SPC** 5 November 1996

**Legal category** POM

## CAPOZIDE* TABLETS

**Presentation**
*Capozide 50 mg/25 mg:* White, biconvex, round tablets with possible slight mottling, each containing captopril 50 mg and hydrochlorothiazide 25 mg. Engraved with 'Squibb' and 390 on one side with a bisect bar on the other.

Other ingredients: lactose, magnesium stearate, maize starch, microcrystalline cellulose, stearic acid.

**Uses**
*Actions:* Captopril, designated chemically as l-[(2S)-3-mercapto-2-methyl-propionyl]-L-proline, is a specific competitive inhibitor of angiotensin I-converting enzyme, and hydrochlorothiazide is a diuretic-antihypertensive agent.

Captopril and hydrochlorothiazide lower blood pressure by different, though complementary, mechanisms. With diuretic treatment, blood pressure and blood volume fall resulting in a rise in angiotensin II levels which tend to blunt the hypotensive effect. Captopril blocks this rise in angiotensin II. The anti-hypertensive effects of captopril and hydrochlorothiazide are additive.

*Indications:* For the treatment of mild to moderate hypertension in patients who have been stabilised on the individual components given in the same proportions.

**Dosage and administration**
*Adults:* The usual dose of Capozide is one tablet daily. A daily dose of two tablets should not be exceeded.

*Elderly:* The dose should be kept as low as possible to achieve adequate blood pressure control. In some patients half a tablet daily may be sufficient.

*Children:* Safety and effectiveness of Capozide has not been established.

*Patients with renal failure:* Capozide is not recommended for use in patients with significant renal impairment.

**Contra-indications, warnings, etc**
*Contra-indications:* Capozide is contra-indicated in patients with anuria or hyper-sensitivity to captopril, thiazides, or any sulphonamide-derived drug.

*Pregnancy:* Captopril has been shown to be lethal to rabbit and sheep foetuses. There were no foetotoxic effects to hamster or rat foetuses.

Capozide is contra-indicated in pregnancy and should not be used in women of childbearing potential unless protected by effective contraception.

Exposure of the mother in the second and third trimesters of pregnancy has been associated with oligohydramnios and neonatal hypotension and/or anuria.

*Precautions:* Capozide should not be used in patients with aortic stenosis or outflow tract obstruction.

*Warnings*
*Haematological:* Neutropenia/agranulocytosis, thrombocytopenia and anaemia have been reported in patients receiving captopril.

In patients with normal renal function and no other complicating factors, neutropenia occurs rarely.

Captopril should not be used routinely in patients with pre-existing impaired renal function, collagen vascular disease, immunosuppressant therapy, treatment with allopurinol or procainamide, or a combination of these complicating factors. Some of these patients developed serious infections which in a few instances did not respond to intensive antibiotic therapy.

During treatment, all patients should be instructed to report any sign of infection (e.g. persistent sore throat, fever), when a differential white blood cell count should be performed. Capozide and other concomitant medication should be withdrawn if neutropenia (neutrophils less than 1000/mm³) is detected or suspected.

In most patients neutrophil counts rapidly returned to normal upon discontinuing captopril.

*Renal:* Proteinuria is a rare complication of captopril therapy.

Some patients with renal disease, particularly those with bilateral renal artery stenoses or unilateral renal artery stenoses in a single functioning kidney, have developed increased concentrations of blood urea and serum creatinine. Discontinuation of Capozide may be required.

Recent clinical observations have shown a high incidence of anaphylactoid-like reactions during haemodialysis with high-flux dialysis membranes (e.g. AN69) in patients receiving ACE inhibitors (See 'Contra-indications').

*Hepatic:* Capozide should be used with caution in patients with impaired hepatic function or progressive liver disease because of the known risks associated with alterations in fluid and electrolyte balance resulting from thiazide treatment in such patients.

*Electrolyte imbalance:* Patients receiving Capozide, should be observed for clinical signs of thiazide-induced fluid or electrolyte imbalance. In such patients periodic determinations of serum electrolytes should be performed. Because captopril reduces the production of aldosterone, its combination with hydrochlorothiazide may minimise diuretic-induced hypokalaemia. However, some patients may still require potassium supplements. Potassium-sparing diuretics should not be used in conjunction with Capozide.

*Nursing mothers:* Capozide should not be used in nursing mothers.

*Surgery/anaesthesia:* In patients undergoing major surgery, or during anaesthesia with agents which produce hypotension, captopril will block angiotensin II formation secondary to compensatory renin release. This may lead to hypotension which can be corrected by volume expansion.

Thiazides may decrease the arterial response to noradrenaline. In emergency surgery, pre-anaesthetic and anaesthetic agents should be administered in reduced doses. Thiazides may increase the response to tubocurarine.

*Metabolic disorders:* Hyperuricaemia may occur, or frank gout be precipitated by thiazides in certain patients. Insulin requirements in diabetic patients may be altered by thiazides and latent diabetes mellitus may emerge. The captopril component of Capozide has been shown to ameliorate these effects of thiazides.

*Clinical chemistry:* Capozide may cause a false-positive urine test for acetone.

*Side-effects*
*Haematological:* With captopril, neutropenia, anaemia and thrombocytopenia have been reported (see 'Warnings').

With thiazides, leucopenia, agranulocytosis, thrombocytopenia and aplastic anaemia have occurred.

*Renal:* Proteinuria, elevated blood urea and creatinine, elevated serum potassium and acidosis (see 'Warnings').

*Cardiovascular:* Hypotension has been reported in volume depleted patients. Tachycardia.

*Skin:* With captopril, rashes, usually pruritic, may occur. They are usually mild, transient and maculopapular, rarely urticarial. In a few cases the rash has been associated with fever and some patients have developed angio-neurotic oedema. Pruritus, flushing, vesicular rash, and photosensitivity have been reported.

With thiazides, purpura, photosensitivity, rash, urticaria, necrotising angiitis, Stevens-Johnson syndrome and other hypersensitivity reactions have been observed.

*Gastro-intestinal:* Reversible and usually self-limiting taste impairment has been reported. Weight loss may be associated with the loss of taste. Stomatitis, resembling aphthous ulcers, has been reported. Elevation of liver enzymes has been noted in a few patients receiving captopril. Rare cases of hepatocellular injury and cholestatic jaundice have been reported. Gastric irritation and abdominal pain may occur. Pancreatitis has been reported rarely in patients treated with ACE Inhibitors; in some cases this has proved fatal.

*Other:* Paraesthesias of the hands, serum sickness, cough, bronchospasm and lymphadenopathy have been reported.

With thiazides, dizziness, vertigo, headache, xanthopsia, hyperglycaemia, hypokalaemia, glycosuria, hyperuricaemia, hypercalcaemia, muscle spasm, weakness and restlessness have been reported.

*Overdosage:* In the event of overdosage, blood pressure should be monitored and if hypotension develops volume expansion is the treatment of choice.

Captopril is removed by dialysis.

*Drug interactions: Diuretics:* Potassium-sparing diuretics (triamterene, amiloride and spironolactone), or potassium supplements may cause significant increase in serum potassium. *Indomethacin:* A reduction of anti-hypertensive effectiveness may occur. This is probably also the case with other non-steroidal anti-inflammatory drugs. *Vasodilators:* Capozide has been reported to act synergistically with peripheral vasodilators such as minoxidil. This may improve blood pressure control, and awareness of this interaction may avert an initial hypotensive response. *Clonidine:* It has been suggested that the anti-hypertensive effect of captopril can be delayed whe patients treated with clonidine are changed to Capoz ide. *Allopurinol and procainamide:* There have bee reports of neutropenia and/or Stevens-Johnson syn drome in patients on captopril plus either allopurin or procainamide. Although a causal relationship ha not been established, these combinations should onl be used with caution, especially in patients wit impaired renal function. *Immunosuppressants:* Aza thioprine and cyclophosphamide have been assoc ated with blood dyscrasias in patients with rena failure who were also taking captopril. *Probeneci* The renal clearance of captopril is reduced in th presence of probenecid.

**Pharmaceutical precautions** Do not store above 30° (86°F). Keep bottles tightly closed to protect th contents from moisture.

**Legal category** POM.

**Package quantities** Capozide: Calendar packs of 2 tablets (OP).

**Further information** Capozide is designed to ai drug compliance by providing a convenient once dail preparation of captopril combined with hydrochlor thiazide for the treatment of mild to moderate hype tension. Significant anti-hypertensive activity i detectable throughout a 24 hour period following ora therapy.

By combining lower doses than might be require if each component were used alone, side effect especially the hypokalaemia associated with diuretic can be minimised.

**Product licence number**
Capozide Tablets 50 mg/25 mg 0034/0263

## CAPOZIDE* LS TABLETS

**Qualitative and quantitative compostiion** Eac tablet contains: Captopril 25 mg and Hydrochlorothia zide 12.5 mg.

**Pharmaceutical form** Tablets.

**Clinical particulars**

*Therapeutic indications:* For the treatment of mild t moderate hypertension in patients who have bee stabilised on the individual components given in th same proportions. Capozide LS is particularly suitab for older patients and others requiring lower doses c the components.

*Posology and method of administration:*
*Adults including the elderly:* One tablet daily.

*Children:* Safety and effectiveness of Capozide L have not been established.

*Patients with renal failure:* Capozide LS is no recommended for use in patients with significar renal impairment.

*Contra-indications:* Capozide LS is contra indicated i patients with anuria or hypersensitivity to captopr thiazides, or any sulphonamide derived drug.

*Pregnancy:* Captopril has been shown to be lethal t rabbit and sheep foetuses. There were no foetotox effects to hamster or rat foetuses.

Capozide ls is contra indicated in pregnancy an should not be used in women of child bearing potenti unless protected by effective contraception.

Exposure of the mother in the second and thir trimesters of pregnancy has been associated wit oligohydramnios and neonatal hypertension and c anuria.

*Special warnings and special precautions for use:*
*Precautions:* Capozide LS should not be used i patients with aortic stenosis or outflow tract obstru tion.

*Warnings:*
*Haematological:* Neutropenia agranulocytosis, throm bocytopenia and anaemia have been reported i patients receiving captopril.

In patients with normal renal function and no othe complicating factors, neutropenia occurs rarely.

Captopril should not be used routinely in patien with pre existing impaired renal function, collage vascular disease, immunosuppressant therapy, trea ment with allopurinol or procainamide, or a comb nation of these complicating factors. Some of thes patients developed serious infections which in a fe instances did not respond to intensive antibiot therapy.

During treatment, all patients should be instructe to report any sign of infection (e.g. persistent so throat, fever), when a differential white blood ce count should be performed. Capozide LS and othe concomitant medication should be withdrawn if ne tropenia (neutrophils less than 1000 mm³) is detecte or suspected.

In most patients neutrophil counts rapidly returne to normal upon discontinuing captopril.

*Renal:* Proteinuria is a rare complication of captopril therapy.

Some patients with renal disease, particularly those with bilateral renal artery stenoses or unilateral renal artery stenoses in a single functioning kidney, have developed increased concentrations of blood urea and serum creatinine. Discontinuation of Capozide LS may be required.

*Renal:* Recent clinical observations have shown a high incidence of anaphylactoid like reactions during haemodialysis with high flux dialysis membranes, (e.g. AN69) in patients receiving ACE Inhibitors (see *Contra indications*).

*Hepatic:* Capozide LS should be used with caution in patients with impaired hepatic function or progressive liver disease because of the known risks associated with alterations in fluid and electrolyte balance resulting from thiazide treatment in such patients.

*Electrolyte imbalance:* Patients receiving Capozide LS should be observed for clinical signs of thiazide induced fluid or electrolyte imbalance. In such patients periodic determinations of serum electrolytes should be performed. Because captopril reduces the production of aldosterone, its combination with hydrochlorothiazide may minimise diuretic induced hypokalaemia. However, some patients may still require potassium supplements. Potassium sparing diuretics should not be used in conjunction with Capozide LS.

*Surgery anaesthesia:* In patients undergoing major surgery, or during anaesthesia with agents which produce hypotension, captopril will block angiotensin IIformation secondary to compensatory renin release. This may lead to hypotension which can be corrected by volume expansion.

Thiazides may decrease the arterial response to noradrenaline. In emergency surgery, pre anaesthetic and anaesthetic agents should be administered in reduced doses. Thiazides may increase the response to tubocurarine.

*Metabolic disorders:* Hyperuricaemia may occur, or frank gout be precipitated by thiazides in certain patients. Insulin requirements in diabetic patients may be altered by thiazides and latent diabetes mellitus may emerge. The captopril component of Capozide LS has been shown to ameliorate these effects of thiazides.

*Clinical chemistry:* Capozide LS may cause a false positive urine test for acetone.

*Interactions with other medicaments and other forms of interaction:*

Diuretics: Potassium sparing diuretics (triamterene, amiloride and spironolactone), or potassium supplements may cause significant increase in serum potassium.

Indomethacin: A reduction of anti hypertensive effectiveness may occur. This is probably also the case with other non steroidal anti inflammatory drugs.

Vasodilators: Capozide LS has been reported to act synergistically with peripheral vasodilators such as minoxidil. This may improve blood pressure control and awareness of this interaction may avert an initial hypotensive response.

Clonidine: It has been suggested that the anti hypertensive effect of captopril can be delayed when patients treated with clonidine are changed to Capozide LS.

Allopurinol and procainamide: There have been reports of neutropenia and or Stevens Johnson syndrome in patients on captopril plus either allopurinol or procainamide. Although a causal relationship has not been established, these combinations should only be used with caution, especially in patients with impaired renal function.

Immunosuppressants: Azathioprine and cyclophosphamide have been associated with blood dyscrasias in patients with renal failure who were also taking captopril.

Probenecid: The renal clearance of captopril is reduced in the presence of probenecid.

*Pregnancy and lactation:* Captopril has been shown to be lethal to rabbit and sheep foetuses. There were no foetotoxic effects to hamster or rat foetuses.

Capozide LS is contra indicated in pregnancy and should not be used in women of child bearing potential unless protected by effective contraception.

Exposure of the mother in the second and third trimesters of pregnancy has been associated with oligohydramnios and neonatal hypertension and or anuria.

Capozide LS should not be used in nursing mothers.

*Effects on ability to drive and use machines:* Not applicable.

*Undesirable effects:*
*Haematological:* With captopril, neutropenia, anaemia and thrombocytopenia have been reported (see *Warnings*).

With thiazides, leucopenia, agranulocytosis, thrombocytopenia and aplastic anaemia have occurred.

*Renal:* Proteinuria, elevated blood urea and creatinine, elevated serum potassium and acidosis. (see *Warnings*)

*Cardiovascular:* Hypotension has been reported in volume depleted patients. Tachycardia.

*Skin:* With captopril, rashes, usually pruritic, may occur. They are usually mild, transient and maculopapular, rarely urticarial. In a few cases the rash has been associated with fever and some patients have developed angio neurotic oedema. Pruritus, flushing, vesicular rash, and photosensitivity have been reported.

With thiazides, purpura, photosensitivity, rash, urticaria, necrotising angiitis, Stevens Johnson syndrome and other hypersensitivity reactions have been observed.

*Gastrointestinal:* Reversible and usually self limiting taste impairment has been reported. Weight loss may be associated with the loss of taste. Stomatitis, resembling aphthous ulcers, has been reported. Elevation of liver enzymes has been noted in a few patients receiving captopril. Rare cases of hepatocellular injury and cholestatic jaundice have been reported. Gastric irritation and abdominal pain may occur. Pancreatitis has been reported rarely in patients treated with ACE Inhibitors; in some cases this has proved fatal.

*Other:* Paraesthesias of the hands, serum sickness, cough, bronchospasm and lymphadenopathy have been reported.

With thiazides, dizziness, vertigo, headache, xanthopsia, hyperglycaemia, hypokalaemia, glycosuria, hyperuricaemia, hypercalcaemia, muscle spasm, weakness and restlessness have been reported.

*Overdose:* In the event of overdosage, blood pressure should be monitored and if hypotension develops volume expansion is the treatment of choice.

Captopril is removed by dialysis.

**Pharmacological properties**

*Pharmacodynamic properties:* Captopril inhibits angiotension converting enzyme which is responsible for the conversion of Angiotensin I to the pressor substance Angiotensin II.

Hydrochloride is a diuretic which increases the excretion of sodium and chloride ions. The resulting fall in blood pressure and blood volume results in an increase in angiotension II levels which tend to reduce the hypotensive effect.

*Pharmacokinetic properties:*
Captopril: After oral administration of therapeutic doses of captopril rapid absorption occurs with peak blood levels at about one hour. Average minimal absorption is approximately 75%. In a 24 hour period over 95% of the absorbed dose is eliminated in the urine; 40 to 50% is unchanged drug; most of the remainder is the disulphide dimer of captopril and captopril cysteine disulphide.

Approximately 25 to 30% of the circulating drug is bound to plasma proteins. The apparent elimination half life for total radioactivity in blood is probably less than 3 hours. An accurate determination of half life of unchanged captopril is not, at present, possible but it is probably less than 2 hours. In patients with renal impairment, however, retention of captopril occurs (see posology and method of administration).

*Hydrochlorothiazide:* The mean plasma half life of hydrochlorothiazide in fasted individuals has been reported to be approximately 2.5 hours. Onset of diuresis occurs in 2 hours and the peak effect at about 4 hours. Its action persists for approximately 6 to 12 hours. Hydrochlorothiazide is eliminated rapidly by the kidney.

**Pharmaceutical particulars**

*List of excipients:* Lactose, magnesium stearate, maize starch, microcrystalline cellulose, stearic acid.

*Incompatibilities:* None.

*Shelf life:* 36 months.

*Special precautions for storage:* Store below 30°C. Protect from moisture

*Nature and contents of container:*
PVC/PVDC Blister
Foil strips

*Instructions for use/handling:* No special instructions.

**Marketing authorisation number**  0034 0279

**Date of approval/revision of SPC**  March 1995

**Legal category**  POM

## ECONACORT* CREAM

**Presentation**  White cream containing 1% w/w econazole nitrate and 1% w/w hydrocortisone.

Other ingredients: Benzoic acid, butylated hydroxyanisole, liquid paraffin, ethoxylated oleic acid glycerides, stearate esters of ethylene glycol and polyoxyethylene glycol, water.

**Uses**  *Actions:* Econazole nitrate is a broad spectrum antifungal and antibiotic agent, active against dermatophytes (*Trichophyton rubrum, Trichophyton mentagrophytes, Epidermophyton floccosum* and *Malassezia furfur*); pathogenic yeasts; *Candida albicans* and other *Candida* species. It is also active against Gram-positive bacteria.

Hydrocortisone is a widely used topical anti-inflammatory agent of value in the treatment of inflammatory skin conditions including atopic and infantile eczema, contact sensitivity reactions and intertrigo.

*Indications:* Econacort is indicated for the topical treatment of inflammatory dermatoses where infection by susceptible organisms co-exist.

**Dosage and administration**
*Adults and children:* To be massaged gently into the affected and surrounding skin area morning and evening. The cream is particularly suitable for moist and weeping lesions.

*Elderly:* Natural thinning of the skin occurs in the elderly, hence corticosteroids should be used sparingly and for short periods of time.

**Contra-indications, warnings, etc**
*Contra-indications:* Hypersensitivity to either of the active ingredients.

In tuberculous and most viral lesions of the skin, particularly herpes simplex, vaccinia and varicella.

Should not be used for facial rosacea, acne vulgaris and perioral dermatitis.

*Precautions:* Econacort cream should not be used in or near the eyes.

If used in infants and children, or on the face, courses should be limited to 5 days and occlusion should not be used.

*Pregnancy:* Topical administration of corticosteroids to pregnant animals can cause abnormalities of foetal development including cleft palate and intra-uterine growth retardation. There may, therefore, be a very small risk of such effects in the human foetus.

*Side-effects:* Econazole nitrate and hydrocortisone are well tolerated. Where adverse reactions occur they are usually reversible on cessation of therapy.

Side-effects of econazole nitrate are limited to occasional local irritation manifested by erythema, burning or stinging sensation, and pruritis, but these may be minimised by the hydrocortisone component.

The possibility of the systemic effects which are associated with all steroid therapy should be considered. These effects may be enhanced with occlusive dressings.

*Overdosage:* Topically applied corticosteroids can be absorbed in sufficient amounts to produce systemic effects.

In the event of accidental ingestion, the patient should be observed and treated symptomatically.

**Pharmaceutical precautions**  Store below 25°C. Avoid freezing.

**Legal category**  POM.

**Package quantities**  Tubes of 30 g (OP).

**Further information**  Nil.

**Product licence number**  0034/0249.

## ECOSTATIN* CREAM

**Presentation**
Ecostatin Cream is a white, vanishing-type cream containing 1% w/w econazole nitrate in a cream base.

Other ingredients: Benzoic acid, butylated hydroxyanisole, liquid paraffin, ethoxylated oleic acid glycerides, stearate esters of ethylene glycol and polyoxyethylene, perfume, water.

**Uses**  *Actions:* Econazole nitrate is a broad spectrum antifungal agent, active against dermatophytes (*Trichophyton rubrum, Trichophyton mentagrophytes, Epidermophyton floccosum* and *Malassezia furfur*); pathogenic yeasts; *Candida albicans* and other *Candida* species. Also active against some Gram-positive bacteria, e.g. staphylococci and streptococci.

**Indications**  All fungal skin infections due to dermatophytes (e.g. *Trichophyton* species), yeasts (e.g. *Candida* species), moulds and other fungi. These include ringworm (tinea) infections, athlete's foot, paronychia, pityriasis versicolor, erythrasma, intertrigo, fungal nappy rash, candidal vulvitis and candidal balanitis. Bacterial skin infections due to Gram-positive organisms.

**Dosage and administration**
*Adults and children:* Ecostatin Cream should be massaged gently into the affected and surrounding skin area morning and evening. The cream is particularly suitable for moist or weeping lesions.

Clinical improvement usually occurs promptly; however, complete disappearance of the symptoms of the disease may require prolonged treatment. Therapy should continue for several days following both clinical and mycological cure in order to prevent relapse.

*Elderly:* No specific dosage recommendations.

**Contra-indications, warnings, etc**
*Contra-indications:* Patients with a history of sensitivity to any of the components of this preparation.

*Precautions:* Ecostatin Cream should not be used in or near the eyes. Avoid contact with diaphragms and condoms.

*Pregnancy:* No specific precautions apply; systemic absorption is likely to be negligible.

*Side-effects:* Ecostatin Cream is well tolerated. Side-effects are limited to occasional local irritation manifested by erythema, burning or stinging sensations and pruritus.

**Pharmaceutical precautions** Ecostatin Cream should be stored below 25°C. Avoid freezing.

**Legal category** P.

**Package quantities** Tubes of 30 g and 15 g (OP).

**Further information** Nil.

**Product licence number** 0034/0231.

## ECOSTATIN* PESSARIES AND TWIN PACK

**Presentation**
*Pessaries:* White, opaque, oval pessaries each containing 150 mg econazole nitrate in an hydrogenated vegetable oil base. 3 pessary treatment pack.

Other ingredients: Hard fat.

*Twin pack:* Three Ecostatin pessaries with applicator plus 15 g Ecostatin Cream (containing 1% w/w econazole nitrate).

The Cream also contains: benzoic acid, butylated hydroxyanisole, liquid paraffin, ethoxylated oleic acid glycerides, stearate esters of ethylene glycol and polyoxyethylene, perfume, water.

**Uses** *Actions:* Econazole nitrate has a broad spectrum of antifungal activity. It is highly active against *Candida albicans* and other *Candida* species and is effective in controlling infections of the vagina and vulva caused by such organisms (thrush).

*Indications:* Vulvovaginal candidosis. In addition to vaginal treatment the Twin Pack contains cream for topical application to the anogenital area.

**Dosage and administration** *Adults:* Pessaries: One pessary to be inserted at bedtime for three consecutive nights. Administration should be continued even if menstruation occurs and despite the disappearance of signs and symptoms of the infection.

The pessary should be inserted high into the vagina while the patient is supine.

*Cream:* The cream is applied twice daily, in the morning and evening, to the anogenital area.

*Note:* To prevent re-infection with *Candida*, the male consort should be treated concurrently with Ecostatin Cream, applied twice daily to the external genital area during the treatment period.

Although a three day course of therapy usually suffices, it may be necessary to institute a second course of therapy.

*Children:* Vulvovaginal candidosis is not normally a problem in children, therefore there are no specific dosage recommendations.

*Elderly:* No specific dosage recommendations or precautions apply.

**Contra-indications, warnings, etc**
*Contra-indications:* Patients with a history of sensitivity to any of the components of this preparation.

*Precautions:* Avoid contact between contraceptive diaphragms and condoms and this product since the rubber may be damaged by the preparation.

*Pregnancy:* Ecostatin pessaries are effective in the candidal vaginitis associated with pregnancy. Safety of systemic econazole has not been established but percutaneous absorption following topical application is likely to be low. However, as with other agents, Ecostatin should not be used during the first trimester of pregnancy unless the physician deems its use essential for the welfare of the patient. In pregnancy, extra care should be taken in using an applicator to prevent the possibility of mechanical trauma.

*Side-effects:* Patients may rarely complain of discomfort; this is usually transitory and disappears with continued treatment. Seldom is it necessary to discontinue econazole pessary treatment.

Ecostatin Cream is well tolerated. Side-effects are limited to occasional local irritation manifested by erythema, burning or stinging sensation, and pruritus.

**Pharmaceutical precautions** *Storage:* Store below 25°C.

**Legal category** Cream P.
Pessaries POM.

**Package quantities** *Pessaries:* Pack of three pessaries with applicator (OP).
*Twin pack:* Three pessaries with applicator plus 15 g cream (OP).

**Further information** Nil.

**Product licence numbers**
Ecostatin Pessaries    0034/0233
Ecostatin Cream        0034/0231

## ECOSTATIN* -1 PESSARY

**Qualitative and quantitative composition** Ecostatin-1 Pessary contains Econazole Nitrate 150 mg.

**Pharmaceutical form** Pessary

**Clinical particulars**
*Therapeutic indications:* The treatment of vaginitis due to *Candida albicans* and other yeasts.

*Posology and method of administration:*
*Adults:* The recommended dose is one pessary inserted at bedtime. The pessary should be inserted as high as possible into the vagina, using the applicator, with the patient in the supine position.

Although one course of therapy usually suffices, it may be necessary to institute a second course of therapy.

*Elderly:* No specific dosage recommendations or precautions apply.

*Children:* Vulvovaginal candidosis is not normally a problem in children, therefore there are no specific dosage recommendations.

*Contra-indications:* Patients with a known history of sensitivity to any of the components of the preparation.

*Special warnings and special precautions for use:* Avoid contact between this product and contraceptive diaphragms and condoms since the rubber may be damaged by the preparation. To prevent re-infection with *Candida*, the male consort should be treated concurrently with Ecostatin Cream. Although one course of therapy usually suffices, it may be necessary to institute a second course of therapy.

*Interactions with other medicaments and other forms of interaction:* None known.

*Pregnancy and lactation:* Ecostatin-1 Pessaries are effective in the candidal vaginitis associated with pregnancy. Safety of systemic econazole has not been established but percutaneous absorption following topical application is likely to be low. However, as with other agents, Ecostatin should not be used during the first trimester of pregnancy unless the physician deems its use essential for the welfare of the patient. In pregnancy, extra care should be taken in using an applicator, to prevent the possibility of mechanical trauma.

*Effects on ability to drive and use machines:* None known.

*Undesirable effects:* Patients may rarely complain of transitory discomfort.

*Overdose:* There have been no recorded cases of overdose.

**Pharmacological properties**
*Pharmacodynamic properties:* Econazole nitrate has a broad spectrum of antifungal activity. It is highly active against *Candida albicans* and other *Candida* species and is effective in controlling infections of the vagina and vulva caused by such organisms (thrush).

*Pharmacokinetic properties:* Not applicable.

**Pharmaceutical particulars**
*List of excipients:* Colloidal silicon dioxide, hard fat, natural polysaccharides, stearyl heptanoate.

*Incompatibilities:* None known.

*Shelf life:* 60 months.

*Special precautions for storage:* Store below 25°C.

*Nature and contents of container:* Pre-formed PVC mould packed in a cardboard carton. The carton includes an applicator with directions for use.

*Instructions for use/handling:* No special instructions apply.

**Marketing authorisation number** 0034/0266

**Date of approval/revision of SPC** January 1997

**Legal category** POM

## FLORINEF* TABLETS

**Presentation** Round, pale pink tablets, scored on one side and engraved Squibb and 429 on reverse, containing 0.1 mg fludrocortisone acetate.

Other ingredients: Dicalcium phosphate, erythrosin, lactose, magnesium stearate, maize starch, sodium benzoate, talc.

**Uses** *Actions:* Qualitatively, the physiological action of fludrocortisone acetate is similar to hydrocortisone. In very small doses, fludrocortisone maintains life in adrenalectomised animals, enhances the deposition of liver glycogen and produces thymic involution, eosinopenia, retention of sodium and increased urinary excretion of potassium.

*Indications:* For partial replacement therapy for primary and secondary adrenocortical insufficiency in Addison's disease and for the treatment of salt-losing adrenogenital syndrome.

**Dosage and administration**
*Adult dosage:* A daily dosage range of 0.05–0.3 mg Florinef tablets orally. Supplementary parenteral administration of sodium-retaining hormones is not necessary. When an enhanced glucocorticoid effect is desirable, cortisone or hydrocortisone by mouth should be given concomitantly with Florinef tablets.

*Children:* May be used adjusted to the age and weight of the child according to the severity of the condition (see 'Precautions').

*Elderly:* No specific dosage recommendations or precautions.

**Contra-indications, warnings, etc**
*Contra-indications:* Hypersensitivity to any of the ingredients.

Systemic infections unless specific anti-infective therapy is employed.

Because of its marked effect on sodium retention, the use of Florinef in the treatment of conditions other than those indicated, is not advised.

Since Florinef is a potent mineralocorticoid both the dosage and salt intake should be carefully monitored to avoid the development of hypertension, oedema or weight gain. Periodic checking of serum electrolyte levels is advisable during prolonged therapy.

*Precautions:* Florinef is a potent mineralocorticoid and is used predominantly for replacement therapy. Although glucocorticoid side effects may occur, these can be reduced by reducing the dosage.

Undesirable effects may be minimised using the lowest effective dose for the minimum period. Frequent patient review is required to titrate the dose appropriately against disease activity (see Dosage section).

Adrenal cortical atrophy develops during prolonged therapy and may persist for years after stopping treatment. Withdrawal of corticosteroids after prolonged therapy must, therefore, always be gradual to avoid acute adrenal insufficiency and should be tapered off over weeks or months according to the dose and duration of treatment. Patients on long-term systemic therapy with Florinef may require supportive corticosteroid therapy in times of stress (such as trauma, surgery or severe illness) both during the treatment period and up to a year afterwards. If corticosteroids have been stopped following prolonged therapy they may need to be reintroduced temporarily.

Patients should carry steroid treatment cards which give clear guidance on the precautions to be taken to minimise risk and which provides details of prescriber, drug, dosage and the duration of treatment.

*Anti-inflammatory/immunosuppressive effects:* Suppression of the inflammatory response and immune function increases the susceptibility to infections and their severity. The clinical presentation may often be atypical and serious infections such as septicaemia and tuberculosis may be masked and may reach an advanced stage before being recognised.

Chickenpox is of particular concern since this normally minor illness may be fatal in immunosuppressed patients. Patients (or parents of children receiving Florinef tablets) without a definite history of chickenpox should be advised to avoid close personal contact with chickenpox or herpes zoster. If exposed they should seek urgent medical attention. Passive immunisation with varicella zoster immunoglobulin (VZIG) is needed by exposed non-immune patients who are receiving systemic corticosteroids or who have used them within the previous 3 months; this should be given within 10 days of exposure to chickenpox. If a diagnosis of chickenpox is confirmed the illness warrants specialist care and urgent treatment. Corticosteroids should not be stopped and the dose may need to be increased.

During corticosteroid therapy antibody response will be reduced and therefore affect the patient's response to vaccines. Live vaccines should not be administered.

*Special precautions:* Particular care is required when

considering use of systemic corticosteroids in patients with the following conditions and frequent patient monitoring is necessary.

Recent intestinal anastomoses, diverticulitis, thrombophlebitis, existing or previous history of severe affective disorders (especially previous steroid psychosis), exanthematous disease, chronic nephritis, or renal insufficiency, metastatic carcinoma, osteoporosis (post-menopausal females are particularly at risk); in patients with an active peptic ulcer (or a history of peptic ulcer). Myasthenia gravis. Latent or healed tuberculosis; in the presence of local or systemic viral infection, systemic fungal infections or in active infections not controlled by antibiotics. In acute psychoses; in acute glomerulonephritis. Hypertension; congestive heart failure; glaucoma (or a family history of glaucoma), previous steroid myopathy or epilepsy. Liver failure.

Corticosteroid effects may be enhanced in patients with hypothyroidism or cirrhosis.

Diabetes may be aggravated, necessitating a higher insulin dosage. Latent diabetes mellitus may be precipitated.

Menstrual irregularities may occur, and this possibility should be mentioned to female patients.

Rare instances of anaphylactoid reactions have occurred in patients receiving corticosteroids, especially when a patient has a history of drug allergies.

Aspirin should be used cautiously in conjunction with corticosteroids in patients with hypoprothrombinaemia.

*Children:* Growth and development of children on prolonged corticosteroid therapy should be carefully observed. Corticosteroids cause dose-related growth retardation in infancy, childhood and adolescence which may be irreversible.

*Elderly:* The common adverse effects on systemic corticosteroids may be associated with more serious consequences in old age, especially osteoporosis, hypertension, hypokalaemia, diabetes, susceptibility to infection and thinning of the skin. Close clinical supervision is required to avoid life-threatening reactions.

*Pregnancy and nursing mothers:* It may be decided to continue a pregnancy in a woman requiring replacement mineralocorticoid therapy, despite the risk to the foetus. When corticosteroids are essential however, patients with normal pregnancies may be treated as though they were in the non-gravid state.

There is evidence of harmful effects in pregnancy in animals. There may be a small risk of cleft palate and intra-uterine growth retardation. Hypoadrenalism may occur in the neonate. Patients with pre-eclampsia or fluid retention require close monitoring.

Corticosteroids are found in breast milk.

Infants born of mothers who have received substantial doses of corticosteroids during pregnancy or during breast feeding should be carefully observed for signs of hypoadrenalism. Maternal treatment should be carefully documented in the infant's medical records to assist in follow up.

*Drug interactions:* Barbiturates, phenytoin, rifampicin, rifabutin, carbamazepine, primidone and aminoglutethimide may enhance the metabolic clearance of corticosteroids, resulting in decreased therapeutic effects.

Corticosteroids antagonise the effects of hypoglycaemic agents (including insulin), anti-hypertensives and diuretics. The hypokalaemic effects of acetazolamide, loop diuretics, thiazide diuretics and carbenoxolone are enhanced.

The efficacy of coumarin anticoagulants may be enhanced by concurrent corticosteroid therapy and close monitoring of the INR or prothombin time is required to avoid spontaneous bleeding.

The renal clearance of salicylates is increased by corticosteroids and steroid withdrawal may result in salicylate intoxication.

*Side-effects:* Where adverse reactions occur they are usually reversible on cessation of therapy. The incidence of predictable side-effects, including hypothalamic-pituitary-adrenal suppression correlate with the relative potency of the drug, dosage, timing of administration and duration of treatment (see Warnings and Precautions).

Patients should be watched closely for the following adverse reactions which may be associated with any corticosteroid therapy.

*Anti-inflammatory and immunosuppressive effects:* Increased susceptibility and severity of infections with suppression of clinical symptoms and signs, opportunistic infections, recurrence of dormant tuberculosis (see Warnings and Precautions).

*Fluid and electrolyte disturbances:* sodium retention, fluid retention, congestive heart failure in susceptible patients, potassium loss, cardiac arrhythmias or ECG changes due to potassium deficiency, hypokalaemic alkalosis, increased calcium excretion and hypertension.

*Musculoskeletal:* muscle weakness, fatigue, steroid myopathy, loss of muscle mass, osteoporosis, avascular osteonecrosis, vertebral compression fractures, delayed healing of fractures, aseptic necrosis of femoral and humeral heads, pathological fractures of long bones and spontaneous fractures, tendon rupture.

*Gastrointestinal:* dyspepsia, peptic ulcer with possible subsequent perforation and haemorrhage, pancreatitis, abdominal distension and ulcerative oesophagitis, candidiasis.

*Dermatologic:* impaired wound healing, thin fragile skin, petechiae and ecchymoses, facial erythema, increased sweating, purpura, striae, hirsutism, acneiform eruptions, lupus erythematous-like lesions and suppressed reactions to skin tests.

*Neurological:* euphoria, psychological dependence, depression, insomnia, convulsions, increased intracranial pressure with papilloedema (pseudo-tumour cerebri) usually after treatment, vertigo, headache, neuritis or paraesthesias and aggravation of pre-existing psychiatric conditions and epilepsy.

*Endocrine/metabolic:* menstrual irregularities and amenorrhoea; development of the Cushingoid state; suppression of growth in childhood and adolescence; secondary adrenocortical and pituitary unresponsiveness, particularly in times of stress (e.g. trauma, surgery or illness); decreased carbohydrate tolerance; manifestations of latent diabetes mellitus and increased requirements for insulin or oral hypoglycaemic agents in diabetes, weight gain. Negative protein and calcium balance. Increased appetite.

*Ophthalmic:* posterior subcapsular cataracts, increased intraocular pressure, glaucoma, exophthalmos, papilloedema, corneal or scleral thinning, exacerbation of ophthalmic viral or fungal diseases.

*Others:* necrotising angiitis, thrombophlebitis, thrombo-embolism, leucocytosis, insomnia, syncopal episodes and anaphylactoid reactions, particularly where there is a history of drug allergies.

*Withdrawal symptoms and signs:* On withdrawal, fever, myalgia, arthralgia, rhinitis, conjunctivitis, painful itchy skin nodules and weight loss may occur. Too rapid a reduction in dose following prolonged treatment can lead to acute adrenal insufficiency, hypotension and death (see Warnings and Precautions).

*Overdosage:* A single large dose should be treated with plenty of water by mouth. Careful monitoring of serum electrolytes is essential, with particular consideration being given to the need for administration of potassium chloride and restriction of dietary sodium intake.

**Pharmaceutical precautions** *Storage:* Below 25°C.

**Legal category** POM.

**Package quantities** Bottles of 56 tablets.

**Further information** Nil.

**Product licence numbers**
Florinef Tablets 0.1 mg 0034/5027R.

# FUNGILIN* LOZENGE
# FUNGILIN* ORAL SUSPENSION
# FUNGILIN* ORAL TABLETS

**Qualitative and quantitative composition**

*Fungilin Lozenge:* Round, pale yellow, engraved '929' and 'Squibb' containing 10,000 units (10 mg) amphotericin.

*Fungilin Oral Suspension:* Orange-flavoured, viscous suspension containing 100,000 units (100 mg) amphotericin per ml.

*Fungilin Oral Tablets:* Yellow to tan, scored one side and engraved 'Squibb' and '430' on reverse, containing 100,000 (100 mg) amphotericin.

**Pharmaceutical form**
Oral Lozenge
Oral Suspension
Oral Tablets.

**Clinical particulars**

***Therapeutic indications:***
*Lozenge/Suspension:* For the treatment of candidal lesions (thrush) of the oral and perioral areas. The suspension may be used in the treatment of denture stomatitis.

*Suspension/Tablets:* For the treatment of intestinal candidosis and the suppression of the intestinal reservoir of *C. albicans* which may precipitate cutaneous or vaginal candidosis.

*Posology and method of administration:*
*Adults:*
*Lozenge:* Dissolve one lozenge slowly in the mouth four times a day. Depending on the severity of infection, the dose may be increased to 8 lozenges daily.

To clear the condition fully may require 10-15 days' treatment.

*Suspension:* For denture stomatitis and oral infections caused by *C. albicans*, 1 ml should be placed in the mouth four times daily; it should be kept in contact with lesions for as long as possible.

For the treatment of suppression of intestinal candidosis, 2 ml four times daily.

*Tablets:* 1 or 2 tablets four times daily.

Administration of Fungilin for oral and intestinal candidosis should be continued for 48 hours after clinical cure to prevent relapse.

*Infants and children:*
*Lozenge:* Not recommended
*Suspension:* For intestinal and oral candidosis, 1 ml should be dropped into the mouth four times daily. The suspension should be held in contact with oral lesions for as long as possible before swallowing.

For prophylaxis in the newborn, the suggested dose is 1 ml daily.

*Tablets:* Not recommended

*Elderly:* No specific dosage recommendations or precautions.

*Contra-indications:* There are no known contra-indications to the use of these products.

*Special warnings and special precautions for use:* No specific warnings or precautions apply.

*Interactions with other medicaments and other forms of interaction:* None known.

*Pregnancy and lactation:* No special precautions apply; absorption of amphotericin from the gastro-intestinal tract is negligible.

*Effects on ability to drive and use machines:* Not applicable.

*Undesirable effects:* Gastro-intestinal side-effects have occasionally been reported following continuous administration of amphotericin for several months in daily doses in excess of 3 g. These have been mild in nature and have readily cleared on cessation of treatment. No systemic toxic effects or allergic reactions have been associated with its oral use.

*Overdose:* Since absorption of amphotericin from the gastro-intestinal tract is negligible, overdosage causes no systemic toxicity.

**Pharmacological properties**

*Pharmacodynamic properties:*
*Actions:* Amphotericin is an antifungal antibiotic active against a wide range of yeasts and yeast-like fungi including *Candida albicans*. Extensive clinical experience has not shown problems of toxicity or sensitisation.

*Pharmacokinetic properties:* Absorption from the gastro-intestinal tract is negligible even with very large doses.

*Preclinical safety data:* No further relevant information.

**Pharmaceutical particulars**

*List of excipients:*
*Lozenge:* Acacia powder, d-mannitol, flavours, magnesium stearate, polyvinyl alcohol, talc.

*Suspension:* Citric acid, ethanol, flavours, glycerol, methyl and propyl parahydroxybenzoates, potassium chloride, sodium benzoate, sodium carboxymethylcellulose, sodium phosphate, sodium metabisulphite, water.

*Tablets:* Ethyl cellulose, lactose, maize starch, magnesium stearate, talc.

*Incompatibilities:* None known

*Shelf life:*
*Lozenge:* 18 months
*Suspension:* 48 months
*Tablets:* 24 months

*Special precautions for storage:*
*Lozenge/Tablets:* Store below 25°C.
*Suspension:* Store below 25°C, protect from direct sunlight. Discard any unused suspension 4 days after opening.

*Dilution:* Fungilin Suspension should not be diluted prior to use; it is formulated to coat and adhere to the oral lesions being treated.

*Nature and contents of container:*
*Lozenge:* Aluminium tube, foil or blister pack of 60 lozenges.
*Suspension:* 12 ml bottles with graduated dropper.
*Tablets:* Bottles of 56 tablets.

*Instructions for use/handling:* No special handling instructions.

**Marketing authorisation numbers**
Lozenge: 0034/5034R
Suspension: 0034/5038R
Tablets: 0034/5039R

**Date of approval/revision of SPC**
Lozenge: November 1995
Suspension/Tablets January 1996

**Legal category** POM

## FUNGIZONE* INTRAVENOUS

**Qualitative and quantitative composition** Each vial contains as a yellow, fluffy powder: amphotericin 50,000 units (50 mg).

**Pharmaceutical form** Powder for Injection

**Clinical particulars**

*Therapeutic indications:* Fungizone Intravenous should be administered primarily to patients with progressive, potentially fatal infections. This potent drug should not be used to treat the common forms of fungal disease which show only positive skin or serological tests.

Fungizone Intravenous is specifically intended to treat cryptococcosis (torulosis); North American blastomycosis; the disseminated forms of candidosis, coccidioidomycosis and histoplasmosis; mucormycosis (phycomycosis) caused by species of the genera *Mucor, Rhizopus, Absidia, Entomophthora,* and *Basidiobolus* sporotrichosis (*Sporotrichum schenckii*), aspergillosis (*Aspergillus fumigatus*).

Amphotericin may be helpful in the treatment of American mucocutaneous leishmaniasis but is not the drug of choice in primary therapy.

*Posology and method of administration:*
*Adults and children:* Fungizone should be administerd by intravenous infusion over a period of 2-4 hours. Reduction of the infusion rate may reduce the incidence of side-effects. In rare instances infusion times of up to 6 hours may be necessary. Initial daily dose should be 0.25 mg/kg of body weight gradually increasing to a level of 1.0 mg/kg of body weight depending on individual response and tolerance. Within the range of 0.25-1.0 mg/kg the daily dose should be maintained at the highest level which is not accompanied by unacceptable toxicity.

In seriously ill patients the daily dose may be gradually increased up to a total of 1.5 mg/kg. Since amphotericin is excreted slowly, therapy may be given on alternate days in patients on the higher dosage schedule. Several months of therapy are usually necessary; a shorter period of therapy may produce an inadequate response and lead to relapse.

When commencing all new courses of treatment, it is advisable to administer a test dose immediately preceding the first dose. A volume of the infusion containing 1 mg (i.e. 10 ml) should be infused over 20-30 minutes and the patient carefully observed for at least a further 30 minutes. It should be noted that patient responses to the test dose may not be predictive of subsequent severe side effects.

Whenever medication is interrupted for a period longer than seven days, therapy should be resumed by starting with the lowest dosage level, i.e. 0.25 mg/kg of body weight and increased gradually.

*CAUTION:* Under no circumstances should a total daily dose of 1.5 mg/kg be exceeded. The recommended concentration for intravenous infusion is 10 mg/100 ml.

*Elderly:* No specific dosage recommendations or precautions.

*Preparation of solutions:* Reconstitute as follows: An initial concentrate of 5 mg amphotericin per ml is first prepared by rapidly expressing 10 ml sterile water for injection, without a bacteriostatic agent, directly into the lyophilized cake, using a sterile needle (minimum diameter: 20 gauge) and syringe. Shake the vial immediately until the colloidal solution is clear. The infusion solution, providing 10 mg/100 ml is obtained by further dilution (1:50) with 5% Glucose Injection of pH above 4.2. The pH of each container of Glucose Injection should be ascertained before use. Commercial Glucose Injection usually has a pH above 4.2; however, if it is below 4.2 then 1 or 2 ml of buffer should be added to the Glucose Injection before it is used to dilute a concentrated solution of amphotericin. The recommended buffer has the following composition:

Dibasic sodium phosphate (anhydrous) 1.59 g
Monobasic sodium phosphate (anhydrous) 0.96 g
Water for Injections BP q.s. to 100 ml

The buffer should be sterilised before it is added to the Glucose Injection, either by filtration through a bacterial filter, or by autoclaving for 30 mins at 15lb pressure (121°C).

*CAUTION:* Aseptic technique must be strictly observed in all handling, since no preservative or bacteriostatic agent is present. Do not reconstitute with saline solutions. The use of any diluent other than the ones recommended or the presence of a bacteriostatic agent in the diluent may cause precipitation of the amphotericin. Do not use the initial concentrate or the infusion solution if there is any evidence of precipitation of foreign matter.

An in-line membrane filter may be used for intravenous infusion of amphotericin; however the mean pore diameter of the filter should not be less than 1.0 micron in order to assure passage of the amphotericin dispersion.

Other preparations for injection should not be added to the infusion solution or administered via the cannula being used to administer Fungizone Intravenous.

The use of Fungizone Intravenous by other routes has been documented in the published literature:

*Bladder irrigation/instillation (e.g. candiduria):* Continuous irrigation with 50 mg Fungizone in 1 litre sterile water each day until urinary cultures are negative. Intermittent use of volumes of 100-400 ml (concentrations of 37.5-200 mcg/ml) has also been reported. The urine should be alkalinized (with potassium citrate) and antifungal ointment applied to the perineal area.

*Lung inhalation (e.g. pulmonary aspergillosis):* 8-40 mg amphotericin (nebulized in sterile water or 5% Glucose) has been given daily in divided doses. Concurrent eradication of oral and intestinal yeast reservoirs is recommended.

*Intrathecal (e.g. coccidiodal meningitis):* Current published dosage recommendations are for maintenance 0.25-1.0 mg amphotericin 2-4 times weekly following intitiation with a low dose (0.025 mg) and cautious increases. Amphotericin is irritating when injected into the CSF.

*Other:* Other uses of solutions prepared using Fungizone Intravenous include local instillations for the treatment of fungal infections of the ear, eye, peritoneum, lung cavities and joint spaces.

*Contra-indications:* Those patients who are hypersensitive to amphotericin, unless, in the opinion of the physician, the condition requiring treatment is life-threatening and amenable only to such therapy.

*Special warnings and special precautions for use:* Prolonged therapy with amphotericin is usually necessary. Unpleasant reactions are quite common when the drug is given parenterally at therapeutic dosage levels. Some of these reactions are potentially dangerous. Hence amphotericin should be used parenterally only in hospitalised patients, or those under close clinical observation. If BUN or serum creatinine exceeds twice the upper limit of normal the drug should be discontinued or the dosage markedly reduced until renal function is improved. Weekly blood counts and serum potassium determinations are also advisable. Low serum magnesium levels have also been noted during treatment with amphotericin. Therapy should be discontinued if liver function test results (elevated bromsulphalein, alkaline phosphatase and bilirubin) are abnormal.

Leucoencephalopathy has been reported very occasionally following the use of amphotericin injection in patients who received total body irradiation. Most of these patients received high cumulative doses of amphotericin.

Rapid intravenous infusion, over less than one hour, particularly in patients with renal insufficiency, has been associated with hyperkalaemia and arrhythmias and should therefore be avoided.

Corticosteroids should not be administered concomitantly unless they are necessary to control drug reactions. Other nephrotoxic antibiotics and antineoplastic agents should not be given concomitantly except with great caution.

*Interactions with other medicaments and other forms of interaction:* Concomitant administration of nephrotoxic drugs or antineoplastics should be avoided if at all possible.

The hypokalaemia following amphotericin therapy may potentiate the toxicity of digitalis glycosides or enhance the curariform actions of skeletal muscle relaxants.

Corticosteroids may increase the potassium loss due to amphotericin.

Flucytosine toxicity may be enhanced during concomitant administration, possibly due to an increase in its cellular uptake and/or impairment of its renal excretion.

Acute pulmonary reactions have occasionally been observed in patients given amphotericin during or shortly after leukocyte transfusions. It is advisable to separate these infusions as far as possible and to monitor pulmonary function.

*Pregnancy and lactation:* Safety for use in pregnancy has not been established; therefore it should be used during pregnancy only if the possible benefits to be derived outweigh the potential risks involved.

*Effects on ability to drive and use machines:* Not applicable.

*Undesirable effects:* While some patients may tolerate full intravenous doses of amphotericin without difficulty, most will exhibit some intolerance. In patients experiencing adverse reactions these may be made less severe by giving aspirin, antihistamines or anti-emetics. Febrile reactions may be decreased by the intravenous administration of small doses of adrenal corticosteroids, e.g. 25 mg hydrocortisone. This may be administered just prior to or during amphotericin infusion. The dosage and duration of such corticosteroid therapy should be kept to a minimum. Administration of the drug on alternate days may decrease anorexia and phlebitis. Adding a small amount of heparin to the infusion may lessen the incidence of thrombophlebitis and coagulation problems. Extravasation may cause chemical irritation. The adverse reactions that are most commonly observed are: fever (sometimes with shaking chills), headache, anorexia, weight loss, nausea and vomiting, malaise, muscle and joint pains, dyspepsia, cramping epigastric pain, diarrhoea, local venous pain at the injection site with phlebitis and thrombophlebitis, normochromic normocytic anaemia and hypokalaemia. Abnormal renal function including hypokalaemia, azotaemia, hyposthenuria, renal tubular acidosis or nephrocalcinosis, is also commonly observed and usually improves upon interruption of therapy; however, some permanent impairment often occurs, especially in those patients receiving large amounts (over 5 g) of amphotericin.

The following adverse reactions occur less frequently or rarely; anuria (oliguria); cardiovascular toxicity including arrhythmias, ventricular fibrillation, cardiac arrest, hypotension, hypertension; coagulation defects; thrombocytopenia; leucopenia; agranulocytosis; eosinophilia; leucocytosis; melaena or haemorrhagic gastroenteritis; maculopapular rash and pruritus; hearing loss, tinnitus; transient vertigo, blurred vision, or diplopia; encephalopathy (see precautions); peripheral neuropathy, convulsions and other neurologic symptoms; anaphylactoid reactions, acute liver failure and flushing.

*Overdose:* Amphotericin overdoses can result in cardio-respiratory arrest. If an overdose is suspected, discontinue therapy and monitor the patient's clinical status (e.g., cardio-respiratory, renal, and liver function, haematologic status serum electrolytes) and administer supportive therapy as required. Amphotericin is not haemodialysable. Prior to reinstituting therapy, the patient's condition should be stabilised (including correction of electrolyte deficiencies, etc.)

**Pharmacological properties**

*Pharmacodynamic properties:* Amphotericin is a polyene antifungal antibiotic active against a wide range of yeasts and yeast-like fungi including *Candida albicans.* Crystalline amphotericin is insoluble in water; therefore, the antibiotic is solubilised by the addition of sodium desoxycholate to form a mixture which provides a colloidal dispersion for parenteral administration. Amphotericin is fungistatic rather than fungicidal in concentrations obtainable in body fluids. It probably acts by binding to sterols in the fungal cell membrane with a resultant change in membrane permeability which allows leakage of intracellular components. Mammalian cell membranes also contain sterols and it has been suggested that the damage to human and fungal cells may share common mechanisms. No strains of Candida resistant to amphotericin have been reported in clinical use, and although in vitro testing does produce a small number of resistant isolates this occurs only following repeated subcultures.

*Pharmacokinetic properties:* An initial intravenous infusion of 1 to 5 mg of amphotericin per day gradually increased to 0.65 mg/kg daily, produces peak plasma concentrations of approximately 2 to 4 mg/l which can persist between doses since the plasma half-life of amphotericin is about 24 hours. It has been reported that amphotericin is highly bound (more than 90%) to plasma proteins and is poorly dialysable.

Amphotericin is excreted very slowly by the kidney with 2 to 5% of a given dose being excreted in biologically active form. After treatment is discontinued the drug can be detected in the urine for at least seven weeks. The cumulative urinary output over a seven day period amounts to approximately 40% of the amount of drug infused.

Details of tissue distribution and possible metabolic pathways are not known.

*Preclinical safety data:* No further relevant data.

**Pharmaceutical particulars**

*List of excipients:* Other ingredients: sodium desoxycholate and sodium phosphate buffer.

*Incompatibilities:* None known.

*Shelf life:* 24 months

*Special precautions for storage:* Vials of powder for reconstitution should be stored in a refrigerator. The concentrate (5 mg per ml after reconstitution with 10 ml sterile Water for Injections) should be stored protected from light. The absence of any microbial preservative and the risk of contamination during reconstitution mean that the product should be stored for no more than 8 hours at room temperature (25°C) or 24 hours in a refrigerator (2-8°C). Should the need arise and a validated aseptic reconstitution technique is applied, the product is chemically stable when stored for 24 hours at room temperature or one week in a refrigerator. It is not intended as a multidose vial. Any unused material should be discarded. Solutions prepared for intravenous infusion (i.e. 10 mg or less amphotericin per 100 ml) should be used promptly after preparation and should be protected from light during administration.

*Nature and contents of container:* Amber glass vials closed with a grey butyl rubber stopper. Vials of 50 mg

*Instructions for use/handling:* See *Posology and method of administration.* Aseptic technique must be strictly observed during the preparation of the concentrate, the buffer and the infusion.

**Marketing authorisation number** 0034/5041R

**Date of approval/revision of SPC** 30 July 1996

**Legal category** POM

## GRANEODIN* OINTMENT

**Qualitative and quantitative composition** Soft, slightly opaque, colourless ointment, containing neomycin (as sulphate) 1625 units (0.25%) and gramicidin 0.025% in Plastibase* (liquid paraffin and polyethylene resin).

**Pharmaceutical form** Ointment

**Clinical particulars**

*Therapeutic indications:* Superficial bacterial infections such as impetigo; impetiginised eczema; infected eczema; bacterial infections of the ear (see *Contra-indications*).

**Posology and method of administration**

*Adults and children:* To be applied two to four times a day. Any crusts should be removed and the ointment rubbed well in.

*Elderly:* No specific dosage recommendations or precautions.

If a satisfactory response has not been achieved after 7 days, treatment should be stopped and the organism identified.

In cases of sycosis barbae a longer period of therapy may be necessary to treat the deep infection in the follicle.

*Contra-indications:* Fungal or viral infections of the skin or for the treatment of deep-seated infections.

Persons with known sensitivity to neomycin.

Should not be applied to the external auditory canal in patients with perforated eardrums.

Should not be used for extensive areas because of possible risk of systemic absorption and neomycin-induced ototoxicity.

*Special warnings and special precautions for use:* The possibility of sensitivity to neomycin should be taken into consideration during treatment. Since the use of occlusive dressings may increase the risk of sensitivity reactions, such dressings should be avoided.

*Children:* No specific precautions apply.

*Interaction with other medicaments and other forms of interaction:* None stated.

*Pregnancy and lactation:* There are theoretical risks of neomycin-induced foetal ototoxicity; therefore the product should be used with caution only when the benefit outweighs the potential risk.

*Effects on ability to drive and use machines:* None stated.

*Undesirable effects:*

*Neomycin:* Sensitivity reactions may occur especially with prolonged use. Ototoxicity and nephrotoxicity have been reported. The product should be used with caution and in small amounts in the treatment of skin infections following extensive burns, open lesion and other conditions where absorption of neomycin is possible particulary in children and elderly. The product should also be used with care in patients with established hearing loss and those with renal impairment.

*Gramicidin:* Sensitivity has occasionally been reported.

*Overdose:* In the event of accidental ingestion, the patient should be observed and treated symptomatically.

**Pharmacological properties**

*Pharmacodynamic properties:*

*Actions: Neomycin* is active against a wide range of Gram-positive and Gram-negative bacteria, including many of the organisms responsible for bacterial skin infections.

*Gramicidin* is active against Gram-positive bacteria and supplements the action of neomycin against the many common skin pathogens found in this group.

*Pharmacokinetic properties:* Not applicable.

*Preclinical safety data:* No further relevant data.

**Pharmaceutical particulars**

*List of excipients:* Liquid paraffin and polyethylene resin.

*Incompatibilities:* None known.

*Shelf life:* 48 months

*Special precautions for storage:*
*Storage:* Store below 25°C.
*Dilution:* Not recommended.

*Nature and contents of container:* Aluminium tubes of 25 g

*Instructions for use/handling:* Not applicable.

**Marketing authorisation number** 0034/5042R

**Date of approval/revision of SPC** 21 August 1996

**Legal category** POM

## HALCIDERM* TOPICAL

**Presentation** A white topical preparation containing halcinonide 0.1% in a water-miscible base.

Other ingredients: Benzyl alcohol, castor oil, silicone fluid, macrogol ether, propylene glycol, stearates, water, white soft paraffin.

**Uses** *Actions:* Halcinonide is a potent corticosteroid with rapid anti-inflammatory, antipruritic and anti-allergic actions.

Halciderm is suitable for both wet and dry lesions.

*Indications:* Halciderm is indicated in acute and chronic corticosteroid-responsive conditions which may include: psoriasis, atopic eczema, contact eczema, follicular eczema, infantile eczema, neurodermatitis, anogenital eczema, nummular eczema, seborrhoeic or flexural eczema, otitis externa without frank infection.

**Dosage and administration** *Adults:* Halciderm should be applied to the affected area two, or occasionally three, times daily. In long-term therapy, or where lower strength preparations are required, do not dilute but use intermittently.

*Children:* In infants, long-term continuous topical steroid therapy should be avoided. Courses should be limited to 5 days and occlusion should not be used.

*Elderly:* Natural thinning of the skin occurs in the elderly; hence corticosteroids should be used sparingly and for short periods of time.

**Contra-indications, warnings, etc**

*Contra-indications:* Contra-indicated in patients with a history of hypersensitivity to the product components.

Halciderm is not intended for ophthalmic use, nor should it be applied in the external auditory canal of patients with perforated eardrums.

Halciderm is contra-indicated in tuberculous and most viral lesions of the skin, particularly herpes simplex, vaccinia, varicella. The product should not be used in fungal or bacterial skin infections without suitable concomitant anti-infective therapy.

It should not be used for facial rosacea, acne vulgaris, perioral dermatitis or napkin eruptions.

*Precautions:* Adrenal suppression can occur with prolonged use of topical corticosteroids or treatment of extensive areas. These effects are more likely to occur in infants and children and if occlusive dressings are used. If used in childhood, or on the face, courses should be limited to 5 days and occlusion should not be used.

Topical corticosteroids may be hazardous in psoriasis for a number of reasons including rebound relapses following development of tolerance, risk of generalised pustular psoriasis and local and systemic toxicity due to impaired barrier function of the skin. Steroids may have a place in psoriasis of the scalp and chronic plaque psoriasis of the hands and feet. Careful patient supervision is important.

*Pregnancy:* There is inadequate evidence of safety in human pregnancy. Topical administration of corticosteroids to pregnant animals can cause abnormalities of foetal development including cleft palate and intrauterine growth retardation. There may, therefore, be a very small risk of such effects in the human foetus. Caution should be exercised when topical corticosteroids are administered to nursing women.

*Side-effects:* Halcinonide is well tolerated. Where adverse reactions occur they are usually reversible on cessation of therapy. However the following side-effects have been reported usually with prolonged usage:

Dermatologic – impaired wound healing, thinning of the skin, petechiae and ecchymoses, facial erythema and telangiectasia, increased sweating, purpura, striae, hirsutism, acneiform eruptions, lupus erythematosus-like lesions and suppressed reaction to skin tests. These effects may be enhanced with occlusive dressings.

Oedema and electrolyte imbalance have not been observed even when high topical dosage has been used. The possibility of the systemic effects which are associated with all steroid therapy should be considered.

*Overdosage:* Topically applied corticosteroids can be absorbed in sufficient amounts to produce systemic effects (see Side-effects).

In the event of accidental ingestion, the patient should be observed and treated symptomatically.

**Pharmaceutical precautions** *Storage:* Halciderm should be stored below 25°C.

*Dilution:* Due to special formulation of topical Halciderm, normal dermatological diluents should not be used. For further information consult the manufacturer.

**Legal category** POM.

**Package quantities** Tubes containing 30 g.

**Further information** Halciderm contains halcinonide 0.1%, dissolved in the non-aqueous phase of the formulation.

**Product licence number** 0034/0160.

## HYDREA* CAPSULES

**Qualitative and quantitative composition** Pink, opaque capsule body with green, opaque cap, printed in black with 'BMS 303' containing 500 mg of hydroxyurea

**Pharmaceutical form** Hard gelatin capsule.

**Clinical particulars**

*Therapeutic indications:* The treatment of chronic myeloid leukaemia.

The treatment of cancer of the cervix in conjunction with radiotherapy.

*Posology and method of administration:*

*Adults:* Treatment regimens can be continuous or intermittent. The continuous regimen is particularly suitable for chronic myeloid leukaemia, while the intermittent regimen, with its diminished effect on the bone marrow, is more satisfactory for the management of cancer of the cervix.

Hydrea should be started 7 days before concurrent irradiation therapy. If Hydrea is used concomitantly with radiotherapy, adjustment of radiation dosage is not usually necessary.

An adequate trial period for determining the antineoplastic effect of Hydrea is six weeks. Where there is a significant clinical response therapy may be continued indefinitely, provided that the patient is kept under adequate observation and shows no unusual or severe reactions. Therapy should be interrupted if the white cell count drops below $2.5 \times 10^9$L or the platelet count below $100 \times 10^9$/L.

*Continuous therapy:* Hydrea 20-30 mg/kg should be given daily in single doses. Dosage should be based on the patient's actual or ideal weight, whichever is the less. Therapy should be monitored by repeat blood counts.

*Intermittent therapy:* Hydrea 80 mg/kg in single doses should be given every third day. Using the intermittent regimes the likelihood of WBC depression is diminished, but if low counts are produced, 1 or more doses of Hydrea should be omitted.

Concurrent use of Hydrea with other myelosuppressive agents may require adjustments of dosages.

*Children:* Because of the rarity of these conditions in children, dosage regimens have not been established.

*Elderly:* Elderly patients may be more sensitive to the effects of hydroxyurea, and may require a lower dosage regimen.

*NB:* If the patient prefers, or is unable to swallow capsules, the contents of the capsules may be emptied into a glass of water and taken immediately. The contents of capsules should not be inhaled or allowed to come into contact with the skin or mucous membranes. Spillages must be wiped immediately.

*Contra-indications:* Marked leucopenia ($<2.5$wbcx$10^9$ /L), thrombocytopenia ($< 100 \times 10^9$ /L), or severe anaemia and those who have previously shown hypersensitivity to Hydrea.

*Special warnings and special precautions for use:* The complete status of the blood, including bone marrow examination, if indicated, as well as kidney function and liver function should be determined prior to, and repeatedly during, treatment. The determination of haemoglobin level, total leukocyte counts, and platelet counts should be performed at least once a week throughout the course of hydroxyurea therapy. If WBC falls below $2.5 \times 10^9$/L or platelet count to $<100 \times 10^9$/L, therapy should be interrupted. Counts should be rechecked after 3 days and treatment resumed when they rise significantly towards normal.

Severe anaemia must be corrected with whole blood replacement before initiating therapy with Hydroxyurea. If, during treatment, anaemia occurs, correct without interrupting Hydrea therapy. Erythrocytic abnormalities; megaloblastic erythropoeisis, which is self-limiting, is often seen early in the course of hydroxyurea therapy. The morphologic change resembles pernicious anaemia, but is not related to vitamin $B_{12}$ or folic acid deficiency. Hydroxyurea may also delay plasma iron clearance and reduce the rate of iron utilization by erythrocytes but it does not appear to alter the red blood cell survival time.

Hydroxyurea should be used with caution in patients with marked renal dysfunction.

In patients receiving long-term therapy with hydroxyurea for myeloproliferative disorders, such as polycythemia, secondary leukaemia has been reported. It is unknown whether this leukaemogenic effect is secondary to hydroxyurea or associated with the patient's underlying disease.

The possibility of an increase in serum uric acid, resulting in the development of gout or, at worst, uric acid nephropathy, should be borne in mind in patients treated with hydroxyurea, especially when used with other cytotoxic agents. It is therefore important to monitor uric acid levels regularly and maintain a high fluid intake during treatment.

*Interaction with other medicaments and other forms of interaction:* The myelosuppressive activity may be potentiated by previous or concomitant radiotherapy or cytotoxic therapy.

*Pregnancy and lactation:* Drugs which affect DNA synthesis, such as hydroxyurea, may be potent mutagenic agents. The physician should carefully consider this possibility before administering this drug to male or female patients who may contemplate conception. Since Hydrea is a cytotoxic agent it has produced a teratogenic effect in some animal species.

In rats and dogs, high doses of hydroxyurea reduced sperm production. Hydroxyurea is excreted in human breast milk.

Hydrea should not normally be administered to patients who are pregnant, or to mothers who are breast feeding, unless the potential benefits outweigh the possible hazards.

When appropriate both male and female patients should be counselled concerning the use of contraceptive measures before and during treatment with Hydrea.

*Effects on ability to drive and use machines:* Not applicable.

*Undesirable effects:* Bone-marrow suppression is the major toxic effect of Hydrea, while leucopenia, thrombocytopenia and anaemia may occur in that order. Other side-effects are generally rare, but the following have been reported; anorexia, nausea, vomiting, diarrhoea, constipation, headache, drowsiness, dizziness, stomatitis, alopecia, skin rash, melaena, abdominal pain, disorientations, pulmonary oedema, hallucinations, convulsions, potentiation of the erythema caused by irradiation, skin ulceration, dysuria and impairment of renal tubular function accompanied by elevation in serum uric acid, blood urea nitrogen, and creatinine levels. Fever, chills, malaise, asthenia and elevation of hepatic enzymes have been reported. Acute pulmonary reactions consisting of diffuse pulmonary infiltrates/fibrosis, and dyspnoea have been rarely reported. Skin cancer has also been rarely reported.

In some patients, hyperpigmentation, erythema, atrophy of skin and nails, scaling, violet papules and alopecia have been observed following several years of long-term daily maintenance therapy with hydroxyurea.

*Overdose:* Immediate treatment consists of gastric lavage, followed by supportive therapy for the cardio-respiratory systems if required. In the long term, careful monitoring of the haemopoietic system is essential and, if necessary, blood should be transfused.

Acute mucocutaneous toxicity has been reported in patients receiving hydroxyurea at a dosage several times greater than that recommended. Soreness, violet erythema, oedema on palms and foot soles followed by scaling of hands and feet, intense generalised hyperpigmentation of skin, and severe acute stomatitis were observed.

**Pharmacological properties**

*Pharmacodynamic properties:* Hydroxyurea is an orally active antineoplastic agent. Although the mechanism of action has not yet been clearly defined, hydroxyurea appears to act by interfering with synthesis of DNA.

*Pharmacokinetic properties:* After oral administration hydroxyurea is readily absorbed from the gastro-intestinal tract. Peak plasma concentrations are reached in 2 hours; by 24 hours the serum concentrations are virtually zero. Approximately 80% of an oral or intravenous dose of 7 to 30 mg/kg may be recovered from the urine within 12 hours. Hydroxyurea crosses the blood-brain barrier. Hydroxyurea is well distributed throughout the body.

*Preclinical safety data:* No further relevant data.

**Pharmaceutical particulars**

*List of excipients:* Citric acid, erythrosine, gelatin, indigotine, lactose, magnesium stearate, sodium lauryl sulphate, sodium phosphate, titanium dioxide, yellow iron oxide, opacode S-1-8100 HV black, purified water.

*Incompatibilities:* None known

*Shelf life:* Blister packs–24 months
Amber glass bottles–60 months

*Special precautions for storage:* Store below 25°C. Keep tightly closed.

*Nature and contents of container:* 100 capsules may be packaged in any of the following: amber glass bottles, PVC/PVDC blisters or PVC/ aluminum blisters.

*Instructions for use/handling:* Procedures for proper handling and disposal of anticancer drugs should be considered.

**Date of approval/revision of SPC** 4 January 1997

**Legal category** POM

## IPRAL* TABLETS

**Presentation**
*Tablets:* Round, white tablets engraved Squibb and 513, containing 100 mg trimethoprim.

Round, white tablets engraved Squibb and 514, containing 200 mg trimethoprim.

Other ingredients: Gelatin, lactose, magnesium stearate, maize starch, talc.

**Uses** *Actions:* Trimethoprim is bactericidal in-vitro against most pathogenic Gram-positive and Gram-negative bacteria. Exceptions are *Nocardia* species, *Treponema pallidum, Pseudomonas aeruginosa,* anaerobic bacteria and possibly *Mycobacterium* and *Neisseria* species and *Brucella abortus.*

*Indications: Urinary tract:* In the treatment of acute and chronic urinary tract infections and for prophylactic treatment of patients with a tendency to recurrent urinary infections.

*Respiratory tract:* In the treatment of acute and chronic bronchitis, bronchopneumonia and lobar pneumonia.

Ipral is particularly useful for patients sensitive to sulphonamides.

**Dosage and administration**
*Ipral Tablets: Adults and Children over 12 years:* For acute urinary tract and respiratory tract infections, 200 mg twice daily. For long-term and prophylactic therapy of urinary tract infections, 100 mg at night.

*6 to 12 years:* 100 mg twice daily

*Elderly:* There are no specific dosage recommendations or precautions for use in the elderly except, as with other drugs, to monitor those patients with impaired renal or hepatic function.

**Contra-indications, warnings, etc**
*Contra-indications:* Ipral should not be given to patients with severe renal insufficiency where blood levels cannot be monitored regularly. Trimethoprim should not be given to patients with a history of sensitivity to the drug, or used in patients with megaloblastic anaemia and other blood dyscrasias. It should not be administered to pregnant women, premature infants nor during the first two months of life.

*Precautions:* Care is necessary in administration to patients with impaired renal function. Regular haematological examinations should be performed during long-term therapy. Special precautions should be exercised in patients with a predisposition to folate deficiency. Ipral should be used with caution in patients with severe hepatic impairment.

*Pregnancy and nursing mothers:* Contra-indicated during pregnancy and in nursing mothers. Trimethoprim is excreted in breast milk.

*Side-effects:* Ipral is well tolerated at therapeutic doses with few side-effects. Nausea, vomiting, gastro-intestinal upset and dermatological reactions such as pruritus and rash have been reported. Erythema multiforme (Stevens Johnson Syndrome) has occurred in association with trimethoprim and toxic epidermal necrolysis (Lyell Syndrome), which is associated with a high mortality, has occurred rarely. Given over a prolonged period, Ipral may depress haemopoiesis due to an effect on folic acid metabolism. This effect may be reversed by calcium folinate.

*Drug interactions:* Trimethoprim may increase serum levels of digoxin, phenytoin and procainamide. Concurrent use of trimethoprim and bone marrow depressants may increase the likelihood of myelo suppression. The anti-folate effect of other folat inhibitors such as methotrexate, pyrimethamine ma be increased. An increased risk of nephrotoxicity ha been reported with the use of trimethoprim an cyclosporin.

Trimethoprim may interfere with diagnostic test including serum methotrexate assay where dihydro folate reductase is used and the Jaffé reaction fo creatinine.

*Treatment of overdosage:* Symptoms of overdosag include diarrhoea and vomiting. Treatment i symptomatic and gastric lavage and forced diuresi may be used. Calcium folinate may be used t counteract any effect of Ipral on bone-marrow.

**Pharmaceutical precautions** *Storage:* Ipral tablet should be stored in closed containers at roon temperature.

**Legal category** POM.

**Package quantities**
100 mg Tablets: Packs of 100 and 500 tablets.
200 mg Tablets: Packs of 100 tablets.

**Further information** Absorption from the oral rout is rapid, and peak plasma levels are obtained betwee one and four hours. Ipral is well distributed througl out the tissues and is excreted, predominantl unchanged, in the urine.

Nearly all of an oral dose of trimethoprim is excrete within 48 hours both unchanged and as metabolites

**Product licence numbers**

| | |
|---|---|
| Ipral Tablets 100 mg | 0034/0190. |
| Ipral Tablets 200 mg | 0034/0204. |

## KENALOG* INTRA-ARTICULAR / INTRAMUSCULAR INJECTION

**Qualitative and quantitaive composition** Kenalo Intra-articular / Intramuscular Injection contair triamcinolone acetonide 40 mg per ml of sterile sus pension.

**Pharmaceutical form** Sterile aqueous suspensic for injection.

**Clinical particulars**

*Therapeutic indications:*
*Intra-articular use:* for alleviating the joint pain, swel ing and stiffness associated with rheumatoid arthrit and osteoarthrosis, with an inflammatory componen also for bursitis, epicondylitis, and tenosynovitis.

*Intramuscular use:* Where sustained system corticosteroid treatment is required: *Allergic state* e.g. bronchial asthma, seasonal or perennial allerg rhinitis. In seasonal allergies, patients who do n respond to conventional therapy may achieve remission of symptoms over the entire period with single intramuscular injection (see *Dosage*); *End crine disorders,* e.g. primary or secondary adren cortical insufficiency. *Collagen disorders,* e.g. durin an exacerbation of maintenance therapy of selecte cases of SLE or acute rheumatic carditis; *Dermatolo ical diseases,* e.g. pemphigus, severe dermatitis an Stevens Johnson Syndrome; *Rheumatic, Gastrointe tinal or Respiratory disorders*–as an adjunctive, shor term therapy; *Haematological disorders,* e.g. acquire (autoimmune) haemolytic anaemia; *Neoplastic di eases,* e.g. palliative management of leukaemia an lymphomas; *Renal disease,* such as acute interstiti nephritis, minimal change nephrotic syndrome lupus nephritis.

*Posology and method of administration:* Kenalo Intra-articular/Intramuscular Injection is for intr articular or intramuscular use only and should not b administered via intravenous, epidural, intrathecal any other unapproved route of administration. Stri aseptic precautions should be observed. Since th duration of effect is variable, subsequent doses shoul be given when symptoms recur and not at s intervals.

*Intra-articular Injection:* For intra-articular administr tion or injection into tendon sheaths and bursae, th dose of Kenalog Injection may vary from 5 mg 10 mg (0.125–0.25 ml) for smaller joints and up 40 mg (1.0 ml) for larger joints, depending on th specific disease entity being treated. Single injectio into several sites for multiple joint involvement, up a total of 80 mg, have been given without und reactions.

It is recommended that, when injections are give into the sheaths of short tendons, Adcortyl Injectic (triamcinolone acetonide 10 mg/ml) should be use (see under *Precautions,* re Achilles tendon).

*Intramuscular injection:* to avoid the danger of su cutaneous fat atrophy, it is important to ensure th deep intramuscular injection is given into the glute site. The deltoid should not be used. Alternate sides should be used for subsequent injections.

*Adults and children over 12 Years:* The suggested initial dose is 40 mg (1.0 ml) injected deeply into the upper, outer quadrant of the gluteal muscle. Subsequent dosage depends on the patient's response and period of relief. Patients with hay fever or pollen asthma who do not respond to conventional therapy may obtain a remission of symptoms lasting throughout the pollen season after a single dose of 40-100 mg given when allergic symptoms appear (see *Warnings* and *Precautions*.)

*Elderly:* Treatment of elderly patients, particularly if long term, should be planned bearing in mind the more serious consequences of the common side effects of corticosteroids in old age, especially osteoporosis, diabetes, hypertension, susceptibility to infection and thinning of the skin. Close clinical supervision is required to avoid life-threatening reactions.

*Children from 6-12 years of age:* The suggested initial dose of 40 mg (1.0 ml injected deeply into the gluteal muscle should be scaled according to the severity of symptoms and the age and weight of the child. Kenalog is not recommended for children under six years. Growth and development of children on prolonged corticosteroid therapy should be carefully observed (see *Warnings* and *Precautions*).

*Contra-indications:* Hypersensitivity to any of the ingredients.

Systemic infections unless specific anti-infective therapy is employed.

*Special warnings and special precautions for use:*
*Warnings – Intra-articular injection:* Patients should be specifically warned to avoid over-use of joints in which symptomatic benefit has been obtained. Severe joint destruction with necrosis of bone may occur if repeated intra-articular injections are given over a long period of time. Care should be taken if injections are given into tendon sheaths to avoid injection into the tendon itself.

Due to the absence of a true tendon sheath, the Achilles tendon should not be injected with depot corticosteroids.

*Intramuscular injection:* During prolonged therapy a liberal protein intake is essential to counteract the tendency to gradual weight loss sometimes associated with negative nitrogen balance and wasting of skeletal muscle.

*Precautions:* Administration by non-approved routes (see *Posology and method of administration*).

Intra-articular injection should not be carried out in the presence of active infection in or near joints. The preparation should not be used to alleviate joint pain arising from infectious states such as gonococcal or tubercular arthritis.

Undesirable effects may be minimised using the lowest effective dose for the minimum period, and by administering the daily requirement, whenever possible, as a single morning dose on alternate days. Frequent patient review is required to titrate the dose appropriately against disease activity (see dosage section).

Adrenal cortical atrophy develops during prolonged therapy and may persist for years after stopping treatment. Withdrawal of corticosteroids after prolonged therapy must, therefore, always be gradual to avoid acute adrenal insufficiency and should be tapered off over weeks or months according to the dose and duration of treatment. During prolonged therapy any intercurrent illness, trauma or surgical procedure will require a temporary increase in dosage. If corticosteroids have been stopped following prolonged therapy they may need to be reintroduced temporarily.

Patients should carry steroid treatment cards which give clear guidance on the precautions to be taken to minimise risk and which provide details of prescriber, drug, dosage and the duration of treatment.

Suppression of the inflammatory response and immune function increases the susceptibility to infections and their severity. The clinical presentation may often be atypical and serious infections such as septicaemia and tuberculosis may be masked and may reach an advanced stage before being recognised.

Chickenpox is of particular concern since this normally minor illness may be fatal in immunosuppressed patients. Patients (or parents of children receiving Kenalog Injection) without a definite history of chickenpox should be advised to avoid close personal contact with chickenpox or herpes zoster. If exposed they should seek urgent medical attention. Passive immunisation with varicella zoster immunoglobulin (VZIG) is needed by exposed non-immune patients who are receiving systemic corticosteroids or who have used them within the previous 3 months; this should be given within 10 days of exposure to chickenpox. If a diagnosis of chickenpox is confirmed, the illness warrants specialist care and urgent treat-

ment. Corticosteroids should not be stopped and the dose may need to be increased.

During corticosteroid therapy antibody response will be reduced and therefore affect the patient's response to vaccines. Live vaccines should not be administered.

*Special precautions:* Particular care is required when considering use of systemic corticosteroids in patients with the following conditions and frequent patient monitoring is necessary.

Recent intestinal anastomoses, diverticulitis, thrombophlebitis, existing or previous history of severe affective disorders (especially previous steroid psychosis), exanthematous disease, chronic nephritis, or renal insufficiency, metastatic carcinoma, osteoporosis (post-menopausal females are particularly at risk); in patients with an active peptic ulcer (or a history of peptic ulcer). Myasthenia gravis. Latent or healed tuberculosis; in the presence of local or systemic viral infection, systemic fungal infections or in active infections not controlled by antibiotics. In acute psychoses; in acute glomerulonephritis. Hypertension; congestive heart failure; glaucoma (or a family history of glaucoma), previous steroid myopathy or epilepsy. Liver failure.

Corticosteroid effects may be enhanced in patients with hypothyroidism or cirrhosis.

Diabetes may be aggravated, necessitating a higher insulin dosage. Latent diabetes mellitus may be precipitated.

Menstrual irregularities may occur, and this possibility should be mentioned to female patients.

Rare instances of anaphylactoid reactions have occurred in patients receiving corticosteroids, especially when a patient has a history of drug allergies.

All corticosteroids increase calcium excretion

Aspirin should be used cautiously in conjunction with corticosteroids in patients with hypoprothrombinaemia.

*Use in children:* Kenalog is not recommended for children under six years. Corticosteroids cause dose-related growth retardation in infancy, childhood and adolescence which may be irreversible, therefore growth and development of children on prolonged corticosteroid therapy should be carefully observed.

*Use in elderly:* The common adverse effects of systemic corticosteroids may be associated with more serious consequences in old age, especially osteoporosis, hypertension, hypokalaemia, diabetes, susceptibility to infection and thinning of the skin. Close clinical supervision is required to avoid life-threatening reactions.

*Interactions with other medicaments and other forms of interaction:* Barbiturates, phenytoin, rifampicin, rifabutin, carbamazepine, primidone and aminoglutethimide may enhance the metabolic clearance of corticosteroids, resulting in decreased therapeutic effects.

Corticosteroids antagonise the effects of hypoglycaemic agents (including insulin), anti-hypertensives and diuretics. The hypokalaemic effects of acetazolamide, loop diuretics, thiazide diuretics and carbenoxolone are enhanced.

The efficacy of coumarin anticoagulants may be enhanced by concurrent corticosteroid therapy and close monitoring of the INR or prothrombin time is required to avoid spontaneous bleeding.

The renal clearance of salicylates is increased by corticosteroids and steroid withdrawal may result in salicylate intoxication.

*Pregnancy and lactation:* Corticosteroids are not recommended for pregnant patients, particularly in the first trimester, or for nursing mothers, except when the disease for which they are indicated warrants their use. When corticosteroids are essential however, patients with normal pregnancies may be treated as though they were in the non-gravid state.

There is evidence of harmful effects in pregnancy in animals. There may be a small risk of cleft palate and intra-uterine growth retardation. Hypoadrenalism may occur in the neonate. Patients with pre-eclampsia or fluid retention require close monitoring.

Corticosteroids are found in breast milk.

Infants born of mothers who have received substantial doses of corticosteroids during pregnancy or during breast feeding should be carefully observed for signs of hypoadrenalism. Maternal treatment should be carefully documented in the infant's medical records to assist in follow up.

*Effects on ability to drive and use machines:* None known.

*Undesirable effects:* Where adverse reactions occur they are usually reversible on cessation of therapy. The incidence of predictable side-effects, including hypothalamic-pituitary-adrenal suppression correlate with the relative potency of the drug, dosage, timing of administration and duration of treatment (see *Warnings* and *Precautions*).

Absorption of triamcinolone following injection by the intra-articular route is rare. However, patients

should be watched closely for the following adverse reactions which may be associated with any corticosteroid therapy:

*Anti-inflammatory and immunosuppressive effects:* Increased susceptibility and severity of infections with suppression of clinical symptoms and signs, opportunistic infections, recurrence of dormant tuberculosis (see *Warnings* and *Precautions*).

*Fluid and electrolyte disturbances:* sodium retention, fluid retention, congestive heart failure in susceptible patients, potassium loss, cardiac arrhythmias or ECG changes due to potassium deficiency, hypokalaemic alkalosis, increased calcium excretion and hypertension.

*Musculoskeletal:* muscle weakness, fatigue, steroid myopathy, loss of muscle mass, osteoporosis, avascular osteonecrosis, vertebral compression fractures, delayed healing of fractures, aseptic necrosis of femoral and humeral heads, pathological fractures of long bones and spontaneous fractures, tendon rupture.

*Gastrointestinal:* dyspepsia, peptic ulcer with possible subsequent perforation and haemorrhage, pancreatitis, abdominal distension and ulcerative oesophagitis, candidiasis.

*Dermatological:* impaired wound healing, thin fragile skin, petechiae and ecchymoses, facial erythema, increased sweating, purpura, striae, hirsutism, acneiform eruptions, lupus erythematous-like lesions and suppressed reactions to skin tests.

*Neurological:* euphoria, psychological dependence, depression, insomnia, convulsions, increased intracranial pressure with papilloedema (pseudo-tumour cerebri) usually after treatment, vertigo, headache, neuritis or paraesthesias and aggravation of pre-existing psychiatric conditions and epilepsy.

*Endocrine:* menstrual irregularities and amenorrhoea; development of the Cushingoid state; suppression of growth in childhood and adolescence; secondary adrenocortical and pituitary unresponsiveness, particularly in times of stress (e.g. trauma, surgery or illness); decreased carbohydrate tolerance; manifestations of latent diabetes mellitus and increased requirements for insulin or oral hypoglycaemic agents in diabetes, weight gain. Negative protein and calcium balance. Increased appetite.

*Ophthalmic:* posterior supcapsular cataracts, increased intraocular pressure, glaucoma, exophthalmos, papilloedema, corneal or scleral thinning, exacerbation of ophthalmic viral or fungal diseases.

*Others:* necrotising angiitis, thrombophlebitis, thromboembolism, leucocytosis, insomnia, syncopal episodes and anaphylactoid reactions, particularly where there is a history of drug allergies.

*Withdrawal symptoms and signs:* On withdrawal, fever, myalgia, arthralgia, rhinitis, conjunctivitis, painful itchy skin nodules and weight loss may occur. Too rapid a reduction in dose following prolonged treatment can lead to acute adrenal insufficiency, hypotension and death (see *Warnings* and *Precautions*).

*Intra-articular injection:* Reactions following intraarticular administration have been rare. In a few instances, transient flushing and dizziness have occurred. Pain and other local symptoms may continue for a short time before effective relief is obtained, but an increase in joint discomfort has seldom occurred. Local fat atrophy may occur if the injection is not given into the joint space, but is temporary and disappears within a few weeks to months.

*Overdose:* Not applicable.

**Pharmacological properties**

*Pharmacodynamic properties:* Triamcinolone acetonide is a synthetic glucocorticoid with marked anti-inflammatory and anti-allergic actions.
*Intra-articular injection:* Following local injection, relief of pain and swelling and greater freedom of movement are usually obtained within a few hours.

*Intramuscular injection:* Provides an extended duration of therapeutic effect and fewer side effects of the kind associated with oral corticosteroid therapy, particularly gastro-intestinal reactions such as peptic ulceration. Studies indicate that, following a single intramuscular dose of 80 mg triamcinolone acetonide, adrenal suppression occurs within 24–48 hours and then gradually returns to normal, usually in approximately three weeks. This finding correlates closely with the extended duration of therapeutic action of triamcinolone acetonide.

*Pharmacokinetic properties:* Triamcinolone acetonide may be absorbed into the systemic circulation from synovial spaces. However clinically significant systemic levels after intra-articular injection are unlikely to occur except perhaps following treatment of large joints with high doses. Systemic effects do not ordinarily occur with intra-articular injections when the proper techniques of administration and the recommended dosage regimens are observed.

Triamcinolone acetonide is absorbed slowly, though almost completely, following depot administration by deep intramuscular injection; biologically active levels are achieved systemically for prolonged periods (weeks to months). In common with other corticosteroids, triamcinolone is metabolised largely hepatically but also by the kidney and is excreted in urine. The main metabolic route is 6-beta-hydroxylation; no significant hydrolytic cleavage of the acetonide occurs.

In view of the hepatic metabolism and renal excretion of triamcinolone acetonide, functional impairments of the liver or kidney may affect the pharmacokinetics of the drug.

*Preclinical safety data:* See *Pregnancy and lactation.*

## Pharmaceutical particulars

*List of excipients:* Benzyl alcohol. polysorbate 80, sodium carboxymethylcellulose, sodium chloride, water.

*Incompatibilities:* The injection should not be physically mixed with other medicinal products.

*Shelf life:* 36 months

*Special precautions for storage:* In an upright position below 25°C: avoid freezing.

*Nature and contents of container:* Carton containing 5 x 1 ml glass vials or individually cartoned 1 ml and 2 ml syringes.

*Instructions for use/handling:* No special handling instructions.

**Marketing authorisation number** 0034/5045R

**Date of approval/revision of SPC** March 1997

**Legal category** POM

## NYSTADERMAL* CREAM

**Qualitative and quantitative composition** A yellow to light buff cream containing in each gram nystatin 100,000 units and triamcinolone acetonide 0.1% w/w.

**Pharmaceutical form** Topical cream.

**Clinical particulars**

*Therapeutic indications:* Nystadermal Cream is indicated for those cases of cutaneous candidosis where the addition of a corticosteroid to the antifungal antibiotic may be beneficial in controlling the commonly associated inflammation and pruritus.

Nystadermal Cream will also be of benefit in those cases of eczema where *Candida* is either the precipitating cause, or present as a secondary invader.

*Posology and method of administration:*

*Adults and children:* To be applied to moist, weeping lesions two to four times daily.

*Elderly:* Corticosteroids should be used sparingly and for short periods of time, as natural thinning of the skin occurs in the elderly; hence, if, after about 7 days application, little or no improvement has occurred, cultural isolation of the offending organism should be followed by appropriate local or systemic antimicrobial therapy.

*Contra-indications:* There are no known contraindications or special precautions for topical application of nystatin.

Corticosteroids are contra-indicated in tuberculous and most viral lesions of the skin, particularly herpes simplex and varicella. The products should not be used in fungal lesions not susceptible to nystatin or bacterial skin infections without suitable concomitant anti-infective therapy.

In patients with hypersensitivity to any of the components.

Should not be used for facial rosacea, acne vulgaris or perioral dermatitis.

*Special warnings and special precautions for use:* Adrenal suppression can occur, even without occlusion. The use of occlusive dressings should be avoided because of the increased risk of sensitivity reactions and increased percutaneous absorption.

If used in childhood, or on the face, courses should be limited to 5 days and occlusion should not be used.

*Children:* In infants, long-term continuous topical steroid therapy should be avoided. Courses should be limited to 5 days and occlusion should not be used.

*Interactions with other medicaments and other forms of interaction:* None known.

*Pregnancy and lactation:* There is inadequate evidence of safety in human pregnancy. Topical administration of corticosteroids to pregnant animals can cause abnormalities of foetal development including cleft palate and intra-uterine growth retardation. There may, therefore, be a very small risk of such effects in the human foetus.

*Effects on ability to drive and use machines:* None known.

*Undesirable effects:* There have been no substantiated reports of sensitivity associated with topical nystatin.

Triamcinolone acetonide is well tolerated. Where adverse reactions occur they are usually reversible on cessation of therapy. However the following side

effects have been reported usually with prolonged usage:

Dermatologic – impaired wound healing, thinning of the skin, petechiae and ecchymoses, facial erythema and telangiectasia, increased sweating, purpura, striae, hirsutism, acneiform eruptions, lupus erythematosus-like lesions and suppressed reactions to skin tests.

These effects may be enhanced with occlusive dressings.

Signs of systemic toxicity such as oedema and electrolyte imbalance have not been observed even when high topical dosage has been used. The possibility of the systemic effects which are associated with all steroid therapy should be considered.

*Overdose:* Topically applied corticosteroids can be absorbed in sufficient amounts to produce systemic effects (see Side-Effects).

In the event of accidental ingestion, the patient should be observed and treated symptomatically.

## Pharmacological properties

*Pharmacodynamic properties:*

*Actions:* Triamcinolone acetonide is a potent fluorinated corticosteroid with anti-inflammatory, antipruritic and anti-allergic actions. Nystatin is an antifungal antibiotic active against a wide range of yeasts and yeast-like fungi including *Candida albicans.*

The cream is formulated for use on moist, weeping lesions.

*Pharmacokinetic properties:* In common with other corticosteroids, triamcinolone is absorbed from sites of local application. When administered under occlusive dressings, or when the skin is broken, a sufficient amount may be absorbed to produce systemic effects.

Nystatin is formulated in oral and topical dosage forms and is not systemically absorbed from any of these preparations.

*Preclinical safety data:* No further relevant information.

## Pharmaceutical particulars

*List of excipients:* Aluminium hydroxide, antifoam emulsion, benzyl alcohol, macrogol ether, perfume, propylene glycol, sorbitol, titanium dioxide, white soft paraffin, water.

*Incompatibilities:* None known.

*Shelf life:* 24 months.

*Special precautions for storage:* Store below 25°C. Avoid freezing.

*Nature and contents of container:* Aluminium tubes of 15 g.

*Instructions for use/handling:* Not applicable.

**Marketing authorisation number** 0034/0131R.

**Date of approval/revision of SPC** 29 November 1995.

**Legal category** POM.

## NYSTAN* CREAM, GEL AND OINTMENT

**Qualitative and quantitative composition**

*Cream:* Pale buff, containing 100,000 units per gram nystatin in a vanishing-cream base.

*Ointment:* Yellow to amber, containing 100,000 units per gram nystatin in plastibase.

*Gel:* Yellow to amber, opaque gel containing 100,000 units nystatin per gram.

**Pharmaceutical form** Topical cream, gel, ointment.

**Clinical particulars**

*Therapeutic indications:* For the treatment of cutaneous and mucocutaneous mycoses, particularly those caused by *Candida albicans.*

*Posology and method of administration:*

*Adults and children:* To be applied two to four times daily.

*Elderly:* No specific dosage recommendations or precautions.

*Contra-indications:* There are no known contraindications or special precautions for topical application of nystatin.

*Special warnings and special precautions for use:*

*Children:* No specific precautions apply; systemic absorption is negligible.

*Interactions with other medicaments and other forms of interaction:* None known.

*Pregnancy and lactation:* No specific precautions apply; systemic absorption is negligible.

*Effects on ability to drive and use machines:* None known.

*Undesirable effects:* There have been no substantiated reports of sensitivity associated with topical nystatin.

*Overdose:* Since absorption of nystatin from the gastro-intestinal tract is negligible, accidental ingestion causes no systemic toxicity.

## Pharmacological properties

*Pharmacodynamic properties:*

*Actions:* Nystatin is a polyene, antifungal antibiotic active against a wide range of yeasts and yeast-like fungi, including *Candida albicans.*

*Pharmacokinetic properties:* Nystatin is formulated in oral and topical dosage forms and is not systemically absorbed from any of these preparations.

*Preclinical safety data:* No further relevant information.

## Pharmaceutical particulars

*List of excipients:*

*Cream:* Aluminium hydroxide, antifoam emulsion, benzyl alcohol, macrogol ether, perfume, propylene glycol, sorbitol, titanium dioxide, white soft paraffin, water.

*Ointment:* Liquid paraffin and polyethylene resin.

*Gel:* Carbopol, chlorocresol, perfume, potassium phosphates, sodium hydroxide, water.

*Incompatibilities:* None known.

*Shelf life:* 48 months.

*Special precautions for storage:*
Cream and Gel: Store below 25°C. Avoid freezing.
Ointment: Store below 25°C.

*Nature and contents of container:*
Cream and Ointment: Aluminium tubes of 30 g.
Gel: Aluminium tubes of 30 g.

*Instructions for use/handling:* Not applicable.

**Marketing authorisation numbers**
Cream       0034/5058R
Ointment    0034/0161R
Gel           0034/0142R

**Date of approval/revision of SPC**
Cream       22 November 1995
Ointment    30 November 1995
Gel           28 November 1995

**Legal category** POM.

## NYSTAN* ORAL SUSPENSION
## NYSTAN* FOR SUSPENSION
## NYSTAN* TABLETS

**Qualitative and quantitative composition**

*Nystan Oral Suspension:* Ready mixed oral suspension containing 100,000 units nystatin per ml.

*Nystan for Suspension:* Powder for reconstitution to provide oral suspension containing 100,000 units nystatin per ml.

*Nystan Tablets:* Tablets containing 500,000 units nystatin.

**Pharmaceutical form** Oral suspension, Granules for the preparation of oral suspension and oral tablets.

**Clinical particulars**

*Therapeutic indications:*

*Suspension:* The prevention and treatment of candidal infections of the oral cavity, oesophagus and intestinal tract. The suspension provides effective prophylaxis against oral candidosis in those born of mothers with vaginal candidosis.

*Tablets:* Tablets for intestinal candidosis. Also for use in patients who may be susceptible to candida overgrowth, e.g. patients with malignant disease especially if receiving cytotoxic drugs, and those patients receiving high doses or prolonged courses of antibiotics or corticosteroids.

*Posology and method of administration:*

*Reconstitution of granules for suspension:* Add 23 ml water to the bottle and shake vigorously.

*Adults:* For the treatment of denture sores, and oral infections in adults caused by *C. albicans*, 1 ml of the suspension should be dropped into the mouth four times daily; it should be kept in contact with the affected areas as long as possible.

*Tablets:* For the treatment of intestinal candidosis 1 tablet four times daily, but this dose may be doubled. For prophylaxis a total daily dosage of 1 million units has been found to suppress the overgrowth of *C. albicans* in patients receiving broad-spectrum antibiotic therapy.

Administration should be continued for 48 hours after clinical cure to prevent relapse.

*Children: Suspension:* In intestinal and oral candidosis (thrush) in infants and children, 1 ml should be dropped into the mouth four times a day. The longer the suspension is kept in contact with the affected area in the mouth, before swallowing, the greater will be its effect.

For prophylaxis in the newborn the suggested dose is 1 ml once daily.

*Elderly:* No specific dosage recommendations or precautions.

*Contra-indications:* Contra-indicated in patients with a history of hypersensitivity to any of the components.

*Special warnings and special precautions for use:*

ystan Oral Suspension contains sugar. For children ith disaccharide intolerance the sugar-free formulaon, Nystan For Suspension, is recommended.

Nystan oral preparations should not be used for eatment of systemic mycoses.

*teractions with other medicaments and other forms f interaction:* None known.

*regnancy and lactation:* Animal reproductive studies ave not been conducted with nystatin.

It is not known whether nystatin can cause foetal arm when administered to a pregnant woman, owever absorption of nystatin from the gastrotestinal tract is negligible. Nystatin should be rescribed during pregnancy only if the potential enefits to be derived outweigh the possible risks volved.

*Nursing mothers:* Though gastro-intestinal absorpon is insignificant, it is not known whether nystatin excreted in human breast milk and caution should e exercised when nystatin is prescribed for nursing omen.

*ffects on ability to drive and use machines:* None nown.

*ndesirable effects:* Nystatin is generally well tolered by all age groups, even during prolonged use. arely, oral irritation or sensitisation may occur. ausea has been reported occasionally during therpy.

Large oral doses of Nystatin have occasionally roduced diarrhoea, gastro-intestinal distress, nausea nd vomiting. Rash, including urticaria, has been ported rarely. Steven-Johnson Syndrome has been ported very rarely.

*verdose:* Since the absorption of nystatin from the astro-intestinal tract is negligible, overdosage or ccidental ingestion causes no systemic toxicity.

**harmacological properties**

*harmacodynamic properties:* Nystatin is an antifunal antibiotic active against a wide range of yeasts nd yeast-like fungi, including *Candida albicans.*

*harmacokinetic properties:* Nystatin is formulated in ral and topical dosage forms and is not systemically bsorbed from any of these preparations.

*reclinical safety data:* No further relevant informaon.

**harmaceutical particulars**

*st of excipients*

*Nystan Oral Suspension:* Ethanol, flavours, glycerin, ethyl parahydroxybenzoate, pH adjusters (hydrochric acid, sodium hydroxide), propyl parahydroxynzoate, sodium carboxymethylcellulose, sodium hosphate, sucrose, water.

*Nystan for Suspension:* Methyl parahydroxybenate, propyl parahydroxybenzoate, saccharin, sacharin sodium, sodium benzoate, sodium rboxymethylcellulose, water, wood cellulose.

*Nystan Tablets:* Carnauba wax, castor oil, chalk, on oxide, lactose, magnesium stearate, maize starch, icrocrystalline cellulose, polysorbate 20, polyvione, shellac, sorbic acid, stearic acid, sucrose, talc, hite beeswax.

*compatibilities:* None known.

*helf life:*

eady-mixed suspension: 36 months.

ranules for suspension: 12 months.

econstituted suspension: 7 days.

ablets: 36 months.

*pecial precautions for storage:*

ystan Suspension: Store below 25°C.

ystan for Suspension: Store the dry powder below °C.

ablets: Store below 25°C.

*ature and contents of container:*

*Nystan Oral Suspension:* 30 ml amber glass bottle, acked in a cardboard carton with a graduated, olyethylene dropper.

*Nystan For Suspension:* 24 ml amber glass bottle, acked in a cardboard carton with a graduated, olyethylene dropper.

*Tablets:* Amber glass bottle of 56 tablets, packed in cardboard carton.

*structions for use/handling:*

*Suspension:* Shake well before use.

Dilution is not recommended as this may reduce erapeutic efficacy.

**arketing authorisation numbers**

ystan Oral Suspension    0034/0130R

ystan for Suspension    0034/5061R

ystan Tablets    0034/5063R

**ate of approval/revision of SPC**

ystan Oral suspension    28 November 1995

ystan for Suspension    30 November 1995

ystan Tablets    12 March 1996

**egal category**    POM.

## NYSTAN* PASTILLES

**Presentation** Yellow-brown, aniseed flavoured soft pastille providing 100,000 units nystatin per pastille; containing sugar and cinnamon.

Other ingredients: Aniseed oil, cinnamon oil, dextrose monohydrate, gelatin, liquid glucose, pH adjusters (hydrochloric acid/potassium hydroxide), silicone antifoam emulsion, sucrose, water.

**Uses** *Actions:* Nystatin is an antifungal antibiotic active against a wide range of yeasts and yeast-like fungi, including *Candida albicans.*

*Indications:* For the treatment of oral candidosis.

**Dosage and administration** No food or drink should be taken for five minutes before or one hour after consumption of the pastille. The pastilles should be sucked slowly and retained in the mouth for as long as possible in accordance with the doctors instructions.

*Adults and children:* One pastille to be sucked slowly, four times a day for 7–14 days.

*Elderly:* No specific dosage recommendations or precautions.

**Contra-indications, warnings, etc**

*Contra-indications:* Contra-indicated in patients with a history of hypersensitivity to any of its components.

*Precautions:* The pastilles contain sugar and should be administered with caution to patients with disaccharide intolerance.

Nystan pastilles should not be used for the treatment of systemic mycoses.

*Pregnancy and lactation:* Animal reproductive studies have not been conducted with nystatin.

It is not known whether nystatin can cause foetal harm when administered to a pregnant woman, however absorption of nystatin from the gastrointestinal tract is negligible. Nystatin should be prescribed during pregnancy only if the potential benefits to be derived outweigh the possible risks involved.

Though gastrointestinal absorption is insignificant, it is now known whether nystatin is excreted in human breast milk and caution should be exercised when nystatin is prescribed for nursing women.

*Side-effects:* Nystatin is generally well tolerated by all age groups, even during prolonged use. Rarely, oral irritation or sensitisation may occur. Nausea has been reported occasionally during therapy.

Large oral doses of nystatin have occasionally produced diarrhoea, gastrointestinal distress, nausea and vomiting. Rash, including urticaria, has been reported rarely. Stevens-Johnson Syndrome has been reported very rarely.

*Overdosage:* Since the absorption of nystatin from the gastro-intestinal tract is negligible, overdosage causes no systemic toxicity.

**Pharmaceutical precautions** *Storage:* Store below 25°C.

**Legal category** POM.

**Package quantities** Packs of 28 pastilles.

**Further information** The pastille allows longer contact of the active ingredient nystatin with the mucous membrane than liquid formulations.

Successful treatment of oral candidosis also includes good oral hygiene. Patients with dentures are advised to remove them whilst sucking the pastilles.

**Product licence number** 0034/0248.

## NYSTAN* PESSARIES
## NYSTAN* VAGINAL CREAM

**Qualitative and quantitative composition**

*Pessaries:* Each pessary contains 100,000 units nystatin.

*Cream:* Each 4 g application contains 100,000 units nystatin.

**Pharmaceutical form**

Vaginal tablet.

Cream.

**Clinical particulars**

*Therapeutic indications:* The treatment of candidal vaginitis.

*Posology and method of administration:*

*Adults:*

*Pessaries:* 1 or 2 pessaries should be inserted high into the vagina for 14 consecutive nights, or longer, regardless of any intervening menstrual period.

*Cream:* Insert 1 or 2 applications (of 4 g each) high into the vagina for 14 consecutive nights, or longer, regardless of any intervening menstrual period.

*Children:*

*Cream:* Vulvovaginal candidosis is rarely a problem

in children. It is suggested that the vaginal cream is the most acceptable formulation for children.

*Pessaries:* Not recommended for children under 12 years.

*Elderly:* No specific dosage recommendations or precautions.

*Contra-indications:* There are no known contra-indications to the use of nystatin.

*Special warnings and special precautions for use:* Avoid contact between the cream and contraceptive diaphragms and condoms, since the rubber may be damaged by the preparation.

*Interactions with other medicaments and other forms of interaction:* None known.

*Pregnancy and lactation:* There is no evidence that nystatin is absorbed systemically from the vagina. However, as with all drugs, caution should be exercised in pregnancy. Care should be taken while using an applicator to prevent the possibility of mechanical trauma.

*Effects on ability to drive and use machines:* None known.

*Undesirable effects:* Nystan is well tolerated and no substantiated sensitivity reactions have been associated with its use. Some transient local discomfort may be experienced.

*Overdose:* Since the absorption of nystatin from the gastro-intestinal tract is negligible, overdosage or accidental ingestion causes no systemic toxicity.

**Pharmacological properties**

*Pharmacodynamic properties:* Nystatin is an antifungal antibiotic active against a wide range of yeasts and yeast-like fungi, including *Candida albicans.*

*Pharmacokinetic properties:* Nystatin is formulated in oral and topical dosage forms and is not systemically absorbed from any of these preparations.

*Preclinical safety data:* No further relevant information.

**Pharmaceutical particulars**

*List of excipients*

*Pessaries:* Lactose, magnesium stearate, maize starch, microcrystalline cellulose.

*Cream:* Aluminium hydroxide, antifoam emulsion, benzyl alcohol, macrogol ether, pH adjusters (hydrochloric acid, sodium hydroxide), propylene glycol, sorbitol, water, white soft paraffin.

*Incompatibilities:* None known.

*Shelf life*

Pessaries: 12 months.

Cream: 24 months.

*Special precautions for storage:*

Pessaries: Store below 25°C.

Cream: Store below 25°C. Avoid freezing.

*Nature and contents of container*

Pessaries: Foil strip, packed in a carton with an applicator, in packs of 28 pessaries.

Cream: 60 g aluminium tube, packed in a cardboard carton with a vaginal applicator.

*Instructions for use/handling:* Dilution of the vaginal cream is not recommended as this may reduce therapeutic efficacy.

**Marketing authorisation numbers**

Pessaries    0034/5062R

Cream    0034/0137R

**Date of approval/revision of SPC**

Pessaries    6 September 1996

Cream    22 November 1995

**Legal category** POM

## OPHTHAINE* SOLUTION

**Qualitative and quantitative composition** Ophthaine Solution contains proxymetacaine hydrochloride 0.5%, chlorbutol 0.2%, benzalkonium chloride 0.01%, glycerol, pH modifiers, water.

**Pharmaceutical form** Sterile, aqueous ophthalmic solution

**Clinical particulars**

*Therapeutic indications:* Topical anaesthesia in ophthalmic practice.

*Posology and method of administration:*

*Adults and children:* Administered by topical instillation into the eye. The recommended doses are as follows:

Deep anaesthesia: Instil 1 drop every five to ten minutes for 5-7 doses.

Removal of sutures: Instil 1 or 2 drops two or three minutes before removal of stitches.

Removal of foreign bodies: Instil 1 or 2 drops prior to operating.

Tonometry: Instil 1 or 2 drops immediately before measurement.

*Elderly:* No specific dosage recommendations or precautions.

*Contra-indications:* Patients with known hypersensitivity to proxymetacaine or any of the other components.

*Special warnings and special precautions for use:*
*Precautions:* Ophthaine solution is not intended for long-term use.

Ophthaine Solution is not miscible with fluorescein. However, the eye can be anaesthetised with Ophthaine Solution before fluorescein is administered.

Use cautiously and sparingly in patients with known allergies, cardiac disease, or hyperthyroidism.

Regular and prolonged use of a topical ocular anaesthetic, e.g. in conjunction with contact lens insertion, may cause softening and erosion of the corneal epithelium, which could produce corneal opacification with accompanying loss of vision.

Protection of the eye from irritating chemicals, foreign bodies and rubbing during the period of anaesthesia is very important. Tonometers soaked in sterilising or detergent solutions should be thoroughly rinsed with sterile distilled water prior to use. Patients should be advised to avoid touching the eye until the anaesthesia has worn off.

*Interactions with other medicaments and other forms of interaction:* None known.

*Pregnancy and lactation:* Not applicable.

*Effect on ability to drive and use machines:* Not applicable.

*Undesirable effects:* Pupillary dilatation or cycloplegic effects have rarely been observed with Ophthaine Solution. Irritation of the conjunctiva or other toxic reactions attributable to the preparation have occurred only rarely. A severe, immediate-type apparently hyperallergic corneal reaction may rarely occur which includes acute, intense and diffuse epithelial keratitis; a grey ground-glass appearance; sloughing of large areas of necrotic epithelium; corneal filaments and sometimes, iritis with descemetitis.

*Overdose:* None known.

**Pharmacological properties**

*Pharmacodynamic properties:* Proxymetacaine hydrochloride is a rapidly acting local anaesthetic. With a single drop the onset of anaesthesia occurs in an average of 13 seconds and will persist for an average of 15 minutes.

*Pharmacokinetic properties:* No detectable systemic concentration of proxymetacaine has been recorded in patients following ocular administration of Ophthaine Solution.

*Preclinical safety data:* Minimal absorption with rapid hydrolysis of proxymetacaine.

**Pharmaceutical particulars**

*List of excipients:* Glycerol, pH modifiers, water.

*Incompatibilities:* None known.

*Shelf life:* 24 months.

*Special precautions for storage:* Store in a refrigerator (2-8°C). Do not freeze. Protect from light. If solution shows more than a very pale yellow colour, it should be discarded. The product should not be used one month after first opening the container.

*Nature and contents of container:* Bottles of 15 ml.

*Instructions for use/handling:* None.

**Marketing authorisation number** 0034/5064R

**Date of approval/revision of SPC** October 1996

**Legal category** POM

## PRONESTYL* TABLETS

**Presentation**

*Tablets:* White, engraved Squibb and 754 on one side and scored on reverse, containing 250 mg procainamide hydrochloride.

Other ingredients: Ethylcellulose, lactose, magnesium stearate, maize starch, stearic acid, sucrose.

**Uses**

*Actions:* Procainamide is a class I antiarrhythmic agent (Vaughan Williams classification). Abnormal automaticity and excitability are reduced: the former by a slowing of the rate of diastolic phase 4 depolarisation; the latter by a reduction of the rate of rise of phase 0 depolarisation.

Action potention duration is prolonged but the effect on refractory period is greater.

These actions are apparent throughout the myocardium, and are most pronounced within the atria. Abnormal ectopic foci may be suppressed by the slowing of phase 4 depolarisation, while re-entrant tachyarrhythmias may be inhibited both by the reduced excitability of the myocardium and by the prolongation of the refractory period. In those arrhythmias not fully suppressed, procainamide is likely to slow the tachycardia.

Following oral administration therapeutic levels (3–10 mcg/ml) are usually obtained by 30 minutes, with maximal levels occurring after 60 minutes.

*Indications:* The treatment of atrial tachycardia.

The treatment of symptomatic or potentially malignant ventricular arrhythmias (i.e. extrasystoles or tachycardia).

The treatment or prophylaxis of symptomatic or potentially malignant ventricular arrhythmias following acute myocardial infarction.

**Dosage and administration**

*Children:* Pronestyl is not recommended.

*Adults:* Oral Pronestyl can be used for maintenance therapy once control of arrhythmias is achieved. Intravenous therapy is available for more serious tachyarrhythmias.

Plasma concentrations correlate well with therapeutic and toxic effects; consequently plasma level assays should be carried out if facilities are available. The usual effective antiarrhythmic serum concentration is 3–10 mcg/ml. Toxic manifestations are rare in concentrations less than 12 mcg/ml.

Oral therapy is preferred for treatment of arrhythmias which do not require immediate suppression, and for prevention of recurrence of serious arrhythmias after initial control by cardioversion, by intravenous Pronestyl Injection or by other antiarrhythmic therapy. Ideally, the oral dose and interval of administration should be adjusted for the individual patient, based on clinical assessment of the degree of underlying myocardial disease, the patient's age, and renal function.

As a general guide, for younger patients with normal renal function, an initial total daily oral dose of up to 50 mg/kg of body weight of Pronestyl Tablets may be used, given in divided doses, every three hours, to maintain therapeutic blood levels. For older patients, especially those over 50 years of age, or for patients with renal, hepatic, or cardiac insufficiency, lesser amounts or longer intervals may produce adequate blood levels. The initial total daily dose should be divided for administration at three, four, or six hour intervals as estimated for the patient's needs; then, the dose and interval should be adjusted for the individual.

To provide up to 50 mg per kg of body weight per day:

| *Patients weighing* | |
|---|---|
| 40–50 kg | 250 mg 3 hrly to 500 mg 6 hrly |
| 60–70 kg | 375 mg 3 hrly to 750 mg 6 hrly |
| 80–90 kg | 500 mg 3 hrly to 1 g 6 hrly |
| More than 100 kg | 625 mg 3 hrly to 1.25 g 6 hrly |

*Atrial arrhythmias:* Higher dosages, than for ventricular arrhythmias, may be required (see 'Warnings and precautions').

*Elderly:* Reduction in dose or increase in dosage interval may be necessary to maintain constant blood levels without accumulation (see Dosage).

*Patients with renal or hepatic impairment:* Dose reduction or increase in dosage interval may be necessary to produce adequate blood levels without accumulation.

**Contra-indications, warnings, etc**

*Contra-indications:* Hypersensitivity to the drug is an absolute contra-indication. In this connection, cross sensitivity to procaine and related drugs must be borne in mind.

Procainamide should not be administered to patients with complete atrioventricular heart block or a high degree of A-V block or bifascicular block unless an electrical pacemaker is operative.

Systemic lupus erythematosus:

'Torsade de Pointes', a variant form of ventricular tachycardia associated with a prolonged QT interval, should not be treated with Pronestyl which may aggravate rather than suppress this arrhythmia.

*Warnings and precautions:* Myasthenia gravis: Patients with myasthenia gravis may show worsening of symptoms from procainamide due to its procaine-like effect on diminishing acetylcholine release at skeletal muscle motor nerve endings, so that procainamide administration may be hazardous without optimal adjustment of anticholinesterase medications and other precautions.

Digitalis intoxication: Procainamide may further depress conduction and ventricular asystole or fibrillation may result.

If the patient develops first degree heart block, dosage reduction and/or discontinuation of procainamide should be considered.

Caution in patients with congestive heart failure, acute ischaemic heart disease, cardiogenic shock or cardiomyopathy as even slight depression in myocardial contractility may reduce the cardiac outp of the damaged heart.

Cardiotoxicity may be reflected by hypotensio excessive widening of the QRS complex prolongation of the PR interval or the appearance proarrhythmic effects.

In patients with significant impairment of renal hepatic function, accumulation of Pronestyl m occur, leading to drug toxicity.

The electrophysiological action of procainami may be affected by electrolyte imbalance.

*Pregnancy and nursing mothers:* Safety has not bee established; therefore, Pronestyl should be us during pregnancy only if the possible benefits o weigh the potential risks involved. Procainami crosses the placenta but the extent is unknow Procainamide is excreted in breast milk; therefore, should not be given to nursing mothers because the potential risk of adverse reactions in the infant.

*Side-effects:* A lupus-like syndrome has been reporte after prolonged courses of Pronestyl. The lupus-li syndrome seldom appears in less than two month but is very common after six months. It is virtual completely reversible and tests for antinuclear facto are usually positive before clinical signs appear. It perhaps more often observed in patients who a slow acetylators. If long-term treatment is considere desirable, it is advisable to undertake serological tes at no less than monthly intervals and to contin treatment for no longer than absolutely necessary.

Agranulocytosis is a rare side effect of prolong procainamide therapy. Susceptibility to this is great in the period following coronary bypass surgery. T patient should be instructed to report any soreness the mouth, throat, or gums, unexplained fever or a symptoms of upper respiratory tract infection. If a of these should occur, and leucocyte counts indica cellular depression, Pronestyl therapy should discontinued, and appropriate treatment should instituted immediately.

Nausea, vomiting, diarrhoea, abdominal pain, an rexia, bitter taste, mental depression, psychoses wi hallucinations, dizziness, headache, pruritus, chil fever, hepatitis and allergic reactions (such as vasc litis, eosinophilia, skin reactions or angioneuro oedema) may occur infrequently. They are usually n sufficiently severe to discontinue treatment.

Neutropenia, thrombocytopenia or haemoly anaemia may rarely be encountered.

As with all other class 1 agents, proarrhythm effects may occur.

*Drug interactions:*

*Amiodarone:* Concomitant use of amiodarone m result in increased plasma procainamide concent tions and subsequent toxicity.

*Other antiarrhythmic drugs:* Additive effects c occur and dosage reduction may be necessary.

*Antihypertensive agents:* Procainamide m produce an additive effect and dosage adjustme may be necessary.

*Anticholinergic drugs:* Additive antivagal effects A-V nodal conduction may occur.

*Neuromuscular blocking agents:* Possibly redu dosage of neuromuscular blocking drugs, procainamide may reduce acetylcholine release.

*Captopril:* There have been reports of neutroper and/or Stevens-Johnson syndrome in patients procainamide plus captopril. Although a caus relationship has not been established, th combination should only be used with cautio especially in patients with impaired renal function.

*Sulphonamides:* p-amino benzoic acid is metabolite of procainamide and can inhibit the acti of sulphonamides.

*Trimethoprim:* The renal clearance of procainami is reduced by trimethoprim resulting in increas pharmacodynamic response.

*Pharmacokinetic interactions:* The elimination procainamide may be decreased by cimetidine propranolol, and increased by alcohol.

*Overdosage:* After intravenous administration, b seldom after oral, hypotension may occ Progressive widening of the QRS or A-V conducti block may be seen as may increased ventricul extrasystoles or even ventricular tachycardia or fib lation. Procainamide and n-acetyl procainamide a removed by haemodialysis but not by peritone dialysis. No specific antidote is known.

Overdosage should be managed by gene supportive measures and close observation. Flu expansion and the infusion of noradrenaline micrograms/ml in Sodium Chloride Injection BP) m be useful for hypotension; insertion of a tempora ventricular pacing system may be beneficial.

**Pharmaceutical precautions**

*Storage:* Store below 25°C.

Dispense only in dry, well-sealed containers.

**Legal category** POM.

**Package quantities** Bottles of 100.

**ırther information** Procainamide is less readily ·drolysed than procaine and plasma levels decline owly – about 10–20% per hour. The drug is excreted imarily in the urine, about 10% as free and njugated p-aminobenzoic acid and about 60% in e unchanged form. The remainder is mainly exeted as n-acetyl procainamide.

The formation of n-acetyl procainamide will depend on the acetylator status of the patient. As this etabolite also has significant antiarrhythmic activity d a somewhat slower renal clearance than ocainamide, both acetylation rate capability and nal function will affect the duration of action.

**oduct licence number** 0034/5066R.

## RONESTYL* SOLUTION FOR JJECTION

**esentation**

*olution for Injection:* A sterile, aqueous solution ntaining 100 mg/ml procainamide hydrochloride. ther ingredients: Benzyl alcohol, sodium hydroxide, dium metabisulphite, water.

**ses**

*ctions:* Procainamide is a class I antiarrhythmic ent (Vaughan Williams classification). Abnormal tomaticity and excitability are reduced: the former a slowing of the rate of diastolic phase 4 polarisation; the latter by a reduction of the rate of se of phase 0 depolarisation.

Action potention duration is prolonged but the fect on refractory period is greater.

These actions are apparent throughout the yocardium, and are most pronounced within the ria. Abnormal ectopic foci may be suppressed by e slowing of phase 4 depolarisation, while re-entrant chyarrhythmias may be inhibited both by the reced excitability of the myocardium and by the olongation of the refractory period. In those rhythmias not fully suppressed, procainamide is ely to slow the tachycardia.

The action of procainamide begins almost mediately after intravenous administration with aximal effects being observed at 30 minutes.

*dications:* The treatment of symptomatic or otentially malignant ventricular arrhythmias (i.e. trasystoles or tachycardia).

The treatment or prophylaxis of symptomatic or otentially malignant ventricular arrhythmias llowing acute myocardial infarction.

**osage and administration**

*ildren:* Pronestyl is not recommended.

*dults:* Intravenous therapy should be reserved for ore serious tachyarrhythmias, in which case lministration should be under continuous ECG onitoring. Once control is achieved oral Pronestyl n be substituted (see data sheet for Pronestyl blets).

Plasma concentrations correlate well with therautic and toxic effects; consequently plasma level says should be carried out if facilities are available. e usual effective antiarrhythmic serum concentran is 3–10 mcg/ml. Toxic manifestations are rare in ncentrations less than 12 mcg/ml.

*dministration:* To initiate therapy, the dose should diluted in 5% Dextrose Injection BP immediately ior to administration to facilitate control of dosage te; the dose should be given at a rate no greater an 50 mg per minute under ECG control, and blood essure must be taken before each dose (see ecautions). Slow administration allows for some itial tissue distribution.

*cute control of tachyarrhythmia:* 100 mg may be ven every 5 minutes by slow injection, at a rate not ceeding 50 mg in any one minute, until the rhythmia is suppressed or a maximum dosage of 1 am has been administered.

Some effects may be seen after the first 100 or 0 mg and it is unusual to require more than 500 to 0 mg to achieve satisfactory antiarrhythmic effects.

*ronic suppression of arrhythmias:* An alternative proach to achieving and then maintaining a erapeutic plasma concentration is to infuse 500 to 0 mg of procainamide at a constant rate over a riod of 25 to 30 minutes and then change to another fusion for maintenance at a rate of 2 to 6 mg/min ee Table below).

Intravenous therapy should be terminated as soon the patient's basic cardiac rhythm appears to be abilized and, if indicated, the patient should be aced on oral antiarrhythmic maintenance therapy. period of 3 to 4 hours (one half-life) should elapse ter the last intravenous dose of procainamide before lministering the first oral dose of procainamide.

*Dilutions and rates for intravenous infusions†*

| *Approximate final concentration* | *Infusion bottle size (ml)* | *ml of Pronestyl (100 mg/ml) to be added* | *Infusion rate* |
|---|---|---|---|
| 0.2% (2 mg/ml) | 500<br>250 | 10<br>5 | 1–3 ml/min |
| 0.4% (4 mg/ml) | 500<br>250 | 20<br>10 | 0.5–1.5 ml/min |

†*Caution:* The flow rate of all intravenous infusion solutions must be closely monitored. These dilutions are calculated to deliver 2–6 mg per minute at the infusion rates listed.

*Elderly:* Reduction in dose or increase in dosage interval may be necessary to maintain constant blood levels without accumulation (see Dosage).

*Patients with renal or hepatic impairment:* Dose reduction or increase in dosage interval may be necessary to produce adequate blood levels without accumulation.

**Contra-indications, warnings, etc**

*Contra-indications:* Hypersensitivity to the drug is an absolute contra-indication. In this connection, cross sensitivity to procaine and related drugs must be borne in mind.

Procainamide should not be administered to patients with complete atrioventricular heart block or a high degree of A-V block or bifasicular block unless an electrical pacemaker is operative.

'Torsade de Pointes', a variant form of ventricular tachycardia associated with a prolonged QT interval, should not be treated with Pronestyl which may aggravate rather than suppress this arrhythmia.

*Warnings and precautions:* Myasthenia gravis: Patients with myasthenia gravis may show worsening of symptoms from procainamide due to its procaine-like effect on diminishing acetylcholine release at skeletal muscle motor nerve endings, so that procainamide administration may be hazardous without optimal adjustment of anticholinesterase medications and other precautions.

Digitalis intoxication: Procainamide may further depress conduction and ventricular asystole or fibrillation may result.

If the patient develops first degree heart block, dosage reduction and/or discontinuation of procainamide should be considered.

Caution in patients with congestive heart failure, acute ischaemic heart disease, cardiogenic shock or cardiomyopathy as even slight depression in myocardial contractility may reduce the cardiac output of the damaged heart.

Hypotension may occur when Pronestyl is administered intravenously. Patients should be kept in a supine position and blood pressure readings made frequently. If hypotension occurs the rate of injection should be reduced or temporarily discontinued and, if necessary, a vasopressor agent administered cautiously.

Intravenous administration should be monitored by ECG. Excessive widening of the QRS complex or prolongation of the P-R interval suggests the occurrence of myocardial toxicity and Pronestyl administration should be stopped. Cardiotoxicity may also be reflected by the appearance of proarrhythmic effects.

In patients with significant impairment of renal or hepatic function, accumulation of Pronestyl may occur, leading to drug toxicity.

The electrophysiological action of procainamide may be affected by electrolyte imbalance.

*Pregnancy and nursing mothers:* Safety has not been established: therefore, Pronestyl should be used during pregnancy only if the possible benefits outweigh the potential risks involved. Procainamide crosses the placenta but the extent is unknown. Procainamide is excreted in breast milk; therefore, it should not be given to nursing mothers because of the potential risk of adverse reactions in the infant.

*Side-effects:* A lupus-like syndrome has been reported after prolonged courses of Pronestyl. The lupus-like syndrome seldom appears in less than two months, but is very common after six months. It is virtually completely reversible and tests for antinuclear factors are usually positive before clinical signs appear. It is perhaps more often observed in patients who are slow acetylators. If long-term treatment is considered desirable, it is advisable to undertake serological tests at no less than monthly intervals and to continue treatment for no longer than absolutely necessary.

Agranulocytosis is a rare side effect of prolonged procainamide therapy. Susceptibility to this is greater in the period following coronary bypass surgery. The patient should be instructed to report any soreness of the mouth, throat, or gums, unexplained fever or any symptoms of upper respiratory tract infection. If any of these should occur, and leucocyte counts indicate cellular depression, Pronestyl therapy should be discontinued, and appropriate treatment should be instituted immediately.

Nausea, vomiting, diarrhoea, abdominal pain, anorexia, bitter taste, mental depression, psychoses with hallucinations, dizziness, headache, pruritus, chills, fever, hepatitis and allergic reactions (such as vasculitis, eosinophilia, skin reactions or angioneurotic oedema) may occur infrequently. They are usually not sufficiently severe to discontinue treatment.

Neutropenia, thrombocytopenia or haemolytic anaemia may rarely be encountered.

As with all other class 1 agents, proarrhythmic effects may occur.

Pronestyl injection contains sodium metabisulphite. This ingredient has been associated with allergic reactions in sensitive individuals.

*Drug interactions:*

*Amiodarone:* Concomitant use of amiodarone may result in increased plasma procainamide concentrations and subsequent toxicity. The dosage of intravenous procainamide should be reduced by 20% to 30% during concomitant administration.

*Other antiarrhythmic drugs:* Additive effects can occur and dosage reduction may be necessary.

*Antihypertensive agents:* Procainamide may produce an additive effect and dosage adjustment may be necessary.

*Anticholinergic drugs:* Additive antivagal effects on A-V nodal conduction may occur.

*Neuromuscular blocking agents:* Possibly reduce dosage of neuromuscular blocking drugs as procainamide may reduce acetylcholine release.

*Captopril:* There have been reports of neutropenia and/or Stevens-Johnson syndrome in patients on procainamide plus captopril. Although a causal relationship has not been established, this combination should only be used with caution, especially in patients with impaired renal function.

*Sulphonamides:* p-amino benzoic acid is a metabolite of procainamide and can inhibit the action of sulphonamides.

*Trimethoprim:* The renal clearance of procainamide is reduced by trimethoprim resulting in increased pharmacodynamic response.

*Pharmacokinetic interactions:* The elimination of procainamide may be decreased by cimetidine or propranolol, and increased by alcohol.

*Overdosage:* After intravenous administration, but seldom after oral, hypotension may occur. Progressive widening of the QRS or A-V conduction block may be seen as may increased ventricular extrasystoles or even ventricular tachycardia or fibrillation. Procainamide and n-acetyl procainamide are removed by haemodialysis but not by peritoneal dialysis. No specific antidote is known.

Overdosage should be managed by general supportive measures and close observation. Fluid expansion and the infusion of noradrenaline (8 micrograms/ml in Sodium Chloride Injection BP) may be useful for hypotension; insertion of a temporary ventricular pacing system may be beneficial.

**Pharmaceutical precautions**

*Storage:* Store below 25°C.

**Legal category** POM.

**Package quantities** Solution 100 mg/ml: 10 ml multidose vials.

**Further information** Procainamide is less readily hydrolysed than procaine and plasma levels decline slowly – about 10–20% per hour. The drug is excreted primarily in the urine, about 10% as free and conjugated p-aminobenzoic acid and about 60% in the unchanged form. The remainder is mainly excreted as n-acetyl procainamide.

The formation of n-acetyl procainamide will depend upon the acetylator status of the patient. As this metabolite also has significant antiarrhythmic activity and a somewhat slower renal clearance than procainamide, both acetylation rate capability and renal function will affect the duration of action.

**Product licence number** 0034/5065R.

## STARIL* TABLETS

**Qualitative and quantitative composition** Staril tablets contain 10 mg or 20 mg fosinopril sodium.

**Pharmaceutical form** Tablets.

**Clinical particulars**

*Therapeutic indications:*

*Hypertension:* Staril is indicated in the treatment of hypertension. Staril may be used alone as initial therapy or in combination with other antihypertensive agents. The antihypertensive effects of Staril and diuretics used concomitantly are approximately additive.

*Heart failure:* Staril is indicated for the treatment of heart failure in combination with a diuretic. In these patients, Staril improves symptoms and exercise tolerance, reduces severity of heart failure and decreases the frequency of hospitalisation for heart failure.

*Posology and method of administration:*
*Adults and children over 12 years*

*Hypertensive patients not being treated with diuretics:* The dose range is 10 to 40 mg per day administered in a single dose and without regard to meals. The normal starting dose for patients is 10 mg once a day. Dosage may need to be adjusted after approximately 4 weeks according to blood pressure response. No additional blood pressure lowering is achieved with doses greater than 40 mg daily. If blood pressure is not adequately controlled with Staril alone, a diuretic can be added.

*Hypertensive patients being treated with concomitant diuretic therapy:* The diuretic should preferably be discontinued for several days prior to beginning therapy with Staril to reduce the risk of an excessive hypotensive response. If blood pressure is inadequately controlled after an observation period of approximately 4 weeks, diuretic therapy may be resumed. Alternatively, if diuretic therapy cannot be discontinued, an initial dose of 10 mg of Staril should be used with careful medical supervision for several hours, until blood pressure has stabilised. In diuretic treated hypertensive patients, mean cerebral blood flow is maintained between 4 and 24 hours after Staril, despite significant reduction in blood pressure.

*Heart failure:* The recommended initial dose is 10 mg once daily, initiated under close medical supervision. If the initial dose is well tolerated patients should be titrated to a dose of up to 40 mg once daily. The appearance of hypotension after the initial dose should not preclude careful dose titration of Staril, following effective management of the hypotension. Staril should be used in conjunction with a diuretic.

*Heart failure – high risk patients:* It is recommended that treatment is initiated in hospital for patients with severe cardiac failure (NYHA IV) and those at particular risk of first dose hypotension, i.e. patients on multiple or high dose diuretics (e.g. >80 mg frusemide), patients with hypovolaemia, hyponatraemia (serum sodium <130 meq/l), pre-existing hypotension (systolic blood pressure <90 mmHg), patients with unstable cardiac failure and those on high-dose vasodilator therapy.

*Children:* The paediatric use of Staril has not been established.

*Elderly:* No dosage reduction is necessary in patients with clinically normal renal and hepatic function as no significant differences in the phamacokinetic parameters or antihypertensive effect of fosinoprilat have been found compared with younger subjects.

*Impaired hepatic function:* Treatment should be initiated at a dose of 10 mg. Although the rate of hydrolysis may be slowed, the extent of hydrolysis is not appreciably reduced in patients with hepatic impairment. In this group of patients, there is evidence of reduced hepatic clearance of fosinoprilat with compensatory increase in renal excretion.

*Renal impairment:* Treatment should be initiated at a dose of 10 mg. Depending on the response, the dose should then be titrated to achieve the desired therapeutic effect.

Absorption, bioavailability, protein binding, biotransformation and metabolism are not appreciably altered by reduced renal function. In patients with impaired renal function, the total body clearance of fosinoprilat is approximately 50% slower than that in patients with normal renal function. However, since hepatobiliary elimination compensates at least partially for diminished renal elimination, the body clearance of fosinoprilat is not appreciably different over a wide range of renal insufficiency (creatinine clearances ranging from < 10 to 80 ml/min/1.73 m², i.e. including end-stage renal failure).

Clearance of fosinoprilat by haemodialysis and peritoneal dialysis averages 2% and 7%, respectively, of urea clearances.

*Contra-indications:* A history of hypersensitivity to fosinopril or any of the tablet excipients.

Pregnancy: Staril is contra-indicated in pregnancy. It has been shown to be lethal to rabbit foetuses at doses that were maternally toxic. Oligohydramnios and neonatal hypotension and/or anuria have been reported following use of ACE inhibitors in the second and third trimester of pregnancy.

Nursing mothers: Staril should not be given to nursing mothers as fosinoprilat has been detected in human breast milk.

*Special warnings and special precautions for use:*
*Warnings:*

*Hypotension:* As with all ACE inhibitors, a hypotensive response may be observed. If this occurs it is usually associated with the first dose and in most instances, symptoms are relieved simply by the patient lying down. A transient, hypotensive episode is not a contra-indication to continuing therapy once the patient's blood pressure has been stabilised.

As with other ACE inhibitors, patients at risk of an excessive hypotensive response, sometimes associated with renal dysfunction, include those with: congestive heart failure, renovascular hypertension, renal dialysis, or volume and/or salt depletion of any aetiology. In patients with any one of these risk factors, it may be prudent to discontinue or reduce the dose of diuretic therapy or take other measures to ensure adequate hydration prior to initiating fosinopril treatment. Treatment of these high risk patients should be initiated under careful medical supervision and they should be followed closely, particularly if it becomes necessary to resume or increase the dose of diuretic or Staril.

*Impaired renal function:* When treated with ACE inhibitors, patients with pre-existing congestive heart failure, renovascular hypertension (especially renal artery stenosis), and salt or volume depletion of any aetiology are at increased risk of developing findings indicative of renal dysfunction, including: increases in BUN and serum creatinine and potassium; proteinuria; changes in urine volume (including oliguria/anuria); and an abnormal urinalysis. Dosage reduction and/or discontinuation of diuretic and/or fosinopril may be required.

*Anaphylactoid-like reactions:* Recent clinical observations have shown a high incidence of anaphylactoid-like reactions during haemodialysis with high-flux dialysis membranes (e.g. AN69) in patients receiving ACE inhibitors. Therefore, this combination should be avoided. Similar reactions during LDL aphoresis with dextran sulphate absorption have been observed. Rare instances of anaphylactoid reactions during desensitisation treatment (hymenoptera venom) have been recorded with other ACE inhibitors.

*Idiosyncratic:* Angioedema involving the extremities, face, lips, mucous membranes, tongue, glottis or larynx has been seen in patients treated with ACE inhibitors. If such symptoms occur during treatment with Staril, therapy should be discontinued.

*Liver function:* Rare potentially fatal cases of cholestatic jaundice and hepatocellular injury have been reported with ACE inhibitors. Patients who develop jaundice or marked elevations of hepatic enzymes should discontinue ACE inhibitor treatment.

*Hyperkalaemia:* When treated with ACE inhibitors, patients at risk of developing hyperkalaemia include those with renal insufficiency, diabetes mellitus, and those using concomitant potassium-sparing diuretics, potassium supplements and/or potassium-containing salt substitutes.

*Neutopenia:* ACE inhibitors have been reported rarely to cause agranulocytosis and bone marrow depression; these occur more frequently in patients with renal impairment, especially if they also have a collagen-vascular disease such as systemic lupus erythematosus or scleroderma. Monitoring of white blood cell counts should be considered in such patients.

*Surgery/anaesthesia:* ACE inhibitors may augment the hypotensive effects of anaesthetics and analgesics. If hypotension occurs in patients undergoing surgery/anaesthesia and concomitantly receiving ACE inhibitors, it can usually be corrected by intravenous administration of fluid.

*Precautions:*

*Pretreatment assessment of renal function:* Evaluation of the hypertensive patient should include assessment of renal function prior to initiation of therapy and during treatment where appropriate.

*Interactions with other medicaments and other forms of interaction:*

*Potassium supplements and potassium-sparing diuretics:* Fosinopril can attenuate potassium loss caused by a thiazide diuretic. Potassium-sparing diuretics or potassium supplements can increase the risk of hyperkalaemia. Therefore, if concomitant use of such agents is indicated, they should be given with caution and the patient's serum potassium should be monitored frequently.

*Antacids:* Antacids may impair absorption of fosinopril. Administration of Staril and antacids should be separated by at least 2 hours.

*NSAIDs:* Non-steroidal anti-inflammatory drugs may interefere with the anti-hypertensive effect. However, the concomitant use of fosinopril and NSAIDs (including aspirin) is not associated with an increase in clinically significant adverse reactions.

*Lithium:* Concomitant therapy with lithium may increase the serum lithium concentration.

*Other anti-hypertensive agents:* Combination with other anti-hypertensive agents such as beta blockers, methyldopa, calcium antagonists, and diuretics may increase the anti-hypertensive efficacy.

*Other drugs:* In pharmacokinetic studies with nifedipine, propranolol, cimetidine, metoclopramide and propantheline the bioavailability of fosinoprilat was not altered by coadministration of Staril with any one of these drugs.

Staril has been used concomitantly with paracetamol, antihistamines, hypoglycaemic agents, insuli lipid-lowering agents or oestrogen without eviden of clinically important adverse events.

*Laboratory tests:* Staril may cause a false lo measurement of serum digoxin levels with assa using the charcoal absorption method for digoxi Other kits which use the antibody coated-tube metho may be used.

*Pregnancy and lactation:* See Contra-indications.

*Effect on ability to drive and use machines:* N applicable.

*Undesirable effects:* In placebo controlled studie there were no significant differences in clinical advers experiences.

The most commonly reported side-effects wi Staril were dizziness, cough, upper respirato symptoms, nausea/vomiting, diarrhoea and abdom nal pain, palpitations/chest pain, rash/pruritu musculoskeletal pain/paraesthesia, fatigue and tas disturbance.

As with other ACE-inhibitors, hypotension, inclu ing orthostatic hypotension, has been reported Staril heart failure trials. Pancreatitis has been r ported rarely in patients treated with ACE inhibitor in some cases this has proved fatal.

The incidence and type of side-effects did not diff between elderly and younger patients.

Laboratory test findings showed some mode usually transient, decreases in haemoglobin a haematocrit values and, infrequently, small increas in blood urea.

*Overdose:* Blood pressure should be monitored and hypotension develops, volume expansion is the tre ment of choice. Fosinoprilat cannot be removed fro the body by dialysis.

**Pharmacological properties**

*Pharmacodynamic properties:* Fosinopril, {(4S)-4-C clohexyl-1-[(RS)-2-methyl-1-(propionyloxy)propox (4-phenylbutyl)=phosphinoylacetyl}-L-proline; s dium salt, is the ester prodrug of an angiotens converting enzyme (ACE) inhibitor, fosinoprilat. A giotensin converting enzyme is a peptidyl dipeptida enzyme that catalyses a number of peptide conve sions. These include the conversion of decapepti Angiotensin I to the octapeptide, Angiotensin II. Sta also inhibits kininase, the enzyme that degrad bradykinin.

*Pharmacokinetic properties:* The absolute absorpti of fosinopril averaged 36% of an oral dose, and w not affected by the presence of food. Rapid a complete hydrolysis to active fosinoprilat occurs the gastrointestinal mucosa and liver.

The time to reach $C_{max}$ is independent of dos achieved in approximately three hours and consiste with peak inhibition of the angiotensin I press response 3 to 6 hours following administration.

In hypertensive patients with normal renal a hepatic function who received repeated doses fosinopril, the effective $T_{\frac{1}{2}}$ for accumulation of fosin prilat averaged 11.5 hours. In patients with hea failure, the effective $T_{\frac{1}{2}}$ was 14 hours. Fosinoprilat highly protein bound (> 95%), has a relatively sm volume of distribution and negligible binding cellular components in blood. The elimination fosinopril is by both hepatic and renal routes. Unli other ACE-inhibitors, there is compensatory excreti by the alternative route in patients with renal hepatic insufficiency.

*Preclinical safety data:* Animal studies indicate toxicity profile which is an extension of the pharm cological effects of fosinopril. It has shown no e dence of carcinogenicity in rodent studies and potential for mutagenicity in either *in vitro* or *in vi* tests.

**Pharmaceutical particulars**

*List of excipients:*

*Staril Tablets 10 mg:* White, flat end, diamo tablets each containing fosinopril sodium 10 m Engraved with Squibb and unilog number 158 on o face and a star design on the other.

*Staril Tablets 20 mg:* White, round biconvex table each containing fosinopril sodium 20 mg. Engrav with Squibb and unilog number 609 on one face a a star design on the other.

Other ingredients: Crospovidone, lactose, sodiu stearyl fumarate, microcrystalline cellulose, povidor

*Incompatibilities:* None known.

*Shelf life:* 36 months.

*Special precautions for storage:* Store below 30°C ir dry place.

*Nature and contents of container:* Cartons containi blister packs of 28 tablets.

*Instructions for use/handling:* No special handli instructions.

**larketing authorisation numbers**
taril Tablets 10 mg 0034/0293
taril Tablets 20 mg 0034/0294

**ate of approval/revision of SPC** November 1995.

**egal category** POM.

## 'RI-ADCORTYL* CREAM
## RI-ADCORTYL* OINTMENT

**ualitative and quantitative composition** Contain-g in each gram the following:Triamcinolone aceton-le 0.1%, Neomycin (as sulphate) 0.25%, Gramicidin .025%, Nystatin100,000 units.

**harmaceutical form**
Topical Cream
Topical Ointment

**linical particulars**

*herapeutic indications:* The topical treatment of uperficial bacterial infections, cutaneous candidosis nd dermatological conditions, threatened or compli-ated by bacterial or candidal superinfections, which re known to respond to topical steroid therapy. These aclude: atopic eczema, contact eczema, follicular czema, infantile eczema, otitis externa without frank ıfection, anogenital pruritus, nummular eczema, ost-traumatic infective eczema, seborrhoeic eczema, ıtertrigo, neurodermatitis and infected insect bites.

*osology and method of administration:*
*.dults and children:* Apply to the affected area two to our times daily.

*Elderly:* Corticosteroids should be used sparingly nd for short periods of time, as natural thinning of ıe skin occurs in the elderly.

If, after about 7 days application, little or no nprovement has occurred, cultural isolation of the ffending organism should be followed by appropri-te local or systemic antimicrobial therapy.

*'ontra-indications:* In tuberculous and most viral esions of the skin, particularly herpes simplex and aricella. Also in fungal lesions not susceptible to ystatin.

In patients with hypersensitivity to any of the omponents.

Should not be used for facial rosacea, acne vulgaris r perioral dermatitis.

Should not be applied to the external auditory canal ı patients with perforated eardrums.

The products should not be used for extensive areas ecause of possible risk of systemic absorption and eomycin-induced ototoxicity.

*'pecial warnings and special precautions for use:* .drenal suppression can occur, even without occlu-ion. The use of occlusive dressings should be avoided ecause of the increased risk of sensitivity reactions nd increased percutaneous absorption. The ossibility of sensitivity to neomycin should be taken ıto consideration especially in the treatment of atients suffering from leg ulcers.

Steroid-antibiotic combinations should not be con-nued for more than 7 days in the absence of any linical improvement, since in this situation occult xtension of infection may occur due to the masking ffect of the steroid.

Extended or recurrent application may increase the sk of contact sensitisation and should be avoided.

If used on the face, courses should be limited to 5 ays and occlusion should not be used.

*Children:* In infants, long-term continuous topical teroid therapy should be avoided. Courses should be mited to 5 days and occlusion should not be used.

*ıteractions with other medicaments and other forms f interaction:* Not applicable

*'regnancy and lactation:* There is inadequate evidence f safety in human pregnancy. Topical administration f corticosteroids to pregnant animals can cause bnormalities of foetal development including cleft alate and intra-uterine growth retardation. There ıay, therefore, be a very small risk of such effects in ıe human foetus. There are theoretical risks of eomycin-induced foetal ototoxicity; therefore the roduct should be used with caution only when the enefit outweighs the potential risk.

*'ffects on ability to drive and use machines:* Not pplicable.

*Indesirable effects:*
*'riamcinolone Acetonide:* The following side effects ave been reported. Usually with prolonged usage: ermatologic–impaired wound healing, thinning of ıe skin, petechiae and ecchymoses, facial erythema nd telangiectasia, increased sweating, purpura, triae, hirsutism, acneiform eruptions, lupus rythematosus-like lesions and suppressed reactions ɔ skin tests. These effects may be enhanced with cclusive dressings.

The possibility of the systemic effects which are associated with all steroid therapy should be considered.

*Neomycin:* Sensitivity reactions may occur especially with prolonged use. Ototoxicity and nephrotoxicity have been reported. The product should be used with caution and in small amounts in the treatment of skin infections following extensive burns, trophic ulceration and other conditions where absorption of neomycin is possible. The product should be used with care in patients with established hearing loss.

*Gramicidin:* Sensitivity has occasionally been reported.

*Nystatin:* There have been no substantiated reports of sensitivity associated with topical nystatin.

*Overdose:* Topically applied corticosteroids can be absorbed in sufficient amounts to produce systemic effects (see *Side effects*).

In the event of accidental ingestion, the patient should be observed and treated symptomatically.

**Pharmacological properties**

*Pharmacodynamic properties:* Triamcinolone acetonide is a potent fluorinated corticosteroid with rapid anti- inflammatory, antipruritic and anti-allergic actions.

The combined action of the antibiotics neomycin and gramicidin provides comprehensive antibacterial therapy against a wide range of gram-positive and gram-negative bacteria, including those micro-organisms responsible for most bacterial skin infections.

Nystatin is an antifungal antibiotic, active against a wide range of yeasts and yeast-like fungi, including candida albicans.

*Pharmacokinetic properties:* Not applicable.

*Preclinical safety data:* No further relevant data

**Pharmaceutical particulars**

*List of excipients:*
*Cream:* Aluminium hydroxide, antifoam emulsion, benzyl alcohol, ethanol, ethylenediamine, hydrochloric acid, macrogol ether, perfume, polysorbate 60, propylene glycol, sorbitol, titanium dioxide, white soft paraffin, water.
*Ointment:* Polyethylene resin, liquid paraffin.

*Incompatibilities:* None known.

*Shelf life:* 24 months.

*Special precautions for storage:*
*Cream:* Store below 25°C. Avoid freezing.
*Ointment:* Store below 25°C.

*Nature and contents of container:* Aluminium tubes.

*Instruction for use/handling:* None.

**Marketing authorisation numbers**
Cream 0034/5093R
Ointment 0034/5094R

**Date of approval/revision of SPC**
Cream: October 1995
Ointment: January 1996

**Legal category** POM

## TRI-ADCORTYL* OTIC OINTMENT

**Qualitative and quantitative composition** Containing in each gram the following:Triamcinolone acetonide 0.1%, Neomycin (as sulphate) 0.25%, Gramicidin 0.025%, Nystatin 100,000 units.

**Pharmaceutical form** Aural Ointment.

**Clinical particulars**

*Therapeutic indications:* For the topical treatment of otitis externa, known to respond to topical steroid therapy, complicated by superficial bacterial or fungal infections.

*Posology and method of administration:*
*Adults and children:* Apply a small amount directly from the tube into the aural canal two to four times daily.

*Elderly:* Corticosteroids should be used sparingly and for short periods of time, as natural thinning of the skin occurs in the elderly.

If, after about 7 days application, little or no improvement has occurred, cultural isolation of the offending organism should be followed by appropriate local or systemic antimicrobial therapy.

*Contra-indications:* In tuberculous and most viral lesions of the skin, particularly herpes simplex and varicella. Also in fungal lesions not susceptible to nystatin.

In patients with hypersensitivity to any of the components.

Should not be used for facial rosacea, acne vulgaris or perioral dermatitis.

Should not be applied to the external auditory canal in patients with perforated eardrums.

The products should not be used for extensive areas because of possible risk of systemic absorption and neomycin-induced ototoxicity.

*Special warnings and special precautions for use:* Adrenal suppression can occur, even without occlusion. The use of occlusive dressings should be avoided because of the increased risk of sensitivity reactions and increased percutaneous absorption. The possibility of sensitivity to neomycin should be taken into consideration especially in the treatment of patients suffering from leg ulcers.

Steroid-antibiotic combinations should not be continued for more than 7 days in the absence of any clinical improvement, since in this situation occult extension of infection may occur due to the masking effect of the steroid.

Extended or recurrent application may increase the risk of contact sensitisation and should be avoided.

If used in childhood, or on the face, courses should be limited to 5 days and occlusion should not be used.

Not for ophthalmic use.

*Children:* In infants, long-term continuous topical steroid therapy should be avoided. Courses should be limited to 5 days and occlusion should not be used.

*Interactions with other medicaments and other forms of interaction:* Not applicable

*Pregnancy and laction:* There is inadequate evidence of safety in human pregnancy. Topical administration of corticosteroids to pregnant animals can cause abnormalities of foetal development including cleft palate and intra-uterine growth retardation. There may, therefore, be a very small risk of such effects in the human foetus. There are theoretical risks of neomycin-induced foetal ototoxicity; therefore the product should be used with caution only when the benefit outweighs the potential risk.

*Effects on ability to drive and use machines:* Not applicable.

*Undesirable effects:*
*Triamcinolone acetonide:* Triamcinolone acetonide is well tolerated. Where adverse reactions occur they are usually reversible on cessation of therapy. However the following side effects have been reported usually with prolonged usage:

Dermatologic–impaired wound healing, thinning of the skin, petechiae and ecchymoses, facial erythema and telangiectasia, increased sweating, purpura, striae, hirsutism, acneiform eruptions, lupus erythematosus-like lesions and suppressed reactions to skin tests.

These effects may be enhanced with occlusive dressings.

Signs of systemic toxicity such as oedema and electrolyte imbalance have not been observed even when high topical dosage has been used. The possibility of the systemic effects which are associated with all steroid therapy should be considered.

*Neomycin:* Sensitivity reactions may occur especially with prolonged use. Ototoxicity and nephrotoxicity have been reported. The product should be used with caution and in small amounts in the treatment of skin infections following extensive burns, trophic ulceration and other conditions where absorption of neomycin is possible. The product should be used with care in patients with established hearing loss.

*Gramicidin:* Sensitivity has occasionally been reported.

*Nystatin:* There have been no substantiated reports of sensitivity associated with topical nystatin.

*Overdose:* Topically applied corticosteroids can be absorbed in sufficient amounts to produce systemic effects (see side effects).

In the event of accidental ingestion, the patient should be observed and treated symptomatically.

**Pharmacological properties**

*Pharmacodynamic properties:* Triamcinolone acetonide is a potent fluorinated corticosteroid with rapid anti- inflammatory, antipruritic and anti-allergic actions.

The combined action of the antibiotics neomycin and gramicidin provides comprehensive antibacterial therapy against a wide range of gram-positive and gram-negative bacteria, including those micro-organisms responsible for most bacterial skin infections.

Nystatin is an antifungal antibiotic, active against a wide range of yeasts and yeast-like fungi, including *candida albicans.*

Pharmacokinetic properties: Not applicable.

*Preclinical safety data:* No further relevant data

**Pharmaceutical particulars**

*List of excipients:* Polylethylene resin and liquid paraffin

*Incompatibilites:* None known.

*Shelf life:* 48 months.

*Special precautions for storage:* Store below 25°C.

*Nature and contents of container:* Aluminium tubes.

*Instructions for use/handling:* None.

**Marketing authorisation number** 0034/5095R

**Date of approval/revision of SPC** January 1996

**Legal category** POM

## VELOSEF* CAPSULES 250MG AND 500MG
## VELOSEF* SYRUP 250MG/5ML

**Qualitative and quantitative composition**

*Capsules 250 mg:* Opaque, orange body with opaque blue cap printed Squibb and 113 in white on each half. Each capsule contains 250 mg cephradine.

*Capsules 500 mg:* Opaque blue printed in white with Squibb and 114 on each half. Each capsule contains 500 mg cephradine.

*Syrup 250 mg:* When reconstituted contains 250 mg cephradine per 5 ml.

**Pharmaceutical form**

Oral tablets.
Oral powder for reconstitution.

**Clinical particulars**

*Therapeutic indications:* In the treatment of infections of the urinary and respiratory tracts and of the skin and soft tissues. These include:

Upper respiratory infections–pharyngitis, sinusitis, otitis media, tonsillitis, laryngo-tracheo bronchitis.

Lower respiratory infections–acute and chronic bronchitis, lobar and bronchopneumonia.

Urinary tract infections–cystitis, urethritis, pyelonephritis.

Skin and soft tissue infections–abscess, cellulitis, furunculosis, impetigo.

Cephradine has been shown to be effective in reducing the incidence of postoperative infections in patients undergoing surgical procedures associated with a high risk of infection. It is also of value where postoperative infections would be disastrous and where patients have a reduced host resistance to bacterial infection. Protection is best ensured by achieving adequate local tissue concentrations at the time contamination is likely to occur. Thus, cephradine should be administered immediately prior to surgery and continued during the postoperative period.

Bacteriology studies to determine the causative organisms and their sensitivity to cephradine should be performed. Therapy may be instituted prior to receiving the results of the sensitivity test.

*Posology and method of administration:* Cephradine may be given without regard to meals.

*Adults:* For urinary tract infections the usual dose is 500 mg four times daily or 1 g twice daily; severe or chronic infections may require larger doses. Prolonged intensive therapy is needed for complications such as prostatitis and epididymitis. For respiratory tract infections and skin and soft tissue infections the usual dose is 250 mg or 500 mg four times daily or 500 mg or 1 g twice daily depending on the severity and site of infections.

*Children:* The usual dose is from 25 to 50 mg/kg/day total, given in two or four equally divided doses.

For otitis media daily doses from 75 to 100 mg/kg in divided doses every 6 to 12 hours are recommended. Maximum dose 4 g per day.

*Elderly:* There are no specific dosage recommendations or precautions for use in the elderly except, as with other drugs, to monitor those patients with impaired renal or hepatic function.

*All patients, irrespective of age and weight:* Larger doses (up to 1 g four times daily) may be given for severe or chronic infections. Therapy should be continued for a minimum of 48-72 hours after the patient becomes asymptomatic or evidence of bacterial eradication has been obtained. In infections caused by haemolytic strains of streptococci, a minimum of 10 days treatment is recommended to guard against the risk of rheumatic fever or glomerulonephritis. In the treatment of chronic urinary tract infections, frequent bacteriological and clinical appraisal is necessary during therapy and may be necessary for several months afterwards. Persistent infections may require treatment for several weeks. Smaller doses than those indicated above should not be used. Doses for children should not exceed doses recommended for adults. As cephradine is available in both injectable and oral form, patients may be changed from the cephradine injectable to cephradine oral at the same dosage level.

*Renal impairment dosage:*

*Patients not on dialysis:* The following dosage schedule is suggested as a guideline based on a dosage of 500 mg Q6H and on creatinine clearance. Further modification in the dosage schedule may be required because of the dosage selected and individual variation.

| Creatinine Clearance | Dose | Time Interval |
|---|---|---|
| more than 20 ml/min | 500 mg | 6 hours |
| 5-20 ml/min | 250 mg | 6 hours |
| less than 5 ml/min | 250 mg | 50-70 hours |

*Patients on chronic, intermittent haemodialysis:*

| | |
|---|---|
| 250 mg | At start of haemodialysis |
| 250 mg | 6-12 hours after start |
| 250 mg | 36-48 hours after start |
| 250 mg | At start of next haemodialysis if >30 hours after previous dose. |

Further modification of the dosage schedule may be necessary in children.

*Contra-indications:* Patients with known hypersensitivity to the cephalosporin antibiotics.

*Special warnings and special precautions for use:* After treatment with cephradine, a false positive reaction for glucose in the urine may occur with Benedict's or Fehling's solution or with reagent tablets such as Clinitest*, but not with enzyme-based tests such as Clinistix* or Diastix*.

As with all antibiotics, prolonged use may result in overgrowth of non-susceptible organisms.

*Interactions with other medicaments and other forms of interaction:* There is evidence of partial cross-allergenicity between the penicillins and the cephalosporins. Therefore cephradine should be used with caution in those patients with known hypersensitivity to penicillins. There have been instances of patients who have had reactions to both drug classes (including anaphylaxis).

*Pregnancy and lactation:* Although animal studies have not demonstrated any teratogenicity, safety in pregnancy has not been established. Cephradine is excreted in breast milk and should be used with caution in lactating mothers.

*Effects on ability to drive and use machines:* None known

*Undesirable effects:* Limited essentially to gastrointestinal disturbances and on occasion to hypersensitivity phenomena. The latter are more likely to occur in individuals who have previously demonstrated hypersensitivity and those with a history of allergy, asthma, hay fever or urticaria. The majority of reported side-effects have been mild and are rare, and include glossitis, heartburn, dizziness, tightness in the chest, nausea, vomiting, diarrhoea, abdominal pain, vaginitis, candidal overgrowth. Skin and hypersensitivity reactions include urticaria, skin rashes, joint pains, oedema.

As with other cephalosporins, mild transient eosinophilia, leucopenia and neutropenia, positive direct Coombs tests and pseudomembraneous colitis have been reported.

*Clinical Chemistry:* Elevations of BUN and Serum Creatinine have been reported. In clinical trials, elevations of SGOT, SGPT, total bilirubin and alkaline phosphates were observed.

*Overdose:* None known.

**Pharmacological properties**

*Pharmacodynamic properties:*

*Actions:* Cephradine is a broad-spectrum, bactericidal antibiotic active against both Gram-positive and Gram-negative bacteria. It is also highly active against most strains of penicillinase-producing Staphylococci.

*Microbiology:* The following organisms have shown in vitro sensitivity to cephradine.

Gram-positive–Staphylococci (both penicillin sensitive and resistant strains), Streptococci, *Streptococcus pyogenes* (beta haemolytic) and *streptococcus pneumoniae.*

Gram-negative–*Escherichia coli, Klebsiella*, spp, *Proteus mirabilis, Haemophilus influenzae, Shigella* spp., *Salmonella* spp. (including *Salmonella typhi*) and *Neisseria* spp.

Because cephradine is unaffected by penicillinase, many strains of *Escherichia coli* and *Staphylococcus aureus* which produce this enzyme are susceptible to cephradine but resistant to ampicillin.

*Pharmacokinetic properties:* Cephradine has a high degree of stability to many beta-lactamases. It has a low degree of protein-binding and a large volume of distribution. Therefore, tissue levels are generally found to be high. Oral cephradine can be given twice or four times daily, and is well absorbed.

*Human pharmacology:* Cephradine is acid stable and is rapidly absorbed following oral administration in the fasting state. Following doses of 250 mg, 500 mg and 1000 mg average peak serum levels of approximately 9, 16.5, and 24.2 micrograms/ml, respectively, were obtained at one hour. The presence of food in the gastrointestinal tract delays the absorption but does not affect the total amount of cephradine absorbed. Measurable serum levels are present six hours after administration. Over 90% of the drug is excreted unchanged in the urine within 6 hours. Peak urine concentrations are approximately 1600 micrograms/ml following a 250 mg dose, 3200 micrograms/ml following a 500 mg dose, and 4000 microgram ml following a 1000 mg dose. After 48 hours' admi istration of 100 mg/kg/day of cephradine for th treatment of otitis media, cephradine has been meas ured in the middle ear exudate at an average level 3.6 microgram/ml.

*Preclinical safety data:* No relevant further dat available.

**Pharmaceutical particulars**

*List of excipients:*

*Capsules 250 mg:* Erythrosine, gelatin capsules, i digo carmine, iron oxide, lactose, magnesium ste rate, titanium dioxide.

*Capsules 500 mg:* Gelatin capsules, indigo carmin lactose, magnesium stearate, titanium dioxide.

*Syrup:* Citric acid, flavours, guar gum, methylcell lose, sodium citrate, sucrose.

*Incompatibilities:* None known

*Shelf life:* Capsules: 36 months.
Syrup: 48 months.

*Special precautions for storage:*
*Capsules:* Store below 25°C.
*Syrup:* Store below 25°C.

After reconstitution; discard unused syrup after days if stored in refrigerator, or seven days at belo 25°C.

*Nature and contents of container:*

Capsules: Blister packs of 20 or 100 capsules.
Syrup: Bottles of 100 ml.

*Instructions for use/handling:* Not applicable

**Marketing authorisation numbers**

| | |
|---|---|
| Velosef Capsules 250 mg | 0034/0133R |
| Velosef Capsules 500 mg | 0034/0134R |
| Velosef Syrup 250 mg/5 ml | 0034/0136R |

**Date of approval/revision of SPC** 4 February 1997

**Legal category** POM.

## VELOSEF* FOR INJECTION

**Presentation** Velosef for Injection is a sterile powd blend of cephradine and L-arginine. Aft reconstitution, Velosef for Injection 500 mg and 1.0 vials provide 500 mg and 1.0 g of cephradine activit respectively.

**Uses** *Actions:* Cephradine is a broad-spectru bactericidal antibiotic active against both Gran positive and Gram-negative bacteria. It is also high active against most strains of penicillinase-producir staphylococci.

*Microbiology:* The following organisms have show *in vitro* sensitivity to cephradine:

Gram-positive – *Staphylococci* (both penicill sensitive and resistant strains), *Streptococ Streptococcus pyogenes* (beta haemolytic) an *Streptococcus pneumoniae.*

Gram-negative – *E. coli, Klebsiella, P. mirabil Haemophilus influenzae, Shigella* spp., *Salmonel* spp. (including *Salmonella typhi*) and *Neisseria* spp.

Because cephradine is unaffected by penicillinas many strains of *E. coli* and *Staphylococcus aure* which produce this enzyme are susceptible cephradine but resistant to ampicillin.

*Indications:* The treatment of infections of the urina and respiratory tracts and of the skin and soft tissue bones and joints; also septicaemia and endocarditi These include:

Upper respiratory infections – pharyngitis, sinusiti otitis media, tonsillitis, laryngo-tracheo-bronchitis.

Lower respiratory infections – acute and chron bronchitis, lobar and bronchopneumonia.

Urinary tract infections – cystitis, urethritis, pyel nephritis.

Skin and soft tissue infections – abscess, celluliti furunculosis, impetigo.

Velosef has been shown to be effective in reducir the incidence of postoperative infections in patien undergoing surgical procedures associated with high risk of infection. It is also of value where pos operative infection would be disastrous and whe patients have a reduced host resistance to bacteri infection. Protection is best ensured by achievin adequate local tissue concentrations at the tim contamination is likely to occur. Thus, Velosef shou be administered immediately prior to surgery ar continued during the postoperative period.

Bacteriological studies to determine the causativ organisms and their sensitivity to cephradine shou be performed. Therapy may be instituted prior t receiving the results of the sensitivity test.

Sterile Velosef for injection is indicated primari for those patients unable to tolerate oral medicatio It is also indicated for intravenous use either by dire injection or by intravenous infusion for the treatme of serious and life-threatening infections.

**osage and administration** Intramuscular or intra-
enous injection and intravenous infusion.

*dults: Treatment:* The usual dose range of Velosef
•r injection is 2-4 g daily in four equally divided
oses. This may be increased up to 8 g a day for
evere infections, e.g. septicaemia and endocarditis.
or the majority of infections, the usual dose is 500 mg
i.d. in equally spaced doses; severe or chronic
ifections may require larger doses. Prolonged
itensive therapy is needed for complications such as
rostatitis and epididymitis. Patients who are severely
 and who require high serum levels of cephradine
•r treating their infections should be started on
travenous therapy.

Limited experience indicates that intraperitoneal
dministration of Velosef may be effective after
urgery in cases of peritonitis where a surgical
rainage system has been established.

*rophylaxis:* The recommended dose for surgical
rophylaxis is a single, pre-operative 1–2 g IM or IV
ose. Subsequent parenteral or oral doses can be
dministered as appropriate.

*hildren:* The usual dose is 50-100 mg/kg/day total
iven in four equally divided doses. More serious
nesses (e.g. typhoid fever) may require 200-300 mg/
g/day.

*Iderly:* There are no specific dosage recom-
endations or precautions for use in the elderly
xcept, as with other drugs, to monitor those patients
ith impaired renal or hepatic function.

*Il patients, regardless of age and weight:* Therapy
hould be continued for a minimum of 48-72 hours
fter the patient becomes asymptomatic or evidence
f bacterial eradication has been obtained. In
ifections caused by haemolytic strains of
treptococci, a minimum of 10 days of treatment is
ecommended to guard against the risk of rheumatic
ever or glomerulonephritis. In the treatment of
hronic urinary tract infections, frequent bacterio-
gical and clinical appraisal is necessary during
erapy and may be necessary for several months
fterwards. Persistent infections may require treat-
ent for several weeks. Smaller doses than those
dicated above should not be used. Doses for children
hould not exceed doses recommended for adults. As
elosef is available in both injectable and oral form,
atients may be changed from Velosef injectable to
elosef oral at the same dosage level.

*enal impairment dosage:*
*atients not on dialysis:* The following dosage sched-
le is suggested as a guideline based on a dosage of
00 mg Q6H and on creatinine clearance. Further
odification in the dosage schedule may be required
ecause of the dosage selected and individual varia-
on.

| *reatinine clearance* | *Dose* | *Time interval* |
|---|---|---|
| ore than 20 ml/min | 500 mg | 6 hours |
| 5–20 ml/min | 250 mg | 6 hours |
| ss than 5 ml/min | 250 mg | 50–70 hours |

*atients on chronic intermittent haemodialysis:*
50 mg At start of haemodialysis
50 mg 6–12 hours after start
50 mg 36–48 hours after start
50 mg At start of next haemodialysis >30 hours
 after previous dose

Further modification of the dosage schedule may
e necessary in children.

*econstitution: For intramuscular use:* Aseptically add
terile water for injection or 0.9% sodium chloride
jection according to the following table:

| *Single dose* vial size* | *Volume of diluent to be added* |
|---|---|
| 500 mg | 2.0 ml |
| 1 g | 4.0 ml |

\* Preparation contains no bactericide and is not
intended for multiple dose use.

Shake to effect solution and withdraw the entire
contents. Intramuscular solutions should be used
within 2 hours at room temperature; when stored in a
refrigerator at 5°C, solutions retain full potency for 12
hours. Reconstituted solutions may vary in colour
from light to straw yellow; however, this does not
affect the potency.

*For intravenous use:* Velosef for injection may be
administered by direct intravenous injection or by
infusion. A 3 microgram/ml serum concentration can
be maintained for each milligram of cephradine per
kg body weight per hour of infusion.

*For direct intravenous administration:* Suitable
intravenous injection solutions are Sterile Water for
Injection, 5% Glucose Injection or 0.9% Sodium
Chloride Injection.

Aseptically add 5 ml of diluent to the 500 mg vial or
10 ml to the 1 g vial. Shake to effect solution and
withdraw the entire contents. The solution may be
slowly injected directly into a vein over a 3 to 5 minute
period. The solution should be used within 2 hours
when kept at room temperature; if stored at 5°C,
solutions retain full potency for 12 hours.

*For continuous or intermittent intravenous infusion:*
Suitable intravenous infusion solutions are Sterile
Water for Injection (50 mg/ml cephradine solutions
are approximately isotonic); 5% or 10% Glucose
Injection; 0.9% Sodium Chloride Injection; Sodium
Lactate Injection (M/6 sodium lactate); Glucose and
Sodium Chloride Injection; Lactated Ringer's Injection;
Ringer's Injection; 5% Glucose in Lactated Ringer's
Injection; 5% Glucose in Ringer's Injection.

Aseptically add 10 ml of the diluent to the 1 g vial
and shake to effect solution. Aseptically transfer the
entire contents to the IV infusion diluent. Intravenous
infusions prepared remain potent for 24 hours at
room temperature or 1 week at 5°C at concentrations
up to 10 mg/ml (1%), and for 10 hours at room
temperature or 48 hours at 5°C at concentrations up
to 50 mg/ml (5%). For prolonged infusion, replace 5%
infusions every 10 hours and 1% infusions every 24
hours with freshly-prepared solutions.

*N.B. Only cephradine solubilised with arginine may
be reconstituted with solutions containing calcium
salts, such as Ringer's Solutions.*

For further information on compatibilities consult
the manufacturer.

Protect solutions of cephradine from concentrated
light or direct sunlight.

**Contra-indications, warnings, etc**
*Contra-indications:* Patients with known hypersensitivity to the cephalosporin antibiotics.

*Precautions:* After treatment with Velosef a false
positive reaction for glucose in the urine may occur
with Benedict's solution or Fehling's solution or with
reagent tablets such as Clinitest\*, but not with
enzyme-based tests such as Clinistix\* or Diastix\*.

As with all antibiotics, prolonged use may result in
overgrowth of non-susceptible organisms.

*Administration in renal impairment:* A modified
dosage schedule in patients with decreased renal
function is necessary (see Dosage).

*Drug interactions:* There is evidence of partial cross-
allergenicity between the penicillins and the
cephalosporins. Therefore Velosef should be used
with caution in those patients with known hypersensitivity to penicillins.

*Pregnancy and breast feeding:* Although animal

studies have not demonstrated any teratogenicity,
safety in pregnancy has not been established.
Cephradine is excreted in breast milk and should be
used with caution in lactating mothers.

*Side-effects:* Limited essentially to gastro-intestinal
disturbances and on occasion to hypersensitivity
phenomena. The latter are more likely to occur in
individual's who have previously demonstrated
hypersensitivity and those with a history of allergy,
asthma, hay fever or urticaria. The majority of reported
side-effects have been mild and are rare, and include
glossitis, heartburn, headache, dizziness, dyspnoea,
paraesthesia, nausea, vomiting, diarrhoea, abdominal
pain, candidal overgrowth, vaginitis. Skin and hypersensitivity reactions include urticaria, skin rashes,
joint pains, oedema.

As with other cephalosporins, mild transient
eosinophilia, leucopenia and neutropenia, rarely
positive direct Coombs tests and pseudomembranous
colitis have been reported.

*Clinical chemistry:* Elevations of BUN and Serum
Creatinine have been reported. In clinical trials, elevations of SGOT, SGPT, total bilirubin and alkaline
phosphates were observed.

*Injection:* As with other parenterally administered
antibiotics, transient pain may be experienced at the
injection site, but is seldom the cause for discontinuing
treatment. Thrombophlebitis has been reported
following intravenous injection.

Since sterile abscesses have been reported
following accidental subcutaneous injection, the
preparation should be administered by deep intramuscular injection.

**Pharmaceutical precautions** *Storage (before
reconstitution):* At room temperature. Not for
multidose use.

**Legal category** POM.

**Package quantities** *500 mg single-dose vials:* Pack
of 5.
*1 g single-dose vials:* Single-vial pack.

**Further information** Cephradine has a high degree
of stability to beta-lactamases. It has a low degree of
protein binding and a large volume of distribution.
Therefore, tissue levels are generally found to be high.

*Human pharmacology:* Following intramuscular
administration of a single 0.5 g dose of cephradine to
normal volunteers, the average peak serum
concentration was 8.41 microgram/ml with the time
to peak concentration being 0.93 hours. The serum
half-life averaged 1.25 hours. A single 1 g intravenous
dose resulted in serum concentrations of 86 micro-
gram/ml at 5 minutes and 12 microgram/ml at 1 hour;
these concentrations declined to 1 microgram/ml at 4
hours. Continuous infusion of 500 mg per hour into a
70 kg man maintained a concentration of about
21.4 microgram/ml cephradine activity; this study
showed that a serum concentration of approximately
3 microgram/ml can be obtained for each milligram
of cephradine administered per kg of body weight per
hour of infusion.

Cephradine is excreted unchanged in the urine. The
kidneys excrete 57% to 80% of an intramuscular dose
in the first six hours; this results in a high urine
concentration, e.g. 880 microgram/ml of urine after a
500 mg intramuscular dose. Probenecid slows tubular
secretion and almost doubles peak serum
concentration.

Assays of bone obtained at surgery have shown
that cephradine penetrates bone tissue.

**Product licence numbers**
Velosef Injection 500 mg    0034/0198
Velosef Injection 1 g    0034/0199

\**Trade Mark*

# Stafford-Miller Ltd
45 Broadwater Road
Welwyn Garden City
Herts AL7 3SP

## ALPHOSYL* LOTION AND CREAM

**Presentation** The lotion is a light, free-flowing emulsion and the cream is smooth and homogenous. Both are light tan in colour and contain: alcoholic extract of coal tar 5% w/w and allantoin 2% w/w.

**Uses** The treatment of psoriasis and psoriasis of the scalp.

*Alphosyl lotion:* For the treatment of psoriasis of the body and scalp.

*Alphosyl cream:* For the treatment of psoriasis, its moisturising capability makes it particularly useful on flexures.

**Dosage and administration**
*Lotion and cream:* Apply liberally two to four times daily, rub vigorously into the affected areas. Alphosyls do not stain, and can be applied freely, even to the scalp. Where hard scales exist, apply after a hot bath. Optimum results may take several weeks of daily application. After the lesions have been brought under control continue use to help prevent recurrence.

**Contra-indications, warnings, etc** Alphosyl lotion and cream are contra-indicated in patients with acute psoriasis, and those with a known sensitivity to coal tar. Skin irritation, acne-like eruptions or photosensitivity may occur in patients who are sensitive to coal tar. These undesirable effects resolve when treatment is stopped.

*Use in pregnancy and lactation:* Safety in pregnancy and lactation has not been established, and hence, use in the first trimester of pregnancy is best avoided.

*Special warnings and precautions:* For external use only. Discontinue if irritation occurs or in cases of sensitivity to coal tar.

**Pharmaceutical precautions** Store at room temperature. Do not refrigerate.

**Legal category** P

**Package quantities**
*Alphosyl Lotion:* Bottles of 250 ml.
*Alphosyl Cream:* Tube of 100 g.

**Product licence numbers**
Alphosyl lotion   0036/5008
Alphosyl cream   0036/5006

## ALPHOSYL* HC CREAM

**Presentation** A cream containing refined alcoholic extract of coal tar 5% w/w, allantoin 2% w/w and hydrocortisone PhEur 0.5% w/w in a greaseless aqueous cream base. The cream is smooth, homogeneous and light tan in colour.

**Uses** The treatment of psoriasis. The anti-inflammatory action of the hydrocortisone in Alphosyl HC cream enhances the basic Alphosyl action.

**Dosage and administration**
*Adults, including elderly:* Apply cream sparingly twice daily to psoriatic plaques. Rub in well. Not recommended for children under 5 years. Six years and over as above.

**Contra-indications, warnings, etc**
*Contra-indications:* Tuberculosis or fungal lesions of the skin, herpes simplex, vaccinia or varicella, and a history of hypersensitivity to any of the ingredients.

*Other undesirable effects:* Hypersensitivity reactions may occasionally occur. See special warnings below.

*Use in pregnancy and lactation:* Topical administration of corticosteroids to pregnant animals can cause abnormality of foetal development. Topical steroids should not be used extensively in pregnancy, i.e., in large amounts or for long periods because of the risk of teratogenic effects or significant absorption causing suppression of the HPA axis.

*Other special warnings and precautions:* For external use only. Avoid contact with the eyes. Use sparingly. Discontinue use if sensitivity occurs.
  The following results of steroid use are uncommon at this dosage, however:
- When used over large areas or for prolonged periods systemic side effects can result.
- Under occlusive dressings or in intertriginous areas,

topical steroids may cause skin atrophy manifesting as striae, thinning and telangiectasia.
- Viral, bacterial or fungal infection of the skin may be substantially exacerbated by topical steroid treatment unless accompanied by appropriate therapy.
- Wound healing can be significantly retarded.

**Pharmaceutical precautions** Store between 4°C and 25°C

**Legal category** POM

**Package quantities** Tubes of 30 g and 100 g.

**Further information** Nil.

**Product licence number** 0036/0026

## ALPHOSYL* 2 IN 1 SHAMPOO

**Presentation** Alphosyl 2 in 1 Shampoo is a green pearlescent lotion shampoo with a herbal fragrance containing alcoholic extract of coal tar 5% w/w.

**Uses** Alphosyl 2 in 1 Shampoo is indicated for the treatment of psoriasis, seborrhoeic dermatitis, scaling and itching (often associated with eczema) and dandruff.

**Dosage and administration** Wet hair thoroughly then briskly rub a liberal amount of Alphosyl 2 in 1 Shampoo into the hair and scalp. Rinse thoroughly and repeat the procedure massaging the scalp for several minutes and working the shampoo into a rich lather. Rinse thoroughly.

*Dandruff:* Use once or twice weekly as necessary, or as directed by a physician.

*Psoriasis, seborrhoeic dermatitis, scaling and itching:* Use every two or three days, or as directed by a physician.

**Contra-indications, warnings, etc** Sensitivity to coal tar. Skin irritation or photosensitivity may occur in some patients who are sensitive to coal tar. These undesirable effects resolve when treatment is stopped. Avoid contact with eyes. If necessary rinse out with warm water. Keep out of reach of children.

*Use during pregnancy and lactation:* There is no or inadequate evidence of safety of coal tar in human pregnancy but it has been in wide use for many years without apparent ill consequence. However, use in the first trimester of pregnancy is best avoided.

**Legal category** GSL

**Package quantities** Bottles of 125 ml and 250 ml.

**Further information** Alphosyl 2 in 1 Shampoo also contains a conditioning agent, Guar Hydroxypropyltrimonium Chloride. Alphosyl 2 in 1 Shampoo is also of value in the removal of ointments and pastes used in the treatment of psoriasis of the scalp.

**Product licence number** 0036/0052.

## COLIFOAM*

**Presentation** An aerosol can releasing a white odourless foam containing Hydrocortisone Acetate PhEur 10% w/w.

**Uses** Anti-inflammatory corticosteroid therapy for the topical treatment of ulcerative colitis, proctosigmoiditis and granular proctitis. For rectal administration.

**Dosage and administration** One applicatorful inserted into the rectum once or twice daily for two or three weeks and every second day thereafter.

**Contra-indications, warnings, etc**
*Contra-indications:* Local contra-indications to the use of intrarectal steroids include obstruction, abscess, perforation, peritonitis, fresh intestinal anastomoses, extensive fistulae, and tuberculous, fungal or viral infections.

*Pregnancy:* Systemic and topical administration of corticosteroids to pregnant animals can cause abnormalities of foetal development. The relevance of this finding to human beings has not been established, but at present steroids should not be used extensively in pregnancy, that is in large amounts or for prolonged periods.

*Warnings:* General precautions common to all corti-

costeroid therapy should be observed during trea ment with Colifoam especially in the case of your children. Treatment should be administered wi caution in patients with severe ulcerative disea because of their predisposition to perforation of th bowel wall. Although uncommon at this dosage, loc irritation may occur. For external use only.

**Pharmaceutical precautions** Pressurised contain containing flammable propellant. Protect from su light and do not expose to temperatures above 50° Do not spray on a naked flame or any incandesce material. Keep away from sources of ignition–r smoking. Do not pierce or burn even after use. Sto below 25°C. Do not refrigerate.

**Legal category** POM.

**Package quantities** Aerosol canister containi 20.8 g of foam (approximately 14 applications), plus plastic applicator.

**Further information** An illustrated instruction leafl is enclosed with each pack.

**Product licence number** 0036/0021.

## NYTOL*

**Presentation** Each white uncoated biconvex tabl scored with an 'N' contains 25 mg of Diphenhydr mine Hydrochloride BP.

**Uses** An aid to the relief of temporary sle disturbance.

**Dosage and administration** Two tablets to be take 20 minutes before going to bed, or as directed by physician. Not recommended for children under years.

**Contra-indications, warnings, etc** Nytol is contrainc cated in patients who are hypersensitive to diphe hydramine and in those with the following condition asthma, narrow angle glaucoma, prostatic hype trophy, stenosing peptic ulcer, pyloroduodenal o struction, or bladder neck obstruction.

*Interactions:* Diphenhydramine has additive effec with alcohol and other CNS depressants (hypnotic sedatives, tranquilisers). Monoamine oxidase (MA( inhibitors prolong and intensify the anticholinerg effects of diphenhydramine. Diphenhydramine shou not be used in patients receiving one of these drug unless directed by a doctor.

*Effects on ability to drive and to use machines:* Nyt is a hypnotic and will produce drowsiness or sedatic soon after the dose has been taken. This will affe the patient's ability to drive and to use machines.

*Other undesirable effects:* Dizziness, drowsiness ar grogginess are the undesirable effects most fr quently reported by Nytol users. The frequencies these are approximately 6%, 4.5% and 7% respe tively. These effects are mild and wear off about eig hours after taking medication. Dryness of mout nausea and nervousness have also been reporte with diphenhydramine. The antihistamines have bee reported rarely to cause thrombocytopaenia.

*Use in pregnancy and lactation:* Diphenhydramii crosses the placenta. Because animal reproductic studies are not always predictive of human respons and since there is inadequate experience with use diphenhydramine in pregnant women, this drug not recommended during pregnancy. Diphenhydr mine has been detected in milk. Because of high risks of antihistamines for infants, diphenhydrami is not recommended in nursing mothers.

*Other special warnings and precautions:* Nytol shou be used with caution in patients with myasthen gravis or seizure disorders. Tolerance may develo with continuous use.

*Overdose:* Overdosage causes CNS depression ar CNS stimulation. Treatment should be supportive ar directed towards specific symptoms. Convulsions ar marked CNS stimulation should be treated wi parenteral diazepam.

**Pharmaceutical precautions** Store in a dry place.

**Legal category** P.

**Package quantities** Bottles of 20 tablets.

**urther information** Nil.

**roduct licence number** 0036/0050.

## IYTOL ONE-A-NIGHT*

**ualitative and quantitative composition** Nytol One--Night contains 50 mg Diphenhydramine Hydrochlo-de BP per tablet.

**harmaceutical form** Tablets to be taken orally.

**linical particulars**

*herapeutic indication:* An aid to the relief of tempo-ry sleep disturbance.

*osology and method of administration:* One tablet to e taken 20 minutes before going to bed, or as directed y a physician. Not recommended for children under 6 years.

*ontra-indications:* Nytol One-A-Night is contraindi-ated in patients who are hypersensitive to diphen-ydramine and in those with the following conditions: sthma, narrow angle glaucoma, prostatic hyper-ophy, stenosing peptic ulcer, pyloroduodenal ob-truction or bladder neck obstruction.

*pecial warnings and precautions for use:* Nytol One--Night should be used with caution in patients with iyasthenia gravis or seizure disorders. Tolerance ay develop with continuous use.

*nteraction with other drugs and other forms of nteraction:* Diphenhydramine has additive effects vith alcohol and other CNS depressants (hypnotics, edatives, tranquillisers). Monoamine oxidase (MAO) hibitors prolong and intensify the anticholinergic ffects of diphenhydramine. Diphenhydramine should ot be used in patients receiving one of these drugs nless directed by a doctor.

*regnancy and lactation:* Diphenhydramine crosses ne placenta. Because animal reproduction studies re not always predictive of human response and nce there is inadequate experience with use of phenhydramine in pregnant women, this drug is ot recommended during pregnancy. Diphenhydra-ine has been detected in milk. Because of higher sks of antihistamines for infants, Nytol One-A-Night not recommended in nursing mothers.

*ffects on ability to drive and use machines:* Nytol ne-A-Night is a hypnotic and will produce drowsi-ess or sedation soon after the dose has been taken. his will affect the patient's ability to drive and use nachines.

*ndesirable effects:* Dizziness, drowsiness and grog-ness are the undesirable effects most frequently eported by Nytol One-A-Night users. The frequency f these are approximately 6%, 4.5% and 7% respec-vely. These effects are mild and wear off about 8 ours after taking the medication. Dryness of mouth, ausea and nervousness have also been reported vith diphenhydramine. The antihistamines have been eported rarely to cause thrombocytopaenia.

*verdose:* Overdosage causes CNS depression and NS stimulation. Treatment should be supportive and irected towards specific symptoms. Convulsions and arked CNS stimulation should be treated with arenteral diazepam.

**harmacological properties** Diphenhydramine hydro-hloride is the active ingredient in Nytol One-A-Night, is an antihistamine with well known pharmacologi-al activities. As with most of the older antihistamines, phenhydramine hydrochloride has a pronounced edative effect. Diphenhydramine hydrochloride has een formulated into Nytol One-A-Night, a tablet for se as an aid to the relief of temporary sleep isturbance.

*harmacodynamic properties:* Diphenhydramine is n ethanolamine-derivative antihistamine. It is an ntihistamine with anticholinergic and marked seda-ve effects. It acts by inhibiting the effects on H1-eceptors. Diphenhydramine is effective in reducing leep onset (i.e., time to fall asleep) and increasing ne depth and quality of sleep.

*harmacokinetic properties:* Diphenhydramine hydro-hloride is rapidly absorbed following oral administra-on. Apparently it undergoes first-pass metabolism the liver and only about 40-60% of an oral dose eaches systemic circulation as unchanged diphen-ydramine. It is rapidly distributed throughout the hole body. Peak plasma concentration are attained vithin 1-4 hours. The sedative effect also appears to e maximal within 1-3 hours after administration of a ngle dose. It is positively correlated with the plasma rug concentration.

Diphenhydramine is approximately 80-85% bound plasma proteins. Diphenhydramine is rapidly and lmost completely metabolised. The drug is metabol-ed principally to diphenylmethoxyacetic acid and is lso dealkylated. The metabolites are conjugated with lycine and glutamine and excreted in urine. Only about 1% of a single dose is excreted unchanged in urine. The elimination half-life ranges from 2.4-9.3 hours in healthy adults. The terminal elimination half-life is prolonged in liver cirrhosis.

**Pharmaceutical particulars**

*List of excipients:* Anhydrous Lactose USNF, Stearic Acid Powder USP, Microcrystalline Cellulose PhEur, Silicon Dioxide USNF, Maize Starch PhEur.

*Incompatibilities:* None known.

*Shelf-life:* Nytol One-A-Night has a shelf-life of 2 years in Aclar/PE/PVC blister packs.

*Special precautions for storage:* Store in a dry place.

*Nature and contents of container:* Aclar/polyethylene/PVC strip with a heat sealable aluminium foil. Blister strips of 20 tablets.

*Instructions for use/handling:* Not appropriate.

**Marketing authorisation number** 0036/0069

**Date of approval/revision of SPC** 15 September 1995

**Legal category** P

## OTOMIZE* EAR SPRAY

**Presentation** A non-pressurised pump action aerosol spray containing Dexamethasone PhEur 0.1% w/w, Neomycin Sulphate PhEur 3250 IU/ml and Acetic Acid (glacial) BP 2% w/w as a mobile milky aqueous suspension.

**Uses** Otomize is indicated for the treatment of otitis externa.

**Dosage and administration**
*Adults, children and the elderly:* One metered dose (60 mg) to be administered directly into each affected ear three times daily. Treatment should be continued until two days after symptoms have disappeared. Discontinue treatment if there is no clinical improvement after 7 days.

Before using the product for the first time, prime the pump by depressing actuator 6-10 times until a fine spray is obtained. Use within 1 month of first actuation. If more than one week has elapsed since the last use, dispose of the contents of the pump chamber by 1 or 2 depressions of the actuator.

**Contra-indications, warnings, etc**
*Contra-indications:* The product should not be used in patients with a known sensitivity to neomycin.

*Special precautions:* The topical application of neomycin, as with other aminoglycosides, to patients where a perforated ear drum has been diagnosed or is suspected carries a risk of ototoxicity. The benefits of treatment with neomycin should be weighed against the risk of infection itself causing hearing loss.

The CSM has warned that when otitis externa is treated topically with preparations containing aminoglycosides, in patients who have a perforation of the tympanic membrane, there is an increased risk of drug-induced deafness. It is therefore important to ensure that there is no perforation in such patients. However, in the presence of a perforation many specialists do use such agents cautiously in patients with otitis media.

*Other undesirable effects:* Some patients may experience a transient stinging or burning sensation for the first few days of treatment.

*Use in pregnancy and lactation:* There is inadequate evidence of safety in human pregnancy. Topical administration of corticosteroids to pregnant animals can cause abnormalities of foetal development including cleft palate and intra-uterine growth retardation. There may therefore be a very small risk of such effects in the human foetus.

**Pharmaceutical precautions** Store upright in the carton below 25°C. Do not freeze.

**Further information** The product provides a rapid and convenient means of treatment. It is also easy to administer because of its unique spray form.

**Legal category** POM.

**Package quantities** 5 ml bottles

**Product licence number** 0036/0042

## PIRITON* INJECTION

**Presentation** Piriton (Chlorphenamine Maleate BP) is a potent antihistamine.

Each 1 ml of Piriton Injection contains Chlorphenamine Maleate BP 10 mg. It is coulourless. Other ingredients: Sodium chloride, Water for Injections.

**Uses** Piriton Injection is indicated for acute urticaria, control of allergic reactions to insect bites and stings, angioneurotic oedema, drug and serum reactions, desensitisation reactions, hayfever, vasomotor rhinitis, severe pruritus of non-specific origin.

**Dosage and administration** The usual dose of Piriton Injection for adults is 10 to 20 mg, but not more than 40 mg should be given per 24 hours. The injection may be subcutaneous, intramuscular or intravenous.

When a rapid effect is desired, as in anaphylactic reactions, the intravenous route is recommended in addition to emergency therapy with adrenalin, corticosteroids, oxygen and supportive therapy as required. In this case Piriton Injection should be injected slowly over a period of one minute, using the smallest adequate syringe. Any drowsiness, giddiness or hypotension which may follow is usually transitory.

Chlorophenamine in common with other drugs having anticholinergic effects, should be used with caution in epilepsy, raised intra-ocular pressure including glaucoma, prostatic hypertrophy; severe hypertension or cardiovascular disease; bronchitis, bronchiectasis and asthma; hepatic disease and thyrotoxicosis. Children and the elderly are more likely to experience the neurological anticholinergic effects.

The effects of alcohol may be increased.

*Drug interactions:* Concurrent use of chlorphenamine and hypnotics or anxiolytics may potentiate drowsiness. Concurrent use of alcohol may have a similar effect.

Chlorphenamine inhibits phenytoin metabolism and can lead to phenytoin toxicity.

The anticholinergic effects of chlorphenamine are intensified by MAOIs (see *Contra-indications*).

*Pregnancy:* There is inadequate evidence of safety in human pregnancy. Piriton Injection should only be used during pregnancy when clearly needed and when the potential benefits outweigh the potential unknown risks to the foetus. Use during the third trimester may result in reactions in neonates.

In the event of a blood transfusion reaction, a dose of 10 to 20 mg of Piriton should be given by the subcutaneous route. This can be repeated to a total of 40 mg per 24 hours, or oral forms of Piriton may be given until the symptoms subside.

Piriton Injection may be helpful in the prevention of delayed reactions to penicillin and other drugs when given separately by intramuscular injection immediately prior to administration of the other drug. The usual dose is 10 mg.

Piriton Injection cannot, however, be relied on to prevent anaphylactic reactions in patients known to be allergic to a particular drug.

**Contra-indications, warnings, etc**
*Contra-indications:* Piriton Injection is contra-indicated in patients who are hypersensitive to antihistamines or to any of the other ingredients.

The anticholinergic properties of chlorphenamine are intensified by monoamine oxidase inhibitors (MAOIs). Piriton Injection is therefore contra-indicated in patients who have been treated with MAOIs within the last fourteen days.

*Precautions:* The anticholinergic properties of chlorphenamine may cause drowsiness, dizziness, blurred vision and psychomotor impairment which may seriously hamper patients' ability to drive and use machinery.

*Lactation:* It is reasonable to assume that chlorphenamine maleate may inhibit lactation and may be secreted in breast milk. The use of Piriton preparations in mothers breast feeding their babies requires that the therapeutic benefits of the drug should be weighed against the potential hazards to the mother and baby.

*Side-effects:* Sedation varying from slight drowsiness to deep sleep. The following may also occasionally occur; inability to concentrate; lassitude; blurred vision; gasto-intestinal disturbances such as anorexia, dyspepsia, nausea, vomiting, diarrhoea and abdominal pain; hepatitis including jaundice; urinary retention; headaches; dry mouth; dizziness; palpitations; tachycardia; arrhythmias; hypotension; chest tightness; thickening of bronchial secretions; haemolytic anaemia and other blood dyscrasias; allergic reactions including exfoliative dermatitis, photosensitivity and urticaria, twitching, muscular weakness and incoordination; tinnitus; depression, irritability and nightmares.

Children and the elderly are more likely to experience the neurological anticholinergic effects.

Some patients have reported a stinging or burning sensation at the site of injection. Rapid intravenous injection may cause transitory hypotension or CNS stimulation.

*Overdosage:* The estimated lethal dose of chlorphenamine is 25 to 50 mg per kg body weight. Symptoms and signs include sedation, paradoxical stimulation of CNS, toxic psychosis, seizures, apnoea, convulsions, anticholinergic effects, dystonic reactions and cardiovascular collapse including arrhythmias.

Symptomatic and supportive measures should be provided with special attention to cardiac, respiratory, renal and hepatic functions, and fluid and electrolyte balance.

Treat hypotension and arrhythmias vigorously, CNS convulsions may be treated with i.v. diazepam or phenytoin. Haemoperfusion may be used in severe cases.

**Pharmaceutical precautions** Piriton Injection should be stored below 25°C and protected from light.

**Legal category** POM.

**Package quantities** Piriton Injection is supplied in boxes of 5 ampoules.

**Further information** Nil.

**Product licence number** 0036/0087.

## PIRITON* SYRUP

**Presentation** Piriton Syrup is a colourless syrup containing 4 mg Chlorphenamine Maleate BP in 10 ml.

*Other ingredients:* Sugar, glycerol, alcohol, tingle flavour, peppermint oil, water, and as preservative, a mixture of methyl, ethyl and propyl parahydroxybenzoates.

**Uses** Piriton Syrup is indicated for symptomatic control of all allergic conditions responsive to antihistamines, including hayfever, vasomotor rhinitis, urticaria, angioneurotic oedema, food allergy, drug and serum reactions, insect bites.

**Dosage and administration**

*Adults:* 10 ml every 4 to 6 hours (daily max. 24 mg i.e. 60 ml).

*Children aged 6–12 years:* 5 ml every 4 to 6 hours (daily max. 12 mg i.e. 30 ml).

*Children aged 2–5 years:* 2.5 ml every 4 to 6 hours (daily max. 6 mg i.e. 15 ml).

*Children aged 1–2 years:* 2.5 ml twice daily. Not recommended in children below 1 year.

*Elderly:* As in adults but such patients are prone to confusional psychosis and other neurological anticholinergic effects.

**Contra-indications, warnings, etc**

*Contra-indications:* Piriton Syrup is contra-indicated in patients who are hypersensitive to antihistamines or to any of the syrup ingredients.

The anticholinergic properties of chlorphenamine are intensified by monoamine oxidase inhibitors (MAOIs). Piriton Syrup is therefore contra-indicated in patients who have been treated with MAOIs within the last fourteen days.

*Precautions:* The anticholinergic properties of chlorphenamine may cause drowsiness, dizziness, blurred vision and psychomotor impairment which may seriously affect patients' ability to drive and use machinery.

Chlorphenamine in common with other drugs having anticholinergic effects, should be used with caution in epilepsy, raised intra-ocular pressure including glaucoma, prostatic hypertrophy; severe hypertension or cardiovascular disease; bronchitis, bronchiectasis and asthma; hepatic disease and thyrotoxicosis. Children and the elderly are more likely to experience the neurological anticholinergic effects.

The effects of alcohol may be increased.

Piriton Syrup contains sugar. It should be administered with care to patients with diabetes mellitus. Long-term use increases the risk of dental caries and it is essential that adequate dental hygiene is maintained.

*Drug interactions:* Concurrent use of chlorphenamine and hypnotics or anxiolytics may potentiate drowsiness. Concurrent use of alcohol may have a similar effect.

Chlorphenamine inhibits phenytoin metabolism and can lead to phenytoin toxicity.

The anticholinergic effects of chlorphenamine are intensified by MAOIs (see *Contra-indications*).

*Pregnancy:* There is inadequate evidence of safety in human pregnancy. Piriton Syrup should only be used during pregnancy when clearly needed and when the potential benefits outweigh the potential unknown risks to the foetus. Use during the third trimester may result in reactions in neonates.

*Lactation:* It is reasonable to assume that chlorphenamine maleate may inhibit lactation and may be secreted in breast milk. The use of Piriton preparations in mothers breast feeding their babies requires that the therapeutic benefits of the drug should be weighed against the potential hazards to the mother and baby.

*Side-effects:* Sedation varying from slight drowsiness to deep sleep. The following may also occasionally occur; inability to concentrate; lassitude; blurred vision; gastro-intestinal disturbances such as anorexia, dyspepsia, nausea, vomiting, diarrhoea and abdominal pain; hepatitis including jaundice; urinary retention; headaches; dry mouth; dizziness; palpitations; tachycardia; arrhythmias; hypotension; chest tightness; thickening of bronchial secretions; haemolytic anaemia and other blood dyscrasias; allergic reactions including exfoliative dermatitis, photosensitivity and urticaria, muscular weakness and incoordination; tinnitus; depression, irritability and nightmares.

Children and the elderly are more likely to experience the neurological anticholinergic effects.

*Overdosage:* The estimated lethal dose of chlorphenamine is 25 to 50 mg per kg body weight. Symptoms and signs include sedation, paradoxical stimulation of CNS, toxic psychosis, seizures, apnoea, convulsions, anticholinergic effects, dystonic reactions and cardiovascular collapse including arrhythmias.

Symptomatic and supportive measures should be provided with special attention to cardiac, respiratory, renal and hepatic functions, and fluid and electrolyte balance.

Treatment of overdosage should include gastric lavage or induced emesis using Syrup of Ipecacuanha. Following these measures activated charcoal and cathartics may be administered to minimise absorption.

Hypotension and arrhythmias should be treated vigorously. CNS convulsions may be treated with i.v. diazepam or phenytoin. Haemoperfusion may be used in severe cases.

**Pharmaceutical precautions** Piriton Syrup should be stored at a temperature not exceeding 25°C and protected from light. Piriton Syrup may be diluted with Syrup BP. The resultant mixture should be used within fourteen days.

**Legal category** P.

**Package quantities** Piriton Syrup is supplied in 150 ml amber glass bottles.

**Further information** Nil.

**Product licence number** 0036/0088.

## PIRITON* TABLETS

**Presentation** Piriton Tablets are round, biconvex, yellow tablets with a P to one side of the breakline, the reverse face being blank. Each tablet contains 4 mg of the potent antihistamine Chlorphenamine Maleate BP.

*Other ingredients:* Lactose, maize starch, magnesium stearate, colour, yellow iron oxide (E172).

**Uses** Piriton Tablets are indicated for symptomatic control of all allergic conditions responsive to antihistamines, including hayfever, vasomotor rhinitis, urticaria, angioneurotic oedema, food allergy, drug and serum reactions, insect bites.

**Dosage and administration**

*Adults:* 4 mg 4 to 6 hourly (daily max. 24 mg).

*Children aged 6 to 12 years:* 2 mg 4 to 6 hourly (daily max. 12 mg).

*Elderly:* As in adults but such patients are prone to confusional psychosis and other neurological anticholinergic effects.

**Contra-indications, warnings, etc**

*Contra-indications:* Piriton Tablets are contra-indicated in patients who are hypersensitive to antihistamines or to any of the other ingredients.

The anticholinergic properties of chlorphenamine are intensified by monoamine oxidase inhibitors (MAOIs). Piriton Tablets are therefore contra-indicated in patients who have been treated with MAOIs within the last fourteen days.

*Precautions:* The anticholinergic properties of chlorphenamine may cause drowsiness, dizziness, blurred vision and psychomotor impairment which may seriously affect patients ability to drive and use machinery.

Chlorphenamine in common with other drugs having anticholinergic effects, should be used with caution in epilepsy, raised intra-ocular pressure including glaucoma, prostatic hypertrophy; severe hypertension or cardiovascular disease; bronchitis, bronchiectasis and asthma; hepatic disease and thyrotoxicosis. Children and the elderly are more likely to experience the neurological anticholinergic effects.

The effects of alcohol may be increased.

*Drug interactions:* Concurrent use of chlorphenamine and hypnotics or anxiolytics may potentiate drowsiness. Concurrent use of alcohol may have a similar effect.

Chlorphenamine inhibits phenytoin metabolism and can lead to phenytoin toxicity.

The anticholinergic effects of chlorphenamine are intensified by MAOIs (see *Contra-indications*).

*Pregnancy:* There is inadequate evidence of safety in human pregnancy. Piriton Tablets should only be used during pregnancy when clearly needed and when the potential benefits outweigh the potential unknown risks to the foetus. Use during the thi trimester may result in reactions in neonates.

*Lactation:* It is reasonable to assume that chlorphe amine maleate may inhibit lactation and may b secreted in breast milk. The use of Piriton preparation in mothers breast feeding their babies requires tha the therapeutic benefits of the drug should be weighe against the potential hazards to the mother and baby

*Side-effects:* Sedation varying from slight drowsines to deep sleep. The following may also occasionall occur; inability to concentrate; lassitude; blurre vision; gastro-intestinal disturbances such as an rexia, dyspepsia, nausea, vomiting, diarrhoea an abdominal pain; hepatitis including jaundice; urinar retention; headaches; dry mouth; dizziness; palpit tions; tachycardia; arrhythmias; hypotension; ches tightness; thickening of bronchial secretions; haemo lytic anaemia and other blood dyscrasias; allergi reactions including exfoliative dermatitis, photoser sitivity and urticaria, twitching, muscular weakne and inco-ordination; tinnitus; depression, irritabilit and nightmares.

Children and the elderly are more likely to exper ence the neurological anticholinergic effects.

*Overdosage:* The estimated lethal dose of chlorpher amine is 25 to 50 mg per kg body weight. Symptom and signs include sedation, paradoxical stimulatio of CNS, toxic psychosis, seizures, apnoea, convu sions, anticholinergic effects, dystonic reactions an cardiovascular collapse including arrhythmias.

Symptomatic and supportive measures should b provided with special attention to cardiac, respirator renal and hepatic functions, and fluid and electroly balance.

Treatment of overdosage should include gastri lavage or induced emesis using Syrup of Ipecacuanh Following these measures activated charcoal an cathartics may be administered to minimise absorp tion.

Hypotension and arrhythmias should be treate vigorously, CNS convulsions may be treated with i.v diazepam or phenytoin. Haemoperfusion may be use in severe cases.

**Pharmaceutical precautions** Piriton Tablets shoul be stored below 30°C.

**Legal category** P.

**Package quantities** Piriton Tablets are supplied i packs of 500.

**Further information** Nil.

**Product licence number** 0036/0090.

## PROCTOFOAM* HC

**Presentation** An aerosol can releasing a mucoadhe ent, white, odourless foam containing Hydrocortison Acetate PhEur 1% w/w and Pramoxine Hydrochlorid USP 1% w/w.

**Uses** For the short term (not more than 5-7 days relief of the symptoms of itching, irritation, discomfo or pain associated with local, noninfective anal o perianal conditions.

**Dosage and administration** One applicatorful pe rectum 2 or 3 times daily, and after each bowe evacuation (up to a maximum of 4 times daily). Fo perianal administration, apply a small quantity on fingers. Not recommended in children.

**Contra-indications, warnings, etc**

*Contra-indications:* Hypersensitivity to pramoxine hy drochloride or to any component of the preparatio Bacterial, viral or fungal infection.

*Other undesirable effects:* Although uncommon a this dosage, local burning, itching, irritation, allergi dermatitis, secondary infection and skin atrophy ma occur. Systemic absorption of topical corticosteroi has produced reversible suppression of the hypotha lamic–pituitary–adrenal axis and manifestations o Cushing's Syndrome.

*Use in pregnancy and lactation:* Safety for use i pregnancy and lactation has not been establishe There is inadequate evidence of safety in huma pregnancy. Topical administration of corticosteroi to pregnant animals can cause abnormalities of foet development including cleft palate and intra-uterin growth retardation. There may be a very small risk such effects in the human foetus.

No data is available on the use of topical corticoste roids and local anaesthetic agents in nursing mother However, the product has been used by nursin mothers for many years without apparent ill cons quence.

*Other special warnings and precautions:* Not fo prolonged use. Contact sensitisation to local anaest etics is common following prolonged applicatio Seek medical advice if symptoms worsen or do no improve within 7 days, or if bleeding occurs. Keep o of the reach of children. For external use only. Rect examination must be performed to exclude serious pathology before initiating treatment with Proctofoam HC.

*Overdosage:* Excess use of topical corticosteroids may produce systemic adverse effects.

*Incompatibilities:* Compatibility with barrier methods of contraception has not been demonstrated.

**Pharmaceutical precautions** Pressurised container containing flammable propellant. Protect from sunlight and do not expose to temperatures above 50°C. Do not spray on a naked flame or any incandescent material. Keep away from sources of ignition–no smoking. Do not pierce or burn even after use. Do not refrigerate. Store below 25°C

**Legal category** POM.

**Package quantities** Aerosol canister containing 20 g of foam (approximately 40 doses), plus a plastic applicator.

**Further information** An illustrated instruction leaflet is enclosed with each pack. Shake canister vigorously before use.

**Product licence number** 0036/5002.

## QUELLADA-M* CREAM SHAMPOO

**Qualitative and quantitative composition** Malathion USP 1.0% w/w

**Pharmaceutical form** Cream shampoo

**Clinical particulars**

*Therapeutic indications:* For the treatment of head lice and pubic lice infestation. Family members and close contacts should also be treated.

*Posology and method of administration:* For topical external use only.
As this product does not contain alcohol, it may be more suitable for those with asthma or eczema.

*Adults, the elderly and children aged 6 months and over:*

*For head lice:*

1. Wet the hair thoroughly with warm water and apply sufficient shampoo to work up a rich lather and ensure that no part of the scalp is uncovered. Pay special attention to the back of the neck and the area behind the ears. Take care to avoid the eyes.
2. Leave for at least five minutes.
3. Rinse thoroughly with clean warm water and repeat procedure.
4. While hair is still wet, comb with an ordinary comb. A fine-toothed louse comb can then be used to remove the dead lice and eggs.
5. This treatment should be carried out a total of three times at three day intervals.

*For pubic lice:* Application and dosage are as for the head. Apply the lotion to the pubic hair and the hair between the legs and arms.

*Contra-indications:* None stated.

*Special warnings and precautions for use:* As with all shampoos, avoid contact with the eyes. Children under six months should only be treated under medical supervision.
When Quellada-M cream shampoo is used by a school nurse or other health officer in the mass treatment of large numbers of children, it is advisable that protective plastic or rubber gloves be worn. Keep out of the reach of children.
Continued prolonged treatment with this product should be avoided. It should be used for not more than three times at three day intervals then not repeated within a three week period.

*Interactions with other medicaments and other forms of interaction:* None stated

*Pregnancy and lactation:* Quellada-M cream shampoo is not known to have any effect on fertility, pregnancy and lactation. Its use in pregnant or lactating women is not recommended unless there is an overdue need.

*Effects on ability to drive and use machines:* None stated.

*Undesirable effects:* None stated.

*Overdose:* In the event of deliberate or accidental ingestion, empty stomach contents by gastric lavage and keep patient warm. In the event of massive ingestion, atropine and pralidoxime may be required to counteract cholinesterase inhibition.

**Pharmacological properties**

*Pharmacodynamic properties:* Quellada-M cream shampoo contains malathion, a widely used organophosphorous insecticide which is active by cholinesterase inhibition. It is effective against a wide range of insects, but is one of the least toxic organophosphorous insecticides since it is rapidly detoxified by plasma carboxylesterases.

*Pharmacokinetic properties:* Quellada-M cream shampoo is applied topically to the affected area.

*Preclinical safety data:* None stated.

**Pharmaceutical particulars**

*List of excipients:* Sodium lauryl sulphate paste; cetostearyl alcohol; lauric diethanolamide; ethoxylated lanolin (50%); methyl hydroxybenzoate; propyl hydroxybenzoate; hydrochloric acid; citric acid (anhydrous); dibasic sodium phosphate; colour yellow (E110); sodium edetate; perfume M&B 1658; purified water.

*Incompatibilities:* None stated.

*Shelf life:* 18 months.

*Special precautions for storage:* Store at or below 20°C.

*Nature and contents of container:* Boxed, internally lacquered aluminium tube with polyethylene cap containing 40 g of product.

*Instructions for use/handling:* None stated

*Marketing authorisation holder:* Ultra Chemical Limited, Tubiton House, Oldham, Lancashire, OL1 3HS.

**Marketing authorisation number** 14236/0005

**Date of approval/revision of SPC** July 1995

**Legal category** P

## QUELLADA-M* LIQUID

**Qualitative and quantitative composition** Malathion 0.5% w/w

**Pharmaceutical form** Liquid emulsion

**Clinical particulars**

*Therapeutic indications:* Eradication of head lice, pubic lice and their eggs. Treatment of scabies.

*Posology and method of administration:* For topical external use only.
As this product does not contain alcohol, it may be more suitable for those with asthma or eczema.

*Adults, the elderly and children aged 6 months and over:*

*Treatment of headlice:* Rub the liquid into the scalp until all the hair and scalp is thoroughly moistened. Leave the hair to dry naturally in a warm but well ventilated room. After 12 hours, or the next day, if preferred, shampoo hair in the normal way. Rinse the hair and comb whilst wet to remove dead lice and eggs (nits) using the louse comb.

*Treatment of crab (pubic) lice:* Apply Quellada-M liquid to the entire skin surface. Pay particular attention to all hairy areas including beards and moustaches. Avoid any other areas above the neck. Leave on for at least one hour before washing but preferably Quellada-M liquid should be left on overnight. Wash off in the usual manner.

*Treatment of scabies:* Apply Quellada-M liquid to the entire skin surface. In adults it may not be necessary to apply above the neck but children under the age of two years should have a thin film of Quellada-M liquid applied to the scalp, face and ears, avoiding the eyes and mouth. Do not wash off or bathe for 24 hours. If hands or any other parts must be washed during this period, the treatment must be re-applied to those areas immediately.
No special sterilisation of clothing is necessary, ordinary laundering or dry-cleaning with hot-iron pressing is sufficient. The infestation is cleared by the treatment. However, the itching and rash may persist for up to 7 days. An anti-irritant cream can be applied if necessary. Family members and close contacts should also be treated simultaneously.

*Children aged 6 months and under:* On medical advice only.

*Contra-indications:* Known sensitivity to malathion. Not to be used on infants less than 6 months except on medical advice.

*Special warnings and precautions for use:* Avoid contact with the eyes. For external use only. Keep out of the reach of children. If inadvertently swallowed, a doctor or casualty department should be contacted at once.
When Quellada-M liquid is used by a school nurse or other health officers in the mass treatment of large numbers of children, it is advisable that protective plastic or rubber gloves be worn.

Continued prolonged treatment with this product should be avoided. It should be used not more than once a week and for not more than three consecutive weeks.

*Interactions with other medicaments and other forms of interaction:* None stated.

*Pregnancy and lactation:* No known effects in pregnancy and lactation. However, as with all medicines, use with caution.

*Effects on ability to drive and use machines:* None stated.

*Undesirable effects:* Very rarely skin irritation has been reported.

*Overdose:* It is most unlikely that a toxic dose of malathion will be ingested. Treatment consists of gastric lavage, assisted respiration and if necessary in the event of massive ingestion, administration of atropine and pralidoxime.

**Pharmacolgical properties**

*Pharmacodynamic properties:* Quellada-M liquid contains malathion, a widely used organophosphorous insecticide which is active by cholinesterase inhibition. It is effective against a wide range of insects, but is one of the least toxic organophosphorous insecticides since it is rapidly detoxified by plasma carboxylesterases.

*Pharmacokinetic properties:* None stated. Quellada-M liquid is applied topically to the affected area.

*Preclinical safety data:* None stated.

**Pharmaceutical particulars**

*List of excipients:* Methyl hydroxybenzoate; propyl hydroxybenzoate; lanette wax SX,; potassium citrate; citric acid; perfume HT 52; water.

*Incompatibilities:* None stated.

*Shelf life:* Two and a half years.

*Special precautions for storage:* Store at or below 25°C. Protect from sunlight.

*Nature and contents of container:* Boxed, clear or amber glass bottles with polyethylene caps and polypropylene faced wads containing either 50 ml or 200 ml of product.

*Instructions for use/handling:* None stated.

*Marketing authorisation holder:* Ultra Chemical, Tubiton House, Oldham, Lancashire, OL1 3HS

**Marketing authorisation number** 14236/0004

**Date of approval/revision of SPC** October 1995

**Legal category** P

## ROZEX* GEL

**Qualitative and quantitative composition** Metronidazole PhEur 0.75% w/w.

**Pharmaceutical form** Gel

**Clinical particulars**

*Therapeutic indications:* Indicated in the treatment of inflammatory papules, pustules and erythema of rosacea.

*Posology and method of administration:* For topical administration only.

*Adults:* Apply and rub in a film of gel twice daily, morning and evening, to entire affected area after washing.

*Elderly:* The dosage recommended in the elderly is the same as that recommended in adults.

*Children:* Not recommended.

*Contra-indications:* Contraindicated in individuals with a history of hypersensitivity to metronidazole, parabens or other ingredients in the formulation.

*Special warnings and special precautions for use:* Rozex Gel has been reported to cause lacrimation of the eyes, therefore, contact with the eyes should be avoided. If a reaction suggesting local irritation occurs patients should be directed to use the medication less frequently, discontinue use temporarily or discontinue use until further instructions. Metronidazole is a nitroimidazole and should be used with care in patients with evidence of, or history of, blood dyscrasia. Exposure of treated sites to ultraviolet or strong sunlight should be avoided during use of metronidazole.

*Interaction with other medicaments and other forms of interaction:* Drug interactions are less likely with topical administration but should be kept in mind when Rozex Gel is prescribed for patients receiving anticoagulant treatment. Oral metronidazole has been reported to potentiate the anti-coagulant effect of dicoumarin and warfarin, resulting in a prolongation of prothrombin time.

*Pregnancy and lactation:* There is no experience to

date with the use of Rozex Gel in pregnancy. Metronidazole crosses the placental barrier and rapidly enters the foetal circulation. There is inadequate evidence of the safety of metronidazole in human pregnancy. In animals, metronidazole was not teratogenic or embryotoxic unless administered at extremely high doses. Rozex Gel should only be used in pregnancy when there is no safer alternative.

After oral administration, metronidazole is excreted in breast milk in concentrations similar to those found in the plasma, metronidazole blood levels from topical administration are significantly lower than those achieved after oral administration. A decision should be made to discontinue nursing or to discontinue the drug, taking into account the importance of the drug to the mother.

*Effects on ability to drive and use machines:* Not applicable.

*Undesirable effects:* Because of the minimal absorption of metronidazole and consequently its insignificant plasma concentration after topical administration, the adverse experiences reported with the oral form of the drug have not been reported with Rozex Gel. Adverse reactions reported with Rozex Gel include watery (tearing) eyes if the gel is applied too closely to this area, transient redness and mild dryness, burning and skin irritation.

*Overdosage:* There is no human experience with overdosage of Rozex Gel. The acute oral toxicity of Rozex Gel was determined to be greater than 5 g/kg (the highest dose given) in albino rats.

### Pharmacological properties

*Pharmacodynamic properties:* Metronidazole is an antiprotozoal and antibacterial agent which is active against a wide range of pathogenic micro-organisms. The mechanisms of action of metronidazole in rosacea are unknown but available evidence suggests that the effects may be antibacterial and/or anti-inflammatory.

*Pharmacokinetic properties:* Metronidazole is rapidly and nearly totally absorbed after oral administration. The drug is not significantly bound to serum proteins and distributes well to all body compartments with the lowest concentration found in the fat. Metronidazole is excreted primarily in the urine as parent drug, oxidative metabolites and conjugates.

Bioavailability studies with Rozex Gel in rosacea patients treated with 7.5 mg metronidazole applied topically to the face resulted in a maximum serum concentration of 66 nanograms/ml which is approximately 100 times less than those attained after a single oral dose of 250 mg. In most patients at most time points after Rozex Gel application, serum concentrations of metronidazole were below the detectable limits of the assay (25 nanograms/ml).

*Preclinical safety data:* The toxicity studies conducted with the metronidazole 0.75% topical Gel formulation demonstrate that the product is non-toxic in rats after acute oral administration of 5 g/kg and produced no ocular irritation in rabbit eyes. The formulation produced no observable effects in rabbits after dermal application of 13 mg/kg for 90 days.

No compound-related dermal or systemic effects were observed in a 13-week cutaneous route toxicity study, in which Rozex gel containing Metronidazole 0.75% w/w was applied daily to rabbits at doses ranging between 0.13 and 13 mg/kg.

Metronidazole has shown evidence of carcinogenic activity in a number of studies involving chronic, oral administration in mice and rats but not in studies involving hamsters.

One study showed a significant enhancement of UV induced skin tumours in hairless mice treated with Metronidazole intraperitoneally (15 micrograms per g body weight and per day for 28 weeks). Although the significance of these studies to man is not clear patients should be advised to avoid or minimise exposure of Metronidazole treated sites to sun.

Metronidazole has shown mutagenic activity in several in vitro bacterial assay systems. In addition, a dose-response increase in the frequency of micronuclei was observed in mice after intraperitoneal injection and an increase in chromosome aberrations have been reported in patients with Crohn's disease who were treated with 200 to 1200 mg/day of metronidazole for 1 to 24 months. However, no excess chromosomal aberrations in circulating human lymphocytes have been observed in patients treated for 8 months.

### Pharmaceutical particulars

*List of excipients:* Carbomer (Carbopol 940) BP; Disodium Edetate PhEur; Methyl Hydroxybenzoate PhEur; Propyl Hydroxybenzoate PhEur; Propylene Glycol PhEur; Sodium Hydroxide PhEur; Purified Water PhEur.

*Incompatibilities:* None known

*Shelf life:* Rozex Gel has a shelf life when unopened of 36 months.

*Special precautions for storage:* Store at a temperature not exceeding 25°C, away from direct heat. Do not freeze.

*Nature and contents of container:* Aluminium tubes with epoxy phenolic lining; pack sizes: 5 g or 30 g.

*Instructions for use/handling:* Not applicable.

*Marketing authorisation holder:* Galderma (UK) Ltd, Leywood House, Woodside Road, Amersham, Buckinghamshire, HP6 6AA.

**Marketing authorisation number** 10590/0016

**Date of approval/revision of SPC** 4 January 1996

**Legal category** POM

## TARCORTIN*

**Presentation** Hydrocortisone PhEur 0.5% w/w ar refined alcoholic extract of coal tar 5% w/w in vanishing cream base. It is a light tan, homogeneou cream.

**Uses** Tarcortin cream is a stimulating antipruritic. It indicated for sub-acute and chronic eczema, localise neurodermatitis, seborrhoea, dermatitis venenata ar psoriasis, excluding widespread plaque psoriasis.

**Dosage and administration** Tarcortin is applie topically. Apply twice daily or more frequently to th affected area by gentle massage until the cream ha vanished into the skin. No dressing is needed. Lor term use in children is not advised.

**Contra-indications, warnings, etc**

*Contra-indications:* The use of Tarcortin is contr indicated in the presence of viral or fungal infection tubercular or syphilitic lesions, and in bacterial infe tions, unless used in conjunction with appropria chemotherapy.

*Interactions:* None known.

*Other undesirable effects:* The use of coal tar ca cause skin irritation, acne-like eruptions and phot sensitivity.

*Use in pregnancy and lactation:* There is inadequa evidence of the safety of topical steroids in huma pregnancy. Topical administration of corticosteroi to pregnant animals can cause abnormalities of foet development, including cleft palate and intra-uteri growth retardation. There may, therefore, be a ve small risk of such effects in the human foetus.

*Other special warnings and precautions:* The crea should be massaged well into the affected area prevent a temporary discolouration of skin, hair fabric. Although generally regarded as safe, even f long term administration in adults, there is a potent for overdose in infancy. Extreme caution is require in dermatoses of infancy including napkin eruptio In such patients, courses of treatment should n normally exceed 7 days.

Topical corticosteroids may be hazardous in pso asis for a number of reasons, including rebour relapse following development of tolerance, risk generalised pustular psoriasis and local system toxicity due to impaired barrier function of the ski Careful patient supervision is important.

**Pharmaceutical precautions** Do not refrigerate. Sto at room temperature.

**Legal category** POM

**Package quantities** Tubes of 100 g.

**Product licence number** 0036/5007

*Trade Mark

# STD Pharmaceutical Products Ltd
Fields Yard, Plough Lane
Hereford HR4 0EL

## FIBRO-VEIN* 3.0%,1.0%,0.5% and 0.2%

**Qualitative and quantitative composition**

Fibro-vein 3.0%: Sodium Tetradecyl Sulphate BP 3.0% w/v.

Fibro-vein 1.0%: Sodium Tetradecyl Sulphate BP 1.0% w/v

Fibro-vein 0.5%: Sodium Tetradecyl Sulphate BP 0.5% w/v

Fibro-vein 0.2%: Sodium Tetradecyl Sulphate BP 0.2% w/v

**Pharmaceutical form** Intravenous injection

**Clinical particulars**

*Therapeutic indications:* Fibro-vein 3% & 1%; For the treatment of varicose veins of the leg by injection sclerotherapy. Fibro-vein 0.5%; For the treatment of varicose veins and venous flares of the leg by injection sclerotherapy. Fibro-vein 0.2%; For the treatment of minor venules and spider veins (venous flares) by injection sclerotherapy.

*Posology and method of administration:*

*Route of administration:* For intravenous administration into the lumen of an isolated segment of emptied vein followed by immediate continuous compression.

*Recommended doses and dosage schedules:* Adults: Fibro-vein 3.0%; 0.5 to 1.0 ml of 3.0% Fibro-vein injected intravenously at a maximum of 4 sites (maximum 4 ml).

Fibro-vein 1.0%: 0.25 to 1.0 ml of 1.0% Fibro-vein injected intravenously into the lumen of an isolated segment of emptied superficial vein, followed by immediate compression. A maximum of 10 sites (10 ml total) may be injected during one treatment session.

Fibro-vein 0.5%: 0.25 to 1.0 ml of 0.5% Fibro-vein injected intravenously into the lumen of an isolated segment of emptied superficial vein, followed by immediate compression. A maximum of 10 sites (10 ml total) may be injected during one treatment session.

Fibro-vein 0.2%: 0.1 to 1.0 ml of 0.2% Fibro-Vein injected intravenously at a maximum of 10 sites (maximum 10 ml).

The smallest of needles (30 gauge) should be used to perform the injection which should be made slowly so that the blood content of these veins is expelled. In the treatment of spider veins an air block technique may be used.

*Children:* all strengths: not recommended in children

*The elderly:* As for adults

*Contra-indications:*

1. Allergy to sodium tetradecyl sulphate or to any component of the preparation.
2. Patients unable to walk due to any cause.
3. Patients currently taking oral contraceptives.
4. Significant obesity.
5. Acute superficial thrombophlebitis.
6. Local or systemic infection.
7. Varicosities caused by pelvic or abdominal tumours.

8. Uncontrolled systemic disease e.g. diabetes mellitus.
9. Surgical valvular incompetence requiring surgical treatment.

*Special warnings and special precautions for use:*

1. Fibro-vein should only be administered by practitioners familiar with an acceptable injection technique. Thorough pre-injection assessment for valvular competence and deep vein patency must be carried out. Extreme care in needle placement and slow injection of the minimal effective volume at each injection site are essential for safe and efficient use.
2. A history of allergy should be taken from all patients prior to treatment. Where special caution is indicated a test dose of 0.25 to 0.5 ml Fibro-vein should be given up to 24 hours before any further therapy.
3. Treatment of anaphylaxis may require, depending on the severity of attack, some or all of the following: injection of adrenaline, injection of hydrocortisone, injection of antihistamine, endotracheal intubation with use of a laryngoscope and suction. The treatment of varicose veins by fibro-vein should not be undertaken in clinics where these items are not readily available.
4. Extreme caution in use is required in patients with arterial disease such as severe peripheral atherosclerosis or thromboangiitis obliterans (Buerger's Disease).
5. Special care is required when injecting above and posterior to the medial malleolus where the posterior tibial artery may be at risk.
6. Pigmentation may be more likely to result if blood is extravasated at the injection site (particularly when treating smaller surface veins) and compression is not used.

*Interaction with other medicaments and other forms of interaction:* Do not use with heparin in the same syringe.

*Pregnancy and lactation:* Safety for use in pregnancy has not been established. Use only when clearly needed for symptomatic relief and when the potential benefits outweigh the potential hazards to the foetus. It is not known whether sodium tetradecyl sulphate is excreted in human milk. Caution should be exercised when used in nursing mothers.

*Effects on ability to drive and to use machines:* None known.

*Undesirable effects:*

1. Local: Pain or burning. Skin pigmentation. Tissue necrosis and ulceration may occur with extravasation. Paraesthesia and anaesthesia may occur if an injection effects a cutaneous nerve.
2. Vascular: Superficial thrombophlebitis. Deep vein thrombosis and pulmonary embolism are very rare. Inadvertent intra-arterial injection is very rare but may lead to gangrene. Most cases have involved the posterior tibial artery above the medial malleolus.
3. Systemic reactions: Allergic reactions are rare, presenting as local or generalised rash, urticaria, nausea or vomiting, asthma, vascular collapse. Ana-

phylactic shock, which may potentially be fatal, is extremely rare.

*Overdose:* Not applicable.

**Pharmacological properties**

*Pharmacodynamic properties:* Sodium tetradecyl sulphate damages the endothelium cells within the lumen of the injected vein. The object of compression sclerotherapy is then to compress the vein so that the resulting thrombus is kept to the minimum and the subsequent formation of scar tissue within the vein produces a fibrous cord and permanent obliteration. Non-compressed veins permit the formation of a large thrombus and produce less fibrosis within the vein.

*Pharmacokinetic properties:* Not applicable.

*Preclinical safety data:* Not applicable

**Pharmaceutical particulars**

*List of excipients:* All strengths: Benzyl Alcohol BP, Disodium Hydrogen Phosphate BP, potassium di-hydrogen phosphate analar, Water for Injections BP

*Incompatibilities:* Do not use with heparin in the same syringe

*Shelf life:* 36 months

*Special precautions for storage:* Store below 25° away from direct sunlight.

*Nature and contents of containers:* Fibro-vein 3.0%: 2 ml ampoules and 5 ml vials; Fibro-vein 1.0%: 2 ml ampoules; Fibro-vein 0.5%: 2 ml ampoules; Fibro-vein 0.2%: 5 ml vials

2 ml ampoules type 1 neutral hydrolytic glass conforming with PhEur requirements for injectable preparations.

5 ml glass vials type 1 neutral hydrolytic glass conforming with PhEur requirements for injectable preparations. Sealed with a chlorobutyl rubber bung and silver aluminium 'tear off' seal conforming with the PhEur requirements

*Instructions for use/handling:* Each 2 ml glass ampoule is for single use only.

The in use period of each 5 ml multidose vial is a single session of therapy and for use in the treatment of a single patient. Unused vial contents should be discarded immediately afterwards.

**Marketing authorisation numbers**
Fibro-vein 3.0%  0398/5000R
Fibro-vein 1.0%  0398/0003
Fibro-vein 0.5%  0398/0002
Fibro-vein 0.2%  0398/0004

**Date of approval/revision of SPC**
Fibro-vein 3.0%:  24 October 1995.
Fibro-vein 1.0%:  17 April 1996.
Fibro-vein 0.5%:  17 April 1996.
Fibro-vein 0.2%:  27 March 1995

**Legal category**  POM

*Trade Mark

# Stiefel Laboratories (UK) Limited
Holtspur Lane
Wooburn Green
High Wycombe
Buckinghamshire HP10 0AU

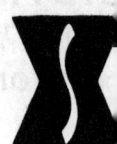

## BRĀSIVOL* 1 FINE
## BRĀSIVOL* 2 MEDIUM

**Presentation** Brāsivol is an abrasive cleansing paste in two grades, each containing graded particles of fused synthetic aluminium oxide in a non-irritant soap-detergent base.

*Brāsivol No. 1 Fine* is an off-white paste containing 38% aluminium oxide.

*Brāsivol No. 2 Medium* is a light-blue paste containing 52% aluminium oxide.

Excipients: glycerol, polyethylene glycol, stearic acid, lauric acid, myristic acid, quaternium 15, bentonite, sodium lauryl sulphate, colour: fine E172, medium E131, fragrance BV-2, purified water.

**Uses** Brāsivol is a cleansing and abrading agent which effectively removes debris from blocked pores. It is used in the management of acne vulgaris, either as a sole agent or as an adjunct to other treatment.

**Dosage and administration** The product is intended for use in adults and children over 12 years of age. The patient should commence treatment with Brāsivol No. 1 Fine. The product should be applied to wetted skin and rubbed gently but firmly over the affected area with a circular motion for 15–20 seconds, then rinsed off thoroughly with water. This routine may be repeated 2 or 3 times daily, replacing ordinary soap and water.

If the condition does not improve after 2 to 3 weeks, the treatment should be repeated using Brāsivol No. 2 Medium in place of Brāsivol No. 1.

Once you have established the most suitable grade for your condition and skin type, continue treatment for 2 to 3 months.

**Contra-indications, warnings, etc** Brāsivol is contra-indicated in the presence of superficial venules, telangiectasia, cystic acne and rosacea.

Care should be taken to avoid using Brāsivol close to the eyes or mouth and male patients using an electric razor should shave before applying Brāsivol.

A degree of dryness and redness will be seen during the first few days of treatment. Over-enthusiastic use, however, can cause irritation and, if this occurs, treatment should be interrupted for a day or two and then resumed.

There is no experimental evidence of the safety of the drug in human pregnancy but it has been in wide use for many years without ill consequence.

**Pharmaceutical precautions** Nil.

**Legal category** GSL.

**Package quantities**
*Brāsivol No. 1 Fine.* 75 g.
*Brāsivol No. 2 Medium.* 75 g.

**Further information** Brāsivol assists in the treatment of acne by exerting a debrading effect on the skin surface, unblocking the follicles, thus allowing the removal of retained sebum and permitting the sebaceous glands to return to normal size and activity.

**Product licence numbers**
Brāsivol No. 1 Fine      0174/5000R
Brāsivol No. 2 Medium    0174/5001R

## DRICLOR*

**Presentation** Driclor is a clear colourless alcoholic solution containing Aluminium Chloride Hexahydrate PhEur 20% w/w.

Excipients: ethanol, purified water.

**Uses** Driclor is indicated for the treatment of hyperhidrosis.

**Dosage and administration** Apply Driclor last thing at night after drying the affected areas carefully. Wash off in the morning. Do not re-apply the product during the day.

Initially the product may be applied each night until sweating stops during the day. The frequency of application may then be reduced to twice a week or less.

**Contra-indications, warnings, etc** Ensure that the affected areas to be treated are completely dry before application.

Do not apply Driclor to broken, irritated, or recently shaven skin.

Driclor may cause irritation which may be alleviated by the use of a weak, corticosteroid cream.

Avoid contact with the eyes.

There are no restrictions on the use of Driclor during pregnancy and lactation.

Avoid direct contact with clothing and polished metal surfaces.

**Pharmaceutical precautions** Store upright in a cool place.

Replace cap tightly after use.

Inflammable – keep away from naked flame.

**Legal category** P.

**Package quantities** 60ml in roll-on applicator plastic bottle.

**Further information** Aluminium chloride hexahydrate acts locally, in the stratum corneum and in the terminal duct, to relieve hyperhidrosis.

**Product licence number** 0174/0044.

## DUOFILM*

**Presentation** Duofilm is a clear mobile liquid containing:

Salicylic Acid BP      16.7% w/w
Lactic Acid BP         16.7% w/w
in Flexible Collodion BP.

**Uses** Duofilm is for topical application only and is indicated in the treatment of warts.

**Dosage and administration** For application to the affected areas on the surface of the skin.

*Adults (including the elderly):* Apply daily to the affected areas only.

*Children under 12:* Children over two years are to be treated under supervision, but treatment of infants is not recommended.

**Contra-indications, warnings, etc** Avoid applying to normal skin.

Duofilm should not be used on the face or anogenital regions.

There are no restrictions on the use of Duofilm during pregnancy and lactation.

**Pharmaceutical precautions** Store upright in a cool place.

Replace cap tightly after use.

Highly inflammable – keep away from naked flame.

**Legal category** P.

**Package quantities** Duofilm is available in an amber screw-capped applicator bottle containing 15 ml.

**Further information** Lactic acid affects the keratinisation process, reducing the hyperkeratosis which is characteristic of warts. It is caustic, leading to the destruction of the keratotic tissue of the wart and of the causative virus. Salicylic acid is keratolytic, producing desquamation by solubilising the intercellular cement in the stratum corneum.

**Product licence number** 0174/0025R.

## ISOTREX* GEL

**Qualitative and quantitative composition** Isotretinoin 0.05%.

**Pharmaceutical form** Gel for cutaneous use.

### Clinical particulars
*Therapeutic indications:* Isotrex Gel is indicated for the topical treatment of mild to moderate inflammatory and non-inflammatory acne vulgaris.

*Posology and method of administration:* Apply Isotrex Gel sparingly over the whole affected area once or twice daily.

Patients should be advised that 6–8 weeks of treatment may be required before a therapeutic effect is observed.

*Paediatric use:* The safety and efficacy of Isotrex G has not been established in children since acn vulgaris rarely presents in this age group.

*Elderly patients:* There are no specific recommenda tions. Acne vulgaris does not present in the elderly.

*Contra-indications:* Isotrex Gel should not be used patients with known hypersensitivity to any of th ingredients.

*Special warnings and special precautions for us* Contact with the eyes, mouth and mucous membrane and with abraded or eczematous skin should b avoided. Care should be taken not to let the medicatio accumulate in skin fold areas and in the angles of th nose.

Application to sensitive areas of skin, such as th neck, should be made with caution.

Although tretinoin has not been shown to initiate promote carcinogenesis in humans, tretinoin applie topically to albino hairless mice had resulted in a dos related acceleration in ultraviolet-β radiation induce cutaneous tumours. The same author also observe the opposite effect in another study of low, non irritating concentrations of tretinoin. The significanc of these findings as related to man is unknow however, caution should be observed in patients wit a personal or family history of cutaneous epitheliom Exposure to sunlight of areas treated with Isotrex G should be avoided or minimised. When exposure t strong sunlight cannot be avoided a sunscreen pro uct and protective clothing should be used. Patient with sunburn should not use Isotrex Gel due to th possibility of increased sensitivity to sunlight. The us of sunlamps should be avoided during treatment.

*Interactions with other medicaments and other form of interaction:* Concomitant topical medication shoul be used with caution during therapy with Isotrex Ge Particular caution should be exercised when usin preparations containing a peeling agent (for examp Benzoyl Peroxide) or abrasive cleansers.

*Pregnancy and lactation:* Category B1. There is inad equate evidence of the safety of topically applie isotretinoin in human pregnancy.

Isotretinoin has been associated with teratogenicit in humans when administered systemically. Repro duction studies conducted in rabbits using Isotrex G applied topically at up to 60 times the human dos have, however, revealed no harm to the foetus. Th use of Isotrex gel should be avoided during pregnanc

*Use during lactation:* Percutaneous absorption o isotretinoin from Isotrex Gel is negligible. It is no known, however, whether isotretinoin is excreted i human milk. Isotrex Gel should not be used durin lactation.

*Effects on ability to drive and use machines:* Isotre Gel is presumed to be safe or unlikely to produce a effect on ability to drive or use machines.

*Undesirable effects:* In normal use, Isotrex Gel ma cause stinging, burning or irritation; erythema an peeling at the site of application may occur.

If undue irritation occurs, treatment should b interrupted temporarily and resumed once the reac tion subsides. If irritation persists, treatment shoul be discontinued. Reactions will normally resolve o discontinuation of therapy.

*Overdosage:* Acute overdosage of Isotrex Gel has ne been reported to date. Accidental ingestion of Isotre Gel resulting in overdosage of isotretinoin could b expected to induce symptoms of hypervitaminosis A These include severe headaches, nausea or vomiting drowsiness, irritability and pruritus.

### Pharmacological properties
*Pharmacodynamic properties:* Isotretinoin is structu ally and pharmacologically related to Vitamin A whic regulates epithelial cell growth and differentiation.

The Pharmacological action of isotretinoin remain to be fully elucidated. When used systemically suppresses sebaceous gland activity and reduce sebum production; it also affects comedogenesi suppresses *Propionibacterium acnes* and reduce inflammation.

When applied topically, the mode of action o isotretinoin may be comparable with its stereoisome tretinoin. Tretinoin stimulates mitosis in the epidermi

›d reduces intercellular cohesion in the stratum rneum; it contests the hyperkeratosis characteristic acne vulgaris and aids desquamation, preventing e formation of lesions. Tretinoin also mediates an creased production of less cohesive epidermal baceous cells, this appears to promote the initial pulsion and subsequent prevention of comedones.

Animal studies have demonstrated that topical otretinoin elicits epidermal hyperplasia reduces perkeratosis and suppresses sebum production d sebaceous gland size. The anti-inflammatory tion of isotretinoin when applied topically has been nfirmed in man.

*armacokinetic properties:* Percutaneous absorption isotretinoin from the gel is negligible. After applying g per day of isotretinoin 0.05% gel to acne of the ce, chest and back for 30 days, HPLC assays for otretinoin and tretinoin demonstrated non-detectae levels in the plasma samples (0.02 μg/ml). Applyg $^{14}$C isotretinoin in a cream base on the healthy skin human volunteers resulted in only 0.03% of the pically applied dose being recovered through estiating the radioactivity of blood, urine and faecal mples.

*eclinical safety data:* Not applicable. The relevant formation is given in Clinical Paticulars.

**armaceutical particulars**

*st of excipients:* Butylated hydroxytoluene; hyoxypropylcellulose; ethanol.

*compatibilities:* Not applicable.

*elf life:* (a) For the product as packaged for sale – ree years.

(b) After first opening the container – Two months.

*ecial precautions for storage:* Store below 25°C.

*ature and contents of container:* Aluminium tube of g, fitted with a screw cap.

*structions for use/handling:* There are no special structions for use or handling of Isotrex Gel.

**arketing authorisation number** 0174/0073.

**ate of approval/revision of SPC** April 1997.

**gal category** POM.

## SOTREXIN*

**ualitative and quantitative composition**

*ctive ingredients:* Isotretinoin PhEur 0.05% w/w and ythromycin PhEur 2.00% w/w.

**armaceutical form** Gel for cutaneous use.

**inical particulars**

*erapeutic indications:* Isotrexin is indicated for the pical treatment of mild to moderate acne vulgaris d is effective in treating both inflammatory and n-inflammatory lesions.

*osology and method of administration:*

*dults:* Apply Isotrexin sparingly over the entire fected area once or twice daily.

Patients should be advised that, in some cases, six eight weeks of treatment may be required before e full therapeutic effect is observed.

*se in children:* Not established for prepubescent ildren, in whom acne vulgaris rarely presents.

*se in the elderly:* No specific recommendations as ne vulgaris does not present in the elderly.

*ontra-indications:* Isotrexin should not be used in tients with known hypersensitivity to any of the gredients.

*ecial warnings and precautions for use:* Contact ith the mouth, eyes and mucous membranes and ith abraded or eczematous skin should be avoided. pplication to sensitive areas of skin, such as the eck, should be made with caution. As Isotrexin may use increased sensitivity to sunlight, deliberate or olonged exposure to sunlight or sunlamps should avoided or minimised. Concomitant topical meditions should be used with caution because a cumutive irritant effect may occur.

*teractions with other medicaments and other forms interaction:* None known.

*egnancy and lactation:* Category B1. The safety of otrexin for use in human pregnancy has not been tablished. An evaluation of experimental animal udies does not indicate direct or indirect harmful fects with respect to the development of the embryo foetus, the course of gestation and peri- and posttal development.

Isotretinoin has been associated with teratogenicity humans when administered systemically. However, production studies conducted in rabbits using topil isotretinoin applied at up to 60 times the human erapeutic dose have revealed no harm to the foetus. ere is no evidence of risk from the erythromycin mponent in human pregnancy.

The use of Isotrexin should be avoided by women ho are pregnant or intending to conceive.

*Use during lactation:* Percutaneous absorption of isotretinoin from Isotrexin is negligible. However, as it is not known if isotretinoin is excreted in human milk, Isotrexin should not be used during lactation.

*Effects on ability to drive and use machines:* None.

*Undesirable effects:* Isotrexin may cause stinging, burning or irritation; erythema and peeling at the site of application may occur. These local effects usually subside with continued treatment. If undue irritation occurs, treatment should be interrupted temporarily and resumed once the reaction subsides. If irritation persists, treatment should be discontinued. Reactions will usually resolve on discontinuation of therapy.

*Overdose:* Acute overdosage of Isotrexin has not been reported to date. The isotretinoin and erythromycin components are not expected to cause problems on ingestion of the topical gel.

**Pharmacological properties**

*Pharmacodynamic properties:* Isotretinoin is structurally and pharmacologically related to vitamin A, which regulates epithelial cell growth and differentiation. The pharmacological action of isotretinoin has not been fully determined. When used systemically, it suppresses sebaceous gland activity and reduces sebum production; it also affects comedogenesis, inhibits follicular keratinisation, suppresses *Propionibacterium acnes* and reduces inflammation. It is thought that topically applied isotretinoin stimulates mitosis in the epidermis and reduces intercellular cohesion in the stratum corneum; contests the hyperkeratosis characteristic of acne vulgaris and aids desquamation, preventing the formation of lesions. It is also thought that it mediates an increased production of less cohesive epidermal sebaceous cells. This appears to promote the initial expulsion and subsequent prevention of comedones.

Studies in animal models have shown similar activity when isotretinoin is applied topically. Inhibition of sebum production by topical isotretinoin has been demonstrated in the ears and flank organs of the Syrian hamster. Application of isotretinoin to the ear for 15 days led to a 50% reduction in sebaceous gland size, and application to the flank organ resulted in a 40% reduction. Topical application of isotretinoin has also been shown to have an effect on the epidermal differentiation of rhino mouse skin. Reduction in the size of the utriculi or superficial cysts leading to normal looking follicles was a predominant feature of isotretinoin treatment and has been used to quantify the antikeratinising effects of isotretinoin.

Isotretinoin has topical anti-inflammatory actions. Topically applied isotretinoin inhibits luekotriene-$B_4$-induced migration of polymorphonuclear leukocytes, which accounts for topical isotretinoin's anti-inflammatory action. A significant inhibition was produced by topically applied isotretinoin but only a weak inhibition by topical tretinoin. This may account for the reduced rebound effect seen with topical isotretinoin when compared with topical tretinoin.

Erythromycin is a macrolide antibiotic which acts by interfering with bacterial protein synthesis by reversibly binding to ribosomal subunits, thereby inhibiting translocation of aminoacyl transfer-RNA and inhibiting polypeptide synthesis. In the treatment of acne, it is effective through reduction in the population of *Propionibacterium acnes* and through prevention of release of inflammatory mediators by the bacteria. Resistance of *P. acnes* to topical erythromycin can occur, but evidence exists that the combination of erythromycin and isotretinoin in Isotrexin is effective against erythromycin-resistant strains of *P. acnes*.

The isotretinoin component of Isotrexin is very useful in treating the comedonal phase of the disease, while the erythromycin component is effective in the treatment of mild to moderate inflammatory acne vulgaris. Since most cases of acne consist of a combination of comedonal and inflammatory disease, combination topical therapy involving erythromycin and isotretinoin represents a logical approach to treatment.

*Pharmacokinetic properties:* Percutaneous absorption of isotretinoin and erythromycin from Isotrexin is negligible. In a maximised study of the topical absorption of the two components from Isotrexin in patients suffering from widespread acne, isotretinoin levels were shown to be only slightly raised from baseline levels (isotretinoin is normally present in plasma). Levels remained below 5 ng/ml, and were not increased in the presence of erythromycin when compared to topical isotretinoin alone. The levels of erythromycin were not detectable.

Under conditions of normal use in patients with acne, percutaneous absorption of the active components was negligible.

*Preclinical safety data:* Isotretinoin and erythromycin, the active ingredients in Isotrexin are well-established pharmacopoeial substances which are regularly used in the topical and systemic treatment of acne vulgaris. Preclinical safety studies have not been conducted on Isotrexin, as an extensive range of toxicological studies has been conducted on isotretinoin and erythromycin as well as their respective topical formulations. A human patch tests for irritation has shown the combination to be comparable to the application of either component alone, with an acceptably low potential for irritation.

**Pharmaceutical particulars**

*List of excipients:* Hydroxypropylcellulose USNF; Butylated Hydroxytoluene (BHT) PhEur; Ethanol BP.

*Incompatibilities:* None known.

*Shelf life:* (a) For the product packaged for sale – two years.

(b) After first opening the container – comply with expiry date.

*Special precautions for storage:* Store below 25°C.

*Nature and contents of container:* Internally lacquered membrane-sealed aluminium tubes fitted with a polypropylene screw-cap, packed into a carton. Pack size 30 grammes.

*Instructions for use/handling:* None.

**Marketing authorisation number** 00174/0200.

**Date of approval/revision of SPC** October 1996.

**Legal category** POM.

## LACTICARE*

**Qualitative and quantitative composition** Lactic acid 5% w/w, sodium pyrrolidone carboxylate 2.5% w/w.

**Pharmaceutical form** Lotion for cutaneous use.

**Clinical particulars**

*Therapeutic indications:* LactiCare is indicated for the symptomatic relief of hyperkeratotic and other chronic dry skin conditions, and for dry skin conditions caused by low humidity or the use of detergents.

*Posology and method of administration:* Use as required on affected areas or as directed by a doctor.

*Contra-indications:* None.

*Special warnings and special precautions for use:* Keep away from the eyes and mucous membranes. Should contact with the eyes occur, remove with water.

Keep out of reach of children.

*Interactions with other medicaments and other forms of interaction:* None known.

*Pregnancy and lactation:* Although there is no experimental evidence to support the safety of the drug during pregnancy and lactation, no adverse effects have been reported.

*Effects on ability to drive and use machines:* None.

*Undesirable effects:* Occasionally a transient mild stinging sensation may occur. Should prolonged irritation develop when used on abraded or inflamed skin, discontinue use.

*Overdose:* Not applicable.

**Pharmacological properties**

*Pharmacodynamic properties:* Both lactic acid and sodium pyrrolidone carboxylic acid are hygroscopic. They enhance the ability of the stratum corneum to retain water and counteract the tendency of the skin to dry out. Lactic acid also modulates epidermal keratinisation and increases skin extensibility.

*Pharmacokinetic properties:* Not applicable.

*Preclinical safety data:* There are no preclinical data of any relevance additional to that already included in other sections of the SPC.

**Pharmaceutical particulars**

*List of excipients:* Carbomer 940; imidurea; dehydroacetic acid; sodium hydroxide; polyethylene glycol ether complex; glyceryl monostearate; cetyl alcohol; isopropyl palmitate; light liquid paraffin; myristyl lactate; antaria essence 73/82; purified water.

*Incompatibilities:* None.

*Shelf life:* (a) For the product as packaged for sale – 3 years.

(b) After first opening the container – Comply with expiry date.

*Special precautions for storage:* None.

*Nature and contents of container:* High density polyethylene bottle containing 150 ml.

*Instructions for use/handling:* There are no special instructions for use or handling of LactiCare.

**Marketing authorisation number** 0174/0038.

**Date of approval/revision of SPC** 5 April 1995.

**Legal category** GSL.

## OILATUM* CREAM

**Qualitative and quantitative composition** Arachis oil 21.0% w/w.

**Pharmaceutical form** Oil in water for cutaneous use.

**Clinical particulars**

*Therapeutic indications:* Oilatum Cream is indicated in the treatment of dry, sensitive skin, ichthyosis and similar conditions. The use of Oilatum Cream in such conditions reduces moisture loss from the stratum corneum and thus restores skin flexibility.

*Posology and method of administration:* Oilatum Cream may be used as often as required. Apply to the affected areas and rub in well.

It is especially effective after washing when the normal acid condition of the skin may be disturbed and when the sebum content of the stratum corneum may be depleted.

The product is suitable for use in adults, children and the elderly.

*Contra-indications:* None.

*Special warnings and special precautions for use:* Patients with a known hypersensitivity to any of the ingredients should not use the product.

*Interactions with other medicaments and other forms of interaction:* None known.

*Pregnancy and lactation:* There are no restrictions on the use of Oilatum Cream during pregnancy or lactation.

*Effects on ability to drive and use machines:* None.

*Undesirable effects:* None.

*Overdose:* Not applicable.

**Pharmacological properties**

*Pharmacodynamic properties:* Arachis oil exerts an emollient effect by forming an occlusive film which reduces trans-epidermal water loss, thus restoring normal skin humidity levels.

*Pharmacokinetic properties:* Not applicable.

*Preclinical safety data:* Not applicable.

**Pharmaceutical particulars**

*List of excipients:* Polyvinyl pyrrolidone; propylene glycol; glyceryl monostearate; macrogol monostearate; stearic acid; isopropyl palmitate; quaternium 15; potassium sorbate; fragrance 2174 H; purified water.

*Incompatibilities:* None.

*Shelf life:* (a) For the product as packaged for sale – Three years.

(b) After first opening the container – Comply with expiry date.

*Special precautions for storage:* None.

*Nature and contents of container:* Internally lined aluminium tubes of 40 g and 80 g.

*Instructions for use/handling:* There are no special instructions for use or handling of Oilatum Cream.

**Marketing authorisation number** 0174/5014R.

**Date of approval/revision of SPC** 23 March 1995.

**Legal category** GSL.

## OILATUM* EMOLLIENT

**Presentation** Oilatum Emollient is a liquid bath additive. Active ingredient: Liquid paraffin 63.4% w/w.

Excipients: acetylated wool alcohols, isopropyl palmitate, macrogol 400 dilaurate, macrogol ester, fragrance floral spice.

**Uses** Oilatum Emollient is indicated in the treatment of contact dermatitis, atopic dermatitis, senile pruritus, ichthyosis and related dry skin conditions. Oilatum Emollient replaces oil and water and hydrates the keratin. Oilatum Emollient is particularly suitable for infant bathing. The preparation also overcomes the problem of cleansing the skin in conditions where the use of soaps, soap substitutes and colloid or oat-meal baths proves irritating.

**Dosage and administration** Oilatum Emollient should always be used with water, either added to water or applied to wet skin.

*Adult bath:* Add 1–3 capfuls to an 8 inch bath of water. Soak for 10–20 minutes. Pat dry.

*Infant bath:* Add ½–2 capfuls to a basin of water. Apply gently over entire body with a sponge. Pat dry.

*Skin cleansing:* Rub a small amount of oil into wet skin. Rinse and pat dry.

Where conditions permit, and particularly in cases of extensive areas of dry skin, Oilatum Emollient should be used as a bath oil, ensuring complete coverage by immersion. In addition to the therapeutic benefits, this method of use provides a means of sedating tense patients, particularly relevant in cases of acute pruritic dermatoses where relaxation of tension appears to relieve symptoms.

The product is suitable for use in adults, children and the elderly.

**Contra-indications, warnings, etc** The patient should be advised to use care to avoid slipping in the bath. If a rash or skin irritation occurs, stop using the product and consult your doctor.

Contains acetylated lanolin alcohols; avoid use in individuals with known lanolin hypersensitivity.

There is no evidence of the safety of Oilatum Emollient in human pregnancy or lactation, but it has been in wide use for many years without ill consequence.

**Pharmaceutical precautions** Nil.

**Legal category** GSL.

**Package quantities** Oilatum Emollient is available in bottles containing 250 ml and 500 ml.

**Further information** Light liquid paraffin exerts an emollient effect by forming an occlusive film in the stratum corneum. This prevents excessive evaporation of water from the skin surface and aids in the prevention of dryness.

**Product licence number** 0174/5010R.

## OILATUM* GEL

**Presentation** Oilatum Gel is an emollient shower gel containing Light Liquid Paraffin BP 70% w/w.

Other ingredients: Polyethylene, macrogol 400 dilaurate, macrogol ester, 2-octadodecanol, macrogol myristyl ether propionate, polyphenylmethylsiloxane copolymer, fragrance floral spice.

**Uses** Oilatum Gel is indicated in the treatment of contact dermatitis, atopic eczema, senile pruritus, ichthyosis and related dry skin conditions.

**Dosage and administration** Oilatum Gel should be used as frequently as necessary. Daily application is recommended.

Oilatum Gel should always be applied to wet skin, normally as a shower gel.

Shower as usual. Apply Oilatum Gel to wet skin and massage gently. Rinse briefly and lightly pat the skin dry.

**Contra-indications, warnings, etc** Use care to avoid slipping in the shower.

**Pharmaceutical precautions** Store below 25°C.

**Legal category** GSL.

**Package quantities** Oilatum Gel is supplied in tubes of 65 g and 125 g.

**Further information** Oilatum Gel exerts an emollient effect through deposition of an occlusive film of light liquid paraffin on the stratum corneum. This prevents excessive evaporation of moisture from the skin, thus improving hydration, reducing roughness and scaling and relieving discomfort and itching.

**Product licence number** 0174/0072.

## OILATUM* PLUS

**Qualitative and quantitative composition** Light liquid paraffin 52.5% w/w, benzalkonium chloride 6.0% w/w, triclosan 2.0% w/w.

**Pharmaceutical form** Solution.

**Clinical particulars**

*Therapeutic indications:* For the prophylactic treatment of eczemas at risk from infection.

*Posology and method of administration:* Oilatum Plus should always be diluted with water. It is an effective cleanser and should not be used with soap.

*Adults and children:* In an eight inch bath add 2 capfuls, in a four inch bath add 1 capful.

*Infants:* Add 1 ml (just sufficient to cover the bottom of the cap) and mix well with water.

Not recommended for babies younger than 6 months.

*Contra-indications:* Patients with a known hypersensitivity to any of the ingredients should not use the product.

*Special warnings and special precautions for use:* Avoid contact of the undiluted product with the eyes and the skin. If the undiluted product comes into contact with the eye, reddening and watering may occur. Eye irrigation should be performed for 15 minutes and the eye examined under fluorescein stain. If there is persistent irritation or any uptake of fluorescein, the patient should be referred for ophthalmological opinion.

Take care to avoid slipping in the bath.

*Interactions with other medicaments and other forms of interaction:* None known.

*Pregnancy and lactation:* There are no restrictions on the use of Oilatum Plus during pregnancy or lactation.

*Effects on ability to drive and use machines:* None.

*Undesirable effects:* None known.

*Overdosage:* Oilatum Plus is intended for topical use only. Ingestion may cause gastro intestinal irritation with vomiting and diarrhoea. Vomiting may result in foam aspiration. In the case of accidental ingestion give 1 to 2 glasses of milk or water. If a large quantity of the product is ingested, the patient should be observed in hospital and the use of activated charcoal may be considered.

**Pharmacological properties**

*Pharmacodynamic properties:* Benzalkonium chloride and triclosan are anti-bacterial agents with proven efficacy against *Staphylococcus aureus*, the principal causative organism in infected eczemas.

Light liquid paraffin is an emollient widely used in the treatment of eczema.

*Pharmacokinetic properties:* Not applicable.

*Preclinical safety data:* Not applicable.

**Pharmaceutical particulars**

*List of excipients:* Acetylated lanolin alcohols; isopropyl palmitate; oleyl alcohol; polyoxyethylene lauryl ether.

*Incompatibilities:* None known.

*Shelf life:* (a) For the product as packaged for sale Three years.

(b) After first opening the container – Comply with expiry date.

*Special precautions for storage:* None.

*Nature and contents of container:* White high density polyethylene bottle containing 500 ml.

*Instructions for use/handling:* There are no special instructions for use or handling of Oilatum Plus.

**Marketing authorisation number** 0174/0070.

**Date of approval/revision of SPC** 30 March 1995.

**Legal category** GSL.

## PANOXYL* Acne Gel 5
## PANOXYL* Acne Gel 10

**Presentation** White viscous gels containing benzoyl peroxide 5 and 10% w/w in an ethanolic base.

Excipients: magnesium aluminium silicate, hypromellose, macrogol lauryl ether, ethanol, citric acid, fragrance 6565A, purified water.

**Uses** PanOxyl 5 and 10 are each indicated for use in the treatment of acne vulgaris.

**Dosage and administration**

*Adults, the elderly and children over 12 years:* Treatment should normally commence with PanOxyl 5. Apply the gel to the affected areas once daily. Washing prior to application greatly enhances the efficacy of the preparation. The reaction of the skin to benzoyl peroxide differs in individual patients, and for this reason the higher percentage of benzoyl peroxide PanOxyl 10 may be required in order to provide satisfactory drying and desquamative action.

*Children under 12 years:* Not recommended.

**Contra-indications, warnings, etc** Avoid contact with eyes, mouth and mucous membranes. Take care when applying to the neck and other sensitive areas. Do not use in patients with known hypersensitivity to benzoyl peroxide.

In normal use, a mild burning sensation will probably be felt on first application and a moderate reddening and peeling of the skin will occur within a few days. During the first few weeks of treatment a sudden increase in peeling will occur in most patients.

There are no restrictions on the use of PanOxyl 5 and PanOxyl 10 during pregnancy and lactation.

PanOxyl 5 and PanOxyl 10 may bleach dyed fabrics.

**Pharmaceutical precautions** Store in a cool place.

**Legal category** P.

**Package quantities** PanOxyl 5 and PanOxyl 10 are supplied in tubes each containing 40 g.

**Further information** Benzoyl peroxide has sebostatic and keratolytic activity coupled with antibacterial activity against Propionibacterium acnes, the organism implicated in acne vulgaris. Its use in the treatment of acne is well established.

**Product licence numbers**
PanOxyl 5   0174/0019R
PanOxyl 10  0174/0020R

# ANOXYL* AQUAGEL* 2.5
# ANOXYL* AQUAGEL* 5
# ANOXYL* AQUAGEL* 10

**Presentation** White viscous gels containing benzoyl peroxide 2.5, 5 and 10% w/w in an aqueous, non alcoholic base.

Excipients: carbomer, diisopropanolamine, propylene glycol, macrogol lauryl ether, sodium lauryl sulphate, purified water.

**Uses** PanOxyl Aquagel 2.5, 5 and 10 are each indicated for use in the topical treatment of acne vulgaris.

**Dosage and administration** Treatment should normally begin with PanOxyl Aquagel 2.5. Apply to the affected areas once daily. Washing prior to application enhances the efficacy of the preparation.

The reaction of the skin to benzoyl peroxide differs in individual patients. The higher concentration in PanOxyl Aquagel 5 or 10 may be required to produce a satisfactory response.

**Contra-indications, warnings, etc** PanOxyl Aquagel should not be prescribed for patients with a known hypersensitivity to benzoyl peroxide.

Avoid contact with the eyes, mouth and mucous membranes. Care should be taken when applying the product to the neck and other sensitive areas. In normal use, a mild burning sensation will probably be felt on first application and a moderate reddening and peeling of the skin will occur within a few days. During the first weeks of treatment a sudden increase in peeling will occur in most patients, this is not harmful and will normally subside within a day or two if treatment is temporarily discontinued. If excessive irritation, redness or peeling occurs discontinue use.

There are no restrictions on the use of PanOxyl Aquagel during pregnancy and lactation.

These products may bleach dyed fabrics.

**Pharmaceutical precautions** Store in a cool place.

**Legal category** P.

**Package quantities** Tubes of 40 g.

**Further information** Benzoyl peroxide has sebostatic and keratolytic activity coupled with antibacterial activity against Propionibacterium acnes, the organism implicated in acne vulgaris. Its use in the treatment of acne is well established.

**Product licence numbers**
PanOxyl Aquagel 2.5    0174/0049
PanOxyl Aquagel 5      0174/0050
PanOxyl Aquagel 10     0174/0051

# PANOXYL* CREAM 5
# PANOXYL* LOTION 5
# PANOXYL* LOTION 10

**Presentation** Panoxyl 5 is available as a white lotion or cream containing benzoyl peroxide 5% w/w.

Panoxyl 10 is a white lotion containing benzoyl peroxide 10% w/w.

Excipients: macrogol 1000 monostearate, stearic acid, glyceryl monostearate, isopropyl palmitate, propylene glycol, zinc caproate, zinc laurate, zinc myristate, purified water.

**Uses** Panoxyl 5 and 10 are each indicated for use in the treatment of acne vulgaris.

**Dosage and administration** Treatment should normally commence with Panoxyl 5. Apply the lotion or cream to the affected areas once daily. Washing with soap and water prior to application greatly enhances the efficacy of the preparation.

The reaction of the skin to benzoyl peroxide differs in individual patients. The higher concentration in Panoxyl 10 may be required to ensure a satisfactory response.

**Contra-indications, warnings, etc** Panoxyl should not be prescribed for patients with a known hypersensitivity to benzoyl peroxide.

Avoid contact with the eyes, mouth and other mucous membranes. Care should be taken when applying the product to the neck and other sensitive areas. In normal use, a mild burning sensation will probably be felt on first application and a moderate reddening and peeling of the skin will occur within a few days. During the first weeks of treatment a sudden increase in peeling will occur in most patients, this is not harmful and will normally subside within a day or two if treatment is temporarily discontinued.

There are no restrictions on the use of the product during pregnancy and lactation.

Panoxyl may bleach dyed fabrics.

**Pharmaceutical precautions** Store in a cool place.

**Legal category** P.

**Package quantities** Lotion: Bottles of 30 ml.

Cream: Tubes of 40 g.

**Further information** Benzoyl peroxide has sebostatic and keratolytic activity coupled with antibacterial activity against Propionibacterium acnes, the organism implicated in acne vulgaris. Its use in the treatment of acne is well established.

**Product licence numbers**
Panoxyl Lotion 5     0174/5003R
Panoxyl Cream 5      0174/5007R
Panoxyl Lotion 10    0174/0034

# PANOXYL* WASH 10%

**Qualitative and quantitative composition** Benzoyl peroxide 10.0% w/w.

**Pharmaceutical form**    Lotion for cutaneous use.

**Clinical particulars**
*Therapeutic indications:* Panoxyl Wash 10% is indicated for the treatment of acne vulgaris.

*Posology and method of administration*
*Adults:* Wet the affected area with water and wash thoroughly with Panoxyl Wash. Rinse well with warm water, then rinse with cold water. Pat dry with a clean towel. Use once a day.

*Elderly patients:* There are no specific recommendations. Acne vulgaris does not present in the elderly.

*Paediatric use:* The product is not intended for use in pre-pubescent children since acne vulgaris rarely presents in this age group.

*Contra-indications:* Patients with a known hypersensitivity to any of the ingredients should not use the product.

*Special warnings and special precautions for use:* Avoid contact with the eyes, mouth and other mucous membranes. Care should be taken when applying the product to the neck and other sensitive areas.

The product may bleach dyed fabrics.

Keep out of the reach of children.

*Interactions with other medicaments and other forms of interaction:* None.

*Pregnancy and lactation:* There are no restrictions on the use of the product during pregnancy or lactation.

*Effects on ability to drive and use machines:* None.

*Undesirable effects:* In normal use, a mild burning sensation will probably be felt on first application and a moderate reddening and peeling of the skin will occur within a few days. During the first few weeks of treatment a sudden increase in peeling will occur in most patients; this is not harmful and will normally subside in a day or two if treatment is temporarily discontinued.

*Overdose:* Not applicable.

**Pharmacological properties**
*Pharmacodynamic properties:* Benzoyl peroxide has antibacterial activity against *Propionibacterium acnes*, the organism implicated in acne vulgaris. It has keratolytic activity and is sebostatic, counteracting the hyperkeratinisation and excessive sebum production associated with acne.

*Pharmacokinetic properties:* Not applicable.

*Preclinical safety data:* Not applicable. Benzoyl peroxide has been in widespread use for many years.

**Pharmaceutical particulars**
*List of excipients:* Magnesium aluminium silicate; citric acid monohydrate; sodium alkyl aryl polyether sulphonate; sodium dihexyl sulphosuccinate; sodium lauryl sulphoacetate; hydroxypropylmethylcellulose; polyoxyethylene lauryl ether; imidurea; purified water.

*Incompatibilities:* None.

*Shelf life:* (a) For the product as packaged – 2 years.
(b) After first opening the container – Comply with expiry date.

*Special precautions for storage:* Store at room temperature.

*Nature and contents of container:* Flip top polyethylene bottle containing 150 ml.

*Instructions for use/handling:* There are no special instructions for use or handling of Panoxyl Wash 10%.

**Marketing authorisation number**    0174/0048.

**Date of approval/revision of SPC**    23 March 1995.

**Legal category**    P.

# POLYTAR* AF

**Presentation** Polytar AF is a medicated scalp treatment containing the following active ingredients: Tar blend[†] 1% w/w, Zinc pyrithione 1% w/w in a shampoo base.

([†]Tar blend consists of Pine Tar BP, 30% w/w; Cade Oil BPC, 30% w/w; Coal Tar Solution BP, 10% w/w; Arachis Oil Extract of Coal Tar BP, 30% w/w).

Excipients: coconut diethanolamide, triethanolamine lauryl sulphate, carbomer, hypromellose, octoxinol, glycerol, imidurea, purified water.

**Uses** Polytar AF is indicated in the topical treatment of scalp disorders such as dandruff, seborrhoeic dermatitis and psoriasis.

Polytar AF has antibacterial and antifungal properties. It is fungicidal against the pathogenic yeasts of the pityrosporum genus which are implicated in dandruff and seborrhoeic dermatitis.

Polytar AF suppresses DNA synthesis in hyperplastic skin; this inhibits mitotic activity and protein synthesis. The product decreases epidermal proliferation and promotes a return to normal keratinisation.

Polytar AF relieves the scaling and pruritus normally associated with seborrhoeic dermatitis and dandruff.

**Dosage and administration** Adults, children and the elderly: Shake the bottle before use. Wet the hair and massage Polytar AF into the hair, scalp and surrounding skin. Leave for 2–3 minutes, then rinse thoroughly.

Treatment: Use two or three times weekly for at least 3 weeks or until the condition clears.

Prophylaxis for seborrhoeic dermatitis and dandruff: use Polytar AF weekly.

**Contra-indications, warnings, etc**
*Contra-indications:* Polytar AF should not be used by patients with known hypersensitivity to any of the ingredients.

*Precautions:* Avoid contact with the eyes. Tar products may cause skin irritation, rashes and, rarely, photosensitivity. Zinc pyrithione may cause dermatitis, should this occur, Polytar AF should be discontinued.

*Pregnancy and lactation:* The safety of Polytar AF in human pregnancy or lactation has not been established.

**Pharmaceutical precautions**    Store below 25°C.

**Legal category**    GSL.

**Package quantities** Polytar AF is available in bottles of 150 ml.

**Further information**    Nil.

**Product licence number**    0174/0071.

# POLYTAR* EMOLLIENT

**Presentation** Polytar Emollient is a liquid bath additive. The active ingredients are as follows:

Tar blend[†]                25% w/w
Light Liquid Paraffin       35% w/w
([†]Tar blend consists of: Pine Tar BP, 30% w/w; Cade Oil BPC, 30% w/w; Coal Tar Solution BP, 10% w/w; Arachis Oil Extract of Coal Tar BP, 30% w/w.)

Excipients: octoxinol, sorbitan mono-oleate, polysorbate 80, isopropyl palmitate, macrogol 400 dilaurate, purified water.

**Uses** Polytar Emollient is indicated in the treatment of psoriasis, eczema, atopic and pruritic dermatoses. The use of Polytar Emollient may be combined with ultraviolet radiation and other adjunctive therapy.

Polytar Emollient is also of value in removing loose psoriatic scales and paste following dithranol treatment.

**Dosage and administration** 15–30 mls (2–4 capfuls) of Polytar Emollient should be added to an 8 inch bath and the patient instructed to soak for 20 minutes.

**Contra-indications, warnings, etc** Patients should be instructed to guard against slipping when entering or leaving the bath.

Tar products may cause skin irritation, rashes and rarely, photosensitivity. In the event of such a reaction, discontinue use and consult your doctor. Tar products may stain baths and fabrics.

There is no evidence of the safety of Polytar Emollient in human pregnancy but it has been in wide use for many years without apparent ill consequence.

**Pharmaceutical precautions**    Nil.

**Legal category**    GSL.

**Package quantities** Polytar Emollient is available in bottles of 350 ml.

**Further information** Tar preparations have keratoplastic and antipruritic activity and are widely used as topical therapy for a range of dermatoses. The use of emollient bath oils in the management of dry and itching skin is well established. Mineral oil exerts its emollient effect by skin absorption.

Polytar Emollient is prescribable on FP10 for the treatment of psoriasis, eczema, atopic and pruritic dermatoses.

**Product licence number**    0174/5011R.

## POLYTAR* LIQUID

**Qualitative and quantitative composition** Tar Blend 1% w/w. Tar Blend comprises: Pine tar, cade oil, coal tar solution, arachis oil extract of coal tar.

**Pharmaceutical form** Medicated shampoo.

**Clinical particulars**
*Therapeutic indications:* Polytar Liquid is indicated in the treatment of scalp disorders including psoriasis, dandruff, seborrhoea, eczema and pruritus. Polytar Liquid is also of value in the removal of ointments and pastes used in the treatment of psoriasis.

*Posology and method of administration:* The hair should be wetted and sufficient Polytar Liquid applied to produce an abundant lather. The scalp and adjacent areas should be vigorously massaged with the fingertips. The hair should then be thoroughly rinsed and the procedure repeated.

Polytar Liquid should be used once or twice weekly.

*Contra-indications:* Patients with a known hypersensitivity to any of the ingredients should not use the product.

*Special warnings and special precautions for use:* There are no special warnings or precautions.

*Interactions with other medicaments and other forms of interaction:* There are no known interactions with other medicaments or other forms of interaction.

*Pregnancy and lactation:* There is no, or inadequate evidence of the safety of Polytar Liquid in human pregnancy and lactation, but it has been in wide use for many years without apparent ill consequence.

*Effects on ability to drive and use machines:* The use of this product will not affect the ability to drive and to use machines.

*Undesirable effects:* Tar products may cause skin irritation, rashes and rarely, photosensitivity. If irritation occurs and persists, treatment should be discontinued.

*Overdose:* The product is intended for external use only. It is applied to the scalp and rinsed off. Use of an excessive quantity is not a cause for concern.

**Pharmacological properties**
*Pharmacodynamic properties:* Tars suppress DNA synthesis in hyperplastic skin, inhibiting mitotic activity and protein synthesis. They decrease epidermal proliferation and dermal infiltration and thus promote a return to normal keratinisation.

Tars also have vasoconstrictor, antipruritic and antiseptic properties.

*Pharmacokinetic properties:* The product is applied topically and acts at the site of application. The potential for systemic absorption from a wash-off shampoo is extremely low.

*Preclinical safety data:* Tar preparations have been in widespread use for many years and their safety in humans has been established.

**Pharmaceutical particulars**
*List of excipients:* Oleyl alcohol; coconut diethanolamide; hexylene glycol; polysorbate 80; triethanolamine lauryl sulphate; sodium chloride; citric acid; octylphenoxypolyethoxy ethanol; imidurea; fragrance 5412; purified water.

*Incompatibilities:* There are no known incompatibilities.

*Shelf life:* (a) For the product as packaged for sale – 3 years.

(b) After first opening the container – Comply with expiry date.

*Special precautions for storage:* There are no special precautions for storage.

*Nature and contents of container:* High density polyethylene bottles of 150 ml and 250 ml.

*Instructions for use/handling:* There are no special instructions for use or handling of Polytar Liquid.

**Marketing authorisation number** 0174/5016R.

**Date of approval/revision of SPC** 18 September 1995.

**Legal category** GSL.

## POLYTAR PLUS*

**Presentation** Polytar Plus is a concentrated antiseptic, tar medicated scalp cleanser adjusted to pH 5.5, containing the hair conditioners: Polypeptide and oleyl alcohol and the active ingredient: Tar blend† 1% w/w.

(†Tar blend consists of: Pine Tar BP, 30% w/w; Cade Oil BPC, 30% w/w; Coal Tar Solution BP, 10% w/w; Arachis Oil Extract of Coal Tar BP, 30% w/w.)

Excipients: coconut diethanolamide, hexylene glycol, macrogol oleyl ether, polysorbate 80, triethanolamine lauryl sulphate, citric acid, octoxinol, imidurea, fragrance 5412, purified water.

**Uses** Polytar Plus is indicated in the treatment of scalp disorders such as dandruff, psoriasis, seborrhoea, eczema and pruritus. Polytar Plus is also of value in the removal of ointments and pastes used in the treatment of psoriasis. Polytar Plus is especially suitable for dry hair.

**Dosage and administration**
*Aduts, children and the elderly:* The hair should be wetted and sufficient Polytar Plus applied to produce an abundant lather. The scalp and adjacent areas should be vigorously massaged with the fingertips. The hair should then be thoroughly rinsed and the procedure repeated.

Polytar Plus should be used once or twice weekly.

**Contra-indications, warnings, etc** Tar products may cause skin irritation, rashes and rarely, photosensitivity. In the event of such a reaction, discontinue use and consult your doctor.

There are no restrictions on the use of Polytar Plus during pregnancy or lactation.

**Pharmaceutical precautions** Nil.

**Legal category** GSL.

**Package quantities** Polytar Plus is available in bottles of 350 ml.

**Further information** Tars suppress DNA synthesis in hyperplastic skin, this inhibits mitotic activity and protein synthesis. By decreasing epidermal proliferation and dermal infiltration, they promote a return to normal keratinisation. Tars also have vasoconstricting, astringent and antipruritic properties.

Polytar Plus is prescribable on FP10 for psoriasis, eczema and seborrhoea of the scalp and for dandruff.

**Product licence number** 0174/0037.

## SPECTRABAN* LOTION 25

**Presentation** SpectraBAN Lotion contains Padimate O 3.2% w/w and Para Aminobenzoic Acid USP 5% w/w in an ethanolic base. The product, which is non-greasy and invisible on the skin, is pink in colour.

Excipients: ethanol, carbomer, polyoxyethylene cocoamine, colour E122, oleyl alcohol, fragrance A3012, purified water.

**Uses** SpectraBAN Lotion is a protective sunscreen lotion indicated in patients at risk from exposure to ultraviolet light within the UVB wavelength range (280–315 nanometres). It is this narrow waveband of ultraviolet light which is responsible for burning and tanning of the skin in man. The product has a UVB Sun Protection Factor 25, thus it should allow 25 times normal exposure to sunlight before burning.

SpectraBAN Lotion is indicated for protection from UV radiation in abnormal cutaneous photosensitivity resulting from genetic disorders or photodermatoses, including those resulting from radiotherapy; chronic or recurrent herpes simplex labialis.

**Dosage and administration** Apply carefully and evenly to areas to be exposed or protected only by light clothing. Allow to dry before dressing. Allow 45 minutes before swimming or sweat producing exercise. A single application may give day long protection but the product should be re-applied frequently during prolonged sunning or after swimming or excessive sweating.

**Contra-indications, warnings, etc** Sunscreen preparations occasionally produce a sensitivity reaction. Treatment should be discontinued if a skin rash or irritation develops. Do not apply to broken skin. Avoid contact with the eyes, mouth and other mucous membranes.

The product can stain clothing and other items permanently.

There is no evidence of the safety of the drug in human pregnancy but it has been in wide use for many years without apparent ill consequence.

**Pharmaceutical precautions** Avoid flame.

**Legal category** GSL.

**Package quantities** SpectraBAN Lotion is available in bottles containing 150 ml.

**Further information** SpectraBAN Lotion is prescribable on FP10.

**Product licence number** 0174/0035.

## STIEDEX* LOTION

**Presentation** Stiedex Lotion contains desoxymethasone USP 0.25% w/w, Salicylic Acid PhEur 1.0% w/w.

Excipients: Polyol fatty acid ester, 1,2-propylene glycol, ethanol, sodium hydroxide, disodium edetate, purified water.

**Uses** Stiedex Lotion contains a potent corticosteroid and is indicated for the treatment of psoriasis, particularly of the scalp (but excluding widesprea plaque psoriasis), seborrhoeic eczema, chron lichenified eczema, lichen planus, lichen simplex, no bullous ichthyosiform erythroderma.

Stiedex Lotion is especially suitable for use in hai regions such as scalp, cheeks, neck and chest and f skin areas difficult to reach such as the audito meatus.

**Dosage and administration** Stiedex Lotion shou be applied to the affected areas once or twice dai preferably morning and/or night. When the sk condition improves, application may be reduced once daily. In order to prevent recurrence, treatme with Stiedex Lotion should be continued for son days after complete control of the condition. If th lotion is being used on the face or in children, cours should be limited to five days duration.

**Contra-indications, warnings, etc** *Contra-indic tions:* Stiedex Lotion is contra-indicated in infants ar young children, in facial rosacea, acne vulgari perioral dermatitis, perianal and genital pruritis, na kin eruptions, bacterial (e.g. impetigo), viral (e. Herpes simplex), and fungal (e.g. Candida or de matophyte) infections.

Stiedex Lotion contains propylene glycol ar should not be used in patients with a known hyperse sitivity to this, or any of the other ingredients.

*Precautions:* The continuous administration of topic steroids over prolonged periods may result in adren suppression; in infants and children, this may caus growth retardation. The use of occlusive dressin enhances the absorption of the steroid, and consequence, systemic effects are more likely occur. Salicyclic acid may enhance absorption of th steroid or itself be absorbed. Adrenal suppression unlikely in short courses of treatment or with dos not exceeding 10 g daily.

Long term continuous therapy should be avoid in all patients irrespective of age. The lotion shou not be applied to extensive skin surfaces and applic tion under occlusion should be restricted to de matoses involving limited areas.

The use of topical corticosteroids may be hazardo in psoriasis for a number of reasons including rebou relapses following development of tolerance, risk generalised pustular psoriasis and local and system toxicity due to impaired barrier function of the ski Careful patient supervision is important if Stied Lotion is used in psoriasis.

Prolonged administration of potent corticosteroi has been shown also to cause a thinning in sk collagen and subcutaneous atrophy, resulting striae, thinning and dilation of superficial bloo vessels. These changes are particularly liable to occ on the face.

Percutaneous absorption of salicylic acid due extensive use could lead to salicylism.

Salicylic acid may alter the permeability of the sk to other substances applied simultaneously. The u of other preparations, cosmetics etc., on skin treat with Stiedex Lotion should be avoided.

Stiedex Lotion should not be applied to or near th eye.

*Use in pregnancy:* There is inadequate evidence safety in human pregnancy. Topical administration corticosteroids to pregnant animals can cause abno malities of foetal development including cleft pala and intra-uterine growth retardation. There may the fore be a very small risk of such effects in the huma foetus.

**Pharmaceutical precautions** Stiedex Lotion shou be protected from heat and stored below 25°C.

**Legal category** POM.

**Package quantities** 50 ml.

**Further information** Nil.

**Product licence number** 0174/0062.

## STIEDEX* LP

**Presentation** Stiedex LP contains 0.05% w/w desox methasone in an oily cream base.

Excipients: isopropyl myristate, wool alcohols oi ment, edetic acid, purified water.

**Uses** Stiedex LP contains a potent corticosteroid a is indicated for the treatment of a wide range of acu inflammatory and allergic conditions, and chronic sk disorders.

Stiedex LP is specifically indicated for the treatme of eczema (including atopic, seborrhoeic and nu mular eczema), intertrigo, psoriasis, pompholyx, chen planus and discoid lupus erythematosus; acu and chronic allergic dermatoses, neurodermatit erythroderma, and may also be used in the no specific treatment of sunburn and insect bites.

**Dosage and administration** Stiedex LP should applied sparingly to the affected area and rubb gently into the skin. Initially, application should be made 2–3 times daily and the frequency of administration reduced as the condition subsides.

Stiedex LP may be applied under an occlusive dressing. The affected area should be thoroughly cleansed prior to administration of cream and dressing to prevent infection.

### Contra-indications, warnings, etc

*Contra-indications:* Stiedex LP is not suitable for infants and young children. Stiedex LP is contra-indicated in facial rosacea, acne vulgaris, perioral dermatitis, perianal and genital pruritus, napkin eruptions, bacterial (e.g. impetigo), viral (e.g. *Herpes simplex*) and fungal (e.g. *Candida* and dermatophyte) infections.

Stiedex LP is contra-indicated in patients with hypersensitivity to the preparation.

Stiedex LP is not suitable for use in the treatment of inflammatory disorders of the eye.

There is inadequate evidence of safety in human pregnancy. Topical administration of corticosteroids to pregnant animals can cause abnormalities of foetal development including cleft palate and intra-uterine growth retardation. There may therefore be a very small risk of such effects in the human foetus.

*Precautions:* The continuous administration of topical steroids over prolonged periods may result in adrenal suppression; in infants and children, this may cause growth retardation. The use of occlusive dressings enhances the absorption of the active substance, desoxymethasone, and in consequence systemic effects are more likely to occur. Adrenal suppression is unlikely in short courses of treatment or with doses not exceeding 10 g daily.

Prolonged administration of potent corticosteroids has been shown also to cause a reduction in skin collagen and subcutaneous atrophy, resulting in striae, thinning and dilation of superficial blood vessels. These changes are particularly liable to occur on the face.

### Pharmaceutical precautions
Stiedex LP should be stored in a cool, dry place.

**Legal category** POM.

**Package quantities** Stiedex LP is available in tubes of 30 g and 100 g.

**Further information** Stiedex LP contains no preservative. Stiedex LP may be diluted by admixture with Oily Cream BP.

**Product licence number** 0174/0053.

## STIEMYCIN*

**Presentation** A clear colourless solution in an amber glass screw-capped applicator bottle. The applicator allows the product to be applied directly to the involved skin.

Each ml contains 20 mg erythromycin base PhEur in an amount equivalent to 20 mg of erythromycin base 1st International Standard, in an ethanol base also containing propylene glycol and Laureth 4.

**Uses** Stiemycin is indicated for use in the topical treatment of acne vulgaris.

**Dosage and administration** To be applied to the affected area twice daily after washing.

**Contra-indications, warnings, etc** Stiemycin is contra-indicated in patients with known sensitivity to any of the ingredients.

Concomitant topical acne therapy should be used with caution because a cumulative irritant effect may occur.

Avoid contact with eyes and other mucous membranes.

This product is for external use only.

There is no evidence of hazard from erythromycin in human pregnancy. It has been in wide use for many years without apparent ill consequence.

**Pharmaceutical precautions** Store in a cool place.

**Legal category** POM.

**Package quantity** 50 ml.

**Further information** Nil.

**Product licence number** 0174/0047.

## ZEASORB* POWDER

**Presentation** ZeaSORB is an off-white, highly absorbent, soft, antiseptic dusting powder containing the following:

| | |
|---|---|
| Chloroxylenol BPC | 0.5% w/w |
| Aluminium dihydroxyallantoinate | 0.2% w/w |

Excipients: talc, fragrance 6A, microcrystalline cellulose.

**Uses** Intertrigo, hyperhidrosis, bromidrosis, prevention of tinea pedis and related conditions.

**Dosage and administration** The affected areas should be dried as thoroughly as possible before applying ZeaSORB Powder. The powder should be smoothed over the surface of the skin, between joints and in folds.

ZeaSORB is intended for use in adults, the elderly and, with supervision, in children. Special care should be taken when using the product in children to avoid inhalation.

**Contra-indications, warnings, etc** Can be irritant to the eyes. Problems of granuloma have been associated with contact of talc with broken skin. As with all powders, take care to avoid inhalation.

There are no restrictions on the use of ZeaSORB in pregnancy and lactation.

**Pharmaceutical precautions** Store in a cool dry place.

**Legal category** P.

**Package quantities** ZeaSORB Powder is available in sifter-top plastic containers of 50 g.

**Further information** ZeaSORB Powder is non-caking and remains soft on saturation, preventing irritation.

**Product licence number** 0174/5015R.

*Trade Mark

# Thames Laboratories Ltd
Abbey Road
The Industrial Estate
Wrexham
LL13 9PW

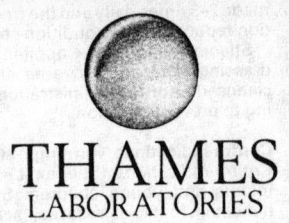

## BIOPLEX* MOUTHWASH

**Qualitative and quantitative composition** Carbenoxolone Sodium BP 1% ᵐ/ₘ. USAN, INNM: Carbenoxolone disodium. INN: Carbenoxolone sodium.

**Pharmaceutical form** Granules.

**Clinical particulars**

*Therapeutic indications:* The treatment of mouth ulcers.

*Posology and method of administration:* To be used topically in the mouth. Adults, children and elderly: 2 g of the granules to be dissolved in 30 to 50 ml warm water and used as a mouthwash 3 times a day and once at night until the ulcers have healed. The mouthwash is to be spat out and not swallowed.

*Contra-indications:* None known.

*Special warnings and special precautions for use:* No special warnings or precautions are necessary for the small dose of carbenoxolone in Bioplex Mouthwash.

*Interactions with other medicaments and other forms of interaction:* Spironoloactone and amiloride inhibit the healing of gastric ulcers by carbenoxolone but their effect on Bioplex Mouthwash is unknown.

*Pregnancy and lactation:* No teratogenic effects have been reported with carbenoxolone but, in common with other drugs, Bioplex Mouthwash should be used with caution in patients who may become pregnant.

*Effects on ability to drive and use machines:* None known.

*Undesirable effects:* Undesirable effects of carbenoxolone are exceedingly rare with the low local dose applied as Bioplex Mouthwash. When given by mouth in larger doses (80 to 300 mg/day) carbenoxolone can produce a mineralocorticoid-like hypernatræmia with hypokalæmia and occasional hypertension with oedema.

*Overdose:* Unlikely, even if the total daily dose were ingested.

**Pharmacological properties**

*Pharmacodynamic properties:* Carbenoxolone Sodium BP is an ulcer healing agent whose exact mechanism of action is unknown. In the stomach carbenoxolone is cytoprotective and associated with increased mucus production.

*Pharmacokinetic properties:*
(a) General characteristics: Carbenoxolone is readily absorbed from the gastric mucosa (and presumably from other mucosae). The carbenoxolone circulates reversibly bound to plasma proteins, is conjugated in the liver to mono- and diglucuronides and excreted via the bile. Enterohepatic recirculation may occur.
(b) Characteristics in patients: Absorption of carbenoxolone from Bioplex Mouthwash is low.

*Preclinical safety data:* No additional data are available for Carbenoxolone Sodium BP.

**Pharmaceutical particulars**

*List of excipients:* Inactive ingredients in Bioplex Mouthwash are; Sodium Citrate BP, Lactose BP, Disodium Edetate BP and Peppermint Oil BP.

*Incompatibilities:* None known.

*Shelf life:* Three years.

*Special precautions for storage:* Store in a dry place.

*Nature and contents of container:* Paper 44 gsm/polythene 10–12 gsm/aluminium foil 0.008 mm/polythene 23–25 gsm.

*Instructions for handling:* None.

*Marketing authorisation holder:* Biorex Laboratories Limited, 2 Crossfield Chambers, Gladbeck Way, Enfield, Middlesex, EN2 7HT.

**Marketing authorisation number** 0181/0029

**Date of approval/revision of SPC** August 1996

**Legal category** POM

## BRITIAZIM*

**Presentation** White flat tablets scored on one side. Each tablet contains 60 mg Diltiazem Hydrochloride USP. Other ingredients include lactose.

**Uses**

*Actions:* Diltiazem is a calcium antagonist. It inhibits the slow channel entry of extracellular calcium during membrane depolarisation of cardiac and vascular smooth muscle. The resulting reduction in intracellular calcium modifies myocardial contractility, thus reducing myocardial oxygen demand. This increases exercise capacity. The inhibition of calcium entry into the smooth muscle of vascular tissue causes vasodilatation, particularly of the coronary blood vessels. This increases blood supply to the myocardium and relieves coronary artery spasm.

*Indications:* For the prophylaxis and treatment of angina pectoris.

**Dosage and administration**

*Adults:* The usual dose is one tablet (60 mg) three times daily. However, patient responses may vary and dosage requirements can differ significantly between individual patients. If necessary the dose can be increased to 360 mg daily in divided doses. High doses up to 480 mg/day have been used with benefit in some patients especially in unstable angina. There is no evidence of any decrease in efficacy at these high doses. Diltiazem has not been reported to precipitate angina.

*Elderly patients and patients with impaired hepatic or renal function:* Treatment should be started with one tablet (60 mg) twice daily. Heart rate should be monitored regularly. The dose should not be increased if the heart rate falls below 50 beats per minute.

*Children:* not recommended.

**Contra-indications, warnings, etc**

*Contra-indications:* Britiazim is contra-indicated in patients with bradycardia, second or third degree heart block, left ventricular failure or sick sinus syndrome. Britiazim should not be used in pregnant women or in women of child-bearing potential.

*Warnings and precautions:* Britiazim should be used with caution in patients with reduced left ventricular function. Patients with first degree heart block should be observed closely.

*Drug interactions:* Diltiazem may increase the blood levels of beta blockers with low bioavailability and the doses of both diltiazem and beta blockers should be reduced when both drugs are used concurrently.

The blood levels of carbamazepine, cyclosporin and theophylline may be increased by diltiazem.

Diltiazem may cause small increases in the plasma levels of digitalis.

$H_2$ antagonists may increase the plasma levels of diltiazem. Care should be taken when alpha blockers are used concurrently as pronounced falls in blood pressure may occur.

*Pregnancy:* Britiazim should not be used in pregnancy or in women of child bearing potential.

*Nursing mothers:* Diltiazem hydrochloride is excreted in breast milk and if administration of Britiazim is considered essential, an alternative method of infant feeding should be instituted.

*Side effects:* Flushing, ankle oedema, headache, nausea, malaise and rashes; occasionally severe. Allergic skin reactions including erythema multiforme and vasculitis have been reported. Bradycardia and heart block. Hepatitis has occasionally been reported.

*Overdosage:* Severe hypotension and sinus bradycardia leading to AV conduction defects may occur.

If overdose should occur, the patient should be observed in a coronary care unit. It is reported that spontaneous recovery usually occurs.

**Pharmaceutical precautions** Protect from light.

**Legal category** POM

**Package quantity** Blister packs of 100 tablets.

**Further information** There is little information on the pharmacokinetics of diltiazem. Due to a first pass hepatic effect the bioavailability of Britiazim is variable

and about 50%. A mean half life of 4–6 hours has been reported and diltiazem is 80–85% protein bound. Extensive metabolism occurs in the liver and little of the unchanged drug is excreted in the urine.

**Product licence number** 4408/0023

## CALCEOS*

**Qualitative and quantitative composition** Each tablet contains 1250 mg calcium carbonate PhEur (equivalent to 500 mg elemental calcium) plus 400 IU vitamin $D_3$ PhEur (10 mcg cholecalciferol).

**Pharmaceutical form** Greyish white square chewable tablets, with a lemon flavour.

**Clinical particulars**

*Therapeutic indications:* Vitamin D and calcium deficiency correction in the elderly. Vitamin and calcium supplement as an adjunct to specific therapy for osteoporosis.

*Posology and method of administration:* For adults only. One tablet, twice per day. Chew the tablets and take with a glass of water.

*Contra-indications:* Hypersensitivity to one of the constituents. Hypercalcaemia as a result of hyperparathyroidism (primary or secondary). Hypercalciuria, calcium lithiasis, tissue calcification (nephrocalcinosis). Vitamin D overdose. Myeloma and bone metastases. Renal insufficiency (creatinin clearance less than 20 ml/min). Calceos is also contra-indicated in patients where prolonged immobilisation is accompanied by hypercalcaemia and/or hypercalciuria. In these cases, treatment should only be resumed when the patient becomes mobile.

*Special warnings and special precautions for use:* Calculate the total vitamin D intake in case of treatment with another drug containing this vitamin.

Plasma and urinary calcium levels should be monitored regularly.

In the elderly, renal function must be monitored regularly.

In patients with renal failure, dosage has to be adapted according to the creatinine clearance.

In case of long term treatment, the urinary calcium excretion must be monitored and treatment must be reduced or momentarily suspended if urinary calcium exceeds 7.5 to 9 mmol/24 h (300 to 360 mg/24 h).

*Interaction with other medicaments and other forms of interaction:*
- In case of treatment with digitalis glycosides: risk of cardiac arrhythmias. Clinical surveillance is required and possibly electrocardiographic and serum calcium monitoring are recommended.
- Associations to be taken into account in the case of treatment with thiazide diuretics: Risk of hypercalcaemia by decreasing urinary calcium excretion.
- Calcium may impair the absorption of tetracyclines, etidronate, iron or fluoride. At least 3 hours should intervene between taking Calceos and these agents.

*Pregnancy and lactation:* Normal requirements for calcium and vitamin D are raised during pregnancy and lactation. If supplementation is necessary, it should be given at a different time to iron supplements. Calcium is excreted in breast milk but not sufficiently to produce an adverse effect in the infant.

*Effects on ability to drive and use machines:* None known.

*The following side effects have been observed:*
- Hypercalciuria in cases of prolonged treatment at high doses, exceptionally hypercalcaemia.
- Hypophosphateamia.
- Nausea.
- Mild gastro-intestinal disturbances such as constipation can occur but are infrequent.

*Overdose:* The most serious consequence of acute or chronic overdosage would be hypercalcaemia due to vitamin D toxicity.

Clinical signs: anorexia, intense thirst, nausea, vomiting, polyuria, polydipsia, dehydration, hypertension, vasomotor disorders, constipation.

Laboratory signs: hypercalcaemia, hypercalciuria, npaired renal function tests.

Emergency treatment: Calcium and vitamin D treatnent must be stopped. Rehydration and, according the severity, isolated or combined use of diuretics, orticosteriods, calcitonin, peritoneal dialysis may be ecessary in severe cases.

**harmacological properties**

*harmacodynamic properties:* Calceos is a fixed ombination of calcium and vitamin D. The high alcium and vitamin D concentration in each dose nit facilitates absorption of a sufficient quantity of alcium, with a limited number of doses. Vitamin D is volved in calcium-phosphorus metabolism. It allows ctive absorption of calcium and phosphorus from ne intestine and their uptake by bone.

*harmacokinetic properties:*

*alcium carbonate:* Absorption: In the stomach, calium carbonate releases calcium ion as a function of H. Calcium is essentially absorbed in the proximal art of the small intestine. The rate of absorption of alcium in the gastrointestinal tract is of the order of 0% of the dose ingested.

Elimination: Calcium is eliminated in sweat and astrointestinal secretions. The urinary calcium excreon depends on the glomerular filtration and rate of ubular resorption of calcium.

*Vitamin $D_3$:* Vitamin $D_3$ is absorbed from the intestine nd transported by protein binding in the blood to the ver (first hydroxylation) and to the kidney (2nd ydroxylation).

Non-hydroxylated vitamin $D_3$ is stored in reserve ompartments such as muscle and adipose tissues.

Its plasma half-life is of the order of several days; it s eliminated in faeces and urine.

**harmaceutical particulars**

*ist of excipients:* Xylitol, Sorbitol, Polyvinylpyrrolione, Lemon flavouring*, Magnesium stearate.

*Composition of the lemon flavouring: essential ils of lemon, orange, litsea cubeba, maltodextrin, cacia gum, sodium citrate.

*ncompatibilities:* None known.

*helf life:* 36 months.

*pecial precautions of storage:* None.

*lature and contents of container:* Polypropylene ubes containing 15 chewable tablets. Cartons of 1, 2 r 4 tubes may be available.

*nstructions for use/handling:* None.

*Marketing authorisation holder:* Laboratoire Innothra, 10 av. Paul Vaillant-Couturier, BP 35–94111 Arcueil edex, France.

**larketing authorisation number** 5856/0001

**ate of approval/revision of SPC** November 1996.

**egal category** P.

## HENOFALK*

**ualitative and quantitative composition** Each capule of Chenofalk contains the following active ingreient: Chenodeoxycholic acid 250 mg.

**harmaceutical form** White, opaque, hard gelatin apsules.

**linical particulars**

*herapeutic indications:* For the dissolution of radiolcent gallstones in patients with a functioning gall ladder. Chenodeoxycholic acid is a naturally occurng bile acid which reduces the cholesterol level in iliary fluid.

*osology and method of administration:* Oral.

*dults:* 3–5 capsules daily or 15 mg Chenodeoxycholic cid (CDCA)/kg body weight per day in two divided oses. The following dosage regimen is recomnended:

| *ody weight kg)* | Capsules daily (in 2 doses) | mg (CDCA/kg/ day) |
|---|---|---|
| 5–57 | 3 | 13.2–16.6 |
| 8–75 | 4 | 13.3–17.2 |
| 6–95 | 5 | 13.2–16.5 |

doses are unequal the larger dose should be taken late evening to counteract the rise in biliary holesterol saturation which occurs in the early orning. The late evening dose may usefully be taken ith food to help maintain bile flow overnight.

The time required for dissolution of gallstones is kely to range from 6 to 24 months depending on tone size and composition. Follow-up cholecystorams or ultrasound investigation may be useful at month intervals until the gallstones have disapeared.

Treatment should be continued until 2 successive holecystograms and/or ultrasound 4–12 weeks apart ave failed to demonstrate gallstones. This is because iese techniques do not permit reliable visualisation f stones less than 2 mm in diameter.

The likelihood of recurrence of gallstones after dissolution by bile acid treatment has been estimated as up to 50% at 5 years.

The efficiency of Chenofalk in treating radio-opaque or partially radio-opaque gallstones has not been tested but these are generally thought to be less soluble than radiolucent stones.

Non-cholesterol stones account for 10–15% of radiolucent stones and may not be dissolved by bile acids.

*Elderly:* There is no evidence to suggest that any alteration in the adult dose is needed but the relevant precautions should be taken into account.

*Children:* Cholesterol rich gallstones are rare in children but when they occur, dosage should be related to bodyweight.

*Contra-indications:* Chenofalk is not suitable for the dissolution of radio-opaque gallstones. It should not be used in patients with a non-functioning gallbladder, biliary cholic, complete or incomplete biliary obstruction, chronic liver disease, liver cirrhosis, gastric or duodenal ulcer, inflammatory bowel disease.

*Special warnings and special precautions for use:* Chenodeoxycholic acid given in long-term studies at doses of 600 mg/kg/day to rats and 1,000 mg/kg/day to mice, induced malignant liver cell tumours in female rats and benign liver cell tumours in female rats and male mice. The clinical significance of these findings is not known.

*Interactions with other medicaments and other forms of interactions:* Some drugs such as cholestyramine, charcoal, colestipol and certain antacids (e.g. aluminium hydroxide) bind bile acids *in vitro*. They could therefore have a similar effect *in vivo* and may interfere with the absorption of Chenofalk.

*Use during pregnancy:* The safety of this medicinal product for use in human pregnancy has not been established. Chenodeoxycholic acid has been shown to cause liver damage in the foetuses of certain species of experimental animals when given in doses equivalent to 5–10 times that normally recommended for use in humans. A toxic metabolite of chenodeoxycholic acid has been found in these species which does not arise in humans.

If chenodeoxycholic acid is given to women of childbearing age, measures should be taken to prevent pregnancy. A non-hormonal contraceptive method is indicated. Should pregnancy occur treatment should be immediately discontinued.

*Effects on ability to drive and use machines:* Chenofalk is not expected to affect ability to drive and use machines.

*Undesirable effects:* Chenodeoxycholic acid is generally well tolerated. In some patients diarrhoea may occur at the start of treatment, but this can usually be controlled by a slight dosage reduction and the dose can subsequently be gradually increased again to an optimum level. Some instances of pruritus and transient rises in liver transaminases have been reported.

*Overdosage:* Serious adverse effects are unlikely to occur in overdosage. However, liver function should be monitored. If necessary, ion-exchange resins may be used to bind acids in the intestines.

**Pharmacological properties**

*Pharmacodynamic properties:* Chenodeoxycholic acid is a bile acid which effects a reduction in cholesterol in biliary fluid primarily by solubilising cholesterol.

*Pharmacokinetic particulars:* Chenodeoxycholic acid occurs naturally in the body. When given orally it is rapidly and completely absorbed from the jejunum and efficiently extracted by the liver. Glycine and taurine conjugates are excreted in the bile. In the intestine some of the conjugates are reabsorbed and some deconjugated. The liberated CDCA is in part reabsorbed and partly biotransformed by bacteria. Most of the CDCA absorbed is dehydroxylated to lithocholic acid. This is conjugated and sulphated and excreted.

**Pharmaceutical particulars**

*List of excipients:* Chenofalk contains the following excipients: Maize starch, silicon dioxide, magnesium stearate, gelatin, titanium dioxide.

*Incompatibilities:* None known.

*Shelf life:* 3 years.

*Special precautions for storage:* None.

*Nature and contents of container:* Clear PVC blister strips with aluminium foil backing packed in cardboard cartons. Each carton contains six blister strips of 10 capsules.

*Instructions for use/handling:* None.

**Marketing authorisation number** 4408/0002.

**Date of approval/revision of SPC** March 1995.

**Legal category** POM.

## CLOTAM* CAPSULES 200 MG

**Qualitative and quantitative composition** Tolfenamic acid 200 mg.

**Pharmaceutical form** Capsules for oral administration.

**Clinical particulars**

*Therapeutic indications:* Migraine.

*Posology and method of administration:*
*Adults:* Migraine – acute attacks: 200 mg when the first symptoms of migraine appear. The treatment can be repeated once after 2–3 hours if a satisfactory response is not obtained.

*Children:* A paediatric dosage regimen has not yet been established.

*Elderly:* Normal adult dose.

*Contra-indications:* Active peptic ulceration. Significantly impaired kidney or liver function. Tolfenamic acid is contraindicated in patients in whom attacks of asthma, urticaria or acute rhinitis are precipitated by aspirin or other non-steroidal anti-inflammatory agents.

*Special warnings and precautions for use:* As is the case with other NSAIDs, tolfenamic acid should be used with caution in patients with a history of gastrointestinal ulceration, or impaired liver or kidney function.

*Interaction with other medicaments and other forms of interaction: Anticoagulants:* In patients treated with anticoagulants, close monitoring of blood coagulation is recommended.

*Diuretics:* The effect of loop diuretics may be reduced.

*Pregnancy and lactation: Pregnancy:* Reproduction studies in animals have not shown any signs of foetal damage. Controlled studies in pregnant women are not available. As is the case with the use of other NSAIDs, tolfenamic acid should not be given in the last trimester, due to risks of premature closure of the ductus arteriosus and prolonged parturition.

*Lactation:* Tolfenamic acid is excreted to such a very small extent in mothers' milk that it should be without risk to the breast-fed baby.

*Effects on ability to drive and use machines:* Tolfenamic acid does not have any effect on the ability to drive or use machines.

*Undesirable effects:* Tolfenamic acid is well tolerated at the recommended dosage. The following side effects have been observed:

*Gastrointestinal tract:* Diarrhoea, nausea, epigastric pain, vomiting, dyspepsia. (Gastrointestinal ulceration has been reported in only 6 patients in 13 years.)

*Allergic skin reactions:* Drug exanthema, erythema, pruritus, urticaria.

*Urinary tract:* Harmless dysuria in the form of smarting during urination may occur occasionally, most commonly in males. The occurrence is correlated with the concentration of a metabolite and is most probably due to local irritation of the urethra. Increased consumption of liquid or reduction of the dose diminishes the risk of smarting. The urine may, due to coloured metabolites, become a little more lemon-coloured.

As is the case with the use of other NSAIDs, the side effects listed below have occasionally been observed:

*Central nervous system:* Headache, vertigo, tremor, euphoria, fatigue.

*Respiratory tract:* Isolated cases of dyspnoea, pulmonary infiltration, bronchospasm and asthma attack.

*Haematology:* Isolated cases of thrombocytopenia, anaemia and leucopenia.

*Liver:* Isolated cases of reversible liver function disturbances and toxic hepatitis.

*Overdose:* No symptoms of overdosage are known in man. In cases where treatment is required, this should be symptomatic. There is no specific antidote to tolfenamic acid.

**Pharmacological properties**

*Pharmacodynamic properties:* NSAID with anti-inflammatory, analgesic and antipyretic effects. Tolfenamic acid is a prostaglandin synthesis inhibitor.

*Pharmacokinetic properties:* Tolfenamic acid is absorbed quickly and almost completely after oral administration. Hepatic first pass metabolism is as low as 15% (bioavailability 85%). Maximum plasma concentrations are reached after about 2 hours. The half-life in plasma is about 2 hours. Tolfenamic acid is extensively bound to plasma proteins (99%). It is metabolised in the liver and tolfenamic acid, as well as the metabolites are conjugated with glucuronic acid. About 90% of a given dose of tolfenamic acid is excreted in the urine as glucuronic acid conjugates, and about 10% is excreted in the faeces. Enterohepatic circulation exists.

*Preclinical safety data:* The therapeutic index for

tolfenamic acid is high, and gastrointestinal ulceration and kidney changes have only been seen with oral doses approximately 6–10 times the maximum therapeutic dose recommended for tolfenamic acid. In human volunteers, tolfenamic acid did not affect renal function.

**Pharmaceutical particulars**

*List of excipients:* Wheat starch, Lactose monohydrate, Macrogol 6000, Povidone K 30, Talc, (Gelatin capsules: Gelatin, Titanium dioxide (E171), Opacode S-1-9005 Red (E172)).

*Incompatibilities:* None.

*Shelf-life:* Five years.

*Special precautions for storage:* None.

*Nature and contents of container:* Al/PVC strip. HDPE tablet container with LDPE closure. Pack sizes: 3, 6, 10 and 30 capsules.

*Instructions for use/handling:* The capsules are to be swallowed whole.

*Marketing authorisation holder:* A/S GEA Farmaceutisk Fabrik, Holger Danskes Vej 89, DK-2000 Frederiksberg, Denmark.

**Marketing authorisation number** 4012/0036.

**Date of approval/revision of SPC** August 1996.

**Legal category** POM

## COLGEN*

**Presentation** Creamy white powder or compress of sterile non denatured collagen. The powder is presented in a plastic screw capped vial fitted with a sprinkler top containing 400 mg collagen. Compresses measure 7 cm x 5 cm and contain 300 mg collagen. Both presentations are double wrapped in sachets.

**Uses** For use in surgical procedures to assist in the control of capillary, venous and small arterial bleeding when ligation and other methods of control are impractical or ineffective.

**Dosage and administration** *Adults, children and the elderly:* Use the smallest quantity of Colgen necessary to achieve haemostasis. The quantity required will vary. Use dry and handle with dry instruments. Apply to site of bleeding with or without pressure.

**Contra-indications, warnings, etc**
*Contra-indications:* Colgen is contra-indicated for use in patients sensitive to collagen. The product should not be used for packing or implantation in fracture sites or laminectomy sites. The product should not be used for control of haemorrhage for large arteries or for use around the optic nerve and chiasma. The product should not be used for non-haemorrhagic serious oozing surfaces.

*Warnings and precautions:* Do not use large amounts of Colgen for packing.

Use of Colgen should be avoided in infected and contaminated wounds, if used, any visible excess product should be removed prior to closure.

Care should be taken not to apply the product too tightly when used during vascular surgery.

In urological procedures minimal amounts of Colgen should be used and care must be exercised to prevent blockage of ureter, urethra or a catheter, by dislodged portions of the product. The use of Colgen Compress but not Colgen Powder has been investigated in clinical trials in urological surgery.

Colgen Compress should not be used as a surface dressing except for immediate control of bleeding.

Colgen should be applied with or without pressure against the bleeding surface. Avoid packing tightly, especially within the bony enclosure of the CNS or within other relatively rigid cavities where swelling may interfere with normal function or possibly cause necrosis. The use of Colgen Powder but not Colgen Compress has been investigated in clinical trials in neurosurgery.

No clinical trials investigating the use of Colgen in ENT surgery have been undertaken. If used in ENT surgery (e.g. controlling epistaxis in nasal surgery or controlling haemorrhage in tonsillectomy) care must be taken that none of the material is aspirated by the patient.

*Interactions:* Since absorption of Colgen could be impaired in chemically cauterised areas, its use should not be preceded by application of silver nitrate or any other escharotic chemicals.

*Side-effects:* No side-effects have been reported in clinical practice. Although no cases have been reported, the possibility of foreign body reactions and encapsulation of fluid with or without infection may exist and the use of Colgen in certain situations may lead to obstruction or stenosis.

*Use in pregnancy or lactation:* Safety of use in pregnancy and lactation has not been established.

**Pharmaceutical precautions** Check the integrity of the sachet before use, do not re-sterilise. Discard any unused portion. Use dry, as moistening with saline or thrombin impairs haemostatic activity. Do not handle with wet instruments.

**Legal category** P

**Package quantities** Cartons, each containing 10 individually wrapped vials or compresses.

**Further information** Nil.

**Product licence numbers**
Powder          4408/0015
Compress        4408/0016

## PSORIN* OINTMENT

**Presentation** A sand-coloured ointment containing Dithranol BP (0.11% w/w), Coal Tar BP (1% w/w) and Salicylic Acid BP (1.6% w/w) in a high density emollient vanishing base. Other ingredients are yellow beeswax, white soft paraffin, cod liver oil, lanolin, zinc oxide and corn starch.

**Uses** The topical treatment of sub-acute and chronic (stable) psoriasis. Dithranol and coal tar both suppress the proliferation of psoriatic tissue. Salicylic acid acts as a keratolytic. The emollient base helps to promote healing of psoriatic areas.

**Dosage and administration** *Adults, children and elderly:* Following a 24 hour skin test, a small quantity of Psorin should be applied to the affected areas morning and evening for seven days. If no redness occurs, it may then be applied more liberally twice daily.

**Contra-indications, warnings etc** Psorin should not be used to treat patients with unstable psoriasis which tends to deteriorate in the sunlight and where the skin is hot to the touch and itchy.

Patients sensitive to dithranol, coal tar or salicylic acid should not be treated with Psorin; a 24-hour skin test is recommended prior to treatment.

Contact with the eyes should be avoided.

It is not recommended that users of Psorin should spend long periods in direct sunlight.

Use should be discontinued if irritation of the skin occurs.

There is no evidence to support the safe use of Psorin in pregnant or lactating women.

**Pharmaceutical precautions** Store in a cool place away from light.

**Legal category** P.

**Package quantities** Tubes of 50 g and 100 g.

**Further information** The concentration of both dithranol and coal tar is low in Psorin which helps to minimise problems of staining commonly caused by these substances.

**Product licence number** 4408/0008.

## PSORIN* SCALP GEL

**Presentation** Dithranol BP 0.25% and Salicylic Acid BP 1.6% in a pale yellow gel containing methyl salicylate, white soft paraffin and light liquid paraffin. The gel has a distinct characteristic smell of oil of wintergreen.

**Uses** For the topical treatment of psoriasis of the scalp.

**Dosage and administration** Before beginning regular treatment a small area of affected skin should be treated. The gel should be left on the skin for 10–20 minutes and then washed off with an appropriate shampoo. If there is no major reaction within 24 hours then full treatment can be instituted.

Psorin Scalp Gel is applied to areas of the scalp affected by psoriasis avoiding spread to healthy skin. The gel should be left on the affected area for 10–20 minutes and then removed with an appropriate shampoo. Treatment should be repeated initially on alternate days and then daily until the lesions have resolved. As treatment progresses, the gel can be left on the scalp for periods of up to one hour. Several weeks of treatment may be necessary.

**Contra-indications, warnings, etc**
*Contra-indications:* Psorin Scalp Gel should not be used in patients who are known to be sensitive to dithranol or salicyclic acid. It should not be used in unstable psoriasis where the skin is hot to touch, itchy and deteriorates in the sun.

*Precautions:* Avoid contact with the eyes, nose and mucous membranes.

*Side-effects:* The treatment may include a feeling of warmth. If there is a prolonged or severe burning sensation the contact time should be reduced. Normally this sensation resolves within 3–4 days and the full treatment regimen can be resumed. In extreme

cases it may be necessary to stop treatment. Dithran may cause staining of skin, hair and clothing. Stainin of healthy skin will be more marked and will resolv after cessation of treatment.

*Use in pregnancy and lactation:* Although there is n experimental evidence to support the safety of th product in pregnancy, the active ingredients hav been in widespread use for many years witho apparent ill-effect.

*Overdose:* If excess gel is applied, it should b removed with neutral or slightly acidic shampoo.

*Interactions:* Dithranol preparations should not b used within two weeks of withdrawing potent topic steroids.

**Pharmaceutical precautions** Store at 25°C or belo protected from light.

**Legal category** P.

**Package quantities** Psorin Scalp Gel is supplied 50 g tubes.

**Further information** Nil.

**Product licence number** 4408/0024.

## SALOFALK* ENEMA 2 g

**Qualitative and quantitative composition** Each enem contains the following active ingredient: Mesalazi 2 g in 59 ml of suspension.

**Pharmaceutical form** Enema.

**Clinical particulars**
*Therapeutic indications:* Therapeutic and prophylax of acute attacks of mild ulcerative colitis, especially the rectum and sigmoid colon and also in th descending colon.

*Posology and method of administration:*
Method of administration: Rectal.
Adults and the elderly: 1 enema once a day bedtime. The action of Salofalk is enhanced if th patient lies on the left side when introducing th enema. The dosage should be adjusted to suit th progress of the condition. Do not discontinue trea ment suddenly.
Children: There is no recommended dose f children. Mesalazine should not be used in babies ar infants.

*Contra-indications:* Severe renal and hepatic functi disturbances. Active gastrointestinal ulcers. Hype sensitivity to salicylates.

*Special warnings and special precautions for use:* Th drug should not be prescribed for infants or your children. Special caution is advised in patients wi an increased bleeding tendency. Regular checks the blood count and renal function are recommende especially during long-term treatment.

*Interactions with other medicaments and other form of interactions:* Although the following interactio are theoretically possible, owing to the low degree absorption of the rectally administered mesalazin the risk of their onset is extremely low: mesalazi may potentiate the actions of sulphonylureas. Inte actions with coumarin, methotrexate, probenic sulphinpyrazone, spironolactone, frusemide and fampicin cannot be excluded. Mesalazine can theore ically potentiate the side effects of glucocorticoids the stomach.

*Use during pregnancy and lactation:* Animal expe ments on mesalazine have produced no evidence embryonic effects. No untoward effects were seen a reproductive and fertility study with mesalazin breast-fed rat pups. Mesalazine is acetylated in t body and passes in this form into breast milk. Limit use of mesalazine in pregnancy has shown untoward effect on the foetus: however, it should b used with caution during pregnancy and only if th potential benefits outweigh the potential risk.

*Effects on ability to drive and use machines:* Salofa Enema is not expected to affect ability to drive a use machines.

*Undesirable effects:* Theoretically, hypersensitiv reactions such as allergic exanthema, bronchospas and a drug-induced lupus erythematosus-like sy drome can occur. Reduced erythrocytic oxygenati is also hypothetically possible. Headache and dige tive disturbances such as nausea and diarrhoea m occur. Isolated cases of hair loss have been reporte

*Overdose:* Symptoms of renal disturbances have be reported in the course of studies on animals dosages considerably higher than those used human medicine (a factor in the order of magnitu of 28).

**Pharmacological properties**
*Pharmacodynamic properties:* Mesalazine is the b logically active metabolite of salicylazosulphapyridi

that is used in the treatment of certain chronic inflammatory conditions of the intestine.

*Pharmacokinetic particulars:* Following rectal administration the major fraction is recovered from the faeces, a small percentage (approximately 15%) is absorbed; the absorbed mesalazine is excreted mainly in the urine; biliary excretion is secondary. The acetylated and the non-acetylated forms of mesalazine bind slightly to plasma proteins.

## Pharmaceutical particulars

*List of excipients:* Salofalk Enemas contain the following excipients: Carbomer, disodium edetate, potassium acetate, potassium metabisulphite, purified water, sodium benzoate, xanthan gum.

*Incompatibilities:* None known.

*Shelf-life:* 24 months.

*Special precautions for storage:* Store at room temperature (15-25°C) and protect from light.

*Nature and contents of container:* Low density concertina shaped polythene bottle with a low density polythene application nozzle packed in cartons containing seven individually blister packed bottles.

*Instructions for use/handling:* None.

**Marketing authorisation number** 4408/0035

**Date of approval/revision of SPC** January 1996

**Legal category** POM

## SALOFALK SUPPOSITORIES 500 mg

**Qualitative and quantitative composition** Each suppository contains the following active ingredient: Mesalazine 500 mg.

**Pharmaceutical form** Suppository.

## Clinical particulars

*Therapeutic indications:* Management of mild and moderate attacks of ulcerative colitis, especially in the rectum and sigmoid colon and also in the descending colon.

*Posology and method of administration:* Method of administration: Rectal.

Adults and the elderly: 1 to 2 suppositories, 2 to 3 times daily. The action of Salofalk is enhanced if the patient lies on the left side when introducing the suppository. The dosage should be adjusted to suit the progress of the condition. Do not discontinue treatment suddenly.

Children: There is no recommended dose for children. Mesalazine should not be used in babies and infants.

*Contra-indications:* Severe renal and hepatic function disturbances. Active gastrointestinal ulcers. Hypersensitivity to salicylates.

*Special warnings and special precautions for use:* The drug should not be prescribed for infants or young children. Special caution is advised in patients with an increased bleeding tendency. Regular checks of the blood count and renal function are recommended especially during long-term treatment.

*Interactions with other medicaments and other forms of interactions:* Although the following interactions are theoretically possible, owing to the low degree of absorption of the rectally administered mesalazine, the risk of their onset is extremely low: mesalazine may potentiate the actions of sulphonylureas. Interactions with coumarin, methotrexate, probenicid, sulphinpyrazone, spironolactone, frusemide and rifampicin cannot be excluded. Mesalazine can theoretically potentiate the side effects of glucocorticoids on the stomach.

*Use during pregnancy and lactation:* Animal experiments on mesalazine have produced no evidence of embryonic effects. No untoward effects were seen in a reproductive and fertility study with mesalazine in breast-fed rat pups. Mesalazine is acetylated in the body and passes in this form into breast milk. Limited use of mesalazine in pregnancy has shown no untoward effect on the foetus: however, it should be used with caution during pregnancy and only if the potential benefits outweigh the potential risks.

*Effects on ability to drive and use machines:* Salofalk suppositories are not expected to affect ability to drive and use machines.

*Undesirable effects:* Theoretically, hypersensitivity reactions such as allergic exanthema, bronchospasm and a drug-induced lupus erythematosus-like syndrome can occur. Reduced erythrocytic oxygenation is also hypothetically possible. Headache and digestive disturbances such as nausea and diarrhoea may occur. Elevated methaemoglobin values are theoretically possible.

*Overdose:* Symptoms of renal disturbances have been reported in the course of studies on animals at dosages considerably higher than those used in

human medicine (a factor in the order of magnitude of 28).

## Pharmacological properties

*Pharmacodynamic properties:* Mesalazine is the biologically active metabolite of salicylazosulphapyridine that is used in the treatment of certain chronic inflammatory conditions of the intestine.

*Pharmacokinetic particulars:* Following rectal administration the major fraction is recovered from the faeces, a small percentage (approximately 15%) is absorbed; the absorbed mesalazine is excreted mainly in the urine; biliary excretion is secondary. The acetylated and the non-acetylated forms of mesalazine bind slightly to plasma proteins.

## Pharmaceutical particulars

*List of excipients:* Salofalk Suppositories contain the following excipients: Hard fat, docusate sodium, cetyl alcohol.

*Incompatibilities:* None known.

*Shelf-life:* 36 months.

*Special precautions for storage:* Store at room temperature (15–25°C) and protect from light.

*Nature and contents of container:* Cartons of ten or thirty suppositories in white, opaque PVC/PE moulded strips. Each strip contains five suppositories.

*Instructions for use/handling:* None.

**Marketing authorisation number** 4408/0034

**Date of approval/revision of SPC** January 1996

**Legal category** POM

## SALOFALK* TABLETS

**Presentation** Yellow, oval tablets containing 250 mg mesalazine (5-aminosalicylic acid) coated with an acrylic based resin (Eudragit L) formulated to release the active ingredient in the terminal ileum and colon.

**Uses** For the treatment of mild to moderate acute exacerbations of ulcerative colitis. For the maintenance of remission of ulcerative colitis.

## Dosage and administration

*Adults:* Maintenance treatment: 3 to 6 tablets daily in divided doses. Acute treatment: 6 tablets daily in three divided doses.

*Elderly:* Salofalk tablets should be used with caution in elderly patients and only in patients with normal kidney function.

*Children:* There is no recommended doses for children. Mesalazine should not be used in babies and infants.

## Contra-indications, warnings etc

*Contra-indications:* Known hypersensitivity to salicylates, severe hepatic and renal disease, active peptic ulcer, blood clotting abnormalities. Mesalazine should not be used in the case of pathological propensity to bleeding.

*Precautions:* Mesalazine is rapidly excreted by the kidney as the acetylated metabolite N-acetyl-5-aminosalicylic acid. It is recommended that in patients with renal impairment, Salofalk tablets should be used with caution and only after a careful evaluation of the potential benefit versus risk of treatment. Serious blood dyscrasias have been reported very rarely with mesalazine. Haematological investigations should be performed if the patient develops unexplained bleeding, bruising, purpura, anaemia, fever or sore throat. Treatment should be stopped if there is suspicion or evidence of blood dyscrasia.

*Use during pregnancy and lactation:* Animal experiments on mesalazine have produced no evidence of embryonic effects. No untoward effects were seen in a reproductive and fertility study with mesalazine in breast-fed rat pups. Mesalazine is acetylated in the body and passes in this form into breast milk. Limited use of mesalazine in pregnancy has shown no untoward effect on the foetus; however, mesalazine should be used with caution during pregnancy and only if the potential benefits outweigh the potential risks.

*Side effects:* Salofalk may cause hypersensitivity reactions. Mesalazine may be associated with an exacerbation of the symptoms of colitis in those patients who have previously had such problems with sulphasalazine. There have been rare reports of leucopenia, neutropenia, agranulocytosis, aplastic anaemia and thrombocytopenia, pancreatitis, hepatitis, allergic lung reactions, lupus erythematosus-like reactions and rash (including urticaria), interstitial nephritis and nephrotic syndrome with oral mesalazine treatment, usually reversible on withdrawal. Renal failure has been reported. Mesalazine-induced nephrotoxicity should be suspected in patients developing renal dysfunction during treatment. Increased methaemoglobin levels may occur.

*Interactions:* The hypoglycaemic action of sulphonureas can be intensified, as can gastrointestinal haemorrhage caused by coumarins. The toxicity of methotrexate can be increased. The uricosuric action of probenecid and sulphinpyrazone can be decreased, as can the diuretic action of frusemide and the action of spironolactone. The antituberculosis action of rifampicin can also be diminished.

*Treatment of overdose:* There is no specific antidote to mesalazine. In many cases of overdosage, gastric lavage and intravenous transfusion of electrolytes to promote diuresis should be implemented.

**Pharmaceutical precautions** None.

**Package Quantities** Blister packs of 100 tablets.

**Legal category** POM

**Further information** The active ingredient of Salofalk tablets is 5-aminosalicylic acid (mesalazine). Sulphasalazine is made up of two components, 5-aminosalicylic acid and sulphapyridine linked by an azo bond. The former is the active moeity in the treatment of inflammatory bowel disease. Since Salofalk tablets contain only the active component, mesalazine, the sulphapyridine associated side effects are absent. The enteric coating of Salofalk Tablets disintegrates above pH6 and releases the active ingredient in the terminal ileum.

**Product licence number** 10341/0004

## SOLVAZINC*

**Qualitative and quantitative composition** Each Solvazinc tablet contains the following active ingredient: Zinc sulphate monohydrate: 125 mg.

**Pharmaceutical form** Effervescent tablet.

## Clinical particulars

*Therapeutic indications:* Zinc sulphate is a source of zinc which is an essential trace element and involved in a number of body enzyme systems.
   Indications: For the treatment of zinc deficiency.

*Posology and method of administration:* Method of administration: oral after dissolution in water.
   Adults: One tablet, dissolved in water, once to three times daily after meals.
   Children: More than 30 kg: One tablet, dissolved in water, once to three times daily after meals.
   10-30 kg: ½ tablet, dissolved in water, once to three times daily after meals.
   Less than 10 kg: ½ tablet, dissolved in water, once daily after meals.

*Contra-indications:* None.

*Special warnings and precautions for use:* Accumulation of zinc may occur in cases of renal failure.

*Interactions with other medicaments and other forms of interaction:* Zinc may inhibit the absorption of concurrently administered tetracyclines; when both are being given an interval of at least 3 hours should be allowed.

*Pregnancy and lactation:* The safety of this product in human pregnancy has not been established. Zinc crosses the placenta and is present in breast milk.

*Effects on ability to drive and use machines:* Solvazinc is not expected to affect ability to drive and use machines.

*Undesirable effects:* Zinc salts may cause abdominal pain and dyspepsia.

*Overdose:* Zinc sulphate is corrosive in overdosage. Symptoms are corrosion and inflammation of the mucous membrane of the mouth and stomach; ulceration of the stomach followed by perforation may occur. Gastric lavage and emesis should be avoided. Demulcents such as milk should be given. Chelating agents such as sodium edetate may be useful.

## Pharmacological properties

*Pharmacodynamic properties:* Zinc is an essential trace element involved in many enzyme systems. Severe deficiency causes skin lesion, alopecia, diarrhoea, increased susceptibility to infections and failure to thrive in children. Symtoms of less severe deficiency include distorted or absent perceptions of taste and smell and poor wound healing.

*Pharmacokinetic properties:* Zinc is absorbed from the gastrointestinal tract and distributed throughout the body. The highest concentrations occur in hair, eyes, male reproductive organs and bone. Lower levels are present in liver, kidney and muscle.
   In blood 80% is found in erythrocytes. Plasma zinc levels range from 70 to 110 µg per dl and about 50% of this is loosely bound to albumin. About 7% is amino-acid bound and the rest is tightly bound to alpha 2-macroglobulins and other proteins.

## Pharmaceutical particulars

*List of excipients:* Solvazinc contains the following

excipients: Sorbitol, polyethylene glycol, sodium hydrogen carbonate, citric acid, saccharin sodium, liquid paraffin.

*Incompatibilities:* None.

*Shelf-life:* 5 years.

*Special precautions for storage:* Store below 25°C, protect from moisture.

*Nature and contents of container:* Aluminium tubes with polythene caps containing a desiccant capsule and packed in cardboard cartons. Each carton contains 3 tubes of 30 tablets.

*Instruction for use/handling:* None.

**Marketing authorisation number** 4408/0004

**Date of approval/revision of SPC** October 1996

**Legal category** P

# URSOFALK*

**Qualitative and quantitative composition** Each capsule of Ursofalk contains the following active ingredient: ursodeoxycholic acid 250 mg.

**Pharmaceutical form** White, opaque, hard gelatin capsules.

### Clinical particulars
*Therapeutic indications:* Ursofalk is indicated in the treatment of primary biliary cirrhosis (PBC) and for the dissolution of radiolucent gallstones in patients with a functioning gall bladder.

*Posology and method of administration:* Method of administration: Oral.

*Primary biliary cirrhosis*
*Adults and the elderly:* 10–15 mg ursodeoxycholic acid (UDCA) per kg per day in two to four divided doses. The following dosage regimen is recommended:

| Body Weight (kg) | Capsules Daily (in 2–4 divided doses) | mg (UDCA)/kg/ day |
|---|---|---|
| 50–62 | 2–4 | 10.0–16.1 |
| 63–85 | 3–5 | 11.9–14.7 |
| 86–120 | 4–7 | 11.6–14.6 |

*Children:* Dosage should be related to bodyweight.

*Dissolution of gallstones*
*Adults:* 8–12 mg ursodeoxycholic acid (UDCA) per kg per day in two divided doses. The following dosage regime is recommended:

| Body weight (kg) | Capsules daily (in 2 divided doses) | mg (UDCA)/kg/ day |
|---|---|---|
| 50–62 | 2 | 8.1–10.0 |
| 63–85 | 3 | 8.8–11.9 |
| 86–120 | 4 | 8.3–11.6 |

If doses are unequal the larger dose should be taken in late evening to counteract the rise in biliary cholesterol saturation which occurs in the early morning. The late evening dose may usefully be taken with food to help maintain bile flow overnight.

The time required for dissolution of gallstones is likely to range from 6 to 24 months depending on stone size and composition. Follow-up cholecystograms or ultrasound investigation may be useful at 6 month intervals until the gallstones have disappeared.

Treatment should be continued until 2 successive cholecystograms and/or ultrasound investigations 4–12 weeks apart have failed to demonstrate gallstones. This is because these techniques do not permit reliable visualisation of stones less than 2 mm in diameter.

The likelihood of recurrence of gallstones after dissolution by bile acid treatment has been estimated as up to 50% at 5 years.

The efficiency of Ursofalk in treating radio-opaque or partially radio-opaque gallstones has not been tested but these are generally thought to be less soluble than radiolucent stones.

Non-cholesterol stones account for 10–15% of radiolucent stones and may not be dissolved by bile acids.

*Elderly:* There is no evidence to suggest that any alteration in the adult dose is needed but the relevant precautions should be taken into account.

*Children:* Cholesterol rich gallstones are rare in children but when they occur, dosage should be related to bodyweight.

*Contra-indications:* Ursofalk is not suitable for the dissolution of radio-opaque gallstones and should not be used in patients with non-functioning gall bladder.

*Special warnings and precautions for use:* A product of this class has been found to be carcinogenic in animals. The relevance of these findings to the clinical use of Ursofalk has not been established.

*Interactions with other medicaments and other forms of interaction:* Some drugs, such as cholestyramine, charcoal, colestipol and certain antacids (e.g. aluminium hydroxide) bind bile acids *in vitro* and may interfere with the absorption of Ursofalk.

Drugs which increase cholesterol elimination in bile, such as oestrogenic hormones, oestrogen-rich contraceptive agents and certain blood cholesterol lowering agents, such as clofibrate, should not be taken with Ursofalk.

UDCA may increase the absorption of cyclosporin in transplantation patients.

*Pregnancy and lactation:* Ursofalk should not be used in pregnancy. When treating women of childbearing potential, non-hormonal or low oestrogen oral contraceptive measures are recommended.

*Effects on ability to drive and use machines:* Ursofalk is not expected to affect ability to drive and use machines.

*Undesirable effects:* Diarrhoea may occur rarely.

*Overdose:* Serious adverse effects are unlikely to occur in overdosage, however, liver function should be monitored. If necessary, ion-exchange resins may be used to bind bile acids in the intestines.

### Pharmacological properties

*Pharmacodynamic properties:* UDCA is a bile acid which effects a reduction in cholesterol in biliary fluid primarily by dispersing the cholesterol and forming a liquid-crystal phase.

UDCA affects the enterohepatic circulation of bile salts by reducing the ileal reabsorption of endogenous more hydrophobic and potentially toxic salts such as cholic and chenodeoxycholic acids.

*In-vitro* studies show that UDCA has a direct hepatoprotective effect and reduces the hepatoxicity of hydrophobic bile salts. Immunological effects have also been demonstrated with a reduction in abnormal expression of HLA Class I antigens on hepatocytes as well as suppression of cytokine and interleukin production.

*Pharmacokinetic properties:* Ursodeoxycholic acid occurs naturally in the body. When given orally it is rapidly and completely absorbed. It is 96–98% bound to plasma proteins and efficiently extracted by the liver and excreted in the bile as glycine and taurine conjugates. In the intestine some of the conjugates are deconjugated and reabsorbed. The conjugates may also be dehydroxylated to lithocholic acid, part of which is absorbed, sulphated by the liver and excreted via the biliary tract.

### Pharmaceutical particulars
*List of excipients:* Ursofalk contains the following excipients: Maize starch, colloidal anhydrous silica, magnesium stearate, gelatin, titanium dioxide.

*Incompatibilities:* None known.

*Shelf-life:* 36 months.

*Special precautions for storage:* None.

*Nature and contents of container:* Clear PVC blister strips with aluminium foil backing packed in cardboard cartons. Each carton contains six blister strips of ten capsules.

*Instructions for handling:* None.

**Marketing authorisation number** 4408/0001

**Date of approval/revision of SPC** October 1996

**Legal category** POM

*Trade Mark

# Tillomed Laboratories Ltd
## Unit 2, Campus 5
## Letchworth Business Park
## Letchworth Garden City
## Hertfordshire SG6 2JF

## BETA-PROGRANE*

**Qualitative and quantitative composition** Propranolol Hydrochloride BP 160 mg.

**Pharmaceutical form** Gastro-resistant capsules.

### Clinical particulars

*Therapeutic indications:* Control of hypertension, management of angina, anxiety and essential tremor, adjunctive management of thyrotoxicosis, prophylaxis of migraine.

*Posology and method of administration:*
*Hypertension:* One 160 mg capsule daily taken either morning or evening. If necessary, it can be increased to 2 capsules daily. A further reduction in blood pressure can be attained if a diuretic or other antihypertensive agent is given in addition.

*Angina, anxiety, essential tremor, thyrotoxicosis, prophylaxis of migraine.* One capsule daily.

*Children:* Not intended for use in children.

*Elderly patients:* The usual dose is one 160 mg capsule daily.

*Contra-indications:* Beta-Prograne should not be used: In the presence of second or third degree heart block, if there is a history of wheezing or asthma, after prolonged fasting, in metabolic acidosis.

*Special warnings and precautions for use:* This medicine should not be taken if there is a history of wheezing or asthma, until a doctor or pharmacist has been consulted.

Special care should be taken with patients whose cardiac reserve is poor. Myocardial contractility must be maintained and signs of failure controlled with digitalis and diuretics.

Beta-Prograne modifies the tachycardia of hypoglycaemia. In patients suffering from ischaemic heart disease treatments should not be discontinued abruptly.

Caution should be exercised when transferring patients from clonidine to beta adrenoceptor blocking drugs. If clonidine and beta adrenoceptor blocking drugs are given concurrently, clonidine should not be discontinued until several days after withdrawal of the adrenoceptor blocking drug.

Care should be taken in prescribing a beta adrenoceptor blocking drug with class 1 antidysrhythmic agents such as disopyramide.

Beta adrenoceptor blocking drugs should be used with caution in combination with verapamil in patients with impaired ventricular function. The combination should not be given to patients with conduction abnormalities. Neither drug should be administered intravenously within 48 hours of discontinuing the other.

Anaesthesia: As with all beta adrenoceptor blocking drugs it may be decided to withdraw Beta-Prograne before surgery. In this case 48 hours should be allowed to elapse between the last dose and anaesthesia. If treatment is continued care should be taken when using anaesthetic agents such as ether, cyclopropane and trichlorethylene. Vagal dominance, if it occurs, may be corrected with atropine (1–2 mg I.V.).

Cessation of therapy with a beta adrenergic blocker should be gradual.

*Interactions with other medicaments and other forms of interaction:* The pharmacokinetics of propranolol are affected by the following drugs:
Cimetidine: Increased plasma concentration of propranolol.
Rifampicin: Reduced plasma concentration of propranolol.
Adverse effects may occur if beta-blockers are administered concurrently with the following drugs:
Adrenaline – severe hypotension.
Amphetamines, phenylephrine, phenylpropanolamine and other sympathomimetic amines – severe hypotension, rarely.
Ergotamine – increased peripheral vasoconstriction.
Indomethacin – antagonism of hypertensive effect.
Lignocaine and similar anti-arrhythmics – increased risk of myocardial depression and bradycardia.

Nifedipine – severe hypotension and heart failure occasionally in susceptible patients.
Prenylamine – increased myocardial depression.
Beta adrenoceptor blocking agents can potentiate the effect of anti-diabetic drugs, and potentiate the hypotensive effect of general anaesthetics.
Administration of propranolol to patients on chlorpromazine therapy can result in raised levels of chlorpromazine.

*Pregnancy and lactation:* As with all drugs Beta-Prograne should not be given in pregnancy unless its use is essential. The use of propranolol in the lactating mother should be avoided unless essential, in order to protect the neonate. Beta blockers have been known to cause bradycardia in the foetus, and this may persist after birth.

*Effects on ability to drive and use machines:* None known.

*Undesirable effects:* Beta-Prograne is usually well tolerated.
Minor side effects, such as cold extremities, nausea, insomnia, lassitude and diarrhoea are usually transient.
Isolated cases of paraesthesia of the hands have been reported.
There have been reports of skin rashes and/or dry eyes.

*Overdose:* Excessive bradycardia can be countered with atropine 1-2 mg intravenously, followed, if necessary, by a beta adrenoceptor stimulant such as Isoprenaline 25 micrograms initially, or orciprenaline 0.5 mg given by slow intravenous injection. Glucagon has been reported to be useful as a cardiac stimulant in a dose of 10 mg intravenously.

### Pharmacological properties

*Pharmacodynamic properties:* Beta adrenoceptor blocking drug.

*Pharmacokinetic properties:* Sustained release form. The coating of the multiple microgranules provides a sustained release of the active principle, propranolol, and allows a 24 hours sustained action.

*Preclinical safety data:* There is no evidence of teratogenicity with propranolol.

### Pharmaceutical particulars
*List of excipients:* Neutral Microgranules HSE, Povidone FP, Ethylcellulose HSE, Talc PhEur. Capsule components: Gelatine HSE, Titanium Dioxide HSE, Sulphur Dioxide HSE.

*Incompatibilities:* None known

*Shelf life:* 60 months

*Special precautions for storage:* Store at room temperature below 25° C. Protect from light and moisture.

*Nature and contents of container: Blister packs:* PVC: Colourless 250 micron thickness. Aluminium: 32 microns thickness, 28 capsules per pack, 14 capsules per blister strip.

*Securitainer:* Polypropylene body, polyethylene cap with a tear strip closure, 100 capsules per pack.

*Instruction for use/handling:* Not applicable.

**Marketing authorisation number** 11311/0001

**Date of approval/revision of SPC** 7 November 1995

**Legal category:** POM

## HALF BETA-PROGRANE*

**Qualitative and quantitative composition** Propranolol Hydrochloride BP 80 mg.

**Pharmaceutical form** Gastro-resistant capsules.

### Clinical particulars

*Therapeutic indications:* Control of hypertension, management of angina, anxiety and essential tremor, adjunctive management of thyrotoxicosis, prophylaxis of migraine, prophylaxis of upper gastro-intestinal bleeding in patients with portal hypertension and oesophageal varices.

*Posology and method of administration:*
*Hypertension:* An adequate response is seen in most patients at the usual starting dose of one Beta-Prograne capsule per day, 160 mg (taken either morning or evening). Blood pressure can be further reduced by raising the dose in 80 mg increments using Half Beta-Prograne up to 320 mg per day.
A further reduction in BP can be attained if a diuretic is given in addition.
*Angina, essential tremor, thyrotoxicosis, prophylaxis of migraine:* Adequate control is gained in most patients on one Half Beta-Prograne capsule per day (either morning or evening). If necessary, further control may be gained by increasing the dose in 80 mg increments (one Half Beta-Prograne) to a maximum of 240 mg per day, taken either morning or evening, which may be administered in the most convenient form using either Beta-Prograne or Half Beta-Prograne capsules.
*Portal hypertension:* Since portal blood pressure cannot normally be monitored directly, the therapeutic objective should be reduction of resting heart rate by approximately 25 %. Initial dosing should commence with one 80 mg Half Beta-Prograne capsule daily increasing by 80 mg increments to a maximum dose of 320 mg per day which may be administered in the most convenient form using either Beta-Prograne or Half Beta-Prograne capsules.
*Anxiety:* Start patients on a single Half Beta-Prograne per day, and increase to a single Beta-Prograne for further control. Review patients after 6 to 12 months.

*Children:* Not intended for use in children.

*Elderly patients:* The usual starting dose is one Half Beta-Prograne capsule daily, increasing as appropriate.

*Contra-indications:* Half Beta-Prograne should not be used: In the presence of second or third degree heart block, if there is a history of wheezing or asthma, after prolonged fasting, in metabolic acidosis and in patients with cardiogenic shock.

*Special warnings and precautions for use:* This medicine should not be taken if there is a history of wheezing or asthma, until a doctor or pharmacist has been consulted.
Special care should be taken with patients whose cardiac reserve is poor. Beta-adrenoceptor blocking drugs should be avoided in overt heart failure. However, they may be used in patients whose signs of failure have been controlled.
Heart failure due to thyrotoxicosis often responds to propranolol alone but if other adverse factors coexist myocardial contractility must be maintained and signs of failure controlled with digitalis and diuretics.
One of the pharmacological actions of propranolol is to reduce the heart rate. In the rare instance when symptoms are attributable to the slow heart rate the dose may be reduced. Propranolol modifies the tachycardia of hypoglycaemia.
In patients suffering from ischaemic heart disease, treatments should not be discontinued abruptly.
Liver function will deteriorate in patients with portal hypertension and hepatic encephalopathy may develop. There have been some reports suggesting that treatment with propranolol may increase the risk of developing hepatic encephalopathy.
Anaesthesia: Care should be taken when using anaesthetic agents with propranolol. The anaesthetist should be informed and the choice of anaesthetic should be the agent with as little negative inotropic activity as possible.

*Interference with laboratory tests:* Propranolol has been reported to interfere with the estimation of serum bilirubin by the diazo method and with the determination of catecholamines by methods using fluorescence. Cessation of therapy with a beta-adrenoceptor blocker should be gradual.
Caution should be exercised when transferring patients from clonidine to beta-adrenoceptor blocking drugs. If clonidine and beta-adrenoceptor drugs are given concurrently, clonidine should not be discontinued until several days after withdrawal of the adrenoceptor blocking drug.
Care should be taken in prescribing a beta-adreno-

ceptor blocking drug with class 1 antidysrhythmic agents such as disopyramide.

Beta-adrenoceptor blocking drugs should be used with caution in combination with verapamil in patients with impaired ventricular function. The combination should not be given to patients with conduction abnormalities. Neither drug should be administered intravenously within 48 hours of discontinuing the other.

*Interaction with other medicaments and other forms of interaction*: The pharmacokinetics of propranolol are affected by the following drugs:

Cimetidine: Increased plasma concentration of propranolol.

Rifampicin: Reduced plasma concentration of propranolol.

Adverse effects may occur if beta-blockers are administered concurrently with the following drugs:

Adrenaline – severe hypotension.

Amphetamines, phenylephrine, phenylpropanololamine and other sympathomimetic amines – severe hypotension, rarely.

Ergotamine – increased peripheral vasoconstriction.

Indomethacin – antagonism of hypertensive vasoconstriction.

Lignocaine and similar anti-arrhythmics – increased risk of myocardial depression and bradycardia.

Nifedipine – severe hypotension and heart failure occasionally in susceptible patients.

Prenylamine – increased myocardial depression.

Beta-adrenoceptor blocking agents can potentiate the effect of anti-diabetic drugs and potentiate the hypotensive effect of general anaesthetics.

Administration of propranolol to patients on chlorpromazine therapy can result in raised levels of propranolol.

*Pregnancy and lactation:* As with all drugs, propranolol should not be given in pregnancy unless its use is essential. The use of propranolol in the lactating mother should be avoided.

*Effects on ability to drive and use machines:* None known.

*Undesirable effects:* Half Beta-Prograne is usually well tolerated.

Minor side effects, such as cold extremities, nausea, sleep disturbances, lassitude, muscle fatigue and diarrhoea are usually transient.

Isolated cases of paraesthesia of the hands have been reported.

There have been reports of skin rashes and/or dry eyes.

Thrombocytopenia and purpura may occur as may bradycardia.

*Overdose:* Excessive bradycardia can be countered with atropine 1-2 mg intravenously. If necessary, this may be followed by a bolus dose of glucagon 10 mg intravenously. If required this may be repeated or followed by an intravenous infusion of glucagon 1-10 mg/HR I.V. depending on response. If no response to glucagon occurs, or if glucagon is unavailable, a beta-adrenoceptor stimulant such as isoprenaline 25 micrograms initially or orciprenaline 0.5 mg may be given by slow intravenous injection.

**Pharmacological properties**

*Pharmacodynamic properties*: Beta-adrenoceptor blocking drug.

*Pharmacokinetic properties:* Sustained release form. The coating of the multiple microgranules provides a sustained release of the active principle, propranolol, and allows a 24 hours sustained action.

*Preclinical safety data:* There is no evidence of teratogenicity with propranolol.

**Pharmaceutical particulars**

*List of excipients:* Neutral Microgranules HSE, Povidone FP, Ethylcellulose HSE, Talc PhEur. Capsule components: Gelatine HSE, Titanium Dioxide HSE, Sulphur Dioxide HSE.

*Incompatibilities:* None known.

*Shelf life:* 60 months.

*Special precautions for storage:* Store at room temperature below 25°C. Protect from light and moisture.

*Nature and contents of container:* Blister packs: PVC: Colourless 250 micron thickness. Aluminium: 25 microns thickness, 28 capsules per pack, 14 capsules per blister strip.

*Instruction for use/handling:* Not applicable.

**Marketing authorisation number** 11311/0017

**Date of approval/revision of SPC** 7/11/95

**Legal category** POM

## NIFEREX* ELIXIR

**Qualitative and quantitative composition** Each 5 ml of elixir contains 217.40 mg polysaccharide-iron complex (equivalent to 100 mg elemental iron).

**Pharmaceutical form** Oral solution.

**Clinical particulars**

*Therapeutic indications:* The prophylaxis and treatment of uncomplicated iron-deficiency anaemia.

*Posology and method of administration:* The method of administration is by oral use.

*Adults:*

Prophylactic dose: 2.5 ml daily (50 mg elemental iron daily).

Therapeutic dose: 5 ml once or twice daily (100–200 mg elemental iron daily).

*Children (therapeutic dose):*

6–12 years: 5 ml daily (100 mg elemental iron daily).

2–5 years: 2.5 ml daily (50 mg elemental iron daily).

*Infants (including premature babies):* One drop of elixir (from paediatric dropper) per 0.45 kg body weight, three times daily (3.33 mg elemental iron per kg body weight daily). One drop contains approximately 500 micrograms elemental iron.

*Elderly patients:* The normal adult dose is appropriate.

*Pregnancy (during second and third trimester):* 5 ml daily (100 mg elemental iron daily).

*Contra-indications:*

Known iron overload.

Hypersensitivity to the product or ingredients.

Haemosiderosis and haemochromatosis.

Active peptic ulcer.

Repeated blood transfusion.

Regional enteritis and ulcerative colitis.

Haemolytic anaemias.

*Special warnings and special precautions for use:* Patients post-gastrectomy have poor absorption of iron. Caution is advised when prescribing iron preparations to individuals with history of peptic ulcer.

Duration of treatment should generally not exceed 3 months *after* correction of anaemia.

Co-existing of deficiency of Vitamin $B_{12}$ or folic acid should be ruled out since combined deficiencies produce microcytic blood film.

Iron deficiency in a male patient warrants careful investigation to determine its cause which forms the basis of primary treatment.

Patients suffering from iron overload are particularly susceptible to infection. Treatment of iron overload should be with caution.

*Interaction with other medicaments and other forms of interaction:* Iron and tetracyclines interfere with absorption of each other.

Iron and zinc interfere with absorption of each other.

Absorption of iron is impaired by magnesium trisilicate, trientine, antacids, neomycin, cholestyramine, tea, eggs or milk.

Absorption of penicillamine, levodopa, bisphosphonates, ciprofloxacin, norfloxacin and ofloxacin is reduced by iron.

Chloramphenicol delays plasma clearance of iron and incorporation of iron into red blood cells by interfering with erythropoiesis.

*Pregnancy and lactation:* Administration of drugs during the first trimester of pregnancy requires careful assessment of potential risks versus benefits to be gained and should not be administered unless clearly indicated. For the remainder of the pregnancy, iron therapy may be indicated but only on advice of a physician. Iron is excreted in breast milk but not in clinically significant concentrations (about 0.5 mg/day).

*Effects on ability to drive and use machines:* None known.

*Undesirable effects:* Anorexia, nausea, vomiting, gastro-intestinal discomfort, constipation, diarrhoea, dark stools and allergic reactions. These side-effects may be minimised by taking the elixir after food.

*Overdosage:* Iron overdosage is an acute emergency requiring urgent medical attention. An acute intake of 75 mg/kg of elemental iron is considered extremely dangerous in young children.

*Symptoms:* Initial symptoms of iron overdosage include, nausea, vomiting, diarrhoea, abdominal pain, haematemesis, rectal bleeding, lethargy and circulatory collapse. Hyperglycaemia and metabolic acidosis may also occur. However, if overdosage is suspected, treatment should be implemented immediately. In severe cases, after a latent phase, relapse may occur after 24–48 hours, manifested by hypotension, coma, hypothermia, hepatocellular necrosis, renal failure, pulmonary oedema, diffuse vascular congestion, coagulopathy and/or convulsions. In many cases, full recovery may be complicated by long-term effects such as hepatic necrosis, toxic encephalitis, CNS damage and pyloric stenosis.

*Treatment:* The following steps are recommended to minimise or prevent further absorption of the medication.

*Children:* 1. Administer an emetic such as syrup of ipecac.

2. Emesis should be followed by gastric lavage with desferrioxamine solution (2 g/l). This should then be followed by the installation of desferrioxamine 5 mg in 50–100 ml water, to be retained in the stomach. Inducing diarrhoea in children may be dangerous and should not be undertaken in young children. Keep the patient under constant surveillance to detect possible aspiration of vomitus, maintain suction apparatus and standby emergency oxygen in case of need.

3. Severe poisoning: In the presence of shock and/or coma with high serum iron levels (serum iron >90 micromol/l) immediate supportive measures plus I.V infusion of desferrioxamine should be instituted. Desferrioxamine 15 mg/kg body weight should be administered every hour by slow I.V. infusion to a maximum 80 mg/kg/24 hours.

Warning: Hypotension may occur if the infusion is too rapid.

4. Less severe poisoning: I.M. desferrioxamine 1 g 4–6 hourly is recommended.

5. Serum iron levels should be monitored throughout.

*Adults:* 1. Administer an emetic.

2. Gastric lavage may be necessary to remove drug already released into the stomach. This should be undertaken using a desferrioxamine solution (2 g/l).

Desferrioxamine 5 g in 50–100 ml water should be introduced into the stomach following gastric emptying. Keep the patient under constant surveillance to detect possible aspiration of vomitus, maintain suction apparatus and standby emergency oxygen in case of need.

3. A drink of mannitol or sorbitol should be given to induce small bowel emptying.

4. Severe poisoning: In the presence of shock and/or coma with high serum iron levels (>142 micromol/l), immediate supportive measures plus I.V. infusion of desferrioxamine should be instituted. The recommended dose of desferrioxamine is 5 mg/kg/h by slow I.V. infusion up to a maximum of 80 mg/kg/24 hours.

Warning: Hypotension may occur if the infusion rate is too rapid.

5. Less severe poisoning: I.M. desferrioxamine 50 mg/kg up to a maximum dose of 4 g should be given.

6. Serum iron levels should be monitored throughout.

**Pharmacological properties**

*Pharmacodynamic properties:* Niferex (polysaccharide-iron complex) is a source of iron which is an essential constituent of the body being necessary for haemoglobin formation and for the oxidative processes of living tissues.

*Pharmacokinetic properties:* Niferex is a highly water soluble polysaccharide-iron complex which is stable in the range pH 4.5 to 11.0 and which disassociates only after leaving the stomach.

The iron is released for absorption from the intestinal tract over a period of one hour, with subsequent significant and effective plasma levels.

Pharmacokinetic study of oral polysaccharide-iron complex in rats shows absorption rate constant (Ka) of 2.33 hours, 19 fold greater than elimination rate constant as obtained from the terminal exponential fraction (Kel – 0.12 hours$^{-1}$). A lag time before absorption of 12 minutes was observed.

t max. = 60 minutes

c max. = 200 micrograms Fe/100 ml

$t^{1/2}$ = 5.8 hours

*Pre-clinical safety data:* Not applicable.

**Pharmaceutical particulars**

*List of excipients:* Ethyl alcohol (96%); sorbitol solution 70% (non-crystallising); caramel; hydrochloric acid; purified water.

*Incompatibilities:* No known incompatibilities other than those stated under *Interactions* above.

*Shelf life:* The shelf life of Niferex Elixir, as packaged for sale, is three years.

There are no recommendations for dilution or reconstitution of the product.

There is no information on the shelf life of the product after first opening the container.

*Special precautions for storage:* Store below 25°C.

*Nature and contents of container*

*(a) 30 ml paediatric dropper bottle:* Plastic (low density polyethylene) bottle with a plastic dropper applicator. The screw cap is composed of high density polyethylene.

*(b) 240 ml bottle:* Glass bottle with a plastic screw cap closure.

*Instructions for use/handling:* No special instructions.

**Marketing authorisation number** 11311/0023.

**Date of revision/approval of SPC** February 1995.

**Legal category** P.

# NIFEREX-150* CAPSULES

**Qualitative and quantitative composition** Each capsule contains 326.10 mg polysaccharide-iron complex equivalent to 150 mg of elemental iron).

**Pharmaceutical form** Capsule (oral).

**Clinical particulars**

*Therapeutic indications:* The treatment of uncomplicated iron-deficiency anaemia.

*Posology and method of administration:* The method of administration is by oral use.

*Adults:* One capsule daily.

*Children:* Not recommended for children under 12 years of age.

*Elderly:* One capsule daily.

*Contra-indications:*

Known iron overload.

Hypersensitivity to the product or ingredients.

Haemosiderosis and haemochromatosis.

Active peptic ulcer.

Repeated blood transfusion.

Regional enteritis and ulcerative colitis.

Haemolytic anaemias.

*Special warnings and special precautions for use:* Patients post-gastrectomy have poor absorption of iron. Caution is advised when prescribing iron preparations to individuals with history of peptic ulcer. Duration of treatment should generally not exceed 3 months *after* correction of anaemia.

Co-existing deficiency of Vitamin $B_{12}$ or folic acid should be ruled out since combined deficiencies produce microcytic blood film.

Iron deficiency in a male patient warrants careful investigation to determine its cause which forms the basis of primary treatment.

Patients suffering from iron overload are particularly susceptible to infection. Treatment of iron overload should be with caution.

*Interaction with other medicaments and other forms of interaction:* Iron and tetracyclines interfere with absorption of each other.

Iron and zinc interfere with absorption of each other.

Absorption of iron is impaired by magnesium trisilicate, trientine, antacids, neomycin, cholestyramine, tea, eggs or milk.

Absorption of penicillamine, levodopa, bisphosphonates, ciprofloxacin, norfloxacin and ofloxacin is reduced by iron.

Chloramphenicol delays plasma clearance of iron and incorporation of iron into red blood cells by interfering with erythropoiesis.

*Pregnancy and lactation:* Administration of drugs during the first trimester of pregnancy requires careful assessment of potential risks versus benefits to be gained and should not be administered unless clearly indicated. For the remainder of the pregnancy, iron therapy may be indicated but only on advice of a physician. Iron is excreted in breast milk but not in clinically significant concentrations (about 0.5 mg/day).

*Effects on ability to drive and use machines:* None known.

*Undesirable effects:* Anorexia, nausea, vomiting, gastro-intestinal discomfort, constipation, diarrhoea, dark stools and allergic reactions. These side-effects may be minimised by taking the capsules after food.

*Overdosage:* Iron overdosage is an acute emergency requiring urgent medical attention. An acute intake of 75 mg/kg of elemental iron is considered extremely dangerous in young children.

*Symptoms:* Initial symptoms of iron overdosage include nausea, vomiting, diarrhoea, abdominal pain, haematemesis, rectal bleeding, lethargy and circulatory collapse. Hyperglycaemia and metabolic acidosis may also occur. However, if overdosage is suspected, treatment should be implemented immediately. In severe cases, after a latent phase, relapse may occur after 24–48 hours, manifested by hypotension, coma, hypothermia, hepatocellular necrosis, renal failure, pulmonary oedema, diffuse vascular congestion, coagulopathy and/or convulsions. In many cases, full recovery may be complicated by long-term effects such as hepatic necrosis, toxic encephalitis, CNS damage and pyloric stenosis.

*Treatment*

*Children:* 1. Administer an emetic such as syrup of ipecac.

2. Emesis should be followed by gastric lavage with desferrioxamine solution (2 g/l). This should then be followed by the installation of desferrioxamine 5 mg in 50–100 ml water, to be retained in the stomach. Inducing diarrhoea in children may be dangerous and should not be undertaken in young children. Keep the patient under constant surveillance to detect possible aspiration of vomitus, maintain suction apparatus and standby emergency oxygen in case of need.

3. Severe poisoning: In the presence of shock and/or coma with high serum iron levels (serum iron >90

micromol/l) immediate supportive measures plus I.V. infusion of desferrioxamine should be instituted. Desferrioxamine 15 mg/kg body weight should be administered every hour by slow I.V. infusion to a maximum 80 mg/kg/24 hours.

Warning: Hypotension may occur if the infusion is too rapid.

4. Less severe poisoning: I.M. desferrioxamine 1 g 4–6 hourly is recommended.

5. Serum iron levels should be monitored throughout.

*Adults:* 1. Administer an emetic.

2. Gastric lavage may be necessary to remove drug already released into the stomach. This should be undertaken using a desferrioxamine solution (2 g/l). Desferrioxamine 5 g in 50–100 ml water should be introduced into the stomach following gastric emptying. Keep the patient under constant surveillance to detect possible aspiration of vomitus, maintain suction apparatus and standby emergency oxygen in case of need.

3. A drink of mannitol or sorbitol should be given to induce small bowel emptying.

4. Severe poisoning: In the presence of shock and/or coma with high serum iron levels (>142 micromol/l), immediate supportive measures plus I.V. infusion of desferrioxamine should be instituted. The recommended dose of desferrioxamine is 5 mg/kg/h by slow I.V. infusion up to a maximum of 80 mg/kg/24 hours.

Warning: Hypotension may occur if the infusion rate is too rapid.

5. Less severe poisoning: I.M. desferrioxamine 50 mg/kg to a maximum dose of 4 g should be given.

6. Serum iron levels should be monitored throughout.

**Pharmacological properties**

*Pharmacodynamic properties:* Niferex (polysaccharide-iron complex) is a source of iron which is an essential constituent of the body being necessary for haemoglobin formation and for the oxidative processes of living tissues.

*Pharmacokinetic properties:* Niferex is a highly water-soluble polysaccharide-iron complex which is stable in the range pH 4.5 to 11.0 and which disassociates only after leaving the stomach.

The iron is released for absorption from the intestinal tract over a period of one hour, with subsequent significant and effective plasma levels.

Pharmacokinetic study of oral polysaccharide-iron complex in rats shows absorption rate constant (Ka) of 2.33 hours, 19 fold greater than elimination rate constant as obtained from the terminal exponential fraction (Kel – 0.12 hours⁻¹). A lag time before absorption of 12 minutes was observed.

t max. = 60 minutes

c max. = 200 micrograms Fe/100 ml

$t^{1/2}$ = 5.8 hours

*Pre-clinical safety data:* Not applicable.

**Pharmaceutical particulars**

*List of excipients:* Nu-pareil PG 30–35 mesh; povidone; shellac solids (pharmaceutical glaze); hydrogenated castor oil; indigo carmine (E132); erythrosine (E127); sunset yellow (E110); titanium dioxide (E171); purified shellac; gelatine; methylene chloride*; isobutanol*.

* not detectable in the final formulation.

*Incompatibilities:* No known incompatibilities other than those stated under *Interactions* above.

*Shelf life:* The shelf life of Niferex-150 capsules, as packaged for sale, is three years.

There are no recommendations for dilution or reconstitution of the product.

There is no information on the shelf life of the product after first opening the container.

*Special precautions for storage:* Store below 25˚C.

*Nature and contents of container:* Securitainer of pigmented polypropylene each fitted with a tamper-evident closure (tear-strip) of polyethylene. Each pack contains 100 capsules.

*Instructions for use/handling:* No special instructions.

**Marketing authorisation number** 11311/0024.

**Date of approval/revision of SPC** February 1995.

**Legal category** P.

# NORIMODE*

**Qualitative and quantitative composition** Loperamide hydrochloride 2.0 mg per unit dose.

**Pharmaceutical form** Tablets for oral administration.

**Clinical particulars**

*Therapeutic indications:* Symptomatic treatment of acute diarrhoea of any aetiology.

Symptomatic treatment of acute exacerbations of chronic diarrhoea for periods of up to 5 days, in adults and children over 9 years.

Symptomatic treatment of chronic diarrhoea in adults.

*Posology and method of administration:* Tablets to be taken orally.

*Adults:* (i) *Acute diarrhoea:* Two tablets initially, followed by one tablet after every loose stool, for up to five days.

The usual dosage is 3 to 4 tablets a day; the maximum daily dose should not exceed 8 tablets.

(ii) *Chronic diarrhoea:* The starting dosage should be between 2 and 4 tablets per day in divided doses, depending on severity. The dose may be titrated according to clinical response. Studies have demonstrated large individual patient variation. Once the maintenance dose is established, the tablets may be given on a twice daily regimen.

*Children:* Acute diarrhoea only.

9–12 years: one tablet four times daily until diarrhoea is controlled, for up to five days.

Under 9 years: not recommended.

*Use in elderly:* As for adults.

*Contra-indications:* When inhibition of peristalsis must be avoided, particularly when ileus or constipation are present.

When abdominal distension develops, particularly in severely dehydrated children.

In patients with acute ulcerative colitis, or pseudo-membranous colitis associated with broad spectrum antibiotics.

*Special warnings and special precautions for use:* Loperamide should not be used for prolonged periods until the underlying cause of the diarrhoea has been investigated, as persistent diarrhoea can be an indicator of potentially more serious conditions.

In patients with diarrhoea, especially children, fluid and electrolyte depletion may occur. Use of loperamide does not preclude the administration of appropriate fluid and electrolyte replacement therapy.

Loperamide should be used with caution in patients with hepatic dysfunction which because of considerable first-pass metabolism in the liver could result in relative overdosage.

Patients with inflammatory bowel disease receiving loperamide should be carefully observed for signs of toxic megacolon.

*Interactions with other medicaments and other forms of interaction:* None known.

*Use during pregnancy and lactation:* Safety in pregnancy has not been established, although studies in animals have not demonstrated any teratogenic effects. As with other drugs it is not advisable to administer loperamide during pregnancy.

Although the level of loperamide secreted in human milk is extremely low, caution is advised if loperamide is to be administered to a nursing mother.

*Effects on ability to drive and use machines:* None known.

*Undesirable effects:* Abdominal cramps, skin reactions (including urticaria), and less frequently paralytic ileus and abdominal bloating have been reported.

*Overdose:* In cases of overdosage the following effects may be observed – constipation, ileus and neurological symptoms (CNS depression – miosis, muscular hypertonia, somnolence and bradypnoea). If intoxication is suspected naloxone may be given as an antidote. Since the duration of action of loperamide is longer than that of naloxone, the patient should be kept under constant observation for at least 48 hours in order to detect any possible depression of the central nervous system.

**Pharmacological properties** Loperamide binds to the opiate receptor in the gut wall, reducing propulsive peristalsis, increasing intestinal transit times and enhancing resorption of water and electrolytes. Loperamide increases the tone of the anal sphincter.

Loperamide does not act centrally because, due to its high affinity for the gut wall, and its high first-pass metabolism, very little reaches the systemic circulation.

The half-life of loperamide in man is 10.8 hours with a range of 9–14 hours. Studies on distribution in rats show high affinity for the gut wall with preference for binding to receptors in the longitudinal muscle layer. Loperamide is well absorbed from the gut, but is almost completely extracted and metabolised by the liver where it is conjugated and excreted via the bile. Due to this very high first-pass effect, plasma concentrations of unchanged drug remain extremely low.

Excretion occurs mainly through the faeces.

**Pharmaceutical particulars**

*List of excipients:* Ludipress (consisting of lactose monohydrate 94%, polyvinylpyrollidone 6%), magnesium stearate.

*Incompatibilities (major):* None.

*Shelf life:* Four years.

*Special precautions for storage:* Store below 25˚C; protect from light and moisture.

*Nature and contents of container:* PVC/Aluminium foil blister pack containing 30 tablets (10 tablets per blister strip) in an outer cardboard carton. A patient information leaflet will be enclosed.

**Marketing authorisation number** 11311/0016.

**Date of approval/revision of SPC** March 1994.

**Legal category** POM.

## RONICOL*

**Presentation** Round, white tablets with RONICOL imprinted across one face and a single break-bar on the other, containing 60.88 mg nicotinyl alcohol tartrate (equivalent to 25 mg nicotinyl alcohol).

**Uses**
*Properties:* Ronicol is the alcohol corresponding to nicotinic acid. Ronicol is rapidly absorbed and metabolised to nicotinic acid. Peak plasma levels of nicotinic acid are reached at about 30 minutes with a subsequent decline in baseline values. Ronicol exerts a direct vasodilator action on the walls of small arteries and arterioles; there is a slight transient tendency towards a fall in blood pressure and slowing of the pulse.

*Indications:* Treatment of circulatory disorders including peripheral vascular disease without intraluminal obstruction.

**Dosage and administration** Ronicol tablets are for oral administration.

*Adults:* 1–2 tablets four times daily.

*Children:* No dosage recommendations are made for the administration of Ronicol to children.

*Use in elderly:* Many studies of Ronicol have included a high proportion of elderly patients. Dosage should be as for younger adults.

**Contra-indications, warnings, etc**
*Use in pregnancy:* There is inadequate evidence of safety of Ronicol in human pregnancy but it has been in wide use for many years without apparent ill consequence, animal studies have shown no hazard. The established medical principle of only administering drugs in early pregnancy when considered absolutely necessary should be observed.

*Precautions:* Care should be taken in the administration of Ronicol in patients with pre-diabetic or diabetic metabolic disorders as this may lead to an increase in the insulin needs of the patient.

*Side-effects:* At optimal doses it is common for the patient to experience mild, transient flushing of the face and a feeling of warmth in the region of the head. More severe symptoms such as sustained flushing, hypotension, faintness or dizziness due to vasodilation may respond to a reduction in dose. Rashes and symptoms of gastric irritation resolve on discontinuation of treatment. Transient elevations of transaminases and alkaline phosphatase are frequently seen and do not normally require dosage adjustment. However, isolated cases of hepatocellular injury have been reported, in some instances associated with reversible nodular changes in the liver. In patients receiving high doses for long periods, liver function should be closely monitored.

*Treatment of overdosage:* Acute overdosage should be treated by gastric lavage and appropriate symptomatic therapy.

**Pharmaceutical precautions**
*Storage:* No special storage precautions are required.

**Legal category** P.

**Package quantities** Ronicol tablets in packs of 100.

**Further information** Nil.

**Product licence number** 11311/0020.

## TILORYTH* 250 mg

**Qualitative and quantitative composition** Per capsule: Erythromycin base 250 mg.

**Pharmaceutical form** Gastro-resistant capsules.

**Clinical particulars**
*Therapeutic indications:* These are based on the antibacterial activity and pharmacokinetic characteristics of erythromycin. They take account both of the clinical studies carried out with this drug and of its place in the range of antibacterial products on the market.

Erythromycin is an antibiotic effective in the treatment of bacterial disease caused by susceptible organisms.

Examples of its use include:

- Ear, nose and throat, stomatological.
- Upper and lower respiratory tract infections of mild to moderate severity.
- Skin and soft tissue infections including pustular acne.
- Dental infections.
- Osteoarticular.
- Genito-urinary infections, including gonorrhoea, syphilis and chlamydia infections.
- Chemoprophylaxis of acute articular rheumatism relapse in the case of contra-indication to penicillin G or V.

Erythromycin is usually active against the following organisms *in vitro* and in clinical infection: *Streptococcus pyogenes,* Alpha haemolytic streptococci, *Staphylococcus aureus, Streptococcus pneumoniae, Mycoplasma pneumoniae, Treponema pallidum, Corynebacterium diptheriae, Corynebacterium minutissimum, Entamoeba histolytica, Listeria monocytogenes, Neisseria gonorrhoea, Bordetella pertussis, Legionella pneumophila, Haemophilus influenzae, Chlamydia trachomatis, Propionibacterium acnes.*

*Posology and method of administration:* Oral. The capsules must be swallowed whole and not chewed.

*Adults:* 250 mg every six hours just before or with meals. 500 mg every twelve hours may be given if desired. When justified by the severity of the infection the dosage can be augmented by increasing the number of doses (500 mg three to four times a day). For severe infections the dose may be increased up to 4 g daily in divided doses.

*Elderly:* As for adults.

*Children:* Age, weight and severity of infection are important factors in determining the correct dosage. 30–50 mg/kg/day in divided doses given every six hours or twice daily. For the treatment of more severe infections, this dose may be doubled; elevated doses should be given every six hours. The drug should be given just before or with meals. This product may be given to children of any age group who can swallow the intact capsules.

*Streptococcal infections:* For active infection – a full therapeutic dose is given for at least ten days. In continuous prophylaxis against recurrences of streptococcal infections in patients with evidence of rheumatic fever heart disease, the dose is 250 mg twice daily. For the prevention of bacterial endocarditis in patients with valvular disease scheduled for dental or surgical procedures of the upper respiratory tract, adult dose is 1.0 gram (children 20 mg/kg) 2 hours before surgery. Following surgery, 500 mg for adults (children 10 mg/kg) orally every six hours for 8 doses.

*Primary syphilis:* 30–40 grams given in divided doses over a period of 10–16 days.

*Amoebic dysentery:* Dosage for adults is 250 mg four times daily for 10 to 14 days; for children 30–50 mg/kg/day in divided doses for 10 to 14 days.

*Legionnaires' disease:* 1–4 g daily in divided doses until clinical signs and symptoms indicate a clinical cure. Prolonged treatment may be required.

*Pertussis:* 30–50 mg/kg/day given in divided doses for 5–14 days, depending upon eradication of a positive culture.

*Acne:* Initially, one capsule (250 mg) twice daily, which may be reduced to a maintenance dose of one capsule (250 mg) once daily after one month according to response. Prolonged treatment may be required.

*Contra-indications:* Allergy to erythromycin.

Association with the vasoconstrictor ergot alkaloids, notably ergotamine and dihydroergotamine (cf. interaction with other medicaments).

Severe liver insufficiency.

Migraine crisis treated with ergot derivatives (cf. interaction with other medicaments).

Association with astemizole, terfenadine (cf. interaction with other medicaments).

*Special warnings and special precautions for use:* In cases of hepatic insufficiency the administration of erythromycin is not recommended. If it is necessary, then regular supervision with hepatic tests and eventually a reduced dosage regimen is necessary.

Prolonged or repeated administration of erythromycin could favour the growth of non susceptible organisms or the appearance of mycoses.

Asthmatic subjects treated with theophylline should be subject to special control for clinical symptoms of intoxication and eventually to drug monitoring for plasma concentrations of theophylline (cf. Interaction with other medicaments).

*Interaction with other medicaments and other forms of interaction:* Ergotism manifestations with the possibility of necrosis of the extremities has been reported after the simultaneous use of erythromycin and of products with ergotamine or other vasoconstrictor ergot derivatives. Concomitant usage is contra-indicated.

Astemizole, terfenadine: risk of ventricular rhythm disorders, notably 'torsades de pointe': reduction of astemizole liver metabolism by erythromycin. Concomitant usage is contra-indicated.

In a few patients receiving high doses of theophylline, concomitant use of erythromycin has caused a increase of serum theophylline levels and signs c toxicity.

Concomitant use with carbamazepine should b avoided as increased serum levels of this drug hav been reported together with symptoms of toxicity.

In the case of combination with bromocriptine, will be necessary to take into account the possibl increase of bromocriptine plasma levels, with possibl increase of anti-parkinsonian activity, or the appeai ance of overdose dopaminergic signs (dyskinesia).

Erythromycin increases circulating cyclosporin lev els (inhibition of cyclosporin catabolism) and creat nine levels.

Combination with digoxin: precaution of use. Eryth romycin can increase digoxin serum levels to toxi values. Clinical and electrocardiographic supervisio are recommended together with eventual adaptatio of the digoxin dosage regimen.

Combination with warfarin: precaution of use. Ris of haemorrhage. Increase of the anticoagulant effec of warfarin. Mechanism invoked: decrease of hepati catabolism of warfarin. More frequent control c prothrombin level and adaptation of the dosag regimen of oral anticoagulant during treatment wit macrolide and 8 days following its discontinuation.

The administration of an antibiotic so-called bacte riostatic like erythromycin, can counter the bacter cidal effect of other antibiotics such as the beta lactamines.

Erythromycin presents a microbiological antagc nism with lincomycin and with clindamycin.

*Pregnancy and lactation*
*Pregnancy:* Erythromycin should be used in preg nancy only when clearly indicated.

*Breast-feeding:* Erythromycin is found in the moth er's milk at concentrations which can be superior t maternal serum concentrations, and can cause mil gastro-intestinal symptoms in breast-fed infants. Cau tion should be exercised when erythromycin is admi istered to a nursing mother.

*Effects on ability to drive and use machines:* Non known.

*Undesirable effects:* Digestive manifestations: nause vomiting, gastralgia, diarrhoea.

Rare skin allergy reactions.

Transitory increases of transaminases and choles tatic hepatitis have been reported with erythromyci derivatives.

Very rare reversible auditive disturbances hav been reported in particular with aged patients or wit patients with renal insufficiency, or with patient having received high doses.

*Overdose:* Overdosage symptoms are nausea, hea ing loss, vomiting and diarrhoea. Recommende treatment is gastric lavage and/or administration c activated charcoal together with general supportiv measures.

Neither haemodialysis nor peritoneal dialysis ar capable of extracting erythromycin.

**Pharmacological properties** Erythromycin is a ma crolide antibiotic.

*Pharmacodynamic properties:*
*Distribution:* Erythromycin diffuses well into th tissues, notably in the lungs, the tonsils and th prostate.

Erythromycin diffuses only slightly into the cerebr spinal fluid.

Erythromycin traverses the placental barrier. concentrates in the milk.

Binding with plasma proteins: the binding of eryth romycin base with plasma proteins is about 65%, wi a predominance for alpha 1 acid glycoprotein (appro imately 55%). (Study with erythromycin C14).

*Biotransformation:* Erythromycin is partly metabo ised by the liver.

*Excretion:* Erythromycin concentrates in the live and is eliminated in active form, principally by th bile, at concentrations superior to those of serum.

Renal elimination is in the order of 2 to 5% for th unchanged form.

*Antibacterial activity:* The natural antibacterial spe trum of erythromycin is as follows:

| *Species normally susceptible* | *MIC (mcg/m* |
|---|---|
| Streptococcus pyogenes (group A, beta hemolytic) | 0.005–0.2 |
| Streptococcus sanguis | 0.02–3.1 |
| Bordetella pertussis | 0.02–1.6 |
| Corynebacterium diptheriae | 0.006–3.1 |
| Listeria monocytogenes | 0.1–0.3 |
| Clostridium perfringens | 0.1–6 |
| Mycoplasma pneumoniae | 0.001–0.02 |
| Chlamydia trachomatis | 0.1–0.5 |
| Legionella pneumophila | 0.06–0.5 |
| Treponema pallidum | — |
| Leptospira | — |
| Campylobacter jejuni | 0.05–>50 |
| Ureaplasma urealyticum | 2–>4 |

| Non-constantly susceptible species | MIC (mcg/ml) |
|---|---|
| Streptococcus pneumoniae (pneumococcus) | 0.001–0.2 |
| Neisseria meningitidis (meningococcus) | 0.1–1.6 |
| Neisseria gonorrhoea (gonococcus) | 0.005–0.4 |
| Haemophilus influenzae | 0.1–6 |
| Bacteroides fragilis | 0.1–>100 |
| Vibrio cholerae | — |
| Staphylococcus aureus | 0.005–>100 |

| Resistant species | MIC>4 mcg/ml |
|---|---|
| Enterobacteriaceae | 0.1–>100 |
| Pseudomonas | — |

When constant strain susceptibility has not been established for a certain species, in vitro testing of the strain is the only method of establishing whether it is sensitive, intermediary or resistant.

Among the streptococcus pyogenes of Group A a few rare strains are resistant.

A microbiological antagonism exists between erythromycin and lincomycin and clindamycin.

Cross resistance is usual between the various macrolides.

Micro-organisms having an MIC less than 1 or possibly 2 mcg/ml are usually considered as susceptible.

For micro-organisms with an MIC situated between 2 and 4 mcg/ml the failure frequency increases depending on the site of infection.

*Pharmacokinetic properties:* In healthy subjects, following administration of 2 capsules before meals, the concentration peak was attained at a mean of 2.9 hours, the apparent half-life of elimination was 1.9 hours, the mean maximum concentration being 2.47 mg/l.

*Preclinical safety data:* Animal studies have revealed no evidence of impaired fertility or foetal harm related to erythromycin. However, there are no adequate studies in pregnant women. Because animal studies are not always predictive of human response, this drug should be used during pregnancy only if clearly needed.

## Pharmaceutical particulars

*List of excipients:* Neutral microgranules (sucrose 75%, corn starch 25%); hydroxypropylmethylcellulose; triacetin; methacrylic acid and ethyl acrylic copolymer; talc; hard gelatin capsules.

*Incompatibilities:* None known.

*Shelf life:* 36 months.

*Special precautions for storage:* Keep bottles tightly closed. Protect from light. Store below 25°C.

*Nature and contents of container:* Cardboard boxes of 30 capsules containing enteric coated microgranules in doses of 250 mg of erythromycin, in thermoformed PVC/aluminium blisters. Polypropylene bottles of 100 capsules.

*Instructions for use/handling:* The capsules must be swallowed whole and not chewed.

**Marketing authorisation number**   11311/0028.

**Date of approval/revision of SPC**   October 1995.

**Legal category**   POM.

*Trade Mark

**Trinity Pharmaceuticals Ltd**
Tuition House
27/37 St George's Road
London SW19 4EU

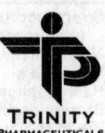

TRINITY
PHARMACEUTICALS

## ADIPINE* MR 10
## ADIPINE* MR 20

### Qualitative and quantitative composition
Adipine MR 10: each modified release tablet contains 10 mg of Nifedipine.
Adipine MR 20: each modified release tablet contains 20 mg of Nifedipine.

**Pharmaceutical form**  Modified release tablets for oral use.

### Clinical particulars
*Therapeutic indications:* Hypertension. Prophylaxis of chronic stable angina pectoris.

*Posology and method of administration:* The treatment should be as individual as possible according to the seriousness of the disease and the responsiveness of the patient.

Dependent on the respective clinical picture stabilisation with reference to the final dose should be made slowly.

Nifedipine should be taken with a little water.

The recommended starting dose of nifedipine is 10 mg every 12 hours swallowed with water with subsequent titration of dosage according to response. The dose may be adjusted to 40 mg every 12 hours.

The pharmacokinetics of nifedipine are altered in the elderly so that lower maintenance doses of nifedipine may be required compared to younger patients.

Nifedipine is metabolised primarily by the liver and therefore patients with liver dysfunction should be carefully monitored. Patients with renal impairment should not require adjustment of dosage.

Nifedipine is not recommended for use in children.

The simultaneous intake of food delays, but does not reduce overall absorption.

The intervals between the recommended individual maximal daily doses of nifedipine should be not less than 4 hours. Discontinuation of Adipine MR especially from high doses should be made gradually.

Treatment may be continued indefinitely.

*Contra-indications:* Hypersensitivity to nifedipine or other dihydropyridines because of the theoretical risk of cross reactivity.

Nifedipine should not be used in clinically significant aortic stenosis, unstable angina, or during or within one month of a myocardial infarction.

Nifedipine must not be administered in cases of cardiogenic shock.

Nifedipine should not be used for the treatment of acute attacks of angina.

The safety of nifedipine in malignant hypertension has not been established.

Nifedipine should not be used for secondary prevention of myocardial infarction.

Nifedipine should not be administered concomitantly with rifampicin since effective plasma levels of nifedipine may not be achieved owing to enzyme induction.

Caution is required in cases of markedly low blood-pressure (severe hypotension with less than 90 mm Hg systolic) as well as in cases of cardiac failure.

*Special warnings and special precautions for use:* None.

*Interaction with other medicaments and other forms of interaction:* The hypotensive effect of Nifedipine can be increased by other hypotensive drugs as well as by tricyclic antidepressants. When combined with nitrates the effects on blood-pressure and heart rate increase.

When administering Nifedipine and beta receptor blockers at the same time, careful surveillance of the patient is necessary as this might produce a major lowering of the blood-pressure; occasional cardiac failure has also been observed.

Adipine MR is not a beta blocker and therefore gives no protection against the dangers of abrupt beta blocker withdrawal. Any such withdrawal should be a gradual reduction of the dose of the beta blocker preferably over 8 to 10 days. Adipine MR will not prevent possible rebound effects after cessation of other hypertensive therapy.

Certain calcium antagonists may increase the negatively inotropic effect of antiarrhythmics such as amiodarone and quinidine. In this connection, no observations were made with Nifedipine. In individual cases, Nifedipine causes a drop of the quinidine plasma level or after discontinuation of Nifedipine a marked increase of the quinidine plasma level so that in combined therapy the control of the quinidine plasma level is recommended.

Nifedipine may cause an increase of theophylline plasma levels so that the control of the latter is recommended.

Cimetidine and, to a lesser extent, ranitidine may lead to an increase in the Nifedipine plasma level and thus to a more intensive action of Nifedipine.

As with other dihydropyridines, nifedipine should not be taken with grapefruit juice because bioavailability is increased.

The simultaneous administration of nifedipine and digoxin may lead to reduced digoxin clearance and hence an increase in the plasma digoxin. Digoxin levels should be monitored and, if necessary, the digoxin dose reduced.

Nifedipine should not be administered concomitantly with rifampicin since effective plasma levels of nifedipine may not be achieved owing to enzyme induction (see *Contra-indications*).

*Pregnancy and lactation:* Nifedipine must not be administered during the entire pregnancy as experimental studies have shown foetal deformities. There is no information on humans. Nifedipine penetrates into the mother's milk. As there is no information with respect to possible effects on babies, the child should be weaned, if treatment with Nifedipine should be necessary during the lactation period.

*Effects on ability to drive and use machines:* The treatment of high blood-pressure with this therapy requires regular medical control. Due to different reactions occurring in individual cases, the ability to drive or of operating machines might be affected. This happens much more at the start of treatment and when changing preparations and is increased by co-administration of alcohol.

*Undesirable effects:* Especially at the beginning of therapy Nifedipine often might cause temporary headaches and flushing with a sensation of warmth (erythema, erythromelalgia).

Occasionally, tachycardia, palpitations as well as lower leg oedema due to vasodilatation may occur. Furthermore, vertigo and fatigue have been observed. Also occasionally, there may be paraesthesia and a drop in blood-pressure.

In rare cases, treatment with Nifedipine may cause gastro-intestinal disturbances such as nausea, a sensation of fullness and diarrhoea. Furthermore, hypersensitivity reactions of the skin such as pruritis, urticaria and rashes, and in individual cases exfoliative dermatitis, have been observed.

Reductions in the blood count such as anaemia, leucopenia, thrombopenia, thrombocytic purpura after the administration of Nifedipine have been described.

Very rarely, after long-term treatment, alterations of the gingiva (hyperplasia of the gingiva) might occur which disappear completely after stopping treatment.

In individual cases, liver dysfunctions (intrahepatic cholestasis, increases of transaminases) have been observed which disappear after stopping treatment.

Rarely, especially in elderly patients, gynaecomastia has been described in connection with long-term therapy which so far has disappeared in all cases after discontinuation of the treatment.

In individual cases – especially with higher doses – courbature, trembling of the fingers (tremor) as well as a minor temporary alteration of optical perception have been observed.

In individual cases an increase in the blood sugar level in the serum (hyperglycaemia) has been observed. This should be taken into account above all with patients suffering from diabetes mellitus.

Exacerbation of angina pectoris may occur frequently at the start of treatment with sustained release formulations of nifedipine. The occurrence of myocardial infarction has been described although it is not possible to distinguish such an event from the natural couse of ischaemic heart disease.

In dialysis patients with malignant hypertension and hypovolaemia, caution is required as due to vasodilatation a marked drop in the blood-pressure may be produced. Also, during the first weeks of therapy, daily urine volume may be increased.

In case of renal insufficiency during the administration of Nifedipine renal function may be temporarily impaired.

*Overdosage:*
*Symptoms of intoxication:* Clouding of consciousness and even coma, a fall in blood pressure, tachycardia, bradycardia, hyperglycaemia, metabolic acidosis, hypoxia and cardiogenic shock with pulmonary oedema have been described.

*Therapy for intoxications:* The most important therapeutic objectives are the elimination of the drug and the restoration of a stable circulation.

After oral ingestion, a thorough stomach lavage and charcoal instillation if need be, in combination with a lavage of the small intestine are indicated.

Especially, in the case of an overdose with the controlled release preparation, an elimination as complete as possible, including also from the small intestine, should be aimed at in order to avoid the inevitable re-absorption of the drug.

When administering laxatives, however, the reduction of the muscular tone of the intestines and even intestinal atony due to the effect of a calcium antagonist must be taken into account. As haemodialysis is not recommended since Nifedipine cannot be dialysed (high plasma protein bound, relatively low distribution volume) plasmapheresis, however, is recommended.

Bradycardia is symptomatically treated with atropine and/or beta-sympathomimetics, in cases of very serious bradycardia a temporary pacemaker therapy will be necessary.

Low blood-pressure as a consequence of cardiogenic shock and arterial vasodilatation can be treated with calcium (1–2 g of calcium gluconate administered intravenously), dopamine (up to 25 mcg for each kilogram of weight per minute), dobutamine (up to 15 mcg for each kilogram of weight per minute), adrenaline and/or noradrenaline. The dosage of these drugs can be titrated according to the effect obtained on the blood-pressure. The serum-calcium level should be kept at the upper limit of the normal range.

Additional intake of fluid should be monitored carefully to prevent overload.

### Pharmacological properties
*Pharmacodynamic properties:* Nifedipine is a calcium antagonist of the 1,4-dihydro-pyridine type. Calcium antagonists exert an inhibitory effect on the calcium ion inflow through the slow calcium channel in the cell. Nifedipine acts primarily on the smooth muscle cells of the coronary arteries and the peripheral resistance vessels. This effect causes a vasodilatation. Administered in therapeutic doses, Nifedipine has virtually no direct effect on the myocardium.

In the heart, Nifedipine mainly dilates the large coronary arteries. Furthermore, Nifedipine reduces the muscle tone of the conorary arteries, which may produce an improvement in blood circulation. At the same time, Nifedipine, due to vasodilatation, reduces the peripheral resistance (afterload).

At the start of treatment with this calcium antagonist, the heart rate and the cardiac output will be increased by a reflex action. This increase, however, is not sufficient to compensate the vasodilatation.

In long-term treatment with Nifedipine, the cardiac output increases at first and then returns to the initial value. A particularly marked decrease in blood-pressure after the administration of Nifedipine can be observed with concurrent use of anti-hypertensive agents.

*Pharmacokinetic properties:* The active substance Nifedipine is rapidly and almost completely absorbed from the gastro-intestinal tract after oral administration on an empty stomach. Nifedipine is subject to a 'first pass metabolism' in the liver, resulting in a systemic availability of orally administered Nifedipine of between 50 to 70%. Following administration of a Nifedipine-containing solution maximum serum concentrations are reported to occur after approx. 15 minutes. After the administration of other preparations having an immediate release peak serum concentrations are attained after 15 to 75 minutes.

Approx. 95% of Nifedipine is bound to plasma proteins.

Nifedipine is almost completely metabolised in the liver by oxidative and hydrolytic processes. These metabolites do not show any pharmacodynamic activity.

About 70 to 80% of a Nifedipine dose is excreted in the urine in the form of its metabolites, the main metabolite (M-I) accounts for about 60 to 80% of the administered Nifedipine dose. The rest is excreted in the form of metabolites with the faeces. The unaltered substance is found only in traces (less than 0.1%) in the urine.

The elimination half-life is about 2 to 5 hours.

A cumulation of the substance during permanent therapy with usual doses has not been described.

In cases of reduced hepatic function, the elimination half-life is markedly prolonged and total clearance is reduced. In some cases dose reduction may be necessary.

*Bioavailability:* A bioavailability study with Adipine MR 20 made in the year 1991 with 24 volunteers showed the following results compared to the reference preparation:

| | *Test preparation* | *Reference preparation* |
|---|---|---|
| Maximum steady-state plasma concentration (0–12 h) ($C_{ss,max1}$) (ng/ml): | 36.3±12.1 | 39.8±15.9 |
| Maximum steady-state plasma concentration (12–24 h) ($C_{ss,max2}$) (ng/ml): | 39.1±15.4 | 50.3±19.6 |
| Area under the concentration-time-curve (24 h) ($AUC_{ss}$) (ng/ml*h): | 394.3±165.7 | 435.6±194.6 |
| Plateau time (0–24 h) (h): | 3.67±1.37 | 3.68±1.97 |
| Peak-trough-fluctuation (0–12 h) (PTF1) (1%): | 182.1±40.3 | 204.6±66.7 |
| Peak-trough-fluctuation (12–24 h) (PTF2) (%): | 206.4±48.2 | 246.6±85.6 |

Values as mean values ±SD.

*Preclinical safety data:*

*Acute toxicity:* Acute toxicity has been studied on various species of animals. No specific sensibility was found.

*Subchronic and chronic toxicity:* Studies on rats and dogs did not show any toxic effect of Nifedipine.

*Tumorigenicity:* A long-time study (2 years) on the rat did not yield any indications for oncogenous effects of Nifedipine.

*Mutagenicity:* The studies in vivo and in vitro were negative without exception so that any mutagenic action in human beings can be excluded sufficiently.

*Reproductive toxicology:* Experimental studies carried out with three species of animals brought about indications for teratogenous effects (cleft palate, cardiovascular anomalies) in two species of animals. There is no experience with the application to human beings during the first six months of pregnancy. The administration of Nifedipine without detrimental consequences during the last three months has been described for a small number of cases. Nifedipine has a tocolytical effect.

Nifedipine penetrates into the mother's milk. For its administration during the nursing period the experience gathered is not sufficient.

**Pharmaceutical particulars**

*List of excipients:* Lactose, microcrystalline cellulose, macrogol 6000, magnesium stearate, maize starch, hydroxypropylmethylcellulose, polysorbate 80 (Tween 80), talc, colourants E171, E172.

*Incompatibilities:* None known.

*Shelf life:* 2 years. The medication should not be used after the printed expiration date.

*Special precautions for storage:* To be kept protected from light.

Store below 25°C (Adipine MR 10).

Note: The active substance Nifedipine is light-sensitive and is protected by special packaging.

When modified release tablets are taken out, they should not be exposed unnecessarily to intensive light for a prolonged period of time.

*Nature and contents of container:* The modified release tablets are sealed in blister packages made of aluminium foil and PVC film. The blisters are packed, along with the package leaflet, in a folded cardboard box.

Packs containing 56 modified release tablets.

*Instructions for use/handling:* None.

*Marketing authorisation holder:* STADA Arzneimittel AG, Stadastrasse 2-18, 61118 Bad Vilbel, FRG.

**Marketing authorisation numbers**

Adipine MR 10 11204/0038
Adipine MR 20 11204/0005

**Date of approval/revision of SPC** March 1997.

**Legal category** POM.

# ANGITIL* SR 90
# ANGITIL* SR 120
# ANGITIL* SR 180

**Presentation**

*Angitil SR 90* capsules are white and transparent, printed '90 mg'. Each capsule contains 90 mg Diltiazem Hydrochloride USP.

*Angitil SR 120* capsules are brown and transparent, printed '120 mg'. Each capsule contains 120 mg Diltiazem Hydrochloride USP.

*Angitil SR 180* capsules are pale brown and transparent, printed '180 mg'. Each capsule contains 180 mg Diltiazem Hydrochloride USP.

The capsules also contain the following inactive ingredients: sucrose, maize starch, povidone, ethylcellulose, talc, dibutyl sebacate, cetyl alcohol, sodium lauryl sulphate, gelatin and the colourings E171 and E172. The 120 mg and 180 mg capsules also contain the colour E132.

**Uses**

*Actions:* Diltiazem hydrochloride is a calcium antagonist. It selectively restricts calcium entry through voltage-dependent calcium channels into vascular smooth muscle cells and myocardial cells. This results in a reduction in the amount of intra-cellular calcium available to activate contractile proteins. This leads to a reduction of myocardial oxygen consumption, dilation of coronary arteries, mild peripheral vasodilation, negative dromotrophic effects, and reflex positive chronotropic and inotropic effects due to reflex sympathetic activity being partially inhibited, with a slight reduction or no change in heart rate.

*Indications:* Management of angina pectoris and treatment of mild to moderate hypertension.

**Dosage and administration** Dosage may be taken with or without food, and should be swallowed whole and not chewed.

*Angina:*

*Adults:* The usual initial dose is 90 mg twice daily. Dosage may be increased to 120 mg or 180 mg twice daily, if required.

*Elderly and patients with impaired renal of hepatic function:* In the elderly, dosage should commence at one diltiazem 60 mg tablet twice daily and the dose carefully titrated as required.

*Hypertension:*

*Adults:* The usual initial dose is 90 mg twice daily. Dosage may be increased to 120 mg or 180 mg twice daily.

*Elderly and patients with impaired renal or hepatic function:* The starting dose should be one diltiazem 60 mg tablet twice daily, increasing to one 90 mg capsule twice daily and then to one 120 mg capsule twice daily if clinically indicated.

*Children:* Diltiazem preparations are not recommended for children. Safety and efficacy in children have not been established.

In order to avoid confusion, it is suggested that patients once titrated to an effective dose using either tablets or capsules should remain on this treatment and should not be changed between different presentations.

**Contra-indications, warnings, etc**

*Contra-indications:* Pregnancy and in women of child bearing capacity. Patients with bradycardia (less than 50 bpm), second or third degree heart block, sick sinus syndrome, decompensated cardiac failure, patients with left ventricular dysfunction following myocardial infarction. Concurrent use with dantrolene infusion because of the risk of ventricular fibrillation.

*Warnings and precautions:* The product should be used with caution in patients with reduced left ventricular function. Patients with mild bradycardia, first degree AV block or prolonged PR interval should be observed closely. Diltiazem is considered unsafe in patients with acute porphyria.

*Drug interactions:* Due consideration should be given to the possibility of an additive effect when diltiazem is prescribed with drugs which may induce bradycardia or other anti-arrhythmic drugs.

Diltiazem hydrochloride has been used safely in combination with beta-blockers, diuretics, ACE-inhibitors and other anti-hypertensive agents. It is recommended that patients receiving these combinations should be regularly monitored. Concomitant use with alpha-blockers such as prazosin should be strictly monitored because of the possible synergistic hypotensive effect of this combination. Patients with pre-existing conduction defects should not receive the combination of diltiazem and beta-blockers.

Case reports have suggested that blood levels of carbamazepine, cyclosporin and theophylline may be increased when given concurrently with diltiazem hydrocholoride. Care should be exercised in patients taking these drugs. In common with other calcium antagonists diltiazem hydrocholoride may cause small increases in plasma levels of digoxin.

Concurrent use with $H_2$-antagonists may increase serum levels of diltiazem.

Treatment with diltiazem has been continued without problem during anaesthesia, but the anaesthetist should be made aware of the treatment regimen.

*Pregnancy and lactation:* Diltiazem hydrochloride is contra-indicated in pregnant women or women of child bearing potential, and is not recommended in nursing mothers.

*Side-effects:* Diltiazem is generally well tolerated. Occasional undesirable effects are nausea, gastrointestinal disturbances, headache, skin rashes, oedema of the legs, flushing, hypotension and fatigue which disappear on cessation of treatment. Diltiazem may cause depression of atrioventricular nodal conduction and bradycardia. Changes in liver function tests and renal function have been reported in a few cases.

*Overdosage:* The clinical symptoms of acute intoxication may include pronounced hypotension or even collapse and sinus bradycardia with or without atrioventricular conduction defects.

The patient should be closely monitored in hospital to exclude arrhythmias or atrioventricular conduction defects. Gastric lavage and osmotic diuresis should be undertaken when considered appropriate. Symptomatic bradycardia and high grade atrioventricular block may respond to atropine, isoprenaline or occasionally temporary cardiac pacing.

Hypotension may require correction with plasma volume expanders, intravenous calcium gluconate and positive inotropic agents. The formulation employs a controlled release system which will continue to release diltiazem for some hours.

**Pharmaceutical precautions** Store in a dry place.

**Legal category** POM.

**Package quantities** Blister packs containing 28 or 56 capsules.

**Further information** Nil.

**Product licence numbers**

Angitil SR 90 capsules 06934/0010
Angitil SR 120 capsules 06934/0011
Angitil SR 180 capsules 06934/0012.

*Product licence holder:* Laboratoires Ethypharm, 21 Rue Saint Matthieu, 78550 Houdan, France.

# ARTRACIN* SR

**Presentation** Blue/colorless capsules containing white sustained release beads. Each capsule containing 75 mg Indomethacin BP.

The capsules also contain the following inactive ingredients: sucrose, corn starch, lactose, povidone, talc, magnesium stearate, polymers of methacrylic acid, acrylic acid esters and methacrylic acid esters. The capsule shell contains gelatin and E171, E127, E132 and E172 as colourants.

**Uses** Non steroidal analgesic and anti-inflammatory agent indicated in active rheumatoid arthritis, osteoarthritis, ankylosing spondylitis, degenerative joint disease of the hip, acute musculo-skeletal disorders and low back pain. Also indicated in periarticular disorders, such as bursitis, tendinitis, synovitis, tenosynovitis and capsulitis. Also indicated in inflammation, pain and oedema following orthopaedic procedures and the treatment of pain and associated symptoms of primary dysmenorrhoea.

**Dosage and administration** Artracin SR capsules should always be given with food or milk to reduce the chance of gastro-intestinal disturbance.

*Adults:* One capsule once or twice daily, depending on patient needs and response.

*Children:* Safety in children has not been established.

*Elderly:* Particular care should be taken with older patients who are more susceptible to side-effects from indomethacin.

To minimise the evolution of unwanted reactions, it is helpful in chronic conditions to start the therapy with a low dosage, increasing as required.

*Dysmenorrhoea:* One capsule a day, starting with the onset of cramps or bleeding, and continuing for as long as symptoms usually last.

**Contra-indications, warnings, etc**

*Contra-indications:* Patients with angioneurotic oedema or who have, with aspirin or other non-steroidal anti-inflammatory drugs, experienced acute asthmatic attacks, urticaria or rhinitis.

Active peptic ulcer, a history of recurrent gastro-intestinal lesions, sensitivity to indomethacin or to aspirin.

*Interactions:* Co-administration of diflunisal with indomethacin increases the plasma level of indomethacin by about a third, with a concomitant decrease in renal clearance. Fatal gastro-intestinal haemorrhage has occurred. The combination should not be used.

Use of Artracin SR with aspirin or other salicylates is not recommended because there is no enhancement of therapeutic effect while the incidence of gastro-intestinal side-effects is increased. Moreover, co-administration of aspirin may decrease the blood concentration of indomethacin.

Artracin SR may decrease the tubular secretion of methotrexate, thus potentiating toxicity; simultaneous use should be undertaken with caution.

Patients receiving anticoagulants should be observed carefully for alteration of prothrombin time, even though clinical studies suggest no influence from indomethacin on hypoprothrombinaemia induced by anticoagulants.

Indomethacin can inhibit platelet aggregation – an effect which disappears within 24 hours of discontinuation; the bleeding time may be prolonged and this effect may be exaggerated in patients with an underlying haemostatic defect.

Artracin SR and triamterene should not be administered together, since reversible renal failure may be induced.

Co-administration of probenecid may increase plasma levels of indomethacin.

Because indomethacin may reduce the antihypertensive effect of beta-blockers, patients receiving dual therapy should have the antihypertensive effect of their therapy reassessed.

If the patient is receiving corticosteroids concomitantly, a reduction in dosage of these may be possible, but should only be effected slowly under supervision.

Indomethacin is an inhibitor of prostaglandin synthesis and, therefore, the following drug interactions may occur: indomethacin may raise plasma lithium levels and reduce renal lithium clearance in subjects with steady state plasma lithium concentrations. At the onset of such combined therapy, plasma lithium concentration should be monitored more frequently.

Artracin SR may reduce the diuretic and antihypertensive effect of thiazides and frusemide in some patients. Indomethacin may cause blocking of the frusemide-induced increase in plasma renin activity.

It is reported that a few patients receiving non-steroidal anti-inflammatory drugs manifest borderline elevations in liver function test results; if these persist or worsen or symptoms of liver disease, a rash or eosinophilia develop, treatment with Artracin SR should be stopped. Periodic assessments to detect, at an early stage, unwanted effects on peripheral blood (anaemia) and liver function are advisable. The dexamethasone suppression test may give false negative results. An increase in plasma potassium concentration (including hyperkalaemia) has been reported, even in the absence of renal impairment. Since indomethacin is eliminated primarily by the kidney, patients with impaired renal function should be monitored closely and a lower daily dosage may be needed to avoid accumulation.

*Effects on ability to drive and use machines:* Patients should be warned that they may experience dizziness and should therefore avoid driving or undertaking other activities which require full alertness.

*Warnings and adverse effects:* The most common side-effects are headache, dizziness and dyspepsia; patients should be warned that they may experience dizziness and should therefore avoid untaking activities which require full alertness. If headache persists even after dosage reduction, Artracin SR should be withdrawn.

Gastro-intestinal disorders which occur can be reduced by giving Artracin SR with food, milk or antacids. Ulceration of the oesophagus, stomach or duodenum may also occur, accompanied by haemorrhage and perforation (a few fatalities have been reported).

Intestinal ulceration has rarely been associated with stenosis and obstruction. Also, bleeding without obvious ulceration and perforation of pre-existing sigmoid lesions (such as a diverticulum or carcinoma) have occurred; and increased abdominal pain in patients with ulcerative colitis (or the development of this condition) and regional ileitis have been rarely reported. If gastro-intestinal bleeding does occur, treatment with Artracin SR should be discontinued.

Blood dyscrasias, particularly thrombocytopenia, have been reported.

Oedema and increased blood pressure also sometimes occur, as does haematuria.

Hypersensitivity reactions include pruritus, urticaria, angiitis erythema nodosum. Skin rash and hair loss may also occur.

Acute respiratory distress, including sudden dyspnoea and asthma, have been reported on rare occasions. Bronchospasm may be precipitated in patients suffering from, or with a previous history of, bronchial asthma or allergic disease.

Artracin SR should be used with caution in patients with hepatic or renal dysfunction. Hepatitis and jaundice have been reported rarely.

Non-steroidal anti-inflammatory drugs may precipitate renal decompensation in those with renal or hepatic dysfunction, diabetes mellitus, advanced age, extracellular volume depletion, congestive cardiac failure, sepsis or concomitant use of other nephrotoxic drugs. Also, there have been reports of acute interstitial nephritis with haematuria, proteinuria and occasionally the nephrotic syndrome in long term therapy with indomethacin.

In common with other anti-inflammatory analgesic antipyretic agents, Artracin SR may mask the signs and symptoms of infectious disease and this should be borne in mind in order to avoid delay in starting treatment for infection.

Artracin SR should be used with caution in patients with an existing, albeit controlled infection.

Particular care should be taken with older patients who are more susceptible to side-effects from indomethacin.

*CNS:* Headache, dizziness or lightheadedness, depression, vertigo and fatigue are not uncommon; infrequently there may be confusion, anxiety or other psychiatric disturbance, drowsiness, convulsions, neuropathy or paraesthesia, involuntary movements, insomnia, aggravation of epilepsy or Parkinsonism. All are often transient and likely to abate or disappear with reduced or ceased dosage.

*Gastro-intestinal:* Nausea, anorexia, vomiting, epigastric discomfort or abdominal pain, constipation or diarrhoea all have been reported; more rarely, stomatitis, flatulence, ulceration at any point in the gastro-intestinal tract (even with resultant stenosis and obstruction), bleeding (even without obvious ulceration or from a diverticulum) and perforation of pre-existing sigmoid lesions have all been reported.

*Hepatic:* Rarely, hepatitis and jaundice (some fatalities have been reported).

*Cardiovascular/renal:* Oedema, increased blood pressure, hypotension, tachycardia, chest pain, arrhythmia, palpitations, congestive cardiac failure, elevation of blood urea and haematuria all have been reported infrequently.

In patients with renal, cardiac or hepatic impairment, caution is required since the use of non-steroidal anti-inflammatory drugs may result in deterioration of renal function. The dose should be kept as low as possible and renal function should be monitored.

Non-steroidal anti-inflammatory drugs have been reported to cause nephrotoxicity in various forms and their use can lead to interstitial nephritis, nephrotic syndrome and renal failure.

*Dermatological/hypersensitivity:* Itching, urticaria, angioneurotic oedema, angiitis, erythema nodosum, rash and exfoliative dermatitis all have been reported infrequently – as have Stevens-Johnson syndrome, erythema multiforme, toxic epidermal necrolysis, hair loss, acute anaphylaxis (including acute loss of blood pressure) and acute respiratory distress (including sudden dyspnoea, asthma and pulmonary oedema). There may be bronchospasm in patients with a history of bronchial asthma or other allergic disease.

*Haematological:* Blood dyscrasias (thrombocytopenia, leucopenia, petechiae, ecchymosis, purpura, aplastic or haemolytic anaemia, agranulocytosis and bone marrow depression, disseminated intravascular coagulation) may occur infrequently.

*Ocular:* Blurred vision and orbital and peri-orbital pain are seen infrequently. Corneal deposits and retinal disturbances have been reported in some patients with rheumatoid arthritis on prolonged therapy with indomethacin, and ophthalmic examinations are desirable in patients given prolonged treatment.

*Aural:* Tinnitus, or hearing disturbances (rarely deafness) have been reported.

*Genito-urinary:* Proteinuria, nephrotic syndrome, interstitial nephritis, renal insufficiency or failure all have been reported.

*Other:* Hyperglycaemia, glycosuria, hyperkalaemia, vaginal bleeding, epistaxis, breast changes (enlargement, tenderness, gynaecomastia), flushing, sweating and ulcerative stomatitis all have been reported rarely.

*Use in pregnancy and lactation:* Artracin SR should not be used during pregnancy, or during lactation as indomethacin is secreted in breast milk.

*Overdose:* Many of the unwanted symptoms associated with indomethacin therapy may be seen. Treatment is symptomatic and supportive – emptying the stomach by induction of vomiting and/or lavage and use of activated charcoal. Antacid therapy may be useful. Close monitoring thereafter is required because intestinal ulceration may develop. It can be noted that indomethacin has a biphasic plasma elimination with the terminal phase showing a half-life ranging between 2 and 12 hours.

**Pharmaceutical precautions**　　Store in a cool, dry place and protect from light.

**Legal category**　　POM.

**Package quantities**　　Packs of 100 capsules.

**Further information**　　Nil.

**Product licence number**　　4416/0066.

*Product licence holder:* Lagap Pharmaceuticals Limited, Woolmer Way, Bordon, Hampshire GU35 9QE.

# KETOCID* 200

**Qualitative and quantitative composition**　　Each capsule contains 200 mg Ketoprofen BP.

**Pharmaceutical form**　　Modified release capsule.

**Clinical particulars**

*Therapeutic indications:* Ketoprofen is an analgesic anti-inflammatory and antipyretic; recommended for the treatment of rheumatoid arthritis, osteoarthritis ankylosing spondylitis and other musculoskeletal conditions including bursitis, capsulitis, synovitis tendinitis, fibrositis and low back pain. It is also useful to relieve the pain of sciatica, acute gout and dysmenorrhoea.

*Posology and method of administration:*
*Adults:* One 200 mg capsule to be taken orally once daily with a little food.

*Elderly:* As for adult dosage as there is no evidence that the pharmacokinetics of ketoprofen are altered in the elderly.

*Children:* There are no recommendations for the use of this product in children.

*Contra-indications:* Ketoprofen should not be given to patients with active peptic ulceration or a history of recurrent peptic ulceration or chronic dyspepsia known hypersensitivity to ketoprofen, aspirin or other non-steroidal anti-inflammatory agents or with severe renal dysfunction.

*Special warnings and precautions for use:* Some patients with a history of bronchial asthma or allergic disease may suffer bronchospasm, particularly those with a history of allergy to ketoprofen and related compounds. As non-steroidal anti-inflammatory agents can inhibit renal prostaglandin synthesis and interfere with renal function, care should be taken in patients with renal impairment. NSAIDs have been reported to cause nephrotoxicity in various forms interstitial nephritis, nephrotic syndrome and renal failure. In patients with renal, cardiac, or hepatic impairment caution is required since the use of NSAIDs may result in deterioration of renal function the dose should be kept as low as possible and renal function should be monitored. As with other drugs in the same therapeutic category, patients should be advised to take ketoprofen with food, to minimise gastric intolerance.

*Interactions with other medicaments and other forms of interaction:* The active ingredient, ketoprofen, is highly protein bound. Therefore alteration of the dosage of other protein bound drugs such as anticoagulants, sulphonamides and hydantoins such as phenytoin may be necessary when taken together Serious interactions have been reported with methotrexate, digoxin, lithium and diuretics. To avoid the risk of increased side effects, ketoprofen should not be given with other non-steroidal anti-inflammatory agents.

*Pregnancy and lactation:* There is no evidence of teratogenic effects of ketoprofen but as with all drugs administration during pregnancy should be avoided unless essential. Because ketoprofen interferes with prostaglandin synthesis, there may be premature closure of the ductus arteriosus or persistent pulmonary hypertension in the neonate, or delay in labour if administered within a few days before delivery. Small amounts of ketoprofen are excreted in breast milk so use in nursing mothers should be avoided.

*Effects on ability to drive and use machines:* Ketoprofen can cause nausea, dizziness, confusion and drowsiness, therefore patients should be warned of these effects and advised to be careful if driving or operating machinery.

*Undesirable effects:* The most common adverse effects relate to the gastrointestinal tract, mainly indigestion, dyspepsia, heartburn, various types of abdominal discomfort, nausea, constipation and diarrhoea. Other effects such as headache, dizziness confusion, drowsiness, oedema, change of mood and insomnia occur less commonly. Peptic ulceration perforation and gastrointestinal haemorrhage may rarely occur. Other rare adverse events reported include haematological reactions such as thrombocytopenia, hepatic or renal damage, dermatological reactions, bronchospasm and anaphylaxis. Should any severe adverse event occur, treatment should be stopped immediately.

*Overdose:* As with other propionic acid derivatives ketoprofen demonstrates less toxicity than aspirin or paracetamol. The most likely symptoms of overdosage are drowsiness, abdominal pain and vomiting but hypotension, bronchospasm and gastro-intestinal haemorrhage may occur. Since this is a controlled release (modified release) preparation, continued absorption from capsules in the gastrointestinal tract may be expected. Treatment should be symptomatic and may include gastric washout and the use of activated charcoal.

**Pharmacological properties**
*Pharmacodynamic properites:* Ketoprofen is a propionic acid derivative which has analgesic, anti-pyretic and anti-inflammatory properties. It is a strong inhibitor of prostaglandin synthetase.

*Pharmacokinetic properties:* This controlled release (modified release) ketoprofen formulation is designed to release ketoprofen over a period of time. Following a pharmacokinetic study in volunteers it was found that the average time to achieve maximum plasma concentration was 6.9 hours. The average half-life was found to be 7.4 hours, with a range of 5.5 to 8.0 hours. The average mean residence time was about 14 hours with an average clearance of 2.4 litres per hour. The study carried out over a five day period at the proposed dosage of once daily indicates that there is no accumulation on continued daily dosing. Ketoprofen is very highly bound to plasma protein.

*Preclinical safety data:* None provided.

**Pharmaceutical particulars**
*List of excipients:* Polyethylene Glycol 4000 BP, Ethylcellulose USP, Stearic Acid (purified) USP, Talc PhEur, Eudragit 'RS' HSE.

Neutral pellets: Sucrose PhEur, Corn Starch PhEur.

Ingredients removed during manufacturing process: Ethanol 96% BP, Acetone BP, Purified Water PhEur.

Capsule shell: Erythrosine E127 HSE, Titanium dioxide E171 HSE, Gelatin BP.

*Incompatibilities:* None reported.

*Shelf life:* 48 months.

*Special precautions for storage:* Store in a dry place below 25°C. Protect from light.

*Nature and contents of container:* Blister packs composed of PVC-PVdC/Aluminium-PVdC, containing 28 capsules.

*Instruction for use/handling:* Not applicable.

**Marketing authorisation number** 08829/0041

**Date of approval/revision of SPC** 23 January 1996.

**Legal category** POM.

## MONOMAX* SR 40
## MONOMAX* SR 60

**Qualitative and quantitative composition**
Monomax SR 40: Isosorbide Mononitrate 40 mg.
Monomax SR 60: Isosorbide Mononitrate 60 mg.

**Pharmaceutical form** Modified release capsules.

**Clinical particulars**
*Therapeutic indications:* For the prophylaxis of angina pectoris.

*Posology and method of administration*
*Dosage recommendations:* Dosage may be taken with or without food, and should be swallowed whole and not chewed.

*Prophylaxis of angina: Adults:* Usual adult dose is 40 mg per day. The daily dose may be increased to 60 mg.

*Children:* Safety and efficacy in children has not been established.

*Elderly:* There is no evidence of a need for routine dosage adjustment in the elderly, but special care may be needed in those with increased susceptibility to hypotension or marked hepatic or renal insufficiency.

*Contra-indications:* This product should not be given to patients with a known sensitivity to nitrates.

Isosorbide-5-Mononitrate should not be used in patients with acute myocardial infarction with low filling pressure, marked anaemia, head trauma, cerebral haemorrhage, severe hypotension or hypovolaemia.

*Special warnings and special precautions for use:* Isosorbide-5-Mononitrate should be used with caution in patients who are predisposed to closed angle glaucoma.

Isosorbide-5-Mononitrate should be used with caution in patients suffering from hypothyroidism, hypothermia, malnutrition, severe liver or renal disease. Monomax SR capsules are not indicated for relief of acute angina attacks; in the event of an acute attack, sublingual or buccal glyceryl trinitrate tablets/sprays should be used.

*Interaction with other medicaments and other forms of interaction:* Some of the effects of alcohol may be potentiated by this agent.

Vasodilators, antihypertensives and diuretics may potentiate the hypotension caused by nitrates particularly in the elderly.

There is no evidence of interaction with food.

*Pregnancy and lactation:* This product should not be used during pregnancy or lactation unless considered essential by the physician.

*Effects on ability to drive and use machines:* Since postural hypotension with symptoms such as dizziness has been reported, patients should be advised to be careful when driving or operating machinery if they suffer from these symptoms.

*Undesirable effects:* Side-effects including flushing, postural hypotension and dry skin rashes may occur occasionally. Headache may occur at the onset of treatment but may be minimised by commencing with low doses and gradually increasing the dose.

Using the recommended dosage schedules there is no evidence of development of nitrate tolerance.

*Overdose:* Treatment should be symptomatic. The main symptom is likely to be hypotension.

**Pharmacological properties**
*Pharamacodynamic properties:* Nitrate compounds relax smooth muscle causing dilatation of the veins and arteries, and to a lesser extent of the arterioles. The result is a very marked reduction of preload, accompanied by lowering of right heart pressures and left ventricular and diastolic pressure.

The dimensions of the right and left ventricles and ejection volumes are reduced but the reflex increase of heart rate prevents any reduction of cardiac output. Myocardial oxygen consumption may thus fall by more than 50% in parallel with the reduction of left ventricular preload. At higher doses, afterload is also decreased by arterial and arteriolar dilatation; this also helps to improve cardiac function.

Nitrate compounds exert a dilatory and antispasmodic effect on the coronary vessels; they are effective against both spontaneous and induced spasms.

*Pharmacokinetic properties:* In man, Isosorbide-5-Mononitrate is absorbed completely and rapidly following oral administration.

Isosorbide-5-Mononitrate is not subject to the 'hepatic first-pass' effect, and provides a low degree of inter-individual variation of blood levels.

Monomax SR capsules have all the pharmackonetic characteristics of a true sustained-release dosage form. Compared with an immediate-release dosage form, the peak plasma concentration obtained is lower and occurs later, while the apparent elimination half-life is unchanged; there is less fluctuation between $C_{max}$ and $C_{min}$.

The slow continuous diffusion of the active ingredient from the sustained-release microgranules makes it possible, at steady state, to maintain plasma concentrations above the putative effective level of 100 ng/ml for a period of about 16 hours for the 40 mg capsules and 20 hours for the 60 mg capsules.

*Preclinical safety data:* Isosorbide-5-Mononitrate produces very few toxic effects and is less toxic than isosorbide dinitrate. After chronic adminstration at high doses (60 mg/kg), signs of toxicity have been detected in canine liver and kidneys. Tests conducted have shown no evidence of a teratogenic or mutagenic potential.

**Pharmaceutical particulars**
*List of excipients:* Lactose PhEur; sucrose and maize starch microgranules; Shellac FRP; Eudragit L100; Eudragit RS100; Talc PhEur; Gelatin; E171; Ethyl alcohol 95% FRP (ND†); Acetone BP (ND†); E172 (ND†).

† *Not detected in the finished product.*

*Incompatibilities:* None known.

*Shelf life:* 2 years.

*Special precautions for storage:* Store in a dry place below 25°C.

*Nature and contents of container:* Blister packs (20 μm aluminium/250 μm PVC) – boxed in cardboard cartons containing 28 capsules.

*Instructions for use/handling:* Not applicable.

**Marketing authorisation numbers**
40 mg 8829/0029
60 mg 8829/0030.

**Date of approval/revision of SPC** 2 April 1996

**Legal category** POM.

## PROBETA* LA

**Presentation** Sustained release capsules containing 160 mg Propranolol Hydrochloride BP. The capsules are presented as a transparent pink body with an opaque white cap printed with 160 SR 45.

The capsules also contain the following inactive ingredients: sucrose, corn starch, shellac and talc. The capsule shells contain gelatin and E171 and E127 as colourants.

**Uses** Propranolol hydrochloride acts as a competitive blocking agent of β-adrenergic receptor sites. It is used in the treatment of hypertension and angina.

**Dosage and administration**
*Adults:*
*Hypertension:* The initial dose is one capsule taken orally in the morning or evening. An adequate response is seen by most patients at this dosage. If necessary, the dose can be increased to two capsules. A further reduction in blood pressure may be achieved by combining propranolol hydrochloride with other anti-hypertensive agents.

*Angina:* Most patients will respond to one capsule daily taken orally in the morning or evening.

*Children:* Probeta LA is not intended for use in children.

*Elderly:* The evidence concerning the relationship between blood level and age is conflicting. For patients already established on 160 mg propranolol daily, one capsule of Probeta LA may be given. It is suggested that elderly patients being started off on propranolol treatment may need smaller initial doses and in these circumstances an alternative preparation should be used.

**Contra-indications, warnings, etc**
*Contra-indications:* Propranolol hydrochloride should not be used in the presence of second or third degree heart block; in patients with cardiogenic shock; if there is a history of bronchospasm; after prolonged fasting and in metabolic acidosis.

*Precautions:* Withdrawal of the drug for any reason should be gradual.

Propranolol hydrochloride should be used with caution in patients whose cardiac reserve is poor. It should be avoided in overt heart failure but may be used where the signs of heart failure are controlled.

One of the pharmacological actions of propranolol is to reduce the heart rate. In the rare instance when symptoms may be attributable to the slow heart rate, the dose may be reduced.

In patients with ischaemic heart disease treatment should not be discontinued abruptly. Either the equivalent dose of another β-blocker may be substituted or the withdrawal of Probeta LA should be gradual. This can be done by substituting the equivalent dose in propranolol 40 mg tablets and then reducting the dose.

Care should be exercised when treating patients with renal impairment as it has been suggected that a reduced initial dosage is given.

Hepatic metabolism is a major route of elimination and therefore patients with liver disease may need to be given a reduced dosage. In these circumstances this preparation is not recommended.

In patients with portal hypertension, liver function will deteriorate and there is a risk of developing hepatic encephalopathy.

Caution should be exercised when transferring patients from clonidine to β-adrenoceptor blocking drugs.

Probeta LA should not impair ability to drive and use machines.

*Interactions:* If propranolol hydrochloride and clonidine are given concurrently, clonidine should not be discontinued until several days after withdrawal of the β-blocker.

Propranolol modifies the tachycardia of hypoglycaemia. Caution should be exercised in the concurrent use of proprranolol hydrochloride and hypoglycaemia therapy in diabetic patients. Propranolol may prolong the hypoglycaemic response to insulin.

Care should be taken in the parenteral administration of preparations containing adrenaline to patients taking β-adrenoceptor blocking drugs as, in rare cases, vasoconstriction, hypertension and bradycardia may result.

Care should be taken in prescribing a β-adrenoceptor blocking drug with Class 1 antidysrhythmic agents such as disopyramide.

β-adrenoceptor blocking drugs should be used with caution in combination with verapamil in patients with impaired ventricular function. The combination should not be given to patients with conduction abnormalities. Neither drug should be administered intravenously within 48 hours of discontinuing the other.

As with all β-blocking drugs it may be necessary to withdraw propranolol hydrochloride before surgery. Twenty-four hours should be allowed to elapse between the last dose and anaesthesia. If propranolol hydrochloride treatment is continued throughout surgery the anaesthetist. should be informed and care should be taken when using anaesthetic agents such as ether, cyclopropane and trichloroethylene. Vagal dominance if it occurs may be corrected by 1–2 mg I.V. atropine.

*Use in pregnancy and lactation:* Although there is no evidence that propranolol is teratogenic, Probeta LA should not be used in pregnancy unless absolutely necessary. It is excreted in breast milk but the quantity is small and should not affect the infant.

*Side-effects:* Minor side-effects such as cold extremities, nausea, insomnia, lassitude, diarrhoea and muscle fatigue are usually transient. Isolated cases of paraesthesia of the hands have been reported. There have been reports of skin rashes and/or dry eyes associated with the use of β-adrenergic blocking drugs. The reported incidence is small and in most cases, the symptoms have cleared when treatment is withdrawn. Cases of bradycardia, thrombocytopenia and purpura have rarely been recorded. A low incidence of CNS symptoms, including hallucinations have been reported. If these symptoms are not attributed to some other cause, Probeta LA should be withdrawn.

Rare cases of blood dyscrasias have been reported. Bradycardia and hypotension are usually a sign of overdosage but may rarely be due to intolerance of the drug in which case it should be withdrawn.

*Overdose:* Excessive bradycardia can be countered with 1–2 mg I.V. atropine, followed if necessary by a bolus dose of glucagon 10 mg I.V. This may be repeated if necessary or followed by an intravenous infusion of glucagon 1–10 mg/hour depending on response. If glucagon is unavailable a β-receptor stimulant such as isoprenaline 25 micrograms I.V. or orciprenaline 500 micrograms I.V. may be given by slow intravenous injection.

**Pharmaceutical precautions** Store in a cool dry place and protect from light.

**Legal category** POM.

**Package quantities** Packs of 100 capsules.

**Further information** Interference with laboratory tests: Propranolol has been reported to interfere with the estimation of serum bilirubin by the diazo method and with the determination of catecholamines by methods using fluorescence.

**Product licence number** 4416/0068.

*Product licence holder:* Lagap Pharmaceuticals Limited, Woolmer Way, Bordon, Hampshire GU35 9QE.

# VOLSAID* RETARD 75
# VOLSAID* RETARD 100

**Qualitative and quantitative composition** Each controlled release tablet of Volsaid Retard 75 contains 75 mg Diclofenac Sodium BP.

Each controlled release tablet of Volsaid Retard 100 contains 100 mg Diclofenac Sodium BP.

**Pharmaceutical form** Modified release tablets.

**Clinical particulars**

*Therapeutic indications:* Diclofenac sodium is a non-steroidal anti-inflammatory drug (NSAID); recommended for the treatment of rheumatoid arthritis; osteoarthritis; ankylosing spondylitis; acute gout; low back pain, relief of pain in fractures; acute musculoskeletal disorders and trauma including periarthritis (particularly frozen shoulder), bursitis, tendinitis, tenosynovitis, dislocations, sprains and strains; and the control of pain and inflammation in orthopaedic, dental and other minor surgery.

*Posology and method of administration*

*Adults:* Volsaid Retard 75: One tablet to be taken orally once or twice a day, swallowed whole preferably with food.

Volsaid Retard 100: One tablet to be taken orally once a day, swallowed whole preferably with food.

*Children:* Not suitable for use in children.

*Elderly:* Care should be used when treating patients who are frail or have a low body weight as they will in general be more susceptible to adverse reactions. The lowest effective dose should be used in these patients. The standard adult dose may be used for other elderly patients.

*Contra-indications:* Diclofenac sodium should not be given to patients who are hypersensitive to diclofenac sodium, with active or suspected peptic ulcers, gastro-intestinal bleeding and who when taking aspirin or other NSAIDs suffer attacks of asthma, urticaria or acute rhinitis.

*Special warnings and precautions for use:* Patients with a history of gastro-intestinal ulceration, haematemesis, or melaena, should be carefully observed, and care should be taken when treating patients with ulcerative colitis, Crohn's disease, haematological abnormalities, or bleeding diathesis. Elderly patients and those with renal, hepatic or cardiac impairment should also be carefully monitored as renal function may be reduced by NSAID therapy. Renal function should be monitored and the lowest effective dose used.

In patients with impairment of cardiac or renal function, those recovering from major surgery or those being treated with diuretics, prostaglandins are important for the maintenance of renal blood flow. The possibility of inhibition of prostaglandin synthetase should be considered when giving diclofenac to these patients. On stopping diclofenac, effects on renal function are usually reversible.

Diclofenac should be stopped if liver function tests show abnormalities which persist or worsen, or if liver disease develops of if other symptoms such as eosinophilia or rash occur.

Diclofenac sodium may trigger an attack in patients with hepatic porphyria.

Monitoring of renal function, hepatic function (elevation of liver enzymes may occur) and blood counts should be performed on long-term NSAID patients, as a precautionary measure.

*Interactions with other medicaments and other forms of interaction:* Diclofenac may increase plasma concentrations of lithium (by the impairment of its excretion from the kidneys) and digoxin.

Methotrexate and NSAIDs should only be administered within 24 hours of each other if given with extreme caution. NSAIDs are reported to increase the plasma levels of methotrexate resulting in increased toxicity.

If other systemic NSAIDs are given concomitantly with diclofenac sodium the frequency of side-effects may be increased.

NSAIDs may increase cyclosporin nephrotoxicity as a result of their effect on renal prostaglandins.

There is an increased risk of convulsions if quinolone antibiotics are given while NSAIDs are being taken, and caution is advised when considering their use.

The activity of diuretics may be inhibited by some NSAIDs. Increased serum potassium levels may result when diclofenac is given concomitantly with potassium-sparing diuretics. Serum potassium levels should therefore be monitored.

Care is required when giving anticoagulants with NSAIDs as diclofenac may reversibly inhibit platelet aggregation. Monitoring is recommended to ensure the desired response to the anticoagulants is maintained as there are rare reports of increased risk of haemorrhage with combined diclofenac and anti-coagulant therapy.

It has been reported that hypo- and hyperglycaemic effects have occurred rarely when diclofenac and oral antidiabetic agents have been given together and adjustment of the hypoglycaemic may be required.

*Pregnancy and lactation:* Diclofenac sodium should only be used during pregnancy or lactation if considered essential.

Diclofenac sodium is reported to cross the placenta in mice and rats but there have not been any studies reported for humans.

*Effects on ability to drive and use machines:* Patients should not drive or operate machinery if they experience dizziness or other central nervous system disturbances.

*Undesirable effects:* Common side-effects include nausea, headache, diarrhoea, epigastric pain, anorexia, dyspepsia, flatulence, abdominal cramps, vertigo and dizziness. Serious effects such as peptic ulcer, gastro-intestinal bleeding and bloody diarrhoea have occasionally been reported, and there are reports of isolated cases of lower gut disorders (exacerbations of ulcerative colitis or Crohn's procotocolitis and non-specific haemorrhagic colitis), glossitis, constipation, pancreatitis, oesophageal lesions and aphthous stomatitis.

Skin rashes and eruptions have occasionally been reported and rarely urticaria. There are also rare reports of erythema multiforme, Stevens-Johnson syndrome, Lyell's syndrome, bullous reactions, eczema, erythroderma, hair loss, photosensitivity reactions and purpura.

Isolated effects on the central nervous system include drowsiness, tiredness, impaired hearing, insomnia, convulsions, irritability, anxiety, depression, psychotic reactions, tremors, memory disturbance, vertigo, disturbance of sensation, disorientation, disturbance of vision, tinnitus, nightmares and taste alterations.

Occasional effects on the kidney include acute renal insufficiency, urinary abnormalities (e.g. haematuria, proteinuria), nephrotic syndrome, papillary necrosis and interstitial nephritis.

Effects on the live include occasional reports of elevation of serum aminotransferase enzymes (ALT ST) and rarely, liver function disorders including hepatitis with or without jaundice.

Leucopenia, haemolytic anaemia, thrombocytopenia, aplastic anaemia and agranulocytosis have rarely been reported. Other rarely reported reactions include hypersensitivity reactions (anaphylactic/anaphylactoid systemic reactions, hypotension, bronchspasm), oedema, palpitation, impotence, chest pain and hypertension.

*Overdose:* Gastric lavage and treatment with activated charcoal should be used as soon as possible after overdosage in order to prevent absorption of the drug.

Further treatment is supportive and symptomatic Complications that might be encountered include renal failure, hypotension, convulsions, respiratory depression, and gastro-intestinal irritation.

**Pharmacological properties**

*Pharmacodynamic properties:* Diclofenac sodium is a non-steroidal anti-inflammatory drug (NSAID) with analgesic and antipyretic properties. It is an inhibitor of prostaglandin synthetase.

*Pharmacokinetic properties:* This extended release diclofenac formulation is designed to release diclofenac over a period of time. Following a pharmacokinetic study with the 100 mg tablet in volunteers, it was found that the average time to reach maximum plasma concentrations was 6.05 hours. The average elimination half-life was found to be 6.75 hours. The average maximum plasma concentrations were found to be 262 ng/ml.

*General characteristics of the active substance:* Diclofenac sodium is almost totally absorbed after oral administration, and it is subject to significant first-pass metabolism with only approximately 60% of an oral dose reaching the systemic circulation.

Diclofenac sodium is highly protein bound (>99%). It is mainly excreted in the form of metabolites via the urine but also in the bile.

The main metabolite has a minimal anti-inflammatory activity compared to the parent drug.

*Characteristics in patients:* Plasma concentrations of unchanged diclofenac are not reported to be significantly affected by age, renal or hepatic impairment The metabolite concentations may be increased by severe renal impairment.

*Preclinical safety data:* None provided.

**Pharmaceutical particulars**

*List of excipients:* Talc PhEur; Ethylcellulose PhEur Magnesium Stearate PhEur; Povidone PhEur; Stearic Acid USP.

*Coating ingredients:* Hydroxypropyl methylcellulose PhEur; Ethylcellulose PhEur; Diethylphthalate USP, Titanium Dioxide (E171) PhEur; Polyethylene glyco 4000 BP; Red iron oxide (E172) USP (100 mg tablet only); Yellow iron oxide (E172) USP (100 mg tablet only).

*Incompatibilities:* None reported.

*Shelf life:* 18 months.

*Special precautions for storage:* Store in a dry place below 25˚C. Protect from light.

*Nature and contents of container:* Blister composed of PVC – PVdC/aluminium-PVdC containing 28 and 56 tablets.

*Instruction for use/handling:* Not applicable.

**Marketing authorisation numbers**
Volsaid Retard 75　　8829/0045
Volsaid Retard 100　　8829/0046.

**Date of approval/revision of SPC** 22 January 1996.

**Legal category** POM.

*Trade Mark

# Typpharm Limited
14 Parkstone Road
Poole
Dorset

## EFFERCITRATE* TABLETS

**Qualitative and quantitative composition**
*Active constituents*

| | |
|---|---|
| Potassium Citrate BP | 1.5 g |
| Citric Acid BP | 0.25 g |

*Other constituents*

| | |
|---|---|
| Saccharin Sodium BP | 5.0 mg |
| Lemon Flavour (Givaudan 84260B) | 7.5 mg |
| Lime Flavour (Givaudan 84278B) | 7.5 mg |
| Polyethylene Glycol 6000 | 100.0 mg |
| Dioctyl Sodium Sylphosuccinate BPC | 1.0 mg |
| Polyvinylpyrrolidone BPC | 65.0 mg |
| Magnesium Stearate BP | 10.0 mg |

**Pharmaceutical form** Effervescent tablets.

**Clinical particulars**
*Therapeutic indications:* For the treatment of cystitis, symptoms of cystitis and as initial therapy in mild symptomatic cystitis prior to an MSU result. Confirmed bacterial infections should then be treated with an appropriate course of an antibacterial agent.

*Posology and method of administration*
Adults and children over 6 years: Two tablets dissolved in a glass of water up to three times daily.

*Children: 1–6 years:* One tablet dissolved in a glass of water up to three times daily.

*Under one year:* Not recommended.

*Elderly:* As adult dose.

Sufficient should be given to render and maintain the urine alkaline.

*Contra-indications:* None.

*Special warnings and special precautions for use:* Caution should be observed in patients with kidney disease, hypertension of heart disease.

If symptoms persist or worsen, patients should seek medical advice.

*Interactions with other medicaments and other forms of interaction:* None known.

*Pregnancy and lactation:* Patients should consult a doctor before taking Effercitrate in pregnancy or lactation.

*Effects on ability to drive and use machines:* Not applicable.

*Undesirable effects:* Gastric irritation may occur. The tablets should always be well diluted with water. Gastric effects may be minimised by taking with or after meals.

*Overdose:* Hyperkalaemia may occur. Below 6.5 mmol/litre poisoning is minimal, moderate up to 8 mmol/litre and severe above 8 mmol/litre. Absolute toxicity is governed by pH and sodium levels. Hyperkalaemia symptoms may be transiently controlled with calcium gluconate, glucose or glucose and insulin, sodium bicarbonate or hypertonic sodium infusions, cationic exchange resins or haemo and peritoneal dialysis. Patients who are digitalised may experience acute digitalis intoxication during potassium removal.

**Pharmacological properties**
*Pharmacodynamic properties:* Potassium citrate renders the urine alkaline.

*Pharmacokinetic properties:* Alkalisation of the urine affects the growth of pathogens. The growth of E. coli is inhibited at a pH above 7.5. Alkalised urine is soothing to the epithelium of the bladder and uretha unlike the natural acid urine (symptoms of cystitis).

*Preclinical safety data:* The active ingredients of Effercitrate tablets are simple compounds with a well established medicinal use and recognised efficacy and an acceptable level of safety.

**Pharmaceutical particulars**
*List of excipients:* Saccharin Sodium BP; Lemon Flavour (Givaudan 84260B); Lime Flavour (Givaudan 84278B); Polyethylene Glycol 6000; Dioctyl Sodium Sulphosuccinate BPC; Polyvinylpyrrolidone BPC; Magnesium Stearate BP.

*Incompatibilities:* None known.

*Shelf life:* Three years.

*Special precautions for storage:* Store in a cool dry place below 20°C.

*Nature and contents of container:* Aluminium tubes with plastic cap containing desiccant of 12 tablets.

*Instructions for use/handling:* Not applicable.

**Marketing authorisation number** 0551/0002

**Date of approval/revision of SPC** May 1995

**Legal category** P.

## GOLDEN* EYE DROPS

**Qualitative and quantitative composition** 0.1% w/v propamidine isethionate.

**Pharmaceutical form** A clear colourless solution practically free from particles.

**Clinical particulars**
*Therapeutic indications:* Indicated for the treatment of minor eye and eyelid infections such as conjunctivitis and blepharitis.

*Posology and method of administration:* For topical ophthalmic administration.

*Adults (elderly and children):* One or two drops up to four times daily. Medical advice should be obtained if there has been no significant improvement after two days.

*Contra-indications:*
i. Hypersensitivity to propamidine or any component of the preparation.
ii. Soft or gas permeable contact lenses.

*Special warnings and precautions for use:*
i. If vision is disturbed or symptoms become worse during therapy, discontinue use and consult a physician.
ii. If there is no significant improvement after two days therapy, discontinue use and consult a physician.

*Interactions with other medicaments and other forms of interaction:* None known.

*Pregnancy and lactation:* Safety of use in pregnancy and lactation has not been established. Use during pregnancy and lactation only if considered essential by a physician.

*Effects on ability to drive and use machines:* May cause transient blurring of vision on instillation. Patients should be warned not to drive or operate machinery unless vision is clear.

*Undesirable effects:* Hypersensitivity may occur, in which case treatment should be discontinued immediately.

*Overdose:* Topical overdose not applicable. Oral ingestion of a full 10 ml bottle is unlikely to cause any toxic effects.

**Pharmacological properties**
*Pharmacodynamic properties:* Propamidine is a member of the aromatic diamidine class of compounds which possess bacteriostatic properties against a wide range of organisms.

These diamidines exert antibacterial action against pyogenic cocci, antibiotic resistant staphylococci and some gram negative bacilli. The activity of the diamidines is retained in the presence of organic matter such as tissue fluids, pus and serum.

*Pharmacokinetic properties:* No data available.

*Preclinical safety data:* Not applicable.

**Pharmaceutical particulars**
*List of excipients:* Sodium chloride, benzalkonium chloride solution, purified water.

*Incompatibilities:* None known.

*Shelf life:* 48 months unopened and 28 days after opening.

*Special precautions for storage:* Store below 25°C.

*Nature and contents of container:* Polypropylene dropper bottle (10 ml) fitted with a low density polyethylene nozzle and a high density polyethylene tamper evident cap.

*Instructions for use/handling:* Not applicable.

**Marketing authorisation number** 0551/0003

**Date of approval/revision of SPC** November 1996.

**Legal category** P.

## GOLDEN* EYE OINTMENT

**Qualitative and quantitative composition** 0.15% w/w Dibromopropamidine Isethionate BP.

**Pharmaceutical form** A smooth uniform off white translucent greasy ointment.

**Clinical particulars**
*Therapeutic indications:* Indicated for the treatment of minor eye and eyelid infections such as conjunctivitis and blepharitis.

*Posology and method of administration:* For topical ophthalmic administration.

*Adults (elderly and children):* Apply topically once or twice daily. Medical advice should be obtained if there has been no significant improvement after two days.

*Contra-indications:* Hypersensitivity to dibromopropamidine or to any component of the preparation.

*Special warnings and precautions for use:*
i. If vision is disturbed or symptoms become worse during therapy, discontinue use and consult a physician.
ii. If there is no significant improvement after two days therapy, discontinue use and consult a physician.

*Interactions with other medicaments and other forms of interaction:* None known.

*Pregnancy and lactation:* Safety of use in pregnancy and lactation has not been established. Use during pregnancy and lactation only if considered essential by a physician.

*Effects on ability to drive and use machines:* Eye Ointment will cause blurring of vision on application. Patients should be warned not to drive or operate machinery unless vision is clear.

*Undesirable effects:* Hypersensitivity may occur, in which case treatment should be discontinued immediately.

*Overdose:* Topical overdose not applicable. Oral ingestion of a full 5 gram tube is unlikely to cause any toxic effects.

**Pharmacological properties**
*Pharmacodynamic properties:* Dibromopropamidine is a member of the aromatic diamidine class of compounds which possess bacteriostatic properties against a wide range of fungi and bacteria.

These diamidines exert antibacterial action against pyogenic cocci, antibiotic resistant staphylococci and some gram negative bacilli. The activity of the diamidines is retained in the presence of organic matter such as pus and blood.

*Pharmacokinetic properties:* No data available.

*Preclinical safety data:* Not applicable.

**Pharmaceutical particulars**
*List of excipients:* Liquid paraffin and plastibase 30W.

*Incompatibilities:* None known.

*Shelf life:* 60 months unopened and 28 days after opening.

*Special precautions for storage:* Store below 25°C.

*Nature and contents of container:* A white pigmented, collapsible multi laminate tube (5 gram) incorporating an aluminium foil barrier with inner polyethylene coating with a polyethylene elongated nozzle with a screw cap.

*Instruction for use/handling:* Not applicable.

**Marketing authorisation number** 0551/0004

**Date of approval/revision of SPC** November 1996.

**Legal category** P.

## VERACUR* GEL

**Qualitative and quantitative composition**
*Active constituents:* Formaldehyde (as Formaldehyde Solution BP) 0.75% w/w.

**Pharmaceutical form** Clear colourless gel.

**Clinical particulars**
*Therapeutic indications:* For the treatment of warts, particularly plantar warts (verrucae).

*Posology and method of administration*
Adults: Apply directly on to the wart or verruca and

cover with a plaster, twice daily. Remove scale and dead tissue from the top of the wart with an emery board or pumice stone.

Correct application technique is essential. Treatment may need to be continued for eight weeks or more.

*Children:* As adult dose.

*Elderly:* As adult dose.

*Contra-indications:* Application to broken skin.

*Special warnings and special precautions for use:* Do not apply to broken skin. For external use only. Keep out of reach of children.

If required, protect surrounding skin with a thin film of vaseline petroleum jelly before application.

*Interactions with other medicaments and other forms of interaction:* None known.

*Pregnancy and lactation:* The safety for use in pregnancy has not been established. Use only when considered essential by a physician.

*Effects on ability to drive and use machines:* Not applicable.

*Undesirable effects:* Formaldehyde vapour is irritant to the eyes, nose and respiratory tract and may cause coughing, dysphagia, spasm of the larynx, bronchitis and pneumonia. Asthma has been reported after repeated exposure. Concentrated solutions applied to the skin cause whitening and hardening. Contact dermatitis and sensitivity reactions have occurred after the use of conventional concentrations.

*Overdose:* Contaminated skin should be washed with soap and water. If accidentally ingested, avoid gastric lavage or emesis, but give water, milk or charcoal. Treat for shock and acidosis if necessary.

**Pharmacological properties**

*Pharmacodynamic properties:* Formaldehyde solution is a disinfectant effective against vegetative bacteria, fungi and many viruses.

*Pharmacokinetic properties:* If ingested, formaldehyde is rapidly metabolised to formic acid in the tissues, especially liver and erythrocytes. The formic acid may then be excreted as carbon dioxide and water excreted in the urine as formate, or metabolised to labile methyl groups.

*Preclinical safety data:* Formaldehyde solution has a well established medicinal use, recognised efficacy and an acceptable level of safety for topical use at appropriate concentrations.

**Pharmaceutical particulars**

*List of excipients*

| | |
|---|---|
| Carbopol 940 | 1.0% w/w |
| Sodium Hydroxide BP | 0.105% w/w |
| Deionised water | 97.30% w/w |

*Incompatibilities:* None known.

*Shelf life:* Five years.

*Special precautions for storage:* Store in a cool dry place.

*Nature and contents of container:* Aluminium tubes, epoxy resin lined, enclosed in cardboard cartons.

*Instructions for use/handling:* Not applicable.

**Marketing authorisation number**   0551/5000R

**Date of approval/revision of SPC**   March 1995.

**Legal category**   GSL.

*\*Trade Mark*

# UCB Pharma Limited
## Star House
## 69 Clarendon Road
## Watford WD1 1DJ

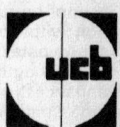

## NOOTROPIL* TABLETS 800 mg ▼
## NOOTROPIL* TABLETS 1200 mg ▼
## NOOTROPIL* SOLUTION 33% ▼

### Presentation
*Tablets:* White, oblong, scored, film coated tablets containing 800 mg or 1200 mg piracetam marked N on either side of the break line.

*Solution:* A clear and colourless solution containing 333.3 mg piracetam per ml is also available for patients suffering with dysphagia.

### Uses
Nootropil is indicated for patients suffering from myoclonus of cortical origin, irrespective of aetiology, and should be used in combination with other anti-myoclonic therapies.

### Dosage and administration
*Adults:* The dosage regimen shows an important inter-individual variability, requiring an individualised dose-finding approach: a reasonable protocol would be to introduce piracetam in a dosage of 7.2 g/day, increasing by 4.8 g/day every 3 to 4 days up to a maximum of 20 g/day, given in 2 or 3 divided doses, while keeping other anti-myoclonic drugs unchanged in optimal dosage. If possible, depending upon clinical benefit, an attempt should be made to reduce the dosage of other anti-myoclonic drugs subsequently.

*Solution:* It is advisable to follow each dose with a drink of water or soft drink to reduce the bitter taste of the solution.

### Contra-indications, warnings, etc
Piracetam is contra-indicated in patients with severe renal insufficiency (renal creatinine clearance of less than 20 ml per minute), hepatic impairment and those under 16 years of age.

*Pregnancy and lactation:* In animal studies piracetam was not teratogenic and had no effect on fertility at the maximal tested dose of 2.7 g/kg/day for the rabbit and 4.8 g/kg/day for rats and mice. Piracetam readily crosses the placental barrier and, very probably, passes into the mother's milk. Since the safety of use in human pregnancy is not established, Nootropil is to be avoided during pregnancy and lactation. Young women using the product should be receiving adequate contraceptive precautions.

*Precautions:* Abrupt discontinuation of treatment should be avoided as this may, in some myoclonic patients, induce myoclonic or generalised seizures.

As piracetam is almost exclusively excreted by the kidneys, caution should be exercised in treating patients with known renal impairment. In renally impaired and elderly patients, the increase in terminal half-life is directly related to renal function as measured by creatinine clearance. Dosage adjustment is therefore required in those with mild to moderate renal impairment and elderly patients with diminished renal function. The dosage should be modified according to the following scheme if creatinine clearance is between 20 and 60 ml/min or serum creatinine is between 1.25 and 3 mg/100 ml (112–270 µmol/litre).

| Creatinine clearance | Serum creatinine | Dosage |
|---|---|---|
| 60–40 ml/min | 1.25–1.7 mg/100 ml (112–153 µmol/l) | ½ usual dose |
| 40–20 ml/min | 1.7–3 mg/100 ml (153–270 µmol/l) | ¼ usual dose |

*Side-effects:* In placebo-controlled trials covering a range of doses between 1.6 and 15 grams daily undesirable effects reported with an incidence of more than one per cent but less than three per cent are; hyperkinesia, insomnia, weight increase, somnolence, nervousness and depression. Reported effects of less than one per cent are diarrhoea and rash.

*Drug interactions:* In a single case, confusion, irritability and sleep disorders were reported in concomitant use with thyroid extract (T3+T4). At present, based on a small number of studies, no interaction has been found with the following anti-epileptic medications: clonazepam, carbamazepine, phenytoin, phenobarbitone and sodium valproate. To date, there are no known interactions with other drugs.

*Driving:* In clinical studies, at dosages between 1.6 and 15 grams per day, hyperkinesia, somnolence, nervousness and depression were reported more frequently in patients on piracetam than on placebo. There is no experience on driving ability in dosages

between 15 and 20 grams daily. Caution should therefore be exercised by patients intending to drive or use machinery whilst taking piracetam.

*Overdosage:* Acute toxicological studies in animals showed lethal doses were obtained in mice (18.2 g/kg and higher) but not in rats and dogs dosed respectively at 21 g/kg or 10 g/kg.

No specific measure is indicated. The pateints' general condition should be closely monitored. Close attention should be given to keeping the patient well hydrated and monitoring the urine flow.

**Pharmaceutical precautions** The product should be stored at room temperature.

**Legal category** POM.

**Package quantities**

| | |
|---|---|
| Tablets 800 mg: | A box of 90 tablets with 15 tablets to a blister pack. |
| Tablets 1200 mg: | A box of 56 tablets with 14 tablets to a blister pack. |
| Solution 33% | Brown glass bottles containing 300 ml of solution. |

**Further information** Piracetam is rapidly and almost completely absorbed, and peak plasma levels are reached within 1.5 hours after administration. The extent of oral bio-availability, assessed from Area Under Curve (AUC), is close to 100% for capsules, tablets and solution. Peak levels and AUC are proportional to the dose given. The volume of distribution of piracetam is 0.7 l/kg and the plasma half-life is 5.0 hours in young adult men. Piracetam crosses the blood-brain and the placental barriers and diffuses across membranes used in renal dialysis. Up to now, no metabolite of piracetam has been found. Piracetam is excreted nearly completely in urine and urinary excretion is dose-independent. Excretion half-life values are consistent with those calculated from plasma/ blood data. Clearance of the compound is highly dependent on the renal creatinine clearance and would be expected to diminish in renal insufficiency.

**Product licence numbers**
Nootropil Tablets 800 mg   8972/0011
Nootropil Tablets 1200 mg   8972/0012
Nootropil Solution 33%   8972/0013

## PRESERVEX* TABLETS ▼

### Qualitative and quantitative composition

| | mg per tablet |
|---|---|
| Aceclofenac | 100.0 |
| Microcrystalline cellulose | 89.2 |
| Sodium croscarmellose | 6.6 |
| Glyceryl palmitostearate | 2.6 |
| Povidone (polyvidone) | 6.6 |
| **Tablet core weight** | **205.0** |
| *Film coating* | |
| Sepifilm 752 White, composed of: | |
| Hydroxypropyl methylcellulose | 6.2[1] |
| Polyoxyethylene 40 stearate | 0.9[1] |
| Titanium dioxide | 1.9[1] |
| **Total tablet weight** | **214.0** |

[1] Approximate quantities.

**Pharmaceutical form** Preservex tablets 100 mg are presented as white round film-coated tablets, 8 mm in diameter, with an 'A' embosssed on one side.

### Clinical particulars
*Therapeutic indications:* Preservex is indicated for the relief of pain and inflammation in osteoarthritis, rheumatoid arthritis and ankylosing spondylitis.

*Posology and method of administration:* Preservex tablets are supplied for oral administration and should be swallowed whole with a sufficient quantity of liquid. When Preservex was administered to fasting and fed healthy volunteers only the rate and not the extent of aceclofenac absorption was affected and as such Preservex can be taken with food.

*Adults:* The recommended dose is 200 mg daily, taken as two separate 100 mg doses, one tablet in the morning and one in the evening.

*Children:* There are no clinical data on the use of Preservex in children.

*Elderly:* The pharmacokinetics of Preservex are not altered in elderly patients, therefore it is not considered necessary to modify the dose or dose frequency.

As with other non-steroidal anti-inflammatory drugs (NSAIDs), caution should be exercised in the treatment of elderly patients, who are generally more prone to adverse reactions, and who are more likely to be suffering from impaired renal, cardiovascular or hepatic function and receiving concomitant medication.

*Renal insufficiency:* There is no evidence that the dosage of Preservex needs to be modified in patients with mild renal impairment, but as with other NSAIDs caution should be exercised (see also Precautions).

*Hepatic insufficiency:* There is some evidence that the dose of Preservex should be reduced in patients with hepatic impairment and it is suggested that an initial daily dose of 100 mg be used.

*Contra-indications:* Preservex should not be administered to patients with active or suspected peptic ulcer or gastro-intestinal bleeding.

Preservex should not be given to patients with moderate to severe renal impairment.

Preservex should not be prescribed during pregnancy, unless there are compelling reasons for doing so. The lowest effective dosage should be used.

Preservex should not be administered to patients previously sensitive to aceclofenac or in whom aspirin or NSAIDs precipitate attacks of asthma, acute rhinitis or urticaria or who are hypersensitive to these drugs.

*Special warnings and special precautions for use:*
*Warnings:* Gastro-intestinal: Close medical surveillance is imperative in patients with symptoms indicative of gastro-intestinal disorders, with a history suggestive of gastro-intestinal ulceration, with ulcerative colitis or with Crohn's disease, bleeding diathesis or haematological abnormalities.

Gastro-intestinal bleeding or ulcerative perforation, haematemesis and melaena have in general more serious consequences in the elderly. They can occur at any time during treatment, with or without warning symptoms or a previous history. In the rare instances where gastro-intestinal bleeding or ulceration occurs in patients receiving Preservex, the drug should be withdrawn.

Hepatic: Close medical surveillance is also imperative in patients suffering from severe impairment of hepatic function.

Hypersensitivity reactions: As with other NSAIDs, allergic reactions, including anaphylactic/anaphylactoid reactions, can also occur without earlier exposure to the drug.

*Precautions:*
Renal: Patients with mild renal or cardiac impairment and the elderly should be kept under surveillance, since the use of NSAIDs may result in deterioration of renal function. The lowest effective dose should be used and renal function monitored regularly.

The importance of prostaglandins in maintaining renal blood flow should be taken into account in patients with impaired cardiac or renal function, those being treated with diuretics or recovering from major surgery. Effects on renal function are usually reversible on withdrawal of Preservex.

Hepatic: If abnormal liver function tests persist or worsen, clinical signs or symptoms consistent with liver disease develop or if other manifestations occur (eosinophilia, rash), Preservex should be discontinued. Hepatitis may occur without prodromal symptoms.

Use of Preservex in patients with hepatic porphyria may trigger an attack.

Haematological: Preservex may reversibly inhibit platelet aggregation (see anticoagulants under Interactions).

Long term treatment: All patients who are receiving NSAIDs should be monitored as a precautionary measure e.g. renal function, hepatic function (elevation of liver enzymes may occur) and blood counts.

*Interactions:*
Lithium and digoxin: Preservex, like many NSAIDs, may increase plasma concentrations of lithium and digoxin.

Diuretics: Preservex, like other NSAIDs, may inhibit the activity of diuretics. Although it was not shown to affect blood pressure control when co-administered with bendrofluazide, interactions with other diuretics cannot be ruled out. When concomitant administration with potassium-sparing diuretics is employed, serum potassium should be monitored.

Anticoagulants: Like other NSAIDs, Preservex may enhance the activity of anticoagulants. Close monitoring of patients on combined anticoagulant and Preservex therapy should be undertaken.

Antidiabetic agents: Clinical studies have shown that diclofenac can be given together with oral antidiabetic agents without influencing their clinical effect. However, there have been isolated reports of hypoglycaemic and hyperglycaemic effects. Thus with Preservex, consideration should be given to adjustment of the dosage of hypoglycaemic agents.

Methotrexate: Caution should be exercised if NSAIDs and methotrexate are administered within 24 hours of each other, since NSAIDs may increase methotrexate plasma levels, resulting in increased toxicity.

Other NSAIDs and steroids: Concomitant therapy with aspirin, other NSAIDs and steroids may increase the frequency of side effects.

Cyclosporin: Cyclosporin nephrotoxicity may be increased by the effect of NSAIDs on renal prostaglandins.

Quinolone antimicrobials: Convulsions may occur due to an interaction between quinolones and NSAIDs. This may occur in patients with or without a previous history of epilepsy or convulsions. Therefore, caution should be exercised when considering the use of a quinolone in patients who are already receiving a NSAID.

*Use during pregnancy and lactation:*

*Pregnancy:* There is no information on the use of Preservex during pregnancy. The regular use of NSAIDs during the last trimester of pregnancy may increase uterine tone and contraction. NSAID use may also result in premature closure of the fetal ductus arteriosus *in utero* and possibly persistent pulmonary hypertension of the new born, delay onset and increase duration of labour.

Animal studies indicate that there was no evidence of teratogenesis in rats although the systemic exposure was low and in rabbits, treatment with aceclofenac (10 mg/kg/day) resulted in a series of morphological changes in some fetuses.

*Lactation:* There is no information on the secretion of Preservex to breast milk; there was however no notable transfer of radio-labelled ($^{14}C$) aceclofenac to the milk of lactating rats.

The use of Preservex should therefore be avoided in pregnancy and lactation unless the potential benefits to the mother outweigh the possible risks to the fetus.

*Effects of ability to drive and use machines:* Patients suffering from dizziness, vertigo, or other central nervous system disorders whilst taking NSAIDs should refrain from driving or handling dangerous machinery.

*Undesirable effects:* The majority of side-effects observed have been reversible and of a minor nature and include gastro-intestinal disorders (dyspepsia, abdominal pain, nausea and diarrhoea) and occasional occurrence of dizziness. Dermatological complaints including pruritus and rash and abnormal hepatic enzyme levels and raised serum creatinine have occasionally been reported.

If serious side-effects occur, Preservex should be withdrawn.

The following adverse events (described as most frequent ≥5%, occasional <5% or rare cases <0.1%) were reported during all clinical trials.

*Gastro-intestinal system disorders:* Most frequent: dyspepsia (7.5%), abdominal pain (6.2%). Occasional: nausea (1.5%), diarrhoea (1.5%), flatulence (0.8%), gastritis (0.6%), constipation (0.5%), vomiting (0.5%), ulcerative stomatitis (0.1%). Rare cases: (all <0.1%) pancreatitis, melaena, stomatitis.

*Central and peripheral nervous system:* Occasional: dizziness (1%), vertigo (0.3%). Rare cases: (all <0.1%) paraesthesia, tremor.

*Psychiatric:* Rare cases: (all <0.1%) depression, abnormal dreaming, somnolence, insomnia.

*Skin and appendages:* Occasional: pruritus (0.9%), rash (0.5%), dermatitis (0.2%). Rare cases: (all <0.1%) eczema.

*Liver and biliary:* Occasional: hepatic enzymes increased (2.5%).

*Metabolic:* Occasional: BUN increased (0.4%), blood creatinine increased (0.3%). Rare cases: (all <0.1%) alkaline phosphatase increased, hyperkalaemia.

*Cardiovascular:* Rare cases: (all <0.1%) oedema (dependent), palpitation, leg cramps flushing, purpura.

*Respiratory:* Rare cases: (all <0.1%) dyspnoea, stridor.

*Blood:* Rare cases: (all <0.1%) anaemia, granulocytopenia, thrombocytopenia.

*Body as a whole, general:* Rare cases (all <0.1%) headache, fatigue, face oedema, hot flushes, allergic reaction, weight increase.

*Others:* Rare cases (all <0.1%) abnormal vision, abnormal taste.

*Overdose:* Management of acute poisoning with NSAIDs essentially consists of supportive and symptomatic measures.

There are no human data available on the consequences of Preservex overdosage. The therapeutic measures to be taken are: absorption should be prevented as soon as possible after overdosage by means of gastric lavage and treatment with activated charcoal; supportive and symptomatic treatment should be given for complications such as hypotension, renal failure, convulsions, gastro-intestinal irritation, and respiratory depression; specific therapies such as forced diuresis, dialysis or haemoperfusion are probably of no help in eliminating NSAIDs due to their high rate of protein binding and extensive metabolism.

**Pharmacological properties**

*Pharmacodynamic properties:* Aceclofenac is a non-steroidal agent with marked anti-inflammatory and analgesic properties.

The mode of action of aceclofenac is largely based on the inhibition of prostaglandin synthesis. Aceclofenac is a potent inhibitor of the enzyme cyclo-oxygenase, which is involved in the production of prostaglandins.

*Pharmacokinetic properties:* After oral administration, aceclofenac is rapidly and completely absorbed as unchanged drug. Peak plasma concentrations are reached approximately 1.25 to 3.00 hours following ingestion. Aceclofenac penetrates into the synovial fluid, where the concentrations reach approximately 57% of those in plasma. The volume of distribution is approximately 25 L.

The mean plasma elimination half-life is around 4 hours. Aceclofenac is highly protein-bound (>99%). Aceclofenac circulates mainly as unchanged drug. 4'-Hydroxyaceclofenac is the main metabolite detected in plasma. Approximately two-thirds of the administered dose is excreted via the urine, mainly as hydroxymetabolites.

No changes in the pharmacokinetics of aceclofenac have been detected in the elderly.

*Preclinical safety data:* The results from preclinical studies conducted with aceclofenac are consistent with those expected for NSAIDs. The principal target organ was the gastro-intestinal tract. No unexpected findings were recorded.

Aceclofenac was not considered to have any mutagenic activity in three *in vitro* studies and an *in vivo* study in the mouse.

Aceclofenac was not found to be carcinogenic in either the mouse or rat.

**Pharmaceutical particulars**

*List of excipients:* The excipients used in Preservex tablets 100 mg are those commonly recommended for use in pharmaceutical preparations. These are microcrystalline cellulose, sodium croscarmellose, povidone, glyceryl palmitosterate and the film coat, containing partially substituted hydroxypropyl methylcellulose, polyoxyethylene 40 stearate and titanium dioxide.

*Incompatibilities:* None known.

*Shelf life:* The shelf-life for this product shall not exceed three years from the date of manufacture.

*Special precautions for storage:* The tablets are to be stored at 25°C or below.

*Nature and contents of container:* The immediate container for Preservex tablets 100 mg is a laminated aluminium/aluminium foil pack. Each foil strip contains either 10 or 14 tablets. One, two, four or six foil strips will be provided with a patient information leaflet inside a carton.

*Instructions for use/handling:* None.

*Marketing authorisation holder:* Prodesfarma SA, Carrer del Pont Reixat No 5, Apartado PO Box 26, 08960 Sant Just Desvern, Barcelona, Spain.

**Marketing authorisation number** 08448/0001.

**Date of approval/revision of SPC** November 1995.

**Legal category** POM.

## ZIRTEK* TABLETS 10mg
## ZIRTEK* SOLUTION 1 mg/1 ml

**Presentation**

*Tablets:* White, oblong, film-coated tablets containing 10 mg cetirizine dihydrochloride. Each tablet is scored and bears the code Y/Y.

*Solution:* A clear, colourless, banana flavoured, sugar free solution with a slightly sweet taste containing 1 mg/1 ml cetirizine dihydrochloride.

**Uses** Cetirizine is a potent antihistamine with a low potential for drowsiness at pharmacologically active doses and with additional anti-allergic properties. It is a selective $H_1$ antagonist with negligible effects on other receptors and is therefore virtually free from anti-cholinergic and anti-serotonin effects. Cetirizine inhibits the histamine-mediated 'early' phase of the allergic reaction and also reduces the migration of inflammatory cells and the release of mediators associated with the 'late' allergic response. Zirtek is indicated for the treatment of perennial rhinitis, seasonal allergic rhinitis (hay fever) and chronic idiopathic urticaria in adults and children aged 6 years and over, and for seasonal rhinitis (hay fever) in children aged between 2 to 6 years.

**Dosage and administration**

*Tablets*

*Adults and children 6 years and over:* One 10 mg tablet daily.

*Solution*

*Adults and children 6 years and over:* Either 10 ml (10 mg) once daily, or 5 ml (5 mg) twice daily.

*Children aged between 2 to 6 years:* Either 5 ml (5 mg) once daily, or 2.5 ml (2.5 mg) twice daily.

At present there are no data to suggest that the recommended dose needs to be reduced in elderly patients. However, in patients with renal insufficiency dosage should be reduced to half the daily dose of either tablets or drinkable solution.

**Contra-indications, warnings, etc**

*Contra-indications:* Zirtek is contra-indicated in patients with a history of hypersensitivity to any constituent in tablet or solution.

Zirtek is contra-indicated in lactating women as the active ingredient, cetirizine, is excreted in breast milk.

*Precautions:* Studies conducted with healthy volunteers at doses of 20 and 25 mg/day have not revealed effects on alertness or reaction time, however, patients are advised not to exceed the recommended dose if driving or operating machinery.

*Pregnancy:* No adverse effects have been reported from animal studies. There has been little or no use of Zirtek in pregnancy. As with other drugs the use of Zirtek in pregnancy should be avoided.

*Drug interactions:* To date, there are no known interactions with any other drugs. Studies with diazepam and cimetidine have revealed no evidence of interactions. As with other antihistamines it is advisable to avoid excessive alcohol consumption.

*Side-effects:* In objective tests of psychomotor function, the incidence of sedation with cetirizine was similar to that of placebo.

There have been occasional reports of mild and transient side effects such as headaches, dizziness, drowsiness, agitation, dry mouth and gastro-intestinal discomfort. If affected the dose may be taken as 5 mg in the morning and 5 mg in the evening.

*Overdosage:* Drowsiness can be a symptom of overdosage in adults; in children, agitation can occur. In the case of massive overdosage, gastric lavage should be performed together with the usual supportive measures. To date, there is no specific antidote.

**Pharmaceutical precautions** Store below 30°C.

**Legal category** POM.

**Package quantities** Zirtek tablets are supplied in cartons containing 30 tablets in 3 blister packs of 10.

Zirtek solution is available in 200 ml amber coloured glass bottles.

**Further information** Peak blood levels of the order of 0.3 micrograms/ml are reached between thirty and sixty minutes after administration of a 10 mg dose of cetirizine. The terminal half-life is approximately 1[illegible] hours in adults and 6 hours in children aged between 6 and 12 years and 5 hours in children aged between 2 to 6 years. This data is consistent with the urinary excretion half-life of the drug. The cumulative urinary excretion represents two thirds of the dose given in either adults or children. Consequently, the apparent plasma clearance in children is higher than that measured in adults. Cetirizine is strongly bound to plasma proteins.

**Product licence numbers**

Tablets 5221/0001

Solution 5221/0002

**Trade Mark*

# Warner Lambert Consumer Healthcare
Lambert Court
Chestnut Avenue
Eastleigh
Hampshire SO53 3ZQ

**WARNER LAMBERT**

**CONSUMER HEALTHCARE**

## ABIDEC DROPS*

**Presentation** A clear yellow liquid, with a characteristic odour and taste. Each 0.6 ml contains:

| | |
|---|---|
| Vitamin A PhEur | 4000 units |
| Vitamin B₁ (Thiamine Hydrochloride PhEur) | 1 mg |
| Vitamin B₂ (Riboflavine PhEur) | 400 micrograms |
| Vitamin B₆ (Pyridoxine Hydrochloride PhEur) | 500 micrograms |
| Vitamin C (Ascorbic Acid PhEur) | 50 mg |
| Vitamin D₂ (Ergocalciferol PhEur) | 400 units |
| Nicotinamide PhEur | 5 mg |

**Uses** The prevention of vitamin deficiencies and for the maintenance of normal growth and health during the early years of infancy and childhood; multivitamin supplement.

**Dosage and administration**
*Infants less than one year old:* 0.3 ml daily.

*Older children:* 0.6 ml daily.

*Adults:* Not appropriate.

**Contra-indications, warnings, etc**
*Contra-indications:* Abidec Drops are contra-indicated in individuals with known hypersensitivity to the product or any of it's components.

*Interactions with other medicaments and other forms of interaction:* None.

*Effects on ability to drive and use machines:* Unlikely to produce an effect.

*Other undesirable effects:*
*Ascorbic acid (C), Nicotinamide, Pyridoxine (B₆), Riboflavine (B₂) and Thiamine (B₁):* These water soluble vitamins are generally non-toxic compounds with a wide margin of safety, the excess amounts being rapidly excreted in the urine. Adverse effects are not anticipated at the quantities present in Abidec Drops.

*Ergocalciferol (D₂):* The only known adverse effects of Vitamin D occur when excessive doses are taken. Adverse effects are not anticipated at the quantity present in Abidec Drops.

*Vitamin A palmitate:* Adverse effects are extremely rare at daily doses of less than 9 mg.

*Use in pregnancy and lactation:* Not appropriate.

*Other special warnings and precautions:* When prescribing Abidec drops, as with all multi-vitamin preparations, allowance should be made for vitamins obtained from other sources to prevent hypervitaminosis occurring.

*Overdosage (symptoms and signs):* Abidec Drops contain levels of vitamins which present little risk in overdosage.
*Ascorbic acid (C):* Ascorbic acid is not stored to a great extent by the body, any excess amounts are eliminated in the urine. Ascorbic acid is thought to become toxic at chronic doses in excess of 6 g.
*Ergocalciferol:* Excessive doses of Vitamin D, 60,000 units per day, can result in hypercalcaemia and hypercalciuria. Adverse effects of hypercalcaemia may include muscle weakness, apathy, headache, anorexia, nausea and vomiting, hypertension and cardiac arrhythmia's.
*Nicotinamide:* A single large dose of Nicotinamide is unlikely to have serious ill effects, though transient abnormalities of liver function might occur.
*Pyridoxine hydrochloride:* Acute doses less than 500 mg per day appear to be safe. Excessive doses may lower serum folate concentrations. Sensory neuropathy has been described with chronic dosing of 200 mg daily.
*Riboflavine:* Riboflavine has been found to be practically non-toxic.
*Thiamine hydrochloride:* When taken orally, Thiamine is non-toxic. If large doses are ingested they are not stored by the body but excreted unchanged by the kidneys.
*Vitamin A palmitate:* Acute administration of high doses of Vitamin A, nausea, vomiting and irritability. In infants acute toxicity can lead to transient hydrocephalus. All these effects disappear within 24 hours of taking retinol.

*Treatment:* Treatment should be supportive and symptomatic.

*Pharmacological particulars:*
*Ascorbic acid (Vitamin C):* Ascorbic acid is a water soluble vitamin and a powerful antioxidant. It is a cofactor in numerous biological processes, such as the metabolism of folic acid, amino acid oxidation and the absorption and transport of iron. It is also required for the formation, maintenance and repair of intercellular cement material. Ascorbic acid is important in the defence against infection, the normal functioning of T-lymphocytes and for effective phagocytic activity of leucocytes. It also protects cells against oxidation damage to essential molecules.
*Ergocalciferol (Vitamin D₂):* Vitamin D is a regulator of both calcium and phosphate homeostasis.
*Nicotinamide:* Nicotinamide is an essential component of co-enzymes responsible for proper tissue respiration.
*Pyridoxine hydrochloride (Vitamin B₆):* Vitamin B₆ is a constituent of the co-enzymes, pyridoxal pyrophosphate and pyridoxamine phosphate, both of which play an important role in protein metabolism.
*Riboflavine (Vitamin B₂):* Riboflavine is essential for the utilisation of energy from food. It is a component of co-enzymes which play an essential role in oxidative/reductive metabolic reactions. Riboflavine is also necessary for the functioning of pyridoxine and nicotinic acid.
*Thiamine hydrochloride (Vitamin B₁):* Vitamin B₁ is essential for proper carbohydrate metabolism and plays an essential role in the decarboxylation of alpha keto acids.
*Vitamin A palmitate:* Vitamin A plays an essential role in the function of the retina, the growth and function of epithelial tissue, bone growth, reproduction and embryonic development.

*Pharmacokinetic properties:*
*Absorption:* Vitamin A, B₁, B₂, B₆, C, D₂ and Nicotinamide are well absorbed from the gastro-intestinal tract.
*Distribution:* The vitamins present in Abidec Drops are widely distributed to all tissues in the body.
*Metabolism and elimination: Ascorbic acid (Vitamin C):* Ascorbic acid reaches a maximum plasma concentration after 4 hours following oral administration after which there is rapid urinary excretion. Following oral administration 60% of the dose is excreted in 24 hours either as ascorbic acid or it's metabolite dihydroascorbic acid.
*Ergocalciferol (Vitamin D₂):* Vitamin D circulates in the blood associated with Vitamin D binding protein. It is stored in fat deposits. Ergocalciferol is hydroxylated in the liver and gut to 25-hydroxy cholecalciferol which is then further metabolised in the kidney to the active form 1,25-dihydroxycholecalciferol and other metabolites. Ergocalciferol and it's metabolites are excreted largely in the bile with eventual elimination in the faeces, with only a small amount of some of the metabolites appearing in the urine.
*Nicotinamide:* Nicotinamide is readily taken up into tissues and utilised for the synthesis of the co-enzyme forms Nicotinamide adenine dinucleotide (NAD) and Nicotinamide adenine dinucleotide phosphate (NADP). Nicotinamide is degraded in the liver and other organs to a number of products that are excreted in the urine, the major metabolites being N-methyl-2-pyridone-5-carboxamide and n-methylnicotinamide.
*Pyridoxine hydrochloride (Vitamin B₆):* The half life of pyridoxine ranges from 15–20 days. Once absorbed vitamin B₆ is converted to it's active co-enzyme form pyridoxal 5-phosphate. Muscle is the major storage site for pyridoxal 5-phosphate. It is degraded in the liver to 4-pyridoxic acid which is eliminated by the kidneys.
*Riboflavine (Vitamin B₂):* Following absorption Riboflavine is converted into the coenzymes: flavin mononucleotide (FMN) and flavin adenine dinucleotide (FAD). Riboflavine is not stored in the body tissues to any great extent and amounts in excess of the body's requirements are excreted in the urine largely unchanged.
*Thiamine hydrochloride (Vitamin B₁):* Thiamine has a plasma half life of 24 hours and is not stored to any great extent in the body. Excess ingested thiamine is excreted in the urine as either the free vitamin or as the metabolite, pyrimidine.
*Vitamin A palmitate:* Vitamin A palmitate is hydrolysed in the intestinal lumen to retinol which is then absorbed. Retinol circulates in the blood bound to retinol binding protein which protects it from glomerular filtration. The complex circulates to target tissues where the vitamin is released, permeates the cell and binds intracellularly to cellular retinol binding protein. Of the absorbed retinol 20–50% is either conjugated or oxidised to various products and excreted over a matter of days in the urine and faeces, while the remainder is stored. This stored retinol is gradually metabolised by the liver and peripheral tissues.

**Pharmaceutical precautions** When stored at a temperature not exceeding 25°C and out of direct sunlight, this product is expected to have a shelf life of 2 years.

**Legal category** GSL

**Package quantities** 50 ml pack (2 x 25 ml + 2 droppers graduated at 0.3 ml and 0.6 ml). 25 ml pack (1 x 25 ml + 1 dropper graduated at 0.3 ml and 0.6 ml).

**Further information** Nil.

**Product licence number:** 15513/0036

## ANUSOL* CREAM

**Qualitative and quantitative composition** Each 100 g of cream contains: Bismuth Oxide 2.14 g, Balsam Peru 1.80 g, Zinc Oxide 10.75 g.

**Pharmaceutical form** A buff coloured cream.

**Clinical particulars**
*Therapeutic indications:* Symptomatic relief of uncomplicated internal and external haemorrhoids, pruritus ani, proctitis and fissures. Also indicated postoperatively in ano-rectal surgical procedures and after incision of thrombosed or sclerosed ano-rectal veins.

*Posology and method of administration:* Topical.

*Adults and elderly (over 65 years):* Apply to the affected area at night, in the morning and after each evacuation until the condition is controlled. Thoroughly cleanse the affected area, dry and apply cream. Anusol Cream is prepared in a vanishing cream base and may be gently smoothed onto the affected area without the need to apply a gauze dressing. For internal conditions use rectal nozzle provided and clean it after each use. Not to be taken orally.
*Children:* Not recommended.

*Contra-indications:* Known hypersensitivity to any of the constituents.

*Special warnings and precautions for use:* None known.

*Interaction with other medicaments and other forms of interaction:* None known.

*Pregnancy and lactation:* Whilst formal studies on the effect of this product during human pregnancy have not been conducted, there is no epidemiological evidence of adverse effect, either to the pregnant mother or foetus.

*Effects on ability to drive and use machines:* None known.

*Undesirable effects:* Rarely, sensitivity reactions. Patients may occasionally experience transient burning on application, especially if the anoderm is not intact.

*Overdose:* Treatment of a large acute overdose should include gastric lavage, purgation with magnesium sulphate and complete bed rest. If necessary, apply oxygen and give general supportive measures.

**Pharmacological properties**
*Pharmacodynamic properties:* Anusol Cream provides antiseptic, astringent and emollient properties

which help to relieve discomfort associated with minor ano-rectal conditions. It also provides lubricating properties for use with suppositories.

Bismuth oxide is weakly astringent with supposed antiseptic properties and has a protective action on mucous membranes and raw surfaces. Zinc oxide is an astringent and mild antiseptic and probably owes its actions to the ability of the zinc ion to precipitate protein but other mechanisms may be involved. Zinc oxide is also used to absorb skin moisture and decrease friction and discourage growth of certain bacteria. Balsam Peru has a very mild antiseptic action by virtue of it's content of cinnamic and benzoic acids. It is believed to promote the growth of epithelial cells.

*Pharmacokinetic properties:* The active ingredients exert their therapeutic effect without being absorbed into the systemic circulation. These observations are supported by evidence from various studies and reviews.

*Pre-clinical safety data:* The active ingredients of Anusol are well known constituents of medicinal products and their safety profile is well documented

**Pharmaceutical particulars**
*List of excipients:* Anusol Cream contains Glycerol monostearate, Liquid paraffin, Propylene glycol, Polysorbate 60, Sorbitan monostearate, Titanium dioxide, Methyl p-hydroxybenzoate, Propyl p-hydroxybenzoate, Purified water.

*Incompatibilities:* None known.

*Shelf life:* 3 years when stored in the original packaging.

*Special precautions for storage:* Store at a temperature not exceeding 25°C.

*Nature and contents of container:* Pack size 23 g, externally printed and internally lacquered aluminium tube with plastic cap.

*Instructions for use/handling:* No special requirements.

**Marketing authorisation number** 15513/0041

**Date of approval/revision of SPC** 27 March 1996

**Legal category:** GSL

## ANUSOL* OINTMENT

**Presentation** A light buff coloured ointment having the characteristic odour of Balsam Peru. Each 100 g of ointment contains: bismuth subgallate 2.25 g, bismuth oxide 0.875 g, balsam Peru 1.875 g and zinc oxide 10.75 g.

**Uses** Anusol Ointment provides antiseptic, astringent and emollient properties which help to relieve discomfort associated with minor ano-rectal conditions. It is indicated for the symptomatic relief of uncomplicated internal and external haemorrhoids, pruritus ani, proctitis and fissures. Also indicated postoperatively in ano-rectal surgical procedures and after incision of thrombosed or sclerosed ano-rectal veins.

**Dosage and administration** Topical.

*Adults:* Apply to the affected area at night, in the morning and after each evacuation until the condition is controlled. Thoroughly cleanse the affected area, dry and apply cream or ointment. It should be applied on a gauze dressing. For internal conditions use rectal nozzle provided and clean it after each use. Not to be taken orally.

*Elderly (over 65 years):* As for adults.

*Children:* Not recommended.

**Contra-indications, warnings, etc** History of sensitivity to any of the constituents.

*Pregnancy:* Whilst formal studies on the effect of this product during human pregnancy have not been conducted, there is no epidemiological evidence of adverse effect, either to the pregnant mother or the foetus.

*Precautions:* None applicable.

*Side-effects:* Rarely, sensitivity reactions. Patients may occasionally experience transient burning on application, especially if the anoderm is not intact.

*Overdose:* Treatment of a large acute overdose should include gastric lavage, purgation with magnesium sulphate and complete bed rest. If necessary, apply oxygen and give general supportive measures.

**Pharmaceutical precautions** Store at a temperature not exceeding 25°C

**Legal category** GSL

**Package quantity** tubes of 25 g

**Product licence number** 15513/0042

## ANUSOL* SUPPOSITORIES

**Presentation** White torpedo shaped suppositories with a characteristic odour of Balsam Peru enclosed in a moulded strip pack.

Each 2.8 g suppository contains:
Bismuth Subgallate BP    59 mg
Bismuth Oxide            24 mg
Balsam Peru PhEur        49 mg
Zinc Oxide PhEur         296 mg

**Uses** For the relief of internal haemorrhoids (piles), and other related ano-rectal conditions.

**Dosage and administration**
*Adults:* Remove wrapper and insert one suppository into the anus at night, in the morning and after each evacuation. Not to be taken orally.

*Elderly (over 65 years):* As for adults.

*Children:* Not recommended.

**Contra-indications, warnings, etc**
*Contra-indications:* History of sensitivity to any of the constituents.

*Pregnancy and lactation:* Whilst formal studies on the effect of this product during human pregnancy have not been conducted, there is no epidemiological evidence of adverse effect, either to the pregnant mother or the foetus.

*Precautions:* None applicable.

*Other undesirable effects:* Rarely, sensitivity reactions. Patients may occasionally experience transient burning on application, especially if the anoderm is not intact.

*Overdosage:* Treatment of a large acute overdose should include gastric lavage, purgation with magnesium sulphate and complete bed rest. If necessary, give oxygen and general supportive measures.

**Pharmaceutical precautions** Store at a temperature not exceeding 25°C.

**Legal category** GSL.

**Package quantities** Box of 12 and 24 suppositories.

**Product licence number** 15513/0043

## CALADRYL* LOTION AND CREAM

**Presentation**
*Lotion:* A smooth, pink, viscous suspension with a characteristic odour.

*Cream:* A smooth, pink cream with a characteristic odour.

*Composition:* Caladryl Lotion and Cream: Zinc oxide 8.0%, Diphenhydramine hydrochloride 1.0%, Racemic camphor 0.1%.

*Action:* Caladryl combines the cooling and soothing effects of calamine and camphor with the powerful antihistaminic and antipruritic effects of Diphenhydramine hydrochloride.

**Uses** For relief of irritation associated with urticaria, herpes zoster and other minor skin affections, to alleviate the discomforts of sunburn, prickly heat, insect bites and nettle stings. In infants it may be used for hives.

**Dosage and administration** Topical application to skin only.

*Adults:* Apply to affected area three or four times daily.

*Elderly (over 65 years):* As for adults.

*Children and infants of all age groups:* As for adults.

Caladryl lotion may be dabbed on the affected part using a pad of cotton wool. The cream may be lightly smoothed on.

**Contra-indications, warnings etc** Do not use on chicken pox or measles or exudative dermatoses, unless supervised by a doctor. Do not use on extensive areas of the skin except as directed by a doctor. Do not use any other drugs containing Diphenhydramine while using this product.

*Pregnancy and lactation:* The safety of Caladryl in pregnancy and lactation has not been established. Like any medicine, Caladryl should only be used if the possible benefits outweigh the potential risks involved. Diphenhydramine is known to be absorbed through the skin. Diphenhydramine crosses the placental barrier and is secreted in breast milk.

*Precautions and warnings:* Caladryl should not be applied to raw, or broken surfaces or mucous membranes as this may result in percutaneous absorption giving rise to systemic effects. Avoid contact with the eyes.

If a burning sensation or rash develops or if the condition persists, treatment should be discontinued. If necessary remove by washing with soap and water.

*Side-effects:* Rarely, sensitivity, eczematous reactions and photosensitivity have been reported after topical application of antihistamines. If this occurs, treatment should be discontinued.

*Overdose:* Accidental ingestion or excessive absorption of Caladryl may lead to dose-related signs of Diphenhydramine toxicity. These include drowsiness and sedation with anticholinergic symptoms prevailing. Camphor may produce nausea, vomiting and dizziness. At higher doses, delirium leading to coma, ataxia, increased muscle reflexes and cloniform convulsions may appear.

*Treatment of overdose:* The stomach should be emptied by lavage and aspiration. In cases of acute poisoning, activated charcoal may be useful. A Sodium sulphate purgative may be given. Convulsions may be controlled with diazepam or Thiopentone sodium. In the case of camphor poisoning, lipid haemodialysis or resin haemoperfusion may be useful.

**Pharmaceutical precautions** Lotion: Store at a temperature not exceeding 30°C
　Cream: Store at a temperature not exceeding 25°C

**Legal category** P.

**Package quantities** Lotion: 125 ml. Cream: 42 g.

**Further information** Nil

**Product licence numbers**
Lotion:　0018/5092R
Cream:　0018/5093R

## CALGEL* TEETHING GEL

**Presentation** Calgel Teething Gel contains Lignocaine hydrochloride BP 0.33% w/w and Cetylpyridinium chloride BP 0.1% w/w in a clear yellow, water soluble sugar-free base. It has a herbal flavour.

**Uses** Calgel Teething Gel is indicated for use in teething. Calgel Teething Gel acts quickly to help relieve teething pain and soothe infants' gums. It also has mild antiseptic properties.

**Dosage and administration** Calgel Teething Gel is suitable for babies from the age of 3 months. A small quantity of Calgel Teething Gel, approximately one-third of an inch (7.5 mm), should be squeezed onto the tip of a clean finger and rubbed gently onto the affected area of the gum. Application may be repeated after an interval of 20 minutes if necessary, with up to six applications in one day.

**Contra-indications, warnings, etc**
*Contra-indications:* None.

*Precautions:* The recommended dosage should not be exceeded. Keep out of reach of children.

*Side-effects:* When used according to instructions side effects would not be expected. However, isolated cases of hypersensitivity to lignocaine hydrochloride have been reported in adults and in a child over 12 years following local injection. Hypersensitivity presented in these cases as localised oedema with slight difficulty in breathing or as generalised rash.

Chamomile, a minor ingredient in the herbal flavouring agent, has been documented as causing allergic reactions. Hypersensitivity to Chamomile normally manifests as breathing difficulties in atopic individuals. Anaphylactic reactions have been reported in individuals drinking herbal tea infusions containing Chamomile (herbal tea asthma). Sensitised individuals may demonstrate positive skin reactions to preparations containing Chamomile.

In the event of any unwanted side effects, use should be discontinued and a doctor consulted.

*Drug Interactions:* No drug interactions with Calgel Teething Gel are known. Drug interactions between intravenously administered Lignocaine and oral Procainamide, oral Phenytoin alone or in combination with Phenobarbitone, Primidone or Carbamazepine, oral Propanolol, and non-potassium sparing diuretics including Bumetanide, Frusemide and Thiazide have been reported. These drug effects are unlikely to be relevant to the use of Calgel Teething Gel.

*Toxicity and treatment of overdosage:* Suppression of pharyngeal sensation with concomitant effects on swallowing may theoretically result from excessive topical oral use of Calgel Teething Gel. Such an effect has been reported in an adult who gargled and swallowed 5 ml of a 2% Lignocaine hydrochloride solution (equivalent to 100 mg Lignocaine). However assuming proportionality of body surface area and pharyngeal surface area, this dose would be equivalent to a single dose of 5.4 g of Calgel Teething Gel for a 3 month old child.

It is most unlikely, even with misuse or excessive application of Calgel Teething Gel, that the large amounts of Lignocaine hydrochloride or Cetylpyridinium chloride required to produce clinically-relevant toxic effects would be reached. In the event of overdose, use should be discontinued and a doctor consulted.

**Pharmaceutical precautions** Store below 25°C.

**Legal category** GSL.

**Package quantities** Single packs of 10 g

**Further information** Calgel Teething Gel is considered to be of low cariogenic potential since the sweetening agents are sorbitol, xylitol and saccharin sodium.

**Product licence number** 15513/0015

## CALPOL* PAEDIATRIC
## CALPOL* PAEDIATRIC SUGAR FREE

**Presentation** Calpol Paediatric and Calpol Paediatric Sugar Free: Each 5 ml dose of viscous, pink, strawberry flavoured suspension contains 120 mg Paracetamol BP.

**Uses** Calpol products are indicated for the treatment of mild to moderate pain (including teething pain), and as antipyretics.

**Dosage and administration**
*Children 1 to under 6 years:* 5 to 10 ml Calpol Paediatric (120 mg to 240 mg paracetamol).

*3 months to under 1 year:* 2.5 to 5 ml Calpol Paediatric (60 mg to 120 mg paracetamol).

*Infants under 3 months:* A 2.5 ml dose of Calpol Paediatric is suitable for babies who develop a fever following vaccination at 2 months. In other cases, use only under medical supervision. Repeat every 4 hours, if necessary, up to a maximum of 4 doses per 24 hours.

*Use in the elderly:* In the elderly the rate and extent of paracetamol absorption is normal but plasma half-life is longer and paracetamol clearance is lower than in young adults.

*Dilution:* Calpol Paediatric may be diluted 1:1 with Syrup BP. Calpol Paediatric Sugar Free may be diluted 1:1 with either Sorbitol Solution BPC (non-crystallising) or Glycerol BP. In all cases dilutions should be freshly-prepared, stored below 25°C and used within 28 days.

**Contra-indications, warnings, etc**
*Contra-indications:* Calpol is contra-indicated in patients with known hypersensitivity to paracetamol.

*Precautions:* Calpol should be used with caution in the presence of severe hepatic or renal dysfunction.

*Side-effects:* Paracetamol has been widely used and when taken at the usual recommended dosage, side-effects are mild and infrequent and reports of adverse reactions are rare. Skin rashes and other allergic reactions occur rarely.

Most reports and adverse reactions to paracetamol relate to overdosage with the drug.

Isolated cases of thrombocytopenic purpura, haemolytic anaemia and agranulocytosis have been recorded.

Chronic hepatic necrosis has been reported in a patient who took daily therapeutic doses of paracetamol for about a year and liver damage has been reported after daily ingestion of excessive amounts for shorter periods. A review of a group of patients with chronic active hepatitis failed to reveal differences in the abnormalities of liver function in those who were long-term users of paracetamol nor was the control of their disease improved after paracetamol withdrawal.

Nephrotoxicity following therapeutic doses of paracetamol is uncommon, but papillary necrosis has been reported after prolonged administration.

*Drug interactions:* Patients who have taken barbiturates, tricyclic antidepressants and alcohol may show diminished ability to metabolise large doses of paracetamol, the plasma half-life of which can be prolonged.

Alcohol can increase the hepatotoxicity of paracetamol overdosage and may have contributed to the acute pancreatitis reported in one patient who had taken an overdose of paracetamol.

Chronic ingestion of anticonvulsants or oral steroid contraceptives induce liver enzymes and may prevent attainment of therapeutic paracetamol levels by increasing first pass metabolism or clearance.

*Use in pregnancy and lactation:* Data are not available on the use of Calpol during pregnancy. There is epidemiological evidence of safety of paracetamol in human pregnancy.

A Pharmacokinetic study in 12 nursing mothers revealed that less than 1% of the dose ingested by a nursing mother appears in human milk, therefore maternal ingestion of therapeutic doses does not present a risk to the infant.

*Toxicity and treatment of overdosage:* Pallor, anorexia, nausea and vomiting are frequent early symptoms of paracetamol overdosage. Hepatic necrosis is a dose-related complication of paracetamol overdosage. Hepatic enzymes may become elevated and prothrombin time prolonged within 12 to 48 hours but clinical symptoms may not be apparent until 1 to 6 days after ingestion. Toxicity is likely in adults who have taken more than 10 g.

To protect the patient against delayed hepatoxicity, paracetamol overdosage should be treated promptly by gastric lavage followed by intravenous N-acetylcysteine or oral Methionine. Additional therapy (further Methionine or intravenous cysteamine or intravenous N-acetylcysteine) is normally considered in the light of blood paracetamol content and the time elapsed since ingestion. Fulminant hepatic failure which may follow paracetamol overdosage requires specialised management.

In paracetamol overdosage with liver cell damage paracetamol half life is often prolonged from around 2 hours in normal adults to 4 hours or longer. However liver cell damage has been found in patients with a paracetamol half life less than 4 hours. Diminution in $^{14}CO_2$ excretion after oral $^{14}C$-aminopyrine has been reported to correlate better with liver cell damage in paracetamol overdosage than do plasma paracetamol concentration or half life or conventional liver function test measurements. Concomitant renal failure due to acute tubular necrosis may accompany paracetamol-induced fulminant hepatic failure. The incidence is, however, no more frequent in these patients than in others with fulminant hepatic failure from other causes.

**Pharmaceutical precautions** Store below 25°C. Protect from light.

**Legal category** P.

**Package quantities** Calpol Paediatric: Bottles of 1 litre. Calpol Paediatric Sugar Free: Bottles of 1 litre.

**Further information** The viscous consistency of Calpol Paediatric and Calpol Paediatric Sugar Free helps keep the medicine on the spoon and so makes it easier to administer.

Paracetamol does not cause the gastro-intestinal side-effects that may be seen after standard doses of aspirin.

70 ml and 140 ml bottles of Calpol Infant Suspension (120 mg Paracetamol BP/5 ml), and 140 ml bottles of Calpol Sugar Free Infant Suspension (120 mg Paracetamol BP/5 ml) are also available over the counter from pharmacies.

**Product licence numbers**

| | |
|---|---|
| Calpol Paediatric | 15513/0007 |
| Calpol Paediatric Sugar Free | 15513/0008 |

## DRAPOLENE* CREAM

**Presentation** Drapolene Cream is a pink, water-miscible preparation available in tubs containing 75 g, 150 g, 350 g or 500 g of cream. Drapolene Cream contains:

| | |
|---|---|
| Benzalkonium Chloride | 0.01% w/w |
| Cetrimide BP | 0.2% w/w |
| White Soft Paraffin | 10% w/w |
| Wool Fat (Purified lanolin) | 2% w/w |
| Cetyl Alcohol | 5% w/w |
| Polawax | 5% w/w |
| Chlorocresol | 0.1% w/w |
| Amaranth | 0.002% w/w |
| Purified Water | |

The components benzalkonium chloride and cetrimide are quaternary ammonium compounds used topically for their antiseptic and disinfectant properties. White Soft Paraffin, wool fat and cetyl alcohol are emollient, protective and hydrating. These properties are useful in dry skin conditions.

**Uses** Drapolene is indicated for the relief of nappy rash and for use as an adjunct to baby care hygiene for the prevention of nappy rash.

Drapolene is indicated for the relief of urinary dermatitis in adults, and as an adjunct to patient care hygiene for the prevention of urinary dermatitis.

Drapolene is indicated for the symptomatic relief of minor burns, limited sunburn and the effects of weather.

**Dosage and administration**
*Babies:* The nappy area should be washed then dried thoroughly at each change of nappy. Drapolene Cream should be applied, paying particular attention to folds in the skin.

*Adults:* The affected area (or the area of application) should be washed and dried thoroughly before applying Drapolene. Regular routine application is advised.

Drapolene should be applied as required for minor burns, sunburn and the effects of weather.

**Contra-indications, warnings, etc**
*Precautions:* For external use only. Keep out of the reach of children. It is inadvisable to apply Drapolene Cream to a baby or adult who has an established hypersensitivity to Benzalkonium chloride, Cetrimide or lanolin. Use should be discontinued if an allergic hypersensitivity reaction is suspected.

*Side and adverse effects:* Allergic hypersensitivity reactions may occur in individuals who are sensitive to one or several components of Drapolene Cream.

Hypersensitivity to lanolin is recognised but rare. In a few individuals, Benzalkonium chloride, used as a preservative in ophthalmic solutions, was associated with oedema and conjunctivitis. Dermatitis as a result of contact allergy to Benzalkonium chloride in plaster of Paris, has also been reported.

Hypersensitivity to Cetrimide is also known to occur, presenting as a localised contact dermatitis. In severe cases the rash may be generalised.

*Toxicity and treatment of overdosage:* There are no reports of adverse events resulting from excessive application or ingestion of Drapolene Cream..

**Pharmaceutical precautions** Store below 25°C.

**Legal category** GSL.

**Package quantities** Tubs of 75 g, 150 g, 350 g and 500 g.

**Further information** Nil

**Product licence number** 15513/0016

## LYCLEAR* CREME RINSE

**Presentation** Lyclear Creme Rinse contains 1% w/w Permethrin plus 20% w/w Isopropanol in a creme rinse base. It is orange in colour.

**Uses** Lyclear Creme Rinse is indicated for the treatment of infections with the head louse *Pediculus humanus capitis.*

**Dosage and administration**
*Adults and children 6 months of age and over:* Lyclear Creme Rinse should be used after hair has been washed with a mild proprietary shampoo and towelled dry. The bottle should be shaken thoroughly and enough Lyclear Creme Rinse applied to saturate the hair and scalp. Particular attention should be given to the areas behind the ears and at the nape of the neck.

Lyclear Creme Rinse should be left on the hair for 10 minutes before rinsing the hair thoroughly with water. The hair should then be dried in the usual way.

One bottle of Lyclear Creme Rinse is sufficient for shoulder-length hair of average thickness. More may be applied if required and, although no maximum dose has been defined, it is most unlikely that more than two bottles will be required for any one course of treatment.

97–99% of individuals with head lice are successfully treated with a single application of Lyclear Creme Rinse. Residual activity may persist for up to six weeks.

It is not necessary to remove dead eggs or nits except for cosmetic purposes. A fine-toothed comb may be used if desired.

*Use in the elderly:* Lyclear Creme Rinse is suitable for use in the elderly.

*Pharmacology:* Permethrin is rapidly absorbed across the insect cuticle. The principal physiological lesion is the induction of electrochemical abnormalities across the membranes of excitable cells, leading to sensory hyperexcitability, inco-ordination and prostration. When presented in an aqueous base the ovicidal activity of permethrin is increased by the addition of an alcohol.

*Pharmacokinetics:* Permethrin is rapidly metabolised by ester hydrolysis to inactive metabolites which are excreted primarily in the urine. The application of creme rinse to the hair of volunteers for the recommended application time resulted in extremely low or undetectable levels of permethrin metabolites in plasma and urine samples. *In vitro* studies have shown that permethrin levels on hair were not affected by chlorine in concentrations used in swimming pools.

**Contra-indications, warnings, etc**
*Contra-indications:* The use of Lyclear Creme Rinse is contra-indicated in individuals with a known hypersensitivity to the product, its components, other pyrethroids or pyrethrins.

*Precautions:* For external use only. Keep out of reach of children.

Nursing staff who routinely use Lyclear Creme Rinse may wish to wear gloves to avoid any possible irritation to the hands.

Children under 6 months of age should be treated on the advice of a doctor.

Neither Permethrin or Lyclear Creme Rinse are irritants to the eyes. However, should Lyclear Creme Rinse be accidentally introduced into the eyes, rinse immediately with plenty of water.

*Side- and adverse effects*: Lyclear Creme Rinse is generally well-tolerated with a low potential for inducing skin reactions. In a few individuals erythema, rash, and/or irritation of the scalp has been reported following application of the Creme Rinse, but as an infection with head lice is often associated with such scalp irritation it is difficult in most instances to determine the underlying cause.

If severe or prolonged signs and symptoms of scalp irritation, skin discomfort, or other undesirable effects occur in association with the use of Lyclear Cream Rinse it should be brought to the attention of a doctor or pharmacist.

*Use during pregnancy and lactation*: Reproduction studies have been performed in mice, rats and rabbits (200–400 mg/kg/day orally) and have revealed no evidence of impaired fertility or harm to the foetus due to Permethrin. There are however, only very limited data on the use of Permethrin in pregnant women. Because animal reproduction studies are not always predictive of the human response, treatment should be considered during pregnancy only if clearly needed.

Studies following oral administration of Permethrin in cattle have indicated that very low concentrations of Permethrin are excreted in milk. However it is not known whether Permethrin is excreted in human milk. Whilst it is unlikely that the concentrations of Permethrin in the milk will present any risk to the infant, consideration should be given to withholding treatment during nursing or temporarily discontinuing nursing.

*Drug interactions*: No interactions are known.

*Toxicity and treatment of overdosage*: There are no reports of overdosage with Lyclear Creme Rinse. On the basis of animal and human-volunteer studies, it is extremely unlikely, even with misuse or excessive application, that the amount of Permethrin needed to produce clinically–relevant toxic effects would be reached. The most likely symptoms and signs following repeated, excessive application would be hypersensitivity-type reactions.

Symptomatic treatment is indicated should hypersensitivity-type reactions occur.

Theoretically if swallowed by a small child, alcoholic intoxication may occur due to the Isopropanol content of Lyclear Creme Rinse.

In the event of accidental ingestion of the contents of a bottle by a child, a doctor should be consulted immediately. Gastric lavage should be considered within two hours of ingestion and management should relate to treatment of alcoholic intoxication.

**Pharmaceutical precautions**   Shake well before use. Store below 25°C. Protect from light. Keep out of the reach of children.

**Legal category**   P

**Package quantities**   Plastic bottle of 59 ml.

**Further information**   Permethrin is not affected by the chlorine in swimming baths, so normal swimming activities may continue after use. Lyclear Creme Rinse may be used as normal in asthmatics, however, contact your doctor or pharmacist before commencing treatment if you have any particular concerns.

**Product licence number** 15513/0019

## LYCLEAR* DERMAL CREAM

**Qualitative and quantitative composition**   Permethrin, Medical Grade 5.0% w/w (Cis/Trans Isomers 25/75).

**Pharmaceutical form**   Cream for topical application.

**Clinical particulars**

*Therapeutic indications*: Lyclear Dermal Cream is indicated for the treatment of scabies.

*Posology and method of administration*: Lyclear Dermal Cream is suitable for use by adults and children of 2 months of age and above. Lyclear Dermal Cream is also suitable for use by the elderly.

Lyclear Dermal Cream should be applied to clean, dry, cool skin. If the patient has taken a warm bath prior to treatment the skin should be allowed to cool before the cream is applied.

Lyclear Dermal Cream is a vanishing cream and when rubbed gently into the skin it will disappear. Therefore, there is no need to continue to apply cream to the skin until it remains detectable on the surface.

Older children should be supervised by an adult when applying the cream to ensure that a thorough treatment is administered.

The whole body should be washed thoroughly 8–12 hours after treatment.

*Use in adults and children over 2 months of age*: In view of the great individual variability in body area and skin types precise recommendations are not possible. For adults and children over 12 years of age up to one 30 g tube may be used as a single application. A few adults may need to use more than one tube to ensure total body coverage, but not more than two tubes (60 g in total) should be used for a single application. For children 12 years and under the following table indicates the approximate amount of cream to be used as a single application. These drug recommendations are only approximate and are intended to serve as a guide. (Recommendations are based on the use of a 30 g tube).

Children aged

| | |
|---|---|
| 2 months to 1 year | up to 1/8 of a tube |
| 1–5 years | up to 1/4 of a tube |
| 6–12 years | up to 1/2 of a tube |

In cases where the head, neck, scalp and ears are treated (see below) the dosage may be increased to ensure total body coverage.

In adults and children over 2 years of age Lyclear Dermal cream should be applied to the whole body excluding the head and paying particular attention to the areas between the fingers and toes, wrists, axillae, external genitalia, buttocks and under finger and toe nails. In women, the whole body application should include the breasts.

During the treatment period, Lyclear Dermal Cream should be re-applied to the hands if they are washed with soap and water.

Children between 2 months and 2 years should be treated under medical supervision. Lyclear Dermal Cream should be applied over the whole body as directed for adults and children over 2 years, but should include the palms, soles, face, neck, scalp and ears. Care must be taken to avoid the vicinity of the mouth where it could be licked off, and areas close to the eyes.

Approximately 90% of individuals are cured with a single application of cream. If necessary, a second application may be given not less than 7 days after the initial application, if there are no signs of the original lesions healing or if new lesions are present.

*Use in the elderly*: In the elderly Lyclear Dermal Cream should be used as directed for adults and children over 12 years but should also include the head, neck, scalp and ears. Care must be taken to avoid applying Lyclear Dermal Cream to areas close to the eyes.

*Contra-indications*: Lyclear Dermal Cream is contra-indicated in subjects with known hypersensitivity to the product, its components, other pyrethroids or pyrethrins.

*Special warnings and special precautions for use*: Lyclear Dermal Cream is for external use only and should be kept out of the reach of children.

Permethrin is not an eye irritant but contact of Lyclear Dermal Cream with the eyes should be avoided because the cream itself may cause marked irritation. In the event of inadvertent eye contamination, the affected area should be rinsed immediately with plenty of water or, if readily available, normal saline.

Nursing staff who routinely apply Lyclear Dermal Cream may wish to wear gloves to avoid any possible irritation to the hands.

There is an increasing body of data specifically relating to the use of Lyclear Dermal Cream for the treatment of scabies in the elderly and in view of these data it is considered that there is no need for any special precautions for use in this age group.

*Interaction with other medicaments and other forms of interaction*: No interactions are known. The treatment of eczematous-like reactions with corticosteroids should be withheld prior to treatment with Lyclear Dermal Cream, as there is a risk of exacerbating the scabies infestation by reducing the immune response to the mite. The likelihood of interactions between the two treatments leading to potentiated adverse reactions or reduced efficacy is, however, small.

*Pregnancy and lactation*: There are limited data on the use of Lyclear Dermal Cream in pregnancy which provide no indication of any risk to the foetus. Furthermore the amount of permethrin absorbed systemically following a whole body application is extremely low. Some permethrin may cross the placental barrier. The negative mutagenicity tests and the very low mammalian toxicity would suggest that any risk to the foetus following treatment with Lyclear Dermal Cream is minimal.

Studies, following oral administration of Permethrin in cattle have indicated that very low concentrations of Permethrin are excreted in milk. It is not known whether Permethrin is excreted in human breast milk. However because only extremely small amounts of Permethrin are absorbed systemically following treatment with Lyclear Dermal Cream and in theory only a very small percentage of this systemic Permethrin may pass into the breast milk, it is unlikely that the

concentrations of Permethrin in the milk will present any risk to the neonate/infant.

Reproduction studies in mice, rats and rabbits given oral dosage of 200 to 400 mg/kg bodyweight/day revealed no evidence of impaired fertility. In addition Permethrin did not show any adverse effects on the reproductive function of rats given an oral dosage of 180 mg/kg bodyweight/day in a three generation study.

There was no evidence of teratogenicity in reproduction studies in mice, rats and rabbits.

*Effects on ability to drive and use machines*: None known.

*Undesirable effects*: In scabies patients, skin discomfort, usually described as burning, stinging or tingling, occurs in a few individuals soon after Lyclear Dermal Cream is applied. This occurs more frequently in patients with severe scabies and is usually mild and transient.

Other transient signs and symptoms of irritation, including erythema, oedema, eczema, rash and pruritus which may follow the treatment of scabies with Lyclear Dermal Cream are generally considered to be part of the natural history of scabies.

In patients treated for scabies, itching may persist for up to 4 weeks post-treatment. This is generally regarded as due to an allergic reaction to the dead mites under the skin and is not necessarily indicative of a treatment failure.

*Overdose*: There are no reports of overdosage with Lyclear Dermal Cream. Application of a full tube of cream to a 2 month old would result in a dose of approximately 350 mg/kg bodyweight to the skin. It is unlikely that such a dose would cause overt signs of systemic toxicity even if 100% of the Permethrin was absorbed.

It is possible that excessive application of Lyclear Dermal Cream might result in localised adverse reactions or more severe skin reactions. Symptomatic treatment is indicated should hypersensitivity-type reactions occur.

In the event of accidental ingestion of the contents of a tube of Lyclear Dermal Cream by a child, gastric lavage should be considered if consultation is within 2 hours of ingestion.

**Pharmacological properties**

*Pharmacodynamic properties*: The principle physiological action in insects (lice) exposed to Permethrin is induction of electrochemical abnormalities across the membranes of excitable cells, leading to sensory hyperexcitability, inco-ordination and prostration. It is assumed that the mode of action against arachnids (mites) is similar.

*Pharmacokinetic properties*: Permethrin is rapidly metabolised in mammals by ester hydrolysis to inactive metabolites which are excreted primarily in the urine. The principal metabolites of Permethrin are detectable in the urine within hours of a whole body application of the cream to healthy volunteers or scabies patients. The highest levels of excretion are detectable within the first 48 hours, but very low levels of metabolite are still detectable in the urine of some individuals 28 days after treatment. The overall pattern of excretion indicates a mean of approximately 0.5% of applied Permethrin is absorbed during the first 48 hours.

*Preclinical safety data*: In vitro and in vivo genetic toxicity studies were all negative, revealing no potential for Permethrin to induce mutagenic changes.

In repeated long-term bioassays for carcinogenic potential performed in rats, no evidence of oncogenicity was observed. Similar studies in mice have shown species specific increases in pulmonary adenomas, a common benign tumour of mice of high spontaneous background incidence. In one of these studies, there was an increased incidence of benign liver adenomas and of pulmonary alveolar cell carcinomas only in female mice when Permethrin was given in their food at 1:5000 parts per million (approximately 750 mg/kg bodyweight/day) for two years. It is considered that these findings do not indicate a significant oncogenic potential for Permethrin in humans.

**Pharmaceutical particulars**

*List of excipients*:

| | |
|---|---|
| Fractionated coconut oil BP | 11.0% w/w |
| Glyceryl monostearate PhEur | 4.50% w/w |
| Macrogol (2) cetyl ether | 2.59% w/w |
| Cetomacrogol 1000 BP | 0.91% w/w |
| Isopropyl myristate BP | 1.0% w/w |
| Lanolin alcohols/liquid paraffin Mixture (amerchol 1-101) | 1.0% w/w |
| Butylated hydroxytoluene BP | 0.02% w/w |
| Glycerol PhEur | 2.0% w/w |
| Formaldehyde solution BP | 0.278% w/w |
| Carbomer 934p | 0.1% w/w |
| Sodium hydroxide BP | 0 034% w/w |
| Purified water PhEur to | 100.0% w/w |

*Incompatibilities*: None known.

*Shelf life:* 60 months.

*Special precautions for storage:* Store below 25°C. Do not freeze.

*Nature and contents of container:* Plastic foil laminate ointment tubes (30 g) with polyolefin screw caps.

*Instructions for use/handling:* Not applicable.

**Marketing authorisation number** 15513/0033

**Date of approval/revision of SPC** August 1996

**Legal category** P

## ORALDENE*

**Presentation** Oraldene contains 0.1% w/v hexetidine. It is a clear red solution.

**Uses** Oraldene is indicated for use in minor mouth infections including thrush, as an aid in the prevention and treatment of gingivitis and in the management of sore throat and recurrent aphthous ulcers. Oraldene is also of value in the alleviation of halitosis and pre and post dental surgery to aid decontamination of the oral cavity thereby aiding the healing process.

### Dosage and administration

*Adults and children 12 years and over:* Topical administration to the oral and pharyngeal cavity. Rinse the mouth or gargle with at least 15 ml of undiluted solution, two or three times a day. Do not swallow. Oraldene should not be diluted prior to use. Oraldene should not be swallowed in large quantities.

*Children aged 6 to 11 years:* As recommended for adults.

*Children under 6 years:* Not recommended.

*The elderly:* As recommended for adults.

*Hepatic/renal dysfunction:* Not applicable.

### Contra-indications, warnings, etc

*Contra-indications:* None known.

*Special warnings and special precautions for use:* None known.

*Interaction with other medicaments and other forms of interaction:* No interactions are known.

*Pregnancy and lactation:* No formal studies have been conducted in man. However, on the basis of animal studies and, in theory, the negligible systemic absorption it is considered highly unlikely that the use of Oraldene during pregnancy will present a risk to the foetus.

It is not known whether hexetidine is excreted in human breast milk, however, in view of the negligible amount of hexetidine which could be predicted to be systemically absorbed, it is unlikely that concentrations of hexetidine in the milk will present any risk to the neonate/infant.

*Effects on ability to drive and operate machinery:* No special comment–unlikely to produce an effect.

*Other undesirable effects:* Oraldene is generally very well-tolerated with a low potential for causing irritation, or sensitisation reactions. Prolonged use of Oraldene is also well-tolerated.

Patch testing with hexetidine containing ointment was negative for irritation or sensitisation potential.

In a few individuals mild irritation (described as sore mouth, burning or itching), of the tongue and/or buccal tissues has been reported. Other side effects which are reported very rarely include transient anaesthesia and taste impairment.

*Overdosage:*

*Signs and symptoms of overdosage:* Alcohol intoxication. There are no reports of overdosage with Oraldene. Hexetidine, at the strength present in Oraldene is non-toxic.

Acute alcoholic intoxication is extremely unlikely, however, it is theoretically possible that, if a massive dose were swallowed by a small child, alcoholic intoxication may occur due to the ethanol content. There is no evidence to suggest that repeated, excessive administration of hexetidine would lead to hypersensitivity-type reactions.

*Treatment of overdosage:* Treatment of overdose is symptomatic but rarely required. In the event of accidental ingestion of the contents of a bottle by a child, a doctor should be consulted immediately. Gastric lavage should be considered within two hours of ingestion and management should relate to treatment of alcoholic intoxication.

*Pharmacodynamics:* Hexetidine is a broad spectrum antimicrobial. It is active both *in vivo* and *in vitro*, against gram positive and negative bacterium, as well as yeasts (*Candida albicans*) and fungi. Oraldene against oral pathogens has been widely studied. Hexetidine has no known pharmacological effects in man.

*Pharmacokinetic properties:* Specific Pharmacodynamic studies have not been carried out on Oraldene in man.

The oral retention of hexetidine to mucous membranes and dental plaque has been observed. In studies using radiolabelled hexetidine it has been shown that retention on buccal tissues can extend to between 8 and 10 hours after a single oral rinse and in some cases hexetidine has been detected on oral tissues up to 65 hours post-treatment.

No absorption studies following the topical application of Oraldene have been performed in man.

*Pharmacokinetics in renal impairment:* There have been no specific studies of Oraldene or hexetidine in hepatic impairment.

*Pharmacokinetics in elderly:* There have been no specific studies of Oraldene or hexetidine in the elderly.

*Pre-clinical safety data:*

*Mutagenicity:* Hexetidine did not produce a significant increase in mutagenesis when studied in vitro using the standard Ames test.

*Carcinogenicity:* No specific Carcinogenicity studies using hexetidine have been performed.

*Teratogenicity:* No teratogenic effects were observed in New Zealand white rabbits orally dosed with 5, 10 and 20 mg hexetidine/kg/day from day 6 through day 18 of gestation.

A small number of does died as a result of the toxic effects of hexetidine, but no other clinical signs or behavioural changes were observed during the study.

Hexetidine was considered embryofetotoxic as manifest by a small number of abortions, a significant increase in the number of reabsorptions and post-implantation losses observed in the those does receiving 10 and 20 mg hexetidine/kg/day, and a significant reduction in foetal weight in the 20 mg/kg/day treatment group.

*Fertility:* Hexetidine administered orally, after mating, in New Zealand white rabbits had no apparent effect on fertility when compared to the control group.

**Pharmaceutical precautions** Store below 25°C. Protect from light. Shake well before use.

*Shelf life:* 2 years.

**Legal category** GSL.

**Package quantities** Oraldene is presented in clear 100 ml and 200 ml glass bottles, with white aluminium ROPP cap.

**Further information**

*List of excipients:* Polysorbate 80, citric acid, saccharin sodium, peppermint oil, anise oil, methyl salicylate, levomenthol, clove oil, eucalyptol, ethanol 96%, carmoisine (E122), Ponceau 4R (E124), purified water.

**Product licence number** 15513/0067

## SUDAFED* TABLETS AND ELIXIR

**Presentation** Each brownish red, biconvex, film coated tablet contains 60 mg Pseudoephedrine hydrochloride BP and is imprinted 'WELLCOME SUDAFED' on one side.

Each 5 ml of red elixir contains 30 mg Pseudoephedrine Hydrochloride BP and has a raspberry flavour.

**Uses** Sudafed is a decongestant of the mucous membranes of the upper respiratory tract, especially the nasal mucosa and sinuses, and is indicated for the symptomatic relief of conditions such as allergic rhinitis, vasomotor rhinitis, the common cold and influenza.

### Dosage and administration

*Adults and children over 12 years:* 1 tablet or 10 ml elixir every 4–6 hours up to 4 times a day.

*Children 6 to 12 years:* 5 ml elixir every 4–6 hours up to 4 times a day.

*2 to 5 years:* 2.5 ml elixir every 4–6 hours up to 4 times a day.

Sudafed Elixir may be diluted 1:1 (1 in 2) or 1:3 (1 in 4) with syrup BP. These dilutions are stable for 4 weeks if stored at 25°C.

*Use in the elderly:* There have been no specific studies of Sudafed in the elderly. Experience has indicated that normal adult dosage is appropriate.

*Hepatic dysfunction:* Caution should be exercised when administering Sudafed to patients with severe hepatic impairment.

*Renal dysfunction:* Caution should be exercised when administering Sudafed to patients with moderate to severe renal impairment.

*Pharmacology:* Pseudoephedrine has direct and indirect sympathomimetic activity and is an orally effective upper respiratory tract decongestant. Pseudoephedrine is substantially less potent than Ephedrine in producing both tachycardia and elevation in systolic blood pressure and considerably less potent in causing stimulation of the central nervous system.

### Contra-indications, warnings, etc

*Contra-indications:* Sudafed is contra-indicated in individuals with known hypersensitivity to the product or any of its components.

Sudafed is contra-indicated in individuals with severe hypertension or coronary artery disease.

Sudafed is contra-indicated in individuals who are taking or have taken monoamine oxidase inhibitors within the preceding two weeks. The concomitant use of Sudafed and this type of product may occasionally cause a rise in blood pressure.

*Precautions:* Although Sudafed has virtually no pressor effects in normotensive patients, Sudafed should be used with caution in patients suffering mild to moderate hypertension.

As with other sympathomimetic agents, Sudafed should be used with caution in patients with hypertension, heart disease, diabetes, hyperthyroidism, elevated intraocular pressure and prostatic enlargement.

Caution should be exercised when using the product in the presence of severe hepatic impairment or moderate to severe renal impairment (particularly if accompanied by cardiovascular disease).

*Interactions with other medicaments and other forms of interaction:* Concomitant use of Sudafed with tricyclic antidepressants, sympathomimetic agents (such as decongestants, appetite suppressants and amphetamine-like psychostimulants) or with monoamine oxidase inhibitors, which interferes with the catabolism of sympathomimetic amines, may occasionally cause a rise in blood pressure.

Because of its Pseudoephedrine content, Sudafed may partially reverse the hypotensive action of drugs which interfere with sympathetic activity including Bretylium, Bethanidine, Guanethidine, Debrisoquine, Methyldopa, alpha- and beta-adrenergic blocking agents.

*Side and adverse effects:* Serious adverse effects associated with the use of Pseudoephedrine are rare. Symptoms of central nervous system excitation may occur, including sleep disturbances and, rarely, hallucinations have been reported.

Skin rashes, with or without irritation, have occasionally been reported. Urinary retention has been reported occasionally in men receiving Pseudoephedrine; prostatic enlargement could have been an important predisposing factor.

*Use in pregnancy and lactation:* Although Pseudoephedrine has been in widespread use for many years without apparent ill consequence, there are no specific data on its use during pregnancy. Caution should therefore be exercised by balancing the potential benefit of treatment to the mother against any possible hazards to the developing foetus.

Systemic administration of Pseudoephedrine, up to 50 times the human daily dosage in rats and up to 35 times the human daily dosage in rabbits, did not produce teratogenic effects.

Pseudoephedrine is excreted in breast milk in small amounts but the effect of this on breast-fed infants is not known. It has been estimated that 0.5–0.7% of a single dose of Pseudoephedrine ingested by a mother will be excreted in the breast milk over 24 hours.

*Toxicity and treatment of overdosage:* As with other sympathomimetic agents, symptoms of overdosage include irritability, restlessness, tremor, convulsions, palpitations, hypertension and difficulty in micturition.

Necessary measures should be taken to maintain and support respiration and control convulsions. Gastric lavage should be performed if indicated. Catheterisation of the bladder may be necessary. If desired, the elimination of Pseudoephedrine can be accelerated by acid diuresis or by dialysis.

**Pharmaceutical precautions**

*Tablets:* Store below 30°C. Keep dry. Protect from light. *Elixir:* Store below 25°C. Protect from light.

**Legal category** P

**Package quantities** Sudafed Tablets: Container of 100 tablets. Pack containing a blister strip of 12 or 24 tablets. Sudafed Elixir: Bottles of 100 ml and 1 litre.

**Product licence numbers**

Tablets 15513/0024

Elixir 15513/0023.

## SUDAFED* PLUS TABLETS AND SYRUP

**Presentation** Each tablet contains 2.5 mg Triprolidine hydrochloride BP and 60 mg Pseudoephedrine hydrochloride BP. Scored and coded 'WELLCOME M2A'. White in colour.

Each 5 ml of clear, golden-yellow syrup contains 1.25 mg Triprolidine hydrochloride BP and 30 mg Pseudoephedrine hydrochloride BP, and has a pleasant flavour.

**Uses** Symptomatic relief of allergic rhinitis

**Dosage and administration**
*Adults and children over 12 years:* 1 tablet or 10 ml every 4–6 hours up to 4 times a day.

*Children 6 to 12 years:* 5 ml every 4–6 hours up to 4 times a day.

*2 to 5 years:* 2.5 ml every 4–6 hours up to 4 times a day.

*Use in the elderly:* No specific studies have been carried out in the elderly, but Triprolidine and Pseudoephedrine have been widely used in older people.

*Hepatic dysfunction:* Caution should be exercised when administering Sudafed Plus to patients with severe hepatic impairment.

*Renal dysfunction:* Caution should be exercised when administering Sudafed Plus to patients with moderate to severe renal impairment.

*Pharmacology:* Triprolidine provides symptomatic relief in conditions believed to depend wholly or partly upon the triggered release of histamine. It is a potent competitive histamine H1- receptor antagonist of the pyrrolidine class with mild central nervous system depressant properties which may cause drowsiness. Pseudoephedrine has direct and indirect sympathomimetic activity and is an effective upper respiratory decongestant. Pseudoephedrine is substantially less potent than ephedrine in producing both tachycardia and elevation of systolic blood pressure and considerably less potent in causing stimulation of the central nervous system.

**Contra-indications, warnings, etc**
*Contra-indications:* Sudafed Plus is contra-indicated in individuals with known hypersensitivity to Pseudoephedrine or Triprolidine.

Sudafed Plus is contra-indicated in patients who are taking or have taken monoamine oxidase inhibitors within the preceding two weeks. The concomitant use of Pseudoephedrine and this type of product may occasionally cause a rise in blood pressure

Sudafed Plus is contra-indicated in patients with severe hypertension or severe coronary artery disease.

*Precautions:* Sudafed Plus may cause drowsiness and impair performance in tests of auditory vigilance. Patients should not drive or operate machinery until they have determined their own response.

Although there are no objective data, users of Sudafed Plus should avoid the concomitant use of alcohol or other centrally acting sedatives.

Although Pseudoephedrine has virtually no pressor effects in normotensive patients, Sudafed Plus should be used with caution in patients suffering mild to moderate hypertension. As with other sympathomimetic agents, Sudafed Plus should be used with caution in patients with hypertension, heart disease, diabetes, hyperthyroidism, elevated intraocular pressure and prostatic enlargement. Sudafed Plus may cause drowsiness and impair performance in tests of auditory vigilance. There is individual variation in response to antihistamines.

Caution should be exercised when using the product in the presence of severe hepatic impairment or moderate or severe renal impairment (particularly if accompanied by cardiovascular disease).

There is insufficient information available to determine whether Triprolidine or Pseudoephedrine have mutagenic or carcinogenic potential.

*Interactions with other medicaments and other forms of interaction:* Although there is no objective data, users of Sudafed Plus should avoid concomitant use of alcohol or other centrally acting sedatives. Concomitant use of Sudafed Plus with tricyclic antidepressants, sympathomimetic agents (such as decongestants, appetite suppressants and amphetamine-like psychostimulants, or with monoamine oxidase inhibitors which interfere with sympathetic activity including Bretylium Bethanide, Guanethidine, Debrisoquine, Methyldopa, alpha- and beta-adrenergic blocking agents.

*Side-effects:* Central nervous system (CNS) excitation may occur, drowsiness being reported most frequently. Sleep disturbance and, rarely, hallucinations have been reported.

Skin rashes with or without irritation, tachycardia, dryness of mouth, nose and throat have occasionally been reported. Urinary retention has been reported occasionally in men receiving Pseudoephedrine; prostatic enlargement could have been an important predisposing factor.

*Use in pregnancy and lactation:* Although Pseudoephedrine has been in widespread use for many years without apparent ill-consequence, there are no specific data on their use during pregnancy. Caution should therefore be exercised by balancing the potential benefit of treatment to the mother against any possible hazards to the developing foetus.

In rats and rabbits systemic administration of Triprolidine up to 75 times the human dose did not produce teratogenic effects.

Systemic administration of Pseudoephedrine, up to 50 times the human dose in rats and up to 35 times the human dose in rabbits, did not produce teratogenic effects.

Pseudoephedrine is excreted in breast milk in small amounts but the effect of this on breast-fed infants is not known. It has been estimated that 0.5 to 0.7% of a single dose of Pseudoephedrine ingested by a mother will be excreted in the breast milk over 24 hours.

*Toxicity and treatment of overdosage:* The effects from acute toxicity from Sudafed Plus may include drowsiness, lethargy, dizziness, ataxia, weakness, hypotonicity, respiratory depression, dryness of the skin and mucous membranes, tachycardia, hypertension, hyperpyrexia, hyperactivity, irritability, convulsions and difficulty with micturition.

Necessary measures should be taken to maintain and support respiration and control convulsions. Gastric lavage should be performed up to 3 hours after ingestion if indicated. Catheterisation of the bladder may be necessary. If desired, the elimination of Pseudoephedrine can be accelerated by acid diuresis or by dialysis.

**Pharmaceutical precautions** Tablets: Store below 25°C in a dry place. Protect from light. Syrup: Store below 25°C. Protect from light.

**Legal category** P

**Package quantities** Sudafed Plus Tablets: Packs of 100 tablets. Sudafed Plus Syrup: Bottles of 100 ml and 1 litre.

**Product licence numbers**
Tablets　　　15513/0029
Syrup　　　　15513/0030

## ZOVIRAX* COLD SORE CREAM

**Presentation** Zovirax Cold Sore Cream is a smooth white cream and contains 5% w/w Aciclovir in a water miscible base containing propylene glycol. It is supplied in tubes containing 2 g.

**Uses** Zovirax Cold Sore Cream is indicated for the treatment of herpes simplex virus infections of the lips and face.

*Immunocompromised patients:* Zovirax Cold Sore Cream is not recommended for use in immunocompromised patients. Such patients must be advised to consult a physician concerning the treatment of any infection.

**Dosage and administration** Zovirax Cold Sore Cream should be applied five times daily at approximately four hourly intervals, omitting the night time application. It is important to start treatment as early as possible after the start of an infection, ideally during the prodromal period. Treatment should be continued for 5 days. If healing has not occurred, treatment may be continued for up to an additional 5 days. Patients should wash their hands before and after applying the cream, and avoid unnecessary rubbing of the lesions or touching them with a towel, to avoid aggravating or transferring the infection.

*Ocular herpes:* Zovirax Cold Sore Cream must not be used for treatment of ocular herpes infections.

*Genital herpes:* Zovirax Cold Sore Cream must not be used for treatment of genital herpes without prior medical advice.

*Use in the elderly:* No special comment.

*Pharmacology:* Aciclovir is an antiviral agent which is highly active *in vitro* against herpes simplex virus (HSV) types I and II. Toxicity to mammalian host cells is low.

Aciclovir is phosphorylated after entry into herpes infected cells to the active compound Aciclovir tri-

phosphate. The first step in this process is dependent on the presence of the HSV-coded thymidine kinase. Aciclovir triphosphate acts as an inhibitor of, and substrate for, the herpes-specified DNA polymerase, preventing further viral DNA synthesis without affecting normal cellular processes.

**Contra-indications, warnings, etc**
*Contra-indications:* Zovirax Cold Sore Cream is contra-indicated in patients known to be hypersensitive to Aciclovir or propylene glycol.

*Precautions:* Zovirax Cold Sore Cream should only be used on cold sores on the lips and face. It is not recommended for application to mucous membranes, such as in the mouth or eye. Particular care should be taken to avoid contact with the eye.

In severely immune-compromised patients (e.g. AIDS patients or bone marrow transplant recipients) oral dosing should be considered. The results of a wide range of mutagenicity tests *in vitro* and *in vivo* indicate that Aciclovir does not pose a genetic risk to man.

Aciclovir was not found to be carcinogenic in long term studies in the rat and the mouse. Largely reversible adverse effects on spermatogenesis in association with overall toxicity in rats and dogs have been reported only at systemic doses of Aciclovir greatly in excess of those employed therapeutically. Two-generation studies in mice did not reveal any effect of orally administered Aciclovir on fertility.

There is no experience of the effect of Zovirax Cold Sore Cream on human female fertility. Zovirax (Aciclovir) Tablets have been shown to have no definitive effect upon sperm count, morphology or motility in man.

*Side-effects:* Transient burning or stinging may follow application of Zovirax Cold Sore Cream in some patients. Mild drying or flaking of the skin has occurred in about 5% of patients. Erythema and itching have been reported in a small proportion of patients.

Contact dermatitis has been reported rarely following application. Where sensitivity tests have been conducted, the reactive substances have most often been shown to be components of the cream base rather than Aciclovir.

*Drug interactions:* Probenecid increases the mean half-life and area under the plasma concentration curve of systematically administered aciclovir. However, this is likely to be of little relevance to the topical application of Aciclovir.

*Use in pregnancy and lactation:* Systemic administration of Aciclovir in internationally accepted standard tests did not produce embryotoxic or teratogenic effects in rats, rabbits or mice.

In a non-standard test in rats, foetal abnormalities were observed, but only following such high subcutaneous doses that maternal toxicity was produced. The clinical relevance of these findings is uncertain.

Following oral administration of 200 mg Aciclovir five times a day, the drug has been detected in human breast milk at concentrations ranging from 0.6 to 4.1 times the corresponding plasma concentrations. These concentrations would potentially expose nursing infants to Aciclovir dosages of up to 0.3 mg/kg/day. The dosage received by a nursing infant following maternal use of Zovirax Cold Sore Cream would be insignificant.

*Toxicity and treatment of overdosage:* No untoward effects would be expected if the entire contents of a 2 g tube of Zovirax Cold Sore Cream containing 100 mg of Aciclovir were ingested orally. Oral doses of 800 mg five times daily (4 g per day), have been administered for seven days without adverse effects.

Single intravenous doses of up to 80 mg/kg have been inadvertently administered without adverse effects. Aciclovir is dialysable.

**Pharmaceutical precautions** Store below 25°C. Do not refrigerate.

**Legal category** P

**Package quantities** Tubes of 2 g.

**Further information** Patients should ensure that they avoid the potential of virus transmission, particularly when active lesions are present.

**Product licence number** 0003/0304
*Product licence holder:* The Wellcome Foundation Limited, Greenford, Middlesex, UB6 0NN.

*Trade Mark

# Wellcome UK
## The Wellcome Foundation Limited
## Stockley Park
## Middlesex
## UB11 1BT

THE QUEEN'S AWARD
FOR TECHNOLOGICAL ACHIEVEMENT TO THE
WELLCOME RESEARCH LABORATORIES
OF THE WELLCOME FOUNDATION LTD

THE QUEEN'S AWARD
FOR EXPORT ACHIEVEMENT

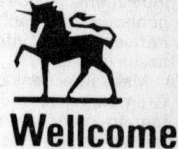
Wellcome

## BRETYLATE* INJECTION

**Qualitative and quantitative composition** Bretylium Tosylate HSE 5.0% w/v.

**Pharmaceutical form** Injection.

**Clinical particulars**

*Therapeutic indications:* Bretylate Injection is indicated primarily for the treatment of ventricular fibrillation and has often proved effective in ventricular fibrillation resistant to direct current countershock, with or without additional use of other anti-arrhythmic drugs such as lignocaine. Consideration should be given at an early stage to the use of Bretylate Injection in resuscitation from ventricular fibrillation.

Bretylate Injection is also indicated for ventricular tachycardia and has proved successful in restoring sinus rhythm where other anti-arrhythmics have failed.

Anti-arrhythmic effectiveness of Bretylate Injection has been demonstrated in:

- Acute myocardial infarction or chronic ischaemic heart disease;
- Ventricular fibrillation complicating severe hypothermia;
- and, ventricular arrhythmias following cardiac surgery.

*Posology and method of administration*

*Adults:* For ventricular fibrillation or ventricular tachycardia with associated haemodynamic disturbance, the minimal suggested initial dose is 5 mg/kg bodyweight administered undiluted by rapid intravenous injection. Resuscitation should be continued with further attempts at electrical cardioversion. The anti-fibrillatory effect in responding patients will usually be apparent within 5 to 15 minutes.

If no response is evident after 5 minutes, the dose of bretylium may be repeated or increased to 10 mg/kg by bolus injection. There is little experience with total dosages greater than 40 mg/kg, although with such dosage, adverse effects have not been apparent. In some patients the full anti-arrhythmic effect of Bretylate Injection may require several hours to develop.

If Bretylate Injection is to be used for less serious ventricular rhythm disturbances, it should be given more slowly and in diluted form to reduce the risk of vomiting.

*Dilution:* Bretylate Injection should be diluted with one of the recommended infusion fluids (see below) in the ratio of 1 part Bretylate Injection added to not less than 4 parts of infusion fluid, i.e. to give a final concentration of not more than 10 mg/ml.

When diluted with either Glucose Intravenous Infusion BP (5% w/v) or Sodium Chloride Intravenous Infusion BP (0.9% w/v) in the ratios recommended, Bretylate Injection is stable for up to 24 hours.

*Administration by infusion:* The diluted solution (prepared as recommended above) should be infused initially over a period of at least 8 minutes, preferably over 15 to 30 minutes, so as to provide a total dose of 5 to 10 mg/kg bodyweight. If the arrhythmia persists, this initial dose may be repeated at one to two hour intervals.

Once control of the arrhythmia has been established, maintenance therapy using the diluted solution can be given either as a continuous infusion at the rate of 1 to 2 mg per minute, or with a dosage of 5 to 10 mg/kg bodyweight infused over a period of 15 to 30 minutes every 6 hours.

*Intramuscular administration:* Bretylate Injection has been administered by intramuscular injection. A dose of 5 to 10 mg/kg bodyweight is recommended and this is administered undiluted at intervals of 6 to 8 hours. The site of injection should be varied on repeated injection and not more than 5 ml given into any one site.

*Dosage in renal impairment:* With repeated bolus doses or continuous intravenous infusions of Bretylate Injection in patients with impaired renal function, it is necessary to reduce the dosage in proportion to the reduction in creatinine clearance. The use of a nomogram is recommended for administration of Bretylate Injection as an infusion to patients with renal impairment, and the literature should be consulted for details.

The following table is intended to be used as a guide for administering Bretylate Injection by continuous infusion.

| Creatinine clearance (ml/minute) | Rate of infusion (mg/hour) |
|---|---|
| 40–<90 | 10–40 |
| 10–<40 | 2–10 |
| 1–<10 | 0.6–2 |

*Children:* Information on the use of Bretylate Injection as an anti-arrhythmic agent in children is sparse and there are no data on its use in doses in excess of 5 mg/kg/bodyweight.

*Use in the elderly:* The decision to treat with Bretylate rests on the balance between the expected anti-arrhythmic effect and the disadvantages of inappropriate dosing, taking into account the degree of reduction in cardiac and renal function.

*Monitoring:* It is recommended that heart rate and blood pressure are monitored during the administration of Bretylate.

*Route of administration:* Intravenous injection or infusion or intramuscular injection.

*Contra-indications:* Bretylate Injection is likely to cause a severe hypertensive response in patients with phaeochromocytoma and is therefore contra-indicated in this condition.

*Special warnings and precautions for use:* Bretylate Injection is not recommended as a prophylactic agent to prevent serious ventricular arrhythmias, but data are conflicting.

Orthostatic hypotension may occur 20 to 30 minutes after acute administration of Bretylate Injection, and in patients with poor cardiac function clinically significant hypotension may occur even in the supine position. An asymptomatic fall in blood pressure usually need not be treated unless the systolic pressure falls below 75 to 80 mm Hg. Hypotension may also be troublesome after cardiac surgery.

Hypovolaemia will augment the hypotensive response to Bretylate Injection. If the blood pressure does not respond to simple postural manoeuvres intravenous fluid should be given. Hypotension requiring such treatment may also respond to vasopressors. Hypersensitivity to infused catecholamines must, however, be anticipated and caution exercised.

Intramuscular administration of bretylium may cause tissue necrosis at the site of injection; this is rare if the site of injection is varied and the injected volume limited to 5 ml.

*Interaction with other medicaments and other forms of interaction:* Parenteral administration of bretylium may exacerbate ventricular tachyarrhythmias caused by digitalis toxicity.

Hypersensitivity to infused catecholamines would be expected after Bretylate administration because it blocks their normal mechanism of metabolism, namely neuronal uptake and subsequent degradation by monoamine oxidase. For this reason, when it is necessary to increase perfusion pressure to vital organs after bretylium-induced hypotension, noradrenaline or other sympathomimetics should only be given under expert supervision.

The hypotension resulting from adrenergic neurone blockade has been prevented by inhibition of the noradrenaline uptake mechanism, principally by tricyclic antidepressants.

*Pregnancy and lactation:* There is no reference to the use of bretylium as an anti-arrhythmic in pregnancy in the published literature.

No information is available on the excretion of bretylium into breast milk nor, therefore, on its effects on the breastfed infant.

*Effect on ability to drive and use machines:* None known.

*Undesirable effects:* The most common side effect following the administration of bretylium is hypotension, especially in patients whose initial haemodynamic state and/or cardiac function are poor.

Hypotension with increased pulmonary vascular resistance has also been reported.

Immediately after commencement of bretylium administration, more ectopic beats may arise, but this effect does not usually lead to serious problems.

Nausea and vomiting may occur following rapid intravenous administration of bretylium.

Moderate increases in blood pressure, heart rate and a positive inotropic effect may occur on commencement of bretylium administration.

*Overdose:* Bretylium overdose has been reported in a patient with recurrent ventricular fibrillation and tachycardia who was inadvertently given an intravenous bolus of 2 g (approximately 30 mg/kg bodyweight). The authors reported ultimately successful control of the ventricular tachyarrhythmias but the patient exhibited marked hypertension with peak blood pressure of 310/90 mm Hg, followed within an hour or so by marked hypotension refractory to intravenous dobutamine and volume-expansion therapy.

Bretylate can be eliminated by haemodialysis.

**Pharmacological properties**

*Pharmacodynamic properties:* Bretylium is a Class III anti-arrhythmic agent. It may produce pharmacological defibrillation, but more usually it facilitates electrical conversion to sinus rhythm in patients with ventricular fibrillation.

Acute administration of bretylium in both animals and man leads to a biphasic cardiovascular response. Monitoring of heart rate and blood pressure is therefore recommended. An initial release or noradrenaline from adrenergic nerve endings is accompanied by an acute rise in systemic arterial pressure and heart rate, followed within 20 to 30 minutes by reductions in vascular resistance, systemic arterial pressure and heart rate. The hypotension caused by Bretylate is orthostatic and was found to occur rarely in recumbent patients with acute myocardial infarction receiving the drug in a coronary care unit.

*Pharmacokinetic properties:* The anti-arrhythmic effects of a single dose of bretylium last for up to 12 hours. After a single intravenous dose bretylium appears to be eliminated from serum with an elimination half-life of about 13.5 hours. Apart from the particular effect of the drug on ventricular fibrillation, which seems to be exerted within 5 to 15 minutes of initial intravenous bolus administration, the anti-arrhythmic effects of bretylium seem to be related to tissue concentrations rather than serum or plasma concentrations of the drug and the latter are therefore probably not useful indicators during acute treatment.

*Preclinical safety data:* There are no preclinical data of relevance to the prescriber which are additional to that in other sections of the SPC.

**Pharmaceutical particulars**

*List of excipients:* Water for Injections PhEur.

*Incompatibilities:* None known.

*Shelf life:* 60 months.

*Special precautions for storage:* Store below 25°C. Do not freeze. Protect from light.

*Nature and contents of container* Neutral glass ampoules 2 ml and 10 ml. Nominal fill volume. Pack sizes: 2, 10 ml.

*Instructions for use/handling:* Not applicable.

**Marketing authorisation number** 0003/0038R.

**Date of approval/revision of SPC** February 1997.

**Legal category** POM.

## CEFIZOX* INJECTION

**Presentation** Vials containing 1 g of ceftizoxime as its sterile sodium salt. Ceftizoxime sodium is a white to pale yellow crystalline powder. For each gram of ceftizoxime there is approximately 60 mg (2.6 mmol) of sodium.

**Uses** Broad-spectrum, bactericidal, cephalosporin antibiotic indicated for the treatment of infections either before the infecting organism has been identified, or when caused by bacteria of known sensitivity. Indications include lower respiratory tract infections, genito-urinary tract infections including gonorrhoea, intra-abdominal infections, septicaemia, skin and soft tissue infections.

Many infections caused by aerobic and anaerobic, Gram-negative and Gram-positive organisms resistant to other cephalosporins, aminoglycosides, or penicillins, have responded to treatment with Cefizox. Cefizox has been effective in the treatment of seriously ill, immunocompromised patients e.g. those with neutropenia and granulocytopenia.

*Bacteriology:* Cefizox is active *in vitro* against a wide range of Gram-positive and Gram-negative organisms. These include the following:

*Gram-positive aerobes – staphylococci including Staph. pyogenes* and *Staph. epidermidis*, streptococci including *Strep. pneumoniae* and *Strep. pyogenes*, *Corynebacterium diphtheriae*. Most strains of enterococci are resistant.

*Gram-negative aerobes – Esch. coli,* Klebsiella spp., Proteus spp, both indole positive and negative, Serratia spp, Enterobacter spp, Providencia spp, many strains of Pseudomonas spp., Citrobacter spp., *Haemophilus influenzae* including ampicillin-resistant strains, Neisseria spp including β-lactamase-producing strains, Salmonella spp, Shigella spp, *Aeromonas hydrophila, Yersinia enterocolitica.*

*Anaerobes*– Bacteroides spp. including many, but not all strains of *B.fragilis.*, Peptococcus spp., Eubacterium spp., Clostridium spp.

Cefizox is stable to a broad spectrum of β-lactamases produced by both aerobic and anaerobic organisms.

**Dosage and administration** Cefizox may be given by slow intravenous injection, by continuous or intermittent intravenous infusion or by deep intramuscular injection. Dosage and route of administration should be determined by the condition of the patient, severity of the infection and susceptibility of the causative organisms.

*General guidelines: Adults:*

| Type of infection | Dosage | Route |
|---|---|---|
| Urinary tract | 0.5–1 g 12–hourly | i.m. or i.v. |
| Gonorrhoea | 1 g single dose | i.m. |
| Other infections | 1–2 g 8–12 hourly | i.m.* or i.v. |
| Severe or life-threatening infections | 2–3 g 8–hourly | i.m.* or i.v. |

* When administering 2 g intramuscularly, the dose should be divided and given in different large muscle masses.

Dosages in excess of 4 g daily are rarely necessary but, exceptionally, dosages up to 8 g per day have been given and were well tolerated.

*Children over the age of 3 months:* 30 to 60 mg/kg bodyweight/day in 2 to 4 divided doses, increased in severe or life-threatening infections to 100 to 150 mg/kg bodyweight/day. The total dose should not exceed the adult dose.

*Children under the age of 3 months:* There are insufficient data to recommend the use of Cefizox.

*Dosage in renal impairment:* Modification of dosage is necessary in patients with impaired renal function. For an adult, following an initial loading dose of 500 mg to 1.0 g, i.m. or i.v., the maintenance dosing schedule shown below should be followed (no data are available for children):

| *Creatinine clearance ml/min.* | *Less severe infections* | *Severe or life-threatening infections* |
|---|---|---|
| 50–79 | 500 mg 8–hourly | 0.75–1.5 g 8–hourly |
| 5–49 | 250-500 mg 12–hourly | 0.5–1.0 g 12–hourly |
| 0–4 (dialysis patients) | 500 mg 48–hourly or 250 mg 24–hourly | 0.5–1.0 g 48–hourly or 0.5 g 24–hourly |

In patients undergoing haemodialysis, no additional supplemental dosing is required following haemodialysis; however, dosing should be timed so that the patient receives the dose (according to the table above), at the end of the dialysis.

*Preparation of parenteral solutions:* Reconstitute with 3 ml Water for Injections BP. Shake well. Further dilutions may be used. See '*Administration*'.

These solutions are stable for 8 hours at 25°C and for 24 hours at 5°C. When freshly reconstituted, Cefizox is a colourless to pale yellow solution with a pH of 6.0 to 8.0. Reconstituted solutions may discolour. Yellow discoloration will not alter potency or therapeutic efficacy. Discard solution if markedly discoloured.

*Administration: i.m. injection:* Inject deep within the body of a relatively large muscle. When administering 2 g, the dose should be divided and given in different large muscle masses. For intramuscular injection, Cefizox may be diluted with 0.5% lignocaine.

*i.v. injection:* Inject slowly over 3 to 5 mins. either directly or *via* the tubing of an established intravenous infusion (see below).

*i.v. infusion:* For intermittent or continuous infusion, dilute Cefizox reconstituted with Water for Injections BP, or Sodium Chloride Injection BP in 50 to 100 ml of one of the following solutions:

Glucose Intravenous Infusion BP (5% w/v and 10% w/v)
Sodium Chloride Intravenous Infusion BP
Sodium Chloride and Glucose Intravenous Infusion BP (0.18% and 4% w/v, 0.45% or 0.9% and 5% w/v)
Compound Sodium Chloride Injection BPC 1959 (Ringer's Solution for Injection)
Compound Sodium Lactate Intravenous Infusion BP.

Cefizox in these fluids is stable for 8 hours at 25°C and for 24 hours at 5°C.

*Use in the elderly:* It is recommended that the dose is reduced even though the serum creatinine level shows a normal value. In the presence of renal impairment doses should be reduced according to the table above, on the basis of creatinine clearance values.

**Contra-indications, warnings, etc**

*Contra-indications:* Hypersensitivity to cephalosporin antibiotics.

*Precautions:* Cefizox should be given cautiously to penicillin-sensitive patients. Although cephalosporin antibiotics may usually be given safely to such patients, cross reactions have been reported. Special care is required in patients who have had an anaphylactic reaction to penicillin.

Patients with impaired renal function– see *Dosage and administration.*

Cefizox has not been shown to alter renal function, but renal status should be monitored, especially in seriously ill patients receiving maximum dose therapy and co-administration of aminoglycoside antibiotics. Although the occurrence has not been reported with Cefizox, nephrotoxicity has been reported following concomitant administration of other cephalosporins and aminoglycosides.

As with any antibiotic, prolonged use may result in overgrowth of non-susceptible organisms.

*Side- and adverse effects:* Cefizox is generally well tolerated. The most common adverse reactions have been local, following i.m. or i.v. injection. These include burning, cellulitis, pain, induration, tenderness, paraesthesia and phlebitis. Other adverse reactions include hypersensitivity reactions (rash, pruritus, fever), gastro-intestinal disturbance (diarrhoea, nausea and vomiting), vaginitis, transient eosinophilia, and thrombocytosis. Neutropenia, leucopenia and thrombocytopenia have been reported rarely. Some individuals have developed a positive Coombs' test. Transient elevation in SGOT, SGPT, alkaline phosphatase, BUN and serum creatinine have occasionally been observed.

*Use in pregnancy and lactation:* Animal studies have not revealed evidence of an adverse effect on the developing fetus but there are no data in pregnant women. Thus, the benefit of using Cefizox in pregnancy should be weighed against the possible hazard. Ceftizoxime is excreted in human milk in low concentrations. Caution should therefore be exercised if Cefizox is administered to a nursing mother.

*Toxicity:* None has been reported.

*Treatment of overdosage:* Not applicable.

**Pharmaceutical precautions** Store below 25°C. Protect from light.

**Legal category** POM

**Package quantities** Single vials.

**Further information** Ceftizoxime is not metabolised and is excreted virtually unchanged by the kidneys within 24 hours, thus providing high urinary concentrations. It passes readily into various body fluids and tissues including those of the full-term fetus.

*Interference with laboratory tests:* A false-positive reaction to glucose may occur with reducing substances but not with the use of specific glucose oxidase methods.

**Product licence number** 0003/0175

## CICATRIN* POWDER
## CICATRIN* CREAM

**Presentation** Each gram of powder/cream contains:

| | |
|---|---|
| Neomycin Sulphate BP | 3,300 units |
| Zinc Bacitracin BP | 250 units |
| l-Cysteine | 2 mg |
| Glycine | 10 mg |
| dl-Threonine | 1 mg |

**Uses** Topical broad-spectrum antibacterial. Super ficial bacterial infection of skin, such as impetigc varicose ulcers, pressure sores, trophic ulcers an burns.

**Dosage and administration** *Adults:* Before use, th area for application should be cleaned gently. Debri such as pus or crusts should be removed from th affected area.

A light dusting of the powder or thin film of th cream should be applied to the affected area up t three times/day, depending on the clinical conditior Treatment should not be continued for more than days without medical supervision. See *Contra indications, warnings, etc.*

*Children:* The adult dose is suitable for use in olde children, however in infants dosage should b reduced.

A possibility of increased absorption exists in ver young children, thus Cicatrin Cream and Powder ar not recommended for use in neonates.

*Use in the elderly:* No specific studies have bee carried out in the elderly. However, Cicatrin Crear and Powder are suitable for use in the elderly (se *Dosage in renal impairment* and *Precautions an warnings*).

*Dosage in renal impairment:* Dosage should b reduced in patients with reduced renal function (se *Precautions and warnings*).

**Contra-indications, warnings, etc**

*Contra-indications:* The use of Cicatrin Cream c Powder is contra-indicated in patients who hav demonstrated allergic hypersensitivity to the produ or any of its constituents, or to cross-sensitisir substances such as framycetin, kanamycin, gent micin and other related antibiotics.

The use of Cicatrin Cream or Powder is contr indicated in circumstances where significant system absorption could occur, e.g. application of larg amounts, treatment of large areas or chronic wound or prolonged treatment.

The presence of pre-existing nerve deafness is contra-indication to the use of Cicatrin Cream an Powder in circumstances in which significant system absorption could occur.

Cicatrin Cream or Powder should not be used c pre-term infants and are not recommended for use neonates.

Cicatrin Cream or Powder should not be applied the eyes.

*Precautions:* Caution should be exercised so that th recommended dosage is not exceeded (see *Dosag and administration* and *Contra-indications*).

Following significant systemic absorption, amin glycosides such as neomycin can cause irreversib ototoxicity (and exacerbate existing partial nerv deafness); both neomycin sulphate and bacitracin zi have nephrotoxic potential.

After a treatment course, administration should n be repeated for at least three months.

In neonates and infants, absorption by immatu skin may be enhanced and renal function may immature (see *Contra-indications*).

In renal impairment the plasma clearance of ne mycin is reduced, this is associated with an increas risk of ototoxicity; therefore, a reduction in do should be made that relates to the degree of rer impairment.

As with other antibacterial preparations, prolong use may result in overgrowth by non-susceptib organisms, including fungi.

Concurrent administration of other amin glycosides is not recommended.

*Mutagenicity:* There is insufficient informati available to determine whether the active ingredier have mutagenic potential.

*Carcinogenicity:* There is insufficient informati available to determine whether the active ingredier have carcinogenic potential.

*Teratogenicity:* There is insufficient informati available to determine whether the active ingredie have teratogenic potential.

Neomycin present in maternal blood can cross t placenta and may give rise to a theoretical risk of fe ototoxicity.

*Fertility:* There is insufficient information availat to determine whether any of the active ingredie can affect fertility.

*Side- and adverse effects:* The incidence of allerg hypersensitivity to neomycin sulphate in the gene population is low. However, there is an increas incidence of sensitivity to neomycin in certain select groups of patients in dermatological practi particularly those with venous stasis eczema a ulceration.

Allergic hypersensitivity to neomycin following topical application may manifest itself as a reddening and scaling of the affected skin, as an eczematous exacerbation of the lesion, or as a failure of the lesion to heal.

Allergic hypersensitivity, following topical application of bacitracin zinc has been reported but is rare.

Anaphylactic reactions following the topical administration of bacitracin zinc have been reported but are rare.

*Drug interactions:* Following significant systemic absorption, neomycin sulphate can intensify and prolong the respiratory depressant effect of neuro-muscular blocking agents.

*Use in pregnancy and lactation:* There is little information to demonstrate the possible effect of topically applied neomycin in pregnancy and lactation, therefore the use of Cicatrin is not recommended.

No information is available regarding the excretion of the active ingredients in human milk.

*Toxicity and treatment of overdosage:* No specific symptoms or signs have been associated with excessive use of Cicatrin Powder or Cream. However, consideration should be given to significant systemic absorption (see *Precautions and warnings*).

Use of the product should be stopped and the patient's general status, hearing acuity, renal and neuromuscular functions should be monitored. Blood levels of neomycin sulphate and bacitracin zinc should be determined, and haemodialysis may reduce the serum level of neomycin sulphate.

**Pharmaceutical precautions** Store below 25°C. Keep dry.

**Legal category** POM

**Package quantities** *Cicatrin Powder:* Puffer packs of 15 g (OP) and 50 g (OP). *Cicatrin Cream:* Tubes of 15 g (OP) and 30 g (OP).

**Further information** Cicatrin Powder should not be diluted.

**Product licence numbers**
Cicatrin Powder: 0003/5081
Cicatrin Cream: 0003/5082

# DIGIBIND*
## Digoxin-specific antibody fragments (Fab)

**Presentation** Each vial of Digibind contains a sterile, lyophilised, crystalline off-white powder, comprising 38 mg of antigen-binding fragments (Fab) derived from specific anti-digoxin antibodies raised in sheep; approximately 75 mg Sorbitol BP and approximately 28 mg Sodium Chloride BP.

**Uses** Digibind is indicated for the treatment of known or strongly suspected digoxin or digitoxin toxicity, where measures beyond the withdrawal of the digitalis glycoside and correction of any serum electrolyte abnormality are felt to be necessary.

## Dosage and administration
*Dosage:* The dosage of Digibind varies according to the amount of digoxin (or digitoxin) to be neutralised. The average dose used during clinical testing was 10 vials. When determining the dose for Digibind, the following guidelines should be considered:

Dosage estimates are based on a steady-state volume of distribution of 5 l/kg for digoxin (0.5 l/kg for digitoxin) to convert serum digitalis concentration to the amount of digitalis in the body. These volumes are population averages and vary widely among individuals. Many patients may require higher doses for complete neutralisation. Doses should ordinarily be rounded up to the next whole vial.

Erroneous calculations may result from inaccurate estimates of the amount of digitalis ingested or absorbed or from non steady-state serum digitalis concentrations. Inaccurate serum digitalis concentration measurements are a possible source of error; this is especially so for very high values, since most digoxin assay kits are not designed to measure values above 5 nanogram/ml.

If, after several hours, toxicity has not adequately reversed or appears to recur, re-administration of Digibind at a dose guided by clinical judgement may be required.

*Acute ingestion of unknown amount of glycoside: Adults and children over 20 kg:* If a patient presents with potentially life-threatening digitalis toxicity after acute ingestion of an unknown amount of digoxin or digitoxin, and neither a serum digoxin concentration nor an estimate of the ingested amount is available, 10 vials of Digibind can be administered. This amount will be adequate to treat most life-threatening ingestions in adults and large children.

As an alternative, the physician may consider administering 10 vials of Digibind, observing the patient's response, and following with an additional 10 vials if clinically indicated.

*Infants and children ≤ 20 kg:* In infants and small children (≤ 20 kg) with potentially life-threatening digitalis toxicity after acute ingestion of an unknown amount of digoxin or digitoxin, when neither a serum concentration nor an estimate of the ingested amount is available, clinical judgement must be exercised to estimate an appropriate number of vials of Digibind to administer.

This estimate should be based on the maximum likely total body load of glycoside and the neutralising capacity of Digibind (one vial of Digibind per 0.5 mg of digoxin or digitoxin). It is important to monitor for volume overload during administration of Digibind.

*Acute ingestion of known amount of glycoside:* Each vial of Digibind contains 38 mg of purified digoxin-specific Fab fragments which will bind approximately 0.5 mg of digoxin. Thus one can calculate the total number of vials required by dividing the total digitalis body load in mg by 0.5 (see Formula 1).

Formula 1

$$\text{Dose (in number of vials)} = \frac{\text{Total body load (mg)}}{0.5}$$

For toxicity from an acute ingestion, total body load in milligrams will be approximately equal to the amount ingested in milligrams for digitoxin, or the amount ingested in milligrams multiplied by 0.80 (to account for incomplete absorption) for digoxin. Table 1 gives Digibind doses based on an estimate of the number of digoxin tablets (0.25 mg) ingested as a single dose and is applicable to children or adults.

TABLE 1 *Approximate Digibind Dose for Reversal of a Single Large Digoxin Overdose*

| Number of digoxin tablets* | Digibind Dose (number of vials) |
|---|---|
| 25 | 10 |
| 50 | 20 |
| 75 | 30 |
| 100 | 40 |
| 150 | 60 |
| 200 | 80 |

* 0.25 mg tablets with 80% bioavailability.

*Toxicity during chronic therapy: Adults and children over 20 kg:* In adults and children over 20 kg with digitalis toxicity resulting from chronic digoxin or digitoxin therapy and for whom a steady-state serum concentration is not available, a dose of 6 vials of Digibind will usually be adequate to reverse toxicity.

Table 2 (see below) gives dosage estimates in number of vials for adult patients for whom a steady-state serum digoxin concentration is known. The Digibind dose (in number of vials) represented in Table 2 can be approximated using the following formula:

Formula 2

Dose (in number of vials)
$$= \frac{(\text{serum digoxin concentration in ng/ml} \times \text{weight in kg})}{100}$$

In patients for whom a steady-state serum digoxin concentration is known the Digibind dose (in number of vials) can be approximated using the following formula:

Formula 3

Dose (in number of vials)
$$= \frac{\text{serum digitoxin concentration in ng/ml} \times \text{weight in kg}}{1000}$$

*Infants and children ≤ 20 kg:* In infants and small children with toxicity resulting from chronic digoxin or digitoxin therapy and for whom a steady-state serum concentration is not available, a dose of one vial of Digibind will usually suffice.

Clinical experience in children has indicated that the calculation of dose of Digibind from steady-state serum digoxin concentration may be carried out as for adults.

Table 3 gives dosage estimates in milligrams for infants and small children based on the steady-state serum digoxin concentration. The Digibind dose represented in Table 3 can be estimated by multiplying the dose (in number of vials) calculated from Formula 2 by the amount of Digibind contained in a vial (38 mg/vial).

Formula 4

Dose (in mg) = 38 x dose (in number of vials)

For very small doses, it may be necessary to dilute the reconstituted vial with sterile isotonic saline to achieve a concentration of 1 mg/ml, and to administer the dose with a tuberculin syringe.

*Use in the elderly:* Clinical experience has indicated that Digibind is effective and that calculation of dose may be carried out as for adults.

*Use in renal impairment:* See *Precautions*.

*Administration:* The contents of each vial to be used should be dissolved in 4 ml of sterile Water for Injection BP, by gentle mixing, thus producing an approximately isosmotic solution with a protein concentration of between 8.5 and 10.5 mg/ml. This may be diluted further to any convenient volume with sterile saline suitable for infusion.

The final solution of Digibind should be infused intravenously over a 30 minute period. Infusion through a 0.22 micron membrane filter is recommended to remove any incompletely dissolved aggregates of Digibind. If cardiac arrest seems imminent, Digibind can be given as a bolus intravenous injection.

*Pharmacology:* The affinity constant ($K_D$) of Fab for digoxin is high ($10^{11}M^{-1}$) and greater than that of digoxin for its receptor (Na-K ATPase). The affinity constant of Fab for digitoxin is also high (fifteen fold lower than for digoxin). Digoxin and digitoxin are therefore attracted away from the receptor on heart tissue (and presumably other tissues as well, though this has not been studied) and their rate of elimination is changed from that governed by the kinetics of receptor binding to that governed by the kinetics of access and elimination of Fab.

In dogs, anti-digoxin Fab reverses arrhythmic manifestations of digoxin toxicity much more quickly than does IgG. There is a suggestion that reversal of inotropy with Fab lags behind reversal of cardiac electrophysiological effects.

The plasma elimination (β) half-life of ovine digoxin-specific Fab in the baboon is 9 to 13 h and that of the parent IgG antibody is 61h. The total volume of distribution of Digibind in the baboon appears to be about 9 times greater than that of IgG and more ready diffusion of the smaller moiety sufficiently accounts for this.

About 93% of radioactively labelled Fab, injected into baboons, was recovered in the urine within 24h and the corresponding amount of recoverable

TABLE 2: *Adult Dose Estimate of Digibind (in number of vials) from Steady-State Serum Digoxin Concentration*

| Patient Weight (kg) | Serum Digoxin Concentration (ng/ml) | | | | | | |
|---|---|---|---|---|---|---|---|
| | 1 | 2 | 4 | 8 | 12 | 16 | 20 |
| 40 | 0.5ᵛ | 1ᵛ | 2ᵛ | 3ᵛ | 5ᵛ | 7ᵛ | 8ᵛ |
| 60 | 0.5ᵛ | 1ᵛ | 3ᵛ | 5ᵛ | 7ᵛ | 10ᵛ | 12ᵛ |
| 70 | 1ᵛ | 2ᵛ | 3ᵛ | 6ᵛ | 9ᵛ | 11ᵛ | 14ᵛ |
| 80 | 1ᵛ | 2ᵛ | 3ᵛ | 7ᵛ | 10ᵛ | 13ᵛ | 16ᵛ |
| 100 | 1ᵛ | 2ᵛ | 4ᵛ | 8ᵛ | 12ᵛ | 16ᵛ | 20ᵛ |

ᵛ=vials

TABLE 3: *Infants and Small Children Dose Estimates of Digibind (in mg) from Steady-State Serum Digoxin Concentration*

| Patient Weight (kg) | Serum Digoxin Concentration (ng/ml) | | | | | | |
|---|---|---|---|---|---|---|---|
| | 1 | 2 | 4 | 8 | 12 | 16 | 20 |
| 1 | 0.4 mg* | 1 mg* | 1.5 mg* | 3 mg | 5 mg | 6 mg | 8 mg |
| 3 | 1 mg* | 2 mg* | 5 mg | 9 mg | 14 mg | 18 mg | 23 mg |
| 5 | 2 mg* | 4 mg | 8 mg | 15 mg | 23 mg | 30 mg | 38 mg |
| 10 | 4 mg | 8 mg | 15 mg | 30 mg | 46 mg | 61 mg | 76 mg |
| 20 | 8 mg | 15 mg | 30 mg | 61 mg | 91 mg | 122 mg | 152 mg |

* Dilution of reconstituted vial to 1 mg/ml may be desirable.

digoxin-specific IgG was less than 1%. Much of the urinary Fab was not intact; after glomerular filtration, low molecular weight proteins are taken into proximal renal tubular cells and catabolised.

Corresponding information on human patients is sparse, but the close relationship of therapeutic performance to predictions suggest that the animal data will be helpful. The human plasma elimination half-life after intravenous administration of Digibind is about l6 to 20h with good renal function.

Ordinarily, following administration of Digibind, improvements in signs and symptoms begin within 30 minutes.

### Contra-indications, warnings, etc
*Contra-indications:* None known.

*Precautions:* Failure to respond to Digibind raises the possibility that the clinical problem is not caused by digitalis intoxication. If there is no response to an adequate dose of Digibind, the diagnosis of digitalis toxicity should be questioned.

Although allergic reactions have been reported rarely, the possibility of anaphylactic, hypersensitive or febrile reactions should be borne in mind. The likelihood of an allergic reaction is distinctly greater where there is a history of allergy to antibiotics or asthma. Since papain is used to cleave the whole antibody into Fab and Fc fragments, and traces of papain or inactivated papain residues may be present in Digibind, patients with known allergies to papain, chymopapain or other papaya extracts would be at particular risk, as would those allergic to ovine proteins. However, as the Fab fragment of the antibody lacks the antigenic determinants of the Fc fragment it should present less of an immunogenic threat to patients than does an intact immunoglobulin molecule.

Many patients with mild or moderate renal dysfunction and some with severe renal dysfunction have been treated successfully with Digibind. There has been no evidence that administration of Digibind to patients with renal dysfunction will exacerbate that dysfunction; the dominant pattern of serial serum creatinine measurements has been one of stable or improved renal function after Digibind administration. The time course and general pattern of therapeutic effect have not been different in patients with severe renal dysfunction, although excretion of the Fab-digoxin complexes from the body is slowed in this situation. A theoretical possibility exists that digoxin could be released after some days from Fab-digoxin complexes which remained in the circulation because their excretion was prevented by renal failure. However, this phenomenon has proved to be rare.

Patients previously dependent on the inotropism of digoxin may develop signs of heart failure when treated with Digibind. After successful management of poisoning, digoxin has had to be reinstituted in some cases. If deemed absolutely necessary, additional inotropic support can be obtained from a non-glycoside inotropic drug such as dopamine or dobutamine, but caution is required as catecholamines and catecholamine analogues can aggravate arrhythmias caused by cardiac glycosides.

Parenteral drug products should be inspected visually for particulate matter and discoloration prior to administration, whenever solution and container permit.

*Monitoring and laboratory tests:* Patients should have continuous electrocardiographic monitoring during and for at least 24 hours after administration of Digibind.

Presence of the exogenous antibody fragments will interfere with radioimmunoassay measurements of digoxin.

The total serum digoxin concentration may rise precipitously following administration of Digibind, but this will be almost entirely bound to the Fab fragment and therefore not able to react with receptors in the body.

Serum potassium concentrations should be followed carefully. Since severe digitalis intoxication can cause life-threatening elevation in serum potassium concentration by shifting it from within the cells. When the effect of digitalis is reversed by Digibind, potassium returns to the cell causing the serum potassium concentrations to fall. It is possible for there to be a total body deficit of potassium in the presence of digitalis toxicity-induced hyperkalaemia and Digibind treatment could result in a significant hypokalaemia.

*Side- and adverse effects:* Allergic responses are possible or probable attribution to Digibind have been reported rarely. The development of a pruritic rash (either with or without facial flushing and swelling) or shaking or chills without fever, have occurred on the day of treatment. Urticaria and thrombocytopenia have occurred up to 16 days post treatment. There are no reports of any allergic reactions to re-administra-

tion of Digibind in the same patient, but there are few instances on which information is available.

*Use in pregnancy and lactation:* To date there is no evidence that Digibind administered during human pregnancy causes foetal abnormalities; however, the use of Digibind should be considered only if the expected clinical benefit of treatment to the mother outweighs any possible risk to the developing foetus.

*Carcinogenesis, mutagenesis, impairment of fertility:* There have been no long-term studies performed in animals to evaluate carcinogenic or mutagenic potential or effects on fertility.

*Drug interactions:* No drug interactions have been identified.

*Toxicity and treatment of overdosage:* Not relevant.

**Pharmaceutical precautions** Store at 2 to 8˚C. Protect from light. After reconstitution store between 2 and 8˚C for up to 4 hours.

Reconstituted product should be used promptly. If it is not used immediately, it may be stored under refrigeration between 2 and 8˚C for up to 4 hours. The reconstituted product may be diluted with sterile isotonic saline to a convenient volume.

**Legal category** POM

**Package quantities** Single vial of lyophilised powder containing 38 mg of antigen-binding fragments (Fab).

**Further information** Digoxin-specific antibody Fab fragments have been used successfully to treat a case of lanatoside C intoxication. Reversal of β-methyl digoxin and β-acetyl digoxin-induced arrhythmias by Digibind has been verified in guinea-pigs.

**Product licence number** 0003/0207

## EXOSURF* NEONATAL

**Presentation** Exosurf Neonatal is supplied as a vial of sterile powder together with a vial of sterile diluent.

Each vial of powder contains 108 mg colfosceril palmitate as a sterile, white, freeze-dried powder together with hexadecanol, tyloxapol and sodium chloride. It contains no preservative.

Each vial of diluent provides sufficient Water for Injections BP for reconstitution of the powder.

The reconstituted product is an opaque, white suspension.

**Uses** Exosurf Neonatal is indicated for the treatment of newborn infants with or at risk of respiratory distress syndrome, who are undergoing mechanical ventilation and whose heart rate and arterial oxygenation are continuously monitored.

**Dosage and administration** A dose of 5 ml per kg birth weight reconstituted Exosurf Neonatal should be given via the endotracheal tube. A second equal dose should be given by the same route approximately 12 hours later if the baby is still intubated.

Each dose corresponds to 67.5 mg of colfosceril palmitate per kg birth weight.

*Reconstitution:* The contents of each vial of Exosurf Neonatal should be reconstituted with the diluent supplied. If this is not available use 8 ml of Water for Injections BP (i.e. sterile, preservative-free water). This gives a white suspension containing 13.5 mg per ml colfosceril palmitate.

Exosurf Neonatal is physically and chemically stable for 24 hours after reconstitution if stored between 2˚C and 30˚C. Exosurf Neonatal contains no antimicrobial preservative. Reconstitution should therefore be performed, either immediately before use, or, if storage is required, under sterile conditions. In either case, any unused suspension should be discarded.

Carry out the reconstitution as follows:

1. Fill a sterile syringe with 8 ml of diluent.
2. Allow the vacuum in the vial of Exosurf Neonatal to draw the diluent into the vial through a sterile needle.
3. Aspirate the resulting suspension back into the syringe and then release the syringe plunger to allow the suspension to return into the Exosurf Neonatal vial.
4. Repeat aspiration and return three or four times to ensure adequate mixing of the vial contents. If the suspension appears to separate, gently shake or swirl the vial to resuspend.
5. Withdraw the required volume of Exosurf Neonatal suspension from the vial with the tip of the withdrawing needle well below the froth on the surface of the suspension.

*Administration:* Exosurf Neonatal should be administered only by those trained and experienced in the care and resuscitation of pre-term infants (see *Precautions*).

Exosurf Neonatal can only be administered to endotracheally intubated infants undergoing mechanical ventilation. Infants should NOT be intubated solely for the administration of Exosurf Neonatal.

The infant's airway should be cleared by suction prior to the administration of Exosurf Neonatal.

Exosurf Neonatal is administered from a syringe into the endotracheal tube via the side-port on a special endotracheal adaptor, without interrupting mechanical ventilation. The part of the endotracheal tube outside the infant should be aligned vertically during administration (see diagram below).

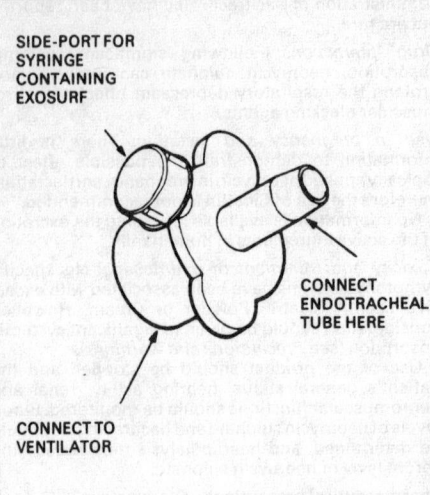

SIDE-PORT FOR SYRINGE CONTAINING EXOSURF

CONNECT ENDOTRACHEAL TUBE HERE

CONNECT TO VENTILATOR

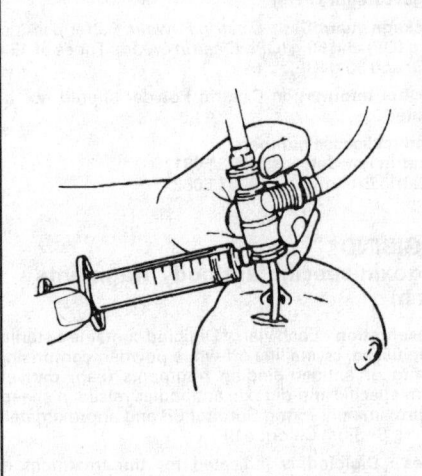

The total dose should be administered at a rat slow enough to allow the reconstituted Exosu Neonatal suspension to pass into the lungs throug the endotracheal tube without accumulation. Th minimum recommended time for administration o the full dose is 4 minutes.

Dosing should be slowed or interrupted if th infant's skin colour deteriorates, the heart rate slow arterial oxygen monitors indicate more than transitor depression of arterial oxygen concentration or Exosu Neonatal accumulates in the endotracheal tube (se *Precautions*).

### Contra-indications, warnings, etc
*Contra-indications:* There are no known contra-ind cations to treatment with Exosurf Neonatal.

*Precautions:* Exosurf Neonatal should only be admin istered with adequate facilities for ventilation an monitoring of babies with RDS.

Preterm birth is hazardous. Surfactant administra tion can be expected to diminish the severity of RD and hence to diminish complications of the intensiv care, especially of the ventilatory support required fo the treatment of RDS, but cannot be expected t eliminate entirely the mortality and morbidity assoc ated with preterm delivery. Infants who but for th administration of surfactant might have died fro RDS may be exposed to other complications of the immaturity.

As a consequence of the surfactant properties Exosurf Neonatal, chest expansion may impro rapidly after dosing . To avoid the risk of pneumoth rax and other forms of pulmonary air leak, rap reduction in peak ventilatory pressure may therefo be necessary.

The improvement in lung mechanics resulting fro Exosurf Neonatal administration may result in rap improvement in arterial oxygen concentration. Aft any appropriate reduction in ventilator pressure, rap reduction in inspired oxygen concentration may be needed to avoid hyperoxaemia.

Infants no longer requiring positive pressure ventilation may require treatment for apnoea of prematurity. In clinical trials, infants treated with Exosurf Neonatal had a higher incidence of apnoea, probably as a consequence of earlier ending of positive pressure ventilation. There were no adverse consequences in terms of increased mortality or long-term morbidity associated with this increased incidence.

Problems encountered during dosing in the clinical trials included reflux of Exosurf and changes in arterial oxygen pressure (rises and falls of greater than 20 mmHg). These should be managed by careful attention to the dosing instructions (see *Administration*).

Exosurf Neonatal was non-mutagenic in the Ames Salmonella test.

No studies have been performed to determine whether Exosurf Neonatal has carcinogenic potential.

The effects of Exosurf Neonatal on fertility have not been studied.

*Side- and adverse effects:* Pulmonary haemorrhage, the incidence of which increases the more immature the infant, is a rare but sometimes fatal complication of preterm delivery. In a placebo-controlled trial of single dose Exosurf Neonatal prophylaxis in babies with birth weight 500 to 700 g, the incidence of pulmonary haemorrhage was significantly increased in the Exosurf group (11% versus 2% in the placebo group). Although no other single trial of Exosurf Neonatal has demonstrated a significant increase in pulmonary haemorrhage, cross study analyses suggest that Exosurf Neonatal administration may be associated with an increase from 1% to 2% in the incidence of pulmonary haemorrhage. As might be expected, this association appears to be more marked the more immature the infant. In an open uncontrolled study of Exosurf Neonatal administration in 11,455 infants the reported incidence of pulmonary haemorrhage was 4%.

Pulmonary haemorrhage after surfactant administration is believed to be a consequence of increased pulmonary blood flow in the presence of a patent ductus arteriosus. Preventative measures, early diagnosis and treatment of patent ductus arteriosus, especially during the first three days of life, may reduce the incidence of pulmonary haemorrhage.

In occasional infants (approximately three per thousand) Exosurf Neonatal administration has been associated with obstruction of the endotracheal tube by mucous secretions. If endotracheal tube obstruction is suspected this should be treated, according to normal practice, by suction of the tube, or by replacement of the tube if suction is unsuccessful.

*Pregnancy and lactation:* Not relevant with this product.

*Drug interactions:* No specific drug interactions have been identified.

*Toxicity and treatment of overdosage:* There have been no reports of overdosage with Exosurf Neonatal. In case of accidental overdosage, as much as possible of the suspension should be aspirated and the baby should then be managed with supportive treatment, with particular attention to fluid and electrolyte balance.

**Pharmaceutical precautions** Store below 30°C. Do not freeze.

**Legal category** POM

**Package quantities**
Vial of freeze-dried powder
Vial of preservative-free sterile Water for Injections BP.
Five sterile endotracheal tube adaptors (2.5, 3.0, 3.5, 4.0 and 4.5 mm I.D.)

**Further information**
Infants with mature lungs, major congenital abnormalities, chromosomal abnormalities, hydrops fetalis, or suspected of having congenital infection were excluded from the clinical trials. The safety and efficacy of Exosurf Neonatal in these infants is therefore unknown.

**Product licence numbers**
Exosurf Neonatal: 0003/0283
Preservative-free sterile Water for Injections BP: 0003/0284

# FLOLAN*

**Presentation** Each vial contains 500 micrograms (500,000 nanogram (ng)) sterile, freeze-dried epoprostenol (formerly known as prostacyclin) as the sodium salt supplied as a sterile, white to off-white freeze-dried powder. The sodium content is approximately 1 mg per vial.

Each 50 ml vial of sterile diluent for Flolan contains Sodium Chloride BP 0.147% w/v and Glycine BP 0.188% w/v in clear solution. The alkalinity of the diluent has been adjusted to pH 10.5 ± 0.3 by the addition of sodium hydroxide.

A filter unit is provided for use during reconstitution.

**Uses** Flolan is indicated as an alternative to heparin during renal dialysis, especially when a high risk of bleeding problems due to heparin exists.

*Pharmacology:* Epoprostenol is a naturally occurring prostaglandin produced by the intima of blood vessels and is the most potent inhibitor of platelet aggregation known. The inhibition is dose-related. Unlike many other prostaglandins, it is not metabolised during passage through the pulmonary circulation.

Epoprostenol sodium is a potent vasodilator. The cardiovascular effects disappear within 30 minutes of the end of infusion.

It inhibits platelet aggregation by elevating platelet cyclic adenosine monophosphate. The action is dose-related above 2 nanogram/kg/min, following intravenous administration. Significant inhibition of aggregation induced by adenosine diphosphate is observed after intravenous administration of 4 or more nanogram/kg/min. Effects on platelets usually disappear within 30 minutes of discontinuing infusion of epoprostenol sodium.

Higher doses of epoprostenol sodium (20 nanogram/kg/min) disperse circulating platelet aggregates and increase by up to two-fold the cutaneous bleeding time.

Epoprostenol sodium reduces platelet procoagulant activity and the release of heparin neutralising factor.

The fate of epoprostenol sodium in man is not fully established. At normal physiological pH and temperature, epoprostenol sodium is hydrolysed with a half-life of 2 to 3 minutes to 6-keto prostaglandin $F_{1\alpha}$.

**Dosage and administration** Flolan is suitable for continuous infusion only, either intravascularly or into the blood supplying the dialyser.

The following schedule of infusion has been found effective in adults:
*Prior to dialysis:* 5 nanogram/kg/min intravenously.
*During dialysis:* 5 nanogram/kg/min into the arterial inlet of the dialyser.

The infusion should be stopped at the end of dialysis.

The recommended doses should be exceeded only with appropriate patient monitoring.

*Use in children:* There is no specific information on the use of Flolan in children.

*Use in the elderly:* There is no specific information available on the use of Flolan in elderly patients.

*Reconstitution:* Only the diluent provided for the purpose should be used. The enclosed filter unit must be used once only and then discarded after use.

To reconstitute Flolan, a strict aseptic technique must be used. **Particular care should be taken in calculating dilutions**, and in diluting Flolan the following procedure is recommended:
1. Withdraw approximately 10 ml of the sterile diluent into a sterile syringe.
2. Inject the contents of the syringe into the vial containing Flolan and dissolve the contents completely.
3. Draw up all the Flolan solution into the syringe.
4. Re-inject the entire contents into the residue of the original 50 ml of sterile diluent.
5. Mix well. This solution is now referred to as the *concentrated solution* and contains Flolan 10,000 nanograms per millilitre. The *concentrated solution* is normally further diluted before use. It may be diluted with physiological saline (0.9%),

provided a ratio of 6 volumes of saline to 1 volume of *concentrated solution* is not exceeded; e.g. 50 ml of *concentrated solution* further diluted with a maximum of 300 ml saline. Other common intravenous fluids are unsatisfactory for the dilution of the *concentrated solution* as the required pH is not attained. Flolan solutions are less stable at low pH. For administration using a pump capable of delivering small volume constant infusions, suitable aliquots of concentrated solution may be diluted with sterile physiological saline.
6. Before further dilution, draw up the *concentrated solution* into a larger syringe.
7. The filter provided should then be attached to the syringe and the *concentrated solution* is dispensed by filtration using firm but not excessive pressure. The typical time taken for filtration of 50 ml of solution is 70 seconds.

When reconstituted and diluted as directed, Flolan infusion solutions have a pH of approximately 10 and will retain 90% of their initial potency for approximately 12 hours at 25°C.

*Infusion rate guidance:* In general, the infusion rate may be calculated by the following formula:

$$\text{Infusion rate (ml/min)} = \frac{\text{Dosage (ng/kg/min)} \times \text{bodyweight (kg)}}{\text{Concentration of infusion (ng/ml)}}$$

Examples:
Flolan may be administered in diluted form (1) or as the *concentrated solution* (2) (see Tables below).

**Contra-indications, warnings, etc**
*Contra-indications:* There are no recognised contra-indications to the administration of Flolan in renal dialysis.

*Precautions:* Because of the high pH of the final infusion solutions, care should be taken to avoid extravasation during their administration and consequent risk of tissue damage.

Flolan is a potent vasodilator. The cardiovascular effects during infusion disappear within 30 minutes of the end of administration.

Flolan is not a conventional anticoagulant. Flolan has been successfully used instead of heparin in renal dialysis, but in a small proportion of dialyses clotting has developed in the dialysis circuit, requiring termination of dialysis.

Haemorrhagic complications have not been encountered with Flolan but the possibility should be considered when the drug is administered to patients with spontaneous or drug-induced haemorrhagic diatheses.

Blood pressure and heart rate should be monitored during administration of Flolan. Tachycardia, bradycardia and hypotension may occur during infusions of Flolan.

The effects of Flolan on heart-rate may be masked by concomitant use of drugs which affect cardiovascular reflexes.

If excessive hypotension occurs during administration of Flolan, the dose should be reduced or the infusion discontinued.

The hypotensive effect of Flolan may be enhanced by the use of acetate buffer in the dialysis bath during renal dialysis.

Elevated serum glucose levels have been reported during infusion of Flolan in man but these are not inevitable.

*Drug interactions:* Flolan may potentiate the action of heparin, and standard anticoagulant monitoring is advisable when Flolan is administered to patients receiving concomitant anticoagulants.

---

1. *Diluted:* A commonly used dilution is: 10 ml *concentrated solution* + 40 ml physiological saline (0.9%). Resultant concentration = 2,000 nanogram/ml epoprostenol.

| | | Body weight (kilograms) | | | | | | | |
|---|---|---|---|---|---|---|---|---|---|
| | | 30 | 40 | 50 | 60 | 70 | 80 | 90 | 100 |
| Dosage (ng/kg/min) | 1 | 0.90 | 1.20 | 1.50 | 1.80 | 2.10 | 2.40 | 2.70 | 3.00 |
| | 2 | 1.80 | 2.40 | 3.00 | 3.60 | 4.20 | 4.80 | 5.40 | 6.00 |
| | 3 | 2.70 | 3.60 | 4.50 | 5.40 | 6.30 | 7.20 | 8.10 | 9.00 |
| | 4 | 3.60 | 4.80 | 6.00 | 7.20 | 8.40 | 9.60 | 10.80 | 12.00 |
| | 5 | 4.50 | 6.00 | 7.50 | 9.00 | 10.50 | 12.00 | 13.50 | 15.00 |

Flow rates in mls/hr

2. Using *concentrated solution,* i.e. 10,000 nanogram/ml epoprostenol:

| | | Body weight (kilograms) | | | | | | | |
|---|---|---|---|---|---|---|---|---|---|
| | | 30 | 40 | 50 | 60 | 70 | 80 | 90 | 100 |
| Dosage (ng/kg/min) | 1 | 0.18 | 0.24 | 0.30 | 0.36 | 0.42 | 0.48 | 0.54 | 0.60 |
| | 2 | 0.36 | 0.48 | 0.60 | 0.72 | 0.84 | 0.96 | 1.08 | 1.20 |
| | 3 | 0.54 | 0.72 | 0.90 | 1.08 | 1.26 | 1.44 | 1.62 | 1.80 |
| | 4 | 0.72 | 0.96 | 1.20 | 1.44 | 1.68 | 1.92 | 2.16 | 2.40 |
| | 5 | 0.90 | 1.20 | 1.50 | 1.80 | 2.10 | 2.40 | 2.70 | 3.00 |

Flow rates in mls/hr

The vasodilator effect of Flolan may augment or be augmented by concomitant use of other vasodilators.

*Use in pregnancy and lactation:* In the absence of adequate experience of administration of Flolan to pregnant women, the potential benefit to the mother must be weighed against the unknown risks to the fetus.

There is no information on the use of Flolan during lactation.

*Side- and adverse effects:* Facial flushing is commonly seen, even in the anaesthetised patient.

Headache and gastro-intestinal symptoms including nausea, vomiting and abdominal colic have occurred in some conscious individuals.

Jaw pain, dry mouth, lassitude, reddening over the infusion site, chest pain and tightness have been reported with varying frequency.

Bradycardia, accompanied by pallor, nausea, sweating and sometimes abdominal discomfort and orthostatic hypotension, have occurred in healthy volunteers at doses of epoprostenol sodium greater than 5 nanogram/kg/min. Bradycardia associated with a considerable fall in systolic and diastolic blood pressure has followed intravenous administration of a dose of epoprostenol sodium equivalent to 30 nanogram/kg/min in healthy conscious volunteers.

*Toxicity and treatment of overdosage:* The main feature of overdosage is likely to be hypotension.

Reduce the dose or discontinue the infusion and initiate appropriate supportive measures as necessary; for example, plasma volume expansion and/or adjustment to pump flow.

**Pharmaceutical precautions**

Store Flolan vials at a temperature below 25°C. Protect from light. Keep dry. Do not freeze.

Under these conditions, freeze-dried Flolan in an unopened vial should not be affected by moisture present in the atmosphere.

Store the sterile glycine buffer diluent at a temperature below 25°C. Do not freeze. Protect from light.

The stability of solutions of Flolan is pH dependent. Only the diluent supplied should be used for reconstitution of freeze-dried Flolan and only the recommended infusion solutions, in the stated ratio, should be used for further dilution, otherwise the required pH may not be maintained.

The reconstituted ***concentrated solution*** when prepared as directed using the sterile glycine buffer provided, contains 10,000 nanograms epoprostenol per ml and is suitable for further dilution as recommended.

Reconstitution and dilution should be carried out immediately prior to use (see *Reconstitution and dilution*).

Glycine buffer diluent contains no preservative, consequently a vial should be used once only and then discarded.

**Legal category** POM

**Package quantities** 1 vial of 500 micrograms epoprostenol with 1 50 ml vial of sterile diluent.

**Further information** Nil.

**Product licence numbers**
Flolan Freeze-Dried Powder: 0003/0151
Glycine Buffer Diluent: 0003/0276

## KEMADRIN* INJECTION

**Qualitative and quantitative composition** Procyclidine Hydrochloride BP 5 mg/ml.

**Pharmaceutical form** Injection.

**Clinical particulars**

*Therapeutic indications:* Kemadrin is indicated in all forms of Parkinson's Disease (Paralysis Agitans), postencephalitic and arteriosclerotic.

Symptoms often responding well to Kemadrin include: rigidity, akinesia, tremor, speech and writing difficulties; gait; sialorrhoea and drooling; sweating; oculogyric crises and depressed mood.

Kemadrin is also used to control troublesome extrapyramidal symptoms induced by neuroleptic drugs including Pseudo-Parkinsonism, acute dystonic reactions and akathisia.

*Posology and method of administration:*

*Adults:* The variation in optimum dosage from one patient to another should be taken into consideration by the physician. Treatment is usually started at 2.5 mg three times a day, increasing by 2.5–5 mg daily at intervals of two or three days until the optimum clinical response is achieved. The usual maximum total daily dose is 30 mg. However, at the discretion of the attending physician where appropriate this total may be as high as 60 mg.

The daily dosage used in the control of neuroleptic-induced extrapyramidal symptoms is usually not more than 20 mg daily. After a period of 3–4 months, Kemadrin should be stopped and the patient observed to see if the neuroleptic-induced extrapyramidal symptoms recur. Cessation of treatment periodically is to be recommended even in patients who appear to require the drug for longer periods.

Avoid abrupt discontinuation of treatment.

Kemadrin may be combined with levodopa or amantadine in patients who are inadequately controlled on a single agent.

In acute dystonia 5 mg Kemadrin intravenously is frequently effective within 5 minutes. An occasional patient may need 10 mg or more and may require up to half an hour to obtain relief.

Kemadrin Injection may be given intramuscularly in doses of 5–10 mg repeated after 20 minutes if necessary, up to a daily maximum of 20 mg.

*Children:* Not applicable.

*Use in the elderly:* Elderly patients are more sensitive to anticholinergics, and a reduced dose may be required.

*Contra-indications:* Tardive dyskinesias.

*Special warnings and special precautions for use:* As with all anticholinergics such as Kemadrin, cautious prescribing is indicated in patients predisposed to glaucoma, obstructive disease of the gastro-intestinal tract, those with urinary symptoms associated with prostatic hypertrophy and in hepatic and renal impairment.

In a proportion of patients undergoing neuroleptic treatment, tardive dyskinesias will occur. While anticholinergic agents do not cause this syndrome, when given in combination with neuroleptics they may reduce the threshold at which dyskinesias appear in patients predisposed to this abnormality. In such individuals subsequent adjustment of neuroleptic therapy is indicated.

*Interaction with other medicaments and other forms of interaction:* The anticholinergic activity of Kemadrin may be increased by agents having anticholinergic activity, e.g. antidepressants (e.g. Amitriptyline), phenothiazines (e.g. Thioridazine), amantadine and disopyramide. The absorption of ketoconazole may be reduced by concomitant administration of Kemadrin.

*Pregnancy and lactation:* The safety of using Kemadrin during pregnancy has not been established. However, extensive clinical use has not given any evidence that it in any way compromises the normal course of pregnancy. No data are available on the excretion of this drug in breast milk.

*Effects on ability to drive and use machines:* Blurring of vision. At higher doses dizziness, mental confusion and hallucinations may occur.

*Undesirable effects:* The main side-effects are those to be expected from any anticholinergic agent. Dry mouth, blurring of vision and constipation are most commonly recorded. At higher doses dizziness, mental confusion and hallucinations may occur. The unwanted anticholinergic effects are easily reversed by reducing the dosage.

In rare instances, Kemadrin administered for the treatment of neuroleptic-induced symptoms was associated with an apparent worsening of the patient's state.

*Overdose:* Reports of overdosage are relatively rare. Symptoms of overdosage are agitation, restlessness and confusion with severe sleeplessness lasting up to 24 hours or more. Visual and occasionally auditory hallucinations are likely. Most subjects are euphoric but the occasional patient may be anxious and aggressive. The pupils are widely dilated and unreactive to light. In recorded cases, the disorientation has lasted 1 to 4 days and ended in recuperative sleep.

If procyclidine has been ingested within the previous hour or two (or possibly longer in view of its likely effects on gastric motility) then gastric lavage is probably indicated. Other active measures such as the use of cholinergic agents or haemodialysis are extremely unlikely to be of clinical value, although if convulsions occur they should be controlled by injections of diazepam.

**Pharmacological properties**

*Pharmacodynamic properties:* Procyclidine is a synthetic anticholinergic agent which blocks the excitatory effects of acetycholine at the muscarinic receptor.

Idiopathic Parkinson's Disease is now thought to result from degeneration of neurones in the substantia nigra whose axons project and inhibit cells in the corpus striatum. Blockade by neuroleptic drugs of the dopamine released by these terminals produces a similar clinical picture. The cell bodies in the corpus striatum also receive cholinergic innervation which is excitatory. Relief of the Parkinsonian syndrome can be achieved either by potentiation of the dopaminergic system or blockade of the cholinergic input by anticholinergics. It is by a central action of this latter type that procyclidine exerts its effect.

*Pharmacokinetic properties:* Procyclidine is adequately absorbed from the gastro-intestinal tract and disappears rapidly from the tissues. After intravenous administration it acts within 5 to 20 minutes with a duration of up to 4 hours. After both oral and IV dosing the mean values for volume of distribution, total body clearance and plasma elimination half-life of procyclidine were of the order of 1 litre/kg, 68 ml/min and 12 hours respectively.

*Preclinical safety data:* There are no pre-clinical data of relevance to the prescriber which are additional to that alrady included in other sections of the SPC.

**Pharmaceutical particulars**

*List of excipients:* Lactic acid 10 mcg. Lactic acid for pH 3.9 to 4.5 (quantity not fixed). Water for Injections to 2 ml.

*Incompatibilities:* None known.

*Shelf life:* 5 years.

*Special precautions for storage:* Store below 25°C.

*Nature and contents of container:* 2 ml neutral glass ampoules.

*Instructions for use/handling:* No special instructions.

**Marketing authorisation number** 0003/5256R

**Date of approval/revision of SPC** November 1996.

**Legal category** POM.

## KEMADRIN* TABLETS

**Qualitative and quantitative composition** Procyclidine Hydrochloride 5 mg per tablet.

**Pharmaceutical form** Tablet.

**Clinical particulars**

*Therapeutic indications:* Kemadrin is indicated in all forms of Parkinson's Disease (Paralysis Agitans), postencephalitic and arteriosclerotic.

Symptoms often responding well to Kemadrin include: rigidity, akinesia, tremor, speech and writing difficulties, gait, sialorrhoea and drooling, sweating, oculogyric crises and depressed mood.

Kemadrin is also used to control troublesome extrapyramidal symptoms induced by neuroleptic drugs including Pseudo-Parkinsonism, acute dystonic reactions and akathisia.

*Posology and method of administration:*

*Adults:* The variation in optimum dosage from one patient to another should be taken into consideration by the physician. Treatment is usually started at 2.5 mg three times a day, increasing by 2.5–5 mg daily at intervals of two or three days until the optimum clinical response is achieved. The usual maximum total daily dose is 30 mg. However, at the discretion of the attending physician where appropriate this total may be as high as 60 mg.

The daily dosage used in the control of neuroleptic-induced extrapyramidal symptoms is usually not more than 20 mg daily. After a period of 3–4 months Kemadrin should be stopped and the patient observed to see if the neuroleptic-induced extrapyramidal symptoms recur. Cessation of treatment periodically is to be recommended even in patients who appear to require the drug for longer periods.

Avoid abrupt discontinuation of treatment.

Kemadrin may be combined with levodopa or amantadine in patients who are inadequately controlled on a single agent.

*Children:* Not applicable.

*Use in the elderly:* Elderly patients are more sensitive to anticholinergics, and a reduced dose may be required.

*Contra-indications:* Tardive dyskinesias.

*Special warnings and special precautions for use:* As with all anticholinergics such as Kemadrin, cautious prescribing is indicated in patients predisposed to glaucoma, obstructive disease of the gastro-intestinal tract, those with urinary symptoms associated with prostatic hypertrophy and in hepatic and renal impairment.

In a proportion of patients undergoing neuroleptic treatment, tardive dyskinesias will occur. While anticholinergic agents do not cause this syndrome, when given in combination with neuroleptics they may reduce the threshold at which dyskinesias appear in patients predisposed to this abnormality. In such individuals subsequent adjustment of neuroleptic therapy is indicated.

*Interaction with other medicaments and other forms of interaction:* The anticholinergic activity of Kemadrin may be increased by agents having anticholinergic activity, e.g. antidepressants (e.g. amitriptyline), phenothiazines (e.g. thioridazine), amantadine and disopyramide. The absorption of ketoconazole may be reduced by concomitant administration of Kemadrin.

*Pregnancy and lactation:* The safety of using Kemadrin

uring pregnancy has not been established. However, xtensive clinical use has not given any evidence that in any way compromises the normal course of regnancy. No data are available on the excretion of is drug in breast milk.

*ffects on ability to drive and use machines:* Blurring f vision. At higher doses dizziness, mental confusion nd hallucinations may occur.

*ndesirable effects:* The main side-effects are those be expected from any anticholinergic agent. Dry outh, blurring of vision and constipation are most ommonly recorded. At higher doses dizziness, ental confusion and hallucinations may occur. The nwanted anticholinergic effects are easily reversed y reducing the dosage.

In rare instances, Kemadrin administered for the eatment of neuroleptic-induced symptoms was as- ociated with an apparent worsening of the patient's ate.

*verdose:* Reports of overdosage are relatively rare. ymptoms of overdosage are agitation, restlessness nd confusion with severe sleeplessness lasting up to 4 hours or more. Visual and occasionally auditory allucinations are likely. Most subjects are euphoric ut the occasional patient may be anxious and ggressive. The pupils are widely dilated and unreac- ve to light. In recorded cases, the disorientation has sted 1 to 4 days and ended in recuperative sleep.

If procyclidine has been ingested within the previous our or two (or possibly longer in view of its likely fects on gastric motility) then gastric lavage is robably indicated. Other active measures such as e use of cholinergic agents or haemodialysis are xtremely unlikely to be of clinical value, although if onvulsions occur they should be controlled by jections of diazepam.

**harmacological properties**

*harmacodynamic properties:* Procyclidine is a syn- etic anticholinergic agent which blocks the excita- ry effects of acetylcholine at the muscarinic receptor.

Idiopathic Parkinson's Disease is now thought to sult from degeneration of neurones in the substantia gra whose axons project and inhibit cells in the orpus striatum. Blockade by neuroleptic drugs of the opamine released by these terminals produces a milar clinical picture. The cell bodies in the corpus riatum also receive cholinergic innervation which is xcitatory. Relief of the Parkinsonian syndrome can e achieved either by potentiation of the dopaminergic ystem or blockade of the cholinergic input by ticholinergics. It is by a central action of this latter pe that procyclidine exerts its effect.

*harmacokinetic properties:* Procyclidine is ade- uately absorbed from the gastro-intestinal tract and sappears rapidly from the tissues. After intravenous dministration it acts within 5 to 20 minutes with a uration of up to 4 hours. After both oral and IV osing the mean values for volume of distribution, tal body clearance and plasma elimination half-life procyclidine were of the order of 1 litre/kg, 68 ml/ in and 12 hours respectively.

*eclinical safety data:*

*Mutagenicity:* No data are available regarding the utagenic potential of procyclidine hydrochloride.

*Carcinogenicity:* There are no data on the carcino- enic potential of procyclidine hydrochloride.

*Teratogenicity:* No teratogenic effects were seen rats dosed subcutaneously with 10, 30 or 100 mg/ /day on days 8 to 16 of pregnancy. Maternal odyweight gain was reduced at doses of 30 or 0 mg/kg/day, and a 10% reduction in fetal weight as seen at 100 mg/kg/day.

*Fertility:* A three generation study in rats dosed at mg/kg/day via the diet before and during pregnancy owed only that the number of viable pups was ightly decreased from the second mating. No other arameters were affected.

**armaceutical particulars**

*st of excipients:* Lactose; sodium starch glycollate; vidone; magnesium stearate.

*compatibilities:* None.

*helf life:* 5 years.

*oecial precautions for storage:* Store below 25°C.

*ature and contents of container:* Amber glass bottles th low density polyethylene snap-fit closures.

Polypropylene containers with polyethylene snap-lids. Round enamelled tins with lever lids.

*ck sizes:* Bottles of 100 and 500 tablets.

*structions for use/handling:* See *Posology and ethod of administration.*

**arketing authorisation number** 0003/5255R

**ate of approval/revision of SPC** October 1995.

**gal category** POM

## LAMICTAL* TABLETS ▼
## LAMICTAL* Dispersible ▼

**Presentation** Lamictal Tablets 25 mg are pale-yellow, rounded-square tablets, multifaceted on one side and flat with 'LAMICTAL 25' on the other, each containing 25 mg lamotrigine.

Lamictal Tablets 50 mg are pale-yellow, rounded-square tablets, multifaceted on one side and flat with 'LAMICTAL 50' on the other, each containing 50 mg lamotrigine.

Lamictal Tablets 100 mg are pale-yellow, rounded-square tablets, multifaceted on one side and flat with 'LAMICTAL 100' on the other, each containing 100 mg lamotrigine.

Lamictal Tablets 200 mg are pale-yellow, rounded-square tablets, multifaceted on one side and flat with 'LAMICTAL 200' on the other, each containing 200 mg lamotrigine.

Lamictal Dispersible 5 mg are white, elongated, biconvex tablets, with 'LAMICTAL 5' on one side and scored on the other and contain 5 mg lamotrigine in each tablet.

Lamictal Dispersible 25 mg are white, rounded-square tablets, multifaceted on one side and flat with 'LAMICTAL 25' on the other and contain 25 mg lamotrigine in each tablet.

Lamictal Dispersible 100 mg are white, rounded-square tablets, multifaceted on one side and flat with 'LAMICTAL 100' on the other and contain 100 mg lamotrigine in each tablet.

**Uses**

*Therapeutic indications:* Epilepsy.

*Monotherapy in adults and children over 12 years of age:*

1. simple partial seizures
2. complex partial seizures
3. secondarily generalised tonic clonic seizures
4. primary generalised tonic-clonic seizures.

Monotherapy in children under 12 years of age is not recommended until such time as adequate information is made available from controlled trials in this particular target population.

*Add-on therapy in adults and children over 2 years of age:*

1. simple partial seizures
2. complex partial seizures
3. secondarily generalised tonic clonic seizures.
4. primary generalised tonic-clonic seizures.

Lamictal is also indicated for the treatment of seizures associated with Lennox-Gastaut syndrome.

*Mode of action:* The results of pharmacological studies suggest that lamotrigine is a use-dependent blocker of voltage gated sodium channels. It produces a use and voltage-dependent block of sustained repetitive firing in cultured neurones and inhibits pathological release of glutamate (the amino acid which plays a key role in the generation of epileptic seizures), as well as inhibiting glutamate-evoked bursts of action potentials.

*Pharmacokinetics:* Lamotrigine is rapidly and completely absorbed from the gut with no significant first pass metabolism. Peak plasma concentrations occur approximately 2.5 hours after oral drug administration. Time to maximum concentration is slightly delayed after food but the extent of absorption is unaffected. The pharmacokinetics are linear up to 450 mg, the highest single dose tested. There is considerable inter-individual variation in steady state maximum concentrations but within and individual concentrations vary very little.

Binding to plasma proteins is about 55%. It is very unlikely that displacement from plasma proteins would result in toxicity, The volume of distribution is 0.92 to 1.22 l/kg.

The mean steady state clearance in healthy adults is 39 ± 14 ml/min. Clearance of lamotrigine is primarily metabolic with subsequent elimination of glucuronide-concentrated materials in urine. Less than 10% is excreted unchanged in the urine. Only about 2% of drug-related material is excreted in faeces. Clearance and half-life are independent of dose. The mean elimination half-life in healthy adults is 24 to 35 hours. Up-glucuronyl transferases have been identified as the enzymes responsible for metabolism of lamotrigine. In a study of subjects with Gilbert's syndrome, mean apparent clearance was reduced by 32% compared with normal controls but the values are within the range for the general population.

Lamotrigine induces its own metabolism to a modest extent depending on dose. However, there is no evidence that lamotrigine affects the pharmacokinetics of other AED's and data suggests that interactions between lamotrigine and drugs metabolised by cytochrome P450 enzymes are unlikely to occur.

The half-life of lamotrigine is greatly affected by concomitant medication. Mean half-life is reduced to approximately 14 hours when given with enzyme-inducing drugs such as carbamazepine and phenytoin and is increased to a mean of approximately 70 hours when co-administered with sodium valproate alone.

Clearance adjusted for bodyweight is higher in children aged 12 years and under than in adults, with the highest values in children under 5 years. The half-life of lamotrigine is generally shorter in children than in adults with a mean value of approximately 7 hours when given with enzyme inducing drugs such as carbamazepine and phenytoin, and increasing to mean values of approximately 45 to 55 hours when co-administered with sodium valproate alone (see *Dosage and administration).*

To date there have been no specific studies of lamotrigine pharmacokinetics in elderly patients with epilepsy. However, a single-dose study in 12 healthy volunteers aged 65 to 76 years and a population analysis of 144 patients including 25 patients aged 65 years and over indicated that no dosage adjustment is required for the elderly.

There is no experience of treatment with lamotrigine of patients with renal failure. Pharmacokinetic studies using single doses in subjects with renal failure indicate that lamotrigine pharmacokinetics are little affected but plasma concentrations of the major glucuronide metabolite increase almost eight-fold due to reduced renal clearance.

*Pharmacodynamics:* In tests designed to evaluate the central nervous system effects of drugs, the results obtained using doses of 240 mg lamotrigine administered to healthy adult volunteers did not differ from placebo, whereas both 1000 mg phenytoin and 10 mg diazepam each significantly impaired fine visual motor co-ordination and eye movements, increased body sway and produced subjective sedative effects.

In another study, single oral doses of 600 mg carbamazepine significantly impaired fine visual motor co-ordination and eye movements, while increasing both body sway and heart rate, whereas results with lamotrigine at doses of 150 mg and 300 mg did not differ from placebo.

**Dosage and administration**

*Dosage in monotherapy:*

*Adults and children over 12 years:* The initial Lamictal dose in monotherapy is 25 mg once a day for two weeks, followed by 50 mg once a day for two weeks. Thereafter, the dose should be increased by a maximum of 50 mg–100 mg every 1–2 weeks until the optimal response is achieved. The usual maintenance dose to achieve optimal response is 100–200 mg/day given once a day or as two divided doses. Some patients have required 500 mg/day of Lamictal to achieve the desired response.

*Recommended dose escalation of Lamictal for ADULTS AND CHILDREN OVER 12 YEARS on monotherapy*

| *Weeks 1–2* | *Weeks 3–4* | *Usual maintenance dose* |
|---|---|---|
| 25 mg (once a day) | 50 mg (once a day) | 100–200 mg (once a day or two divided doses)<br>To achieve maintenance, doses may be increased by 50–100 mg every 1–2 weeks. |

The initial dose and subsequent dose escalation should not be exceeded to minimise the risk of rash (see *Special warnings and special precautions for use*).

*Children aged 2 to 12 years:* There was insufficient evidence available from appropriate studies in children, upon which to base dosage recommendations for monotherapy use in children under the age of 12 years (see *Uses*).

*Dosage in add-on therapy:*

*Adults and children over 12 years:* In patients taking valproate with/without any other anti-epileptic drug (AED) the initial Lamictal dose is 25 mg every alternate day for two weeks, followed by 25 mg once a day for two weeks. Thereafter, the dose should be increased by a maximum of 25–50 mg every 1–2 weeks until the optimal response is achieved. The usual maintenance dose to achieve optimal response is 100–200 mg/day given once a day or in two divided doses.

In those patients taking enzyme inducing AEDs with/without other AEDs (except valproate) the initial Lamictal dose is 50 mg once a day for two weeks, followed by 100 mg/day given in two divided doses for two weeks. Thereafter, the dose should be increased by a maximum of 100 mg every 1–2 weeks until the optimal response is achieved. The usual maintenance dose to achieve optimal response is 200–400 mg/day given in two divided doses. Some patients have required 700 mg/day of Lamictal to achieve the desired response.

In patients taking AEDs where the pharmacokinetic interaction with lamotrigine is currently not known, the dose escalation as recommended for lamotrigine with concurrent valproate should be used, thereafter, the dose should be increased until optimal response is achieved.

*Recommended dose escalation of Lamictal for ADULTS AND CHILDREN OVER 12 YEARS on combined drug therapy*

| Concomitant medication | Weeks 1–2 | Weeks 3–4 | Usual maintenance dose |
|---|---|---|---|
| Valproate with/without any other AEDs | 12.5 mg (given as 25 mg on alternate days) | 25 mg (once a day) | 100–200 mg (once a day or two divided doses) To achieve maintenance, doses may be increased by 25–50 mg every 1–2 weeks. |
| Enzyme inducing AEDs† with/ without other AEDs (except valproate) | 50 mg (once a day) | 100 mg (two divided doses) | 200–400 mg (two divided doses) To achieve maintenance, doses may be increased by 100 mg every 1–2 weeks. |

† e.g. phenytoin, carbamazepine, phenobarbitone and primidone

Note: In patients taking AEDs where the pharmacokinetic interaction with lamotrigine is currently not known, the dose escalation as recommended for lamotrigine with concurrent valproate should be used. Thereafter, the dose should be increased until optimal response is achieved.

The initial dose and subsequent dose escalation should not be exceeded to minimise the risk of rash (see *Special warnings and precautions for use*).

*Children aged 2 to 12 years:* In patients taking valproate with/without any other anti-epileptic drug (AED), the initial Lamictal dose is 0.2 mg/kg bodyweight/day given once a day for two weeks, followed by 0.5 mg/kg/day given once a day for two weeks. Thereafter, the dose should be increased by a maximum of 0.5–1 mg/kg every 1–2 weeks until the optimal response is achieved. The usual maintenance dose to achieve optimal response is 1–5 mg/kg/day given once a day or in two divided doses.

In those patients taking enzyme inducing AEDs with/without other AEDs (except valproate) the initial Lamictal dose is 2 mg/kg bodyweight/day given in two divided doses for two weeks, followed by 5 mg/kg/day for two weeks. Thereafter, the dose should be increased by a maximum of 2–3 mg/kg every 1–2 weeks until the optimal response is achieved. The usual maintenance dose to achieve optimal response is 5–15 mg/kg/day given in two divided doses.

In patients taking AEDs where the pharmacokinetic interaction with lamotrigine is currently not known, the dose escalation as recommended for lamotrigine with concurrent valproate should be used, thereafter, the dose should be increased until optimal response is achieved.

*Recommended dose escalation of Lamictal for children aged 2–12 years on combined drug therapy (Total daily dose in mg/kg bodyweight/day).*

| Concomitant medication | Weeks 1–2 | Weeks 3–4 | Maintenance dose |
|---|---|---|---|
| Valproate with/without any other AEDs | 0.2 mg/kg‡ (once a day) | 0.5 mg/kg (once a day) | 1-5 mg/kg (once a day or two divided doses) To achieve maintenance, doses may be increased by 0.5–1 mg/kg every 1–2 weeks. |
| Enzyme inducing AEDs† with/ without other AEDs (except valproate) | 2 mg/kg (two divided doses) | 5 mg/kg (two divided doses) | 5–15 mg/kg (two divided doses) To achieve maintenance, doses may be increased by 2–3 mg/kg every 1–2 weeks. |

† e.g. phenytoin, carbamazepine, phenobarbitone and primidone.

Note: In patients taking AEDs where the pharmacokinetic interaction with lamotrigine is currently not known, the dose escalation as recommended for lamotrigine with concurrent valproate should be used, thereafter, the dose should be increased until optimal response is achieved.

‡ If the calculated daily dose is 2.5–5 mg, then 5 mg Lamictal may be taken on alternate days for the first two weeks. If the calculated daily dose is less then 2.5 mg, then Lamictal should not be administered.

The initial dose and subsequent dose escalation should not be exceeded to minimise the risk of rash (see *Special warnings and special precautions for use*).

It is likely that patients aged 2–6 years will require a maintenance dose at the higher end of the recommended range.

*Children aged less than 2 years:* There is insufficient information on the use of Lamictal in children aged less than 2 years.

*Use in the elderly:* There is limited information on the use of Lamictal in elderly patients. To date, there is no evidence to suggest that the response of this age group differs from that in the young. However, elderly patients should be treated cautiously.

*Administration:* Lamictal tablets should be swallowed whole with a little water.

Lamictal Dispersible Tablets may be chewed or dispersed in a small volume of water (at least enough to cover the whole tablet) or swallowed whole with a little water.

To ensure a therapeutic dose is maintained, the weight of a child must be monitored and the dose reviewed as weight changes occur. If the doses calculated for children, according to bodyweight, do not equate to whole tablets the dose to be administered is that equal to the lower number of whole tablets.

**Contra-indications, warnings, etc**

*Contra-indications:* Lamictal is contra-indicated in individuals with known hypersensitivity to lamotrigine.

Lamictal is cleared primarily by metabolism in the liver. No studies have been carried out in patients with significant impairment of hepatic function. Until such data become available Lamictal is contra-indicated in this condition.

*Special warnings and special precautions for use:* There have been reports of adverse skin reactions, which have generally occurred within the first 8 weeks after initiation of lamotrigine (Lamictal) treatment. The majority of rashes are mild and self limiting. However, rarely, serious potentially life threatening skin rashes including Stevens Johnson syndrome (SJS) and toxic epidermal necrolysis (TEN) have been reported (see *Undesirable effects*).

The approximate incidence of serious skin rashes in adults and children over the age of 12 is 1 in 1000. The risk is higher in children under the age of 12 than in adults. Available data from a number of studies suggest the incidence in children under the age of 12 requiring hospitalisation due to rash ranges from 1 in 300 to 1 in 100 (see *Undesirable effects*).

In children, the initial presentation of a rash can be mistaken for an infection, physicians should consider the possibility of a drug reaction in children that develop symptoms of rash and fever during the first eight weeks of therapy.

Additionally the overall risk of rash appears to be strongly associated with:

- High initial doses of lamotrigine and exceeding the recommended dose escalation of lamotrigine therapy (see *Dosage and method of administration*).
- Concomitant use of valproate, which increases the mean half-life of lamotrigine nearly two fold (see *Dosage and method of administration*).

All patients (adults and children) who develop a rash should be promptly evaluated and lamotrigine withdrawn immediately unless the rash is clearly not drug related.

Rash has also been reported as part of a hypersensitivity syndrome associated with a variable pattern of systemic symptoms including fever, lymphadenopathy, facial oedema and abnormalities of the blood and liver. The syndrome shows a wide spectrum of clinical severity and may, rarely, lead to disseminated intravascular coagulation (DIC) and multiorgan failure. It is important to note that early manifestations of hypersensitivity (e.g. fever, lymphadenopathy) may be present even though rash is not evident. Patients should be warned to seek immediate medical advice if signs and symptoms develop. If such signs and symptoms are present the patient should be evaluated immediately and Lamictal discontinued if an alternative aetiology cannot be established.

As with other AEDs, abrupt withdrawal of Lamictal may provoke rebound seizures. Unless safety concerns (for example rash) require an abrupt withdrawal, the dose of Lamictal should be gradually decreased over a period of 2 weeks.

When concomitant antiepileptic drugs (AEDs) are withdrawn to achieve Lamictal monotherapy or other antiepileptic drugs (AEDs) are added-on to Lamictal monotherapy consideration should be given to the effect this may have on lamotrigine pharmacokinetics (see *Interaction with other drugs and other forms of interaction*).

During clinical experience with lamotrigine used as add-on therapy, there have been, rarely, deaths following rapidly progressive illnesses with status epilepticus, rhabdomyolysis, multiorgan dysfunction and disseminated intravascular coagulation (DIC). The contribution of lamotrigine to these events remain to be established.

Lamictal is a weak inhibitor of dihydrofolate reduc tase hence there is a possibility of interference wit folate metabolism during long-term therapy. How ever, during prolonged human dosing, lamotrigin did not induce significant changes in the haemoglobi concentration, mean corpuscular volume, or serur or red blood cell folate concentrations up to 1 year c red blood cell folate concentrations for up to 5 years

In single dose studies in subjects with end-stag renal failure, plasma concentrations of lamotrigin were not significantly altered. However, accumulatic of the glucuronide metabolite is to be expecte caution should therefore be exercised in treatin patients with renal failure.

*Interaction with other drugs and other forms interaction:* Antiepileptic agents which induce dru metabolising enzymes (such as phenytoin, carbama zepine, phenobarbitone and primidone) enhance th metabolism of lamotrigine and may increase dos requirements.

Sodium valproate, which competes with lamotr gine for hepatic drug-metabolising enzymes, reduce the metabolism of lamotrigine.

There is no evidence that lamotrigine cause clinically significant induction or inhibition of hepat oxidative drug-metabolising enzymes. Lamotrigin may induce its own metabolism but the effect modest and unlikely to have significant clinic consequences.

Although changes in the plasma concentratior of other antiepileptic drugs have been reporte controlled studies have shown no evidence th lamotrigine affects the plasma concentrations concomitant anti-epileptic drugs. Evidence from *vitro* studies indicates that lamotrigine does n displace other antiepileptic drugs from protei binding sites.

There have been reports of central nervous syste events including headache, nausea, blurred visio dizziness, diplopia and ataxia in patients taking ca bamazepine following the introduction of lamotrigin These events usually resolve when the dose carbamazepine is reduced.

In a study of 12 female volunteers, lamotrigine d not affect plasma concentrations of ethinyloestradi and levonorgestrel following the administration of th oral contraceptive pill. However, as with the intr duction of other chronic therapy in patients takir oral contraceptives, any change in the menstru bleeding pattern should be reported to the patien physician.

*Undesirable effects:* Adverse experiences reporte during Lamictal monotherapy trials include headach tiredness, rash, nausea, dizziness, drowsiness ar insomnia.

In double-blind, add-on clinical trials, skin rashe occurred in up to 10% of patients taking lamotrigir and in 5% of patients taking placebo. The skin rashe led to the withdrawal of lamotrigine treatment in 2 of patients. The rash, usually maculopapular appearance, generally appears within eight weeks starting treatment and resolves on withdrawal lamotrigine (see *Special warnings and special preca tions for use*).

Rarely, serious potentially life threatening sk rashes, including Stevens Johnson syndrome ar toxic epidermal necrolysis (Lyell Syndrome) hav been reported. Although the majority recover on dru withdrawal, some patients experience irreversib scarring and there have been rare cases of associate death (see *Special warnings and special precautio for use*).

The approximate incidence of serious skin rash in adults and children over the age of 12 is 1 in 1,00 The risk is higher in children under the age of 12 th in adults. Available data from a number of studi suggest the incidence in children under the age of requiring hospitalisation due to rash ranges from 1 300 to 1 in 100 (see *Special warnings and spec precautions for use*).

In children, the initial presentation of a rash can mistaken for an infection, physicians should consid the possibility of a drug reaction in children th develop symptoms of rash and fever during the fir eight weeks of therapy.

Additionally the overall risk of rash appears to strongly associated with:

- High initial doses of lamotrigine and exceeding t recommended dose escalation of lamotrigine the apy (see *Dosage and administration*).
- Concomitant use of valproate, which increases t mean half life of lamotrigine nearly two fold (s *Dosage and administration*).

All patients (adults and children) who develop rash should be promptly evaluated and lamotrigi withdrawn immediately unless the rash is clearly n drug related.

Rash has also been reported as part of a hyperse

sitivity syndrome associated with a variable pattern of systemic symptoms including fever, lymphadenopathy, facial oedema and abnormalities of the blood and liver. The syndrome shows a wide spectrum of clinical severity and may, rarely, lead to disseminated intravascular coagulation (DIC) and multiorgan failure. It is important to note that early manifestations of hypersensitivity (e.g. fever, lymphadenopathy) may be present even though rash is not evident. Patients should be warned to seek immediate medical advice if signs and symptoms develop. If such signs and symptoms are present the patient should be evaluated immediately and Lamictal discontinued if an alternative aetiology cannot be established.

Other adverse experiences reported when lamotrigine is added-on to standard antiepileptic drug regimens have included diplopia, blurred vision, conjunctivitis, dizziness, drowsiness, headache, unsteadiness, tiredness, gastrointestinal disturbance (including vomiting), irritability/aggression, tremor, agitation, confusion and haematological abnormalities (including neutropenia, leucopenia and thrombocytopenia).

*Use in pregnancy and lactation:*

*Fertility:* Administration of Lamictal did not impair fertility in animal reproductive studies. There is no experience of the effect of Lamictal on human fertility.

*Teratogenicity:* Lamotrigine is a weak inhibitor of dihydrofolate reductase. There is a theoretical risk of human foetal malformations when the mother is treated with a folate inhibitor during pregnancy. However, reproductive toxicology studies with lamotrigine in animals at doses in excess of the human therapeutic dosage showed no teratogenic effects.

*Pregnancy:* There are insufficient data available on the use of lamotrigine in human pregnancy to evaluate its safety. Lamotrigine should not be used in pregnancy unless, in the opinion of the physician, the potential benefits of treatment to the mother outweigh any possible risks to the developing foetus.

*Lactation:* Preliminary data indicate that lamotrigine passes into breast milk in concentrations usually of the order of 40-45% of the plasma concentration.

In the small number of infants known to have been breastfed, the dose of lamotrigine received was calculated to be approximately 0.06-0.75 mg/kg/24 hours, and no adverse experiences were reported.

*Effects on ability to drive and use machines:* Two volunteer studies have demonstrated that the effect of lamotrigine on fine visual motor co-ordination, eye movements, body sway and subjective sedative effects did not differ from placebo.

In clinical trials with lamotrigine adverse events of a neurological character such as dizziness and diplopia have been reported. As there is individual variation in response to all antiepileptic drug therapy patients should consult their physician on the specific issues of driving and epilepsy.

*Toxicity and treatment of overdosage: Symptoms and signs:* Ingestion of between 1.35 and 4 g lamotrigine has been reported in a few patients. Clinical consequences were not severe, signs and symptoms included nystagmus, ataxia, dizziness, somnolence, headache and vomiting.

A patient who ingested a dose calculated to be between 4 and 5 g lamotrigine was admitted to hospital with coma lasting 8-12 hours followed by recovery over the next 2 to 3 days. A further patient who ingested 5.6 g lamotrigine was found unconscious. Following treatment with activated charcoal for suspected intoxication the patient recovered after sleeping for 16 hours.

*Treatment:* In the event of overdosage, the patient should be admitted to hospital and given appropriate supportive therapy. Gastric lavage should be performed if indicated.

**Pharmaceutical precautions** Lamictal Tablets (non-dispersible): Store below 30°C. Keep dry.

Lamictal Dispersible: Store below 30°C. Protect from light. Keep dry.

**Legal category** POM

**Package quantities**

| | |
|---|---|
| Lamictal Tablets 25 mg: | Blister pack of 3 x 7 tablets |
| Lamictal Tablets 25 mg: | Blister pack of 3 x 14 tablets |
| Lamiictal Tablets 25 mg: | Blister pack of 4 x 14 tablets |
| Lamictal Tablets 50 mg: | Blister pack of 3 x 14 tablets |
| Lamictal Tablets 50 mg: | Blister pack of 4 x 14 tablets |
| Lamictal Tablets 100 mg: | Blister pack of 4 x 14 tablets |
| Lamictal Tablets 200 mg: (Calendar pack) | Blister pack of 4 x 14 tablets |
| Lamictal Dispersible 5 mg: | Blister pack of 2 x 14 tablets |
| Lamictal Dispersible 25 mg: | Blister pack of 4 x 14 tablets |
| Lamictal Dispersible 100 mg: | Blister pack of 4 x 14 tablets |

**Further information** Nil.

**Product licence numbers**

| | |
|---|---|
| Lamictal Tablets 25 mg: | 0003/0272 |
| Lamictal Tablets 50 mg: | 0003/0273 |
| Lamictal Tablets 100 mg: | 0003/0274 |
| Lamictal Tablets 200 mg: | 0003/0297 |
| Lamictal Dispersible 5 mg: | 0003/0346 |
| Lamictal Dispersible 25 mg: | 0003/0347 |
| Lamictal Dispersible 100 mg: | 0003/0348 |

# LANOXIN* TABLETS
# LANOXIN-125* TABLETS
# LANOXIN-PG* TABLETS
# LANOXIN-PG* ELIXIR
# LANOXIN* INJECTION

**Presentation** Lanoxin Tablets each contain 250 micrograms (0.25 mg) of Digoxin BP, scored and coded 'WELLCOME X3A', white in colour.

Lanoxin-125 Tablets each contain 125 micrograms (0.125 mg) of Digoxin BP, coded 'WELLCOME Y3B', white in colour.

Lanoxin-PG (Paediatric/Geriatric) Tablets each contain 62.5 micrograms (0.0625 mg) of Digoxin BP, coded 'WELLCOME U3A' and coloured blue.

Lanoxin-PG (Paediatric/Geriatric) Elixir contains 50 micrograms (0.050 mg) of Digoxin BP in each ml. Clear, bright yellow in colour and lime-flavoured.

Lanoxin Injection is a clear, colourless, sterile aqueous solution containing 250 micrograms (0.25 mg) of Digoxin BP per ml in each 2 ml ampoule.

**Uses** Lanoxin is indicated in the management of chronic cardiac failure. Its therapeutic benefit is greatest in those patients with ventricular dilatation.

Lanoxin is specifically indicated where cardiac failure is accompanied by atrial fibrillation.

Lanoxin is indicated in the management of certain supraventricular arrhythmias, particularly atrial flutter and fibrillation, where its major beneficial effect is reduction of the ventricular rate.

**Dosage and administration** The dose of Lanoxin for each patient has to be tailored individually according to age, lean body weight and renal function. Suggested doses are intended only as an initial guide.

Lanoxin PG Elixir, 50 micrograms in 1 ml, is supplied with a graduated pipette and this should be used for measurement of all doses.

*Adults and children over 10 years:* Rapid oral loading: 750 to 1500 micrograms (0.75 to 1.5 mg) as a single dose.

Where there is less urgency, or a greater risk of toxicity e.g. in the elderly, the oral loading dose should be given in divided doses 6 hours apart, assessing clinical response before giving each additional dose (see *Precautions*).

*Slow Oral Loading:*

250 to 750 micrograms (0.25 to 0.75 mg) should be given daily for 1 week followed by an appropriate maintenance dose. A clinical response should be seen within one week.

NOTE: The choice between slow and rapid oral loading depends on the clinical state of the patient and the urgency of the condition.

*Maintenance:*

The maintenance dosage should be based upon the percentage of the peak body stores lost each day through elimination. The following formula has had wide clinical use:

$$\text{Maintenance dose} = \frac{\text{Peak body stores} \times \%\ \text{daily loss}}{100}$$

Where: peak body stores = loading dose % daily loss = 14 + creatinine clearance ($C_{cr}$)/5.

$C_{cr}$ is creatinine clearance corrected to 70 kg bodyweight or 1.73 m² body surface area. If only serum creatinine ($S_{cr}$) concentrations are available, a $C_{cr}$ (corrected to 70 kg bodyweight) may be estimated in men as:

$$C_{cr} = \frac{(140\text{–age})}{S_{cr}\ (\text{in mg/100 ml})}$$

*NOTE:* Where serum creatinine values are obtained in micromol/l, these may be converted to mg/100 ml (mg %) as follows:

$$S_{cr}\ (\text{mg/100 ml}) = \frac{S_{cr}\ (\text{micromol/l}) \times 113.12}{10{,}000} = \frac{S_{cr}\ (\text{micromol/l})}{88.4}$$

Where 113.12 is the molecular weight of creatinine.

*For women,* this result should be multiplied by 0.85.

*NOTE:* These formulae cannot be used for creatinine clearance in children.

In practice, this will mean that most patients will be maintained on 0.125 to 0.75 mg digoxin daily; however, in those who show increased sensitivity to the adverse effects of digoxin, a dosage of 62.5 microgram (0.0625 mg) daily or less may suffice.

*Emergency parenteral loading: (In patients who have not been given cardiac glycosides within the preceding two weeks):* The loading of parenteral Lanoxin is 500 to 1,000 micrograms (0.5 to 1.0 mg) depending on age, lean body weight and renal function.

The loading dose should be administered in divided doses with approximately half of the total dose given as the first dose and further fractions of the total dose given at intervals of 4 to 8 hours, assessing clinical response before giving each additional dose. Each dose should be given by intravenous infusion (see *Dilution*) over 10 to 20 minutes.

*Neonates, infants and children up to 10 years of age (if cardiac glycosides have not been given in the preceding two weeks):* The *intravenous loading dose* in the above groups should be administered in accordance with the following schedule:

| | |
|---|---|
| Pre-term neonates < 1.5 kg | 20 microgram/kg over 24 hours |
| Pre-term neonates 1.5 kg–2.5 kg | 30 microgram/kg over 24 hours |
| Term neonates up to 2 years | 35 microgram/kg over 24 hours |
| 2 to 5 years | 35 microgram/kg over 24 hours |
| 5 to 10 years | 25 microgram/kg over 24 hours |

The loading dose should be administered in divided doses with approximately half the total dose given as the first dose and further fractions of the total dose given at intervals of 4 to 8 hours, assessing clinical response before giving each additional dose. Each dose should be given by intravenous infusion (see *Dilution*) over 10 to 20 minutes.

*Oral loading dose:* This should be administered in accordance with the following schedule:

| | |
|---|---|
| Pre-term neonates < 1.5 kg | 25 microgram/kg over 24 hours |
| Pre-term neonates 1.5 kg–2.5 kg | 30 microgram/kg over 24 hours |
| Term neonates up to 2 years | 45 microgram/kg over 24 hours |
| 2 to 5 years | 35 microgram/kg over 24 hours |
| 5 to 10 years | 25 microgram/kg over 24 hours |

The loading dose should be administered in divided doses with approximately half the total dose given as the first dose and further fractions of the total dose given at intervals of 4 to 8 hours, assessing clinical response before giving each additional dose.

*Maintenance:*

The maintenance dose should be administered in accordance with the following schedule:

Pre-term neonates: daily dose = 20% of 24–hour loading dose (intravenous or oral)

Term neonates and children up to 10 years: daily dose = 25% of 24–hour loading dose (intravenous or oral)

These dosage schedules are meant as guidelines and careful clinical observation and monitoring of serum digoxin levels (see *Monitoring*) should be used as a basis for adjustment of dosage in these paediatric patient groups.

If cardiac glycosides have been given in the two weeks preceding commencement of Lanoxin therapy, it should be anticipated that optimum loading doses of Lanoxin will be less than those recommended above.

*Use in the elderly:* The tendency to impaired renal function and low lean body mass in the elderly influences the pharmacokinetics of Lanoxin, such that high serum digoxin levels and associated toxicity can occur quite readily, unless doses of Lanoxin lower than those in non-elderly patients are used. Serum digoxin levels should be checked regularly and hypokalaemia avoided.

*Dose recommendations in renal disorder or with diuretic therapy:* See *Precautions.*

*Dilution:* Lanoxin Injection, 250 micrograms per ml when diluted in the ratio of 1 to 250 (i.e. One 2 ml ampoule containing 500 micrograms added to 500 ml of infusion solution) is known to be compatible with the following infusion solutions and stable for up to 48 hours at room temperature (20 to 25°C):

Sodium Chloride Intravenous Infusion BP 0.9% w/v

Sodium Chloride (0.18% w/v) and Glucose (4% w/v) Intravenous Infusion BP

Glucose Intravenous Infusion BP 5% w/v

Dilution should be carried out either under full aseptic conditions or immediately before use. Any unused solution should be discarded.

*Monitoring:* Serum concentrations of digoxin may be

expressed in Conventional Units of nanogram/ml or SI Units of nanoMol/l. To convert ng/ml to nmol/l, multiply ng/ml by 1.28.

The serum concentration of digoxin can be determined by radioimmunoassay. Blood should be taken 6 hours or more after the last dose of Lanoxin. There are no rigid guidelines as to the range of serum concentrations that are most efficacious but most patients will benefit, with little risk of toxic symptoms developing, with digoxin concentrations from 0.8 nanogram/ml, ng/ml (1.02 nanoMol/litre, nM/L) to 2.0 ng/ml (2.56 nM/L). Above this range toxic symptoms and signs become more frequent and levels above 3.0 ng/ml (3.84 nM/L) are quite likely to be toxic. However, in deciding whether a patient's symptoms are due to digoxin, the patient's clinical state together with the serum potassium level and thyroid function are important factors.

Other glycosides, including metabolites of digoxin, can interfere with the assays that are available and one should always be wary of values which do not seem commensurate with the clinical state of the patient.

### Contra-indications, warnings, etc

*Contra-indications:* Lanoxin is contra-indicated in intermittent complete heart block or second degree atrioventricular block, especially if there is a history of Stokes-Adams attacks.

Lanoxin is contra-indicated in arrhythmias caused by cardiac glycoside intoxication.

Lanoxin is contra-indicated in supraventricular arrhythmias associated with an accessory atrioventricular pathway, as in the Wolff-Parkinson-White syndrome unless the electrophysiological characteristics of the accessory pathway and any possible deleterious effect of digoxin on these characteristics has been evaluated. If an accessory pathway is known or suspected to be present and there is no history of previous supraventricular arrhythmias, Lanoxin is similarly contra-indicated.

Lanoxin is contra-indicated in hypertrophic obstructive cardiomyopathy, unless there is concomitant atrial fibrillation and heart failure, but even then caution should be exercised if digoxin is to be used.

Lanoxin is contra-indicated in patients known to be hypersensitive to digoxin or other digitalis glycosides.

*Precautions:* Arrhythmias may be precipitated by digoxin toxicity, some of which can resemble arrhythmias for which the drug could be advised. For example, atrial tachycardia with varying atrioventricular block requires particular care as clinically the rhythm resembles atrial fibrillation.

In some cases of sinoatrial disorder (i.e. Sick Sinus syndrome) digoxin may cause or exacerbate sinus bradycardia or cause sinoatrial block.

Determination of the serum digoxin concentration may be very helpful in making a decision to treat with further digoxin, but toxic doses of other glycosides may cross-react in the assay and wrongly suggest apparently satisfactory measurements. Observations during the temporary withholding of digoxin might be more appropriate.

In cases where cardiac glycosides have been taken in the preceding two weeks, the recommendations for initial dosing of a patient should be reconsidered and a reduced dose is advised.

The dosing recommendations should be reconsidered if patients are elderly or there are other reasons for the renal clearance of digoxin being reduced. A reduction in both initial and maintenance doses should be considered.

Hypokalaemia sensitises the myocardium to the actions of cardiac glycosides.

Hypomagnesaemia and marked hypercalcaemia increase myocardial sensitivity to cardiac glycosides.

Rapid intravenous injection can cause vasoconstriction producing hypertension and/or reduced coronary flow. A slow injection rate is therefore important in hypertensive heart failure and acute myocardial infarction.

Administering Lanoxin to a patient with thyroid disease requires care. Initial and maintenance doses of Lanoxin should be reduced when thyroid function is subnormal. In hyperthyroidism there is relative digoxin resistance and the dose may have to be increased. During the course of treatment of thyrotoxicosis, dosage should be reduced as the thyrotoxicosis comes under control.

Patients with malabsorption syndrome or gastrointestinal reconstructions may require larger doses of digoxin.

The risk of provoking dangerous arrhythmias with direct current cardioversion is greatly increased in the presence of digitalis toxicity and is in proportion to the cardioversion energy used.

For elective direct current cardioversion of a patient who is taking digoxin, the drug should be withheld for 24 hours before cardioversion is performed. In emergencies, such as cardiac arrest, when attempting cardioversion, the lowest effective energy should be applied.

Direct current cardioversion is inappropriate in the treatment of arrhythmias thought to be caused by cardiac glycosides.

Many beneficial effects of digoxin on arrhythmias result from a degree of atrioventricular conduction blockade. However, when incomplete atrioventricular block already exists the effects of a rapid progression in the block should be anticipated. In complete heart block the idioventricular escape rhythm may be suppressed.

The administration of digoxin in the period immediately following myocardial infarction is not contra-indicated. However, the possibility of arrhythmias arising in patients who may be hypokalaemic after myocardial infarction and are likely to be cardiologically unstable must be borne in mind. The limitations imposed thereafter on direct current-cardioversion must also be remembered.

Although many patients with chronic congestive cardiac failure benefit from acute administration of digoxin, there are some in whom it does not lead to constant, marked or lasting haemodynamic improvement. It is therefore important to evaluate the response of each patient individually when Lanoxin is continued long-term.

The intramuscular route is painful and is associated with muscle necrosis. This route cannot be recommended.

Patients with severe respiratory disease may have an increased myocardial sensitivity to digitalis glycosides.

No data are available on whether or not digoxin has mutagenic, carcinogenic or teratogenic effects; however, maternally-administered digoxin has been used to treat fetal tachycardia and congestive heart failure.

There is no information available on the effect of digoxin on human fertility.

*Drug interactions:* These may arise from effects on the renal excretion, tissue binding, plasma protein binding, distribution within the body, gut absorptive capacity and sensitivity to Lanoxin. Consideration of the possibility of an interaction whenever concomitant therapy is contemplated is the best precaution and a check on serum digoxin concentration is recommended when any doubt exists.

Agents causing hypokalaemia or intracellular potassium deficiency may cause increased sensitivity to Lanoxin; they include diuretics, lithium salts, corticosteroids and carbenoxolone.

Serum levels of digoxin may be *INCREASED* by concomitant administration of the following: amiodarone; captopril; flecainide; prazosin; propafenone; quinidine; spironolactone; tetracycline; erythromycin (and possibly other antibiotics); and propantheline.

Serum levels of digoxin may be *REDUCED* by concomitant administration of the following: antacids; kaolin-pectin; some bulk laxatives and cholestyramine, diphenoxylate; sulphasalazine; neomycin; rifampicin; cytostatics; phenytoin; metoclopramide; and penicillamine.

Calcium channel blocking agents may either increase or cause no change in serum digoxin levels. Verapamil increases serum digoxin levels. Nifedipine and diltiazem may increase or have no effect on serum digoxin levels. Isradipine causes no change in serum digoxin levels.

Milrinone does not alter steady-state serum digoxin levels.

*Side- and adverse effects: Non-cardiac:* These are principally associated with overdosage but may occur from a temporarily high serum concentration due to rapid absorption. They include anorexia, nausea and vomiting and usually disappear within a few hours of taking the drug. Diarrhoea can also occur. It is inadvisable to rely on nausea as an early warning of excessive digoxin dosage.

Gynaecomastia can occur with long-term administration.

Weakness, apathy, fatigue, malaise, headache, visual disturbances, depression and even psychosis have been reported as adverse central nervous system effects.

Oral digoxin has also been associated with intestinal ischaemia and, rarely, with intestinal necrosis.

Skin rashes of urticarial or scarlatiniform character are rare reactions to digoxin, and may be accompanied by pronounced eosinophilia.

Very rarely, digoxin can cause thrombocytopenia.

*Cardiac:* Digoxin toxicity can cause various arrhythmias and conduction disturbances. Usually an early sign is the occurrence of ventricular premature contractions; they can proceed to bigeminy or even trigeminy. Atrial tachycardias, frequently an indication for digoxin, may nevertheless occur with excessive dosage of the drug. Atrial tachycardia with some degree of atrioventricular block is particularly characteristic, and the pulse rate may not necessarily be fast (see also *Precautions*).

*Use in pregnancy and lactation:* The use of digoxin in pregnancy is not contra-indicated, although the dosage and control may be less predictable in pregnant than in non-pregnant women with some requiring an increased dosage of digoxin during pregnancy. As with all drugs, use should be considered only when the expected clinical benefit of treatment to the mother outweighs any possible risk to the developing fetus.

Although digoxin is excreted in breast milk, the quantities are minute and breast feeding is not contra-indicated.

*Toxicity and treatment of overdosage:* For symptoms and signs see *Side-and adverse effects*.

After recent ingestion, such as accidental or deliberate self-poisoning, the load available for absorption may be reduced by gastric lavage.

An overdosage of digoxin of 10 to 15 mg in adults without heart disease and of 6 to 10 mg in children aged 1 to 3 years without heart disease appeared to be the dose resulting in death in half of the patients. If more than 25 mg of digoxin was ingested by an adult without heart disease, death or progressive toxicity responsive only to digoxin-binding Fab antibody fragments (Digibind*) resulted. If more than 10 mg of digoxin was ingested by a child aged 1 to 3 years without heart disease, the outcome was uniformly fatal when Fab fragment treatment was not given.

If hypokalaemia is present, it should be corrected with potassium supplements either orally or intravenously depending on the urgency of the situation. In cases where a large amount of Lanoxin has been ingested, hyperkalaemia may be present due to release of potassium from skeletal muscle. Before administering potassium in digoxin overdose the serum potassium level must be known.

Bradyarrhythmias may respond to atropine but temporary cardiac pacing may be required. Ventricular arrhythmias may respond to lignocaine or phenytoin.

Dialysis is not particularly effective in removing digoxin from the body in potentially life-threatening toxicity.

Rapid reversal of the complications that are associated with serious poisoning by digoxin, digitoxin and related glycosides has followed intravenous administration of digoxin-specific (ovine) antibody fragments (Fab) when other therapies have failed. Digibind* is the only specific treatment for digoxin toxicity and is very effective. For details consult the literature supplied with Digibind*.

### Pharmaceutical precautions
Tablets: Store below 25°C.
Elixir: Store below 25°C. Do not dilute.
Injection: Store below 25°C. Protect from light.
Dilution should be carried out either under full aseptic conditions or immediately before use. Any unused solution should be discarded.

### Legal category POM

### Package quantities
| | |
|---|---|
| Lanoxin Tablets: | Bottle of 500 |
| Lanoxin-125 Tablets: | Bottle of 500 |
| Lanoxin-PG Tablets: | Bottle of 500 |
| Lanoxin-PG Elixir: | Bottle of 60 ml |
| Lanoxin Injection: | Ampoule of 2 ml; box of 5 ampoules |

**Further information** Intravenous administration of a loading dose produces an appreciable pharmacological effect within 5 to 30 minutes; this reaches a maximum in 1 to 5 hours.

Using the oral route, the onset of effect occurs in 0.5 to 2 hours and reaches its maximum at 2 to 6 hours.

The terminal elimination half-life of digoxin in patients with normal renal function is 30 to 40 hours. It will be prolonged in patients with impaired renal function, and in anuric patients will be of the order of 100 hours.

### Product licence numbers
| | |
|---|---|
| Lanoxin Tablets: | 0003/0090R |
| Lanoxin 125 Tablets: | 0003/0102R |
| Lanoxin PG Tablets: | 0003/0091R |
| Lanoxin PG Elixir: | 0003/5260R |
| Lanoxin Injection: | 0003/5259R |

## MALOPRIM* TABLETS

**Presentation** Each white tablet is scored and contains 12.5 mg Pyrimethamine BP and 100 mg Dapsone BP, coded 'WELLCOME H9A'.

**Uses** Maloprim is indicated as a causal prophylactic and suppressive agent against malaria caused by *Plasmodium falciparum*. Maloprim is particularly recommended when resistance to pyrimethamine or other anti-folate preparation is known or suspected. It is also effective in chloroquine-resistant areas.

## osage and administration

dults and children over 10 years: 1 tablet once
weekly.

hildren 5 to 10 years: ½ tablet once weekly.

Under 5 years: Formulation not applicable.
THE RECOMMENDED DOSE MUST NOT BE
XCEEDED.

The constituents are rapidly absorbed and prophy-
ctic cover can be expected shortly after taking the
rst dose. Prophylaxis should commence before
rrival in an endemic area and be continued once
weekly. On returning to a non-malarious area dosage
hould be maintained for a further four weeks.

Use in the elderly: No specific studies have been
arried out in the elderly. It is advisable to assess renal
nd hepatic function and if there is serious impairment
aution should be exercised. (See Precautions.)

At the doses recommended for the prevention of
nalaria, Maloprim is unlikely to have any adverse
ffect on older people normally in good health.

## ontra-indications, warnings, etc

ontra-indications: Maloprim should not be given to
dividuals with a known history of hypersensitivity
 sulphonamides, sulphones or pyrimethamine.

recautions: Maloprim should not be used for the
eatment of acute attacks of malaria.

Subjects taking malaria prophylaxis should be
arned that no antimalarial agent gives complete
rotection. Further precautionary measures, such as
overing exposed areas of the body, application of
sect repellents and use of mosquito nets should be
dvised. Malaria should be considered in the differ-
ntial diagnosis of any pyrexial illness. Such measures
re particularly important in rural areas of East Africa.

Short term usage of Maloprim is unlikely to carry
xcess risk in patients with renal or hepatic impair-
ent. However, patients with significant kidney or
ver disease taking Maloprim for prolonged periods
hould be monitored regularly for signs of bone
arrow depression.

Maloprim may exacerbate folate deficiency in indi-
iduals predisposed to this condition through disease
r malnutrition. Accordingly, a folic acid supplement
hould be given to such individuals.

At high doses (100 mg/kg 5 times a week for 104
eeks), dapsone has been reported to be carcinogenic
 male rats but not female rats, nor in mice of either
ex. The clinical significance of this finding is not
nown. However, cancer mortality among American
prosy patients receiving long-term dapsone therapy
as no greater over a 40–year period than that
xpected from population statistics.

Five intraperitoneal doses of 125 mg pyrimetham-
e/kg bodyweight, administered over a period of 24
eeks to mice, were associated with an increase in
ng tumours. Doses of 62.5 mg and 31.25 mg/kg
odyweight did not induce a statistically significant
crease in tumour numbers. Both higher doses were
xic and led to death of more than half of the treated
nimals before the end of the study period.

Pyrimethamine was not mutagenic in the Ames
st. Chromosome abnormalities have been reported
 bone marrow cells from patients with P.falciparum
alaria given total doses of 200 and 300 mg pyrime-
amine. There are no data available on whether or
ot dapsone has mutagenic potential.

ide- and adverse effects: Side effects caused by
aloprim at the recommended doses are rare.

Severe bone marrow depression leading to agran-
ocytosis or red cell hypoplasia has been reported,
articularly in association with doses of one tablet
wice weekly.

There have been rare instances of pneumonia,
ssociated with eosinophilic pulmonary infiltration,
eveloping soon after initiation of prophylaxis.

Cyanosis, attributable to methaemoglobinaemia,
as been reported, usually following doses higher
an those recommended.

Administration of excessive doses over a prolonged
eriod may produce haemolytic or megaloblastic
naemia.

The haemolytic effect of dapsone is dose-related
nd greater in glucose-6–phosphate dehydrogenase
eficiency. The dosage of dapsone as used in
aloprim is insufficient to cause clinically apparent
sease in the majority of individuals. However, rare
ses of haemoglobinuria have been reported in
ucose-6–phosphate dehydrogenase-deficient indi-
duals following Maloprim administration.

Insomnia has been reported when pyrimethamine
as been given at weekly doses above those recom-
ended.

Other reactions associated on rare occasions with
yrimethamine or dapsone, usually at higher doses,
clude: after short-term dosage– rash and other skin
sorders; thrombocytopenia; a mononucleosis-like
ndrome; jaundice and psychosis; and after long
rm dosage– motor neuropathy and hypoalbuminae-
ia.

A dapsone (or sulphone) syndrome, a form of
hypersensitivity reaction, has been rarely reported
and may occur during the first 6 weeks of therapy. Its
most common features are hepatitis (most prominent), fever and rash (often an exfoliative dermatitis),
which may be accompanied by hepatosplenomagaly,
renal papillary necrosis and by those reactions
described in the sections on short- and long-term
dosage. Patients usually improve on dapsone withdrawal, however may require steroid treatment. Fatalities have been reported.

Drug interactions: Maloprim, through its mode of
action, may depress folate metabolism in patients
already receiving treatment with other folate inhibitors, or agents associated with myelosuppression,
including co-trimoxazole, trimethoprim, proguanil
and zidovudine.

In vitro data suggest that antacid salts and antidiarrhoeal earths reduce the absorption of pyrimethamine.

Probenecid may reduce renal excretion of dapsone
and its metabolites leading to a rise in serum levels.

Rifampicin may shorten the plasma half-life of
dapsone.

Use in pregnancy and lactation: The safety of
Maloprim in human pregnancy has not been
established. In view of the theoretical risk of fetal
malformation with all folate inhibitors, caution should
be exercised in the administration of Maloprim during
pregnancy, particularly in the first trimester.

Pregnant women should be advised against making
unnecessary visits to endemic areas. In addition,
consideration should be given to the likelihood of
contracting malaria in the area to be visited. Maloprim
should only be advised during pregnancy if an
unavoidable visit to a hyper-endemic area of known
or suspected chloroquine-resistant malaria is to be
undertaken.

A folate supplement, preferably as folinic acid or
calcium folate, should be given to all pregnant women
taking Maloprim.

The amount of Maloprim constituents excreted in
breast milk is insufficient to contra-indicate its use in
lactating mothers, but breast-fed infants should not
receive other anti-folate agents.

Toxicity and treatment of overdosage: Acute overdosage: The most commonly observed effects of acute
overdosage are methaemoglobinaemia, and in
extreme cases, convulsions. There is a possibility of
anaemia developing due to the haemolytic effect of
dapsone and inhibition of folate metabolism following
large doses of pyrimethamine.

In view of the rapid absorption of both constituents
of Maloprim, gastric lavage should only be considered
within the first 2 hours of ingestion. Oral administration of activated charcoal over several days has been
shown to decrease the plasma half-life of dapsone.
As there is evidence to suggest enterohepatic circulation of pyrimethamine, this measure may also be of
value in its elimination. In addition, adequate fluids
should be given to ensure optimal diuresis.

Routine supportive measures, including maintenance of a clear airway and control of convulsions
should be given. Methaemoglobinaemia should be
treated by oral administration of ascorbic acid, 200 mg
three times daily, or by intravenous administration of
methylene blue according to the level of methaemoglobin. (Methylene blue should not be given to
patients with G-6–PD deficiency.) To counteract
possible folate deficiency, calcium folinate should be
given for 3 days in a dose of 9 to 15 mg, 6–hourly.

Chronic overdosage: The most likely effects of chronic
overdosage are methaemoglobinaemia, haemolytic
anaemia and megaloblastic anaemia.

Maloprim administration should be discontinued.
Ascorbic acid or methylene blue is of value in the
treatment of methaemoglobinaemia. (Methylene blue
should not be given to patients with G-6–PD deficiency.) Calcium folinate is of value in the treatment
of megaloblastic anaemia.

Pharmaceutical precautions    Store below 25°C.
Protect from light.

Legal category    POM

Package quantities    Strip pack of 30 tablets as 5 foil
strips of 6 tablets.

Further information    Nil.

Product licence number    0003/5117R.

## MIGRIL* TABLETS

Presentation    White, round, biconvex, compression-
coated tablets with a pink core, scored and impressed
'WELLCOME A4A', with each tablet containing 2 mg
Ergotamine Tartrate BP, 50 mg Cyclizine Hydro-
chloride BP and Caffeine BP equivalent to 100 mg
Caffeine Hydrate BP.

Uses    Migril is indicated for the relief of the acute
migraine attack.

### Dosage and administration

Adults: Migril should be taken as soon as possible
after the first warning of an attack of migraine and
repeated if necessary at the prescribed intervals.

The usual initial dose is one tablet.

Additional doses of a half to one tablet may then be
required at half-hourly intervals.

No more than 4 tablets (8 mg ergotamine) should
be taken in any one attack.

No more than 6 tablets (12 mg ergotamine) should
be given in any one week.

Children: There is no absolute contra-indication to the
use of Migril in children but its use is not
recommended.

Use in the elderly: There are no absolute contra-
indications to the use of Migril in the elderly, but see
Contra-indications and Precautions.

### Contra-indications, warnings, etc

Contra-indications: Migril is contra-indicated during
pregnancy because of a direct effect of ergotamine on
the uterus. In animals, ergotamine has been reported
to inhibit implantation, cause peri-natal mortality and
fetal retardation.

Migril is contra-indicated during lactation and
breast-feeding; it may suppress milk production and
may also be excreted in milk at levels high enough to
cause pharmacological effects in breast-fed infants.

Migril is contra-indicated in pre-existing vascular
disease including coronary disease, obliterative
vascular disease, angina, claudication, peripheral
ischaemia, Raynaud's syndrome and hypertension.

Migril should not be taken if there is a hypersensitivity to any of its constituents.

Precautions: Migril should not be used for migraine
prophylaxis because of the risk of inducing ergotism.

The use of ergotamine-containing compounds
carries the risk of precipitating arterial constriction
and other manifestations of ergotism.

Use the minimum effective dosage of Migril necessary since individual sensitivity to the arterial effects
of ergotamine varies considerably.

Discontinue the use of Migril if symptoms of arterial
insufficiency develop, including coldness, numbness
or tingling of the extremities.

Doses of ergotamine as small as 2 mg have caused
signs of arterial insufficiency but this is a very rare
occurrence.

Migril should be used with caution in patients with
infective hepatitis because of an increased risk of
precipitating peripheral ischaemia.

Repeated doses of ergotamine have occasionally
been associated with renal artery spasm and loss of
renal function.

Alcohol and Migril should not be taken concurrently.

Ergotamine should be used with care when hyperthyroidism, sepsis or anaemia are present.

Cyclizine, in common with other antihistamines,
may cause sedation; patients should be cautioned
about driving or operating machinery.

Drug interactions: The concomitant use of ergot
alkaloids and β-blocking agents increases the risks of
peripheral vasoconstriction.

Vomiting and peripheral ischaemia have been
reported after concomitant use of ergot alkaloids and
the antibiotics erythromycin and oleandomycin.

Side- and adverse effects: Habitual use of ergotamine-
containing preparations can produce a syndrome of
non-migrainous rebound headaches, in which case
Migril should be discontinued.

Side-effects seen with Migril are usually due to the
ergotamine components of the preparation and are
more common if the dosage recommendations are
exceeded. They include intermittent claudication,
coldness and whiteness of the extremities, dysaesthesia, paraesthesia, formication and precordial pain.

Other side-effects seen with ergotamine include
muscle cramps, joint pains, raised blood pressure,
pulselessness, cyanosis, thrombophlebitis, peripheral
arterial thrombosis, gangrene, abdominal pain,
coronary infarction, cerebral thrombosis, nausea,
dyspnoea, decreased visual acuity, vertigo and
diarrhoea. These effects have mostly occurred following habitual chronic use exceeding the recommended
dose; they may occasionally occur however at the
therapeutic dose.

Arterial vasospasm severe enough to threaten the
viability of the limbs has been reported after routine
therapy but it is more normally to be expected after
prolonged overdosage.

Use in pregnancy and lactation: See Contra-
indications.

Toxicity and treatment of overdosage:

Acute overdosage: Symptoms: Acute overdosage
with an ergotamine-containing preparation is characterised by nausea, vomiting, tachycardia, hypotonia
and peripheral ischaemia. Blood pressure may be
difficult to measure.

Treatment: If vomiting has not occurred, efforts should

be made to clear the stomach contents. General supportive measures should be applied and intravenous vasodilators may be necessary to relieve vasospasm.

Peritoneal dialysis and forced diuresis may help to eliminate ergotamine from the body.

*Chronic overdosage: Symptoms*: Chronic overdosage with ergotamine-containing preparations usually presents as peripheral ischaemia threatening the viability of the affected limb.

*Treatment:* Withdraw Migril immediately.

Intravenous vasodilators such as nitroprusside and nitroglycerin may be used to re-establish normal blood flow. Captopril has also been used to reverse the effects of chronic overdosage with ergotamine.

Re-establishment of blood flow may be associated with intense burning sensations in the affected areas but these usually resolve after several weeks.

**Pharmaceutical precautions** Store below 25°C. Keep dry. Protect from light.

**Legal category** POM

**Package quantities** Bottle of 100 tablets.

**Further information** Nil.

**Product licence number** 0003/5114R

## OTOSPORIN* EAR DROPS

**Presentation** Each ml of milky-white liquid contains 10,000 Units Polymyxin B Sulphate BP, 3,400 Units Neomycin Sulphate BP, and 1% w/v Hydrocortisone BP, in an aqueous base.

**Uses** Otosporin Ear Drops are indicated for the treatment of otitis externa due to, or complicated by, bacterial infection.

*In vitro activity:* Otosporin Ear Drops are active against a wide range of bacterial pathogens. The range of activity includes:

GRAM-POSITIVE ORGANISMS:
*Staphylococcus epidermidis* and *Staphylococcus aureus*;
GRAM-NEGATIVE ORGANISMS:
Enterobacter spp.
Escherichia spp.
Haemophilus spp.
Klebsiella spp.
Proteus spp.
*Pseudomonas aeruginosa*

Otosporin Ear Drops are not expected to be active against streptococci, including *Streptococcus pyogenes*.

Hydrocortisone possesses anti-inflammatory, anti-allergic and antipruritic activity.

**Dosage and administration**
*Adults:* Following cleansing and drying of the external auditory meatus and canal as appropriate, three drops should be instilled into the affected ear three or four times daily. Alternatively, a gauze wick may be introduced into the external auditory canal and kept saturated with the solution; the wick may be left in place for 24 to 48 hours.

Soap should not be used for cleansing of the external auditory meatus and canal as it may inactivate the antibiotics.

*Children:* As for adults.

*Use in the elderly:* As for adults.

**Contra-indications, warnings, etc**
*Contra-indications:* The use of Otosporin Ear Drops is contra-indicated in patients in whom perforation of the tympanic membrane is known or suspected.

The use of Otosporin Ear Drops is contra-indicated in patients who have demonstrated allergic hypersensitivity to any of the components of the preparation or to cross-sensitising substances such as framycetin, kanamycin, gentamicin and other related antibiotics.

The use of Otosporin Ear Drops is contra-indicated in the presence of untreated viral, fungal and tubercular infections.

*Precautions:* Occasionally, delayed hypersensitivity to corticosteroids may occur. Treatment with topical steroid antibiotic combinations should not be continued for more than seven days in the absence of any clinical improvement, since prolonged use may lead to occult extension of infection due to the masking effect of the steroid. Prolonged use may also lead to skin sensitisation and the emergence of resistant organisms.

All topically active corticosteroids possess the potential to suppress the pituitary-adrenal axis following systemic absorption. Development of adverse systemic effects due to the hydrocortisone component of Otosporin Ear Drops is considered to be unlikely, although the recommended dosage should not be exceeded, particularly in infants.

Prolonged, unsupervised use should be avoided as it may lead to irreversible partial or total deafness, especially in the elderly and in patients with impaired renal function.

Use in the immediate pre- and post-operative period is not advised as neomycin may rarely cause neuromuscular block; because it potentiates skeletal muscle relaxant drugs, it may cause respiratory depression and arrest.

*Side- and adverse effects:* The incidence of allergic hypersensitivity reactions to neomycin sulphate in the general population is low. There is, however, an increased incidence of hypersensitivity to neomycin in certain selected groups of patients in dermatological practice, particularly those with venous stasis eczema and ulceration, and chronic otitis externa.

Allergic hypersensitivity reactions following topical application of polymyxin B sulphate and hydrocortisone are rare.

Allergic hypersensitivity to neomycin following topical use may manifest itself as an eczematous exacerbation with reddening, scaling, swelling and itching or as a failure of the lesion to heal.

Stinging and burning have occasionally been reported when Otosporin Ear Drops gained access to the middle ear.

Otosporin Ear Drops should only be used in the ear and are not suitable for use in the eye.

*Use in pregnancy and lactation:* Safety for use in pregnancy and lactation has not been established. There is inadequate evidence of safety in human pregnancy. Topical administration of corticosteroids to pregnant animals can cause abnormalities of fetal development, including cleft palate and intra-uterine growth retardation. There may be a very small risk of such effects in the human fetus.

As well as suppression of the neonatal HPA axis, there is a risk of fetal toxicity if aminoglycoside antibiotic preparations are administered during pregnancy.

No information is available regarding the excretion of polymyxin B sulphate and neomycin or their metabolites in human breast milk, following the use of Otosporin Ear Drops.

There is no information available on the levels of hydrocortisone which may appear in human breast milk following topical administration. When Otosporin Ear Drops are used as recommended, it is unlikely that sufficient hydrocortisone would be absorbed to produce detectable levels in breast milk.

*Toxicity and treatment of overdosage:* There is no experience of overdosage with Otosporin.

**Pharmaceutical precautions** Store below 15°C. Protect from light. Shake before use.

**Legal category** POM

**Package quantities** Plastic drop-dose bottles of 5 ml and 10 ml.

**Further information** Nil.

**Product licence number** 0003/5106R

## PENTOSTAM* INJECTION

**Presentation** Pentostam is a faintly yellow, sterile, aqueous solution containing Sodium Stibogluconate BP equivalent to 100 mg pentavalent antimony in each ml.

**Uses** Pentostam is indicated for the following diseases: Visceral leishmaniasis (kala azar); cutaneous leishmaniasis; South American mucocutaneous leishmaniasis. Note: Cutaneous and diffuse cutaneous leishmaniasis caused by *Leishmania aethiopica* infections are unresponsive to treatment with pentavalent antimony compounds, including Pentostam, at conventional dosage, but may respond slowly at higher dosage.

*Mode of action:* The mode of action of Pentostam is unknown. *In vitro* exposure of amastigotes to 500 mg $Sb^{5+}$/ml results in a greater than 50% decrease in parasite DNA, RNA protein and purine nucleoside triphosphate levels. It has been postulated that the reduction in ATP (adenosine triphosphate) and GTP (guanosine triphosphate) synthesis contributes to decreased macromolecular synthesis.

*Pharmacokinetics:* Following intravenous or intramuscular administration of sodium stibogluconate, antimony is excreted rapidly *via* the kidneys, the majority of the dose being detected in the first 12–hour urine collection. This rapid excretion is reflected by a marked fall in serum or whole blood antimony levels to approximately 1 to 4% of the peak level by 8 hours after an intravenous dose. During daily administration, there is a slow accumulation of sodium stibogluconate into the central compartment so that tissue concentrations reach a theoretical maximum level after at least 7 days.

**Dosage and administration** Except where otherwise stated, all doses should be given by the intravenous or intramuscular route (see *Precautions*).

All dosage recommendations are based on th findings of the WHO Expert Committee on leish maniasis which met in 1984. There are no speci recommendations for different age groups.

*Visceral leishmaniasis:* 10 to 20 mg $Sb^{5+}$ (0.1 to 0.2 m Pentostam)/kg bodyweight to a maximum of 850 m (8.5 ml Pentostam) daily for a minimum period of 2 days. Patients should be examined for evidence o relapse after 2 and 6 months, and in Africa aft 12 months.

*Cutaneous leishmaniasis NOT caused by aethiopica:* The dosage regimen outlined for viscer leishmaniasis is recommended. Alternatively, singl non-inflamed nodular lesions known not to be due t *L. braziliensis* may be treated with intralesion injections of 100 to 300 mg $Sb^{5+}$ (1 to 3 ml Pentostan repeated once or twice if necessary at intervals of 1 t 2 days. Infiltration must be thorough and produc complete blanching of the base of the lesion.

Individuals with cutaneous leishmaniasis due to *braziliensis* should be treated systemically for sever days after the lesion is healed.

Note: After successful treatment of *L. braziliensi* anti-leishmania antibody titres decline steadily over to 24 months.

*Muco-cutaneous leishmaniasis:* Patients with paras tologically confirmed leishmaniasis should be treate with 20 mg $Sb^{5+}$ (0.2 ml Pentostam)/kg bodyweight t a maximum of 850 mg (8.5 ml Pentostam) dail continuing this dosage for several days longer than takes to achieve parasitological and clinical cure.

In the event of relapse, a further course should b given for at least twice the previous duration.

*Diffuse cutaneous leishmaniasis in the New Wor and leishmaniasis recidivans:* Owing to the rarity o these conditions, precise data on dosage are n available. A dose of 10 to 20 mg $Sb^{5+}$ (0.1 to 0.2 r Pentostam)/kg bodyweight to a maximum of 850 m (8.5 ml Pentostam) may be given daily for 2 to weeks. If there is a response, then treatment shou be maintained until several days after clinical cure a leishmaniasis recidivans and for several months aft clinical and parasitological cure of diffuse cutaneo leishmaniasis.

*Use in the elderly:* There is little information on th effects of Pentostam on elderly individuals. If trea ment of cutaneous leishmaniasis is necessary the local infiltration is preferred. The normal precautio should be strictly adhered to when treating old patients for visceral leishmaniasis.

**Contra-indications, warnings, etc**
*Contra-indications:* Pentostam should not be given t any patient with significantly impaired renal functio Pentostam should not be given to any patient wh has experienced a serious adverse reaction to previous dose.

*Precautions:* Intravenous injection should be admi istered very slowly over 5 minutes to reduce the ri of local thrombosis. In the unlikely event of coughin vomiting or substernal pain occurring, administrati should be discontinued immediately. In such case extreme care should be taken if Pentostam is r administered by this route.

Successful treatment of mucocutaneous leishma iasis may induce severe inflammation around th lesion. In cases of pharyngeal or tracheal involveme this may be life-threatening. Under such circur stances, corticosteroids may be used.

Very rarely, anaphylactic shock may develop duri treatment for which adrenaline injection ar appropriate supportive measures should be give immediately.

Pentostam should be used cautiously in patien with heart disease.

Electrocardiographic changes, notably alteratio in T wave amplitude, may be expected in the major of patients given Pentostam and are not of serio significance. Where electrocardiograms have be done in patients receiving doses in excess of 20 m kg bodyweight/day, modest increases in the rat corrected QT interval have been observed. There no firm evidence of drug-induced arrhythmias patients receiving Pentostam, but it is recommende that treatment is withdrawn if conducti disturbances occur.

Patients who have recently received other an monial drugs should be monitored closely for sig of antimony intoxication such as bradycardia a cardiac arrhythmias during administration Pentostam.

Intercurrent infections, such as pneumonia, shou be sought and treated concomitantly.

High concentrations of antimony are found in th livers of animals after repeated dosage with pen valent antimony. Pentostam should therefore be us with caution in patients with hepatic diseas However, some abnormalities of liver function m be expected in cases of visceral leishmaniasis. In su patients the benefit of pentavalent antimony treatme utweighs the risk. Pentostam may induce mild evation of hepatic enzymes in serum which later turn to normal; in these cases, treatment should not e stopped.

*rug interactions:* No interactions with Pentostam ave been reported.

*ide- and adverse effects:* The majority of side-effects re transitory in nature.

Approximately 1 to 2% of patients complain of ausea, vomiting and/or diarrhoea and a slightly gher number of abdominal pain.

Other common side-effects include anorexia, alaise, myalgia, headache and lethargy.

Transient coughing immediately following injection as reported with varying frequency during several ials.

Intravenous injection of Pentostam may cause ansient pain along the course of the vein and ventually thrombosis of that vein.

During some early trials of sodium stibogluconate, neumonia occurred in a small number of patients eated for visceral leishmaniasis and this occasionally roved fatal. Pneumonia is a feature of the visceral ishmaniasis disease process; however, it has been ssociated with the toxicity profile of trivalent antiony. It is, therefore, not possible to determine hether these cases were due to the disease or to entostam.

Other (rarely reported) side-effects include fever, gor, sweating, vertigo, facial flushing, worsening of sions on the cheek, bleeding from the nose or gum, ubsternal pain, jaundice and rash.

*se in pregnancy and lactation:* Although no effects n the fetus have been reported, Pentostam should e withheld during pregnancy unless the potential enefits to the patient outweigh the possible risk to e fetus.

Children should not be breast-fed by mothers eceiving Pentostam.

*oxicity and treatment of overdosage:* Main ymptoms of antimony overdosage are gastrotestinal disturbances (nausea, vomiting and severe arrhoea). Haemorrhagic nephritis and hepatitis may so occur.

There is only limited information on the use of elating agents in the treatment of intoxication with ntimony compounds. Dimercaprol has been reported be effective: a dose of 200 mg by intramuscular jection, every six hours until recovery is complete, suggested. 2,3-dimercaptosuccinic acid (DMSA) ay also be effective treatment.

**harmaceutical precautions** Store below 25°C and rotect from light.

The contents should not be used more than one onth after removing the first dose.

**egal category** POM

**ackage quantities** Rubber-capped bottle of 100 ml.

**urther information** There is no information on hether Pentostam interferes with the accuracy of outine biochemical tests.

**roduct licence number** 0003/5105R.

## EMPREX* CAPSULES

**resentation** Each opaque white capsule contains mg acrivastine. Markings include 'WELLCOME' and unicorn printed in black, and 'SEMPREX' printed in ddish-brown.

**ses** Antihistamine. Semprex is indicated for the mptomatic relief of allergic rhinitis, including hay ver. Semprex is also indicated for chronic idiopathic ticaria, symptomatic dermographism, cholinergic ticaria and idiopathic acquired cold urticaria.

**osage and administration**

*dults, and children over 12 years:* One 8 mg capsule ree times a day.

*se in the elderly:* As yet, no specific studies have en carried out in the elderly. Until further information is available, Semprex should not be given to derly patients.

*harmacology:* Acrivastine provides symptomatic lief in conditions believed to depend wholly or partly on the triggered release of histamine.

It is a potent competitive histamine $H_1$-antagonist hich lacks significant anticholinergic effects, and has low potential to penetrate the central nervous stem.

After oral administration of a single dose of 8 mg rivastine to adults, the onset of action, as deterined by the ability to antagonise histamine-induced eals and flares in the skin, is within 1 hour. Peak fects occur at 2 hours, and although activity declines owly thereafter, significant inhibition of histamineduced weals and flares still occurs 8 hours after se.

In patients, relief from the symptoms of allergic rhinitis is apparent within 1 hour after the systemic administration of the drug.

*Pharmacokinetics:* Acrivastine is well absorbed from the gut. In healthy adult volunteers, the peak plasma concentration (Cmax) is approximately 150 nanogram/ml, occurring at about 1.5 hours (Tmax) after the administration of 8 mg acrivastine. The plasma half-life is approximately 1.5 hours. In multiple dose studies over 6 days, no accumulation of acrivastine was observed.

**Contra-indications, warnings, etc** Semprex is contra-indicated in individuals with known hypersensitivity to acrivastine or triprolidine. Renal excretion is the principal route of elimination of acrivastine. Until specific studies have been carried out Semprex should not be given to patients with significant renal impairment (creatinine clearance less than 50 ml per minute or serum creatinine greater than 150 micromoles per litre).

*Precautions:* Most patients do not experience drowsiness with Semprex. Nevertheless, as there is individual variation in response to all medication, it is sensible to caution all patients about engaging in activities requiring mental alertness, such as driving a car or operating machinery, until patients are familiar with their own response to the drug.

It is usual to advise patients not to undertake tasks requiring mental alertness whilst under the influence of alcohol and other CNS depressants. Concomitant administration of acrivastine may, in some individuals, produce additional impairment.

*Side- and adverse effects:* Reports of drowsiness directly attributable to Semprex are extremely rare. Indeed, for the great majority of patients, treatment with Semprex is not associated with clinically significant anticholinergic or sedative side-effects.

*Use in pregnancy and lactation:* No data are available on the use of Semprex during pregnancy, therefore caution should be exercised by balancing the potential benefits of treatment against any possible hazard. Systemic administration of acrivastine in animal reproductive studies did not produce embryotoxic or teratogenic effects and did not impair fertility.

There is no information on the levels of acrivastine which may appear in human breast milk after administration of Semprex.

*Toxicity and treatment of overdosage:* There is no experience of overdosage with Semprex. Appropriate supportive therapy, including gastric lavage, should be initiated if indicated.

**Pharmaceutical precautions** Protect from light. Keep dry. Store below 25°C.

**Legal category** POM

**Package quantities** 84 capsules as 4 blister strips of 21 tablets.

**Further information** Nil.

**Product licence number** 0003/0254.

## VALOID* TABLETS
## VALOID* INJECTION

**Presentation** Valoid Tablets each contain 50 mg Cyclizine Hydrochloride BP, scored, coded 'WELLCOME T4A', white in colour.

Valoid Injection contains 50 mg cyclizine lactate in each 1 ml ampoule.

**Uses** Valoid is indicated for the prevention and treatment of nausea and vomiting including motion sickness, nausea and vomiting caused by narcotic analgesics and by general anaesthetics in the postoperative period and radiotherapy, especially for breast cancer since cyclizine does not elevate prolactin levels.

Valoid may be of value in relieving vomiting and attacks of vertigo associated with Meniere's disease and other forms of vestibular disturbance when the oral route cannot be used.

Valoid Injection, by the intravenous route, is also indicated pre-operatively in patients undergoing emergency surgery in order to reduce the hazard of regurgitation and aspiration of gastric contents during induction of general anaesthesia.

*Pharmacology:* Cyclizine is a histamine $H_1$-receptor antagonist of the piperazine class which is characterised by a low incidence of drowsiness. It possesses anticholinergic and anti-emetic properties. The exact mechanism by which cyclizine can prevent or suppress both nausea and vomiting from various causes is unknown. Cyclizine increases lower oesophageal sphincter tone and reduces the sensitivity of the labyrinthine apparatus. It may inhibit the part of the midbrain known collectively as the emetic centre.

In healthy adult volunteers the administration of a single oral dose of 50 mg cyclizine resulted in a peak plasma concentration of approximately 70 nanogram/ml occurring at about 2 hours after drug administration. The plasma elimination half-life was approximately 20 hours.

Cyclizine produces its anti-emetic effect within 2 hours and lasts approximately 4 hours.

The N-demethylated derivative, norcyclizine, has been identified as a metabolite of cyclizine.

Norcyclizine has little antihistamine ($H_1$) activity compared to cyclizine and has a plasma elimination half-life of approximately 20 hours. After a single oral dose of 50 mg cyclizine given to a single adult male volunteer, urine collected over the following 24 hours contained less than 1% of the total dose administered.

**Dosage and administration**

*Valoid Tablets:*

*Adults and children over 12 years:* 1 tablet up to three times daily.

*Children 6 to 12 years:* ½ tablet, up to three times daily.

*Under 6 years:* Formulation not applicable.

*Valoid Injection*

*Adults*: 50 mg intramuscularly or intravenously up to three times daily. When used intravenously, Valoid should be injected slowly into the bloodstream, with only minimal withdrawal of blood into the syringe.

For the prevention of postoperative nausea and vomiting, administer the first dose by slow intravenous injection 20 minutes before the anticipated end of surgery.

Cyclizine given intravenously, in half the recommended dose, increases the lower oesophageal sphincter tone and thereby reduces the hazard of regurgitation and aspiration of gastric contents if given to patients, undergoing emergency surgery, before induction of general anaesthesia.

*Use in the elderly*: There have been no specific studies of Valoid in the elderly. Experience has indicated that normal adult dosage is appropriate.

**Contra-indications, warnings, etc**

*Contra-indications*: Valoid should not be given to individuals with known hypersensitivity to cyclizine.

*Precautions*: Although studies designed to detect drowsiness did not reveal sedation in healthy adults who took a single *oral* therapeutic dose (50 mg) of cyclizine, sedation of short duration was reported by subjects receiving intravenous cyclizine. Patients should not drive or operate machinery until they have determined their own response.

Although there are no data available, patients should be cautioned that Valoid may have additive effects with alcohol and other central nervous system depressants, e.g. hypnotics and tranquillisers.

As with other anticholinergic agents, Valoid should be used with caution and appropriate monitoring in patients with glaucoma, obstructive disease of the gastrointestinal tract and in males with possible prostatic hypertrophy. Valoid Injection may have a hypotensive effect.

Cyclizine should be used with caution in patients with severe heart failure. In such patients, cyclizine may cause a fall in cardiac output associated with increases in heart rate, mean arterial pressure and pulmonary wedge pressure.

There have been no specific studies in hepatic and/or renal dysfunction.

Cyclizine was not mutagenic in a full Ames test, including use of S9-microsomes.

No long-term studies have been conducted in animals to determine whether cyclizine has a potential for carcinogenesis.

*Side- and adverse effects*: Urticaria, drug rash, drowsiness, dryness of the mouth, nose and throat, blurred vision, tachycardia, urinary retention, constipation, restlessness, nervousness, insomnia and auditory and visual hallucinations have been reported, particularly when dosage recommendations have been exceeded. Cholestatic jaundice has occurred in association with cyclizine. Single case reports have been documented of fixed drug eruption, generalised chorea, hypersensitivity hepatitis and agranulocytosis.

A single case of anaphylaxis has been recorded following intravenous administration of cyclizine coadministered with propanidid in the same syringe. An increase in excitatory phenomena (tremor and muscle movements) has been reported when cyclizine has been given before propanidid and methohexitone anaesthesia.

*Use in pregnancy and lactation*: Some animal studies are interpreted as indicating that cyclizine may be teratogenic.

In a study involving prolonged administration of cyclizine to male and female rats there was no evidence of impaired fertility after continuous treatment for 90 to 100 days. There is no experience of the effect of Valoid on human fertility.

In the absence of any definitive human data, the use of Valoid in pregnancy is not advised.

It is not known whether cyclizine or its metabolite are excreted in human milk.

*Drug interactions*: Valoid may have additive effects with alcohol and other central nervous system depressants e.g. hypnotics, tranquillisers. Valoid enhances the soporific effect of pethidine. Because of its anticholinergic activity cyclizine may enhance the side-effects of other anticholinergic drugs.

*Toxicity and treatment of overdosage*: *Symptoms*: Symptoms of acute toxicity from cyclizine arise from peripheral anticholinergic effects and effects on the central nervous system.

Peripheral anticholinergic symptoms include dry mouth, nose and throat, blurred vision, tachycardia and urinary retention. Central nervous system effects include drowsiness, dizziness, inco-ordination, ataxia, weakness, hyperexcitability, disorientation, impaired judgement, hallucinations, hyperkinesia, extrapyramidal motor disturbances, convulsions, hyperpyrexia and respiratory depression.

An oral dose of 5 mg/kg is likely to be associated with at least one of the clinical symptoms stated above. Younger children are more susceptible to convulsions. The incidence of convulsions, in children less than 5 years, is about 60% when the oral dose ingested exceeds 40 mg/kg.

*Treatment*: In the management of acute overdosage with Valoid, gastric lavage and supportive measures for respiration and circulation should be performed if necessary. Convulsions should be controlled in the usual way with parenteral anticonvulsant therapy.

**Pharmaceutical precautions**
Injection: Store below 25°C. Protect from light.
Tablets: Store below 25°C.

**Legal category**
Injection: POM
Tablets: P

**Package quantities**
Injection: Box of 5 ampoules
Tablets: Bottle of 100.

**Further information** Nil.

**Product licence numbers**
Injection: 0003/5212R
Tablets: 0003/5213R

## VALTREX* ▼

**Presentation** Each white tablet is marked 'VALTREX' and '500' and contains 500 mg valaciclovir as valaciclovir hydrochloride (556 mg).

Also contains: microcrystalline cellulose; crospovidone; povidone K90; magnesium stearate; colloidal anhydrous silica; white colour concentrate; carnauba wax and acid brilliant green BS.

**Uses** Valtrex is indicated for the treatment of herpes zoster (shingles).

Valtrex is indicated for the treatment of herpes simplex infections (HSV) of the skin and mucous membranes, including initial and recurrent genital herpes.

*Mode of action:* Valaciclovir, an antiviral, is the L-valine ester of aciclovir. Aciclovir is a purine (guanine) nucleoside analogue.

Valaciclovir is rapidly and almost completely converted in man to aciclovir and valine, probably by the enzyme valaciclovir hydrolase. Aciclovir is a specific inhibitor of herpes viruses with *in vitro* activity against herpes simplex viruses (HSV) type 1 and type 2, varicella zoster virus (VZV), cytomegalovirus (CMV), Epstein-Barr Virus (EBV), and human herpes virus 6 (HHV-6). Aciclovir inhibits herpes virus DNA synthesis once it has been phosphorylated to the active triphosphate form. The first stage of phosphorylation requires the activity of a virus-specific enzyme. In the case of HSV, VZV and EBV this enzyme is the viral thymidine kinase (TK), which is only present in virus infected cells. Selectivity is maintained in CMV with phosphorylation, at least in part, being mediated through the phosphotransferase gene product of UL97. This requirement for activation of aciclovir by a virus specific enzyme largely explains its unique selectivity. The phosphorylation process is completed (conversion from mono- to triphosphate) by cellular kinases. Aciclovir triphosphate competitively inhibits the virus DNA polymerase and incorporation of this nucleoside analogue results in obligate chain termination, halting virus DNA synthesis and thus blocking virus replication.

Extensive monitoring of clinical isolates from patients receiving aciclovir therapy or prophylaxis has revealed that virus with reduced sensitivity to aciclovir is extremely rare in the immunocompetent, and is only found infrequently in severely immunocompromised individuals e.g. solid organ or bone marrow transplant recipients, patients receiving chemotherapy for malignant disease and people infected with human immunodeficiency virus (HIV). Resistance is normally due to a thymidine kinase deficient phenotype which results in a virus which is profoundly disadvantaged in the natural host. Infrequently, reduced sensitivity to aciclovir has been described as a result of subtle alterations in either the virus thymidine kinase or DNA polymerase. The virulence of these variants resembles that of wild-type virus.

*Pharmacokinetics:* After oral administration, valaciclovir is well absorbed and rapidly and almost completely converted to aciclovir and valine. This conversion is probably mediated by valaciclovir hydrolase, an enzyme isolated from human liver. Mean peak aciclovir concentrations are 15 to 25 micromolar (3.3 to 5.7 microgram/ml) following single doses of 500 to 1,000 mg valaciclovir, and occur at a median time of 1.50 hours post dose. The bioavailability of aciclovir from 1,000 mg valaciclovir is 54% and is not reduced by food. Peak plasma concentrations of valaciclovir are only 4% of aciclovir levels, occur at a median time of 45 to 60 minutes post dose, and are below measurable concentrations 3 hours after dosing. The valaciclovir and aciclovir pharmacokinetic profiles are similar after single and repeat dosing. Binding of aciclovir to plasma proteins is very low (15%).

The elimination plasma half-life of aciclovir after both single and multiple dosing with aciclovir is approximately 3 hours. Less than 1% of the administered dose of valaciclovir is recovered in the urine. Valaciclovir is eliminated principally as aciclovir and the known aciclovir metabolite, 9-carboxymethoxymethylguanine (CMMG) in the urine.

Herpes zoster and herpes simplex do not significantly alter the pharmacokinetics of valaciclovir and aciclovir after oral administration of Valtrex.

**Dosage and administration**
*Dosage in adults:* For treatment of herpes zoster, 1,000 mg Valtrex to be taken three times per day for seven days.

For treatment of herpes simplex, 500 mg of Valtrex to be taken twice daily. For recurrent episodes, treatment should be for five days. For initial episodes, which can be more severe, treatment may have to be extended to 10 days.

Dosing should begin as early as possible. For recurrent episodes of herpes simplex, this should ideally be during the prodromal period or immediately the first signs or symptoms appear. Valtrex can prevent lesion development when taken at the first signs and symptoms of an HSV recurrence.

*Dosage in children:* No data are available.

*Dosage in the elderly*: Dosage modification is not required unless renal function is significantly impaired (see *Dosage in renal impairment*). Adequate hydration should be maintained.

*Dosage in renal impairment*: The dose of Valtrex should be modified as follows in patients with significantly impaired renal function:

| *Creatinine Clearance* | *Valtrex Dose* *Herpes zoster* | *Herpes simplex* |
|---|---|---|
| 15 to 30 ml/min | 1,000 mg twice a day | No modification |
| <15 ml/min | 1,000 mg once a day | 500 mg once a day |

In patients on haemodialysis the Valtrex dose recommended for patients with a creatinine clearance of less than 15 ml/min should be used, but the dose should be administered after the haemodialysis has been performed.

*Dosage in hepatic impairment:* Dose modification is not required in patients with mild or moderate cirrhosis (hepatic synthetic function maintained). Pharmacokinetic data in patients with advanced cirrhosis (impaired hepatic synthetic function and evidence of portal-systemic shunting) do not indicate the need for dosage adjustment; however, clinical experience is limited.

**Contra-indications, warnings, etc**
*Contra-indications:* Valtrex is contra-indicated in patients known to be hypersensitive to valaciclovir, aciclovir or any component of their formulations.

*Precautions:* The valaciclovir dose should be adjusted in patients with significant renal impairment (see *Dosage in renal impairment*).

The results of mutagenicity tests *in vitro* and *in vivo* indicate that valaciclovir is unlikely to pose a genetic risk to humans.

Valaciclovir was not carcinogenic in bio-assays performed in mice and rats.

Valaciclovir was not teratogenic in rats or rabbits.

Subcutaneous administration of aciclovir in internationally accepted tests did not produce teratogenic effects in rats or rabbits. In additional studies in rats, fetal abnormalities were observed at subcutaneous doses that produced plasma levels of 100 microgram/ml and maternal toxicity.

Valaciclovir did not affect fertility in male or fema rats dosed by the oral route.

*Use in pregnancy and lactation:* There are no data the use of Valtrex in pregnancy. Valtrex should or be used in pregnancy if the potential benefit outweig the potential risk.

In prospective studies there has not been increased incidence of birth defects in approximate 300 women exposed to systemic aciclovir (most oral doses of 800 to 1,000 mg per day), during the fi trimester of pregnancy, as compared with t incidence in the general population. The report defects show no uniqueness or pattern to sugges common aetiology. The daily aciclovir area under t plasma concentration versus time curve (AUC) follo ing Valtrex 1,000 mg and 3,000 mg per day would 2 to 4 times greater than that expected with o Zovirax* 1,000 mg per day.

No data are available on valaciclovir excretion human breast milk. Caution is therefore advised Valtrex is given to breast feeding mothers.

A study in lactating rats given radiolabell valaciclovir orally, demonstrated the presence drug-related substance in milk.

Aciclovir has been detected in human breast milk concentrations ranging from 0.6 to 4.1 times t corresponding aciclovir plasma concentrations. The levels would potentially expose nursing infants aciclovir doses of up to 0.3 mg/kg/day. Howev aciclovir is used for the treatment of neonatal herp simplex at intravenous doses of 30 mg/kg/day.

*Drug interactions:* Cimetidine and probene increase the area under the plasma concentrati time curve of aciclovir by reducing its renal clearan however, no dosage adjustment is necessary due the wide therapeutic index of aciclovir. Other dru which affect renal physiology could affect plasr levels of aciclovir.

*Side- and adverse effects:* In clinical trials for t treatment of herpes zoster or herpes simplex the m commonly reported adverse experiences were m headache and nausea. These were reported in similar proportion of patients on valaciclovir, aciclo and placebo.

There have been reports of renal insufficien microangiopathic haemolytic anaemia and thromb cytopenia (sometimes in combination) in sever immunocompromised patients receiving high dos (8 g daily) of valaciclovir for prolonged periods clinical trials. These findings have been observed patients not treated with valaciclovir who have t same underlying or concurrent conditions.

*Toxicity and treatment of overdosage:* There are present no data available on overdosage with Valtr

A dose equivalent to the aciclovir exposure fro approximately 15 g Valtrex has been inadverten administered as a single intravenous dose of aciclo (up to 80 mg/kg) without adverse effects.

In the event of a symptomatic Valtrex overdo occurring, aciclovir is removable by haemodialysis

**Pharmaceutical precautions** Store below 30°C.

**Legal category** POM

**Package quantities**
Shingles Treatment Pack: 42 tablets (OP).
HS Treatment Pack: 10 tablets (OP)

**Further information** In patients with HIV infection, t disposition and pharmacokinetic characteristics aciclovir after oral administration of single or multi doses of 1,000 mg or 2,000 mg valaciclovir are ur tered compared with healthy subjects.

In the over 50's, Valtrex shortened the med duration of the pain of shingles to 38 days, compa with Zovirax (51 days) p=0.001. (Beutner KR. *et* Antimicrob Ag Chemother 1995; 39:1546–1553.) the under 50's there was no significant difference pain duration compared with placebo.)

**Product licence number** 0003/0352

## ZOVIRAX* CREAM

**Presentation** Zovirax Cream is white and contains w/w aciclovir in an aqueous cream base. It is suppl in tubes containing 2 g or 10 g.

**Uses** Zovirax Cream is indicated for the treatmen herpes simplex virus infections of the skin includ initial and recurrent genital herpes and herpes labia

Do not use in eyes.

**Dosage and administration** Zovirax Cream should applied five times daily at approximately four ho intervals, omitting the night time application. Tre ment should be continued for 5 days. If, after 5 da healing is not complete then treatment may continued for up to an additional 5 days. Zovi Cream should be applied to the lesion or impend lesion as early as possible after the start of an infecti It is particularly important to start treatment recurrent episodes during the prodromal period or when lesions first appear.

*Use in the elderly:* No special comment.

*Pharmacology:* Aciclovir is an antiviral agent which is highly active *in vitro* against herpes simplex virus (HSV) types I and II and varicella zoster virus. Toxicity to mammalian host cells is low.

Aciclovir is phosphorylated after entry into herpes infected cells to the active compound aciclovir triphosphate. The first step in this process is dependent on the presence of the HSV-coded thymidine kinase. Aciclovir triphosphate acts as an inhibitor of, and substrate for, the herpes-specified DNA polymerase, preventing further viral DNA synthesis without affecting normal cellular processes.

**Contra-indications, warnings, etc**

*Contra-indications:* Zovirax Cream is contra-indicated in patients known to be hypersensitive to aciclovir or propylene glycol.

*Precautions:* In severely immunocompromised patients (e.g. AIDS patients or bone marrow transplant recipients) oral Zovirax dosing should be considered. Such patients should be encouraged to consult a physician concerning the treatment of any infection.

Zovirax Cream is not recommended for application to mucous membranes such as in the mouth, eye or vagina, as it may be irritant.

Particular care should be taken to avoid accidental introduction into the eye.

The results of a wide range of mutagenicity tests *in vitro* and *in vivo* indicate that aciclovir does not pose a genetic risk to man. Aciclovir was not found to be carcinogenic in long-term studies in the rat and the mouse.

Largely reversible adverse effects on spermatogenesis in association with overall toxicity in rats and dogs have been reported only at doses of aciclovir greatly in excess of those employed therapeutically. There has been no experience of the effect of Zovirax Cream on human fertility. Two generation studies in mice did not reveal any effect of (orally administered) aciclovir on fertility. Zovirax Tablets have been shown to have no definite effect upon sperm count, morphology or motility in man.

*Side- and adverse effects:* Transient burning or stinging following application of Zovirax Cream may occur in some patients. Mild drying or flaking of the skin has occurred in about 5% of patients. Erythema and itching have been reported in a small proportion of patients.

Contact dermatitis has been reported rarely following application. Where sensitivity tests have been conducted, the reactive substances have most often been shown to be components of the cream base rather than aciclovir.

*Use in pregnancy and lactation:* Systemic administration of aciclovir in internationally accepted standard tests did not produce embryotoxic or teratogenic effects in rats, rabbits or mice.

In a non-standard test in rats, fetal abnormalities were observed, but only following such high subcutaneous doses that maternal toxicity was produced. The clinical relevance of these findings is uncertain.

Experience in humans is limited, so use of Zovirax Cream should be considered only when the potential benefits outweigh the possibility of unknown risks.

Limited human data show that the drug does pass into breast milk following systemic administration.

*Drug interactions:* Probenecid increases the mean half-life and area under the plasma concentration curve of systemically administered aciclovir. However, this is likely to be of little relevance to the topical application of aciclovir.

*Toxicity and treatment of overdosage:* No untoward effects would be expected if the entire contents of a Zovirax Cream 10 g tube containing 500 mg of aciclovir were ingested orally. Oral doses of 800 mg five times daily (4 g per day), have been administered for seven days without adverse effects. Single intravenous doses of up to 80 mg/kg have been inadvertently administered without adverse effects. Aciclovir is dialysable.

**Pharmaceutical precautions** Store below 25°C. Do not refrigerate.

Zovirax Cream contains a specially formulated base and should not be diluted or used as a base for the incorporation of other medicaments.

**Legal category** POM

**Package quantities** Tubes of 2 g (OP) and 10 g (OP).

**Further information** Nil.

**Product licence number** 0003/0180.

## ZOVIRAX* EYE OINTMENT

**Qualitative and quantitative composition** Aciclovir 3.0% w/w.

**Pharmaceutical form** Ophthalmic ointment.

**Clinical particulars**

*Therapeutic indications:* Treatment of herpes simplex keratitis.

*Posology and method of administration:* Topical administration to the eye.

*Adults:* 1 cm ribbon of ointment should be placed inside the lower conjunctival sac five times a day at approximately four hourly intervals, omitting the night time application. Treatment should continue for at least 3 days after healing is complete.

*Children:* As for adults.

*Use in the elderly:* As for adults.

*Contra-indications:* Zovirax Eye Ointment is contra-indicated in patients with a known hypersensitivity to aciclovir.

*Special warnings and precautions for use:* None.

*Interaction with other medicaments and other forms of interaction:* Probenecid increases the aciclovir mean half-life and area under the plasma concentration curve of systemically administered aciclovir. Other drugs affecting renal physiology could potentially influence the pharmacokinetics of aciclovir. However, clinical experience has not identified other drug interactions with aciclovir.

*Pregnancy and lactation:* Experience in humans is limited, so the use of Zovirax Eye Ointment should be considered only when the potential benefits outweigh the possibility of unknown risks. Systemic administration of aciclovir in internationally accepted standard tests did not produce embryotoxic or teratogenic effects in rats, rabbits or mice.

In a non-standard test in rats, foetal abnormalities were observed, but only following such high subcutaneous doses that maternal toxicity was produced. The clinical relevance of these findings is uncertain.

There is no information on the effect of Zovirax Eye Ointment on human female fertility. Two-generation studies in mice did not reveal any effect of (orally administered) aciclovir on fertility.

Limited human data show that the drug does pass into breast milk.

*Effect on ability to drive and use machines:* Not applicable.

*Undesirable effects:* Transient mild stinging immediately following application may occur in a small proportion of patients. Superficial punctate keratopathy has been reported but has not resulted in patients being withdrawn from therapy, and healing has occurred without apparent sequelae. Local irritation and inflammation such as blepharitis and conjunctivitis have also been reported.

The results of a wide range of mutagenicity tests *in vitro* and *in vivo* indicate that aciclovir does not pose a genetic risk to man. Aciclovir was not found to be carcinogenic in long-term studies in the rat and the mouse. Largely reversible adverse effects on spermatogenesis in association with overall toxicity in rats and dogs have been reported only at doses of aciclovir greatly in excess of those employed therapeutically. Zovirax Tablets have been shown to have no definite effect upon sperm count, morphology or motility in man.

*Overdose:* No untoward effects would be expected if the entire contents of the tube containing 135 mg of aciclovir were ingested orally. Oral doses of 800 mg five times daily (4 g per day) have been administered for seven days without adverse effects.

Single intravenous doses of up to 80 mg/kg have been inadvertently administered without adverse effects. Aciclovir is dialysable by haemodialysis.

**Pharmacological properties**

*Pharmacodynamic properties:* Aciclovir is an antiviral agent which is highly active *in vitro* against herpes simplex (HSV) types I and II, but its toxicity to mammalian cells is low.

Aciclovir is phosphorylated to the active compound aciclovir triphosphate after entry into a herpes infected cell. The first step in this process requires the presence of the HSV coded thymidine kinase. Aciclovir triphosphate acts as an inhibitor of, and substrate for, herpes specified DNA polymerase, preventing further viral DNA synthesis without affecting normal cellular processes.

*Pharmacokinetic properties:* Aciclovir is rapidly absorbed from the ophthalmic ointment through the corneal epithelium and superficial ocular tissues, achieving antiviral concentrations in the aqueous humor. It has not been possible by existing methods to detect aciclovir in the blood after topical application to the eye. However, trace quantities are detectable in the urine. These levels are not therapeutically significant.

*Preclinical safety data:* There are no preclinical data of relevance to the prescriber which are additional to that in other sections of the SPC.

**Pharmaceutical particulars**

*List of excipients:* White petroleum USP.

*Incompatibilities:* None known.

*Shelf life:* 5 years.

*Special precautions for storage:* Store below 25°C.

*Nature and contents of container:* Laminate ophthalmic ointment tubes closed with high-density polyethylene screw caps. Pack size 4.5 g.

*Instructions for use/handling:* No special instructions.

**Marketing authorisation number** 0003/0150.

**Date of approval/revision of SPC** 17 May 1996.

**Legal category** POM.

## ZOVIRAX* TABLETS
## ZOVIRAX* SUSPENSION
## ZOVIRAX* DOUBLE-STRENGTH SUSPENSION

**Presentation** Each blue, film-coated, biconvex, shield-shaped, dispersible tablet is impressed with 'ZOVIRAX 200' on one side and a triangle on the obverse and contains 200 mg aciclovir.

Each pale pink, film-coated, biconvex, shield-shaped, dispersible tablet is impressed with 'ZOVIRAX 400' on one side and a triangle on the obverse and contains 400 mg aciclovir.

Each white, film-coated, biconvex, elongated, dispersible tablet is impressed with the words 'ZOVIRAX 800' on one side, is scored on the other side, and contains 800 mg aciclovir.

Zovirax Suspension is an off-white suspension with a banana odour and taste and contains 200 mg aciclovir per 5 ml.

Zovirax Double-Strength Suspension is an off-white viscous suspension with an orange odour and taste and contains 400 mg aciclovir per 5 ml.

**Uses** Zovirax Tablets and Zovirax Suspensions are indicated for the treatment of herpes simplex virus infections of the skin and mucous membranes including initial and recurrent genital herpes.

Zovirax Tablets and Zovirax Suspensions are indicated for the suppression (prevention of recurrences) of recurrent herpes simplex infections in immunocompetent patients.

Zovirax Tablets and Zovirax Suspensions are indicated for the prophylaxis of herpes simplex infections in immunocompromised patients.

Zovirax Tablets and Zovirax Suspensions are indicated for the treatment of varicella (chickenpox) and herpes zoster (shingles) infections.

*Mode of action:* Aciclovir is a synthetic purine nucleoside analogue with *in vitro* and *in vivo* inhibitory activity against human herpes viruses, including herpes simplex virus (HSV) types I and II and varicella zoster virus (VZV).

The inhibitory activity of aciclovir for HSV I, HSV II and VZV is highly selective. The enzyme thymidine kinase (TK) of normal, uninfected cells does not use aciclovir effectively as a substrate, hence toxicity to mammalian host cells is low. However, TK encoded by HSV and VZV converts aciclovir to aciclovir monophosphate, a nucleoside analogue which is further converted to the diphosphate and finally to the triphosphate by cellular enzymes. Aciclovir triphosphate interferes with the viral DNA polymerase and inhibits viral DNA replication with resultant chain termination following its incorporation into the viral DNA.

Prolonged or repeated courses of aciclovir in severely immunocompromised individuals may result in the selection of virus strains with reduced sensitivity, which may not respond to continued aciclovir treatment. Most of the clinical isolates with reduced sensitivity have been relatively deficient in viral TK; however, strains with altered viral TK or viral DNA polymerase have also been reported. *In vitro* exposure of HSV isolates to aciclovir can also lead to the emergence of less sensitive strains. The relationship between the *in vitro*-determined sensitivity of HSV isolates and clinical response to aciclovir therapy is not clear.

*Pharmacokinetics:* Aciclovir is only partially absorbed from the gut. Mean steady-state peak plasma concentrations ($C^{ss}$max) following doses of 200 mg aciclovir administered four-hourly were 3.1 microMol (0.7 micrograms/ml) and the equivalent trough plasma levels ($C^{ss}$min) were 1.8 microMol (0.4 micrograms/ml). Corresponding steady-state plasma concentrations following doses of 400 mg and 800 mg aciclovir administered four-hourly were 5.3 microMol (1.2

micrograms/ml) and 8 microMol (1.8 micrograms/ml) respectively, and equivalent trough plasma levels were 2.7 microMol (0.6 micrograms/ml) and 4 microMol (0.9 micrograms/ml).

In adults the terminal plasma half-life after administration of intravenous aciclovir is about 2.9 hours. Most of the drug is excreted unchanged by the kidney. Renal clearance of aciclovir is substantially greater than creatinine clearance, indicating that tubular secretion, in addition to glomerular filtration, contributes to the renal elimination of the drug.

9-carboxymethoxymethylguanine is the only significant metabolite of aciclovir, and accounts for 10-15% of the dose excreted in the urine. When aciclovir is given one hour after 1 gram of probenecid the terminal half-life and the area under the plasma concentration time curve is extended by 18% and 40% respectively.

In adults, mean steady state-peak plasma concentrations ($C^{ss}max$) following a one hour infusion of 2.5 mg/kg, 5 mg/kg and 10 mg/kg were 22.7 microMol (5.1 micrograms/ml), 43.6 microMol (9.8 micrograms/ml) and 92 microMol (20.7 micrograms/ml), respectively. The corresponding trough levels ($C^{ss}min$) 7 hours later were 2.2 microMol (0.5 micrograms/ml), 3.1 microMol (0.7 micrograms/ml) and 10.2 microMol (2.3 micrograms/ml), respectively. In children over 1 year of age similar mean peak ($C^{ss}max$) and trough ($C^{ss}min$) levels were observed when a dose of 250 mg/m² was substituted for 5 mg/kg and a dose of 500 mg/m² was substituted for 10 mg/kg. In neonates and young infants (0 to 3 months of age) treated with doses of 10 mg/kg administered by infusion over a one-hour period every 8 hours the $C^{ss}max$ was found to be 61.2 microMol (13.8 micrograms/ml) and $C^{ss}min$ to be 10.1 microMol (2.3 micrograms/ml). The terminal plasma half-life in these patients was 3.8 hours. In the elderly, total body clearance falls with increasing age associated with decreases in creatinine clearance although there is little change in the terminal plasma half-life.

In patients with chronic renal failure the mean terminal half-life was found to be 19.5 hours. The mean aciclovir half-life during haemodialysis was 5.7 hours. Plasma aciclovir levels dropped approximately 60% during dialysis.

Cerebrospinal fluid levels are approximately 50% of corresponding plasma levels. Plasma protein binding is relatively low (9 to 33%) and drug interactions involving binding site displacement are not anticipated.

**Dosage and administration**

*Dosage in adults: Treatment of herpes simplex infections:* 200 mg Zovirax should be taken five times daily at approximately four-hourly intervals omitting the night time dose. Treatment should continue for 5 days, but in severe initial infections this may have to be extended.

In severely immunocompromised patients (e.g. after marrow transplant) or in patients with impaired absorption from the gut the dose can be doubled to 400 mg Zovirax or, alternatively, intravenous dosing could be considered.

Dosing should begin as early as possible after the start of an infection; for recurrent episodes this should preferably be during the prodromal period or when lesions first appear.

*Suppression of herpes simplex infections in immunocompetent patients:* 200 mg Zovirax should be taken four times daily at approximately six-hourly intervals.

Many patients may be conveniently managed on a regimen of 400 mg Zovirax twice daily at approximately twelve-hourly intervals.

Dosage titration down to 200 mg Zovirax taken thrice daily at approximately eight-hourly intervals or even twice daily at approximately twelve-hourly intervals, may prove effective.

Some patients may experience break-through infections on total daily doses of 800 mg Zovirax.

Therapy should be interrupted periodically at intervals of six to twelve months, in order to observe possible changes in the natural history of the disease.

*Prophylaxis of herpes simplex infections in immunocompromised patients:* 200 mg Zovirax should be taken four times daily at approximately six-hourly intervals.

In severely immunocompromised patients (e.g. after marrow transplant) or in patients with impaired absorption from the gut, the dose can be doubled to 400 mg Zovirax or, alternatively, intravenous dosing could be considered.

The duration of prophylactic administration is determined by the duration of the period at risk.

*Treatment of varicella and herpes zoster infections:* 800 mg Zovirax should be taken five times daily at approximately four-hourly intervals, omitting the night time dose. Treatment should continue for seven days.

In severely immunocompromised patients (e.g. after marrow transplant) or in patients with impaired absorption from the gut, consideration should be given to intravenous dosing.

Dosing should begin as early as possible after the start of an infection: treatment of herpes zoster yields better results if initiated as soon as possible after the onset of the rash. Treatment of chickenpox in immunocompetent patients should begin within 24 hours after onset of the rash.

*Dosage in children:*
*Treatment of herpes simplex infections, and prophylaxis of herpes simplex infections in the immunocompromised:* Children aged two years and over should be given adult dosages and children below the age of two years should be given ***half*** the adult dose.

*Treatment of varicella infections:*
*6 years and over:* 800 mg Zovirax four times daily.
*2 to 5 years:* 400 mg Zovirax four times daily.
*Under 2 years:* 200 mg Zovirax four times daily.
Treatment should continue for five days.

Dosing may be more accurately calculated as 20 mg/kg bodyweight (not to exceed 800 mg) Zovirax four times daily.

No specific data are available on the suppression of *herpes simplex* infections or the treatment of *herpes zoster* infections in immunocompetent children.

Zovirax Suspension may be diluted with an equal volume of either Syrup BP or Sorbitol Solution (70%) (non-crystallising) BP. The diluted product is stable for 4 weeks at 25°C but it is recommended that all dilutions are freshly prepared.

*Dosage in the elderly:* In the elderly, total aciclovir body clearance declines along with creatinine clearance. Adequate hydration of elderly patients taking high oral doses of Zovirax should be maintained. Special attention should be given to dosage reduction in elderly patients with impaired renal function.

*Dosage in renal impairment:* In the management of *herpes simplex* infections in patients with impaired renal function, the recommended oral doses will not lead to accumulation of aciclovir above levels that have been established by intravenous infusion. However, for patients with severe renal impairment (creatinine clearance less than 10 ml/minute) an adjustment of dosage to 200 mg aciclovir twice daily at approximately twelve-hourly intervals is recommended.

In the treatment of *varicella* and *herpes zoster* infections it is recommended to adjust the dosage to 800 mg aciclovir twice daily at approximately twelve-hourly intervals for patients with severe renal impairment (creatinine clearance less than 10 ml/minute), and to 800 mg aciclovir three times daily at intervals of approximately six to eight hours for patients with moderate renal impairment (creatinine clearance in the range 10 to 25 ml/minute).

*Administration:* Zovirax Dispersible Tablets may be dispersed in a minimum of 50 ml of water or swallowed whole with a little water.

**Contra-indications, warnings, etc**

*Contra-indications:* Zovirax Tablets and Zovirax Suspensions are contra-indicated in patients known to be hypersensitive to aciclovir.

*Precautions:* The data currently available from clinical studies is not sufficient to conclude that treatment with Zovirax reduces the incidence of chickenpox-associated complications in immunocompetent patients.

The results of a wide range of mutagenicity tests *in vitro* and *in vivo* indicate that aciclovir is unlikely to pose a genetic risk to man. Aciclovir was not found to be carcinogenic in long-term studies in the rat and the mouse. Largely reversible adverse effects on spermatogenesis in association with overall toxicity in rats and dogs have been reported only at doses of aciclovir greatly in excess of those employed therapeutically. Zovirax Tablets have been shown to have no definitive effect upon sperm count, morphology or motility in man.

*Side- and adverse effects:* Skin rashes have been reported in a few patients receiving Zovirax Tablets; the rashes have resolved on withdrawal of the drug.

Gastrointestinal effects including nausea, vomiting, diarrhoea and abdominal pains have been reported in some patients receiving Zovirax Tablets. In double-blind, placebo-controlled trials the incidence of gastrointestinal events has not been found to differ between placebo and aciclovir recipients.

Reversible neurological reactions, notably dizziness, confusional states, hallucinations and somnolence, have occasionally been reported, usually in patients with renal impairment or other predisposing factors.

Occasional reports of accelerated diffuse hair loss have been received. As this type of hair loss has been associated with a wide variety of disease processes and medicines, the relationship of the event to aciclovir therapy is uncertain.

Other events reported rarely in patients receiving oral formulations of Zovirax include mild, transient rises in bilirubin and liver-related enzymes, small increases in blood urea and creatinine, small decreases in haematological indices, headaches.

*Use in pregnancy and lactation:* Experience in humans is limited so the use of Zovirax Tablets or Zovirax Suspensions should be considered only when the potential benefits outweigh the possibility of unknown risks. Systemic administration of aciclovir in internationally accepted standard tests did not produce embryotoxic or teratogenic effects in rats, rabbits or mice.

In a non-standard test in rats, fetal abnormalities were observed, but only following such high subcutaneous doses that maternal toxicity was produced. The clinical relevance of these findings is uncertain.

There is no experience of the effect of Zovirax Tablets or Zovirax Suspensions on human female fertility. Two-generation studies in mice did not reveal any effect of aciclovir on fertility.

Following oral administration of 200 mg Zovirax five times a day, aciclovir has been detected in breast milk at concentrations ranging from 0.6 to 4.1 times the corresponding plasma levels. These levels would potentially expose nursing infants to aciclovir dosages of up to 0.3 mg/kg/day. Caution is therefore advised if Zovirax is to be administered to a nursing woman.

*Drug interactions:* Probenecid increases the aciclovir mean half-life and area under the plasma concentration curve. Other drugs affecting renal physiology could potentially influence the pharmacokinetics of aciclovir. However, clinical experience has not identified other drug interactions with aciclovir.

*Toxicity and treatment of overdosage:* Aciclovir is only partly absorbed in the gastrointestinal tract. It is unlikely that serious toxic effects would occur if a dose of up to 5 g were taken on a single occasion. No data are available on the consequences of the ingestion of higher doses; such an occurrence warrants close observation of the patient.

Single intravenous doses of up to 80 mg/kg have been inadvertently administered without adverse effects. Aciclovir is dialysable by haemodialysis.

**Pharmaceutical precautions**

Zovirax Tablets 200 mg: Store below 30°C. Protect from light. Keep dry.

Zovirax Tablets 400 mg: Store below 30°C. Protect from light. Keep dry.

Zovirax Tablets 800 mg: Store below 30°C. Protect from light. Keep dry.

Zovirax Suspension: Store below 25°C.

Zovirax Double-Strength Suspension: Store below 30°C.

**Legal category** POM

**Package quantities**

| | |
|---|---|
| Zovirax Tablets 200 mg: | Pack of 25 tablets (OP) |
| Zovirax Tablets 400 mg: | Pack of 56 tablets (OP) |
| Zovirax Tablets 800 mg (Shingles Treatment Pack): | Pack of 35 tablets (OP) |
| Zovirax Suspension: | Bottle of 125 ml (OP) |
| Zovirax Double-Strength Suspension (Chickenpox Treatment Pack): | 50 ml bottle (OP) |

**Further information** Nil.

**Product licence numbers**

| | |
|---|---|
| Zovirax Tablets 200 mg: | 0003/0344 |
| Zovirax Tablets 400 mg: | 0003/0345 |
| Zovirax Tablets 800 mg: | 0003/0299 |
| Zovirax Suspension: | 0003/0202 |
| Zovirax Double-Strength Suspension: | 0003/0264 |

## ZOVIRAX* I.V. for Intravenous Infusion

**Presentation** Vials containing the equivalent o 250 mg and 500 mg sterile aciclovir as the freeze dried sodium salt, a white to off-white powder. Whe reconstituted as directed, Zovirax I.V. has a pH c about 11. The sodium ion content is approximatel 26 mg and 52 mg per vial, respectively.

**Uses**

Zovirax I.V. is indicated for the treatment of *Herpe simplex* infections in immunocompromised patien and severe initial genital herpes in the non-immun compromised.

Zovirax I.V. is indicated for the prophylaxis c *Herpes simplex* infections in immunocompromise patients.

Zovirax I.V. is indicated for the treatment of *Varice zoster* infections.

Zovirax I.V. is indicated for the treatment of herpe encephalitis.

Zovirax I.V. is indicated for the treatment of *Herp simplex* infections in the neonate and infant up 3 months of age.

*Mode of action:* Aciclovir is a synthetic purine nucl oside analogue with *in vitro* and *in vivo* inhibito ctivity against human herpes viruses, including *Ierpes simplex* virus types 1 and 2 and *Varicella oster* virus (VZV), Epstein Barr virus (EBV) and ytomegalovirus (CMV). In cell culture aciclovir has ie greatest antiviral activity against HSV-1, followed n decreasing order of potency) by HSV-2, VZV, EBV, nd CMV.

The inhibitory activity of aciclovir for HSV-1, HSV-2, ZV and EBV is highly selective. The enzyme thymi-ine kinase (TK) of normal, uninfected cells does not se aciclovir effectively as a substrate, hence toxicity ) mammalian host cells is low; however, TK encoded y HSV, VZV and EBV converts aciclovir to aciclovir onophosphate, a nucleoside analogue, which is irther converted to the diphosphate and finally to the iphosphate by cellular enzymes. Aciclovir triphos-nate interferes with the viral DNA polymerase and hibits viral DNA replication with resultant chain ermination following its incorporation into the viral NA.

*harmacokinetics:* In adults, the terminal plasma half-fe of aciclovir after administration of Zovirax I.V. is bout 2.9 hours. Most of the drug is excreted un-nanged by the kidney. Renal clearance of aciclovir is ubstantially greater than creatinine clearance, indi-ating that tubular secretion, in addition to glomerular tration, contributes to the renal elimination of the rug. 9-carboxymethoxymethylguanine is the only gnificant metabolite of aciclovir and accounts for 10 15% of the dose excreted in the urine.

When aciclovir is given one hour after 1 gram of robenecid the terminal half-life and the area under e plasma concentration time curve, are extended by 3% and 40% respectively.

In adults, mean steady-state peak plasma concen-ations ($C^{ss}max$) following a one-hour infusion of .5 mg/kg, 5 mg/kg, 10 mg/kg and 15 mg/kg were 22.7 iicromolar (5.1 microgram/ml), 43.6 micromolar .8 microgram/ml), 92 micromolar (20.7 microgram/ l) and 105 micromolar (23.6 microgram/ml), respec-vely. The corresponding trough levels ($C^{ss}min$) 7 ours later were 2.2 micromolar (0.5 microgram/ml), 1 micromolar (0.7 microgram/ml), 10.2 micromolar .3 microgram/ml), and 8.8 micromolar (2.0 micro-ram/ml), respectively. In children over 1 year of age milar mean peak ($C^{ss}max$) and trough ($C^{ss}min$) levels ere observed when a dose of 250 mg/m² was ubstituted for 5 mg/kg and a dose of 500 mg/m² was ubstituted for 10 mg/kg. In neonates (0 to 3 months f age) treated with doses of 10 mg/kg administered y infusion over a one-hour period every 8 hours the $^{ss}max$ was found to be 61.2 micromolar (13.8 micro-ram/ml) and the $C^{ss}min$ to be 10.1 micromolar ..3 microgram/ml).

The terminal plasma half-life in these patients was 8 hours. In the elderly, total body clearance falls with creasing age and is associated with decreases in eatinine clearance although there is little change in e terminal plasma half-life.

In patients with chronic renal failure the mean rminal half-life was found to be 19.5 hours. The ean aciclovir half-life during haemodialysis was 5.7 ours. Plasma aciclovir levels dropped approximately )% during dialysis.

Cerebrospinal fluid levels are approximately 50% of orresponding plasma levels.

Plasma protein binding is relatively low (9 to 33%) d drug interactions involving binding site displace-ent are not anticipated.

**osage and administration** A course of treatment ith Zovirax I.V. usually lasts 5 days, but this may be ljusted according to the patient's condition and sponse to therapy. Treatment for herpes encephali-s and neonatal *Herpes simplex* infections usually sts 10 days.

The duration of prophylactic administration of ovirax I.V. is determined by the duration of the eriod at risk.

*osage in adults:* Patients with *Herpes simplex* (except erpes encephalitis) or *Varicella zoster* infections iould be given Zovirax I.V. in doses of 5 mg/kg odyweight every 8 hours.

Immunocompromised patients with *Varicella zoster* fections or patients with herpes encephalitis should given Zovirax I.V. in doses of 10 mg/kg bodyweight very 8 hours provided renal function is not impaired ee *Dosage in renal impairment*).

*osage in children:* The dose of Zovirax I.V. for iildren aged between 3 months and 12 years is lculated on the basis of body surface area.

iildren with *Herpes simplex* (except herpes enceph-itis) or *Varicella zoster* infections should be given ovirax I.V. in doses of 250 mg per square metre of ody surface area every 8 hours.

In immunocompromised children with *Varicella ster* infections or children with herpes encephalitis, ovirax I.V. should be given in doses of 500 mg per uare metre body surface area every 8 hours if renal nction is not impaired.

Children with impaired renal function require an appropriately modified dose, according to the degree of impairment.

The dosage of Zovirax I.V. in neonates and infants up to 3 months of age is calculated on the basis of bodyweight.

Neonates and infants up to 3 months of age with *Herpes simplex* infections should be given Zovirax I.V. in doses of 10 mg/kg/bodyweight every 8 hours. Treatment for neonatal herpes simplex infections usually lasts 10 days.

*Dosage in the elderly:* In the elderly, total aciclovir body clearance declines in parallel with creatinine clearance. Special attention should be given to dosage reduction in elderly patients with impaired creatinine clearance.

*Dosage in renal impairment:* Caution is advised when administering Zovirax I.V. to patients with impaired renal function. The following adjustments in dosage are suggested:

| *Creatinine Clearance* | *Dosage* |
|---|---|
| 25 to 50 ml/min | The dose recommended above (5 or 10 mg/kg bodyweight or 500 mg/m²) should be given every 12 hours. |
| 10 to 25 ml/min | The dose recommended above (5 or 10 mg/kg bodyweight or 500 mg/m²) should be given every 24 hours. |
| 0(anuric) to 10 ml/min | In patients receiving continuous ambulatory peritoneal dialysis (CAPD) the dose recommended above (5 or 10 mg/kg bodyweight or 500 mg/m²) should be halved and administered every 24 hours. In patients receiving haemodialysis the dose recommended above (5 or 10 mg/kg bodyweight or 500 mg/m²) should be halved and administered every 24 hours and after dialysis. |

*Reconstitution:* Zovirax I.V. should be reconstituted using the following volumes of either Water for Injections BP or Sodium Chloride Intravenous Injection BP (0.9% w/v) to provide a solution containing 25 mg aciclovir per ml:

| *Formulation* | *Volume of fluid for reconstitution* |
|---|---|
| *250 mg vial* | *10 ml* |
| *500 mg vial* | *20 ml* |

*From the calculated dose, determine the appropriate number and strength of vials to be used. To reconstitute each vial add the recommended volume of infusion fluid and shake gently until the contents of the vial have dissolved completely.*

*Administration:* The required dose of Zovirax I.V. should be administered by slow intravenous infusion over a one-hour period.

After reconstitution Zovirax I.V. may be administered by a controlled-rate infusion pump.

Alternatively, the reconstituted solution may be further diluted to give an aciclovir concentration of not greater than 5 mg/ml (0.5% w/v) for administration by infusion:

Add the required volume of reconstituted solution to the chosen infusion solution, as recommended below, and shake well to ensure adequate mixing occurs.

For children and neonates, where it is advisable to keep the volume of infusion fluid to a minimum, it is recommended that dilution is on the basis of 4 ml reconstituted solution (100 mg aciclovir) added to 20 ml of infusion fluid.

For adults, it is recommended that infusion bags containing 100 ml of infusion fluid are used, even when this would give an aciclovir concentration substantially below 0.5% w/v. Thus, one 100 ml infusion bag may be used for any dose between 250 mg and 500 mg aciclovir (10 and 20 ml of reconstituted solution) but a second bag must be used for doses between 500 and 1,000 mg.

When diluted in accordance with the recommended schedules, Zovirax I.V. is known to be compatible with the following infusion fluids and stable for up to 12 hours at room temperature (15°C to 25°C):

Sodium Chloride Intravenous Infusion BP (0.45% and 0.9% w/v);

Sodium Chloride (0.18% w/v) and Glucose (4% w/v) Intravenous Infusion BP;

Sodium Chloride (0.45% w/v) and Glucose (2.5% w/v) Intravenous Infusion BP;

Compound Sodium Lactate Intravenous Infusion BP (Hartmann's Solution).

Zovirax I.V. when diluted in accordance with the above schedule will give an aciclovir concentration not greater than 0.5% w/v.

Since no antimicrobial preservative is included, reconstitution and dilution must be carried out under full aseptic conditions, immediately before use, and any unused solution discarded.

Should any visible turbidity or crystallisation appear in the solution before or during infusion, the preparation should be discarded.

**Contra-indications, warnings, etc.**

*Contra-indications:* Zovirax I.V. is contra-indicated in patients known to be previously hypersensitive to aciclovir.

*Precautions:* The dose of Zovirax I.V. must be adjusted in patients with impaired renal function in order to avoid accumulation of aciclovir in the body (see *Dosage in renal impairment*).

In patients receiving Zovirax I.V. at higher doses (e.g. for herpes encephalitis), specific care regarding renal function should be taken, particularly when patients are dehydrated or have any renal impairment.

Reconstituted Zovirax I.V. has a pH of approximately 11.0 and should not be administered by mouth.

The results of a wide range of mutagenicity tests *in vitro* and *in vivo* indicate that aciclovir is unlikely to pose a genetic risk to man.

Aciclovir was not found to be carcinogenic in long-term studies in the rat and the mouse.

Systemic administration of aciclovir in internationally accepted standard tests did not produce embryotoxic or teratogenic effects in rabbits, rats or mice.

In a non-standard test in rats, fetal abnormalities were observed but only following such high subcutaneous doses that maternal toxicity was produced. The clinical relevance of these findings is uncertain.

Largely reversible adverse effects on spermatogenesis in association with overall toxicity in rats and dogs have been reported only at doses of aciclovir greatly in excess of those employed therapeutically. Two-generation studies in mice did not reveal any effect of (orally administered) aciclovir on fertility.

There is no experience of the effect of Zovirax I.V. on human fertility. Zovirax Tablets have been shown to have no definitive effect upon sperm count, morphology or motility in man.

*Side- and adverse effects:* Rapid increases in blood urea and creatinine levels may occasionally occur in patients given Zovirax I.V. This is believed to be related to peak plasma levels and the state of hydration of the patient. To avoid this effect the drug should not be given as an intravenous bolus injection but by slow infusion over a one hour period. Adequate hydration of the patient should be maintained.

Renal impairment developing during treatment with Zovirax I.V. usually responds rapidly to rehydration of the patient and/or dosage reduction or withdrawal of the drug. Progression to acute renal failure, however, can occur in exceptional cases.

Severe local inflammatory reactions, sometimes leading to breakdown of the skin, have occurred when Zovirax I.V. has been inadvertently infused into extravascular tissues.

Reversible neurological reactions such as confusion, hallucinations, agitation, tremors, somnolence, psychosis, convulsions and coma have been associated with Zovirax I.V. therapy, usually in medically complicated cases.

Nausea and vomiting have been reported in patients receiving therapy with Zovirax I.V.

Other events reported in patients receiving Zovirax I.V. include increases in liver-related enzymes, rashes and fevers and decreases in haematological indices (anaemia, thrombocytopenia, leucopenia).

*Use in pregnancy and lactation:* Limited data are available on the use of aciclovir during pregnancy. Caution should therefore be exercised by balancing the potential benefits of treatment against any possible hazard.

Following oral administration of 200 mg five times a day, aciclovir has been detected in human breast milk at concentrations ranging from 0.6 to 4.1 times the corresponding plasma levels. These levels would potentially expose nursing infants to aciclovir dosages of up to 0.3 mg/kg bodyweight/day. Caution is therefore advised if Zovirax is to be administered to a nursing woman.

*Drug interactions:* Probenecid increases the aciclovir mean half-life and area under the plasma concentration-time curve. Other drugs affecting renal physiology could potentially influence the pharmacokinetics of aciclovir. However, clinical experience has not identified other drug interactions with aciclovir.

*Toxicity and treatment of overdosage:* Single doses of Zovirax I.V. up to 80 mg/kg bodyweight have been inadvertently administered without adverse effects. Aciclovir is dialysable.

**Pharmaceutical precautions** Store below 25°C.

Zovirax I.V. contains no antimicrobial preservative. Reconstitution or dilution should therefore be carried out under full aseptic conditions immediately before use and any unused solution discarded. Reconstituted or diluted solutions should not be refrigerated.

**Legal category** POM.

**Package quantities**
250 mg: pack of 5 vials
500 mg: pack of 5 vials

**Further information** Nil.

**Product licence number** 0003/0159

## ZYLORIC* TABLETS
## ZYLORIC-300* TABLETS

**Presentation** Zyloric Tablets–white, round, biconvex tablets, scored and impressed 'WELLCOME' and 'U4A' and containing 100 mg Allopurinol BP.

Zyloric-300 Tablets–white, round, biconvex tablets, scored and impressed 'WELLCOME' and 'C9B' and containing 300 mg Allopurinol BP.

**Uses** Zyloric is indicated for the main clinical manifestations of urate/uric acid deposition. These are gouty arthritis, skin tophi and/or renal involvement through crystal deposition or stone formation. The main clinical manifestations occur in: idiopathic gout; uric acid lithiasis; acute uric acid nephropathy; neoplastic disease and myeloproliferative disease with high cell turnover rates, in which high urate levels occur either spontaneously, or after cytotoxic therapy; certain enzyme disorders which lead to overproduction of urate and involve: hypoxanthine guanine phosphoribosyltransferase, including Lesch-Nyhan syndrome; glucose-6-phosphatase including glycogen storage disease, phosphoribosylpyrophosphate synthetase; adenine phosphoribosyltransferase; glutathione reductase.

Zyloric is indicated for the management of 2,8-dihydroxyadenine (2,8-DHA) renal stones related to deficient activity of adenine phosphoribosyltransferase.

Zyloric is indicated for the management of recurrent calcium oxalate renal stones in the presence of hyperuricosuria, when fluid, dietary and similar measures have failed.

*Mode of action:* Allopurinol inhibits xanthine oxidase (XO), the enzyme which catalyses the following reaction:

$$\text{hypoxanthine} \xRightarrow{XO} \text{xanthine} \xRightarrow{XO} \text{urate/uric acid}$$

Allopurinol decreases urate formation in two ways:
1. The inhibition of XO reduces the amount of hypoxanthine and xanthine converted to urate/uric acid;
2. This action makes more hypoxanthine and xanthine available for re-utilisation in the purine metabolic cycle, which in turn, by a feedback mechanism, decreases overall *de novo* purine formation.

Since allopurinol decreases urate formation, it reduces urate/uric acid concentrations in both body fluids and urine. In contrast, the uricosuric agents which increase urate/uric acid excretion *via* the kidney will reduce the urate concentration in body fluids, but increase urate/uric acid concentrations in urine. Reduction of the urate concentrations in body fluids by allopurinol permits mobilisation and dissolution of urate deposits anywhere in the body, the commonest sites being those in the skin, bones, joints and kidney interstitial tissue.

Therapeutic effects therefore include:

The resolution of skin tophi and the healing of urate sinuses; eventual reduction in the frequency of attacks of acute gouty arthritis; improvement in joint mobility; reduction of the urate load to be excreted *via* the kidney; prevention and treatment of acute uric acid nephropathy; and, in the long term, reduced risk of renal impairment by urate/uric acid and prevention and dissolution of uric acid renal stones.

**Dosage and administration** The dosage should be adjusted by monitoring serum urate concentrations and urinary urate/uric acid levels at appropriate intervals.

*Dose frequency*: Zyloric may be taken orally once a day after a meal. It is well tolerated, especially after food. Should the daily dosage exceed 300 mg and gastrointestinal intolerance be manifested, a divided doses regimen may be appropriate.

*Adults:* 2 to 10 mg/kg bodyweight/day or: 100 to 200 mg daily in mild conditions; 300 to 600 mg daily in moderately severe conditions; or 700 to 900 mg daily in severe conditions.

The initial dosage should be in the range of 100 to 300 mg per day which may be taken as a single dose, preferably after food.

*Children under 15 years*: 10 to 20 mg/kg bodyweight/day, or 100 to 400 mg daily.

Use in children is rarely indicated, except in malignant conditions (especially leukaemia), and certain enzyme disorders such as Lesch-Nyhan syndrome.

*Use in the elderly*: In the absence of specific data, the lowest dosage which produces satisfactory urate reduction should be used. Particular attention should be paid to dosage advice in *Dosage recommendations in renal disorder* and *Precautions*.

*Dosage recommendations in renal disorder*: Since allopurinol and its metabolites are excreted by the kidney, impaired renal function may lead to retention of the drug and/or its metabolites with consequent prolongation of plasma half lives. In the presence of impaired renal function, serious consideration should be given to initiating treatment with a maximum dose of 100 mg/day and increasing it only if the serum and/or urinary urate response is unsatisfactory. In severe renal insufficiency, it may be advisable to use less than 100 mg per day or to use single doses of 100 mg at longer intervals than one day.

Alternative schedules based on creatinine clearances are unsatisfactory because of the imprecision of low clearance values.

If facilities are available to monitor plasma oxipurinol concentrations, the dose should be adjusted to maintain plasma oxipurinol levels below 100 micromol/litre (15.2 micrograms/ml).

*Dosage recommendations in renal dialysis:* Allopurinol and its metabolites are removed by renal dialysis. If dialysis is required two to three times a week, consideration should be given to an alternative dosage schedule of 300 to 400 mg Zyloric immediately after each dialysis with none in the interim.

*Treatment of high urate turnover conditions, e.g. neoplasia, Lesch-Nyhan syndrome*: It is advisable to correct existing hyperuricaemia and/or hyperuricosuria with Zyloric before starting cytotoxic therapy. It is important to ensure adequate hydration to maintain optimum diuresis and to attempt alkalinisation of urine to increase solubility of urinary urate/uric acid. Dosage of Zyloric should be in the lower range.

If urate nephropathy or other pathology has compromised renal function, the advice given in *Dosage recommendations in renal disorder* should be followed.

These steps may reduce the risk of xanthine and/or oxipurinol deposition complicating the clinical situation. See also *Drug interactions* and *Side and adverse effects*.

**Contra-indications, warnings, etc**

*Contra-indications*: Known intolerance of allopurinol. Zyloric is contra-indicated as a treatment for the acute attack of gout. Prophylactic therapy may be started when the acute attack has completely subsided, provided anti-inflammatory agents are also taken.

*Precautions:* Zyloric should be withdrawn IMMEDIATELY when a skin rash or other evidence of sensitivity occurs.

Dosage reduction should be considered in the presence of severe hepatic or renal disorder.

Asymptomatic hyperuricaemia *per se* is NOT an indication for use of Zyloric. Fluid and dietary modification with management of the underlying cause may correct the condition. If other clinical conditions suggest a need for Zyloric it must be introduced at low dosage (50 to 100 mg/day) to reduce the risk of adverse reactions and increased only if the serum urate response is unsatisfactory. Extra caution should be exercised if renal function is poor (see also *Dosage recommendations in renal disorder*). Zyloric must be withdrawn IMMEDIATELY and PERMANENTLY at the first signs of intolerance.

*Acute gouty attacks:* In the early stages of treatment with Zyloric, as with the uricosuric agents, an acute attack of gouty arthritis may be precipitated. Therefore, it is advisable to give prophylaxis with a suitable anti-inflammatory agent or colchicine (0.5 mg three times a day) for at least one month.

*Xanthine deposition*: In conditions where the rate of urate formation is greatly increased (e.g. malignant disease and its treatment, Lesch-Nyhan syndrome), the absolute concentration of xanthine in urine could, in rare cases, rise sufficiently to allow deposition in the urinary tract. This risk may be minimised by adequate hydration to achieve optimal urine dilution.

*Impaction of uric acid renal stones*: Adequate therapy with Zyloric will lead to dissolution of large uric acid renal pelvic stones with the remote possibility of impaction in the ureter.

*Use in pregnancy and lactation:* There is inadequate evidence of safety of Zyloric in human pregnancy, although it has been in wide use for many years without apparent ill consequence.

One study in mice receiving a high intraperitoneal dose on days 10 or 13 of pregnancy resulted in fetal abnormalities but extensive studies of high oral doses in mice, rats and rabbits during days 8 to 16 produced none.

Use in pregnancy only when there is no safer alternative and when the disease itself carries ris for the mother or child.

Based on data from a single individual, oxipurin (126 micromol/l, 19.2 microgram/ml), allopurin (4.4 micromol/l, 0.6 microgram/ml) and allopurin riboside (5.6 micromol/l, 1.5 microgram/ml) ha been demonstrated in human breast milk four hou after a single dose of allopurinol 300 mg. There a no data concerning the effects of these metabolit on the breast-fed baby.

*Drug interactions: 6-mercaptopurine and azath prine*: When 6-mercaptopurine or azathioprine given by mouth concurrently with Zyloric, only on quarter of the usual dose of 6-mercaptopurine azathioprine should be given because inhibition xanthine oxidase will prolong their activity.

Adenine arabinoside: Evidence suggests that t plasma half-life of adenine arabinoside is increased the presence of allopurinol. When the two produc are used concomitantly extra vigilance is necessa to recognise enhanced toxic effects.

*Salicylates and uricosuric agents*: Oxipurinol, t major metabolite of allopurinol and itself therapeu cally active, is excreted by the kidney in a similar w to urate. Hence drugs with uricosuric activity such probenecid or large doses of salicylate may accelera the excretion of oxipurinol. This may decrease t therapeutic activity of Zyloric, but the significan needs to be assessed in each case.

*Chlorpropamide*: If Zyloric is given concomitantly wi chlorpropamide when renal function is poor, the may be an increased risk of prolonged hypoglycaen activity.

*Coumarin anticoagulants*: There is no evidence th interaction between allopurinol and the coumari seen under experimental conditions has any clinic significance. However, all patients receiving an coagulants must be carefully monitored.

*Phenytoin*: Allopurinol may inhibit hepatic oxidati of phenytoin but the clinical significance has not be demonstrated.

*Theophylline*: Experimental studies of the effect allopurinol on theophylline metabolism have p duced contradictory findings. There have been clinical reports of interactions.

*Side- and adverse effects*: Adverse reactions association with Zyloric are rare in the overall treat population and mostly of a minor nature. T incidence is higher in the presence of renal and/ hepatic disorder.

*Skin reactions*: These are the most common reactio and may occur at any time during treatment. Th may be pruritic, maculopapular, sometimes sca sometimes purpuric and rarely exfoliative. Zylo should be withdrawn IMMEDIATELY should su reactions occur. After recovery from mild reactio Zyloric may, if desired, be reintroduced at a sm dose (e.g. 50 mg/day) and gradually increased. If t rash recurs, Zyloric should be PERMANENTLY wi drawn.

*Generalised hypersensitivity*: Skin reactio associated with exfoliation, fever, lymphadenopat arthralgia and/or eosinophilia resembling Steve Johnson and/or Lyell syndrome occur rare Associated vasculitis and tissue response may manifested in various ways including hepatitis, int stitial nephritis and, very rarely, epilepsy. If su reactions do occur, it may be at any time during tre ment. Zyloric should be withdrawn IMMEDIATE and PERMANENTLY.

Corticosteroids may be beneficial in overcomi them. When generalised hypersensitivity reactio have occurred, renal and/or hepatic disorder h usually been present particularly when the outcor has been fatal.

*Angioimmunoblastic lymphadenopathy*: Ang immunoblastic lymphadenopathy has been describ rarely following biopsy of a generalised lymphade pathy. It appears to be reversible on withdrawal Zyloric.

*Granulomatous hepatitis*: Very rarely granulomato hepatitis, without overt evidence of more generalis hypersensitivity, has been described. It appears to reversible on withdrawal of Zyloric.

*Gastrointestinal disorder*: In early clinical studi nausea and vomiting were reported. Further repo suggest that this reaction is not a significant probl and can be avoided by taking Zyloric after mea Recurrent haematemesis has been reported as extremely rare event, as has steatorrhoea.

*Blood and lymphatic system*: Occasional reports ha been received of thrombocytopenia, agranulocyto and aplastic anaemia, particularly in individuals w impaired renal function, reinforcing the need particular care in this group of patients.

*Miscellaneous*: The following complaints have be

eported occasionally: fever; general malaise; asthenia; headache; vertigo; ataxia; somnolence; coma;
depression; paralysis; paraesthesiae; neuropathy;
visual disorder; cataract; macular changes; taste
perversion; stomatitis; changed bowel habit; infertility; impotence; nocturnal emission; diabetes mellitus;
hyperlipaemia; furunculosis; alopecia; discoloured
hair; angina; hypertension; bradycardia; oedema;
uraemia; haematuria; gynaecomastia.

*Toxicity and treatment of overdosage:* Accidental or
deliberate ingestion of up to 5 g allopurinol, or very
rarely 20 g, has been reported. Symptoms and signs
included nausea, vomiting, diarrhoea and dizziness.
Recovery followed general supportive measures.
Massive absorption of Zyloric may lead to considerable inhibition of xanthine oxidase activity, which
should have no untoward effects unless 6-mercapto-
purine and/or azathioprine is being taken concomitantly. Adequate hydration to maintain optimum
diuresis facilitates excretion of allopurinol and its
metabolites. If considered necessary haemodialysis
may be used.

**Pharmaceutical precautions** Store below 25°C. Keep
dry.

**Legal category** POM

**Package quantities**
Zyloric Tablets:    Bottle of 100 tablets.
Zyloric-300 Tablets:   Calendar pack of 2 x 14 tablets.

**Further information** Nil.

**Product licence numbers**
Zyloric Tablets     0003/5207
Zyloric-300 Tablets   0003/0092

*Trade Mark

# Windsor Healthcare Limited
Ellesfield Avenue
Bracknell
Berkshire RG12 8YS

## DULCO-LAX*

### Qualitative and quantitative composition
*Dulco-lax:* Circular, biconvex, yellow, sugar-coated and enteric-coated tablets each containing 5 mg of bisacodyl.

*Dulco-lax Suppositories for Children 5 mg:* Smooth white torpedo shaped suppositories, each containing 5 mg of bisacodyl.

*Dulco-lax Suppositories 10 mg:* Smooth white torpedo shaped suppositories, each containing 10 mg of bisacodyl.

### Pharmaceutical form
Tablets for oral administration.
Suppositories for rectal administration.

### Clinical particulars
*Therapeutic indications:* Constipation, either chronic or of recent onset, whenever a stimulant laxative is required.

Bowel clearance before surgery or radiological investigation. Replacement of the evacuant enema in all its indications.

**Posology and method of administration** Dulco-lax is suitable for routine use in adults of all ages, and in children over 10 years of age. Children under 10 years should not take Dulco-lax without medical advice. Unless otherwise prescribed by the doctor, the following dosages are recommended:

*1. For constipation*
*Sugar-coated tablets (5 mg)*
Adults and children over 10 years: One to two tablets at night (5–10 mg).

Children under 10 years should not take Dulco-lax without medical advice.

Children aged 4 to 10 years: One tablet (5 mg) at night.

Children under 4 years: Paediatric suppositories (5 mg) are recommended.

Sugar-coated tablets should be taken at night to produce evacuation the following morning. The tablets have a special coating and should, therefore, not be taken together with milk or antacids. The tablets should be swallowed whole with adequate fluid.

*Suppositories (5 & 10 mg)*
Adults and children over 10 years: One 10 mg suppository to be administered in the morning.

Children under 10 years: One 5 mg suppository to be administered under medical supervision only.

Suppositories are usually effective in about 30 minutes. A suppository should be unwrapped and inserted into the rectum pointed end first.

*2. For preparation for diagnostic procedures and preoperatively*
When using Dulco-lax to prepare the patient for radiographic examination of the abdomen or employing it preoperatively, tablets should be combined with suppositories in order to achieve complete evacuation of the intestine.

Adults and children over 10 years: Two to four tablets the night before and insert one 10 mg suppository the following morning.

Children aged 4–10 years: One tablet the night before and insert one 5 mg suppository the following morning.

No specific information on the use of this product in the elderly is available. Clinical trials have included patients over 65 years and no adverse reactions specific to this age group have been reported.

*Contra-indications:* Dulco-lax must not be used in patients with ileus, intestinal obstruction, acute surgical abdominal conditions such as acute appendicitis, acute inflammatory bowel diseases, and in severe dehydration.

Dulco-lax suppositories should not be used when anal fissures or ulcerative proctitis with mucosal damage are present.

*Special warnings and special precautions for use:* As with all laxatives, Dulco-lax should not be used on a continuous daily basis for long periods.

If laxatives are needed every day, the cause of constipation should be investigated. Prolonged excessive use may lead to electrolyte imbalance and hypokalaemia, and may precipitate the onset of rebound constipation.

The use of suppositories may lead to painful sensations and local irritation, especially in anal fissures and ulcerative proctitis.

Children under 10 years should not take Dulco-lax without medical advice.

*Interaction with other medicaments and other forms of interaction:* The concomitant use of antacids and milk products may reduce the resistance of the coating of the tablets and result in dyspepsia and gastric irritation.

The concomitant use of diuretics or adreno-corticosteroids may increase the risk of electrolyte imbalance. However, this situation only arises if excessive doses of Dulco-lax are taken (see *Overdose* section).

*Pregnancy and lactation:* There are no reports of undesirable or damaging effects during pregnancy or to the foetus attributable to the use of Dulco-lax. Nevertheless, medicines should not be used in pregnancy, especially the first trimester, unless the expected benefit is thought to outweigh any possible risk to the foetus.

Although the active ingredient of Dulco-lax is not known to be excreted in breast milk, its use during breast feeding is not recommended.

*Effects on ability to drive and use machines:* Dulco-lax has no effect on ability to drive and use machinery.

*Undesirable effects:* Abdominal discomfort and diarrhoea may occasionally occur. Local irritation has been reported when the suppository formulation has been administered.

*Overdose: Symptoms:* If high doses are taken diarrhoea, abdominal cramps and a clinically significant loss of potassium and other electrolytes can occur. This may also lead to increased sensitivity to cardiac glycosides.

*Therapy:* Within a short time after ingestion of oral forms of Dulco-lax, absorption can be minimised or prevented by inducing vomiting. Otherwise, gastric lavage should be performed. Replacement of fluids and correction of electrolyte imbalance (particularly hypokalaemia) may be required. This is especially important in the elderly and the young. Administration of antispasmodics may be of some value.

### Pharmacological properties
*Pharmacodynamic properties:* Bisacodyl is a locally acting laxative from the triarylmethane group, which, after metabolism by hydrolysis, stimulates the mucosa of the large intestine causing peristalsis of the colon.

*Pharmacokinetic properties:* Hydrolysis of bisacodyl by enzymes of the enteric mucosa forms desacetylbisacodyl which is absorbed and excreted partly via urine and bile as glucuronide. By bacterial cleavage the active form, the free diphenol, is formed in the colon. Formulations of bisacodyl which are resistant to gastric and small intestinal juice, like Dulco-lax sugar-coated tablets, reach the colon without any appreciable absorption and therefore avoid enterohepatic circulation. Consequently, these oral forms have an onset of action between 6–12 hours after administration.

Suppository formulations of bisacodyl have an onset of action within 15–30 minutes, although in some cases it may be prolonged to 15–60 minutes. The onset of action is determined by the release of the active substance from the preparation.

After administration, only small amounts of the drug are systemically available. Urinary excretion reflects low systemic burden after oral and rectal administraiton.

There is no relationship between the laxative effect and plasma levels of the active diphenol.

*Preclinical safety data:* There are no preclinical data of relevance to the prescriber which are additional to that already included in other sections of the SPC.

### Pharmaceutical particulars
*List of excipients: Tablets:* Lactose, maize starch (dried), soluble maize starch, glycerol (85%), magnesium stearate, sucrose, talc, acacia (powered), titanium dioxide, eudragit L, eudragit S, dibutyl phthalate, macrogol 6000, yellow iron oxide, white beeswax, carnauba wax.

*Suppositories:* Hard fat (Adeps solidus).

*Incompatibilities:* None stated.

*Shelf life:* 5 years.

*Special precautions for storage:* Store below 25°C.

*Nature and contents of container:* Dulco-lax Table are presented in aluminium foil blister strips coate with PVC film or combination lacquer.

Dulco-lax Suppositories and Dulco-lax Supposit ries for Children are presented in aluminium f blister strips coated with polyethylene.

Dulco-lax Tablets are available in packs of 10, and 60 (Packs of 10 are available for general sale the UK). Dulco-lax Suppositories are available in pac of 10 and 20, and Dulco-lax Suppositories for Childre are available in packs of 5.

*Instructions for use/handling:* None stated.

### Marketing authorisation numbers
| | |
|---|---|
| Dulco-lax Tablets | 6772/0007 |
| Dulco-lax Suppositories | 6772/0009 |
| Dulco-lax Suppositories for Children | 6772/0008 |

**Date of approval/revision of SPC** May 1997.

**Legal category** P.

## LAXOBERAL*

**Presentation** A clear, yellowish orange, fruit-fl voured liquid containing sodium picosulphate 5 n per 5 ml.

### Uses
*Action:* Laxoberal contains a synthetic laxative, s dium picosulphate, which is broken down by bacte in the large intestine to the active substance, bis-( hydroxyphenyl)-2-pyridylmethane. A predictab evacuation of soft formed stools occurs usually 10– hours after administration.

*Indications:* Constipation, either recent or chron whenever a stimulant laxative is required. Bow clearance before surgery, labour or radiological inve tigations.

Laxoberal is suitable for routine use in both adu and children.

### Dosage and administration
*Adults:* 5-15 ml at night.

*Children:* 5-10 years: 2.5-5 ml at night.
2-5 years: 2.5 ml at night.

*Diluent:* Laxoberal may be diluted with purified wate

### Contra-indications, warnings, etc
*Contra-indications:* As with any laxative, Laxobe should not be given to patients with undiagnos abdominal pain, or where intestinal obstruction suspected.

*Precautions:* It is generally recommended that lax tives should not be given to patients being prepare for barium enema examinations where inflammato bowel disease, such as ulcerative colitis, is suspecte This recommendation applies also to Laxoberal.

As Laxoberal is broken down by bacteria in t large intestine, it is possible that in patients taki broad-spectrum antibiotics there may be some lo of laxative action.

Although Laxoberal has been in wide general u for many years, there is no evidence of ill-consequer during human pregnancy. Only in doses much high than the equivalent maximum therapeutic dose man were effects on foetal development seen animals. Drug-induced foetal malformations did n occur.

Medicines should not be used in pregnancy, esp cially the first trimester, unless the expected benefit thought to outweigh any possible risk to the foetus

*Side-effects:* As with most laxatives of this gro there have been occasional reports of mild abdomir discomfort following Laxoberal administration.

*Overdosage:* Colicky lower abdominal pain and po sible signs of dehydration may be expected partic larly in the elderly and the very young. Gastric lava should be performed where appropriate. Adequa hydration must be maintained and the serum pota sium should be measured. Antispasmodics may value. Particular care about fluid balance should taken in the elderly and young.

**Pharmaceutical precautions** Laxoberal should stored at room temperature and protected from lig

**Legal category** P.

**Pack size** 100 ml. 300 ml.

**urther information** Laxoberal is also available as a ml presentation under the trade name Dulco-lax quid.

**oduct licence number** 6772/0011

# HARMATON* CAPSULES

**ialitative and quantitative composition** Each cap-le contains:

| tive ingredients | | Declaration per capsule |
|---|---|---|
| andardised Panax ginseng extract | | 40.0 mg |
| 15 Pharmaton | | 41.0 |
| amin A Palmitate | (Vit.A) | 2667 IU |
| olecalciferol | (Vit.D3) | 200 IU |
| _-α-Tocopherol acetate | (Vit.E) | 10 mg |
| iamine mononitrate | (Vit.B1) | 1.4 mg |
| ooflavine | (Vit.B2) | 1.6 mg |
| ridoxine hydrochloride | (Vit.B6) | 2.0 mg |
| anocobalamine | (Vit.B12) | 1.0 mcg |
| otin | | 150.0 mcg |
| cotinamide | | 18.0 mg |
| corbic acid | | 60.0 mg |
| lic acid | | 0.1 mg |
| pper(II) sulphate dried | (Cu: 2.0 mg) | 5.6 mg |
| dium selenite, dried | (Se: 50.0 mcg) | 111.0 mcg |
| anganese(II) sulphate monohydrate | (Mn: 2.5 mg) | 7.75 mg |
| agnesium sulphate, dried | (Mg: 10.0 mg) | 71.0 mg |
| n(II) sulphate, dried | (Fe: 10.0 mg) | 33.0 mg |
| nc sulphate, monohydrate | (Zn: 1.0 mg) | 2.75 mg |
| basic calcium phosphate, anhydrous | (Ca: 100.0 mg) | 340.0 mg |
| cithin | | 100.0 mg |

**armaceutical form** Soft gelatin capsules for oral se.

**inical particulars**

**erapeutic indications:** Pharmaton Capsules contain amins, minerals and standardised Ginseng Extract 15 in amounts which suit the body's daily require-ents. The capsules are indicated for:
States of exhaustion (eg caused by stress), tired-ss, feeling of weakness, vitality deficiency.
Prevention and treatment of symptoms caused by balanced or deficient nutrition.

**osology and method of administration:**
*Adults:* The recommended daily dosage is one to vo capsules per day. The first capsule should eferably be taken with breakfast and the second th lunch.
*Children:* Not recommended for use in children.
*Elderly:* There no special dosage recommendations r the elderly.

**ontra-indications:** Hypersensitivity to any of the gredients. Hypercalcaemia and/or hypercalciuria, emochromatosis, iron overload syndrome, hyper-taminosis A or D, concomitant retinoid (eg against ne) or vitamin D therapy, renal insufficiency, preg-ncy.

**ther special warnings and precautions:** An allowance ould be made for vitamins or minerals obtained om other sources.

**teraction with other medicaments and other forms interaction:** There is no evidence from clinical perience that Pharmaton Capsules interacts with her medications.

**egnancy and lactation:** Reproduction studies with imals using the standardised Panax ginseng extract 115 Pharmaton showed no adverse effects on rtility, nor any teratogenic effects. However, con-olled studies with pregnant women are not available. Controlled studies with women using multivitamin-ineral preparations at the usual dosage during the urse of the first trimester resulted in no fetal risks. ere are no signs indicating a risk if this type of eparation is taken during the second and third

trimesters, and probability of injuring the fetus ap-pears to be very low.
Large doses of vitamin A (10,000 IU per day) have been found to be teratogenic if administered during the first trimester of pregnancy. Vitamin D given during the last trimester of pregnancy may cause hypercalcaemia in infants. As with many other medi-cines an assessment of benefits versus risks should be made before this product is administered during this period.
WARNING: Do not take Vitamin A supplements if you are pregnant or likely to become pregnant except on the advice of a doctor or ante-natal clinic.

*Effects on ability to drive and use machines:* None known.

*Undesirable effects:* Gastrointestinal reactions (eg abdominal pain, nausea) have been reported rarely.

*Overdose:* Nervousness may occur following an overdose of the product.
The toxicity of the product in large overdoses is caused by the toxicity of the liposoluble vitamins A and D. A *safe dose* for both vitamins is considered to be 5-10 x RDA (each capsule contains the EU %RDA for vitamins A and D).
Prolonged supply of larger amounts (40-55 x RDA for Vitamin A; 10-25 x RDA for Vitamin D) can cause symptoms of chronic toxicity. Acute toxic symptoms are only seen at even higher doses.
*Iron:* Severe acute toxicity in man has been reported from doses of iron ranging from 12-1500 x RDA (each capsule contains the UK %RDA for iron). Most incidents of acute iron toxicity have resulted from accidental oral ingestion of iron pills by children. Longer-term doses of iron up to 6-7 x RDA have been reported to have no toxic effect.
*Symptoms:* Initial symptoms include nausea, vom-iting, diarrhoea, abdominal pain, haematemesis, rec-tal bleeding, lethargy and circulatory collapse. Hyperglycaemia and metabolic acidosis may also occur.
*Treatment:* To minimise or prevent further absorp-tion of the medication, as follows:
– Induce vomiting eg by administration of an emetic
– Gastric lavage with desferrioxamine solution (2 g/l). Then desferrioxamine (5–10 g in 50-100 ml water) should be introduced into the stomach to be retained.
– Severe poisoning: Shock and/or coma with high iron levels (serum iron >90 µmol/l in children, >142 µmol/l in adults); immediate supportive meas-ures plus i.v. infusion of desferrioxamine should be instituted.
– Less severe poisoning: i.m. desferrioxamine is recommended (1 g 4-6 hourly in children; 50 mg/kg up to a maximum dose of 4 g in adults).

**Pharmacological properties**

*Pharmacodynamic properties:* Pharmaton Capsules exert a stimulant effect at physical and psychological levels through the combined action of various sub-stances on the basic metabolic processes.
The standardised ginseng extract G115 raises the general level of cellular activity, which is expressed by a pronounced increase in the physical and mental capacity.
In animal experiments, it caused a reduction of lactic acid concentration in muscles during exercise. An increase in the dopamine and noradrenaline content and a reduction in the serotonin content in the brain stem could be observed.
Vitamins, minerals and trace elements correct and prevent impairment of the cell metabolism in situa-tions with increased demands. Low supply of vita-mins, minerals, and trace elements may cause disturbances, such as debility, tiredness, decrease in vitality, reduced force of resistance, and decelerated convalescence. The composition and dosages of the preparation were chosen according to the European RDA-requirements for food supplements.
Choline, inositol, linoleic acid and linolenic acid, in

the form of lecithin, improve energy output and lipid metabolism.

*Pharmacokinetic properties:* Pharmacokinetic studies of Pharmaton Capsules have not been carried out, because of the complex composition of the product and the small quantities of the active ingredients contained. Moreover, these substances are well known.
Pharmacokinetic studies of the standardised gin-seng extract G115 are not possible, because it is a complex extract. In the ginseng root more than 200 substances have been identified to date. Pharmacoki-netic studies of individual purified ginsenosides have been carried out in various animal species:
Using radioactively labelled ($^{14}$C) Ginsenoside Rgl, originated from the standarised Panax ginseng extract G115 Pharmaton, a bioavailability of 30% was deter-mined in mice.
With intraperitoneal application, depending on the tested animal species and the Ginsenoside type, a half-life of between 27 minutes and 14.5 hours was measured.

*Preclinical safety data*
*Acute toxicity:* The oral $LD_{50}$ of the standardized Panax ginseng extract G115 Pharmaton is more than 5 g/kg of body weight in the mouse and the rat, and more than 2 g/kg in the mini-pig.

*Reproduction toxicity:* The effect of standardised Panax ginseng extract G115 Pharmaton on reproduc-tive performance was studied in two generations of Sprague-Dawley rats. Animals of both sexes were fed either control diet or diet supplemented with the standardised Panax ginseng extract G115 Pharmaton at dose levels of 1.5, 5 or 15 mg/kg body weight/day. Parameters of reproduction and lactation in the treated groups were comparable to those of the controls for two generations of dams and pups. No treatment-related effects were seen in weekly body weights and food consumption, haematological and blood chem-istry parameters, and ophthalmic, macroscopic and histopathological examinations.

*Fetal toxicity:* The standardised Panax ginseng extract G115 Pharmaton, administered to pregnant Wistar rats and pregnant New Zealand rabbits, caused no abnormality in the foetal development.
The rats were treated with 40 mg/kg/day from the 1st to the 15th day after mating.
The rabbits were treated with 20 mg/kg/day from the 7th to the 16th day after mating.
The fetuses were removed by caesarean section on the 21st day in the rats and on the 27th day in the rabbits.

**Pharmaceutical particulars**

*List of excipients:*
*Capsule:* Rape oil; hard fat; ethyl vanillin; arachis oil; gelatin powder.
*Capsule shell:* Gelatin; glycerol 85%; iron oxide red (E172); iron oxide black (E172).

*Incompatibilities:* None stated.

*Shelf-life:* Two years

*Special precautions for storage:* Pharmaton Capsules should be kept tightly closed in a dry place below 25°C.

*Nature and contents of container:* Brown glass bottles (hydrolytical class III, PhEur) with pilfer proof alumin-ium caps (with rubber inserts) containing either 30 or 100 capsules.
or
Aluminium foil/polyvinylchloride/polyvinylidench-loride blister packs of 4, 30, 90 and 100 capsules.

*Instructions for use/handling:* None stated.

**Marketing authorisation number** 6772/0014

**Date of approval/revision of SPC** 27 March 1997.

**Legal category** P.

*Trade Mark

# Wyeth Laboratories
## incorporating A. H. Robins and Lederle Laboratories
Huntercombe Lane South
Taplow
Maidenhead, Berks SL6 0PH

 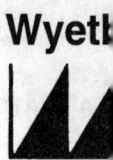

## ACHROMYCIN* CAPSULES

**Presentation** *Capsules 250 mg:* Each opaque, orange capsule printed 'Lederle 4874' contains 250 mg tetracycline hydrochloride.

**Uses** Achromycin is a broad-spectrum antibiotic used for the treatment of infections caused by tetracycline-sensitive organisms.

For example, Achromycin is highly effective in the treatment of infections caused by *Borrellia recurrentis* (relapsing fever), *Calymmatobacterium granulomatis* (granuloma inguinale), *Chlamydia* species (psittacosis, lymphogranuloma venereum, trachoma, inclusion conjunctivitis), *Francisella tularensis* (tularaemia), *Haemophilus ducreyi* (chancroid), *Leptospira* ( meningitis, jaundice), *Mycoplasma pneumoniae* (nongonococcal urethritis) *Pseudomonas mallei* and *pseudomallei* (glanders and melioidosis), *Rickettsiae* (typhus fever, Q fever, rocky mountain spotted fever), *Vibrio* species (cholera). It is also highly effective, alone or in combination with streptomycin, in the treatment of infections due to *Brucella* species (brucellosis), and *Yersinia pestis* (bubonic plague). Severe acne vulgaris.

Other sensitive organisms include: *Actinomyces israelii, Bacillus anthracis* (pneumonia), *Clostridium* species (gas gangrene, tetanus), *Entamoeba histolytica* (dysentery), *Neisseria gonorrhoeae*, and anaerobic species, *Treponema pallidum* and *pertenue* (syphillis and yaws).

**Dosage and administration** *Adults:* 1 capsule four times a day. This may be increased to 6 or 8 capsules daily in severe infections.

*Children:* Not recommended for children under 12 years of age. For children above the age of 12 years, the dose is 25–50 mg/kg divided in 2 or 4 equal doses. The maximum dose should not exceed the recommended adult dosage.

*Elderly:* Achromycin should be used with caution in the treatment of elderly patients where accumulation is a possibility.

*Administration:* Achromycin should be swallowed whole with plenty of fluid while sitting or standing. Doses should be taken an hour before or two hours after meals and therapy should be continued for up to three days after characteristic symptoms of the infection have subsided.

### Contra-indications, warnings, etc.

*Contra-indications:* A history of hypersensitivity to tetracyclines. Overt renal insufficiency. Children under 12 years of age.

*Warnings:* The use of tetracyclines during tooth development in children under the age of 12 years may cause permanent discolouration. Enamel hypoplasia has also been reported.

Achromycin should be used with caution in patients with renal or hepatic dysfunction or in conjunction with other potentially hepatotoxic or nephrotoxic drugs. Concurrent use with the anaesthetic methoxyflurane increases the risk of kidney failure. The anti-anabolic action of the tetracyclines may cause an increase in BUN.

Lower doses are indicated in cases of renal impairment to avoid excessive systemic accumulation, and if therapy is prolonged, serum level determinations are advisable. Patients who have known liver disease should not receive more than 1 g daily. In long term therapy, periodic laboratory evaluation of organ systems, including haematopoietic, renal and hepatic studies should be performed.

Cross resistance between tetracyclines may develop in micro-organisms and cross-sensitisation in patients. Achromycin should be discontinued if there are signs/symptoms of overgrowth of resistant organisms including candida, enteritis, glossitis, stomatitis, vaginitis, pruritus ani or staphylococcal enterocolitis.

Patients taking oral contraceptives should be warned that if diarrhoea or breakthrough bleeding occur, there is a possibility of contraceptive failure.

*Interactions:* Achromycin should not be used with penicillins. Tetracyclines depress plasma prothrombin activity and reduced doses of concomitant anticoagulants may be required.

Absorption of Achromycin is impaired by the concomitant administration of iron, calcium, zinc, magnesium and particularly aluminium salts commonly used as antacids.

The concomitant use of tetracyclines may reduce the efficacy of oral contraceptives; an increased incidence of breakthrough bleeding may also be experienced (see statement under *Warnings*).

*Use in pregnancy:* Results of animal studies indicate that tetracyclines cross the placenta, are found in foetal tissues, and can have toxic effects on the developing foetus (often related to retardation of skeletal development). Evidence of embryotoxicity has also been noted in animals treated early in pregnancy.

Achromycin therefore, should not be used in pregnancy unless considered essential in which case the maximum daily dose should be 1 g.

The use of drugs of the tetracycline class during tooth development (last half of pregnancy) may cause permanent discolouration of the teeth (yellow-grey-brown). This adverse reaction is more common during long term use of the drugs but has been observed following repeated short term courses. Enamel hypoplasia has also been reported.

*Use in lactation:* Tetracyclines have been found in the milk of lactating women who are taking a drug in this class. Permanent tooth discolouration may occur in the developing infant, and enamel hypoplasia has been reported. Therefore, Achromycin should not be administered to lactating women.

*Side-effects:* Gastro-intestinal disturbances including nausea, vomiting and diarrhoea may occur and as with all antibiotics overgrowth of resistant organisms may cause glossitis, stomatitis, vaginitis, or staphylococcal enterocolitis. Photosensitivity and dermatological reactions are rare. Bulging fontanelles in infants and benign intracranial hypertension in adults have been reported. Treatment should cease if evidence of raised intracranial pressure develops. Hypersensitivity reactions, including urticaria, angioneurotic oedema, anaphylaxis, anaphylactoid purpura, pericarditis and exacerbation of systemic lupus erythematosus may occur. Haemolytic anaemia, thrombocytopenia, neutropenia and eosinophilia have been reported. When given over prolonged periods, tetracyclines have been reported to produce brown-black microscopic discolouration of the thyroid gland. No abnormalities of thyroid function are known to occur.

*Overdosage:* No specific antidote. Gastric lavage plus oral administration of milk or antacids.

**Pharmaceutical precautions** Achromycin Capsules should be stored at controlled room temperature (15–30°C) in the original pack.

**Legal category** POM

**Package quantity** Bottles of 100

**Further information** Nil

**Product licence number** 0095/0041

## ACHROMYCIN* INTRAVENOUS/INTRAPLEURAL

**Presentation** Achromycin Intravenous 250 mg and 500 mg. Each vial contains tetracycline hydrochloride 250 mg or 500 mg buffered with 625 mg or 1,250 mg of ascorbic acid respectively.

**Uses** Achromycin is a broad spectrum antibiotic indicated alone or adjunctively in the treatment of infections caused by tetracycline-sensitive organisms.

For example, Achromycin is highly effective in the treatment of infections caused by *Borrellia recurrentis* (relapsing fever), *Calymmatobacterium granulomatis* (granuloma inguinale), *Chlamydia* species (psittacosis, lymphogranuloma venereum, trachoma, inclusion conjunctivitis), *Francisella tularensis* (tularaemia), *Haemophilus ducreyi* (chancroid), *Leptospira* (meningitis, jaundice), *Mycoplasma pneumoniae* (nongonococcal urethritis) *Pseudomonas mallei* and *pseudomallei* (glanders and melioidosis), *Rickettsiae* (typhus fever, Q fever, rocky mountain spotted fever), *Vibrio* species (cholera). It is also highly effective,

alone or in combination with streptomycin, in the treatment of infections due to *Brucella* species (brucellosis), and *Yersinia pestis* (bubonic plague).

Other sensitive organisms include: *Actinomyces israelii, Bacillus anthracis* (pneumonia), *Clostridium* species (gas gangrene, tetanus), *Entamoeba histolytica* (dysentery), *Neisseria gonorrhoeae*, and anaerobic species, *Treponema pallidum* and *pertenue* (syphilis and yaws).

The treatment of recurrent pleural effusions, secondary to neoplastic disease or end stage cirrhosis by intrapleural administration.

### Dosage and administration
*For antibiotic use by intravenous infusion:*
*Adults:* 500 mg every 12 hours by intravenous infusion. Maximum daily dosage should not exceed 2 g.

*Children over the age of twelve years:* Up to 10 mg/kg body weight per day in divided doses by intravenous infusion.

*Elderly:* Achromycin should be used with caution in the treatment of elderly patients where accumulation is a possibility.

*Administration:* Achromycin should be reconstituted and diluted immediately before administration by intravenous infusion. The use of a terminal filter (suitable pore size 0.22 micron) in line with the giving set is recommended. Reconstitute the injection by adding 5 ml of Water for Injection to the 250 mg vial, or 10 ml Water for Injection to the 500 mg vial and then dilute the resulting solution (50 mg/ml) to at least 100 ml (up to 1,000 ml) with any of the following diluents immediately before administration by intravenous infusion at a rate not exceeding 100 ml in five minutes: Sodium Chloride Intravenous Infusion BP 0.9%, Glucose Intravenous Infusion BP, Sodium Chloride and Glucose Intravenous Infusion BP, Compound Sodium Lactate Intravenous Infusion BP.

Oral Achromycin medication should replace parenteral as soon as practical, and be continued for up to three days after characteristic symptoms of the infection have subsided.

*For pleural effusions by intrapleural administration.*

*Adults:* A single dose of 500 mg by intrapleural administration.

*Administration:* The pleural space should first be completely drained with a thoracostomy tube which should be positioned to give optimum drainage. 500 mg of Achromycin in 30–50 ml of sterile saline is then instilled through the tube into the pleural space followed by flushing of the thoracostomy tube with more saline. The patient's position must then be altered frequently to ensure contact of the Achromycin with both the visceral and parietal pleural surfaces. It is recommended that initially the patient should be rotated to the left and right lateral decubitus, prone and supine positions for intervals of 2–3 minutes and then left in each of these positions for 30 minutes with the tube clamped. The thoracostomy tube should then be reconnected to negative pressure and the tube removed when drainage is complete or minimal. This can take up to 48–72 hours.

This procedure has been reported to produce pleural symphysis in up to 90% of cases.

### Contra-indications, warnings, etc
*Contra-indications:* A history of hypersensitivity to tetracyclines. Overt renal insufficiency. Children under twelve years of age.

*Warnings and precautions:* Achromycin should be used with caution in patients with renal or hepatic dysfunction or in conjunction with other potentially hepatotoxic or nephrotoxic drugs. Concurrent use with the anaesthetic methoxyflurane increases the risk of kidney failure. The anti-anabolic action of the tetracyclines may cause an increase in BUN.

Lower doses are indicated in cases of renal impairment to avoid excessive systemic accumulation, and if therapy is prolonged, serum level determinations are advisable. Patients who have known liver disease should not receive more than 1 g daily. In long term therapy, periodic laboratory evaluation of organ systems, including haematopoietic, renal and hepatic studies should be performed.

Cross-resistance between tetracyclines may d

op in micro-organisms and cross-sensitisation in :ients. Achromycin should be discontinued if there signs/symptoms of overgrowth of resistant organ-ıs including candida, enteritis, glossitis, stomatitis, initis, pruritus ani or staphylococcal enterocolitis. 'atients taking oral contraceptives should be rned that if diarrhoea or breakthrough bleeding ur there is a possibility of contraceptive failure.

*eractions:* Achromycin should not be used with nicillins. Tetracyclines depress plasma prothrombin ivity and reduced dosages of concurrent anticoag-nts may be required.

'he concomitant use of tetracyclines may reduce efficacy of oral contraceptives; an increased idence of breakthrough bleeding may also be perienced (see statement under Warnings and cautions).

*e in pregnancy:* Results of animal studies indicate t tetracyclines cross the placenta, are found in tal tissues and can have toxic effects on the veloping foetus (often related to retardation of letal development). Evidence of embryotoxicity s also been noted in animals treated early in gnancy. Achromycin therefore, should not be used pregnancy unless considered essential in which e the maximum daily dose should be 1 g.

'he use of drugs of the tetracycline class during th development (last half of pregnancy) may cause rmanent discolouration of the teeth (yellow-grey-own). This adverse reaction is more common during g term use of the drugs but has been observed lowing repeated short term courses.

:namel hypoplasia has also been reported.

*e in lactation:* Tetracyclines have been found in the k of lactating women who are taking a drug in this ss. Permanent tooth discolouration may occur in developing infant and enamel hypoplasia has en reported. Therefore, Achromycin should not be ministered to lactating women.

*e in children:* The use of tetracyclines during tooth velopment in children under the age of 12 years y cause permanent discolouration. Enamel hypo-sia has also been reported.

*le-effects:* Gastro-intestinal disturbances including usea, vomiting and diarrhoea may occur and as h all antibiotics overgrowth of resistant organisms y cause glossitis, stomatitis, vaginitis, or staphylo-ccal enterocolitis. Photosensitivity and dermatolog-l reactions are rare. Bulging fontanelles in infants d benign intracranial hypertension in adults has en reported. Treatment should cease if evidence of sed intracranial pressure develops. Hypersensitiv-reactions including urticaria, angioneurotic oe-ma, anaphylaxis, anaphylactoid purpura, ricarditis and exacerbation of systemic lupus ery-matosus may occur. Haemolytic anaemia, throm-cytopenia, neutropenia and eosinophilia have been orted. When given over prolonged periods, tetra-lines have been reported to produce brown-black croscopic discolouration of the thyroid gland. No normalities of thyroid function are known to occur. ntrapleural administration may be associated with nsient local pain (which can be controlled by algesics) and/or pyrexia.

*erdosage:* No specific antidote. Use appropriate pportive treatment.

**armaceutical precautions** Store in the original pack controlled room temperature (15–30°C) and protect m light. Achromycin should be reconstituted and uted immediately before administration by intra-nous infusion. The increase in injection volume, used by displacement, during dissolution of the wder with Water for Injection, is clinically insignifi-nt when calculating dosage and volume to be ected. The brown appearance of the vial is produced en the injection is sterilised by irradiation and does t indicate any degradation.

The following substances are incompatible in solu-n with Achromycin Intravenous, and should not be ministered in the same drip:

Aminophylline, amphotericin, barbiturates, cephal-in, chloramphenicol, chlorothiazide, chlorproma-e, cyanocobalamin, dimenhydrinate, erythromycin, parin, hydrocortisone, methicillin, methohexitone, thyldopa, nitrofurantoin, novobiocin, penicillins, enytoin, polymixin B, prochlorperazine, riboflavine, dium bicarbonate, sulphadiazine, sulphafurazole, opentone sodium, vitamin B complex, warfarin, rious inorganic ions (Ca, Mg, Al, Mn, Fe) and donor od.

*ote:* The use of solutions containing calcium should avoided as these tend to form precipitates (espe-lly in neutral to alkaline solution) and therefore ould not be used unless necessary. However, mpound Sodium Lactate Intravenous Infusion BP y be used with caution since the calcium ion ntent in this diluent does not normally precipitate racycline in an acid medium.

**Legal category** POM

**Package quantities**
Achromycin Intravenous 250 mg: 6 X 250 mg vials
Achromycin Intravenous 500 mg: 6 X 500 mg vials.

**Further information** Nil

**Product licence numbers**
Achromycin Intravenous 250 mg 0095/5034
Achromycin Intravenous 500 mg 0095/5035

## ACHROMYCIN* OINTMENT

**Presentation** *Achromycin Ointment 3%:* Each gram of yellow ointment contains tetracycline hydrochloride 30 mg, in a white soft paraffin and wool-fat base.

**Uses** Achromycin is a broad-spectrum antibiotic.

Achromycin Ointment 3% is indicated for the treatment of superficial pyogenic infections of the skin. It is indicated for local infections caused by both susceptible Gram-positive and Gram-negative organisms including Streptococci, Staphylococci and the Coli-aerogenes group.

**Dosage and administration** *Adults, including the elderly and children over 8 years of age:* Apply the ointment directly to the involved area, preferably on sterile gauze once or more daily as the condition indicates. In severe local infections, local treatment should be supplemented by oral therapy.

**Contra-indications, warnings, etc**
*Contra-indications:* Achromycin Ointment is contra-indicated in patients with a history of hypersensitivity to tetracycline hydrochloride or any other ingredient.

*Use in pregnancy and lactation:* The use of drugs of the tetracycline class during tooth development (last half of pregnancy through early childhood) may cause permanent discoloration of the teeth (yellow-grey-brown). This adverse reaction is more common during long-term oral or otherwise systemic use of the drugs and the risk of such effects from topical usage is considered negligible. However, to reduce the theoretical risk of damage to permanent dentition, topical tetracyclines should not be used during the last half of pregnancy or during lactation, unless, other drugs are unlikely to be effective or are contraindicated.

*Precautions:* The use of antibiotics may result in overgrowth of non-susceptible organisms. Constant observation of the patient is essential. If new infections appear during therapy, appropriate measures should be taken.

To reduce the theoretical risk of damage to permanent dentition, topical tetracyclines should not be used in children under 8 years of age, unless other drugs are unlikely to be effective or are contraindicated.

The concomitant use of oral tetracyclines may reduce the efficacy of oral contraceptives. An increased incidence of breakthrough bleeding may also be experienced.

*Side-effects:* Some patients may be allergic to any of the components.

If adverse reaction or idiosyncrasy occurs, discontinue medication.

**Pharmaceutical precautions** The product should be stored in a cool place (8°–15°C) in the original pack.

Dilution is not recommended.

Achromycin Ointment may cause a yellow staining of clothes. Following extended use, a similar local staining of the skin may occur which disappears on cessation of treatment.

**Legal category** POM.

**Package quantities** Tubes of 30 g.

**Further information** Nil.

**Product licence number** 0095/5031

## ANTEPSIN* TABLETS AND SUSPENSION

**Qualitative and quantitative composition** Each Antepsin (1 g) tablet contains 1 gram of the active ingredient sucralfate.

*Antepsin Suspension:* each 5 ml dose contains 1 gram sucralfate.

**Pharmaceutical form** Antepsin Tablets 1 gram are white, oblong biconvex, uncoated tablets engraved 'Antepsin' on one side and 'WY' breakbar '39' on the other.

Antepsin Suspension is a white to off-white viscous suspension with an odour of aniseed/caramel.

**Clinical particulars**

*Therapeutic indications:*
*Antepsin Tablets*: Treatment of duodenal ulcer, gastric ulcer, chronic gastritis.
*Antepsin Suspension*: Treatment of duodenal ulcer, gastric ulcer, chronic gastritis, and the prophylaxis of gastrointestinal haemorrhage from stress ulceration in seriously ill patients.

*Posology and method of administration:* For oral administration
*Duodenal ulcer, gastric ulcer, chronic gastritis:*
*Adults:* The usual dose is 2 grams twice daily to be taken on rising and at bedtime, or 1 gram 4 times a day to be taken 1 hour before meals and at bedtime. Maximum daily dose: 8 grams. For ease of administration Antepsin Tablets may be dispersed in 10–15 ml of water.

Four to six weeks' treatment is usually needed for ulcer healing, but up to twelve weeks may be necessary in resistant cases.

Antacids may be used as required for relief of pain, but should not be taken half an hour before or after Antepsin.

*Children and elderly:* see below
*Prophylaxis of gastrointestinal haemorrhage from stress ulceration:*
*Adults:* The usual dose is 1 gram six times a day. A maximum dose of 8 grams daily should not be exceeded. Antacids may be used as required for relief of pain, but should not be taken half an hour before or after Antepsin.

*Elderly:* There are no special dosage requirements for elderly patients but as with all medicines, the lowest effective dose should be used.

*Children:* Safety and effectiveness in children has not been established.

*Contra-indications:* Contraindicated in individuals who are hypersensitive to any of the ingredients of Antepsin.

*Special warnings and special precautions:* The product should only be used with caution in patients with renal dysfunction, due to the possibility of increased aluminium absorption.

In patients with severe renal impairment or on dialysis, Antepsin should be used with extreme caution and only for short-term treatment. The concomitant use of other aluminium containing medications is not recommended in view of the enhanced potential for aluminium absorption and toxicity.

*Interaction with other medicaments and other forms of interaction*: Concomitant administration of Antepsin may reduce the bioavailability of certain drugs including tetracycline, ciprofloxacin, norfloxacin, ketoconazole, digoxin, warfarin, phenytoin, and $H_2$ antagonists. The bioavailability of these agents may be restored by separating the administration of these agents from Antepsin by two hours. This interaction appears to be non systemic in origin presumably resulting from these agents being bound by Antepsin in the gastrointestinal tract. Because of the potential of Antepsin to alter the absorption of some drugs from the gastrointestinal tract, the separate administration of Antepsin from that of other agents should be considered when alterations in bioavailability are felt to be critical for concomitantly administered drugs.

The administration of Antepsin Suspension and enteral feeds by nasogastric tube should be separated by one hour in patients receiving Antepsin Suspension for the prophylaxis of stress ulceration. In rare cases bezoar formation has been reported when Antepsin and enteral feeds have been given too closely together.

*Pregnancy and lactation:* Teratogenicity studies in mice, rats, and rabbits at doses up to 50 times the human dose have revealed no evidence of harm to the foetus. Safety in pregnant women has not been established and Antepsin should be used during pregnancy only if clearly needed.

It is not known whether this drug is excreted in human milk. Caution should be exercised when Antepsin is administered to nursing women.

*Effects on ability to drive and use machines:* None stated (presumed to be safe or unlikely to produce any effect).

*Undesirable effects:* Adverse reactions to Antepsin in clinical trials were minor and only rarely led to discontinuation of the drug. Adverse events seen during use of Antepsin have included constipation, diarrhoea, nausea, vomiting, gastric discomfort, indigestion, flatulence, dry mouth, rash, back pain, dizziness, headache, vertigo, drowsiness and hypersensitivity reactions including pruritus, oedema and urticaria.

*Overdose:* There is no experience in humans with overdosage. Acute oral toxicity studies in animals, however, using doses up to 12 g/kg body weight, could not find a lethal dose. Risks associated with overdosage, should, therefore, be minimal.

**Pharmacological properties**

*Pharmacodynamic properties:* The action of Antepsin is non-systemic as the drug is only minimally absorbed from the gastro-intestinal tract. The small amounts that are absorbed are excreted primarily in the urine. Antepsin exerts a generalized cytoprotective effect by preventing gastro-intestinal mucosal injury.

Studies in humans and animal models show that Antepsin forms an ulcer adherent complex with the proteinaceous exudate of the ulcer site. This property enables Antepsin to form a protective barrier over the ulcer lesion giving sustained protection against the penetration and action of gastric acid, pepsin and bile. Studies both in humans and animals demonstrate that Antepsin protects the gastric mucosa against various irritants such as alcohol, acetylsalicylic acid and sodium taurocholate.

Antepsin also directly inhibits pepsin activity and absorbs bile salts. It has only weak antacid activity. It does not alter gastric emptying time, nor normal digestive function. Antepsin has no demonstrated pharmacological effect on the cardiovascular or central nervous systems.

*Pharmacokinetic properties:* Sucralfate is only minimally absorbed from the gastro-intestinal tract. The small amounts that are absorbed are excreted primarily in the urine. Absorption of aluminium from sucralfate may be increased in patients on dialysis or with renal dysfunction (see also 'other special warnings and precautions')

*Preclinical safety data:* There was no evidence of carcinogenesis in mice and rats receiving oral sucralfate in dosages of up to 1 g/kg daily (12 times the usual human dosage) for 2 years. In animal studies there was no evidence of impaired fertility. The effect of sucralfate on human fertility is not known.

**Pharmaceutical particulars**

*List of excipients: Antepsin 1 g:* Polyethylene glycol 8000, microcrystalline cellulose, calcium carboxymethyl cellulose, magnesium stearate.

*Antepsin Suspension:* Sodium saccharin, sodium dihydrogen phosphate, glycerol, E217, E219, xanthan gum, aniseed flavour and caramel flavour.

*Incompatibilities:* None known

*Shelf life:*
Antepsin 1 g 36 months.
Antepsin Suspension 36 months

*Special precautions for storage:* Antepsin Tablets and Suspension: Store below 25°C.

*Nature and contents of container: Antepsin 1 g:* Polypropylene containers (pack size 112). *Antepsin suspension:* HDPE bottle (pack size 560 ml)

*Instructions for use/handling:* None stated.

**Marketing authorisation numbers**
Antepsin Suspension 0011/0160
Antepsin Tablets (1 g) 0011/0176

**Date of approval/revision of SPC** 31 May 1995.

**Legal category** POM

## ASENDIS*

**Presentation** *25 mg Tablets:* Cream, flat, heptagonal-shaped tablets, engraved on one side with 'LL25', each containing 25 mg of amoxapine.

*50 mg Tablets:* Orange, flat, heptagonal-shaped tablets, scored on one side and engraved 'LL50' on the other, each containing 50 mg of amoxapine.

*100 mg Tablets:* Mottled blue, flat, heptagonal-shaped tablets, scored on one side with 'LL100' on the other side, each containing 100 mg of amoxapine.

**Uses** Asendis is an anti-depressant indicated for the symptomatic treatment of depressive illness.

**Dosage and administration**

*Adults:* Initially 100–150 mg daily increasing slowly according to clinical response up to 300 mg daily, in divided doses or one dose which may be given at night.

*Usual maintenance dose:* 150–250 mg daily.

*Elderly:* An initial dose of 25 mg twice a day is recommended. If necessary, the dosage may be increased under close supervision after 5 to 7 days to a maximum of 50 mg three times daily. Less than the normal dose may be sufficient to produce satisfactory clinical response.

*Children (under 16 years):* Not recommended.

Studies have demonstrated that the initial clinical effect of Asendis can occur within four to seven days. Treatment should be maintained for a minimum period of one month, and current psychiatric practice suggests that several months treatment may be necessary after initial clinical improvement.

**Contra-indications, warnings, etc**

*Contra-Indications:* Recent myocardial infarction or coronary artery insufficiency. Heartblock or other cardiac arrhythmias. Mania. Severe liver disease. Use in patients hypersensitive to dibenzoxazepines, or in patients who are currently receiving, or have received, monoamine oxidase inhibitors in the preceding two weeks.

*Precautions and warnings:* In common with other drugs of this class, caution should be exercised when using in patients with any of the following conditions: urinary retention, narrow angle glaucoma, hyperthyroidism, cardiovascular disorders, blood dyscrasias and hepatic or renal impairment. Asendis should only be used with particular caution in patients with a history of epilepsy or recent convulsions.

Psychotic manifestations may be exacerbated during treatment with tri/tetracyclic anti-depressants.

A minority of patients may not improve during the first 2–4 weeks of treatment. Patients should be closely monitored during this period, especially those posing a high suicidal risk.

As with many other anti-depressants, Asendis may initially impair alertness. Patients should be warned of the possible hazard when driving or operating machinery.

Concurrent administration with electroconvulsive therapy may increase the hazards associated with such therapy.

Withdrawal symptoms may occur on abrupt cessation of therapy and include insomnia, irritability, and excessive perspiration. The dosage of Asendis should be reduced gradually upon the discontinuation of therapy.

In common with other anti-depressants, the elderly are more prone to experiencing adverse reactions, especially agitation and confusion, hence the importance of initiating treatment at a lower dose (see *Dosage*).

*Interactions:* The drug interactions experienced with Asendis are those that could be expected from a drug of this class and include the following:

Asendis may decrease the anti-hypertensive effect of guanethidine, debrisoquine, bethanidine and possibly clonidine. It would be advisable to review all such anti-hypertensive therapy during treatment.

Asendis should not be given with sympathomimetic agents such as adrenaline, ephedrine, isoprenaline, noradrenaline, phenylephrine and phenylpropanolamine.

Asendis may potentiate the effects of drugs having an anticholinergic action, ethchlorvynol, thyroid hormone therapy, and the central nervous depressant action of alcohol.

Barbiturates may increase the metabolism of tri/tetracyclic anti-depressants.

Anaesthetics given during tri/tetracyclic anti-depressant therapy may increase the risk of arrhythmias and hypotension. If surgery is necessary, the anaesthetist should be informed that a patient is being so treated.

Caution should be exercised if Asendis is given concomitantly with Lithium.

Serum levels of several tricyclic anti-depressants have been reported to be significantly increased when cimetidine is administered concurrently; although such an interaction has not been reported to date with Asendis.

*Adverse effects:* In common with certain other drugs of this class, the following adverse effects have been reported with Asendis. These have been categorised according to incidence.

*Incidence greater than 1%:* The most frequent types of adverse reactions occurring in clinical trials were sedative and anticholinergic, these included; drowsiness (14%), dry mouth (14%), constipation (12%), and blurred vision (7%).

*Less frequently reported reactions:*

*CNS and neuromuscular:* anxiety, insomnia, restlessness, nervousness, palpitations, tremors, confusion, excitement, nightmares, ataxia, alterations in EEG patterns.

*Allergic:* oedema, skin rash.

*Endocrine:* elevation of prolactin levels.

*Gastrointestinal:* nausea.

*Other:* dizziness, headache, fatigue, weakness, excessive appetite, increased perspiration.

*Incidence less than 1%:*

*Anticholinergic:* disturbances of accommodation, mydriasis, urinary retention, nasal stuffiness.

*Cardiovascular:* hypotension, hypertension, syncope, tachycardia.

*Allergic:* drug fever, urticaria, photosensitisation, pruritis, rarely vasculitis, hepatitis.

*CNS and neuromuscular:* tingling, paraesthesia of the extremities, tinnitus, disorientation, seizures, hypomania, numbness, inco-ordination, disturbed concentration, hyperthermia, extrapyramidal symptoms including rarely tardive dyskinesia. Neuroleptic malignant syndrome (see below).

*Haematological:* leukopenia, agranulocytosis.

*Gastrointestinal:* epigastric distress, vomiting, flatulence, abdominal pain, peculiar taste, diarrhoea.

*Endocrine:* increased or decreased libido, impotence, menstrual irregularity, breast enlargement and galactorrhoea in the female, syndrome of inapprop ate antidiuretic hormone secretion.

*Other:* lacrimation, weight loss or gain, altered li function, painful ejaculation.

Following the use of Asendis worldwide, isolat cases of Neuroleptic Malignant Syndrome have be reported. This syndrome is potentially fatal a presents with symptoms of hyperpyrexia, mus rigidity, altered mental status, and evidence of au nomic instability. If a patient is diagnosed as sufferi from Neuroleptic Malignant Syndrome, the manag ment should include: (1) immediate discontinuat of antipsychotic drugs and other drugs not essen to concurrent therapy (2) symptomatic treatment a monitoring of vital signs and (3) treatment of a concomitant serious medical problems.

*Use in pregnancy and lactation:* There are not a quately well controlled studies in pregnant wom Asendis should therefore be used during pregnan only if the potential benefit justifies the potential r to the foetus. Asendis like many other systemic dru is excreted in human milk. The effects of the drug infants are unknown, and hence the administration nursing mothers cannot be recommended.

*Overdosage:* Toxic manifestations of Asendis ov dose differ significantly from those of other tricy antidepressants. The risk of cardiotoxicity is low a tends to be limited to sinus tachycardia. Howev convulsions may occur frequently (40–50%) in th taking substantial overdoses and status epilepticus not uncommon. Respiratory and/or metabolic acido may develop, usually in association with repeat seizures. Acute renal failure or transient impairm in renal function may develop 2–5 days after subst tial overdose of Asendis. There is a rare potential inducing permanent neurological damage.

There is no specific antidote for Asendis; treatm should be symptomatic and supportive with spec attention to prevention or control of seizures. If patient is conscious, emesis should be induced soon as possible, followed by gastric lavage. Adm istration of activated charcoal after gastric lavage m reduce absorption and facilitate drug elimination. adequate airway should be established in unc scious patients, who may also need full support vital functions and cardiac monitoring. Convulsio when they occur, typically begin within 12 hours ingestion and may respond to standard anticonv sant therapy such as intravenous diazepam and phenytoin. More rigorous treatment is requi should status epilepticus develop. Drugs which known to potentiate respiratory depression should avoided. Treatment for renal impairment, shoul occur, is the same as for non-drug-induced re dysfunction.

**Pharmaceutical precautions** Store at controlled ro temperature (15–30°C).

**Legal category** POM

**Package quantities** Bottles containing 100 tablets.

**Further information** Nil.

**Product licence numbers**
Asendis 25 mg tablets 0095/0056
Asendis 50 mg tablets 0095/0057
Asendis 100 mg tablets 0095/0058

## ATIVAN* INJECTION

**Presentation** Ativan injection is a clear, colourl solution containing lorazepam BP at a concentrat of 4 mg/ml supplied in 1 ml quantities in clear gl ampoules.

**Uses** Ativan injection is indicated for: Pre-operat medication or premedication for uncomfortable prolonged investigations e.g. bronchoscopy, art ography, endoscopy. The treatment of acute anx states, acute excitement or acute mania. The con of status epilepticus.

**Dosage and administration** *Route of administrati* Ativan injection can be given intravenously or int muscularly. However, the intravenous route is to preferred. Care should be taken to avoid injection i small veins and intra-arterial injection.

Absorption from the injection site is considera slower if the intramuscular route is used and as ra an effect may be obtained by oral administration Ativan tablets.

Ativan should not be used for long term chro treatment.

*Preparation of the injection* Ativan injection is slig viscid when cool. To facilitate injection it may diluted 1:1 with normal Saline or Water for inject BP immediately before administration. If given int muscularly it should always be diluted.

Ativan injection is presented as a 1 ml solution i 2 ml ampoule to facilitate dilution.

Ativan injection should not be mixed with ot drugs in the same syringe.

*sage:*

*.Premedication: Adults:* 0.05 mg/kg (3.5 mg for an rage 70 kg man) By the intravenous route the ction should be given 30–45 minutes before sur-y when sedation will be evident after 5–10 minutes I maximal loss of recall will occur after 30–minutes. By the intramuscular route the injection uld be given 1–1½ hours before surgery when ation will be evident after 30–45 minutes and ximal loss of recall will occur after 60–90 minutes. *Children:* Ativan injection is not recommended in dren under 12.

*.Acute Anxiety: Adults:* 0.025–0.03 mg/kg (1.75– mg for an average 70 kg man). Repeat 6 hourly. *Children:* Ativan injection is not recommended in dren under 12.

*.Status epilepticus: Adults:* 4 mg intravenously dren: 2 mg intravenously.

*Elderly:* The elderly may respond to lower doses d half the normal adult dose may be sufficient.

**ntra-indications, warnings, etc.**

*ntra-indications:*

. Ativan injection should not be given to patients h a previous history of sensitivity to benzodiaze-es or any of the vehicle constituents (polyethylene col, propylene glycol, benzyl alcohol), or to patients h acute pulmonary insufficiency.

. Ativan injection is not recommended for -patient use unless the patient is accompanied.

*e in pregnancy:* Safety for use in pregnancy has not en established. Ativan injection should not be ministered during pregnancy or lactation unless in judgement of the physician such administration is ically justifiable. Ativan injection is not recom-nded for use in the first three months of pregnancy. e during the late phase of pregnancy or at delivery y require ventilation of the infant at birth.

*cautions and warnings:*

. Patients should remain under observation for at st eight hours and preferably overnight.

. Patients should not drive or operate machinery hin 24–48 hours of administration of Ativan injec-n and should be advised not to take alcohol.

. The addition of scopolamine to Ativan injection not recommended, since their combination has en observed to cause an increased incidence of dation, hallucination and irrational behaviour.

. The effects of centrally acting cerebral depressant ugs may be potentiated.

. This product should be used with caution in tients with impairment of renal or hepatic function.

. The injection should be given slowly except in control of status epilepticus where rapid injection required.

. Airway obstruction may occur in heavily sedated ients and therefore equipment necessary to main-n a patent airway and to support respiration/ ntilation should be available.

. Extreme care must be taken in administering van injection to elderly or very ill patients and to se with limited pulmonary reserve, because of the ssibility that apnoea and/or cardiac arrest may cur. Care should also be exercised when administ-ing Ativan injection to a patient with status epilep-us, especially when the patient has received other ntral nervous system depressants.

. Elderly patients may require a lower dosage.

10. There is no evidence to support the use of Ativan ection in coma or shock.

11. There is insufficient data regarding obstetrical fety of parenteral Ativan, including use in cesarean ction. Respiratory depression, poor sucking and pothermia in the neonate after delivery have occa-nally been reported, especially in infants who are risk. Such use, therefore, is not recommended.

12. As with all benzodiazepines doctors should be are of the possibility of dependence and withdrawal mptoms in certain patients. In normal acute usage pendence is unlikely to occur but the risk increases h higher doses and longer-term use and is further reased in patients with a history of alcoholism, ug abuse or in patients with marked personality sorders.

Symptoms such as anxiety, depression, headache, somnia, tension and sweating have been reported lowing abrupt discontinuation of benzodiazepines. her symptoms such as persistent tinnitus, involun-y movements, paraesthesia, perceptual changes, nfusion, convulsions, abdominal and muscle amps and vomiting may be characteristic of benzo-zepine withdrawal syndrome.

13. The use of benzodiazepines may release suicidal ndencies in depressed patients. Lorazepam should t be used alone to treat depression or anxiety sociated with depression. Other rarely reported haviitiour effects of the benzodiazepines include radoxical aggressive outbursts, excitement and nfusion.

*de effects:* Lorazepam is well tolerated and imbal-ce or ataxia are signs of excessive dosage. Drowsi-

ness may occur. Occasional confusion, hangover, headache on waking, dizziness, blurred vision, nau-sea, vomiting, restlessness, depression, crying, sob-bing, hallucinations and diplopia have been reported. In addition blood dyscrasias and increased liver enzymes have occasionally been reported. On rare occasions visual disturbances, hypotension, hyper-tension, gastro-intestinal disturbances and mild tran-sient skin rashes have also been reported.

*Overdosage:* As with other benzodiazepines, overdos-age should not present a threat to life unless combined with other CNS depressants (including alcohol). Gen-eral supportive measures should be used and the treatment of overdosage is symptomatic. The patient is likely to sleep and a clear airway should be maintained.

**Pharmaceutical precautions** Store in a refrigerator between 0°C and 4°C. Protect from light.

**Legal category** CD (Sch 4), POM

**Package quantities** 10 x 1 ml solution (in 2 ml am-poules) per pack.

**Further information** Ativan is metabolised by a simple one-step process to a pharmacologically inac-tive glucuronide. There is minimal risk of accumula-tion after repeated doses, giving a wide margin of safety. Ativan injection can be administered concur-rently with a wide range of other drugs and has minimal effect on blood pressure. Tolerance at the injection site is generally good although, rarely, pain and redness have been reported.

**Product licence number** 0011/0051

# AUDICORT* EAR DROPS

**Qualitative and quantitative composition**

| Active constituent | per ml | Specification reference |
|---|---|---|
| Triamcinolone acetonide | 1.0 mg | BP |
| Neomycin base in propylene glycol equivalent to neomycin base | 3.5 mg | HSE |

**Pharmaceutical form** Audicort is a clear, pale yellow to yellow solution for topical application to the ear.

**Clinical particulars**

*Therapeutic indications:* Audicort is anti-inflammatory and antibacterial. The preparation is indicated in the treatment of acute and chronic otitis externa due to or complicated by bacterial infection.

*Posology and method of administration:* Adults and the elderly. After careful cleansing of the ear, admin-ister 2–5 drops of Audicort topically to the ear, usually three or four times daily. If desired, the drops may be used to saturate a gauze or cotton wick placed in the ear. This wick should be kept saturated by instilling 2–5 drops, three to four times a day, and should be replaced every 24–48 hours. Treatment should be reviewed after seven days with continuation of ther-apy up to 14 days if resolution has not occurred.

*Contra-indications:* Audicort is contraindicated in in-fants and children and in patients with perforated tympanic membrane. Hypersensitivity to triamcino-lone acetonide, neomycin or propylene glycol. The preparation should not be used in the eyes.

*Special warnings and special precautions for use:* The tympanic membrane should be checked for integrity before Audicort drops are prescribed.

Use of an antibiotic may occasionally result in an overgrowth of non-susceptible micro-organisms, while the presence of an anti-inflammatory steroid may encourage their spread. If superinfection does occur, the drug should be stopped and appropriate therapy instituted.

Unlikely to produce any serious toxic effects if ingested.

*Interaction with other medicaments and other forms of interaction:* None.

*Pregnancy and lactation:* Topical administration of corticosteroids to pregnant animals can cause abnor-malities of foetal development including cleft palate and intra-uterine growth retardation. There may there-fore be a very small risk of such effects in the human foetus. Audicort should only be used in pregnancy when there is no safer alternative.

Although corticosteroids appear in breast milk, the absorption of triamcinolone acetonide from Audicort is expected to be minimal so the risk to the baby is considered to be small.

*Effects on ability to drive and operate machines:* None

*Undesirable effects:* Side-effects from triamcinolone and neomycin in otic drops are rare, but neomycin has occasionally been responsible for localised skin sensitisation. Discomfort (stinging) may be experi-enced by some patients on application of the drops. If

local reactions such as irritation or erythema occur, medication should be discontinued.

If absorbed systemically, neomycin is known to be ototoxic. However, during the course of treatment with Audicort, the maximum total exposure to neo-mycin is 35 mg and this is not thought to pose a significant clinical risk.

*Overdose:* Overdose of triamcinolone acetonide and neomycin undecylenate otic drops has not been reported. Excess drops can be removed from the ear by gentle washing.

**Pharmacological properties**

*Pharmacodynamic properties:*
1. Neomycin (antibiotic) as neomycin undecylenate.
2. Triamcinolone acetonide (corticosteroid with anti-inflammatory action)

*Pharmacokinetic properties:* Audicort Ear Drops are recommended for topical administration.

Absorption of triamcinolone acetonide by this route of administration is usually minimal. However, when applied topically, particularly to large areas, when the skin is broken, or under occlusive dressings, cortico-steroids may be absorbed in sufficient quantities to cause systemic effects.

Absorption of neomycin after topical application is also likely to be minimal. However, absorption has been reported to occur from inflamed skin.

**Pharmaceutical particulars**

*List of excipients:* Undecylenic acid PhEur; Trome-thamine USP; Disodium edetate BP; Sodium metabi-sulphite BP; Benzoic acid BP; Water (purified) BP; Propylene glycol BP.

*Incompatibilities:* None

*Shelf life:* 18 months.

*Special precautions for storage:* Audicort Ear Drops should be stored in a refrigerator (2–8°C) in the original container. Do not freeze. Excessive heating of the solution should be avoided. Audicort should not be diluted.

*Nature and contents of container:* Plastic dropper bottles containing 10 ml of solution.

*Instructions for use and handling:* None

**Marketing authorisation number** 0095/5069R

**Date of approval/revision of SPC** November 1996

**Legal category** POM

# AUREOCORT* OINTMENT

**Qualitative and quantitative composition** Aureocort Ointment is a topical preparation containing the active ingredients chlortetracycline hydrochloride 3.09% w/w and triamcinolone acetonide 0.1% w/w.

**Pharmaceutical form** Ointment for topical administra-tion.

**Clinical particulars**

*Therapeutic indications:* Aureocort combines the anti-inflammatory action of triamcinolone acetonide with the anti-infective properties of chlortetracycline.

It is indicated in the treatment of secondarily infected atopic dermatitis, contact dermatitis, eczema, neurodermatitis, otitis externa, seborrhoeic dermati-tis, varicose eczema and vesiculo–pustular dermatitis. It may also be used in the treatment of infected insect bites.

*Posology and method of administration:*

*Adults, children over 8 years and the elderly:* Aureo-cort Ointment should be applied sparingly to the affected area, either directly or on sterile gauze, two or three times daily.

Please refer to the 'Special warnings and precau-tions for use' section.

*Contra-indications:* The use of Aureocort is contra-indicated in tuberculous, fungal or viral lesions of the skin (herpes simplex, vaccinia and varicella), and primary bacterial infections, e.g. impetigo, pyoderma and furunculosis.

Aureocort Topical preparations are also contra-indicated in patients with a history of hypersensitivity to tetracyclines, corticosteroids, or any other ingredi-ent in the preparation.

*Special warnings and precautions for use:* To reduce the theoretical risk of damage to permanent dentition by tetracyclines, Aureocort Topical preparations should not be used in children under 8 years of age unless other drugs are unlikely to be effective or are contra-indicated.

Use of antibiotics topically may result in overgrowth of non-susceptible organisms; if new infections ap-pear during therapy, appropriate measures should be taken.

The use of corticosteroids on infected areas should be continuously and carefully observed, bearing in mind the potential spreading of infections (caused by organisms not sensitive to chlortetracycline) by anti-inflammatory corticosteroids. It may be advisable to discontinue corticosteroid therapy and/or initiate alternative antibacterial measures in these circumstances. Generalised dermatological conditions may require systemic corticosteroid therapy.

Steroid-antibiotic combinations should not be continued for more than 7 days in the absence of any clinical improvement, since in this situation, occult extension of infection may occur due to the masking effect of the steroid. Extended or recurrent application may increase the risk of contact sensitisation, and should be avoided. Occlusion should not be used when treating conditions of the face.

*Interactions with other medicaments and other forms of interactions:* Not applicable.

*Pregnancy and lactation:* Topical administration of corticosteroids to pregnant rabbits has been reported to cause abnormalities of foetal development, including cleft palate and intrauterine growth retardation at relatively low doses. The relevance of this finding to human beings has not been established. However, topical corticosteroids should not be used extensively (large amounts or for long periods) in early pregnancy. The use of corticosteroid/antibiotic preparations, containing drugs of the tetracyclines class, during tooth development (last half of pregnancy through early childhood) may cause permanent discolouration of the teeth (yellow-grey-brown). This adverse reaction, related only to tetracyclines, is more common during long-term oral or otherwise systemic use of tetracyclines and the risk of such effects from topical usage is considered negligible. However, to reduce the theoretical risk of damage to permanent dentition by tetracyclines, and the risk of any abnormalities of foetal development by corticosteroids, topical corticosteroid / tetracycline combinations should not be used during pregnancy or lactation unless other drugs are unlikely to be effective, or are contra-indicated.

*Effects on ability to drive and use machinery:* Not applicable.

*Undesirable effects:* A few patients may be allergic to any of the components. If adverse reaction or idiosyncrasy occurs, medication should be discontinued.

Systemic absorption of corticosteroids may occur if they are used over extensive body areas, with or without occlusive non-permeable dressings. When occlusive non-permeable dressings are used, miliaria, folliculitis and pyoderma may sometimes develop beneath the occlusive material.

Localised atrophy and striae have been reported with the use of corticosteroids by the occlusive technique.

*Overdosage:* Not applicable.

**Pharmacological properties**

*Pharmacodynamic properties:* Aureocort ointment contains two active ingredients:

(i) Chlortetracycline is a broad spectrum antibiotic. It is active against a large number of gram-positive and gram-negative bacteria, including some which are resistant to penicillin.
(ii) Triamcinolone acetonide is a corticosteroid with anti-inflammatory, anti-pruritis and anti-allergic effects.

*Pharmacokinetic properties:* Topically applied tetracycline preparations are not absorbed into the general circulation to any significant degree.

Absorption of triamcinolone acetonide from topically applied preparations is usually minimal. However, corticosteroids may be absorbed in sufficient amount to cause systemic effects if applied to large areas, when the skin is broken, or under occlusive dressings.

*Pre-clinical safety data:* Nothing of any relevance to the prescriber.

**Pharmaceutical particulars**

*List of excipients:* White Petroleum Jelly, Anhydrous Lanolin.

*Incompatibilities:* None known.

*Shelf-life:* 36 months.

*Special precautions for storage:* Store at a controlled room temperature (15–30°C) in the original pack.

*Nature and contents of container:* Collapsible aluminium tubes with crocus yellow, low density polythene caps.

**Marketing authorisation number** 0095/5076R

**Date of approval/revision of SPC** December 1995

**Legal category** POM

## AUREOMYCIN* OINTMENT AUREOMYCIN* OPHTHALMIC OINTMENT

**Presentation**

*Aureomycin Ointment 3%:* Each gram of yellow ointment contains chlortetracycline hydrochloride 30 mg in a greasy base of anhydrous lanolin and white petroleum jelly.

*Aureomycin Ophthalmic Ointment 1%:* Each gram of yellow ointment contains 10 mg chlortetracycline hydrochloride in a greasy base of anhydrous lanolin, liquid paraffin and white petroleum jelly.

**Uses** Aureomycin is a broad-spectrum antibiotic.

*Aureomycin Ointment 3%:* Aureomycin topical preparations are indicated for the treatment of superficial pyogenic infections of the skin caused by susceptible Gram-positive cocci (Streptococci, Staphylococci and Pneumococci) and Gram-negative bacteria (Coli-aerogenes group).

*Aureomycin Ophthalmic Ointment 1%:* Aureomycin Ophthalmic Ointment 1% is indicated for the treatment of superficial eye infections caused by organisms sensitive to chlortetracycline hydrochloride including trachoma.

**Dosage and administration** *Adults, children over 8 years, and the elderly:*

*Aureomycin Ointment 3%:* In the treatment of local skin infections apply the preparation directly to the involved area, preferably on sterile gauze once or more daily as the condition warrants. In severe local infection, topical application should be supplemented by oral administration.

*Aureomycin Ophthalmic Ointment 1%:* Aureomycin Ophthalmic Ointment should be applied to the infected eye up to three times daily or more frequently if required.

*Recommended dosage in the treatment of Trachoma:* Trachoma may require oral systemic therapy in addition to topical ophthalmic therapy.

Topical chemotherapy for trachoma must be intensive and prolonged, six weeks being the minimum recommended duration for continuous intensive treatment.

If less frequent or intermittent applications are used, the duration of treatment must be further prolonged. The recommended intermittent applications of chlortetracycline for 5 consecutive days (or once daily for 10 days), each month for six months each year, to be repeated as necessary.

**Contra-indications, warnings, etc**
*Contra-indications:* Aureomycin Topical Preparations are contra-indicated in patients with a history of hypersensitivity to chlortetracycline hydrochloride or any other ingredient in the preparation.

*Use in pregnancy and lactation:* The use of drugs of the tetracycline class during tooth development (last half of pregnancy through early childhood) may cause permanent discoloration of the teeth (yellow-grey-brown). This adverse reaction is more common during long-term oral or otherwise systemic use of the drugs and the risk of such effects from topical usage is considered negligible.

However, to reduce the theoretical risk of damage to permanent dentition, topical tetracyclines should not be used during the last half of pregnancy or during lactation unless other drugs are unlikely to be effective or are contra-indicated.

*Precautions:* The use of antibiotics may result in overgrowth of non-susceptible organisms. If new infections appear during therapy, appropriate measures should be taken.

To reduce the theoretical risk of damage to permanent dentition, topical tetracyclines should not be used in children under 8 years of age unless other drugs are unlikely to be effective or are contra-indicated.

*Interactions:* The concomitant use of oral tetracyclines may reduce the efficacy of oral contraceptives; an increased incidence of breakthrough bleeding may also be experienced.

*Side-effects:* Some patients may be allergic to any of the components. If adverse reaction or idiosyncrasy occurs, discontinue medication.

**Pharmaceutical precautions** *Aureomycin Ointment 3%:* The product should be stored in a cool place (8°–15°C). The ointment may be diluted with a base of 10% lanolin and white petroleum jelly.
*Aureomycin Ophthalmic Ointment 1%:* The product should be stored in a cool place (8°–15°C). Dilution of Aureomycin Ophthalmic Ointment is not recommended.

Aureomycin Ointment may cause a yellow staining of clothes. Following extended use a similar local staining of the skin may occur which disappears cessation of treatment.

**Legal category** POM

**Package quantities**
Aureomycin Ointment 3%: Tubes of 30 g
Aureomycin Ophthalmic Ointment 1%: Tubes of 3

**Further information** Nil

**Product licence numbers**
Aureomycin Ointment 3% 0095/5019
Aureomycin Ophthalmic Ointment 1% 0095/5020

## BEGRIVAC*

**Presentation** Begrivac is a colourless to sligh opalescent suspension for injection. Each 0.5 contains 15 micrograms of each of three purif influenza antigens prepared from the strains of vi recommend by the WHO.

**Uses** Active immunisation against influenza (genu virus influenza) from 9 years of age onwards advisable particularly in the following groups:-

Adults and children at risk of infection, with dise of the heart and/or circulatory system, or chro diseases of the respiratory tract or kidney.

Diabetics and persons with other chronic metab disease.

Persons with congenital, acquired or iatroge immunodeficiency.

Residents of nursing homes, old peoples hom and other long stay facilities where rapid spreac likely to follow introduction of infection.

**Dosage and administration** Intramuscular or de subcutaneous injection.

*Adults and children over 12 years:* single dose 0.5

*Children 9 to 12 years:* single dose 0.5 ml followed a second dose after 4–6 weeks if not vaccinated influenza in previous 4 years.

Reimmunisation should be considered annually.

**Contra-indications, warnings, etc** The vaccinat should be postponed in the case of persons who acutely ill, convalescing or thought to be in incubation phase of an illness.

Begrivac is contraindicated in patients known develop severe allergic reactions to constituents the vaccine.

Vaccination with Begrivac should be avoided persons who are classed as 'allergic to chicken prote on the basis of history-taking, or who are classed suffering from chicken protein allergy on the basis a positive skin test. If the vaccination is absolut indicated consideration can be given to carrying an allergy test and, if the result is negative, vaccination against influenza.

*Warnings and precautions:* Unintentional intravas lar administration may result in reactions extendi as far as shock. Immediate measures depending degree of severity: Adrenaline, high doses of corti steroids, volume replacement, oxygen.

The vaccine may contain traces of Polysorb (Tween) 80, and Polymyxin B from the manufacturi process.

*Pregnancy and lactation:* Pregnancy and breast fe ing are not contra-indications to vaccination w Begrivac.

*Side effects:* Local reactions may occur in the form transient reddening (especially after subcutanec injection), swelling and pain, occasionally accom nied by swelling of regional Lymph nodes.

Generalised reactions such as fatigue, headac cardiovascular reactions, outbreaks of sweati chills, elevations in temperature, myalgia, arthral or gastrointestinal complaints occur in occasio cases. These symptoms require treatment in exc tional cases only.

Allergic reactions have been observed; in very r cases these have developed as far as shock.

In rare cases neuralgia and paresthesia may occ Isolated cases of inflammatory diseases of the cent or peripheral nervous system have been report These have included ascending paralysis through respiratory paralysis (e.g. Guillain-Barré-Syndrom

*Drug interactions:* Vaccinations given during imm nosuppressive therapy as well as in cases of cong ital or acquired immunodeficiency may be of limi or uncertain success.

No intervals are necessary with regard to ot vaccinations.

*Overdose:* Not applicable.

**Pharmaceutical precautions** Begrivac should stored at 2–8°C.

*List of excipients:* sodium timerfonate, formaldehy ether, sodium chloride, potassium chloride, mag sium chloride, sodium hydrogen phosphate, pot sium hydrogenphosphate, water for injections.

**al category** POM

**kage quantities** Packs of 1 or 10 prefilled syringes

**ther information** The protective effect commences ut 10 days after vaccination. Generally, protection sists for about one year. The vaccine induced nunity should be renewed every year, especially ne at risk groups.

rotective levels of antibody are formed against the uenza virus types included in the vaccine in up to 5 of individuals vaccinated.

**duct licence number** 0086/0179

## LCIUM LEUCOVORIN

**sentation** *Powder for Injection 15 mg, 30 mg:* Vials taining a lyophilised powder of 15 mg or 30 mg nic acid as the calcium salt.

*ution for Injection 350 mg in 35 ml (Lederfolin ution):* Vial containing a solution of 350 mg folinic I as the calcium salt.

*lets 15 mg:* Each yellowish-white scored tablet tains 15 mg folinic acid respectively as the calcium .

**es** Calcium leucovorin is the calcium salt of a formyl ivative of tetra-hydrofolic acid, the metabolite of c acid, and an essential coenzyme for nucleic acid thesis.

*Calcium leucovorin rescue:* Calcium leucovorin is d to diminish the toxicity and counteract the action folic acid antagonists such as methotrexate in otoxic therapy. This procedure is commonly known Calcium Leucovorin Rescue.

*Advanced colorectal cancer–Enhancement of 5-orouracil (5-FU) Cytotoxicity:* Calcium leucovorin reases the thymine depleting effects of 5-FU ulting in enhanced cytotoxic activity. Clinical stud- in advanced colorectal cancer show greater effi-y for combination regimens of 5-FU with covorin compared to 5-FU given alone.

*Treatment of folate deficiency:* Calcium leucovorin also been demonstrated to be effective in produc- amelioration of the blood picture in a number of galoblastic anaemias due to folate deficiency.

**sage and administration**

*Calcium leucovorin rescue: Adults, children and the erly:* Calcium Leucovorin Rescue therapy should nmence 24 hours after the beginning of methotrex- infusion. Dosage regimes vary depending upon dose of methotrexate administered. In general, calcium leucovorin should be administered at a se of 15 mg (approximately 10 mg/m²) every 6 irs for 10 doses either parenterally by intramuscu- injection, bolus intravenous injection or intra- ous infusion, (refer to (ii) for information ncerning use of calcium leucovorin with infusion ds), or orally using calcium leucovorin tablets. Do administer calcium leucovorin intrathecally.

Where overdosage of methotrexate is suspected, dose of calcium leucovorin should be equal to or her than the offending dose of methotrexate and uld be administered in the first hour. In the sence of gastrointestinal toxicity, nausea or vom-g, calcium leucovorin should be administered enterally. Do not administer calcium leucovorin rathecally. Further, oral administration of doses ater than 50 mg is not recommended since the sorption of calcium leucovorin is saturable. In the e of intravenous administration, no more than ) mg of calcium leucovorin should be injected per nute due to the calcium content of the solution.

n addition to calcium leucovorin administration, asures to ensure the prompt excretion of metho-xate are important as part of Calcium Leucovorin scue therapy. These measures include:

. Alkalinisation of urine so that the urinary pH is ater than 7.0 before methotrexate infusion (to rease solubility of methotrexate and its metabo-s).

). Maintenance of urine output of 1800–2000 cc/m²/ hr by increased oral or intravenous fluids on days 3 and 4 following methotrexate therapy.

. Plasma methotrexate concentration, BUN and atinine should be measured on days 2, 3 and 4.

These measures must be continued until the plasma thotrexate level is less than $10^{-7}$ molar (0.1μM).

Delayed methotrexate excretion may be seen in me patients. This may be caused by a third space cumulation (as seen in ascites or pleural effusion example), renal insufficiency or inadequate hydra-n. Under such circumstances, higher doses of cium leucovorin or prolonged administration may indicated. Dosage and administration guidelines these patients are given in Table 1. Patients who perience delayed early methotrexate elimination likely to develop reversible renal failure.

ch vial of Calcium Leucovorin Powder for Injection 15 mg or 30 mg should be reconstituted with 3 ml of water for injection to produce a solution for intramuscular or intravenous administration.

*Table 1: Dosage and Administration Guidelines for Calcium Leucovorin Rescue:*

| *Clinical Situation* | *Laboratory Findings* | *Leucovorin Dosage and Duration* |
|---|---|---|
| Normal Methotrexate Elimination | Serum methotrexate level approximately 10μM at 24 hours after administration, 1μM at 48 hours and less than 0.2μM at 72 hours. | 15 mg PO, IM or IV every 6 hours for 60 hours (10 doses starting at 24 hours after start of methotrexate infusion). |
| Delayed Late Methotrexate Elimination | Serum methotrexate level remaining above 0.2μM at 72 hours, and more than 0.05μM at 96 hours after administration. | Continue 15 mg PO, IM or IV every 6 hours, until methotrexate level is less than 0.05μM. |
| Delayed Early Methotrexate Elimination and/or Evidence of Acute Renal Injury | Serum methotrexate level of 50μM or more at 24 hours or 5μM or more at 48 hours after administration, OR; a 100% or greater increase in serum creatinine level at 24 hours after methotrexate administration. | 150 mg IV every 3 hours, until methotrexate level is less than 1 micromolar; then 15 mg IV every 3 hours until methotrexate level is less than 0.05μM. |

(ii) *Colorectal cancer: Enhancement of 5-FU cytotoxicity: Adults and the elderly: Administration:* The 350 mg vial of Calcium Leucovorin Solution for Injection (Lederfolin Solution) should be used to administer the high doses of calcium leucovorin required in combination regimens.

When used in combination regimens with 5-FU, calcium leucovorin should only be given by the intravenous route. The agents should not be mixed together.

Each vial of Calcium Leucovorin 350 mg (Lederfolin Solution) contains 1.4 mEq (0.7 mmol) of calcium per vial and it is recommended that the solution is administered over not less than 3–5 minutes.

For intravenous infusion, the 350 mg in 35 ml Solution for Injection (Lederfolin Solution) may be diluted with any of the following infusion fluids before use: Sodium Chloride 0.9%; Glucose 5%; Glucose 10%; Glucose 10% and Sodium Chloride 0.9% Injection; Compound Sodium Lactate Injection.

Calcium leucovorin should not be mixed together with 5-FU in the same infusion.

*Dosage:* Various combination regimens have been studied and based on the available clinical evidence the following regimen has been found to be effective in advanced colorectal carcinoma:

Calcium leucovorin given at a dose of 200 mg/m² by slow intravenous injection, followed immediately by 5-FU at an initial dose of 370 mg/m² by intravenous injection. The injection of leucovorin should not be given more rapidly than over 3–5 minutes because of the calcium content of the solution. This treatment is repeated daily for 5 consecutive days. Subsequent courses may be given after a treatment-free interval of 21–28 days.

For the above regimen, modification of the 5-FU dosage and the treatment-free interval may be necessary depending on patient condition, clinical response and dose limiting toxicity. A reduction of Calcium leucovorin dosage is not required. The number of repeat cycles used is at the discretion of the clinician.

On the basis of the available data, no specific dosage modifications are recommended in the use of the combination regimen with 5-FU in the elderly. However, particular care should be taken when treating elderly or debilitated patients as these patients are at increased risk of severe toxicity with this therapy (see *Warnings and Precautions*).

*Children:* There are no data available on the use of this combination in children.

(iii) *Treatment of folate deficiency: Children up to 12 years of age:* 0.25 mg/kg/day.

*Adults and the elderly:* 10–20 mg daily. Oral therapy with one tablet (15 mg) of calcium leucovorin daily is more usual.

**Contra-indications, warnings, etc**

*Contra-indications:* Calcium leucovorin should not be used for the treatment of pernicious anaemia or other megaloblastic anaemias where vitamin $B_{12}$ is deficient.

*Warnings and precautions:* Calcium leucovorin should only be used with methotrexate or 5-FU under the direct supervision of a clinician experienced in the use of cancer chemotherapeutic agents. When calcium leucovorin has been administered intrathecally following intrathecal overdose of methotrexate, a death has been reported.

Calcium leucovorin should not be given simultaneously with an anti-neoplastic folic acid antagonist, (e.g. methotrexate), to modify or abort clinical toxicity, as the therapeutic effect of the antagonist may be nullified. Concomitant calcium leucovorin will not however inhibit the antibacterial activity of other folic acid antagonists such as trimethoprim and pyrimethamine.

Folinates given in large amounts may counteract the antiepileptic effect of phenobarbitone, phenytoin and primidone and increase the frequency of seizures in susceptible patients.

Seizures and/or syncope have been reported rarely in cancer patients receiving leucovorin, usually in association with fluoropyrimidine administration, and most commonly in those with CNS metastases or other predisposing factors; however a causal relationship has not been established.

In the combination regimen with 5-FU, the toxicity profile of 5-FU is enhanced by calcium leucovorin. The commonest manifestations are leucopenia, mucositis, stomatitis and/or diarrhoea which may be dose limiting. When calcium leucovorin and 5-FU are used in the treatment of colorectal cancer, the 5-FU dosage must be reduced more in cases of toxicity than when 5-FU is used alone. Toxicities observed in patients treated with the combination are qualitatively similar to those observed in patients treated with 5-FU alone. Gastrointestinal toxicities are observed more commonly and may be more severe or even life threatening. In severe cases, treatment is withdrawal of 5-FU and calcium leucovorin, and supportive intravenous therapy. Elderly or debilitated patients are at a greater risk of severe toxicity with this therapy.

Each vial of Lederfolin Solution contains 4.6 mEq (4.6 mmol) of sodium. This and the use of diluting infusion fluids containing sodium should be borne in mind when treating patients requiring a restricted sodium intake.

*Side effects:* Adverse reactions to calcium leucovorin are rare, but occasional pyrexial reactions have been reported following parenteral administration.

*Overdosage:* There have been no reported sequelae in patients who have received significantly more calcium leucovorin than the recommended dosage. There is no specific antidote. In cases of overdosage, patients should be given appropriate supportive care. Should overdosage of the combination of 5-FU with calcium leucovorin occur, the overdosage instructions for 5-FU should be followed.

*Use in pregnancy and lactation:* Reproduction studies have been performed in rats and rabbits at doses of at least 50 times the human dose. These studies have revealed no evidence of harm to the foetus due to calcium leucovorin. There are, however, no adequate and well controlled studies in pregnant women. Because animal reproduction studies are not always predictive of human response, calcium leucovorin should only be used in pregnant women if the potential benefit justifies the potential risk to the foetus.

It is not known whether calcium leucovorin is excreted in human milk. Because many drugs are excreted in human milk, caution should be exercised when calcium leucovorin is administered to a nursing mother.

**Pharmaceutical precautions** Store Calcium Leucovorin Solution for Injection (Lederfolin Solution) under refrigerated conditions (2°–8°C) in original containers. Protect from light.

Store all other presentations at controlled room temperature (15°–30°C) in original containers.

The reconstituted solutions of the Calcium Leucovorin Powder for Injection presentations are intended for immediate administration but may be stored for up to 24 hours under refrigeration (2°–8°C) if necessary.

When the 350 mg in 35 ml Calcium Leucovorin Solution for Injection (Lederfolin Solution) is diluted with the recommended infusion fluids (see Dosage and Administration), the resulting solutions are intended for immediate use but may be stored for up to 24 hours under refrigerated conditions (2°–8°C) prior to use if necessary.

Calcium leucovorin should not be mixed together with 5-FU in the same intravenous injection or infusion.

**Legal category** POM

**Package quantities**
Powder for Injection 15 mg, 30 mg Boxes of one vial.
Solution for Injection 350 mg in 35 ml Boxes of one vial.
Tablets 15 mg Bottles of 10 tablets.

**Further information** Further information, particularly on high-dosage regimens in conjunction with methotrexate, is available on request.

**Product licence numbers**
Powder for injection 15 mg and 30 mg 0095/0087
Tablets 15 mg 0095/0033
Solution for injection 350 mg 0095/0274

## CALCIUM LEUCOVORIN INJECTION 3 mg/ml

**Qualitative and quantitative composition** Calcium Leucovorin equivalent to Leucovorin (free acid) 3.0 mg/ml

**Pharmaceutical form** Sterile solution for injection

**Clinical particulars**

*Therapeutic indications:* Calcium Leucovorin is the calcium salt of a formyl derivative of tetrahydrofolic acid, the metabolite of folic acid and an essential coenzyme for nucleic acid synthesis.

*Calcium Leucovorin rescue:* Calcium Leucovorin is used to diminish the toxicity and counteract the action of folic acid antagonists such as methotrexate in cytotoxic therapy. This procedure is commonly known as Calcium Leucovorin Rescue.

*Treatment of folate deficiency:* Calcium Leucovorin has also been demonstrated to be effective in producing amelioration of the blood picture in a number of megaloblastic anaemias due to folate deficiency.

*Posology and method of administration:*
*Method of administration:* Intramuscular injection, bolus intravenous injection or intravenous infusion.

*Dosage:* Adults, children and the elderly
*Calcium Leucovorin rescue:* Calcium Leucovorin Rescue therapy should commence 24 hours after the beginning of methotrexate infusion. Dosage regimes vary depending upon the dose of methotrexate administered. In general, the Calcium Leucovorin should be administered at a dose of 15 mg (approximately 10 mg/m²) every 6 hours for 10 doses, either parenterally by intramuscular injection, bolus intravenous injection or intravenous infusion or orally using Calcium Leucovorin tablets. Do not administer Calcium Leucovorin intrathecally.

Where overdosage of methotrexate is suspected, the dose of Calcium Leucovorin should be equal to or higher than the offending dose of methotrexate and should be administered in the first hour. In the presence of gastrointestinal toxicity, nausea or vomiting, Calcium Leucovorin should be administered parenterally. Do not administer Calcium Leucovorin intrathecally. Further, oral administration of doses greater than 50 mg is not recommended since the absorption of Calcium Leucovoin is saturable. In the case of intravenous administration, no more than 160 mg of Calcium Leucovorin should be injected per minute due to the calcium content of the solution.

In addition to Calcium Leucovorin administration, measures to ensure the prompt excretion of methotrexate are important as part of Calcium Leucovorin Rescue Therapy. These measures include:
(a) Alkalinisation of urine so that the urinary pH is greater than 7.0 before methotrexate infusion (to increase solubility of methotrexate and its metabolites).
(b) Maintenance of urine output of 1800–2000 cc/m²/24hr by increased oral or intravenous fluids on days 2,3 and 4 following methotrexate therapy.
(c) Plasma methotrexate concentration, BUN and creatinine should be measured on days 2,3 and 4.

These measures must be continued until the plasma methotrexate level is less than $10^{-7}$ molar (0.1μM).

Delayed methotrexate excretion may be seen in some patients. This may be caused by a third space accumulation (as seen in ascites or pleural effusion for example), renal insufficiency of inadequate hydration. Under such circumstances, higher doses of Calcium Leucovorin or prolonged administration may be indicated. Dosage and administration guidelines for these patients are given in Table 1. Patients who experience delayed early methotrexate elimination are likely to develop reversible renal failure.

*Treatment of folate deficiency:*
Children up to 12 years: 0.25 mg/kg/day
Adults and the elderly: 10-20 mg daily. Oral therapy with one tablet (15 mg) of Calcium Leucovorin daily is more usual.

*Contra-indications:* Calcium Leucovorin should not be used for the treatment of pernicious anaemia or other megaloblastic anaemias where Vitamin $B_{12}$ is deficient.

*Special warnings and special precautions for use:* Calcium Leucovorin should only be used with methotrexate or 5-FU under the direct supervision of a clinician experienced in the use of cancer chemotherapeutic agents.

When Calcium Leucovorin has been administered intrathecally following intrathecal overdose of methotrexate, a death has been reported.

Seizures and/or syncope have been reported rarely in cancer patients receiving leucovorin, usually in association with fluoropyrimidine administration and most commonly in those with CNS metastases or other predisposing factors; however a causal relationship has not been established.

*Interactions with other medicaments and other forms of interaction:* Calcium Leucovorin should not be given simultaneously with an anti-neoplastic folic acid antagonist, eg methotrexate, to modify or abort clinical toxicity, as the therapeutic effect of the antagonist may be nullified. Concomitant Calcium Leucovorin will not inhibit the anti-bacterial activity of other folic acid antagonists such as trimethoprim and pyrimethamine.

Folinates given in large amounts may counteract the anti-epileptic effect of phenobarbitone, phenytoin and primidone and increase the frequency of seizures in susceptible patients.

*Pregnancy and lactation:* Reproduction studies have been performed in rats and rabbits at doses of at least 50 times the human dose. These studies have revealed no evidence of harm to the foetus due to Calcium Leucovorin. There are, however, no adequate and well-controlled studies in pregnant women, because animal studies are not always predictive of human response. Calcium Leucovorin should only be used in pregnant women if the potential benefit justifies the potential risk to the foetus.

It is not known whether Calcium Leucovorin is excreted in human milk. As many drugs are excreted in human milk, caution should be exercised when Calcium Leucovorin is administered to a nursing mother.

*Effects on ability to drive and use machines:* None.

*Undesirable effects:* Adverse reactions to Calcium Leucovorin are rare, but occasional pyrexial reactions have been reported following parenteral administration.

*Overdose:* There have been no reported sequelae in patients who have received significantly more Calcium Leucovorin than the recommended dosage. There is no specific antidote. In cases of overdosage, patients should be given appropriate supportive care. Should overdosage of the combination of 5-FU with Calcium Leucovorin occur, the overdosage instructions for 5-FU should be followed.

**Pharmacological properties**

*Pharmacodynamic properties:* Calcium Leucovorin is the calcium salt of a formyl tetrahydrofolic acid, the metabolite of folic acid and an essential coenzyme for nucleic acid synthesis. Calcium Leucovorin is used therefore to diminish the toxicity and counteract the action of folic acid antagonists such as methotrexate in cytotoxic therapy (Calcium Leucovorin Rescue).

Calcium Leucovorin is also effective in the treatment of megaloblastic anaemia.

*Pharmacokinetic properties:* Parenteral administration of Calcium Leucovorin gives higher peak plasma levels than oral administration, but the total plasma folate pool (folinic acid plus its metabolite ($N^5$-methyl $H_4$-folate) remains unchanged.)

$N^5$-methyl-$H_4$-folate rapidly disperses into the extracellular fluids within 10 minutes following intravenous dosage.

Folinic acid in the plasma compartment is rapidly cleared by renal excretion.

*Preclinical safety data:* Nothing of relevance to prescriber.

**Pharmaceutical particulars**

*List of excipients:* Water for Injection, sodium hydroxide and hydrochloric acid.

*Incompatibilities:* None.

*Shelf life:* 24 Months

*Special precautions for storage:* Store at controlled room temperature (15° to 25°C) in the original container.

*Nature and contents of container:* 1 ml amber glass ampoules

*Instructions for use/handling:* Use within 24 hours of opening.

**Marketing authorisation number** 0095/5053R

**Date of approval/revision of SPC** April 1996

**Legal category** POM

## CRINONE* 4% AND 8% PROGESTERONE VAGINAL GEL

**Qualitative and quantitative composition**

| Active Ingredient | 4% gel mg/dose | 8% gel % w/w | mg/dose | % w/w |
|---|---|---|---|---|
| Progesterone | 45 | 4.0 | 90 | 8.0 |

**Pharmaceutical form** Vaginal gel.

**Clinical particulars**
*Therapeutic indications:* Treatment of disorders associated with progesterone deficiency, such as:
Premenstrual syndrome
Menstrual irregularities, dysmenorrhoea, secondary amenorrhoea
Dysfunctional (anovulatory) uterine bleeding occurring before menopause
Menopausal disorders (in combination with oestrogen therapy)
Infertility due to inadequate luteal phase
For use during in-vitro fertilisation, where infertility is mainly due to tubal, idiopathic or endometriosis linked sterility associated with normal ovulatory cycle

*Posology and method of administration:* Intravaginal application.
Treatment of progesterone deficiency: one application (1.125 g 4% gel) every other day, preferably in the morning, from day 15 to day 25 of the cycle.
Maintenance therapy can be achieved with an every other day application from day 15 to day 25 of the cycle.
Treatment of menopausal disorders: one application (1.125 g 4% gel) every other day for the last days of each oestrogenic sequence.
Treatment of infertility due to inadequate luteal phase: one application (1.125 g 8% gel) every day starting after documented ovulation or arbitrarily the 18th-21st day of the cycle.
When used during in-vitro fertilisation, daily application

**Table 1: Dosage and Administration Guidelines for Calcium Leucovorin Rescue:**

| Clinical Situation | Laboratory Findings | Leucovorin Dosage and Duration |
|---|---|---|
| Normal methotrexate elimination | Serum methotrexate level approx. 10μM 24 hours after administration, 1μM at 48 hours and less than 0.2μM at 72 hours. | 15 mg, PO, IM or IV every 6 hours for 60 hours (10 doses starting 24 hours after start of methotrexate infusion). |
| Delayed late methotrexate elimination | Serum methotrexate level remaining above 0.2μM at 72 hours and more than 0.05μM at 96 hours after administration. | Continue 15 mg PO, IM or IV every 6 hours, until methotrexate level is less than 0.05μM. |
| Delayed early methotrexate elimination and /or evidence of acute renal injury | Serum methotrexate level of 50μM or more at 24 hours or 5μM or more at 48 hours after administration, OR; a 100% or greater increase in serum creatinine level at 24 hours after methotrexate administration. | 150 mg IV every 3 hours until methotrexate level is less than 1 micromolar; then 15 mg IV every 3 hours until methotrexate level is less than 0.05μM. |

ion of Crinone 8% gel should be continued for 30 ys if there is laboratory evidence of pregnancy.
*Children:* not applicable.

*ntra-indications:* Known allergy to any of the cipients. Undiagnosed uterine bleeding. Porphyria

*ecial warnings and special precautions for use:* utious use in severe hepatic insufficiency. The oduct should not be used concurrently with other al intravaginal therapy.

*eraction with other medicaments and other forms interaction:* No interaction reported.

*egnancy and lactation:* In case of corpus luteum ficiency, Crinone can be used during the first month pregnancy.
Do not use during lactation.

*fects on ability to drive and use machines:* Drivers d users of machines are warned that risk of mnolence may occur.

*ndesirable effects:* Rare cases of somnolence. Occsional spotting.

*verdose:* Not applicable.

**armacological properties**

*armacodynamic properties:* Those of the naturally curring progesterone with induction of a full secrey endometrium.

*armacokinetic properties:* The progesterone vagil gel is based on a polycarbophil delivery system hich attaches to the vaginal mucosa and provides a olonged release of progesterone for at least three ys.

*eclinical safety data:* In rabbits, Crinone was an eye itant categorised class IV (minimal effects clearing less than 24 hours), but not a dermal irritant.
A moderate vaginal irritation was found in rabbits ter application of 2.0 ml/day of 8% gel for 5 days.

**armaceutical particulars**

*st of excipients:* Glycerin, light liquid paraffin, drogenated palm oil glyceride, carbomer 974P, rbic acid, polycarbophil, sodium hydroxide, purified ater.

*compatibilities:* No incompatibilities were found th the usual contraceptive devices.

*elf life:* 24 months.

*ecial precautions for storage:* Store below 25°C.

*ature and contents of container:* A single use, one ece, white polyethylene applicator with a twist-off p, designed for intravaginal application.
Each applicator contains 2.6 g of gel and delivers 125 g of gel. Each one is wrapped up and sealed in paper/aluminium/polyethylene foil overwrap.
The applicators are packed in cardboard boxes ntaining 2 (sample pack) and 6 units of Crinone 4% ogesterone vaginal gel, and 15 units of Crinone 8% ogesterone vaginal gel.

*structions for use/handling:* Crinone is applied dictly from the specially designed sealed applicator to the vagina. Remove the applicator from the aled wrapper. DO NOT remove the twist-off cap at is time.

Grip the applicator firmly by the thick end. Shake down like a thermometer to ensure that the contents are at the thin end.
Twist off the tab and discard.
The applicator may be inserted while you are in a sitting position or when lying on your back with the knees bent. Gently insert the thin end of applicator well into the vagina.
Press the thick end of the applicator firmly to deposit gel. Remove the applicator and discard in a waste container.
Crinone coats the vaginal mucosa to provide long-lasting release of progesterone.

**arketing authorisation numbers**
rinone 4% progesterone vaginal gel 11764/0004
rinone 8% progesterone vaginal gel 11764/0005

**ate of approval/revision of SPC** September 1996

**egal category** POM

## ETECLO* TABLETS

**resentation** Tablets 300 mg: Each blue, film-coated blet, embossed 'LL' on one side and '5422' on the verse side, contains:
etracycline hydrochloride 115.4 mg
hlortetracycline hydrochloride 115.4 mg
emeclocycline hydrochloride 69.2 mg

**ses** For the treatment of infections caused by tracycline-sensitive organisms. For example, Deteo is highly effective in the treatment of infections aused by *Borrellia recurrentis* (relapsing fever), *alymmatobacterium granulomatis* (granuloma inuinale), *Chlamydia* species (psittacosis, lymphogranuloma venereum, trachoma, inclusion conjunctivitis), *Francisella tularensis* (tularaemia), *Haemophilus ducreyi* (chancroid), *Leptospira* (meningitis, jaundice), *Mycoplasma pneumoniae* (non-gonococcal urethritis), *Pseudomonas mallei* and *pseudomallei* (glanders and melioidosis), *Rickettsiae* (typhus fever, Q fever, rocky mountain spotted fever), *Vibrio* species (cholera). It is also highly effective, alone or in combination with streptomycin, in the treatment of infections due to *Brucella* species (brucellosis), and *Yersinia pestis* (bubonic plague). Severe acne vulgaris.

Other sensitive organisms include: *Actinomyces israelii*, *Bacillus anthracis* (pneumonia), *Clostridium* species (gas gangrene, tetanus), *Entamoeba histolytica* (dysentery), *Neisseria gonorrhoeae*, and anaerobic species, *Treponema pallidum* and *pertenue* (syphilis and yaws).

**Dosage and administration** *Dosage: Adults only:* One tablet every 12 hours.

This may be increased to 3 or 4 tablets daily for short periods in more severe infections.

*Gonorrhoea:* 1,200 mg (4 tablets) followed by a similar dose six hours later.

*Non-gonococcal urethritis:* One tablet twice daily for 10–21 days.

*Children:* Not recommended for children under 12 years of age.

*Elderly:* Deteclo should be used with caution in the treatment of elderly patients where accumulation is a possibility.

*Administration:* Deteclo should be swallowed whole with plenty of fluid while sitting or standing. Deteclo should be taken an hour before or two hours after meals and therapy should be continued for up to three days after characteristic symptoms of the infection have subsided.

**Contra-indications, warnings etc**
*Contra-indications:* A history of hypersensitivity to tetracyclines. Overt renal insufficiency. Children under twelve years of age.

*Warnings and precautions:* Deteclo should be used with caution in patients with renal or hepatic dysfunction or in conjunction with other potentially hepatotoxic or nephrotoxic drugs. Concurrent use with the anaesthetic methoxyflurane increases the risk of kidney failure. The anti-anabolic action of the tetracyclines may cause an increase in BUN.

Lower doses are indicated in cases of renal impairment to avoid excessive systemic accumulation, and if therapy is prolonged, serum level determinations are advisable. Patients who have known liver disease should not receive more than 1 g daily. In long term therapy, periodic laboratory evaluation of organ systems, including haematopoietic, renal and hepatic studies should be performed.

Photoallergic reactions may occur in hypersensitive persons and such patients should be warned to avoid direct exposure to natural or artificial sunlight and to discontinue treatment at the first sign of skin discomfort.

Cross-resistance between tetracyclines may develop in micro-organisms and cross-sensitisation in patients. Deteclo should be discontinued if there are signs/symptoms of overgrowth of resistant organisms including candida, enteritis, glossitis, stomatitis, vaginitis, pruritus ani or staphylococcal enterocolitis.

Patients taking oral contraceptives should be warned that if diarrhoea or breakthrough bleeding occur there is a possibility of contraceptive failure.

*Interactions:* Deteclo should not be used with penicillins. Tetracyclines depress plasma prothrombin activity and reduced doses of concomitant anticoagulants may be required.

Absorption of Deteclo is impaired by the concomitant administration of iron, calcium, zinc, magnesium and particularly aluminium salts commonly used as antacids.

The concomitant use of tetracyclines may reduce the efficacy of oral contraceptives; an increased incidence of breakthrough bleeding may also be experienced (see statement under Warnings and Precautions).

*Use in pregnancy:* Results of animal studies indicate that tetracyclines cross the placenta, are found in foetal tissues and can have toxic effects on the developing foetus (often related to retardation of skeletal development). Evidence of embryotoxicity has also been noted in animals treated early in pregnancy. Deteclo therefore, should not be used in pregnancy unless considered essential, in which case the maximum daily dose should be 1 g.

The use of drugs of the tetracycline class during tooth development (last half of pregnancy) may cause permanent discolouration of the teeth (yellow-grey-brown). This adverse reaction is more common during long term use of the drugs but has been observed following repeated short term courses. Enamel hypoplasia has also been reported.

*Use in lactation:* Tetracyclines have been found in the milk of lactating women who are taking a drug in this class. Permanent tooth discolouration may occur in the developing infant and enamel hypoplasia has been reported. Therefore, Deteclo should not be administered to lactating women.

*Use in children:* The use of tetracyclines during tooth development in children under the age of 12 years may cause permanent discolouration. Enamel hypoplasia has also been reported.

*Side-effects:* Gastro-intestinal disturbances including nausea, vomiting and diarrhoea may occur and, as with all antibiotics, overgrowth of resistant organisms may cause glossitis, stomatitis, vaginitis, or staphylococcal enterocolitis. Dermatological reactions are rare. Bulging fontanelles in infants and benign intracranial hypertension in adults have been reported. Treatment should cease if evidence of raised intracranial pressure develops. Hypersensitivity reactions including: urticaria, angioneurotic oedema, anaphylaxis, anaphylactoid purpura, pericarditis and exacerbation of systemic lupus erythematosus may occur. Haemolytic anaemia, thrombocytopenia, neutropenia and eosinophilia have been reported. When given over prolonged periods tetracyclines have been reported to produce brown-black microscopic discolouration of the thyroid gland. No abnormalities of thyroid function are known to occur.

*Overdosage:* No specific antidote. Gastric lavage plus oral administration of milk or antacids.

**Pharmaceutical precautions** Store at controlled room temperature (15–30°C) in the original pack or in containers which prevent access of light and moisture.

**Legal category** POM

**Package quantities** Bottles of 100 and 500

**Further information** Deteclo is a unique combination of three effective tetracycline broad-spectrum antibiotics. The ratio of the different tetracyclines has been carefully chosen to ensure that high therapeutic blood levels are rapidly realised and maintained with a reduced potential for side-effects, on a twice daily dosage regime, because of their different rates of absorption and excretion.

**Product licence number** 0095/5070R

## DIAMOX*

***Presentation*** *Tablets 250 mg:* Each white tablet coded "Lederle 4395" contains acetazolamide 250 mg. *Sodium Parenteral 500 mg:* Each vial contains an amount of sterile acetazolamide sodium equivalent to 500 mg of acetazolamide. The pH has been adjusted to approximately 9.2 with sodium hydroxide and, if necessary, hydrochloric acid.

**Uses** Diamox is an enzyme inhibitor which acts specifically on carbonic anhydrase. It is indicated in the treatment of:

(i) *Glaucoma:* Diamox is useful in glaucoma (chronic simple (open angle) glaucoma, secondary glaucoma, and perioperatively in acute angle closure glaucoma where delay of surgery is desired in order to lower intraocular pressure) because it acts on inflow, decreasing the amount of aqueous secretion.

(ii) *Abnormal retention of fluids:* Diamox is a diuretic whose effect is due to the effect on the reversible hydration of carbon dioxide and dehydration of carbonic acid reaction in the kidney. The result is renal loss of $HCO_3$-ion which carries out sodium, water and potassium. Diamox can be used in conjunction with other diuretics when effects on several segments of the nephron are desirable in the treatment of fluid retaining states.

(iii) *Epilepsy:* In conjunction with other anticonvulsants best results with Diamox have been seen in petit mal in children. Good results, however, have been seen in patients, both children and adults, with other types of seizures such as grand mal, mixed seizure patterns, myoclonic jerk patterns etc.

**Dosage and administration**
*Tablets 250 mg:*

(i) *Glaucoma (simple acute congestive and secondary): Adults:* 250–1,000 mg (1–4 tablets) per 24 hours, usually in divided doses for amounts over 250 mg daily.

(ii) *Abnormal retention of fluid:* Congestive heart failure, drug-induced oedema.

*Adults:* For diuresis, the starting dose is usually 250–375 mg (1–1½ tablets) once daily in the morning. If, after an initial response, the patient fails to continue to lose oedema fluid, do not increase the dose but allow for kidney recovery by omitting a day. Best results are often obtained on a regime of 250–375 mg (1–1½ tablets) daily for two days, rest a day, and repeat, or merely giving the Diamox every other day. The use of Diamox does not eliminate the need for other therapy, eg. digitalis, bed rest and salt restriction in congestive heart failure and proper supplementation with elements such as potassium in drug-induced oedema.

For cases of fluid retention associated with premenstrual tension, a daily dose (single) of 125–375 mg is suggested.

iii) *Epilepsy: Adults:* 250–1,000 mg daily in divided doses.

*Children:* 8–30 mg/kg in daily divided doses and not to exceed 750 mg/day.

The change from other medication to Diamox should be gradual.

*Sodium Parenteral 500 mg:* Intravenous or intramuscular administration may be employed in the same dosage as indicated for oral use. The direct intravenous route is preferred as the intramuscular use is limited by the alkaline pH of the solution.

Each vial should be reconstituted with at least 5 ml of Water for Injection prior to use.

*Elderly:* Diamox should only be used with particular caution in elderly patients or those with potential obstruction in the urinary tract or with disorders rendering their electrolyte balance precarious or with liver dysfunction.

**Contra-indications, warnings, etc** *Contra-indications:* Acetazolamide therapy is contra-indicated in situations in which sodium and/or potassium blood serum levels are depressed, in cases of marked kidney and liver disease or dysfunction, suprarenal gland failure, and hyper-chloremic acidosis.

Long-term administration of Diamox is contra-indicated in patients with chronic non-congestive angle-closure glaucoma since it may permit organic closure of the angle to occur while the worsening glaucoma is masked by lowered intraocular pressure.

Diamox should not be used in patients hypersensitive to sulphonamides.

*Warnings: Use in pregnancy:* Acetazolamide has been reported to be teratogenic and embryotoxic in rats, mice, hamsters and rabbits at oral or parenteral doses in excess of ten times those recommended in human beings. Although there is no evidence of these effects in human beings, there are no adequate and well-controlled studies in pregnant women. Therefore, Diamox should not be used in pregnancy, especially during the first trimester.

*Use in lactation:* Diamox has been detected in low levels in the milk of lactating women who have taken Diamox. Although it is unlikely that this will lead to any harmful effects in the infant, extreme caution should be exercised when Diamox is administered to lactating women.

*Precautions:* Increasing the dose does not increase the diuresis and may increase the incidence of drowsiness and/or paraesthesia.

Increasing the dose often results in a decrease in diuresis. Under certain circumstances, however, very large doses have been given in conjunction with other diuretics in order to secure diuresis in complete refractory failure.

When Diamox is prescribed for long-term therapy, special precautions are advisable. The patient should be cautioned to report any unusual skin rash. Periodic blood cell counts and electrolyte levels are recommended. A precipitous drop in formed blood cell elements or the appearance of toxic skin manifestations should call for diminution or cessation of Diamox therapy.

In patients with pulmonary obstruction or emphysema where alveolar ventilation may be impaired, Diamox may aggravate acidosis and should be used with caution.

The pH of parenteral acetazolamide is 9.1. Care should be taken during intravenous administration of alkaline preparations to avoid extravasation and possible development of skin necrosis.

*Effects on ability to drive and use machines:* Increasing the dose does not increase the diuresis and may increase the incidence of drowsiness and/or paraesthesia. Less commonly, fatigue, dizziness and ataxia have been reported. Disorientation has been observed in a few patients with oedema due to hepatic cirrhosis. Such cases should be under close supervision. Transient myopia has been reported.

These conditions invariably subside upon diminution or discontinuance of the medication.

*Side-effects:* Adverse reactions during short-term therapy are usually non-serious. Those effects which have been noted include: paraesthesias, particularly a 'tingling' feeling in the extremities; some loss of appetite; taste disturbance, polyuria, flushing, thirst, headache, dizziness, fatigue, irritability, depression, reduced libido and occasional instances of drowsiness and confusion. Rarely, photosensitivity has been reported.

During long-term therapy, metabolic acidosis and electrolyte imbalance may occasionally occur. This can usually be corrected by the administration of bicarbonate.

Transient myopia has been reported. This condition invariably subsides upon diminution or withdrawal of the medication.

Gastro-intestinal disturbances such as nausea, vomiting and diarrhoea.

Diamox is a sulphonamide derivative and therefore some side-effects similar to those caused by sulphonamides have occasionally been reported. These include fever, agranulocytosis, thrombocytopenia, thrombocytic purpura, leukopenia, and aplastic anaemia, bone marrow depression, pancytopenia, rash (including erythema multiforme, Stevens-Johnson Syndrome, toxic epidermal necrolysis), anaphylaxis, crystalluria, calculus formation, renal and ureteral colic, and renal lesions have been reported.

Other occasional adverse reactions include: urticaria, melaena, haematuria, glycosuria, impaired hearing and tinnitus, abnormal liver function and rarely, hepatitis or cholestatic jaundice, flaccid paralysis, and convulsions.

*Drug interactions:* Diamox is a sulphonamide derivative. Sulphonamides may potentiate the effects of folic acid antagonists. Possible potentiation of the effects of folic acid antagonists, hypoglycaemics and oral anti-coagulants may occur. Concurrent administration of acetazolamide and aspirin may result in severe acidosis and increase central nervous system toxicity. Adjustment of dose may be required when Diamox is given with cardiac glycosides or hypertensive agents.

When given concomitantly, acetazolamide modifies the metabolism of phenytoin, leading to increased serum levels of phenytoin. Severe osteomalacia has been noted in a few patients taking acetazolamide in combination with other anticonvulsants. There have been isolated reports of reduced primidone and increased carbamazepine serum levels with concurrent administration of acetazolamide.

*Overdosage:* No specific antidote. Supportive measure with correction of electrolyte and fluid balance. Force fluids.

**Pharmaceutical precautions** The products should be stored at controlled room temperature (15°–25°C).

Reconstituted solutions contain no preservative and should be used immediately or within 24 hours if stored in a refrigerator (2°–8°C).

**Legal category** POM

**Package quantities**
Tablets 250 mg: Bottles of 100 and 1,000
Sodium Parenteral 500 mg: Vials of 500 mg

**Further information** Diamox Acetazolamide Sodium Parenteral contains 2.36 millimoles of sodium per vial.

**Product licence numbers**
Tablets 250 mg 0095/5075R
Sodium Parenteral 500 mg 0095/5073R

## DIAMOX* SR

**Presentation** Diamox SR is a two tone orange capsule containing orange film coated pellets designed to deliver 250 mg of acetazolamide as a sustained release preparation.

**Uses** Diamox is an enzyme inhibitor which acts specifically on carbonic anhydrase which affects the reversible hydration of carbon dioxide and dehydration of carbonic acid in the kidney and other sites. The result is renal loss of $HCO_3$-ion which carries out sodium, water and potassium.

*Indication:* Glaucoma: Diamox SR acts on inflow, decreasing the amount of aqueous secretion. For chronic simple (open angle) glaucoma, secondary glaucoma, and perioperatively in acute angle closure glaucoma where delay of surgery is desired in order to lower intra-ocular pressure.

**Dosage and administration**
*Adults:* One or two 250 mg capsules a day.

*Children:* This product is not intended for administration to children.

*Elderly:* Diamox SR should be used with particular caution in elderly patients or those with potential obstruction in the urinary tract or with disorders rendering their electrolyte balance precarious or with liver dysfunction.

Capsules should be swallowed whole. Do not chew or crush.

**Contra-indications, warnings, etc**
*Contra-indications:* Diamox SR therapy is contra-indicated in situations in which sodium and/or potassium blood serum levels are depressed, in cases of marked kidney and liver dysfunction, suprarenal gland failure and hyperchloraemic acidosis.

Long-term administration of Diamox SR is contra-indicated in patients with chronic non-congestive angle-closure glaucoma since it may permit organic closure of the angle to occur while the worseni glaucoma is masked by lowered intra-ocular pressu

Diamox SR should not be used in patients hypers sitive to sulphonamides.

*Warnings: use in pregnancy:* Acetazolamide has be reported to be teratogenic and embryotoxic in ra mice, hamsters and rabbits at oral or parenteral do in excess of ten times those recommended in hum beings. Although there is no evidence of these effe in human beings, there are no adequate and w controlled studies in pregnant women. Therefo Diamox SR should not be used in pregnancy, es cially during the first trimester.

*Use in lactation:* Diamox has been detected in l levels in the milk of lactating women who have ta Diamox. Although it is unlikely that this will lead any harmful effects in the infant, extreme cauti should be exercised when Diamox SR is administe to lactating women.

*Precautions:* Increasing the dose does not increa the diuresis and may increase the incidence drowsiness and/or paraesthesia.

When Diamox SR is prescribed for long-te therapy, special precautions are advisable. The patie should be cautioned to report any unusual skin ra Periodic blood cell counts and electrolyte levels a recommended. A precipitous drop in formed blo cell elements or the appearance of toxic skin manif tations should call for diminution or cessation Diamox SR therapy.

In patients with pulmonary obstruction or emp sema where alveolar ventilation may be impair Diamox SR may aggravate acidosis and should used with caution.

*Effects on ability to drive and use machines:* Increasi the dose does not increase the diuresis and m increase the incidence of drowsiness and/or para thesia. Less commonly, fatigue, dizziness and ata have been reported. Disorientation has been observ in a few patients with oedema due to hepatic cirrho Such cases should be under close supervision. Tra sient myopia has been reported.

These conditions invariably subside upon dimir tion or discontinuance of the medication.

*Side-effects:* Adverse reactions during short-te therapy are usually non-serious. Those effects wh have been noted include: paraesthesias, particularl 'tingling' feeling in the extremities, some loss appetite, taste disturbance, polyuria, flushing, thir headache, dizziness, fatigue, irritability, depressi reduced libido and occasional instances of drowsine and confusion. Rarely, photosensitivity has be reported.

During long-term therapy, metabolic acidosis a electrolyte imbalance may occasionally occur. T can usually be corrected by the administration bicarbonate.

Transient myopia has been reported. This conditi invariably subsides upon diminution or discontin ance of the medication.

Gastro-intestinal disturbances such as nausea, vo iting and diarrhoea.

Diamox is a sulphonamide derivative and therefo some side-effects similar to those caused by sulpho amides have occasionally been reported. These clude fever, agranulocytosis, thrombocytope thrombocytic purpura, leukopenia, and aplastic an mia, bone marrow depression, pancytopenia, ra (including erythema multiforme, Stevens-Johns Syndrome, toxic epidermal necrolysis), anaphyla crystalluria, calculus formation, renal and urete colic and renal lesions.

Other occasional adverse reactions include: u caria, melaena, haematuria, glycosuria, impair hearing and tinnitus, abnormal liver function a rarely, hepatitis or cholestatic jaundice, flaccid par ysis and convulsions.

*Drug interactions:* Diamox SR is a sulphonami derivative. Sulphonamides may potentiate the effe of folic acid antagonists. Possible potentiation of t effects of folic acid antagonists, hypoglycaemics a oral anti-coagulants. Concurrent administration acetazolamide and aspirin may result in severe a dosis and increase central nervous system toxici Adjustment of dose may be required when Diam SR is given with cardiac glycosides or hypertens agents.

When given concomitantly, Diamox SR modifi the metabolism of phenytoin, leading to increas serum levels of phenytoin. Severe osteomalacia h been noted in a few patients taking acetazolamide combination with other anticonvulsants. There ha been isolated reports of reduced primidone a increased carbamazepine serum levels with conc rent administration of acetazolamide.

*Overdosage:* No specific antidote. Supportive mea ures with correction of electrolyte and fluid balanc Force fluids.

**armaceutical precautions** Store at controlled room
mperature (15°–25°C) in the original pack or in well
led dispensing containers which prevent access of
t and moisture.

**gal category** POM

**kage quantities**
lister pack of 28 capsules
ottles of 100 or 500 capsules

**ther information** Nil

**duct licence number** 0095/0239

# MOTANE* TABLETS
# MOTANE* LA
# MOTANE* ELIXIR

**alitative and quantitative composition** Dimotane
lets: Tablet containing Brompheniramine Maleate
4.0 mg.
imotane LA: Tablet containing Brompheniramine
leate BP 12.0 mg (one-third of active ingredient in
ting for immediate release; two-thirds of active
redient in delayed-release core)
imotane Elixir: Elixir containing Brompheniramine
leate BP 2.0 mg per 5 ml

**armaceutical form** Dimotane Tablets: Round peach-
oured tablet for oral use. One side is engraved
R', the other side is scored with a breakline.
imotane LA: Peach coloured, sugar coated, modi-
d release tablet for oral use
imotane Elixir: A clear pale yellow-green liquid
h an odour and taste of cola.

**nical particulars**

*erapeutic indications:* Antihistamine in the treat-
nt of allergic conditions and reactions such as
yfever and urticaria.

*sology and method of administration:*

*motane Tablets*
Adults and older patients: 1–2 tablets 3 or 4 times
ly.
Children 6–12 years: ½–1 tablet 3 or 4 times daily.
Under 6 years: Not recommended.

*motane LA*
Adults and older patients: 1–2 tablets night and
orning.
Children 6–12 years: 1 tablet at night at retiring. A
ther tablet may be taken in the morning if neces-
ry.
Under 6 years: Not recommended.

*motane Elixir*
Adults and older patients: 10–20 ml 3 or 4 times
ly.
Children 6–12 years: 5–10 ml 3 or 4 times daily.
Children 3–6 years: 5 ml 3 or 4 times daily.
Children under 3 years: 0.4–1 mg/kg per 24 hours in
ur divided doses or at the discretion of the physician

*ntra-indications:* Hypersensitivity to any of the
gredients.

*ecial warnings and special precautions for use:* In
mmon with many other antihistamines, bromphen-
mine has an anticholinergic action and should
erefore be used with caution in patients with asthma
specially children), closed-angle glaucoma and pro-
tic disease.
Brompheniramine maleate may act as a cerebral
mulant in children and the elderly. If this occurs, it
possible that insomnia, nervousness, pyrexia and
mors may occur, and, very rarely, hallucinations
d convulsions. It is advisable that children receiving
ompheniramine should not be left unattended for
g periods. This product should be used with care
epileptic patients.

*eractions with other medicaments and other forms
interaction:* This product may potentiate the seda-
e effects of CNS depressants including alcohol,
rbiturates, hypnotics, opioid analgesics, anxiolytics
d neuroleptics.
Antihistamines exhibit an additive anticholinergic
tion with other anticholinergic drugs, such as
enothiazines and tricyclic antidepressants.
Monoamine oxidase inhibitors prolong and inten-
y the anticholinergic effects of antihistamines.

*egnancy and lactation:* Safety for the use of Dimo-
ne during pregnancy has not been established.
erefore, this product should not be used during
egnancy unless considered essential by the physi-
an.

*fects on the ability to drive and use machines:*
owsiness may occur. Patients receiving bromphen-
mine should not drive or operate machinery unless
has been shown that their physical and mental
pacity remains unaffected.

*ndesirable effects:* The most common side effect is
sedation which may diminish after a few days of
treatment.
Anticholinergic effects such as blurred vision, dry
mouth, tachycardia and urinary retention may occur.
Other side effects which have been reported rarely
are nervousness, urticaria, constipation, pyrexia, dizziness, hallucinations and convulsions.

*Overdose:* Overdose may be fatal especially in infants
and children. The patient may be unconscious, and
shows hypotension, coma and occasionally convulsions. Initial excitement is often seen in children.
Management of overdose consists of gastric lavage
together with appropriate supportive therapy dependent upon individual symptoms.

**Pharmacological properties**

*Pharmacodynamic properties:* Brompheniramine belongs to the alkylamine group of $H_1$-antihistamines. It
competitively antagonises the effects of histamine on
$H_1$ receptors and blocks the constrictor responses to
histamine of intestinal and bronchial smooth muscle.
Within the vascular tree, brompheniramine inhibits
both the vasoconstrictor and the vasodilator effects
of histamine. Secondary to injury, antigens or histamine-releasing pharmacological agents, brompheniramine counteracts both oedema and wheal
formation. It also blocks the increased nasal secretion
and impaired airflow following nasal histamine challenge.
Single doses of 4–12 mg of brompheniramine have
produced CNS depression in terms of subjective
sedation and objective impairment of skilled performance which lasts for 5–7 hours.

*Pharmacokinetic properties:* (a) General characteristics: Following oral administration, brompheniramine
is readily absorbed and distributed into the tissues;
peak plasma concentrations are seen at approximately
3 hours after a single oral dose of 10 mg to fasting
subjects. Following administration of a controlled
release tablet peak plasma levels occur between 3 and
5 hours. An elimination half life of about 25 hours has
been reported.
Brompheniramine appears to undergo moderate
first pass metabolism.
The major route of elimination is hepatic metabolism with unchanged drug and metabolites being
excreted primarily in the urine. Less than 3% is
excreted in the faeces.
(b) Characteristics in patients: Effective anti-allergic
doses of brompheniramine (8 mg) have produced
plasma concentrations of 8–16 microgram/litre over
several hours.
Oral brompheniramine 10 mg produced drowsiness
in all of a group of adult volunteers, peaking at around
3–4 hours after administration, coinciding with peak
plasma concentrations.

**Pharmaceutical particulars**

*List of excipients:* Dimotane Tablets: Maize starch,
dibasic calcium phosphate dihydrate, magnesium
stearate, iron oxide red and iron oxide yellow (E172).
Dimotane LA: Magnesium stearate, sucrose, calcium sulphate, talc, maize starch, zein, stearic acid,
glycol monosterate, guar gum, acacia gum, gelatin,
carnauba wax, beeswax, titanium dioxide (E171), iron
oxide red and iron oxide yellow.
Dimotane Elixir: Sodium benzoate, citric acid anhydrous, sucrose, quinoline yellow (E104), cola flavour,
ethanol (96%), water.

*Incompatibilities:* Incompatibility has been reported
with some diatrizoate, iodipamide and iothalamate
salts.

*Shelf life:* Dimotane Tablets, Dimotane Elixir: Three
years. Dimotane LA: Four years.

*Special precautions for storage:* Dimotane Tablets:
Store below 25°C. Protect from light. Dimotane LA:
Supplied in amber glass bottles, therefore no special
storage precautions are required, however the tablets
may discolour on exposure to strong sunlight. Dimotane Elixir: None

*Nature and contents of container:* Dimotane Tablets:
Amber glass screw cap bottle containing 28 tablets.
Dimotane LA: Amber glass screw cap bottle containing 28 tablets. Dimotane Elixir: Amber glass bottle
containing 500 ml

*Instructions for use/handling:* Not applicable.

**Marketing authorisation numbers**
Dimotane Tablets 0100/5004
Dimotane LA 0100/5006
Dimotane Elixir 0100/5005

**Date of approval/revision of the SPC** September
1996

**Legal category** P

# DIMOTANE* PLUS PAEDIATRIC
# DIMOTANE* PLUS

**Qualitative and quantitative composition** Dimotane
Plus Paediatric is a liquid preparation containing two
active ingredients, Brompheniramine Maleate BP
2.0 mg per 5 ml and Pseudoephedrine Hydrochloride
BP 5.0 mg per 5 ml.
This product also contains ethanol and sodium
benzoate.
Dimotane Plus is a liquid preparation containing
two active ingredients, Brompheniramine Maleate BP
4.0 mg per 5 ml and Pseudoephedrine Hydrochloride
BP 30.0 mg per 5 ml.
This product also contains ethanol and sodium
benzoate.

**Pharmaceutical form** Oral liquid.

**Clinical particulars**

*Therapeutic indications:* Symptomatic relief of allergic
rhinitis.

*Posology and method of administration:*

*Dimotane Plus Paediatric:* This product is recommended for paediatric use only:
Children:
6–12 years: 10 ml three times daily.
2–5 years: 5 ml three times daily.
Children under 2 years: not recommended.
The dosage interval should not be less than four
hours.
Do not exceed three doses per day.

*Dimotane Plus:*
Adults and older patients: 10 ml three times daily.
Children 6–12 years: 5 ml three times daily.
Children 2–5 years: 2.5 ml three times daily. Dimo-
tane Plus Paediatric is recommended.
Children under 2 years: not recommended.
The dosage interval should not be less than four
hours. Do not exceed three doses per day.

*Contra-indications:* Hypersensitivity to the active ingredients. Coma or pre-coma states. Known brain
disease or epilepsy. Use in patients with acute
ischaemic heart disease. Thyrotoxicosis. Glaucoma or
urinary retention. Patients currently receiving or who
have within two weeks received, monoamine oxidase
inhibitors or tricyclic antidepressants. Patients receiving other sympathomimetic drugs. Hypertension or
patients receiving antihypertensive therapy.

*Special warnings and precautions for use:* In common
with many other antihistamines, brompheniramine
has an atropine-like action and should therefore be
used with caution in patients with bronchial asthma,
especially children. May act as a cerebral stimulant in
children and occasionally in adults. If this occurs it is
possible that insomnia, nervousness, hyperpyrexia or
tremor may occur and very rarely epileptiform convulsions. Therefore children taking this product
should not be left unattended for long periods. Should
be used in caution in patients receiving digitalis,
adrenergic blockers or non-steroidal anti-inflammatory drugs.

*Interactions with other medicaments and other forms
of interaction:* May potentiate the effects of CNS
depressants including alcohol. The effects of anticholinergic drugs may be potentiated.

*Pregnancy and lactation:* This product should not be
used in pregnancy unless considered essential by the
physician.

*Effects on the ability to drive and use machines:*
Drowsiness may occur. Patients receiving this product
should not drive or operate machinery unless it has
been shown that their physical and mental capability
remains unaffected.

*Undesirable effects:* None known

*Overdose:* Gastric lavage together with appropriate
supporting therapy dependent upon individual response to the constituents of the preparation.

**Pharmacological properties**

*Pharmacodynamic properties:* Dimotane Plus and
Dimotane Plus Paediatric have been formulated to
combine an anti-histamine (brompheniramine maleate) and a decongestant (pseudoephedrine hydrochloride) for use in allergic rhinitis for paediatric use only.

*Pharmacokinetic properties:* Dimotane Plus Paediatric
is a liquid preparation containing two active ingredients, (Brompheniramine Maleate 2.0 mg/5 ml and
Pseudoephedrine Hydrochloride 15.0 mg/5 ml).
Dimotane Plus is a liquid preparation containing
two active ingredients, (Brompheniramine Maleate
4.0 mg/5 ml and Pseudoephedrine Hydrochloride
30.0 mg/5 ml).
The pharmacokinetic characteristics of both active
ingredients are well documented in the standard
reference texts, such as 'Martindale–The Extra Pharmacopoeia, 29th Edition'. The dosage regime com-

plies with the requirements of the text and the BNF for both active ingredients.

**Pharmaceutical particulars**

*List of excipients:* Glycerol, sodium carboxymethyl cellulose, saccharin sodium, sodium benzoate, disodium edetate, Lycasin, ethanol, citric acid, purified water, caramel (E150), grape flavour, Hyflo Supercel.

*Incompatibilities:* None known

*Shelf life:* Two years.

*Special precautions for storage:* There are no special storage precautions for this product

*Nature and contents of container:* This product will be presented in amber glass bottles with screw caps or jay caps. Bottles size 500 ml.

*Instructions for use/handling:* Not applicable.

**Marketing authorisation numbers**
Dimotane Plus Paediatric 0100/0086
Dimotane Plus 0100/0085

**Date of approval/revision of SPC** October 1995

**Legal category** POM

## EFEXOR* ▼

**Presentation** Efexor are peach coloured, shield-shaped tablets impressed with the tablet strength and embossed with the Wyeth logo on one side, and plain on the other.

Efexor Tablets are available containing 37.5, 50 or 75 mg of venlafaxine as hydrochloride.

**Uses** Efexor is indicated for the treatment of depressive illness in both hospitalised patients and outpatients.

**Dosage and administration**

*Adults:* The usual recommended dose is 75 mg per day given in two divided doses (37.5 mg twice daily). If, after several weeks, further clinical improvement is required, the dose may be increased to 150 mg per day given in two divided doses (75 mg twice daily).

If, in the judgement of the physician, a higher dose is required, for example in more severely depressed or hospitalised patients, a starting dose of 150 mg per day may be given in two divided doses (75 mg twice daily). The daily dose may then be increased by up to 75 mg every two or three days until the desired response is achieved. The maximum recommended dose is 375 mg per day. The dose should then be gradually reduced to the usual dosage, consistent with patient response and tolerance.

It is recommended that Efexor be taken with food.

*Patients with renal or hepatic impairment:* For patients with mild renal impairment (GFR >30 ml/minute) or mild hepatic impairment (PT <14 seconds), no change in dosage is necessary.

For patients with moderate renal impairment (GFR 10–30 ml/minute) or moderate hepatic impairment (PT 14–18 seconds), the dose should be reduced by 50%. This dose may be given once daily due to the longer half-lives of venlafaxine and O-desmethylvenlafaxine in these patients.

Insufficient data are available to support the use of Efexor in patients with severe renal impairment (GFR <10 ml/minute) or severe hepatic impairment (PT >18 seconds).

*Elderly patients:* No adjustment in the usual dosage is recommended for elderly patients.In a trial investigating the kinetics of venlafaxine in the elderly, the half-life (at steady-state conditions) was prolonged by 1–2 hours, mainly in the male subjects. This was apparently due to an 18% reduction in the clearance of venlafaxine and O-desmethylvenlafaxine. The small increase in steady-state plasma levels of venlafaxine and O-desmethylvenlafaxine which resulted, was not judged to be clinically significant; no adjustment in dosage is necessary. However, as with any therapy, caution should be exercised in treating the elderly (eg. due to the possibility of renal impairment. See also dosage recommendations for renal impairment). The lowest effective dose should always be used and patients should be carefully monitored when an increase in the dose is required.

*Maintenance/continuation/extended treatment:* The physician should periodically re-evaluate the usefulness of long-term treatment with Efexor for the individual patient. It is generally agreed that acute episodes of major depression require several months or longer of sustained therapy. Efexor has been shown to be efficacious during long-term (up to 12 months) treatment.

*Discontinuing Efexor:* No definitive withdrawal syndrome has been observed with Efexor. During clinical trials, symptoms reported on abrupt discontinuation of Efexor from daily doses of 150 mg or more included fatigue, nausea and dizziness and one episode of hypomania. Discontinuation effects are well known to occur with antidepressants; therefore, when Efexor has been administered for more than one week and is then stopped, it is generally recommended that the dose be reduced gradually over a few days and the patient monitored in order to minimise the risk of discontinuation symptoms. Patients who have received Efexor for six weeks or more should have their dose reduced gradually over at least a one-week period.

*Children:* Safety and effectiveness in individuals below 18 years of age have not been established and such use is not recommended.

**Contra-indications, warnings, etc**

*Contra-indications:*

(1) Known or suspected pregnancy.

(2) Insufficient data are available to support the use of Efexor in lactating women. Therefore, such use is contra-indicated.

(3) Known hypersensitivity to venlafaxine or any other component of the product.

(4) Concomitant use of Efexor with monoamine oxidase inhibitors.

(5) Safety and effectiveness in individuals below 18 years of age have not been established and such use is not recommended.

*Pregnancy and lactation:* The safety of Efexor for use during human pregnancy has not been established. Therefore, the use of Efexor during known or suspected pregnancy is contra-indicated. Patients should be advised to notify their physician if they become pregnant or intend to become pregnant during therapy.

Insufficient data are available to support the use of Efexor in lactating women. Therefore, such use is contra-indicated.

*Precautions and warnings:*

(1) The risk of suicide must be considered in all depressed patients. The smallest quantity of tablets should be prescribed consistent with good patient management in order to reduce the possibility of overdose.

(2) During the development of Efexor, 0.2% of patients had a convulsion or event described as possibly having been a seizure. Although this rate was low and all the patients recovered, Efexor (as with all antidepressants) should be introduced with caution in patients with a history of epilepsy and should be discontinued in any patient developing a seizure whilst taking Efexor.

(3) During clinical trials, rash developed in 4% of patients given Efexor. Patients should be advised to notify their physician if they develop a rash, urticaria, or a related allergic phenomenon.

(4) Three percent (3%) of the 2,181 patients who received Efexor in clinical trials were judged to have clinically significant blood pressure increases. The increases were dose-related. In general, patients treated with 200 mg/day or less, showed minor increases, while in a short-term dose-ranging study, the highest dose (300 to 375 mg/day) was associated with mean increases in supine and diastolic blood pressure of approximately 4 mm Hg by week 4, and 7 mm Hg by week 6. The presence of treated hypertension or elevated blood pressure at baseline did not seem to predispose patients to further increases during Efexor therapy. For patients treated with doses greater than 200 mg/day routine blood pressure monitoring may be advisable.

(5) Due to the possibility of drug abuse with CNS active drugs, physicians should evaluate patients for a history of drug abuse and follow such patients closely. Clinical studies have shown no evidence of drug-seeking behaviour, development of tolerance, or dose escalation over time among patients taking Efexor.

(6) Efexor has not been evaluated or used to any appreciable extent in patients with a recent history of myocardial infarction or unstable heart disease and, therefore, should be used with caution in these patients. No serious arrhythmias were observed in patients treated with venlafaxine, and mean PR, QRS or QTc intervals were not significantly prolonged. The mean heart rate was increased by approximately 4 beats/minute during treatment.

(7) The clearances of venlafaxine and its active metabolite are decreased and half-lives increased in patients with moderate to severe renal impairment or cirrhosis of the liver. Therefore, Efexor should be used with caution in these patients. A lower or less frequent dose may be necessary in such patients as indicated in the Dosage and Administration Section.

(8) Although Efexor has been shown not to affect psychomotor, cognitive, or complex behaviour performance in healthy volunteers, any psychoactive drug may impair judgement, thinking or motor skills and therefore patients should be cautioned about their ability to drive a car or operate hazardous machinery.

(9) Postural hypotension has been observed occasionally during Efexor treatment. Patients, especially the elderly, should be alerted to the possibility dizziness or unsteadiness.

(10) Women of childbearing potential should ploy adequate contraception whilst taking Efexor.

*Interactions:* Adverse reactions, some serious, h been reported when Efexor therapy has been initia soon after discontinuation of an MAOI and when MAOI has been initiated soon after discontinuatio Efexor. Given these reactions as well as the seri sometimes fatal interactions reported with conco tant or immediately consecutive administration MAOIs and other antidepressants with pharmaco ical properties similar to Efexor, do not use Efexo combination with an MAOI or within at least 14 d of discontinuing MAOI treatment. Allow at leas days after stopping Efexor before starting an MAO

The risk of using Efexor in combination with ot CNS-active drugs has not been systematically ev ated, except in the case of lithium and diazep Consequently, caution is advised if the concomit administration of Efexor and other such drugs required.

In an interaction study, although lithium sign cantly reduced the renal clearance of venlafaxine effect on the renal clearance of the active metabol O-desmethylvenlafaxine, was small. Therefore, si the major route of elimination of venlafaxine is metabolism to O-desmethylvenlafaxine, and not re excretion, the total clearance values for venlafax and its metabolite were not significantly affected was also found that venlafaxine itself had no sign cant effect on the kinetics of lithium.

The pharmacokinetic profiles of venlafaxine and desmethylvenlafaxine were not significantly alte by the administration of diazepam. Venlafaxine no effect on the pharmacokinetic profile of diazep or on the psychomotor or psychometric effe induced by diazepam.

Cimetidine inhibited the first-pass metabolism venlafaxine but had no significant effect on formation or elimination of O-desmethylvenlafax which is present in much greater quantities in systemic circulation. No dosage adjustment theref seems necessary when Efexor is coadministered w cimetidine. For elderly patients or patients w hepatic dysfunction, the interaction could potenti be more pronounced. Therefore, clinical monitor is recommended when Efexor is administered w cimetidine in these patients.

The pharmacokinetic profiles of venlafaxine, desmethylvenlafaxine, and ethanol were not alte when venlafaxine and ethanol were administe together to healthy volunteers who consumed alco on an occasional basis (equivalent to 3 to 30 oun of ethanol per month). The administration of venlaf ine in a stable regimen did not potentiate the psyc motor and psychometric effects induced by etha in these same social drinkers when they were receiving venlafaxine.

There is no evidence suggesting incompatib between treatment with Efexor and treatment w either antihypertensives, (including β-blockers, A inhibitors and diuretics) or hypoglycaemic agents.

*Side-effects:* In clinical studies the following adve events occurred most frequently with Efexor a occurred more frequently than placebo; naus headache, insomnia, somnolence, dry mouth, di ness, constipation, asthenia, sweating and nervo ness.

The occurrence of most of these adverse eve was dose-related and the majority of them decreas in intensity and frequency over time. They gener did not lead to cessation of treatment.

Other adverse events which occurred less of were, in order of decreasing frequency: anore dyspepsia, abdominal pain, anxiety, impotence, normality of accommodation, vasodilation, vomiti tremor, paraesthesia, abnormal ejaculation/orgas chills, hypertension, palpitation, weight gain , ag tion, decreased libido.

Clinically significant weight change was seen in l than 1% of patients treated with Efexor in clin trials.

The adverse events, nausea and impotence are w known to be associated with drugs having sero nergic activity.

The overall incidence of nausea associated w Efexor in placebo-controlled studies was 36% co pared to 12% in placebo-treated patients. This in dence decreased with time reducing to a le comparable with placebo after 3 weeks. The naus experienced was usually mild to moderate, a infrequently resulted in vomiting or withdrawal.

The incidence of nausea is also dose related wit reduced incidence being shown at the usual dose 75 mg/day. The incidence is likely to increase at higher end of the dose range, particularly when dos are increased rapidly.

The overall incidence of impotence in clinical tri was 7%.

Treatment with Efexor was associated with

crease in blood pressure in some patients during nical trials (see *Precautions and warnings*).

Postural hypotension has been observed occasion- y during Efexor treatment.

Reversible increases of liver enzymes were seen in small number (0.5%) of patients during clinical trials ith Efexor.

Alterations in serum cholesterol have been seen in me patients treated with Efexor. A mean increase approximately 0.07 mmol/litre from baseline was oserved in patients treated with Efexor. The clinical gnificance of this is not known.

Cases of hyponatraemia have rarely been reported ith antidepressants, including SSRIs, usually in the derly and in patients taking diuretics and/or other- se volume depleted. Similarly cases of hyponatrae- ia have rarely been reported with Efexor, usually in e elderly, which have resolved upon discontinuation the drug.

*verdose:* In post-marketing experience, electrocar- ogram changes (e.g. prolongation of QT interval, undle branch block, QRS prolongation), sinus and ntricular tachycardia, bradycardia and seizures have een reported in association with overdosage of enlafaxine, usually when in combination with over- ose of this drug and/or alcohol. Such events are rare nd usually resolve spontaneously.

anagement of Overdosage; Ensure an adequate rway, oxygenation and ventilation. Monitoring of rdiac rhythm and vital signs is recommended as are eneral supportive and symptomatic measures. Use activated charcoal, induction of emesis or gastric vage should be considered. No specific antidotes r Efexor are known.

The haemodialysis clearance of venlafaxine and its ain active metabolite are low, therefore, they are ot considered dialysable.

**harmaceutical particulars**

*st of ingredients:* The active constituent is venlafax- e as hydrochloride. Other constituents are micro- ystalline cellulose, lactose, sodium starch glycollate, agnesium stearate, yellow and brown iron oxide.

*helf-life:* Three years

*pecial precautions for storage:* Store in a dry place room temperature (at or below 30°C)

**egal category** POM

**ackage quantities**

37.5 and 75 mg tablets: Blister packs containing 56 blets.

50 mg tablets: Blister packs containing 42 tablets

**urther information** Efexor is a structurally novel ntidepressant which is chemically unrelated to tri- yclic, tetracyclic, or other available antidepressant gents. It is a racemate with two active enantiomers.

The mechanism of Efexor's antidepressant action humans is believed to be associated with its otentiation of neurotransmitter activity in the central ervous system. Preclinical studies have shown that enlafaxine and its major metabolite, O-desmethyl- enlafaxine, are potent neuronal serotonin and norad- naline re-uptake inhibitors (SNRI) and weak hibitors of dopamine reuptake. In addition, venlafax- e and O-desmethylvenlafaxine reduce β-adrenergic sponsiveness in animals after both acute (single ose) and chronic administration. Venlafaxine and its ajor metabolite appear to be equipotent with respect their overall action on neurotransmitter re-uptake.

Venlafaxine has virtually no affinity for rat brain uscarinic, histaminergic or adrenergic receptors *in itro*. Pharmacologic activity at these receptors may e related to various side-effects seen with other ntidepressant drugs, such as anticholinergic, seda- ve and cardiovascular effects.

*harmacokinetic properties:* Venlafaxine is well ab- orbed and undergoes extensive first-pass metabo- sm. Mean peak plasma concentrations of venlafaxine ange from approximately 33 to 172ng/ml after 25 to 50 mg single doses, and are reached in approxi- ately 2.4 hours. Venlafaxine is extensively metabol- ed in the liver. O-desmethylvenlafaxine is the major ctive metabolite of venlafaxine. The mean disposition alf-life of venlafaxine and O-desmethylvenlafaxine is pproximately 5 and 11 hours, respectively. Mean eak O-desmethyl venlafaxine plasma concentrations ange from approximately 61 to 325ng/ml and are eached in approximately 4.3 hours. Plasma concen- ations of venlafaxine and O-desmethylvenlafaxine enerally correlated well with dose levels. Venlafaxine nd O-desmethylvenlafaxine are 27% and 30% bound plasma proteins respectively. O-desmethylvenla- axine, other minor venlafaxine metabolites, and non- etabolised venlafaxine are excreted primarily rough the kidneys.

**roduct licence numbers**

7.5 mg 0011/0199
0 mg 0011/0200
5 mg 0011/0201

# EFEXOR* XL ▼

**Qualitative and quantitative composition** There are two strengths of Efexor XL capsules, containing 84.4 mg or 168.8 mg of venlafaxine hydrochloride, equivalent to 75 mg or 150 mg of venlafaxine free base, in an extended release formulation. Venlafaxine is chemically defined as (R/S)-1-[(2-dimethylamino)-1-(4-methoxy phenyl)ethyl]cyclohexanol hydrochloride.

**Pharmaceutical form** Efexor XL 75 mg capsules are opaque peach modified release capsules printed in red with 'W' and '75'. Efexor XL 150 mg capsules are opaque dark orange modified release capsules printed in white with 'W' and '150'.

**Clinical particulars**

*Therapeutic indications:* Efexor XL is indicated for the treatment of depressive illness.

*Posology and method of administration:* The recommended dose for Efexor XL is 75 mg, given once daily. If after 2 weeks further clinical improvement is required, the dose may be increased to 150 mg once daily. If needed, the dose can be further increased up to 225 mg once daily. Dose increments should be made at intervals of approximately 2 weeks or more, but not less than 4 days. Antidepressant activity with the 75 mg dose was observed after 2 weeks of treatment.

Efexor XL should be taken with food. Each capsule should be swallowed whole with fluid. Do not divide, crush, chew, or place the capsule in water. Efexor XL should be administered once daily, at approximately the same time, either in the morning or in the evening.

Depressed patients who are currently being treated with Efexor Tablets may be switched to Efexor XL. For example, a patient receiving Efexor Tablets 37.5 mg b.d. would receive Efexor XL 75 mg o.d. When switching, individual dosage adjustments may be necessary.

*Patients with renal or hepatic impairment:* The half lives of venlafaxine and O-desmethylvenlafaxine are increased in patients with renal and hepatic impairment.

For patients with mild renal impairment (GFR > 30 ml/minute) or mild hepatic impairment, no change in dosage is necessary.

For patients with moderate renal impairment (GFR 10-30 ml/minute) or moderate hepatic impairment, the dose should be reduced by 50%. For patients requiring a lower daily dose than 75 mg, treatment may be provided with Efexor Tablets.

Insufficient data are available to support the use of Efexor XL in patients with severe renal impairment (GFR < 10 ml/minute) or severe hepatic impairment.

*Elderly patients:* No adjustment from the usual dosage is recommended for elderly patients. However, as with any therapy, caution should be exercised in treating the elderly (e.g. due to the possibility of renal impairment. See also dosage recommendations for renal impairment). The lowest effective dose should always be used, and patients should be carefully monitored when an increase in the dose is required.

*Paediatric use:* Safety and effectiveness in individuals below 18 years of age have not been established, and such use is not recommended.

*Maintenance/continuation/extended treatment:* The physician should periodically re-evaluate the usefulness of long-term Efexor XL treatment for the individual patient. It is generally agreed that acute episodes of major depression require several months or longer of sustained pharmacological therapy.

Venlafaxine has been shown to be efficacious during long-term (up to 12 months) treatment.

*Discontinuing Efexor XL:* Patients who have received Efexor XL at a dosage of 150 mg/day or greater for more than 1 week, or who have received a lower dose of Efexor XL for 6 weeks or more, should have their dose reduced gradually over at least a 1-week period to minimise the risk of discontinuation symptoms.

*Contra-indications:*

1. Known or suspected pregnancy.
2. Insufficient data are available to support the use of Efexor XL in lactating women. Therefore, such use is contra-indicated.
3. Known hypersensitivity to venlafaxine or any other component of the product.
4. Concomitant use of venlafaxine with monoamine oxidase inhibitors.
5. Paediatric Use–Safety and effectiveness in individuals below 18 years of age have not been established, and such use is not recommended.

*Special warnings and precautions for use:* Women of childbearing potential should employ adequate contraception whilst taking Efexor XL.

The risk of suicide attempt must be considered in all depressed patients. Prescriptions for Efexor XL should be written for the smallest quantity of capsules consistent with good patient management in order to reduce the possibility of overdose.

In clinical trials with venlafaxine, seizures were reported in 0.2% of all venlafaxine-treated patients. All patients recovered. No seizures occurred in Efexor XL-treated patients during clinical trials. However, as with all antidepressants, Efexor XL should be introduced with care in patients with a history of seizure and should be discontinued in any patient who develops seizures.

During clinical trials, rash developed in 3% of patients treated with venlafaxine. Patients should be advised to notify their physician if they develop a rash, urticaria or related allergic phenomenon.

Clinical studies have shown no evidence of drug-seeking behaviour, development of tolerance, or dose escalation over time among patients taking venlafaxine. However, physicians should evaluate patients for a history of drug abuse, and follow such patients closely, observing them for signs of misuse or abuse of Efexor XL.

The clearances of venlafaxine and its active metabolite are decreased and half-lives increased in patients with moderate to severe renal impairment or cirrhosis of the liver. Therefore, Efexor XL should be used with caution in these patients. A lower daily dose might be necessary in such patients and treatment may be provided with Efexor Tablets as indicated above under 'Posology and Method of Administration'.

Venlafaxine has not been evaluated or used to any appreciable extent in patients with a recent history of myocardial infarction or unstable heart disease. Therefore, it should be used with caution in these patients. Clinically significant electrocardiogram findings were observed in 1% of the venlafaxine-treated patients compared with 0.2% of the placebo-treated patients. Clinically significant changes in PR, QRS or QTc intervals were rarely observed in patients treated with venlafaxine during clinical trials. The mean heart rate was increased by approximately 4 beats/minute during treatment with venlafaxine.

Increases in blood pressure have been reported in patients treated with high doses of venlafaxine. Blood pressure monitoring is advisable in patients receiving daily doses of >200 mg.

*Interactions with other medicaments and other forms of interaction:* Adverse reactions, some serious, have been reported when venlafaxine therapy is initiated soon after discontinuation of an MAOI, and when an MAOI is initiated soon after discontinuation of venlafaxine. Given these reactions as well as the serious, sometimes fatal interactions reported with concomitant or immediately consecutive administration of MAOIs and other antidepressants with pharmacological properties similar to Efexor XL, do not use Efexor XL in combination with an MAOI, or within at least 14 days of discontinuing MAOI treatment. Allow at least 7 days after stopping Efexor XL before starting an MAOI.

The risk of using venlafaxine in combination with other CNS-active drugs has not been systematically evaluated, except in the case of lithium, imipramine and diazepam. Caution is advised if the concomitant administration of Efexor XL and other CNS-active drugs is required.

The pharmacokinetic profiles of venlafaxine and its active metabolite O-desmethylvenlafaxine (ODV) were not altered when Efexor Tablets and diazepam, Efexor Tablets and lithium, or Efexor Tablets and ethanol (0.5 g/kg/day) were administered together to healthy volunteers. Venlafaxine had no effect on the pharmacokinetic profiles of diazepam, lithium or ethanol in these studies. Administration of Efexor Tablets did not affect the psychomotor and psychometric effects induced by diazepam or ethanol.

Venlafaxine did not affect the hepatic metabolism of the tricyclic antidepressant, imipramine or its active metabolite, desipramine. However, the renal clearance of 2-hydroxy desipramine was reduced with coadministration of Efexor Tablets. Imipramine partially inhibited the formation of ODV. However, no dosage adjustment of either drug is necessary when Efexor XL and imipramine are given concomitantly.

Cimetidine inhibited the first-pass metabolism of venlafaxine, but had no apparent effect on the formation or elimination of ODV, which is present in much greater quantities in the systemic circulation. Therefore, no dosage adjustment seems necessary when Efexor XL is coadministered with cimetidine. For elderly patients, or patients with hepatic dysfunction, the interaction could potentially be more pronounced, and for such patients, clinical monitoring is indicated when Efexor XL is administered with cimetidine.

Venlafaxine is primarily metabolised to its equally active metabolite, ODV, by the cytochrome P450 enzyme CYP2D6. However, unlike many other antidepressants, no dosage adjustment is necessary when Efexor XL is administered concomitantly with drugs which inhibit CYP2D6, or when used in patients who are poor CYP2D6 metabolisers, since the total concentration of active compound (venlafaxine and ODV) is not affected.

Venlafaxine is a relatively weak inhibitor of CYP2D6, and does not inhibit CYP1A2, CYP2C9 or CYP3A4. Therefore, Efexor XL is not expected to interact with other drugs metabolised by these hepatic enzymes.

The major elimination pathways for venlafaxine are through CYP2D6 and CYP3A4. Therefore, caution should be used with concomitant intake of drugs which inhibit both of these enzymes. Such interactions have not been studied to date.

Venlafaxine and ODV are 27% and 30% bound to plasma proteins. Therefore, drug interactions due to protein binding of venlafaxine and the major metabolite are not expected.

There is no evidence suggesting incompatibility between treatment with venlafaxine and treatment with either antihypertensives (including β-blockers, ACE inhibitors and diuretics) or hypoglycaemic agents.

There are no clinical studies to evaluate the benefit of combined use of Efexor XL with another antidepressant or electroconvulsive therapy (ECT).

*Pregnancy and lactation:* The safety of Efexor XL for use during human pregnancy has not been established. Therefore, the use of Efexor XL during known or suspected pregnancy is contra-indicated. Patients should be advised to notify their physician if they become pregnant, or intend to become pregnant during therapy.

Insufficient data are available to support the use of venlafaxine in lactating women. In preclinical studies, venlafaxine and ODV were found to pass into maternal milk. It is not known whether venlafaxine or its metabolites are excreted in human milk. Therefore, such use is contra-indicated.

*Effects on ability to drive and use machines:* Although venlafaxine has been shown not to affect psychomotor, cognitive or complex behaviour performance in healthy volunteers, any psychoactive drug may impair judgement, thinking or motor skills. Therefore, patients should be cautioned about their ability to drive or operate hazardous machinery.

*Undesirable effects:* The most commonly observed adverse events associated with the use of venlafaxine in clinical trials, which were not seen at an equivalent incidence in placebo-treated patients, were:- nausea, insomnia, dry mouth, somnolence, dizziness, constipation, sweating, nervousness, asthenia and abnormal ejaculation/orgasm.

Other adverse events occurring in at least 3% of patients and more frequently (greater than 1% difference) with venlafaxine than with placebo, were:- anorexia, abnormal vision/accommodation, impotence, vomiting, tremor, abnormal dreams, vasodilatation, hypertension, rash, agitation, hypertonia and paraesthesia.

The occurrence of most of these adverse events was dose-related, and the majority of them decreased in intensity and frequency over time. They generally did not lead to cessation of treatment.

In clinical studies the incidence of nausea was lower, and the adaptation to nausea appeared to be improved, with Efexor XL compared with Efexor Tablets. A two- to three-fold reduction in the incidence and severity of nausea was observed with Efexor XL when compared with Efexor Tablets in studies with non-depressed subjects.

Of the patients who received venlafaxine in all premarketing trials, 2.2% were judged to have had clinically significant blood pressure increases compared with 0.4% of placebo-treated patients. In studies with Efexor Tablets, the increases in blood pressure were dose-related. In general, patients treated with ≤200 mg per day showed minor increases, while in a short-term dose ranging study, the highest dose (300-375 mg/day) was associated with mean increases in supine diastolic blood pressure of approximately 4 mm Hg by week 4, and 7 mm Hg by week 6. The presence of treated hypertension or elevated blood pressure at baseline did not seem to predispose patients to further increases during venlafaxine therapy.

Postural hypotension was observed, and considered clinically significant in 0.4% of patients treated with Efexor Tablets and 0.8% of comparator-treated patients. As with other antidepressants, this effect may be more apparent in the elderly.

Reversible increases in liver enzymes were seen during clinical trials in a small number of patients (0.5%) treated with Efexor Tablets.

Alterations in serum cholesterol are seen in some patients treated with venlafaxine. A mean increase of 0.07 mmol/litre from baseline was observed in patients treated with Efexor Tablets, a change of unknown clinical significance.

Clinically significant weight gain or loss was seen in less than 1% of patients treated with venlafaxine during all premarketing trials.

Cases of hyponatraemia have rarely been reported with antidepressants including SSRIs, usually in the elderly and in patients taking diuretics or who are otherwise volume depleted. Similarly, cases of hyponatraemia have been reported rarely with Efexor Tablets, usually in the elderly, which have resolved on discontinuation of the drug.

During clinical trials, symptoms reported on abrupt cessation of Efexor Tablets included fatigue, nausea, dizziness, and one episode of hypomania. In addition, during dose reduction or following discontinuation of Efexor XL, the following events occurred at two or more times the placebo incidence: dizziness, dry mouth, insomnia, nausea, nervousness and sweating. Discontinuation effects are well known to occur with antidepressants. Therefore, it is recommended that the dosage of Efexor XL is reduced gradually and the patient monitored.

*Overdose:* Among the patients treated with Efexor XL in premarketing evaluations, there were 2 reports of acute overdosage, either alone or in combination with other drugs. One patient took a combination of 6 g of Efexor XL and 2.5 mg of lorazepam. This patient was hospitalised, treated symptomatically, and recovered without any untoward effects. The other patient took 2.85 g of Efexor XL. This patient reported paraesthesia in all four limbs, but recovered without sequelae.

In post-marketing experience with Efexor Tablets, electrocardiogram changes (e.g. prolongation of QT interval, bundle branch block, QRS prolongation), sinus and ventricular tachycardia, bradycardia and seizures have been reported in association with overdosage of Efexor Tablets, either alone or in combination with other drugs and/or alcohol. Such events are rare and usually resolve spontaneously.

*Management of overdosage:* Ensure an adequate airway, oxygenation and ventilation. Monitoring of cardiac rhythm and vital signs is recommended. General supportive and symptomatic measures are also recommended. Use of activated charcoal, induction of emesis, or gastric lavage should be considered. No specific antidotes for venlafaxine are known.

The haemodialysis clearance of venlafaxine and its main metabolite, ODV, are low. Therefore, they are not considered dialysable.

**Pharmacological properties** Venlafaxine is a structurally novel antidepressant which is chemically unrelated to tricyclic, tetracyclic, or other available antidepressants. It is a racemate with two active enantiomers.

*Pharmacodynamic properties:* The mechanism of venlafaxine's antidepressant action in humans is believed to be associated with its potentiation of neurotransmitter activity in the central nervous system. Preclinical studies have shown that venlafaxine and its major metabolite, ODV, are potent inhibitors of serotonin and noradrenaline reuptake. Venlafaxine also weakly inhibits dopamine uptake. Studies in animals show that tricyclic antidepressants may reduce β-adrenergic responsiveness following chronic administration. In contrast, venlafaxine and ODV reduce β-adrenergic responsiveness after both acute (single dose) and chronic administration. Venlafaxine and ODV are very similar with respect to their overall action on neurotransmitter reuptake.

Venlafaxine has virtually no affinity for rat brain muscarinic cholinergic, $H_1$ histaminergic or $\alpha_1$-adrenergic receptors *in vitro*. Pharmacological activity at these receptors may be related to various side effects seen with other antidepressant drugs, such as anticholinergic, sedative and cardiovascular side effects.

Venlafaxine does not possess monoamine oxidase (MAO) inhibitory activity.

*In vitro* studies revealed that venlafaxine has virtually no affinity for opiate, benzodiazepine, phencyclidine (PCP), or N-methyl-d-aspartic acid (NMDA) receptors. It has no significant central nervous system (CNS) stimulant activity in rodents. In primate drug discrimination studies, venlafaxine showed no significant stimulant or depressant abuse liability.

*Pharmacokinetic properties:* At least 92% of a single oral dose of venlafaxine is absorbed. After administration of Efexor XL, the peak plasma concentrations of venlafaxine and ODV are attained within 6.0 ± 1.5 and 8.8 ± 2.2 hours, respectively. The rate of absorption of venlafaxine from the Efexor XL capsules is slower than its rate of elimination. Therefore, the apparent elimination half-life of venlafaxine following administration of Efexor XL capsules (15 ± 6 hours) is actually the absorption half-life instead of the true disposition half-life (5 ± 2 hours) observed following administration of an immediate release tablet.

When equal daily doses of venlafaxine were administered as either the immediate release tablet, or the extended release capsule, the exposure (AUC, area under the concentration curve) to both venlafaxine and ODV was similar for the two treatments, and the fluctuation in plasma concentrations was slightly lower following treatment with the Efexor XL capsule. Therefore, the Efexor XL capsule provides a slower rate of absorption, but the same extent of absorptic (i.e. AUC), as the Efexor immediate release tablet.

Venlafaxine undergoes extensive first-pass meta olism in the liver, primarily by CYP2D6, to the maj metabolite ODV. Venlafaxine is also metabolised N-desmethylvenlafaxine, catalysed by CYP3A3/4, ar to other minor metabolites.

Venlafaxine and its metabolites are excreted p marily through the kidneys. Approximately 87% of venlafaxine dose is recovered in the urine within 4 hours as either unchanged venlafaxine, unconjugate ODV, conjugated ODV, or other minor metabolites.

Administration of Efexor XL with food has no effe on the absorption of venlafaxine, or on the subseque formation of ODV.

Subject age and sex do not significantly affect th pharmacokinetics of venlafaxine. No accumulation venlafaxine or ODV has been observed during chron administration in healthy subjects.

*Preclinical safety data:* Studies with venlafaxine in ra and mice revealed no evidence of carcinogenesi Venlafaxine was not mutagenic in a wide range of *in vitro* and *in vivo* tests.

**Pharmaceutical particulars**

*List of excipients:* Microcrystalline cellulose, ethylce lulose, hydroxypropyl methylcellulose, gelatin, re and yellow iron oxides (E172), titanium dioxide (E17 and printing ink.

*Incompatibilities:* None known.

*Shelf Life:* Two years.

*Special precautions for storage:* Store in a dry plac at room temperature (at or below 25°C).

*Nature and contents of container:* PVC/aluminium fc blister packs of 28 capsules.

*Instructions for use/handling:* Not applicable

**Marketing authorisation numbers**

Efexor XL 75 mg: 00011/0223
Efexor XL 150 mg: 00011/0224

**Date of first authorisation** 5 August 1997

**Date of approval/revision of SPC** May 1997

**Legal category** POM

## EQUAGESIC*

**Presentation** Equagesic tablets are three layer, fl bevel-edged tablets, 12.0 mm in diameter. A whi layer is sandwiched between a yellow layer and a pir layer. The yellow face is marked WYETH and the pir face is plain.

Each tablet contains:
Ethoheptazine citrate 75 mg
Meprobamate BP 150 mg
Aspirin BP 250 mg

**Uses** Equagesic is an analgesic with muscle-relaxa properties indicated for short-term symptomatic trea ment of pain occurring in musculoskeletal disorders

**Dosage and administration** *Route of administratio* Oral

*Dosage: Adults:* Two tablets three or four times dai as needed for the relief of pain .

*Elderly:* The elderly may respond to lower doses ar half the normal adult dose or less may be sufficient.

*Children:* Not recommended for children.

**Contra-indications, warnings, etc**

*Contra-indications:*

1. Equagesic should not be used in patients know to be hypersensitive to the active ingredients or t compounds related to meprobamate such as carisc prodol or carbromal.

2. Meprobamate should not be used in patients wi a known propensity for dependence on drugs incluc ing alcohol and in patients susceptible to attacks acute intermittent porphyria.

3. Aspirin should not be used in patients with activ peptic ulceration, haemophilia or in renal disease.

4. Equagesic should not be used during lactation.

5. Equagesic should not be used concurrently wi coumarin-type anticoagulants.

6. Pregnancy: there is no evidence as to drug safe in human pregnancy nor is there evidence that it free from hazard. Do not use during pregnanc especially during the first three months, unless the are compelling reasons.

7. Do not give to children under 12 unless yo doctor tells you to, because of a possible associatic of aspirin with Reye's Syndrome.

*Precautions and warnings:*

1. This product may cause drowsiness. Patien receiving this medication should not drive or operat machinery unless the drug has been shown not t interfere with physical or mental ability.

2. Meprobamate may increase the effects of concu

ntly administered central nervous system depres- nts including alcohol.
3. The concurrent use of CNS depressant drugs ould be avoided in hepatic or renal insufficiency.
4. Meprobamate may induce seizures in epileptic tients, and meprobamate withdrawal may precipi- :e convulsions.
5. Like barbiturates, meprobamate causes induction liver enzymes, so that the availability and blood vels of drugs given concurrently that are metabol- ed in the liver may be affected. These include the llowing: systemic steroids (including oral contracep- 'es), phenytoin, griseofulvin, rifampicin, phenothia- es (such as chlorpromazine) and tricyclic tidepressants. The clinical importance of the effect enzyme induction by meprobamate on concurrently ministered agents has not been established.
6. Individual response in overdosage with mepro- mate is variable but in some cases the symptoms ay be severe. It is therefore advisable that caution ould be observed in prescribing drugs which ntain meprobamate to patients with depression or others who may be liable to suicidal ideation or ent.
7. Some degree of dependence may occasionally cur with meprobamate in certain cases if dosage commendations are exceeded with withdrawal mptoms on sudden discontinuation. This is more ely in individuals with emotionally unstable person- ties if the drug is taken over long periods, or in hers liable to alcohol or other drug dependence. eatment in these cases should be withdrawn grad- lly.
Equagesic is recommended for use for short periods ly and therefore the risk of dependence occurring ith this product is very small.

*spirin:* 8.(a) Aspirin may prolong labour and contrib- e to maternal and neonatal bleeding and is best oided at term. It may precipitate bronchospasm and ay induce attacks of asthma in susceptible subjects. spirin should only be used with great caution in tients with a history of peptic ulceration.
(b) Concomitant administration with certain other edications such as corticosteroids or oral hypogly- emics may require adjustment of dosage of the rious drugs. The action of uricosuric agents may be hibited.

*verdosage: Meprobamate:* Acute poisoning with eprobamate produces coma, shock, vasomotor and spiratory collapse. Very few suicide attempts have oved successful and documented fatal doses have nged from 12 g to 47.6 g. Recovery has occurred ter ingestion of similar large amounts (20–40 g). astric lavage is only effective within a short period drug ingestion as meprobamate is rapidly absorbed om the gastrointestinal tract. Blood concentrations ay be reduced by a regime of forced alkaline diuresis haemodialysis. Respiration may require assistance.
*spirin:* Overdosage with aspirin will result in the pearance of the signs and symptoms of salicylism. eatment of aspirin poisoning is largely symptomatic d directed towards correction of the acid-base lance and electrolyte balance of the plasma.

*de effects:* Drowsiness, dizziness and nausea may experienced with Equagesic but these symptoms ually disappear as treatment continues. Ataxia, miting, hypotension, paraesthesia and paradoxical citement may also occur.
Hypersensitivity reactions have been reported in out 2% of patients being treated with meprobamate. ese reactions include skin rashes, and may arise ter one to four doses of the drug. They may be eneralised or local, and include urticaria, itchy aculopapular rashes or erythema. Severe systemic actions with shaking, chills and fever, nausea and miting, hypotension and collapse have occasionally curred.
Blood disorders, including non-thrombocytopenic urpura, and rarely, thrombocytopenia, agranulocy- sis, aplastic anaemia and pancytopenia have oc- rred. Rarely reported reactions, usually occurring part of a generalised hypersensitivity reaction, clude hyperpyrexia, angioneurotic oedema, bron- ospasm, oliguria and anuria. Anaphylaxis, ery- ema multiforme, exfoliative dermatitis, stomatitis, octitis, Stevens Johnson syndrome and bullous ermatitis have also been reported.
Hypersensitivity reactions to aspirin may manifest emselves as asthma, skin reactions and shock. spirin may induce gastrointestinal haemorrhage, hich is occasionally severe but in most cases blood ss is not significant.

**harmaceutical precautions** Store in a cool dry place. eep tightly closed. Where necessary dispense Equa- esic tablets into suitable well-closed glass bottles.

**egal category** CD (Sch 3), POM

**ackage quantities** Bottles of 100 tablets

**Further information** Safety and efficacy have not been established beyond short-term use.

**Product licence number** 0011/5009R

## HibTITER*

**Presentation** HibTITER is a clear, colourless solution presented in single dose vials. Each vial contains 0.72 ml to allow easy withdrawal of the 0.5 ml dose. 0.5 ml contains 10 µg of purified Haemophilus b polysaccharide and approximately 25 µg of $CRM_{197}$ protein.

**Uses** HibTITER Haemophilus b Conjugate Vaccine (Diphtheria $CRM_{197}$ Protein Conjugate) is indicated for the immunisation of children from 2 months of age to prevent invasive diseases caused by *Haemophilus influenzae* type b.

**Dosage and administration** HibTITER is indicated for children from 2 months of age for the prevention of invasive Haemophilus b disease.

Immunisation against Haemophilus b disease is not normally required in children over 48 months of age. However, they may receive HibTITER if they are considered to be at increased risk of invasive Haemophilus b disease.

For infants 2 to 12 months of age, the immunising dose is three separate injections of 0.5 ml given at a minimum of one monthly intervals intramuscularly, preferably in the outer aspect of the *vastus lateralis* (mid-thigh). Children 13 months of age and over who have not been vaccinated previously should receive one intramuscular injection.

| *Age at first Immunisation (months)* | *Number of doses* |
|---|---|
| 2–12 | 3 |
| 13 and over | 1 |

HibTITER may be given to premature infants according to their chronological age.

HibTITER and Haemophilus type b polysaccharide conjugated to tetanus toxoid (PRP-T) vaccine may be used interchangeably in the UK primary immunisation schedule.

HibTITER may be administered in the same syringe as Trivax-AD† (Adsorbed Diphtheria, Tetanus and Pertussis vaccine (DTP)). No other DTP vaccine should be used.

*Instructions for mixing HibTITER and DTP vaccine:* Draw 0.5 ml of each vaccine into a syringe. Shake well. The vaccines should be administered within 30 minutes of mixing. If administration is delayed for over 30 minutes then the mixed vaccines and the syringe should be discarded in the normal way.

**Contra-indications, warnings, etc**
*Contra-indications:* Hypersensitivity to any component of the vaccine, including diphtheria toxoid. Acute infectious illness.

*Warnings:* HibTITER is not contraindicated in patients with impaired immune responsiveness, whether due to the use of immunosuppressive therapy, a genetic defect, human immunodeficiency virus (HIV) infection, or other causes. If the vaccine is used in persons deficient in producing antibody, the expected immune response may not be obtained. Deferral of administration of vaccine may be considered in individuals receiving immunosuppressive therapy.

*Pregnancy and lactation:* HibTITER is not recommended for use in pregnant or lactating women. No reproduction studies have been conducted with HibTITER in animals. It is not known whether HibTITER can cause foetal abnormalities when administered to pregnant women or affect reproduction capacity.

*Precautions:* HibTITER is for intramuscular use only. The vaccine should not be injected intradermally or intravenously, since the safety and immunogenicity of these routes have not been evaluated. As with the injection of any biological material, Adrenaline Injection (1:1000) should be available for immediate use should an anaphylactic or other allergic reaction occur.

HibTITER will not protect against *Haemophilus influenzae* other than b strains or other microorganisms that cause meningitis or septic disease.

If a child presents with acute febrile illness, the vaccination should be delayed.

As with any vaccine HibTITER may not protect 100% of individuals receiving the vaccine. Cases of Hib disease, although rare, may occur after vaccination.

As with any intramuscular injection, HibTITER should be given with caution to infants or children with thrombocytopenia or any condition that would contra-indicate intramuscular injection.

Antigenuria has been detected following receipt of Haemophilus b conjugate vaccine and therefore antigen detection in urine may not have diagnostic value in suspected Haemophilus b disease within two weeks of immunisation.

Immunisation with HibTITER does not substitute for routine diphtheria immunisation.

*Side-effects:* Local erythema, warmth or swelling (≥ 2 cm) have been reported at the site of injection.

Systemic effects which have been reported following the administration of HibTITER include fever, headache, malaise, irritability, prolonged crying, loss of appetite, vomiting, diarrhoea and rash including urticaria. Seizures and erythema multiforme have been reported more rarely.

Children 2–6 months of age who received HibTITER at the same time (but at a separate injection site) as Diphtheria and Tetanus Toxoid and Pertussis Vaccine Adsorbed (DTP) and Oral Polio Vaccine (OPV) or DTP and Inactivated Polio Vaccine (IPV) showed no difference in the rate and type of reactions seen when DTP or DTP-IPV was administered alone.

*Drug interactions:* No impairment of the antibody response to the individual antigens has been seen when HibTITER is mixed and administered in the same syringe as Trivax-AD† (diphtheria and tetanus toxoid and pertussis vaccine adsorbed).

No impairment of the antibody response to the individual antigens has been seen when HibTITER is given at the same time but at separate sites as diphtheria and tetanus toxoid and pertussis vaccine adsorbed (DTP) plus oral polio vaccine (OPV) to children 2–20 months of age or measles, mumps and rubella vaccine (MMR) to children of 14 to 16 months of age.

*Overdose:* There is no experience with overdoses of HibTITER.

**Pharmaceutical precautions** HibTITER should be stored at 2–8°C. The vaccine should not be frozen.

**Legal category** POM

**Package quantities** Packs containing 1 and 10 monodose vials.

**Further information** None.

**Product licence number** 0095/0266

## LEDERFEN*

**Presentation**

*Lederfen 300 mg Tablets:* Light blue, film coated, capsule shaped tablets, each containing 300 mg of fenbufen and engraved 'WY050' on one side.

*Lederfen 300 mg Capsules:* Dark blue capsules, each containing 300 mg of fenbufen and printed 'WY052' on both the cap and body.

*Lederfen 450 mg Tablets:* Light blue, film coated, lozenge shaped tablets each containing 450 mg of fenbufen and engraved 'WY051' on one side.

**Uses** Lederfen is a non-steroidal, anti-inflammatory drug (NSAID) indicated for the symptomatic treatment of rheumatoid arthritis, osteoarthritis, ankylosing spondylitis and acute musculoskeletal disorders.

**Dosage and administration** *Adults: 300 mg Tablets or Capsules:* One in the morning and two at night.

*450 mg Tablets:* one in the morning and one at night.

*Elderly:* Clinical studies conducted in elderly patients and patients with mild to moderate renal impairment have shown that the pharmacokinetics of Lederfen are not affected to any clinically relevant extent and the standard adult dose may be used (also see 'Precautions').

*Children:* Not recommended for administration to children under the age of 14.

**Contra-indications, warnings, etc**
*Contra-indications:* Active or suspected peptic ulcer or a history of peptic ulceration.

Hypersensitivity to propionic acid anti-inflammatory drugs, or aspirin.

Since the potential exists for cross-sensitivity, Lederfen should not be used in patients in whom attacks of asthma, urticaria or acute rhinitis are precipitated by aspirin or other NSAIDs.

*Precautions:* As with other NSAIDs, Lederfen should be used with great caution in patients with a history of peptic or intestinal ulceration, and only after other forms of treatment have been carefully considered. Gastrointestinal ulceration, haematemesis or melaena may occur with or without warning symptoms or a previous history.

It is unnecessary to modify the dosage of Lederfen in mild to moderate renal impairment, however, in common with other NSAIDs, there have been a few reports of deterioration in renal function associated with Lederfen therapy. In view of this, doses in patients with pre-existing renal disease or impaired cardiac or hepatic function should be kept to the minimum necessary to achieve the desired therapeutic effect and renal function should be monitored.

See *Interactions* section for precautions on use with other drugs.

*Use in pregnancy and lactation:* Lederfen should not

be prescribed during pregnancy or lactation, unless there are compelling reasons for doing so and only after careful consideration of the risk/benefit ratio. If absolutely necessary, the lowest effective dose should be used.

*Warnings and adverse effects:* Skin rashes including erythema, maculo-papular, morbilliform and urticaria are the most commonly encountered adverse reactions. Stevens-Johnson syndrome has occasionally been reported. Angioedema, facial oedema, erythema multiforme, epidermal necrolysis, periorbital oedema, pupura, and photosensitivity reactions have all been occasionally reported.

Lederfen treatment should be discontinued immediately on appearance of a rash. Anti-histamine therapy may help any pruritis associated with the rash. The rash is more common in women and in patients with the rare diagnoses of sero-negative rheumatoid arthritis and psoriatic arthritis. If rash does occur, it will most commonly be seen within the second week of therapy but is very unlikely to occur after two weeks of therapy. The median duration of therapy before a rash occurs is ten days. 80% of eruptions will have resolved after one week of discontinuation of therapy and by two weeks nearly 100% of eruptions will have resolved.

NSAIDs have been reported to cause nephrotoxicity in various forms and their use can lead to interstitial nephritis, nephrotic syndrome and renal failure.

In common with other NSAIDs, allergic interstitial lung disorders (allergic alveolitis, or pulmonary eosinophilia) have been reported rarely; these reactions have resolved within 4-6 weeks of discontinuing therapy.

Vomiting, dyspepsia and nausea are the most commonly encountered gastrointestinal effects. Abdominal pain, diarrhoea, gastritis, haematemesis, gastrointestinal haemorrhage, melaena, constipation, stomatitis, ulcerative stomatitis and anorexia have also occasionally been reported.

Oedema, dizziness, depression, sleep disturbances including vivid dreams, paraesthesia, headache, drowsiness, fatigue, fever and malaise have also occasionally been reported. Increased perspiration and flushing occur rarely. Hypersensitivity reaction such as anaphylaxis and bronchospasm have been reported rarely.

In common with other NSAID's, disturbances of vision and tinnitus have occasionally been reported.

Slight decreases in blood leucocytes, haemoglobin and haematocrit as well as slight increases in prothrombin time and eosinophils have occasionally been recorded. Haematological effects such as agranulocytosis, thrombocytopenia, granulocytopenia, aplastic anaemia, pancytopenia and haemolytic anaemia have been reported rarely. Transient elevations in values of liver function tests have occurred in some patients. Hepatic disorders including hepatitis and jaundice have been reported rarely.

*Drug interactions:* Lederfen is strongly protein bound–prescribers should be aware of the consequences of increased or decreased blood levels of either drug if Lederfen is administered with other protein bound drugs such as sulphonylureas, methotrexate, salicylates, hypoglycaemics etc.

Caution should be exercised if NSAIDs and methotrexate are administered within 24 hours of each other, since NSAIDs may increase methotrexate plasma levels resulting in increased toxicity.

In common with other NSAIDs, fenbufen when administered concurrently with quinolone antibiotics may cause an increased incidence of quinolone CNS side-effects such as convulsions.

Quinolones should not be administered concurrently with Lederfen.

Lederfen produces minor prolongation of prothrombin time in patients taking warfarin. These changes are unlikely to be clinically significant, but patients previously stabilised on oral anticoagulant therapy should be monitored for changes in prothrombin time.

Increases in serum lithium have been reported with some NSAIDs. Serum lithium levels should be monitored if Lederfen is added to therapy for patients previously stabilised on lithium.

*Overdosage:* Experience of Lederfen overdosage is limited. There is no specific antidote. Gastric lavage should be performed if appropriate. Otherwise, management should be symptomatic and supportive.

**Pharmaceutical precautions** Store in the original container at room temperature (below 25°C).

**Legal category** POM

**Package quantities**
300 mg Tablets and Capsules: Blister packs of 84 tablets/capsules designated Lederfen CP.
450 mg Tablets: Blister packs of 56 tablets.

**Further information** Fenbufen is a pro-drug. It is converted into active metabolites following absorption.

**Product licence numbers**
Lederfen 300 mg Tablets 0095/0081
Lederfen 300 mg Capsules 0095/0043
Lederfen 450 mg Tablets 0095/0092

## LEDERMYCIN*

**Presentation** *Capsules 150 mg:* Each two-piece, hard shell capsule, with a peach coloured body and a dark red cap, printed Lederle 9123 contains 150 mg of demeclocycline hydrochloride.

**Uses**
1. For the treatment of infections caused by tetracycline-sensitive organisms. For example, Ledermycin is highly effective in the treatment of infections caused by *Borrellia recurrentis* (relapsing fever), *Calymmatobacterium granulomatis* (granuloma inguinale), *Chlamydia* species (psittacosis, lymphogranuloma venereum, trachoma, inclusion conjunctivitis), *Francisella tularensis* (tularaemia), *Haemophilus ducreyi* (chancroid), *Leptospira* (meningitis, jaundice), *Mycoplasma pneumoniae* (non-gonococcal urethritis), *Pseudomonas mallei* and *Pseudomallei* (glanders and melioidosis), *Rickettsiae* (typhus fever, Q fever, rocky mountain spotted fever), *Vibrio* species (cholera). It is also highly effective, alone or in combination with streptomycin, in the treatment of infections due to *Brucella* species (brucellosis), and *Yersinia pestis* (bubonic plague). Severe acne vulgaris.

Other sensitive organisms include: *Actinomyces israelii, Bacillus anthracis* (pneumonia), *Clostridium* species (gas gangrene, tetanus), *Entamoeba histolytica* (dysentery), *Neisseria gonorrhoeae*, and anaerobic species, *Treponema pallidum* and *pertenue* (syphilis and yaws).

2. For the treatment of chronic hyponatraemia associated with the syndrome of inappropriate secretion of antidiuretic hormone (SIADH) secondary to malignant disease, where water restriction is ineffective, and the patient does not have concomitant cirrhosis.

**Dosage and administration**

1. *For antibiotic use: Adults:* 600 mg daily in two or four divided doses. For primary atypical pneumonia the average daily dose is 900 mg in three divided doses for six days.

*Elderly:* Use with caution in elderly patients. See Contra-indications and Warnings.

*Children:* Not recommended for children under 12 years of age.

2. *For the treatment of chronic hyponatraemia due to SIADH: (Adults only)*
Initially: 900–1,200 mg daily in divided doses.
Maintenance dose: 600–900 mg daily in divided doses.

Ledermycin should be swallowed whole with plenty of fluid while sitting or standing. Doses should be taken an hour before or two hours after meals and antibiotic therapy should be continued for one to three days after characteristic symptoms or fever have subsided. The incidence of rheumatic fever or glomerulonephritis following streptococcal infections suggests that therapy of a streptococcal infection should be continued for eight full days even though symptoms have subsided.

Ledermycin therapy in the treatment of chronic hyponatraemia due to SIADH should not be withdrawn without commencing other methods of control.

**Contra-indications, warnings, etc**
*Contra-indications:* A history of hypersensitivity to tetracyclines. Overt renal insufficiency. Children under twelve years of age.

*Warnings and precautions:* Ledermycin should be used with caution in patients with renal or hepatic dysfunction, or in conjunction with other potentially hepatotoxic or nephrotoxic drugs. Concurrent use with the anaesthetic methoxyflurane increases the risk of kidney failure. The anti-anabolic action of the tetracyclines may cause an increase in BUN. The treatment of chronic hyponatraemia may necessitate the administration of high doses of Ledermycin for prolonged periods, so increasing the potential for nephrotoxicity (manifested by rises in plasma urea and creatinine) and photo-allergic reactions.

Cross-resistance between tetracyclines may develop in micro-organisms and cross-sensitisation in patients. Ledermycin should be discontinued if there are signs/symptoms of overgrowth of resistant organisms including candida, enteritis, glossitis, stomatitis, vaginitis, pruritus ani or staphylococcal enterocolitis.

Lower doses are indicated in cases of renal impairment to avoid excessive systemic accumulation, and if therapy is prolonged, serum level determinations are advisable. Patients who have known liver disease should not receive more than 1 g daily. In long term therapy, periodic laboratory evaluation of organ systems, including haematopoietic, renal and hepa studies should be performed.

Ledermycin has the greatest potential of the tet cycline analogues for causing photo-allergic reactio in hypersensitive persons. Such patients should warned to avoid direct exposure to natural or artific sunlight and to discontinue therapy at the first sign skin discomfort.

Patients taking oral contraceptives should warned that if diarrhoea or breakthrough bleedi occur there is a possibility of contraceptive failure.

*Interactions:* Ledermycin should not be used w penicillins. Tetracyclines depress plasma prothromb activity and reduced doses of concomitant ar coagulants may be required.

Absorption of Ledermycin is impaired by the co comitant administration of iron, calcium, zinc, ma nesium and particularly aluminium salts commor used as antacids.

The concomitant use of tetracyclines may redu the efficacy of oral contraceptives; an increas incidence of breakthrough bleeding may also experienced (see statement under *Warnings a precautions*).

*Use in pregnancy:* Results of animal studies indica that tetracyclines cross the placenta, are found foetal tissues and can have toxic effects on t developing foetus (often related to retardation skeletal development). Evidence of embryotoxic has also been noted in animals treated early pregnancy. Ledermycin, therefore, should not be us in pregnancy unless considered essential.

The use of tetracyclines during tooth developme (last half of pregnancy and children to the age of years) may cause permanent discolouration of t teeth. This adverse reaction is more common duri long term use of the drugs but has been observ following repeated short term courses. Enamel hyp plasia has also been reported.

*Use in lactation:* Tetracyclines have been found in t milk of lactating women who are taking a drug in th class. Permanent tooth discolouration may occur the developing infant and enamel hypoplasia h been reported. Therefore, Ledermycin should not administered to lactating women.

*Side-effects:* Gastro-intestinal disturbances includi nausea, vomiting and diarrhoea may occur and, with all antibiotics, overgrowth of resistant organisn may cause glossitis, stomatitis, vaginitis, or staphyl coccal enterocolitis. Dermatological reactions are ra Bulging fontanelles in infants and benign intracran hypertension in adults have been reported. Treatme should cease if evidence of raised intracranial pressu develops. Hypersensitivity reactions including ur caria, angioneurotic oedema, anaphylaxis, anaphyla toid purpura, pericarditis and exacerbation systemic lupus erythymatosus may occur.

Haemolytic anaemia, thrombocytopenia, neut penia and eosinophilia have been reported. Wh given over prolonged periods, tetracyclines have be reported to produce brown black microscopic disc ouration of the thyroid gland. No abnormalities thyroid function are known to occur. Reversib nephrogenic diabetes insipidus can occur especia if treatment is prolonged and/or at high dosages.

*Overdosage:* No specific antidote. Gastric lavage pl oral administration of milk or antacids. Maintain flu and electrolyte balance.

**Pharmaceutical precautions** Ledermycin Capsul should be stored at controlled room temperature (1 30°C), in either the original pack or in containers whic prevent access of light and moisture.

**Legal category** POM

**Package quantities** Bottles of 100

**Further information** Nil

**Product licence number** 0095/0052

## LEDERSPAN* INJECTION 20 mg/ml
## LEDERSPAN* INJECTION 5 mg/ml

**Presentation** *Suspension 20 mg/ml:* Vials containi a sterile suspension of 20 mg or 100 mg of micronis triamcinolone hexacetonide in 1 ml or 5 ml respe tively of an aqueous vehicle with 0.9% benzyl alcoh as preservative.

*Suspension 5 mg/ml:* Vials containing a sterile su pension of 25 mg of micronised triamcinolone he acetonide in 5 ml of an aqueous vehicle with 0.9 benzyl alcohol as preservative.

**Uses** Triamcinolone hexacetonide is a relatively inso uble corticosteroid (0.0003% at 25°C in water). It has prolonged effect on tissue at the local injection sit the duration usually ranging from a few weeks several months.

*Lederspan 20 mg/ml (for intra-articular and intr*

ˊnovial administration): is indicated in the treatment ˋ rheumatoid arthritis; osteoarthritis; synovitis and ɹrsitis; tendinitis and tenosynovitis; and epicondyli-s.

ederspan 5 mg/ml (for intra-lesional and sub-lesional dministration): is indicated in the treatment of cystic ɜne; alopecia areata, nummular and dyshydrotic zema; granuloma annulare; keloids; lichen planus; scoid lupus erythematosus; localised neuroderma-tis.

**osage and administration** *Adults (including the derly): For intra-articular and intra-synovial use:* mg–30 mg (0.1–1.5 ml), depending on the size of int (or synovial space) to be injected, the degree of flammation and the amount of fluid present. In eneral, large joints (such as knee, hips, shoulder) quire 10–30 mg, whereas small joints (such as terphalangeal, metacarpophalangeal) require 2-mg. When much synovial fluid is present, aspiration ay be performed before administering Lederspan. ubsequent dosage and frequency of injection can est be judged by clinical response. Since Lederspan ovides prolonged activity, injections into a single int or synovial space more frequently than every ree to four weeks are not recommended. Repeated tra-articular injections should be as infrequent as ossible, consistent with adequate patient care.

Strict asepsis is mandatory during administration. opical ethyl chloride spray may be used locally efore injection. Since micronised triamcinolone hex-etonide has been designed for ease of administra-on, a small-bore needle (including 24 gauge needles) ay be used. The vial should be gently agitated to hieve uniform suspension before each use.

Lederspan triamcinolone hexacetonide 20 mg/ml erile suspension is formulated to be diluted prior to tra-articular or intra-synovial injection. Sterile sus-ensions of Lederspan may be diluted with a local naesthetic such as 1% or 2% lidocaine hydrochloride sing formulations which do not contain parabens ior to intra-articular or intra-synovial injections. The ptimum dilution for injection into a joint, 1:1, 1:2 or 4 should be determined depending on the dose to e administered. This dose is dependant on the size f the joint, degree of inflammation and amount of uid present.

Lederspan may be administered by Dermojet and e Porton Injector.

*or intra-lesional and sub-lesional use:* The dosage is 5 mg or less per square inch of affected skin. No ore than 5 mg should be injected at any one site, nd no more than a total dosage of 30 mg should be xceeded regardless of the number of sites injected. required, the injection can be repeated at one or two eek intervals.

Strict asepsis is mandatory during administration. opical ethyl chloride spray may be used locally efore injection. Since micronised triamcinolone hex-etonide has been designed for ease of administra-on, a small-bore needle (including 24 gauge needles) ay be used. The vial should be gently agitated to hieve uniform suspension before each use.

Lederspan triamcinolone hexacetonide 5 mg/ml erile suspension is formulated to be diluted prior to tra-lesional injection. Sterile suspension of Leder-pan may be diluted with a local anaesthetic such as % or 2% lidocaine hydrochloride using formulations hich do not contain parabens prior to intralesional jections. Intralesional injections may also be diluted ith aqueous vehicles such as Sodium Chloride jection BP, Dextrose (5% and 10%) in Sodium hloride for Injection, or Water for Injection BP. These olutions are used as isotonic vehicles. The additional smotic effect of the drug when added to these ehicles should not be enough to produce any iscomfort or tissue irritation when administered. The ptimum dilution for intra-lesional use 1:1, 1:2 or 1:4 hould be determined by the nature of the lesion, its ze, the depth of injection, the volume needed, and e location of the lesion. In general, more superficial jections should be performed with a dilution of 1:4. ertain conditions, such as keloids, require a concen-ated suspension (5 mg/ml), with variation in dose nd dilution as dictated by the condition of the dividual patient. Subsequent dosage, dilution and equency of injections are best judged by the clinical esponse.

Lederspan may be administered by Dermojet and e Porton Injector.

*hildren:* Not recommended.

**ontra-indications, warnings, etc.**
*Contra-indications:* Although active, latent or ques-onably healed tuberculosis, ocular herpes simplex nd acute psychosis are generally considered to be bsolute contra-indications to glucocorticoid therapy, e minimal systemic activity of triamcinolone hex-cetonide after local injection might permit cautious se when indicated. The drug should not be used hen there is history of hypersensitivity to any of the omponents of the formulation or when previous injections have produced local atrophy. Infected joints should not be injected with corticosteroids.

As with other glucocorticoid agents, relative contra-indications are active peptic ulcer, acute glomerulo-nephritis, myasthenia gravis, osteoporosis, fresh in-testinal anastomoses, diverticulitis, thrombophlebitis, psychic disturbances, pregnancy, diabetes mellitus, hyperthyroidism, acute coronary artery disease, hy-pertension, limited cardiac reserve and local or sys-temic infections, including fungal and exanthematous diseases. The minimal systemic activity of this prepa-ration, however, reduces the risks involved in its use in the presence of these conditions.

*Precautions and side-effects:* As with all glucocorti-coids, an exacerbation of symptoms or 'flare-up' may occur following intra-articular or intra-synovial injec-tions. Local atrophy, burning, flushing, pain and swelling may occur. Other local effects include ab-scess, erythema, skin discolouration or depigmenta-tion and necrosis at the injection site. Anaphylactic reactions are very rare.

In addition, prolonged and repeated use in weight-bearing joints may result in further joint degeneration. This is probably related to premature use of still-diseased joints following relief of pain and other symptoms. Not more than two or three large joints should be treated simultaneously in the same patient.

Systemic effects are rare with Lederspan due its slow release from the injection site. In addition to those common to all glucocorticoids, some effects particularly associated with triamcinolone therapy are anorexia, myopathy and depression of mood.

In treating conditions such as tendinitis or tenosyn-ovitis, care should be taken that Lederspan is injected into the space between tendon sheath and tendon and not into the tendon itself.

If severe reactions occur or an acute infection develops during therapy, use of the drug should be discontinued and appropriate measures taken.

*Use in pregnancy and lactation:* Lederspan should not be administered to patients who are pregnant or to mothers who are breast feeding.

*Overdose:* Overdosage or excessive frequency of intralesional injections into the same site may produce local subcutaneous atrophy. If this occurs, recovery may be delayed for several months because of the prolonged action of the drug.

**Pharmaceutical precautions** Lederspan should be stored at room temperature (15–30°C). Do not freeze. It may be diluted with Water for Injection BP, Sodium Chloride Injection BP, Sodium Chloride and Dextrose Injection BP, Lignocaine Hydrochloride Injection BP, immediately prior to injection.

Fluids containing methyl or propyl hydroxyben-zoates or phenol should be avoided since these tend to cause flocculation of the steroid.

**Legal category** POM

**Package quantities**
20 mg/ml: Single vials containing 20 mg in 1 ml and 100 mg in 5 ml.
5 mg/ml: Single vials containing 25 mg in 5 ml.

**Further information** Nil

**Product licence numbers**
Lederspan 20 mg/ml 0095/0008
Lederspan 5 mg/ml 0095/0009

## LOXAPAC*

**Presentation** *10 mg Capsules:* Two piece, hard shell, opaque capsules with a yellow body and a green cap, printed with script 'Lederle' over 'L2' on one half and '10 mg' on the other in grey ink, containing 10 mg loxapine as loxapine succinate. The capsules have a locking feature.

*25 mg Capsules:* Two piece, hard shell, opaque capsules with a light green body and a dark green cap, printed with script 'Lederle' over 'L3' on one half and '25 mg' on the other in grey ink, containing 25 mg loxapine as loxapine succinate. The capsules have a locking feature.

*50 mg Capsules:* Two piece, hard shell, opaque capsules with a blue body and a dark green cap, printed with script 'Lederle' over 'L4' on one half and '50 mg' on the other in white ink, containing 50 mg loxapine as loxapine succinate. The capsules have a locking feature.

**Uses** The treatment of acute and chronic psychotic states.

**Dosage and administration** *Adults:* Initially 20–50 mg/day in two doses. Dosage is then increased over 7–10 days to the range 60–100 mg/day in 2–4 doses, until there is effective control of psychotic symptoms.

Maximum daily dose: 250 mg.

Maintenance doses should be adjusted to the needs of the patient, usually in the range of 20–100 mg/day in divided doses.

*Children:* Not recommended for use in children.

**Contra-indications, warnings, etc.**
*Contra-indications:* Use in comatose or semi-coma-tose patients or in severe drug-induced depressed states (alcohol, barbiturates, narcotics). In individuals with known hypersensitivity to the drug.

*Drug interactions:* Loxapac may increase the CNS depression produced by drugs such as alcohol, hypnotics, sedatives, antihistamines, strong analge-sics or other anti-psychotics. There have been reports of respiratory depression with concurrent use of loxapine and lorazepam.

The anticholinergic effect of loxapine may be enhanced by other anticholinergic drugs. The possi-bility of occurrence of heat stroke, severe constipation, paralytic ileus and atropine-like psychoses should be noted. Neuroleptics may impair the anti-parkinsonian effect of l-dopa, while therapeutic efficacy of the neuroleptic may be reduced. Concurrent use of neuroleptics and tricyclic antidepressants may con-tribute to increased incidence of tardive dyskinesia.

Loxapine may reduce serum levels of phenytoin.

There have been rare reports of patients developing neurotoxicity when treated concurrently with lithium; lithium serum levels were within normal limits and the mechanism of action is unknown.

*Precautions:* Loxapac may impair mental and/or phys-ical abilities, especially during the first few days of therapy. Therefore, ambulatory patients should be warned about activities requiring alertness, (e.g. operating machinery or vehicles) and about concom-itant use of alcohol and other CNS depressants.

Loxapac should be used with extreme caution in patients with a history of convulsive disorders, since it lowers the convulsive threshold. Seizures have been reported in epileptic patients receiving Loxapac at antipsychotic dose levels, and may occur even with maintenance of routine anticonvulsant drug therapy.

Loxapac has an antiemetic effect in animals. Since this effect may also occur in man, Loxapac may mask signs of overdosage of toxic drugs and may obscure conditions such as intestinal obstruction and brain tumour.

Loxapac should be used with caution in patients with cardiovascular disease. Increased pulse rates have been reported in the majority of patients receiv-ing antipsychotic doses; transient hypotension has been reported. In the presence of severe hypotension requiring vasopressor therapy, the preferred drugs may be noradrenaline or angiotensin. Usual doses of adrenaline may be ineffective because of inhibition of its vasopressor effect by Loxapac.

The possibility of ocular toxicity from Loxapac cannot be excluded at this time. Therefore, careful observation should be made for pigmentary retinop-athy and lenticular pigmentation, since these have been observed in some patients receiving certain other antipsychotic drugs for prolonged periods.

Because of possible anticholinergic action, the drug should be used cautiously in patients with glaucoma or a tendency to urinary retention, particularly with concomitant administration of anticholinergic type anti-Parkinson medication.

*Warnings and adverse effects: CNS effects:* Manifes-tations of adverse effects on the central nervous system other than extrapyramidal effects, have been seen infrequently. Drowsiness usually mild, may occur at the beginning of therapy or when dosage is increased and usually subsides with continued Loxa-pac therapy. Dizziness, faintness, staggering gait, muscle twitching, weakness, confusional states and seizures have been reported.

Extrapyramidal (Neuromuscular) reactions during the administration of Loxapac have been reported frequently, often during the first few days of treatment. In most patients, these reactions involved Parkinson-like symptoms such as tremor, rigidity, excessive salivation, and a mask like face. Also, akathisia (motor restlessness) has been reported relatively frequently. These symptoms are usually not severe and can be controlled by reduction of dosage or by administration of anti-Parkinson drugs in usual dosage. Dystonias include spasms of muscles of the neck and face, tongue protrusion, and oculogyric choreo-athetoid movements. These reactions sometimes require re-duction or temporary withdrawal of Loxapac dosage in addition to appropriate counteractive drugs.

As with all antipsychotic agents, persistent tardive dyskinesia may appear in some patients on long term therapy or may appear after drug therapy has been discontinued. The risk appears to be greater in elderly patients on high-dose therapy, especially females. The symptoms are persistent and in some patients appear to be irreversible. The syndrome is character-ised by rhythmical involuntary movement of the tongue, face, mouth or jaw (e.g. protrusion of tongue, puffing of cheeks, puckering of mouth, chewing movements). Sometimes these may be accompanied by involuntary movements of extremities.

There is no known effective treatment for tardive dyskinesia; anti-Parkinson agents usually do not alleviate the symptoms of this syndrome. It is suggested that all antipsychotic agents be discontinued if these symptoms appear.

Should it be necessary to reinstitute treatment, or increase the dose of the agent, or switch to a different antipsychotic agent, the syndrome may be masked. It has been suggested that fine vermicular movements of the tongue may be an early sign of the syndrome, and, if the medication is stopped at that time, the syndrome may not develop.

*Cardiovascular effects:* Tachycardia, hypotension, hypertension, lightheadedness, and syncope have been reported. A few cases of ECG changes similar to those seen with phenothiazines have been reported. It is not known whether these were related to administration.

*Skin:* Dermatitis, oedema (puffiness of face), pruritis, and seborrhoea have been reported with Loxapac. The possibility of photosensitivity and/or phototoxicity occurring has not been excluded; skin rashes of uncertain aetiology have been observed in a few patients during hot summer months.

*Endocrine effects:* Hormonal effects of anti-psychotic neuroleptic drugs include hyperprolactinaemia. Galactorrhoea, hyperprolactinaemia and amenorrhoea have been reported rarely.

*Anticholinergic effects:* Dry mouth, nasal congestion, constipation, and blurred vision have occurred; these are more likely to occur with concomitant use of anti-Parkinson agents.

*Other adverse reactions:* Nausea, vomiting, weight gain, weight loss, dyspnoea, ptosis, hyperpyrexia, flushed facies, headache, paraesthesia, and polydipsia have been reported in some patients. Transient abnormalities of liver function tests have been reported rarely. Jaundice has been reported in patients taking neuroleptic medication.

Neuroleptic Malignant Syndrome has been reported rarely following the use of Loxapac. This syndrome is potentially fatal and presents with symptoms of hyperpyrexia, muscle rigidity, altered mental status and evidence of autonomic instability. If a patient is diagnosed as suffering from Neuroleptic Malignant Syndrome, the management should include: (1) immediate discontinuation of antipsychotic drugs and other drugs not essential to concurrent therapy (2) symptomatic treatment and monitoring of vital signs and (3) treatment of any concomitant serious medical problems.

*Use in pregnancy and lactation:* Loxapac should not be used during pregnancy or lactation unless considered essential by the physician. Studies in animals do not indicate a teratogenic effect but there is no information on uses during human pregnancy. Loxapac crosses the placenta and is excreted in breast milk.

*Overdosage:* Signs and symptoms of overdosage might be expected to include convulsive seizures and range from mild depression of the CNS and cardiovascular systems to profound hypotension, respiratory depression and unconsciousness. Renal failure has been reported following Loxapac administration. Severe extrapyramidal reactions should be treated with anticholinergic anti-Parkinson agents or diphenhydramine hydrochloride, and anticonvulsant therapy should be initiated as indicated.

The treatment of overdosage would be essentially symptomatic and supportive. Early gastric lavage and extended dialysis might be expected to be beneficial. Centrally acting emetics may have little effect because of the antiemetic action of loxapine. Avoid analeptics, such as picrotoxin and pentylenetetrazole, which may cause convulsions. Severe hypotension might be expected to respond to the administration of levarterenol or phenylephrine. ADRENALINE SHOULD NOT BE USED SINCE ITS USE IN A PATIENT WITH PARTIAL ADRENERGIC BLOCKADE MAY FURTHER LOWER THE BLOOD PRESSURE. Additional measures include oxygen and intravenous fluids.

**Pharmaceutical precautions** Store at controlled room temperature (15–30°C).

**Legal category** POM

**Package quantities** Bottles containing 100 capsules.

**Product licence numbers**
Loxapac 10 mg Capsules 0095/0036
Loxapac 25 mg Capsules 0095/0037
Loxapac 50 mg Capsules 0095/0038

## METHOTREXATE SODIUM TABLETS METHOTREXATE INJECTION

**Presentation** *Tablets 2.5 mg:* Round convex, scored, uncoated, yellow tablets embossed '2.5' and 'MI', containing Methotrexate Sodium equivalent to 2.5 mg of Methotrexate per tablet.

*Injection:* A clear, yellow, sterile, aqueous, isotonic solution containing Methotrexate Sodium equivalent to 50 mg, 200 mg, 500 mg, 1 g or 5 g of Methotrexate per vial together with sodium chloride and sodium hydroxide or hydrochloric acid to adjust the pH to approximately 8.5. The injection does not contain an antimicrobial preservative.

**Uses** *Properties:* Methotrexate, a derivative of folic acid, belongs to the class of cytotoxic agents known as antimetabolites. It acts principally during the 'S' phase of cell division, by the competitive inhibition of the enzyme dihydrofolate reductase, thus preventing the reduction of dihydrofolate to tetrahydrofolate, a necessary step in the process of DNA synthesis and cellular replication. Actively proliferating tissues such as malignant cells, bone marrow, foetal cells, buccal and intestinal mucosa, and cells of the urinary bladder are generally more sensitive to the effects of Methotrexate. When cellular proliferation in malignant tissues is greater than in most normal tissues, Methotrexate may impair malignant growth without irreversible damage to normal tissues.

The mechanism of action in rheumatoid arthritis is unknown; it may effect immune function. Clarification of the effect of Methotrexate on immune activity and its relation to rheumatoid immunopathogenesis await further investigation.

In psoriasis, the rate of production of epithelial cells in the skin is greatly increased over normal skin. This differential in proliferation rates is the basis for the use of Methotrexate to control the psoriatic process.

*Indications:* The treatment of neoplastic disease. The treatment of severe cases of uncontrolled psoriasis, unresponsive to conventional therapy.

The treatment of adults with severe, active, classical or definite rheumatoid arthritis who are unresponsive or intolerant to conventional therapy.

**Dosage and administration** *Adults and children:* Methotrexate may be given by oral, intramuscular, intravenous (bolus injection or infusion), intrathecal, intra-arterial and intraventricular routes of administration. Dosages are based on the patient's body weight or surface area except in the case of intrathecal or intraventricular administration when a maximum dose of 15 mg is recommended. Doses should be reduced in cases of haematological deficiency and hepatic or renal impairment. Larger doses (greater than 100 mg) are usually given by intravenous infusion over periods not exceeding 24 hours. Part of the dose may be given in an initial rapid intravenous injection.

Methotrexate has been used with beneficial effects in a wide variety of neoplastic diseases, alone and in combination with other cytotoxic agents, hormones, radiotherapy or surgery. Dosage schedules therefore vary considerably, depending on the clinical use, particularly when intermittent high-dose regimes are followed by the administration of Calcium Leucovorin (calcium folinate) to rescue normal cells from toxic effects.

Dosage regimes for Calcium Leucovorin rescue are discussed under *Further information.*

Examples of doses of Methotrexate that have been used for particular indications are given below.

*Choriocarcinoma and other trophoblastic tumours:* Non-metastatic gestational trophoblastic neoplasms have been treated successfully with 0.25–1 mg/kg up to a maximum of 60 mg intramuscularly every 48 hours for four doses, followed by Calcium Leucovorin Rescue. This course of treatment is repeated at seven day intervals until levels of urinary chorionic gonadotrophin hormone return to normal. Not less than four courses of treatment are usually necessary. Patients with complications, such as extensive metastases, may be treated with Methotrexate in combination with other cytotoxic drugs.

Methotrexate has also been used in similar doses for the treatment of hydatidiform mole and chorioadenoma destruens.

*Leukaemia in children:* In acute lymphocytic leukaemia remissions are usually best induced with a combination of corticosteroids and other cytotoxic agents.

Methotrexate 15 mg/m², given parenterally or orally once weekly, in combination with other drugs appears to be the treatment of choice for maintenance of drug-induced remissions.

*Meningeal leukaemia in children:* Doses up to 15 mg, intrathecally, at weekly intervals, until the CSF appears normal (usually two to three weeks), have been found useful for the treatment of meningeal leukaemia.

Although intravenous doses of the order of 50 mg/m² of Methotrexate do not appreciably penetrate the CSF, larger doses of the order of 500 mg/m² or greater do produce cytotoxic levels of Methotrexate in the CSF. This type of therapy has been used in short courses, followed by administration of Calcium Leucovorin, as initial maintenance therapy to preve leukaemic invasion of the central nervous system children with poor prognosis lymphocytic leukaemi

*Lymphoma:* Non-Hodgkin's lymphoma, eg. childho lymphosarcoma has recently been treated with 30 mg/kg (approximately 90–900 mg/m²) of Meth trexate given by intravenous injection and infusi followed by administration of Calcium Leucovor with the higher doses. Some cases of Burkit lymphoma, when treated in the early stages wi courses of 15 mg/m² daily orally for five days, ha shown prolonged remissions. Combination chem therapy is also commonly used in all stages of th disease.

*Breast cancer:* Methotrexate, in intravenous doses 10–60 mg/m², is commonly included in cyclical cor bination regimes with other cytotoxic drugs in th treatment of advanced breast cancer. Similar regim have also been used as adjuvant therapy in ear cases following mastectomy and/or radiotherapy.

*Osteogenic sarcoma:* The use of Methotrexate alo and in cyclical combination regimes has recently bee introduced as an adjuvant therapy to the prima treatment of osteogenic sarcoma by amputation wi or without prosthetic bone replacement. This h involved the use of intravenous infusions of 2 300 mg/kg (approximately 600–9,000 mg/m²) of Met otrexate followed by Calcium Leucovorin rescu Methotrexate has also been used as the sole treatme in metastatic cases of osteogenic sarcoma.

*Bronchogenic carcinoma:* Intravenous infusions 20–100 mg/m² of Methotrexate have been included cyclical combination regimes for the treatment advanced tumours. High doses with Calcium Leuc vorin rescue have also been employed as the so treatment.

*Head and neck cancer:* Intravenous infusions of 24 1,080 mg/m² with Calcium Leucovorin rescue ha been used both as pre-operative adjuvant therapy ar in the treatment of advanced tumours. Intra-arteri infusions of Methotrexate have been used in th treatment of head and neck cancers.

*Bladder carcinoma:* Intravenous injections or inf sions of Methotrexate in doses up to 100 mg eve one or two weeks have been used in the treatment bladder carcinoma with promising results, varyir from only symptomatic relief to complete thoug unsustained regressions. The use of high doses Methotrexate with Calcium Leucovorin rescue currently being evaluated.

*Elderly:* Methotrexate should be used with extrem caution in elderly patients, a reduction in dosag should be considered.

Assessment of renal function, liver function ar blood elements should be made by history, physic examination and laboratory tests before beginnir Methotrexate, periodically during Methotrexate the apy, and before reinstituting Methotrexate after a re period.

Particular attention should be given to the appea ance of liver toxicity by carrying out liver functic tests before starting Methotrexate treatment ar repeating these at two to four month intervals durir therapy. Treatment should not be instituted or shoul be discontinued if any abnormality of liver functic tests, or liver biopsy, is present or develops durir therapy.

Such abnormalities should return to normal with two weeks after which treatment may be recomm enced at the discretion of the physician.

*Dosage and administration with reference to psorias and rheumatoid arthritis:*

*Adults: Psoriasis:* In most cases of severe uncontrolle psoriasis, unresponsive to conventional therapy, 1 25 mg orally once a week and adjusted by the patient response is recommended.

The use of Methotrexate in psoriasis may perm the return to conventional topical therapy whic should be encouraged.

*Rheumatoid arthritis:* In adults with severe, acut classical or definite rheumatoid arthritis who a unresponsive or intolerant to conventional therap 7.5 mg orally once weekly or divided oral doses 2.5 mg at 12 hour intervals for 3 doses (7.5 mg) as course once weekly. The schedule may be adjuste gradually to achieve an optimal response but shoul not exceed a total weekly dose of 20 mg. Onc response has been achieved, the schedule should b reduced to the lowest possible effective dose.

*Elderly:* Methotrexate should be used with extrem caution in elderly patients, a reduction in dosag should be considered.

*Children:* Safety and effectiveness in children hav not been established, other than in cancer chem therapy.

**Contra-indications, warnings, etc**

*Contra-indications:* Profound impairment of renal

epatic function or haematological impairment. Liver isease including fibrosis, cirrhosis, recent or active epatitis; active infectious disease; and overt or aboratory evidence of immunodeficiency syndrome(s). Serious cases of anaemia, leucopenia, or rrombocytopenia. Methotrexate is contra-indicated n pregnant patients. Because of the potential for erious adverse reactions from Methotrexate in breast ed infants, breast feeding is contra-indicated in omen taking Methotrexate. Patients with a known llergic hypersensitivity to Methotrexate should not eceive Methotrexate.

*Warnings:* Methotrexate has been shown to be teragenic; it has been reported to cause foetal death nd/or congenital abnormalities. Therefore, it is not ecommended in women of childbearing potential nless the benefits can be expected to outweigh the onsidered risks. If this drug is used during pregnancy or antineoplastic indications, or if the patient becomes pregnant while taking this drug, the patient hould be appraised of the potential hazard to the oetus.

Methotrexate should be used with extreme caution n patients with haematological depression, renal npairment, peptic ulcer, ulcerative colitis, ulcerative tomatitis, diarrhoea, debility and in young children nd the elderly. (See Dosage and Administration).

Patients with pleural effusions or ascites should ave these drained if appropriate before treatment or eatment should be withdrawn.

Deaths have been reported with the use of Methoexate. Serious adverse reactions including deaths ave been reported with concomitant administration f Methotrexate (usually in high doses) along with ome non-steroidal anti-inflammatory drugs NSAIDs).

Concomitant administration of folate antagonists uch as Trimethoprim/Sulphamethoxazole has been eported to cause an acute megaloblastic pancytoenia in rare instances.

Symptoms of gastro-intestinal toxicity, usually first nanifested by stomatitis, indicate interruption of herapy otherwise haemorrhagic enteritis and death om intestinal perforation may occur.

Methotrexate affects spermatogenesis and oogensis during the period of its administration which may esult in decreased fertility. To date, this effect appears o be reversible on discontinuing therapy. Conception hould be avoided for at least six months after reatment with Methotrexate has ceased. Patients eceiving Methotrexate and their partners should be dvised appropriately.

Methotrexate has some immunosuppressive activy and therefore the immunological response to oncurrent vaccination may be decreased. In addition, oncomitant use of a live vaccine could cause a severe ntigenic reaction.

*Precautions:* Methotrexate should only be used by linicians who are familiar with the various characterstics of the drug and its mode of action. Before eginning Methotrexate therapy or reinstituting Methtrexate after a rest period, assessment of renal unction, liver function and blood elements should be nade by history, physical examination and laboratory ests. Patients undergoing therapy should be subject o appropriate supervision so that signs of possible oxic effects or adverse reactions may be detected nd evaluated with minimal delay.

It is essential that the following laboratory tests are ncluded regularly in the clinical evaluation and nonitoring of patients receiving Methotrexate: comlete haematological analysis, urinalysis, renal funcion tests, liver function tests and, when high doses re administered, determination of plasma levels of Methotrexate.

Particular attention should be given to the appearnce of liver toxicity which may occur without orrelative changes in liver function tests. Treatment hould not be instituted, or should be discontinued, if ny abnormality in liver function tests or liver biopsy s present or develops during therapy. Such abnornalities should return to normal within two weeks, fter which treatment may be recommenced at the iscretion of the physician.

When to perform a liver biopsy in rheumatoid rthritis patients has not been established either in erms of a cumulative Methotrexate dose or duration f therapy.

Pleuropulmonary manifestation of rheumatoid arhritis have been reported in the literature. In patients vith rheumatoid arthritis, the physician should be pecifically alerted to the potential for Methotrexate nduced adverse effects in the pulmonary system. Patients should be advised to contact their physicians mmediately should they develop a cough or dypnoea (see *Side-effects*).

Haemopoietic suppression caused by Methotrexate nay occur abruptly and with apparently safe dosages. ny profound drop in white-cell or platelet counts ndicate immediate withdrawal of the drug and approriate supportive therapy (see *Side effects*).

It should be noted that intrathecal doses are transported into the cardiovascular system and may give rise to systemic toxicity. Systemic toxicity of Methotrexate may also be enhanced in patients with renal dysfunction, ascites or other effusions due to prolongation of serum half life.

High doses may cause the precipitation of Methotrexate or its metabolites in the renal tubules. A high fluid throughput and alkalinisation of the urine to pH 6.5–7.0 by oral or intravenous administration of sodium bicarbonate (5 x 625 mg tablets every three hours) or Diamox* (500 mg orally four times a day) is recommended as a preventive measure.

*Carcinogenesis, mutagenesis, and impairment of fertility:* Animal carcinogenicity studies have demonstrated Methotrexate to be free of carcinogenic potential. Although Methotrexate has been reported to cause chromosomal damage to animal somatic cells and bone marrow cells in humans, these effects are transient and reversible. In patients treated with Methotrexate, evidence is insufficient to permit conclusive evaluation of any increased risk of neoplasia.

Methotrexate has been reported to cause impairment of fertility, oligospermia, menstrual dysfunction and amenorrhoea in humans, during and for a short period after cessation of therapy. In addition, Methotrexate causes embryotoxicity, abortion and foetal defects in humans. Therefore, the possible risks of effects on reproduction should be discussed with patients of child-bearing potential (see *Warnings*).

*Drug interactions:* Methotrexate is extensively protein bound and may be displaced by certain drugs such as salicylates, sulphonamides, diuretics, hypoglycaemics, diphenylhydantoins, tetracyclines, chloramphenicol, p-aminobenzoic acid, and the acidic anti-inflammatory drugs, so causing a potential for increased toxicity when used concurrently. Concomitant use of other drugs with nephrotoxic or hepatotoxic potential (including alcohol) should be avoided.

Caution should be used when NSAIDs and salicylates are administered concomitantly with Methotrexate. These drugs have been reported to reduce the tubular secretion of Methotrexate in an animal model and thereby may enhance its toxicity. Renal tubular transport is also diminished by probenecid and penicillins; use of Methotrexate with these drugs should be carefully monitored.

Patients using constant dosage regimens of NSAIDs have received concurrent doses of Methotrexate without problems observed. Therefore, until more is known about the NSAIDs/Methotrexate interaction, it is recommended that Methotrexate dosage be carefully controlled during treatment with NSAIDs.

Methotrexate should be used with caution in patients taking drugs known to have an antifolate potential including nitrous oxide.

Vitamin preparations containing folic acid or its derivatives may alter response to Methotrexate.

Serum levels of Methotrexate may be increased by etretinate and severe hepatitis has been reported following concurrent use.

*Side-effects:* The most common adverse reactions include ulcerative stomatitis, leucopenia, nausea and abdominal distress. Although very rare, anaphylactic reactions to Methotrexate have occurred. Others reported are eye irritation, malaise, undue fatigue, chills and fever, dizziness, loss of libido/impotence and decreased resistance to infection. Opportunistic infections such as herpes zoster have been reported in relation to or attributed to the use of Methotrexate. In general, the incidence and severity of side effects are considered to be dose-related. Adverse reactions for the various systems are as follows:

*Integument:* Erythematous rashes, pruritus, urticaria, photosensitivity, pigmentary changes, alopecia, ecchymosis, telangiectasia, acne, furunculosis. Lesions of psoriasis may be aggravated by concomitant exposure to ultraviolet radiation. Skin ulceration has been reported in psoriatic patients. The recall phenomenon has been reported in both radiation and solar damaged skin.

*Haematopoietic:* Bone marrow depression is most frequently manifested by leukopenia, but thrombocytopenia, anaemia, or any combination may occur. Infection or septicaemia and haemorrhage from various sites may result. Hypogammaglobulinaemia has been reported.

*Alimentary system:* Mucositis (most frequently stomatitis although gingivitis, pharyngitis and even enteritis, intestinal ulceration and bleeding) may occur. In rare cases the effect of Methotrexate on the intestinal mucosa has led to malabsorption or toxic megacolon. Nausea, anorexia and vomiting and/or diarrhoea may also occur.

*Hepatic:* Hepatic toxicity resulting in significant elevations of liver enzymes, acute liver atrophy, necrosis, fatty metamorphosis, periportal fibrosis or cirrhosis or death may occur, usually following chronic administration.

*Urogenital system:* Renal failure and uraemia may

follow Methotrexate administration, usually in high doses. Vaginitis, vaginal ulcers, cystitis, haematuria and nephropathy have also been reported.

*Pulmonary system:* Infrequently an acute or chronic interstitial pneumonitis, often associated with blood eosinophilia, may occur and deaths have been reported. Acute pulmonary oedema has also been reported after oral and intrathecal use. Pulmonary fibrosis is rare. A syndrome consisting of pleuritic pain and pleural thickening has been reported following high doses.

In the treatment of rheumatoid arthritis, Methotrexate induced lung disease is a potentially serious adverse drug reaction which may occur acutely at any time during therapy. It is not always fully reversible. Pulmonary symptoms (especially a dry, non productive cough) may require interruption of treatment and careful investigation.

*Central nervous system:* Headaches, drowsiness and blurred vision have occurred. Following low doses of Methotrexate, transient subtle cognitive dysfunction, mood alteration, or unusual cranial sensations have been reported occasionally. Aphasia, paresis, hemiparesis, and convulsions have also occurred following administration of higher doses.

There have been reports of leukoencephalopathy following intravenous Methotrexate in high doses, or low doses following cranial-spinal radiation.

*Adverse reactions following intrathecal Methotrexate* are generally classified into three groups, acute, subacute, and chronic. The acute form is a chemical arachnoiditis manifested by headache, back or shoulder pain, nuchal rigidity, and fever. The subacute form may include paresis, usually transient, paraplegia, nerve palsies, and cerebellar dysfunction. The chronic form is a leukoencephalopathy manifested by irritability, confusion, ataxia, spasticity, occasionally convulsions, dementia, somnolence, coma, and rarely, death. There is evidence that the combined use of cranial radiation and intrathecal Methotrexate increases the incidence of leukoencephalopathy.

Additional reactions related to or attributed to the use of Methotrexate such as osteoporosis, abnormal (usually 'megaloblastic') red cell morphology, precipitation of diabetes, other metabolic changes, and sudden death have been reported.

*Overdosage:* Calcium Leucovorin is the antidote for neutralising the immediate toxic effects of Methotrexate on the haemopoietic system. It may be administered orally, intramuscularly, or by an intravenous bolus injection or infusion. In cases of accidental overdosage, a dose of Calcium Leucovorin equal to or higher than the offending dose of Methotrexate should be administered within one hour and dosing continued until the serum levels of Methotrexate are below $10^{-7}$M. Other supporting therapy such as a blood transfusion and renal dialysis may be required.

**Pharmaceutical precautions** Parenteral Methotrexate preparations do not contain an antimicrobial preservative. Any unused injection should be discarded.

Parenteral Methotrexate preparations are stable for 24 hours when diluted with the following intravenous infusion fluids: 0.9% Sodium Chloride; Glucose; Sodium Chloride and Glucose; Compound Sodium Chloride (Ringers Injection); Compound Sodium Lactate (Lactated Ringers Injection).

Methotrexate preparations should be stored at controlled room temperature (15˚–30˚C) and protected from direct sunlight. Other drugs should not be mixed with Methotrexate in the same infusion container.

*Handling of cytotoxic drugs:* Cytotoxic drugs should only be handled by trained personnel in a designated area. The work surface should be covered with disposable plastic-backed absorbent paper.

Protective gloves and goggles should be worn to avoid the drug accidentally coming into contact with the skin or eyes.

Methotrexate is not vesicant and should not cause harm if it comes in contact with the skin. It should, of course, be washed off with water immediately. Any transient stinging may be treated with bland cream. If there is any danger of systemic absorption of significant quantities of Methotrexate, by any route, Calcium Leucovorin cover should be given.

Cytotoxic preparations should not be handled by pregnant staff.

Any spillage or waste material may be disposed of by incineration. We do not make any specific recommendations with regard to the temperature of the incinerator.

**Legal category** POM

**Package quantities**
Tablets 2.5 mg: Bottles of 100.
Injection 50 mg in 2 ml: Boxes of 1 Vial.
Injection 200 mg in 8 ml: Boxes of 1 Vial.
Injection 500 mg in 20 ml: Boxes of 1 Vial.
Injection 1 g in 40 ml: Boxes of 1 Vial.
Injection 5 g in 200 ml: Boxes of 1 Vial.

**Further information** Dosage regimes for Calcium

Leucovorin rescue vary, depending upon the dose of Methotrexate administered. In general, up to 150 mg are usually given in divided doses, over 12–24 hours, by intramuscular injection, bolus intravenous injection or intravenous infusion or orally, followed by 12–15 mg intramuscularly, IV, or 15 mg (one tablet) orally, every six hours for the next 48 hours. Rescue therapy is usually started following a delay of 8 to 24 hours from the beginning of the Methotrexate infusion. One tablet (15 mg) of Calcium Leucovorin every six hours for 48–72 hours may be sufficient when lower doses (less than 100 mg) of Methotrexate have been given.

Calcium Leucovorin is available as an injection (3 mg/ml) in 1 ml ampoules, as a vial of powder for injection (15 mg and 30 mg), and as tablets (15 mg) in bottles of 10.

Further information on other formulations of Methotrexate, on results with particular cyclical regimes of combinations of cytotoxic drugs and other aspects of cancer chemotherapy with Methotrexate is available on request.

**Product licence numbers**
Tablets 2.5 mg 0095/5079R
Injection 25 mg/ml 0095/0016

## MICROVAL*

**Presentation** Microval tablets are round white lustrous coated, convex tablets 5.0 mm in diameter. Each tablet contains 30 micrograms levonorgestrel.

**Uses** Oral contraception. Microval is particularly indicated for the older woman changing from combined oral contraceptives and for women for whom oestrogen treatment is considered unsuitable.

**Dosage and administration** The tablets are started on the first day of menstruation and taken daily without interruption for as long as contraception is desired. They should be taken at the same time each day, preferably after the evening meal or at bedtime so that the interval between tablets is always about 24 hours. Protection may be reduced when the interval increases beyond 27 hours.

During the first cycle additional contraceptive precautions should be taken for the first 14 days.

If a tablet is not taken at the usual time it should be taken as soon as possible and the next tablet taken at the usual time. If the interval between tablets is more than 27 hours protection may be impaired. The patient should take one tablet as soon as she remembers and thereafter one tablet daily as before but should use additional contraceptive measures until the tablets have been taken regularly for 14 days. If a tablet is missed the patient should take one tablet daily as before but should use additional contraceptive measures until the tablets have been taken regularly for 14 days

If vomiting occurs shortly after a tablet has been taken contraceptive protection can be maintained by taking another tablet, provided that it is taken within three hours of the normal time. The last tablet in the pack may be used for this purpose. If repeated vomiting or diarrhoea endanger absorption additional contraceptive precautions should be used for 14 days after the symptoms have disappeared.

Irregular spotting or bleeding may occur with a proportion of women initially but menstrual regularity is usually re-established after the first few cycles. Those patients whose menstrual patterns do not become reasonably regular after three to four cycles or who have prolonged bleeding or amenorrhoea lasting for two months should be instructed to return for advice.

Women who change from a combined oral contraceptive to Microval should stop taking the previous product, leave seven clear days and take the first Microval tablet on the eighth day, then continue to take 1 tablet daily. Additional contraceptive precautions should be taken until the fourteenth tablet has been taken.

Microval does not diminish the yield of breast milk and can be used from the seventh post-partum day.

**Contra-indications, warnings, etc**
*Contra-indications:* Microval should not be given:

1. To patients with established hepatic disease or to those in whom there is evidence of persistently abnormal liver function such as the Dubin-Johnson and Rotor syndromes, or to those who have a history during pregnancy of idiopathic jaundice or severe pruritus.

2. To patients with a history of infectious hepatitis until the liver function tests have returned to normal values.

3. To patients with abnormal vaginal bleeding of unknown aetiology.

4. To patients with suspected pregnancy.

5. Although the risk of thromboembolism has not been associated with progestogen-only contraceptives, it is at present required that a history of thromboembolic disorders should be regarded as a contra-indication.

*Precautions:*

1. Oral contraceptive medication should be discontinued if there is a gradual or sudden, partial or complete loss of vision, proptosis or diplopia, papilloedema or any evidence of retinal or vascular lesions.

2. Caution should be observed in prescribing oral contraceptives for any patients with a history of migraine, or if migraine is being treated with vasoconstrictor drugs. If migraine worsens or migraine or severe headache develops for the first time during treatment, medication should be discontinued immediately.

3. Women with hypertension who are taking Microval require careful observation and their blood pressure should be monitored regularly.

4. A small fraction of the progestogen has been identified in the milk of mothers receiving the drug. The long-range effects to the nursing infant are currently unknown.

5. Examination of the pelvic organs, breasts and blood pressure should precede prescription of Microval and should be repeated regularly.

6. Ectopic pregnancies appear to occur more frequently on progestogen-only oral contraceptives.

*Side-effects:* Microval is well tolerated but certain endocrine effects which are also characteristic of ovulatory cycles may occur. Those noted are headache, slight weight gain, nausea, skin disorders, breast tenderness and spotting between periods. The incidence of such effects with Microval is low and tends to decrease as treatment continues.

*Drug interactions:* Caution should be observed in prescribing oral contraceptives for patients taking other drugs since various interactions have been reported. Pregnancies have been reported in women taking oral contraceptives concurrently with rifampicin and other antibiotics, anti-epileptic drugs, barbiturates and other sedative drugs.

Steroids affect drug metabolism and the therapeutic or toxic effects of other drugs may be modified. Interactions have been reported between oral contraceptives and tricyclic antidepressants, anti-coagulants and corticosteroids.

*Overdosage:* No reports of serious ill-effects from overdosage with oral contraceptives have been reported. In general, therefore, treatment of overdosage is not necessary. If overdosage is, however, discovered within one hour and is so large that treatment seems desirable, gastric lavage or a suitable dose of ipecacuanha can be used. There are no specific antidotes and further treatment should be symptomatic.

**Pharmaceutical precautions** Store at or below room temperature.

**Legal category** POM

**Package quantities** Microval tablets are supplied in memo packs of 35 tablets.

**Further information** Estimates from clinical trials show that, if the tablets are taken correctly, out of 100 women taking them for one year, on average one woman may become pregnant during that year. Microval, although not quite as effective as combined oral contraceptives, provides an extremely high degree of protection and is very much more effective than withdrawal, condom, rhythm method or chemicals and comparable to the I.U.C.D. and diaphragm.

Levonorgestrel is a totally synthetic progestogen which possesses no inherent oestrogenicity. It has anti-oestrogenic properties and has minimal effects on metabolic functions.

**Product licence number** 0011/0040

## MINOCIN 50*
## MINOCIN* 100 mg TABLETS

**Presentation** *Tablets 50 mg:* Each beige film-coated tablet, embossed M/50 on one face, contains Minocycline hydrochloride equivalent to 50 mg Minocycline base.

*Tablets 100 mg:* Each orange, film-coated tablet, embossed M/100 on one face, contains Minocycline hydrochloride equivalent to 100 mg Minocycline base.

**Uses** Minocycline is a broad spectrum antibiotic used for the treatment of infections caused by tetracycline-sensitive organisms. Some tetracycline-resistant strains of Staphylococci are also sensitive.

*Typical indications include:* Gonorrhoea. Non-gonococcal urethritis. Prostatitis. Acne. Acute and chronic bronchitis. Bronchiectasis. Lung abscess. Pneumonia. Ear, nose and throat infections. Urinary tract infections. Pelvic inflammatory disease (eg salpingitis, oophoritis). Skin and soft tissue infections caused by minocycline sensitive organisms. Ophthalmological infections. Nocardiosis. Prophylactic treatment of asymptomatic meningococcal carriers. Pre- and pos operative prophylaxis of infection.

**Dosage and administration** *Adults:*

1. *Routine antibiotic use:* 200 mg daily in divide doses.

2. *Acne:* 50 mg twice daily, for a minimum of weeks.

3. *Gonorrhoea:* In adult males: 200 mg initiall followed by 100 mg every 12 hours for a minimum 4 days with post-therapy cultures within 2–3 day Adult females may require more prolonged therapy

4. *Prophylaxis of asymptomatic meningococc carriers:* 100 mg bid for five days, usually followed b a course of rifampicin.

*Children:* For children above 12 years of age th recommended dosage for Minocin is one 50 mg tabl every 12 hours. Minocin is not recommended f children under 12 years old.

*Elderly:* Minocin may be used at the normal recon mended dosage in elderly patients even with mild moderate renal impairment, however caution is a vised in patients with severe renal impairment.

*Administration:* To reduce the risk of oesophage irritation and ulceration, the tablets should be swa lowed whole with plenty of fluid, while sitting standing. Unlike earlier tetracyclines, absorption Minocin is not significantly impaired by food moderate amounts of milk.

Treatment of acne should be continued for minimum of six weeks. If, after six months, there no satisfactory response Minocin should be disconti ued and other therapies considered. If Minocin is be continued for longer than six months, patien should be monitored at least three monthly thereaft for signs and symptoms of hepatitis or SLE (se warnings and precautions).

**Contra-indications, warnings, etc**
*Contra-indications:* Known hypersensitivity to tetr cyclines. Use in pregnancy, lactation, children und the age of 12 years, complete renal failure.

*Warnings and precautions:* Minocin should be use with caution in patients with hepatic dysfunction an in conjunction with alcohol and other hepatotox drugs. Rare cases of auto-immune hepatotoxicity an isolated cases of systemic lupus erythematosus (SL and also exacerbation of pre-existing SLE have bee reported. If patients develop signs or symptoms SLE or hepatotoxicity, or suffer exacerbation of pr existing SLE, minocycline should be discontinue Clinical studies have shown that there is no significa drug accumulation in patients with renal impairme when they are treated with Minocin in the recon mended doses. In cases of severe renal insufficienc reduction of dosage and monitoring of renal functio may be required.

Cross-resistance between tetracyclines may d velop in micro-organisms and cross-sensitisation patients. Minocin should be discontinued if there a signs/symptoms of overgrowth of resistant orga isms, eg enteritis, glossitis, stomatitis, vaginitis, pr ritus ani or staphylococcal enteritis.

Patients taking oral contraceptives should b warned that if diarrhoea or breakthrough bleedir occur there is a possibility of contraceptive failure.

*Interactions:* Minocin should not be used with penici lins. Tetracyclines depress plasma prothrombin acti ity and reduced doses of concomitant anticoagulan may be necessary.

Absorption of Minocin is impaired by the concom tant administration of antacids, iron, calcium, mag nesium, aluminium and zinc salts. Unlike earli tetracyclines, absorption of Minocin is not signi cantly impaired by food or moderate amounts of mil

*Use in pregnancy:* Results of animal studies indica that tetracyclines cross the placenta, are found foetal tissues and can have toxic effects on th developing foetus (often related to retardation skeletal development). Evidence of embryotoxici has also been noted in animals treated early pregnancy. Minocin therefore, should not be used pregnancy unless considered essential.

The use of drugs of the tetracycline class durir tooth development (last half of pregnancy) may caus permanent discolouration of the teeth (yellow-gre brown). This adverse reaction is more common durin long term use of the drugs but has been observe following repeated short term courses. Enamel hyp plasia has also been reported.

*Use in lactation:* Tetracyclines have been found in th milk of lactating women who are taking a drug in th class. Permanent tooth discolouration may occur the developing infant and enamel hypoplasia ha been reported.

*Use in children:* The use of tetracyclines during too development in children under the age of 12 yea may cause permanent discolouration (see above Enamel hypoplasia has also been reported.

'de-effects: In common with other tetracyclines astrointestinal disturbances including nausea, ano- xia, vomiting and diarrhoea may occur. Dermatolog- al reactions such as erythema multiforme, Stevens ohnson syndrome, exfoliative dermatitis and photo- nsitivity have been reported, as well as maculopa- ular and erythematous rashes and, rarely, fixed drug uptions. Hypersensitivity reactions can include urti- ria, fever, arthralgia, pulmonary infiltration, angi- neurotic oedema, anaphylaxis and anaphylactoid urpura. Rarely pericarditis and renal failure including terstitial nephritis have been reported. Isolated cases f systemic lupus erythematosus (SLE) and also kacerbation of pre-existing SLE have been reported.

Headache, lightheadedness, dizziness, vertigo and, rely, impaired hearing have occurred with Minocin nd patients should be warned about the possible azards of driving or operating machinery during eatment.

As with other tetracyclines bulging fontanelles in fants and benign intracranial hypertension in juve- iles and adults have been reported. Treatment should ease if evidence of raised intracranial pressure evelops.

Blood: haemolytic anaemia, thrombocytopenia, eutropenia and eosinophilia have been reported with tracyclines.

In common with other tetracyclines, transient in- reases in liver function test values and rarely hepatitis nd acute liver failure have been reported. Some epatic reactions have an auto-immune basis, and ay occur after several months of Minocin treatment see dosage and administration). There have been olated incidences of pancreatitis.

When given over prolonged periods, tetracyclines ave been reported to produce brown-black micro- opic discolouration of thyroid tissue. Hyperpigmen- tion of skin, nails or discolouration of teeth and uccal mucosa have been reported occasionally. hese are generally reversible on cessation of therapy. here are isolated cases of discolouration of conjunc- va, lacrimal secretions, breast secretions and perspi- tion. See also Uses in Pregnancy and Lactation.

*verdosage:* No specific antidote. Gastric lavage plus ppropriate supportive treatment.

**harmaceutical precautions** The product should be ored at controlled room temperature (below 30°C) the original pack or in containers which prevent ccess of moisture.

Protect from light.

**egal category** POM

**ackage quantities**
50 mg Tablets: Blister packs of 84
100 mg Tablets: Bottles of 20 and 50

**urther information** Nil

**roduct licence numbers**
0 mg Tablets 0095/0062
00 mg Tablets 0095/0006

## MINOCIN MR*

**resentation** Minocin MR is a two piece hard shell apsule with an orange body and brown opaque cap, ontaining a mixture of yellow and off-white round ellets. The capsule is marked in white with Lederle nd the number 8560.

Each capsule contains minocycline hydrochloride quivalent to 100 mg minocycline.

**ses** Minocin MR capsules are indicated for the eatment of acne.

**osage and administration** *Adults:* One capsule very 24 hours.

*hildren over 12 years:* One capsule every 24 hours.

*lderly:* No special dosing requirements.

*dministration:* To reduce the risk of oesophageal ritation and ulceration, the capsules should be wallowed whole with plenty of fluid, while sitting or tanding. Unlike earlier tetracyclines, absorption of linocin MR is not significantly impaired by food or oderate amounts of milk.

Treatment of acne should be continued for a inimum of six weeks. If, after six months, there is o satisfactory response Minocin MR should be iscontinued and other therapies considered. If Min- cin MR is to be continued for longer than six months, atients should be monitored at least three monthly ereafter for signs and symptoms of hepatitis or SLE see warnings and precautions)

**ontra-indications, warnings, etc**

*ontra-indications:* Known hypersensitivity to tetra- yclines. Use in pregnancy, lactation, children under ne age of 12 years, complete renal failure.

*Varnings, precautions:* Minocin MR should be used vith caution in patients with hepatic dysfunction and conjunction with alcohol and other hepatotoxic drugs. Rare cases of auto-immune hepatotoxicity and isolated cases of systemic lupus erythmatosus (SLE) and also exacerbation of pre-existing SLE have been reported. If patients develop signs or symptoms of SLE or hepatotoxicity, or suffer exacerbation of pre-existing SLE, minocycline should be discontinued. Clinical studies have shown that there is no significant drug accumulation in patients with renal impairment when they are treated with Minocin MR in the recommended doses. In cases of severe renal insufficiency, reduction of dosage and monitoring of renal function may be required.

Cross-resistance between tetracyclines may develop in micro-organisms and cross-sensitisation in patients. Minocin MR should be discontinued if there are signs/symptoms of overgrowth of resistant organisms, eg enteritis, glossitis, stomatitis, vaginitis, pruritus ani or staphylococcal enteritis.

Women taking oral contraceptives should be warned that if diarrhoea or breakthrough bleeding occur there is a possibility of contraceptive failure.

*Interactions:* Minocin MR should not be used with penicillins. Tetracyclines depress plasma prothrombin activity and reduced doses of concomitant anticoagulants may be necessary.

Absorption of Minocin MR is impaired by the concomitant administration of antacids, iron, calcium, magnesium, aluminium and zinc salts. Unlike earlier tetracyclines, absorption of Minocin MR is not significantly impaired by food or moderate amounts of milk.

*Use in pregnancy:* Results of animal studies indicate that tetracyclines cross the placenta, are found in foetal tissues and can have toxic effects on the developing foetus (often related to retardation of skeletal development). Evidence of embryotoxicity has also been noted in animals treated early in pregnancy. Minocin MR therefore, should not be used in pregnancy unless considered essential.

The use of drugs of the tetracycline class during tooth development (last half of pregnancy) may cause permanent discolouration of the teeth (yellow-grey-brown). This adverse reaction is more common during long term use of the drugs but has been observed following repeated short term courses. Enamel hypoplasia has also been reported.

*Use in lactation:* Tetracyclines have been found in the milk of lactating women who are taking a drug in this class. Permanent tooth discolouration may occur in the developing infant and enamel hypoplasia has been reported.

*Use in children:* The use of tetracyclines during tooth development in children under the age of 12 years may cause permanent discolouration (see above). Enamel hypoplasia has also been reported.

*Side-effects:* In common with other tetracyclines gastrointestinal disturbances including nausea, anorexia, vomiting and diarrhoea may occur. Dermatological reactions such as erythema multiforme, Stevens Johnson syndrome, exfoliative dermatitis and photosensitivity have been reported, as well as maculopapular and erythematous rashes and, rarely, fixed drug eruptions. Hypersensitivity reactions can include urticaria, fever, arthralgia, pulmonary infiltration, angioneurotic oedema, anaphylaxis and anaphylactoid purpura. Rarely pericarditis and renal failure including interstitial nephritis have been reported. Isolated cases of systemic lupus erythematosus (SLE) and also exacerbation of pre-existing SLE have been reported. (see also warnings and precautions)

Headache, light-headedness, dizziness, vertigo and, rarely, impaired hearing have occurred with Minocin MR and patients should be warned about the possible hazards of driving or operating machinery during treatment.

As with other tetracyclines bulging fontanelles in infants and benign intracranial hypertension in juveniles and adults have been reported. Treatment should cease if evidence of raised intracranial pressure develops.

Blood: haemolytic anaemia, thrombocytopenia, neutropenia and eosinophilia have been reported with tetracyclines.

In common with other tetracyclines, transient increases in liver function test values and rarely hepatitis, and acute liver failure have been reported. Some hepatic reactions have an auto-immune basis, and may occur after several months of Minocin MR treatment (see *Dosage and administration*). There have been isolated incidences of pancreatitis.

When given over prolonged periods, tetracyclines have been reported to produce brown-black microscopic discolouration of thyroid tissue. Hyperpigmentation of skin, nails or discolouration of teeth and buccal mucosa have been reported occasionally. These are generally reversible on cessation of therapy. There are isolated cases of discolouration of conjunctiva, lacrimal secretions, breast secretions and perspiration. See also Uses in Pregnancy and Lactation.

*Overdosage:* No specific antidote. Gastric lavage plus appropriate supportive treatment.

**Pharmaceutical precautions** The product should be stored at controlled room temperature (15–25°C) in the original container. Protect from light.

**Legal category** POM

**Package quantities** Minocin MR is available in calendar packs of 56 capsules.

**Further information** Minocin MR capsules have been formulated as a 'double pulse' delivery system in which a portion of the minocycline is delivered in the stomach, and a second dose is available for absorption in the duodenum and upper GI tract.

**Product licence number** 0095/0240

## MINULET*

**Presentation** Each white sugar coated tablet contains 30 micrograms ethinyloestradiol and 75 micrograms gestodene.

**Uses** Oral contraception and the recognised gynaecological indications for such oestrogen-progestogen combinations. The mode of action includes the inhibition of ovulation by suppression of the mid-cycle surge of luteinising hormone, the inspissation of cervical mucus so as to constitute a barrier to sperm, and the rendering of the endometrium unreceptive to implantation.

**Dosage and administration**

*First treatment cycle:* 1 tablet daily for 21 days, starting with the tablet marked number 1, on the first day of the menstrual cycle. Additional contraception (barriers and spermicides) is not required.

*Subsequent cycles:* Each subsequent course is started when 7 tablet-free days have followed the preceding course. A withdrawal bleed should occur during the 7 tablet-free days.

*Changing from another 21 day combined oral contraceptive:* The first tablet of Minulet should be taken on the first day immediately after the end of the previous oral contraceptive course. Additional contraception is not required. A withdrawal bleed should not be expected until the end of the first pack of Minulet.

*Changing from an Every Day (ED) 28 day combined oral contraceptive:* The first tablet of Minulet should be taken on the day immediately after the day on which the last active pill in the ED pack has been taken. The remaining tablets in the ED pack should be discarded. Additional contraception is not required. A withdrawal bleed should not be expected until the end of the first pack of Minulet.

*Changing from a Progestogen-only-Pill (POP):* The first tablet of Minulet should be taken on the first day of menstruation even if the POP for that day has already been taken. The remaining tablets in the POP pack should be discarded. Additional contraception is not required.

*Post-partum and post-abortum use:* After pregnancy combined oral contraception can be started in non-lactating women 21 days after a vaginal delivery, provided that the patient is fully ambulant and there are no puerperal complications.

If the pill is started later than 21 days after delivery, then alternative contraception (barriers and spermicides) should be used until oral contraception is started and for the first 7 days of pill-taking. If unprotected intercourse has taken place after 21 days post partum, then oral contraception should not be started until the first menstrual bleed after childbirth. After a miscarriage or abortion oral contraception may be started immediately.

*Special circumstances requiring additional contraception:*

*Missed pills:* If a tablet is delayed it should be taken as soon as possible and if it is taken within 12 hours of the correct time, additional contraception is not needed. Further tablets should then be taken at the usual time. If the delay exceeds 12 hours, the last missed pill should be taken when remembered, the earlier missed pills left in the pack and normal pill-taking resumed. If one or more tablets are omitted from the 21 days of pill-taking, additional contraception (barriers and spermicides) should be used for the next 7 days of pill-taking. In addition, if one or more pills are missed during the last 7 days of pill-taking, the subsequent pill-free interval should be disregarded and the next pack started the day after taking the last tablet from the previous pack. In this case, a withdrawal bleed should not be expected until the end of the second pack. If the patient does not have a withdrawal bleed at the end of the second pack she must return to her doctor to exclude the possibilty of pregnancy.

*Gastro-intestinal upset:* Vomiting or diarrhoea may

reduce the efficacy by preventing full absorption. Additional contraception (barriers and spermicides) should be used during the upset and for the 7 days following the upset. If these 7 days overrun the end of a pack, the next pack should be started without a break. In this case, a withdrawal bleed should not be expected until the end of the second pack. If the patient does not have a withdrawal bleed at the end of the second pack she must return to her doctor to exclude the possibility of pregnancy.

Mild laxatives do not impair contraceptive action.

*Interaction with other drugs:* Some drugs accelerate the metabolism of oral contraceptives when taken concurrently and these include barbiturates, phenytoin, phenylbutazone and rifampicin. Other drugs suspected of having the capacity to reduce the efficacy of oral contraceptives include ampicillin and other antibiotics. It is, therefore, advisable to use non-hormonal methods of contraception (barriers and spermicides) in addition to the oral contraceptive as long as an extremely high degree of protection is required during treatment with such drugs. The additional contraception should be used while the concurrent medication continues and for 7 days afterwards. If these extra precautions overrun the end of the pack, the next pack should be started without a break. In this case, a withdrawal bleed should not be expected until the end of the second pack. If the patient does not have a withdrawal bleed at the end of the second pack she must return to her doctor to exclude the possibility of pregnancy.

**Contra-indications, warnings, etc**

*Contra-indications:*

1. Suspected pregnancy.
2. Thrombotic disorders and a history of these conditions, sickle-cell anaemia, disorders of lipid metabolism and other conditions in which, in individual cases, there is known or suspected to be a much increased risk of thrombosis.
3. Acute or severe chronic liver diseases. Dubin-Johnson syndrome. Rotor syndrome. History, during pregnancy, of idiopathic jaundice or severe pruritus.
4. History of herpes gestationis.
5. Mammary or endometrial carcinoma, or a history of these conditions.
6. Abnormal vaginal bleeding of unknown cause.
7. Deterioration of otosclerosis during pregnancy.

*Warnings:*

1. There is a general opinion, based on statistical evidence, that users of combined oral contraceptives experience, more often than non-users, venous thromboembolism, arterial thrombosis, including cerebral and myocardial infarction, and subarachnoid haemorrhage. Full recovery from such disorders does not always occur, and it should be realised that in a few cases they are fatal. How often these disorders occur in users of the modern low-dose pills is not known, but there are reasons for suggesting that they may occur less often than with older pills containing more oestrogen. Certain factors may entail some risk of thrombosis, e.g. smoking, obesity, varicose veins, cardiovascular diseases, diabetes and migraine. The suitability of a combined oral contraceptive should be judged according to the severity of such conditions in the individual case, and should be discussed with the patient before she decides to take it.
2. The risk of arterial thrombosis associated with combined oral contraceptives increases with age, and this risk is aggravated by cigarette smoking. The use of combined oral contraceptives by women in the older age group, especially those who are cigarette smokers, should therefore be discouraged and alternative methods used.
3. The possibility cannot be ruled out that certain chronic diseases may occasionally deteriorate during the use of combined oral contraceptives (see *Precautions*).
4. The combination of ethinyloestradiol and gestodene, like other contraceptive steroids, is associated with an increased incidence of neoplastic nodules in the rat liver, the relevance of which to man is unknown.
5. Malignant liver tumours have been reported on rare occasions in long-term users of oral contraceptives. Benign hepatic tumours have also been associated with oral contraceptive usage. A hepatic tumour should be considered in the differential diagnosis when upper abdominal pain, enlarged liver or signs of intra-abdominal haemorrhage occur.
6. Numerous epidemiological studies have been reported on the risks of ovarian, endometrial, cervical and breast cancer in women using combined oral contraceptives. The evidence is clear that combined oral contraceptives offer substantial protection against both ovarian and endometrial cancer.

An increased risk of cervical cancer in long term users of combined oral contraceptives has been reported in some studies, but there continues to be controversy about the extent to which this is attributable to the confounding effects of sexual behaviour and other factors.

The evidence linking combined oral contraceptive use and breast cancer remains inconclusive. The results of some studies suggest an increased risk of breast cancer presenting below the age of about 35, the risk rising with duration of use. Any possible increased risk of breast cancer with combined oral contraceptives is however likely to be small and may be expected to be less with low dosage pills. This possible risk should be weighed against the many benefits of combined oral contraceptives, including their protective effects against ovarian and endometrial cancers.

*Reasons for stopping oral contraception immediately:*

1. Occurrence of migraine in patients who have never previously suffered from it. Exacerbation of pre-existing migraine. Any unusually frequent or unusually severe headaches.
2. Any kind of acute disturbance of vision.
3. Suspicion of thrombosis or infarction.
4. Six weeks before elective operations and during immobilisation, e.g. after accidents, etc.
5. Significant rise in blood-pressure.
6. Jaundice.
7. Clear exacerbation of conditions known to be capable of deteriorating during oral contraception or pregnancy.
8. Pregnancy is a reason for stopping immediately because it has been suggested by some investigations that oral contraceptives taken in early pregnancy may slightly increase the risk of foetal malformations. Other investigations have failed to support these findings. The possibility therefore cannot be excluded, but it is certain that if a risk exists at all, it is very small.

*Precautions:*

1. Examination of the pelvic organs, breasts and blood-pressure should precede the prescribing of any combined oral contraceptive and should be repeated regularly.
2. Before starting treatment, pregnancy must be excluded.
3. The following conditions require careful observation during medication: a history of severe depressive states, varicose veins, diabetes, hypertension, epilepsy, otosclerosis, multiple sclerosis, porphyria, tetany, disturbed liver function, gall-stones, cardiovascular diseases, renal diseases, chloasma, uterine fibroids, asthma, the wearing of contact lenses, or any disease that is prone to worsen during pregnancy. The first appearance or deterioration of any of these conditions may indicate that the oral contraceptive should be stopped.
4. The risk of the deterioration of chloasma, which is often not fully reversible, is reduced by the avoidance of excessive exposure to sunlight.

*Side-effects:* Occasional side-effects may include nausea, vomiting, headaches, breast tenderness, changed body weight or libido, depressive moods and chloasma.

*Menstrual changes:*

1. *Reduction of menstrual flow:* This is not abnormal and it is to be expected in some patients. Indeed, it may be beneficial where heavy periods were previously experienced.
2. *Missed menstruation:* Occasionally, withdrawal bleeding may not occur at all. If the tablets have been taken correctly, pregnancy is very unlikely, but should be ruled out before a new course of tablets is started.

*Intermenstrual bleeding:* Very light 'spotting' or heavier 'breakthrough bleeding' may occur during tablet-taking, especially in the first few cycles. It appears to be generally of no significance, except where it indicates errors of tablet-taking, or where the possibility of interaction with other drugs exists (q.v.). However, if irregular bleeding is persistent, an organic cause should be considered.

*Effect on adrenal and thyroid glands:* Oral contraceptives have no significant influence on adrenocortical function. The ACTH function test for the adrenal cortex remains unchanged. The reduction in corticosteroid excretion and the elevation of plasma corticosteroids are due to an increased cortisol-binding capacity of the plasma proteins.

The response to metyrapone is less pronounced than in untreated women and is thus similar to that during pregnancy.

The radio-iodine uptake shows that thyroid function is unchanged. There is a rise in serum protein-bound iodine, similar to that in pregnancy and during the administration of oestrogens. This is due to the increased capacity of the plasma proteins for binding thyroid hormones, rather than to any change in glandular function. In women taking oral contraceptives, the content of protein-bound iodine in blood serum should therefore, not be used for evaluation of thyroid function.

*Effect on blood chemistry:* Oral contraceptives may accelerate erythrocyte sedimentation in the absence of any disease. This effect is due to a change in the proportion of the plasma protein fractions. Increases in plasma copper, iron and alkaline phosphatase ha also been recorded.

*Overdosage:* There have been no reports of serio ill-effects from overdosage, even when a considerab number of tablets have been taken by a small child. general, it is, therefore, unnecessary to treat overdo age. However, if overdosage is discovered within tw or three hours and is so large that treatment seen desirable, gastric lavage can be safely used.

There are no specific antidotes and further tre ment should be symptomatic.

**Pharmaceutical precautions** Store in cool, dry co ditions. Shelf-life five years.

**Legal category** POM

**Package quantities** Individual packs containi 3 months' supply.

**Further information** Nil.

**Product licence number** 0011/0135

## MONOCOR* TABLETS

**Presentation**

*Tablets 5 mg:* Pink, round, scored, biconvex fil coated tablets marked 'LL' on one side and '5' reverse, each containing 5 mg bisoprolol fumara (2:1).

*Tablets 10 mg:* White, round biconvex film-coat tablets marked 'LL' on one side and '10' on revers each containing 10 mg bisoprolol fumarate (2:1).

**Uses**

*Indications:* The management of hypertension. Th management of angina pectoris.

*Mode of action:* Monocor is a potent, highly cardi selective $B_1$-adrenoceptor blocking agent devoid intrinsic sympathomimetic activity and without rel vant membrane stabilising activity.

As with other beta-blocking agents, the mode action in hypertension is not clear but it is known th Monocor reduces the heart rate and depresses plasm renin activity.

In patients with angina, blocking of cardiac receptors causes a diminished cardiac oxygen d mand because of the resulting reduced heart actio This makes Monocor effective in eliminating reducing the symptoms.

**Dosage and administration**

*Adults*: The usual adult dose is 10 mg once daily wi a maximum recommended dose of 20 mg per day. some patients, 5 mg per day may be adequate.

It is not necessary to alter the dose in patients wi mild to moderate hepatic or renal dysfunction. patients with severe renal failure (creatinine clearan less than 20 ml/min) or in patients with severe hepa dysfunction, the dosage should not exceed 10 m Monocor once daily.

Experience of use of Monocor in renal dialys patients is limited. However, there is no evidence th the dosage regimen needs to be altered.

*Elderly:* No dosage adjustment is normally requir but 5 mg per day may be adequate in some elde patients; as for other adults, the dosage may have be reduced in cases of severe renal or hepa dysfunction.

*Children:* There is no paediatric experience wi bisoprolol, therefore its use cannot be recommend for children.

**Contra-indications, warnings etc**

*Contra-indications*: As with other beta-adrenocept antagonists, Monocor should not be used in cases untreated cardiac failure, cardiogenic shock, sinoatr block, second or third degree AV block, mark bradycardia (less than 50 beats per minute) or extren hypotension or severe asthma.

*Precautions:* Monocor should be used with care patients with a prolonged PR conduction interv poor cardiac reserve and peripheral circulatory distu bances, such as Raynaud's phenomena.

In patients suffering ischaemic heart disease trea ment should not be discontinued abruptly.

Due to the low affinity of Monocor for $B_2$-recepto the drug does not appear to have a hypoglycaem effect. However, it should be used with caution diabetic patients since the symptoms of hypoglyca mia (in particular tachycardia) may be masked.

Although Monocor is a highly selective $B_1$-adren ceptor blocking agent, it should be used with cauti in patients with chronic obstructive airways disea or a family history of asthma. In some asthma patients some increase in airways resistance m occur and this may be regarded as a signal discontinue therapy. Bronchospasm can usually reversed by commonly used bronchodilators such salbutamol.

*regnancy and lactation:* No teratogenic effects have een demonstrated in animal studies but the safety of Ionocor during human pregnancy has not been stablished. Like other beta-blockers, the benefits of se during pregnancy should be weighed against the ossible hazards to mother and foetus. Beta-blockers dministered in late pregnancy may cause bradycar-ia or hypotension in the foetus/neonate.

Studies in animals suggest that no clinically relevant evels of Monocor reach the breast milk. However, as n pregnancy, caution should be exercised for use uring lactation.

*ide-effects:* Monocor is usually well tolerated. The eported side-effects are generally attributable to the harmacological activity of a beta-blocker and include assitude, fatigue, dizziness, mild headache, muscle nd joint ache, perspiration, aggravation of intermit-ent claudication or Raynaud's disease, paraesthesia nd coldness of the extremities, bronchospasm, edema and occasional gastro-intestinal side effects uch as nausea/vomiting and diarrhoea. A marked ecrease in blood pressure and pulse rate or a isturbance of AV conduction may be observed ccasionally. As with other beta-blockers, skin rashes, ruritis and dry eyes have been reported although the ncidence is low. Sleep disturbances, including vivid reams, of a type noted with other beta blockers have ccasionally been reported. Discontinuation of the rug is recommended if any such reaction is not therwise explicable.

*rug interactions:* Monocor may potentiate the effect f other concurrently administered anti-hypertensive rugs. Concomitant treatment with reserpine, alpha-nethyldopa and clonidine may cause an exaggerated ecrease in heart rate. In particular, if clonidine is to e discontinued this should not be done until Monocor reatment has been discontinued for several days.

Monocor should also be used with care when nyocardial depressants, inhibitors of AV conduction uch as calcium antagonists of the verapamil and iltiazem type, or Class I antidysrrhythmic agents uch as disopyramide are used concurrently.

The intravenous administration of calcium antago-ists and antiarrhythmic agents is not recommended uring Monocor therapy.

The concurrent use of rifampicin can reduce the limination half-life of Monocor, although an increase n dose is generally not necessary. The effects of nsulin or oral hypoglycaemic agents may be poten-ated when used concurrently with Monocor.

*naesthesia:* Prior to anaesthesia, the anaesthetist hould be informed if the patient is taking Monocor. n cases of severe ischaemic heart disease the risk/ enefit of continuing treatment should be evaluated. are should be taken when using either cyclopropane r trichloroethylene.

*verdosage:* In the case of overdosage or a precipitous rop in pulse rate and/or blood pressure, treatment vith Monocor must be discontinued. Excessive brad-cardia may be countered by atropine 0.5–2.0 mg ntravenously. If necessary this may be followed by a eta stimulant such as orciprenaline by slow intra-enous injection. Glucagon may also be useful as a ardiac stimulant in a dose of 1 to 5 mg intravenously.

**harmaceutical precautions** No special require-nents.

**egal category** POM

**ackage quantities** Calenderised blister packs of 28 ablets in strips of 14. White plastic bottles containing 00 tablets.

**urther information** Monocor is absorbed almost ompletely from the gastrointestinal tract. Together vith the very small first past effect in the liver, this esults in a high bioavailability of approximately 90% he drug is cleared equally by the liver and kidneys. he high bioavailability and the dual pathway of learance lead to predictable blood levels. The long lasma half-life (10–12 hours) provides 24 hour fficacy following a once daily dosage. About 95% of he drug substance is excreted through the kidneys, alf of this as unchanged Monocor. There are no ctive metabolites in man.

**roduct licence numbers**
ablets 5 mg 0095/0177
ablets 10 mg 0095/0178

## ONOZIDE*10

**resentation** White, round, biconvex, film coated ablets marked B-14 on one side and LL on the other, ach containing 10 mg bisoprolol fumarate (2:1), and .25 mg hydrochlorothiazide.

**ses** Management of hypertension.

*lode of Action:* Bisoprolol is a potent, highly cardi-selective $\beta_1$-adrenoreceptor antagonist devoid of intrinsic sympathomimetic activity and without relevant membrane stabilising activity.

As with other $\beta_1$-antagonists, the mode of action in hypertension is not clear but it is known that bisoprolol reduces the heart rate and markedly depresses plasma renin activity.

Hydrochlorothiazide is a thiazide diuretic which has an antihypertensive action. It exerts its diuretic effect by inhibiting the resorption of sodium and chloride ions in the loop of Henle and distal tubule. It also appears to decrease peripheral resistance. Hydrochlorothiazide is frequently used in combination with a $\beta$-adrenoceptor antagonist where an additional antihypertensive effect is required.

**Dosage and administration** *Adults:* One tablet daily. No dose reduction is needed in patients with mild to moderate hepatic or renal dysfunction.

*Elderly:* As for adults.

*Children:* There is no paediatric experience with bisoprolol and it is not therefore recommended for children.

**Contra-indications, warnings, etc**
*Contra-indications:* As with other $\beta$-adrenoceptor antagonist diuretic combinations, Monozide 10 should not be used in cases of untreated or decompensated cardiac failure, cardiogenic shock, sinoatrial block, second or third degree AV block, marked bradycardia (heart rate less than 50 beats/min), extreme hypotension, acute myocardial infarction, and severe asthma. It should not be used in patients with a known allergic hypersensitivity to thiazides or sulphonamides, with severe renal or hepatic failure, as well as in patients with severe hypokalaemia or hyponatraemia.

*Precautions:* Monozide 10 tablets should be used with care in patients with prolonged PR conduction interval, poor cardiac reserve and peripheral circulatory disturbances, such as Raynaud's phenomenon.

In patients with ischaemic heart disease, treatment should not be withdrawn abruptly.

Since bisoprolol is a highly selective $\beta_1$-adrenoceptor antagonist, Monozide 10 may be used with caution in patients with a medical history of chronic obstructive airways disease or a family history of asthma. However, in some patients an increase in airways resistance may occur and this may be regarded as a signal to discontinue therapy. This bronchospasm can usually be reversed by commonly used bronchodilators such as salbutamol.

Due to the low affinity of bisoprolol for $\beta_2$-receptors, Monozide 10 does not appear to have a hypoglycaemic effect. However, it should be used with caution in diabetic patients since the symptoms of hypoglycaemia (in particular, tachycardia) may be masked and hydrochlorothiazide may impair glucose tolerance further.

Clinical trials have shown that the low dose of hydrochlorothiazide in this formulation reduces the elevation in uric acid levels normally associated with higher doses of hydrochlorothiazide. However, care should be taken in patients with a predisposition to gout or hyperuricaemia.

The particularly low dose of hydrochlorothiazide in this formulation (6.25 mg) reduces the possibility of significant electrolyte imbalance occurring. However, all patients treated with diuretics should receive periodic monitoring for signs of fluid or electrolyte imbalance. Hypokalaemia can be induced as a result of thiazide therapy and potassium levels should be checked; particularly in older patients, those receiving digitalis preparations for heart failure, those on diets low in potassium and patients suffering from gastro-intestinal complaints.

*Pregnancy and lactation:* No teratogenic effects have been demonstrated with bisoprolol in animal studies, but thiazide diuretics are not generally recommended for use during pregnancy. Beta-blockers administered in late pregnancy may cause bradycardia or hypotension in the foetus/neonate. Like other anti-hypertensive therapy, the benefits of use during pregnancy should be weighed against the possible hazard to mother and foetus. Whilst clinically relevant levels of bisoprolol may not appear in breast milk, hydrochlorothiazide does appear in the milk and if treatment is essential the patient should stop breast feeding.

*Drug interactions:* Bisoprolol may potentiate the effect of other concurrently administered antihypertensive drugs. Concomitant treatment with reserpine, a-methlydopa and clonidine may cause an exaggerated decrease in heart rate and blood pressure. In particular, if clonidine is to be discontinued, this should not be done until treatment with Monozide 10 has been discontinued for several days.

Monozide 10 should also be used with care when myocardial depressants, inhibitors of AV conduction such as calcium antagonists of the verapamil and diltiazem type, or class I antidysrhythmic agents such as disopyramide are used concurrently.

The intravenous administration of calcium antagonists and antiarrhythmic agents is not recommended during therapy with Monozide 10.

Lithium should not generally be administered with diuretics as lithium clearance may be significantly reduced.

The concurrent use of rifampicin can reduce the elimination half-life of bisoprolol, although an increase in dose is generally not necessary. The effects of insulin or oral hypoglycaemic agents may be potentiated when used concurrently with bisoprolol.

*Anaesthesia:* Prior to anaesthesia, the anaesthetist should be informed if the patient is taking Monozide 10. In cases of severe ischaemic heart disease, the risk/benefit of continuing treatment should be evaluated. Care should be taken when using volatile anaesthetics because of an increased hypotensive effect. Hydrochlorothiazide may increase the responsiveness to agents of the tubocurarine type.

*Side-effects:* Monozide 10 is usually well tolerated with reported side-effects generally attributable to its pharmacological effects and reflects those of other drugs in the same classes. These include lassitude, fatigue,dizziness, mild headache,muscle and joint ache, perspiration, aggravation of intermittent claudication or Raynaud's disease, paraesthesia and coldness of the extremities,bronchospasm, oedema, pruritus and occasional G.I. side effects such as nausea/vomiting and diarrhoea and sleep disturbances. Occasionally a marked decrease in blood pressure and pulse rate or a disturbance of AV conduction may be observed. Dry eyes noted with other $\beta$-blockers have not been reported for patients treated with Monozide 10 but may rarely occur.

Skin rashes, photosensivity, anaphylactic reactions and blood dyscrasias including thrombocytopenia have been associated with hydrochlorothiazide therapy, but occur only rarely. There are no reports of similar reactions associated with Monozide 10 therapy.

*Overdosage:* In the case of overdosage or a precipitous drop in pulse rate and/or blood pressure, treatment with Monozide 10 must be discontinued. If necessary, the following antidotes should be administered alone or consecutively: intravenous atropine 0.5–2.0 mg, intravenous orciprenaline 0.5 mg by slow intravenous injection; also glucagon may be given at a dose level of 1 to 5 mg.

**Pharmaceutical precautions** No special requirement.

**Legal category** POM

**Package quantities** Calendar packs of 28

**Further information** The particularly low dose of hydrochlorothiazide used in this formulation has been shown to reduce the incidence/severity of side effects such as hypokalaemia and hyperuricaemia when compared to therapy using standard doses of the drug (25 mg). When combined with bisoprolol, a potent $\beta_1$ selective adrenoceptor antagonist, the tablet provides a convenient combination which should help the patient with its single daily dose, whilst minimising side-effects.

**Product licence number** 0095/0269

## MUCAINE*

**Presentation** Mucaine Suspension is a white suspension with the odour and flavour of peppermint. *Each 5 ml contains:*
Oxethazaine 10 mg
Magnesium Hydroxide BP 100 mg
Aluminium Hydroxide Mixture BP 4.75 ml

**Uses** Mucaine is an antacid mixture containing a topical anaesthetic and is indicated for oesophagitis whatever its cause, including peptic oesophagitis with or without hiatus hernia, radiation oesophagitis and the heartburn of late pregnancy.

The relief obtained in the symptomatic treatment of oesophagitis is due to the surface anaesthetic, oxethazaine, aided by the physical and antacid properties of the vehicle. Oxethazaine is stable at the levels of acidity or alkalinity found in the upper gastrointestinal tract and has relatively prolonged action.

**Dosage and administration** *Route of Administration:* Oral

*Adults:* One to two 5 ml doses should be taken three or four times daily, 15 minutes before meals, and at bedtime, or as required. The dose should not be washed down with a drink.

*The elderly:* The adult dosage schedule can be used in the elderly.

*Children:* Not recommended for children.

**Contra-indications, warnings, etc**
*Contra-indications:* The aluminium ion combines with phosphate to form an insoluble complex which is not absorbed. When high doses are given together with a low phosphorus diet, phosphate depletion occurs.

Phosphate depletion does not occur in patients on a normal diet. Mucaine is contra-indicated in patients with hypophosphataemia.

The use of magnesium containing antacids is contraindicated in patients with severe renal impairment because hypermagnesaemia is more likely to occur.

*Use in pregnancy and lactation:* A rabbit study has shown a dose related reduction in litter size although the relevance of these findings to man is unknown. There is no evidence of safety of oxethazaine in human pregnancy, therefore the product should not be used during the first trimester of pregnancy or during lactation.

*Precautions:*

1. The use of magnesium containing antacids in patients with mild to moderate renal impairment should be carefully observed due to the increased risk of hypermagnesaemia.
2. In patients with chronic renal failure, hyperaluminaemia may occur.

*Interactions:* The rate and/or extent of absorption of many drugs may be increased or decreased when they are used concurrently with aluminium-magnesium hydroxide containing antacids. Therefore, as a general rule, medication should not be taken within one to two hours of an antacid, if possible.

This includes: tetracycline, iron salts, chlorpromazine, levodopa, isoniazid, digoxin, $H_2$-antagonists, indomethacin, nitrofurantoin, and dicoumarol.

*Side effects:* Mucaine is well tolerated and the side effects which have been reported are almost invariably mild and transient in nature, consisting principally of constipation, dryness of mouth, and nausea. Hypersensitivity reactions including skin eruptions (dermatitis urticaria), pruritus, glossitis and angioedema have been reported on rare occasions.

*Action in case of overdosage:* Not reported. Treatment should be symptomatic.

**Pharmaceutical precautions** Store in a cool place and discard contents of opened bottle after 14 days.

**Legal category** POM

**Package quantities** Polypropylene bottles of 200 ml (OP)

**Further information** It is important to stress that Mucaine should not be washed down with a drink because maximal relief depends on good contact between the affected mucosal surface and the suspension as it passes down the oesophagus.

**Product licence number** 0011/5014

## NIPENT* ▼

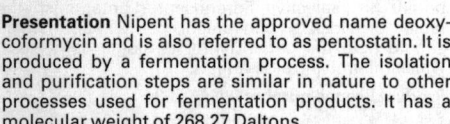

**Presentation** Nipent has the approved name deoxycoformycin and is also referred to as pentostatin. It is produced by a fermentation process. The isolation and purification steps are similar in nature to other processes used for fermentation products. It has a molecular weight of 268.27 Daltons.

Nipent is provided as a sterile lyophilised apyrogenic powder for reconstitution in single dose vials.

*Composition:* Each vial contains 10 mg Nipent, 50 mg mannitol and sufficient sodium hydroxide or hydrochloric acid to maintain the pH at 7.0–8.2. The powder is reconstituted by adding 5 ml of sterile water for injection and given intravenously as a bolus or further diluted with 5% dextrose injection or 0.9% sodium chloride injection and given over 20–30 minutes. (Nipent solution when so diluted does not interact with PVC infusion containers or administration sets at a concentration of 0.18 mg/ml to 0.33 mg/ml.)

*Action:* Nipent is a potent transition state inhibitor of the enzyme adenosine deaminase (ADA). The greatest activity of ADA is found in cells of the lymphoid system with T-cells having higher activity than B-cells and T-cell malignancies having higher activity than B-cell malignancies. Nipent inhibition of ADA, as well as direct inhibition of RNA synthesis and increased DNA damage, may contribute to the overall cytotoxic effect of Nipent. The precise mechanism of Nipent's antitumour effect, however, in hairy cell leukaemia is not known.

Nipent has been shown to have activity against a variety of lymphoid malignancies but is most active against indolent cancers with lower ADA concentration, such as hairy cell leukaemia.

*Indications:* Nipent is indicated as single agent therapy for the treatment of adults with hairy cell leukaemia.

**Dosage and administration**

*Adults:* It is recommended that patients receive hydration with 500 to 1,000 ml of 5% dextrose in 0.5 normal saline or equivalent before Nipent administration. An additional 500 ml of 5% dextrose or equivalent should be administered after Nipent is given.

The recommended dosage of Nipent for the treatment of hairy cell leukaemia is 4 mg/m² in a single administration every other week. Nipent may be given intravenously by bolus injection or diluted in a larger volume (25 to 50 ml) with 5% dextrose injection PhEur or 0.9% sodium chloride injection PhEur and given over 20 to 30 minutes. Dilution of the entire contents of a reconstituted vial with 25 ml or 50 ml provides a Nipent concentration of 0.33 mg/ml or 0.18 mg/ml respectively for the diluted solutions. Caution in the handling and preparation of the solution should be exercised, and the use of polythene gloves is recommended. If the solution contacts the skin or mucosae immediately wash thoroughly with soap and water.

Higher doses are not recommended.

No extravasation injuries were reported in clinical studies.

The optimal duration of treatment has not been determined. In the absence of major toxicity and with observed continuing improvement, the patient should be treated until a complete response has been achieved. Although not established as required, the administration of two additional doses has been recommended following the achievement of a complete response.

All patients receiving Nipent at 6 months should be assessed for response to treatment. If the patient has not achieved a complete or partial response, treatment with Nipent should be discontinued.

If the patient has achieved a partial response, Nipent treatment should be continued in an effort to achieve a complete response. At anytime thereafter that a complete response is achieved two additional doses of Nipent are recommended. Nipent treatment should then be stopped. If the best response to treatment at the end of 12 months is a partial response, it is recommended that treatment with Nipent be stopped.

Withholding or discontinuation of individual doses may be needed when severe adverse reactions occur. Drug treatment should be withheld in patients with severe rash, and withheld or discontinued in patients showing evidence of nervous system toxicity.

Nipent treatment should be withheld in patients with active infection occurring during the treatment but may be resumed when the infection is controlled.

*Dosage adjustment in renal insufficiency:* There is limited experience in patients with impaired renal function (creatinine clearance less than 60 ml/min). Two patients with impaired renal function (creatinine clearances 50 to 60 ml/min) achieved complete response without unusual adverse events when treated with 2 mg/m². Given this limited data, Nipent is contraindicated in patients whose creatinine clearance is <60 ml/min.

*Dosage adjustments in patients with cytopenias:* No dosage reduction is recommended at the start of therapy with Nipent in patients with anaemia, neutropenia, or thrombocytopenia. In addition, dosage reductions are not recommended during treatment in patients with anaemia and thrombocytopenia. Nipent should be temporarily withheld if the absolute neutrophil count falls during treatment below 200 cells/mm³ in a patient who had an initial neutrophil count greater than 500 cells/mm³ and may be resumed when the count returns to predose levels.

*Liver impairment:* Because of limited experience treating patients with abnormal liver function, treatment of such patients should be done with caution.

*Elderly over 65 years:* The recommended dosage of Nipent for the treatment of hairy cell leukaemia in the elderly is 4 mg/m² in a single administration every other week. Clinical trials have included patients over 65 years old and no adverse reactions specific to this age group have been reported.

*Children under 12 years:* Hairy cell leukaemia is a disease affecting adults, most commonly in the sixth decade of life. Safety and effectiveness of Nipent in children have not been established.

*Laboratory tests:* Prior to initiating therapy with Nipent, renal function should be assessed with a serum creatinine and/or a creatinine clearance assay. Complete blood counts, serum creatinine and BUN should be performed before each dose of Nipent and at other appropriate periods during therapy. Severe neutropenia has been observed following the early courses of treatment with Nipent and therefore frequent monitoring of complete blood counts is recommended during this time. If haematologic parameters do not improve with subsequent courses, patients should be evaluated for disease status, including a bone marrow examination. Periodic monitoring of the peripheral blood for hairy cells should be performed to assess the response to treatment.

In addition, bone marrow aspirates and biopsies may be required at 2 to 3 month intervals to assess the response to treatment.

**Contra-indications, warnings, etc**

*Contra-indications:* Nipent is contra-indicated in patients who have demonstrated hypersensitivity t Nipent.

Nipent is contra-indicated in patients with impaire renal function.

Nipent is contra-indicated in patients with acti infection.

Nipent is contra-indicated in pregnancy.

*Precautions:* Nipent should be administered under th supervision of a physician qualified and experience in the use of anticancer chemotherapeutic agents. Th use of higher doses than those specified are n recommended. Dose-limiting severe renal, liver, pu monary and CNS toxicities occurred in phase I studi using Nipent at higher dose (20–25 mg/m²) tha recommended.

Patients with hairy cell leukaemia may experien myelosuppression primarily during the first fe courses of treatment. Patients with infections prior t Nipent treatment have, in some cases, develope worsening of their condition leading to death, where others have achieved complete response. Patien with infection should be treated only when th potential benefit of treatment justifies the potenti risk to the patient. Efforts should be made to contr the infection before treatment is initiated or resume

In patients with progressive hairy cell leukaemi the initial courses of Nipent treatment were associate with worsening of neutropenia. Therefore, freque monitoring of complete blood counts during this tim is necessary. If severe neutropenia continues beyor the initial cycles, patients should be evaluated f disease status, including a bone marrow examinatio Therapy with Nipent requires regular patient obse vation and monitoring of haematologic paramete and blood chemistry values. If severe adverse rea tions occur, the drug should be withheld and appr priate corrective measures should be taken accordir to the clinical judgement of the physician.

Extra care should be taken in treating patien beginning therapy with poor performance.

Renal toxicity was observed at higher doses in ear studies; however, in patients treated at the recon mended dose, elevations in serum creatinine we usually minor and reversible. There were som patients who began treatment with normal ren function who had evidence of mild to modera toxicity at a final assessment.

Rashes, occasionally severe, were commonly r ported and may worsen with continued treatmer Withholding of treatment may be required.

Nipent treatment should be withheld or disconti ued in patients showing evidence of nervous syste toxicity.

Nipent may have harmful effects on the genotyp Therefore it is recommended that men undergoir treatment with Nipent should not father a child durir the treatment and up to 6 months thereafter. Contr ception is to be guaranteed for women of childbearir age. Should a pregnancy occur during treatment, th possibility of a genetic consultation is to be consi ered.

*Drug interactions:* The use of Nipent in combinatic with fludarabine phosphate is not recommended. In clinical investigation in patients with refracto chronic lymphocytic leukaemia using Nipent at th recommended dose in combination with fludarabir phosphate, 4 of 6 patients on the study had severe fatal pulmonary toxicity.

Allopurinol and Nipent are both associated wi skin rashes. Based on clinical studies in 25 refracto patients who received both Nipent and allopurin the combined use of Nipent and allopurinol did n appear to produce a higher incidence of skin rashe than observed with Nipent alone. There has been report of one patient who received both drugs an experienced a hypersensitivity vasculitis that resulte in death. It was unclear whether this adverse eve and subsequent death resulted from the drug comb nation.

Biochemical studies have demonstrated that Nipe enhances the effects of vidarabine, a purine nucle side with antiviral activity. The combined use vidarabine and Nipent may result in an increase adverse reactions associated with each drug. Th therapeutic benefit of the drug combination has n been established.

*Use in pregnancy:* Nipent must not be used durir pregnancy. Women of childbearing potential recei ing Nipent should be advised not to become pregnar

No fertility studies have been conducted in anima Incompletely reversible seminiferous tubular atroph and degeneration in rats and in dogs may be indicati of potential effects on male fertility. The possib adverse effects on human fertility have not bee determined.

Nipent is teratogenic in mice and rats. There are n adequate and well-controlled studies in pregna women.

It is not known whether Nipent is excreted in huma milk. Because many drugs are excreted in human mi

ınd because of the potential for serious adverse eactions from Nipent in nursing infants, nursing is ıot recommended.

*ıdverse reactions:* The following adverse events were eported during clinical studies in patients with hairy ell leukaemia who were refractory to alpha-interferon ır were treated as frontline therapy. Most patients xperienced an adverse event. The drug association ıf these adverse events has not been established. lowever some of these adverse events can in many ases be attributed to Nipent administration whereas ıthers may be associated with the disease itself. 12% ıf patients withdrew from treatment due to an adverse vent.

Nipent is lymphotoxic. Aside from myelosuppresion, Nipent is immunosuppressive in particular by uppression of the CD4+ lymphocyte subset. CD4+ ounts smaller than 200 per ml are usually seen during reatment with Nipent and CD4+ count suppression an outlast the end of treatment by more than months. With the exception of frequent herpes oster infections, the clinical consequences of the uppression of CD4+ counts in hairy cell leukaemia re not well understood yet. Long term consequences re not predictable but currently there is no evidence ır higher frequency of secondary malignancies or pportunistic infections.

The most commonly reported adverse events in inical studies in patients with hairy cell leukaemia vere abdominal pain, asthenia, chills, fatigue, fever, eadache, infection, allergic reaction and pain. Many atients experienced nausea and vomiting and some ave experienced anorexia, weight loss, weight gain, iarrhoea and liver damage. Less frequently cellulitis, hotosensitivity reaction, sepsis and malaise were ecorded.

The most frequently observed laboratory abnoralities include leucopenia, anaemia and thrombocytopenia and blood dyscrasias. Less frequently osinophilia, hypochromic anaemia, pancytopenia, etechiae and splenomegaly have been noted along ith ecchymosis and lymphadenopathy. Electrolyte isturbance has resulted in peripheral oedema. Less equently bilirubinaemia, hyperglycaemia, increased UN, LDH, creatinine and SGOT were observed.

The elevations in liver function tests that occurred uring treatment with Nipent were generally reversile.

Adverse events involving the respiratory system ıcluded cough and pneumonia and less frequently sthma, dyspnea, pharyngitis, rhinitis, sinusitis and pper respiratory tract infection.

Less frequent events of the cardiovascular system ere atrial fibrillation, congestive heart failure, flushıg, haemorrhage, shock and thrombophlebitis. These ccurred in less than 10% of patients receiving Nipent.

Disturbances of the nervous system have also been eported (see Precautions). Anxiety, depression, dizıess, insomnia and paresthesia have all been deribed.

Less severe but no less frequent were adverse vents involving the skin and appendages eg dry skin, erpes infections, rash and pruritus. Conjunctivitis as also been reported as has acne, alopecia, exfoliave dermatitis and skin discolouration less frequently.

Minor digestive disorders have been reported eg onstipation, dyspepsia, dysphagia and flatulence. ore severe but less frequently jaundice has been bserved.

Less frequently observed effects on the musculoceletal system are arthralgia, bone disorder, joint sorder and myalgia.

Disturbance of the urinary system was a less equent event with the exception of dysuria and aematuria.

*eatment of overdosage:* No specific antidote for ipent is known. Nipent administered at higher doses an recommended (20–50 mg/m²/5 days) was assoated with deaths due to severe renal, hepatic and ılmonary and CNS toxicity. In overdose, management would include general supportive measures rough any period of toxicity that occurs.

**armaceutical precautions** Store under refrigerated orage conditions between 2–8°C.

Caution in handling and preparation of solution ould be exercised, and the use of polyethylene oves is recommended. If the solution of Nipent ıntacts the skin or mucosae, immediately wash oroughly with soap and water.

The solution when diluted for infusion should be ed immediately or failing this, stored in a refrigeraır at 2–8°C for no more than 8 hours. Any unused lution should be discarded.

There are no incompatibilities but acidic solution ould be avoided.

**gal category** POM.

**ckage quantities** Nipent is supplied in single dose mg glass vials packaged in an individual carton.

**Further information** Nil.

**Product licence number** 0018/0199

## NOVANTRONE* INJECTION

**Presentation** *Novantrone injection (2 mg/ml):* Glass vials containing a sterile, dark blue aqueous isotonic solution of mitozantrone hydrochloride equivalent to 20 mg, 25 mg and 30 mg mitozantrone, together with sodium chloride and a buffer of sodium acetate and acetic acid to approximately pH3.

**Uses** Novantrone is an antineoplastic agent.

Novantrone is indicated in the treatment of advanced breast cancer, non-Hodgkin's lymphoma and adult acute non-lymphocytic leukaemia.

Novantrone has also been used in the palliation of non-resectable primary hepatocellular carcinoma.

**Dosage and administration**

*Dosage:*

*1. Advanced Breast Cancer, Non-Hodgkin's Lymphoma, Hepatoma:*

(a) *Single Agent Dosage:* The recommended initial dosage of Novantrone used as a single agent is 14 mg/m² of body surface area, given as a single intravenous dose which may be repeated at 21–day intervals. A lower initial dosage (12 mg/m² or less) is recommended in patients with inadequate bone marrow reserves. e.g. due to prior chemotherapy or poor general condition.

Dosage modification and the timing of subsequent dosing should be determined by clinical judgement depending on the degree and duration of myelosuppression. For subsequent courses the prior dose can usually be repeated if white blood cell and platelet counts have returned to normal levels after 21 days. The following table is suggested as a guide to dosage adjustment, in the treatment of advanced breast cancer, non-Hodgkin's lymphoma and hepatoma according to haematological nadir (which usually occurs about 10 days after dosing).

| Nadir after Prior Dose WBC (per mm³) | | Platelets (per mm³) | Time to Recovery | Subsequent dose after adequate haematological recovery |
|---|---|---|---|---|
| >1,500 | AND | >50,000 | ≤21 days | Repeat prior dose after recovery, or increase by 2 mg/m² if myelosuppression is not considered adequate. |
| >1,500 | AND | >50,000 | >21 days | Withhold until recovery then repeat prior dose. |
| <1,500 | OR | <50,000 | Any duration | Decrease by 2 mg/m² from prior dose after recovery. |
| <1,000 | OR | <25,000 | Any duration | Decrease by 4 mg/m² from prior dose after recovery. |

(b) *Combination Therapy:* Novantrone has been given as part of combination therapy. In advanced breast cancer, combinations of Novantrone with other cytotoxic agents including cyclophosphamide and 5-fluorouracil or methotrexate and mitomycin C have been shown to be effective. Reference should be made to the published literature for information on dosage modifications and administration. Novantrone has also been used in various combinations for non-Hodgkin's lymphoma, however data are presently limited and specific regimens cannot be recommended.

As a guide, when Novantrone is used in combination chemotherapy with another myelosuppressive agent, the initial dose of Novantrone should be reduced by 2-4 mg/m² below the doses recommended for single agent usage; subsequent dosing, as outlined in the table above, depends on the degree and duration of myelosuppression.

*2. Acute Non-Lymphocytic Leukaemia:*

(a) *Single Agent Dosage in Relapse:* The recommended dosage for remission induction is 12 mg/m² of body surface area, given as a single intravenous dose daily for five consecutive days (total of 60 mg/m²). In clinical studies with a dosage of 12 mg/m² daily for 5 days, patients who achieved a complete remission did so as a result of the first induction course.

(b) *Combination Therapy:* Novantrone has been used in combination regimens for the treatment of ANLL. Most clinical experience has been with Novantrone combined with cytosine arabinoside. This combination has been used successfully for primary treatment of ANLL as well as in relapse.

An effective regimen for induction in previously untreated patients has been Novantrone 10-12 mg/m² IV for 3 days combined with cytosine arabinoside 100 mg/m² IV for 7 days (by continuous infusion). This is followed by second induction and consolidation courses as thought appropriate by the treating clinician. In clinical studies, duration of therapy in induction and consolidation courses with Novantrone have been reduced to 2 days and that of cytosine arabinoside to 5 days. However, modification to the above regimen should be carried out by the treating clinician depending on individual patient factors.

Efficacy has also been demonstrated with Novantrone in combination with Etoposide in patients who had relapsed or who were refractory to primary conventional chemotherapy. The use of Novantrone in combination with Etoposide as with other cytotoxics may result in greater myelosuppression than with Novantrone alone.

Reference should be made to the published literature for information on specific dosage regimens. Novantrone should be used by clinicians experienced in the use of chemotherapy regimens. Dosage adjustments should be made by the treating clinician as appropriate, taking into account toxicity, response and individual patient characteristics. As with other cytotoxic drugs, Novantrone should be used with caution in combination therapy until wider experience is available.

(c) *Paediatric Leukaemia:* As experience with Novantrone in paediatric leukaemia is limited, dosage recommendations in this patient population cannot at present be given.

*Method of intravenous administration:* **NOT FOR INTRATHECAL USE** Syringes containing this product should be labelled 'NOVANTRONE NOT FOR INTRATHECAL USE'

Care should be taken to avoid contact of Novantrone with the skin, mucous membranes, or eyes: see Pharmaceutical precautions for further directions on handling. Vials should be dispensed in the upright position in order to prevent drops of Novantrone collecting in the stopper during preparation and leading to potential aerosolization of the solution.

Dilute the required volume of Novantrone injection to at least 50 ml in either of the following intravenous infusions: Sodium Chloride 0.9%, Glucose 5%, or Sodium Chloride 0.18% and Glucose 4%. Use Luer-lock fittings on all syringes and sets. Large bore needles are recommended to minimise pressure and the possible formation of aerosols. The latter may also be reduced by the use of a venting needle. Administer the resulting solution over not less than 3 minutes via the tubing of freely running intravenous infusion of the above fluids. Novantrone should not be mixed with other drugs in the same infusion.

If extravasation occurs the administration should be stopped immediately and restarted in another vein. The non-vesicant properties of Novantrone minimise the possibility of severe local reaction following extravasation.

**Contra-indications, warnings etc.**

*Contra-indications:* **NOT FOR INTRATHECAL USE.** Demonstrated hypersensitivity to the drug.

*Warnings:* Novantrone should be used with caution in patients with myelosuppression (see Dosage section) or poor general condition.

Cases of functional cardiac changes, including congestive heart failure and decreases in left ventricular ejection fraction have been reported. The majority of these cardiac events have occurred in patients who have had prior treatment with anthracyclines, prior mediastinal/thoracic radiotherapy, or with pre-existing heart disease. It is recommended that patients in these categories are treated with Novantrone at full cytotoxic dosage and schedule. However, added caution is required in these patients and careful regular cardiac examinations are recommended from the initiation of treatment.

As experience of prolonged treatment with Novantrone is presently limited, it is suggested that cardiac examinations also be performed in patients without identifiable risk factors during therapy exceeding a cumulative dose of 160 mg/m².

Careful supervision is recommended when treating patients with severe hepatic insufficiency.

The effects of Novantrone on human fertility or pregnancy have not been established. As with other antineoplastic agents, patients and their partners should be advised to avoid conception for at least six months after cessation of therapy. Novantrone should not normally be administered to patients who are pregnant or to mothers who are breast feeding.

Novantrone is mutagenic in vitro and in vivo in the rat. In the same species there was a possible association between administration of the drug and development of malignant neoplasia. The carcinogenic potential in man is unknown.

There is no experience with the administration of Novantrone other than by the intravenous route. Safety for intrathecal use has not been established.

*Precautions:* Novantrone is an active cytotoxic drug which should be used by clinicians familiar with the use of antineoplastic agents, and having the facilities for regular monitoring of clinical, haematological and biochemical parameters during and after treatment.

Full blood counts should be undertaken serially during a course of treatment. Dosage adjustments may be necessary based on these counts (see Dosage section).

*Side-effects:* Novantrone is clinically well tolerated demonstrating a low overall incidence of adverse events particularly those of a severe, irreversible, or life-threatening nature.

Some degree of leucopenia is to be expected following recommended doses of Novantrone. With the single dose every 21 days, suppression of WBC count below 1000/mm$^3$ is infrequent; leucopenia is usually transient reaching its nadir at about 10 days after dosing with recovery usually occurring by the 21st day. Thrombocytopenia can occur and anaemia occurs less frequently. Myelosuppression may be more severe and prolonged in patients having had extensive prior chemotherapy or radiotherapy or in debilitated patients.

When Novantrone is used as a single injection given every 21 days in the treatment of advanced breast cancer and lymphomas, the most commonly encountered side effects are nausea and vomiting, although in the majority of cases these are mild and transient. Alopecia may occur, but is most frequently of minimal severity and reversible on cessation of therapy.

Other side effects which have occasionally been reported include allergic reactions, amenorrhoea, anorexia, constipation, diarrhoea, dyspnoea, fatigue and weakness, fever, gastrointestinal bleeding, stomatitis/mucositis/conjunctivitis and non-specific neurological side effects such as somnolence, confusion, anxiety and mild paraesthesia. Tissue necrosis following extravasation has been reported rarely. In patients with leukaemia, the pattern of side effects is generally similar, although there is an increase in both frequency and severity, particularly of stomatitis and mucositis.

Changes in laboratory test values have been observed infrequently e.g. elevated serum creatinine and blood urea nitrogen levels, increased liver enzyme levels (with occasional reports of severe impairment of hepatic function in patients with leukaemia).

Cardiovascular effects, which have occasionally been of clinical significance, include decreased left ventricular ejection fraction, ECG changes and acute arrhythmia. Congestive heart failure has been reported and has generally responded well to treatment with digitalis and/or diuretics. In patients with leukaemia an increase in the frequency of adverse cardiac events has been observed; the direct role of Novantrone in these cases is difficult to assess as most patients had received prior therapy with anthracyclines and since the clinical course in leukaemic patients is often complicated by anaemia, fever, sepsis and intravenous fluid therapy.

Novantrone may impart a blue-green coloration to the urine for 24 hours after administration and patients should be advised that this is to be expected. Blue discoloration of skin and nails has been reported occasionally. Nail dystrophy or reversible blue coloration of the sclerae may be seen very rarely.

*Overdosage:* There is no known specific antidote for Novantrone. Haemopoietic, gastrointestinal, hepatic or renal toxicity may be seen depending on dosage given and the physical condition of the patient. In cases of overdosage the patient should be monitored closely and management should be symptomatic and supportive.

**Pharmaceutical precautions** Store at controlled room temperature (15°–25°C). Do not freeze.

Novantrone injection does not contain an antimicrobial preservative. Therefore, in accordance with normal practice, dilutions for infusion should be used or discarded within 24 hours. Novantrone dilutions will maintain potency for 24 hours at room temperature in PVC or glass containers.

Novantrone must not be mixed in the same infusion as heparin since a precipitate may form. Because specific compatibility data are not available it is recommended that Novantrone should not be mixed in the same infusion with other drugs.

*Handling of cytotoxic drugs:* Novantrone, in common with other potentially hazardous cytotoxic drugs, should only be handled by adequately trained personnel. Pregnant staff should not be involved in the reconstitution or administration of Novantrone.

Care should be taken to avoid contact of Novantrone with the skin, mucous membranes, or eyes. The use of goggles, gloves and protective gowns is recommended during preparation, administration and disposal and the work surface should be covered with disposable plastic-backed absorbent paper.

Aerosol generation should be minimised. Novantrone can cause staining. Skin accidentally exposed to Novantrone should be rinsed copiously with warm water and if the eyes are involved standard irrigation techniques should be used.

*Spillage disposal:* The following clean-up procedure is recommended if Novantrone is spilled on equipment or environmental surfaces. Prepare a 50% solution of fresh concentrated bleach (any recognised proprietary brand containing either sodium or calcium hypochlorite) in water. Wet absorbent tissues in the bleach solution and apply the wetted tissues to the spillage. The spillage is deactivated when the blue colour has been fully discharged. Collect up the tissues with dry tissues. Wash the area with water and soak up the water with dry tissues. Appropriate protective equipment should be worn during the clean-up procedure. All Novantrone contaminated items (eg, syringes, needles, tissues, etc) should be treated as toxic waste and disposed of accordingly. Incineration is recommended.

**Legal category** POM

**Package quantities** Novantrone injection is a sterile aqueous solution of mitozantrone hydrochloride, equivalent to 2 mg/ml mitozantrone. It is available in the following vial sizes:

20 mg in 10 ml: packs of 1 vial.
25 mg in 12.5 ml: packs of 1 vial.
30 mg in 15 ml: packs of 1 vial.

**Further information** Although its mechanism of action has not been determined, Novantrone is a DNA-reactive agent. It has a cytocidal effect on proliferating and non-proliferating cultured human cells, suggesting activity against rapidly proliferating and slow-growing neoplasms.

Animal pharmacokinetic studies in rats, dogs and monkeys given radiolabelled Novantrone indicate rapid, extensive dose proportional distribution into most tissues. Novantrone does not cross the blood-brain barrier to any appreciable extent. Distribution into testes is relatively low. In pregnant rats the placenta is an effective barrier. Plasma concentrations decrease rapidly during the first two hours and slowly thereafter. Animal data established biliary excretion as the major route of elimination. In rats, tissue elimination half-life of radioactivity ranged from 20 days to 25 days as compared with plasma half-life of 12 days. Novantrone is not absorbed significantly in animals following oral administration.

Pharmacokinetic studies in patients following intravenous administration of Novantrone demonstrated a triphasic plasma clearance. Distribution to tissues is rapid and extensive. Elimination of the drug is slow with a mean half-life of 12 days (range 5—18) and persistent tissue concentrations. Similar estimates of half-life were obtained from patients receiving a single dose of Novantrone every 21 days and patients dosed on 5 consecutive days every 21 days.

Novantrone is excreted via the renal and hepatobiliary systems. Only 20–32% of the administered dose was excreted within the first five days after dosing (urine 6–11%, faeces 13–25%). Of the material recovered in the urine 65% was unchanged mitozantrone and the remaining 35% is primarily comprised of two inactive metabolites and their glucuronide conjugates. Approximately two thirds of the excretion occurred during the first day.

**Product licence number** 0095/0088

# OVRAN*
# OVRAN 30*
# OVRANETTE*

**Presentation** Ovran tablets are round, white, sugar coated tablets. Each tablet contains 250 micrograms Levonorgestrel (d-norgestrel) BP and 50 micrograms Ethinyloestradiol PhEur.

Ovran 30 tablets are round, white sugar coated tablets, 5.7 mm in diameter. Each tablet contains 250 micrograms Levonorgestrel (d-norgestrel) BP and 30 micrograms Ethinyloestradiol PhEur.

Ovranette tablets are round, beige sugar coated tablets, 5.7 mm in diameter. Each tablet contains 150 micrograms Levonorgestrel (d-norgestrel) BP and 30 micrograms Ethinyloestradiol PhEur

**Uses** Oral contraception. Treatment of endometriosis, spasmodic dysmenorrhoea, premenstrual tension, oligomenorrhoea. Treatment of abnormal uterine bleeding such as menorrhagia, metropathia haemorrhagica. Emergency treatment of acute uterine bleeding.

**Dosage and administration**
*First treatment cycle:* 1 tablet daily for 21 days, starting with the tablet marked number 1, on the first day of the menstrual cycle. Additional contraception (barriers and spermicides) is not required.

*Subsequent cycles:* Each subsequent course is started when seven tablet-free days have followed the preceding course. A withdrawal bleed should occur during the 7 tablet-free days.

*Changing from another 21 day combined oral contraceptive:* The first tablet of Ovran, Ovran 30 or Ovranette should be taken on the first day immediately after the end of the previous oral contraceptive course. Additional contraception is not required. A withdrawal bleed should not be expected until the end of the fir[st] pack.

*Changing from an Every Day (ED) 28 day combine[d] oral contraceptive:* The first tablet of Ovran, Ovran 3[0] or Ovranette should be taken on the day immediate[ly] after the day on which the last active pill in the E[D] pack has been taken. The remaining tablets in the E[D] pack should be discarded. Additional contraception [is] not required. A withdrawal bleed should not b[e] expected until the end of the first pack.

*Changing from a Progestogen-only-Pill (POP):* Th[e] first tablet of Ovran, Ovran 30 or Ovranette should b[e] taken on the first day of menstruation even if the PO[P] for that day has already been taken. The remaini[ng] tablets in the POP pack should be discarded. Add[i]tional contraception is not required.

*Post-partum and post-abortum use:* After pregnan[cy] combined oral contraception can be started in no[n-]lactating women 21 days after a vaginal deliver[y] provided that the patient is fully ambulant and the[re] are no puerperal complications.

If the pill is started later than 21 days after deliver[y] then alternative contraception (barriers and sperm[i]cides) should be used until oral contraception [is] started and for the first 7 days of pill-taking. [If] unprotected intercourse has taken place after 21 da[ys] post partum, then oral contraception should not b[e] started until the first menstrual bleed after childbirt[h].

After a miscarriage or abortion oral contracepti[on] may be started immediately.

*Other indications:* Ovran and Ovranette can be us[ed] for the indications listed below, but Ovran usual[ly] provides the more convenient dosage unit.

*Endometriosis:* Treatment should be continuous wi[th] 1 Ovran tablet daily. If spotting or breakthroug[h] bleeding occurs it may be necessary to give 2 table[ts] daily or rarely 3 tablets daily in divided doses.

*Spasmodic dysmenorrhoea, premenstrual tensi[on,] oligomenorrhoea:* Dosage as for oral contraception.

*Functional uterine bleeding:* When the diagnosis h[as] been established, dosage is similar to the dosage f[or] oral contraception, but in the first one or two cycle[s] it may be necessary to give 2 Ovran tablets (or [in] exceptional cases), 3 tablets daily in order to contr[ol] the regularity of the cycle.

*Emergency treatment of the acute uterine bleeding:* [4] Ovran tablets are given immediately. If bleedi[ng] continues, medication is continued at a dose of [4] tablets daily in divided doses. This can usually [be] reduced to 2 tablets within two to four days. Treatme[nt] should continue for 10 days and after this time it c[an] either be discontinued to be followed after seven da[ys] by a complete course of 1 tablet daily for 21 days (s[ee] 'Functional uterine bleeding') or it can be continu[ed] for one to three months to inhibit the menses. In t[he] latter case, it should be possible to reduce the dosa[ge] to 1 tablet daily.

*Special circumstances requiring additional contrace[p]tion:*

*Missed pills:* If a tablet is delayed it should be taken [as] soon as possible and if it is taken within 12 hours [of] the correct time, additional contraception is n[ot] needed. Further tablets should then be taken at t[he] usual time. If the delay exceeds 12 hours, the la[st] missed pill should be taken when remembered, t[he] earlier missed pills left in the pack and normal p[ill] taking resumed. If one or more tablets are omitt[ed] from the 21 days of pill-taking, additional contrace[p]tion (barriers and spermicides) should be used for t[he] next 7 days of pill-taking. In addition, if one or mo[re] pills are missed during the last 7 days of pill-taki[ng] the subsequent pill-free interval should be dis[re]garded and the next pack started the day after taki[ng] the last tablet from the previous pack. In this case [a] withdrawal bleed should not be expected until t[he] end of the second pack. If the patient does not hav[e a] withdrawal bleed at the end of the second pack s[he] must return to her doctor to exclude the possibility [of] pregnancy.

*Gastro-intestinal upset:* Vomiting or diarrhoea m[ay] reduce the efficacy by preventing full absorpti[on]. Additional contraception (barriers and spermicid[es]) should be used during the stomach upset and for t[he] 7 days following the upset. If these 7 days overrun t[he] end of a pack, the next pack should be started with[out] a break. In this case, a withdrawal bleed should [not] be expected until the end of the second pack. If t[he] patient does not have a withdrawal bleed at the e[nd] of the second pack she must return to her doctor [to] exclude the possibility of pregnancy.

Mild laxatives do not impair contraceptive actio[n].

*Interaction with other drugs:* Some drugs acceler[ate] the metabolism of oral contraceptives when ta[ken] concurrently and these include barbiturates, phe[ny]toin, phenylbutazone and rifampicin. Other dru[gs] suspected of having the capacity to reduce the effic[acy] of oral contraceptives include ampicillin and ot[her] ntibiotics. It is, therefore, advisable to use non-ormonal methods of contraception (barriers and permicides) in addition to the oral contraceptive as ong as an extremely high degree of protection is equired during treatment with such drugs. The dditional contraception should be used while the oncurrent medication continues and for 7 days fterwards. If these extra precautions overrun the end f the pack, the next pack should be started without a reak. In this case, a withdrawal bleed should not be xpected until the end of the second pack. If the atient does not have a withdrawal bleed at the end f the second pack she must return to her doctor to xclude the possibility of pregnancy.

**ontra-indications, warnings, etc**

*ontra-indications:*

1. Suspected pregnancy.
2. Thrombotic disorders and a history of these onditions, sickle-cell anaemia, disorders of lipid etabolism and other conditions in which, in individ-al cases, there is known or suspected to be a much creased risk of thrombosis.
3. Acute or severe chronic liver diseases. Du-in-Johnson syndrome. Rotor syndrome. History, uring pregnancy, of idiopathic jaundice or severe ruritus.
4. History of herpes gestationis.
5. Mammary or endometrial carcinoma, or a history f these conditions.
6. Abnormal vaginal bleeding of unknown cause.
7. Deterioration of otosclerosis during pregnancy.

*/arnings:*

1. There is a general opinion, based on statistical vidence, that users of combined oral contraceptives xperience, more often than non-users, venous romboembolism, arterial thrombosis, including cer-oral and myocardial infarction, and subarachnoid aemorrhage. Full recovery from such disorders does ot always occur, and it should be realised that in a w cases they are fatal. How often these disorders ccur in users of the low-dose pills is not known, but ere are reasons for suggesting that they may occur ss often than with older pills containing more estrogen. Certain factors may entail some risk of rombosis, e.g. smoking, obesity, varicose veins, ardiovascular diseases, diabetes and migraine. The itability of a combined oral contraceptive should be dged according to the severity of such conditions in e individual case, and should be discussed with the atient before she decides to take it.
2. The risk of arterial thrombosis associated with ombined oral contraceptives increases with age, and is risk is aggravated by cigarette smoking. The use combined oral contraceptives by women in the der age group, especially those who are cigarette nokers, should therefore be discouraged and alter-ative methods used.
3. The possibility cannot be ruled out that certain ronic diseases may occasionally deteriorate during e use of combined oral contraceptives (see *Precau-ons*).
4. Malignant liver tumours have been reported on re occasions in long-term users of oral contracep-es. Benign hepatic tumours have also been associ-ed with oral contraceptive usage. A hepatic tumour ould be considered in the differential diagnosis hen upper abdominal pain, enlarged liver or signs intra-abdominal haemorrhage occur.
5. Numerous epidemiological studies have been ported on the risks of ovarian, endometrial, cervical d breast cancer in women using combined oral ntraceptives. The evidence is clear that combined al contraceptives offer substantial protection ainst both ovarian and endometrial cancer.

An increased risk of cervical cancer in long term ers of combined oral contraceptives has been ported in some studies, but there continues to be ntroversy about the extent to which this is attribut-le to the confounding effects of sexual behaviour d other factors.

The evidence linking combined oral contraceptive e and breast cancer remains inconclusive. The sults of some studies suggest an increased risk of east cancer presenting below the age of about 35, e risk rising with duration of use. Any possible creased risk of breast cancer with combined oral ntraceptives is however likely to be small and may expected to be less with low dosage pills. This ossible risk should be weighed against the many nefits of combined oral contraceptives, including eir protective effects against ovarian and endo-etrial cancers.

*easons for stopping oral contraception immediately:*

1. Occurrence of migraine in patients who have ever previously suffered from it. Exacerbation of pre-isting migraine. Any unusually frequent or unusu-y severe headaches.
2. Any kind of acute disturbance of vision.
3. Suspicion of thrombosis or infarction.
4. Six weeks before elective operations, or treatment of varicose veins by sclerotherapy and during immo-bilisation, e.g. after accidents, etc.
5. Significant rise in blood-pressure.
6. Jaundice.
7. Clear exacerbation of conditions known to be capable of deteriorating during oral contraception or pregnancy.
8. Pregnancy is a reason for stopping immediately because it has been suggested by some investigations that oral contraceptives taken in early pregnancy may slightly increase the risk of foetal malformations. Other investigations have failed to support these findings. The possibility therefore cannot be excluded, but it is certain that if a risk exists at all, it is very small.

*Precautions:*

1. Examination of the pelvic organs, breasts and blood-pressure should precede the prescribing of any combined oral contraceptive and should be repeated regularly.
2. Before starting treatment, pregnancy must be excluded.
3. The following conditions require careful obser-vation during medication: a history of severe depres-sive states, varicose veins, diabetes, hypertension, epilepsy, otosclerosis, multiple sclerosis, porphyria, tetany, disturbed liver function, gall-stones, cardio-vascular diseases, renal diseases, chloasma, uterine fibroids, asthma, the wearing of contact lenses, or any disease that is prone to worsen during pregnancy. The first appearance or deterioration of any of these conditions may indicate that the oral contraceptive should be stopped.
4. The risk of the deterioration of chloasma, which is often not fully reversible, is reduced by the avoidance of excessive exposure to sunlight.

*Side-effects:* Occasional side-effects may include nau-sea, vomiting, headaches, breast tenderness, changed body weight or libido, depressive moods, chloasma and altered serum lipid profile.

*Menstrual changes:*

1. Reduction of menstrual flow: This is not abnormal and it is to be expected in some patients. Indeed, it may be beneficial where heavy periods were previ-ously experienced.
2. Missed menstruation: Occasionally, withdrawal bleeding may not occur at all. If the tablets have been taken correctly, pregnancy is very unlikely, but should be ruled out before a new course of tablets is started.

*Intermenstrual bleeding:* Very light 'spotting' or heav-ier 'breakthrough bleeding' may occur during tablet-taking, especially in the first few cycles. It appears to be generally of no significance, except where it indicates errors of tablet-taking, or where the possi-bility of interaction with other drugs exists (q.v.). However, if irregular bleeding is persistent, an organic cause should be considered.

*Effect on adrenal and thyroid glands:* Oral contracep-tives have no significant influence on adrenocortical function. The ACTH function test for the adrenal cortex remains unchanged. The reduction in corticosteroid excretion and the elevation of plasma corticosteroids are due to an increased cortisol-binding capacity of the plasma proteins.

The response to metyrapone is less pronounced than in untreated women and is thus similar to that during pregnancy.

The radio-iodine uptake shows that thyroid function is unchanged. There is a rise in serum protein-bound iodine, similar to that in pregnancy and during the administration of oestrogens. This is due to the increased capacity of the plasma proteins for binding thyroid hormones, rather than to any change in glandular function. In women taking oral contracep-tives, the content of protein-bound iodine in blood serum should therefore, not be used for evaluation of thyroid function.

*Effect on blood chemistry:* Oral contraceptives may accelerate erythrocyte sedimentation in the absence of any disease. This effect is due to a change in the proportion of the plasma protein fractions. Increases in plasma copper, iron and alkaline phosphatase have also been recorded.

*Overdosage:* There have been no reports of serious ill-effects from overdosage, even when a considerable number of tablets have been taken by a small child. In general, it is, therefore, unnecessary to treat overdos-age. However, if overdosage is discovered within two or three hours and is so large that treatment seems desirable, gastric lavage can be safely used.

There are no specific antidotes and further treat-ment should be symptomatic.

**Pharmaceutical precautions** Store in cool, dry con-ditions. Shelf-life three years

**Legal category** POM

**Package quantities** Ovran and Ovran 30 are supplied in memo packs of 21 tablets. Ovranette is supplied in triple packs containing 3 months supply

**Further information** Pearl Index: Ovran, 0.19, Ovran 30, 0.13. Ovranette, 0.35.

**Product licence numbers**
Ovran 0011/0015
Ovran 30 0011/0050
Ovranette 0011/0041

## PIPRIL* INJECTION

**Presentation** Vials containing 1 g or 2 g of piperacillin as piperacillin sodium.

Infusion bottles containing 4 g of piperacillin as piperacillin sodium.

Infusion pack containing a 4 g piperacillin infusion bottle, a bottle of Water for Injection BP 50 ml, and a sterile, pyrogen free, transfer needle.

Each 1 g of Pipril contains 1.85 mEq (42.6 mg) of sodium.

**Uses** Pipril is a broad spectrum bactericidal penicillin antibiotic indicated for the treatment of infections caused by sensitive organisms, and for peri-operative prophylaxis; for example in patients undergoing abdominal surgery, vaginal hysterectomy, caesarian section.

Pipril is highly active against the following clinically important bacteria:

*Gram-negative:* Acinetobacter species; Citrobacter species; Enterobacter species; *Escherichia coli; Haemophilus influenzae; Klebsiella pneumoniae* and other species; *Neisseria gonorrhoeae; Neisseria meningitidis* †; *Proteus mirabilis;* Proteus sp (indole positive); Providencia species; *Pseudomonas aeruginosa* and other species; *Serratia marcescens* and other species; Shigella species †. *Anaerobes: Bacteroides fragilis;* Bacteroides species; Clostridium species; Fusobacterium species; Peptococcus species; Peptostreptococcus species; Veillonella species.

*Gram-positive:* Streptococcus species; Enterococci; *Streptococcus (Diplococcus) pneumoniae;* B-haemolytic streptococci including Group A (*S. pyogenes*) Group B (*S. agalactiae*); *Staphylococcus aureus* ‡; *Staphylococcus epidermidis* ‡.

† While piperacillin is active in vitro against these organisms, clinical efficacy has not yet been established.
‡ Methicillin-susceptible, beta-lactamase-negative organisms only.

Because of its broad spectrum of activity, Pipril is indicated for the treatment of the following systemic and/or local infections in which one or more suscep-tible organisms have been detected or are suspected. Systemic infections including bacterial septicaemia and endocarditis. Urogenital tract infections including gonorrhoea. Respiratory tract infections. Ear, nose and throat and oral cavity infections. Intra-abdominal infections including those of the biliary tract. Gynae-cological and obstetric infections. Skin and soft tissue infections including infected wounds and burns. Bone and joint infections. Proven or suspected infections in patients with impaired or suppressed immunological status. Peri-operative prophylaxis.

**Dosage and administration** Pipril may be given by slow intravenous injection, by intravenous infusion or by intramuscular injection.

For infants and children, intravenous administration of Pipril is recommended.

*Intravenous injection:* Each gram of Pipril should be reconstituted with at least 5 ml of Water for Injection. The reconstituted solution should be given by slow intravenous injection over three to five minutes.

*Intravenous infusion:* Each gram of Pipril should be reconstituted with at least 5 ml of Water for Injection. The total dose should then be further diluted to at least 50 ml before infusion over 20–40 minutes. Suit-able diluents are listed under Pharmaceutical Precau-tions.

*Intramuscular injection:* Each gram of Pipril should be reconstituted with at least 2 ml of Water for Injection or 0.5–1.0% lignocaine. Administration should be by deep intramuscular injection. A single dose in adults should not exceed 2 g. A single dose in children should not exceed 0.5 g.

*Adult dosage: Patients with normal renal function: Serious and complicated infections:* 200–300 mg/kg/day. The usual dose is therefore 4 g every six or eight hours by IV administration. In life-threatening infec-tions, particularly those caused by Pseudomonas and Klebsiella species a dosage of not less than 16 g/day is recommended.

*Mild and uncomplicated infections:* 100–150 mg/kg/day. The usual dose is therefore 2 g IV every six or eight hours; 4 g IV every twelve hours or 2 g IM every eight or twelve hours.

*For peri-operative prophylaxis:* 2 g just prior to surgery (or, in caesarian section, when the umbilical cord is clamped) followed by at least two doses of 2 g at four or six hour intervals within 24 hours of surgery.

*Acute gonorrhoea:* a single dose of 2 g IM.

| Renal function | Creatinine clearance (ml/min) | Serum level (mg %) | Maximum daily dosage (in divided doses) | Dose schedule |
|---|---|---|---|---|
| Mild impairment | 40–80 | 1.5–3.0 | 16 grams | 4 g q 6h |
| Moderate impairment | 20–40 | 3.1–5.0 | 12 grams | 4 g q 8h |
| Severe impairment | <20 | >5 | 8 grams | 4 g q 12h |
| Patients on haemodialysis* | — | — | 6 grams | 2 g q 8h |

*Haemodialysis removes 30% to 50% of drug in four hours; an additional dose of 1 g of Pipril should be administered following each dialysis period.

Dosages for children over one month of age with renal impairment:

| Creatinine clearance ml/min* | Urinary tract infection (uncomplicated) | Urinary tract infection (complicated) | Serious systemic infection |
|---|---|---|---|
| >40 | No adjustment necessary | | |
| 20–40 | No adjustment | 150 mg/kg/day | 200 mg/kg/day |
| <20 | 75 mg/kg/day | 100 mg/kg/day | 133 mg/kg/day |

* adjusted for body surface, 1.73 M (squared).

*Patients with renal insufficiency:* In adults with renal impairment, intravenous or intramuscular dosage should be adjusted. Given below are the recommended maximum daily dosages of Pipril according to the degree of renal impairment as assessed by the physician. Regular monitoring is advised to ensure that adequate serum concentrations are achieved.

*Duration of therapy:* Pipril treatment in acute infections should be continued for three to four days after the disappearance of clinical signs and symptoms of the disease. However, the duration of treatment should be determined by the physician on the basis of the clinical course of infection.

*Elderly:* Pipril may be used at the same dose levels as adults except in cases of renal impairment when the dosage should be reduced.

*Paediatric dosage:*

*Infants and children (under 12 years of age) with normal renal function:*

*Less serious and uncomplicated infections:* 100–200 mg/kg/day intravenously, in 3 or 4 divided doses.

*Serious and complicated infections:* 200–300 mg/kg/day, intravenously, in 3 or 4 divided doses.

*Neonates:*
*Dosages for children 0–1 month of age:*

| | |
|---|---|
| <7 days old or >7 days old but less than 2000 g: | 150 mg/kg/day intravenously in 3 divided doses. |
| >7 days old and over 2000 g: | 300 mg/kg/day intravenously in 3 or 4 divided doses. |

*Infants (over 1 month of age) and children (under 12 years) with renal impairment:* In paediatric patients with renal impairment, the dosage should be adjusted according to age and degree of that impairment.

*Dosages for children over one month of age with renal impairment:*

**Contra-indications, warnings, etc**
*Contra-indications:* Penicillin hypersensitivity or severe cephalosporin hypersensitivity.

*Precautions:* Use with caution in patients with infectious mononucleosis.

Bleeding manifestations have occurred in some patients receiving beta-lactam antibiotics. These reactions have sometimes been associated with abnormalities of coagulation tests such as clotting time, platelet aggregation and prothrombin time and are much more likely to occur in patients with renal failure. If bleeding manifestations occur as a result of antibiotic therapy, the antibiotic should be discontinued and appropriate therapy instituted.

As with other antibiotics, overgrowth of non-susceptible organisms may cause superinfections, especially during prolonged treatment. The possibility of antibiotic-induced pseudomembranous colitis should be considered in cases of severe persistent diarrhoea.

Neuromuscular excitability or convulsions have been known to occur following large intravenous doses of penicillins.

Pipril is a monosodium compound containing 1.85 mEq (42.6 mg) of sodium per gram. This should be borne in mind if used in patients with sodium and fluid retention.

*Use in pregnancy and lactation:* The product has been in clinical use since 1982 and the limited number of reported cases of use in human pregnancy have shown no evidence of untoward effect. The benefits of use during pregnancy should be weighed against possible hazards to mother and foetus. Piperacillin is licensed for use in neonates.

Piperacillin is excreted in low concentrations in breast milk.

*Warnings and side-effects:* Serious and occasionally fatal anaphylactic reactions have been reported in patients receiving therapy with penicillins. Before initiating therapy with piperacillin, careful inquiry should be made concerning previous hypersensitivity reactions to penicillins, cephalosporins and other allergens. If an allergic reaction occurs during therapy with piperacillin, the antibiotic should be discontinued. Serious hypersensitivity reactions may require adrenaline and other emergency measures.

Side effects are uncommon and typical of the injectable penicillins.

In common with other penicillins, anaphylactic reactions have occasionally been reported in patients receiving piperacillin. Mild allergic reactions such as rash, pruritus, urticaria and fever may occur. These occur more frequently in patients with cystic fibrosis. Rarely, interstitial nephritis has been reported.

Hepatitis and cholestatic jaundice have been reported rarely with some penicillins.

Gastrointestinal disturbances have been reported. Transient increases in liver function test values may be observed.

Transient leucopenia, neutropenia, thrombocytopenia and/or eosinophilia may occur.

Rarely, significant leucopenia may be associated with prolonged therapy.

Dermatological manifestations such as erythema multiforme and Stevens-Johnson syndrome have been reported on rare occasions.

In vitro, Pipril can be inactivated by β-lactamases produced by some strains of gram-negative and gram-positive bacteria.

Prolonged use of an anti-infective may result in the development of superinfection due to organisms resistant to that anti-infective.

Cross-resistance between piperacillin and other β-lactam antibiotics e.g. carbenicillin and ampicillin is possible.

Pain after intramuscular injections (rarely accompanied by induration) has been observed infrequently. This can be minimised by reconstituting Pipril with 0.5–1.0% lignocaine.

*Interactions:* Pipril acts synergistically with aminoglycosides. Concurrent therapy with both drugs given in full therapeutic doses may be used in the treatment of life-threatening infections or in patients with impaired immune status. Pipril and aminoglycosides should not, however, be mixed in the same solution but administered separately.

Pipril may be used in combination with β-lactamase resistant penicillins in proven or suspected mixed infections involving β-lactamase producing *Staphylococcus aureus.*

Pipril may be administered (separately) with metronidazole in the treatment of mixed aerobic/anaerobic infections.

Cefoxitin should not be given with Pipril when Pseudomonas infections are suspected or confirmed as in vitro data have shown possible antagonism. However, Pipril may be administered concomitantly with other β-lactam antibiotics provided that an additive or synergistic antibacterial action is first ascertained through in vitro tests where appropriate.

During simultaneous administration of high doses of heparin, oral anticoagulants and other drugs which may affect the blood coagulation system and/or thrombocyte function, the coagulation parameters should be tested more frequently and monitored regularly.

The ureidopenicillins including piperacillin have been reported to prolong the action of vecuronium. Caution is indicated when piperacillin is used perioperatively with vecuronium and similar neuromuscular blocking agents.

Penicillins may reduce the excretion of methotrexate. Serum levels of methotrexate should be monitored in patients on high dose methotrexate therapy.

*Overdosage:* Other than general supportive treatment no specific antidote is known. Excessive serum levels of piperacillin may be reduced by dialysis. In cases of motor excitability or convulsions administration of appropriate anticonvulsant drugs, such as diazepam or barbiturates, may be indicated. Daily doses of piperacillin of 24 grams and above have been administered in man without observation of adverse effects.

**Pharmaceutical precautions** Pipril should be stored in a dry place at room temperature. Pipril should be freshly prepared prior to administration, any unused solution being discarded.

However, Pipril solutions are chemically stable for at least 24 hours at room temperature or 48 hours at 4°C.

Pipril may be administered in all commonly used intravenous infusion fluids including:

Dextrose 5%, Sodium Chloride 0.9%, Dextrose 5% and Sodium Chloride 0.9%, Lactated Ringer's Injection. The above fluids admixed with 40 mEq Potassium Chloride and/or 30 mEq Sodium Bicarbonate, Dextran 6% in Sodium Chloride 0.9%, Dextrose 30%, Mannitol 20%, Water for Injection.

Because of chemical instability, Pipril should not be diluted with solutions containing only sodium bicarbonate.

Pipril should not be added to blood products or protein hydrolysates.

Pipril has also been shown to be compatible over 24 hours at room temperature when mixed with cephazolin sodium, flucloxacillin sodium, cephamandole nafate, or cefoxitin sodium in either Dextrose 5% or Saline 0.9% or when piperacillin is diluted with Lactated Ringer's Injection. The diluted solution must be administered within 2 hours.

Pipril should not be mixed in the same solution with aminoglycosides and should be administered separately from any drugs unless compatibility is proven.

**Legal category** POM

**Package quantities**
Vials containing 1 g or 2 g Pipril boxed singly.
Infusion bottles containing 4 g Pipril, boxed singly.
Pipril 4 g Infusion Packs containing a 4 g infusion bottle, a 50 ml bottle of Water for Injection BP and transfer needle.

**Further information** Pipril is widely distributed following parenteral administration into human tissues and body fluids, particularly bile. Pipril penetrates into cerebrospinal fluid in the presence of meningitis. It is not absorbed when given orally. As with other penicillins, Pipril is rapidly excreted, unchanged by glomerular filtration and tubular secretion achieving high urinary concentrations for up to 12 hours after dosing. The binding of piperacillin to human serum protein is low (16%).

**Product licence number** 0095/0073

# PNU-IMUNE*

**Qualitative and quantitative composition** Each 0.5 ml of Pnu-Imune contains 25µg of antigen to each of the 23 most prevalent or invasive pneumococcal types (see table below).

*Antigens present in Pnu-Imune according to Danish Nomenclature [25µg of each per 0.5 ml dose]:*

| 1 | 2 | 3 | 4 | 5 | 6B | 7F | 8 | | 9N | 9V | 10A | 11A |
| 12F | 14 | | 15B | 17F | 18C | 19A | 19F | 20 | | 22F | 23F | 33F |

**Pharmaceutical form** Pnu-Imune is a clear, colourless to very light amber sterile solution for injection.

**Clinical particulars**

*Therapeutic indications:* Pnu-Imune vaccine consists of a mixture of highly purified capsular polysaccharides from the 23 most prevalent types of *Streptococcus pneumoniae* (pneumococcus) which account for at least 90% of pneumococcal blood isolates. Pnu-Imune is indicated for immunisation against pneumococcal disease caused by those pneumococcal types included in the vaccine.

*Adults:* Pnu-Imune vaccine should be considered in all those aged over two years in whom pneumococcal infection is likely to be more common and/or dangerous such as immunocompetent individuals who are at increased risk of pneumococcal disease or its complications because of chronic illnesses (e.g.

cardiovascular or pulmonary disease, diabetes mellitus, alcoholism or cirrhosis); and for immunocompromised individuals at increased risk of pneumococcal disease or its complications (e.g., splenic dysfunction or anatomical asplenia including sickle cell disease, Hodgkin's disease, lymphoma, multiple myeloma, chronic renal failure, nephrotic syndrome, or conditions such as organ transplantation and Human Immunodeficiency Virus (HIV) associated with immunosuppression).

*Children:* Not recommended in children less than 2 years.

*Posology and method of administration:* A single dose of 0.5 ml is given subcutaneously or intramuscularly (preferably in the deltoid muscle or lateral mid-thigh). Intradermal administration should be avoided. The vaccine should not be injected intravenously.

Individuals with HIV should be immunised as early as possible in the disease process.

Pnu-Imune should be inspected visually for particulate matter and discoloration prior to administration.

*Simultaneous administration with other vaccines:* Pneumococcal vaccine may be given at the same time as influenza vaccine at a different site as there is no antigenic competition. Pnu-Imune, unlike influenza vaccine, is not required annually and therefore the need for simultaneous administration is not always present.

A possible attenuation of the response to Pnu-Imune may be seen in immunocompromised individuals when co-administered influenza vaccine. This effect has not been seen in clinical studies involving other patient groups.

*Re-immunisation:* Re-immunisation should be considered after 5 years in individuals at highest risk of pneumococcal infection or where antibody levels are likely to have declined rapidly such as those with no spleen, with splenic dysfunction or with nephrotic syndrome or transplant patients. Re-immunisation before 5 years may cause increased incidence and severity of local reactions.

As antibody levels may decline more rapidly in children, re-immunisation should be carefully considered after 3 to 5 years for children with nephrotic syndrome, asplenia, or sickle cell anaemia who would be 10 years old or younger at the time of re-immunisation.

Persons who received the 14 valent vaccine should not be routinely re-vaccinated with the 23 valent vaccine, as increased coverage is modest and duration of protection is not well defined.

*Contra-indications:* Hypersensitivity to any component of the vaccine, including thiomersal, a mercury derivative. The occurrence of any type of neurological symptoms or signs following administration of this product is a contra-indication to further use. The vaccine should not be administered to persons with acute febrile illnesses until their temporary symptoms and/or signs have abated.

Persons who have received any pneumococcal vaccine in the last three years.

Persons who are receiving immunosuppressive therapy or who have received it in the last 10 days.

Patients with Hodgkin's Disease who have received extensive chemotherapy and/or nodal irradiation.

Pregnant or lactating women.

*Special warnings and special precautions:* As with the injection of any biological material, Adrenaline Injection (1:1000) should be available for immediate use should an anaphylactic or other allergic reaction occur. Pnu-Imune is not an effective agent for prophylaxis against pneumococcal disease caused by types not present in the vaccine.

The expected serum antibody response may not be obtained in patients with impaired immune responsiveness, whether due to the use of immunosuppressive therapy, a genetic defect, HIV infection, or other causes. In order to maximise the benefits of vaccination, patients with HIV should be vaccinated as early as possible in the disease process.

At least 2 weeks should elapse between immunisation and the initiation of chemotherapy or immunosuppressive therapy to allow development of adequate antibody response.

Defer immunisation if acute febrile illness is present.

Patients who have had episodes of pneumococcal pneumonia or other pneumococcal infection may have high levels of pre-existing pneumococcal antibodies that may result in increased reactions to Pnu-Imune, mostly local, but occasionally systemic. Caution should be exercised if such patients are considered for immunisation with Pnu-Imune.

Where required prophylactic antibiotic therapy against pneumococcal infection should not be stopped after immunisation with Pnu-Imune.

Because antibody response to capsular types that most often cause pneumococcal disease in children less than 2 years may be poor Pnu-Imune vaccine

may not be effective and is not generally recommended in this group.

To avoid accidental re-vaccination, a clear note of vaccination should be kept in the patient's records.

*Interaction with other medicaments and other forms of interaction:* When Pnu-Imune is given with an unrelated vaccine, such as vaccine against influenza virus, there is no antigenic competition.

*Pregnancy and lactation:* Animal reproduction studies to evaluate teratology and embryotoxicity have not been conducted with Pnu-Imune. It is not known whether Pnu-Imune can cause foetal harm when administered to a pregnant woman or can affect reproduction capacity. Pnu-Imune is not recommended for use in pregnant women.

It is not known whether the vaccine is excreted in human milk. Because many drugs are excreted in human milk, caution should be exercised if Pnu-Imune is administered to a nursing woman.

*Effects on ability to drive and use machines:* Pnu-Imune is not known to affect the ability to drive or operate machines.

*Undesirable effects:* Mild side effects, such as erythema and pain at the injection site occur in approximately 50% of persons given pneumococcal vaccine. Fever, myalgia, and severe local reactions have been reported in less than 1% of those vaccinated.

Fever and myalgia are usually confined to the 24 hour period following immunisation. Rash and arthralgia have been reported infrequently.

Although rare, fever over 38.9°C and marked local swelling have been reported with pneumococcal polysaccharide vaccine. Rash, urticaria, arthritis, arthralgia, adenitis, and anaphylactoid reactions have been reported rarely.

Patients with otherwise stabilised idiopathic thrombocytopenic purpura have, on rare occasions, experienced a relapse in their thrombocytopenia, occurring 2 to 14 days after immunisation, and lasting up to 2 weeks.

Reactions of greater severity or extent are unusual. Temporal association of neurological disorders such as paraesthesia and acute radiculoneuropathy, including Guillain-Barre syndrome, have been reported rarely following parenteral injections of biological products including pneumococcal vaccine.

*Overdose:* There is no experience with overdosage of Pnu-Imune.

**Pharmacological properties** Pneumococci are surrounded by a polysaccharide capsule, which make the bacteria resistant to attack by white blood cells. However, human blood serum may contain antibodies, which render the bacteria vulnerable to attack. Pnu-Imune vaccine, composed of the purified polysaccharides from bacterial cells, stimulates production of these antibodies and provides active immunity to the 23 types of pneumococcal bacteria represented in the vaccine.

*Pharmacodynamic properties:* In clinical studies with polyvalent pneumococcal vaccines, more than 90% of all adults showed twofold or greater increase in geometric mean antibody titre for each capsular type contained in the vaccine (data on file, Lederle Laboratories). Patients over the age of 2 years with anatomical or functional asplenia and otherwise intact lymphoid function generally respond to pneumococcal vaccines with a serological conversion comparable to that observed in healthy individuals of the same age.

Most healthy adults, including the elderly, demonstrate at least a twofold rise in type-specific antibodies within 2 to 3 weeks of immunisation. Similar antibody responses have been reported in patients with alcoholic cirrhosis and insulin-dependent diabetes mellitus. In contrast, elderly individuals with chronic pulmonary disease failed to mount a comparable immune response. In immunocompromised patients, the response to immunisation may also be lower. Children under 2 years of age respond poorly to most capsular polysaccharide types. Further, response to some pneumococcal types (e.g., 6A and 14) that are important in paediatric infection is decreased in children less than 5 years of age.

Following immunisation of healthy adults, antibody levels remain elevated for at least 5 years, but in some individuals these may fall to pre-immunisation levels within 10 years. A more rapid decline in antibodies may occur in children, particularly those who have undergone a splenectomy and those with sickle cell disease, in whom antibodies for some types can fall to pre-immunisation levels 3 to 5 years after immunisation. Similar rates of decline can occur in children with nephrotic syndrome.

Patients with AIDS may have an impaired antibody response to pneumococcal vaccine. However, HIV-infected adults show a normal immune response to the 23 valent vaccine when the circulating level of CD4 cells is above 500/µL, but a reduced response when the cell population falls below that threshold.

*Pharmacokinetic properties:* The capsule of the pneumococcus, despite its lack of toxicity, is the major bacterial structure responsible for the virulence of the organism. The polysaccharide capsule has an anti-phagocytic effect, interrupting phagocytic activity elicited by activation of complement and permitting the establishment and progression of infection in the non-immune host. Opsonisation of pneumococci is required for their phagocytosis. Identified as complex polysaccharides, the capsules of the pneumococcus were the first non-protein substances shown to be antigenic in humans, which laid the basis for the subsequent use of pneumococcal capsular polysaccharides as vaccines. Induction of anticapsular polysaccharide antibodies in the host mediate immunity through activation of complement for effective opsonisation. IgM and IgG antibodies confer protection by altering the surface properties of the pneumococcal cell, which facilitates phagocytosis.

*Preclinical safety data:* Not applicable.

**Pharmaceutical particulars**

*List of excipients:* Thiomersal, sodium phosphate buffer.

*Incompatibilities:* None.

*Shelf life:* Pnu-Imune may be stored at 2° to 8°C for up to 2 years.

*Special precautions for storage:* Pnu-Imune should not be frozen. Storage should be under refrigeration, away from the freezer compartment at 2–8°C.

*Nature and contents of container:* Pnu-Imune is supplied in a 0.5 ml single dose vial for use with a syringe only.

*Instructions for use/handling:* There are no special instructions for use/handling.

**Marketing authorisation number**  0095/0292

**Date of approval/revision of SPC**  6 January 1997

**Legal category**  POM

# PREMARIN* TABLETS

**Presentation** Premarin Tablets contain naturally conjugated oestrogens.

Premarin Tablets 0.625 mg are maroon, oval, sugar-coated tablets.

Premarin Tablets 1.25 mg are yellow, oval, sugar-coated tablets.

Premarin Tablets 2.5 mg are purple, oval, sugar-coated tablets.

**Uses** Menopausal and postmenopausal oestrogen therapy in women without a uterus for:

1. Vasomotor symptoms such as sweating and flushes.

2. Allied disorders of the menopause such as atrophic vaginitis, kraurosis vulvae, atrophic urethritis.

3. Prophylaxis of osteoporosis in women at risk of developing fractures.

**Dosage and administration**

*Adults:* Premarin 0.625–1.25 mg daily is the usual starting dose. Continuous administration is recommended. For maintenance, the lowest effective dose should be used.

*Vasomotor symptoms:* 0.625–1.25 mg daily depending on the response of the individual.

*Atrophic vaginitis, kraurosis vulvae, atrophic urethritis:* 0.625–1.25 mg daily depending on the response of the individual.

*Prophylaxis of osteoporosis:* the minimum effective dose is 0.625 mg daily for most patients. Hormone replacement therapy has been found to be effective in the prevention of osteoporosis when started soon after the menopause and used for 5 years and probably up to 10 years. Treatment should start as soon as possible after the onset of the menopause and certainly within 2 to 3 years. Protection appears to be effective for as long as treatment is continued, however data beyond 10 years are limited. A careful re-appraisal of the risk-benefit ratio should be undertaken before treating for longer than 5 to 10 years. For long term use see also Precautions and Warnings.

At present there is no established screening programme for determining women at risk of developing osteoporotic fractures. Epidemiological studies suggest a number of individual risk factors which contribute to the development of postmenopausal osteoporosis. These include: early menopause; family history of osteoporosis; thin, small frame; cigarette use; recent prolonged systemic corticosteroid use.

If several of these risk factors are present in a patient consideration should be given to oestrogen replacement therapy.

*Concomitant progestogen use:* In women with an intact uterus the addition of a progestogen for 12–14 days per cycle is essential. See also *Precautions and Warnings.*

For most postmenopausal women therapy may be commenced at any convenient time.

Before therapy commences it is recommended that the patient is fully informed of all likely benefits and potential risks. She should have a full physical and gynaecological examination with special emphasis on blood pressure, breasts, abdomen and pelvic organs, and endometrial assessment carried out if appropriate. Follow-up examinations are recommended every 6–12 months.

*Elderly:* There are no special dosage requirements for elderly patients, but as with all medicines, the lowest effective dose should be used.

*Children:* Not recommended.

**Contra-indications, warnings etc**

*Contra-indications:*

1. Known or suspected pregnancy.
2. History of, known or suspected cancer of the breast.
3. Known or suspected oestrogen-dependent neoplasia. Undiagnosed abnormal genital bleeding.
4. Active thrombophlebitis or thromboembolic disorders. See also *Warnings and precautions* number 4.
5. Acute or chronic liver disease or history of liver disease where the liver function tests have failed to return to normal. Rotor syndrome or Dubin-Johnson syndrome.
6. Severe cardiac or renal disease.
7. Hypersensitivity to the components of Premarin tablets.

*Pregnancy and lactation:* Premarin is contra-indicated in the event of known or suspected pregnancy and during lactation.

*Warnings and precautions:*

1. In the female there is an increased risk of endometrial hyperplasia and carcinoma associated with unopposed oestrogens administered long-term (for more than one year). However, the appropriate addition of a progestogen to an oestrogen regimen lowers this additional risk.

2. There is suggestive evidence of a small increased risk of breast cancer with oestrogen replacement therapy used for long term (greater than 5 years). Some studies have reported an increased risk in long-term users, others, however, have not shown this relationship. It is not known whether concurrent progestogen use influences the risk of breast cancer in post menopausal women taking hormone replacement therepy. Women on long-term therapy should have regular breast examinations, should be instructed in self-breast examination and mammographic investigations conducted where considered appropriate.

There is a need for caution when prescribing oestrogens in women who have a history of, or known breast nodules or fibrocystic disease. Breast status should be closely monitored, supported by regular mammography.

3 Certain diseases may be made worse by hormone replacement therapy and patients with these conditions should be closely monitored. These include otosclerosis, multiple sclerosis, systemic lupus erythematosis, porphyria, melanoma, epilepsy, migraine and asthma. In addition pre-existing uterine fibroids may increase in size during oestrogen therapy and symptoms associated with endometriosis may be exacerbated.

4. Studies to date do not indicate that there is an increased risk of thromboembolic disease, including stroke, myocardial infarction and thrombophlebitis with oestrogen replacement therapy at the current recommended low dosages in apparently normal women.

If an acute vascular thromboembolic event occurs coincidentally during therapy, current opinion suggests that treatment should be discontinued. However,there is no evidence that a history of deep vein thrombosis, pulmonary embolism, stroke or myocardial infarction should be a contra-indication to oestrogen replacement therapy, but in the absence of sufficient data Premarin should be used with caution in these patients.

5. Oestrogens may cause fluid retention and therefore patients with cardiac or renal dysfunction should be carefully observed.

6. If jaundice, migraine-like headaches, visual disturbances, thromboembolic phenomena or a significant increase in blood pressure develop after initiating therapy, the medication should be discontinued while the cause is investigated.

7. Premarin is not an oral contraceptive neither will it restore fertility. If Premarin is administered together with a progestogen to women with an intact uterus of child-bearing potential they should be advised to adhere to non-hormonal contraceptive methods.

8. Most studies indicate that oestrogen replacement therapy has little effect on blood pressure and some indicate that oestrogen use may be associated with a small decrease. In addition, most studies on combined therapy indicate that the addition of a progestogen also has little effect on blood pressure. Rarely, idiosyncratic hypertension may occur.

When oestrogens are administered to hypertensive women, supervision is necessary and blood pressure should be monitored at regular intervals.

9. Changed oestrogen levels may affect certain endocrine and liver function tests.

10. Consideration should be given to discontinue treatment at least four weeks prior to surgery or during periods of prolonged immobilisation.

11. It has been reported that there is an increase in the risk of surgically confirmed gallbladder disease in women receiving postmenopausal oestrogens.

12. A worsening of glucose tolerance may occur in patients taking oestrogens and therefore diabetic patients should be carefully observed while receiving hormone replacement therapy.

13. As larger doses of oestrogen may increase thyroid binding globulin leading to increased circulating total thyroid hormone, care should be taken in providing oestrogens for patients with thyrotoxicosis.

14 Administration of oestrogens may lead to hypercalcaemia in patients with breast cancer and bone metastases. If this occurs, the drug should be stopped and appropriate measures taken to reduce the calcium level.

*Side-effects:* The following side-effects have been reported with oestrogen therapy.

1. Genitourinary system - premenstrual-like syndrome, increase in size of uterine fibromyomata, vaginal candidiasis, change in cervical erosion and in degree of cervical secretion, cystitis-like syndrome.
2. Breasts - Tenderness, enlargement, secretion.
3. Gastrointestinal - Nausea, vomiting abdominal cramps, bloating, cholestatic jaundice.
4. Skin - Chloasma or melasma which may persist when drug is discontinued, erythema multiforme, erythema nodosum, haemorrhagic eruption, loss of scalp hair, hirsutism.
5. Eyes - Steepening of corneal curvature, intolerance to contact lenses.
6. CNS - Headaches, migraine, dizziness, mental depression, chorea.
7. Miscellaneous - Increase or decrease in weight, reduced carbohydrate tolerance, aggravation of porphyria, oedema, changes in libido, leg cramps.

*Acute overdosage:* Numerous reports of ingestion of large doses of oestrogen-containing oral contraceptives by young children indicate that acute serious ill effects do not occur. Overdosage of oestrogen may cause nausea, and withdrawal bleeding may occur in females.

**Pharmaceutical precautions** No special requirements for storage are necessary.

**Legal category** POM

**Package quantities** Triple packs with 3 blister strips of 28 tablets

**Further information** After the menopause the protective effect that endogenous oestrogens appear to have on the female cardiovascular system is lost, and the risk of women developing cardiovascular disease rises to become similar to that of men.

Most studies show that oral administration of conjugated equine oestrogens to postmenopausal women increase serum high density lipoprotein (HDL-cholesterol) and decrease the potentially atherogenic low density lipoprotein (LDL-cholesterol) levels. This improves the lipid profile and is recognised as a factor contributing to the beneficial effect of conjugated equine oestrogens on the risk of coronary heart disease in post menopausal women.

Premarin tablets contain the following excipients: lactose, methylcellulose, magnesium stearate, syrup, glucose, glyceryl mono-oleate, polyethylene glycol, carnauba wax, calcium sulphate anhydrous, microcrystalline cellulose.

**Product licence numbers**
Premarin Tablets 0.625 mg 0011/0165
Premarin Tablets 1.25 mg 0011/0166
Premarin Tablets 2.5 mg 0011/0167

## PREMARIN* VAGINAL CREAM

**Qualitative and quantitative composition** Each 1 gram of the cream contains 0.625 mg conjugated oestrogens USP.

**Pharmaceutical form** Cream for intravaginal or topical administration.

**Clinical particulars**

*Therapeutic indication:* Short-term treatment of atrophic vaginitis and post-menopausal atrophic urethritis, Kraurosis vulvae.

*Posology and method of administration:*

*Adults:* The usual recommended dose is 1 to 2 g daily administered intravaginally or topically to the vaginal area, depending on the severity of the condition. Administration should be cyclic (e.g. three weeks on and one week off). It should start on the fifth day of bleeding in the patient who is menstruating and arbitrarily if not.

The lowest effective dose which will control symptoms should be used and the need for continuing treatment should be reviewed periodically. Should long-term therapy be considered in women with an intact uterus, an oral progestogen for 10–14 days at the end of each cycle is essential.

Before therapy commences it is recommended that the patient is fully informed of all the likely benefits and potential risks. She should have a full physical and gynaecological examination, with special emphasis on blood pressure, breasts, abdomen and pelvic organs, and endometrial assessment, carried out if appropriate. Follow-up examinations are recommended every 6–12 months. Any break-through bleeding is an indication for endometrial evaluation.

*Elderly:* There are no special dosage requirements for elderly patients, but as with all medicines, the lowest effective dose should be used.

*Children:* Not recommended.

*Contra-indications:*

1. Known or suspected pregnancy.
2. History of, known or suspected cancer of the breast.
3. Known or suspected oestrogen-dependent neoplasia. Undiagnosed abnormal genital bleeding.
4. Active thrombophlebitis or thromboembolic disorders. See also Warnings and precautions number 4.
5. Acute or chronic liver disease or history of liver disease where the liver function tests have failed to return to normal. Rotor syndrome or Dubin-Johnson syndrome.
6. Severe cardiac or renal disease.

*Special warnings and precautions for use:* Due to oestrogen absorption following the application of Premarin Vaginal Cream, prolonged administration might result in systemic effects. Therefore, the following warnings and precautions should be considered.

1. In the female there is an increased risk o endometrial hyperplasia and carcinoma associatec with unopposed oestrogens administered long-term (for more than one year). However, the appropriate addition of a progestogen to an oestrogen regimen lowers this additional risk.

2. There is suggestive evidence of a small increased risk of breast cancer with oestrogen replacemen therapy used for long-term (greater than 5 years). Some studies have reported an increased risk in long term users, others, however, have not shown thi relationship. It is not known whether concurrer progestogen use influences the risk of breast cance in post-menopausal women taking hormone replace ment therapy. Women on long-term therapy shoul have regular breast examinations, should be ir structed in self-breast examination and mamm graphic investigations conducted where considere appropriate.

There is a need for caution when prescribin oestrogens in women who have a history of, or know breast nodules or fibrocystic disease. Breast statu should be closely monitored, supported by regul mammography.

3. Certain diseases may be made worse by hormor replacement therapy and patients with these conc tions should be closely monitored. These inclu ostosclerosis, multiple sclerosis, systemic lupus er thematosus, porphyria, melanoma, epilepsy, n graine and asthma. In addition pre-existing uteri fibroids may increase in size during oestrogen thera and symptoms associated with endometriosis m be exacerbated.

4. Studies to date do not indicate that there is increased risk of thromboembolic disease, includi stroke, myocardial infarction and thrombophleb with oestrogen replacement therapy at the curre recommended low dosages in apparently norn women.

If an acute vascular thromboembolic event occu coincidentally during therapy, current opinion su gests that treatment should be discontinued. Ho ever, there is no evidence that a history of deep v thrombosis, pulmonary embolism, stroke or myoc dial infarction should be a contra-indication to oest gen replacement therapy, but in the absence sufficient data Premarin should be used with cauti in these patients.

5. Oestrogens may cause fluid retention and the fore patients with cardiac or renal dysfunction sho be carefully observed.

6. If jaundice, migraine-like headaches, visual turbances, thromboembolic phenomena or a sign cant increase in blood pressure develop after initiat therapy, the medication should be discontinued w the cause is investigated.

7. Women with an intact uterus of child-bear

›tential should be advised to adhere to non-hor-
onal contraceptive methods.
8. Most studies indicate that oestrogen replacement erapy has little effect on blood pressure and some dicate that oestrogen use may be associated with a nall decrease. In addition, most studies on combined erapy indicate that the addition of a progestogen so has little effect on blood pressure. Rarely, iosyncratic hypertension may occur.
When oestrogens are administered to hypertensive omen, supervision is necessary and blood pressure ould be monitored at regular intervals.
9. Changed oestrogen levels may affect certain docrine and liver function tests.
10. Consideration should be given to discontinue atment at least four weeks prior to surgery or ring periods of prolonged immobilisation.
11. It has been reported that there is an increase in e risk of surgically confirmed gall bladder disease women receiving postmenopausal oestrogens.
12. A worsening of glucose tolerance may occur in tients taking oestrogens and therefore diabetic tients should be carefully observed while receiving rmone replacement therapy.

*teraction with other medicaments and other forms interaction:* None known.

*egnancy and lactation:* Premarin Vaginal Cream is ntra-indicated in the event of known or suspected egnancy and during lactation.

*fects on ability to drive and use machines:* Not plicable.

*ndesirable effects:* The following side effects have en reported with oestrogen therapy.
1. Genitourinary system–Premenstrual-like syn- ome, increase in size of uterine fibromyomata, ginal candidiasis, change in cervical erosion and in gree of cervical secretion, cystitis-like syndrome.
2. Breasts–Tenderness, enlargement, secretion.
3. Gastrointestinal–Nausea, vomiting, abdominal amps, bloating, cholestatic jaundice.
4. Skin–Chloasma or melasma which may persist nen drug is discontinued, erythema multiforme, ythema nodosum, haemorrhagic eruption, loss of alp hair, hirsutism.
5. Eyes–Steepening of corneal curvature, intoler- ce to contact lenses.
6. CNS–Headaches, migraine, dizziness, mental pression, chorea.
7. Miscellaneous–Increase or decrease in weight, duced carbohydrate tolerance, aggravation of por- yria, oedema, changes in libido, leg cramps.

*erdose:* Numerous reports of ingestion of large ses of oestrogen-containing oral contraceptives by ung children indicate that acute serious ill effects not occur. Overdosage of oestrogen may cause usea, and withdrawal bleeding may occur in fe- ales.

**armacological properties**

*armacodynamic properties:* Conjugated oestrogen am has identical pharmacological actions to en- genous oestrogens. In this preparation the oestro- nic action is utilised to restore levels and thus event the symptoms of postmenopausal oestrogen ficiency.

*armacokinetic properties:* As a topical preparation information is included.

*eclinical safety data:* There are no pre-clinical data relevance to the prescriber which are additional to at already included in other sections of the SPC.

**armaceutical particulars**

*st of excipients:* Mineral oil, glyceryl monostearate, tyl alcohol, cetyl esters wax, white wax, methyl arate, sodium lauryl sulphate, phenyl ethyl alcohol, cerin, propylene glycol monostearate, purified ter

*compatibilities:* not applicable.

*elf life:* 2 years.

*ecial precautions for storage:* Store at room tem- rature (approx. 25°C).

*ture and contents of container:*

*mary container:* Aluminium tube with a white ew-on cap, containing 42.5 g of cream.

*condary container:* Cardboard carton.

*structions for use/handling:* Not applicable.

**arketing authorisation number** 0011/0163.

**te of approval/revision of SPC** October 1995

**gal category** POM

## REMIQUE*

**esentation** Premique is a light blue oval biconvex gar coated tablet. Each tablet contains conjugated oestrogens 0.625 mg and medroxyprogesterone acetate (MPA) 5.0 mg.

**Uses** Menopausal and postmenopausal oestrogen therapy in women with an intact uterus for:
1. Vasomotor symptoms associated with oestrogen deficiency
2. Atrophic vaginitis.
3. Atrophic urethritis.
4. Prevention and management of osteoporosis associated with oestrogen deficiency, in women at risk of developing fractures.

Epidemiological studies suggest a number of individual risk factors which contribute to the development of post-menopausal osteoporosis. These include: early menopause; family history of osteoporosis; thin, small frame; cigarette use; recent prolonged systemic corticosteroid use. If several of the risk factors are present in a patient, consideration should be given to oestrogen replacement therapy.

**Dosage and administration**

*Adults:* Premique is taken orally, in a continuous 28-day regimen of one tablet taken daily. There should be no break between packs.

Before therapy commences it is recommended that the patient is fully informed of all likely benefits and potential risks. She should have a full physical and gynaecological examination, with special emphasis on blood pressure, breasts, abdomen, pelvic organs and endometrial assessment carried out if appropriate.

For most postmenopausal women therapy may be commenced at any convenient time although if the patient is still menstruating commencement on first day of bleeding is recommended.

Since progestogens are only administered to reduce the risk of endometrial hyperplasia and endometrial carcinoma, patients without a uterus do not require Premique.

*Vasomotor symptoms, atrophic vaginitis, and atrophic urethritis:* The usual starting dose is one tablet 0.625 mg/5.0 mg daily.

*Prevention and management of osteoporosis:* The usual starting dose is one tablet daily. For prevention and treatment of osteoporosis, Premique should be used for at least 5 years and probably up to 10 years. It has been shown that bone mass conservation is sustained only as long as conjugated oestrogen therapy is administered, however data beyond 10 years are limited. Treatment should start as soon as possible after the onset of the menopause and certainly within 2–3 years.

*Maintenance/continuation/extended treatment:* The continuous regimen of oestrogen plus MPA for 28 days without a break is frequently associated with the development of an atrophic endometrium. However, breakthrough bleeding and spotting may occur in the early stages of Premique therapy. To reduce the likelihood of breakthrough bleeding/spotting occurring and to achieve amenorrhoea a starting dose of 5.0 mg is appropriate.

If breakthrough bleeding persists and endometrial abnormality has been ruled out, cyclic therapy should be considered as an alternative therapy.

Follow-up examinations are recommended every 6–12 months; all patients using Premique should be monitored at least annually for symptoms of endometrial abnormality. For long term use, see also warnings and precautions No.2.

*Elderly:* There are no special dosage requirements for elderly patients, but, as with all medicines, the lowest effective dose should be used.

*Children:* Not recommended

**Contra-indications, warnings, etc**

*Contra-indications:*
1. Known or suspected pregnancy.
2. Known or suspected cancer of the breast.
3. Known or suspected oestrogen-dependent neoplasia.
4. Undiagnosed abnormal genital bleeding.
5. Active thrombophlebitis or thromboembolic disorders.
6. Acute or chronic liver disease where the LFTs have failed to return to normal. Rotor or Dubin Johnson syndrome.
7. Severe cardiac or renal disease.
8. Hypersensitivity to any of the components of Premique tablets.

*Use in pregnancy and lactation:* Premique is contra-indicated in the event of known or suspected pregnancy and during lactation.

*Warnings and precautions:*
1. In the female there is an increased risk of endometrial hyperplasia and carcinoma associated with the administration of unopposed oestrogens. However, the appropriate addition of a progestogen to an oestrogen regimen lowers this additional risk.
2. There is suggestive evidence of a small increased risk of breast cancer with oestrogen replacement therapy used for long-term (greater than 5 years). Some studies have reported an increased risk for long term users, others, however, have not shown this relationship. It is not known whether concurrent progestogen use influences the risk of breast cancer in post menopausal women taking hormone replacement therapy. Women on long term therapy should have regular breast examinations, should be instructed in self-breast examination and mammographic investigations conducted where considered appropriate.

There is a need for caution when prescribing oestrogens in women who have a history of or known breast nodules or fibrocystic disease. Breast status should be closely monitored, supported by regular mammography.

3. Studies to date do not indicate that there is an increased risk of thromboembolic disease, including stroke, myocardial infarction and thrombophlebitis with oestrogen replacement therapy at the current recommended low dosages in apparently normal women.

If an acute vascular thromboembolic event occurs coincidentally during therapy, current opinion suggests that treatment should be discontinued. However, there is no evidence that a past history of deep vein thrombosis, pulmonary embolism, stroke or myocardial infarction associated with known risk factors (such as prolonged immobilisation, post-trauma or post-operatively) should be a contra-indication to oestrogen replacement therapy, but in the absence of sufficient data Premique should be used with caution in these patients.

If there is any sudden loss of vision, or there is a sudden onset of proptosis, diplopia or migraine, or if thromboembolic phenomena develop after initiating therapy the drug should be discontinued while the cause is investigated.

Consideration should be given to discontinuing treatment at least four weeks prior to surgery and during periods of prolonged immobilisation.

4. If jaundice develops, therapy should be discontinued.

5. An increase in the risk of surgically confirmed gallbladder disease has been reported in women receiving postmenopausal oestrogens.

6. Certain patients may develop undesirable manifestations of excessive oestrogenic/progestogenic stimulation such as abnormal uterine bleeding, mastodynia, etc. In the event of abnormal vaginal bleeding, adequate diagnostic measures, including endometrial sampling when indicated, should be undertaken to rule out malignancy.

7. Most studies indicate that oestrogen replacement therapy has little effect on blood pressure and some indicate that oestrogen use may be associated with a small decrease. In addition, most studies on combined therapy indicate that the addition of a progestogen has little effect on blood pressure. During trials with Premarin/MPA a few patients had a rise in blood pressure; these changes were mostly judged not to be of clinical significance.

When oestrogens are administered to hypertensive women, supervision is necessary, and blood pressure should be monitored at regular intervals.

If a significant increase in blood pressure develops after initiating therapy, treatment should be discontinued while the cause is investigated. Rarely, idiosyncratic hypertension may occur.

8. Oestrogens/progestogens may cause some degree of fluid retention and therefore patients with cardiac or renal dysfunction should be monitored.

9. Changes in glucose tolerance have been observed in some patients on oestrogen/progestogen. Decreased endogenous insulin levels during hormone replacement therapy have been observed. Diabetic patients should be carefully observed while receiving Premique.

10. Patients should be advised that Premique is not an oral contraceptive, neither will it restore fertility. Women of child-bearing potential should be advised to adhere to non-hormonal contraceptive methods.

11. Patients who have a history of depression should be observed and therapy discontinued if the depression recurs to a serious degree.

12. Certain diseases may be made worse by hormone replacement therapy and patients with these conditions should be closely monitored. These include otosclerosis, multiple sclerosis, systemic lupus erythematosis, porphyria, melanoma, epilepsy, migraine and asthma. In addition pre-existing uterine fibroids may increase in size during oestrogen therapy and symptoms associated with endometriosis may be exacerbated.

*Interactions with other medicines:* Rifampicin reportedly decreases oestrogenic activity during concomitant use with ethinyloestradiol in oral contraceptives. This effect has been attributed to increased metabolism of oestrogen, presumably by induction of hepatic microsomal enzymes. It is not known whether there are similar effects on conjugated oestrogens. Phenytoin may also decrease oestrogen levels by a similar mechanism.

Changed oestrogen levels may affect certain endocrine and liver function tests.

*Sid- effects*: The following side-effects have been reported with oestrogen/progestogen therapy.

1. Genitourinary system: PMS-like syndrome,vaginal bleeding, increase in size of uterine fibromyomata.
2. Breasts: Pain, tenderness, enlargement, secretion.
3. Gastrointestinal: Nausea, abdominal cramps, flatulence, bloating, cholelithiasis, cholestatic jaundice.
4. Skin: Alopecia, rash, pruritis, hirsutism. Chloasma or melasma, which may continue after the drug is discontinued.
5. Eyes: Visual disturbance.
6. CNS: Headache, nervousness.
7. Miscellaneous: Increase or decrease in weight, oedema, aggravation of porphyria, reduction in carbohydrate tolerance, leg cramps.

*Acute overdosage:* Numerous reports of ingestion of large doses of oestrogen/progestogen-containingoral contraceptives by young children indicate that acute serious ill effects have not been observed. Overdosage of oestrogens may cause nausea, and withdrawal bleeding may occur in females.

Should large overdoses occur and medical concerns arise, the standard practices of gastric evacuation, activated charcoal administration, and general supportive therapy may be applicable.

**Pharmaceutical precautions** Store in a dry place below (25°C).

**Legal category** POM

**Package quantities** A 28-day pack containing one wallet holding 28 tablets containing conjugated oestrogens 0.625 mg and medroxyprogesterone acetate 5.0 mg. A carton containing three wallets (3 x 28 days) of tablets.

**Further information** After the menopause, the protective effect that endogenous oestrogens appear to have on the female cardiovascular system is lost, and the risk of women developing cardiovascular disease rises to become similar to that of men.

A decreased risk of coronary heart disease in postmenopausal women taking oestrogen replacement therapy has been observed. Oral administration of conjugated oestrogens alone to postmenopausal women increased serum high density lipoprotein cholesterol (HDL-C) levels and decreased low density lipoprotein cholesterol (LDL-C) levels. These changes improve the lipid profile and are recognised as a contributory factor to the reduced risk of coronary heart disease in women. Although some of the effects may be modified by the addition of MPA, clinical trial results suggest that the combination of conjugated oestrogens with MPA show similar beneficial effects on lipid parameters to that seen during treatment with conjugated oestrogen therapy alone.

Premique contains the following excipients: calcium phosphate tribasic, calcium sulphate, carnauba wax, microcrystalline cellulose, glyceryl mono-oleate, lactose, magnesium stearate, methyl cellulose, polyethylene glycol, pharmaceutical glaze, sucrose, titanium dioxide (E171) and colour (E132).

**Product licence number** 0011/0212

## PREMIQUE* CYCLE

**Presentation** Premique Cycle is composed of two separate lots of tablets presented in a 28 day calendar pack. Each calendar pack contains 28 conjugated oestrogen tablets and 14 MPA tablets.

The conjugated oestrogen tablets are maroon, biconvex, sugar-coated, and contain 0.625 mg conjugated oestrogens.

The MPA tablets are round, white, imprinted '10' on one side and contain 10.0 mg of the progestogen, medroxyprogesterone acetate (MPA).

**Uses** Treatment of the following conditions in women with an intact uterus:

1. Vasomotor symptoms associated with oestrogen deficiency.
2. Atrophic vaginitis
3. Atrophic urethritis
4. Prevention and management of osteoporosis associated with oestrogen deficiency, in women at risk of developing fractures.

Epidemiological studies suggest a number of individual risk factors which contribute to the development of post-menopausal osteoporosis. These include: early menopause; family history of osteoporosis; thin, small frame; cigarette use; recent prolonged systemic corticosteroid use. If several of the risk factors are present in a patient, consideration should be given to oestrogen replacement therapy.

**Dosage and administration**
*Adults:* Premique Cycle is available for oral use in a sequential regimen. That is, 28 days of oestrogen therapy 0.625 mg, with 14 days of MPA tablets taken with the oestrogen tablet on days 15–28. There should be no break between packs.

Before therapy commences it is recommended that the patient is fully informed of all likely benefits and potential risks. She should have a full physical and gynaecological examination, with special emphasis on blood pressure, breasts, abdomen, pelvic organs and endometrial assessment carried out if appropriate.

For most postmenopausal women therapy may be commenced at any convenient time although if the patient is still menstruating commencement on first day of bleeding is recommended.

Since progestogens are only administered to reduce the risk of endometrial hyperplasia and endometrial carcinoma, patients without a uterus will not require Premique Cycle.

Patients should be advised that a regular withdrawal bleed will usually occur at the end of one cycle of Premique Cycle and the beginning of the next.

*Vasomotor symptoms, atrophic vaginitis, atrophic urethritis:* One oestrogen tablet 0.625 mg daily for 28 days. One MPA tablet is also taken daily on days 15–28.

*Prevention and management of osteoporosis:* One oestrogen tablet 0.625 mg daily for 28 days. One MPA tablet is taken daily on days 15–28. For prevention and treatment of osteoporosis Premique Cycle should be used for at least 5 years, and probably up to 10 years. It has been shown that bone mass conservation is sustained only as long as conjugated oestrogen therapy is administered, however data beyond 10 years are limited. Treatment should start as soon as possible after the onset of the menopause and certainly within 2–3 years.

*Maintenance/continuation/extended treatment:* Follow up examinations are recommended every 6–12 months; all patients using Premique Cycle should be monitored at least annually for symptoms of endometrial abnormality. For prevention and treatment of osteoporosis long term treatment is necessary. For long term use, see also Warnings and Precautions No.2.

*Elderly:* There are no special dosage requirements for elderly patients, but, as with all medicines the lowest effective dose should be used.

*Children:* Not recommended

**Contra-indications, warnings, etc.**
*Contra-indications:*

1. Known or suspected pregnancy.
2. Known or suspected cancer of the breast.
3. Known or suspected oestrogen-dependent neoplasia.
4. Undiagnosed abnormal genital bleeding.
5. Active thrombophlebitis or thromboembolic disorders.
6. Acute or chronic liver disease where the LFTs have failed to return to normal. Rotor or Dubin Johnson Syndrome
7. Severe cardiac or renal disease
8. Hypersensitivity to any of the components in the conjugated oestrogen or MPA tablets.

*Use in pregnancy and lactation:* Premique Cycle is contra-indicated in the event of known or suspected pregnancy and during lactation.

*Warnings and precautions:*

1. In the female there is an increased risk of endometrial hyperplasia and carcinoma associated with the administration of unopposed oestrogens. However, the appropriate addition of a progestogen to an oestrogen regimen lowers this additional risk.

2. There is suggestive evidence of a small increased risk of breast cancer with oestrogen replacement therapy used for long-term (greater than 5 years). Some studies have reported an increased risk for long term users, others, however, have not shown this relationship. It is not known whether concurrent progestogen use influences the risk of breast cancer in post menopausal women taking hormone replacement therapy. Women on long term therapy should have regular breast examinations, should be instructed in self-breast examination and mammographic investigations conducted where considered appropriate.

There is a need for caution when prescribing oestrogens in women who have a history of or known breast nodules or fibrocystic disease. Breast status should be closely monitored, supported by regular mammography.

3. Studies to date do not indicate that there is an increased risk of thromboembolic disease, including stroke, myocardial infarction and thrombophlebitis with oestrogen replacement therapy at the curre recommended low dosages in apparently norm women.

If an acute vascular thromboembolic event occu coincidentally during therapy, current opinion su gests that treatment should be discontinued. Ho ever, there is no evidence that a past history of de vein thrombosis, pulmonary embolism, stroke myocardial infarction associated with known r factors (such as prolonged immobilisation, po trauma or post-operatively) should be a cont indication to oestrogen replacement therapy, but the absence of sufficient data Premique Cycle shou be used with caution in these patients.

If there is any sudden loss of vision, or there is sudden onset of proptosis, diplopia or migraine, o thromboembolic phenomena develop after initiati therapy the drug should be discontinued while t cause is investigated.

Consideration should be given to discontinui treatment at least four weeks prior to surgery a during periods of prolonged immobilisation.

4. If jaundice develops, therapy should be discont ued.

5. An increase in the risk of surgically confirm gallbladder disease has been reported in wom receiving postmenopausal oestrogens.

6. Certain patients may develop undesirable ma festations of excessive oestrogenic/progestoge stimulation, such as abnormal uterine bleeding, m todynia, etc. In the event of abnormal vaginal bleedi adequate diagnostic measures, including endomet sampling when indicated, should be undertaken rule out malignancy.

7. Most studies indicate that oestrogen replacem therapy has little effect on blood pressure and so indicate that oestrogen use may be associated wit small decrease. In addition, most studies on combin therapy indicate that the addition of a progestog has little effect on blood pressure. During trials w Premique Cycle a few patients had a rise in blo pressure; these changes were mostly judged not be of clinical significance.

When oestrogens are administered to hypertens women, supervision is necessary, and blood press should be monitored at regular intervals.

If a significant increase in blood pressure develo after initiating therapy treatment should be discont ued while the cause is investigated. Rarely, idios cratic hypertension may occur.

8. Oestrogens/progestogens may cause some gree of fluid retention and therefore patients w cardiac or renal dysfunction should be monitored.

9. Changes in glucose tolerance have been observ in some patients on oestrogen/progestogen. [ creased endogenous insulin levels during hormo replacement therapy have been observed. Diabe patients should be carefully observed while receivi Premique Cycle.

10. Patients should be advised that the resumpti of menses associated with hormone replacem therapy is not indicative of fertility. There is no data support Premique Cycle as an appropriate form contraception. Women of child-bearing potential t ing Premique Cycle require contraception and sho be advised to adhere to non-hormonal contracept methods.

11. Patients who have a history of depress should be observed and therapy discontinued if depression recurs to a serious degree.

12. Certain diseases may be made worse hormone replacement therapy and patients with th conditions should be closely monitored. These inclu otosclerosis, multiple sclerosis, systemic lupus e thematosus, melanoma, porphyria, epilepsy, graine and asthma. In addition pre-existing ute fibroids may increase in size during oestrogen thera and symptoms associated with endometriosis m be exacerbated.

*Interactions with other medicines:* Rifampicin rep edly decreases oestrogenic activity during conco tant use with ethinyloestradiol in oral contraceptiv This effect has been attributed to increased meta lism of oestrogen, presumably by induction of hep microsomal enzymes. It is not known whether th are similar effects on conjugated oestrogens. Phe toin may also decrease oestrogen levels by a sim mechanism.

Changed oestrogen levels may affect certain en crine and liver function tests.

*Side-effects:* The following side-effects have b reported with oestrogen/progestogen therapy.

1. Genitourinary system: PMS-like s drome,vaginal bleeding, increase in size of ute fibromyomata.
2. Breasts: Pain, tenderness, enlargement, sec tion.
3. Gastrointestinal: Nausea, abdominal cram flatulence, bloating, cholelithiasis, cholestatic ja dice.
4. Skin: Alopecia, rash, pruritis, hirsutism. Chloas

or melasma, which may continue after the drug is discontinued.

5. Eyes: Visual disturbance.

6. CNS: Headache, nervousness.

7. Miscellaneous: Increase or decrease in weight, oedema, aggravation of porphyria, reduction in carbohydrate tolerance, leg cramps.

*Acute overdosage:* Numerous reports of ingestion of large doses of oestrogen/progestogen-containing oral contraceptives by young children indicate that acute serious ill effects have not been observed. Overdosage of oestrogens may cause nausea, and withdrawal bleeding may occur in females.

Should large overdoses occur and medical concerns arise, the standard practices of gastric evacuation, activated charcoal administration, and general supportive therapy may be applicable.

**Pharmaceutical precautions** Store in a dry place below 25°C.

**Legal category** POM

Pharmaceutical excipients in the oestrogen tablets are: lactose, methylcellulose, magnesium stearate. Coating ingredients are syrup, sucrose, glyceryl mono-oleate, polyethylene glycol, carnauba wax, calcium sulphate, shellac solution, microcrystalline cellulose, titanium dioxide (E171) and colours E110, E132 and E127. Pharmaceutical excipients in the progestogen tablets are: lactose, microcrystalline cellulose, methylcellulose and magnesium stearate.

**Package quantities** A 28-day calendar pack containing 28 oestrogen tablets 0.625 mg and 14 medroxyprogesterone acetate tablets 10.0 mg. A carton containing three calendar packs of 28 oestrogen and 14 MPA tablets.

**Further information** After the menopause, the protective effect that endogenous oestrogens appear to have on the female cardiovascular system is lost, and the risk of women developing cardiovascular disease rises to become similar to that of men.

A decreased risk of coronary heart disease in postmenopausal women taking oestrogen replacement therapy has been observed. Oral administration of conjugated oestrogens alone to postmenopausal women increased serum high density lipoprotein cholesterol (HDL-C) levels and decreased low density lipoprotein cholesterol (LDL-C) levels. These changes improve the lipid profile and are recognised as a contributory factor to the reduced risk of coronary heart disease in women. Although some of the effects may be modified by the addition of MPA, clinical trial results suggest that the combination of conjugated oestrogens with MPA show similar beneficial effects on lipid parameters to that seen during treatment with conjugated oestrogen therapy alone.

**Product licence number** 0011/0205

# PREMPAK*-C

**Presentation** Prempak-C 0.625 consists of 28 maroon tablets containing natural conjugated oestrogens 0.625 mg plus 12 light brown tablets containing norgestrel 0.15 mg.

Prempak-C 1.25 consists of 28 yellow tablets containing natural conjugated oestrogens 1.25 mg plus 12 light brown tablets containing norgestrel 0.15 mg.

**Uses** Menopausal and postmenopausal oestrogen therapy in women with an intact uterus for:

1. Vasomotor symptoms such as sweating and hot flushes

2. Allied disorders of the menopause such as atrophic vaginitis, kraurosis vulvae, atrophic urethritis

3. Prophylaxis of osteoporosis in women at risk of developing fractures.

**Dosage and administration**

*Adults:* Conjugated oestrogens 0.625 mg–1.25 mg daily. One norgestrel tablet should be taken daily from day 17 to day 28 of oestrogen therapy. Continuous oestrogen administration is recommended. For maintenance, the lowest effective dose should be used.

*Vasomotor symptoms:* 0.625–1.25 mg conjugated oestrogens daily depending on the response of the individual. One norgestrel tablet should be taken daily from day 17 to day 28 of oestrogen therapy.

*Atrophic vaginitis, kraurosis vulvae, atrophic urethritis:* 0.625–1.25 mg conjugated oestrogens daily depending on the response of the individual. One norgestrel tablet should be taken daily from day 17 to day 28 of oestrogen therapy.

*Prophylaxis of osteoporosis:* The minimum effective dose is 0.625 mg daily for most patients. One norgestrel tablet should be taken daily from day 17 to day 28 of oestrogen therapy. Hormone replacement therapy has been found to be effective in the prevention of osteoporosis when started soon after the menopause and used for 5 years and probably up to 10 years. Treatment should start as soon as possible after the

onset of the menopause and certainly within 2 to 3 years. Protection appears to be effective for as long as treatment is continued, however data beyond 10 years are limited. A careful re-appraisal of the risk-benefit ratio should be undertaken before treating for longer than 5 to 10 years. For long term use see also precautions and warnings.

At present there is no established screening programme for determining women at risk of developing osteoporotic fractures. Epidemiological studies suggest a number of individual risk factors which contribute to the development of postmenopausal osteoporosis. These include: early menopause; family history of osteoporosis; thin, small frame; cigarette use; recent prolonged systemic corticosteroid use.

If several of these risk factors are present in a patient, consideration should be given to oestrogen replacement therapy.

For most postmenopausal women therapy may be commenced at any convenient time although if the patient is still menstruating, commencement on first day of bleeding is recommended. Withdrawal bleeding usually occurs within three to seven days after the last norgestrel tablet.

Since progestogens are only administered to protect against hyperplastic changes of the endometrium, patients without a uterus will not require a progestogen.

Before therapy commences it is recommended that the patient is fully informed of all the likely benefits and potential risks. She should have a full physical and gynaecological examination, with special emphasis on blood pressure, breasts, abdomen and pelvic organs, and endometrial assessment carried out if indicated. Follow-up examinations are recommended every 6–12 months.

Breakthrough bleeding may occasionally occur in the first few weeks after initiating treatment and will usually settle. It can also be the result of poor compliance, or concurrent antibiotic use. It may however indicate endometrial pathology and therefore any doubt as to the cause of breakthrough bleeding is an indication for endometrial evaluation including endometrial biopsy.

*Elderly:* There are no special dosage requirements for elderly patients, but as with all medicines, the lowest effective dose should be used.

*Children:* Not recommended.

**Contra-indications, warnings etc**
*Contra-indications:*

1. Known or suspected pregnancy.

2. History of, known or suspected cancer of the breast.

3. Known or suspected oestrogen-dependent neoplasia. Undiagnosed abnormal genital bleeding.

4. Active thrombophlebitis or thromboembolic disorders. See also *Warnings and Precautions number 4.*

5. Acute or chronic liver disease or history of liver disease where the liver function tests have failed to return to normal. Rotor syndrome or Dubin-Johnson syndrome.

6. Severe cardiac or renal disease.

*Use in pregnancy and lactation:* Prempak-C is contra-indicated in the event of known or suspected pregnancy and during lactation.

*Warnings and precautions:*

1. In the female there is an increased risk of endometrial hyperplasia and carcinoma associated with unopposed oestrogen administered long-term (for more than one year). However, the appropriate addition of a progestogen to an oestrogen regimen lowers this additional risk.

2. There is suggestive evidence of a small increased risk of breast cancer with oestrogen replacement therapy used for long term (greater than 5 years). Some studies have reported an increased risk of breast cancer in long-term users, others however, have not shown this relationship. It is not known whether concurrent progestogen use influences the risk of breast cancer in postmenopausal women taking hormone replacement therapy. Women on long-term therapy should have regular breast examinations, and should be instructed in self-breast examination. Regular mammographic investigations should be conducted where considered appropriate.

There is a need for caution when prescribing oestrogens in women who have a history of, or known breast nodules, or fibrocystic disease. Breast status should be closely monitored, supported by regular mammography.

3. Certain diseases may be made worse by hormone replacement therapy and patients with these conditions should be closely monitored. These include otosclerosis, multiple sclerosis, systemic lupus erythematosis, porphyria, melanoma, epilepsy, migraine and asthma. In addition pre-existing uterine fibroids may increase in size during oestrogen therapy and symptoms associated with endometriosis may be exacerbated.

4. Studies to date do not indicate that there is an increased risk of thromboembolic disease, including stroke, myocardial infarction and thrombophlebitis, with oestrogen replacement therapy, at the current recommended low dosages in apparently normal women.

If an acute vascular thromboembolic event occurs coincidentally during therapy, current opinion suggests that treatment should be discontinued.

However, there is no evidence that a past history of deep vein thrombosis, pulmonary embolism, stroke or myocardial infarction should be a contra-indication to hormone replacement therapy, but in the absence of sufficient data Prempak-C should be used with caution in these patients.

5. Oestrogens may cause fluid retention and therefore patients with cardiac or renal dysfunction should be carefully observed.

6. If jaundice, migraine-like headaches, visual disturbance, thromboembolic phenomena or a significant increase in blood pressure develop after initiating therapy, the medication should be discontinued while the cause is investigated.

7. Prempak-C is not an oral contraceptive neither will it restore fertility. Women of child-bearing potential should be advised to adhere to non-hormonal contraceptive methods.

8. Most studies indicate that oestrogen replacement therapy has little effect on blood pressure and some indicate that oestrogen use may be associated with a small decrease. In addition, most studies on combined therapy indicate that the addition of a progestogen also has little effect on blood pressure. Rarely, idiosyncratic hypertension may occur.

When oestrogens are administered to hypertensive women, supervision is necessary and blood pressure should be monitored at regular intervals.

9. Changed oestrogen levels may affect certain endocrine and liver function tests.

10. Consideration should be given to discontinue treatment at least four weeks prior to surgery or during periods of prolonged immobilisation.

11. It has been reported that there is an increase in the risk of surgically confirmed gallbladder disease in women receiving postmenopausal oestrogens.

12. A worsening of glucose tolerance may occur in patients taking oestrogens and therefore diabetic patients should be carefully observed while receiving hormone replacement therapy.

*Side-effects:* The following side effects have been reported with oestrogen/progestogen therapy:

1. Genitourinary system - Breakthrough bleeding, spotting, change in menstrual flow, dysmenorrhoea, premenstrual-like syndrome, amenorrhoea, increase in size of uterine fibromyomata, vaginal candidiasis, change in cervical erosion and in degree of cervical secretion, cystitis-like syndrome.

2. Breasts - Tenderness, enlargement, secretion.

3. Gastrointestinal - Nausea, vomiting, abdominal cramps, bloating, cholestatic jaundice.

4. Skin - Chloasma or melasma which may persist when drug is discontinued, erythema multiforme, erythema nodosum, haemorrhagic eruption, loss of scalp hair, hirsutism.

5. Eyes - Steepening of corneal curvature, intolerance to contact lenses.

6. CNS - Headaches, migraine, dizziness, mental depression, chorea.

7. Miscellaneous - Increase or decrease in weight, reduced carbohydrate tolerance, aggravation of porphyria, oedema, changes in libido, leg cramps.

*Acute overdosage:* Numerous reports of ingestion of large doses of oestrogen-containing oral contraceptives by young children indicate that acute serious ill effects do not occur. Overdosage of oestrogen may cause nausea, and withdrawal bleeding may occur in females.

**Pharmaceutical precautions** No special requirements for storage are necessary.

**Legal category** POM

**Package quantities** Triple packs with 3 blister strips of 28 oestrogen tablets 0.625 mg or 1.25 mg and 12 norgestrel tablets 0.15 mg.

**Further information** After the menopause the protective effect that endogenous oestrogens appear to have on the female cardiovascular system is lost, and the risk of women developing cardiovascular disease rises to become similar to that of men.

Most studies show that oral administration of conjugated equine oestrogens to post menopausal women increase serum high density lipoprotein (HDL-cholesterol) and decrease the potentially atherogenic low density lipoprotein (LDL-cholesterol) levels. This improves the lipid profile and is recognised as a factor contributing to the beneficial effect of conjugated equine oestrogens on the risk of coronary heart disease in post menopausal women. A possible attenuation of these effects may occur with the addition of a progestogen. However epidemiologic data on combined oestrogen and progestogen therapy are limited.

Prempak-C provides oestrogen/progestogen therapy for the menopausal syndrome and associated disorders. The blister strip contains 28 oestrogen tablets. From day 17 to day 28 inclusive each bubble contains in addition one norgestrel 0.15 mg tablet. The two tablets should be taken together for these twelve days.

**Product licence numbers**
Prempak-C 0.625 0011/0161
Prempak-C 1.25 0011/0162

## PROSTAP* 3 Leuprorelin Acetate Depot Injection 11.25 mg

**Qualitative and quantitative composition** *Prostap 3 Powder:* 11.25 mg leuprorelin acetate (equivalent to 10.72 mg base).
*Sterile vehicle:* Each ml contains sodium carboxymethyl cellulose 5 mg, mannitol 50 mg, polysorbate 80 1 mg in water for injection.

**Pharmaceutical form** *Prostap 3 Powder 11.25 mg:* A sterile, lyophilised, white, odourless PLA (poly DL-lactic acid) microsphere powder for subcutaneous injection after reconstitution with the sterile vehicle to provide a 3 month depot injection.
*Sterile vehicle:* Prefilled syringes containing 2 ml of clear, colourless, slightly viscous, sterile vehicle for reconstitution of the powder.

**Clinical particulars**
*Therapeutic indications:* Prostap 3 is indicated for use in the management of advanced prostatic cancer.

*Posology and method of administration:*
*Dosage:*
*Male adults:* The usual recommended dose is 11.25 mg presented as a three month depot injection and administered as a single subcutaneous injection at intervals of three months. The majority of patients will respond to this dosage. Prostap therapy should not be discontinued when remission or improvement occurs. As with other drugs administered regularly by injection, the injection site should be varied periodically.

Response to Prostap 3 therapy should be monitored by clinical parameters and by measuring prostate-specific antigen (PSA) serum levels. Clinical studies have shown that testosterone levels increased during the first 4 days of treatment in the majority of non-orchidectomised patients. They then decreased and reached castrate levels by 2–4 weeks. Once attained, castrate levels were maintained as long as drug therapy continued. If a patient's response appears to be sub-optimal, then it would be advisable to confirm that serum testosterone levels have reached or are remaining at castrate levels. Transient increases in acid phosphatase levels sometimes occur early in the treatment period but usually return to normal or near normal values by the 4th week of treatment.

*Elderly men:* as for adults.

*Women and children:* the use of Prostap 3 in women and children is not recommended.

*Administration:* The vial of Prostap 3 microsphere powder should be reconstituted immediately prior to administration by subcutaneous injection. However, the suspension is considered stable for up to 24 hours. Remove flip-cap from vial of Prostap 3 Powder and cap from pre-filled syringe containing 2 ml Sterile Vehicle. Ensure 23 gauge needle is fixed securely by screwing needle hub onto the syringe and inject whole contents of syringe into vial of Prostap 3 Powder using an aseptic technique. Remove the syringe/needle and keep aseptic. Shake the vial gently for 15–20 seconds to produce a uniform cloudy suspension of Prostap. Immediately draw up suspension into syringe taking care to exclude air bubbles. Change the needle on syringe using a 23 gauge needle. Having cleaned an appropriate injection site and ensured that the needle is fixed securely, administer the suspension by subcutaneous injection taking care not to enter a blood vessel. Apply sterile dressing to injection site if required.

The injection should be given as soon as possible after mixing. If any settling of suspension occurs in vial or syringe, re-suspend by gentle shaking and administer immediately.

No other fluid can be used for reconstitution of Prostap 3 Powder.

*Contra-indications:* There are no known contra-indications to the use of Prostap 3 in men.

The use of Prostap 3 is not indicated in women.

*Special warnings and special precautions for use:*
*Men:* In the initial stages of therapy, a transient rise in levels of testosterone, dihydro-testosterone and acid phosphatase may occur. In some cases, this may be associated with a 'flare' or exacerbation of the tumour growth resulting in temporary deterioration of the patient's condition. These symptoms usually subside on continuation of therapy. 'Flare' may manifest itself as systemic or neurological symptoms in some cases.

In order to reduce the risk of flare, an anti-androgen may be administered beginning 3 days prior to leuprorelin therapy and continuing for the first two to three weeks of treatment. This has been reported to prevent the sequelae of an initial rise in serum testosterone.

Patients at risk of ureteric obstruction or spinal cord compression should be considered carefully and closely supervised in the first few weeks of treatment. These patients should be considered for prophylactic treatment with anti-androgens. Should urological/neurological complications occur, these should be treated by appropriate specific measures.

If an anti-androgen is used over a prolonged period, due attention should be paid to the contraindications and precautions associated with its extended use.

Whilst the development of pituitary adenomas has been noted in chronic toxicity studies at high doses in some animal species, this has not been observed in long term clinical studies with leuprorelin acetate.

*Precautions:*
*Men:* Patients with urinary obstruction and patients with metastatic vertebral lesions should begin Prostap 3 therapy under close supervision for the first few weeks of treatment.

*Interaction with other medicaments and other forms of interaction:* None have been reported.

*Pregnancy and lactation:* The use of Prostap 3 is not indicated in women. However, leuprorelin acetate is contraindicated in women who are or may become pregnant while receiving the drug. Leuprorelin acetate should not be used in women who are breast-feeding.

*Effects on ability to drive and operate machines:* None reported.

*Undesirable effects:* Many side effects seen during treatment with Prostap 3 are due to the specific pharmacological action or the disease condition itself.

The administration of Prostap is often associated with hot flushes and sometimes sweating. Impotence and decreased libido will be expected with Prostap therapy. Gynaecomastia has been reported occasionally.

In cases where a 'tumour flare' occurs after Prostap therapy, an exacerbation may occur in any symptoms or signs due to disease, for example, bone pain, urinary obstruction etc. These symptoms subside on continuation of therapy.

Adverse events which have been reported include peripheral oedema, fatigue, nausea, headache (occasionally severe), arthralgia, dizziness, insomnia, paraesthesia, visual disturbances, weight changes and irritation at the injection site. Hypersensitivity reactions including rash, pruritis, urticaria and, rarely, wheezing have also been reported. Anaphylactic reactions are rare.

*Overdose:* There is no clinical experience with the effects of an acute overdose of leuprorelin acetate. In animal studies, doses of up to 500 times the recommended human dose resulted in dyspnoea, decreased activity and local irritation at the injection site. In cases of overdosage, the patients should be monitored closely and management should be symptomatic and supportive.

**Pharmacological properties**
*Pharmacodynamic properties:* Prostap 3 contains leuprorelin acetate, a synthetic nonapeptide analogue of naturally occurring gonadotrophin releasing hormone (GnRH) which possesses greater potency than the natural hormone. Leuprorelin acetate is a peptide and therefore unrelated to the steroids. Chronic administration results in an inhibition of gonadotrophin production and subsequent suppression of ovarian and testicular steroid secretion. This effect is reversible on discontinuation of therapy.

Administration of leuprorelin acetate results in an initial increase in circulating levels of gonadotrophins which leads to a transient increase in gonadal steroid levels in both men and women. Continued administration of leuprorelin acetate results in a decrease of gonadotrophin and sex steroid levels. In men serum testosterone levels, initially raised in response to early luteinising hormone (LH) release, fall to castrate levels in about 2–4 weeks.

Prostap 3 is inactive when given orally.

*Pharmacokinetic properties:* Leuprorelin acetate is well absorbed after subcutaneous injection. It binds to the luteinising hormone releasing hormone (LHRH) receptors and is rapidly degraded. An initially high plasma level of leuprorelin peaks at around 3 hours after Prostap 3 injection, followed by a decrease to maintenance levels in 7 to 14 days. Prostap 3 provides continuous plasma levels for up to 117 days resulting in suppression of testosterone to below castrati level within 4 weeks of the first injection in the major of patients.

The metabolism, distribution and excretion of le prorelin acetate in humans have not been fu determined.

*Preclinical safety data:* Animal studies have show that leuprorelin acetate has a high acute safety fact No major overt toxicological problems have be seen during repeated administration. Whilst the c velopment of pituitary adenomas has been noted chronic toxicity studies at high doses in some anin species, this has not been observed in long-te clinical studies. No evidence of mutagenicity teratogenicity has been shown. Animal reproducti studies showed increased foetal mortality and c creased foetal weights reflecting the pharmacologic effects of this LHRH antagonist.

**Pharmaceutical particulars**
*List of excipients:* Poly (D-L lactic acid), Mannitol.

*Incompatibilities:* No other fluid other than the Ster Vehicle provided for Prostap 3 can be used for t reconstitution of Prostap 3 Powder.

*Shelf life:* 36 months unopened. Once reconstitut with sterile vehicle, the suspension should be adm istered immediately.

*Special precautions for storage:* Store at or bel room temperature (25°C), in the original contain Protect from light.

*Nature and contents of container:* Vials containi 11.25 mg leuprorelin acetate as microsphere powd Prefilled syringes containing 2 ml of Sterile Vehicle

*Instructions for use and handling:* See above.

**Marketing authorisation numbers**
Prostap 3: 0095/0311
Sterile Vehicle: 0095/0220

**Date of approval/revision of SPC** December 1996

**Legal category** POM

## PROSTAP* SR

**Qualitative and quantitative composition**
*Prostap SR Powder:* 3.75 mg leuprorelin acet (equivalent to 3.57 mg base).

*Sterile Vehicle:* Each ml contains sodium carbo methyl cellulose 5 mg, mannitol 50 mg, polysorb 80 1 mg in water for injection.

**Pharmaceutical form** *Prostap SR Powder 3.75 mg:* sterile, lyophilised, white odourless PLGA† mic sphere powder for subcutaneous or intramuscu injection after reconstitution with the sterile vehicle week depot injection).

†PLGA = Copoly (DL-lactic acid/glycolic acid) 75:25 mol%.

*Sterile vehicle:* Prefilled syringes containing 1 m clear, colourless, slightly viscous, sterile vehicle reconstitution of the microsphere.

**Clinical particulars**
*Therapeutic indications:*
(I) Treatment of advanced prostatic cancer.
(ii) Management of endometriosis, including p relief and reduction of endometriotic lesions.
(iii) Endometrial preparation prior to intrauter surgical procedures including endometrial ablation resection.

*Posology and method of administration:*
*Dosage:*
*Advanced prostatic cancer:* The usual recommenc dose is 3.75 mg administered as a single subcuta ous or intramuscular injection every month. T majority of patients will respond to a 3.75 mg do Prostap therapy should not be discontinued wh remission or improvement occurs. As with ot drugs administered chronically by injection, the in tion site should be varied.

Response to Prostap therapy may be monitored clinical parameters and by measuring serum levels testosterone and acid phosphatase. Clinical stud have shown that testosterone levels increased dur the first 4 days of treatment in the majority of n orchidectomised patients. They then decreased a reached castrate levels by 2–4 weeks. Once attain castrate levels were maintained as long as d therapy continued. Transient increases in acid ph phatase levels sometimes occur early in the treatm period but usually return to normal or near norr values by the 4th week of treatment.

*Endometriosis:* The recommended dose is 3.75 administered as a single subcutaneous or intram cular injection every month for a maximum perio 6 months. Treatment should be initiated during first 5 days of the menstrual cycle.

*Endometrial preparation prior to intrauterine surg* A single 3.75 mg subcutaneous or intramusc ection 5–6 weeks prior to surgery. Therapy should initiated during days 3 to 5 of the menstrual cycle.

*derly:* As for adults.

*ildren:* Safety and efficacy in children have not been tablished.

*dministration:* The vial of Prostap SR microsphere wder should be reconstituted immediately prior to ministration by subcutaneous or intramuscular ection. Remove flip-cap from vial of Prostap SR wder and cap from prefilled syringe containing nl of Sterile Vehicle. Ensure 23 gauge needle is ed securely to the syringe and inject whole contents syringe into vial of Prostap SR Powder using an eptic technique. Remove the syringe/needle and ep aseptic. Shake vial gently for 15–20 seconds to oduce a uniform cloudy suspension of Prostap.

Immediately draw up suspension into syringe taking re to exclude air bubbles. Change the needle on ringe using a 23 gauge needle if the suspension is be administered subcutaneously or alternatively a gauge needle for intramuscular administration. ving cleaned an appropriate injection site and sured that the needle is fixed securely, administer suspension by subcutaneous or intramuscular ection as appropriate taking care not to enter a ood vessel. Apply sterile dressing to injection site if quired.

The injection should be given as soon as possible er mixing. If any settling of suspension occurs in l or syringe, re-suspend by gentle shaking and minister immediately.

*No other fluid can be used for reconstitution of ostap SR Powder.*

*ntra-indications:*

*omen:* Prostap is contra-indicated in women who e or may become pregnant while receiving the drug. ostap should not be used in women who are eastfeeding or have undiagnosed abnormal vaginal eeding.

*en:* There are no known contra-indications to the e of Prostap in men.

*ecial warnings and special precautions for use:*

*en:* In the initial stages of therapy, a transient rise in els of testosterone, dihydro-testosterone and acid osphatase may occur. In some cases, this may be sociated with a 'flare' or exacerbation of the tumour owth resulting in temporary deterioration of the tient's condition. These symptoms usually subside continuation of therapy. 'Flare' may manifest itself systemic or neurological symptoms in some cases.

n order to reduce the risk of flare, an anti-androgen ay be administered beginning 3 days prior to prorelin therapy and continuing for the first two to ee weeks of treatment. This has been reported to event the sequelae of an initial rise in serum stosterone.

Patients at risk of ureteric obstruction or spinal cord mpression should be considered carefully and sely supervised in the first few weeks of treatment. ese patients should be considered for prophylactic atment with anti-androgens. Should urological or urological complications occur, these should be ated by appropriate specific measures.

f an anti-androgen is used over a prolonged period, e attention should be paid to the contra-indications d precautions associated with its extended use.

Whilst the development of pituitary adenomas has en noted in chronic toxicity studies at high doses in me animal species, this has not been observed in ng term clinical studies with Prostap.

*omen:* During the early phase of therapy, sex roids temporarily rise above baseline because of physiological effect of the drug. Therefore, an rease in clinical signs and symptoms may be served during the initial days of therapy, but these ll dissipate with continued therapy.

Prostap may cause an increase in uterine cervical sistance, which may result in difficulty in dilating e cervix for intrauterine surgical procedures.

*ecautions:*

*en:* Patients with urinary obstruction and patients th metastatic vertebral lesions should begin Prostap erapy under close supervision for the first few weeks treatment.

*Women:* Since menstruation should stop with ective doses of Prostap, the patient should notify r physician if regular menstruation persists.

*eraction with other medicaments and other forms interaction:* None have been reported.

*egnancy and lactation:* Safe use of leuprorelin etate in pregnancy has not been established clinily. Before starting treatment with Prostap, pregncy must be excluded.

Prostap should not be used in women who are eastfeeding.

When used monthly at the recommended dose, ostap usually inhibits ovulation and stops menstruon. Contraception is not ensured, however, by taking Prostap and therefore patients should use non-hormonal methods of contraception during treatment.

Patients should be advised that if they miss successive doses of Prostap, breakthrough bleeding or ovulation may occur with the potential for conception. Patients should be advised to see their physician if they believe they may be pregnant. If a patient becomes pregnant during treatment, the drug must be discontinued. No teratological effect has been demonstrated in rats and rabbits. The patient must be appraised of this evidence and the potential for an unknown risk to the foetus.

*Effects on ability to drive and operate machines:* None reported.

*Undesirable effects:* Side-effects seen with Prostap are due mainly to the specific pharmacological action, namely increases and decreases in certain hormone levels. Adverse events which have been reported infrequently include peripheral oedema, fatigue, nausea, headache (occasionally severe), arthralgia, dizziness, insomnia, paraesthesia, visual disturbances, weight changes and irritation at the injection site. Hypersensitivity reactions including rash, pruritus, urticaria and, rarely, wheezing have also been reported. Anaphylactic reactions are rare.

*Men:* In cases where a 'tumour flare' occurs after Prostap therapy, an exacerbation may occur in any symptoms or signs due to disease, for example, bone pain, urinary obstruction etc. These symptoms subside on continuation of therapy.

Impotence and decreased libido will be expected with Prostap therapy.

The administration of Prostap is often associated with hot flushes and sometimes sweating.

Gynaecomastia has been reported occasionally.

*Women:* Those adverse events occurring most frequently with Prostap are associated with hypo-oestrogenism; the most frequently reported are hot flushes, mood swings including depression (occasionally severe), and vaginal dryness. Oestrogen levels return to normal after treatment is discontinued.

Breast tenderness or change in breast size may occur occasionally. Hair loss has also been reported occasionally.

The induced hypo-oestrogenic state results in a small loss in bone density over the course of treatment, some of which may not be reversible. The extent of bone demineralisation due to hypo-oestrogenaemia is proportional to time and, consequently, is the adverse event responsible for limiting the duration of therapy to 6 months. The generally accepted level of bone loss with LHRH analogues such as Prostap is 5%. In clinical studies the levels varied between 2.3% and 15.7% depending on the method of measurement. During one six-month treatment period, this bone loss should not be important. In patients with major risk factors for decreased bone mineral content such as chronic alcohol and/or tobacco use, strong family history of osteoporosis, or chronic use of drugs that can reduce bone mass such as anticonvulsants or corticosteroids, Prostap therapy may pose an additional risk. In these patients, the risks and benefits must be weighed carefully before therapy with Prostap is instituted.

*Overdose:* There is no clinical experience with the effects of an acute overdose of Prostap. In animal studies, doses of up to 500 times the recommended human dose resulted in dyspnoea, decreased activity and local irritation at the injection site. In cases of overdosage, the patients should be monitored closely and management should be symptomatic and supportive.

**Pharmacological properties**

*Pharmacodynamic properties:* Prostap is a synthetic nonapeptide analogue of naturally occurring gonadotrophin releasing hormone (GnRH) which possesses greater potency than the natural hormone. Prostap is a peptide and therefore unrelated to the steroids. Chronic administration results in an inhibition of gonadotrophin production and subsequent suppression of ovarian and testicular steroid secretion. This effect is reversible on discontinuation of therapy.

Administration of leuprorelin acetate results in an initial increase in circulating levels of gonadotrophins which leads to a transient increase in gonadal steroid levels in both men and women. Continued administration of leuprorelin acetate results in a decrease of gonadotrophin and sex steroid levels. In men serum testosterone levels, initially raised in response to early luteinising hormone (LH) release, fall to castrate levels in about 2–4 weeks. Oestradiol levels will decrease to postmenopausal levels in premenopausal women within one month of initiating treatment.

The drug is well absorbed from the subcutaneous or intramuscular route, binds to luteinising hormone releasing hormone (LHRH) receptors and is rapidly degraded. In this dose form, an initial high level of leuprorelin in the plasma is achieved within 3 hours followed by a drop over 24–48 hours to maintenance levels of 0.3–0.8ng/ml and a slow decline thereafter. Effective levels persist for 30–40 days after a single dose. Prostap is inactive when given orally.

*Pharmacokinetic properties:* Studies submitted show that single intramuscular or subcutaneous doses of leuprorelin acetate over the dose range 3.75 to 15 mg results in detectable levels of leuprorelin for more than 28 days, good bioavailability, a consistent and predictable pharmacokinetic profile, and biological efficacy at plasma levels of less than 0.5ng/ml. The pharmacokinetic profile is similar to that seen in animal studies using the compound, with an initial high level of drug released from the microcapsules during reconstitution and injection followed by a plateau over a 2–3 week period before levels gradually become undetectable. There appears to be no significant difference between the routes of administration (im vs sc) in biological effectiveness or pharmacokinetics.

The metabolism, distribution and excretion of leuprorelin acetate in humans have not been fully determined.

**Pharmaceutical particulars**

*List of excipients:* Gelatin. Copoly (DL-lactic acid/glycolic acid) 75:25 mol%. Mannitol.

*Incompatibilities:* None reported.

*Shelf life:* 36 months unopened.

Once reconstituted with sterile vehicle, the suspension should be administered immediately.

*Special precautions for storage:* Store at room temperature (15–25°C), in the original container. Protect from light.

*Nature and contents of container:* Vials containing 3.75 mg leuprorelin acetate as microsphere powder.

Prefilled syringes containing 1 ml of Sterile Vehicle.

*Instructions for use and handling:* None.

**Marketing authorisation numbers**
Prostap SR 0095/0218
Sterile Vehicle 0095/0220

**Date of approval/revision of SPC** June 1996

**Legal category** POM

## RHEUMOX* 600
## RHEUMOX* CAPSULES

**Presentation** *Rheumox 600:* Pale orange, film coated, capsule shaped tablets. One side scored with a breakline and the other engraved 'WYETH', containing Azapropazone Dihydrate 600 mg. This product also contains sunset yellow (E110) and quinoline yellow (E104).

*Rheumox Capsules:* Two-tone orange size 1 capsule, monogrammed 'WYETH Rheumox' containing Azapropazone Dihydrate 300 mg. This product also contains sunset yellow (E110) and erythrosine lake (E127).

**Uses** Rheumox is a non-steroidal anti-inflammatory analgesic agent indicated in the treatment of rheumatoid arthritis, ankylosing spondylitis and attacks of acute gouty arthritis in patients for whom other therapy has been ineffective.

Rheumox should be used in suitable low-risk patients (see *Contra-indications, warnings, etc*).

**Dosage and administration**
*Route of administration:* Oral.

The lowest effective dose of Rheumox should be used for the shortest duration.

Dosage recommendations for Rheumox are lower for patients older than 60 years and for patients of any age who have reduced renal function. Rheumox is contraindicated in severe renal insufficiency. If any abnormality is suspected, renal function should be investigated before commencing treatment with Rheumox.

*Rheumatoid arthritis and ankylosing spondylitis:*
*Adults under 60 years with adequate renal function:*
Rheumox 600 Tablets: One 600 mg tablet night and morning.

Rheumox 300 mg Capsules: One 300 mg capsule four times daily or two 300 mg capsules night and morning.

*Adults over 60 years:*
Rheumox 300 mg capsules: One 300 mg capsule twice daily.

*Adults of any age with reduced renal function:* Please follow dosage instructions for adults over 60 years, given above.

*Acute gout:*
*Adults under 60 years with adequate renal function:* 1800 mg per day in divided doses until the acute symptoms subside, normally by the fourth day, after which 1200 mg per day in divided doses is taken until symptoms have resolved. If symptoms persist then appropriate alternative therapy for chronic gout should be considered. In treating acute gout, it is good

practice to ensure that the patient increases their fluid intake.

*Adults over 60 years:* Rheumox is not recommended in acute gout in patients with a creatinine clearance of less than 60 ml per minute.

1800 mg in divided doses during the first 24 hours followed by 1200 mg per day in divided doses. A maximum maintenance dose of 600 mg per day in divided doses should be achieved as early as possible, preferably by the fourth day. Treatment with Rheumox should only be continued until the acute symptoms resolve. If symptoms persist then appropriate alternative therapy for chronic gout should be considered. In treating acute gout, it is good practice to ensure that the patient increases their fluid intake.

*Adults of any age with reduced renal function:* Please follow dosage instructions for adults over 60 years, given above.

*Children:* Not recommended.

**Contra-indications, warnings etc**

*Contra-indications:*

1. Use in patients with a history or evidence of peptic ulceration or ulcerative colitis.
2. Use in patients with severe renal insufficiency.
3. Rheumox should not be given to patients known to be hypersensitive to this drug or to other non-steroidal anti-inflammatory drugs (NSAIDs).
4. Use in patients with a history or evidence of blood dyscrasia.
5. Use in patients with severe hepatic insufficiency.
6. Rheumox significantly potentiates the action of warfarin in many patients and must not be used with this or other oral anticoagulants.
7. Rheumox increases the plasma concentration of phenytoin and should not be given to patients taking this drug.
8. Rheumox should not be given to patients taking methotrexate.
9. Rheumox, as with other Non-Steroidal Anti-Inflammatory Drugs (NSAIDs) should not be used in patients suffering from porphyria.

*Precautions and warnings:*

1. Rheumox should only be considered for use in rheumatoid arthritis, ankylosing spondylitis and attacks of acute gouty arthritis in patients for whom other therapy has been ineffective.
2. Azapropazone should not be used in patients who are at a high risk of developing serious adverse events known to be associated with NSAID therapy, for example, patients who are suffering from gastro-intestinal, severe renal or heart disease, or who are taking diuretics. This would include elderly patients and particularly those who already have or are suspected to have any of these conditions. In addition, patients who are on long-term therapy or multiple therapies should be carefully evaluated before treatment with Rheumox is initiated.
3. Serious gastrointestinal adverse effects such as bleeding, ulceration and perforation can occur at any time with or without warning symptoms in patients treated with Rheumox. Although this applies to all patients, elderly or debilitated patients are less able to tolerate serious ulceration or bleeding events. If any sign of gastrointestinal bleeding occurs, Rheumox should be stopped immediately.
4. Azapropazone is excreted unchanged mainly by the kidney and should therefore be used with caution in older patients and in adults with any reduced renal function. NSAIDs in general inhibit renal prostaglandin synthesis and in patients with reduced renal function this action may result in overt renal decompensation. In such cases, the reduced dosage recommendations for the treatment of adults over 60 years should be followed. If any abnormality is suspected, renal function should be fully investigated before commencing therapy with Rheumox. See also *Contra-indications.*
5. A large number of photosensitivity reactions have been reported in association with Rheumox. Patients taking azapropazone should be advised to avoid direct exposure to sunlight or to use sunblock preparations.
6. Rheumox can cause fluid retention. It should therefore be used with caution in patients with fluid retention, hypertension or heart failure.
7. If abnormal liver function tests occur, persist or worsen, or if clinical signs and symptoms indicate the development of liver disease, Rheumox should be discontinued.
8. Inhibition of renal lithium clearance by Rheumox has not been reported but the possibility of this occurring should be borne in mind.
9. Rheumox may precipitate bronchospasm in patients with bronchial asthma or allergic disease.
10. The concomitant administration of corticosteroids with Rheumox may increase the risk of gastro-intestinal bleeding and ulceration.
11. Patients on long-term treatment with Rheumox should be carefully monitored and regularly reviewed. Haematological effects associated with chronic NSAID therapy should be borne in mind.

*Use in pregnancy and lactation:* Animal reproduction studies did not result in foetal abnormalities but safety in human pregnancy cannot be assumed and its use should be avoided in pregnancy whenever possible. Azapropazone is excreted in small quantities in breast milk and should not therefore be used in breast feeding women.

*Interactions:*

1. Consult the section 'Contraindications' with phenytoin, warfarin and methotrexate.
2. Since azapropazone is highly protein bound, it may possibly displace other protein bound drugs. It may therefore interfere with the blood sugar lowering effect of oral hypoglycaemic agents. Concurrent use of these drugs is not recommended.
3. Concomitant use with azapropazone of lithium or digoxin may cause an increase in serum levels of these compounds. Concomitant use of cimetidine may cause an increase in azapropazone and decrease in cimetidine plasma levels respectively.

*Side-effects:* See also *Contra-indications, warnings, etc.*

1. Serious gastrointestinal events including bleeding, gastric and duodenal ulceration, perforation and haemorrhage have been reported. Epidemiological studies show that these reactions occur more frequently than for other NSAIDs. In addition diarrhoea, dyspepsia, nausea, vomiting, melaena, and stomatitis have also been reported.
2. Blood disorders including thrombocytopenia, pancytopenia, neutropenia and leucopenia have been reported. Anaemia and haemolytic anaemia have also been reported and some patients may develop a positive direct Coombs test without haemolytic anaemia. Rheumox should be discontinued in the presence of haemolytic anaemia or a positive direct Coombs test.
3. NSAIDs have been reported to cause nephrotoxicity in various forms and their use can lead to interstitial nephritis, nephrotic syndrome and renal failure. Renal impairment and renal failure have been reported in association with Rheumox.
4. Oedema and angioneurotic oedema.
5. Occasional central nervous system effects including dizziness, headache, and fatigue.
6. Skin rashes including a high frequency of photosensitivity reactions.
7. Allergic alveolitis, pulmonary fibrosis and fibrosing alveolitis has been reported rarely and if this occurs Rheumox should be discontinued. Many NSAIDs may precipitate bronchospasm in patients with bronchial asthma or allergic disease, and this has been reported in association with Rheumox.
8. Hepatic side-effects including jaundice and hepatitis have been reported rarely.

*Treatment of overdosage:* If overdosage should occur, two specific courses of action are suggested on theoretical grounds. Since Rheumox is poorly soluble in gastric juice, stomach lavage should recover any gastric residue of the drug, provided of course that it is done early enough. Since Rheumox is predominantly excreted by the kidney, forced alkaline diuresis is theoretically indicated.

In addition to the above mentioned treatment, patients should be managed with symptomatic and supportive care.

**Pharmaceutical precautions** Protect from light.

**Legal category** POM

**Package quantities**

Rheumox 600 Tablets: Amber glass bottles of 100 tablets.

Rheumox Capsules: Amber glass bottles of 100 capsules.

**Further information** Nil

**Product licence numbers**

Rheumox 600 Tablets 0100/0059

Rheumox Capsules 0100/0037

## TAZOCIN*

**Presentation** Vials containing a white to off-white sterile, lyophilised powder of piperacillin and tazobactam as the sodium salts. The product contains no excipients or preservatives.

*2.25 g Tazocin:* Each vial contains sterile piperacillin sodium equivalent to 2 grams piperacillin and sterile tazobactam sodium equivalent to 250 milligrams tazobactam. Each 2.25 g vial contains 4.69 mEq (108.0 mg) sodium.

*4.5 g Tazocin:* Each vial contains sterile piperacillin sodium equivalent to 4 grams piperacillin and sterile tazobactam sodium equivalent to 500 milligrams tazobactam. Each 4.5 g vial contains 9.37 mEq (216.0 mg) sodium.

**Uses** Piperacillin, a broad spectrum, semi-synthetic penicillin active against many gram-positive and gram-negative aerobic and anaerobic bacteria, exe bactericidal activity by inhibition of both septum a cell wall synthesis. Tazobactam, a triazolylmet penicillanic acid sulphone, is a potent inhibitor many β-lactamases, in particular the plasmid me ated enzymes which commonly cause resistance penicillins and cephalosporins including the thi generation cephalosporins. The presence of tazob tam in the piperacillin/tazobactam formulation hances and extends the antibiotic spectrum piperacillin to include many β-lactamase produc bacteria normally resistant to it and other β-lact antibiotics. Thus, piperacillin/tazobactam combi the properties of a broad-spectrum antibiotic and a lactamase inhibitor.

Piperacillin/tazobactam is highly active against peracillin-sensitive micro-organisms as well as ma β-lactamase producing, piperacillin-resistant mic organisms.

*Gram-negative bacteria:* most plasmid mediatec lactamase producing and non-β-lactamase produc strains of *Escherichia coli, Klebsiella* spp. (includ *K. oxytoca, K. pneumoniae*), *Proteus* spp. (includ *Proteus vulgaris , Proteus mirabilis*), *Salmonella* s *Shigella* spp., *Neisseria gonorrhoeae, Neisseria m ingitidis, Moraxella* spp. (including *M. catarrha Haemophilus* spp. *(including H. influenzae, H. pa fluenzae), Pasteurella multocida, Yersinia* spp., *Ca pylobacter* spp., *Gardnerella vaginalis.* Ma chromosomally mediated β-lactamase producing a non-β-lactamase producing strains of *Enterobac* spp. (including *E. cloacae, E. aerogenes*), *Citrobac* spp (including *C. freundii, C. diversus*), *Providen* spp., *Morganella morganii, Serratia* spp. (including *marcescens, S. liquifaciens*), *Pseudomonas aeru nosa* and other *Pseudomonas* spp. (including *cepacia, P. fluorescens*), *Xanthamonas maltoph Acinetobacter* spp.

*Gram-positive bacteria:* β-lactamase producing a non-β-lactamase producing strains of streptococci *pneumoniae, S. pyogenes, S. bovis, S. agalact S. viridans,* Group C, Group G), enterococci *(E. calis)* , *Staphylococcus aureus* (not methicillin-re tant *S. aureus*), *S. saprophyticus, S. epiderm* (coagulase-negative staphylococci), corynebacte *Listeria monocytogenes.*

*Anaerobic bacteria:* β-lactamase producing a non-β-lactamase producing anaerobes such as *B teroides* spp. (including *B. bivius, B. disiens, capillosus, B. melaninogenicus, B. oralis*), the *Bac oides fragilis* group (including *B. fragilis, B. vulga B. distasonis, B. ovatus, B. thetaiotaomicron, uniformis, B. asaccharolyticus*), as well as *Peptostr tococcus* spp., *Fusobacterium* spp., *Eubacteri* group, *Clostridia* spp. (including *C. difficile, C. perf gens*), *Veillonella* spp., and *Actinomyces* spp.

*Indications:* Piperacillin/tazobactam is indicated the treatment of the following systemic and/or lo bacterial infections in which susceptible organis have been detected or are suspected:

Lower respiratory tract infections; urinary tr infections (complicated and uncomplicated); in abdominal infections; skin and skin structure in tions; bacterial septicaemia; polymicrobic infectio

Polymicrobic Infections: Piperacillin/tazobacta indicated for polymicrobic infections including th where aerobic and anaerobic organisms are s pected (intra-abdominal, skin and skin structure, lov respiratory tract).

While piperacillin/tazobactam is indicated only the conditions listed above, infections caused piperacillin susceptible organisms are also amena to piperacillin/tazobactam treatment due to its pip acillin content. Therefore, the treatment of mi infections caused by piperacillin susceptible org isms and β-lactamase producing organisms susce ble to piperacillin/tazobactam should not require addition of another antibiotic.

Piperacillin/tazobactam is particularly useful in treatment of mixed infections and in presump therapy prior to the availability of the results sensitivity tests because of its broad-spectrum activity.

Piperacillin/tazobactam acts synergistically v aminoglycosides against certain strains of *Pseu monas aeruginosa.* Combined therapy has b successful, especially in patients with impaired h defences. Both drugs should be used in full therape doses. As soon as results of culture and susceptib test become available, antimicrobial therapy sho be adjusted.

**Dosage and administration**

*Dosage:*

*Adults and children over 12 years:* The usual dos for adults and children over 12 years with nor renal function is 4.5 g piperacillin/tazobactam gi every eight hours.

The total daily dose depends on the severity localisation of the infection and can vary from 2.2 to 4.5 g piperacillin/tazobactam administered ev six or eight hours.

*ildren under the age of 12 years:* Until further perience is available, piperacillin/tazobactam ould not be used in children under the age of 12 ars.

*derly:* Piperacillin/tazobactam may be used at the me dose levels as adults except in cases of renal pairment (see below).

*nal insufficiency:* In patients with renal insuffi- ncy, the intravenous dose should be adjusted to e degree of actual renal function impairment.

The suggested daily doses are as follows:

ravenous dosage schedule for adults with impaired nal function:

| eatinine earance l/min) | Recommended Piperacillin/Tazobactam Dosage |
|---|---|
| -80 | 12 g/1.5 g/day Divided Doses 4 g/500 mg q8H |
| 20 | 8 g/1 g/day Divided Doses 4 g/500 mg 12H |

r patients on haemodialysis, the maximum daily se is 8 g/1 g piperacillin/tazobactam. In addition, cause haemodialysis removes 30%–50% of pipera- lin in 4 hours, one additional dose of 2 g/250 mg peracillin/tazobactam should be administered fol- wing each dialysis period. For patients with renal lure and hepatic insufficiency, measurement of rum levels of piperacillin/tazobactam will provide ditional guidance for adjusting dosage.

*ration of therapy:* In acute infections, treatment th piperacillin/tazobactam should be continued for ty-eight hours beyond resolution of clinical symp- ms or the fever.

*lministration:* Piperacillin/tazobactam may be given slow intravenous injection (3–5 minutes) or by usion (20–30 minutes).

*constitution directions:*

*ravenous injection:* Each vial of 2.25 g Tazocin ould be reconstituted with 10 ml of one of the lowing diluents. Each vial of 4.5 g Tazocin should reconstituted with 20 ml of one of the following uents. Shake gently until dissolved. The total IV ection should be given over 3–5 minutes.

*luents for reconstitution:* Sterile Water for Injection; dium Chloride Injection; Bacteriostatic Water for ection.

*ravenous infusion:* Each vial of 2.25 g Tazocin ould be reconstituted with 10 ml of one of the onstitution diluents. Each vial of 4.5 g Tazocin ould be reconstituted with 20 ml of one of the constitution diluents. The reconstituted solution ould be further diluted to at least 50 ml with one of reconstitution diluents, or with Dextrose 5% in ater or Dextrose 5% and 0.9% Sodium Chloride.

**ntra-indications, warnings, etc**

*ntra-indications:* The use of piperacillin/tazobactam contra-indicated in patients with a history of allergic actions to any of the penicillins and/or cephalospo- s or β-lactamase inhibitors.

*arnings:* Serious and occasionally fatal anaphylactic actions have been reported in patients receiving erapy with penicillins. These reactions are more apt occur in persons with a history of sensitivity to ultiple allergens. There have been reports of patients th a history of penicillin hypersensitivity who have perienced severe hypersensitivity reactions when ated with a cephalosporin. Before initiating therapy th piperacillin/tazobactam, careful inquiry should made concerning previous hypersensitivity reac- ns to penicillins, cephalosporins, and other aller- ns. If an allergic reaction occurs during therapy with peracillin/tazobactam, the antibiotic should be dis- ntinued. Serious hypersensitivity reactions may quire adrenaline and other emergency measures.

*ecautions:* While piperacillin/tazobactam possesses characteristic low toxicity of the penicillin group antibiotics, periodic assessment of organ system nctions including renal, hepatic, and haematopoietic ring prolonged therapy is advisable.

Bleeding manifestations have occurred in some tients receiving β-lactam antibiotics. These reac- ns have sometimes been associated with abnor- alities of coagulation tests such as clotting time, telet aggregation and prothrombin time and are ore likely to occur in patients with renal failure. If eding manifestations occur as a result of antibiotic erapy, the antibiotic should be discontinued and propriate therapy instituted.

n case of severe, persistent diarrhoea, the possibil- of antibiotic-induced pseudomembranous colitis st be taken into consideration.

As with other antibiotics, the possibility of emergence of resistant organisms which might cause superinfections should be kept in mind, particularly during prolonged treatment. If this occurs, appropriate measures should be taken.

As with other penicillins, patients may experience neuromuscular excitability or convulsions if higher than recommended doses are given intravenously.

Periodic electrolyte determinations should be made in patients with low potassium reserves, and the possibility of hypokalaemia should be kept in mind with patients who have potentially low potassium reserves and who are receiving cytotoxic therapy or diuretics. Modest elevation of indices of liver function may be observed.

Antimicrobials used in high doses for short periods to treat gonorrhoea may mask or delay the symptoms of incubating syphilis. Therefore, prior to treatment, patients with gonorrhoea should also be evaluated for syphilis. Specimens for darkfield examination should be obtained from patients with any suspected primary lesion, and serologic tests should be made for a minimum of 4 months.

*Interactions with other drugs:* Concurrent administration of probenecid and piperacillin/tazobactam produced a longer half life and lower renal clearance for both piperacillin and tazobactam, however, peak plasma concentrations of either drug are unaffected. No interaction is found between piperacillin/tazobactam and either vancomycin or tobramycin.

Whenever piperacillin/tazobactam is used concurrently with another antibiotic, especially an aminoglycoside, the drugs must not be mixed in intravenous solutions or administered concurrently due to physical incompatibility.

During simultaneous administration of high doses of heparin, oral anticoagulants and other drugs which may affect the blood coagulation system and/or the thrombocyte function, the coagulation parameters should be tested more frequently and monitored regularly.

The ureidopenicillins including piperacillin have been reported to prolong the action of vecuronium. Caution is indicated when piperacillin is used perioperatively with vecuronium and similar neuromuscular blocking agents.

Penicillins may reduce the excretion of methotrexate. Serum levels of methotrexate should be monitored in patients on high dose methotrexate therapy.

*Use during pregnancy and lactation:* Adequate studies on the use of piperacillin/tazobactam during pregnancy and the period of breast feeding are not yet available. Piperacillin/tazobactam did not affect fertility in rats and was not teratogenic in mice or rats. Until further experience is available, however, pregnant or nursing women should be treated only if the therapeutic benefit outweighs the risk to the patient and the foetus.

*Side-effects:* Rarely, significant leucopenia may be associated with prolonged therapy. Very rarely, interstitial nephritis may occur.

Hepatitis and cholestatic jaundice have been reported rarely with some penicillins and β-lactamase inhibitors.

Many of the patients treated in clinical trials were severely ill and had multiple underlying diseases and physiological impairments, making it difficult to determine causal relationship of adverse experiences to therapy with piperacillin/tazobactam.

Adverse local reactions that were reported as possibly, probably or definitely related to therapy with piperacillin/tazobactam therapy were phlebitis (0.2%) and thrombophlebitis (0.3%).

The most frequently reported systemic adverse clinical reactions that were reported as possibly, probably, or definitely related to piperacillin/tazobactam were diarrhoea (3.8%), rash (0.6%), erythema (0.5%), pruritus (0.5%), vomiting (0.4%), allergic reactions (0.4%), nausea (0.3%), urticaria (0.2%) and superinfection (0.2%).

Additional adverse systemic clinical reactions reported as possibly, probably or definitely drug related occurring in less than 0.1% of the patients were: skin reactions, eruption, increased sweating, erythema multiforme, eczema, exanthema, maculo-papular rash, soft/loose stools, stomatitis, constipation, muscular weakness, hallucination, dry mouth, hypotension, muscle pain, superficial phlebitis, fever, hot flushes, oedema, tiredness. Local reactions included injection site inflammation and injection site pain when solution was not prepared according to recommendations (see Dosage and administration).

Adverse laboratory changes without regard to drug relationship that were reported during clinical trials were: transient reduction in the white blood cell count (leukopenia), eosinophilia, thrombocytosis, thrombocytopaenia, positive Coombs test, hypokalaemia, transient rise in the serum levels of liver enzymes (SGOT, SGPT, alkaline phosphatase), bilirubin. Rarely, increased levels of renal function parameters (urea, creatinine) have been detected in serum.

*Overdosage:* No specific antidote is known.

There is no specific experience with overdose of Tazocin however in the event of an emergency, all required intensive medical measures are indicated as in the case of piperacillin. Excessive serum levels of Piperacillin may be reduced by dialysis. However, daily doses of 24 g piperacillin and above have been administered in man without observation of adverse effects.

In case of motor excitability or convulsions, anticonvulsive agents (e.g. diazepam or barbiturates) may be indicated.

In case of severe, anaphylactic reactions, the usual counter measures are to be initiated.

**Pharmaceutical precautions** *Lyophilized powder:* Vials containing sterile piperacillin/tazobactam lyophilized powder may be stored at controlled room temperature (15–25°C) for up to 3 years.

*Solutions:* When reconstituted as directed, solutions are stable for 24 hours when stored under refrigeration (2–8°C).

Tazocin should be administered through an infusion set separately from any other drugs unless compatibility is proven.

Diluted solutions are stable for 24 hours when stored under refrigeration (2–8°C) in IV. bags or syringes. Unused solution should be discarded.

Piperacillin/tazobactam should not be mixed with other drugs in a syringe or infusion bottle since compatibility has not been established. Whenever piperacillin/tazobactam is used concurrently with another antibiotic, the drugs must be administered separately.

Because of chemical instability, piperacillin/tazobactam should not be used with solutions containing only sodium bicarbonate.

Piperacillin/tazobactam should not be added to blood products or albumin hydrolysates.

**Legal category** POM

**Package quantities** Vials containing 2.25 g Tazocin, boxed singly.

Vials containing 4.5 g Tazocin, boxed singly.

Tazocin 4.5 g Infusion Packs containing a 4.5 g infusion bottle, a 50 ml bottle of Water for Injection BP and a transfer needle.

**Product licence numbers**
2.25 g 0095/0252
4.5 g 0095/0254

## THIOTEPA INJECTION

**Qualitative and quantitative composition** Thiotepa 15 mg

**Pharmaceutical form** Sterile powder for injection

**Clinical particulars**

*Therapeutic indications:* Thiotepa (N,N',N'' triethylenethiophosphoramide) is a polyfunctional alkylating agent used alone or in combination with other cytotoxic drugs, or in surgery in the treatment of neoplastic diseases. It is believed to exert its cytotoxic effects by the alkylation of DNA.

*Posology and method of administration:* Thiotepa (15 mg) should be reconstituted with 1.5 ml Water for Injection immediately prior to use. Reconstituted solutions should be clear to slightly opaque. Solutions that are grossly opaque or precipitated should be discarded.

Thiotepa may be given by intravenous, intramuscular and intrathecal routes of injection; it may be given directly into pleural, pericardial or peritoneal cavities and as a bladder instillation.

Use Luer-Lock fittings on all syringes and sets. Large bore needles are recommended to minimise pressure and possible formation of aerosols. The latter may also be reduced by the use of a venting needle.

*For intramuscular injection, bladder and intracavitary instillations:*

*Dosage: Adults and the elderly:* Up to 60 mg in single or divided doses. Doses should be reduced in cases of leucopenia as indicated in Table 1. Single dose administration of 90 mg Thiotepa as a bladder instillation is described under 'Bladder Cancer'.

Table 1

| *WBC Count Cells/mm³* | *Dose of Thiotepa Adults and Children over 12 years* |
|---|---|
| 6000 | 60 mg |
| 5000–6000 | 45 mg |
| 4500–5000 | 30 mg |
| 4000–4500 | 20 mg |
| 3500–4000 | 10 mg |
| 3000–3500 | 5 mg |
| below 3000 | omit dose |

*Children:* Use in children is not recommended.

*Intrathecal injection:* Up to a maximum of 10 mg.

It is essential that a complete blood count should be performed 12–24 hours before each dose of Thiotepa. Thrombocytopenia in the absence of leucopenia has been noted.

Dosage schedules of Thiotepa vary widely according to the route of administration and the indication.

Examples of dosage schedules used according to specific tumour types are given below:

*Breast cancer:* Patients with advanced breast cancer have been treated with Thiotepa as part of a combination regime, given intramuscularly in divided doses of 15–30 mg three times weekly for two weeks; this representing one course of treatment. An interval of six to eight weeks is recommended between courses to allow bone marrow recovery.

An alternative schedule employs Thiotepa as part of a combination regime, given as an initial priming dose of 15 mg intramuscularly or intravenously each day for four days. This may be followed in three weeks by maintenance doses of 15 mg I.M. every 14–21 days.

*Bladder cancer:* Instillations of Thiotepa have been used to treat multiple superficial tumours of the bladder, resulting in a complete clinical response in about one third of patients. Patients are dehydrated for 8–12 hours prior to treatment. Up to 60 mg Thiotepa dissolved in 60 ml sterile water is instilled into the bladder by catheter once a week for four weeks. During removal of the catheter following instillation, Thiotepa injection is continued to ensure bathing of the prostatic and pendulous urethra . The solution should be retained for up to two hours and the patient should be frequently repositioned to ensure maximum contact with the urothelium.

Patients are generally cytoscoped two weeks after a course of four instillations. If a response is observed a second course of four Thiotepa instillations may be given, generally at a reduced dosage, eg. 15–60 mg with intervals of one to two weeks between instillations.

Instillations of Thiotepa have been used prophylactically as an adjunct to surgical resection of superficial tumours of the bladder, resulting in a marked decrease in the recurrence rate. It is recommended that there should be a minimum interval of one week between tumour resection and the commencement of prophylactic instillation of Thiotepa. 30–60 mg Thiotepa dissolved in 60 ml sterile water is instilled into the bladder for two hours and repeated at intervals of one to two weeks for a total of 4–8 instillations. This initial course may be followed by instillations of Thiotepa, 30–60 mg every four to six weeks for one year or longer.

Single dose Thiotepa instillations have been used prophylactically as an adjunct of surgical resection in the treatment of superficial tumours of the bladder. 90 mg Thiotepa dissolved in 100 mg sterile water is instilled into the bladder with the patient in the left lateral position. After 15 minutes the patient is transferred to the right lateral postion and after a further 15 minutes the bladder is emptied. It is felt that such single dose administration may decrease the incidence of systemic toxicity by decreasing the extent of systemic absorption of the drug.

*Note:* Patients who have had previous radiotherapy to the bladder are at increased risk of drug toxicity.

*Malignant meningeal disease:* Intrathecal injections of Thiotepa have been found to be useful for the palliative treatment of cases of meningeal infiltration by leukaemia and lymphoma. Clinical experience has shown Thiotepa to be effective in carcinomatous involvement of the meninges, but published data is limited. Thiotepa, at a concentration of 1 mg/ml in sterile water is administered by injection through a lumbar theca in doses of up to 10 mg on alternate days until there is clearance of malignant cells from the cerebrospinal fluid (CSF). It is recommended that if no improvement occurs in the CSF after three courses of treatment, that treatment should be changed. Not more than four injections should be given on alternative days. Routine blood counts should be performed prior to each dose of Thiotepa.

*Ovarian cancer:* Ovarian cancer has been treated with Thiotepa as a single agent or as part of a combination regime in a variety of schedules. For example, 15 mg Thiotepa IV or IM may be given daily for four days initially and then continued with single doses administered at weekly or two weekly intervals.

*Intracavitary instillation of Thiotepa:* Instillations of Thiotepa have been used to treat malignant pleural effusions and abdominal ascites. The procedure recommended, is first to aspirate as much fluid as possible and then to instil the dose of Thiotepa, 10–60 mg in 20–60 ml sterile water. This may be repeated at weekly or two weekly intervals.

*Prevention of recurrences of Pterygium:* A 1:2,000 solution of Thiotepa in sterile Ringer's solution (ie 15 mg powder in 30 ml Ringer's), applied topically as eye drops, at three hourly intervals daily for up to six weeks after surgical removal of the pterygium, is effective in reducing the recurrence rate following surgery.

*Condyloma acuminata:* Thiotepa applied topically or instilled intraurethrally in a gel, has been successfully used to eradicate condyloma acuminata. The drug may be administered by first reconstituting 60 mg Thiotepa with 5 ml sterile water. This is diluted to 15 ml, using a sterile mixture of water and lubricating jelly made to a consistency viscous enough to remain in the urethra and fluid enough to allow easy injection. This therapy may be repeated at weekly intervals.

*Contra-indications:* Thiotepa administration is contra-indicated in patients with a WBC count below 3,000 and/or platelet count below 100,000.

*Special warnings and precautions:* Thiotepa must be stored in a refrigerator (2–8°C). The occurence of a precipitate on reconstitution (with 1.5 ml of Water for Injection) indicates that polymerisation has occured with the formation of less active constituents and the injection must be discarded.

Reconstituted solutions may be stored in a refrigerator (2–8°C) for 24 hours. However, if a precipitate forms, the solution must be discarded.

Thiotepa may be mixed in the same syringe with Procaine Hydrochloride 2% or with adrenaline 1 in 1,000 or with both.

Trained personnel should reconstitute Thiotepa in a designated area. Adequate protective gloves and goggles should be worn and the work surface should be covered with plastic-backed absorbent paper. Thiotepa is not a vesicant and should not cause harm if it comes in contact with the skin. It should, of course be washed off with water immediately. Any transient stinging may be treated with bland cream. The cytotoxic preparation should not be handled by pregnant staff.

Any spillage or waste material may be disposed of by incineration. We do not make any specific recommendations with regard to the temperature of the incinerator.

Thiotepa has been reported to possess mutagenic activity on the basis of bacterial, plant and mammalian mutagenicity tests. It has also been reported to be carcinogenic in mice and rats. These effects are consistent with its activity as an alkylating agent. The carcinogenic potential in humans has not been clearly established.

Thiotepa should only be used by clinicians who are familiar with the various characteristics of cytotoxic drugs and their clinical toxicity. WBC and platelet counts are recommended 12–24 hours before each dose of Thiotepa regardless of route of administration, except when used topically as eye drops or in the treatment of condyloma acuminata. Dosage should be reduced as indicated above, in the presence of a compromised bone marrow, as manifested by a reduced WBC count or platelet count. Safe use in children has not been established.

*Interaction with other medicaments and other forms of interaction:* See dosage schedules for special tumour types, for usage with concomitant surgery or radiotherapy.

*Pregnancy and lactation:* Thiotepa is teratogenic and embryotoxic in mice and rats following intraperitoneal administration. In addition, it has been reported to interfere with spermatogenesis and ovarian function in rodent species. The drug therefore, should not normally be administered to patients who are pregnant or to mothers who are breast feeding unless the benefit outweighs the risk to the foetus or child.

*Effects on ability to drive and use machines:* None.

*Undesirable effects:* The most serious side-effect is upon the blood forming elements and is a direct consequence of the cytotoxic effect of the drug. In addition, Thiotepa may occasionally cause vomiting, headache and anorexia. Alopecia has been reported as a rare complication of therapy with Thiotepa. Local irritation comparable to a mild radiation cystitis, may follow bladder instillations of Thiotepa, while haemorrhagic cystitis is rare. Depigmentation of periorbital skin has been reported rarely following the use of Thiotepa eye drops.

*Overdose:* There is no specific antidote. Gastric lavage, forced fluids and general supportive measures are recommended. Blood counts should be carried out to estimate damage to the haematopoietic system and blood transfusions should be given as required.

**Pharmacological properties**

*Pharmacodynamic properties:* Thiotepa is an ethyleneimine compound whose antineoplastic effect is related to its alkylating action. It is not a vesicant and may be given by all parenteral routes, as well as directly into tumour masses.

*Pharmacokinetic properties:* Variable absorption occurs from intramuscular injection sites. Absorption through serous membranes such as the bladder and pleura occurs to some extent. Only traces of changed thiotepa and triethylene phosphoramide excreted in the urine, together with a large proport of metabolites.

*Preclinical Safety Data:* Nothing of relevance to prescriber.

**Pharmaceutical particulars**

*List of excipients:* Water for Injection.

*Incompatabilities:* None

*Shelf life:* 18 months

*Special precautions for storage:* Thiotepa must stored in a refrigerator (2–8°C). Reconstituted solutic may be stored in a refrigerator (2–8°C) for up to hours.

*Nature and contents of container:* Flint glass vial w butyl rubber stopper. Pack size: 15 mg

*Instructions for use/handling:* See *Special warni and precautions.*

**Marketing authorisation number** 0095/0234

**Date of approval/revision of SPC** 26 July 1996

**Legal category** POM

## TRAXAM* FOAM

**Presentation** Aerosol canister which dispenses white 'quick break' type foam containing 3.17% w felbinac upon actuation. The propellant used in ca is a non-chlorofluorocarbon, Butane 40 (5% w/w).

**Uses** Traxam Foam is a topical anti-inflammatory a analgesic. It is indicated for the relief of sympto associated with soft tissue injuries such as sprai strains and contusions.

**Dosage and administration** The foam should dispensed onto the hand and rubbed lightly into affected area(s). Traxam Foam is formulated to bre down into a clear liquid when warmed by contact w the skin.

Gently rub a golf-ball sized quantity of foam (1 inches or 4 cm in diameter) into the affected area( to 4 times a day.

The total daily dose should not exceed 25 g of fo irrespective of the number of affected areas; a g ball size aliquot of foam weighs approximately 1 g

If symptoms do not resolve within 14 days, i advisable to review the patient to assess whet continued treatment is appropriate.

*Elderly:* No special dosage recommendations made for elderly patients.

*Children:* Safe use of felbinac in early childhood not been established.

Hands should be washed following application Traxam Foam unless they are the treatment site.

**Contra-indications, warnings, etc**

*Contra-indications:* Hypersensitivity to the ingre ents. Patients in whom attacks of asthma, urticaria acute rhinitis are precipitated by aspirin or other n steroidal anti-inflammatory agents.

*Warnings:* Use of Traxam Foam should be limitec intact and non-diseased skin. Contact with muc membranes and the eyes should be avoided. Patie should avoid actuation of the aerosol can near th face or eyes. Traxam Foam should not be applied w occlusive dressings or simultaneously to the sa site as other topical preparations.

*Pregnancy and lactation:* As the safety of felbinac human pregnancy and lactation has not been est lished, its use in these circumstances is not recc mended.

As with other non-steroidal anti-inflammat agents which inhibit prostaglandin synthesis, dysto and delayed parturition were observed when felbi was administered subcutaneously in animal studie

*Interactions:* Felbinac is highly protein bound. Ho ever, serum levels following topical application Traxam Foam are extremely low therefore clini drug interactions are unlikely.

*Side effects:* A low incidence of mild local irritati erythema, dermatitis, pruritus and paraesthe which recovers spontaneously upon cessation treatment, may be expected with Traxam Foa Systemic side-effects are rare; gastro-intestinal dis bances and hypersensitivity reactions such as wi spread rashes including urticaria and bronchospa have been reported with felbinac.

*Overdosage:* It is unlikely that Traxam Foam wo cause adverse systemic effects even if accide ingestion should occur. Patients should consu doctor if ingestion is suspected.

**Pharmaceutical precautions** Traxam Foam is pac in a pressurised canister. Protect the canister fr sunlight and do not expose to temperatures ab 50°C. Extremes of temperature can occur in mo 's. Do not pierce or burn the canister even when ɪpty. Do not refrigerate. Do not spray or use near y ignition source (eg. naked flame, open fire) or ile smoking.

Traxam Foam should be stored below 25°C.

**gal category** POM

**ckage quantities** Aerosol canister dispensing 100 g Traxam Foam.

**oduct licence number** 0095/0238

## RAXAM* GEL

**esentation** Clear, non-greasy, non staining gel ntaining 30 mg felbinac in each gram.

**es** Traxam Gel is a topical anti-inflammatory and algesic. It is indicated for the relief of symptoms sociated with soft tissue injuries such as sprains, ains and contusions.

**sage and administration** Rub 1 g of Traxam Gel pproximately 1 inch (2.5cm)) lightly into the affected ea 2 to 4 times a day. If symptoms do not resolve thin 14 days, the patient should be reviewed to sess whether continued treatment is appropriate.

The total dose should not exceed 25 g per day gardless of the number of affected areas.

*derly:* No special dosage recommendations are ade for elderly patients.

*ildren:* Safe use of felbinac in early childhood has t been established.

Hands should be washed following application of axam Gel unless they are the treatment site.

**ntra-indications, warnings, etc**

*ntra-indications:* Hypersensitivity to the ingredi-ts. Patients in whom attacks of asthma, urticaria or ute rhinitis are precipitated by aspirin or other non-eroidal anti-inflammatory agents.

*arnings:* Use of Traxam Gel should be limited to act and non-diseased skin. Contact with mucous embranes and the eyes should be avoided. Traxam l should not be applied with occlusive dressings or nultaneously to the same site as other topical eparations.

*egnancy and lactation:* As the safety of felbinac in man pregnancy and lactation has not been estab-hed, its use in these circumstances is not recom-ended.

As with other non-steroidal anti-inflammatory ents which inhibit prostaglandin synthesis, dystocia d delayed parturition were observed when felbinac s administered subcutaneously in animal studies.

*eractions:* Felbinac is highly protein bound. How-er, serum levels following topical application of axam Gel are extremely low therefore clinical drug eractions are unlikely.

*de effects:* The overall incidence of side effects orted with Traxam Gel is low (less than 2%). Local ects such as mild local erythema, irritation, derma-s, pruritis, and paraesthesia, which recover spon-eously on cessation of treatment, are the most mmon reactions. Systemic side-effects are rare; stro-intestinal disturbances and hypersensitivity ctions, such as widespread rashes including urti-ia and bronchospasm, have been reported with binac.

*erdosage:* It is unlikely that Traxam Gel would use adverse systemic effects even if accidental estion should occur. Patients should consult a ctor if ingestion is suspected.

**armaceutical precautions** Replace the tube cap er use. Dilution is not recommended.

Store below 25°C.

**gal category** POM

**ckage quantities** Tubes containing 100 g of gel

**oduct licence number** 0095/0119

## RI-MINULET*

**esentation** The memo pack holds six beige tablets ntaining 30 micrograms ethinyloestradiol and micrograms gestodene, five dark brown tablets ntaining 40 micrograms ethinyloestradiol and micrograms gestodene, and ten white tablets ntaining 30 micrograms ethinyloestradiol and 0 micrograms gestodene.

All tablets have a lustrous, sugar-coating.

**es** Oral contraception and the recognised gynae-logical indications for such oestrogen-progestogen mbinations. The mode of action includes the inhi-ion of ovulation by suppression of the mid-cycle rge of luteinising hormone, the inspissation of vical mucus so as to constitute a barrier to sperm, and the rendering of the endometrium unreceptive to implantation.

**Dosage and administration**

*First treatment cycle:* 1 tablet daily for 21 days, starting with the tablet marked number 1, on the first day of the menstrual cycle.

Additional contraception (barriers and spermicide) is not required.

*Subsequent cycles:* Each subsequent course is started when seven tablet-free days have followed the preceding course. A withdrawal bleed should occur during the 7 tablet-free days.

*Changing from another 21 day combined oral contraceptive:* The first tablet of Tri-Minulet should be taken on the first day immediately after the end of the previous oral contraceptive course. Additional contraception is not required. A withdrawal bleed should not be expected until the end of the first pack of Tri-Minulet.

*Changing from an Every Day (ED) 28 day combined oral contraceptive:* The first tablet of Tri-Minulet should be taken on the day immediately after the day on which the last active pill in the ED pack has been taken. The remaining tablets in the ED pack should be discarded. Additional contraception is not required. A withdrawal bleed should not be expected until the end of the first pack of Tri-Minulet.

*Changing from a Progestogen-only-Pill (POP):* The first tablet of Tri-Minulet should be taken on the first day of menstruation even if the POP for that day has already been taken. The remaining tablets in the POP pack should be discarded. Additional contraception is not required.

*Post-partum and post-abortum use:* After pregnancy combined oral contraception can be started in non-lactating women 21 days after a vaginal delivery, provided that the patient is fully ambulant and there are no puerperal complications.

If the pill is started later than 21 days after delivery, then alternative contraception (barriers and spermicides) should be used until oral contraception is started and for the first 7 days of pill-taking. If unprotected intercourse has taken place after 21 days post partum, then oral contraception should not be started until the first menstrual bleed after childbirth.

After a miscarriage or abortion oral contraception may be started immediately.

*Special circumstances requiring additional contraception:*

*Missed pills:* If a tablet is delayed it should be taken as soon as possible and if it is taken within 12 hours of the correct time, additional contraception is not needed. Further tablets should then be taken at the usual time. If the delay exceeds 12 hours, the last missed pill should be taken when remembered, the earlier missed pills left in the pack and normal pill-taking resumed. If one or more tablets are omitted from the 21 days of pill-taking, additional contraception (barriers and spermicides) should be used for the next 7 days of pill-taking. In addition, if one or more pills are missed during the last 7 days of pill-taking, the subsequent pill-free interval should be disregarded and the next pack started the day after taking the last tablet from the previous pack. In this case, a withdrawal bleed should not be expected until the end of the second pack. If the patient does not have a withdrawal bleed at the end of the second pack she must return to her doctor to exclude the possibility of pregnancy.

*Gastro-intestinal upset:* Vomiting or diarrhoea may reduce the efficacy by preventing full absorption. Additional contraception (barriers and spermicides) should be used during the stomach upset and for the 7 days following the upset. If these 7 days overrun the end of a pack, the next pack should be started without a break. In this case, a withdrawal bleed should not be expected until the end of the second pack. If the patient does not have a withdrawal bleed at the end of the second pack she must return to her doctor to exclude the possibility of pregnancy.

Mild laxatives do not impair contraceptive action.

*Interaction with other drugs:* Some drugs accelerate the metabolism of oral contraceptives when taken concurrently and these include barbiturates, phenytoin, phenylbutazone and rifampicin. Other drugs suspected of having the capacity to reduce the efficacy of oral contraceptives include ampicillin and other antibiotics. It is, therefore, advisable to use non-hormonal methods of contraception (barriers and spermicides) in addition to the oral contraceptive as long as an extremely high degree of protection is required during treatment with such drugs. The additional contraception should be used while the concurrent medication continues and for 7 days afterwards. If these extra precautions overrun the end of the pack, the next pack should be started without a break. In this case, a withdrawal bleed should not be expected until the end of the second pack. If the patient does not have a withdrawal bleed at the end of the second pack she must return to her doctor to exclude the possibility of pregnancy.

**Contra-indications, warnings, etc**

*Contra-indications:*

1. Suspected pregnancy.
2. Thrombotic disorders and a history of these conditions, sickle-cell anaemia, disorders of lipid metabolism and other conditions in which, in individual cases, there is known or suspected to be a much increased risk of thrombosis.
3. Acute or severe chronic liver diseases. Dubin-Johnson syndrome. Rotor syndrome. History, during pregnancy, of idiopathic jaundice or severe pruritus.
4. History of herpes gestationis.
5. Mammary or endometrial carcinoma, or a history of these conditions.
6. Abnormal vaginal bleeding of unknown cause.
7. Deterioration of otosclerosis during pregnancy.

*Warnings:*

1. There is a general opinion, based on statistical evidence, that users of combined oral contraceptives experience, more often than non-users, venous thromboembolism, arterial thrombosis, including cerebral and myocardial infarction, and subarachnoid haemorrhage. Full recovery from such disorders does not always occur, and it should be realised that in a few cases they are fatal. How often these disorders occur in users of the modern low-dose pills is not known, but there are reasons for suggesting that they may occur less often than with older pills containing more oestrogen. Certain factors may entail some risk of thrombosis, e.g. smoking, obesity, varicose veins, cardiovascular diseases, diabetes and migraine. The suitability of a combined oral contraceptive should be judged according to the severity of such conditions in the individual case, and should be discussed with the patient before she decides to take it.
2. The risk of arterial thrombosis associated with combined oral contraceptives increases with age, and this risk is aggravated by cigarette smoking. The use of combined oral contraceptives by women in the older age group, especially those who are cigarette smokers, should therefore be discouraged and alternative methods used.
3. The possibility cannot be ruled out that certain chronic diseases may occasionally deteriorate during the use of combined oral contraceptives (see *Precautions*).
4. The combination of ethinyloestradiol and gestodene, like other contraceptive steroids, is associated with an increased incidence of neoplastic nodules in the rat liver, the relevance of which to man is unknown.
5. Malignant liver tumours have been reported on rare occasions in long-term users of oral contraceptives. Benign hepatic tumours have also been associated with oral contraceptive usage. A hepatic tumour should be considered in the differential diagnosis when upper abdominal pain, enlarged liver or signs of intra-abdominal haemorrhage occur.
6. Numerous epidemiological studies have been reported on the risks of ovarian, endometrial, cervical and breast cancer in women using combined oral contraceptives. The evidence is clear that combined oral contraceptives offer substantial protection against both ovarian and endometrial cancer.

An increased risk of cervical cancer in long term users of combined oral contraceptives has been reported in some studies, but there continues to be controversy about the extent to which this is attributable to the confounding effects of sexual behaviour and other factors.

The evidence linking combined oral contraceptive use and breast cancer remains inconclusive. The results of some studies suggest an increased risk of breast cancer presenting below the age of about 35, the risk rising with duration of use. Any possible increased risk of breast cancer with combined oral contraceptives is however likely to be small and may be expected to be less with low dosage pills. This possible risk should be weighed against the many benefits of combined oral contraceptives, including their protective effects against ovarian and endometrial cancers.

*Reasons for stopping oral contraception immediately:*

1. Occurrence of migraine in patients who have never previously suffered from it. Exacerbation of pre-existing migraine. Any unusually frequent or unusually severe headaches.
2. Any kind of acute disturbance of vision.
3. Suspicion of thrombosis or infarction.
4. Six weeks before elective operations and during immobilisation, e.g. after accidents, etc.
5. Significant rise in blood-pressure.
6. Jaundice.
7. Clear exacerbation of conditions known to be capable of deteriorating during oral contraception or pregnancy.
8. Pregnancy is a reason for stopping immediately

because it has been suggested by some investigations that oral contraceptives taken in early pregnancy may slightly increase the risk of foetal malformations. Other investigations have failed to support these findings. The possibility therefore cannot be excluded, but it is certain that if a risk exists at all, it is very small.

*Precautions:*
1. Examination of the pelvic organs, breasts and blood-pressure should precede the prescribing of any combined oral contraceptive and should be repeated regularly.
2. Before starting treatment, pregnancy must be excluded.
3. The following conditions require careful observation during medication: a history of severe depressive states, varicose veins, diabetes, hypertension, epilepsy, otosclerosis, multiple sclerosis, porphyria, tetany, disturbed liver function, gall-stones, cardiovascular diseases, renal diseases, chloasma, uterine fibroids, asthma, the wearing of contact lenses, or any disease that is prone to worsen during pregnancy. The first appearance or deterioration of any of these conditions may indicate that the oral contraceptive should be stopped.
4. The risk of the deterioration of chloasma, which is often not fully reversible, is reduced by the avoidance of excessive exposure to sunlight.

*Side-effects:* Occasional side-effects may include nausea, vomiting, headaches, breast tenderness, changed body weight or libido, depressive moods and chloasma.

*Menstrual changes:*
1. *Reduction of menstrual flow:* This is not abnormal and it is to be expected in some patients. Indeed, it may be beneficial where heavy periods were previously experienced.
2. *Missed menstruation:* Occasionally, withdrawal bleeding may not occur at all. If the tablets have been taken correctly, pregnancy is very unlikely, but should be ruled out before a new course of tablets is started.

*Intermenstrual bleeding:* Very light 'spotting' or heavier 'breakthrough bleeding' may occur during tablet-taking, especially in the first few cycles. It appears to be generally of no significance, except where it indicates errors of tablet-taking, or where the possibility of interaction with other drugs exists (q.v.). However, if irregular bleeding is persistent, an organic cause should be considered.

*Effect on adrenal and thyroid glands:* Oral contraceptives have no significant influence on adrenocortical function. The ACTH function test for the adrenal cortex remains unchanged. The reduction in corticosteroid excretion and the elevation of plasma corticosteroids are due to an increased cortisol-binding capacity of the plasma proteins.

The response to metyrapone is less pronounced than in untreated women and is thus similar to that during pregnancy.

The radio-iodine uptake shows that thyroid function is unchanged. There is a rise in serum protein-bound iodine, similar to that in pregnancy and during the administration of oestrogens. This is due to the increased capacity of the plasma proteins for binding thyroid hormones, rather than to any change in glandular function. In women taking oral contraceptives, the content of protein-bound iodine in blood serum should therefore, not be used for evaluation of thyroid function.

*Effect on blood chemistry:* Oral contraceptives may accelerate erythrocyte sedimentation in the absence of any disease. This effect is due to a change in the proportion of the plasma protein fractions. Increases in plasma copper, iron and alkaline phosphatase have also been recorded.

*Overdosage:* There have been no reports of serious ill-effects from overdosage, even when a considerable number of tablets have been taken by a small child. In general, it is, therefore, unnecessary to treat overdosage. However, if overdosage is discovered within two or three hours and is so large that treatment seems desirable, gastric lavage can be safely used.

There are no specific antidotes and further treatment should be symptomatic.

**Pharmaceutical precautions** Store in cool, dry conditions. Shelf-life five years

**Legal category** POM

**Package quantities** Individual packs containing 3 months' supply.

**Further information** NIL

**Product licence number** 0011/0140

# TRINORDIOL*

**Presentation** The memo pack holds six light brown tablets, containing 50 micrograms Levonorgestrel BP and 30 micrograms Ethinyloestradiol PhEur, five white tablets containing 75 micrograms Levonorgestrel BP and 40 micrograms Ethinyloestradiol PhEur and ten ochre tablets containing 125 micrograms Levonorgestrel BP and 30 micrograms Ethinyloestradiol PhEur.

All tablets are round 5.6 mm in diameter with a lustrous sugar coating.

**Uses** Oral contraception

**Dosage and administration**
*First treatment cycle:* 1 tablet daily for 21 days, starting with the tablet marked number 1, on the first day of the menstrual cycle.

Additional contraception (barriers and spermicide) is not required.

*Subsequent cycles:* Each subsequent course is started when seven tablet-free days have followed the preceding course. A withdrawal bleed should occur during the 7 tablet-free days.

*Changing from another 21 day combined oral contraceptive:* The first tablet of Trinordiol should be taken on the first day immediately after the end of the previous oral contraceptive course. Additional contraception is not required. A withdrawal bleed should not be expected until the end of the first pack of Trinordiol.

*Changing from an Every Day (ED) 28 day combined oral contraceptive:* The first tablet of Trinordiol should be taken on the day immediately after the day on which the last active pill in the ED pack has been taken. The remaining tablets in the ED pack should be discarded. Additional contraception is not required. A withdrawal bleed should not be expected until the end of the first pack of Trinordiol.

*Changing from a Progestogen-only-Pill (POP):* The first tablet of Trinordiol should be taken on the first day of menstruation even if the POP for that day has already been taken. The remaining tablets in the POP pack should be discarded. Additional contraception is not required.

*Post-partum and post-abortum use:* After pregnancy combined oral contraception can be started in non-lactating women 21 days after a vaginal delivery, provided that the patient is fully ambulant and there are no puerperal complications.

If the pill is started later than 21 days after delivery, then alternative contraception (barriers and spermicides) should be used until oral contraception is started and for the first 7 days of pill-taking. If unprotected intercourse has taken place after 21 days post partum, then oral contraception should not be started until the first menstrual bleed after childbirth.

After a miscarriage or abortion oral contraception may be started immediately.

*Special circumstances requiring additional contraception:*
*Missed pills:* If a tablet is delayed it should be taken as soon as possible and if it is taken within 12 hours of the correct time, additional contraception is not needed. Further tablets should then be taken at the usual time. If the delay exceeds 12 hours, the last missed pill should be taken when remembered, the earlier missed pills left in the pack and normal pill-taking resumed. If one or more tablets are omitted from the 21 days of pill-taking, additional contraception (barriers and spermicides) should be used for the next 7 days of pill-taking. In addition, if one or more pills are missed during the last 7 days of pill-taking, the subsequent pill-free interval should be disregarded and the next pack started the day after taking the last tablet from the previous pack. In this case, a withdrawal bleed should not be expected until the end of the second pack. If the patient does not have a withdrawal bleed at the end of the second pack she must return to her doctor to exclude the possibility of pregnancy.

*Gastro-intestinal upset:* Vomiting or diarrhoea may reduce the efficacy by preventing full absorption. Additional contraception (barriers and spermicides) should be used during the stomach upset and for the 7 days following the upset. If these 7 days overrun the end of a pack, the next pack should be started without a break. In this case, a withdrawal bleed should not be expected until the end of the second pack. If the patient does not have a withdrawal bleed at the end of the second pack she must return to her doctor to exclude the possibility of pregnancy.

Mild laxatives do not impair contraceptive action.

*Interaction with other drugs:* Some drugs accelerate the metabolism of oral contraceptives when taken concurrently and these include barbiturates, phenytoin, phenylbutazone and rifampicin. Other drugs suspected of having the capacity to reduce the efficacy of oral contraceptives include ampicillin and other antibiotics. It is, therefore, advisable to use non-hormonal methods of contraception (barriers and spermicides) in addition to the oral contraceptive as long as an extremely high degree of protection is required during treatment with such drugs. The additional contraception should be used while concurrent medication continues and for 7 da afterwards. If these extra precautions overrun the e of the pack, the next pack should be started witho break. In this case, a withdrawal bleed should not expected until the end of the second pack. If patient does not have a withdrawal bleed at the e of the second pack she must return to her docto exclude the possibility of pregnancy.

**Contra-indications, warnings, etc**
*Contra-indications:*
1. Suspected pregnancy.
2. Thrombotic disorders and a history of th conditions, sickle-cell anaemia, disorders of li metabolism and other conditions in which, in indiv ual cases, there is known or suspected to be a mc increased risk of thrombosis.
3. Acute or severe chronic liver diseases. bin-Johnson syndrome. Rotor syndrome. Histc during pregnancy, of idiopathic jaundice or sev pruritus.
4. History of herpes gestationis.
5. Mammary or endometrial carcinoma, or a hist of these conditions.
6. Abnormal vaginal bleeding of unknown cause
7. Deterioration of otosclerosis during pregnanc

*Warnings:*
1. There is a general opinion, based on statisti evidence, that users of combined oral contracepti experience, more often than non-users, vene thromboembolism, arterial thrombosis, including c ebral and myocardial infarction, and subarachnc haemorrhage. Full recovery from such disorders dc not always occur, and it should be realised that i few cases they are fatal. How often these disord occur in users of the low-dose pills is not known, there are reasons for suggesting that they may oc less often than with older pills containing m oestrogen. Certain factors may entail some risk thrombosis, e.g. smoking, obesity, varicose vei cardiovascular diseases, diabetes and migraine. suitability of a combined oral contraceptive should judged according to the severity of such condition the individual case, and should be discussed with patient before she decides to take it.
2. The risk of arterial thrombosis associated v combined oral contraceptives increases with age, a this risk is aggravated by cigarette smoking. The of combined oral contraceptives by women in older age group, especially those who are cigare smokers, should therefore be discouraged and alt native methods used.
3. The possibility cannot be ruled out that cert chronic diseases may occasionally deteriorate dur the use of combined oral contraceptives (see *Prec tions*).
4. Malignant liver tumours have been reported rare occasions in long-term users of oral contrac tives. Benign hepatic tumours have also been asso ated with oral contraceptive usage. A hepatic tum should be considered in the differential diagnc when upper abdominal pain, enlarged liver or sig of intra-abdominal haemorrhage occur.
5. Numerous epidemiological studies have be reported on the risks of ovarian, endometrial, cervi and breast cancer in women using combined c contraceptives. The evidence is clear that combi oral contraceptives offer substantial protect against both ovarian and endometrial cancer.

An increased risk of cervical cancer in long te users of combined oral contraceptives has be reported in some studies, but there continues to controversy about the extent to which this is attrib able to the confounding effects of sexual behavi and other factors.

The evidence linking combined oral contracept use and breast cancer remains inconclusive. results of some studies suggest an increased risk breast cancer presenting below the age of about the risk rising with duration of use. Any possi increased risk of breast cancer with combined c contraceptives is however likely to be small and n be expected to be less with low dosage pills. T possible risk should be weighed against the ma benefits of combined oral contraceptives, includ their protective effects against ovarian and en metrial cancers.

*Reasons for stopping oral contraception immediat*

1. Occurrence of migraine in patients who h never previously suffered from it. Exacerbation of existing migraine. Any unusually frequent or unu ally severe headaches.
2. Any kind of acute disturbance of vision.
3. Suspicion of thrombosis or infarction.
4. Six weeks before elective operations or treatm of varicose veins by sclerotherapy and during imr bilisation, e.g. after accidents, etc.
5. Significant rise in blood-pressure.
6. Jaundice.

Clear exacerbation of conditions known to be able of deteriorating during oral contraception or gnancy.

Pregnancy is a reason for stopping immediately ause it has been suggested by some investigations oral contraceptives taken in early pregnancy may htly increase the risk of foetal malformations. er investigations have failed to support these ings. The possibility therefore cannot be excluded, it is certain that if a risk exists at all, it is very small.

*cautions:*

Examination of the pelvic organs, breasts and od-pressure should precede the prescribing of any nbined oral contraceptive and should be repeated ularly.

Before starting treatment, pregnancy must be luded.

The following conditions require careful obser- on during medication: a history of severe depres- states, varicose veins, diabetes, hypertension, epsy, otosclerosis, multiple sclerosis, porphyria, ny, disturbed liver function, gall-stones, cardio- cular diseases, renal diseases, chloasma, uterine oids, asthma, the wearing of contact lenses, or any ase that is prone to worsen during pregnancy. first appearance or deterioration of any of these ditions may indicate that the oral contraceptive uld be stopped.

The risk of the deterioration of chloasma, which often not fully reversible, is reduced by the idance of excessive exposure to sunlight.

*e-effects:* Occasional side-effects may include nau- , vomiting, headaches, breast tenderness, changed y weight or libido, depressive moods, chloasma altered serum lipid profile.

*nstrual changes:*

*Reduction of menstrual flow:* This is not abnormal it is to be expected in some patients. Indeed, it y be beneficial where heavy periods were previ- ly experienced.

*Missed menstruation:* Occasionally, withdrawal eding may not occur at all. If the tablets have been en correctly, pregnancy is very unlikely, but should ruled out before a new course of tablets is started.

*ermenstrual bleeding:* Very light 'spotting' or heav- 'breakthrough bleeding' may occur during tablet- ing, especially in the first few cycles. It appears to generally of no significance, except where it icates errors of tablet-taking, or where the possi- ty of interaction with other drugs exists (q.v.). wever, if irregular bleeding is persistent, an organic se should be considered.

*ect on adrenal and thyroid glands:* Oral contracep- s have no significant influence on adrenocortical ction. The ACTH function test for the adrenal cortex nains unchanged. The reduction in corticosteroid retion and the elevation of plasma corticosteroids due to an increased cortisol-binding capacity of plasma proteins.

he response to metyrapone is less pronounced n in untreated women and is thus similar to that ing pregnancy.

he radio-iodine uptake shows that thyroid function nchanged. There is a rise in serum protein-bound ine, similar to that in pregnancy and during the ninistration of oestrogens. This is due to the reased capacity of the plasma proteins for binding roid hormones, rather than to any change in ndular function. In women taking oral contracep- s, the content of protein-bound iodine in blood um should therefore, not be used for evaluation of roid function.

*ect on blood chemistry:* Oral contraceptives may elerate erythrocyte sedimentation in the absence any disease. This effect is due to a change in the portion of the plasma protein fractions. Increases plasma copper, iron and alkaline phosphatase have o been recorded.

*erdosage:* There have been no reports of serious effects from overdosage, even when a considerable mber of tablets have been taken by a small child. In neral, it is, therefore, unnecessary to treat overdos- e. However, if overdosage is discovered within two three hours and is so large that treatment seems sirable, gastric lavage can be safely used.

here are no specific antidotes and further treat- nt should be symptomatic.

**armaceutical precautions** Store in cool, dry con- ions. Shelf-life five years

**al category** POM

**ckage quantities** Individual packs containing nonths' supply.

**rther information** Nil.

**duct licence number** 0011/0066

## VARIDASE* TOPICAL 125,000 UNITS PER VIAL

**Qualitative and quantitative composition** Varidase Topical contains the active ingredients Streptokinase HSE 100,000 IU and Streptodornase HSE 25,000 IU.

**Pharmaceutical form** Sterile powder for topical use.

**Clinical particulars**

*Therapeutic indications:* Varidase Topical is indicated wherever removal of clotted blood, fibrinous or purulent accumulations is required.

It is indicated in the treatment of suppurative surface lesions such as ulcers, pressure sores, amputation sites, diabetic gangrene, radiation necrosis, infected wounds and surgical incisions, until the wound is thoroughly cleansed of clots, fibrinous exudates and pus.

It is also indicated in the treatment of burns and may be used prior to skin grafting.

Varidase Topical can be used to dissolve clots in the bladder or in urinary catheters.

*Posology and method of administration:*

*Adults, children and the elderly:* Directions for use in the cleansing of necrotic infected and sloughy wounds.

*Reconstitution: Single vial:* The contents should be gently mixed with 20 ml of sterile physiological saline or, if unavailable, 20 ml of Water for Injection until the powder is completely dissolved. The resulting clear solution can then be withdrawn into a syringe.

*Combi-Pack:* Insert one end of the sterile transfer needle into the diluent vial and push the Varidase vial down onto the outer end of the needle.

(Ensure that the transfer needle goes centrally through the upraised circle on the stoppers).

Invert the vials so that the Varidase vial is under the diluent vial and allow the full 20 ml of diluent to run into the Varidase vial to dissolve the powder. Remove the empty diluent vial and discard. If necessary, gently agitate the Varidase vial until the powder is completely dissolved. The resulting clear solution can then be poured from the transfer needle.

As Varidase Topical is packed under vacuum, care should be taken when inserting a needle into the vial.

Excess agitation of the vial should be avoided to prevent frothing and denaturing of the enzymes.

As Varidase Topical does not contain a preservative, multidose use is not recommended.

*Standard methods of application:* Pre-soak gauze with Varidase Topical solution then apply to the wound. Following application, a semi-occlusive dressing is necessary to prevent drying out of the wound, e.g. a polyethylene film taped on two sides. Alternatively the wound may be packed with dry gauze which is then soaked with Varidase Topical solution and dressed with a semi-occlusive dressing.

*Alternative method of application:* Where wounds are covered by a thick dry eschar it is usually necessary to cross hatch the eschar into approximately 3–5 mm squares and to a sufficient depth to allow the access of the enzymes to the underlying fibrinous purulent material.

Alternatively, Varidase Topical may be introduced under the eschar, taking care that the solution enters only the cavity beneath and that the volume is not sufficient to cause pain through increased pressure. Introducing Varidase Topical in this way often results in the eschar becoming partly detached thus facilitating its mechanical removal.

*Special technique of application:* Varidase Topical may be applied in jelly form. This can be prepared by dissolving the contents of one vial in 5 ml of sterile water and mixing the resulting solution thoroughly, but gently, with 15 ml of inert jelly, such as K-Y or carboxymethylcellulose (CMC) jelly. This method can be particularly useful in cases of burns where dressings are not employed.

*Frequency of application:* Varidase Topical treatment should be repeated once or twice a day. Care should be taken to irrigate the lesion thoroughly with physiological saline to remove loosened material prior to the next application.

*Duration of treatment:* Treatment should be continued until healthy granulations are present and re-epithelialisation has begun, usually within one to two weeks. In mixed wounds, where granulation has started in some areas, Varidase use can continue until the entire wound is clean and granulating without any harmful effects to the healthy tissues.

*Contra-indications:* Active haemorrhage. Known hypersensitivity to streptokinase and/or streptodornase.

*Special warnings and precautions for use:* Varidase Topical is intended for local use only. *It should not be used intramuscularly or intravenously.* This product contains streptokinase, which when used systemically is known to be antigenic. However, if used as recommended, there is no evidence to suggest that Varidase Topical is antigenic.

In order to avoid cross-infection, a new vial of Varidase Topical and a separate sterile syringe and needle should be used for each individual patient.

Varidase Topical has been shown to be a sensitiser when administered at relatively low intradermal doses to guinea pigs. The relevance of these findings to humans is considered important only where prolonged repetitive treatment is anticipated. Under such circumstances, the potential to induce allergic reactions may be minimised as described under *Undesirable effects.*

*Interactions with other medicaments and other forms of interaction:* The preparation is buffered to physiological pH. The enzymes of Varidase Topical can be inactivated by the concomitant use of other preparations of an acidic or alkaline pH. Aluminium reacts with Varidase Topical. If the reconstituting fluid has a high calcium content, the solution becomes opalescent, but this does not affect the potency of the enzymes.

*Pregnancy and lactation:* Safe use of Varidase Topical during pregnancy and lactation has not been established. Use in these circumstances should be avoided unless considered essential by the physician.

*Effects on the ability to drive and use machines:* None known.

*Undesirable effects:* Allergic reactions to the application of Varidase Topical are infrequent and may be minimised by careful and frequent removal of exudate followed by thorough irrigation using physiological saline prior to retreatment with Varidase Topical. Transient slight burning pain has been reported rarely after application of Varidase Topical.

*Overdose:* There is no specific antidote. Removal of the preparation by careful washing or by irrigation/suction drainage is recommended.

**Pharmacological properties**

*Pharmacodynamic properties:* Streptokinase acts indirectly upon a substrate of fibrin or fibrinogen by activating a fibrinolytic enzyme in human serum. Upon application of streptokinase in situ, the activation of this fibrinolytic system brings about rapid dissolution of blood clots and the fibrinous portion of exudates. Streptodornase liquifies the viscous nucleoprotein of dead cells or pus. Thus the action of the enzymes results in the liquefaction of the two main viscous substances resulting from inflammatory or infectious processes thereby facilitating cleansing and desloughing of wounds.

Varidase Topical has no effect on collagen, living cells or healthy tissue.

*Pharmacokinetic properties:* There are no published reports concerning the pharmacokinetics of Varidase.

**Pharmaceutical particulars**

*List of excipients:* Sodium phosphate monobasic, sodium phosphate dibasic.

*Incompatibilities:* None known.

*Shelf life:* 18 months (unopened).

1 day (reconstituted solution stored in a refrigerator at 2–8°C).

*Special precautions for storage:* The unreconstituted and reconstituted product should be stored in a refrigerator (2–8°C).

*Nature and contents of container:* 25cc borosilicate Type 1 glass vial with butyl rubber stopper and metal seal with pull tab.

The product is available in:

Boxes containing a single vial of Varidase Topical sterile powder.

Combi-packs containing 1 vial of Varidase Topical sterile powder, 1 vial of Diluent (20 ml of sterile sodium chloride 0.9% solution BP) and 1 sterile transfer needle.

*Instructions for use/handling:* Refer to section 4.2 ('Posology and method of administration').

**Marketing authorisation numbers**

| | |
|---|---|
| Varidase Topical 125,000 units per vial | 0095/5038R |
| Diluent for Varidase Topical (Combi-Pack) | 1502/0006R |

**Date of approval/revision of SPC** 15 March 1996

**Legal category** POM

## ZOTON*

**Presentation**

*Zoton Capsules 15 mg:* Opaque yellow capsules for oral administration. Each capsule contains 15 mg lansoprazole as enteric coated granules.

*Zoton Capsules 30 mg:* Two tone lilac/purple capsules

for oral administration. Each capsule contains 30 mg lansoprazole as enteric coated granules.

**Uses** Zoton is effective in the treatment of acid-related disorders of the upper gastro-intestinal tract, with the benefit of rapid symptom relief. Zoton is also effective in combination with antibiotics in the eradication of *Helicobacter pylori* (*H. pylori*).

*Indications:* Healing and long term management of gastro oesophageal reflux disease (GORD).

Healing and maintenance therapy for patients with duodenal ulcer.

Relief of reflux-like symptoms (eg. heartburn) and/or ulcer-like symptoms (eg. upper epigastric pain) associated with acid-related dyspepsia.

Healing of benign gastric ulcer.

Zoton is also effective in patients with benign peptic lesions, including reflux oesophagitis, unresponsive to H2 receptor antagonists.

Eradication of *H. pylori* from the upper gastrointestinal tract in patients with duodenal ulcer or gastritis when used in combination with appropriate antibiotics.

### Dosage and administration
*Dosage:*

*Gastro oesophageal reflux disease:* Zoton 30 mg once daily for 4 weeks. The majority of patients will be healed after the first course. For those patients not fully healed at this time, a further 4 weeks treatment at the same dosage should be given.

For long term management, a maintenance dose of Zoton 15 mg or 30 mg once daily can be used dependant upon patient response.

*Duodenal ulcer:* The recommended dose is Zoton 30 mg once daily for 4 weeks.

For prevention of relapse, the recommended maintenance dose is Zoton 15 mg once daily.

*Acid-related dyspepsia:* Zoton 15 mg or 30 mg once daily for 2–4 weeks depending on the severity and persistence of symptoms. Patients who do not respond after 4 weeks, or who relapse shortly afterwards, should be investigated.

*Benign gastric ulcer:* Zoton 30 mg once daily for 8 weeks.

*Eradication of H. pylori:* The following combinations have been shown to be effective when given for 7 days;

Zoton 30 mg twice daily plus two of the following antibiotics; clarithromycin 250 mg twice daily, amoxycillin 1 g twice daily, or metronidazole 400 mg twice daily.

The best eradication results are obtained when clarithromycin is combined with either amoxycillin or metronidazole. When used in combination with the recommended antibiotics, Zoton is associated with *H. pylori*-eradication rates of up to 90%.

Zoton should be taken once daily, except when used to eradicate *H. pylori*. To achieve the optimal acid inhibitory effect, and hence most rapid healing and symptom relief, Zoton should be administered in the morning before food.

The capsules should be swallowed whole. Do not crush or chew.

*Elderly:* Dose adjustment is not required in the elderly. The normal daily dosage should be given.

*Children:* There is no experience with Zoton in children.

*Impaired hepatic and renal function:* Lansoprazole is metabolised substantially by the liver. Clinical trials in patients with liver disease indicate that metabolism of lansoprazole is prolonged in patients with severe hepatic impairment. However, no dose adjustment is necessary; the recommended dose should not be exceeded.

There is no need to alter the dosage in patients with impaired renal function.

### Contra-indications, warnings, etc
*Contra-indications:* The use of Zoton is contra-indicated in patients with a history of hypersensitivity to any of the ingredients of Zoton capsules.

*Warnings and precautions:* In common with other anti-ulcer therapies, the possibility of malignancy should be excluded when gastric ulcer is suspected, as symptoms may be alleviated and diagnosis delayed. Similarly, the possibility of serious underlying disease such as malignancy should be excluded before treatment for dyspepsia commences, particularly in patients of middle age or older who have new or recently changed dyspeptic symptoms.

Before using Zoton with antibiotics to eradicate *H. pylori*, prescribers should refer to the full prescribing information of the respective antibiotics for guidance.

Zoton is not known to affect ability to drive or operate machines.

*Use in pregnancy and lactation:* There is insufficient experience to recommend the use of Zoton in pregnancy. Animal studies do not reveal any teratogenic effect. Reproduction studies indicate slightly reduced litter survival and weights in rats and rabbits given very high doses of lansoprazole. The use of Zoton in pregnancy should be avoided.

Animal studies indicate that lansoprazole is secreted in breast milk. There is no information on the secretion of lansoprazole into breast milk in humans. The use of Zoton during breast feeding should be avoided unless considered essential.

*Side effects:* Zoton is well-tolerated, with adverse events generally being mild and transient.

The most commonly reported adverse events are headache, dizziness, fatigue and malaise.

Gastrointestinal effects include diarrhoea, constipation, abdominal pain, dyspepsia, nausea, vomiting, flatulence and dry or sore mouth or throat.

Alterations in liver function test values and, rarely, jaundice or hepatitis, have been reported.

Dermatological reactions include skin rashes, urticaria and pruritus. These generally resolve on discontinuation of drug therapy.

Other hypersensitivity reactions include angioedema, wheezing, and very rarely, anaphylaxis. A few cases of interstitial nephritis have been reported in association with proton pump inhibitors.

Haematological effects (thrombocytopenia, eosinophilia and leucopenia) have occurred rarely. Bruising, purpura and petechiae have also been reported.

Other reactions include arthralgia, myalgia, depression, peripheral oedema and, rarely, paraesthesia or blurred vision.

*Interactions:* Lansoprazole is hepatically metabolised and studies indicate that it is a weak inducer of Cytochrome P450. There is the possibility of interaction with drugs which are metabolised by the liver. Caution should be exercised when oral contraceptives and preparations such as phenytoin, theophylline, or warfarin are taken concomitantly with the administration of Zoton.

No clinically significant effects on NSAIDs or diazepam have been found.

Antacids and sucralfate may reduce the bioavailability of lansoprazole and should, therefore, not taken within an hour of Zoton.

*Animal toxicology:* Gastric tumours have been served in life-long studies in rats.

An increased incidence of spontaneous ret atrophy has been observed in life-long studies in r These lesions which are common to albino laborat rats have not been observed in monkeys or dog life-long studies in mice. They are considered to rat specific. No such treatment related changes h been observed in patients treated continuously long periods.

*Overdosage:* There is no information on the effec overdosage. However, Zoton has been given at do up to 120 mg/day without significant adverse effe Symptomatic and supportive therapy should be gi as appropriate.

**Pharmaceutical precautions** Zoton Capsules sho be stored at room temperature (15–25°C) in a place.

**Legal category** POM

### Package quantities
Zoton Capsules 30 mg: Blister packs of 56, 28, 1 7 capsules.

Zoton Capsules 15 mg: Blister packs of 56 or capsules.

**Further information** Lansoprazole is a member class of drugs called proton pump inhibitors. Its m of action is to inhibit specifically the H⁺ / K⁺ ATP (proton pump) of the parietal cell in the stomach, terminal step in acid production, thus reducing gas acidity, a key requirement for healing of acid-rela disorders such as gastric ulcer, duodenal ulcer reflux oesophagitis. A single dose of 30 mg inhi pentagastrin-stimulated acid secretion by appr mately 80%, indicating effective acid inhibition fr the first day of dosing.

Lansoprazole exhibits high (80–90%) bioavailab with a single dose. As a result, effective acid inhibi is achieved rapidly. Peak plasma levels occur wit 1.5 to 2.0 hours. The plasma elimination half-ranges from 1 to 2 hours following single or mult doses in healthy subjects. The plasma protein bind is 97%.

Lansoprazole has a prolonged pharmacolog action providing effective acid suppression over hours, thereby promoting rapid healing and sympt relief.

*Helicobacter pylori* is the cause of the vast majo of cases of non-immune gastritis, and is implicated the cause of a very high proportion of gastric duodenal ulcers. There is evidence that *H. pylori* m also be associated with gastric carcinoma.

By reducing gastric acidity, Zoton creates an e ronment in which appropriate antibiotics can effective against *H. pylori*. *In vitro* studies have sho that lansoprazole has a direct antimicrobial effect *H. pylori*.

The eradication of *H. pylori* results in the cure high proportion of patients with peptic ulcer disea thus reducing the need for long term anti-secret therapy, and preventing complications such as gast intestinal haemorrhage.

**Marketing authorisation numbers**
Zoton Capsules 15 mg 0095/0302
Zoton Capsules 30 mg 0095/0264

*Trade Mark

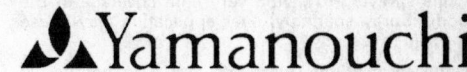
## CILLIN* INJECTION

**alitative and quantitative composition** Procaine icillin PhEur 300 mg (300,000 units) and Benzyl-icillin Sodium PhEur 60 mg (100,000 units) per ml on constitution.

**armaceutical form** Powder for constitution.

**ical particulars**
*erapeutic indications:* For the treatment of infec-ns due to penicillin sensitive organisms.

*osology and method of administration:*
*ults and the elderly:* Usually 1 ml 24 hourly or 12 urly, or as directed by the physician.
*ildren:* Over 25 kg – as for adults. Under 25 kg – portionally to body weight.
*acute uncomplicated gonorrhoea:* Up to 12 ml as a gle dose, or as directed by the physician.
*early syphilis:* 3 ml (4 ml in heavier patients) daily 10 days, or as directed by the physician.
*ntra-indications:* Hypersensitivity to penicillin or caine.
*ecial warnings and precautions for use:* None.
*eraction with other medicaments and other forms interaction:* Probenecid delays the excretion of icillin.
*egnancy and lactation:* The safety of Bicillin Injection hese circumstances has not been established.
*ects on ability to drive and use machines:* None own.
*desirable effects:* Skin reactions may occur but ually resolve on cessation of therapy. Generalised, stemic reactions are rare and usually associated h a history of allergy or penicillin intolerance.
*erdose:* General supportive measures.

**armacological properties**
*armacodynamic properties:* The penicillin constit-nts of Bicillin are bactericidal, inhibiting the struc-al cross linkages in the bacterial cell wall. Whilst the sodium penicillin component offers an mediate but short acting effect, the procaine peni-in component provides a depot effect, often pro-cing therapeutic blood levels for 24 hours following ection.
*armacokinetic properties:* After an intramuscular se of 300,000 units of procaine penicillin, a peak um concentration of benzylpenicillin of about units/ml is attained in 1 to 3 hours falling to unit/ml at 6 hours; serum concentrations are lower n those achieved after an equivalent dose of nzylpenicillin.
*eclinical safety data:* There is no relevant preclinical fety data.

**armaceutical particulars**
*t of excipients:* Polysorbate 80 NF, Sodium Citrate hydrous) USP, Citric Acid PhEur.
*compatibilities:* None known.
*elf life:* 5 years.
*ecial precautions for storage:* Not more than 15°C en unconstituted. Upon constitution the prepara-n is for single-dose use only. It may be kept at 2°C–C for up to 24 hours after constitution but must be carded after the first usage or at the end of that riod of 24 hours.
*ture and contents of container:* Glass multi-dose ection vial, with rubber stopper and aluminium al. Each vial contains 1.8 g (1,800,000 units Procaine nicillin PhEur and 360 mg (600,000 units) Benzyl-nicillin Sodium PhEur and on constitution provides ml of an injection containing in each ml 300 mg 0,000 units) Procaine Penicillin PhEur and 60 mg 0,000 units) Benzylpenicillin Sodium PhEur.
*structions for use/handling:* For constitution, add ml water for injections to each vial, to produce nl injection, equivalent to Fortified Procaine Penicil-Injection BP.

**arketing authorisation number** 0166/0147.

**te of approval/revision of SPC** October 1995.

**gal category** POM.

## CONOTRANE*

**Presentation** A white cream containing 0.1% w/w benzalkonium chloride and 22% w/w Dimethicone 350 BP.

**Uses** *Action:* Conotrane combines the water repel-lent properties of dimethicone with the antiseptic activity of benzalkonium chloride.
*Indications:* Conotrane is used for protection of the skin from moisture, irritants, chafing and contamina-tion with bacteria or yeasts; as in the prevention and treatment of napkin rash, in the prevention of pressure sores, and in the management of incontinence.

**Dosage and administration** The cream should be applied to the affected area several times a day as necessary or after every napkin change.

**Contra-indications, warnings, etc**
*Contra-indications:* Known hypersensitivity to benzal-konium chloride.
*Side-effects:* Local hypersensitivity to benzalkonium chloride is rare.

**Pharmaceutical precautions** Store in a cool place.

**Legal category** GSL.

**Package quantities** 100 g tube; 500 g jar.

**Further information** Nil.

**Product licence number** 0015/0113.

*Product licence holder:* Boehringer Ingelheim Limited, Bracknell, Berkshire

## DE-NOL*

**Presentation** De-Nol is presented as a clear red liquid containing 120 mg tri-potassium di-citrato bis-muthate (calculated as $Bi_2O_3$) in each 5 ml. The inactive ingredients in De-Nol include ethanol and sucrose.

**Uses** Ulcer healing agent. For the treatment of gastric and duodenal ulcers.

**Dosage and administration** By oral administration. Each dose is to be diluted with 15 ml of water.
*Adults and the elderly:* Two 5 ml spoonsful twice daily (half an hour before breakfast and half an hour before the evening meal). Alternatively, one 5 ml spoonful four times a day (half an hour before each of the three main meals of the day and two hours after the evening meal). The treatment course should be taken for the full 28-day period and it is important that a dose is not missed. If necessary, one further course of therapy may be given. Maintenance therapy with De-Nol is not indicated, but treatment may be repeated after an interval of one month.
*Children:* Not recommended.
   Milk should not be drunk by itself during the course of treatment as this can prevent the medicine from working properly. Small quantities of milk on breakfast cereal or in tea or coffee taken with meals are permissible. Antacids should not be taken for half an hour before or half an hour after taking a dose of De-Nol as these can interfere with the action of the drug.

**Contra-indications, warnings, etc**
*Contra-indications:* De-Nol should not be adminis-tered to patients with renal disorders, and on theoret-ical grounds is contra-indicated in pregnancy.
*Interactions:* De-Nol may inhibit the efficacy of orally administered tetracyclines.
*Side effects:* Blackening of the stool usually occurs; darkening of the tongue, nausea and vomiting have been reported.
*Overdosage:* Extremely few cases of overdosage have occurred; contact the company for further informa-tion.

**Pharmaceutical precautions** Normal pharmaceutical storage and handling are indicated.

**Legal category** P.

**Package quantities** Treatment pack of 560 ml as an original pack (OP).

**Further information** Some patients with an associ-ated gastritis may experience an initial discomfort whilst taking De-Nol. Each 5 ml dose contains ca 100 mg ethanol and 500 mg sucrose.

**Product licence number** 0166/5024.

## DE-NOLTAB*

**Qualitative and quantitative composition** Tri-potas-sium di-citrato bismuthate HSE 120 mg (as $Bi_2O_3$).

**Pharmaceutical form** Tablet.

**Clinical particulars**
*Therapeutic indications:* For the treatment of gastric and duodenal ulcers.
*Posology and method of administration:*
*For adults and the elderly:* One tablet to be taken four times a day, half an hour before each of the three main meals and two hours after the last meal of the day, or two tablets to be taken twice daily, half an hour before breakfast and half an hour before the evening meal, or as directed by the physician.
   The maximum duration for one course of treatment is two months; De-Noltab should not be used for maintenance therapy.
*For children:* Not recommended.
*Contra-indications:* In cases of severe renal insuffici-ency.
*Special warnings and precautions for use:* None stated.
*Interactions with other medicaments and other forms of interaction:* The efficacy of oral tetracyclines may be inhibited.
*Pregnancy and lactation:* On theoretical grounds De-Noltab is contraindicated in pregnancy. No informa-tion is available on excretion in breast milk.
*Effects on ability to drive and use machines:* None reported.
*Undesirable effects:* Blackening of the stool usually occurs; nausea and vomiting have been reported.
*Overdose:* Extremely few cases of overdosage have been reported; contact the company for further information.

**Pharmacological properties**
*Pharmacodynamic properties:* The active constituent exerts a local healing effect at the ulcer site, and by eradication or reduction of *Helicobacter pylori* defers relapse.
*Pharmacokinetic properties:* The action is local in the gastro-intestinal tract.
*Preclinical safety data:* No relevant pre-clinical safety data has been generated.

**Pharmaceutical particulars**
*List of excipients:* potassium citrate, ammonium citrate, povidone K 30, amberlite IRP-S8, polyethylene glycol 6000, magnesium stearate, maize starch, hypro-mellose.
*Incompatibilities:* None.
*Shelf life:* Four years.
*Special precautions for storage:* None.
*Nature and contents of container:* Amber glass bottles and/or aluminium foil strips, containing 112 tablets.
*Instructions for use/handling:* None.

**Marketing authorisation number** 0166/0124.

**Date of approval/revision of SPC** 20 January 1997.

**Legal category** P.

## DERMAMIST*

**Presentation** A pressurised aerosol delivering White Soft Paraffin BP 10% as a clear colourless spray. Dermamist also contains Liquid Paraffin BP and Fractionated Coconut Oil BP, with butane/isobutane/propane as propellant.

**Uses** Dermamist is indicated for the treatment of dry skin conditions including pruritus of the elderly, eczema and ichthyosis by topical application.

**Dosage and administration**
*For adults, children and the elderly:* Shake before use. Bathe or shower for not more than ten minutes. Pat

dry and apply spray without delay. Do not spray on face. Spray from a distance of approximately 8 inches. Spray away from the face and move the can quickly while spraying to give a very light coverage of the body. Spray sparingly; over application may cause the skin to feel oily.

**Contra-indications, warnings, etc** Do not use if sensitive to any of the ingredients. For external use only. Keep out of reach of children. Do not spray on face. Use in a ventilated area. Avoid inhalation. Guard against slipping. Do not apply to broken skin. Discontinue use if the condition is made worse. Do not spray on a naked flame or incandescent material.

**Pharmaceutical precautions** Store below 25°C. Highly flammable; pressurised container. Protect from sunlight. Do not puncture, burn or expose to temperature over 50°C (122°F) even when empty.

**Legal category** P.

**Package quantities** 250 ml canister.

**Further information** Nil.

**Product licence number** 13147/0001

*Product licence holder:* Caraderm Ltd, Pine Valley, Rostrevor, Co. Down, Northern Ireland BT34 3DE.

# DISIPAL* TABLETS

**Presentation** Disipal Tablets are presented as yellow sugar-coated tablets each containing 50 mg Orphenadrine Hydrochloride BP, imprinted 'Disipal'. Disipal Tablets comply with the monograph for Orphenadrine Hydrochloride Tablets BP. The inactive ingredients in Disipal Tablets include lactose, sucrose, amaranth, tartrazine and sunset yellow.

**Uses** Anticholinergic, for the treatment of all forms of Parkinsonism, including drug-induced (neuroleptic syndrome).

**Dosage and administration** *By oral administration: Adults and the elderly:* Initially 150 mg daily in divided doses, increasing by 50 mg every two or three days until maximum benefit is obtained. Optimal dosage is usually 250–300 mg daily in divided doses in idiopathic and post-encephalitic Parkinsonism, 100–150 mg daily in divided doses in arteriosclerotic Parkinsonism, and 150–300 mg daily in divided doses in the neuroleptic syndrome. Maximal dosage, 400 mg daily in divided doses. The elderly may be more susceptible to side-effects at doses which are clinically optimal.

*Children:* A dosage for children has not been established.

**Contra-indications, warnings, etc**
*Contra-indications:* Contra-indicated in patients with tardive dyskinesia, glaucoma or prostatic hypertrophy.

*Special precautions:* Use with caution in patients with micturition difficulties or in pregnancy, and in the presence of cardiovascular disease and hepatic or renal impairment. Avoid abrupt discontinuation of treatment. For some patients orphenadrine may be a drug of abuse.

*Side-effects:* Occasionally dry mouth, disturbances of visual accommodation, gastro-intestinal disturbances, dizziness and micturition difficulties may occur; these usually disappear spontaneously or may be controlled by a slight reduction in dosage. Less commonly, tachycardia, hypersensitivity, nervousness, euphoria and insomnia may be seen.

*Overdosage:* Toxic effects are anticholinergic in nature and the treatment is gastric lavage, cholinergics such as carbachol, anticholinesterases such as physostigmine and general non-specific treatment.

**Pharmaceutical precautions** Normal pharmaceutical storage and handling are indicated.

**Legal category** POM.

**Package quantities** 250×50 mg, 1,000×50 mg.

**Further information** Although very rarely reported, there may be provocation of dextropropoxyphene side-effects when that drug is administered concurrently with orphenadrine. Patients on Disipal may show spuriously elevated values for the $T_3$ test using a Sephadex method, but these are not indicative of hyperthyroidism. Each tablet contains ca 60 mg sucrose.

**Product licence number** 0166/5001

# FLOMAX MR*

**Qualitative and quantitative composition** Each capsule contains as active ingredient tamsulosin hydrochloride 400 microgram, equivalent to 367 microgram tamsulosin.

**Pharmaceutical form** Capsule, modified release.

**Clinical particulars**
*Therapeutic indications:* Treatment of functional symptoms of benign prostatic hyperplasia (BPH).

*Posology and method of administration:* One capsule daily, to be taken after breakfast.

The capsule should be swallowed whole with a drink of water (about 150 ml) in the standing or sitting position.

The capsules should not be crunched or chewed, as this will interfere with the modified release of the active ingredient.

*Contra-indications:* Hypersensitivity to tamsulosin hydrochloride or any other component of the product; severe hepatic insufficiency.

*Special warnings and precautions for use:* Rarely, transient postural symptoms have occurred during orthostatic provocation testing after the first dose.

Use in patients with micturition syncope is not advised.

*Interactions with other medicaments and other forms of interaction:* Concurrent administration of other $\alpha_1$-adrenoceptor antagonists could lead to hypotensive effects.

No interactions have been seen when Flomax MR was given concomitantly with either atenolol, enalapril or nifedipine. Concomitant cimetidine brings about a rise and frusemide a fall in plasma levels of tamsulosin, but as levels remain within the normal range posology need not be changed.

No interactions at the level of hepatic metabolism have been seen during in vitro studies with liver microsomal fractions (representative of the cytochrome $P_{450}$-linked drug metabolising enzyme system), involving amitriptyline, salbutamol, glibenclamide and finasteride. Diclofenac and warfarin, however, may increase the elimination rate of tamsulosin.

*Pregnancy and lactation:* Not applicable as Flomax MR is intended for male patients only.

*Effects on ability to drive and use machines:* No data is available on whether Flomax MR adversely affects the ability to drive or operate machines. However, in this repect, patients should be aware of the fact that dizziness can occur.

*Undesirable effects:* The following adverse reactions have been reported during the use of Flomax MR: dizziness, abnormal ejaculation and, less frequently headache, asthenia, postural hypotension and palpitations.

*Overdose:* No cases of acute overdosage have been reported. However, acute hypotension is likely to occur after overdosage in which case cardiovascular support should be given. Blood pressure can be restored and heart rate brought back to normal by lying the patient down. If this does not help then volume expanders, and when necessary, vasopressors could be employed. Renal function should be monitored and general supportive measures applied. Dialysis is unlikely to be of help as tamsulosin is very highly bound to plasma proteins.

Measures, such as emesis, can be taken to impede absorption. When large quantities are involved, gastric lavage can be applied and activated charcoal and an osmotic laxative, such as sodium sulphate, can be administered.

**Pharmacological properties**
*Pharmacodynamic properties: Pharmacotherapeutic group:* Alpha$_1$-adrenoceptor antagonist. Preparations for the exclusive treatment of prostatic disease.

*Mechanism of action:* Tamsulosin binds selectively and competitively to postsynaptic alpha$_1$-receptors, in particular to the subtype alpha$_{1A}$. Antagonism of these receptors, which mediate smooth muscle contractility in the prostate and urethra, reduces outflow resistance.

*Pharmacodynamic effects:* Flomax MR increases maximum urinary flow rate by reducing smooth muscle tension in prostate and urethra and thereby relieving obstruction.

It also improves the complex of irritative and obstructive symptoms in which bladder instability and tension of the smooth muscles of the lower urinary tract play an important role.

Alpha-blockers can reduce blood pressure by lowering peripheral resistance. No reduction in blood pressure of any clinical significance was observed during studies with Flomax MR.

*Pharmacokinetic properties: Absorption:* Tamsulosin is absorbed from the intestine and is almost completely bioavailable.

Absorption of tamsulosin is reduced by a recent meal.

Uniformity of absorption can be promoted by the patient always taking Flomax MR after the usual breakfast.

Tamsulosin shows linear kinetics.

After a single dose of Flomax MR in the fed state,

plasma levels of tamsulosin peak at around 6 h and, in the steady state, which is reached by day multiple dosing, $C_{max}$ in patients is about two th higher than that reached after a single dose. Altho this was seen in elderly patients, the same find would also be expected in young ones.

There is a considerable inter-patient variatio plasma levels both after single and multiple dosin

*Distribution:* In man, tamsulosin is about 99% bo to plasma proteins and volume of distribution is s (about 0.2 l/kg).

*Biotransformation:* Tamsulosin has a low first p effect, being metabolised slowly. Most tamsulos present in plasma in the form of unchanged drug. metabolised in the liver.

In rats, hardly any induction of microsomal l enzymes was seen to be caused by tamsulosin.

No dose adjustment is warranted in mode hepatic insufficiency.

None of the metabolites are more active than original compound.

*Excretion:* Tamsulosin and its metabolites mainly excreted in the urine with about 9% of a d being present in the form of unchanged drug.

After a single dose of Flomax MR in the fed st and in the steady state in patients, elimination h lives of about 10 and 13 hours respectively have b measured.

The presence of renal impairment does not warr lowering the dose.

*Preclinical safety data:* As is also the case with ot alpha$_1$-blockers, tamsulosin (at doses expected to g exposure equivalent to 6 times that seen in m suppressed mating behaviour and/or ejaculation fu tion in male rats and, as a result, inhibited their ferti

**Pharmaceutical particulars**
*List of excipients:* Flomax MR modified release c sules contain the following excipients: microcrys line cellulose, methylacrylic acid copolyn polysorbate 80, sodium lauryl sulphate, triacetin, cium stearate, talc, hard gelatin, indigotine E1 titanium dioxide E171, yellow iron oxide E172 and iron oxide E172.

*Incompatibilities:* None known.

*Shelf life:* As packaged for sale, Flomax MR modif release capsules can be used up to two years a manufacture. The expiry date is printed on package.

*Special precautions for storage:* None.

*Nature and contents of container:* Strips contain 10 capsules per strip; three strips or one strip i cardboard box.

*Instructions for use/handling:* No special instructio

**Marketing authorisation number** 00166/0171.

**Date of approval/revision of SPC** 14 March 1996.

**Legal category** POM.

# HERPID*

**Presentation** A clear, colourless solution contain Idoxuridine BP 5% in dimethyl sulphoxide, of spect scopic quality.

**Uses** *Action:* The antiviral agent idoxuridine arre replication of DNA viruses, e.g. varicella/zoster; h pesvirus hominis; vaccinia. The idoxuridine is c solved in dimethyl sulphoxide which penetrates skin and carries the antiviral agent to the deeper lev of the epidermis where the virus is replicating.

*Indications:* Cutaneous herpes simplex and herp zoster (shingles).

**Dosage and administration** Herpid should painted on the lesions and their erythematous ba 4 times daily for four days. Treatment should start soon as the condition has been diagnosed, idea within two to three days after the rash appears. Go results are less likely if treatment is not started with seven days.

No specific information on the use of this prod in the elderly is available. Clinical trials have inclu patients over 65 years and no adverse reactic specific to this age group have been reported.

**Contra-indications, warnings, etc**
*Contra-indications:* Animal studies have shown id uridine to be teratogenic. Consequently, Her should not be prescribed for women who are pregna or at risk of becoming pregnant. In a small number cases of women who used Herpid inadvertently early pregnancy and who were followed to term, infant was normal in each case.

Known hypersensitivity to either idoxuridine dimethyl sulphoxide.

Dermographia.

*Side-effects:* Patients often experience stinging wh applying Herpid and a distinctive taste during a cou of treatment; both effects are transient.

Skin reactions have occasionally been reported. Over-usage of the solution may lead to maceration the skin.

*arning:* Herpid in the eye causes stinging: treat by ashing out with water.

*verdosage:* There is no clinical experience of over-sage. Standard supportive measures should be opted.

**armaceutical precautions** Herpid should be stored its box at room temperature. Do not refrigerate as e contents of the bottle may solidify. If crystals do rm, allow to redissolve before use by warming the ttle gently (in the palm of the hand) until the lution is clear. Because the solution is hygroscopic, y remaining after completion of treatment should discarded.

**gal category** POM.

**ckage quantities** 5 ml bottle, with brush (OP).

**rther information** Herpid can damage some syn-etic materials (e.g. artificial silk and Terylene) and inted cotton fabrics. Contact between Herpid and ese materials should therefore be avoided.

The use of Herpid in children with malignant disease ight be justified but, although not a contra-indica-n, its use in children under the age of 12 years is t recommended.

**oduct licence number** 1416/0001.

*oduct licence holder:* Boehringer Ingelheim Limited, acknell, Berkshire.

## POBASE*

**esentation** Lipobase is the bland cream base as ed in Locoid Lipocream. The inactive constituents Lipobase are cetostearyl alcohol, cetomacrogol, uid paraffin, white soft paraffin, methyl paraben, dium citrate, citric acid, and purified water.

**ses** For topical use where it is desired by the ysician to reduce gradually the topical dosage of coid Lipocream. It may also be used where a ntinuously alternating application of the active oduct and the base is required e.g. in prophylactic erapy. Application of Lipobase is also recommended here it is felt by the physician that the use of a bland nollient base is preferable to the cessation of therapy th the active product. Lipobase may also be used diluent for the active product in those cases where lution is regarded as necessary by the prescriber.

Lipobase may also be used, other than in conjunc-on with a topical corticosteroid, for its emollient tion, and for the treatment of mild skin lesions such pruritus or dry, scaly skin, where topical corticoste-id therapy is not warranted.

**osage and administration**
*dults, children and the elderly:* Lipobase may be ed either by replacing an application of the active oduct or alternating the application of the active oduct and the base, gradually diminishing the plication of active product until therapy ceases.

When used for its emollient activity or for the eatment of mild skin lesions such as pruritus or dry, aly skin, the product should be applied three or four nes a day or as directed by the physician.

**ontra-indications, warnings, etc** None.

**armaceutical precautions** Store at room temper-ure (15–25°C).

**gal category** P.

**ckage quantities** Tubes of 50 g as an original pack P).

**rther information** Lipobase is a high fat content l in water emulsion, the oily phase constituting 70% weight of the finished product.

**oduct licence number** 0166/0125.

## OCOID* CREAM
## OCOID* OINTMENT

**esentation** Locoid Cream, containing 0.1% hydro-rtisone 17-butyrate in a cream base. The inactive onstituents in Locoid Cream are cetostearyl alcohol, tomacrogol, liquid paraffin, white soft paraffin, opyl paraben, butyl paraben, citric acid, sodium trate, and purified water.

Locoid Ointment, containing 0.1% hydrocortisone 7-butyrate in an ointment base. The inactive constit-ents in Locoid Ointment are liquid paraffin and olyethylene.

**ses** Eczema and dermatitis of all types including opic eczema, photodermatitis, primary irritant and lergic dermatitis, lichen planus, lichen simplex, urigo nodularis, discoid lupus erythematosus, nec-biosis lipoidica, pretibial myxoedema and erythe-matosus psoriasis of the scalp, chronic plaque psoriasis of the palms and soles, and other forms of psoriasis (excluding widespread plaque psoriasis).

**Dosage and administration** Apply a small quantity to the affected part two or three times daily. Application may be made under occlusion in the more resistant lesions such as thickened psoriatic plaques on elbows and knees.

**Contra-indications, warnings, etc**
*Contra-indications:* Facial rosacea, acne vulgaris, perioral dermatitis, perianal and genital pruritus, napkin eruptions, bacterial (e.g. impetigo), viral (e.g. herpes simplex) and fungal (e.g. candida or dermatophyte) infections.

*Side-effects:* Local and systemic toxicity is common especially following long continued use on large areas of damaged skin, in flexures and with polythene occlusion. If used in childhood, or on the face, courses should be limited to 5 days and occlusion should not be used. Local irritation may occur in those with a hypersensitivity to parabens.

*Use in pregnancy and lactation:* There is inadequate evidence of safety in human pregnancy. Topical administration of corticosteroids to pregnant animals can cause abnormalities of fetal development including cleft plate and intra-uterine growth retardation. There may therefore be a very small risk of such effects in the human fetus.

*Other warnings and precautions:* Long term continuous therapy should be avoided in all patients irrespective of age. Application under occlusion should be restricted to dermatoses involving limited areas.

Topical corticosteroids may be hazardous in psoriasis for a number of reasons including rebound relapses following development of tolerance, risk of generalised pustular psoriasis and local and systemic toxicity due to impaired barrier function of the skin. Steroids may have a place in psoriasis of the scalp and chronic plaque psoriasis of the hands and feet. Careful patient supervision is important.

*Overdosage:* Overdosage would result in the topical and systemic signs and symptoms associated with high corticosteroid dosage. If overdosage should occur, treatment should not stop immediately but be gradually withdrawn. Adrenal insufficiency may need therapy with intravenous hydrocortisone. It should be noted that overdosage of this topical corticosteroid product would be unlikely to occur other than as a result of severe and prolonged abuse of product.

**Pharmaceutical precautions** Store at room temperature (15–25°C).

**Legal category** POM.

**Package quantities** *Locoid Cream:* Tubes of 30 g and 100 g as original packs (OP).

*Locoid Ointment:* Tubes of 30 g and 100 g as original packs (OP).

**Further information** Locoid is a non-fluorinated topical steroid. Whilst clinical trials have shown it to be as effective as the potent fluorinated steroids, in clinical practice there is a low incidence of reported clinical side-effects.

**Product licence numbers**
Locoid Cream 0166/0058
Locoid Ointment 0166/0059

## LOCOID CRELO*

**Qualitative and quantitative composition** Hydrocortisone butyrate 0.1% (w/w).

**Pharmaceutical form** Topical emulsion.

**Clinical particulars**
*Therapeutic indications:* The product is recommended for clinical use in the treatment of conditions responsive to topical corticosteroids, e.g. eczema, dermatitis and psoriasis. The product is intended for topical application especially to the scalp, hirsute or facial skin.

*Posology and method of administration:* Adults, children and the elderly: A small quantity to be applied two or three times a day, only sufficient to cover the affected area. The formulation of the product makes it suitable for use in both scaly lesions and for moist, weeping lesions. Replace the cap firmly after use.

*Contra-indications:* Contra-indicated in the presence of bacterial (e.g. impetigo), viral (e.g. herpes simplex), fungal (e.g. candida or dermatophyte), infections.

*Special warnings and special precautions for use:* Avoid contact with the eyes. Although generally regarded as safe, even for long-term administration in adults, there is a potential for overdosage in infancy. Extreme caution is required in dermatoses of infancy including napkin eruption. In such patients, courses of treatment should not normally exceed 7 days.

*Interactions with other medicaments and other forms of interaction:* None known.

*Pregnancy and lactation:* There is inadequate evidence of safety in human pregnancy. Topical administration of corticosteroids to pregnant animals can cause abnormalities of fetal development including cleft palate and intra-uterine growth retardation. There may therefore be a very small risk of such effects in the human fetus. The use of topical corticosteroids during lactation is unlikely to present a hazard to infants being breast-fed.

*Effects on ability to drive and use machines:* None known.

*Undesirable effects:* Locoid Crelo is usually well tolerated; if signs of hypersensitivity do occur, treatment should be ceased.

In naturally occluded or moist areas of the skin, especially in small children, where absorption may be favoured, unduly prolonged therapy may give rise to systemic side-effects.

*Overdose:* Overdosage would result in the topical and systemic signs and symptoms associated with high corticosteroid dosage. If overdosage should occur, treatment should not stop immediately but be gradually withdrawn. Adrenal insufficiency may need therapy with intravenous hydrocortisone. It should be noted that overdosage of this topical corticosteroid product would be unlikely to occur other than as a result of severe and prolonged abuse of the product.

**Pharmacological properties**
*Pharmacodynamic properties:* The active constituent, hydrocortisone butyrate, is an established topical corticosteroid, equi-efficacious with those corticosteroids classified as potent.

*Pharmacokinetic properties:* In human in-vivo studies, the potency of this form of active ingredient has been shown to be of the same order as other topical corticosteroids classed as potent. The active ingredient metabolises to hydrocortisone and butyric acid.

*Preclinical safety data:* The well-established use of hydrocortisone 17-butyrate topical preparations over many years does not warrant further safety evaluation studies in animals.

**Pharmaceutical particulars**
*List of excipients:* Cetomacrogol 1000 BP, Cetostearyl Alcohol PhEur, White Soft Paraffin BP, Hard Paraffin HSE, Borage Oil HSE, Butylhydroxytoluene PhEur, Propyleneglycol PhEur, Sodium Citrate HSE, Anhydrous Citric Acid PhEur, Propyl Parahydroxybenzoate PhEur, Butyl Hydroxybenzoate BP, Purified Water PhEur.

*Incompatibilities:* None known.

*Shelf life:* 2 years.

*Special precautions for storage:* Room temperature (15°C–25°C).

*Nature and contents of container:* White opaque low density polyethylene bottles of 100 g capacity, equipped with a natural low density polyethylene dropper applicator, closed with a white polypropylene screw cap.

*Instructions for use/handling:* No special instructions.

**Marketing authorisation number** 0166/0170

**Date of approval/revision of SPC** April 1995.

**Legal category** POM.

## LOCOID LIPOCREAM*

**Presentation** Locoid Lipocream, containing 0.1% hydrocortisone 17-butyrate in a high fat content cream base. The inactive constituents in Locoid Lipocream are cetostearyl alcohol, cetomacrogol, liquid paraffin, white soft paraffin, methyl paraben, sodium citrate, citric acid, and purified water.

**Uses** The product is recommended for clinical use in the treatment of conditions responsive to topical corticosteroids, e.g. eczema, dermatitis and psoriasis. The product is intended for topical application.

**Dosage and administration**
*Adults, children and the elderly:* A small quantity to be applied two or three times a day, only sufficient to cover the affected area. The formulation of the product makes it suitable for use in both for scaly lesions and for moist, weeping lesions.

**Contra-indications, warnings, etc**
*Contra-indications:* Contra-indicated in the presence of bacterial (e.g. impetigo), viral (e.g. herpes simplex), or fungal (e.g. candida or dermatophyte), infections.

*Side-effects:* Locoid Lipocream is usually well tolerated; if signs of hypersensitivity do occur, treatment should be ceased.

In naturally occluded or moist areas of the skin, especially in small children, where absorption may be favoured, unduly prolonged therapy may give rise to systemic side-effects.

*Use in pregnancy and lactation:* There is inadequate evidence of safety in human pregnancy. Topical administration of corticosteroids to pregnant animals can cause abnormalities of fetal development including cleft palate and intra-uterine growth retardation. There may therefore be a very small risk of such effects in the human fetus. The use of topical corticosteroids during lactation is unlikely to present a hazard to infants being breast-fed.

*Other warnings and precautions:* Although generally regarded as safe, even for long-term administration in adults, there is a potential for overdosage in infancy. Extreme caution is required in dermatoses of infancy including napkin eruption. In such patients, courses of treatment should not normally exceed 7 days.

*Overdosage:* Overdosage would result in the topical and systemic signs and symptoms associated with high corticosteroid dosage. If overdosage should occur, treatment should not stop immediately but be gradually withdrawn. Adrenal insufficiency may need therapy with intravenous hydrocortisone. It should be noted that overdosage of this topical corticosteroid product would be unlikely to occur other than as a result of severe and prolonged abuse of the product.

**Pharmaceutical precautions** Store at room temperature (15–25°C).

**Legal category** POM.

**Package quantities** Tubes of 30 g and 100 g as original packs (OP).

**Further information** Locoid, a non-fluorinated topical steroid has been shown to be as effective as the potent fluorinated steroids, yet in clinical practice there is a low incidence of reported side-effects. The oily phase constitutes 70% by weight of the product.

**Product licence number** 0166/0112.

## LOCOID* SCALP LOTION

**Presentation** Locoid Scalp Lotion contains 0.1% hydrocortisone 17-butyrate in an alcohol/water base, specially formulated for the treatment of skin disorders of the scalp. The inactive constituents of Locoid Scalp Lotion are glycerin, povidone, citric acid, sodium citrate, iso-propyl alcohol, and purified water.

**Uses** In the treatment of steroid-responsive dermatoses of the scalp, including seborrhoea capitis with or without an associated severe dandruff; psoriasis of the scalp (excluding widespread plaque psoriasis).

**Dosage and administration**
*Adults, children and the elderly:* Apply a small quantity 2 to 3 times daily to the affected area of the scalp, or as directed.

**Contra-indications, warnings, etc** *Contra-indications:* Facial rosacea, acne vulgaris, perioral dermatitis, perianal and genital pruritus, napkin eruptions, bacterial (e.g. impetigo), viral (e.g. herpes simplex) and fungal (e.g. candida or dermatophyte) infections, known hypersensitivity to the product.

*Side-effects:* Local and systemic toxicity is common especially following long continued use on large areas. Local irritation may occur.

*Use in pregnancy and lactation:* There is inadequate evidence of safety in human pregnancy. Topical administration of corticosteroids to pregnant animals can cause abnormalities of fetal development including cleft palate and intra-uterine growth retardation. There may therefore be a very small risk of such effects in the human fetus.

*Other warnings and precautions:* Long term continuous therapy should be avoided in all patients irrespective of age. Application under occlusion should be restricted to dermatoses involving limited areas.

Topical corticosteroids may be hazardous in psoriasis for a number of reasons including rebound relapses following development of tolerance, risk of generalised pustular psoriasis and local and systemic toxicity due to impaired barrier function of the skin. Steroids may have a place in psoriasis of the scalp and chronic plaque psoriasis of the hands and feet. Careful patient supervision is important.

*Overdosage:* Overdosage would result in the topical and systemic signs and symptoms associated with high corticosteroid dosage. If overdosage should occur, treatment should not stop immediately but be gradually withdrawn. Adrenal insufficiency may need therapy with intravenous hydrocortisone. It should be noted that overdosage of this topical corticosteroid product would be unlikely to occur other than as a result of severe and prolonged abuse of product.

**Pharmaceutical precautions** Store at room temperature (15–25°C).

**Legal category** POM.

**Package quantities** Plastic squeeze bottles of 30 ml and 100 ml as original packs (OP).

**Further information** Locoid lotion should be kept away from the eyes, and not used near a fire or naked flame.

**Product licence number** 0166/0060.

## LOCOID* C CREAM

**Qualitative and quantitative composition** Hydrocortisone 17-butyrate 0.1% and Chlorquinaldol 3%.

**Pharmaceutical form** Cream.

**Clinical particulars**
*Therapeutic indications:* The product is recommended for clinical use in the treatment of conditions responsive to topical corticosteroids, e.g. eczema, dermatitis and psoriasis, where there is concurrent infection by a micro-organism susceptible to chlorquinaldol, or where such infection is to be prevented.

*Posology and method of administration:* To be applied to the affected part two to four times a day, or as directed by the prescriber. Where necessary, application may be made under an occlusive dressing.

*Contra-indications:* This preparation is contra-indicated in the presence of viral or fungal infections, tubercular or syphilitic lesions, and in bacterial infections (other than those at the site of inunction responsive to topical chlorquinaldol) unless used in connection with appropriate chemotherapy.

*Special warnings and special precautions for use:* Contact with the eyes should be avoided.

*Interaction with other medicaments and other forms of interaction:* None stated.

*Pregnancy and lactation:* This preparation should not be applied extensively, i.e. in large amounts or for prolonged periods, in pregnancy.

*Effects on ability to drive and use machines:* None stated.

*Undesirable effects:* In infants, long-term continuous topical therapy should be avoided. Adrenal suppression can occur, even without occlusion.

*Overdose:* No details stated.

**Pharmacological properties**
*Pharmacodynamic properties:* The active substance is a well-established topical corticosteroid, with an activity classified at potent.

Chlorquinaldol is an established anti-infectious agent with an anti-bacterial and anti-fungal activity.

*Pharmacokinetic properties:* In-vivo studies have demonstrated the topical activity of the product, e.g. by the McKenzie-Stoughton test.

Chlorquinaldol acts topically at the site of application.

*Preclinical safety data:* No relevant preclinical safety data has been generated.

**Pharmaceutical particulars**
*List of excipients:* Cetostearyl Alcohol BP, Cetomacrogol 1000 BP, Liquid Paraffin BP, White Soft Paraffin BP, Sodium citrate (anhydrous) USP, Citric Acid (anhydrous) PhEur, Purified Water PhEur.

*Incompatibilities:* None stated.

*Shelf life:* 4 years.

*Special precautions for storage:* Store at room temperature (not more than 25°C).

*Nature and contents of container:* Collapsible aluminium tube with plastic screw cap containing 30 g or 50 g.

*Instructions for use/handling:* Not applicable.

**Marketing authorisation number** 0166/0056

**Date of approval/revision of SPC** 15 March 1995.

**Legal category** POM.

## LOCOID* C OINTMENT

**Qualitative and quantitative composition** Hydrocortisone 17-butyrate 0.1% and Chlorquinaldol 3%.

**Pharmaceutical form** Ointment.

**Clinical particulars**
*Therapeutic indications:* The product is recommended for clinical use in the treatment of conditions responsive to topical corticosteroids, e.g. eczema, dermatitis and psoriasis, where there is concurrent infection by a micro-organism susceptible to chlorquinaldol, or where such infection is to be prevented.

*Posology and method of administration:* To be applied to the affected part two to four times a day, or as directed by the prescriber. Where necessary, application may be made under an occlusive dressing.

*Contra-indications:* This preparation is contra-indicated in the presence of viral or fungal infections, tubercular or syphilitic lesions, and in bacterial inf tions (other than those at the site of inunct responsive to topical chlorquinaldol) unless used connection with appropriate chemotherapy.

*Special warnings and special precautions for u* Contact with the eyes should be avoided.

*Interaction with other medicaments and other for of interaction:* None stated.

*Pregnancy and lactation:* This preparation should be applied extensively, i.e. in large amounts or prolonged periods, in pregnancy.

*Effects on ability to drive and use machines:* No stated.

*Undesirable effects:* In infants, long-term continuc topical therapy should be avoided. Adrenal suppr sion can occur, even without occlusion.

*Overdose:* No details stated.

**Pharmacological properties**
*Pharmacodynamic properties:* The active substar is a well-established topical corticosteroid, with activity classified at potent.

Chlorquinaldol is an established anti-infectic agent with an anti-bacterial and anti-fungal activity

*Pharmacokinetic properties:* In-vivo studies have de onstrated the topical activity of the product, e.g. the McKenzie-Stoughton test.

Chlorquinaldol acts topically at the site of appli tion.

*Preclinical safety data:* No relevant preclinical saf data has been generated.

**Pharmaceutical particulars**
*List of excipients:* Plastibase 50 W.

*Incompatibilities:* None stated.

*Shelf life:* 5 years.

*Special precautions for storage:* Store at room te perature (not more than 25°C).

*Nature and contents of container:* Collapsible alum ium tube with plastic screw cap containing 30 g 50 g.

*Instructions for use/handling:* Not applicable.

**Marketing authorisation number** 0166/0057

**Date of approval/revision of SPC** 15 March 1995.

**Legal category** POM.

## MILDISON* LIPOCREAM

**Presentation** Mildison Lipocream is presented as oil-in-water high-lipid content emollient base conta ing Hydrocortisone BP 1% w/w. The inactive ingre ents of Mildison Lipocream are cetostearyl alcoh cetomacrogol, liquid paraffin, white soft paraff methyl paraben, citric acid, sodium citrate, and pu fied water.

**Uses** By topical administration in the treatment eczema and dermatitis of all types, including atop eczema, photodermatitis, otitis externa, primary ir tant and allergic dermatitis, intertrigo, prurigo nod laris, seborrhoeic dermatitis, and insect bite reactio

**Dosage and administration**
*For adults, children and the elderly:* Apply a sm quantity only sufficient to cover the affected area tv or three times a day. The formulation of the produ makes it suitable for use both for dry scaly lesio and for moist or weeping lesions.

**Contra-indications, warnings, etc**
*Contra-indications:* Contra-indicated in the presen of bacterial (e.g. impetigo), viral (e.g. herpes simple: or fungal (e.g. candida or dermatophyte), infections

*Side-effects:* Mildison 1% is usually well tolerated. signs of hypersensitivity do occur, treatment shou cease.

In naturally occluded or moist areas of the sk especially in small children, where absorption may favoured, unduly prolonged therapy may give rise systemic side-effects.

*Use in pregnancy and lactation:* There is inadequa evidence of safety in human pregnancy. Topic administration of corticosteroids to pregnant anima can cause abnormalities of fetal development inclu ing cleft palate and intra-uterine growth retardatio There may therefore be a very small risk of su effects in the human fetus. The use of topical cortic steroids during lactation is unlikely to present a haza to infants being breast-fed.

*Other warnings and precautions:* Although general regarded as safe, even for long-term administrati in adults, there is a potential for overdosage in infanc Extreme caution is required in dermatoses of infan including napkin eruption. In such patients, cours of treatment should not normally exceed 7 days.

*Overdosage:* Overdosage would result in the topic and systemic signs and symptoms associated wi

gh corticosteroid dosage. If overdosage should
cur, treatment should not stop immediately but be
adually withdrawn. Adrenal insufficiency may need
erapy with intravenous hydrocortisone. It should be
ted that overdosage of this topical corticosteroid
oduct would be unlikely to occur other than as a
sult of severe and prolonged abuse of the product.

**armaceutical precautions** Store at room temper-
ure (15–25°C).

**gal category** POM.

**ckage quantities** Tubes of 30 g as an original pack
P).

**rther information** Hydrocortisone is a topical
eroid well known for its efficacy and safety. The
pocream base promotes both hydration of the
ratum corneum and suppleness of dry, scaly, exco-
ted skin, with greater patient acceptability than an
dinary ointment. The product is particularly suited
r use on dry, subacute and chronic lesions and for
ose patients presenting with mixed lesions.

**oduct licence number** 0166/0131.

## INERYT*

**ualitative and quantitative composition** Erythro-
ycin PhEur 40 mg and Zinc Acetate USP 12 mg per
l on constitution.

**armaceutical form** Dry powder bottle and solvent
ottle to be admixed on dispensing.

## Clinical particulars

*Therapeutic indications:* Topical treatment of acne
vulgaris.

*Posology and method of administration:* For children,
adults, and the elderly. Apply twice daily over the
whole of the affected area for a period of 10 to 12
weeks.

*Contra-indications:* Zineryt is contra-indicated in patients who are hypersensitive to erythromycin or other
macrolide antibiotics, or to zinc, di-isopropyl sebacate
or ethanol.

*Special warnings and special precautions for use:*
Cross resistance may occur with other antibiotics of
the macrolide group and also with lincomycin and
clindamycin. Contact with the eyes or the mucous
membranes of the nose and mouth should be avoided.

*Interaction with other medicaments and other forms
of interaction:* None known.

*Pregnancy and lactation:* There is no contraindication
to the use of Zineryt in pregnancy or lactation.

*Effects on ability to drive and use machines:* None.

*Undesirable effects:* Occasionally a burning sensation
or a slight redness of the skin may be observed; this
is due to the alcohol base of Zineryt and is transient
and of minor clinical significance.

*Overdose:* It is not expected that overdosage would
occur in normal use. Patients showing idiosyncratic
hypersensitivity should wash the treated area with
copious water and simple soap.

## Pharmacological properties

*Pharmacodynamic properties:* Erythromycin is known
to be efficacious, at 4%, in the topical treatment of
acne vulgaris. Zinc, topically, is established as an aid
to wound healing. The zinc acetate is solubilised by
complexing with the erythromycin, and delivery of
the complex is enhanced by the chosen vehicle.

*Pharmacokinetic properties:* The complex does not
survive in the skin, and erythromycin and zinc penetrate independently. The erythromycin penetrates,
and is partially systemically absorbed (0–10% in vitro,
40–50% in animal studies); that portion absorbed is
excreted in 24–72 hours. The zinc is not absorbed
systemically.

*Preclinical safety data:* No relevant pre-clinical safety
data has been generated.

## Pharmaceutical particulars

*List of excipients:* Di-isopropyl sebacate, ethanol.

*Incompatibilities:* None known.

*Shelf life:* 2 years; 5 weeks after constitution.

*Special precautions for storage:* None. Store at room
temperature (15°C–25°C).

*Nature and contents of container:* Screw-capped HDPE
bottles; an applicator cap is fitted when dispensed.
When constituted packs are of 30 ml and 90 ml.

*Instructions for use/handling:* None.

**Marketing authorisation number** 0166/0109

**Date of approval/revision of SPC** 27 January 1995.

**Legal category** POM.

*Trade Mark

# ZENECA Pharma
King's Court
Water Lane
Wilmslow, Cheshire SK9 5AZ

ZENECA

## AMPHOCIL*

**Qualitative and quantitative composition**

| *Ingredient* | *Specification reference* | *Quantity (W/W)* |
|---|---|---|
| Amphotericin | USP | 5.060 |
| Sodium cholesteryl sulphate | House | 2.672 |
| Tromethamine | USP | 0.571 |
| Disodium edetate | PhEur | 0.034 |
| Lactose, monohydrate | PhEur | 91.311 |
| Hydrochloric acid | PhEur | 0.353[a] |
| Water for injection | PhEur | [b] |
| Nitrogen | NF | [c] |

[a] HCl qs to a target pH of 7.0±0.5.
[b] Mean NMT 2.0% residual moisture and no individual vial greater than 2.5%.
[c] Used to fill vial headspace.

**Pharmaceutical form** Amphotericin B USP, 5% (W/W), lyophilisate for reconstitution. Each vial contains either 50 mg (50,000 IU) or 100 mg (100,000 IU) of Amphotericin B USP as a complex with sodium cholesteryl sulphate.

**Clinical particulars**
*Therapeutic indications:* Amphocil is indicated for the treatment of severe systemic and/or deep mycoses in cases where toxicity or renal failure precludes the use of conventional amphotericin B in effective doses, and in cases where prior systemic antifungal therapy has failed. Fungal infections successfully treated with Amphocil include disseminated candidiasis and aspergillosis. Amphocil has been used successfully in severely neutropenic patients.

Amphocil is not intended for use in common, clinically inapparent fungal diseases diagnosed only by skin tests or serological determinations.

*Posology and method of administration:*
*Dosage:* Therapy may begin at a daily dose of 1.0 mg/kg of body weight, increasing to the recommended dose of 3.0–4.0 mg/kg as required. Doses as high as 6 mg/kg have been used in patients. Dosage should be adjusted to the individual requirements of each patient. The median cumulative dose in clinical studies was 3.5 g and the medial treatment duration was 16 days. Ten percent (10%) of patients received 13 g or more of Amphocil over a period of 27 to 409 days.

*Administration:* Amphocil is administered by intravenous infusion at a rate of 1 to 2 mg/kg/hour. If the patient experiences acute reactions or cannot tolerate the infusion volume, the infusion time may be extended. Pre-medication (e.g. paracetamol, antihistamines, antiemetics) may be administered to patients who have previously suffered infusion related adverse reactions.

*Paediatric patients:* A limited number of paediatric patients have been treated with Amphocil at daily doses (mg/kg) similar to those in adults. No unusual adverse events were reported.

*Elderly patients:* A limited number of elderly patients have been treated with Amphocil; available data do not indicate the need for specific dose recommendations or precautions in elderly patients.

*Contra-indications:* Amphocil should not be administered to patients who have documented hypersensitivity to any of its components, unless, in the opinion of the physician, the advantages of using Amphocil outweigh the risks of hypersensitivity.

*Special warnings and special precautions for use:* A test dose which is advisable when commencing all new courses of treatment should immediately precede the first dose; a small amount of drug (e.g. 20 ml of a solution containing 0.1 g per litre) should be infused over 10 minutes and the patient carefully observed for the next 30 minutes.
*In the treatment of diabetic patients:* It should be noted that each vial of Amphocil contains lactose monohydrate.

*In the treatment of renal dialysis patients:* Amphocil should be administered only at the end of each dialysis period. Serum electrolytes, particularly potassium and magnesium, should be regularly monitored.
*Interaction with other medicaments and other forms of interaction:* There have been no reported interactions between Amphocil and other drugs including cyclosporine. However, caution should be used in patients receiving concomitant therapy with drugs known to interact with conventional amphotericin B such as nephrotoxic drugs (aminoglycosides, cisplatin and pentamidine), corticosteroids and corticotropin (ACTH) that may potentiate hypokalaemia and digitalis glycosides, muscle relaxants and antiarrhythmic agents whose effects may be potentiated in the presence of hypokalaemia.

The use of flucytosine with Amphocil has not been studied. While the synergy between amphotericin B and flucytosine has been reported, amphotericin B may enhance the toxicity of flucytosine by increasing its cellular uptake and impeding its renal excretion.

*Pregnancy and use during lactation:*
*Pregnancy:* Animal reproductive toxicology studies with Amphocil have shown no evidence of harm to the foetus. Although the active ingredient, amphotericin B, has been in wide use for many years without apparent ill consequence, there is inadequate evidence of safety of Amphocil in human pregnancy. Therefore it is recommended that administration of Amphocil is avoided in pregnancy unless the anticipated benefit to the patient outweighs the potential risk to the foetus.

*Nursing mothers:* It is not known whether amphotericin B is excreted in human milk. Consideration should be given to discontinuation of nursing during treatment with Amphocil.

*Effects on the ability to drive and use machines:* Not applicable to current indication or expected use.

*Undesirable effects:* In general, the physician should monitor the patient for any type of adverse event associated with conventional amphotericin B. The appearance of adverse reactions does not generally prevent the patient completing the course of treatment. Caution should be exercised when high doses or prolonged therapy is indicated.

Acute reactions including fever, chills and rigours may occur. Anaphylactoid reactions including hypotension, tachycardia, bronchospasm, dyspnoea, hypoxia and hyperventilation have also been reported. Most acute reactions are successfully treated by reducing the rate of infusion and prompt administration of anti-histamines and adrenal corticosteroids. Serious anaphylactoid effects may necessitate discontinuation of Amphocil and treatment with additional supportive therapy (e.g. adrenaline).

Clinical studies conducted so far have shown Amphocil to be less nephrotoxic than conventional amphotericin B. Serum creatinine levels tend to remain consistent throughout the course of therapy even in patients with renal insufficiency. Patients who developed renal insufficiency during treatment with conventional amphotericin B, were stabilised or improved when Amphocil was substituted. Decreases in renal function attributable to Amphocil treatment were rare. However, as with conventional amphotericin B, renal function should be monitored with particular attention to those patients receiving concomitant therapy with nephrotoxic drugs.

There have been no reports of unequivocal hepatic toxicity of Amphocil. Changes in alkaline phosphatase and bilirubin levels were infrequent.

Changes in coagulation, thrombocytopenia and hypomagnesemia were sometimes observed on Amphocil. Anaemia, which is a very common adverse event during treatment with conventional amphotericin B, developed in only 2.5% of the patients treated with Amphocil.

Other reported events include nausea, vomiting, hypertension, headache, backache, diarrhoea and abdominal pain.

*Overdose:* In case of overdose, stop administration immediately and carefully monitor the patient's clinical status (renal, liver and cardiac function, haematological status, serum electrolytes) and institute symptomatic treatment.

**Pharmacological properties**
*Pharmacodynamic properties:* Amphotericin B is a macrocyclic polyene antibiotic isolated from *Streptomyces nodosus*. Amphotericin B has a high affinity for ergosterol, the primary sterol in fungal cell membranes, and a lesser affinity for cholesterol, the predominant sterol of mammalian cell membranes. Binding of amphotericin B to ergosterol results in damage to the fungal cell membrane, enhanc membrane permeability and eventual cell deat Mammalian cell membranes also contain sterols, a it has been suggested that the damage caused amphotericin B to human cells follows a similar mo of action to that of fungal cells. Amphocil is conside to have the same mode of action as convention amphotericin B, but with reduced toxicity.

Amphocil is a novel formulation of amphotericin based on its unique affinity for sterols. Amphocil is stable complex of amphotericin B and sodium chole teryl sulphate, a naturally occurring cholesterol m tabolite. Amphotericin B and sodium choleste sulphate are complexed in a near equimolar ratio form uniform disc-shaped microparticles. Amphо is not a liposomal formulation but a colloidal dispe sion of amphotericin B and sodium cholesteryl su phate.

Pharmacological studies indicated that overall, Ar phocil is essentially equivalent, *in vitro*, to conve tional amphotericin B against a variety of fung pathogens. Higher doses of Amphocil are tolerate thus it is generally more effective in eradicating fung infections than conventional amphotericin B in seve *in vivo* models.

*Pharmacokinetic properties:* Pharmacokinetic studi in animals demonstrate that the distribution of Ar phocil and conventional amphotericin B are notab different. Lower peak plasma levels of amphoteric B and greater total area under the curve values aft Amphocil treatment, compared to comparable dos of conventional amphotericin B have been observe Higher concentrations of amphotericin B measured the liver, spleen and bone marrow after Ampho administration were not accompanied by evidence increased toxicity in these organ systems. Levels the kidney, a primary site of toxicity of convention amphotericin B, were 4- to 5-fold lower after treatme with Amphocil and correlated with reduced nephr toxicity compared to conventional amphotericin. Ma imum plasma concentrations of amphotericin B we lower in Amphocil treated animals. The terminal ha life was longer in the Amphocil treated animals owi to the accumulation of amphotericin B in the liver ar its subsequent slow release.

In bone marrow transplant patients administer Amphocil at doses of 0.5 to 8.0 mg/kg/day, there wa an increase in both the volume of distribution ($V_{ss}$ and the total plasma clearance ($Cl_t$) as the dos escalated. The mean values of $V_{ss}$, $Cl_t$ and termin half-life for doses ≤2.0 mg/kg were 2.25 l/kg, 0.0855 h/kg and 22.1 hours, respectively. The mean valu for doses >2.0 mg/kg were 3.61 l/kg, 0.116 l/h/kg ar 27.2 hours respectively. The maximum steady-sta concentrations achievable after multiple dosir ranged from 658 to 6212 µg/l for doses of 0.5 8.0 mg/kg respectively. There was no evidence continued accumulation of Amphocil at doses 8.0 mg/kg/day. Thee was no net change in ren function over the duration of Amphocil treatme (range from 1 to 108 days, median 28 days).

*Preclinical safety data:* Amphocil was found to generally less toxic than conventional amphotericin in a series of acute and repeat dose studies, with a to 5-fold increased margin of safety. There were n unique toxicities observed following treatment wi Amphocil relative to conventional amphotericin Nephrotoxicity was diminished during Amphoc treatment even at dose levels 4- to 5-fold higher tha toxic doses of conventional amphotericin B. Acc mulation of amphotericin B in the liver followir Amphocil administration was observed; howeve there were no associated signs of increased hepato icity relative to conventional amphotericin B. *In-vit* and *in-vivo* tests on induction of gene and chrom some mutations were negative for amphotericin Carcinogenicity studies have not been conducted wi amphotericin B or Amphocil. To date there have bee no clinical reports of carcinogenicity associated wit the use of amphotericin B. Embryo-foetal studies rats and rabbits, at doses of 2.5 mg/kg/day or great showed maternal toxicity i.e. reduced weight gain ar loss of appetite. There were no adverse effects c embryo-foetal development up to 10 mg/kg/da There are no specific data for the effect of Amphoc on human fertility, but in multiple dose toxicity studie of up to 13 weeks (in rats and dogs) there was n ffect on ovarian or testicular histology. Although mphotericin B has not been associated with peri- or ost-natal effects, no studies with Amphocil are vailable.

**harmaceutical particulars**

*ist of excipients:* The following excipients are conained in each vial of lyophilised product: Sodium holesteryl sulphate; Tromethamine USP; Edetate )isodium PhEur; Hydrochloric Acid PhEur; Water for njection PhEur; Lactose Monohydrate PhEur.

*ncompatibilities:* Do not reconstitute lyophilised pow-ler/cake with saline or dextrose solutions. Do not add aline or electrolytes to the reconstituted concentrate, r mix with other drugs.

If administered through an existing intravenous ine, flush with 5% Dextrose for Injection prior to nfusion of Amphocil, otherwise administer via a eparate line.

The use of any solution other than those recomnended, or the presence of a bacteriostatic agent (e.g. enzyl alcohol) in the solution may cause precipitation of Amphocil.

Do not use material that shows evidence of precipitation or any other particulate matter. Strict aseptic echnique should always be followed during reconstiution and dilution since no preservatives are present n the lyophilised drug or in the solutions used for econstitution and dilution.

*Shelf life:* Unopened vials of lyophilised material have shelf-life of 36 months and should be stored below 30°C (86°F). After reconstitution, the drug should be efrigerated at 2–8°C (36–46°F) and used within 24 ours. Do not freeze. After further dilution with 5% )extrose for Injection, the infusion should be stored n a refrigerator (2–8°C) and used within 24 hours. Partially used vials should be discarded.

*Special precautions for storage:* Store below 30°C 86°F).

*Nature and contents of container:* The container is a Type I moulded glass vial, the stopper is a grey butyl yophilisation type stopper, and the cap is an aluminum ring with either a green or yellow polypropylene lip-off top.

*nstructions for use/handling:* Directions for reconstiution and dilution: Amphocil must be reconstituted by addition of sterile Water for Injection, PhEur, using sterile syringe and a 20-gauge needle.

Rapidly inject into the vial:
50 mg/vial – 10 ml sterile Water for Injection
100 mg/vial – 20 ml sterile Water for Injection.

Shake gently by hand, rotating the vial, until the yellow fluid becomes clear. Note that the fluid may be opalescent. The liquid in each reconstituted vial will contain 5 mg of amphotericin B per ml. For infusion, further dilute to a final concentration of 0.625 mg/ml by diluting 1 volume of the reconstituted Amphocil with 7 volumes of 5% Dextrose for Injection.

*Market authorisation holder:* Sequus Pharmaceuticals ncorporated, 1050 Hamilton Court, Menlo Park, CA 94025, USA.

**Marketing authorisation number** 11866/0002–3.

**Date of approval/revision of SPC** 21 December 1995.

**Legal category** POM.

## ARIMIDEX* ▼

**Qualitative and quantitative composition** Each tablet contains 1 mg anastrozole.

**Pharmaceutical form** Tablet.

**Clinical particulars**

*Therapeutic indication:* Treatment of advanced breast cancer in post-menopausal women whose disease progressed following treatment with tamoxifen or other anti-oestrogens. Efficacy has not been demonstrated in oestrogen receptor negative patients unless they had a previous positive clinical reponse to tamoxifen.

*Posology and method of administration*

*Adults including the elderly:* One 1 mg tablet to be taken orally once a day.

*Children:* Not recommended for use in children.

*Renal impairment:* No dose change is recommended in patients with mild or moderate renal impairment.

*Hepatic impairment:* No dose change is recommended in patients with mild hepatic disease.

*Contra-indications:* Arimidex is contra-indicated in: pre-menopausal women; pregnant or lactating women; patients with severe renal impairment (creatinine clearance less than 20 ml/min); patients with moderate or severe hepatic disease; patients with known hypersensitivity to anastrozole or to any of the excipients as referenced in the list of excipients.

Oestrogen-containing therapies should not be coadministered with Arimidex as they would negate its pharmacological action.

*Special warnings and special precautions for use:* Arimidex is not recommended for use in children as safety and efficacy have not been established in this group of patients.

The menopause should be defined biochemically in any patient where there is doubt about hormonal status.

There are no data to support the safe use of Arimidex in patients with moderate or severe hepatic impairment, or patients with severe impairment of renal function (creatinine clearance less than 20 ml/min).

*Interaction with other medicaments and other forms of interaction:* Antipyrine and cimetidine clinical interaction studies indicate that the co-administration of Arimidex with other drugs is unlikely to result in clinically significant drug interactions mediated by cytochrome P450.

A review of the clinical trial safety database did not reveal evidence of clinically significant interaction in patients treated with Arimidex who also received other commonly prescribed drugs.

There is no clinical information to date on the use of Arimidex in combination with other anti-cancer agents.

Oestrogen-containing therapies should not be coadministered with Arimidex as they would negate its pharmacological action.

*Pregnancy and lactation:* Arimidex is contra-indicated in pregnant or lactating women

*Effects on ability to drive and use machines:* Arimidex is unlikely to impair the ability of patients to drive and operate machinery. However, asthenia and somnolence have been reported with the use of Arimidex and caution should be observed when driving or operating machinery while such symptoms persist.

*Undesirable effects:* Arimidex has generally been well tolerated. Adverse events have usually been mild to moderate with only few withdrawals from treatment due to undesirable events.

The pharmacological action of Arimidex may give rise to certain expected effects. These include hot flushes, vaginal dryness and hair thinning. Arimidex may also be associated with gastro-intestinal disturbances (anorexia, nausea, vomiting, and diarrhoea), asthenia, somnolence, headache or rash.

Vaginal bleeding has been reported infrequently, mainly in patients during the first few weeks after changing from existing hormonal therapy to treatment with Arimidex. If bleeding persists, further evaluation should be considered.

A causal relationship between anastrozole and thromboembolic events is not established. In clinical trials the frequency of thromboembolic events was not significantly different between anastrozole 1 mg and megestrol acetate, although the incidence with anastrozole 10 mg was lower.

Hepatic changes (elevated gamma-GT or less commonly alkaline phosphatase) have been reported in patients with advanced breast cancer, many of whom had liver and/or bone metastases. A causal relationship for these changes has not been established. Slight increases in total cholesterol have also been observed in clinical trials with Arimidex.

*Overdose:* There is no clinical experience of accidental overdosage. In animal studies, anastrozole demonstrated low acute toxicity. Clinical trials have been conducted with various dosages of Arimidex, up to 60 mg in a single dose given to healthy male volunteers and up to 10 mg daily given to post-menopausal women with advanced breast cancer; these dosages were well tolerated. A single dose of Arimidex that results in life-threatening symptoms has not been established. There is no specific antidote to overdosage and treatment must be symptomatic.

In the management of an overdose, consideration should be given to the possibility that multiple agents may have been taken. Vomiting may be induced if the patient is alert. Dialysis may be helpful because Arimidex is not highly protein bound. General supportive care, including frequent monitoring of vital signs and close observation of the patient, is indicated.

**Pharmacological properties**

*Pharmacodynamic properties:* Arimidex is a potent and highly selective non-steroidal aromatose inhibitor. In post-menopausal women, oestradiol is produced primarily from the conversion of androstenedione to oestrone through the aromatase enzyme complex in peripheral tissues. Oestrone is subsequently converted to oestradiol. Reducing circulating oestradiol levels has been shown to produce a beneficial effect in women with breast cancer. In post-menopausal women, Arimidex at a daily dose of 1 mg produced oestradiol suppression of greater than 80% using a highly sensitive assay.

In controlled clinical trials, Arimidex at the daily dose of 1 mg has demonstrated comparable clinical efficacy to a standard hormonal treatment with megestrol acetate.

Arimidex does not possess any progestogenic, androgenic or oestrogenic activity.

Daily doses of Arimidex up to 10 mg do not have any effect on cortisol or aldosterone secretion, measured before or after standard ACTH challenge testing. Corticoid supplements are therefore not needed.

*Pharmacokinetic properties:* Absorption of anastrozole is rapid and maximum plasma concentrations typically occur within two hours of dosing (under fasted conditions). Anastrozole is eliminated slowly with a plasma elimination half-life of 40 to 50 hours. Food slightly decreases the rate but not the extent of absorption. The small change in the rate of absorption is not expected to result in a clinically significant effect on steady-state plasma concentrations during once daily dosing of Arimidex tablets. Approximately 90 to 95% of plasma anastrozole steady-state concentrations are attained after 7 daily doses. There is no evidence of time or dose-dependency of anastrozole pharmacokinetic parameters.

Anastrozole pharmacokinetics are independent of age in post-menopausal women.

Pharmacokinetics have not been studied in children.

Anastrozole is only 40% bound to plasma proteins.

Anastrozole is extensively metabolised by post-menopausal women less than 10% of the dose excreted in the urine unchanged within 72 hours of dosing. Metabolism of anastrozole occurs by N-dealkylation, hydroxylation and glucuronidation. The metabolites are excreted primarily via the urine. Triazole, the major metabolite in plasma, does not inhibit aromatase.

The apparent oral clearance of anastrozole in volunteers with stable hepatic cirrhosis or renal impairment was in the range observed in healthy volunteers.

*Preclinical safety data:*

*Acute toxicity:* In acute toxicity studies in rodents the median lethal dose of anastrozole was greater than 100 mg/kg/day by the oral route and greater than 50 mg/kg/day by the intraperitoneal route.

*Chronic toxicity:* Multiple dose toxicity studies utilised rats and dogs. No no-effect levels were established for anastrozole in the toxicity studies, but those effects that were observed at the low doses (1 mg/kg/day) and mid doses (dog 3 mg/kg/day; rat 5 mg/kg/day) were related to either the pharmacological or enzyme inducing properties of anastrozole and were unaccompanied by toxic or degenerative changes.

*Mutagenicity:* Genetic toxicology studies with anastrozole show that it is not a mutagen or a clastogen.

*Reproductive toxicology:* Oral administration of anastrozole to pregnant rats and rabbits caused no teratogenic effects at doses up to 1.0 and 0.2 mg/kg/day respectively. Those effects that were seen (placental enlargement in rats and pregnancy failure in rabbits) were related to the pharmacology of the compound.

*Carcinogenicity:* No carcinogenicity studies have been conducted using anastrozole.

**Pharmaceutical particulars**

*List of excipients:* Lactose PhEur; Polyvidone PhEur; Sodium Starch Glycollate BP; Magnesium Stearate PhEur; Methylhydroxypropylcellulose PhEur; Macrogol 300 PhEur; Titanium Dioxide PhEur.

*Incompatibilities:* Nil.

*Shelf life:* The shelf life of Arimidex is 3 years when stored below 30°C.

*Special precautions for storage:* Nil.

*Nature and contents of container:* PVC blister/aluminium foil packs of 28 and 84 tablets contained in a carton.

*Instructions for use/handling:* Nil.

**Marketing authorisation number** 12619/0106.

**Date of approval/revision of SPC** December 1996.

**Legal category** POM.

## ATROMID*-S

**Qualitative and quantitative composition** Clofibrate PhEur 500 mg.

**Pharmaceutical form** Capsules.

**Clinical particulars**

*Therapeutic indications:* Atromid-S is indicated in the treatment of severe hyperlipoproteinaemia where full investigation has been performed to define the abnormality. It should be used in conjunction with appropriate dietary measures and after diet alone has failed to produce an adequate response. Other risk factors such as hypertension and smoking should be dealt with. Examples of abnormal lipid patterns are:

| Frederickson type | Lipoprotein elevated | Major lipid elevations |
|---|---|---|
| I (very rare) | Chylomicrons | Triglycerides |
| IIa | β(LDL) | Cholesterol |
| IIb | pre-β+β (LDL+VLDL) | Cholesterol+ Triglycerides |
| III (rare) | abnormal β(LDL) | Chol.+TG |
| IV | pre-β(VLDL) | Triglycerides |
| V (rare) | Chylomicrons +pre-β(VLDL) | Triglycerides+ Cholesterol |

Atromid-S is effective in patients with Type III hyperlipidaemia and in patients with severe hypertriglyceridaemia found in some patients in Types IIB, IV and V.

*Posology and method of administration:*
*Route of administration:* Oral.

*Adults:* A dose of 20–30 mg/kg body weight is given daily. This should be divided into 2 or 3 doses after meals. The effective dose level must be maintained. Examples of dosage:

Patients over 65 kg: 2 g daily (4 x 500 mg capsules).
Patients 50–65 kg: 1.5 g daily (3 x 500 mg capsules).

The biochemical response to clofibrate is variable and it is not always possible to predict from lipoprotein type or other factors which patients will obtain favourable results. It is essential that lipid levels be measured and that the drug be discontinued in any patient in whom lipids do not show significant improvement within three months of initiating therapy.

*Children:* Atromid-S would not normally be given to children, but if it were necessary, the dosage should be calculated from body weight (20–30 mg/kg).

*Elderly patients:* There are no special dosage recommendations for the elderly, but it may be advisable to monitor elderly patients so that optimum dosage can be individually determined.

*Contra-indications:* The significance of the rise in maternal cholesterol levels during late pregnancy is unclear. Similarly, the effect of Atromid-S, which is present in breast milk, on the infant has not been studied. Because of this, Atromid-S should not be given during pregnancy or lactation.

Atromid-S is contraindicated in patients with acute impairment of renal, biliary or hepatic function.

Because of its effect on cholesterol metabolism, Atromid-S may increase the lithogenicity of bile and raise the frequency of gallstone formation. Accordingly, Atromid-S should not be used in patients with a history of, or existing, gall bladder disease or stones.

*Special warnings and special precautions for use:* In patients with low serum albumin levels, for example those with nephrotic syndrome, high levels of unbound drug may give rise to myalgia with increased creatinine kinase levels. Such patients must be treated with caution.

*Interactions with other medicaments and other forms of interaction:* Atromid-S displaces the oral anticoagulants from protein binding sites and this potentiates their activity. Patients receiving anticoagulants should have their dosage halved when treated with Atromid-S. The anticoagulant dose can be adjusted later if necessary.

Atromid-S may also displace other acidic drugs, such as phenytoin or sulphonylureas eg tolbutamide, from protein binding sites and thereby potentiate the effect of such drugs.

*Pregnancy and lactation:* The significance of the rise in maternal cholesterol levels during late pregnancy is unclear. Similarly, the effect of Atromid-S, which is present in breast milk, on the infant has not been studied. Because of this, Atromid-S should not be given during pregnancy or lactation.

*Effect on ability to drive and use machines:* Clofibrate does not enter the Central Nervous System and therefore Atromid-S is unlikely to have any effect on the ability to drive or operate machinery.

*Undesirable effects:* Clofibrate has been shown to produce liver tumours in rats and mice. The liver changes found in rodents have not been seen in other species, including sub-human primates and man. The relevance of this finding to man has not been established.

Side effects are seldom seen but include transient slight upper abdominal discomfort, nausea and looseness of the bowels and impotence. It is usually unnecessary to discontinue treatment. Infrequently headache, fatigue, drowsiness, skin rashes, pruritus, alopecia and weight gain have been reported. Rarely dizziness, cardiac arrhythmia and a myositis-like syndrome comprising myalgia, myopathy, muscle cramps and sometimes rhabdomyolysis have been reported. Patients who develop signs of muscle toxicity should be monitored closely and CPK levels checked. Treatment with Atromid-S should be stopped if myopathy is suspected or if CPK rises to ≥ 10 times the upper limit of normal. The risk of serious muscle toxicity is increased if Atromid-S is used concomitantly with HMG-CoA reductase inhibitors or other fibrates. Combination therapy should be used with caution and patients monitored closely for signs of muscle toxicity. Due to its action on bile there is an increased incidence of gallstones.

At therapeutic doses Atromid-S does not enter the liver cell. In some cases slight and usually transient increases in serum transaminase levels have been observed. It is considered that these reflect adaptive responses of the liver. In large, long term studies, even transient increases in transaminase levels have seldom been reported. Atromid-S has not been shown to affect serum bilirubin or bromosulphthalein tests. Very occasional liver dysfunction and hepatomegaly have been reported. Serial liver biopsy studies in patients undergoing long-term treatment have confirmed the absence of hepatotoxicity in man. The liver changes found in rodents are species specific and are not seen in the human.

Atromid-S normally has no effect on the blood parameters. Isolated cases of adverse effects include slight fluctuation in haemoglobin values and occasional reduction in white cell counts. Agranulocytosis and neutropenia have been reported extremely rarely in patients with other predisposing factors who were concurrently receiving Atromid-S.

*Overdose:* No adverse biochemical or clinical effects have been observed upon overdosage with Atromid-S, but should these occur, symptomatic treatment should be administered.

**Pharmacological properties**

*Pharmacodynamic properties:* Atromid-S is a lipid lowering drug, being a member of the fibric acid class of hypolipidaemic agents. It lowers serum cholesterol and triglyceride levels by reducing very low density lipoprotein (VLDL) and low-density lipoprotein (LDL). It also increases high density lipoprotein (HDL).

*Pharmacokinetic properties:* Atromid-S is readily absorbed following oral dosage and is hydrolysed to the active acid. The plasma half-life is approximately 16 hours and the drug is excreted via the kidneys. In patients with renal failure the half-life may increase to 60–190 hours. Some 91–97% is bound to serum albumin, and may displace other similarly bound drugs. The volume of distribution is 5-9 litres; none enters the cerebrospinal fluid. Concomitant administration of cholestyramine does not impair absorption of Atromid-S.

*Pre-clinical safety data*: The liver changes found in rodents are species specific and are not seen in the human.

Clofibrate is a drug on which extensive clinical experience has been obtained. All relevant information for the prescriber is provided elsewhere in the Prescribing Information.

**Pharmaceutical particulars**

*List of excipients:* Gelatin PhEur; Glycerol PhEur; Ponceau 4R (E124); Purified Water; Sodium Ethyl Hydroxybenzoate; Sodium Propyl Hydroxybenzoate BP.

*Incompatibilities:* See *Interactions.*

*Shelf life:* 5 years.

*Special precautions for storage*: Store below 25°C. Protect from light and moisture.

*Nature and contents of container*: HDPE bottle, with plastic screw cap, containing 100 capsules.

*Instructions for use/handling:* Not applicable.

**Marketing authorisation number** 12619/0001.

**Date of approval/revision of SPC** April 1996

**Legal category** POM

## AVLOCLOR* TABLETS

**Qualitative and quantitative composition** Tablets containing 250 mg chloroquine phosphate which is equivalent to 155 mg chloroquine base.

**Pharmaceutical form** Tablets.

**Clinical particulars**

*Therapeutic indications*

(a) Treatment of malaria.
(b) Prophylaxis and suppression of malaria.
(c) Treatment of amoebic hepatitis and abscess.
(d) Treatment of discoid and systemic lupus erythematosus.
(e) Treatment of rheumatoid arthritis.

*Posology and method of administration* The dose should be taken after food.

*(a) Treatment of malaria*

*P. falciparum and P. malariae infections*

*Adults:* A single dose of four tablets, followed by two tablets six hours later and then two tablets a day for two days.

*Children:* A single dose of 10 mg base/kg, followed by 5 mg base/kg six hours later and then 5 mg base/kg a day for two days.

| Age (years) | Initial dose | Second dose 6 hrs after first | Dose on each of the two subsequent days |
|---|---|---|---|
| 1–4 | 1 tablet | ½ tablet | ½ tablet |
| 5–8 | 2 tablets | 1 tablet | 1 tablet |
| 9–14 | 3 tablets | 1½ tablets | 1½ tablets |

*P. vivax and P. ovale infections*

*Adults:* A single dose of four tablets, followed by two tablets six hours later and then two tablets a day for two days. Follow with a course of treatment with primaquine if a radical cure is required.

*Children:* A single dose of 10 mg base/kg, followed by 5 mg base/kg six hours later and then 5 mg base/kg a day for two days. Follow with a course of treatment with primaquine if a radical cure is required.

*Elderly patients:* There are no special dosage recommendations for the elderly, but it may be advisable to monitor elderly patients so that optimum dosage can be individually determined.

*Hepatic or renally impaired patients:* Caution is necessary when giving Avloclor to patients with renal disease or hepatic disease.

*(b) Prophylaxis and suppression of malaria*

*Adults:* Two tablets taken once a week, on the same day each week. Start one week before exposure to risk and continue until four weeks after leaving the malarious area.

*Children:* A single dose of 5 mg chloroquine base/kg per week on the same day each week. Start one week before exposure to risk and continue until four weeks after leaving the malarious area.

For practical purposes, children aged over 14 years may be treated as adults. The dose given to infants and children should be calculated on their body weight and must not exceed the adult dose regardless of weight.

1–4 years: ½ tablet
5–8 years: 1 tablet
9–14 years: 1½ tablets

*Elderly patients:* There are no special dosage recommendations for the elderly, but it may be advisable to monitor elderly patients so that optimum dosage can be individually determined.

*Hepatic or renally impaired patients:* Caution is necessary when giving Avloclor to patients with renal disease or hepatic disease.

*(c) Amoebic hepatitis*

*Adults:* Four tablets daily for two days followed by one tablet twice daily for two or three weeks.

*Elderly patients:* There are no special dosage recommendations for the elderly, but it may be advisable to monitor elderly patients so that optimum dosage can be individually determined.

*Hepatic or renally impaired patients*: Caution is necessary when giving Avloclor to patients with renal disease or hepatic disease.

*(d) Lupus erythematosus*

*Adults:* One tablet twice daily for one to two weeks followed by a maintenance dosage of one tablet daily.

*Elderly patients:* There are no special dosage recommendations for the elderly, but it may be advisable to monitor elderly patients so that optimum dosage can be individually determined.

*Hepatic or renally impaired patients:* Caution is necessary when giving Avloclor to patients with renal disease or hepatic disease.

*(e) Rheumatoid arthritis*

*Adults:* The usual dosage is one tablet daily.

*Elderly patients:* There are no special dosage recommendations for the elderly, but it may be advisable to monitor elderly patients so that optimum dosage can be individually determined.

*Hepatic or renally impaired patients:* Caution is necessary when giving Avloclor to patients with renal disease or hepatic disease.

*Contra-indications*: There are no absolute contra-indications to the use of Avloclor.

*Warnings and precautions for use:* In any locality where drug resistant malaria is known or suspected it is essential to take professional advice on what prophylactic regimen or treatment regimen is appropriate.

Caution is necessary when giving Avloclor to patients with impaired hepatic function, particularly when associated with cirrhosis. Caution is also necessary in patients with porphyria. Avloclor may precipitate severe constitutional symptoms and an increase in the amount of porphyrins excreted in the urine. This reaction is especially apparent in patients with high alcohol intake.

Caution is necessary when giving Avloclor to patients with renal disease.

Avloclor should be used with care in patients with a history of epilepsy.

Prolonged therapy with high doses may lead to ccasional development of irreversible retinal damge.

Considerable caution is needed in the use of vloclor for long-term high dosage therapy and such se should only be considered when no other drug is vailable.

Patients receiving Avloclor continuously at higher ose levels for periods longer than 12 months should ndergo ophthalmic examination before treatment nd at three monthly intervals. This also applies to atients receiving Avloclor at weekly intervals for a eriod of more than 3 years as a prophylactic against alarial attacks or if the total consumption exceeds .6 g/kg.

Full blood counts should be carried out regularly uring extended treatment as bone marrow suppreson may occur rarely.

The use of Avloclor in patients with psoriasis may recipitate a severe attack.

*teractions with other medicaments and other forms f interaction:* None have been reported or are known.

*regnancy and lactation:*

*regnancy:* Pregnancy increases the risks from maria. As with all drugs, the use of Avloclor during regnancy should be avoided if possible unless, in e case of life threatening infections, in the judgement f the physician, potential benefit outweighs the risk. here is evidence to suggest that Avloclor given to omen in high doses throughout pregnancy can give se to foetal abnormalities including ocular or cochar damage.

*Lactation:* Although Avloclor is excreted in breast ilk, the amount is insufficient to confer any benefit n the infant. Separate chemoprophylaxis for the nfant is required.

*ffect on ability to drive and use machinery:* Defects visual accommodation may occur on first taking vloclor and patients should be warned regarding riving or operating machinery.

*ossible adverse reactions:* The adverse reactions hich may occur at doses used in the prophylaxis or eatment of malaria are generally not of a serious ature. Where prolonged high dosage is required, ie the treatment of rheumatoid arthritis, adverse eactions can be of a more serious nature.

Adverse reactions reported after Avloclor use are: eadache, gastro-intestinal disturbances, skin erupons, pruritus, occasional depigmentation or loss of air, difficulty in accommodation, blurring of vision, orneal opacities, retinal degeneration, electrocardioraphic changes, neurological and psychiatric hanges, including convulsions and psychosis, thromocytopenia, agranulocytosis, aplastic anaemia, allerc reactions, erythema multiforme, Stevens-Johnson yndrome, cardiomyopathy.

Changes in liver function, including hepatitis and bnormal liver function tests, have been reported arely.

*verdose:* Chloroquine is highly toxic in overdose nd children are particularly susceptible. The chief ymptoms of overdosage include circulatory collapse ue to a potent cardiotoxic effect, respiratory arrest nd coma. Symptoms may progress rapidly after itial nausea and vomiting. Cardiac complications ay occur without progressively deepening coma.

Death may result from circulatory or respiratory ailure or cardiac arrhythmia. If there is no demonstrale cardiac output due to arrhythmias, asystole or lectromechanical dissociation, external chest comression should be persisted with for as long as ecessary, or until adrenaline and diazepam can be iven (see below).

Gastric lavage should be carried out urgently, first rotecting the airway and instituting artificial ventilaon where necessary. There is a risk of cardiac arrest ollowing aspiration of gastric contents in more erious cases. Activated charcoal left in the stomach ay reduce absorption of any remaining chloroquine om the gut. Circulatory status (with central venous ressure measurement), respiration, plasma electroytes and blood gases should be monitored, with orrection of hypokalaemia and acidosis if indicated. ardiac arrhythmias should not be treated unless life reatening; drugs with quinidine-like effects should e avoided. Intravenous sodium bicarbonate 1-mmol/kg over 15 minutes may be effective in conuction disturbances, and DC shock is indicated for entricular tachycardia and ventricular fibrillation.

Early administration of the following has been hown to improve survival in cases of serious poisonng:

1. Adrenaline infusion 0.25 micrograms/kg/min inially, with increments of 0.25 micrograms/kg/min ntil adequate systolic blood pressure (more than 00 mm/Hg) is restored; adrenaline reduces the effects f chloroquine on the heart through its inotropic and asoconstrictor effects.

2. Diazepam infusion (2 mg/kg over 30 minutes as a loading dose, followed by 1-2 mg/kg/day for up to 2-4 days). Diazepam may minimise cardiotoxicity.

Acidification of the urine, haemodialysis, peritoneal dialysis or exchange transfusion have not been shown to be of value in treating chloroquine poisoning. Chloroquine is excreted very slowly, therefore cases of overdosage require observation for several days.

**Pharmacological properties**

*Pharmacodynamic properties:* The mode of action of chloroquine on plasmodia has not been fully elucidated. Chloroquine binds to and alters the properties of DNA. Chloroquine also binds to ferriprotoporphyrin IX and this leads to lysis of the plasmodial membrane.

In suppressive treatment, chloroquine inhibits the erythrocytic stage of development of plasmodia. In acute attacks of malaria, it interrupts erythrocytic schizogony of the parasite. Its ability to concentrate in parasitised erythrocytes may account for the selective toxicity against the erythrocytic stages of plasmodial infection.

*Pharmacokinetic properties:* Studies in volunteers using single doses of chloroquine phosphate equivalent to 300 mg base have found peak plasma levels to be achieved within one to six hours. These levels are in the region of 54-102 microgram/litre, the concentration in erythrocytes being some 4.8 times higher. The elimination half-life of chloroquine is dose dependent and is approximately one hundred hours. Following a single dose, chloroquine may be detected in plasma for more than four weeks. Mean bioavailability from tablets of chloroquine phosphate is 89%. Chloroquine is widely distributed in body tissues such as the eyes, kidneys, liver, and lungs where retention is prolonged.

The principal metabolite is monodesethylchloroquine, which reaches a peak concentration of 10-20 microgram/litre within a few hours. Mean urinary recovery, within 3-13 weeks, is approximately 50% of the administered dose, most being unchanged drug and the remainder as metabolite. Chloroquine may be detected in urine for several months.

*Pre-clinical safety data*

Avloclor has been widely used for many years in clinical practice. There is no animal data which adds significant information relevant to the prescriber, to that covered elsewhere in this document.

**Pharmaceutical particulars**

*List of excipients:* Magnesium stearate PhEur; Maize starch PhEur.

*Incompatibilities:* None have been reported or are known.

*Shelf life:* 5 years.

*Special precautions for storage:* Store below 30°C. Protect from light and moisture.

*Nature and contents of container:* HDPE bottle of 100's and PVC/Aluminium Foil Blister Pack of 20's

*Instructions for use/handling:* No special instructions.

**Marketing authorisation number** 12619/0002

**Date of approval/revision of SPC** October 1996

**Legal category** POM.

P. for prevention of malaria.

## CASODEX* TABLETS 50 mg ▼

**Qualitative and quantitative composition** Each tablet contains 50 mg bicalutamide (INN)

**Pharmaceutical form** White film-coated tablet

**Clinical particulars**

*Therapeutic indication:* Treatment of advanced prostate cancer in combination with LHRH analogue therapy or surgical castration.

*Posology and method of administration:*

*Adult males including the elderly:* One tablet (50 mg) once a day.

Treatment with Casodex should be started at least 3 days before commencing treatment with an LHRH analogue, or at the same time as surgical castration.

*Children:* Casodex is contra-indicated in children.

*Renal impairment:* no dosage adjustment is necessary for patients with renal impairment.

*Hepatic impairment:* no dosage adjustment is necessary for patients with mild hepatic impairment. Increased accumulation may occur in patients with moderate to severe hepatic impairment (see *Special warnings and special precautions for use*).

*Contra-indications:* Casodex is contra-indicated in females and children.

Casodex must not be given to any patient who has shown a hypersensitivity reaction to its use.

*Special warnings and special precautions for use:* Casodex is extensively metabolised in the liver. Data suggests that its elimination may be slower in subjects with severe hepatic impairment and this could lead to some accumulation of Casodex. Therefore, Casodex should be used with caution in patients with moderate to severe hepatic impairment.

*Interaction with other medicaments and other forms of interaction:* There is no evidence of any pharmacodynamic or pharmacokinetic interactions between Casodex and LHRH analogues.

Although Casodex does not appear to interact with commonly co-prescribed drugs, formal interaction studies have not been undertaken. Therefore caution should be exercised when prescribing Casodex with other drugs which may inhibit drug oxidation e.g. cimetidine and ketoconazole. In theory, this could result in increased plasma concentrations of Casodex which theoretically could lead to an increase in side effects.

Casodex has shown no evidence of causing enzyme induction during dosing up to 150 mg daily.

In vitro studies have shown that Casodex can displace the coumarin anticoagulant, warfarin, from its protein binding sites. It is therefore recommended that if Casodex is started in patients who are already receiving coumarin anticoagulants, prothrombin time should be closely monitored.

*Pregnancy and lactation:* Casodex is contra-indicated in females and must not be given to pregnant women or nursing mothers.

*Effects on ability to drive and use machines:* Casodex is unlikely to impair the ability of patients to drive or operate machinery. However, it should be noted that occasionally somnolence may occur. Any affected patients should exercise caution.

*Undesirable effects:* Casodex in general, has been well tolerated with few withdrawals due to adverse events.

The pharmacological action of Casodex may give rise to certain expected effects. These include hot flushes, pruritus and in addition, breast tenderness and gynaecomastia which may be reduced by concomitant castration. Casodex may also be associated with the occurrence of diarrhoea, nausea, vomiting, asthenia and dry skin.

Hepatic changes (elevated levels of transaminases, cholestasis and jaundice) have been observed in clinical trials with Casodex. The changes were frequently transient, resolving or improving despite continued therapy or following cessation of therapy. Hepatic failure has occurred very rarely in patients treated with Casodex, but a causal relationship has not been established with certainty. Periodic liver function testing should be considered.

Rare cardiovascular effects such as angina, heart failure, conduction defects including PR and QT interval prolongations, arrhythmias and non-specific ECG changes have been observed.

Thrombocytopenia has been reported rarely.

In addition, the following adverse experiences were reported in clinical trials (as possible adverse drug reactions in the opinion of investigating clinicians, with a frequency of ≥ 1%) during treatment with Casodex plus an LHRH analogue. No causal relationship of these experiences to drug treatment has been made and some of the experiences reported are those that commonly occur in elderly patients:

Cardiovascular system: heart failure.

Gastrointestinal system: anorexia, dry mouth, dyspepsia, constipation, flatulence.

Central nervous system: dizziness, insomnia, somnolence, decreased libido.

Respiratory system: dyspnoea.

Urogenital: impotence, nocturia.

Haematological : anaemia.

Skin and appendages: alopecia, rash, sweating, hirsutism.

Metabolic and nutritional: diabetes mellitus, hyperglycaemia, oedema, weight gain, weight loss.

Whole body: abdominal pain, chest pain, headache, pain, pelvic pain, chills.

*Overdose:* There is no human experience of overdosage. There is no specific antidote; treatment should be symptomatic. Dialysis may not be helpful, since Casodex is highly protein bound and is not recovered unchanged in the urine. General supportive care, including frequent monitoring of vital signs, is indicated.

**Pharmacological properties**

*Pharmacodynamic properties:* Casodex is a non-steroidal anti-androgen, devoid of other endocrine activity. It binds to androgen receptors without activating gene expression, and thus inhibits the androgen stimulus. Regression of prostatic tumours results from this inhibition.

Casodex is a racemate with its antiandrogenic activity being almost exclusively in the (R)-enantiomer.

*Pharmacokinetic properties:* Casodex is well absorbed following oral administration. There is no evidence of any clinically relevant effect of food on bioavailability.

The (S)-enantiomer is rapidly cleared relative to the

(R)-enantiomer, the latter having a plasma elimination half-life of about 1 week.

On daily administration of Casodex, the (R)-enantiomer accumulates about 10 fold in plasma as a consequence of its long half-life.

Steady state plasma concentrations of the (R)-enantiomer of approximately 9 µg per ml are observed during daily administration of 50 mg doses of Casodex. At steady state the predominantly active (R)-enantiomer accounts for 99% of the total circulating enantiomers.

The pharmacokinetics of the (R)-enantiomer are unaffected by age, renal impairment or mild to moderate hepatic impairment. There is evidence that for subjects with severe hepatic impairment, the (R)-enantiomer is more slowly eliminated from plasma.

Casodex is highly protein bound (96%) and extensively metabolised (via oxidation and glucuronidation): Its metabolites are eliminated via the kidneys and bile in approximately equal proportions.

*Preclinical safety data*: Casodex is a potent antiandrogen and a mixed function oxidase enzyme inducer in animals. Target organ changes, including tumour induction, in animals, are related to these activities. None of the findings in the preclinical testing is considered to have relevance to the treatment of advanced prostate cancer patients.

**Pharmaceutical particulars**
*List of excipients:* Casodex includes the following excipients: Lactose PhEur; Magnesium Stearate PhEur; Methylhydroxypropylcellulose PhEur; Polyethylene Glycol 300 PhEur; Polyvidone PhEur; Sodium Starch Glycollate BP; Titanium Dioxide PhEur.

*Incompatibilities:* None known.

*Shelf life:* 3 years

*Special precautions for storage:* Store below 30°C

*Nature and contents of container:* PVC blister/aluminium foil packs.

*Instructions for use/handling:* No special precautions required.

**Marketing authorisation number** 12619/0102

**Date of apporval/revision of SPC** March 1996

**Legal category** POM

## CETAVLEX* CREAM

**Presentation** A white water-miscible cream containing 0.5% w/w cetrimide (incorporated as Strong Cetrimide Solution BP). Inactive ingredients are cetostearyl alcohol, liquid paraffin, methylparahydroxybenzoate, propylparahydroxybenzoate and water.

**Uses** Cetavlex is an antiseptic cream for skin disorders such as minor wounds, burns, abrasions and napkin rash.

*Mode of action:* Studies with cetrimide have shown it to be active against a wide range of vegetative bacteria, both Gram positive and Gram negative, including *Staph. aureus* the commonest cause of infection in wounds and burns. Certain Gram negative bacteria, particularly strains of *Pseudomonas* and *Proteus* remain the least susceptible of the pathogenic bacteria to cetrimide, requiring a higher concentration than other species to produce an effective kill.

Cetrimide is cationic in nature, binding strongly to skin and other tissue, and thus absorption is negligible.

**Dosage and administration** Apply liberally to the affected area. In some cases it may be necessary to cover the wound or burn with a clean dressing.

**Contra-indications, warnings, etc** Cetavlex is contra-indicated for patients who have previously shown a hypersensitivity reaction to cetrimide preparations.

For topical application only. Keep out of the eyes and ears.

*Side-effects:* Irritative skin reactions can occasionally occur. Hypersensitivity to cetrimide preparations has been reported, usually developing after repeated applications, but is rare. Should such a reaction occur stop application of the product.

*Accidental ingestion:* The toxicity of Cetavlex arises from the content of cetrimide. It seems unlikely that systemic toxicity will occur from accidental ingestion of the cream. However, in the event of large quantities being swallowed carry out gastric lavage with milk, raw egg, gelatin or mild soap. Do not induce vomiting.

Central paralysis cannot be countered by curare antagonists or CNS stimulants but sympathomimetic drugs have been given.

Mechanically assisted ventilation with oxygen may be necessary. Persistent convulsions may be controlled with cautious doses of diazepam or a short-acting barbiturate. Do not give alcohol in any form.

**Pharmaceutical precautions** Store below 30°C and use undiluted. Cetrimide is incompatible with soap and other anionic agents.

**Legal category** GSL.

**Package quantities** Tubes of 50 g (OP).

**Further information** Nil.

**Product licence number** 12619/0003.

## CORWIN*

**Presentation** Corwin tablets containing xamoterol fumarate equivalent to 200 mg xamoterol are round, biconvex, dark yellow, film coated tablets impressed with 'CORWIN' on one face and with an 'S' logo on the reverse. The impressions are highlighted in white. The inactive ingredients are calcium phosphate, gelatin, iron oxide, lactose, macrogol, magnesium carbonate, magnesium stearate, methylhydroxypropylcellulose, sodium starch glycollate and titanium dioxide.

**Uses** Chronic mild heart failure: Corwin is recommended for the treatment of patients who are not breathless at rest but who are limited by symptoms on exertion (eg breathlessness and fatigue). Treatment with Corwin should be initiated under hospital supervision only after the patient has been fully assessed [see 'Initiation of treatment' below]. After initiation of treatment the appropriate follow-up should be provided by hospital or general practitioners.

Corwin is contra-indicated in patients with moderate to severe heart failure. Some patients with moderate to severe heart failure have shown deterioration on Corwin. See 'Contra-indications' below.

*Mode of action:* Corwin is a beta$_1$-selective partial agonist. At rest and under conditions of low sympathetic drive Corwin acts predominantly as a beta adrenoceptor agonist. On exercise and under conditions of increased sympathetic drive, eg severe heart failure, Corwin acts as a beta adrenoceptor antagonist. In mild heart failure, Corwin improves cardiac efficiency by modestly increasing myocardial contractility, improving diastolic relaxation and lowering left ventricular filling pressure. The improved ventricular function results in increased cardiac output with no attendant increase in myocardial oxygen demand. This improvement in myocardial performance is maintained on exercise.

Many heart failure patients suffer from concomitant ischaemic heart disease. In patients with angina pectoris, a reduction in myocardial ischaemia on exercise has been demonstrated with Corwin at the dose levels recommended for heart failure.

**Dosage and administration**
*Adults:* Treatment should be started with 200 mg once a day for a week; dosage should then be increased to 200 mg twice daily provided that there are no adverse effects. The usual effective dose is 200 mg twice daily (but see renal impairment warning below). Improvement in symptoms of heart failure (eg dyspnoea, fatigue) may be progressive over a period of several weeks.

*Elderly patients:* No specific dosage reduction is necessary except in those with suspected or established renal impairment (see below).

*Initiation of treatment:* Treatment should be initiated under hospital supervision after full assessment of the patient who has completed an exercise test which excludes diagnosis of moderate or severe heart failure. In addition to other exclusion criteria under 'Contra-indications' and depending on the method used, the patient should be able to complete one of the following exercise tests (equivalent to 3.6 kilojoules).

- For a bicycle ergometer; two minutes of exercise starting with a load of 20 W for the first minute and at a load of 40 W for the second minute.
- For an exercise treadmill; two minutes of exercise at a treadmill speed of 4 km/h with the treadmill level (ie 0% incline).
- For a corridor walk test; 150 yards on the level in two minutes.
- Alternatively, any other standardised exercise test in which the patient achieves a basal workload equivalent to one of the tests defined above (equivalent to 3.6 kilojoules).

Patients who are unable to complete the minimum of two minutes exercise on the bicycle ergometer or equivalent should not be given Corwin. Assessment of the patient's heart failure status should also include such tests as an ECG and a chest X-ray. Additional investigations such as an echocardiogram may be necessary.

*Children:* There is no paediatric experience with Corwin and for this reason it is not recommended for use in children.

**Contra-indications, warnings, etc**
*Contra-indications:* Corwin is contra-indicated in p tients with moderate to severe heart failure becau some patients with moderate to severe heart failu have shown deterioration on Corwin.

Corwin should, therefore, not be used in patie with the following features:

- Those who are short of breath or fatigued at rest limited on minimal exercise.
- Those who have a resting tachycardia (>90 bea per minute) or hypotension (systo BP<100 mmHg).
- Those who present with acute pulmonary oeder or who have a history of repeated episodes of acu pulmonary oedema.
- Those with peripheral oedema, a raised jugul venous pressure, an enlarged liver or a third hea sound.
- Those who require treatment with doses of diureti in excess of frusemide 40 mg per day or equivale
- Those who require treatment with an ACE inhibit

*Precautions:* Deterioration of disease: Corwin shou be withdrawn from patients whose mild heart failu deteriorates whilst on the drug, for example, if t patient develops worsening symptoms (shortness breath and/or fatigue), diminishing effort toleranc or the appearance of signs such as peripheral oedem a raised jugular venous pressure, an enlarged liver a third heart sound. If Corwin is withdrawn, the patie should be carefully observed.

Renal impairment: Since Corwin is excreted by t kidneys, dosage should be adjusted in cases of seve impairment of renal function. No significant accum lation of Corwin occurs at a GFR greater than 35 n min/1.73 m². Significant accumulation of Corwin c curs only when GFR decreases to 15–35 ml/m 1.73 m². This level of renal impairment is usual clinically evident and approximates to a doubling the serum creatinine (eg greater than 250 micromc or 3 mg/dl). The dose of Corwin is 200 mg daily wh clinical evidence indicates suspected or establish renal impairment (approximate doubling of seru creatinine value or a GFR of 15–35 ml/min/1.73 m²).

Obstructive airways disease: Due to the beta adre oceptor antagonist effects of Corwin, an increase airways resistance may be provoked in patients wi asthma or chronic obstructive airways disease. such an event, Corwin should be withdrawn a increased airways resistance may be reversed by t use of inhaled bronchodilator preparations such salbutamol. Corwin should be used with caution patients with co-existing obstructive airways diseas

Liver function: Elevations of liver enzymes ha been reported rarely in patients receiving Corwin b in such cases no relationship to the drug has be established.

Aortic stenosis/hypertrophic obstructive cardiom opathy: As with other drugs which increase the for of myocardial contraction, Corwin should be us with caution in patients with outflow obstruction.

Cardiac arrhythmias: Cardiac arrhythmias are co mon in patients with heart failure. Occasional cas of ventricular arrhythmias have been reported duri Corwin therapy and, in some patients, Corwin cann be excluded as a contributory factor. Ambulato (Holter) ECG monitoring studies have not shown a evidence that Corwin therapy promotes arrhythmia In patients with atrial fibrillation, concurrent thera with a cardiac glycoside must be maintained.

*Pregnancy and lactation:* There is no evidence for t safety of the drug in human pregnancy. When hi doses of Corwin were given to rats and rabbits duri the second half of pregnancy, the cardiovascu effects of the drug led to deformations. It is recor mended, therefore, that administration of the drug avoided in pregnancy unless the condition its carries sufficient risks to the mother and foetus warrant use.

Studies in rats show that Corwin is excreted in t breast milk of lactating females. Its use in lactati women who are breast feeding should be avoided.

*Side-effects:* Rarely bronchospasm, worsening obstructive airways disease and hypotension ha been observed after introduction of Corwin.

Adverse experiences in controlled studies showe a small excess in incidence over placebo of gastroi testinal complaints, headache and dizziness.

Although there was also an apparent excess angina/chest pain such events are not uncommon ar are to be expected in heart failure patients. Oth controlled studies with Corwin in patients with angi pectoris showed reduced incidence of myocardi ischaemia during exercise.

Rash, palpitations and muscle cramp were al reported.

*Overdosage:* There is no experience of overdosa with Corwin. Effects are unlikely to be life threatenin symptomatic conservative management is recor mended.

**armaceutical precautions** Corwin tablets should stored at room temperature.

**gal category** POM.

**ckage quantities** Corwin tablets (200 mg) in cal-dar packs of 56 tablets (OP).

**rther information** Corwin should not be co-ministered with other beta$_1$ adrenoceptor agonists antagonists because of competition between these ugs and Corwin for the beta$_1$ adrenoceptor.

Corwin has been co-administered without evidence incompatibility with a range of other therapies luding thiazide and potassium-sparing diuretics, rdiac glycosides, warfarin, antiplatelet drugs and n-steroidal anti-inflammatory drugs.

**oduct licence number** 12619/0009.

## IPRIVAN* 1%

**esentation** White, aqueous and isotonic emulsion intravenous injection containing 10 mg propofol r 1 ml. The vehicle contains glycerol, purified egg osphatide, sodium hydroxide, soybean oil and ater.

**es** Diprivan 1% is a short-acting intravenous aesthetic agent suitable for induction and mainte-nce of general anaesthesia.

Diprivan 1% may also be used for sedation of ntilated patients receiving intensive care, for a riod of up to three days.

Diprivan 1% may also be used for sedation for rgical and diagnostic procedures.

*armacodynamic properties:* Propofol (2, 6-diisopro-lphenol) is a short-acting general anaesthetic agent th a rapid onset of action of approximately 30 conds. Recovery from anaesthesia is usually rapid. e mechanism of action, like all general anaesthetics, poorly understood.

n general, falls in mean arterial blood pressure and ght changes in heart rate are observed when privan 1% is administered for induction and main-nance of anaesthesia. However, the haemodynamic rameters normally remain relatively stable during aintenance and the incidence of untoward haemo-namic changes is low.

Although ventilatory depression can occur follow-administration of Diprivan 1%, any effects are alitatively similar to those of other intravenous aesthetic agents and are readily manageable in nical practice.

Diprivan 1% reduces cerebral blood flow, intracra-al pressure and cerebral metabolism. The reduction intracranial pressure is greater in patients with an evated baseline intracranial pressure.

Recovery from anaesthesia is usually rapid and ar headed with a low incidence of headache and st-operative nausea and vomiting.

In general, there is less post-operative nausea and miting following anaesthesia with Diprivan 1% than llowing anaesthesia with inhalational agents. There evidence that this may be related to a reduced netic potential of propofol.

Diprivan 1%, at the concentrations likely to occur nically, does not inhibit the synthesis of adrenocort-al hormones.

*armacokinetic properties:* The decline in propofol ncentrations following a bolus dose or following termination of an infusion can be described by a ree compartment open model with very rapid stribution (half-life 2 to 4 minutes) rapid elimination alf-life 30 to 60 minutes) and a slower final phase, presentative of redistribution of propofol from orly perfused tissue.

Propofol is extensively distributed and rapidly ared from the body (total body clearance 1.5 to 2 res/minute). Clearance occurs by metabolic proc-sses, mainly in the liver, to form inactive conjugates propofol and its corresponding quinol, which are creted in urine.

When Diprivan 1% is used to maintain anaesthesia, ood concentrations asymptotically approach the eady-state value for the given administration rate. e pharmacokinetics are linear over the recom-ended range of infusion rates of Diprivan 1%.

**osage and administration** For specific guidance lating to the administration of Diprivan 1% using e Diprifusor target controlled infusion (TCI) system, ich incorporates Diprifusor TCI Software, see Ad-nistration Section below. Such use is restricted to duction and maintenance of anaesthesia in adults. e Diprifusor TCI system is not recommended for e in ICU sedation or sedation for surgical and agnostic procedures, or in children.

*duction of general anaesthesia:*

*dults:* In unpremedicated and premedicated patients, s recommended that Diprivan 1% should be titrated oproximately 4 ml [40 mg] every 10 seconds in an erage healthy adult by bolus injection or infusion) against the response of the patient until the clinical signs show the onset of anaesthesia. Most adult patients aged less than 55 years are likely to require 1.5 to 2.5 mg/kg of Diprivan 1%. The total dose required can be reduced by lower rates of administra-tion [2 to 5 ml/min (20 to 50 mg/min)]. Over this age, the requirement will generally be less. In patients of ASA Grades 3 and 4, lower rates of administration should be used (approximately 2 ml [20 mg] every 10 seconds).

*Elderly patients:* Diprivan 1% should be titrated against the response of the patient. Patients over the age of about 55 years may require lower doses of Diprivan 1% for induction of anaesthesia.

*Children:* Diprivan 1% is not recommended for induction of anaesthesia in children less than 3 years of age.

When used to induce anaesthesia in children, it is recommended that Diprivan 1% be given slowly until the clinical signs show the onset of anaesthesia. The dose should be adjusted for age and/or weight. Most patients over 8 years of age are likely to require approximately 2.5 mg/kg of Diprivan 1% for induction of anaesthesia. Under this age the requirements may be more. Lower dosage is recommended for children of ASA grades 3 and 4.

Administration of Diprivan 1% by a Diprifusor TCI system is not recommended for induction of general anaesthesia in children.

*Maintenance of general anaesthesia:*

*Adults (including elderly patients):* Anaesthesia can be maintained by administering Diprivan 1% either by continuous infusion or by repeat bolus injections to prevent the clinical signs of light anaesthesia. Recov-ery from anaesthesia is typically rapid and it is therefore important to maintain Diprivan 1% admin-istration until the end of the procedure.

*Continuous infusion:* The required rate of adminis-tration varies considerably between patients, but rates in the region of 4 to 12 mg/kg/hr usually maintain satisfactory anaesthesia.

*Repeat bolus injections:* If a technique involving repeat bolus injections is used, increments of 25 mg (2.5 ml) to 50 mg (5.0 ml) may be given according to clinical need.

*Children:* Diprivan 1% is not recommended for maintenance of anaesthesia in children less than 3 years of age.

Anaesthesia can be maintained by administering Diprivan 1% by infusion or repeat bolus injection to prevent the clinical signs of light anaesthesia. The required rate of administration varies considerably between patients, but rates in the region of 9 to 15 mg/kg/hr usually achieve satisfactory anaesthesia.

Administration of Diprivan 1% by a Diprifusor TCI system is not recommended for maintenance of general anaesthesia in children.

*Sedation during intensive care*

*Adults (including elderly patients):* When used to provide sedation for ventilated patients undergoing intensive care, it is recommended that Diprivan 1% be given by continuous infusion. The infusion rate should be adjusted according to the depth of sedation required but rates in the region of 0.3 to 4.0 mg/kg/hr should achieve satisfactory sedation. Rates of infusion greater than 4.0 mg/kg/hr are not recommended. Diprivan 1% may be diluted with 5% Dextrose (see *Dilution and Co-administration table* below).

It is recommended that blood lipid levels be monitored should Diprivan 1% be administered to patients thought to be at particular risk of fat overload. Administration of Diprivan 1% should be adjusted appropriately if the monitoring indicates that fat is being inadequately cleared from the body. If the patient is receiving other intravenous lipid concur-rently, a reduction in quantity should be made in order to take account of the amount of lipid infused as part of the Diprivan 1% formulation; 1.0 ml of Diprivan 1% contains approximately 0.1 g of fat.

Administration of Diprivan 1% by a Diprifusor TCI system is not recommended for sedation during intensive care.

*Children:* Diprivan 1% is not recommended for sedation in children as safety and efficacy have not been demonstrated. Although no causal relationship has been established, serious adverse events (includ-ing fatalities) have been observed from spontaneous reports of unlicensed use. These events were seen most often in children with respiratory tract infections given doses in excess of those recommended for adults.

*Sedation for surgical and diagnostic procedures*

*Adults:* To provide sedation for surgical and diagnostic procedures, rates of administration should be indivi-dualised and titrated to clinical response.

Most patients will require 0.5 to 1 mg/kg over 1 to 5 minutes for onset of sedation.

Maintenance of sedation may be accomplished by titrating Diprivan 1% infusion to the desired level of sedation – most patients will require 1.5 to 4.5 mg/kg/hr. In addition to the infusion, bolus administration of 10 to 20 mg may be used if a rapid increase in the depth of sedation is required. In patients of ASA Grades 3 and 4 the rate of administration and dosage may need to be reduced.

Administration of Diprivan 1% by a Diprifusor TCI system is not recommended for sedation for surgical and diagnostic procedures.

*Elderly patients:* Diprivan 1% should be titrated against the response of the patient. Patients over the age of about 55 years may require lower doses of Diprivan 1% for sedation for surgical and diagnostic procedures.

*Children:* Diprivan 1% is not recommended for sedation in children as safety and efficacy have not been demonstrated.

*Administration:* Diprivan 1% has no analgesic prop-erties and therefore supplementary analgesic agents are generally required in addition to Diprivan 1%. Diprivan 1% has been used in association with spinal and epidural anaesthesia and with commonly used premedicants, neuromuscular blocking drugs, inha-lation agents and analgesic agents; no pharmacolog-ical incompatibility has been encountered. Lower doses of Diprivan 1% may be required where general anaesthesia is used as an adjunct to regional anaes-thetic techniques.

Diprivan 1% can be used for infusion undiluted from glass containers, plastic syringes or Diprivan 1% pre-filled syringes or diluted with 5% Dextrose (Intra-venous Infusion BP) only, in PVC infusion bags or glass infusion bottles. Dilutions, which must not exceed 1 in 5 (2 mg propofol per ml) should be prepared aseptically immediately before administra-tion and must be used within 6 hours of preparation.

It is recommended that, when using diluted Diprivan 1% the volume of 5% Dextrose removed from the infusion bag during the dilution process is totally replaced in volume by Diprivan 1% emulsion (see *Dilution and Co-administration table* below).

The dilution may be used with a variety of infusion control techniques, but a giving set used alone will not avoid the risk of accidental uncontrolled infusion of large volumes of diluted Diprivan 1%. A burette, drop counter or volumetric pump must be included in the infusion line. The risk of uncontrolled infusion must be taken into account when deciding the maximum amount of Diprivan 1% in the burette.

When Diprivan 1% is used undiluted to maintain anaesthesia, it is recommended that equipment such as syringe pumps or volumetric infusion pumps should always be used to control infusion rates.

Diprivan 1% may be administered via a Y-piece close to the injection site, into infusions of Dextrose 5% Intravenous Infusion BP, Sodium Chloride 0.9% Intravenous Infusion BP or Dextrose 4% with Sodium Chloride 0.18% Intravenous Infusion BP.

The glass pre-filled syringe (PFS) has a lower frictional resistance than plastic disposable syringes and operates more easily. Therefore, if Diprivan 1% is administered using a hand held pre-filled syringe, the line between the syringe and the patient must not be left open if unattended.

When the pre-filled syringe presentation is used in a syringe pump appropriate compatibility should be ensured. In particular, the pump should be designed to prevent syphoning and should have an occlusion alarm set no greater than 1000 mm Hg. If using a programmable or equivalent pump that offers options for use of different syringes then choose only the B-D 50/60 ml PLASTIPAK setting when using the Diprivan 1% pre-filled syringe.

Diprivan 1% may be premixed with alfentanil injection containing 500 micrograms/ml alfentanil in the ratio of 20:1 to 50:1 v/v. Mixtures should be prepared using sterile technique and used within 6 hours of preparation.

In order to reduce pain on initial injection, Diprivan 1% may be mixed with preservative free Lignocaine Injection 0.5% or 1%; (see *Dilution and Co-administra-tion table* below).

*Target controlled infusion–Administration of Dipri-van 1% by a Diprifusor TCI system* Administration of Diprivan 1% by a Diprifusor TCI system is restricted to induction and maintenance of general anaesthesia in adults. It is not recommended for use in ICU sedation or sedation for surgical and diagnostic procedures, or in children.

To achieve induction and maintenance of anaesthe-sia in adults, Diprivan 1% may be administered with the assistance of a Target Controlled Infusion (TCI) system. Such systems allow the anaesthetist to achieve and control a desired speed of induction and depth of anaesthesia by setting and adjusting target (predicted) blood concentrations of propofol. Diprivan 1% may be administered by TCI only with a Diprifusor TCI system incorporating Diprifusor TCI software. Such systems will operate only on recognition of electronically tagged pre-filled syringes containing Diprivan 1% or 2% Injection. The Diprifusor TCI system will automatically adjust the infusion rate for the concentration of Diprivan recognised. Users must be familiar with the infusion pump users' manual, and with the administration of Diprivan 1% by TCI and with the correct use of the syringe identification system, all of which are set out in the Diprifusor training manual, available from Zeneca at the address below.

Guidance on propofol target concentrations is given below. In view of interpatient variability in propofol pharmacokinetics and pharmacodynamics, in both premedicated and unpremedicated patients the target propofol concentration should be titrated against the response of the patient in order to achieve the depth of anaesthesia required.

In adult patients under 55 years of age anaesthesia can usually be induced with target propofol concentrations in the region of 4 to 8 mcg/ml. An initial target of 4 mcg/ml is recommended in premedicated patients and in unpremedicated patients an initial target of 6 mcg/ml is advised. Induction time with these targets is generally within the range of 60 to 120 seconds. Higher targets will allow more rapid induction of anaesthesia but may be associated with more pronounced haemodynamic and respiratory depression.

A lower initial target concentration should be used in patients over the age of about 55 years and in patients of ASA grades 3 and 4. The target concentration can then be increased in steps of 0.5 to 1.0 mcg/ml at intervals of 1 minute to achieve a gradual induction of anaesthesia.

Supplementary analgesia will generally be required and the extent to which target concentrations for maintenance of anaesthesia can be reduced will be influenced by the amount of concomitant analgesia administered. Target propofol concentrations in the region of 3 to 6 mcg/ml usually maintain satisfactory anaesthesia.

The predicted propofol concentration on waking is generally in the region of 1.0 to 2.0 mcg/ml and will be influenced by the amount of analgesia given during maintenance.

**Contra-indications, warnings, etc**

*Contra-indications:* Diprivan 1% is contra-indicated in patients with a known allergy to Diprivan.

*Precautions:* Diprivan 1% should be given by those trained in anaesthesia or, where appropriate, doctors trained in the care of patients in Intensive Care. Patients should be constantly monitored and facilities for maintenance of a patent airway, artificial ventilation, oxygen enrichment and other resuscitative facilities should be readily available at all times. Diprivan 1% should not be administered by the person conducting the diagnostic or surgical procedure.

When Diprivan 1% is administered for sedation for surgical and diagnostic procedures patients should be continually monitored for early signs of hypotension, airway obstruction and oxygen desaturation.

As with other intravenous anaesthetic and sedative agents, patients should be instructed to avoid alcohol before and for at least 8 hours after administration of Diprivan 1%.

Diprivan 1% should be used with caution when used to sedate patients undergoing some procedures where spontaneous movements are particularly undesirable, such as ophthalmic surgery.

As with other intravenous sedative agents, when Diprivan 1% is given along with central nervous system depressants, such as potent analgesics, the sedative effect may be intensified and the possibility of severe respiratory or cardiovascular depression should be considered.

During bolus administration for operative procedures, extreme caution should be exercised in patients with acute pulmonary insufficiency or respiratory depression.

Concomitant use of central nervous system depressants e.g. alcohol, general anaesthetics, narcotic analgesics will result in accentuation of their sedative effects. When Diprivan 1% is combined with centrally depressant drugs administered parenterally severe respiratory and cardiovascular depression may occur. It is recommended that Diprivan 1% is administered following the analgesic and the dose should be carefully titrated to the patient's response.

During induction of anaesthesia, hypotension and transient apnoea may occur depending on the dose and use of premedicants and other agents.

Occasionally, hypotension may require use of intravenous fluids and reduction of the rate of administration of Diprivan 1% during the period of anaesthetic maintenance.

An adequate period is needed prior to discharge of the patient to ensure full recovery after general anaesthesia.

*Dilution and co-administration of Diprivan 1% with other drugs or infusion fluids:*

(see also *Additional precautions* section)

| *Co-administration technique* | *Additive or diluent* | *Preparation* | *Precautions* |
|---|---|---|---|
| Pre-mixing | Dextrose 5% Intravenous Infusion BP | Mix 1 part of Diprivan1% with up to 4 parts of Dextrose 5% Intravenous Infusion BP in either PVC infusion bags or glass infusion bottles. When diluted in PVC bags it is recommended that the bag should be full and that the dilution be prepared by withdrawing a volume of infusion fluid and replacing it with an equal volume of Diprivan1%. | Prepare aseptically immediately before administration. The mixture is stable for up to 6 hours. |
| | Lignocaine Hydrochloride Injection. (0.5% or 1% without preservatives) | Mix 20 parts of Diprivan1% with up to 1 part of either 0.5% or 1% Lignocaine Hydrochloride Injection. | Prepare mixture aseptically immediately prior to administration. Use for induction only. |
| | Alfentanil injection (500 microgram/ml) | Mix Diprivan 1% with alfentanil injection in a ratio of 20:1 to 50:1 v/v. | Prepare mixture aseptically; use within 6 hours of preparation. |
| Co-administration via a Y-piece connector | Dextrose 5% Intravenous Infusion BP | Co-administer via a Y-piece connector. | Place the Y-piece connector close to the injection site. |
| | Sodium Chloride 0.9% Intravenous Infusion BP | As above. | As above. |
| | Dextrose 4% with Sodium Chloride 0.18% Intravenous Infusion BP | As above. | As above. |

When Diprivan 1% is administered to an epileptic patient, there may be a risk of convulsion.

As with other intravenous anaesthetic agents, caution should be applied in patients with cardiac, respiratory, renal or hepatic impairment or in hypovolaemic, elderly or debilitated patients.

The risk of relative vagal overactivity may be increased because Diprivan 1% lacks vagolytic activity; it has been associated with reports of bradycardia, (occasionally profound) and also asytole. The intravenous administration of an anticholinergic agent before induction, or during maintenance of anaesthesia should be considered, especially in situations where vagal tone is likely to predominate or when Diprivan 1% is used in conjunction with other agents likely to cause a bradycardia.

Appropriate care should be applied in patients with disorders of fat metabolism and in other conditions where lipid emulsions must be used cautiously.

Use is not recommended with electroconvulsive treatment.

As with other anaesthetics, sexual disinhibition may occur during recovery.

*Obstetrics:* Diprivan 1% crosses the placenta and may be associated with neonatal depression. It should not be used for obstetric anaesthesia.

*Pregnancy:* Teratology studies in rats and rabbits showed no teratogenic effects. Diprivan 1% has been used during termination of pregnancy in the first trimester. It should not be used in pregnancy.

*Lactation:* Safety to the neonate has not been established following the use of Diprivan 1% in mothers who are breast feeding.

*Effect on ability to drive or operate machinery:* Patients should be advised that performance at skilled tasks, such as driving and operating machinery, may be impaired for some time after general anaesthesia.

*Additional precautions:* Diprivan 1% contains no antimicrobial preservatives and supports growth of micro-organisms. When Diprivan 1% is to be aspirated, it must be drawn aseptically into a sterile syringe or giving set immediately after opening the ampoule or breaking the vial seal. Administration must commence without delay. Asepsis must be maintained for both Diprivan 1% and infusion equipment throughout the infusion period. Any drugs or fluids added to the Diprivan 1% line must be adm
istered close to the cannula site. Diprivan 1% m
not be administered via a microbiological filter.

Diprivan 1% and any syringe containing Dipriv
1% are for single use in an individual patient. For u
in long term maintenance of anaesthesia or sedati
in intensive care it is recommended that the infusi
line and reservoir of Diprivan 1% be discarded a
replaced at regular intervals.

*Side-effects:* General: Induction of anaesthesia
generally smooth with minimal evidence of excitati
Side-effects during induction, maintenance and rec
ery occur uncommonly. Changes in cardiovascu
parameters are usually slight but such changes m
be important in patients with impaired myocard
oxygen delivery capacity and hypovolaemia. Wh
Diprivan 1% is administered, convulsions, myoclon
and opisthotonos may occur, usually after terminati
of administration of the product and occasiona
delayed. Spontaneous movements and pulmon
oedema have been observed. During the recove
phase nausea, vomiting and headache occur in onl
small proportion of patients. Rarely, discolouration
urine has been reported following prolonged adm
istration of Diprivan 1%. Rarely, clinical features
anaphylaxis, which may include angioedema, bro
chospasm, erythema and hypotension, occur follo
ing Diprivan 1% administration. There have be
reports of post-operative fever.

Local. The local pain which may occur during
induction phase of Diprivan 1% anaesthesia can
minimised by the co-administration of lignocaine (s
*Dosage and administration*) and by the use of t
larger veins of the forearm and antecubital fos
Thrombosis and phlebitis are rare. Accidental clini
extravasation and animal studies showed minin
tissue reaction. Intra-arterial injection in animals
not induce local tissue effects.

*Overdosage:* Accidental overdosage is likely to cau
cardiorespiratory depression. Respiratory depressi
should be treated by artificial ventilation with oxyg
Cardiovascular depression would require lowering
the patient's head and, if severe, use of plas
expanders and pressor agents.

**Pharmaceutical precautions**

*Storage precautions:* Diprivan 1% should be stor
between 2°C and 25°C; it must not be frozen.

*In-use precautions:* Containers should be shak
before use.

Any portion of the contents remaining after u
should be discarded.

Diprivan 1% should not be mixed prior to admin
tration with injections or infusion fluids other than
Dextrose or Lignocaine Injection (see *Dosage a*
*administration*).

The neuromusculat blocking agents, atracuri
and mivacurium should not be given through
same intravenous line as Diprivan 1% without pr
flushing.

**Legal category** POM.

**Package quantities** Ampoules of 20 ml in boxes
5. Vials of 50 ml and 100 ml. Pre-filled syringes
50 ml.

**Further information** Nil.

**Product licence number** 12619/0010.

## DIPRIVAN* 2%

**Qualitative and quantitative composition** Wh
aqueous and isotonic emulsion for intravenous inj
tion containing 20 mg propofol per 1 ml.

**Pharmaceutical form** Oil-in-water emulsion for int
venous injection.

**Clinical particulars**

*Therapeutic indications:* Diprivan 2% is a short-acti
intravenous anaesthetic agent suitable for inducti
and maintenance of general anaesthesia.

Diprivan 2% may also be used for sedation
ventilated patients receiving intensive care, for
period of up to 3 days.

*Posology and method of administration:*

*Induction of general anaesthesia:*

*Adults:* Diprivan 2% may be used to induce anaest
sia by infusion.

Administration of Diprivan 2% by bolus injectior
not recommended.

Diprivan 2% may be used to induce anaesthesia
infusion but only in those patients who will rece
Diprivan 2% for maintenance of anaesthesia.

In unpremedicated and premedicated patients, i
recommended that Diprivan 2% should be titrat
(approximately 2 ml (40 mg) every 10 seconds in
average healthy adult by infusion) against the
sponse of the patient until the clinical signs show
onset of anaesthesia. Most adult patients aged le
than 55 years are likely to require 1.5 to 2.5 mg/kg

Diprivan 2%. The total dose required can be reduced by lower rates of administration (1 to 2.5 ml/min (20 to 50 mg/min). Over this age, the requirement will generally be less. In patients of ASA Grades 3 and 4, lower rates of administration should be used (approximately 1 ml (20 mg every 10 seconds).

*Elderly patients:* Diprivan 2% should be titrated against the response of the patient. Patients over the age of about 55 years may require lower doses of Diprivan 2% for induction of anaesthesia.

*Children:* Diprivan 2% is not recommended for induction of anaesthesia in children less than 3 years of age.

When used to induce anaesthesia in children, it is recommended that Diprivan 2% be given by slow infusion until the clinical signs show the onset of anaesthesia. The dose should be adjusted for age and/or weight. Most patients over 8 years of age are likely to require approximately 2.5 mg/kg of 'Diprivan' 2% for induction of anaesthesia. Under this age the requirement may be more. Lower dosage is recommended for children of ASA grades 3 and 4.

*Maintenance of general anaesthesia:* Anaesthesia can be maintained by administering Diprivan 2% by continuous infusion to prevent the clinical signs of light anaesthesia. Administration of Diprivan 2% by bolus injection is not recommended. Recovery from anaesthesia is typically rapid and it is therefore important to maintain Diprivan 2% administration until the end of the procedure.

*Adults (including elderly patients):* The required rate of administration varies considerably between patients, but rates in the region of 4 to 12 mg/kg/h usually maintain satisfactory anaesthesia.

*Children:* Diprivan 2% is not recommended for maintenance of anaesthesia in children less than 3 years of age.

The required rate of administration varies considerably between patients but rates in the region of 9 to 15 mg/kg/h usually achieve satisfactory anaesthesia.

*Sedation during intensive care:*

*Adults (including elderly patients):* When used to provide sedation for ventilated patients undergoing intensive care, it is recommended that Diprivan 2% be given by continuous infusion.

The infusion rate should be adjusted according to the depth of sedation required, but rates in the region of 0.3 to 4.0 mg/kg/h should achieve satisfactory sedation. Rates of infusion greater than 4.0 mg/kg/h are not recommended.

It is recommended that blood lipid levels be monitored should Diprivan 2% be administered to patients thought to be at particular risk of fat overload.

Administration of Diprivan 2% should be adjusted appropriately if the monitoring indicates that fat is being inadequately cleared from the body. If the patient is receiving other intravenous lipid concurrently, a reduction in quantity should be made in order to take account of the amount of lipid infused as part of the Diprivan 2% formulation: 1.0 ml of Diprivan 2% contains approximately 0.1 g of fat.

*Children:* Diprivan 2% is not recommended for sedation in children as safety and efficacy have not been demonstrated. Although no causal relationship has been established, serious adverse events (including fatalities) have been observed from spontaneous reports of unlicensed use of Diprivan. These events were seen most often in children with respiratory tract infections given doses in excess of those recommended for adults.

*Administration:* Diprivan 2% has no analgesic properties and therefore supplementary analgesic agents are generally required in addition to Diprivan 2%.

Diprivan has been used in association with spinal and epidural anaesthesia and with commonly used premedicants, neuromuscular blocking drugs, inhalational agents and analgesic agents; no pharmacological incompatibility has been encountered. Lower doses of Diprivan 2% may be required where general anaesthesia is used as an adjunct to regional anaesthetic techniques.

Diprivan 2% should not be diluted.

When Diprivan 2% is used to maintain anaesthesia, it is recommended that equipment such as syringe pumps or volumetric infusion pumps should always be used to control infusion rates.

Diprivan 2% should not be mixed prior to administration with injections or infusion fluids. However, Diprivan 2% may be co-administered via a Y-piece connector close to the injection site with the following:

Dextrose 5% Intravenous Infusion BP.
Sodium Chloride 0.9% Intravenous Infusion BP.
Dextrose 4% with Sodium Chloride 0.18% Intravenous Infusion BP.

*Contra-indications:* Diprivan 2% is contra-indicated in patients with a known allergy to Diprivan 1% or Diprivan 2%.

*Special warnings and special precautions for use:* Diprivan 2% should be given by those trained in anaesthesia, or where appropriate, doctors trained in the care of patients in Intensive Care. Facilities for maintenance of a patent airway, artificial ventilation and oxygen enrichment should be available.

During induction of anaesthesia, hypotension and transient apnoea may occur depending on the dose and use of premedicants and other agents.

Occasionally, hypotension may require use of intravenous fluids and reduction of the rate of administration of Diprivan 2% during the period of anaesthetic maintenance.

An adequate period is needed prior to discharge of the patient to ensure full recovery after general anaesthesia.

When Diprivan 2% is administered to an epileptic patient, there may be a risk of convulsion.

As with other intravenous anaesthetic agents, caution should be applied in patients, with cardiac, respiratory, renal or hepatic impairment or in hypovolaemic or debilitated patients.

The risk of relative vagal overactivity may be increased because Diprivan 2% lacks vagolytic activity. Diprivan has been associated with reports of bradycardia (occasionally profound) and also asystole. The intravenous administration of an anticholinergic agent before induction, or during maintenance of anaesthesia should be considered, especially in situations where vagal tone is likely to predominate or when Diprivan 2% is used in conjunction with other agents likely to cause a bradycardia.

Appropriate care should be applied in patients with disorders of fat metabolism and in other conditions where lipid emulsions must be used cautiously.

Use is not recommended with electroconvulsive treatment.

As with other anaesthetics sexual disinhibition may occur during recovery.

*Additional precautions:* Diprivan 2% contains no antimicrobial preservatives and supports growth of micro-organisms. Asepsis must be maintained for both Diprivan 2% and infusion equipment throughout the infusion period. Any drugs or fluids added to the Diprivan 2% infusion line must be administered close to the cannula site. Diprivan 2% must not be administered via a microbiological filter.

Diprivan 2% and any syringe containing Diprivan 2% are for single use in an individual patient. For use in long-term maintenance of anaesthesia or sedation in intensive care it is recommended that the infusion line and reservoir of Diprivan 2% be discarded and replaced at regular intervals.

*Interaction with other medicaments and other forms of interaction:* see *Administration.*

*Pregnancy and lactation:*

*Pregnancy:* Teratology studies in rats and rabbits showed no teratogenic effects. Diprivan has been used during termination of pregnancy in the first trimester. Diprivan 2% should not be used in pregnancy.

*Obstetrics:* Diprivan crosses the placenta and may be associated with neonatal depression. It should not be used for obstetric anaesthesia.

*Lactation:* Safety to the neonate has not been established following the use of Diprivan 2% in mothers who are breast feeding. Diprivan 2% should be avoided, or mothers should stop breast feeding.

*Effects on ability to drive and use machines:* Patients should be advised that performance at skilled tasks, such as driving and operating machinery, may be impaired for some time after general anaesthesia.

*Undesirable effects:*

*General:* Induction of anaesthesia is generally smooth with minimal evidence of excitation. Side effects during induction, maintenance and recovery occur uncommonly. When Diprivan 2% is administered convulsions, myoclonus and opisthotonus may occur, usually after termination of administration of the product and occasionally delayed. Pulmonary oedema has been observed. During the recovery phase, nausea, vomiting and headache occur in only a small proportion of patients. Rarely, discolouration of urine has been reported following prolonged administration with Diprivan. Rarely, clinical features of anaphylaxis, which may include angioedema, bronchospasm, erythema and hypotension, occur following Diprivan administration. There have been reports of post-operative fever.

*Local:* The local pain which may occur during the induction phase can be minimised by the use of the larger veins of the forearm and anticubital fossa. Thrombosis and phlebitis are rare. Accidental clinical extravasation and animal studies showed minimal tissue reaction. Intra-arterial injection in animals did not induce local tissue effects.

*Overdose:* Accidental overdosage is likely to cause cardiorespiratory depression. Respiratory depression should be treated by artificial ventilation with oxygen. Cardiovascular depression would require lowering of the patient's head and, if severe, use of plasma expanders and pressor agents.

**Pharmacological properties**

*Pharmacodynamic properties:* Propofol (2, 6-diisopropylphenol) is a short-acting general anaesthetic agent with a rapid onset of action of approximately 30 seconds. Recovery from anaesthesia is usually rapid. The mechanism of action, like all general anaesthetics, is poorly understood.

In general, falls in mean arterial blood pressure and slight changes in heart rate are observed when Diprivan 2% is administered for induction and maintenance of anaesthesia. However, the haemodynamic parameters normally remain relatively stable during maintenance and the incidence of untoward haemodynamic changes is low.

Although ventilatory depression can occur following administration of Diprivan 2%, any effects are qualitatively similar to those of other intravenous anaesthetic agents and are readily manageable in clinical practice.

Diprivan 2% reduces cerebral blood flow, intracranial pressure and cerebral metabolism. The reduction in intracranial pressure is greater in patients with an elevated baseline intracranial pressure.

Recovery from anaesthesia is usually rapid and clear headed with a low incidence of headache and post-operative nausea and vomiting.

In general, there is less post-operative nausea and vomiting following anaesthesia with Diprivan 2% than following anaesthesia with inhalational agents. There is evidence that this may be related to a reduced emetic potential of propofol.

Diprivan 2%, at the concentrations likely to occur clinically, does not inhibit the synthesis of adrenocortical hormones.

*Pharmacokinetic properties:* The decline in propofol concentrations following a bolus dose or following the termination of an infusion can be described by a three compartment open model with very rapid distribution (half-life 2 to 4 minutes), rapid elimination (half-life 30 to 60 minutes), and a slower final phase, representative of redistribution of propofol from poorly perfused tissue.

Propofol is extensively distributed and rapidly cleared from the body (total body clearance 1.5 to 2 litres/minute). Clearance occurs by metabolic processes, mainly in the liver, to form inactive conjugates of propofol and its corresponding quinol, which are excreted in urine.

When Diprivan 2% is used to maintain anaesthesia, blood concentrations asymptotically approach the steady-state value for the given administration rate. The pharmacokinetics are linear over the recommended range of infusion rates of Diprivan 2%.

*Preclinical safety data:* Propofol is a drug on which extensive clinical experience has been obtained. All relevant information for the prescriber is provided elsewhere in the Summary of Product Characteristics.

**Pharmaceutical particulars**

*List of excipients:* Glycerol PhEur; Nitrogen USNF; Purified Egg Phosphatide; Sodium Hydroxide PhEur; Soybean Oil USP; Water for Injections PhEur.

*Incompatibilities:* The neuromuscular blocking agents, atracurium and mivacurium should not be given through the same intravenous line as Diprivan 2% without prior flushing.

*Shelf life:*

*Shelf life of the product as packaged for sale:* 2 years.

*Shelf life after dilution:* Diprivan 2% should not be diluted.

*Special precautions for storage:* Storage Precautions: Diprivan 2% should be stored between 2°C and 25°C; it must not be frozen.

*Nature and contents of container:* Emulsion for injection: 50 ml vial containing propofol 20 mg/ml.

*Instructions for use/handling:* In-use precautions Containers should be shaken before use.

Any portion of the contents remaining after use should be discarded.

Diprivan 2% should not be mixed prior to administration with injections or infusion fluids.

**Marketing authorisation number** 12619/0110

**Date of approval/revision of SPC** June 1997

**Legal category** POM.

## EXELDERM* CREAM

**Qualitative and quantitative composition** Sulconazole nitrate 1.0% w/w.

**Pharmaceutical form** Cream.

**Clinical particulars**

*Therapeutic indications:* Exelderm Cream is indicated in the management of dermatophyte infections resulting in tinea pedis, tinea corporis and tinea cruris, pityriasis versicolor and candidiasis.

*Posology and method of administration*
*Adults:* Exelderm Cream should be gently massaged into the affected and surrounding skin areas twice daily (morning and evening). For less severe cases only once daily administration may be sufficient.

Often, clinical improvement with relief of symptoms occurs within one week. However, treatment should be continued for 2–3 weeks after clinical cure to prevent relapse.

*Children and elderly patients:* No special precautions are required.

*Contra-indications:* Exelderm is contra-indicated in patients with hypersensitivity to the formulated product or imidazoles.

*Special warnings and special precautions for use:* Treatment should be discontinued if a reaction suggesting sensitivity or irritation occurs. If the patient shows no clinical improvement after 4 weeks of treatment the diagnosis should be reviewed. Avoid the introduction of Exelderm into the eyes. Lens changes were seen in one animal species following very high repeated oral doses.

*Interactions with other medicaments and other forms of interaction:* None have been reported or are known.

*Pregnancy and lactation:* This product should not be used in pregnancy unless considered essential to the welfare of the patient.

*Effects on ability to drive and use machines:* There is no evidence to suggest that sulconazole will affect the ability to drive or operate machinery.

*Undesirable effects:* Occasional itching, burning, erythema, stinging and blistering have been reported.

*Overdosage:* The 30 g tube of Exelderm contains 300 mg of sulconazole nitrate. Toxic effects are very unlikely even if the full contents are ingested but if they occur symptomatic treatment should be given.

**Pharmacological properties**
*Pharmacodynamic properties:* Sulconazole is a substituted imidazole antimicrobial agent. Its primary site of action is the fungal cell membrane. At low concentrations, sulconazole is primarily fungistatic and acts by inhibiting the biosynthesis of ergosterol and other sterols which are essential membrane components. At higher concentrations sulconazole is fungicidal and causes direct damage to cell membranes by allowing a build up of toxic concentrations of hydrogen peroxide.

*Pharmacokinetic properties:* There is a limited amount of data available on the pharmacokinetic properties of sulconazole. From one study, it was estimated that about 12% of the dose was absorbed through the skin regardless of whether or not the stratum corneum has been removed. Absorption from the gastro-intestinal tract is unlikely to be high since most drugs of this type are poorly absorbed.

**Pharmaceutical particulars**
*List of excipients:* Propylene Glycol PhEur; Stearyl Alcohol USF; Isopropyl Myristrate USF; Cetyl Alcohol USF; Polysorbate 60 PhEur; Sorbitan Monostearate BP; Glyceryl Stearate and PEG 100 Stearate; Sodium Hydroxide BP; Ascorbyl Palmitate USF; Purified Water; Sodium Hydroxide Solution/Nitric Acid Solution may be added to adjust pH.

*Incompatibilities:* None stated.

*Shelf life:* 3 years.

*Special precautions for storage:* Store below 30°C.

*Nature and contents of container:* Internally lacquered aluminium tubes (30 g).

*Instructions for use/handling:* For topical application only. Keep out of the eyes.

**Marketing authorisation number** 12619/0013.

**Date of approval/revision of SPC** January 1995.

**Legal category** POM.

## FLUOTHANE*

**Presentation** Fluothane is a colourless, volatile liquid, non-explosive and non-flammable in the concentrations usually used. Chemically it is 2-bromo-2-chloro-1,1,1-trifluoroethane stabilised with thymol 0.01% w/w (Halothane PhEur).

**Uses** Fluothane is a volatile anaesthetic which is suitable for the induction and maintenance of anaesthesia for all types of surgery and in patients of all ages.

*Mode of action:* When inhaled, Fluothane is absorbed through the alveoli into the bloodstream. In the bloodstream Fluothane circulates through the body to the principal site of action, the brain. Here Fluothane causes a progressive depression of the central nervous system, beginning with the higher centres (cerebral cortex) and spreading to the vital centres in the medulla. This depression is reversible. However, its mode of action, like all anaesthetic agents, is unknown.

Fluothane may cause bronchodilation. Bronchial relaxation is usually dose-related and may be due to blockage of pathways, causing bronchoconstriction or depression of bronchial muscular tone.

Fluothane causes a reversible, dose-related decline in renal blood flow, glomerular filtration rate and urinary flow.

Fluothane may be absorbed by the rubber used in some anaesthetic circuits. The rubber/gas partition coefficient at 20°C is 120.

Fluothane has a relatively low solubility in blood and therefore alveoli/blood concentrations equilibrate rapidly. The triexponential decline in Fluothane blood concentrations following the end of administration is thought to represent distribution into three compartments; the vessel rich group (brain/heart/liver), the musculature and adipose tissue. Approximately 80% of the inhaled Fluothane is eliminated unchanged by the lungs. The remaining 20% is metabolised in the liver by oxidative and, under hypoxic conditions, reductive pathways. The main metabolites are trifluoroacetic acid, bromide and chloride salts (via the oxidative pathway) and fluoride salts (via the reductive pathway). The concentrations of metabolites peak 24 hours post-operatively and are eliminated by renal excretion during the following week.

**Dosage and administration** A number of anaesthetic vaporisers specially designed for use with Fluothane are available. Open, semi-open, semi-closed and closed circuit systems have all been used with good results.

For induction of anaesthesia in the adult patient a concentration of 2–4% Fluothane in oxygen or oxygen/nitrous oxide may be used. In children a concentration of 1.5–2% Fluothane in oxygen or oxygen/nitrous oxide is used. A concentration of 0.5–2% is usually adequate for maintenance of anaesthesia in both adults and children. The lower concentration is usually most suitable for elderly patients.

**Contra-indications, warnings, etc** Fluothane can induce liver damage; however, the incidence of severe liver damage (jaundice, which may lead to hepatic failure as a consequence of massive hepatic cell necrosis) is unknown. The risk of developing hepatic failure appears to be increased by repeated exposure. Although short intervals of time between exposures are likely to increase the risk of hepatotoxicity, even long intervals between exposure may not eliminate the risks, since some patients have developed severe reactions following Fluothane given many years after the previous exposure. On the information which is available at the present time, it is advised that the following precautions be taken:

i. A careful anaesthetic history should be taken prior to use, to determine previous exposure and previous reactions following Fluothane anaesthesia.
(ii) Repeated exposure to Fluothane within a period of at least 3 months should be avoided unless there are overriding clinical circumstances.
(iii) History of unexplained jaundice and pyrexia in a patient following exposure to Fluothane is a contra-indication to its future use in that patient unless absolutely essential.
(iv) Patients should be informed if they have developed a reaction possibly related to Fluothane anaesthesia; such patients should be provided with a medical alert card stating the problem.

Fluothane is contra-indicated in patients with a previous history of malignant hyperpyrexia or those susceptible to maligant hyperpyrexia.

As Fluothane causes relaxation of the uterine muscle it is advisable that anaesthesia should be maintained in the lightest plane possible during obstetric operations. Obstetric use, especially at high concentrations, may result in post partum haemorrhage.

The role of Fluothane in liver damage occasionally observed after anaesthesia has not been definitely established. However, as such cases appear more frequently after repeated anaesthetic administration, the appearance of unexplained jaundice and pyrexia following exposure to Fluothane should be regarded as a contra-indication to its later use. Repeat exposure within a period of three months should be avoided in all patients. Further risk factors, (other than repeated exposure) appear to be female gender, obesity and middle age.

Halothane is a potent cerebral vasodilator. Increases in cerebral blood flow and/or intracranial pressure may be observed during anaesthesia with Fluothane. These may be more marked in the presence of intracranial space-occupying lesions. The use of a moderate hyperventilation during neurosurgery in recommended to counteract the rise in intracranial fluid pressure which may occur with Fluothane.

Malignant hyperpyrexia has been reported in some patients receiving Fluothane, more commonly when co-administered with suxamethonium. This syndrome occurs with other anaesthetic agents, and may respond to intravenous dantrolene sodium.

During the induction of Fluothane anaesthesia a moderate fall in blood pressure commonly occurs. (Halothane lowers arterial blood pressure in a dose-dependent manner). The pressure tends to rise when the vapour concentration is reduced to maintenance levels, but it usually remains steady below the pre-operative level. This hypotensive effect is useful in providing a clear operating field and a reduction in haemorrhage. However, if necessary, intravenous doses of methoxamine (5 mg are usually adequate) can be given to counteract the fall in blood pressure.

Anaesthesia with Fluothane may be associated with bradycardia, which may augment its hypotensive effect. The intravenous administration of an anticholinergic agent before induction or during maintenance of anaesthsia should be considered, especially in situations where vagal tone is likely to be predominant or when Fluothane is used in conjunction with other agents likely to cause a bradycardia.

Cardiac arrhythmias have been reported during anaesthesia with Fluothane. Caution is required with regard to the administration of Fluothane to patients with phaeochromocytoma, as it is possible that this may lead to an increased likelihood of intra-operative arrhythmias.

Fluothane may cause respiratory depression, particularly at higher concentrations.

Halothane causes relaxation of skeletal muscle. Caution is required when using Fluothane in patients with myasthenia gravis or those co-administered aminoglycoside antibiotics.

Caution should be exercised during the administration of adrenaline to patients anaesthetised with Fluothane as arrhythmias may be precipitated. For this reason the dose of adrenaline should be restricted and an antiarrhythmic agent administered as appropriate. Caution should also be applied for other sympathomimetics, and for aminophylline, theophylline and tricyclic antidepressants, which may also precipitate arrhythmias.

Fluothane augments the action of non-depolarising muscle relaxants and the muscle relaxant effects of aminoglycosides.

Fluothane may augment the hypotension caused by the ganglionic-blocking effect of tubocurarine.

Bradycardia and/or hypotension may occur during Fluothane anaesthesia. Hypotension may occur particularly during induction.

Shivering may be observed during recovery from anaesthesia, especially if the patient is in cool surroundings.

Post-operative nausea and vomiting may occu after Fluothane anaesthesia.

Ensure adequate room ventilation when Fluothane is being used. Keep the concentration of Fluothane in air as low as possible.

Halothane is absorbed by the rubber used in some anaesthetic circuits. This is of clinical importance when halothane-free circuits are required for patients susceptible to malignant hyperpyrexia, or who have demonstrated hypersensitivity to previous administration of halothane. If rubber circuits are used, and a patient with known sensitivity is next on the list, the a new circuit should be set up.

*Pregnancy:* Data from animal experiments have indicated that halothane may have teratogenic potentia in some species. Although these findings cannot b directly related to man, it would be prudent to avoi general anaesthesia with Fluothane during ear pregnancy, except where such use is essential.

*Lactation:* There are no well controlled studies wit Fluothane in lactating women. Fluothane has bee detected in breast milk of lactating women, but th effects of Fluothane on breast fed neonates has n been established. However, Fluothane has been i wide use for over 30 years without apparent consequence.

*Effect on ability to drive or operate machinery:* Patien should be advised that performance at skilled task such as driving and operating machinery, may b impaired for some time after general anaesthesia.

*Accidental ingestion:* Cases of ingestion must b treated symptomatically.

**Pharmaceutical precautions** Bottles of Fluothar must be securely closed and stored below 25° protected from light. Fluothane must be kept in th original container until immediately prior to its use.

Whilst in the liquid phase, Fluothane must not b diluted or contaminated; however, in the vapo phase it may be administered together with oxyge or a mixture of nitrous oxide and oxygen.

**Legal category** P.

**Package quantities** Fluothane is supplied in bottl of 250 ml.

**Further information** *Spillage:* Absorb spillage usi a suitable absorbent material and transfer to a clos container for disposal. In case of insufficient venti tion wear suitable respiratory equipment. *Dispos*

Disposal is normally carried out by incineration under carefully controlled conditions.

**Product licence number** 12619/0014.

# FULCIN* 500 TABLETS
# FULCIN* 125 TABLETS
# FULCIN* ORAL SUSPENSION

**Presentation** Fulcin is griseofulvin in a fine-particle form designed to give optimal absorption when taken orally.

Fulcin 500 is presented as white, bi-convex tablets, one side plain, the obverse marked with 'F'. Each contains 500 mg Griseofulvin PhEur. Inactive ingredients are calcium carboxymethylcellulose, magnesium stearate, maize starch and povidone. Fulcin 125 Tablets are white, bi-convex, plain on one face and a bisecting line on the reverse face with 'F' imprinted either side of the breakline. Each contains 125 mg Griseofulvin PhEur. Inactive ingredients are calcium carboxymethylcellulose, magnesium stearate, maize starch and povidone.

Fulcin Oral Suspension is a brown aqueous suspension which contains 2.5% w/v Griseofulvin PhEur. Inactive ingredients are calcium chloride, chocolate flavour, cocoa powder, methylhydroxybenzoate, peppermint oil, propyl hydroxybenzoate, sodium alginate, sodium carboxymethylcellulose, sodium citrate, sucrose, vanillin and water.

**Uses** Fulcin is effective against the dermatophytes causing ringworm (tinea), including *Microsporum canis, Trichophyton rubrum, Trichophyton verrucosum* and *Epidermophyton* spp.

Fulcin is indicated for the treatment of fungal infections of the skin, hair and nails when topical therapy has failed or is considered inappropriate.

*Mode of action:* Griseofulvin inhibits fungal cell mitosis by causing disruption of the mitotic spindle structure, thereby arresting the metaphase of cell division. It is deposited in varying degrees in the keratin precursor cells of skin, hair and nails, rendering the keratin resistant to fungal invasion. As the infected keratin is shed, it is replaced with healthy tissue.

Fulcin is not effective in infections caused by candida albicans (monilia), aspergilli, malassezia furfur (pityriasis versicolor) and nocardia species.

Following oral administration, griseofulvin is absorbed principally from the duodenum. Peak plasma concentrations of the drug (approx 1–2 microgram/ml) occur about 4 hours after dosing. Concentrations of approximately 12–25 microgram/g are maintained in skin during long term administration, whilst concurrent serum levels remain at 1–2 microgram/ml. When the drug is discontinued, the drug is not detectable after 2 days in the skin and after 4 days in the plasma. The drug has an elimination half-life of 9–24 hours and it is metabolised in the liver, the major metabolite being 6-demethylgriseofulvin which is microbiologically inactive. The metabolites are excreted mainly in the urine whilst unchanged griseofulvin is excreted mainly in the faeces. Griseofulvin is also excreted in sweat.

**Dosage and administration** The adult dosage is normally 500 mg daily, but in severe conditions up to twice this amount may be given, reducing to the lower level when a clinical response has occurred. The normal dosage may be given as one 125 mg tablet or 5 ml of suspension four times a day, or as one 500 mg tablet once daily after food.

For children the most suitable form is the pleasantly flavoured Fulcin Oral Suspension. The daily dosage is 10 mg griseofulvin per kg body weight daily, i.e. 5 ml of suspension for every 12.5 kg in single or divided doses after food.

There are no special dosage recommendations for the elderly, but it may be advisable to monitor elderly patients so that optimum dosage can be individually determined.

The duration of treatment depends on the type of infection and the time required for normal replacement of infected tissues.

For complete eradication of the infection, Fulcin treatment should be combined with general measures of care and hygiene. Reservoirs of infection may include clothing, footwear and bedding as well as the patient's hair.

**Contra-indications, warnings, etc** Fulcin should not be used for prophylaxis.

Fulcin should not be administered to patients who have established porphyria or hepatocellular failure or to patients with lupus erythematosus and related conditions.

Fulcin is contra-indicated in pregnancy. Griseofulvin administered to rats during pregnancy has been associated with foetotoxicity and tail deformities at high dosages. Some case reports of human foetal abnormalities have been observed. There is no evidence of safety in human pregnancy and some case

reports suggest that griseofulvin may produce human foetal abnormalities. Women should not become pregnant during or within one month of treatment with griseofulvin; if they do, they should seek genetic advice.

Fulcin may decrease the response to coumarin anticoagulants administered concomitantly.

Liver enzyme inducing drugs, such as barbiturates, may reduce the effectiveness of Fulcin therapy.

Barbiturates can reduce the effectiveness of Fulcin therapy by interfering with gastrointestinal absorption of the drug.

Breakthrough bleeding and amenorrhoea have been reported in patients taking griseofulvin and oral contraceptive steroids. Since failures of oral contraceptive therapy have been reported whilst receiving 'Fulcin' additional contraceptive precautions should be taken during and for one month after treatment.

Griseofulvin is capable of producing aneuploidy (abnormal segregation of chromosomes following cell division) in mammalian cells exposed to the compound *in vitro* and *in vivo*.

Griseofulvin may damage sperm cells; males should not father children within 6 months of treatment.

Patients should be warned that an enhancement of the effects of alcohol by griseofulvin has been reported.

Long-term administration of high doses of griseofulvin with food has been reported to induce hepatomas in mice and thyroid tumours in rats but not in hamsters. The clinical significance of this finding for man is not known. In view of these data, Fulcin should not be used prophylactically.

Griseofulvin may falsely elevate urinary levels of VMA.

*Lactation:* It is not known if griseofulvin is excreted in breast milk. Safety in children of nursing mothers has not been established.

*Effect on ability to drive or operate machinery:* Fulcin may impair the ability of some individuals to drive and operate machinery. There have been occasional reports of dizziness and confusion with impaired coordination and griseofulvin has been reported to enhance the effects of alcohol.

*Side-effects:* Fulcin is generally well tolerated. Urticarial reactions and skin rashes have been noted in a few cases. There have been occasional complaints of headache and gastric discomfort which, in most cases, have regressed during treatment. Dizziness, fatigue, granulocytopenia and leucopenia have also been reported. Photosensitivity associated with griseofulvin therapy has been recorded and there have been rare reports of precipitation of lupus erythematosus and related conditions, erythema multiforme, toxic epidermal necrolysis and related conditions, peripheral neuropathy, confusion with impaired co-ordination and of oral candidiasis.

*Overdosage:* Treatment of overdosage should be symptomatic.

**Pharmaceutical precautions** *Fulcin tablets:* Store below 25°C, protected from moisture.
*Fulcin Oral Suspension:* Store below 25°C.

**Legal category** POM.

**Package quantities** *Fulcin 500 tablets:* Containers of 100 tablets (OP).
*Fulcin 125 Tablets:* Containers of 100 tablets (OP).
*Fulcin Oral Suspension:* Bottles of 100 ml (OP).

**Further information** A suitable diluent for Fulcin Oral Suspension is Syrup BP which has been preserved with methylhydroxybenzoate. The dilution should be used within 14 days of preparation.

**Product licence numbers**
Fulcin 500 Tablets     12619/0017
Fulcin 125 Tablets     12619/0016
Fulcin Oral Suspension   12619/0015

# HIBICET* HOSPITAL CONCENTRATE

**Qualitative and quantitative composition** Chlorhexidine Gluconate 1.5% w/v. (incorporated as Chlorhexidine Gluconate Solution PhEur 7.5% v/v) Cetrimide 15% w/v (incorporated as Strong Cetrimide Solution BP.)

**Pharmaceutical form** Liquid.

**Clinical particulars**
*Therapeutic indications:* Hibicet Hospital Concentrate is an antimicrobial preparation with cleansing properties for general antiseptic purposes.

*Posology and method of administration:* For external use only.
Dilute as follows:

| Method of preparation | Dilution rate | Use |
|---|---|---|
| 10 ml made up to 1 litre with water | 1 in 100 (1%) Aqueous | Cleansing/antiseptic treatment of wounds and burns.† Swabbing in obstetrics, gynaecology and urology. Cleansing/disinfectant soak for used metal instruments. Clean instrument disinfection where no means of sterilisation is available (30 minutes immersion).‡ Cleansing/disinfection of equipment, furniture and fittings in the vicinity of the patient. Storage of clinical thermometers and sterile instruments. |
| 35 ml made up to 1 litre with water | 1 in 30 (approx) Aqueous | Cleansing/antiseptic treatment of wounds and burns where greater cleansing/antisepsis is required. † Cleansing/disinfectant soak for soiled instruments. |
| 35 ml with 200 ml water made up to 1 litre with 95% alcohol | 1 in 30 (approx) in 70% Alcohol | Rapid skin antisepsis before operation and other invasive procedures. Disinfection of clean instruments and equipment (two minutes immersion). † Disinfection of clinical thermometers. |

† Sterilise the dilution by autoclaving at 115–116°C for 30 minutes or 121–123°C for 15 minutes.
‡ Endoscopes should not be placed in solution of Hibicet.

*Children and elderly patients:* There are no special dosage recommendations for either elderly patients or children. The normal adult dose is appropriate unless otherwise recommended by the physician.

*Contra-indications:* Hibicet preparations are contraindicated for patients who have previously shown a hypersensitivity reaction to either chlorhexidine or cetrimide. However, such reactions are extremely rare.

*Special warnings and special precautions for use:* For external use only. Dilute before use. Avoid contact with the brain, meninges and ears. Not for injection. Do not use in body cavities or as an enema.

The concentrated solution is irritant to eyes and mucous membranes. Keep all solutions out of the eyes. If solutions do come into contact with eyes, wash out promptly and thoroughly with water.

If concentrated cetrimide solutions come into contact with the skin, rinse promptly and thoroughly with water.

Prolonged skin contact with alcoholic solutions should be avoided. Allow to dry before proceeding.

Solutions applied to wounds, burns or broken skin should be sterilised according to BP recommendations.

Syringes and needles which have been immersed in Hibicet solutions should be thoroughly rinsed in sterile water or saline before use.

Hibicet solutions may affect glass cement and therefore are not suitable for the disinfection of endoscopes.

*Interactions with other medicaments and other forms of interaction:* See *Incompatibilities*.

*Pregnancy and lactation:* There is no evidence of any adverse effects on the foetus arising from the use of Hibicet Hospital Concentrate during pregnancy. Therefore no special precautions are recommended.

*Effects on ability to drive and use machines:* None have been reported or are known.

*Undesirable effects:* Irritative skin reactions can occasionally occur and rare hypersensitivity to cetrimide preparations, usually developing after repeated application, has been reported.

There have been rare reports of severe burn-like reactions to concentrated cetrimide solutions. Should such a reaction occur treat as a chemical burn.

Generalised allergic reactions to chlorhexidine have also been reported but are extremely rare.

In all these cases, stop application of the product.

*Overdose:* This has not been reported.
*Accidental oral or rectal administration:* If the product is swallowed give large quantities of milk, raw egg, gelatin or mild soap. Avoid vomiting or lavage if it is believed that a concentrated solution has been ingested.

Central paralysis cannot be countered by curare antagonists or CNS stimulants but sympathomimetic drugs have been given.

Mechanically assisted ventilation with oxygen may be necessary. Persistent convulsions may be controlled with cautious doses of diazepam or a short-acting barbiturate. Do not give alcohol in any form.

*Accidental intravenous infusion:* Massive haemolysis can occur which will require blood transfusion.

*Accidental intra-uterine administration:* Introduction into the uterus can lead to haemolysis and pulmonary embolism.

**Pharmacological properties**

*Pharmacodynamic properties:* Hibicet Hospital Concentrate is a topical antiseptic for external use only and is not intended to be administered orally or parentally. The active agents, chlorhexidine gluconate and cetrimide are strongly cationic, binding to skin, mucosa and exposed tissues, thus percutaneous absorption is poor. There are, as a consequence, no general pharmacological studies available on the effects of Hibicet Hospital Concentrate or other topically administered chlorhexidine/cetrimide formulations.

If chlorhexidine is systemically absorbed there is no evidence of metabolic cleavage of the drug, however, animal studies suggest that systemically absorbed cetrimide may be metabolised to some extent.

Both active agents have a broad spectrum of antimicrobial activity and are bacteriostatic at low concentrations whilst at higher concentrations their activity is rapidly bactericidal. They are both active against dermatophytic fungi (including the yeast *C. Albicans*) and enveloped viruses such as HIV.

*Pharmacokinetic properties:* Percutaneous absorption of the active agents in Hibicet Hospital Concentrate is poor. Studies in animals using $^{14}$C-Labelled cetrimide have shown that even after oral dosing only small amounts were found in the blood plasma and approximately 2% was excreted in the bile during the first 12 hours after treatment: only small amounts of radioactivity were found in the liver, kidneys, spleen, heart, lungs and skeletal muscle and tissue radioactivity declined rapidly.

Similarly, attempts to detect percutaneous absorption of chlorhexidine gluconate in man have shown that, if it occurs at all, the level is exceedingly small and insignificant–the limit of detection used being of the order of 0.005 mg/litre.

Furthermore, it is very unlikely that the pharmacokinetic properties of either chlorhexidine gluconate or cetrimide will be altered significantly in special situations, such as hepatic failure, renal failure, treatment of children, the elderly, in pregnancy or nursing mothers.

*Preclinical safety data:* Chlorhexidine and cetrimide are drugs on which extensive clinical experience has been obtained. All relevant information for the prescriber is provided elsewhere in the Summary of Product Characteristics.

**Pharmaceutical particulars**

*List of excipients:* Benzyl Benzoate BP; industrial methylated spirit; D-gluconolactone; Isopropyl Alcohol BP; liquid deodoriser; Purified Water PhEur; Sodium Hydroxide BP; Sunset yellow FCF (E110); Terpineol BP.

*Incompatibilities:* Hypochlorite bleaches may cause brown stains to develop in fabrics which have previously been in contact with preparations containing chlorhexidine.

Chlorhexidine and cetrimide are incompatible with soap and other anionic agents.

*Shelf life:* 4 years.

*Special precautions for storage:* Store below 30°C.

*Nature and contents of container:* White HDPE bottle (5 litres).

*Instructions for use/handling:* Dilute before use.

Dilute with tap water of an acceptable bacteriological standard or alcohol (ethanol, industrial methylated spirits or isopropanol). Add diluent slowly to prevent excessive foaming.

As a precaution against bacterial contamination, aqueous stock solutions should contain at least 4% v/v of isopropanol or 7% v/v of ethanol which may be denatured (ie industrial methylated spirit).

Hibicet solutions used for instrument storage should contain 0.4% w/v sodium nitrite to inhibit metal corrosion. Such solutions must be changed every 7 days. Prolonged immersion of rubber appliances in Hibicet solutions is undesirable.

As cork may protect certain Gram-negative organisms from the action of antiseptics, Hibicet solutions must be stored in bottles with glass, plastic or rubber closures.

See also *Posology and method of administration* and *Special warnings and special precautions for use.*

**Marketing authorisation number** 12619/0054.

**Date of approval/revision of SPC** January 1997

**Legal category** GSL

## HIBISCRUB*

**Presentation** Hibiscrub is presented as a red, detergent solution containing 4% w/v chlorhexidine gluconate (equivalent to 20% v/v Chlorhexidine Gluconate Solution PhEur). Inactive ingredients are d-gluconolactone, isopropyl alcohol, lauryl dimethylamine oxide, perfume, polyoxyethylene-polyoxypropylene block copolymer, Ponceau 4R and water.

**Uses** Hibiscrub is an antimicrobial preparation for pre-operative surgical hand disinfection, antiseptic handwashing on the ward and pre-operative and post-operative skin antisepsis for patients undergoing elective surgery.

*Mode of action:* Chlorhexidine is effective against a wide range of Gram negative and Gram positive vegetative bacteria, yeasts, dermatophyte fungi and lipophilic viruses. It is inactive against bacterial spores except at elevated temperatures.

Because of its cationic nature, chlorhexidine binds strongly to skin, mucosa and other tissues and is thus very poorly absorbed. No detectable blood levels have been found in man following oral use and percutaneous absorption, if it occurs at all, is insignificant.

**Dosage and administration** *Pre-operative surgical hand disinfection:* Wet the hands and forearms, apply 5 ml of Hibiscrub and wash for one minute cleaning the fingernails with a brush or scraper. Rinse, apply a further 5 ml of Hibiscrub and continue washing for a further two minutes. Rinse thoroughly and dry.

*Antiseptic handwash on the ward:* Wet the hands and forearms, apply 5 ml of Hibiscrub and wash for one minute. Rinse thoroughly and dry.

*Pre-operative skin antisepsis for the patient:* The patient washes his whole body in the bath or shower on at least two occasions, usually the day before and the day of operation as follows:

The day before the operation, the patient washes with 25 ml of Hibiscrub beginning with the face and working downwards paying particular attention to areas around the nose, axillae, umbilicus, groin and perineum. The body is then rinsed and the wash repeated with a further 25 ml, this time including the hair. Finally the patient rinses his entire body thoroughly and dries on a clean towel. This procedure should be repeated the following day. Patients confined to bed can be washed with Hibiscrub using a standard bed-bath technique.

Conventional disinfection of the operation site will then be performed when the patient is in theatre.

*Post-operative skin antisepsis for the patient:* The patient washes his whole body, excluding the operation wound, in the bath or shower usually on the third day after the operation using the procedure described above.

**Contra-indications, warnings, etc** Hibiscrub is contra-indicated for persons who have previously shown a hypersensitivity reaction to chlorhexidine. However, such reactions are extremely rare.

For external use only. Avoid contact with brain, meninges and middle ear. In patients with head or spinal injuries or perforated ear drum, the benefit of use in pre-operative preparation should be evaluated against the risk of contact.

Not for injection or use in body cavities.

Keep out of the eyes. If chlorhexidine solutions come into contact with eyes, wash out promptly and thoroughly with water.

*Side-effects:* Irritative skin reactions can occasionally occur. Generalised allergic reactions to chlorhexidine have also been reported but are extremely rare.

*Accidental ingestion:* Chlorhexidine taken orally is poorly absorbed. Treat with gastric lavage using milk, raw egg, gelatin or mild soap. Employ supportive measures as appropriate.

**Pharmaceutical precautions** Hypochlorite bleaches may cause brown stains to develop in fabrics which have previously been in contact with preparations containing chlorhexidine.

Chlorhexidine is incompatible with soap and other anionic agents.

Store below 25°C, protect from light.

**Legal category** GSL.

**Package quantities** Containers of 250 ml (OP), 500 ml, 5 litres. Dispensing brackets and pumps are available.

**Further information** Nil.

**Product licence number** 12619/0020.

## HIBISOL*

**Presentation** Hibisol is presented as an alcoholic solution containing 0.5% w/v chlorhexidine gluconate (equivalent to 2.5% v/v Chlorhexidine Gluconate Solution PhEur) in 70% w/w Isopropyl Alcohol BP wi emollients. Inactive ingredients are castor oil, glycerc isopropyl alcohol and water.

**Uses** Hibisol is a rapid-acting antimicrobial prepar tion for the disinfection of clean intact skin. It is use for pre-operative surgical hand disinfection, han disinfection on the ward prior to aseptic procedure or after handling contaminated material, and f disinfection of patients' skin prior to surgery or othe invasive procedures.

*Mode of action:* Chlorhexidine is effective against wide range of Gram negative and Gram positiv vegetative bacteria, yeasts, dermatophyte fungi an lipophilic viruses. It is inactive against bacterial spore except at elevated temperatures.

Because of its cationic nature, chlorhexidine bind strongly to skin, mucosa and other tissues and is thu very poorly absorbed. No detectable blood level have been found in man following oral use an percutaneous absorption, if it occurs at all, is insigni icant.

**Dosage and administration**

*Pre-operative surgical hand disinfection:* Dispens 5 ml of Hibisol and spread thoroughly over both hand and forearms, rubbing vigorously. When dry apply further 5 ml and repeat the procedure.

*NB.* Before the first operation on a list or subse quently when hands are soiled the hands should b cleansed and disinfected with an effective antisepti detergent handwash.

*Antiseptic hand disinfection on the ward:* Dispens 3 ml of Hibisol and spread thoroughly over the hand and wrists rubbing vigorously until dry.

*NB.* If the hands are soiled, cleanse and *dry* befor using Hibisol or alternatively use an effective antise tic/detergent handwash.

*Disinfection of patients' skin:* Prior to surgery, app Hibisol to a sterile swab and rub vigorously over th operation site for a minimum of two minutes. Hibis is also used for preparation of the skin prior to invasiv procedures such as venepuncture.

**Contra-indications, warnings, etc** Hibisol is contra indicated for persons who have previously shown hypersensitivity reaction to chlorhexidine. Howeve such reactions are extremely rare.

For external use only. Avoid contact with the brai meninges and middle ear. Not for injection. Do nc use in body cavities.

The solution is irritant to eyes and mucous mem branes. Keep out of the eyes. If the solution doe come into contact with eyes, wash out promptly an thoroughly with water.

Flammable. This preparation contains alcoho When use is to be followed by diathermy do not allov pooling of the fluid to occur, and ensure that the ski and surrounding drapes are dry.

Prolonged skin contact with alcoholic solution should be avoided. Allow to dry before proceeding.

*Side-effects:* Irritative skin reactions can occasionall occur. Generalised allergic reactions to chlorhexidin have also been reported but are extremely rare.

*Accidental ingestion:* Chlorhexidine taken orally i poorly absorbed. Treat with gastric lavage using mil raw egg, gelatin or mild soap avoiding pulmonar aspiration. Do not use apomorphine. Assist respira tion if necessary and keep patient warm. Intravenou laevulose can accelerate alcohol metabolism. In se vere cases, haemodialysis or peritoneal dialysis ma be necessary.

**Pharmaceutical precautions** Flammable.

Hypochlorite bleaches may cause brown stains t develop in fabrics which have previously been i contact with preparations containing chlorhexidine.

Chlorhexidine is incompatible with soaps and othe anionic agents.

Store below 25°C.

**Legal category** GSL.

**Package quantities** Containers of 500 ml.

**Further information** A suitable antiseptic-deterger preparation which is compatible with Hibisol is Hibis crub.

**Product licence number** 12619/0021.

## HIBITANE* OBSTETRIC CREAM

**Qualitative and quantitative composition** Chlorhexi dine Gluconate 1% w/w (incorporated as Chlorhexi dine Gluconate Solution PhEur 5.0% v/w).

**Pharmaceutical form** Cream

**Clinical particulars**

*Therapeutic indications* Hibitane Obstetric Cream i an antimicrobial preparation for use as an antisepti and lubricant in obstetric and gynaecological practice osology and method of administration:

dults: Apply liberally to the skin around the vulva
d perineum of the patient, and to the gloved hands
the midwife or doctor.

Elderly and children: There are no special dosage
commendations for either elderly patients or chil-
en.

ontra-indications: Hibitane preparations are contra-
dicated for patients who have previously shown a
persensitivity reaction to chlorhexidine. However,
ch reactions are extremely rare.

pecial warnings and special precautions for use: For
pical application only. Keep out of the eyes and
rs. Avoid contact with the brain and meninges.

teractions with other medicaments and other forms
interaction: See Incompatibilities.

regnancy and lactation: There is no evidence of any
dverse effects on the foetus arising from the use of
ibitane Obstetric Cream during pregnancy and laction. Therefore no special precautions are recom-
ended.

ffects on ability to drive and use machines: None
ave been reported or are known.

ndesirable effects: Irritative skin reactions can occa-
onally occur. Generalised allergic reactions to chlor-
exidine have also been reported but are extremely
re.

verdose
ccidental ingestion: Chlorhexidine taken orally is
oorly absorbed. Treat with gastric lavage using milk,
w egg, gelatin or mild soap. Employ supportive
easures as appropriate.

harmacological properties
harmacodynamic properties: Chlorhexidine is effec-
ve against a wide range of Gram negative and Gram
ositive vegetative bacteria, yeasts, dermatophyte
ngi and lipophilic viruses. It is inactive against
acterial spores except in elevated temperatures.

harmacokinetic properties: Because of its cationic
ature, chlorhexidine binds strongly to skin, mucosa
nd other tissues and is thus very poorly absorbed.
here are, as a consequence, no general pharmaco-
gical studies on chlorhexidine available and its
fects on internal organs are minimal. No detectable
ood levels have been found in man following oral
se and percutaneous absorption, if it occurs at all, is
significant.

reclinical safety data: Chlorhexidine is a drug on
hich extensive clinical experience has been ob-
ined. All relevant information for the prescriber is
rovided elsewhere in the Summary of Product
haracteristics.

harmaceutical particulars
st of excipients: Cetostearyl Alcohol PhEur; Cetos-
aryl Alcohol/Ethylene Oxide Condensate; Isopropyl
cohol BP; Linalyl Acetate; Liquid Paraffin PhEur;
hite Soft Paraffin BP; Purified Water PhEur.

compatibilities: Hypochlorite bleaches may cause
rown stains to develop in fabrics which have previ-
usly been in contact with preparations containing
lorhexidine.
Chlorhexidine is incompatible with soap and other
nionic agents.

helf life: 3 years.

pecial precautions for storage: Store below 30°C

ature and contents of container: White HDPE bottle
50 ml).

structions for use/handling: Use undiluted.

arketing authorisation number 12619/0024

ate of approval/revision of spc February 1997

egal category GSL

# IBITANE* 5% CONCENTRATE

ualitative and quantitative composition Chlorhexi-
ne gluconate 5% w/v (incorporated as Chlorhexidine
luconate Solution PhEur)

harmaceutical form Liquid

linical particulars

herapeutic indications: Hibitane 5% Concentrate is
n antimicrobial agent for general antiseptic purposes.
surface active agent is present to inhibit precipitation
hen dilutions are made with hard water.

osology and method of administration: For external
opical) use only.
No special dosages or indications are specified for
se of this product for children or the elderly.
Dilute before use with freshly distilled water, tap
ater of an acceptable bacteriological standard or
lcohol (ethanol, Industrial Methylated Spirit or iso-
ropanol).

| Method of preparation | Concentration of active ingredient required (chlorhexidine gluconate) | Use |
|---|---|---|
| 10 ml made up to 1 litre with water (1 in 100) | 1 in 2,000 (0.05%) aqueous | Swabbing in obstetrics, wounds and burns. † Storage of sterile instruments |
| 10 ml with 15 ml water made up to 100 ml with 95% alcohol (1 in 10) | 1 in 200 (0.5%) in 70% Alcohol | Pre-operative skin disinfection. Emergency instrument disinfection (2 minutes' immersion). (Excluding endoscopes containing cemented glass components) |

† Sterilise the dilution by autoclaving at 115–116°C for 30 minutes or 121–123°C for 15 minutes.

Contra-indications: Hibitane preparations are contra-
indicated for patients who have previously shown a
hypersensitivity reaction to chlorhexidine. However,
such reactions are extremely rare.

Special warnings and special precautions for use: For
external use only.
Dilute before use.
Solutions applied to wounds, burns or broken skin
should be sterile.
Syringes, needles or instruments which have been
immersed in Hibitane solutions should be thoroughly
rinsed in sterile water or saline before use.
Avoid contact with the brain, meninges and middle
ear.
Not for injection.
Do not use in body cavities.
The concentrated solution is irritant to eyes and
mucous membranes. Keep all solutions out of the
eyes.
If chlorhexidine solutions come into contact with
the eyes, wash out promptly and thoroughly with
water.
Prolonged skin contact with alcoholic solutions
should be avoided. Allow to dry before proceeding.
As with any other antiseptic agent, antimicrobial
activity may be diminished through incompatibility or
in the presence of significant quantities of organic
matter.

Interactions with other medicaments and other forms
of interaction: Hibitane 5% Concentrate contains a
surfactant and therefore instruments containing ce-
mented glass components should not be disinfected
with solutions prepared from Hibitane 5% Concentrate.
The low solubility of inorganic salts of chlorhexidine
may cause precipitation and consequent loss of
activity if Hibitane 5% Concentrate is diluted with a
solution containing inorganic anions, for example,
saline or peritoneal dialysis fluid. This precipitation
may occur when Hibitane 5% Concentrate is used to
disinfect catheters intended for use in peritoneal
dialysis. Inadvertent repeated exposure of peritoneal
membranes to precipitated material has been claimed
as a possible predisposing factor for peritoneal
fibrosis.

Pregnancy and lactation: There is no evidence of any
adverse effects from the use of Hibitane 5% Concentrate during pregnancy and lactation therefore no
special precautions are recommended.

Effects on ability to drive and use machines: None
have been reported or are known.

Undesirable effects: Irritative skin reactions can occasionally occur. Generalised allergic reactions to chlorhexidine have also been reported but are extremely
rare.

Overdose: This has not been reported.
Accidental ingestion: Chlorhexidine taken orally is
poorly absorbed. Treat with gastric lavage with milk,
raw egg, gelatin or mild soap. Employ supportive
measures as appropriate.
Accidental intravenous infusion: Blood transfusion
may be necessary to counteract haemolysis.

Pharmacological properties
Pharmacodynamic properties: Chlorhexidine is effective against a wide range of Gram negative and Gram
positive vegetative bacteria, yeasts, dermatophyte
fungi and lipophilic viruses. It is inactive against
bacterial spores except at elevated temperatures.

Pharmacokinetic properties: Because of its cationic
nature, chlorhexidine binds strongly to skin, mucosa
and other tissues and is thus very poorly absorbed.
No detectable blood levels have been found in man
following oral use and percutaneous absorption, if it
occurs at all, is insignificant.

Preclinical safety data: Chlorhexidine is a drug on
which extensive clinical experience has been obtained. All relevant information for the prescriber is

provided elsewhere in the Summary of Product
Characteristics.

Pharmaceutical particulars
List of excipients: Carmoisine E122; D-gluconolactone;
Isopropyl Alcohol BP; Linalyl acetate; Nonylphenol/
ethylene oxide condensate; Purified Water PhEur.

Incompatibilities: Hypochlorite bleaches may cause
brown stains to develop in fabrics which have previously been in contact with preparations containing
chlorhexidine.
Chlorhexidine is incompatible with soap and other
anionic agents.

Shelf life: 4 years

Special precautions for storage: Store below 30°C

Nature and contents of container HDPE bottle (5 litres)

Instructions for use/handling: As cork may protect
certain Gram-negative organisms from the action of
antiseptics, Hibitane solutions must be stored in
bottles with glass, plastic or rubber closures.
As a precaution against bacterial contamination,
stock aqueous solutions should contain at least 4% v/
v of isopropanol or 7% v/v of ethanol which may be
denatured (for example, Industrial Methylated Spirit).
Aqueous dilutions of Hibitane used for instrument
storage should contain 0.1% w/v sodium nitrite to
inhibit metal corrosion. Such solutions must be
changed every 7 days.
See Special warnings and special precautions for
use.

Marketing authorisation number 12619/0022

Date of approval/revision of SPC January 1997

Legal category GSL

# INDERAL* TABLETS AND INJECTION

Presentation
1. Tablets each containing 10 mg Propranolol Hydrochloride PhEur. Pink, round, bi-convex, film coated
tablets, impressed with the legend 'INDERAL' 10 on
one face. The impressions are highlighted in white.
2. Tablets each containing 40 mg Propranolol Hydrochloride PhEur. Pink, round, bi-convex, film coated
tablets, impressed with the legend 'INDERAL' 40 on
one face. The impressions are highlighted in white.
3. Tablets each containing 80 mg Propranolol Hydrochloride PhEur. Pink, round, bi-convex, film coated
tablets, impressed with the legend 'INDERAL' 80 on
one face. The impressions are highlighted in white.
Inactive ingredients of Inderal tablets are calcium
carboxymethylcellulose, carmine, gelatin, glycerol,
lactose, magnesium carbonate, magnesium stearate,
methylhydroxypropyl cellulose and titanium dioxide.
4. Injection – a solution containing Propranolol
Hydrochloride PhEur. 1 mg per 1 ml in glass ampoules
of 1 ml. Inactive ingredients are citric acid and water.

Uses Inderal, a beta-adrenoceptor blocking drug, is
indicated in:

a. the control of hypertension
b. the management of angina pectoris
c. the long term prophylaxis against reinfarction after
   recovery from acute myocardial infarction
d. the control of most forms of cardiac arrhythmia
e. the prophylaxis of migraine
f. the management of essential tremor
g. relief of situational anxiety and generalised anxiety
   symptoms, particularly those of somatic type
h. prophylaxis of upper gastro-intestinal bleeding in
   patients with portal hypertension and oesophageal
   varices
i. the adjunctive management of thyrotoxicosis and
   thyrotoxic crisis
j. management of hypertrophic obstructive cardiomyopathy
k. management of phaeochromocytoma perioperatively (with an alpha-adrenoceptor blocking drug).

The intravenous injection is intended for the emergency treatment of cardiac arrhythmias and thyrotoxic
crisis.

Mode of action: Propranolol is a competitive antagonist at both beta$_1$ and beta$_2$-adrenoceptors. It has no
agonist activity at the beta-adrenoceptor, but has
membrane stabilising activity at concentrations exceeding 1–3 mg/litre, though such concentrations are
rarely achieved during oral therapy. Competitive beta-
adrenoceptor blockade has been demonstrated in
man by a parallel shift to the right in the dose-heart
rate response curve to beta-agonists such as isoprenaline.
Propranolol, as with other beta-adrenoceptor blocking drugs, has negative inotropic effects, and is
therefore contra-indicated in uncontrolled heart failure.
Propranolol is a racemic mixture and the active
form is the S (–) isomer. With the exception of
inhibition of the conversion of thyroxine to triiodothyronine it is unlikely that any additional ancillary

properties possessed by R (+) propranolol, in comparison with the racemic mixture will give rise to different therapeutic effects.

Propranolol is effective and well tolerated in most ethnic populations, although the response may be less in black patients.

Following intravenous administration the plasma half-life of propranolol is about 2 hours and the ratio of metabolites to parent drug in the blood is lower than after oral administration. In particular 4-hydroxypropranolol is not present after intravenous administration. Propranolol is completely absorbed after oral administration and peak plasma concentrations occur 1–2 hours after dosing in fasting patients. The liver removes up to 90% of an oral dose with an elimination half-life of 3 to 6 hours. Propranolol is widely and rapidly distributed throughout the body with highest levels occurring in the lungs, liver, kidney, brain and heart. Propranolol is highly protein bound (80–95%).

## Dosage and administration

*Adults: Oral:*

*Hypertension:* A starting dose of 80 mg twice a day may be increased at weekly intervals according to response. The usual dose range is 160–320 mg per day. With concurrent diuretic or other antihypertensive drugs a further reduction of blood pressure is obtained.

*Angina, migraine and essential tremor:* A starting dose of 40 mg two or three times daily may be increased by the same amount at weekly intervals according to patient response. An adequate response in migraine and essential tremor is usually seen in the range 80–160 mg/day and in angina in the range 120–240 mg/day.

*Situational and generalised anxiety:* A dose of 40 mg daily may provide short term relief of acute situational anxiety. Generalised anxiety, requiring longer term therapy, usually responds adequately to 40 mg twice daily which, in individual cases, may be increased to 40 mg three times daily. Treatment should be continued according to response. Patients should be reviewed after six to twelve months' treatment.

*Arrhythmias, anxiety tachycardia, hypertrophic obstructive cardiomyopathy and thyrotoxicosis:* A dosage range of 10–40 mg three or four times a day usually achieves the required response.

*Post myocardial infarction:* Treatment should start between days 5 and 21 after myocardial infarction, with an initial dose of 40 mg four times a day for 2 or 3 days. In order to improve compliance the total daily dosage may thereafter be given as 80 mg twice daily.

*Portal hypertension:* Dosage should be titrated to achieve approximately 25% reduction in resting heart rate. Dosing should begin with 40 mg twice daily, increasing to 80 mg twice daily depending on heart rate response. If necessary, the dose may be increased incrementally to a maximum of 160 mg twice daily.

*Phaeochromocytoma:* (Used only with an alpha-receptor blocking drug). Pre-operative: 60 mg daily for three days is recommended. Non-operable malignant cases: 30 mg daily.

*Intravenou:* The intravenous injection is intended for the emergency treatment of cardiac arrhythmias and thyrotoxic crisis. The initial dose of Inderal is 1 mg (1 ml) injected over one minute. This may be repeated at two minute intervals until a response is observed or to a maximum dose of 10 mg in conscious patients or 5 mg in patients under anaesthesia.

*Children: Arrhythmias, phaeochromocytoma, thyrotoxicosis;* Dosage should be individually determined and the following is only a guide: *Oral:* 250–500 micrograms/kg three or four times daily as required. *Intravenous:* 25–50 micrograms/kg injected slowly under ECG control and repeated three or four times daily as required.

*Migraine: Oral: Under the age of 12:* 20 mg two or three times daily. *Over the age of 12:* the adult dose.

*Fallot's Tetralogy:* The value of Inderal in this condition is confined mainly to the relief of right-ventricular outflow tract shut-down. It is also useful for treatment of associated arrhythmias and angina. Dosage should be individually determined and the following is only a guide: *Oral:* Up to 1 mg/kg repeated three or four times daily as required. *Intravenous:* Up to 100 micrograms/kg injected slowly under ECG control, repeated three or four times daily as required.

*Elderly patients:* Evidence concerning the relation between blood level and age is conflicting. With regard to the elderly, the optimum dose should be individually determined according to clinical response.

**Contra-indications, warnings, etc** Inderal must not be used if there is a history of bronchial asthma or bronchospasm.

Bronchospasm can usually be reversed by beta₂-agonist bronchodilators such as salbutamol. Large doses of the beta₂-agonist bronchodilator may be required to overcome the beta-blockade produced by propranolol and the dose should be titrated according to the clinical response; both intravenous and inhalational administration should be considered. The use of intravenous aminophylline and/or the use of ipratropium (given by nebuliser), may also be considered. Glucagon (1 to 2 mg given intravenously) has also been reported to produce a bronchodilator effect in asthmatic patients. Oxygen or artifical ventilation may be required in severe cases.

Inderal, as with other beta-adrenoceptor blocking drugs, must not be used in patients with any of the following conditions: known hypersensitivity to the substance, bradycardia, cardiogenic shock, hypotension, metabolic acidosis, after prolonged fasting, severe peripheral arterial circulatory disturbances, second or third degree heart block, sick sinus syndrome, untreated phaeochromocytoma, uncontrolled heart failure or Prinzmetal's angina.

Inderal as with other beta-adrenoceptor blocking drugs:

– although contra-indicated in uncontrolled heart failure (see *Contra-indications*), may be used in patients whose signs of heart failure have been controlled. Caution must be exercised in patients whose cardiac reserve is poor.
– although contra-indicated in severe peripheral arterial circulatory disturbances (see *Contra-indications*), may also aggravate less severe peripheral arterial circulatory disturbances.
– due to its negative effect on conduction time, caution must be exercised if it is given to patients with first degree heart block.
– may modify the tachycardia of hypoglycaemia.
– may mask the signs of thyrotoxicosis.
– will reduce heart rate, as a result of its pharmacological action. In the rare instances when a treated patient develops symptoms which may be attributable to a slow heart rate, the dose may be reduced.
– should not be discontinued abruptly in patients suffering from ischaemic heart disease. Either the equivalent dosage of another beta-adrenoceptor blocking drug may be substituted or the withdrawal of Inderal should be gradual.
– may cause a more severe reaction to a variety of allergens, when given to patients with a history of anaphylactic reaction to such allergens. Such patients may be unresponsive to the usual doses of adrenaline used to treat the allergic reactions.

Since the half-life may be increased in patients with significant hepatic or renal impairment, caution must be exercised when starting treatment and selecting the initial dose.

Inderal must be used with caution in patients with decompensated cirrhosis.

In patients with portal hypertension, liver function may deteriorate and hepatic encephalopathy may develop. There have been reports suggesting that treatment with propranolol may increase the risk of developing hepatic encephalopathy.

Inderal modifies the tachycardia of hypoglycaemia. Caution must be exercised in the concurrent use of Inderal and hypoglycaemic therapy in diabetic patients. Inderal may prolong the hypoglycaemic response to insulin.

Caution must be exercised when prescribing a beta-adrenoceptor blocking drug with Class 1 antiarrhythmic agents such as disopyramide.

Combined use of beta-adrenoceptor blocking drugs and calcium channel blockers with negative inotropic effects e.g. verapamil, diltiazem can lead to an exaggeration of these effects, particularly in patients with impaired ventricular function and/or sino-atrial or atrio-ventricular conduction abnormalities. This may result in severe hypotension, bradycardia and cardiac failure. Neither the beta-adrenoceptor blocking drug nor the calcium channel blocker should be administered intravenously within 48 hours of discontinuing the other.

Concomitant therapy with dihydropyridines e.g. nifedipine, may increase the risk of hypotension, and cardiac failure may occur in patients with latent cardiac insufficiency.

Beta-adrenoceptor blocking drugs may exacerbate the rebound hypertension which can follow the withdrawal of clonidine. If the two drugs are co-administered, the beta-adrenoceptor blocking drug should be withdrawn several days before discontinuing clonidine. If replacing clonidine by beta-adrenoceptor blocking drug therapy, the introduction of beta-adrenoceptor blocking drugs should be delayed for several days after clonidine administration has stopped.

Digitalis glycosides, in association with beta-adrenoceptor blocking drugs, may increase atrio-ventricular conduction time.

Concomitant use of sympathomimetic agents, e.g. adrenaline, may counteract the effect of beta-adrenoceptor blocking drugs. Caution must be exercised in the parenteral administration of preparations containing adrenaline to patients taking beta-adrenoceptor blocking drugs as, in rare cases, vasoconstrictio hypertension and bradycardia may result.

Administration of propranolol during infusion lignocaine may increase the plasma concentration lignocaine by approximately 30%. Patients alrea receiving propranolol tend to have higher lignocai levels than controls. The combination should avoided.

Caution must be exercised if ergotamine, dihydroc gotamine or related compounds are given in comi nation with propranolol since vasospastic reactio have been reported in a few patients.

Concomitant use of prostaglandin synthetase inhi iting drugs, e.g. ibuprofen or indomethacin, ma decrease the hypotensive effects of propranolol.

Concomitant administration of propranolol a chlorpromazine may result in an increase in plasm levels of both drugs. This may lead to an enhance antipsychotic effect for chlorpromazine and an i creased antihypertensive effect for propranolol.

Concomitant use of cimetidine or hydralazine w increase, whereas concomitant use of alcohol w decrease, the plasma levels of propranolol.

*Anaesthesia:* Caution must be exercised when usir anaesthetic agents with Inderal. The anaesthet should be informed and the choice of anaesthe should be the agent with as little negative inotrop activity as possible. Use of beta-adrenoceptor bloc ing drugs with anaesthetic drugs may result attenuation of the reflex tachycardia and increase t risk of hypotension. Anaesthetic agents causing m ocardial depression are best avoided.

*Interference with laboratory tests:* Inderal has bee reported to interfere with the estimation of seru bilirubin by the diazo method and with the determ nation of catecholamines by methods using fluore cence.

*Pregnancy:* As with all drugs, Inderal should not b given during pregnancy unless its use is essenti. There is no evidence of teratogenicity with Indera However beta-adrenoceptor blocking drugs redu placental perfusion, which may result in intra-uteri foetal death, immature and premature deliveries. addition, adverse effects (especially hypoglycaem and bradycardia in the neonate and bradycardia in t foetus) may occur. There is an increased risk of cardi and pulmonary complications in the neonate in t post-natal period.

*Lactation:* Most beta-adrenoceptor blocking dru particularly lipophilic compounds, will pass into brea milk although to a variable extent. Breast feeding therefore not recommended following administratic of these compounds.

*Effect on ability to drive or operate machinery:* Th use of Inderal is unlikely to result in any impairme of the ability of patients to drive or operate machiner However, it should be taken into account that occ sionally dizziness or fatigue may occur.

*Undesirable events:* Inderal is usually well tolerate In clinical studies, the undesired events reported a usually attributable to the pharmacological actions propranolol.

The following undesired events, listed by boc system, have been reported.

Cardiovascular: bradycardia, heart failure deterie ration, postural hypotension which may be associate with syncope, cold extremities. In susceptible patient precipitation of heart block, exacerbation of interm tent claudication, Raynaud's phenomenon.

CNS: confusion, dizziness, mood changes, nigh mares, psychoses and hallucinations, sleep distu bances.

Endocrine: hypoglycaemia in children.

Gastrointestinal: gastrointestinal disturbance.

Haematological: purpura, thrombocytopenia.

Integumentary: alopecia, dry eyes, psoriasiforr skin reactions, exacerbation of psoriasis, skin rashes

Neurological: paraesthesia.

Respiratory: bronchospasm may occur in patien with bronchial asthma or a history of asthmat complaints, sometimes with fatal outcome (see Co tra-indications).

Special senses: visual disturbances.

Others: fatigue and/or lassitude (often transient), a increase in ANA (antinuclear antibodies) has bee observed, however the clinical relevance of this is n clear; isolated reports of myasthenia gravis lik syndrome or exacerbation of myasthenia gravis hav been reported.

Discontinuance of the drug should be considered according to clinical judgement, the well-being of th patient is adversely affected by any of the abov reactions. Cessation of therapy with a beta-adrenocep tor blocking drug should be gradual. In the rare even of intolerance manifested as bradycardia and hyp tension, the drug should be withdrawn and, if neces sary, treatment for overdosage instituted.

*Overdosage:* The symptoms of overdosage may include bradycardia, hypotension, acute cardiac insufficiency and bronchospasm.

General treatment should include: close supervision, treatment in an intensive care ward, the use of gastric lavage, activated charcoal and a laxative to prevent absorption of any drug still present in the gastrointestinal tract, the use of plasma or plasma substitutes to treat hypotension and shock.

Excessive bradycardia can be countered with atropine 1–2 mg intravenously and/or a cardiac pacemaker. If necessary, this may be followed by a bolus dose of glucagon 10 mg intravenously. If required, this may be repeated or followed by an intravenous infusion of glucagon 1–10 mg/hour depending on response. If no response to glucagon occurs or if glucagon is unavailable, a beta-adrenoceptor stimulant such as dobutamine 2.5 to 10 micrograms/kg/minute by intravenous infusion may be given. Dobutamine, because of its positive inotropic effect could also be used to treat hypotension and acute cardiac insufficiency. It is likely that these doses would be inadequate to reverse the cardiac effects of beta-blockade if a large overdose has been taken. The dose of dobutamine should therefore be increased if necessary to achieve the required response according to the clinical condition of the patient.

**Pharmaceutical precautions** Inderal tablets should be stored below 30°C, protected from light and moisture.

Inderal injection should be stored below 30°C, protected from light.

**Legal category** POM.

**Package quantities**

*Tablets 10 mg:* Containers of 100 (OP).

*Tablets 40 mg:* Containers of 100 (OP).

*Tablets 80 mg:* Containers of 100 (OP).

*Injection:* 1 ml ampoules in boxes of 10.

**Further information** *Compatibility with intravenous infusion fluids:* Inderal Injection is compatible with 0.9% w/v sodium chloride and 5% w/v dextrose.

**Product licence numbers**

| | |
|---|---|
| Inderal Tablets 10 mg | 12619/0030 |
| Inderal Tablets 40 mg | 12619/0031 |
| Inderal Tablets 80 mg | 12619/0032 |
| Inderal Injection | 12619/0027 |

# INDERAL* LA
# HALF-INDERAL* LA

**Presentation** Inderal LA and Half-Inderal LA capsules contain spheroids of the beta-adrenoceptor blocking drug propranolol hydrochloride which have a sustained release coating to provide long action.

*Inderal LA capsules* each contain 160 mg Propranolol Hydrochloride PhEur. Inderal LA is presented as size 1 gelatin capsules with a clear pink body and opaque, lavender cap marked Inderal LA in white.

*Half-Inderal LA capsules* each contain 80 mg Propranolol Hydrochloride PhEur. Half-Inderal LA is presented as size 3 gelatin capsules with a clear pink body and opaque, pale lavender cap and marked Half-Inderal LA in black.

Inactive ingredients are erythrosine, ethylcellulose, gelatin, glycerol, iron oxide, methylhydroxypropylcellulose, microcrystalline cellulose, and titanium dioxide.

**Uses** Inderal LA and Half-Inderal LA are indicated in the management of angina, essential tremor, relief of situational anxiety and generalised anxiety symptoms, particularly those of somatic type, prophylaxis of upper gastro-intestinal bleeding in patients with portal hypertension and oesophageal varices, the adjunctive management of thyrotoxicosis, and the prophylaxis of migraine.

Inderal LA is indicated in the control of hypertension.

One Half-Inderal LA capsule daily is unlikely on its own to be sufficient to treat hypertension, but it may be used as a starting dose in appropriate patients (e.g. the elderly) or to provide a convenient method of gradual dosage alteration.

*Mode of action:* Propranolol is a competitive antagonist at both $beta_1$ and $beta_2$-adrenoceptors. It has no agonist activity at the beta-adrenoceptor, but has membrane stabilising activity at concentrations exceeding 1–3 mg/litre, though such concentrations are rarely achieved during oral therapy. Competitive beta-adrenoceptor blockade has been demonstrated in man by a parallel shift to the right in the dose-heart rate response curve to beta-agonists such as isoprenaline.

Propranolol, as with other beta-adrenoceptor blocking drugs, has negative inotropic effects, and is therefore contra-indicated in uncontrolled heart failure.

Propranolol is a racemic mixture and the active form is the S (–) isomer. With the exception of inhibition of the conversion of thyroxine to triiodothyronine it is unlikely that any additional ancillary properties possessed by R (+) propranolol, in comparison with the racemic mixture will give rise to different therapeutic effects.

Propranolol is effective and well tolerated in most ethnic populations, although the response may be less in black patients.

The sustained release preparation of propranolol maintains a higher degree of $beta_1$-blockade 24 hours after dosing compared with conventional propranolol.

Propranolol is completely absorbed after oral administration. Following oral dosing with the sustained release preparation of propranolol the blood profile is flatter than after conventional Inderal but the half-life is increased to between 10 and 20 hours. The liver removes up to 90% of an oral dose with an elimination half-life of 3 to 6 hours. Propranolol is widely and rapidly distributed throughout the body with highest levels occurring in the lungs, liver, kidney, brain and heart. Propranolol is highly protein bound (80–95%).

**Dosage and administration** *Adults: Hypertension:* The usual starting dose is one 160 mg Inderal LA capsule daily, taken either morning or evening. An adequate response is seen in most patients at this dosage. If necessary, it can be increased in 80 mg Half-Inderal LA increments until an adequate response is achieved. A further reduction in blood pressure can be obtained if a diuretic or other antihypertensive agent is given in addition to Inderal LA and Half-Inderal LA.

*Angina, essential tremor, thyrotoxicosis and the prophylaxis of migraine:* One Half-Inderal LA capsule daily taken either morning or evening may be sufficient to provide adequate control in many patients. If necessary the dose may be increased to one Inderal LA capsule per day and an additional Half-Inderal LA increment may be given.

*Situational and generalised anxiety:* One Half-Inderal LA capsule taken daily should be sufficient to provide short term relief of acute situational anxiety. Generalised anxiety, requiring longer term therapy, usually responds adequately at the same dosage. In individual cases, the dosage may be increased to one Inderal LA capsule per day. Treatment should be continued according to response. Patients should be reviewed after six to twelve months' treatment.

*Portal hypertension:* Dosage should be titrated to achieve approximately 25% reduction in resting heart rate. Dosing should begin with one 80 mg Half-Inderal LA capsule daily, increasing to one 160 mg Inderal LA capsule daily depending on heart rate response. Further 80 mg Half-Inderal LA increments may be added up to a maximum dose of 320 mg once daily.

Patients who are already established on equivalent daily doses of Inderal tablets should be transferred to the equivalent doses of Half-Inderal LA or Inderal LA daily taken either morning or evening.

*Children:* Inderal LA and Half-Inderal LA are not intended for use in children.

*Elderly patients:* Evidence concerning the relation between blood level and age is conflicting. It is suggested that treatment should start with one Half-Inderal LA capsule once daily. The dose may be increased to one Inderal LA capsule daily or higher as appropriate.

**Contra-indications, warnings, etc** Inderal LA and Half-Inderal LA must not be used if there is a history of bronchial asthma or bronchospasm.

Bronchospasm can usually be reversed by $beta_2$-agonist bronchodilators such as salbutamol. Large doses of the $beta_2$-agonist bronchodilator may be required to overcome the beta-blockade produced by propranolol and the dose should be titrated according to the clinical response; both intravenous and inhalational administration should be considered. The use of intravenous aminophylline and/or the use of ipratropium (given by nebuliser), may also be considered. Glucagon (1 to 2 mg given intravenously) has also been reported to produce a bronchodilator effect in asthmatic patients. Oxygen or artifical ventilation may be required in severe cases.

Inderal LA and Half-Inderal LA, as with other beta-adrenoceptor blocking drugs, must not be used in patients with any of the following conditions: known hypersensitivity to the substance, bradycardia, cardiogenic shock, hypotension, metabolic acidosis, after prolonged fasting, severe peripheral arterial circulatory disturbances, second or third degree heart block, sick sinus syndrome, untreated phaeochromocytoma, uncontrolled heart failure or Prinzmetal's angina.

Inderal LA and Half-Inderal LA as with other beta-adrenoceptor blocking drugs:

- although contra-indicated in uncontrolled heart failure (see *Contra-indications*), may be used in patients whose signs of heart failure have been controlled. Caution must be exercised in patients whose cardiac reserve is poor.
- although contra-indicated in severe peripheral arterial circulatory disturbances (see *Contra-indications*), may also aggravate less severe peripheral arterial circulatory disturbances.
- due to its negative effect on conduction time, caution must be exercised if it is given to patients with first degree heart block.
- may modify the tachycardia of hypoglycaemia.
- may mask the signs of thyrotoxicosis.
- will reduce heart rate, as a result of its pharmacological action. In the rare instances when a treated patient develops symptoms which may be attributable to a slow heart rate, the dose may be reduced.
- should not be discontinued abruptly in patients suffering from ischaemic heart disease. Either the equivalent dosage of another beta-adrenoceptor blocking drug may be substituted or the withdrawal of Inderal LA should be gradual. This can be achieved by first substituting the daily Inderal LA dose by the equivalent in Half-Inderal LA capsules and then gradually reducing the number of capsules.
- may cause a more severe reaction to a variety of allergens, when given to patients with a history of anaphylactic reaction to such allergens. Such patients may be unresponsive to the usual doses of adrenaline used to treat the allergic reactions.

Since the half-life may be increased in patients with significant hepatic or renal impairment, caution must be exercised when starting treatment and selecting the initial dose.

Inderal LA and Half-Inderal LA must be used with caution in patients with decompensated cirrhosis.

In patients with portal hypertension, liver function may deteriorate and hepatic encephalopathy may develop. There have been reports suggesting that treatment with propranolol may increase the risk of developing hepatic encephalopathy.

Inderal LA and Half-Inderal LA modify the tachycardia of hypoglycaemia. Caution must be exercised in the concurrent use of Inderal LA or Half-Inderal LA and hypoglycaemic therapy in diabetic patients. Propranolol may prolong the hypoglycaemic response to insulin.

Caution must be exercised when prescribing a beta-adrenoceptor blocking drug with Class 1 antiarrhythmic agents such as disopyramide.

Combined use of beta-adrenoceptor blocking drugs and calcium channel blockers with negative inotropic effects e.g. verapamil, diltiazem can lead to an exaggeration of these effects, particularly in patients with impaired ventricular function and/or sino-atrial or atrio-ventricular conduction abnormalities. This may result in severe hypotension, bradycardia and cardiac failure. Neither the beta-adrenoceptor blocking drug nor the calcium channel blocker should be administered intravenously within 48 hours of discontinuing the other.

Concomitant therapy with dihydropyridines e.g. nifedipine, may increase the risk of hypotension, and cardiac failure may occur in patients with latent cardiac insufficiency.

Beta-adrenoceptor blocking drugs may exacerbate the rebound hypertension which can follow the withdrawal of clonidine. If the two drugs are co-administered, the beta-adrenoceptor blocking drug should be withdrawn several days before discontinuing clonidine. If replacing clonidine by beta-adrenoceptor blocking drug therapy, the introduction of beta-adrenoceptor blocking drugs should be delayed for several days after clonidine administration has stopped.

Digitalis glycosides, in association with beta-adrenoceptor blocking drugs, may increase atrio-ventricular conduction time.

Concomitant use of sympathomimetic agents, e.g. adrenaline, may counteract the effect of beta-adrenoceptor blocking drugs. Caution must be exercised in the parenteral administration of preparations containing adrenaline to patients taking beta-adrenoceptor blocking drugs as, in rare cases, vasoconstriction, hypertension and bradycardia may result.

Administration of propranolol during infusion of lignocaine may increase the plasma concentration of lignocaine by approximately 30%. Patients already receiving propranolol tend to have higher lignocaine levels than controls. The combination should be avoided.

Caution must be exercised if ergotamine, dihydroergotamine or related compounds are given in combination with propranolol since vasospastic reactions have been reported in a few patients.

Concomitant use of prostaglandin synthetase inhibiting drugs, e.g. ibuprofen or indomethacin, may decrease the hypotensive effects of propranolol.

Concomitant administration of propranolol and chlorpromazine may result in an increase in plasma levels of both drugs. This may lead to an enhanced antipsychotic effect for chlorpromazine and an increased antihypertensive effect for propranolol.

Concomitant use of cimetidine will increase,

whereas concomitant use of alcohol will decrease, the plasma levels of propranolol.

*Anaesthesia:* Caution must be exercised when using anaesthetic agents with Inderal LA and Half-Inderal LA. The anaesthetist should be informed and the choice of anaesthetic should be the agent with as little negative inotropic activity as possible. Use of beta-adrenoceptor blocking drugs with anaesthetic drugs may result in attenuation of the reflex tachycardia and increase the risk of hypotension. Anaesthetic agents causing myocardial depression are best avoided.

*Interference with laboratory tests:* Inderal LA and Half-Inderal LA have been reported to interfere with the estimation of serum bilirubin by the diazo method and with the determination of catecholamines by methods using fluorescence.

*Pregnancy:* As with all drugs, Inderal LA and Half-Inderal LA should not be given during pregnancy unless their use is essential. There is no evidence of teratogenicity with Inderal. However beta-adrenoceptor blocking drugs reduce placental perfusion, which may result in intra-uterine foetal death, immature and premature deliveries. In addition, adverse effects (especially hypoglycaemia and bradycardia in the neonate and bradycardia in the foetus) may occur. There is an increased risk of cardiac and pulmonary complications in the neonate in the post-natal period.

*Lactation:* Most beta-adrenoceptor blocking drugs particularly lipophilic compounds, will pass into breast milk although to a variable extent. Breast feeding is therefore not recommended following administration of these compounds.

*Effect on ability to drive or operate machinery:* The use of Inderal LA or Half-Inderal LA is unlikely to result in any impairment of the ability of patients to drive or operate machinery. However, it should be taken into account that occasionally dizziness or fatigue may occur.

*Undesirable events:* Inderal LA and Half-Inderal LA are usually well tolerated. In clinical studies, the undesired events reported are usually attributable to the pharmacological actions of propranolol.

The following undesired events, listed by body system, have been reported.

Cardiovascular: bradycardia, heart failure deterioration, postural hypotension which may be associated with syncope, cold extremities. In susceptible patients: precipitation of heart block, exacerbation of intermittent claudication, Raynaud's phenomenon.

CNS: confusion, dizziness, mood changes, nightmares, psychoses and hallucinations, sleep disturbance.

Gastrointestinal: gastrointestinal disturbance.

Haematological: purpura, thrombocytopenia.

Integumentary: alopecia, dry eyes, psoriasiform skin reactions, exacerbation of psoriasis, skin rashes.

Neurological: paraesthesia.

Respiratory: bronchospasm may occur in patients with bronchial asthma or a history of asthmatic complaints, sometimes with fatal outcome (see *Contra-indications*).

Special senses: visual disturbances.

Others: fatigue and/or lassitude (often transient), an increase in ANA (antinuclear antibodies) has been observed, however the clinical relevance of this is not clear; isolated reports of myasthenia gravis like syndrome or exacerbation of myasthenia gravis have been reported in patients administered propranolol.

Discontinuance of the drug should be considered if, according to clinical judgement, the well-being of the patient is adversely affected by any of the above reactions. Cessation of therapy with a beta-adrenoceptor blocking drug should be gradual. In the rare event of intolerance manifested as bradycardia and hypotension, the drug should be withdrawn and, if necessary, treatment for overdosage instituted.

*Overdosage:* The symptoms of overdosage may include bradycardia, hypotension, acute cardiac insufficiency and bronchospasm.

General treatment should include: close supervision, treatment in an intensive care ward, the use of gastric lavage, activated charcoal and a laxative to prevent absorption of any drug still present in the gastrointestinal tract, the use of plasma or plasma substitutes to treat hypotension and shock.

Excessive bradycardia can be countered with atropine 1–2 mg intravenously and/or a cardiac pacemaker. If necessary, this may be followed by a bolus dose of glucagon 10 mg intravenously. If required, this may be repeated or followed by an intravenous infusion of glucagon 1–10 mg/hour depending on response. If no response to glucagon occurs or if glucagon is unavailable, a beta-adrenoceptor stimulant such as dobutamine 2.5 to 10 micrograms/kg/minute by intravenous infusion may be given. Dobutamine, because of its positive inotropic effect could also be used to treat hypotension and acute cardiac insufficiency. It is likely that these doses would be inadequate to reverse the cardiac effects of beta-blockade if a large overdose has been taken. The dose of dobutamine should therefore be increased if necessary to achieve the required response according to the clinical condition of the patient.

**Pharmaceutical precautions** Store below 30°C, protected from light and moisture.

**Legal category** POM.

**Package quantities** Patient Calendar Pack of 28 capsules (OP).

**Further information** Inderal LA and Half-Inderal LA capsules provide controlled release of propranolol hydrochloride such that blood levels are maintained for over 24 hours following a single oral dose and, unlike therapy with conventional tablets, irregular peaks and troughs of blood level are avoided.

**Product licence numbers**
Inderal LA 12619/0028
Half-Inderal LA 12619/0029

## INDERETIC*

**Presentation** White, opaque capsules, printed with Inderetic. Each capsule contains 80 mg Propranolol Hydrochloride PhEur and 2.5 mg Bendrofluazide PhEur. Inactive ingredients are gelatin, lactose, magnesium stearate and titanium dioxide.

**Uses** The management of hypertension.

*Mode of action:* Propranolol is a competitive antagonist at both the beta$_1$ and beta$_2$-adrenoceptors. It has no agonist activity at the beta-adrenoceptor, but has membrane stabilising activity at concentrations exceeding 1–3 mg/litre, though such concentrations are rarely achieved during oral therapy. Competitive beta-adrenoceptor blockade has been demonstrated in man by a parallel shift to the right in the dose-heart rate response curve to beta-agonists such as isoprenaline.

Propranolol, as with other beta-adrenoceptor blocking drugs, has negative inotropic effects, and is therefore contra-indicated in uncontrolled heart failure.

Propranolol is a racemic mixture and the active form is the S (−) isomer. With the exception of inhibition of the conversion of thyroxine to triiodothyronine it is unlikely that any additional ancillary properties possessed by R (+) propranolol, in comparison with the racemic mixture will give rise to different therapeutic effects.

Bendrofluazide causes diuresis by inhibiting sodium and water reabsorption in the proximal part of the distal tubule of the kidney. The consequences of this are a lowering in plasma volume and therefore cardiac output. However the main mechanism by which bendrofluazide lowers blood pressure is by its vasodilatory property which results in a lowering of peripheral resistance.

Propranolol is effective and well tolerated in most ethnic populations. Black patients respond better to the combination of propranolol and diuretics than to propranolol alone.

Propranolol is completely absorbed after oral administration and peak plasma concentrations occur 1–2 hours after dosing in fasting patients. The liver removes up to 90% of an oral dose with an elimination half-life of 3 to 6 hours. Propranolol is widely and rapidly distributed throughout the body with highest levels occurring in the lungs, liver, kidney, brain and heart. Propranolol is highly protein bound (80–95%).

Bendrofluazide is readily absorbed after oral administration and peak plasma concentrations occur 2–3 hours after dosing. Approximately 70% of the administered dose is metabolised and the remainder is recovered as unchanged drug in the urine. The elimination half-life is between 3 and 9 hours. Bendrofluazide has a high oral bioavailability and the drug distributes to extracellular spaces. Bendrofluazide is 94% bound to human serum albumin. There are no pharmacokinetic interactions between bendrofluazide and propranolol.

**Dosage and administration** *Adults:* One capsule twice daily should prove effective in most cases.

For new patients a maximum response is achieved usually within two weeks. If a greater antihypertensive effect is desired, Inderetic is compatible with most other antihypertensives which may be added (see *Warnings* below).

*Children:* There is no paediatric experience with Inderetic and for this reason it is not recommended for children.

*Elderly patients:* Evidence concerning the relation between blood level and age is conflicting. The optimum dose should be individually determined.

**Contra-indications, warnings, etc** Inderetic must not be used if there is a history of bronchial asthma or bronchospasm. The product label states the following warning: Do not take Inderetic if you have a history of asthma or wheezing. A similar warning appears in the Patient Information Leaflet.

Bronchospasm can usually be reversed by beta$_2$ agonist bronchodilators such as salbutamol. Large doses of the beta$_2$-agonist bronchodilator may be required to overcome the beta-blockade produced by propranolol and the dose should be titrated according to the clinical response; both intravenous and inhalational administration should be considered. The use of intravenous aminophylline and/or the use of ipratropium (given by nebuliser), may also be considered. Glucagon (1 to 2 mg given intravenously) has also been reported to produce a bronchodilator effect in asthmatic patients. Oxygen or artifical ventilation may be required in severe cases.

Inderetic must not be used in patients with any of the following conditions: known hypersensitivity to either component (or other thiazides), bradycardia, cardiogenic shock, hypotension, metabolic acidosis, after prolonged fasting, severe peripheral arterial circulatory disturbances, second or third degree heart block, sick sinus syndrome, untreated phaeochromocytoma, uncontrolled heart failure, Prinzmetal's angina, anuria or renal failure.

Due to its beta-adrenoceptor blocking drug component, Inderetic:

– although contra-indicated in uncontrolled heart failure (see *Contra-indications*), may be used in patients whose signs of heart failure have been controlled. Caution must be exercised in patients whose cardiac reserve is poor.
– although contra-indicated in severe peripheral arterial circulatory disturbances (see *Contra-indications*), may also aggravate less severe peripheral arterial circulatory disturbances.
– due to its negative effect on conduction time, caution must be exercised if it is given to patients with first degree heart block.
– may modify the tachycardia of hypoglycaemia.
– may mask the signs of thyrotoxicosis.
– will reduce heart rate, as a result of its pharmacological action. In the rare instances when a treated patient develops symptoms which may be attributable to a slow heart rate, the dose may be reduced.
– should not be discontinued abruptly in patients suffering from ischaemic heart disease.
– may cause a more severe reaction to a variety of allergens, when given to patients with a history of anaphylactic reaction to such allergens. Such patients may be unresponsive to the usual doses of adrenaline used to treat the allergic reactions.

Since the half-life may be increased in patients with significant hepatic or renal impairment, caution must be exercised when starting treatment and selecting the initial dose.

Inderetic must be used with caution in patients with decompensated cirrhosis.

In patients with portal hypertension, liver function may deteriorate and hepatic encephalopathy may develop. There have been reports suggesting that treatment with propranolol may increase the risk of developing hepatic encephalopathy.

As with other combinations of beta-adrenoceptor blocking drugs and diuretics and due to it bendrofluazide component, Inderetic:

– may be associated with minor changes in potassium status. Potassium depletion may be dangerous in patients receiving digitalis or those with hepatic cirrhosis with ascites.
– may decrease glucose tolerance. Caution must be exercised when administered to patients with a known predisposition to diabetes.

Inderetic modifies the tachycardia of hypoglycaemia. Caution should be exercised in the concurrent use of Inderetic and hypoglycaemic therapy in diabetic patients. Inderetic may prolong the hypoglycaemic response to insulin.

Caution must be exercised when prescribing a beta-adrenoceptor blocking drug with Class 1 antiarrhythmic agents such as disopyramide.

Combined use of beta-adrenoceptor blocking drugs and calcium channel blockers with negative inotropic effects e.g. verapamil, diltiazem can lead to an exaggeration of these effects, particularly in patients with impaired ventricular function and/or sino-atrial or atrio-ventricular conduction abnormalities. This may result in severe hypotension, bradycardia and cardiac failure. Neither the beta-adrenoceptor blocking drug nor the calcium channel blocker should be administered intravenously within 48 hours of discontinuing the other.

Concomitant therapy with dihydropyridines e.g. nifedipine, may increase the risk of hypotension, and cardiac failure may occur in patients with latent cardiac insufficiency.

Beta-adrenoceptor blocking drugs may exacerbate the rebound hypertension which can follow the withdrawal of clonidine. If the two drugs are co-administered, the beta-adrenoceptor blocking drug should be withdrawn several days before discontinu ing clonidine. If replacing clonidine by beta-adrenoceptor blocking drug therapy, the introduction of beta-adrenoceptor blocking drugs should be delayed for several days after clonidine administration has stopped.

Digitalis glycosides, in association with beta-adrenoceptor blocking drugs, may increase atrio-ventricular conduction time.

Concomitant use of sympathomimetic agents, e.g. adrenaline, may counteract the effect of beta-adrenoceptor blocking drugs. Caution must be exercised in the parenteral administration of preparations containing adrenaline to patients taking beta-adrenoceptor blocking drugs as, in rare cases, vasoconstriction, hypertension and bradycardia may result.

Administration of propranolol during infusion of lignocaine may increase the plasma concentration of lignocaine by approximately 30%. Patients already receiving propranolol tend to have higher lignocaine levels than controls. The combination should be avoided.

Caution must be exercised if ergotamine, dihydroergotamine or related compounds are given in combination with propranolol since vasospastic reactions have been reported in a few patients.

Concomitant use of prostaglandin synthetase inhibiting drugs, e.g. ibuprofen or indomethacin, may decrease the hypotensive effects of propranolol.

Concomitant administration of propranolol and chlorpromazine may result in an increase in plasma levels of both drugs. This may lead to an enhanced antipsychotic effect for chlorpromazine and an increased antihypertensive effect for propranolol.

Concomitant use of cimetidine or hydralazine will increase, whereas concomitant use of alcohol will decrease, the plasma levels of propranolol.

Preparations containing lithium generally should not be given with diuretics because they may reduce its renal clearance.

*Anaesthesia:* Caution must be exercised when using anaesthetic agents with Inderetic. The anaesthetist should be informed and the choice of anaesthetic should be the agent with as little negative inotropic activity as possible. Use of beta-adrenoceptor blocking drugs with anaesthetic drugs may result in attenuation of the reflex tachycardia and increase the risk of hypotension. Anaesthetic agents causing myocardial depression are best avoided.

*Interference with laboratory tests:* Inderetic has been reported to interfere with the estimation of serum bilirubin by the diazo method and with the determination of catecholamines by methods using fluorescence.

*Pregnancy:* Inderetic must not be given during pregnancy.

*Lactation:* As diuretics pass into breast milk, they should be avoided in mothers who wish to breast feed. Similarly, breast feeding is not recommended following administration of lipophilic beta-adrenoceptor blocking drugs.

*Effect on ability to drive or operate machinery:* The use of Inderetic is unlikely to result in any impairment of the ability of patients to drive or operate machinery. Studies to investigate these effects of bendrofluazide have not been carried out. When driving vehicles or operating machinery, it should be taken into account that occasional dizziness or fatigue may occur.

*Undesirable events:* Inderetic is usually well tolerated. In clinical studies, the undesired events reported are usually attributable to the pharmacological actions of propranolol or bendrofluazide.

Possible undesired events, listed by body system, include:

Cardiovascular: bradycardia, heart failure deterioration, postural hypotension which may be associated with syncope, cold extremities. In susceptible patients: precipitation of heart block, exacerbation of intermittent claudication, Raynaud's phenomenon.

CNS: confusion, dizziness, mood changes, nightmares, psychoses and hallucinations, sleep disturbances.

Gastrointestinal: gastrointestinal disturbance.

Haematological: purpura, thrombocytopenia.

Integumentary: alopecia, dry eyes, psoriasiform skin reactions, exacerbation of psoriasis, skin rashes.

Neurological: paraesthesia.

Respiratory: bronchospasm may occur in patients with bronchial asthma or a history of asthmatic complaints, sometimes with fatal outcome (see *Contra-indications*).

Special senses: visual disturbances.

Others: fatigue and/or lassitude (often transient), an increase in ANA (antinuclear antibodies) has been observed, however the clinical relevance of this is not clear; isolated reports of myasthenia gravis like syndrome or exacerbation of myasthenia gravis have been reported in patients administered propranolol.

Adverse effects of bendrofluazide are uncommon in the dose contained in Inderetic.

Hypokalaemia may occur and may be dangerous in patients receiving digitalis or in those with hepatic cirrhosis when coma may be precipitated.

Hyperuricaemia sometimes occurs, but an attack of gout is rare.

The thiazide diuretics increase blood urea and they should be used with care in patients with renal failure.

Reports of other adverse reactions to thiazides include skin rashes with associated photosensitivity, necrotising vasculitis, acute pancreatitis, blood dyscrasias and aggravation of pre-existing myopia.

Discontinuance of Inderetic should be considered if, according to clinical judgement, the well-being of the patient is adversely affected by any of the above reactions, bearing in mind that cessation of therapy with a beta-adrenoceptor blocking drug should be gradual.

*Overdosage:* The symptoms of overdosage may include bradycardia, hypotension, acute cardiac insufficiency and bronchospasm.

General treatment should include: close supervision, treatment in an intensive care ward, the use of gastric lavage, activated charcoal and a laxative to prevent absorption of any drug still present in the gastrointestinal tract, the use of plasma or plasma substitutes to treat hypotension and shock.

Excessive bradycardia can be countered with atropine 1–2 mg intravenously and/or a cardiac pacemaker. If necessary, this may be followed by a bolus dose of glucagon 10 mg intravenously. If required, this may be repeated or followed by an intravenous infusion of glucagon 1–10 mg/hour depending on response. If no response to glucagon occurs or if glucagon is unavailable, a beta-adrenoceptor stimulant such as dobutamine 2.5 to 10 micrograms/kg/minute by intravenous infusion may be given. Dobutamine, because of its positive inotropic effect could also be used to treat hypotension and acute cardiac insufficiency. It is likely that these doses would be inadequate to reverse the cardiac effects of beta-blockade if a large overdose has been taken. The dose of dobutamine should therefore be increased if necessary to achieve the required response according to the clinical condition of the patient.

Excessive diuresis should be countered by maintaining normal fluid and electrolyte balance.

**Pharmaceutical precautions** Store below 25°C, protected from light and moisture.

**Legal category** POM.

**Package quantities** Containers of 60 capsules (OP).

**Further information** Inderetic is designed to aid drug compliance by providing a convenient presentation of the standard beta-adrenoceptor blocking drug Inderal, propranolol hydrochloride, with the diuretic bendrofluazide for the treatment of hypertension. Concurrent use of propranolol and bendrofluazide produces a more pronounced and consistent antihypertensive response than when either component is used alone.

**Product licence number** 12619/0033.

## INDEREX*

**Presentation** Capsules, having opaque pink caps and opaque grey bodies printed with the name Inderex. Each capsule contains 160 mg Propranolol Hydrochloride PhEur in the form of spheroids having a sustained release coating to provide long action and 5 mg Bendrofluazide PhEur. Inactive ingredients are erythrosine, ethylcellulose, gelatin, iron oxide, lactose, maize starch, methylhydroxypropylcellulose, microcrystalline cellulose, Patent Blue V, stearic acid, talc and titanium dioxide.

**Uses** The management of hypertension.

*Mode of action:* Propranolol is a competitive antagonist at both the $beta_1$ and $beta_2$-adrenoceptors. It has no agonist activity at the beta-adrenoceptor, but has membrane stabilising activity at concentrations exceeding 1–3 mg/litre, though such concentrations are rarely achieved during oral therapy. Competitive beta-adrenoceptor blockade has been demonstrated in man by a parallel shift to the right in the dose-heart rate response curve to beta-agonists such as isoprenaline. The sustained release preparation of propranolol maintains a higher degree of $beta_1$ – blockade 24 hours after dosing compared with conventional propranolol.

Propranolol, as with other beta-adrenoceptor blocking drugs, has negative inotropic effects, and is therefore contra-indicated in uncontrolled heart failure.

Propranolol is a racemic mixture and the active form is the S (–) isomer. With the exception of inhibition of the conversion of thyroxine to triiodothyronine it is unlikely that any additional ancillary properties possessed by R (+) propranolol, in comparison with the racemic mixture will give rise to different therapeutic effects.

Bendrofluazide causes diuresis by inhibiting sodium and water reabsorption in the proximal part of the distal tubule of the kidney. The consequences of this are a lowering in plasma volume and therefore cardiac output. However the main mechanism by which bendrofluazide lowers blood pressure is by its vasodilatory property which results in a lowering of peripheral resistance.

Propranolol is effective and well tolerated in most ethnic populations. Black patients respond better to the combination of propranolol and diuretics than to propranolol alone.

Propranolol is completely absorbed after oral administration. Following oral dosing with the sustained release preparation of propranolol the blood profile is flatter than after conventional Inderal but the half-life is increased to between 10 and 20 hours. The liver removes up to 90% of an oral dose with an elimination half-life of 3 to 6 hours. Propranolol is widely and rapidly distributed throughout the body with highest levels occurring in the lungs, liver, kidney, brain and heart. Propranolol is highly protein bound (80–95%).

Bendrofluazide is readily absorbed after oral administration and peak plasma concentrations occur 2–3 hours after dosing. Approximately 70% of the administered dose is metabolised and the remainder is recovered as unchanged drug in the urine. The elimination half-life is between 3 and 9 hours. Bendrofluazide has a high oral bioavailability and the drug distributes to extracellular spaces. Bendrofluazide is 94% bound to human serum albumin. There are no pharmacokinetic interactions between bendrofluazide and propranolol.

**Dosage and administration** *Adults:* One capsule daily should prove effective in most cases.

For new patients a maximum response is achieved usually within two weeks. If a greater antihypertensive effect is desired, Inderex is compatible with most other antihypertensives which may be added (see *Warnings* below).

*Children:* There is no paediatric experience with Inderex and for this reason it is not recommended for children.

*Elderly patients:* Evidence concerning the relation between blood level and age is conflicting. The optimum dose should be individually determined.

**Contra-indications, warnings, etc** Inderex must not be used if there is a history of bronchial asthma or bronchospasm.

Bronchospasm can usually be reversed by $beta_2$-agonist bronchodilators such as salbutamol. Large doses of the $beta_2$-agonist bronchodilator may be required to overcome the beta-blockade produced by propranolol and the dose should be titrated according to the clinical response; both intravenous and inhalational administration should be considered. The use of intravenous aminophylline and/or the use of ipratropium (given by nebuliser), may also be considered. Glucagon (1 to 2 mg given intravenously) has also been reported to produce a bronchodilator effect in asthmatic patients. Oxygen or artifical ventilation may be required in severe cases.

Inderex must not be used in patients with any of the following conditions: known hypersensitivity to either component (or other thiazides), bradycardia, cardiogenic shock, hypotension, metabolic acidosis, after prolonged fasting, severe peripheral arterial circulatory disturbances, second or third degree heart block, sick sinus syndrome, untreated phaeochromocytoma, uncontrolled heart failure, Prinzmetal's angina, anuria or renal failure.

Due to its beta-adrenoceptor blocking drug component, Inderex:

- although contra-indicated in uncontrolled heart failure (see *Contra-indications*), may be used in patients whose signs of heart failure have been controlled. Caution must be exercised in patients whose cardiac reserve is poor.
- although contra-indicated in severe peripheral arterial circulatory disturbances (see *Contra-indications*), may also aggravate less severe peripheral arterial circulatory disturbances.
- due to its negative effect on conduction time, caution must be exercised if it is given to patients with first degree heart block.
- may modify the tachycardia of hypoglycaemia.
- may mask the signs of thyrotoxicosis.
- will reduce heart rate, as a result of its pharmacological action. In the rare instances when a treated patient develops symptoms which may be attributable to a slow heart rate, the dose may be reduced.
- should not be discontinued abruptly in patients suffering from ischaemic heart disease.
- may cause a more severe reaction to a variety of allergens, when given to patients with a history of anaphylactic reaction to such allergens. Such patients may be unresponsive to the usual doses of adrenaline used to treat the allergic reactions.

Since the half-life may be increased in patients with significant hepatic or renal impairment, caution must be exercised when starting treatment and selecting the initial dose.

Inderex must be used with caution in patients with decompensated cirrhosis.

In patients with portal hypertension, liver function may deteriorate and hepatic encephalopathy may develop. There have been reports suggesting that treatment with propranolol may increase the risk of developing hepatic encephalopathy.

As with other combinations of beta-adrenoceptor blocking drugs and diuretics and due to its bendrofluazide component, Inderex:

- may be associated with minor changes in potassium status. Potassium depletion may be dangerous in patients receiving digitalis or those with hepatic cirrhosis with ascites.
- may decrease glucose tolerance. Caution must be exercised when administered to patients with a known predisposition to diabetes.

Inderex modifies the tachycardia of hypoglycaemia. Caution must be exercised in the concurrent use of Inderex and hypoglycaemia therapy in diabetic patients. Inderex may prolong the hypoglycaemic response to insulin.

Caution must be exercised when prescribing a beta-adrenoceptor blocking drug with Class 1 antiarrhythmic agents such as disopyramide.

Combined use of beta-adrenoceptor blocking drugs and calcium channel blockers with negative inotropic effects e.g. verapamil, diltiazem can lead to an exaggeration of these effects, particularly in patients with impaired ventricular function and/or sino-atrial or atrio-ventricular conduction abnormalities. This may result in severe hypotension, bradycardia and cardiac failure. Neither the beta-adrenoceptor blocking drug nor the calcium channel blocker should be administered intravenously within 48 hours of discontinuing the other.

Concomitant therapy with dihydropyridines e.g. nifedipine, may increase the risk of hypotension, and cardiac failure may occur in patients with latent cardiac insufficiency.

Beta-adrenoceptor blocking drugs may exacerbate the rebound hypertension which can follow the withdrawal of clonidine. If the two drugs are co-administered, the beta-adrenoceptor blocking drug should be withdrawn several days before discontinuing clonidine. If replacing clonidine by beta-adrenoceptor blocking drug therapy, the introduction of beta-adrenoceptor blocking drugs should be delayed for several days after clonidine administration has stopped.

Digitalis glycosides, in association with beta-adrenoceptor blocking drugs, may increase atrio-ventricular conduction time.

Concomitant use of sympathomimetic agents, e.g. adrenaline, may counteract the effect of beta-adrenoceptor blocking drugs. Caution must be exercised in the parenteral administration of preparations containing adrenaline to patients taking beta-adrenoceptor blocking drugs as, in rare cases, vasoconstriction, hypertension and bradycardia may result.

Administration of propranolol during infusion of lignocaine may increase the plasma concentration of lignocaine by approximately 30%. Patients already receiving propranolol tend to have higher lignocaine levels than controls. The combination should be avoided.

Caution must be exercised if ergotamine, dihydroergotamine or related compounds are given in combination with propranolol since vasospastic reactions have been reported in a few patients.

Concomitant use of prostaglandin synthetase inhibiting drugs, e.g. ibuprofen or indomethacin, may decrease the hypotensive effects of propranolol.

Concomitant administration of propranolol and chlorpromazine may result in an increase in plasma levels of both drugs. This may lead to an enhanced antipsychotic effect for chlorpromazine and an increased antihypertensive effect for propranolol.

Concomitant use of cimetidine or hydralazine will increase, whereas concomitant use of alcohol will decrease, the plasma levels of propranolol.

Preparations containing lithium generally should not be given with diuretics because they may reduce its renal clearance.

*Anaesthesia:* Caution must be exercised when using anaesthetic agents with Inderex. The anaesthetist should be informed and the choice of anaesthetic should be the agent with as little negative inotropic activity as possible. Use of beta-adrenoceptor blocking drugs with anaesthetic drugs may result in attenuation of the reflex tachycardia and increase the risk of hypotension. Anaesthetic agents causing myocardial depression are best avoided.

*Interference with laboratory tests:* Inderex has been reported to interfere with the estimation of serum bilirubin by the diazo method and with the determination of catecholamines by methods using fluorescence.

*Pregnancy:* Inderex must not be given in pregnancy.

*Lactation:* As diuretics pass into breast milk, they should be avoided in mothers who wish to breast feed. Similarly, breast feeding is not recommended following administration of lipophilic beta-adrenoceptor blocking drugs.

*Effect on ability to drive or operate machinery:* The use of Inderex is unlikely to result in any impairment of the ability of patients to drive or operate machinery. Studies to investigate the effects of bendrofluazide have not been carried out. When driving vehicles or operating machinery, it should be taken into account that occasional dizziness or fatigue may occur.

*Undesirable events:* Inderex is usually well tolerated. In clinical studies, the undesired events reported are usually attributable to the pharmacological actions of propranolol or bendrofluazide.

Possible undesired events, listed by body system, include:

Cardiovascular: bradycardia, heart failure deterioration, postural hypotension which may be associated with syncope, cold extremities. In susceptible patients: precipitation of heart block, exacerbation of intermittent claudication, Raynaud's phenomenon.

CNS: confusion, dizziness, mood changes, nightmares, psychoses and hallucinations, sleep disturbance.

Gastrointestinal: gastrointestinal disturbance.

Haematological: purpura, thrombocytopenia.

Integumentary: alopecia, dry eyes, psoriasiform skin reactions, exacerbation of psoriasis, skin rashes.

Neurological: paraesthesia.

Respiratory: bronchospasm may occur in patients with bronchial asthma or a history of asthmatic complaints, sometimes with fatal outcome (see *Contra-indications*).

Special senses: visual disturbances.

Others: fatigue and/or lassitude (often transient), an increase in ANA (antinuclear antibodies) has been observed, however the clinical relevance of this is not clear; isolated reports of myasthenia gravis like syndrome or exacerbation of myasthenia gravis have been reported in patients administered propranolol.

Adverse effects of bendrofluazide are uncommon in the dose contained in Inderex.

Hypokalaemia may occur and may be dangerous in patients receiving digitalis or in those with hepatic cirrhosis when coma may be precipitated.

Hyperuricaemia sometimes occurs, but an attack of gout is rare.

The thiazide diuretics increase blood urea and they should be used with care in patients with renal failure.

Reports of other adverse reactions to thiazides include skin rashes with associated photosensitivity, necrotising vasculitis, acute pancreatitis, blood dyscrasias and aggravation of pre-existing myopia.

Discontinuance of Inderex should be considered if, according to clinical judgement, the well-being of the patient is adversely affected by any of the above reactions, bearing in mind that cessation of therapy with a beta-adrenoceptor blocking drug should be gradual.

*Overdosage:* The symptoms of overdosage may include bradycardia, hypotension, acute cardiac insufficiency and bronchospasm.

General treatment should include: close supervision, treatment in an intensive care ward, the use of gastric lavage, activated charcoal and a laxative to prevent absorption of any drug still present in the gastrointestinal tract, the use of plasma or plasma substitutes to treat hypotension and shock.

Excessive bradycardia can be countered with atropine 1–2 mg intravenously and/or a cardiac pacemaker. If necessary, this may be followed by a bolus dose of glucagon 10 mg intravenously. If required, this may be repeated or followed by an intravenous infusion of glucagon 1–10 mg/hour depending on response. If no response to glucagon occurs or if glucagon is unavailable, a beta-adrenoceptor stimulant such as dobutamine 2.5 to 10 micrograms/kg/minute by intravenous infusion may be given. Dobutamine, because of its positive inotropic effect could also be used to treat hypotension and acute cardiac insufficiency. It is likely that these doses would be inadequate to reverse the cardiac effects of beta-blockade if a large overdose has been taken. The dose of dobutamine should therefore be increased if necessary to achieve the required response according to the clinical condition of the patient.

Excessive diuresis should be countered by maintaining normal fluid and electrolyte balance.

**Pharmaceutical precautions** Store below 25°C, protected from light and moisture.

**Legal category** POM.

**Package quantities** Patient calendar pack of 28 capsules (OP).

**Further information** Inderex is designed to aid dru compliance by providing a convenient presentatio of a sustained release formulation of propranolc hydrochloride with the diuretic bendrofluazide for th treatment of hypertension. Concurrent use of proprar olol and bendrofluazide produces a more pronounce and consistent antihypertensive response than whe either component is used alone.

**Product licence number** 12619/0034.

## KALTEN*

**Presentation** Hard gelatin capsules with opaque re caps and opaque cream bodies. Each capsule imprinted KALTEN and with an 'S' logo in black. Eac capsule contains Atenolol PhEur 50 mg, Hydrochlc rothiazide PhEur 25 mg and Amiloride Hydrochlorid PhEur (dihydrate) 2.84 mg (equivalent to amilorid hydrochloride 2.5 mg). The inactive ingredients ar gelatin, iron oxide, lactose, magnesium stearat maize starch, sodium lauryl sulphate, sodium starc glycolate and titanium dioxide.

**Uses** Management of hypertension.

*Mode of action:* Kalten combines the antihypertensiv activity of a beta-adrenoceptor blocking drug, atenc lol, and a potassium sparing diuretic preparatior hydrochlorothiazide and amiloride.

Atenolol is a beta-adrenoceptor blocking drug whic is $beta_1$-selective (i.e. acts preferentially on beta adrenergic receptors in the heart). Selectivity de creases with increasing dose. Atenolol is withou intrinsic sympathomimetic and membrane stabilisin activities, and, as with other beta-adrenoceptor block ing drugs, has negative inotropic effects (and i therefore contra-indicated in uncontrolled heart fai ure). As with other beta-adrenoceptor blocking drugs its mode of action in the treatment of hypertension i unclear. It is unlikely that any additional ancillar properties possessed by S (–) atenolol, in compariso with the racemic mixture, will give rise to differer therapeutic effects.

Atenolol is effective and well tolerated in mos ethnic populations although the response may be les in black patients.

Hydrochlorothiazide is a thiazide diuretic acting o the distal tubule. It exerts its effect on sodium an water excretion by inhibiting sodium absorptio thereby impeding the capacity of the kidneys t concentrate the urine. It has a relatively flat dose response curve.

Amiloride is a potassium sparing diuretic whic although having a mild antihypertensive effect is use primarily for its potassium conserving effects. It act on the early distal tubule. Studies show that th combination of hydrochlorothiazide and amiloride i the ratio of 10 to 1 is optimal to achieve these effects

Absorption of atenolol following oral dosing i consistent but incomplete (approximately 40–50% with peak plasma concentrations occurring 2–4 hour after dosing. Atenolol blood levels are consistent an subject to little variability. There is no significar hepatic metabolism of atenolol and more than 90% o that absorbed reaches the systemic circulation unal tered. The plasma half-life is about 6 hours but thi may rise in severe renal impairment since the kidne is the major route of elimination. Atenolol penetrate tissues poorly due to its low lipid solubility and it concentration in brain tissue is low. Plasma protei binding is low (approximately 3%).

Absorption of hydrochlorothiazide following ora dosing is rapid but incomplete. The hydrochlorothia zide blood levels are consistent and subject to littl variability. There is no significant hepatic metabolisr of hydrochlorothiazide. The plasma half-life is be tween 6 and 10 hours and the kidney is the main rout of elimination.

Absorption of amiloride following oral dosing i rapid but incomplete. The amiloride blood levels ar inconsistent and subject to moderate variability. Ther is no significant hepatic metabolism of amiloride an the plasma half-life is about 6 hours.

Thus, atenolol, hydrochlorothiazide and amilorid have compatible pharmacokinetics and when give together, no clinically significant pharmacokineti interactions occur.

**Dosage and administration**
*Adults including the elderly:* One capsule daily. Kalte is recommended for use in hypertensive patient where monotherapy with a beta-adrenoceptor block ing drug or diuretic proves inadequate. Where neces sary another antihypertensive drug, such as vasodilator, can be added. Patients can be transferre to preparations containing beta-adrenoceptor block ing drugs from other antihypertensive treatment with the exception of clonidine (see 'Warnings' below

Kalten contains low effective doses of both a beta adrenoceptor blocking drug and a combination c diuretics with a potassium-sparing action, and ma be suited to older patients where higher doses of these drugs may be considered inappropriate.

*Children:* There is no paediatric experience with Kalten; therefore this is not recommended for use in children.

**Contra-indications, warnings, etc** Kalten should not be used in patients with any of the following conditions: known hypersensitivity to any of the components, bradycardia, cardiogenic shock, hypotension, metabolic acidosis, severe peripheral arterial circulatory disturbances, second or third degree heart block, sick sinus syndrome, untreated phaeochromocytoma, uncontrolled heart failure, hyperkalaemia (serum potassium greater than 5.5 mmol/l), those receiving concomitant therapy with potassium-sparing diuretics or potassium supplements, anuria, acute renal failure, severe progressive renal disease, diabetic nephropathy, blood urea over 10 mmol/l or serum creatinine over 130 micromol/l in whom serum electrolyte and blood urea levels cannot be monitored carefully and frequently.

In renal impairment, use of a potassium-conserving agent may result in the rapid development of hyperkalaemia (see *Warnings*).

Kalten must not be given during pregnancy or lactation.

Due to its beta-adrenoceptor blocking drug component, Kalten:

- although contra-indicated in uncontrolled heart failure (see *Contra-indications*), may be used in patients whose signs of heart failure have been controlled. Caution must be exercised in patients whose cardiac reserve is poor.
- may increase the number and duration of angina attacks in patients with Prinzmetal's angina due to unopposed alpha receptor mediated coronary artery vasoconstriction. Atenolol is a beta₁-selective beta-adrenoceptor blocking drug; consequently, the use of Kalten may be considered although utmost caution must be exercised.
- although contra-indicated in severe peripheral arterial circulatory disturbances (see *Contra-indications*), may also aggravate less severe peripheral arterial circulatory disturbances.
- due to its negative effect on conduction time, caution must be exercised if it is given to patients with first degree heart block.
- may modify the tachycardia of hypoglycaemia.
- may mask the signs of thyrotoxicosis.
- will reduce heart rate, as a result of its pharmacological action. In the rare instances when a treated patient develops symptoms which may be attributable to a slow heart rate, the dose may be reduced.
- should not be discontinued abruptly in patients suffering from ischaemic heart disease.
- may cause a more severe reaction to a variety of allergens, when given to patients with a history of anaphylactic reaction to such allergens. Such patients may be unresponsive to the usual doses of adrenaline used to treat the allergic reactions.

Kalten contains the cardioselective beta-adrenoceptor blocking drug atenolol. Although cardioselective (beta₁) beta-adrenoceptor blocking drugs may have less effect on lung function than non-selective beta-adrenoceptor blocking drugs, as with all beta-adrenoceptor blocking drugs, these should be avoided in patients with reversible obstructive airways disease, unless there are compelling clinical reasons for their use. Where such reasons exist, Kalten may be used with caution. Occasionally, some increase in airways resistance may occur in asthmatic patients, however, and this may usually be reversed by commonly used dosage of bronchodilators such as salbutamol or isoprenaline.

The label and patient information leaflet for this product state the following warning: "If you have ever had asthma or wheezing, you should not take this medicine unless you have discussed these symptoms with the prescribing doctor".

Due to its diuretic component, caution must be exercised if Kalten is used in:

- severely ill patients in whom metabolic or respiratory acidosis may occur (e.g. decompensated diabetes or cardiopulmonary disease) or in whom fluid and electrolyte balance is critical. Acidosis may be associated with rapid increases in serum potassium.
- patients with hepatic impairment. Amiloride has been reported to precipitate hepatic encephalopathy and deepening jaundice has also occurred in cirrhotic patients.
- diabetic patients, or those with a known predisposition to diabetes, particularly those with abnormal renal function. Hyperkalaemia has commonly occurred in diabetic patients on amiloride, especially those with chronic renal disease or pre-renal azotemia. The status of renal function should therefore be determined before Kalten is given to known or suspected diabetics. Lowering of glucose tolerance may occur and the insulin dosage of the diabetic patient may require adjustment. Kalten should be discontinued at least 3 days before glucose tolerance testing.
- patients with renal impairment (see *Contra-indications*) since the use of potassium conserving diuretics may result in the rapid development of hyperkalaemia. Caution is also necessary to avoid the cumulative or toxic effects due to a reduced excretion of the components of Kalten. Azotaemia may be precipitated or increased by hydrochlorothiazide. If increasing azotaemia and oliguria occur, treatment should be discontinued. Changes in plasma potassium have been observed in patients receiving amiloride and hydrochlorothiazide particularly in: the elderly; diabetics; patients with hepatic cirrhosis or congestive heart failure who had known renal impairment, were seriously ill, or were undergoing vigorous diuretic therapy; those receiving digitalis for heart failure; those taking an abnormal (low in potassium) diet and those suffering from gastro-intestinal complaints. The measurement of potassium levels are especially appropriate in these patients.
- Patients should be carefully observed for clinical, laboratory and ECG evidence of hyperkalaemia (not always associated with an abnormal ECG). Should hyperkalaemia develop, discontinue treatment immediately and if necessary, take active measures to reduce the serum potassium to normal. Hypokalaemia although less likely to occur may predispose to arrhythmias in patients receiving digitalis.

Hyponatraemia and hypochloraemia may occur with Kalten. Any chloride deficiency may be corrected by ammonium chloride (except in hepatic disease) and is largely prevented by a normal salt intake.

Kalten may be associated with hyperuricaemia.

Combined use of beta-adrenoceptor blocking drugs and calcium channel blockers with negative inotropic effects e.g. verapamil, diltiazem can lead to an exaggeration of these effects, particularly in patients with impaired ventricular function and/or sino-atrial or atrio-ventricular conduction abnormalities. This may result in severe hypotension, bradycardia and cardiac failure. Neither the beta-adrenoceptor blocking drug nor the calcium channel blocker should be administered intravenously within 48 hours of discontinuing the other.

Concomitant therapy with dihydropyridines e.g. nifedipine, may increase the risk of hypotension, and cardiac failure may occur in patients with latent cardiac insufficiency.

Beta-adrenoceptor blocking drugs may exacerbate the rebound hypertension which can follow the withdrawal of clonidine. If the two drugs are co-administered, the beta-adrenoceptor blocking drug should be withdrawn several days before discontinuing clonidine. If replacing clonidine by beta-adrenoceptor blocking drug therapy, the introduction of beta-adrenoceptor blocking drugs should be delayed for several days after clonidine administration has stopped.

Caution must be exercised when prescribing a beta-adrenoceptor blocking drug with Class 1 antiarrhythmic agents such as disopyramide.

Digitalis glycosides, in association with beta-adrenoceptor blocking drugs, may increase atrio-ventricular conduction time.

Concomitant use of sympathomimetic agents, e.g. adrenaline, may counteract the effect of beta-adrenoceptor blocking drugs.

Concomitant use with insulin and oral antidiabetic drugs may lead to the intensification of the blood sugar lowering effects of these drugs.

Concomitant use of prostaglandin synthetase inhibiting drugs, e.g. ibuprofen or indomethacin, may decrease the hypotensive effects of beta-adrenoceptor blocking drugs.

Preparations containing lithium should not generally be given with diuretics because they may reduce its renal clearance.

*Anaesthesia:* Caution must be exercised when using anaesthetic agents with Kalten. The anaesthetist should be informed and the choice of anaesthetic should be the agent with as little negative inotropic activity as possible. Use of beta-adrenoceptor blocking drugs with anaesthetic drugs may result in attenuation of the reflex tachycardia and increase the risk of hypotension. Anaesthetic agents causing myocardial depression are best avoided.

*Effect on ability to drive or operate machinery:* The use of Kalten is unlikely to result in any impairment of the ability of patients to drive or operate machinery. However, it should be taken into account that occasionally dizziness or fatigue may occur.

*Undesirable events:* Kalten is well tolerated. In clinical studies, the undesired events reported are usually attributable to the pharmacological actions of its components.

The following undesired events, listed by body system, have been reported:

*Atenolol monotherapy:* Cardiovascular: bradycardia, heart failure deterioration, postural hypotension which may be associated with syncope, cold extremities. In susceptible patients: precipitation of heart block, intermittent claudication, Raynaud's phenomenon.

CNS: confusion, dizziness, headache, mood changes, nightmares, psychoses and hallucinations, sleep disturbances of the type noted with other beta-adrenoceptor blocking drugs.

Gastrointestinal: dry mouth, gastrointestinal disturbances.

Haematological: purpura, thrombocytopenia.

Integumentary: alopecia, dry eyes, psoriasiform skin reactions, exacerbation of psoriasis, skin rashes.

Neurological: paraesthesia.

Respiratory: bronchospasm may occur in patients with bronchial asthma or a history of asthmatic complaints.

Special senses: visual disturbances.

Others: fatigue, an increase in ANA (antinuclear antibodies) has been observed, however the clinical relevance of this is not clear.

*Amiloride and hydrochlorothiazide:* Biochemical: electrolyte imbalance, glycosuria, hyperglycaemia, hyperuricaemia.

Cardiovascular: necrotising vasculitis, orthostatic hypotension secondary to diuresis.

CNS: dizziness, headache, vertigo.

Gastrointestinal: acute pancreatitis, anorexia, constipation, cramps, diarrhoea, dry mouth, gastric irritation, jaundice, nausea, pain, salivary gland inflammation, thirst, vomiting.

Haematological: blood dyscrasias, purpura.

Integumentary: skin rashes with associated photosensitivity, urticaria.

Musculoskeletal: muscle cramps.

Neurological: paraesthesia.

Respiratory: pneumonitis, respiratory distress.

Special senses: transient blurred vision, xanthopsia.

Others: fatigue, fever, restlessness. Hypersensitivity reactions, including pulmonary oedema with symptoms of shock, have been reported with hydrochlorothiazide.

Discontinuance of Kalten should be considered if, according to clinical judgement, the well being of the patient is adversely affected by any of the above reactions.

*Overdosage:* The symptoms of overdosage may include bradycardia, hypotension, acute cardiac insufficiency and bronchospasm.

General treatment should include: close supervision, treatment in an intensive care ward, the use of gastric lavage, activated charcoal and a laxative to prevent absorption of any drug still present in the gastrointestinal tract, the use of plasma or plasma substitutes to treat hypotension and shock. The possible use of haemodialysis or haemoperfusion may be considered.

Dehydration, electrolyte imbalance and hepatic coma are treated by the established procedures. If hyperkalaemia occurs, active measures should be taken to reduce the serum potassium levels. For respiratory impairment, oxygen or artificial respiration should be administered. Bronchospasm can usually be reversed by bronchodilators.

Excessive diuresis should be countered by maintaining normal fluid and electrolyte balance.

Excessive bradycardia can be countered with atropine 1–2 mg intravenously and/or a cardiac pacemaker. If necessary, this may be followed by a bolus dose of glucagon 10 mg intravenously. If required, this may be repeated or followed by an intravenous infusion of glucagon 1–10 mg/hour depending on response. If no response to glucagon occurs or if glucagon is unavailable, a beta-adrenoceptor stimulant such as dobutamine 2.5 to 10 micrograms/kg/minute by intravenous infusion may be given. Dobutamine, because of its positive inotropic effect could also be used to treat hypotension and acute cardiac insufficiency. It is likely that these doses would be inadequate to reverse the cardiac effects of beta-adrenoceptor blockade if a large overdose has been taken. The dose of dobutamine should therefore be increased if necessary to achieve the required response according to the clinical condition of the patient.

**Pharmaceutical precautions** Kalten capsules should be stored below 25°C, protected from light and moisture.

**Legal category** POM.

**Package quantities** Calendar packs of 28 (OP).

**Further information** When the combined antihypertensive effect of a beta-adrenoceptor blocking drug and a potassium-conserving diuretic is required, Kalten is a simple, convenient and acceptable therapy which may be expected to improve patient compliance.

The effect of Kalten following a one capsule oral dose is sustained for at least 24 hours.

**Product licence number** 12619/0035.

## MERONEM*

**Qualitative and quantitative composition:** Vial for i.v. injection or infusion

| | *Meronem 250 mg* | *Meronem 500 mg* | *Meronem 1000 mg* |
|---|---|---|---|
| *Active ingredient:* | | | |
| Meropenem trihydrate | 285 mg | 570 mg | 1140 mg |
| equivalent to anhydrous meropenem | 250 mg | 500 mg | 1000 mg |
| *Excipient:* | | | |
| Anhydrous sodium carbonate | 52 mg | 104 mg | 208 mg |

For each gram of meropenem (anhydrous potency) the vial contains 90 mg (3.9 mmol) of sodium.

Infusion Kits are also available containing either a 500 mg or 1 g vial together with a 100 ml bag of 0.9% w/v sodium chloride intravenous infusion.

**Pharmaceutical form:** Powder for constitution for intravenous administration.

**Clinical particulars**

*Therapeutic indications:* Meronem IV is indicated for treatment, in adults and children, of the following infections caused by single or multiple bacteria sensitive to meropenem:

- Pneumonias and nosocomial pneumonias
- Urinary tract infections
- Intra-abdominal infections
- Gynaecological infections, such as endometritis. Skin and skin structure infections
- Meningitis
- Septicaemia
- Empiric treatment, for presumed infections in adult patients with febrile neutropenia, used as monotherapy or in combination with anti-viral or anti-fungal agents.

Meronem has proved efficacious alone or in combination with other antimicrobial agents in the treatment of polymicrobial infections.

Intravenous meropenem has been used effectively in patients with cystic fibrosis and chronic lower respiratory tract infections, either as monotherapy or in combination with other antibacterial agents. Eradication of the organism was not always established.

There is no experience in paediatric patients with neutropenia or primary or secondary immunodeficiency.

*Posology and method of administration:*

*Adults:* The dosage and duration of therapy shall be established depending on type and severity of infection and the condition of the patient.

The recommended daily dosage is as follows:

– 500 mg IV every 8 hours in the treatment of pneumonia, UTI, gynaecological infections such as endometritis, skin and skin structure infections.

– 1 g IV every 8 hours in the treatment of nosocomial pneumonias, peritonitis, presumed infections in neutropenic patients, septicaemia.

In cystic fibrosis, doses up to 2 g every 8 hours have been used; most patients have been treated with 2 g every 8 hours.

In meningitis the recommended dosage is 2 g every 8 hours.

As with other antibiotics, particular caution is recommended in using meropenem as monotherapy in critically ill patients with known or suspected Pseudomonas aeruginosa lower respiratory tract infection.

Regular sensitivity testing is recommended when treating Pseudomonas aeruginosa infection.

*Dosage schedule for adults with impaired renal function:* Dosage should be reduced in patients with creatinine clearance less than 51 ml/min, as scheduled below.

| *Creatinine clearance (ml/min)* | *Dose (based on unit doses of 500 mg, 1 g, 2 g)* | *Frequency* |
|---|---|---|
| 26–50 | one unit dose | every 12 hours |
| 10–25 | one-half unit dose | every 12 hours |
| <10 | one-half unit dose | every 24 hours |

Meropenem is cleared by haemodialysis; if continued treatment with Meronem is necessary, it is recommended that the unit dose (based on the type and severity of infection) is administered at the completion of the haemodialysis procedure to restore therapeutically effective plasma concentrations.

There is no experience with the use of Meronem in patients under peritoneal dialysis.

*Dosage in adults with hepatic insufficiency:* No dosage adjustment is necessary in patients with hepatic insufficiency (See *Warnings and Precautions*).

*Elderly patients:* No dosage adjustment is required for the elderly with normal renal function or creatinine clearance values above 50 ml/min.

*Children:* For children over 3 months and up to 12 years of age the recommended dose is 10–20 mg/kg every 8 hours depending on type and severity of infection, susceptibility of the pathogen and the condition of the patient. In children over 50 kg weight, adult dosage should be used.

For children aged 4 to 18 years with cystic fibrosis, doses ranging from 25 to 40 mg/kg every 8 hours have been used to treat acute exacerbations of chronic lower respiratory tract infections.

In meningitis the recommended dose is 40 mg/kg every 8 hours.

There is no experience in children with renal impairment.

*Method of administration:* Meronem IV can be given as an intravenous bolus injection over approximately 5 minutes or by intravenous infusion over approximately 15 to 30 minutes using the specific available presentations.

Meronem IV to be used for bolus intravenous injection should be constituted with sterile Water for Injections (5 ml per 250 mg Meropenem). This provides an approximate concentration of 50 mg/ml. Constituted solutions are clear and colourless or pale yellow.

Meronem IV for intravenous infusion may be constituted with compatible infusion fluids (50 to 200 ml) (see *Incompatibilities* and *Special precautions for storage*).

*Contra-indications:* Meronem is contra-indicated in patients who have demonstrated hypersensitivity to this product.

*Special warnings and special precautions for use:* There is some clinical and laboratory evidence of partial cross-allergenicity between other carbapenems and beta-lactam antibiotics, penicillins and cephalosporins. Severe reactions (including anaphylaxis) have been reported with most beta-lactam antibiotics. Before initiating therapy with meropenem, careful inquiry should be made concerning previous hypersensitivity reactions to beta-lactam antibiotics. Meronem should be used with caution in patients with such a history. If an allergic reaction to meropenem occurs, the drug should be discontinued and appropriate measures taken.

Use of Meronem in patients with hepatic disease should be made with careful monitoring of transaminase and bilirubin levels.

As with other antibiotics, overgrowth of non-susceptible organisms may occur and, therefore, continuous monitoring of each patient is necessary.

Use in infections caused by methicillin resistant staphylococci is not recommended.

Rarely, pseudomembranous colitis has been reported on Meronem as with practically all antibiotics and may vary in severity from slight to life-threatening. Therefore, antibiotics should be prescribed with care for individuals with a history of gastro-intestinal complaints, particularly colitis.

It is important to consider the diagnosis of pseudomembranous colitis in the case of patients who develop diarrhoea in association with the use of Meronem. Although studies indicate that a toxin produced by Clostridium difficile is one of the main causes of antibiotic-associated colitis, other causes should be considered.

The co-administration of Meronem with potentially nephrotoxic drugs should be considered with caution. For dosage see *Posology and method of administration.*

*Paediatric use:* Efficacy and tolerability in infants under 3 months old have not been established; therefore, Meronem is not recommended for use below this age. There is no experience in children with altered hepatic or renal function.

Keep all medicines away from children.

*Interactions with other medicaments and other forms of interaction:* Probenecid competes with meropenem for active tubular secretion and thus inhibits the renal excretion, with the effect of increasing the elimination half-life and plasma concentration of meropenem. As the potency and duration of action of Meronem dosed without probenecid are adequate, the co-administration of probenecid with Meronem is not recommended.

The potential effect of Meronem on the protein binding of other drugs or metabolism has not been studied. The protein binding of Meronem is low (approximately 2%) and, therefore, no interactions with other compounds based on displacement from plasma proteins would be expected. Meronem has been administered concomitantly with other medications without adverse pharmacological interactions. However, no specific data regarding potential drug interactions is available.

*Pregnancy and lactation*

*Pregnancy:* The safety of Meronem in human pregnancy has not been evaluated. Animal studies have not shown any adverse effect on the developing foetus. The only adverse effect observed in animal reproductive studies was an increased incidence of abortions in monkeys at 13 times the expected exposure in man. Meronem should not be used in pregnancy unless the potential benefit justifies the potential risk to the foetus. In every case, it should be used under the direct supervision of the physician.

*Lactation:* Meropenem is detectable at very low concentrations in animal breast milk. Meronem should not be used in breast-feeding women unless the potential benefit justifies the potential risk to the baby.

*Effects on ability to drive and use machines:* No data is available, but it is not anticipated that Meronem will affect the ability to drive and use machines.

*Undesirable effects:* Serious adverse events are rare. During the clinical trials the following adverse events have been reported:

*Local intravenous injection site reactions:* inflammation, thrombophlebitis, pain at the site of injection

*Skin reactions:* rash, pruritus, urticaria

*Gastro-intestinal:* abdominal pain, nausea, vomiting, diarrhoea. Pseudomembranous colitis has been reported.

*Blood:* Reversible thrombocythaemia, eosinophilia, thrombocytopenia and neutropenia. A positive direct or indirect Coombs test may develop in some subjects; there have been reports of reduction in partial thromboplastin time.

*Liver function:* Increases in serum concentrations of bilirubin, transaminases, alkaline phosphatase and lactic dehydrogenase alone or in combination have been reported.

*Central nervous system:* headache, paraesthesiae. Convulsions have been reported but a causal link with Meronem has not been established.

*Other:* Oral and vaginal candidosis.

*Overdose:* Accidental overdosage could occur during therapy, particularly in patients with renal impairment. Treatment of overdosage should be symptomatic. In normal individuals rapid renal elimination will occur; in subjects with renal impairment haemodialysis will remove meropenem and its metabolite.

**Pharmacological properties**

*Pharmacodynamic properties:* Meropenem is a carbapenem antibiotic for parenteral use, that is relatively stable to human dehydropeptidase-1 (DHP-1) and therefore, does not require the addition of an inhibitor of DHP-1.

Meropenem exerts its bactericidal action by interfering with vital bacterial cell wall synthesis. The ease with which it penetrates bacterial cell walls, its high level of stability to all serine β-lactamases and its marked affinity for the Penicillin Binding Proteins (PBPs) explain the potent bactericidal action of meropenem against a broad spectrum of aerobic and anaerobic bacteria. Minimum bactericidal concentrations (MBC) are commonly the same as the minimum inhibitory concentrations (MIC). For 76% of the bacteria tested, the MBC:MIC ratios were 2 or less.

Meropenem is stable in susceptibility tests and these tests can be performed using normal routine methods. In vitro tests show that meropenem acts synergistically with various antibiotics. It has been demonstrated both in vitro and in vivo that meropenem has a post-antibiotic effect.

A single set of meropenem susceptibility criteria are recommended based on pharmacokinetics and correlation of clinical and microbiological outcomes with zone diameter and minimum inhibitory concentrations (MIC) of the infecting organisms.

| *CATEGORISATION* | *METHOD OF ASSESSMENT* Zone Diameter (mm) | MIC breakpoints (mg/L) |
|---|---|---|
| Susceptible | ≥14 | ≤4 |
| Intermediate | 12 to 13 | 8 |
| Resistant | ≤11 | ≥16 |

The in vitro antibacterial spectrum of meropenem includes the majority of clinically significant Gram-positive and Gram-negative, aerobic and anaerobic strains of bacteria, as shown below:

*Gram-positive aerobes:* Bacillus spp, *Corynebacterium diphtheriae, Enterococcus liquifaciens, Enterococcus avium, Listeria monocytogenes,* Lactobacillus spp, *Nocardia asteroides, Staphylococcus aureus* (penicillinase negative and positive), Staphylococci-coagulase negative; including, *Staphylococcus saprophyticus, Staphylococcus capitis, Staphylococcus cohnii, Staphylococcus xylosus, Staphylococcus warneri, Staphylococcus hominis, Staphylococcus simulans, Staphylococcus intermedius, Staphylococcus sciuri, Staphylococcus lugdunensis, Streptococcus pneumoniae* (penicillin susceptible and resistant), *Streptococcus agalactiae, Streptococcus pyogenes, Streptococcus equi, Streptococcus bovis, Streptococcus mitis, Streptococcus mitior, Streptococcus milleri, Streptococcus sanguis, Streptococcus viridans, Streptococcus salivarius, Streptococcus morbillorum,* Streptococcus Group G, Streptococcus Group F, Rhodococcus equi.

*Gram-negative aerobes:* Achromobacter

xylosoxidans, Acinetobacter anitratus, Acinetobacter lwoffii, Acinetobacter baumannii, Aeromonas hydrophila, Aeromonas sorbria, Aeromonas caviae, Alcaligenes faecalis, Bordetella bronchiseptica, Brucella melitensis, Campylobacter coli, Campylobacter jejuni, Citrobacter freundii, Citrobacter diversus, Citrobacter koseri, Citrobacter amalonaticus, Enterobacter aerogenes, Enterobacter (Pantoea) agglomerans, Enterobacter cloacae, Enterobacter sakazakii, Escherichia coli, Escherichia hermannii, Gardnerella vaginalis, Haemophilus influenzae (including β-lactamase positive and ampicillin resistant strains), Haemophilus parainfluenzae, Haemophilus ducreyi, Helicobacter pylori, Neisseria meningitidis, Neisseria gonorrhoeae (including β-lactamase positive, penicillin resistant and spectinomycin resistant strains), Hafnia alvei, Klebsiella pneumoniae, Klebsiella aerogenes, Klebsiella ozaenae, Klebsiella oxytoca, Moraxella (Branhamella) catarrhalis, Morganella morganii, Proteus mirabilis, Proteus vulgaris, Proteus penneri, Providencia rettgeri, Providencia stuartii, Providencia alcalifaciens, Pasteurella multocida, Plesiomonas shigelloides, Pseudomonas aeruginosa, Pseudomonas putida, Pseudomonas alcaligenes, Burkholderia (Pseudomonas) cepacia, Pseudomonas fluorescens, Pseudomonas stutzeri, Pseudomonas pseudomallei, Pseudomonas acidovorans, Salmonella spp including Salmonella enteritidis/typhi, Serratia marcescens, Serratia liquefaciens, Serratia rubidaea, Shigella sonnei, Shigella flexneri, Shigella boydii, Shigella dysenteriae, Vibrio cholerae, Vibrio parahaemolyticus, Vibrio vulnificus, Yersinia enterocolitica.

Anaerobic bacteria: Actinomyces odontolyticus, Actinomyces meyeri, Bacteroides-Prevotella-Porphyromonas spp, Bacteroides fragilis, Bacteroides vulgatus, Bacteroides variabilis, Bacteroides pneumosintes, Bacteroides coagulans, Bacteroides uniformis, Bacteroides distasonis, Bacteroides ovatus, Bacteroides thetaiotaomicron, Bacteroides eggerthii, Bacteroides capsillosis, Prevotella buccalis, Prevotella corporis, Bacteroides gracilis, Prevotella melaninogenica, Prevotella intermedia, Prevotella bivia, Prevotella splanchnicus, Prevotella oralis, Prevotella disiens, Prevotella rumenicola, Bacteroides ureolyticus, Prevotella oris, Prevotella buccae, Prevotella denticola, Bacteroides levii, Porphyromonas asaccharolytica, Bifidobacterium spp, Bilophila wadsworthia, Clostridium perfringens, Clostridium bifermentans, Clostridium ramosum, Clostridium sporogenes, Clostridium cadaveris, Clostridium sordellii, Clostridium butyricum, Clostridium clostridiiformis, Clostridium innocuum, Clostridium subterminale, Clostridium tertium, Eubacterium lentum, Eubacterium aerofaciens, Fusobacterium mortiferum, Fusobacterium necrophorum, Fusobacterium nucleatum, Fusobacterium varium, Mobiluncus curtisii, Mobiluncus mulieris, Peptostreptococcus anaerobius, Peptostreptococcus micros, Peptostreptococcus saccharolyticus, Peptococcus saccharolyticus, Peptostreptococcus asaccharolyticus, Peptostreptococcus magnus, Peptostreptococcus prevotii, Propionibacterium acnes, Propionibacterium avidum, Propionibacterium granulosum. Stenotrophomonas maltophilia, Enterococcus faecium and methicillin-resistant staphylococci have been found to be resistant to meropenem.

Pharmacokinetic properties: A 30 minute intravenous infusion of a single dose of Meronem in healthy volunteers results in peak plasma levels of approximately 11 microgram/ml for the 250 mg dose, 23 microgram/ml for the 500 mg dose and 49 microgram/ml for the 1 g dose.

However, there is no absolute pharmacokinetic proportionality with the administered dose both as regards Cmax and AUC. Furthermore, a reduction in plasma clearance from 287 to 205 ml/min for the range of dosage 250 mg to 2 g has been observed.

A 5 minute intravenous bolus injection of Meronem in healthy volunteers results in peak plasma levels of approximately 52 microgram/ml for the 500 mg dose and 112 microgram/ml for the 1 g dose.

Intravenous infusions of 1 g over 2 minutes, 3 minutes and 5 minutes were compared in a three-way crossover trial. These durations of infusion resulted in peak plasma levels of 110, 91 and 94 microgram/ml, respectively.

After an IV dose of 500 mg, plasma levels of meropenem decline to values of 1 microgram/ml or less, 6 hours after administration.

When multiple doses are administered at 8 hourly intervals to subjects with normal renal function, accumulation of meropenem does not occur.

In subjects with normal renal function, meropenem's elimination half-life is approximately 1 hour.

Plasma protein binding of meropenem is approximately 2%.

Approximately 70% of the administered dose is recovered as unchanged meropenem in the urine over 12 hours, after which little further urinary excretion is detectable. Urinary concentrations of meropenem in excess of 10 microgram/ml are maintained for up to 5 hours after the administration of a 500 mg dose. No accumulation of meropenem in plasma or urine was observed with regimens using 500 mg administered every 8 hours or 1 g administered every 6 hours in volunteers with normal renal function.

The only metabolite of meropenem is microbiologically inactive.

Meropenem penetrates well into most body fluids and tissues including cerebrospinal fluid of patients with bacterial meningitis, achieving concentrations in excess of those required to inhibit most bacteria.

Studies in children have shown that the pharmacokinetics of Meronem in children are similar to those in adults. The elimination half-life for meropenem was approximately 1.5 to 2.3 hours in children under the age of 2 years and the pharmacokinetics are linear over the dose range of 10 to 40 mg/kg.

Pharmacokinetic studies in patients with renal insufficiency have shown the plasma clearance of meropenem correlates with creatinine clearance. Dosage adjustments are necessary in subjects with renal impairment.

Pharmacokinetic studies in the elderly have shown a reduction in plasma clearance of meropenem which correlated with age-associated reduction in creatinine clearance.

Pharmacokinetic studies in patients with liver disease have shown no effects of liver disease on the pharmacokinetics of meropenem.

Pre-clinical safety data: Animal studies indicate that meropenem is well tolerated by the kidney. In animal studies meropenem has shown nephrotoxic effects, only at high dose levels (500 mg/kg).

Effects on the CNS; convulsions in rats and vomiting in dogs, were seen only at high doses (>2000 mg/kg).

For an IV dose the $LD_{50}$ in rodents is greater than 2000 mg/kg. In repeat dose studies (up to 6 months) only minor effects were seen including a small decrease in red cell parameters and an increase in liver weight in dogs treated with doses of 500 mg/kg.

There was no evidence of mutagenic potential in the 5 tests conducted and no evidence of reproductive and teratogenic toxicity in studies at the highest possible doses in rats and monkeys; the no effect dose level of a (small) reduction in $F_1$ body weight in rat was 120 mg/kg. There was an increased incidence of abortions at 500 mg/kg in a preliminary study in monkeys.

There was no evidence of increased sensitivity to meropenem in juveniles compared to adult animals. The intravenous formulation was well tolerated in animal studies.

The sole metabolite of meropenem had a similar profile of toxicity in animal studies.

**Pharmaceutical particulars**

List of excipients: Meronem for i.v. injection and infusion includes the excipient anhydrous sodium carbonate.

Incompatibilities: Meronem should not be mixed with or added to other drugs.

Meronem is compatible with the following infusion fluids:

0.9% Sodium Chloride solution
5% or 10% Glucose solution
5% Glucose solution with 0.02% Sodium Bicarbonate
0.9% Sodium Chloride and 5% Glucose solution
5% Glucose with 0.225% Sodium Chloride solution
5% Glucose with 0.15% Potassium Chloride solution
Mannitol 2.5% or 10% solution.

For reconstitution instructions using the Meronem Infusion Kit see leaflet enclosed in the carton.

Shelf-life: Meronem has a shelf life of 3 years.

Special precautions for storage: Store below 25°C.

It is recommended to use freshly prepared solutions of Meronem for i.v. injection and infusion. Reconstituted product should be used immediately and must be stored for no longer than 24 hours under refrigeration, only if necessary.

| Diluent | Hours stable up to 25°C | 4°C |
|---|---|---|
| Solution (1–20 mg/ml) prepared with: | | |
| 0.9% sodium chloride | 8 | 48 |
| 5% glucose | 3 | 14 |
| 5% glucose and 0.225% sodium chloride | 3 | 14 |
| 5% glucose and 0.9% sodium chloride | 3 | 14 |
| 5% glucose and 0.15% potassium chloride | 3 | 14 |

| Diluent | Hours stable up to 25°C | 4°C |
|---|---|---|
| 2.5% or 10% mannitol intravenous infusion | 3 | 14 |
| 10% glucose | 2 | 8 |
| 5% glucose and 0.02% sodium bicarbonate intravenous infusion | 2 | 8 |

Solutions of Meronem should not be frozen.

Nature and contents of containers: Type 1 glass vials closed with halobutilic rubber stopper and sealed with an aluminium cap.

Packs for intravenous administration: Pack of 10 vials containing 250 mg, 500 mg or 1 g meropenem.

Infusion kits containing one vial of either 500 mg or 1 g meropenem together with a 100 ml bag of 0.9% w/v sodium chloride intravenous infusion.

Instructions for use/handling: Refer to Posology and method of administration. Standard aseptic technique should be employed during constitution. Shake constituted solution before use.

All vials are for single use only.

**Marketing authorisation numbers**
250 mg    12619/0097
500 mg    12619/0098
1 g       12619/0099

**Date of approval/revision of SPC** July 1997

**Legal category** POM

## METOSYN* FAPG CREAM
## METOSYN* OINTMENT

**Presentation** Metosyn consists of the corticosteroid fluocinonide presented as FAPG Cream and as Ointment. In Metosyn FAPG Cream, fluocinonide 0.05% w/w is dissolved completely in propylene glycol with fatty alcohols added to produce a white, homogeneous, semi-solid preparation. Inactive ingredients in Metosyn FAPG Cream are citric acid, hexanetriol, polyethylene glycol, propylene glycol, and stearyl alcohol. Metosyn Ointment contains fluocinonide 0.05% w/w completely dissolved in a petroleum base. Inactive ingredients contained in Metosyn ointment are amerchol CAB, propylene carbonate, propylene glycol and white soft paraffin.

**Uses** Metosyn is suitable for treating a wide variety of local inflammatory, pruritic and allergic disorders of the skin. It is indicated for topical application in the following conditions:

Eczema and dermatitis, atopic eczema, seborrhoeic dermatitis, discoid eczema, contact dermatitis, neurodermatitis. Prurigo. Psoriasis (excluding widespread plaque psoriasis). Lichen planus. Discoid lupus erythematosus.

Metosyn FAPG Cream may be used for wet or dry lesions. Metosyn Ointment, with its emollient effects, is particularly suitable for dry scaly lesions.

Mode of action: Fluocinonide is a synthetic anti-inflammatory corticosteroid. Its mechanisms of action are related to vasoconstriction and suppression of membrane permeability, mitotic activity, the immune response and release of inflammatory mediators.

The extent of percutaneous absorption of fluocinonide is determined by many factors including the vehicle, the integrity of the epidermal barrier and the use of occlusive dressings. Following absorption, fluocinonide is metabolised primarily in the liver and excreted by the kidneys.

**Dosage and administration** Adults: A small quantity of Metosyn FAPG Cream or Metosyn Ointment should be applied three to four times daily to the affected area and massaged well in.

Once improvement is apparent, usage may be reduced to twice or even once daily.

Children: Under one year: Metosyn preparations are not advised in the treatment of children under one year of age.

Over one year: As adult dose, however it is recommended that treatment should not normally be extended beyond five days and occlusion in such cases should not be used.

Elderly: As adult dose.

It is recommended that Metosyn is used undiluted (see Pharmaceutical precautions).

**Contra-indications, warnings, etc** Metosyn is contra-indicated in rosacea, acne and peri-oral dermatitis. As with all topical steroids, Metosyn is contra-indicated in tuberculous, syphilitic, fungal and viral infections of the skin. The product should not be used for napkin eruptions or anogenital pruritus.

The eyes should be avoided.

Long-term continuous topical steroid therapy can produce atrophic skin changes and dilatation of the superficial blood vessels particularly when occlusive dressings are used or where skin folds are involved. Prolonged use of topical steroids or treatment of extensive areas, even without occlusion, can result in sufficient absorption of the steroid to produce the features of hypercorticalism and underlying adrenal suppression, especially in infants and children.

It is recommended that treatment on the face should not normally be extended beyond five days, and occlusion in such cases should not be used.

Where there is bacterial infection associated with an inflammatory skin condition, Metosyn should only be administered if adequate antibacterial cover is also given.

When using topical corticosteroids to treat psoriasis there are risks of rebound relapse following the development of tolerance, and of generalised pustular psoriasis. Impairment of the barrier function of the skin may lead to local and systemic toxicity. Careful patient supervision is important.

Treatment should be discontinued if unfavourable reactions are seen.

*Pregnancy:* There is inadequate evidence of safety in human pregnancy. Topical administration of steroids to pregnant animals can cause abnormalities of foetal development, including cleft palate and intra-uterine growth retardation. There may therefore be a very small risk of such effects on the human foetus.

*Lactation:* Topical steroids should not be applied to the breasts prior to nursing. When topical steroid treatment is considered necessary for other parts of the body both the amount applied and the length of treatment should be minimised.

*Side-effects:* With Metosyn, side-effects are extremely rare, but, as with all topical steroids, the occasional patient may show an adverse reaction such as hypersensitivity. Irritation at the site of application may occur infrequently. Extensive treatment, particularly involving occlusive dressings or where skin folds are involved, can result in both local atrophic changes, such as striae, skin thinning and telangiectasia, and systemic effects such as adrenal suppression.

The use of topical steroids on infected lesions, without the addition of appropriate anti-infective therapy, can result in the spread of opportunist infections.

*Overdosage:* A 25 g tube of Metosyn FAPG Cream or Ointment contains 12.5 mg of fluocinonide. Toxic effects are not likely to occur following accidental ingestion. Similarly, the components of the vehicles, singly or collectively, have not been shown to produce toxic effects in these quantities.

**Pharmaceutical precautions** Metosyn FAPG Cream should be stored in its original tube below 30°C.

Metosyn Ointment should be stored in its original tube below 25°C.

It is recommended that the product be used undiluted. However, if dilution of Metosyn Ointment is required, white soft paraffin should be used and special FAPG diluent should be used to dilute Metosyn FAPG Cream.

**Legal category** POM.

**Package quantities** Tubes of 25 g (OP) and 100 g FAPG Cream.

Tubes of 25 g (OP) and 100 g Ointment.

**Further information** Effect on ability to drive or operate machinery: no precautions are necessary.

Metosyn FAPG Cream and Metosyn Ointment do not contain lanolin or parabens.

**Product licence numbers**
Metosyn FAPG Cream    12619/0039
Metosyn Ointment    12619/0041

# METOSYN* SCALP LOTION

**Presentation** Metosyn Scalp Lotion is a clear, colourless, slightly viscous solution containing 0.05% w/v fluocinonide in a vehicle containing citric acid, ethanol, di-isopropyladipate and propylene glycol.

**Uses** Steroid-responsive dermatoses of the scalp such as psoriasis (excluding widespread plaque psoriasis), seborrhoeic dermatitis and severe dandruff.

*Mode of action:* Fluocinonide is a synthetic anti-inflammatory corticosteroid. Its mechanisms of action are related to vasoconstriction and suppression of membrane permeability, mitotic activity, the immune response and release of inflammatory mediators.

The extent of percutaneous absorption of fluocinonide is determined by many factors including the vehicle, the integrity of the epidermal barrier and the use of occlusive dressings. Following absorption, fluocinonide is metabolised primarily in the liver and excreted by the kidneys.

**Dosage and administration** *All age groups:* A small quantity of Metosyn Scalp Lotion should be applied to the scalp morning and night until improvement is noticeable. Improvement may then be maintained with application once a day or less frequently. However, Metosyn Scalp Lotion should be prescribed for short courses of therapy and not used by patients on

a continuous basis. In childhood, courses should be limited to five days.

**Contra-indications, warnings, etc**
*Contra-indications:* Metosyn is contra-indicated in infections of the scalp and hypersensitivity to the preparation. Metosyn preparations are not advised in the treatment of children under one year of age.

Care must be taken to keep Metosyn Scalp Lotion away from the eyes and it must not be used near a naked flame.

If hypersensitivity develops treatment should be discontinued.

Long-term continuous topical steroid therapy can produce atrophic skin changes and dilatation of the superficial blood vessels particularly when occlusive dressings are used or where skin folds are involved. Prolonged use of topical steroids or treatment of extensive areas, even without occlusion, can result in sufficient absorption of the steroid to produce the features of hypercorticalism and underlying adrenal suppression, especially in infants and children.

It is recommended that treatment on the face and for children should not normally be extended beyond five days, and occlusion in such cases should not be used.

Metosyn Scalp Lotion with rare exceptions (for example in a heavily bearded area where other formulations may not be suitable) should not be applied to the face.

Development of secondary infection requires withdrawal of therapy and commencement of appropriate antimicrobial therapy.

When using topical corticosteroids to treat psoriasis there are risks both of rebound relapse following the development of tolerance, and of generalised pustular psoriasis. Impairment of the barrier function of the skin may lead to local and systemic toxicity. Careful patient supervision is important.

*Pregnancy:* There is inadequate evidence of safety in human pregnancy. Topical administration of steroids to pregnant animals can cause abnormalities of foetal development, including cleft palate and intra-uterine growth retardation. There may therefore be a very small risk of such effects on the human foetus.

*Lactation:* When topical steroid treatment is considered necessary during breast feeding, both the amount applied and the length of treatment should be minimised.

*Side-effects:* With Metosyn, side effects are extremely rare, but, as with all topical steroids, the occasional patient may show an adverse reaction such as hypersensitivity. Irritation at the site of application may occur infrequently. Treatment of large areas such as the scalp can result in local atrophic changes such as striae, skin thinning and telangiectasia and systemic effects such as adrenal suppression.

The use of topical steroids on infected lesions, without the addition of appropriate anti-infective therapy, can result in the spread of opportunist infections.

A burning feeling may be noticed on application and this may, on occasion, warrant discontinuation of therapy.

*Overdosage:* A 30 ml bottle of Metosyn Scalp Lotion contains 15 mg of fluocinonide and 30% w/v ethanol. Toxic effects are unlikely to occur following accidental ingestion.

**Pharmaceutical precautions** Metosyn Scalp Lotion should be stored in its original bottle below 25°C. The bottle should not be stored or opened near a naked flame. Use undiluted.

**Legal category** POM.

**Package quantities** Glass bottles containing 30 ml with plastic applicator (OP).

**Further information** Effect on ability to drive or operate machinery: No precautions are necessary.

**Product licence number** 12619/0040.

# MYSOLINE* TABLETS
# MYSOLINE* ORAL SUSPENSION

**Presentation** Mysoline tablets are round, white, biconvex, plain on one face and with a bisecting line on the reverse face with 'M' imprinted either side of the break-line, and contain 250 mg Primidone PhEur. Inactive ingredients are calcium carboxymethylcellulose, gelatin, magnesium stearate, povidone and stearic acid.

Mysoline Oral Suspension is a white, pleasantly flavoured aqueous suspension which contains 250 mg Primidone PhEur per 5 ml. Inactive ingredients are aluminium magnesium silicate, cetostearyl alcohol/ethylene oxide condensate, methyl hydroxybenzoate, propyl hydroxybenzoate, sodium carboxymethylcellulose, sucrose, vanilla flavouring and water.

**Uses** Mysoline is indicated in the management of

grand mal and psychomotor (temporal lobe) epilepsy. It is also of value in the management of focal or Jacksonian seizures, myoclonic jerks and akinetic attacks.

Mysoline is also indicated in the management of essential tremor.

*Mode of action:* The activity of Mysoline is due to the anticonvulsant properties of three active moieties namely primidone itself and its two major metabolites phenobarbitone and phenylethylmalonamide. The relative contribution of these three moieties to the clinical anticonvulsant effect has not been firmly established. Although the precise mode of action of Mysoline is unknown, in common with other anticonvulsants, effects on the neuronal membrane particularly with respect to alteration of ionic fluxes are likely to play a fundamental role.

Mysoline, as with other anticonvulsants, can induce liver enzymes, and although there is insufficient evidence to suggest a causal relationship, there is a theoretical risk of hepatic damage.

Mysoline may also affect vitamin D metabolism which may predispose to the development of bone disease.

Mysoline is absorbed rapidly from the gastrointestinal tract, peak plasma levels being attained approximately 3 hours after ingestion. Primidone is well distributed in all organs and tissues: it crosses the blood-brain and placental barriers and is excreted in breast milk. The pharmacokinetics of primidone are complex because of biotransformation into two metabolites, phenobarbitone and phenylethylmalonamide, that have anticonvulsant activity and complex pharmacokinetic properties. Primidone has a plasma half-life of approximately 10 hours which is considerably shorter than those of its principal metabolites. Primidone and phenylethylmalonamide are bound to plasma proteins to only a small extent, whereas approximately half of phenobarbitone is bound. Approximately 40% of the drug is excreted unchanged in urine.

**Dosage and administration** *Epilepsy:* Treatment must always be planned on an individual basis. In many patients it will be possible to use Mysoline alone, but in some, Mysoline will need to be combined with other anticonvulsants or with supporting therapy

Mysoline is usually given twice daily. Begin with 125 mg once daily late in the evening. Every three days increase the daily dosage by 125 mg until the patient is receiving 500 mg daily. Thereafter, every three days increase the daily dosage by 250 mg in adults or 125 mg in children under 9 years – until control is obtained or the maximum tolerated dosage is being given. This may be as much as 1.5 g a day in adults; 1 g a day in children.

Average daily maintenance doses:

| | Tablets (250 mg) or 5 ml measures of suspension (250 mg/5 ml) | Milligrams |
|---|---|---|
| Adults and children over 9 years | 3–6 | 750–1,500 |
| Children 6–9 years | 3–4 | 750–1,000 |
| Children 2–5 years | 2–3 | 500–750 |
| Children up to 2 years | 1–2 | 250–500 |

The total daily dose is usually best divided and given in two equal amounts, one in the morning and the other in the evening. In certain patients, it may be considered advisable to give a larger dose when the seizures are more frequent. For instance: 1) if the attacks are nocturnal then all or most of the day's dose may be given in the evening; 2) if the attacks are associated with some particular event such as menstruation, a slight increase in the appropriate dose is often beneficial.

*Elderly patients:* It is advisable to monitor elderly patients with reduced renal function who are receiving primidone.

*Patients on other anticonvulsants:* Where a patient's attacks are not sufficiently well controlled with other anticonvulsants, or disturbing side effects have arisen Mysoline may be used to augment or replace existing treatment. First add Mysoline to the current anticonvulsant treatment by the method of gradual introduction described previously. When a worthwhile effect has been achieved and the amount of Mysoline being given has been built up to at least half the estimated requirement, withdrawal of the previous treatment can then be attempted. This should be done gradually over a period of two weeks, during which time it may be necessary to increase the Mysoline dosage to maintain control. Withdrawal of previous treatment should not be too rapid or status epilepticus may occur. Where phenobarbitone formed the major part of the previous treatment, however, both its withdrawal and Mysoline substitution should be made earlier, so as to prevent excessive drowsiness from interfering with accurate assessment of the optimum dosage of Mysoline.

*Essential tremor:* Initially a dose of 50 mg daily should be introduced using Mysoline Suspension. The daily dose should be increased gradually over a 2–3 week period until remission of symptoms or the highest dose tolerated up to a maximum of 750 mg daily.

Patients with essential tremor who have not previously been exposed to anticonvulsants, or other drugs known to induce increased hepatic enzyme activity, may experience acute symptoms of intolerance to Mysoline, frequently characterised by vertigo, unsteadiness and nausea. It is, therefore, essential to start such patients at a low dosage (initially 50 mg daily) increasing very slowly up to the maximum tolerated dose or that which produces remission of tremor (up to 750 mg daily).

**Contra-indications, warnings, etc** Patients who exhibit hypersensitivity or an allergic reaction to primidone should not receive the drug. Primidone should not be administered to patients with acute intermittent porphyria.

Mysoline should be given with caution, and may be required in reduced dosage, in children, the elderly, debilitated patients or those with impaired renal, hepatic or respiratory function.

Primidone is a potent CNS depressant and is partially metabolised to phenobarbitone. After prolonged administration there is a potential for tolerance, dependence and a withdrawal reaction on abrupt cessation of treatment.

The effects of other CNS depressants such as alcohol and barbiturates may be enhanced by the administration of 'Mysoline'.

Both primidone and its major metabolite phenobarbitone induce liver enzyme activity. This may lead to altered pharmacokinetics in concomitantly administered drugs including other anticonvulsants such as phenytoin and coumarin anticoagulants. Blood levels of both Mysoline and any additional anticonvulsant agent may be altered by concomitant administration.

Breakthrough bleeding and failure of contraceptive therapy have been noted in patients taking anticonvulsant drugs and oral contraceptive steroids. This is usually assumed to be due to induction of liver enzymes by the anticonvulsant with accelerated breakdown of the hormones.

As with most other anticonvulsants, patients who drive vehicles or operate machinery should be aware of the possibility of impaired reaction time.

*Pregnancy:* There is some evidence of a higher than average incidence of congenital abnormalities in infants born of epileptic mothers. The factors influencing this are unknown, but the possibility that anticonvulsant therapy may be involved and the very slight risk of an abnormal foetus must be weighed against the risks of withholding treatment during pregnancy.

Withdrawal symptoms may occur in the newly born whose mothers have received Mysoline during late pregnancy.

Long-term anticonvulsant therapy can be associated with decreased serum folate levels. As folic acid requirements are also increased during pregnancy, regular screening of patients at risk is advised, and treatment with folic acid and vitamin $B_{12}$, although controversial, should be considered.

Anticonvulsant therapy in pregnancy has occasionally been associated with coagulation disorders in the neonates. For this reason pregnant patients should be given vitamin $K_1$ through the last month of pregnancy up to the time of delivery. In the absence of such pre-treatment, 10 mg vitamin $K_1$ may be given to the mother at the time of delivery, and 1 mg should be given immediately to the neonate at risk.

During breast feeding the baby should be monitored for sedation.

*Side-effects:* If side-effects do appear they are generally confined to the early stages of treatment when patients frequently feel drowsy and listless.

Visual disturbances, nausea, headache, dizziness, vomiting, nystagmus and ataxia have been reported but these are usually transient even when pronounced. On occasions an idiosyncratic reaction may occur which involves these symptoms in an acute and severe form necessitating withdrawal of treatment.

Dermatological reactions including severe skin eruptions and rarely systemic conditions such as systemic lupus erythematosus have been reported. Occasional cases of arthralgia and rarely, personality changes, which may include psychotic reactions, have been reported.

Exceptionally, as with phenytoin and phenobarbitone, megaloblastic anaemia may develop requiring discontinuation of primidone. This condition may respond to treatment with folic acid and/or vitamin $B_{12}$. There have been isolated reports of other blood dyscrasias.

*Overdosage:* Primidone is metabolised extensively to phenobarbitone and overdosage leads to varying degrees of CNS depression which, depending on the dose ingested, may include ataxia, loss of consciousness, respiratory depression and coma. Treatment should include aspiration of stomach contents and general supportive measures. There is no specific antidote.

**Pharmaceutical precautions** Store below 25°C.

**Legal category** POM.

**Package quantities** *Tablets 250 mg:* Containers of 100 (OP).
*Suspension (250 mg/5 ml):* Bottles of 250 ml (OP).

**Further information** Nil.

**Product licence numbers**
Mysoline Tablets        12619/0046
Mysoline Oral Suspension   12619/0045

## NASEPTIN*

**Qualitative and quantitative composition** Chlorhexidine Hydrochloride PhEur 0.1%w/w Neomycin Sulphate PhEur 0.5%w/w.

**Pharmaceutical form** Cream.

**Clinical particulars**
*Therapeutic indications:* Naseptin is an antimicrobial cream, intended for application to the nares. It is used for eradicating nasal infection with, and carriage of, staphylococci.

*Posology and method of administration:* A small amount of Naseptin is placed on the little finger and applied to the inside of each nostril.
*For prophylaxis:* Naseptin is applied as above, twice daily, to prevent patients from becoming carriers and to inhibit the dispersion of staphylococci.

*For eradication of infection:* Naseptin is applied four times daily for 10 days to eliminate organisms from the nares.

*Children and elderly patients:* There are no special dosage recommendations for either elderly patients or children.

*Contra-indications:* Naseptin is contra-indicated for patients who have previously shown a hypersensitivity reaction to neomycin. Naseptin is contra-indicated for patients who have previously shown a hypersensitivity reaction to chlorhexidine. However, such reactions are extremely rare.

*Special warnings and special precautions for use:* For nasal application only. Keep out of the eyes and ears.

Irritative skin reaction can occasionally occur. Prolonged used of neomycin can lead to skin sensitisation, ototoxicity and nephrotoxicity.

*Interaction with other medicaments and other forms of interaction:* See *Incompatibilities.*

*Pregnancy and lactation:* Chlorhexidine and neomycin cannot be detected in the blood following application of Naseptin. Consequently, the use of Naseptin is unlikely to have any effect on the foetus or on breast feeding.

*Effects on ability to drive and use machines:* Naseptin has no effect on the ability to drive and operate machinery.

*Undesirable effects:* Irritative skin reactions can occasionally occur.

Topical application of neomycin preparations can lead to skin sensitisation in a small number of patients. Prolonged use of neomycin can lead to ototoxicity and nephrotoxicity. Therefore, use with caution in children, elderly patients and patients with impaired hearing.

*Overdose:*
*Accidental ingestion:* Accidental ingestion of the contents of a Naseptin tube is not likely to have any adverse effects on the patient.

**Pharmacological properties**
*Pharmacodynamic properties:* Chlorhexidine is effective against a wide range of Gram negative and Gram positive vegetative bacteria, yeasts, dermatophyte fungi and lipophilic viruses. It is inactive against bacterial spores except at elevated temperatures.

Neomycin is a rapidly bactericidal aminoglycoside antibiotic effective against Gram positive organisms including staphylococci and a wide range of Gram negative organisms. Strains of *Pseudomonas aeruginosa* are resistant to neomycin, as are fungi and viruses.

*Pharmacokinetic properties:* Because of its cationic nature, chlorhexidine binds strongly to skin, mucosa and other tissues and is thus very poorly absorbed. No detectable blood levels have been found in man following oral use and percutaneous absorption, if it occurs at all, is insignificant.

Neomycin is either not absorbed or is absorbed only minimally through intact skin. Any neomycin which is absorbed will be rapidly excreted by the kidneys in an unchanged state.

**Pharmaceutical particulars**
*List of excipients:* Arachis Oil PhEur; Cetostearyl Alcohol PhEur; Cetostearyl Alcohol/Ethylene Oxide Condensate HSE; Purified Water PhEur.

*Incompatibilities:* Hypochlorite bleaches may cause brown stains to develop in fabrics which have previously been in contact with preparations containing chlorhexidine.

Chlorhexidine is incompatible with soap and other anionic agents.

*Shelf life:* 3 years.

*Special precautions for storage:* Store below 30°C.

*Nature and contents of container:* Collapsible, internally lacquered aluminium tubes with a white food-grade polypropylene screw cap (15 grammes).

*Instructions for use/handling:* For nasal application only.

**Marketing authorisation number** 12619/0047.

**Date of approval/revision of SPC** September 1996.

**Legal category** POM.

## NOLVADEX*
## NOLVADEX-D TABLETS
## NOLVADEX-FORTE TABLETS

**Presentation** *Nolvadex:* White, round, bi-convex tablets, each containing Tamoxifen Citrate PhEur equivalent to 10 mg of tamoxifen, marked with Nolvadex 10 on one face.

*Nolvadex-D:* White, octagonal, bi-convex tablets, each containing Tamoxifen Citrate PhEur equivalent to 20 mg of tamoxifen, marked with Nolvadex-D on one face.

*Nolvadex-Forte:* White, elongated octagonal tablets, each containing Tamoxifen Citrate PhEur equivalent to 40 mg of tamoxifen, marked with Nolvadex Forte on one face and bisected on the other side.

Inactive ingredients are croscarmellose sodium, gelatin, lactose, macrogol, magnesium stearate, maize starch, methylhydroxypropylcellulose, and titanium dioxide.

**Uses** At the recommended dosage Nolvadex has anti-oestrogenic properties and competes with oestrogen for binding sites in target organs. It does not have androgenic properties.

Nolvadex is indicated for:

1. The treatment of breast cancer. The proportion of patients with breast cancer who respond to Nolvadex is similar to that seen with oestrogens or androgens. However, because Nolvadex produces fewer serious undesirable events it is more acceptable to the patient.
2. The treatment of anovulatory infertility.

*Mode of action:* Nolvadex (tamoxifen) is a non-steroidal antioestrogen. In man Nolvadex acts primarily as an antioestrogen, inhibiting the effects of endogenous oestrogen, probably by binding with oestrogen receptors. However, clinical results have shown some benefit in oestrogen receptor negative tumours which may indicate other mechanisms of action. It is recognised that tamoxifen also displays oestrogenic-like effects on several body systems including the endometrium, bone and blood lipids.

After oral administration, tamoxifen is absorbed rapidly with maximum serum concentrations attained within 4–7 hours. Steady state concentrations (about 300 ng/ml) are achieved after four weeks treatment with 40 mg daily. The drug is highly protein bound to serum albumin (>99%). Metabolism is by hydroxylation, demethylation and conjugation, giving rise to several metabolites which have a similar pharmacological profile to the parent compound and thus contribute to the therapeutic effect. Excretion occurs primarily via the faeces and an elimination half-life of approximately seven days has been calculated for the drug itself, whereas that for N-desmethyltamoxifen, the principal circulating metabolite, is 14 days.

**Dosage and administration**
1. *Breast cancer:* The recommended daily dose of tamoxifen is normally 20 mg. No additional benefit, in terms of delayed recurrence or improved survival in patients, has been demonstrated with higher doses. Substantive evidence supporting the use of treatment with 30–40 mg per day is not available, although these doses have been used in some patients with advanced disease.

*Elderly patients:* Similar dosage regimens of Nolvadex have been used in elderly patients with breast cancer and in some of these patients it has been used as sole therapy.

2. *Infertility:* Before commencing any course of treat-

ment, whether initial or subsequent, the possibility of pregnancy must be excluded. In women who are menstruating regularly, but with anovular cycles, the initial course of treatment consists of 20 mg of Nolvadex daily on the second, third, fourth and fifth days of the menstrual cycle. If unsatisfactory basal temperature records or poor pre-ovulatory cervical mucus indicate that this initial course of treatment has been unsuccessful, further courses may be given during subsequent menstrual periods, increasing the dosage to 40 mg and then to 80 mg daily.

In women who are not menstruating regularly the initial course may begin on any day. If no signs of ovulation are demonstrable then a subsequent course of treatment may start 45 days later, with dosage increased as above. If a patient responds with menstruation, then the next course of treatment is commenced on the second day of the cycle.

**Contra-indications, warnings, etc** *Pregnancy:* Nolvadex must not be administered during pregnancy. There have been a small number of reports of spontaneous abortions, birth defects and foetal deaths after women have taken Nolvadex, although no causal relationship has been established.

Reproductive toxicology studies in rats, rabbits and monkeys have shown no teratogenic potential.

In rodent models of foetal reproductive tract development, tamoxifen was associated with changes similar to those caused by oestradiol, ethynyloestradiol, clomiphene and diethylstilboestrol (DES). Although the clinical relevance of these changes is unknown, some of them, especially vaginal adenosis, are similar to those seen in young women who were exposed to DES *in utero* and who have a 1 in 1000 risk of developing clear-cell carcinoma of the vagina or cervix. Only a small number of pregnant women have been exposed to tamoxifen. Such exposure has not been reported to cause subsequent vaginal adenosis or clear-cell carcinoma of the vagina or cervix in young women exposed *in utero* to tamoxifen.

Women should be advised not to become pregnant whilst taking Nolvadex and should use barrier or other non-hormonal contraceptive methods if sexually active. Pre-menopausal patients must be carefully examined before treatment to exclude pregnancy. Women should be appraised of the potential risks to the foetus, should they become pregnant whilst taking Nolvadex or within two months of cessation of therapy.

Menstruation is suppressed in a proportion of premenopausal women receiving Nolvadex for the treatment of breast cancer.

Cystic ovarian swellings have occasionally been observed in premenopausal women receiving Nolvadex.

A small number of patients with bony metastases have developed hypercalcaemia on initiation of therapy.

When Nolvadex is used in combination with coumarin-type anticoagulants, a significant increase in anticoagulant effect may occur. Where such co-administration is initiated, careful monitoring of the patient is recommended.

When Nolvadex is used in combination with cytotoxic agents, there is increased risk of thromboembolic events occurring.

An increased incidence of endometrial changes, including hyperplasia, polyps and cancer, has been reported in association with Nolvadex treatment. The incidence and pattern of this increase suggest that the underlying mechanism is related to the oestrogenic properties of Nolvadex. Any patients receiving or having previously received Nolvadex who report abnormal vaginal bleeding, or who presents with menstrual irregularities, vaginal discharge and symptoms such as pelvic pain or pressure should be promptly investigated.

Tamoxifen was not mutagenic in a range of *in vitro* and *in vivo* mutagenicity tests. Tamoxifen was genotoxic in some *in vitro* tests and *in vivo* genotoxicity tests in rodents. Gonadal tumours in mice and liver tumours in rats receiving tamoxifen have been reported in long-term studies. The clinical relevance of these findings has not been established.

A number of second primary tumours, occurring at sites other than the endometrium and the opposite breast, have been reported in clinical trials, following the treatment of breast cancer patients with tamoxifen. No causal link has been established and the clinical significance of these observations remains unclear.

*Lactation:* It is not known if Nolvadex is excreted in human milk and therefore the drug is not recommended during lactation. The decision either to discontinue nursing or discontinue Nolvadex should take into account the importance of the drug to the mother.

*Undesirable events:* During long-term treatment undesirable events are not as numerous or as serious with Nolvadex as with the androgens and oestrogens which are also used to treat breast cancer. Those that have been reported can be classified as either due to the anti-oestrogenic action of the drug, e.g. hot flushes, vaginal bleeding, vaginal discharge and pruritus vulvae, or as more general effects, e.g. gastro-intestinal intolerance, tumour flare, light-headedness, skin rash and, occasionally, fluid retention and alopecia.

When undesirable events are severe it may be possible to control them by a simple reduction of dosage without loss of control of the disease. If undesirable events do not respond to this measure, it may be necessary to stop the treatment.

Falls in platelet count, usually only to 80,000–90,000 per cu mm but occasionally lower, have been reported in patients taking tamoxifen for breast cancer.

A number of cases of visual disturbance including corneal changes, cataracts and retinopathy, have been described mainly in patients treated with exceptionally high doses for long periods of time.

Uterine fibroids have been reported.

Leucopenia has been observed following the administration of Nolvadex, sometimes in association with anaemia and/or thrombocytopenia. Neutropenia has been reported on rare occasions; this can sometimes be severe.

There have been infrequent reports of venous thromboembolic events occurring during Nolvadex therapy. There is evidence of a small increased risk of these events during Nolvadex therapy, especially when used in combination with cytotoxic agents.

Nolvadex has been associated with changes in liver enzyme levels and on rare occasions with a spectrum of more severe liver abnormalities, including fatty liver, cholestasis and hepatitis.

*Overdosage:* On theoretical grounds overdosage would be expected to cause enhancement of the anti-oestrogenic side-effects mentioned above. Observations in animals show that extreme overdosage (100–200 times recommended daily dose) may produce oestrogenic effects.

There is no specific antidote to overdosage, and treatment must be symptomatic.

**Pharmaceutical precautions** Store below 30°C, protected from light.

**Legal category** POM.

**Package quantities** Nolvadex tablets are blister packed in containers of 30 tablets (OP).

Nolvadex-D tablets are blister packed in containers of 30 tablets (OP).

Nolvadex-Forte tablets are blister packed in containers of 30 tablets (OP).

**Further information** *Effect on ability to drive or operate machinery:* There is no evidence that Nolvadex results in impairment of these activities.

**Product licence numbers**

| | |
|---|---|
| Nolvadex | 12619/0048 |
| Nolvadex-D | 12619/0049 |
| Nolvadex-Forte | 12619/0050 |

## PALUDRINE* TABLETS

**Qualitative and quantitative composition** Proguanil hydrochloride BP 100 mg.

**Pharmaceutical form** Tablets for oral administration.

**Clinical particulars**
*Therapeutic indications:* Paludrine is an effective antimalarial agent. It is recommended for the prevention and suppression of malaria.

Paludrine is effective against the tissue forms of some strains of *P. falciparum* and acts through an active metabolite cycloguanil. The mechanism of action is probably due to inhibition of dihydrofolate reductase. The effect of this action is to prevent schizogony and its main effect is against the developing primary tissue schizonts.

Proguanil is well absorbed in man with peak plasma concentrations of approximately 140 ng/ml occurring around 4 hours after an oral dose of 200 mg to an adult. The active triazine metabolite cycloguanil peaks at approximately 75 ng/ml 1 hour later. The elimination half-lives for proguanil and cycloguanil are reported to be of the order of 20 hours.

There is a low degree of drug accumulation after repeat doses, leading to steady state conditions after approximately 3 days. When daily doses are not taken, blood levels fall sharply but do not disappear completely until at least two or three doses are missed.

*Posology and method of administration:* Non-immune subjects entering a malarious area are advised to begin treatment with Paludrine 1 week before, or if this is not possible, then at least 24 hours before arrival. The daily dose of Paludrine should be continued throughout exposure to risk and for 4 weeks after leaving the area.

*Adults:* Two tablets (200 mg) daily

*Children: Under 1 year:* ¼ tablet (25 mg) daily

*1 to 4 years:* ½ tablet (50 mg) daily

*5 to 8 years:* 1 tablet (100 mg) daily

*9 to 14 years:* 1½ tablets (150 mg) daily

*Over 14 years:* Adult daily dose

The daily dose is best taken with water, after fooc at the same time each day.

Provided the tablet fragment gives the minimun amount specified, precise accuracy in children's dos age is not essential since the drug possesses a wid safety margin.

For a young child, the dose may be administere crushed and mixed with milk, honey or jam.

*Elderly patients:* There are no special dosage rec ommendations for the elderly, but it may be advisabl to monitor elderly patients so that optimum dosag can be individually determined.

*Renal impairment:* Based on a theoretical mode derived from a single dose pharmacokinetic study the following guidance is given for adults with rena impairment. (See *Contra-indications* and *Specia warnings and special precautions for use.*)

| *Creatinine clearance ml/min/1.73 m²* | *Dosage* |
|---|---|
| ≥60 | 200 mg once daily (standard dose) |
| 20 to 59 | 100 mg once daily |
| 10 to 19 | 50 mg every second day |
| <10 | < 50 mg once weekly |

The grade of renal impairment and/or the serur creatinine concentration may be approximatel equated to creatinine clearance levels as indicate below.

| *Creatinine clearance ml/min/1.73 m²* | *Approx* serum creatinine (micromol/l)* | *Renal impairment grade (arbitrarily divided for dosage purposes)* |
|---|---|---|
| ≥ 60 | - | - |
| 20 to 59 | 150 to 300 | Mild |
| 10 to 19 | 300 to 700 | Moderate |
| < 10 | > 700 | Severe |

* Serum creatinine concentration is only an approx mate guide to renal function unless corrected for age weight and sex.

*Contra-indications:* Paludrine should be used wit caution in patients with severe renal impairment. (Se *Posology and method of administration* and *Specia warnings and special precautions for use.*)

*Special warnings and special precautions for use* Paludrine should be used with caution in patients wit severe renal impairment. (See *Posology and metho of administration*). There have been rare reports c haematological changes in such patients.

In any locality where drug-resistant malaria i known or suspected, it is essential to take loca medical advice on what prophylactic regimen i appropriate. Prophylactic use of Paludrine alone ma not be sufficient.

*Interactions with other medicaments and other form of interaction:* None have been reported or are known

*Pregnancy and lactation:*
*Pregnancy:* Pregnancy increases the risks from ma laria. It is generally accepted that all drug treatmer should be avoided if possible during the first trimeste of pregnancy. Paludrine has been widely used fc over 40 years and a causal connection between it use and any adverse effect on mother or foetus ha not been established.

*Lactation:* Although Paludrine is excreted in breas milk, the amount is insufficient to confer any benef on the infant. Separate chemoprophylaxis for th infant is required.

*Effects on ability to drive and use machines:* There i no evidence to suggest that Paludrine causes sedatio or is likely to affect concentration.

*Undesirable effects:* At normal dosage levels the sid effect most commonly encountered is mild gastri intolerance. This usually subsides as treatment i continued.

Mouth ulceration and stomatitis have on occasio been reported. Isolated cases of skin reactions an reversible hair loss have been reported in associatio with the use of proguanil.

Haematological changes in patients with sever renal impairment have been reported.

*Overdose:* The following effects have been reporte in cases of overdosage:

Haematuria, renal irritation, epigastric discomfo and vomiting. There is no specific antidote an symptoms should be treated as they arise.

**Pharmacological properties**
*Pharmacodynamic properties:* Proguanil is an ant

malarial drug and dihydrofolate reductase inhibitor. It acts like the other antifolate antimalarials by interfering with the folic-folinic acid systems and thus exerts its effect mainly at the time the nucleus is dividing. Since its activity is dependent on its metabolism, proguanil has a slow schizonticidal effect in the blood. It also has some schizonticidal activity in the tissues.

Proguanil is effective against the exoerythrocytic forms of some strains of *Plasmodium falciparum* but it has little or no activity against the exoerythrocytic forms of *P. vivax*. It has a marked sporonticidal effect against some strains *P. falciparum*; it does not kill the gametocytes, but renders them non-infective for the mosquito while the drug is present in the blood. Malaria parasites in the red blood cells are killed more rapidly by chloroquine or quinine than by proguanil, which is therefore not the best drug to use for the treatment of acute malaria. Reynolds (1982).

Soon after proguanil was introduced, it was observed that the drug was inactive as an inhibitor of the in vitro growth of *P.gallinaceum* and *P. cynomolgi*, but that sera from dosed monkeys were active against *P. cynomolgi* in vitro. These findings suggested that proguanil was activated in vivo.

Since that time it has been accepted by most investigators in this field that cycloguanil is the active metabolite of proguanil and that parent compound is inactive per se. Ferone (1984).

Cycloguanil acts by binding to the enzyme dihydrofolate reductase in the malaria parasite. The effect of this action is to prevent the completion of schizogony. This is seen in the asexual blood stages as an arrest of maturation of the developing schizonts and an accumulation of large, abnormal looking trophozoites.

Proguanil is highly active against the primary exoerythocytic forms of *P. falciparum* and it has a fleeting inhibiting action on those of *P. vivax*. Proguanil is therefore a valuable drug for causal prophylaxis in falciparum malaria.

*Pharmacokinetic properties:* Proguanil is absorbed from the gastro-intestinal tract and peak concentrations in the circulation are attained about 3 hours after the dose is taken; about 65% in the plasma is bound to proteins and high concentrations occur in erythrocytes. The blood concentration rapidly diminishes and about 60% of a dose is excreted unchanged in the urine and about 30% as the active metabolite cycloguanil. Reynolds (1982).

About 10% of the drug is excreted in the faeces.

Work in volunteers showed that up to 66% of single 300 mg dose was recovered from urine over a 4 day period. Of this, up to 76% was proguanil, up to 43% was cycloguanil and up to 11% was 4-chlorophenyl-biguanide (4-CPB). Smith et al (1961).

Proguanil is well absorbed in man. Peak concentrations of approximately 170 ng/ml (plasma) and 1000 ng/ml (whole blood) occur approximately 5 hours after an oral dose of 200 mg. The active triazine metabolite cycloguanil peaks 1 hour later, and the inactive metabolite 4-chlorophenylbiguanide (4-CPB) a further hour later. Proguanil and 4-CPB are concentrated in red cells but cycloguanil is not. Elimination of the parent drug is the rate-limiting factor determining whole blood and plasma concentration of the metabolites. The elimination half-life is approximately 16 hours. White (1988).

The mean elimination half-life of cycloguanil is approximately 11 hours. Watkins (1987).

There is a low degree of drug accumulation after repeat doses, leading to steady state conditions after approximately 3 days. When daily doses are not taken, blood levels fall sharply but do not disappear completely until at least 2 or 3 doses are missed. Kelly and Fletcher (1986).

There have been no recent pharmacokinetic studies of proguanil reported in children, the elderly, pregnant women or patients with renal and hepatic impairment. White (1985).

Proguanil is active against the asexual blood forms of all species of the human malaria parasite. It achieves clinical cure in all forms of malaria and radical cure in most falciparum infections. However, the clinical response is slow and its use for the treatment of an acute malarial attack is not recommended. Proguanil is a good suppressive of all forms of malaria, often with suppressive cure in falciparum infection.

Proguanil has little apparent effect on the production, number or morphology of the gametocytes of *P. falciparum*, but in appropriate doses inhibits the later development of sporogonic forms in the mosquito. Mosquitoes fed on gametocyte carriers receiving therapeutic doses do not become infective. Sporogony in *P. vivax* is similarly affected. Proguanil is therefore a valuable drug for sporonticidal prophylaxis. Bruce-Chwatt (1986).

*Pre-clinical safety data:* Proguanil is a drug on which extensive clinical experience has been obtained. All relevant information for the prescriber is provided elsewhere in the Summary of Product Characteristics.

**Pharmaceutical particulars**

*List of excipients:* Calcium carbonate PhEur; Gelatin PhEur; Magnesium Stearate PhEur; Maize Starch PhEur.

*Incompatibilities:* None known.

*Shelf life:* 5 years.

*Special precautions for storage:* Store below 30 °C.

*Nature and contents of container:* HDPE bottles (100) and blister packs (98).

*Instructions for use/handling:* Use as directed by the prescriber.

**Marketing authorisation number** 12619/0051

**Date of approval/revision of SPC** September 1996

**Legal category** P

# PEPTAVLON* INJECTION

**Qualitative and quantitative composition** Pentagastrin BP 0.025% w/v.

**Pharmaceutical form** Solution for injection.

**Clinical particulars**

*Therapeutic indications:* Peptavlon is used for the diagnostic testing of gastric secretion.

*Posology and method of administration:* For administration either subcutaneously or by continuous intravenous infusion.

*Adults (including the elderly) and children:* The following procedure is adopted for testing gastric secretion with Peptavlon.

The patient receives no medication (e.g. antacids, etc.) that might affect the results of the test for 24 hours and no food for 12 hours before the test. On the morning of the test a radio-opaque tube (Leven No. 7 or Ryle's 12-16Fr.) is passed into the patient's stomach by way of the nose. Radiological observation is used to ensure that the tube is correctly positioned in the lower part of the body of the stomach.

The tube is securely fastened to the patient's nose and forehead with adhesive tape to ensure that it is not displaced. The patient lies on his left side.

The gastric juices are then collected by applying continuous suction (at 30–50 mm Hg below atmospheric pressure) to this tube, supplemented by manual suction. The patient takes occasional deep breaths to improve collection. The basal secretion is obtained by collecting samples at 15 minute intervals over an hour.

Peptavlon is then given, either at a dose of:

a. 6 micrograms/kg/body weight subcutaneously, or
b. 0.6 micrograms/kg/hour as a continuous intravenous infusion. A Tuberculin syringe is used to give a dose correct to 0.01 ml.

If dilution is required normal saline may be used.

Specimens of the gastric juices are again collected over periods of 10 or 15 minutes. The volume of the sample is measured and it is immediately filtered through gauze into a bottle. The acidity of each sample is determined by titration.

*Contra-indications:* When the patient has previously shown a severe idiosyncratic response to the drug, Peptavlon should not be administered.

*Special warnings and special precautions for use:* As pentagastrin stimulates gastric acid secretion it should be used with caution in patients with acute or bleeding peptic ulcer disease, though there is no clinical evidence to contra-indicate use.

*Interactions with other medicaments and other forms of interaction:* None known.

*Pregnancy and lactation*
*Pregnancy:* Peptavlon should not be administered during pregnancy.
*Lactation:* No special precautions are required.

*Effects on ability to drive and use machines:* No precautions are required.

*Undesirable effects:* At the recommended dosage the incidence of side-effects is extremely small, although very occasionally an individual may respond with hypotension and associated dizziness and faintness. Other unwanted effects reported are mild abdominal discomfort, abdominal cramps, nausea, vomiting, flushing, sweating, headaches, drowsiness or exhaustion, heaviness or weakness of the legs, allergic reactions, bradycardia, tachycardia. These effects disappear once administration of Peptavlon has ceased.

*Overdosage:* The form of presentation makes it unlikely that overdosage will occur, and no such occurrence has been reported. As maximal secretory response is produced by the normal dosage, increased dosage would be expected to have no sequel other than an accentuation of the known side-effects.

**Pharmacological properties**

*Pharmacodynamic properties:* Pentagastrin is a synthetic pentapeptide containing the carboxyl terminal tetrapeptide responsible for the actions of natural gastrins. The most prominent action of pentagastrin is to stimulate the secretion of gastric acid, pepsin and intrinsic factor. Additionally, it stimulates pancreatic secretion, inhibits absorption of water and electrolytes from the ileum, contracts the smooth muscle of the lower oesophageal sphincter and stomach (but delays gastric emptying time), relaxes the sphincter of Oddi and increases blood flow in the gastric mucosa.

*Pharmacokinetic properties:* Pentagastrin stimulates gastric acid secretion approximately ten minutes after subcutaneous injection, with peak response occurring in most cases twenty to thirty minutes after administration. Duration of activity is usually between sixty and eighty minutes.

Pentagastrin is rapidly absorbed after administration. Pentagastrin has a short half-life (10 minutes or less) in the circulation. It is metabolised primarily in the liver and excretion is mainly by the kidneys.

*Preclinical safety data:* Pentagastrin is a drug on which extensive clinical experience has been obtained. All relevant information for the prescriber is provided elsewhere in the Summary of Product Characteristics.

**Pharmaceutical particulars**

*List of excipients:* Sodium chloride, ammonium chloride, water.

*Incompatibilities:* None known.

*Shelf life:* 24 months.

*Special precautions for storage:* Store away from light, below 4°C but above freezing.

*Nature and contents of container:* 2 ml glass ampoules in boxes of 5.

*Instructions for use/handling:* If dilution is required Sodium Chloride Injection BP may be used. This solution should be prepared immediately before it is required for use.

**Marketing authorisation number** 12619/0052.

**Date of approval/revision of SPC** July 1995.

**Legal category** POM.

# SEROQUEL* ▼

**Qualitative and quantitative composition**

*25 mg tablet:* Each tablet contains 25 mg quetiapine (as 28.78 mg quetiapine fumarate).
*100 mg tablet:* Each tablet contains 100 mg quetiapine (as 115.13 mg quetiapine fumarate).
*200 mg tablet:* Each tablet contains 200 mg quetiapine (as 230.26 mg quetiapine fumarate).

**Pharmaceutical form** Film-coated tablets.

**Clinical particulars**

*Therapeutic indications:* Seroquel is indicated for the treatment of schizophrenia.

*Posology and method of administration:* Seroquel should be administered twice daily, with or without food.

*Adults:* The total daily dose for the first 4 days of therapy is 50 mg (Day 1), 100 mg (Day 2), 200 mg (Day 3) and 300 mg (Day 4).

From Day 4 onwards, the dose should be titrated to the usual effective dose range of 300 to 450 mg/day. Depending on the clinical response and tolerability of the individual patient, the dose may be adjusted within the range 150 to 750 mg/day.

*Elderly:* As with other antipsychotics, Seroquel should be used with caution in the elderly, especially during the initial dosing period. Elderly patients should be started on Seroquel 25 mg/day. The dose should be increased daily, in increments of 25 to 50 mg, to an effective dose, which is likely to be lower than that in younger patients.

*Children and adolescents:* The safety and efficacy of Seroquel have not been evaluated in children and adolescents.

*Renal and hepatic impairment:* The oral clearance of quetiapine is reduced by approximately 25% in patients with renal or hepatic impairment. Quetiapine is extensively metabolised by the liver, and therefore should be used with caution in patients with known hepatic impairment.

*Patients with renal or hepatic impairment:* Should be started on Seroquel 25 mg/day. The dose should be increased daily, in increments of 25 to 50 mg, to an effective dose.

*Contra-indications:* Seroquel is contra-indicated in

*Table 1 Adverse events that occurred in at least 1% of patients treated with Seroquel in the placebo-controlled Phase-II/III trials[a]*

| Body system and COSTART Term | Number (%) of patients with adverse events | |
|---|---|---|
| | Seroquel (n = 510) | Placebo (n = 206) |
| Total number (%) of patients with adverse events[b] | 406 (79.6) | 155 (75.2) |
| **Body as a whole** | | |
| Headache | 99 (19.4) | 36 (17.5) |
| Asthenia | 18 (3.5) | 6 (2.9) |
| Abdominal pain | 16 (3.1) | 1 (0.5) |
| Back pain | 10 (2.0) | 1 (0.5) |
| Fever | 8 (1.6) | 2 (1.0) |
| Chest pain | 9 (1.8) | 3 (1.5) |
| **Cardiovascular system** | | |
| Postural hypotension | 36 (7.1) | 5 (2.4) |
| Tachycardia | 36 (7.1) | 10 (4.9) |
| Hypertension | 9 (1.8) | 3 (1.5) |
| **Digestive system** | | |
| Constipation | 44 (8.6) | 10 (4.9) |
| Dry mouth | 33 (6.5) | 6 (2.9) |
| Dyspepsia | 32 (6.3) | 5 (2.4) |
| Diarrhoea | 10 (2.0) | 4 (1.9) |
| GGT increased | 8 (1.6) | 1 (0.5) |
| **Haemic and lymphatic system** | | |
| Leucopenia | 8 (1.6) | 0 |
| **Metabolic and nutritional disorders** | | |
| ALT (SGPT) increased | 31 (6.1) | 3 (1.5) |
| AST (SGOT) increased | 18 (3.5) | 2 (1.0) |
| Weight gain | 10 (2.0) | 0 |
| **Musculoskeletal system** | | |
| Myalgia | 6 (1.2) | 1 (0.5) |
| **Nervous system** | | |
| Somnolence | 89 (17.5) | 22 (10.7) |
| Dizziness | 49 (9.6) | 9 (4.4) |
| Anxiety | 16 (3.1) | 6 (2.9) |
| **Respiratory system** | | |
| Rhinitis | 17 (3.3) | 1 (0.5) |
| **Skin and appendages** | | |
| Rash | 22 (4.3) | 6 (2.9) |
| Dry skin | 6 (1.2) | 2 (1.0) |
| **Special senses** | | |
| Ear pain | 6 (1.2) | 0 |
| **Urogenital system** | | |
| Urinary tract infection | 7 (1.4) | 1 (0.5) |

[a] Only adverse events that occurred in a higher proportion of patients treated with Seroquel than with placebo are presented. Adverse events for which the incidence with Seroquel was equal to or less than that with placebo included the following: pain, infection, hostility, accidental injury, hypotension, nausea, vomiting, agitation, insomnia, nervousness, akathisia, hypertonia, tremor, depression, paraesthesia, pharyngitis, amblyopia. Patients may have had more than one adverse event.

patients who are hypersensitive to any component of this product.

*Special warnings and special precautions for use:*
*Cardiovascular disease:* Seroquel may induce orthostatic hypotension, especially during the initial dose-titration period; this is more common in elderly patients than in younger patients.

In clinical trials, quetiapine was not associated with a persistent increase in QT$_c$ intervals. However, as with other antipsychotics, caution should be exercised when quetiapine is prescribed with drugs known to prolong the QT$_c$ interval, especially in the elderly.

Seroquel should be used with caution in patients with known cardiovascular disease, cerebrovascular disease, or other conditions predisposing to hypotension.

*Seizures:* In controlled clinical trials there was no difference in the incidence of seizures in patients treated with Seroquel or placebo. As with other antipsychotics, caution is recommended when treating patients with a history of seizures.

*Neuroleptic malignant syndrome:* Neuroleptic malignant syndrome has been associated with antipsychotic treatment. Clinical manifestations include hyperthermia, altered mental status, muscular rigidity, autonomic instability, and increased creatine phosphokinase. In such an event, Seroquel should be discontinued and appropriate medical treatment given.

*Tardive dyskinesia:* As with other antipsychotics, there is a potential for Seroquel to cause tardive dyskinesia after long-term treatment. If signs and symptoms of tardive dyskinesia appear, dose reduction or discontinuation of Seroquel should be considered.

*Interactions with other medicaments and other forms of interaction:* Given the primary central nervous system effects of quetiapine, Seroquel should be used with caution in combination with other centrally acting drugs and alcohol.

The pharmacokinetics of lithium were not altered when co-administered with Seroquel.

Quetiapine did not induce the hepatic enzyme systems involved in the metabolism of antipyrine.

Co-administration of Seroquel and phenytoin (microsomal enzyme inducer) caused increases in clearance of quetiapine. Increased doses of Seroquel may be required to maintain control of psychotic symptoms in patients co-administered Seroquel and phen-

ytoin, or other hepatic enzyme inducers (eg, carbamazepine, barbiturates, rifampicin). The dose of Seroquel may need to be reduced if phenytoin is withdrawn and replaced with a non-inducer (e.g. sodium valproate).

The pharmacokinetics of quetiapine were not significantly altered following co-administration with the antipsychotics risperidone or haloperidol. However, co-administration of Seroquel and thioridazine caused increases in clearance of quetiapine.

The pharmacokinetics of quetiapine were not significantly altered following co-administration with the antidepressants imipramine (a known CYP2D6 inhibitor) or fluoxetine (a known CYP3A4 and CYP2D6 inhibitor).

CYP3A4 is the primary enzyme responsible for cytochrome P450 mediated metabolism of quetiapine. The pharmacokinetics of quetiapine were not altered following co-administration with cimetidine or fluoxetine, both of which are known P450 enzyme inhibitors. However, caution is recommended when Seroquel is co-administered with potent CYP3A4 inhibitors (such as systemic ketoconazole or erythromycin).

*Pregnancy and lactation:* The safety and efficacy of Seroquel during human pregnancy have not been established (see *Pre-clinical safety data, Reproduction studies,* for animal reproductive toxicology data). Therefore, Seroquel should only be used during pregnancy if the benefits justify the potential risks.

The degree to which quetiapine is excreted into human milk is unknown. Women who are breast feeding should therefore be advised to avoid breast feeding while taking Seroquel.

*Effect on ability to drive and use machines:* Because Seroquel may cause somnolence, patients should be cautioned about operating hazardous machines, including motor vehicles.

*Undesirable effects:* The most frequent and significant adverse events reported from short-term controlled trials of Seroquel were somnolence (17.5%), dizziness (10%), constipation (9%), postural hypotension (7%), dry mouth (7%), and liver enzyme abnormalities (6%).

Table 1 lists the adverse events that occurred in at least 1% of patients treated with Seroquel in the placebo-controlled Phase-II/III trials.

Seroquel may be associated with mild asthenia, rhinitis and dyspepsia. As with other antipsychotics,

Seroquel may also be associated with limited weight gain, predominantly during the early weeks of treatment.

As with other antipsychotics with $\alpha_1$ adrenergic blocking activity, Seroquel may induce orthostatic hypotension (associated with dizziness), tachycardia and, in some patients, syncope; these events occur especially during the initial dose-titration period (see *Special warnings and special precautions for use*).

There have been occasional reports of seizures in patients administered Seroquel, although the frequency was no greater than that observed in patients administered placebo in controlled clinical trials (see *Special warnings and special precautions for use*).

As with other antipsychotic agents, rare cases of possible neuroleptic malignant syndrome have been reported in patients treated with Seroquel (see *Special warnings and special precautions for use*).

As with other antipsychotic agents, Seroquel has been associated with variations in white blood cell count. Transient asymptomatic leucopenia and/or neutropenia have been observed in patients administered Seroquel, recorded at an incidence of 1.6% in placebo-controlled clinical trials. Occasionally, eosinophilia has been observed.

Asymptomatic elevations in serum transaminase (ALT, AST) or GGT levels have been observed in some patients administered Seroquel. These elevations were usually reversible on continued Seroquel treatment.

Small elevations in non-fasting serum triglyceride levels and total cholesterol have been observed during treatment with Seroquel.

Seroquel treatment was associated with small dose-related decreases in thyroid hormone levels, particularly total T$_4$ and free T$_4$. The reduction in total and free T$_4$ was maximal within the first 2 to 4 weeks of quetiapine treatment, with no further reduction during long-term treatment. There was no evidence of clinically significant changes in TSH concentration over time. In nearly all cases, cessation of quetiapine treatment was associated with a reversal of the effects on total and free T$_4$, irrespective of the duration of treatment.

As with other antipsychotics, Seroquel may cause prolongation of the QT$_c$ interval, but in clinical trials this was not associated with a persistent increase (see *Special warnings and special precautions for use*).

*Overdose:* In clinical trials, experience with Seroquel in overdosage is limited. Estimated doses of Seroquel in excess of 10 g have been taken; no fatalities were reported and patients recovered without sequelae.

In general, reported signs and symptoms were those resulting from an exaggeration of the drug's known pharmacological effects, ie, drowsiness and sedation, tachycardia and hypotension.

There is no specific antidote to quetiapine. In cases of severe intoxication, the possibility of multiple drug involvement should be considered, and intensive care procedures are recommended, including establishing and maintaining a patent airway, ensuring adequate oxygenation and ventilation, and monitoring and support of the cardiovascular system.

Close medical supervision and monitoring should be continued until the patient recovers.

**Pharmacological properties** Therapeutic classification: N05A

*Pharmacodynamic properties:* Quetiapine is an atypical antipsychotic agent which interacts with a broad range of neurotransmitter receptors. Quetiapine exhibits a higher affinity for serotonin (5HT$_2$) receptors in the brain than it does for dopamine D$_1$ and D$_2$ receptors in the brain. Quetiapine also has high affinity at histaminergic and adrenergic $\alpha_1$ receptors, with a lower affinity at adrenergic $\alpha_2$ receptors, but no appreciable affinity at cholinergic muscarinic or benzodiazepine receptors. Quetiapine is active in tests for antipsychotic activity, such as conditioned avoidance.

The results of animal studies predictive of EPS liability revealed that quetiapine causes only weak catalepsy at effective dopamine D$_2$ receptor blocking doses, that quetiapine causes selective reduction in the firing of mesolimbic A10 dopaminergic neurones versus the A9 nigrostriatal neurones involved in motor function, and that quetiapine exhibits minimal dystonic liability in neuroleptic-sensitised monkeys. The results of three placebo-controlled clinical trials, including one that used a dose range of Seroquel of 75 to 750 mg/day, identified no difference between Seroquel and placebo in the incidence of EPS or use of concomitant anticholinergics.

Seroquel does not produce sustained elevations in prolactin. In a multiple fixed-dose clinical trial, there were no differences in prolactin levels at study completion between Seroquel, across the recommended dose range, and placebo.

In clinical trials, Seroquel has been shown to be effective in the treatment of both positive and negative symptoms of schizophrenia. In one trial against

·hlorpromazine, and two against haloperidol, Sero-
uel showed similar short-term efficacy.

*Pharmacokinetic properties:* Quetiapine is well ab-orbed and extensively metabolised following oral dministration. The principal human plasma metabo-ites do not have significant pharmacological activity.

The bioavailability of quetiapine is not significantly ffected by administration with food. The elimination alf-life of quetiapine is approximately 7 hours. Quetiapine is approximately 83% bound to plasma roteins.

Clinical trials have demonstrated that Seroquel is ffective when given twice a day. This is further upported by data from a positron emission tomog-aphy (PET) study which identified that $5HT_2$ and $D_2$ eceptor occupancy are maintained for up to 12 hours fter dosing with quetiapine.

The pharmacokinetics of quetiapine are linear, and o not differ between men and women.

The mean clearance of quetiapine in the elderly is pproximately 30 to 50% lower than that seen in dults aged 18 to 65 years.

The mean plasma clearance of quetiapine was educed by approximately 25% in subjects with severe enal impairment (creatinine clearance less than 0 ml/min/1.73 m²) and in subjects with hepatic im-airment (stable alcoholic cirrhosis), but the individual learance values are within the range for normal ubjects.

Quetiapine is extensively metabolised, with parent ompound accounting for less than 5% of unchanged rug-related material in the urine or faeces, following ne administration of radiolabelled quetiapine. Ap-roximately 73% of the radioactivity is excreted in the rine and 21% in the faeces.

*In vitro* investigations established that CYP3A4 is ne primary enzyme responsible for cytochrome 450 mediated metabolism of quetiapine.

Quetiapine and several of its metabolites were ound to be weak inhibitors of human cytochrome 450 1A2, 2C9, 2C19, 2D6 and 3A4 activities, but only t concentrations at least 10- to 50-fold higher than nose observed in the usual effective dose range of 00 to 450 mg/day in humans. Based on these *in vitro* esults, it is unlikely that co-administration of quetia-ine with other drugs will result in clinically significant rug inhibition of cytochrome P450 mediated metab-lism of the other drug.

*re-clinical safety data:*

*cute toxicity studies:* Quetiapine has low acute oxicity. Findings in mice and rats after oral (500 mg/ g) or intraperitoneal (100 mg/kg) dosing were typical f an effective neuroleptic agent and included de-reased motor activity, ptosis, loss of righting reflex, uid around the mouth and convulsions.

*Repeat-dose toxicity studies:* In multiple-dose stud-s in rats, dogs and monkeys, anticipated central ervous system effects of an antipsychotic drug were bserved with quetiapine (eg, sedation at lower doses nd tremor, convulsions or prostration at higher xposures).

Hyperprolactinaemia, induced through the dopa-ine $D_2$ receptor antagonist activity of quetiapine or s metabolites, varied between species but was most arked in the rat, and a range of effects consequent this were seen in the 12-month study, including ammary hyperplasia, increased pituitary weight, ecreased uterine weight and enhanced growth of males.

Reversible morphological and functional effects on e liver, consistent with hepatic enzyme induction, ere seen in mouse, rat and monkey.

Thyroid follicular cell hypertrophy and concomitant anges in plasma thyroid hormone levels occurred rat and monkey.

Pigmentation of a number of tissues, particularly e thyroid, was not associated with any morphologi-al or functional effects.

Transient increases in heart rate, unaccompanied y an effect on blood pressure, occurred in dogs.

Posterior triangular cataracts seen after 6 months dogs at 100 mg/kg/day were consistent with inhibi-on of cholesterol biosynthesis in the lens. No ataracts were observed in Cynomolgus monkeys osed up to 225 mg/kg/day, nor in rodents. Monitoring clinical studies did not reveal drug-related corneal pacities in man.

No evidence of neutrophil reduction or agranulo-tosis was seen in any of the toxicity studies.

*Carcinogenicity studies:* In the rat study (doses 0, ), 75 and 250 mg/kg/day) the incidence of mammary lenocarcinomas was increased at all doses in female ts, consequential to prolonged hyperprolactinae-ia.

In male rat (250 mg/kg/day) and mouse (250 and 0 mg/kg/day), there was an increased incidence of yroid follicular cell benign adenomas, consistent ith known rodent-specific mechanisms resulting om enhanced hepatic thyroxine clearance.

*Reproduction studies:* Effects related to elevated prolactin levels (marginal reduction in male fertility and pseudopregnancy, protracted periods of diestrus, increased precoital interval and reduced pregnancy rate) were seen in rats, although these are not directly relevant to humans because of species differences in hormonal control of reproduction.

Quetiapine had no teratogenic effects.

*Mutagenicity studies:* Genetic toxicity studies with quetiapine show that it is not a mutagen or clastogen.

**Pharmaceutical particulars**

*List of excipients:* Core: Povidone PhEur; Calcium Hydrogen Phosphate PhEur; Microcrystalline Cellulose PhEur; Sodium Starch Glycollate Type A PhEur; Lactose Monohydrate PhEur; Magnesium Stearate PhEur.

Coating: Hydroxypropyl Methylcellulose 2910 PhEur; Macrogol 400 PhEur; Titanium Dioxide PhEur (E171); Ferric Oxide, Yellow PhFr (E172) (25 mg and 100 mg tablets); Ferric Oxide, Red PhFr (E172) (25 mg tablets).

*Incompatibilities:* None known

*Shelf life:* The shelf life of Seroquel is 24 months when stored below 30°C.

*Special precautions for storage:* None stated.

*Nature and contents of container:*

*25 mg tablet:* The tablets are round, 6 mm, peach coloured, bi-convex and film-coated.

*100 mg tablet:* The tablets are round, 8.5 mm, yellow coloured, bi-convex and film-coated.

*200 mg tablet:* The tablets are round, 11 mm, white, bi-convex and film-coated.

The tablets are packed into PVC aluminium foil blister strips. The blister strips are themselves packed into cartons.

25 mg tablets, 60 tablets in 6 strips of 10 blisters.

100 mg and 200 mg tablets, 60 tablets in 6 strips of 10 blisters and 90 tablets in 9 strips of 10 blisters.

Mixed pack, 8 tablets 1 strip containing 6 x 25 mg and 2 x 100 mg tablets.

*Instructions for use/handling:* Nil

**Marketing authorisation numbers**

| | |
|---|---|
| 25 mg tablet | 12619/0112 |
| 100 mg tablet | 12619/0113 |
| 200 mg tablet | 12619/0114 |

**Date of approval/revision of SPC** July 1997

**Legal category** POM

## SIOPEL* CREAM

**Qualitative and quantitative composition** Strong Cetrimide Solution B.P. 0.75% v/w and Dimethicone 1000 Ph. Eur. 10% w/w

**Pharmaceutical form** A smooth, white homogenous cream.

**Clinical particulars**

*Therapeutic indication:* An effective water-repellant barrier cream with antiseptic properties, useful whenever the skin needs to be protected from water-soluble irritants.

*Posology and method of administration:* Wash and dry the skin. Apply the cream sparingly and massage well into the skin. Apply three to five times daily for three to four days then once or twice daily.

*Contra-indications:* Siopel cream is contra-indicated for patients who have previously shown a hypersensitivity reaction to cetrimide preparations .

*Special warnings and special precautions for use:* For topical application only. Keep out of the eyes and avoid contact with the brain, meninges and middle ear. Do not use in body cavities or as an enema.

Do not use on skin that is acutely inflamed or weeping, or before the skin has been cleansed of contaminating irritants.

*Interaction with other medicaments and other forms of interaction:* None have been reported or are known.

*Pregnancy and lactation:* There is no evidence of any adverse effects on the foetus arising from the use of Siopel cream during pregnancy and therefore no special precautions are recommended.

*Effects on ability to drive and use machines:* None have been reported or are known.

*Undesirable events:* Irritative skin reactions can occasionally occur and hypersensitivity to cetrimide preparations has been reported, usually developing after repeated application, but is rare. Should such reactions occur, stop application of the product.

*Overdose:* It seems unlikely that systemic toxicity will occur from accidental ingestion of the cream. However, in the event of large quantities being swallowed, carry out gastric lavage with milk, raw egg, gelatin or mild soap, and apply supportive measures as appropriate. Do not induce vomiting.

Central paralysis cannot be countered by curare antagonists or CNS stimulants but sympathomimetic drugs have been given.

Mechanically assisted ventilation with oxygen may be necessary. Persistent convulsions may be controlled with cautious doses of diazepam or a short-acting barbiturate. Do not give alcohol in any form.

**Pharmacological properties**

*Pharmacodynamic properties:* Siopel cream is a topical agent for application to intact skin only, and is not intended to be administered by any other route.

Dimethicone 1000 is strongly substantive, binding firmly to the skin surface. There is no evidence of percutaneous absorption and in common with other silicone fluids, is considered to be physiologically inert. There are, as a consequence, no general pharmacological or pharmacokinetic studies available on dimethicone.

Studies with cetrimide have shown it to be active against a wide range of vegetative bacteria, both Gram positive and Gram negative, including *Staph. aureus* the commonest cause of infection in wounds and burns. Certain Gram negative bacteria, particularly strains of Pseudomonas and Proteus remain the least susceptible of the pathogenic bacteria to cetrimide, requiring a higher concentration than other species to produce an effective kill.

Cetrimide is cationic in nature, binding strongly to skin and other tissue and thus absorption is negligible.

*Pharmacokinetic properties:* Dimethicone 1000–see *Pharmacodynamic properties.*

Cetrimide–Isomaa has studied the absorption, distribution and excretion of orally administered $^{14}C$-labelled cetrimide in female rats. Approximately 80% of the dose of radioactivity was found in the gastro-intestinal tract 8 hours after administration. Only small amounts were found in the blood plasma and approximately 2% was excreted in the bile during the first 12 hours after treatment. The low levels of radioactivity in the serum and bile, together with the large amounts of the antiseptic found in the gastro-intestinal tract, indicate poor intestinal absorption of cetrimide. Only small amounts of radioactivity were found in the liver, kidneys, spleen, heart, lungs and skeletal muscle, and the tissue radioactivity decline rapidly, only traces being found in the tissues 4 days after administration. Within 3 days of ingestion, 92% of the administered radioactivity had been excreted in the faeces and 1% in the urine. No radioactivity was found in the expired $CO_2$ collected during day 1 after administration. Thin-layer chromatography of bile and urine samples indicated that cetrimide was metabolised to some extent in the rat.

**Pharmaceutical particulars**

*List of excipients:* Arachis Oil PhEur; Butylated Hydroxytoluene BP; Cetostearyl Alcohol BP; Anhydrous Citric Acid PhEur; Methyl Parahydroxybenzoate PhEur; Purified Water PhEur.

*Incompatibilities:* Cetrimide is incompatible with soap and other anionic agents.

*Shelf life:* 4 years.

*Special precautions for storage:* Store below 25°C

*Nature and content of container:* Aluminium tube (50 g); White polypropylene jar (250 g and 500 g)

*Instructions for use/handling:* For topical application only. See also *Special warnings and special precautions for use.*

**Marketing authorisation number** 12619/0055

**Date of approval/revision of spc:** August 1995

**Legal category** GSL.

## SORBICHEW*

**Presentation** Sorbichew tablets contain isosorbide dinitrate.

The chewable tablets are round, green, scored tablets marked 'S' on one face and marked 810 on the reverse, each containing 5 mg isosorbide dinitrate. The inactive ingredients are D & C yellow No. 10, F D & C Blue No. 1, hydrogenated vegetable oil, lime flavour, magnesium stearate, mannitol, povidone, starch, sugar and water.

**Uses** Sorbichew is indicated in the management of angina pectoris to prevent or abort the acute attack.

*Mode of action:* Isosorbide dinitrate acts predominantly as a vasodilator with effects on both veins and arteries.

Following systemic absorption isosorbide dinitrate is metabolised by the liver to isosorbide-2-mononitrate and isosorbide-5-mononitrate. The elimination half-life of isosorbide dinitrate is approximately 0.8 hours. The bioavailability is 22±14% after oral administration because of significant first-pass metabolism. The volume of distribution is 1.5±0.8 l/kg with around 30% binding to plasma proteins. Clearance has been shown to be 45±20 ml/min/kg. Isosorbide-2-mononitrate has a half-life of approximately 2 hours with that of isosorbide-5-mononitrate being 5 hours.

**Dosage and administration** *Adults including the elderly:*

*Treatment of the acute attack:* Either one or two Sorbichew tablets should be chewed until dissolved completely and swallowed.

*Prevention of an expected attack:* Immediately prior to the stressful event either one or two Sorbichew tablets should be chewed until dissolved completely and swallowed.

No dosage reduction is necessary in patients with renal or hepatic impairment.

Sorbichew tablets are scored for easier dose adjustment.

*Children:* The safety and efficacy of Sorbichew in children has not been established.

**Contra-indications, warnings, etc** Sorbichew is contra-indicated in patients with a known sensitivity to the drug or to isosorbide-5-mononitrate and in cases of marked low blood pressure, shock and acute myocardial infarction with low left ventricular filling pressure.

*Pregnancy and lactation:* Animal studies have shown no adverse effects on the foetus, however since its safety and efficacy during pregnancy and lactation have not been established, Sorbichew like other drugs should not be administered to pregnant women and nursing mothers unless considered essential. No data are available on the presence of isosorbide mononitrate in breast milk.

The hypotensive effects of other drugs may be potentiated.

*Side-effects:* A number of nitrate-related adverse effects may occur during treatment, including flushing, headache, dizziness and weakness. The incidence of such effects is normally highest at the commencement of treatment and tends to decline with time. If headache is a problem, a temporary lowering of the dose may be necessary. Nausea and vomiting may occur occasionally. Postural hypotension may occur, especially with high doses. Dry rash and/or exfoliative dermatitis have been described rarely with isosorbide dinitrate and similar reactions might be expected.

*Overdosage:* Overdosage should be treated symptomatically. The main symptom is likely to be hypotension and this may be treated by elevation of the legs to promote venous return. Symptomatic and supportive treatment e.g. plasma expanders and if necessary the careful use of vasopressor agents to counterbalance the hypotensive effects may be necessary. Methaemoglobinaemia will normally respond to methylene blue infusion.

**Pharmaceutical precautions** Store below 25°C, protect from moisture.

**Legal category** P.

**Package quantities** Sorbichew: 5 mg chewable tablets are supplied in containers of 100 (OP).

**Further information** *Effect on ability to drive or operate machinery:* The effect of isosorbide dinitrate upon an individual's performance of skilled and potentially dangerous tasks, such as car driving and the operation of machinery, has not been evaluated. However, there have been no published reports of impaired performance of such tasks.

Unlike glyceryl trinitrate, Sorbichew tablets are stable and therefore loss of potency when carried by the patient does not normally occur.

Sorbichew has an approximate onset of action of two minutes and duration of action up to two hours.

**Product licence number** 12619/0056.

## SORBID*-20 SA

**Qualitative and quantitative composition** Isosorbide Dinitrate 20 mg

**Pharmaceutical form** Sustained release capsules.

**Clinical particulars**
*Therapeutic indications:* Sorbid-20 SA is indicated in the prophylaxis of angina pectoris.

*Posology and method of administration:*
*Adult:* 1 - 2 Sorbid-20 SA capsules should be swallowed twice daily.

Patients already accustomed to prophylactic nitrate therapy may normally be transferred directly to a therapeutic dose of Sorbid-20 SA. For patients not receiving prophylactic nitrate therapy, it is recommended that they are started with a low dose, which should be increased gradually.

No dosage reduction is necessary in patients with renal or hepatic impairment.

The capsules should be swallowed whole with a little fluid.

*Children:* The safety and efficacy of Sorbid-20 SA in children has not been established.

*Elderly patients:* There is no evidence to suggest that an adjustment of dose is necessary. However, caution may be required in elderly patients who are known to be susceptible to the effects of hypotensive medication.

*Contra-indications:* Sorbid-20 SA is contraindicated in patients with a known sensitivity to the drug or to isosorbide 5-mononitrate and in cases of marked low blood pressure, shock and acute myocardial infarction with low left ventricular filling pressure.

*Special warnings and special precautions for use:* Sorbid-20 SA is not indicated for the relief of acute anginal attacks. In the event of an acute attack, sublingual or buccal glyceryl trinitrate or sprays should be used.

*Interactions with other medicaments and other forms of interaction:* The hypotensive effects of other drugs may be potentiated.

Beta-adrenoceptor blocking drugs have a different pharmacological action in angina and may have a complementary effect when administered with Sorbid-20 SA.

*Pregnancy and lactation:* Animal studies have shown no adverse effects on the foetus, however since its safety and efficacy during pregnancy and lactation have not been established, Sorbid-20 SA like other drugs should not be administered to pregnant women and nursing mothers unless considered essential. No data are available on the presence of isosorbide mononitrate in breast milk.

*Effects on ability to drive and use machines:* The effect of isosorbide dinitrate upon an individual's performance of skilled and potentially dangerous tasks, such as car driving and the operation of machinery, has not been evaluated. However, there have been no published reports of impaired performance of such tasks.

*Undesirable effects:* A number of nitrate-related adverse effects may occur during treatment, including flushing, headache, dizziness and weakness. The incidence of such effects is normally highest at the commencement of treatment and tends to decline with time. If headache is a problem, a temporary lowering of the dose may be necessary.

Nausea and vomiting may occur occasionally.

Postural hypotension may occur, especially with high doses.

Dry rash and/or exfoliative dermatitis have been described rarely with isosorbide dinitrate and similar reactions might be expected.

*Overdose:* Overdosage should be treated symptomatically. The stomach should be aspirated to remove any remaining tablets.

The main symptom is likely to be hypotension and this may be treated by elevation of the legs to promote venous return. Symptomatic and supportive treatment e.g. plasma expanders and if necessary the careful use of vasopressor agents to counterbalance the hypotensive effects may be necessary. Methaemoglobinaemia will normally respond to methylene blue infusion.

**Pharmacological properties**
*Pharmacodynamic properties:* Isosorbide dinitrate acts predominantly as a vasodilator with effects on both veins and arteries.

*Pharmacokinetic properties:* Following oral dosing with Sorbid-20 SA, the peak blood level of isosorbide dinitrate is approximately 8 ng/ml. Isosorbide dinitrate is metabolised by the liver to isosorbide 2-mononitrate and isosorbide 5-mononitrate. The corresponding values for the peak blood level of the 2-mononitrate is approximately 25 ng/ml and for the 5-mononitrate 135 ng/ml. The elimination half-life of isosorbide dinitrate is 2 - 3 hours, the half-life of isosorbide 2-mononitrate is 4 - 5 hours and the half-life of isosorbide 5-mononitrate is 5 - 6 hours.

*Preclinical safety data:* Isosorbide dinitrate is a drug on which extensive clinical experience has been obtained. Relevant information for the prescriber is provided elsewhere in the Summary of Product Characteristics.

**Pharmaceutical particulars**
*List of excipients:* Black Iron Oxide (E172); Erythrosine (E127); Gelatin USNF; Maize Starch PhEur; Quinoline Yellow (E104); Shellac USNF; Sucrose PhEur; Ta PhEur.

*Incompatibilities:* Nil.

*Shelf life:* 3 years.

*Special precautions for storage:* Store below 25°C Protect from light and moisture.

*Nature and contents of container:* Blister pack contai ing 56 capsules.

*Instructions for use/handling:* Use as directed by th prescriber.

**Marketing authorisation number** 12619/0057

**Date of approval/revision of SPC** April 1996

**Legal category** P

## SORBID*-40 SA

**Qualitative and quantitative composition** Isosorbic Dinitrate 40 mg

**Pharmaceutical form** Sustained release capsules.

**Clinical particulars**
*Therapeutic Indications:* Sorbid-40 SA is indicated the prophylaxis of angina pectoris.

*Posology and method of administration:*

*Adults:* 1 - 2 Sorbid-40 SA capsules should swallowed twice daily.

Patients already accustomed to prophylactic nitra therapy may normally be transferred directly to therapeutic dose of Sorbid-40 SA. For patients n receiving prophylactic nitrate therapy, it is recor mended that they are started with a low dose, whi should be increased gradually.

No dosage reduction is necessary in patients wi renal or hepatic impairment.

The capsules should be swallowed whole with little fluid.

*Children:* The safety and efficacy of Sorbid-40 SA children has not been established.

*Elderly patients:* There is no evidence to suggest th an adjustment of dose is necessary. However, cauti may be required in elderly patients who are known be susceptible to the effects of hypotensive medic tion.

*Contra-indications:* Sorbid-40 SA is contraindicated patients with a known sensitivity to the drug or isosorbide 5-mononitrate and in cases of marked lo blood pressure, shock and acute myocardial infarcti with low left ventricular filling pressure.

*Special warnings and special precautions for us* Sorbid-40 SA is not indicated for the relief of acu anginal attacks. In the event of an acute attac sublingual or buccal glyceryl trinitrate or spra should be used.

*Interactions with other medicaments and other forr of interaction:* The hypotensive effects of other dru may be potentiated.

Beta-adrenoceptor blocking drugs have a differe pharmacological action in angina and may have complementary effect when administered with S bid-40 SA.

*Pregnancy and lactation:* Animal studies have sho no adverse effects on the foetus, however since safety and efficacy during pregnancy and lactati have not been established, Sorbid-40 SA like oth drugs should not be administered to pregnant wom and nursing mothers unless considered essential. data are available on the presence of isosorbi mononitrate in breast milk.

*Effects on ability to drive and use machines:* The eff of isosorbide dinitrate upon an individual's perfor ance of skilled and potentially dangerous tasks, su as car driving and the operation of machinery, has r been evaluated. However, there have been no pu lished reports of impaired performance of such tas

*Undesirable effects:* A number of nitrate-related verse effects may occur during treatment, includi flushing, headache, dizziness and weakness. T incidence of such effects is normally highest at commencement of treatment and tends to decl with time. If headache is a problem a tempor lowering of the dose may be necessary.

Nausea and vomiting may occur occasionally.

Postural hypotension may occur, especially w high doses.

Dry rash and/or exfoliative dermatitis have be described rarely with isosorbide dinitrate and simi reactions might be expected.

*Overdose:* Overdosage should be treated symptom ically. The stomach should be aspirated to remo any remaining tablets.

The main symptom is likely to be hypotension a this may be treated by elevation of the legs to prom venous return. Symptomatic and supportive tre ment e.g. plasma expanders and if necessary the careful use of vasopressor agents to counterbalance the hypotensive effects may be necessary. Methaemoglobinaemia will normally respond to methylene blue infusion.

### Pharmacological properties

*Pharmacodynamic properties:* Isosorbide dinitrate acts predominantly as a vasodilator with effects on both veins and arteries.

*Pharmacokinetic properties:* Following oral dosing with Sorbid-40 SA, the peak blood level of isosorbide dinitrate is approximately 15 ng/ml. Isosorbide dinitrate is metabolised by the liver to isosorbide 2-mononitrate and isosorbide 5-mononitrate. The corresponding values for the peak blood level of the 2-mononitrate is approximately 45 ng/ml and for the 5-mononitrate 286 ng/ml. The elimination half-life of isosorbide dinitrate is 2 - 3 hours, the half-life of isosorbide 2-mononitrate is 4 - 5 hours and the half-life of isosorbide 5-mononitrate is 5 - 6 hours.

*Preclinical safety data:* Isosorbide dinitrate is a drug on which extensive clinical experience has been obtained. Relevant information for the prescriber is provided elsewhere in the Summary of Product Characteristics.

### Pharmaceutical particulars

*List of excipients:* Black Iron Oxide (E172); Erythrosine (E127); Gelatin USNF; Maize Starch PhEur; Shellac USNF; Sucrose PhEur; Talc PhEur.

*Incompatibilities:* Nil.

*Shelf life:* 3 years.

*Special precautions for storage:* Store below 25°C. Protect from light and moisture.

*Nature and contents of container:* Blister pack containing 56 capsules.

*Instructions for use/handling:* Use as directed by the prescriber.

**Marketing authorisation number** 12619/0058

**Date of approval/revision of spc** April 1996

**Legal category** P

## SORBITRATE*

**Presentation** Sorbitrate tablets contain isosorbide dinitrate. Sorbitrate tablets are available containing 10 mg and 20 mg isosorbide dinitrate. The 10 mg tablets are oval, yellow, scored tablets marked 'S' on one face and marked '780' on the reverse. Inactive ingredients in Sorbitrate Tablets 10 mg are D & C Yellow No. 10, lactose, magnesium stearate, starch, pregelatinised starch and water. The 20 mg tablets are oval, blue, scored tablets marked 'S' on one face and marked '820' on the reverse. Inactive ingredients in Sorbitrate Tablets 20 mg are FD & C Blue No. 1, lactose, magnesium stearate, starch, pregelatinised starch and water.

**Uses** Sorbitrate is indicated for:
a. prophylaxis of angina pectoris
b. congestive cardiac failure – as adjunctive therapy in the management of severe acute or chronic congestive cardiac failure.

*Mode of action:* Isosorbide dinitrate acts predominantly as a vasodilator with effects on both veins and arteries.

Following systemic absorption isosorbide dinitrate is metabolised by the liver to isosorbide-2-mononitrate and isosorbide-5-mononitrate. The elimination half-life of isosorbide dinitrate is approximately 0.8 hours. The bioavailability is 22±14% after oral administration because of significant first-pass metabolism. The volume of distribution is 1.5±0.8 l/kg with around 30% binding to plasma proteins. Clearance has been shown to be 45±20 ml/min/kg. Isosorbide-2-mononitrate has a half-life of approximately 2 hours with that of isosorbide-5-mononitrate being 5 hours.

**Dosage and administration** *Adults:Angina Prophylaxis: 10–40 mg, three to four times daily depending on individual requirement.*

Patients already accustomed to prophylactic nitrate therapy may normally be transferred directly to a therapeutic dose of Sorbitrate. For patients not receiving prophylactic nitrate therapy, it is recommended that they are started with a low dose, which should be increased gradually.

*Congestive Cardiac Failure:* In severe congestive cardiac failure Sorbitrate tablets may be taken in doses of 10–40 mg three to four times daily depending on patient requirements. In this situation optimal individual dose is best determined by continuous haemodynamic monitoring. The use of Sorbitrate in severe congestive cardiac failure should be considered adjunctive therapy to more conventional treatment (e.g. digitalis, diuretics, etc.).

No dosage reduction is necessary in patients with renal or hepatic impairment.

The tablets should be swallowed whole with a little fluid.

*Elderly patients:* There is no evidence to suggest that an adjustment of dose is necessary. However, caution may be required in elderly patients who are known to be susceptible to the effects of hypotensive medication.

*Children:* The safety and efficacy of Sorbitrate in children has not been established.

**Contra-indications, warnings, etc** Sorbitrate is contra-indicated in patients with a known sensitivity to the drug or to isosorbide-5-mononitrate and in cases of marked low blood pressure, shock and acute myocardial infarction with low left ventricular filling pressure.

Sorbitrate is not indicated for the relief of acute anginal attacks. In the event of an acute attack, sublingual or buccal glyceryl trinitrate or sprays should be used.

*Pregnancy and lactation:* Animal studies have shown no adverse effects on the foetus, however, since its safety and efficacy during pregnancy and lactation have not been established, Sorbitrate like other drugs should not be administered to pregnant women and nursing mothers unless considered essential. No data are available on the presence of isosorbide mononitrate in breast milk.

The hypotensive effects of other drugs may be potentiated.

*Side-effects:* A number of nitrate related adverse effects may occur during treatment, including flushing, headache, dizziness and weakness. The incidence of such effects is normally highest at the commencement of treatment and tends to decline with time. If headache is a problem, a temporary lowering of the dose may be necessary. Nausea and vomiting may occur occasionally. Postural hypotension may occur, especially with high doses. Dry rash and/or exfoliative dermatitis have been described rarely with isosorbide dinitrate and similar reactions might be expected.

*Overdosage:* Overdosage should be treated symptomatically. The stomach should be aspirated to remove any remaining tablets. The main symptom is likely to be hypotension and this may be treated by elevation of the patient's legs to promote venous return. Symptomatic and supportive treatment e.g. plasma expanders and if necessary the careful use of vasopressor agents to counterbalance the hypotensive effects may be necessary. Methaemoglobinaemia will normally respond to methylene blue infusion.

**Pharmaceutical precautions** Store below 25°C; protect from moisture.

**Legal category** P.

**Package quantities** Sorbitrate tablets: 20 mg tablets are supplied in containers of 100 (OP).

10 mg tablets are supplied in containers of 100 (OP) and 500.

**Further information** *Effect on ability to drive or operate machinery:* The effect of isosorbide dinitrate upon an individual's performance of skilled and potentially dangerous tasks, such as car driving and the operation of machinery, has not been evaluated. However, there have been no published reports of impaired performance of such tasks.

Unlike glyceryl trinitrate, Sorbitrate tablets are stable and therefore loss of potency when carried by the patient does not normally occur. The duration of action of the tablets is estimated to be four to six hours.

Beta-adrenoceptor blocking drugs have a different pharmacological action in angina and may have a complementary effect when administered with Sorbitrate.

**Product licence numbers**

| | |
|---|---|
| Sorbitrate Tablets 20 mg | 12619/0060 |
| Sorbitrate Tablets 10 mg | 12619/0059 |

## SYNALAR* CREAM
## SYNALAR* OINTMENT

**Presentation** Synalar is presented as a white, water-miscible cream and a greasy ointment. Both preparations contain 0.025% w/w Fluocinolone Acetonide PhEur. The inactive ingredients in Synalar Cream are benzyl alcohol, cetostearyl alcohol, citric acid, liquid paraffin, polysorbate 60, propylene glycol, purified water and sorbitan monostearate. The inactive ingredients in Synalar Ointment are citric acid, lanolin, propylene glycol and white soft paraffin.

**Uses** Synalar Cream and Ointment contain an effective topical steroid and are suitable for treating a wide variety of inflammatory, pruritic and allergic

disorders of the skin. Synalar is particularly suitable for topical application in:

Eczema and dermatitis; atopic eczema, seborrhoeic eczema, discoid eczema, otitis externa, contact dermatitis, neurodermatitis.

Prurigo.

Psoriasis (excluding widespread plaque psoriasis). Lichen planus. Discoid lupus erythematosus.

*Mode of action:* Fluocinolone acetonide is a synthetic anti-inflammatory steroid. Its mechanisms of action are related to vasoconstriction and suppression of membrane permeability, mitotic activity, the immune response and release of inflammatory mediators.

The extent of percutaneous absorption of fluocinolone acetonide is determined by many factors including the vehicle, the integrity of the epidermal barrier and the use of occlusive dressings. Following absorption, fluocinolone acetonide is metabolised primarily in the liver and excreted by the kidneys.

**Dosage and administration** A small quantity of Synalar is applied lightly to the affected area two or three times a day, and massaged gently and thoroughly into the skin. These recommendations apply to both children and adults, including the elderly.

When an occlusive dressing is required, the affected area should first be thoroughly cleansed. Synalar is then applied and covered with a suitable dressing. Occlusion should not be used for children or for the face.

In some cases the application of hot, moist compresses may be an advantage. The cream is particularly suitable for moist or weeping surfaces and for flexures of the body. The ointment is suitable for dry, scaly lesions.

**Contra-indications, warnings, etc** Synalar is contra-indicated in primary infections of the skin caused by bacteria, fungi or viruses and in rosacea, acne, perioral dermatitis, anogenital pruritus and napkin eruption.

Synalar preparations are not advised in the treatment of children under one year of age. The eyes should be avoided.

Long-term continuous topical steroid therapy can produce local atrophic skin changes, and dilatation of the superficial blood vessels particularly when occlusive dressings are used or where skin folds are involved. Prolonged use of topical steroids or treatment of extensive areas, even without occlusion, can result in sufficient absorption of the steroid to produce the features of hypercorticalism and underlying adrenal suppression, especially in infants and children.

It is recommended that treatment on the face and for children should not normally be extended beyond five days, and occlusion in such cases should not be used.

When there is an infection associated with an inflammatory skin condition, Synalar should only be administered if adequate anti-infective cover is given.

When using topical steroids to treat psoriasis there are risks both of rebound relapse following the development of tolerance, and of generalised pustular psoriasis. Impairment of the barrier function of the skin may lead to local and systemic toxicity. Careful patient supervision is important.

Treatment should be discontinued if unfavourable reactions are seen.

*Pregnancy:* There is inadequate evidence of safety in human pregnancy. Topical administration of steroids to pregnant animals can cause abnormalities of foetal development, including cleft palate and intrauterine growth retardation. There may therefore be a very small risk of such effects on the human foetus.

*Lactation:* Topical steroids should not be applied to the breasts prior to nursing. When topical steroid treatment is considered necessary during breast feeding, both the amount applied and the length of treatment should be minimised.

*Side-effects:* With Synalar, side-effects are extremely rare, but, as with all topical steroids, the occasional patient may show an adverse reaction such as hypersensitivity. Irritation at the site of application may occur infrequently. Extensive treatment particularly involving occlusive dressings or where skin folds are involved, can result in both local atrophic changes, such as striae, skin thinning and telangiectasia and systemic effects such as adrenal suppression.

The use of topical steroids on infected lesions, without the addition of appropriate anti-infective therapy, can result in the spread of opportunist infections.

*Accidental ingestion:* The 30 g tube of Synalar contains 7.5 mg of the steroid. No toxic effects are likely to occur even if the full contents of a 30 g tube are ingested. Similarly the ingredients of the base are unlikely to have any toxic effect in the quantities in which they occur. Therefore no remedial action is required in the event of accidental ingestion.

**Pharmaceutical precautions** Store below 25°C.

**Legal category** POM.

**Package quantities** Synalar Cream and Ointment are supplied in tubes of 30 g (OP).

**Further information** *Effect on ability to drive or operate machinery:* No precautions are necessary.

**Product licence numbers**

| | |
|---|---|
| Synalar Cream | 12619/0063 |
| Synalar Ointment | 12619/0069 |

## SYNALAR* CREAM 1 IN 4 DILUTION SYNALAR* OINTMENT 1 IN 4 DILUTION

**Presentation** Synalar Cream 1 in 4 dilution is presented as a white, water-miscible cream. Synalar Ointment 1 in 4 dilution is a greasy ointment. Both contain 0.00625% w/w Fluocinolone Acetonide PhEur. The inactive ingredients of Synalar Ointment 1 in 4 dilution are citric acid, lanolin, propylene glycol and white soft paraffin. The inactive ingredients of Synalar Cream 1 in 4 dilution are benzyl alcohol, cetostearyl alcohol, citric acid, liquid paraffin, polysorbate, propylene glycol, sorbitan monostearate and water.

**Uses** Synalar Cream and Ointment dilutions contain an effective topical steroid and are suitable for treating the milder forms of a wide variety of inflammatory, pruritic and allergic disorders of the skin. Synalar Cream and Ointment dilutions are particularly suitable for topical application in:

Eczema and dermatitis: atopic eczema, seborrhoeic eczema, discoid eczema, otitis externa, contact dermatitis, neurodermatitis.

Prurigo.

Psoriasis (excluding widespread plaque psoriasis).

Lichen planus. Discoid lupus erythematosus.

Synalar Cream and Ointment dilutions are indicated for milder forms of these conditions; for maintenance therapy when control has been achieved with Synalar; for use under occlusive dressings; and for paediatric dermatology, e.g.: infantile eczema.

*Mode of action:* Fluocinolone acetonide is a synthetic anti-inflammatory corticosteroid. Its mechanisms of action are related to vasoconstriction and suppression of membrane permeability, mitotic activity, the immune response and release of inflammatory mediators.

The extent of percutaneous absorption of fluocinolone acetonide is determined by many factors including the vehicle, the integrity of the epidermal barrier and the use of occlusive dressings. Following absorption, fluocinolone acetonide is metabolised primarily in the liver and excreted by the kidneys.

**Dosage and administration** A small quantity of the Synalar Cream or Ointment dilution is applied lightly to the affected area two or three times a day, and massaged gently and thoroughly into the skin. These recommendations apply to both children and adults, including the elderly.

When an occlusive dressing is required, the affected area should first be thoroughly cleansed. Synalar Cream or Ointment dilution is then applied and covered with a suitable dressing. Occlusion should not be used for children or for the face.

The Cream dilution is particularly suitable for moist or weeping surfaces and for flexures of the body. The Ointment dilution is suitable for dry, scaly lesions.

**Contra-indications, warnings, etc** Synalar Cream and Ointment dilutions are contra-indicated in primary infections of the skin caused by bacteria, fungi or viruses and in rosacea, acne, perioral dermatitis, anogenital pruritus and napkin eruption.

Synalar preparations are not advised in the treatment of children under one year of age. The eyes should be avoided.

Long-term continuous topical steroid therapy can produce local atrophic skin changes and dilatation of the superficial blood vessels, particularly when occlusive dressings are used or where skin folds are involved. Prolonged use of topical steroids or treatment of extensive areas, even without occlusion, can result in sufficient absorption of the steroid to produce the features of hypercorticalism and underlying adrenal suppression, especially in infants and children.

It is recommended that treatment on the face and for children should not normally be extended beyond five days, and occlusion in such cases should not be used.

When there is an infection associated with an inflammatory skin condition, Synalar preparations should only be administered if adequate anti-infective cover is given.

When using topical steroids to treat psoriasis there are risks both of rebound relapse following the development of tolerance, and of generalised pustular psoriasis. Impairment of the barrier function of the skin may lead to local and systemic toxicity. Careful patient supervision is important.

Treatment should be discontinued if unfavourable reactions are seen.

*Pregnancy:* There is inadequate evidence of safety in human pregnancy. Topical administration of steroids to pregnant animals can cause abnormalities of foetal development, including cleft palate and intra-uterine growth retardation. There may therefore be a very small risk of such effects on the human foetus.

*Lactation:* Topical steroids should not be applied to the breasts prior to nursing. When topical steroid treatment is considered necessary during breast feeding, both the amount applied and the length of treatment should be minimised.

*Side-effects:* With Synalar preparations, side-effects are extremely rare, but, as with all topical steroids, the occasional patient may show an adverse reaction such as hypersensitivity. Irritation at the site of application may occur infrequently. Extensive treatment particularly involving occlusive dressings or where skin folds are involved, can result in both local atrophic changes, such as striae, skin thinning and telangiectasia, and systemic effects such as adrenal suppression.

The use of topical steroids on infected lesions, without the addition of appropriate anti-infective therapy, can result in the spread of opportunist infections.

*Accidental ingestion:* Toxic effects are not likely to occur following accidental ingestion of the contents of a 50 g tube. If greater quantities are ingested and toxicity develops, symptomatic treatment should be given.

**Pharmaceutical precautions** Store below 25°C.

**Legal category** POM.

**Package quantities** Synalar Cream and Ointment 1 in 4 dilutions are supplied in 50 g tubes (OP).

**Further information** *Effect on ability to drive or operate machinery:* No precautions are necessary.

**Product licence numbers**

| | |
|---|---|
| Synalar Cream 1 in 4 dilution | 12619/0064 |
| Synalar Ointment 1 in 4 dilution | 12619/0070 |

## SYNALAR* CREAM 1 IN 10 DILUTION

**Presentation** Synalar Cream 1 in 10 dilution is presented as a white, water-miscible cream which contains 0.0025% w/w Fluocinolone Acetonide PhEur. The inactive ingredients in Synalar Cream 1 in 10 dilution are benzyl alcohol, cetostearyl alcohol, citric acid, liquid paraffin, polysorbate 60, propylene glycol, purifed water and sorbitan monostearate.

**Uses** Synalar Cream 1 in 10 dilution contains an effective topical steroid and is suitable for treating the milder forms of a wide variety of inflammatory, pruritic and allergic disorders of the skin. Synalar Cream 1 in 10 dilution is particularly suitable for topical application in:

Eczema and dermatitis; atopic eczema, seborrhoeic eczema, discoid eczema, otitis externa, contact dermatitis, neurodermatitis.

Prurigo.

Psoriasis (excluding widespread plaque psoriasis).

Lichen planus. Discoid lupus erythematosus.

Synalar Cream 1 in 10 dilution is indicated for milder forms of these conditions; for maintenance therapy when control has been achieved with Synalar; for use under occlusive dressings; and for paediatric dermatology, e.g. infantile eczema.

*Mode of action:* Fluocinolone acetonide is a synthetic anti-inflammatory corticosteroid. Its mechanisms of action are related to vasoconstriction and suppression of membrane permeability, mitotic activity, the immune response and release of inflammatory mediators.

The extent of percutaneous absorption of fluocinolone acetonide is determined by many factors including the vehicle, the integrity of the epidermal barrier and the use of occlusive dressings. Following absorption, fluocinolone acetonide is metabolised primarily in the liver and excreted by the kidneys.

**Dosage and administration** A small quantity of Synalar Cream 1 in 10 dilution is applied lightly to the affected area two or three times a day, and massaged gently and thoroughly into the skin. These recommendations apply to both children and adults, including the elderly.

When an occlusive dressing is required, the affected area should first be thoroughly cleansed; Synalar Cream 1 in 10 dilution is then applied and covered with a suitable dressing. Synalar Cream 1 in 10 dilution is particularly suitable for moist and weeping surfaces and for flexures of the body.

**Contra-indications, warnings, etc** Synalar Cream 1 in 10 dilution is contra-indicated in primary infections of the skin caused by bacteria, fungi or viruses and in rosacea, acne, perioral dermatitis, anogenital pruritus and napkin eruption.

Synalar preparations are not advised in the treatment of children under one year of age. The eyes should be avoided.

Long-term continuous topical steroid therapy ca produce local atrophic skin changes and dilatation o the superficial blood vessels, particularly when occlu sive dressings are used or where skin folds ar involved. Prolonged use of topical steroids or treat ment of extensive areas, even without occlusion, ca result in sufficient absorption of the steroid to produc the features of hypercorticalism and underlying adre nal suppression, especially in infants and children.

It is recommended that treatment on the face an for children should not normally be extended beyon five days and occlusion in such cases should not b used.

When there is an infection associated with a inflammatory skin condition, Synalar preparation should only be administered if adequate anti-infectiv cover is given.

When using topical steroids to treat psoriasis ther are risks both of rebound relapse following th development of tolerance, and of generalised pustula psoriasis. Impairment of the barrier function of th skin may lead to local and systemic toxicity. Carefu patient supervision is important.

Treatment should be discontinued if unfavourabl reactions are seen.

*Pregnancy:* There is inadequate evidence of safety i human pregnancy. Topical administration of steroid to pregnant animals can cause abnormalities of foeta development, including cleft palate and intra-uterin growth retardation. There may therefore be a ver small risk of such effects on the human foetus.

*Lactation:* Topical steroids should not be applied t the breasts prior to nursing. When topical steroi treatment is considered necessary during breas feeding, both the amount applied and the length c treatment should be minimised.

*Side-effects:* With Synalar preparations, side-effect are extremely rare, but, as with all topical steroid the occasional patient may show an adverse reactio such as hypersensitivity. Irritation at the site c application may occur infrequently. Extensive trea ment particularly involving occlusive dressings o where skin folds are involved, can result in both loca atrophic changes, such as striae, skin thinning an telangiectasia, and systemic effects such as adren suppression.

The use of topical steroids on infected lesion without the addition of appropriate anti-infectiv therapy, can result in the spread of opportunis infections.

*Accidental ingestion:* Toxic effects are not likely t occur following accidental ingestion of the content of a 50 g tube. If greater quantities are ingested an toxicity develops, symptomatic treatment should b given.

**Pharmaceutical precautions** Store below 25°C.

**Legal category** POM.

**Package quantities** Synalar Cream 1 in 10 dilution i supplied in 50 g tubes (OP).

**Further information** *Effect on ability to drive c operate machinery:* No precautions are necessary.

**Product licence number** 12619/0065.

## SYNALAR* GEL

**Presentation** Synalar Gel consists of Fluocinolon Acetonide PhEur 0.025% w/w, presented as a clea water-miscible gel. The inactive ingredients are ca boxypolymethylene, citric acid, disodium edetat industrial methylated spirits, methylparahydroxybe zoate, propylene glycol, propylparahydroxybenzoat purified water and triethanolamine.

**Uses** Synalar Gel is an effective topical stero formulated as a clear, non-greasy gel. It is designe for application to the scalp and other hairy region but can equally well be applied elsewhere on th body. Specific indications for Synalar Gel are sebo rhoea, seborrhoeic dermatitis and psoriasis of th scalp, but it may be applied satisfactorily to inflan matory dermatoses on other parts of the body.

*Mode of action:* Fluocinolone acetonide is a synthet anti-inflammatory corticosteroid. Its mechanisms action are related to vasoconstriction and suppressic of membrane permeability, mitotic activity, the ir mune response and release of inflammatory medi tors.

The extent of percutaneous absorption of fluocin lone acetonide is determined by many factors inclu ing the vehicle, the integrity of the epidermal barri and the use of occlusive dressings. Following absor tion, fluocinolone acetonide is metabolised primari in the liver and excreted by the kidneys.

**Dosage and administration** A small quantity Synalar Gel is massaged into the scalp night ar morning using the finger tips. For maintenance therapy, treatment should be repeated once or twice weekly.

These recommendations apply to both children and adults, including the elderly.

**Contra-indications, warnings, etc** Synalar Gel is contra-indicated in primary infections of the skin caused by bacteria, fungi or viruses and in rosacea, acne, perioral dermatitis, anogenital pruritus and napkin eruption.

Synalar preparations are not advised in the treatment of children under one year of age. The eyes should be avoided.

Long term continuous topical steroid therapy can produce local atrophic skin changes and dilatation of the superficial blood vessels, particularly when occlusive dressings are used or where skin folds are involved. Prolonged use of topical steroids or treatment of extensive areas, even without occlusion, can result in sufficient absorption of the steroid to produce the features of hypercorticalism and underlying adrenal suppression, especially in infants and children.

It is recommended that treatment on the face and for children should not normally be extended beyond five days, and occlusion in such cases should not be used.

When there is an infection associated with an inflammatory skin condition, Synalar preparations should only be administered if adequate anti-infective cover is given.

When using topical steroids to treat psoriasis there are risks both of rebound relapse following the development of tolerance, and of generalised pustular psoriasis. Impairment of the barrier function of the skin may lead to local and systemic toxicity. Careful patient supervision is important.

Treatment should be discontinued if unfavourable reactions are seen.

*Pregnancy:* There is inadequate evidence of safety in human pregnancy. Topical administration of steroids to pregnant animals can cause abnormalities of foetal development, including cleft palate and intrauterine growth retardation. There may therefore be a very small risk of such effects on the human foetus.

*Lactation:* Topical steroids should not be applied to the breasts prior to nursing. When topical steroid treatment is considered necessary during breast feeding, both the amount applied and the length of treatment should be minimised.

*Side-effects:* With Synalar preparations, side-effects are extremely rare, but, as with all topical steroids, the occasional patient may show an adverse reaction such as hypersensitivity. Irritation at the site of application may occur infrequently. Extensive treatment, particularly involving occlusive dressings or where skin folds are involved, can result in both local atrophic changes, such as striae, skin thinning and telangiectasia and systemic effects such as adrenal suppression.

The use of topical steroids on infected lesions, without the addition of appropriate anti-infective therapy, can result in the spread of opportunist infections.

*Accidental ingestion:* The 30 g tube of Synalar Gel contains 7.5 mg of the steroid. No toxic effects are likely to occur, even if the full contents of a 30 g tube are ingested. Similarly the ingredients of the base are unlikely to have any toxic effects in the quantities in which they occur. Therefore no remedial action is required in the event of ingestion.

**Pharmaceutical precautions** Store below 25°C.

**Legal category** POM.

**Package quantities** Synalar Gel is supplied in 30 g tubes (OP).

**Further information** *Effect on ability to drive or operate machinery:* No precautions are necessary.

**Product licence number** 12619/0066.

## SYNALAR* C CREAM AND OINTMENT

**Presentation** These products contain 0.025% w/w of the steroid Fluocinolone Acetonide PhEur and 3% w/w Clioquinol BP (chinoform, iodochlorhydroxyquinoline). Synalar C is presented as an off-white, water-miscible cream and as a greasy ointment. The inactive ingredients of Synalar C Cream are cetostearyl alcohol, citric acid, disodium edetate, liquid paraffin, methylparahydroxybenzoate, polysorbate, propylparahydroxybenzoate, propylene glycol, sorbitan monostearate and water. The inactive ingredients of Synalar C Ointment are citric acid, lanolin, liquid paraffin, propylene glycol and white soft paraffin.

**Uses** Synalar C combines the effective topical steroid Synalar with the effective antibacterial and antifungal agent Clioquinol BP.

It is indicated for inflammatory dermatoses – including eczema, dermatitis, seborrhoea and intertrigo – where secondary bacterial and/or fungal infection is present or is likely to occur.

*Mode of action:* Fluocinolone acetonide is a synthetic anti-inflammatory corticosteroid. Its mechanisms of action are related to vasoconstriction and suppression of membrane permeability, mitotic activity, the immune response and release of inflammatory mediators.

Clioquinol is a broad-spectrum antibacterial and antifungal agent. Its precise mechanism of action is unknown.

The extent of percutaneous absorption of fluocinolone acetonide is determined by many factors including the vehicle, the integrity of the epidermal barrier and the use of occlusive dressings. Following absorption, fluocinolone acetonide is metabolised primarily in the liver and excreted by the kidneys.

A significant amount of clioquinol applied to the skin may be absorbed. Excretion is via the faeces and urine.

**Dosage and administration** A small quantity of the Synalar C preparation is applied lightly to the affected area two or three times a day, and massaged gently and thoroughly into the skin. These recommendations apply to both children and adults, including the elderly.

Treatment should not normally be for longer than seven days and it is preferable to identify the causative organism.

If used in childhood or on the face, courses should be limited to five days, and occlusion should not be used.

If an occlusive dressing is indicated, the affected area is first thoroughly cleansed. The Synalar C preparation is then applied and covered with a suitable dressing. Synalar C Cream is particularly suitable for very inflamed or weeping surfaces and for flexures of the body, whilst Synalar C Ointment is more suitable for dry scaly lesions.

**Contra-indications, warnings, etc** Synalar C preparations are contra-indicated in primary infections of the skin caused by bacteria, fungi or viruses and in rosacea, acne, perioral dermatitis and napkin eruptions.

Synalar C preparations are not advised in the treatment of children under one year of age. The eyes should be avoided.

Long-term continuous topical steroid therapy can produce local atrophic skin changes and dilatation of the superficial blood vessels, particularly when occlusive dressings are used or where skin folds are involved. Prolonged use of topical steroids or treatment of extensive areas, even without occlusion, can result in sufficient absorption of the steroid to produce the features of hypercorticalism and underlying adrenal suppression, especially in infants and children.

In the presence of a viral infection, the use of an appropriate agent should be instituted. If a favourable response does not occur promptly Synalar C should be discontinued until the infection has been adequately controlled.

Treatment should be discontinued if unfavourable reactions are seen. This product should not be used by patients with known iodine-sensitivity.

*Pregnancy:* There is inadequate evidence of safety in human pregnancy. Topical administration of steroids to pregnant animals can cause abnormalities of foetal development, including cleft palate and intra-uterine growth retardation. There may therefore be a very small risk of such effects on the human foetus.

*Lactation:* Topical steroids should not be applied to the breasts prior to nursing. When topical steroid treatment is considered necessary during breast feeding, both the amount applied and the length of treatment should be minimised.

*Side-effects:* With Synalar preparations, side-effects are extremely rare, but, as with all topical steroids, the occasional patient may show an adverse reaction such as hypersensitivity. Irritation at the site of application may occur infrequently. Extensive treatment, particularly involving occlusive dressings or where skin folds are involved, can result in both local atrophic changes, such as striae, skin thinning and telangiectasia and systemic effects such as adrenal suppression.

Local application of clioquinol in creams or ointments may occasionally cause severe irritation, which may be less marked because of the fluocinolone acetonide.

Staining may occur due to breakdown of the clioquinol. A protective covering may be placed over the application to prevent staining of clothing or linen.

*Accidental ingestion:* The 15 g tube of Synalar C contains 3.75 mg of steroid and 0.45 g of Clioquinol BP. No toxic effects are likely to occur, even if the full contents of a tube are ingested. Similarly the ingredients of the base are unlikely to have any toxic effects in the quantities in which they occur. Therefore no remedial action is required in the event of ingestion.

**Pharmaceutical precautions** Store below 25°C.

**Legal category** POM.

**Package quantities** Synalar C Cream and Ointment are available in tubes of 15 g (OP).

**Further information** *Effect on ability to drive or operate machinery:* No precautions are necessary.

**Product licence numbers**

| | |
|---|---|
| Synalar C Ointment | 12619/0062 |
| Synalar C Cream | 12619/0061 |

## SYNALAR* N CREAM

**Qualitative and quantitative composition** Fluocinolone Acetonide PhEur 0.025% w/w and Neomycin Sulphate PhEur 3250 IU/g.

**Pharmaceutical form** Cream.

**Clinical particulars**

*Therapeutic indications:* Synalar N combines the effective topical corticosteroid Synalar with an effective antibacterial agent Neomycin Sulphate PhEur. It is indicated for inflammatory dermatoses including eczema, dermatitis, seborrhoea and intertrigo, where secondary bacterial infection is present or is likely to occur.

*Posology and method of administration*

*Adults (including the elderly) and children:* A small quantity of the Synalar N preparation is applied lightly to the affected area two or three times a day, and massaged gently and thoroughly into the skin. These recommendations apply to both children and adults, including the elderly.

Treatment should not normally be for longer than seven days and it is preferable to identify the causative organism.

It is recommended that treatment on the face and for children should not normally be extended beyond five days and occlusion in such cases should not be used.

If an occlusive dressing is indicated, the affected area is first thoroughly cleansed. The Synalar N preparation is then applied and covered with a suitable dressing.

Synalar N Cream is particularly suitable for very inflamed or weeping surfaces and for flexures of the body.

*Contra-indications:* Synalar N is contra-indicated in primary infections of the skin caused by bacteria, fungi or viruses and in rosacea, acne, perioral dermatitis, and napkin eruption.

Synalar preparations are not advised in the treatment of children under one year of age.

Synalar N is contra-indicated in patients with a history of hypersensitivity to neomycin.

Topical neomycin preparations should not be applied to the external auditory canal of patients with perforated eardrums.

The eyes should be avoided.

*Special warnings and special precautions for use:* Long-term continuous topical steroid therapy can produce local atrophic skin changes and dilatation of the superficial blood vessels, particularly when occlusive dressings are used or where skin folds are involved. Prolonged use of topical steroids or treatment of extensive areas, even without occlusion, can result in sufficient absorption of the steroid to produce the features of hypercorticalism and underlying adrenal suppression, especially in infants and children.

In the presence of a viral or fungal infection, the use of an appropriate agent should be instituted. If a favourable response does not occur promptly, Synalar N should be discontinued until the infection has been adequately controlled.

Because of the potential hazard of nephrotoxicity and ototoxicity associated with neomycin, prolonged use or use of large amounts of the product should be avoided in conditions where absorption of neomycin is possible. Care is particularly needed in elderly or renally-impaired patients.

Not for ophthalmic use.

Treatment should be discontinued if unfavourable reactions are seen.

*Interactions with other medicaments and other forms of interaction:* None known.

*Pregnancy and lactation:*

*Pregnancy:* There is inadequate evidence of safety in human pregnancy. Topical administration of steroids to pregnant animals can cause abnormalities of foetal development, including cleft palate and intra-uterine growth retardation. There may therefore be a very small risk of such effects on the human foetus.

*Lactation:* Topical steroids should not be applied to the breasts prior to nursing. When topical steroid treatment is considered necessary during breast feeding, both the amount applied and the length of treatment should be minimised.

*Effects on ability to drive and use machines:* No precautions are necessary.

*Undesirable effects:* With Synalar preparations, side-effects are extremely rare, but, as with all topical steroids, the occasional patient may show an adverse reaction such as hypersensitivity. Irritation at the site of application may occur infrequently. Extensive treatment, particularly involving occlusive dressings or where skin folds are involved, can result in both local atrophic changes, such as striae, skin thinning and telangiectasia, and systemic effects such as adrenal suppression.

*Overdosage:* Accidental ingestion: The 30 g tube of Synalar N contains 7.5 mg of steroid and 150 mg of neomycin. No toxic effects are likely to occur, even if the full contents of a 30 g tube are ingested. Similarly the ingredients of the base are not likely to have any toxic effects in the quantities in which they occur. Therefore no remedial action is required in the event of ingestion.

**Pharmacological properties**
*Pharmacodynamic properties:* Fluocinolone acetonide is a synthetic anti-inflammatory corticosteroid. Its mechanisms of action are related to vasoconstriction and suppression of membrane permeability, mitotic activity, the immune response and release of inflammatory mediators.

Neomycin sulphate is an aminoglycoside antibacterial agent which inhibits bacterial protein synthesis.

*Pharmacokinetic properties:* The extent of percutaneous absorption of fluocinolone acetonide is determined by many factors including the vehicle, the integrity of the epidermal barrier and the use of occlusive dressings. Following absorption, fluocinolone acetonide is metabolised primarily in the liver and excreted by the kidneys.

Neomycin sulphate is not absorbed through intact skin. It is readily absorbed from large denuded, burned or granulating areas. Excretion is then as unchanged drug.

*Preclinical safety data:* Fluocinolone acetonide and neomycin sulphate are drugs on which extensive clinical experience has been obtained. All relevant information for the prescriber is provided elsewhere in the summary of product characteristics.

**Pharmaceutical particulars**
*List of excipients:* Propylene Glycol PhEur; Cetostearyl Alcohol PhEur; Liquid Paraffin PhEur; Polysorbate 60 PhEur; Sorbitan Monostearate BP; Methyl Parahydroxybenzoate PhEur; Propyl Parahydroxybenzoate PhEur; Purified Water PhEur.

*Incompatibilities:* None known.

*Shelf life:* 3.5 years.

*Special precautions for storage:* Store below 25°C.

*Nature and contents of container:* Collapsible aluminium tubes (30 g).

*Instructions for use/handling:* Not applicable.

**Marketing authorisation number** 12619/0067.

**Date of approval/revision of SPC** September 1995.

**Legal category** POM.

## SYNALAR* N OINTMENT

**Qualitative and quantitative composition** Fluocinolone Acetonide PhEur 0.025% w/w and Neomycin Sulphate PhEur 3250 IU/g.

**Pharmaceutical form** Ointment.

**Clinical particulars**
*Therapeutic indications:* Synalar N combines the effective topical corticosteroid Synalar with an effective antibacterial agent Neomycin Sulphate PhEur.

It is indicated for inflammatory dermatoses – including eczema, dermatitis, seborrhoea and intertrigo where secondary bacterial infection is present or is likely to occur.

*Posology and method of administration:* A small quantity of the Synalar N preparation is applied lightly to the affected area two or three times a day, and massaged gently and thoroughly into the skin. These recommendations apply to both children and adults, including the elderly.

If an occlusive dressing is indicated, the affected area is first thoroughly cleansed. The Synalar N preparation is then applied and covered with a suitable dressing.

Synalar N Cream is particularly suitable for very inflamed or weeping surfaces and for flexures of the body, whilst Synalar N Ointment is more suitable for dry scaly lesions.

Treatment should not normally be for longer than seven days and it is preferable to identify the causative organism.

If used in childhood or on the face, courses should be limited to five days and occlusion in such cases should not be used.

*Contra-indications:* Synalar N preparations are contra-indicated in primary infections of the skin caused by bacteria, fungi or viruses and in rosacea, acne, perioral dermatitis and napkin eruption.

Synalar preparations are not advised in the treatment of children under one year of age. The eyes should be avoided.

Synalar N is contra-indicated in those patients with a history of hypersensitivity to neomycin.

Topical neomycin preparations should not be applied to the external auditory canal of patients with perforated eardrums.

*Special warnings and special precautions for use:* Long-term continuous topical steroid therapy can produce local atrophic skin changes and dilation of the superficial blood vessels, particularly when occlusive dressings are used or where skin folds are involved. Prolonged use of topical steroids or treatment of extensive areas, even without occlusion, can result in sufficient absorption of the steroid to produce the features of hypercorticalism and underlying adrenal suppression, especially in infants and children.

In the presence of a viral or fungal infection, the use of an appropriate agent should be instituted. If a favourable response does not occur promptly, Synalar N should be discontinued until the infection has been adequately controlled.

Because of the potential hazard of nephrotoxicity and ototoxicity associated with neomycin, prolonged use or use of large amounts of the product should be avoided in conditions where absorption of neomycin is possible. Care is particularly needed in elderly or renally-impaired patients.

These preparations are not for ophthalmic use.

Treatment should be discontinued if unfavourable reactions are seen.

*Pregnancy and lactation*

Pregnancy: There is inadequate evidence of safety in human pregnancy. Topical administration of steroids to pregnant animals can cause abnormalities of foetal development, including cleft palate and intra-uterine growth retardation. There may therefore be a very small risk of such effects on the human foetus.

*Lactation:* Topical steroids should not be applied to the breasts prior to nursing. When topical steroid treatment is considered necessary during breast feeding, both the amount applied and the length of treatment should be minimised.

*Effects on ability to drive and use machines:* No precautions are necessary.

*Undesirable effects:* With Synalar preparations, side-effects are extremely rare, but, as with all topical steroids, the occasional patient may show an adverse reaction such as hypersensitivity. Irritation at the site of application may occur infrequently. Extensive treatment, particularly involving occlusive dressings or where skin folds are involved, can result in both local atrophic changes, such as striae, skin thinning and telangiectasia, and systemic effects such as adrenal suppression.

*Overdosage: Accidental ingestion:* The 30 g tube of Synalar N contains 7.5 mg of steroid and 150 mg of neomycin. No toxic effects are likely to occur, even if the full contents of a 30 g tube are ingested. Similarly the ingredients of the base are not likely to have any toxic effects in the quantities in which they occur. Therefore no remedial action is required in the event of ingestion.

**Pharmacological properties**
*Pharmacodynamic properties:* Fluocinolone acetonide is a synthetic anti-inflammatory corticosteroid. Its mechanisms of action are related to vasoconstriction and suppression of membrane permeability, mitotic activity, the immune response and release of inflammatory mediators.

Neomycin sulphate is an aminoglycoside antibacterial agent which inhibits bacterial protein synthesis.

*Pharmacokinetic properties:* The extent of percutaneous fluocinolone acetonide is determined by many factors including the vehicle, the integrity of the epidermal barrier and the use of occlusive dressings. Following absorption, fluocinolone acetonide is metabolised primarily in the liver and excreted by the kidneys.

Neomycin is not absorbed through intact skin. It is readily absorbed from large denuded, burned or granulating areas. Excretion is then as unchanged drug.

**Pharmaceutical particulars**
*List of excipients:* Propylene Glycol PhEur; Lanolin; Liquid Paraffin PhEur; White Soft Paraffin BP.

*Incompatibilities:* None known.

*Shelf life:* 42 months.

*Special precautions for storage:* Store below 25°C.

*Nature and contents of container:* Unlacquered, late banded collapsible aluminium tubes (30 g).

**Marketing authorisation number** 12619/0068.

**Date of approval/revision of SPC** September 1995

**Legal category** POM.

## TENIF*

**Presentation** Tenif is presented as reddish brow capsules bearing the name Tenif and an 'S' logo. Eac capsule contains Atenolol PhEur 50 mg and a su tained release formulation of nifedipine 20 mg. Th inactive ingredients are gelatin, iron oxide, lactos macrogol, magnesium carbonate, magnesium ste rate, maize starch, methylhydroxypropylcellulose, m crocrystalline cellulose, polysorbate, sodium laur sulphate and titanium dioxide.

**Uses** Management of hypertension where therap with either a calcium channel blocker or a bet adrenoceptor blocking drug proves inadequate.

Management of chronic stable angina pecto where therapy with either a calcium channel block or a beta-adrenoceptor blocking drug proves inad quate.

*Mode of action:* Atenolol is a beta-adrenocept blocking drug which is beta$_1$-selective (i.e. acts pre erentially on beta$_1$-adrenergic receptors in the hea Selectivity decreases with increasing dose. Atenol is without intrinsic sympathomimetic and membra stabilising activities, and, as with other beta-adren ceptor blocking drugs, has negative inotropic effec (and is therefore contra-indicated in uncontroll heart failure). As with other beta-adrenoceptor bloc ing drugs, its mode of action in the treatment hypertension is unclear. It is probably the action atenolol in reducing cardiac rate and contractil which makes it effective in eliminating or reducing th symptoms of patients with angina. It is unlikely th any additional ancillary properties possessed by S ( atenolol, in comparison with the racemic mixture, w give rise to different therapeutic effects.

Atenolol is effective and well tolerated in mo ethnic populations although the response may be le in black patients.

Nifedipine is a calcium channel blocker. It is powerful coronary and peripheral vasodilator whi increases myocardial oxygen supply and reduc blood pressure (afterload) and peripheral resistanc Concomitant use of beta$_1$-adrenergic blockade the fore, ameliorates the reflex sympathetic response nifedipine monotherapy by blocking the rise in he rate, while atenolol's tendency to increase periphe resistance is balanced by the vasodilatation a increased sympathetic tone induced by the calciu antagonist. Consequently, greater antihypertensive antianginal efficacy is achieved by the concomita use of nifedipine and atenolol than either drug alo This beneficial pharmacodynamic interaction a results in fewer side effects when lower dosages the two drugs are used in combination.

Absorption of atenolol following oral dosing consistent but incomplete (approximately 40–50 with peak plasma concentrations occurring 2–4 hou after dosing. Atenolol blood levels are consistent a subject to little variability. There is no significa hepatic metabolism of atenolol and more than 90% that absorbed reaches the systemic circulation un tered. The plasma half-life is about 6 hours but t may rise in severe renal impairment since the kidn is the major route of elimination. Atenolol penetra tissues poorly due to its low lipid solubility and concentration in brain tissue is low. Plasma prote binding is low (approximately 3%).

Absorption of nifedipine following oral dosing complete with peak plasma concentrations occurri about every 3 hours after dosing. Nifedipine is > 9 plasma protein bound. There is significant hepa metabolism of nifedipine. The plasma half-life between 6 and 11 hours for the sustained formulati of nifedipine.

Co-administration of atenolol and nifedipine h little effect on the pharmacokinetics of either. In t elderly, the systemic bioavailability and eliminat half-life of both components are increased.

**Dosage and administration**
*Adults: Hypertension:* One capsule daily swallow with water. If necessary, the dosage may be increas to one capsule dosed every 12 hours. Patients can transferred to the combination from other antihyp tensive treatments with the exception of clonid (see 'Precautions' below).

*Angina:* One capsule every 12 hours swallowed w water. Where additional efficacy is necessary, prop lactic nitrate therapy or additional nifedipine may of benefit.

*Elderly patients:* Dosage should not exceed one capsule daily in hypertension or one capsule twice daily in angina.

The pharmacokinetics of nifedipine are altered in the elderly so that lower maintenance doses of nifedipine may be required compared to younger patients.

*Children:* There is no paediatric experience with Tenif and therefore Tenif should not be used in children.

**Contra-indications, warnings, etc** Tenif should not be used in patients with any of the following conditions: known hypersensitivity to either component or other dihydropyridines because of the theoretical risk of cross-reactivity; bradycardia; cardiogenic shock; hypotension; metabolic acidosis; severe peripheral arterial circulatory disturbances; second or third degree heart block; sick sinus syndrome; untreated phaeochromocytoma; uncontrolled heart failure; women capable of childbearing or during pregnancy or during lactation; patients with clinically significant aortic stenosis; patients with marked renal impairment i.e. creatinine clearance below 15 ml/min/1.73 m²; serum creatinine greater than 600 micromol/litre); patients receiving calcium channel blockers with negative inotropic effects e.g. verapamil and diltiazem; unstable angina; or during or within one month of a myocardial infarction.

Tenif should not be used for the treatment of acute attacks of angina.

The safety of Tenif in malignant hypertension has not been established.

Tenif should not be used for secondary prevention of myocardial infarction.

Tenif should not be administered concomitantly with rifampicin since effective plasma levels of nifedipine may not be achieved owing to enzyme induction.

Due to its beta-adrenoceptor blocking drug component, Tenif:

- although contra-indicated in uncontrolled heart failure (see *Contra-indications*), may be used in patients whose signs of heart failure have been controlled. Caution must be exercised in patients whose cardiac reserve is poor.
- may increase the number and duration of angina attacks in patients with Prinzmetal's angina due to unopposed alpha receptor mediated coronary artery vasoconstriction. Atenolol is a $beta_1$-selective beta-adrenoceptor blocking drug; consequently, the use of Tenif may be considered although utmost caution must be exercised.
- although contra-indicated in severe peripheral arterial circulatory disturbances (see *Contra-indications*), may also aggravate less severe peripheral arterial circulatory disturbances.
- due to its negative effect on conduction time, caution must be exercised if it is given to patients with first degree heart block.
- may modify the tachycardia of hypoglycaemia.
- may mask the signs of thyrotoxicosis.
- will reduce heart rate, as a result of its pharmacological action. In the rare instances when a treated patient develops symptoms which may be attributable to a slow heart rate, the dose may be reduced.
- should not be discontinued abruptly in patients suffering from ischaemic heart disease.
- may cause a more severe reaction to a variety of allergens, when given to patients with a history of anaphylactic reaction to such allergens. Such patients may be unresponsive to the usual doses of adrenaline used to treat the allergic reactions.

Tenif contains the cardioselective beta-adrenoceptor blocking drug atenolol. Although cardioselective ($beta_1$) beta-adrenoceptor blocking drugs may have less effect on lung function than non-selective beta-adrenoceptor blocking drugs, as with all beta-adrenoceptor blocking drugs, these should be avoided in patients with reversible obstructive airways disease, unless there are compelling clinical reasons for their use. Where such reasons exist, Tenif may be used with caution. Occasionally, some increase in airways resistance may occur in asthmatic patients, however, and this may usually be reversed by commonly used dosage of bronchodilators such as salbutamol or isoprenaline.

The label and patient information leaflet for this product state the following warning: "If you have ever had asthma or wheezing, you should not take this medicine unless you have discussed these symptoms with the prescribing doctor".

Due to its nifedipine component it should be noted that:

- in rare cases, a transient increase in blood glucose has been observed with nifedipine in acute studies. This should be considered in patients suffering from diabetes mellitus. Nifedipine has no diabetogenic effect.
- ischaemic pain occurs in a small proportion of patients following introduction of nifedipine monotherapy. Although a 'steal' effect has not been demonstrated, patients experiencing this effect should discontinue nifedipine therapy.

Hypertensive or anginal patients with clinically significant liver disease have not been studied and no dosage adjustment is suggested from the systemic availability of the monocomponents in patients with cirrhosis. However nifedipine is metabolised primarily by the liver and therefore patients with liver dysfunction should be carefully monitored. As a precaution, it is recommended that the dose should not exceed one capsule daily.

Tenif must not be used in conjunction with calcium channel blockers with negative inotropic effects, e.g. verapamil, diltiazem since this can lead to an exaggeration of these effects particularly in patients with impaired ventricular function and/or sino-atrial or atrio-ventricular conduction abnormalities. This may result in severe hypotension, bradycardia and cardiac failure (see *Contra-indications*).

Concomitant therapy with additional dihydropyridines e.g. nifedipine, may increase the risk of hypotension, and cardiac failure may occur in patients with latent cardiac insufficiency.

*Atenolol monotherapy:* Digitalis glycosides, in association with beta-adrenoceptor blocking drugs, may increase atrio-ventricular conduction time.

Beta-adrenoceptor blocking drugs may exacerbate the rebound hypertension which can follow the withdrawal of clonidine. If the two drugs are co-administered, the beta-adrenoceptor blocking drug should be withdrawn several days before discontinuing clonidine. If replacing clonidine by beta-adrenoceptor blocking drug therapy, the introduction of beta-adrenoceptor blocking drugs should be delayed for several days after clonidine administration has stopped.

Caution must be exercised when prescribing a beta-adrenoceptor blocking drug with Class 1 antiarrhythmic agents such as disopyramide.

Concomitant use of sympathomimetic agents, e.g. adrenaline, may counteract the effect of beta-adrenoceptor blocking drugs.

Concomitant use with insulin and oral antidiabetic drugs may lead to the intensification of the blood sugar lowering effects of these drugs.

Concomitant use of prostaglandin synthetase inhibiting drugs, e.g. ibuprofen or indomethacin, may decrease the hypotensive effects of beta-adrenoceptor blocking drugs.

*Anaesthesia:* Caution must be exercised when using anaesthetic agents with Tenif. The anaesthetist should be informed and the choice of anaesthetic should be the agent with as little negative inotropic activity as possible. Use of beta-adrenoceptor blocking drugs with anaesthetic drugs may result in attenuation of the reflex tachycardia and increase the risk of hypotension. Anaesthetic agents causing myocardial depression are best avoided.

*Nifedipine monotherapy:* The antihypertensive effect of nifedipine can be potentiated by simultaneous administration of cimetidine.

The simultaneous administration of nifedipine and quinidine may lead to serum quinidine levels being suppressed regardless of dosage of quinidine.

The simultaneous administration of nifedipine and digoxin may lead to reduced digoxin clearance and hence an increase in the plasma digoxin level. Patients' plasma digoxin levels should be monitored and, if necessary, the digoxin dose reduced.

As with other dihydropyridines, nifedipine should not be taken with grapefruit juice because bioavailability is increased.

Nifedipine should not be administered concomitantly with rifampicin since effective plasma levels of nifedipine may not be achieved owing to enzyme induction.

*Pregnancy and lactation:* Tenif is contra-indicated in women capable of childbearing or during pregnancy or during lactation (see *Contra-indications*).

*Effect on ability to drive or operate machinery:* The use of Tenif is unlikely to result in any impairment of the ability of patients to drive or operate machinery. However, it should be taken into account that occasionally dizziness or fatigue may occur.

*Undesirable events:* Tenif is well tolerated. In clinical studies, the undesired events reported are usually attributed to the pharmacological actions of its components.

The following undesired events, listed by body system, have been reported:

*Tenif*

Cardiovascular: flushing, oedema.

CNS: dizziness, headache.

Gastrointestinal: gastrointestinal disturbance.

Others: fatigue.

*Atenolol monotherapy*

Cardiovascular: bradycardia, heart failure deterioration, postural hypotension which may be associated with syncope, cold extremities. In susceptible patients: precipitation of heart block, intermittent claudication, Raynaud's phenomenon.

CNS: confusion, mood changes, nightmares, psychoses and hallucinations, sleep disturbances of the type noted with other beta-blockers.

Gastrointestinal: dry mouth.

Haematological: purpura, thrombocytopenia.

Integumentary: alopecia, dry eyes, psoriasiform skin reactions, exacerbation of psoriasis, skin rashes.

Neurological: paraesthesia.

Respiratory: bronchospasm may occur in patients with bronchial asthma or a history of asthmatic complaints.

Special senses: visual disturbances.

Others: an increase in ANA (antinuclear antibodies) has been observed, however the clinical relevance of this is not clear.

*Nifedipine monotherapy*

Cardiovascular: palpitations, tachycardia, gravitational oedema, marked reduction in blood pressure in dialysis patients with malignant hypertension and hypovolaemia.

Neurological: paraesthesia.

Gastrointestinal: gingival hyperplasia, hypersensitivity type jaundice and disturbances of liver function such as increased transaminase or intra-hepatic cholestasis which regress after discontinuing therapy.

Integumentary: skin reactions such as pruritus, urticaria, exanthema and exfoliative dermatitis.

Musculoskeletal: myalgia, tremor (both after high doses).

Urogenital: increased frequency of micturition, gynaecomastia (in older men on long term therapy, which usually regresses on withdrawal of therapy).

As with other sustained release dihydropyridines, exacerbation of angina pectoris may occur rarely at the start of treatment with sustained release formulations of nifedipine. The occurrence of myocardial infarction has been described although it is not possible to distinguish such an event from the natural course of ischaemic heart disease.

Discontinuance of Tenif should be considered if, according to clinical judgement, the well-being of the patient is adversely affected by any of the above reactions.

*Overdosage:* The symptoms of overdosage may include bradycardia, hypotension, acute cardiac insufficiency and bronchospasm.

General treatment should include: close supervision, treatment in an intensive care ward, the use of gastric lavage, activated charcoal and a laxative to prevent absorption of any drug still present in the gastrointestinal tract, the use of plasma or plasma substitutes to treat hypotension and shock. The possible use of haemodialysis or haemoperfusion may be considered.

Excessive bradycardia can be countered with atropine 1–2 mg intravenously and/or a cardiac pacemaker. If necessary, this may be followed by a bolus dose of glucagon 10 mg intravenously. If required, this may be repeated or followed by an intravenous infusion of glucagon 1–10 mg/hour depending on response. Intravenous calcium gluconate combined with metaraminol may be beneficial for hypotension induced by nifedipine. If no response to glucagon occurs or if glucagon is unavailable, a beta-adrenoceptor stimulant such as dobutamine 2.5 to 10 micrograms/kg/minute by intravenous infusion may be given. Dobutamine, because of its positive inotropic effect could also be used to treat hypotension and acute cardiac insufficiency. It is likely that these doses would be inadequate to reverse the cardiac effects of beta-blockade if a large overdose has been taken. The dose of dobutamine should therefore be increased if necessary to achieve the required response according to the clinical condition of the patient.

In severe cases of hypotension cardiac pacing with appropriate cardiorespiratory support may be necessary.

Bronchospasm can usually be reversed by bronchodilators.

**Pharmaceutical precautions** Tenif capsules should be stored below 30°C, protected from light and moisture.

**Legal category** POM.

**Package quantities** Calendar packs of 28 capsules (OP).

**Further information** When the combined antihypertensive effect or antianginal effect of a beta-adrenoceptor blocking drug and calcium antagonist is required, Tenif is a convenient and acceptable therapy. The combination of atenolol and the slow release formulation of nifedipine, given once daily, provides control of raised blood pressure over a 24 hour period and may be expected to improve patient compliance. Given twice daily the combination provides control of angina.

**Product licence number** 12619/0071.

# TENORETIC*

**Qualitative and quantitative composition** Atenolol PhEur 100 mg, Chlorthalidone PhEur 25 mg

**Pharmaceutical form** Brown film coated tablets.

**Clinical particulars**

*Therapeutic indications:* Management of hypertension.

*Posology and method of administration:*
*Adults:* One tablet daily. Most patients with hypertension will give a satisfactory response to a single tablet daily of Tenoretic. There is little or no further fall in blood pressure with increased dosage and, where necessary, another antihypertensive drug, such as a vasodilator, can be added.

*Elderly:* Dosage requirements are often lower in this age group.

*Children:* There is no paediatric experience with Tenoretic, therefore this preparation is not recommended for children.

*Renal impairment:* In patients with severe renal impairment, a reduction in the daily dose or in frequency of administration may be necessary.

*Contra-indications:* Tenoretic should not be used in patients with any of the following: known hypersensitivity to either component; bradycardia; cardiogenic shock; hypotension; metabolic acidosis; severe peripheral arterial circulatory disturbances; second or third degree heart block; sick sinus syndrome; untreated phaeochromocytoma; uncontrolled heart failure.

Tenoretic must not be given during pregnancy or lactation.

*Special warnings and special precautions for use:* Due to its beta-adrenoceptor blocking drug component Tenoretic:

- although contra-indicated in uncontrolled heart failure (see *Contra-indications*) may be used in patients whose signs of heart failure have been controlled. Caution must be exercised in patients whose cardiac reserve is poor.
- may increase the number and duration of angina attacks in patients with Prinzmetal's angina due to unopposed alpha receptor mediated coronary artery vasoconstriction. Atenolol is a beta$_1$-selective beta-adrenoceptor blocking drug; consequently the use of Tenoretic may be considered although utmost caution must be exercised.
- although contraindicated in severe peripheral arterial circulatory disturbances (see *Contra-indications*) may also aggravate less severe peripheral arterial circulatory disturbances.
- due to its negative effect on conduction time, caution must be exercised if it is given to patients with first degree heart block.
- may modify the tachycardia of hypoglycaemia.
- may mask the signs of thyrotoxicosis.
- will reduce heart rate, as a result of its pharmacological action. In the rare instances when a treated patient develops symptoms which may be attributable to a slow heart rate, the dose may be reduced.
- should not be discontinued abruptly in patients suffering from ischaemic heart disease.
- may cause a more severe reaction to a variety of allergens, when given to patients with a history of anaphylactic reaction to such allergens. Such patients may be unresponsive to the usual doses of adrenaline used to treat the allergic reactions.

Tenoretic contains the cardioselective beta adrenoceptor blocking drug atenolol. Although cardioselective (beta$_1$) beta-adrenoceptor blocking drugs may have less effect on lung function than non-selective beta-adrenoceptor blocking drugs, as with all beta-adrenoceptor blocking drugs, these should be avoided in patients with reversible obstructive airways disease, unless there are compelling clinical reasons for their use. Where such reasons exist, Tenoretic may be used with caution. Occasionally, some increase in airways resistance may occur in asthmatic patients, however, and this may usually be reversed by commonly used dosage of bronchodilators such as salbutamol or isoprenaline.

The label and patient information leaflet for this product state the following warning: "If you have ever had asthma or wheezing, you should not take this medicine unless you have discussed these symptoms with the prescribing doctor".

Due to its chlorthalidone component:

- hypokalaemia may occur. Measurement of potassium levels is appropriate, especially in the older patient, those receiving digitalis preparations for cardiac failure, those taking an abnormal (low in potassium) diet or those suffering from gastrointestinal complaints. Hypokalaemia may predispose to arrhythmias in patients receiving digitalis.
- caution must be exercised in patients with severe renal failure (see *Posology and method of administration*).
- impaired glucose tolerance may occur and caution must be exercised if chlorthalidone is administered to patients with a known pre-disposition to diabetes mellitus.
- hyperuricaemia may occur. Only a minor increase in serum uric acid usually occurs but in cases of prolonged elevation, the concurrent use of a uricosuric agent will reverse the hyperuricaemia.

*Interactions with other medicaments and other forms of interaction:* Combined use of beta-adrenoceptor blocking drugs and calcium channel blockers with negative inotropic effects eg verapamil, diltiazem, can lead to an exaggeration of these effects particularly in patients with impaired ventricular function and/or sino-atrial or atrio-ventricular conduction abnormalities. This may result in severe hypotension, bradycardia and cardiac failure. Neither the beta-adrenoceptor blocking drug nor the calcium channel blocker should be administered intravenously within 48 hours of discontinuing the other.

Concomitant therapy with dihydropyridines eg nifedipine, may increase the risk of hypotension, and cardiac failure may occur in patients with latent cardiac insufficiency.

Digitalis glycosides, in association with beta-adrenoceptor blocking drugs, may increase atrio-ventricular conduction time.

Beta-adrenoceptor blocking drugs may exacerbate the rebound hypertension which can follow the withdrawal of clonidine. If the two drugs are co-administered, the beta-adrenoceptor blocking drug should be withdrawn several days before discontinuing clonidine. If replacing clonidine by beta-adrenoceptor blocking drug therapy, the introduction of beta-adrenoceptor blocking drugs should be delayed for several days after clonidine administration has stopped.

Caution must be exercised when prescribing a beta-adrenoceptor blocking drug with Class 1 antiarrhythmic agents such as disopyramide.

Concomitant use of sympathomimetic agents, eg adrenaline, may counteract the effect of beta-adrenoceptor blocking drugs.

Concomitant use with insulin and oral antidiabetic drugs may lead to the intensification of the blood sugar lowering effects of these drugs.

Concomitant use of prostaglandin synthetase inhibiting drugs (eg ibuprofen, indomethacin) may decrease the hypotensive effects of beta-adrenoceptor blocking drugs.

Preparations containing lithium should not be given with diuretics because they may reduce its renal clearance.

Caution must be exercised when using anaesthetic agents with Tenoretic. The anaesthetist should be informed and the choice of anaesthetic should be an agent with as little negative inotropic activity as possible. Use of beta-adrenoceptor blocking drugs with anaesthetic drugs may result in attenuation of the reflex tachycardia and increase the risk of hypotension. Anaesthetic agents causing myocardial depression are best avoided.

*Pregnancy and lactation:*

*Pregnancy:* Tenoretic must not be given during pregnancy.

*Lactation:* Tenoretic must not be given during lactation.

*Effects on ability to drive and use machines:* Use is unlikely to result in any impairment of the ability of patients to drive or operate machinery. However, it should be taken into account that occasionally dizziness or fatigue may occur.

*Undesirable effects:* Tenoretic is well tolerated. In clinical studies, the undesired events reported are usually attributable to the pharmacological actions of its components.

The following undesired events, listed by body system, have been reported with Tenoretic or either of its components:

Biochemical: hyperuricaemia, hypokalaemia, impaired glucose tolerance (see *Special warnings and special precautions for use*).

Cardiovascular: bradycardia; heart failure deterioration; postural hypotension which may be associated with syncope; cold extremities. In susceptible patients: precipitation of heart block; intermittent claudication; Raynaud's phenomenon.

CNS: confusion; dizziness; headache; mood changes; nightmares; psychoses and hallucinations; sleep disturbances of the type noted with other beta-adrenoceptor blocking drugs.

Gastrointestinal: dry mouth, gastrointestinal disturbances; nausea.

Haematological: leucopenia; purpura; thrombocytopenia.

Integumentary: alopecia; dry eyes; psoriasiform skin reactions; exacerbation of psoriasis; skin rashes.

Neurological: paraesthesia.

Respiratory: bronchospasm may occur in patient with bronchial asthma or a history of asthmati complaints.

Special senses: visual disturbances.

Others: fatigue; an increase in ANA (Antinuclea Antibodies) has been observed, however the clinica relevance of this is not clear.

Discontinuance of Tenoretic should be considere if, according to clinical judgement, the well-being c the patient is adversely affected by any of the abov reactions.

*Overdose:* The symptoms of overdosage may includ bradycardia, hypotension, acute cardiac insufficienc and bronchospasm.

General treatment should include: close superv sion, treatment in an intensive care ward, the use c gastric lavage, activated charcoal and a laxative t prevent absorption of any drug still present in th gastrointestinal tract, the use of plasma or plasm substitutes to treat hypotension and shock. Th possible use of haemodialysis or haemoperfusio may be considered.

Excessive bradycardia may be countered wit atropine 1-2 mg intravenously and/or a cardiac pac maker. If necessary, this may be followed by a bolu dose of glucagon 10 mg intravenously. If require this may be repeated or followed by an intravenou infusion of glucagon 1-10 mg/hour depending o response. If no response to glucagon occurs or glucagon is unavailable, a beta-adrenoceptor stim lant such as dobutamine 2.5 to 10 micrograms/k minute by intravenous infusion may be given. Dob tamine, because of its positive inotropic effects cou be used to treat hypotension and acute cardia insufficiency. It is likely that these doses would b inadequate to reverse the cardiac effects of bet adrenoceptor blockade if a large overdose has bee taken. The dose of dobutamine should therefore b increased if necessary to achieve the required r sponse according to the clinical condition of th patient.

Bronchospasm can usually be reversed by bro chodilators.

Excessive diuresis should be countered by mai taining normal fluid and electolyte balance.

**Pharmacological properties**

*Pharmacodynamic properties:* Tenoretic combine the antihypertensive activity of two agents, a bet adrenoceptor blocking drug (atenolol) and a diuret (chlorthalidone).

Atenolol is beta$_1$-selective (ie acts preferentially c beta$_1$-adrenergic receptors in the heart). Selectivi decreases with increasing dose.

Atenolol is without intrinsic sympathomimetic an membrane stabilising activities and, as with oth beta-adrenoceptor blocking drugs, has negative in tropic effects (and is therefore contraindicated uncontrolled heart failure).

As with other beta-adrenoceptor blocking drug the mode of action of atenolol in the treatment hypertension is unclear.

It is unlikely that any additional ancillary properti possessed by S (–) atenolol, in comparison with th racemic mixture, will give rise to different therapeut effects.

Chlorthalidone, a monosulfonamyl diuretic, i creases excretion of sodium and chloride. Natriures is accompanied by some loss of potassium. Th mechanism by which chlorthalidone reduces bloc pressure is not fully known but may be related to th excretion and redistribution of body sodium.

Atenolol is effective and well-tolerated in mo ethnic populations. Black patients respond better the combination of atenolol and chlorthalidone, th to atenolol alone.

The combination of atenolol with thiazide-like di retics has been shown to be compatible and genera more effective than either drug used alone.

*Pharmacokinetic properties:* Absorption of ateno following oral dosing is consistent but incomple (approximately 40-50%) with peak plasma concentr tions occurring 2-4 hours after dosing. The ateno blood levels are consistent and subject to lit variability. There is no significant hepatic metabolis of atenolol and more than 90% of that absorb reaches the systemic circulation unaltered. T plasma half-life is about 6 hours but this may rise severe renal impairment since the kidney is the maj route of elimination. Atenolol penetrates tissu poorly due to its low lipid solubility and its concentr tion in brain tissue is low. Plasma protein binding low (approximately 3%).

Absorption of chlorthalidone following oral dosi is consistent but incomplete (approximately 60%) wi peak plasma concentrations occuring about 12 hou after dosing. The chlorthalidone blood levels a consistent and subject to little variability. The plasn half-life is about 50 hours and the kidney is the maj oute of elimination. Plasma protein binding is high pproximately 75%).

Co-administration of chlorthalidone and atenolol as little effect on the pharmacokinetics of either.

Tenoretic is effective for at least 24 hours after a ngle oral daily dose. This simplicity of dosing acilitates compliance by its acceptability to patients.

*reclinical safety data:* Atenolol and Chlorthalidone re drugs on which extensive clinical experience has een obtained. Relevant information for the prescriber provided elsewhere in the Summary of Product haracteristics.

**harmaceutical particulars**

*ist of excipients:* Heavy Magnesium Carbonate hEur; Maize Starch PhEur; Sodium Lauryl Sulphate hEur; Gelatin PhEur; Magnesium Stearate PhEur; lethylhydroxypropylcellulose PhEur; Macrogol 300 P; Iron Oxide yellow E172; Iron Oxide red E172; lagnesium Carbonate PhEur.

*compatibilities:* None known.

*helf life:* 4 years.

*pecial precautions for storage:* Store below 25°C. rotect from light and moisture.

*ature and contents of container:* Calendar packs of 3 tablets.

*structions for use/handling:* Use as directed by the rescriber.

**larket authorisation number** 12619/0073

**ate of approval/revision of SPC** February 1997.

**egal category** POM

## ENORET* 50

**resentation** Tenoret 50 tablets are round, bi-onvex, brown, film-coated tablets impressed TEN-RET 50 on one face and with an 'S' logo on the everse. The impressions are highlighted in white. ach tablet contains 50 mg Atenolol PhEur and 2.5 mg Chlorthalidone PhEur. The inactive ingredi-nts are gelatin, iron oxide, macrogol, magnesium arbonate, magnesium stearate, methylhydroxypro-ylcellulose, sodium lauryl sulphate and maize starch.

**ses** *Hypertension:* Particularly suited to the older atient. The combination of low effective doses of a eta-adrenoceptor blocking drug and diuretic may be uited to older patients where full doses of both may e considered inappropriate.

*lode of action:* Tenoret 50 combines the antihyper-nsive activity of two agents, a beta-adrenoceptor locking drug (atenolol) and a diuretic (chlorthali-one).

Atenolol is beta$_1$-selective (i.e. acts preferentially on eta$_1$-adrenergic receptors in the heart). Selectivity ecreases with increasing dose. Atenolol is without trinsic sympathomimetic and membrane stabilising ctivities and, as with other beta-adrenoceptor block-g drugs, has negative inotropic effects (and is erefore contra-indicated in uncontrolled heart fail-e). As with other beta-adrenoceptor blocking drugs, e mode of action of atenolol in the treatment of ypertension is unclear. It is unlikely that any addi-onal ancillary properties possessed by S (–) atenolol, comparison with the racemic mixture, will give rise different therapeutic effects.

Chlorthalidone, a monosulfonamyl diuretic, in-eases excretion of sodium and chloride. Natriuresis accompanied by some loss of potassium. The echanism by which chlorthalidone reduces blood ressure is not fully known but may be related to the xcretion and redistribution of body sodium. Chlor-alidone usually does not decrease normal blood ressure.

The combination of atenolol with thiazide-like diu-tics has been shown to be compatible and generally ore effective than either drug used alone as an ntihypertensive agent.

Atenolol is effective and well-tolerated in most hnic populations. Black patients respond better to e combination of atenolol and chlorthalidone, than atenolol alone.

Co-administration of chlorthalidone and atenolol as little effect on the pharmacokinetics of either.

Absorption of atenolol following oral dosing is onsistent but incomplete (approximately 40–50%) ith peak plasma concentrations occurring 2–4 hours ter dosing. Atenolol blood levels are consistent and ubject to little variability. There is no significant epatic metabolism of atenolol and more than 90% of at absorbed reaches the systemic circulation unal-red. The plasma half-life is about 6 hours but this ay rise in severe renal impairment since the kidney the major route of elimination. Atenolol penetrates ssues poorly due to its low lipid solubility and its oncentration in brain tissue is low. Plasma protein nding is low (approximately 3%).

Absorption of chlorthalidone following oral dosing is consistent but incomplete (approximately 60%) with peak plasma concentrations occurring about 12 hours after dosing. The chlorthalidone blood levels are consistent and subject to little variability. The plasma half-life is about 50 hours and the kidney is the major route of elimination. Plasma protein binding is high (approximately 75%).

**Dosage and administration** *Adults including the elderly:* One tablet daily. Older patients with hypertension who do not respond to low dose therapy with a single agent should have a satisfactory response to a single tablet daily of Tenoret 50. Where hypertensive control is not achieved addition of a small dose of a third agent, e.g. a vasodilator, may be appropriate.

*Children:* There is no paediatric experience with Tenoret 50, therefore this preparation is not recommended for children.

*Renal failure:* In patients with renal impairment a reduction in daily dose or in frequency of administration may be necessary.

**Contra-indications, warnings, etc** Tenoret 50 should not be used in patients with any of the following conditions: known hypersensitivity to either component, bradycardia, cardiogenic shock, hypotension, metabolic acidosis, severe peripheral arterial circulatory disturbances, second or third degree heart block, sick sinus syndrome, untreated phaeochromocytoma or uncontrolled heart failure.

Tenoret 50 must not be given during pregnancy or lactation.

Due to its beta-adrenoceptor blocking drug component, Tenoret 50:

- although contra-indicated in uncontrolled heart failure (see *Contra-indications*), may be used in patients whose signs of heart failure have been controlled. Caution must be exercised in patients whose cardiac reserve is poor.
- may increase the number and duration of angina attacks in patients with Prinzmetal's angina due to unopposed alpha receptor mediated coronary artery vasoconstriction. Atenolol is a beta$_1$-selective beta-adrenoceptor blocking drug; consequently, the use of Tenoret 50 may be considered although utmost caution must be exercised.
- although contra-indicated in severe peripheral arterial circulatory disturbances (see *Contra-indications*), may also aggravate less severe peripheral arterial circulatory disturbances.
- due to its negative effect on conduction time, caution must be exercised if it is given to patients with first degree heart block.
- may modify the tachycardia of hypoglycaemia.
- may mask the signs of thyrotoxicosis.
- will reduce heart rate, as a result of its pharmacological action. In the rare instances when a treated patient develops symptoms which may be attributable to a slow heart rate, the dose may be reduced.
- should not be discontinued abruptly in patients suffering from ischaemic heart disease.
- may cause a more severe reaction to a variety of allergens, when given to patients with a history of anaphylactic reaction to such allergens. Such patients may be unresponsive to the usual doses of adrenaline used to treat the allergic reactions.

Tenoret 50 contains the cardioselective beta-adrenoceptor blocking drug atenolol. Although cardioselective (beta$_1$) beta-adrenoceptor blocking drugs may have less effect on lung function than non-selective beta-adrenoceptor blocking drugs, as with all beta-adrenoceptor blocking drugs, these should be avoided in patients with reversible obstructive airways disease, unless there are compelling clinical reasons for their use. Where such reasons exist, Tenoret 50 may be used with caution. Occasionally, some increase in airways resistance may occur in asthmatic patients, however, and this may usually be reversed by commonly used dosage of bronchodilators such as salbutamol or isoprenaline.

The label and patient information leaflet for this product state the following warning: "If you have ever had asthma or wheezing, you should not take this medicine unless you have discussed these symptoms with the prescribing doctor".

Due to its chlorthalidone component:

- hypokalaemia may occur. Measurement of potassium levels is appropriate, especially in the older patient, those receiving digitalis preparations for cardiac failure, those taking an abnormal (low in potassium) diet or those suffering from gastrointestinal complaints. Hypokalaemia may predispose to arrhythmias in patients receiving digitalis.
- caution must be exercised in patients with severe renal failure (see *Dosage and administration*).
- impaired glucose tolerance may occur and caution must be exercised if chlorthalidone is administered to patients with a known pre-disposition to diabetes mellitus.
- hyperuricaemia may occur. Only a minor increase in serum uric acid usually occurs but in cases of prolonged elevation, the concurrent use of a uricosuric agent will reverse the hyperuricaemia.

Combined use of beta-adrenoceptor blocking drugs and calcium channel blockers with negative inotropic effects e.g. verapamil, diltiazem can lead to an exaggeration of these effects particularly in patients with impaired ventricular function and/or sino-atrial or atrio-ventricular conduction abnormalities. This may result in severe hypotension, bradycardia and cardiac failure. Neither the beta-adrenoceptor blocking drug nor the calcium channel blocker should be administered intravenously within 48 hours of discontinuing the other.

Concomitant therapy with dihydropyridines e.g. nifedipine, may increase the risk of hypotension, and cardiac failure may occur in patients with latent cardiac insufficiency.

Beta-adrenoceptor blocking drugs may exacerbate the rebound hypertension which can follow the withdrawal of clonidine. If the two drugs are co-administered, the beta-adrenoceptor blocking drug should be withdrawn several days before discontinuing clonidine. If replacing clonidine by beta-adrenoceptor blocking drug therapy, the introduction of beta-adrenoceptor blocking drugs should be delayed for several days after clonidine administration has stopped.

Caution must be exercised when prescribing a beta-adrenoceptor blocking drug with Class 1 antiarrhythmic agents such as disopyramide.

Digitalis glycosides, in association with beta-adrenoceptor blocking drugs, may increase atrio-ventricular conduction time.

Concomitant use of sympathomimetic agents, e.g. adrenaline, may counteract the effect of beta-adrenoceptor blocking drugs.

Concomitant use with insulin and oral antidiabetic drugs may lead to the intensification of the blood sugar lowering effects of these drugs.

Concomitant use of prostaglandin synthetase inhibiting drugs, e.g. ibuprofen or indomethacin, may decrease the hypotensive effects of beta-adrenoceptor blocking drugs.

Preparations containing lithium should not be given with diuretics because they may reduce its renal clearance.

*Anaesthesia:* Caution must be exercised when using anaesthetic agents with Tenoret 50. The anaesthetist should be informed and the choice of anaesthetic should be the agent with as little negative inotropic activity as possible. Use of beta-adrenoceptor blocking drugs with anaesthetic drugs may result in attenuation of the reflex tachycardia and increase the risk of hypotension. Anaesthetic agents causing myocardial depression are best avoided.

*Effect on ability to drive or operate machinery:* The use of Tenoret 50 is unlikely to result in any impairment of the ability of patients to drive or operate machinery. However, it should be taken into account that occasionally dizziness or fatigue may occur.

*Undesirable events:* Tenoret 50 is well tolerated. In clinical studies, the undesired events reported are usually attributable to the pharmacological actions of its components.

The following undesired events, listed by body system, have been reported with Tenoret 50 or either of its components.

Biochemical: hyperuricaemia, hypokalaemia, impaired glucose tolerance (see *Contra-indications, warnings etc*).

Cardiovascular: bradycardia, heart failure deterioration, postural hypotension which may be associated with syncope, cold extremities. In susceptible patients: precipitation of heart block, intermittent claudication, Raynaud's phenomenon.

CNS: confusion, dizziness, headache, mood changes, nightmares, psychoses and hallucinations, sleep disturbances of the type noted with other beta-adrenoceptor blocking drugs.

Gastrointestinal: dry mouth, gastrointestinal disturbances, nausea.

Haematological: leucopenia, purpura, thrombocytopenia.

Integumentary: alopecia, dry eyes, psoriasiform skin reactions, exacerbation of psoriasis, skin rashes.

Neurological: paraesthesia.

Respiratory: bronchospasm may occur in patients with bronchial asthma or a history of asthmatic complaints.

Special senses: visual disturbances.

Others: fatigue, an increase in ANA (antinuclear antibodies) has been observed, however the clinical relevance of this is not clear.

Discontinuance of Tenoret 50 should be considered if, according to clinical judgement, the well-being of the patient is adversely affected by any of the above reactions.

*Overdosage:* The symptoms of overdosage may

include bradycardia, hypotension, acute cardiac insufficiency and bronchospasm.

General treatment should include: close supervision, treatment in an intensive care ward, the use of gastric lavage, activated charcoal and a laxative to prevent absorption of any drug still present in the gastrointestinal tract, the use of plasma or plasma substitutes to treat hypotension and shock. The possible use of haemodialysis or haemoperfusion may be considered.

Excessive bradycardia can be countered with atropine 1–2 mg intravenously and/or a cardiac pacemaker. If necessary, this may be followed by a bolus dose of glucagon 10 mg intravenously. If required, this may be repeated or followed by an intravenous infusion of glucagon 1–10 mg/hour depending on response. If no response to glucagon occurs or if glucagon is unavailable, a beta-adrenoceptor stimulant such as dobutamine 2.5 to 10 micrograms/kg/minute by intravenous infusion may be given. Dobutamine, because of its positive inotropic effect could also be used to treat hypotension and acute cardiac insufficiency. It is likely that these doses would be inadequate to reverse the cardiac effects of beta-adrenoceptor blockade if a large overdose has been taken. The dose of dobutamine should therefore be increased if necessary to achieve the required response according to the clinical condition of the patient.

Bronchospasm can usually be reversed by bronchodilators.

Excessive diuresis should be countered by maintaining normal fluid and electrolyte balance.

**Pharmaceutical precautions** Tenoret 50 should be stored below 25°C, protected from light and moisture.

**Legal category** POM.

**Package quantities** Calendar packs of 28 tablets (OP).

**Further information** When the combined antihypertensive effect of a beta-adrenoceptor blocking drug and a diuretic is required, Tenoret 50 one tablet daily is a simple, convenient and acceptable therapy which may be expected to improve patient compliance.

**Product licence number** 12619/0072.

# TENORMIN* TABLETS
# TENORMIN* LS TABLETS
# TENORMIN* 25 TABLETS

**Presentation** Tenormin tablets, containing Atenolol PhEur 100 mg are round, biconvex, orange, film-coated tablets impressed with TENORMIN on one face and an 'S' logo on the reverse. The impressions are highlighted in white.

Tenormin LS tablets, containing Atenolol PhEur 50 mg are round, biconvex, orange, film-coated tablets impressed with TENORMIN LS on one face and bisected on the reverse. The impressions are highlighted in white.

Tenormin 25 tablets, containing Atenolol PhEur 25 mg, are round, biconvex, white, film-coated tablets impressed with TENORMIN 25 on one face and an 'S' logo on the reverse.

The inactive ingredients are gelatin, magnesium carbonate, magnesium stearate, methylhydroxypropylcellulose, sodium lauryl sulphate, maize starch and titanium dioxide. In addition, Tenormin 25 contains glycerol and Tenormin and Tenormin LS contain macrogol, sunset yellow lake and talc.

## Uses

i) Management of hypertension
ii) Management of angina pectoris
iii) Management of cardiac arrhythmias
iv) Myocardial infarction: early intervention in the acute phase.

*Mode of action:* Tenormin (atenolol) is a beta-adrenoceptor blocking drug which is beta$_1$-selective (i.e. acts preferentially on beta$_1$-adrenergic receptors in the heart). Selectivity decreases with increasing dose. It is without intrinsic sympathomimetic and membrane stabilising activities, and, as with other beta-adrenoceptor blocking drugs, has negative inotropic effects (and is therefore contra-indicated in uncontrolled heart failure). As with other beta-adrenoceptor blocking drugs, its mode of action in the treatment of hypertension is unclear. It is probably the action of Tenormin in reducing cardiac rate and contractility which makes it effective in eliminating or reducing the symptoms of patients with angina. It is unlikely that any additional ancillary properties possessed by S (–) atenolol, in comparison with the racemic mixture, will give rise to different therapeutic effects.

Tenormin is effective and well tolerated in most ethnic populations although the response may be less in black patients. Tenormin is compatible with diuretics, other antihypertensive agents and antianginal agents (see *Warnings*).

Early intervention with Tenormin in acute myocardial infarction reduces infarct size and decreases morbidity and mortality. Fewer patients with a threatened infarction progress to frank infarction; the incidence of ventricular arrhythmias is decreased and marked pain relief may result in reduced need of opiate analgesics. Early mortality is decreased. Tenormin is an additional treatment to standard coronary care.

Absorption of atenolol following oral dosing is consistent but incomplete (approximately 40–50%) with peak plasma concentrations occurring 2–4 hours after dosing. Atenolol blood levels are consistent and subject to little variability. There is no significant hepatic metabolism of atenolol and more than 90% of that absorbed reaches the systemic circulation unaltered. The plasma half-life is about 6 hours but this may rise in severe renal impairment since the kidney is the major route of elimination. Atenolol penetrates tissues poorly due to its low lipid solubility and its concentration in brain tissue is low. Plasma protein binding is low (approximately 3%).

**Dosage and administration** *Adults: Hypertension:* One tablet daily. Most patients respond to 100 mg daily given orally as a single dose. Some patients, however, will respond to 50 mg given as a single daily dose. The effect will be fully established after one to two weeks. A further reduction in blood pressure may be achieved by combining Tenormin with other antihypertensive agents. For example, co-administration of Tenormin with a diuretic, as in Tenoretic, provides a highly effective and convenient antihypertensive therapy.

*Angina:* Most patients with angina pectoris will respond to 100 mg given orally once daily or 50 mg given twice daily. It is unlikely that additional benefit will be gained by increasing the dose.

*Arrhythmias:* A suitable initial dose of Tenormin is 2.5 mg (5 ml) injected intravenously over a 2.5 minute period (i.e. 1 mg/minute). (See also prescribing information for Tenormin Injection.) This may be repeated at 5 minute intervals until a response is observed up to a maximum dosage of 10 mg. If Tenormin is given by infusion, 150 micrograms/kg bodyweight may be administered over a 20 minute period. If required, the injection or infusion may be repeated every 12 hours. Having controlled the arrhythmias with intravenous 'Tenormin', a suitable oral maintenance dosage is 50–100 mg daily, given as a single dose.

*Myocardial infarction:* For patients suitable for treatment with intravenous beta-adrenoceptor blockade and presenting within 12 hours of the onset of the chest pain, Tenormin 5–10 mg should be given by slow intravenous injection (1 mg/minute) followed by Tenormin 50 mg orally about 15 minutes later provided no untoward effects occur from the intravenous dose. This should be followed by a further 50 mg orally 12 hours after the intravenous dose and then 12 hours later by 100 mg orally to be given once daily. If bradycardia and/or hypotension requiring treatment, or any other untoward effects occur, Tenormin should be discontinued.

*Elderly patients:* Dosage requirements may be reduced, especially in patients with impaired renal function.

*Children:* There is no paediatric experience with Tenormin and for this reason it is not recommended for use in children.

*Renal failure:* Since Tenormin is excreted via the kidneys dosage should be adjusted in cases of severe impairment of renal function. No significant accumulation of Tenormin occurs in patients who have a creatinine clearance greater than 35 ml/min/1.73 m² (normal range is 100–150 ml/min/1.73 m²). For patients with a creatinine clearance of 15–35 ml/min/1.73 m² (equivalent to serum creatinine of 300–600 micromol/litre) the oral dose should be 50 mg daily and the intravenous dose should be 10 mg once every two days. For patients with a creatinine clearance of <15 ml/min/1.73 m² (equivalent to serum creatinine of >600 micromol/litre) the oral dose should be 25 mg daily or 50 mg on alternate days and the intravenous dose should be 10 mg once every four days.

Patients on haemodialysis should be given 50 mg orally after each dialysis; this should be done under hospital supervision as marked falls in blood pressure can occur.

**Contra-indications, warnings, etc** Tenormin as with other beta-adrenoceptor blocking drugs, should not be used in patients with any of the following conditions: known hypersensitivity to the substance, bradycardia, cardiogenic shock, hypotension, metabolic acidosis, severe peripheral arterial circulatory disturbances, second or third degree heart block, sick sinus syndrome, untreated phaeochromocytoma or uncontrolled heart failure.

Tenormin as with other beta-adrenoceptor blocking drugs:

– although contra-indicated in uncontrolled hea[rt] failure (see *Contra-indications*), may be used i[n] patients whose signs of heart failure have bee[n] controlled. Caution must be exercised in patient[s] whose cardiac reserve is poor.
– may increase the number and duration of angin[a] attacks in patients with Prinzmetal's angina due t[o] unopposed alpha receptor mediated coronary a[r]tery vasoconstriction. Tenormin is a beta$_1$-selectiv[e] beta-adrenoceptor blocking drug; consequently, i[ts] use may be considered although utmost cautio[n] must be exercised.
– although contra-indicated in severe peripheral a[r]terial circulatory disturbances (see *Contra-indic[a]tions*), may also aggravate less severe peripher[al] arterial circulatory disturbances.
– due to its negative effect on conduction tim[e] caution must be exercised if it is given to patient[s] with first degree heart block.
– may modify the tachycardia of hypoglycaemia.
– may mask the signs of thyrotoxicosis.
– will reduce heart rate, as a result of its pharmaco[-] logical action. In the rare instances when a treate[d] patient develops symptoms which may be attribu[t-] able to a slow heart rate, the dose may be reduce[d]
– should not be discontinued abruptly in patient[s] suffering from ischaemic heart disease.
– may cause a more severe reaction to a variety [of] allergens, when given to patients with a history [of] anaphylactic reaction to such allergens. Such pa[-] tients may be unresponsive to the usual doses [of] adrenaline used to treat the allergic reactions.

Although cardioselective (beta$_1$) beta-adrenocept[or] blocking drugs may have less effect on lung functio[n] than non-selective beta-adrenoceptor blocking drug[s] as with all beta-adrenoceptor blocking drugs, thes[e] should be avoided in patients with reversible obstru[c-] tive airways disease, unless there are compellin[g] clinical reasons for their use. Where such reason[s] exist, Tenormin may be used with caution. Occasion[-] ally, some increase in airways resistance may occ[ur] in asthmatic patients, however, and this may usual[ly] be reversed by commonly used dosage of broncho[d]ilators such as salbutamol or isoprenaline.

The label and patient information leaflet for th[e] product state the following warning: "If you have ev[er] had asthma or wheezing, you should not take th[is] medicine unless you have discussed these symptom[s] with the prescribing doctor".

Caution must be exercised when prescribing a bet[a-] adrenoceptor blocking drug with Class 1 antia[r-] rhythmic agents such as disopyramide.

Combined use of beta-adrenoceptor blocking drug[s] and calcium channel blockers with negative inotrop[ic] effects e.g. verapamil, diltiazem can lead to a[n] exaggeration of these effects, particularly in patien[ts] with impaired ventricular function and/or sino-atri[al] or atrio-ventricular conduction abnormalities. Th[is] may result in severe hypotension, bradycardia an[d] cardiac failure. Neither the beta-adrenoceptor bloc[k]ing drug nor the calcium channel blocker should b[e] administered intravenously within 48 hours of disco[n-] tinuing the other.

Concomitant therapy with dihydropyridines e.[g.] nifedipine, may increase the risk of hypotension, an[d] cardiac failure may occur in patients with latent cardi[ac] insufficiency.

Beta-adrenoceptor blocking drugs may exacerba[te] the rebound hypertension which can follow th[e] withdrawal of clonidine. If the two drugs are c[o-] administered, the beta-adrenoceptor blocking dru[g] should be withdrawn several days before discontin[u-] ing clonidine. If replacing clonidine by beta-adren[o-] ceptor blocking drug therapy, the introduction of bet[a-] adrenoceptor blocking drugs should be delayed f[or] several days after clonidine administration ha[s] stopped.

Digitalis glycosides, in association with beta-adre[n-] oceptor blocking drugs, may increase atrio-ventricul[ar] conduction time.

Concomitant use of sympathomimetic agents, e.[g.] adrenaline, may counteract the effect of beta-adren[o-] ceptor blocking drugs.

Concomitant use with insulin and oral antidiabet[ic] drugs may lead to the intensification of the bloo[d] sugar lowering effects of these drugs.

Concomitant use of prostaglandin synthetase inhi[b-] iting drugs, e.g. ibuprofen or indomethacin, m[ay] decrease the hypotensive effects of beta-adrenocept[or] blocking drugs.

*Anaesthesia:* Caution must be exercised when usin[g] anaesthetic agents with Tenormin. The anaesthet[ist] should be informed and the choice of anaesthet[ic] should be the agent with as little negative inotrop[ic] activity as possible. Use of beta-adrenoceptor block[-] ing drugs with anaesthetic drugs may result [in] attenuation of the reflex tachycardia and increase [the] risk of hypotension. Anaesthetic agents causing m[y-] ocardial depression are best avoided.

*Pregnancy:* Tenormin crosses the placental barri[er]

ɒd appears in the cord blood. No studies have been ɾrformed on the use of Tenormin in the first trimester ɒd the possibility of foetal injury cannot be excluded. ɘnormin has been used under close supervision for e treatment of hypertension in the third trimester. dministration of Tenormin to pregnant women in e management of mild to moderate hypertension s been associated with intra-uterine growth retar- ɒtion.

The use of Tenormin in women who are, or may come pregnant, requires that the anticipated benefit weighed against the possible risks, particularly in e first and second trimesters, since beta-adrenocep- r blocking agents, in general, have been associated th a decrease in placental perfusion which may sult in intra-uterine deaths, immature and premature liveries.

*ctation:* There is significant accumulation of Tenor- n in breast milk. Caution should be exercised when ɘnormin is administered to a nursing woman.

*fect on ability to drive or operate machinery:* The e of Tenormin is unlikely to result in any impairment the ability of patients to drive or operate machinery. owever, it should be taken into account that occa- onally dizziness or fatigue may occur.

*ndesirable events:* Tenormin is well tolerated. In nical studies, the undesired events reported are ually attributable to the pharmacological actions of enolol.

The following undesired events, listed by body stem, have been reported.

Cardiovascular: bradycardia, heart failure deterio- tion, postural hypotension which may be associated th syncope, cold extremities. In susceptible patients: ecipitation of heart block, intermittent claudication, ynaud's phenomenon.

CNS: confusion, dizziness, headache, mood anges, nightmares, psychoses and hallucinations, ep disturbances of the type noted with other beta- renoceptor blocking drugs.

Gastrointestinal: dry mouth, gastrointestinal distur- nces.

Haematological: purpura, thrombocytopenia.

Integumentary: alopecia, dry eyes, psoriasiform n reactions, exacerbation of psoriasis, skin rashes.

Neurological: paraesthesia.

Respiratory: bronchospasm may occur in patients th bronchial asthma or a history of asthmatic mplaints.

Special senses: visual disturbances.

Others: fatigue, an increase in ANA (antinuclear tibodies) has been observed, however the clinical evance of this is not clear.

Discontinuance of the drug should be considered if, cording to clinical judgement, the well-being of the tient is adversely affected by any of the above actions.

*erdosage:* The symptoms of overdosage may clude bradycardia, hypotension, acute cardiac insuf- ency and bronchospasm.

General treatment should include: close supervi- n, treatment in an intensive care ward, the use of stric lavage, activated charcoal and a laxative to event absorption of any drug still present in the strointestinal tract, the use of plasma or plasma ostitutes to treat hypotension and shock. The ssible uses of haemodialysis or haemoperfusion ay be considered.

Excessive bradycardia can be countered with atro- e 1–2 mg intravenously and/or a cardiac pace- aker. If necessary, this may be followed by a bolus se of glucagon 10 mg intravenously. If required, s may be repeated or followed by an intravenous usion of glucagon 1–10 mg/hour depending on ponse. If no response to glucagon occurs or if cagon is unavailable, a beta-adrenoceptor stimu- t such as dobutamine 2.5 to 10 micrograms/kg/ nute by intravenous infusion may be given. Dobu- nine, because of its positive inotropic effect could o be used to treat hypotension and acute cardiac ufficiency. It is likely that these doses would be dequate to reverse the cardiac effects of beta- ckade if a large overdose has been taken. The dose dobutamine should therefore be increased if cessary to achieve the required response according the clinical condition of the patient.

Bronchospasm can usually be reversed by bron- odilators.

**armaceutical precautions** Tenormin, Tenormin and Tenormin 25 Tablets should be stored below C, protected from light and moisture.

**gal category** POM.

**ckage quantities** Tenormin Tablets: 100 mg in endar packs of 28 (OP). Tenormin LS Tablets: mg in Calendar packs of 28 (OP). Tenormin 25 blets: 25 mg in Calendar packs of 28 (OP).

**ther information** Tenormin is effective for at least hours after a single oral dose. The drug facilitates compliance by its acceptability to patients and simplicity of dosing. The narrow dose range and early patient response ensure that the effect of the drug in individual patients is quickly demonstrated. Tenormin is compatible with diuretics, other hypotensive agents and antianginals (but see *Warnings*). Since it acts preferentially on beta-adrenergic receptors in the heart, Tenormin may, with care, be used successfully in the treatment of patients with respiratory disease who cannot tolerate non-selective beta-adrenoceptor blocking drugs.

**Product licence numbers**

| | |
|---|---|
| Tenormin Tablets | 12619/0078 |
| Tenormin LS Tablets | 12619/0077 |
| Tenormin 25 Tablets | 12619/0076 |

## TENORMIN* INJECTION

**Presentation** Tenormin Injection contains 5 mg Atenolol PhEur in 10 ml isotonic, citrate buffered aqueous solution. The inactive ingredients are citric acid/sodium citrate, sodium chloride and water.

**Uses** Management of arrhythmias and for the early intervention treatment of acute myocardial infarction.

*Mode of action:* Tenormin (atenolol) is a beta-adrenoceptor blocking drug which is $beta_1$-selective (i.e. acts preferentially on $beta_1$-adrenergic receptors in the heart). Selectivity decreases with increasing dose. Atenolol is without intrinsic sympathomimetic and membrane stabilising activities, and, as with other beta-adrenoceptor blocking drugs, has negative inotropic effects (and is therefore contra-indicated in uncontrolled heart failure). As with other beta-adrenoceptor blocking drugs, its mode of action in the treatment of hypertension is unclear. It is probably the action of Tenormin in reducing cardiac rate and contractility which makes it effective in eliminating or reducing the symptoms of patients with angina. It is unlikely that any additional ancillary properties possessed by S (–) atenolol, in comparison with the racemic mixture, will give rise to different therapeutic effects.

Tenormin is effective and well tolerated in most ethnic populations although the response may be less in black patients. Tenormin is compatible with diuretics, other antihypertensive agents and antianginal agents (see *Warnings*).

Early intervention with Tenormin in acute myocardial infarction reduces infarct size and decreases morbidity and mortality. Fewer patients with a threatened infarction progress to frank infarction; the incidence of ventricular arrhythmias is decreased and marked pain relief may result in reduced need of opiate analgesics. Early mortality is decreased.

Tenormin is an additional treatment to standard coronary care.

Following intravenous administration, the blood levels of atenolol decay tri-exponentially with an elimination half-life of about 6 hours. Throughout the intravenous dose range of 5–10 mg the blood level profile obeys linear pharmacokinetics and beta-blockade is still measurable 24 hours after a 10 mg intravenous dose. The plasma half-life is about 6 hours but this may rise in severe renal impairment since the kidney is the major route of elimination. Atenolol penetrates tissues poorly due to its low lipid solubility and its concentration in brain tissue is low. Plasma protein binding is low (approximately 3%).

**Dosage and administration** *Adults: Arrhythmias:* A suitable initial dose of Tenormin is 2.5 mg (5 ml) injected intravenously over a 2.5 minute period (i.e. 1 mg/minute). This may be repeated at 5 minute intervals until a response is observed up to a maximum dosage of 10 mg. If Tenormin is given by infusion, 150 micrograms/kg bodyweight may be administered over a 20 minute period. If required, the injection or infusion may be repeated every 12 hours. Having controlled the arrhythmias with intravenous Tenormin, a suitable oral maintenance dosage is 50–100 mg daily (see prescribing information for Tenormin and Tenormin LS Tablets).

*Myocardial infarction:* For patients suitable for treatment with intravenous beta-adrenoceptor blockade and presenting within 12 hours of the onset of the chest pain, Tenormin 5–10 mg should be given by slow intravenous injection (1 mg/minute) followed by Tenormin 50 mg orally about 15 minutes later provided no untoward effects occur from the intravenous dose. This should be followed by a further 50 mg orally 12 hours after the intravenous dose and then 12 hours later by 100 mg orally to be given once daily. If bradycardia and/or hypotension requiring treatment or any other untoward effects occur, Tenormin should be discontinued.

*Elderly patients:* Dosage requirements may be reduced, especially in patients with impaired renal function.

*Children:* There is no paediatric experience with Tenormin and for this reason it is not recommended for children.

*Renal failure:* Since Tenormin is excreted via the kidneys, dosage should be adjusted in cases of severe impairment of renal function. No significant accumulation of Tenormin occurs in patients who have a creatinine clearance greater than 35 ml/min/1.73 m² (normal range is 100–150 ml/min/1.73 m²). For patients with a creatinine clearance of 15–35 ml/min/1.73 m² (equivalent to serum creatinine of 300–600 micromol/litre) the oral dose should be 50 mg daily and the intravenous dose should be 10 mg once every two days. For patients with a creatinine clearance of <15 ml/min/1.73 m² (equivalent to serum creatinine of >600 micromol/litre) the oral dose should be 25 mg daily or 50 mg on alternate days; and the intravenous dose should be 10 mg once every four days.

Patients on haemodialysis should be given 50 mg orally after each dialysis; this should be done under hospital supervision as marked falls in blood pressure can occur.

**Contra-indications, warnings, etc** Tenormin as with other beta-adrenoceptor blocking drugs, should not be used in patients with any of the following conditions: known hypersensitivity to the substance, bradycardia, cardiogenic shock, hypotension, metabolic acidosis, severe peripheral arterial circulatory disturbances, second or third degree heart block, sick sinus syndrome, untreated phaeochromocytoma or uncontrolled heart failure.

Tenormin as with other beta-adrenoceptor blocking drugs:

- although contra-indicated in uncontrolled heart failure (see *Contra-indications*), may be used in patients whose signs of heart failure have been controlled. Caution must be exercised in patients whose cardiac reserve is poor.
- may increase the number and duration of angina attacks in patients with Prinzmetal's angina due to unopposed alpha receptor mediated coronary artery vasoconstriction. Tenormin is a $beta_1$-selective beta-adrenoceptor blocking drug; consequently, its use may be considered although utmost caution must be exercised.
- although contra-indicated in severe peripheral arterial circulatory disturbances (see *Contra-indications*), may also aggravate less severe peripheral arterial circulatory disturbances.
- due to its negative effect on conduction time, caution must be exercised if it is given to patients with first degree heart block.
- may modify the tachycardia of hypoglycaemia.
- may mask the signs of thyrotoxicosis.
- will reduce heart rate, as a result of its pharmacological action. In the rare instances when a treated patient develops symptoms which may be attributable to a slow heart rate, the dose may be reduced.
- should not be discontinued abruptly in patients suffering from ischaemic heart disease.
- may cause a more severe reaction to a variety of allergens, when given to patients with a history of anaphylactic reaction to such allergens. Such patients may be unresponsive to the usual doses of adrenaline used to treat the allergic reactions.

Although cardioselective ($beta_1$) beta-adrenoceptor blocking drugs may have less effect on lung function than non-selective beta-adrenoceptor blocking drugs, as with all beta-adrenoceptor blocking drugs, these should be avoided in patients with reversible obstructive airways disease, unless there are compelling clinical reasons for their use. Where such reasons exist, Tenormin may be used with caution. Occasionally, some increase in airways resistance may occur in asthmatic patients, however, and this may usually be reversed by commonly used dosage of bronchodilators such as salbutamol or isoprenaline.

The label and patient information leaflet for this product state the following warnings:

Label: "Tenormin Injection should be used with caution in patients with a history of asthma or wheezing."

Patient Information Leaflet: "If you have ever had asthma or wheezing, you should not be given this medicine unless you have discussed these symptoms with the prescribing doctor."

Caution must be exercised when prescribing a beta-adrenoceptor blocking drug with Class 1 antiarrhythmic agents such as disopyramide.

Combined use of beta-adrenoceptor blocking drugs and calcium channel blockers with negative inotropic effects e.g. verapamil, diltiazem can lead to an exaggeration of these effects, particularly in patients with impaired ventricular function and/or sino-atrial or atrio-ventricular conduction abnormalities. This may result in severe hypotension, bradycardia and cardiac failure. Neither the beta-adrenoceptor blocking drug nor the calcium channel blocker should be administered intravenously within 48 hours of discontinuing the other.

Concomitant therapy with dihydropyridines e.g.

nifedipine, may increase the risk of hypotension, and cardiac failure may occur in patients with latent cardiac insufficiency.

Beta-adrenoceptor blocking drugs may exacerbate the rebound hypertension which can follow the withdrawal of clonidine. If the two drugs are co-administered, the beta-adrenoceptor blocking drug should be withdrawn several days before discontinuing clonidine. If replacing clonidine by beta-adrenoceptor blocking drug therapy, the introduction of beta-adrenoceptor blocking drugs should be delayed for several days after clonidine administration has stopped.

Digitalis glycosides, in association with beta-adrenoceptor blocking drugs, may increase atrio-ventricular conduction time.

Concomitant use of sympathomimetic agents, e.g. adrenaline, may counteract the effect of beta-adrenoceptor blocking drugs.

Concomitant use with insulin and oral antidiabetic drugs may lead to the intensification of the blood sugar lowering effects of these drugs.

Concomitant use of prostaglandin synthetase inhibiting drugs, e.g. ibuprofen or indomethacin, may decrease the hypotensive effects of beta-adrenoceptor blocking drugs.

*Anaesthesia:* Caution must be exercised when using anaesthetic agents with Tenormin. The anaesthetist should be informed and the choice of anaesthetic should be the agent with as little negative inotropic activity as possible. Use of beta-adrenoceptor blocking drugs with anaesthetic drugs may result in attenuation of the reflex tachycardia and increase the risk of hypotension. Anaesthetic agents causing myocardial depression are best avoided.

*Pregnancy:* Tenormin crosses the placental barrier and appears in the cord blood. No studies have been performed on the use of Tenormin in the first trimester and the possibility of foetal injury cannot be excluded. Tenormin has been used under close supervision for the treatment of hypertension in the third trimester. Administration of Tenormin to pregnant women in the management of mild to moderate hypertension has been associated with intra-uterine growth retardation.

The use of Tenormin in women who are, or may become pregnant, requires that the anticipated benefit be weighed against the possible risks, particularly in the first and second trimesters, since beta-andrenoceptor blocking agents, in general, have been associated with a decrease in placental perfusion which may result in intra-uterine deaths, immature and premature deliveries.

*Lactation:* There is significant accumulation of Tenormin in breast milk. Caution should be exercised when Tenormin is administered to a nursing woman.

*Effect on ability to drive or operate machinery:* The use of Tenormin is unlikely to result in any impairment of the ability of patients to drive or operate machinery. However, it should be taken into account that occasionally dizziness or fatigue may occur.

*Undesirable events:* Tenormin is well tolerated. In clinical studies, the undesired events reported are usually attributable to the pharmacological actions of atenolol.

The following undesired events, listed by body system, have been reported.

Cardiovascular: bradycardia, heart failure deterioration, postural hypotension which may be associated with syncope, cold extremities. In susceptible patients: precipitation of heart block, intermittent claudication, Raynaud's phenomenon.

CNS: confusion, dizziness, headache, mood changes, nightmares, psychoses and hallucinations, sleep disturbances of the type noted with other beta-adrenoceptor blocking drugs.

Gastrointestinal: dry mouth, gastrointestinal disturbances.

Haematological: purpura, thrombocytopenia.

Integumentary: alopecia, dry eyes, psoriasiform skin reactions, exacerbation of psoriasis, skin rashes.

Neurological: paraesthesia.

Respiratory: bronchospasm may occur in patients with bronchial asthma or a history of asthmatic complaints.

Special senses: visual disturbances.

Others: fatigue, an increase in ANA (antinuclear antibodies) has been observed, however the clinical relevance of this is not clear.

Discontinuance of the drug should be considered if, according to clinical judgement, the well-being of the patient is adversely affected by any of the above reactions.

*Overdosage:* The symptoms of overdosage may include bradycardia, hypotension, acute cardiac insufficiency and bronchospasm.

General treatment should include: close supervision, treatment in an intensive care ward, the use of gastric lavage, activated charcoal and a laxative to prevent absorption of any drug still present in the gastrointestinal tract, the use of plasma or plasma substitutes to treat hypotension and shock. The possible use of haemodialysis or haemoperfusion may be considered.

Excessive bradycardia can be countered with atropine 1–2 mg intravenously and/or a cardiac pacemaker. If necessary, this may be followed by a bolus dose of glucagon 10 mg intravenously. If required, this may be repeated or followed by an intravenous infusion of glucagon 1–10 mg/hour depending on response. If no response to glucagon occurs or if glucagon is unavailable, a beta-adrenoceptor stimulant such as dobutamine 2.5 to 10 micrograms/kg/minute by intravenous infusion may be given. Dobutamine, because of its positive inotropic effect could also be used to treat hypotension and acute cardiac insufficiency. It is likely that these doses would be inadequate to reverse the cardiac effects of beta-blockade if a large overdose has been taken. The dose of dobutamine should therefore be increased if necessary to achieve the required response according to the clinical condition of the patient.

Bronchospasm can usually be reversed by bronchodilators.

**Pharmaceutical precautions** Tenormin Injection should be stored below 25°C, protected from light.

Dilutions of Tenormin Injection in Dextrose Injection BP, Sodium Chloride Injection BP, or Sodium Chloride and Dextrose Injection BP may be used.

**Legal category** POM.

**Package quantities** 10 ml ampoules in boxes of 10.

**Further information** The narrow dose range and early patient response to Tenormin ensure that the effect of the drug in individual patients is quickly demonstrated. Tenormin is fully compatible with diuretics, other hypotensive agents and antianginals (but see *Warnings*). Since it acts preferentially on beta-adrenergic receptors in the heart, Tenormin may, with care, be used successfully in the treatment of patients with respiratory disease who cannot tolerate non selective beta-adrenoceptor blocking drugs.

**Product licence number** 12619/0074.

## TENORMIN* SYRUP

**Presentation** Tenormin Syrup is a clear, colourless, lemon and lime flavoured syrup containing 0.5% w/v Atenolol PhEur (equivalent to 25 mg/5 ml). The inactive ingredients are citric acid, flavour, methylhydroxybenzoate, propylhydroxybenzoate, saccharin sodium, sodium citrate, sorbitol and water.

**Uses**

(a) Management of hypertension.
(b) Management of angina.
(c) Management of cardiac arrhythmias.
(d) Myocardial infarction: early intervention in the acute phase.

*Mode of action:* Tenormin (atenolol) is a beta-adrenoceptor blocking drug which is $beta_1$-selective (i.e. acts preferentially on $beta_1$-adrenergic receptors in the heart). Selectivity decreases with increasing dose. Atenolol is without intrinsic sympathomimetic and membrane stabilising activities, and, as with other beta-adrenoceptor blocking drugs, has negative inotropic effects (and is therefore contra-indicated in uncontrolled heart failure). As with other beta-adrenoceptor blocking drugs, its mode of action in the treatment of hypertension is unclear. It is probably the action of Tenormin in reducing cardiac rate and contractility which makes it effective in eliminating or reducing the symptoms of patients with angina. It is unlikely that any additional ancillary properties possessed by S (–) atenolol, in comparison with the racemic mixture, will give rise to different therapeutic effects.

Tenormin is effective and well tolerated in most ethnic populations although the response may be less in black patients. Tenormin is compatible with diuretics, other antihypertensive agents and antianginal agents (see *Warnings*).

Early intervention with Tenormin in acute myocardial infarction reduces infarct size and decreases morbidity and mortality. Fewer patients with a threatened infarction progress to frank infarction; the incidence of ventricular arrhythmias is decreased and marked pain relief may result in reduced need of opiate analgesics. Early mortality is decreased. Tenormin is an additional treatment to standard coronary care.

Absorption of atenolol following oral dosing is consistent but incomplete (approximately 40–50%) with peak plasma concentrations occurring 2–4 hours after dosing. Atenolol blood levels are consistent and subject to little variability. There is no significant hepatic metabolism of atenolol and more than 90% of that absorbed reaches the systemic circulation unaltered. The plasma half-life is about 6 hours but th may rise in severe renal impairment since the kidn is the major route of elimination. Atenolol penetrat tissues poorly due to its low lipid solubility and concentration in brain tissue is low. Plasma prote binding is low (approximately 3%).

**Dosage and administration**

*Adults: Hypertension:* Two or four 5 ml spoonfu daily i.e. 50 mg or 100 mg in patients unable to ta 50 mg or 100 mg tablets.

Most patients respond to 100 mg once daily. Son patients, however, will respond to 50 mg given as single daily dose. The effect will be fully establish after one to two weeks. A further reduction in bloo pressure may be achieved by combining Tenorm with other antihypertensive agents.

*Angina:* Most patients with angina pectoris w respond to 100 mg (four 5 ml spoonfuls) given ora once a day or 50 mg (two 5 ml spoonfuls) given twi daily. It is unlikely that additional benefit will be gain by increasing the dose.

*Arrhythmias:* A suitable initial dose of Tenorm Injection is 2.5 mg (5 ml) given intravenously ove 2.5 minute period (i.e. 1 mg/minute). (See prescribi information for Tenormin Injection). This may repeated at 5 minute intervals until a response observed up to a maximum dosage of 10 mg. Tenormin Injection is given by infusion, 150 micr grams/kg bodyweight may be administered over 20 minute period. If required, the injection or infusi may be repeated every 12 hours. Having controll the arrhythmias, a suitable oral maintenance dosa is 50–100 mg (two to four 5 ml spoonfuls) of Tenorm Syrup daily given as a single dose.

*Myocardial infarction:* For patients suitable for tre ment with intravenous beta-adrenoceptor blocka and presenting within 12 hours of the onset of t chest pain, Tenormin Injection 5–10 mg should given by slow intravenous administration (1 m minute) followed by Tenormin Syrup 50 mg (two 5 spoonfuls) orally about 15 minutes later provided untoward effects occur from the intravenous dos This should be followed by a further 50 mg orally hours after the intravenous dose and then 12 hou later by 100 mg (four 5 ml spoonfuls) orally to given once daily. If bradycardia and/or hypotensi requiring treatment, or any other untoward effe occur, Tenormin should be discontinued.

*Elderly patients:* Dosage requirements may be duced, especially in patients with impaired re function.

*Children:* There is no paediatric experience w Tenormin and for this reason it is not recommend for use in children.

*Renal failure:* Since Tenormin is excreted via t kidneys dosage should be adjusted in cases of seve impairment of renal function. No significant accum lation of Tenormin occurs in patients who have creatinine clearance greater than 35 ml/min/1.73 (normal range is 100–150 ml/min/1.73 $m^2$). For p tients with a creatinine clearance of 15–35 ml/m 1.73 $m^2$ (equivalent to serum creatinine of 300–600 cromol/litre) the oral dose should be 50 mg daily a the intravenous dose should be 10 mg once every tw days. For patients with a creatinine clearance <15 ml/min/1.73 $m^2$ (equivalent to serum creatinine >600 micromol/litre) the oral dose should be 25 r daily or 50 mg on alternate days and the intravenc dose should be 10 mg once every four days.

Patients on haemodialysis should be given 50 r orally after each dialysis: this should be done unc hospital supervision as marked falls in blood press can occur.

**Contra-indications, warnings, etc** Tenormin as w other beta-adrenoceptor blocking drugs, should r be used in patients with any of the following con tions: known hypersensitivity to the substance, bra ycardia, cardiogenic shock, hypotension, metabc acidosis, severe peripheral arterial circulatory dist bances, second or third degree heart block, sick sin syndrome, untreated phaeochromocytoma or unco trolled heart failure.

Tenormin as with other beta-adrenoceptor blocki drugs:

- although contra-indicated in uncontrolled he failure (see *Contra-indications*), may be used patients whose signs of heart failure have be controlled. Caution must be exercised in patie whose cardiac reserve is poor.
- may increase the number and duration of ang attacks in patients with Prinzmetal's angina due unopposed alpha receptor mediated coronary tery vasoconstriction. Tenormin is a $beta_1$-select beta-adrenoceptor blocking drug; consequently, use may be considered although utmost cauti must be exercised.
- although contra-indicated in severe peripheral terial circulatory disturbances (see *Contra-indi*

tions), may also aggravate less severe peripheral arterial circulatory disturbances.
due to its negative effect on conduction time, caution must be exercised if it is given to patients with first degree heart block.
may modify the tachycardia of hypoglycaemia.
may mask the signs of thyrotoxicosis.
will reduce heart rate, as a result of its pharmacological action. In the rare instances when a treated patient develops symptoms which may be attributable to a slow heart rate, the dose may be reduced.
should not be discontinued abruptly in patients suffering from ischaemic heart disease.
may cause a more severe reaction to a variety of allergens, when given to patients with a history of anaphylactic reaction to such allergens. Such patients may be unresponsive to the usual doses of adrenaline used to treat the allergic reactions.

Although cardioselective ($beta_1$) beta-adrenoceptor ocking drugs may have less effect on lung function ıan non-selective beta-adrenoceptor blocking drugs, s with all beta-adrenoceptor blocking drugs, these ıould be avoided in patients with reversible obstrucve airways disease, unless there are compelling inical reasons for their use. Where such reasons xist, Tenormin may be used with caution. Occasionly, some increase in airways resistance may occur asthmatic patients, however, and this may usually e reversed by commonly used dosage of bronchodators such as salbutamol or isoprenaline.

The label and patient information leaflet for this roduct state the following warning: "If you have ever ad asthma or wheezing, you should not take this edicine unless you have discussed these symptoms ith the prescribing doctor".

Caution must be exercised when prescribing a betadrenoceptor blocking drug with Class 1 antiarythmic agents such as disopyramide.

Combined use of beta-adrenoceptor blocking drugs nd calcium channel blockers with negative inotropic ffects e.g. verapamil, diltiazem can lead to an xaggeration of these effects, particularly in patients ith impaired ventricular function and/or sino-atrial r atrio-ventricular conduction abnormalities. This ay result in severe hypotension, bradycardia and ardiac failure. Neither the beta-adrenoceptor blockg drug nor the calcium channel blocker should be dministered intravenously within 48 hours of disconnuing the other.

Concomitant therapy with dihydropyridines e.g. fedipine, may increase the risk of hypotension, and ardiac failure may occur in patients with latent cardiac sufficiency.

Beta-adrenoceptor blocking drugs may exacerbate e rebound hypertension which can follow the ithdrawal of clonidine. If the two drugs are coministered, the beta-adrenoceptor blocking drug ıould be withdrawn several days before discontinug clonidine. If replacing clonidine by beta-adrenoptor blocking drug therapy, the introduction of betadrenoceptor blocking drugs should be delayed for everal days after clonidine administration has opped.

Digitalis glycosides, in association with beta-adrenceptor blocking drugs, may increase atrio-ventricular onduction time.

Concomitant use of sympathomimetic agents, e.g. drenaline, may counteract the effect of beta-adrenoptor blocking drugs.

Concomitant use with insulin and oral antidabetic ugs may lead to the intensification of the blood gar lowering effects of these drugs.

Concomitant use of prostaglandin synthetase inhibng drugs, e.g. ibuprofen or indomethacin, may ecrease the hypotensive effects of beta-adrenoceptor ocking drugs.

naesthesia: Caution must be exercised when using ıaesthetic agents with Tenormin. The anaesthetist ould be informed and the choice of anaesthetic ould be the agent with as little negative inotropic tivity as possible. Use of beta-adrenoceptor blockg drugs with anaesthetic drugs may result in tenuation of the reflex tachycardia and increase the sk of hypotension. Anaesthetic agents causing mycardial depression are best avoided.

egnancy: Tenormin crosses the placental barrier d appears in the cord blood. No studies have been rformed on the use of Tenormin in the first trimester d the possibility of foetal injury cannot be excluded. enormin has been used under close supervision for e treatment of hypertension in the third trimester. dministration of Tenormin to pregnant women in e management of mild to moderate hypertension as been associated with intra-uterine growth retaration.

e use of Tenormin in women who are, or may come pregnant, requires that the anticipated benefit e weighed against the possible risks, particularly in e first and second trimesters, since beta-adrenocepr blocking agents in general have been associated with a decrease in placental perfusion which may result in intra-uterine deaths, immature and premature deliveries.

*Lactation:* There is significant accumulation of Tenormin in breast milk. Caution should be exercised when Tenormin is administered to a nursing woman.

*Effect on ability to drive or operate machinery:* The use of Tenormin is unlikely to result in any impairment of the ability of patients to drive or operate machinery. However, it should be taken into account that occasionally dizziness or fatigue may occur.

*Undesirable events:* Tenormin is well tolerated. In clinical studies, the undesired events reported are usually attributable to the pharmacological actions of atenolol.

The following undesired events, listed by body system, have been reported.

Cardiovascular: bradycardia, heart failure deterioration, postural hypotension which may be associated with syncope, cold extremities. In susceptible patients: precipitation of heart block, intermittent claudication, Raynaud's phenomenon.

CNS: confusion, dizziness, headache, mood changes, nightmares, psychoses and hallucinations, sleep disturbances of the type noted with other beta-adrenoceptor blocking drugs.

Gastrointestinal: dry mouth, gastrointestinal disturbances.

Haematological: purpura, thrombocytopenia.

Integumentary: alopecia, dry eyes, psoriasiform skin reactions, exacerbation of psoriasis, skin rashes.

Neurological: paraesthesia.

Respiratory: bronchospasm may occur in patients with bronchial asthma or a history of asthmatic complaints.

Special senses: visual disturbances.

Others: fatigue, an increase in ANA (antinuclear antibodies) has been observed, however the clinical relevance of this is not clear.

Discontinuance of the drug should be considered if, according to clinical judgement, the well-being of the patient is adversely affected by any of the above reactions.

*Overdosage:* The symptoms of overdosage may include bradycardia, hypotension, acute cardiac insufficiency and bronchospasm.

General treatment should include: close supervision, treatment in an intensive care ward, the use of gastric lavage, activated charcoal and a laxative to prevent absorption of any drug still present in the gastrointestinal tract, the use of plasma or plasma substitutes to treat hypotension and shock. The possible use of haemodialysis or haemoperfusion may be considered.

Excessive bradycardia can be countered with atropine 1–2 mg intravenously and/or a cardiac pacemaker. If necessary, this may be followed by a bolus dose of glucagon 10 mg intravenously. If required, this may be repeated or followed by an intravenous infusion of glucagon 1–10 mg/hour depending on response. If no response to glucagon occurs or if glucagon is unavailable, a beta-adrenoceptor stimulant such as dobutamine 2.5 to 10 micrograms/kg/minute by intravenous infusion may be given. Dobutamine, because of its positive inotropic effect could also be used to treat hypotension and acute cardiac insufficiency. It is likely that these doses would be inadequate to reverse the cardiac effects of beta-blockade if a large overdose has been taken. The dose of dobutamine should therefore be increased if necessary to achieve the required response according to the clinical condition of the patient.

Bronchospasm can usually be reversed by bronchodilators.

**Pharmaceutical precautions** Tenormin Syrup should be stored below 25°C, protected from light.

**Legal category** POM.

**Package quantities** 300 ml bottle (OP).

**Further information** Tenormin Syrup is intended for patients unable to swallow Tenormin tablets. Tenormin is effective for at least 24 hours after once daily dosing with 10 ml or 20 ml Tenormin Syrup. Tenormin Syrup facilitates compliance by its acceptability to patients and the once-daily dosing regimen. The narrow dose range and early patient response ensure that the effect of the drug in individual patients is quickly demonstrated. Tenormin is compatible with diuretics, other hypotensive agents and antianginals (but see *Warnings*). Since it acts preferentially on beta-adrenergic receptors in the heart, Tenormin may, with care, be used successfully in the treatment of patients with respiratory disease who cannot tolerate non-selective beta-adrenoceptor blocking drugs.

**Product licence number** 12619/0075.

## TOMUDEX* ▼

**Qualitative and quantitative composition** Tomudex contains 2 mg raltitrexed in each vial.

**Pharmaceutical form** Powder for intravenous injection.

**Clinical particulars**

*Therapeutic indications:* The palliative treatment of advanced colorectal cancer where 5-fluorouracil and folinic acid based regimens are either not tolerated or in appropriate.

*Posology and method of administration*

*Adults:* The dose of Tomudex is calculated on the basis of the body surface area. The recommended dose is 3 mg/m² given intravenously, as a single short, intravenous infusion in 50 to 250 ml of either 0.9% sodium chloride solution or 5% dextrose (glucose) solution. It is recommended that the infusion is given over a 15 minute period. Other drugs should not be mixed with Tomudex in the same infusion container. In the absence of toxicity, treatment may be repeated every 3 weeks.

Dose escalation above 3 mg/m² is not recommended, since higher doses have been associated with an increased incidence of life-threatening or fatal toxicity.

Prior to the initiation of treatment and before each subsequent treatment a full blood count (including a differential count and platelets), liver transaminases, serum bilirubin and serum creatinine measurements should be performed. The total white cell count should be greater than 4,000/mm³, the neutrophil count greater than 2,000/mm³ and the platelet count greater than 100,000/mm³ prior to treatment. In the event of toxicity the next scheduled dose should be withheld until signs of toxic effects regress. In particular, signs of gastrointestinal toxicity (diarrhoea or mucositis) and haematological toxicity (neutropenia or thrombocytopenia) should have completely resolved before subsequent treatment is allowed. Patients who develop signs of gastrointestinal toxicity should have their full blood counts monitored at least weekly for signs of haematological toxicity.

Based on the worst grade of gastrointestinal and haematological toxicity observed on the previous treatment and provided that such toxicity has completely resolved, the following dose reductions are recommended for subsequent treatment:

*25% dose reduction:* in patients with WHO grade 3 haematological toxicity (neutropenia or thrombocytopenia) or WHO grade 2 gastrointestinal toxicity (diarrhoea or mucositis).

*50% dose reduction:* in patients with WHO grade 4 haematological toxicity (neutropenia or thrombocytopenia) or WHO grade 3 gastrointestinal toxicity (diarrhoea or mucositis).

Once a dose reduction has been made, all subsequent doses should be given at the reduced dose.

Treatment should be discontinued in the event of any WHO grade 4 gastrointestinal toxicity (diarrhoea or mucositis) or in the event of a WHO grade 3 gastrointestinal toxicity associated with WHO grade 4 haematological toxicity. Patients with such toxicity should be managed promptly with standard supportive care measures including i.v. hydration and bone marrow support. In addition pre-clinical data suggest that consideration should be given to the administration of folinic acid. From clinical experience with other antifolates folinic acid may be given at a dose of 25 mg/m² i.v. every 6 hours until the resolution of symptoms. Further use of Tomudex in such patients is not recommended.

It is essential that the dose reduction scheme should be adhered to since the potential for life threatening and fatal toxicity increases if the dose is not reduced or treatment not stopped as appropriate.

*Elderly:* Dosage and administration as for adults. However, as with other cytotoxics, Tomudex should be used with caution in elderly patients (see *Warnings/Precautions*).

*Children:* Tomudex is not recommended for use in children as safety and efficacy have not been established in this group of patients.

*Renal impairment:* For patients with abnormal serum creatinine, before the first or any subsequent treatment, a creatinine clearance should be performed or calculated. If creatinine clearance is ≤65 ml/min, the following dose modifications are recommended:

Dose modification in the presence of renal impairment

| *Creatinine clearance* | *Dose as % of 3.0 mg/m²* | *Dosing interval* |
|---|---|---|
| >65 ml/min | Full dose | 3-weekly |
| 25 to 65 ml/min | 50% | 4-weekly |
| <25 ml/min | No therapy | Not applicable |

See Contra-indications for use in patients with severe renal impairment.

*Hepatic impairment:* No dosage adjustment is recommended for patients with mild to moderate hepatic impairment. However, given that a proportion of the drug is excreted via the faecal route (see *Pharmacokinetic properties*), and that these patients usually form a poor prognosis group, patients with mild to moderate hepatic impairment need to be treated with caution. (See *Warnings and precautions for use.*) Tomudex has not been studied in patients with severe hepatic impairment, clinical jaundice or decompensated liver disease and its use in such patients is not recommended.

*Contra-indications:* Tomudex should not be used in pregnant women, in women who may become pregnant during treatment or women who are breast feeding. Pregnancy should be excluded before treatment with Tomudex is commenced (see *Pregnancy* section).

Tomudex is contra-indicated in patients with severe renal impairment.

*Special warnings and special precautions for use:* It is recommended that Tomudex is only given by or under the supervision of a physician who is experienced in cancer chemotherapy, and in the management of chemotherapy-related toxicity. Patients undergoing therapy should be subject to appropriate supervision so that signs of possible toxic effects or adverse reactions may be detected and treated promptly (see *Posology and method of administration*).

In common with other cytotoxic agents of this type, caution is necessary in patients with depressed bone marrow function, poor general condition, or prior radiotherapy.

Patients whose disease progressed on previous treatment for advanced disease with 5-fluorouracil based regimens may also be resistant to the effects of Tomudex.

Elderly patients are more vulnerable to the toxic effects of Tomudex. Extreme care should be taken to ensure adequate monitoring of adverse reactions especially signs of gastrointestinal toxicity (diarrhoea or mucositis).

A proportion of the Tomudex is excreted via the faecal route (see *Pharmacokinetic properties*), therefore, patients with mild to moderate hepatic impairment should be treated with caution.

Treatment with Tomudex in patients with severe hepatic impairment is not recommended.

It is recommended that pregnancy should be avoided during treatment and for at least 6 months after cessation of treatment if either partner is receiving Tomudex (see also *Pregnancy and lactation*).

There is no clinical experience with extravasation. However, perivascular tolerance studies in animals did not reveal any significant irritant reaction.

Tomudex is a cytotoxic agent and should be handled according to normal procedures adopted for such agents (see *Instructions for use/handling*).

*Interaction with other medicaments and other forms of interaction:* No specific interaction studies have been conducted in man.

Folinic acid, folic acid or vitamin preparations containing these agents must not be given immediately prior to or during administration of Tomudex, since they may interfere with its action.

There is no experience to date in relation to the combined use of Tomudex with other cytotoxic agents.

Tomudex is 93% protein bound and while it has the potential to interact with similarly highly protein bound drugs, no displacement interaction with warfarin has been observed *in vitro.* Data suggest that active tubular secretion may contribute to the renal excretion of raltitrexed, indicating a potential interaction with other actively secreted drugs such as non-steroidal anti-inflammatory drugs (NSAIDs). However, a review of the clinical trial safety database did not reveal evidence of clinically significant interaction in patients treated with Tomudex who also received concomitant NSAIDs, warfarin and other commonly prescribed drugs.

*Pregnancy and lactation:* Pregnancy should be avoided if either partner is receiving Tomudex. It is also recommended that conception should be avoided for at least 6 months after cessation of treatment.

Tomudex should not be used during pregnancy or in women who may become pregnant during treatment (see the *Pre-clinical Safety Data*). Pregnancy should be excluded before treatment with Tomudex is started. Tomudex should not be given to women who are breast feeding.

Fertility studies in the rat indicate that Tomudex can cause impairment of male fertility. Fertility returned to normal three months after dosing ceased. Tomudex caused embryolethality and foetal abnormalities in pregnant rats.

*Effects on ability to drive and use machines:* Tomudex may cause malaise or asthenia following infusion and the ability to drive/use machinery could be impaired whilst such symptoms continue.

*Undesirable effects:* As with other cytotoxic drugs, Tomudex may be associated with certain adverse drug reactions. These mainly include reversible effects on the haemopoietic system, liver enzymes and gastrointestinal tract.

The following effects were reported as possible adverse drug reactions. The incidences represent those that were reported in the colorectal cancer clinical trials irrespective of the clinician's assessment of causality.

*Gastrointestinal system:* The most frequent effects were nausea in 57% of patients, diarrhoea (37%), vomiting (35%) and anorexia (27%). The incidences of severe (WHO Grade 3 and 4) gastrointestinal adverse events were 12% for nausea and vomiting, 12% for diarrhoea and 2% for mucositis. Other effects include mouth ulceration, dyspepsia and constipation. Severe diarrhoea may be associated with concurrent haematological suppression, especially leucopenia. Subsequent treatment may need to be discontinued or the dose reduced according to the grade of toxicity (see *Posology and method of administration*). Nausea and vomiting are usually responsive to antiemetics.

*Haemopoietic system:* Leucopenia (23%), anaemia (21%) and thrombocytopenia (4%) have been reported in clinical trials. They are usually mild to moderate, reaching nadir in the first and second week after treatment and recover by the third week. The incidence of severe (WHO Grade 4) leucopenia or thrombocytopenia was 5% and 1% respectively. These may be potentially life-threatening or fatal especially if associated with signs of gastrointestinal toxicity (see *Posology and method of administration*).

*Metabolic and nutritional:* Reversible increases in AST and ALT have been commonly reported in clinical trials (16% and 13% of patients respectively). Such changes have usually been asymptomatic and self-limiting when not associated with progression of the underlying malignancy. Other effects were weight loss, dehydration, peripheral oedema and increases in alkaline phosphatase.

*Musculoskeletal and nervous system:* Arthralgia and hypertonia (usually muscular cramps) have each been reported in less than 5% of patients.

*Skin, appendages and special senses:* Rash was commonly reported in clinical trials (15% of patients) sometimes associated with pruritus. Other effects were desquamation, alopecia, sweating, taste perversion and conjunctivitis each in less than 5% of patients.

*Whole body:* The most frequent effects were asthenia (45%) and fever (30%) which were usually mild to moderate and reversible. Severe asthenia can occur and may be associated with malaise and a flu-like syndrome. Other effects were abdominal pain (23%), pain (8%), headache (7%) and infection (5%). Cellulitis and sepsis were also reported each in less than 5% of patients.

*Overdose:* There is no clinically proven antidote available. In the case of inadvertent or accidental administration of an overdose, preclinical data suggest that consideration should be given to the administration of folinic acid. From clinical experience with other antifolates folinic acid may be given at a dose of 25 mg/m² i.v. every 6 hours. As the time interval between Tomudex administration and folinic acid rescue increases, its effectiveness in counteracting toxicity may diminish.

The expected manifestations of overdose are likely to be an exaggerated form of the adverse drug reactions anticipated with the administration of the drug. Patients should, therefore, be carefully monitored for signs of gastrointestinal and haematological toxicity. Symptomatic treatment and standard supportive care measures for the management of this toxicity should be applied.

**Pharmacological properties**

*Pharmacodynamic properties:* Raltitrexed is a folate analogue belonging to the family of anti-metabolites and has potent inhibitory activity against the enzyme thymidylate synthase (TS). Compared to other anti-metabolites such as 5-fluorouracil or methotrexate, raltitrexed acts as a direct and specific TS inhibitor. TS is a key enzyme in the *de novo* synthesis of thymidine triphosphate (TTP), a nucleotide required exclusively for deoxyribonuleic acid (DNA) synthesis. Inhibition of TS leads to DNA fragmentation and cell death. Raltitrexed is transported into cells via a reduced folate carrier (RFC) and is then extensively polyglutamated by the enzyme folyl polyglutamate synthetase (FPGS) to polyglutamate forms that are retained in cells and are even more potent inhibitors of TS. Raltitrexed polyglutamation enhances TS inhibitory potency and increases the duration of TS inhibition in cells which may improve antitumour activity. Polyglutamation could also contribute to increased toxicity due to drug retention in normal tissues.

In clinical trials, Tomudex at the dose of 3 mg/m² i.v. every 3 weeks has demonstrated clinical antitumour activity with an acceptable toxicity profile in patients with advanced colorectal cancer.

Four large clinical trials have been conducted with Tomudex in advanced colorectal cancer. Of the three comparative trials, two showed no statistical difference between Tomudex and the combination of 5-fluorouracil plus folinic acid for survival while one trial showed a statistically significant difference favour of the combination of 5-fluorouracil plus folin acid. Tomudex as a single agent was as effective the combination of 5-fluorouracil and folinic acid terms of objective response rate in all trials.

*Pharmacokinetic properties:* Following intraveno administration at 3.0 mg/m², the concentration-tin profile in patients was triphasic: Peak concentration found at the end of the infusion, were followed by rapid initial decline in concentration. This was fo lowed by a slow elimination phase. The key pharm cokinetic parameters are presented below:

*Summary of mean pharmacokinetic parameters patients administered 3.0 mg/m² Raltitrexed by intr venous infusion*

| $C_{max}$ (ng/ml) | $AUC_{0-\infty}$ (ng.h/ml) | $CL$ (ml/min) | $CL_r$ (ml/min) | $V_{SS}$ (l) | $t_{1/2}\beta$ (h) | $t_{1/2}Y$ (h) |
|---|---|---|---|---|---|---|
| 656 | 1856 | 51.6 | 25.1 | 548 | 1.79 | 198 |

Key: $C_{max}$: Peak plasma concentration.
$AUC$: Area under plasma concentration-time curve.
$CL$: Clearance. $CL_r$: Renal clearance.
$V_{SS}$: Volume of distribution at steady state.
$t_{1/2}\beta$: Half life of the second ($\beta$) phase.
$t_{1/2}Y$: Terminal half life.

The maximum concentrations of raltitrexed i creased linearly with dose over the clinical dose ran tested.

During repeated administration at three week inte vals, there was no clincally significant plasma acc mulation of raltitrexed in patients with normal ren function.

Apart from the expected intracellular polyglutam tion, raltitrexed was not metabolised and was excrete unchanged mainly in the urine, 40–50%. Raltitrexe was also excreted in the faeces with approximate 15% of the radioactive dose being eliminated over 10 day period. In the ¹⁴C-raltitrexed trial approximate half of the radiolabel was not recovered during th study period. This suggests that a proportion of th raltitrexed dose is retained within tissues, perhaps raltitrexed polyglutamates, beyond the end of th measurement period (29 days). Trace levels of radi abel were detected in red blood cells on Day 29.

Raltitrexed pharmacokinetics are independent age and gender. Pharmacokinetics have not bee evaluated in children.

Mild to moderate hepatic impairment led to a sma reduction in plasma clearance of less than 25%.

Mild to moderate renal impairment (creatinir clearance of 25 to 65 ml/min) led to a significa reduction (approximately 50%) in raltitrexed plasn clearance.

*Pre-clinical safety data:* Perivascular tolerance studies in animals did not reveal any significa irritant reaction.

*Acute toxicity:* The approximate $LD_{50}$ values for th mouse and rat are 875–1249 mg/kg and >500 mg/ respectively. In the mouse, levels of 750 mg/kg a above caused death by general intoxication.

*Chronic toxicity:* In one month continuous and s month intermittent dosing studies in the rat, toxic was related entirely to the cytotoxic nature of th drug. Principal target organs were the gastrointesti tract, bone marrow and the testes. In similar studi in the dog, cumulative dose levels similar to that us clinically, elicited only pharmacologically-relat changes to proliferating tissue. Target organs in th dog were therefore similar to the rat.

*Mutagenicity:* Tomudex was not mutagenic in th Ames test or in supplementary tests using *E. coli* chinese hamster ovary cells. Tomudex caused i creased levels of chromosome damage in an *in vit* assay of human lymphocytes. This effect was ameli rated by the addition of thymidine, thus confirming to be due to the anti-metabolic nature of the drug. *in vivo* micronucleus study in the rat indicated that cytotoxic dose levels, Tomudex is capable of causi chromosome damage in the bone marrow.

*Reproductive toxicology:* Fertility studies in the r indicate that Tomudex can cause impairment of ma fertility. Fertility returned to normal three months aft dosing ceased. Tomudex caused embryolethality a foetal abnormalities in pregnant rats.

*Carcinogenicity:* The carcinogenic potential of T mudex has not been evaluated.

**Pharmaceutical particulars**

*List of excipients:* Mannitol PhEur, USP; Dibas Sodium Phosphate Heptahydrate USP; Sodium H droxide PhEur, USNF.

*Incompatibilities:* There is no information on inco patibilities at present and therefore Tomudex shou not be mixed with any other drug.

*Shelf life:* The expiry life of Tomudex is 18 mont when stored at 2 to 8°C protected from light.

Once reconstituted, Tomudex is chemically stab for 24 hours at 25°C exposed to ambient light. F ɔrage recommendation, see Instructions for use/ ındling.

*ecial precautions for storage:* Refrigerate at 2–8°C, otected from light.

*ature and contents of container:* Tomudex is packed 5 ml clear neutral type I glass vials, with a omobutyl rubber closure and an aluminium crimp al with a plastic flip-off cover.

The vials are packed in individual cartons to protect e product from light.

*structions for use/handling:* Each vial, containing ng of raltitrexed, should be reconstituted with 4 ml sterile water for injections to produce a 0.5 mg/ml lution.

The appropriate dose of solution is diluted in 50–0 ml of either 0.9% sodium chloride or 5% glucose extrose) injection and administered by a short travenous infusion over a period of 15 minutes.

There is no preservative or bacteriostatic agent esent in Tomudex or the materials specified for constitution or dilution. Tomudex must therefore be constituted and diluted under aseptic conditions d it is recommended that solutions of Tomudex ould be used as soon as possible. Reconstituted mudex solution may be stored refrigerated (2–8°C) up to 24 hours.

In accordance with established guidelines, when uted in 0.9% sodium chloride of 5% glucose extrose) solution, it is recommended that adminis-tion of the admixed solution should commence as on as possible after admixing. The admixed solution ust be completely used or discarded within 24 hours reconstitution of Tomudex intravenous injection.

Reconstituted and diluted solutions do not need to protected from light.

Do not store partially used vials or admixed solu-ns for future patient use.

Any unused injection or reconstituted solution ould be discarded in a suitable manner for cytotox-.

Tomudex should be reconstituted for injection by ained personnel in a designated area for the recon-tution of cytotoxic agents. Cytotoxic preparations ch as Tomudex should not be handled by pregnant omen.

Reconstitution should normally be carried out in a rtial containment facility with extraction e.g. a minar air flow cabinet, and work surfaces should be vered with disposable plastic-backed absorbent per.

Appropriate protective clothing, including normal rgical disposable gloves and goggles, should be orn. In case of contact with skin, immediately wash oroughly with water. For splashes in the eye irrigate th clean water, holding the eyelids apart, for at least minutes. Seek medical attention.

Any spillages should be cleared up using standard ocedures.

Waste material should be disposed of by incinera-n in a manner consistent with the handling of totoxic agents.

**arketing authorisation number** 12619/0107.

**te of approval/revision of SPC** March 1997.

**gal category** POM.

## IVALAN*

**alitative and quantitative composition** Viloxazine drochloride equivalent to 50 mg Viloxazine

**armaceutical form** Tablet

**nical particulars**

*erapeutic indications:* Vivalan is indicated in the atment of symptoms of depressive illness espe-lly where sedation is not required.

*sology and method of administration:*

*lults:* Most patients respond to 300 mg/day prefer-ly taken as 200 mg in the morning and 100 mg at nchtime. Total daily dose should not exceed 400 mg d the last dose of the day should not be taken later an 6.00 pm.

*Elderly:* 100 mg/day initially. The initial dose should increased with caution under close supervision. If the normal maintenance dose may be sufficient produce a satisfactory clinical response.

*Children:* Vivalan is not recommended in children der 14 years of age.

*ntra-indications:* Mania, severe liver disease, his-y of peptic ulcer, recent myocardial infarction and ring breast feeding.

*ecial warnings and special precautions for use:* valan should be used with caution in patients with haemic heart disease and congestive cardiac fail-e, or any degree of heart block.

Caution is advised when administering Vivalan to tients with epilepsy, especially those receiving enytoin.

Patients posing a high suicidal risk require close initial supervision.

If surgery is necessary during therapy, the anaesthetist should be informed that the patient has received Vivalan.

*Interactions with other medicaments and other forms of interaction:* Vivalan should not be given concurrently with, or within 2 weeks of cessation of therapy with monoamine oxidase inhibitors.

Vivalan may decrease the antihypertensive effect of guanethidine, debrisoquine, bethanidine and possibly clonidine.

When Vivalan is co-administered with drugs which undergo hepatic metabolism via oxidative pathways, there is a possibility of an interaction. It may be necessary therefore to adjust the dose of such coadministered drugs which have narrow therapeutic margins, for example the dosage of phenytoin, carbamazepine and theophylline may need to be reduced.

On theoretical grounds, caution is advised when patients receiving L-DOPA are treated with Vivalan.

Most antidepressants have been shown to potentiate the central nervous depressant action of alcohol, and, therefore, patients should be advised of the risks involved in drinking alcohol whilst on antidepressant medication.

*Pregnancy and lactation:*

*Pregnancy:* There is no evidence as to the drug's safety in human pregnancy; do not use during pregnancy, especially during the first and third trimesters, unless there are compelling reasons.

*Lactation:* Vivalan should not be used during lactation.

*Effects on ability to drive and use machines:* Vivalan initially may impair alertness, and patients should be advised of the possible hazard when driving or operating machinery.

*Undesirable effects:* Nausea is frequently observed but may be transient. Headache and vomiting may also occur.

As improvement may not occur during the first 2 weeks of treatment, patients should be closely monitored during this period.

Anticholinergic side effects, such as dry mouth, disturbance of accommodation, tachycardia, constipation and hesitancy of micturition have been reported less frequently with viloxazine than with tricyclic antidepressants.

Cardiac arrhythmias and severe hypotension are less likely to occur with viloxazine than with tricyclic antidepressants in high dosage or in deliberate overdosage.

Adverse effects which have been reported rarely with viloxazine include exacerbation of anxiety and agitation, drowsiness, confusion, ataxia, dizziness, insomnia, tremor, paresthesia, sweating, musculoskeletal pain, mild hypertension and skin rashes.

Psychotic manifestations, including hypomania and aggressive behaviour may be exacerbated.

Two serious adverse effects possibly associated with Vivalan have been reported:

(a) Isolated cases of liver damage and jaundice associated with elevated transaminases.
(b) Convulsions

Withdrawal symptoms are rare but may include malaise, headache and vomiting.

*Overdose:* Vivalan is rapidly absorbed and gastric lavage should be carried out with minimum of delay. Overdosage should be treated on general principles with careful monitoring of vital functions, together with intensive supportive therapy where necessary. As the drug is almost exclusively excreted in urine, forced diuresis may be performed to reduce blood levels. There is no specific antidote.

**Pharmacological properties**

*Pharmacodynamic properties:* Vivalan belongs to a class of psychotropic agents, the bicyclics. It is well established that Vivalan selectively inhibits noradrenaline uptake at central and peripheral sites and there is some evidence that Vivalan facilitates release of neuronal stores of 5-hydroxytryptamine. However, the precise relationship of these properties to the clinical antidepressant activity of Vivalan is unclear. The overall profile of Vivalan is quite atypical and different from the classical tricyclic antidepressant drugs. In particular, Vivalan produces fewer significant central effects, has little anticholinergic activity and less sympathomimetic activity.

*Pharmacokinetic properties:* The plasma half-life of viloxazine following administration is in the region of 2 to 5 hours. Viloxazine is rapidly and extensively metabolised by two major metabolic pathways. One involves hydroxylation in the aromatic ring, the other hydroxylation in both aromatic and heterocyclic rings. None of the metabolites identified in man has any significant pharmacological activity in animals. Therefore, it seems likely that the parent compound alone is responsible for the observed antidepressant properties in man. The metabolites of viloxazine are almost exclusively eliminated by the kidneys as glucuronide conjugates. Viloxazine is not highly protein bound.

*Preclinical safety data:* None stated

**Pharmaceutical particulars**

*List of excipients:* Calcium phosphate BP; Glycerol PhEur; Magnesium stearate PhEur; Maize starch PhEur; Methyl hydroxypropylcellulose PhEur; Microcrystalline cellulose PhEur; Sodium starch glycollate BP; Titanium dioxide PhEur (E171).

*Incompatibilities:* Vivalan should not be given concurrently with, or within 2 weeks of cessation of therapy with monoamine oxidase inhibitors.

*Shelf life:* 5 years

*Special precautions for storage:* Store below 25°C

*Nature and contents of container:* HDPE bottle (100); Carton containing blister strips (10x10)

*Instructions for use/handling:* Use as directed by the prescriber.

**Marketing authorisation number** 12619/0081

**Date of approval/revision of SPC** 11 March 1997

**Legal category** POM

## ZESTORETIC* 20
## ZESTORETIC* 10

**Presentation** Zestoretic 20: White, round, biconvex, uncoated tablets containing 20 mg lisinopril as the dihydrate and 12.5 mg Hydrochlorothiazide PhEur. The inactive ingredients are calcium hydrogen phosphate, magnesium stearate, maize starch, pregelatinised maize starch and mannitol. The tablet is plain on one face and marked 'Zestoretic' on the reverse.

Zestoretic 10: Peach, round, biconvex, uncoated tablets containing 10 mg lisinopril as the dihydrate and 12.5 mg Hydrochlorothiazide PhEur. The inactive ingredients are calcium hydrogen phosphate, iron oxide, magnesium stearate, maize starch, pregelatinised maize starch and mannitol. The tablet is plain on one face and marked 'Zt 10' on the reverse.

**Uses** Zestoretic 20 and Zestoretic 10 are indicated in the management of mild to moderate hypertension in patients who have been stabilised on the individual components given in the same proportions.

*Mode of action:* Zestoretic is a fixed dose combination product containing lisinopril, an inhibitor of angiotensin converting enzyme (ACE) and hydrochlorothiazide, a thiazide diuretic. Both components have complementary modes of action and exert an additive antihypertensive effect.

Lisinopril is a peptidyl dipeptidase inhibitor. It inhibits the angiotensin converting enzyme (ACE) that catalyses the conversion of angiotensin I to the vasoconstrictor peptide, angiotensin II. Angiotensin II also stimulates aldosterone secretion by the adrenal cortex. Inhibition of ACE results in decreased concentrations of angiotensin II which results in decreased vasopressor activity and reduced aldosterone secretion. The latter decrease may result in an increase in serum potassium concentration.

While the mechanism through which lisinopril lowers blood pressure is believed to be primarily suppression of the renin-angiotensin-aldosterone system, lisinopril is antihypertensive even in patients with low-renin hypertension. ACE is identical to kininase II, an enzyme that degrades bradykinin. Whether increased levels of bradykinin, a potent vasodilatory peptide, play a role in the therapeutic effects of lisinopril remains to be elucidated.

Hydrochlorothiazide is a diuretic and an antihypertensive agent. It affects the distal renal tubular mechanism of electrolyte reabsorption and increases excretion of sodium and chloride in approximately equivalent amounts. Natriuresis may be accompanied by some loss of potassium and bicarbonate. The mechanism of the antihypertensive effect of the thiazides is unknown. Thiazides do not usually affect normal blood pressure.

When combined with other antihypertensive agents, additive falls in blood pressure may occur.

Concomitant administration of lisinopril and hydrochlorothiazide has little or no effect on the bioavailability of either drug. The combination tablet is bioequivalent to concomitant administration of the separate entities.

*Lisinopril:* Following oral administration of lisinopril, peak serum concentrations occur within about 7 hours. On multiple dosing lisinopril has an effective half life of accumulation of 12.6 hours. Declining serum concentrations exhibit a prolonged terminal phase which does not contribute to drug accumulation. This terminal phase probably represents saturable binding to ACE and is not proportional to dose. Lisinopril does not appear to bind to other serum proteins.

Impaired renal function decreases elimination of lisinopril, which is excreted via the kidneys, but this decrease become clinically important only when the glomerular filtration rate is below 30 ml/min. Older patients have higher blood levels and higher values for the area under the plasma concentration time curve than younger patients. Lisinopril can be removed by dialysis.

Based on urinary recovery, the mean extent of absorption of lisinopril is approximately 25%, with interpatient variability (6–60%) at all doses tested (5–80 mg).

Lisinopril does not undergo metabolism and absorbed drug is excreted unchanged entirely in the urine. Lisinopril absorption is not effected by the presence of food in the gastrointestinal tract.

Studies in rats indicate that lisinopril crosses the blood-brain barrier poorly.

*Hydrochlorothiazide:* When plasma levels have been followed for at least 24 hours, the plasma half-life has been observed to vary between 5.6 and 14.8 hours. At least 61% of the dose is eliminated unchanged within 24 hours. After oral hydrochlorothiazide, diuresis begins within 2 hours, peaks in about 4 hours and lasts 6 to 12 hours. Hydrochlorothiazide crosses the placental but not the blood-brain barrier.

**Dosage and administration**

*Adults:*

*Essential hypertension:* The usual dosage of Zestoretic 20 and Zestoretic 10 is one tablet, administered once daily. As with all other medication taken once daily, Zestoretic should be taken at approximately the same time each day.

In general, if the desired therapeutic effect cannot be achieved in a period of 2 to 4 weeks at this dose level, the dose can be increased in two tablets administered once daily.

*Dosage in renal insufficiency:* Thiazides may not be appropriate diuretics for use in patients with renal impairment and are ineffective at creatinine clearance values of 30 ml/min or below (i.e. moderate or severe renal insufficiency).

Zestoretic 20 and Zestoretic 10 are not to be used as initial therapy in any patient with renal insufficiency.

In patients with creatinine clearance of >30 and <80 ml/min, Zestoretic 20 or Zestoretic 10 may be used, but only after titration of the individual components.

*Prior diuretic therapy:* Symptomatic hypotension may occur following the initial dose of Zestoretic; this is more likely in patients who are volume and/or salt depleted as a result of prior diuretic therapy. If possible, the diuretic therapy should be discontinued for 2–3 days prior to initiation of therapy with lisinopril alone, in a 2.5 mg dose.

*Use in the elderly:* In clinical studies the efficacy and tolerability of lisinopril and hydrochlorothiazide, administered concomitantly, were similar in both elderly and younger hypertensive patients.

Lisinopril was equally effective in elderly (65 years or older) and non-elderly hypertensive patients. In elderly hypertensive patients, monotherapy with lisinopril was as effective in reducing diastolic blood pressure as monotherapy with either hydrochlorothiazide or atenolol. In clinical studies, age did not affect the tolerability of lisinopril.

*Paediatric use:* Safety and effectiveness in children have not been established.

**Contra-indications, warnings, etc**

*Contra-indications:* Zestoretic is contra-indicated in patients with anuria.

Zestoretic is contra-indicated in patients who are hypersensitive to any component of the product and in patients with a history of angioneurotic oedema relating to previous treatment with an angiotensin-converting enzyme inhibitor and in patients with hereditary or idiopathic angioedema.

Zestoretic is contra-indicated in patients who are hypersensitive to other sulphonamide-derived drugs.

Zestoretic is contra-indicated in pregnancy and treatment should be stopped if pregnancy is suspected. See also *Pregnancy and lactation* under *Precautions*.

*Precautions:*

*Hypotension and electrolyte/fluid imbalance:* As with all antihypertensive therapy, symptomatic hypotension may occur in some patients. This was rarely seen in uncomplicated hypertensive patients but is more likely in the presence of fluid or electrolyte imbalance, e.g. volume depletion, hyponatraemia, hypochloraemic alkalosis, hypomagnesaemia or hypokalaemia which may occur from prior diuretic therapy, dietary salt restriction, dialysis, or during intercurrent diarrhoea or vomiting. Periodic determination of serum electrolytes should be performed at appropriate intervals in such patients.

In patients at increased risk of symptomatic hypotension, initiation of therapy and dose adjustment should be monitored under close medical supervision.

Particular consideration should be given when therapy is administered to patients with ischaemic heart or cerebrovascular disease because an excessive fall in blood pressure could result in a myocardial infarction or cerebrovascular accident.

If hypotension occurs, the patient should be placed in the supine position and, if necessary, should receive an intravenous infusion of normal saline. A transient hypotensive response is not a contra-indication to further doses. Following restoration of effective blood volume and pressure, reinstitution of therapy at reduced dosage may be possible; or either of the components may be used appropriately alone.

As with other vasodilators, Zestoretic should be given with caution to patients with aortic stenosis or hypertrophic cardiomyopathy.

*Renal function impairment:* Thiazides may not be appropriate diuretics for use in patients with renal impairment and are ineffective at creatinine clearance values of 30 ml/min or below (i.e. moderate or severe renal insufficiency).

Zestoretic should not be administered to patients with renal insufficiency (creatinine clearance ≤80 ml/min) until titration of the individual components has shown the need for the doses present in the combination tablet.

In some patients with bilateral renal artery stenosis or stenosis of the artery to a solitary kidney, who have been treated with angiotensin converting enzyme inhibitors, increases in blood urea and serum creatinine, usually reversible upon discontinuation of therapy, have been seen. This is especially likely in patients with renal insufficiency. If renovascular hypertension is also present there is an increased risk of severe hypotension and renal insufficiency. In these patients, treatment should be started under close medical supervision with low doses and careful dose titration. Since treatment with diuretics may be a contributory factor to the above, renal function should be monitored during the first few weeks of Zestoretic therapy.

Some hypertensive patients with no apparent pre-existing renal disease have developed usually minor and transient increases in blood urea and serum creatinine when lisinopril has been given concomitantly with a diuretic. If this occurs during therapy with Zestoretic, the combination should be discontinued. Reinstitution of therapy at reduced dosage may be possible, or either of the components may be used appropriately alone.

The use of Zestoretic is not indicated in patients requiring dialysis for renal failure. A high incidence of anaphylactoid reactions has been reported in patients dialysed with high-flux membranes (e.g. AN69) and treated concomitantly with an ACE inhibitor. This combination should therefore be avoided.

*Hepatic disease:* Thiazides should be used with caution in patients with impaired hepatic function or progressive liver disease, since minor alterations of fluid and electrolyte balance may precipitate hepatic coma.

*Surgery/anaesthesia:* In patients undergoing major surgery or during anaesthesia with agents that produce hypotension, lisinopril may block angiotensin II formation secondary to compensatory renin release. If hypotension occurs and is considered to be due to this mechanism, it can be corrected by volume expansion.

*Metabolic and endocrine effects:* Thiazide therapy may impair glucose tolerance. Dosage adjustment of antidiabetic agents, including insulin, may be required.

Thiazides may decrease urinary calcium excretion and may cause intermittent and slight elevation of serum calcium. Marked hypercalcaemia may be evidence of hidden hyperparathyroidism. Thiazides should be discontinued before carrying out tests for parathyroid function.

Increases in cholesterol and triglyceride levels may be associated with thiazide diuretic therapy.

Thiazide therapy may precipitate hyperuricaemia and/or gout in certain patients. However, lisinopril may increase urinary uric acid and thus may attenuate the hyperuricaemic effect of hydrochlorothiazide.

*Hypersensitivity/angioneurotic oedema:* Angioneurotic oedema of the face, extremities, lips, tongue, glottis and/or larynx has been reported rarely in patients treated with angiotensin-converting enzyme inhibitors, including lisinopril. In such cases, Zestoretic should be discontinued promptly and appropriate monitoring should be instituted to ensure complete resolution of symptoms prior to dismissing the patient.

In those instances where swelling has been confined to the face and lips the condition generally resolved without treatment, although antihistamines have been useful in relieving symptoms.

Angioneurotic oedema associated with laryngeal oedema may be fatal. Where there is involvement of the tongue, glottis or larynx, likely to cause airway obstruction, appropriate emergency therapy should be administered promptly. This may include the administration of adrenaline and/or the maintenan of a patent airway. The patient should be under clo medical supervision until complete and sustain resolution of symptoms has occurred.

Angiotensin converting enzyme inhibitors cause higher rate of angioedema in black patients than non-black patients.

Patients with a history of angioedema unrelated ACE inhibitor therapy may be at increased risk angioedema while receiving an ACE inhibitor (s also *Contra-indications*).

In patients receiving thiazides, sensitivity reactic may occur with or without a history of allergy bronchial asthma. Exacerbation or activation of sy temic lupus erythematosus has been reported w the use of thiazides.

*Race:* Angiotensin converting enzyme inhibitors cau a higher rate of angioedema in black patients than non-black patients.

*Cough:* Cough has been reported with the use of A inhibitors. Characteristically, the cough is non-prod tive, persistent and resolves after discontinuation therapy. ACE inhibitor-induced cough should considered as part of the differential diagnosis cough.

*Pregnancy and lactation:* Zestoretic is contra-indicat in pregnancy and treatment should be stopped pregnancy is suspected.

ACE inhibitors can cause foetal and neonatal m bidity and mortality when administered to pregna women during the second and third trimesters. U of ACE inhibitors during this period has been asso ated with foetal and neonatal injury including hyp tension, renal failure, hyperkalaemia and/or sk hypoplasia in the newborn. Maternal oligohydra nios, presumably representing decreased foetal re function, has occurred and may result in limb contr tures, craniofacial deformations and hypoplastic lu development.

These adverse effects to the embryo and foetus not appear to have resulted from intrauterine A inhibitor exposure limited to the first trimester.

Infants whose mothers have taken lisinopril shou be closely observed for hypotension, oliguria a hyperkalaemia. Lisinopril, which crosses the placen has been removed from the neonatal circulation peritoneal dialysis with some clinical benefit, a theoretically may be removed by exchange tra fusion. There is no experience with the removal hydrochlorothiazide, which also crosses the placen from the neonatal circulation.

It is not known whether lisinopril is secreted human milk; however, thiazides do appear in hum milk. Because of the potential for serious reactions breast-fed infants, a decision should be made wheth to discontinue breast feeding or to discontin Zestoretic, taking into account the importance of drug to the mother.

*Serum potassium:* The potassium losing effect thiazide diuretics is usually attenuated by the pot sium conserving effect of lisinopril. The use potassium supplements, potassium-sparing age or potassium-containing salt substitutes, particula in patients with impaired renal function, may lead a significant increase in serum potassium. If conco itant use of Zestoretic and any of these agents deemed appropriate, they should be used with cauti and with frequent monitoring of serum potassium.

*Desensitisation:* Patients receiving ACE inhibit during desensitisation treatment (e.g. Hymenopte venom) have sustained anaphylactoid reactions. the same patients, these reactions have been avoid when ACE inhibitors were temporarily withheld b they reappeared upon inadvertent rechallenge.

*Lithium:* Lithium generally should not be given w diuretics or ACE inhibitors. Diuretic agents and A inhibitors reduce the renal clearance of lithium a add a high risk of lithium toxicity. Refer to prescribing information for lithium preparations fore use of such preparations.

*Other agents:* Indomethacin may diminish the a hypertensive effect of concomitantly-administe Zestoretic. In some patients with compromised re function who are being treated with non-steroi anti-inflammatory drugs (NSAIDs), the co-administ tion of lisinopril may result in a further deteriorat of renal function. The antihypertensive effect Zestoretic may be potentiated when given conco tantly with other agents likely to cause postu hypotension.

Thiazides may increase the responsiveness to t ocurarine.

*Side-effects:* Zestoretic is usually well tolerated. clinical studies, side effects have usually been m and transient, and in most instances have not requi interruption of therapy. The side effects that ha een observed have been limited to those reported reviously with lisinopril or hydrochlorothiazide.

One of the most common clinical side effects was izziness, which generally responded to dosage re-uction and seldom required discontinuation of ther-py.

Other side effects were headache, dry cough, fatigue nd hypotension including orthostatic hypotension.

Less common were diarrhoea, nausea, vomiting, ry mouth, rash, gout, palpitations, chest discomfort, nuscle cramps and weakness, paraesthesia, asthenia nd impotence.

Pancreatitis has been reported rarely with lisinopril nd with hydrochlorothiazide and, therefore, is a otential side effect of Zestoretic.

*lypersensitivity/angioneurotic oedema:* Angioneu-otic oedema of the face, extremities, lips, tongue, lottis and/or larynx has been reported rarely (see 'recautions').

A symptom complex has been reported which may nclude one or more of the following: fever, vasculitis, nyalgia, arthralgia/arthritis, a positive ANA, elevated SR, eosinophilia and leucocytosis; rash, photosensi-vity, or other dermatological manifestations may ccur.

*aboratory test findings:* Laboratory side effects have arely been of clinical importance. Occasional hyper-lycaemia, hyperuricaemia and hyper- or hypokalae-ia have been noted. Usually minor and transient ncreases in blood urea nitrogen and serum creatinine ave been seen in patients without evidence of pre-xisting renal impairment. If such increases persist, ey are usually reversible upon discontinuation of estoretic. Bone marrow depression, manifest as naemia and/or thrombocytopenia and/or leucopenia as been reported. Agranulocytosis has been rarely eported. Small decreases in haemoglobin and hae-natocrit have been reported frequently in hyperten-ve patients treated with Zestoretic but were rarely of linical importance unless another cause of anaemia o-existed. Rarely, elevations of liver enzymes and/or erum bilirubin have occurred, but a causal relation-hip to Zestoretic has not been established.

Other side-effects reported with the individual omponents alone, and which may be potential side-ffects with Zestoretic, are:

*lydrochlorothiazide:* Anorexia, gastric irritation, con-ipation, jaundice (intrahepatic cholestatic jaundice), ancreatitis, sialoadenitis, vertigo, xanthopsia, leuco-enia, agranulocytosis, thrombocytopenia, aplastic naemia, haemolytic anaemia, purpura, photosensi-vity, urticaria, necrotizing angiitis (vasculitis) (cuta-eous vasculitis), fever, respiratory distress including neumonitis and pulmonary oedema, anaphylactic eactions, hyperglycaemia, glycosuria, hyperuricae-ia, electrolyte imbalance including hyponatraemia, nuscle spasm, restlessness, transient blurred vision, enal failure, renal dysfunction and interstitial nephri-s.

*isinopril:* myocardial infarction or cerebrovascular ccident possibly secondary to excessive hypotension high risk patients, tachycardia, abdominal pain and ndigestion, mood alterations, mental confusion, ertigo have occurred; as with other angiotensin onverting enzyme inhibitors, taste disturbance and eep disturbance have been reported; bronchos-asm, rhinitis, sinusitis, alopecia, urticaria, diaphore-s, pruritus, psoriasis and severe skin disorders, ncluding pemphigus, toxic epidermal necrolysis, tevens-Johnson Syndrome and erythema multi-rme), have been reported; hyponatraemia, uraemia, iguria/anuria, renal dysfunction, acute renal failure, epatitis (hepatocellular or cholestatic), jaundice, and aemolytic anaemia.

*verdosage:* No specific information is available on e treatment of overdosage with Zestoretic. Treat-ent is symptomatic and supportive. Therapy with estoretic should be discontinued and the patient nould be kept under very close supervision. Thera-eutic measures depend on the nature and severity f the symptoms. Measures to prevent absorption nd methods to speed elimination should be em-loyed.

*Lisinopril:* The most likely features of overdosage ould be hypotension, electrolyte disturbance and enal failure. If severe hypotension occurs, the patient nould be placed in the shock position and an travenous infusion of normal saline should be given apidly. Treatment with angiotensin II (if available) ay be considered. Angiotensin converting enzyme hibitors may be removed from the general circula-on by haemodialysis. The use of high-flux polyacry-nitrile dialysis membranes should be avoided. erum electrolytes and creatinine should be moni-red frequently.

*Hydrochlorothiazide:* The most common signs and mptoms observed are those caused by electrolyte epletion (hypokalaemia, hypochloraemia, hypona-aemia) and dehydration resulting from excessive diuresis. If digitalis has also been administered hypo-kalaemia may accentuate cardiac arrhythmias.

**Pharmaceutical precautions** Zestoretic 20: Store below 30°C. Zestoretic 10: Store below 30°C, protected from light.

**Legal category** POM.

**Package quantities** Zestoretic 10 and Zestoretic 20: Calendar packs of 28 tablets (OP).

**Further information** Nil.

**Product licence numbers**
Zestoretic 20: 12619/0083
Zestoretic 10: 12619/0091

## ZESTRIL*

**Presentation** White, round, biconvex uncoated tab-lets, impressed with a heart shape plus a number denoting tablet strength on one side, containing 2.5 mg lisinopril as the dihydrate. The inactive ingre-dients are calcium hydrogen phosphate, magnesium stearate, maize starch and mannitol.

Pink, round, biconvex uncoated tablets, impressed with a heart shape plus a number denoting the tablet strength on one side and a bisecting line impressed on the other, containing 5 mg lisinopril as the dihy-drate. The inactive ingredients are calcium hydrogen phosphate, iron oxide, magnesium stearate, maize starch and mannitol.

Pink, round, biconvex uncoated tablets, impressed with a heart shape plus a number denoting the tablet strength and the trademark on one side, containing 10 mg lisinopril as the dihydrate. The inactive ingre-dients are calcium hydrogen phosphate, iron oxide, magnesium stearate, maize starch and mannitol.

Red, round, biconvex uncoated tablets, impressed with a heart shape plus a number denoting the tablet strength and the trademark on one side, containing 20 mg lisinopril as the dihydrate. The inactive ingre-dients are calcium hydrogen phosphate, iron oxide, magnesium stearate, maize starch and mannitol.

**Uses** *Indications:*
*Hypertension:* Zestril is indicated in the treatment of all grades of essential hypertension and renovascular hypertension. Zestril may be used alone or with other anti-hypertensive agents.

*Congestive heart failure:* Zestril is also indicated in the treatment of congestive heart failure as adjunctive therapy with non-potassium sparing diuretics and, where appropriate, digitalis. Treatment with Zestril should be initiated under close medical supervision (in hospital for severe heart failure).

*Acute myocardial infarction:* Zestril is indicated for the treatment of haemodynamically stable patients, de-fined as patients who are not in cardiogenic shock and who have a systolic blood pressure greater than 100 mmHg. Zestril may be initiated within 24 hours of the acute myocardial infarction to prevent the subse-quent development of left ventricular dysfunction or heart failure and to improve survival. Patients should receive, as appropriate, the standard recommended treatments such as thrombolytics, aspirin and beta-blocker.

Administration is by the oral route.

*Mode of action:* Lisinopril is a peptidyl dipeptidase inhibitor. It inhibits the angiotensin-converting en-zyme (ACE) that catalyses the conversion of angioten-sin I to the vasoconstrictor peptide, angiotensin II. Angiotensin II also stimulates aldosterone secretion by the adrenal cortex. Inhibition of ACE results in decreased concentrations of angiotensin II which results in decreased vasopressor activity and reduced aldosterone secretion. The latter decrease may result in an increase in serum potassium concentration.

While the mechanism through which lisinopril lowers blood pressure is believed to be primarily suppression of the renin-angiotensin-aldosterone-system, lisinopril is antihypertensive even in patients with low-renin hypertension. ACE is identical to kininase II, an enzyme that degrades bradykinin. Whether increased levels of bradykinin, a potent vasodilatory peptide, play a role in the therapeutic effects of lisinopril remains to be elucidated.

Angiotensin converting enzyme inhibitors may have a lesser effect on blood pressure in black hypertensive patients than in non-black hypertensive patients.

Following oral administration of lisinopril, peak serum concentrations occur within about 7 hours, although there was a trend to a small delay in time taken to reach peak serum concentrations in acute myocardial infarction patients. On multiple dosing lisinopril has an effective half life of accumulation of 12.6 hours.

Declining serum concentrations exhibit a prolonged terminal phase which does not contribute to drug accumulation. This terminal phase probably repre-sents saturable binding to ACE and is not proportional to dose. Lisinopril does not appear to bind to other serum proteins.

Impaired renal function decreases elimination of lisinopril, which is excreted via the kidneys, but this decrease becomes clinically important only when the glomerular filtration rate is below 30 ml/min. Older patients have higher blood levels and higher values for the area under the plasma concentration time curve than younger patients. Lisinopril can be re-moved by dialysis.

Based on urinary recovery, the mean extent of absorption of lisinopril is approximately 25%, with interpatient variability (6–60%) at all doses tested (5–80 mg).

Lisinopril does not undergo metabolism and ab-sorbed drug is excreted unchanged entirely in the urine. Lisinopril absorption is not affected by the presence of food in the gastrointestinal tract.

Studies in rats indicate that lisinopril crosses the blood-brain barrier poorly.

**Dosage and administration** Since absorption of Zestril tablets is not affected by food, the tablets may be administered before, during or after meals. Zestril should be administered in a single daily dose. As with all other medication taken once daily, Zestril should be taken at approximately the same time each day.

*Hypertension:* The need for dosage titration should be determined by measurement of the blood pressure just before the next dose.

*Essential and Renovascular Hypertension:* Treatment should be started with 2.5 mg once daily and adjusted to achieve optimal blood pressure control. For essen-tial hypertension, in general, if the desired therapeutic effect cannot be achieved in a period of 2 to 4 weeks on a certain dose level, the dose can be further increased.

A 2.5 mg dose seldom achieves a therapeutic response. The usual effective dose range is 10–20 mg once daily. The maximum recommended dose is 40 mg once daily.

*Diuretic treated patients:* If possible, the diuretic should be discontinued, or the dose reduced, 2 to 3 days before beginning therapy with Zestril (see 'Precautions') and may be resumed later if required.

*Use in the elderly:* Age alone does not appear to affect the efficacy or safety profile of Zestril. Thus, elderly patients should start treatment with Zestril as directed above.

*Congestive heart failure:* Zestril may be used as adjunctive therapy with non-potassium sparing diu-retics with or without digitalis.

*Initial dosage:* Treatment should be initiated under close medical supervision, with a recommended starting dose of 2.5 mg with subsequent dose titration.

In the treatment of severe or unstable congestive heart failure, Zestril should always be initiated in hospital under close medical supervision. Other pa-tients who may also be considered to be at higher risk should also have treatment initiated in hospital. These include patients who are on high dose loop diuretics (e.g. >80 mg frusemide) or on multiple diuretic ther-apy, have hypovolaemia, hyponatraemia (serum so-dium <130 mEq/l) or systolic blood pressure <90 mm Hg, are on high dose vasodilator therapy, have a serum creatinine >150 μmol/l or are aged 70 years or over.

If possible, the dose of diuretic should be reduced before beginning treatment. Blood pressure and renal function should be monitored closely both before and during treatment because severe hypotension and, more rarely, consequent renal failure have been reported with angiotensin-converting enzyme (ACE) inhibitors. The appearance of hypotension after the initial dose of Zestril does not preclude subsequent careful dose adjustment with the drug, following effective treatment of the hypotension.

*Maintenance dosage:* The dose should be gradually increased, depending on the patient's response, to the usual maintenance dose (5–20 mg). In clinical trials doses were adjusted at 4 week intervals in patients requiring an additional therapeutic effect. Dose adjustment should be based on the clinical response of individual patients.

*Acute myocardial infarction:* Treatment with Zestril may be started within 24 hours of the onset of symptoms. The first dose of Zestril is 5 mg given orally, followed by 5 mg after 24 hours, 10 mg after 48 hours and then 10 mg once daily thereafter. Patients with a low systolic blood pressure (120 mmHg or less) should be given a lower dose – 2.5 mg orally (see *Precautions*). If hypotension occurs (systolic blood pressure less than or equal to 100 mmHg), a daily maintenance dose of 5 mg may be given with temporary reductions to 2.5 mg if needed. If prolonged hypotension occurs (systolic blood pressure less than 90 mmHg for more than 1 hour), Zestril should be withdrawn.

Dosing should continue for six weeks. The benefit

appears to be greatest in patients with large myocardial infarctions and evidence of impaired left ventricular function. Patients who develop symptoms of heart failure, should continue with Zestril (see *Dosage and administration* for congestive heart failure).

Zestril is compatible with intravenous or transdermal glyceryl trinitrate.

*Impaired renal function:* Zestril is excreted by the kidney and should be used with caution in patients with renal insufficiency.

Zestril is dialysable (see *Precautions*). Dialysis patients may be given the usual dose of Zestril on dialysis days. On the days when patients are not on dialysis the dosage should be tailored to the blood pressure response.

*Paediatric use:* Zestril has not been studied for use in children.

## Contra-indications, warnings, etc

*Contra-indications:* Zestril is contra-indicated in pregnancy and treatment should be stopped if pregnancy is suspected. ACE inhibitors can cause foetal and neonatal morbidity and mortality when administered to pregnant women during the second and third trimesters. Use of ACE inhibitors during this period has been associated with foetal and neonatal injury including hypotension, renal failure, hyperkalaemia and/or skull hypoplasia in the newborn. Maternal oligohydramnios, presumably representing decreased foetal renal function, has occurred and may result in limb contractures, craniofacial deformations and hypoplastic lung development.

These adverse effects to the embryo and foetus do not appear to have resulted from intrauterine ACE inhibitor exposure limited to the first trimester.

Infants whose mothers have taken lisinopril should be closely observed for hypotension, oliguria and hyperkalaemia. Lisinopril which crosses the placenta, has been removed from the neonatal circulation by peritoneal dialysis with some clinical benefit, and theoretically may be removed by exchange transfusion.

Zestril is contra-indicated in patients who are hypersensitive to any component of this product, in patients with a history of angioneurotic oedema relating to previous ACE-inhibitor therapy and in patients with hereditary or idiopathic angioedema.

*Precautions:*
*Assessment of renal function:* Evaluation of the patient should include assessment of renal function prior to initiation of therapy and during treatment.

*Impaired renal function:* Zestril should be used with caution in patients with renal insufficiency, as they may require reduced or less frequent doses (see 'Dosage and Administration'). Close monitoring of renal function during therapy should be performed as deemed appropriate in those with renal insufficiency. In the majority, renal function will not alter, or may improve.

Renal failure has been reported in association with ACE inhibitors and has been mainly in patients with severe congestive heart failure or underlying renal disease, including renal artery stenosis. If recognised promptly and treated appropriately, renal failure is usually reversible.

In some patients with bilateral renal artery stenosis or stenosis of the artery to a solitary kidney, who have been treated with angiotensin converting enzyme inhibitors, increases in blood urea and serum creatinine, usually reversible upon discontinuation of therapy, have been seen. This is especially likely in patients with renal insufficiency. If renovascular hypertension is also present there is an increased risk of severe hypotension and renal insufficiency. In these patients, treatment should be started under close medical supervision with low doses and careful dose titration. Since treatment with diuretics may be a contributory factor to the above, they should be discontinued and renal function should be monitored during the first weeks of Zestril therapy.

Some hypertensive patients, with no apparent preexisting renal disease, have developed increases in blood urea and creatinine when Zestril has been given concurrently with a diuretic. Dosage reduction of Zestril and/or discontinuation of the diuretic may be required. This situation should raise the possibility of underlying renal artery stenosis.

*In acute myocardial infarction:* Treatment with lisinopril should not be initiated in patients with evidence of renal dysfunction, defined as serum creatinine concentration exceeding 177 μmol/l and/or proteinuria exceeding 500 mg/24 h. If renal dysfunction develops during treatment with Zestril (serum creatinine concentrations exceeding 265 μmol/l or a doubling from the pre-treatment value) then the physician should consider withdrawal of Zestril.

*Haemodialysis patients:* A high incidence of anaphylactoid relations has been reported in patients dialysed with high-flux membranes (e.g. AN69) and treated

concomitantly with an ACE inhibitor. This combination should therefore be avoided.

*Symptomatic hypotension:* Symptomatic hypotension was seen rarely in uncomplicated hypertensive patients. It is more likely to occur in patients who have been volume-depleted by diuretic therapy, dietary salt restriction, dialysis, diarrhoea, or vomiting. In these patients, by discontinuing diuretic therapy or significantly reducing the diuretic dose 2 to 3 days prior to initiating Zestril, the possibility of this occurrence is reduced.

Severe hypotension has been reported with ACE inhibitors mainly in patients with severe heart failure. Many of these patients were on high doses of loop diuretics, and some had hyponatraemia or functional renal impairment. In patients at risk, initiation of therapy and dose adjustment should be monitored under close medical supervision. If hypotension develops, the patient should be placed in a supine position. Volume repletion with oral fluids or intravenous normal saline may be required. Intravenous atropine may be necessary if there is associated bradycardia. Treatment with Zestril may be restarted with careful dose titration following restoration of effective blood volume and pressure.

Similar caution and close supervision may apply also to patients with ischaemic heart or cerebrovascular disease in whom severe hypotension could result in a myocardial infarct or cerebrovascular accident.

As with other vasodilators, Zestril should be given with caution to patients with aortic stenosis or hypertrophic cardiomyopathy.

In some patients with congestive heart failure who have normal or low blood pressure, additional lowering of systemic blood pressure may occur with Zestril. If such hypotension becomes symptomatic, a reduction of dose or discontinuation of Zestril may become necessary.

The appearance of hypotension after the initial dose of Zestril does not preclude subsequent careful dose adjustment with the drug after effective management of hypotension.

*Hypotension in acute myocardial infarction:* Treatment with lisinopril must not be initiated in acute myocardial infarction patients who are at risk of further serious haemodynamic deterioration after treatment with a vasodilator. These are patients with systolic blood pressure of 100 mmHg or lower or cardiogenic shock. During the first 3 days following the infarction, the dose should be reduced if the systolic blood pressure is 120 mmHg or lower. Maintenance doses should be reduced to 5 mg or temporarily to 2.5 mg if systolic blood pressure is 100 mmHg or lower. If hypotension persists (systolic blood pressure less than 90 mmHg for more than 1 hour) then Zestril should be withdrawn.

*Angioneurotic oedema:* has been reported with ACE inhibitors, including Zestril. In such cases, Zestril should be discontinued immediately and the patient observed. Where swelling is confined to the face, lips and mouth, the condition will usually resolve without further treatment, although antihistamines may be useful in relieving symptoms. These patients should be followed carefully until the swelling has resolved. However, angioedema associated with laryngeal oedema may be fatal. Where there is involvement of the tongue, glottis or larynx, likely to cause airways obstruction, emergency therapy should be administered promptly. This may include the administration of adrenaline and/or the maintenance of a patent airway. The patient should be under close medical supervision until complete and sustained resolution of symptoms has occurred.

Angiotensin converting enzyme inhibitors cause a higher rate of angioedema in black patients than in non-black patients.

Patients with a history of angioedema unrelated to ACE inhibitor therapy may be at increased risk of angioedema while receiving an ACE inhibitor (see also *Contra-indications*).

*Race:* Angiotensin converting enzyme inhibitors cause a higher rate of angioedema in black patients than in non-black patients.

*Cough:* Cough has been reported with the use of ACE inhibitors. Characteristically, the cough is non-productive, persistent and resolves after discontinuation of therapy. ACE inhibitor-induced cough should be considered as part of the differential diagnosis of cough.

*Surgery/anaesthesia:* In patients undergoing major surgery or during anaesthesia with agents that produce hypotension, Zestril blocks angiotensin II formation secondary to compensatory renin release. This may lead to hypotension which can be corrected by volume expansion.

*General:* Zestril should not be used in patients with aortic stenosis, cor pulmonale or outflow tract obstruction.

Where Zestril is used as a single agent in hypertension, Afro-Caribbean patients may show a reduce therapeutic response.

*Drug interactions:* Combination with other antihype tensive agents such as beta-blockers and diureti may increase the antihypertensive efficacy. Zest minimises the development of thiazide-induced h pokalaemia and hyperuricaemia. Indomethacin m reduce the antihypertensive efficacy of Zestril. some patients with compromised renal function w are being treated with non steroidal anti-inflammato drugs (NSAIDs), the co-administration of lisinopr may result in a further deterioration in renal functio

Zestril has been used with nitrates without signi cant clinical interaction.

As Zestril may reduce the elimination of lithiu serum levels of lithium should be monitored if lithiu salts are administered.

*Plasma potassium:* Usually remains within norm limits. If Zestril is given with a diuretic, the likeliho of diuretic-induced hypokalaemia may be lessene Zestril may elevate plasma potassium levels in p tients with renal failure. Potassium supplemen potassium-sparing diuretics and potassium conta ing salt substitutes are not recommended.

*Breast-feeding mothers:* Caution should be exercis if Zestril is given to breast-feeding mothers because is not known whether Zestril is excreted in hum milk.

*Side-effects:* Hypotension has occurred in associati with therapy with Zestril. This appears to occur certain specific sub-groups (see *Precautions*).

Angioneurotic oedema of the face, extremities, lip tongue, glottis and/or larynx has been reported rar (see *Precautions*).

Other hypersensitivity reactions have been ported.

*Other adverse reactions:* Dizziness, headache, di rhoea, cough, nausea and fatigue are the mo frequent. Other less frequent side effects include ra and asthenia. Rare side-effects include:

*Cardiovascular:* Myocardial infarction or cereb vascular accident possibly secondary to excessi hypotension in high risk patients (see *Precaution* palpitations, tachycardia.

*Digestive:* Abdominal pain and indigestion; mouth; hepatitis (hepatocellular or cholestatic); ja dice; pancreatitis; vomiting.

*Nervous system:* Mental confusion; mood alte tions; paraesthesia; vertigo. As with other angioten converting enzyme inhibitors, taste disturbance a sleep disturbances have been reported.

*Respiratory:* Bronchospasm; rhinitis; sinusitis.

*Skin:* Alopecia; diaphoresis; pruritus; urtica psoriasis and severe skin disorders have been ported, including pemphigus; toxic epidermal nec lysis; Stevens-Johnson Syndrome and erythe multiforme.

*Urogenital:* Impotence, oliguria/anuria, acute re failure, renal dysfunction, uraemia. There have be reports of haemolytic anaemia in patients taki lisinopril although no causal relationship has be established.

A symptom complex has been reported which m include one or more of the following: fever, vasculi myalgia, arthralgia/arthritis, a positive ANA, eleva ESR, eosinophilia and leucocytosis. Rash, photos sitivity or other dermatological manifestations m occur.

*Laboratory test findings:* Clinically important chang in standard laboratory parameters were rarely as ciated with administration of Zestril. Increases blood urea, serum creatinine, liver enzymes a serum bilirubin, usually reversible upon discontin tion of Zestril, have been seen.

Bone marrow depression, manifest as anaem and/or thrombocytopenia and or leucopenia has be reported. Agranulocytosis has been rarely reporte

Small decreases in haemoglobin and haematoc rarely of clinical importance unless another cause anaemia coexisted, have occurred.

Hyperkalaemia has occurred.

Hyponatraemia has occurred.

Patients receiving ACE inhibitors during desensi ation treatment (e.g. hymenoptera venom) have s tained anaphylactoid reactions. In the same patie these reactions have been avoided when ACE inh tors were temporarily withheld but they reappea on inadvertent rechallenge.

*Overdosage:* The symptoms of overdosage m include severe hypotension, electrolyte disturba and renal failure. After ingestion of an overdose, patient should be kept under very close supervisi Therapeutic measures depend on the nature a severity of the symptoms. Measures to prev absorption and methods to speed elimination sho e employed. If severe hypotension occurs, the patient ould be placed in the shock position and an travenous infusion of normal saline should be given pidly. Treatment with angiotensin II (if available) ay be considered. Angiotensin converting enzyme hibitors may be removed from the circulation by aemodialysis. The use of high-flux polyacrylonitrile ialysis membranes should be avoided. Serum elec-olytes and creatinine should be monitored fre-uently.

**narmaceutical precautions** Store below 30°C.

**egal category** POM.

**ackage quantities**
Tablets 20 mg: Calendar packs of 28 tablets (OP).
Tablets 10 mg: Calendar packs of 28 tablets (OP).
Tablets 5 mg: Calendar packs of 28 tablets (OP).
Tablets 2.5 mg: Calendar packs of 28 tablets (OP).

**urther information** Nil.

**oduct licence numbers**

| | |
|---|---|
| estril Tablets 2.5 mg | 12619/0084 |
| estril Tablets 5 mg | 12619/0085 |
| estril Tablets 10 mg | 12619/0086 |
| estril Tablets 20 mg | 12619/0087 |

## OLADEX* 3.6 mg

**ualitative and quantitative composition** Goserelin etate (equivalent to 3.6 mg goserelin).

**harmaceutical form**
Sterile depot.

**linical particulars**
*herapeutic indications:*
Prostate Cancer: Zoladex is indicated in the management of prostate cancer suitable for hormonal manipulation.
) Advanced breast cancer in pre- and peri-menopausal women suitable for hormonal manipulation.
i) Endometriosis: In the management of endometriosis, Zoladex alleviates symptoms, including pain, and reduces the size and number of endometrial lesions.
/) Endometrial thinning: Zoladex is indicated for the prethinning of the uterine endometrium prior to endometrial ablation or resection.
) Uterine fibroids: In conjunction with iron therapy in the haematological improvement of anaemic patients with fibroids prior to surgery.

*osology and method of administration:*
*dults:* One 3.6 mg depot of Zoladex injected subcu-neously into the anterior abdominal wall, every 28 ays. No dosage adjustment is necessary for patients ith renal or hepatic failure or in the elderly.

Endometriosis should be treated for a period of six onths only, since at present there are no clinical ata for longer treatment periods. Repeat courses ould not be given due to concern about loss of bone ineral density.

For use in endometrial thinning, four or eight weeks eatment. The second depot may be required for the atients with a large uterus or to allow flexible surgical ning.

For women who are anaemic as a result of uterine roids, Zoladex 3.6 mg depot with supplementary on may be administered for up to three months efore surgery.

*Children:* Zoladex is not indicated for use in children.

*ontra-indications:* Zoladex should not be given to atients with a known hypersensitivity to Zoladex or LHRH analogues. Zoladex should not be used in egnancy (see *Pregnancy and lactation* section).

*pecial warnings and special precautions for use:*
Zoladex is not indicated for use in children, as safety d efficacy have not been established in this group patients.

*Males:* The use of Zoladex in men at particular risk developing ureteric obstruction or spinal cord ompression should be considered carefully and the atients monitored closely during the first month of erapy. Consideration should be given to the initial se of an anti-androgen (e.g. cyproterone acetate 0 mg daily for three days before and three weeks ter commencement of Zoladex) at the start of LHRH alogue therapy since this has been reported to event the possible sequelae of the initial rise in rum testosterone. If spinal cord compression or nal impairment due to ureteric obstruction are esent or develop, specific standard treatment of ese complications should be instituted.

*Females:* The use of LHRH agonists in women may use a loss of bone mineral density. Currently ailable data on Zoladex indicate a mean loss of 6% in vertebral bone mineral density following a six onth course of treatment with progressive recovery a mean loss compared to baseline of 2.6% six onths after cessation of treatment.

Zoladex should be used with caution in women with known metabolic bone disease.

Zoladex may cause an increase in uterine cervical resistance, which may result in difficulty in dilating the cervix.

Currently, there are no clinical data on the effect of treating benign gynaecological conditions with Zoladex for periods in excess of six months.

*Interactions with other medicaments and other forms of interaction:* None known.

*Pregnancy and lactation:*
*Pregnancy:* Although reproductive toxicity in animals gave no evidence of teratogenic potential, Zoladex should not be used in pregnancy as there is a theoretical risk of abortion or foetal abnormality if LHRH agonists are used during pregnancy. Potentially fertile women should be examined carefully before treatment to exclude pregnancy. Non hormonal methods of contraception should be employed during therapy and in the case of endometriosis should be continued until menses are resumed.

*Lactation:* The use of Zoladex during breast feeding is not recommended.

*Effects on ability to drive and use machines:* There is no evidence that Zoladex results in impairment of these activities.

*Undesirable events:*
*General:* Rare incidences of hypersensitivity reactions, which may include some manifestations of anaphylaxis have been reported. Arthralgia has been reported. Skin rashes have been reported which are generally mild, often regressing without discontinuation of therapy. Changes in blood pressure, manifest as hypotension or hypertension, have been occasionally observed in patients administered Zoladex. These changes are usually transient, resolving either during continued therapy or after cessation of therapy with Zoladex. Rarely, such changes have been sufficent to require medical intervention including withdrawal of treatment from Zoladex.

Occasional local reactions include mild bruising at the subcutaneous injection site.

*Males:* Pharmacological effects in men include hot flushes and a decrease in libido, seldom requiring withdrawal of therapy. Breast swelling and tenderness have been noted infrequently. Initially, prostate cancer patients may experience a temporary increase in bone pain, which can be managed symptomatically. Isolated cases of ureteric obstruction and spinal cord compression have been recorded.

*Females:* Pharmacological effects in women include hot flushes and sweating, and loss in libido, seldom requiring withdrawal of therapy. Headaches, mood changes including depression, vaginal dryness and change in breast size have been noted.

Initially breast cancer patients may experience a temporary increase in signs and symptoms, which can be managed symptomatically. In women with fibroids, degeneration may occur.

Rarely, breast cancer patients with metastases have developed hypercalcaemia on initiation of therapy.

Rarely, some women may enter the menopause during treatment with LHRH analogues and do not resume menses on cessation of therapy. This may simply be a physiological change.

*Overdosage:* There is no human experience of overdosage. Animal tests suggest that no effect other than the intended therapeutic effects on sex hormone concentration and on the reproductive tract will be evident with higher doses of Zoladex. If overdosage occurs, this should be managed symptomatically.

**Pharmacological properties**
*Pharmacodynamic properties:* Zoladex (D-Ser(Bu$^t$)$^6$ Azgly$^{10}$ LHRH) is a synthetic analogue of naturally occurring LHRH. On chronic administration Zoladex results in inhibition of pituitary LH secretion leading to a fall in serum testosterone concentrations in males and serum oestradiol concentrations in females. This effect is reversible on discontinuation of therapy. Initially, Zoladex, like other LHRH agonists, may transiently increase serum testosterone concentration in men and serum oestradiol concentration in women.

During early treatment with Zoladex some women may experience vaginal bleeding of variable duration and intensity. Such bleeding probably represents oestrogen withdrawal bleeding and is expected to stop spontaneously.

In men by around 21 days after the first depot injection testosterone concentrations have fallen to within the castrate range and remain suppressed with continuous treatment every 28 days. This inhibition leads to prostate tumour regression and symptomatic improvement in the majority of patients.

In women serum oestradiol concentrations are suppressed by around 21 days after the first depot injection and, with continuous treatment every 28 days, remain suppressed at levels comparable with those observed in postmenopausal women. This suppression is associated with a response in hormone dependent advanced breast cancer, uterine fibroids and endometriosis. It will produce endometrial thinning and will result in amenorrhoea in the majority of patients.

Zoladex in combination with iron has been shown to induce amenorrhoea and improve haemoglobin concentrations and related haematological parameters in women with fibroids who are anaemic. The combination produced a mean haemoglobin concentration 1 g/dl above that achieved by iron therapy alone.

*Pharmacokinetic properties:* The bioavailability of Zoladex is almost complete. Administration of a depot every four weeks ensures that effective concentrations are maintained with no tissue accumulations. Zoladex is poorly protein bound and has a serum elimination half-life of two to four hours in subjects with normal renal function. The half-life is increased in patients with impaired renal function. For the compound given monthly in a depot formulation, this change will have minimal effect. Hence, no change in dosing is necessary in these patients. There is no significant change in pharmacokinetics in patients with hepatic failure.

*Preclinical safety data:* Following long-term repeated dosing with Zoladex, an increased incidence of benign pituitary tumours has been observed in male rats. Whilst this finding is similar to that previously noted in this species following surgical castration, any relevance to man has not been established.

In mice, long term repeated dosing with multiples of the human dose produced histological changes in some regions of the digestive system manifested by pancreatic islet cell hyperplasia and a benign proliferative condition in the pyloric region of the stomach, also reported as a spontaneous lesion in this species. The clinical relevance of these findings is unknown.

**Pharmaceutical particulars**
*List of excipients:* lactide/glycolide co-polymer.

*Incompatibilities:* None known.

*Shelf life:* 2 years.

*Special precautions for storage:* Store below 25°C.

*Nature and contents of container:* Single dose syringe applicator.

*Instructions for use handling:* Use as directed by the prescriber. Use only if pouch is undamaged. Use immediately after opening pouch.

**Marketing authorisation number** 12619/0088.

**Date of approval/revision of SPC** May 1996.

**Legal category** POM.

## ZOLADEX* LA

**Qualitative and quantitative composition** Each depot contains goserelin acetate equivalent to 10.8 mg goserelin.

**Pharmaceutical form** Sustained release sterile depot.

**Clinical particulars**
*Therapeutic indication:* Zoladex LA is indicated for prostate cancer suitable for hormonal manipulation.

*Posology and method of administration:*

*Adult males (including the elderly):* One depot of Zoladex LA injected subcutaneously into the anterior abdominal wall every 12 weeks.

*Children:* Zoladex LA is not indicated for use in children.

*Renal impairment:* No dosage adjustment is necessary for patients with renal impairment.

*Hepatic impairment:* No dosage adjustment for patients with hepatic impairment.

*Contra-indications:* Zoladex LA should not be given to patients with a known hypersensitivity to Zoladex or to other LHRH analogues.

*Special warnings and special precautions for use:* Zoladex LA is not indicated for use in females, since there is insufficient evidence of reliable suppression of serum oestradiol. For female patients requiring treatment with goserelin, refer to the prescribing information for Zoladex 3.6 mg.

Zoladex LA is not indicated for use in children, as safety and efficacy have not been established in this group of patients.

The use of Zoladex LA in patients at particular risk of developing ureteric obstruction or spinal cord compression should be considered carefully and the patients monitored closely during the first month of therapy. Consideration should be given to the initial use of an antiandrogen (e.g. cyproterone acetate 300 mg daily for three days before and three weeks after commencement of Zoladex) at the start of LHRH analogue therapy since this has been reported to prevent the possible sequelae of the initial rise in serum testosterone. If spinal cord compression or renal impairment due to ureteric obstruction are present or develop, specific standard treatment of these complications should be instituted.

*Interaction with other medicaments and other forms of interaction:* None known.

*Pregnancy and lactation:* Zoladex LA is not indicated for use in females.

*Effects on ability to drive and use machinery:* There is no evidence that Zoladex LA results in impairment of ability to drive or operate machinery.

*Undesirable effects:* Rare incidences of hypersensitivity reactions, which may include some manifestations of anaphylaxis, have been reported. Pharmacological effects in men include hot flushes and a decrease in libido, seldom requiring withdawal of therapy. Breast swelling and tenderness have been noted infrequently. Initially, prostate cancer patients may experience a temporary increase in bone pain, which can be managed symptomatically. Isolated cases of spinal cord compression have been recorded.

Changes in blood pressure, manifest as hypotension or hypertension, have been occasionally observed in patients administered Zoladex. The changes are usually transient, resolving either during continued therapy or after cessation of therapy with Zoladex. Rarely, such changes have been sufficient to require medical intervention, including withdrawal of treatment from Zoladex.

Although not reported by patients in the clinical trial program of Zoladex LA, following the administration of Zoladex 3.6 mg, arthralgia, skin rashes which are generally mild and often regress without discontinuation of therapy, and isolated cases of ureteric obstruction have been recorded.

*Overdose:* There is no human experience of overdosage. Animal tests suggest that no effect other than the intended therapeutic effects on sex hormone concentrations and on the reproductive tract will be evident with higher doses of Zoladex LA. If overdosage occurs, this should be managed symptomatically.

### Pharmacological properties

*Pharmacodynamic properties:* Zoladex (D-Ser(Bu$^t$)$^6$ Azgly$^{10}$ LHRH) is a synthetic analogue of naturally occurring luteinising-hormone releasing hormone (LHRH). On chronic administration Zoladex LA results in inhibition of pituitary luteinising hormone secretion leading to a fall in serum testosterone concentrations in males. Initially, Zoladex LA like other LHRH agonists transiently increases serum testosterone concentrations.

In men by around 21 days after the first depot injection, testosterone concentrations have fallen to within the castrate range and remain suppressed with treatment every 12 weeks.

*Pharmacokinetic properties:* Administration of Zoladex LA every 12 weeks ensures that exposure to goserelin is maintained with no clinically significant accumulation. Zoladex is poorly protein bound and has a serum elimination half-life of two to four hours in subjects with normal renal function. The half-life is increased in patients with impaired renal function. For the compound given in a 10.8 mg depot formulation every 12 weeks this change will not lead to any accumulation. Hence, no change in dosing is necessary in these patients. There is no significant change in pharmacokinetics in patients with hepatic failure.

*Preclinical safety data:* Following long-term repeated dosing with Zoladex, an increased incidence of benign pituitary tumours has been observed in male rats. Whilst this finding is similar to that previously noted in this species following surgical castration, any relevance to humans has not been established.

In mice, long term repeated dosing with multiples of the human dose produced histological changes in some regions of the digestive system. This is manifested by pancreatic islet cell hyperplasia and a benign proliferative condition in the pyloric region of the stomach, also reported as a spontaneous lesion in this species. The clinical relevance of these findings is unknown.

### Pharmaceutical particulars

*List of excipients:* A blend of high and low molecular weight lactide/glycolide copolymers.

*Incompatibilities:* None known.

*Shelf life:* 24 months.

*Special precautions for storage:* Store below 25˚C.

*Nature and contents of container:* Zoladex LA is supplied as a single dose syringe applicator in a sealed pouch which contains a desiccant.

*Instructions for use/handling:* Use as directed by the prescriber. Use only if pouch is undamaged. Use immediately after opening pouch.

**Marketing authorisation number** 12619/0103.

**Date of approval/revision of SPC** 9 May 1995.

**Legal category** POM.

## ZOMIG* ▼

**Qualitative and quantitative composition** Tablets for oral administration containing 2.5 mg of zolmitriptan.

**Pharmaceutical form** Tablets.

### Clinical particulars

*Therapeutic indications:* Zomig is indicated for the acute treatment of migraine with or without aura.

*Posology and method of administration:* The recommended dose of Zomig to treat a migraine attack is 2.5 mg.

If symptoms persist or return within 24 hours, a second dose has been shown to be effective. If a second dose is required, it should not be taken within 2 hours of the initial dose.

If a patient does not achieve satisfactory relief with 2.5 mg doses, subsequent attacks can be treated with 5 mg doses of Zomig.

In those patients who respond, significant efficacy is apparent within 1 hour of dosing.

Zomig is equally effective whenever the tablets are taken during a migraine attack; although it is advisable that Zomig tablets are taken as early as possible after the onset of migraine headache.

In the event of recurrent attacks, it is recommended that the total intake of Zomig in a 24 hour period should not exceed 15 mg.

Zomig is not indicated for prophylaxis of migraine.

*Use in children:* Safety and efficacy of Zomig in paediatric patients have not been established.

*Use in patients aged over 65 years:* Safety and efficacy of Zomig in individuals aged over 65 years have not been systematically evaluated.

*Patients with hepatic impairment:* There is no clinical or pharmacokinetic experience in patients with hepatic impairment treated with Zomig.

*Patients with renal impairment:* No dosage adjustment required (see *Pharmacokinetic properties*).

*Contra-indications:* Zomig is contra-indicated in patients with known hypersensitivity to any component of the product.

Zomig must not be given to patients with uncontrolled hypertension.

*Special warnings and special precautions for use:* Zomig should only be used where a clear diagnosis of migraine has been established. Care should be taken to exclude other potentially serious neurological conditions. There are no data on the use of Zomig in hemiplegic or basilar migraine.

Zomig should not be given to patients with symptomatic Wolff-Parkinson-White syndrome or arrhythmias associated with other cardiac accessory conduction pathways.

This class of compounds (5HT$_{1D}$ agonists) has been associated with coronary vasospasm, as a result, patients with ischaemic heart disease were excluded from clinical trials. Zomig is, therefore, not recommended in this patient group. In patients in whom unrecognised coronary artery disease is likely, cardiovascular evaluation prior to commencement of treatment with 5HT$_{1D}$ agonists is recommended.

As with other 5HT$_{1D}$ agonists, atypical sensations over the precordium (see *Undesirable effects*) have been reported after the administration of zolmitriptan, but in clinical trials these have not been associated with arrhythmias or ischaemic changes on ECG. Zomig may cause mild, transient increases in blood pressure (which may be more pronounced in the elderly), however, this has not been associated with clinical sequelae in the clinical trial programme.

*Interactions with other medicaments and other forms of interaction:* There is no evidence that concomitant use of migraine prophylactic medications has any effect on the efficacy or unwanted effects of Zomig (for example beta blockers, oral dihydroergotamine, pizotifen).

The pharmacokinetics and tolerability of Zomig were unaffected by acute symptomatic treatments such as paracetamol, metoclopramide and ergotamine. However, it is recommended that patients should leave at least 6 hours between taking an ergotamine preparation and starting Zomig, and vice versa. Concomitant administration of other 5HT$_{1D}$ agonists within 12 hours of Zomig treatment should be avoided.

Following administration of moclobemide, a specific MAO-A inhibitor, there was a small increase (26%) in AUC for zolmitriptan and a 3-fold increase in AUC of the active metabolite. Therefore, a maximum intake of 7.5 mg Zomig in 24 hours is recommended in patients taking an MAO-A inhibitor.

*Pregnancy and lactation:*
*Pregnancy:* Zomig should be used in pregnancy only if the benefits to the mother justify potential risk to the foetus. There are no studies in pregnant women, but there is no evidence of teratogenicity in animal studies. (See *Preclinical safety data*).

*Lactation:* Studies have shown that zolmitriptan passes into the milk of lactating animals. No data exist

for passage of zolmitriptan into human breast m Therefore, caution should be exercised when adm istering Zomig to women who are breast-feeding

*Effects on ability to drive and use machines:* Th was no significant impairment of performance psychomotor tests with doses up to 20 mg Zom Use is unlikely to result in an impairment of the abi of patients to drive or operate machinery. Howeve should be taken into account that somnolence m occur.

*Undesirable effects:* Zomig is well tolerated. Adve reactions are typically mild/moderate, transient, serious and resolve spontaneously without additio treatment. Possible adverse reactions tend to oc within 4 hours of dosing and are no more frequ following repeated dosing.

The following adverse reactions have been the m commonly reported: nausea; dizziness; somnolen warm sensation; asthenia; dry mouth.

Abnormalities or disturbances of sensation ha been reported; heaviness, tightness or pressure m occur in the throat, neck, limbs and chest (with evidence of ischaemic changes on ECG), as m myalgia, muscle weakness, paraesthesia and dysa thesia.

*Overdose:* Volunteers receiving single oral doses 50 mg commonly experienced sedation.

The elimination half-life of zolmitriptan tablets is to 3 hours, (see *Pharmacokinetic properties*) a therefore monitoring of patients after overdose w Zomig tablets should continue for at least 15 hours while symptoms or signs persist.

There is no specific antidote to zolmitriptan . cases of severe intoxication, intensive care procedu are recommended, including establishing and ma taining a patent airway, ensuring adequate oxyge tion and ventilation, and monitoring and support the cardiovascular system.

### Pharmacological properties

*Pharmacodynamic properties:* In pre-clinical studi zolmitriptan has been demonstrated to be a select agonist for the vascular human recombinant 5HT and 5HT$_{1D\beta}$ receptor subtypes. Zolmitriptan is a h affinity 5HT$_{1D}$ receptor agonist with modest affinity 5HT$_{1A}$ receptors. Zolmitriptan has no significant af ity (as measured by radioligand binding assays) pharmacological activity at 5HT$_2$-, 5HT$_3$-, 5HT$_4$-, alph , alpha$_2$-, or beta$_1$-, adrenergic; H$_1$-, H$_2$-, histamin muscarinic; dopaminergic$_1$, or dopaminergic$_2$ rec tors. The 5HT$_{1D\alpha}$ receptor is predominately loca presynaptically at both the peripheral and cent synapses of the trigeminal nerve and preclini studies have shown that zolmitriptan is able to ac both these sites.

*Pharmacokinetic properties:* Zolmitriptan is rapi and well absorbed (at least 64%) after oral administ tion to man. The mean absolute bioavailability of parent compound is approximately 40%. There is active metabolite (183C91, the N-desmethyl meta lite) which is also a 5HT$_{1D}$ agonist and is 2 to 6 tim as potent, in animal models, as zolmitriptan.

In healthy subjects, when given as a single do zolmitriptan and its active metabolite 183C91, disp dose-proportional AUC and C$_{max}$ over the dose ran 2.5 to 50 mg. Absorption is rapid with 75% of C achieved within 1 hour and plasma concentratio are sustained subsequently for 4 to 6 hours. Zolmit tan absorption is unaffected by the presence of fo There is no evidence of accumulation on multi dosing of zolmitriptan.

Zolmitriptan is eliminated largely by hepatic b transformation followed by urinary excretion of metabolites. There are three major metabolites: indole acetic acid, (the major metabolite in plas and urine), the N-oxide and N-desmethyl analogu The N-desmethylated metabolite (183C91) is act whilst the others are not. Plasma concentrations 183C91 are approximately half those of the par drug, hence it would therefore be expected to cont ute to the therapeutic action of Zomig. Over 60% single oral dose is excreted in the urine (mainly as indole acetic acid metabolite) and about 30% in faec mainly as unchanged parent compound.

Following intravenous administration, the me total plasma clearance is approximately 10 ml/min of which one third is renal clearance. Renal cleara is greater than glomerular filtration rate suggesti renal tubular secretion. The volume of distribut following intravenous administration is 2.4 L Plasma protein binding is low (approximately 25 The mean elimination half-life of zolmitriptan is 2.5 3 hours. The half-lives of its metabolites are simi suggesting their elimination is formation-rate limit

Renal clearance of zolmitriptan and all its meta lites is reduced (7 to 8 fold) in patients with moder to severe renal impairment compared to heal subjects, although the AUC of the parent compou and the active metabolite were only slightly hig (16 and 35% respectively) with a 1 hour increase f-life to 3 to 3.5 hours. These parameters are within e ranges seen in healthy volunteers.

n a small group of healthy individuals there was no armacokinetic interaction with ergotamine. Con- mitant administration of Zomig with ergotamine/ ffeine was well tolerated and did not result in any crease in adverse events or blood pressure changes compared with Zomig alone.

Selegiline, an MAO-B inhibitor, and fluoxetine (a ective serotonin reuptake inhibitor; SSRI) had no ect on the pharmacokinetic parameters of zolmitrip-

The pharmacokinetics of zolmitriptan in healthy erly subjects were similar to those in healthy young unteers.

clinical safety data: An oral teratology study of mig has been conducted. At the maximum tolerated ses of Zomig, 1200 mg/kg/day (AUC 605 μg/ml.h : prox. 3700 x AUC of the human maximum recom- mended daily intake of 15 mg) and 30 mg/kg/day (AUC 4.9 μg/ml.h : approx. 30 x AUC of the human maximum recommended daily intake of 15 mg) in rats and rabbits, respectively, no signs of teratogenicity were apparent.

Five genotoxicity tests have been performed. It was concluded that Zomig is not likely to pose any genetic risk in humans.

Carcinogenicity studies in rats and mice were conducted at the highest feasible doses and gave no suggestion of tumorogenicity.

Reproductive studies in male and female rats, at dose levels limited by toxicity, revealed no effect on fertility.

**Pharmaceutical particulars**

*List of excipients:* The following excipients are con- tained in each tablet as indicated: hydroxypropyl methylcellulose; iron oxide–yellow; lactose; magne- sium stearate; microcrystalline cellulose; polyethyl- ene glycol (400 and 8000); sodium starch glycollate; titanium dioxide.

*Incompatibilities:* None known

*Shelf-life:* 24 months when stored below 30°C.

*Special precautions for storage:* Store below 30°C.

*Nature and contents of container:* carton containing a strip of 3 tablets; carton containing 2 strips of 3 tablets (with wallet).

*Instructions for use/handling:* No specific instructions.

**Marketing authorisation number** 12619/0116

**Date of approval/revision of SPC** 7 March 1997

**Legal Category** POM

*Trade Mark*

# ODE OF PRACTICE FOR THE PHARMACEUTICAL INDUSTRY

**erative Date: 1 January 1996**

**RODUCTION**

**omoting Health**

he commitment of Britain's pharmaceutical ustry to providing high quality effective medicines ngs major benefits to both the health of the nation the country's economy.

he National Health Service spends over £4 billion ear on medicines yet this represents less than 11 cent of its total expenditure. Medicine exports are rth nearly £4 billion a year – the United Kingdom's ond largest foreign exchange earner in nufactured goods. Five of the top twenty prescribed dicines worldwide were discovered in Britain.

nvestment into researching and developing new ducts in the UK is now running at around £1.5 ion a year and each new medicine takes an average welve years to develop before it is licensed for use doctors, with no guarantee of commercial success.

s vital therefore that the pharmaceutical industry eps the medical profession informed about its ducts and promotes their rational use.

**e Association of the British Pharmaceutical lustry and its Code of Practice**

he Association of the British Pharmaceutical lustry (ABPI) is the trade association representing nufacturers of prescription medicines. It was med in 1930 and now represents more than 100 mpanies which produce 95 per cent of the dicines supplied to the National Health Service.

he ABPI Code of Practice for the Pharmaceutical ustry has been regularly revised since its inception 1958 and is drawn up in consultation with the British dical Association, the Royal Pharmaceutical ciety of Great Britain and the Medicines Control ency of the Department of Health.

t is a condition of membership of the ABPI to abide the Code in both the spirit and the letter. Companies ich are not members of the Association may give ir formal agreement to abide by the Code and cept the jurisdiction of the Prescription Medicines de of Practice Authority and about fifty have done Thus the Code is accepted by virtually all armaceutical companies operating in the UK.

**suring High Standards**

The aim of the Code of Practice for the armaceutical Industry is to ensure that the omotion of medicines to members of the health fessions and to administrative staff is carried out a responsible, ethical and professional manner. The de recognises and seeks to achieve a balance tween the needs of patients, industry, health fessionals and the general public, bearing in mind political and social environment within which the ustry operates and the statutory controls covering dicines.

Strong support is given to the Code by the industry h all companies devoting considerable resources ensure that their promotional activities comply with Any complaint made against a company under the de is regarded as a serious matter by both that mpany and the industry as a whole. A number of nctions may be applied against a company ruled in each of the Code.

Companies must ensure that all relevant personnel appropriately trained in the requirements of the de and have strict internal procedures under which promotional material and activities are reviewed to sure compliance with the Code and the appropriate al requirements. The Code reflects and extends ll beyond the legal requirements controlling the vertising of medicines.

The Code incorporates the principles set out in:

- the International Federation of Pharmaceutical Manufacturers Associations' (IFPMA) Code of Pharmaceutical Marketing Practices
- the European Federation of Pharmaceutical Industries' Associations' (EFPIA) European Code of Practice for the Promotion of Medicines
- the European Community Directive on the advertising of medicinal products for human use (92/28/EEC) and
- the World Health Organisation (WHO) Ethical criteria for medicinal drug promotion.

**onitoring the Code of Practice**

The Code is administered by the Prescription edicines Code of Practice Authority which is sponsible for the provision of advice, guidance, nciliation and training on the Code as well as for complaints procedure. Complaints which are ade under the Code about promotional material or promotional activities of companies are nsidered by the Code of Practice Panel and, where quired, by the Code of Practice Appeal Board. ports on completed cases are published quarterly the Authority and are available on request.

Complaints about the promotion of medicines should be submitted to the Director of the Prescription Medicines Code of Practice Authority, 12 Whitehall, London SW1A 2DY, telephone 0171 930 9677, facsimile 0171 930 4554.

**Guidance on the interpretation of the Code appears as supplementary information to the text in italics.**

## PROVISIONS OF THE CODE OF PRACTICE

**Clause 1 Scope of Code and Definition of Certain Terms**

**1.1** This Code applies to the promotion of medicines to members of the United Kingdom health professions and to appropriate administrative staff and to information made available to the general public about medicines so promoted.

It does not apply to the promotion of over-the-counter medicines to members of the health professions when the object of that promotion is to encourage their purchase by members of the general public.

*Clause 1.1 Scope of the Code*

*For the purposes of the application of the Code, the United Kingdom includes the Channel Islands and the Isle of Man.*

*The Code applies to the promotion of medicines to members of the health professions and to appropriate administrative staff as specified in Clause 1.1. This includes promotion at meetings for UK residents held outside the UK. It also applies to promotion to UK health professionals and to administrative staff at international meetings held outside the UK, except that the promotional material distributed at such meetings will need to comply with local requirements.*

*The Code does not apply to the promotion of over-the-counter medicines to members of the health professions when the object of that promotion is to encourage their purchase by members of the general public as specified in Clause 1.1. Thus, for example an advertisement to doctors for an over-the-counter medicine does not come within the scope of the Code if its purpose is to encourage doctors to recommend the purchase of the medicine by patients. Where the advertisement is designed to encourage doctors to prescribe the medicine, then it comes within the scope of the Code.*

*Advertisements for over-the-counter medicines to pharmacists are outside the scope of the Code. Advertisements to pharmacists for other medicines come within the scope of the Code.*

*Clause 1.1 Journals with an International Distribution*

*The Code applies to the advertising of medicines in professional journals which are published in the UK and/or intended for a UK audience.*

*International journals which are produced in English in the UK are subject to the Code even if only a small proportion of their circulation is to a UK audience. It is helpful in these circumstances to indicate that the information in the advertisement is consistent with the UK marketing authorisation.*

*Where a journal is published in the UK but intended for distribution solely to overseas countries local requirements and/or the requirements of the International Federation of Pharmaceutical Manufacturers Associations' (IFPMA) Code of Pharmaceutical Marketing Practices should be borne in mind.*

*Clause 1.1 Advertising to the Public and Advertising Over-the-Counter Medicines to Health Professionals and the Retail Trade*

*The promotion of medicines to the general public for self medication is covered by the Code of Standards of Advertising Practice for Over-the-Counter Medicines of the Proprietary Association of Great Britain (PAGB). The PAGB also has a Code of Practice for Advertising Over-the-Counter Medicines to Health Professionals and the Retail Trade.*

*Clause 1.1 Promotion to Administrative Staff*

*The provisions of the Code apply in their entirety to the promotion of medicines to appropriate administrative staff except where the text indicates otherwise. For example, the prescribing information required under Clause 4 must be included in promotional material provided to administrative staff but it is not permissible to provide samples of medicines to them as this is proscribed by Clause 17.1.*

*Particular attention is drawn to the provisions of Clause 12.1 and the supplementary information to that Clause, which concerns the appropriateness of promotional material to those to whom it is addressed.*

**1.2** The term 'promotion' means any activity undertaken by a pharmaceutical company or with its authority which promotes the prescription, supply, sale or administration of its medicines.

It includes:

- journal and direct mail advertising
- the activities of representatives including detail aids and other printed material used by representatives
- the supply of samples
- the provision of inducements to prescribe, supply or buy medicines by the gift, offer or promise of any benefit or bonus, whether in money or in kind
- the provision of hospitality for promotional purposes
- the sponsorship of promotional meetings
- the sponsorship of scientific meetings including payment of travelling and accommodation expenses in connection therewith
- the provision of information to the general public either directly or indirectly, and
- all other sales promotion in whatever form, such as participation in exhibitions, the use of audio-cassettes, films, records, tapes, video recordings, electronic media, interactive data systems and the like.

It does not include:

- replies made in response to individual enquiries from members of the health professions or in response to specific communications whether of enquiry or comment, including letters published in professional journals, but only if they relate solely to the subject matter of the letter or enquiry and are not promotional in nature
- factual, accurate, informative announcements and reference material relating, for example, to pack changes, adverse-reaction warnings, trade catalogues and price lists, provided they include no product claims
- measures or trade practices relating to prices, margins or discounts which were in existence on 1 January 1993
- data sheets, the contents of which are determined by regulations made under the Medicines Act 1968 and summaries of product characteristics as provided for in EC Directive 65/65
- the labelling on medicines and accompanying package leaflets insofar as they are not promotional for the medicines concerned; the contents of labels and package leaflets are covered by regulations
- statements relating to human health or diseases provided there is no reference, either direct or indirect, to specific medicines.

*Clause 1.2 Replies Intended for Use in Response to Individual Enquiries*

*Replies intended for use in response to enquiries which are received on a regular basis may be drafted in advance provided that they are used only when they directly and solely relate to the particular enquiry. Documents must not have the appearance of promotional material.*

**1.3** The term 'medicine' means any branded or unbranded medicine intended for use in humans which requires a marketing authorization.

**1.4** The term 'health profession' includes members of the medical, dental, pharmacy or nursing professions and any other persons who in the course of their professional activities may prescribe, supply or administer a medicine.

**1.5** The term 'over-the-counter medicine' means those medicines or particular packs of medicines which are primarily advertised to the general public for use in self medication.

**1.6** The term 'representative' means a representative calling on members of the health professions and administrative staff in relation to the promotion of medicines.

*Clause 1.6 Representatives*

*'Medical representatives' and 'generic sales representatives' are distinguished in Clause 16.3 relating to examinations for representatives.*

**Clause 2 Methods of Promotion**

Methods of promotion must never be such as to bring discredit upon, or reduce confidence in, the pharmaceutical industry.

*Clause 2 Discredit to and Reduction of Confidence in the Industry*

*A ruling in breach of this Clause is a sign of particular censure and is reserved for such circumstances.*

## Clause 3 Martketing Authorization.

**3.1** A medicine must not be promoted prior to the grant of the marketing authorization which permits its sale or supply.

**3.2** The promotion of a medicine must be in accordance with the terms of its marketing authorization and must not be inconsistent with the particulars listed in its summary of product characteristics or data sheet.

### Clause 3 Marketing Authorization

*The legitimate exchange of medical and scientific information during the development of a medicine is not prohibited provided that any such information or activity does not constitute promotion which is prohibited under this or any other Clause.*

### Clause 3 Promotion at International Conferences

*The promotion of medicines at international meetings held in the UK may on occasion pose certain problems with regard to medicines or indications for medicines which do not have a marketing authorization in the UK although they are so authorized elsewhere.*

*The display and provision of promotional material for such medicines is permitted at international meetings in the UK provided that the following conditions are met:*

- *the meeting must be a truly international meeting of high scientific standing with a significant proportion of delegates from outside the UK*
- *any promotional material for medicines or for indications which do not have a UK marketing authorization must be clearly and prominently labelled as such*
- *the material is certified in accordance with Clause 14, except that the signatories need certify only that in their belief the material is a fair and truthful presentation of the facts about the medicine.*

### Clause 3.1 Advance Notification of New Products or Product Changes

*Health authorities and trust hospitals etc, need to estimate their likely budgets two or three years in advance in order to meet Treasury requirements and there is a need for them to receive advance information about the introduction of new medicines, or changes to existing medicines, which may significantly affect their level of expenditure during future years.*

*At the time of this information is required, the medicines concerned (or the changes to them) will not be the subject of marketing authorizations (though applications will often have been made) and it would thus be contrary to the Code for them to be promoted. Information may, however, be provided on the following basis:*

*(i) the information must relate to:*

- *(a) a product which contains a new active substance, or*
- *(b) a product which contains a newly synthesized active substance, or*
- *(c) a product which is to have a significant addition to the existing range of authorized indications, or*
- *(d) a product which has a novel and innovative means of administration*

*(ii) there must be significant budgetary implications*
*(iii) only factual information must be provided, including an indication of the likely cost, and it must not be presented in the style of promotional material*
*(iv) information should not be directed to those who would be expected to prescribe the product, but to those concerned with budgets*
*(v) if requested, further information may be supplied or a presentation made.*

### Clause 3.2 Unauthorized Indications

*The promotion of indications not covered by the marketing authorization for a medicine is prohibited by this Clause.*

## Clause 4 Prescribing Information and other Obligatory Information

**4.1** The prescribing information listed in Clause 4.2 must be provided in a clear and legible manner in all promotional material for a medicine except for abbreviated advertisements (see Clause 5) and for promotional aids which meet the requirements of Clause 18.3.

The prescribing information must form part of the promotional material and must not be separate from it.

### Clause 4.1 Prescribing Information, Summaries of Product Characteristics and Data Sheets

*Each promotional item for a medicine must be able to stand alone. For example when a 'Dear Doctor' letter on a medicine is sent in the same envelope with a brochure about the same medicine, each item has to include the prescribing information. It does not suffice to have the prescribing information on only one of the items. The inclusion of a summary of product characteristics or data sheet moreover does not suffice to conform with the provisions of this Clause.*

*The prescribing information must be consistent with the summary of product characteristics or data sheet for the medicine.*

### Clause 4.1 Advertisements for Devices

*Where an advertisement relates to the merits of a device used for administering medicines, such as an inhaler, which is supplied containing a variety of medicines, the prescribing information for one only need be given if the advertisement makes no reference to any particular medicine.*

*Full prescribing information must, however, be included in relation to each particular medicine which is referred to.*

### Clause 4.1 Prescribing Information at Exhibitions

*The prescribing information for medicines promoted on posters and exhibition panels at meetings must either be provided on the posters or panels themselves or must be available at the company stand. If the prescribing information is made available at the company stand, this should be referred to on the posters or panels.*

### Clause 4.1 Legibility of Prescribing Information

*The prescribing information is the essential information which must be provided in promotional material. It follows therefore that the information must be given in a clear and legible manner which assists readability.*

*Legibility is not simply a question of type size. The following recommendations will help to achieve clarity:*

- *type size should be such that a lower case letter 'x' is no less than 1 mm in height*
- *lines should be no more than 100 characters in length, including spaces*
- *sufficient space should be allowed between lines to facilitate easy reading*
- *a clear style of type should be used*
- *there should be adequate contrast between the colour of the text and the background*
- *dark print on a light background is preferable*
- *emboldening headings and starting each section on a new line aids legibility.*

**4.2** The prescribing information consists of the following:

- the name of the medicine (which may be either a brand name or a generic name)
- a quantitative list of the active ingredients, using approved names where such exist, or other non-proprietary names; alternatively, the non-proprietary name of the product if it is the subject of an accepted monograph
- at least one authorised indication for use consistent with the summary of product characteristics or data sheet
- a succinct statement of the information in the summary of product characteristics or data sheet relating to the dosage and method of use relevant to the indications quoted in the advertisement and, where not otherwise obvious, the route of administration
- a succinct statement of the side-effects, precautions and contra-indications relevant to the indications in the advertisement, giving, in an abbreviated form, the substance of the relevant information in the summary of product characteristics or data sheet
- any warning issued by the Medicines Commission, a committee appointed under Section 4 of the Medicines Act 1968 or the licensing authority, which is required to be included in advertisements
- the cost (excluding VAT) of either a specified package of the medicine to which the advertisement relates, or a specified quantity or recommended daily dose, calculated by reference to any specified package of the product except in the case of advertisements in journals printed in the UK which have more than 15 per cent of their circulation outside the UK and audio-visual advertisements and prescribing information provided in association with them
- the legal classification of the product
- the number of the relevant marketing authorization and the name and address of the holder of the authorization or the name and address of the part of the business responsible for its sale or supply.

In addition the non-proprietary name of the

medicine or a list of the active ingredients us approved names where such exist must app immediately adjacent to the most prominent disp of the brand name in not less than 10 point bold o a type size which occupies a total area no less t that taken by the brand name.

The information specified above in relation dosage, method of use, side effects, precautions contra-indications and any warning which is requi to be included in advertisements, must be place such a position in the advertisement that relationship to the claims and indications for product can be appreciated by the reader.

### Clause 4.2 Black Triangle Symbol

*Certain newly marketed medicines are require show an inverted black triangle on their promotic material, other than promotional aids, to denote special reporting is required in relation to adve reactions. This is not a Code of Practice or a statu requirement.*

*The agreement between the Committee on Sa of Medicines and the ABPI on the use of the b triangle is that:*

*The symbol should always be black and its should normally be not less than 5 mm per side with a smaller size of 3 mm per side for A5 advertisements and a larger size of 7.5 mm per s for A3 size advertisements:*

- *the symbol should appear once and be loca adjacent to the most prominent display of name of the product*
- *no written explanation of the symbol is necess.*

### Clause 4.2 Non-Proprietary Name

*'Immediately adjacent to . . .' means immedia before, immediately after, immediately above immediately below.*

**4.3** In the case of audio-visual material such as fil video recordings and such like and in the case of in active data systems, the prescribing information n be provided either:

- by way of a document which is made available all persons to whom the material is shown or se or
- by inclusion on the audio-visual recording or the interactive data system itself.

When the prescribing information is included in interactive data system instructions for accessing must be clearly displayed.

### Clause 4.3 Prescribing Information on Audio-Vis Material

*Where prescribing information is shown in the au visual material as part of the recording, it must be sufficient clarity and duration so that it is ea readable. The prescribing information must be integral part of the advertisement and must app with it. It is not acceptable for the advertisement a the prescribing information to be separated by other material.*

**4.4** In the case of audio material, ie. material w consists of sound only, the prescribing informat must be provided by way of a document which made available to all persons to whom the materia played or sent.

**4.5** In the case of a journal advertisement where prescribing information appears overleaf, a referer to where it can be found must appear on the ou edge of the initial page of the advertisement in at le 8 point type.

**4.6** In the case of printed promotional mate consisting of more than four pages, a clear referer must be given to where the prescribing informat can be found.

**4.7** Promotional material other than advertiseme appearing in professional publications must inclu the date on which the promotional material w drawn up or last revised.

### Clause 4.7 Dates on Loose Inserts

*A loose insert is not regarded for this purpose appearing in the professional publication with wh it is sent and must therefore bear the date on whic was drawn up or last revised.*

## Clause 5 Abbreviated Advertisements

**5.1** Abbreviated advertisements are advertiseme which are exempt from the requirement to inclu prescribing information for the advertised medici provided that they meet with the requirements of Clause.

**5.2** Abbreviated advertisements may only appea professional publications i.e. publications sent delivered wholly or mainly to members of the health professions and/or appropriate administrative staff. A loose insert in such a publication cannot be an abbreviated advertisement. Abbreviated advertisements are not permissible in relation to any medicine where the licensing authority has issued a direction that abbreviated advertisements must not be issued.

## Clause 5.2 Abbreviated Advertisements–Professional Publications

*Abbreviated advertisements are largely restricted to journals and other such professional publications sent or delivered wholly or mainly to members of the health professions etc. A promotional mailing or representative leave piece cannot be an abbreviated advertisement and an abbreviated advertisement cannot appear as part of another promotional item, such as in a brochure consisting of a full advertisement for another of the company's medicines.*

*Diaries and desk pads bearing a number of advertisements are considered to be professional publications and may include abbreviated advertisements for medicines. Similarly, video programmes and such like sent to doctors etc may be considered professional publications and an abbreviated advertisement may be affixed to the side of the video cassette or included on the box containing the video. The prescribing information must, however, be made available for any advertisement for a medicine appearing on audio-visual material or in an interactive data system. Such advertisements cannot be deemed abbreviated advertisements.*

5.3 Abbreviated advertisements must be no larger than 420 square centimetres in size.

5.4 Abbreviated advertisements must contain the following information:
- the name of the medicine (which may be either a brand name or a generic name)
- the non-proprietary name of the medicine or a list of the active ingredients using approved names where such exist
- at least one indication for use consistent with the summary of product characteristics or the data sheet
- the legal classification of the product
- any warning issued by the Medicines Commission, a committee appointed under Section 4 of the Medicines Act 1968 or the licensing authority which is required to be included in advertisements
- the name and address of the holder of the marketing authorization or the name and address of the part of the business responsible for its sale or supply
- a statement that further information is available on request to the holder of the marketing authorization or that it may be found in the data sheet.

The non-proprietary name of the medicine or the list of the active ingredients, using approved names where such exist, must appear immediately adjacent to the most prominent display of the brand name in not less than 10 point bold or in a type size which occupies a total area no less than that taken by the brand name.

5.5 Abbreviated advertisements may in addition contain a concise statement consistent with the summary of product characteristics or data sheet, giving the reason why the medicine is recommended for the indication or indications given.

## Clause 5.4 Non-Proprietary Name

*'immediately adjacent to . . .' means immediately before, immediately after, immediately above or immediately below.*

## Clauses 5.4 and 5.5 Abbreviated Advertisements–Permitted Information

*The contents of abbreviated advertisements are restricted as set out in Clauses 5.4 and 5.5 and the following information should not therefore be included in abbreviated advertisements:*
- *marketing authorization numbers*
- *references*
- *dosage particulars*
- *details of pack sizes*
- *cost*
- *quantitative particulars, unless the quantitative information forms part of the licensed name of the medicine.*

*There may be exceptions to the above if the information provided, for example the cost of the medicine or the frequency of its dosage or its availability as a patient pack, is given as the reason why the medicine is recommended for the indication or indications referred to in the advertisement.*

*Artwork used in abbreviated advertisements must not convey any information about a medicine which*

is additional to that permitted under Clauses 5.4 and 5.5.

*Telephone numbers may be included in abbreviated advertisements.*

## Clause 6 Journal Advertising

6.1 No single advertisement included in a journal may consist of more than two consecutive pages.

6.2 Where the two pages of an advertisement are not facing, neither must be false or misleading when read in isolation.

6.3 No advertisement taking the form of a loose insert in a journal may consist of more than a single sheet of a size no larger than the page size of the journal itself, printed on one or both sides.

6.4 No issue of a journal may bear advertising for a particular product on more than three pages.

## Clause 6 Journal Advertisements

*See Clause 4 and in particular Clause 4.5 regarding the requirements for prescribing information in journal advertisements*

*A two page journal advertisement is one where the pages follow on continuously without interruption by intervening editorial text or other copy. Thus, for example, promotional material on two successive right hand pages cannot be a single advertisement. Each such page would need to be treated as a separate advertisement for the purposes of prescribing information.*

*Similarly, if promotional material appears on the outer edges of the left and right hand pages of a double page spread, and the promotional material is separated by intervening editorial matter then again each page would need to be treated as a separate advertisement.*

## Clause 6.3 Advertising on the Outside of Journals

*Advertising such as cards stapled to a journal and 'wraparounds' must not have a greater surface area than that outlined for loose inserts under Clause 6.3.*

## Clause 6.4 Limitation on Number of Pages of Advertising

*To conform with Clause 6.4 there can be no more than three one page advertisements for a product in a journal. Alternatively there can be one double page advertisement and another separate one page advertisement. Advertisements consisting of three consecutive pages are not permitted. Advertisements taking the form of inserts, whether loose or bound in, count towards the three pages allowed. A loose insert printed on both sides counts as two pages.*

*A summary of product characteristics or a data sheet is permitted as an insert in addition to the three pages of advertising which is allowed.*

*Inserts and supplements which are not advertisements as such, though they may be regarded as promotional material, for example reports of conference proceedings, are not subject to the restrictions of Clauses 6.3 and 6.4.*

## Clause 7 Information, Claims and Comparisons
### Clause 7 General

*The application of this clause is not limited to information or claims of a medical or scientific nature. It includes, inter alia, information or claims relating to pricing and market share. Thus, for example, any claim relating to the market share of a product must be substantiated without delay upon request as required under Clause 7.4.*

7.1 Upon reasonable request, companies must promptly provide members of the health professions and appropriate administrative staff with accurate and relevant information about the medicines which the company markets.

7.2 Information, claims and comparisons must be accurate, balanced, fair, objective and unambiguous and must be based on an up-to-date evaluation of all the evidence and reflect that evidence clearly. They must not mislead either directly or by implication.

## Clause 7.2 Misleading Information, Claims and Comparisons

*The following are areas where particular care should be taken by companies:*
- **claims for superior potency in relation to weight** are generally meaningless and best avoided unless they can be linked with some practical advantage, for example, reduction in side-effects or cost of effective dosage
- **the use of data derived from in-vitro studies, studies in healthy volunteers and in animals.** *Care must be taken with the use of such data so as not to mislead as to its significance. The extrapolation of such data to the clinical situation should only*

be made where there is data to show that it is of direct relevance and significance
- **economic evaluation of medicines.** *The economic evaluation of medicines is a relatively new science. Care must be taken that any claim involving the economic evaluation of a medicine is borne out by the data available and does not exaggerate its significance.*

*To be acceptable as the basis of promotional claims, the assumptions made in an economic evaluation must be clinically appropriate and consistent with the marketing authorization.*

*Attention is drawn to guidance on good practice in the conduct of economic evaluation of medicines which has been given by the Department of Health and the ABPI and which is available upon request from the Prescription Medicines Code of Practice Authority.*
- **emerging clinical or scientific opinion.** *Where a clinical or scientific issue exists which has not been resolved in favour of one generally accepted viewpoint, particular care must be taken to ensure that the issue is treated in a balanced manner in promotional material*
- **hanging comparisons** *whereby a medicine is described as being better or stronger or suchlike without stating that with which the medicine is compared must not be made*
- **price comparisons.** *Price comparisons, as with any comparison, must be accurate, fair and must not mislead. Valid comparisons can only be made where like is compared with like. It follows therefore that in making a price comparison it should be made on the basis of the equivalent dosage requirement for the same indications. For example, to compare the cost per ml for topical preparations is likely to mislead unless it can be shown that their usage rates are similar or, where this is not possible, for the comparison to be qualified in such a way as to indicate that usage rates may vary*
- **statistical information.** *Care must be taken to ensure that there is a sound statistical basis for all information, claims and comparisons in promotional material. Differences which do not reach statistical significance must not be presented in such a way as to mislead.*

*Instances have occurred where claims have been based on published papers in which the arithmetic and/or statistical methodology was incorrect. Accordingly, before statistical information is included in promotional material it must have been subjected to statistical appraisal.*

7.3 Any information, claim or comparison must be capable of substantiation.

7.4 Substantiation for any information, claim or comparison must be provided without delay at the request of members of the health professions or appropriate administrative staff. It need not be provided, however, in relation to the validity of indications approved in the marketing authorization.

7.5 When promotional material refers to published studies, clear references must be given.

7.6 All artwork including illustrations, graphs and tables must conform to the letter and spirit of the Code. Graphs and tables must be presented in such a way as to give a clear, fair, balanced view of the matters with which they deal, and must not be included unless they are relevant to the claims or comparisons being made.

## Clause 7.6 Artwork, Illustrations, Graphs and Tables

*Care must be taken to ensure that artwork does not mislead as to the nature of a medicine or any claim or comparison and that it does not detract from any warnings or contra-indications. For example, anatomical drawings used to show results from a study must not exaggerate those results and depictions of children should not be used in relation to products not licensed for use in childen in any way which might encourage such use.*

*Particular care should be taken with graphs and tables to ensure that they do not mislead, for example by their incompleteness or by the use of suppressed zeros or unusual scales. Differences which do not reach statistical significance must not be presented in such a way as to mislead.*

*Graphs and tables must be adequately labelled so that the information presented can be readily understood. If a graph, table or suchlike is taken from a published paper but has not been reproduced in its entirety, the graph must clearly be labelled as having been adapted from the paper in question (see also Clause 7.5). Any such adaptation must not distort or mislead as to the significance of that graph, table etc. It should also be noted that if a table, graph etc in a paper is unacceptable in terms of the requirements of the Code, because, for example, it gives a visually* misleading impression as to the data shown, then it must not be used or reproduced in promotional material.

**7.7** Information and claims about side-effects must reflect available evidence or be capable of substantiation by clinical experience. It must not be stated that a product has no side-effects, toxic hazards or risks of addiction. The word 'safe' must not be used without qualification.

*Clause 7.7 Use of the Word 'Safe'*

The restrictions on the word 'safe' apply equally to grammatical derivatives of the word such as safety. For example, 'demonstrated safety' or 'proven safety' are prohibited under this Clause.

**7.8** Exaggerated or all-embracing claims must not be made and superlatives must not be used except for those limited circumstances where they relate to a clear fact about a medicine. Claims should not imply that a medicine or an active ingredient has some special merit, quality or property unless this can be substantiated.

*Clause 7.8 Superlatives*

Superlatives are those grammatical expressions which denote the highest quality or degree such as best, strongest, widest etc. A claim that a product was 'the best' treatment for a particular condition for example could not be substantiated as there are too many variables to enable such a sweeping claim to be proven. The use of a superlative which could be substantiated is a simple statement of fact which can be very clearly demonstrated, such as that a particular medicine is the most widely prescribed in the UK for a certain condition, if this is not presented in a way which misleads as to its significance.

*Clause 7.8 Use of the Words 'The' and 'Unique'*

In certain circumstances the use of the word 'the' can imply a special merit, quality or property for a medicine which is unacceptable under this clause if it cannot be substantiated. For example, a claim that a product is 'The analgesic' implies that it is in effect the best, and might not be acceptable under this clause.

Similarly, great care needs to be taken with the use of the word 'unique'. Although in some circumstances the word unique may be used to describe some clearly defined special feature of a medicine, in many instances it may simply imply a general superiority. In such instances it is not possible to substantiate the claim as the claim itself is so ill defined.

**7.9** The word 'new' must not be used to describe any product or presentation which has been generally available, or any therapeutic indication which has been generally promoted, for more than twelve months in the UK.

**7.10** Brand names of other companies' products must not be used unless the prior consent of the proprietors has been obtained.

**Clause 8 Disparaging References**

**8.1** The medicines, products and activities of other pharmaceutical companies must not be disparaged.

*Clause 8.1 Disparaging References*

Much pharmaceutical advertising contains comparisons with other products and, by the nature of advertising, such comparisons are usually made to show an advantage of the advertised product over its comparator. Provided that such critical references to another company's products are accurate, balanced, fair etc, and can be substantiated, they are acceptable under the Code.

Unjustified knocking copy in which the products or activities of a competitor are unfairly denigrated is prohibited under this Clause.

**8.2** The clinical and scientific opinions of members of the health professions must not be disparaged.

**Clause 9 Format, Suitability and Causing Offence, Sponsorship**

**9.1** All material and activities must recognise the special nature of medicines and the professional standing of the audience to which they are directed and must not be likely to cause offence. High standards must be maintained at all times.

*Clause 9.1 Suitability and Taste*

The special nature of medicines and the professional audience to which the material is directed require that the standards set for the promotion of medicines are higher than those which might be acceptable for general commodity advertising.

It follows, therefore, that certain types, styles and methods of promotion even where they might be acceptable for the promotion of products other than medicines are unacceptable. These include:

- the display of naked or partially naked people for the purpose of attracting attention to the material or the use of sexual imagery for that purpose
- 'teaser' advertising whereby promotional material is intended to 'tease' the recipient by eliciting an interest in something which will be following or will be available at a later date without providing any actual information about it
- the provision of rubber stamps to doctors for use as aids to prescription writing
- the provision of private prescription forms preprinted with the name of a medicine.

**9.2** The name or photograph of a member of a health profession must not be used in any way that is contrary to the conventions of that profession.

**9.3** Promotional material must not imitate the devices, copy slogans or general layout adopted by other companies in a way that is likely to mislead or confuse.

**9.4** Promotional material must not include any reference to the Medicines Commission, a committee appointed under Section 4 of the Medicines Act 1968, or the licensing authority, unless this is specifically required by the licensing authority.

**9.5** Reproductions of official documents must not be used for promotional purposes unless permission has been given in writing by the appropriate body.

**9.6** Extremes of format, size or cost of promotional material must be avoided.

**9.7** Postcards, other exposed mailings, envelopes or wrappers must not carry matter which might be regarded as advertising to the general public, contrary to Clause 20.1.

*Clause 9.7 Reply Paid Cards*

Reply paid cards which are intended to be returned to companies through the post and which relate to a medicine which may not legally be advertised to the general public should not bear both the name of the medicine and information as to its usage but may bear one or the other.

**9.8** The telephone, telemessages, e-mail, telex and facsimile machines must not be used for promotional purposes except with the prior permission of the recipient.

**9.9** All material relating to medicines and their uses which is sponsored by a pharmaceutical company must clearly indicate that it has been sponsored by that company.

**Clause 10 Disguised Promotion**

**10.1** Promotional material and activities must not be disguised.

*Clause 10.1 Disguised Promotional Material*

Promotional material sent in the guise of personal communications, for example by using envelopes or postcards addressed in real or facsimile handwriting is inappropriate. Envelopes must not be used for the dispatch of promotional material if they bear words implying that the contents are non-promotional, for example that the contents provide information relating to safety.

Advertisements in journals must not resemble editorial matter. Care must also be taken with company sponsored reports on meetings and the like to ensure that they are not disguised promotion. Sponsorship must be declared in accordance with Clause 9.9.

**10.2** Market research activities, post-marketing surveillance studies, clinical assessments and the like must not be disguised promotion.

*Clause 10.2 Guidelines for Company Sponsored Safety Assessment of Marketed Medicines*

Attention is drawn to the Guidelines for Company Sponsored Safety Assessment of Marketed Medicines (SAMM) which have been produced jointly by the ABPI, the British Medical Association, the Committee on Safety of Medicines, the Medicines Control Agency and the Royal College of General Practitioners. These state that SAMM studies should not be undertaken for the purposes of promotion.

*Clause 10.2 Market Research*

Market research is the collection and analysis of information and must be unbiased and non-promotional. The use to which the statistics or information is put may be promotional. The two phases must be kept distinct.

Attention is drawn to the Guidelines Pharmaceutical Market Research Practice produ by the British Pharmaceutical Market Research Gr and the ABPI.

**Clause 11 Provision of Reprints and the Use Quotations**

**11.1** Reprints of articles in journals must not provided unsolicited unless the articles have be refereed.

*Clause 11.1 Provision of Reprints*

The provision of an unsolicited reprint of an art about a medicine constitutes promotion of medicine and all relevant requirements of the C must therefore be observed. Particular attention m be paid to the requirements of Clause 3.

When sending an unsolicited reprint of an art about a medicine, it should be accompanied prescribing information.

**11.2** Quotations from medical and scient literature, or from personal communications m accurately reflect the meaning of the author.

*Clause 11.2 Quotations*

Any quotation chosen by a company for use promotional material must comply with requirements of the Code itself. For example, to qu from a paper which stated that a certain medicine v 'safe and effective' would not be acceptable even was an accurate reflection of the meaning of author of the paper, as it is prohibited under Cla 7.7 of the Code to state without qualification promotional material that a medicine is safe.

Care should be taken in quoting from any study the like to ensure that it does not mislead as to overall significance. (See Clause 7.2 which prohi misleading information, claims etc in promotic material.) Attention is drawn to the provisions Clause 7.5 which requires that when promotic material refers to published studies clear referen must be given to where they can be found.

**11.3** Quotations relating to medicines taken fr public broadcasts, for example on radio and televisi and from private occasions, such as med conferences or symposia, must not be used with the formal permission of the speaker.

**11.4** The utmost care must be taken to avoid ascrib claims or views to authors when these no lon represent the current views of the authors concern

*Clause 11.4 Current Views of Authors*

If there is any doubt as to the current view of author, companies should check with the author p to its use in promotional material.

**Clause 12 Distribution of Promotional Material**

**12.1** Promotional material should only be sent distributed to those categories of persons whose ne for, or interest in, the particular information c reasonably be assumed.

*Clause 12.1 Distribution of Promotional Material*

Promotional material should be tailored to whom directed. For example, promotional material devis for general practitioners might not be appropriate hospital doctors and, similarly, material devised clinicians might not be appropriate for use w National Health Service administrative staff.

**12.2** Restraint must be exercised on the frequer of distribution and on the volume of promotio material distributed.

*Clause 12.2 Frequency of Mailings*

The style of mailings is relevant to their acceptab to doctors and criticism of their frequency is m likely to arise where their informational content limited or where they appear to be elaborate a expensive. A higher frequency rate will be accep for mailings on new products than for others.

**12.3** Mailing lists must be kept up-to-date. Reque from health professionals to be removed fr promotional mailing lists must be complied w promptly and no name may be restored except their request or with their permission.

**Clause 13 Scientific Service Responsible Information**

Companies must have a scientific service to comp and collate all information, whether received fr medical representatives or from any other sour about medicines which they market.

**use 14 Certification of Promotional Material**

**1** Promotional material must not be issued unless final form, to which no subsequent amendments be made, has been certified by two persons on alf of the company in the manner provided by this use. One of the two persons must be a doctor. The er must be a pharmacist or some other ropriately qualified person or a senior official of company or an appropriately qualified person ose services are retained for that purpose.

*use 14.1 Certification*

*acceptable way to comply with Clause 14.1 is for final proof to be certified but this is not obligatory vided that that which is certified is in its final form vhich no subsequent amendments will be made.*

*ll promotional material must be certified in this y including promotional aids, audio-visual material, motional material on databases and resentatives' technical briefing materials.*

*)ther material issued by companies which relates nedicines but which is not intended as promotional terial for those medicines per se, for example porate advertising, press releases and educational terial for patients etc, should be examined to ure that it does not contravene the Code or the evant statutory requirements.*

*n certifying audio, audio-visual material and terial used on interactive data systems, companies st ensure that a written transcript of the material is tified including reproductions of any graphs, tables d the like that appear in the recording. In the event a complaint, a copy of the written transcript of the terial will be requested.*

*See also the supplementary information to Clause n promotion at international conferences regarding certification of such material.*

*use 14.1 Joint Ventures and Co-Promotion*

*a joint venture in which a third party provides a vice on behalf of a number of pharmaceutical npanies, the pharmaceutical companies involved responsible for any activity carried out by that d party on their behalf.*

*t follows therefore that the pharmaceutical npanies involved should be aware of all aspects of service carried out on their behalf and take this o account when certifying the material or activity olved. Similarly if two or more pharmaceutical npanies organize a joint meeting each company ould ensure that the arrangements for the meeting acceptable.*

*Under co-promotion arrangements whereby npanies jointly promote the same medicine and promotional material bears both company names, ch company should certify the promotional material olved as they will be held jointly responsible for it der the Code.*

**2** The names of those nominated, together with ir qualifications, shall be notified in advance to the oduct Information and Assessment Unit of the Post ensing Division of the Medicines Control Agency d to the Prescription Medicines Code of Practice thority. The names and qualifications of designated ernative signatories must also be given. Changes the names of nominees must be promptly notified.

**.3** The certificate must certify that the signatories ve examined the final proof of the material and that their belief it is in accordance with the requirements the relevant advertising regulations and this Code, not inconsistent with the marketing authorization d the summary of product characteristics or data eet and is a fair and truthful presentation of the ts about the medicine.

Material which is still in use must be recertified at ervals of no more than two years to ensure that it ntinues to conform with the relevant advertising gulations and the Code.

**.4** Companies shall preserve all certificates, gether with the material in the form certified and ormation indicating the persons to whom it was dressed, the method of dissemination and the date first dissemination, for not less than three years er its final use and produce them upon request m the Medicines Control Agency or the Prescription edicines Code of Practice Authority.

*ause 14.4 Retention of Documentation*

*mpanies should note that the Medicines Control ency is entitled to request particulars of an vertisement, including particulars as to the content d form of the advertisement, the method of ssemination and the date of the first dissemination, d such a request is not subject to any time limit. is does not apply to the certificates themselves in spect of which the three year limit in Clause 14.4 is plicable.*

**Clause 15 Representatives**

*Clause 15 Representatives*

*All provisions in the Code relating to the need for accuracy, balance, fairness, good taste etc apply equally to oral representations as well as printed material. Representatives must not make claims or comparisons which are in any way inaccurate, misleading, disparaging, in poor taste etc, or which are outside the terms of the marketing authorization for the medicine or are inconsistent with the data sheet. Indications for which the medicine does not have a marketing authorization must not be promoted.*

*Attention is also drawn to the provisions of Clause 9.8 which prohibits the use of the telephone, telemessages, e-mail and telex and facsimile machines for promotional purposes except with the prior permission of the recipient.*

*Clause 15 Contract Representatives*

*Companies employing contract representatives are responsible for their conduct and must ensure that they comply with the provisions of this and all other relevant clauses in the Code, and in particular the training requirements under Clauses 15.1, 16.1, 16.2 and 16.3.*

**15.1** Representatives must be given adequate training and have sufficient scientific knowledge to enable them to provide full and accurate information about the medicines which they promote.

**15.2** Representatives must at all times maintain a high standard of ethical conduct in the discharge of their duties and must comply with all relevant requirements of the Code.

**15.3** Representatives must not employ any inducement or subterfuge to gain an interview. No fee should be paid or offered for the grant of an interview.

*Clause 15.3 Hospitality and Payments for Meetings*

*Attention is drawn to the requirements of Clauses 18 and 19 which prohibit the provision of any financial inducement for the purposes of sales promotion and require that any hospitality provided is secondary to the purpose of a meeting, is not out of proportion to the occasion and does not extend beyond members of the health professions or appropriate administrative staff.*

*Meetings organised for groups of doctors, other health professionals and/or appropriate administrative staff which are wholly or mainly of a social or sporting nature are unacceptable.*

*Representatives organising meetings are permitted to provide appropriate hospitality and/or to meet any reasonable, actual costs which may have been incurred. For example, if the refreshments have been organised and paid for by a medical practice the cost may be reimbursed as long as it is reasonable in relation to what was provided and the refreshments themselves were appropriate for the occasion.*

*Donations in lieu of hospitality are unacceptable as they are inducements for the purpose of holding a meeting. If hospitality is not required at a meeting there is no obligation or right to provide some benefit of an equivalent value.*

*Clause 15.3 General Medical Council*

*The General Medical Council is the regulatory body for the medical profession and is responsible for giving advice on standards of professional conduct and on medical ethics. This guidance is set out in 'Duties of a doctor', a series of four booklets, one of which 'Good medical practice' covers a number of aspects of relationships with the pharmaceutical industry. In relation to representatives, doctors are advised that 'You must not ask for or accept fees for agreeing to meet sales representatives'.*

**15.4** Representatives must ensure that the frequency, timing and duration of calls on health professionals, administrative staff in hospitals and health authorities and the like, together with the manner in which they are made, do not cause inconvenience. The wishes of individuals on whom representatives wish to call and the arrangements in force at any particular establishment must be observed.

*Clause 15.4 Frequency and Manner of Calls on Doctors*

*The number of calls made on a doctor and the intervals between successive visits are relevant to the determination of frequency.*

*Companies should arrange that intervals between visits do not cause inconvenience. The number of calls made on a doctor by a representative each year should not normally exceed three on average. This does not include the following which may be additional to those three visits:*

- *attendance at group meetings, including audio-visual presentations and the like*
- *a visit which is requested by a doctor or a call which is made in order to respond to a specific enquiry*
- *a visit to follow up a report of an adverse reaction.*

*Representatives must always endeavour to treat doctors' time with respect and give them no cause to believe that their time might have been wasted. If for any unavoidable reasons, an appointment cannot be kept, the longest possible notice must be given.*

**15.5** In an interview, or when seeking an appointment for one, representatives must at the outset take reasonable steps to ensure that they do not mislead as to their identity or that of the company they represent.

**15.6** Representatives must transmit forthwith to the scientific service referred to in Clause 13 any information which they receive in relation to the use of the medicines which they promote, particularly reports of side-effects.

**15.7** Representatives must be paid a fixed basic salary and any addition proportional to sales of medicines must not constitute an undue proportion of their remuneration.

**15.8** Representatives must provide, or have available to provide if requested, a copy of the summary of product characteristics, or where one does not exist, a copy of the data sheet or a document with a similar content, when initiating a discussion on a medicine.

*Clause 15.8 Provision of Summary of Product Characteristics/Data Sheet*

*If discussion on a medicine is initiated by the person or persons on whom a representative calls, the representative is not obliged to have available the information on that medicine referred to in this clause.*

**15.9** Companies must prepare detailed briefing material for medical representatives on the technical aspects of each medicine which they will promote. A copy of such material must be made available to the Medicines Control Agency and the Prescription Medicines Code of Practice Authority on request. Briefing material must comply with the relevant requirements of the Code, with the exception of Clause 7.10, and, in particular, is subject to the certification requirements of Clause 14.

Briefing material must not advocate, either directly or indirectly, any course of action which would be likely to lead to a breach of the Code.

*Clause 15.9 Briefing Material*

*The detailed briefing material referred to in this clause consists of both the training material used to instruct medical representatives about a medicine and the instructions given to them as to how the product should be promoted.*

**15.10** Companies are responsible for the activities of their representatives if these are within the scope of their employment even if they are acting contrary to the instructions which they have been given.

**Clause 16 Training**

**16.1** All relevant personnel including members of staff concerned in any way with the preparation or approval of promotional material or of information to be provided to members of the UK health professions and to appropriate administrative staff or of information to be provided to the public, must be fully conversant with the requirements of the Code.

*Clause 16.1 Training*

*Extensive in house training on the Code is carried out by companies and by the Prescription Medicines Code of Practice Authority.*

*In addition, the Authority runs seminars on the Code which are open to all companies and personnel from advertising agencies, public relations agencies and the like which act for the pharmaceutical industry. Details of these seminars can be obtained from the Authority.*

**16.2** Representatives must pass the appropriate ABPI representatives examination, as specified in Clause 16.3, within two years of starting such employment.

*Clause 16.2 Time Allowed to Pass Examination*

*Representatives must pass the appropriate examination within two years of starting employment as a representative irrespective of whether those two years have been spent with one company or with more than one company. A representative cannot, for example, do eighteen months with one company and* eighteen months with another and so on and thus avoid the examination entirely.

In the event of extenuating circumstances, such as prolonged illness, the Director of the Prescription Medicines Code of Practice Authority may agree to the continued employment of a person as a respresentative past the end of the two year period, subject to the representative passing the examination within a reasonable time.

**16.3** The Medical Representatives Examination is appropriate for, and must be taken by, representatives whose duties comprise or include one or both of:
– calling upon doctors and/or dentists
– the promotion of medicines on the basis, *inter alia*, of their particular therapeutic properties.

The Generic Sales Representatives Examination is appropriate for, and must be taken by, representatives who promote medicines primarily on the basis of price, quality and availability.

*Clause 16.3 Medical Representatives and Generic Sales Representatives*

*The ABPI examinations for medical representatives and generic sales representatives are based on a syllabus published by the ABPI which covers, as appropriate, subjects such as body systems, disease processes and pharmacology, the classification of medicines and pharmaceutical technology. Information on the National Health Service and pharmaceutical industry forms an additional core part of the syllabus. The syllabus is complementary to, and may be incorporated within, the company's induction training which is provided to representatives as a pre-requisite to carrying out their function. Normally representatives should be entered for the appropriate ABPI examination within their first year of employment.*

**16.4** The following exemptions apply in relation to Clause 16.2:
– persons who were employed as medical representatives on 1 October 1979 are exempt from the need to take the Medical Representatives Examination
– persons with an acceptable professional qualification, for example in pharmacy, medicine or nursing, who were employed as medical representatives at any time before 1 October 1984, are exempt from the need to take the Medical Representatives Examination
– persons who were employed as Generic Sales Representatives on 1 January 1993 are exempt from the need to take the Generic Sales Representatives Examination
– persons who were employed as representatives on 1 January 1996 who had not previously been required to take an examination because they neither promoted generic medicines nor called on doctors and/or dentists are exempt from the need to take either examination.

**16.5** Persons who have passed the Medical Representatives Examination whose duties change so as to become those specified in Clause 16.3 as being appropriate to the Generic Sales Representatives Examination are exempt from the need to take that examination.

Persons who have passed the Generic Sales Representatives Examination whose duties change so as to become those specified in Clause 16.3 as being appropriate to the Medical Representatives Examination must pass that examination within two years of their change of duties.

**16.6** Details of the numbers of medical and generic sales representatives who have passed the respective examinations above together with the examination status of others, must be provided to the Prescription Medicines Code of Practice Authority on request.

**Clause 17 Samples**

*Clause 17 Definition of Sample*

*A sample is a small supply of a medicine provided to members of the health professions in order that they may familiarise themselves with it and acquire experience in dealing with it. This includes samples provided for identification purposes for which the provisions of Clause 17 equally apply.*

*Titration packs, free goods or bonus stock provided to pharmacists and others are not samples. Neither are starter packs classified as samples. This is because they are not for the purposes described above. Starter packs are small packs designed to provide sufficient medicine for a doctor to initiate treatment in such circumstances as a call out in the night or in other instances where there might be some undesirable but unavoidable delay in filling a prescription. It follows therefore that the types of medicines for which starter packs are appropriate are limited.*

**17.1** Samples may only be provided to health professionals and must not be provided to administrative staff.

**17.2** No more than ten samples of a particular medicine may be provided to an individual health professional during the course of a year.

**17.3** Samples may only be supplied in response to written requests which have been signed and dated.

*Clause 17.3 Sample Requests*

*This Clause does not preclude the provision of a preprinted sample request form bearing the name of the product for signing and dating by the applicant.*

*All signed and dated written requests for samples should be retained for not less than one year.*

**17.4** A sample of a medicine must be no larger than the smallest presentation of the medicine on the market.

**17.5** Each sample must be marked 'free medical sample–not for resale' or words to that effect and must be accompanied by a copy of the summary of product characteristics, or where one does not exist, a copy of the data sheet or a document with a similar content.

**17.6** Samples of medicines which are controlled under the Misuse of Drugs Act 1971 are prohibited except for those medicines coming within Schedule 5 to the Misuse of Drugs Regulations 1985.

**17.7** Samples distributed by representatives must be handed direct to the health professionals requesting them or persons authorised to receive them on their behalf.

**17.8** The distribution of samples in hospitals must comply with individual hospital requirements.

**17.9** Companies must have an adequate system of accountability for samples of medicines which they distribute.

**17.10** Samples which are sent by post must be packed so as to be reasonably secure against being opened by young children. No unsolicited medicine must be sent through the post.

**17.11** Unsolicited medicines must not be supplied to the general public.

**Clause 18 Gifts and Inducements**

**18.1** No gift, benefit in kind or pecuniary advantage shall be offered or given to members of the health professions or to administrative staff as an inducement to prescribe, supply, administer or buy any medicine, subject to the provisions of Clause 18.2.

*Clause 18.1 Provision of Medical and Educational Goods and Services*

*Clause 18.1 does not prevent the provision of medical and educational goods and services which will enhance patient care or benefit the National Health Service. The provision of such goods or services must not be done in such a way as to be an inducement to prescribe, supply, administer or buy any medicine. They must not bear the name of any medicine but may bear a corporate name.*

*Clause 18.1 General Medical Council*

*In its publication 'Good medical practice' which is referred to in the supplementary information to Clause 15.3, the General Medical Council advises doctors that 'You should not ask for or accept any material rewards, except those of insignificant value, from companies that sell or market drugs or appliances'.*

*Clause 18.1 Terms of Trade*

*Measures or trade practices relating to prices, margins and discounts which were in existence on 1 January 1993 are outside the scope of the Code (see Clause 1.2) and are excluded from the provisions of this clause.*

*Trade practices which have been developed subsequent to 1 January 1993 are subject to the Code.*

*Clause 18.1 Package Deals*

*Clause 18.1 does not prevent the offer of package deals whereby the purchaser of particular medicines receives with them other associated benefits, such as apparatus for administration, provided that the transaction as a whole is fair and reasonable.*

*Clause 18.1 Donations to Charities*

*Donations to charities made by companies in return for health professionals' attendance at company stands at meetings or offered as rewards for completing and returning quiz cards in mailings and such like are not unacceptable under this clause provided that the level of donation for each individual is modest, the money is for a reputable charity and any action required of the health professional is not inappropriate. Any donation to a charity must not*

constitute a payment that would otherwise unacceptable under the Code. For example, it wo not be acceptable for a representative to pay int practice equipment fund set up as a charity as would be a financial inducement prohibited un Clause 18.1. Donations to charities in return representatives gaining interviews are also prohib under Clause 15.3 of the Code.

Any offer by a company of a donation to a cha which is conditional upon some action by a hea professional must not place undue pressure on health professional to fulfil that condition. At all tir the provisions of Clauses 2 and 9.1 must be kep mind.

**18.2** Gifts in the form of promotional aids and pri whether related to a particular product or of gene utility, may be distributed to members of the hea professions and to appropriate administrative st provided that the gift or prize is inexpensive a relevant to the practice of their profession employment.

*Clause 18.2 Gifts*

*Items provided on long term or permanent loan t doctor or a practice are regarded as gifts and subject to the requirements of this clause.*

*Gifts must be inexpensive and relevant to recipients' work. An 'inexpensive' gift means which has cost the donor company no more than excluding VAT.*

*Items of general utility which have been held to acceptable gifts to doctors as being inexpensive a of relevance to their work include pens, pads, diar nail brushes, surgical gloves, desk trays, calendar low value phone card, a peak flow whistle, walk sticks and desk clocks.*

*Items which are for use in the home, and have use in the ordinary course of the practice of medic or any other health profession, such as table ma are unacceptable. Other examples of items wh have been found unacceptable are plant seeds a compact discs of music which were not conside relevant items and an x-ray light box and an age-s register on grounds of costs.*

*Names of medicines should not be used promotional aids when it would be inappropriate do so, for example when it might mislead as to nature of the item.*

*Clause 18.2 Competitions and Quizzes*

*The use of competitions, quizzes and suchlike for purposes of sales promotion are not necessarily unacceptable form of promotion. Any competiti must, however, be in good taste and must not invo any subject matter which is inappropriate for promotion of a medicine as required under Clau 9.1. A competition is more likely to be consider acceptable if its subject matter is clearly related to practice of medicine and pharmacy.*

*Any competition used for promotional purpos must be a bona fide test of skill and must recogn the professional standing of the recipients.*

*The provisions of Clause 18.2 apply to the provis of competition prizes. Prizes of a higher value th would ordinarily be acceptable for a promotional a are acceptable where the competition is a serious c and the prizes are few in number, relevant to t potential recipient's work and not out of proportion the skill required in the competition. The maximu acceptable cost to the donor of a prize in a promotio competition is £100, excluding VAT.*

*Gladstone bags, a desk clock and a business ca holder are examples of prizes which have been fou acceptable in particular competitions or quizzes.*

*Computer equipment and a substantial travel awa offered as a prize in a promotional competition examples of prizes which have been found u acceptable on grounds of cost.*

*Attention is drawn to the fact that the items list above as acceptable competition prizes or gifts a instances where the particular examples in questi were found acceptable. It does not mean that a such item is automatically acceptable under the Coc*

*Clause 18.2 Gifts to or for use by Patients*

*Some items distributed as promotional aids a intended for use by patients and these are r generally unacceptable provided that they meet t requirements of Clause 18.2, for example, sm inexpensive puzzles and toys for a young child to pl with during a visit to the doctor.*

*Other items which may be made available patients, for example by completing a request ca enclosed with a medicine, should meet the releva principles set out in Clause 18.2, that is they shou be inexpensive and related to either the conditi under treatment or general health. Care must be tak that any such activity meets all the requirements the Code and in particular Clause 20.*

*No gift or promotional aid for use by patients mu*

*given for the purpose of encouraging patients to quest a particular medicine.*

3 The prescribing information for a medicine as quired under Clause 4 does not have to be included a promotional aid if the promotional aid includes more than the following about the medicine:
the name of the medicine
an indication that the name of the medicine is a trade mark
the name of the company responsible for marketing the product.

*ause 18.3 Promotional Aids–Name of the Medicine*

*e name of the medicine means the brand name or e non-proprietary name. Both names may be luded but it is not obligatory to include both. A omotional aid may bear the names of more than e medicine.*

*ause 18.3 Prescribing Information on Note Pads and lendars*

*promotional aid consists of a note pad or calendar which the individual pages bear advertising aterial, there is no need for the individual pages to mply with Clause 4 provided that the information quired by that Clause is given elsewhere; for ample, on the cover.*

**ause 19 Hospitality and Meetings**

**.1** Companies are permitted to provide appropriate spitality to members of the health professions and propriate administrative staff in association with entific and promotional meetings, scientific con-esses and other such meetings. Hospitality must be condary to the purpose of the meeting. The level of spitality offered must be appropriate and not out of oportion to the occasion and the costs involved ust not exceed that level which the recipients would rmally adopt when paying for themselves. It must t extend beyond members of the health professions appropriate administrative staff.

*ause 19.1 Hospitality and Meetings*

*e provision of hospitality includes the payment of asonable, actual travel costs which a company may ovide to sponsor a delegate to attend a meeting. e payment of travel expenses and the like for rsons accompanying the delegate is not permitted.*

*The payment of reasonable honoraria and mbursement of out of pocket expenses, including vel, for speakers, is permissible.*

*Pharmaceutical companies may appropriately onsor a wide range of meetings. These range from nall lunchtime audio-visual presentations in a group actice, hospital meetings and meetings at stgraduate education centres, launch meetings for w products, management training courses, eetings of clinical trialists, patient support group eetings, satellite symposia through to large ernational meetings organised by independent dies with sponsorship from pharmaceutical mpanies.*

*With any meeting, certain basic principles apply:*

- *the meeting must have a clear educational content*
- *the hospitality associated with the meeting must be secondary to the nature of the meeting, must be appropriate and not out of proportion to the occasion and*
- *any hospitality provided must not extend to spouses and other persons unless that person is a member of the health professions or appropriate administrative staff and qualifies as a proper delegate or participant at the meeting in their own right. It follows therefore that spouses and other such persons must not otherwise be invited to meetings.*

*Administrative staff may be invited to meetings here appropriate. For example, receptionists might invited to a meeting in a general practice when the bject matter related to practice administration.*

*A useful criterion in determining whether the rangements for any meeting are acceptable is to oply the question 'would you and your company be lling to have these arrangements generally known?' e impression that is created by the arrangements any meeting must always be kept in mind.*

*Meetings organised for groups of doctors, other alth professionals and/or for administrative staff hich are wholly or mainly of a social or sporting ture are unacceptable.*

*Clause 19.1 General Medical Council*

*In its publication 'Good medical practice' which is referred to in the supplementary information to Clause 15.3, the General Medical Council advises doctors that 'You may accept personal travel grants and hospitality from companies for conferences or educational meetings, as long as the main purpose of the event is educational. The amount you receive must not be more than you would normally spend if you were paying for yourself'.*

*Clause 19.1 Postgraduate Education Allowance (PGEA) Approved Courses*

*The provisions of this and all other relevant clauses in the Code apply equally to meetings organized or sponsored by pharmaceutical companies which are PGEA approved. The fact that a course is PGEA approved does not mean that the arrangements for the meeting are automatically acceptable under the Code. The relevant provisions of the Code, and in particular, those relating to hospitality, must be observed.*

**19.2** Payments may not be made to doctors or groups of doctors, either directly or indirectly, for rental for rooms to be used for meetings.

*Clause 19.2 Payment of Room Rental*

*This provision does not preclude the payment of room rental to postgraduate medical centres and the like.*

*Payment of room rental to doctors or groups of doctors is not permissible even if such payment is made to equipment funds or patients' comforts funds and the like or to charities or companies.*

**19.3** When meetings are sponsored by pharmaceutical companies, that fact must be disclosed in the papers relating to the meetings and in any published proceedings.

*Clause 19.3 Sponsorship and Reports of Meetings*

*Attention is drawn to Clause 9.9 which requires that all material relating to medicines and their uses which is sponsored by a pharmaceutical company must clearly indicate that it has been sponsored by that company.*

*It should be noted that where companies are involved in the sponsorship and/or distribution of reports on meetings or symposia etc these reports may constitute promotional material and thus be fully subject to the requirements of the Code.*

**Clause 20 Relations with the General Public and the Media**

**20.1** Medicines must not be advertised to the general public if they are prescription only medicines or are medicines which, though not prescription only, may not legally be advertised to the general public. This prohibition does not apply to vaccination campaigns carried out by companies and approved by the health ministers.

*Clause 20.1 Advertising of Medicines to the General Public*

*The advertising of prescription only medicines to the general public is also prohibited by regulations.*

*The promotion of medicines to the general public for self medication purposes is covered by the Code of Standards of Advertising Practice for Over-the-Counter Medicines of the Proprietary Association of Great Britain (PAGB).*

*Methods of sale of medicines through pharmacies are also covered by the Code of Ethics of the Royal Pharmaceutical Society of Great Britain.*

**20.2** Information about medicines which is made available to the general public either directly or indirectly must be factual and presented in a balanced way. It must not raise unfounded hopes of successful treatment or be misleading with respect to the safety of the product.

Statements must not be made for the purpose of encouraging members of the public to ask their doctors to prescribe a specific medicine.

*Clause 20.2 Information to the General Public*

*This clause allows for the provision of non promotional information about prescription medicines to the general public either in response to a direct inquiry from an individual, including inquiries from journalists, or by dissemination of such information via press conferences, press announcements, television and radio reports, public relations activities and the like. It also includes information provided by means of posters distributed for display in surgery waiting rooms etc.*

*Any information so provided must observe the principles set out in this clause, that is, it should be factual, balanced and must not be made for the purpose of encouraging members of the public to ask their doctors to prescribe a specific medicine. It must not constitute the advertising of medicines to the general public prohibited under Clause 20.1. The provisions of Clause 20.3 must be observed if an inquiry is from an individual member of the public.*

*Particular care must be taken in responding to approaches from the media to ensure that the provisions of this clause are upheld.*

*In the event of a complaint which relates to the provisions of this clause, companies will be asked to provide copies of any information supplied, including copies of any relevant press releases and the like. This information will be assessed to determine whether it fulfils the requirements of this clause.*

*Summaries of product characteristics or data sheets for medicines may be provided to members of the public on request.*

*Companies may provide members of the health professions with leaflets concerning a medicine with a view to their provision to patients to whom the medicine has already been prescribed, provided that such a leaflet is factual and non-promotional in nature.*

*Clause 20.2 Financial Information*

*Information made available in order to inform shareholders, the Stock Exchange and the like by way of annual reports and announcements etc. may relate to both existing medicines and those not yet marketed. Such information must be factual and presented in a balanced way.*

*Clause 20.2 Approval of Information*

*Information on medicines made available under this Clause should be examined to ensure that it does not contravene the Code or the relevant statutory requirements.*

**20.3** Requests from individual members of the public for information or advice on personal medical matters must be refused and the enquirer recommended to consult his or her own doctor.

*Clause 20.3 Requests for Information or Advice on Personal Medical Matters*

*This clause prohibits the provision of information or advice on personal medical matters to individual members of the general public requesting it. The intention behind this prohibition is to ensure that companies do not intervene in the patient/doctor relationship by offering advice or information which properly should be in the domain of the doctor. However, information may be given, including information on medicines prescribed for the enquirer, provided that it complies with the requirements of Clauses 20.1 and 20.2 and does not impinge on the principle behind this clause. For example, answering requests by members of the public as to whether a particular medicine contains sucrose or some other inactive ingredient, or whether there would be problems associated with drinking alcohol whilst taking the medicine or whether the medicine should be taken before or after a meal, is acceptable. The situation with enquiries relating to side-effects, the indications for a medicine and such like is not as clear cut and particular caution is required in dealing with them.*

*All requests from members of the general public need to be handled with great care and a decision taken as to whether the company can responsibly answer the inquiry.*

*Requests from patients for information may in some instances best be handled by passing the information to the patients' doctors for discussion with them rather than providing the information direct to the patients concerned.*

**20.4** The introduction of a new medicine must not be made known to the general public until reasonable steps have been taken to inform the medical and pharmaceutical professions of its availability.

**20.5** Companies are responsible for information about their products which is issued by their public relations agencies.

**Clause 21 Compliance with Undertakings**

When an undertaking has been given in relation to a ruling under the Code, the company concerned must ensure that it complies with that undertaking.

# PRESCRIPTION MEDICINES CODE OF PRACTICE AUTHORITY: CONSTITUTION AND PROCEDURE

## INTRODUCTION

The Code of Practice for the Pharmaceutical Industry is administered by the Prescription Medicines Code of Practice Authority. The Authority is responsible for the provision of advice, guidance and training on the Code of Practice as well as for the complaints procedure. It is also responsible for arranging for conciliation between companies when requested to do so and for scrutinising journal advertising on a regular basis. Complaints made under the Code about promotional material or the promotional activities of companies are considered by the Code of Practice Panel and, where required, by the Code of Practice Appeal Board. Reports on cases are published quarterly by the Authority and are available on request.

The names of individuals complaining from outside the pharmaceutical industry are kept confidential. In exceptional cases it may be necessary for a company to know the identity of the complainant so that the matter can be properly investigated. Even in these instances, the name of the complainant is only disclosed with the complainant's permission.

Complaints about the promotion of medicines should be submitted to the Director of the Prescription Medicines Code of Practice Authority, 12 Whitehall, London SW1A 2DY; telephone 0171 930 9677; facsimile 0171 930 4554.

## STRUCTURE AND RESPONSIBILITIES

### 1 Prescription Medicines Code of Practice Authority

**1.1** The Prescription Medicines Code of Practice Authority is responsible for the administration of the Code of Practice for the Pharmaceutical Industry including the provision of advice, guidance and training on the Code. It is also responsible for arranging for conciliation between companies when requested to do so and for scrutinising journal advertising on a regular basis.

**1.2** The Authority also administers the complaints procedure by which complaints made under the Code are considered by the Code of Practice Panel and, where required, by the Code of Practice Appeal Board.

**1.3** The Authority is appointed by and reports to the Board of Management of The Association of the British Pharmaceutical Industry (ABPI) and consists of the Director, Secretary and Deputy Secretary.

**1.4** The Director has the authority to request copies of any relevant material from a pharmaceutical company, including copies of the certificates authorizing any such material and copies of relevant briefing material for representatives.

**1.5** The Authority may consult the Code of Practice Appeal Board upon any matter concerning the Code of Practice or its administration.

### 2 Code of Practice Panel – Constitution and Procedure

**2.1** The Code of Practice Panel consists of members of the Prescription Medicines Code of Practice Authority and meets as business requires to consider complaints made under the Code.

**2.2** Two members of the Authority form a quorum for a meeting of the Panel. Decisions are made by majority voting. The Director or, in his absence, the Secretary, acts as Chairman of the Panel and has both an original and a casting vote.

**2.3** The Director of the Authority may obtain expert assistance in any field. Expert advisers who are consulted may be invited to attend a meeting of the Panel but have no voting rights.

### 3 Code of Practice Appeal Board – Constitution

**3.1** The Code of Practice Appeal Board and its Chairman are appointed by the Board of Management of the ABPI. The appointment of independent members to the Appeal Board is made following consultation with the Medicines Control Agency.

**3.2** The Appeal Board comprises:

- an independent, legally qualified Chairman;
- three independent medical members appointed in consultation with the British Medical Association, one with recent experience as a general practitioner and one with recent experience as a hospital consultant;
- four medical directors or medically qualified senior executives from pharmaceutical companies;
- one independent pharmacist appointed following consultation with the Royal Pharmaceutical Society of Great Britain;
- one member from an independent body involved in providing information on medicines;
- eight directors or senior executives from pharmaceutical companies.

**3.3** The Chairman of the Appeal Board is appointed for a term of five years which may be renewed. Members of the Appeal Board are each appointed for a term of three years which may be renewed.

**3.4** The Director, Secretary and Deputy Secretary of the Code of Practice Authority comprise the secretariat to the Appeal Board. The secretariat attend meetings of the Appeal Board as observers and provide administrative support to the Appeal Board as appropriate.

### 4 Code of Practice Appeal Board – Procedure

**4.1** The Code of Practice Appeal Board meets as business requires to consider appeals under the Code and any other matter which relates to the Code. The Appeal Board receives reports on all complaints which have been submitted under the Code and details of the action taken on them.

**4.2** The Chairman and seven members of the Appeal Board constitute a quorum. Two of those present must be independent members, at least one of whom must be medically qualified, and there must also be present at least one medically qualified member from a pharmaceutical company.

In the event that a quorum cannot be attained for the consideration of a case because of the number of members barred under Paragraph 4.4 below, or for any other reason, the Chairman may co-opt appropriate persons to the Appeal Board so as to enable a quorum to be achieved.

**4.3** Decisions are made by majority voting. The Chairman has both an original and a casting vote.

**4.4** If a member of the Appeal Board is concerned in a case either as complainant or respondent, that member does not receive copies of the papers circulated in connection with the case and is required to withdraw from the Appeal Board during its consideration.

Members of the Appeal Board are also required to declare any other interest in a case prior to its consideration. The Chairman determines whether it is appropriate for that member to remain for the consideration of the case.

**4.5** The Chairman may obtain expert assistance in any field. Expert advisers may be invited to attend a meeting of the Appeal Board but have no voting rights.

**4.6** When appeals are considered by the Appeal Board, the respondent company is entitled to have a representative or representatives appear before the Appeal Board to state the company's case.

**4.7** Where an appeal is brought which is concerned with an issue of fact between a complainant and the company concerned which cannot be properly resolved without the oral evidence of the persons directly involved, the Chairman may invite such persons to attend and give evidence.

## COMPLAINTS PROCEDURE

### 5 Action on Complaints

**5.1** When the Director receives information from which it appears that a company may have contravened the Code, the chief executive of the company concerned is requested to comment on the matters of complaint.

If a complaint concerns a matter closely similar to one which has been the subject of a previous adjudication, it may be allowed to proceed at the discretion of the Director if new evidence is adduced by the complainant or if the passage of time or a change in circumstances raises doubts as to whether the same decision would be made in respect of the current complaint. The Director should normally allow a complaint to proceed if it covers matters similar to those in a decision of the Code of Practice Panel which was not the subject of appeal to the Code of Practice Appeal Board.

If a complainant does not accept a decision of the Director that a complaint should not be proceeded with because a similar complaint has been adjudicated upon previously and nothing has changed in the meantime, then the matter is referred to the Chairman of the Appeal Board for his decision which is final.

**5.2** When the complaint is from a pharmaceutical company, the complaint must be signed or authorised in writing by the company's chief executive and must state those clauses of the Code which are alleged to have been breached.

**5.3** Upon receipt of a complaint, the company c cerned has ten working days in which to submi comments in writing.

### 6 Establishment of *Prima Facie Case* and Consid tion by the Code of Practice Panel

**6.1** Upon receipt of the comments from the responc company, the Director must determine whether th is a *prima facie* case to answer under the Code. I the view of the Director, no *prima facie* case has b established the complainant and the responc company are so advised. If the complainant does accept that view, the matter is referred to the Chairr of the Code of Practice Appeal Board for his decis which is final.

**6.2** Once it has been determined that a *prima f* case exists, the case is referred to the Code of Prac Panel to determine whether or not there has bee breach of the Code.

### 7 Code of Practice Panel: Rulings

**7.1** Where the Code of Practice Panel rules that th is a breach of the Code, the company concerned is advised and is given the reasons for the decision.

The respondent company has ten working day provide a written undertaking that the promotic activity or use of the material in question (if already discontinued or no longer in use) will ce forthwith and that all possible steps will be take avoid a similar breach of the Code in the future. T undertaking must be signed by the chief executiv the company or with his or her authority and must accompanied by details of the actions taken by company to implement the undertaking, including date on which the promotional material was fin used or appeared and/or the last date on which promotional activity took place.

The company must also pay within twenty work days an administrative charge based on the num of matters ruled in breach of the Code.

**7.2** Where the Panel rules that there is no breach the Code, the complainant and respondent comp are so advised. Where the complaint is from pharmaceutical company, the complainant must within twenty working days an administrative cha based on the number of matters alleged and ruled to be in breach of the Code.

When advised of the outcome, the complainant be sent a copy of the comments and enclosu submitted by the respondent in relation to complaint. If the respondent objects to this becaus regards part of the material as being confidential, the matter cannot be settled by the Director, the will be referred to the Chairman of the Code of Prac Appeal Board for his decison which is final.

**7.3** The complainant or the respondent company m appeal against rulings of the Panel to the Code Practice Appeal Board. Appeals must be lodged wi ten working days of the notification of the ruling the Panel and must be accompanied by reasons as why the Panel's ruling is not accepted. These reas will be circulated to the Appeal Board.

**7.4** Where an appeal is lodged by the complain the respondent company has ten working days comment on the reasons given by the complain for the appeal and these comments will be circula to the Appeal Board.

The complainant has five working days to comm on the respondent company's comments upon reasons given by the complainant for the appeal a these comments also will be circulated to the App Board.

In the event that the respondent objects to cert of its comments being made available to the compla ant on the grounds of confidentiality, and the ma cannot be settled by the Director, then the matter be referred to the Chairman of the Code of Prac Appeal Board who will decide whether those partic comments can be included in the evidence wh goes before the Code of Practice Appeal Board.

### 8 Code of Practice Panel: Reports to the Appeal Bo

**8.1** Refusal to comply with the procedures set ou Paragraphs 5, 6 and 7 above shall be reported to Code of Practice Appeal Board for consideration relation to the provisions of Paragraph 11.1 below.

**8.2** The Code of Practice Panel may also report to Appeal Board any company whose conduct in relat to the Code, or in relation to a particular case bef it, warrants consideration by the Appeal Board relation to the provisions of Paragraphs 10.3 and 1 below. Such a report to the Appeal Board may made notwithstanding the fact that a company h provided an undertaking requested by the Panel.

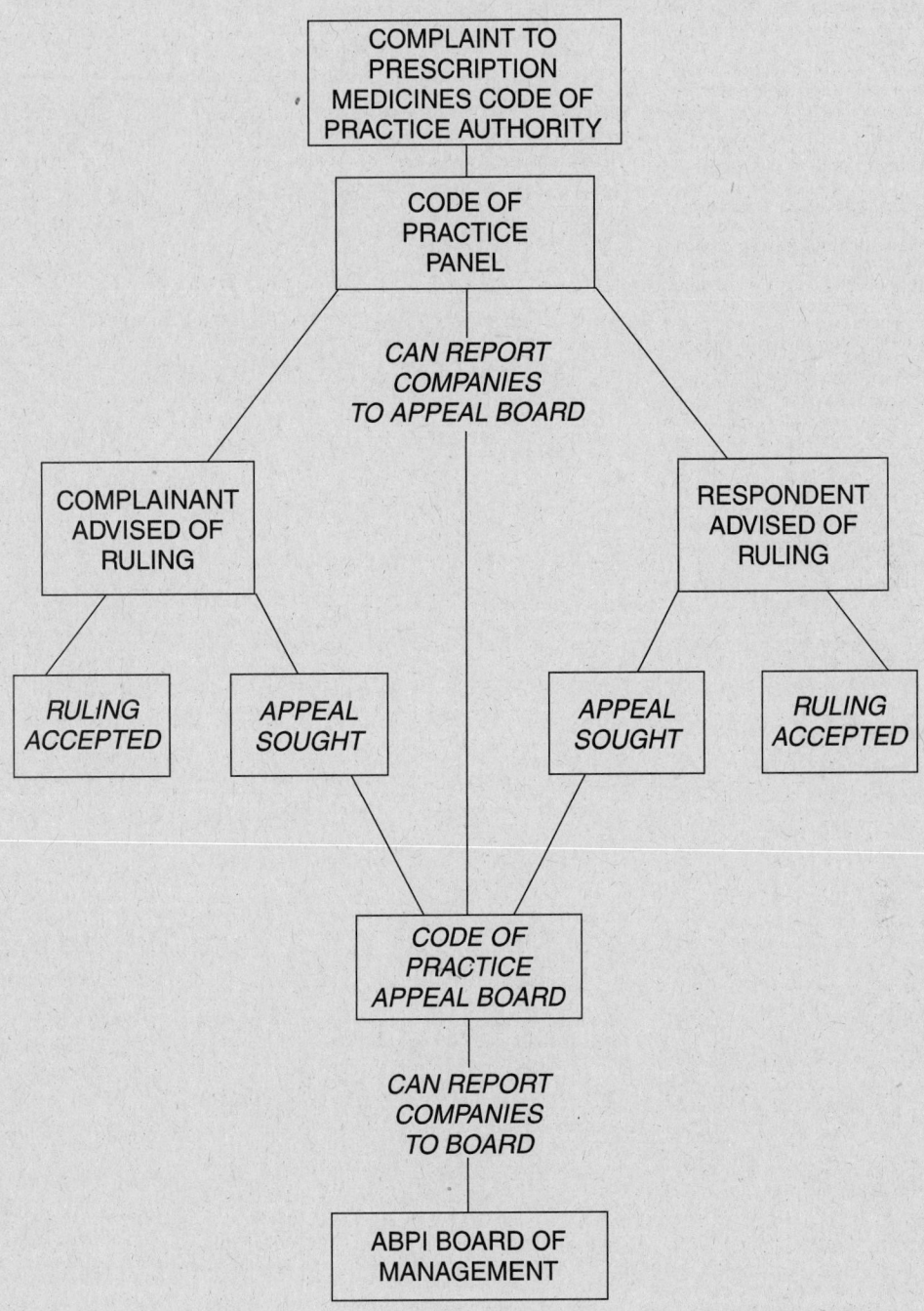

**8.3** Where the Panel reports a company to the Appeal Board under the provisions of Paragraphs 8.1 and 8.2 above, the company concerned is provided with a copy of the report prior to its consideration and is entitled to have a representative or representatives appear before the Appeal Board to state the company's case.

## 9 Action on Complaints about Safety from the Medicines Control Agency

**9.1** In the event of the Medicines Control Agency making a complaint which relates to the safety or proper use of a medicine, and requesting that an advertisement be withdrawn, the respondent company has five working days to respond with its comments.

**9.2** If the Code of Practice Panel upholds the complaint, the company is required to suspend the advertisement or practice forthwith pending the final outcome of the case.

## 10 Code of Practice Appeal Board: Rulings

**10.1** Where the Code of Practice Appeal Board rules that there is no breach of the Code, the complainant and the respondent company are so advised.

Where a complainant pharmaceutical company appeals and the Appeal Board upholds the ruling that there was no breach of the Code, the complainant pharmaceutical company must pay within twenty working days an administrative charge based on the number of matters taken to appeal on which no breach is ruled.

Where a respondent company appeals and the Appeal Board rules that there was no breach of the Code, the complainant pharmaceutical company must pay within twenty working days an administrative charge based on the number of matters taken to appeal on which no breach is ruled.

**10.2** Where the Appeal Board rules that there is a breach of the Code, the respondent company is so advised in writing and is given the reasons for the decision. The respondent company then has five working days to provide a written undertaking providing the information specified in Paragraph 7.1.

The company must also pay within twenty working days an administrative charge based on the number of matters ruled in breach of the Code.

**10.3** A company ruled in breach of the Code may also be required by the Appeal Board to take steps to recover items given in connection with the promotion of a medicine. Details of the action taken must be provided in writing to the Appeal Board.

**10.4** Where a company is ruled in breach of the Code the Appeal Board may require an audit of the company's procedures in relation to the Code to be carried out by the Prescription Medicines Code of Practice Authority.

## 11 Code of Practice Appeal Board: Reports to the Board of Management

**11.1** Where the Code of Practice Appeal Board considers that the conduct of a company in relation to the Code or a particular case before it warrants such action, it may report the company to the Board of Management of the ABPI for it to consider whether further sanctions should be applied against that company. Such a report may be made notwithstanding the fact that the company has provided an undertaking requested by either the Code of Practice Panel or the Appeal Board.

**11.2** Where such a report is made to the Board of Management, the Board of Management may decide:
- to reprimand the company and publish details of that reprimand;
- to require an audit of the company's procedures in relation to the Code to be carried out by the Prescription Medicines Code of Practice Authority and following that audit, decide whether to impose requirements on the company concerned to improve its procedures in relation to the Code;
- to require the company to publish a corrective statement;
- to suspend or expel the company from the ABPI; or
- in the case of companies not in membership of the ABPI, to remove the company from the list of non member companies which have agreed to abide by the Code and to advise the Medicines Control Agency that responsibility for that company under the Code can no longer continue to be accepted.

**11.3** Where a report is made to the Board of Management under Paragraph 11.1 above, the company concerned is provided with a copy of the report prior to its consideration and is entitled to have a representative or representatives appear before the Board of Management to state the company's case.

## 12 Case Reports

**12.1** At the conclusion of any case under the Code, the complainant is advised of the outcome and a report is published summarising the details of the case.

**12.2** The respondent company and the medicine concerned are named in the report.

In a case where the complaint was initiated by a company or by an organisation or official body, that company or organisation or official body are named in the report. The information given must not, however, be such as to identify any individual person.

**12.3** A copy of the report on a case is made available to the respondent company prior to publication. Any amendments to the report suggested by the respondent company are considered by the Director, consulting with the other party where appropriate. If either party does not accept the Director's decision as to whether or not a report should be amended, the matter is referred to the Chairman of the Code of Practice Appeal Board for his decision which is final.

**12.4** Copies of all case reports are submitted to the Code of Practice Appeal Board and to the Board of Management for information prior to publication.

Copies of the published reports are sent to the Medicines Control Agency, the Office of Fair Trading, the British Medical Association, the Royal Pharmaceutical Society of Great Britain, and the editors of the British Medical Journal and the Pharmaceutical Journal. Copies of the published reports are also available to anyone on request.

# GENERAL PROVISIONS

## 13 Time Periods for Responding to Matters under the Code

The number of working days within which companies or complainants must respond to enquiries etc, from the Prescription Medicines Code of Practice Authority, as referred to in the above procedures, are counted from the date of receipt of the notification in question.

An extension in time to respond to such notifications may be granted at the discretion of the Director of the Authority.

## 14 Withdrawal of Complaints and Notices of Appeal

**14.1** A complaint may be withdrawn by a complainant with the consent of the respondent company up until such time as the respondent company's comments on the complaint have been received by the Prescription Medicines Code of Practice Authority, but not thereafter.

**14.2** Notice of appeal may be withdrawn by a complainant with the consent of the respondent company up until such time as the respondent company's comments on the reasons for the appeal have been received by the Authority, but not thereafter.

**14.3** Notice of appeal may be withdrawn by a respondent company at any time but if notice is given after the papers relating to its appeal have been circulated to the Code of Practice Appeal Board, then the higher administrative charge will be payable.

## 15 Code of Practice Levy and Administrative Charges

**15.1** An annual Code of Practice levy is paid by members of the ABPI. The levy together with the administrative charges referred to in Paragraphs 7 and 10 above are determined by the Board of Management subject to approval at a General Meeting of the ABPI by a simple majority of those present and voting.

**15.2** Administrative charges are payable only by pharmaceutical companies and companies are liable for such charges whether they are members of the ABPI or not.

There are two levels of administrative charge.

The lower level is payable by a company which accepts either a ruling of the Code of Practice Panel that it was in breach of the Code or a rejection by the Panel of its allegation against another company. The lower level is also payable by a complainant company if a ruling of the Panel that there was a breach of Code is subsequently overturned by the Code Practice Appeal Board.

The higher level is paid by a company wh unsuccessfully appeals a decision of the Panel.

**15.3** Where two or more companies are ruled breach of the Code in relation to a matter involv co-promotion, each company shall be separat liable to pay an administrative charge.

**15.4** The number of administrative charges wh apply in a case is determined by the Director of Prescription Medicines Code of Practice Authority a company does not agree with the Director's decisi the matter is referred to the Chairman of the Code Practice Appeal Board for his decision which is fin

## 16 Possible Breaches identified by the Code of Pr tice Panel or Code of Practice Appeal Board

**16.1** Where the Code of Practice Panel or Code Practice Appeal Board identifies a possible breach the Code of Practice which has not been address by the complainant in a case, the respondent compa is invited to comment. The company has ten work days to respond in writing.

**16.2** If the company accepts there is a breach of Code of Practice, the company is requested to prov an undertaking providing the information specifie Paragraph 7.1 above. No administrative charge sh be payable in these circumstances and there shall no case report on the matter in question.

**16.3** If the company does not accept there is a bre of the Code of Practice the procedures under Pa graph 6 above onwards shall be followed.

## 17 Scrutiny of Advertisements

**17.1** A sample of advertisements issued by pharn ceutical companies is scrutinised by the Prescript Medicines Code of Practice Authority in relation to requirements of the Code on a continuing basis.

**17.2** Where a *prima facie* breach of the Code identified under this procedure, the company c cerned is requested to comment in writing within working days of receipt of the notification.

**17.3** If the company accepts there is a breach of Code, the company is requested to provide undertaking providing the information specified Paragraph 7.1 above. No administrative charge payable in these circumstances.

**17.4** If the company does not accept there is a bre of the Code, the procedures under Paragraph 6 abc onwards is followed.

## 18 Provision of Advice and Conciliation

**18.1** The Prescription Medicines Code of Pract Authority is available to provide informal guidar and advice in relation to the requirements of the Co and, where appropriate, may seek the views of Code of Practice Appeal Board.

**18.2** Companies wishing to seek the assistance o conciliator with the view to reaching agreement inter-company differences about promotion may c tact the Director of the Authority for advice a assistance.

## 19 Amendments to the Code of Practice

**19.1** The Code of Practice for the Pharmaceuti Industry and this Constitution and Procedure may amended by a simple majority of those present a voting at a General Meeting of the ABPI.

**19.2** The views of the Prescription Medicines Code Practice Authority, the Code of Practice Panel and Code of Practice Appeal Board must be sought on a proposal to amend the Code or this Constitution a Procedure. The views of the Medicines Cont Agency, the British Medical Association and the Ro Pharmaceutical Society of Great Britain must also invited.

**19.3** The Prescription Medicines Code of Pract Authority, the Code of Practice Panel and the Code Practice Appeal Board may, in the light of th experience, make recommendations for amendme of the Code and this Constitution and Procedure.

## 20 Annual Report

An annual report of the Prescription Medicines Co of Practice Authority is published each year with approval of the Code of Practice Appeal Board. T report includes details of the work of the Author the Code of Practice Panel and the Code of Pract Appeal Board during that year.

# INDEX

# Guidelines for company-sponsored safety assessment of marketed medicines (SAMM)

**Introduction**

It is well-recognised that there is a continuous need to monitor the safety of medicines as they are used in clinical practice. Spontaneous reporting schemes (*e.g.* the UK yellow card system) provide important early warning signals of potential drug hazards and also provide a means of continuous surveillance. Formal studies to evaluate safety may also be necessary, particularly in the confirmation and characterisation of possible hazards identified at an earlier stage of drug development. Such studies may also be useful in identifying previously unsuspected reactions.

**Scope of guidelines**

These guidelines apply to the conduct of all company-sponsored studies which evaluate the safety of marketed products. They take the place of previous guidelines on post-marketing surveillance which were published in 1988 (BMJ, 296: 399–400). Studies performed under those guidelines were found to have some notable limitations (BMJ, 1992, 304: 1470–1472) and these new guidelines have been prepared in response to the problems identified. The major changes may be summarised as follows:

(1) The scope of the guidelines has been expanded to include all company-sponsored studies which are carried out to evaluate safety of marketed medicines. It should be emphasised that this includes both studies conducted in general practice and in the hospital setting. The name of the guidelines has been changed to reflect the emphasis on safety assessment rather than merely surveillance.

(2) The guidelines have been developed to provide a framework on which a variety of data collection methods can be used to improve the evaluation of the safety of marketed medicines. Whilst it is recognised that the design used needs to be tailored to particular drugs and hazards, the guidelines define the essential principles which may be applied in a variety of situations. The study methods in this field continue to develop and therefore there will be a need to review regularly these guidelines to ensure that they reflect advances made in the assessment of drug safety.

The guidelines have been formulated and agreed by a Working Party which includes representation from the Medicines Control Agency (MCA), Committee on Safety of Medicines (CSM), Association of the British Pharmaceutical Industry (ABPI), British Medical Association (BMA) and the Royal College of General Practitioners (RCGP). Other guidelines exists for the conduct of 'Phase IV clinical trials' where the medication is provided by the sponsoring company (see section 2(b) below). Some of these studies will also meet the definition of a SAMM study (see below) and should therefore also comply with the present guidelines.

**1. Definition of Safety Assessment of Marketed Medicines**

(a) Safety assessment of marketed medicines (SAMM) is defined as 'a formal investigation conducted for the purpose of assessing the clinical safety of marketed medicine(s) in clinical practice'.

(b) Any study of a marketed drug which has the evaluation of clinical safety as a specific objective should be included. Safety evaluation will be a specific objective in post-marketing studies either when there is a known safety issue under investigation and/or when the numbers of patients to be included will add significantly to the existing safety data for the product(s). Smaller studies conducted primarily for other purposes should not be considered as SAMM studies. However, if a study which is not conducted for the purpose of evaluating safety unexpectedly identifies a hazard, the manufacturer would be expected to inform the MCA immediately and the section of these guidelines covering liaison with regulatory authorities would thereafter apply.

(c) In cases of doubt as to whether or not a study comes under the scope of the guidelines the sponsor should discuss the intended study plan with the MCA.

**2. Scope and Objectives of SAMM**

(a) SAMM may be conducted for the purpose of identifying previously unrecognised safety issues (hypothesis-generation) or to investigate possible hazards (hypothesis-testing).

(b) A variety of designs may be appropriate including observational cohort studies, case-surveillance or case-control studies. Clinical trials may also be used to evaluate the safety of marketed products, involving systematic allocation of treatment (for example randomisation). Such studies must also adhere to the current guidelines for Phase IV clinical trials.

(c) The design to be used will depend on the objectives of the study, which must be clearly defined in the study plan. Any specific safety concerns to be investigated should be identified in the study plan and explicitly addressed by the proposed methods.

**3. Design of studies**

*Observational cohort studies*

(a) The population studied should be as representative as possible of the general population of users, and be unselected unless specifically targeted by the objectives of the study (for example a study of the elderly). Exclusion criteria should be limited to the contraindications stated in the data sheet or summary of product characteristics (SPC). The prescriber should be provided with a data sheet or SPC for all products to be used. Where the product is prescribed outside the indications on the data sheet, such patients should be included in the analysis of the study findings.

(b) Observational cohort studies should normally include appropriate comparator group(s). The comparator group(s) will usually include patients with the disease/indication(s) relevant to the primary study drug and such patients will usually be treated with alternative therapies.

(c) The product(s) should be prescribed in the usual manner, for example on an FP10 form written by the general practitioner or through the usual hospital procedures.

(d) Patients must not be prescribed particular medicines in order to include them in observational cohort studies since this is unethical (see section 15 of the 'Guidelines on the Practices of Ethics Committees in Medical Research involving Human Subjects', Royal College of Physicians, 1990).

(e) The prescribing of a drug and the inclusion of the patient in a study are two issues which must be clearly separated. Drugs must be prescribed solely as a result of a normal clinical evaluation, and since such indications may vary from doctor to doctor a justification for the prescription should be recorded in the study documents. In contrast, the inclusion of the patient in the study must be solely dependent upon the criteria for recruitment which have been specifically identified in the study procedures. Any deviation from the study criteria for recruitment could lead to selection bias.

(f) The study plan should stipulate the maximum number of patients to be entered by a single doctor. No patient should be prospectively entered into more than one study simultaneously.

*Case-control studies*

(g) Case-control studies are usually conducted retrospectively. In case-control studies comparison is made between the history of drug exposure of cases with the disease of interest and appropriate controls without the disease. The study design should attempt to account for known sources of bias and confounding.

*Case-surveillance*

(h) The purpose of case-surveillance is to study patients with diseases which are likely to be drug-related and to ascertain drug exposure. Companies who sponsor such studies should liaise particularly closely with the MCA in order to determine the most appropriate arrangements for the reporting of cases.

*Clinical trials*

(i) Large clinical trials are sometimes useful in the investigation of post-marketing safety issues and these may involve random allocation to treatment. In other respects, an attempt should be made to study patients under as normal conditions as possible. Exclusion criteria should be limited to the contraindications in the data sheet or SPC unless they are closely related to the particular objectives of the study. Clinical trials must also adhere to the current guidelines for Phase IV clinical trials (see 2(b) above). Studies which fulfil the definition of SAMM but are performed under a clinical trial exemption (CTX) or under the clinical trial on a marketed product (CTMP) scheme are within the scope of these guidelines.

**4. Conduct of studies**

(a) Responsibility for the conduct and quality of company-sponsored studies shall be vested in the company's medical department under the supervision of a named medical practitioner registered in the United Kingdom, and whose name shall be recorded in the study documents.

(b) Where a study is performed for a company by an agent, a named medical practitioner registered in the United Kingdom shall be identified by the agent to supervise the study and liaise with the compar medical department.

(c) Consideration should be given to the appointm of an independent advisory group(s) to monitor safety information and oversee the study.

**5. Liaison with regulatory authorities**

(a) Companies proposing to perform a SAMM stu are encouraged to discuss the draft study plan w the Medicines Control Agency (MCA) at an early sta Particular consideration should be given to spec safety issues which may require investigation.

(b) Before the study commences a study plan sho be finalised which explains the aims and objectives the study, the methods to be used (including statist analysis) and the record keeping which is to maintained. The company shall submit the study p plus any proposed initial communications to doct to the MCA at least one month before the plann start of the study. The MCA will review the propos study and may comment. The responsibility for conduct of the study will, however, rest with sponsoring pharmaceutical company.

(c) The company should inform the MCA when study has commenced and will normally provide brief report on its progress at least every six mont or more frequently if requested by MCA.

(d) The regulatory requirements for reporting of s pected adverse reactions must be fulfilled. Compan should endeavour to ensure that they are notified serious suspected adverse reactions and sho report these to the MCA within 15 days of rece Events which are not suspected by the investigato be adverse reactions should not be reported indiv ually as they occur. These and minor adverse reactic should be included in the final report.

(e) A final report on the study should be sent to MCA within 3 months of follow-up being complet Ideally this should be a full report but a brief rep within 3 months followed by a full report withi months of completion of the study would normally acceptable. The findings of the study should submitted for publication.

(f) Companies are encouraged to follow MCA gui lines on the content of progress reports and fi reports.

**6. Promotion of medicines**

(a) SAMM studies should not be conducted for purposes of promotion.

(b) Company representatives should not be involv in SAMM studies in such a way that it could be se as a promotional exercise.

**7. Doctor Participation**

(a) Subject to the doctor's terms of service, paym may be offered to the doctor in recompense for time and any expenses incurred according to suggested scale of fees published by the BMA.

(b) No inducement for a doctor to participate ir SAMM study should be offered, requested or give

**8. Ethical Issues**

(a) The highest possible standards of professio conduct and confidentiality must always be ma tained. The patient's right to confidentiality is pa mount. The patient's identity in the study docume should be codified and only his or her doctor sho be capable of decoding it.

(b) Responsibility for the retrieval of information fr personal medical records lies with the consultant general practitioner responsible for the patient's ca Such information should be directed to the medi practitioner nominated by the company or agent, w is thereafter responsible for the handling of su information.

(c) Reference to a Research Ethics Committee required if patients are to be approached for inforn tion, additional investigations are to be performed if it is proposed to allocate patients systematically treatments.

**9. Procedure for complaints**

A study which gives cause for concern on scienti ethical or promotional grounds should be referred the MCA, ABPI and the company concerned. Conce regarding possible scientific fraud should be refer to the ABPI. They will be investigated and, if appro ate, referred to the General Medical Council.

**10. Review of Guidelines**

The Working Party will review these guidelines necessary.

# Poisons Information Services

**BELFAST**
Director: Professor D G Johnson
Address: National Poisons Information
Service (Belfast)
Royal Victoria Hospital
Grosvenor Road
Belfast
BT12 6BA
Telephone: 01232 240503 (24-hour service)
01232 248095 (Regional Drug and Poisons
Information Service)
Fax: 01232 248030

**BIRMINGHAM**
Director: Dr J A Vale
Address: National Poisons Information
Service (Birmingham Centre)
West Midlands Poisons Unit
City Hospital NHS Trust
Dudley Road
Birmingham
B18 7QH
Telephone: 0121 507 5588/5599 (24-hour service)
Fax: 0121 507 5580

**CARDIFF**
Director: Professor P A Routledge
Address: Welsh National Poisons Unit
Therapeutics and Toxicology Centre,
Academic Centre,
Llandough Hospital
Penarth
Cardiff
CF64 2XX
Telephone: 01222 709901 (24-hour service)
Fax: 01222 704357

**DUBLIN**
Director: Dr J A Tracey
Address: Poisons Information Centre
Beaumont Hospital
PO Box 1297
Beaumont Road
Dublin 9
Eire
Telephone: 00 353 1 8379966
00 353 1 8379964
Fax: 00 353 1 8376982

**EDINBURGH**
Director: Dr A T Proudfoot
Address: Scottish Poisons Information Bureau
The Royal Infirmary of Edinburgh NHS Trust
Lauriston Place
Edinburgh
EH3 9YW
Telephone: 0131 536 2300 (24-hour service)
Fax: 0131 536 2304
TOXBASE: For access contact 0131 5362298

**LEEDS**
Director: Dr A Judd
Address: National Poisons Information Service (Leeds)
Pharmacy Department
The General Infirmary
Great George Street
Leeds
LS1 3EX
Telephone: 0113 243 0715 (24-hour service)
Fax: 0113 244 5849

**LONDON**
Director: Dr G N Volans
Address: National Poisons Information Service (London)
Medical Toxicology Unit
Guy's & St Thomas' Hospital Trust
Avonley Road
London SE14 5ER
Telephone: 0171 635 9191 (24-hour emergency service)
0171 771 5370 (laboratory enquiries and Unit
Staff)
Fax: 0171 771 5309

**NEWCASTLE**
Director: Dr D N Bateman
Address: National Poisons Information Service (Newcastle)
Regional Drug and Therapeutics Centre
Wolfson Unit
Claremont Place
Newcastle upon Tyne
NE2 4HH
Telephone: 0191 232 1525 (Direct line, normal office hours)
0191 232 5131 (24-hour service)
Fax: 0191 261 5733

## Monitoring of drug overdoses

The poisons information service monitors reports of drug overdosage in a similar manner to the monitoring of adverse reactions by the Committee on Safety of Medicines. Doctors are encouraged to report unusual or severe cases to this service (whether or not they need to use the service for information or advice). In particular, the service would be keen to hear reports of overdose of those drugs also highlighted by the CSM, using the black triangle, since experience of overdose with these drugs is bound to be limited.

## Overdose in pregnancy

All National Poisons Information Service (NPIS) Centres are able to advise on patients who take overdoses while pregnant, however the Newcastle Centre of the NPIS has been designated as the National Co-ordinating Centre for enquiries about poisoning in pregnancy. This service includes the follow up of the outcome of patients exposed to potential overdose in pregnancy. Enquiries about poisoning in pregnancy can, therefore, be directed to any NPIS centre, or to the Newcastle Centre directly on the telephone numbers above, or in writing.

# Products new to this edition

*The following list comprises products which are the subject of data sheets or summaries of product characteristics (SPCs) in this edition of the Compendium but which were not included in the 1996–97 edition. It does not necessarily follow that they are recently introduced products.*

Aciclovir I.V. 348
Aclarubicin medac Injection 704
ACT-HIB DTP dc 948
Actidose-Aqua 220
Actrapid Penfill 890
Acular 54
Aldactide 1273
Aldactone 1273
Alphagan 54
Alphanate 60
Aricept 308
Asmasal Clickhaler 322
Atracurium Besylate Injection 350

Baclofen Tablets 601
Becloforte Easi-Breathe Inhaler 31
Becotide Easi-Breathe Inhalers 35
Begrivac 1464
Betagan 55
Botox 55

Cabaser 977
Cacit D3 1066
Caelyx 1248
Calceos 1414
Calcium Leucovorin 352
Campto 1083
Canesten Hydrocortisone 132
Captopril Tablets BP 407
CCNU Capsules 705
Cefuroxime 631
Ciproxin I.V. Flexibag 134
Clotam Capsules 1415
Co-amilofruse Tablets BP 603
Cobalin-H 662
Colazide 88
Corlan Pellets 330
Cozaar-Comp 727
Creon 1000 1357
Crixivan 729
Cromogen Easi-Breathe Inhaler 119

Dermestril 1185
Dermol 500 Lotion 268
Diazepam Rectubes 2.5 mg and
     20 mg 254
Diazepam Rectubes 5 mg and
     10 mg 254
Dicobalt Edetate Injection 221
Differin Gel 404
Digenac XL 315

Diovan 813
Dramamine 1277

Edronax 997
Efalith Ointment 1277
Elleste Duet 1 mg 1279
Entocort Enema 91
Epaderm 159
Epinephrine Injection 1:1000 526
Epivir Solution 430
Epivir Tablets 431
Erecnos 396
Evorel Conti 540
Evorel Sequi 540

Fareston 925
Femapak 40 1360
Femara 818
Fenbufen 410
Fentanyl Citrate Injection 365
Flomax MR 1502
Fortipine LA40 900
Fragmin Multi-Dose Vial 1001
Fraxiparine 1191
Frusene 924
Fybozest Orange 1077

Gaviscon Advance 1078
GelTears 238
Gestronol Hexanoate Ampoules 223
Glucagen 1 mg 894
Granocyte 246

Human Mixtard 891
Hypurin Bovine in Cartridges 256
Hypurin Bovine in Vials 256
Hypurin Porcine in Cartridges 257
Hypurin Porcine in Vials 257

Imigran Nasal Spray 436
Imunovir 786
Innohep Syringe 20,000 IU/ml 622
Insulatard Penfill 890
Intal Spincaps 1092
Invirase 1135
Isocard Transdermal Spray 306
Isotrexin 1409

Ketoprofen Capsules 608
Klaricid XL 15

Lacrilube 57
Lipitor 941
Lipobay 137
Liquifilm 57
Lodine 768
Lomotil 1281
Lubri-Tears 27
Lyclear Dermal Cream 1436

Malarone 441
Menophase 1282
Meprobamate Tablets 413
Metronidazole Tablets 291
Micanol Cream 335
Minims Proxymetacaine and
     Fluorescein 243
Minitran 139
Minocycline Tablets 412
Mirena 1232
Mitomycin for Injection 377
Mixtard Penfill 890
MMR II 954
Modisal 610
Monovent 610
Morcap 1200

Naramig 445
Naropin 99
Nasacort 1098
Nasobec Aqueous 121
Nasonex 1258
Natrilix SR 1305
Nitromin 286
Norimin 1284
Norinyl-1 1285
Nozinan 662
Nu-Seals Cardio 75 653
Nuvelle TS 1238
Nystatin Oral Suspension 1394

OncoTICE 921
OPV Poliomyelitis Vaccine 336
Oramorph SR 187
Oxis Turbohaler 101

Pabrinex 662
Palladone Capsules 781
Palladone-SR Capsules 782
Persantin Retard 178
Phenylephrine Injection 592
Plendil 103

Pnu-imune 1486
Posicor 1151
Predsol suppositories 340
Protamine Sulphate Injection 593
Protium 594
Pylorid 450

Rapilysin 195
Rehidrat Multipack 1287
Rheomacrodex in Dextrose 227
Rheomacrodex in Normal Saline 228
Rilutek 1105
Rinatec Nasal Spray 0.03% 179
Rubilin 342

Sandrena 913
Seroquel 1529
Sporanox Liquid 569
Suprax 1112
Synphase 1288
Syscor MR 142
Sytron 663

Tasmar 1163
Telfast 517
Temazepam Tablets 10 mg and
     20 mg 612
Tensipine MR 315
Testosterone Enanthate
     Ampoules 229
Timolol Eye Drops 702

Ultiva 461

Ventolin Easi-Breathe Inhaler 47
Vesanoid 1169
Viazem XL 303
Vistide 1054

Wellvone 466

Xalatan 1057

Zamadol Capsules 77
Zipzoc 960
Zispin 916
Zomig 1550
Zorac 57
Zumenon Tablets 1 mg 1370
Zyprexa 660

# Directory of participants

This directory is included in the Compendium so that doctors and other professional people may obtain additional information about products from participating companies.

Medical Information
**Abbott Laboratories Ltd**
Abbott House
Norden Road
Maidenhead
Berkshire SL6 4XE

*Telephone:*
Maidenhead (01628) 773355

*Facsimile:* (01628) 644185

**Alcon Laboratories (UK) Ltd**
Pentagon Park
Boundary Way
Hemel Hempstead
Hertfordshire HP2 7UD

*Telephone:* (01442) 341234

*Facsimile:* (01442) 341200

Medical Information
**Allen & Hanburys Ltd**
Stockley Park West
Uxbridge
Middlesex UB11 1BT

*Telephone:* (0181) 990 3001 or
FREEFONE 0800 371891 (including 24-hour emergency service)

*Facsimile:* (0181) 990 4372

Customer Services
*Telephone:* FREEFONE 0800
371441

*Facsimile:* (0181) 990 4328

Medical Information
**Allergan Ltd**
Coronation Road
High Wycombe
Buckinghamshire HP12 3SH

*Telephone:* (01494) 427026

*Facsimile:* (01494) 473593

**Alpha Therapeutic UK Ltd**
Howlett Way
Thetford
Norfolk IP24 1HZ

*Telephone:*
Thetford (01842) 761942

*Facsimile:* (01842) 766661

**Amersham International plc**
White Lion Road
Amersham
Buckinghamshire HP7 9LL

*Telephone:* (01494) 543973 or
543637

*Facsimile:* (01494) 543821

Medical Information
**Approved Prescription
Services Ltd**
Brampton Road
Hampden Park
Eastbourne
East Sussex BN22 9AG

*Telephone:* (01323) 501111

*Facsimile:* (01323) 520306

**ASTA Medica Ltd**
168 Cowley Road
Cambridge CB4 4DL

*Telephone:*
Medical Information (including 24-hour emergency service)
(01223) 428811
All other enquiries (01223) 423434

*Facsimile:* (01223) 420943

Medical Information Department
**Astra Pharmaceuticals Ltd**
Home Park
Kings Langley
Hertfordshire WD4 8DH

*Telephone:*
Kings Langley (01923) 266191 (including 24-hour emergency service)

*Facsimile:* (01923) 261416

**Baker Norton**
Gemini House
Flex Meadow
Harlow
Essex CM19 5TJ

*Telephone:* 01279 426666

*Facsimile:* 01279 432110

**Bayer plc**
Pharmaceutical Division
Bayer House
Strawberry Hill
Newbury
Berkshire RG14 1JA

*Telephone:* (01635) 563000

*Facsimile:* (01635) 563616

**Bayer Bridgend**
Bayer House
Strawberry Hill
Newbury
Berkshire RG14 1JA

*Telephone:* (01635) 563000

*Facsimile:* (01635) 563616

Medical Information Department
**Beecham Research**
Welwyn Garden City
Hertfordshire AL7 1EY

*Telephone*
Welwyn Garden (01707) 325111
or FREEFONE (0800) 616482
(including 24-hour emergency service)

*Facsimile:* (0181) 913 4560

Medical Information Department
**Bencard**
Welwyn Garden City
Hertfordshire AL7 1EY

*Telephone*
Welwyn Garden (01707) 325111
or FREEFONE (0800) 616482
(including 24-hour emergency service)

*Facsimile:* (0181) 913 4560

Medical Information
**Berk Pharmaceuticals Limited**
Brampton Road
Hampden Park
Eastbourne
East Sussex BN22 9AG

*Telephone:* (01323) 501111

*Facsimile:* (01323) 520306

Medical Information
**Biogen**
Ocean House
The Ring
Bracknell
Berkshire RG12 1AX

*Telephone:* (01344) 867033

*Facsimile:* (01344) 867416

Medical Information
**Bioglan Laboratories Ltd**
5 Hunting Gate
Hitchin
Hertfordshire SG4 0TJ

*Telephone:*
Hitchin (01462) 438444

Emergency Medical Information:
Dr R. Mason
(01767) 627085

*Facsimile:* (01462) 421242

Information Services
**Boehringer Ingelheim Ltd**
Ellesfield Avenue
Bracknell
Berkshire RG12 8YS

*Telephone:* (01344) 424600 (including 24-hour emergency service)

*Facsimile:* (01344) 741444

Information Services
**Boehringer Ingelheim Hospital Division**
Ellesfield Avenue
Bracknell
Berkshire RG12 8YS

*Telephone:*
Bracknell (01344) 424600 (including 24-hour emergency service)

*Facsimile:* (01344) 741444

Medical Information Department
**Boehringer Mannheim UK Ltd**
Simpson Parkway
Kirkton Campus
Livingston
West Lothian EH54 7BH

*Telephone:*
Livingston (01506) 412512

*Facsimile:* (01506) 411395

**Bristol-Myers
Pharmaceuticals**
Bristol-Myers Squibb House
141-149 Staines Road
Hounslow
Middlesex TW3 3JA

*Telephone:*
Medical Information Only: (0181) 754 3740
BMS House and emergencies: (0181) 572 7422 and FREEFONE 0800 7311736

*Facsimile:* (0181) 754 3789

**Bristol-Myers Squibb
Pharmaceuticals Ltd**
Bristol-Myers Squibb House
Staines Road
Hounslow TW3 3JA

*Telephone:*
Medical Information Only: (0181) 754 3740 and FREEFONE 0800 7311736
BMS House and emergencies: (0181) 572 7422

*Facsimile:* (0181) 754 3789

**Britannia Pharmaceuticals Ltd**
41–51 Brighton Road
Redhill
Surrey RH1 6YS

*Telephone:*
Redhill (01737) 773741

*Facsimile:* (01737) 762672

**Cambridge Laboratories**
Richmond House
Old Brewery Court
Sandyford Road
Newcastle upon Tyne NE2 1XG

*Telephone:* (0191) 261 5950

*Facsimile:* (0191) 261 5915

**Centeon Ltd**
RPR House
52 St Leonards Road
Eastbourne
East Sussex BN21 3YG

*Telephone:* (01323) 410200

*Facsimile:* (01323) 410306

**Chauvin Pharmaceuticals Ltd**
Ashton Road
Harold Hill
Romford
Essex RM3 8SL

*Telephone:* 01708 383838

*Facsimile:* 01708 371316

**Chugai Pharma UK Limited**
Mulliner House
Flanders Road
Turnham Green
London W4 1NN

*Telephone:* (0181) 987 5680

*Facsimile:* (0181) 987 5661

**CIBA Laboratories**
See **Novartis Pharmaceuticals
UK Ltd**

**CIBA Vision Ophthalmics**
Flanders Road
Hedge End
Southampton SO30 2LG

*Telephone:* (01489) 775534

*Facsimile:* (01489) 798074

Technical Department
**Cox Pharmaceuticals**
A. H. Cox & Co Limited
Whiddon Valley
Barnstaple
North Devon EX32 8NS

*Telephone:*
Medical information (including 24-hour emergency service) (01271) 311257
All other enquiries (01271) 311200

*Facsimile:* (01271) 311329

Medical Information
**CP Pharmaceuticals Ltd**
Ash Road North
Wrexham LL13 9UF

*Telephone:* (01978) 661261
Direct Line (08.30–16.30 hours): (01978) 666172

*Facsimile:* (01978) 661702

**DBL (David Bull Laboratories)**
See **Faulding Pharmaceuticals**

Medical Information Department
**Delandale Laboratories Ltd**
Foundation Park
Roxborough Way
Maidenhead
Berkshire SL6 3UD

*Telephone:* (01628) 501200

*Facsimile:* (01628) 501278

Medical Information
**Dermal Laboratories Ltd**
Tatmore Place
Gosmore
Hitchin
Hertfordshire SG4 7QR

*Telephone:*
Hitchin (01462) 458866
Emergency Medical Information
Telephone: Dr M. Whitefield
0181-455 4998

*Facsimile:* (01462) 422128

**E. C. DeWitt & Company Ltd**
Tudor Road
Manor Park
Runcorn
Cheshire WA7 1SZ

*Telephone:* (01928) 579029

*Facsimile:* (01928) 579712

Medical Information and Drug Surveillance Department.
**Dista Products Ltd**
**(a subsidiary of Eli Lilly and Company Limited)**
Dextra Court
Chapel Hill
Basingstoke
Hampshire RG21 5SY

*Telephone:*
Direct Lines (08.30–17.30 hours) for medical information on:
• Antimicrobial and Oncology: (01256) 315246
• Cardiology: (01256) 315244
• Endocrine & Gastroenterology: (01256) 315245
• Neurology: (01256) 315264
• Psychiatric: (01256) 315264, (01256) 315907 or (01256) 315249
• Other products (including 24 hour Emergency Service): Basingstoke (01256) 315000 or Basingstoke (01256) 52011

*Facsimile:* (01256) 315569

**Dominion Pharma Ltd**
Dominion House
Lion Lane
Haslemere
Surrey GU27 1JL

*Telephone:* (01428) 661078
*Facsimile:* (01428) 661075

**Dumex Ltd**
Tring Business Centre
Upper Icknield Way
Tring
Hertfordshire HP23 4JX

*Telephone:* (01442) 890090
*Facsimile:* (01442) 890899

Medical Information Department
**Du Pont Pharmaceuticals Ltd**
Avenue One
Letchworth Garden City
Herts SG6 2HU

*Telephone:* (01462) 488200
*Facsimile:* (01462) 488319

**Eastern Pharmaceuticals Ltd**
Coomb House
7 St John's Road
Isleworth
Middlesex TW7 6NA

*Telephone:* (0181) 569 8174
*Facsimile:* (0181) 569 8175

**Eisai Ltd**
3 Shortlands
Hammersmith
London W6 8EE

*Telephone:* (0181) 600 1400
*Facsimile:* (0181) 600 1401

Medical Information Department
**Elan Pharma**
Lambert Court
Chestnut Avenue
Eastleigh
Hants SO53 3ZQ

*Telephone:* (01703) 620500
*Facsimile:* (01703) 629819

**Ethical Generics Ltd**
West Point
46–48 West Street
Newbury
Berkshire RG14 1BD

*Telephone:* (01635) 568400
*Facsimile:* (01635) 568401

**Euroderma Limited**
The Old Coach House
34 Elm Road
Chessington
Surrey KT9 1AW

*Telephone:* (0181) 974 2266
*Facsimile:* (0181) 974 2005

**Evans Medical Ltd**
Evans House
Regent Park
Kingston Road
Leatherhead
Surrey KT22 7PQ

*Telephone:* (01372) 364000
*Facsimile:* (01372) 364190

Medical Information
**Faulding Pharmaceuticals Plc**
Spartan Close
Tachbrook Park
Warwick CV34 6RS

*Telephone:* (01926) 821010 (direct line)
*Facsimile:* (01926) 821041

**Ferring Pharmaceuticals Ltd**
Greville House
Hatton Road
Feltham
Middlesex TW14 9PX

*Telephone:* (0181) 831 4600
*Emergency service:* 0850 437 854
*Facsimile:* (0181) 893 1577

**Forley Ltd**
54 Hillbury Avenue
Harrow
Middlesex HA3 8EW

*Telephone:* (0181) 665 9169
*Facsimile:* (0181) 665 9616

**Fournier Pharmaceuticals Ltd**
22–23 Progress Business Centre
Whittle Parkway
Slough SL1 6DG

*Telephone:* (01753) 740400
*Facsimile:* (01753) 740444

**Fujisawa Ltd**
8th Floor, CP House
97–107 Uxbridge Road
London W5 5TL

*Telephone:* (0181) 840 9520 (including 24-hour emergency service)
*Facsimile:* (0181) 840 9521

**Galderma (UK) Ltd**
Leywood House
Woodside Road
Amersham
Bucks HP6 6AA

*Telephone:*
(01494) 432606
*Facsimile:* (01494) 432607

**Geigy Pharmaceuticals**
See **Novartis Pharmaceuticals UK Ltd**

Medical Information Department
**Genus Pharmaceuticals**
Huntercombe Lane South
Taplow
Maidenhead
Berkshire SL6 0PH

*Telephone:* (01628) 604377 (including 24-hour emergency service)
*Facsimile:* (01628) 666368

**Glaxo Laboratories**
See **Glaxo Wellcome**

Medical Information
**Glaxo Wellcome**
Stockley Park West
Uxbridge
Middlesex UB11 1BT

*Telephone enquiries* (including 24 hour emergency service):
Asthma & Allergy Products (0181) 990 3001 or FREEFONE 0800 371891
Gastrointestinal and Dermatology Products (0181) 990 4951 or FREEFONE 0800 318319
Herpes, Epilepsy & Migraine Products (0181) 990 4876 or FREEFONE 0800 413828
Hospital & Other products (0181) 990 4877 or FREEFONE 0800 413524

*Facsimile:* (0181) 990 4372

Customer Services
*Telephone:* FREEFONE 0800 221441
*Facsimile:* (0181) 990 4328

**Glenwood Laboratories Ltd**
Unit D
Jenkins Dale
Chatham
Kent ME4 5RD

*Telephone:* (01634) 830535
*Facsimile:* (01634) 831345

**Goldshield Healthcare**
NLA Tower
12–16 Addiscombe Road
Croydon CR9 6BP

*Telephone:* (0181) 649 8500
*Facsimile:* (0181) 686 0807

Medical Information Department
**Hoechst Marion Roussel Ltd**
Broadwater Park
Denham
Uxbridge
Middlesex UB9 5HP

*Telephone:* (01895) 834343 or FREEFONE 0800 282833

24-hour emergency service (01895) 837586

*Facsimile:* (01895) 834479

**ICN Pharmaceuticals Ltd**
1 Elmwood
Chineham Business Park
Crockford Lane
Basingstoke
Hampshire RG24 8WG

*Telephone:* (01256) 707744
*Facsimile:* (01256) 707334

Medical Information
**Immuno Ltd**
(A division of Baxter Healthcare Ltd)
Wallingford Road
Compton
Newbury
Berkshire RG20 7QW

*Telephone:* (01635) 206265
*Facsimile:* (01635) 206126

**International Medication Systems (UK) Ltd**
Evans House
Regent Park
Kingston Road
Leatherhead
Surrey KT22 7PQ

*Telephone:* (01372) 364000
*Facsimile:* (01372) 364190

Medical Information
**Invicta Pharmaceuticals**
A Division of Pfizer Ltd
Sandwich
Kent CT13 9NJ

*Telephone:*
Sandwich (01304) 616161 (including 24-hour emergency service)
Sandwich (01304) 625210 (medical information only)

The Medical Information Department
**Janssen-Cilag Ltd**
Saunderton
High Wycombe
Buckinghamshire HP14 4HJ

*Telephone:* FREEFONE 0800 7318450 (including 24-hour emergency service)
*Facsimile:* (01494) 567445

**JHC Healthcare Ltd**
The Maltings
Bridge Street
Hitchin
Herts SG5 2DE

*Telephone:* (01462) 432533
*Facsimile:* (01462) 432535

Medical Information Department
**Knoll Ltd**
9 Castle Quay
Castle Boulevard
Nottingham NG7 1FW

*Telephone:* (0115) 912 5000
*Facsimile:* (0115) 912 5069

**Kyowa Hakko UK Ltd**
CP House
97–107 Uxbridge Road
Ealing
London W5 5TL

*Telephone:* (0181) 840 4600
*Facsimile:* (0181) 567 3250

Medical Department
**Laboratories for Applied Biology Ltd**
91 Amhurst Park
London N16 5DR

*Telephone:* (0181) 800 2252
*Facsimile:* (0181) 809 6884

**Lagap Pharmaceuticals Ltd**
Woolmer Way
Bordon
Hampshire GU35 9QE

*Telephone:*
Bordon (01420) 478301
*Facsimile:* (01420) 487073
(01420) 474427

**Lederle Laboratories**
See **Wyeth Laboratories**

Medical Department
**Leo Laboratories Ltd**
Longwick Road
Princes Risborough
Buckinghamshire HP27 9RR

*Telephone:*
Princes Risborough (01844) 347333
*Facsimile:* (01844) 342278

Medical Information and Drug Surveillance Department
**Eli Lilly and Company Limited**
Dextra Court
Chapel Hill
Basingstoke
Hampshire RG21 5SY

*Telephone:*
Direct Lines (08.30–17.30 hours) for medical information on:

Antimicrobial and Oncology:
(01256) 315246
Cardiology: (01256) 315244
Endocrinology and Gastroenterology: (01256) 315245
Neurology: (01256) 315264
Psychiatric: (01256) 315264,
(01256) 315907 or (01256)
315249
Other products (including 24
hour Emergency Service): Basingstoke (01256) 315000 or Basingstoke (01256) 52011

Facsimile: (01256) 315569

**...nk Pharmaceuticals Ltd**
8 Sterling Buildings
Carfax
Horsham
West Sussex RH12 1DR

Telephone: (01403) 272451

Facsimile: (01403) 272455

**...pha Pharmaceuticals Ltd**
Harrier House
...gh Street
West Drayton
Middlesex UB7 7QG

Telephone:
Medical Information Department
(9.00 to 17.00 hours): (01895)
52258
24-hour Emergency Service:
(01895) 452200

Facsimile: (01895) 452296

**...he Liposome Company Ltd**
Shortlands
Hammersmith International Cen-
...e
London W6 8EH

Telephone: (0181) 324 0058

Facsimile: (0181) 563 1653

Medical Information Department
**...orex Synthelabo Ltd**
Foundation Park
Roxborough Way
Maidenhead
Berkshire SL6 3UD

Telephone: (01628) 501200

Facsimile: (01628) 501278

**...orex Synthelabo UK & Ireland
Ltd**
Foundation Park
Roxborough Way
Maidenhead
Berkshire SL6 3UD

Telephone: (01628) 501200

Facsimile: (01628) 501278

**...RC Products Ltd**
London International House
Burnford Place
Broxbourne
Hertfordshire EN10 6LN

Telephone: (01992) 451111

Facsimile: (01992) 470133

Medical Department
**...undbeck Ltd**
Sunningdale House
Caldecotte Lake Business Park
Caldecotte
Milton Keynes MK7 8LF

Telephone: (01908) 649966

Facsimile: (01908) 647888

Regulatory and Professional
Services Department
**3M Health Care Limited**
3M House
Morley Street
Loughborough
Leicestershire LE11 1EP

Telephone:
Loughborough (01509) 611611
(including 24-hour emergency
service)

Facsimile: (01509) 237288

**Marion Merrell Ltd**
See **Hoechst Marion Roussel Ltd**

Medical Information Department
**Martindale Pharmaceuticals**
Bampton Road
Harold Hill
Romford
Essex RM3 8UG

Telephone: (01708) 386660

Facsimile: (01708) 384032

**medac Gesellschaft für klinische
Spezialpräparate mbH**
Fehlandtstrasse 3
20354 Hamburg
Germany

Telephone: +49(0)40 350 91-0

Facsimile: +49(0)40 350 91-300

Medical Department
**E. Merck Pharmaceuticals**
(A Division of Merck Ltd)
Harrier House
West Drayton
Middlesex UB7 7QG

Telephone: Medical Information
Department (0900 to 1700 hours):
(01895) 452258

24-hour Emergency Service:
(01895) 452200

Facsimile: (01895) 452296

Medical Department
**Merck Sharp & Dohme Ltd**
Hertford Road
Hoddesdon
Hertfordshire EN11 9BU

Telephone:
Hoddesdon (01992) 467272
(including 24-hour emergency
service)

Facsimile: (01992) 451066

**Monmouth Pharmaceuticals
Ltd**
3 & 4 Huxley Road
Surrey Research Park
Guildford
Surrey GU2 5RE

Telephone: (01483) 565299

Facsimile: (01483) 563658

Medical Information Department
**Napp Laboratories Ltd**
(A member of Napp
Pharmaceutical Group)
Cambridge Science Park
Milton Road
Cambridge CB4 4GW

Telephone:
Cambridge (01223) 424444
(including 24-hour emergency
service)

Telex: 817805

Facsimile: (01223) 424441

**Newport Synthesis Ltd**
Baldoyle Industrial Estate
Baldoyle
Dublin 13
Ireland

Telephone: 00353-1-8320020

Facsimile: 00353-1-8320026

UK Distributor:
Nycomed (UK) Ltd
Telephone: (0121) 7422444
Facsimile: (0121) 7222190

**Nexstar Pharmaceuticals Ltd**
The Quorum
Barnwell Road
Cambridge CB5 8RE

Telephone: (01223) 571400

Facsimile: (01223) 571444

The Medical Department
**Norgine Ltd**
Chaplin House
Widewater Place
Moorhall Road
Harefield
Middlesex UB9 6NS

Telephone: (01895) 826600

Facsimile: (01895) 825865

**Novartis Consumer Health**
Mill Road
Holmwood
Nr Dorking
Surrey RH5 4NU

Telephone: (01306) 742800

Facsimile: (01306) 743995

**Novartis Pharmaceuticals UK Ltd**
Frimley Business Park
Frimley
Camberley
Surrey GU16 5SG

Telephone: (01276) 698370

Facsimile: (01276) 698449

**Novex Pharma Ltd**
Innovex House
Marlow Park
Marlow
Bucks SL7 1TB

Telephone: (01628) 491500

Facsimile: (01628) 487799

Medical Information
**Novo Nordisk Pharmaceuticals
Ltd**
Novo Nordisk House
Broadfield Park
Brighton Road
Pease Pottage
Crawley
West Sussex RH11 9RT

Telephone: (01293) 613555

Facsimile: (01293) 613535

Medical Department
**Nycomed (UK) Ltd**
Nycomed House
2111 Coventry Road
Sheldon
Birmingham B26 3EA

Telephone: (0121) 742 2444

Facsimile: (0121) 722 2190

The Medical Information Officer
**Organon Laboratories Limited**
Cambridge Science Park
Milton Road
Cambridge CB4 4FL

Telephone: Daytime and Emergency Cambridge (01223) 423445

Facsimile: (01223) 424368

Mr C. Ponty
Business Manager
**Organon Teknika Ltd**
Science Park
Milton Road
Cambridge CB4 4FL

Telephone: Daytime and Emergency Cambridge (01223) 423650

Facsimile: (01223) 420264

**Orion Pharma (UK) Ltd**
1st Floor, Leat House
Overbridge Square
Hambridge Lane
Newbury
Berkshire RG14 5UX

Telephone: (01635) 520300

Facsimile: (01635) 520319

The Information Department
**Paines & Byrne Ltd**
Yamanouchi House
Pyrford Road
West Byfleet
Surrey KT14 6RA

Telephone: (01932) 355405

Facsimile: (01932) 353458

Medical Information Department
**Parke-Davis**
Lambert Court
Chestnut Avenue
Eastleigh
Hampshire SO53 3ZQ

Telephone:
Eastleigh (01703) 620500

Facsimile: (01703) 629819

**Pasteur Merieux MSD Ltd**
Clivemont House
Clivemont Road
Maidenhead
Berkshire SL6 7BU

Telephone:
Maidenhead (01628) 785291

Facsimile: (01628) 671722

**Penn Pharmaceuticals Ltd**
Tafarnaubach
Industrial Estate
Tredegar
Gwent NP2 3AA

Telephone: (01495) 711222

Facsimile: (01495) 711225/718285

**Perstorp Pharma**
A division of Perstorp Ltd
Intec 2
Wade Road
Basingstoke
Hampshire RG24 8NE

Telephone:
Basingstoke (01256) 477868

Facsimile: (01256) 321508

Medical Information
**Pfizer Ltd**
Sandwich
Kent CT13 9NJ

Telephone:
Sandwich (01304) 616161
(including 24-hour emergency
service)
Sandwich (01304) 625210
(medical information only)

**Pfizer Consumer Healthcare**
Wilsom Road
Alton
Hampshire GU34 2TJ

Telephone: (01420) 84801

Facsimile: (01420) 89376

Medical Information Department
**Pharmacia & Upjohn**
Davy Avenue
Knowlhill
Milton Keynes MK5 8PH

Telephone: (01908) 661101

Facsimile: (01908) 603051

Medical Department
**Pharmax Limited**
Bourne Road
Bexley
Kent DA5 1NX
*Telephone:* (01322) 550550
*Facsimile:* (01322) 558776


**Procter & Gamble Pharmaceuticals UK Ltd**
Lovett House
Lovett Road
Staines
Middlesex TW18 3AZ
*Telephone:* (01784) 495000
*Facsimile:* (01784) 495297


Medical Information Department
**Quinoderm Ltd**
Manchester Road
Oldham
Lancashire OL8 4PB
*Telephone:* (0161) 624 9307
*Facsimile:* (0161) 627 0928


Medical Information Unit
**Reckitt & Colman Products Ltd**
Dansom Lane
Hull HU8 7DS
*Telephone:* (01482) 326151 (including 24-hour emergency service)
*Facsimile:* (01482) 582526


**Rhône-Poulenc Rorer Ltd**
RPR House
50 Kings Hill Avenue
West Malling
Kent ME19 4AH
*Telephone:* (01732) 584493
            (0990) 239604
*Facsimile:* (01732) 584086


Medical Information
**Richborough Pharmaceuticals**
A Division of Pfizer Ltd
Sandwich
Kent CT13 9NJ
*Telephone:*
Sandwich (01304) 616161 (including 24-hour emergency service)
Sandwich (01304) 625210 (medical information only)


Drug Information
**Roche Products Ltd**
PO Box 8
Welwyn Garden City
Hertfordshire AL7 3AY
*Telephone:*
Welwyn Garden (01707) 366000
*Facsimile:* (01707) 390378


**Roussel Laboratories Ltd**
See **Hoechst Marion Roussel Ltd**


**Rybar Laboratories Ltd**
East Anton
Andover
Hants SP10 5RG
*Telephone:* (01264) 333455
*Facsimile:* (01264) 333460


**Sandoz Pharmaceuticals (UK) Ltd**
See **Novartis Pharmaceuticals UK Ltd**


Medical Affairs Department
**Sankyo Pharma UK Limited**
Sankyo House
Repton Place
White Lion Road
Amersham
Buckinghamshire HP7 9LP
*Telephone:* (01494) 766866
*Facsimile:* (01494) 766557


Medical Information Services
**Sanofi Winthrop Ltd**
One Onslow Street
Guildford
Surrey GU1 4YS
*Telephone:* (01483) 505515 (including 24-hour emergency service)
*Facsimile:* (01483) 535432


Medical Information Department
**Schering Health Care Limited**
The Brow
Burgess Hill
West Sussex RH15 9NE
*Telephone:*
Burgess Hill (01444) 232323
*Facsimile:* (01444) 246613


Medical Information
**Schering-Plough Ltd**
Schering-Plough House
Shire Park
Welwyn Garden City
Herts AL7 1TW
*Telephone:* (01707) 363636
*Facsimile:* (01707) 363692


Medical Information Department
**Schwarz Pharma Limited**
Schwarz House
East Street
Chesham
Buckinghamshire HP5 1DG
*Telephone:*
Chesham (01494) 772071
*Facsimile:* (01494) 773934


**Searle**
Division of Monsanto plc
PO Box 53
Lane End Road
High Wycombe
Buckinghamshire HP12 4HL
*Telephone:*
High Wycombe (01494) 521124 (including 24-hour emergency service)
*Facsimile:* (01494) 447872


**Serono Laboratories (U.K.) Ltd**
99 Bridge Road East
Welwyn Garden City
Hertfordshire AL7 1BG
*Telephone:*
Welwyn Garden (01707) 331972
*Facsimile:* (01707) 371873


Medical Department
**Servier Laboratories Ltd**
Fulmer Hall
Windmill Road
Fulmer
Slough
Buckinghamshire SL3 6HH
*Telephone:*
Slough (01753) 662744
*Facsimile:* (01753) 663456


**Seton Healthcare Group plc**
Tubiton House
Medlock Street
Oldham OL1 3HS
*Telephone:*
Medical information (9.00–17.00)+24-hour emergency service: (0161) 652 2222
Customer care (sales enquiries): (0161) 654 3000
*Facsimile:* (0161) 626 9090


**Shire Pharmaceuticals Ltd**
East Anton
Andover
Hants SP10 5RG
*Telephone:* (01264) 333455
*Facsimile:* (01264) 333460


Technical Services Department
**Smith & Nephew
Healthcare Ltd**
Healthcare House
Goulton Street
Hull HU3 4DJ
*Telephone:* (01482) 222200
*Facsimile:* (01482) 222211


Medical Information Department
**SmithKline Beecham
Pharmaceuticals**
Welwyn Garden City
Hertfordshire AL7 1EY
*Telephone:*
Welwyn Garden (01707) 325111 or FREEFONE (0800) 616482 (including 24-hour emergency service)
*Facsimile:* (0181) 913 4560


**Solvay Healthcare Ltd**
Hamilton House
Gaters Hill
West End
Southampton
Hampshire SO18 3JD
*Telephone:* (01703) 472281
*Facsimile:* (01703) 465350


**Speywood Pharmaceuticals Ltd**
1 Bath Road
Maidenhead
Berkshire SL6 4UH
*Telephone:* (01628) 771417
*Facsimile:* (01628) 770211


**E. R. Squibb & Sons Ltd**
Bristol-Myers Squibb House
141–149 Staines Road
Hounslow
Middlesex TW3 3JA
*Telephone:*
Medical Information Only: (0181) 754 3740 and FREEFONE 0800 7311736
BMS House and emergencies (0181) 572 7422
*Facsimile:* (0181) 754 3789


Medical Information
**Stafford-Miller Ltd**
45 Broadwater Road
Welwyn Garden City
Hertfordshire AL7 3SP
*Telephone:* (01707) 331001
*Facsimile:* (01707) 373370


**STD Pharmaceutical Products Ltd**
Fields Yard
Plough Lane
Hereford HR4 0EL
*Telephone:*
Hereford (01432) 353684
*Facsimile:* (01432) 342383


**Stiefel Laboratories (UK) Ltd**
Holtspur Lane
Wooburn Green
High Wycombe
Buckinghamshire HP10 0AU
*Telephone:*
Bourne End (01628) 524966
*Facsimile:* (01628) 810021


**Thames Laboratories Ltd**
Abbey Road
Wrexham Industrial Estate
Wrexham LL13 9PW
*Telephone:* (01978) 661351
*Facsimile:* (01978) 661673

Medical Information
*Telephone:* (01244) 288888
*Facsimile:* (01244) 280299


**Tillomed Laboratories Ltd**
Unit 2, Campus 5
Letchworth Business Park
Letchworth Garden City
Herts SG6 2JF
*Telephone:* (01462) 480344
*Facsimile:* (01462) 482213


Medical Information
**Trinity Pharmaceuticals Ltd**
The Old Exchange
12 Compton Road
London SW19 7QD
*Telephone:* (0181) 944 9443
*Facsimile:* (0181) 947 9325


**Typharm Ltd**
14 Parkstone Road
Poole
Dorset BH15 2PG
*Telephone:*
Poole (01202) 666626
*Facsimile:* (01202) 666309


**UCB Pharma Ltd**
Star House
69 Clarendon Road
Watford
Hertfordshire WD1 1DJ
*Telephone:* (01923) 211811
*Facsimile:* (01923) 229002


**Warner-Lambert Consumer
Healthcare**
Lambert Court
Chestnut Avenue
Eastleigh
Hampshire SO53 3ZQ
*Telephone:* (01703) 641400
*Facsimile:* (01703) 629816


**Wellcome UK**
See **Glaxo Wellcome**


Information Services
**Windsor Healthcare Ltd**
Ellesfield Avenue
Bracknell
Berkshire RG12 8YS
*Telephone:* (01344) 484448 (including 24-hour emergency service)
*Facsimile:* (01344) 741444


Medical Information Department
**Wyeth Laboratories**
Huntercombe Lane South
Taplow
Maidenhead
Berkshire SL6 0PH
*Telephone:*
Burnham (Bucks) (01628) 604377 (including 24-hour emergency service)
*Facsimile:* (01628) 666368


Medical Information Officer
**Yamanouchi Pharma Limited**
Yamanouchi House
Pyrford Road
West Byfleet
Surrey KT14 6RA
*Telephone:* (01932) 345535/342291
*Facsimile:* (01932) 353458


Medical Information
**Zeneca Pharma**
King's Court
Water Lane
Wilmslow
Cheshire SK9 5AZ
*Telephone:* (01625) 712712 or FREEFONE 0800 200123 (both include 24-hour emergency service)
*Facsimile:* (01625) 712581

*Brand names are in ordinary type, generic names in italics. *Under the generic entry, products with an asterisk contain a number of active ingredients and may be available in more than one formulation; products without an asterisk contain a single active ingredient. In certain instances such products may also be available with added constituents and these formulations are often designated by the principal brand name with the addition of a suffix or other mark of distinction. Where several presentations of a product bear the same proprietary name, the page number given below is that of the first of the respective entries. It should be noted that although different products may contain the same active ingredient this does not imply that they are equivalent in regard to bio-availability or therapeutic activity.*

## IN CONFIDENCE – COMMITTEE ON SAFETY OF MEDICINES
## REPORT ON SUSPECTED ADVERSE DRUG REACTION
**(For advice on reporting reactions see The Reporting of Adverse Reactions section in this book)**

| NAME OF PATIENT (To allow for linkage with other reports for same patient. Please give record number for hospital patients) | Family name | | | Sex | AGE or DATE OF BIRTH | WEIGHT (Kg.) |
|---|---|---|---|---|---|---|
| | Forename | | | | | |

| SUSPECT DRUG (Please give brand name if known) | ROUTE | DAILY DOSE | DATE STARTED | DATE STOPPED | INDICATION | |
|---|---|---|---|---|---|---|
| | | | | | | |

**SUSPECTED REACTION**

DATE OF ONSET _____ DATE STOPPED _____

OUTCOME (eg fatal, recovered) _____

**REPORTING DOCTOR (BLOCK LETTERS)**

Name: _____

Address: _____

Tel. No: _____ Specialty _____

Signature: _____ Date: _____

**SEND TO CSM, FREEPOST, London SW8 5BR**
**OR if you are in one of the following NHS regions:**
**TO CSM West Midlands, FREEPOST, Birmingham B18 7BR**
**OR CSM Northern, FREEPOST, Newcastle upon Tyne NE1 1BR**
**OR CSM Wales, FREEPOST, Cardiff CF4 1ZZ**
**OR CSM Mersey, FREEPOST, Liverpool L3 3AB**

If you would like information about other reports associated with the suspected drug, please tick box

---

✂ - - - - - - - - - - - - - - - - - - - - - - - - - - - - - - - - - - - - - - - - - - - - - - - - - - -

---

## IN CONFIDENCE – COMMITTEE ON SAFETY OF MEDICINES
## REPORT ON SUSPECTED ADVERSE DRUG REACTION
**(For advice on reporting reactions see The Reporting of Adverse Reactions section in this book)**

| NAME OF PATIENT (To allow for linkage with other reports for same patient. Please give record number for hospital patients) | Family name | | | Sex | AGE or DATE OF BIRTH | WEIGHT (Kg.) |
|---|---|---|---|---|---|---|
| | Forename | | | | | |

| SUSPECT DRUG (Please give brand name if known) | ROUTE | DAILY DOSE | DATE STARTED | DATE STOPPED | INDICATION | |
|---|---|---|---|---|---|---|
| | | | | | | |

**SUSPECTED REACTION**

DATE OF ONSET _____ DATE STOPPED _____

OUTCOME (eg fatal, recovered) _____

**REPORTING DOCTOR (BLOCK LETTERS)**

Name: _____

Address: _____

Tel. No: _____ Specialty _____

Signature: _____ Date: _____

**SEND TO CSM, FREEPOST, London SW8 5BR**
**OR if you are in one of the following NHS regions:**
**TO CSM West Midlands, FREEPOST, Birmingham B18 7BR**
**OR CSM Northern, FREEPOST, Newcastle upon Tyne NE1 1BR**
**OR CSM Wales, FREEPOST, Cardiff CF4 1ZZ**
**OR CSM Mersey, FREEPOST, Liverpool L3 3AB**

If you would like information about other reports associated with the suspected drug, please tick box

**OTHER DRUGS**
(Please record all other drugs, including self-medication, taken during the last 3 months, and give brand name if known)

| DRUG | ROUTE | DAILY DOSE | DATE STARTED | DATE STOPPED | INDICATION |
|------|-------|-----------|--------------|--------------|------------|
|      |       |           |              |              |            |
|      |       |           |              |              |            |
|      |       |           |              |              |            |
|      |       |           |              |              |            |
|      |       |           |              |              |            |

ADDITIONAL NOTES _____

_____

_____

_____

_____

✂ - - - - - - - - - - - - - - - - - - - - - - - - - - - - - - - - - - - - - - - - - - - - - - -

**OTHER DRUGS**
(Please record all other drugs, including self-medication, taken during the last 3 months, and give brand name if known)

| DRUG | ROUTE | DAILY DOSE | DATE STARTED | DATE STOPPED | INDICATION |
|------|-------|-----------|--------------|--------------|------------|
|      |       |           |              |              |            |
|      |       |           |              |              |            |
|      |       |           |              |              |            |
|      |       |           |              |              |            |
|      |       |           |              |              |            |

ADDITIONAL NOTES _____

_____

_____

_____

_____

## IN CONFIDENCE – COMMITTEE ON SAFETY OF MEDICINES
## REPORT ON SUSPECTED ADVERSE DRUG REACTION
### (For advice on reporting reactions see The Reporting of Adverse Reactions section in this book)

| NAME OF PATIENT (To allow for linkage with other reports for same patient. Please give record number for hospital patients) | Family name | | | Sex | AGE or DATE OF BIRTH | WEIGHT (Kg.) |
|---|---|---|---|---|---|---|
| | Forename | | | | | |

| SUSPECT DRUG (Please give brand name if known) | ROUTE | DAILY DOSE | DATE STARTED | DATE STOPPED | INDICATION | |
|---|---|---|---|---|---|---|
| | | | | | | |

SUSPECTED REACTION

_____

_____

DATE OF ONSET _____  DATE STOPPED _____

OUTCOME  (eg fatal, recovered) _____

**REPORTING DOCTOR (BLOCK LETTERS)**

Name: _____

Address: _____

Tel. No: _____  Specialty _____

**SEND TO CSM, FREEPOST, London SW8 5BR**
**OR if you are in one of the following NHS regions:**
**TO CSM West Midlands, FREEPOST, Birmingham B18 7BR**
**OR CSM Northern, FREEPOST, Newcastle upon Tyne NE1 1BR**
**OR CSM Wales, FREEPOST, Cardiff CF4 1ZZ**
**OR CSM Mersey, FREEPOST, Liverpool L3 3AB**

Signature: _____  Date: _____

If you would like information about other reports associated with the suspected drug, please tick box

- - - - - - - - - - - - - - - - - - - - - - - - - - - - - - - - - - - - - - - - - - ✂ - - - - - -

## IN CONFIDENCE – COMMITTEE ON SAFETY OF MEDICINES
## REPORT ON SUSPECTED ADVERSE DRUG REACTION
### (For advice on reporting reactions see The Reporting of Adverse Reactions section in this book)

| NAME OF PATIENT (To allow for linkage with other reports for same patient. Please give record number for hospital patients) | Family name | | | Sex | AGE or DATE OF BIRTH | WEIGHT (Kg.) |
|---|---|---|---|---|---|---|
| | Forename | | | | | |

| SUSPECT DRUG (Please give brand name if known) | ROUTE | DAILY DOSE | DATE STARTED | DATE STOPPED | INDICATION | |
|---|---|---|---|---|---|---|
| | | | | | | |

SUSPECTED REACTION

_____

_____

DATE OF ONSET _____  DATE STOPPED _____

OUTCOME  (eg fatal, recovered) _____

**REPORTING DOCTOR (BLOCK LETTERS)**

Name: _____

Address: _____

Tel. No: _____  Specialty _____

**SEND TO CSM, FREEPOST, London SW8 5BR**
**OR if you are in one of the following NHS regions:**
**TO CSM West Midlands, FREEPOST, Birmingham B18 7BR**
**OR CSM Northern, FREEPOST, Newcastle upon Tyne NE1 1BR**
**OR CSM Wales, FREEPOST, Cardiff CF4 1ZZ**
**OR CSM Mersey, FREEPOST, Liverpool L3 3AB**

Signature: _____  Date: _____

If you would like information about other reports associated with the suspected drug, please tick box

**OTHER DRUGS**
(Please record all other drugs, including self-medication, taken during the last 3 months, and give brand name if known)

| DRUG | ROUTE | DAILY DOSE | DATE STARTED | DATE STOPPED | INDICATION |
|------|-------|------------|--------------|--------------|------------|
|      |       |            |              |              |            |
|      |       |            |              |              |            |
|      |       |            |              |              |            |
|      |       |            |              |              |            |
|      |       |            |              |              |            |

ADDITIONAL NOTES

--------------------✂--------------------------------------------------------------------

**OTHER DRUGS**
(Please record all other drugs, including self-medication, taken during the last 3 months, and give brand name if known)

| DRUG | ROUTE | DAILY DOSE | DATE STARTED | DATE STOPPED | INDICATION |
|------|-------|------------|--------------|--------------|------------|
|      |       |            |              |              |            |
|      |       |            |              |              |            |
|      |       |            |              |              |            |
|      |       |            |              |              |            |
|      |       |            |              |              |            |

ADDITIONAL NOTES

**IN CONFIDENCE – COMMITTEE ON SAFETY OF MEDICINES**
**REPORT ON SUSPECTED ADVERSE DRUG REACTION**
**(For advice on reporting reactions see The Reporting of Adverse Reactions section in this book)**

| NAME OF PATIENT (To allow for linkage with other reports for same patient. Please give record number for hospital patients) | Family name | | | Sex | AGE or DATE OF BIRTH | WEIGHT (Kg.) |
|---|---|---|---|---|---|---|
| | Forename | | | | | |

| SUSPECT DRUG (Please give brand name if known) | ROUTE | DAILY DOSE | DATE STARTED | DATE STOPPED | INDICATION | |
|---|---|---|---|---|---|---|
| | | | | | | |

SUSPECTED REACTION

REPORTING DOCTOR (BLOCK LETTERS)

Name: _____

Address: _____

DATE OF ONSET _____ DATE STOPPED _____

OUTCOME (eg fatal, recovered) _____

Tel. No: _____ Specialty _____

**SEND TO CSM, FREEPOST, London SW8 5BR**
**OR if you are in one of the following NHS regions:**
**TO CSM West Midlands, FREEPOST, Birmingham B18 7BR**
**OR CSM Northern, FREEPOST, Newcastle upon Tyne NE1 1BR**
**OR CSM Wales, FREEPOST, Cardiff CF4 1ZZ**
**OR CSM Mersey, FREEPOST, Liverpool L3 3AB**

Signature: _____ Date: _____

If you would like information about other reports associated with the suspected drug, please tick box

------------------------------✂------------------------------

**IN CONFIDENCE – COMMITTEE ON SAFETY OF MEDICINES**
**REPORT ON SUSPECTED ADVERSE DRUG REACTION**
**(For advice on reporting reactions see The Reporting of Adverse Reactions section in this book)**

| NAME OF PATIENT (To allow for linkage with other reports for same patient. Please give record number for hospital patients) | Family name | | | Sex | AGE or DATE OF BIRTH | WEIGHT (Kg.) |
|---|---|---|---|---|---|---|
| | Forename | | | | | |

| SUSPECT DRUG (Please give brand name if known) | ROUTE | DAILY DOSE | DATE STARTED | DATE STOPPED | INDICATION | |
|---|---|---|---|---|---|---|
| | | | | | | |

SUSPECTED REACTION

REPORTING DOCTOR (BLOCK LETTERS)

Name: _____

Address: _____

DATE OF ONSET _____ DATE STOPPED _____

OUTCOME (eg fatal, recovered) _____

Tel. No: _____ Specialty _____

**SEND TO CSM, FREEPOST, London SW8 5BR**
**OR if you are in one of the following NHS regions:**
**TO CSM West Midlands, FREEPOST, Birmingham B18 7BR**
**OR CSM Northern, FREEPOST, Newcastle upon Tyne NE1 1BR**
**OR CSM Wales, FREEPOST, Cardiff CF4 1ZZ**
**OR CSM Mersey, FREEPOST, Liverpool L3 3AB**

Signature: _____ Date: _____

If you would like information about other reports associated with the suspected drug, please tick box

**OTHER DRUGS**
(Please record all other drugs, including self-medication, taken during the last 3 months, and give brand name if known)

| DRUG | ROUTE | DAILY DOSE | DATE STARTED | DATE STOPPED | INDICATION |
|---|---|---|---|---|---|
| | | | | | |
| | | | | | |
| | | | | | |
| | | | | | |
| | | | | | |
| | | | | | |

ADDITIONAL NOTES _____

_____

_____

_____

_____

- - - - - - - - - ✂ - - - - - - - - - - - - - - - - - - - - - - - - - - - - - - - - - - - - - - - - - - - - - - -

**OTHER DRUGS**
(Please record all other drugs, including self-medication, taken during the last 3 months, and give brand name if known)

| DRUG | ROUTE | DAILY DOSE | DATE STARTED | DATE STOPPED | INDICATION |
|---|---|---|---|---|---|
| | | | | | |
| | | | | | |
| | | | | | |
| | | | | | |
| | | | | | |
| | | | | | |

ADDITIONAL NOTES _____

_____

_____

_____

_____

**IN CONFIDENCE – COMMITTEE ON SAFETY OF MEDICINES**
**REPORT ON SUSPECTED ADVERSE DRUG REACTION**
**(For advice on reporting reactions see The Reporting of Adverse Reactions section in this book)**

| NAME OF PATIENT (To allow for linkage with other reports for same patient. Please give record number for hospital patients) | Family name | | | | Sex | AGE or DATE OF BIRTH | WEIGHT (Kg.) |
|---|---|---|---|---|---|---|---|
| | Forename | | | | | | |

| SUSPECT DRUG (Please give brand name if known) | ROUTE | DAILY DOSE | DATE STARTED | DATE STOPPED | INDICATION | | |
|---|---|---|---|---|---|---|---|
| | | | | | | | |

SUSPECTED REACTION

_____

_____

DATE OF ONSET _____ DATE STOPPED _____

OUTCOME (eg fatal, recovered) _____

REPORTING DOCTOR (BLOCK LETTERS)

Name: _____

Address: _____

Tel. No: _____ Specialty _____

**SEND TO CSM, FREEPOST, London SW8 5BR**
**OR if you are in one of the following NHS regions:**
**TO CSM West Midlands, FREEPOST, Birmingham B18 7BR**
**OR CSM Northern, FREEPOST, Newcastle upon Tyne NE1 1BR**
**OR CSM Wales, FREEPOST, Cardiff CF4 1ZZ**
**OR CSM Mersey, FREEPOST, Liverpool L3 3AB**

Signature: _____ Date: _____

If you would like information about other reports associated with the suspected drug, please tick box

------------------------------✂------------------------------

**IN CONFIDENCE – COMMITTEE ON SAFETY OF MEDICINES**
**REPORT ON SUSPECTED ADVERSE DRUG REACTION**
**(For advice on reporting reactions see The Reporting of Adverse Reactions section in this book)**

| NAME OF PATIENT (To allow for linkage with other reports for same patient. Please give record number for hospital patients) | Family name | | | | Sex | AGE or DATE OF BIRTH | WEIGHT (Kg.) |
|---|---|---|---|---|---|---|---|
| | Forename | | | | | | |

| SUSPECT DRUG (Please give brand name if known) | ROUTE | DAILY DOSE | DATE STARTED | DATE STOPPED | INDICATION | | |
|---|---|---|---|---|---|---|---|
| | | | | | | | |

SUSPECTED REACTION

_____

_____

DATE OF ONSET _____ DATE STOPPED _____

OUTCOME (eg fatal, recovered) _____

REPORTING DOCTOR (BLOCK LETTERS)

Name: _____

Address: _____

Tel. No: _____ Specialty _____

**SEND TO CSM, FREEPOST, London SW8 5BR**
**OR if you are in one of the following NHS regions:**
**TO CSM West Midlands, FREEPOST, Birmingham B18 7BR**
**OR CSM Northern, FREEPOST, Newcastle upon Tyne NE1 1BR**
**OR CSM Wales, FREEPOST, Cardiff CF4 1ZZ**
**OR CSM Mersey, FREEPOST, Liverpool L3 3AB**

Signature: _____ Date: _____

If you would like information about other reports associated with the suspected drug, please tick box

**OTHER DRUGS**
(Please record all other drugs, including self-medication, taken during the last 3 months, and give brand name if known)

| DRUG | ROUTE | DAILY DOSE | DATE STARTED | DATE STOPPED | INDICATION |
|------|-------|-----------|--------------|--------------|------------|
|      |       |           |              |              |            |
|      |       |           |              |              |            |
|      |       |           |              |              |            |
|      |       |           |              |              |            |
|      |       |           |              |              |            |

ADDITIONAL NOTES _____

_____

_____

_____

_____

- - - - - - ✂ - - - - - - - - - - - - - - - - - - - - - - - - - - - - - - - - - - - - - - - - - - - - - - - - - - - -

**OTHER DRUGS**
(Please record all other drugs, including self-medication, taken during the last 3 months, and give brand name if known)

| DRUG | ROUTE | DAILY DOSE | DATE STARTED | DATE STOPPED | INDICATION |
|------|-------|-----------|--------------|--------------|------------|
|      |       |           |              |              |            |
|      |       |           |              |              |            |
|      |       |           |              |              |            |
|      |       |           |              |              |            |
|      |       |           |              |              |            |

ADDITIONAL NOTES _____

_____

_____

_____

_____

## IN CONFIDENCE – COMMITTEE ON SAFETY OF MEDICINES
## REPORT ON SUSPECTED ADVERSE DRUG REACTION
### (For advice on reporting reactions see The Reporting of Adverse Reactions section in this book)

| NAME OF PATIENT (To allow for linkage with other reports for same patient. Please give record number for hospital patients) | Family name | | | Sex | AGE or DATE OF BIRTH | WEIGHT (Kg.) |
|---|---|---|---|---|---|---|
| | Forename | | | | | |

| SUSPECT DRUG (Please give brand name if known) | ROUTE | DAILY DOSE | DATE STARTED | DATE STOPPED | INDICATION | |
|---|---|---|---|---|---|---|
| | | | | | | |

**SUSPECTED REACTION**

DATE OF ONSET _____ DATE STOPPED _____

OUTCOME (eg fatal, recovered) _____

**REPORTING DOCTOR (BLOCK LETTERS)**

Name: _____

Address: _____

Tel. No: _____ Specialty _____

Signature: _____ Date: _____

**SEND TO CSM, FREEPOST, London SW8 5BR**
**OR if you are in one of the following NHS regions:**
**TO CSM West Midlands, FREEPOST, Birmingham B18 7BR**
**OR CSM Northern, FREEPOST, Newcastle upon Tyne NE1 1BR**
**OR CSM Wales, FREEPOST, Cardiff CF4 1ZZ**
**OR CSM Mersey, FREEPOST, Liverpool L3 3AB**

If you would like information about other reports associated with the suspected drug, please tick box

- - - - - - - - - - - - - - - - - - - - - - - ✂ - - - - - - - - - - - - -

## IN CONFIDENCE – COMMITTEE ON SAFETY OF MEDICINES
## REPORT ON SUSPECTED ADVERSE DRUG REACTION
### (For advice on reporting reactions see The Reporting of Adverse Reactions section in this book)

| NAME OF PATIENT (To allow for linkage with other reports for same patient. Please give record number for hospital patients) | Family name | | | Sex | AGE or DATE OF BIRTH | WEIGHT (Kg.) |
|---|---|---|---|---|---|---|
| | Forename | | | | | |

| SUSPECT DRUG (Please give brand name if known) | ROUTE | DAILY DOSE | DATE STARTED | DATE STOPPED | INDICATION | |
|---|---|---|---|---|---|---|
| | | | | | | |

**SUSPECTED REACTION**

DATE OF ONSET _____ DATE STOPPED _____

OUTCOME (eg fatal, recovered) _____

**REPORTING DOCTOR (BLOCK LETTERS)**

Name: _____

Address: _____

Tel. No: _____ Specialty _____

Signature: _____ Date: _____

**SEND TO CSM, FREEPOST, London SW8 5BR**
**OR if you are in one of the following NHS regions:**
**TO CSM West Midlands, FREEPOST, Birmingham B18 7BR**
**OR CSM Northern, FREEPOST, Newcastle upon Tyne NE1 1BR**
**OR CSM Wales, FREEPOST, Cardiff CF4 1ZZ**
**OR CSM Mersey, FREEPOST, Liverpool L3 3AB**

If you would like information about other reports associated with the suspected drug, please tick box

**OTHER DRUGS**
(Please record all other drugs, including self-medication, taken during the last 3 months, and give brand name if known)

| DRUG | ROUTE | DAILY DOSE | DATE STARTED | DATE STOPPED | INDICATION |
|---|---|---|---|---|---|
| | | | | | |
| | | | | | |
| | | | | | |
| | | | | | |
| | | | | | |
| | | | | | |

ADDITIONAL NOTES _____

_____

_____

_____

_____

✂ - - - - - - - - - - - - - - - - - - - - - - - - - - - - - - - - - - - - - - - - - - - - - - - - - - - - -

**OTHER DRUGS**
(Please record all other drugs, including self-medication, taken during the last 3 months, and give brand name if known)

| DRUG | ROUTE | DAILY DOSE | DATE STARTED | DATE STOPPED | INDICATION |
|---|---|---|---|---|---|
| | | | | | |
| | | | | | |
| | | | | | |
| | | | | | |
| | | | | | |
| | | | | | |

ADDITIONAL NOTES _____

_____

_____

_____

_____

**IN CONFIDENCE – COMMITTEE ON SAFETY OF MEDICINES**
**REPORT ON SUSPECTED ADVERSE DRUG REACTION**
**(For advice on reporting reactions see The Reporting of Adverse Reactions section in this book)**

| NAME OF PATIENT (To allow for linkage with other reports for same patient. Please give record number for hospital patients) | Family name | | | Sex | AGE or DATE OF BIRTH | WEIGHT (Kg.) |
|---|---|---|---|---|---|---|
| | Forename | | | | | |

| SUSPECT DRUG (Please give brand name if known) | ROUTE | DAILY DOSE | DATE STARTED | DATE STOPPED | INDICATION | |
|---|---|---|---|---|---|---|
| | | | | | | |

SUSPECTED REACTION

DATE OF ONSET _____ DATE STOPPED _____

OUTCOME (eg fatal, recovered) _____

**SEND TO CSM, FREEPOST, London SW8 5BR**
**OR if you are in one of the following NHS regions:**
**TO CSM West Midlands, FREEPOST, Birmingham B18 7BR**
**OR CSM Northern, FREEPOST, Newcastle upon Tyne NE1 1BR**
**OR CSM Wales, FREEPOST, Cardiff CF4 1ZZ**
**OR CSM Mersey, FREEPOST, Liverpool L3 3AB**

REPORTING DOCTOR (BLOCK LETTERS)

Name: _____

Address: _____

Tel. No: _____ Specialty _____

Signature: _____ Date: _____

If you would like information about other reports associated with the suspected drug, please tick box

---

**IN CONFIDENCE – COMMITTEE ON SAFETY OF MEDICINES**
**REPORT ON SUSPECTED ADVERSE DRUG REACTION**
**(For advice on reporting reactions see The Reporting of Adverse Reactions section in this book)**

| NAME OF PATIENT (To allow for linkage with other reports for same patient. Please give record number for hospital patients) | Family name | | | Sex | AGE or DATE OF BIRTH | WEIGHT (Kg.) |
|---|---|---|---|---|---|---|
| | Forename | | | | | |

| SUSPECT DRUG (Please give brand name if known) | ROUTE | DAILY DOSE | DATE STARTED | DATE STOPPED | INDICATION | |
|---|---|---|---|---|---|---|
| | | | | | | |

SUSPECTED REACTION

DATE OF ONSET _____ DATE STOPPED _____

OUTCOME (eg fatal, recovered) _____

**SEND TO CSM, FREEPOST, London SW8 5BR**
**OR if you are in one of the following NHS regions:**
**TO CSM West Midlands, FREEPOST, Birmingham B18 7BR**
**OR CSM Northern, FREEPOST, Newcastle upon Tyne NE1 1BR**
**OR CSM Wales, FREEPOST, Cardiff CF4 1ZZ**
**OR CSM Mersey, FREEPOST, Liverpool L3 3AB**

REPORTING DOCTOR (BLOCK LETTERS)

Name: _____

Address: _____

Tel. No: _____ Specialty _____

Signature: _____ Date: _____

If you would like information about other reports associated with the suspected drug, please tick box

**OTHER DRUGS**
(Please record all other drugs, including self-medication, taken during the last 3 months, and give brand name if known)

| DRUG | ROUTE | DAILY DOSE | DATE STARTED | DATE STOPPED | INDICATION |
|------|-------|-----------|--------------|--------------|------------|
|  |  |  |  |  |  |
|  |  |  |  |  |  |
|  |  |  |  |  |  |
|  |  |  |  |  |  |
|  |  |  |  |  |  |
|  |  |  |  |  |  |

ADDITIONAL NOTES

_____

_____

_____

_____

- - - - - - - - - - ✂ - - - - - - - - - - - - - - - - - - - - - - - - - - - - - - - - - - - - - - - - -

**OTHER DRUGS**
(Please record all other drugs, including self-medication, taken during the last 3 months, and give brand name if known)

| DRUG | ROUTE | DAILY DOSE | DATE STARTED | DATE STOPPED | INDICATION |
|------|-------|-----------|--------------|--------------|------------|
|  |  |  |  |  |  |
|  |  |  |  |  |  |
|  |  |  |  |  |  |
|  |  |  |  |  |  |
|  |  |  |  |  |  |
|  |  |  |  |  |  |

ADDITIONAL NOTES

_____

_____

_____

_____

# IN CONFIDENCE – COMMITTEE ON SAFETY OF MEDICINES
## REPORT ON SUSPECTED ADVERSE DRUG REACTION
### (For advice on reporting reactions see The Reporting of Adverse Reactions section in this book)

| NAME OF PATIENT (To allow for linkage with other reports for same patient. Please give record number for hospital patients) | Family name | | | Sex | AGE or DATE OF BIRTH | WEIGHT (Kg.) |
|---|---|---|---|---|---|---|
| | Forename | | | | | |

| SUSPECT DRUG (Please give brand name if known) | ROUTE | DAILY DOSE | DATE STARTED | STOPPED | INDICATION | |
|---|---|---|---|---|---|---|
| | | | | | | |

**SUSPECTED REACTION**

DATE OF ONSET _____ DATE STOPPED _____

OUTCOME (eg fatal, recovered) _____

**REPORTING DOCTOR (BLOCK LETTERS)**

Name: _____

Address: _____

Tel. No: _____ Specialty _____

Signature: _____ Date: _____

If you would like information about other reports associated with the suspected drug, please tick box

SEND TO CSM, FREEPOST, London SW8 5BR
OR if you are in one of the following NHS regions:
TO CSM West Midlands, FREEPOST, Birmingham B18 7BR
OR CSM Northern, FREEPOST, Newcastle upon Tyne NE1 1BR
OR CSM Wales, FREEPOST, Cardiff CF4 1ZZ
OR CSM Mersey, FREEPOST, Liverpool L3 3AB

--------------------------------✂--------------------------------

# IN CONFIDENCE – COMMITTEE ON SAFETY OF MEDICINES
## REPORT ON SUSPECTED ADVERSE DRUG REACTION
### (For advice on reporting reactions see The Reporting of Adverse Reactions section in this book)

| NAME OF PATIENT (To allow for linkage with other reports for same patient. Please give record number for hospital patients) | Family name | | | Sex | AGE or DATE OF BIRTH | WEIGHT (Kg.) |
|---|---|---|---|---|---|---|
| | Forename | | | | | |

| SUSPECT DRUG (Please give brand name if known) | ROUTE | DAILY DOSE | DATE STARTED | STOPPED | INDICATION | |
|---|---|---|---|---|---|---|
| | | | | | | |

**SUSPECTED REACTION**

DATE OF ONSET _____ DATE STOPPED _____

OUTCOME (eg fatal, recovered) _____

**REPORTING DOCTOR (BLOCK LETTERS)**

Name: _____

Address: _____

Tel. No: _____ Specialty _____

Signature: _____ Date: _____

If you would like information about other reports associated with the suspected drug, please tick box

SEND TO CSM, FREEPOST, London SW8 5BR
OR if you are in one of the following NHS regions:
TO CSM West Midlands, FREEPOST, Birmingham B18 7BR
OR CSM Northern, FREEPOST, Newcastle upon Tyne NE1 1BR
OR CSM Wales, FREEPOST, Cardiff CF4 1ZZ
OR CSM Mersey, FREEPOST, Liverpool L3 3AB

**OTHER DRUGS**
(Please record all other drugs, including self-medication, taken during the last 3 months, and give brand name if known)

| DRUG | ROUTE | DAILY DOSE | DATE STARTED | DATE STOPPED | INDICATION |
|------|-------|-----------|--------------|--------------|------------|
|      |       |           |              |              |            |
|      |       |           |              |              |            |
|      |       |           |              |              |            |
|      |       |           |              |              |            |
|      |       |           |              |              |            |
|      |       |           |              |              |            |

ADDITIONAL NOTES

---

✂ - - - - - - - - - - - - - - - - - - - - - - - - - - - - - - - - - - - - - - - - - -

---

**OTHER DRUGS**
(Please record all other drugs, including self-medication, taken during the last 3 months, and give brand name if known)

| DRUG | ROUTE | DAILY DOSE | DATE STARTED | DATE STOPPED | INDICATION |
|------|-------|-----------|--------------|--------------|------------|
|      |       |           |              |              |            |
|      |       |           |              |              |            |
|      |       |           |              |              |            |
|      |       |           |              |              |            |
|      |       |           |              |              |            |
|      |       |           |              |              |            |

ADDITIONAL NOTES

## IN CONFIDENCE – COMMITTEE ON SAFETY OF MEDICINES
## REPORT ON SUSPECTED ADVERSE DRUG REACTION
### (For advice on reporting reactions see The Reporting of Adverse Reactions section in this book)

| NAME OF PATIENT (To allow for linkage with other reports for same patient. Please give record number for hospital patients) | Family name | | | Sex | AGE or DATE OF BIRTH | WEIGHT (Kg.) |
|---|---|---|---|---|---|---|
| | Forename | | | | | |

| SUSPECT DRUG (Please give brand name if known) | ROUTE | DAILY DOSE | DATE STARTED | STOPPED | INDICATION | |
|---|---|---|---|---|---|---|
| | | | | | | |

**SUSPECTED REACTION**

DATE OF ONSET _____ DATE STOPPED _____

OUTCOME  (eg fatal, recovered) _____

**REPORTING DOCTOR (BLOCK LETTERS)**

Name: _____

Address: _____

Tel. No: _____ Specialty _____

Signature:                                        Date:

**SEND TO CSM, FREEPOST, London SW8 5BR**
**OR if you are in one of the following NHS regions:**
**TO CSM West Midlands, FREEPOST, Birmingham B18 7BR**
**OR CSM Northern, FREEPOST, Newcastle upon Tyne NE1 1BR**
**OR CSM Wales, FREEPOST, Cardiff CF4 1ZZ**
**OR CSM Mersey, FREEPOST, Liverpool L3 3AB**

If you would like information about other reports associated with the suspected drug, please tick box

---

## IN CONFIDENCE – COMMITTEE ON SAFETY OF MEDICINES
## REPORT ON SUSPECTED ADVERSE DRUG REACTION
### (For advice on reporting reactions see The Reporting of Adverse Reactions section in this book)

| NAME OF PATIENT (To allow for linkage with other reports for same patient. Please give record number for hospital patients) | Family name | | | Sex | AGE or DATE OF BIRTH | WEIGHT (Kg.) |
|---|---|---|---|---|---|---|
| | Forename | | | | | |

| SUSPECT DRUG (Please give brand name if known) | ROUTE | DAILY DOSE | DATE STARTED | STOPPED | INDICATION | |
|---|---|---|---|---|---|---|
| | | | | | | |

**SUSPECTED REACTION**

DATE OF ONSET _____ DATE STOPPED _____

OUTCOME  (eg fatal, recovered) _____

**REPORTING DOCTOR (BLOCK LETTERS)**

Name: _____

Address: _____

Tel. No: _____ Specialty _____

Signature:                                        Date:

**SEND TO CSM, FREEPOST, London SW8 5BR**
**OR if you are in one of the following NHS regions:**
**TO CSM West Midlands, FREEPOST, Birmingham B18 7BR**
**OR CSM Northern, FREEPOST, Newcastle upon Tyne NE1 1BR**
**OR CSM Wales, FREEPOST, Cardiff CF4 1ZZ**
**OR CSM Mersey, FREEPOST, Liverpool L3 3AB**

If you would like information about other reports associated with the suspected drug, please tick box

**OTHER DRUGS**
**(Please record all other drugs, including self-medication, taken during the last 3 months, and give brand name if known)**

| DRUG | ROUTE | DAILY DOSE | DATE STARTED | DATE STOPPED | INDICATION |
|---|---|---|---|---|---|
| | | | | | |
| | | | | | |
| | | | | | |
| | | | | | |
| | | | | | |
| | | | | | |

ADDITIONAL NOTES _____

_____

_____

_____

------------------------ ✂ ------------------------------------------------------------

**OTHER DRUGS**
**(Please record all other drugs, including self-medication, taken during the last 3 months, and give brand name if known)**

| DRUG | ROUTE | DAILY DOSE | DATE STARTED | DATE STOPPED | INDICATION |
|---|---|---|---|---|---|
| | | | | | |
| | | | | | |
| | | | | | |
| | | | | | |
| | | | | | |
| | | | | | |

ADDITIONAL NOTES _____

_____

_____

_____